Goodman & Gilman's The PHARMACOLOGICAL BASIS OF THERAPEUTICS

EDITORS

Joel G. Hardman, Ph.D.

Professor of Pharmacology, Emeritus
Vanderbilt University Medical Center
Nashville, Tennessee

Lee E. Limbird, Ph.D.

Professor of Pharmacology
Associate Vice Chancellor for Research
Vanderbilt University Medical Center
Nashville, Tennessee

CONSULTING EDITOR

Alfred Goodman Gilman, M.D., Ph.D., D.Sc. (Hon.)

Raymond and Ellen Willie Distinguished Chair in Molecular Neuropharmacology
Regental Professor and Chairman, Department of Pharmacology
University of Texas Southwestern Medical Center
Dallas, Texas

GOODMAN & GILMAN'S The PHARMACOLOGICAL BASIS OF THERAPEUTICS

Tenth Edition

McGraw-Hill
MEDICAL PUBLISHING DIVISION

New York   Chicago   San Francisco   Lisbon   London   Madrid   Mexico City
Milan   New Delhi   San Juan   Seoul   Singapore   Sydney   Toronto

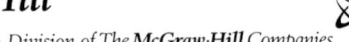

McGraw-Hill

A Division of The McGraw·Hill Companies

Goodman and Gilman's THE PHARMACOLOGICAL BASIS OF THERAPEUTICS, 10/e

1234567890 DOWDOW 0987654321

ISBN 0-07-135469-7

This book was set in Times Roman by York Graphic Services, Inc. The editors were Martin J. Wonsiewicz and John M. Morriss; the production supervisor was Philip Galea; and the cover designer was Marsha Cohen/Parallelogram. The index was prepared by Irving Condé Tullar and Coughlin Indexing Services, Inc.
R.R. Donnelley and Sons Company was printer and binder.

This book is printed on acid-free paper.

Library of Congress Cataloging-in-Publication Data

Goodman and Gilman's the pharmacological basis of therapeutics.—10th ed. / [edited by]
    Joel G. Hardman, Lee E. Limbird, Alfred Goodman Gilman.
        p. ; cm.
    Includes bibliographical references and index.
    ISBN 0-07-135469-7
    1. Pharmacology.   2. Chemotherapy.   I. Title: Pharmacological basis of therapeutics.
II. Goodman, Louis Sanford   III. Gilman, Alfred   IV. Hardman, Joel G.
V. Limbird, Lee E.   VI. Gilman, Alfred Goodman
    [DNLM: 1. Pharmacology.   2. Drug Therapy.   QV 4 G6532 2002]
RM300 G644   2001
615′.7—dc21   2001030728

Contents

S E C T I O N   I

GENERAL PRINCIPLES   1

S E C T I O N   I I

DRUGS ACTING AT SYNAPTIC AND NEUROEFFECTOR JUNCTIONAL SITES   113

A P P E N D I C E S

Contributors

Contributors*

Huda Akil, Ph.D. [23]
Codirector and Senior Research Scientist, Mental Health Research Institute, and Gardner Quatron Distinguished Professor of Neuroscience in Psychiatry, University of Michigan, Ann Arbor, Michigan

Ross J. Baldessarini, M.D. [19, 20]
Professor of Psychiatry and Neuroscience, Harvard Medical School; Director, Laboratories for Psychiatric Research, Mailman Research Center; Director, Bipolar and Psychiatric Disorders Program, McLean Division of Massachusetts General Hospital, Belmont, Massachusetts

Charles Beattie, M.D., Ph.D. [13]
Professor and Chair, Department of Anesthesiology, Vanderbilt University School of Medicine, Nashville, Tennessee

John E. Bennett, M.D. [49]
Head, Clinical Mycology Section, National Institutes of Health, Bethesda, Maryland

Thomas P. Bersot, M.D., Ph.D. [36]
Professor of Medicine, University of California, San Francisco; Associate Investigator, Gladstone Institute of Cardiovascular Disease; Chief, Lipid Clinic, San Francisco General Hospital, San Francisco, California

Floyd E. Bloom, M.D. [12]
Chair, Department of Neuropharmacology, The Scripps Research Institute, La Jolla, California

Jeffrey A. Bluestone, Ph.D. [53]
A.W. and Mary Margaret Clausen Distinguished Professor of Medicine, and Director, University of California San Francisco Diabetes Center, Metabolic Research Unit and Hormone Research Institute, San Francisco, California

Lewis E. Braverman, M.D. [57]
Professor of Medicine and Chief, Section of Endocrinology, Diabetes, and Nutrition, Boston University Medical Center, Boston, Massachusetts

Joan Heller Brown, Ph.D. [7]
Professor of Pharmacology, School of Medicine, University of California San Diego, La Jolla, California

Nancy J. Brown, M.D. [25, 33]
Associate Professor of Medicine and Pharmacology, Vanderbilt University School of Medicine, Nashville, Tennessee

Paul Calabresi, M.D. [52]
Professor and Chair Emeritus, Department of Medicine, Brown University School of Medicine, Providence, Rhode Island

William A. Catteral, Ph.D. [15]
Professor and Chair, Department of Pharmacology, University of Washington School of Medicine, Seattle, Washington

Bruce A. Chabner, M.D. [52]
Chief, Division of Hematology and Oncology, Massachusetts General Hospital, and Professor of Medicine, Harvard Medical School, Boston, Massachusetts

Henry F. Chambers, III, M.D. [43, 46, 47]
Professor of Medicine, University of California, San Francisco, School of Medicine, and Chief, Infectious Diseases, San Francisco General Hospital, San Francisco, California

Dennis S. Charney, M.D. [17]
Chief, Mood and Anxiety Disorder Research Program, National Institutes of Mental Health, Bethesda, Maryland

Wilson Colucci, M.D. [34]
Professor of Medicine and Physiology, Boston University School of Medicine, and Chief, Cardiovascular Medicine, Boston University Medical Center, Boston, Massachusetts

Ann M. Coulston, M.S., R.D. [63, 64]
Nutrition Consultant, Hartner/Coulston Nutrition Associates, Stanford University Medical School, Woodside, California

C. Michael Crowder, M.D., Ph.D. [14]
Assistant Professor, Departments of Anesthesiology and Molecular Biology and Pharmacology, Washington University School of Medicine, St. Louis, Missouri

Stephen N. Davis, M.D. [61]
Rudolph Kampmeier Professor of Medicine and Molecular Physiology and Biophysics, and Chief, Division of Diabetes and Endocrinology, Vanderbilt University School of Medicine, Nashville, Tennessee

*The numbers in brackets following each contributor's name indicate the chapters written or co-written by that contributor.

Lynn A. Drake, M.D. [65]
Lecturer, Department of Dermatology, Harvard Medical School, Boston, Massachusetts

Lauralea Edwards, D.Ph. [Appendix I]
Pharmaceutical Consultant, Mill Creek, Washington

Alex S. Evers, M.D. [14]
Henry Mallinckrodt Professor of Anesthesiology and Professor of Molecular Biology and Pharmacology, Washington University School of Medicine, St. Louis, Missouri

Alan P. Farwell, M.D. [57]
Associate Professor of Medicine, Division of Endocrinology, University of Massachusetts Medical Center, Worcester, Massachusetts

Michael F. Fleming, M.D., MPH [18]
Professor of Family Medicine, University of Wisconsin Medical School, Madison, Wisconsin

Rocio Garcia-Carbonero, M.D. [52]
Visiting Fellow, Massachusetts General Hospital and Dana Farber Cancer Institute, Boston, Massachusetts

Alfred L. George, Jr., M.D [5]
Professor of Medicine and Pharmacology, and Director, Division of Genetic Medicine, Vanderbilt University School of Medicine, Nashville, Tennessee

Alfred Goodman Gilman, M.D., Ph.D., D.Sc. (Hon.) [Introduction to Section I]
Raymond and Ellen Willie Distinguished Chair in Molecular Neuropharmacology, Regental Professor and Chair, Department of Pharmacology, University of Texas Southwestern Medical Center, Dallas, Texas

Daryl K. Granner, M.D. [61]
Professor of Molecular Physiology and Biophysics, and Director, Vanderbilt Diabetes Center, Vanderbilt University School of Medicine, Nashville, Tennessee

Howard B. Gutstein, M.D. [23]
Director of Research, Division of Anesthesiology, Critical and Palliative Care, and Associate Professor, Departments of Anesthesiology and Molecular Genetics, MD Anderson Cancer Center, University of Texas, Houston, Texas

David W. Haas, M.D. [51]
Associate Professor of Medicine, Division of Infectious Diseases, Vanderbilt University School of Medicine, Nashville, Tennessee

R. Adron Harris, Ph.D. [17, 18]
Professor, Section on Neurobiology, Colleges of Natural Sciences and Pharmacy, and Director, Waggoner Center for Alcohol and Addiction Research, University of Texas at Austin, Austin, Texas

Frederick G. Hayden, M.D. [50]
Stuart S. Richardson Professor of Clinical Virology, Professor of Internal Medicine and Pathology, and Associate Director, Clinical Microbiology Laboratory, University of Virginia Health Sciences Center, Charlottesville, Virginia

Robert S. Hillman, M.D. [54]
Professor of Medicine, University of Vermont College of Medicine, Burlington, Vermont

Brian B. Hoffman, M.D. [6, 10]
Professor of Medicine, Stanford University School of Medicine, Geriatrics Research, Education and Clinical Center, Veterans Affairs Medical Center, Palo Alto, California

Willemijntje A. Hoogerwerf, M.D. [37]
Assistant Professor of Medicine, University of Texas Medical Branch, Galveston, Texas

Edwin K. Jackson, Ph.D. [29, 30, 31]
Professor of Pharmacology and Medicine, and Associate Director, Center for Clinical Pharmacology, University of Pittsburgh Medical Center, Pittsburgh, Pennsylvania

Syed Fazle-Ali Jafri, M.D. [39]
Assistant Professor of Internal Medicine and Clinical Associate Director, Division of Gastroenterology, University of Texas Medical Branch, Galveston, Texas

Roger A. Johns, M.D. [16]
Mark C. Rogers Professor and Chair, Department of Anesthesiology and Critical Care Medicine, The Johns Hopkins University School of Medicine, Baltimore, Maryland

Terry P. Kenakin, Ph.D. [2]
Principal Research Scientist, Glaxo Wellcome Research and Development, Research Triangle Park, North Carolina

David M. Kerins, M.D. [32]
Assistant Professor of Medicine, Vanderbilt University School of Medicine, Nashville, Tennessee

Curtis D. Klaassen, Ph.D. [4, 67, 68]
Professor of Pharmacology and Toxicology, University of Kansas Medical Center, Kansas City, Kansas

Alan M. Krensky, M.D. [53]
Shelagh Galligan Professor of Pediatrics and Chief, Division of Immunology & Transplantation Biology, Stanford University School of Medicine, Palo Alto, California

Lawrence M. Lichtenstein, M.D., Ph.D. [28]
Professor of Medicine and Director, Division of Clinical Immunology. The Johns Hopkins University School of Medicine, Director, Johns Hopkins Asthma and Allergy Center, Baltimore, Maryland

Paul R. Lichter, M.D. [66]
F. Bruce Fralick Professor of Ophthalmology and Chair, Department of Ophthalmology and Visual Sciences, University of Michigan, W.K. Kellogg Eye Center, Ann Arbor, Michigan

David S. Loose-Mitchell, Ph.D. [58]
Associate Professor of Integrative Biology and Pharmacology, University of Texas Health Science Center at Houston, Houston, Texas

Kenneth Mackie, M.D. [15]
Associate Professor of Anesthesiology and of Physiology and Biophysics, University of Washington School of Medicine, Seattle, Washington

Robert W. Mahley, M.D., Ph.D. [36]
Professor of Pathology and Medicine, University of California, San Francisco, and Director, Gladstone Institute of Cardiovascular Disease, San Francisco, California

Philip W. Majerus, M.D. [55]
Professor of Medicine and Biochemistry, Division of Hematology, Washington University School of Medicine, St. Louis, Missouri

Robert Marcus, M.D. [62, 63, 64]
Professor of Medicine, Stanford University School of Medicine, and Director, Aging Study Unit, Geriatrics Research, Education and Clinical Center, Veterans Affairs Medical Center, Palo Alto, California

Steven E. Mayer, Ph.D. [11]
Professor Emeritus of Pharmacology, University of California San Diego, La Jolla, California

James O. McNamara, M.D. [21]
Carl R. Deane Professor of Neuroscience in the Departments of Medicine (Neurology), Neurobiology, and Pharmacology, Duke University Medical Center, Durham, North Carolina

S. John Mihic, Ph.D. [17, 18]
Associate Professor, Section of Neurobiology, College of Natural Sciences, Waggoner Center for Alcohol and Addiction Research, University of Texas at Austin, Austin, Texas

Eric J. Moody, M.D. [16]
Associate Professor of Anesthesiology and Critical Care Medicine, The Johns Hopkins University School of Medicine, Baltimore, Maryland

Sayoko E. Moroi, M.D., Ph.D. [66]
Assistant Professor of Ophthalmology, Department of Ophthalmology and Visual Sciences, University of Michigan, W.K. Kellogg Eye Center, Ann Arbor, Michigan

Jason D. Morrow, M.D. [26, 27]
F. Tremaine Billings Professor of Medicine and Pharmacology, Vanderbilt University School of Medicine, Nashville, Tennessee

Alan S. Nies, M.D. [3]
Senior Vice President, Clinical Sciences, Merck Research Laboratories, Rahway, New Jersey

John A. Oates, M.D. [33]
Thomas F. Frist Sr. Professor of Medicine and Professor of Pharmacology, Vanderbilt University School of Medicine, Nashville, Tennessee

Charles P. O'Brien, M.D., Ph.D. [24]
Professor and Vice Chair, Department of Psychiatry, University of Pennsylvania School of Medicine, and Chief of Psychiatry, Veterans Administration Medical Center, Philadelphia, Pennsylvania

Henry Ooi, M.B., M.R.C.P.I. [34]
Cardiomyopathy Fellow, Section of Cardiology, Boston University Medical Center, Boston, Massachusetts

Keith L. Parker, M.D., Ph.D. [56, 60]
Wilson Distinguished Professor of Biomedical Research, Departments of Internal Medicine and Pharmacology, University of Texas Southwestern Medical Center, Dallas, Texas

Pankaj J. Pasricha, M.D. [37, 38, 39]
Associate Professor of Medicine, Anatomy and Neuroscience; Senior Scientist, Department of Biomedical Engineering; Chief, Division of Gastroenterology and Hepatology, University of Texas Medical Branch, Galveston, Texas

Luiz Paz-Ares, M.D. [52]
Department of Medical Oncology, Hospital Universitario Doce de Octubre, Madrid, Spain

William A. Petri Jr., M.D., Ph.D. [44, 45, 48]
Professor of Internal Medicine, Pathology, and Microbiology, Division of Infectious Diseases, University of Virginia Health Sciences Center, Charlottesville, Virginia

Stephen Paul Raffanti, M.D. [51]
Associate Professor of Medicine, Division of Infectious Diseases, Vanderbilt University School of Medicine, Nashville, Tennessee

L. Jackson Roberts, II, M.D. [25, 26, 27]
Professor of Pharmacology and Medicine, Vanderbilt University School of Medicine, Nashville, Tennessee

David Robertson, M.D. [32]
Professor of Medicine, Pharmacology, and Neurology, and Director, Clinical Research Center, Vanderbilt University School of Medicine, Nashville, Tennessee

Rose Marie Robertson, M.D. [32]
Professor and Vice Chair for Special Projects, Department of Medicine, Vanderbilt University School of Medicine, Nashville, Tennessee

Dan Roden, M.D., C.M. [35, Appendix I]
Professor of Medicine and Pharmacology, and Director, Division of Clinical Pharmacology, Vanderbilt University School of Medicine, Nashville, Tennessee

Christopher S. Rogers, B.S. [5]
Graduate Student, Department of Pharmacology, Vanderbilt University School of Medicine, Nashville, Tennessee

Elliott M. Ross, Ph.D. [2]
Professor of Pharmacology, University of Texas Southwestern Medical Center, Dallas, Texas

David Ryan, M.D. [52]
Instructor in Medicine, Harvard Medical School, Boston, Massachusetts

Elaine Sanders-Bush, Ph.D. [11]
Professor of Pharmacology and Psychiatry, Vanderbilt University School of Medicine, Nashville, Tennessee

Bernard P. Schimmer, Ph.D. [56, 60]
Professor of Medical Research and Pharmacology, Banting & Best Department of Medical Research, University of Toronto, Toronto, Ontario, Canada

Danny D. Shen, Ph.D. [Appendix II]
Professor and Chair, Department of Pharmacy, University of Washington School of Pharmacy, Seattle, Washington

Brett A. Simon, M.D., Ph.D. [16]
Associate Professor of Anesthesiology and Critical Care Medicine, The Johns Hopkins University School of Medicine, Baltimore, Maryland

Peter J. Snyder, M.D. [59]
Professor of Medicine, University of Pennsylvania School of Medicine, Philadelphia, Pennsylvania

George M. Stancel, Ph.D. [58]
Dean, Graduate School of Biomedical Sciences, and Professor of Integrative Biology and Pharmacology, University of Texas Health Science Center at Houston, Houston, Texas

David G. Standaert, M.D., Ph.D. [22]
Associate Professor of Neurology, Harvard Medical School and Massachusetts General Hospital, Neurology, Boston, Massachusetts

Terry B. Strom, M.D. [53]
Professor of Medicine, Harvard Medical School, Beth Israel Deaconess Medical Center, Boston, Massachusetts

Bruce A. Sullenger, Ph.D. [5]
Vice Chair, Department of Surgery, Duke University Medical Center, Durham, North Carolina

Steven H. Sutter, M.D. [65]
Assistant Professor of Dermatology, University of Oklahoma College of Medicine, Oklahoma City, Oklahoma

Frank I. Tarazi, Ph.D. [20]
Assistant Professor of Psychiatry and Neuroscience, Harvard Medical School, and Associate Neuropharmacologist, Mailman Research Center, McLean Division of Massachusetts General Hospital, Boston, Massachusetts

Palmer Taylor, Ph.D. [6, 7, 8, 9]
Sandra and Monroe Trout Professor and Chair, Department of Pharmacology, School of Medicine, University of California San Diego, La Jolla, California

Kenneth E. Thummel, Ph.D. [Appendix II]
Associate Professor of Pharmaceutics, University of Washington School of Pharmacy, Seattle, Washington

Douglas M. Tollefsen, M.D., Ph.D. [55]
Professor of Medicine, Division of Hematology, Washington University School of Medicine, St. Louis, Missouri

James W. Tracy, Ph.D. [40, 41, 42]
Professor of Comparative Biosciences and Pharmacology, Associate Dean for Research and Graduate Training, School of Veterinary Medicine, University of Wisconsin, Madison, Wisconsin

Bradley J. Undem, Ph.D. [28]
Professor of Medicine, The Johns Hopkins University School of Medicine, Johns Hopkins Asthma and Allergy Center, Baltimore, Maryland

Leslie T. Webster, Jr., M.D., Sc.D. (Hon.) [40, 41, 42]
John H. Hord Professor of Pharmacology, Emeritus, Case Western Reserve University School of Medicine, Cleveland, Ohio

Grant R. Wilkinson, Ph.D., D.Sc. [1]
Professor of Pharmacology, Vanderbilt University School of Medicine, Nashville, Tennessee

Eric L. Wyatt, M.D. [65]
Dermatologist in private practice, Oklahoma City, Oklahoma

Anne B. Young, M.D., Ph.D. [22]
Julieanne Dorn Professor of Neurology, Harvard Medical School, and Chief, Department of Neurology, Massachusetts General Hospital, Boston, Massachusetts

Consultants to the Editors

Consultants to the Editors

Joseph Awad, M.D.
Jeffrey Balser, M.D., Ph.D.
Douglas H. Brown, M.D.
Brian M. Cox, Ph.D.
Lauralea Edwards, D.Ph.

Raymond C. Harris, Jr., M.D.
J. Harold Helderman, M.D.
Christopher D. Lind, M.D.
Denis M. O'Day, M.D.
Paul Ragan, M.D.

William Schaffner, M.D.
Richard G. Shelton, M.D.
Douglas E. Vaughan, M.D.
Ronald G. Wiley, M.D., Ph.D.
Alastair Wood, M.D.

Preface

The tenth edition of *Goodman and Gilman's The Pharmacological Basis of Therapeutics* marks the sixtieth anniversary of this book. The objectives that guided the two original authors in writing the first edition have continued to guide authors and editors of subsequent editions, including this one. These objectives—stated in the preface to the first edition, which is reprinted herein—are: correlation of pharmacology with related medical sciences, reinterpretation of the actions and uses of drugs from the viewpoint of important advances in medicine, and placing of emphasis on the application of pharmacodynamics to therapeutics.

We are indebted to the new and returning contributors to this edition, who worked diligently to revise and update their chapters in a field that is undergoing change at a remarkable pace, and we are grateful to our consultants, who reviewed and made suggestions for improving many chapters. We also are pleased to acknowledge three other individuals who played indispensable roles in the preparation of this edition. Lauralea Edwards, D.Ph., provided thorough and well-researched reviews of the text for accuracy of pharmaceutical information and in addition assisted the editors in the early planning of the edition. Tracy Shields as editorial assistant worked tenaciously and efficiently and with much initiative in preparing the final chapter manuscripts submitted to the publisher and in documenting the accuracy of references. Lynne Hutchison served as managing editor for this edition. Her superb organization and management of the editorial office, effective and diplomatic interactions with contributors and the publisher, well-developed literary skills, and enthusiasm for the project made the many pieces of the book come together in a timely and accurate fashion. The completion of this edition would not have been possible, much less pleasurable, without the dedicated work of these talented women. We also appreciate the help of John Morriss and Kathleen McCullough of McGraw-Hill.

The timing of the publication of the tenth edition of this book, the first edition of the new millennium, is significant. We witness a spectacular revolution in biology and biomedical science that is coupled inexorably with unparalleled access to information. We are struck by a profound tension between knowledge and wisdom. We earnestly seek both. But they fight with each other, particularly when we teach, write, and reason. How do we transmit our intellectual heritage while sustaining the necessary context of insight and applicability? What is the next-generation biomedical textbook to be? Certainly not just a database; print pages will retain their place as a necessary medium of analysis and reason.

Our history provides guidance to meet this challenge. The first edition of this book often is credited with establishing pharmacology as a discipline. This accolade was not earned because of organized exposition of facts, but rather because of synthesis of pharmacological information and application of this synthesis to clinical science. The original authors of this book, Louis S. Goodman and Alfred Gilman, made many contributions as researchers, teachers, and sage advisors, but commentators note the creation of this work as their most notable accomplishment. This opinion is borne out by the continuation of the book through ten editions. The careful reader can find many scholarly passages in this edition that appeared in the first and second editions of this book. The seventh edition of this book (1985) was dedicated to Alfred Gilman shortly after his death. The eighth edition (1990) was dedicated to Louis Goodman as he retired from an active editorial role. Louis Goodman, the founder of this book, died on November 19, 2000. He is remembered fondly for his wisdom, scholarship, gruff sense of humor, impeccable sense of perfection, and infuriatingly successful motivational orations for those who would rise to the challenge.

We rededicate this edition to Louis S. Goodman and Alfred Gilman in recognition of their vision and many contributions and with the hope that the need met by the first edition of this book will be met by this and subsequent editions. A book such as this will remain extraordinarily valuable if its heritors adhere to its founding precepts envisioned by these two men.

ALFRED GOODMAN GILMAN
JOEL G. HARDMAN
LEE E. LIMBIRD

June 5, 2001

Preface to the First Edition

Three objectives have guided the writing of this book—the correlation of pharmacology with related medical sciences, the reinterpretation of the actions and uses of drugs from the viewpoint of important advances in medicine, and the placing of emphasis on the applications of pharmacodynamics to therapeutics.

Although pharmacology is a basic medical science in its own right, it borrows freely from and contributes generously to the subject matter and technics of many medical disciplines, clinical as well as preclinical. Therefore, the correlation of strictly pharmacological information with medicine as a whole is essential for a proper presentation of pharmacology to students and physicians. Furthermore, the reinterpretation of the actions and uses of well-established therapeutic agents in the light of recent advances in the medical sciences is as important a function of a modern textbook of pharmacology as is the description of new drugs. In many instances these new interpretations necessitate radical departures from accepted but outworn concepts of the actions of drugs. Lastly, the emphasis throughout the book, as indicated in its title, has been clinical. This is mandatory because medical students must be taught pharmacology from the standpoint of the actions and uses of drugs in the prevention and treatment of disease. To the student, pharmacological data per se are valueless unless he/she is able to apply this information in the practice of medicine. This book has also been written for the practicing physician, to whom it offers an opportunity to keep abreast of recent advances in therapeutics and to acquire the basic principles necessary for the rational use of drugs in his/her daily practice.

The criteria for the selection of bibliographic references require comment. It is obviously unwise, if not impossible, to document every fact included in the text. Preference has therefore been given to articles of a review nature, to the literature on new drugs, and to original contributions in controversial fields. In most instances, only the more recent investigations have been cited. In order to encourage free use of the bibliography, references are chiefly to the available literature in the English language.

The authors are greatly indebted to their many colleagues at the Yale University School of Medicine for their generous help and criticism. In particular they are deeply grateful to Professor Henry Gray Barbour, whose constant encouragement and advice have been invaluable.

LOUIS S. GOODMAN
ALFRED GILMAN

New Haven, Connecticut
November 20, 1940

S E C T I O N   I

GENERAL PRINCIPLES

INTRODUCTION
Alfred Goodman Gilman

Publication of the tenth edition of *Goodman and Gilman's The Pharmacological Basis of Therapeutics,* the first new-millennium edition of a textbook that has documented six decades of spectacular progress in both the basic and applied aspects of pharmacology, provokes both retrospection and thoughts of the future.

Some things do not change. The first (1941) edition of this textbook began: "The subject of pharmacology is a broad one and embraces the knowledge of the source, physical and chemical properties, compounding, physiological actions, absorption, fate, and excretion, and therapeutic uses of drugs. A *drug* may be broadly defined as any chemical agent which affects living protoplasm, and few substances would escape inclusion by this definition." It is a tribute to both the original authors and to the validity of their definition of the discipline that this paragraph has appeared virtually unchanged in every subsequent edition of this work.

Most things do change. Comparison of the table of contents of the first and current edition of this textbook offers a concise but amazing view of progress during a single lifetime. For example, in the first edition, the section entitled *Chemotherapy of Infectious Diseases* spans 182 pages, but there is no mention of an antibiotic; instead there are four chapters on syphilotherapy and four more on the sulfonamides. *Cancer* is not found in the index, and *carcinoma* provides only cursory references to pain relief. Antihypertensives, antipsychotics, and antidepressants are not present in 1941, and the list goes on and on.

This progress, so evident, has many mothers, particularly chemistry, all of the basic biomedical disciplines, and all of the clinical specialties. Techniques of chemical synthesis have improved enormously and now include the powerful approach of combinatorial chemistry; these provide the raw materials for the pharmacopoeia. Detailed understanding of both normal and pathological physiology and biochemistry bring mechanistic insight into disease. Molecular biology and genetics offer powerful DNA-based technologies for decoding the blueprints for all organisms, assigning functions to unknown genes, identifying inherited contributions to disease, and synthesizing human proteins in cultured microbes or mammalian cells for use as therapeutic agents. Equally critical are appropriate experimental and statistical approaches to therapy; the double-blind, placebo-controlled clinical trial is the *sine qua non.* Pharmacology draws on all of these disciplines and their techniques to identify disease-relevant targets (receptors) for drug actions, select the chemicals best suited to manipulate each target, understand in detail the consequences of the drug–receptor interaction, maximize the specificity of drug interaction, minimize toxicity, optimize and vary the pharmacokinetic profiles of drugs, and prove that the agents identified are in fact appropriate for clinical use.

The chapters included in Section I of this book provide understanding of the basic principles that underlie both current therapy and the advances that will be witnessed by all interested in pharmacology and medicine. In brief, *pharmacokinetics* (Chapter 1) explores the factors that determine the relationship between drug dosage and the time-varying concentration of drug at its site(s) of action. The practical importance of these relationships is enormous, and the critical pharmacokinetic parameters that dictate the use of many important therapeutic agents are tabulated in Appendix II. *Pharmacodynamics* (Chapter 2) is, in turn, concerned with the relationships between the concentration of drugs at its site(s) of action and the magnitude of effect that is achieved. Included in this discussion is consideration of mechanism of drug action, the most basic aspect of pharmacology. A push-button physician does not understand *how* a drug works and thus ignores an opportunity to individualize therapy for each patient. A curious and thoughtful physician will use such understanding to build a rational framework for optimal and individualized use of drugs. Appreciation of pharmacodynamics, coupled with knowledge of normal and pathological function, permits wise choices for specific situations, to say nothing of the satisfaction that comes from best practice.

The concepts of pharmacokinetics and pharmacodynamics, together with those of *toxicology* (Chapter 4), come to focus in Chapter 3, *Principles of Therapeutics.* The introduction to this chapter contains a truly important statement: "Because all patients differ in their responses to drugs, *each therapeutic encounter* must be considered an experiment with a hypothesis that can be tested." The discussion provides the basis for such critical behavior. The push-button physician does not appreciate the opportunity that such behavior affords.

Chapter 5, *Gene Therapy,* offers a view of a future in which physicians practice molecular surgery to replace genes whose products are not expressed or whose functions have been lost (*e.g.,* in cystic fibrosis, muscular dystrophy, primary hypercholesterolemia), to repair genes whose functions have been altered (*e.g.,* with ribozymes), or to silence aberrant dominant genes (*e.g.,* with antisense oligonucleotides or ribozymes). The capacity to detect *in utero* mutations transmitted in germ cells will have a major impact on inherited genetic disease. The hoped-for ability to replace or repair defective genes in somatic cells offers enormous promise for acquired (or inherited) genetic disease—cancer being the superlative example.

Sequencing of the genomes of many species, including the human genome and those of a variety of human pathogens, is a true landmark in biology—one that will likely remain at or near the top of the list forever. The coincidence of these events with the arrival of a new century will make easy the ultimate designation of 20th-century biomedicine as pregenome practice and 21st-century biomedicine as a new era. The information in the genomes enables not only the discussion of gene therapy and selection of new targets for chemotherapy of infectious disease, but also much more. The path is visible to knowledge of the expression of every exon in the human genome in every cell type in a wide variety of normal and pathological situations. We have nonbiased, broadly applicable approaches to discover the functions of thousands of genes that are still mysterious. Knowledge of the molecular basis of normal and abnormal function is thus exploding, as will ways to exploit such knowledge. We have acquired simultaneously the means to express in heterologous systems and therefore interrogate the products of human genes. We will learn all of their secrets—for example, their catalytic activities and the identities of their interacting partners. Additional knowledge of the atomic structures of these molecules and the precise bases for their interactions with other cellular players will permit manipulation of these activities with ever more specific drugs designed to have one action and only that action.

In the current political environment, we hear alarm that the cost of drugs is rising, constituting an ever-increasing fraction of healthcare expenditures. Although the cost of drug discovery is extremely high, drug therapy usually is very inexpensive, in terms of overall healthcare costs, if it obviates or shortens hospitalization. We should look forward with joy to an era when the cost of drug therapy, including gene therapy, constitutes the vast majority of the healthcare budget, when hospitals exist only as trauma centers, and when life is not compromised by long-term disability or ended prematurely by disease.

PHARMACOKINETICS

The Dynamics of Drug Absorption, Distribution, and Elimination

Grant R. Wilkinson

To produce its characteristic effects, a drug must be present in appropriate concentrations at its sites of action. Although obviously a function of the amount of drug administered, the concentrations of active, unbound (free) drug attained also depend upon the extent and rate of its absorption, distribution (which mainly reflects relative binding to plasma and tissue proteins), metabolism (biotransformation), and excretion. These disposition factors are depicted in Figure 1–1 and are described in this chapter.

PHYSICOCHEMICAL FACTORS IN TRANSFER OF DRUGS ACROSS MEMBRANES

The absorption, distribution, metabolism, and excretion of a drug all involve its passage across cell membranes. Mechanisms by which drugs cross membranes and the physicochemical properties of molecules and membranes that influence this transfer are, therefore, important. The determining characteristics of a drug are its molecular size and shape, degree of ionization, relative lipid solubility of

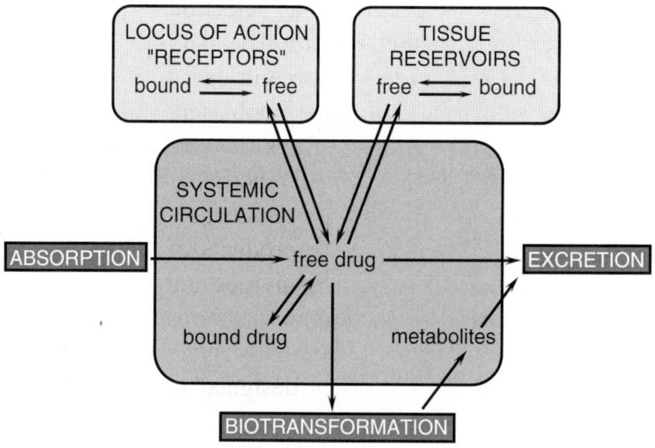

Figure 1–1. Schematic representation of the interrelationship of the absorption, distribution, binding, metabolism, and excretion of a drug and its concentration at its locus of action.

Possible distribution and binding of metabolites are not depicted.

its ionized and nonionized forms, and its binding to tissue proteins.

When a drug permeates a cell, it obviously must traverse the cellular plasma membrane. Other barriers to drug movement may be a single layer of cells (intestinal epithelium) or several layers of cells (skin). Despite such structural differences, the diffusion and transport of drugs across these various boundaries have many common characteristics, since drugs in general pass through cells rather than between them. The plasma membrane thus represents the common barrier.

Cell Membranes. The plasma membrane consists of a bilayer of amphipathic lipids, with their hydrocarbon chains oriented inward to form a continuous hydrophobic phase and their hydrophilic heads oriented outward. Individual lipid molecules in the bilayer vary according to the particular membrane and can move laterally, endowing the membrane with fluidity, flexibility, high electrical resistance, and relative impermeability to highly polar molecules. Membrane proteins embedded in the bilayer serve as receptors, ion channels, or transporters to elicit electrical or chemical signaling pathways and provide selective targets for drug actions.

Most cell membranes are relatively permeable to water either by diffusion or by flow resulting from hydrostatic or osmotic differences across the membrane, and bulk flow of water can carry with it drug molecules. Such transport is the major mechanism by which drugs pass across most capillary endothelial membranes. However, proteins and drug molecules bound to them are too large and polar for this type of transport to occur; thus, transcapillary movement is limited to unbound drug. Paracellular transport through intercellular gaps is sufficiently large that passage across most capillaries is limited by blood flow and not by other factors (*see* below). As described later, this type of transport is an important factor in filtration across glomerular membranes in the kidney. Important exceptions exist in such capillary diffusion, however, since "tight" intercellular junctions are present in specific tissues and paracellular transport in them is limited. Capillaries of the central nervous system (CNS) and a variety of epithelial tissues have tight junctions (*see* below). Although bulk flow of water can carry with it small, water-soluble substances, if the molecular mass of these compounds is greater than 100 to 200 daltons, such transport is limited. Accordingly, most large lipophilic drugs must pass through the cell membrane itself by one or more processes.

Passive Membrane Transport.   Drugs cross membranes either by passive processes or by mechanisms involving the active participation of components of the membrane. In the former, the drug molecule usually penetrates by passive diffusion along a concentration gradient by virtue of its solubility in the lipid bilayer. Such transfer is directly proportional to the magnitude of the concentration gradient across the membrane, the lipid:water partition coefficient of the drug, and the cell surface area. The greater the partition coefficient, the higher is the concentration of drug in the membrane and the faster is its diffusion. After a steady state is attained, the concentration of the unbound drug is the same on both sides of the membrane if the drug is a nonelectrolyte. For ionic compounds, the steady-state concentrations will be dependent on differences in pH across the membrane, which may influence the state of ionization of the molecule on each side of the membrane and on the electrochemical gradient for the ion.

Weak Electrolytes and Influence of pH.   Most drugs are weak acids or bases that are present in solution as both the nonionized and ionized species. The nonionized molecules are usually lipid-soluble and can diffuse across the cell membrane. In contrast, the ionized molecules are usually unable to penetrate the lipid membrane because of their low lipid solubility.

   Therefore, the transmembrane distribution of a weak electrolyte usually is determined by its pK_a and the pH gradient across the membrane. The pK_a is the pH at which half of the drug (weak electrolyte) is in its ionized form. To illustrate the effect of pH on distribution of drugs, the partitioning of a weak acid ($pK_a = 4.4$) between plasma (pH = 7.4) and gastric juice (pH = 1.4) is depicted in Figure 1–2. It is assumed that the gastric mucosal membrane behaves as a simple lipid barrier that is permeable only to the lipid-soluble, nonionized form of the acid. The ratio of nonionized to ionized drug at each pH is readily calculated from the Henderson–Hasselbalch equation. Thus, in plasma, the ratio of nonionized to ionized drug is 1:1000; in gastric juice, the ratio is 1:0.001. These values are given in brackets in Figure 1–2. The total concentration ratio between the plasma and the gastric juice would therefore be 1000:1 if such a system came to a steady state. For a weak base with a pK_a of 4.4, the ratio would be reversed, as would the thick horizontal arrows in Figure 1–2, which indicate the predominant species at

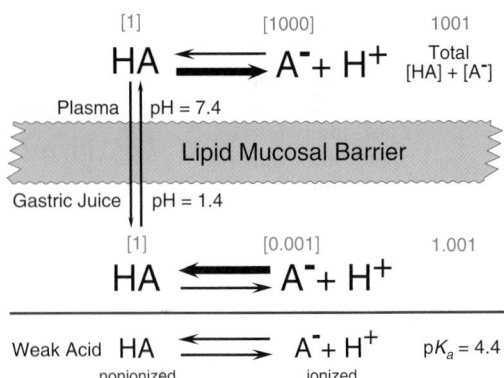

Figure 1–2. Influence of pH on the distribution of a weak acid between plasma and gastric juice, separated by a lipid barrier.

each pH. Accordingly, at steady state, an acidic drug will accumulate on the more basic side of the membrane and a basic drug on the more acidic side—a phenomenon termed *ion trapping*. These considerations have obvious implications for the absorption and excretion of drugs, as discussed more specifically below. The establishment of concentration gradients of weak electrolytes across membranes with a pH gradient is a purely physical process and does not require an active transport system. All that is necessary is a membrane preferentially permeable to one form of the weak electrolyte and a pH gradient across the membrane. The establishment of the pH gradient is, however, an active process.

Carrier-Mediated Membrane Transport.   While passive diffusion through the bilayer is dominant in the disposition of most drugs, carrier-mediated mechanisms also can play an important role. *Active transport* is characterized by a requirement for energy, movement against an electrochemical gradient, saturability, selectivity, and competitive inhibition by cotransported compounds. The term *facilitated diffusion* describes a carrier-mediated transport process in which there is no input of energy and therefore enhanced movement of the involved substance is down an electrochemical gradient. Such mechanisms, which may be highly selective for a specific conformational structure of a drug, are involved in the transport of endogenous compounds whose rate of transport by passive diffusion otherwise would be too slow. In other cases, they function as a barrier system to protect cells from potentially toxic substances.

   The responsible transporter proteins often are expressed within cell membranes in a domain-specific fashion such that they mediate either drug uptake or efflux, and often such an arrangement facilitates vectorial transport across cells. Thus, in the liver, a number of basolaterally localized transporters with different substrate specificities are involved in the uptake of bile acids and amphipathic organic anions and cations into the hepatocyte, and a similar variety of ATP-dependent transporters in the canalicular membrane export such compounds into the bile. Analogous situations also are present in intestinal and renal tubular membranes. An important efflux transporter present at these sites and also in the capillary endothelium of brain capillaries is P-glycoprotein, which is encoded by the multidrug resistance-1 (*MDR1*) gene, important in resistance to cancer chemotherapeutic agents (Chapter 52). P-glycoprotein localized in the enterocyte also limits the oral absorption of transported drugs since it exports the compound back into the intestinal tract subsequent to its absorption by passive diffusion.

DRUG ABSORPTION, BIOAVAILABILITY, AND ROUTES OF ADMINISTRATION

Absorption describes the rate at which a drug leaves its site of administration and the extent to which this occurs. However, the clinician is concerned primarily with a parameter designated as *bioavailability,* rather than absorption. *Bioavailability* is a term used to indicate the fractional extent to which a dose of drug reaches its site of action or a biological fluid from which the drug has access to its site of action. For example, a drug given orally must be absorbed first from the stomach and intestine, but this may be limited by the characteristics of the dosage form and/or the drug's physicochemical properties. In addition, drug then passes through the liver, where metabolism and/or biliary excretion may occur before it reaches the systemic circulation. Accordingly, a fraction of the administered and absorbed dose of drug will be inactivated or diverted before it can reach the general circulation and be distributed to its sites of action. If the metabolic or excretory capacity of the liver for the agent in question is large, bioavailability will be substantially reduced (the so-called *first-pass effect*). This decrease in availability is a function of the anatomical site from which absorption takes place; other anatomical, physiological, and pathological factors can influence bioavailability (*see* below), and the choice of the route of drug administration must be based on an understanding of these conditions.

Oral (Enteral) *versus* Parenteral Administration. Often there is a choice of the route by which a therapeutic agent may be given, and a knowledge of the advantages and disadvantages of the different routes of administration is then of primary importance. Some characteristics of the major routes employed for systemic drug effect are compared in Table 1–1.

Oral ingestion is the most common method of drug administration. It also is the safest, most convenient, and most economical. Disadvantages to the oral route include limited absorption of some drugs because of their physical characteristics (*e.g.,* water solubility), emesis as a result of irritation to the gastrointestinal mucosa, destruction of some drugs by digestive enzymes or low gastric pH,

irregularities in absorption or propulsion in the presence of food or other drugs, and necessity for cooperation on the part of the patient. In addition, drugs in the gastrointestinal tract may be metabolized by the enzymes of the intestinal flora, mucosa, or the liver before they gain access to the general circulation.

The parenteral injection of drugs has certain distinct advantages over oral administration. In some instances, parenteral administration is essential for the drug to be delivered in its active form. Availability is usually more rapid, extensive, and predictable than when a drug is given by mouth. The effective dose therefore can be more accurately delivered. In emergency therapy and when a patient is unconscious, uncooperative, or unable to retain anything given by mouth, parenteral therapy may be a necessity. The injection of drugs, however, has its disadvantages: asepsis must be maintained; pain may accompany the injection; it is sometimes difficult for patients to perform the injections themselves if self-medication is necessary; and there is the risk of inadvertent administration of a drug when it is not intended. Expense is another consideration.

Oral Ingestion. Absorption from the gastrointestinal tract is governed by factors such as surface area for absorption, blood flow to the site of absorption, the physical state of the drug (solution, suspension, or solid dosage form), its water solubility, and concentration at the site of absorption. For drugs given in solid form, the rate of dissolution may be the limiting factor in their absorption, especially if they have low water solubility. Since most drug absorption from the gastrointestinal tract occurs *via* passive processes, absorption is favored when the drug is in the nonionized and more lipophilic form. Based on the pH-partition concept presented in Figure 1–2, it would be predicted that drugs that are weak acids would be better absorbed from the stomach (pH 1 to 2) than from the upper intestine (pH 3 to 6), and *vice versa* for weak bases. However, the epithelium of the stomach is lined with a thick mucous layer, and its surface area is small; by contrast, the villi of the upper intestine provide an extremely large surface area ($\sim$200 m^2). Accordingly, the rate of absorption of a drug from the intestine will be greater than that from the stomach even if the drug is predominantly ionized in the intestine and largely nonionized in the stomach. Thus, any factor that accelerates gastric emptying will be likely to increase the rate of drug absorption, while any factor that delays gastric emptying will probably have the opposite effect, regardless of the characteristics of the drug.

Drugs that are destroyed by gastric juice or that cause gastric irritation sometimes are administered in dosage forms with a coating that prevents dissolution in the acidic gastric contents. However, some enteric-coated

Table 1–1

Some Characteristics of Common Routes of Drug Administration*

ROUTE	ABSORPTION PATTERN	SPECIAL UTILITY	LIMITATION AND PRECAUTIONS
Intravenous	Absorption circumvented Potentially immediate effects	Valuable for emergency use Permits titration of dosage Usually required for high-molecular-weight protein and peptide drugs Suitable for large volumes and for irritating substances, when diluted	Increased risk of adverse effects Must inject solutions *slowly,* as a rule Not suitable for oily solutions or insoluble substances
Subcutaneous	Prompt, from aqueous solution Slow and sustained, from repository preparations	Suitable for some insoluble suspensions and for implantation of solid pellets	Not suitable for large volumes Possible pain or necrosis from irritating substances
Intramuscular	Prompt, from aqueous solution Slow and sustained, from repository preparations	Suitable for moderate volumes, oily vehicles, and some irritating substances	Precluded during anticoagulant medication May interfere with interpretation of certain diagnostic tests (*e.g.,* creatine kinase)
Oral ingestion	Variable; depends upon many factors (*see* text)	Most convenient and economical; usually more safe	Requires patient cooperation Availability potentially erratic and incomplete for drugs that are poorly soluble, slowly absorbed, unstable, or extensively metabolized by the liver and/or gut

*See text for more complete discussion and for other routes.

preparations of a drug also may resist dissolution in the intestine, and very little of the drug may be absorbed.

Controlled-Release Preparations. The rate of absorption of a drug administered as a tablet or other solid oral-dosage form is partly dependent upon its rate of dissolution in the gastrointestinal fluids. This factor is the basis for the so-called *controlled-release, extended-release, sustained-release,* or *prolonged-action* pharmaceutical preparations that are designed to produce slow, uniform absorption of the drug for 8 hours or longer. Potential advantages of such preparations are reduction in the frequency of administration of the drug as compared with conventional dosage forms (possibly with improved compliance by the patient), maintenance of a therapeutic effect overnight, and decreased incidence and/or intensity of undesired effects by elimination of the peaks in drug concentration that often occur after administration of immediate-release dosage forms.

Many controlled-release preparations fulfill these expectations. However, such products have some drawbacks. Generally, interpatient variability, in terms of the systemic concentration of the drug that is achieved, is greater for controlled-release

than for immediate-release dosage forms. During repeated drug administration, trough drug concentrations resulting from controlled-release dosage forms may not be different from those observed with immediate-release preparations, although the time interval between trough concentrations is greater for a well-designed controlled-release product. It is possible that the dosage form may fail, and "dose-dumping" with resultant toxicity can occur, since the total dose of drug ingested at one time may be several times the amount contained in the conventional preparation. Controlled-release dosage forms are most appropriate for drugs with short half-lives (less than 4 hours). So-called controlled-release dosage forms are sometimes developed for drugs with long half-lives (greater than 12 hours). These usually more expensive products should not be prescribed unless specific advantages have been demonstrated.

Sublingual Administration. Absorption from the oral mucosa has special significance for certain drugs, despite the fact that the surface area available is small. For example, nitroglycerin is effective when retained sublingually because it is nonionic and has a very high lipid solubility. Thus, the drug is absorbed very rapidly. Nitroglycerin also is very potent; relatively few molecules need to be absorbed to produce the therapeutic effect. Since venous drainage from the mouth is to the superior vena cava, the drug also is protected from rapid hepatic first-pass metabolism, which is sufficient to prevent the appearance of any active nitroglycerin in the systemic circulation if the sublingual tablet is swallowed.

Rectal Administration.   The rectal route often is useful when oral ingestion is precluded because the patient is unconscious or when vomiting is present—a situation particularly relevant to young children. Approximately 50% of the drug that is absorbed from the rectum will bypass the liver; the potential for hepatic first-pass metabolism is thus less than that for an oral dose. However, rectal absorption often is irregular and incomplete, and many drugs cause irritation of the rectal mucosa.

Parenteral Injection.   The major routes of parenteral administration are intravenous, subcutaneous, and intramuscular. Absorption from subcutaneous and intramuscular sites occurs by simple diffusion along the gradient from drug depot to plasma. The rate is limited by the area of the absorbing capillary membranes and by the solubility of the substance in the interstitial fluid. Relatively large aqueous channels in the endothelial membrane account for the indiscriminate diffusion of molecules regardless of their lipid solubility. Larger molecules, such as proteins, slowly gain access to the circulation by way of lymphatic channels.

Drugs administered into the systemic circulation by any route, excluding the intraarterial route, are subject to possible first-pass elimination in the lung prior to distribution to the rest of the body. The lungs serve as a temporary storage site for a number of agents, especially drugs that are weak bases and are predominantly nonionized at the blood pH, apparently by their partition into lipid. The lungs also serve as a filter for particulate matter that may be given intravenously, and, of course, they provide a route of elimination for volatile substances.

Intravenous.   Factors relevant to absorption are circumvented by intravenous injection of drugs in aqueous solution, because bioavailability is complete and rapid. Also, drug delivery is controlled and achieved with an accuracy and immediacy not possible by any other procedure. In some instances, as in the induction of surgical anesthesia, the dose of a drug is not predetermined but is adjusted to the response of the patient. Also, certain irritating solutions can be given only in this manner, since the blood vessel walls are relatively insensitive, and the drug, if injected slowly, is greatly diluted by the blood.

As there are advantages to the use of this route of administration, so are there liabilities. Unfavorable reactions are likely to occur, since high concentrations of drug may be attained rapidly in both plasma and tissues.

Because of this, it is advisable to intravenously administer a drug slowly by infusion rather than by rapid injection, and with close monitoring of the patient's response. Furthermore, once the drug is injected there is no retreat. Repeated intravenous injections are dependent upon the ability to maintain a patent vein. Drugs in an oily vehicle or those that precipitate blood constituents or hemolyze erythrocytes should not be given by this route.

Subcutaneous.   Injection of a drug into a subcutaneous site often is used. It can be used only for drugs that are not irritating to tissue; otherwise, severe pain, necrosis, and tissue sloughing may occur. The rate of absorption following subcutaneous injection of a drug often is sufficiently constant and slow to provide a sustained effect. Moreover, it may be varied intentionally. For example, the rate of absorption of a suspension of insoluble insulin is slow compared with that of a soluble preparation of the hormone. The incorporation of a vasoconstrictor agent in a solution of a drug to be injected subcutaneously also retards absorption. Absorption of drugs implanted under the skin in a solid pellet form occurs slowly over a period of weeks or months; some hormones are effectively administered in this manner.

Intramuscular.   Drugs in aqueous solution are absorbed quite rapidly after intramuscular injection, depending upon the rate of blood flow to the injection site. This may be modulated to some extent by local heating, massage, or exercise. For example, jogging may cause a precipitous drop in blood sugar when insulin is injected into the thigh, rather than into the arm or abdominal wall, since running markedly increases blood flow to the leg. Generally, the rate of absorption following injection of an aqueous preparation into the deltoid or vastus lateralis is faster than when the injection is made into the gluteus maximus. The rate is particularly slower for females after injection into the gluteus maximus. This has been attributed to the different distribution of subcutaneous fat in males and females, since fat is relatively poorly perfused. Very obese or emaciated patients may exhibit unusual patterns of absorption following intramuscular or subcutaneous injection. Very slow, constant absorption from the intramuscular site results if the drug is injected in solution in oil or suspended in various other repository vehicles. Antibiotics often are administered in this manner. Substances too irritating to be injected subcutaneously sometimes may be given intramuscularly.

Intraarterial.   Occasionally a drug is injected directly into an artery to localize its effect in a particular tissue or organ—for example, in the treatment of liver tumors and head/neck cancers. Diagnostic agents are sometimes administered by this route. Intraarterial injection requires great care and should be reserved for experts. The first-pass and cleansing effects of the lung are not available when drugs are given by this route.

Intrathecal. The blood-brain barrier and the blood–cerebrospinal fluid barrier often preclude or slow the entrance of drugs into the CNS. Therefore, when local and rapid effects of drugs on the meninges or cerebrospinal axis are desired, as in spinal anesthesia or acute CNS infections, drugs are sometimes injected directly into the spinal subarachnoid space. Brain tumors also may be treated by direct intraventricular drug administration.

Pulmonary Absorption.   Provided that they do not cause irritation, gaseous and volatile drugs may be inhaled and absorbed through the pulmonary epithelium and mucous membranes of the respiratory tract. Access to the circulation is rapid by this route, because the lung's surface area is large. The principles governing absorption and excretion of anesthetic and other therapeutic gases are discussed in Chapters 13, 14, and 16.

In addition, solutions of drugs can be atomized and the fine droplets in air (aerosol) inhaled. Advantages are the almost instantaneous absorption of a drug into the blood, avoidance of hepatic first-pass loss, and, in the case of pulmonary disease, local application of the drug at the desired site of action. For example, drugs can be given in this manner for the treatment of bronchial asthma (*see* Chapter 28). Past disadvantages, such as poor ability to regulate the dose and cumbersomeness of the methods of administration, have to a large extent been overcome by technological advances, including metered-dose inhalers and more reliable aerolizers.

Pulmonary absorption is an important route of entry of certain drugs of abuse and of toxic environmental substances of varied composition and physical states. Both local and systemic reactions to allergens may occur subsequent to inhalation.

Topical Application.   ***Mucous Membranes.*** Drugs are applied to the mucous membranes of the conjunctiva, nasopharynx, oropharynx, vagina, colon, urethra, and urinary bladder primarily for their local effects. Occasionally, as in the application of synthetic antidiuretic hormone to the nasal mucosa, systemic absorption is the goal. Absorption through mucous membranes occurs readily. In fact, local anesthetics applied for local effect sometimes may be absorbed so rapidly that they produce systemic toxicity.

Skin.   Few drugs readily penetrate the intact skin. Absorption of those that do is dependent on the surface area over which they are applied and to their lipid solubility, since the epidermis behaves as a lipid barrier (*see* Chapter 65). The dermis, however, is freely permeable to many solutes; consequently, systemic absorption of drugs occurs much more readily through abraded, burned, or denuded skin. Inflammation and other conditions that increase cutaneous blood flow also enhance absorption. Toxic effects sometimes are produced by absorption through the skin of highly lipid-soluble substances (*e.g.,* a lipid-soluble insecticide in an organic solvent). Absorption through the skin can be enhanced by suspending the drug in an oily vehicle and rubbing the resulting preparation into the skin. Because hydrated skin is more permeable than dry skin, the dosage form may be modified or an occlusive dressing may be used to facilitate absorption. Controlled-release topical patches are becoming increasingly available. A patch containing scopolamine, placed behind the ear where body temperature and blood flow enhance absorption, releases sufficient drug to the systemic circulation to protect the wearer from motion sickness. Transdermal estrogen replacement therapy yields low maintenance levels of estradiol while minimizing the high estrone metabolite levels observed following oral administration.

Eye.   Topically applied ophthalmic drugs are used primarily for their local effects (*see* Chapter 66). Systemic absorption that results from drainage through the nasolacrimal canal is usually undesirable. In addition, drug that is absorbed after such drainage is not subject to first-pass hepatic elimination. Unwanted systemic pharmacological effects may occur for this reason when β-adrenergic receptor antagonists are administered as ophthalmic drops. Local effects usually require absorption of the drug through the cornea; corneal infection or trauma thus may result in more rapid absorption. Ophthalmic delivery systems that provide prolonged duration of action (*e.g.,* suspensions and ointments) are useful additions to ophthalmic therapy. Ocular inserts, developed more recently, provide continuous delivery of low amounts of drug. Very little is lost through drainage; hence, systemic side effects are minimized.

Bioequivalence.   Drugs are not administered as such; instead, they are formulated into drug dosage forms. Drug products are considered to be pharmaceutical equivalents if they contain the same active ingredients and are identical in strength or concentration, dosage form, and route of administration. Two pharmaceutically equivalent drug products are considered to be bioequivalent when the rates and extents of bioavailability of the active ingredient in the two products are not significantly different under suitable test conditions. In the past, dosage forms of a drug from different manufacturers and even different lots of preparations from a single manufacturer sometimes differed in their bioavailability. Such differences were seen primarily among oral dosage forms of poorly soluble, slowly absorbed drugs. They result from differences in crystal form, particle size, or other physical characteristics of the drug that are not rigidly controlled in formulation and manufacture of the preparations. These factors affect disintegration of the dosage form and dissolution of the drug and hence the rate and extent of drug absorption.

The potential nonequivalence of different drug preparations has been a matter of concern. Strengthened regulatory requirements have resulted in few, if any, documented cases of nonequivalence between approved drug products. The significance of possible nonequivalence of drug preparations is further discussed in connection with drug nomenclature and the choice of drug name in writing prescription orders (*see* Appendix I).

DISTRIBUTION OF DRUGS

Following absorption or administration into the systemic blood, a drug distributes into interstitial and intracellular fluids. This process reflects a number of physiological factors and the particular physicochemical properties of the individual drug. Cardiac output, regional blood flow, and tissue volume determine the rate of delivery and potential amount of drug distributed into tissues. Initially, liver, kidney, brain, and other well-perfused organs receive most of the drug, whereas delivery to muscle, most viscera, skin, and fat is slower. This second distribution phase may require minutes to several hours before the concentration of drug in tissue is in distribution equilibrium with that in blood. The second phase also involves a far larger fraction of body mass than does the initial phase and generally accounts for most of the extravascularly distributed drug. With exceptions such as the brain, diffusion of drug into the interstitial fluid occurs rapidly because of the highly permeable nature of the capillary endothelial membrane. Thus, tissue distribution is determined by the partitioning of drug between blood and the particular tissue. Lipid solubility is an important determinant of such uptake as is any pH gradient between intracellular and extracellular fluids for drugs that are either weak acids or bases. However, in general, ion trapping associated with the latter factor is not large, since the pH difference (7.0 *versus* 7.4) is small. The more important determinant of blood:tissue partitioning is the relative binding of drug to plasma proteins and tissue macromolecules.

Plasma Proteins. Many drugs are bound to plasma proteins, mostly to plasma albumin for acidic drugs and to α_1-acid glycoprotein for basic drugs; binding to other plasma proteins generally occurs to a much smaller extent. The binding is usually reversible; covalent binding of reactive drugs such as alkylating agents occurs occasionally.

The fraction of total drug in plasma that is bound is determined by the drug concentration, its affinity for the binding sites, and the number of binding sites. Simple mass-action relationships determine the unbound and bound concentrations (*see* Chapter 2). At low concentrations of drug (less than the plasma-protein binding dissociation constant), the fraction bound is a function of the concentration of binding sites and the dissociation constant. At high drug concentrations (greater than the dissociation constant), the fraction bound is a function of the number of binding sites and the drug concentration. Therefore, plasma binding is a saturable and nonlinear process. For most drugs, however, the therapeutic range of plasma concentrations is limited; thus, the extent of binding and the unbound fraction is relatively constant. The percentage values listed in Appendix II refer only to this situation unless otherwise indicated. The extent of plasma binding also may be affected by disease-related factors. For example, hypoalbuminemia secondary to severe liver disease or the nephrotic syndrome results in reduced binding and an increase in the unbound fraction. Also, conditions resulting in the acute phase reaction response (cancer, arthritis, myocardial infarction, Crohn's disease) lead to elevated levels of α_1-acid glycoprotein and enhanced binding of basic drugs.

Because binding of drugs to plasma proteins is rather nonselective, many drugs with similar physicochemical characteristics can compete with each other and with endogenous substances for these binding sites. For example, displacement of unconjugated bilirubin from binding to albumin by the sulfonamides and other organic anions is known to increase the risk of bilirubin encephalopathy in the newborn. Concern for drug toxicities based on a similar competition between drugs for binding sites has, in the past, been overemphasized. Since drug responses, both efficacious and toxic, are a function of unbound concentrations, steady-state unbound concentrations will change only when either drug input (dosing rate) or clearance of unbound drug is changed [*see* Equation (1–1) and discussion later in this chapter]. Thus, steady-state unbound concentrations are independent of the extent of protein binding. However, for narrow-therapeutic-index drugs, a transient change in unbound concentrations occurring immediately following the dose of a displacing drug could be of concern. A more common problem resulting from competition of drugs for plasma-protein binding sites is misinterpretation of measured concentrations of drugs in plasma, since most assays do not distinguish free drug from bound drug.

Importantly, binding of a drug to plasma proteins limits its concentration in tissues and at its locus of action, since only unbound drug is in equilibrium across membranes. Accordingly, after distribution equilibrium is achieved, the concentration of active, unbound drug in intracellular water is the same as that in plasma except when carrier-mediated transport is involved. Binding also limits glomerular filtration of the drug, since this process does not immediately change the concentration of free drug in the plasma (water is also filtered). However, plasma-protein binding generally does not limit renal tubular secretion or biotransformation, since these processes lower the free drug concentration, and this is rapidly followed by dissociation of the drug–protein complex. Drug transport and metabolism also are limited by plasma binding except when these are especially efficient and drug clearance, calculated on the basis of unbound drug, exceeds organ plasma flow. In this situation, binding of the drug to plasma protein may be viewed as a transport mechanism that fosters drug elimination by delivering drug to sites for elimination.

Tissue Binding. Many drugs accumulate in tissues at higher concentrations than those in the extracellular fluids and blood. For example, during long-term administration of the antimalarial agent quinacrine, the concentration of drug in the liver may be several thousandfold higher than that in the blood. Such accumulation may be a result of active transport or, more commonly, binding. Tissue binding of drugs usually occurs with cellular constituents such as proteins, phospholipids, or nuclear proteins and generally is reversible. A large fraction of drug in the body may be bound in this fashion and serve as a reservoir that prolongs drug action in that same tissue or at a distant site reached through the circulation.

Fat as a Reservoir.   Many lipid-soluble drugs are stored by physical solution in the neutral fat. In obese persons, the fat content of the body may be as high as 50%, and even in starvation it constitutes 10% of body weight; hence, fat can serve as an important reservoir for lipid-soluble drugs. For example, as much as 70% of the highly lipid-soluble barbiturate thiopental may be present in body fat 3 hours after administration. However, fat is a rather stable reservoir because it has a relatively low blood flow.

Bone.   The tetracycline antibiotics (and other divalent-metal-ion chelating agents) and heavy metals may accumulate in bone by adsorption onto the bone-crystal surface and eventual incorporation into the crystal lattice. Bone can become a reservoir for the slow release of toxic agents such as lead or radium into the blood; their effects can thus persist long after exposure has ceased. Local destruction of the bone medulla also may lead to reduced blood flow and prolongation of the reservoir effect, since the toxic agent becomes sealed off from the circulation; this may further enhance the direct local damage to the bone. A vicious cycle results, whereby the greater the exposure to the toxic agent, the slower is its rate of elimination.

Redistribution.   Termination of drug effect usually is by metabolism and excretion, but it also may result from redistribution of the drug from its site of action into other tissues or sites. Redistribution is a factor in terminating drug effect primarily when a highly lipid-soluble drug that acts on the brain or cardiovascular system is administered rapidly by intravenous injection or by inhalation. A good example of this is the use of the intravenous anesthetic thiopental, a highly lipid-soluble drug. Because blood flow to the brain is so high, the drug reaches its maximal concentration in brain within a minute after it is injected intravenously. After injection is concluded, the plasma concentration falls as thiopental diffuses into other tissues, such as muscle. The concentration of the drug in brain follows that of the plasma, because there is little binding of the drug to brain constituents. Thus, onset of anesthesia is rapid, but so is its termination. Both are directly related to the concentration of drug in the brain.

Central Nervous System and Cerebrospinal Fluid.   The distribution of drugs into the CNS from the blood is unique, because functional barriers are present that restrict entry of drugs into this critical site. One reason for this is that the brain capillary endothelial cells have continuous tight junctions; therefore, drug penetration into the brain depends on transcellular rather than paracellular transport between cells. The unique characteristics of pericapillary glial cells also contribute to the blood–brain barrier. At the choroid plexus, a similar blood–cerebrospinal fluid (CSF) barrier is present except that it is epithelial cells that are joined by tight junctions rather than endothelial cells. As a result, the lipid solubility of the nonionized and unbound species of the drug is an important determinant of its uptake by the brain; the more lipophilic it is, the more likely it is to cross the blood–brain barrier. This situation often is used in drug design to alter brain distribution; for example, nonsedating antihistamines achieve far lower brain concentrations than do other agents in this class. Increasing evidence also indicates that drugs may penetrate into the CNS by specific uptake transporters normally involved in the transport of nutrients and endogenous compounds from blood into the brain and CSF. Recently, it has been discovered that another important factor in the functional blood–brain barrier also involves membrane transporters which are, in this case, efflux carriers present in the brain capillary endothelial cell. P-glycoprotein is the most important of these and functions by a combination of not allowing drug to even translocate across the endothelial cell and also by exporting any drug that enters the brain by other means. Such transport may account for the brain, and other tissues where P-glycoprotein is similarly expressed (*e.g.,* the testes), being pharmacological sanctuary sites where drug concentrations are below those necessary to achieve a desired effect even though blood levels are adequate. This situation apparently occurs with HIV protease inhibitors (Kim *et al.,* 1998) and also with loperamide—a potent, systemically active opioid that lacks any central effects characteristic of other opioids (*see* Chapter 23). Efflux transporters that actively secrete drug from the CSF into the blood also are present in the choroid plexus. Regardless of whether a drug is pumped out of the CNS by specific transporters or diffuses back into the blood, drugs also exit the CNS along with the bulk flow of CSF through the arachnoid villi. In general, the blood–brain barrier's function is well maintained; however, meningeal and encephalic inflammation increase the local permeability. There also is the potential that the blood–brain barrier may be advantageously modulated to enhance the treatment of infections or tumors in the brain. To date, however, such an approach has not been shown to be clinically useful.

Placental Transfer of Drugs.   The potential transfer of drugs across the placenta is important, since drugs may cause congenital anomalies. Administered immediately before delivery, they also may have adverse effects on the neonate. Lipid solubility, extent of plasma binding, and degree of ionization of weak acids and bases are important general determinants, as previously discussed. The fetal plasma is slightly more acidic than that of the mother (pH 7.0 to 7.2 *versus* 7.4), so that ion-trapping of basic drugs occurs. As in the brain, P-glycoprotein is present in the placenta and functions as an export transporter to limit fetal exposure to potentially toxic agents. But the view that the placenta is an absolute barrier to drugs is inaccurate. A more appropriate approximation is that the fetus is to at least some extent exposed to essentially all drugs taken by the mother.

EXCRETION OF DRUGS

Drugs are eliminated from the body either unchanged by the process of excretion or converted to metabolites. Excretory organs, the lung excluded, eliminate polar compounds more efficiently than substances with high lipid solubility. Lipid-soluble drugs thus are not readily eliminated until they are metabolized to more polar compounds.

The kidney is the most important organ for excreting drugs and their metabolites. Substances excreted in the feces are mainly unabsorbed, orally ingested drugs or metabolites excreted either in the bile or secreted directly into the intestinal tract and, subsequently, not reabsorbed. Excretion of drugs in breast milk is important, not because of the amounts eliminated, but because the excreted drugs are potential sources of unwanted pharmacological effects in the nursing infant. Pulmonary excretion is important mainly for the elimination of anesthetic gases and vapors (*see* Chapters 13, 14, and 16); occasionally, small quantities of other drugs or metabolites are excreted by this route.

Renal Excretion. Excretion of drugs and metabolites in the urine involves three processes: glomerular filtration, active tubular secretion, and passive tubular reabsorption. Changes in overall renal function generally affect all three processes to a similar extent. Renal function is low compared to body size in neonates but rapidly matures within the first few months after birth. During adulthood there is a slow decline in renal function, about 1% per year, so that in the elderly a substantial degree of impairment is usually present.

The amount of drug entering the tubular lumen by filtration is dependent on the glomerular filtration rate and the extent of plasma binding of the drug; only unbound drug is filtered. In the proximal renal tubule, active, carrier-mediated tubular secretion also may add drug to the tubular fluid. Transporters such as P-glycoprotein and the multidrug resistance–associated protein-type 2 (MRP2) localized in the apical, brush-border membrane are largely responsible for the secretion of amphipathic anions and conjugated metabolites (such as glucuronides, sulfates, and glutathione adducts), respectively. Transport systems that are similar but more selective for organic cationic drugs (OCDs) are involved in the secretion of organic bases. Membrane transporters, mainly located in the distal renal tubule, also are responsible for any active reabsorption of drug from the tubular lumen back into the systemic circulation. However, most of such reabsorption occurs by nonionic diffusion.

In the proximal and distal tubules, the nonionized forms of weak acids and bases undergo net passive reabsorption. The concentration gradient for back-diffusion is created by the reabsorption of water with Na^+ and other inorganic ions. Since the tubular cells are less permeable to the ionized forms of weak electrolytes, passive reabsorption of these substances is pH-dependent. When the tubular urine is made more alkaline, weak acids are excreted more rapidly and to a greater extent, primarily because they are more ionized and passive reabsorption is decreased. When the tubular urine is made more acidic, the excretion of weak acids is reduced. Alkalinization and acidification of the urine have the opposite effects on the excretion of weak bases. In the treatment of drug poisoning, the excretion of some drugs can be hastened by appropriate alkalinization or acidification of the urine. Whether or not alteration of urine pH results in a significant change in drug elimination depends upon the extent and persistence of the pH change and the contribution of pH-dependent passive reabsorption to total drug elimination. The effect is greatest for weak acids and bases with pK_a values in the range of urinary pH (5 to 8). However, alkalinization of urine can produce a fourfold to sixfold increase in excretion of a relatively strong acid such as salicylate when urinary pH is changed from 6.4 to 8.0. The fraction of nonionized drug would decrease from 1% to 0.04%.

Biliary and Fecal Excretion. Transport systems analogous to those in the kidney also are present in the canalicular membrane of the hepatocyte, and these actively secrete drugs and metabolites into bile. P-glycoprotein transports a plethora of amphipathic, lipid-soluble drugs, whereas MRP2 is mainly involved in the secretion of conjugated metabolites of drugs (glutathione conjugates, glucuronides, and some sulfates). MRP2 also is involved in the excretion of endogenous compounds, and the Dubin-Johnson syndrome is caused by a genetically determined absence of this transporter. Active biliary secretion of organic cations also involves transporters. Ultimately, drugs and metabolites present in bile are released into the intestinal tract during the digestive process. Because secretory transporters such as P-glycoprotein also are expressed on the apical membrane of enterocytes, direct secretion of drugs and metabolites may occur from the systemic circulation into the intestinal lumen. Subsequently, drugs and metabolites can be reabsorbed back into the body from the intestine which, in the case of conjugated metabolites like glucuronides, may require their enzymatic hydrolysis by the intestinal microflora. Such enterohepatic recycling, if extensive, may prolong significantly the presence of a drug and its effects within the body prior to elimination by other pathways.

Excretion by Other Routes.   Excretion of drugs into sweat, saliva, and tears is quantitatively unimportant. Elimination by these routes is dependent mainly upon diffusion of the nonionized, lipid-soluble form of drugs through the epithelial cells of the glands and is pH-dependent. Drugs excreted in the saliva enter the mouth, where they are usually swallowed. The concentration of some drugs in saliva parallels that in plasma. Saliva therefore may be a useful biological fluid in which to determine drug concentrations when it is difficult or inconvenient to obtain blood. The same principles apply to excretion of drugs in breast milk. Since milk is more acidic than plasma, basic compounds may be slightly concentrated in this fluid, and the concentration of acidic compounds in the milk is lower than in plasma. Nonelectrolytes, such as ethanol and urea, readily enter breast milk and reach the same concentration as in plasma, independent of the pH of the milk. Although excretion into hair and skin also is quantitatively unimportant, sensitive methods of detection of drugs in these tissues have forensic significance.

METABOLISM OF DRUGS

The lipophilic characteristics of drugs that promote their passage through biological membranes and subsequent access to their site of action hinder their excretion from the body. Renal excretion of unchanged drug plays only a modest role in the overall elimination of most therapeutic agents, since lipophilic compounds filtered through the glomerulus are largely reabsorbed back into the systemic circulation during passage through the renal tubules. The metabolism of drugs and other xenobiotics into more hydrophilic metabolites is therefore essential for the elimination of these compounds from the body and termination of their biological activity. In general, biotransformation reactions generate more polar, inactive metabolites that are readily excreted from the body. However, in some cases, metabolites with potent biological activity or toxic properties are generated. Many of the metabolic biotransformation reactions leading to inactive metabolites of drugs also generate biologically active metabolites of endogenous compounds. The following discussion focuses on the biotransformation of drugs but is generally applicable to the metabolism of all xenobiotics as well as a number of endogenous compounds, including steroids, vitamins, and fatty acids.

Phase I and Phase II Metabolism.   Drug biotransformation reactions are classified as either phase I functionalization reactions or phase II biosynthetic (conjugation) reactions. Phase I reactions introduce or expose a functional group on the parent compound. Phase I reactions generally result in the loss of pharmacological activity, although there are examples of retention or enhancement of activity. In rare instances, metabolism is associated with an altered pharmacological activity. Prodrugs are pharmacologically inactive compounds, designed to maximize the amount of the active species that reaches its site of action. Inactive prodrugs are converted rapidly to biologically active metabolites, often by the hydrolysis of an ester or amide linkage. If not rapidly excreted into the urine, the products of phase I biotransformation reactions can then react with endogenous compounds to form a highly water-soluble conjugate.

Phase II conjugation reactions lead to the formation of a covalent linkage between a functional group on the parent compound or phase I metabolite with endogenously derived glucuronic acid, sulfate, glutathione, amino acids, or acetate. These highly polar conjugates are generally inactive and are excreted rapidly in the urine and feces. An example of an active conjugate is the 6-glucuronide metabolite of morphine, which is a more potent analgesic than its parent compound.

Site of Biotransformation.   The metabolic conversion of drugs generally is enzymatic in nature. The enzyme systems involved in the biotransformation of drugs are localized in the liver, although every tissue examined has some metabolic activity. Other organs with significant metabolic capacity include the gastrointestinal tract, kidneys, and lungs. Following nonparenteral administration of a drug, a significant portion of the dose may be metabolically inactivated in either the intestinal epithelium or the liver before it reaches the systemic circulation. This first-pass metabolism significantly limits the oral availability of highly metabolized drugs. Within a given cell, most drug-metabolizing activity is found in the endoplasmic reticulum and the cytosol, although drug biotransformations also can occur in the mitochondria, nuclear envelope, and plasma membrane. Upon homogenization and differential centrifugation of tissues, the endoplasmic reticulum breaks up, and fragments of the membrane form microvesicles, referred to as microsomes. The drug-metabolizing enzymes in the endoplasmic reticulum therefore often are classified as microsomal enzymes. The enzyme systems involved in phase I reactions are located primarily in the endoplasmic reticulum, while the phase II conjugation enzyme systems are mainly cytosolic. Often drugs biotransformed through a phase I reaction in the endoplasmic reticulum are conjugated at this same site or in the cytosolic fraction of the same cell.

Cytochrome P450 Monooxygenase System.   The cytochrome P450 enzymes are a superfamily of heme-thiolate proteins widely distributed across all living kingdoms. The enzymes are involved in the metabolism of a plethora of chemically diverse, endogenous and exogenous compounds, including drugs, environmental chemicals, and other xenobiotics. Usually they function as a terminal oxidase in a multicomponent electron-transfer chain that introduces a single atom of molecular oxygen into the substrate with the other atom being incorporated into water. In microsomes, the electrons are supplied from NADPH *via* cytochrome P450 reductase, which is closely associated with cytochrome P450 in the lipid membrane of the smooth endoplasmic reticulum. Cytochrome P450 catalyzes many reactions, including aromatic and side-chain hydroxylation; *N*-, *O*- and *S*-dealkylation; *N*-oxidation; *N*-hydroxylation; sulfoxidation; deamination; dehalogenation; and desulfuration. Details and examples of cytochrome P450–mediated metabolism are shown in Table 1–2. A number of reductive reactions also are catalyzed by these enzymes, generally under conditions of low oxygen tension.

Of the approximately 1000 currently known cytochrome P450s, about 50 are functionally active in human beings. These are categorized into 17 families and many subfamilies according to the amino acid–sequence similarities of the predicted proteins; the abbreviated term *CYP* is used for identification. Sequences that are greater than 40% identical belong to the same family, identified by an Arabic number; within a family, sequences greater than 55% identical are in the same subfamily, identified by a letter; and different individual isoforms within the subfamily are identified by an Arabic number. About 8 to 10 isoforms in the CYP1, CYP2, and CYP3 families primarily are involved in the majority of all drug metabolism reactions in human beings; members of the other families are important in the biosynthesis and degradation of steroids, fatty acids, vitamins, and other endogenous compounds. Each individual CYP isoform appears to have a characteristic substrate specificity based on structural features of the substrate; considerable overlap, however, often is present. As a result, two or more CYP isoforms and other drug-metabolizing enzymes often are involved in a drug's overall metabolism, leading to the formation of many primary and secondary metabolites. The various isoforms also have characteristic inhibition and induction profiles, as described later. Additionally, CYP-catalyzed metabolism is often regio- and stereoselective; the latter characteristic may be important if the administered drug

is a racemate and the enantiomers have different pharmacological activities.

The relative contributions of the various CYP isoforms in the metabolism of drugs is illustrated in Figure 1–3. CYP3A4 and CYP3A5, which are very similar isoforms, together are involved in the metabolism of about 50% of drugs; moreover, CYP3A is expressed in both the intestinal epithelium and the kidney. It is now recognized that metabolism by CYP3A during absorption through the intestinal enterocyte is a significant factor, along with hepatic first-pass metabolism, in the poor oral bioavailability of many drugs. Isoforms in the CYP2C family and CYP2D6 subfamily also are involved to a large extent in the metabolism of drugs. Although isoforms such as CYP1A1/2, CYP2A6, CYP2B1, and CYP2E1 are not involved to any major extent in the metabolism of therapeutic drugs, they do, however, catalyze the activation of many procarcinogenic environmental chemicals to the ultimate carcinogenic form. Accordingly, they are considered to be important in susceptibility to various cancers, such as tobacco smoking–associated lung cancer.

Other oxidative enzymes such as dehydrogenases and flavin-containing monooxygenases also are capable of catalyzing the metabolism of specific drugs, but, in general, such enzymes are of minor overall importance.

Hydrolytic Enzymes.   The reactions of the major hydrolytic enzymes are illustrated in Table 1–2. A number of nonspecific esterases and amidases have been identified in the endoplasmic reticulum of human liver, intestine, and other tissues. The alcohol and amine groups exposed following hydrolysis of esters and amides are suitable substrates for conjugation reactions. Microsomal epoxide hydrolase is found in the endoplasmic reticulum of essentially all tissues and is in close proximity to the cytochrome P450 enzymes. Epoxide hydrolase generally is considered a detoxification enzyme, hydrolyzing highly reactive arene oxides generated from cytochrome P450 oxidation reactions to inactive, water-soluble transdihydrodiol metabolites. Protease and peptidase enzymes are widely distributed in many tissues and are involved in the biotransformation of polypeptide drugs. Delivery of such drugs across biological membranes requires the inhibition of these enzymes or the development of stable analogs.

Conjugation Reactions.   Both an activated form of an endogenous compound and an appropriate transferase enzyme are necessary for the formation of a conjugated metabolite. In the case of glucuronidation—the most important conjugation reaction (Figure 1–3)—uridine diphosphate glucuronosyltransferases (UGTs) catalyze the transfer of glucuronic acid to aromatic and aliphatic alcohols, carboxylic acids, amines, and free sulfhydryl groups of both exogenous and endogenous compounds to form *O*-, *N*-, and *S*-glucuronides, respectively. Glucuronidation also is important in the elimination of endogenous steroids, bilirubin, bile acids, and fat-soluble vitamins. The increased water solubility of a glucuronide conjugate promotes its elimination in the urine or bile. Unlike most phase II reactions, which are localized in the cytosol, UGTs are microsomal enzymes. This location facilitates direct access of phase I metabolites formed at the same site. In addition to the liver, UGTs also are found in the intestinal epithelium, kidney, and skin. About 15 human UGTs have been identified, and, based on amino acid similarity (>50% identity), two main families have been categorized. Members of the

Table 1–2
Major Reactions Involved in Drug Metabolism

Reaction		Examples
I. OXIDATIVE REACTIONS		
N-Dealkylation	$RNHCH_3 \rightarrow RNH_2 + CH_2O$	Imipramine, diazepam, codeine, erythromycin, morphine, tamoxifen, theophylline, caffeine
O-Dealkylation	$ROCH_3 \rightarrow ROH + CH_2O$	Codeine, indomethacin, dextromethorphan
Aliphatic hydroxylation	$RCH_2CH_3 \rightarrow RCHCH_3$ (OH)	Tolbutamide, ibuprofen, pentobarbital, meprobamate, cyclosporine, midazolam
Aromatic hydroxylation	(benzene → arene oxide → phenol)	Phenytoin, phenobarbital, propanolol, phenylbutazone, ethinylestradiol, amphetamine, warfarin
N-Oxidation	$RNH_2 \rightarrow RNHOH$	Chlorpheniramine, dapsone, meperidine
	$R_1R_2NH \rightarrow R_1R_2N{-}OH$	Quinidine, acetaminophen
S-Oxidation	$R_1R_2S \rightarrow R_1R_2S{=}O$	Cimetidine, chlorpromazine, thioridazine, omeprazole
Deamination	$RCHCH_3(NH_2) \rightarrow R{-}C(OH)(NH_2){-}CH_3 \rightarrow R{-}C({=}O){-}CH_3 + NH_2$	Diazepam, amphetamine
II. HYDROLYSIS REACTIONS		
	$R_1COR_2 \rightarrow R_1COOH + R_2OH$	Procaine, aspirin, clofibrate, meperidine, enalapril, cocaine
	$R_1CNR_2 \rightarrow R_1COOH + R_2NH_2$	Lidocaine, procainamide, indomethacin
III. CONJUGATION REACTIONS		
Glucuronidation	UDP-glucuronic acid $+ R{-}OH \rightarrow$ (glucuronide-O-R) $+ UDP$	Acetaminophen, morphine, oxazepam, lorazepam
Sulfation	$ROH + $ 3′-phosphoadenosine-5′-phosphosulfate (PAPS) $\rightarrow R{-}O{-}S({=}O)_2{-}OH + $ 3′-phosphoadenosine-5′-phosphate	Acetaminophen, steroids, methyldopa
Acetylation	acetyl-coenzyme A ($CoAS{-}C({=}O){-}CH_3$) $+ RNH_2 \rightarrow RNH{-}C({=}O){-}CH_3 + CoA{-}SH$	Sulfonamides, isoniazid, dapsone, clonazepam

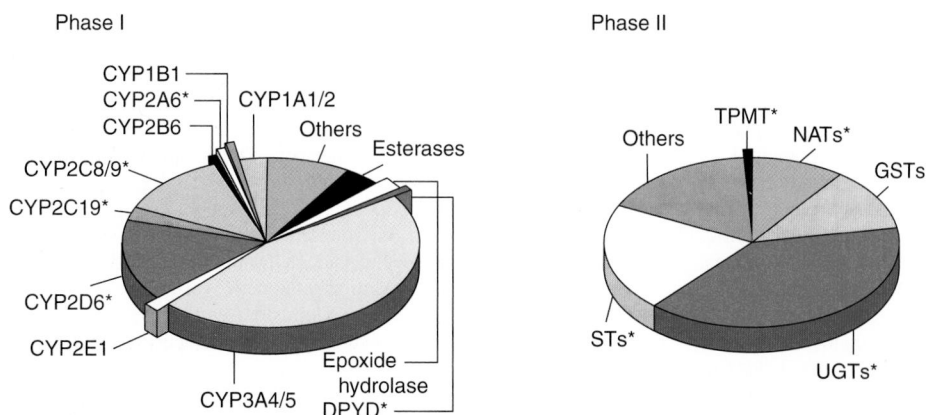

Figure 1–3. The proportion of drugs metabolized by the major phase I and phase II enzymes.

The relative size of each pie section indicates the estimated percentage of phase I (*left panel*) or phase II (*right panel*) metabolism that each enzyme contributes to the metabolism of drugs based on literature reports. Enzymes that have functional allelic variants are indicated by an asterisk. In many cases, more than one enzyme is involved in a particular drug's metabolism: CYP, cytochrome P450; DPYD, dihydropyrimidine dehydrogenase; GST, glutathione *S*-transferases; NAT, *N*-acetyltransferases; ST, sulfotransferases; TPMT, thiopurine methyltransferase; UGT, UDP-glucuronosyltransferases.

human UGT1A family are all encoded by a complex gene, and individual isoforms are produced by alternative splicing of 12 promoters/exon 1 with common exons 2 to 5 to produce multiple different proteins. By contrast, UGT2 contains only three subfamilies: 2A, 2B, and 2C. While it appears that individual UGTs have characteristic substrate specificities, there is considerable overlap, so that multiple isoforms may be responsible for formation of a particular glucuronide metabolite. Cytosolic sulfation also is an important conjugation reaction that involves the catalytic transfer by sulfotransferases (STs) of inorganic sulfur from activated 3′-phosphoadenosine-5′-phosphosulfate to the hydroxyl group of phenols and aliphatic alcohols. Therefore, drugs and primary metabolites with a hydroxyl group often form both glucuronide and sulfate metabolites. Two *N*-acetyltransferases (NAT1 and NAT2) are involved in the acetylation of amines, hydrazines, and sulfonamides. In contrast to most drug conjugates, acetylated metabolites often are less water-soluble than the parent drug, and this may result in crystalluria unless a high urine flow rate is maintained.

Factors Affecting Drug Metabolism.   A hallmark of drug metabolism is a large interindividual variability that often results in marked differences in the extent of metabolism and, as a result, the drug's rate of elimination and other characteristics of its plasma concentration–time profile. Such variability is a major reason why patients differ in their responses to a standard dose of a drug and it must be considered in optimizing a dosage regimen for a particular individual. A combination of genetic, environmental, and disease-state factors affect drug metabolism, with the relative contribution of each depending on the specific drug. *Genetic Variation.*   Advances in molecular biology have shown that genetic diversity is the rule rather than the

exception with all proteins, including enzymes that catalyze drug-metabolism reactions. For an increasing number of such enzymes, allelic variants with different catalytic activities from that of the wild-type form have been identified. The differences involve a variety of molecular mechanisms leading to a complete lack of activity, a reduction in catalytic ability, or, in the case of gene duplication, enhanced activity. Furthermore, these traits are generally inherited in an autosomal, Mendelian recessive fashion and, if sufficiently prevalent, result in subpopulations with different drug-metabolizing abilities, *i.e., genetic polymorphism*. In addition, the frequency of specific allelic variants often varies according to the racial ancestry of the individual. It is possible to phenotype or genotype a person with respect to a particular genetic variant, and it is likely that such characterization will become increasingly useful in individualizing drug therapy, especially for drugs with a narrow therapeutic index. Accumulating evidence also suggests that individual susceptibility to diseases associated with environmental chemicals, such as cancer, may reflect genetic variability in drug-metabolizing enzymes.

A number of genetic polymorphisms are present in several cytochrome P450s that lead to altered drug metabolizing ability. The best characterized of these is that associated with CYP2D6. About 70 *single nucleotide polymorphisms* (SNPs) and other genetic variants of functional importance have been identified in the CYP2D6 gene, many of which result in an inactive enzyme while others reduce catalytic activity; gene duplication also occurs. As a result, four phenotypic subpopulations of metabolizers exist: poor (PM), intermediate (IM), extensive (EM), and ultrarapid (UM). Some of the variants are relatively rare, whereas others are more common, and importantly, their frequency varies according to racial background. For example, 5% to 10% of Caucasians of European ancestry are PMs, whereas the frequency of this homozygous phenotype in individuals of Southeast Asian origin is only about 1% to 2%. More than 65 commonly used drugs are metabolized by CYP2D6, including tricyclic antidepressants, neuroleptic agents, selective serotonin reuptake inhibitors, some antiarrhythmic agents, β-adrenergic receptor antagonists, and certain opiates. The clinical importance of the CYP2D6 polymorphism is mainly in the greater likelihood of an adverse reaction in PMs when the affected metabolic pathway is a major contributor to the drug's overall elimination. Also, in UMs, usual drug doses may be inefficacious, or in the case where an active metabolite is formed, for example, the CYP2D6-catalyzed formation of morphine from codeine, an exaggerated response occurs. Inhibitors of CYP2D6, such as quinidine and selective serotonin reuptake inhibitors, may convert a genotypic EM into a phenotypic PM, a phenomenon termed *phenocopying* that is an important aspect of drug interactions with this particular CYP isoform.

CYP2C9 catalyzes the metabolism of some 16 commonly used drugs, including that of warfarin and phenytoin, both of which have a narrow therapeutic index. The two most common allelic CYP2C9 variants have markedly reduced catalytic activity (5% to 12%) compared to the wild-type enzyme. As a consequence, patients who are heterozygous or homozygous for the mutant alleles require a lower anticoagulating dose of warfarin, especially the latter group, relative to homozygous, wild-type individuals. Also, initiating warfarin therapy is more difficult, and there is an increased risk of bleeding complications. Similarly, high plasma concentrations of phenytoin and associated adverse effects occur in patients with variant CYP2C9 alleles. Genetic polymorphism also occurs with CYP2C19, where 8 allelic variants have been identified that result in a catalytically inactive protein. About 3% of Caucasians are phenotypically PMs, whereas the frequency is far higher in Southeast Asians, 13% to 23%. Proton-pump inhibitors such as omeprazole and lansoprazole are among the 18 or so drugs importantly metabolized by CYP2C19 to an extent determined by the gene dose. The efficacy of the recommended 20-mg dose of omeprazole in combination with amoxicillin in eradicating *Helicobacter pylori* is markedly reduced in patients of the homozygous wild-type genotype compared with the 100% cure rate in homozygous PMs, reflecting differences in the drug's effect on gastric acid secretion. Although CYP3A activity shows marked interindividual variability (>10-fold), no significant functional polymorphisms have been found in the gene's coding region; it is, therefore, likely that unknown regulatory factors primarily determine such variability. Genetic variability also is present with dihydropyrimidine dehydrogenase (DPYD), which is a key enzyme in the metabolism of 5-fluorouracil. Accordingly, there is a marked risk of developing severe drug-induced toxicity in the 1% to 3% of cancer patients treated with this antimetabolite who have substantially reduced DPYD activity compared to the general population.

A polymorphism in a conjugating drug-metabolizing enzyme, namely that in NAT2, was one of the first to be found to have a genetic basis some 50 years ago. This isoform is involved in the metabolism of about 16 common drugs including isoniazid, procainamide, dapsone, hydralazine, and caffeine.

About 15 allelic variants have been identified, some of which are without functional effect, but others are associated with either reduced or absent catalytic activity. Considerable heterogeneity is present in the worldwide population frequency of these alleles, so that the slow-acetylator phenotype frequency is about 50% in American whites and blacks, 60% to 70% in North Europeans, but only 5% to 10% in Southeast Asians. It has been speculated that acetylator phenotype may be associated with environmental agent–induced disease such as bladder and colorectal cancer; however, definitive evidence is not yet available. Similarly, genetic variability in the catalytic activity of glutathione S-transferases may be linked to individual susceptibility to such diseases. Thiopurine methyltransferase (TPMT) is critically important in the metabolism of 6-mercaptopurine, the active metabolite of azathioprine. As a result, homozygotes for alleles encoding inactive TPMT (0.3% to 1% of the population) predictably exhibit severe pancytopenia if given standard doses of azathioprine; such patients typically can be treated with 10% to 15% of the usual dose.

Environmental Determinants. The activity of most drug-metabolizing enzymes may be modulated by exposure to certain exogenous compounds. In some instances, this may be a drug, which, if concomitantly administered with a second agent, results in a drug:drug interaction. Additionally, dietary micronutrients and other environmental factors can up- or down-regulate the enzymes, termed *induction* and *inhibition,* respectively. Such modulation is thought to be a major contributor to interindividual variability in the metabolism of many drugs.

Inhibition of Drug Metabolism. A consequence of inhibiting drug-metabolizing enzymes is an increase in the plasma concentration of parent drug and a reduction in that of metabolite, exaggerated and prolonged pharmacological effects, and an increased likelihood of drug-induced toxicity. These changes occur rapidly and with essentially no warning and are most critical for drugs that are extensively metabolized and have a narrow therapeutic index. Knowledge of the cytochrome-P450 isoforms that catalyze the main pathway of metabolism of a drug provides a basis for predicting and understanding inhibition, especially with regard to drug-drug interactions. This is because many inhibitors are more selective for some isoforms than others. Often, inhibition occurs because of competition between two or more substrates for the same active site of the enzyme, the extent of which depends on the relative concentrations of the substrates and their affinities for the enzyme. In certain instances, however, the enzyme may be irreversibly inactivated; for example, the substrate or a metabolite forms a tight complex with the heme iron of cytochrome P450 (cimetidine, ketoconazole) or the heme group may be destroyed (norethindrone, ethinylestradiol). A common mechanism of inhibition for some phase II enzymes is the depletion of necessary cofactors.

Inhibition of the CYP3A-catalyzed mechanism is both common and important. Because of the high expression level of CYP3A in the intestinal epithelium and the fact that oral ingestion is the most common route of entry of drugs and environmental agents into the body, inhibition of the isoform's activity at this site is often particularly consequential, even if that in the liver is unaffected. This is because of the potential, large increase in bioavailability associated with the reduction in first-pass metabolism for drugs that usually exhibit this effect to a substantial extent. The antifungal agents ketoconazole and itraconazole, HIV protease inhibitors (especially ritonavir), macrolide antibiotics such as erythromycin and clarithromycin but not azithromycin, are all potent CYP3A inhibitors. Certain calcium channel blockers such as diltiazem, nicardipine, and verapamil also inhibit CYP3A, as does a constituent of grapefruit juice. Many inhibitors of CYP3A also reduce P-glycoprotein function, so that drug-drug interactions may involve a dual mechanism. Also, the disposition of drugs that are not significantly metabolized but are eliminated by P-glycoprotein–mediated transport also may be affected by a CYP3A inhibitor. For example, the impaired excretion of digoxin by quinidine and a large number of other unrelated drugs is caused by inhibition of P-glycoprotein. With CYP2D6, quinidine and selective serotonin reuptake inhibitors are potent inhibitors that may produce phenocopying. On the other hand, other drugs are more general inhibitors of cytochrome P450–catalyzed metabolism. For example amiodarone, cimetidine (but not ranitidine), paroxitene, and fluoxetine reduce the metabolic activity of several CYP isoforms. Phase I metabolic enzymes other than cytochrome P450 also may be inhibited by drug administration, as exemplified by the potent effect of valproic acid on microsomal epoxide hydrolase, and the inhibition of xanthine oxidase by allopurinol, which can result in life-threatening toxicity in patients concurrently receiving 6-mercaptopurine.

Induction of Drug Metabolism. Up-regulation of drug-metabolizing activity usually occurs by enhanced gene transcription following prolonged exposure to an inducing agent, although with CYP2E1 stabilization of the protein against degradation is the major mechanism. As a result, the consequences of induction take considerable time to be fully exhibited, *c.f.,* inhibition of metabolism. Moreover, the consequences of induction are an increased rate of metabolism, enhanced oral first-pass metabolism and reduced bioavailability, and a corresponding decrease in the drug's plasma concentration, all factors that reduce drug exposure. By contrast, for drugs that are metabolized to an active or reactive metabolite, induction may be associated with increased drug effects or toxicity, respectively. In some cases, a drug can induce both the metabolism of other compounds and its own metabolism; such *autoinduction* occurs with the anticonvulsant carbamazepine. In many cases involving induction, the dosage of an affected drug must be increased to maintain the therapeutic effect. This is particularly the case when induction is extensive following administration of a highly effective inducer; in fact, women are advised to use an alternative to oral contraceptives for birth control during rifampin therapy because efficacy cannot be assured. The therapeutic risk associated with metabolic induction is most critical when administration of the inducing agent is stopped while maintaining the same dose of a drug that has been previously given. In this case, as the inducing effect wears off, plasma concentrations of the second drug will rise unless the dose is reduced, with an increase in the potential for adverse effects.

Inducers generally are selective for certain CYP subfamilies and isoforms, but at the same time, multiple other enzymes may be simultaneously up-regulated through a common molecular mechanism. For example, polycyclic aromatic hydrocarbons derived from environmental pollutants, cigarette smoke, and charbroiled meats produce marked induction of the CYP1A subfamily of enzymes both in the liver and extrahepatically. This involves activation of the cytosolic arylhydrocarbon receptor (AhR), which interacts with another regulatory protein, the AhR nuclear translocator (Arnt); the complex functions as a transcription factor to up-regulate CYP1A expression. In addition, the expression of phase II enzymes such as UGTs, GSTs, and NAD(P)H:quinone oxidoreductase are simultaneously increased. A similar type of receptor mechanism involving the pregnane X receptor (PXR) is involved in the induction of CYP3A by a wide variety of diverse chemicals, including drugs such as rifampin and rifabutin, barbiturates and other anticonvulsants, some glucocorticoids, and even alternative medicines such as St. John's wort. These latter drugs also can affect other CYP isoforms; for example, rifampin and carbamazepine induce CYP1A2, CYP2C9, and CYP2C19. Chronic alcohol use also results in enzyme induction, especially with CYP2E1; the risk of hepatotoxic adverse effects of acetaminophen is higher in alcoholics because of increased CYP2E1-mediated formation of a reactive metabolite, *N*-acetyl-*p*-benzoquinoneimine.

Disease Factors. Since the liver is the major location of drug-metabolizing enzymes, dysfunction in this organ in patients with hepatitis, alcoholic liver disease, biliary cirrhosis, fatty liver, and hepatocarcinomas potentially can lead to impaired drug metabolism. In general, the severity of the liver damage determines the extent of reduced metabolism; unfortunately, common clinical tests of liver function are of little value in assessing this. Moreover, even in severe cirrhosis, the extent of impairment is only to about 30% to 50% of the activity in non-liver-diseased patients. However, with drugs that undergo substantial hepatic first-pass metabolism, oral bioavailability may be increased two- to fourfold in liver disease which, coupled with the prolonged presence of drugs in the body, increases the risk of exaggerated pharmacological responses and adverse effects. It appears that cytochrome-P450 isoforms are affected to a greater extent by liver disease than are those that catalyze phase II reactions such as glucuronosyltransferases.

Severe cardiac failure and shock can result in both decreased perfusion of the liver and impaired metabolism. The best example of this is the almost twofold reduction in lidocaine metabolism in cardiac failure, which also is accompanied by a change in distribution to a similar extent. As a result, the loading and maintenance doses of lidocaine used to treat cardiac arrhythmias in such patients are substantially different from those used in patients without this condition.

Age and Sex. Functional cytochrome P450 isoforms and to a lesser degree phase II drug-metabolizing enzymes develop early in fetal development, but the levels, even at birth, are lower than those found postnatally. Both phase I and phase II enzymes begin to mature gradually following the first 2 to 4 weeks postpartum, although the pattern of development is variable for the different enzymes. Thus, newborns and infants are able to metabolize drugs relatively efficiently but generally at a slower rate than are adults. An exception to this is the impairment of bilirubin glucuronidation at birth, which contributes to the hyperbilirubinemia of newborns. Full maturity appears to occur in the second decade of life with a subsequent slow decline in function associated with aging. Unfortunately, few generalizations are possible regarding the extent or clinical importance of such age-related changes in an individual patient. This is particularly true for elderly patients who, because of multiple diseases, may be taking a large number of drugs, many of which may produce drug-drug interactions. In addition, increased sensitivity of target organs and impairment of physiological control mechanisms further complicate the use of drugs in the elderly population. Phase I drug-metabolizing enzymes appear to be affected to a greater extent than are those that catalyze phase II reactions. However, the changes are often modest relative to other causes of interindividual variability in metabolism. On the other hand, for drugs exhibiting a high first-pass effect, even a small reduction in metabolizing ability may significantly increase oral bioavailability. Drug use in the elderly, therefore, generally requires moderate reductions in drug dose and awareness of the possibility of exaggerated pharmacodynamic responsiveness.

A number of examples indicate that drug treatment and/or responsiveness of men and women may be different for certain drugs. Some sex-related differences in drug-metabolizing activity, especially that catalyzed by CYP3A, also have been noted. However, such differences are minor and unimportant relative to other factors involved in interindividual variability in metabolism. One exception to this generalization is pregnancy, where induction of certain drug-metabolizing enzymes occurs in the second and third trimesters. As a result, drug dosage may have to be increased during this period and returned to its previous level postpartum. This situation is particularly important in the treatment of patients with seizures using phenytoin during their pregnancy. Many oral contraceptive agents also are potent irreversible inhibitors of CYP isoforms through a suicide-inactivation mechanism.

CLINICAL PHARMACOKINETICS

A fundamental hypothesis of clinical pharmacokinetics is that a relationship exists between the pharmacological effects of a drug and an accessible concentration of the drug (*e.g.,* in blood or plasma). This hypothesis has been documented for many drugs, although for some drugs no clear or simple relationship has been found between pharmacological effect and concentration in plasma. In most cases, as depicted in Figure 1–1, the concentration of drug in the systemic circulation will be related to the concentration of drug at its sites of action. The pharmacological effect that results may be the clinical effect desired, a toxic effect, or, in some cases, an effect unrelated to therapeutic efficacy or toxicity. Clinical pharmacokinetics attempts to provide both a quantitative relationship between dose and effect and a framework with which to interpret measurements of concentrations of drugs in biological fluids. The importance of pharmacokinetics in patient care is based on the improvement in therapeutic efficacy that can be attained by application of its principles when dosage regimens are chosen and modified.

The various physiological and pathophysiological variables that dictate adjustment of dosage in individual patients often do so as a result of modification of pharma-

cokinetic parameters. The four most important parameters are *clearance,* a measure of the body's efficiency in eliminating drug; *volume of distribution,* a measure of the apparent space in the body available to contain the drug; *elimination half-life,* a measure of the rate of removal of drug from the body; and *bioavailability,* the fraction of drug absorbed as such into the systemic circulation. Of lesser importance are the *rates* of availability and distribution of the agent.

Clearance

Clearance is the most important concept that needs to be considered when a rational regimen for long-term drug administration is to be designed. The clinician usually wants to maintain steady-state concentrations of a drug within a *therapeutic window* associated with therapeutic efficacy and a minimum of toxicity. Assuming complete bioavailability, the steady state will be achieved when the rate of drug elimination equals the rate of drug administration:

$$\text{Dosing rate} = CL \cdot C_{ss} \qquad (1\text{–}1)$$

where CL is clearance from the systemic circulation and C_{ss} is the steady-state concentration of drug. Thus, if the desired steady-state concentration of drug in plasma or blood is known, the rate of clearance of drug by the patient will dictate the rate at which the drug should be administered.

The concept of clearance is extremely useful in clinical pharmacokinetics, because its value for a particular drug usually is constant over the range of concentrations encountered clinically. This is true because systems for elimination of drugs such as metabolizing enzymes and transporters usually are not saturated, and thus the *absolute* rate of elimination of the drug is essentially a linear function of its concentration in plasma. A synonymous statement is that the elimination of most drugs follows first-order kinetics—a constant *fraction* of drug in the body is eliminated per unit of time. If mechanisms for elimination of a given drug become saturated, the kinetics approach zero-order—a constant *amount* of drug is eliminated per unit of time. Under such a circumstance, clearance will vary with the concentration of drug, often according to the following equation:

$$CL = v_m / (K_m + C) \qquad (1\text{–}2)$$

where K_m represents the concentration at which half of the maximal rate of elimination is reached (in units of mass/volume) and v_m is equal to the maximal rate of elimination (in units of mass/time). This equation is analogous to the Michaelis–Menten equation for enzyme kinetics. Design of dosage regimens for such drugs is more complex than when elimination is first-order and clearance is independent of the drug's concentration (*see* below).

Principles of drug clearance are similar to those of renal physiology, where, for example, creatinine clearance is defined as the rate of elimination of creatinine in the urine relative to its concentration in plasma. At the simplest level, clearance of a drug is its rate of elimination by all routes normalized to the concentration of drug, *C*, in some biological fluid:

$$CL = \text{rate of elimination}/C \qquad (1\text{–}3)$$

Thus, when clearance is constant, the rate of drug elimination is directly proportional to drug concentration. It is important to note that clearance does not indicate how much drug is being removed but, rather, the volume of biological fluid such as blood or plasma from which drug would have to be completely removed to account for the elimination. Clearance is expressed as a volume per unit of time. Clearance usually is further defined as blood clearance (CL_b), plasma clearance (CL_p), or clearance based on the concentration of unbound drug (CL_u), depending on the concentration measured (C_b, C_p, or C_u).

Clearance by means of various organs of elimination is additive. Elimination of drug may occur as a result of processes that occur in the kidney, liver, and other organs. Division of the rate of elimination by each organ by a concentration of drug (*e.g.*, plasma concentration) will yield the respective clearance by that organ. Added together, these separate clearances will equal systemic clearance:

$$CL_{renal} + CL_{hepatic} + CL_{other} = CL \qquad (1\text{–}4)$$

Other routes of elimination could include that in saliva or sweat, secretion into the intestinal tract, and metabolism at other sites.

Systemic clearance may be determined at steady state by using Equation (1–1). For a single dose of a drug with complete bioavailability and first-order kinetics of elimination, systemic clearance may be determined from mass balance and the integration of Equation (1–3) over time.

$$CL = \text{Dose}/AUC \qquad (1\text{–}5)$$

where *AUC* is the total area under the curve that describes the concentration of drug in the systemic circulation as a function of time (from zero to infinity).

Examples. In Appendix II, the plasma clearance for cephalexin is reported as 4.3 ml · min^{-1} · kg^{-1}, with 90% of the drug excreted unchanged in the urine. For a 70-kg man, the clearance from plasma would be 300 ml/minute, with renal clearance accounting for 90% of this elimination. In other words, the kidney is able to excrete cephalexin at a rate such that it is completely removed (cleared) from approximately 270 ml of plasma per minute. Because clearance usually is assumed to remain constant in a stable patient, the rate of elimination of cephalexin will depend on the concentration of drug in the plasma [Equation (1–3)]. Propranolol is cleared from the blood at a rate of 16 ml · min^{-1} · kg^{-1} (or 1120 ml/minute in a 70-kg man), almost exclusively by the liver. Thus, the liver is able to remove the amount of drug contained in 1120 ml of blood per minute. Even though the liver is the dominant organ for elimination, the plasma clearance of some drugs exceeds the rate of plasma (and blood) flow to this organ. Often this is because the drug partitions readily into red blood cells, and the rate of drug delivered to the eliminating organ is considerably higher than suspected from measurement of its concentration in plasma. The relationship between plasma and blood clearance at steady state is given by:

$$\frac{CL_p}{CL_b} = \frac{C_b}{C_p} = 1 + H\left[\frac{C_{rbc}}{C_p} - 1\right] \qquad (1\text{–}6)$$

Clearance from the blood, therefore, may be estimated by dividing the plasma clearance by the drug's blood to plasma concentration ratio, obtained from knowledge of the hematocrit ($H = 0.45$) and the red cell to plasma concentration ratio. In most instances the blood clearance will be less than liver blood flow (1.5 liters/minute) or, if renal excretion also is involved, the sum of the two eliminating organs' blood flows. For example, the plasma clearance of tacrolimus, about 2 liters/minute, is more than twofold higher than the hepatic plasma flow rate and even exceeds the organ's blood flow, despite the fact that the liver is the predominant site of this drug's extensive metabolism. However, after taking into account the extensive distribution of tacrolimus into red cells, its clearance from the blood is only about 63 ml/minute, and it is actually a low- rather than high-clearance drug, as might be interpreted from the plasma clearance value. Sometimes, however, clearance from the blood by metabolism exceeds liver blood flow, and this indicates extrahepatic metabolism. In the case of esmolol (11.9 liters/minute), the blood clearance value is greater than cardiac output, because the drug is efficiently metabolized by esterases present in red blood cells.

A further definition of clearance is useful for understanding the effects of pathological and physiological variables on drug elimination, particularly with respect to an individual organ. The rate of presentation of drug to the organ is the product of blood flow (Q) and the arterial drug concentration (C_A), and the rate of exit of drug from the organ is the product of blood flow and the venous drug concentration (C_V). The difference between these rates at steady state is the rate of drug elimination:

$$\text{Rate of elimination} = Q \cdot C_A - Q \cdot C_V$$
$$= Q(C_A - C_V) \qquad (1\text{–}7)$$

Division of Equation (1–7) by the concentration of drug entering the organ of elimination, C_A, yields an expression for clearance of the drug by the organ in question:

$$CL_{organ} = Q\left[\frac{C_A - C_V}{C_A}\right] = Q \cdot E \qquad (1\text{–}8)$$

The expression $(C_A - C_V)/C_A$ in Equation (1–8) can be referred to as the extraction ratio for the drug (E).

Hepatic Clearance. The concepts developed in Equation (1–8) have important implications for drugs that are eliminated by the liver. Consider a drug that is efficiently removed from the blood by hepatic processes—metabolism and/or excretion of drug into the bile. In this instance, the concentration of drug in the blood leaving the liver will be low, the extraction ratio will approach unity, and the clearance of the drug from blood will become limited by hepatic blood flow. Drugs that are cleared efficiently by the liver (*e.g.,* drugs in Appendix II with systemic clearances greater than $6 \text{ ml} \cdot \text{min}^{-1} \cdot \text{kg}^{-1}$, such as diltiazem, imipramine, lidocaine, morphine, and propranolol) are restricted in their rate of elimination, not by intrahepatic processes, but by the rate at which they can be transported in the blood to the liver.

Additional complexities also have been considered. For example, the equations presented above do not account for drug binding to components of blood and tissues, nor do they permit an estimation of the intrinsic ability of the liver to eliminate a drug in the absence of limitations imposed by blood flow, termed *intrinsic clearance.* In biochemical terms and under first-order conditions, intrinsic clearance is a measure of the ratio of the Michaelis–Menten kinetic parameters for the eliminating process, *i.e.,* v_m/K_m. Extensions of the relationships of Equation (1–8) to include expressions for protein binding and intrinsic clearance have been proposed for a number of models of hepatic elimination (*see* Morgan and Smallwood, 1990). All of these models indicate that, when the capacity of the eliminating organ to metabolize the drug is large in comparison with the rate of presentation of drug, clearance will approximate the organ's blood flow. In contrast, when the metabolic capability is small in comparison to the rate of drug presentation, clearance will be proportional to the unbound fraction of drug in blood and the drug's intrinsic clearance. Appreciation of these concepts allows understanding of a number of possibly puzzling experimental results. For example, enzyme induction or hepatic disease may change the rate of drug metabolism in an isolated hepatic microsomal enzyme system but not change clearance in the whole animal. For a drug with a high extraction ratio, clearance is limited by blood flow, and changes in intrinsic clearance due to enzyme induction or hepatic disease should have little effect. Similarly, for drugs with high extraction ratios, changes in protein binding due to disease or competitive binding interactions should have little effect on clearance. In contrast, changes in intrinsic clearance and protein binding will affect the clearance of drugs with low intrinsic clearances and, thus, extraction ratios, but changes in blood flow should have little effect (Wilkinson and Shand, 1975).

Renal Clearance. Renal clearance of a drug results in its appearance as such in the urine; changes in the pharmacokinetic properties of drugs due to renal disease also may be explained in terms of clearance concepts. However, the complications that relate to filtration, active secretion, and reabsorption must be considered. The rate of filtration of a drug depends on the volume of fluid that is filtered in the glomerulus and the unbound concentration of drug in plasma, since drug bound to protein is not filtered. The rate of secretion of drug by the kidney will depend on the drug's intrinsic clearance by the transporters involved in active secretion as affected by the drug's binding to plasma proteins, the degree of saturation of these transporters, and the rate of delivery of the drug to the secretory site. In addition, processes involved in drug reabsorption from the tubular fluid must be considered. The influences of changes in protein binding, blood flow, and the number of functional nephrons are analogous to the examples given above for hepatic elimination.

Distribution

Volume of Distribution. Volume is a second fundamental parameter that is useful in considering processes of drug disposition. The volume of distribution (V) relates the amount of drug in the body to the concentration of drug (C) in the blood or plasma, depending upon the fluid measured. This volume does not necessarily refer to an identifiable physiological volume, but merely to the fluid volume that would be required to contain all of the drug in the body at the same concentration as in the blood or plasma:

$$V = \text{amount of drug in body}/C \qquad (1\text{–}9)$$

A drug's volume of distribution, therefore, reflects the extent to which it is present in extravascular tissues. The plasma volume of a typical 70-kg man is 3 liters, blood volume is about 5.5 liters, extracellular fluid volume outside the plasma is 12 liters, and the volume of total body water is approximately 42 liters. However, many drugs exhibit volumes of distribution far in excess of these values. For example, if 500 μg of digoxin were in the body of a 70-kg subject, a plasma concentration of approximately 0.75 ng/ml would be observed. Dividing the amount of drug in the body by the plasma concentration yields a volume of distribution for digoxin of about 650 liters, or a value almost ten times greater than the total body volume of a 70-kg man. In fact, digoxin distributes preferentially to muscle and adipose tissue and to its specific receptors, leaving a very small amount of drug in the plasma. For drugs that are extensively bound to plasma proteins but that are not bound to tissue components, the volume of distribution will approach that of the plasma volume. In contrast, certain drugs have high volumes of distribution even though most of the drug in the

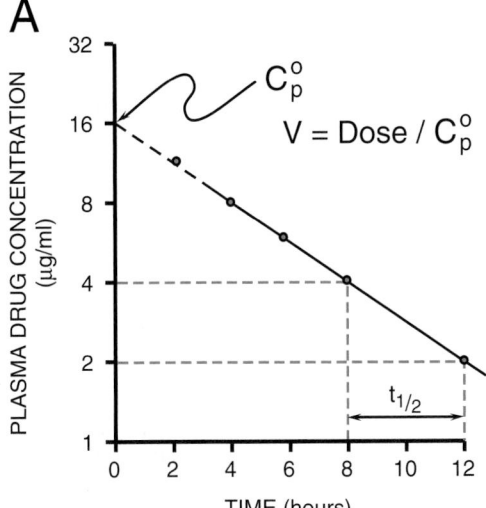

A

C_p^o

$V = Dose / C_p^o$

PLASMA DRUG CONCENTRATION (μg/ml)

TIME (hours)

$t_{1/2}$

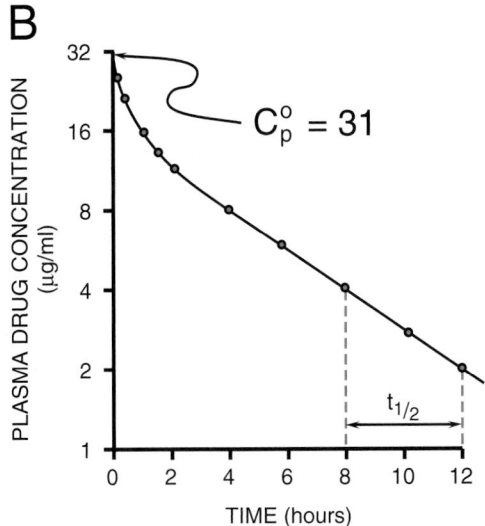

B

$C_p^o = 31$

PLASMA DRUG CONCENTRATION (μg/ml)

TIME (hours)

$t_{1/2}$

Figure 1–4. Plasma concentration–time curves following intravenous administration of a drug (500 mg) to a 70-kg man.

A. In this example, drug concentrations are measured in plasma from 2 hours after the dose is administered. The semilogarithmic plot of plasma concentration *versus* time appears to indicate that the drug is eliminated from a single compartment by a first-order process [Equation (1–10)] with a half-life of 4 hours ($k = 0.693/t_{1/2} = 0.173$ h^{-1}). The volume of distribution (V) may be determined from the value of C_p obtained by extrapolation to $t = 0$ ($C_p^o = 16$ μg/ml). Volume of distribution [Equation (1–9)] for the one-compartment model is 31.3 liters or 0.45 liter/kg ($V = $ dose/C_p^o). The clearance for this drug is 90 ml/min; for a one-compartment model, $CL = kV$. **B.** Sampling before 2 hours indicates that, in fact, the drug follows multiexponential kinetics. The terminal disposition half-life is 4 hours, clearance is 84 ml/min [Equation (1–5)], V_{area} is 29 liters [Equation (1–11)], and V_{ss} is 26.8 liters. The initial or "central" distribution volume for the drug ($V_1 = $ dose/C_p^o) is 16.1 liters. The example chosen indicates that multicompartment kinetics may be overlooked when sampling at early times is neglected. In this particular case, there is only a 10% error in the estimate of clearance when the multicompartment characteristics are ignored. For many drugs multicompartment kinetics may be observed for significant periods of time, and failure to consider the distribution phase can lead to significant errors in estimates of clearance and in predictions of the appropriate dosage. Also, the difference between the "central" distribution volume and other terms reflecting wider distribution is important in deciding a loading dose strategy.

circulation is bound to albumin, because these drugs are also sequestered elsewhere.

The volume of distribution may vary widely depending on the relative degrees of binding to plasma and tissue proteins, the partition coefficient of the drug in fat, and so forth. As might be expected, the volume of distribution for a given drug can differ according to patient's age, gender, body composition, and presence of disease.

Several volume terms commonly are used to describe drug distribution, and they have been derived in a number of ways. The volume of distribution defined in Equation (1–9) considers the body as a single homogeneous compartment. In this *one-compartment model,* all drug administration occurs directly into the central compartment and distribution of drug is instantaneous throughout the volume (V). Clearance of drug from this compartment occurs

in a first-order fashion, as defined in Equation (1–3); that is, the amount of drug eliminated per unit of time depends on the amount (concentration) of drug in the body compartment. Figure 1–4A and Equation (1–10) describe the decline of plasma concentration with time for a drug introduced into this compartment.

$$C = (\text{dose}/V) \cdot exp(-kt) \qquad (1-10)$$

where k is the rate constant for elimination that reflects the fraction of drug removed from the compartment per unit of time. This rate constant is inversely related to the half-life of the drug ($k = 0.693/t_{1/2}$).

The idealized one-compartment model discussed above does not describe the entire time course of the plasma concentration. That is, certain tissue reservoirs can be distinguished from the central compartment, and the drug concentration appears to decay in a manner that can be described by multiple exponential terms (*see* Figure 1–4B). Nevertheless, the one-compartment model is sufficient to apply to most clinical situations for most drugs.

Rate of Drug Distribution. The multiple exponential decay observed for a drug that is eliminated from the body with first-order kinetics results from differences in the rates at which the drug equilibrates with tissues. The rate of equilibration will depend upon the ratio of the perfusion of the tissue to the partition of drug into the tissue. In many cases, groups of tissues with similar perfusion/partition ratios all equilibrate at essentially the same rate, such that only one apparent phase of distribution (rapid initial fall of concentration, as in Figure 1–4*B*) is seen. It is as though the drug starts in a "central" volume, which consists of plasma and tissue reservoirs that are in rapid equilibrium with it, and distributes to a "final" volume, at which point concentrations in plasma decrease in a log-linear fashion with a rate constant of k (*see* Figure 1–4*B*).

If the pattern or ratio of blood flows to various tissues changes within an individual or differs among individuals, rates of drug distribution to tissues also will change. However, changes in blood flow also may cause some tissues that were originally in the "central" volume to equilibrate sufficiently more slowly so as to appear only in the "final" volume. This means that central volumes will appear to vary with disease states that cause altered regional blood flow. After an intravenous bolus dose, drug concentrations in plasma may be higher in individuals with poor perfusion (*e.g.,* shock) than they would be if perfusion were better. These higher systemic concentrations may, in turn, cause higher concentrations (and greater effects) in tissues such as brain and heart, whose usually high perfusion has not been reduced by the altered hemodynamic state. Thus, the effect of a drug at various sites of action can be variable, depending on perfusion of these sites.

Multicompartment Volume Terms. Two different terms have been used to describe the volume of distribution for drugs that follow multiple exponential decay. The first, designated V_{area}, is calculated as the ratio of clearance to the rate of decline of concentration during the elimination (final) phase of the logarithmic concentration *versus* time curve:

$$V_{area} = \frac{CL}{k} = \frac{\text{dose}}{k \cdot AUC} \qquad (1\text{–}11)$$

The estimation of this parameter is straightforward, and the volume term may be determined after administration of a single dose of drug by intravenous or oral routes (where the dose used must be corrected for bioavailability). However, another multicompartment volume of distribution may be more useful, especially when the effect of disease states on pharmacokinetics is to be determined. The volume of distribution at steady state (V_{ss}) represents the volume in which a drug would appear to be distributed during steady state if the drug existed throughout that volume at the same concentration as that in the measured fluid (plasma or blood). Following intravenous dosing, estimation of V_{ss} is more complicated than Equation (1–11), but feasible (Benet and Galeazzi, 1979). It is more difficult to estimate V_{ss} following oral dosing. Although V_{area} is a convenient and easily calculated parameter, it varies when the rate constant for drug elimination changes, even when there has been no change in the distribution space. This is because the terminal rate of decline of the concentration of drug in blood or plasma depends not only on clearance but also on the rates of distribution of drug between the "central" and "final"

volumes. V_{ss} does not suffer from this disadvantage. When using pharmacokinetics to make drug dosing decisions, the differences between V_{area} and V_{ss} usually are not clinically significant. Nonetheless, both are quoted in the table of pharmacokinetic data in Appendix II, depending upon availability in the published literature.

Half-Life

The half-life ($t_{1/2}$) is the time it takes for the plasma concentration or the amount of drug in the body to be reduced by 50%. For the simplest case, the one-compartment model (Figure 1–4*A*), half-life may be determined readily and used to make decisions about drug dosage. However, as indicated in Figure 1–4*B*, drug concentrations in plasma often follow a multiexponential pattern of decline; two or more half-life terms may thus be calculated.

In the past, the half-life that was usually reported corresponded to the terminal log-linear phase of elimination. However, as greater analytical sensitivity has been achieved, the lower concentrations measured appeared to yield longer and longer terminal half-lives. For example, a terminal half-life of 53 hours is observed for gentamicin (*versus* the more clinically relevant 2- to 3-hour value in Appendix II), and biliary cycling is probably responsible for the 120-hour terminal value for indomethacin (as compared with the 2.4-hour half-life listed in Appendix II). The relevance of a particular half-life may be defined in terms of the fraction of the clearance and volume of distribution that is related to each half-life and whether plasma concentrations or amounts of drug in the body are best related to measures of response. The single half-life values given for each drug in Appendix II are chosen to represent the most clinically relevant half-life.

Early studies of pharmacokinetic properties of drugs in disease were compromised by their reliance on half-life as the sole measure of alterations of drug disposition. It is now appreciated that half-life is a derived parameter that changes as a function of both clearance and volume of distribution. A useful approximate relationship between the clinically relevant half-life, clearance, and volume of distribution at steady state is given by:

$$t_{1/2} \cong 0.693 \cdot V_{ss}/CL \qquad (1\text{–}12)$$

Clearance is the measure of the body's ability to eliminate a drug; thus, as clearance decreases, due to a disease process, for example, half-life would be expected to increase. However, this reciprocal relationship is valid only when the disease does not change the volume of distribution. For example, the half-life of diazepam increases with increasing age; however, it is not clearance that changes as a function of age, but the volume of distribution (Klotz *et al.,* 1975). Similarly, changes in protein binding of the drug may affect its clearance as well as its volume of distribution, leading to unpredictable changes in half-life as a function of disease. The half-life of tolbutamide, for example, decreases in patients with acute viral hepatitis, exactly the opposite from what one might expect. The disease alters the drug's protein binding in both plasma and tissues, causing no change in volume of distribution but an increase in clearance, because higher concentrations of unbound drug are present (Williams *et al.,* 1977).

Although it can be a poor index of drug elimination, half-life does provide a good indication of the time required to reach steady state after a dosage regimen is initiated or changed (*i.e.,* four half-lives to reach approximately 94% of a new steady state), the time for a drug to be removed from the body, and a means to estimate the appropriate dosing interval (*see* below).

Steady State.

Equation (1–1) indicates that a steady-state concentration eventually will be achieved when a drug is administered at a constant rate. At this point, drug elimination [the product of clearance and concentration; Equation (1–3)] will equal the rate of drug availability. This concept also extends to intermittent dosage (*e.g.,* 250 mg of drug every 8 hours). During each interdose interval, the concentration of drug rises and falls. At steady state, the entire cycle is repeated identically in each interval. Equation (1–1) still applies for intermittent dosing, but it now describes the average drug concentration (C_{ss}) during an interdose interval. Steady-state dosing is illustrated in Figure 1–5.

Extent and Rate of Bioavailability

Bioavailability. It is important to distinguish between the rate and extent of drug absorption and the amount of drug that ultimately reaches the systemic circulation, as discussed above. The amount of the drug that reaches the systemic circulation depends not only on the administered dose but also on the fraction of the dose, *F*, which is absorbed and escapes any first-pass elimination. This fraction often is called *bioavailability.* Reasons for incomplete absorption have been discussed above. Also, as noted previously, if the drug is metabolized in the intestinal epithelium or the liver, or excreted in bile, some of the active drug absorbed from the gastrointestinal tract will be eliminated before it can reach the general circulation and be distributed to its sites of action.

Knowing the extraction ratio (E_H) for a drug across the liver [*see* Equation (1–8)], it is possible to predict the maximum oral

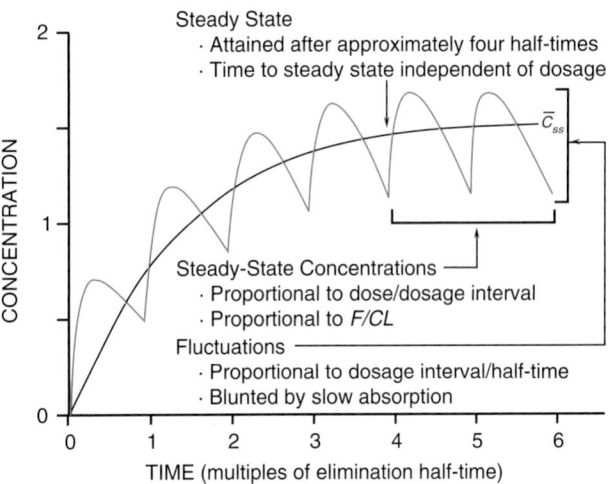

Figure 1–5. Fundamental pharmacokinetic relationships for repeated administration of drugs.

The blue line is the pattern of drug accumulation during repeated administration of a drug at intervals equal to its elimination half-time, when drug absorption is 10 times as rapid as elimination. As the rate of absorption increases, the concentration maxima approach 2 and the minima approach 1 during the steady state. The black line depicts the pattern during administration of equivalent dosage by continuous intravenous infusion. Curves are based upon the one-compartment model.

Average concentration ($\overline{C}_{ss}$) when the steady state is attained during intermittent drug administration:

$$\overline{C}_{ss} = \frac{F \cdot \text{dose}}{CL \cdot T}$$

where *F* = fractional bioavailability of the dose and *T* = dosage interval (time). By substitution of infusion rate for *F* · dose/*T*, the formula is equivalent to Equation (1–1) and provides the concentration maintained at steady state during continuous intravenous infusion.

availability (F_{max}), assuming hepatic elimination follows first-order processes:

$$F_{max} = 1 - E_H = 1 - (CL_{hepatic} / Q_{hepatic}) \qquad (1-13)$$

Thus, if the hepatic blood clearance for the drug is large relative to hepatic blood flow, the extent of availability will be low when it is given orally (*e.g.,* lidocaine). This reduction in availability is a function of the physiological site from which absorption takes place, and no modification of dosage form will improve the availability under conditions of linear kinetics. Incomplete absorption and/or intestinal metabolism following oral dosing will, in practice, reduce this predicted maximal value of *F*.

When drugs are administered by a route that is subject to first-pass loss, the equations presented previously that contain the terms *dose* or *dosing rate* [Equations (1–1), (1–5), (1–10), and (1–11)] also must include the bioavailability term F, such that the available dose or dosing rate is used. For example, Equation (1–1) is modified to:

$$F \cdot \text{dosing rate} = CL \cdot C_{ss} \qquad (1\text{–}14)$$

Rate of Absorption. Although the rate of drug absorption does not, in general, influence the average steady-state concentration of the drug in plasma, it may still influence drug therapy. If a drug is absorbed rapidly (*e.g.*, a dose given as an intravenous bolus) and has a small "central" volume, the concentration of drug initially will be high. It will then fall as the drug is distributed to its "final" (larger) volume (*see* Figure 1–4*B*). If the same drug is absorbed more slowly (*e.g.*, by slow infusion), it will be distributed while it is being given, and peak concentrations will be lower and will occur later. Controlled-release preparations are designed to provide a slow and sustained rate of absorption in order to produce a less fluctuating plasma concentration–time profile during the dosage interval compared to more immediate-release formulations. A given drug may act to produce both desirable and undesirable effects at several sites in the body, and the rates of distribution of drug to these sites may not be the same. The relative intensities of these different effects of a drug may thus vary transiently when its rate of administration is changed.

Nonlinear Pharmacokinetics

Nonlinearity in pharmacokinetics (*i.e.*, changes in such parameters as clearance, volume of distribution, and half-life as a function of dose or concentration of drug) usually is due to saturation of protein binding, hepatic metabolism, or active renal transport of the drug.

Saturable Protein Binding. As the molar concentration of drug increases, the unbound fraction eventually also must increase (as all binding sites become saturated). This usually occurs only when drug concentrations in plasma are in the range of tens to hundreds of micrograms per milliliter. For a drug that is metabolized by the liver with a low intrinsic clearance/extraction ratio, saturation of plasma-protein binding will cause both V and clearance to increase as drug concentrations increase; half-life may thus remain constant [*see* Equation (1–12)]. For such a drug, C_{ss} will not increase linearly as the rate of drug administration is increased. For drugs that are cleared with high intrinsic clearances/extraction ratios, C_{ss} can remain linearly proportional to the rate of drug administration. In this case, hepatic clearance would not change, and the increase in V would increase the half-time of disappearance by reducing the fraction of the total drug in the body that is delivered to the liver per unit of time. Most drugs fall between these two extremes, and the effects of nonlinear protein binding may be difficult to predict.

Saturable Elimination. In this situation, the Michaelis–Menten equation [Equation (1–2)] usually describes the nonlinearity. All active processes are undoubtedly saturable, but they will appear to be linear if values of drug concentrations encountered in practice are much less than K_m. When they exceed K_m, nonlinear kinetics is observed. The major consequences of saturation of metabolism or transport are the opposite of those for saturation of protein binding. When both conditions are present simultaneously, they may virtually cancel each others' effects, and surprisingly linear kinetics may result; this occurs over a certain range of concentrations for salicylic acid.

Saturable metabolism causes oral first-pass metabolism to be less than expected (higher F), and there is a greater fractional increase in C_{ss} than the corresponding fractional increase in the rate of drug administration. The latter can be seen most easily by substituting Equation (1–2) into Equation (1–1) and solving for the steady-state concentration:

$$C_{ss} = \frac{\text{dosing rate} \cdot K_m}{v_m - \text{dosing rate}} \qquad (1\text{–}15)$$

As the dosing rate approaches the maximal elimination rate (v_m), the denominator of Equation (1–15) approaches zero and C_{ss} increases disproportionately. Because saturation of metabolism should have no effect on the volume of distribution, clearance and the relative rate of drug elimination decrease as the concentration increases; therefore, the log plasma level-time curve is concave-decreasing until metabolism becomes sufficiently desaturated and first-order elimination is present. Thus, the concept of a constant half-life is not applicable to nonlinear metabolism occurring in the usual range of clinical concentrations. Consequently, changing the dosing rate for a drug with nonlinear metabolism is difficult and unpredictable, since the resulting steady state is reached more slowly, and, importantly, the effect is disproportionate to the alteration in the dosing rate.

Phenytoin provides an example of a drug for which metabolism becomes saturated in the therapeutic range of concentrations (*see* Appendix II). K_m (5 to 10 mg per liter) is typically near the lower end of the therapeutic range (10 to 20 mg per liter). For some individuals, especially children, K_m may be as low as 1 mg per liter. If, for such an individual, the target concentration is 15 mg per liter, and this is attained at a dosing rate of 300 mg per day, then, from Equation (1–15), v_m equals 320 mg per day. For such a patient, a dose 10% less than optimal (*i.e.*, 270 mg per day) will produce a C_{ss} of 5 mg per liter, well below the desired value. In contrast, a dose 10% greater than optimal (330 mg per day) will exceed metabolic capacity (by 10 mg per day) and cause a long and slow but unending climb in concentration until toxicity occurs. Dosage cannot be controlled so precisely (less than 10% error). Therefore, for those patients in whom the target concentration for phenytoin is more than tenfold greater than the K_m, alternating inefficacious therapy and toxicity is almost unavoidable. For a drug like phenytoin that has a narrow therapeutic index and exhibits nonlinear metabolism, therapeutic drug monitoring (*see* below) is most important.

Design and Optimization of Dosage Regimens

Following administration of a dose of drug, its effects usually show a characteristic temporal pattern (Figure 1–6). Onset of the effect is preceded by a lag period, after which the magnitude of the effect increases to a maximum and then declines; if a further dose is not administered, the effect eventually disappears. This time-course reflects changes in the drug's concentration as determined by the pharmacokinetics of its absorption, distribution, and elimination. Accordingly, the intensity of a drug's effect is related to its concentration above a minimum effective concentration, whereas the duration of this effect is a reflection of the length of time the drug level is above this value. These considerations, in general, apply to both desired and undesired (adverse) drug effects and, as a re-

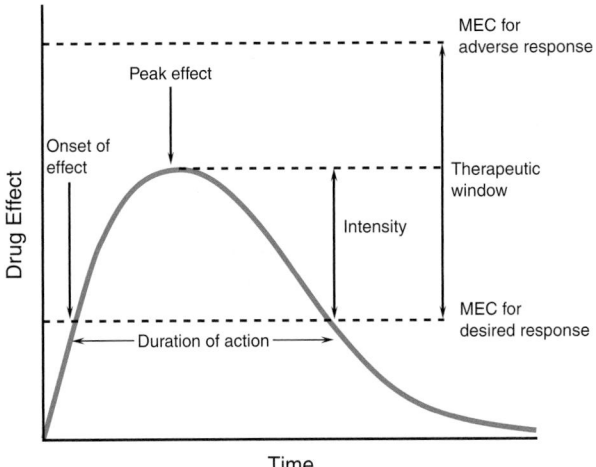

Figure 1–6. Temporal characteristics of drug effect and relationship to the therapeutic window.

A lag period is present before the drug concentration exceeds the minimum effective concentration (MEC) for the desired effect. Following onset of the response, the intensity of the effect increases as the drug continues to be absorbed and distributed. This reaches a peak, after which drug elimination results in a decline in the effect's intensity that disappears when the drug concentration falls back below the MEC. Accordingly, the duration of a drug's action is determined by the time period over which concentrations exceed the MEC. A similar MEC exists for each adverse response, and if drug concentration exceeds this, toxicity will result. Thus, the therapeutic goal should be to obtain and maintain concentrations within the therapeutic window for the desired response with a minimum of toxicity. Drug response below the MEC for the desired effect will be subtherapeutic, whereas above the MEC for an adverse effect, the probability of toxicity will increase. Increasing or decreasing drug dosage shifts the response curve up or down the intensity scale and is used to modulate the drug's effect. Increasing the dose also prolongs a drug's duration of action but at the risk of increasing the likelihood of adverse effects. Accordingly, unless the drug is nontoxic (e.g., penicillins), increasing the dose is not a useful strategy for extending a drug's duration of action. Instead, another dose of drug should be given to maintain concentrations within the therapeutic window.

sult, a *therapeutic window* exists reflecting a concentration range that provides efficacy without unacceptable toxicity. Similar considerations apply after multiple dosing associated with long-term therapy; therefore they determine the amount and frequency of drug administration to achieve an optimal therapeutic effect. In general, the lower limit of the therapeutic range appears to be approximately equal to the drug concentration that produces about half of the greatest possible therapeutic effect, and the upper limit of the therapeutic range is such that no more than 5% to 10% of patients will experience a toxic effect. For some drugs, this may mean that the upper limit of the range is no more than twice the lower limit. Of course, these figures can be highly variable, and some patients may benefit greatly from drug concentrations that exceed the therapeutic range, while others may suffer significant toxicity at much lower values.

For a limited number of drugs, some effect of the drug is easily measured (e.g., blood pressure, blood glucose), and this can be used to optimize dosage, using a trial-and-error approach. Even in this ideal case, certain quantitative issues arise, such as how often to change dosage and by how much. These usually can be settled with simple rules of thumb based on the principles discussed (e.g., change dosage by no more than 50% and no more often than every three to four half-lives). Alternatively, some drugs have very little dose-related toxicity, and maximum efficacy is usually desired. For these drugs, doses well in excess of the average required will both ensure efficacy (if this is possible) and prolong drug action. Such a "maximal dose" strategy typically is used for penicillins and most β-adrenergic receptor antagonists.

For many drugs, however, the effects are difficult to measure (or the drug is given for prophylaxis), toxicity and lack of efficacy are both potential dangers, and/or the therapeutic index is narrow. In these circumstances, doses must be titrated carefully, and drug dosage is limited by toxicity rather than efficacy. Thus, the therapeutic goal is to maintain steady-state drug levels within the *therapeutic window*. For most drugs, the actual concentrations associated with this desired range are not and need not be known. It is sufficient to understand that efficacy and toxicity are generally concentration-dependent, and how drug dosage and frequency of administration affect the drug level. However, for a small number of drugs, where there is a small (two- to threefold) difference between concentrations resulting in efficacy and toxicity (e.g., digoxin, theophylline, lidocaine, aminoglycosides, cyclosporine, and anticonvulsants), a plasma-concentration range associated with effective therapy has been defined. In this case, a target level strategy is reasonable, wherein a desired (target) steady-state concentration of the drug (usually in plasma) associated with efficacy and minimal toxicity is chosen, and a dosage is computed that is expected to achieve this value. Drug concentrations are subsequently measured, and dosage is adjusted if necessary to approximate the target more closely (*see also* Chapter 3).

Maintenance Dose.   In most clinical situations, drugs are administered in a series of repetitive doses or as a continuous infusion to maintain a steady-state concentration of drug associated with the therapeutic window. Thus, calculation of the appropriate maintenance dosage is a primary goal. To maintain the chosen steady-state or target concentration, the rate of drug administration is adjusted such that the rate of input equals the rate of loss. This relationship was defined previously in Equations (1–1) and (1–14) and is expressed here in terms of the desired target concentration:

$$\text{Dosing rate} = \text{target } C_p \cdot CL/F \qquad (1\text{--}16)$$

If the clinician chooses the desired concentration of drug in plasma and knows the clearance and bioavailability for that drug in a particular patient, the appropriate dose and dosing interval can be calculated.

Example.   Oral digoxin is to be used as a maintenance dose to gradually "digitalize" a 69-kg patient with congestive heart failure. A steady-state plasma concentration of 1.5 ng/ml is selected as an appropriate target. Based on the fact that the patient's creatinine clearance (CL_{CR}) is 100 ml/min, digoxin's clearance may be estimated from data in Appendix II.

$$
\begin{aligned}
CL &= 0.88\ CL_{CR} + 0.33\ \text{ml} \cdot \text{min}^{-1} \cdot \text{kg}^{-1} \\
&= 0.88 \times 100/69 + 0.33\ \text{ml} \cdot \text{min}^{-1} \cdot \text{kg}^{-1} \\
&= 1.6\ \text{ml} \cdot \text{min}^{-1} \cdot \text{kg}^{-1} \\
&= 110\ \text{ml} \cdot \text{min}^{-1} = 6.6\ \text{liters} \cdot \text{hr}^{-1}
\end{aligned}
$$

Equation (1–16) is then used to calculate an appropriate dosing rate knowing that the oral bioavailability of digoxin is 70% ($F = 0.7$)

$$
\begin{aligned}
\text{Dosing rate} &= \text{Target } C_p \cdot CL/F \\
&= 1.5\ \text{ng} \cdot \text{ml}^{-1} \times 1.6/0.7\ \text{ml} \cdot \text{min}^{-1} \cdot \text{kg}^{-1} \\
&= 3.43\ \text{ng} \cdot \text{min}^{-1} \cdot \text{kg}^{-1} \\
&= 236\ \text{ng} \cdot \text{min}^{-1} \text{ for a 69-kg patient} \\
&= 236\ \text{ng} \cdot \text{min}^{-1} \times 60\ \text{min} \times 24\ \text{hr} \\
&= 340\ \mu\text{g} = 0.34\ \text{mg/24 hr}
\end{aligned}
$$

In practice, the dose rate would be rounded to the closest dosage size, either 0.375 mg/24 hr, which would result in a steady-state plasma concentration of 1.65 ng/ml (1.5 × 375/340), or 0.25 mg/24 hr, which would provide a value of 1.10 ng/ml (1.5 × 250/340).

Dosing Interval for Intermittent Dosage.   In general, marked fluctuations in drug concentrations between doses are not desirable. If absorption and distribution were instantaneous, fluctuation of drug concentrations between doses would be governed entirely by the drug's elimination half-life. If the dosing interval (T) was chosen to be equal to the half-life, then the total fluctuation would be twofold; this is often a tolerable variation.

Pharmacodynamic considerations modify this. If a drug is relatively nontoxic, such that a concentration many times that necessary for therapy can be tolerated easily, the maximal dose strategy can be used, and the dosing interval can be much longer than the elimination half-life (for convenience). The half-life of amoxicillin is about 2 hours, but it is often given in large doses every 8 or 12 hours.

For some drugs with a narrow therapeutic range, it may be important to estimate the maximal and minimal concentrations that will occur for a particular dosing interval. The minimal steady-state concentration $C_{ss,\ min}$ may be reasonably determined by the use of Equation (1–17):

$$C_{ss,min} = \frac{F \cdot \text{dose}/V_{ss}}{1 - exp(-kT)} \cdot exp(-kT) \qquad (1\text{--}17)$$

where k equals 0.693 divided by the clinically relevant plasma half-life and T is the dosing interval. The term $exp(-kT)$ is, in fact, the fraction of the last dose (corrected for bioavailability) that remains in the body at the end of a dosing interval.

For drugs that follow multiexponential kinetics and that are administered orally, the estimation of the maximal steady-state concentration $C_{ss,\ max}$ involves a complicated set of exponential constants for distribution and absorption. If these terms are ignored for multiple oral dosing, one may easily predict a maximal steady-state concentration by omitting the $exp(-kT)$ term in the numerator of Equation (1–17) [see Equation (1–18), below]. Because of the approximation, the predicted maximal concentration from Equation (1–18) will be greater than that actually observed.

Example.   In the patient with congestive heart failure discussed above, an oral maintenance dosing of 0.375 mg/24 hr of digoxin was calculated to achieve an average plasma concentration of 1.65 ng/ml during the dosage interval. Digoxin has a narrow therapeutic index, and plasma levels between 0.8 and 2.0 ng/ml are usually associated with efficacy and minimal toxicity. It is, therefore, important to know what maximum and minimum plasma concentrations would be predicted with the above regimen. This first requires estimation of digoxin's volume of distribution based on data in Appendix II.

$$
\begin{aligned}
V_{ss} &= 3.12\ CL_{CR} + 3.84\ \text{liters} \cdot \text{kg}^{-1} \\
&= 3.12 \times (100/69) + 3.84\ \text{liters} \cdot \text{kg}^{-1} \\
&= 8.4\ \text{liters} \cdot \text{kg}^{-1} \\
&= 580\ \text{liters for a 69-kg patient}
\end{aligned}
$$

Combining this value with that of digoxin's clearance provides an estimate of digoxin's elimination half-life in the patient [Equations (1–1) through (1–12)].

$$
\begin{aligned}
t_{1/2} &= 0.693\ V_{ss}/CL \\
&= \frac{0.693 \times 580\ \text{liters}}{6.6\ \text{liters} \cdot \text{hr}^{-1}} \\
&= 61\ \text{hr}
\end{aligned}
$$

Accordingly, the fractional rate constant of elimination is equal to 0.01136 hr^{-1} (0.693/61 hr). Maximum and minimum digoxin plasma concentrations may then be predicted depending upon the dosage interval. If this were every 2 days:

$$C_{ss,max} = \frac{F \cdot \text{dose}/V_{ss}}{1 - exp(-kT)}$$
$$= \frac{0.7 \times 0.375 \times 2 \text{ mg}/580 \text{ liters}}{0.42} \quad (1\text{--}18)$$
$$= 2.15 \text{ ng/ml}$$

$$C_{ss,min} = C_{ss,max} \cdot exp(-kT)$$
$$= (2.15 \text{ ng/ml})(0.58) \quad (1\text{--}19)$$
$$= 1.25 \text{ ng/ml}$$

Accordingly, the plasma concentrations would fluctuate about twofold, consistent with the similarity of the dosage interval to digoxin's half-life. Also, the peak concentration would be above the upper value of the therapeutic range, exposing the patient to possible adverse effects, and at the end of the dosing interval the concentration would be above but close to the lower limit. By using the same dosing rate but decreasing the frequency of dosing, a much smoother plasma concentration *versus* time profile would be obtained while still maintaining an average steady-state value of 1.65 ng/ml. For example, with a 0.375-mg dose every 24 hours, the predicted maximum and minimum plasma concentrations would be 1.90 and 1.44 ng/ml, respectively, which are in the upper portion of the therapeutic window. By contrast, administering a more conservative dosing rate of 0.25 every 24 hours would produce peak and trough values of 1.26 and 0.96 ng/ml, respectively, that would be associated with a steady-state value of 1.10 ng/ml. Of course the clinician must balance the problem of compliance with regimens that involve frequent dosage against the problem of periods when the patient may be subjected to concentrations of the drug that could be too high or too low.

Loading Dose. The "loading dose" is one or a series of doses that may be given at the onset of therapy with the aim of achieving the target concentration rapidly. The appropriate magnitude for the loading dose is:

$$\text{Loading dose} = \text{target } C_p \cdot V_{ss}/F \quad (1\text{--}20)$$

A loading dose may be desirable if the time required to attain steady state by the administration of drug at a constant rate (four elimination half-lives) is long relative to the temporal demands of the condition being treated. For example, the half-life of lidocaine is usually 1 to 2 hours. Arrhythmias encountered after myocardial infarction obviously may be life threatening, and one cannot wait 4 to 8 hours to achieve a therapeutic concentration of lidocaine by infusion of the drug at the rate required to attain this concentration. Hence, use of a loading dose of lidocaine in the coronary care unit is standard.

The use of a loading dose also has significant disadvantages. First, the particularly sensitive individual may be exposed abruptly to a toxic concentration of a drug. Moreover, if the drug involved has a long half-life, it will take a long time for the concentration to fall if the level achieved was excessive. Loading doses tend to be large, and they are often given parenterally and rapidly; this can be particularly dangerous if toxic effects occur as a result of actions of the drug at sites that are in rapid equilibrium with plasma. This occurs because the loading dose calculated on the basis of V_{ss} subsequent to drug distribution is initially constrained within the initial and smaller "central" volume of distribution. It is, therefore, usually advisable to divide the loading dose into a number of smaller fractional doses that are administered over a period of time. Alternatively, the loading dose should be administered as a continuous intravenous infusion over a period of time. Ideally this should be given in an exponentially decreasing fashion to mirror the concomitant accumulation of the maintenance dose of the drug, and this is now technically feasible using computerized infusion pumps.

Example. "Digitalization," in the patient described above, is gradual if only a maintenance dose is administered (for at least 10 days based on a half-life of 61 hours). A more rapid response could be obtained (if deemed necessary by the physician; *see* Chapter 34) by using a loading dose strategy and Equation (1–20):

$$\text{Loading dose} = 1.5 \text{ ng} \cdot \text{ml}^{-1} \times 580 \text{ liters}/0.7$$
$$= 1243 \ \mu\text{g} \sim 1 \text{ mg}$$

To avoid toxicity, this oral loading dose, which also could be intravenously administered, would be given as an initial 0.5-mg dose followed by a 0.25-mg dose at 6 to 8 hours later along with careful monitoring of the patient. It also would be prudent to give the final 0.25-mg fractional dose, if necessary, in two 0.125-mg divided doses separated by 6 to 8 hours to avoid overdigitalization, particularly if there were a plan to initiate an oral maintenance dose within 24 hours of beginning digoxin therapy.

Individualizing Dosage. A rational dosage regimen is based on knowledge of *F, CL, V_{ss},* and *$t_{1/2}$,* and some information about rates of absorption and distribution of the drug. Recommended dosage regimens generally are designed for an "average" patient; usual values for the important determining parameters and appropriate adjustments that may be necessitated by disease or other factors are presented in Appendix II. This "one size fits all" approach, however, overlooks the considerable and unpredictable interpatient variability that usually is present in these pharmacokinetic parameters. For many drugs, one standard deviation in the values observed for *F, CL,* and *V_{ss}* is about

20%, 50%, and 30%, respectively. This means that 95% of the time the C_{ss} that is achieved will be between 35% and 270% of the target; this is an unacceptably wide range for a drug with a low therapeutic index. Individualization of the dosage regimen to a particular patient is, therefore, critical for optimal therapy. The pharmacokinetic principles, described above, provide a basis for modifying the dosage regimen to obtain a desired degree of efficacy with a minimum of unacceptable adverse effects. In situations where the drug's plasma concentration can be measured and related to the therapeutic window, additional guidance for dosage modification is obtained. Such measurement and adjustment are appropriate for many drugs with low therapeutic indices (*e.g.,* cardiac glycosides, antiarrhythmic agents, anticonvulsants, theophylline, and others).

Therapeutic Drug Monitoring

The major use of measured concentrations of drugs (at steady state) is to refine the estimate of CL/F for the patient being treated [using Equation (1–14) as rearranged below]:

$$CL/F(\text{patient}) = \text{dosing rate}/C_{ss}(\text{measured}) \qquad (1\text{–}21)$$

The new estimate of CL/F can be used in Equation (1–16) to adjust the maintenance dose to achieve the desired target concentration.

Certain practical details and pitfalls associated with therapeutic drug monitoring should be kept in mind. The first of these relates to the time of sampling for measurement of the drug concentration. If intermittent dosing is used, when during a dosing interval should samples be taken? It is necessary to distinguish between two possible uses of measured drug concentrations to understand the possible answers. A concentration of drug measured in a sample taken at virtually any time during the dosing interval will provide information that may aid in the assessment of drug toxicity. This is one type of therapeutic drug monitoring. It should be stressed, however, that such use of a measured concentration of drug is fraught with difficulties because of interindividual variability in sensitivity to the drug. When there is a question of toxicity, the drug concentration can be no more than just one of many items that serve to interpret the clinical situation.

Changes in the effects of drugs may be delayed relative to changes in plasma concentration because of a slow rate of distribution or pharmacodynamic factors. Concentrations of digoxin, for example, regularly exceed 2 ng/ml (a potentially toxic value) shortly after an oral dose, yet these peak concentrations do not cause toxicity; indeed, they occur well before peak effects. Thus, concentrations of drugs in samples obtained shortly after administration can be uninformative or even misleading.

When concentrations of drugs are used for purposes of adjusting dosage regimens, samples obtained shortly after administration of a dose are almost invariably misleading. The

purpose of sampling during supposed steady state is to modify the estimate of CL/F and thus the choice of dosage. Early postabsorptive concentrations do not reflect clearance; they are determined primarily by the rate of absorption, the "central" (rather than the steady-state) volume of distribution, and the rate of distribution, all of which are pharmacokinetic features of virtually no relevance in choosing the long-term maintenance dosage. When the goal of measurement is adjustment of dosage, the sample should be taken well after the previous dose—as a rule of thumb just before the next planned dose, when the concentration is at its minimum. There is an exception to this approach: some drugs are nearly completely eliminated between doses and act only during the initial portion of each dosing interval. If it is questionable whether or not efficacious concentrations of such drugs are being achieved, a sample taken shortly after a dose may be helpful. On the other hand, if a concern is whether or not low clearance (as in renal failure) may cause accumulation of drug, concentrations measured just before the next dose will reveal such accumulation and are considerably more useful for this purpose than is knowledge of the maximal concentration. For such drugs, determination of both maximal and minimal concentrations is thus recommended.

A second important aspect of the timing of sampling is its relationship to the beginning of the maintenance dosage regimen. When constant dosage is given, steady state is reached only after four half-lives have passed. If a sample is obtained too soon after dosage is begun, it will not accurately reflect this state and the drug's clearance. Yet, for toxic drugs, if sampling is delayed until steady state is ensured, the damage may have been done. Some simple guidelines can be offered. When it is important to maintain careful control of concentrations, the first sample should be taken after two half-lives (as calculated and expected for the patient), assuming no loading dose has been given. If the concentration already exceeds 90% of the eventual expected mean steady-state concentration, the dosage rate should be halved, another sample obtained in another two (supposed) half-lives, and the dosage halved again if this sample exceeds the target. If the first concentration is not too high, the initial rate of dosage is continued; even if the concentration is lower than expected, it is usually reasonable to await the attainment of steady state in another two estimated half-lives and then proceed to adjust dosage as described above.

If dosage is intermittent, there is a third concern with the time at which samples are obtained for determination of drug concentrations. If the sample has been obtained just prior to the next dose, as recommended, concentration will be a minimal value, not the mean. However, as discussed above, the estimated mean concentration may be calculated by using Equation (1–14).

If a drug follows first-order kinetics, the average, minimum, and maximum concentrations at steady state are linearly related to dose and dosing rate [*see* Equations (1–14), (1–17), and (1–18)]. Therefore, the ratio between the measured and the desired concentrations can be used to adjust the dose, consistent with available dosage sizes:

$$\frac{C_{ss}(\text{measured})}{C_{ss}(\text{desired})} = \frac{\text{dose (previous)}}{\text{dose (new)}} \qquad (1\text{–}22)$$

In the previously described patient given 0.375 mg digoxin every 24 hours, for example, if the measured steady-state concentration was found to be 1.65 ng/ml rather than a desired level of 1.3 ng/ml, an appropriate, practical change in the dosage regimen would be to reduce the daily dose to 0.25 mg digoxin.

$$\text{Dose (new)} = \frac{C_{ss} \text{ (desired)}}{C_{ss} \text{ (measured)}} \times \text{dose (previous)}$$

$$= \frac{1.3}{1.65} \times 0.375 = 0.295 \sim 0.25 \text{ mg/24 hr}$$

Compliance

Ultimately, therapeutic success is dependent on the patient's actually taking the drug according to the prescribed dosage regimen—"Drugs don't work if you don't take them." Noncompliance with the dosing schedule is a major and often unappreciated reason for therapeutic failure, especially in the long-term treatment of disease using antihypertensive, antiretroviral, and anticonvulsant agents. When no special efforts are made to address this issue, only about 50% of patients follow the prescribed dosage regimen in a reasonably satisfactory fashion; approximately one-third only partly comply; and about 1 in 6 patients is essentially noncompliant. Missed doses are more common than too many doses. The number of drugs does not appear to be as important as the number of times a day doses must be remembered (Farmer, 1999). Reducing the number of required dosing occasions will improve adherence to a prescribed dosage regimen. Equally important is the need to involve patients in the responsibility for their own health, using a variety of strategies based on improved communication regarding the nature of the disease and the overall therapeutic plan.

BIBLIOGRAPHY

Benet, L.Z., and Galeazzi, R.L. Noncompartmental determination of the steady-state volume of distribution. *J. Pharm. Sci.,* **1979,** *68*:1071–1074.

Farmer, K.C. Methods for measuring and monitoring medication regimen adherence in clinical trials and clinical practice. *Clin. Ther.,* **1999,** *21*:1074–1090.

Kim, R.B., Fromm, M.F., Wandel, C., Leake, B., Wood, A.J.J., Roden, D.M., and Wilkinson, G.R. The drug transporter P-glycoprotein limits oral absorption and brain entry of HIV-1 protease inhibitors. *J. Clin. Invest.,* **1998,** *101*:289–294.

Klotz, U., Avant, G.R., Hoyumpa, A., Schenker, S., and Wilkinson, G.R. The effects of age and liver disease on the disposition and elimination of diazepam in adult man. *J. Clin. Invest.,* **1975,** *55*:347–359.

Morgan, D.J., and Smallwood, R.A. Clinical significance of pharmacokinetic models of hepatic elimination. *Clin. Pharmacokinet.,* **1990,** *18*:61–76.

Wilkinson, G.R., and Shand, D.G. Commentary: a physiological approach to hepatic drug clearance. *Clin. Pharmacol. Ther.,* **1975,** *18*:377–390.

Williams, R.L., Blaschke, T.F., Meffin, P.J., Melmon, K.L., and Rowland, M. Influence of acute viral hepatitis on disposition and plasma binding of tolbutamide. *Clin. Pharmacol. Ther.,* **1977,** *21*:301–309.

Wormhoudt, L.W., Commandeur, J.N., and Vermeulen, N.P. Genetic polymorphisms of human *N*-acetyltransferase, cytochrome P450, glutathione-S-transferase, and epoxide hydrolase enzymes: relevance to xenobiotic metabolism and toxicity. *Crit. Rev. Toxicol.,* **1999,** *29*:59–124.

MONOGRAPHS AND REVIEWS

Birkett, D.J. *Pharmacokinetics Made Easy.* McGraw-Hill, Sydney, Australia, **1998.**

Carruthers, S.G., Hoffman, B.B., Melmon, K.L., and Nierenberg, D.W., eds. *Melmon and Morelli's Clinical Pharmacology,* 4th ed. McGraw-Hill, New York, **2000.**

Evans, W.E., Schentag, J.J., and Jusko, W.J., eds. *Applied Pharmacokinetics: Principles of Therapeutic Drug Monitoring,* 3rd ed. Applied Therapeutics Inc., Vancouver, WA, **1992.**

Levy, R.H., Thummel, K.E., Trager, W.F., Hansten, P.D., and Eichelbaum, M., eds. *Metabolic Drug Interactions.* Lippincott Williams & Wilkins, Philadelphia, **2000.**

Parkinson, A. Biotransformation of xenobiotics. In, *Casarett & Doull's Toxicology: The Basic Science of Poisons,* 5th ed. McGraw-Hill, New York, **1996.**

Pratts, W.B., and Taylor, P., eds. *Principles of Drug Action: The Basis of Pharmacology,* 3rd ed. Churchill Livingstone, New York, **1990.**

Rowland, M., and Tozer, T.N., eds. *Clinical Pharmacokinetics: Concepts and Applications,* 3rd ed. Williams & Wilkins, Philadelphia, **1995.**

Acknowledgment

The author wishes to acknowledge Drs. Leslie Z. Benet, Deanna L. Kroetz, and Lewis B. Sheiner, authors of this chapter in the ninth edition of *Goodman and Gilman's The Pharmacological Basis of Therapeutics,* some of whose text has been retained in this edition.

CHAPTER 2

PHARMACODYNAMICS

Mechanisms of Drug Action and the Relationship
Between Drug Concentration and Effect

Elliott M. Ross and Terry P. Kenakin

This chapter provides an introduction to the concept of receptors, the structural and functional families of receptors, and the interplay among the diverse signaling pathways activated by receptor occupancy. These introductory concepts are amplified in subsequent chapters detailing the structure and function of receptors for individual drug groups. The latter part of the chapter presents means for quantifying receptor activation by agonists and blockade by antagonists. The functional relevance of partial agonists and inverse antagonists also is described as a prelude to the intentional development of mechanistically diverse drugs via *classical or new combinatorial strategies.*

Pharmacodynamics can be defined as the study of the biochemical and physiological effects of drugs and their mechanisms of action. The objectives of the analysis of drug action are to delineate the chemical or physical interactions between drug and target cell and to characterize the full sequence and scope of actions of each drug. Such a complete analysis provides the basis for both the rational therapeutic use of a drug and the design of new and superior therapeutic agents. Basic research in pharmacodynamics also provides fundamental insights into biochemical and physiological regulation.

MECHANISMS OF DRUG ACTION

The effects of most drugs result from their interaction with macromolecular components of the organism. These interactions alter the function of the pertinent component and thereby initiate the biochemical and physiological changes that are characteristic of the response to the drug. The term *receptor* denotes the component of the organism with which the chemical agent was presumed to interact. The statement that the receptor for a drug can be any functional macromolecular component of the organism has several fundamental corollaries. One is that a drug potentially is capable of altering the rate at which any bodily function proceeds. Another is that drugs do not create effects, but instead modulate intrinsic physiological functions.

Drug Receptors

At least from a numerical standpoint, proteins form the most important class of drug receptors. Examples are the receptors for hormones, growth factors, and neurotransmitters, the enzymes of crucial metabolic or regulatory pathways (*e.g.,* dihydrofolate reductase, acetylcholinesterase), proteins involved in transport processes (*e.g.,* Na^+,K^+-ATPase), or structural proteins (*e.g.,* tubulin). Specific binding properties of other cellular constituents also can be exploited. Thus, nucleic acids are important drug receptors, particularly for cancer chemotherapeutic agents.

A particularly important group of drug receptors are proteins that normally serve as receptors for endogenous regulatory ligands (*e.g.,* hormones, neurotransmitters). Many drugs act on such physiological receptors and are often particularly selective, because physiological receptors are specialized to recognize and respond to individual signaling molecules with great selectivity. Drugs that bind to physiological receptors and mimic the regulatory effects of the endogenous signaling compounds are termed *agonists*. Other drugs bind to receptors without regulatory effect, but their binding blocks the binding of the endogenous agonist. Such compounds, which may still produce useful effects by inhibiting the action of an agonist (*e.g.,* by competition for agonist binding sites), are termed *antagonists*. Agents that are only partly as effective as agonists are termed *partial agonists*, and those that stabilize the receptor in its inactive conformation are termed *inverse agonists*. (*See* below, "Quantitation of Drug–Receptor Interactions and Elicited Effect.")

The binding of drugs to receptors can involve all known types of interactions—ionic, hydrogen bonding, hydrophobic, van der Waals, and covalent. In most interactions between drugs and receptors, it is likely that bonds of multiple types are important. If binding is covalent, the duration of drug action is frequently, but not necessarily, prolonged. Noncovalent interactions of high affinity also may appear to be essentially irreversible.

Structure–Activity Relationship and Drug Design. Both the affinity of a drug for its receptor and its intrinsic activity are determined by its chemical structure. This relationship is frequently quite stringent. Relatively minor modifications in the drug molecule may result in major changes in pharmacological properties.

Exploitation of structure–activity relationships has on many occasions led to the synthesis of valuable therapeutic agents. Because changes in molecular configuration need not alter all actions and effects of a drug equally, it is sometimes possible to develop a congener with a more favorable ratio of therapeutic to toxic effects, enhanced selectivity among different cells or tissues, or more acceptable secondary characteristics than those of the parent drug. Therapeutically useful antagonists of hormones or neurotransmitters have been developed by chemical modification of the structure of the physiological agonist. Minor modifications of structure also can have profound effects on the pharmacokinetic properties of drugs.

Given adequate information about both the molecular structures and the pharmacological activities of a relatively large group of congeners, it should be possible to identify those chemical properties that are required for optimal action at the receptor—size, shape, the position and orientation of charged groups or hydrogen bond donors, and so on. Advances in computational chemistry, structural analysis of organic compounds, and the biochemical measurement of the primary actions of drugs at their receptors have enriched the quantitation of structure–activity relationships and its use in drug design (Kuntz, 1992; Schreiber, 1992). The importance of specific drug–receptor interactions can be evaluated further by analyzing the responsiveness of receptors that have been selectively mutated at individual amino acid residues. Such information is increasingly allowing the optimization or design of chemicals that can bind to a receptor with improved affinity, selectivity, or regulatory effect. Similar structure-based approaches also are used to improve pharmacokinetic properties of drugs (*see* Chapter 1). Knowledge of the structures of receptors and of drug-receptor complexes, determined at atomic resolution by X-ray crystallography or nuclear magnetic resonance (NMR) spectroscopy, is even more helpful in the design of ligands.

Ironically, advances in molecular biology that contribute to structure-motivated drug design also have spawned powerful but entirely random searches for new drugs. In this approach, huge libraries of randomly synthesized chemicals are generated either by synthetic chemistry or by genetically engineered microbes. A library then is screened for pharmacologically active agents using mammalian cells or microorganisms that have been engineered to express the receptor of therapeutic interest and the associated biochemical machinery necessary for detection of the receptor's response. Active compounds initially discovered by such random screens then can be modified and improved using knowledge of their structure–function relationships.

Cellular Sites of Drug Action. Because drugs act by altering the activities of their receptors, the sites at which a drug acts and the extent of its action are determined by the location and functional capacity of its receptors. Selective localization of drug action within the organism is therefore not necessarily dependent upon selective distribution of the drug. If a drug acts on a receptor that serves functions common to most cells, its effects will be widespread. If the function is a vital one, the drug may be particularly difficult or dangerous to use. Nevertheless, such a drug may be clinically important. Digitalis glycosides, important in the treatment of heart failure, are potent inhibitors of an ion transport process that is vital to most cells. As such, they can cause widespread toxicity, and their margin of safety is dangerously low. Other examples could be cited, particularly in the area of cancer chemotherapy. If a drug interacts with receptors that are unique to only a few types of differentiated cells, its effects are more specific. Hypothetically, the ideal drug would cause its therapeutic effect by such an action. Side effects would be minimized, but toxicity might not be. If the differentiated function were a vital one, this type of drug also could be very dangerous. Some of the most lethal chemical agents known (*e.g.*, botulinum toxin) show such specificity. Note also that, even if the primary action of a drug is localized, the consequent physiological effects of the drug may be widespread.

Receptors for Physiological Regulatory Molecules

The term *receptor* has been used operationally to denote any cellular macromolecule to which a drug binds to initiate its effects. Among the most important drug receptors are cellular proteins, whose normal function is to act as receptors for endogenous regulatory ligands—particularly hormones, growth factors, and neurotransmitters. The function of such physiological receptors consists of binding the appropriate ligand and, in response, propagating its regulatory signal in the target cell.

Identification of the two functions of a receptor, ligand binding and message propagation, correctly suggests the existence of functional domains within the receptor: a *ligand-binding domain* and an *effector domain*. The structure and function of these domains often can be deduced from high-resolution structures of receptor proteins and/or by analysis of the behavior of intentionally mutated receptors. Increasingly, the mechanism of intramolecular coupling of ligand binding with functional activation also can be learned. The biological importance of these functional domains is further indicated by the evolution both of different receptors for diverse ligands that act by similar biochemical mechanisms and of multiple receptors for a single ligand that act by unrelated mechanisms.

The regulatory actions of a receptor may be exerted directly on its cellular target(s), *effector protein(s)*, or may be conveyed by intermediary cellular signaling molecules called *transducers*. The receptor, its cellular target, and any intermediary molecules are referred to as a *receptor-effector system* or *signal transduction pathway*. Frequently, the proximal cellular effector protein is not the ultimate physiological target, but rather is an enzyme or transport protein that creates, moves, or degrades a small molecule metabolite or ion known as a *second messenger*. Second messengers can diffuse through a cell and convey information to a wide variety of targets, which can respond simultaneously to the output of a single receptor.

Receptors and their associated effector and transducer proteins also act as integrators of information as they coordinate signals from multiple ligands with each other and with the metabolic activities of the cell (*see* below). This integrative function is particularly evident when one considers that the different receptors for scores of chemically unrelated ligands utilize relatively few biochemical mechanisms to exert their regulatory functions, and that even these few pathways may share common signaling molecules.

An important property of physiological receptors, which also makes them excellent targets for drugs, is that they act catalytically and hence are biochemical signal amplifiers. The catalytic nature of receptors is obvious when the receptor itself is an enzyme, but all known physiological receptors are formally catalysts. For example, when a single agonist molecule binds to a receptor that is an ion channel, many ions flow through the channel. Similarly, a single steroid hormone molecule binds to its receptor and initiates the transcription of many copies of specific mRNAs, which in turn can give rise to multiple copies of a single protein.

A Framework for Considering Agonist Activity. If two drugs bind to the same receptor at the same site, why can one be an agonist and the other an antagonist? This question, more broadly stated, is also central to understanding the dynamics of protein structure and protein–ligand interactions. At a detailed level, the atomic interactions that allow a bound ligand to alter

the structure of the protein to which it binds are increasingly well understood. High-resolution structures of liganded and unliganded proteins combined with increasingly accurate theoretical structural modeling and functional studies of mutant proteins are clarifying how we can think about induced conformational changes.

From a functional perspective, however, the question of agonist action can be restated as: How does a receptor use the free energy of ligand binding to shift its conformation to the active state? A receptor, by definition, exists in at least two conformational states, active (**a**) and inactive (**i**).

$$R_i \rightleftharpoons R_a$$
$$\Updownarrow \qquad \Updownarrow$$
$$D{\cdot}R_i \rightleftharpoons D{\cdot}R_a$$

These conformations might correspond to the open and closed states of an ion channel, the active and inactive states of a protein tyrosine kinase, or the productive *versus* nonproductive conformations of a receptor for coupling to G proteins. If these states are in equilibrium and the inactive state predominates in the absence of drug, then the basal signal output will be low. The *extent* to which the equilibrium is shifted toward the active state is determined by the *relative* affinity of the drug for the two conformations (Figure 2–1). A drug that has a higher affinity for the active conformation than for the inactive conformation will drive the equilibrium to the active state and thereby activate the receptor. Such a drug will be an agonist. A full agonist is sufficiently selective for the active conformation that, at a saturating concentration, it will drive the receptor essentially

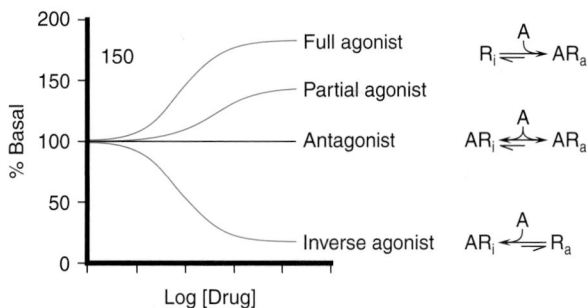

Figure 2–1. Regulation of the activity of a receptor with conformation-selective drugs.

The ordinate is the regulatory activity of the receptor produced by R_a, the active conformation as shown in scheme 1. If drug A selectively binds to R_a, it will shift the equilibrium toward net accumulation of R_a and produce a response. If drug A has equal affinity for R_i and R_a, it will not perturb the equilibrium between them and have no effect on net activity. If the drug selectively binds to R_i, then the net amount of R_a will be diminished. If there is sufficient R_a to produce an elevated basal response in the absence of ligand (agonist-independent constitutive activity), then activity will be observably inhibited; drug A will be an inverse agonist.

completely to the active state (*see* Figure 2–1). If a different but perhaps structurally similar compound binds to the same site on R but with only moderately greater affinity for R_a than for R_i, its effect will be less, even at saturating concentrations. A drug that displays such intermediate effectiveness is referred to as a *partial agonist*. Note that, in an absolute sense, all agonists are partial; selectivity for R_a over R_i cannot be total. A drug that binds with equal affinity to either conformation will not alter the activation equilibrium and will act as a competitive antagonist. Last, a drug with preferential affinity for R_i will actually produce an effect opposite to that of an agonist; examples of such *inverse agonists* do exist (*see* Chapters 11 and 17). If the *preexisting* equilibrium for unliganded receptors lies far in the direction of R_i, negative antagonism may be difficult to observe and to distinguish from simple competitive antagonism.

Careful biochemical studies of receptor–drug interactions, coupled with the analysis of receptors in which the intrinsic R_a/R_i equilibrium has been shifted by mutation, have supported this general model of drug action. The model is readily applicable to experimental data through the use of appropriate computer-assisted analysis and is frequently used as a guide to understanding drug action.

Physiological Receptors: Structural and Functional Families.   The last two decades have witnessed both an explosion in our appreciation of the number of physiological receptors and, in parallel, the development of our understanding of the fundamental structural motifs and biochemical mechanisms that characterize them. Molecular cloning has identified both completely novel receptors (and their regulatory ligands) and numerous isoforms of previously known receptors. There now exist data banks devoted exclusively to structures of single classes of receptors. Members of various classes of receptors, transducers, and effector proteins have been purified, and their mechanisms of action are understood in considerable biochemical detail. Receptors, transducers, and effectors can be expressed *via* molecular genetic strategies and studied in cultured cells. Alternatively, they can be expressed in large amounts in cells of convenience (bacteria, yeast, *etc.*) to facilitate their purification.

Receptors for physiological regulatory molecules can be assigned to a relatively few functional families whose members share both common mechanisms of action and similar molecular structures (Figure 2–2). For each receptor family, there is now at least a rudimentary understanding of the structures of ligand-binding domains and effector domains and of how agonist binding influences the regulatory activity of the receptor. The relatively small number of biochemical mechanisms and structural formats used for cellular signaling is fundamental to the ways in which target cells integrate signals from multiple receptors to produce additive, synergistic, or mutually

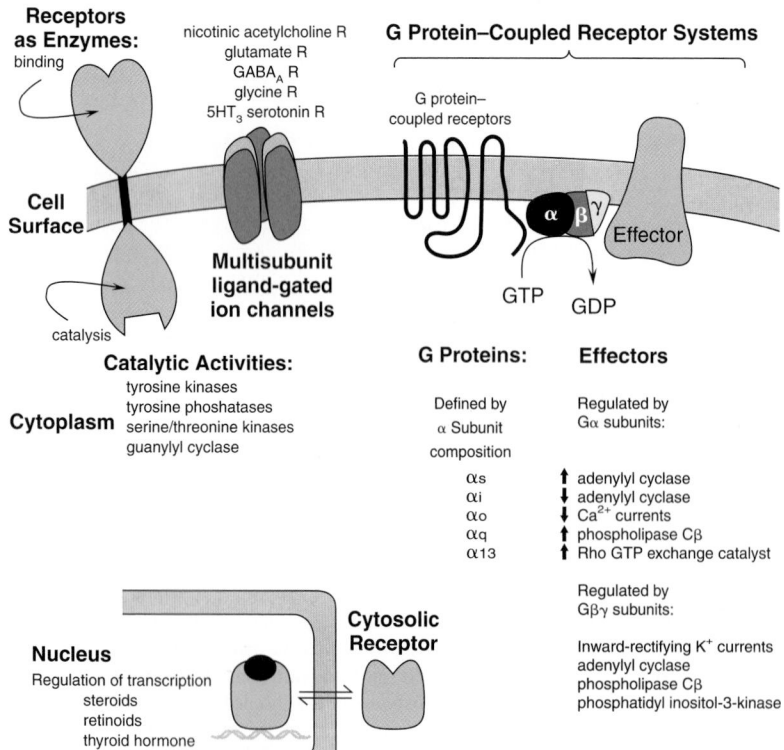

Figure 2–2. Structural motifs of physiological receptors and their relationships to signaling pathways.

Schematic diagram of the diversity of mechanisms for control of cell function by receptors for endogenous agents acting *via* the cell surface or in the nucleus.

inhibitory responses. Figure 2–1 provides a schematic diagram of various receptor families and their transducer and effector molecules.

Receptors as Enzymes: Receptor Protein Kinases. The largest group of receptors with intrinsic enzymatic activity are cell surface protein kinases, which exert their regulatory effects by phosphorylating diverse effector proteins at the inner face of the plasma membrane. Phosphorylation can alter the biochemical activities of an effector or its interactions with other proteins. Most receptor protein kinases target tyrosine residues in their substrates; these include receptors for insulin, many cytokines and diverse peptides, and proteins that direct growth or differentiation. A few receptor protein kinases also phosphorylate serine or threonine residues. The structurally most simple receptor protein kinases are composed of an agonist-binding domain on the extracellular surface of the plasma membrane, a single membrane-spanning element, and a protein kinase domain on the inner membrane face. Many variations on this basic plan exist, including obligate oligomerization and the addition of multiple regulatory or protein-binding domains to the intracellular protein kinase domain.

Another family of receptors that are functionally protein kinases contains a modification of the structure described above. Protein kinase–associated receptors lack the intracellular enzymatic domains but, in response to agonists, bind and/or activate distinct protein kinases on the cytoplasmic face of the plasma membrane. Receptors of this group include several receptors for neurotrophic peptides and the multisubunit antigen receptors on T and B lymphocytes. The antigen receptors also involve tyrosine protein phosphatases in their cellular regulatory activity, and it is plausible that other receptors that apparently lack cytoplasmic effector domains may recruit still other effector proteins.

Receptors with Other Enzymatic Activity. The domain structure just described for cell surface protein kinases is varied in other receptors to utilize other signaling outputs. A family of protein tyrosine phosphatases has extracellular domains with a sequence reminiscent of cellular adhesion molecules. Although the extracellular ligands for many of these phosphatases are not yet known, the importance of their enzymatic activity has been demonstrated through genetic and biochemical experiments in multiple cell types. In the receptors for atrial natriuretic peptides and the peptide guanylin, the intracellular domain is not a protein kinase but a guanylyl cyclase, which synthesizes the second messenger, cyclic GMP. Receptors with guanylyl cyclase activity also serve as pheromone receptors in invertebrates. There may be other variations on this transmembrane topology.

Ion Channels. Receptors for several neurotransmitters form agonist-regulated, ion-selective channels in the plasma membrane, termed *ligand-gated ion channels,* which convey their signals by altering the cell's membrane potential or ionic composition. This group includes the nicotinic cholinergic receptor; the $GABA_A$ receptor for gamma-aminobutyric acid; and receptors for glutamate, aspartate, and glycine (*see* Chapters 9, 12, and 17). They are all multisubunit proteins, with each subunit predicted to span the plasma membrane several times. Symmetrical association of the subunits allows each to form a segment of the channel wall and to cooperatively control channel opening and closing.

G Protein–Coupled Receptors. A large family of receptors use distinct heterotrimeric GTP-binding regulatory proteins, known as G proteins, as transducers to convey signals to their effector proteins. G protein–coupled receptors include those for many biogenic amines, eicosanoids, and other lipid signaling molecules as well as numerous peptide and protein ligands. G protein–regulated effectors include enzymes such as adenylyl cyclase and phospholipase C and plasma membrane ion channels selective for Ca^{2+} and K^+ (Figure 2–2). Because of their number and physiological importance, G protein–coupled receptors are widely used targets for drugs; it has been estimated that about half of all nonantibiotic prescription drugs are directed toward these receptors.

G protein–coupled receptors span the plasma membrane as a bundle of seven alpha helices. Agonists bind to a cleft within the extracellular face of the bundle or to a globular ligand-binding domain sometimes found at the amino terminus. G proteins bind to the cytoplasmic face of the receptors. Receptors in this family respond to agonists by promoting the binding of GTP to the G protein. GTP activates the G protein and allows it in turn to activate the effector protein. The G protein remains active until it hydrolyzes bound GTP to GDP, which does not activate. G proteins are composed of a GTP-binding α subunit, which confers specific recognition by receptor, and an associated dimer of β and γ subunits. Activation of the $G\alpha$ subunit by GTP allows it to both regulate an effector protein and drive the release of $G\beta\gamma$ subunits, which can regulate their own group of effectors.

A cell may express as many as twenty G protein–coupled receptors, each with distinctive specificity for one or several of its half-dozen G proteins. Each $G\alpha$ can regulate one or more effectors. Receptors for multiple ligands can thus integrate their signals through a single G protein. A receptor also may generate multiple signals by activating more than one G protein species. Similarly, a $G\alpha$ subunit can regulate the activities of more than one effector. Thus, the receptor–G protein effector systems are complex networks of convergent and divergent interactions that permit extraordinarily versatile regulation of cell function (Ross, 1992).

Transcription Factors. Receptors for steroid hormones, thyroid hormone, vitamin D, and the retinoids are soluble DNA-binding proteins that regulate the transcription of specific genes (Mangelsdorf *et al.*, 1994). They are part of a larger family of transcription factors whose members may be regulated by phosphorylation, association with other cellular proteins, or by binding to metabolites or cellular regulatory ligands. These receptors act as dimers—some as homodimers and some as heterodimers—with homologous cellular proteins, but they may be regulated by higher-order oligomerization with other regulating molecules. They provide striking examples of conservation of structure and mechanism, in part because they are assembled as three largely independent domains. The region nearest the carboxyl terminus binds hormone and serves a negative regulatory role; that is, removal of this domain leaves a constitutively active fragment that may be nearly as effective in regulating transcription as is the intact hormone-liganded receptor. Hormone binding presumably also relieves this inhibitory constraint. The central region of the receptor mediates binding to specific sites on nuclear DNA to activate or inhibit transcription of the nearby gene. These regulatory sites in DNA are likewise receptor-specific: the sequence of a "glucocorticoid-responsive element," with only slight variation, is associated with each glucocorticoid-responsive gene. The function of the amino-terminal region of the receptor is less well defined, but its loss decreases the receptor's regulatory activity. The activity of each domain is largely independent, a phenomenon best demonstrated by the construction of chimeric receptors that reflect the hormone binding or DNA regulatory activity characteristic of the "parent" receptor contributing that domain.

Cytoplasmic Second Messengers.   *Cyclic AMP.* Physiological signals also are integrated within the cell as a result of interactions between second-messenger pathways. Compared with the number of receptors and cytosolic signaling proteins, there are relatively few recognized cytoplasmic second messengers. However, their synthesis or release and degradation or excretion reflect the activities of many pathways. Well-studied second messengers include cyclic AMP and cyclic GMP, Ca^{2+}, inositol phosphates, diacylglycerol, and nitric oxide; our list of this diverse group of molecules is still growing. Second messengers influence each other both directly, by altering the other's metabolism, and indirectly, by sharing intracellular targets. This superficially confusing pattern of regulatory pathways allows the cell to respond to agonists, singly or in combination, with an integrated array of cytoplasmic second messengers and responses. Cyclic AMP, the prototypical second messenger, remains a good example for understanding the regulation and function of most second messengers. It is synthesized by adenylyl cyclase under the control of many G protein–coupled receptors; stimulation is mediated by G_s and inhibition by G_i.

There are at least ten tissue-specific adenylyl cyclase isozymes, each with its unique pattern of regulatory responses. Several adenylyl cyclase isozymes are either stimulated or inhibited by G protein $\beta\gamma$ subunits, which allows G proteins other than G_s to modulate cyclase activity. Some isozymes are stimulated by Ca^{2+} or Ca^{2+}–calmodulin complexes. Each of the isozymes has its own pattern of enhancement or attenuation by phosphorylation and other regulatory influences, providing a broad array of regulatory features to individual target cells. Cyclic AMP is eliminated by a combination of hydrolysis, catalyzed by cyclic nucleotide phosphodiesterases, and extrusion by several plasma membrane transport proteins. Phosphodiesterases form yet another family of important signaling proteins whose activities are regulated by controlled transcription as well as by second messengers (cyclic nucleotides and Ca^{2+}) and interactions with yet other signaling proteins.

In most cases, cyclic AMP functions by activating cyclic AMP–dependent protein kinases, a relatively small group of closely related proteins. However, these protein kinases phosphorylate both final physiological targets (metabolic enzymes or transport proteins) and numerous protein kinases and other regulatory proteins. This latter group includes transcription factors that allow cyclic AMP to regulate gene expression in addition

to more acute cellular events. In addition to activating a protein kinase, cyclic AMP also directly regulates the activity of plasma membrane cation channels, which are particularly important in olfactory neurons. Cyclic AMP signals are thus propagated throughout the biochemical behavior of the target cell.
Calcium. Intracellular Ca^{2+}, another particularly well-studied second messenger, offers several interesting comparisons with cyclic AMP. The release of Ca^{2+} into the cytoplasm is mediated by diverse channels: plasma membrane channels regulated by G proteins, membrane potential, K^+ or Ca^{2+} itself, and channels in specialized regions of endoplasmic reticulum that respond to the second messenger inositol trisphosphate (IP_3), or, in muscle, to cell depolarization. Ca^{2+} is removed both by extrusion and by reuptake into the endoplasmic reticulum. Ca^{2+} propagates its signals through a much wider range of proteins than does cyclic AMP, including metabolic enzymes, protein kinases, and Ca^{2+}-binding regulatory proteins that regulate still other ultimate and intermediary effectors.

Regulation of Receptors

Receptors not only initiate regulation of physiological and biochemical function but also are themselves subject to many regulatory and homeostatic controls. These controls include regulation of the synthesis and degradation of the receptor by multiple mechanisms, covalent modification, association with other regulatory proteins, and/or relocalization within the cell. Transducer and effector proteins similarly are regulated. Modulating inputs may come from other receptors, directly or indirectly, and receptors are almost always subject to feedback regulation by their own signaling outputs.

Continued stimulation of cells with agonists generally results in a state of *desensitization* (also referred to as *refractoriness* or *down-regulation*), such that the effect that follows continued or subsequent exposure to the same concentration of drug is diminished (Figure 2–3). This phenomenon is very important in therapeutic situations; an example is attenuated response to the repeated use of β-adrenergic agonists as bronchodilators for the treatment of asthma (*see* Chapter 10).

Feedback inhibition of signaling may be limited to output only from the stimulated receptor, a situation known as *homologous desensitization*. Attenuation also may extend to the action of all receptors that share a common signaling pathway, *heterologous desensitization* (Figure 2–3). Homologous desensitization indicates feedback directed to the receptor molecule itself (phosphorylation, proteolysis, decreased synthesis, *etc.*), whereas heterologous desensitization may involve inhibition or loss of one or more downstream proteins that participate in signaling from other receptors. Mechanisms involved in homologous and heterologous desensitization of specific receptors and signaling pathways are discussed in greater detail in later chapters related to individual receptor families.

Predictably, supersensitivity to agonists also frequently follows chronic reduction of receptor stimulation. Such situations can result, for example, from the long-term administration of β-adrenergic antagonists such as propranolol (*see* Chapter 10).

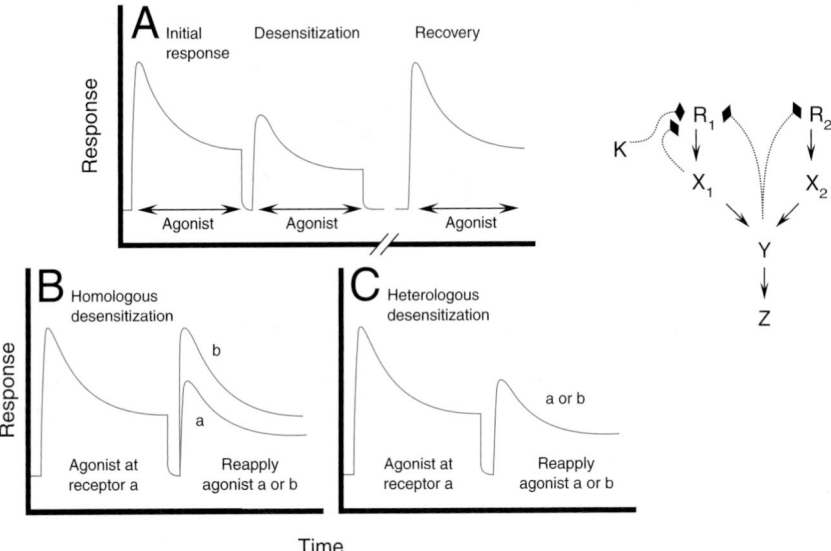

Figure 2–3. Desensitization in response to an agonist.

A. Upon exposure to an agonist, the *initial response* usually peaks and then decreases to approach some tonic level, elevated but below the maximum. If the drug is removed for a brief period, the state of *desensitization* is maintained, such that a second addition of agonist also provokes a diminished response. Removal of the drug for a more extended period allows the cell to "reset" its capacity to respond, and *recovery* of response usually is complete. *B* and *C*. Desensitization may be *homologous (B)*, affecting responses elicited only by the stimulated receptor, or *heterologous (C)*, acting on several receptors or on a pathway that is common to many receptors. Agonist a acts at receptor a and agonist b at receptor b. Homologous desensitization can reflect feedback from a transducer (or effector) unique to the pathway of the receptor (X_1) or from an off-pathway component (K) that is sensitive to the activation state of the receptor. Heterologous desensitization is initiated by transducers or effectors common to multiple receptor signaling pathways (Y or Z).

Diseases Resulting from Receptor Malfunction.   In addition to variability among individuals in their responses to drugs (*see* Chapter 3), several definable diseases arise from disorders in receptors or receptor–effector systems. The loss of a receptor in a highly specialized signaling system may cause a relatively limited phenotypic disorder, such as the genetic deficiency of the androgen receptor in the testicular feminization syndrome (Griffin *et al.*, 1995). Deficiencies of more widely used signaling systems have a broader spectrum of effects, as are seen in myasthenia gravis or some forms of insulin-resistant diabetes mellitus, which result from autoimmune depletion of nicotinic cholinergic receptors (*see* Chapter 9) or insulin receptors (*see* Chapter 61), respectively. A lesion in a component of a signaling pathway that is used by many receptors can cause a generalized endocrinopathy. Heterozygous deficiency of G_s, the G protein that activates adenylyl cyclase in all cells, causes multiple endocrine disorders (Spiegel and Weinstein, 1995). Homozygous deficiency in G_s presumably would be lethal.

The expression of aberrant or ectopic receptors, effectors, or coupling proteins potentially can lead to supersensitivity, subsensitivity, or other untoward responses. Among the most interesting and significant events is the appearance of aberrant receptors as products of *oncogenes,* which transform otherwise normal cells into malignant cells. Virtually any type of

signaling system may have oncogenic potential. The *erb*A oncogene product is an altered form of a receptor for thyroid hormone, constitutively active because of the loss of its ligand-binding domain (Mangelsdorf *et al.*, 1994). The *ros* and *erb*B oncogene products are activated, uncontrolled forms of the receptors for insulin and epidermal growth factor, respectively, both known to enhance cellular proliferation (Yarden and Ulrich, 1988). The *mas* oncogene product (Young *et al.*, 1986) is a G protein–coupled receptor, probably the receptor for a peptide hormone. Constitutive activation of G protein–coupled receptors due to subtle mutations in receptor structure has been shown to give rise to retinitis pigmentosa, precocious puberty, and malignant hyperthyroidism (reviewed in Clapham, 1993). G proteins can themselves be oncogenic when either overexpressed or constitutively activated by mutation (Lyons *et al.*, 1990).

Mutation of receptors can alter either acute responsiveness to drug therapy or its continuing efficacy. For example, a mutation of β-adrenergic receptors, which mediate airway smooth muscle relaxation and bronchial airflow, accelerates desensitization to β-adrenergic agonists used to treat asthma (Turki *et al.*, 1995; *see* Chapter 28). As the mutations that mediate these pathologies are discovered, they can be replicated using the cloned genes, so as to allow development of suitable drugs to target them specifically.

Classification of Receptors and Drug Effects

Traditionally, drug receptors have been identified and classified primarily on the basis of the effect and relative potency of selective agonists and antagonists. For example, the effects of acetylcholine that are mimicked by the alkaloid muscarine and that are selectively antagonized by atropine are termed *muscarinic effects*. Other effects of acetylcholine that are mimicked by nicotine are described as *nicotinic effects*. By extension, these two types of cholinergic effects are said to be mediated by muscarinic or nicotinic receptors. Although it frequently contributes little to delineation of the mechanism of drug action, such categorization provides a convenient basis for summarizing drug effects. A statement that a drug activates a specified type of receptor is a succinct summary of its spectrum of effects and of the agents that will regulate it. However, the accuracy of this statement may be altered when new receptors or receptor subtypes are identified or additional drug mechanisms or side effects are revealed.

Significance of Receptor Subtypes. As the diversity and selectivity of drugs increased, it became clear that multiple subtypes of receptors exist within many previously defined classes of receptors. Molecular cloning further accelerated discovery of novel receptor subtypes, and their expression as recombinant proteins has facilitated discovery of subtype-selective drugs. Distinct but related receptors may, but need not, display distinctive patterns of selectivity among agonist or antagonist ligands. When selective ligands are not known, the receptors are more commonly referred to as *isoforms* rather than as *subtypes*. Receptor subtypes may display different mechanisms of signal output. For example, M_1- and M_3-muscarinic receptors activate G_q to initiate Ca^{2+} signaling, and M_2- and M_4-muscarinic receptors activate G_i to activate other signaling pathways. The distinction between classes and subtypes of receptors is, however, often arbitrary and/or historical. The α_1-, α_2-, and β-adrenergic receptors differ from each other both in selectivity among drugs and in their choice of G protein transducers (G_i, G_q, and G_s, respectively), yet α and β are considered receptor classes and α_1 and α_2 are considered subtypes. The α_{1A}, α_{1B}, and α_{1C} receptor isoforms differ little in their biochemical properties; the same is nearly true for the β_1, β_2, and β_3 subtypes.

Pharmacological differences among receptor subtypes are exploited therapeutically through the development and use of receptor-selective drugs. Such drugs may be used to elicit different responses from a single tissue when receptor subtypes initiate different intracellular signals, or they may serve to differentially modulate different cells or tissues that express one or another receptor subtype. Increasing the selectivity of a drug among tissues or among responses elicited from a single tissue may determine whether the drug's therapeutic benefits outweigh its unwanted effects.

The molecular biological search for novel receptors has moved well beyond the search for isoforms of known receptors toward the discovery of hundreds of genes for completely novel human receptors. Many of these receptors can be assigned to known families based on sequence, and their functions can be confirmed with appropriate ligands. However, many are "orphans," the designation give to receptors whose ligands are unknown. Discovery of the endogenous ligands and physiological functions of orphan receptors is widely hoped to lead to new drugs that can modulate currently intractable disease states.

The discovery of numerous receptor isoforms raises the question of their importance to the organism, particularly when their signaling mechanisms and specificity for endogenous ligands are indistinguishable. Perhaps this multiplicity of genes facilitates the independent, cell-specific, and temporally controlled expression of receptors according to the developmental needs of the organism. Regardless of their mechanistic implications (or lack thereof), discovery of isoform-selective ligands may substantially improve our targeting of therapeutic drugs.

Actions of Drugs Not Mediated by Receptors

If one restricts the definition of receptors to macromolecules, then several drugs may be said not to act upon receptors as such. Some drugs specifically bind small molecules or ions that are normally or abnormally found in the body. One example is the therapeutic neutralization of gastric acid by a base (antacid). Another example is the use of mesna, a free radical scavenger rapidly eliminated by the kidneys, to bind to reactive metabolites associated with some cancer chemotherapeutic agents and thus minimize their untoward effects on the urinary tract (*see* Chapter 52). Other agents act according to colligative effects without a requirement for highly specific chemical structure. For example, certain relatively benign compounds, such as mannitol, can be administered in quantities sufficient to increase the osmolarity of various body fluids and thereby cause appropriate changes in the distribution of water (*see* Chapter 29). Depending on the agent and route of administration, this effect can be exploited to promote diuresis, catharsis, expansion of circulating volume in the vascular compartment, or reduction of cerebral edema.

Certain drugs that are structural analogs of normal biological chemicals may be incorporated into cellular components and thereby alter their function. This property has been termed a "counterfeit incorporation mechanism," and has been particularly useful with analogs of pyrimidines and purines that can be incorporated into nucleic acids; such drugs have clinical utility in antiviral and cancer chemotherapy (*see* Chapters 50 and 52).

QUANTITATION OF DRUG–RECEPTOR INTERACTIONS AND ELICITED EFFECT

Receptor Pharmacology

The major aim of receptor pharmacology is to understand and quantify the effects of chemicals (drugs) on biological systems. This is important in the therapeutic arena because drugs are nearly always used therapeutically in systems different from those in which they were discovered and tested. Biological systems interpret the effects of drugs in different ways, and these interpretations can be confusing. What is needed is a standard scale of drug activity that transcends biological systems and can be used to predict the effects of the drug in all systems. Receptor pharmacology strives to furnish the tools to accomplish this goal.

The basic currency of receptor pharmacology is the dose–response curve, a depiction of the observed effect of a drug as a function of its concentration in the receptor compartment. Figure 2–4A shows a typical dose–response curve; it reaches a maximal asymptote value when the drug occupies all of the receptor sites. The range of concentrations needed to fully depict the dose–response relationship usually is too wide to be useful in the format shown in Figure 2–4A. Most dose–response curves are therefore plotted with the logarithm of the concentration as the x axis (see Figure 2–4B). Dose–response curves have three basic properties: threshold, slope, and maximal asymptote; these parameters characterize and quantitate the activity of the drug.

In general, drugs can do two things to receptors: (1) bind to them and (2) possibly change their behavior

toward the host cell system. The first function is governed by the chemical property of *affinity,* ruled by the chemical forces that cause the drug to associate with the receptor. The second is governed by a quantity referred to as *efficacy.* Efficacy is the information encoded in a drug's chemical structure that causes the receptor to change accordingly when the drug is bound. Historically, efficacy has been treated operationally as a proportionality constant that quantifies the extent of functional change imparted to a receptor upon binding a drug.

Classical Receptor Theory. Receptor occupancy theory, in which it is assumed that response emanates from a receptor occupied by a drug, has its basis in the law of mass action, with modifying constants added to accommodate experimental findings. Agonism was described by modification of this model by Ariëns (1954), Stephenson (1956), and Furchgott (1966). Stephenson introduced another important concept, *stimulus,* which is the initial effect of drug upon the receptor itself; stimulus is then processed by the system to yield the observable response. Antagonism was modeled by Gaddum (1937, 1957) and Schild (1957) to determine the affinity of antagonists.

The basic components of drug receptor–mediated response are shown in Figure 2–5. Affinity is measured by the equilibrium

classical receptor occupancy theory

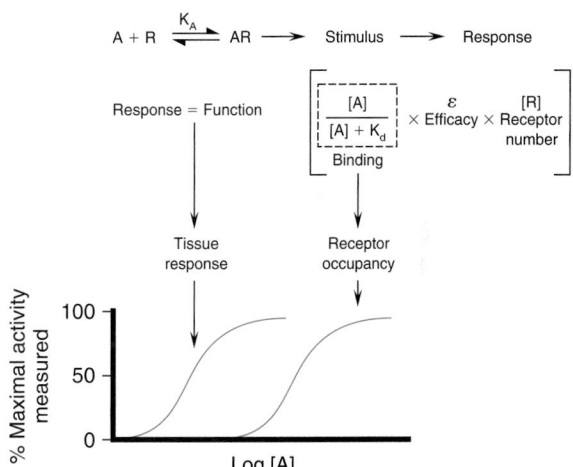

Figure 2–5. Classical receptor occupancy theory.

Drug A binds to receptor R to form a complex AR, the proximal signal from which is then processed by the cell to produce an observable response. Occupancy of the receptor is given by the Langmuir adsorption isotherm: $[A]/([A] + K_d)$. The amplitude of the signal for each bound receptor is determined by the efficacy ε, which is multiplied by receptor concentration $[R]$ to yield the total receptor-mediated stimulus. A cascade of biochemical events in the cell processes this stimulus to produce the response. Fractional receptor binding and fractional final response are shown as functions of drug concentration, $[A]$.

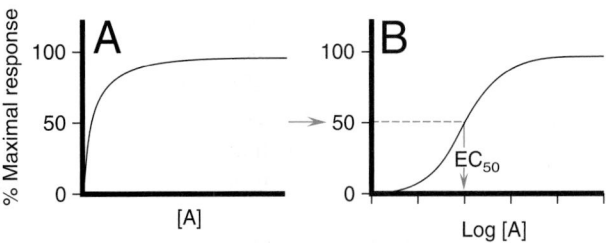

Figure 2–4. Graded responses (y axis as a percent of maximal response) expressed as a function of the concentration of drug A present at the receptor.

The hyperbolic shape of the curve in panel A becomes sigmoid when plotted semilogarithmically, as in panel B. The concentration of drug that produces 50 percent of the maximal response quantifies drug activity and is referred to as the EC_{50} (effective concentration for 50 percent response).

dissociation constant of the drug–receptor complex (denoted K_d); the fraction of receptors occupied by the drug is determined by the concentration of drug and K_d, as shown (*see* Figure 2–5). Intrinsic efficacy is a proportionality constant (denoted ε) that defines the power of the drug to induce response. The product of occupancy, intrinsic efficacy, and receptor number yields the total receptor-mediated stimulus given to the system. Stimulus is conveyed to physiological effectors by biochemical reactions to produce the response. It should be noted that efficacy is a function of occupancy and the stimulus–response function (comprising all of the biochemical reactions that take place to translate agonist binding into response) and amplifies stimulus. Therefore, the location of the dose–response curves for response is shifted to the left of the receptor occupancy curve (Figure 2–5).

Before discussion of the quantitation of drug–receptor effects, it is worth considering this amplification process further because it can control the observed response to a drug.

Transmission of Receptor Stimulus by the Target Tissue. The activation of a receptor by a drug can be thought of as an initial signal that is then amplified by the cell. Different cells have different amplification properties; thus a weak receptor signal may produce no visible response in one cell type and a powerful signal in another. The amplification properties of the cell (referred to as the *stimulus-response capability*) control the observed outcome of drug–receptor interaction, as shown in Figure 2–6 for three hypothetical drugs and three different cell types. In cell I, which amplifies a stimulus relatively

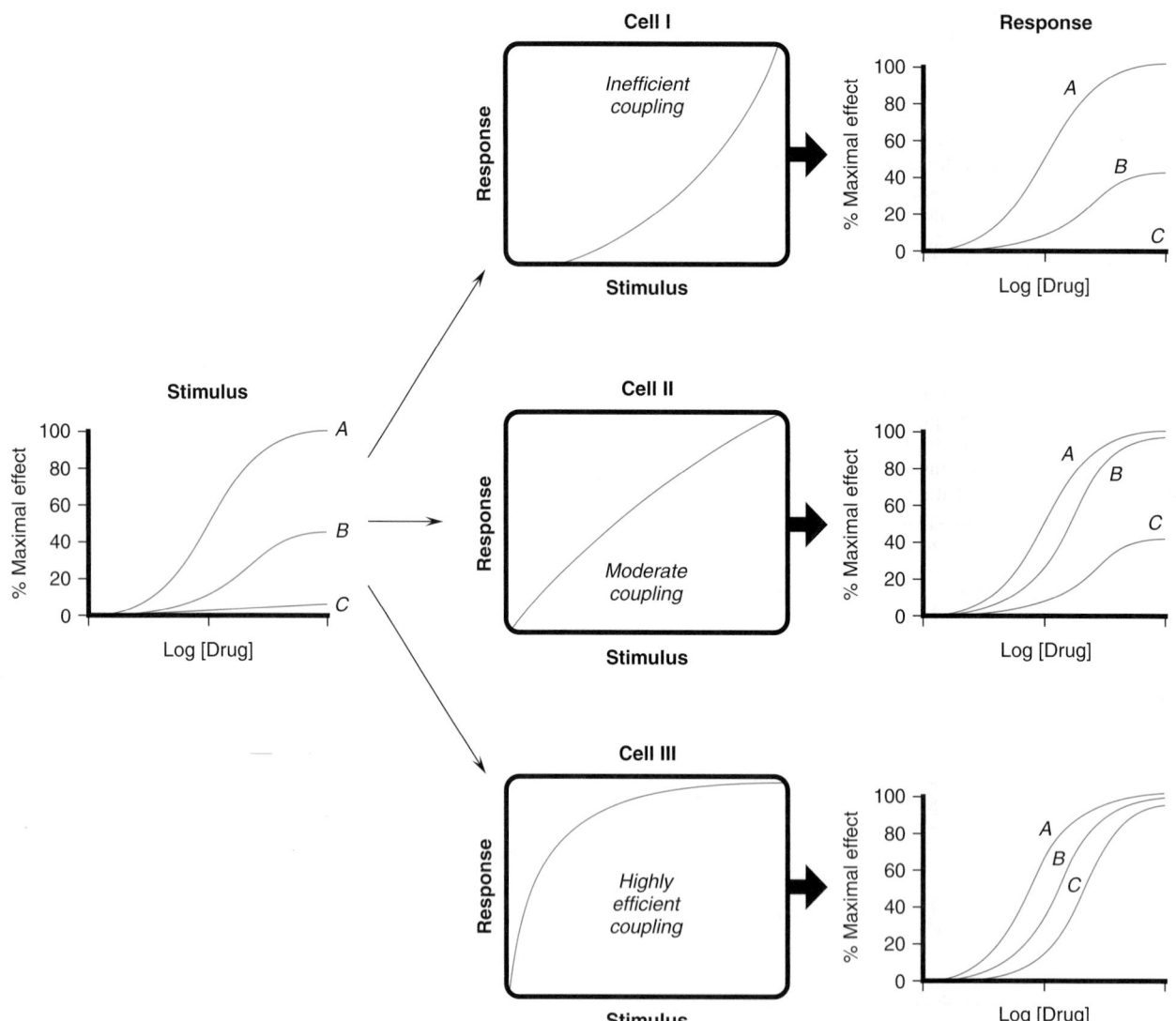

Figure 2–6. Different efficiencies of cellular stimulus-response processing can produce different levels of response for three agonists of differing efficacies.

See text for details.

weakly, drug A produces a full tissue response and would be labeled a full agonist. Drug B produces a partial (submaximal) tissue response and would be a partial agonist. Drug C produces no response, but nevertheless occupies the receptor and therefore would antagonize the effects of either drug A or drug B; it would be referred to as an antagonist. When these same drugs are tested on cell II, which has a more efficiently coupled stimulus-response mechanism, drug A remains a full agonist, drug B is now also a full agonist, and drug C, which had insufficient efficacy to cause a physiological response in cell I, is now a partial agonist. The properties of these drugs have not changed; only the efficiency of the signaling system has changed. Thus, the labels for these drugs change as well. Drug B goes from a partial agonist to a full agonist and drug C goes from an antagonist to a partial agonist. This progression continues when these drugs are tested in cell III, which has even more efficient signaling machinery. Now all three drugs act as full agonists (Figure 2–6). This example illustrates the potential fallacy of classifying drugs on the basis of what they do rather than what they are. What drugs do depends on the receptor and its associated signaling proteins; classification by magnitude of physiological effect can be seriously misleading when drugs are tested in one cellular format for therapeutic use in another. The alternative is to classify drugs according to the magnitude of their two molecular properties: affinity for the receptor and efficacy once bound. By quantifying these system-independent properties, drug activity can be predicted in all systems as long as the identity of the receptor is known.

Quantifying Agonism. Drugs have two observable properties in biological systems: potency and magnitude of effect (when a biological response is produced). Potency is controlled by four factors: two relate to the biological system containing the receptors (receptor density and efficiency of the stimulus–response mechanisms of the tissue) and two relate to the interaction of drug with its receptor (affinity and efficacy). When the relative potency of two agonists of equal efficacy is measured in the same biological system, downstream signaling effects cancel and the comparison yields a relative measure of the affinity and efficacy of the two agonists (*see* Figure 2–7A). Thus, measuring agonist potency ratios is one method of measuring the capability of different agonists to induce a response in a test system and for predicting comparable activity in another. Another method

of estimating agonist activity is to compare maximal asymptotes in systems where the agonists do not produce system maximal response (Figure 2–7B). The advantage of using maxima is that this property is solely dependent upon efficacy, whereas potency is a mixed function of both affinity and efficacy.

Quantifying Antagonism. Characteristic patterns of antagonism are associated with certain mechanisms of blockade of receptors. One is simple competitive antagonism, whereby a drug that lacks intrinsic efficacy but retains affinity competes with the agonist for the binding site. The characteristic pattern of such antagonism is the concentration-dependent production of a parallel shift to the right of the agonist dose–response curve with no change in the maximal asymptotic response (Figure 2–8A). The magnitude of the rightward shift of the curve depends only upon the concentration of the antagonist and its affinity for the receptor. The affinity of a competitive antagonist for its receptor can therefore be determined according to its concentration-dependent ability to shift the dose–response curve for an agonist rightward, as first noted by Schild (1957). Note that a partial agonist similarly can compete with a "full" agonist for binding to the receptor. However, increasing concentrations of a partial agonist will inhibit response to a finite level characteristic of the drug's intrinsic efficacy; a competitive antagonist will reduce the response to zero. Partial agonists thus can be used therapeutically to buffer a response by inhibiting untoward stimulation without totally abolishing the stimulus from the receptor.

An antagonist may dissociate so slowly from the receptor as to be essentially irreversible in its action. Under these circumstances, the maximal response to the agonist will be depressed at some antagonist concentrations (Figure 2–8B). Operationally, this is referred to as *noncompetitive antagonism,* although the molecular mechanism of action really cannot be unequivocally inferred from the effect. An irreversible antagonist competing for the same binding site as the agonist also can produce the pattern of antagonism shown in Figure 2–8B.

Noncompetitive antagonism can be produced by another type of drug, referred to as an *allosteric antagonist.* This type of drug produces its effect by binding a site on the receptor distinct from that of the primary agonist and thereby changing the affinity of the receptor for the agonist (*see* Figure 2–8). In the case of an allosteric antagonist, the affinity of the receptor for the agonist is decreased by the antagonist (*see* Figure 2–8C). In

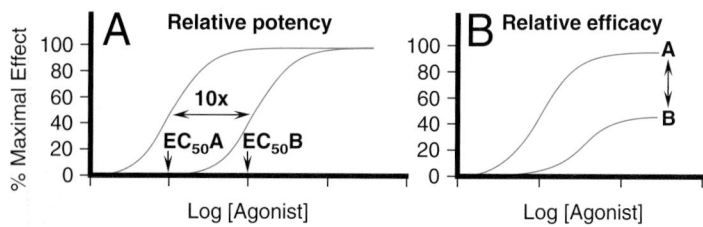

Figure 2–7. Two ways of quantifying agonism.

A. The relative potency of two agonists, when obtained in the same tissue, is a function of their relative affinities and intrinsic efficacies. *B.* In systems where the two drugs do not both produce the maximal response characteristic of the tissue, the observed maximal response is a nonlinear function of their relative intrinsic efficacies.

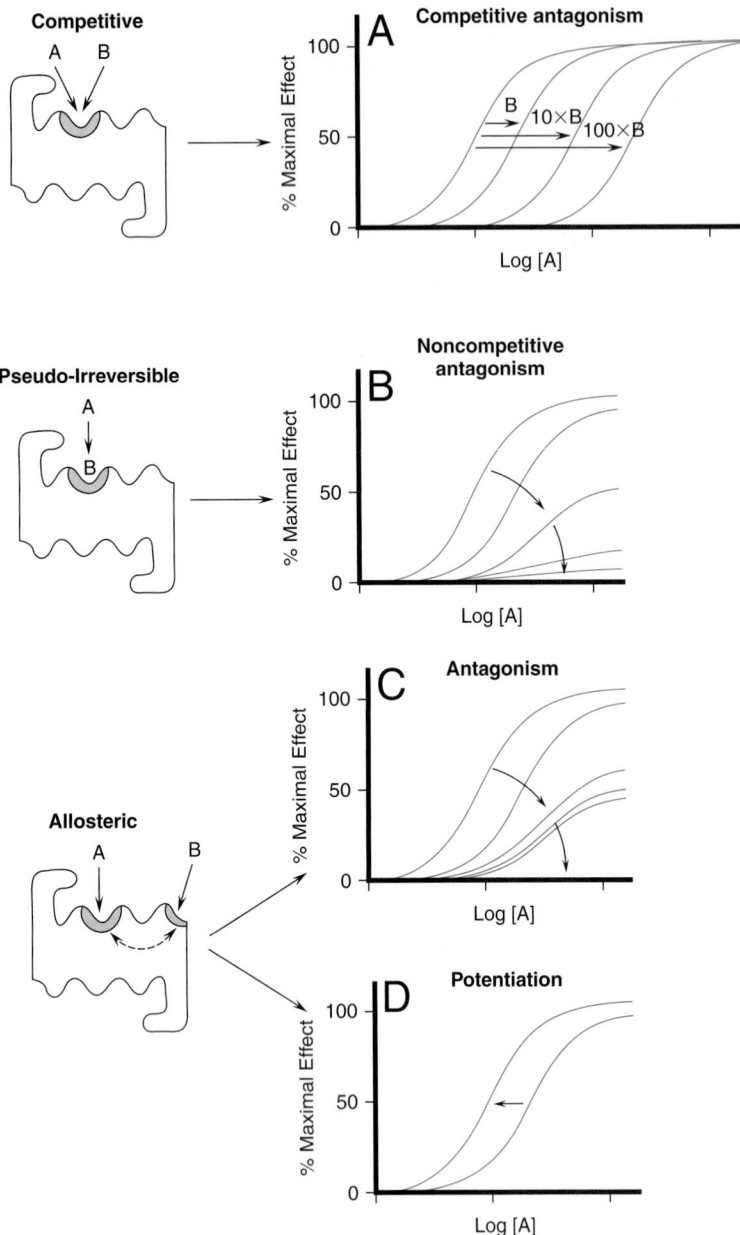

Figure 2–8. Mechanisms of receptor antagonism.

A. Competitive antagonism occurs when the agonist A and antagonist B compete for the same binding site on the receptor. Response curves for the agonist are shifted to the right in a concentration-related manner by the antagonist such that the EC_{50} for the agonist increases linearly with the concentration of the antagonist. *B.* If the antagonist binds to the same site as the agonist but does so irreversibly or pseudoirreversibly (slow dissociation but no covalent bond), it causes a shift of the dose–response curve to the right, with further depression of the maximal response. Allosteric effects occur when the ligand B binds to a different site on the receptor to either inhibit response (see panel *C*) or potentiate response (see panel *D*). This effect is saturable; inhibition reaches a limiting value when the allosteric site is fully occupied.

contrast, some allosteric effects potentiate the effects of agonists (Figure 2–8D). Thus, in cases where the pathology may involve a failing agonist system (*i.e.,* myasthenia gravis, Alzheimer's disease), an allosteric potentiator of the endogenous response would strengthen the signal and, importantly, preserve the natural pattern of response.

By allowing both the overexpression of wild-type receptors and the creation (and discovery) of constitutively active mutant receptors, molecular genetic technology has facilitated the study of a novel class of functional antagonists, the inverse agonists. As discussed above, receptors spontaneously can adopt active

conformations that produce a cellular response. The fraction of unoccupied receptors in the active conformation usually is too low to allow observation of their agonist-independent activity; but this activity can be observed readily, either when the receptor is expressed at heterologously high levels or when mutation shifts the conformational equilibrium toward the active form. In these situations, the tissue behaves as if there were an agonist present, and a conventional competitive antagonist has no effect. However, because inverse agonists selectively bind to the inactive form of the receptor and shift the conformational equilibrium toward the inactive state, these agents are capable of inhibiting agonist-independent or constitutive signaling. In systems that are not constitutively active, inverse agonists will behave exactly like competitive antagonists, which in part explains why the properties of inverse agonists and the number of such agents previously described as competitive antagonists were not appreciated until recently.

It is not known to what extent constitutive receptor activity is a pathologically important phenomenon, and it is therefore unclear to what extent inverse agonism is a therapeutically relevant property. In some cases, however, the preferability of an inverse agonist over a competitive antagonist is obvious. For example, the human herpesvirus KSHV encodes a constitutively active chemokine receptor that generates a second messenger that drives cell growth and viral replication (Arvanitakis *et al.,* 1997). Clearly, in such a case a conventional antagonist would not be useful as the chemokine agonist is not involved, and an inverse agonist would be the only viable intervention.

PROSPECTUS

The continuing identification and expansion of molecular families for receptors, especially at the advent of the human genome era, coupled with the enormous potential for generating new molecules with combinatorial chemistry or recombinant DNA strategies, forecast a new era of diversity and specificity in therapeutic intervention.

BIBLIOGRAPHY

Ariëns, E.J. Affinity and intrinsic activity in the theory of competitive inhibition. I. Problems and theory. *Arch. Int. Pharmacodyn.,* **1954,** *99:*32–49.

Arvanitakis, L., Geras-Raaka, E., Varma, A., Gershengorn, M.C., Cesarman, E. Human herpesvirus KSHV encodes a constitutively active G protein–coupled receptor linked to cell proliferation. *Nature,* **1997,** *385:*347–350.

Clapham, D.E. Mutations in G protein–linked receptors: novel insights on disease. *Cell,* **1993,** *75:*1237–1239.

Furchgott, R.F. The use of β-haloalkylamines in the differentiation of receptors and in the determination of dissociation constants of receptor-agonist complexes. In, *Advances in Drug Research,* Vol. 3 (Harper, N.J., and Simmonds, A.B., eds.) Academic Press, London, New York, **1966,** pp. 21–55.

Gaddum, J.H. The quantitative effects of antagonistic drugs. *J. Physiol.,* London, **1937,** *89:*7P–9P.

Gaddum, J.H. Theories of drug antagonism. *Pharmacol. Rev.,* **1957,** *9:*211–218.

Griffin, J.E., McPhaul, M.J., Russell, D.W., Wilson, J.D. The androgen resistance syndromes. In, *The Metabolic and Molecular Bases of Inherited Disease,* 7th ed. (Scriver, C.R., Beaudet, A.L., Sly, W.L., and Valle, D., eds.) McGraw-Hill, New York, **1995,** pp. 2967–2998.

Kuntz, I.D. Structure-based strategies for drug design and discovery. *Science,* **1992,** *257:*1078–1082.

Lyons, J., Landis, C.A., Harsh, G., Vallar, L., Grünewald, K., Feichtinger, H., Duh, A.Y., Clark, O.H., Kawasaki, E., Bourne, H.R., and McCormick, F. Two G protein oncogenes in human endocrine tumors. *Science,* **1990,** *249:*655–659.

Mangelsdorf, D.J., Umesono, K., Evans, R.M. The retinoid receptors. In, *The Retinoids: Biology, Chemistry, and Medicine,* 2nd ed. (Sporn, M.B., Roberts, A.B., and Goodman, D.S., eds.) Raven Press, New York, **1994,** pp. 319–349.

Ross, E.M. G proteins and receptors in neuronal signaling. In, *An Introduction to Molecular Neurobiology.* (Hall, Z.W., ed.) Sinauer Associates, MA, **1992,** pp. 181–206.

Schild, H.O. Drug antagonism and pAx. *Pharmacol. Rev.,* **1957,** *9:*242–246.

Schreiber, S.L. Using the principles of organic chemistry to explore cell biology. *Chem. & Eng. News,* **1992,** *70*(43):22–32.

Spiegel, A.M., and Weinstein, L.S. Pseudohypoparathyroidism. In, *The Metabolic and Molecular Bases of Inherited Disease,* 7th ed. (Scriver, C.R., Beaudet, A.L., Sly, W.L., and Valle, D., eds.) McGraw-Hill, New York, **1995,** pp. 3073–3089.

Stephenson, R.P. A modification of receptor theory. *Br. J. Pharmacol.,* **1956,** *11:*379–393.

Turki, J., Pak, J., Green, S.A., Martin, R.J., and Liggett, S.B. Genetic polymorphisms of the beta(2)-adrenergic receptor in nocturnal and non-nocturnal asthma: evidence that GLY16 correlates with the nocturnal phenotype. *J. Clin. Invest.,* **1995,** *95:*1635–1641.

Yarden, Y., and Ulrich, A. Growth factor receptor tyrosine kinases. *Annu. Rev. Biochem.,* **1988,** *57:*443–478.

Young, D., Waitches, G., Birchmeier, C., Fasano, O., Wigler, M. Isolation and characterization of a new cellular oncogene encoding a protein with multiple potential transmembrane domains. *Cell,* **1986,** *45:*711–719.

C H A P T E R   3

PRINCIPLES OF THERAPEUTICS

Alan S. Nies

The regulations governing the development of new drugs have evolved over the past century to assure the safety and efficacy of new medications for the population. The safety or efficacy of a drug in an individual patient is never assured. Because all patients differ in their responses to drugs, each therapeutic encounter must be considered an experiment with a hypothesis that can be tested. The scientific basis of the hypothesis derives from the database generated from controlled clinical trials during drug development and the experience obtained postmarketing. Well-defined endpoints must be established prior to therapy. These may be clinical endpoints, such as reduction of fever or pain, or they may be surrogate markers, such as reduction of blood cholesterol or blood pressure, that are correlated with the clinical outcome. Individualization of therapy for a particular patient requires a basic understanding of pharmacokinetics and pharmacodynamics. Many factors can influence that patient's response to a drug, including the age of the patient; disease of the organs of drug elimination (kidney, liver); the concurrent use of other drugs, foods, and chemicals (drug interactions); previous therapy with the same or similar drugs (tolerance); and a variety of genetic factors that can influence the kinetics and toxicity of drugs (pharmacogenetics). For a limited number of drugs, monitoring of the concentration of the drug in plasma can be useful to control for pharmacokinetic variability. Monitoring of pharmacodynamic variability requires close attention to the patient's responses, using predefined goals for acceptable efficacy and toxicity. Some adverse events are extensions of the drug's pharmacological effect and often are avoidable if therapy is individualized. However, other serious adverse reactions are related to an interaction of the drug with variables unique to the individual patient. When a drug is first marketed, it has been tested in only a limited number of well-characterized patients. Adverse events that occur as commonly as 1 per 1000 patients may not be discovered prior to marketing, and rare events may not be discovered for several years after a drug is on the market. It is the responsibility of all health care professionals to monitor the effects of drugs postmarketing and to report serious adverse events that may be drug-related to the FDA and/or the drug manufacturer. In the future, it is likely that the genetic and environmental bases of interindividual variation and of rare, adverse drug reactions will be discovered and that screening techniques will be applied to individualize therapy and assess individual risk. This would improve the overall safety of pharmacotherapy.

THERAPY AS A SCIENCE

Over a century ago, Claude Bernard formalized criteria for gathering valid information in experimental medicine. However, application of these criteria to therapeutics and to the process of making decisions about therapeutics has, until recently, been slow and inconsistent. Although the diagnostic aspects of medicine are approached with scientific sophistication, therapeutic decisions often are made on the basis of impressions and traditions. Over the past three decades, the principles of human experimentation have been defined, and the techniques for evaluation of therapeutic interventions have progressed to the point that it should now be considered absolutely unethical to apply the *art*, as opposed to the *science*, of therapeutics to any patient who directly (the adult or child) or indirectly (the fetus) receives drugs for therapeutic purposes. Therapeutics must now be dominated by objective evaluation of an adequate base of factual knowledge. This philosophy has been popularized recently under the terminology of "evidence-based medicine."

Conceptual Barriers to Therapeutics as a Science. The most important barrier that inhibited the development of therapeutics as a science seems to have been the belief that multiple variables in diseases and in the effects of drugs are uncontrollable. If this were true, the scientific method would not be applicable to the study of pharmacotherapy. In fact, therapeutics is the aspect of patient care that is most amenable to the acquisition of useful data, since it involves an intervention and provides an opportunity to observe a response. Recently, it has become evident that many of the important aspects of disease cannot be adequately assessed by objective data. For instance, dyspnea may not be predicted by measures of pulmonary function with spirometry, and the pain of angina pectoris often is not well correlated with ST-segment depression on the electrocardiogram. Nonetheless, there is a tendency to ignore or denigrate the subjective, symptomatic "soft" data in favor of the objective "hard" endpoints. The challenge for clinical investigators has been to objectify or "harden" subjective measures so that they are useful for quantifying drug responses. It is now appreciated that clinical phenomena that are important to patients—such as dyspnea, pain, and ability to function—can be defined, described, and quantified with some precision. The approach to complex clinical data has been artfully discussed by Feinstein (1983, 1999).

Another barrier to the realization of therapeutics as a science was overreliance on traditional diagnostic labels for disease. This encouraged the physician to think of a disease as static rather than dynamic, to view patients with the same "label" as a homogeneous rather than a heterogeneous population, and to consider a disease as a single entity even when information about pathogenesis was not available. If diseases are not considered to be dynamic, "standard" therapies in "standard" doses will be the order of the day; decisions will be reflexive. Needed instead is an attitude that makes the physician responsible for recognition of and compensation for changes that occur in pathophysiology as the underlying process evolves. For example, the term *myocardial infarction* refers to localized destruction of myocardial cells caused by interruption of the blood supply; however, decisions about therapy must take into account a variety of autonomic, hemodynamic, and electrophysiological variables that change as a function of the time, size, and location of the infarction. Failure to take all such variables into account while planning a therapeutic maneuver may result in ineffective therapy in some patients while exposing others to avoidable toxicity. A diagnosis or label of a disease or syndrome usually indicates a spectrum of possible causes and outcomes. Therapeutic experiments that fail to control for the known variables that affect prognosis yield uninterpretable data. Often, if not usually, not all of the relevant variables are known. In such cases, the response to a therapeutic intervention can be a clue to sort out the parameters that contribute to the response and may be a way to discover the underlying variables that contribute to the disease.

A third conceptual barrier was the incorrect notion that data derived empirically are useless, because they are not generated by application of the scientific method. Empiricism often is defined as the practice of medicine founded on mere experience, without the aid of science or a knowledge of principles. The connotations of this definition are misleading; empirical observations need not be scientifically unsound. In fact, concepts of therapeutics have been greatly advanced by the clinical observer who makes careful and controlled observations of the outcome of a therapeutic intervention. The results, even when the mechanisms of disease and their interactions with the effects of drugs are not understood, are nevertheless often crucial to appropriate therapeutic decisions. Frequently, the initial suggestion that a drug may be efficacious in one condition arises from careful, empirical observations that are made while the drug is being used for another purpose. Examples of valid empirical observations that have resulted in new uses of drugs include the use of *penicillamine* to treat arthritis, *lidocaine* to treat cardiac arrhythmias, *propranolol* and *clonidine* to treat hypertension, and *sildenafil* for male erectile dysfunction. Conversely, empiricism, when not coupled with appropriate observational methods and statistical techniques, often results in findings that are invalid or misleading.

Clinical Trials. Application of the scientific method to experimental therapeutics is exemplified by a well-designed and well-executed clinical trial. Clinical trials form the basis for therapeutic decisions by all physicians, and it is therefore essential that they be able to evaluate the results and conclusions of such trials critically. To maximize the likelihood that useful information will result from the experiment, testable hypotheses of the study must be clearly defined, homogeneous populations of patients must be selected, appropriate control groups must be found, meaningful and sensitive indices of drug effects must be chosen for observation, and the observations must be converted into data and then into valid conclusions. The *sine qua non* of any clinical trial is its controls. Many different types of controls may be used, and the term *controlled clinical trial* is not synonymous with *randomized, double-blind, placebo-controlled trial.* Selection of a proper control group is as critical to the eventual utility of an experiment as the selection of the experimental group. Although the randomized, double-blind controlled trial is the most effective design for avoiding bias and distributing unknown variables between the "treatment" and "control" groups, it is not necessarily the optimal design for all studies. It may be impossible to use this design to study disorders that occur rarely, disorders in patients who cannot—by regulation, ethics, or both—be studied (*e.g.,* children, fetuses, or some patients with psychiatric diseases), or disorders with a typically fatal outcome (*e.g.,* rabies), where historical controls can be used.

There are several requirements in the design of clinical trials to test the relative effects of alternative therapies. (1) *Specific outcomes* of therapy that are clinically relevant and quantifiable must be measured. These may include subjective assessments, which are important in determining whether a therapy improves the patient's well-being. Quality of life can be assessed by the experimental subject and can be tabulated objectively and incorporated into evaluation of a therapy (Guyatt *et al.,* 1993). Wherever possible, well-defined clinical endpoints, *i.e.,* survival or pain relief, should be used, rather than an intermediate endpoint or "surrogate" marker (Fleming and DeMets, 1996; Bucher *et al.,* 1999). A surrogate marker is a clinical sign or laboratory test that correlates with the clinical outcome of a disease. Blood pressure, blood cholesterol, CD4 lymphocyte count in acquired immunodeficiency syndrome (AIDS), and premature ventricular complexes are examples of surrogate markers that have been used as endpoints in clinical trials. Although surrogate markers often are useful to reduce the length and sample size of a clinical trial, the results of such trials may be misleading, as the Cardiac Arrhythmia Suppression Trial (CAST) demonstrated (Echt *et al.,* 1991). In CAST, the antiarrhythmic drugs *encainide, flecainide,* and *moricizine* were effective in suppressing ventricular arrhythmias (the surrogate marker) in patients following a myocardial infarction, but the drugs nonetheless increased mortality. The ultimate test of a drug's efficacy must rest with actual clinical outcomes. (2) The *accuracy of diagnosis* and the *severity of the disease* must be comparable in the groups being contrasted; otherwise, false-positive and false-negative errors may occur. This is a particular issue in developing therapies for poorly understood syndromes, such as fibromyalgia and chronic fatigue syndrome. (3) The *dosages* of the drugs must be chosen and individualized in a manner that allows relative efficacy to be compared at equivalent toxicities or allows relative toxicities to be compared at equivalent efficacies. (4) *Placebo effects,* which occur in a large percentage of patients, can confound many studies—particularly those that involve subjective responses; controls must take this into account (Temple, 1997). (5) *Compliance* with the experimental regimens should be assessed before subjects are assigned to experimental or control groups. The drug-taking behavior of the subjects should be reassessed during the course of the trial. Noncompliance, even if randomly distributed between both groups, may cause falsely low estimates of the true potential benefits or toxicity of a particular treatment. (6) *Sample size* should be estimated prior to beginning a clinical trial so that the trial has the power to detect a statistically significant effect if, in fact, such an effect exists. Depending upon such factors as the overall prognosis and variability of the disease and the anticipated improvement and variability in outcome or toxicity from the new treatment, very large numbers of subjects may be needed; otherwise, the possibility of a false-negative result is high (*i.e.,* no statistically significant differences between the two treatments will be found, even though differences actually exist). It may be very difficult to determine whether or not a new therapy is equivalent to existing therapy without the use of a placebo. Even with large sample sizes, there can be uncertainty. Unless there is a substantial effect of therapy that has been consistently demonstrated in previous trials, it may be impossible to assure that either the standard therapy or the new therapy has a significant effect, *i.e.,* is better than a putative placebo, even if the two are shown to be statistically equivalent. (7) *Ethical considerations* may be major determinants of the types of controls that can be used and must be evaluated explicitly (Passamani, 1991). For example, in therapeutic trials that involve life-threatening diseases for which there already is an effective therapy, the use of a placebo is unethical, and new treatments must be compared with "standard" therapies.

The results of clinical trials of new therapeutic agents or of old agents for new indications may have severe limitations in terms of what can be expected of drugs when they are used in an office practice (Feinstein, 1994). To reduce variability, patients for experimental trials often are selected to eliminate coexisting diseases and concomitant therapy. Such trials usually assess the effect of only one or two drugs, not the many that might be given to or taken by the same patient under the care of a physician. Clinical trials usually are performed with relatively small numbers of patients for periods of time that may be shorter than are necessary in practice, and compliance may be better controlled than it can be in practice. These factors lead to several inescapable conclusions:

1. Even if the result of a valid clinical trial of a drug is thoroughly understood, the physician can only develop a hypothesis about what the drug might do to any particular patient. In effect, the physician uses the results of a clinical trial to establish an experiment in each patient. The detection of anticipated and unanticipated effects and the determination of whether or not they are due to the drug(s) being used are important responsibilities of the physician during the supervision of a therapeutic regimen. If an effect of a drug is not seen in a clinical trial, it may still be revealed in the setting of clinical practice. About one-half or more of both useful and adverse effects of drugs that were not recognized in the initial formal

trials subsequently were discovered and reported by practicing physicians.

2. If an anticipated effect of a drug has not occurred in a patient, this does not mean that the effect cannot occur in that patient or in others. Many factors in the individual patient may contribute to lack of efficacy of a drug. They include, for example, misdiagnosis, poor compliance by the patient to the regimen, poor choice of dosage or dosage intervals, coincidental development of an undiagnosed separate illness that influences the outcome, the use of other agents that interact with primary drugs to nullify or alter their effects, undetected genetic or environmental variables that modify the disease or the pharmacological actions of the drug, or unknown therapy by another physician who is caring for the same patient. Of equal importance, even when a regimen appears to be efficacious and innocuous, a physician should not attribute all improvement to the therapeutic regimen chosen, nor should a physician assume that a deteriorating condition reflects only the natural course of the disease. This is particularly a problem if the adverse effect of the drug mimics a common manifestation of the disease being treated (*e.g.,* sudden death produced by an antiarrhythmic drug). Similarly, if an anticipated untoward or toxic effect is not seen in a particular patient, it still can occur in others. Physicians who use only their own experience with a drug to make decisions about its use expose their patients unduly to unjustifiable risk. For example, simply because a doctor has not seen a case of chloramphenicol-induced aplastic anemia in practice does not mean that such a disaster may not occur; the drug still should be used only for the proper indications.

3. Rational therapy is based on observations that have been evaluated critically. It is no less crucial to have a scientific approach to the treatment of an individual patient than to use this approach when investigating drugs in a research setting. In both instances, it is the patient who benefits. Such an approach can be formalized in the practice setting by performing a randomized, controlled trial in an individual patient who has stable clinical symptomatology. With this strategy, a specific therapy of uncertain efficacy can be compared with a placebo or alternative therapy in a double-blind design with well-defined endpoints that are tailored to the individual patient. The outcome of such an "*n* of 1" trial is immediately relevant to the particular patient, although it may not apply to all other patients (Guyatt *et al.,* 1986).

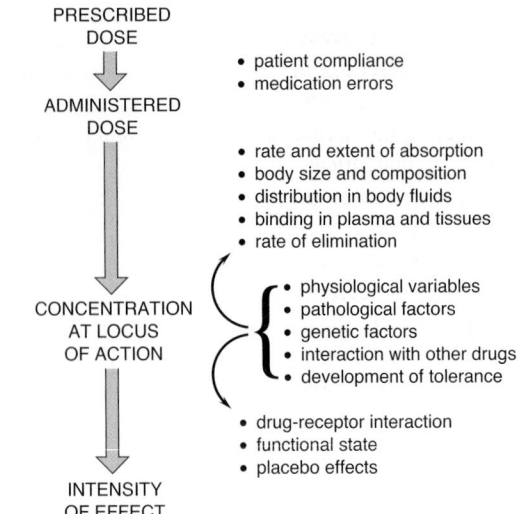

Figure 3–1. Factors that determine the relationship between prescribed drug dosage and drug effect. (Modified from Koch-Weser, 1972.)

INDIVIDUALIZATION OF DRUG THERAPY

As has been implied above, therapy as a science does not apply simply to the evaluation and testing of new, investigational drugs in animals and human beings. It applies with equal importance to the treatment of each patient as an individual. Therapists of every type have long recognized and acknowledged that individual patients show wide variability in response to the same drug or treatment method. Progress has been made in identifying the sources of variability. Important factors are presented in Figure 3–1; the basic principles that underlie these sources of variability have been presented in Chapters 1 and 2. The following discussion relates to the strategies that have been developed to deal with variability in the clinical setting. (*See also* Appendix II.)

Pharmacokinetic Considerations

Interpatient and intrapatient variation in disposition of a drug must be taken into account in choosing a drug regimen. For a given drug, there may be wide variation in its pharmacokinetic properties among individuals. For some drugs, this variability may account for one-half or more of the total variation in eventual response. The relative importance of the many factors that contribute to these differences depends in part on the drug itself and on its usual route of elimination. Drugs that are excreted primarily unchanged by the kidney tend to have smaller differences in disposition among patients with similar renal function than do drugs that are inactivated by metabolism. Of drugs that are extensively metabolized, those with high metabolic clearance and large presystemic (first-pass) elimination have marked differences in bioavailability, whereas those with slower biotransformation tend to have the largest variation in elimination rates among individuals. Studies in identical and nonidentical twins have revealed that genotype is a very important determinant of differences in the rates of metabolism (Penno and Vesell, 1983). For many drugs, physiological and pathological variations in organ function are major determinants of their rate of disposition. For example, the clearance of digoxin and gentamicin is related to the rate of glomerular filtration, whereas that of lidocaine and propranolol is dependent primarily on the rate of hepatic blood flow. The effect of diseases that involve the kidneys or liver is to impair elimination and to increase the variability in the disposition of drugs. In such settings, measurements of concentrations of drugs in biological fluids can be used to assist in the individualization of drug therapy. Since old age and renal or hepatic diseases also may affect the responsiveness of target tissues (*e.g.,* the brain), the physician should be alert to the possibility of a shift in the range of therapeutic concentrations.

A test should not be performed simply because an assay is available. More assays of drugs are available than are generally useful. Determinations of concentrations of drug in blood, serum, or plasma are particularly useful when well-defined criteria are fulfilled: (1) There must be a demonstrated relationship between the concentration of the drug in plasma and the eventual therapeutic effect that is desired and/or the toxic effect that must be avoided. (2) There should be substantial interpatient variability in disposition of the drug (and small intrapatient variation). Otherwise, concentrations of drug in plasma could be predicted adequately from dose alone. (3) It should be difficult to monitor intended or unintended effects of the drug. Whenever clinical effects or minor toxicity are measured easily (*e.g.,* the effect of a drug on blood pressure or blood coagulation), such assessments should be preferred in the decision to make any necessary adjustment of dosage of the drug. However, the effects of some drugs in certain settings are not easily monitored. For example, the effect of Li$^+$ on manic-depressive illness may be delayed and difficult to quantify. For some drugs, the initial manifestation of toxicity may be serious (*e.g.,* digitalis-induced arrhythmias or theophylline-induced seizures). The same concepts apply to a number of agents used for cancer chemotherapy. Other drugs (*e.g.,* antiarrhythmic agents) produce toxic effects that mimic symptoms or signs of the disease being treated. Many drugs are used for prophylaxis of an intermittent, potentially dangerous event; examples include anticonvulsants and antiarrhythmic agents. In each of these situations, titration of drug dosage may be aided

by measurements of concentrations of the drug in blood (4). The concentration of drug required to produce therapeutic effects should be close to the value that causes substantial toxicity (*see* below). If this circumstance does not apply, patients could simply be given the largest dose known to be necessary to treat a disorder, as is commonly done with penicillin. However, if there is an overlap in the concentration–response relationship for desirable and undesirable effects of the drug, as is true for theophylline, determinations of concentration of drug in plasma may allow the dose to be optimized. All four of the above-described criteria should be met if the measurement of drug concentrations is to be of significant value in the adjustment of dosage. Knowledge of concentrations of drugs in plasma or urine also is particularly useful for the detection of therapeutic failures that are due to lack of patient compliance with a medical regimen or for identification of patients with unexpected extremes in the rate of drug disposition.

Assay of drugs to assist the physician in achieving a desired concentration of drug in blood or plasma (*i.e.,* "targeting" the dose) is another example of the use of an intermediate or surrogate endpoint of therapy in place of the ultimate clinical goal. Surrogate markers also can be applied in other ways; one is to provide an indication for a change in the choice of drug therapy. Measurements of concentrations of drugs in plasma and/or measurements of one or more pharmacological effects of the drug can provide an indication of probable lack of efficacy. Other issues of importance with regard to the measurement and interpretation of drug concentrations are discussed in Chapter 1 and Appendix II.

Pharmacodynamic Considerations

Considerable interindividual variation in the response to drugs remains after the concentration of the drug in plasma has been adjusted to a target value; for some drugs, this pharmacodynamic variability accounts for much of the total variation in responsiveness among patients. As discussed in Chapter 2, the relationship between the concentration of a drug and the magnitude of the observed response may be complex, even when responses are measured in simplified systems *in vitro,* although typical sigmoidal concentration–effect curves usually are seen (*see* Chapter 2). When drugs are administered to patients, however, there is no single characteristic relationship between the drug concentration in plasma and the measured effect; the concentration–effect curve may be concave upward, concave downward, linear, sigmoid, or an inverted-U shape. Moreover, the concentration–effect relationship may

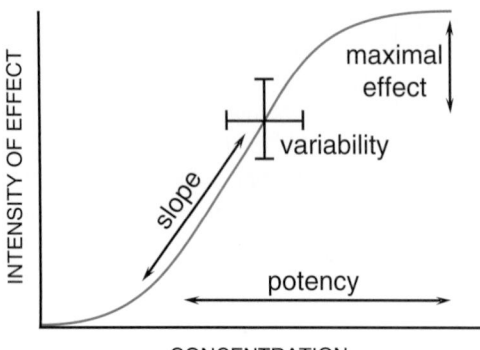

Figure 3–2. The log concentration–effect relationship.

Representative log concentration–effect curve, illustrating its four characterizing variables. Here, the effect is measured as a function of increasing drug concentration in the plasma. Similar relationships also can be plotted as a function of the dose of drug administered. These plots are referred to as dose–effect curves. (*See* text for further discussion.)

be distorted if the response being measured is a composite of several effects, such as the change in blood pressure produced by a combination of cardiac, vascular, and reflex effects. However, such a composite concentration–effect curve often can be resolved into simpler curves for each of its components. These simplified concentration–effect relationships, regardless of their exact shape, can be viewed as having four characteristic variables: potency, slope, maximal efficacy, and individual variation. These are illustrated in Figure 3–2 for the common sigmoidal log dose–effect curve.

Potency. The location of the concentration–effect curve along the *concentration axis* is an expression of the *potency* of a drug. Although often related to the dose of a drug required to produce an effect, potency is more properly related to the concentration of the drug in plasma to approximate more closely the situation in isolated systems *in vitro* and to avoid the complicating factors of pharmacokinetic variables. Although potency obviously affects drug dosage, potency *per se* is relatively unimportant in the clinical use of drugs as long as the required dose can be given conveniently and there is no toxicity related to the chemical structure of the drug rather than to its mechanism. There is no justification for the view that more potent drugs are superior therapeutic agents. However, if the drug is to be administered by transdermal absorption, a highly potent drug is required, since the capacity of the skin to absorb drugs is limited.

Maximal Efficacy. The maximal effect that can be produced by a drug is its *maximal,* or *clinical, efficacy* (which

is related to, but not precisely the same as, the term *efficacy* as discussed in Chapter 2). Maximal efficacy is determined principally by the properties of the drug and its receptor–effector system and is reflected in the plateau of the concentration–effect curve. In clinical use, however, a drug's dosage may be limited by undesired effects, and the true maximal efficacy of the drug may not be achievable. The maximal efficacy of a drug is clearly a major characteristic—of much greater clinical importance than its potency. Furthermore, the two properties are not related and should not be confused. For instance, although some thiazide diuretics have similar or greater potency than the loop diuretic furosemide, the maximal efficacy of furosemide is considerably greater.

Slope. The slope of the concentration–effect curve reflects the mechanism of action of a drug, including the shape of the curve that describes drug binding to its receptor (*see* Chapter 2). The steepness of the curve dictates the range of doses that are useful for achieving a clinical effect. Aside from this fact, the slope of the concentration–effect curve has more theoretical than practical usefulness.

Biological Variability. Different individuals vary in the magnitude of their response to the same concentration of a single drug or to similar drugs when the appropriate correction has been made for differences in potency, maximal efficacy, and slope. In fact, a single individual may not always respond in the same way to the same concentration of drug. A concentration–effect curve applies only to a single individual at one time or to an average individual. The intersecting brackets in Figure 3–2 indicate that an effect of varying intensity will occur in different individuals at a specified concentration of a drug or that a range of concentrations is required to produce an effect of specified intensity in all of the patients.

Attempts have been made to define and measure individual "sensitivity" to drugs in the clinical setting, and progress has been made in understanding some of the determinants of sensitivity to drugs that act at specific receptors. For example, responsiveness to β-adrenergic receptor agonists may change because of disease (*e.g.,* thyrotoxicosis or heart failure) or because of prior administration of either β-adrenergic agonists or antagonists that can cause changes in the concentration of the β-adrenergic receptor and/or coupling of the receptor to its effector systems (Iaccarino *et al.,* 1999; *see also* Chapter 10). Receptors are not static components of the cell; they are in a dynamic state that is influenced by both endogenous and exogenous factors.

Concentration–Percent or Quantal Concentration–Effect Curve. The concentration of a drug that produces a specified effect in a single patient is termed the *individual effective concentration*. This is a *quantal* response, since the defined effect is either present or absent. Individual effective concentrations usually are lognormally distributed, which means that a normal variation curve is the result of plotting the logarithms of the concentration against the frequency of patients achieving the defined effect (Figure 3–3A). A cumulative frequency distribution of individuals achieving the defined effect as a function of drug concentration is the *concentration–percent curve* or the *quantal concentration–effect curve*. This curve resembles the sigmoid shape of the graded concentration–effect curve discussed above (Figure 3–2), but the slope of the concentration–percent curve is an expression of the pharmacodynamic variability in the population rather than an expression of the concentration range from a threshold to a maximal effect in the individual patient.

The dose of a drug required to produce a specified effect in 50% of the population is the *median effective dose,* abbreviated as the ED_{50} (Figure 3–3B). In preclinical studies of drugs, the *median lethal dose,* as determined in experimental animals, is abbreviated as LD_{50}. The ratio of the LD_{50} to the ED_{50} is an indication of the *therapeutic index,* which is a statement of how *selective* the drug is in producing its desired *versus* its adverse effects. In clinical studies, the dose, or preferably the concentration, of a drug required to produce toxic effects can be compared to the concentration required for the therapeutic effects in the population to evaluate the clinical therapeutic index. However, since pharmacodynamic variation in the population may be marked, the concentration or dose of drug required to produce a therapeutic effect in most of the population will usually overlap the concentration required to produce toxicity in some of the population, even though the drug's therapeutic index in an individual patient may be large. Also, the concentration–percent curves for efficacy and toxicity need not be parallel, adding yet another complexity to the determination of the therapeutic index in patients. Finally, *no drug produces a single effect,* and, depending on the effect being measured, the therapeutic index for a drug will vary. For example, much less codeine is required for cough suppression than for control of pain in 50% of the population, and thus the margin of safety, selectivity, or therapeutic index of codeine is much greater as an antitussive than as an analgesic.

Other Factors That Affect Therapeutic Outcome

The variation in pharmacokinetic and pharmacodynamic parameters that accounts for much of the need to

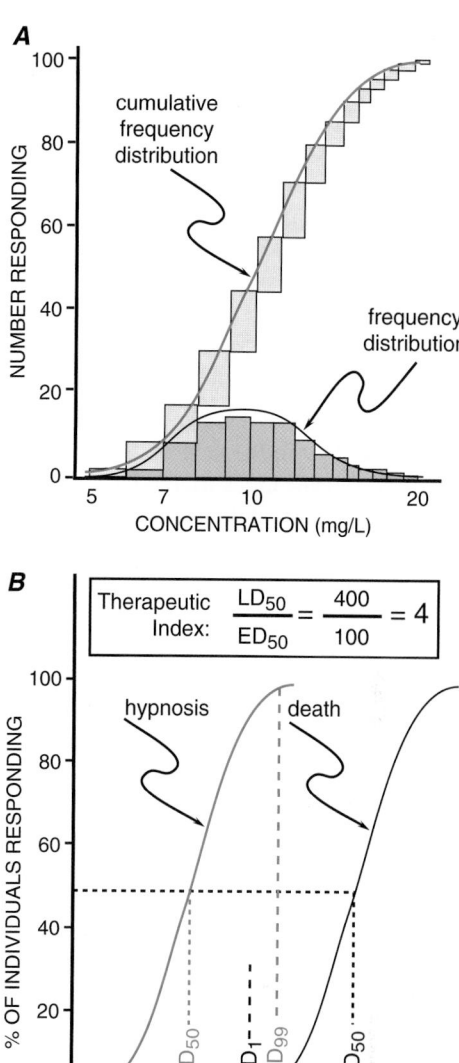

Figure 3–3.   Frequency distribution curves and quantal concentration–effect and dose–effect curves.

A. *Frequency distribution curves.* An experiment was performed on 100 subjects, and the effective plasma concentration that produced a quantal response was determined for each individual. The number of subjects who required each dose is plotted, giving a lognormal frequency distribution (*colored bars*). The gray bars demonstrate that the normal frequency distribution, when summated, yields the cumulative frequency distribution—a sigmoidal curve that is a quantal concentration–effect curve. **B.** *Quantal dose–effect curves.* Animals were injected with varying doses of sedative-hypnotic, and the responses were determined and plotted. The calculation of the therapeutic index, the ratio of the LD_{50} to the ED_{50}, is an indication of how selective a drug is in producing its desired effects relative to its toxicity. (*See* text for additional explanation.)

individualize therapy has been discussed. Other factors, listed in Figure 3–1, also should be considered as potential determinants of success or failure of therapy. The following presentation serves as an introduction to these subjects, some of which also are discussed in Chapter 1 and Appendix II.

Age. Most drugs are developed and tested in young to middle-aged adults. At each extreme of the age spectrum, individuals differ both in the way they handle drugs (pharmacokinetics) and in their response to drugs (pharmacodynamics). These differences may require substantial alterations in the dose or dose regimen to produce the desired effect in the young or in the very old.

Children. Most medications have not been developed or specifically evaluated in children, and formulations often are inadequate for proper administration. Thus, development of new drugs for children and rational use of old compounds require an integrated approach to pharmacokinetic, pharmacodynamic, and formulation issues. There is no reliable, broadly applicable principle or formula for converting doses of drugs used in adults to doses that are safe and effective in children. When the drug manufacturer does not provide adequate information about pediatric dosage, there can be substantial risk in deriving a dose for children and infants from an adult dose by, for example, simply reducing the dose based upon body weight or surface area. In general, pathways of drug clearance (hepatic and renal) are limited in the newborn, particularly the premature infant. The unique physiology of the newborn has led to past therapeutic disasters, such as gray-baby syndrome (inadequate glucuronidation of chloramphenicol with drug accumulation) and sulfonamide-induced kernicterus (displacement of bilirubin from plasma proteins in the face of increased bilirubin production from fetal erythrocyte turnover, decreased bilirubin conjugation, acidosis, and decreased blood-brain barrier). Careful pharmacokinetic studies in the newborn coupled with clinical therapeutic drug monitoring have markedly improved our knowledge of neonatal developmental pharmacology and resulted in safe therapeutics.

Pathways of drug clearance develop variably over the first year of life and may be influenced by induction of drug-metabolizing enzymes (*e.g.,* phenobarbital exposure). Precise developmental patterns have not been mapped out for most isoforms of cytochrome P450. For CYP1A2, studies using caffeine as a model substrate have revealed the pattern shown in Figure 3–4 (Lambert *et al.,* 1986). Such a pattern has been noted for many compounds (*e.g.,* theophylline, anticonvulsants) where a very limited metabolic clearance in the newborn matures dur-

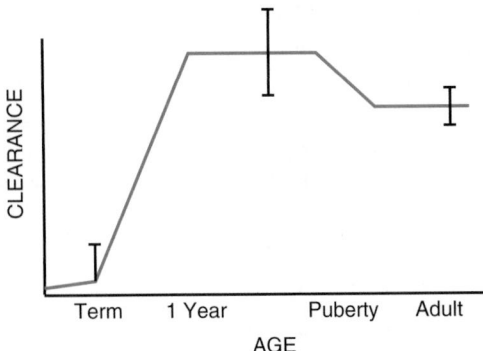

Figure 3–4. Representative developmental changes in drug clearance.

ing the first year of life (albeit with considerable intersubject and metabolic pathway variability) and ultimately achieves weight-adjusted clearance values that exceed those of adults. At puberty, clearance begins to decline, earlier in girls than in boys, to adult levels. The mechanisms regulating such developmental changes are uncertain, and other pathways of drug clearance likely mature with different patterns (deWildt *et al.,* 1999). The critical point is that, at times of physiological change (the premature, the neonate, puberty), major changes in pharmacokinetics are likely to occur, variability is likely to be greatest (both within the same patient over time and among patients), and dosing adjustment, often aided by therapeutic drug monitoring for drugs with narrow therapeutic indices, becomes critical to safe, effective therapeutics. The 7-day-old neonate may be very different pharmacokinetically from the same patient as a newborn, and doses that were appropriate for a 10-year-old on a weight-adjusted basis might well result in overdose for the same patient at age 14.

Pharmacodynamic differences between children and adults have led to unexpected outcomes of therapy and adverse effects. For example, while antihistamines and barbiturates generally sedate adults, these drugs cause many children to become "hyperactive." Of great concern are the effects of medications, particularly when used chronically, on physical and cognitive development. Chronic therapy with phenobarbital can have a significant effect on learning and behavior in children. Tetracyclines deposit in developing teeth, with resultant permanent staining. While children are at risk for all the side effects of chronic corticosteroid therapy seen in adults, such drugs will also stunt linear growth. Children, however, are not always at increased risk for adverse drug effects. For example, while young children appear to be at higher risk for hepatotoxicity from valproic acid than are adults, they are at much lower risk for hepatotoxicity from isoniazid and possibly acetaminophen overdose.

In 1997 Congress passed the Food and Drug Administration Modernization Act (FDAMA). One of this act's aims is to enhance the amount of available information on drug use in children. FDAMA and the Final Rule that followed give the FDA the ability to request information on marketed drugs and reward pharmaceutical companies with 6 months of additional marketing exclusivity for studies that adequately address the request. For drugs in development, a plan to obtain data in children must be negotiated with the FDA prior to the drug's approval for marketing. The data required for children depend on the disease being studied. If the disease is similar in adults and children and there is no known reason to suspect the drug to behave differently in children, then the bulk of the adult efficacy data can be extrapolated to children if similar drug exposure in children and adults can be assured. Thus, pharmacokinetic data in children are required along with adequate exposure for safety assessment, but the FDA efficacy standard for adequate and well-controlled trials prior to approval of the drug for children may not be required. This approach by the FDA is novel and has already resulted in the accumulation of much new data in children. The rest of the world has its eyes on this initiative, and discussions are under way in Europe regarding the requirements for approval of drugs for children (Conroy *et al.*, 2000).

Pediatric formulations of old and new drugs remain a problem for practical therapeutics. While toxicity of the vehicles used to administer drugs (*e.g.*, diethylene glycol toxicity from elixir of sulfanilamide) led to the Pure Food and Drug Act of 1938, the "gasping syndrome" associated with excess administration of drugs preserved with benzyl alcohol was described in the newborn as recently as the 1980s. For intravenous medications, formulations are often too concentrated for proper measurement of the tiny doses required for newborns. Oral formulations frequently present major problems with palatability and possible adverse reactions to flavoring and coloring agents. Particularly for pediatric suspensions, syrups, and chewable tablets, different preparations of the same drugs, while being equivalent from the point of view of bioavailability, may differ in acceptability to a specific patient.

The Elderly. As adults age, gradual changes in drug kinetics and effects result in an increase in the interindividual variability of doses required for a given effect. The pharmacokinetic changes result from changes in body composition and the function of drug-eliminating organs. The reduction in lean body mass, serum albumin, and total body water and the increase in percentage of body fat result in changes in the distribution of drugs depending on their lipid solubility and protein binding. The clearance of many drugs is reduced in the elderly. Renal function declines at a variable rate to about 50% of that in the young

adult. Hepatic blood flow and the function of some of the drug-metabolizing enzymes also is reduced in the elderly, but the variability of this change is great. In general, the activities of cytochrome P450 enzymes are reduced, but conjugation mechanisms are relatively well maintained. Frequently, the elimination half-life of drugs is increased as a consequence of a larger apparent volume of distribution (of lipid-soluble drugs) and/or a reduction of the renal or metabolic clearance.

Changes in pharmacodynamics also are important factors in treating the elderly. Drugs that depress the central nervous system produce increased effects at any given plasma concentration. Physiological changes and loss of homeostatic resilience can result in increased sensitivity to unwanted effects of drugs, such as hypotension from psychotropic medications and hemorrhage from anticoagulants, even if dosage is appropriately adjusted to account for the age-related pharmacokinetic changes.

The proportion of our population in the elderly and very old age groups is increasing. These individuals have more illnesses than younger people and consume a disproportionate share of prescription and over-the-counter drugs. These factors, combined with the changes in pharmacokinetics and pharmacodynamics that occur with aging, make the elderly age group a population in whom drug use is likely to be marred by serious adverse drug effects and drug interactions. It is a population that should receive drugs only when absolutely necessary for well-defined indications and at the lowest effective doses. Prospectively defined endpoints, appropriate use of therapeutic drug monitoring, and frequent reviews of the patient's drug history—with discontinuation of those drugs that did not achieve the endpoint desired or are no longer required—would greatly improve the health of the elderly population. On the other hand, appropriate therapy should not be withheld because of these concerns. Outcomes data with a number of drug interventions have proven that the elderly can benefit at least as much as, and often more than, the young in the treatment of chronic diseases such as hypertension and hypercholesterolemia (LaRosa *et al.*, 1999). Furthermore the natural history of chronic diseases of the elderly, such as osteoporosis and prostate hyperplasia, can be halted or reversed by appropriate drug therapy.

Gender. Although there may be some pharmacokinetic or pharmacodynamic differences between the sexes, early drug development until recently has been performed exclusively in males because of FDA guidelines that prohibited the participation of women of childbearing potential. In the 1990s, the FDA readdressed the importance of including women in early clinical trials, and the previous guidelines were revised to allow the participation of women in all phases of drug development. It is expected that at the time of drug approval, the database will be sufficiently complete to allow a rational assessment of the pharmacokinetic, pharmacodynamic, and safety issues in each sex (Sherman *et al.,* 1995; Harris *et al.,* 1995).

Drug–Drug Interactions. The use of several drugs often is essential to obtain a desired therapeutic objective or to treat coexisting diseases. Examples abound, and the choice of drugs to be employed concurrently can be based on sound pharmacological principles. In the treatment of hypertension, a single drug is effective in only a modest percentage of patients. In the treatment of heart failure, the concurrent use of a diuretic with a vasodilator and/or a cardiac glycoside often is essential to achieve an adequate cardiac output and to keep the patient free from edema. Multiple-drug therapy is the norm in cancer chemotherapy and for the treatment of certain infectious diseases. The goals in these cases usually are to improve therapeutic effectiveness and to delay the emergence of malignant cells or of microorganisms that are resistant to the effects of available drugs. When physicians use several drugs concurrently, they face the problem of knowing whether a specific combination in a given patient has the potential to result in an interaction, and if so, how to take advantage of the interaction if it leads to improvement in therapy or how to avoid the consequences of an interaction if they are adverse.

A *potential drug interaction* refers to the possibility that one drug may alter the intensity of pharmacological effects of another drug given concurrently. The net result may be enhanced or diminished effects of one or both of the drugs or the appearance of a new effect that is not seen with either drug alone.

The frequency of significant beneficial or adverse drug interactions is unknown. Surveys that include data obtained *in vitro,* in animals, and in case reports tend to predict a frequency of interactions that is higher than actually occurs. While such reports have contributed to skepticism about the overall importance of drug interactions, there are potential interactions of definite clinical importance, and the physician must be alert to the possibility of their occurrence. Estimates of the incidence of clinical drug–drug interactions range from 3% to 5% in patients taking a few drugs to 20% in patients who are receiving 10 to 20 drugs. Because most hospitalized patients receive at least six drugs, the scope of the problem clearly is significant. The recent successful treatment

of AIDS with multiple drugs, including several that have potent effects to alter the activity of drug-metabolizing enzymes, has heightened the public awareness of drug interactions. Recognition of beneficial effects and recognition and prevention of adverse drug interactions require a thorough knowledge of the intended and possible effects of drugs that are prescribed, an inclination to attribute unusual events to drugs rather than to disease, and adequate observation of the patient. Automated monitoring of prescription orders in the hospital or outpatient pharmacy may decrease the physician's need to memorize potential interactions. Nevertheless, knowledge of likely mechanisms of drug interactions is the only way the clinician can be prepared to analyze new findings systematically. It is incumbent upon the physician to be familiar with the basic principles of drug–drug interactions in planning a therapeutic regimen. Such reactions are discussed for individual drugs throughout this textbook.

Interactions may be either pharmacokinetic (alteration of the absorption, distribution, or elimination of one drug by another) or pharmacodynamic (*e.g.,* interactions between agonists and antagonists at drug receptors). The most important adverse drug–drug interactions occur with drugs that have serious toxicity and a low therapeutic index, such that relatively small changes in drug level can have significant adverse consequences. Additionally, drug–drug interactions can be clinically important if the disease being controlled with the drug is serious or potentially fatal if undertreated.

Pharmacokinetic Drug–Drug Interactions. Drugs may interact at any point during their absorption, distribution, metabolism, or excretion; the result may be an increase or decrease in the concentration of drug at the site of action. As individuals vary in their rates of disposition of any given drug, the magnitude of an interaction that alters pharmacokinetic parameters is not always predictable, but it can be very significant.

The delivery of drug into the circulation may be altered by physicochemical interactions that occur prior to absorption. For example, drugs may interact in an intravenous solution to produce an insoluble precipitate that may or may not be obvious. In the gut, drugs may chelate with metal ions or adsorb to medicinal resins. Thus, Ca^{2+} and other metallic cations contained in antacids are chelated by tetracycline, and the complex is not absorbed. Cholestyramine adsorbs and inhibits the absorption of thyroxine, cardiac glycosides, warfarin, corticosteroids, and probably other drugs. The rate and sometimes the extent of absorption can be affected by drugs that alter gastric motility, but this is usually of little clinical consequence. Interactions within the gut may be indirect and complex. Antibiotics that alter the gastrointestinal flora can reduce the rate of bacterial synthesis of vitamin K such that the effect of oral anticoagulants, which compete with vitamin K, will be enhanced. If a drug is metabolized by the gastrointestinal microorganisms, antibiotic therapy may result in an increase in the absorption of the drug, as has been demonstrated for some patients receiving digoxin (Lindenbaum *et al.,* 1981).

Recently, it has become evident that a number of drugs are substrates for various promiscuous transport systems that are present in many cells. P-glycoprotein (PGP) is the best studied of these systems, but many other systems are being discovered, such as the family of organic anion transporter systems. PGP is present in intestinal cells, renal tubular cells, biliary canalicular cells, and cells making up the blood-brain barrier. In the gut, PGP pumps drug into the lumen and thereby limits absorption. In the blood-brain barrier, PGP eliminates drug from the central nervous system (CNS), thus altering drug distribution. In the liver and kidney, PGP transports drug into the biliary canalicula and tubular lumen, thereby enhancing drug elimination. Inhibition of PGP therefore can alter the absorption, distribution, and elimination of drugs and is a topic of much current investigation. Cyclosporin A, quinidine, verapamil, itraconazole, and clarithromycin are examples of drugs that can inhibit PGP, whereas rifampin apparently can induce PGP. It is curious that inhibitors and inducers of CYP3A4 often appear to have similar effects on PGP, although this is not always true (Kim *et al.,* 1999). Much as there has been an explosion of information in the past decade about the CYP drug-metabolizing enzymes, the next decade promises a rich yield of information on PGP and similar transport systems.

Many drugs are extensively bound to plasma albumin (acidic drugs) or α_1-acid glycoprotein (basic drugs). In general, only unbound drug is free to exert an effect or to be distributed to the tissues. Thus, displacement of one drug from its binding site by another might be expected to result in a change in drug effects. Although such binding/displacement interactions occur, they are rarely of clinical significance. This is because the displaced drug distributes rapidly into the tissues: the larger the apparent volume of distribution of the drug, the less is the rise in the concentration of free drug in the plasma. Furthermore, following the displacement, more free drug is available for metabolism and excretion. Thus, the body's clearance processes eventually reduce the free drug concentration to that which existed prior to the drug displacement interaction. As a result, the effect of such an interaction is usually small, transient, and frequently unrecognized. However, the relationship of free drug to the total (bound plus free) drug is changed, and the interpretation of plasma drug assays that measure total drug concentration must be altered.

A few drugs are actively transported to their site of action. For instance, the antihypertensive drugs *guanethidine* and *guanadrel* inhibit sympathetic nervous system function after being transported into adrenergic neurons by the norepinephrine-uptake mechanism. Inhibition of this neuronal uptake system by tricyclic antidepressants and some sympathomimetic amines will inhibit the sympathetic blockade and reduce the antihypertensive effects of guanethidine and guanadrel. More drugs may be transported away from their site of action by PGP or other transporters. For example, cancer chemotherapy may be limited by transport of anticancer drugs out of tumor cells by PGP. Attempts have been made to block PGP in order to enhance chemotherapy, thus making use of a drug–drug interaction to enhance clinical efficacy (Krishan *et al.,* 1997).

Interactions involving drug metabolism can increase or decrease the amount of drug available for action by inhibition or induction of metabolism, respectively (*see also* Chapter 1). Interactions may occur among administered drugs or between drugs and dietary substances [*e.g.,* grapefruit juice (a CYP3A4 inhibitor)], herbal remedies [*e.g.,* St. John's wort (a CYP3A inducer); *see* Fugh-Berman, 2000], or other chemicals [*e.g.,* alcohol; other organic solvents (CYP2E1 inducers); cigarette smoke; polychlorinated biphenyls (CYP1A2 inducers)]. The effects of enzyme induction or inhibition are most obvious when drugs are given orally, because all of the absorbed compound must pass through the liver prior to reaching the systemic circulation. Additionally, the intestinal mucosa contains substantial amounts of CYP3A4, which can metabolize some drugs before they reach the portal circulation. Therefore, even for drugs that have a systemic clearance that is mainly dependent on hepatic blood flow (*e.g.,* propranolol), the amount of drug that escapes metabolism on the first pass will be influenced by enzyme induction or inhibition. Examples of drugs that are affected by enzyme inducers are oral anticoagulants, quinidine, corticosteroids, low-dose estrogen contraceptives, theophylline, mexiletine, methadone, HIV protease inhibitors, and some β-adrenergic blocking agents. Knowledge of the specific pathways of metabolism of a drug and of the molecular mechanisms of enzyme induction can help in planning studies of possible drug interactions, and preclinical drug development commonly includes studies to determine pathways of drug metabolism (Yuan *et al.,* 1999). Thus, if a compound is found to be metabolized by CYP3A4 in *in vitro* studies, the potential for clinically significant interactions can be focused on studies with commonly used drugs that can either inhibit (*e.g.,* ketoconazole) or induce (*e.g.,* rifampin) this enzyme. Probes for the evaluation of potential drug–drug interactions by the different CYP isoforms in human beings are being developed (*e.g.,* midazolam or erythromycin for CYP3A and dextromethorphan for CYP2D6). The example of arrhythmias triggered by a combination of terfenadine (which has been withdrawn from the market) and ketoconazole highlights the need for such studies in early drug development. In this interaction, ketoconazole inhibits the metabolism of terfenadine (by CYP3A4) to its active metabolite, resulting in high concentrations of unmetabolized terfenadine, which is toxic (Peck, 1993).

The ability of one drug to inhibit the renal excretion of another is dependent on an interaction at active transport sites. Many of the reported interactions occur at the anion transport site, where, for example, probenecid inhibits the excretion of penicillin to cause the desirable effects of elevated plasma concentrations of the antibiotic and a longer half-life. Similarly, the renal elimination of methotrexate is inhibited by probenecid, salicylates, and phenylbutazone, but in this case methotrexate toxicity may result from the interaction. Interactions at the transport site for basic drugs include the inhibition of excretion of procainamide by cimetidine and amiodarone. An interaction at renal tubular PGP causes inhibition of the excretion of digoxin by quinidine, verapamil, and amiodarone. Finally, the excretion of Li^+ can be affected by drugs that alter the ability of the proximal renal tubule to reabsorb Na^+. Thus, clearance of Li^+ is reduced and concentrations of Li^+ in plasma are increased by diuretics that cause volume depletion and by nonsteroidal anti-inflammatory drugs that enhance proximal tubular reabsorption of Na^+.

Pharmacodynamic Drug–Drug Interactions.   There are numerous examples of drugs that interact at a common receptor site or that have additive or inhibitory effects due to actions at different sites in an organ. Such interactions are described throughout this textbook. Frequently overlooked is the multiplicity of effects of many drugs. Thus, phenothiazines are effective α-adrenergic antagonists; many antihistamines and tricyclic antidepressants are potent antagonists at muscarinic receptors. These "minor" actions of drugs may be the cause of drug interactions.

Other interactions of an apparently pharmacodynamic nature are poorly understood or are mediated indirectly. Halogenated hydrocarbons, including many general anesthetics, sensitize the myocardium to the arrhythmogenic actions of catecholamines. This effect may result from an action on the pathway that leads from adrenergic receptor to effector, but the details are unclear. The striking interaction between meperidine and monoamine oxidase inhibitors to produce seizures and hyperpyrexia may be related to excessive amounts of an excitatory neurotransmitter, but the mechanism has not been elucidated.

One drug may alter the normal internal milieu, thereby augmenting or diminishing the effect of another agent. A well-known example of such an interaction is the enhancement of the toxic effects of digoxin as a result of diuretic-induced hypokalemia.

Summary: Drug–Drug Interactions.   Drug–drug interactions are only one of the many factors discussed in this chapter that can alter the patient's response to therapy. The major task of the physician is to determine if an interaction has occurred and the magnitude of its effect. When unexpected effects are seen, a drug interaction should be suspected. Careful drug histories are important, because patients may take over-the-counter drugs or herbal products, take drugs prescribed by another physician, or take drugs prescribed for another patient. Care must be exercised when major changes are made in a drug regimen, and drugs that are not necessary should be discontinued. When an interaction is discovered, the interacting drugs often may be used effectively with adjustment of dosage or other therapeutic modifications.

Fixed-Dose Combinations.   The concomitant use of two or more drugs adds to the complexity of individualization of drug therapy. The dose of each drug should be adjusted to achieve optimal benefit. Thus, patient compliance is essential yet more difficult to achieve. To obviate the latter problem, many fixed-dose drug combinations are marketed. The use of such combinations is advantageous only if the ratio of the fixed doses corresponds to the needs of the individual patient.

In the United States, a fixed-dose combination of drugs is considered a "new drug" and as such must be approved by the FDA before it can be marketed, even though the individual drugs are available for concurrent use. For such drugs to be approved, they must meet certain conditions. The two drugs must act to achieve a better therapeutic response than either drug alone, so that additional efficacy is achieved or the same effect is achieved with less toxicity (*e.g.,* many antihypertensive drug combinations); or one drug must act to reduce the incidence of adverse effects caused by the other (*e.g.,* a diuretic that promotes the urinary excretion of K^+ combined with a K^+-sparing diuretic).

Placebo Effects.   The net effect of drug therapy is the sum of the pharmacological effects of the drug and the nonspecific placebo effects associated with the therapeutic effort. Although identified specifically with administration of an inert substance in the guise of medication, placebo effects are associated with the taking of any drug, active or inert.

Placebo effects result presumably from the physician–patient relationship, the significance of the therapeutic effort to the patient, or the mental set imparted by the therapeutic setting and by the physician. They vary significantly in different individuals and in any one patient at different times. Placebo effects commonly are manifested as alterations of mood, other subjective effects, and objective effects that are under autonomic or voluntary control. They may be favorable or unfavorable relative to the therapeutic objectives. Exploited to advantage, placebo effects can significantly supplement pharmacological effects and can represent the difference between success and failure of therapy.

A placebo (in this context, better termed *dummy medication*) is an indispensable element of many controlled clinical trials. In contrast, a placebo has only a limited role in the routine practice of medicine. A supportive physician–patient relationship generally is preferable to the use of a placebo for promoting therapeutic benefits. Relief or lack of relief of symptoms upon administration of a placebo is not a reliable basis for determining whether the symptoms have a "psychogenic" or "somatic" origin.

Tolerance.   Tolerance may be acquired to the effects of many drugs, especially the opioids, various CNS depressants, and organic nitrates. When this occurs, *cross-tolerance* may develop to the effects of pharmacologically related drugs, particularly those acting at the same receptor site, and drug dosage must be increased to maintain a given therapeutic effect. Since tolerance does not usually develop equally to all effects of a drug, the therapeutic index may decrease. However, there also are examples of the development of tolerance to the undesired effects of a drug and a resultant increase in its therapeutic index (*e.g.*, tolerance to sedation produced by phenobarbital when used as an anticonvulsant).

The mechanisms involved in the development of tolerance are only partially understood. Tolerance may occur as the result of induced synthesis of the hepatic microsomal enzymes involved in drug biotransformation. Another example of *pharmacokinetic tolerance* is the development of resistance of cancer cells to drug-induced cytotoxicity due to the induction of PGP, which transports drug out of the cell, thereby reducing the intracellular concentration of the chemotherapeutic agent. The most important factor in the development of tolerance to the opioids, barbiturates, ethanol, and organic nitrates is a type of cellular adaptation referred to as *pharmacodynamic tolerance*; multiple mechanisms are involved, including changes in the number, affinity, or function of drug receptors. Tachyphylaxis, such as that to histamine-releasing agents and to the sympathomimetic amines that act indirectly by releasing norepinephrine, has been attributed to depletion of available mediator, but other mechanisms also may contribute. The subject of tolerance is discussed in more detail in Chapter 24.

Genetic Factors.   Genetic factors are the major determinants of the normal variability of drug effects and are responsible for a number of striking quantitative and qualitative differences in pharmacological activity. Basic principles of human genetics apply to genetic loci coding for proteins involved in handling of drugs, *e.g.*, drug metabolizing enzymes, carrier proteins, and receptors. Thus (1) allelic variation is common; (2) there are often several different alleles producing variant proteins at a given locus; (3) some allelic variants are "silent," with no functional consequences, while others may markedly alter the handling of foreign compounds; (4) gene frequencies for different alleles are likely to vary among different human populations, suggesting the need for vigilance in extrapolation of kinetic and safety data from one population to another; (5) some allelic variants are classified as "polymorphisms," variant alleles with a frequency of at least 1%, while other, less common variants are classified as "rare inborn errors of metabolism." The consequences of pharmacogenetic variation include: (1) altered clearance of drugs, resulting in a "functional overdose" in those individuals unable to metabolize the compound; (2) failure to convert a prodrug to an active drug; (3) altered pharmacodynamics (*e.g.*, hemolytic anemia secondary to

glucose-6-phosphate dehydrogenase deficiency); and (4) idiosyncratic drug reactions, such as aplastic anemia or hepatotoxicity.

The superfamily of cytochrome P450 enzymes has been extensively investigated for pharmacogenetic variants (Ingelman-Sundberg *et al.*, 1999). For example, an abnormality in CYP2D6 (present in 3% to 10% of various populations) results in deficient metabolism of many compounds. For some of these drugs—for example, the tricyclic antidepressants—toxicity of "standard" doses may result from accumulation when used in CYP2D6-deficient patients, while for other drugs, either because of a wide therapeutic index (*e.g.*, dextromethorphan) or because multiple pathways are involved in clearance (*e.g.*, propranolol), no dosage adjustment is required.

During drug development, compounds may be screened *in vitro* with human tissue preparations or recombinantly expressed human cytochrome P450 enzymes to ascertain if pharmacogenetic polymorphisms are likely to be involved in metabolism of the drug. Single-dose studies in subjects genotyped for various polymorphisms may help clarify whether the potential for altered drug handling is clinically relevant. For pharmacogenetics to become clinically useful, molecular diagnostic tests for pharmacogenetic variants, done in routine clinical laboratories, must become available, so that a physician can individualize choice of medication or dose regimen based on each specific patient's drug metabolism profile. If a relatively rare but severe adverse reaction to a drug (*e.g.*, a 1 in 5000 risk of hepatotoxicity) is strongly linked to a given pharmacogenetic polymorphism, such pharmacogenetic "prescreens" could markedly decrease the risk for individual patients and the population as a whole.

Approach to Individualization

After it has been determined that pharmacotherapy is necessary to modify the symptoms or outcome of a disease, the therapist is faced with two types of decisions: the first is qualitative (the initial choice of a specific drug) and the second is quantitative (the initial dosage regimen). Optimal treatment will result only when the physician is aware of the sources of variation in response to drugs and when the dosage regimen is designed on the basis of the best available data about the diagnosis, severity, and stage of the disease, presence of concurrent diseases or drug treatment, and predefined goals of acceptable efficacy and limits of acceptable toxicity. If objectively assessable expectations of drug therapy are not set before therapy is initiated, therapy is likely to be ineffective and continued longer than necessary unless an obvious adverse effect occurs.

In most clinical settings, the decision about the choice of drug is influenced substantially by the confidence the physician has in the accuracy of the diagnosis and estimates of the extent and severity of disease. Based on the best available information, the physician must decide on an initial drug from a group of reasonable alternatives. The extent of this evaluation is itself dependent on many factors, including a cost-benefit analysis of diagnostic tests, and this must be based on the availability and specificity of alternative therapies and the likelihood of a reduction in future utilization of expensive health care. The initial dosage regimen is determined by estimation, if possible, of the pharmacokinetic properties of the drug in the individual patient. The estimate must be based on an appreciation of the variables that are most likely to affect the disposition of the particular drug. These variables have been discussed above (*see* Figure 3–1 and Appendix II). Subsequent adjustments may be aided in some instances by measurement of drug concentrations but must ultimately be based on whether the regimen is efficacious, either without adverse effects or at an acceptable level of toxicity.

It has been stated above that every therapeutic plan is and should be treated as an experiment. As such, most of the considerations that were specified in the discussion of clinical trials must be applied to individual patients. Of utmost importance is the definition of specific goals of treatment and the means to assess whether or not these goals are being achieved. Whenever possible, the objective endpoint should be related as closely as possible to the clinical goals of therapy (*e.g.,* shrinkage of a tumor or eradication of an infection). Many clinical goals are, however, difficult to assess (*e.g.,* the prevention of cardiovascular complications associated with hypertension and diabetes). In such cases, it is necessary to use surrogate markers, such as a reduction in blood pressure or the concentration of glucose or cholesterol in plasma. These intermediate endpoints are based on demonstrated (in clinical trials) or assumed correlation of the surrogate marker with the ultimate clinical benefit. In many cases—such as improvement of exercise tolerance in patients with congestive heart failure, the elimination of asymptomatic ventricular arrhythmias, or the change in CD4 lymphocyte count in AIDS—the link between the surrogate marker and the ultimate goal is controversial (Fleming and DeMets, 1996).

The value or utility of each regimen must be assessed at intervals during the course of therapy. The utility of a regimen can be defined as the benefit it produces plus the dangers of not treating the disease minus the sum of the adverse effects of therapy. Another common expression of the usefulness of a regimen is its ratio of risks to benefits (representing a balance between the efficacious and toxic effects of the drug). A definitive evaluation of the utility of a drug is not easy; nevertheless, some sense of the value of a regimen must be established in the minds of the physician and the patient. Knowledge of the usefulness of a given regimen may be a critical determinant of protracted compliance by the patient to a long-term regimen or logical discontinuation by the physician of a marginally efficacious and risky therapy. It must be remembered that the physician, the patient, and the patient's family may have disparate opinions of the utility of a therapeutic regimen. In one study of antihypertensive therapy in which all patients were judged to be improved by the physician, only 48% of the patients considered themselves improved and 8% felt worse. Relatives thought that only 1% of the patients were improved and that 99% had evidence of adverse effects of therapy (Jachuck *et al.,* 1982).

DRUG REGULATION AND DEVELOPMENT

Drug Regulation.   The history of drug regulation in the United States reflects the growing involvement of governments in most countries to ensure some degree of efficacy and safety in marketed medicinal agents. The first legislation, the Federal Food and Drug Act of 1906, was concerned with the interstate transport of adulterated or misbranded foods and drugs. There were no obligations to establish drug efficacy and safety. The federal act was amended in 1938, following the deaths of 105 children that resulted from the marketing of a solution of sulfanilamide in diethylene glycol, an excellent but highly toxic solvent. The amended act, the enforcement of which was entrusted to the FDA, was concerned primarily with the truthful labeling and safety of drugs. Toxicity studies were required, as well as approval of a new drug application (NDA), before a drug could be promoted and distributed. However, no proof of efficacy was required, and extravagant claims for therapeutic indications were commonly made (Wax, 1995).

In this relatively relaxed atmosphere, research in basic and clinical pharmacology burgeoned in both industrial and academic laboratories. The result was a flow of new drugs, called "wonder drugs" by the lay press, for the treatment of both infectious and organic disease. Because efficacy was not rigorously defined, a number of therapeutic claims could not be supported by data. The risk-to-benefit ratio was seldom mentioned, but it emerged in dramatic fashion early in the 1960s. At that time, thalidomide, a hypnotic with no obvious advantage over other drugs in its class, was introduced in Europe. After a short period, it became apparent that the incidence of a relatively rare birth defect, phocomelia, was increasing. It soon reached epidemic proportions, and retrospective epidemiological research firmly established the causative agent to be thalidomide taken early in the course of pregnancy. The reaction to the dramatic demonstration of the teratogenicity of a needless drug was worldwide. In the United States, it resulted in the Harris-Kefauver Amendments to the Food, Drug, and Cosmetic Act in 1962.

The Harris-Kefauver Amendments are sound legislation. They require sufficient pharmacological and toxicological research in animals before a drug can be tested in human beings.

The data from such studies must be submitted to the FDA in the form of an application for an investigational new drug (IND) before clinical studies can begin. Three phases of clinical testing (*see* below) have evolved to provide the data that are used to support an NDA. For drugs introduced after 1962, proof of efficacy is required, as is documentation of relative safety in terms of the risk-to-benefit ratio for the disease entity to be treated. The 1962 amendments also required manufacturers to provide data to support the claims of efficacy for all drugs marketed between 1938 and 1962.

To demonstrate efficacy, "adequate and well-controlled investigations" must be performed. This generally has been interpreted to mean two replicate clinical trials that are usually, but not always, randomized, double blind, and placebo controlled. Safety is demonstrated by having a sufficiently large database of patients/subjects who have received the drug at the time of filing an NDA with the FDA for approval. As a result of these requirements, the number of patients on the drug, the number of studies, the development cost, and the time required for the clinical studies to complete the NDA have increased. The regulatory review time also increased as a result of the mass and complexity of the data, so that by 1990 the average review time was approaching three years. This increased the inherent tension that exists between the FDA, which is motivated to protect the public health, and the drug developers, who are motivated to market effective and profitable drugs. Competing pressures also exist in the community, where medical practitioners and patient activist groups have criticized the FDA for delaying approval, while some "watchdog" groups criticize the FDA for allowing drugs on the market that occasionally cause unexpected problems after they are marketed. The FDA has the difficult task of balancing the requirement that drugs be safe and effective and yet allowing useful medications to be made available in a timely manner.

Beginning in the late 1980s with pressure from AIDS activists, the FDA undertook a number of initiatives that have had profound effects in streamlining the process of regulatory approval. These initiatives have all but eliminated the concern about the "drug lag," where drugs were available in other countries significantly sooner than in the United States (Kessler *et al.*, 1996). First, the FDA initiated new "treatment" IND regulations that allow patients with life-threatening diseases for which there is no satisfactory alternative treatment to receive drugs for therapy prior to general marketing if there is limited evidence of drug efficacy without unreasonable toxicity (Figure 3–5). Second, the agency has established expedited reviews for drugs used to treat life-threatening diseases. Congress has enacted the Prescription Drug User Fee Act (PDUFA), whereby the FDA collects a fee from drug manufacturers that is to be used to help fund the personnel required to speed the review process (Shulman and Kaitin, 1996). Finally, the FDA is becoming involved more actively in the drug-development process in order to facilitate the approval of drugs. A priority review system has been established for drugs in new therapeutic classes and drugs for the treatment of life-threatening or debilitating diseases. By working with the pharmaceutical industry throughout the period of clinical drug development, the FDA attempts to reduce the time from submission of an IND application to the approval of an NDA. This streamlining process is accomplished by the interactive design of well-planned,

focused clinical studies using validated surrogate markers or clinical endpoints other than survival or irreversible morbidity. Sufficient data then will be available earlier in the development process to allow a risk-benefit analysis and a possible decision for approval. In some cases, this system may reduce or obviate the need for phase 3 testing prior to approval. Coupled with this expedited development process is the requirement, when appropriate, for restricted distribution to certain specialists or facilities and for postmarketing studies to answer remaining issues of risks, benefits, and optimal uses of the drug. If postmarketing studies are inadequate or demonstrate lack of safety or clinical benefit, approval for the new drug may be withdrawn. In 1997, these changes were codified in the FDA Modernization Act (FDAMA) (Suydam and Elder, 1999). As a result of these initiatives, the review time at the FDA has been dramatically reduced to a period of less than one year, with an ultimate goal of ten months. Details of this act, which includes a variety of other initiatives, such as those discussed above for pediatric drug development, are available on the Internet at www.fda.gov/opacom/7modact.html. These new initiatives by the FDA are based on the assumption that society is willing to accept unknown risks from drugs used to treat life-threatening or debilitating diseases. Some worry that such shortcuts in the drug approval process will result in the release of drugs without sufficient information to determine their utility and proper use. However, as long as the patient's safety can be reasonably ensured, the new plans to accelerate the drug-development process should prove beneficial to patients with such illnesses.

A seemingly contradictory directive to the FDA also is contained in the Food, Drug, and Cosmetic Act—that is, the FDA cannot interfere with the practice of medicine. Thus, once the efficacy of a new agent has been proven in the context of acceptable toxicity, the drug can be marketed. The physician then is allowed to determine its most appropriate use. However, physicians must realize that new drugs are inherently more risky because of the relatively small amount of data about their effects. Yet there is no practical way to increase knowledge about a drug before it is marketed. A systematic method for postmarketing surveillance is an indispensable requirement for early optimization of drug use.

Before a drug can be marketed, a package insert for use by physicians must be prepared. This is a cooperative effort between the FDA and the pharmaceutical company. The insert usually contains basic pharmacological information as well as essential clinical information in regard to approved indications, contraindications, precautions, warnings, adverse reactions, usual dosage, and available preparations. Promotional materials cannot deviate from information contained in the insert.

One area in which the FDA does not have clear authority is in the regulation of "dietary supplements," including vitamins, minerals, proteins, and herbal preparations. Until 1994, the FDA regulated such supplements as either food additives or drugs, depending on the substance and the indications that were claimed. However, in 1994, Congress passed the Dietary Supplement Health and Education Act (DSHEA), which weakened the authority of the FDA. The Act defined *dietary supplement* as a product intended to supplement the diet that contains "(A) a vitamin; (B) a mineral; (C) an herb or other botanical;

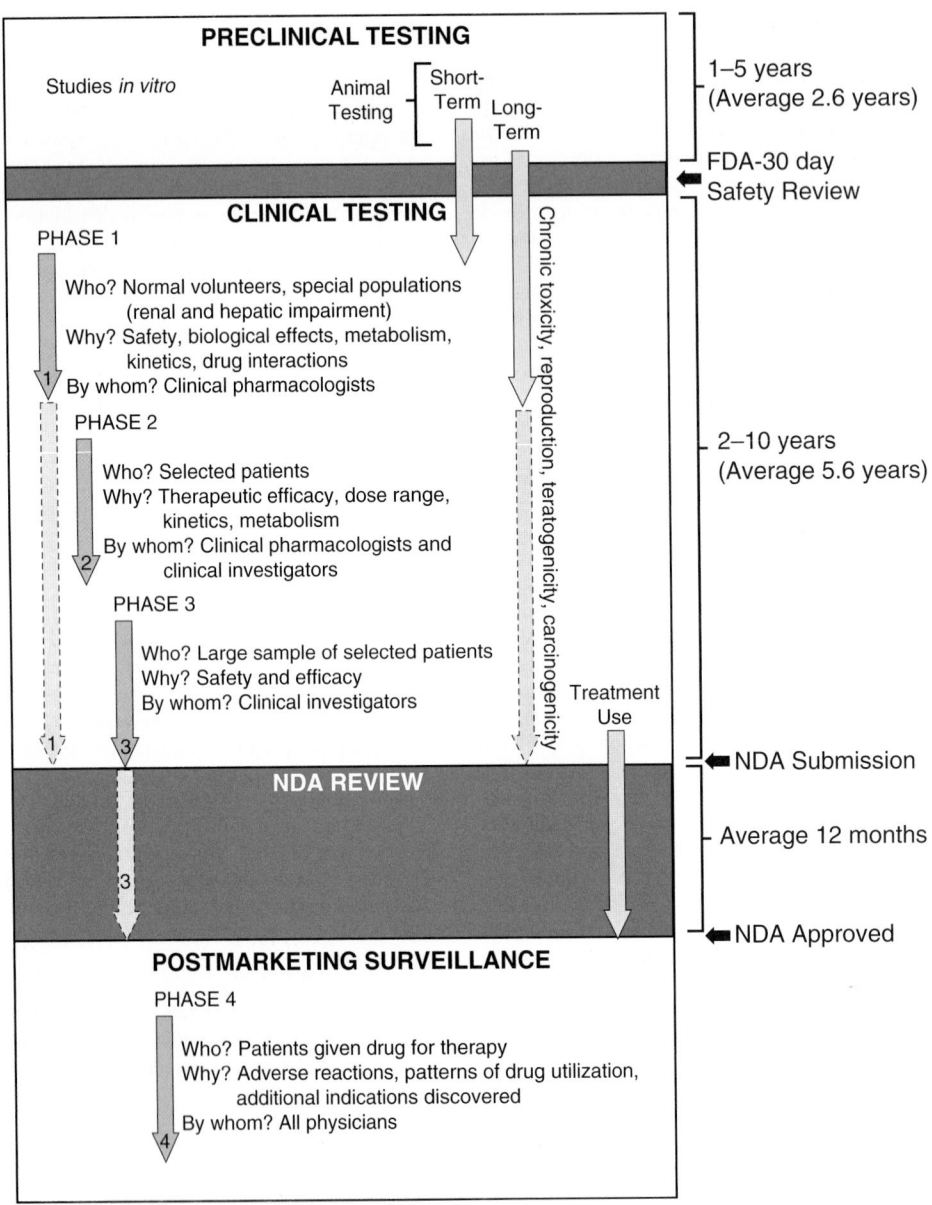

PRECLINICAL TESTING

Studies *in vitro*

Animal Testing {Short-Term, Long-Term}

1–5 years
(Average 2.6 years)

FDA-30 day
Safety Review

CLINICAL TESTING

PHASE 1

Who? Normal volunteers, special populations
(renal and hepatic impairment)
Why? Safety, biological effects, metabolism,
kinetics, drug interactions
By whom? Clinical pharmacologists

PHASE 2

Who? Selected patients
Why? Therapeutic efficacy, dose range,
kinetics, metabolism
By whom? Clinical pharmacologists and
clinical investigators

PHASE 3

Who? Large sample of selected patients
Why? Safety and efficacy
By whom? Clinical investigators

Chronic toxicity, reproduction, teratogenicity, carcinogenicity

Treatment Use

2–10 years
(Average 5.6 years)

NDA REVIEW

NDA Submission

Average 12 months

NDA Approved

POSTMARKETING SURVEILLANCE

PHASE 4

Who? Patients given drug for therapy
Why? Adverse reactions, patterns of drug utilization,
additional indications discovered
By whom? All physicians

Figure 3–5. The phases of drug development in the United States.

(D) an amino acid; (E) a dietary substance for use by man to supplement the diet by increasing the total daily intake; or (F) a concentrate, metabolite, constituent, extract or combination of an ingredient described in clause (A), (B), (C), (D), or (E)." Such products must be labeled as "dietary supplement." The FDA does not have the authority to require approval prior to marketing of such supplements unless the supplements make specific claims relating to the diagnosis, treatment, prevention, or cure of a disease. However, the common conditions associated with natural states—such as pregnancy, menopause, aging, and adolescence—will not be treated as diseases by the FDA. Treatment of hot flashes, symptoms of the menstrual cycle, morning sickness associated with pregnancy, mild memory problems associated with aging, hair loss, and noncystic acne are examples of claims that can be made without prior FDA approval. Also, health maintenance and other "nondisease" claims such as "helps you relax" or "maintains a healthy circulation" are allowed without approval. Many supplements with such claims are labeled as follows: "This statement has not been evaluated by the FDA. This product is not intended to diagnose, treat, cure, or prevent any disease." The FDA cannot remove such products from the market unless they can prove that there is a "significant or unreasonable risk of illness or injury" when the product is used as directed or under normal conditions of use. It is the manufacturer's responsibility to ensure that its products are safe.

As a result of the DSHEA legislation, a large number of unregulated products that have not been demonstrated to be safe or effective are widely available. There have been several occasions where such products have been associated with serious adverse effects or have been shown to interact with prescription drugs (*see* Fugh-Berman, 2000). Under these circumstances, the FDA can act, but the burden is on the FDA to prove the supplements are unsafe. In many ways this situation is analogous to the lack of regulation of drugs that existed prior to the 1938 disaster involving elixir of sulfanilamide, described above. Physicians and patients alike should be aware of the lack of regulation of dietary supplements. Adverse reactions or suspected interactions with such substances should be reported to the FDA using the same mechanisms as for adverse drug reactions (*see* below).

Drug Development. Except for concern about governmental interference with the practice of medicine, the average physician has not considered it important to understand the process of drug development. Yet, an appreciation of this process is necessary to estimate the risk-to-benefit ratio of a drug and to realize the limitations of the data that support the efficacy and safety of a marketed product.

By the time an IND application has been initiated and a drug reaches the stage of testing in human beings, its pharmacokinetic, pharmacodynamic, and toxic properties have been evaluated *in vitro* and in several species of animals in accordance with regulations and guidelines published by the FDA. Although the value of many requirements for preclinical testing is self-evident, such as those that screen for direct toxicity to organs and characterize dose-related effects, the value of others is controversial, particularly because of the well-known interspecies variation in the effects of drugs. Interestingly, although many of the preclinical tests have not been convincingly shown to predict effects that are eventually observed in human beings, the risk of cautious testing of a new drug is surprisingly low.

Trials of drugs in human beings in the United States are generally conducted in three phases, which must be completed before an NDA can be submitted to the FDA for review; these are outlined in Figure 3–5. Although assessment of risk is a major objective of such testing, this is far more difficult than is the determination of whether or not a drug is efficacious for a selected clinical condition. Usually about two to three thousand carefully selected patients receive a new drug during phase 3 clinical trials. At most, only a few hundred are treated for more than 3 to 6 months, regardless of the likely duration of therapy that will be required in practice. Thus, the most profound and overt risks that occur almost immediately after the drug is given can be detected in a phase 3 study if these occur more often than once per 100 administrations. Risks that are medically important but delayed or less frequent than 1 in 1000 administrations may not be revealed prior to marketing. It is thus obvious that a number of unanticipated adverse and beneficial effects of drugs are detectable only after the drug is used broadly. The same can be more convincingly stated about most of the effects of drugs on children or the fetus, where premarketing experimental studies are restricted. It is for these reasons that many countries, including the United States, have established systematic methods for the surveillance of the effects of drugs after they have been approved for distribution (Brewer and Colditz, 1999; *see also* below).

ADVERSE DRUG REACTIONS AND DRUG TOXICITY

Any drug, no matter how trivial its therapeutic actions, has the potential to do harm. Adverse reactions are a cost of modern medical therapy. Although the mandate of the FDA is to ensure that drugs are safe and effective, both of these terms are relative. The anticipated benefit from any therapeutic decision must be balanced by the potential risks. Patients, to a greater extent than physicians, are unaware of the limitations of the premarketing phase of drug development in defining even relatively common risks of new drugs. Since only a few thousand patients are exposed to experimental drugs in more or less controlled and well-defined circumstances during drug development, adverse drug effects that occur as frequently as 1 in 1000 patients may not be detected prior to marketing. Postmarketing surveillance of drug usage is thus imperative to detect infrequent but significant adverse effects.

"Mechanism-based" adverse drug reactions (extensions of the principal pharmacological action of the drug) are relatively easily predicted by preclinical and clinical pharmacology studies. For "idiosyncratic" adverse reactions, which result from an interaction of the drug with unique host factors that are unrelated to the principal action of the drug, current approaches to "safety assessment," both preclinically and in clinical trials, are problematic. The relative rarity of severe idiosyncratic reactions (*e.g.,* severe dermatological, hematological, or hepatological toxicities) presents epidemiological ascertainment issues. In addition, it is clear that a population risk of 1 in 1000 is not distributed evenly across the population; some patients, because of unique genetic or environmental factors, are at an extremely high risk, while the remainder of the population may be at low or no risk. In contrast to the human heterogeneity underlying idiosyncratic risk, the standard process of drug development—particularly the preclinical safety assessment using inbred healthy animals maintained in a defined environment on a defined diet and manifesting predictable habits—limits the identification of risk for idiosyncratic adverse drug reactions in the human population. Understanding the genetic and environmental bases of idiosyncratic adverse events holds the promise of assessing individual rather than population risk, thereby improving the overall safety of pharmacotherapy.

Postmarketing Detection of Adverse Reactions. Several strategies exist to detect adverse reactions after marketing of a drug, but debate continues about the most efficient and effective method. Formal approaches for estimation of the magnitude of an adverse drug effect are the follow-up or "cohort" study of patients who are receiving a particular drug, the "case-control" study, where the potential for a drug to cause a particular disease is assessed, and meta-analysis of pre- and postmarketing studies. Cohort studies can estimate the incidence of an adverse reaction, but they cannot, for practical reasons, discover rare events. To have any significant advantage over the premarketing studies, a cohort study must follow at least 10,000 patients who are receiving the drug to detect with 95% confidence one event that occurs at a rate of 1 in 3300, and the event can be attributed to the drug only if it does not occur spontaneously in the control population. If the adverse event occurs spontaneously in the control population, substantially more patients and controls must be followed to establish the drug as the cause of the event (Strom and Tugwell, 1990). Meta-analyses combine the data from several studies in an attempt to discern benefits or risks that are sufficiently uncommon that an individual study lacks the power to discover them (Temple, 1999). Case-control studies also can discover rare drug-induced events. However, it may be difficult to establish the appropriate control group (Feinstein and Horwitz, 1988), and a case-control study cannot establish the incidence of an adverse drug effect. Furthermore, the suspicion of a drug as a causative factor in a disease must be the impetus for the initiation of such case-control studies.

The magnitude of the problem of adverse reactions to marketed drugs is difficult to quantify. It has been estimated that 3% to 5% of all hospitalizations can be attributed to adverse drug reactions, resulting in 300,000 hospitalizations annually in the United States. Once hospitalized, patients have about a 30% chance of an untoward event related to drug therapy, and the risk attributable to each course of drug therapy is about 5%. The chance of a life-threatening drug reaction is about 3% per patient in the hospital and about 0.4% per each course of therapy (Jick, 1984). Adverse reactions to drugs are the most common cause of iatrogenic disease (Leape *et al.,* 1991).

Because of the shortcomings of cohort and case-control studies and meta-analyses, other approaches must be used. Spontaneous reporting of adverse reactions has proven to be an effective way to generate an early signal that a drug may be causing an adverse event. It is the only practical way to detect rare events, events that occur after prolonged use of drug, adverse effects that are delayed in appearance, and many drug–drug interactions. In the past few years, considerable effort has gone into improving the reporting system in the United States, which is now called MEDWATCH (Brewer and Colditz, 1999). Still, the voluntary reporting system in the United States is deficient as compared with the legally mandated systems of the United

Kingdom, Canada, New Zealand, Denmark, and Sweden. Most physicians feel that detecting adverse reactions is a professional obligation, but relatively few actually report such reactions. Many physicians are not aware that the FDA has a reporting system for adverse drug reactions, even though the system has been repeatedly publicized in major medical journals.

The most important spontaneous reports are those that describe serious reactions, whether they have been described previously or not. Reports on newly marketed drugs (within the past 3 years) are the most significant, even though the physician may not be able to attribute a causal role to a particular drug. The major use of this system is to provide early warning signals of unexpected adverse effects that can then be investigated by more formal techniques. However, the system also serves to monitor changes in the nature or frequency of adverse drug reactions due to aging of the population, changes in the disease itself, or the introduction of new, concurrent therapies. The primary sources for the reports are responsible, alert physicians; other potentially useful sources are nurses, pharmacists, and students in these disciplines. In addition, hospital-based pharmacy and therapeutics committees and quality assurance committees frequently are charged with monitoring adverse drug reactions in hospitalized patients, and reports from these committees should be forwarded to the FDA. The simple forms for reporting may be obtained 24 hours a day, 7 days a week by calling (800)-FDA-1088, or reporting can be done directly on the Internet (www.fda.gov/medwatch). Additionally, health professionals may contact the pharmaceutical manufacturer, who is legally obligated to file reports with the FDA.

GUIDE TO THE "THERAPEUTIC JUNGLE"

The flood of new drugs in recent years has provided many dramatic improvements in therapy, but it also has created a number of problems of equal magnitude. Not the least of these is the "therapeutic jungle," the term used to refer to the combination of the overwhelming number of drugs, the confusion over nomenclature, and the associated uncertainty of the status of many of these drugs. A reduction in the marketing of close congeners and drug mixtures and an improvement in the quality of advertising are important ingredients in the remedy for the therapeutic jungle. However, physicians also can contribute to the remedy by employing nonproprietary rather than proprietary names whenever appropriate, by using prototypes both as an instructional device and in clinical practice, by adopting a properly critical attitude toward new drugs, and by knowing and making use of reliable sources of pharmacological information. Most important, they should develop a "way of thinking about drugs" based upon pharmacological principles.

Drug Nomenclature. The existence of many names for each drug, even when the names are reduced to a minimum, has led to a lamentable and confusing situation in drug nomenclature. In addition to its formal *chemical* name, a new drug is usually assigned a *code* name by the pharmaceutical manufacturer. If the drug appears promising and the manufacturer wishes to place it on the market, a United States Adopted Name (USAN) is selected by the USAN Council, which is jointly sponsored by the American Medical Association, the American Pharmaceutical Association, and the United States Pharmacopeial Convention, Inc. This *nonproprietary* name often is referred to as the *generic* name. If the drug is eventually admitted to the *United States Pharmacopeia* (*see* below), the USAN becomes the *official* name. However, the nonproprietary and official names of an older drug may differ. Subsequently, the drug also will be assigned a *proprietary* name or *trademark* by the manufacturer. If the drug is marketed by more than one company, it may have several proprietary names. If mixtures of the drug with other agents are marketed, each such mixture also may have a separate proprietary name.

There is increasing worldwide adoption of the same name for each therapeutic substance. For newer drugs, the USAN is usually adopted for the nonproprietary name in other countries, but this is not true for older drugs. International agreement on drug names is mediated through the World Health Organization and the pertinent health agencies of the cooperating countries.

One area of continued confusion and ambiguity is the designation of the stereochemical composition in the name of a drug. The nonproprietary names usually give no indication of the drug's stereochemistry except for a few drugs such as levodopa and dextroamphetamine. Even the chemical names cited by the USAN Council often are ambiguous. Physicians and other medical scientists are frequently ignorant about drug stereoisomerism and are likely to remain so until the system of nonproprietary nomenclature incorporates stereoisomeric information (Gal, 1988).

The nonproprietary or official name of a drug should be used whenever possible, and such a practice has been adopted in this textbook. The use of the nonproprietary name is clearly less confusing when the drug is available under multiple proprietary names and when the nonproprietary name more readily identifies the drug with its pharmacological class. The best argument for the proprietary name is that it is frequently more easily pronounced and remembered as a result of advertising. **For purposes of identification, representative proprietary names, designated by** SMALLCAP TYPE, **appear throughout the text as well as in the index.** Not all proprietary names for drugs are included, because the number of proprietary names for a single drug may be large and because proprietary names differ from country to country.

The Drug Price Competition and Patent Term Restoration Act of 1984 allows more generic versions of brand-name drugs to be approved for marketing. When the physician prescribes drugs, the question arises as to whether the nonproprietary name or a proprietary name should be employed. A pharmacist may substitute a preparation that is equivalent unless the physician indicates "no substitution" or specifies the manufacturer on the prescription. In view of the discussion above on the individualization of drug therapy, it is understandable why a physician who has carefully adjusted the dose of a drug to a patient's individual requirements for chronic therapy may be reluctant to surrender control over the source of the drug that the patient receives (Burns, 1999).

Based on a number of considerations—such as the frequency of use of a drug that is available from only a single manufacturer, the cost of filling a prescription, and the markup of the pharmacist—it appears as though the overall savings to society of prescribing the least expensive nonproprietary preparation is about 5% (*see* Trout and Lee, 1981). Of course, savings in individual situations can be very much greater. On the other hand, the lower wholesale cost of the nonproprietary preparation sometimes is not passed on to the consumer (Bloom *et al.*, 1986). More importantly, prescribing by nonproprietary name could result in the patient receiving a preparation of inferior quality or of uncertain bioavailability, and therapeutic failures due to decreased bioavailability have been reported (Hendeles *et al.*, 1993). To address this issue, the FDA has established standards for bioavailability and compiled information about the interchangeability of drug products, which are published annually (*Approved Drug Products with Therapeutic Equivalence Evaluations*). Because of potential cost savings to the individual patient and simplification of the "therapeutic jungle," nonproprietary names should be used when prescribing except for drugs with a low therapeutic index and known differences in bioavailability among marketed products (Hendeles *et al.*, 1993).

Use of Prototypes. It is obviously crucial for the physician to be thoroughly familiar with the pharmacological properties of a drug before it is administered. It follows that the patient will benefit if the physician avoids the temptation to choose from many different drugs for the patient's regimen. A physician's needs for therapeutic agents usually can be satisfied by thorough knowledge of one or two drugs in each therapeutic category. Inevitably, a small number of drugs can be used more effectively. When the clinical setting calls for a drug that the physician uses infrequently, he or she should feel obligated to learn about its effects, to use great caution in its administration, and to apply appropriate procedures in monitoring its effects.

For teaching purposes in this textbook, the confusion created by the welter of similar drugs is reduced by restricting major attention to prototypes in each pharmacological class. A teaching prototype is often the agent most likely to be employed in clinical use, but this is not always true. A particular drug may be retained as the prototype, even though a new congener is clinically superior, either because more is known about the older drug or because it is more illustrative for the entire class of agents.

Attitude Toward New Drugs. A reasonable attitude toward new drugs is summarized by the adage that advises the physician to be "neither the first to use a new drug nor the last to discard the old." Only a minor fraction of new drugs represents a significant therapeutic advance. The limitation of information about toxicity and efficacy at the time of release of a drug has been emphasized above, and this is particularly pertinent to comparisons with older agents in the same therapeutic class. Nevertheless, the important advances in therapeutics in the last fifty years emphasize the obligation to keep abreast of significant advances in pharmacotherapy.

SOURCES OF DRUG INFORMATION

The physician's need for objective, concise, and well-organized information on drugs is obvious. Among the available sources are textbooks of pharmacology and therapeutics, leading medical journals, drug compendia, professional seminars and meetings, and advertising. Despite this cornucopia of information, responsible medical spokespeople insist that most practicing physicians are unable to extract the objective and unbiased data required for the practice of rational therapeutics (Woosley, 1994).

Depending on their aim and scope, pharmacology textbooks provide (in varying proportions) basic pharmacological principles, critical appraisal of useful categories of therapeutic agents, and detailed descriptions of individual drugs or prototypes that serve as standards of reference for assessing new drugs. In addition, pharmacodynamics and pathological physiology are correlated. Therapeutics is considered in virtually all textbooks of medicine, but often superficially.

The source of information described as most often used by physicians in an industry survey is the *Physicians' Desk Reference* (PDR). The brand-name manufacturers whose products appear support this book. No comparative data on efficacy, safety, or cost are included. The information is identical to that contained in drug package inserts, which are largely based on the results of phase 3 testing; its primary value is thus in learning what indications for use of a drug have been approved by the FDA.

There are, however, several inexpensive, unbiased sources of information on the clinical uses of drugs that provide balanced comparative data. All recognize that the physician's legitimate use of a drug in a particular patient is not limited by FDA-approved labeling in the package insert. The *United States Pharmacopeia Dispensing Information* (USPDI), first published in 1980, comes in two volumes. One, *Drug Information for the Health Care Professional,* consists of drug monographs that contain practical, clinically significant information aimed at minimizing the risks and enhancing the benefits of drugs. Monographs are developed by USP staff and are reviewed

by advisory panels and other reviewers. The *Advice for the Patient* volume is intended to reinforce, in lay language, the oral consultation provided by the therapist, and this may be provided to the patient in written form. These volumes are published frequently. *AMA Drug Evaluations,* compiled by the American Medical Association Department of Drugs in cooperation with the American Society for Clinical Pharmacology and Therapeutics, includes general information on the use of drugs in special settings (*e.g.,* pediatrics, geriatrics, renal insufficiency, *etc.*) and reflects the consensus of a panel on the effective clinical use of therapeutic agents. *Facts and Comparisons* also is organized by pharmacological classes and is updated monthly. Information in monographs is presented in a standard format and incorporates FDA-approved information, which is supplemented with current data obtained from the biomedical literature. A useful feature is the comprehensive list of preparations with a "Cost Index," an index of the average wholesale price for equivalent quantities of similar or identical drugs. Many of these publications are available on diskette or CD-ROM for personal computers.

Industry promotion—in the form of direct-mail brochures, journal advertising, displays, professional courtesies, or the detail person or pharmaceutical representative—is intended to be persuasive rather than educational. The pharmaceutical industry cannot, should not, and indeed does not purport to be responsible for the education of physicians in the use of drugs.

Over 1500 medical journals are published regularly in the United States. However, of the two to three dozen medical publications with circulations in excess of 70,000 copies, the great majority are sent to physicians free of charge and paid for by the industry. In addition, special supplements of some peer-reviewed journals are entirely supported by a single drug manufacturer whose product is prominently featured and favorably described. Objective journals, which are not supported by drug manufacturers, include *Clinical Pharmacology and Therapeutics,* which is devoted to original articles that evaluate the actions and effects of drugs in human beings, and *Drugs,* which publishes timely reviews of individual drugs and drug classes. The *New England Journal of Medicine, Annals of Internal Medicine, Journal of the American Medical Association, Archives of Internal Medicine, British Medical Journal, Lancet,* and *Postgraduate Medicine* offer timely therapeutic reports and reviews. The *Prescriber's Letter* (www.prescribersletter.com) is a newsletter that gives alerts and practical advice on old and new drugs. The *Medical Letter* (www.medletter.com) provides objective summaries, in a biweekly newsletter, of scientific reports and consultants' evaluations of the safety, efficacy, and rationale for use of a drug.

The *United States Pharmacopeia* (USP) and *National Formulary* (NF) were recognized as "official compendia" by the Federal Food and Drug Act of 1906. The approved therapeutic agents used in medical practice in the United States are described and defined with respect to source, chemistry, physical properties, tests for identity and purity, assay, and storage. The two official compendia are now published in a single volume.

BIBLIOGRAPHY

Bloom, B.S., Wierz, D.J., and Pauly, M.V. Cost and price of comparable branded and generic pharmaceuticals. *JAMA,* **1986,** *256*:2523–2530.

deWildt, S.N., Kearns, G.L., Leeder, J.S., and van den Anker, J.N. Cytochrome P450 3A: ontogeny and drug disposition. *Clin. Pharmacokinet.,* **1999,** *37*:485–505.

Echt, D.S., Liebson, P.R., Mitchell, L.B., Peters, R.W., Obias-Manno, D., Barker, A.H., Arensberg, D., Baker, A., Friedman, L., Greene, H.L., Huther, M.L., and Richardson, D.W. Mortality and morbidity in patients receiving encainide, flecainide, or placebo. The Cardiac Arrhythmia Suppression Trial. *N. Engl. J. Med.,* **1991,** *324*:781–788.

Feinstein, A.R. An additional basic science for clinical medicine. *Ann. Intern. Med.,* **1983,** *99*:393–397, 544–550, 705–712, 843–848.

Fugh-Berman, A. Herb-drug interactions. *Lancet,* **2000,** *355*:134–138.

Guyatt, G., Sackett, D., Taylor, D.W., Chong, J., Roberts, R., and Pugsley, S. Determining optimal therapy—randomized trials in individual patients. *N. Engl. J. Med.,* **1986,** *314*:889–892.

Jachuck, S.J., Brierley, H., Jachuck, S., and Wilcox, P.M. The effect of hypotensive drugs on the quality of life. *J.R. Coll. Gen. Pract.,* **1982,** *32*:103–105.

Kim, R.B., Wandel, C., Leake, B., Cvetkovic, M., Fromm, M.F., Dempsey, P.J., Roden, M.M., Belas, F., Chaudhary, A.K., Roden, D.M., Wood, A.J., and Wilkinson, G.R. Interrelationship between substrates and inhibitors of human CYP3A and P-glycoprotein. *Pharm. Res.,* **1999,** *16*:408–414.

Krishan, A., Fitz, C.M., and Andritsch, I. Drug retention, efflux, and resistance in tumor cells. *Cytometry,* **1997,** *29*:279–285.

Lambert, G.H., Schoeller, D.A., Kotake, A.N., Flores, C., and Hay, D. The effect of age, gender, and sexual maturation on the caffeine breath test. *Dev. Pharmacol. Ther.,* **1986,** *9*:375–388.

LaRosa, J.C., He, J., and Vupputuri, S. Effect of statins on risk of coronary disease: a meta-analysis of randomized controlled trials. *JAMA,* **1999,** *282*:2340–2346.

Leape, L.L., Brennan, T.A., Laird, N., Lawthers, A.G., Localio, A.R., Barnes, B.A., Hebert, L., Newhouse, J.P., Weiler, P.C., and Hiatt, H. The nature of adverse events in hospitalized patients. Results of the Harvard Medical Practice Study II. *N. Engl. J. Med.,* **1991,** *324*:377–384.

Lindenbaum, J., Rund, D.G., Butler, V.P. Jr., Tse-Eng, D., and Saha, J.R. Inactivation of digoxin by the gut flora: reversal by antibiotic therapy. *N. Engl. J. Med.,* **1981,** *305*:789–794.

Penno, M.B., and Vesell, E.S. Monogenic control of variations in antipyrine metabolite formation. New polymorphism of hepatic drug oxidation. *J. Clin. Invest.,* **1983,** *71*:1698–1709.

Young, F.E., Norris, J.A., Levitt, J.A., and Nightingale, S.L. The FDA's new procedure for the use of investigational drugs in treatment. *JAMA,* **1988,** *259*:2267–2270.

Yuan, R., Parmelee, T., Balian, J.D., Uppoor, R.S., Ajayi, F., Burnett, A., Lesko, L.J., and Marroum, P. In vitro metabolic interaction studies: experience of the Food and Drug Administration. *Clin. Pharmacol. Ther.,* **1999,** *66*:9–15.

MONOGRAPHS AND REVIEWS

Brewer, T., and Colditz, G.A. Postmarketing surveillance and adverse drug reactions: current perspectives and future needs. *JAMA,* **1999,** *281*:824–829.

Bucher, H.C., Guyatt, G.H., Cook, D.J., Holbrook, A., and McAlister, F.A. Users' guides to the medical literature: XIX. Applying clinical trial results A. How to use an article measuring the effect of an intervention on surrogate endpoints. Evidence-Based Medicine Working Group. *JAMA,* **1999,** *282*:771–778.

Burns, M. Management of narrow therapeutic index drugs. *J. Thromb. Thrombolysis,* **1999,** *7*:137–143.

Conroy, S., McIntyre, J., Choonara, I., and Stephenson, T. Drug trials in children: problems and the way forward. *Br. J. Clin. Pharmacol.,* **2000,** *49*:93–97.

Feinstein, A.R. "Clinical judgment" revisited: the distraction of quantitative models. *Ann. Intern. Med.,* **1994,** *120*:799–805.

Feinstein, A.R. Statistical reductionism and clinicians' delinquencies in humanistic research. *Clin. Pharmacol. Ther.,* **1999,** *66*:211–217.

Feinstein, A.R., and Horwitz, R.I. Choosing cases and controls: the clinical epidemiology of "clinical investigation." *J. Clin. Invest.,* **1988,** *81*: 1–5.

Fleming, T.R., and DeMets, D.L. Surrogate end points in clinical trials: are we being misled? *Ann. Intern. Med.,* **1996,** *125*:605–613.

Gal, J. Stereoisomerism and drug nomenclature. *Clin. Pharmacol. Ther.,* **1988,** *44*:251–253.

Guyatt, G.H., Feeny, D.H., and Patrick, D.L. Measuring health-related quality of life. *Ann. Intern. Med.,* **1993,** *118*:622–629.

Harris, R.Z., Benet, L.Z., and Schwartz, J.B. Gender effects in pharmacokinetics and pharmacodynamics. *Drugs,* **1995,** *50*:222–239.

Hendeles, L., Hochhaus, G., and Kazerounian, S. Generic and alternative brand-name pharmaceutical equivalents: select with caution. *Am. J. Hosp. Pharm.,* **1993,** *50*:323–329.

Iaccarino, G., Lefkowitz, R.J., and Koch, W.J. Myocardial G protein-coupled receptor kinases: implications for heart failure therapy. *Proc. Assoc. Am. Physicians,* **1999,** *111*:399–405.

Ingelman-Sundberg, M., Oscarson, M., and McLellan, R.A. Polymorphic human cytochrome P450 enzymes: an opportunity for individualized drug treatment. *Trends Pharmacol. Sci.,* **1999,** *20*:342–349.

Jick, H. Adverse drug reactions: the magnitude of the problem. *J. Allergy Clin. Immunol.,* **1984,** *74*:555–557.

Kaitin, K.I., Richard, B.W., and Lasagna, L. Trends in drug development: the 1985–86 new drug approvals. *J. Clin. Pharmacol.,* **1987,** *27*:542–548.

Kessler, D.A., Hass, A.E., Feiden, K.L., Lumpkin, M., and Temple, R. Approval of new drugs in the United States. Comparison with the United Kingdom, Germany, and Japan. *JAMA,* **1996,** *276*:1826–1831.

Koch-Weser, J. Serum drug concentrations as therapeutic guides. *N. Engl. J. Med.,* **1972,** *287*:227–231.

Passamani, E. Clinical trials—are they ethical? *N. Engl. J. Med.,* **1991,** *324*:1589–1592.

Peck, C.C. Understanding consequences of concurrent therapies. *JAMA,* **1993,** *269*:1550–1552.

Sherman, L.A., Temple, R., and Merkatz, R.B. Women in clinical trials: an FDA perspective. *Science,* **1995,** *269*:793–795.

Shulman, S.R., and Kaitin, K.I. The Prescription Drug User Fee Act of 1992: A 5-year experiment for industry and the FDA. *Pharmacoeconomics,* **1996,** *9*:121–133.

Smith, W.M. Drug choice in disease states. In, *Clinical Pharmacology: Basic Principles in Therapeutics,* 2nd ed. (Melmon, K.L., and Morelli, H.F., eds.) Macmillan, New York, **1978,** pp. 3–24.

Strom, B.L., and Tugwell, P. Pharmacoepidemiology: current status, prospects, and problems. *Ann. Intern. Med.,* **1990,** *113*:179–181.

Suydam, L.A., and Elder, D.K. FDAMA update. *Food Drug Law J.,* **1999,** *54*:21–33.

Temple, R. Meta-analysis and epidemiologic studies in drug development and postmarketing surveillance. *JAMA,* **1999,** *281*:841–844.

Temple, R.J. When are clinical trials of a given agent vs. placebo no longer appropriate or feasible? *Control. Clin. Trials,* **1997,** *18*:613–620.

Trout, M.E., and Lee, A.M. Generic substitution: a boon or a bane to the physician and the consumer? In, *Drug Therapeutics: Concepts for Physicians.* (Melmon, K.L., ed.) Elsevier North-Holland, Inc., New York, **1981.**

Wax, P.M. Elixirs, diluents, and the passage of the 1938 Federal Food, Drug, and Cosmetic Act. *Ann. Intern. Med.,* **1995,** *122*:456–461.

Woosley, R.L. Centers for education and research in therapeutics. *Clin. Pharmacol. Ther.,* **1994,** *55*:249–255.

PRINCIPLES OF TOXICOLOGY AND TREATMENT OF POISONING

Curtis D. Klaassen

Chemicals that are developed into drugs must have therapeutic efficacy and be safe. Unfortunately, all chemicals have the potential to produce unwanted effects. Therefore, in the development of drugs, it is essential to select chemicals that have a margin of safety between the dose that produces the desired (therapeutic) effect and the dose that produces undesired (toxic) effects. The margin of safety for some drugs is small, and some people intentionally overdose themselves. As a result, toxic effects of drugs often are observed.

The physician must be aware that the symptoms a patient manifests might be due to chemical exposure, either to a drug or another chemical. This chapter summarizes the principles of how chemicals produce toxic effects as well as the principles for the treatment of poisoning.

PRINCIPLES OF TOXICOLOGY

Toxicology is the science of the adverse effects of chemicals on living organisms. The discipline often is divided into several major areas. The *descriptive toxicologist* performs toxicity tests (*described below*) to obtain information that can be used to evaluate the risk that exposure to a chemical poses to human beings and to the environment. The *mechanistic toxicologist* attempts to determine how chemicals exert deleterious effects on living organisms. Such studies are essential for the development of tests for the prediction of risks, for facilitating the search for safer chemicals, and for rational treatment of the manifestations of toxicity. The *regulatory toxicologist* judges whether or not a drug or other chemical has a low enough risk to justify making it available for its intended purpose.

The Food and Drug Administration (FDA) regulates drugs, medical devices, cosmetics, and food additives in interstate commerce. For food additives, the FDA attempts to determine the acceptable daily intake (ADI) that can be consumed over an entire lifetime without any appreciable risk. The Environmental Protection Agency (EPA) is responsible for regulation of pesticides, toxic chemicals, hazardous wastes, and toxic pollutants in water and air. The Occupational Safety and Health Administration (OSHA) determines whether or not employers are providing working conditions that are safe for employees. Employers must keep the concentration of each chemical in the air of the workplace below a threshold limit value (TLV). The Consumer Products Safety Commission regulates all articles sold for use in homes, in schools, or for recreation except those products regulated by the FDA and the EPA.

Two specialized areas of toxicology are particularly important for medicine. *Forensic toxicology,* which combines analytical chemistry and fundamental toxicology, is concerned with the medicolegal aspects of chemicals. Forensic toxicologists assist in postmortem investigations to establish the cause or circumstances of death. *Clinical toxicology* focuses on diseases that are caused by or are uniquely associated with toxic substances. Clinical toxicologists treat patients who are poisoned by drugs and other chemicals and develop new techniques for the diagnosis and treatment of such intoxications.

The physician must evaluate the possibility that a patient's signs and symptoms might be caused by toxic chemicals present in the environment or administered as therapeutic agents. Many of the adverse effects of drugs mimic symptoms of disease. Appreciation of the principles of toxicology is necessary for the recognition and management of such clinical problems.

DOSE–RESPONSE RELATIONSHIP

Evaluation of the dose–response or the dose–effect relationship is crucially important to toxicologists. There is a graded dose–response relationship in an *individual* and a quantal dose–response relationship in the *population* (*see* Chapter 3). Graded doses of a drug given to an individual usually result in a greater magnitude of response as the dose is increased. In a quantal dose–response relationship, the percentage of the population affected increases as the dose is raised; the relationship is quantal in that the effect is specified to be either present or absent in a given individual (*see* Figure 3–3). This quantal dose–response phenomenon is extremely important in toxicology and is used to determine the *median lethal dose* (LD$_{50}$) of drugs and other chemicals.

The LD$_{50}$ is determined experimentally. The chemical being evaluated usually is administered to mice or rats (orally or intraperitoneally) at several doses (usually four or five) in the lethal range (Figure 4–1*A*). To linearize such data, the response (death) can be converted to units of *deviation from the mean,* or *probits* (from the contraction of *probability units*). The probit designates the deviation from the median; a probit of 5 corresponds to a 50% response, and, because each probit equals one standard deviation, a probit of 4 equals 16% and a probit of 6 equals 84%. A plot of percent of population responding, in probit units, against log dose yields a straight line (Figure 4–1*B*). The LD$_{50}$ is determined by drawing a vertical line from the point on the line where the probit unit equals 5 (50% mortality). The slope of the dose–effect curve also is important. The LD$_{50}$ for both compounds depicted in Figure 4–1 is the same (10 mg/kg). However, the slopes of the dose–response curves are quite different. At a dose equal to one half of the LD$_{50}$ (5 mg/kg), less than 5% of the animals exposed to compound B would die, but 30% of the animals given compound A would die.

The quantal, or "all-or-none," response is not limited to lethality. As described in Chapter 3, similar dose–effect curves can be constructed for any effect produced by chemicals.

RISK AND ITS ASSESSMENT

There are marked differences in the LD$_{50}$'s of various chemicals. Some result in death at doses of a fraction of a microgram (LD$_{50}$ for botulinum toxin equals 10 pg/kg); others may be relatively harmless in doses of several grams or more. While categories of toxicity that are of some practicality have been devised, based on the amount required to produce death, often it is not easy to distinguish between toxic and nontoxic chemicals. Paracelsus (1493–1541) noted that "All substances are poisons; there is none which is not a poison. The right dose differentiates a poison and a remedy." Although society wants the toxicologist to categorize all chemicals as either safe or toxic,

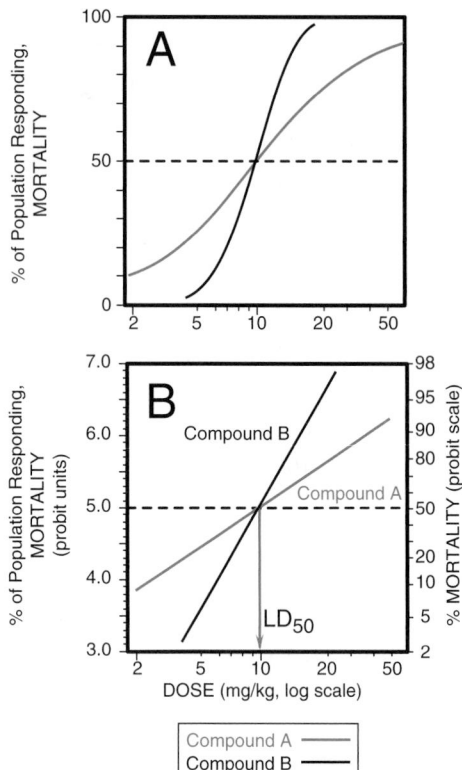

Figure 4–1. Dose–response relationships.

A. The toxic response to a chemical is evaluated at several doses in the toxic or lethal range. The midpoint of the curve representing percent of population responding (response here is DEATH) *versus* dose (log scale) represents the LD$_{50}$, or the concentration of drug that is lethal in 50% of the population. *B.* A linear transformation of the data in *A* is provided by plotting the log of the dose administered *versus* the percent of the population killed in probit units.

this is not possible. The real concern is the *risk* associated with use of the chemical, not whether or not a chemical is toxic. In the assessment of risk, one also must consider the harmful effects of the chemical accrued directly or indirectly through adverse effects on the environment when used in the quantity and in the manner proposed. Depending on the use and disposition of a chemical, a very toxic compound ultimately may be less harmful than a relatively nontoxic one.

At present there is much concern about the risk from exposure to chemicals that have produced cancer in laboratory animals. For most of these chemicals, it is not known if they also produce cancer in human beings. The regulatory agencies take one of three approaches to potential chemical carcinogens. For food additives, the FDA is very cautious, as large numbers of people are likely to be exposed to the chemicals, and they are not likely to have beneficial effects to individuals. For drugs, the FDA weighs the relative risks and benefits of the drugs for patients. Thus, it is unlikely that the FDA will approve the use of a drug that produces tumors in laboratory animals for a mild ailment, but it may approve its use for a serious disease. In fact, most cancer chemotherapeutic drugs also are chemical carcinogens.

In the regulation of environmental carcinogens, the EPA attempts to limit lifetime exposure such that the incidence of cancer due to the chemical would be no more than one in a million people. To determine the daily allowable exposure for human beings, mathematical models are used to extrapolate doses of chemicals that produce a particular incidence of tumors in laboratory animals (often in the range of 10% to 20%) to those that should produce cancer in no more than one person in a million. The models used are conservative and are thought to provide adequate protection from undue risks from exposure to potential carcinogens.

Acute versus Chronic Exposure.   Effects of acute exposure to a chemical often differ from those that follow subacute or chronic exposure. Acute exposure occurs when a dose is delivered as a single event. Chronic exposure is likely to be to small quantities of a substance over a long period of time, which often results in the slow accumulation of the compound in the body. Evaluation of *cumulative* toxic effects is receiving increased attention because of chronic exposure to low concentrations of various natural and synthetic chemical substances in the environment.

Chemical Forms of Drugs That Produce Toxicity.   The "parent" drug administered to the patient often is the chemical form producing the desired therapeutic effect. Similarly, the toxic effects of drugs often are due to deleterious effects of the parent drug. However, toxic effects of drugs (as well as therapeutic effects) and other chemicals also can be due to metabolites of the drug produced by enzymes, light, or reactive oxygen species.

Toxic Metabolites.   The metabolites of many chemicals are responsible for their toxicities. Most organophosphate insecticides are biotransformed by the cytochrome P450 system to produce their toxicities; for example, parathion is biotransformed to paraoxon (*see* Figure 4–2). Paraoxon is a stable metabolite that binds to and inactivates cholinesterase. Some metabolites of drugs are not chemically stable and are referred to as *reactive intermediates*. An example of a toxic reactive intermediate is the metabolite of acetaminophen (*see* Figure 4–3), which is very reactive and binds to nucleophiles such as glutathione; when cellular glutathione is depleted, the metabolite binds to cellular macromolecules, the mechanism by which acetaminophen

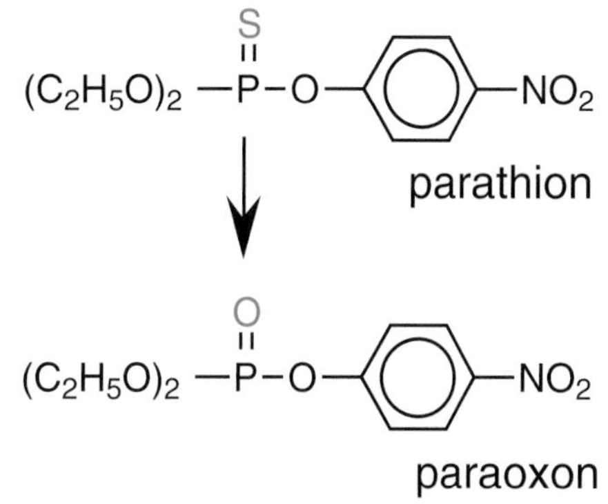

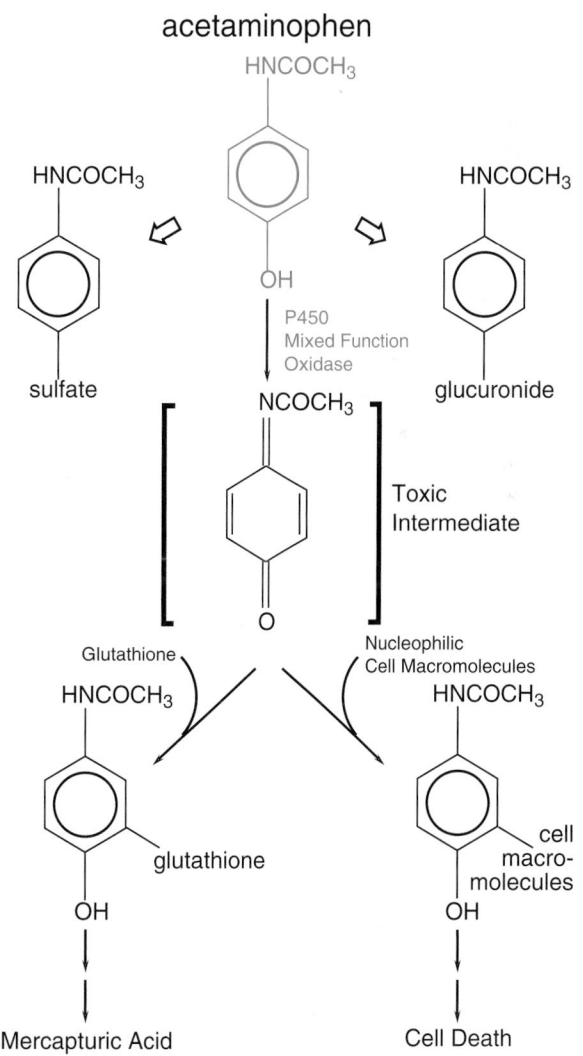

Figure 4–2. Biotransformation of parathion.

Figure 4–3. Pathways of acetaminophen metabolism.

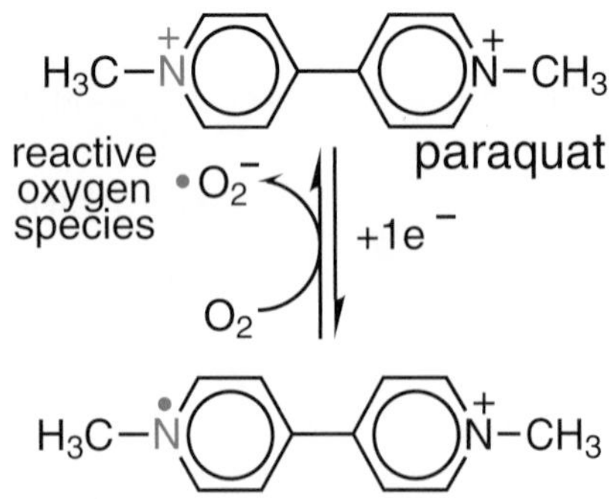

Figure 4–4. Biotransformation of paraquat.

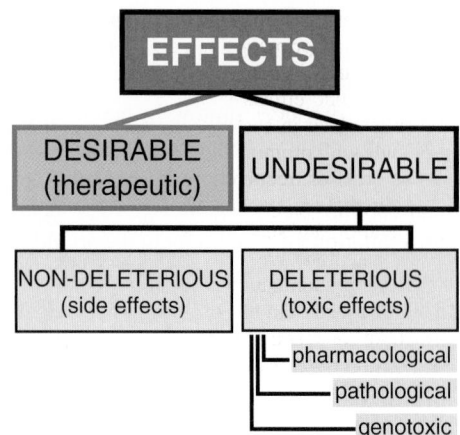

Figure 4–5. Classification of the effects of chemicals.

kills liver cells. Both parathion and acetaminophen are more toxic under conditions in which the cytochrome P450 enzymes are increased, such as following ethanol or phenobarbital exposure, because these are responsible for the production of the toxic metabolites (*see* Chapter 1).

Phototoxic and Photoallergic Reactions. Many chemicals are activated to toxic metabolites by hepatic enzymatic biotransformation. However, some chemicals can be activated in the skin by ultraviolet and/or visible radiation. In photoallergy, radiation absorbed by a drug, such as a sulfonamide, results in its conversion to a product that is a more potent allergen than the parent compound. Phototoxic reactions to drugs, in contrast to photoallergic ones, do not have an immunological component. Drugs, either absorbed locally into the skin or that have reached the skin through the systemic circulation, may be the object of photochemical reactions within the skin; this can lead directly either to chemically induced photosensitivity reactions or to enhancement of the usual effects of sunlight. Tetracyclines, sulfonamides, chlorpromazine, and nalidixic acid are examples of phototoxic chemicals; generally, they are innocuous to skin if not exposed to light.

Reactive Oxygen Species. Paraquat is an herbicide that produces severe lung injury. Its toxicity is not due to paraquat or its metabolites but rather to reactive oxygen species formed during one-electron reduction of paraquat paired with electron donation to oxygen (*see* Figure 4–4).

SPECTRUM OF UNDESIRED EFFECTS

The spectrum of undesired effects of chemicals may be broad and ill-defined (*see* Figure 4–5). In therapeutics, a drug typically produces numerous effects, but usually only one is sought as the primary goal of treatment; most of the other effects are referred to as *undesirable effects* of that drug for that therapeutic indication. *Side effects* of drugs usually are nondeleterious; they include effects such as dry mouth occurring with tricyclic antidepressant therapy. Mechanistic categorization of *toxic* effects is a necessary

prelude to their avoidance or, if they occur, to their rational and successful management.

Types of Toxic Reactions. Toxic effects of drugs may be classified as pharmacological, pathological, or genotoxic (alterations of DNA), and their incidence and seriousness are related, at least over some range, to the concentration of the toxic chemical in the body. An example of a pharmacological toxicity is excessive depression of the central nervous system (CNS) by barbiturates; an example of a pathological effect is hepatic injury produced by acetaminophen; an example of a genotoxic effect is a neoplasm produced by a nitrogen mustard. If the concentration of chemical in the tissues does not exceed a critical level, the effects usually will be reversible. The pharmacological effects usually disappear when the concentration of drug or chemical in the tissues is decreased by biotransformation or excretion from the body. Pathological and genotoxic effects may be repaired. If these effects are severe, death may ensue within a short time; if more subtle damage to DNA is not repaired, cancer may appear in a few months or years in laboratory animals or in a decade or more in human beings.

Local versus Systemic Toxicity. Local toxicity is the effect that occurs at the site of first contact between the biological system and the toxicant. Local effects can be caused by ingestion of caustic substances or inhalation of irritant materials. Systemic toxicity requires absorption and distribution of the toxicant; most substances, with the exception of highly reactive chemical species, produce systemic toxic effects. The two categories are not mutually exclusive. Tetraethyllead, for example, injures skin at the site of contact and deleteriously affects the CNS after it is absorbed into the circulation.

Most systemic toxicants affect one or a few organs predominantly. The target organ of toxicity is not necessarily the site of accumulation of the chemical. For example, lead is concentrated in bone, but its primary toxic action is on soft tissues; DDT (chlorophenothane) is concentrated in adipose tissue but produces no known toxic effects there.

The CNS is involved in systemic toxicity most frequently, as many compounds with prominent effects elsewhere also affect the brain. Next in order of frequency of involvement in systemic toxicity are the circulatory system; the blood and hematopoietic system; visceral organs such as liver, kidney, and lung; and the skin. Muscle and bone are least often affected. With substances that have a predominantly local effect, the frequency of tissue reaction depends largely on the portal of entry (skin, gastrointestinal tract, or respiratory tract).

Reversible and Irreversible Toxic Effects.   The effects of drugs on human beings must, whenever possible, be reversible; otherwise, the drugs would be prohibitively toxic. If a chemical produces injury to a tissue, the capacity of the tissue to regenerate or recover will largely determine the reversibility of the effect. Injuries to a tissue such as liver, which has a high capacity to regenerate, usually are reversible; injury to the CNS is largely irreversible, because the highly differentiated neurons of the brain have an extremely limited ability to divide and regenerate.

Delayed Toxicity.   Most toxic effects of drugs occur at a predictable (usually short) time after administration. However, such is not always the case. For example, aplastic anemia caused by chloramphenicol may appear weeks after the drug has been discontinued. Carcinogenic effects of chemicals usually have a long latency period, and 20 to 30 years may pass before tumors are observed. Because such delayed effects cannot be assessed during any reasonable period of initial evaluation of a chemical, there is an urgent need for reliably predictive, short-term tests for such toxicity as well as for systematic surveillance of the long-term effects of marketed drugs and other chemicals (*see* Chapter 3).

Chemical Carcinogens.   Chemical carcinogens are classified into two major groups, *genotoxic* and *nongenotoxic*. Genotoxic carcinogens interact with DNA, whereas nongenotoxic carcinogens do not. Chemical carcinogenesis is a multistep process. Most genotoxic carcinogens are themselves unreactive (*procarcinogens* or *proximate carcinogens*) but are converted to *primary* or *ultimate carcinogens* in the body. The drug-metabolizing enzymes (phase I and phase II) often convert the proximate carcinogens to reactive electron-deficient intermediates (electrophiles). These reactive intermediates can interact with electron-rich (nucleophilic) centers in DNA to produce a mutation. Such interaction of the ultimate carcinogen with DNA in a cell is thought to be the initial step in chemical carcinogenesis. The DNA may revert to normal if DNA repair mechanisms operate successfully; if not, the transformed cell may grow into a tumor that becomes apparent clinically.

Nongenotoxic carcinogens, also referred to as *promoters,* do not produce tumors alone but do potentiate the effects of genotoxic carcinogens. Promotion involves facilitation of the growth and development of so-called dormant or latent tumor cells. The time from initiation to the development of a tumor probably depends on the presence of such promoters; for many human tumors, the latent period is 15 to 45 years.

To determine whether or not a chemical is potentially carcinogenic to humans, two main types of laboratory tests are done. One type of study is performed to determine whether or not the chemical is mutagenic, because many carcinogens are also mutagens. These studies are often *in vitro* studies, such as the Ames test using *Salmonella typhimurium* (Ames *et al.,* 1975), which can be completed within a few days. This type of test can detect genotoxic carcinogens but not promoters. The second type of study to detect chemical carcinogens consists of feeding laboratory animals (mice and rats) the chemical at high dosages for their entire life span. Autopsies and histopathological examinations are performed on each animal. The incidence of tumors in control animals and animals fed the chemical are compared to determine whether the chemical produces an increased incidence of tumors. This latter study can detect promoters as well as genotoxic carcinogens.

Allergic Reactions.   *Chemical allergy* is an adverse reaction that results from previous sensitization to a particular chemical or to one that is structurally similar. Such reactions are mediated by the immune system. The terms *hypersensitivity* and *drug allergy* often are used to describe the allergic state.

For a low-molecular-weight chemical to cause an allergic reaction, it or its metabolic product usually acts as a hapten, combining with an endogenous protein to form an antigenic complex. Such antigens induce the synthesis of antibodies, usually after a latent period of at least 1 or 2 weeks. Subsequent exposure of the organism to the chemical results in an antigen–antibody interaction that provokes the typical manifestations of allergy. Dose–response relationships usually are not apparent for the provocation of allergic reactions.

Allergic responses have been divided into four general categories, based on the mechanism of immunological involvement (Coombs and Gell, 1975). Type I, or anaphylactic, reactions in human beings are mediated by IgE antibodies. The Fc portion of IgE can bind to receptors on mast cells and basophils. If the Fab portion of the antibody molecule then binds antigen, various mediators (histamine, leukotrienes, prostaglandins) are released and cause vasodilation, edema, and an inflammatory response. The main targets of this type of reaction are the gastrointestinal tract (food allergies), the skin (urticaria and atopic dermatitis), the respiratory system (rhinitis and asthma), and the vasculature (anaphylactic shock). These responses tend to occur quickly after challenge with an antigen to which the individual has been sensitized and are termed *immediate hypersensitivity reactions.*

Type II, or cytolytic, reactions are mediated by both IgG and IgM antibodies and usually are attributed to their ability to activate the complement system. The major target tissues for cytolytic reactions are the cells in the circulatory system. Examples of type II allergic responses include penicillin-induced hemolytic anemia, methyldopa-induced autoimmune hemolytic anemia, quinidine-induced thrombocytopenic purpura, and sulfonamide-induced granulocytopenia. Fortunately, these autoimmune reactions to drugs usually subside within several months after removal of the offending agent.

Type III, or Arthus, reactions are mediated predominantly by IgG; the mechanism involves the generation of antigen–antibody complexes that subsequently fix complement. The complexes are deposited in the vascular endothelium, where a destructive inflammatory response called *serum sickness* occurs. This phenomenon contrasts with the type II reaction, in which the inflammatory response is induced by antibodies directed against tissue antigens. The clinical symptoms of serum sickness include urticarial skin eruptions, arthralgia or arthritis, lymphadenopathy, and fever. These reactions usually last for 6 to 12 days and then subside after the offending agent is eliminated. Several drugs—such as sulfonamides, penicillins, certain anticonvulsants, and iodides—can induce serum sickness. Stevens–Johnson syndrome, such as that caused by sulfonamides, is a more severe form of immune vasculitis. Symptoms of this reaction include erythema multiforme, arthritis, nephritis, CNS abnormalities, and myocarditis.

Type IV, or delayed-hypersensitivity, reactions are mediated by sensitized T lymphocytes and macrophages. When sensitized cells come in contact with antigen, an inflammatory reaction is generated by the production of lymphokines and the subsequent influx of neutrophils and macrophages. An example of type IV or delayed hypersensitivity is the contact dermatitis caused by poison ivy.

Idiosyncratic Reactions. *Idiosyncrasy* is defined as a genetically determined abnormal reactivity to a chemical. The observed response is qualitatively similar in all individuals, but the idiosyncratic response may take the form of extreme sensitivity to low doses or extreme insensitivity to high doses of chemicals. These genetic polymorphisms can be due to interindividual differences in drug pharmacokinetics, such as phase I and phase II biotransformation enzymes. An example is increased incidence of peripheral neuropathy in patients with inherited deficiencies in acetylation when isoniazid is used for the treatment of tuberculosis. The polymorphisms also can be due to pharmacodynamic factors such as drug-receptor interactions (Evans and Relling, 1999). For example, many black males (about 10%) develop a serious hemolytic anemia when they receive primaquine as an antimalarial therapy. Such individuals have a deficiency of erythrocytic glucose-6-phosphate dehydrogenase (*see* Chapter 40). Genetically determined resistance to the anticoagulant action of warfarin is due to an alteration in the vitamin K epoxide reductase (*see* Chapter 55). The use of genetic information to explain interindividual differences in drug responses or to individualize dosages of drugs for patients with known genetic polymorphisms is referred to as *pharmacogenomics*.

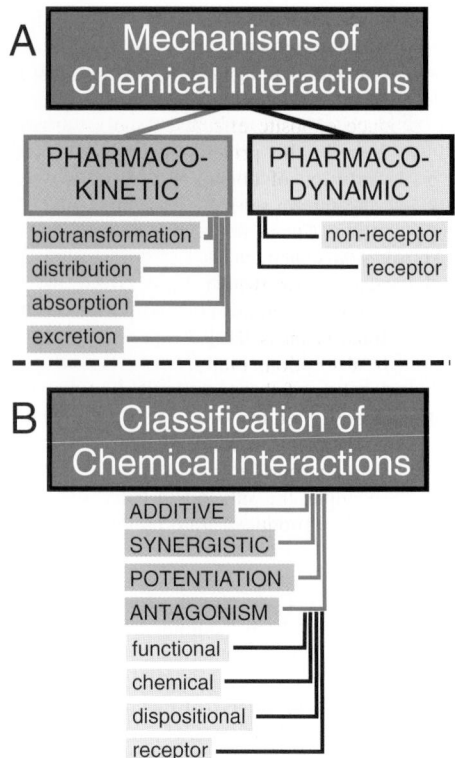

Figure 4–6. Mechanisms and classifications of chemical interactions.

Interactions between Chemicals. The existence of numerous toxicants requires consideration of their potential interactions (*see* Figure 4–6). Concurrent exposures may alter the pharmacokinetics of drugs by changing rates of absorption, the degree of protein binding, or the rates of biotransformation or excretion of one or both interacting compounds. The pharmacodynamics of chemicals can be altered by competition at the receptor; for example, atropine is used to treat organophosphate insecticide toxicity, because it blocks muscarinic cholinergic receptors and prevents their stimulation by excess acetylcholine resulting from inhibition of acetylcholinesterase by the insecticide. Nonreceptor pharmacodynamic drug interactions also can occur when two drugs have different mechanisms of action; for example, aspirin and heparin given together can cause unexpected bleeding. The response to combined toxicants may thus be equal to, greater than, or less than the sum of the effects of the individual agents.

Numerous terms describe pharmacological and toxicological interactions (*see* Figure 4–6B). An *additive* effect describes the combined effect of two chemicals that is equal to the sum of the effect of each agent given alone; the additive effect is the most common. A *synergistic* effect is one in which the combined effect of two chemicals is greater than the sum of the effects of each agent given alone. For example, both carbon tetrachloride and ethanol are hepatotoxins, but together they produce much more injury to the liver than expected from the mathematical sum of their individual effects. *Potentiation* is the increased effect of a toxic agent acting simultaneously with a nontoxic one. Isopropanol alone, for example, is not hepatotoxic; however, it greatly increases the hepatotoxicity of carbon tetrachloride. *Antagonism* is the interference of one chemical with the action of another. An antagonistic agent is often desirable as an antidote. *Functional* or *physiological antagonism* occurs when two chemicals produce opposite effects on the same physiological function. For example, this principle is applied to the ability of an intravenous infusion of dopamine to maintain perfusion of vital organs during certain severe intoxications characterized by marked hypotension. *Chemical antagonism* or *inactivation* is a reaction between two chemicals to neutralize their effects. For example, dimercaprol, or British antilewisite (BAL), chelates with various metals to decrease their toxicity (*see* Chapter 67). *Dispositional antagonism* is the alteration of the disposition of a substance (its absorption, biotransformation, distribution, or excretion) so that less of the agent reaches the target organ or its persistence there is reduced (*see* below). *Antagonism* at the *receptor* for the chemical entails the blockade of the effect of an agonist with an appropriate antagonist that competes for the same site. For example, the antagonist naloxone is used to treat respiratory depression produced by opioids (*see* Chapter 23).

DESCRIPTIVE TOXICITY TESTS IN ANIMALS

Two main principles underlie all descriptive toxicity tests performed in animals. First, effects of chemicals produced in laboratory animals, when properly qualified, apply to toxicity in human beings. When calculated on the basis of dose per unit of body surface, toxic effects in human beings usually are encountered in the same range of concentrations as are those in experimental animals. On the basis of body weight, human beings are generally more vulnerable than experimental animals. Such information is used to select dosages for clinical trials of candidate therapeutic agents and to attempt to set limits on permissible exposure to environmental toxicants.

The second main principle is that exposure of experimental animals to toxic agents in high doses is a necessary and valid method to discover possible hazards to human beings who are exposed to much lower doses. This principle is based on the quantal dose–response concept. As a matter of practicality, the number of animals used in experiments on toxic materials usually will be small compared with the size of human populations potentially at risk. For example, 0.01% incidence of a serious toxic effect (such as cancer) represents 25,000 people in a population of 250 million. Such an incidence is unacceptably high. Yet, detecting an incidence of 0.01% experimentally would probably require a minimum of 30,000 animals. To estimate risk at low dosage, large doses must be given to relatively small groups. The validity of the necessary extrapolation is clearly a crucial question.

Chemicals are first tested for toxicity by estimation of the LD_{50} in two animal species by two routes of administration;

one of these is the expected route of exposure of human beings to the chemical being tested. The number of animals that die in a 14-day period after a single dose is recorded. The animals also are examined for signs of intoxication, lethargy, behavioral modification, and morbidity.

The chemical is next tested for toxicity by subacute exposure, usually for 90 days. The subacute study is performed most often in two species by the route of intended use or exposure, and at least three doses are employed. A variety of parameters are monitored during this period, and, at the end of the study, organs and tissues are examined by a pathologist.

Long-term or chronic studies are carried out in animals at the same time that clinical trials are undertaken (*see* Chapter 3). For drugs, the length of exposure depends somewhat on the intended clinical use. If the drug normally would be used for short periods under medical supervision, as would an antimicrobial agent, a chronic exposure of animals for 6 months might suffice. If the drug would be used in human beings for longer periods, a study of chronic use for 2 years might be required.

Studies of chronic exposure often are used to determine the carcinogenic potential of chemicals. These studies usually are performed in rats and mice for the average lifetime of the species. Other tests are designed to evaluate teratogenicity (congenital malformations), perinatal and postnatal toxicity, and effects on fertility. Teratogenicity studies usually are performed by administering drugs to pregnant rats and rabbits during the period of organogenesis.

In addition to chronic studies for evaluation of carcinogenic potential or teratogenicity, drugs often are tested for *mutagenic* potential. The most popular such test currently available, the reverse mutation test developed by Ames and colleagues (Ames *et al.*, 1975), uses a strain of *S. typhimurium* that has a mutant gene for the enzyme phosphoribosyl adenosine triphosphate (ATP) synthetase. This enzyme is required for histidine synthesis, and the bacterial strain is unable to grow in a histidine-deficient medium unless a reverse mutation is induced. Because many chemicals are not mutagenic or carcinogenic unless activated by enzymes on the endoplasmic reticulum, rat hepatic microsomes usually are added to the medium containing the mutant bacteria and the drug. The Ames test is rapid and sensitive. Its usefulness for the prediction of genotoxic carcinogens is widely accepted, but it does not detect nongenotoxic carcinogens (promoters).

INCIDENCE OF ACUTE POISONING

The true incidence of poisoning in the United States is not known, but in 1998, more than two million cases were voluntarily reported to the American Association of Poison Control Centers. The number of actual poisonings almost certainly exceeds by far the number reported.

Deaths in the United States due to poisoning number more than 775 per year. The incidence of poisoning in children younger than 5 years of age has decreased dramatically over the past 3 decades. For example, there were no reported childhood deaths due to aspirin in 1998, compared to about 140 deaths per year in the early 1960s.

Table 4–1

Substances Most Frequently Involved in Human Poison Exposures

SUBSTANCE	NUMBER	%*
Cleaning substances	229,500	10.2
Analgesics	215,067	9.6
Cosmetics and personal care products	210,224	9.4
Plants	122,578	5.5
Foreign bodies	103,696	4.6
Cough and cold preparations	99,924	4.5
Bites/envenomations	92,182	4.1
Insecticides/pesticides (includes rodenticides)	86,289	3.9
Topicals	83,455	3.7
Food products, food poisoning	78,690	3.5
Sedatives/hypnotics/antipsychotics	70,982	3.2
Antidepressants	67,872	3.0
Hydrocarbons	66,623	3.0
Antimicrobials	62,034	2.8
Chemicals	61,061	2.7
Alcohols	55,246	2.5

*Percentages are based on total number of known ingested substances rather than the total number of human exposure cases.

SOURCE: From Litovitz *et al.,* 1999. Courtesy of the American Journal of Emergency Medicine.

Table 4–2

Categories with Largest Numbers of Deaths

CATEGORY	NUMBER	% OF ALL EXPOSURES IN CATEGORY
Analgesics	264	0.108
Antidepressants	152	0.224
Stimulants and street drugs	118	0.345
Cardiovascular drugs	118	0.279
Sedative/hypnotics/ antipsychotics	89	0.125
Alcohols	56	0.101
Chemicals	45	0.074
Gases and fumes	38	0.092
Cleaning substances	24	0.010
Anticonvulsants	20	0.090
Asthma drugs	18	0.114
Antihistamines	18	0.036
Hydrocarbons	18	0.027
Automotive products	16	0.108
Hormones/hormone antagonists	16	0.043
Insecticides/pesticides (includes rodenticides)	16	0.024

SOURCE: From Litovitz *et al.,* 1999. Courtesy of the American Journal of Emergency Medicine.

This favorable trend probably is due to safety packaging of drugs, drain cleaners, turpentine, and other household chemicals; improved medical training and care; and increased public awareness of potential poisons.

The substances most frequently involved in human poison exposures are shown in Table 4–1. Two of the three categories of substances most frequently responsible for human poisoning are not drugs but cosmetics and cleaning agents. While most drugs are not the most common class of chemicals involved in human poisoning, the top five categories of substances that produce deaths are drugs (Table 4–2). The chemicals most commonly associated with fatalities are tricyclic antidepressants, acetaminophen, salicylates, opiates, cocaine, digoxin, carbon monoxide, and calcium channel blockers. Most of the people who die from poisoning are adults, and the deaths often result from intentional rather than accidental exposure. Children younger than 6 years of age account for 53% of the poisoning incidents reported but only 2% of the deaths. Children between 1 and 2 years of age have the highest incidence of accidental poisoning. Fortunately, most of the substances available to these young children

are not highly toxic. Iron and pesticides are the leading cause of pediatric accidental poisoning fatalities.

It recently has been recognized that the incidence of serious and fatal adverse drug reactions in United States hospitals is extremely high (Lazarou *et al.,* 1998; Institute of Medicine, 1999). It is estimated that each year about 2 million hospitalized patients have serious adverse drug reactions, and about a hundred thousand have fatal adverse drug reactions. If this estimate is correct, then more people die annually from medication errors than from highway accidents, breast cancer, or AIDS.

MAJOR SOURCES OF INFORMATION ON POISONING

Pharmacology textbooks are a good source of information on treatment of poisoning by drugs, but they usually say little about other chemicals. Additional information on drugs and other chemicals can be found in various books on poisoning. (*See* Ellenhorn, 1997; Goldfrank *et al.,* 1998; Haddad *et al.,* 1998; Klaassen, 2001.)

A useful source of information on the treatment of acute poisoning by commercial products is *Clinical Toxicology of Commercial Products* by Gosselin and associates (1984). This book contains seven major sections. One section lists more than 17,500 trade names of products that might be ingested accidentally or suicidally. It lists the manufacturer and ingredients of each commercial product and notes components believed responsible for harmful effects. A popular computerized system for information on toxic substances is POISINDEX (Micromedex, Inc., Denver, Colorado).

There are about 120 poison control centers in the United States, coordinated and served by the FDA's Poisoning Surveillance and Epidemiology Branch, and there are 34 regional poison control centers designated by the American Association of Poison Control Centers. Valuable information can be obtained from these centers by telephone.

PREVENTION AND TREATMENT OF POISONING

Many acute poisonings from drugs could be prevented if physicians provided common-sense instructions about the storage of drugs and other chemicals and if patients or parents of patients accepted this advice. These instructions are so widely publicized that they need not be repeated here.

For clinical purposes, all toxic agents can be divided into two classes: those for which a specific treatment antidote exists and those for which there is no specific treatment. For the vast majority of drugs and other chemicals, there is no specific treatment; symptomatic medical care that supports vital functions is the only strategy.

Supportive therapy, as in other medical emergencies, is the most important aspect of the treatment of drug poisoning. The adage "Treat the patient, not the poison" remains the most basic and important principle of clinical toxicology. Maintenance of respiration and circulation takes precedence. Serial measurement and charting of vital signs and important reflexes help to judge the progress of intoxication, response to therapy, and need for additional treatment. This monitoring usually requires hospitalization. The classification in Table 4–3 often is used to indicate the severity of CNS intoxication. Treatment with large doses of stimulants and sedatives often can cause more harm than the poison. Chemical antidotes should be used judiciously; heroic measures seldom are necessary.

Treatment of acute poisoning must be prompt. The first goal is to maintain the vital functions if their im-

Table 4–3

Signs and Symptoms of CNS Intoxication

DEGREE OF SEVERITY	CHARACTERISTICS
Depressants	
0	Asleep, but can be aroused and can answer questions
I	Semicomatose, withdraws from painful stimuli, reflexes intact
II	Comatose, does not withdraw from painful stimuli, no respiratory or circulatory depression, most reflexes intact
III	Comatose, most or all reflexes absent, but without depression of respiration or of circulation
IV	Comatose, reflexes absent, respiratory depression with cyanosis or circulatory failure and shock, or both
Stimulants	
I	Restlessness, irritability, insomnia, tremor, hyperreflexia, sweating, mydriasis, flushing
II	Confusion, hyperactivity, hypertension, tachypnea, tachycardia, extrasystoles, sweating, mydriasis, flushing, mild hyperpyrexia
III	Delirium, mania, self-injury, marked hypertension, tachycardia, arrhythmias, hyperpyrexia
IV	As in III, plus convulsions, coma, and circulatory collapse

pairment is imminent. The second goal is to keep the concentration of poison in the crucial tissues as low as possible by preventing absorption and enhancing elimination. The third goal is to combat the pharmacological and toxicological effects at the effector sites.

Prevention of Further Absorption of Poison

Emesis. Although emesis is indicated after poisoning by oral ingestion of most chemicals, it is contraindicated in certain situations: (1) If the patient has ingested a corrosive poison, such as a strong acid or alkali (*e.g.,* drain cleaners), emesis increases the likelihood of gastric perforation and further necrosis of the esophagus. (2) If the patient is comatose or in a state of stupor or delirium, emesis may cause aspiration of the gastric contents. (3) If the patient has ingested a CNS stimulant, further stimulation associated with vomiting may precipitate convulsions. (4) If the patient has ingested a petroleum distillate (*e.g.,* kerosene, gasoline, or petroleum-based liquid furniture polish), regurgitated hydrocarbons can be aspirated readily and cause chemical pneumonitis (Ervin, 1983). In contrast, emesis should be considered if the solution that is ingested contains potentially dangerous compounds, such as pesticides.

There are marked differences in the capabilities of various petroleum distillates to produce hydrocarbon pneumonia, which is an acute, hemorrhagic necrotizing process. In general, the ability of various hydrocarbons to produce pneumonitis is inversely proportional to the viscosity of the agent: if the viscosity is high, as with oils and greases, the risk is limited; if the viscosity is low, as with mineral seal oil found in liquid furniture polishes, the risk of aspiration is high.

Vomiting can be induced mechanically by stroking the posterior pharynx. However, this technique is not as effective as the administration of ipecac or apomorphine.

Ipecac.   The most useful household emetic is syrup of ipecac (not ipecac fluid extract, which is 14 times more potent and may cause fatalities). Syrup of ipecac is available in 0.5- and 1-fluid ounce containers (approximately 15 and 30 ml), which may be purchased without prescription. The drug can be given orally, but it takes 15 to 30 minutes to produce emesis; this compares favorably with the time usually required for adequate gastric lavage. The oral dose is 15 ml in children from 6 months to 12 years of age and 30 ml in older children and adults. Because emesis may not occur when the stomach is empty, the administration of ipecac should be followed by a drink of water.

Ipecac acts as an emetic because of its local irritant effect on the enteric tract and its effect on the chemoreceptor trigger zone (CTZ) in the area postrema of the medulla. Syrup of ipecac may be effective even when antiemetic drugs (such as phenothiazines) have been ingested (Thoman and Verhulst, 1966), presumably due to its direct irritant action on the gastrointestinal tract. Ipecac can produce toxic effects on the heart because of its content of emetine, but this usually is not a problem with the dose used for emesis (Manno and Manno, 1977). If emesis does not occur, ipecac should be removed by gastric lavage. Chronic abuse of ipecac for weight reduction can result in cardiomyopathy, ventricular fibrillation, and death.

Apomorphine.   Apomorphine stimulates the CTZ and causes emesis. The drug is unstable in solution and must be prepared just prior to use and thus is not often readily available. Additionally, apomorphine is not effective orally and must be given parenterally, usually by the subcutaneous route—6 mg for adults

and 0.06 mg/kg for children (Goldfrank *et al.,* 1998). However, this can be an advantage over ipecac in that it can be administered to an uncooperative patient and produces vomiting in 3 to 5 minutes. Because apomorphine is a respiratory depressant, it should not be used if the patient has been poisoned by a CNS depressant or if the patient's respiration is slow and labored. At present, apomorphine is rarely used as an emetic.

Gastric Lavage.   Gastric lavage is accomplished by inserting a tube into the stomach and washing the stomach with water, normal saline, or one-half normal saline to remove the unabsorbed poison. The procedure should be performed as soon as possible, but only if vital functions are adequate or supportive procedures have been implemented. The contraindications to this procedure generally are the same as for emesis, and there is the additional potential complication of mechanical injury to the throat, esophagus, and stomach. A position statement has been published by the American Academy of Clinical Toxicology and the European Association of Poison Centres and Clinical Toxicologists (Vale, 1997) on the use of gastric lavage. These groups concluded that gastric lavage should not be used routinely in the management of the poisoned patient but should be reserved for patients who have ingested a potentially life-threatening amount of poison and when the procedure can be undertaken within 60 minutes of ingestion.

The only equipment needed for gastric lavage is a tube and a large syringe. The tube should be as large as possible so that the wash solution, food, and poison (whether in the form of a capsule, pill, or liquid) will flow freely and lavage can be accomplished quickly. A 36-Fr tube or larger should be used in adults and a 24-Fr tube or larger in children. Orogastric lavage is preferred over nasogastric, because a larger tube can be employed. To prevent aspiration, an endotracheal tube with an inflatable cuff should be positioned before lavage is initiated if the patient is comatose, having seizures, or has lost the gag reflex. During gastric lavage, the patient should be placed on his or her left side because of the anatomical asymmetry of the stomach, with the head hanging face down over the edge of the examining table. If possible, the foot of the table should be elevated. This technique minimizes chances of aspiration.

The contents of the stomach should be aspirated with an irrigating syringe and saved for chemical analysis. The stomach then may be washed with saline solution. Saline solution is safer than water in young children because of the risk of water intoxication, manifested by tonic and clonic seizures and coma (Arena, 1975). Only small volumes (120 to 300 ml) of lavage solution should be instilled into the stomach at one time so that the poison is not pushed into the intestine. Lavage should be repeated until the returns are clear, which usually requires 10 to 12 washings and a total of 1.5 to 4 liters of lavage fluid. When the lavage is complete, the stomach may be left empty or an antidote may be instilled through the tube. If no specific antidote is known for the poison, an aqueous suspension of activated charcoal and a cathartic is often given.

Chemical Adsorption. Activated charcoal avidly adsorbs drugs and chemicals on the surfaces of the charcoal particles, thereby preventing absorption and toxicity. Many, but not all, chemicals are adsorbed by charcoal. For example, alcohols, hydrocarbons, metals, and corrosives are not well adsorbed by activated charcoal, and charcoal therefore is of little value in treating these poisonings. The effectiveness of charcoal also is dependent on the time since the ingestion and on the dose of charcoal; one should attempt to achieve a charcoal:drug ratio of at least 10:1. Activated charcoal also can interrupt the enterohepatic circulation of drugs and enhance the net rate of diffusion of the chemical from the body into the gastrointestinal tract. For example, the use of serial doses of activated charcoal has been shown to enhance the elimination of theophylline and phenobarbital (Berg *et al.,* 1982; Berlinger *et al.,* 1983).

During the last two decades, there has been an increase in the use of activated charcoal and a corresponding decrease in the use of ipecac-induced emesis and gastric lavage in the treatment of poisoning. Studies in patients with drug overdoses as well as in normal subjects fail to show a benefit of treatment with ipecac or lavage plus activated charcoal as compared with charcoal alone (Neuvonen *et al.,* 1983; Curtis *et al.,* 1984; Kulig *et al.,* 1985; Albertson *et al.,* 1989). It is concluded generally that adminstration of activated charcoal is the single most important intervention that can be provided to an overdosed patient.

Activated charcoal usually is prepared as a mixture of at least 50 g (about 10 heaping tablespoons) in a glass of water. The mixture is then administered either orally or *via* a gastric tube. Because most poisons do not appear to desorb from the charcoal if charcoal is present in excess, the adsorbed poison need not be removed from the gastrointestinal tract. Activated charcoal should not be used simultaneously with ipecac because charcoal can adsorb the emetic agent in ipecac and thus reduce the drug's emetic effect. Charcoal also may adsorb and decrease the effectiveness of specific antidotes.

Activated charcoal must be distinguished from the so-called universal antidote, which consists of two parts burned toast (not activated charcoal), one part tannic acid (strong tea), and one part magnesium oxide. In practice, the universal antidote is ineffective.

As mentioned, the presence of an adsorbent in the intestine may interrupt enterohepatic circulation of a toxicant, thus enhancing its excretion. Activated charcoal is useful in interrupting the enterohepatic circulation of drugs such as tricyclic antidepressants and glutethimide. A nonabsorbable polythiol resin has been used to treat poisoning by methylmercury due to its ability to bind mercury excreted into the bile (*see* Chapter 67). Cholestyramine hastens the elimination of cardiac glycosides by a similar mechanism.

Chemical Inactivation. Antidotes can change the chemical nature of a poison by rendering it less toxic or preventing its absorption. Formaldehyde poisoning can be treated with ammonia to form hexamethylenetetramine (Goldstein *et al.,* 1974); sodium formaldehyde sulfoxylate can convert mercuric ion to the less soluble metallic mercury (Gosselin *et al.,* 1984); and sodium bicarbonate converts ferrous iron to ferrous carbonate, which is poorly absorbed. Chemical inactivation techniques seldom are used today, however, because valuable time may be lost, whereas emetics, activated charcoal, and gastric lavage are rapid and effective.

In the past, neutralization was the usual treatment of poisoning with acids or bases. Vinegar, orange juice, or lemon juice often has been used for the patient who has ingested alkali, and various antacids often have been advocated for treatment of acid burns. The use of neutralizing agents is controversial, because it may produce excessive heat. Carbon dioxide gas produced from bicarbonates used to treat oral poisoning with acids can cause gastric distention and even perforation. The treatment of choice for ingestion of either acids or alkalis is dilution with water or milk. Similarly, burns produced by acid or alkali on the skin should be treated with copious amounts of water.

Purgation. The rationale for using an osmotic cathartic is to minimize absorption by hastening the passage of the toxicant through the gastrointestinal tract. Few, if any, controlled clinical data are available on the effectiveness of cathartics in the treatment of poisoning. Cathartics generally are considered harmless unless the poison has injured the gastrointestinal tract. Cathartics are indicated after the ingestion of enteric-coated tablets, when the time after ingestion is greater than 1 hour, and for poisoning by volatile hydrocarbons (Rumack and Lovejoy, 1985). Sorbitol is the most effective, but sodium sulfate and magnesium sulfate also are used; all act promptly and usually have minimal toxicity. However, magnesium sulfate should be used cautiously in patients with renal failure or in those likely to develop renal dysfunction, and Na^+-containing cathartics should be avoided in patients with congestive heart failure. Whole-bowel irrigation is a technique that not only promotes defecation, but also eliminates the entire contents of the intestines. This technique uses a high-molecular-weight polyethylene glycol and isosmolar electrolyte solution (PEG-EESS), which does not alter serum electrolytes. It is commercially available as GOLYTELY and COLYTE.

Inhalation and Dermal Exposure to Poisons. When a poison has been inhaled, the first priority is to remove the patient from the source of exposure. Similarly, the skin should be thoroughly washed with water if it has come in contact with a poison. Contaminated clothing should be removed. Initial treatment of all types of chemical injuries to the eye must be rapid; thorough irrigation of the eye with water for 15 minutes should be performed immediately.

Enhanced Elimination of the Poison

Biotransformation. Once a chemical has been absorbed, procedures sometimes can be employed to enhance its rate of elimination. Many drugs are metabolized by the cytochrome P450 system in the endoplasmic reticulum of the liver, and components of this system can be induced by a number of compounds (*see* Chapter 1). However, induction of these oxidative enzymes is too slow (days) to be valuable in the treatment of acute poisoning by most chemical agents.

Many chemicals are toxic because they are biotransformed into more toxic chemicals. Thus, inhibition of biotransformation should decrease the toxicity of such drugs.

For example, ethanol is used to inhibit the conversion of methanol to its highly toxic metabolite, formic acid, by alcohol dehydrogenase (*see* Chapter 68). As discussed earlier in this chapter, acetaminophen is converted by the cytochrome P450 system to an electrophilic metabolite that is detoxified by glutathione, a cellular nucleophile. Acetaminophen does not cause hepatotoxicity until glutathione is depleted, whereupon the reactive metabolite binds to essential macromolecular constituents of the hepatocyte, resulting in cell death. The liver can be protected by maintenance of the concentration of glutathione, and this can be accomplished by the administration of *N*-acetylcysteine (Black, 1980; *see* Chapter 27).

Some drugs are detoxified by conjugation with glucuronic acid or sulfate before elimination from the body, and the availability of the endogenous cosubstrates for conjugation may limit the rate of elimination; such is the case in the detoxication of acetaminophen (Hjelle *et al.*, 1985). When methods become available to replete these compounds, an additional mechanism will be available to treat poisoning. Similarly, detoxication of cyanide by conversion to thiocyanate can be accelerated by the administration of thiosulfate (*see* Chapter 68).

Biliary Excretion. The liver excretes many drugs and other foreign chemicals into bile, but little is known about efficient ways to enhance biliary excretion of xenobiotics for the treatment of acute poisoning. Inducers of microsomal enzyme activity enhance biliary excretion of some xenobiotics, but the effect is slow in onset (Klaassen and Watkins, 1984).

Urinary Excretion. Drugs and poisons are excreted into the urine by glomerular filtration and active tubular secretion (*see* Chapter 1); they can be reabsorbed into the blood if they are in a lipid-soluble form that will penetrate the tubule or if there is an active mechanism for their transport.

There are no methods known to accelerate the active transport of poisons into urine, and enhancement of glomerular filtration is not a practical means to facilitate elimination of toxicants. However, passive reabsorption from the tubular lumen can be altered. Diuretics decrease reabsorption by decreasing the concentration gradient of the drug from the lumen to the tubular cell and by increasing flow through the tubule. Furosemide is used most often, but osmotic diuretics also are employed (*see* Chapter 29). Forced diuresis should be used with caution, especially in patients with renal, cardiac, or pulmonary complications.

Nonionized compounds are reabsorbed far more rapidly than ionized, polar molecules; therefore a shift from the nonionized to the ionized species of the toxicant by alteration of the pH of the tubular fluid may hasten elimination (*see* Chapter 1). Acidic compounds such as phenobarbital and salicylates are cleared much more rapidly in alkaline than in acidic urine. The effect of increasing urine flow and alkalinization of urine on the clearance of phenobarbital is shown in Figure 4–7. Intravenous sodium bicarbonate is used to alkalinize the urine. Renal excretion of basic drugs such as amphetamine theoretically can be enhanced by acidification of the urine. Acidification can be accomplished by the administration of ammonium chloride or ascorbic acid. Urinary excretion of an acidic compound is particularly sensitive to changes in urinary pH if its pKa is within the range of 3.0 to 7.5; for bases the corresponding range is 7.5 to 10.5.

Dialysis. Hemodialysis or hemoperfusion usually has limited use in the treatment of intoxication with chemicals. However, under certain circumstances, such procedures can be lifesaving. The utility of dialysis depends on the amount of poison in the blood relative to the total body burden. Thus, if a poison has a large volume of distribution, as is the case for the tricyclic antidepressants, the plasma will contain too little of the compound for effective removal by dialysis. Extensive binding of the compound to plasma proteins impairs dialysis greatly. The kinetics of elimination of a toxicant by dialysis also is dependent on the rate of dissociation of the compound from binding sites in tissues; for some chemicals, this rate may be slow.

Although peritoneal dialysis requires a minimum of personnel and can be started as soon as the patient is

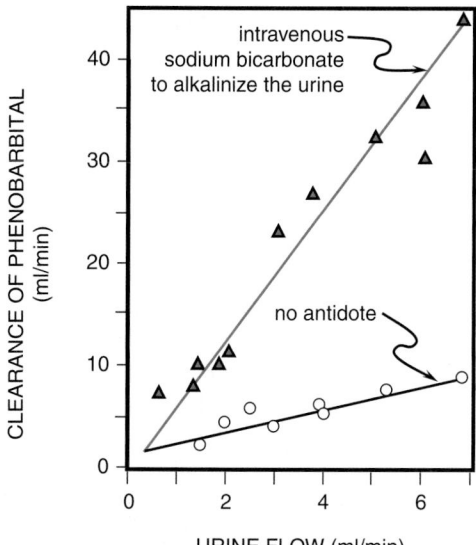

Figure 4–7. Renal clearance of phenobarbital in the dog as related to urinary pH and the rate of urine flow.

The values designated by circles are from experiments in which diuresis was induced by administration of water orally or Na_2SO_4 intravenously and the urinary pH was below 7.0. The values designated by triangles are from experiments in which $NaHCO_3$ was administered intravenously and in which the urinary pH was 7.8 to 8.0. (After Waddell and Butler, 1957. Courtesy of *Journal of Clinical Investigation.*)

admitted to the hospital, it is too inefficient to be of value for the treatment of acute intoxications. Hemodialysis (extracorporeal dialysis) is much more effective than peritoneal dialysis and may be essential in a few life-threatening intoxications, such as with methanol, ethylene glycol, and salicylates.

Passage of blood through a column of charcoal or adsorbent resin (hemoperfusion) is a technique for the extracorporeal removal of a poison (Winchester, 1983). Because of the high adsorptive capacity and affinity of the material in the column, some chemicals that are bound to plasma proteins can be removed. The principal side effect of hemoperfusion is depletion of platelets.

Antagonism or Chemical Inactivation of an Absorbed Poison

The functional and pharmacological antagonism of the effects of absorbed toxicants has been discussed above. If a patient is poisoned with a compound that acts as an agonist at a receptor for which a specific blocking agent is available, administration of the receptor antagonist may be highly effective. Functional antagonism also can be valuable for support of the patient's vital functions. For example, anticonvulsant drugs are used to treat chemically induced convulsions. However, drugs that stimulate antagonistic physiological mechanisms are not always of clinical value and may even decrease the incidence of survival, because it often is difficult to titrate the effect of one drug against another when the two act on opposing systems. An example of such a complication is the use of CNS stimulants to attempt to reverse respiratory depression. Convulsions are a typical complication of such therapy, and mechanical support of respiration is preferred. In addition, the duration of action of the poison and the antidote may differ, sometimes leading to poisoning with the antidote.

Specific chemical antagonists of a toxicant, such as opioid antagonists (*see* Chapter 23) and atropine as an antagonist of pesticide-induced acetylcholine excess (Chapter 7), are valuable but unfortunately rare. Chelating agents with high selectivity for certain metal ions provide such examples (*see* Chapter 67). Antibodies offer the potential for the production of specific antidotes for a host of common poisons and for drugs that frequently are abused or misused. A notable example of such success is the use of purified digoxin-specific Fab fragments of antibodies in the treatment of potentially fatal cases of poisoning with digoxin (*see* Chapter 34). The development of human monoclonal antibodies directed against specific toxins has significant potential therapeutic value.

BIBLIOGRAPHY

Albertson, T.E., Derlet, R.W., Foulke, G.E., Minguillon, M.C., and Tharratt, S.R. Superiority of activated charcoal alone compared with ipecac and activated charcoal in the treatment of acute toxic ingestions. *Ann. Emerg. Med.,* **1989,** *18*:56–59.

Ames, B.N., McCann, J., and Yamasaki, E. Methods for detecting carcinogens and mutagens with the *Salmonella*/mammalian microsome mutagenicity test. *Mutat. Res.,* **1975,** *31*:347–364.

Berg, M.J., Berlinger, W.G., Goldberg, M.J., Spector, R., and Johnson, G.F. Acceleration of the body clearance of phenobarbital by oral activated charcoal. *N. Engl. J. Med.,* **1982,** *307*:642–644.

Berlinger, W.G., Spector, R., Goldberg, M.J., Johnson, G.F., Quee, C.K., and Berg, M.J. Enhancement of theophylline clearance by oral activated charcoal. *Clin. Pharmacol. Ther.,* **1983,** *33*:351–354.

Black, M. Acetaminophen hepatotoxicity. *Gastroenterology,* **1980,** 78:382–392.

Curtis, R.A., Barone, J., and Giacona, N. Efficacy of ipecac and activated charcoal/cathartic. Prevention of salicylate absorption in a simulated overdose. *Arch. Intern. Med.,* **1984,** *144*:48–52.

Evans, W.E., and Relling, M.V. Pharmacogenomics: translating functional genomics into rational therapeutics. *Science,* **1999,** *286*:487–491.

Hjelle, J.J., Hazelton, G.A., and Klaassen, C.D. Acetaminophen decreases adenosine 39′ phosphate 59′ phosphosulfate and uridine diphosphoglucuronic acid in liver. *Drug Metab. Dispos.,* **1985,** 13:35–41.

Kulig, K., Bar-Or, D., Cantrill, S.V., Rosen, P., and Rumack, B.H. Management of acutely poisoned patients without gastric emptying. *Ann. Emerg. Med.,* **1985,** *14*:562–567.

Lazarou, J., Pomeranz, B.H., and Corey, P.N. Incidence of adverse drug reactions in hospitalized patients: a meta-analysis of prospective studies. *J.A.M.A.,* **1998,** *279*:1200–1205.

Litovitz, T.L., Klein-Schwartz, W., Caravati, E.M., Youniss, J., Crouch, B., and Lee, S. 1998 Annual Report of the American Association of Poison Control Centers Toxic Exposure Surveillance System. *Am. J. Emerg. Med.,* **1999,** *17*:435–487.

Neuvonen, P.J., Vartiainen, M., and Tokola, O. Comparison of activated charcoal and ipecac syrup in prevention of drug absorption. *Eur. J. Clin. Pharmacol.,* **1983,** *24*:557–562.

Thoman, M.E., and Verhulst, H.L. Ipecac syrup in antiemetic ingestion. *J.A.M.A.,* **1966,** *196*:433–434.

Waddell, W.J., and Butler, T.C. The distribution and excretion of phenobarbital. *J. Clin. Invest.,* **1957,** *36*:1217–1226.

MONOGRAPHS AND REVIEWS

Arena, J.M. Poisoning and its treatment. In, *Pediatric Therapy,* 5th ed. (Shirkey, H.C., ed.) C. V. Mosby Co., St. Louis, **1975,** pp. 101–136.

Coombs, R.R.A., and Gell, P.G.H. Classification of allergic reactions responsible for clinical hypersensitivity and disease. In, *Clinical Aspects of Immunology.* (Gell, P.G.H., Coombs, R.R.A., and Lachmann, P.J., eds.) Blackwell Scientific Publications, Oxford, U.K., **1975,** pp. 761–781.

Ellenhorn, M.J. *Ellenhorn's Medical Toxicology,* 2nd ed. Williams & Wilkins, Baltimore, **1997.**

Ervin, M.E. Petroleum distillates and turpentine. In, *Clinical Management of Poisoning and Drug Overdose.* (Haddad, L.M., and Winchester, J.F., eds.) W.B. Saunders Co., Philadelphia, **1983,** pp. 771–779.

Goldfrank, L.R., Flomenbaum, N.E., Lewin, N.A., Weisman, R.S., Howland, M.A., and Hoffman, R.S. *Goldfrank's Toxicologic Emergencies,* 6th ed. Appleton & Lange, Stamford, CT, **1998.**

Goldstein, A., Aronow, L., and Kalman, S.M. *Principles of Drug Action: The Basis of Pharmacology,* 2nd ed. John Wiley & Sons, New York, **1974.**

Gosselin, R.E., Smith, R.P., and Hodge, H.C., eds. *Clinical Toxicology of Commercial Products,* 5th ed. Williams & Wilkins, Baltimore, **1984.**

Haddad, L.M., Shannon, M.W., and Winchester, J.F., eds. *Clinical Management of Poisoning and Drug Overdose,* 3rd ed. W.B. Saunders Co., Philadelphia, **1998.**

Institute of Medicine. *To Err Is Human: Building a Safer Health System.* National Academy Press, Washington, DC, **1999.**

Klaassen, C.D., ed. *Casarett and Doull's Toxicology: The Basic Science of Poisons,* 6th ed. McGraw-Hill, Inc., New York, **2001.**

Klaassen, C.D., and Watkins, J.B. III. Mechanisms of bile formation, hepatic uptake, and biliary excretion. *Pharmacol. Rev.,* **1984,** *36*:1–67.

Manno, B.R., and Manno, J.E. Toxicology of ipecac: a review. *Clin. Toxicol.,* **1977,** *10*:221–242.

Rumack, B.H., and Lovejoy, F.H., Jr. Clinical toxicology. In, *Casarett and Doull's Toxicology: The Basic Science of Poisons,* 3rd ed. (Klaassen, C.D., Amdur, M.O., and Doull, J., eds.) Macmillan Publishing Co., New York, **1986,** pp. 879–901.

Vale, J.A. Position statement: gastric lavage. American Academy of Clinical Toxicology; European Association of Poison Centres and Clinical Toxicologists. *J. Toxicol. Clin. Toxicol.,* **1997,** *35*:711–719.

Winchester, J.F. Active methods for detoxification: oral sorbents, forced diuresis, hemoperfusion, and hemodialysis. In, *Clinical Management of Poisoning and Drug Overdose.* (Haddad, L.M., and Winchester, J.F., eds.) W.B. Saunders Co., Philadelphia, **1983,** pp. 154–169.

GENE THERAPY

Christopher S. Rogers, Bruce A. Sullenger, and
Alfred L. George, Jr.

Advances in molecular and cellular biology have described the proteins that mediate many disease processes, while DNA technology provides ready access to the genes that control these events. The size, complexity, and cellular inaccessibility of these proteins make their delivery or modification by conventional pharmacological means impossible. Conceptually, gene therapy can overcome these barriers by the selective introduction of recombinant DNA into tissues so that the biologically active proteins can be synthesized within the cells whose function is to be altered. As such, delivery of recombinant DNA has become a central issue in all gene therapy strategies. Beyond delivery technologies, there exist many therapeutic paradigms that utilize DNA and other nucleic acids as drugs. Although originally envisioned as a treatment for inherited disorders, gene therapy has found applications in acquired illnesses such as cancer and infectious diseases. This chapter provides an introduction to the therapeutic issues and current strategies being explored to apply gene therapy to this wide range of diseases.

The modern era of molecular medicine has been highlighted by revolutionary accomplishments in genetics, genomics, and human molecular biology. There is extraordinary optimism that medicine will soon benefit from the development of new therapeutic technologies to directly target human genes, referred to as *gene therapy*. Growth of this discipline, which has emerged in the past decade, is evidenced by the exponential expansion of the medical and scientific literature devoted to this topic. There are five new biomedical journals that focus exclusively on the subject of gene therapy or nucleic acid drug development, and there are countless books and monographs on the subject. More than 300 clinical trials involving gene transfer in patients have been approved (Rosenberg *et al.*, 2000), and the first nucleic acid drug, an antisense oligonucleotide (*fomivirsen*), has been approved by the United States Food and Drug Administration (FDA).

Despite the tremendous advances over the past decade, gene therapy remains largely investigational. Many substantial obstacles still must be overcome in developing safe and effective nucleic acid delivery strategies that will promote long-lasting, tissue-specific expression of genetic material. This chapter divides the subject of gene therapy into three general themes: technologies for gene delivery, therapeutic paradigms, and disease targets.

GENE TRANSFER TECHNOLOGIES

The ideal DNA delivery system would be one that could accommodate a broad size range of inserted DNA, could be produced easily in a concentrated form, and could be targeted to specific types of cells. Furthermore, such a system would provide long-term gene expression and would be nontoxic and nonimmunogenic. Such a DNA delivery system does not yet exist, and none of the available technologies for *in vivo* gene transfer is without significant limitations. A variety of viral and nonviral technologies are in development for use in human gene therapy. Table 5–1 compares the general features, advantages, and disadvantages of the more commonly employed gene transfer methodologies.

Obstacles to Gene Therapy

The therapeutic applications of gene transfer technology increase with each discovery of a new cellular process. At present, the ability to develop clinically efficacious therapies from scientifically sound principles is limited by several problems that, to some extent, plague all gene therapy strategies. For the foreseeable future, gene therapy is

Table 5–1
Comparison of Gene-Transfer Vectors

VECTOR	CAPACITY (KILOBASES)	HOST RANGE	PERSISTENCE OF EXPRESSION	MAIN ADVANTAGES	MAIN DISADVANTAGES
Retroviruses	<8	Dividing cells only	Stable	Stable expression, low immunogenicity	Use limited to dividing cells, low transfection efficiency, safety concerns over random integration
Adenovirus	<7.5	Most cells	Transient	Wide cell range, infects nondividing cells, high titer production, high transfection efficiency	Transient expression, host immune response
Adeno-associated virus	<5.2	Most cells	Stable	Wide cell range, nonpathogenic and nonimmunogenic, stable expression	Limited carrying capacity, inefficient production
Lentivirus	<8	Dividing, and some nondividing cells	Stable	Stable expression, infects nondividing cells	Safety concerns over HIV-derived vectors, difficult production
Herpes simplex virus	20–30	Many nondividing cells especially neurons		Large carrying capacity	Cytotoxicity, promoter inactivation
Liposomes	>10	Most cells	Transient	Nonpathogenic, inexpensive, simple production, safe	Low efficiency, transient expression
DNA conjugates	>10	Most cells	Transient	Nonpathogenic, inexpensive, simple production, safe	Low efficiency, transient expression

limited to somatic cells (non–germ-line cells). How these cells in a given tissue are targeted by the DNA delivery method has been an area of intense interest. Once the gene has been successfully transferred, the duration of transgene expression becomes important. Finally, the DNA vector itself must be analyzed for its potential to cause unwanted side effects (Jolly, 1994).

DNA Delivery and Pharmacokinetics.   The delivery of exogenous DNA, and its subsequent processing by target cells, require the introduction of new pharmacokinetic paradigms beyond those that describe the conventional medicines in use today (*see* Chapter 1). With *in vivo* gene transfer, one must account for the fate of the DNA vector itself (volume of distribution, rate of clearance into tissues, *etc.*), as well as for the consequences of altered gene expression and protein function. A multicompartmental model to describe these events in a quantitative fashion has been developed (Ledley and Ledley, 1994). Several processes that must be considered include: (1) the distribution of the DNA vector following *in vivo* administration; (2) the fraction of vector taken up by the target cell population; (3) the trafficking of the genetic material within cellular organelles; (4) the rate of degradation of the DNA; (5) the level of mRNA produced; (6) the stability of the mRNA produced; (7) the amount and stability of the protein produced; and (8) the compartmentalization of the transcribed protein within the cell, or its secretory fate. It is conceivable, although yet to be realized, that each of these events may be incorporated into the design of the gene transfer system in a rational way so as to tailor the gene transfer to the specific requirements of the disease being treated.

Duration of Expression of Transferred Gene.   The length of time over which the transferred gene will function is of tremendous importance. In the treatment of inherited diseases, it is desirable to have stable gene expression over many years. In contrast, in the treatment of malignancy, long-term production of a therapeutic protein may be unnecessary and could have deleterious consequences.

Vectors that integrate the transferred DNA into the chromosomes of the recipient cell have the greatest potential for long-term expression. Retroviral vectors and adeno-associated viral vectors have integrating functions. The persistence of the transgene DNA in the genome of the recipient cell does not, however, guarantee long-term gene expression in that cell. The production of the intended mRNA and protein may decline because of inactivation of the transgene promoter even though the DNA persists (Bestor, 2000). In some circumstances, loss of transgene expression may occur because of loss of the transduced cell by host immune processes (*see* Jolly, 1994).

Adverse Consequences of Heterologous Gene Expression. Along with factors that limit gene transfer and expression, there are potential adverse consequences that may arise as a result of successful gene transfer. As with any new drug, it will be impossible to predict these events in advance of more clinical experience. Nonetheless, some specific events can be anticipated independent of the transgene employed. Because, in most circumstances, gene transfer will result in the synthesis of a new protein, the possibility of an immune response must be considered. A severe immune response could inactivate a secreted product (as is seen in hemophilia patients receiving factor VIII replacement therapy) or lead to an "autoimmune" response to transduced tissues. In some circumstances, the DNA vector itself may be immunogenic, as has been demonstrated for adenovirus vectors. An immune response to the vector may limit the duration of its effectiveness or preclude its readministration.

Pathological events may arise from viral vector replication. Significant efforts have been directed toward the design of viral vectors that are unable to replicate (replication-incompetent) in the target cell. This has been achieved by the deletion of specific genes from the viral genome that are necessary for viral replication (*see* Figure 5–1). In order to produce the virus, it must then be grown *in vitro* in a cell specifically designed to provide those functions removed from the virus. By these means, replication-incompetent retroviruses, adenoviruses, adeno-associated viruses, and herpes viruses have been produced. This approach does not completely eliminate replicative potential in all circumstances. The virus may overcome the deletion of replication machinery by the use of unidentified host-cell factors or, theoretically, by recombination in the patient with wild-type viruses. Fortunately, these latter events have not been reported so far.

Ethical and Regulatory Issues. Substantial attention has been directed toward ethical matters associated with gene therapy (Juengst and Walters, 1999). The major issues include concerns regarding the balance of risks and benefits to subjects enrolled in experimental gene transfer research, the selection and protection of research subjects, and the ethics of human germ-line gene transfer. As discussed below, assurance of patient safety has become a central issue in the regulatory process governing gene therapy research. Gene transfer into the human germ line, although potentially feasible, carries great moral implications. The potential to alter the genetic constitution of future generations raises enormous public concern that eugenic practices could evolve by which society selects against individuals with specific genotypes. Concern also has been raised that gene transfer techniques would be used for "frivolous" purposes, such as cosmetic alterations or other enhancements that are unrelated to disease treatment. Continued public debate as well as discussions among scientists and ethicists are critical to the success and widespread acceptance of gene therapy as a standard treatment option.

Arising from public and governmental concern for the safety and ethical implications of gene therapy, strict regulatory processes have evolved (Wivel and Anderson, 1999). In the early 1980s, federal oversight in the United States for gene therapy experimentation in human beings became the responsibility of the National Institutes of Health (NIH) Recombinant DNA Advisory Committee (RAC). The RAC reviews clinical trials involving human gene transfer and provides an important public forum for discussing the scientific and ethical aspects of gene therapy. As with other investigational therapies, clinical gene therapy trials must be reviewed and approved by the FDA prior to commencing. At the local level, gene therapy research involving human beings must be approved by two separate committees in existence at medical centers and other research institutions, the Institutional Review Board (IRB) and the Institutional Biosafety Committee (IBC). The IRB is charged with protecting human subjects from unnecessary risks associated with investigational treatments, while the IBC oversees adherence to the *NIH Guidelines for Research Involving Recombinant DNA Molecules*. These review and oversight mechanisms ensure that the scientific community adheres to stringent safeguards to protect the safety of human subjects participating in gene therapy trials, and they provide reassurance to the public that such experimentation meets strict ethical and professional standards.

Viral Vectors

The natural life cycle of mammalian viruses has made them a logical starting point for the design of therapeutic

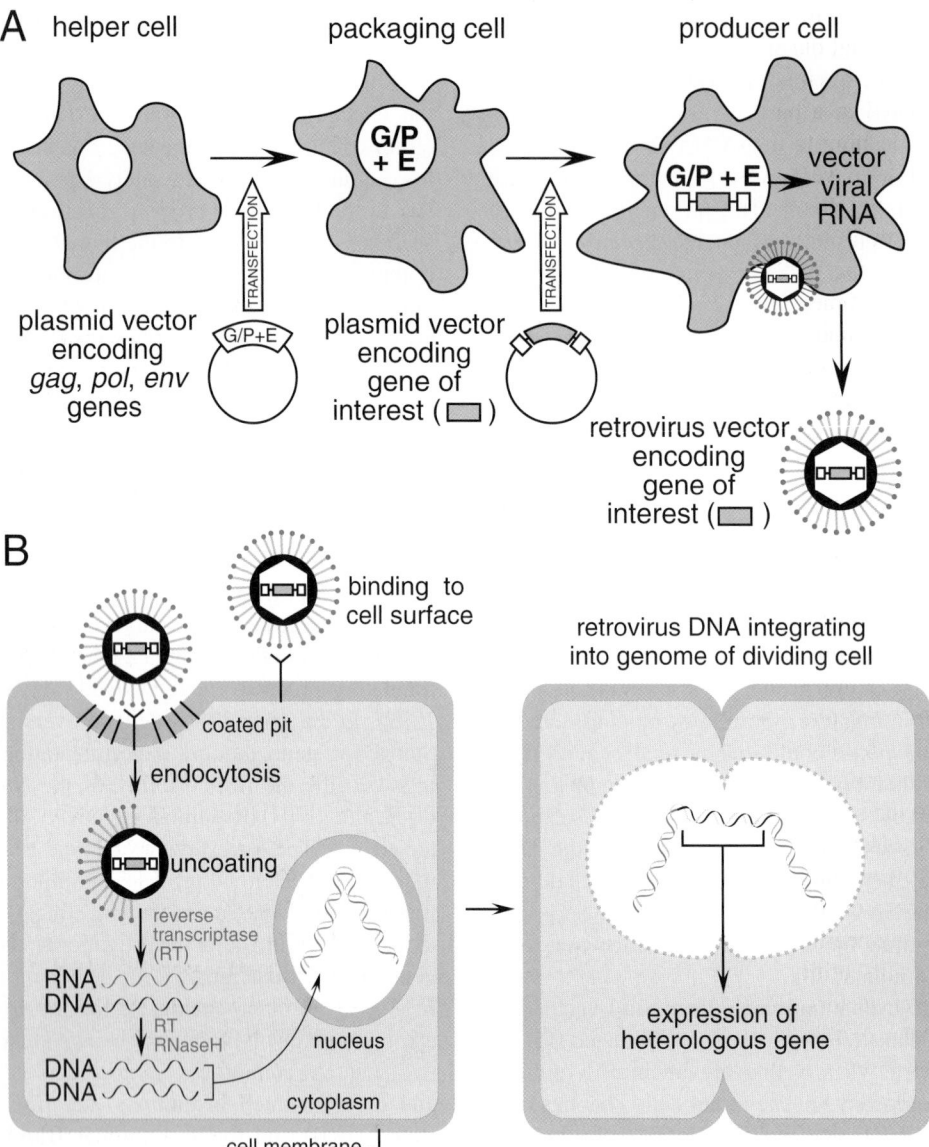

Figure 5–1. Retrovirus-mediated gene transfer.

A. *Overall strategy of retroviral production.* Replication-incompetent retrovirus vectors are produced from a helper cell that is engineered to provide viral functions (DNA) that have been removed from the virus. The *gag* (G), *pol* (P), and *env* (E) DNA sequences are cloned into bacterial plasmids which are then transfected into the helper cell to produce the packaging cell. Packaging cells are able to produce the gag, pol, and envelope proteins required for retroviral replication. A plasmid containing recombinant proviral DNA, but lacking *gag, pol,* and *env* genes, is transfected into the packaging cell line to create the producer cell, which contains all of the molecular machinery necessary to reproduce the recombinant retrovirus that is secreted into the tissue culture medium. Only the recombinant proviral sequence is packaged into the retrovirus. Because the recombinant retrovirus does not contain the *gag, pol,* and *env* genes, cells that this replication-incompetent recombinant retrovirus infects cannot produce additional virions.

B. *Gene expression in target cell following retrovirus-mediated RNA delivery* (*see* retrovirus life-cycle section for a complete explanation).

gene-transfer vehicles. Viruses transfer and express ex-
ogenous genetic material during infection of host cells. In
the simplest analysis, a virus consists of a nucleic acid
genome encapsulated in a particle that can be taken up
by the target cell, leading to the expression of virally encoded genes. For viral vectors to be useful, several viral functions must be altered. In most applications, the
virus is rendered replication-incompetent to prevent uncontrolled spread of the transgene and must have some
element of its own genome removed to allow for insertion
of the transgene. Beyond this, additional modifications
are dependent on the specific virus. Viral vectors have
been used extensively in preclinical research and are the
basis for the majority of gene therapy clinical trials now
under way.

Several important aspects of the viral life cycle and
other biological features must be considered before selecting a vector for a specific application (Robbins and
Ghivizzani, 1998). A critical determinant of the success
of viral-based gene transfer is the ability of the virus to
infect target cells (tropism) and to express a heterologous
gene. Tropism is determined in part by the expression of
specific cell-surface receptors on the host cell that provide
attachment for the infecting virus and facilitate its uptake.
Expression of a heterologous gene requires entry of the
viral genome into the host cell nucleus followed by proper
transcription and translation of its sequences. Several additional factors govern whether expression in the infected
cell will be transient or long lasting. Finally, several aspects of genetic engineering and production of the viral
vector impinge on its utility as a gene transfer vehicle.
The principal viral vectors employed in current clinical
gene transfer trials, or that appear promising for future
trials, are derived from retroviruses, adenovirus, adeno-
associated virus, herpes simplex virus, and lentiviruses.
The following sections describe the basic biological features of each viral vector relevant to their use in gene therapy applications. Specific uses of individual vectors are
described in more detail in later sections of this chapter.

Retroviruses.   Retroviruses are small RNA viruses that
can infect and replicate exclusively within dividing cells
and are capable of integrating their genome into the host
cell DNA. Therefore, retroviral vectors offer the potential for long-term expression in a limited range of target cell types. Most retroviral vectors have been derived
from the Moloney murine leukemia virus (MMLV) and
have been engineered to avoid expression of native viral
genes, thereby preventing host immune responses against
infected cells. Because of their requirement for cell division, retroviral vectors have been mostly used for *ex vivo*

gene transfer (*see* below) or for the investigational treatment of cancer.

Life Cycle.   Retroviruses are composed of an RNA genome that
is packaged in an envelope derived from host cell membrane
along with viral proteins. Three viral genes (*gag, pol, env*) are
required for replication and packaging. For a retrovirus to effect
gene expression, it must first reverse transcribe its positive-
strand RNA genome into double-stranded DNA, which is then
integrated into the host cell DNA. This process is mediated
by the reverse transcriptase and integrase proteins contained
in the retrovirus particle. Breakdown of the host cell nuclear
envelope during mitosis is necessary for entry of the virus into
the nucleus. The integrated provirus is able to use host cell
machinery to carry out transcription of viral mRNAs and their
subsequent processing and translation into viral proteins. The
virus completes its life cycle by synthesizing new positive-strand
RNA genomes from the integrated provirus. An encapsidation
signal (*psi*) within the RNA mediates the organization of the
viral genomic RNA and proteins into particles that bud from
the cell surface.

Vector Design and Production.   Retroviral vectors are constructed from the proviral form of the virus. The *gag, pol,* and
env genes are removed to make room for the gene(s) of therapeutic interest and to eliminate the replicative functions of the
virus (*see* Figure 5–1 for a strategic overview). Up to 8 kb of
heterologous DNA can be incorporated into the retroviral vector. Because all virally encoded mRNAs are eliminated from the
recombinant retrovirus, no viral proteins are produced by retroviral vectors. This removes any potential viral-encoded antigens
that might lead to an immune response to the transduced cells.
Along with the gene of therapeutic interest, sequences containing promoter and enhancer functions also may be included with
the transgene to facilitate its efficient expression and, in some
circumstances, to provide for tissue-specific expression *in vivo*.
Alternatively, the native promoter and enhancer functions contained in the long terminal repeat (LTR) of the virus may be
used for this purpose.

After deletion of the genes encoding viral structural proteins and proteins that mediate viral replication, these viruses
can be produced only in specially engineered viral packaging
cell lines that are capable of providing these proteins (*see* Figure
5–1). The packaging cell line is optimally constructed by stably
inserting the deleted viral genes (*gag, pol,* and *env*) into the cell
in such a manner that these genes will reside on different chromosomes within the packaging cell. This strategy decreases the
likelihood of a recombination event occurring that produces an
intact viral genome that could be packaged into a replication-
competent virus. The packaging cell line is used to construct
a retroviral producer cell line that will generate replication-
incompetent retrovirus containing the gene(s) of interest. This
is done by introducing the recombinant proviral DNA into the
packaging cell line. The recombinant proviral DNA is in the
form of plasmid DNA containing the LTR sequences flanking
a small portion of the *gag* gene that contains the encapsidation
sequence and the genes of interest; this is transfected into the
packaging cell line using standard techniques for DNA transfer.
Several versions of this basic design have been employed to
decrease the likelihood of recombinant events that could lead
to the production of replication-competent virus (Jolly, 1994).

Host Cell Range.   The ability of the virus to infect a specific cell type is determined to a large extent by interactions between the viral envelope protein (encoded by *env*) and a corresponding cell-surface receptor. The MMLV envelope is ecotropic, which means that infection is restricted to the cells of a particular species, in this case mouse. An envelope affording a broader infection range is available by using the *env* gene from the 4070A strain of murine leukemia virus. This envelope gene has amphotropic specificity and can promote the infection of human, murine, and other mammalian cells. Modifications of the envelope protein can be achieved through a phenomenon known as pseudotyping, whereby the retrovirus incorporates alternative envelope proteins during viral packaging. For example, the glycoprotein (dubbed G protein, but not to be confused with G proteins involved in signal transduction; *see* Chapter 2) of vesicular stomatitis virus (VSV-G) has been shown to incorporate efficiently into MMLV retrovirus particles (Chen *et al.,* 1996). Incorporation of VSV-G expands the host range of the vector and improves the efficiency of infection. In addition, pseudotyping with VSV-G improves retroviral vector stability, which allows the pseudotyped virus to be concentrated by ultracentrifugation to higher titers. One drawback of using VSV-G is its toxicity to the mammalian cells that are used for viral packaging. To some extent, this toxicity can be avoided by using packaging cell lines that have inducible VSV-G expression (Iida *et al.,* 1996). Retrovirus vectors pseudotyped with other envelope proteins, such as those derived from the Gibbon ape leukemia virus (Gallardo *et al.,* 1997) and the lymphocytic choriomeningitis virus (Miletic *et al.,* 1999), may be less toxic to mammalian host cells with preservation of the advantages of VSV-G pseudotyping.

General Clinical Applications.   The clinical administration of retroviruses has been accomplished most frequently by the *ex vivo* transduction of patients' cells, and by the direct injection of virus into tissue. The *ex vivo* approach requires the isolation and maintenance in tissue culture of the cells, infection with the viral vector, and subsequent reimplantation into the patient. This approach was used to modify lymphocytes and hematopoietic cells in the treatment of adenosine deaminase deficiency (Parkman *et al.,* 2000) and hyperlipidemia (Grossman *et al.,* 1994); the same strategy also was used to express immune modulatory agents in tumor cells (Lode and Reisfeld, 2000). Direct *in vivo* delivery of retroviral vectors has been utilized largely in the treatment of solid tumors (Gomez-Navarro *et al.,* 1999).

Safety.   The use of retroviral vectors has raised several important safety issues. One concern is that because the virus integrates into the target cell DNA (an attractive feature for long-term expression) and because integration occurs in a nearly random fashion, integration could be mutagenic (insertional mutagenesis). For example, undesired mutations might occur if insertion of the retroviral DNA altered the function of a gene that regulates cell growth. Although replication-competent retroviruses have tumorigenic potential, this has not been observed with the replication-incompetent vectors that are in use as gene transfer agents.

Lentiviruses.   The lentiviruses are a subset of retroviruses that can infect dividing and nondividing cells (Buchschacher, Jr. and Wong-Staal, 2000). The best-studied lentivirus is the human immunodeficiency virus (HIV)-1, and gene transfer vectors derived from this viral genome have

potential advantages over previous retroviral vectors. In particular, they show promise in their ability to efficiently transduce hematopoietic stem cells (Miyoshi *et al.,* 1999). These vectors also are capable of establishing long-term expression. However, because of their lineage, substantial biosafety concerns need to be addressed before lentiviral vectors advance toward use in clinical trials (Amado and Chen, 1999).

Life Cycle.   The biology of lentiviruses is similar to that of retroviruses (Tang *et al.,* 1999). The major difference enabling lentiviruses to infect nondividing cells is the ability of its viral preintegration complex to interact with and be transported by the nuclear membrane. This preintegration complex consists of transcribed viral DNA, integrase, and the matrix protein encoded by the *gag* gene. The matrix protein contains a localization sequence that enables the complex to dock with a nucleopore. Transport into the nucleus of a nondividing cell then provides the viral genome the opportunity to integrate into the host cell DNA.

Vector Design and Production.   Lentiviral vectors derived from HIV-1 are rendered replication-incompetent by deletion of various accessory genes and by the use of packaging cell lines in which components necessary for assembling virus particles are provided by separate genetic elements (Srinivasakumar and Schuening, 1999). This greatly minimizes the possibility of recombination events occurring during vector production that, theoretically, could generate a self-replicating virus. In addition, deletion of the *tat* gene and deletions in the viral LTR region also reduce the likelihood that a replication-competent lentivirus will emerge during production or *in vivo.*

Host Cell Range.   Both actively dividing and nondividing cells can be infected by lentiviral vectors. This includes hematopoietic stem cells and terminally differentiated cells such as muscle, neurons, hepatocytes, and retinal photoreceptors. However, cells may need to be stimulated to enter the G1 phase of the cell cycle before they can be transduced with lentivirus (Park *et al.,* 2000). The lentivirus *env* gene can be replaced by pseudotyping with VSV-G or another appropriate viral envelope protein to facilitate a broader host range (Li *et al.,* 1998). Long-term expression of lentiviral-encoded transgenes has been demonstrated within the central nervous systems of experimental animals. Stable and efficient gene delivery also has been demonstrated in the retina. Expression of lentivirus-encoded transgenes is associated with little or no inflammation or signs of tissue pathology.

Safety.   Given the lineage of lentiviral vectors derived from HIV-1, there has been appropriate concern about the possibility of recombination events leading to the development of a replication-competent virus (Amado and Chen, 1999). Conceivably, a self-replicating lentiviral vector could be harmful by undergoing insertional mutagenesis or by acquiring characteristics of the parent HIV-1. Concerns also have been raised regarding the consequences of HIV infection of an individual treated previously with a lentiviral vector. Theoretically, the wild-type HIV virus could enable mobilization of the gene-transfer vector by acting as a helper virus. This theoretical phenomenon in fact could be an advantage for using lentiviral vectors to treat HIV infection with antiHIV gene therapy. Through improved vector design and production, these and other concerns can be addressed.

Adenoviruses. Adenoviruses are double-stranded, linear DNA viruses that replicate independently of host cell division. Adenoviral vectors possess several attractive features that have encouraged their development for clinical use. They are capable of transducing a broad spectrum of human tissues, including respiratory epithelium, vascular endothelium, cardiac and skeletal muscle, peripheral and central nervous tissue, hepatocytes, the exocrine pancreas, and many tumor types. Over 40 serotypes of human adenoviruses are known, and the clinical spectrum of human adenoviral infections is well described (Horwitz, 1990). Most if not all adults have had prior exposure to adenovirus and are seropositive for antiadenovirus antibodies when tested by sensitive methods.

Efficient gene transfer and transgene expression can be obtained in dividing and nondividing cells. Several routes of administration can be used, including intravenous, intrabiliary, intraperitoneal, intravesicular, intracranial, and intrathecal injection, and direct injection into the target organ parenchyma. The multiple routes of administration provide flexibility in targeting based on anatomical boundaries. There are two significant disadvantages to adenovirus-based vectors. First, because the virus remains episomal after host cell infection, long-term expression generally does not occur. Second, adenoviral infection induces both cellular and humoral immune responses that eliminate virally transduced cells and reduce the efficacy of repeat administration. This immune response also may account for adverse effects of adenoviral gene transfer.

Life Cycle. Infection by adenovirus begins with binding of the fiber protein, which extends from the icosahedral capsid, to the coxsackievirus and adenovirus receptor (CAR) on the host cell surface (Figure 5–2). Following attachment, an interaction between a tripeptide motif (Arg-Gly-Asp) in the penton base occurs with cell-surface integrins ($\alpha v \beta 3$ or $\alpha v \beta 5$), which then leads to receptor-mediated endocytosis and internalization. The virus escapes the endosome prior to its fusion with lysosomal compartments and thus avoids digestion. The viral DNA is able to enter the target cell nucleus and begin transcription of viral mRNA without concomitant cell division. Although integration of viral DNA into the host cell genomic DNA can occur at high levels of infection in dividing cells, this is a relatively infrequent event and does not contribute significantly to the utility of these viruses as gene transfer vectors. Viral gene expression and replication occur in an ordered fashion and are driven in large measure by the *E1A* and *E1B* genes in the 5′ portion of the adenoviral genome. The *E1A* and *E1B* genes provide transactivation functions for transcription of several of the downstream viral genes (*see* Horwitz, 1990).

Since the *E1* genes are involved intimately in adenovirus replication, their removal renders the virus replication-incompetent or, at the very least, severely crippled with respect to replication. Due to the complexity of the virus, it has been more difficult to remove all adenoviral genes, as is done with retroviral vectors. The expression of adenoviral proteins with the currently employed adenoviral vectors leads to both a cellular and a humoral immune response to recombinant adenoviral vectors. In some instances, this may limit the utility of this vector both in terms of host immune response to adenovirally transduced cells and with respect to readministration of the vector.

Vector Design and Production. Although several adenoviral serotypes are known, serotypes 2 and 5 have been used most extensively for vector construction. First-generation adenoviral vectors were engineered by deletion of the E1 and E3 regions in the viral genome. These deletions render the virus replication-incompetent and allow the insertion of foreign DNA of up to 7.5 kb in length. Second-generation adenoviral vectors feature additional deletions of the E2 and E4 regions, modifications that help reduce antigenicity but limit viral gene expression in infected cells. More extensive removal of viral genes results in helper-dependent adenoviral vectors that should be much less likely to induce an immune response and have greatly increased carrying capacity (Kochanek, 1999). However, helper-dependent adenoviral vector systems appear to be less stable *in vivo,* and there are limitations for producing high-titer virus.

Large amounts of adenoviral vector can be produced by growing the recombinant virus in a packaging cell line (typically,

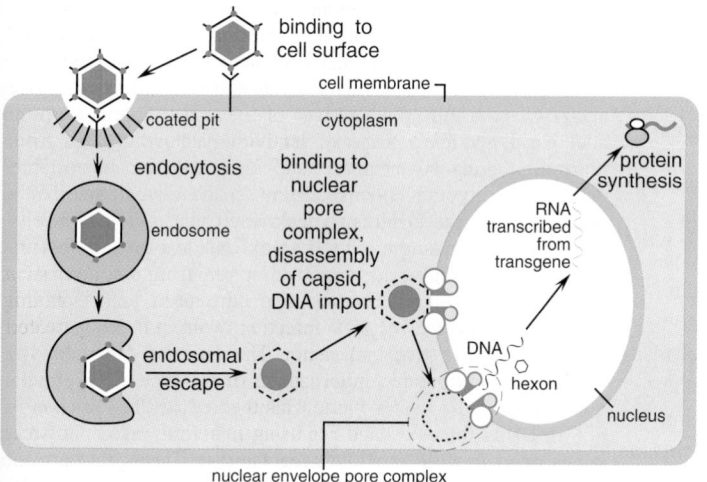

Figure 5–2. Adenovirus-mediated infection of target cells.

Expression of gene of interest in target cell following adenovirus-mediated DNA delivery. A recombinant adenovirus binds to specific receptors on the surface of a target cell and enters the cell by endocytosis. Viral proteins promote the escape of the adenovirus from the endosome prior to its fusion with and destruction by lysosomes. The adenovirus DNA becomes unpackaged and travels to the nucleus where it begins to synthesize new mRNA. The adenovirus-encoded DNA, including the transgene, is not integrated into the genome of the host cell.

human embryonic kidney 293 cells) engineered to express E1 proteins that complement the E1-deficient viral genome. The virus is isolated by lysing the infected packaging cells and purifying the crude lysate by cesium chloride density-gradient centrifugation, a procedure that not only separates the virus from other tissue culture–derived substances but also concentrates the virus to very high titers (over 10^{13} particles per ml). The purified virus is remarkably stable in a variety of aqueous buffers and can be frozen for a prolonged period of time without loss of activity.

Host Cell Range.   Adenoviruses can infect a broad range of dividing and nondividing cells. Their broad host range can be attributed to the near ubiquitous expression of cell-surface receptors that can mediate adenovirus recognition and uptake. However, some cells express low levels of the CAR or present the receptor at an inaccessible cellular location. Modifying the tropism of adenoviral vectors also is feasible (Wickham, 2000). Immunological strategies have been used in which a dual-specific antibody directed at both the viral fiber and a target cell surface protein simultaneously neutralizes the intrinsic targeting of the virus and redirects its attachment to a specific cell type. The fiber protein and its terminal knob domain also can be genetically engineered to redirect or enhance attachment of the virus (Douglas *et al.,* 1999). Finally, an adapter protein strategy can be used in which recombinant CAR is fused to a ligand such as epidermal growth factor (EGF), and the fusion protein facilitates specific attachment of the virus to cells expressing the EGF receptor (Dmitriev *et al.,* 2000).

General Clinical Applications.   There are numerous clinical trials in progress utilizing adenoviral vectors for gene transfer in both inherited and acquired conditions. The lack of long-term expression and resulting immune reaction to infected cells pose substantial obstacles to the treatment of lifelong inherited conditions. The episomal nature of the adenovirus genome ultimately limits the duration of gene expression in tissues with active cell division, such as bone marrow and epithelia, because each round of target cell division after gene transfer is not accompanied by replication of the transgene. The use of replication-incompetent and replication-competent adenoviral vectors also may have utility in the treatment of cancer (*see* below).

Safety.   The main adverse effects of adenoviral vectors relate to the immune reaction elicited by infected cells. Safety concerns over use of adenoviral vectors were heightened following a highly publicized death that occurred during a clinical trial (Marshall, 1999). There also are concerns about the emergence of replication-competent recombinant virus occurring during vector production. There is a need for highly stringent analyses and characterization of recombinant adenoviral vectors intended for clinical use.

Adeno-Associated Viruses.   Adeno-associated viruses (AAV) are small, nonenveloped, single-stranded DNA viruses that have many attributes desirable in a gene-transfer vector. They are nonpathogenic, can stably transduce nondividing cells with high efficiency, and can be engineered to carry heterologous genes without requiring the potential immunogenic expression of viral proteins. The major limitations of AAV as a gene delivery vector are its limited DNA-carrying capacity and shortcomings in producing high-titer virus. Clinical investigations using AAV

vectors are commencing, and there are indications that this gene-transfer vehicle may be well suited to a variety of gene therapy applications (Monahan and Samulski, 2000).

Life Cycle.   Adeno-associated virus has a helper-dependent life cycle, meaning that viral replication requires genetic elements from another viral genome. The virus has two distinct phases to its life cycle. In the absence of helper virus (adenovirus), the wild-type virus will infect a host cell, integrate into the host cell genome, and remain latent for an extended period of time. In the presence of adenovirus, the lytic phase of the virus is induced and leads to active virus replication. Structurally, the AAV genome is composed of two open reading frames (called *rep* and *cap*) flanked by inverted terminal repeat (ITR) sequences. The *rep* region encodes four proteins that mediate AAV replication, viral DNA transcription, and endonuclease functions used in host genome integration. The *rep* genes are the only AAV sequences required for viral replication. The *cap* sequence encodes structural proteins that form the viral capsid. The ITRs contain the viral origins of replication, provide encapsidation signals, and participate in viral DNA integration. The function of many of these proteins and the overall biology of the virus have been studied largely in wild-type viruses (Kotin, 1994).

Infection begins by attachment of the virus to its principal cell-surface receptor, heparan sulfate proteoglycan (Summerford and Samulski, 1998). Additional cofactors, fibroblast growth factor receptor type 1, and $\alpha v \beta 5$ integrin contribute to cellular uptake (Summerford *et al.,* 1999). Internalization of the virus occurs by receptor-mediated endocytosis through clathrin-coated pits (Bartlett *et al.,* 2000a). During the transduction of host cells, the AAV viral genome undergoes circularization and formation of circular concatamers that reside episomally in the host cell (Yang *et al.,* 1999). Generation of these episomal circularized forms of the AAV genome correlate well with long-term transgene expression (Duan *et al.,* 1998). Wild-type AAV can stably integrate into human DNA at a specific location on chromosome 19 (19q13.3-qter); however, recombinant AAV may lose its site-specific integration ability (Rivadeneira *et al.,* 1998).

Vector Design and Production.   Current AAV vectors can be produced using a system of three recombinant plasmids (Xiao *et al.,* 1998). The main vector plasmid contains a transgene located between the two ITRs. A second plasmid provides *rep* and *cap,* and a third plasmid carries essential elements from the adenoviral genome necessary for viral packaging. This triple plasmid strategy obviates the need for coinfection of producer cells by wild-type adenovirus. Because of the small size of the AAV genome, the DNA-carrying capacity is limited to 5.2 kb. This clearly limits the size of the DNA cargo and restricts the capacity of the vector to carry important promoter/enhancer elements to direct gene expression in the target cell. Doubling the vector capacity may be feasible by use of a dual-vector system, in which two halves of a transgene are assembled *in vivo* from two separate AAV vectors that combine into a circular concatamer during transduction (Sun *et al.,* 2000; Yan *et al.,* 2000). Using this approach, it is conceivable to assemble larger genes or to include important regulatory elements that are too large to fit within a single vector molecule (Duan *et al.,* 2000). Currently, the major limitations for production of recombinant

AAV relate to difficulties in obtaining high-titer virus and in quantifying the viral titer.

Host Cell Range.   Recombinant AAV can infect a wide range of host cells. Preclinical studies have demonstrated efficient gene transfer into skeletal muscle, the central nervous system, lung, liver, gastrointestinal tract, and eye.

General Clinical Applications.   The clinical experience with AAV-based gene delivery is growing, and clinical trials exploiting delivery to lung and muscle are in progress. This vector appears to be well suited for establishing long-term expression in muscle, heart, the central nervous system, and other tissues. Early results from clinical trials using AAV vectors to express factor IX ectopically in skeletal muscle for the treatment of hemophilia appear to be successful (*see* below). The ability of this vector system to achieve long-term gene expression without concomitant host immune reactions or cytotoxicity suggests that it may be an appropriate delivery vehicle for the treatment of certain inherited conditions.

Safety.   AAV is a nonpathogenic virus, and early experiences with this viral vector have demonstrated the absence of significant host immune responses. Formerly, there was concern about contamination of AAV vector by the helper adenovirus, but this has been alleviated by newer production schemes (Xiao *et al.,* 1998). Finally, recombinant AAV vectors may integrate randomly into the genome, and there is concern regarding the possibility of insertional mutagenesis. The site-specific integration of wild-type AAV on chromosome 19 may require that specific viral sequences be retained in the vector (Rivadeneira *et al.,* 1998).

Herpes Simplex Virus-1.   The herpes simplex virus (HSV) is a large (152-kb), double-stranded DNA virus that replicates in the nucleus of infected cells and exhibits a broad host cell range. The virus can infect dividing and nondividing cells and persist in a nonintegrated state. Large (20- to 30-kb) sequences of foreign DNA can be inserted into the viral genome by homologous recombination, or through insertion/deletion mutagenesis. Herpes simplex virus-1 has a natural tropism for neuronal tissues, and its potential utility as a gene transfer vehicle for treating neurological conditions including Parkinson's disease and brain cancer has been recognized (Fink and Glorioso, 1997; Simonato *et al.,* 2000). The major drawbacks of using HSV-1 are its cytotoxicity and the occurrence of transgene silencing.

Life Cycle.   The natural biology of HSV-1 infection involves both lytic and latent phases. During primary infection, virus attaches to and penetrates epithelial cells (skin or mucosa) and replicates. Assembled viral capsids exit the infected cell and simultaneously acquire an envelope by budding through the plasma membrane. Virus particles then fuse with peripheral sensory nerves in the vicinity of the primary infection and are transported retrograde in the nerve axon to its cell body. Virus attachment is mediated through heparan sulfate moieties on the target cell surface (Laquerre *et al.,* 1998). Once in the neuronal cell body, the virus can continue in the lytic phase or enter a latent phase. The latent phase is characterized by silencing of lytic genes and expression of a discrete set of latency-associated transcripts (LATs) driven by two latency-associated promoters (LAP1, LAP2). Wild-type virus can reenter the lytic phase and spread viral progeny to the original site of primary infection or into the central nervous system.

Vector Design and Production.   Replication-incompetent HSV-1 has been engineered by deleting several genes essential for the lytic phase, in particular, the immediate-early genes *ICP4, ICP22,* and *ICP27* (Krisky *et al.,* 1998). Deletion of these genes also produces vector that exhibits less cytotoxicity and more prolonged transgene expression in cultured cells. Helper virus-free packaging systems have been developed that permit production of vector capable of transducing neuronal cells *in vivo* without cytopathic effects (Fraefel *et al.,* 1996), although viral titer may be somewhat limited. There are also descriptions of more efficient approaches for engineering recombinant HSV-1 vector that enable insertion of two independent transgene expression cassettes into a single virus (Krisky *et al.,* 1997).

A significant problem with HSV-1 vectors is the difficulty in achieving long-term expression due to transgene silencing. Use of the latency-active promoters to drive gene expression, or linking transgenes to an internal ribosome entry site (IRES) inserted downstream of the latency-associated transcript regulatory sequences, appears to have good prospects for improving the longevity of HSV-1–mediated expression (Goins *et al.,* 1999; Lachmann and Efstathiou, 1997; Marshall *et al.,* 2000).

Host Cell Range.   HSV-1 is capable of infecting a broad range of human cells, but its predilection for neurons is most notable. Modifying the tropism of HSV-1 may permit more specific targeting of the vector. Deletion of viral glycoprotein genes that are responsible for cell attachment produces an entry-incompetent HSV-1, which can be complemented by alternative attachment proteins (Anderson *et al.,* 2000).

General Applications.   Because of their DNA-carrying capacity, HSV-1 vectors may provide a vehicle for delivering particularly large gene cargoes. For example, a complete dystrophin cDNA (14 kb) has been introduced successfully into cultured muscle cells from mice with experimental muscular dystrophy (Akkaraju *et al.,* 1999). Replication-competent HSV-1 vectors are being developed for treatment of brain and other neoplasms (Martuza, 2000).

Safety.   The major safety concern for HSV-1 vectors is their cytotoxicity. Newer production schemes that eliminate helper virus and additional genetic engineering to remove cytopathic genes may reduce this liability.

Nonviral DNA Delivery Strategies

A variety of nonviral approaches to mediate cellular uptake of exogenous DNA have been developed and tested. These include naked plasmid DNA, DNA-liposome complexes, DNA-protein complexes, and DNA-coated gold particles. Production is generally easier and less expensive than with viral vectors. However, in general, low efficiency of transduction and transient expression are substantial limitations to their usefulness in gene therapy. Longer-lasting expression may be possible by engineering the gene of interest with transposons, naturally occurring, mobile genetic elements that can integrate into chromosomal DNA (Yant *et al.,* 2000).

Uncomplexed Plasmid DNA. Surprisingly, purified DNA (or mRNA) can be injected directly into tissues, resulting in transient gene expression. This has been best illustrated in muscle tissue, where direct injection of uncomplexed (naked) DNA is most effective (Wolff *et al.,* 1992). Skin also is capable of expressing plasmid DNA delivered either by direct injection (Hengge *et al.,* 1996) or by other physical methods including ballistic transfection using DNA-coated gold beads (Lin *et al.,* 2000). Expression of an antigenic protein in either skin or muscle using this approach may have utility for immunization (Davis *et al.,* 1995), and clinical trials are addressing the effectiveness and safety of this strategy for vaccination against infectious diseases (Le *et al.,* 2000; Tacket *et al.,* 1999). Plasmid DNA injection of muscle also may prove useful for the ectopic synthesis of therapeutic proteins such as erythropoietin (Tripathy *et al.,* 1996).

DNA-Coated Gold Particles. Plasmid DNA can be affixed to gold particles (approximately 1 micron in diameter) and then "shot" into accessible cells. The DNA is coprecipitated onto the gold particle and then propelled, using an electric spark or pressurized gas as the motive force. This "gene gun" can be used to accelerate the DNA-coated particles into superficial cells of the skin (epidermis) or into skin tumors (melanomas). Gene expression lasts only a few days, which may be more a function of the cells targeted (*e.g.,* skin cells that are sloughed) than the method of delivery. Gene-gun delivery is ideally suited to gene-mediated immunization (Haynes *et al.,* 1996), where only brief expression of antigen is necessary to achieve an immune response.

Liposomes. Liposomes are either unilamellar or multilamellar spheres that are manufactured using a variety of lipids. They are capable of delivering DNA to the interior of cells. The premise is that by surrounding hydrophilic molecules with hydrophobic molecules, agents otherwise impermeable to cell membranes might be escorted into the cell. A diagram illustrating the presumed mechanism for liposome-plasmid transfection is given in Figure 5–3. Proteins and other nonlipid molecules can be incorporated into the lipid membranes. Because the substance to be delivered must be encapsulated within the liposomes, the manufacturing process is complex. Also, most DNA constructs used for gene therapy are large compared to the liposome, so encapsulation efficiency is very low. For convenience, liposomes are classified as either anionic or cationic, based on their net negative or positive charge, respectively.

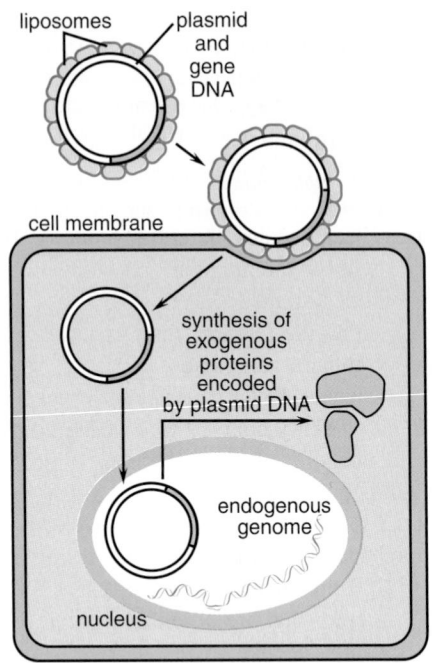

Figure 5–3. Cationic liposome-mediated DNA delivery.

> Liposomes enter cells by fusing with the plasma membrane in a manner that permits their nucleic acid cargo to escape degradation by lysosomes. Plasmid DNA (shown here) must enter the nucleus to be transcribed into mRNA that is then exported to the cytoplasm for translation into protein. Integration of the DNA into the host cell genome is an extremely rare event.

Anionic Liposomes. The first *in vivo* delivery of a gene using liposomes involved transfer of insulin complexed with anionic liposomes into rats (Soriano *et al.,* 1983). The transfected rats had increased circulating levels of insulin and decreased blood glucose concentrations. In spite of this early success, there are significant drawbacks to the use of anionic liposomes for delivering DNA. These structures, when given intravenously, primarily target the reticuloendothelial cells of the liver, making them of little use for other cell targets. Various proteins can be inserted into the external layer of liposomes to alter their *in vivo* behavior, including cell-selective delivery. This approach can enable liposomes given intravenously to evade the reticuloendothelial system. Protein ligands or antibodies to cell surface molecules incorporated into the liposome surface also can target liposomes to specific cell-surface receptors on desired cell populations (Wu and Wu, 1987).

Cationic Liposomes. *In vivo,* cationic liposomes have properties quite different from those of anionic liposomes. Intravenous injection of cationic complexes has been shown to effect transgene expression in most organs if the liposome-DNA complex is injected into the afferent blood supply to the organ. In addition, the liposome-DNA complexes can be administered by intraairway injection or aerosol to target lung epithelium. In experimental animals, neither intravenous injection nor aerosol delivery of cationic liposome-plasmid complexes appears to be toxic (Canonico *et al.,* 1994).

DNA-Protein Conjugates. Cell-specific DNA-delivery systems have been developed that utilize unique cell-surface receptors on the target cell (Michael and Curiel, 1994). By attaching the ligand recognized by such a receptor to the transgene DNA, the DNA-ligand complex becomes selectively bound to and internalized into the target cell (Wu and Wu, 1987). These molecular conjugate vectors are attractive, because they potentially offer cell-specific gene transfer without the attendant problems of viral vectors. Initial model systems focused on developing effective means of attaching the DNA to the ligand using polycations, antibody-antigen complexes, and biotin-streptavidin linkers. Poly-L-lysine (PLL), a polycation, has been widely used, as it can be easily coupled to a variety of protein ligands by chemical cross-linking methods. When the PLL-ligand adduct is mixed with plasmid DNA, macromolecular complexes form in which the DNA is electrostatically bound to the PLL-ligand molecules. These toroidal structures (50 to 100 nm in diameter) present ligands to the cell-surface receptor that are efficiently endocytosed. The transferrin receptor (Zenke *et al.,* 1990), the asialoorosomucoid receptor (Wu and Wu, 1987), and cell-surface carbohydrates (Batra *et al.,* 1994) also have been used to demonstrate the potential of ligand-mediated gene delivery. The asialoorosomucoid receptor is of particular interest, because it is found almost exclusively on hepatocytes and therefore might be useful in mediating gene transfer into the liver.

THERAPEUTIC PARADIGMS

The transfer of nucleic acid molecules into living cells has many diverse clinical applications. Although originally conceived as a treatment of inherited disorders, gene therapy and the use of nucleic acid drugs have been deployed for the treatment of a wide variety of acquired diseases, including cancer and infections. This section contains discussions of many of these different strategies and illustrates their potential applications.

Gene Therapy for Inherited Disorders

Gene therapy can be applied to the treatment of inherited disorders, especially those transmitted by recessive inheritance. In this situation, a genetic defect typically ablates expression of the normal, functional gene product (loss of function). Strategies to restore gene function require high-efficiency delivery of the normal gene sequence to tissues that are affected by the inherited condition. This approach has been referred to as "gene replacement," although gen-

erally no attempt is made to remove the native, mutant gene. A more appropriate term describing this approach might be "gene augmentation." Furthermore, inserting additional copies of a normal gene into a tissue expressing a condition transmitted by a dominant mode of inheritance will not necessarily overcome the cellular defect. This is especially true when a dominant–negative disease mechanism occurs. Use of this paradigm is illustrated for several disease conditions later in this chapter.

Correcting a genetic deficiency requires that the inserted gene product be expressed in sufficient amounts to achieve a therapeutic effect; the threshold for this effect varies widely among genetic diseases. Often, this can be estimated from clinical observations comparing the severity of the disease with the extent of the gene deficiency. This is illustrated by the hemophilias, where the extent of bleeding complications is roughly proportional to the extent of the deficiency in circulating coagulation factors. Such estimates are not possible in other disorders such as cystic fibrosis, where the amount of cystic fibrosis transport regulator (CFTR) gene expression in the airway and in other epithelial cells that is necessary to achieve therapeutic benefit is not known. These issues become more complex in diseases where gene expression must be carried out in a highly regulated fashion. This can be illustrated by the thalassemias, which arise from defects in the synthesis of hemoglobin α or β chains. Excessive production of either subunit chain by an unregulated therapeutic gene transfer could be as harmful as the disease itself.

Genetic Repair Strategies

Several approaches have been developed to repair genetic errors directly rather than complementing the defect with a functional allele. Genetic repair strategies offer several potential advantages, such as a concomitant decrease in the production of deleterious gene products and the increased likelihood that expression of the targeted gene remains under appropriate physiologic control. This paradigm conceptually is well suited for the treatment of inherited conditions arising from dominant-negative mutations.

One strategy is RNA repair, which enlists catalytic RNA molecules (ribozymes) capable of mediating *trans*-splicing reactions. With this approach, a defective portion of an mRNA molecule is replaced with the corresponding wild-type sequence. A second strategy focuses on repairing the mutation at the genomic level by inducing DNA-repair mechanisms using specialized oligonucleotides composed of both RNA and DNA residues. In both cases, the repaired gene or transcript remains under the transcriptional control of the native gene.

RNA Repair by *Trans*-Splicing Ribozymes.   RNA enzymes or ribozymes have been the focus of much study since their discovery in the early 1980s. Numerous biochemical experiments have been performed to elucidate the mechanisms of how certain RNA molecules can form active sites and perform catalysis. More recently, the study of ribozymes has attracted increased attention because of the potential usefulness of these RNA enzymes for a variety of gene therapy applications.

Ribozymes.   The first discovered ribozyme was the self-splicing group I intron from *Tetrahymena thermophila* (*T. thermophila*). The reaction mediated by this RNA enzyme has been extensively characterized, and the mechanism by which it excises itself from precursor ribosomal RNAs (pre-rRNA) without the aid of proteins is well understood (Cech, 1993). The second ribozyme to be recognized was the RNA subunit of RNase P. RNase P catalyzes the removal of upstream sequences on precursor-tRNAs to produce mature 5′ ends on tRNA molecules in a wide variety of cell types (Symons, 1992). A second class of catalytic introns (group II) has been discovered in the organelle genomes of several lower organisms (Frank and Pace, 1998). In addition to the splicing reaction, the group II intron also has the ability to insert itself into double-stranded DNA with assistance from a multifunctional, intron-encoded protein. Several other catalytic RNA motifs have been discovered that naturally are associated with plant and human pathogens. The hammerhead and hairpin ribozymes are derived from satellite RNAs from plant viroid and virusoids, and the hepatitis delta virus (HDV) ribozyme is derived from a short, single-stranded RNA virus found in some patients with hepatitis B virus. Each of these small RNA enzymes catalyzes a self-cleavage reaction that is believed to play a major role in the replication of these single-stranded RNA pathogens (Symons, 1992).

Ribozymes differ in size and catalytic mechanism. Each type of ribozyme adopts a characteristic secondary and tertiary structure that is required for it to assemble a catalytic center and perform catalysis (Cech, 1992). Ribozymes derived from group I introns and RNase P are typically greater than 200 nucleotides in length; both cleave target RNAs to generate products with 3′-hydroxyl and 5′-phosphate termini. By contrast, hammerhead, hairpin, and the HDV ribozymes are only 30 to 80 nucleotides in length and form cleavage products with 2′, 3′ cyclic phosphate and 5′-hydroxyl termini.

All of these self-cleaving ribozymes have been reengineered so that they can cleave other target RNA molecules in *trans* in a sequence-specific manner. This ability to cleave specifically targeted RNAs has led to much speculation about the potential utility of *trans*-cleaving ribozymes as inhibitors of gene expression (Rossi, 1999). Such *trans*-splicing ribozymes may prove to be effective at repairing defective cellular transcripts by cleaving off mutant nucleotides and ligating on functional RNA sequences (*see* Figure 5–4) (Sullenger, 1999).

Ribozyme-mediated RNA repair may be useful for treating a variety of diseases. As mentioned above, the *Tetrahymena* group I ribozyme can catalyze a *trans*-splicing reaction. In the first example of this application, the group I ribozyme from *T. thermophila* was reengineered to repair truncated *lacZ* transcripts *via* targeted *trans*-splicing in *Escherichia coli* (Sullenger and Cech, 1994) and in mammalian cells (Jones *et al.*, 1996). In both settings, the ribozyme spliced restorative sequences onto mutant *lacZ* target RNAs with high fidelity and maintained the open reading frame for translation of the repaired transcripts. In a subsequent study, the efficiency of RNA repair was monitored; the ribozyme was able to revise up to 50% of the truncated *lacZ* transcripts when ribozyme and *lacZ* substrate encoding plasmids were cotransfected into mammalian fibroblasts (Jones and Sullenger, 1997).

More recently, three studies have demonstrated that group I ribozymes can successfully amend faulty transcripts that are associated with common genetic diseases and cancer. In one study, a *trans*-splicing ribozyme was demonstrated capable of repairing transcripts associated with myotonic dystrophy (Phylactou *et al.*, 1998). Other investigations have employed RNA repair to correct sickle β-globin (Lan *et al.*, 1998) and mutant p53 transcripts (Watanabe and Sullenger, 2000).

RNA/DNA Oligonucleotides (Chimeraplasty).   Disease-producing mutations may be repaired by harnessing the DNA mismatch repair machinery in cells. Chimeric RNA/DNA oligonucleotides have been successfully employed to repair mutant sequences at the genomic level in several animal models of disease. Insights gleaned from studies of homologous recombination led Kmiec and colleagues to pioneer this novel form of gene repair, termed chimeraplasty (Yoon *et al.*, 1996). Chimeric oligonucleotides consist of a self-complementary sequence composed of both DNA and modified RNA residues (2′-O-methyl ribonucleotides) that form a duplex structure flanked by two polythymidine hairpin loops (Figure 5–5). The presence of 2′-O-methyl RNA residues provides an increased binding affinity with the target sequence and nuclease resistance.

Design of Chimeric Oligonucleotides.   The conventional chimeric oligonucleotide targeting sequence is made up of two stretches of ten modified ribonucleotide residues interrupted by five deoxynucleotide residues, with the central DNA base designed to mismatch with the targeted mutation (Figure 5–5). At the point of this mismatch, the oligonucleotide sequence serves as a template to guide the DNA repair machinery in correcting the mutation. Chimeric oligonucleotides also can direct the insertion and deletion of single nucleotides. While the typical length for the homologous targeting sequence is 25 bases, it has been shown that the frequency of nucleotide correction increases with the length of this region (Gamper *et al.*, 2000).

Mechanism of Action.   The exact mechanism of action of chimeric RNA/DNA oligonucleotides is not fully understood at this time, but much has been learned using a human cell-free extract assay system (Cole-Strauss *et al.*, 1999; Gamper *et al.*,

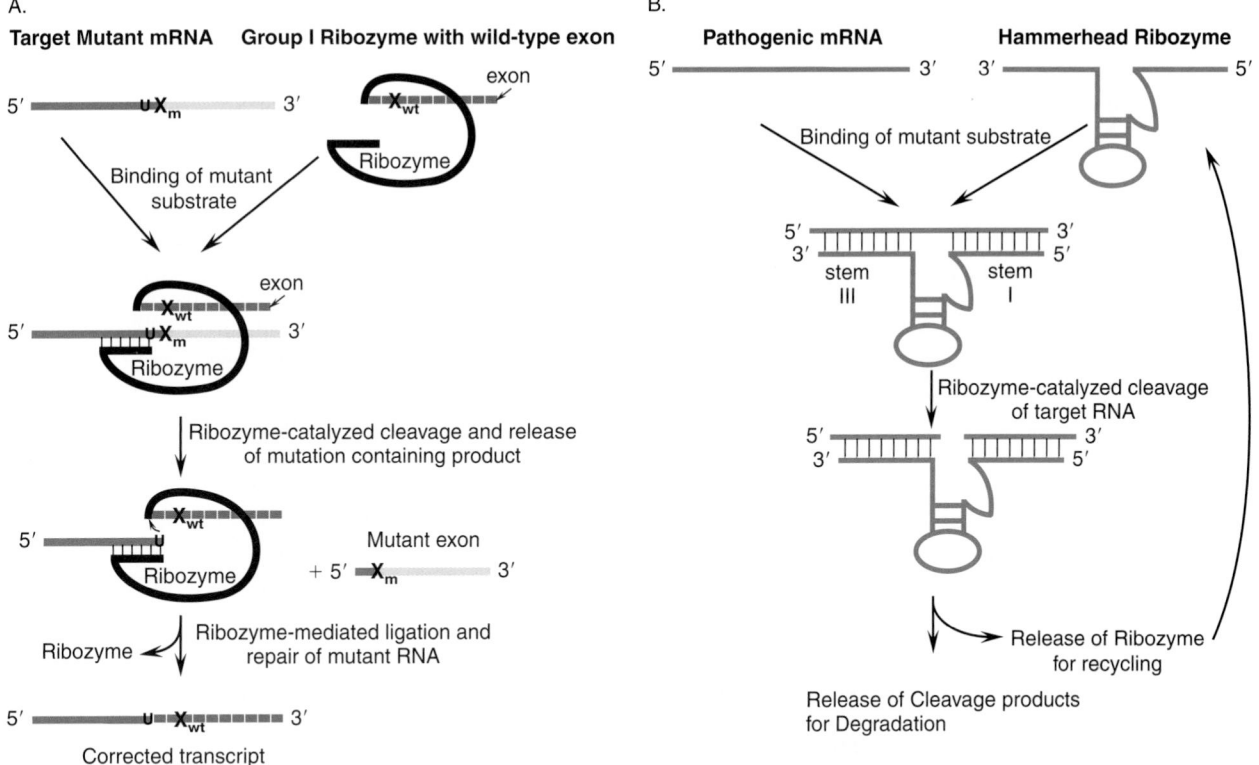

Figure 5–4. Ribozyme-mediated RNA repair and cleavage.

A. Trans-*splicing reaction mediated by a group I intron ribozyme.* The location of the mutant nucleotide in the target mRNA is indicated by X_m and the corresponding base in the wild-type exon is marked by X_{wt}. The *trans*-splicing reaction begins with complementary base-pair formation between the ribozyme and the target mRNA. Sequentially, the ribozyme catalyzes cleavage of the target mRNA and ligation of the wild-type exon to generate a repaired transcript.

B. Trans-*cleavage reaction mediated by a hammerhead ribozyme.* The hammerhead ribozyme first binds to a target RNA through complementary base pairing, and then catalyzes cleavage of the RNA at an unpaired residue positioned between stems I and III. The ribozyme is then released and can mediate another cleavage reaction.

2000). The targeted gene-repair reaction appears to require both the cellular homologous recombination and mismatch repair mechanisms. Studies suggest that the key intermediate is a complement-stabilized D-loop, a four-stranded joint molecule in which the two strands of the chimeric oligonucleotide are base-paired with the complementary target sequence (Figure 5–5). Previous chimeraplasty studies were carried out using a molecule that contained the desired mismatch on both strands of the oligonucleotide. It is now thought that the chimeric RNA/DNA strand stabilizes the interaction with the target sequence, and only the DNA strand serves as a template for mismatch repair; thus, the latter is the only strand requiring the mismatch. It also is believed that the activity of the molecule is increased if the chimeric strand consists of only RNA bases rather than an RNA/DNA mixture.

Chimeric RNA/DNA oligonucleotides were investigated initially by targeting episomally expressed plasmid

DNA, and subsequently were shown to repair genomic DNA mutations in cultured cells. *In vitro* model systems have included the sickle cell hemoglobin β^S allele expressed in lymphoblastoid cells, a defective alkaline phosphatase gene in HuH-7 cells, and the tyrosinase gene in albino mouse melanocytes (Alexeev and Yoon, 1998; Cole-Strauss *et al.,* 1996; Kren *et al.,* 1997).

In vivo gene repair was first demonstrated in the Gunn rat model of Crigler-Najjar syndrome type I, which is caused by a frameshift mutation in the gene encoding UDP-glucuronosyltransferase. The mutation causes loss of enzyme activity and hyperbilirubinemia (Kren *et al.,* 1999). A chimeric oligonucleotide was designed for the site-directed insertion of the missing base in the genomic DNA encoding this protein, and it was delivered intravenously to the liver of affected rats as a complex with

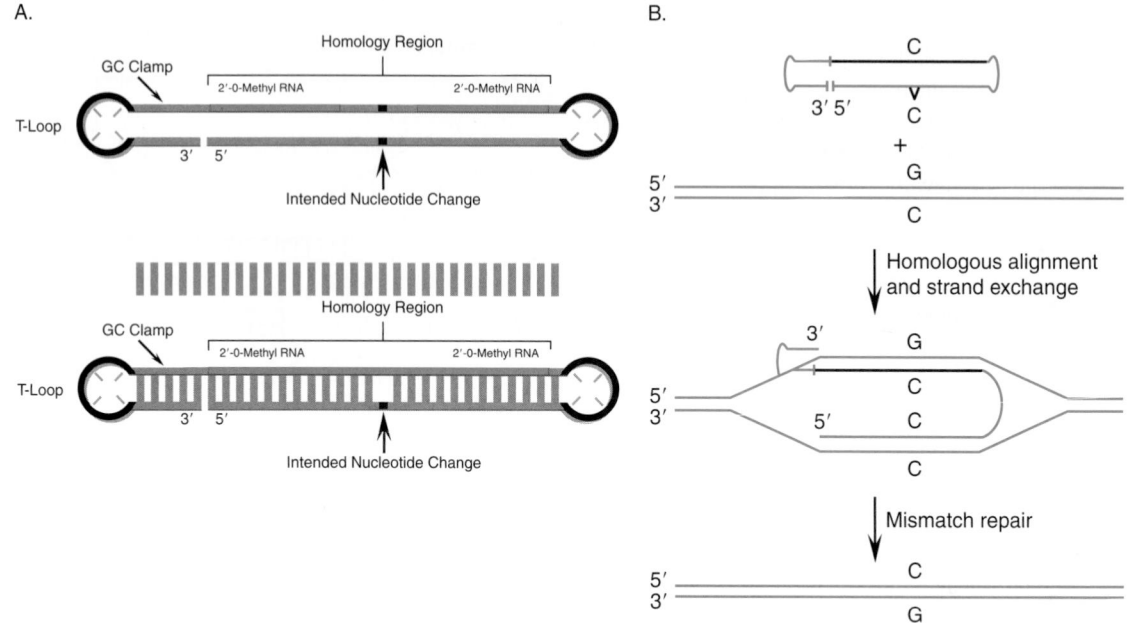

Figure 5–5. Chimeric RNA/DNA oligonucleotide-mediated genetic repair.

A. *Structure of chimeric RNA/DNA oligonucleotides.* The upper strand of a chimeric oligonucleotide shown on top consists of two stretches of 2′-O-methyl RNA residues (*blue*) flanking five DNA residues (*gray*) that form a homology region that is complementary to the target DNA sequence. One position in the sequence (*black arrow*) is designed to form a mismatch with the target sequence. The lower strand is made entirely of DNA and contains the intended nucleotide change. A G-C clamp provides stability and poly-T hairpin loops (T-loop) prevent concatemerization of multiple oligonucleotides. In later generation chimeric RNA/DNA oligonucleotides (*lower structure in A*), the upper strand consists entirely of 2′-O-methyl RNA and only the lower strand provides a mismatch with the target sequence.

B. *Proposed mechanism of chimeric oligonucleotide–mediated DNA repair.* The chimeric oligonucleotide undergoes homologous alignment and strand exchange with the target sequence, forming a complement-stabilized loop. The upper strand (*black*) stabilizes the binding of the oligonucleotide with the target sequence. The lower strand (*blue*) serves as the template for gene repair that is carried out by the cellular mismatch repair machinery.

lactosylated polyethyleneimine (PEI) or encapsulated within anionic liposomes. The mutation was repaired in these experiments with a frequency of 20%, and mRNA transcribed from the repaired gene was translated into functional protein. Serum bilirubin levels fell 25% after the first dose and decreased to nearly 50% of pretreatment levels after a second administration, demonstrating the potential additive effect of repeated chimeric oligonucleotide dosing. Restoration of enzyme activity was confirmed biochemically, and the effects of gene repair persisted for at least six months.

Other investigations have demonstrated the feasibility of *in vivo* chimeraplasty to repair mutations in the tyrosinase gene of albino BALB/c mice, and in the dystrophin genes of both mouse and golden retriever models of Duchenne muscular dystrophy (Alexeev *et al.*, 2000; Bartlett *et al.*, 2000b; Rando *et al.*, 2000).

Current challenges to deploying chimeric RNA/DNA oligonucleotides for human gene therapy include the need for optimal delivery strategies and cost-effective, large-scale synthesis and purification schemes (Ye *et al.*, 1998). Most of the delivery effort has been focused on using charged liposomes and synthetic polymers including PEI and polylysine. The most important concern for optimal activity of the molecule is achieving efficient delivery to the nucleus. Due to the length of the oligonucleotide (typically 68 bases) and the extremely stable secondary structure, synthesis and purification of full-length molecules in sufficient quantities is difficult and costly. By-products of oligonucleotide synthesis could be toxic to cells, and incomplete products may compete with the full-length molecule for target DNA binding. High-performance liquid chromatography and denaturing polyacrylamide gel electrophoresis are the most commonly used purification techniques.

Gene Inactivation Strategies

Approaches for inhibiting the expression of specific genes has become an important therapeutic paradigm for gene-based therapy of many acquired diseases. Antisense oligonucleotides and certain classes of ribozymes are in use or in various stages of development to treat a wide range of disease processes including viral infections and cancer. In fact, a specific antisense oligonucleotide designed for the treatment of ocular cytomegalovirus (CMV) infection was the first nucleic acid drug to receive FDA approval for clinical use.

Antisense Oligonucleotides. Short, synthetic, single-stranded stretches of DNA complementary to an mRNA can block the expression of specific target genes at the level of translation (Galderisi *et al.*, 1999; Ma *et al.*, 2000). First-generation antisense oligonucleotides contained phosphorothioate linkages in which one of the nonbridging oxygen atoms on the phosphate is replaced with sulfur to render the molecule nuclease resistant (*see* structure below). Second-generation antisense oligonucleotides incorporate alternative intramolecular linkages and also feature mixtures of deoxyribonucleotides and chemically substituted ribonucleotides. Newer antisense oligonucleotides may offer improved pharmacokinetic and safety profiles because of reduced nonspecific interactions (Agrawal and Kandimalla, 2000).

Phosphorothioate
oligodeoxynucleotide

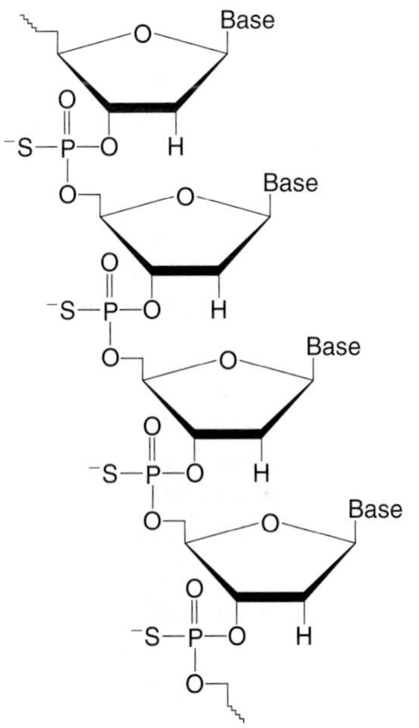

Mechanism of Action. Antisense oligonucleotides exert their effects by sequence-specific and sequence-nonspecific mechanisms (Galderisi *et al.*, 1999; Ma *et al.*, 2000). The principal sequence-specific mechanism involves hybridizing to a target mRNA through Watson-Crick complementary base pairing. This interaction impedes ribosome-mediated translation of mRNA into protein and invites the activity of RNase H, an enzyme that cleaves RNA in the context of an RNA/DNA duplex. The typical length of antisense oligonucleotides (15 to 20 bases) is sufficiently long to achieve highly sequence-specific gene targeting. There also are nonspecific effects of antisense oligonucleotides that are independent of the targeted mRNA sequence. Because of their polyanionic nature, antisense oligonucleotides may bind to a variety of proteins and can activate, complement, or interfere with the coagulation cascade. The latter effects may cause prolongation of plasma clotting times in human subjects (Sheehan and Lan, 1998). Antisense oligonucleotides that contain certain sequence motifs such as cytosine-guanosine dinucleotides (CpG) and guanosine triplets (GGG) can induce significant immune responses, including modulation of T-cell function and the induction of several cytokines, including interleukins, interferon-γ, and tumor necrosis factor-α (Pisetsky, 1999).

Pharmacokinetics. Dose-dependent increases in steady-state plasma levels of antisense oligonucleotides generally have been observed in early-phase clinical trials when the drugs were administered intravenously or subcutaneously (Levin, 1999). Pharmacokinetics are generally independent of the oligonucleotide sequence and length. After intravenous administration, antisense oligonucleotides are excreted mainly in the urine within 24 hours. In experimental animals, detectable levels may be found in most tissues except the brain for up to 48 hours. The elimination half-life of oligonucleotides administered intraocularly is more prolonged (de Smet *et al.*, 1999).

Fomivirsen. Antisense oligonucleotides are primarily in development as antiviral and antineoplastic agents. The first gene-based therapeutic agent to receive FDA approval is *fomivirsen* (VITRAVENE), a 21-base-pair phosphorothioate oligonucleotide targeted to mRNA transcribed from the immediate-early transcriptional unit of human cytomegalovirus (CMV) (Nichols and Boeckh, 2000; Perry and Balfour, 1999). Fomivirsen is indicated for the local (intravitreal) treatment of CMV retinitis for patients with acquired immunodeficiency syndrome. For patients with advanced drug-refractory and sight-threatening disease, weekly fomivirsen treatment can significantly delay disease progression. The most common adverse effects of treatment include increased intraocular pressure and mild to moderate intraocular inflammation, both of which tend to be transient and easily reversible with topical corticosteroids.

Other Antisense Oligonucleotides. Several other antisense oligonucleotides are in early clinical trials for the treatment of various hematologic and solid organ neoplasms (Cotter, 1999; Yuen and Sikic, 2000). Antisense oligonucleotides in development for the treatment of chronic myelogenous leukemia are being targeted to a hybrid mRNA sequence that arises because of a chromosomal translocation resulting in over-expression of mRNA encoding a chimeric oncogene (*bcr/abl*). Other agents in development are designed to block expression of *bcl-2,* a protein that inhibits apoptosis and may play a significant role in the development of various lymphoid malignancies. Additional antineoplastic targets for antisense oligonucleotides include mRNAs encoding protein kinases (*c-raf,* protein kinase C), hematopoietic cell transcription factors (*c-myb*), and other proteins known to be involved in tumorigenesis or tumor suppression (*h-ras,* p53). Results from early clinical trials with these compounds suggest that they are generally well tolerated, and their clinical efficacy is promising.

***Trans*-Cleaving Ribozymes.**   Several investigations have demonstrated the ability of various engineered ribozymes to cleave a specific target RNA sequence *in vitro* (James and Gibson, 1998; Kijima *et al.,* 1995). Most work has been done using hammerhead or hairpin ribozymes, which are considerably smaller than group I intron-derived ribozymes. These molecules can be designed to bind to specific RNA sequences and execute a cleavage reaction that can inactivate the target transcript (Figure 5–4). This strategy for gene inactivation has been applied for the experimental treatment of various viral infections, including HIV-1 and hepatitis B virus (Menke and Hobom, 1997; Wands *et al.,* 1997) and malignant conditions caused by the expression of dominant oncogenes (Irie *et al.,* 1997). *Trans*-cleaving ribozymes have two theoretical advantages compared with other RNA-based inhibition strategies: (1) transcript cleavage results in the direct, irreversible inactivation of the target RNA, and (2) because a single ribozyme can catalyze multiple cleavage reactions and thus destroy multiple transcripts, relatively few ribozyme molecules may be required to inhibit a given target gene effectively.

Inhibition of HIV by Ribozymes.   Ribozymes may be able to cleave viral target RNAs at a number of stages in the viral life cycle. Potential RNA targets include incoming genomic RNAs, early viral mRNAs, late viral mRNAs and full-length genomic RNAs that are being encapsidated. Although cleavage of incoming RNAs would prevent viral integration and therefore be highly effective in protecting cells, the fact that HIV-genomic RNAs are encapsidated within a viral core may make these transcripts difficult for ribozymes to access. Therefore, cleavage of early viral transcripts may prove to be the most attractive strategy for conferring resistance to HIV. Hammerhead and hairpin ribozymes are particularly well suited for this purpose because of their small size, simple secondary structure, and the ease with which they can be manipulated to target specific HIV substrate RNAs for cleavage.

Several studies have suggested that ribozymes can inhibit HIV replication in cell culture experiments when cells are challenged with a very low HIV inoculum. In the first application of this approach to inhibit HIV replication, an anti-*gag* hammerhead ribozyme was generated that specifically cleaved *gag*-encoding RNAs *in vitro* and inhibited HIV replication in a human T-cell line (Sarver *et al.,* 1990). Subsequently, such *trans*-cleaving ribozymes have been designed to target a variety of highly conserved sequences throughout the HIV genome and have been shown to inhibit viral replication to varying degrees in a number of tissue culture studies. Moreover, certain *trans*-cleaving ribozymes have been demonstrated to inhibit the replication of diverse viral strains as well as clinical isolates in primary T-cell cultures (Poeschla and Wong-Staal, 1994). Comparisons between catalytically active and inactive forms of these anti-HIV ribozymes have demonstrated that maximal inhibition of virus replication is usually associated with catalytic activity and is not due simply to the antisense property of these anti-HIV ribozymes.

To assess the activity of ribozymes in more clinically relevant settings, human peripheral blood lymphocytes have been stably transduced with a hairpin ribozyme targeting the U5 region of the HIV genome. These cells were shown to resist challenge by both HIV molecular clones and clinical isolates (Leavitt *et al.,* 1994). More recently, macrophage-like cells that differentiated from hematopoietic stem/progenitor cells from fetal cord blood and were stably transduced with a hairpin ribozyme targeted at the 5′ leader sequence resisted infection by a macrophage-tropic virus (Yu *et al.,* 1995). Transduction of pluripotent hematopoietic stem cells with HIV-resistance genes may represent an avenue to continually generate cells that are resistant to HIV infection. Such stem cells differentiate into monocytes and macrophages, the major targets of HIV infection. Clinical trials to assess the safety and efficacy of this strategy in HIV-infected patients have begun (Wong-Staal *et al.,* 1998).

Cleavage by Ribozymes of Dominant Oncogenes.   Neoplastic transformation often is associated with the expression of mutant oncogenes. Because ribozymes can be designed to inhibit the expression of specific gene products, their potential as antineoplastic agents has been exploited. For example, hammerhead ribozymes have been reported to suppress the tumorigenic properties of various neoplastic cells harboring activated human *ras* genes (Scharovsky *et al.,* 2000), and the *bcr/abl* fusion transcript that arises in chronic myelogenous leukemia (James and Gibson, 1998). *In vitro* experiments have shown that the 8500 nucleotide *bcr/abl* transcript can be cleaved efficiently by a hammerhead ribozyme targeted to the fusion point (James *et al.,* 1996). In CML blast crisis cell lines, expression of ribozymes targeted at *bcr/abl* mRNA has been demonstrated to decrease the production of p210^*bcr/abl*^ and *bcr/abl* transcripts and to reduce cell proliferation (Shore *et al.,* 1993). Similar results have been reported using an anti-*bcr/abl* ribozyme based on the structure of RNase P (Cobaleda and Sanchez-Garcia, 2000).

Insertional Gene Inactivation by Group II Introns.   A recent study suggests that group II introns also are useful for targeted gene inactivation (Guo *et al.,* 2000). Two targets important for HIV infection, the human chemokine receptor CCR5 gene and regions of the HIV-1 proviral DNA, were targeted by a modified group II intron. The coding sequences of both genes could be disrupted in human cells by the insertion of the intron sequence at a defined point. This work, while still preliminary, provides another novel approach for gene inactivation.

Ectopic Synthesis of Therapeutic Proteins

Deficiencies of a variety of growth factors and peptide hormones are potentially amenable to treatment using the paradigm of ectopic gene expression. This approach involves delivery of a gene to evoke expression of a circulating protein from a tissue that normally does not synthesize the product. In experimental animals and early clinical trials, this strategy has been used successfully to induce expression of coagulation factors (factor VIII, IX) growth factors (IGF-1, erythropoietin), and peptide hormones (growth hormone, growth hormone–releasing hormone). In some cases, it is desirable to induce continuous secretion of a therapeutic protein (*e.g.,* factor IX), while in other situations gene expression needs to be under strict regulation (*e.g.,* erythropoietin).

Skeletal muscle has become the most frequently used tissue for ectopic production of therapeutic proteins (MacColl *et al.,* 1999). Skeletal muscle is a large and stable cell mass that can be conveniently accessed by intramuscular injection. In several preclinical studies, both viral and nonviral gene-transfer techniques have been demonstrated to efficiently transduce skeletal muscle with few adverse effects.

There are numerous potential advantages to this strategy of delivering therapeutic proteins using ectopic gene expression. In general, this approach is less expensive and more convenient than delivery of recombinant proteins or plasma-derived concentrates. There also is a greatly reduced risk of transmission of blood-borne diseases, such as hepatitis and HIV infection, that are associated with treatment of hemophilia, for example. Successful use of this paradigm has been demonstrated for the experimental treatment of hemophilia, delivery of human growth hormone for the treatment of congenital dwarfism, and ectopic production of erythropoietin for treatment of chronic anemia, as outlined below.

Factor IX. Hemophilia A and B arise because of congenital deficiency of the coagulation factors VIII and IX, respectively. Preclinical studies using mice and hemophilic dogs have demonstrated the efficacy of an AAV vector encoding factor IX to promote sustained skeletal muscle expression of this coagulation factor sufficient to improve the clinical phenotype (Herzog *et al.,* 1999). Early clinical experience using an AAV vector expressing human factor IX driven by the CMV immediate early promoter in patients with severe hemophilia B has been described (Kay *et al.,* 2000). This study demonstrated modest changes in circulating factor IX and reduced requirement for factor IX protein infusions in a small group of treated patients. Improvements in the attainable expression level may be possible using alternative promoters, including muscle-specific enhancer/promoter sequences (Hagstrom *et al.,* 2000).

Erythropoietin. Erythropoietin (EPO) insufficiency occurs most commonly in chronic renal failure. Frequent injection of recombinant EPO is necessary to maintain adequate hematocrit levels in chronic dialysis patients. The major disadvantage of this therapy is cost. Preclinical studies have demonstrated the utility of inducing erythropoietin production ectopically in skeletal muscle (Tripathy *et al.,* 1996) or skin (Klinman *et al.,* 1999). This has been accomplished by intramuscular or intradermal injection of plasmid DNA or viral vector encoding human EPO under the control of a constitutively active promoter such as the CMV immediate-early promoter. Experimental animals have been shown to maintain elevated plasma EPO levels and elevated hematocrits for several months after treatment.

Under physiological conditions, EPO secretion by the kidney is tightly regulated, and therefore an inducible expression system is desirable for therapeutic applications. Such a system has been developed using an artificial, sirolimus (rapamycin)-regulated transcription factor (Figure 5–6) (Ye *et al.,* 1999). The immunosuppressant sirolimus is an orally administered drug (*see* Chapter 53) capable of interacting with two proteins, FK506 binding protein-12 (FKBP12) and FKBP12-rapamycin-associated protein

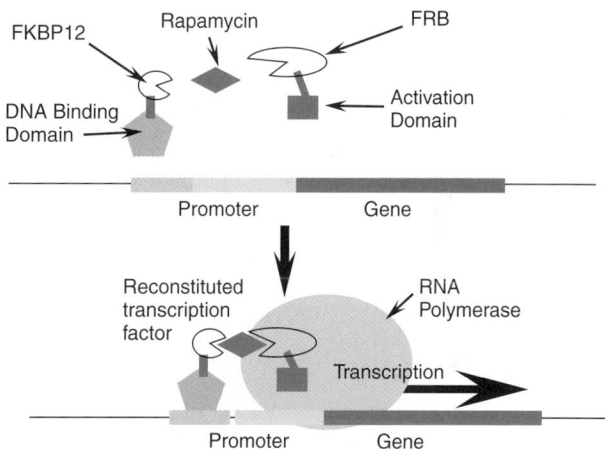

Figure 5–6. Sirolimus (rapamycin)-regulated gene expression system.

Schematic diagram of an expression system used to control ectopic expression of therapeutic proteins. The molecular components illustrated in the upper portion of the figure include (1) an expression vector encoding the gene of interest under the transcriptional control of a promoter, (2) FKBP12 (*see* text) fused to a transcription factor DNA binding domain, (3) the FRB domain of FRAP (*see* text) fused to a transcription factor activation domain, and (4) sirolimus (rapamycin). Sirolimus promotes assembly of a functional transcription factor that activates RNA polymerase to transcribe mRNA from the gene.

(FRAP). The inducible expression system for regulated expression of EPO consists of three molecular components: (1) the transcriptional activation domain from the p65 subunit of nuclear protein kappa B (NFκB) fused to the FKBP12-rapamycin binding (FRB) domain of FRAP; (2) a unique DNA binding domain fused to FKBP12; and (3) a transgene under direct control of the artificial transcription factor. Sirolimus reconstitutes a functional transcription factor by binding both FRB and FKBP12 motifs and bringing the separated activation and DNA binding domains together. The sirolimus-reconstituted transcription factor drives expression of the transgene in a dose-dependent manner. Expression of EPO from skeletal muscle occurs only in the presence of sirolimus, which can be administered orally. This system has been used to induce EPO expression in skeletal muscle of immune competent mice and rhesus monkeys following intramuscular injections of two AAV vectors encoding the separable components of this system.

Other Growth Factors and Hormones. Long-term, regulated expression of human growth hormone has been achieved in mice after intramuscular injection of AAV vectors encoding this gene (Rivera *et al.,* 1999). These studies utilized the sirolimus-inducible system described above for EPO. In these experiments, sirolimus induced significant elevations of serum human growth hormone in a dose-dependent manner with a lag time between drug administration and first measurable serum growth-hormone level of approximately three hours. Growth-hormone levels in blood peaked approximately one day after sirolimus administration in this study. Growth hormone–releasing hormone (GHRH) also can be expressed ectopically in porcine muscle following direct injection of plasmid DNA encoding this peptide under transcriptional control of a skeletal muscle α-actin promoter (Draghia-Akli *et al.,* 1997; Draghia-Akli *et al.,* 1999).

Insulin-like growth factor I (IGF-1) also has been expressed ectopically in skeletal muscle. IGF-1 is critical for the growth of skeletal muscle and other tissues. Intramuscular injection of an AAV virus encoding IGF-l into mice resulted in sustained increases in muscle mass and muscle strength for up to 27 months (Barton-Davis *et al.,* 1998). These effects prevented age-related changes in muscular function, suggesting that this strategy might be of benefit in diseases where skeletal muscle damage secondary to aging is accelerated.

Cancer Gene Therapy

It is generally accepted that cancer arises because of an accumulation of multiple molecular genetic defects that culminate in a cellular phenotype characterized by unregulated growth. Based on this knowledge, a variety of gene therapy strategies have been developed as potential new therapies for cancer (Gomez-Navarro *et al.,* 1999). Indeed, more than half of all approved gene therapy trials relate to cancer treatment. For some neoplastic conditions, gene therapy may provide an effective treatment alternative to conventional therapies, while in other circumstances, it may serve as an adjuvant treatment.

Cancer is an extraordinarily complex disease process, and a variety of gene-based treatment strategies have been conceived (*see* Chapter 52). Current knowledge of the role of protooncogenes and tumor suppressor genes in the genesis of malignancy has stimulated the development of gene therapy tactics directed at ablating or restoring such genes, respectively. In other strategies, cancer cells are endowed with the ability to convert a systemically delivered prodrug to a toxic metabolite (cell-targeted suicide), or are targeted for destruction by replicating viral vectors (viral-mediated oncolysis). Conversely, transfer of drug-resistance genes into normal cells may provide chemoprotection during high-dose antineoplastic drug treatment. Finally, immune system modulation can activate anticancer defense mechanisms. Each of these strategies has advantages and disadvantages as well as unique obstacles to its successful deployment.

The successful development of effective gene-based treatments for cancer faces several challenges. To eradicate a malignancy, any treatment strategy needs to affect every neoplastic cell. Because most cancers exert their morbidity and mortality through metastatic spread, gene delivery methods must be capable of reaching widespread anatomical locations.

Target cell specificity is another important obstacle for gene-based treatment of cancer. An ideal vector would target only malignant cells and have no effect on normal cells. A variety of approaches are under development to exploit unique molecular markers of tumor cells or to use transcriptional targeting strategies through the use of tumor-specific gene promoters (Curiel, 1999; Nettelbeck *et al.,* 2000). Finally, the genetic complexity of cancer implies that multiple approaches may be needed to achieve ultimate success.

Oncogene Inactivation. Several oncogenic proteins have been identified and associated with various malignancies (Park, 1998). A variety of strategies are under development to block expression of these oncogenic proteins in malignant cells by interfering with either transcription or translation. The most commonly applied approach in clinical trials to date has been the use of antisense strategies (*see* above) (Gewirtz *et al.,* 1998). Suboptimal delivery of antisense molecules to malignant cells and the variable efficacy of specific antisense molecules for any given target gene are substantial obstacles to the success of this approach. Transcription of oncogenes also can be inhibited using the adenoviral gene E1A, which interferes with the transcription of *erbB-2,* a strategy useful in treating cancers that overexpress this oncogenic protein, such as breast and ovarian cancers (Gomez-Navarro *et al.,* 1999).

Augmentation of Tumor Suppressor Genes. More than twenty-four tumor-suppressor genes have been identified, and mutations in these genes have been associated with a variety of neoplastic conditions (Fearon, 1998). This knowledge has stimulated efforts to develop techniques to replace or repair defective tumor-suppressor genes in malignant cells. Several clinical trials are under way to deliver p53 using adenoviral vectors to a variety of cancers (Gomez-Navarro *et al.,* 1999). Similarly, viral vectors have been utilized to introduce the retinoblastoma gene and the breast cancer gene BRCA1 into bladder and ovarian cancers, respectively. Preclinical studies have demonstrated success with this approach, but not in all cases. In some situations, this approach will fail, because the mutant gene exhibits a dominant-negative effect on the normal gene. To circumvent this problem for p53 gene therapy, a genetic repair strategy (*see* previous section) rather than a gene-augmentation approach could be more effective (Watanabe and Sullenger, 2000).

Cell-Targeted Suicide.   Conversion of a prodrug to a toxic metabolite by genetically engineering tumor cells is an attractive way to create an artificial difference between normal and neoplastic tissue (Springer and Niculescu-Duvaz, 2000). This can be achieved by the expression of a gene that confers a dominant, negatively selectable phenotype to the cancer cell, such as cell death imparted by expression of a prodrug-metabolizing enzyme. A variety of enzymes are capable of performing such a function, and they typically kill cells by activation of a relatively nontoxic prodrug to a cytotoxic form (Table 5–2). Greater selectivity in killing malignant cells will be obtained by transferring a gene that is not normally found in human beings (*e.g.,* HSV-thymidine kinase), rather than by overexpressing an endogenous gene (*e.g.,* deoxycytidine kinase).

The prototype for this approach utilizes the HSV-1 thymidine kinase gene (HSV-TK) given in combination with the prodrug ganciclovir (Morris *et al.,* 1999). The HSV-TK phosphorylates ganciclovir in a manner distinct from mammalian thymidine kinase. Phosphorylated ganciclovir is ultimately incorporated

Table 5–2

Enzyme-Prodrug Combinations for Cancer Gene Therapy

GENE	PRODRUG
HSV thymidine kinase (HSV-TK)	Ganciclovir Acyclovir
VSV thymidine kinase	Ara-M
Deoxycytidine kinase	Ara-C Fludarabine 2-Chlorodeoxyadenosine Difluorodeoxycytidine
Cytosine deaminase	5-Fluorocytidine
Nucleoside phosphorylase*	MeP-dR

*Nucleoside phosphorylase is encoded by the *E. coli DeoD* gene, the coding sequence used in this therapeutic strategy.

Key: HSV, herpes simplex virus; VSV, vesicular stomatitis virus; Ara-C, cytosine arabinoside or cytarabine; Ara-M, 6-methoxypurine arabinoside; MeP-dR, 6-methylpurine-2'-deoxyriboside.

into DNA and inhibits DNA synthesis and transcription. The efficacy and safety of this approach is being tested in several clinical trials involving multiple malignancies. The major obstacle is selective delivery of HSV-TK to neoplastic cells. Normal cells, especially hepatic cells, also can be rendered ganciclovir-sensitive if transduced by HSV-TK. Another important limitation of this approach is the need to transduce all tumor cells with the prodrug-metabolizing enzyme. This obstacle is circumvented in part due to the "bystander effect," a phenomenon in which generation of the toxic drug by transduced tumor cells facilitates killing of neighboring nontransduced tumor cells by local dissemination of the compound. With the HSV-TK/ganciclovir system, the bystander effect requires functional gap junctions, possibly to enable cell-to-cell spread of the toxic metabolite, which is not diffusable across cell membranes. Combinations of two or more prodrug-metabolizing enzymes may offer enhanced efficacy by virtue of synergy among different toxic metabolites acting through different mechanisms.

The major limitation of this approach has been the requirement to deliver the prodrug-metabolizing enzyme locally at a dose sufficient to transduce most or all tumor cells without systemic dissemination. The emergence of drug-resistant, malignant cell populations also is a potential barrier to this approach.

Chemoprotection.   Gene transfer approaches can be utilized to confer greater drug tolerance to normal bone marrow cells in patients undergoing high-dose chemotherapy. The mechanisms by which cancer cells are able to survive the cytotoxic effects of chemotherapy are well described for a number of chemotherapeutic agents (*see* Chapter 52). Although these genes limit the effectiveness of many chemotherapy regimens, it is possible that they might be exploited to protect normal tissues from the toxic effects of chemotherapy.

The MDR-1 gene encoding the multidrug transporter protein (also known as P-glycoprotein) has received much attention in this regard. This transmembrane protein transports a wide variety of chemotherapeutic agents (*e.g.,* doxorubicin, vinca alkaloids, epipodophyllotoxins, and paclitaxel) and other drugs out of cells, thus protecting them from the agents' toxic effects (Gottesman *et al.,* 1994). Many cancers display a dose-dependent sensitivity to chemotherapy, whereby larger doses of chemotherapy lead to greater tumor regression and improved survival (*see* Chapter 52). This is best illustrated by testicular cancers, which are highly curable when treated aggressively. Unfortunately, toxicity to normal tissues, especially the bone marrow, limits the use of larger doses of chemotherapy in many cancers. To overcome this, autologous bone marrow transplantation has been employed to rescue the bone marrow from the toxic effects of high-dose chemotherapy. Capitalizing on this concept, an investigational gene therapy strategy has been developed whereby the MDR-1 gene would be used to render the bone marrow resistant to the toxic effects of the chemotherapy (Aran *et al.,* 1999).

Clinical trials have demonstrated the safety and feasibility of MDR-1 gene transfer to bone marrow stem cells and peripheral blood hematopoietic progenitor cells in patients undergoing high-dose chemotherapy for advanced cancer (Cowan *et al.,* 1999; Devereux *et al.,* 1998; Hanania *et al.,* 1996; Hesdorffer *et al.,* 1998; Moscow *et al.,* 1999). All studies employed replication-incompetent retroviral vectors to transduce cells *ex vivo* under varying cell culture conditions. In general, the transduction efficiency observed using this approach and the level of engraftment success was low. However, the use of cytokine preconditioning and inclusion of fibronectin cell-adhesion domains in stem-cell cultures prior to viral transfection results in significantly greater transduction efficiency and longer expression in the engrafted marrow cells (Abonour *et al.,* 2000).

Virus-Mediated Oncolysis. Certain viruses, including adenovirus and HSV-1, can infect and lyse tumor cells (Alemany *et al.,* 2000; Heise and Kirn, 2000). In most gene therapy applications, the ability of the virus to replicate in the host cell is disabled. By contrast, oncolysis can be accomplished by enabling the virus to replicate selectively within tumor cells. The use of oncolytic viruses in combination with other gene-based antineoplastic strategies has emerged as a promising addition to the multidimensional treatment of cancer (Hermiston, 2000).

Selective replication of a virus in tumor cells leads to cell lysis and to local dissemination of infective viral progeny to neighboring cancer cells. This phenomenon provides amplification of the initial viral dose. Because cell lysis is the ultimate goal of this treatment, it is not necessary for these viral vectors to establish long-term transgene expression in the targeted host cell. Most investigational uses of this strategy have utilized replication-competent adenovirus and HSV-1.

Two general strategies have been employed to engineer viral vectors capable of replicating in tumor cells and not in normal cells. First, a viral gene required for replication, such as the adenovirus E1A gene, can be driven by a tumor-specific promoter. The other approach involves deleting viral genes whose functions are required for replication in normal cells, but that are not required for replication in neoplastic cells. For example, the adenovirus E1B-55kD gene is required for efficient replication in normal cells expressing an active p53 protein, but virus lacking E1B-55kD (Onxy-015) will replicate within and lyse malignant cells lacking functional p53 (Dix *et al.,* 2000). In a phase I clinical trial using intratumoral injection of Onxy-015 in patients with recurrent head and neck cancer, this viral vector was tolerated well and produced evidence of tumor necrosis at the site of viral injection (Ganly *et al.,* 2000). In a similar strategy, deletion of the gene encoding ribonucleotide reductase in the HSV genome produces a virus that can be replicated selectively in mammalian tumor cells that overexpress this enzyme. Although HSV has a natural tropism for neuronal tissues, studies have demonstrated effectiveness of HSV-based oncolytic vectors for nonneuronal malignancies (Yoon *et al.,* 2000).

Perhaps the greatest utility of replication-selective viruses that target malignant cells will come by coupling this approach with other gene-based cancer treatments. In particular, replication-competent adenoviruses and HSV vectors have been developed that carry one or two prodrug-metabolizing enzymes capable of sensitizing tumor cells to chemotherapy. Aghi *et al.* (1999) have demonstrated that an engineered, replication-competent HSV vector that expresses rat CYP2B1 and HSV-TK confers sensitivity to cyclophosphamide and ganciclovir, respectively, to cultured glioma cells. Similarly, Rogulski *et al.* (2000) utilized double-suicide gene therapy delivered by a replication-competent adenovirus to cervical carcinoma xenografts in mice. In this case, the double-suicide gene combination included HSV-TK/ganciclovir and cytosine deaminase/5-fluorocytosine. This approach dramatically potentiated the efficacy of radiation therapy.

Virus-mediated oncolysis also may enhance antitumor immune responses. These immune responses may include reactions not only to the viral component but also to specific tumor antigens that are released following oncolysis (Agha-Mohammadi and Lotze, 2000). Several observations suggest that these additional immune enhancements may enable eradication of metastases following local tumor treatment. Additional effects on the immune response also can be achieved by engineering the viral vector to direct expression of various cytokines.

Immunomodulation. Most cancer cells exhibit poor immunogenicity, and the neoplastic state itself may be associated with specific impairments in mounting effective antitumor immune responses. Various cytokines can enhance immunity against cancer cells, and this observation has stimulated the development of gene-based approaches to modulate the immune reaction in malignancy (Agha-Mohammadi and Lotze, 2000).

Ectopic Cytokine Expressions. A variety of cytokines have been shown to decrease tumor growth when ectopically expressed in tumor cells or in their microenvironment (Tepper and Mule, 1994). Tumor cells engineered to secrete certain cytokines have been observed to be less able to form tumors when implanted in syngeneic hosts, whereas their *in vitro* growth is unaffected, suggesting that host factors are induced in response to the cytokines that decrease tumorigenicity. Some immunostimulatory agents do not alter the growth rate of the tumor initially, but lead to immunity against tumor growth if the animal is later challenged with wild-type tumor cells. It is apparent that genetically engineered tumor cells elicit a variety of host immune responses depending on the immunomodulatory agent employed. For example, secretion of interleukin-4 (IL-4) by a tumor cell elicits a strong local inflammatory response without any effect on distant tumor cells or on tumor cells administered an exogenous vector at later times. In contrast, granulocyte/macrophage colony-stimulating factor (GM-CSF) has little effect on the tumorigenicity, but evokes a pronounced antitumor immunity (Dranoff *et al.,* 1993). Greater therapeutic efficacy may be achievable by transducing tumor cells with multiple cytokine genes. Various combinations of the interleukins, interferon-γ, and GM-CSF have been demonstrated to elicit antitumor immune responses. As discussed above, delivery of cytokine genes using replication-competent viruses offers great promise for added therapeutic benefits.

Immune Enhancement. Other approaches aimed at increasing the immune response to cancer cells have been developed. One such approach is to express on the surface of cancer cells highly immunogenic molecules, such as allotypic MHC antigens. Alternatively, rather than express an exogenous "rejection" antigen, tumor cells may be modified so that the endogenous, weakly immunogenic, tumor-associated antigens are better recognized. It has been long known that additional "costimulatory" pathways distinct from the T-cell receptor are needed to achieve T-cell activation (*see* Chapter 53). The molecules B7-1 (CD 80) and B7-2 (CD 86) stimulate one such pathway. The B7s, whose expression normally is limited to antigen-presenting cells and other specialized immune effector cells, engage specific receptors (CD-28 and CTLA-4) on the T-cell surface in concert with antigen binding to the T-cell receptor. Subsequently, T-cell activation, cell proliferation, and cytokine production ensue and can lead to the elaboration of antitumor immunity. The absence of a costimulatory signal at the time of T-cell receptor engagement is not a neutral event; rather, it results in the development of tumor-specific anergy, not mere failure to activate the T cell.

Thus, the simple presence of antigens in tumor cells would be expected to produce an immune-tolerant state rather than an immune-responsive state if costimulatory events do not take place. In effect, this is what is seen in most clinical situations where human tumors grow apparently unimpeded by host immune mechanisms. When some tumor cells are provided with costimulatory molecules, effective T-cell activation takes place. This has been demonstrated by ectopic expression of B7 on tumor cells; these genetically engineered tumor cells then are used to stimulate an immune response to the parental tumor cell line.

DNA Vaccines

Vaccination against both infectious and noninfectious diseases is possible using DNA-encoded antigens (Gurunathan *et al.,* 2000; Kowalczyk and Ertl, 1999). Skin or muscle can be inoculated easily with a bacterial plasmid vector carrying a gene coding for an antigenic protein. Following transcription and translation of the gene in host cells, the antigen induces a multifaceted immune reaction featuring both humoral and cell-mediated responses. The ability to stimulate T-helper cell and cytotoxic T-lymphocyte responses provides a potential advantage over conventional protein-based vaccines that do not have these effects. Two additional advantages of DNA vaccines are the relatively low production costs and the lack of risks associated with attenuated pathogens. Furthermore, unmethylated plasmid sequences containing purine-purine-C-G-pyrimidine-pyrimidine sequence motifs stimulate lymphocyte proliferation and cytokine release and thus act as potent adjuvants (Roman *et al.,* 1997; Sato *et al.,* 1996). The major limitations of DNA vaccines include the relatively weak humoral immune response, the theoretical risks of insertional mutagenesis, and provocation of an autoimmune response.

DNA vaccines are being evaluated in both preclinical and clinical studies for the treatment of a wide range of infections (viral, bacterial, parasitic) as well as certain acquired diseases such as malignancy and chronic allergic conditions. The safety and feasibility of using a DNA vaccination strategy to immunize against HIV-1 infection recently has been demonstrated (Boyer *et al.,* 2000).

DISEASE TARGETS FOR GENE THERAPY

This section highlights the use of gene therapy for treatment of various inherited conditions affecting the immune system, hematopoietic system, liver, lung, and skeletal muscle. Many other organ systems and dozens of other genetic disorders that are not discussed also are potential targets for gene therapy. The few topics presented here should illustrate some of the major issues and obstacles facing treatment of other disease targets.

Immunodeficiency Disorders

Gene therapy for the treatment of congenital immunodeficiency disorders illustrates the use of *ex vivo* gene transfer into hematopoietic stem cells. Three distinct immunodeficiency syndromes, adenosine deaminase deficiency (ADA), X-linked severe combined immunodeficiency (SCID-X1), and chronic granulomatous disease (CGD), are current targets of preclinical and clinical gene therapy investigations. Success has been limited by the low efficiency of transducing hematopoietic stem cells, although recent work in SCID-X1 has demonstrated increased effectiveness of retroviral gene transfer using new cell culture techniques (Cavazzana-Calvo *et al.,* 2000).

Adenosine Deaminase Deficiency.   The first genetic disorder to be clinically treated with gene therapy was ADA (Parkman *et al.,* 2000). In children with this disorder, the absence of adenosine deaminase leads to an accumulation of deoxyadenosine triphosphate that is toxic to lymphocytes. Patients with ADA develop recurrent, life-threatening infections due to defective cell-mediated and humoral immune responses. Standard therapy is bone marrow transplantation along with periodic infusions of polyethylene glycol-coupled recombinant enzyme (PEG-ADA). In the first clinical trial, two patients were infused with peripheral blood T lymphocytes that had been transduced with a retroviral vector containing the human ADA gene (Blaese *et al.,* 1995). One of these two patients had long-term persistence of transduced T lymphocytes, while the other had a poor response. The responsive patient experienced amelioration of symptoms of the disease and is living a normal life several years after treatment (Anderson, 2000).

Because of concerns that use of mature T lymphocytes for treatment of ADA would not restore a complete immune-response repertoire, subsequent clinical trials have evaluated the use of *ex vivo* gene therapy utilizing hematopoietic stem cells. Pluripotent hematopoietic stem cells are capable of differentiating into all blood-cell types. Unfortunately, in most studies, the success of transducing hematopoietic stem cells obtained from bone marrow, peripheral blood, or umbilical cord blood has been limited by low transfection efficiency (Halene and Kohn, 2000). Furthermore, transgenes carried by retroviral vectors are poorly expressed in resting, nondividing T lymphocytes (Parkman *et al.,* 2000). Lentiviral vectors may be capable of achieving higher levels of transduction (Case *et al.,* 1999), but significant biosafety concerns exist.

X-linked Severe Combined Immunodeficiency.   In the most common form of SCID, mutations in the gene encoding the cytokine receptor γ-chain (γc) located on the X chromosome confer a lethal immunodeficiency syndrome characterized by impairments in lymphocyte differentiation.

As with ADA, gene therapy approaches utilizing hematopoietic stem cells are envisioned to hold great promise for treating SCID. Results from a recent study demonstrated the use of a retroviral vector to transfer the normal γc gene into stem cells *ex vivo*, which were then reinfused into two infants with SCID-X1 (Cavazzana-Calvo *et al.*, 2000). Ten months after treatment, both patients exhibited normal T-lymphocyte numbers and function associated with detectable expression of the γc protein in circulating lymphocytes. Success in this study has been attributed to improved cell-culture conditions used to maintain and propagate the transduced stem cells. These improvements included cultivating cells on surfaces coated with fibronectin fragments in the presence of a unique blend of cytokines (stem cell factor, megakaryocyte differentiation factor, Flt-3 ligand). Cytokines stimulate stem-cell division and therefore enable retrovirus infection. Fibronectin enhances transduction efficiency by promoting the colocalization of cells with the virus.

Chronic Granulomatous Disease. This disorder is caused by genetic defects in one of four genes encoding subunits of the respiratory-burst oxidase, a superoxide-generating enzyme complex present within phagocytic leukocytes. A defect in this system results in an inability to fight bacterial and fungal infections and can be life threatening. Genetic correction of a small fraction of circulating phagocytes would suffice to provide clinical benefit. This is based on the observation that unaffected female carriers of this X-linked trait have as few as 5% oxidase-positive neutrophils. Allogenic bone marrow transplantation is the standard treatment, although there are many conceivable advantages of a gene-based treatment strategy. Two of the genes that cause CGD (gp91^{phox} and p47^{phox}) are targeted in gene therapy trials (Kume and Dinauer, 2000). In a phase I clinical trial involving five adult patients with p47^{phox} deficiency, intravenous infusions of peripheral blood stem cells transduced *ex vivo* with a retroviral vector carrying normal p47^{phox} were successful in generating functionally corrected granulocytes (Malech *et al.*, 1997). Persistence of the corrected cell phenotype was demonstrated for up to six months after the infusion, although the quantity of functional cells was probably insufficient for clinical benefit. Further work is needed to enhance the efficiency of gene transfer into stem cells and to demonstrate more long-lasting effects.

Liver Disease

The liver can be afflicted with a variety of metabolic, infectious, and neoplastic diseases for which specific molecular interventions can be envisioned. Potential applications are made more feasible by the existence of multiple methods for effecting gene transfer to the liver. Molecular conjugates, adenoviral vectors, liposomes, and retroviral vectors all have been used for hepatocyte gene transfer (Shetty *et al.*, 2000). For *in vivo* gene transfer, the liver is accessible by a number of routes, including direct injection, intravenous, and intrabiliary administration of vectors. *Ex vivo* strategies can be implemented by partial surgical resection of the liver, isolation of hepatocytes, and *in vitro* hepatocyte transduction. The genetically modified cells can then be reimplanted into the liver.

The liver can be targeted selectively for gene transfer by exploiting unique hepatocyte surface receptors that are capable of mediating receptor-mediated endocytosis (Smith and Wu, 1999). Specific ligands that are recognized by the asialoglycoprotein receptor can be coupled to DNA typically in combination with a polymer such as polylysine, or liposomes. Envelope proteins on retroviral vectors also have been genetically modified to incorporate peptide sequences from hepatocyte-targeted proteins such as human hepatocyte growth factor (Nguyen *et al.*, 1998). Some viral vectors may have a natural proclivity to target the liver. Rapid hepatic uptake of adenoviral vectors administered intravenously accounts for approximately 90% of the delivered dose. The adenovirus knob protein (terminal domain of the fiber protein, Figure 5–2) appears responsible for this phenomenon (Zinn *et al.*, 1998).

Familial Hypercholesterolemia. Patients with familial hypercholesterolemia have an inherited deficiency or dysfunction of the low-density lipoprotein (LDL) receptor and, as a consequence, develop extremely high plasma levels of cholesterol and arteriosclerosis at a very early age (*see* Chapter 36). The genetic defect manifests itself as a diminished ability of the liver to clear LDL particles from the blood, and serum lipid levels provide a convenient marker of the disease. Although pharmacological interventions have had limited success, correction of the hepatic dysfunction by orthotopic liver transplantation leads to normalization of blood lipid levels and slowing of arterial disease progression. This clinical observation suggested that if the liver could be genetically modified to express the LDL receptor, the same benefits might be achieved. The Watanabe heritable hyperlipidemic rabbit has served as an ideal animal model, demonstrating that this approach does lead to persistent reductions in serum LDL (Chowdhury *et al.*, 1991). Several patients now have been treated in a clinical trial using an *ex vivo* DNA-delivery approach and retrovirus to introduce the LDL receptor gene into hepatocytes isolated from the patients following partial hepatectomy (Grossman *et al.,* 1994). This study demonstrated the feasibility, safety, and potential efficacy of *ex vivo* hepatic gene therapy.

Hemophilia A.   Inherited deficiency of coagulation factor VIII leads to a lifelong risk of spontaneous hemorrhage that can be debilitating and potentially life-threatening. Standard treatment includes frequent infusions of plasma-derived factor VIII that carries the risk of blood-borne infection as well as significant inconvenience. Hemophilia A is well suited for gene therapy, because factor VIII levels in blood are therapeutic over an extended range, and even modest (5% of normal) levels of the protein can ameliorate the major morbidity associated with this disease (Kay and High, 1999). Unlike hemophilia B and factor IX deficiency, there has been little success in applying the paradigm of ectopic synthesis (*see* above). This is explained by the fact that the full-length factor VIII-coding region is more than 7 kb, and this has restricted vector selection to retroviruses and adenovirus (Balague *et al.,* 2000; VandenDriessche *et al.,* 1999). However, it also is feasible to engineer a recombinant AAV vector carrying a truncated (B domain-deleted) form of factor VIII (Chao *et al.,* 2000). The B domain of factor VIII can be deleted without impairing the pro-coagulant activity of the protein, and the truncated gene (4.4 kb) is well within the carrying capacity of recombinant AAV vectors.

Long-term hepatic expression in experimental animals has been achieved using a variety of viral vectors carrying factor VIII (Kaufman, 1999). Delivery can be achieved intravenously, although gene transfer to organs other than liver, including spleen and lungs, can occur. In addition, *ex vivo* approaches also have been used. Human bone marrow stromal cells have been transduced with factor VIII retroviral vectors and then transplanted into the spleens of immunodeficient mice (Chuah *et al.,* 2000). Although circulating factor VIII levels in the mice rose significantly after engraftment, transgene silencing prevented long-term expression.

A major issue facing gene therapy of hemophilia is the possibility of developing inhibitory antibodies against the transgene. The development of inhibitory antibodies also is a common sequela of protein-based therapy of both hemophilia A and B. Choice of gene transfer vector, dose, and target tissue are likely factors that will influence the propensity for developing antibodies (Kaufman, 1999).

Hemoglobinopathies

Sickle cell disease and the thalassemias are common single-gene disorders associated with substantial morbidity and mortality. In theory, these disorders should be amenable to *ex vivo* gene transfer into hematopoietic stem cells which then would be used to reconstitute a patient's bone marrow with cells expressing a specific transferred gene. However, major challenges remain in developing vectors capable of achieving long-term and therapeutic expression levels of transferred globin genes (Emery and Stamatoyannopoulos, 1999; Persons and Nienhuis, 2000). In addition, gene-repair strategies utilizing either *trans*-splicing ribozymes or chimeric RNA/DNA oligonucleotides have been utilized *in vitro* (*see* above).

The most successful *in vivo* approach to date has been the use of retroviral vectors that carry the β-globin gene with varying segments of its locus control region (LCR), a master switch for controlling the transcription of the entire β-globin gene cluster. Although there have been initial successes in transferring human β-globin gene sequences into hematopoietic stem cells *ex vivo* using retroviral vectors, long-term expression after marrow transplantation in experimental animals has not been observed. Recombinant lentiviruses may be capable of promoting more efficient transfer and integration of the human β-globin gene together with larger segments of its LCR into hematopoietic stem cells (May *et al.,* 2000).

The transient and poor expression of β-globin in hematopoietic stem cells after marrow transplantation has been attributed to transgene silencing and position-effect variegation (Rivella and Sadelain, 1998). Gene silencing is most likely an epigenetic process that results in the silencing of a gene in the progeny of a transduced stem cell. This phenomenon may be caused by sequence motifs in the viral LTR that can be eliminated or modified by reengineering the vector. Position-effect variegation is a phenomenon characterized by highly variable cell-to-cell expression of a gene in red blood cells even when cells are derived from a common progenitor having a single-transgene-integration site. Retroviral vectors carrying very large segments of the LCR also are prone to splicing and other events that affect transgene stability.

Preselection of successfully transduced cells reduces the incidence of gene silencing and of age-dependent reduction in expression levels and may partially circumvent these problems. This approach is presumably successful because hematopoietic stem cells in which the transferred gene is not initially silenced are selected. Two approaches for preselecting transduced stem cells have been conceived. Kalberer *et al.* (2000) have described the successful utilization of *ex vivo* preselection of transduced stem cells on the basis of expression of a marker protein. An alternative approach for preselecting hematopoietic cells capable of longer-term expression of the transgene involves use of a coexpressed drug-resistance gene enabling negative-selection strategies (Emery and Stamatoyannopoulos, 1999).

Lung Diseases

From the perspective of organ specificity, the lung provides an opportunity for highly specific delivery of gene transfer vectors to the respiratory epithelium through the bronchial airways. Clinical trials of gene therapy for lung disease most often have used aerosol systems to achieve topical delivery of gene delivery vectors (Ennist, 1999). However, despite its accessibility, respiratory epithelium strongly resists invasion by foreign particles, including viral and nonviral delivery systems. There are multiple barriers to transducing respiratory epithelial cells by the aerosol route (Boucher, 1999). These barriers include a mucous clearance mechanism that may remove vectors from the airways, a glycocalyx that may block binding to cell surface receptors, and finally an apical cell membrane that expresses a low density of receptors for viral vectors and exhibits a low rate of endocytosis.

Several gene delivery vectors have been applied to treating inherited lung disease (Albelda et al., 2000). Adenoviral vectors are uniquely suited for gene therapy of lung disease because of their natural tropism for respiratory epithelium. However, several studies have demonstrated that adenoviral vectors are inefficient delivery vehicles because of their transient expression and propensity to provoke immune responses (Welsh, 1999). Adeno-associated viral vectors may offer the advantages of more stable expression of the transduced gene and less inflammation.

Cystic Fibrosis. The gene responsible for cystic fibrosis (*CFTR*) was discovered more than ten years ago, and there have been multiple efforts to develop safe and effective vectors for introducing this gene into the respiratory epithelium of patients suffering from this disease (Boucher, 1999). The results from several phase I clinical trials have been published, and most of these involved use of adenoviral vectors to transduce either nasal or pulmonary epithelium. In general, adenoviral vectors are capable of achieving gene transfer, but this is inefficient as judged by the small proportion of transduced cells, and the transient nature of gene expression typically lasting only several days (Grubb et al., 1994; Zuckerman et al., 1999). In addition, immune responses attenuate the effectiveness of subsequent vector administrations (Harvey et al., 1999).

Adeno-associated viral vectors for delivering *CFTR* are now in clinical trials. Preclinical studies demonstrated long-term transgene expression with little immune response in experimental systems. The results of one phase I clinical trial targeting maxillary sinus epithelium in ten cystic-fibrosis patients has been reported (Drapkin et al., 2000). The results from this study are encouraging, but much work remains to evaluate the long-term safety and efficacy of this vector. Liposomal vectors also are under evaluation in cystic fibrosis. The results of three clinical trials have been published and some evidence of effective gene transfer is evident. However, like adenoviral gene transfer in

respiratory epithelium, liposome-mediated gene delivery results in transient expression (Albelda et al., 2000).

Several novel strategies for increasing the efficiency of viral gene transfer to respiratory tissues are being tested. Because most receptors for viral vectors are located on the basolateral membrane of these cells, experimental approaches that disrupt epithelial tight junctions have been tested and demonstrate an increased efficiency of gene transfer applied from the apical cell surface (Boucher, 1999). However, it is unlikely that these strategies can be adopted safely for clinical use. In another approach, modifications of the vector have been engineered to facilitate specific interactions with apical cell-membrane receptors. Modified vectors that target apical purine-nucleotide receptors using monoclonal antibodies (Boucher, 1999), or that target the urokinase/plasminogen-activator receptor by employing small peptide ligands, have been tested and appear to improve gene transfer efficiency *in vitro* (Drapkin et al., 2000).

α_1-Antitrypsin Deficiency. Deficiency of α_1-antitrypsin predisposes individuals to pulmonary emphysema and hepatic cirrhosis. In the lungs, this deficiency renders tissue vulnerable to injury by neutrophilic proteases released at sites of inflammation. Although α_1-antitrypsin is not normally made by respiratory epithelium, gene transfer strategies to achieve expression of the gene in these cells are predicted to have a protective effect on the lung (Albelda et al., 2000).

Currently, recombinant α_1-antitrypsin protein is commercially available for human use and is the standard therapy for this disease. However, this treatment is extremely expensive, intensive, and is associated with exposure risks. Preclinical studies in animals have demonstrated that α_1-antitrypsin can be delivered to the lungs through the bloodstream or the airways in the form of a cationic lipid–DNA complex (Canonico et al., 1994). One clinical study has demonstrated the ability of this plasmid–liposome complex to deliver the α_1-antitrypsin gene to the nasal respiratory epithelium of patients with the disease. In that study, local extracellular concentrations of the expressed protein reached nearly one-third of normal levels (Brigham et al., 2000). In addition, expression of the transgene in the nasal mucosa has a local antiinflammatory effect that does not occur during chronic intravenous treatment with the recombinant protein.

Skeletal Muscle

A variety of inherited disorders of muscle including Duchenne muscular dystrophy and the limb girdle muscular dystrophies are prime targets for the development of gene-based therapies. Mature skeletal muscle presents several unique opportunities and obstacles for gene delivery (Hartigan-O'Connor and Chamberlain, 2000). This tissue can be transduced locally by the direct injection of naked plasmid DNA or DNA carried by viral and nonviral vectors. In addition to these *in vivo* gene transfer methods, myoblast-mediated *ex vivo* gene transfer has been demonstrated to be an alternative delivery strategy (Floyd *et al.,* 1998).

Systemic delivery of genes to muscle is complicated by the large mass of this tissue and a permeability barrier, consisting of the vascular endothelium and extracellular matrix, that blocks access of gene delivery vectors to the myocyte membrane from the vasculature space. A variety of strategies have been developed to breach this permeability barrier. One particularly successful approach has been the employment of the inflammatory mediator histamine. In one study, the hindlimb vasculature of cardiomyopathic hamsters was sequentially perfused with a vasodilator (papaverine), histamine, and an AAV vector carrying either a marker gene (*e.g.,* encoding β-galactosidase) or the gene encoding δ-sarcoglycan (the gene defective in this animal model) (Greelish *et al.,* 1999). Histamine rendered the endothelial barrier in the hindlimb muscles permeable, allowing efficient and widespread transfer of both transgenes.

Skeletal muscle presents other obstacles to infection by certain viral vectors. Adenovirus has a low infectivity of mature skeletal muscle because of the low expression levels of the CAR and integrin molecules that are necessary for attachment and internalization of the virus (Nalbantoglu *et al.,* 1999). This low level of infectivity is maturation-dependent, with transduction being most efficient in immature muscle fibers (Acsadi *et al.,* 1994). By contrast, gene transfer using HSV vectors is not maturation-dependent (van Deutekom *et al.,* 1998). Experimental use of adenovirus to transduce skeletal muscle has been successful, but expression of transgenes has been transient in most cases because of the immune reaction induced by the viral infection. Adeno-associated virus also has been demonstrated to be capable of efficient and stable transduction of adult skeletal muscle (Fisher *et al.,* 1997). In some animal studies, transgene expression was demonstrated to persist for as long as two years.

Duchenne Muscular Dystrophy. Duchenne muscular dystrophy is an X-linked, recessive muscle disease caused by the absence of the cytoskeletal protein, dystrophin. The dystrophin-coding sequence is large (14 kb), precluding the use of viral vectors with limited carrying capacity, such as AAV and first-generation adenoviral vectors. Newer adenoviral vectors capable of carrying the complete dystrophin gene sequence have been tested in experimental models of muscular dystrophy, such as the *mdx* mouse, and have been shown to be effective in transducing muscle cells when delivered locally (Clemens *et al.,* 1996). In addition to the full-length dystrophin gene, viral vectors carrying the related gene for utrophin have been demonstrated to correct the dystrophic phenotype in *mdx* mice (Rafael *et al.,* 1998).

Limb Girdle Muscular Dystrophy. The limb girdle muscular dystrophies are a group of related inherited dis-

orders that include four genetically distinct forms caused by mutations in the α, β, γ, and δ-sarcoglycan genes. The sarcoglycans are putative transmembrane glycoproteins that form a protein complex with dystrophin. Genetic defects in these molecules cause a disease with many similarities to Duchenne dystrophy. Unlike dystrophin, the sarcoglycans are encoded by small gene sequences (less than 2 kb) that can be carried easily by recombinant AAV. Preclinical studies have demonstrated the feasibility of reconstituting sarcoglycan expression in mouse and hamster models of these disorders (Greelish *et al.,* 1999), and a phase I clinical trial is under way to test the safety and efficacy of intramuscular delivery of sarcoglycans using AAV vectors (Stedman *et al.,* 2000).

PROSPECTUS

Human gene therapy remains experimental, but there are several indications that, in the second decade of its evolution, this strategy will emerge as a safe and effective alternative to existing conventional therapies for many inherited and some acquired diseases. Already, some cancer gene therapy protocols are being tested in phase III clinical trials to compare their efficacy and safety with those of standard therapy. Additional antisense oligonucleotide drugs for the treatment of viral infections, including HIV, and possibly for malignancy likely will be approved for clinical use in the near future. The prospects for routine use of gene transfer to achieve ectopic expression of clotting factors and erythropoietin for the treatment of hemophilia and chronic anemia, respectively, in the near future seems promising.

The development of safer, more efficient gene transfer vehicles is critical to the success of most gene therapy paradigms, and advances in this field are tightly coupled to improvements in vector design, manufacture, and efficacy. These advances likely will bring feasibility to other, more heroic, measures such as *in utero* gene therapy. Finally, for progress to be made, it is critical that safety be assured to patients participating in the investigational phases of gene therapy development, and that the ethical concerns of the public be carefully considered and respected.

The demand for gene therapy to treat inherited diseases will certainly grow with the continuing discovery of new genetic conditions and their molecular defects. Gene therapy also could emerge as an important modality for treating more common disorders as we increase our appreciation for the role of allelic variation in conferring disease susceptibility. The need for improved gene transfer technologies and new therapeutic paradigms will only increase as physicians enter the era of genetic medicine.

BIBLIOGRAPHY

Abonour, R., Williams, D.A., Einhorn, L., Hall, K.M., Chen, J., Coffman, J., Traycoff, C.M., Bank, A., Kato, I., Ward, M., Williams, S.D., Hromas, R., Robertson, M.J., Smith, F.O., Woo, D., Mills, B., Srour, E.F., and Cornetta, K. Efficient retrovirus-mediated transfer of the multidrug resistance 1 gene into autologous human long-term repopulating hematopoietic stem cells. *Nat. Med.,* **2000,** *6*:652–658.

Acsadi, G., Jani, A., Massie, B., Simoneau, M., Holland, P., Blaschuk, K., and Karpati, G. A differential efficiency of adenovirus-mediated in vivo gene transfer into skeletal muscle cells of different maturity. *Hum. Mol. Genet.,* **1994,** *3*:579–584.

Aghi, M., Chou, T.C., Suling, K., Breakefield, X.O., and Chiocca, E.A. Multimodal cancer treatment mediated by a replicating oncolytic virus that delivers the oxazaphosphorine/rat cytochrome P450 2B1 and ganciclovir/herpes simplex virus thymidine kinase gene therapies. *Cancer Res.,* **1999,** *59*:3861–3865.

Akkaraju, G.R., Huard, J., Hoffman, E.P., Goins, W.F., Pruchnic, R., Watkins, S.C., Cohen, J.B., and Glorioso, J.C. Herpes simplex virus vector-mediated dystrophin gene transfer and expression in MDX mouse skeletal muscle. *J. Gene Med.,* **1999,** *1*:280–289.

Alexeev, V., Igoucheva, O., Domashenko, A., Cotsarelis, G., and Yoon, K. Localized in vivo genotypic and phenotypic correction of the albino mutation in skin by RNA-DNA oligonucleotide. *Nat. Biotechnol.,* **2000,** *18*:43–47.

Alexeev, V., and Yoon, K. Stable and inheritable changes in genotype and phenotype of albino melanocytes induced by an RNA-DNA oligonucleotide. *Nat. Biotechnol.,* **1998,** *16*:1343–1346.

Anderson, D.B., Laquerre, S., Goins, W.F., Cohen, J.B., and Glorioso, J.C. Pseudotyping of glycoprotein D-deficient herpes simplex virus type 1 with vesicular stomatitis virus glycoprotein G enables mutant virus attachment and entry. *J. Virol.,* **2000,** *74*:2481–2487.

Balague, C., Zhou, J., Dai, Y., Alemany, R., Josephs, S.F., Andreason, G., Hariharan, M., Sethi, E., Prokopenko, E., Jan, H.Y., Lou, Y.C., Hubert-Leslie, D., Ruiz, L., and Zhang, W.W. Sustained high-level expression of full-length human factor VIII and restoration of clotting activity in hemophilic mice using a minimal adenovirus vector. *Blood,* **2000,** *95*:820–828.

Bartlett, J.S., Wilcher, R., and Samulski, R.J. Infectious entry pathway of adeno-associated virus and adeno-associated virus vectors. *J. Virol.,* **2000a,** *74*:2777–2785.

Bartlett, R.J., Stockinger, S., Denis, M.M., Bartlett, W.T., Inverardi, L., Le, T.T., Man, N.T., Morris, G.E., Bogan, D.J., Metcalf-Bogan, J., and Kornegay, J.N. In vivo targeted repair of a point mutation in the canine dystrophin gene by a chimeric RNA/DNA oligonucleotide. *Nat. Biotechnol.,* **2000b,** *18*:615–622.

Barton-Davis, E.R., Shoturma, D.I., Musaro, A., Rosenthal, N., and Sweeney, H.L. Viral mediated expression of insulin-like growth factor I blocks the aging-related loss of skeletal muscle function. *Proc. Natl. Acad. Sci. U.S.A.,* **1998,** *95*:15603–15607.

Batra, R.K., Wang-Johanning, F., Wagner, E., Garver, R.I. Jr., and Curiel, D.T. Receptor-mediated gene delivery employing lectin-binding specificity. *Gene Ther.,* **1994,** *1*:255–260.

Boyer, J.D., Cohen, A.D., Vogt, S., Schumann, K., Nath, B., Ahn, L., Lacy, K., Bagarazzi, M.L., Higgins, T.J., Baine, Y., Ciccarelli, R.B., Ginsberg, R.S., MacGregor, R.R., and Weiner, D.B. Vaccination of seronegative volunteers with a human immunodeficiency virus type 1 env/rev DNA vaccine induces antigen-specific proliferation and lymphocyte production of beta-chemokines. *J. Infect. Dis.,* **2000,** *181*:476–483.

Brigham, K.L., Lane, K.B., Meyrick, B., Stecenko, A.A., Strack, S., Cannon, D.R., Caudill, M., and Canonico, A.E. Transfection of nasal mucosa with a normal alpha 1-antitrypsin gene in alpha 1-antitrypsin-deficient subjects: comparison with protein therapy. *Hum. Gene Ther.,* **2000,** *11*:1023–1032.

Buchschacher, G.L. Jr., and Wong-Staal, F. Development of lentiviral vectors for gene therapy for human diseases. *Blood,* **2000,** *95*:2499–2504.

Canonico, A.E., Conary, J.T., Meyrick, B.O., and Brigham, K.L. Aerosol and intravenous transfection of human alpha 1-antitrypsin gene to lungs of rabbits. *Am. J. Respir. Cell Mol. Biol.,* **1994,** *10*:24–29.

Case, S.S., Price, M.A., Jordan, C.T., Yu, X.J., Wang, L., Bauer, G., Haas, D.L., Xu, D., Stripecke, R., Naldini, L., Kohn, D.B., and Crooks, G.M. Stable transduction of quiescent CD34(+)CD38(−) human hematopoietic cells by HIV-1-based lentiviral vectors. *Proc. Natl. Acad. Sci. U.S.A.,* **1999,** *96*:2988–2993.

Cavazzana-Calvo, M., Hacein-Bey, S., de Saint Basile, G., Gross, F., Yvon, E., Nusbaum, P., Selz, F., Hue, C., Certain, S., Casanova, J.L., Bousso, P., Deist, F.L., and Fischer, A. Gene therapy of human severe combined immunodeficiency (SCID)-X1 disease. *Science,* **2000,** *288*:669–672.

Chao, H., Mao, L., Bruce, A.T., and Walsh, C.E. Sustained expression of human factor VIII in mice using a parvovirus-based vector. *Blood,* **2000,** *95*:1594–1599.

Chen, S.T., Iida, A., Guo, L., Friedmann, T., and Yee, J.K. Generation of packaging cell lines for pseudotyped retroviral vectors of the G protein of vesicular stomatitis virus by using a modified tetracycline inducible system. *Proc. Natl. Acad. Sci. U.S.A.,* **1996,** *93*:10057–10062.

Chowdhury, J.R., Grossman, M., Gupta, S., Chowdhury, N.R., Baker, J.R. Jr., and Wilson, J.M. Long-term improvement of hypercholesterolemia after ex vivo gene therapy in LDLR-deficient rabbits. *Science,* **1991,** *254*:1802–1805.

Chuah, M.K., Van Damme, A., Zwinnen, H., Goovaerts, I., Vanslembrouck, V., Collen, D., and VandenDriessche, T. Long-term persistence of human bone marrow stromal cells transduced with factor VIII-retroviral vectors and transient production of therapeutic levels of human factor VIII in nonmyeloablated immunodeficient mice. *Hum. Gene Ther.,* **2000,** *11*:729–738.

Clemens, P.R., Kochanek, S., Sunada, Y., Chan, S., Chen, H.H., Campbell, K.P., and Caskey, C.T. In vivo muscle gene transfer of full-length dystrophin with an adenoviral vector that lacks all viral genes. *Gene Ther.,* **1996,** *3*:965–972.

Cobaleda, C., and Sanchez-Garcia, I. In vivo inhibition by a site-specific catalytic RNA subunit of RNase P designed against the BCR-ABL oncogenic products: a novel approach for cancer treatment. *Blood,* **2000,** *95*:731–737.

Cole-Strauss, A., Gamper, H., Holloman, W.K., Munoz, M., Cheng, N., and Kmiec, E.B. Targeted gene repair directed by the chimeric RNA/DNA oligonucleotide in a mammalian cell-free extract. *Nucleic Acids Res.,* **1999,** *27*:1323–1330.

Cole-Strauss, A., Yoon, K., Xiang, Y., Byrne, B.C., Rice, M.C., Gryn, J., Holloman, W.K., and Kmiec, E.B. Correction of the mutation responsible for sickle cell anemia by an RNA-DNA oligonucleotide. *Science,* **1996,** *273*:1386–1389.

Cowan, K.H., Moscow, J.A., Huang, H., Zujewski, J.A., O'Shaughnessy, J., Sorrentino, B., Hines, K., Carter, C., Schneider,

E., Cusack, G., Noone, M., Dunbar, C., Steinberg, S., Wilson, W., Goldspiel, B., Read, E.J., Leitman, S.F., McDonagh, K., Chow, C., Abati, A., Chiang, Y., Chang, Y.N., Gottesman, M.M., Pastan, I., and Nienhuis, A. Paclitaxel chemotherapy after autologous stem-cell transplantation and engraftment of hematopoietic cells transduced with a retrovirus containing the multidrug resistance complementary DNA (MDR1) in metastatic breast cancer patients. *Clin. Cancer Res.,* **1999,** 5:1619–1628.

de Smet, M.D., Meenken, C.J., and van den Horn, G.J. Fomivirsen–a phosphorothioate oligonucleotide for the treatment of CMV retinitis. *Ocul. Immunol. Inflamm.,* **1999,** 7:189–198.

Devereux, S., Corney, C., Macdonald, C., Watts, M., Sullivan, A., Goldstone, A.H., Ward, M., Bank, A., and Linch, D.C. Feasibility of multidrug resistance (MDR-1) gene transfer in patients undergoing high-dose therapy and peripheral blood stem cell transplantation for lymphoma. *Gene Ther.,* **1998,** 5:403–408.

Dix, B.R., O'Carroll, S.J., Myers, C.J., Edwards, S.J., and Braithwaite, A.W. Efficient induction of cell death by adenoviruses requires binding of E1B55k and p53. *Cancer Res.,* **2000,** 60:2666–2672.

Dmitriev, I., Kashentseva, E., Rogers, B.E., Krasnykh, V., and Curiel, D.T. Ectodomain of coxsackievirus and adenovirus receptor genetically fused to epidermal growth factor mediates adenovirus targeting to epidermal growth factor receptor-positive cells. *J. Virol.,* **2000,** 74:6875–6884.

Douglas, J.T., Miller, C.R., Kim, M., Dmitriev, I., Mikheeva, G., Krasnykh, V., and Curiel, D.T. A system for the propagation of adenoviral vectors with genetically modified receptor specificities. *Nat. Biotechnol.,* **1999,** 17:470–475.

Draghia-Akli, R., Fiorotto, M.L., Hill, L.A., Malone, P.B., Deaver, D.R., and Schwartz, R.J. Myogenic expression of an injectable protease-resistant growth hormone-releasing hormone augments long-term growth in pigs. *Nat. Biotechnol.,* **1999,** 17:1179–1183.

Draghia-Akli, R., Li, X., and Schwartz, R.J. Enhanced growth by ectopic expression of growth hormone releasing hormone using an injectable myogenic vector. *Nat. Biotechnol.,* **1997,** 15:1285–1289.

Dranoff, G., Jaffee, E., Lazenby, A., Golumbek, P., Levitsky, H., Brose, K., Jackson, V., Hamada, H., Pardoll, D., and Mulligan, R.C. Vaccination with irradiated tumor cells engineered to secrete murine granulocyte-macrophage colony-stimulating factor stimulates potent, specific, and long-lasting anti-tumor immunity. *Proc. Natl. Acad. Sci. U.S.A.,* **1993,** 90:3539–3543.

Drapkin, P.T., O'Riordan, C.R., Yi, S.M., Chiorini, J.A., Cardella, J., Zabner, J., and Welsh, M.J. Targeting the urokinase plasminogen activator receptor enhances gene transfer to human airway epithelia. *J. Clin. Invest.,* **2000,** 105:589–596.

Duan, D., Sharma, P., Yang, J., Yue, Y., Dudus, L., Zhang, Y., Fisher, K.J., and Engelhardt, J.F. Circular intermediates of recombinant adeno-associated virus have defined structural characteristics responsible for long-term episomal persistence in muscle tissue. *J. Virol.,* **1998,** 72:8568–8577.

Duan, D., Yue, Y., Yan, Z., and Engelhardt, J.F. A new dual-vector approach to enhance recombinant adeno-associated virus-mediated gene expression through intermolecular cis activation. *Nat. Med.,* **2000,** 6:595–598.

Fink, D.J., and Glorioso, J.C. Engineering herpes simplex virus vectors for gene transfer to neurons. *Nat. Med.,* **1997,** 3:357–359.

Fisher, K.J., Jooss, K., Alston, J., Yang, Y., Haecker, S.E., High, K., Pathak, R., Raper, S.E., and Wilson, J.M. Recombinant adeno-associated virus for muscle directed gene therapy. *Nat. Med.,* **1997,** 3:306–312.

Floyd, S.S. Jr., Clemens, P.R., Ontell, M.R., Kochanek, S., Day, C.S., Yang, J., Hauschka, S.D., Balkir, L., Morgan, J., Moreland, M.S., Feero, G.W., Epperly, M., and Huard, J. Ex vivo gene transfer using adenovirus-mediated full-length dystrophin delivery to dystrophic muscles. *Gene Ther.,* **1998,** 5:19–30.

Fraefel, C., Song, S., Lim, F., Lang, P., Yu, L., Wang, Y., Wild, P., and Geller, A.I. Helper virus-free transfer of herpes simplex virus type 1 plasmid vectors into neural cells. *J. Virol.,* **1996,** 70:7190–7197.

Gallardo, H.F., Tan, C., Ory, D., and Sadelain, M. Recombinant retroviruses pseudotyped with the vesicular stomatitis virus G glycoprotein mediate both stable gene transfer and pseudotransduction in human peripheral blood lymphocytes. *Blood,* **1997,** 90:952–957.

Gamper, H.B. Jr., Cole-Strauss, A., Metz, R., Parekh, H., Kumar, R., and Kmiec, E.B. A plausible mechanism for gene correction by chimeric oligonucleotides. *Biochemistry,* **2000,** 39:5808–5816.

Ganly, I., Kirn, D., Eckhardt, S.G., Rodriguez, G.I., Soutar, D.S., Otto, R., Robertson, A.G., Park, O., Gulley, M.L., Heise, C., Von Hoff, D.D., and Kaye, S.B. A phase I study of Onyx-015, an E1B attenuated adenovirus, administered intratumorally to patients with recurrent head and neck cancer. *Clin. Cancer Res.,* **2000,** 6:798–806.

Goins, W.F., Lee, K.A., Cavalcoli, J.D., O'Malley, M.E., DeKosky, S.T., Fink, D.J., and Glorioso, J.C. Herpes simplex virus type 1 vector-mediated expression of nerve growth factor protects dorsal root ganglion neurons from peroxide toxicity. *J. Virol.,* **1999,** 73:519–532.

Gottesman, M.M., Germann, U.A., Aksentijevich, I., Sugimoto, Y., Cardarelli, C.O., and Pastan, I. Gene transfer of drug resistance genes. Implications for cancer therapy. *Ann. N.Y. Acad. Sci.,* **1994,** 716:126–138.

Greelish, J.P., Su, L.T., Lankford, E.B., Burkman, J.M., Chen, H., Konig, S.K., Mercier, I.M., Desjardins, P.R., Mitchell, M.A., Zheng, X.G., Leferovich, J., Gao, G.P., Balice-Gordon, R.J., Wilson, J.M., and Stedman, H.H. Stable restoration of the sarcoglycan complex in dystrophic muscle perfused with histamine and a recombinant adeno-associated viral vector. *Nat. Med.,* **1999,** 5:439–443.

Grossman, M., Raper, S.E., Kozarsky, K., Stein, E.A., Engelhardt, J.F., Muller, D., Lupien, P.J., and Wilson, J.M. Successful ex vivo gene therapy directed to liver in a patient with familial hypercholesterolaemia. *Nat. Genet.,* **1994,** 6:335–341.

Grubb, B.R., Pickles, R.J., Ye, H., Yankaskas, J.R., Vick, R.N., Engelhardt, J.F., Wilson, J.M., Johnson, L.G., and Boucher, R.C. Inefficient gene transfer by adenovirus vector to cystic fibrosis airway epithelia of mice and humans. *Nature,* **1994,** 371:802–806.

Guo, H., Karberg, M., Long, M., Jones, J.P. III, Sullenger, B., and Lambowitz, A.M. Group II introns designed to insert into therapeutically relevant DNA target sites in human cells. *Science,* **2000,** 289:452–457.

Hagstrom, J.N., Couto, L.B., Scallan, C., Burton, M., McCleland, M.L., Fields, P.A., Arruda, V.R., Herzog, R.W., and High, K.A. Improved muscle-derived expression of human coagulation factor IX from a skeletal actin/CMV hybrid enhancer/promoter. *Blood,* **2000,** 95:2536–2542.

Halene, S., and Kohn, D.B. Gene therapy using hematopoietic stem cells: sisyphus approaches the crest. *Hum. Gene Ther.,* **2000,** 11:1259–1267.

Hanania, E.G., Giles, R.E., Kavanagh, J., Fu, S.Q., Ellerson, D., Zu, Z., Wang, T., Su, Y., Kudelka, A., Rahman, Z., Holmes, F., Hortobagyi, G., Claxton, D., Bachier, C., Thall, P., Cheng, S., Hester, J., Ostrove, J.M., Bird, R.E., Chang, A., Korbling, M., Seong, D., Cote, R., Holzmayer, T., Deisseroth, A.B., *et al.* Results of MDR-1 vector modification trial indicate that granulocyte/macrophage colony-forming unit cells do not contribute to posttransplant hematopoietic recovery following intensive systemic therapy. *Proc. Natl. Acad. Sci. U.S.A.,* **1996,** *93*:15346–15351.

Harvey, B.G., Leopold, P.L., Hackett, N.R., Grasso, T.M., Williams, P.M., Tucker, A.L., Kaner, R.J., Ferris, B., Gonda, I., Sweeney, T.D., Ramalingam, R., Kovesdi, I., Shak, S., and Crystal, R.G. Airway epithelial CFTR mRNA expression in cystic fibrosis patients after repetitive administration of a recombinant adenovirus. *J. Clin. Invest.,* **1999,** *104*:1245–1255.

Hengge, U.R., Walker, P.S., and Vogel, J.C. Expression of naked DNA in human, pig, and mouse skin. *J. Clin. Invest.,* **1996,** 97:2911–2916.

Herzog, R.W., Yang, E.Y., Couto, L.B., Hagstrom, J.N., Elwell, D., Fields, P.A., Burton, M., Bellinger, D.A., Read, M.S., Brinkhous, K.M., Podsakoff, G.M., Nichols, T.C., Kurtzman, G.J., and High, K.A. Long-term correction of canine hemophilia B by gene transfer of blood coagulation factor IX mediated by adeno-associated viral vector. *Nat. Med.,* **1999,** *5*:56–63.

Hesdorffer, C., Ayello, J., Ward, M., Kaubisch, A., Vahdat, L., Balmaceda, C., Garrett, T., Fetell, M., Reiss, R., Bank, A., and Antman, K. Phase I trial of retroviral-mediated transfer of the human MDR1 gene as marrow chemoprotection in patients undergoing high-dose chemotherapy and autologous stem-cell transplantation. *J. Clin. Oncol.,* **1998,** *16*:165–172.

Iida, A., Chen, S.T., Friedmann, T., and Yee, J.K. Inducible gene expression by retrovirus-mediated transfer of a modified tetracycline-regulated system. *J. Virol.,* **1996,** *70*:6054–6059.

James, H., Mills, K., and Gibson, I. Investigating and improving the specificity of ribozymes directed against the bcr-abl translocation. *Leukemia,* **1996,** *10*:1054–1064.

Jones, J.T., Lee, S.W., and Sullenger, B.A. Tagging ribozyme reaction sites to follow *trans*-splicing in mammalian cells. *Nat. Med.,* **1996,** *2*:643–648.

Jones, J.T., and Sullenger, B.A. Evaluating and enhancing ribozyme reaction efficiency in mammalian cells. *Nat. Biotechnol.,* **1997,** *15*:902–905.

Kalberer, C.P., Pawliuk, R., Imren, S., Bachelot, T., Takekoshi, K.J., Fabry, M., Eaves, C.J., London, I.M., Humphries, R.K., and Leboulch, P. Preselection of retrovirally transduced bone marrow avoids subsequent stem cell gene silencing and age-dependent extinction of expression of human beta-globin in engrafted mice. *Proc. Natl. Acad. Sci. U.S.A.,* **2000,** *97*:5411–5415.

Kay, M.A., Manno, C.S., Ragni, M.V., Larson, P.J., Couto, L.B., McClelland, A., Glader, B., Chew, A.J., Tai, S.J., Herzog, R.W., Arruda, V., Johnson, F., Scallan, C., Skarsgard, E., Flake, A.W., and High, K.A. Evidence for gene transfer and expression of factor IX in haemophilia B patients treated with an AAV vector. *Nat. Genet.,* **2000,** *24*:257–261.

Klinman, D.M., Conover, J., Leiden, J.M., Rosenberg, A.S., and Sechler, J.M. Safe and effective regulation of hematocrit by gene gun administration of an erythropoietin-encoding DNA plasmid. *Hum. Gene Ther.,* **1999,** *10*:659–665.

Kochanek, S. High-capacity adenoviral vectors for gene transfer and somatic gene therapy. *Hum. Gene Ther.,* **1999,** *10*:2451–2459.

Kowalczyk, D.W., and Ertl, H.C. Immune responses to DNA vaccines. *Cell Mol. Life Sci.,* **1999,** *55*:751–770.

Kren, B.T., Cole-Strauss, A., Kmiec, E.B., and Steer, C.J. Targeted nucleotide exchange in the alkaline phosphatase gene of HuH-7 cells mediated by a chimeric RNA/DNA oligonucleotide. *Hepatology,* **1997,** *25*:1462–1468.

Kren, B.T., Parashar, B., Bandyopadhyay, P., Chowdhury, N.R., Chowdhury, J.R., and Steer, C.J. Correction of the UDP-glucuronosyltransferase gene defect in the gunn rat model of Crigler-Najjar syndrome type I with a chimeric oligonucleotide. *Proc. Natl. Acad. Sci. U.S.A.,* **1999,** *96*:10349–10354.

Krisky, D.M., Marconi, P.C., Oligino, T., Rouse, R.J., Fink, D.J., and Glorioso, J.C. Rapid method for construction of recombinant HSV gene transfer vectors. *Gene Ther.,* **1997,** *4*:1120–1125.

Krisky, D.M., Wolfe, D., Goins, W.F., Marconi, P.C., Ramakrishnan, R., Mata, M., Rouse, R.J., Fink, D.J., and Glorioso, J.C. Deletion of multiple immediate-early genes from herpes simplex virus reduces cytotoxicity and permits long-term gene expression in neurons. *Gene Ther.,* **1998,** *5*:1593–1603.

Lachmann, R.H., and Efstathiou, S. Utilization of the herpes simplex virus type 1 latency-associated regulatory region to drive stable reporter gene expression in the nervous system. *J. Virol.,* **1997,** *71*:3197–3207.

Lan, N., Howrey, R.P., Lee, S.W., Smith, C.A., and Sullenger, B.A. Ribozyme-mediated repair of sickle β-globin mRNAs in erythrocyte precursors. *Science,* **1998,** *280*:1593–1596.

Laquerre, S., Argnani, R., Anderson, D.B., Zucchini, S., Manservigi, R., and Glorioso, J.C. Heparan sulfate proteoglycan binding by herpes simplex virus type 1 glycoproteins B and C, which differ in their contributions to virus attachment, penetration, and cell-to-cell spread. *J. Virol.,* **1998,** *72*:6119–6130.

Le, T.P., Coonan, K.M., Hedstrom, R.C., Charoenvit, Y., Sedegah, M., Epstein, J.E., Kumar, S., Wang, R., Doolan, D.L., Maguire, J.D., Parker, S.E., Hobart, P., Norman, J., and Hoffman, S.L. Safety, tolerability and humoral immune responses after intramuscular administration of a malaria DNA vaccine to healthy adult volunteers. *Vaccine,* **2000,** *18*:1893–1901.

Leavitt, M.C., Yu, M., Yamada, O., Kraus, G., Looney, D., Poeschla, E., and Wong-Staal, F. Transfer of an anti-HIV-1 ribozyme gene into primary human lymphocytes. *Hum. Gene Ther.,* **1994,** *5*:1115–1120.

Ledley, T.S., and Ledley, F.D. Multicompartment, numerical model of cellular events in the pharmacokinetics of gene therapies. *Hum. Gene Ther.,* **1994,** *5*:679–691.

Li, X., Mukai, T., Young, D., Frankel, S., Law, P., and Wong-Staal, F. Transduction of CD34+ cells by a vesicular stomach virus protein G (VSV-G) pseudotyped HIV-1 vector. Stable gene expression in progeny cells, including dendritic cells. *J. Hum. Virol.,* **1998,** *1*:346–352.

Lifton, R.P. Molecular genetics of human blood pressure variation. *Science,* **1996,** *272*:676–680.

Malech, H.L., Maples, P.B., Whiting-Theobald, N., Linton, G.F., Sekhsaria, S., Vowells, S.J., Li, F., Miller, J.A., DeCarlo, E., Holland, S.M., Leitman, S.F., Carter, C.S., Butz, R.E., Read, E.J., Fleisher, T.A., Schneiderman, R.D., Van Epps, D.E., Spratt, S.K., Maack, C.A., Rokovich, J.A., Cohen, L.K., and Gallin, J.I. Prolonged production of NADPH oxidase-corrected granulocytes after gene therapy of chronic granulomatous disease. *Proc. Natl. Acad. Sci. U.S.A.,* **1997,** *94*:12133–12138.

Marshall, E. Gene therapy death prompts review of adenovirus vector. *Science,* **1999,** *286*:2244–2245.

Marshall, K.R., Lachmann, R.H., Efstathiou, S., Rinaldi, A., and Preston, C.M. Long-term transgene expression in mice infected with a herpes simplex virus type 1 mutant severely impaired for immediate-early gene expression. *J. Virol.,* **2000,** *74*:956–964.

May, C., Rivella, S., Callegari, J., Heller, G., Gaensler, K.M., Luzzatto, L., and Sadelain, M. Therapeutic haemoglobin synthesis in beta-thalassaemic mice expressing lentivirus-encoded human beta-globin. *Nature,* **2000,** *406*:82–86.

Michael, S.I., and Curiel, D.T. Strategies to achieve targeted gene delivery via the receptor-mediated endocytosis pathway. *Gene Ther.,* **1994,** *1*:223–232.

Miletic, H., Bruns, M., Tsiakas, K., Vogt, B., Rezai, R., Baum, C., Kuhlke, K., Cosset, F.L., Ostertag, W., Lother, H., and von Laer, D. Retroviral vectors pseudotyped with lymphocytic choriomeningitis virus. *J. Virol.,* **1999,** *73*:6114–6116.

Miyoshi, H., Smith, K.A., Mosier, D.E., Verma, I.M., and Torbett, B.E. Transduction of human CD34+ cells that mediate long-term engraftment of NOD/SCID mice by HIV vectors. *Science,* **1999,** *283*:682–686.

Moscow, J.A., Huang, H., Carter, C., Hines, K., Zujewski, J., Cusack, G., Chow, C., Venzon, D., Sorrentino, B., Chiang, Y., Goldspiel, B., Leitman, S., Read, E.J., Abati, A., Gottesman, M.M., Pastan, I., Sellers, S., Dunbar, C., and Cowan, K.H. Engraftment of MDR1 and NeoR gene-transduced hematopoietic cells after breast cancer chemotherapy. *Blood,* **1999,** *94*:52–61.

Nalbantoglu, J., Pari, G., Karpati, G., and Holland, P.C. Expression of the primary coxsackie and adenovirus receptor is downregulated during skeletal muscle maturation and limits the efficacy of adenovirus-mediated gene delivery to muscle cells. *Hum. Gene Ther.,* **1999,** *10*:1009–1019.

Nguyen, T.H., Pages, J.C., Farge, D., Briand, P., and Weber, A. Amphotropic retroviral vectors displaying hepatocyte growth factor-envelope fusion proteins improve transduction efficiency of primary hepatocytes. *Hum. Gene Ther.,* **1998,** *9*:2469–2479.

Park, F., Ohashi, K., Chiu, W., Naldini, L., and Kay, M.A. Efficient lentiviral transduction of liver requires cell cycling in vivo. *Nat. Genet.,* **2000,** *24*:49–52.

Phylactou, L.A., Darrah, C., and Wood, M.J. Ribozyme-mediated *trans*-splicing of a trinucleotide repeat. *Nat. Genet.,* **1998,** *18*:378–381.

Pisetsky, D.S. The influence of base sequence on the immunostimulatory properties of DNA. *Immunol. Res.,* **1999,** *19*:35–46.

Rafael, J.A., Tinsley, J.M., Potter, A.C., Deconinck, A.E., and Davies, K.E. Skeletal muscle-specific expression of a utrophin transgene rescues utrophin-dystrophin deficient mice. *Nat. Genet.,* **1998,** *19*:79–82.

Rando, T.A., Disatnik, M.H., and Zhou, L.Z. Rescue of dystrophin expression in mdx mouse muscle by RNA/DNA oligonucleotides. *Proc. Natl. Acad. Sci. U.S.A.,* **2000,** *97*:5363–5368.

Rivadeneira, E.D., Popescu, N.C., Zimonjic, D.B., Cheng, G.S., Nelson, P.J., Ross, M.D., DiPaolo, J.A., and Klotman, M.E. Sites of recombinant adeno-associated virus integration. *Int. J. Oncol.,* **1998,** *12*:805–810.

Rivella, S., and Sadelain, M. Genetic treatment of severe hemoglobinopathies: the combat against transgene variegation and transgene silencing. *Semin. Hematol.,* **1998,** *35*:112–125.

Rivera, V.M., Ye, X., Courage, N.L., Sachar, J., Cerasoli, F. Jr., Wilson, J.M., and Gilman, M. Long-term regulated expression of growth hormone in mice after intramuscular gene transfer. *Proc. Natl. Acad. Sci. U.S.A.,* **1999,** *96*:8657–8662.

Rogulski, K.R., Wing, M.S., Paielli, D.L., Gilbert, J.D., Kim, J.H., and Freytag, S.O. Double suicide gene therapy augments the antitumor activity of a replication-competent lytic adenovirus through enhanced cytotoxicity and radiosensitization. *Hum. Gene Ther.,* **2000,** *11*:67–76.

Roman, M., Martin-Orozco, E., Goodman, J.S., Nguyen, M.D., Sato, Y., Ronaghy, A., Kornbluth, R.S., Richman, D.D., Carson, D.A., and Raz, E. Immunostimulatory DNA sequences function as T helper-1-promoting adjuvants. *Nat. Med.,* **1997,** *3*:849–854.

Rosenberg, S.A., Blaese, R.M., Brenner, M.K., Deisseroth, A.B., Ledley, F.D., Lotze, M.T., Wilson, J.M., Nabel, G.J., Cornetta, K.,

Economou, J.S., Freeman, S.M., Riddell, S.R., Brenner, M., Oldfield, E., Gansbacher, B., Dunbar, C., Walker, R.E., Schuening, F.G., Roth, J.A., Crystal, R.G., Welsh, M.J., Culver, K., Heslop, H.E., Simons, J., Wilmott, R.W., Boucher, R.C., Siegler, H.F., Barranger, J.A., Karlsson, S., Kohn, D., Galpin, J.E., Raffel, C., Hesdorffer, C., Ilan, J., Cassileth, P., O'Shaughnessy, J., Kun, L.E., Das, T.K., Wong-Staal, F., Sobol, R.E., Haubrich, R., Sznol, M., Rubin, J., Sorcher, E.J., Rosenblatt, J., Walker, R., Brigham, K., Vogelzang, N., Hersh, E., Curiel, D., Evans, C.H., Freedman, R., Liu, J., Simons, J., Flotte, T.R., Holt, J., Lyerly, H.K., Whitley, C.B., Isner, J.M., and Eck, S.L. Human gene marker/therapy clinical protocols. *Hum. Gene Ther.,* **2000,** *11*:919–979.

Sarver, N., Cantin, E.M., Chang, P.S., Zaia, J.A., Ladne, P.A., Stephens, D.A., and Rossi, J.J. Ribozymes as potential anti-HIV-1 therapeutic agents. *Science,* **1990,** *247*:1222–1225.

Sato, Y., Roman, M., Tighe, H., Lee, D., Corr, M., Nguyen, M.D., Silverman, G.J., Lotz, M., Carson, D.A., and Raz, E. Immunostimulatory DNA sequences necessary for effective intradermal gene immunization. *Science,* **1996,** *273*:352–354.

Scharovsky, O.G., Rozados, V.R., Gervasoni, S.I., and Matar, P. Inhibition of *ras* oncogene: a novel approach to antineoplastic therapy. *J. Biomed. Sci.,* **2000,** *7*:292–298.

Sheehan, J.P., and Lan, H.C. Phosphorothioate oligonucleotides inhibit the intrinsic tenase complex. *Blood,* **1998,** *92*:1617–1625.

Shore, S.K., Nabissa, P.M., and Reddy, E.P. Ribozyme-mediated cleavage of the BCRABL oncogene transcript: in vitro cleavage of RNA and in vivo loss of P210 protein-kinase activity. *Oncogene,* **1993,** *8*:3183–3188.

Soriano, P., Dijkstra, J., Legrand, A., Spanjer, H., Londos-Gagliardi, D., Roerdink, F., Scherphof, G., and Nicolau, C. Targeted and nontargeted liposomes for in vivo transfer to rat liver cells of a plasmid containing the preproinsulin I gene. *Proc. Natl. Acad. Sci. U.S.A.,* **1983,** *80*:7128–7131.

Srinivasakumar, N., and Schuening, F.G. A lentivirus packaging system based on alternative RNA transport mechanisms to express helper and gene transfer vector RNAs and its use to study the requirement of accessory proteins for particle formation and gene delivery. *J. Virol.,* **1999,** *73*:9589–9598.

Stedman, H., Wilson, J.M., Finke, R., Kleckner, A.L., and Mendell, J. Phase I clinical trial utilizing gene therapy for limb girdle muscular dystrophy: alpha-, beta-, gamma-, or delta-sarcoglycan gene delivered with intramuscular instillations of adeno-associated vectors. *Hum. Gene Ther.,* **2000,** *11*:777–790.

Sullenger, B.A., and Cech, T.R. Ribozyme-mediated repair of defective mRNA by targeted, *trans*-splicing. *Nature,* **1994,** *371*:619–622.

Summerford, C., Bartlett, J.S., and Samulski, R.J. AlphaVbeta5 integrin: a co-receptor for adeno-associated virus type 2 infection. *Nat. Med.,* **1999,** *5*:78–82.

Summerford, C., and Samulski, R.J. Membrane-associated heparan sulfate proteoglycan is a receptor for adeno-associated virus type 2 virions. *J. Virol.,* **1998,** *72*:1438–1445.

Sun, L., Li, J., and Xiao, X. Overcoming adeno-associated virus vector size limitation through viral DNA heterodimerization. *Nat. Med.,* **2000,** *6*:599–602.

Tacket, C.O., Roy, M.J., Widera, G., Swain, W.F., Broome, S., and Edelman, R. Phase 1 safety and immune response studies of a DNA vaccine encoding hepatitis B surface antigen delivered by a gene delivery device. *Vaccine,* **1999,** *17*:2826–2829.

Tepper, R.I., and Mule, J.J. Experimental and clinical studies of cytokine gene-modified tumor cells. *Hum. Gene Ther.,* **1994,** *5*:153–164.

Tripathy, S.K., Svensson, E.C., Black, H.B., Goldwasser, E., Margalith, M., Hobart, P.M., and Leiden, J.M. Long-term expression of erythropoietin in the systemic circulation of mice after intramuscular injection of a plasmid DNA vector. *Proc. Natl. Acad. Sci. U.S.A.,* **1996,** *93*:10876–10880.

VandenDriessche, T., Vanslembrouck, V., Goovaerts, I., Zwinnen, H., Vanderhaeghen, M.L., Collen, D., and Chuah, M.K. Long-term expression of human coagulation factor VIII and correction of hemophilia A after in vivo retroviral gene transfer in factor VIII-deficient mice. *Proc. Natl. Acad. Sci. U.S.A.,* **1999,** *96*:10379–10384.

Wands, J.R., Geissler, M., Putlitz, J.Z., Blum, H., Weizsacker, F.V., Mohr, L., Yoon, S.K., Melegari, M., and Scaglioni, P.P. Nucleic acid-based antiviral and gene therapy of chronic hepatitis B infection. *J. Gastroenterol. Hepatol.,* **1997,** *12*:S354–S369.

Watanabe, T., and Sullenger, B.A. Induction of wild-type p53 activity in human cancer cells by ribozymes that repair mutant p53 transcripts. *Proc. Natl. Acad. Sci. U.S.A.,* **2000,** *97*:8490–8494.

Wolff, J.A., Ludtke, J.J., Acsadi, G., Williams, P., and Jani, A. Long-term persistence of plasmid DNA and foreign gene expression in mouse muscle. *Hum. Mol. Genet.,* **1992,** *1*:363–369.

Wong-Staal, F., Poeschla, E.M., and Looney, D.J. A controlled, phase 1 clinical trial to evaluate the safety and effects in HIV-1 infected humans of autologous lymphocytes transduced with a ribozyme that cleaves HIV-1 RNA. *Hum. Gene Ther.,* **1998,** *9*:2407–2425.

Wu, G.Y., and Wu, C.H. Receptor-mediated in vitro gene transformation by a soluble DNA carrier system. *J. Biol. Chem.,* **1987,** *262*:4429–4432.

Xiao, X., Li, J., and Samulski, R.J. Production of high-titer recombinant adeno-associated virus vectors in the absence of helper adenovirus. *J. Virol.,* **1998,** *72*:2224–2232.

Yan, Z., Zhang, Y., Duan, D., and Engelhardt, J.F. From the cover: trans-splicing vectors expand the utility of adeno-associated virus for gene therapy. *Proc. Natl. Acad. Sci. U.S.A.,* **2000,** *97*:6716–6721.

Yang, J., Zhou, W., Zhang, Y., Zidon, T., Ritchie, T., and Engelhardt, J.F. Concatamerization of adeno-associated virus circular genomes occurs through intermolecular recombination. *J. Virol.,* **1999,** *73*:9468–9477.

Yant, S.R., Meuse, L., Chiu, W., Ivics, Z., Izsvak, Z., and Kay, M.A. Somatic integration and long-term transgene expression in normal and haemophilic mice using a DNA transposon system. *Nat. Genet.,* **2000,** *25*:35–41.

Ye, X., Rivera, V.M., Zoltick, P., Cerasoli, F. Jr., Schnell, M.A., Gao, G., Hughes, J.V., Gilman, M., and Wilson, J.M. Regulated delivery of therapeutic proteins after in vivo somatic cell gene transfer. *Science,* **1999,** *283*:88–91.

Yoon, K., Cole-Strauss, A., and Kmiec, E.B. Targeted gene correction of episomal DNA in mammalian cells mediated by a chimeric RNA/DNA oligonucleotide. *Proc. Natl. Acad. Sci. U.S.A.,* **1996,** *93*:2071–2076.

Yoon, S.S., Nakamura, H., Carroll, N.M., Bode, B.P., Chiocca, E.A., and Tanabe, K.K. An oncolytic herpes simplex virus type 1 selectively destroys diffuse liver metastases from colon carcinoma. *FASEB J.,* **2000,** *14*:301–311.

Yu, M., Leavitt, M.C., Maruyama, M., Yamada, O., Young, D., Ho, A.D., and Wong-Staal, F. Intracellular immunization of human fetal cord blood stem/progenitor cells with a ribozyme against human immunodeficiency virus type 1. *Proc. Natl. Acad. Sci. U.S.A.,* **1995,** *92*:699–703.

Zenke, M., Steinlein, P., Wagner, E., Cotten, M., Beug, H., and Birnstiel, M.L. Receptor-mediated endocytosis of transferrin-polycation conjugates: an efficient way to introduce DNA into hematopoietic cells. *Proc. Natl. Acad. Sci. U.S.A.,* **1990,** *87*:3655–3659.

Zinn, K.R., Douglas, J.T., Smyth, C.A., Liu, H.G., Wu, Q., Krasnykh, V.N., Mountz, J.D., Curiel, D.T., and Mountz, J.M. Imaging and tissue biodistribution of 99mTc-labeled adenovirus knob (serotype 5). *Gene Ther.,* **1998,** *5*:798–808.

Zuckerman, J.B., Robinson, C.B., McCoy, K.S., Shell, R., Sferra, T.J., Chirmule, N., Magosin, S.A., Propert, K.J., Brown-Parr, E.C., Hughes, J.V., Tazelaar, J., Baker, C., Goldman, M.J., and Wilson, J.M. A phase I study of adenovirus-mediated transfer of the human cystic fibrosis transmembrane conductance regulator gene to a lung segment of individuals with cystic fibrosis. *Hum. Gene Ther.,* **1999,** *10*:2973–2985.

MONOGRAPHS AND REVIEWS

Agha-Mohammadi, S., and Lotze, M.T. Immunomodulation of cancer: potential use of selectively replicating agents. *J. Clin. Invest.,* **2000,** *105*:1173–1176.

Agrawal, S., and Kandimalla, E.R. Antisense therapeutics: is it as simple as complementary base recognition? *Mol. Med. Today,* **2000,** *6*:72–81.

Albelda, S.M., Wiewrodt, R., and Zuckerman, J.B. Gene therapy for lung disease: hype or hope? *Ann. Intern. Med.,* **2000,** *132*:649–660.

Alemany, R., Balague, C., and Curiel, D.T. Replicative adenoviruses for cancer therapy. *Nat. Biotechnol.,* **2000,** *18*:723–727.

Amado, R.G., and Chen, I.S. Lentiviral vectors—the promise of gene therapy within reach? *Science,* **1999,** *285*:674–676.

Anderson, W.F. Gene therapy. The best of times, the worst of times. *Science,* **2000,** *288*:627–629.

Aran, J.M., Pastan, I., and Gottesman, M.M. Therapeutic strategies involving the multidrug resistance phenotype: the MDR1 gene as target, chemoprotectant, and selectable marker in gene therapy. *Adv. Pharmacol.,* **1999,** *46*:1–42.

Bestor, T.H. Gene silencing as a threat to the success of gene therapy. *J. Clin. Invest.,* **2000,** *105*:409–411.

Blaese, R.M., Culver, K.W., Miller, A.D., Carter, C.S., Fleisher, T., Clerici, M., Shearer, G., Chang, L., Chiang, Y., Tolstoshev, P., *et al.* T lymphocyte-directed gene therapy for ADA-SCID: initial trial results after 4 years. *Science,* **1995,** *270*:475–480.

Boucher, R.C. Status of gene therapy for cystic fibrosis lung disease. *J. Clin. Invest.,* **1999,** *103*:441–445.

Cech, T.R. Ribozyme engineering. *Curr. Opin. Struct. Biol.,* **1992,** *2*:605–609.

Cech, T.R. Structure and mechanism of the large catalytic RNAs: group I and II introns and ribonuclease P. In, *The RNA World.* (Gesteland, R.F., and Atkins, J.F., eds.) Cold Spring Harbor Laboratory Press, Cold Spring Harbor, N.Y., **1993,** pp. 239–269.

Cotter, F.E. Antisense therapy of hematologic malignancies. *Semin. Hematol.,* **1999,** *36*:9–14.

Curiel, D.T. Strategies to adapt adenoviral vectors for targeted delivery. *Ann. N.Y. Acad. Sci.,* **1999,** *886*:158–171.

Davis, H.L., Michel, M.L., and Whalen, R.G. Use of plasmid DNA for direct gene transfer and immunization. *Ann. N.Y. Acad. Sci.,* **1995,** *772*:21–29.

Emery, D.W., and Stamatoyannopoulos, G. Stem cell gene therapy for the beta-chain hemoglobinopathies. Problems and progress. *Ann. N.Y. Acad. Sci.,* **1999,** *872*:94–107.

Ennist, D.L. Gene therapy for lung disease. *Trends Pharmacol. Sci.,* **1999,** *20*:260–266.

Fearon, E.R. Tumor suppressor genes. In, *The Genetic Basis of Human Cancer.* (Vogelstein, B., and Kinzler, K.W., eds.) McGraw-Hill, New York, **1998,** pp. 229–236.

Frank, D.N., and Pace, N.R. Ribonuclease P: unity and diversity in a tRNA processing ribozyme. *Annu. Rev. Biochem.,* **1998,** *67*:153–180.

Galderisi, U., Cascino, A., and Giordano, A. Antisense oligonucleotides as therapeutic agents. *J. Cell Physiol.,* **1999,** *181*:251–257.

Gewirtz, A.M., Sokol, D.L., and Ratajczak, M.Z. Nucleic acid therapeutics: state of the art and future prospects. *Blood,* **1998,** *92*:712–736.

Gomez-Navarro, J., Curiel, D.T., and Douglas, J.T. Gene therapy for cancer. *Eur. J. Cancer,* **1999,** *35*:2039–2057.

Gurunathan, S., Klinman, D.M., and Seder, R.A. DNA vaccines: immunology, application, and optimization. *Annu. Rev. Immunol.,* **2000,** *18*:927–974.

Hartigan-O'Connor, D., and Chamberlain, J.S. Developments in gene therapy for muscular dystrophy. *Microsc. Res. Tech.,* **2000,** *48*:223–238.

Haynes, J.R., McCabe, D.E., Swain, W.F., Widera, G., and Fuller, J.T. Particle-mediated nucleic acid immunization. *J. Biotechnol.,* **1996,** *44*:37–42.

Heise, C., and Kirn, D.H. Replication-selective adenoviruses as oncolytic agents. *J. Clin. Invest.,* **2000,** *105*:847–851.

Hermiston, T. Gene delivery from replication-selective viruses: arming guided missiles in the war against cancer. *J. Clin. Invest.,* **2000,** *105*:1169–1172.

Horwitz, M.S. Adenoviruses. In, *Fields Virology.* (Fields, B.N., and Knipe, D.M., eds.) Raven Press, New York, **1990,** pp. 1723–1740.

Irie, A., Kijima, H., Ohkawa, T., Bouffard, D.Y., Suzuki, T., Curcio, L.D., Holm, P.S., Sassani, A., and Scanlon, K.J. Anti-oncogene ribozymes for cancer gene therapy. *Adv. Pharmacol.,* **1997,** *40*:207–257.

James, H.A., and Gibson, I. The therapeutic potential of ribozymes. *Blood,* **1998,** *91*:371–382.

Jolly, D. Viral vector systems for gene therapy. *Cancer Gene Ther.,* **1994,** *1*:51–64.

Juengst, E.T. and Walters, L. Ethical issues in human gene transfer research. In, *The Development of Human Gene Therapy.* (Friedmann, T., ed.) Cold Spring Harbor Laboratory Press, Cold Spring Harbor, N.Y., **1999,** pp. 691–712.

Kaufman, R.J. Advances toward gene therapy for hemophilia at the millennium. *Hum. Gene Ther.,* **1999,** *10*:2091–2107.

Kay, M.A., and High, K. Gene therapy for the hemophilias. *Proc. Natl. Acad. Sci. U.S.A.,* **1999,** *96*:9973–9975.

Kijima, H., Ishida, H., Ohkawa, T., Kashani-Sabet, M., and Scanlon, K.J. Therapeutic applications of ribozymes. *Pharmacol. Ther.,* **1995,** *68*:247–267.

Kotin, R.M. Prospects for the use of adeno-associated virus as a vector for human gene therapy. *Hum. Gene Ther.,* **1994,** *5*:793–801.

Kume, A., and Dinauer, M.C. Gene therapy for chronic granulomatous disease. *J. Lab. Clin. Med.,* **2000,** *135*:122–128.

Levin, A.A. A review of the issues in the pharmacokinetics and toxicology of phosphorothioate antisense oligonucleotides. *Biochim. Biophys. Acta,* **1999,** *1489*:69–84.

Lin, M.T., Pulkkinen, L., Uitto, J., and Yoon, K. The gene gun: current applications in cutaneous gene therapy. *Int. J. Dermatol.,* **2000,** *39*:161–170.

Lode, H.N., and Reisfeld, R.A. Targeted cytokines for cancer immunotherapy. *Immunol. Res.,* **2000,** *21*:279–288.

Ma, D.D., Rede, T., Naqvi, N.A., and Cook, P.D. Synthetic oligonucleotides as therapeutics: the coming of age. *Biotechnol. Annu. Rev.,* **2000,** *5*:155–196.

MacColl, G.S., Goldspink, G., and Bouloux, P.M. Using skeletal muscle as an artificial endocrine tissue. *J. Endocrinol.,* **1999,** *162*:1–9.

Martuza, R.L. Conditionally replicating herpes vectors for cancer therapy. *J. Clin. Invest.,* **2000,** *105*:841–846.

Menke, A., and Hobom, G. Antiviral ribozymes. New jobs for ancient molecules. *Mol. Biotechnol.,* **1997,** *8*:17–33.

Monahan, P.E., and Samulski, R.J. AAV vectors: is clinical success on the horizon? *Gene Ther.,* **2000,** *7*:24–30.

Morris, J.C., Rouraine, T., Wildner, O., and Blaese, R.M. Suicide genes: gene therapy applications using enzyme/prodrug strategies. In, *The Development of Human Gene Therapy.* (Friedmann, T., ed.) Cold Spring Harbor Laboratory Press, Cold Spring Harbor, N.Y., **1999,** pp. 477–526.

Nettelbeck, D.M., Jerome, V., and Muller, R. Gene therapy: designer promoters for tumour targeting. *Trends Genet.,* **2000,** *16*:174–181.

Nichols, W.G., and Boeckh, M. Recent advances in the therapy and prevention of CMV infections. *J. Clin. Virol.,* **2000,** *16*:25–40.

Park, M. Oncogenes. In, *The Genetic Basis of Human Cancer.* (Vogelstein, B., and Kinzler, K.W., eds.) McGraw-Hill, New York, **1998,** pp. 205–228.

Parkman, R., Weinberg, K., Crooks, G., Nolta, J., Kapoor, N., and Kohn, D. Gene therapy for adenosine deaminase deficiency. *Annu. Rev. Med.,* **2000,** *51*:33–47.

Perry, C.M., and Balfour, J.A. Fomivirsen. *Drugs,* **1999,** *57*:375–380.

Persons, D.A., and Nienhuis, A.W. Gene therapy for the hemoglobin disorders: past, present, and future. *Proc. Natl. Acad. Sci. U.S.A.,* **2000,** *97*:5022–5024.

Poeschla, E., and Wong-Staal, F. Antiviral and anticancer ribozymes. *Curr. Opin. Oncol.,* **1994,** *6*:601–606.

Robbins, P.D., and Ghivizzani, S.C. Viral vectors for gene therapy. *Pharmacol. Ther.,* **1998,** *80*:35–47.

Rossi, J.J. Ribozymes, genomics and therapeutics. *Chem. Biol.,* **1999,** *6*:R33–R37.

Shetty, K., Wu, G.Y., and Wu, C.H. Gene therapy of hepatic diseases: prospects for the new millennium. *Gut,* **2000,** *46*:136–139.

Simonato, M., Manservigi, R., Marconi, P., and Glorioso, J. Gene transfer into neurones for the molecular analysis of behaviour: focus on herpes simplex vectors. *Trends Neurosci.,* **2000,** *23*:183–190.

Smith, R.M., and Wu, G.Y. Hepatocyte-directed gene delivery by receptor-mediated endocytosis. *Semin. Liver Dis.,* **1999,** *19*:83–92.

Springer, C.J., and Niculescu-Duvaz, I. Prodrug-activating systems in suicide gene therapy. *J. Clin. Invest.,* **2000,** *105*:1161–1167.

Sullenger, B.A. RNA repair as a novel approach to genetic therapy. *Gene Ther.,* **1999,** *6*:461–462.

Symons, R.H. Small catalytic RNAs. *Annu. Rev. Biochem.,* **1992,** *61*:641–671.

Tang, H., Kuhen, K.L., and Wong-Staal, F. Lentivirus replication and regulation. *Annu. Rev. Genet.,* **1999,** *33*:133–170.

van Deutekom, J.C., Hoffman, E.P., and Huard, J. Muscle maturation: implications for gene therapy. *Mol. Med. Today,* **1998,** *4*:214–220.

Welsh, M.J. Gene transfer for cystic fibrosis. *J. Clin. Invest.,* **1999,** *104*:1165–1166.

Wickham, T.J. Targeting adenovirus. *Gene Ther.,* **2000,** *7*:110–114.

Wivel, N.A., and Anderson, W.F. Human gene therapy: public policy and regulatory issues. In, *The Development of Human Gene Therapy.* (Friedmann, T., ed.) Cold Spring Harbor Laboratory Press, Cold Spring Harbor, N.Y., **1999,** pp. 671–689.

Ye, S., Cole-Strauss, A.C., Frank, B., and Kmiec, E.B. Targeted gene correction: a new strategy for molecular medicine. *Mol. Med. Today,* **1998,** *4*:431–437.

Yuen, A.R., and Sikic, B.I. Clinical studies of antisense therapy in cancer. *Front. Biosci.,* **2000,** *5*:D588–D593.

Acknowledgment

The authors wish to acknowledge Drs. Stephen L. Eck and James M. Wilson, authors of this chapter in the ninth edition of *Goodman and Gilman's The Pharmacological Basis of Therapeutics,* some of whose text has been retained.

SECTION II

DRUGS ACTING AT SYNAPTIC AND NEUROEFFECTOR JUNCTIONAL SITES

NEUROTRANSMISSION

The Autonomic and Somatic Motor Nervous Systems

Brian B. Hoffman and Palmer Taylor

The theory of neurohumoral transmission received direct experimental validation nearly a century ago (see von Euler, 1981), and extensive investigation during the ensuing years led to its general acceptance. Nerves transmit information across most synapses and neuroeffector junctions by means of specific chemical agents known as neurohumoral transmitters or, more simply, neurotransmitters. The actions of many drugs that affect smooth muscle, cardiac muscle, and gland cells can be understood and classified in terms of their mimicking or modifying the actions of the neurotransmitters released by the autonomic fibers at either ganglia or effector cells.

Most of the general principles concerning the physiology and pharmacology of the peripheral autonomic nervous system and its effector organs also apply with certain modifications to the neuromuscular junction of skeletal muscle and to the central nervous system (CNS). In fact, the study of neurotransmission in the CNS has benefited greatly from the delineation of this process in the periphery (see Chapter 12). In both the CNS and the periphery, a series of specializations have evolved to permit the synthesis, storage, release, metabolism, and recognition of transmitters. These specializations govern the actions of the principal autonomic transmitters acetylcholine and norepinephrine. Other neurotransmitters, including several peptides, purines, and nitric oxide, secondarily mediate autonomic function.

A clear understanding of the anatomy and physiology of the autonomic nervous system is essential to a study of the pharmacology of the intervening drugs. The actions of an autonomic agent on various organs of the body often can be predicted if the responses to nerve impulses that reach the organs are known. This chapter covers the anatomy, biochemistry, and physiology of the autonomic and somatic motor nervous systems, with emphasis on sites of action of drugs that are discussed in Chapters 7, 8, 9, and 10.

ANATOMY AND GENERAL FUNCTIONS OF THE AUTONOMIC AND SOMATIC MOTOR NERVOUS SYSTEMS

The autonomic nervous system, as delineated by Langley over a century ago (Langley, 1898), also is called the visceral, vegetative, or involuntary nervous system. In the periphery, its representation consists of nerves, ganglia, and plexuses that provide the innervation to the heart, blood vessels, glands, other visceral organs, and smooth muscle in various tissues. It is therefore widely distributed throughout the body and regulates autonomic functions, which occur without conscious control.

Differences between Autonomic and Somatic Nerves. The efferent nerves of the involuntary system supply all innervated structures of the body except skeletal muscle, which is served by somatic nerves. The most distal synaptic junctions in the autonomic reflex arc occur in ganglia that are entirely outside the cerebrospinal axis. These ganglia are small but complex structures that contain axodendritic synapses between preganglionic and postganglionic neurons. Somatic nerves contain no peripheral ganglia, and the synapses are located entirely within the cerebrospinal axis. Many autonomic nerves form extensive peripheral plexuses, but such networks are absent from the somatic system. Whereas motor nerves to skeletal muscles are myelinated, postganglionic autonomic nerves generally are nonmyelinated. When the spinal efferent nerves are interrupted, the skeletal muscles they innervate lack myogenic tone, are paralyzed, and atrophy, whereas smooth muscles and glands generally show some level of spontaneous activity independent of intact innervation.

Visceral Afferent Fibers. The afferent fibers from visceral structures are the first link in the reflex arcs of the autonomic system. With certain exceptions, such as local axon reflexes, most visceral reflexes are mediated through the central nervous system (CNS). The afferent fibers are, for the most part, non-myelinated and are carried into the cerebrospinal axis by the vagus, pelvic, splanchnic, and other autonomic nerves. For example, about four-fifths of the fibers in the vagus are sensory. Other autonomic afferents from blood vessels in skeletal muscles and from certain integumental structures are carried in somatic nerves. The cell bodies of visceral afferent fibers lie in the dorsal root ganglia of the spinal nerves and in the corresponding sensory ganglia of certain cranial nerves, such as the nodose ganglion of the vagus. The efferent link of the autonomic reflex arc is discussed in the following sections.

The autonomic afferent fibers are concerned with the mediation of visceral sensation (including pain and referred pain); with vasomotor, respiratory, and viscerosomatic reflexes; and with the regulation of interrelated visceral activities. An example of an autonomic afferent system is that arising from the pressoreceptive endings in the carotid sinus and the aortic arch and from the chemoreceptor cells in the carotid and aortic bodies; this system is important in the reflex control of blood pressure, heart rate, and respiration, and its afferent fibers pass in the glossopharyngeal and vagus nerves to the medulla oblongata in the brainstem.

The neurotransmitters that mediate transmission from sensory fibers have not been unequivocally characterized. However, substance P is present in afferent sensory fibers, in the dorsal root ganglia, and in the dorsal horn of the spinal cord, and this peptide is a leading candidate for the neurotransmitter that functions in the passage of nociceptive stimuli from the periphery to the spinal cord and higher structures. Other neuroactive peptides, including somatostatin, vasoactive intestinal polypeptide (VIP), and cholecystokinin, also have been found in sensory neurons (Lundburg, 1996; Hökfelt *et al.*, 2000), and one or more such peptides may play a role in the transmission of afferent impulses from autonomic structures. Enkephalins, present in interneurons in the dorsal spinal cord (within an area termed the *substantia gelatinosa*), have antinociceptive effects that appear to be brought about by presynaptic and postsynaptic actions to inhibit the release of substance P and diminish the activity of cells that project from the spinal cord to higher centers in the CNS. The excitatory amino acids, glutamate and aspartate, also play major roles in transmission of sensory responses to the spinal cord.

Central Autonomic Connections. There probably are no purely autonomic or somatic centers of integration, and extensive overlap occurs. Somatic responses always are accompanied by visceral responses and *vice versa*. Autonomic reflexes can be elicited at the level of the spinal cord. They clearly are demonstrable in the spinal animal, including human beings, and are manifested by sweating, blood pressure alterations, vasomotor

responses to temperature changes, and reflex emptying of the urinary bladder, rectum, and seminal vesicles. Extensive central ramifications of the autonomic nervous system exist above the level of the spinal cord. For example, the integration of the control of respiration in the medulla oblongata is well known. The hypothalamus and the nucleus of the solitary tract (nucleus tractus solitarius) generally are regarded as principal loci of integration of autonomic nervous system functions, which include regulation of body temperature, water balance, carbohydrate and fat metabolism, blood pressure, emotions, sleep, respiration, and sexual responses. Signals are received through ascending spinobulbar pathways. Also, these areas receive input from the limbic system, neostriatum, cortex, and, to a lesser extent, other higher brain centers. Stimulation of the nucleus of the solitary tract and the hypothalamus activates bulbospinal pathways and hormonal output to mediate autonomic and motor responses in the organism (Andresen and Kunze, 1994; Loewy and Spyer, 1990; *see also* Chapter 12). The hypothalamic nuclei that lie posteriorly and laterally are sympathetic in their main connections, while parasympathetic functions evidently are integrated by the midline nuclei in the region of the tuber cinereum and by nuclei lying anteriorly.

Divisions of the Peripheral Autonomic System. On the efferent side, the autonomic nervous system consists of two large divisions: (1) the sympathetic or thoracolumbar outflow and (2) the parasympathetic or craniosacral outflow. A brief outline of those anatomical features necessary for an understanding of the actions of autonomic drugs is given here.

The arrangement of the principal parts of the peripheral autonomic nervous system is presented schematically in Figure 6–1. As discussed below, the neurotransmitter of all preganglionic autonomic fibers, all postganglionic parasympathetic fibers, and a few postganglionic sympathetic fibers is *acetylcholine* (ACh); these so-called cholinergic fibers are depicted in blue. The adrenergic fibers, shown in red, compose the majority of the postganglionic sympathetic fibers; here the transmitter is *norepinephrine* (noradrenaline, levarterenol). The terms *cholinergic* and *adrenergic* were proposed originally by Dale (1954) to describe neurons that liberate ACh and norepinephrine, respectively. As noted above, all of the transmitter(s) of the primary afferent fibers, shown in green, have not been identified conclusively. Substance P and glutamate are thought to mediate many afferent impulses; both are present in high concentrations in the dorsal regions of the spinal cord.

Sympathetic Nervous System. The cells that give rise to the preganglionic fibers of this division lie mainly in the intermediolateral columns of the spinal cord and extend from the first thoracic to the second or third lumbar segment. The axons from these cells are carried in the anterior (ventral) nerve roots and synapse with neurons lying in sympathetic ganglia outside the

cerebrospinal axis. The sympathetic ganglia are found in three locations: paravertebral, prevertebral, and terminal.

The paravertebral sympathetic ganglia consist of 22 pairs that lie on either side of the vertebral column to form the lateral chains. The ganglia are connected to each other by nerve trunks and to the spinal nerves by rami communicantes. The white rami are restricted to the segments of the thoracolumbar outflow; they carry the preganglionic myelinated fibers that exit from the spinal cord by way of the anterior spinal roots. The gray rami arise from the ganglia and carry postganglionic fibers back to the spinal nerves for distribution to sweat glands and pilomotor muscles and to blood vessels of skeletal muscle and skin. The prevertebral ganglia lie in the abdomen and the pelvis near the ventral surface of the bony vertebral column and consist mainly of the celiac (solar), superior mesenteric, aorticorenal, and inferior mesenteric ganglia. The terminal ganglia are few in number, lie near the organs they innervate, and include ganglia connected with the urinary bladder and rectum and the cervical ganglia in the region of the neck. In addition, there are small intermediate ganglia, especially in the thoracolumbar region, that lie outside the conventional vertebral chain. They are variable in number and location but usually are in close proximity to the communicating rami and to the anterior spinal nerve roots.

Preganglionic fibers issuing from the spinal cord may synapse with the neurons of more than one sympathetic ganglion. Their principal ganglia of termination need not correspond to the original level from which the preganglionic fiber exits the spinal cord. Many of the preganglionic fibers from the fifth to the last thoracic segment pass through the paravertebral ganglia to form the splanchnic nerves. Most of the splanchnic nerve fibers do not synapse until they reach the celiac ganglion; others directly innervate the adrenal medulla (*see* below).

Postganglionic fibers arising from sympathetic ganglia innervate visceral structures of the thorax, abdomen, head, and neck. The trunk and the limbs are supplied by means of sympathetic fibers in spinal nerves, as previously described. The prevertebral ganglia contain cell bodies, the axons of which innervate the glands and the smooth muscles of the abdominal and the pelvic viscera. Many of the upper thoracic sympathetic fibers from the vertebral ganglia form terminal plexuses, such as the cardiac, esophageal, and pulmonary plexuses. The sympathetic distribution to the head and the neck (vasomotor, pupillodilator, secretory, and pilomotor) is by way of the cervical sympathetic chain and its three ganglia. All postganglionic fibers in this chain arise from cell bodies located in these three ganglia; all preganglionic fibers arise from the upper thoracic segments of the spinal cord, there being no sympathetic fibers that leave the CNS above the first thoracic level.

The adrenal medulla and other chromaffin tissue are embryologically and anatomically similar to sympathetic ganglia; all are derived from the neural crest. The adrenal medulla differs from sympathetic ganglia in that the principal catecholamine that is released in human beings and many other species is *epinephrine* (adrenaline), whereas norepinephrine is released from postganglionic sympathetic fibers. The chromaffin cells in the adrenal medulla are innervated by typical preganglionic fibers that release acetylcholine.

Parasympathetic Nervous System.   The parasympathetic nervous system consists of preganglionic fibers that originate in

three areas of the CNS and their postganglionic connections. The regions of central origin are the midbrain, the medulla oblongata, and the sacral part of the spinal cord. The midbrain, or tectal, outflow consists of fibers arising from the Edinger-Westphal nucleus of the third cranial nerve and going to the ciliary ganglion in the orbit. The medullary outflow consists of the parasympathetic components of the seventh, ninth, and tenth cranial nerves. The fibers in the seventh cranial, or facial, nerve form the chorda tympani, which innervates the ganglia lying on the submaxillary and sublingual glands. They also form the greater superficial petrosal nerve, which innervates the sphenopalatine ganglion. The ninth cranial, or glossopharyngeal, autonomic components innervate the otic ganglion. Postganglionic parasympathetic fibers from these ganglia supply the sphincter of the iris (pupillae constrictor muscle), the ciliary muscle, the salivary and lacrimal glands, and the mucous glands of the nose, mouth, and pharynx. These fibers also include vasodilator nerves to the organs mentioned. The tenth cranial, or vagus, nerve arises in the medulla and contains preganglionic fibers, most of which do not synapse until they reach the many small ganglia lying directly on or in the viscera of the thorax and abdomen. In the intestinal wall, the vagal fibers terminate around ganglion cells in the plexuses of Auerbach and Meissner. Preganglionic fibers are thus very long, whereas postganglionic fibers are very short. The vagus nerve, in addition, carries a far greater number of afferent fibers (but apparently no pain fibers) from the viscera into the medulla; the cell bodies of these fibers lie mainly in the nodose ganglion.

The parasympathetic sacral outflow consists of axons that arise from cells in the second, third, and fourth segments of the sacral cord and proceed as preganglionic fibers to form the pelvic nerves (nervi erigentes). They synapse in terminal ganglia lying near or within the bladder, rectum, and sexual organs. The vagal and sacral outflows provide motor and secretory fibers to thoracic, abdominal, and pelvic organs, as indicated in Figure 6–1.

Enteric Nervous System.   Stimulation of particular vagal nuclei in the medulla oblongata or certain fibers in the vagal trunk was known for some time to elicit muscle relaxation in certain regions of the stomach or intestine, such as sphincters, instead of the expected and more common contractile response. In the mid-1960s, it became evident that relaxation of the gastrointestinal tract and other visceral organs was not necessarily mediated by adrenergic stimulation; rather, release of other putative transmitters from enteric neurons, located in Auerbach's and Meissner's plexuses, gave rise to hyperpolarization and relaxation of the smooth muscle (Figure 6–1). Over the succeeding years, certain *peptides* (*i.e.,* VIP), *nucleotides* (ATP), and *nitric oxide* (NO) were found to be inhibitory transmitters in the gastrointestinal tract and other visceral organs (*see* Bennett, 1997). Inhibition is achieved either through guanylyl cyclase activation by nitric oxide or hyperpolarization through the activation of K^+ channels. Specific K^+ channel inhibitors such as apamin or inhibitors of nitric oxide synthase can distinguish the inhibitory events and their durations. Noncholinergic excitatory transmitters such as tachykinins (*e.g., substance P*) also are found to be released in regions of the enteric plexus. Substance P is a transmitter of the sensory afferent system, which is released locally or from afferent nerve branches that link to intramural ganglia. The enteric system does not have a unique connection to the CNS. While under the influence of parasympathetic pre-ganglionic nerves, release of transmitters usually is dominated by local control. Coordination of contraction and relaxation at a local level would be expected for regulation of peristaltic waves in the intestine.

Differences among Sympathetic, Parasympathetic, and Motor Nerves.   The sympathetic system is distributed to effectors throughout the body, whereas parasympathetic distribution is much more limited. Furthermore, the sympathetic fibers ramify to a much greater extent. A preganglionic sympathetic fiber may traverse a considerable distance of the sympathetic chain and pass through several ganglia before it finally synapses with a postganglionic neuron; also, its terminals make contact with a large number of postganglionic neurons. In some ganglia, the ratio of preganglionic axons to ganglion cells may be 1:20 or more. In this manner, a diffuse discharge of the sympathetic system is possible. In addition, synaptic innervation overlaps, so that one ganglion cell may be supplied by several preganglionic fibers.

The parasympathetic system, in contrast, has its terminal ganglia very near to or within the organs innervated and thus is more circumscribed in its influences. In some organs a 1:1 relationship between the number of preganglionic and postganglionic fibers has been suggested, but the ratio of preganglionic vagal fibers to ganglion cells in Auerbach's plexus has been estimated as 1:8000. Hence, this distinction between the two systems does not apply to all sites.

The cell bodies of somatic motor neurons are in the ventral horn of the spinal cord; the axon divides into many branches, each of which innervates a single muscle fiber, so that more than 100 muscle fibers may be supplied by one motor neuron to form a motor unit. At each neuromuscular junction, the axonal terminal loses its myelin sheath and forms a terminal arborization that lies in apposition to a specialized surface of the muscle membrane, termed the *motor end-plate.* Mitochondria and a collection of synaptic vesicles are concentrated at the nerve terminal. Through trophic influences of the nerve, those cell nuclei in the multinucleated skeletal muscle cell lying in close apposition to the synapse acquire the capacity to activate specific genes which express synapse-localized proteins (Hall and Sanes, 1993; Sanes and Lichtman, 1999).

Details of Innervation.   The terminations of the postganglionic autonomic fibers in smooth muscle and glands form a rich plexus, or terminal reticulum. The terminal reticulum (sometimes called the autonomic ground plexus) consists of the final ramifications of the postganglionic sympathetic (adrenergic), parasympathetic (cholinergic), and visceral afferent fibers, all

of which are enclosed within a frequently interrupted sheath of satellite or Schwann cells. At these interruptions, varicosities packed with vesicles are seen in the efferent fibers. Such varicosities occur repeatedly but at variable distances along the course of the ramifications of the axon.

"Protoplasmic bridges" occur between the smooth muscle fibers themselves at points of contact between their plasma membranes. They are believed to permit the direct conduction of impulses from cell to cell without the need for chemical transmission. These structures have been termed *nexuses* or *tight junctions,* and they enable the smooth muscle fibers to function as a unit or syncytium.

Sympathetic ganglia are extremely complex, both anatomically and pharmacologically (*see* Chapter 9). The preganglionic fibers lose their myelin sheaths and divide repeatedly into a vast number of end fibers with diameters ranging from 0.1 to 0.3 μm; except at points of synaptic contact, they retain their satellite-cell sheaths. The vast majority of synapses are axodendritic. Apparently, a given axonal terminal may synapse with one or more dendritic processes.

Responses of Effector Organs to Autonomic Nerve Impulses.   From the responses of the various effector organs to autonomic nerve impulses and the knowledge of the intrinsic autonomic tone, one can predict the actions of drugs that mimic or inhibit the actions of these nerves. In most instances, the sympathetic and parasympathetic neurotransmitters can be viewed as physiological or functional antagonists. If one neurotransmitter inhibits a certain function, the other usually augments that function. Most viscera are innervated by both divisions of the autonomic nervous system, and the level of activity at any one moment represents the integration of influences of the two components. Despite the conventional concept of antagonism between the two portions of the autonomic nervous system, their activities on specific structures may be either discrete and independent or integrated and interdependent. For example, the effects of sympathetic and parasympathetic stimulation of the heart and the iris show a pattern of functional antagonism in controlling heart rate and pupillary aperture, respectively. Their actions on male sexual organs are complementary and are integrated to promote sexual function. The control of peripheral vascular resistance is primarily, but not exclusively, due to sympathetic control of arteriolar resistance. The effects of stimulating the sympathetic (adrenergic) and parasympathetic (cholinergic) nerves to various organs, visceral structures, and effector cells are summarized in Table 6–1.

General Functions of the Autonomic Nervous System.   The integrating action of the autonomic nervous system is of vital importance for the well-being of the organism. In general, the autonomic nervous system regulates the activities of structures that are not under voluntary control

Table 6–1

Responses of Effector Organs to Autonomic Nerve Impulses

Effector Organs	Adrenergic Impulses[1]		Cholinergic Impulses[1]
	RECEPTOR TYPE[2]	RESPONSES[3]	RESPONSES[3]
Eye			
Radial muscle, iris	α_1	Contraction (mydriasis) ++	—
Sphincter muscle, iris		—	Contraction (miosis) +++
Ciliary muscle	β_2	Relaxation for far vision +	Contraction for near vision +++
Lacrimal glands	α	Secretion +	Secretion +++
Heart[4]			
SA node	β_1, β_2	Increase in heart rate ++	Decrease in heart rate; vagal arrest +++
Atria	β_1, β_2	Increase in contractility and conduction velocity ++	Decrease in contractility, and shortened AP duration ++
AV node	β_1, β_2	Increase in automaticity and conduction velocity ++	Decrease in conduction velocity; AV block +++
His–Purkinje system	β_1, β_2	Increase in automaticity and conduction velocity +++	Little effect
Ventricles	β_1, β_2	Increase in contractility, conduction velocity, automaticity, and rate of idioventricular pacemakers +++	Slight decrease in contractility
Arterioles			
Coronary	α_1, α_2; β_2	Constriction +; dilation[5] ++	Dilation (constriction with endothelial damage)
Skin and mucosa	α_1, α_2	Constriction +++	Dilation[6]
Skeletal muscle	α; β_2	Constriction ++; dilation[5,7] ++	Dilation[8] +
Cerebral	α_1	Constriction (slight)	Dilation[6]
Pulmonary	α_1; β_2	Constriction +; dilation[5]	Dilation[6]
Abdominal viscera	α_1; β_2	Constriction +++; dilation[7] +	—
Salivary glands	α_1, α_2	Constriction +++	Dilation ++
Renal	α_1, α_2; β_1, β_2	Constriction +++; dilation[7] +	—
Veins (Systemic)	α_1, α_2; β_2	Constriction ++; dilation ++	—
Lung			
Tracheal and bronchial muscle	β_2	Relaxation +	Contraction ++
Bronchial glands	α_1; β_2	Decreased secretion; increased secretion	Stimulation +++
Stomach			
Motility and tone	α_1, α_2; β_2	Decrease (usually)[9] +	Increase[9] +++
Sphincters	α_1	Contraction (usually) +	Relaxation (usually) +
Secretion		Inhibition (?)	Stimulation +++
Intestine			
Motility and tone	α_1, α_2; β_1, β_2	Decrease[9] +	Increase[9] +++
Sphincters	α_1	Contraction (usually) +	Relaxation (usually) +
Secretion	α_2	Inhibition	Stimulation ++
Gallbladder and Ducts	β_2	Relaxation +	Contraction +
Kidney			
Renin secretion	α_1; β_1	Decrease +; increase ++	—
Urinary bladder			
Detrusor	β_2	Relaxation (usually) +	Contraction +++
Trigone and sphincter	α_1	Contraction ++	Relaxation ++

(Continued)

Table 6–1

Responses of Effector Organs to Autonomic Nerve Impulses *(Continued)*

Effector Organs	Adrenergic Impulses[1]			Cholinergic Impulses[1]
	RECEPTOR TYPE[2]	RESPONSES[3]		RESPONSES[3]
Ureter				
Motility and tone	α_1	Increase		Increase (?)
Uterus	α_1; β_2	Pregnant: contraction (α_1); relaxation (β_2). Nonpregnant: relaxation (β_2)		Variable[10]
Sex Organs, Male	α_1	Ejaculation ++		Erection +++
Skin				
Pilomotor muscles	α_1	Contraction ++		—
Sweat glands	α_1	Localized secretion[11] +		Generalized secretion +++
Spleen Capsule	α_1; β_2	Contraction +++; relaxation +		—
Adrenal Medulla		—		Secretion of epinephrine and norepinephrine (primarily nicotinic and secondarily muscarinic)
Skeletal Muscle	β_2	Increased contractility; glycogenolysis; K^+ uptake		—
Liver	α_1; β_2	Glycogenolysis and gluconeogenesis[12] +++		—
Pancreas				
Acini	α	Decreased secretion +		Secretion ++
Islets (β cells)	α_2	Decreased secretion +++		—
	β_2	Increased secretion +		—
Fat Cells	α_2; β_1, β_2, β_3	Lipolysis[12] +++ (thermogenesis); inhibition of lipolysis		—
Salivary Glands	α_1	K^+ and water secretion +		K^+ and water secretion +++
	β	Amylase secretion +		
Nasopharyngeal Glands		—		Secretion ++
Pineal Gland	β	Melatonin synthesis		—
Posterior Pituitary	β_1	Antidiuretic hormone secretion		—

[1] The anatomical classes of adrenergic and cholinergic nerve fibers are depicted in Figure 6–1 in red and blue, respectively. A dash signifies no known functional innervation. Subtypes of muscarinic acetylcholine receptors are not indicated: most glands and smooth muscles appear to contain multiple subtypes with M_3 being dominant, while the heart largely contains M_2-muscarinic receptors (*see* Chapter 7 and Caulfield and Birdsall, 1998).

[2] Where a designation of subtype is not provided, the nature of the subtype has not been determined unequivocally.

[3] Responses are designated 1+ to 3+ to provide an approximate indication of the importance of adrenergic and cholinergic nerve activity in the control of the various organs and functions listed.

[4] β_1-Adrenergic receptors predominate in the human heart, but evidence indicates involvement of β_2-adrenergic receptors in cardiac regulation.

[5] Dilation predominates *in situ* due to metabolic autoregulatory phenomena.

[6] Cholinergic vasodilation at these sites is of questionable physiological significance.

[7] Over the usual concentration range of physiologically released, circulating epinephrine, β-receptor response (vasodilation) predominates in blood vessels of skeletal muscle and liver; α-receptor response (vasoconstriction), in blood vessels of other abdominal viscera. The renal and mesenteric vessels also contain specific dopaminergic receptors, activation of which causes dilation (*see* review by Goldberg *et al.,* 1978).

[8] Sympathetic cholinergic system causes vasodilation in skeletal muscle, but this is not involved in most physiological responses.

[9] While adrenergic fibers terminate at inhibitory β receptors on smooth muscle fibers and at inhibitory α receptors on parasympathetic cholinergic (excitatory) ganglion cells of Auerbach's plexus, the primary inhibitory response is mediated *via* enteric neurons through nitric oxide, purinergic receptors, and peptide receptors.

[10] Uterine responses depend on stage of menstrual cycle, amount of circulating estrogen and progesterone, and other factors.

[11] Palms of hands and some other sites ("adrenergic sweating").

[12] There is significant variation among species in the type of receptor that mediates certain metabolic responses. The human β_3 receptor has been cloned, but its role in lipolysis and/or thermogenesis in human fat cells is uncertain. β receptors also may inhibit leptin release from adipose tissue.

and that function below the level of consciousness. Thus, respiration, circulation, digestion, body temperature, metabolism, sweating, and the secretions of certain endocrine glands are regulated, in part or entirely, by the autonomic nervous system. As Claude Bernard (1878–1879), J.N. Langley (1898, 1901), and Walter Cannon (1929, 1932) emphasized, the constancy of the internal environment of the organism is to a large extent controlled by the vegetative, or autonomic, nervous system.

The sympathetic system and its associated adrenal medulla are not essential to life in a controlled environment. Under circumstances of stress, however, the lack of the sympathoadrenal functions becomes evident. Body temperature cannot be regulated when environmental temperature varies; the concentration of glucose in blood does not rise in response to urgent need; compensatory vascular responses to hemorrhage, oxygen deprivation, excitement, and exercise are lacking; resistance to fatigue is lessened; sympathetic components of instinctive reactions to the external environment are lost; and other serious deficiencies in the protective forces of the body are discernible.

The sympathetic system normally is continuously active; the degree of activity varies from moment to moment and from organ to organ. In this manner, adjustments to a constantly changing environment are accomplished. The sympathoadrenal system also can discharge as a unit. This occurs particularly during rage and fright, when sympathetically innervated structures over the entire body are affected simultaneously. Heart rate is accelerated; blood pressure rises; red blood cells are poured into the circulation from the spleen (in certain species); blood flow is shifted from the skin and splanchnic region to the skeletal muscles; blood glucose rises; the bronchioles and pupils dilate; and, on the whole, the organism is better prepared for "fight or flight." Many of these effects result primarily from, or are reinforced by, the actions of epinephrine, secreted by the adrenal medulla (*see* below). In addition, signals are received in higher brain centers to facilitate purposeful responses or to imprint the event in memory.

The parasympathetic system is organized mainly for discrete and localized discharge. Although it is concerned primarily with conservation of energy and maintenance of organ function during periods of minimal activity, its elimination is not compatible with life. Sectioning the vagus, for example, soon gives rise to pulmonary infection because of the inability of cilia to remove irritant substances from the respiratory tract. The parasympathetic system slows the heart rate, lowers the blood pressure, stimulates gastrointestinal movements and secretions, aids absorption of nutrients, protects the retina from excessive light, and empties the urinary bladder and rectum. Many parasympathetic responses are rapid and reflexive in nature.

NEUROTRANSMISSION

Nerve impulses elicit responses in smooth, cardiac, and skeletal muscles, exocrine glands, and postsynaptic neurons through liberation of specific chemical neurotransmitters. The steps involved and the evidence for them are presented in some detail because the concept of chemical mediation of nerve impulses profoundly affects our knowledge of the mechanism of action of drugs at these sites.

Historical Aspects

The earliest concrete proposal of a neurohumoral mechanism was made shortly after the turn of the twentieth century. Lewandowsky (1898) and Langley (1901) noted independently the similarity between the effects of injection of extracts of the adrenal gland and stimulation of sympathetic nerves. A few years later, in 1905, T.R. Elliott, while a student with Langley at Cambridge, England, extended these observations and postulated that sympathetic nerve impulses release minute amounts of an epinephrine-like substance in immediate contact with effector cells. He considered this substance to be the chemical step in the process of transmission. He also noted that, long after sympathetic nerves had degenerated, the effector organs still responded characteristically to the hormone of the adrenal medulla. In 1905, Langley suggested that effector cells have excitatory and inhibitory "receptive substances" and that the response to epinephrine depended on which type of substance was present. In 1907, Dixon was so impressed by the correspondence between the effects of the alkaloid muscarine and the responses to vagal stimulation that he advanced the important idea that the vagus nerve liberated a muscarine-like substance that acted as a chemical transmitter of its impulses. In the same year, Reid Hunt described the actions of ACh and other choline esters. In 1914, Dale thoroughly investigated the pharmacological properties of ACh along with other esters of choline and distinguished its nicotine-like and muscarine-like actions. He was so intrigued with the remarkable fidelity with which this drug reproduced the responses to stimulation of parasympathetic nerves that he introduced the term *parasympathomimetic* to characterize its effects. Dale also noted the brief duration of the action of this chemical and proposed that an esterase in the tissues rapidly splits ACh to acetic acid and choline, thereby terminating its action.

The studies of Otto Loewi, begun in 1921, provided the first direct evidence for the chemical mediation of nerve impulses by the release of specific chemical agents. Loewi stimulated the vagus nerve of a perfused (donor) frog heart and allowed the perfusion fluid to come in contact with a second (recipient) frog heart used as a test object. The recipient frog heart was found to respond, after a short lag, in the same way as did the donor heart. It was thus evident that a substance was liberated from the first organ that slowed the rate of the second. Loewi referred to this chemical substance as *Vagusstoff* ("vagus substance"; parasympathin); subsequently, Loewi and Navratil (1926) presented evidence to identify it as ACh. Loewi also discovered that an accelerator substance similar to epinephrine and called *Acceleranstoff* was liberated into the perfusion fluid in summer, when the action of the sympathetic fibers in the frog's vagus, a mixed nerve, predominated over that of the inhibitory fibers. Loewi's discoveries eventually were confirmed and became universally accepted. Evidence that the cardiac vagus-substance also is ACh in mammals was obtained in 1933 by Feldberg and Krayer.

In addition to the role of ACh as the transmitter of all postganglionic parasympathetic fibers and of a few postganglionic sympathetic fibers, this substance has been shown to have transmitter function in three additional classes of nerves: preganglionic fibers of both the sympathetic and the parasympathetic systems, motor nerves to skeletal muscle, and certain neurons within the CNS.

In the same year as Loewi's discovery, Cannon and Uridil (1921) reported that stimulation of the sympathetic hepatic nerves resulted in the release of an epinephrine-like substance that increased blood pressure and heart rate. Subsequent experiments firmly established that this substance is the chemical mediator liberated by sympathetic nerve impulses at neuroeffector junctions. Cannon called this substance "sympathin." In many of its pharmacological and chemical properties, "sympathin" closely resembled epinephrine, but also differed in certain important respects. As early as 1910, Barger and Dale noted that the effects of sympathetic nerve stimulation were more closely reproduced by the injection of sympathomimetic primary amines than by that of epinephrine or other secondary amines. The possibility that demethylated epinephrine (norepinephrine) might be "sympathin" had been repeatedly advanced, but definitive evidence for its being the sympathetic nerve mediator was not obtained until specific assays were developed for the determination of sympathomimetic amines in extracts of tissues and body fluids. von Euler in 1946 found that the sympathomimetic substance in highly purified extracts of bovine splenic nerve resembled norepinephrine by all criteria used. Norepinephrine is the predominant sympathomimetic substance in the postganglionic sympathetic nerves of mammals and is the adrenergic mediator liberated by their stimulation (*see* von Euler, 1972). Norepinephrine, its immediate precursor, dopamine, and epinephrine also are neurotransmitters in the CNS (*see* Chapter 12).

Evidence for Neurohumoral Transmission

The concept of neurohumoral transmission or chemical neurotransmission was developed primarily to explain observations relating to the transmission of impulses from postganglionic autonomic fibers to effector cells. The general lines of evidence to support the concept have included (1) demonstration of the presence of a physiologically active compound and its biosynthetic enzymes at appropriate sites; (2) recovery of the compound from the perfusate of an innervated structure during periods of nerve stimulation but not (or in greatly reduced amounts) in the absence of stimulation; (3) demonstration that the compound is capable of producing responses identical with responses to nerve stimulation; and (4) demonstration that the responses to nerve stimulation and to the administered compound are modified in the same manner by various drugs, usually competitive antagonists.

Chemical, rather than electrogenic, transmission at autonomic ganglia and the neuromuscular junction of skeletal muscle

was not generally accepted for a considerable period, because techniques were limited in time and chemical resolution. Techniques of intracellular recording and microiontophoretic application of drugs as well as sensitive analytical assays have overcome these limitations.

Neurotransmission in the peripheral and central nervous systems once was believed to conform to the hypothesis that each neuron contains only one transmitter substance. However, peptides, such as enkephalin, substance P, neuropeptide Y, VIP, and somatostatin; purines such as ATP or adenosine; and small molecules such as nitric oxide, have been found in nerve endings. These substances can depolarize or hyperpolarize nerve terminals or postsynaptic cells. Furthermore, results of histochemical, immunocytochemical, and autoradiographic studies have demonstrated that one or more of these substances is present in the same neurons that contain one of the classical biogenic amine neurotransmitters (Bartfai *et al.*, 1988; Lundberg *et al.*, 1996). For example, enkephalins are found in postganglionic sympathetic neurons and adrenal medullary chromaffin cells. VIP is localized selectively in peripheral cholinergic neurons that innervate exocrine glands, and neuropeptide Y is found in sympathetic nerve endings. These observations suggest that in many instances synaptic transmission may be mediated by the release of more than one neurotransmitter (*see* below).

Steps Involved in Neurotransmission

The sequence of events involved in neurotransmission is of particular importance pharmacologically, since the actions of most drugs modulate the individual steps. The term *conduction* is reserved for the passage of an impulse along an axon or muscle fiber; *transmission* refers to the passage of an impulse across a synaptic or neuroeffector junction. With the exception of the local anesthetics, very few drugs modify axonal conduction in the doses employed therapeutically. Hence, this process is described only briefly.

Axonal Conduction. Current knowledge of axonal conduction stems largely from the investigative work of Hodgkin and Huxley (1952).

At rest, the interior of the typical mammalian axon is approximately 70 mV negative to the exterior. The resting potential is essentially a diffusion potential, based chiefly on the fortyfold higher concentration of K^+ in the axoplasm as compared with the extracellular fluid and the relatively high permeability of the resting axonal membrane to this ion. Na^+ and Cl^- are present in higher concentrations in the extracellular fluid than in the axoplasm, but the axonal membrane at rest is considerably less permeable to these ions; hence their contribution to the resting potential is small. These ionic gradients are maintained by an energy-dependent active transport or pump mechanism, which involves an adenosine triphosphatase (ATPase) activated by Na^+ at the inner and by K^+ at the outer surface of the membrane (*see* Hille, 1992; Hille *et al.*, 1999a).

In response to depolarization to a threshold level, an action potential or nerve impulse is initiated at a local region of the membrane. The action potential consists of two phases. Following a small gating current resulting from depolarization inducing an open conformation of the channel, the initial phase is caused by a rapid increase in the permeability of Na^+ through voltage-sensitive Na^+ channels. The result is inward movement of Na^+ and a rapid depolarization from the resting potential, which continues to a positive overshoot. The second phase results from the rapid inactivation of the Na^+ channel and the delayed opening of a K^+ channel, which permits outward movement of K^+ to terminate the depolarization. Inactivation appears to involve a voltage-sensitive conformational change in which a hydrophobic peptide loop physically occludes the open channel at the cytoplasmic side. Although not important in axonal conduction, Ca^{2+} channels in other tissues (*e.g.*, heart) contribute to the action potential by prolonging depolarization by an inward movement of Ca^{2+}. This influx of Ca^{2+} also serves as a stimulus to initiate intracellular events (Hille, 1992; Catterall, 2000).

The transmembrane ionic currents produce local circuit currents around the axon. As a result of such localized changes in membrane potential, adjacent resting channels in the axon are activated, and excitation of an adjacent portion of the axonal membrane occurs. This brings about the propagation of the action potential without decrement along the axon. The region that has undergone depolarization remains momentarily in a refractory state. In myelinated fibers, permeability changes occur only at the nodes of Ranvier, thus causing a rapidly progressing type of jumping, or saltatory, conduction. The puffer fish poison, tetrodotoxin, and a close congener found in some shellfish, saxitoxin, selectively block axonal conduction; they do so by blocking the voltage-sensitive Na^+ channel and preventing the increase in permeability to Na^+ associated with the rising phase of the action potential. In contrast, batrachotoxin, an extremely potent steroidal alkaloid secreted by a South American frog, produces paralysis through a selective increase in permeability of the Na^+ channel to Na^+, which induces a persistent depolarization. Scorpion toxins are peptides that also cause persistent depolarization, but they do so by inhibiting the inactivation process (*see* Catterall, 2000). Na^+ and Ca^{2+} channels are discussed in more detail in Chapters 15, 32, and 35.

Junctional Transmission.   The arrival of the action potential at the axonal terminals initiates a series of events that trigger transmission of an excitatory or inhibitory impulse across the synapse or neuroeffector junction. These events, diagrammed in Figure 6–2, are as follows.

   1. *Storage and Release of the Transmitter.* The non-peptide (small molecule) neurotransmitters are largely synthesized in the region of the axonal terminals and stored there in synaptic vesicles. Peptide neurotransmitters (or precursor peptides) are found in large dense-core vesicles which are transported down the axon from their site of synthesis in the cell body. During the resting state, there is a continual slow release of isolated quanta of the transmitter; this produces electrical responses at the postjunctional membrane (miniature end-plate potentials, or mepps) that are associated with the maintenance of physiological responsiveness of the effector organ (*see* Katz, 1969). A low level of spontaneous activity within the motor units of skeletal muscle is particularly important, since skeletal muscle lacks inherent tone. The action potential causes the synchronous release of several hundred quanta of neurotransmitter. Depolarization of the axonal terminal triggers this process; a critical step in most but not all nerve endings is the influx of Ca^{2+}, which enters the axonal cytoplasm and promotes fusion between the axoplasmic membrane and those vesicles in close proximity to it (*see* Meir *et al.,* 1999; Hille *et al.,* 1999a). The contents of the vesicles, including enzymes and other proteins, then are discharged to the exterior by a process termed *exocytosis.* Synaptic vesicles may either fully exocytose with complete fusion and subsequent endocytosis or form a transient pore that closes after transmitter has escaped (Murthy and Stevens, 1998).

The presynaptic compartment can be viewed as an autonomous unit containing the components required for vesicle docking, exocytosis, endocytosis, membrane recycling, and recovery of the neurotransmitter (Fernandez-Chacon and Südhof, 1999; Lin and Scheller, 1997). Synaptic vesicles are clustered in discrete areas underlying the presynaptic plasma membrane, termed *active zones;* they often are aligned with the tips of postsynaptic folds. Some 20 to 40 proteins, playing distinct roles as transporter or trafficking proteins, are found in the vesicle. Neurotransmitter transport into the vesicle is driven by an electrochemical gradient generated by the vacuolar proton pump.

The function of the trafficking proteins is less well understood, but the vesicle protein synaptobrevin (VAMP) assembles with the plasma membrane proteins SNAP-25 and syntaxin 1 to form a core complex that initiates or drives the vesicle-plasma membrane fusion process. The submillisecond triggering of exocytosis by Ca^{2+} appears to be mediated by a separate family of proteins, the synaptotagmins.

A family of GTP binding proteins, the Rab 3 family, regulates the fusion process and cycles on and off the vesicle through GTP hydrolysis. Several other regulatory proteins of less well-defined function, synapsin, synaptophysin, and synaptogyrin, also play a role in fusion and exocytosis. So do families of proteins, such as RIM and neurexin, that are found on the active zones of the plasma membrane. Many of the trafficking proteins are homologous to those utilized in vesicular transport in yeast.

Over the last 30 years, an extensive variety of presynaptic receptors have been identified that control the release of neurotransmitters and synaptic strength (Langer, 1997; MacDermott *et al.,* 1999; von Kugelgen *et al.,* 1999). Their diversity nearly parallels that of postsynaptic receptors, and they have the capacity to be inhibitory or excitatory. Such receptors can influence the release of other transmitters from neighboring neurons or actually feed back to influence the subsequent release from the same neuron. The latter receptors are termed *autoreceptors.*

For example, norepinephrine may interact with a presynaptic α_2-adrenergic receptor to inhibit neurally mediated release

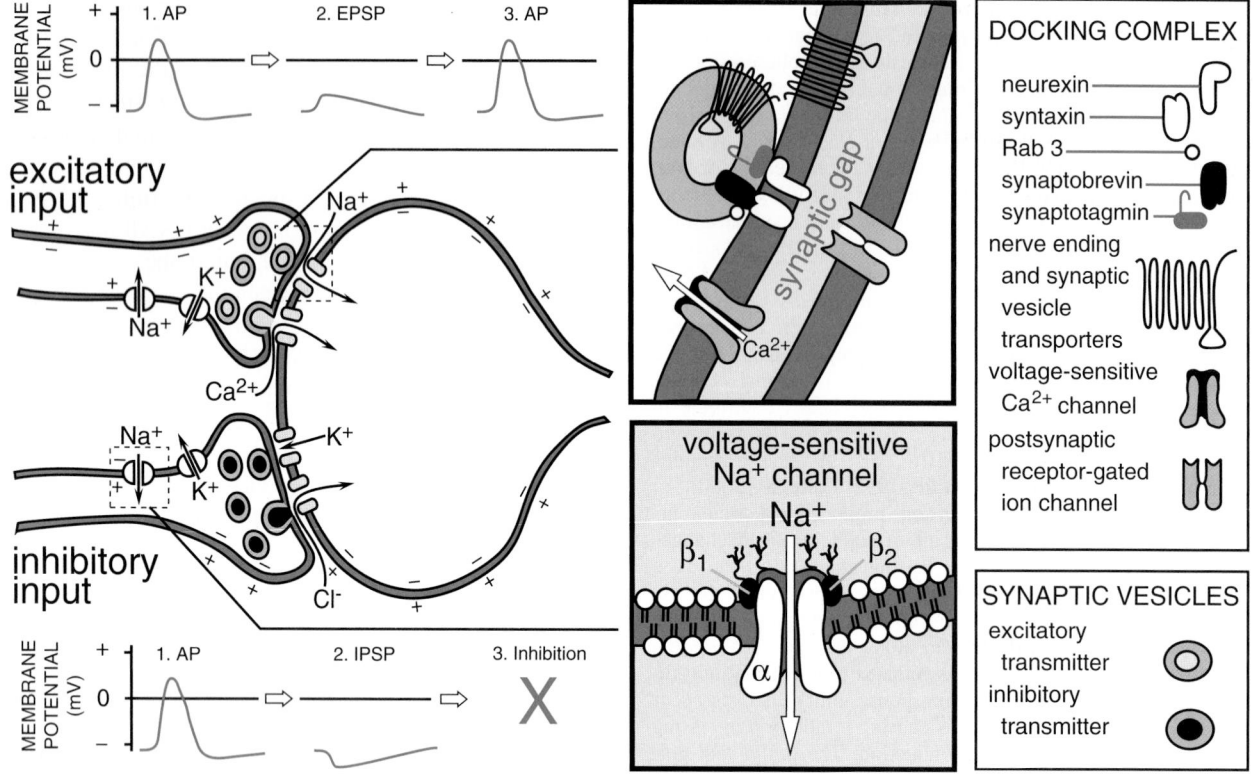

Figure 6–2. Steps involved in excitatory and inhibitory neurotransmission.

1. The nerve action potential (AP) consists of a transient self-propagated reversal of charge on the axonal membrane. (The internal potential, E_i, goes from a negative value, through zero potential, to a slightly positive value primarily through increases in Na^+ permeability and then returns to resting values by an increase in K^+ permeability.) When the action potential arrives at the presynaptic terminal, it initiates release of the excitatory or inhibitory transmitter. Depolarization at the nerve ending and entry of Ca^{2+} initiates docking and then fusion of the synaptic vesicle with membrane of the nerve ending. Docked and fused vesicles are shown. **2.** Combination of the excitatory transmitter with postsynaptic receptors produces a localized depolarization, the excitatory postsynaptic potential (EPSP), through an increase in permeability to cations, most notably Na^+. The inhibitory transmitter causes a selective increase in permeability to K^+ or Cl^-, resulting in a localized hyperpolarization, the inhibitory postsynaptic potential (IPSP). **3.** The EPSP initiates a conducted AP in the postsynaptic neuron; this can be prevented, however, by the hyperpolarization induced by a concurrent IPSP. The transmitter is dissipated by enzymatic destruction, by reuptake into the presynaptic terminal or adjacent glial cells, or by diffusion. (Modified from Eccles, 1964, 1973; Katz, 1966; Catterall, 1992; Jann and Südhof, 1994.)

of norepinephrine. The same subtype of α_2-adrenergic receptor inhibits the release of ACh from cholinergic neurons. Presynaptic muscarinic receptors mediate inhibition of evoked release of acetylcholine (Wessler, 1992) and also influence norepinephrine release in the myocardium and vasculature. Presynaptic nicotinic receptors enhance transmitter release in motor neurons (Bowman *et al.,* 1990) and in a variety of other central and peripheral synapses (MacDermott *et al.,* 1999).

Adenosine, dopamine, glutamate, GABA, prostaglandins, and enkephalins have been shown to influence neurally mediated release of various neurotransmitters. The receptors for these agents exert their modulatory effects, in part, by altering the function of prejunctional ion channels (Tsien *et al.,* 1988; Miller, 1998). A variety of ion channels that directly control transmitter release are found in presynaptic terminals (Meir *et al.,* 1999).

2. *Combination of the Transmitter with Postjunctional Receptors and Production of the Postjunctional Potential.* The transmitter diffuses across the synaptic or junctional cleft and combines with specialized receptors on the postjunctional membrane; this often results in a localized increase in the ionic permeability, or conductance, of the membrane. With certain exceptions, noted below, one of three types of permeability change can occur: (1) a generalized increase in the permeability to cations (notably Na^+, but occasionally Ca^{2+}, resulting in a localized depolarization of the membrane, *i.e.*, an excitatory postsynaptic potential (EPSP); (2) a selective increase in permeability to anions, usually Cl^-, resulting in stabilization or actual hyperpolarization of the membrane, which constitutes an inhibitory postsynaptic potential (IPSP); or (3) an increased permeability to K^+. Because the K^+ gradient is directed out of the cell, hyperpolarization and stabilization of the membrane potential occur (an IPSP).

It should be emphasized that the potential changes associated with the EPSP and IPSP at most sites are the results of passive fluxes of ions down their concentration gradients. The changes in channel permeability that cause these potential changes are specifically regulated by the specialized postjunctional receptors for the neurotransmitter that initiates the response (*see* Chapter 12 and the remainder of this section). These receptors may be clustered on the effector-cell surface, as seen at the neuromuscular junctions of skeletal muscle and other discrete synapses, or distributed in a more uniform fashion, as observed in smooth muscle.

By using microelectrodes that form high-resistance seals on the surface of cells, it is possible to record electrical events associated with a single neurotransmitter-gated channel (*see* Hille, 1992). In the presence of an appropriate neurotransmitter, the channel opens rapidly to a high-conductance state, remains open for about a millisecond, and then closes. A short, square-wave pulse of current is observed as a result of the channel opening and closing. The summation of these microscopic events gives rise to the EPSP. The graded response to a neurotransmitter usually is related to the frequency of opening events rather than to the extent of opening or the duration of opening. High-conductance ligand-gated ion channels usually permit passage of Na^+ or Cl^-; K^+ and Ca^{2+} are involved less frequently. The above ligand-gated channels belong to a large superfamily of ionotropic receptor proteins that includes the nicotinic, glutamate, and certain serotonin (5-HT_3) and purine receptors, which conduct primarily Na^+, cause depolarization, and are excitatory, and gamma-aminobutyric acid (GABA) and glycine receptors, which conduct Cl^-, cause hyperpolarization, and are inhibitory. The nicotinic, GABA, glycine, and 5-HT_3 receptors are closely related, whereas the glutamate and purinergic ionotropic receptors have distinct structures (Karlin and Akabas, 1995). Neurotransmitters also can modulate the permeability of channels for K^+ and Ca^{2+} indirectly. In these cases the receptor and channel are separate proteins, and information is conveyed between them by a G protein (*see* Chapter 2). Other receptors for neurotransmitters act by influencing the synthesis of intracellular second messengers and do not necessarily cause a change in membrane potential. The most widely documented examples of receptor regulation of second-messenger systems

are the activation or inhibition of adenylyl cyclase and the increase in intracellular concentrations of Ca^{2+} that results from release of the ion from internal stores by inositol trisphosphate (*see* Chapter 2).

3. *Initiation of Postjunctional Activity.* If an EPSP exceeds a certain threshold value, it initiates a propagated action potential in a postsynaptic neuron or a muscle action potential in skeletal or cardiac muscle by activating voltage-sensitive channels in the immediate vicinity. In certain smooth muscle types, in which propagated impulses are minimal, an EPSP may increase the rate of spontaneous depolarization, effect the release of Ca^{2+}, and enhance muscle tone; in gland cells, the EPSP initiates secretion through Ca^{2+} mobilization. An IPSP, which is found in neurons and smooth muscle but not in skeletal muscle, will tend to oppose excitatory potentials simultaneously initiated by other neuronal sources. Whether a propagated impulse or other response ensues depends on the summation of all the potentials.

4. *Destruction or Dissipation of the Transmitter.* When impulses can be transmitted across junctions at frequencies up to several hundred per second, it is obvious that there should be an efficient means of disposing of the transmitter following each impulse. At cholinergic synapses involved in rapid neurotransmission, high and localized concentrations of acetylcholinesterase (AChE) are available for this purpose. Upon inhibition of AChE, removal of the transmitter is accomplished principally by diffusion. Under these circumstances, the effects of released ACh are potentiated and prolonged.

Rapid termination of adrenergic transmitters occurs by a combination of simple diffusion and reuptake by the axonal terminals of most of the released norepinephrine (*see* Iversen, 1975). Termination of the action of amino acid transmitters results from their active transport into neurons and surrounding glia. Peptide neurotransmitters are hydrolyzed by various peptidases and dissipated by diffusion; specific uptake mechanisms have not been demonstrated for these substances.

5. *Nonelectrogenic Functions.* The continual quantal release of neurotransmitters in amounts not sufficient to elicit a postjunctional response probably is important in the transjunctional control of neurotransmitter action. The activity and turnover of enzymes involved in the synthesis and inactivation of neurotransmitters, the density of presynaptic and postsynaptic receptors, and other characteristics of synapses probably are controlled by trophic actions of neurotransmitters or other trophic factors released by the neuron or the target cells (Reichardt and Farinas, 1997; Sanes and Lichtman, 1999).

Cholinergic Transmission

Two enzymes, choline acetyltransferase and AChE, are involved in the synthesis and degradation, respectively, of ACh.

Choline Acetyltransferase. Choline acetyltransferase catalyzes the final step in the synthesis of ACh—the acetylation of choline with acetyl coenzyme A (CoA; *see* Wu and Hersh, 1994; Parsons *et al.*, 1993). The primary structure of choline acetyltransferase is known from molecular cloning, and its immunocytochemical localization has proven useful for identification of cholinergic axons and nerve cell bodies.

Acetyl CoA for this reaction is derived from pyruvate *via* the multistep pyruvate dehydrogenase reaction or is synthesized by acetate thiokinase, which catalyzes the reaction of acetate with adenosine triphosphate (ATP) to form an enzyme-bound acyladenylate (acetyl AMP). In the presence of CoA, transacetylation and synthesis of acetyl CoA proceed.

Choline acetyltransferase, like other protein constituents of the neuron, is synthesized within the perikaryon and then is transported along the length of the axon to its terminal. Axonal terminals contain a large number of mitochondria, where acetyl CoA is synthesized. Choline is taken up from the extracellular fluid into the axoplasm by active transport. The final step in the synthesis occurs within the cytoplasm, following which most of the ACh is sequestered within the synaptic vesicles. Although moderately potent inhibitors of choline acetyltransferase exist, they have no therapeutic utility, in part because the uptake of choline is the rate-limiting step in the biosynthesis of ACh.

Choline Transport. Transport of choline from the plasma into neurons is accomplished by distinct high- and low-affinity transport systems. The high-affinity system ($K_m =$ 1 to 5 μM) is unique to cholinergic neurons, is dependent on extracellular Na^+, and is inhibited by hemicholinium. Plasma concentrations of choline approximate 10 μM; thus, the concentration of choline does not limit its availability to cholinergic neurons. Much of the choline formed from AChE-catalyzed hydrolysis of ACh is recycled back into the nerve terminal. The recent cloning of the high-affinity choline transporter found in presynaptic terminals reveals a sequence and structure differing from those of other neurotransmitter transporters, but similar to that of the Na^+-dependent glucose transporter family (Okuda *et al.*, 2000).

Upon acetylation of choline, ACh is transported into and packaged in the synaptic vesicle. The vesicular transporter relies on a proton gradient to drive amine uptake. *Vesamicol* blocks ACh vesicular transport at micromolar concentrations. The genes for choline acetyltransferase and the vesicular transporter are found at the same locus, with the transporter gene positioned in the first intron of the transferase gene. Hence, a common promoter regulates the expression of both genes (Eiden, 1998).

Acetylcholinesterase (AChE). For ACh to serve as a neurotransmitter in the motor system and certain neuronal synapses, it must be removed or inactivated within the time limits imposed by the response characteristics of the synapse. At the neuromuscular junction, immediate removal is required to prevent lateral diffusion and sequential activation of receptors—with "flashlike suddenness," as Dale expressed it. Modern biophysical methods have revealed that the time required for hydrolysis of ACh is less than a millisecond at the neuromuscular junction. Choline has only 10^{-3} to 10^{-5} of the potency of ACh at the neuromuscular junction.

While AChE is found in cholinergic neurons (dendrites, perikarya, and axons), it is more widely distributed than cholinergic synapses. It is highly concentrated at the postsynaptic end-plate of the neuromuscular junction. Butyrylcholinesterase (BuChE; also known as pseudocholinesterase) is present in low abundance in glial or satellite cells but is virtually absent in neuronal elements of the central and peripheral nervous systems. BuChE is synthesized primarily in the liver and is found in liver and plasma; its likely vestigial physiological function is the hydrolysis of ingested esters from plant sources. AChE and BuChE typically are distinguished by the relative rates of ACh and butyrylcholine hydrolysis and by effects of selective inhibitors (*see* Chapter 8). Almost all the pharmacological effects of the anti-ChE agents are due to the inhibition of AChE, with the consequent accumulation of endogenous ACh in the vicinity of the nerve terminal. Distinct, but single, genes encode AChE and BuChE in mammals; the diversity of molecular structures of AChE arise from alternative mRNA processing (Taylor *et al.*, 2000).

Storage and Release of Acetylcholine. Fatt and Katz (1952) recorded at the motor end-plate of skeletal muscle and observed the random occurrence of small (0.1 to 3.0 mV), spontaneous depolarizations at a frequency of approximately one per second. The magnitude of these miniature end-plate potentials (mepps) is considerably below the threshold required to fire a muscle AP; that they are due to the release of ACh is indicated by their enhancement by neostigmine (an anti-ChE agent) and their blockade by *d*-tubocurarine (a competitive antagonist that acts at nicotinic receptors). These results led to the hypothesis that ACh is released from motor-nerve endings in constant amounts, or quanta. The likely morphological counterpart of quantal release was discovered shortly thereafter in the form of synaptic vesicles (De Robertis and Bennett, 1955). Most of the storage and release properties of ACh originally investigated in motor end-plates apply to other fast-responding synapses. When an action potential arrives at the motor-nerve terminal, there is a synchronous release of 100 or more quanta (or vesicles) of ACh (Katz and Miledi, 1965).

Estimates of the ACh content of synaptic vesicles range from 1000 to over 50,000 molecules per vesicle, and it has been calculated that a single motor-nerve terminal contains 300,000 or more vesicles. In addition, an uncertain but possibly significant amount of ACh is present in the extravesicular cytoplasm. Recording the electrical events associated with the opening of single channels at the motor end-plate during continuous application of ACh has permitted estimation of the potential change induced by a single molecule of ACh (3×10^{-7} V); from such calculations, it is evident that even the lower estimate of the ACh content per vesicle (1000 molecules) is sufficient to account for the magnitude of the mepps (Katz and Miledi, 1972).

The release of ACh and other neurotransmitters by exocytosis through the prejunctional membrane is inhibited by botulinum and tetanus toxins from *Clostridium*. Some of the most potent toxins known are produced by these spore-forming anaerobic bacteria (Shapiro *et al.*, 1998). The *Clostridium* toxins, consisting of disulfide-linked heavy and light chains, bind to an as-yet-unidentified receptor on the membrane of the cholinergic nerve terminal. Through endocytosis, they are transported into the cytosol. The light chain is a Zn^{2+}-dependent protease that becomes activated and hydrolyzes components of the core or SNARE complex involved in exocytosis. The various serotypes of botulinum toxin proteolyse selective proteins in the plasma membrane (syntaxin and SNAP-25) and the synaptic vesicle (synaptobrevin). Therapeutic uses of botulinum toxin are described in Chapters 9 and 66.

By contrast, tetanus toxin primarily has a central action, since it is transported in retrograde fashion up the motor neuron to its soma in the spinal cord. From there, the toxin migrates to inhibitory neurons that synapse with the motor neuron and blocks exocytosis in the inhibitory neuron. The block of release of inhibitory transmitter gives rise to tetanus or spastic paralysis. The toxin from the venom of black widow spiders (α-latrotoxin) binds to neurexins, transmembrane proteins that reside on the nerve terminal membrane. This gives rise to massive synaptic vesicle exocytosis (Schiavo *et al.*, 2000).

Characteristics of Cholinergic Transmission at Various Sites. From the comparisons noted above, it is obvious that there are marked differences among various sites of cholinergic transmission with respect to architecture and fine structure, the distributions of AChE and receptors, and the temporal factors involved in normal functioning. For example, in skeletal muscle the junctional sites occupy a small, discrete portion of the surface of the individual fibers and are relatively isolated from those of adjacent fibers; in the superior cervical ganglion, approximately 100,000 ganglion cells are packed within a volume of a few cubic millimeters, and both the presynaptic and postsynaptic neuronal processes form complex networks.

Skeletal Muscle. Stimulation of a motor nerve results in the release of ACh from perfused muscle; close intraarterial injection of ACh produces muscular contraction similar to that elicited by stimulation of the motor nerve. The amount of ACh (10^{-17}mol) required to elicit an EPP following its microiontophoretic application to the motor end-plate of a rat diaphragm muscle fiber is equivalent to that recovered from each fiber following stimulation of the phrenic nerve (Krnjević and Mitchell, 1961).

The combination of ACh with nicotinic acetylcholine receptors at the external surface of the postjunctional membrane induces an immediate, marked increase in permeability to cations. Upon activation of the receptor by ACh, its intrinsic channel opens for about 1 millisecond; during this interval about 50,000 Na^+ ions traverse the channel (Katz and Miledi, 1972). The channel opening process is the basis for the localized depolarizing EPP within the end-plate, which triggers the muscle action potential. The latter, in turn, leads to contraction. Further details concerning these events and their modification by neuromuscular blocking agents are presented in Chapter 9.

Following section and degeneration of the motor nerve to skeletal muscle or of the postganglionic fibers to autonomic effectors, there is a marked reduction in the threshold doses of the transmitters and of certain other drugs required to elicit a response, *i.e.*, denervation supersensitivity has occurred. In skeletal muscle, this change is accompanied by a spread of the receptor molecules from the end-plate region to the adjacent portions of the sarcoplasmic membrane, which eventually involves the entire muscle surface. Embryonic muscle also exhibits this uniform sensitivity to ACh prior to innervation. Hence, innervation represses the expression of the receptor gene by the nuclei that lie in extrajunctional regions of the muscle fiber and directs the subsynaptic nuclei to the expression of the structural and functional proteins of the synapse (Sanes and Lichtman, 1999).

Autonomic Effectors. Stimulation or inhibition of autonomic effector cells occurs upon activation of muscarinic acetylcholine receptors (*see* below). In this case the effector is coupled to the receptor by a G protein (*see* Chapter 2). In contrast to skeletal muscle and neurons, smooth muscle and the cardiac conduction system (SA node, atrium, AV node, and the His-Purkinje system) normally exhibit intrinsic activity, both electrical and mechanical, that is modulated but not initiated by nerve impulses. In the basal condition, unitary smooth muscle exhibits waves of depolarization and/or spikes that are propagated from cell to cell at rates considerably slower than the AP of axons or skeletal muscle. The spikes apparently are initiated by rhythmic fluctuations in the membrane resting potential. In intestinal smooth muscle, the site of the pacemaker activity continually shifts, but in the heart, spontaneous depolarizations normally arise from the SA node; however, when activity of the SA node is repressed or under pathological conditions, they can arise from any part of the conduction system (*see* Chapter 35).

Application of ACh (0.1 to 1 μM) to isolated intestinal muscle causes a decrease in the resting potential (*i.e.*, the membrane potential becomes less negative) and an increase in the frequency of spike production accompanied by a rise in tension. A primary action of ACh in initiating these effects through muscarinic receptors is probably the partial depolarization of the cell membrane, brought about by an increase in Na^+ and, in some instances, Ca^{2+} conductance. ACh also can produce contraction of some smooth muscles when the membrane has been completely depolarized by high concentrations of K^+, provided Ca^{2+}

is present. Hence, ACh stimulates ion fluxes across membranes and/or mobilizes intracellular Ca^{2+} to cause contraction.

In the cardiac conduction system, particularly in the SA and the AV nodes, stimulation of the cholinergic innervation or the direct application of ACh causes inhibition, associated with hyperpolarization of the membrane and a marked decrease in the rate of depolarization. These effects are due, at least in part, to a selective increase in permeability to K^+ (Hille, 1992).

Autonomic Ganglia. The primary pathway of cholinergic transmission in autonomic ganglia is similar to that at the neuromuscular junction of skeletal muscle. Ganglion cells can be discharged by injecting very small amounts of ACh into the ganglion. The initial depolarization is the result of activation of nicotinic ACh receptors, which are ligand-gated cation channels with properties similar to those found at the neuromuscular junction. Several secondary transmitters or modulators either enhance or diminish the sensitivity of the postganglionic cell to ACh. This sensitivity appears to be related to the membrane potential of the postsynaptic nerve cell body or its dendritic branches. Ganglionic transmission is discussed in more detail in Chapter 9.

Actions of Acetylcholine at Prejunctional Sites. Considerable attention has been focused on the possible involvement of prejunctional cholinoceptive sites in both cholinergic and noncholinergic transmission and in the actions of various drugs. Although cholinergic innervation of blood vessels is limited, prejunctional muscarinic receptors appear to be present on sympathetic vasoconstrictor nerves (Steinsland *et al.,* 1973). The physiological role of these receptors is not clear, but their activation causes inhibition of neurally mediated release of norepinephrine (*see* Chapter 7). Because ACh is rapidly hydrolyzed by tissue-localized and circulating esterases, it is unlikely that it plays a role as a circulating hormone analogous to that of epinephrine.

Dilation of blood vessels in response to administered choline esters involves several sites of action, including prejunctional inhibitory synapses on sympathetic fibers and inhibitory cholinergic receptors in the vasculature that are not innervated. The vasodilator effect of ACh on isolated blood vessels requires an intact endothelium. Activation of muscarinic receptors results in the liberation of a vasodilator substance (endothelium-derived relaxing factor or nitric oxide) that diffuses from the endothelium to the adjoining smooth muscle and causes relaxation (*see* below and Chapter 7; *see* also Furchgott, 1999).

Cholinergic Receptors and Signal Transduction. Sir Henry Dale noted that the various esters of choline elicited responses that were similar to those of either nicotine or muscarine, depending on the pharmacological preparation (Dale, 1914). A similarity in response also was noted between muscarine and nerve stimulation in those organs innervated by the craniosacral divisions of the autonomic nervous system. Thus, Dale suggested that ACh or another ester of choline was a neurotransmitter in the autonomic nervous system; he also stated that the compound had dual actions, which he termed a nicotine action (*nicotinic*) and a muscarine action (*muscarinic*).

The capacities of *tubocurarine* and *atropine* to block nicotinic and muscarinic effects of ACh, respectively, provided further support for the proposal of two distinct types of cholinergic receptors. Although Dale had access only to crude plant alkaloids of then-unknown structure from *Amanita muscaria* and *Nicotiana tabacum,* this classification remains as the primary subdivision of cholinergic receptors. Its utility has survived the discovery of several distinct subtypes of nicotinic and muscarinic cholinergic receptors.

Although ACh and certain other compounds stimulate both muscarinic and nicotinic receptors, several other agonists and antagonists are selective for one of the two major types of receptor. ACh itself is a flexible molecule, and indirect evidence suggests that the conformations of the neurotransmitter are distinct when it is bound to nicotinic or muscarinic receptors.

Nicotinic receptors are ligand-gated ion channels, and their activation always causes a rapid (millisecond) increase in cellular permeability to Na^+ and Ca^{2+}, depolarization, and excitation. By contrast, muscarinic receptors belong to the class of G protein–coupled receptors. Responses to muscarinic agonists are slower; they may be either excitatory or inhibitory, and they are not necessarily linked to changes in ion permeability.

The primary structures of various species of nicotinic receptors (Numa *et al.,* 1983; Changeux and Edelstein, 1998) and muscarinic receptors (Bonner, 1989; Caulfield and Birdsall, 1998) have been deduced from the sequences of their respective genes. That these two types of receptor belong to distinct families of proteins is not surprising, retrospectively, in view of their distinct differences in chemical specificity and function.

The nicotinic receptors exist as pentameric arrangements of one to four distinct subunits that are homologous in sequence; the individual subunits are arranged to surround an internal channel. One of the subunits, designated α, is present in at least two copies, and the multiple binding sites for ACh are formed at one of the interfaces of the α-subunit with the neighboring subunit. One α-helical membrane-spanning sequence from each subunit forms the channel boundary (Changeux and Edelstein, 1998; *see* Chapters 9 and 12). The general properties of muscarinic receptor coupling to G proteins and the characteristics of the muscarinic ligand-binding site are described in Chapters 2 and 7.

Subtypes of Nicotinic Receptors. Based on the distinct actions of certain agonists and antagonists that interact with nicotinic receptors from skeletal muscle and ganglia, it long has been evident that not all nicotinic receptors are identical. Heterogeneity of this type of receptor was further revealed by molecular cloning. For example, the muscle nicotinic receptor contains four distinct subunits in a pentameric complex ($\alpha_2\beta\delta\gamma$ or $\alpha_2\beta\delta\varepsilon$). Receptors in embryonic or denervated muscle contain a γ subunit, whereas an ε subunit replaces the γ in adult innervated muscle. This change in expression of the genes encoding the γ and ε subunits gives rise to small differences in ligand selectivity, but the switch may be more important for dictating rates of turnover of the receptors or their tissue localization. Nicotinic receptors in the CNS also exist as pentamers. Because of the diversity of neuronal nicotinic receptor subunits, they have been designated as the α and β subtypes. There are eight subtypes of α ($\alpha2$–$\alpha9$) and three subtypes of β ($\beta2$–$\beta4$) in the mammalian nervous system. Although not all combinations of α and β are functional, the number of permutations of α and β that yield functional receptors is sufficiently large to preclude a pharmacological classification of all subtypes. Homo-oligomeric pentamers of $\alpha7$, $\alpha8$, and $\alpha9$ subunits form functional receptors. Distinctions between nicotinic receptors are listed in Table 6–2; the structure, function, distribution, and subtypes of nicotinic receptors are described in more detail in Chapter 9.

Subtypes of Muscarinic Receptors.   Five subtypes of muscarinic ACh receptors have been detected by molecular cloning. Similar to the different forms of nicotinic receptors, these variants have distinct anatomical localizations and chemical specificities. The muscarinic receptors all act through G-protein signaling systems (*see* discussion below and Table 6–2).

Of the large number of muscarinic antagonists studied over many decades, only pirenzepine, found in the 1970s, showed the unique property of blocking gastric acid secretion at concentrations that did not affect several other responses to muscarinic agonists. These observations and subsequent study of other agonists and antagonists, followed by rapid advances in the cloning of cDNAs that encode muscarinic receptors, led to the identification of five subtypes of muscarinic receptors. They have been designated as M_1 through M_5 based on pharmacological specificity (Bonner, 1989; *see also* Chapter 7).

M_1 receptors are found in ganglia and in some secretory glands; M_2 receptors predominate in the myocardium and also appear to be found in smooth muscle; and M_3 and M_4 receptors are located in smooth muscle and secretory glands. All five subtypes are found in the CNS. Various tissues may contain several subtypes of muscarinic receptors; parasympathetic ganglia in the tissue also contain muscarinic receptors.

The basic functions of muscarinic receptors are mediated by interactions with members of the family of G proteins and thus by G protein–induced changes in the functions of distinct membrane-bound effector molecules. The M_1, M_3, and M_5 subtypes activate a G protein, termed $G_{q/11}$, that is responsible for stimulation of phospholipase C activity; the immediate result is hydrolysis of phosphatidylinositol polyphosphates (which are components of the plasma membrane) to form inositol polyphosphates. Some of the inositol phosphate isomers (chiefly inositol-1,4,5-trisphosphate) cause release of intracellular Ca^{2+} from stores in the endoplasmic reticulum. Thus, these receptors mediate such Ca^{2+}-dependent phenomena as contraction of smooth muscle and secretion (*see* Chapter 2; *see also* Berridge, 1993). The second product of the phospholipase C reaction, diacylglycerol, activates protein kinase C (in conjunction with Ca^{2+}). This arm of the pathway plays a role in modulation of function and in the later phases of the functional response (Dempsey *et al.*, 2000).

A second pathway for mediation of responses to muscarinic agonists is evoked by activation of M_2 and M_4 receptors. These receptors interact with a distinct group of G proteins (in particular those termed G_i and G_o) with resultant inhibition of adenylyl cyclase, activation of receptor-operated K^+ channels (in the heart, for example), and suppression of the activity of voltage-gated Ca^{2+} channels in certain cell types. The functional consequences of these effects are most clear in the myocardium, where inhibition of adenylyl cyclase and activation of K^+ conductances can account for both the negative chronotropic and inotropic effects of ACh.

Other cellular events such as the release of arachidonic acid and the activation of guanylyl cyclase also can result from activation of muscarinic receptors; typically these responses are secondary to the production of other mediators.

Adrenergic Transmission

Under this general heading are included *norepinephrine,* the transmitter of most sympathetic postganglionic fibers and of certain tracts in the CNS, and *dopamine,* the predominant transmitter of the mammalian extrapyramidal system and of several mesocortical and mesolimbic neuronal pathways, as well as *epinephrine,* the major hormone of the adrenal medulla.

A tremendous amount of information about catecholamines and related compounds has accumulated in recent years, partly because of the importance of interactions between the endogenous catecholamines and many of the drugs used in the treatment of hypertension, mental disorders, and a variety of other conditions. The details of these interactions and of the pharmacology of the sympathomimetic amines themselves will be found in subsequent chapters. The basic physiological, biochemical, and pharmacological features are presented here.

Synthesis, Storage, and Release of Catecholamines. *Synthesis.*   The synthesis of epinephrine from tyrosine, by the steps shown in Figure 6–3, was proposed by

Table 6–2

Characteristics of Subtypes of Cholinergic Receptors

RECEPTOR	AGONISTS	ANTAGONISTS	TISSUE	RESPONSES	MOLECULAR MECHANISMS
Nicotinic					
Skeletal muscle (N_M)	Phenyltrimethyl-ammonium[1] Nicotine	d-Tubocurarine Elapid α-Neurotoxins (α-Bungarotoxin)	Neuromuscular junction	End-plate de-polarization, skeletal muscle contraction	Opening of an intrinsic cation channel; compositions of $\alpha1, \beta1, \gamma, \delta$, and ϵ subunits in a stoichiometry of $\alpha_2\beta\gamma\delta$ or $\alpha_2\beta\epsilon\delta$
Neuronal (Peripheral) (N_N)	Dimethylphenyl-piperazinium[1] Epibatidine[1] Nicotine	Trimethaphan	Autonomic ganglia; adrenal medulla	Depolarization and firing of post-ganglionic neuron; depolarization of the medullary cell and secretion of catecholamines	Opening of an intrinsic cation channel; compositions of $\alpha2$ through $\alpha9$ with $\beta2$ through $\beta4$ in the stoichiometry of $\alpha_2\beta_3$
Neuronal (CNS)	Nicotine Cytisine Epibatidine[1]	Several with partial subtype selectivity[2]	Brain and spinal cord	Prejunctional control of neurotransmitter release	Various combinations of $\alpha2$–$\alpha9$ and $\beta2$–$\beta4$
Muscarinic					
M_1	Oxotremorine McN-A-343[1]	Atropine Pirenzepine[1]	Autonomic ganglia CNS[3]	Depolarization (late EPSP) Undefined	Stimulation of PLC through $G_{q/11}$ with formation of IP_3 and DAG; increased cytosolic Ca^{2+}
M_2	—	Atropine Tripitramine[1]	Heart SA node Atrium AV node Ventricle	Slowed spontaneous depolarization; hyperpolarization Shortened duration of action potential; decreased contractile force Decreased conduction velocity Slight decrease in contractile force	Activation of K^+ channels through $\beta\gamma$ subunits of G_i; inhibition of adenylyl cyclase through G_o and G_i; suppression of voltage-gated L-type Ca^{2+} channel activity
M_3	—	Atropine Darifenacin[1]	Smooth muscle Vasculature endothelium Secretory glands	Contraction[4] Dilation of vessels Increased secretion	Similar to M_1 Generation of NO Similar to M_1
M_4	—	Atropine	—	—	Similar to M_2
M_5	—	—	CNS	—	Similar to M_1

Abbreviations: ESPS, excitatory postsynaptic potential; PLC, phospholipase C; IP_3, inositol-1,4,5-trisphosphate; DAG, diacylglycerol.
[1] Denotes the more selective agent.
[2] See Lukas *et al.*, 1999.
[3] The CNS contains all known subtypes of muscarinic receptors (*see* Chapter 7).
[4] Relaxation occurs in sphincters in the urinary and gastrointestinal tracts, but this may result from the release of peptides from intrinsic ganglia or parasympathetic nerves.

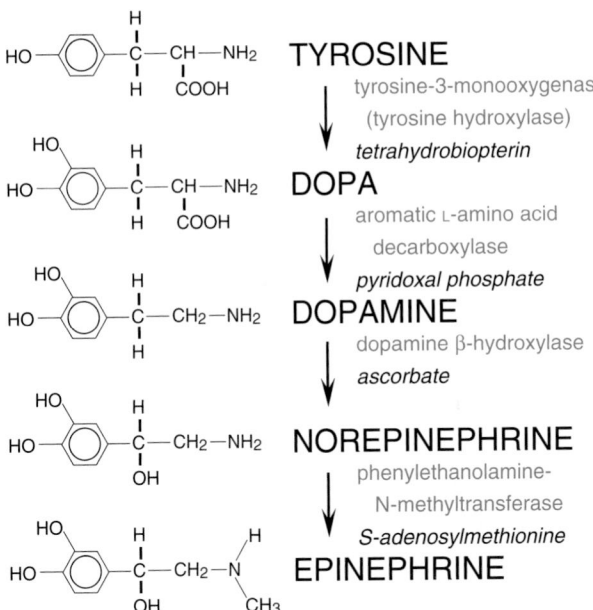

Figure 6–3. Steps in the enzymatic synthesis of dopamine, norepinephrine, and epinephrine.

The enzymes involved are shown in blue; essential cofactors, in italics. The final step occurs only in the adrenal medulla and in a few epinephrine-containing neuronal pathways in the brainstem.

Blaschko in 1939. The enzymes involved have been identified, cloned, and characterized (Nagatsu, 1991). It is important to note that these enzymes are not completely specific; consequently, other endogenous substances as well as certain drugs are similarly acted upon at the various steps. For example, 5-hydroxytryptamine (5-HT, serotonin) can be produced by aromatic L-amino acid decarboxylase (or dopa decarboxylase) from 5-hydroxy-L-tryptophan. Dopa decarboxylase also converts dopa into dopamine, and methyldopa is converted to α-methyldopamine, which, in turn, is converted by dopamine β-hydroxylase to the "false transmitter," α-methylnorepinephrine.

The hydroxylation of tyrosine generally is regarded as the rate-limiting step in the biosynthesis of catecholamines (Zigmond *et al.*, 1989), and tyrosine hydroxylase is activated following stimulation of adrenergic nerves or the adrenal medulla. The enzyme is a substrate for cyclic AMP–dependent and Ca^{2+}-calmodulin-sensitive protein kinase and protein kinase C; kinase-catalyzed phosphorylation may be associated with increased hydroxylase activity (Zigmond *et al.*, 1989; Daubner *et al.*, 1992). This is an important acute mechanism for increasing catecholamine synthesis in response to increased nerve stimulation. In

addition, there is a delayed increase in tyrosine hydroxylase gene expression after nerve stimulation. There is evidence suggesting that this increased expression can occur at multiple levels of regulation, including transcription, RNA processing, regulation of RNA stability, translation, and enzyme stability (Kumer and Vrana, 1996). These mechanisms serve to maintain the content of catecholamines in response to increased release of these transmitters. In addition, tyrosine hydroxylase is subject to feedback inhibition by catechol compounds, an allosteric modulation of enzyme activity. Patients with mutations in the tyrosine hydroxylase gene have been described (Wevers *et al.*, 1999).

Current knowledge concerning the cellular sites and mechanisms of synthesis, storage, and release of catecholamines has been derived from studies of both adrenergically innervated organs and of adrenal medullary tissue. Nearly all the norepinephrine content of the former is confined to the postganglionic sympathetic fibers; it disappears within a few days after section of the nerves. In the adrenal medulla, catecholamines are stored in chromaffin granules (Winkler, 1997; Aunis, 1998). These vesicles contain extremely high concentrations of catecholamines (approximately 21% dry weight), ascorbic acid, and ATP, as well as specific proteins such as chromogranins, the enzyme dopamine β-hydroxylase (DBH), and peptides including enkephalin and neuropeptide Y. Interestingly, vasostatin-1, the N-terminal fragment of chromogranin A, has been found to have antibacterial and antifungal activity (Lugardon *et al.*, 2000). Two types of storage vesicles are found in sympathetic nerve terminals: large dense-core vesicles corresponding to chromaffin granules and small dense-core vesicles containing norepinephrine, ATP, and membrane-bound dopamine β-hydroxylase.

The main features of the mechanisms of synthesis, storage, and release of catecholamines and their modifications by drugs are summarized in Figure 6–4. In the case of adrenergic neurons, the enzymes that participate in the formation of norepinephrine are synthesized in the cell bodies of the neurons and are then transported along the axons to their terminals. In the course of synthesis (*see* Figure 6–3), the hydroxylation of tyrosine to dopa and the decarboxylation of dopa to dopamine take place in the cytoplasm. About half the dopamine formed in the cytoplasm then is actively transported into the DBH-containing storage vesicles, where it is converted to norepinephrine; the remainder, which escaped capture by the vesicles, is deaminated to 3,4-dihydroxyphenylacetic acid (DOPAC) and subsequently *O*-methylated to homovanillic acid (HVA). The adrenal medulla has two distinct catecholamine-containing cell types: those with

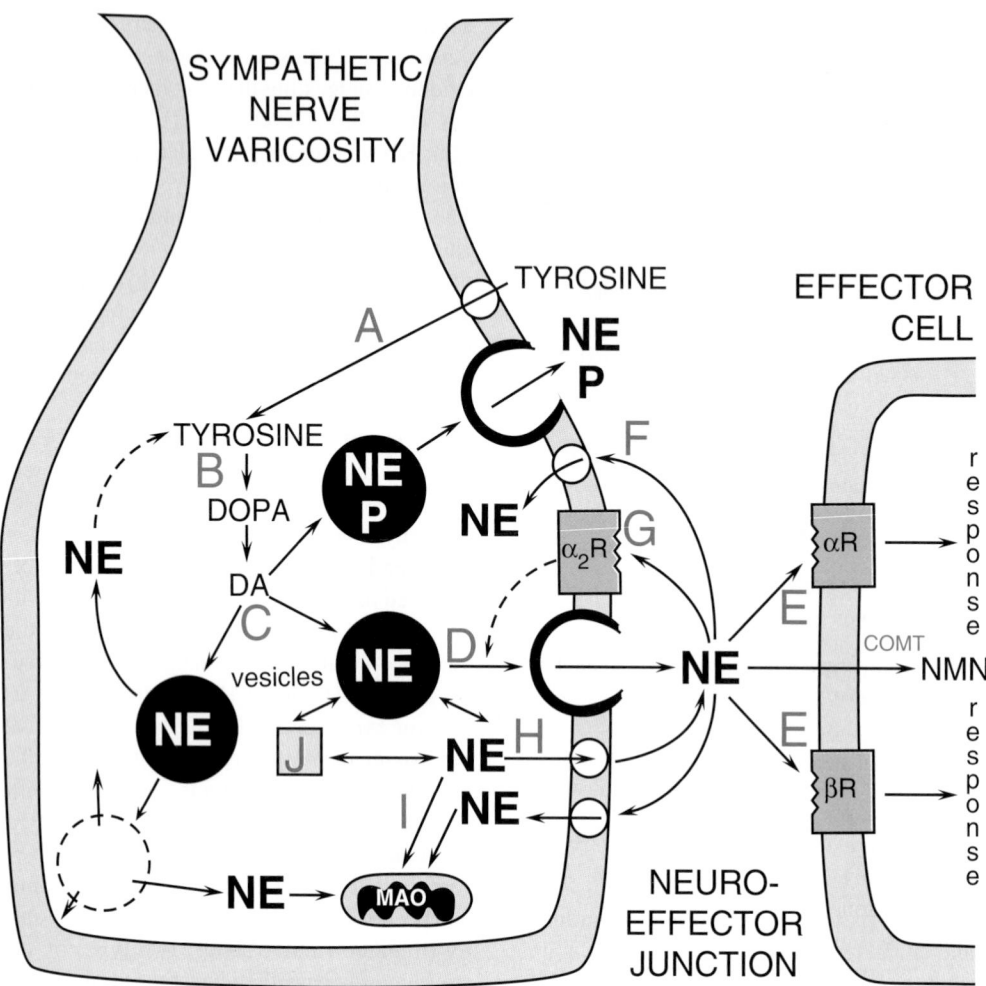

Figure 6–4. Proposed sites of action of drugs on the synthesis, action, and fate of norepinephrine at sympathetic neuroeffector junctions.

The events proposed to occur in this model of a sympathetic neuroeffector junction are as follows. Tyrosine is transported actively into the axoplasm (A) and is converted to DOPA and then to dopamine (DA) by cytoplasmic enzymes (B). Dopamine is transported into the vesicles of the varicosity, where the synthesis and the storage of norepinephrine (NE) take place (C). An action potential causes an influx of Ca^{2+} into the nerve terminal (not shown), with subsequent fusion of the vesicle with the plasma membrane and exocytosis of NE (D). The transmitter then activates α- and β-adrenergic receptors in the membrane of the postsynaptic cell (E). NE that penetrates into these cells (uptake 2) probably is rapidly inactivated by catechol-O-methyltransferase (COMT) to normetanephrine (NMN). The most important mechanism for termination of the action of NE in the junctional space is active reuptake into the nerve (uptake 1) and the storage vesicles (F). Norepinephrine in the synaptic cleft also can activate presynaptic α_2-adrenergic receptors (G), and further inhibit exocytotic release of norepinephrine (dashed line). Other potential neurotransmitters [*e.g.*, ATP and peptides (P)] may be stored in the same or a different population of vesicles.

norepinephrine and those with primarily epinephrine. The latter cell population contains the enzyme phenylethanol-amine-N-methyltransferase. In these cells, the norepineph-rine formed in the granules leaves these structures, pre-

sumably by diffusion, and is methylated in the cytoplasm to epinephrine. Epinephrine then reenters the chromaf-fin granules, where it is stored until released. In adults, epinephrine accounts for approximately 80% of the catecholamines of the adrenal medulla, with norepineph-rine making up most of the remainder (von Euler, 1972).

A major factor that controls the rate of synthesis of epineph-rine, and hence the size of the store available for release from the adrenal medulla, is the level of glucocorticoids secreted by the adrenal cortex. The latter hormones are carried in high con-centration, by the intraadrenal portal vascular system, directly to the adrenal medullary chromaffin cells, where they induce the synthesis of phenylethanolamine-*N*-methyltransferase (*see* Fig-ure 6–3). The activities of both tyrosine hydroxylase and DBH also are increased in the adrenal medulla when the secretion of glucocorticoids is stimulated (Carroll *et al.*, 1991; Viskupic *et al.*, 1994). Thus, any stress that persists sufficiently to evoke an enhanced secretion of corticotropin mobilizes the appropri-ate hormones of both the adrenal cortex (predominantly cortisol) and medulla (epinephrine).

This remarkable relationship is present only in certain mammals, including human beings, for which the adrenal chro-maffin cells are enveloped entirely by steroid-secreting cortical cells. In the dogfish, for example, where the chromaffin cells and steroid-secreting cells are located in independent, noncontigu-ous glands, epinephrine is not formed. Nonetheless, there is ev-idence indicating that phenylethanolamine-*N*-methyltransferase is expressed in mammalian tissues such as brain, heart, and lung, leading to extra-adrenal epinephrine synthesis (Kennedy and Ziegler, 1991; Kennedy *et al.*, 1993).

In addition to its *de novo* synthesis, outlined above, there is a second major mechanism for replenishment of the norepinephrine stored in the terminal portions of the adrenergic fibers—namely, recapture by active transport of norepinephrine previously released to the extracellu-lar fluid. This process is responsible for the termination of the effects of adrenergic impulses in most organs. In blood vessels and in tissues with wide synaptic gaps, re-capture of released norepinephrine is less important. At such sites, a relatively large fraction of the released neu-rotransmitter is inactivated by a combination of extraneu-ronal uptake (*see* below) and enzymatic breakdown and diffusion. To effect the reuptake of norepinephrine into adrenergic nerve terminals and to maintain the concen-tration gradient of norepinephrine within the vesicles, at least two distinct carrier-mediated transport systems are involved: one across the axoplasmic membrane from the extracellular fluid to the cytoplasm and the other from cytoplasm into the storage vesicles.

Storage of Catecholamines. Catecholamines are stored in vesi-cles to ensure their regulated release; this storage decreases in-traneuronal metabolism of these transmitters as well as their leakage outside the cell. The amine transporter has been exten-sively characterized (Schuldiner, 1994). Uptake of catecholamine and ATP into isolated chromaffin granules appears to be driven by pH and potential gradients that are established by an ATP-dependent proton translocase. For every molecule of amine taken up, two H^+ ions are extruded (Brownstein and Hoffman,

1994). Monoamine transporters are relatively promiscuous, ca-pable of transporting dopamine, norepinephrine, epinephrine, and serotonin, for example. Also, meta-iodobenzylguanidine, used clinically to image chromaffin-cell tumors, is a substrate for this transport system (Schuldiner, 1994). Reserpine is a drug that inhibits monoamine transport into these vesicles which ultimately leads to depletion of catecholamine from sympa-thetic nerve endings and in the brain. Several vesicular trans-port cDNAs have been identified with molecular cloning tech-niques; these cDNAs reveal open reading frames predictive of proteins with 12 putative transmembrane domains with struc-tural homology to other transport proteins such as bacterial drug-resistance transporters (Schuldiner, 1994). Regulation of the expression of these various transporters may be important in the regulation of synaptic transmission (Varoqui and Erickson, 1997).

When catecholamines such as norepinephrine are in-jected into the blood of experimental animals, they are rapidly accumulated in tissues with extensive sympathetic innervation, such as heart and spleen; labeled catechol-amines are concentrated in sympathetic nerve endings, and tissue uptake disappears after denervation (reviewed in Brownstein and Hoffman, 1994). This and other evi-dence suggested the presence of transporters on the plasma membrane of sympathetic neurons that could take up cate-cholamines. The amine transport system across the axo-plasmic membranes is Na^+-dependent and is blocked se-lectively by a number of drugs, including cocaine and the tricyclic antidepressants, such as imipramine. This trans-porter has a high affinity for norepinephrine and a some-what lower affinity for epinephrine; the synthetic β-adre-nergic receptor agonist isoproterenol is not a substrate for this system. The neuronal uptake process has been termed *uptake-1* (Iversen, 1975). A number of highly specific neurotransmitter transporters have been identified by pro-tein purification or expression cloning techniques. High-affinity transporters have been identified, for example, for dopamine, norepinephrine, serotonin, and a variety of amino acid transmitters (Amara and Kuhar, 1993; Brownstein and Hoffman, 1994; Masson *et al.*, 1999). These trans-porters are members of an extended family sharing com-mon structural motifs, particularly the putative 12 trans-membrane helices. These plasma membrane transporters appear to have greater substrate specificity than do vesic-ular transporters. Indeed, these transport systems may be viewed as targets ("receptors") for specific drugs such as *cocaine* (dopamine transporter) or *fluoxetine* (serotonin transporter).

Certain sympathomimetic drugs (*e.g., ephedrine, tyra-mine*) produce some of their effects indirectly, chiefly by displacing norepinephrine from the nerve-ending binding sites to the extracellular fluid, where the released endogenous transmitter then acts at receptor sites of the effector cells. The mechanisms by which indirect-acting sympathomimetic amines release norepinephrine from nerve endings are complex. All such agents are substrates for uptake-1. As a result of their transport across the neuronal membrane and release into the axoplasm, they make carrier available at the inner surface of the membrane for the outward transport of norepinephrine ("facilitated exchange diffusion"). In addition, these amines are able to mobilize norepinephrine stored in the vesicles by competing for the vesicular uptake process. Reserpine, which depletes vesicular stores of norepinephrine, also inhibits this uptake mechanism, but, in contrast with the indirect-acting sympathomimetic amines, it enters the adrenergic nerve ending by passive diffusion across the axonal membrane (Bönisch and Trendelenburg, 1988).

These actions of indirect-acting sympathomimetic amines are associated with the phenomenon of *tachyphylaxis*. For example, repeated administration of tyramine results in rapidly decreasing effectiveness, whereas repeated administration of norepinephrine does not reduce effectiveness and, in fact, reverses the tachyphylaxis to tyramine. Although these phenomena have not been explained fully, several hypotheses have been proposed. One possible explanation of tachyphylaxis to tyramine and similarly acting sympathomimetic agents is that the pool of neurotransmitter available for displacement by these drugs is small relative to the total amount stored in the sympathetic nerve ending. This pool is presumed to reside in close proximity to the plasma membrane, and the norepinephrine of such vesicles may be replaced by the less potent amine following repeated administration of the latter substance. In any case, neurotransmitter release by displacement is not associated with the release of dopamine β-hydroxylase and does not require extracellular Ca^{2+}; thus, it is presumed not to involve exocytosis.

There also is an extraneuronal amine transport system, termed *uptake-2*, which exhibits a low affinity for norepinephrine, a somewhat higher affinity for epinephrine, and a still higher affinity for isoproterenol. This uptake process is ubiquitous and is present in glial, hepatic, myocardial, and other cells. Uptake-2 is not inhibited by imipramine or cocaine. It probably is of relatively little physiological importance unless the neuronal uptake mechanism is blocked (Iversen, 1975; Trendelenburg, 1980). It may be of greater importance in the disposition of circulating catecholamines than in the removal of amines that have been released from adrenergic nerve terminals.

Release of Catecholamines.   The full sequence of steps by which the nerve impulse effects the release of norepinephrine from adrenergic fibers is not known. In the adrenal medulla, the triggering event is the liberation of ACh by the preganglionic fibers and its interaction with nicotinic receptors on chromaffin cells to produce a localized depolarization; a succeeding step is the entrance of Ca^{2+} into these cells, which results in the extrusion by exocytosis of the granular contents, including epinephrine, ATP, some neuroactive peptides or their precursors, chromogranins, and DBH. Influx of Ca^{2+} likewise plays an essential role in coupling the nerve impulse, membrane depolarization, and opening of voltage-gated Ca^{2+} channels with the release of norepinephrine at adrenergic nerve terminals. Blockade of N-type Ca^{2+} channels leads to hypotension, likely due to inhibition of norepinephrine release (Bowersox *et al.,* 1992). Ca^{2+}-triggered secretion involves interaction of highly conserved molecular scaffolding proteins leading to docking of granules at the plasma membrane, ultimately leading to secretion (Aunis, 1998). Enhanced activity of the sympathetic nervous system is accompanied by an increased concentration of both DBH and chromogranins in the circulation, supporting the argument that the process of release following adrenergic nerve stimulation also involves exocytosis.

Adrenergic fibers can sustain the output of norepinephrine during prolonged periods of stimulation without exhausting their reserve supply, provided synthesis and uptake of the transmitter are unimpaired. To meet increased needs for norepinephrine, acute regulatory mechanisms come into play that involve activation of tyrosine hydroxylase and dopamine β-hydroxylase (*see* above).

Termination of the Actions of Catecholamines.   The actions of norepinephrine and epinephrine are terminated by (1) reuptake into nerve terminals; (2) dilution by diffusion out of the junctional cleft and uptake at extraneuronal sites; and (3) metabolic transformation. Two enzymes are important in the initial steps of metabolic transformation of catecholamines—monoamine oxidase (MAO) and catechol-*O*-methyltransferase (COMT; *see* Axelrod, 1966; Kopin, 1972). In addition, catecholamines are metabolized by sulfotransferases (Dooley, 1998). However, it is evident that a powerful degradative enzymatic pathway, such as that provided by AChE, is absent from the adrenergic nervous system. The importance of neuronal reuptake of catecholamines is shown by observations that inhibitors of this process (*e.g.,* cocaine, imipramine) potentiate the effects of the neurotransmitter; inhibitors of MAO and COMT have relatively little effect. However, transmitter that is released within the nerve terminal is metabolized by MAO. COMT, particularly in the liver, plays a major role in the metabolism of endogenous circulating and administered catecholamines.

Both MAO and COMT are widely distributed throughout the body, including the brain; the highest concentrations of each are in the liver and the kidney. However, little or no COMT is found in adrenergic neurons. There are distinct differences in the cytological locations of the two enzymes; whereas MAO is associated chiefly with the outer surface of mitochondria, including those within the terminals of adrenergic fibers, COMT is located largely in the cytoplasm. These factors are of importance both in determining the primary metabolic pathways followed by catecholamines in various circumstances and in explaining the effects of certain drugs. Two different isozymes of MAO (MAO-A and MAO-B) are found in widely varying proportions in different cells in the CNS and in peripheral tissues. Selective inhibitors of these two isozymes are available (*see* Chapter 19). Irreversible antagonists of MAO-A enhance the bioavailability of tyramine contained in many foods; tyramine-induced norepinephrine release from sympathetic neurons may lead to markedly increased blood pressure. Selective MAO-B inhibitors (*e.g.,* selegiline) or reversible *MAO-A-selective inhibitors* (moclobemide) are less likely to cause this potential interaction (Volz and Geiter, 1998; Wouters, 1998). MAO inhibitors are useful in the treatment of Parkinson's disease and mental depression (*see* Chapters 19 and 22).

Most of the epinephrine and norepinephrine that enter the circulation—from the adrenal medulla or following administration or that is released by exocytosis from adrenergic fibers—is methylated by COMT to metanephrine or normetanephrine, respectively (Figure 6–5). Norepinephrine that is released intraneuronally by drugs such as reserpine is initially deaminated by MAO to 3,4-dihydroxyphenylglycolaldehyde (DOPGAL; *see* Figure 6–5). The aldehyde is reduced by aldehyde reductase to the glycol, 3,4-dihydroxyphenylethylene glycol (DOPEG), or is oxidized by aldehyde dehydrogenase to form 3,4-dihydroxymandelic acid (DOMA). 3-Methoxy-4-hydroxymandelic acid [generally but incorrectly called vanillylmandelic acid (VMA)] is the major metabolite of catecholamines excreted in the urine. The corresponding product of the metabolic degradation of dopamine, which contains no hydroxyl group in the side chain, is homovanillic acid (HVA). Other metabolic reactions are described in Figure 6–5. Measurement of the concentrations of catecholamines and their metabolites in blood and urine is useful in the diagnosis of pheochromocytoma, a catecholamine-secreting tumor of the adrenal medulla.

Inhibitors of MAO (*e.g., pargyline, nialamide*) can cause an increase in the concentration of norepinephrine, dopamine, and 5-HT in the brain and other tissues accompanied by a variety of pharmacological effects. No striking pharmacological action in the periphery can be attributed to the inhibition of COMT. However, a COMT inhibitor, *entacapone,* has been found to be efficacious in the therapy of Parkinson's disease (Chong and Mersfelder, 2000; *see also* Chapter 22).

Classification of Adrenergic Receptors. Crucial to understanding the remarkably diverse effects of the catecholamines and related sympathomimetic agents is an understanding of the classification and properties of the different types of adrenergic receptors (or adrenoceptors). Elucidation of the characteristics of these receptors and the biochemical and physiological pathways they regu-

late has increased our understanding of the seemingly contradictory and variable effects of catecholamines on various organ systems. Although structurally related (*see* below), different adrenergic receptors regulate distinct physiological processes by controlling the synthesis or release of a variety of second messengers (*see* Tables 6–3 and 6–4).

Ahlquist (1948) first proposed the existence of more than one adrenergic receptor; he based his hypothesis on a study of the abilities of epinephrine, norepinephrine, and other related agonists to regulate various physiological processes. It was known that these drugs could cause either contraction or relaxation of smooth muscle, depending on the site, the dose, and the agent chosen. For example, norepinephrine was known to have potent excitatory effects on smooth muscle and correspondingly low activity as an inhibitor; isoproterenol displayed the opposite pattern of activity. Epinephrine could both excite and inhibit smooth muscle. Thus, Ahlquist proposed the designations α and β for receptors on smooth muscle where catecholamines produce excitatory and inhibitory responses, respectively. An exception is the gut, which generally is relaxed by activation of either α- or β-adrenergic receptors. The rank order of potency of agonists is isoproterenol > epinephrine $\geq$ norepinephrine for β-adrenergic receptors and epinephrine $\geq$ norepinephrine $\gg$ isoproterenol for α-adrenergic receptors (*see* Table 6–3). This initial classification of adrenergic receptors was corroborated by the finding that certain antagonists produce selective blockade of the effects of adrenergic nerve impulses and sympathomimetic agents at α-adrenergic receptors (*e.g.,* phenoxybenzamine), whereas others produce selective β-adrenergic receptor blockade (*e.g.,* propranolol).

β-Adrenergic receptors later were subdivided into β_1 (*e.g.,* those in the myocardium) and β_2 (smooth muscle and most other sites), because epinephrine and norepinephrine essentially are equipotent at the former sites, whereas epinephrine is 10- to 50-fold more potent than norepinephrine at the latter (Lands *et al.,* 1967). Antagonists that discriminate between β_1- and β_2-adrenergic receptors subsequently were developed (*see* Chapter 10). A human gene that encodes a third β-adrenergic receptor (designated β_3) has been isolated (Emorine *et al.,* 1989; Granneman *et al.,* 1993). Since the β_3 receptor is about tenfold more sensitive to norepinephrine than to epinephrine and is relatively resistant to blockade by antagonists such as propranolol, it may mediate responses to catecholamine at sites with "atypical" pharmacological characteristics (*e.g.,* adipose tissue). However, the role of this receptor in regulating lipolysis in human beings remains uncertain (Rosenbaum *et al.,* 1993; Krief *et al.,*

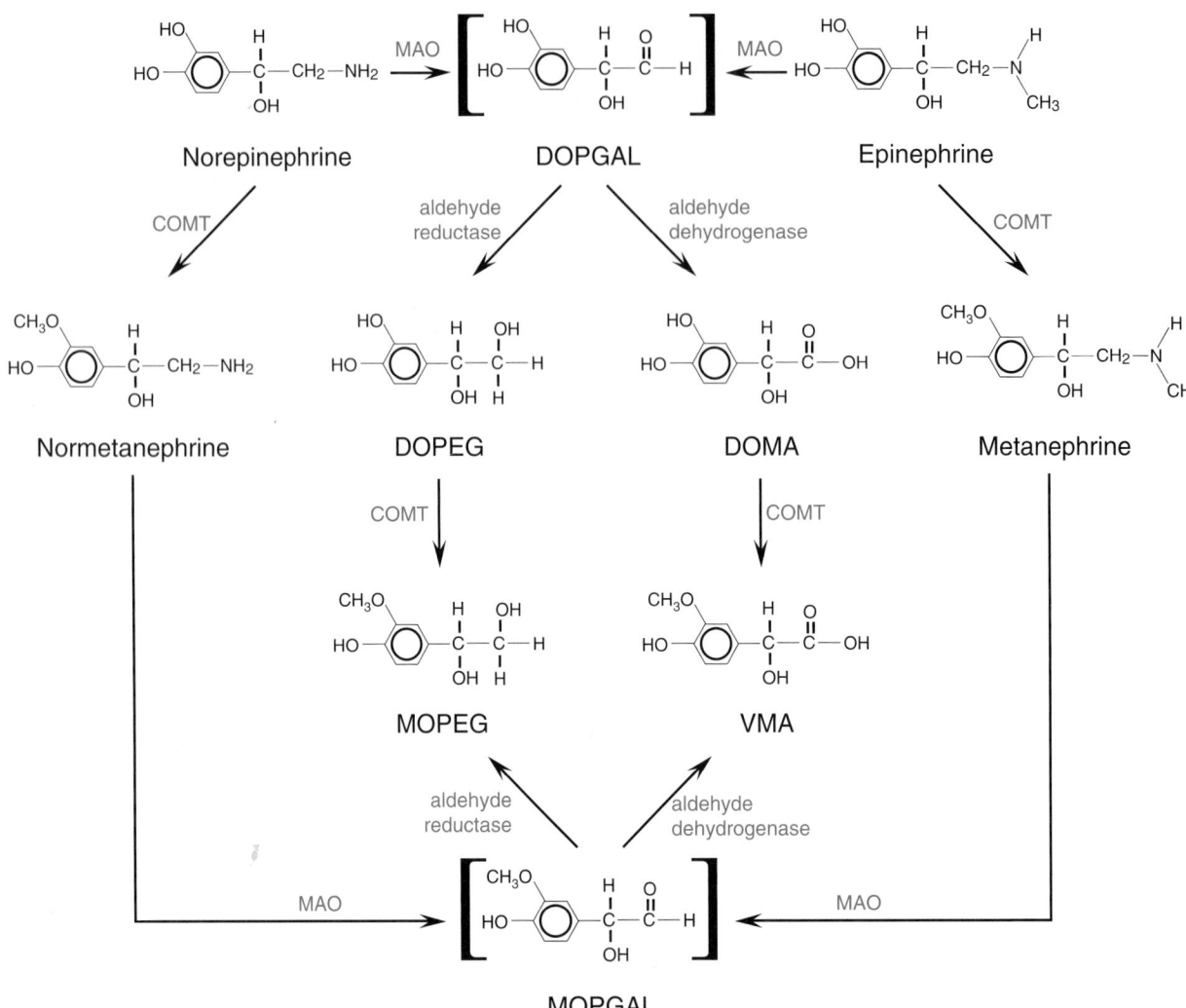

Figure 6–5. Steps in the metabolic disposition of catecholamines.

Both norepinephrine and epinephrine are first oxidatively deaminated by monoamine oxidase (MAO) to 3,4-dihydroxyphenylglycoaldehyde (DOPGAL) and then either reduced to 3,4-dihydroxyphenylethylene glycol (DOPEG) or oxidized to 3,4-dihydroxymandelic acid (DOMA). Alternatively, they can be initially methylated by catechol-O-methyltransferase (COMT) to normetanephrine and metanephrine, respectively. Most of the products of either type of reaction then are metabolized by the other enzyme to form the major excretory products in blood and urine, 3-methoxy-4-hydroxyphenylethylene glycol (MOPEG or MHPG) and 3-methoxy-4-hydroxymandelic acid (VMA). Free MOPEG is largely converted to VMA. The glycol and, to some extent, the O-methylated amines and the catecholamines may be conjugated to the corresponding sulfates or glucuronides. (Modified from Axelrod, 1966; and others.)

1993; Lönnqvist *et al.,* 1993). It has been suggested that polymorphisms in the β_3 receptor gene may be related to risk of obesity or type 2 diabetes in some populations (Arner and Hoffstedt, 1999). Also, there has been interest in the possibility that β_3-receptor-selective agonists might have benefit in treating these disorders (Weyer *et al.,* 1999).

The heterogeneity of α-adrenergic receptors also is now appreciated. The initial distinction was based on functional and anatomical considerations when it was realized that norepinephrine and other α-adrenergic agonists could profoundly inhibit the release of norepinephrine from neurons (*see* Starke, 1987; *see also* Figure 6–4). Indeed, when sympathetic nerves are stimulated in the

Table 6–3
Characteristics of Subtypes of Adrenergic Receptors[1]

RECEPTOR	AGONISTS	ANTAGONISTS	TISSUE	RESPONSES
α_1[2]	Epi $\geq$ NE $\gg$ Iso Phenylephrine	Prazosin	Vascular smooth muscle	Contraction
			Genitourinary smooth muscle	Contraction
			Liver[3]	Glycogenolysis; gluconeogenesis
			Intestinal smooth muscle	Hyperpolarization and relaxation
			Heart	Increased contractile force; arrhythmias
α_2[2]	Epi $\geq$ NE $\gg$ Iso Clonidine	Yohimbine	Pancreatic islets (β cells)	Decreased insulin secretion
			Platelets	Aggregation
			Nerve terminals	Decreased release of NE
			Vascular smooth muscle	Contraction
β_1	Iso $>$ Epi $=$ NE Dobutamine	Metoprolol CGP 20712A	Heart	Increased force and rate of contraction and AV nodal conduction velocity
			Juxtaglomerular cells	Increased renin secretion
β_2	Iso $>$ Epi $\gg$ NE Terbutaline	ICI 118551	Smooth muscle (vascular, bronchial, gastrointestinal, and genitourinary)	Relaxation
			Skeletal muscle	Glycogenolysis; uptake of K^+
			Liver[3]	Glycogenolysis; gluconeogenesis
β_3[4]	Iso $=$ NE $>$ Epi BRL 37344	ICI 118551 CGP 20712A	Adipose tissue	Lipolysis

Abbreviations: Epi, epinephrine; NE, norepinephrine; Iso, isoproterenol.

[1] This table provides examples of drugs that act on adrenergic receptors and of the location of subtypes of adrenergic receptors.

[2] At least three subtypes each of α_1- and α_2-adrenergic receptors are known, but distinctions in their mechanisms of action have not been clearly defined.

[3] In some species (*e.g.*, rat), metabolic responses in the liver are mediated by α_1-adrenergic receptors, whereas in others (*e.g.*, dog) β_2-adrenergic receptors are predominantly involved. Both types of receptors appear to contribute to responses in human beings.

[4] Metabolic responses in adipocytes and certain other tissues with atypical pharmacological characteristics may be mediated by this subtype of receptor. Most β-adrenergic receptor antagonists (including propranolol) do not block these responses.

Table 6–4
Adrenergic Receptors and Their Effector Systems

ADRENERGIC RECEPTOR	G PROTEIN	EXAMPLES OF SOME BIOCHEMICAL EFFECTORS
β_1	G_s	↑ adenylyl cyclase, ↑ L-type Ca^{2+} channels
β_2	G_s	↑ adenylyl cyclase
β_3	G_s	↑ adenylyl cyclase
α_1 Subtypes	G_q	↑ phospholipase C
	G_q	↑ phospholipase D
	G_q, G_i/G_o	↑ phospholipase A_2
	G_q	? ↑ Ca^{2+} channels
α_2 Subtypes	$G_{i\ 1,\ 2,\ or\ 3}$	↓ adenylyl cyclase
	G_i ($\beta\gamma$ subunits)	↑ K^+ channels
	G_o	↓ Ca^{2+} channels (L- and N-type)
	?	↑ PLC, PLA_2

presence of certain α-adrenergic antagonists, the amount of norepinephrine liberated by each nerve impulse increases markedly. This feedback inhibitory effect of norepinephrine on its release from nerve terminals is mediated by α receptors that are pharmacologically distinct from the classical postsynaptic α receptors. Accordingly, these presynaptic α receptors were designated α_2, whereas the postsynaptic "excitatory" α receptors were designated α_1 (*see* Langer, 1997). Compounds such as clonidine are more potent agonists at α_2 than at α_1 receptors; by contrast, phenylephrine and methoxamine selectively activate postsynaptic α_1 receptors. Although there is little evidence to suggest that α_1-adrenergic receptors function presynaptically in the autonomic nervous system, it now is clear that α_2-adrenergic receptors also are present at postjunctional or nonjunctional sites in several tissues. For example, stimulation of postjunctional α_2 receptors in the brain is associated with reduced sympathetic outflow from the CNS and appears to be responsible for a significant component of the antihypertensive effect of drugs such as clonidine (*see* Chapter 10). Thus, the anatomical concept of prejunctional α_2- and postjunctional α_1-adrenergic receptors has been abandoned in favor of a pharmacological and functional classification (*see* Table 6–3).

Cloning revealed additional heterogeneity of both α_1- and α_2-adrenergic receptors (Bylund, 1992). There are three pharmacologically defined α_1-adrenergic receptors (α_{1A}, α_{1B}, and α_{1D}; *see* Table 6–5), with distinct sequences and tissue distributions. Nonetheless, unique functional properties of the different α_1-adrenergic receptor subtypes, for the most part, have not been elucidated. There are three cloned subtypes of α_2-adrenergic receptors (α_{2A}, α_{2B}, α_{2C}; Table 6–5). Distinct patterns of distribution of these subtypes exist in the brain, and it is likely that at least the α_{2A} subtype can serve as a presynaptic autoreceptor (Aantaa *et al.*, 1995; Lakhlani *et al.*, 1997).

Molecular Basis of Adrenergic Receptor Function. The responses that follow activation of all types of adrenergic receptors appear to result from G protein–mediated effects on the generation of second messengers and on the activity of ion channels. As discussed in Chapter 2, these systems involve three interacting proteins—the receptor, the coupling G protein, and effector enzymes or ion channels. The pathways overlap broadly with those discussed for muscarinic receptors and are summarized in Table 6–4.

Structure of Adrenergic Receptors. The adrenergic receptors constitute a family of closely related proteins. They also are related both structurally and functionally to receptors for a wide variety of other hormones and neurotransmitters that are coupled to G proteins (Lefkowitz, 2000). This wider family of receptors includes the muscarinic acetylcholine receptors and even the visual "photon receptor," rhodopsin (*see* Chapter 2). Ligand binding, site-directed labeling, and mutagenesis have revealed that the conserved membrane-spanning regions are crucially involved in the binding of ligands (Strader *et al.*,

Table 6–5

Subtypes of α-Adrenergic Receptors

PHARMACOLOGICAL SUBTYPE	GENE LOCATED ON HUMAN CHROMOSOME NO.	SELECTIVE AGONISTS	SELECTIVE ANTAGONISTS	TISSUE LOCALIZATION
α_{1A}	8	—	5-Methylurapidil (+)-Niguldipine Tamsulosin (compared to α_{1B})	Heart, liver, cerebellum, cerebral cortex, prostate, lung, vas deferens
α_{1B}	5	—	WB4101 (low affinity)	Kidney, spleen, aorta, lung, cerebral cortex
α_{1D}	20	—	—	Aorta, cerebral cortex, prostate, hippocampus
α_{2A}	10	Oxymetazoline	—	Platelet, cerebral cortex, locus ceruleus spinal cord
α_{2B}	2	—	Prazosin*; ARC 239[†]	Liver, kidney
α_{2C}	4	—	Prazosin*; ARC 239[†]	Cerebral cortex

*Prazosin also is a non-subtype selective antagonist at α_1-adrenergic receptors.
[†] ARC 239 blocks the α_{2B} subtype with greater potency than the α_{2C} subtype.

1994; Hutchins, 1994). These regions appear to create a ligand-binding pocket analogous to that formed by the membrane-spanning regions of rhodopsin to accommodate the covalently attached chromophore, retinal, with molecular models placing catecholamines either horizontally (Strader *et al.,* 1994) or perpendicularly (Hutchins, 1994) in the bilayer. The crystal structure of mammalian rhodopsin has been determined and confirms a number of predictions about the structure of G protein–coupled receptors (Palczewski *et al.,* 2000).

β-Adrenergic Receptors.   The three β-adrenergic receptors share approximately 60% amino acid sequence identity within the presumed membrane-spanning domains, where the ligand-binding pocket for epinephrine and norepinephrine is found. Based on results of site-directed mutagenesis, individual amino acids in the β_2-adrenergic receptor that interact with each of the functional groups on the catecholamine agonist molecule have been identified.

All β-adrenergic receptors stimulate adenylyl cyclase *via* interaction with G_s (*see* Chapter 2; *see also* Taussig and Gilman, 1995). Stimulation of the receptor leads to the accumulation of cyclic AMP, activation of the cyclic AMP–dependent protein kinase, and altered function of numerous cellular proteins as a result of their phosphorylation (*see* below). In addition, G_s can enhance directly the activation of voltage-sensitive Ca^{2+} channels in the plasma membrane of skeletal and cardiac muscle; this action provides an additional means of regulating the function of these tissues.

The cyclic AMP–dependent protein kinase (protein kinase A) generally is considered the major intracellular receptor for cyclic AMP. It exists as a tetramer (R_2C_2), consisting of two regulatory (R) and two catalytic (C) subunits. Binding of cyclic AMP causes dissociation of the regulatory subunits, as a result of a 10,000- to 100,000-fold decrease in affinity of R for C, with resultant activation of the catalytic subunits (Francis and Corbin, 1994; Smith *et al.,* 1999). Phosphorylation of various cellular proteins then causes responses that are characteristic of those produced by β-adrenergic agonists. When the stimulus is removed, dephosphorylation of the various protein substrates is catalyzed by phosphoprotein phosphatases. Compartmentalization of protein kinase A is a key determinant in the specificity of responses mediated by this kinase. Localization of protein kinase A is fostered by so-called A-kinase anchoring proteins (AKAPs; Edwards and Scott, 2000).

A well-defined example of these mechanisms is the activation of hepatic glycogen phosphorylase, the enzyme that promotes the rate-limiting step in glycogenolysis, the conversion of glycogen to glucose-1-phosphate. This activation is itself the result of a cascade of phosphorylation reactions. Protein kinase A catalyzes the phosphorylation of phosphorylase kinase, thereby activating it; phosphorylase kinase then phosphorylates and activates phosphorylase. This sequence of successive phosphorylations permits considerable amplification of the initial signal. Thus, only a few receptors need to be stimulated to activate a large number of phosphorylase molecules in a very brief period of time.

Concurrent with the activation of hepatic glycogen phosphorylase, protein kinase A also catalyzes the phosphorylation and inactivation of another enzyme, glycogen synthase, which catalyzes the transfer of glycosyl units from UDP-glucose to glycogen. Phosphorylation decreases the net rate of synthesis of glycogen from glucose. The dual effects of cyclic AMP to enhance conversion of glycogen to glucose and to decrease the synthesis of glycogen from glucose summate to increase the output of glucose from the liver.

Similar types of reactions result in the activation of triglyceride lipase in adipose tissue, with resultant increased release of free fatty acids. The lipase is activated when it is phosphorylated by protein kinase A. Catecholamines provide an increased supply of substrate for oxidative metabolism by this mechanism.

In the heart, stimulation of β-adrenergic receptors leads to positive inotropic and chronotropic responses. Increased intracellular concentrations of cyclic AMP and enhanced phosphorylation of proteins such as troponin and phospholamban are detected after β-adrenergic stimulation. Although these phosphorylation events appear to influence both the actions and the disposition of cellular Ca^{2+}, other events also may contribute to the inotropic response such as direct activation of voltage-sensitive Ca^{2+} channels by G_s.

α-Adrenergic Receptors.

The deduced amino acid sequences from the six α-adrenergic receptor genes, three α_1 genes (α_{1A}, α_{1B}, α_{1D}; Zhong and Minneman, 1999) and three α_2 genes (α_{2A}, α_{2B}, α_{2C}; Bylund, 1992), conform to the well-established paradigm of the seven membrane-spanning G protein–coupled receptors. While not as thoroughly investigated as β-adrenergic receptors, the general structural features and their relation to the functions of ligand binding and G protein activation appear to agree with those set forth in Chapter 2 and above for the β-adrenergic receptors. Within the membrane-spanning domains, the three α_1-adrenergic receptors share approximately 75% identity in amino acid residues, as do the three α_2-adrenergic receptors, but the α_1 and α_2 subtypes are no more similar than are the α and β subtypes (approximately 30% to 40%).

α_2-Adrenergic Receptors.

As shown in Table 6–4, α_2-adrenergic receptors couple to a variety of effectors (Aantaa et al., 1995; Bylund, 1992). Inhibition of adenylyl cyclase activity was the earliest effect observed, but in some systems the enzyme actually is stimulated by α_2 receptors either by G_i $\beta\gamma$ subunits or by weak direct stimulation of G_s. The physiological significance of these latter processes is not currently clear. α_2-Adrenergic receptors activate G protein–gated K^+ channels, resulting in membrane hyperpolarization. In some cases (e.g., cholinergic neurons in the myenteric plexus), this may be Ca^{2+} dependent, whereas in others (e.g., muscarinic acetylcholine receptors in atrial myocytes), it is not and results from direct G protein–mediated coupling of the receptors to the K^+ channels. α_2-Adrenergic receptors also are capable of inhibiting voltage-gated Ca^{2+} channels; this is mediated by G_o proteins. Other second-messenger systems linked to α_2-adrenergic receptor activation include acceleration of Na^+/H^+ exchange, stimulation

of phospholipase $C_{\beta2}$ activity and arachidonic acid mobilization, increased polyphosphoinositide hydrolysis, and increased intracellular availability of Ca^{2+}. The latter is involved in the smooth muscle–contracting effect of α_2 receptor agonists. In addition, it now is clear that α_2 adrenergic receptors activate mitogen-activated protein kinases (MAPKs), likely via $\beta\gamma$ subunits released from pertussis toxin-sensitive G proteins (Della Rocca et al., 1997; Richman and Regan, 1998). This and related pathways lead to activation of a variety of tyrosine kinase–mediated downstream events. These pathways are reminiscent of pathways activated by peptide tyrosine kinase receptors. Although α_2-adrenergic receptors may activate several different signaling pathways, the exact contribution of each to many physiological processes is not clear. The α_{2A}-adrenergic receptor plays a major role in inhibiting norepinephrine release from sympathetic nerve endings and suppressing sympathetic outflow from the brain leading to hypotension (MacMillan et al., 1996; Docherty, 1998; Kable et al., 2000). In addition, the α_{2A}-adrenergic receptor contributes to sedative and anesthetic-sparing effects of α_2-selective agonists (Lakhlani et al., 1997).

α_1-Adrenergic Receptors.

Stimulation of α_1-adrenergic receptors results in the regulation of multiple effector systems. A primary mode of signal transduction involves the mobilization of intracellular Ca^{2+} from endoplasmic stores. This increase in intracellular Ca^{2+} currently is thought to result from activation of phospholipase C_β isoforms through the G_q family of G proteins. The hydrolysis of membrane-bound polyphosphoinositides via phospholipase C results in the generation of two second messengers—diacylglycerol (DAG) and inositol-1,4,5-trisphosphate (IP_3). IP_3 stimulates the release of Ca^{2+} from intracellular stores via a specific receptor-mediated process, while DAG is a potent activator of protein kinase C (see Berridge, 1993). A major component of the responses that follow receptor activation involves regulation of several protein kinases. In addition to protein kinase C, which is activated by Ca^{2+} and diacylglycerol, these include a group of Ca^{2+}- and calmodulin-sensitive protein kinases (Dempsey et al., 2000; Braun and Schulman, 1995). For example, α_1-adrenergic receptors regulate hepatic glycogenolysis in some animal species; this effect results from the activation of phosphorylase kinase by the mobilized Ca^{2+}, aided by the inhibition of glycogen synthase caused by protein kinase C–mediated phosphorylation. Protein kinase C phosphorylates many substrates, including membrane proteins such as channels, pumps, and ion-exchange proteins (e.g., Ca^{2+}-transport ATPase). These effects presumably lead to regulation of various ion conductances.

α_1-Adrenergic stimulation of phospholipase A_2 leads to the release of free arachidonate, which is then metabolized via the cyclooxygenase and lipoxygenase pathways to the bioactive prostaglandins and leukotrienes, respectively (see Chapter 26). Stimulation of phospholipase A_2 activity by various agonists (including epinephrine acting at α_1-adrenergic receptors) is found in many tissues and cell lines, suggesting that this effector is physiologically important. Phospholipase D hydrolyzes phosphatidylcholine to yield phosphatidic acid (PA). Although PA itself may act as a second messenger by releasing Ca^{2+} from intracellular stores, it also is metabolized to the second messenger DAG. Recent studies have demonstrated that phospholipase D is an effector for ADP-ribosylating factor (ARF), suggesting that phospholipase D may play a role in membrane trafficking. Finally, some evidence in vascular smooth muscle suggests that α_1-adrenergic receptors are capable of regulating a Ca^{2+} channel *via* a G protein.

In most smooth muscles, the increased concentrations of intracellular Ca^{2+} ultimately cause contraction as a result of activation of Ca^{2+}-sensitive protein kinases such as the calmodulin-dependent myosin light chain kinase; phosphorylation of the light chain of myosin is associated with the development of tension (Stull *et al.*, 1990). In contrast, the increased concentrations of intracellular Ca^{2+} that result from stimulation of α_1-adrenergic receptors in gastrointestinal smooth muscle cause hyperpolarization and relaxation by activation of Ca^{2+}-dependent K^+ channels (*see* McDonald *et al.*, 1994).

As with α_2 receptors described above, there is considerable evidence demonstrating that α_1 receptors activate MAPKs and other kinases such as PI 3-kinase leading to important effects on cell growth and proliferation (Dorn and Brown, 1999; Gutkind, 1998). For example, prolonged stimulation of α_1 receptors promotes growth of cardiac myocytes and vascular smooth muscle cells.

Localization of Adrenergic Receptors. Presynaptically located α_2- and β_2-adrenergic receptors fulfill important roles in the regulation of neurotransmitter release from sympathetic nerve endings. Presynaptic α_2-adrenergic receptors also may mediate inhibition of release of neurotransmitters other than norepinephrine in the central and peripheral nervous systems. Both α_2- and β_2-adrenergic receptors also are located at postsynaptic sites, *e.g.*, on many types of neurons in the brain. In peripheral tissues, postsynaptic α_2-adrenergic receptors are found in vascular and other smooth muscle cells (where they mediate contraction), adipocytes, and many types of secretory epithelial cells (intestinal, renal, endocrine). Postsynaptic β_2-adrenergic receptors can be found in the myocardium (where they mediate contraction) and also on vascular and other smooth muscle cells (where they mediate relaxation). Both α_2- and β_2-adrenergic receptors may be situated at sites that are relatively remote from nerve terminals releasing norepinephrine. Such extrajunctional receptors typically are found on vascular smooth muscle cells and blood elements (platelets and leukocytes), and may be activated preferentially by circulating catecholamines, particularly epinephrine.

In contrast, α_1- and β_1-adrenergic receptors appear to be located mainly in the immediate vicinity of adrenergic nerve terminals in peripheral target organs, strategically placed to be activated during stimulation of these nerves. These receptors also are widely distributed in the mammalian brain.

The cellular distributions of the three α_1- and three α_2-adrenergic receptor subtypes still are incompletely understood. *In situ* hybridization of receptor mRNA and receptor subtype-specific antibodies indicate that α_{2A}-adrenergic receptors in the brain may be both pre- and postsynaptic. These findings and other studies indicate that this receptor subtype functions as a presynaptic autoreceptor in central noradrenergic neurons (Aantaa *et al.*, 1995; Lakhlani *et al.*, 1997). Using similar approaches, α_{1A} receptor mRNA was found to be the dominant subtype message expressed in prostatic smooth muscle (Walden *et al.*, 1997).

Refractoriness to Catecholamines. Exposure of catecholamine-sensitive cells and tissues to adrenergic ago-

nists causes a progressive diminution in their capacity to respond to such agents. This phenomenon is variously termed *refractoriness, desensitization,* or *tachyphylaxis,* and it significantly limits the therapeutic efficacy and duration of action of catecholamines and other agents (*see* Chapter 2). Although descriptions of such adaptive changes are common, mechanisms are incompletely understood. They have been studied most extensively in cells that synthesize cyclic AMP in response to β-adrenergic receptor agonists.

There is evidence for multiple points of regulation of responsiveness, including the receptors, G proteins, adenylyl cyclase, and cyclic nucleotide phosphodiesterase. The pattern of refractoriness varies according to the extent to which these different components are modified. In some cases, especially when the receptors themselves are altered, desensitization may be limited to the actions of β-adrenergic agents. This often is termed *homologous desensitization*. In other cases, stimulation by a β-adrenergic agonist can cause diminished responsiveness to a wide variety of receptor-mediated stimulators of cyclic AMP synthesis. Although such heterologous desensitization may result from changes in receptors, it also may involve perturbations of more distal elements in the signaling pathway.

One of the most important mechanisms for rapidly regulating β-adrenergic receptor function is agonist stimulation of receptor phosphorylation, which leads to decreased sensitivity to further catecholamine stimulation. The receptors may be phosphorylated by several different protein kinases, but in all cases the end result is the same, decreased coupling to G_s and decreased stimulation of adenylyl cyclase.

Mechanisms for Heterologous Desensitization. One protein kinase that phosphorylates G_s-coupled receptors is protein kinase A, which is stimulated by β-adrenergic receptor-mediated activation of adenylyl cyclase and subsequent elevation of intracellular cyclic AMP levels. This kinase thus enables completion of a negative feedback regulatory loop, phosphorylating and desensitizing the receptor responsible for its stimulation (Hausdorff *et al.*, 1990). The sites of protein kinase A phosphorylation on the β_2-adrenergic receptors have been mapped to the distal portion of the third cytoplasmic loop and the proximal part of the carboxy terminal cytoplasm tail of the receptor, and heterologous desensitization is paralleled by phosphorylation of the residue in the third cytoplasmic loop (Clark *et al.*, 1989; denoted P_2, *see* Figure 6–6). The phosphorylation presumably changes the conformation of the receptor, thereby impairing the coupling to G_s (*see* Figure 6–6).

Mechanisms for Homologous Desensitization. A receptor-directed protein kinase, termed the *β-adrenergic receptor kinase* (βARK), phosphorylates the receptors only when they are occupied by an agonist (Benovic *et al.*, 1986). It subsequently was discovered that βARK is a member of a family of at least

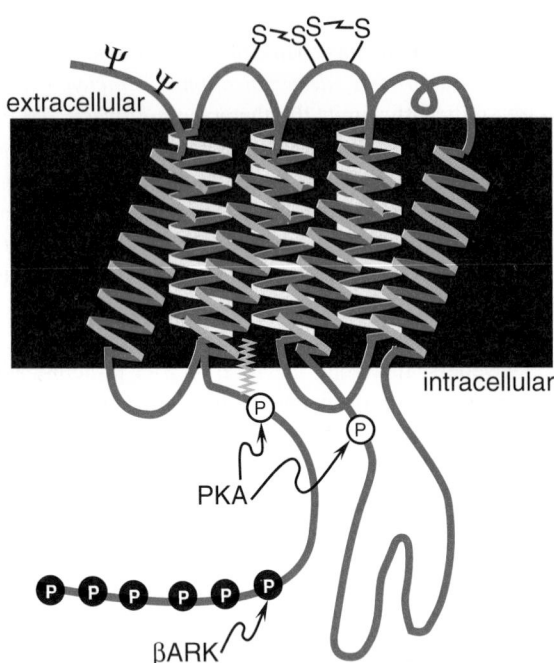

Figure 6–6. Sites of phosphorylation on the β₂-adrenergic receptor.

On the extracellular side of this model of the receptor, S-S represents the proposed disulfide bridges in two extracellular loops. Toward the amino terminus the two consensus sites for *N*-linked glycosylation (Ψ) are shown. On the cytoplasmic side of this model are shown the sites of phosphorylation by the cyclic AMP–dependent protein kinase (PKA; denoted as P in open circles) and β-adrenergic receptor kinase (βARK; denoted as P in black circles). Phosphorylation of the C-terminus of the β-adrenergic receptor by βARK results in subsequent binding of β-arrestin and disruption of functional coupling between β-adrenergic receptors and G_s. Phosphorylation of P by cyclic AMP–dependent protein kinase mediates *heterologous* desensitization of the receptor. The zigzag line indicates the palmitoyl moiety that is covalently attached to Cys-341 in the β₂-adrenergic receptor. (Modified from Collins *et al.*, 1992, with permission.)

six *G protein–coupled receptor kinases* (GRKs) that phosphorylate and regulate a wide variety of G protein–coupled receptors. Because only the agonist-occupied "activated" forms of the β-adrenergic and other receptors are substrates for GRKs, these enzymes provide a mechanism for achieving *homologous* or *agonist-specific* desensitization. GRKs share a similar structural organization (Krupnick and Benovic, 1998; Pitcher *et al.,* 1998). For example, the function of the visual light "receptor" rhodopsin is regulated by a related enzyme, rhodopsin kinase; now called GRK1. While GRK1 is preferentially expressed in retinal rods and cones, GRK2 is broadly expressed in diverse cell types. With the exception of rhodopsin kinase, it is not known with certainty which GRKs regulate which receptors. When β-adrenergic receptors are activated by agonists, they

interact with G_s, dissociating it into α_s and $\beta\gamma$ subunits (*see* Chapter 2). The $G_{\beta\gamma}$-subunit complex, which is attached to the plasma membrane by a lipid group (geranylgeranyl), appears to foster or stabilize βARK (GRK2) association with the plasma membrane, facilitating phosphorylation of the agonist-occupied and activated receptor on multiple serine residues located close to the carboxy terminus of the cytoplasmic tail of the receptor (Figure 6–6).

GRK3 also contains a $\beta\gamma$ binding domain. GRK4 and GRK6 are palmitoylated, and GRK5 contains 2 basic phospholipid-binding domains (Krupnick and Benovic, 1998). GRKs also have been implicated in phosphorylating many other G protein–coupled receptors, including α_{1B} and α_{2A} adrenergic receptors, and receptors for thrombin, angiotensin II, and many other agents. Inhibitors of GRK activity may reduce the development of desensitization. Overexpression of GRK2 in heart cells attenuates β-adrenergic responses in these cells (Koch *et al.,* 1995). Interestingly, there is evidence for increased expression of GRK in the myocardium in patients with congestive heart failure who often have blunted responses to β-adrenergic agonists (Ungerer *et al.,* 1993).

Unlike the situation with protein kinase A-mediated receptor phosphorylation, covalent modification of the G protein–coupled receptor by GRKs alone is not sufficient to fully desensitize receptor function. Rather, a second reaction must occur in which an "arresting" protein binds to the phosphorylated receptor and presumably sterically inhibits its functional coupling to G_s. This protein, called β-arrestin, is one of a family of proteins that fulfills this function in different receptor systems (Krupnick and Benovic, 1998; Lefkowitz, 1998). The homologous protein in the visual system is called arrestin. The arrestin protein binds much more rapidly to the GRK-phosphorylated forms of the receptors than to the nonphosphorylated forms. The binding of an arrestin to the phosphorylated receptor plays a critical role in attenuating receptor signaling in response to agonists.

Agonists also promote a rapid (minutes) and reversible sequestration (internalization) of their receptors and a slower (hours) "down-regulation" of the receptors in which the actual number of receptors in the cell declines. The function of receptor sequestration is not fully understood. Interestingly, there is evidence suggesting that receptor internalization is important for some (Daaka *et al.,* 1998) but not all G protein–coupled receptor-mediated activation of MAP kinase (Schramm and Limbird, 1999; Pierce *et al.,* 2000). Quantitatively, sequestration may not contribute significantly to the mechanisms underlying desensitization, particularly because there is a high degree of amplification between β-adrenergic receptor occupancy and ultimate cyclic AMP–mediated responses in many cells. Nonetheless, some evidence suggests that it may lead to receptor dephosphorylation and resensitization. In addition down-regulation of receptor number contributes to longer-term desensitization of receptor function and undoubtedly is mediated by several distinct processes. These include changes in the rate of receptor turnover, receptor gene transcription, and receptor mRNA turnover. These processes are complex and poorly understood at present (Collins *et al.,* 1992).

There is evidence that sequestration, internalization, and down-regulation may occur for α_2 receptors, although there are important differences among the various subtypes (Saunders and Limbird, 1999; Heck and Bylund, 1998). In addition, some studies have demonstrated phosphorylation and internalization of α_1 receptors after activation by an agonist (Wang *et al.*, 1997; Diviani *et al.*, 1997; Garcia-Sainz *et al.*, 2000).

RELATIONSHIP BETWEEN THE NERVOUS AND THE ENDOCRINE SYSTEMS

The concept that "humours" are secreted at certain sites to act elsewhere in the body can be traced back to Aristotle. In modern terms, the theory of neurohumoral transmission by its very designation implies at least a superficial resemblance between the nervous and the endocrine systems. Yet it should now be clear that the similarities extend considerably deeper, particularly with respect to the autonomic nervous system. In the regulation of homeostasis, the autonomic nervous system is responsible for rapid adjustments to changes in the total environment, which it effects at both its ganglionic synapses and postganglionic terminals by the liberation of chemical agents that act transiently at their immediate sites of release. The endocrine system, in contrast, regulates slower, more generalized adaptations by releasing hormones into the systemic circulation to act at distant, widespread sites over periods of minutes to hours or days. Both systems have major central representations in the hypothalamus, where they are integrated with each other and with subcortical, cortical, and spinal influences. The neurohumoral theory thus may be said to provide a unitary concept of the functioning of the nervous and endocrine systems, in which the differences largely relate to the distances over which the released mediators travel.

PHARMACOLOGICAL CONSIDERATIONS

The foregoing sections contain numerous references to the actions of drugs considered primarily as tools for the dissection and elucidation of physiological mechanisms. This section presents a classification of drugs that act on the peripheral nervous system and its effector organs at some stage of neurotransmission. In the immediately succeeding chapters, as well as elsewhere in the text, the systematic pharmacology of the important members of each of these classes is described.

Each step involved in neurotransmission (*see* Figure 6–2) represents a potential point of therapeutic intervention. This is depicted in the diagram of the adrenergic terminal and its postjunctional site (Figure 6–4). Drugs that affect processes involved in each step of transmission at both cholinergic and adrenergic junctions are summarized in Table 6–6, which lists representative agents that act *via* the mechanisms described below.

Interference with the Synthesis or Release of the Transmitter. *Cholinergic.* Hemicholinium (HC-3), a synthetic compound, blocks the transport system by which choline accumulates in the terminals of cholinergic fibers, thus limiting the synthesis of the ACh store available for release (Birks and MacIntosh, 1957). Vesamicol blocks the transport of ACh into its storage vesicles, preventing its release. The site on the presynaptic nerve terminal for block of ACh release by botulinum toxin was discussed previously; death usually results from respiratory paralysis, unless patients with respiratory failure receive artificial ventilation. Injected locally, botulinum toxin is used in the treatment of muscle dystonias, palsy (*see* Chapter 9), certain ophthalmological conditions associated with spasms of ocular muscles (*see* Chapter 66), or for treatment of anal fissures.

Adrenergic. α-Methyltyrosine (metyrosine) blocks the synthesis of norepinephrine by inhibiting tyrosine hydroxylase, the enzyme that catalyzes the rate-limiting step in catecholamine synthesis. This drug occasionally may be useful in treating selected patients with pheochromocytoma. On the other hand, methyldopa, an inhibitor of aromatic L-amino acid decarboxylase, is—like dopa itself—successively decarboxylated and hydroxylated in its side chain to form the putative "false neurotransmitter" α-methylnorepinephrine. The use of methyldopa in the treatment of hypertension is discussed in Chapter 33. Bretylium, guanadrel, and guanethidine act by preventing the release of norepinephrine by the nerve impulse. However, such agents can transiently stimulate the release of norepinephrine because of their ability to displace the amine from storage sites.

Promotion of the Release of the Transmitter. *Cholinergic.* The ability of cholinergic agents to promote the release of ACh is limited, presumably because ACh and other cholinomimetic agents are quaternary ammonium compounds and do not readily cross the axonal membrane into the nerve ending. The latrotoxins from black widow spider venom and stonefish are known to promote neuroexocytosis by binding to receptors on the neuronal membrane.

Adrenergic. Several drugs that promote the release of the adrenergic mediator lready have been discussed. On the basis of the rate and the duration of the drug-induced release of norepinephrine from adrenergic terminals, one of two opposing effects can predominate. Thus, tyramine, ephedrine, amphetamine, and related drugs cause a

Table 6–6

Type of Action of Representative Agents at Peripheral Cholinergic and Adrenergic Neuroeffector Junctions

MECHANISM OF ACTION	SYSTEM	AGENTS	EFFECT
1. Interference with synthesis of transmitter	Cholinergic	Choline acetyl transferase inhibitors	Minimal depletion of Ach
	Adrenergic	α-Methyltyrosine	Depletion of norepinephrine
2. Metabolic transformation by same pathway as precursor of transmitter	Adrenergic	Methyldopa	Displacement of norepinephrine by false transmitter (α-methylnorepinephrine)
3. Blockade of transport system at nerve terminal membrane	Adrenergic	Cocaine, imipramine	Accumulation of norepinephrine at receptors
	Cholinergic	Hemicholinium	Block of choline uptake with consequent depletion of ACh
4. Blockade of transport system of storage granule (vesicle) membrane	Adrenergic	Reserpine	Destruction of norepinephrine by mitochondrial MAO, and depletion from adrenergic terminals
	Cholinergic	Vesamicol	Block of ACh storage
5. Promotion of neuro-exocytosis or displacement of transmitter from axonal terminal	Cholinergic	Latrotoxins	Cholinomimetic followed by anticholinergic
	Adrenergic	Amphetamine, tyramine	Sympathomimetic
6. Prevention of release of transmitter	Cholinergic	Botulinum toxin	Anticholinergic
	Adrenergic	Bretylium, guanadrel	Antiadrenergic
7. Mimicry of transmitter at postsynaptic receptor	Cholinergic Muscarinic Nicotinic[2]	Muscarine, methacholine[1] Nicotine, epibatidine	Cholinomimetic Cholinomimetic
	Adrenergic α_1 α_2	Phenylephrine Clonidine	Sympathomimetic Sympathomimetic (periphery) Reduced sympathetic outflow (CNS)
	$\beta_{1,2}$	Isoproterenol	Nonselective β-adrenomimetic
	β_1	Dobutamine	Selective cardiac stimulation (but also activates α_1 receptors)
	β_2	Terbutaline	Selective inhibition of smooth muscle contraction

Table 6–6

Types of Action of Representative Agents at Peripheral Cholinergic and Adrenergic Neuroeffector Junctions
(*Continued*)

MECHANISM OF ACTION	SYSTEM	AGENTS	EFFECT
8. Blockade of endogenous transmitter at postsynaptic receptor	Cholinergic Muscarinic Nicotinic, N_M[2] Nicotinic, N_N[3]	Atropine[1] *d*-Tubocurarine Trimethaphan	Muscarinic blockade Neuromuscular blockade Ganglionic blockade
	Adrenergic α $\beta_{1,2}$ β_1 β_2	Phenoxybenzamine Phentolamine Propranolol Metoprolol —	α-Adrenergic blockade (irreversible) α-Adrenergic blockade (reversible) β-Adrenergic blockade Selective adrenergic blockade (cardiac) Selective adrenergic blockade, smooth muscle
9. Inhibition of enzymatic breakdown of transmitter	Cholinergic	Anti-AChE agents (edrophonium, physostigmine, diisopropyl phosphorofluoridate)	Cholinomimetic (muscarinic sites) Depolarization blockade (nicotinic sites)
	Adrenergic	MAO inhibitors (pargyline, nialamine, tranylcypromine)	Little direct effect on norepinephrine or sympathetic responses; potentiation of tyramine

Abbreviations: MAO, monoamine oxidase; ACh, acetylcholine; AChE, acetylcholinesterase.

[1] At least five subtypes of muscarinic receptors exist. Agonists show little selectivity for subtype, whereas several antagonists show partial subtype selectivity.

[2] Two subtypes of muscle nicotinic receptors are known, whereas several subtypes of neuronal nicotinic receptors have been identified.

[3] Multiple neuronal subtypes are found in peripheral ganglia with $\alpha3\beta2$ combinations most prevalent.

relatively rapid, brief liberation of the transmitter and produce a sympathomimetic effect. On the other hand, reserpine, by blocking vesicular uptake of amines, produces a slow, prolonged depletion of the adrenergic transmitter from adrenergic storage vesicles, where it is largely metabolized by intraneuronal MAO. The resultant depletion of transmitter produces the equivalent of adrenergic blockade. Reserpine also causes the depletion of serotonin, dopamine, and possibly other, unidentified amines from central and peripheral sites, and many of its major effects may be a consequence of the depletion of transmitters other than norepinephrine.

A syndrome caused by congenital dopamine-β-hydroxylase deficiency has been described; this syndrome is characterized by the absence of norepinephrine and epinephrine, elevated concentrations of dopamine, intact baroreflex afferent fibers and cholinergic innervation, and undetectable concentrations of plasma dopamine-β-hydroxylase activity (Man in't Veld *et al.*, 1987; Biaggioni and Robertson, 1987). Patients have severe postural hypotension accompanied by other symptoms. *Dihydroxyphenylserine* (L-DOPS) has been shown to improve postural hypotension in this rare disorder. This therapeutic approach cleverly takes advantage of the nonspecificity of aromatic L-amino acid decarboxylase, which synthesizes norepinephrine directly from this drug in the absence of dopamine β-hydroxylase (Man in't Veld *et al.*, 1988; Robertson *et al.*, 1991).

Agonist and Antagonist Actions at Receptors. *Cholinergic.* The nicotinic receptors of autonomic ganglia and skeletal muscle are not identical; they respond differently to certain stimulating and blocking agents and their pentameric structures contain different combinations of homologous subunits (*see* Table 6–2). Dimethylphenylpiperazinium (DMPP) and phenyltrimethylammonium (PTMA) show some selectivity for stimulation of autonomic ganglion cells and end-plates of skeletal muscle, respectively. Trimethaphan and hexamethonium are relatively selective competitive and noncompetitive ganglionic blocking agents. Although tubocurarine effectively blocks transmission at both motor end-plates and autonomic ganglia, its action at the former site predominates. Decamethonium, a depolarizing agent, produces selective neuromuscular blockade. Transmission at autonomic ganglia and the adrenal medulla is complicated further by the presence of muscarinic receptors, in addition to the principal nicotinic receptors (*see* Chapter 9).

Various toxins in snake venoms exhibit a high degree of specificity in the cholinergic nervous system. The α-neurotoxins from the Elapidae family interact with the agonist binding site on the nicotinic receptor. α-Bungarotoxin is selective for the muscle receptor and interacts with only certain neuronal receptors, such as those containing $\alpha7$ through $\alpha9$ subunits. Neuronal bungarotoxin shows a wider range of inhibition of neuronal receptors. A second group of toxins, called the *fasciculins,* inhibit AChE. A third group of toxins, termed the *muscarinic toxins* (MT_1 through MT_4), are partial agonists and antagonists for the muscarinic receptor. Venoms from the Viperidae family of snakes and the fish hunting cone snails also have relatively selective toxins for nicotinic receptors.

Muscarinic receptors, which mediate the effects of ACh at autonomic effector cells, now can be divided into five subclasses. Atropine blocks all the muscarinic responses to injected ACh and related cholinomimetic drugs, whether they are excitatory, as in the intestine, or inhibitory, as in the heart. Newer muscarinic agonists, *pirenzepine* for M_1, *tripitramine* for M_2, and *darifenacin* for M_3, show selectivity as muscarinic blocking agents. Several muscarinic antagonists show sufficient selectivity in clinical setting to minimize the bothersome side effects seen with the nonselective agents at therapeutic doses (*see* Chapter 7).

Adrenergic.   A vast number of synthetic compounds that bear structural resemblance to the naturally occurring catecholamines can interact with α- or β-adrenergic receptors, or both, and produce sympathomimetic effects (*see* Chapter 10). *Phenylephrine* acts selectively at α_1-adrenergic receptor sites, while *clonidine* is a selective α_2-adrenergic agonist. Isoproterenol exhibits agonist activity at both β_1- and β_2-adrenergic receptors. Preferential stimulation of cardiac β_1-adrenergic receptors follows the administration of dobutamine. Terbutaline is an example of a drug with relatively selective action on β_2-adrenergic receptors; it produces effective bronchodilation with minimal effects on the heart. The main features of adrenergic blockade, including the selectivity of various blocking agents for α- and β-adrenergic receptors, have been mentioned (*see also* Chapter 10). Here, too, partial dissociation of effects at β_1- and β_2-adrenergic receptors has been achieved, as exemplified by the β_1-receptor blocking agent metoprolol, which antagonizes the cardiac actions of catecholamines while causing somewhat less antagonism at bronchioles. *Prazosin* and *yohimbine* are representative of α_1- and α_2-adrenergic antagonists, respectively, although prazosin has a relatively high affinity at α_{2B}- and α_{2C}-adrenergic receptor subtypes compared to α_{2A} receptors. Several important drugs that promote the release of norepinephrine or deplete the transmitter resemble, in their effects, activators or blockers of postjunctional receptors (*e.g., tyramine* and *reserpine,* respectively).

Interference with the Destruction of the Transmitter.
Cholinergic.   The anti-ChE agents (Chapter 8) constitute a chemically diverse group of compounds, the primary action of which is inhibition of AChE, with the consequent accumulation of endogenous ACh. At the neuromuscular junction, accumulation of ACh produces depolarization of end-plates and flaccid paralysis. At postganglionic muscarinic effector sites, the response is either excessive stimulation resulting in contraction and secretion or an inhibitory response mediated by hyperpolarization. At ganglia, depolarization and enhanced transmission are observed.

Adrenergic.   The reuptake of norepinephrine by the adrenergic nerve terminals probably is the major mechanism for terminating its transmitter action. Interference with this process is the basis of the potentiating effect of cocaine on responses to adrenergic impulses and injected catecholamines. It also has been suggested that the antidepressant actions and some of the adverse effects of imipramine and related drugs are due to a similar action at adrenergic synapses in the CNS (*see* Chapter 19). Inhibitors of COMT, such as *tolcapone*, enhance dopamine action in the brain of patients with Parkinson's disease (*see* Chapter 22). On the other hand, MAO inhibitors, such as *tranylcypromine*, potentiate the effects of tyramine and may potentiate effects of neurotransmitters.

OTHER AUTONOMIC NEUROTRANSMITTERS

Evidence has accumulated in recent years that the vast majority of neurons in both the central and peripheral nervous systems contain more than one substance with potential or demonstrated activity at relevant postjunctional sites (see Bartfai et al., 1988; Bennett, 1997; Lundberg, 1996; see also Chapter 12). In some cases, especially in peripheral structures, it has been possible to demonstrate that two or more such substances are contained within individual nerve terminals and are released simultaneously upon nerve stimulation. Although the anatomical separation of the parasympathetic and sympathetic components of the autonomic nervous system and the actions of ACh and norepinephrine (their primary neurotransmitters) still provide the essential framework for studying autonomic function, a host of other chemical messengers such as purines, eicosanoids, nitric oxide, and peptides modulate or mediate responses that follow stimulation of the preganglionic neurons of the autonomic nervous system. An expanded view of autonomic neurotransmission has evolved to include instances where substances other than ACh or norepinephrine are released and may function as cotransmitters, neuromodulators, or even primary transmitters. Moreover, vagal fibers innervating the gastrointestinal tract synapse with excitatory and inhibitory postganglionic neurons, allowing for both intrinsic excitation and inhibition during a peristalic wave and inhibition of sphincters.

The evidence for cotransmission, or for so-called nonadrenergic, noncholinergic transmission, in the autonomic nervous system usually encompasses the following considerations: (1) A portion of responses to stimulation of preganglionic or postganglionic nerves or to field stimulation of target structures persists in the presence of concentrations of muscarinic or adrenergic antagonists that completely block their respective agonists. (2) The candidate substance can be detected within nerve fibers that course through target tissues. (3) The substance can be recovered upon microdialysis or in the venous or perfusion effluent following electrical stimulation; such release often can be blocked by tetrodotoxin. (4) Effects of electrical stimulation are mimicked by the application of the substance and are inhibited in the presence of specific antagonists. When such antagonists are not available, reliance often is placed on neutralizing antibodies or selective desensitization produced by prior exposure to the substance. A more recent approach to this challenging problem is the use of "knockout" mice which do not express the putative cotransmitter.

A number of problems confound interpretation of such evidence. It is particularly difficult to establish that substances that fulfill all the listed criteria originate within the autonomic nervous system. In some instances, their origin can be traced to sensory fibers, to intrinsic neurons, or to nerves innervating blood vessels. Also, there may be marked synergism between the candidate sub-

stance and known or unknown transmitters (Lundberg, 1996). In knockout mice, compensatory mechanisms or transmitter redundancy may disguise even well-defined actions (Hökfelt et al., 2000). Finally, it should be recognized that the putative cotransmitter may have primarily a trophic function in maintaining synaptic connectivity or in expressing a particular receptor.

It long has been known that ATP and ACh coexist in cholinergic vesicles (Dowdall et al., 1974) and that ATP and catecholamines both are found within storage granules in nerves and the adrenal medulla (see above). ATP is released along with the transmitters, and either it or its metabolites have a significant function in synaptic transmission in some circumstances (see below). More recently, attention has focused on the growing list of peptides that are found in the adrenal medulla, nerve fibers or ganglia of the autonomic nervous system, or in the structures that are innervated by the autonomic nervous system. This list includes the enkephalins, substance P and other tachykinins, somatostatin, gonadotropin-releasing hormone, cholecystokinin, calcitonin gene–related peptide, galanin, pituitary adenylyl cyclase-activating peptide, VIP, chromogranin, and neuropeptide Y (NPY) (Darlison and Richter, 1999; Lundberg, 1996; Bennett, 1997, Hökfelt et al., 2000). Some of the orphan G protein–coupled receptors discovered in the course of genome sequencing projects may represent receptors for as yet undiscovered peptides or other cotransmitters. The evidence for widespread transmitter function in the autonomic nervous system is substantial for VIP and NPY, and further discussion is confined to these peptides. The possibility that abnormalities in function of neuropeptide cotransmitters, for example in type 2 diabetes, contribute to disease pathogenesis remains of interest (Ahren, 2000).

Cotransmission in the Autonomic Nervous System. Both norepinephrine and ATP elicit excitation when released from certain adrenergic nerve terminals, such as those in the vas deferens and the vasculature. The response to ATP is rapid and that to norepinephrine is slower (Sneddon and Westfall, 1984). Sympathectomy and adrenergic neuron–depleting agents such as reserpine eliminate both phases of the response, consistent with storage of both substances in the same population of vesicles. In other cases, metabolism of ATP to adenosine in the extracellular space results in important modulatory effects. There also is evidence that adenosine exerts inhibitory effects on the release of transmitter, and the administration of adenosine-receptor antagonists such as theophylline results in increased concentrations of norepinephrine and other components of the storage vesicle in the circulation.

The pioneering studies of Hökfelt and coworkers (Lundberg *et al.,* 1979), which demonstrated the existence of VIP and ACh in peripheral autonomic neurons, initiated interest in the possibility of peptidergic cotransmission in the autonomic nervous system. Subsequent work has confirmed the frequent association of these two substances in autonomic fibers, including parasympathetic fibers that innervate smooth muscle and exocrine glands and cholinergic sympathetic neurons that innervate sweat glands (Hökfelt *et al.,* 2000).

The role of VIP in parasympathetic transmission has been most extensively studied in the regulation of salivary secretion. The evidence for cotransmission includes the release of VIP following stimulation of the chorda lingual nerve and the incomplete blockade by atropine of vasodilation when the frequency of stimulation is raised; the latter observation may indicate independent release of the two substances, which is consistent with histochemical evidence for storage of ACh and VIP in separate populations of vesicles. Synergism between ACh and VIP in stimulating vasodilation and secretion also has been described. VIP may be involved in parasympathetic responses in the trachea and the gastrointestinal tract; in the latter it may facilitate sphincter relaxation.

The neuropeptide Y family of peptides is widely distributed in the central and peripheral nervous systems and consists of three members: NPY, pancreatic polypeptide, and peptide YY. In the CNS, NPY function is linked to food and water intake, regulation of mood, and central autonomic control. In the periphery, NPY is found in large vesicles within sympathetic nerve fibers and is involved in the maintenance of vascular tone. NPY and norepinephrine are coreleased, although low-frequency stimulation may favor norepinephrine release. NPY has a potent and prolonged vasoconstrictor action, with small blood vessels being more sensitive. Its activity appears to be synergistic with that of norepinephrine. Multiple subtypes of NPY receptors have been identified and cloned; all appear to function through G proteins (Wahlestedt and Reis, 1993). The role of NPY, especially including its regulation of leptin and regulation of appetite and body weight, offers the potential for discovery of novel drugs for the treatment of obesity (Good, 2000; Poyner *et al.,* 2000; Halford and Blundell, 2000).

Nonadrenergic, Noncholinergic Transmission by Purines.   The smooth muscle of many tissues that are innervated by the autonomic nervous system shows inhibitory junction potentials following stimulation by field electrodes (Bennett, 1997). Since such responses frequently are undiminished in the presence of adrenergic and muscarinic cholinergic antagonists, these observations have been taken as evidence for the existence of nonadrenergic, noncholinergic transmission in the autonomic nervous system.

Burnstock (1969, 1996) and his colleagues have compiled compelling evidence for the existence of purinergic neurotransmission in the gastrointestinal tract, genitouri-

nary tract, and certain blood vessels; ATP has fulfilled all the criteria for a neurotransmitter listed above. However, in at least some circumstances, primary sensory axons may be an important source of ATP (Burnstock, 2000). Although adenosine is generated from the released ATP by ectoenzymes, its primary function appears to be modulatory by causing feedback inhibition of release of the transmitter.

Adenosine can be transported from the cell cytoplasm to activate extracellular receptors on adjacent cells. The efficient uptake of adenosine by cellular transporters and its rapid rate of metabolism to inosine or to adenine nucleotides contribute to its rapid turnover. Several inhibitors of adenosine transport and metabolism are known to influence extracellular adenosine and ATP concentrations (Sneddon *et al.,* 1999).

The purinergic receptors found on the cell surface may be divided into the adenosine (A or P1) and the ATP (P2) receptors (Fredholm *et al.,* 1997). Each of P1 and P2 receptors has been found to have various subtypes. Methylxanthines such as *caffeine* and *theophylline* preferentially block adenosine receptors (*see* Chapter 28). At least seven subtypes of both P1 and P2 receptors have been identified in brain, peripheral tissues, and circulating blood cells. Most mediate their responses *via* G proteins, although the P2X receptors are a subfamily of ion-gated ion channels (Burnstock, 2000). P2Y receptors have been found to activate MAP kinase (Neary, 2000).

Modulation of Vascular Responses by Endothelium-Derived Factors.   Furchgott and colleagues demonstrated that an intact endothelium was necessary to achieve vascular relaxation in response to ACh (*see* Furchgott, 1984, 1999). This inner layer of the blood vessel now is known to modulate autonomic and hormonal effects on the contractility of blood vessels. In response to a variety of vasoactive agents and even physical stimuli, the endothelial cells release a short-lived vasodilator called endothelium-derived relaxing factor (EDRF), now known to be nitric oxide. Less commonly an endothelium-derived hyperpolarizing factor (EDHF) and endothelium-derived contracting factor (EDCF) of as yet undefined compositions are released (Vanhoutte, 1996). EDCF formation is dependent on cyclooxygenase activity.

Products of inflammation and platelet aggregation such as serotonin, histamine, bradykinin, purines, and thrombin exert all or part of their action by stimulating the release of nitric oxide. Endothelial cell-dependent mechanisms of relaxation are important in a variety of vascular beds, including the coronary circulation (Hobbs *et al.,* 1999). Activation of specific G protein–linked receptors on endothelial cells promotes release of nitric oxide. Nitric oxide diffuses readily to the underlying smooth muscle and induces relaxation of vascular smooth muscle by activating guanylyl cyclase, which increases cyclic GMP concentrations. Nitrovasodilating drugs used to lower blood pressure or to treat ischemic heart disease probably act through conversion to or release of nitric oxide (*see* Chapter 32). Nitric oxide also has been shown to be released from certain nerves (*nitrergic*) innervating blood vessels. It has a negative inotropic action on the heart.

Recently, it has become clear that alterations in the release or action of nitric oxide may have importance for a number of major clinical situations such as atherosclerosis (Hobbs *et al.,* 1999; Ignarro, 1999). Furthermore, there is evidence suggesting that the hypotension of endotoxemia or that induced by cytokines is mediated at least in part by induction of enhanced release of nitric oxide; consequently, increased release of nitric oxide may have pathological significance in septic shock. Nitric oxide is synthesized from L-arginine and molecular oxygen by *nitric oxide synthase* (NOS). There are three known forms of this enzyme (Moncada *et al.,* 1997). One form is constitutive, residing in the endothelial cell and releasing nitric oxide over short periods in response to receptor-mediated increases in cellular Ca^{2+} (eNOS) (Michel and Feron, 1997). A second form is responsible for the Ca^{2+}-dependent release from neurons (nNOS). The third form of NOS is induced after activation of cells by cytokines and bacterial endotoxins and, once expressed, synthesizes nitric oxide for long periods of time (iNOS). This Ca^{2+}-independent, high-output form is responsible for the above-mentioned toxic manifestations of nitric oxide. Glucocorticoids inhibit the expression of inducible, but not constitutive, forms of nitric oxide synthase in vascular endothelial cells. However, other endothelium-derived factors also may be involved in vasodilation and hyperpolarization of the smooth muscle cell. There has been considerable interest in the possibility that NOS inhibitors might have therapeutic benefit, for example, in septic shock and neurodegenerative diseases (Hobbs, 1999). Conversely, diminished release of nitric oxide from the endothelial cell layer in atherosclerotic coronary arteries may contribute to the risk of myocardial infarction.

Full contractile responses of cerebral arteries also require an intact endothelium. A family of peptides, termed *endothelins,* are stored in vascular endothelial cells. Their release onto smooth muscle promotes contraction by stimulation of endothelin receptors. Endothelins contribute to the maintenance of vascular homostasis by acting *via* multiple endothelin receptors (Sokolovsky, 1995) to reverse the response to nitric oxide (Rubanyi and Polokoff, 1994).

BIBLIOGRAPHY

Ahlquist, R.P. A study of the adrenotropic receptors. *Am. J. Physiol.,* **1948,** *153*:586–600.

Ahren, B. Autonomic regulation of islet hormone secretion—implications for health and disease. *Diabetologia,* **2000,** *43*:393–410.

Arner, P., and Hoffstedt, J. Adrenoceptor genes in human obesity. *J. Intern. Med.,* **1999,** *245*:667–672.

Benovic, J.L., Strasser, R.H., Caron, M.G., and Lefkowitz, R.J. β-Adrenergic receptor kinase: identification of a novel protein kinase that phosphorylates the agonist-occupied form of the receptor. *Proc. Natl. Acad. Sci. U.S.A.,* **1986,** *83*:2797–2801.

Biaggioni, I., and Robertson, D. Endogenous restoration of noradrenaline by precursor therapy in dopamine-beta-hydroxylase deficiency. *Lancet,* **1987,** *2*:1170–1172.

Bönisch, H., and Trendelenburg, U. The mechanism of action of indirectly acting sympathomimetic amines. In, *Catecholamines I.* (Trendelenburg, U., and Weiner, N., eds.) *Handbook of Experimental Pharmacology.* Vol. 90. Springer-Verlag, Berlin, **1988,** pp. 247–277.

Bowersox, S.S., Singh, T., Nadasdi, L., Zukowska-Grojec, Z., Valentino, K., and Hoffman, B.B. Cardiovascular effects of omega-conopeptides in conscious rats: mechanisms of action. *J. Cardiovasc. Pharmacol.,* **1992,** *20*:756–764.

Cannon, W.B., and Uridil, J.E. Studies on conditions of activity in endocrine glands. VIII. Some effects on the denervated heart of stimulating the nerves of the liver. *Am. J. Physiol.,* **1921,** *58*:353–354.

Carroll, J.M., Evinger, M.J., Goodman, H.M., and Joh, T.H. Differential and coordinate regulation of TH and PNMT mRNAs in chromaffin cell cultures by second messenger system activation and steroid treatment. *J. Mol. Neurosci.,* **1991,** *3*:75–83.

Clark, R.B., Friedman, J., Dixon, R.A.F., and Strader, C.D. Identification of a specific site required for rapid heterologous desensitization of the β-adrenergic receptor by cAMP-dependent protein kinase. *Mol. Pharmacol.,* **1989,** *36*:343–348.

Daaka, Y., Luttrell, L.M., Ahn, S., Della Rocca, G.J., Ferguson, S.S., Caron, M.G., and Lefkowitz, R.J. Essential role for G protein-coupled receptor endocytosis in the activation of mitogen-activated protein kinase. *J. Biol. Chem.,* **1998,** *273*:685–688.

Dale, H.H. The action of certain esters and ethers of choline, and their relation to muscarine. *J. Pharmacol. Exp. Ther.,* **1914,** *6*:147–190.

Daubner, S.C., Lauriano, C., Haycock, J.W., and Fitzpatrick, P.F. Site-directed mutagenesis of serine 40 of rat tyrosine hydroxylase. Effects of dopamine and cAMP-dependent phosphorylation on enzyme activity. *J. Biol. Chem.*, **1992**, *267*:12639–12646.

Della Rocca, G.J., van Biesen, T., Daaka, Y., Luttrell, D.K., Luttrell, L.M., and Lefkowitz, R.J. Ras-dependent mitogen-activated protein kinase activation by G protein–coupled receptors. Convergence of Gi- and Gq-mediated pathways on calcium/calmodulin, Pyk2, and Src kinase. *J. Biol. Chem.*, **1997**, *272*:19125–19132.

Dempsey, E.C., Newton, A.C., Mochly-Rosen, D., Fields, A.P., Reyland, M.E., Insel, P.A., and Messing, R.O. Protein kinase C isozymes and the regulation of diverse cell responses. *Am. J. Physiol. Lung Cell Mol. Physiol.*, **2000**, *279*:L429–L438.

De Robertis, E.D., and Bennett, H.S. Some features of the submicroscopic morphology of synapses in frog and earthworm. *J. Biophys. Biochem. Cytol.*, **1955**, *1*:47–58.

Diviani, D., Lattion, A.L., and Cotecchia, S. Characterization of the phosphorylation sites involved in G protein-coupled receptor kinase- and protein kinase C-mediated desensitization of the alpha1B-adrenergic receptor. *J. Biol. Chem.*, **1997**, *272*:28712–28719.

Dowdall, M.J., Boyne, A.F., and Whittaker, V.P. Adenosine triphosphate, a constituent of cholinergic synaptic vesicles. *Biochem. J.*, **1974**, *140*:1–12.

Emorine, L.J., Marullo, S., Briend-Sutren, M.-M., Patey, G., Tate, K., Delavier-Klutchko, C., and Strosberg, A.D. Molecular characterization of the human β3-adrenergic receptor. *Science*, **1989**, *245*:1118–1121.

Fatt, P., and Katz, B. Spontaneous subthreshold activity at motor nerve endings. *J. Physiol. (Lond.)*, **1952**, *117*:109–128.

Garcia-Sainz, J.A., Vazquez-Prado, J., and del Carmen Medina, L. Alpha₁-adrenoceptors: function and phosphorylation. *Eur. J. Pharmacol.*, **2000**, *389*:1–12.

Granneman, J.G., Lahners, K.N., and Chaudhry, A. Characterization of the human β3-adrenergic receptor gene. *Mol. Pharmacol.*, **1993**, *44*:264–270.

Hille, B., Billiard, J., Babcock, D.F., Nguyen, T., and Koh, D.S. Stimulation of exocytosis without a calcium signal. *J. Physiol.*, **1999a**, *520*(pt 1):23–31.

Hodgkin, A.L., and Huxley, A.F. A quantitative description of membrane current and its application to conduction and excitation in nerve. *J. Physiol. (Lond.)*, **1952**, *117*:500–544.

Kable, J.W., Murrin, L.C., and Bylund, D.B. In vivo gene modification elucidates subtype-specific functions of alpha(2)-adrenergic receptors. *J. Pharmacol. Exp. Ther.*, **2000**, *293*:1–7.

Katz, B., and Miledi, R. The measurement of synaptic delay, and the time course of acetylcholine release at the neuromuscular junction. *Proc. R. Soc. Lond. [Biol.]*, **1965**, *161*:483–495.

Katz, B., and Miledi, R. The statistical nature of the acetylcholine potential and its molecular components. *J. Physiol.*, **1972**, *224*:665–699.

Kennedy, B., Elayan, H., and Ziegler, M.G. Glucocorticoid elevation of mRNA encoding epinephrine-forming enzyme in lung. *Am J Physiol.*, **1993**, *265*:L117–L120.

Kennedy, B., and Ziegler, M.G. Cardiac epinephrine synthesis. Regulation by a glucocorticoid. *Circulation*, **1991**, *84*:891–895.

Koch, W.J., Rockman, H.A., Samama, P., Hamilton, R.A., Bond, R.A., Milano, C.A., and Lefkowitz, R.J. Cardiac function in mice overexpressing the beta-adrenergic receptor kinase or a beta ARK inhibitor. *Science*, **1995**, *268*:1350–1353.

Krief, S., Lönnqvist, F., Raimbault, S., Baude, B., Van Spronsen, A., Arner, P., Strosberg, A.D., Ricquier, D., and Emorine, L.J. Tissue distribution of β3-adrenergic receptor mRNA in man. *J. Clin. Invest.*, **1993**, *91*:344–349.

Krnjević, K., and Mitchell, J.F. The release of acetylcholine in the isolated rat diaphragm. *J. Physiol. (Lond.)*, **1961**, *155*:246–262.

Krupnick, J.G., and Benovic, J.L. The role of receptor kinases and arrestins in G protein-coupled receptor regulation. *Annu. Rev. Pharmacol. Toxicol.*, **1998**, *38*:289–319.

Kumer, S.C., and Vrana, K.E. Intricate regulation of tyrosine hydroxylase activity and gene expression. *J. Neurochem.*, **1996**, *67*:443–462.

Lakhlani, P.P., MacMillan, L.B., Guo, T.Z., McCool, B.A., Lovinger, D.M., Maze, M., and Limbird, L.E. Substitution of a mutant alpha2a-adrenergic receptor via "hit and run" gene targeting reveals the role of this subtype in sedative, analgesic, and anesthetic-sparing responses in vivo. *Proc. Natl. Acad. Sci. U.S.A.*, **1997**, *94*:9950–9955.

Lands, A.M., Arnold, A., McAuliff, J.P., Luduena, F.P., and Brown, T.G. Differentiation of receptor systems activated by sympathomimetic amines. *Nature*, **1967**, *214*:597–598.

Langley, J.N. On the union of cranial autonomic (visceral) fibers with the nerve cells of the superior cervical ganglion. *J. Physiol.*, **1898**, *23*:240–270.

Langley, J.N. Observations on the physiological action of extracts of the supra-renal bodies. *J. Physiol. (Lond.)*, **1901**, *27*:237–256.

Lewandowsky, M. Ueber eine Wirkung des Nebennieren-extractes auf das Auge. *Zentralbl. Physiol.*, **1898**, *12*:599–600.

Lin, R.C., and Scheller, R.C. Structural organization of the synaptic exocytosis core complex. *Neuron*, **1997**, *19*:1087–1094.

Loewi, O., and Navratil, E. Über humorale Übertragbarkeit der Herznervenwirkung. X. Mitteilung. Über das Schicksal des Vagusstoff. *Pflügers Arch. Gesamte Physiol.*, **1926**, *214*:678–688.

Lönnqvist, F., Krief, S., Strosberg, A.D., Nyberg, B., Emorine, L.J., and Arner, P. Evidence for a functional β3-adrenoceptor in man. *Br. J. Pharmacol.*, **1993**, *110*:929–936.

Lugardon, K., Raffner, R., Goumon, Y., Corti, A., Delmas, A., Bulet, P., Aunis, D., and Metz-Boutigue, M.H. Antibacterial and antifungal activities of vasostatin-1, the N-terminal fragment of chromogranin A. *J. Biol. Chem.*, **2000**, *275*:10745–10753.

Lundberg, J.M., Hökfelt, T., Schultzberg, M., Uvnäs-Wallensten, K., Köhler, C., and Said, S.I. Occurrence of vasoactive intestinal polypeptide (VIP)-like immunoreactivity in certain cholinergic neurons of the cat: evidence from combined immunohistochemistry and acetylcholinesterase staining. *Neuroscience*, **1979**, *4*:1539–1559.

MacMillan, L.B., Hein, L., Smith, M.S., Piascik, M.T., and Limbird, L.E. Central hypotensive effects of the alpha2a-adrenergic receptor subtype. *Science*, **1996**, *9*:801–803.

Man in't Veld, A.J., Boomsma, F., Moleman, P., and Schalekamp, M.A.D.H. Congenital dopamine-beta-hydroxylase deficiency. A novel orthostatic syndrome. *Lancet*, **1987**, *1*:183–188.

Moncada, S., Higgs, A., and Furchgott, R. International Union of Pharmacology Nomenclature in Nitric Oxide Research. *Pharmacol. Rev.*, **1997**, *49*:137–142.

Murthy, V.N., and Stevens, C.F. Synaptic vesicles retain their identity through the endocytic cycle. *Nature*, **1998**, *392*:497–501.

Neary, J.T. Trophic actions of extracellular ATP: gene expression profiling by DNA array analysis. *J. Auton. Nerv. Syst.*, **2000**, *81*:200–204.

Okuda, T., Haga, T., Kanai, Y., Endou, H., Ishihara, T., and Katsura, I. Identification and characterization of the high-affinity choline transporter. *Nat. Neurosci.*, **2000**, *3*:120–125.

Palczewski, K., Kumasaka, T., Hori, T., Behnke, C.A., Motoshima, H., Fox, B.A., Le Trong, I., Teller, D.C., Okada, T., Stenkamp, R.E., Yamamoto, M., and Miyano, M. Crystal structure of rhodopsin: A G protein–coupled receptor. *Science*, **2000**, *289*:739–745.

Pierce, K.L., Maudsley, S., Daaka, Y., Luttrell, L.M., and Lefkowitz, R.J. Role of endocytosis in the activation of the extracellular signal-regulated kinase cascade by sequestering and nonsequestering G protein–coupled receptors. *Proc. Natl. Acad. Sci. U.S.A.,* **2000,** *97*:1489–1494.

Pitcher, J.A., Freedman, N.J., and Lefkowitz, R.J. G protein–coupled receptor kinases. *Annu. Rev. Biochem.,* **1998,** *67*:653–692.

Richman, J.G., and Regan, J.W. Alpha₂-adrenergic receptors increase cell migration and decrease F-actin labeling in rat aortic smooth muscle cells. *Am. J. Physiol.,* **1998,** *274*:C654–662.

Rosenbaum, M., Malbon, C.C., Hirsch, J., and Leibel, R.L. Lack of β3-adrenergic effect on lipolysis in human subcutaneous adipose tissue. *J. Clin. Endocrinol. Metab.,* **1993,** *77*:352–355.

Schramm, N.L., and Limbird, L.E. Stimulation of mitogen-activated protein kinase by G protein–coupled alpha(2)-adrenergic receptors does not require agonist-elicited endocytosis. *J. Biol. Chem.,* **1999,** *274*:24935–24940.

Sneddon, P., and Westfall, D.P. Pharmacological evidence that adenosine trisphosphate and noradrenaline are co-transmitters in the guinea-pig vas deferens. *J. Physiol.,* **1984,** *347*:561–580.

Sneddon, P., Westfall, T.D., Todorov, L.D., Mihaylova-Todorova, S., Westfall, D.P., and Kennedy, C. Modulation of purinergic neurotransmission. *Prog. Brain Res.,* **1999,** *120*:11–20.

Steinsland, O.S., Furchgott, R.F., and Kirpekar, S.M. Inhibition of adrenergic neurotransmission by parasympathomimetics in the rabbit ear artery. *J. Pharmacol. Exp. Ther.,* **1973,** *184*:346–356.

Ungerer, M., Bohm, M., Elce, J.S., Erdmann, E., and Lohse, M.J. Altered expression of beta-adrenergic receptor kinase and beta 1-adrenergic receptors in the failing human heart. *Circulation,* **1993,** *87*:454–463.

Varoqui, H., and Erickson, J.D. Vesicular neurotransmitter transporters. Potential sites for the regulation of synaptic function. *Mol. Neurobiol.,* **1997,** *15*:165–191.

Viskupic, E., Kvetnansky, R., Sabban, E.L., Fukuhara, K., Weise, V.K., Kopin, I.J., and Schwartz, J.P. Increase in rat adrenal phenylethanolamine N-methyltransferase mRNA level caused by immobilization stress depends on intact pituitary-adrenocortical axis. *J. Neurochem.,* **1994,** *63*:808–814.

Walden, P.D., Durkin, M.M., Lepor, H., Wetzel, J.M., Gluchowski, C., and Gustafson, E.L. Localization of mRNA and receptor binding sites for the alpha₁ₐ-adrenoceptor subtype in the rat, monkey and human urinary bladder and prostate. *J. Urol.,* **1997,** *157*:1032–1038.

Wang, J., Zheng, J., Anderson, J.L., and Toews, M.L. A mutation in the hamster alpha₁ʙ-adrenergic receptor that differentiates two steps in the pathway of receptor internalization. *Mol. Pharmacol.,* **1997,** *52*:306–313.

Wevers, R.A., de Rijk-van Andel, J.F., Brautigam, C., Geurtz, B., van den Heuvel, L.P., Steenbergen-Spanjers, G.C., Smeitink, J.A., Hoffmann, G.F., and Gabreels, F.J. A review of biochemical and molecular genetic aspects of tyrosine hydroxylase deficiency including a novel mutation (291delC). *J. Inherit. Metab. Dis.,* **1999,** *22*:364–373.

Winkler, H. Membrane composition of adrenergic large and small dense cored vesicles and of synaptic vesicles: consequences for their biogenesis. *Neurochem. Res.,* **1997,** *22*:921–932.

MONOGRAPHS AND REVIEWS

Aantaa, R., Mariamaki, A., and Scheinin, M. Molecular pharmacology of α2-adrenoceptors subtypes. *Ann. Med.,* **1995,** *27*:439–449.

Amara, S.G., and Kuhar, M.J. Neurotransmitter transporters: recent progress. *Annu. Rev. Neurosci.,* **1993,** *16*:73–93.

Andresen, M.C., and Kunze, D.L. Nucleus tractus solitarius—gateway to neural circulatory control. *Annu. Rev. Physiol.,* **1994,** *56*:93–116.

Aunis, D. Exocytosis in chromaffin cells of the adrenal medulla. *Int. Rev. Cytol.,* **1998,** *181*:213–320.

Axelrod, J. Methylation reactions in the formation and metabolism of catecholamines and other biogenic amines. *Pharmacol. Rev.,* **1966,** *18*:95–113.

Bartfai, T., Iverfeldt, K., Fisone, G., and Serfozo, P. Regulation of the release of coexisting neurotransmitters. *Annu. Rev. Pharmacol. Toxicol.,* **1988,** *28*:285–310.

Bennett, M.R. Non-adrenergic non-cholinergic (NANC) transmission to smooth muscle: 35 years on. *Prog. Neurobiol.,* **1997,** *52*:159–195.

Benovic, J.L., Bouvier, M., Caron, M.G., and Lefkowitz, R.J. Regulation of adenylyl cyclase-coupled β-adrenergic receptors. *Annu. Rev. Cell Biol.,* **1988,** *4*:405–428.

Bernard, C. *Leçons sur les phénomènes de la vie communs aux animaux et aux végétaux.* Baillière, Paris, **1878–1879.** (Two volumes.)

Berridge, M.J. Inositol trisphosphate and calcium signalling. *Nature,* **1993,** *361*:315–325.

Birks, R.I., and MacIntosh, F.C. Acetylcholine metabolism at nerve endings. *Br. Med. Bull.,* **1957,** *13*:157–161.

Bonner, T.I. The molecular basis of muscarinic receptor diversity. *Trends Neurosci.,* **1989,** *12*:148–151.

Bowman, W.C., Prior, C., and Marshall, I.G. Presynaptic receptors in the neuromuscular junction. *Ann. N.Y. Acad. Sci.,* **1990,** *604*:69–81.

Braun, A.P., and Schulman, H. The multifunctional calcium/calmodulin-dependent protein kinase: from form to function. *Annu. Rev. Physiol.,* **1995,** *57*:417–445.

Brownstein, M.J., and Hoffman, B.J. Neurotransmitter transporters. *Recent Prog. Horm. Res.,* **1994,** *49*:27–42.

Burnstock, G. Evolution of the autonomic innervation of visceral and cardiovascular systems in vertebrates. *Pharmacol. Rev.,* **1969,** *21*:247–324.

Burnstock, G. Purinergic neurotransmission. *Semin. Neurosci.,* **1996,** *8*:171–257.

Burnstock, G. P2X receptors in sensory neurons. *Br. J. Anaesth.,* **2000,** *84*:476–488.

Bylund, D.B. Subtypes of α1- and α2-adrenergic receptors. *FASEB J.,* **1992,** *6*:832–839.

Cannon, W.B. Organization for physiological homeostasis. *Physiol. Rev.,* **1929,** *9*:399–431.

Cannon, W.B. *The Wisdom of the Body.* Norton, New York, **1932.**

Catterall, W.A. Cellular and molecular biology of voltage-gated sodium channels. *Physiol. Rev.,* **1992,** *72*(suppl 4):S15–S48.

Catterall, W.A. From ionic currents to molecular mechanisms: the structure and function of voltage-gated sodium channels. *Neuron,* **2000,** *26*:13–25.

Caulfield, M.P., and Birdsall, N.J. International Union of Pharmacology: XVII. Classification of muscarinic acetylcholine receptors. *Pharmacol. Rev.,* **1998,** *50*:279–290.

Changeux, J.-P., and Edelstein, S.J. Allosteric receptors after 30 years. *Neuron,* **1998,** *21*:959–980.

Chong, B.S., and Mersfelder, T.L. Entacapone. *Ann. Pharmacother.,* **2000,** *34*:1056–1065.

Collins, S., Caron, M.G., and Lefkowitz, R.J. From ligand binding to gene expression: new insights into the regulation of G-protein–coupled receptors. *Trends Biochem. Sci.,* **1992,** *17*:37–39.

Dale, H.H. The beginnings and the prospects of neurohumoral transmission. *Pharmacol. Rev.,* **1954,** *6*:7–13.

Darlison, M.G., and Richter, D. Multiple genes for neuropeptides and their receptors: co-evolution and physiology. *Trends Neurosci.,* **1999,** 22:81–88.

Docherty, J.R. Subtypes of functional alpha1- and alpha2-adrenoceptors. *Eur. J. Pharmacol.,* **1998,** *361*:1–15.

Dooley, T.P. Cloning of the human phenol sulfotransferase gene family: three genes implicated in the metabolism of catecholamines, thyroid hormones and drugs. *Chem. Biol. Interact.,* **1998,** *109*:29–41.

Dorn, G.W., and Brown, J.H. Gq signaling in cardiac adaptation and maladaptation. *Trends Cardiovasc. Med.,* **1999,** *9*:26–34.

Eccles, J.C. *The Physiology of Synapses.* Springer-Verlag, Berlin; Academic Press, New York, **1964.**

Eccles, J.C. *The Understanding of the Brain.* McGraw-Hill, New York, **1973.**

Edwards, A.S., and Scott, J.D. A-kinase anchoring proteins: protein kinase A and beyond. *Curr. Opin. Cell Biol.,* **2000,** *12*:217–221.

Eiden, L.E. The cholinergic gene locus. *J. Neurochem.,* **1998,** *70*:2227–2240.

Fernandez-Chacon, R., and Südhof, T.C. Genetics of synaptic vesicle function: toward the complete functional anatomy of an organelle. *Annu. Rev. Physiol.,* **1999,** *61*:753–776.

Francis, S.H., and Corbin, J.D. Structure and function of cyclic nucleotide-dependent protein kinases. *Annu. Rev. Physiol.,* **1994,** *56*:237–272.

Fredholm, B.B., Abbracchio, M.P., Burnstock, G., Dubyak, G.R., Harden, T.K., Jacobson, K.A., Schwabe, U., and Williams, M. Towards a revised nomenclature for P1 and P2 receptors. *Trends Pharmacol. Sci.,* **1997,** *18*:79–82.

Furchgott, R.F. The role of endothelium in the responses of vascular smooth muscle to drugs. *Annu. Rev. Pharmacol. Toxicol.,* **1984,** *24*:175–197.

Furchgott, R.F. Endothelium-derived relaxing factor: discovery, early studies, and identification as nitric oxide. *Biosci. Rep.,* **1999,** *19*:235–251.

Goldberg, L.I., Volkman, P.H., and Kohli, J.D. A comparison of the vascular dopamine receptor with other dopamine receptors. *Annu. Rev. Pharmacol. Toxicol.,* **1978,** *18*:57–79.

Good, D.J. How tight are your genes? Transcriptional and posttranscriptional regulation of the leptin receptor, NPY, and POMC genes. *Horm. Behav.,* **2000,** *37*:284–298.

Gutkind, J.S. The pathways connecting G protein-coupled receptors to the nucleus through divergent mitogen-activated protein kinase cascades. *J. Biol. Chem.,* **1998,** *273*:1839–1842.

Halford, J.C., and Blundell, J.E. Pharmacology of appetite suppression. *Prog. Drug Res.,* **2000,** *54*:25–58.

Hall, Z.W., and Sanes, J.R. Synaptic structure and development: the neuromuscular junction. *Cell,* **1993,** 72 (suppl):99–121.

Hausdorff, W.P., Caron, M.G., and Lefkowitz, R.J. Turning off the signal: desensitization of β-adrenergic receptor function. *FASEB J.,* **1990,** *4*:2881–2889.

Heck, D.A., and Bylund, D.B. Differential down-regulation of alpha-2 adrenergic receptor subtypes. *Life Sci.,* **1998,** *62*:1467–1472.

Hille, B. *Ionic Channels of Excitable Membranes.* 2nd ed. Sinauer Associates, Sunderland, MA, **1992.**

Hille, B., Armstrong, C.M., and MacKinnon, R. Ion channels: from idea to reality. *Nat. Med.,* **1999b,** *5*:1105–1109.

Hobbs, A.J., Higgs, A., and Moncada, S. Inhibition of nitric oxide synthase as a potential therapeutic target. *Annu. Rev. Pharmacol. Toxicol.,* **1999,** *39*:191–220.

Hökfelt, T., Broberger, C., Xu, Z.Q., Sergeyev, V., Ubink, R., and Diez, M. Neuropeptides—an overview. *Neuropharmacology,* **2000,** *39*:1337–1356.

Hutchins, C. Three-dimensional models of the D1 and D2 dopamine receptors. *Endocr. J.,* **1994,** *2*:7–23.

Ignarro, L.J. Nitric oxide as a signaling molecule in the vascular system: an overview. *J. Cardiovasc. Pharmacol.,* **1999,** *34*:879–886.

Iversen, L.L. Uptake processes for biogenic amines. In, *Handbook of Psychopharmacology.* Vol. 3. (Iversen, L.L., Iversen, S.D., and Snyder, S.H., eds.) Plenum Press, New York, **1975,** pp. 381–442.

Jahn, R., and Südhof, T.C. Synaptic vesicles and exocytosis. *Annu. Rev. Neurosci.,* **1994,** *17*:219–246.

Karlin, A., and Akabas, M.H. Toward a structural basis for the function of nicotinic acetylcholine receptors and their cousins. *Neuron,* **1995,** *15*:1231–1244.

Katz, B. *Nerve, Muscle, and Synapse.* McGraw-Hill, New York, **1966.**

Katz, B. *The Release of Neural Transmitter Substances.* Charles C Thomas, Springfield, IL, **1969.**

Kelly, R.B. Storage and release of neurotransmitters. *Cell,* **1993,** *72* (*suppl*):43–53.

Kopin, I.J. Metabolic degradation of catecholamines. The relative importance of different pathways under physiological conditions and after administration of drugs. In, *Catecholamines.* (Blaschko, H.K.F., and Muscholl, E., eds.) *Handbuch der Experimentellen Pharmakologie.* Vol. 33. Springer-Verlag, Berlin, **1972,** pp. 271–282.

Langer, S.Z. 25 years since the discovery of presynaptic receptors: present knowledge and future perspectives. *Trends Pharmacol. Sci.,* **1997,** *18*:95–99.

Lefkowitz, R.J. G protein-coupled receptors. III. New roles for receptor kinases and beta-arrestins in receptor signaling and desensitization. *J. Biol. Chem.,* **1998,** *273*:18677–18680.

Lefkowitz, R.J. The superfamily of heptahelical receptors. *Nat. Cell Biol.,* **2000,** *2*:E133–E136.

Lin, R.C., and Scheller, R.H. Structural organization of the synaptic exocytosis core complex. *Neuron,* **1997,** *19*:1087–1094.

Loewy, A.D., and Spyer, K.M., eds. *Central Regulation of Autonomic Functions.* Oxford University Press, New York, **1990.**

Lukas, R.J., Changeux, J.P., Le Novere, N., Albuquerque, E.X., Balfour, D.J., Berg, D.K., Bertrand, D., Chippinelli, V.A., Clarke, P.B., Collins, A.C., Dani, J.A., Grady, S.R., Kellar, K.J., Lindstrom, J.M., Marks, M.J., Quik, M., Taylor, P.W., and Wonnacott, S. International Union of Pharmacology: XX. Current status of the nomenclature for nicotinic acetylcholine receptors and their subunits. *Pharmacol. Rev.,* **1999,** *51*:397–401.

Lundberg, J.M. Pharmacology of cotransmission in the autonomic nervous system: integrative aspects on amines, neuropeptides, adenosine triphosphate, amino acids and nitric oxide. *Pharmacol. Rev.,* **1996,** *48*:113–178.

MacDermott, A.B., Role, L.W., and Siegelbaum, S.A. Presynaptic ionotropic receptors and the control of transmitter release. *Annu. Rev. Neurosci.,* **1999,** *22*:443–485.

Man in't Veld, A., Boomsma, F., Lenders, J., v.d. Meiracker, A., Julien, C., Tulen, J., Moleman, P., Thien, T., Lamberts, S., and Schalekamp, M. Patients with congenital dopamine β-hydroxylase deficiency. A lesson in catecholamine physiology. *Am. J. Hypertens.,* **1988,** *1*:231–238.

Masson, J., Sagn, C., Hamon, M., and Mestikawy, S.E. Neurotransmitter transporters in the central nervous system. *Pharmacol. Rev.*, **1999**, *51*:439–464.

McDonald, T.F., Pelzer, S., Trautwein, W., and Pelzer, D.J. Regulation and modulation of calcium channels in cardiac, skeletal, and smooth muscle cells. *Physiol. Rev.*, **1994**, *74*:365–507.

Meir, A., Ginsburg, S., Butkevich, A., Kachalsky, S.G., Kaiserman, I., Ahdut, R., Demirgoren, S., and Rahamimoff, R. Ion channels in presynaptic nerve terminals and control of transmitter release. *Physiol. Rev.*, **1999**, *79*:1019–1088.

Michel, T., and Feron, O. Nitric oxide synthases: which, where, how, and why? *J. Clin. Invest.*, **1997**, *100*:2146–2152.

Miller, R.J. Presynaptic receptors. *Annu. Rev. Pharmacol. Toxicol.*, **1998**, *38*:201–227.

Nagatsu, T. Genes for human catecholamine-synthesizing enzymes. *Neurosci. Res.*, **1991**, *12*:315–345.

Numa, S., Noda, M., Takahashi, H., Tanabe, T., Toyosoto, M., Furatani, Y., and Kikyotani, S. Molecular structure of the nicotinic acetylcholine receptor. *Cold Spring Harb. Symp. Quant. Biol.*, **1983**, *48*(part 1):57–69.

Parsons, S.M., Prior, C., and Marshall, I.G. Acetylcholine transport, storage, and release. *Int. Rev. Neurobiol.*, **1993**, *35*:279–390.

Poyner, D., Cox, H., Bushfield, M., Treherne, J.M., and Demetrikopoulos, M.K. Neuropeptides in drug research. *Prog. Drug. Res.*, **2000**, *54*:121–149.

Reichardt, L.F., and Farinas, I. Neurotrophic factors and their receptors. In, *Molecular and Cell Approaches to Neural Development.* (Cowan, W.M., Jessel, T.M., and Zipursky, S.L., eds.) Oxford University Press, New York, **1997**, pp. 220–263.

Robertson, D., Haile, V., Perry, S.E., Robertson, R.M., Phillips, J.A., and Biaggioni, I. Dopamine β-hydroxylase deficiency. A genetic disorder of cardiovascular regulation. *Hypertension*, **1991**, *18*:1–8.

Rubanyi, G.M., and Polokoff, M.A. Endothelins: molecular biology, biochemistry, pharmacology, physiology, and pathophysiology. *Pharmacol. Rev.*, **1994**, *46*:325–415.

Sanes, J.R., and Lichtman, J.W. Development of the vertebrate neuromuscular junction. *Annu. Rev. Neurosci.*, **1999**, *22*:389–442.

Saunders, C., and Limbird, L.E. Localization and trafficking of alpha2-adrenergic receptor subtypes in cells and tissues. *Pharmacol. Ther.*, **1999**, *84*:193–205.

Schiavo, G., Matteoli, M., and Montecucco, C. Neurotoxins affecting neuroexocytosis. *Physiol. Rev.*, **2000**, *80*:717–766.

Schuldiner, S. A molecular glimpse of vesicular monoamine transporters. *J. Neurochem.*, **1994**, *62*:2067–2078.

Shapiro, R.L., Hatheway, C., and Swerdlow, D.L. Botulism in the United States: a clinical and epidemiologic review. *Ann. Intern. Med.*, **1998**, *129*:221–228.

Smith, C.M., Radzio-Andzelm, E., Madhusudan, Akamine, P., and Taylor, S.S. The catalytic subunit of cAMP-dependent protein kinase: prototype for an extended network of communication. *Prog. Biophys. Mol. Biol.*, **1999**, *71*:313–341.

Sneddon, P., Westfall, T.D., Todorov, L.D., Mihaylova-Todorova, S., Westfall, D.P., and Kennedy, C. Modulation of purinergic neurotransmission. *Prog. Brain Res.*, **1999**, *120*:11–20.

Sokolovsky, M. Endothelin receptor subtypes and their role in transmembrane signaling mechanisms. *Pharmacol. Ther.*, **1995**, *68*:435–471.

Starke, K. Presynaptic α-autoreceptors. *Rev. Physiol. Biochem. Pharmacol.*, **1987**, *107*:73–146.

Strader, C.D., Fong, T.M., Tota, M.R., Underwood, D., and Dixon, R.A. Structure and function of G protein-coupled receptors. *Annu. Rev. Biochem.*, **1994**, *63*:101–132.

Stull, J.T., Bowman, B.F., Gallagher, P.J., Herring, B.P., Hsu, L.C., Kamm, K.E., Kubota, Y., Leachman, S.A., Sweeney, H.L., and Tansey, M.G. Myosin phosphorylation in smooth and skeletal muscles: regulation and function. *Prog. Clin. Biol. Res.*, **1990**, *327*:107–126.

Taussig, R., and Gilman, A.G. Mammalian membrane-bound adenylyl cyclase. *J. Biol. Chem.*, **1995**, *270*:1–4.

Taylor, P., Luo, Z.D., and Camp, S. The genes encoding the cholinesterases: structure, evolutionary relationships and regulation of their expression. In, *Cholinesterase and Cholinesterase Inhibitors.* (Giacobini, E., ed.) Martin Dunitz, London, **2000**, pp. 63–80.

Trendelenburg, U. A kinetic analysis of the extraneuronal uptake and metabolism of catecholamines. *Rev. Physiol. Biochem. Pharmacol.*, **1980**, *87*:33–115.

Tsien, R.W., Lipscombe, D., Madison, D.V., Bley, K.R., and Fox, A.P. Multiple types of neuronal calcium channels and their selective modulation. *Trends Neurosci.*, **1988**, *11*:431–438.

Vanhoutte, P.M. Endothelium-dependent responses in congestive heart failure. *J. Mol. Cell Cardiol.*, **1996**, *28*:2233–2240.

Volz, H.P., and Gleiter, C.H. Monoamine oxidase inhibitors. A perspective on their use in the elderly. *Drugs Aging*, **1998**, *13*:341–355.

von Euler, U.S. Synthesis, uptake and storage of catecholamines in adrenergic nerves. The effects of drugs. In, *Catecholamines.* (Blaschko, H., and Muscholl, E., eds.) *Handbuch der Experimentellen Pharmakologie.* Vol. 33. Springer-Verlag, Berlin, **1972**, pp. 186–230.

von Euler, U.S. Historical perspective: growth and impact of the concept of chemical neurotransmission. In, *Chemical Neurotransmission—75 Years.* (Stjärne, L., Hedqvist, P., Lagercrantz, H., and Wennmalm, A., eds.) Academic Press, London, **1981**, pp. 3–12.

von Kugelgen, I., Norenberg, W., Koch, H., Meyer, A., Illes, P., and Starke, K. P2-receptors controlling neurotransmitter release from postganglionic sympathetic neurons. *Prog. Brain Res.*, **1999**, *120*:173–182.

Wahlestedt, C., and Reis, D.J. Neuropeptide Y-related peptides and their receptors—are the receptors potential therapeutic drug targets? *Annu. Rev. Pharmacol. Toxicol.*, **1993**, *33*:309–352.

Wessler, I. Acetylcholine at motor nerves: storage, release and presynaptic modulation by autoreceptors and adrenoreceptors. *Int. Rev. Neurobiol.*, **1992**, *34*:283–384.

Weyer, C., Gautier, J.F., and Danforth, E. Development of beta 3-adrenoceptor agonists for the treatment of obesity and diabetes—an update. *Diabetes Metab.*, **1999**, *25*:11–21.

Wouters, J. Structural aspects of monoamine oxidase and its reversible inhibition. *Curr. Med. Chem.*, **1998**, *5*:137–162.

Wu, D., and Hersh, L.B. Choline acetyltransferase: celebrating its fiftieth year. *J. Neurochem.*, **1994**, *62*:1653–1663.

Zhong, H., and Minneman, K.P. Alpha1-adrenoceptor subtypes. *Eur. J. Pharmacol.*, **1999**, *375*:261–276.

Zigmond, R.E., Schwarzschild, M.A., and Rittenhouse, A.R. Acute regulation of tyrosine hydroxylase by nerve activity and by neurotransmitters via phosphorylation. *Annu. Rev. Neurosci.*, **1989**, *12*:415–461.

MUSCARINIC RECEPTOR AGONISTS AND ANTAGONISTS

Joan Heller Brown and Palmer Taylor

Acetylcholine is the endogenous neurotransmitter at cholinergic synapses and neuroeffector junctions in the central and peripheral nervous systems. Its actions are mediated through nicotinic and muscarinic cholinergic receptors, which transduce signals via distinct mechanisms. Muscarinic receptors in the peripheral nervous system primarily are found on the autonomic effector cells that are innervated by postganglionic parasympathetic nerves. Muscarinic receptors also are present in ganglia and on certain cells, such as endothelial cells of blood vessels, that receive little or no cholinergic innervation. Certain brain regions such as the hippocampus, cortex, and thalamus have high densities of muscarinic receptors. Cholinergic agonists mimic the effects of acetylcholine at these sites.

The first section of this chapter describes the pharmacological properties and therapeutic uses of acetylcholine and agonists that stimulate muscarinic receptors; these agonists typically are longer-acting congeners of acetylcholine or natural alkaloids. Several of these agents cross over and confer their cholinomimetic activity by stimulating nicotinic as well as muscarinic receptors. In general, these agonists manifest little selectivity for the various subtypes of muscarinic receptors described below. The clinical uses of the muscarinic receptor agonists, primarily in ophthalmology and to enhance gastrointestinal and bladder tone, are discussed here and also in Chapters 37, 39, and 66.

The last section of this chapter deals with muscarinic receptor antagonists. These drugs inhibit the actions of acetylcholine by blocking receptors at autonomic effector sites innervated by postganglionic cholinergic nerves. They also inhibit the actions of acetylcholine at pre- and postsynaptic muscarinic receptors in ganglia and on central nervous system neurons. Except for the quaternary ammonium-containing compounds, muscarinic receptor antagonists are highly selective for muscarinic over nicotinic receptors. In addition, a growing number of antagonists show selectivity for muscarinic receptor subtypes, thus enhancing selectivity and minimizing unwanted side effects. The therapeutic uses of muscarinic receptor antagonists include treatment of gastrointestinal and urinary tract disorders (see also Chapters 37 and 39), specific respiratory conditions (see also Chapter 28), motion sickness, parkinsonian symptoms (see Chapter 22), and poisoning with cholinesterase inhibitors (see also Chapter 8); their use in ophthalmology is discussed fully in Chapter 66.

I. MUSCARINIC RECEPTOR AGONISTS

Muscarinic cholinergic receptor agonists can be divided into two groups: (1) acetylcholine and several synthetic choline esters and (2) the naturally occurring cholinomimetic alkaloids (particularly pilocarpine, muscarine, and arecoline) and their synthetic congeners. In addition, the anticholinesterase agents (Chapter 8) and the ganglionic stimulants (Chapter 9) have parasympathomimetic actions; their prominent effects may be indirect or can arise from locations other than the postganglionic cholinergic effector site.

ACETYLCHOLINE

Acetylcholine (ACh), first synthesized by Baeyer in 1867, has virtually no therapeutic applications because its actions are diffuse and its hydrolysis, catalyzed by both acetylcholinesterase (AChE) and plasma butyrylcholinesterase, is rapid. Consequently, numerous derivatives have been synthesized in attempts to obtain drugs with more selective and prolonged actions.

Mechanism of Action.   The mechanisms of action of endogenous ACh at the postjunctional membranes of the effector cells and neurons that correspond to the four classes of cholinergic synapses are discussed in Chapter 6. By way of recapitulation, these synapses are found at (1) autonomic effector sites, innervated by postganglionic parasympathetic fibers; (2) sympathetic and parasympathetic ganglion cells and the adrenal medulla, innervated by preganglionic autonomic fibers; (3) motor end-plates on skeletal muscle, innervated by somatic motor nerves; and (4) certain synapses peripherally and within the central nervous system (CNS), where the actions can be either pre- or postsynaptic. When ACh is administered systemically, it has the potential to act at all of these sites; however, as a quaternary ammonium compound, its penetration into the CNS is limited, and butyrylcholinesterase in the plasma reduces the concentrations of ACh that reach areas in the periphery with low blood flow.

The actions of ACh and related drugs at autonomic effector sites are referred to as *muscarinic*, based on the original observation that muscarine acts selectively at those sites and produces the same qualitative effects as ACh. Accordingly, the muscarinic, or parasympathomimetic, actions of the drugs considered in this chapter are practically equivalent to the effects of postganglionic parasympathetic nerve impulses listed in Table 6–1; the differences between the actions of the classical muscarinic agonists are largely quantitative, with limited selectivity for one organ system or another. Muscarinic receptors also are present on autonomic ganglion cells and in the adrenal medulla. Muscarinic stimulation of ganglia and the adrenal medulla usually is thought to be modulatory to nicotinic stimulation. All of the actions of ACh and its congeners at muscarinic receptors can be blocked by atropine. The *nicotinic* actions of cholinergic agonists refer to their initial stimulation, and often in high doses to subsequent blockade, of autonomic ganglion cells, the adrenal medulla, and the neuromuscular junction, actions comparable to those of nicotine.

Properties and Subtypes of Muscarinic Receptors. Muscarinic receptors were characterized initially by analysis of the responses of cells and tissues in the periphery and the CNS. Differential effects of two muscarinic agonists, bethanechol and McN-A-343, on the tone of the lower esophageal sphincter led to the initial designation of muscarinic receptors as M_1 (ganglionic) and M_2 (effector cell) (Goyal and Rattan, 1978; *see also* Chapter 6). The basis for the selectivity of these agonists is unclear, as there is no good evidence that agonists discriminate among the subtypes of muscarinic receptor (*see* Eglen, *et al.,* 1996; Caulfield and Birdsall, 1998). However, subsequent radioligand binding studies definitively revealed the existence of more than a single population of antagonist binding sites (Hammer *et al.,* 1980). In particular, the muscarinic antagonist pirenzepine was shown to bind with high affinity to sites in cerebral cortex and sympathetic ganglia (M_1) but to have lower affinity for sites in cardiac muscle, smooth muscle, and various glands. These data explain the ability of pirenzepine to block agonist-induced responses that are mediated by muscarinic receptors in sympathetic and myenteric ganglia at concentrations considerably lower than those required to block responses that result from direct stimulation of receptors in various effector organs. Newer antagonists that can further discriminate among various subtypes of muscarinic receptors are now available. For example, tripitramine displays selectivity for cardiac M_2- relative to M_3-muscarinic receptors, while darifenacin is relatively selective for antagonizing glandular and smooth muscle M_3 relative to M_2 receptors (*see* Caulfield and Birdsall, 1998; Birdsall *et al.,* 1998; Levine *et al.,* 1999).

The cloning of the cDNAs that encode muscarinic receptors identified five distinct gene products (Bonner *et al.,* 1987), now designated as M_1 through M_5 (*see* Chapter 6). All of the known muscarinic receptor subtypes interact with members of a group of heterotrimeric guanine nucleotide-binding regulatory proteins (G proteins) that, in turn, are linked to various cellular effectors (*see* Chapter 2). Regions within the receptor responsible for the specificity of G protein coupling have been defined, primarily by mutagenesis and receptor subtype chimera studies. In particular, one region at the carboxyl-terminal end of the third intracellular loop of the receptor has been implicated in the specificity of G protein coupling and shows a great deal of homology within M_1, M_3, and M_5 receptors and within M_2 and M_4 receptors (*see* Wess, 1996; Caulfield, 1993; Caulfield and Birdsall, 1998). Conserved regions in the second intracellular loop also confer specificity for proper G protein recognition. Although selectivity is not absolute, stimulation of M_1 or M_3 receptors causes hydrolysis of polyphosphoinositides and mobilization of intracellular Ca^{2+}, as a consequence of interaction with a G protein (G_q) that activates phospholipase C (*see* Chapter 6); this effect in turn results in a variety of Ca^{2+}-mediated events, either directly or as a consequence of the phosphorylation of target proteins. In contrast, M_2- and M_4-muscarinic receptors inhibit adenylyl cyclase and regulate specific ion channels (*e.g.,* enhancement of K^+ conductance in cardiac atrial tissue) through subunits released from pertussis toxin-sensitive G proteins (G_i and G_0) that are distinct from the G proteins used by M_1 and M_3 receptors (*see* Chapters 2 and 12).

Studies using muscarinic receptor subtype-specific antibodies and ligands demonstrate discrete localization of the muscarinic receptor subtypes, for example within brain regions and in different populations of smooth muscle cells (*see* Levey, 1993; Yasuda *et al.,* 1993; Eglen *et al.,* 1996; Caulfield and Birdsall, 1998). The M_1 through M_4 subtypes have been disrupted through gene targeting to create null alleles for each of these genes (Hamilton *et al.,* 1997; Gomeza *et al.,* 1999a and b; Matsui *et al.,* 2000). Altered central responses to cholinergic agonists including seizures, hypothermia, tremors, and analgesia are prominent in the phenotypes of M_1, M_2, and M_4 knockout mice. Mice lacking the M_3 receptor have more obvious peripheral lesions including altered salivation, pupil constriction, and bladder contraction. Minimal phenotypic alteration accompanying specific receptor deletion suggests redundancy in receptor subtypes in various tissue locations.

Pharmacological Properties

Cardiovascular System. ACh has four primary effects on the cardiovascular system: vasodilation, a decrease in cardiac rate (the negative chronotropic effect), a decrease in the rate of conduction in the specialized tissues of the sinoatrial (SA) and atrioventricular (AV) nodes (the negative dromotropic effect), and a decrease in the force of cardiac contraction (the negative inotropic effect). The last-named effect is of lesser significance in ventricular than in atrial muscle. Certain of the above effects can be obscured by the dampening of the direct effects of ACh by baroreceptor and other reflexes.

Although ACh rarely is given systemically, its cardiac actions are of importance because of the involvement of cholinergic vagal impulses in the actions of the cardiac glycosides, antiarrhythmic agents, and many other drugs as well as following afferent stimulation of the viscera during surgical interventions. The intravenous injection of a small dose of ACh produces an evanescent fall in blood pressure owing to generalized vasodilation, accompanied usually by reflex tachycardia. A considerably larger dose is required to elicit bradycardia or block of AV nodal conduction from a direct action of ACh on the heart. If large doses of ACh are injected after the administration of atropine, an increase in blood pressure is observed; the increase is caused by stimulation of the adrenal medulla and sympathetic ganglia to release catecholamines into the circulation and at postganglionic sympathetic nerve endings.

ACh produces dilation of essentially all vascular beds, including those of the pulmonary and coronary vasculature. Vasodilation of coronary beds is mediated through release of nitric oxide and may be elicited by baroreceptor or chemoreceptor reflexes or by direct electrical stimulation of the vagus (Feigl, 1998). However, neither parasympathetic vasodilator nor sympathetic vasoconstrictor tone plays a major role in the regulation of coronary blood flow, in comparison with the effects of local oxygen tension and autoregulatory metabolic factors such as adenosine (Berne and Levy, 1997).

Dilation of vascular beds by acetylcholine is due to the presence of muscarinic receptors, primarily of the M_3 subtype (Bruning *et al.,* 1994; Eglen *et al.,* 1996; Caulfield and Birdsall, 1998), despite the lack of apparent cholinergic innervation of most blood vessels. The muscarinic receptors responsible for relaxation are located on the endothelial cells of the vasculature; when these receptors are stimulated, the endothelial cells release endothelium-derived relaxing factor, or nitric oxide (Moncada and Higgs, 1997), which diffuses to adjacent smooth muscle cells and causes them to relax (Furchgott, 1999; Ignarro *et al.,* 1999; *see* Chapter 6). Vasodilation also may arise secondarily from inhibition by ACh of norepinephrine release from adrenergic nerve endings. If the endothelium is damaged, ACh can stimulate receptors on vascular smooth muscle cells and cause vasoconstriction.

Cholinergic stimulation affects cardiac function directly and by inhibiting the effects of adrenergic activation. The latter depends on the level of sympathetic drive to the heart and results in part from inhibition of cyclic AMP formation and reduction in L-type Ca^{2+} channel activity (*see* Brodde and Michel, 1999). Since cholinergic parasympathetic fibers are distributed extensively to the SA and AV nodes and the atrial muscle, vagal impulses have critical actions on most types of specialized cardiac cells. Cholinergic innervation of the ventricular myocardium is sparse, and the parasympathetic fibers terminate predominantly on specialized conduction tissue such as the Purkinje fibers (Kent *et al.,* 1974; Levy and Schwartz, 1994).

In the SA node, each normal cardiac impulse is initiated by the spontaneous depolarization of the pacemaker cells (*see* Chapter 35). At a critical level—the threshold potential—this depolarization initiates an action potential. The action potential is conducted through the atrial muscle fibers to the AV node and thence through the Purkinje system to the ventricular muscle. ACh slows the heart rate by decreasing the rate of spontaneous diastolic depolarization (the pacemaker current) and by increasing the repolarizing current at the SA node; attainment of the threshold potential and the succeeding events in the cardiac cycle are therefore delayed (DiFrancesco, 1993).

In atrial muscle, ACh decreases the strength of contraction. This direct inhibitory effect of ACh results from M_2 receptor-mediated activation of G protein–regulated K^+ channels (*see* Wickman and Clapham, 1995). Increased K^+ permeability leads to hyperpolarization and shortens the durations of the action potential and the effective refractory period. The rate of impulse conduction in the normal atrium is either unaffected or may increase. The increase is due to the activation of additional Na^+ channels in response to the ACh-induced hyperpolarization. The combination of these factors is the basis for the perpetuation or exacerbation by vagal impulses of atrial flutter or fibrillation arising at an ectopic focus. In contrast, primarily in the AV node and to a much lesser extent in the Purkinje conducting system, ACh slows conduction and increases the refractory period. The decrement in AV nodal conduction usually is responsible for the complete heart block that may be observed when large quantities of cholinergic agonists are administered systemically. With an increase in vagal tone, such as is produced by the digitalis glycosides, the increased refractory period can contribute to the reduction in the frequency with which aberrant atrial impulses are transmitted to the ventricle, and thus decrease the ventricular rate during atrial flutter or fibrillation.

In the ventricle, ACh, whether released by vagal stimulation or applied directly, also has a negative inotropic effect, although it is much smaller than that observed in the atrium. In human beings and most mammals, direct inhibition is not apparent, unless contractility is enhanced by adrenergic stimulation (Higgins *et al.,* 1973; Levy and Schwartz, 1994; Michel and Brodde, 1999). Automaticity of Purkinje fibers is suppressed, and the threshold for ventricular fibrillation is increased (Kent *et al.,* 1974; Kent and Epstein, 1976). Sympathetic and vagal nerve terminals lie in close proximity, and muscarinic receptors are believed to exist at presynaptic as well as postsynaptic sites (Wellstein and Pitschner, 1988). Inhibition of adrenergic stimulation of the heart arises from the capacity of ACh to modulate or depress the myocardial response to catecholamines as well as from a capacity to inhibit the release of norepinephrine from sympathetic nerve endings.

Gastrointestinal and Urinary Tracts. Although stimulation of vagal input to the gastrointestinal tract increases tone, amplitude of contraction, and secretory activity of the stomach and intestine, such responses are inconsistently seen with administered ACh. Poor perfusion and rapid hydrolysis by plasma butyrylcholinesterase limit access of ACh to the muscarinic receptors. Parasympathetic sacral innervation causes detrusor muscle contraction, increased voiding pressure, and ureter peristalsis, but for similar reasons these responses are not evident with administered ACh.

Miscellaneous Effects. The influence of ACh and parasympathetic innervation on various organs and tissues is discussed in detail in Chapter 6. ACh and its analogs stimulate secretion by all glands that receive parasympathetic innervation, including the lacrimal, tracheobronchial, salivary, digestive, and exocrine sweat glands. The effects on the respiratory system, in addition to increased tracheobronchial secretion, include bronchoconstriction and stimulation of the chemoreceptors of the carotid and aortic bodies. When instilled into the eye, they produce miosis (*see* Chapter 66).

Synergisms and Antagonisms. The muscarinic actions of ACh and all the drugs of this class are blocked selectively by atropine, primarily through competitive occupation of muscarinic receptor sites on the autonomic effector cells and secondarily on autonomic ganglion cells. The nicotinic actions of ACh and its derivatives at autonomic ganglia are blocked by hexamethonium and trimethaphan; their actions at the neuromuscular junction of skeletal muscle are antagonized by tubocurarine and other competitive blocking agents (*see* Chapter 9).

CHOLINOMIMETIC CHOLINE ESTERS AND NATURAL ALKALOIDS

Methacholine (acetyl-β-methylcholine) differs from ACh chiefly in its greater duration and selectivity of action. Its action is more prolonged because it is hydrolyzed by AChE at a considerably slower rate than is ACh and is almost totally resistant to hydrolysis by nonspecific cholinesterase or butyrylcholinesterase. Its selectivity is manifested by slight nicotinic and a predominance of muscarinic actions, the latter being the most marked on the cardiovascular system (Table 7–1).

Carbachol (CARBOPTIC, others) and *bethanechol,* which are unsubstituted carbamoyl esters, are resistant to hydrolysis by either AChE or nonspecific cholinesterases; their half-lives are thus sufficiently long that they become distributed to areas of low blood flow. Bethanechol has mainly muscarinic actions, showing some selectivity on gastrointestinal tract and urinary bladder motility. Carbachol retains substantial nicotinic activity, particularly on autonomic ganglia. It is likely that both its peripheral and its ganglionic actions are due, at least in part, to the release of endogenous ACh from the terminals of cholinergic fibers.

The three major natural alkaloids in this group—*pilocarpine, muscarine,* and *arecoline*—have the same principal sites of action as the choline esters discussed above. Muscarine acts almost exclusively at muscarinic receptor sites, and their classification is derived from this fact. Arecoline also acts at nicotinic receptors. Pilocarpine has a dominant muscarinic action, but it causes anomalous

Table 7–1

Some Pharmacological Properties of Choline Esters and Natural Alkaloids

MUSCARINIC AGONIST	SUSCEPTIBILITY TO CHOLINESTERASES	Muscarinic Activity					NICOTINIC ACTIVITY
		CARDIO-VASCULAR	GASTRO-INTESTINAL	URINARY BLADDER	EYE (TOPICAL)	ANTAGONISM BY ATROPINE	
Acetylcholine	+++	++	++	++	+	+++	++
Methacholine	+	+++	++	++	+	+++	+
Carbachol	–	+	+++	+++	++	+	+++
Bethanechol	–	±	+++	+++	++	+++	–
Muscarine	–	++	+++	+++	++	+++	–
Pilocarpine	–	+	+++	+++	++	+++	–

cardiovascular responses, and the sweat glands are particularly sensitive to the drug. Although these naturally occurring alkaloids are of great value as pharmacological tools, present clinical use is restricted largely to the employment of pilocarpine as a sialagogue and miotic agent (*see* Chapter 66).

History and Sources.   Of the several hundred synthetic choline derivatives investigated, only methacholine, carbachol, and bethanechol have had clinical applications. The structures of these compounds are shown in Figure 7–1. Methacholine, the β-methyl analog of ACh, was studied by Hunt and Taveau as early as 1911. Carbachol, the carbamyl ester of choline, and bethanechol, its β-methyl analog, were synthesized and investigated in the 1930s. Pilocarpine is the chief alkaloid obtained from the leaflets of South American shrubs of the genus *Pilocarpus*. Although it was long known by the natives that the chewing of leaves of *Pilocarpus* plants caused salivation, the first experiments were apparently performed in 1874 by a Brazilian physician named Coutinhou. The alkaloid was isolated in

1875, and shortly thereafter the actions of pilocarpine on the pupil and on the sweat and salivary glands were described by Weber.

The poisonous effects of certain species of mushrooms have been known since ancient times, but it was not until Schmiedeberg isolated the alkaloid muscarine from *Amanita muscaria* in 1869 that its properties could be systematically investigated. The role played by muscarine in the development of the neurohumoral theory is recounted in Chapter 6. Arecoline is the chief alkaloid of areca or betel nuts, the seeds of *Areca catechu*. The red-staining betel nut is consumed as a euphoretic by the natives of the Indian subcontinent and East Indies in a masticatory mixture known as betel and composed of the nut, shell lime, and leaves of *Piper betle,* a climbing species of pepper.

Structure–Activity Relationships.   The muscarinic alkaloids show marked differences as well as interesting relationships in structure when compared to the quaternary esters of choline (Figure 7–1). Arecoline and pilocarpine are tertiary amines. *Muscarine,* a quaternary ammonium compound, shows more limited absorption. The chemistry and pharmacology of many

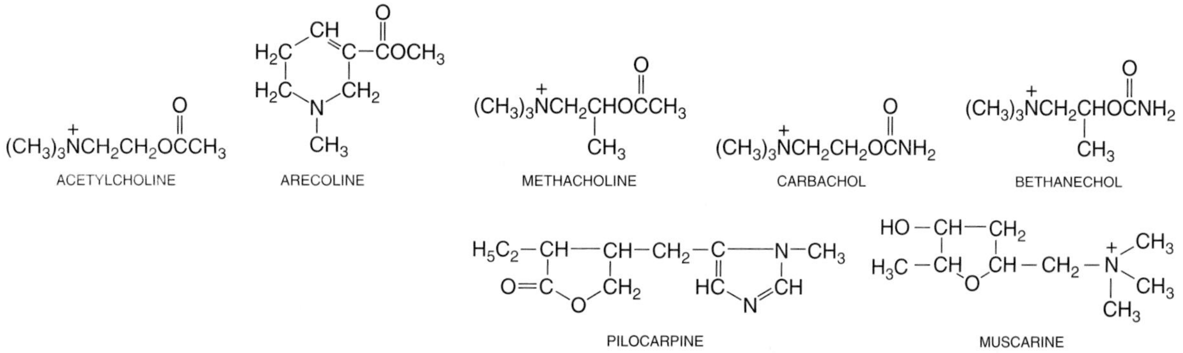

Figure 7–1. Structural formulas of acetylcholine, choline esters, and natural alkaloids that stimulate muscarinic receptors.

natural and synthetic muscarinic compounds have been reviewed by Bebbington and Brimblecombe (1965). McN-A-343 is an agonist that was originally proposed to stimulate M_1 receptors with some selectivity. While it is clear that McN-A-343 can stimulate sympathetic ganglia and inhibitory neurons in myenteric plexus, this is a "functional" rather than a subtype-specific effect. Indeed, no agonists with subtype specificity are known (Caulfield and Birdsall, 1998).

Pharmacological Properties

Gastrointestinal Tract. All of the muscarinic agonists are capable of stimulating smooth muscle of the gastrointestinal tract, thereby increasing tone and motility; large doses will cause spasm and tenesmus. Carbachol, bethanechol, and pilocarpine, in contrast to methacholine, will stimulate the gastrointestinal tract without significant cardiovascular effects.

Urinary Tract. The choline esters and pilocarpine contract the detrusor muscle of the bladder, increase voiding pressure, decrease bladder capacity, and increase ureteral peristalsis. In addition, the trigone and external sphincter muscles relax. Selectivity for bladder stimulation relative to cardiovascular activity is evident for bethanechol. In animals with experimental spinal cord lesions, muscarinic agonists promote evacuation of the bladder.

Exocrine Glands. The choline esters and muscarinic alkaloids stimulate secretion of glands that receive parasympathetic or sympathetic cholinergic innervation, including the lacrimal, salivary, digestive, tracheobronchial, and sweat glands. Pilocarpine (10 mg to 15 mg, subcutaneously), in particular, causes marked diaphoresis in human beings; 2 to 3 liters of sweat may be secreted. Salivation also is increased markedly. Oral pilocarpine appears to cause a more continuous production of saliva. Muscarine and arecoline also are potent diaphoretic agents. Accompanying side effects may include hiccough, salivation, nausea, vomiting, weakness, and, occasionally, collapse. These alkaloids also stimulate the lacrimal, gastric, pancreatic, and intestinal glands, and the mucous cells of the respiratory tract.

Respiratory System. In addition to tracheobronchial secretions, bronchial smooth muscle is stimulated by the muscarinic agonists. Asthmatic patients respond with intense bronchoconstriction and a reduction in vital capacity.

Cardiovascular System. Continuous intravenous infusion of methacholine elicits hypotension and bradycardia just as ACh does, but at 1/200 the dose. Muscarine, at small doses, also leads to a marked fall in the blood pressure and a slowing or temporary cessation of the heartbeat. In contrast, carbachol and bethanechol generally cause only a transient fall in blood pressure at doses that affect the gastrointestinal and urinary tracts. Likewise, pilocarpine produces only a brief fall in blood pressure. However, if this is preceded by an appropriate dose of a nicotinic receptor antagonist, pilocarpine produces a marked rise in pressure. Both the vasodepressor and pressor responses are prevented by atropine; the latter effect also is abolished by α-adrenergic receptor antagonists. These actions of pilocarpine

have not been fully explained, but may arise from ganglionic and adrenomedullary stimulation.

Eye. The muscarinic agonists stimulate the pupillae constrictor and ciliary muscle when applied locally to the eye causing pupil constriction and a loss of accommodation.

Central Nervous System. The intravenous injection of relatively small doses of pilocarpine, muscarine, and arecoline evokes a characteristic cortical arousal or activation response in cats, similar to that produced by injection of anticholinesterase agents or by electrical stimulation of the brainstem reticular formation. The arousal response to all of these drugs is reduced or blocked by atropine and related agents (Krnjević, 1974). The choline esters, being quaternary, do not cross the blood–brain barrier.

Therapeutic Uses

Bethanechol chloride (carbamyl-β-methylcholine chloride; URECHOLINE, others) is available in tablets and as an injection and is used as a stimulant of the smooth muscle of the gastrointestinal tract and, in particular, the urinary bladder. *Pilocarpine hydrochloride* (SALAGEN) is available as 5- or 10-mg oral doses for treatment of xerostomia or as ophthalmic solutions (PILOCAR, others) of varying strength. *Methacholine chloride (acetyl-β-methylcholine chloride;* PROVOCHOLINE) still may be administered for diagnosis of bronchial hyperreactivity and asthmatic conditions. The unpredictability of absorption and intensity of response has precluded its use as a vasodilator or cardiac vagomimetic agent.

Gastrointestinal Disorders. Bethanechol can be of value in certain cases of postoperative abdominal distention and in gastric atony or gastroparesis. The oral route is preferred; the usual dosage is 10 to 20 mg three or four times daily. Bethanechol is given by mouth before each main meal in cases without complete retention; when gastric retention is complete and nothing passes into the duodenum, the subcutaneous route is necessary because the drug is not adequately absorbed from the stomach. Bethanechol likewise has been used to advantage in certain patients with congenital megacolon and with adynamic ileus secondary to toxic states. Prokinetic agents with combined cholinergic-agonist and dopamine-antagonist activity (*metoclopramide*) or serotonin-antagonist activity (*see* Chapter 38) have largely replaced bethanechol in gastroparesis or esophageal reflux disorders.

Urinary Bladder Disorders. Bethanechol may be useful in combating urinary retention and inadequate emptying of the bladder when organic obstruction is absent, as in postoperative and postpartum urinary retention and in certain cases of chronic hypotonic, myogenic, or neurogenic bladder (Wein, 1991). α-Adrenergic-receptor antagonists are useful adjuncts in reducing outlet resistance of the internal sphincter (*see* Chapter 10). Bethanechol may enhance contractions of the detrusor muscle after spinal injury if the vesical reflex is intact, and some benefit has been noted in partial sensory or motor paralysis of the bladder. Catheterization thus can be avoided. For acute retention, multiple subcutaneous doses of 2.5 mg of bethanechol may be administered. The stomach should be empty at the time the drug is injected. In chronic cases, 10 to 50 mg of the drug may be given orally two to four times daily with meals to avoid nausea and vomiting. When voluntary or automatic voiding begins, administration of bethanechol is then slowly withdrawn.

Xerostomia. Pilocarpine is administered orally in 5- to 10-mg doses for the treatment of xerostomia that follows head and neck radiation treatments or that is associated with Sjögren's syndrome (Wiseman and Faulds, 1995). The latter is an autoimmune disorder occurring primarily in women where secretions, particularly salivary and lacrimal, are compromised (Anaya and Talal, 1999; Nusair and Rubinow, 1999). Provided salivary parenchyma maintain a residual function, enhanced salivary secretion, ease of swallowing, and subjective improvement in hydration of the oral cavity are achieved. Side effects typify cholinergic stimulation, with sweating being the most common complaint. Bethanechol offers an alternative oral agent, which some feel produces less diaphoresis (Epstein *et al.,* 1994). *Cevimeline* (EVOXAC) is a newly approved agonist with activity at M_3-muscarinic receptors. These receptors are found on lacrimal and salivary gland epithelia. Cevimeline has a long-lasting sialogogic action and may have fewer side effects than pilocarpine (Anaya and Talal, 1999). Comparative clinical trials with pilocarpine have yet to be conducted.

Ophthalmological. Pilocarpine also is used in the treatment of glaucoma, where it is instilled into the eye usually as a 0.5% to 4.0% solution. It usually is better tolerated than are the anticholinesterases, and pilocarpine is the standard cholinergic agent for initial treatment of open-angle glaucoma. Reduction of intraocular pressure occurs within a few minutes and lasts 4 to 8 hours. The ophthalmic use of pilocarpine alone and in combination with other agents is discussed in Chapter 66. The miotic action of pilocarpine is useful in reversing a narrow-angle glaucoma attack and overcoming the mydriasis produced by atropine; alternated with mydriatics, pilocarpine is employed to break adhesions between the iris and the lens.

CNS. Agonists that show functional selectivity for M_1 and M_2 receptors have been targets of development by drug companies, and some have been in clinical trial for use in treating the intellectual impairment associated with Alzheimer's disease. The potential advantage of such agonists would arise from stimulating postsynaptic M_1 receptors in the CNS without concomitantly stimulating the presynaptic M_2 receptors that inhibit release of endogenous ACh. However, lack of efficacy in improvement of cognitive function has diminished enthusiasm for this approach (Eglen *et al.,* 1999).

Precautions, Toxicity, and Contraindications. Muscarinic agonists are administered subcutaneously to achieve an acute response and orally to treat more chronic conditions. Should serious toxic reactions to these drugs arise, *atropine sulfate* (0.5 mg to 1 mg in adults) should be given subcutaneously or intravenously. *Epinephrine* (0.3 mg to 1 mg, subcutaneously or intramuscularly) also is of value in overcoming severe cardiovascular or bronchoconstrictor responses.

Among the major contraindications to the use of the choline esters are asthma, hyperthyroidism, coronary insufficiency, and acid-peptic disease. Their bronchoconstrictor action is liable to precipitate an asthma attack, and hyperthyroid patients may develop atrial fibrillation. Hypotension induced by these agents can severely reduce coronary blood flow, especially if it is already compromised. Other possible undesirable effects of the cholinergic agents are flushing, sweating, abdominal cramps, belching, a sensation of tightness in the urinary bladder, difficulty in visual accommodation, headache, and salivation.

Toxicology

Poisoning from pilocarpine, muscarine, or arecoline is characterized chiefly by exaggeration of their various parasympathomimetic effects and resembles that produced by consumption of mushrooms of the genus *Inocybe* (*see* below). Treatment consists of the parenteral administration of atropine in doses sufficient to cross the blood–brain barrier and adequate measures to support the respiration and the circulation and to counteract pulmonary edema.

Mushroom Poisoning (Mycetism). Mushroom poisoning has been known for centuries. The Greek poet Euripides (fifth century B.C.) is said to have lost his wife and three children from this cause. In recent years the number of cases of mushroom poisoning has been increasing as the result of the current popularity of the consumption of wild mushrooms. Various species of mushrooms contain many toxins, and species within the same genus may contain distinct toxins.

Although *Amanita muscaria* is the source from which muscarine was isolated, its content of the alkaloid is so low (approximately 0.003%) that muscarine cannot be responsible for the major toxic effects. Much higher concentrations of muscarine are present in various species of *Inocybe* and *Clitocybe*. The symptoms of intoxication attributable to muscarine develop rapidly, within 30 to 60 minutes of ingestion; they include salivation, lacrimation, nausea, vomiting, headache, visual disturbances, abdominal colic, diarrhea, bronchospasm, bradycardia, hypotension, and shock. Treatment with atropine (1 to 2 mg intramuscularly every 30 minutes) effectively blocks these effects (Köppel, 1993; Goldfrank, 1998).

Intoxication produced by *A. muscaria* and related *Amanita* species arises from the neurologic and hallucinogenic properties of muscimol, ibotenic acid, and other isoxazole derivatives. These agents stimulate excitatory and inhibitory amino acid receptors. Symptoms range from irritability, restlessness, ataxia, hallucinations, and delirium to drowsiness and sedation. Treatment is mainly supportive; benzodiazepines are indicated when excitation predominates, whereas atropine often exacerbates the delirium.

Mushrooms from *Psilocybe* and *Panaeolus* species contain psilocybin and related derivatives of tryptamine. They also cause short-lasting hallucinations. *Gyromitra* species (false morels) produce gastrointestinal disorders and a delayed hepatotoxicity. The toxic substance is acetaldehyde methylformylhydrazone, which is converted in the body to reactive hydrazines. Although fatalities from liver and kidney failure have been reported, they are far less frequent than with amatoxin-containing mushrooms discussed below.

The most serious form of mycetism is produced by *Amanita phalloides,* other *Amanita* species, *Lepiota,* and *Galerina* species (Goldfrank, 1998). These species account for more than 90% of all fatal cases. Ingestion of as little as 50 g of *A. phalloides* (deadly nightcap) can be fatal. The principal toxins are the am-atoxins (α- and β-amanitin), a group of cyclic octapeptides that inhibit RNA polymerase II and hence block the synthesis of mRNA. This causes cell death, manifested particularly in the gastrointestinal mucosa, liver, and kidneys. Initial symptoms, which often are unnoticed or, when present, are due to other toxins, include diarrhea and abdominal cramps. A symptom-free period lasting up to 24 hours is followed by hepatic and renal malfunction. Death occurs in 4 to 7 days from renal and he-patic failure (Goldfrank, 1998). Treatment is largely supportive; penicillin, thiotic acid, and silibinin may be effective antidotes, but the evidence is based largely on anecdotal studies (Köppel, 1993).

Because the severity of toxicity and treatment strategies for mushroom poisoning depend on the species ingested, their iden-tification should be sought. Often symptomatology is delayed, causing gastric lavage and administration of activated charcoal to be of limited value. Regional poison control centers in the United States maintain up-to-date information on incidence of poisoning in the region and treatment procedures.

II. MUSCARINIC RECEPTOR ANTAGONISTS

The class of drugs referred to here as muscarinic receptor antagonists includes (1) the naturally occurring alkaloids, *atropine* and *scopolamine;* (2) semisynthetic derivatives of these alkaloids, which primarily differ from the parent compounds in their disposition in the body or their dura-tion of action; and (3) synthetic congeners, some of which show selectivity for particular subtypes of muscarinic re-ceptors. Noteworthy agents among the synthetic deriva-tives include *homatropine* and *tropicamide,* which have a shorter duration of action than atropine, and *methyl-atropine, ipratropium,* and *tiotropium,* which are quater-nized and do not cross the blood–brain barrier. The latter two agents are given by inhalation in the treatment of bronchial asthma and chronic obstructive pulmonary dis-ease. The synthetic derivatives possessing partial recep-tor selectivity include *pirenzepine,* used in the treatment of acid-peptic disease in some countries, and *tolterodine,* used in the treatment of urinary incontinence.

Muscarinic receptor antagonists prevent the effects of ACh by blocking its binding to muscarinic cholinergic receptors at neuroeffector sites on smooth muscle, cardiac muscle, and gland cells; in peripheral ganglia; and in the central nervous system. In general, muscarinic receptor antagonists cause little blockade of the effects of ACh at nicotinic receptor sites. However, quaternary ammonium analogs of atropine and related drugs generally exhibit a greater degree of nicotinic blocking activity and, conse-quently, are more likely to interfere with ganglionic or neuromuscular transmission.

In the CNS, cholinergic transmission appears to be both muscarinic and nicotinic at spinal, subcortical, and cortical levels in the brain (*see* Chapter 12). At high or toxic doses, the central effects of atropine and related drugs generally consist of CNS stimulation followed by depression. Since quaternary compounds penetrate the blood–brain barrier poorly, antagonists of this type have little or no effect on the CNS.

Parasympathetic neuroeffector junctions in different organs are not equally sensitive to even the nonselective muscarinic receptor antagonists (*see* Table 7–2). Small doses of atropine depress salivary and bronchial secretion and sweating. With larger doses, the pupil dilates, accom-modation of the lens to near vision is inhibited, and vagal effects on the heart are blocked so that the heart rate is in-creased. Larger doses inhibit the parasympathetic control of the urinary bladder and gastrointestinal tract, thereby inhibiting micturition and decreasing the tone and motil-ity of the gut. Still larger doses are required to inhibit gastric secretion and motility. Thus, doses of atropine and most related muscarinic receptor antagonists that reduce gastrointestinal tone and depress gastric secretion also al-most invariably affect salivary secretion, ocular accommo-dation, and micturition. This hierarchy of relative sensi-tivities probably is not a consequence of differences in the affinity of atropine for the muscarinic receptors at these sites, because atropine does not show selectivity

Table 7–2
Effects of Atropine in Relation to Dose

DOSE	EFFECTS
0.5 mg	Slight cardiac slowing; some dryness of mouth; inhibition of sweating
1 mg	Definite dryness of mouth; thirst; acceleration of heart, sometimes pre-ceded by slowing; mild dilation of pupils
2 mg	Rapid heart rate; palpitation; marked dryness of mouth; dilated pupils; some blurring of near vision
5 mg	All the above symptoms marked; difficulty in speaking and swallowing; restlessness and fatigue; headache; dry, hot skin; difficulty in micturi-tion; reduced intestinal peristalsis
10 mg and more	Above symptoms more marked; pulse rapid and weak; iris practically obliterated; vision very blurred; skin flushed, hot, dry, and scarlet; ataxia, restlessness, and excitement; hallucinations and delirium; coma

toward different muscarinic receptor subtypes. More likely determinants include the degree to which the functions of various end organs are regulated by parasympathetic tone and the involvement of intramural neurons and reflexes.

The actions of many clinically available muscarinic receptor antagonists differ only quantitatively from those of atropine, considered below as the prototype of the group. No antagonist in the receptor-selective category, including pirenzepine, is completely selective (*i.e.*, has a distinctive affinity for one relative to all other receptor subtypes). In fact, clinical efficacy of some agents may arise from a balance of antagonistic actions on two or more receptor subtypes.

History. The naturally occurring muscarinic receptor antagonists *atropine* and *scopolamine* are alkaloids of the belladonna (Solanaceae) plants. Preparations of belladonna were known to the ancient Hindus and have been used by physicians for many centuries. During the time of the Roman Empire and in the Middle Ages, the deadly nightshade shrub was frequently used to produce obscure and often prolonged poisoning. This prompted Linnaeus to name the shrub *Atropa belladonna,* after Atropos, the oldest of the three Fates, who cuts the thread of life. The name *belladonna* derives from the alleged use of this preparation by Italian women to dilate their pupils; modern-day fashion

photographers are known to use this same device for visual appeal. Atropine (*d,l-hyoscyamine*) also is found in *Datura stramonium,* also known as Jamestown or jimson weed. Scopolamine (*l-hyoscine*) is found chiefly in *Hyoscyamus niger* (henbane). In India, the root and leaves of the jimson weed plant were burned and the smoke inhaled to treat asthma. British colonists observed this ritual and introduced the belladonna alkaloids into western medicine in the early 1800s.

Accurate study of the actions of belladonna dates from the isolation of atropine in pure form by Mein in 1831. In 1867, Bezold and Bloebaum showed that atropine blocked the cardiac effects of vagal stimulation, and 5 years later Heidenhain found that it prevented salivary secretion produced by stimulation of the chorda tympani. Many semisynthetic congeners of the belladonna alkaloids and a large number of synthetic muscarinic receptor antagonists have been prepared, primarily with the objective of altering gastrointestinal or bladder activity without causing dry mouth or pupillary dilation.

Chemistry. Atropine and scopolamine are esters formed by combination of an aromatic acid, tropic acid, and complex organic bases, either tropine (tropanol) or scopine. Scopine differs from tropine only in having an oxygen bridge between the carbon atoms designated as 6 and 7 (Figure 7–2). Homatropine is a semisynthetic compound produced by combining the base tropine with mandelic acid. The corresponding quaternary ammonium derivatives, modified by the addition of a second methyl group to the nitrogen, are methylatropine nitrate, methscopolamine bromide, and homatropine methylbromide.

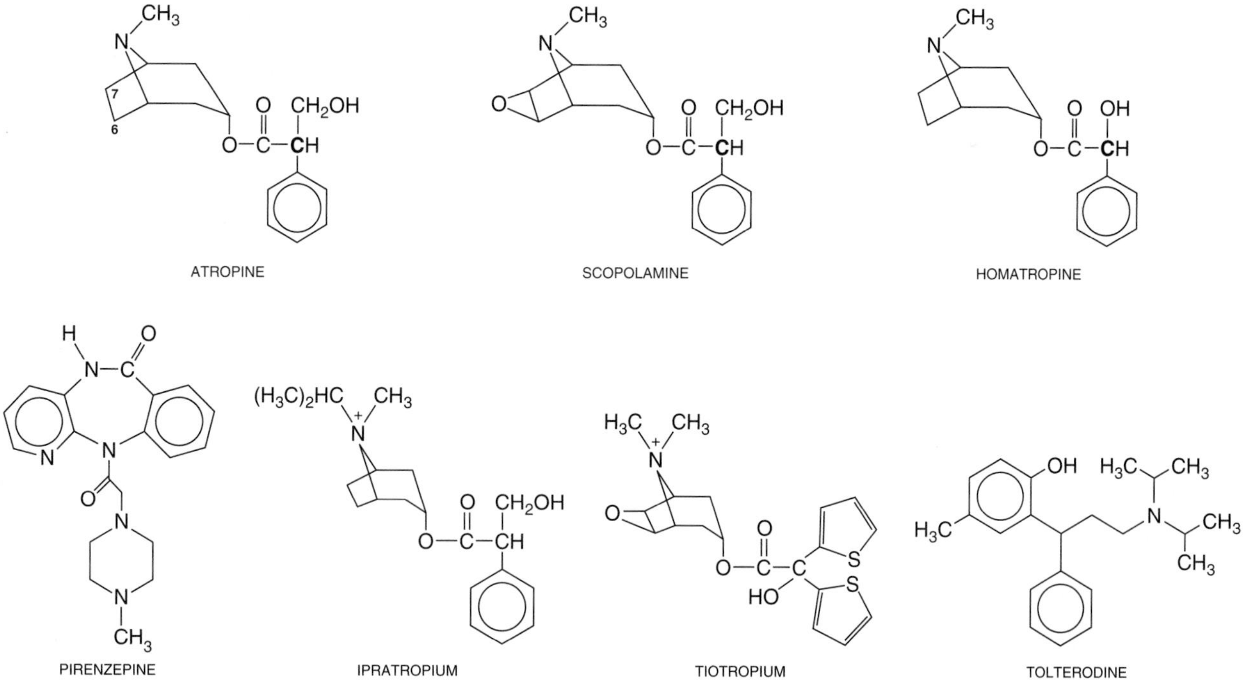

Figure 7–2. Structural formulas of the belladonna alkaloids and semisynthetic and synthetic analogs.

The boldface **C** identifies an asymmetric carbon atom.

Ipratropium and tiotropium also are quaternary tropine analogs esterified with synthetic aromatic acids.

Structure–Activity Relationship. An intact ester of tropine and tropic acid is essential for antimuscarinic action, since neither the free acid nor the base exhibits significant antimuscarinic activity. The presence of a free OH group in the acyl portion of the ester also is important for activity. When given parenterally, quaternary ammonium derivatives of atropine and scopolamine are, in general, more potent than their parent compounds in both muscarinic receptor and ganglionic blocking activities; conversion of the nitrogen from a tertiary to a quaternary group increases blockade at nicotinic receptors. The quaternary derivatives lack CNS activity because of poor penetration into the brain. Given orally, they are poorly and unreliably absorbed.

Both tropic and mandelic acids have an asymmetrical carbon atom (boldface **C** in the formulas in Figure 7–2). Scopolamine is *l*-hyoscine and is much more active than *d*-hyoscine. Atropine is racemized during extraction and consists of *d,l*-hyoscyamine, but antimuscarinic activity is almost wholly due to the naturally occurring *l* form. The synthetic derivatives show a wide latitude of structures that spatially replicate the aromatic acid and the bridged nitrogen of the tropine.

Mechanism of Action. Atropine and related compounds compete with ACh and other muscarinic agonists for a common binding site on the muscarinic receptor. The binding site for competitive antagonists and acetylcholine is in a cleft predicted to be formed by several of the receptor's seven transmembrane helices, as shown recently for the position of retinol in the mammalian rhodopsin structure (Palczewski *et al.*, 2000). An aspartic acid present in the *N*-terminal portion of the third transmembrane helix of all five muscarinic receptor subtypes is believed to form an ionic bond with the cationic quaternary nitrogen in acetylcholine and the tertiary or quaternary nitrogen of the antagonists (*see* Wess, 1996; Caufield and Birdsall, 1998).

Since antagonism by atropine is competitive, it can be overcome if the concentration of ACh at receptor sites of the effector organ is increased sufficiently. Muscarinic receptor antagonists inhibit responses to postganglionic cholinergic nerve stimulation less readily than they inhibit responses to injected choline esters. The difference may be due to release of ACh by cholinergic nerve terminals so close to receptors that very high concentrations of the transmitter gain access to the receptors in the neuroeffector junction.

Pharmacological Properties

Atropine and scopolamine differ quantitatively in antimuscarinic actions, particularly in their ability to affect the CNS. Atropine has almost no detectable effect on the CNS in doses that are used clinically. In contrast, scopolamine has prominent central effects at low therapeutic doses. The

basis for this difference is probably the greater permeation of scopolamine across the blood–brain barrier. Because atropine has limited CNS effects, it is given in preference to scopolamine for most purposes.

Central Nervous System. Atropine in therapeutic doses (0.5 to 1 mg) causes only mild vagal excitation as a result of stimulation of the medulla and higher cerebral centers. With toxic doses of atropine, central excitation becomes more prominent, leading to restlessness, irritability, disorientation, hallucinations, or delirium (*see* discussion of atropine poisoning, below). With still larger doses, stimulation is followed by depression, leading to circulatory collapse and respiratory failure after a period of paralysis and coma.

Scopolamine in therapeutic doses normally causes CNS depression manifested as drowsiness, amnesia, fatigue, and dreamless sleep, with a reduction in rapid eye movement (REM) sleep. It also causes euphoria and is therefore subject to some abuse. The depressant and amnesic effects formerly were sought when scopolamine was used as an adjunct to anesthetic agents or for preanesthetic medication. However, in the presence of severe pain, the same doses of scopolamine can occasionally cause excitement, restlessness, hallucinations, or delirium. These excitatory effects resemble those of toxic doses of atropine. Scopolamine also is effective in preventing motion sickness. This action is probably either on the cortex or more peripherally on the vestibular apparatus.

The belladonna alkaloids and related muscarinic receptor antagonists have long been used in parkinsonism. These agents can be effective adjuncts to treatment with levodopa (*see* Chapter 22). Muscarinic receptor antagonists also are used to treat the extrapyramidal symptoms that commonly occur as side effects of antipsychotic drug therapy (*see* Chapter 20). Certain antipsychotic drugs are relatively potent muscarinic receptor antagonists (Richelson, 1999), and these cause fewer extrapyramidal side effects.

Ganglia and Autonomic Nerves. Cholinergic neurotransmission in autonomic ganglia is mediated primarily by activation of nicotinic acetylcholine receptors, resulting in the generation of action potentials (*see* Chapters 6 and 9). ACh and other cholinergic agonists also cause the generation of slow excitatory postsynaptic potentials that are mediated by ganglionic muscarinic M_1–acetylcholine receptors. This response is particularly sensitive to blockade by pirenzepine. The extent to which the slow excitatory response can alter impulse transmission through the different sympathetic and parasympathetic ganglia is difficult to assess, but the effects of pirenzepine on responses of end organs suggest a physiological modulatory function for the ganglionic M_1 receptor (Caulfield, 1993; Eglen *et al.*, 1996; Birdsall *et al.*, 1998; Caulfield and Birdsall, 1998).

Pirenzepine inhibits gastric acid secretion at doses that have little effect on salivation or heart rate. Since the muscarinic receptors on the parietal cells do not appear to have a high affinity for pirenzepine, the M_1 receptor responsible for alterations in gastric acid secretion is postulated to be localized in intramural ganglia (*see* Eglen *et al.*, 1996). Blockade of ganglionic receptors (rather than those at the neuroeffector junction) also appears to underlie the ability of pirenzepine to inhibit the relaxation of the lower esophageal sphincter. Likewise, blockade of parasympathetic ganglia may contribute to the response to muscarinic antagonists in lung and heart (Barnes, 1993; Wellstein and Pitschner, 1988).

Presynaptic muscarinic receptors also are present on terminals of sympathetic and parasympathetic neurons. Blockade of these presynaptic receptors, which are of variable subtype, generally augments transmitter release. Nonselective muscarinic blocking agents may thus augment ACh release, partially counteracting their effective postsynaptic receptor blockade.

Since muscarinic receptor antagonists can alter autonomic activity at the ganglion and postganglionic neuron, the ultimate response of end organs to blockade of muscarinic receptors is difficult to predict. Thus, while direct blockade at neuroeffector sites predictably reverses the usual effects of the parasympathetic nervous system, concomitant inhibition of ganglionic or presynaptic receptors may produce paradoxical responses.

Eye. The muscarinic receptor antagonists block the responses of the pupillae sphincter muscle of the iris and the ciliary muscle of the lens to cholinergic stimulation (*see* Chapter 66). Thus, they dilate the pupil (mydriasis) and paralyze accommodation (cycloplegia). The wide pupillary dilation results in photophobia; the lens is fixed for far vision, near objects are blurred, and objects may appear smaller than they are. The normal pupillary reflex constriction to light or upon convergence of the eyes is abolished. These effects can occur after either local or systemic administration of the alkaloids. However, conventional systemic doses of atropine (0.6 mg) have little ocular effect, in contrast to equal doses of scopolamine, which cause definite mydriasis and loss of accommodation. Locally applied atropine or scopolamine produces ocular effects of considerable duration; accommodation and pupillary reflexes may not fully recover for 7 to 12 days. The muscarinic receptor antagonists used as mydriatics differ from the sympathomimetic agents in that the latter cause pupillary dilation without loss of accommodation. Pilocarpine, choline esters, physostigmine, and isoflurophate (DFP) in sufficient concentrations can partially or fully reverse the ocular effects of atropine.

Muscarinic receptor antagonists administered systemically have little effect on intraocular pressure except in patients predisposed to narrow-angle glaucoma, where the pressure may occasionally rise dangerously. The rise in pressure occurs when the anterior chamber is narrow and the iris obstructs flow of aqueous humor into the trabeculae. This interferes with drainage of aqueous humor. The drugs may precipitate a first attack in unrecognized cases of this rare condition. In patients with open-

angle glaucoma, an acute rise in pressure is unusual. Atropine-like drugs generally can be used safely in this latter condition, particularly if the patient also is adequately treated with an appropriate miotic agent.

Cardiovascular System. *Heart.* The main effect of atropine on the heart is to alter the rate. Although the dominant response is tachycardia, the heart rate often decreases transiently with average clinical doses (0.4 to 0.6 mg). The slowing is rarely marked, about 4 to 8 beats per minute, and is usually absent after rapid intravenous injection. There are no accompanying changes in blood pressure or cardiac output. This paradoxical effect once was thought to be due to central vagal stimulation; however, cardiac slowing also is seen with muscarinic receptor antagonists that do not readily enter the brain. Studies in human beings show that pirenzepine is equipotent with atropine in decreasing heart rate; its prior administration can prevent any further decrease by atropine. The data suggest that the decreased heart rate may result from blockade of M_1 receptors on postganglionic parasympathetic neurons; this relieves the inhibitory effects of synaptic ACh and increases the release of transmitter (Wellstein and Pitschner, 1988).

Larger doses of atropine cause progressively increasing tachycardia by blocking vagal effects on M_2 receptors on the SA nodal pacemaker. The resting heart rate is increased by about 35 to 40 beats per minute in young men given 2 mg of atropine intramuscularly. The maximal heart rate (*e.g.*, in response to exercise) is not altered by atropine. The influence of atropine is most noticeable in healthy young adults, in whom vagal tone is considerable. In infancy and old age, even large doses of atropine may fail to accelerate the heart. Atropine often produces cardiac arrhythmias, but without significant cardiovascular symptoms.

With low doses of scopolamine (0.1 or 0.2 mg), the cardiac slowing is greater than with atropine. With higher doses, cardioacceleration occurs initially, but it is short lived and is followed within 30 minutes either by a return to the normal rate or by bradycardia.

Adequate doses of atropine can abolish many types of reflex vagal cardiac slowing or asystole—for example, from inhalation of irritant vapors, stimulation of the carotid sinus, pressure on the eyeballs, peritoneal stimulation, or injection of contrast dye during cardiac catheterization. It also prevents or abruptly abolishes bradycardia or asystole caused by choline esters, acetylcholinesterase inhibitors, or other parasympathomimetic drugs, as well as cardiac arrest from electrical stimulation of the vagus.

The removal of vagal influence on the heart by atropine also may facilitate AV conduction. Atropine also shortens the functional refractory period of the AV node and can increase ventricular rate in patients who have atrial fibrillation or flutter. In certain cases of second-degree heart block (*e.g.,* Wenckebach AV block), in which vagal activity is an etiological factor (such as with digitalis toxicity), atropine may lessen the degree of block. In some patients with complete heart block, the idioventricular rate may be accelerated by atropine; in others it is stabilized. Atropine and scopolamine may improve the clinical condition of patients with early myocardial infarction by relieving severe sinus or nodal bradycardia or AV block.

Circulation.   Atropine, in clinical doses, completely counteracts the peripheral vasodilation and sharp fall in blood pressure caused by choline esters. In contrast, when given alone, its effect on blood vessels and blood pressure is neither striking nor constant. This result is expected, because most vascular beds lack significant cholinergic innervation, and the cholinergic sympathetic vasodilator fibers to vessels supplying skeletal muscle do not appear to be involved to any important extent in the normal regulation of tone.

Atropine in toxic, and occasionally therapeutic, doses dilates cutaneous blood vessels, especially those in the blush area (atropine flush). This may be a compensatory reaction permitting the radiation of heat to offset the atropine-induced rise in temperature that can accompany inhibition of sweating.

Respiratory Tract.   The parasympathetic nervous system plays a major role in regulating bronchomotor tone. A diverse set of stimuli cause reflex increases in parasympathetic activity that contribute to bronchoconstriction. Vagal fibers synapse and activate nicotinic and M_1-muscarinic receptors in parasympathetic ganglia located in the airway wall; short postganglionic fibers release acetylcholine, which acts on M_3-muscarinic receptors in airway smooth muscle. The submucosal glands also are innervated by parasympathetic neurons and have predominantly M_3 receptors (*see* Barnes, 2000). Largely owing to the introduction of inhaled ipratropium and tiotropium, anticholinergic therapy of chronic obstructive pulmonary disease and asthma has been revived (Barnes, 2000; Littner *et al.*, 2000).

The belladonna alkaloids inhibit secretions of the nose, mouth, pharynx, and bronchi and thus dry the mucous membranes of the respiratory tract. This action is especially marked if secretion is excessive and is the basis for the use of atropine and scopolamine in preanesthetic medication. The ability of these agents to reduce the occurrence of laryngospasm during general anesthesia appears to be caused by inhibition of respiratory tract secretions that can precipitate reflex laryngospasm. However, the depression of mucous secretion and mucociliary clearance are undesirable side effects of atropine in patients with airway disease.

Inhibition by atropine of bronchoconstriction caused by histamine, bradykinin, and the eicosanoids presumably reflects the participation of parasympathetic efferents in the bronchial reflexes elicited by these agents. The ability to block the indirect bronchoconstrictive effects of inflammatory mediators that are released during attacks of asthma forms the basis for the use of anticholinergic agents, along with β-adrenergic agonists, in the treatment of this disease (*see* Chapter 28).

Gastrointestinal Tract.   Interest in the actions of muscarinic receptor antagonists on the stomach and intestine led to their use as antispasmodic agents for gastrointestinal disorders and in the treatment of peptic ulcer. Although atropine can completely abolish the effects of ACh (and other parasympathomimetic drugs) on the motility and secretions of the gastrointestinal tract, it inhibits only incompletely the effects of vagal impulses. This difference is particularly striking in the effects of atropine on motility of the gut. Preganglionic vagal fibers that innervate the gut synapse not only with postganglionic cholinergic fibers but also with a network of noncholinergic intramural neurons. These neurons, which form the enteric plexus, utilize numerous neurotransmitters including 5-hydroxytryptamine (5-HT) and dopamine. Since therapeutic doses of atropine do not block responses to gastrointestinal hormones or to noncholinergic neurohumoral transmitters, release of these substances from the intramural neurons can still effect changes in motility. Similarly, while vagal activity modulates gastrin-elicited histamine release and gastric acid secretion, the actions of gastrin can occur independent of vagal tone. H_2-histamine receptor antagonists, M_1-muscarinic receptor antagonists, and K^+,H^+-ATPase inhibitors (proton pump inhibitors) have replaced atropine and other nonselective antagonists as inhibitors of acid secretion (*see* Chapter 37).

Secretions.   *Salivary secretion* appears to be mediated through M_3 receptors and is particularly sensitive to inhibition by muscarinic receptor antagonists, which can completely abolish the copious, watery, parasympathetically induced secretion. The mouth becomes dry, and swallowing and talking may become difficult. Gastric secretions during the cephalic and fasting phase are reduced markedly by muscarinic receptor antagonists. In contrast, the intestinal phase of gastric secretion is only partially inhibited. The concentration of acid is not necessarily lowered, because secretion of HCO_3^- as well as of H^+ is blocked. The gastric cells that secrete mucin and proteolytic enzymes are more directly under vagal influence than are the acid-secreting cells, and atropine decreases their secretory function.

Motility. The parasympathetic nerves enhance both tone and motility and relax sphincters, thereby favoring the passage of chyme through the gut. However, the intestine has a complex system of intramural nerve plexuses that regulate motility independent of parasympathetic control; impulses from the CNS only modulate the effects of the intrinsic reflexes (*see* Chapter 6). Both in normal subjects and in patients with gastrointestinal disease, muscarinic antagonists produce prolonged inhibitory effects on the motor activity of the stomach, duodenum, jejunum, ileum, and colon, characterized by a reduction in tone and in amplitude and frequency of peristaltic contractions. Relatively large doses are needed to produce such inhibition.

Other Smooth Muscle.   *Urinary Tract.*   Atropine decreases the normal tone and amplitude of contractions of the ureter and bladder, and often eliminates drug-induced enhancement of ureteral tone. However, this inhibition is not achieved in the absence of inhibition of salivation and lacrimation and blurring of vision. Control of bladder contraction appears to be mediated by multiple muscarinic receptor subtypes. Receptors of the M_2 subtype appear most prevalent in the bladder, yet studies with selective antagonists suggest that the M_3 receptor mediates detrusor muscle contraction. The M_2 receptor may act to inhibit β-adrenergic receptor–mediated relaxation of the bladder and may be involved primarily in the filling stages to diminish urge incontinence (Hegde and Eglen, 1999; Chappel, 2000). In addition, presynaptic M_1 receptors appear to facilitate the release of ACh from parasympathetic nerve terminals (Somogyi and de Groat, 1999).

Biliary Tract.   Atropine exerts a mild antispasmodic action on the gallbladder and bile ducts in human beings. However, this effect usually is not sufficient to overcome or prevent the marked spasm and increase in biliary duct pressure induced by opioids. The nitrites (*see* Chapter 32) are more effective than atropine in this respect.

Sweat Glands and Temperature.   Small doses of atropine or scopolamine inhibit the activity of sweat glands innervated by sympathetic cholinergic fibers, and the skin becomes hot and dry. Sweating may be depressed enough to raise the body temperature, but only notably so after large doses or at high environmental temperatures.

Absorption, Fate, and Excretion.   The belladonna alkaloids and the tertiary synthetic and semisynthetic derivatives are absorbed rapidly from the gastrointestinal tract. They also enter the circulation when applied locally to the mucosal surfaces of the body. Absorption from intact skin is limited, although efficient absorption does occur in the postauricular region. Systemic absorption of inhaled quaternary muscarinic receptor antagonists is minimal. The quaternary ammonium derivatives of the belladonna alkaloids also are poorly absorbed after an oral dose (Ali-Melkkila *et al.,* 1993) and penetrate the conjunctiva of the eye less readily. Central effects are lacking, because these agents do not cross the blood–brain

barrier. Atropine has a half-life of approximately 4 hours; hepatic metabolism accounts for the elimination of about half of a dose, and the remainder is excreted unchanged in the urine. The quaternary agents have somewhat longer durations of action.

Poisoning by Muscarinic Receptor Antagonists and Other Anticholinergic Drugs.   The deliberate or accidental ingestion of belladonna alkaloids or other classes of drugs with atropinic properties is a major cause of poisonings. Many H_1-histamine receptor antagonists, phenothiazines, and tricyclic antidepressants block muscarinic receptors and, in sufficient dosage, produce syndromes that include features of atropine intoxication.

Among the tricyclic antidepressants, *protriptyline* and *amitriptyline* are the most potent muscarinic receptor antagonists, with an affinity for the receptor that is approximately one-tenth that reported for atropine. Since these drugs are administered in therapeutic doses considerably higher than the effective dose of atropine, antimuscarinic effects often are observed clinically (*see* Chapter 19). In addition, overdose with suicidal intent is a danger in the population using antidepressants. Fortunately, most of the newer antidepressants and selective serotonin-reuptake inhibitors are far less anticholinergic (Cusack *et al.,* 1994). In contrast, the newer antipsychotic drugs, classified as "atypical" and characterized by their low propensity for inducing extrapyramidal side effects, include agents that are potent muscarinic receptor antagonists. In particular, *clozapine* binds to human brain muscarinic receptors with only fivefold lower affinity than atropine; *olanzapine* also is a potent muscarinic receptor antagonist (Richelson, 1999). Accordingly, dry mouth is a prominent side effect of these drugs. A paradoxical side effect of clozapine is increased salivation and drooling, possibly the result of selective agonist properties of this drug (Richelson, 1999).

Infants and young children are especially susceptible to the toxic effects of atropinic drugs. Indeed, cases of intoxication in children have resulted from conjunctival instillation of atropinic drugs for ophthalmic refraction and for other ocular effects. Systemic absorption occurs either from the nasal mucosa after the drug has traversed the nasolacrimal duct or from the intestinal tract if it is swallowed. Poisoning with diphenoxylate-atropine (LOMOTIL, others), used to treat diarrhea, has been extensively reported in the pediatric literature. Transdermal preparations of scopolamine used for motion sickness have been noted to cause toxic psychoses, especially in children and in the elderly (Wilkinson, 1987; Ziskind, 1988). Serious intoxication may occur in children who ingest berries or seeds containing belladonna alkaloids. Poisoning from ingestion and smoking of jimson weed, or thorn apple, is not uncommon today.

Table 7–2 shows the oral doses of atropine causing undesirable responses or symptoms of overdosage. These symptoms are predictable from the organs receiving parasympathetic innervation. In cases of full-blown atropine poisoning, the syndrome may last 48 hours or longer. Intravenous injection of the anticholinerase agent *physostigmine* may be used for confirmation. If the typical salivation, sweating, slowing of heart rate, and intestinal hyperactivity do not occur, intoxication with atropine or a related agent is almost certain. Depression and circulatory collapse are evident only in cases of severe intoxication; the blood pressure declines, convulsions may ensue, respiration becomes inadequate, and death due to respiratory failure may follow after a period of paralysis and coma.

Measures to limit intestinal absorption should be initiated without delay if the poison has been taken orally. For symptomatic treatment, slow intravenous injection of physostigmine rapidly abolishes the delirium and coma caused by large doses of atropine but carries some risk of overdose in mild atropine intoxication. Since physostigmine is metabolized rapidly, the patient may again lapse into coma within 1 to 2 hours, and repeated doses may be needed (*see* Chapter 8). If marked excitement is present and more specific treatment is not available, a benzodiazepine is the most suitable agent for sedation and for control of convulsions. Phenothiazines or agents with antimuscarinic activity should not be used, because their antimuscarinic action is likely to intensify toxicity. Support of respiration and control of hyperthermia may be necessary. Ice bags and alcohol sponges help to reduce fever, especially in children.

SYNTHETIC AND SEMISYNTHETIC SUBSTITUTES FOR BELLADONNA ALKALOIDS

Quaternary Ammonium Muscarinic Receptor Antagonists

Ipratropium and Tiotropium. *Ipratropium bromide* (ATROVENT) is a quaternary ammonium compound formed by the introduction of an isopropyl group to the N atom of atropine. A similar agent, *oxitropium bromide,* also is available in Europe; it is an *N*-ethyl-substituted, quaternary derivative of scopolamine. The most recently developed and bronchoselective member of this family is *tiotropium bromide* (SPIRIVA), which has a longer duration of action, but is unavailable in the United States. Ipratropium appears to block all subtypes of muscarinic receptors, whereas tiotropium shows selectivity for M_1 and M_3 receptors by virtue of its slow rate of dissociation. In contrast, it dissociates rapidly from M_2 receptors.

Pharmacological Properties. Ipratropium produces bronchodilation, tachycardia, and inhibition of secretion similar to that of atropine when it is administered parenterally (Gross, 1988). Although somewhat more potent than atropine, ipratropium and tiotropium lack appreciable action on the CNS but have greater inhibitory effects on ganglionic transmission. An unexpected and therapeutically important property of ipratropium and tiotropium, evident upon either local or parenteral administration, is their minimal inhibitory effect on mucociliary clearance, relative to atropine (*see* Gross, 1988). Hence, the use of these agents in patients with airway disease avoids the increased accumulation of lower airway secretions encountered with atropine.

When ipratropium or tiotropium is inhaled, its action is confined almost exclusively to the mouth and airways. Dry mouth is the only side effect reported frequently. Selectivity results from the very inefficient absorption of the drug from the lungs or the gastrointestinal tract. The degree of bronchodilation achieved by these agents is thought to reflect the level of basal parasympathetic tone, supplemented by reflex activation of cholinergic pathways brought about by various stimuli. In normal individuals, inhalation of the drugs can provide virtually complete protection against the bronchoconstriction produced by the subsequent inhalation of such substances as sulfur dioxide, ozone, or cigarette smoke. However, patients with asthma or with demonstrable bronchial hyperresponsiveness are less well protected. Although these drugs cause a marked reduction in sensitivity to methacholine in asthmatic subjects, more modest inhibition of responses to challenge with histamine, bradykinin, or prostaglandin $F_{2\alpha}$ is achieved, and little protection is provided against the bronchoconstriction induced by serotonin or the leukotrienes. The principal clinical use of ipratropium and tiotropium is in the treatment of chronic obstructive pulmonary disease; they are less effective in most asthmatic patients (*see* Gross, 1988; Barnes, 2000; van Noord *et al.,* 2000; Littner *et al.,* 2000). The therapeutic use of ipratropium and tiotropium is discussed further in Chapter 28.

Absorption, Fate, and Excretion. Ipratropium is administered as an aerosol or solution for inhalation whereas tiotropium is administered as a dry powder. As with most drugs administered by inhalation, about 90% of the dose is swallowed. Most of the swallowed drug appears in the feces. After inhalation, maximal responses usually develop over 30 to 90 minutes, with tiotropium having the slower onset. The effects of ipratropium last for 4 to 6 hours, while tiotropium's effects persist for 24 hours, and the drug is amenable to once-daily dosing (Barnes, 1999; van Noord *et al.,* 2000; Littner *et al.,* 2000).

Methscopolamine. *Methscopolamine bromide* (PAMINE) is a quaternary ammonium derivative of scopolamine and therefore lacks the central actions of scopolamine. It is less potent than atropine and is poorly absorbed; however, its action is more prolonged, the usual oral dose (2.5 mg) acting for 6 to 8 hours. Its use has been limited chiefly to gastrointestinal diseases.

Homatropine Methylbromide. *Homatropine methylbromide* is the quaternary derivative of homatropine. It is less potent than atropine in antimuscarinic activity, but it is four times more potent as a ganglionic blocking agent. It is available in a few combination products intended for relief of gastrointestinal spasm.

Propantheline. *Propantheline bromide* (PRO-BANTHINE) has been one of the more widely used of the synthetic muscarinic receptor antagonists lacking receptor selectivity. High doses produce the symptoms of ganglionic blockade, and toxic doses block the skeletal neuromuscular junction. Its duration of action is comparable to that of atropine.

Glycopyrrolate. *Glycopyrrolate* (ROBINUL) is employed orally to inhibit gastrointestinal motility and also is used parenterally to block the effects of vagal stimulation during anesthesia and surgery.

Tertiary-Amine Muscarinic Receptor Antagonists

Agents useful in ophthalmology include *homatropine hydrobromide* (ISOPTO HOMATROPINE) (a semisynthetic derivative of atropine; *see* Figure 7–2), *cyclopentolate hydrochloride* (CYCLOGYL), and *tropicamide* (MYDRIACYL). These agents are preferred to atropine or scopolamine because of their shorter duration of action. Additional information on the ophthalmological properties and preparations of these and other drugs is provided in Chapter 66.

Tertiary-amine muscarinic receptor antagonists gain access to the CNS and are therefore the anticholinergic drugs used to treat parkinsonism and the extrapyramidal side effects of antipsychotic drugs. Specific agents used primarily for these conditions include *benztropine mesylate* (COGENTIN) and *trihexyphenidyl hydrochloride* (ARTANE, others). These drugs are discussed in Chapter 22.

Tertiary amines used for their antispasmodic properties are *dicyclomine hydrochloride* (BENTYL, others), *flavoxate hydrochloride* (URISPAS), and *oxybutynin chloride* (DITROPAN). These agents appear to exert some nonspecific direct relaxant effect on smooth muscle. In therapeutic doses they decrease spasm of the gastrointestinal tract, biliary tract, ureter, and uterus.

Flavoxate, oxybutynin, and its more active enantiomer, (S)-oxybutynin, are indicated for overactive bladder. Side effects of dry mouth and eyes limit the tolerability of these drugs with continued use, and patient acceptance declines. *Tolterodine* (DETROL) is a potent muscarinic antagonist that shows selectivity for the urinary bladder in animal models and in clinical studies.

Its selectivity and greater patient acceptance is surprising, since studies on isolated receptors do not reveal a unique subtype selectivity (Chapple, 2000; Abrams *et al.,* 1998, 1999). Inhibition of a particular complement of receptors in the bladder may give rise to synergism and clinical efficacy. Tolterodine's metabolism depends on CYP2B6 to form the 5-hydroxymethyl metabolite. Since this metabolite possesses similar activity to the parent drug, variations in CYP2B6 levels do not affect the duration of action of the drug.

Selective Muscarinic Receptor Antagonists

Pirenzepine is a tricyclic drug, similar in structure to imipramine. Pirenzepine has selectivity for M_1-, relative to M_2-, and M_3-muscarinic receptors (Caulfield, 1993; Caulfield and Birdsall, 1998). However, pirenzepine's affinities for M_1 and M_4 receptors are comparable, so it does not possess total M_1 selectivity. *Telenzepine* is an analog of pirenzepine that has higher potency and similar selectivity for M_1-muscarinic receptors. Both drugs are used in the treatment of acid-peptic disease in Europe, Japan, and Canada, but not currently in the United States. At therapeutic doses of pirenzepine, the incidence of dry mouth and blurred vision is relatively low. Central effects are not seen because of the drug's low lipid solubility and limited penetration into the CNS. Some studies also have shown pirenzepine and telenzepine to be of therapeutic value in chronic obstructive bronchitis, presumably due to blockade of vagally mediated bronchoconstriction (Cazzola *et al.,* 1990). In both the gastrointestinal tract and airway, the site of M_1 receptor antagonism is believed to be on receptors in ganglia.

Tripitamine and *darifenacin* are selective antagonists for M_2- and M_3-muscarinic receptors, respectively. They are of potential utility in blocking cholinergic bradycardia (M_2) and smooth muscle activity or epithelial secretions (M_3). Darifenacin is in clinical trial for overactive bladder. While not of current therapeutic value, peptide toxins from the venoms of green and black mambas show the greatest selectivity for specific muscarinic receptor subtypes (M_1 and M_4) (Caulfield and Birdsall, 1998).

THERAPEUTIC USES OF MUSCARINIC RECEPTOR ANTAGONISTS

Muscarinic receptor antagonists have been employed in a wide variety of clinical conditions, predominantly to inhibit effects of parasympathetic nervous system activity. The major limitation in the use of the nonselective drugs is often failure to obtain desired therapeutic responses without concomitant side effects. The latter usually are not serious but are sufficiently disturbing to decrease patient compliance, particularly during long-term administration.

Selectivity has been achieved by local administration, either by pulmonary inhalation or instillation in the eye. Minimal systemic absorption and dilution from the site of action minimize systemic effects. Subtype-selective muscarinic receptor antagonists hold the most promise for treating specific clinical symptoms; several are in clinical trials.

Gastrointestinal Tract.   Muscarinic receptor antagonists were once the most widely used drugs for the management of peptic ulcer. Although these drugs can reduce gastric motility and the secretion of gastric acid, antisecretory doses produced pronounced side effects, such as dry mouth, loss of visual accommodation, photophobia, and difficulty in urination. As a consequence, patient compliance in the long-term management of symptoms of acid-peptic disease with these drugs was poor. Because of pirenzepine's relative selectivity for M_1-muscarinic receptors, it clearly offers a marked improvement over atropine. However, the H_2-receptor antagonists and proton pump inhibitors generally are considered to be the drugs of choice to reduce gastric acid secretion (*see* Chapter 37).

Most studies indicate that pirenzepine (100 to 150 mg per day) produces about the same rate of healing of duodenal ulcers as the H_2 receptor antagonists cimetidine or ranitidine; it also may be effective in preventing the recurrence of ulcers (Carmine and Brogden, 1985; Tryba and Cook, 1997). Although less extensive data are available, similar results have been obtained in the treatment of gastric ulcers. Dry mouth occurred in 14% and blurred vision in 2% to 5% of patients treated with pirenzepine, but these side effects necessitated withdrawal of the drug in fewer than 1% of the patients. Studies in human subjects have shown pirenzepine to be more potent in inhibiting gastric acid secretion produced as a result of neural stimuli than that induced by muscarinic agonists, supporting the postulated localization of M_1 receptors at ganglionic sites.

The belladonna alkaloids and their synthetic substitutes also have been used and recommended in a wide variety of conditions known or supposed to involve irritable bowel and increased tone ("spasticity") or motility of the gastrointestinal tract. These agents can reduce tone and motility when administered in maximal tolerated doses, and they might be expected to be efficacious if the condition simply involves excessive smooth muscle contraction, a point that is often in doubt. M_3-selective antagonists might achieve more selectivity, but M_3 receptors also exert a dominant influence on salivation, bronchiolar secretion and contraction, and bladder motility. Alternative agents for treatment of irritable bowel syndrome and its associated diarrhea are discussed in Chapter 38. Diarrhea sometimes associated with irritative conditions of the lower bowel, such as mild dysenteries and diverticulitis, may respond to atropine-like drugs. However, more severe conditions such as salmonella dysenteries, ulcerative colitis, and regional enteritis respond poorly.

The belladonna alkaloids and synthetic substitutes are very effective in reducing excessive salivation, such as that associated with heavy-metal poisoning or parkinsonism and drug-induced salivation.

Uses in Ophthalmology.   Effects limited to the eye are obtained by local administration of muscarinic receptor antagonists to produce mydriasis and cycloplegia. Cycloplegia is not attainable without mydriasis and requires higher concentrations or more prolonged application of a given agent. Mydriasis often is necessary for thorough examination of the retina and optic disc and in the therapy of iridocyclitis and keratitis. The belladonna mydriatics may be alternated with miotics for breaking or preventing the development of adhesions between the iris and the lens. Complete cycloplegia may be necessary in the treatment of iridocyclitis and choroiditis and for accurate measurement of refractive errors. In instances where complete cycloplegia is required, agents such as atropine or scopolamine, which are more effective, are preferred to drugs such as cyclopentolate and tropicamide. Details of the drugs commonly used are given in Chapter 66.

Respiratory Tract.   Atropine and other belladonna alkaloids and substitutes reduce secretion in both the upper and lower respiratory tracts. This effect in the nasopharynx may provide some symptomatic relief of acute rhinitis associated with coryza or hay fever, although such therapy does not affect the natural course of the condition. It is probable that the contribution of antihistamines employed in "cold" mixtures is due primarily to their antimuscarinic properties, except in conditions with an allergic basis.

Systemic administration of belladonna alkaloids or their derivatives for bronchial asthma or obstructive pulmonary disease carries the disadvantage of reducing bronchial secretions and inspissation of the residual secretions. This viscid material is difficult to remove from the respiratory tree, and its presence can dangerously obstruct airflow and predispose to infection.

Ipratropium bromide and tiotropium, administered by inhalation, do not produce adverse effects on mucociliary clearance, in contrast to atropine and other muscarinic antagonists. Thus, their anticholinergic properties can be exploited safely in the treatment of reversible airway disease. These agents often are used with inhalation of long-acting β-adrenergic receptor agonists, although there is little evidence of true synergism. The muscarinic antagonists are more effective in chronic obstructive pulmonary disease, particularly when cholinergic tone is evident. β-Adrenergic agonists control best the intermittent exacerbation of asthma (Barnes, 2000; *see* also Chapter 28).

Cardiovascular System.   The cardiovascular effects of muscarinic-receptor antagonists are of limited clinical application. Generally, these agents are used in coronary care units for short-term interventions or in surgical settings.

Atropine may be considered in the initial treatment of patients with acute myocardial infarction in whom excessive vagal tone causes sinus or nodal bradycardia. Sinus bradycardia is the most common arrhythmia seen during acute myocardial infarction, especially of the inferior or posterior wall. Atropine may prevent further clinical deterioration in cases of high vagal tone or AV block by restoring heart rate to a level sufficient to maintain adequate hemodynamic status and to eliminate AV nodal block. Dosing must be done judiciously; doses that are too low can cause a paradoxical bradycardia (*see* above), while excessive doses will cause tachycardia that may extend the infarct by increasing the demand for oxygen.

Atropine occasionally is useful in reducing the severe bradycardia and syncope associated with a hyperactive carotid sinus reflex. It has little effect on most ventricular rhythms. In some patients, atropine may eliminate premature ventricular contractions associated with a very slow atrial rate. It also may reduce the degree of AV block when increased vagal tone is a major factor in the conduction defect, such as the second-degree AV block that can be produced by digitalis.

Central Nervous System. For many years, the belladonna alkaloids and subsequently the tertiary-amine synthetic substitutes were the only agents helpful in the treatment of parkinsonism. Levodopa or levodopa along with carbidopa now is the treatment of choice, but alternative or concurrent therapy with muscarinic receptor antagonists may be required in some patients (*see* Chapter 22). Centrally acting agents such as benztropine have been shown to be efficacious in preventing dystonias or parkinsonian symptoms in patients treated with antipsychotic drugs (Arana *et al.,* 1988; *see* also Chapter 20).

The belladonna alkaloids were among the first drugs to be used in the prevention of motion sickness. Scopolamine is the most effective prophylactic agent for short (4- to 6-hour) exposures to severe motion, and probably for exposures of up to several days. All agents used to combat motion sickness should be given prophylactically; they are much less effective after severe nausea or vomiting has developed. A preparation for the transdermal administration of scopolamine (TRANSDERM SCOP) has been shown to be highly effective when used prophylactically for the prevention of motion sickness. The drug is incorporated into a multilayered adhesive unit that is applied to the postauricular mastoid region. Absorption of the drug is especially efficient in this area. The duration of action of the preparation is about 72 hours, during which time approximately 0.5 mg of scopolamine is delivered. Dry mouth is common, drowsiness is not infrequent, and blurred vision occurs in some individuals. Rare but severe psychotic episodes have also been reported (Wilkinson, 1987; Ziskind, 1988).

The use of scopolamine to produce tranquilization and amnesia in a variety of circumstances, including labor, is declining. Given alone in the presence of pain or severe anxiety, scopolamine may induce outbursts of uncontrolled behavior.

Uses in Anesthesia. The use of anesthetics that are relatively nonirritating to the bronchi has virtually eliminated the need for prophylactic use of muscarinic receptor antagonists. Atropine commonly is given to prevent vagal reflexes induced by surgical manipulation of visceral organs. Atropine or glycopyrrolate is used with neostigmine to counteract its parasympathomimetic effects when the latter agent is used to reverse muscle relaxation after surgery (*see* Chapter 9). Serious cardiac arrhythmias have occasionally occurred, perhaps because of the initial bradycardia produced by atropine combined with the cholinomimetic effects of neostigmine.

Genitourinary Tract. Atropine often has been given with an opioid in the treatment of renal colic in the hope that it will relax the ureteral smooth muscle; however, as in biliary colic, it probably does not make a major contribution to the relief of pain. Newer synthetic substitutes of atropine, such as tolterodine, can lower intravesicular pressure, increase capacity, and reduce the frequency of urinary bladder contractions by antagonizing the parasympathetic control of this organ without leading to poorly tolerated side effects. This becomes the basis for the use of such agents in enuresis in children, particularly when a progressive increase in bladder capacity is the objective. These agents also are used to reduce urinary frequency in spastic paraplegia and to increase the capacity of the bladder (Chapple, 2000; Goessl *et al.,* 2000).

Anticholinesterase and Mushroom Poisoning. The use of atropine in large doses for the treatment of poisoning by anticholinesterase organophosphorus insecticides is discussed in Chapter 8. Atropine also may be used to antagonize the parasympathomimetic effects of neostigmine or other anticholinesterase agents administered in the treatment of myasthenia gravis. It does not interfere with the salutary effects at the skeletal neuromuscular junction, and it is particularly useful early in therapy, before tolerance to muscarinic side effects has developed. As discussed earlier, atropine is useful as an antidote only for the symptoms of mushroom poisoning by the cholinomimetic alkaloid muscarine, found in certain mushroom species.

PROSPECTUS

The availability of cDNAs encoding five distinct muscarinic receptor subtypes has facilitated the development of subtype-selective agents. Functionally selective muscarinic agonists have been in clinical trial for use in treating intellectual impairment associated with Alzheimer's disease; in theory, these agents lack the unwanted effect of concomitant stimulation of presynaptic muscarinic receptors that inhibit release of endogenous ACh. Subtype-selective muscarinic receptor antagonists show promise in several therapeutic settings—for example, in the treatment of urinary incontinence and for management of irritable bowel syndrome. Therapeutic selectivity may result from targeting unique subsets of receptors that control muscarinic responses within a particular end organ.

BIBLIOGRAPHY

Abrams, P., Freeman, R., Anderstrom, C., and Mattiasson, A. Tolterodine, a new antimuscarinic agent: as effective but better tolerated than oxybutynin in patients with an overactive bladder. *Br. J. Urol.,* **1998,** *81*:801–810.

Ali-Melkkila, A., Kanto, J., and Iisalo, E. Pharmacokinetics and related pharmacodynamics of anticholinergic drugs. *Acta Anaesthesiol. Scand.,* **1993,** *37*:633–642.

Arana, G.W., Goff, D.C., Baldessarini, R.J., and Keepers G.A. Efficacy of anticholinergic prophylaxis for neuroleptic-induced acute dystonia. *Am. J. Psychiatry,* **1988,** *145*:993–996.

Barnes, P.J. Muscarinic receptor subtypes in airways. *Life Sci.,* **1993,** *52:*521–527.

Bonner, T.I., Buckley, N.J., Young, A.C., and Brann, M.R. Identification of a family of muscarinic acetylcholine receptor genes. *Science,* **1987,** *237:*527–532.

Bruning, T.A., Hendriks, M.G., Chang, P.C., Kuypers, E.A., and van Zwieten, P.A. In vivo characterization of vasodilating muscarinic-receptor subtypes in humans. *Circ. Res.,* **1994,** *74:*912–919.

Cazzola, M., D'Amato, G., Guidetti, E., Staudinger, H., Steinijans, V.W., and Kilian, U. An M_1-selective muscarinic receptor antagonist telenzepine improves lung function in patients with chronic obstructive bronchitis. *Pulm. Pharmacol.,* **1990,** *3:*185–189.

Chapple, C.R. Muscarinic receptor antagonists in the treatment of overactive bladder. *Urology,* **2000,** *55:*33–46.

Cusack, B., Nelson, A., and Richelson, E. Binding of antidepressants to human brain receptors: focus on newer generation compounds. *Psychopharmacology (Berl.),* **1994,** *114:*559–565.

Epstein, J.B., Burchell, J.L., Emerton, S., Le, N.D., and Silverman, S. Jr. A clinical trial of bethanechol in patients with xerostomia after radiation therapy. A pilot study. *Oral Surg. Oral Med. Oral Pathol.,* **1994,** *77:*610–614.

Feigl, E.O. Neural control of coronary blood flow. *J. Vasc. Res.,* **1998,** *35:*85–92.

Goessl, C., Sauter, T., Michael, T., Berge, B., Staehler, M., and Miller, K. Efficacy and tolerability of tolterodine in children with detrusor hyperreflexia. *Urology,* **2000,** *55:*414–418.

Gomeza, J., Shannon, H., Kostenis, E., Felder, C., Zhang, L., Brodkin, J., Grinberg, A., Sheng, H., and Wess, J. Pronounced pharmacologic deficits in M_2 muscarinic acetylcholine receptor knockout mice. *Proc. Natl. Acad. Sci. U.S.A.,* **1999,** *96:*1692–1697.

Gomeza, J., Zhang, L., Kostenis, E., Felder, C., Bymaster, F., Brodkin, J., Shannon, H., Xia, B., Deng, C., and Wess, J. Enhancement of D_1 dopamine receptor-mediated locomotor stimulation in M_4 muscarinic acetylcholine receptor knockout mice. *Proc. Natl. Acad. Sci. U.S.A.,* **1999,** *96:*10483–10488.

Hamilton, S.E., Loose, M.D., Qi, M., Levey, A.I., Hille, B., McKnight, G.S., Idzerda, R.L., and Nathanson N.M. Disruption of the M_1 receptor gene ablates muscarinic receptor-dependent M current regulation and seizure activity in mice. *Proc. Natl. Acad. Sci. U.S.A.,* **1997,** *94:*13311–13316.

Hammer, R., Berrie, C.P., Birdsall, N.J., Burgen, A.S., and Hulme, E.C. Pirenzepine distinguishes between different subclasses of muscarinic receptors. *Nature,* **1980,** *283:*90–92.

Kent, K.M., and Epstein, S.E. Neural basis for the genesis and control of arrhythmias associated with myocardial infarction. *Cardiology,* **1976,** *61:*61–74.

Kent, K.M., Epstein, S.E., Cooper, T., and Jacobwitz D.M. Cholinergic innervation of the canine and human ventricular conducting system. Anatomic and electrophysiologic correlations. *Circulation,* **1974,** *50:*948–955.

Levey, A.I. Immunological localization of M1–M5 muscarinic acetylcholine receptors in peripheral tissues and brain. *Life Sci.,* **1993,** *52:*441–448.

Littner, M.R., Ilowite, J.S., Tashkin, D.P., Friedman, M., Serby, C.W., Menjoge, S.S., and Witek, T.J., Jr. Long-acting bronchodilation with once-daily dosing of tiotropium (Spiriva) in stable chronic obstructive pulmonary disease. *Am. J. Respir. Crit. Care Med.,* **2000,** *161:*1136–1142.

Matsui, M., Motomura, D., Karasawa, H., Fujikawa, T., Jiang, J., Komiya, Y., Takahashi, S., and Taketo, M.M. Multiple functional defects in peripheral autonomic organs in mice lacking muscarinic

acetylcholine receptor gene for the M_3 subtype. *Proc. Natl. Acad. Sci. U.S.A.,* **2000,** *97:*9579–9584.

Palczewski, K., Kumasaka, T., Hori, T., Behnke, C.A., Motoshima, H., Fox, B.A., Le Trong, I., Teller, D.C., Okada, T., Stenkamp, R.E., Yamamoto, M., and Miyano, M. Crystal structure of rhodopsin: A G protein–coupled receptor. *Science,* **2000,** *289:*739–745.

Richelson, E. Receptor pharmacology of neuroleptics: relation to clinical effects. *J. Clin. Psychiatry,* **1999,** *60 Suppl. 10:*5–14.

van Noord, J.A., Bantje, T.A., Eland, M.E., Korducki, L., and Cornelissen, P.J. A randomised controlled comparison of tiotropium and ipratropium in the treatment of chronic obstructive pulmonary disease. The Dutch Tiotropium Study Group. *Thorax,* **2000,** *55:*289–294.

Wellstein, A., and Pitschner, H.F. Complex dose-response curves of atropine in man explained by different functions of M_1- and M_2-cholinoceptors. *Naunyn Schmiedebergs Arch. Pharmacol.,* **1988,** *338:*19–27.

Wilkinson, J.A. Side effects of transdermal scopolamine. *J. Emerg. Med.,* **1987,** *5:*389–392.

Yasuda, R.P., Ciesla, W., Flores, L.R., Wall, S.J., Li, M., Satkus, S.A., Weisstein, J.S., Spagnola, B.V., and Wolfe, B.B. Development of antisera selective for M_4 and M_5 muscarinic cholinergic receptors: distribution of M_4 and M_5 receptors in rat brain. *Mol. Pharmacol.,* **1993,** *43:*149–157.

Ziskind, A.A. Transdermal scopolamine-induced psychosis. *Postgrad. Med.,* **1988,** *84:*73–76.

MONOGRAPHS AND REVIEWS

Abrams, P., Larsson, G., Chapple, C., and Wein, A.J. Factors involved in the success of antimuscarinic treatment. *B.J.U. Int.,* **1999,** *83* (Suppl. 2):42–47.

Anaya, J.M., and Talal, N. Sjögren's syndrome comes of age. *Semin. Arthritis Rheum.,* **1999,** *28:*355–359.

Barnes, P.J. Novel approaches and targets for treatment of chronic obstructive pulmonary disease. *Am. J. Respir. Crit. Care Med.,* **1999,** *160:*S72–S79.

Barnes, P.J. The pharmacological properties of tiotropium. *Chest,* **2000,** *117:*63S–66S.

Bebbington, A., and Brimblecombe, R.W. Muscarinic receptors in the peripheral and central nervous systems. *Adv. Drug Res.,* **1965,** *2:*143–172.

Berne, R.M., and Levy, M.N. *Cardiovascular Physiology,* 7th ed. Mosby, St. Louis, **1997.**

Birdsall, N.J.M., Buckley, N.J., Caulfield, M.P., Hammer, R., Kibinger, J.H., Lambrecht, G., Mutschler, E., Nathanson, N.M., and Schwartz, R.D. Muscarinic acetylcholine receptors. In, *The IUPHAR Compendium of Receptor Characterization and Classification.* IUPHAR Media, London **1998,** pp. 36–45.

Brodde, O.E., and Michel, M.C. Adrenergic and muscarinic receptors in the human heart. *Pharmacol. Rev.,* **1999,** *51:*651–690.

Carmine, A.A., and Brogden, R.N. Pirenzepine. A review of its pharmacodynamic and pharmacokinetic properties and therapeutic efficacy in peptic ulcer disease and other allied diseases. *Drugs,* **1985,** *30:*85–126.

Caulfield, M.P. Muscarinic receptors—characterization, coupling and function. *Pharmacol. Ther.,* **1993,** *58:*319–379.

Caulfield, M.P., and Birdsall, N.J. International Union of Pharmacology. XVII. Classification of muscarinic acetylcholine receptors. *Pharmacol. Rev.,* **1998,** *50:*279–290.

DiFrancesco, D. Pacemaker mechanisms in cardiac tissue. *Annu. Rev. Physiol.,* **1993,** *55:*455–472.

Eglen, R.M., Choppin, A., Dillon, M.P., and Hegde, S. Muscarinic receptor ligands and their therapeutic potential. *Curr. Opin. Chem. Biol.,* **1999,** *3:*426–432.

Eglen, R.M., Hedge, S.S., and Watson, N. Muscarinic receptor subtypes and smooth muscle function. *Pharmacol. Rev.,* **1996,** *48:*531–565.

Furchgott, R.F. Endothelium-derived relaxing factor: discovery, early studies, and identification as nitric oxide. *Biosci. Rep.,* **1999,** *19:*235–251.

Goldfrank, L.R. Mushrooms: toxic and hallucinogenic. In, *Goldfrank's Toxicologic Emergencies,* 6th ed. (Goldfrank, L.R., Flomenbaum, N.E., Lewin, N.A., Weisman, R.S., Howland, M.A., and Hoffman, R.S. eds.) Appleton & Lange, Stamford, CT, **1998,** pp. 1207–1220.

Goyal, R.K., and Rattan, S. Neurohumoral, hormonal, and drug receptors for the lower esophageal sphincter. *Gastroenterology,* **1978,** *74:*598–619.

Gross, N.J. Ipratropium bromide. *N. Engl. J. Med.,* **1988,** *319:*486–494.

Hegde, S.S., and Eglen, R.M. Muscarinic receptor subtypes modulating smooth muscle contractility in the urinary bladder. *Life Sci.,* **1999,** *64:*419–428.

Higgins, C.B., Vatner, S.F., and Braunwald, E. Parasympathetic control of the heart. *Pharmacol. Rev.,* **1973,** *25:*119–155.

Ignarro, L.J., Cirino, G., Casini, A., and Napoli, C. Nitric oxide as a signaling molecule in the vascular system: an overview. *J. Cardiovasc. Pharmacol.,* **1999,** *34:*879–886.

Köppel, C. Clinical sympatomatology and management of mushroom poisoning. *Toxicon,* **1993,** *31:*1513–1540.

Krnjevíc, K. Chemical nature of synaptic transmission in vertebrates. *Physiol. Rev.,* **1974,** *54:*418–540.

Levine, R., Birdsall, N.M.J., and Nathanson, N.M., eds. Proceedings of the 8th International Symposium on Subtypes of Muscarinic Receptors. Danvers, MA, August 25–29, 1998. *Life Sci.,* **1999,** *64:*355–596.

Levy, M.N., and Schwartz, P.J., eds. *Vagal Control of the Heart: Experimental Basis and Clinical Implications.* Futura, Armonk NY, **1994.**

Moncada, S., and Higgs, E.A. Molecular mechanisms and therapeutic strategies related to nitric oxide. *FASEB J.,* **1995,** *9:*1319–1330.

Nusair, S., and Rubinow, A. The use of oral pilocarpine in xerostomia and Sjogren's syndrome. *Semin. Arthritis Rheum.,* **1999,** *28:*360–367.

Somogyi, G.T., and de Groat, W.C. Function, signal transduction mechanisms and plasticity of presynaptic muscarinic receptors in the urinary bladder. *Life Sci.,* **1999,** *64:*411–418.

Tryba, M., and Cook, D. Current guidelines on stress ulcer prophylaxis. *Drugs,* **1997,** *54:*581–596.

Wein, A.J. Practical uropharmacology. *Urol. Clin. North Am.,* **1991,** *18:*269–281.

Wess, J. Molecular biology of muscarinic acetylcholine receptors. *Crit. Rev. Neurobiol.,* **1996,** *10:*69–99.

Wickman, K., and Clapham, D.E. Ion channel regulation by G proteins. *Physiol. Rev.,* **1995,** *75:*868–885.

Wiseman, L.R., and Faulds, D. Oral pilocarpine: a review of its pharmacological properties and clinical potential in xerostomia. *Drugs,* **1995,** *49:*143–155.

C H A P T E R 8

ANTICHOLINESTERASE AGENTS

Palmer Taylor

This chapter covers agents that prolong the existence of acetylcholine after it is released from cholinergic nerve terminals. These agents inhibit acetylcholinesterase, which is concentrated in synaptic regions and is responsible for the rapid catalysis of the hydrolysis of acetylcholine. Anticholinesterase agents have therapeutic utility in the treatment of glaucoma and other ophthalmologic conditions (see also Chapter 66), the facilitation of gastrointestinal and bladder motility, and influencing activity at the neuromuscular junction of skeletal muscle to enhance muscle strength in myasthenia gravis. Anticholinesterase agents that cross the blood–brain barrier have shown limited efficacy in the treatment of Alzheimer's disease (see also Chapter 22). Antidotal therapy of the toxic effects of cholinesterase inhibitors used as insecticides and chemical warfare agents is directed to blocking the effects of excessive acetylcholine stimulation and reactivating the phosphorylated, inhibited enzyme. Modification of activity at cholinergic synapses by activation or blockade of muscarinic or nicotinic acetylcholine receptors is discussed in Chapters 7 and 9, respectively.

The function of acetylcholinesterase (AChE) in terminating the action of acetylcholine (ACh) at the junctions of the various cholinergic nerve endings with their effector organs or postsynaptic sites is considered in Chapter 6. Drugs that inhibit AChE are called *anticholinesterase* (anti-ChE) *agents.* They cause ACh to accumulate in the vicinity of cholinergic nerve terminals and thus are potentially capable of producing effects equivalent to excessive stimulation of cholinergic receptors throughout the central and peripheral nervous systems. In view of the widespread distribution of cholinergic neurons, it is not surprising that the anti-ChE agents as a group have received extensive application as toxic agents, in the form of agricultural insecticides and potential chemical warfare "nerve gases." Nevertheless, several members of this class of compounds are widely used as therapeutic agents; others that cross the blood–brain barrier have been approved or are in clinical trial for the treatment of Alzheimer's disease.

Prior to World War II, only the "reversible" anti-ChE agents were generally known, of which physostigmine is the outstanding example. Shortly before and during World War II, a new class of highly toxic chemicals, the organophosphates, was developed chiefly by Schrader, of I. G. Farbenindustrie, first as agricultural insecticides and later as potential chemical warfare agents. The extreme toxicity of these compounds was found to be due to their "irreversible" inactivation of AChE, which resulted in

long-lasting inhibitory activity. Since the pharmacological actions of both classes of anti-ChE agents are qualitatively similar, they are discussed here as a group. Interactions of anti-ChE agents with other drugs acting at peripheral autonomic synapses and the neuromuscular junction are described in Chapters 7 and 9.

History. *Physostigmine*, also called *eserine*, is an alkaloid obtained from the Calabar or ordeal bean, the dried ripe seed of *Physostigma venenosum*, Balfour, a perennial plant found in tropical West Africa. The Calabar bean, also called Eséré nut, chop nut, or bean of Etu Esére, once was used by native tribes of West Africa as an "ordeal poison" in trials for witchcraft.

The Calabar bean was brought to England in 1840 by Daniell, a British medical officer, and early investigations of its pharmacological properties were conducted by Christioson (1855), Fraser (1863), and Argyll-Robertson (1863). A pure alkaloid was isolated by Jobst and Hesse in 1864 and named *physostigmine*. The first therapeutic use of the drug was in 1877 by Laqueur, in the treatment of glaucoma, one of its clinical uses today. Interesting accounts of the history of physostigmine have been presented by Karczmar (1970) and Holmstedt (1972).

As a result of the basic research of Stedman (1929a,b) and associates in elucidating the chemical basis of the activity of physostigmine, others began systematic investigations of a series of substituted aromatic esters of alkyl carbamic acids. *Neostigmine*, a promising member of this series, was introduced into therapeutics in 1931 for its stimulant action on the intestinal tract. It was reported subsequently to be effective in the symptomatic treatment of myasthenia gravis.

It is remarkable that the first account of the synthesis of a highly potent organophosphorus anti-ChE, tetraethyl pyrophosphate (TEPP), was published by Clermont in 1854. More remarkable still is the fact that the investigator survived to report on the compound's taste; a few drops should have been lethal. Modern investigations of the organophosphorus compounds date from the 1932 publication of Lange and Krueger on the synthesis of dimethyl and diethyl phosphorofluoridates. The authors' statement that inhalation of these compounds caused a persistent choking sensation and blurred vision apparently was instrumental in leading Schrader to explore this class for insecticidal activity.

Upon synthesizing approximately 2000 compounds, Schrader (1952) defined the structural requirements for insecticidal (and, as learned subsequently, for anti-ChE) activity (see below; Gallo and Lawryk, 1991). One compound in this early series, *parathion* (a phosphorothioate), later became the most widely used insecticide of this class. *Malathion,* which currently is used extensively, also contains the thionophosphorus bond found in parathion. Prior to and during World War II, the efforts of Schrader's group were directed toward the development of chemical warfare agents. The syntheses of several compounds of much greater toxicity than parathion, such as *sarin, soman,* and *tabun,* were kept secret by the German government. Investigators in the Allied countries also followed Lange and Krueger's lead in the search for potentially toxic compounds; diisopropyl phosphorofluoridate (diisopropyl fluorophosphate; DFP), synthesized by McCombie and Saunders (1946), was studied most extensively by British and American scientists.

In the 1950s, a series of aromatic carbamates was synthesized and found to have a high degree of selective toxicity against insects and to be potent anti-ChE agents (Ecobichon, 2000).

Structure of Acetylcholinesterase. AChE exists in two general classes of molecular forms: simple homomeric oligomers of catalytic subunits (*i.e.,* monomers, dimers, and tetramers) and heteromeric associations of catalytic subunits with structural subunits (Massoulie, 2000; Taylor *et al.,* 2000). The homomeric forms are found as soluble species in the cell, presumably destined for export, or associated with the outer membrane of the cell through either an intrinsic hydrophobic amino acid sequence or an attached glycophospholipid. One heterologous form, largely found in neuronal synapses, is a tetramer of catalytic subunits disulfide-linked to a 20,000-dalton lipid-linked subunit. Similar to the glycophospholipid-attached form, it is found in the outer surface of the cell membrane. The other consists of tetramers of catalytic subunits, disulfide linked to each of three strands of a collagen-like structural subunit. This molecular species, whose molecular mass approaches 10^6 daltons, is associated with the basal lamina of junctional areas of skeletal muscle.

Molecular cloning revealed that a single gene encodes vertebrate AChEs (Schumacher *et al.,* 1986; Taylor *et al.,* 2000). However, multiple gene products are found; this diversity arises from alternative processing of the mRNA. The different forms differ only in their carboxyl-termini; the portion of the gene encoding the catalytic core of the enzyme is invariant. Hence, the individual AChE species can be expected to show identical substrate and inhibitor specificities.

A separate, structurally related gene encodes butyrylcholinesterase, which is synthesized in the liver and is primarily found in plasma (Lockridge *et al.,* 1987). The cholinesterases define a superfamily of proteins whose structural motif is the α, β hydrolase fold (Cygler *et al.,* 1993). The family includes several esterases, other hydrolases not found in the nervous system, and, surprisingly, proteins without hydrolase activity such as thyroglobulin and members of the tactin and neuroligin families of proteins (Taylor *et al.,* 2000).

The three-dimensional structures of AChEs show the active center to be nearly centrosymmetric to each subunit and reside at the base of a narrow gorge about 20 Å in depth (Sussman *et al.,* 1991; Bourne *et al.,* 1995). At the base of the gorge lie the residues of the catalytic triad: serine 203, histidine 447, and glutamate 334 (Figure 8–1). The catalytic mechanism resembles that of other hydrolases, where the serine hydroxyl group is rendered highly nucleophilic through a charge-relay system involving the carboxyl from glutamate, the imidazole on the histidine, and the hydroxyl of the serine (Figure 8–2A).

During enzymatic attack of acetylcholine, an ester with trigonal geometry, a tetrahedral intermediate between enzyme and substrate is formed (Figure 8–2B) that collapses to an acetyl enzyme conjugate with the concomitant release of choline (Figure 8–2C). The acetyl enzyme is very labile to hydrolysis, which results in the formation of acetate and active enzyme (Figure 8–2D; see Froede and Wilson, 1971; Rosenberry, 1975). AChE is one of the most efficient enzymes known and has the capacity to hydrolyze 6×10^5 ACh molecules per molecule of enzyme per minute; this yields a turnover time of 150 microseconds.

Mechanism of Action of AChE Inhibitors. The mechanisms of action of compounds that typify the three classes of anti-ChE agents also are shown in Figure 8–2E to L.

Three distinct domains on AChE constitute binding sites for inhibitory ligands and form the basis for specificity differences between AChE and butyrylcholinesterase: the acyl pocket of the active center, the choline subsite of the active center, and the peripheral anionic site (Taylor and Radić, 1994; Reiner and Radić, 2000). Reversible inhibitors such as edrophonium and tacrine bind to the choline subsite in the vicinity of tryptophan 86 and glutamate 202 (Silman and Sussman, 2000) (Figure 8–2E). *Edrophonium* has a brief duration of action owing to its quaternary structure and the reversibility of its binding to the AChE active center. Additional reversible inhibitors, such as *donepezil,* bind with higher affinity to the active center.

Other reversible inhibitors, such as *propidium* and the peptide toxin *fasciculin,* bind to the peripheral anionic site on AChE. This site resides at the lip of the gorge and is defined by tryptophan 286 and tyrosines 72 and 124 (Figure 8–1).

Drugs that have a carbamoyl ester linkage, such as physostigmine and neostigmine, are hydrolyzed by AChE, but much more slowly than is ACh. Both the quaternary amine neostigmine and the tertiary amine physostigmine exist as cations at physiological pH. By serving as alternate substrates with a similar binding orientation as acetylcholine (*see* Figure 8–2F, G), attack by the active center serine gives rise to the carbamoylated

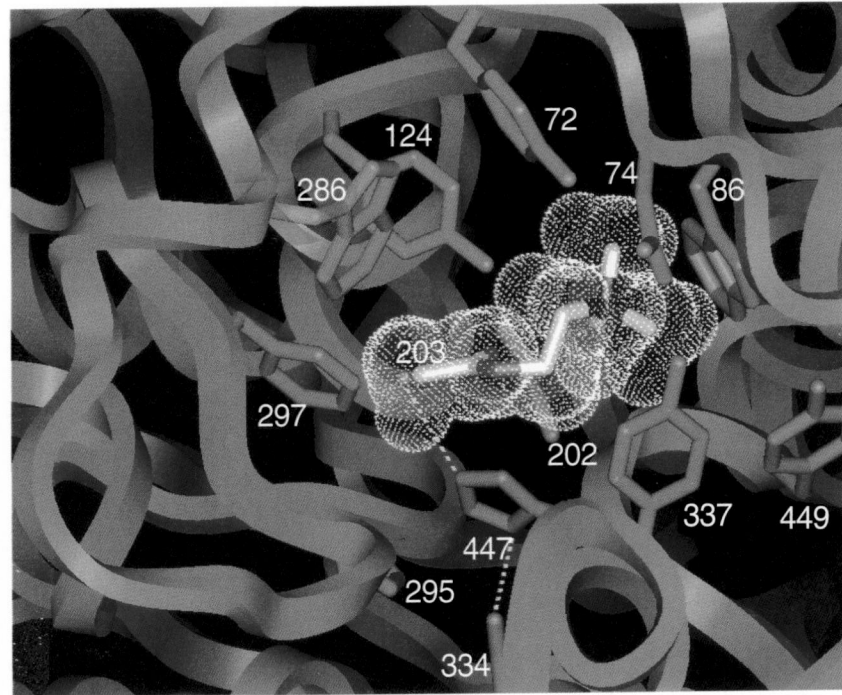

Figure 8–1. The active center gorge of mammalian acetylcholinesterase.

Bound acetylcholine is shown by the dotted structure depicting its van der Waals radii. The crystal structure of mouse cholinesterase active center is shown (Bourne *et al.*, 1995). Included are the side chains of (a) the catalytic triad, Glu_{334}, His_{447}, Ser_{203} (hydrogen bonds are denoted by the dotted lines); (b) acyl pocket, Phe_{295} and Phe_{297}; (c) choline subsite, Trp_{86}, Glu_{202}, and Tyr_{337}; and (d) the peripheral site: Trp_{286}, Tyr_{72}, Tyr_{124}, and Asp_{74}. Tyrosines 337 and 449 are further removed from the active center but likely contribute to stabilization of certain ligands. The catalytic triad, choline subsite, and acyl pocket are located at the base of the gorge, while the peripheral site is at the lip of the gorge. The gorge is 18 to 20 Å deep, with its base centrosymmetric to the subunit.

enzyme. The carbamoyl moiety resides in the acyl pocket outlined by phenylalanines 295 and 297. In contrast to the acetyl enzyme, methylcarbamoyl AChE and dimethylcarbamoyl AChE are far more stable ($t_{1/2}$ for hydrolysis of the dimethylcarbamoyl enzyme is 15 to 30 minutes; *see* Figure 8–2*H*). Sequestration of the enzyme in its carbamoylated form thus precludes the enzyme-catalyzed hydrolysis of ACh for extended periods of time. *In vivo,* the duration of inhibition by the carbamoylating agents is 3 to 4 hours.

The organophosphorus inhibitors, such as *diisopropyl fluorophosphate* (DFP), serve as true hemisubstrates, since the resultant conjugate with the active center serine phosphorylated or phosphonylated is extremely stable (*see* Figure 8–2*I, J, K*). The organophosphorus inhibitors are tetrahedral in configuration, a configuration that resembles the transition state formed in carboxyl ester hydrolysis. Similar to the carboxyl esters, the phosphoryl oxygen binds within the oxyanion hole of the active center. If the alkyl groups in the phosphorylated enzyme are ethyl or methyl, spontaneous regeneration of active enzyme requires several hours. Secondary (as in DFP) or tertiary alkyl groups further enhance the stability of the phosphorylated enzyme, and significant regeneration of active enzyme usually is not observed. Hence, the return of AChE activity depends on synthesis of new enzyme. The stability of the phosphorylated enzyme is enhanced through "aging," which results from the loss of one of the alkyl groups (*see* Figure 8–2*K*; *see also* Aldridge, 1976).

From the foregoing account, it is apparent that the terms *reversible* and *irreversible* as applied to the car-

bamoyl ester and organophosphorus anti-ChE agents, respectively, reflect only quantitative differences in rates of deacylation of the acyl enzyme. Both chemical classes react covalently with the enzyme in essentially the same manner as does ACh.

Action at Effector Organs. The characteristic pharmacological effects of the anti-ChE agents are due primarily to the prevention of hydrolysis of ACh by AChE at sites of cholinergic transmission. Transmitter thus accumulates, and the response to ACh that is liberated by cholinergic impulses or that is spontaneously released from the nerve ending is enhanced. Virtually all the acute effects of moderate doses of organophosphates are attributable to this action. For example, the characteristic miosis that follows local application of DFP to the eye is not observed after chronic postganglionic denervation of the eye because there is no source from which to release endogenous ACh. The consequences of enhanced concentrations of ACh at motor end-plates are unique to these sites and are discussed below.

The tertiary amine and particularly the quaternary ammonium anti-ChE compounds all may have additional direct actions at certain cholinergic receptor sites. For example, the effects of neostigmine on the spinal cord and neuromuscular junction are based on a combination of its anti-ChE activity and direct cholinergic stimulation.

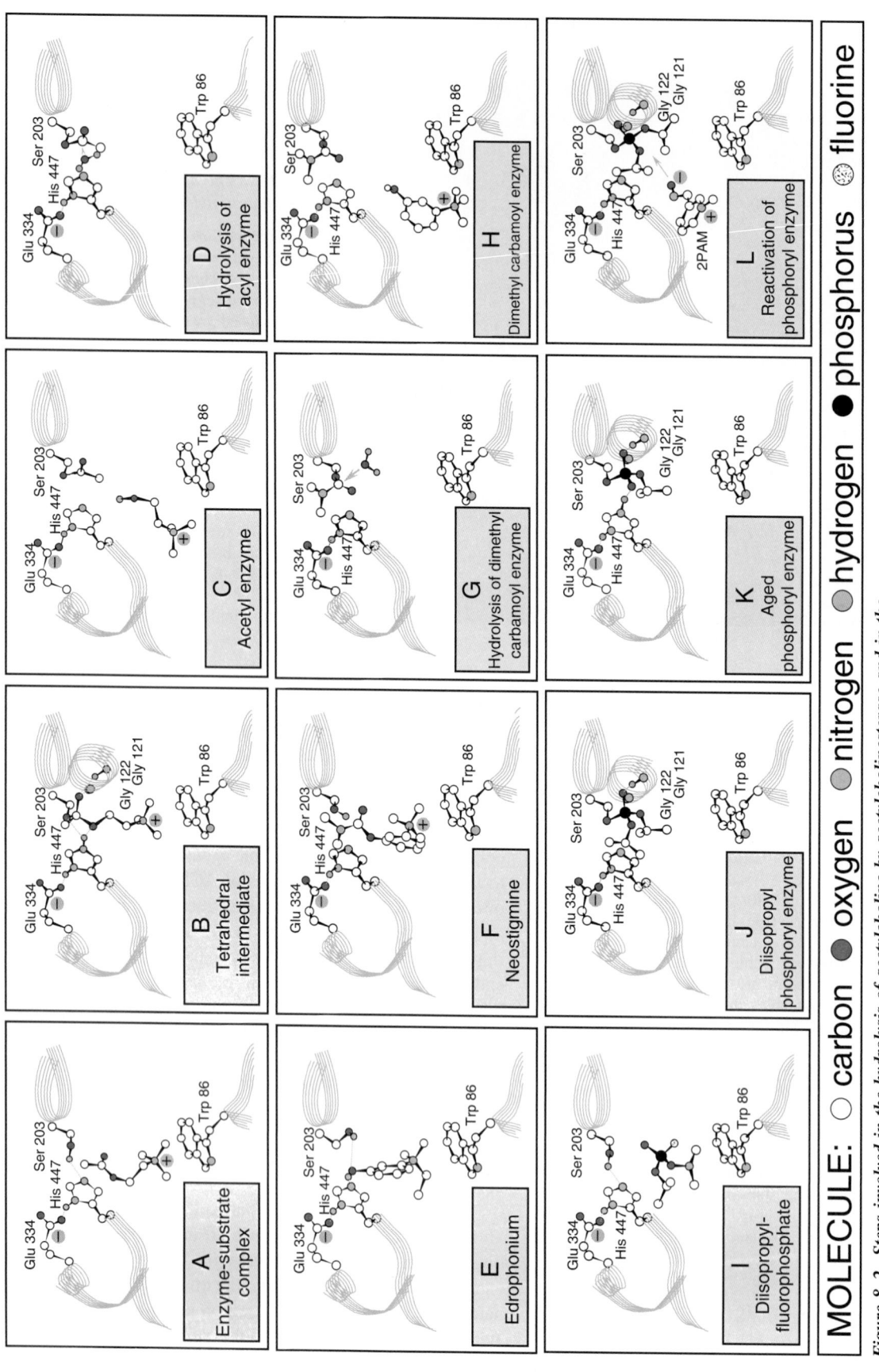

MOLECULE: ○ carbon ● oxygen ○ nitrogen ○ hydrogen ● phosphorus ⊕ fluorine

Figure 8–2. Steps involved in the hydrolysis of acetylcholine by acetylcholinesterase and in the inhibition and reactivation of the enzyme.

The steps shown are as follows: *A.* Binding of substrate acetylcholine. *B.* Attack by the serine hydroxyl with formation of the transient tetrahedral intermediate. *C.* Loss of choline and formation of the acetyl enzyme. *D.* Deacylation of the enzyme by attack with H_2O. *E.* Binding of the reversible inhibitor edrophonium to the active site. *F.* Binding of neostigmine. *G.* Formation of the carbamoylated enzyme. *I.* Binding of diisopropyl fluorophosphate. *J.* Formation *H.* Hydrolysis of the carbamoylated enzyme. *I.* Binding of diisopropyl fluorophosphate. *J.* Formation

178

Chemistry and Structure–Activity Relationships. The structure–activity relationships of anti-ChE drugs have been reviewed extensively (*see* previous editions of this book). Only those agents of general therapeutic or toxicological interest are considered here.

Noncovalent Inhibitors. While drugs of this class interact by reversible and noncovalent association with the active site in AChE, they differ in their disposition in the body and their affinity for the enzyme. *Edrophonium,* a quaternary drug whose activity is limited to peripheral nervous system synapses, has a moderate affinity for AChE. Its volume of distribution is limited and renal elimination is rapid, accounting for its short duration of action. By contrast, *tacrine* and *donepezil* have higher affinities for AChE, are more hydrophobic, and readily cross the blood–brain barrier to inhibit AChE in the central nervous system (CNS). Their partitioning into lipid and their higher affinities for AChE account for their longer durations of action.

"Reversible" Carbamate Inhibitors. Drugs of this class that are of therapeutic interest are shown in Figure 8–3. Stedman's early studies (1929a,b) showed that the essential moiety of the physostigmine molecule was the methyl carbamate of a basically substituted simple phenol. The quaternary ammonium derivative neostigmine is a compound of greater stability and equal or greater potency. *Pyridostigmine* is a close congener that also is employed in the treatment of myasthenia gravis.

An increase in anti-ChE potency and duration of action can result from the linking of two quaternary ammonium moieties. One such example is the miotic agent *demecarium,* which essentially consists of two neostigmine molecules connected by a series of ten methylene groups. The second quaternary group confers additional stability to the interaction by associating with a negatively charged amino side chain, Asp74, near the lip of the gorge. Carbamoylating inhibitors with high lipid solubilities readily cross the blood–brain barrier and have longer durations of action. Such agents (*rivastigmine*) have been approved by the United States Food and Drug Administration (FDA) for the treatment of Alzheimer's disease (Giacobini, 2000; Corey-Bloom *et al.,* 1998; *see* Chapter 22).

The carbamate insecticides, *carbaryl* (SEVIN), *propoxur* (BAYGON), and *aldicarb* (TEMIK), which are used extensively in garden products, inhibit ChE in a fashion identical with other carbamoylating inhibitors. The symptoms of poisoning closely resemble those of the organophosphates (Baron, 1991; Ecobichon, 2000). Carbaryl has a particularly low toxicity from dermal absorption. It is used topically for control of head lice in some countries. Not all carbamates in garden formulations are cholinesterase inhibitors; the dithiocarbamates are fungicidal.

Organophosphorus Compounds. The general formula for this class of cholinesterase inhibitors is presented in Table 8–1. A great variety of substituents is possible: R_1 and R_2 may be alkyl, alkoxy, aryloxy, amido, mercaptan, or other groups, and X, the leaving group, a conjugate base of a weak acid, is found as a halide, cyanide, thiocyanate, phenoxy, thiophenoxy, phosphate, thiocholine, or carboxylate group. For a compilation of the organophosphorus compounds and their toxicity, *see* Gallo and Lawryk (1991).

DFP produces virtually irreversible inactivation of AChE and other esterases by alkylphosphorylation. Its high lipid solubility, low molecular weight, and volatility facilitate inhalation, transdermal absorption, and penetration into the CNS.

The "nerve gases"—tabun, sarin, and soman—are among the most potent synthetic toxic agents known; they are lethal to laboratory animals in submilligram doses. Insidious employment of these agents has occurred in warfare and terrorism attacks (Nozaki and Aikawa, 1995).

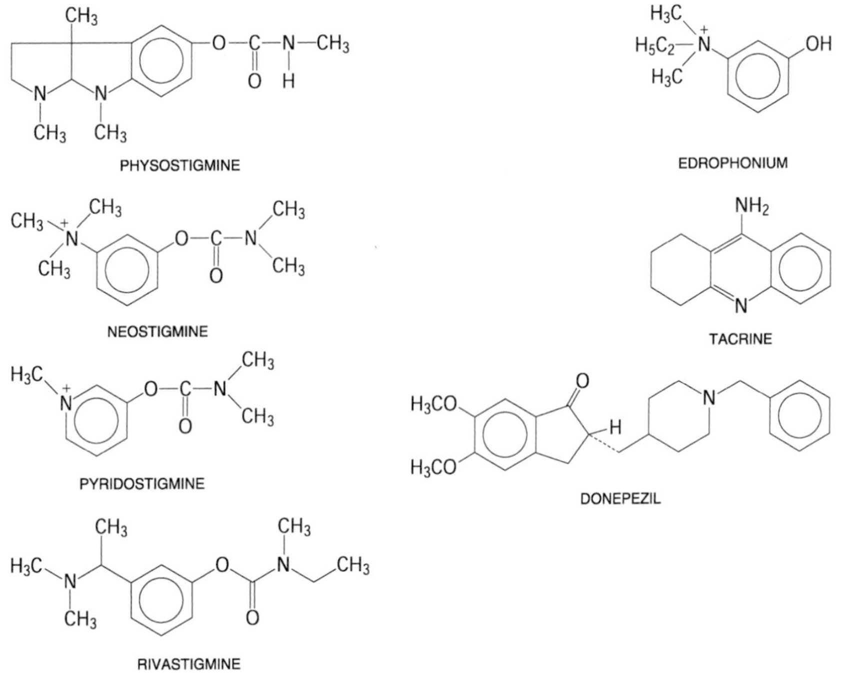

Figure 8–3. Representative "reversible" anticholinesterase agents employed clinically.

Table 8–1

Chemical Classification of Representative Organophosphorus Compounds of Particular Pharmacological or Toxicological Interest

General formula (Schrader, 1952):

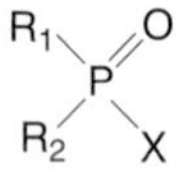

Group A, X = halogen, cyanide, or thiocyanate leaving group; group B, X = alkylthio, arylthio, alkoxy, or aryloxy leaving group; group C, thionophosphorus or thio-thionophosphorus compounds; group D, pyrophosphates and similar compounds; group E, quaternary ammonium leaving group

GROUP	STRUCTURAL FORMULA	COMMON, CHEMICAL, AND OTHER NAMES	COMMENTS
A	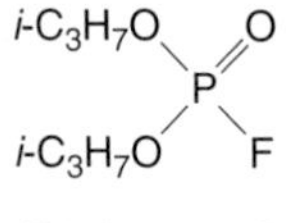	DFP; Isoflurophate; diisopropyl fluorophosphate	Potent, irreversible inactivator
	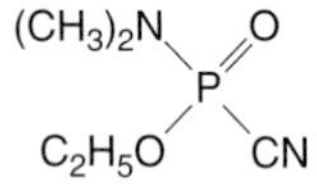	Tabun Ethyl N-dimethylphosphoramido-cyanidate	Extremely toxic "nerve gas"
	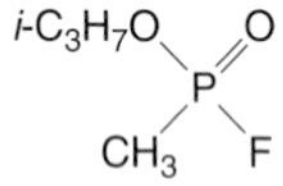	Sarin (GB) Isopropyl methylphosphonofluoridate	Extremely toxic "nerve gas"
	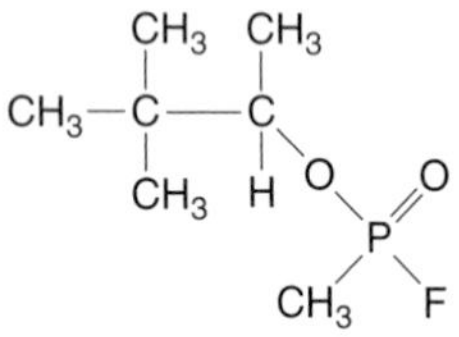	Soman Pinacolyl methylphosphonofluoridate	Extremely toxic "nerve gas"
B	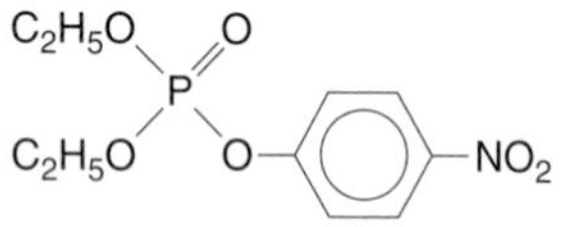	Paraoxon (MINTACOL), E 600 O,O-Diethyl O-(4-nitrophenyl)-phosphate	Active metabolite of parathion
	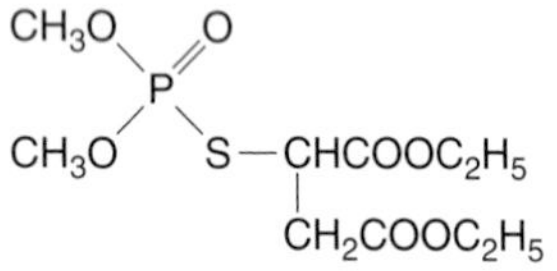	Malaoxon O,O-Dimethyl S-(1,2-dicarboxyethyl)-phosphorothioate	Active metabolite of malathion
C	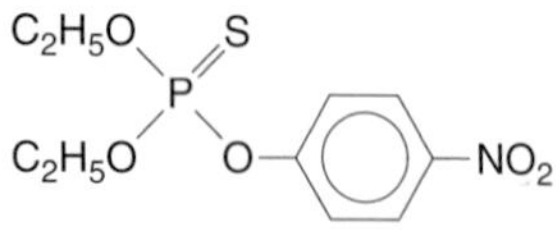	Parathion O,O-Diethyl O-(4-nitrophenyl)-phosphorothioate	Employed as agricultural insecticide, resulting in numerous cases of accidental poisoning. Will be phased out of agricultural use by October, 2003.
	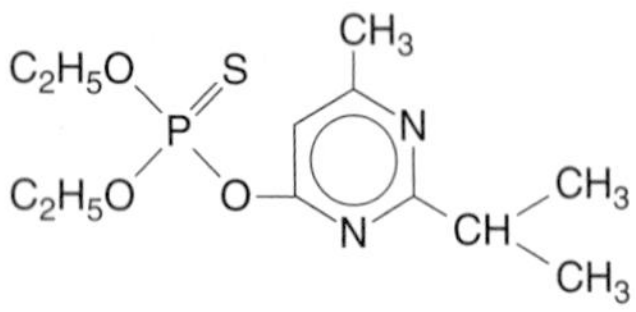	Diazinon, Dimpylate O,O-Diethyl O-(2-isopropyl-6-methyl-4-pyrimidinyl) phosphorothioate	Insecticide in wide use for gardening and agriculture. Now banned for indoor use and being phased out of all outdoor use by 2005
	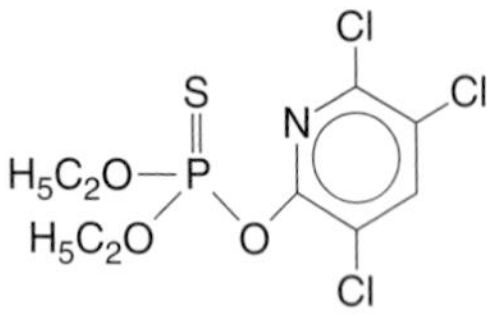	Chlorpyrifos O,O-Diethyl O-(3,5,6-trichloro-2-pyridyl) phosphorothioate	Insecticide with restricted use in consumer products and limited to nonresidential settings

Table 8–1

Chemical Classification of Representative Organophosphorus Compounds of Particular Pharmacological or Toxicological Interest (*Continued*)

General formula (Schrader, 1952):

$$R_1 \diagdown \underset{R_2 \diagup}{\overset{\displaystyle O}{\underset{\displaystyle X}{P}}}$$

Group A, X = halogen, cyanide, or thiocyanate leaving group; group B, X = alkylthio, arylthio, alkoxy, or aryloxy leaving group; group C, thionophosphorus or thio-thionophosphorus compounds; group D, pyrophosphates and similar compounds; group E, quaternary ammonium leaving group

GROUP	STRUCTURAL FORMULA	COMMON, CHEMICAL, AND OTHER NAMES	COMMENTS
	CH_3O S ; CH_3O S—$CHCOOC_2H_5$; $CH_2COOC_2H_5$ (P)	Malathion *O,O*-Dimethyl *S*-(1,2-dicarbethoxy-ethyl) phosphorodithioate	Widely employed insecticide of greater safety than parathion or other agents because of rapid detoxification by higher organisms
D	C_2H_5O O O OC_2H_5 ; C_2H_5O P—O—P OC_2H_5	TEPP Tetraethyl pyrophosphate	Early insecticide
E	C_2H_5O O I^- ; C_2H_5O P $SCH_2CH_3N(CH_3)_3$	Echothiophate (PHOSPHOLINE IODIDE), MI-217 Diethoxyphosphinylthiocholine iodide	Extremely potent choline derivative; employed in treatment of glaucoma; relatively stable in aqueous solution

Because of its low volatility and stability in aqueous solution, parathion (ETILON) became widely used as an insecticide. Its acute and chronic toxicity has limited its agricultural use in the United States and other countries; potentially less hazardous compounds have replaced parathion for home and garden use. Parathion itself is inactive in inhibiting AChE *in vitro; paraoxon* is the active metabolite. The sulfur-for-oxygen substitution is carried out predominantly in the liver by the mixed-function oxidases. This reaction also is carried out in the insect, typically with more efficiency. Parathion probably has been responsible for more cases of accidental poisoning and death than any other organophosphorus compound. The dimethyl congener, methyl parathion, has been put on restricted use limited to non-residential settings. Other insecticides possessing the phosphorothioate structure have been widely employed for home, garden, and agricultural use. These include *diazinon* (SPECTRACIDE, others) and *chlorpyrifos* (DURSBAN, LORSBAN). Chlorpyrifos recently has been placed under restricted use because of evidence of chronic toxicity in the newborn animal. For the same reason, diazinon was banned for indoor use in the United States in 2001 and will be phased out of all outdoor use by 2005.

Malathion (CHEMATHION, MALA-SPRAY) also requires replacement of a sulfur atom with oxygen *in vivo*. This insecticide can be detoxified by hydrolysis of the carboxyl ester linkage by plasma carboxylesterases, and plasma carboxylesterase activity dictates species resistance to malathion. The detoxification reaction is much more rapid in mammals and birds than in insects (*see* Costa *et al.,* 1987). In recent years, malathion has been employed in aerial spraying of relatively populous areas

for control of citrus-orchard-destructive Mediterranean fruit flies and mosquitoes that harbor and transmit viruses harmful to human beings, such as the West Nile encephalitis virus. Evidence of acute toxicity arises only with suicide attempts or deliberate poisoning (Bardin *et al.,* 1994). The lethal dose in mammals is about 1 g/kg. Exposure to the skin results in a small fraction (<10%) of systemic absorption. Malathion is used in the treatment of pediculosis (lice infestations; *see* Chapter 65).

Among the quaternary ammonium organophosphorus compounds (group E in Table 8–1), only *echothiophate* is useful clinically and is limited to ophthalmic administration. Being positively charged, it is not volatile and does not readily penetrate the skin.

Metrifonate is a low-molecular-weight organophosphate that is spontaneously converted to the active phosphoryl ester: dimethyl 2,2-dichlorovinyl phosphate (*DDVP, dichlorvos*). Both metrifonate and DDVP readily cross the blood–brain barrier to inhibit AChE in the CNS. Metrifonate originally was developed for the treatment of schistosomiasis (*see* Chapter 42). Its capacity to inhibit AChE in the CNS and its reported low toxicity led to its clinical trial in Alzheimer's disease (Cummings *et al.,* 1999).

PHARMACOLOGICAL PROPERTIES

Generally, the pharmacological properties of anti-ChE agents can be predicted by knowing those loci where ACh is released physiologically by nerve impulses, the degree of nerve impulse activity, and the responses of the corresponding effector organs to ACh (*see* Chapter 6). The anti-ChE agents potentially can produce all the following effects: (1) stimulation of muscarinic receptor responses at autonomic effector organs; (2) stimulation, followed by depression or paralysis, of all autonomic ganglia and skeletal muscle (nicotinic actions); and (3) stimulation, with occasional subsequent depression, of cholinergic receptor sites in the CNS. Following toxic or lethal doses of anti-ChE agents, most of these effects can be noted (*see* below). However, with smaller doses, particularly those used therapeutically, several modifying factors are significant. In general, compounds containing a quaternary ammonium group do not penetrate cell membranes readily; hence, anti-ChE agents in this category are absorbed poorly from the gastrointestinal tract or across the skin and are excluded from the CNS by the blood–brain barrier after moderate doses. On the other hand, such compounds act preferentially at the neuromuscular junctions of skeletal muscle, exerting their action both as anti-ChE agents and as direct agonists. They have comparatively less effect at autonomic effector sites and ganglia. In contrast, the more lipid-soluble agents are well absorbed after oral administration, have ubiquitous effects at both peripheral and central cholinergic sites, and may be sequestered in lipids for long periods of time. The lipid-soluble organophosphorus agents also are well absorbed through the skin, and the volatile agents are transferred readily across the alveolar membrane (Storm *et al.,* 2000).

The actions of anti-ChE agents on autonomic effector cells and on cortical and subcortical sites in the CNS, where the receptors are largely of the muscarinic type, are blocked by *atropine*. Likewise, atropine blocks some of the excitatory actions of anti-ChE agents on autonomic ganglia, since both nicotinic and muscarinic receptors are involved in ganglionic neurotransmission (*see* Chapter 9).

The sites of action of anti-ChE agents of therapeutic importance are the CNS, eye, intestine, and the neuromuscular junction of skeletal muscle; other actions are of toxicological consequence.

Eye. When applied locally to the conjunctiva, anti-ChE agents cause conjunctival hyperemia and constriction of the sphincter pupillae muscle around the pupillary margin of the iris (miosis) and the ciliary muscle (block of accommodation reflex with resultant focusing to near vision). Miosis is apparent in a few minutes and can last several hours to days. Although the pupil may be "pinpoint" in size, it generally contracts further when exposed to light. The block of accommodation is more transient and

generally disappears before termination of the miosis. Intraocular pressure, when elevated, usually falls as the result of facilitation of outflow of the aqueous humor (*see* Chapter 66).

Gastrointestinal Tract. In human beings, neostigmine enhances gastric contractions and increases the secretion of gastric acid. After bilateral vagotomy, the effects of neostigmine on gastric motility are greatly reduced. The lower portion of the esophagus is stimulated by neostigmine; in patients with marked achalasia and dilation of the esophagus, the drug can cause a salutary increase in tone and peristalsis.

Neostigmine augments the motor activity of the small and large bowel; the colon is particularly stimulated. Atony produced by muscarinic-receptor antagonists or prior surgical intervention may be overcome, propulsive waves are increased in amplitude and frequency, and movement of intestinal contents is thus promoted. The total effect of anti-ChE agents on intestinal motility probably represents a combination of actions at the ganglion cells of Auerbach's plexus and at the smooth muscle fibers, as a result of the preservation of ACh released by the cholinergic preganglionic and postganglionic fibers, respectively.

Neuromuscular Junction. Most of the effects of potent anti-ChE drugs on skeletal muscle can be explained adequately on the basis of their inhibition of AChE at neuromuscular junctions. However, there is good evidence for an accessory direct action of neostigmine and other quaternary ammonium anti-ChE agents on skeletal muscle. For example, the intraarterial injection of neostigmine into chronically denervated muscle, or muscle in which AChE has been inactivated by prior administration of DFP, evokes an immediate contraction, whereas physostigmine does not.

Normally, a single nerve impulse in a terminal motor-axon branch liberates enough ACh to produce a localized depolarization (end-plate potential) of sufficient magnitude to initiate a propagated muscle action potential. The ACh released is rapidly hydrolyzed by AChE, such that the lifetime of free ACh within the synapse ($\sim$200 microseconds) is shorter than the decay of the end-plate potential or the refractory period of the muscle. Therefore, each nerve impulse gives rise to a single wave of depolarization. After inhibition of AChE, the residence time of ACh in the synapse increases, allowing for rebinding of transmitter to multiple receptors. Successive stimulation by diffusion to neighboring receptors in the end plate results in a prolongation of the decay time of the end-plate potential. Quanta released by individual nerve impulses are no longer isolated. This action destroys the synchrony between end-plate depolarizations and the development of the action potentials. Consequently, asynchronous excitation and fibrillation of muscle fibers are observed. With sufficient inhibition of AChE, depolarization of the end-plate predominates, and blockade owing to depolarization ensues (*see* Chapter 9). When ACh persists in the synapse, it also may depolarize the axon terminal, resulting in antidromic firing of the motoneuron; this effect contributes to fasciculations, which involve the entire motor unit.

The anti-ChE agents will reverse the antagonism caused by competitive neuromuscular blocking agents (*see* Chapter 9). Neostigmine normally is not effective against the skeletal muscle paralysis caused by succinylcholine, since this agent also produces neuromuscular blockade by depolarization.

Actions at Other Sites. Secretory glands that are innervated by postganglionic cholinergic fibers include the bronchial, lacrimal, sweat, salivary, gastric (antral G cells and parietal cells), intestinal, and pancreatic acinar glands. Low doses of anti-ChE agents augment secretory responses to nerve stimulation, and higher doses actually produce an increase in the resting rate of secretion.

Anti-ChE agents increase contraction of smooth muscle fibers of the bronchioles and ureters, and the ureters may show increased peristaltic activity.

The cardiovascular actions of anti-ChE agents are complex, since they reflect both ganglionic and postganglionic effects of accumulated ACh on the heart and blood vessels. The predominant effect on the heart from the peripheral action of accumulated ACh is bradycardia, resulting in a fall in cardiac output. Higher doses usually cause a fall in blood pressure, often as a consequence of effects of anti-ChE agents on the medullary vasomotor centers of the CNS.

Anti-ChE agents augment vagal influences on the heart. This shortens the effective refractory period of atrial muscle fibers, and increases the refractory period and conduction time at the SA and AV nodes. At the ganglionic level, accumulating ACh initially is excitatory on nicotinic receptors, but at higher concentrations, ganglionic blockade ensues as a result of persistent depolarization of the cell membrane. The excitatory action on the parasympathetic ganglion cells would tend to reinforce the diminished cardiac output, whereas the opposite sequence would result from the action of ACh on sympathetic ganglion cells. Excitation followed by inhibition also is elicited by ACh at the medullary vasomotor and cardiac centers. All of these effects are complicated further by the hypoxemia resulting from the bronchoconstrictor and secretory actions of increased ACh on the respiratory system; hypoxemia, in turn, would reinforce both sympathetic tone and ACh-induced discharge of epinephrine from the adrenal medulla. Hence, it is

not surprising that an increase in heart rate is seen with severe cholinesterase inhibitor poisoning. Hypoxemia probably is a major factor in CNS depression that appears after large doses of anti-ChE agents. The CNS-stimulant effects are antagonized by atropine, although not as completely as are the muscarinic effects at peripheral autonomic effector sites.

Absorption, Fate, and Excretion. Physostigmine is absorbed readily from the gastrointestinal tract, subcutaneous tissues, and mucous membranes. The conjunctival instillation of solutions of the drug may result in systemic effects if measures (*e.g.,* pressure on inner canthus) are not taken to prevent absorption from the nasal mucosa. Physostigmine, administered parenterally, is largely destroyed in the body within 2 hours, mainly by hydrolytic cleavage by plasma esterases; renal excretion plays only a minor role in its elimination.

Neostigmine and pyridostigmine are absorbed poorly after oral administration, such that much larger doses are needed than by the parenteral route. Whereas the effective parenteral dose of neostigmine is 0.5 to 2 mg, the equivalent oral dose may be 15 to 30 mg or more. Neostigmine and pyridostigmine are destroyed by plasma esterases, and the quaternary alcohols and parent compounds are excreted in the urine; the half-life of these drugs is only 1 to 2 hours (Cohan *et al.,* 1976).

Organophosphorus anti-ChE agents with the highest risk of toxicity are highly lipid-soluble liquids; many have high vapor pressures. The less volatile agents that are commonly used as agricultural insecticides (*e.g.,* parathion, malathion) generally are dispersed as aerosols or as dusts adsorbed to an inert, finely particulate material. Consequently, the compounds are absorbed rapidly through the skin and mucous membranes following contact with moisture, by the lungs after inhalation, and by the gastrointestinal tract after ingestion (Storm *et al.,* 2000).

Following their absorption, most organophosphorus compounds are excreted almost entirely as hydrolysis products in the urine. Plasma and liver esterases are responsible for hydrolysis to the corresponding phosphoric and phosphonic acids. However, the cytochrome P450s are responsible for converting the inactive phosphorothioates containing a phosphorus-sulfur (thiono) bond to phosphorates with a phosphorus-oxygen bond, resulting in their activation. These mixed-function oxidases also play a role in deactivation of certain organophosphorus agents.

The organophosphorus anti-ChE agents are hydrolyzed in the body by two families of enzymes known as the carboxylesterases and the paraoxonases (A-esterases). These enzymes are found in the plasma and liver and scavenge or hydrolyze a large number of organophosphorus compounds (paraoxon, DFP,

TEPP, chlorpyrifos, oxon, tabun, sarin) by cleaving the phospho-ester, anhydride, PF, or PCN bonds. The paraoxonases are metal-loenzymes not related in structure to the cholinesterases and do not appear to form stable intermediates with organophosphates. They are associated with high-density lipoproteins and may prevent oxidation of endogenous lipids (La Du *et al.*, 1999). A genetic polymorphism (Arg192Gln) that governs organophosphate substrate specificity has been found (Furlong *et al.*, 2000). Wide variations in paraoxonase activity exist among animal species. Young animals are deficient in carboxylesterases and paraoxonases, and this may account for age-related toxicities seen in newborn animals and suspected to be a basis for toxicity in human beings (Padilla *et al.*, 2000).

In addition, plasma and hepatic carboxylesterases (aliesterases) and plasma butyrylcholinesterase are inhibited irreversibly by organophosphorus compounds (Lockridge and Masson, 2000); their scavenging capacity for the organophosphates can afford partial protection against inhibition of acetylcholinesterase in the nervous system. The carboxylesterases also catalyze hydrolysis of malathion and other organophosphorus compounds that contain carboxyl-ester linkages, rendering them less active or inactive. Since carboxylesterases are inhibited by organophosphates, toxicity from exposure to two organophosphorus insecticides can be synergistic.

TOXICOLOGY

The toxicological aspects of the anti-ChE agents are of practical importance to the physician. In addition to numerous cases of accidental intoxication from the use and manufacture of organophosphorus compounds as agricultural insecticides (over 40 have been approved for use in the United States), these agents have been used frequently for homicidal and suicidal purposes, largely because of their accessibility. Organophosphorus agents account for as much as 80% of pesticide-related hospital admissions. The World Health Organization documents pesticide toxicity as a widespread global problem; most poisonings occur in developing countries (Bardin *et al.*, 1994; Landrigan *et al.*, 2000). Occupational exposure occurs most commonly by the dermal and pulmonary routes, while oral ingestion is most common in cases of nonoccupational poisoning.

In the United States, the Environmental Protection Agency (EPA), by virtue of revised risk assessments and the Food Quality Protection Act of 1996, has placed several organophosphate insecticides on restricted use or phase-out status in consumer products for home and garden use. A primary concern relates to children, since the developing nervous system may be particularly susceptible to certain of these agents. The Office of Pesticide Programs of the EPA provides continuous reviews of the status of organophosphate pesticides, their tolerance reassessments, and revisions of risk assessments through

their web site (www.epa.gov/pesticides/op/). Public comment is sought prior to decisions on revisions.

Acute Intoxication. The effects of acute intoxication by anti-ChE agents are manifested by muscarinic and nicotinic signs and symptoms and, except for compounds of extremely low lipid solubility, by signs referable to the CNS. Systemic effects appear within minutes after inhalation of vapors or aerosols. In contrast, the onset of symptoms is delayed after gastrointestinal and percutaneous absorption. The duration of effects is determined largely by the properties of the compound: its lipid solubility, whether or not it must be activated to form the oxon, the stability of the organophosphorus-AChE bond, and whether or not "aging" of the phosphorylated enzyme has occurred.

After local exposure to vapors or aerosols or after their inhalation, ocular and respiratory effects generally appear first. Ocular effects include marked miosis, ocular pain, conjunctival congestion, diminished vision, ciliary spasm, and brow ache. With acute systemic absorption, miosis may not be evident due to sympathetic discharge in response to hypotension. In addition to rhinorrhea and hyperemia of the upper respiratory tract, respiratory effects consist of "tightness" in the chest and wheezing respiration, caused by the combination of bronchoconstriction and increased bronchial secretion. Gastrointestinal symptoms occur earliest after ingestion, and include anorexia, nausea and vomiting, abdominal cramps, and diarrhea. With percutaneous absorption of liquid, localized sweating and muscle fasciculations in the immediate vicinity are generally the earliest manifestations. Severe intoxication is manifested by extreme salivation, involuntary defecation and urination, sweating, lacrimation, penile erection, bradycardia, and hypotension.

Nicotinic actions at the neuromuscular junctions of skeletal muscle usually consist of fatigability and generalized weakness, involuntary twitchings, scattered fasciculations, and eventually severe weakness and paralysis. The most serious consequence is paralysis of the respiratory muscles.

The broad spectrum of effects on the CNS includes confusion, ataxia, slurred speech, loss of reflexes, Cheyne–Stokes respiration, generalized convulsions, coma, and central respiratory paralysis. Actions on the vasomotor and other cardiovascular centers in the medulla oblongata lead to hypotension.

The time of death after a single acute exposure may range from less than 5 minutes to nearly 24 hours, depending upon the dose, route, agent, and other factors. The cause of death primarily is respiratory failure, usually accompanied by a secondary cardiovascular component. Peripheral muscarinic and nicotinic as well as central actions all contribute to respiratory embarrassment; effects include laryngospasm, bronchoconstriction, increased tracheobronchial and salivary secretions, compromised voluntary control of the diaphragm and intercostal muscles, and central respiratory depression. Blood pressure may fall to alarmingly low levels and cardiac irregularities intervene. These effects usually result from hypoxemia; they often are reversed by assisted pulmonary ventilation.

Delayed symptoms appearing after one to four days and marked by persistent low blood cholinesterase and severe muscle weakness are termed the *intermediate syndrome* (Marrs, 1993; DeBleecker *et al.*, 1992, 1995). A delayed neurotoxicity also may be evident after severe intoxication (*see* below).

Diagnosis and Treatment. The diagnosis of severe, acute anti-ChE intoxication is made readily from the history of exposure and the characteristic signs and symptoms. In suspected cases of milder acute or chronic intoxication, determination of the ChE activities in erythrocytes and plasma generally will establish the diagnosis (Storm *et al.*, 2000). Although these values vary considerably in the normal population, they usually will be depressed well below the normal range before symptoms are evident.

Treatment is both specific and effective. Atropine in sufficient dosage (*see* below) effectively antagonizes the actions at muscarinic receptor sites, including increased tracheobronchial and salivary secretion, bronchoconstriction, bradycardia, and, to a moderate extent, peripheral ganglionic and central actions. Larger doses are required to get appreciable concentrations of atropine into the CNS. Atropine is virtually without effect against the peripheral neuromuscular compromise. The last-mentioned action of the anti-ChE agents as well as all other peripheral effects can be reversed by *pralidoxime* (2-PAM), a cholinesterase reactivator.

In moderate or severe intoxication with an organophosphorus anti-ChE agent, the recommended adult dose of pralidoxime is 1 to 2 g, infused intravenously within not less than 5 minutes. If weakness is not relieved or if it recurs after 20 to 60 minutes, the dose may be repeated. Early treatment is very important to assure that the oxime reaches the phosphorylated AChE while the latter still can be reactivated. Many of the alkylphosphates are extremely lipid-soluble, and if extensive partitioning into body fat has occurred, toxicity will persist and symptoms may recur after initial treatment. In some cases it has been necessary to continue treatment with atropine and pralidoxime for several weeks.

In addition, general supportive measures are important. These include (1) termination of exposure, by removal of the patient or application of a gas mask if the atmosphere remains contaminated, removal and destruction of contaminated clothing, copious washing of contaminated skin or mucous membranes with water, or gastric lavage; (2) maintenance of a patent airway, including endobronchial aspiration; (3) artificial respiration if required; (4) administration of oxygen; (5) alleviation of persistent convulsions with diazepam (5 to 10 mg, intravenously); and (6) treatment of shock (Marrs, 1993; Bardin *et al.*, 1994).

Atropine should be given in doses sufficient to cross the blood–brain barrier. Following an initial injection of 2 to 4 mg, given intravenously if possible, otherwise intramuscularly, 2 mg should be given every 5 to 10 minutes until muscarinic symptoms disappear, if they reappear, or until signs of atropine toxicity appear. More than 200 mg may be required on the first day. A mild degree of atropine block then should be maintained for up to 48 hours or as long as symptoms are evident. Whereas the AChE reactivators can be of great benefit in the therapy of anti-ChE intoxication (*see* below), their use must be regarded as a supplement to the administration of atropine.

Cholinesterase Reactivators.

Although the phosphorylated esteratic site of AChE undergoes hydrolytic regeneration at a slow or negligible rate, Wilson (1951) found that nucleophilic agents, such as hydroxylamine (NH_2OH), hydroxamic acids (RCONH—OH), and oximes (RCH=NOH), reactivate the enzyme more rapidly than does spontaneous hydrolysis. He reasoned that selective reactivation could

be achieved by a site-directed nucleophile, wherein interaction of a quaternary nitrogen with the negative subsite of the active center would place the nucleophile in close apposition to the phosphorus. This goal was achieved to a remarkable degree by Wilson and Ginsburg with pyridine-2-aldoxime methyl chloride (pralidoxime; *see* Figure 8–2*L* and below); reactivation with this compound occurs at a million times the rate of that with hydroxylamine. The oxime is oriented proximally to exert a nucleophilic attack on the phosphorus; a phosphoryloxime is formed, leaving the regenerated enzyme (Wilson, 1959).

Several *bis*-quaternary oximes were shown subsequently to be even more potent as reactivators for insecticide and nerve gas poisoning (*see* below); an example is HI-6, which is used in Europe as an antidote. The structures of pralidoxime and HI-6 are as follows:

PRALIDOXIME (2-PAM)

HI-6

The velocity of reactivation of phosphorylated AChE by oximes depends on their accessibility to the active center serine (Wong *et al.*, 2000). Furthermore, certain phosphorylated AChEs can undergo a fairly rapid process of "aging," so that within the course of minutes or hours they become completely resistant to the reactivators. "Aging" probably is due to the loss of one alkoxy group, leaving a much more stable monoalkyl- or monoalkoxy-phosphoryl-AChE (Fleisher and Harris, 1965; *see* Figure 8–2*K*). Organophosphorus compounds containing tertiary alkoxy groups are more prone to "aging" than are the congeners containing the secondary or primary alkoxy groups (Aldridge, 1976). The oximes are not effective in antagonizing the toxicity of the more rapidly hydrolyzing carbamoyl ester inhibitors, and since pralidoxime itself has weak anti-ChE activity, they are not recommended for the treatment of overdosage with neostigmine or physostigmine and are contraindicated in poisoning with carbamoylating insecticides such as carbaryl.

Pharmacology, Toxicology, and Disposition.

The reactivating action of oximes *in vivo* is most marked at the skeletal neuromuscular junction. Following a dose of an organophosphorus compound that produces total blockade of transmission, the intravenous injection of an oxime can restore the response to stimulation of the motor nerve within a few minutes. Antidotal effects are less striking at autonomic effector sites, and the quaternary ammonium group restricts entry into the CNS.

High doses of pralidoxime and related compounds can in themselves cause neuromuscular blockade and inhibition of AChE; such actions are minimal at the dose rates recommended as an antidote. If pralidoxime is injected intravenously at a rate more rapid than 500 mg per minute, it can cause mild weakness, blurred vision, diplopia, dizziness, headache, nausea, and tachycardia.

The oximes as a group are metabolized largely by the liver, and the breakdown products are excreted by the kidney.

Delayed Neurotoxicity of Organophosphorus Compounds. Certain fluorine-containing alkylorganophosphorus anti-ChE agents (*e.g.*, DFP, mipafox) have in common with the triarylphosphates, of which *triorthocresylphosphate* (TOCP) is the classical example, the property of inducing delayed neurotoxicity. This syndrome first received widespread attention following the demonstration that TOCP, an adulterant of Jamaica ginger, was responsible for an outbreak of thousands of cases of paralysis that occurred in the United States during Prohibition.

The clinical picture is that of a severe polyneuropathy that begins several days after a single exposure to the toxic compound. It is manifested initially by mild sensory disturbances, ataxia, weakness, muscle fatigue and twitching, reduced tendon reflexes, and tenderness to palpation. In severe cases, the weakness may progress eventually to complete flaccid paralysis, which, over the course of weeks or months, is often succeeded by a spastic paralysis with a concomitant exaggeration of reflexes. During these phases, the muscles show marked wasting. Recovery may require several years and may be incomplete.

Because only certain triarylphosphates and fluorine-containing alkylphosphates have the greatest propensity to produce the organophosphate-induced delayed polyneuropathy (OPIDR), toxicity is not dependent upon inhibition of AChE or other cholinesterases. Evidence points to inhibition of a different esterase, termed a *neurotoxic esterase,* as being linked to the lesions (Johnson, 1993). The enzyme has been isolated and its gene cloned. Its substrate specificity is directed to hydrophobic esters, but its natural substrate and function are unknown (Glynn, 2000). Experimental myopathies that result in generalized necrotic lesions and changes in end-plate cytostructure also are found after long-term exposure to organophosphates (Dettbarn, 1984; DeBleeker *et al.*, 1992).

THERAPEUTIC USES

Although anti-ChE agents have been recommended for the treatment of a wide variety of conditions involving the peripheral nervous system, their widespread acceptability has been established mainly in four areas: atony of the smooth muscle of the intestinal tract and urinary bladder, glaucoma, myasthenia gravis, and termination of the effects of competitive neuromuscular blocking drugs (*see* Chapter 9). Long-acting and hydrophobic cholinesterase inhibitors are the only inhibitors with efficacy, albeit limited, in the treatment of dementia symptoms of Alzheimer's

disease. Physostigmine, with its shorter duration of action, is useful in the treatment of intoxication by atropine and several drugs with anticholinergic side effects (*see* below); it also is indicated for the treatment of Friedreich's or other inherited ataxias. Edrophonium can be used for terminating attacks of paroxysmal supraventricular tachycardia.

Available Therapeutic Agents. The compounds described here are those commonly used as anti-ChE drugs and cholinesterase reactivators in the United States. Preparations used solely for ophthalmic purposes are described in Chapter 66. Conventional dosages and routes of administration are given in the discussion of therapeutic applications of these agents (*see* below).

Physostigmine salicylate (ANTILIRIUM) is available for injection. *Physostigmine sulfate ophthalmic ointment* and *physostigmine salicylate ophthalmic solution* also are available. *Pyridostigmine bromide* is available for oral (MESTINON) or parenteral (REGONOL, MESTINON) use. *Neostigmine bromide* (PROSTIGMIN) is available for oral use. *Neostigmine methylsulfate* (PROSTIGMIN) is marketed for parenteral injection. *Ambenonium chloride* (MYTELASE) is available for oral use. *Edrophonium chloride* (TENSILON, others) is marketed for parenteral injection. *Tacrine* (COGNEX), *donepezil* (ARICEPT), *rivastigmine* (EXELON), and *galantamine* (REMINYL) have been approved for the treatment of Alzheimer's disease.

Pralidoxime chloride (PROTOPAM CHLORIDE) is the only AChE reactivator currently available in the United States and can be obtained in a parenteral formulation.

Paralytic Ileus and Atony of the Urinary Bladder. In the treatment of both these conditions, neostigmine generally is the most satisfactory of the anti-ChE agents. The direct parasympathomimetic agents, discussed in Chapter 7, are employed for the same purposes.

Neostigmine is used for the relief of abdominal distension and acute colonic pseudoobstruction from a variety of medical and surgical causes (Ponec *et al.*, 1999). The usual subcutaneous dose of neostigmine methylsulfate for postoperative paralytic ileus is 0.5 mg, given as needed. Peristaltic activity commences 10 to 30 minutes after parenteral administration, whereas 2 to 4 hours are required after oral administration of neostigmine bromide (15 to 30 mg). A rectal tube should be inserted to facilitate expulsion of gas, and it may be necessary to assist evacuation with a small low enema. The drug should not be used when the intestine or urinary bladder is obstructed, when peritonitis is present, when the viability of the bowel is doubtful, or when bowel dysfunction is a consequence of inflammatory disease.

When neostigmine is used for the treatment of atony of the detrusor muscle of the urinary bladder, postoperative dysuria is relieved, and the time interval between operation and spontaneous urination is shortened. The drug is used in a similar dose and manner as in the management of paralytic ileus.

Glaucoma and Other Ophthalmologic Indications. Glaucoma is a disease complex characterized chiefly by an increase in intraocular pressure that, if sufficiently high and persistent, leads to damage to the optic disc at the juncture of the optic nerve and the retina; irreversible blindness can result. Of the three types of glaucoma—primary, secondary, and congenital—anti-ChE agents are of value in the management of the primary as well as of certain categories of the secondary type (*e.g.,* apha-kic glaucoma, following cataract extraction); the congenital type rarely responds to any therapy other than surgery. Primary glau-coma is subdivided into narrow-angle (acute congestive) and wide-angle (chronic simple) types, based on the configuration of the angle of the anterior chamber where reabsorption of the aqueous humor occurs.

Narrow-angle glaucoma is nearly always a medical emer-gency in which drugs are essential in controlling the acute at-tack, but the long-range management is often surgical (*e.g.,* peripheral or complete iridectomy). Wide-angle glaucoma, on the other hand, has a gradual, insidious onset and is not gener-ally amenable to surgical improvement; in this type, control of intraocular pressure usually is dependent upon continuous drug therapy.

Since the cholinergic agonists and cholinesterase inhibitors also block accommodation and induce myopia, these agents pro-duce transient blurring of far vision and loss of vision at the margin when instilled in the eye. With long-term administration of the cholinergic agonists and anti-ChE agents, the compro-mise of vision diminishes. Nevertheless, other agents without these side effects, such as β-adrenergic receptor antagonists, prostaglandin analogs, or carbonic anhydrase inhibitors, have become the primary topical therapies for open angle glaucoma (Alward, 1998; *see* Chapter 66). Topical treatment with long-acting cholinesterase inhibitors such as *echothiophate* gives rise to symptoms characteristic of systemic cholinesterase inhibi-tion. Echothiophate treatment in advanced glaucoma may be associated with the production of cataracts (Alward, 1998).

Anti-ChE agents have been employed locally in the treat-ment of a variety of other ophthalmologic conditions, including accommodative esotropia and myasthenia gravis confined to the extraocular and eyelid muscles. Adie (or tonic pupil) syndrome results from dysfunction of the ciliary body, perhaps because of local nerve degeneration. Low concentrations of *physostigmine* are reported to decrease the blurred vision and pain associated with this condition. In alternation with a mydriatic drug such as atropine, short-acting anti-ChE agents have proven useful for the breaking of adhesions between the iris and the lens or cornea. (For a complete account of the use of anti-ChE agents in ocular therapy, *see* Chapter 66.)

Myasthenia Gravis. Myasthenia gravis is a neuromuscular disease characterized by weakness and marked fatigability of skeletal muscle (*see* Drachman, 1994); exacerbations and par-tial remissions occur frequently. Jolly (1895) noted the similarity between the symptoms of myasthenia gravis and curare poison-ing in animals and suggested that physostigmine, an agent then known to antagonize curare, might be of therapeutic value. Forty years elapsed before his suggestion was given systematic trial (Walker, 1934).

The defect in myasthenia gravis is in synaptic transmis-sion at the neuromuscular junction. When a motor nerve of a normal subject is stimulated at 25 Hz, electrical and mechan-ical responses are well sustained. A suitable margin of safety exists for maintenance of neuromuscular transmission. Initial responses in the myasthenic patient may be normal, but they diminish rapidly, which explains the difficulty in maintaining voluntary muscle activity for more than brief periods.

The relative importance of prejunctional and postjunctional defects in myasthenia gravis was a matter of considerable de-bate until Patrick and Lindstrom (1973) found that rabbits im-munized with the nicotinic receptor purified from electric eels slowly developed muscular weakness and respiratory difficulties that resembled the symptoms of myasthenia gravis. The rabbits also exhibited decremental responses following repetitive nerve stimulation, enhanced sensitivity to curare, and symptomatic and electrophysiological improvement of neuromuscular trans-mission following administration of anti-ChE agents. Although this experimental allergic myasthenia gravis and the naturally occurring disease differ somewhat, this animal model prompted intense investigation into whether or not the natural disease represented an autoimmune response directed toward the ACh receptor. Antireceptor antibody soon was identified in patients with myasthenia gravis (Almon *et al.,* 1974). Receptor-binding antibodies now are detectable in sera of 90% of patients with the disease, although the clinical status of the patient does not cor-relate precisely with the antibody titer (Drachman *et al.,* 1982; Drachman, 1994; Lindstrom, 2000).

The picture that emerges is that myasthenia gravis is caused by an autoimmune response primarily to the ACh receptor at the postjunctional end-plate. Antibodies, which also are present in plasma, reduce the number of receptors detectable either by snake α-neurotoxin-binding assays (Fambrough *et al.,* 1973) or by electrophysiological measurements of ACh sensitivity (Drachman, 1994). The autoimmune reaction enhances receptor degradation (Drachman *et al.,* 1982). Immune complexes along with marked ultrastructural abnormalities appear in the synaptic cleft. The latter appear to be a consequence of complement-mediated lysis of junctional folds in the end-plate. A related disease that also compromises neuromuscular transmission is Lambert–Eaton syndrome. Here, antibodies are directed against Ca^{2+} channels that are necessary for presynaptic release of ACh (Lang *et al.,* 1998).

In a subset of approximately 10% of patients presenting with a myasthenic syndrome, muscle weakness has a congeni-tal rather than an autoimmune basis. Characterization of bio-chemical and genetic bases of the congenital condition has shown mutations to occur in the acetylcholine receptor which af-fect ligand-binding and channel-opening kinetics (Engel *et al.,* 1998). Other mutations occur as a deficiency in the form of acetylcholinesterase that contains the collagen-like tail unit (Ohno *et al.,* 2000). As expected, following administration of anti-ChE agents (*see* below), subjective improvement is not seen in most congenital myasthenic patients.

Diagnosis. Although the diagnosis of autoimmune myasthe-nia gravis usually can be made from the history, signs, and symptoms, its differentiation from certain neurasthenic, infec-tious, endocrine, congenital, neoplastic, and degenerative neu-romuscular diseases is challenging. However, myasthenia gravis is the only condition in which the aforementioned deficien-cies can be improved dramatically by anti-ChE medication. The edrophonium test for evaluation of possible myasthenia gravis is performed by rapid intravenous injection of 2 mg of edro-phonium chloride, followed 45 seconds later by an additional 8 mg if the first dose is without effect; a positive response consists of brief improvement in strength, unaccompanied by lingual fasciculation (which generally occurs in nonmyasthenic patients).

An excessive dose of an anti-ChE drug results in a choliner-gic crisis. The condition is characterized by weakness resulting from generalized depolarization of the motor end-plate; other features result from overstimulation of muscarinic receptors. The weakness resulting from depolarization block may resemble myasthenic weakness, which is manifest when anti-ChE medication is insufficient. The distinction is of obvious practical importance, since the former is treated by withholding, and the latter by administering, the anti-ChE agent. When the edrophonium test is performed cautiously, limiting the dose to 2 mg and with facilities for respiratory resuscitation immediately available, a further decrease in strength indicates cholinergic crisis, while improvement signifies myasthenic weakness. Atropine sulfate, 0.4 to 0.6 mg or more intravenously, should be given immediately if a severe muscarinic reaction ensues (for complete details, *see* Osserman *et al.,* 1972; Drachman, 1994). Detection of antireceptor antibodies in muscle biopsies or plasma is now widely employed to confirm the diagnosis.

Treatment.   *Pyridostigmine, neostigmine,* and *ambenonium* are the standard anti-ChE drugs used in the symptomatic treatment of myasthenia gravis. All can increase the response of myasthenic muscle to repetitive nerve impulses, primarily by the preservation of endogenous ACh; with equivalent release of ACh, receptors over a greater cross-sectional area of the endplate then presumably are exposed to concentrations of ACh that are sufficient for channel opening and production of a postsynaptic end-plate potential.

When the diagnosis of myasthenia gravis has been established, the optimal single oral dose of an anti-ChE agent can be determined empirically. Baseline recordings are made for grip strength, vital capacity, and a number of signs and symptoms that reflect the strength of various muscle groups. The patient then is given an oral dose of pyridostigmine (30 to 60 mg), neostigmine (7.5 to 15 mg), or ambenonium (2.5 to 5 mg). The improvement in muscle strength and changes in other signs and symptoms are noted at frequent intervals until there is a return to the basal state. After an hour or longer in the basal state, the drug is given again with the dose increased to one and one-half times the initial amount, and the same observations are repeated. This sequence is continued, with increasing increments of one-half the initial dose, until an optimal response is obtained.

The duration of action of these drugs is such that the interval between oral doses required to maintain a reasonably even level of strength usually is 2 to 4 hours for neostigmine, 3 to 6 hours for pyridostigmine, or 3 to 8 hours for ambenonium. However, the dose required may vary from day to day, and physical or emotional stress, intercurrent infections, and menstruation usually necessitate an increase in the frequency or size of the dose. In addition, unpredictable exacerbations and remissions of the myasthenic state may require adjustment of the dosage upward or downward. Although all patients with myasthenia gravis should be seen by a physician at regular intervals, most can be taught to modify their dosage regimens according to their changing requirements. Pyridostigmine is available in sustained-release tablets containing a total of 180 mg, of which 60 mg is released immediately and 120 mg over several hours; this preparation is of value in maintaining patients for 6- to 8-hour periods, but should be limited to use at bedtime. Muscarinic cardiovascular and gastrointestinal side effects of anti-ChE agents generally can be controlled by atropine or other anticholinergic drugs (*see* Chapter 7). However, these anticholinergic drugs mask many side effects of an excessive dose of an anticholinesterase agent. In most patients, tolerance develops eventually to the muscarinic effects, so that anticholinergic

medication is not necessary. A number of drugs, including curariform agents and certain antibiotics and general anesthetics, interfere with neuromuscular transmission (*see* Chapter 9); their administration to patients with myasthenia gravis is hazardous without proper adjustment of anti-ChE dosage and other appropriate precautions.

Other therapeutic measures should be considered as essential elements in the management of this disease. Controlled studies reveal that *corticosteroids* promote clinical improvement in a high percentage of patients. However, when treatment with steroids is continued over prolonged periods, a high incidence of side effects may result (*see* Chapter 60). Gradual lowering of maintenance doses and alternate-day regimens of short-acting steroids are used to minimize side effects. Initiation of steroid treatment augments muscle weakness; however, as the patient improves with continued administration of steroids, doses of anti-ChE drugs can be reduced (Drachman, 1994). Other immunosuppressive agents such as *azathioprine* and *cyclosporine* also have been beneficial in more advanced cases.

Thymectomy should be considered in myasthenia associated with a thymoma or when the disease is not controlled adequately by anti-ChE agents and steroids. The relative risks and benefits of the surgical procedure *versus* anti-ChE and corticosteroid treatment require careful assessment in each case. Since the thymus contains myoid cells with nicotinic receptors (Schluep *et al.,* 1987) and a predominance of patients have thymic abnormalities, the thymus may be responsible for the initial pathogenesis. It also is the source of autoreactive T helper cells. However, the thymus is not required for perpetuation of the condition.

In keeping with the presumed autoimmune etiology of myasthenia gravis, plasmapheresis and immune therapy have produced beneficial results in patients who have remained disabled despite thymectomy and treatment with steroids and anti-ChE agents (Drachman, 1994, 1996). Improvement in muscle strength correlates with the reduction of the titer of antibody directed against the nicotinic cholinergic receptor.

Prophylaxis in Cholinesterase Inhibitor Poisoning. Studies in experimental animals have shown that pretreatment with pyridostigmine reduces the incapacitation and mortality associated with "nerve agent" poisoning, particularly for agents, such as soman, that show rapid aging. The first large-scale administration of pyridostigmine to human beings occurred in 1990 in anticipation of nerve-agent attack in the Persian Gulf. At an oral dose of 30 mg every 8 hours, the incidence of side effects was around 1%, but fewer than 0.1% of the subjects had responses sufficient to warrant discontinuing the drug in the setting of military action (Keeler *et al.,* 1991). Long-term follow-up indicates that veterans of the Persian Gulf Campaign that had received pyridostigmine showed a low incidence of a neurologic syndrome, now termed the *Persian Gulf War syndrome.* It is characterized by impaired cognition, ataxia, confusion, myoneuropathy, adenopathy, weakness, and incontinence (Haley *et al.,* 1997; The Iowa Persian Gulf Study Group, 1997). While pyridostigmine has been implicated by some as the causative agent, the absence of similar neuropathies in pyridostigmine-treated myasthenic patients makes it far more likely that a combination of agents, including combusted organophosphates and insect repellents in addition to pyridostigmine, contributed to this persisting syndrome. It also is difficult to distinguish residual chemical toxicity from posttraumatic stress experienced after combat action.

Intoxication by Anticholinergic Drugs. In addition to atropine and other muscarinic agents, many other drugs, such as the phenothiazines, antihistamines, and tricyclic antidepressants, have central as well as peripheral anticholinergic activity. Physostigmine is potentially useful in reversing the central anticholinergic syndrome produced by overdosage or an unusual reaction to these drugs (Nilsson, 1982). The effectiveness of physostigmine in reversing the anticholinergic effects of these agents has been clearly documented. However, other toxic effects of the tricyclic antidepressants and phenothiazines (*see* Chapters 19 and 20), such as intraventricular conduction deficits and ventricular arrhythmias, are not reversed by physostigmine. In addition, physostigmine may precipitate seizures; hence, its usually small potential benefit must be weighed against this risk. The initial intravenous or intramuscular dose of physostigmine is 2 mg, with additional doses given as necessary. Physostigmine, a tertiary amine, crosses the blood–brain barrier, in contrast to the quaternary anti-AChE drugs. The use of anti-ChE agents to reverse the effects of competitive neuromuscular blocking agents is discussed in Chapter 9.

Alzheimer's Disease. A deficiency of intact cholinergic neurons, particularly those extending from subcortical areas such as the nucleus basalis of Maynert, has been observed in patients with progressive dementia of the Alzheimer's type (Markesbery, 1998). Using a rationale similar to that in other CNS degenerative diseases (*see* Chapter 22), therapy for enhancing concentrations of cholinergic neurotransmitters in the central nervous system was investigated (Mayeux and Sano, 1999). In 1993, the FDA approved *tacrine* (tetrahydroaminoacridine) for use in mild to moderate Alzheimer's disease, but a high incidence of hepatotoxicity and frequent liver function tests limit

the efficacy of this drug. About 30% of the patients receiving low doses of tacrine within three months have alanine aminotransferase values of three times normal; upon discontinuing the drug, liver function values return to normal in 90% of the patients. Other side effects are typical of acetylcholinesterase inhibitors.

More recently, *donepezil* was approved for clinical use. There are efficacy data from multiple trials, most involving several hundred patients (Dooley and Lamb, 2000). At 5- and 10-mg daily oral doses, improved cognition and global clinical function were seen in the 21- to 81-week intervals studied. In long-term studies, the drug delayed symptomatic progression of the disease for periods up to 55 weeks. Side effects are largely attributable to excessive cholinergic stimulation, with nausea, diarrhea, and vomiting being most frequently reported. The drug is well tolerated in single daily doses. Usually, 5-mg doses are administered at night for 4 to 6 weeks; if this dose is well tolerated, the dose can be increased to 10 mg daily.

Rivastigmine, a long-acting carbamoylating inhibitor, recently has been approved for use in the United States and Europe. Although fewer studies have been conducted with it, the drug's efficacy, tolerability, and side effects are similar to those of donepezil (Corey-Bloom *et al.,* 1998; Giacobini, 2000). Eptastigmine, also a carbamoylating inhibitor, was associated with adverse hematologic effects in two studies, resulting in suspension of clinical trials. *Galantamine* is another AChE inhibitor recently approved by the FDA for treating Alzheimer's disease. It has a side-effect profile similar to those of donepezil and rivastigmine.

Therapeutic strategies with new compounds are directed at maximizing the ratio of central to peripheral cholinesterase inhibition and the use of cholinesterase inhibitors in conjunction with selective cholinergic agonists and antagonists. Combination therapy with agents that are directed to slowing the progression of the degenerative disease also are being considered.

BIBLIOGRAPHY

Almon, R.R., Andrew, C.G., and Appel, S.H. Serum globulin in myasthenia gravis: inhibition of α-bungarotoxin binding to acetylcholine receptors. *Science,* **1974,** *186*:55–57.

Argyll-Robertson, D. The Calabar bean as a new agent in ophthalmic practice. *Edinb. Med. J.,* **1863,** *8*:815–820.

Bourne, Y., Marchot, P., and Taylor, P. Acetylcholinesterase inhibition by fasciculin: crystal structure of the complex. *Cell,* **1995,** *83*:493–506.

Christioson, R. On the properties of the ordeal bean of Old Calabar. *Mon. J. Med. (Lond.),* **1855,** *20*:193–204.

Cohan, S.L., Pohlmann, J.L.W., Mikszewki, J., and O'Doherty, D.S. The pharmacokinetics of pyridostigmine. *Neurology,* **1976,** *26*:536–539.

Corey-Bloom, J., Anand, R., and Veach, J. A randomized trial evaluating the efficacy and safety of ENA 713 (rivastigmine tartrate), a new acetylcholinesterase inhibitor, in patients with mild to moderately severe Alzheimer's disease. *Int. J. Psychopharmacol.,* **1998,** *1*:55–65.

Cummings, J.L., Cyrus, P.A., and Bieber, F. Metrifonate treatment of cognitive deficits in Alzheimer's disease. *Neurology,* **1999,** *50*:1214–1221.

Cygler, M., Schrag, J., Sussman, J.L., Harel, M., Silman, I., Gentry, M.K., and Doctor, B.P. Relationship between sequence conservation and three dimensional structure in a large family of esterases, lipases and related proteins. *Protein Sci.,* **1993,** *2*:366–382.

Drachman, D.B., Adams, R.N., Josifek, L.F., and Self, S.G. Functional activities of autoantibodies to acetylcholine receptors and the clinical severity of myasthenia gravis. *N. Engl. J. Med.,* **1982,** *307*:769–775.

Fambrough, D.M., Drachman, D.B., and Satyamurti, S. Neuromuscular junction in myasthenia gravis: decreased acetylcholine receptors. *Science,* **1973,** *182*:293–295.

Fleisher, J.H., and Harris, L.W. Dealkylation as a mechanism for aging of cholinesterase after poisoning with pinacolyl methylphosphonofluoridate. *Biochem. Pharmacol.,* **1965,** *14*:641–650.

Fraser, T.R. On the characters, actions and therapeutical uses of the ordeal bean of Calabar (*Physostigma venenosum,* Balfour). *Edinb. Med. J.,* **1863,** *9*:36–56, 123–132, 235–248.

Furlong, C.E., Li, W.F., Richter, R.J., Shih, D.M., Lusis, A.J., Alleva, E., and Costa, L.G. Genetic and temporal determinants of pesticide sensitivity: role of paroxonase (PON1). *Neurotoxicology,* **2000,** *21*:91–100.

Haley, R.W., Kurt, T.L., and Hom, J. Is there a Gulf War syndrome? *JAMA*, **1997**, *277*:215–222.

The Iowa Persian Gulf Study Group. Self-reported illness and health status among Gulf War veterans. *JAMA*, **1997**, *277*:238–245.

Jolly, F. Pseudoparalysis myasthenica. *Neurol. Zentralbl.*, **1895**, *14*:34.

Keeler, J.R., Hurst, C.G., and Dunn, M.A. Pyridostigmine used as a nerve agent pretreatment under wartime conditions. *JAMA*, **1991**, *266*:693–695.

Lockridge, O., Bartels, C.F., Vaughan, T.A., Wong, C.K., Norton, S.E., and Johnson, L.L. Complete amino acid sequence of human serum cholinesterase. *J. Biol. Chem.*, **1987**, *262*:549–557.

Lockridge, O., and Masson, P. Pesticides and susceptible populations: People with butyrylcholinesterase genetic variants may be at risk. *Neurotoxicology*, **2000**, *21*:113–126.

McCombie, H., and Saunders, B.C. Alkyl fluorophosphonates: preparation and physiological properties. *Nature*, **1946**, *157*:287–289.

Nilsson, E. Physostigmine treatment in various drug-induced intoxications. *Ann. Clin. Res.*, **1982**, *14*:165–172.

Nozaki, H., and Aikawa, N. Sarin poisoning in Tokyo subway. *Lancet*, **1995**, *346*:1446–1447.

Office of Pesticide Programs, Environmental Protection Agency. Available at: www.epa.gov/pesticides/op/. Accessed: Nov. 23, 1999.

Padilla, S., Buzzard, J., and Moser, V.C. Comparison of the role of esterases in the differential age-related sensitivity to chlorpyrifos and methamidophos. *Neurotoxicology*, **2000**, *21*:49–56.

Patrick, J., and Lindstrom, J. Autoimmune response to acetylcholine receptor. *Science*, **1973**, *180*:871–872.

Ponec, R.J., Saunders, M.D., and Kimmey, M.B. Neostigmine for the treatment of acute colonic pseudoobstruction. *N. Engl. J. Med.*, **1999**, *341*:137–141.

Schluep, M., Wilcox, N., Vincent, A., Dhoot, G.K., and Newson-Davis, J. Acetylcholine receptors in human thymic myoid cells in situ: an immunohistological study. *Ann. Neurol.*, **1987**, *22*:212–222.

Schumacher, M., Camp, S., Maulet, Y., Newton, M., MacPhee-Quigley, K., Taylor, S.S., Friedmann, T., and Taylor, P. Primary structure of *Torpedo californica* acetylcholinesterase deduced from its cDNA sequence. *Nature*, **1986**, *319*:407–409.

Stedman, E. III. Studies on the relationship between chemical constitution and physiological action. Part II. The miotic activity of urethanes derived from the isomeric hydroxybenzyldimethylamines. *Biochem. J.*, **1929a**, *23*:17–24.

Stedman, E. Chemical constitution and miotic action. *Am. J. Physiol.*, **1929b**, *90*:528–529.

Sussman, J.L., Harel, M., Frolow, F., Oefner, C., Goldman, A., Toker, L., and Silman, I. Atomic structure of acetylcholinesterase from *Torpedo californica:* a prototypic acetylcholine-binding protein. *Science*, **1991**, *253*:872–879.

Walker, M.B. Treatment of myasthenia gravis with physostigmine. *Lancet*, **1934**, *1*:1200–1201.

Wilson, I.B. Acetylcholinesterase. XI. Reversibility of tetraethyl pyrophosphate inhibition. *J. Biol. Chem.*, **1951**, *190*:111–117.

Wong, L., Radic, Z., Bruggemann, R.J., Hosea, N., Berman, H.A., and Taylor, P. Mechanism of oxime reactivation of acetylcholinesterase analyzed by chirality and mutagenesis. *Biochemistry*, **2000**, *39*:5750–5757.

MONOGRAPHS AND REVIEWS

Aldridge, W.N. Survey of major points of interest about reactions of cholinesterases. *Croat. Chem. Acta*, **1976**, *47*:225–233.

Alward, W.L.M. Medical management of glaucoma. *N. Engl. J. Med.*, **1998**, *339*:1298–1307.

Bardin, P.G., van Eeden, S.F., Moolman, J.A., Foden, A.P., and Joubert, J.R. Organophosphate and carbamate poisoning. *Arch. Intern. Med.*, **1994**, *154*:1433–1441.

Baron, R.L. Carbamate insecticides. In, *Handbook of Pesticide Toxicology.* Vol. 3. (Hayes, W.J., Jr., and Laws, E.R., Jr., eds.) Academic Press, San Diego, CA, **1991**, pp. 1125–1190.

Costa, L.G., Galli, C.L., and Murphy, S.D. (eds.) *Toxicology of Pesticides: Experimental, Clinical, and Regulatory Perspectives. NATO Advanced Study Institute Series H.* Vol. 13. Springer-Verlag, Berlin, **1987.**

De Bleecker, J.L. The intermediate syndrome in organophosphorus poisoning: an overview of experimental and clinical observations. *J. Toxicol.*, **1995**, *33*:683–686.

De Bleecker, J.L., De Reuck, J.L., and Willems, J.L. Neurological aspects of organophosphate poisoning. *Clin. Neurol. Neurosurg.*, **1992**, *94*:93–103.

Dettbarn, W.D. Pesticide induced muscle necrosis: mechanisms and prevention. *Fundam. Appl. Toxicol.*, **1984**, *4*:S18–S26.

Dooley, M., and Lamb, H.M. Donepezil: a review of its use in Alzheimer's disease. *Drugs Aging*, **2000**, *16*:199–226.

Drachman, D.B. Myasthenia gravis. *N. Engl. J. Med.*, **1994**, *330*:1797–1810.

Drachman, D.B. Immunotherapy in neuromuscular disorders: current and future strategies. *Muscle Nerve*, **1996**, *19*:1239–1251.

Ecobichon, D.J. Carbamates. In, *Experimental and Clinical Neurotoxicology*, 2nd ed. (Spencer, P.S., and Schauburg, H.H., eds.). Oxford University Press, New York, **2000.**

Engel, A.G., Ohno, K., Milone, M., and Sine, S.M. Congenital myasthenic syndromes. *Ann. N.Y. Acad. Sci.*, **1998**, *841*:140–156.

Froede, H.C., and Wilson, I.B. Acetylcholinesterase. In, *The Enzymes.* Vol. 5. (Boyer, P.D., ed.) Academic Press, Inc., New York, **1971**, pp. 87–114.

Gallo, M.A., and Lawryk, N.J. Organic phosphorus pesticides. In, *Handbook of Pesticide Toxicology.* Vol. 2. (Hayes, W.J., Jr., and Laws, E.R., Jr., eds.) Academic Press, San Diego, **1991**, pp. 917–1123.

Giacobini, E. Cholinesterase inhibitors: from the Calabar bean to Alzheimer's therapy. In, *Cholinesterases and Cholinesterase Inhibitors.* (Giacobini, E., ed.) Martin Dubitz, London, **2000**, pp. 181–227.

Glynn, P. Neural development and neurodegeneration: two faces of neuropathy target esterase. *Prog. Neurobiol.*, **2000**, *61*:61–74.

Holmstedt, B. The ordeal bean of Old Calabar: the pageant of *Physostigma venenosum* in medicine. In, *Plants in the Development of Modern Medicine.* (Swain, T., ed.) Harvard University Press, Cambridge, MA, **1972**, pp. 303–360.

Johnson, M.K. Symposium introduction: retrospect and prospects for neuropathy target esterase (NTE) and the delayed polyneuropathy (OPIDP) induced by some organophosphorus esters. *Chem. Biol. Interact.*, **1993**, *87*:339–346.

Karczmar, A.G. History of the research with anticholinesterase agents. In, *Anticholinesterase Agents.* Vol. 1. *International Encyclopedia of Pharmacology and Therapeutics.* Sect. 13. (Karczmar, A.G., ed.) Pergamon Press, Ltd., Oxford, **1970**, pp. 1–44.

La Du, B.N., Aviran, M., Billecke, S., Navab, M., Primo-Parmo, S., Sorenson, R.C., and Standiford, T.J. On the physiological roles of the paroxonases. *Chem. Biol. Interact.*, **1999**, *119–120*:379–388.

Landrigan, P.J., Claudio, L., and McConnell, R. Pesticides. In, *Environmental Toxicants: Human Exposures and Their Health Effects.* (Lippman, M., ed.) Wiley, New York, **2000**, pp. 725–739.

Lang, B., Waterman, S., Pinto, A., Jones, D., Moss, S., Boot, J., Brust, P., Williams, M., Stauderman, K., Harpold, M., Motomura, M., Moll, J., Vincent, A., and Newsom-Davis, J. The role of autoantibodies in Lambert-Eaton myasthenic syndrome. *Ann. N.Y. Acad. Sci.,* **1998,** *841*:596–605.

Lindstrom, J.M. Acetylcholine receptors and myasthenia. *Muscle Nerve,* **2000,** *23*:453–477.

Markesbery, W.R. (ed.) *Neuropathology of Dementing Disorders.* Arnold, London, **1998.**

Marrs, T.C. Organophosphate poisoning. *Pharmacol. Ther.,* **1993,** *58*:51–66.

Massoulié, J. Molecular forms and anchoring of acetylcholinesterase. In, *Cholinesterases and Cholinesterase Inhibitors.* (Giacobini, E., ed.) Martin Dunitz, London, **2000,** pp. 81–103.

Mayeux, R., and Sano, M. Treatment of Alzheimer's disease. *N. Engl. J. Med.,* **1999,** *341*:1670–1679.

Ohno, K., Engle, A.G., Brengman, B.S., Shen, X-M, Heidenreich, F., Vincent, A., Milone, M., Tan, E., Demirci, M., Walsh, P., Nakano, S., and Akiguch, I. The spectrum of mutations causing end plate acetylcholinesterase deficiency. *Ann. Neurol.,* **2000,** *47*:162–170.

Osserman, K.E., Foldes, F.F., and Genkins, G. Myasthenia gravis. In, *Neuromuscular Blocking and Stimulating Agents.* Vol. 11. *International Encyclopedia of Pharmacology and Therapeutics,* Sect. 14.

(Cheymol, J., ed.) Pergamon Press, Ltd., Oxford, **1972,** pp. 561–618.

Reiner, E., and Radić, Z. Mechanism of action of cholinesterase inhibitors. In, *Cholinesterases and Cholinesterase Inhibitors.* (Giacobini, E., ed.) Martin Dunitz, London, **2000,** pp. 103–120.

Rosenberry, T.L. Acetylcholinesterase. *Adv. Enzymol. Relat. Areas Mol. Biol.,* **1975,** *43*:103–218.

Schrader, G. *Die Entwicklung neuer Insektizide auf Grundlage von Organischen Fluor- und Phosphorverbindungen.* Monographie No. 62. Verlag Chemie, Weinheim, **1952.**

Silman, I., and Sussman, J.L. Structural studies on acetylcholinesterase. In, *Cholinesterases and Cholinesterase Inhibitors.* (Giacobini, E., ed.) Martin Dunitz, London, **2000,** pp. 9–26.

Storm, J.E., Rozman, K.K., and Doull, J. Occupational exposure limits for 30 organophosphate pesticides based on inhibition of red blood cell acetylcholinesterase. *Toxicology,* **2000,** *150*:1–29.

Taylor, P., Luo, Z.D., and Camp, S. The genes encoding the cholinesterases: structure, evolutionary relationships and regulation of their expression. In, *Cholinesterases and Cholinesterase Inhibitors.* (Giacobini, E., ed.) Martin Dunitz, London, **2000,** pp. 63–80.

Taylor, P., and Radić, Z. The cholinesterases: from genes to proteins. *Annu. Rev. Pharmacol. Toxicol.,* **1994,** *34*:281–320.

Wilson, I.B. Molecular complementarity and antidotes for alkyl phosphate poisoning. *Fed. Proc.,* **1959,** *18*:752–758.

C H A P T E R 9

AGENTS ACTING AT THE NEUROMUSCULAR JUNCTION AND AUTONOMIC GANGLIA

Palmer Taylor

The nicotinic acetylcholine receptor mediates neurotransmission at the neuromuscular junction and peripheral autonomic ganglia; in the central nervous system, it largely controls release of neurotransmitters from presynaptic sites. This chapter focuses on agonists and antagonists at the nicotinic acetylcholine receptor and their clinical utility at the neuromuscular junction or autonomic ganglia. The text begins with an overview of current structural and functional insights regarding the nicotinic acetylcholine receptor and its subtypes. A variety of neuromuscular blocking agents with varying mechanisms of blockade and pharmacokinetic properties are used to produce muscle relaxation during anesthesia (see also Chapter 14). Nicotine transiently stimulates nicotinic receptors on ganglia but is best known for its addictive properties arising from its presynaptic actions influencing neurotransmitter release in the brain (see Chapter 24). The use of ganglionic blocking agents for management of hypertension has been eclipsed by superior agents (see Chapter 33), although these agents are sometimes useful alternatives when other agents fail to control blood pressure in life-threatening circumstances (e.g., in the case of an acute dissecting aortic aneurysm) and in surgery where controlled hypotension is indicated.

Several drugs have as their major action the interruption or mimicry of transmission of the nerve impulse at the neuromuscular junction of skeletal muscle and/or autonomic ganglia. These agents can be classified together, since they interact with a common family of receptors; these receptors are called *nicotinic acetylcholine* (also commonly called *nicotinic cholinergic*) receptors, since they are stimulated by both the neurotransmitter acetylcholine (ACh) and the alkaloid nicotine. Distinct subtypes of nicotinic receptors exist at the neuromuscular junction and the ganglia, and several pharmacological agents that act at these receptors discriminate between them. Neuromuscular blocking agents are distinguished by whether or not they cause depolarization of the motor end plate and, for this reason, are classified either as *competitive (stabilizing)* agents, of which *curare* is the classical example, or as *depolarizing* agents, such as *succinylcholine*. The competitive and depolarizing agents are used widely to achieve muscle relaxation during anesthesia. Ganglionic agents act by stimulating or blocking nicotinic receptors on the postganglionic neuron.

THE NICOTINIC ACETYLCHOLINE RECEPTOR

The concept of the nicotinic acetylcholine receptor, with which ACh combines to initiate the end-plate potential (EPP) in muscle or an excitatory postsynaptic potential (EPSP) in nerve, is introduced in Chapter 6. Classical studies of the actions of curare and nicotine made this the prototypical pharmacological receptor over a century ago. By taking advantage of specialized structures that have evolved to mediate or block cholinergic neurotransmission, peripheral and then central nicotinic receptors have been isolated and characterized over the last 30 years. These accomplishments represent landmarks in the development of molecular pharmacology.

The electric organs from the aquatic species of *Electrophorus* and, especially, *Torpedo* provide rich sources of nicotinic receptor. The electric organ is derived embryologically from myoid tissue; however, in contrast to skeletal muscle, a significant fraction (30% to 40%) of the surface of the membrane is excitable and contains cholinergic receptors. In vertebrate skeletal muscle, motor end plates occupy 0.1% or less of the cell surface. The discovery of seemingly irreversible antagonism of neuromuscular transmission by α toxins from venoms of the krait, *Bungarus multicinctus* (Chang and Lee, 1963), or varieties of the cobra, *Naja naja,* offered suitable markers for identification of the receptor. The α toxins are peptides of about 7000 daltons molecular mass. The interaction of radioisotope-labeled toxins with the receptor initially was applied to an assay for identification of the isolated cholinergic receptor *in vitro* by Changeux and colleagues in 1970 (*see* Changeux and Edelstein, 1998). The α toxins have extremely high affinities and slow rates of dissociation from the receptor, yet the interaction is noncovalent. *In situ* and *in vitro* their behavior resembles that expected for a high-affinity antagonist. Since cholinergic neurotransmission mediates motor activity in marine vertebrates and mammals, a large number of peptide, terpinoid, and alkaloid toxins that block the nicotinic receptors have evolved to enhance predation or protect plant and animal species from predation (Taylor *et al.,* 2000).

Purification of the receptor from *Torpedo* ultimately led to the isolation of complementary DNAs (cDNAs) that encode each of the subunits. These cDNAs, in turn, have permitted the cloning of genes encoding the multiple receptor subunits from mammalian neurons and muscle (Numa *et al.,* 1983). By simultaneously expressing the genes that encode the individual subunits in cellular systems in various permutations and by measuring binding and the electrophysiological events that result from activation by agonists, researchers have been able to correlate functional properties with details of primary structures of the receptor subtypes (Lindstrom, 2000; Karlin and Akabas, 1995; Paterson and Nordberg, 2000).

Nicotinic Receptor Structure. The nicotinic receptor of the electric organ and vertebrate skeletal muscle is a pentamer composed of four distinct subunits (α, β, γ, δ) in the stoichiometric ratio of 2:1:1:1, respectively. In mature innervated muscle end plates, the γ subunit is replaced by ε, a closely related subunit. The individual subunits are about 40% identical in their amino acid sequences, suggesting that they arose from a common primordial gene (Numa *et al.,* 1983).

The nicotinic receptor has become the prototype for other ligand-gated ion channels, which include the receptors for the inhibitory amino acids (gamma-aminobutyric acid and glycine) and certain serotonin (5-HT_3) receptors. The family of ligand-gated ion channels are pentamers of homologous subunits, each having a molecular mass of 40,000 to 60,000 daltons. The aminoterminal 210 residues constitute virtually all of the extracellular domain. This is followed by four transmembrane-spanning domains, with the region between the third and fourth domain forming most of the cytoplasmic component (Figure 9–1).

Each of the subunits within the nicotinic acetylcholine receptor has an extracellular and an intracellular exposure on the postsynaptic membrane. The five subunits are arranged to circumscribe an internally located channel in a fashion similar to petals on a lily (Unwin, 1993; Karlin and Akabas, 1995; Changeux and Edelstein, 1998). The receptor is an asymmetrical molecule (14 nm $\times$ 8 nm) of 250,000 daltons, with the bulk of the nonmembrane-spanning domain on the extracellular surface. In junctional areas (*i.e.,* the motor end plate in skeletal muscle and the ventral surface of the electric organ) the receptor is present at high densities ($10,000/\mu m^2$) in a regular

packing order. This ordering of the receptors has allowed electron microscopy image reconstruction of its molecular structure at a resolution of 10 Å or less (Unwin, 1993; Miyazawa *et al.,* 1999; *see* Figure 9–1).

As is the case for other proteins where cooperativity of both binding and functional responses is evident, the binding sites are found at the subunit interfaces, but of the five interfaces, only two in muscle, $\alpha\gamma$ and $\alpha\delta$, have evolved to bind ligands. The binding of agonists, reversible competitive antagonists, and the elapid α toxins is mutually exclusive and appears to involve overlapping surfaces on the receptor. Both subunits forming the subunit interface contribute to ligand specificity (Taylor *et al.,* 2000).

Measurements of membrane conductances demonstrate that rates of ion translocation are sufficiently rapid (5×10^7 ions per second) to require ion translocation through an open channel, rather than by a rotating carrier of ions. Moreover, agonist-mediated changes in ion permeability (typically an inward movement of primarily Na^+ and secondarily Ca^{2+}) occur through a cation channel intrinsic to the receptor structure. The second transmembrane-spanning region on each of the five subunits forms the internal perimeter of the channel. The agonist-binding site is intimately coupled with an ion channel; simultaneous binding of two agonist molecules in muscle results in a rapid conformational change that opens the channel. Details on the kinetics of channel opening have evolved from electrophysiological patch–clamp techniques that enable one to distinguish the individual opening and closing events of a single receptor molecule (Sakmann, 1992).

Cloning by sequence homology enabled investigators to identify the genes encoding the nicotinic receptor for higher vertebrates, initially in muscle and then in neurons. Neuronal nicotinic receptors found in ganglia and the central nervous system (CNS) also exist as pentamers of subunits composed of one, two, or more subunits. Although only a single subunit of the type sequence α (denoted as $\alpha 1$) is found in abundance in muscle, along with β, δ, and γ or ε, at least eight subtypes of α ($\alpha 2$ through $\alpha 9$) and three of the non-α type (designated as $\beta 2$ through $\beta 4$) are found in neuronal tissues. Although not all permutations of α and β subunits lead to functional receptors, the diversity in subunit composition is large and exceeds the capacity of ligands to distinguish subtypes on the basis of their selectivity. Distinctive selectivities of the receptor subtypes for Na^+ and Ca^{2+} suggest that certain subtypes may possess functions other than rapid transsynaptic signaling. Several congenital myasthenic syndromes recently have been found to arise from mutations in the muscle receptor subunits, and various manifestations of epilepsy arise from mutations of neuronal receptor subunits (Engel *et al.,* 1998; Lindstrom, 2000).

NEUROMUSCULAR BLOCKING AGENTS

History, Sources, and Chemistry. *Curare* is a generic term for various South American arrow poisons. The drug has a long and romantic history. It has been used for centuries by the Indians along the Amazon and Orinoco Rivers for immobilizing and paralyzing wild animals used for food; death results

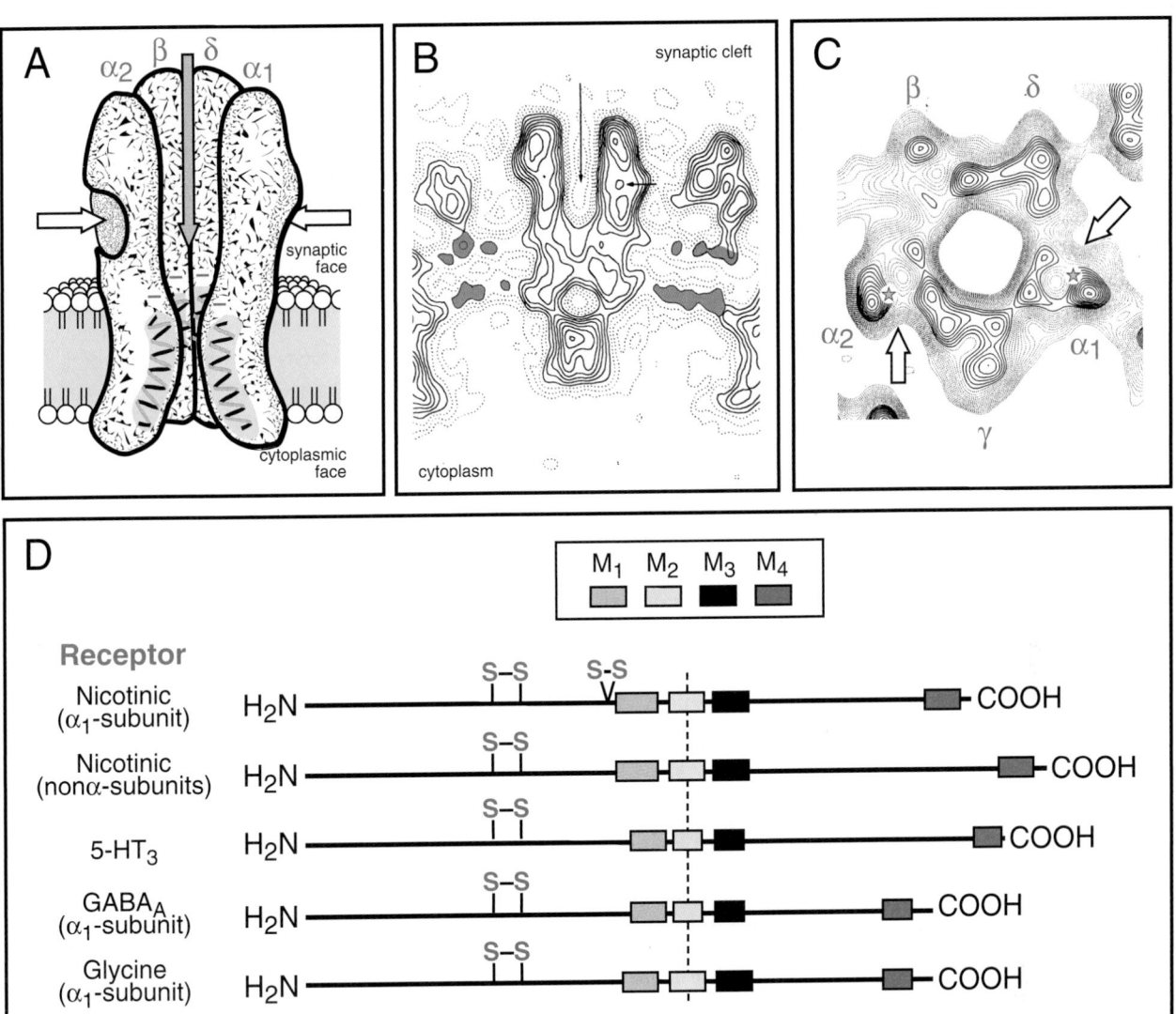

Figure 9–1. Molecular structure of the nicotinic acetylcholine receptor. The structure of the receptor is described in the text.

A. Longitudinal view with the γ subunit removed. The remaining subunits, two copies of α, one of β, and one of δ, are shown to surround an internal channel with an outer vestibule and its constriction located deep in the membrane bilayer region. Spans of α-helices with slightly bowed structures form the perimeter of the channel and come from the M_2 region of the linear sequence (*see* panel **D**). Acetylcholine binding sites, indicated by arrows, are found at the $\alpha\gamma$ and $\alpha\delta$ (not visible) interfaces. Panels **B** and **C** show data on which the structure is based. Panel **D** presents the sequence similarities in ligand-gated ion channel receptors. **B.** Longitudinal view of the electron density of receptor molecules packed in a tubular membrane. Arrows indicate the synaptic surface entry to the pore and agonist site. The additional density in the cytoplasmic region below the receptor arises from an anchoring protein attached to the receptor. **C.** Cross-sectional view of the image reconstructed electron density taken 30 Å above the plane of the membrane. Pseudo-fivefold symmetry is evident. The arrows denote the presumed route of entry of the ligand (ACh) to the binding site shown by the star. $\alpha 1$ and $\alpha 2$ in this panel are identical in sequence; the numeric designations show that there are two copies of the α-subunit in the pentamer. **D.** For each receptor the amino terminal region of about 210 amino acids is found in the extracellular surface. It is then followed by four hydrophobic regions that span the membrane (M_1–M_4), leaving the small carboxyl-terminus on the extracellular surface. The M_2 region is α-helical, and M_2 regions from each subunit of the pentameric receptor line the internal pore of the receptor. Two disulfide loops at positions 128–142 and 192–193 are found in the α-subunit of the nicotinic receptor. The 128–142 motif is conserved in the family of receptors, while the vicinal cysteines at 192 and 193 distinguish α subunits from β, γ, δ, and ε in the nicotinic receptor. (Adapted from Unwin, 1993, with permission.)

from paralysis of skeletal muscles. The preparation of curare was long shrouded in mystery and was entrusted only to tribal witch doctors. Soon after the discovery of the American continent, Sir Walter Raleigh and other early explorers and botanists became interested in curare, and late in the sixteenth century samples of the native preparations were brought to Europe. Following the pioneering work of the scientist/explorer von Humboldt in 1805, the botanical sources of curare became the object of much field search. The curares from eastern Amazonia come from *Strychnos* species. These and other South American species of *Strychnos* examined contain chiefly quaternary neuromuscular blocking alkaloids, whereas the Asiatic, African, and Australian species nearly all contain tertiary, strychnine-like alkaloids.

Curare was the important tool that Claude Bernard used to demonstrate a locus of drug action at or near the nerve terminations of muscle (Bernard, 1856). The modern clinical use of curare apparently dates from 1932, when West employed highly purified fractions in patients with tetanus and spastic disorders.

Research on curare was greatly accelerated by the work of Gill (1940), who, after prolonged and intimate study of the native methods of preparing curare, brought to the United States a sufficient amount of the authentic drug to permit chemical and pharmacological investigations. The first trial of curare for promoting muscular relaxation in general anesthesia was reported by Griffith and Johnson (1942).

Details of the fascinating history of curare, its nomenclature, and the chemical identification of the curare alkaloids are presented in McIntyre, 1947, and Bovet, 1972, and *previous editions* of this textbook.

The essential structure of tubocurarine was established by King in 1935 (Figure 9–2). A synthetic derivative, metocurine (formerly called dimethyl tubocurarine), contains three additional methyl groups, one of which quaternizes the second nitrogen; the other two form methyl ethers at the phenolic hydroxyl groups. This compound possesses two to three times the potency of tubocurarine in human beings.

The most potent of all curare alkaloids are the toxiferines, obtained from *Strychnos toxifera*. A semisynthetic derivative, alcuronium chloride (*N,N'*-diallylnortoxiferinium dichloride), was in wide use clinically in Europe and elsewhere. The seeds of the trees and shrubs of the genus *Erythrina*, widely distributed in tropical and subtropical areas, contain erythroidines that possess curare-like activity.

Gallamine is one of a series of synthetic substitutes for curare described by Bovet and coworkers in 1949 (*see* review by Bovet, 1972). Early structure–activity studies led to the development of the polymethylene *bis*-trimethylammonium series (referred to as the *methonium compounds*) (Barlow and Ing, 1948; Paton and Zaimis, 1952). The most potent agent at the neuromuscular junction was found when the chain contained ten carbon atoms [decamethonium (C10), *see* Figure 9–2]. The member of the series containing six carbon atoms in the chain—hexamethonium (C6)—was found to be essentially devoid of neuromuscular blocking activity but is particularly effective as a ganglionic blocking agent (*see* below).

In 1949, the curariform action of succinylcholine was described, and its clinical application for relaxation of short duration soon followed (*see* Dorkins, 1982).

Classification and Chemical Properties of Neuromuscular Blocking Agents

At present, only a single depolarizing agent, *succinylcholine,* is in general clinical use, whereas multiple competitive or nondepolarizing agents are available (*see* Figure 9–2). Therapeutic selection should be based on achieving a pharmacokinetic profile consistent with the duration of the interventional procedure and minimizing cardiovascular compromise or other side effects (*see* Table 9–1). Two general classifications are useful, since they prove helpful in distinguishing side effects and pharmacokinetic behavior. The first relates to the duration of drug action, and these agents are categorized as long-, intermediate-, and short-acting. The persistent blockade and difficulty in complete reversal after surgery with *d-tubocurarine, metocurine, pancuronium,* and *doxacurium* led to the development of *vecuronium* and *atracurium,* agents of intermediate duration. This was followed by the development of a short-acting agent, *mivacurium.* Often, the long-acting agents are the more potent, requiring the use of low concentrations. The necessity of administering these agents in low concentrations delays their onset. *Rocuronium* and *rapacuronium* are agents of intermediate duration but of rapid onset and lower potency. Their rapid onsets allow them to be used as alternatives to succinylcholine in relaxing the laryngeal and jaw muscles to facilitate tracheal intubation (Bevan, 1994; Savarese *et al.,* 2000).

The second classification is derived from the chemical nature of the agents and includes the natural alkaloids or their congeners, the ammonio steroids, and the benzylisoquinolines (Table 9–1). The natural alkaloid, *d*-tubocurarine, and semisynthetic alkaloid, alcuronium, while of historical importance, seldom are used. Apart from a shorter duration of action, the newer agents exhibit greatly diminished frequency of side effects, chief of which are ganglionic blockade, block of vagal responses, and histamine release. Metocurine shows diminished histamine release and ganglionic blockade when compared with *d*-tubocurarine, but it is not devoid of these side effects. The prototype ammonio steroid, pancuronium, shows virtually no histamine release; however, it blocks muscarinic receptors, and this antagonism primarily is manifested in vagal blockade and tachycardia. Tachycardia is eliminated in the newer ammonio steroids: vecuronium, rocuronium, rapacuronium, and pipecuronium.

The benzylisoquinolines appear to be devoid of vagolytic and ganglionic blocking actions but still show

Competitive Agents

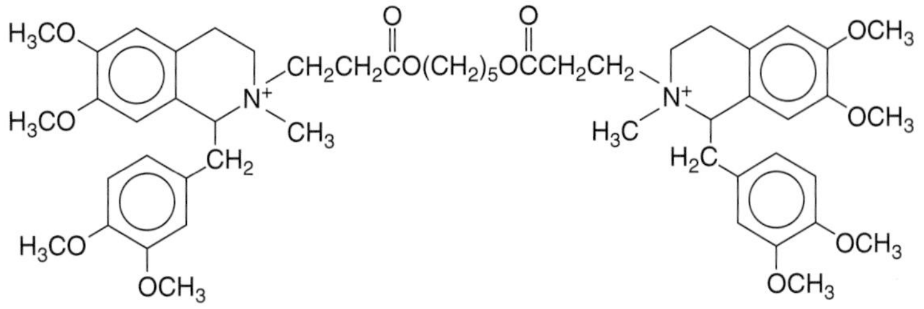

ATRACURIUM

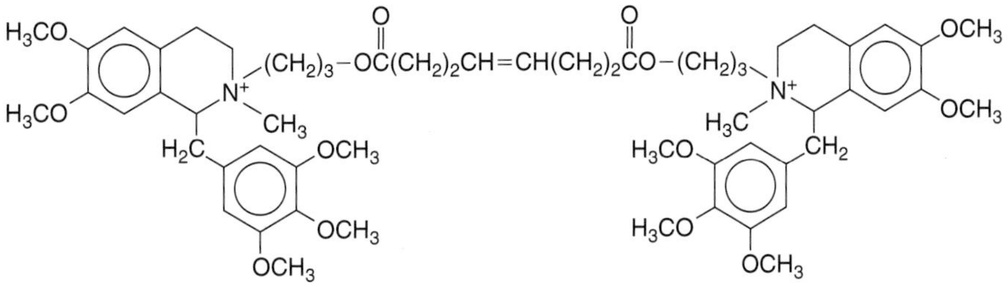

MIVACURIUM

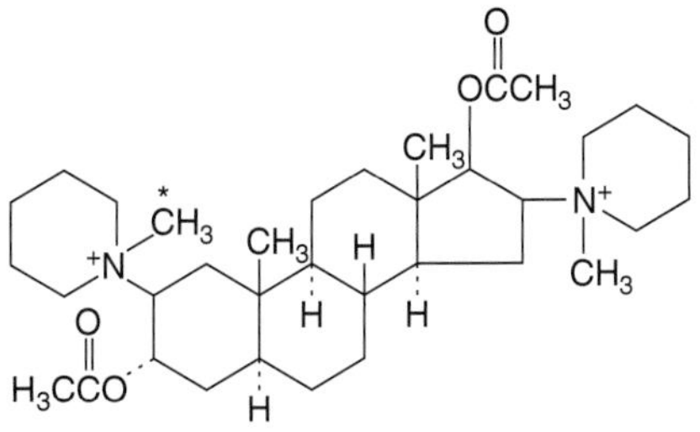

PANCURONIUM

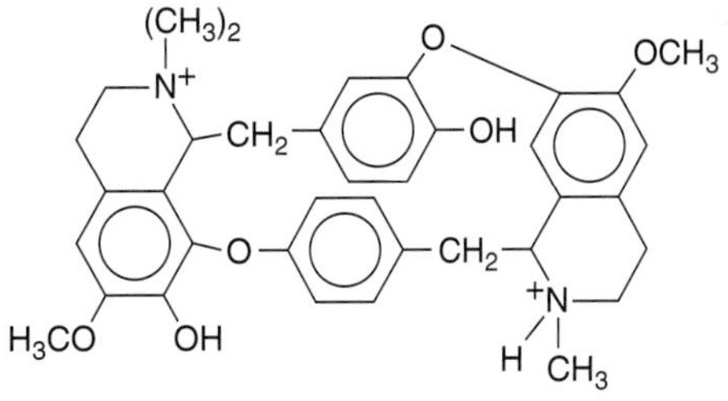

TUBOCURARINE

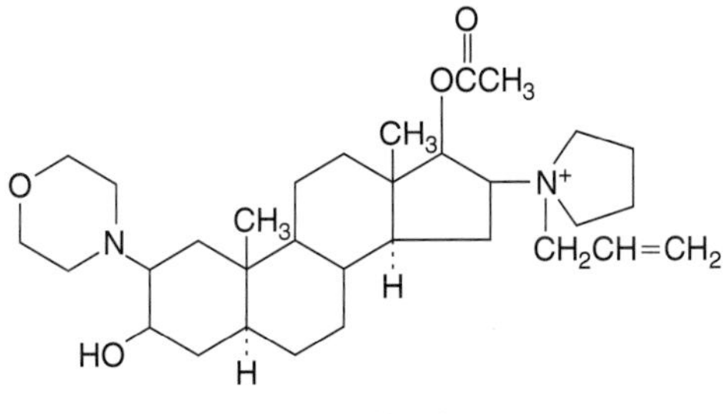

ROCURONIUM

Depolarizing Agents

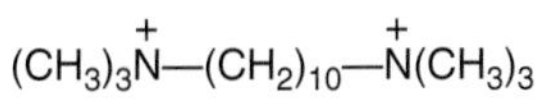

DECAMETHONIUM

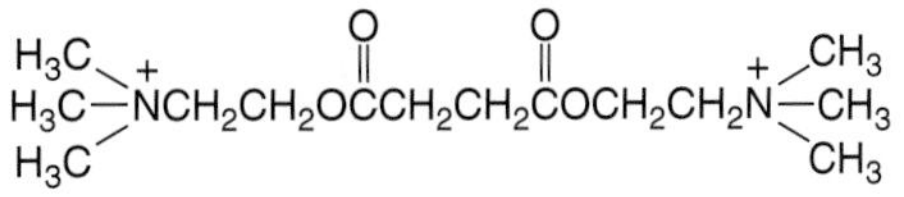

SUCCINYLCHOLINE

*Figure 9–2. Structural formulas of major neuromuscular blocking agents. (*The methyl group is absent in vecuronium.)*

Table 9–1

Classification of Neuromuscular Blocking Agents

AGENT	CHEMICAL CLASS	PHARMACOLOGICAL PROPERTIES	TIME OF ONSET, min	CLINICAL DURATION, min	MODE OF ELIMINATION
Succinylcholine (ANECTINE, others)	Dicholine ester	Ultrashort duration; depolarizing	1–1.5	5–8	Hydrolysis by plasma cholinesterases
d-Tubocurarine	Natural alkaloid (cyclic benzylisoquinoline)	Long duration; competitive	4–6	80–120	Renal elimination; liver clearance
Atracurium (TRACRIUM)	Benzylisoquinoline	Intermediate duration; competitive	2–4	30–60	Hofmann degradation; hydrolysis by plasma esterases; renal elimination
Doxacurium (NUROMAX)	Benzylisoquinoline	Long duration; competitive	4–6	90–120	Renal elimination
Mivacurium (MIVACRON)	Benzylisoquinoline	Short duration; competitive	2–4	12–18	Hydrolysis by plasma cholinesterases
Pancuronium (PAVULON)	Ammonio steroid	Long duration; competitive	4–6	120–180	Renal elimination
Pipecuronium (ARDUAN)	Ammonio steroid	Long duration; competitive	2–4	80–100	Renal elimination; liver metabolism and clearance
Rapacuronium (RAPLON)	Ammonio steroid	Intermediate duration; competitive	1–2	15–30	Liver metabolism and clearance
Rocuronium (ZEMURON)	Ammonio steroid	Intermediate duration; competitive	1–2	30–60	Liver metabolism
Vecuronium (NORCURON)	Ammonio steroid	Intermediate duration; competitive	2–4	60–90	Liver metabolism and clearance; renal elimination

a slight propensity for release of histamine. The unusual metabolism of the prototype compound, atracurium, and its newer congener *mivacurium* confers special indications for use of these compounds. For example, atracurium's disappearance from the body depends on hydrolysis of the ester moiety by plasma esterases and by a spontaneous or Hofmann degradation (cleavage of the *N*-alkyl portion in the benzylisoquinoline). Hence, two routes for degradation are available, both of which remain functional in renal failure. Mivacurium is extremely sensitive

to cholinesterase catalysis, therein accounting for its short duration of action.

Structure–Activity Relationships. Several structural features distinguish competitive and depolarizing neuromuscular blocking agents. The competitive agents are relatively bulky, rigid molecules (*e.g.,* tubocurarine, the toxiferines, the benzylisoquinolines, and the ammonio steroids), whereas the depolarizing agents (*e.g.,* decamethonium, succinylcholine) generally have a more flexible structure that enables free bond rotation (*see* Figure 9–2; *see also* Bovet, 1972). While the distance between quaternary groups in the flexible depolarizing agents can vary up to the limit of the maximal bond distance (1.45 nm for decamethonium), the distance for the rigid competitive blockers is typically 1.0 ± 0.1 nm. *l*-Tubocurarine is considerably less potent than *d*-tubocurarine. While the two enantiomers have similar internitrogen distances, the *d*-isomer has all of the hydrophilic groups localized uniquely to one surface.

Pharmacological Properties

Skeletal Muscle.   A localized paralytic action of curare was first described by Claude Bernard in the 1850s. That the site of action of *d*-tubocurarine and other competitive blocking agents was the motor end plate was subsequently established by modern techniques, including fluorescence and electron microscopy, microiontophoretic application of drugs, patch–clamp analysis of single channels, and intracellular recording. In brief, competitive antagonists combine with the nicotinic acetylcholine receptor at the postjunctional membrane and thereby competitively block the binding of ACh. When the drug is applied directly to the end plate of a single isolated muscle fiber, the muscle cell becomes insensitive to motor-nerve impulses and to directly applied ACh; however, the end-plate region and the remainder of the muscle fiber membrane retain their normal sensitivity to K^+ depolarization, and the muscle fiber still responds to direct electrical stimulation.

To analyze the action of antagonists at the neuromuscular junction further, it is first important to consider certain details of receptor activation by acetylcholine. The steps involved in the release of ACh by the nerve action potential, the development of miniature end-plate potentials (MEPPs), their summation to form a postjunctional end-plate potential, the triggering of the muscle action potential, and contraction are described in Chapter 6. Biophysical experimentation has revealed that the fundamental event elicited by acetylcholine or other agonists is an "all-or-none" opening and closing of the individual receptor channels, which gives rise to a square-wave pulse with an average open-channel conductance of 20 to 30 pS and a duration that is exponentially distributed around a time of about 1 millisecond. The *duration* of channel opening is far more dependent on the nature of the agonist than is the magnitude of the open-channel conductance (*see* Sakmann, 1992).

The influence of increasing concentrations of the competitive antagonist tubocurarine is to diminish progressively the amplitude of the postjunctional end-plate potential. The amplitude of this postjunctional potential may fall to below 70% of its initial value before it is insufficient to initiate the propagated muscle action potential; this provides a safety factor in neuromuscular transmission. Anal-

ysis of the antagonism of tubocurarine on single-channel events shows that, as expected for a competitive antagonist, it reduces the frequency of channel-opening events but does not affect the conductance or duration of opening for a single channel (Katz and Miledi, 1978). At higher concentrations, curare and other competitive antagonists will block the channel directly in a fashion that is noncompetitive with agonists and dependent on membrane potential (Colquhoun *et al.,* 1979).

The decay time of the MEPP is of the same duration as the average lifetime of channel opening (1 to 2 milliseconds). Since the MEPPs are a consequence of the spontaneous release of one or more quanta of ACh ($\sim 10^5$ molecules), individual molecules of ACh released into the synapse have only a transient opportunity to activate the receptor and do not successively rebind to receptors to activate multiple channels before being hydrolyzed by acetylcholinesterase. The concentration of unbound ACh in the synapse from nerve-released ACh diminishes more rapidly than does the decay of the end-plate potential (or current).

If anticholinesterase (anti-ChE) drugs are present, the EPP (or end-plate current) is prolonged up to 25 to 30 milliseconds, which is indicative of the rebinding of transmitter to neighboring receptors before diffusion from the synapse. It is therefore not surprising that anti-ChE agents and tubocurarine act in opposing directions, since increasing the duration of ACh retained in the synapse should favor occupation of the receptor by transmitter and displace tubocurarine.

Simultaneous binding by two agonist molecules at the respective $\alpha\gamma$ and $\alpha\delta$ subunit interfaces of the receptor is required for activation. Activation shows positive cooperativity and thus occurs over a narrow range of concentrations (Sine and Claudio, 1991; Changeux and Edelstein, 1998). Although two competitive antagonist or snake α-toxin molecules can bind to each receptor molecule at the agonist sites, the binding of one molecule of antagonist to each receptor is sufficient to render it nonfunctional (*see* Taylor *et al.,* 1983).

The depolarizing agents, such as succinylcholine and decamethonium, act by a different mechanism. Their initial action is to depolarize the membrane by opening channels in the same manner as ACh. However, they persist for longer durations at the neuromuscular junction, primarily because of their resistance to acetylcholinesterase. The depolarization thus is longer lasting, resulting in a brief period of repetitive excitation that may elicit transient muscle fasciculations. The initial phase is followed by block of neuromuscular transmission and flaccid paralysis. This arises because released acetylcholine binds to receptors on an already depolarized end plate. It is the *change* in end-plate potential elicited by the transient increases in ACh that triggers action potentials. An end plate depolarized from -80 mV to -55 mV by a depolarizing blocking agent is resistant to further depolarization by acetylcholine. In human beings, a sequence of repetitive excitation (fasciculations) followed by block of

Table 9–2

Comparison of Competitive (*d*-Tubocurarine) and Depolarizing (Decamethonium) Blocking Agents

	d-TUBOCURARINE	DECAMETHONIUM
Effect of *d*-tubocurarine chloride administered previously	Additive	Antagonistic
Effect of decamethonium administered previously	No effect, or antagonistic	Some tachyphylaxis; but may be additive
Effect on block of anticholinesterase agents	Reversal of block	No antagonism
Effect on motor end-plate	Elevated threshold to acetylcholine; no depolarization	Partial, persisting depolarization
Initial excitatory effect on striated muscle	None	Transient fasciculations
Character of muscle response to indirect tetanic stimulation during *partial* block	Poorly sustained contraction	Well-sustained contraction

SOURCE: Based on data in Paton and Zaimis, 1952; Zaimis, 1976.

transmission and neuromuscular paralysis is elicited by depolarizing agents; however, this sequence is influenced by such factors as the anesthetic agent used concurrently, the type of muscle, and the rate of drug administration. The different characteristics of depolarization and competitive blockade are listed in Table 9–2.

In other animal species and occasionally in human beings, decamethonium and succinylcholine produce a blockade that has unique features, some of which combine those of the depolarizing and the competitive agents; Zaimis (1976) has termed this type of action a *"dual" mechanism*. In such cases, the depolarizing agents produce initially the characteristic fasciculations and potentiation of the maximal twitch, followed by the rapid onset of neuromuscular block; this block is potentiated by anti-ChE agents. However, following the onset of blockade, there is a poorly sustained response to tetanic stimulation of the motor nerve, intensification of the block by tubocurarine, and usual reversal by anti-ChE agents.

The dual action of the depolarizing blocking agents also is seen in intracellular recordings of membrane potential; when agonist is applied continuously, the initial depolarization is followed by a gradual repolarization. The second phase, repolarization, resembles receptor desensitization (Katz and Thesleff, 1957).

Under clinical conditions, with increasing concentrations of succinylcholine and in time, the block may convert slowly from a depolarizing to a nondepolarizing type, termed *phase I* and *phase II* block (Durant and Katz, 1982). The pattern of neuromuscular blockade produced by depolarizing drugs in anesthetized patients appears to depend, in part, on the anesthetic; fluorinated hydrocarbons may be more apt to predispose the motor end plate to nondepolarization blockade after prolonged use of succinylcholine or decamethonium (*see* Zaimis, 1976;

Fogdall and Miller, 1975). The characteristics of phase I and phase II block are shown in Table 9–3.

During the initial phase of application, depolarizing agents produce channel opening, which can be measured by the statistical analysis of fluctuation of muscle EPPs. The probability of channel opening associated with the binding of drug to the receptor is less with decamethonium than with ACh (Katz and Miledi, 1978). The diminished probability of channel opening would serve to classify decamethonium as a partial agonist at the end plate. Higher concentrations of decamethonium also block the channel directly and thereby interfere with ion permeability (Adams and Sakmann, 1978).

Although the observed fasciculations also may result from stimulation of the prejunctional motor-nerve terminal by the depolarizing agent, giving rise to stimulation of the motor unit in an antidromic fashion, the primary site of action of both competitive and depolarizing blocking agents is the postjunctional membrane. Presynaptic actions of the competitive agents may become significant upon repetitive, high-frequency stimulation, since prejunctional nicotinic receptors may be involved in the mobilization of ACh for release from the nerve terminal (Bowman *et al.*, 1990; Van der Kloot and Molgo, 1994).

Many drugs and toxins block neuromuscular transmission by other mechanisms, such as interference with the synthesis or release of ACh (*see* Van der Kloot and Molgo, 1994; *see also* Chapter 6), but most of these agents are not employed clinically for this purpose. One exception is *botulinum toxin*, which has been administered locally into muscles of the orbit in the management of ocular blepharospasm and strabismus and has been used to control other muscle spasms and to facilitate facial muscle relaxation (*see* Chapters 6 and 66). This toxin also has been injected into the lower esophageal sphincter to treat achalasia (*see* Chapter 38). Another exception is *dantrolene*, which blocks release of Ca^{2+} from the sarcoplasmic reticulum and is used in the treatment of malignant hyperthermia (*see*

Table 9–3

Clinical Responses and Monitoring of Phase I and Phase II Neuromuscular Blockade by Succinylcholine Infusion

RESPONSE	PHASE I	PHASE II
End-plate membrane potential	Depolarized to −55mV	Repolarization towards −80 mV
Onset	Immediate	Slow transition
Dose-dependence	Lower	Ususally higher or follows prolonged infusion
Recovery	Rapid	More prolonged
Train of four and tetanic stimulation	No fade	Fade[†]
Acetylcholinesterase inhibition	Augments	Reverses or antagonizes
Muscle response	Fasciculations → flaccid paralysis	Flaccid paralysis

[†] Posttetanic potentiation follows fade.

below). The sites of action and interrelationship of several agents that serve as pharmacological tools are shown in Figure 9–3.

Sequence and Characteristics of Paralysis. When an appropriate dose of a competitive blocking agent is injected intravenously in human beings, motor weakness gives way to a total flaccid paralysis. Small, rapidly moving muscles such as those of the eyes, jaw, and larynx relax before those of the limbs and trunk. Ultimately the intercostal muscles and finally the diaphragm are paralyzed, and respiration then ceases. Recovery of muscles usually occurs in the reverse order to that of their paralysis, and thus the diaphragm ordinarily is the first muscle to regain function (*see* Feldman and Fauvel, 1994; Savarese *et al.,* 2000).

After a single intravenous dose of 10 to 30 mg of succinylcholine, muscle fasciculations, particularly over the chest and abdomen, occur briefly; then relaxation occurs within 1 minute, becomes maximal within 2 minutes, and disappears as a rule within 5 minutes. Transient apnea usually occurs at the time of maximal effect. Muscle relaxation of longer duration is achieved by continuous intravenous infusion. After infusion is discontinued, the effects of the drug usually disappear rapidly because of its rapid hydrolysis catalyzed by the butyrylcholinesterase of the plasma and liver. Muscle soreness may follow the administration of succinylcholine. Small prior doses of competitive blocking agents have been employed to minimize fasciculations and muscle pain caused by succinylcholine. However, this procedure is controversial, since it increases the requirement for the depolarizing drug.

During prolonged depolarization, muscle cells may lose significant quantities of K^+ and gain Na^+, Cl^-, and Ca^{2+}. In patients in whom there has been extensive injury to soft tissues, the efflux of K^+ following continued administration of succinylcholine can be life-threatening. The life-threatening complications of succinylcholine-induced hyperkalemia are discussed later in this chapter, but it is important to stress that there are many conditions for which succinylcholine administration is contraindicated or must be undertaken with great caution. The change in the nature of the blockade produced by succinylcholine (from phase I to phase II) presents an additional complication with long-term infusions.

Central Nervous System. Tubocurarine and other quaternary neuromuscular blocking agents are virtually devoid of central effects following the intravenous administration of ordinary clinical doses because of their inability to penetrate the blood–brain barrier.

The most decisive experiment performed to resolve whether or not curare significantly affects central functions in the dose range used clinically was that of Smith and associates (1947). Smith (an anesthesiologist) permitted himself to receive intravenously two and one-half times the amount of tubocurarine necessary for paralysis of all skeletal muscles. Adequate respiratory exchange was maintained by artificial respiration. At no time was there any evidence of lapse of consciousness, clouding of sensorium, analgesia, or disturbance of special senses. Despite adequate artificially controlled respiration, "shortness of breath" was experienced, and the accumulation of unswallowed saliva in the pharynx caused the sensation of choking. The experience was decidedly unpleasant. It was concluded that

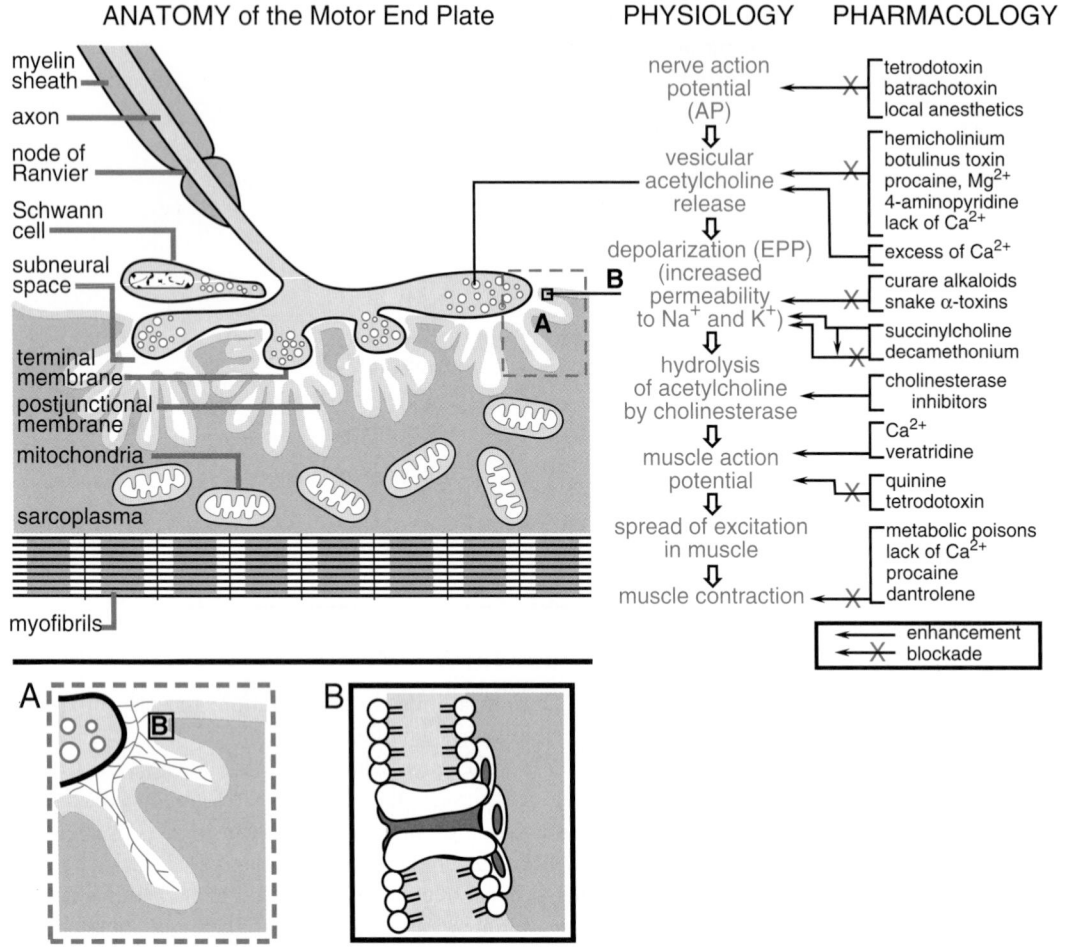

Figure 9–3. Sites of action of agents at the neuromuscular junction and adjacent structures.

The anatomy of the motor end plate, shown at the left, and the sequence of events from liberation of acetylcholine (ACh) by the nerve action potential (AP) to contraction of the muscle fiber, indicated by the middle column, are described in some detail in Chapter 6. The modification of these processes by various agents is shown on the right; an arrow marked with an X indicates inhibition or block; an unmarked arrow indicates enhancement or activation. The insets are enlargements of the indicated structures. The highest magnification depicts the receptor in the bilayer of the postsynaptic membrane. A more detailed view of the receptor is shown in Figure 9–1.

tubocurarine given intravenously even in large doses has no significant central stimulant, depressant, or analgesic effects, and that its sole action in anesthesia is the peripheral paralytic effect on skeletal muscle.

Autonomic Ganglia and Muscarinic Sites. Neuromuscular blocking agents show variable potencies in producing ganglionic blockade. Just as at the motor end plate, ganglionic blockade by tubocurarine and other stabilizing drugs is reversed or antagonized by anti-ChE agents.

At the doses of tubocurarine used clinically, partial blockade probably is produced, both at autonomic ganglia

and at the adrenal medulla, which results in a fall in blood pressure and tachycardia. Pancuronium and metocurine show less ganglionic blockade at common clinical doses. Atracurium, vecuronium, doxacurium, pipecuronium, mivacurium, and rocuronium are even more selective (Pollard, 1994; Savarese *et al.,* 2000). The maintenance of cardiovascular reflex responses usually is desired during anesthesia. Pancuronium has a vagolytic action, presumably from blockade of muscarinic receptors. This leads to tachycardia.

Of the depolarizing agents, succinylcholine at doses causing neuromuscular relaxation rarely causes effects attributable to ganglionic blockade. However, cardiovascular effects are sometimes observed that are probably due to the successive stimulation of vagal ganglia (manifested by bradycardia) and of sympathetic ganglia (resulting in hypertension and tachycardia).

Histamine Release.   Tubocurarine produces typical histamine-like wheals when injected intracutaneously or intraarterially in human beings, and certain clinical responses to tubocurarine (bronchospasm, hypotension, excessive bronchial and salivary secretion) appear to be caused by the release of histamine. Metocurine, succinylcholine, mivacurium, doxacurium, and atracurium also cause histamine release, but to a lesser extent unless administered rapidly. The ammonio steroids, pancuronium, vecuronium, pipecuronium, and rocuronium, have even less tendency to release histamine after intradermal or systemic injection (Basta, 1992; Watkins, 1994). Histamine release typically is a direct action of the muscle relaxant on the mast cell rather than IgE-mediated anaphylaxis (Watkins, 1994).

Actions of Neuromuscular Blocking Agents with Life-Threatening Implications.   The depolarizing agents can release K^+ rapidly from intracellular sites; this may be a factor in production of the prolonged apnea that has been noted in patients who receive these drugs while in electrolyte imbalance (Dripps, 1976). As indicated above, succinylcholine-induced hyperkalemia is a life-threatening complication of the drug. For example, such alterations in the distribution of K^+ are of particular concern in patients with congestive heart failure who are receiving digitalis or diuretics. For the same reason, caution should be used or depolarizing blocking agents should be avoided in patients with extensive soft-tissue trauma or burns. A higher dose of a competitive blocking agent often is indicated in these patients. In addition, succinylcholine administration is contraindicated or should be given with great caution in patients with nontraumatic rhabdomyolysis, ocular lacerations, spinal cord injuries with paraplegia or quadriplegia, or with muscular dystrophies. Succinylcholine no longer is indicated for children 8 years old and younger unless emergency intubation or securing an airway is necessary. Hyperkalemia, rhabdomyolysis, and cardiac arrest have been reported. A subclinical dystrophy frequently is associated with these adverse responses (Savarese *et al.*, 2000). Neonates also may have an enhanced sensitivity to competitive neuromuscular blocking agents.

Synergisms and Antagonisms.   The interactions between the competitive and depolarizing neuromuscular blocking agents already have been considered. From a clinical viewpoint, the most important pharmacological interactions of these drugs are with certain general anesthetics, certain antibiotics, Ca^{2+} channel blockers, and anti-ChE compounds.

Since the anti-ChE agents *neostigmine, pyridostigmine,* and *edrophonium* preserve endogenous ACh and also act directly on the neuromuscular junction, they can be used in the treatment of overdosage with competitive blocking agents. Similarly, upon completion of the surgical procedure many anesthesiologists employ neostigmine or edrophonium to reverse and decrease the duration of competitive neuromuscular blockade. Succinylcholine should never be administered after reversal of competitive blockade with neostigmine; in this circumstance a prolonged and intense blockade often is achieved. A muscarinic antagonist (*atropine* or *glycopyrrolate*) is used concomitantly to prevent stimulation of muscarinic receptors and thereby avoid slowing of the heart rate. The anti-ChE agents, however, are synergistic with the depolarizing blocking agents, particularly in their initial phase of action. Since they will not reverse depolarizing neuromuscular blockade and, in fact, can enhance it, the distinction in the type of neuromuscular blocking agent must be clear.

Many *inhalational anesthetics* (*e.g.,* halothane, isoflurane, and enflurane) exert a stabilizing effect on the postjunctional membrane and therefore act synergistically with the competitive blocking agents. Consequently, when such blocking drugs are used for muscle relaxation as adjuncts to these anesthetics, their doses should be reduced (*see* Fogdall and Miller, 1975).

Aminoglycoside antibiotics produce neuromuscular blockade by inhibiting ACh release from the preganglionic terminal (through competition with Ca^{2+}) and to a lesser extent by noncompetitively blocking the receptor. The blockade is antagonized by calcium salts, but only inconsistently by anti-ChE agents (*see* Chapter 46). The *tetracycline antibiotics* also can produce neuromuscular blockade, possibly by chelation of Ca^{2+}. Additional antibiotics that have neuromuscular blocking action, through both presynaptic and postsynaptic actions, include polymyxin B, colistin, clindamycin, and lincomycin (*see* Pollard, 1994). Ca^{2+} *channel blockers* enhance neuromuscular blockade produced by both competitive and depolarizing antagonists. It is not clear whether this is a result of a diminution of Ca^{2+}-dependent release of transmitter from the nerve ending or is a postsynaptic action. When neuromuscular blocking agents are administered to patients receiving these agents, dose adjustments should be considered; if recovery of spontaneous respiration is delayed, Ca^{2+} salts may facilitate recovery.

Miscellaneous drugs that may have significant interactions with either competitive or depolarizing neuromuscular blocking agents include *trimethaphan, opioid analgesics, procaine, lidocaine, quinidine, phenelzine, phenytoin, propranolol, magnesium salts, corticosteroids, digitalis glycosides, chloroquine, catecholamines,* and *diuretics* (*see* Zaimis, 1976; Pollard, 1994; Savarese *et al.*, 2000).

Toxicology. The important untoward responses of the neuromuscular blocking agents include prolonged apnea, cardiovascular collapse, and those resulting from histamine release.

Failure of respiration to become adequate in the postoperative period may not always be due directly to the drug. An obstruction of the airway, decreased arterial carbon dioxide tension secondary to hyperventilation during the operative procedure, or the neuromuscular depressant effect of excessive amounts of neostigmine used to reverse the action of the competitive blocking drugs also may be implicated. Directly related factors may include alterations in body temperature; electrolyte imbalance, particularly of K^+ (discussed earlier); low plasma butyrylcholinesterase levels, resulting in a reduction in the rate of destruction of succinylcholine; the presence of latent myasthenia gravis or of malignant disease such as small-cell carcinoma of the bronchus (myasthenic syndrome); reduced blood flow to skeletal muscles, causing delayed removal of the blocking drugs; and decreased elimination of the muscle relaxants secondary to reduced renal function. Great care should be taken when administering these agents to dehydrated or severely ill patients.

Malignant Hyperthermia. Malignant hyperthermia is a potentially life-threatening event triggered by the administration of certain anesthetics and neuromuscular blocking agents. The clinical features include contracture, rigidity, and heat production from skeletal muscle resulting in severe hyperthermia, accelerated muscle metabolism, metabolic acidosis, and tachycardia. Uncontrolled release of Ca^{2+} from the sarcoplasmic reticulum of skeletal muscle is the initiating event. Although the halogenated hydrocarbon anesthetics (halothane, isoflurane, and sevoflurane) and succinylcholine alone have been reported to precipitate the response, most of the incidents arise from the combination of depolarizing blocking agent and anesthetic. Susceptibility to malignant hyperthermia, an autosomal dominant trait, is associated with certain congenital myopathies such as *central core disease.* In the majority of cases, however, no clinical signs are visible in the absence of anesthetic intervention.

Determination of susceptibility is made with an *in vitro* contracture test (IVCT) on a fresh biopsy of skeletal muscle, where contractures in the presence of various concentrations of halothane and caffeine are measured. In over 50% of the families, a linkage is found between the IVCT phenotype and a mutation in the gene (*RyR-1*) encoding the skeletal muscle ryanodine receptor (RYR-1). Over 20 mutations in a region of the gene that encodes the cytoplasmic face of the receptor have been described. Other loci have been identified on the L-type Ca^{2+} channel (voltage-gated dihydropyridine receptor) and on other associated proteins or channel subunits. The large size of *RyR-1* and the genetic heterogeneity of the condition have precluded the development of a genotypic determination for malignant hyperthermia (Hopkins, 2000; Jurkat-Rott *et al.,* 2000).

Current treatment entails an intravenous administration of *dantrolene* (DANTRIUM), which blocks Ca^{2+} release and the metabolic sequelae. Dantrolene inhibits Ca^{2+} release from the sarcoplasmic reticulum of skeletal muscle by limiting the capacity of Ca^{2+} and calmodulin to activate RYR-1 (Fruen *et al.,* 1997). RYR-1 and the L-type Ca^{2+} channel are juxtaposed to associate at a triadic junction formed between the T-tubule and sarcoplasmic reticulum. The L-type channel with its T-tubular location serves as the voltage sensor receiving the depolarizing activation signal. The intimate coupling of the two proteins at the triad, along with a host of modulatory proteins in the two organelles and the surrounding cytoplasm, regulate the release of and response to Ca^{2+} (Lehmann-Horn and Jurkat-Rott, 1999).

Rapid cooling, inhalation of 100% oxygen, and control of acidosis should be considered adjunct therapy in malignant hyperthermia. Declining fatality rates for malignant hyperthermia relate to anesthesiologists' awareness of the condition and the efficacy of dantrolene.

Patients with central core disease, so named because of the presence of myofibrillar cores seen upon biopsy of slow-twitch muscle fibers, show muscle weakness in infancy and delayed motor development. These individuals have a high susceptibility to malignant hyperthermia with the combination of an anesthetic and a depolarizing neuromuscular blocker. Central core disease has five allelic variants of *RyR-1* in common with malignant hyperthermia. Patients with other muscle syndromes or dystonias also have an increased frequency of contracture and hyperthermia in the anesthesia setting. Succinylcholine in susceptible individuals also induces *masseter muscle rigidity,* which may complicate endotracheal tube insertion and airway management. This condition has been correlated with a mutation in the gene encoding the α subunit of the voltage-sensitive Na^+ channel (Vita *et al.,* 1995). Masseter muscle rigidity can be an early sign of the onset of malignant hyperthermia if the anesthetic combination is continued (Hopkins, 2000).

Respiratory Paralysis. Treatment of respiratory paralysis arising from an adverse reaction or overdose of a neuromuscular blocking agent should be by positive-pressure artificial respiration with oxygen and maintenance of a patent airway until the recovery of normal respiration is assured. With the competitive blocking agents, this may be hastened by the administration of *neostigmine methylsulfate* (0.5 to 2 mg, intravenously) or *edrophonium* (10 mg, intravenously, repeated as required) (Watkins, 1994).

Interventional Strategies for Other Toxic Effects. Neostigmine antagonizes only the skeletal muscular blocking action of the competitive blocking agents effectively, and it may aggravate such side effects as hypotension or induce bronchospasm. In such circumstances, *sympathomimetic amines* may be given to support the blood pressure. *Atropine* or *glycopyrrolate* is administered to counteract muscarinic stimulation. *Antihistamines* are definitely beneficial to counteract the responses that follow the release of histamine, particularly when administered before the neuromuscular blocking agent.

Absorption, Fate, and Excretion. Quaternary ammonium neuromuscular blocking agents are very poorly and irregularly absorbed from the gastrointestinal tract. This fact was well known to the South American Indians, who ate with impunity the flesh of game killed with curare-poisoned arrows. Absorption is quite adequate from intramuscular sites. Rapid onset is achieved with intravenous administration. The more potent agents, of course, must be given in lower concentrations, and diffusional requirements slow their rate of onset.

When long-acting, competitive blocking agents, such as *d*-tubocurarine and pancuronium, are administered, blockade may diminish after 30 minutes owing to redistribution of the drug, yet residual blockade and plasma levels of the drug persist for longer periods. Subsequent doses show diminished redistribution. Long-acting agents may accumulate with multiple doses.

The ammonio steroids contain ester groups that are hydrolyzed in the liver. Typically, the metabolites have about one-half of the activity of the parent compound and contribute to the total relaxation profile. Ammonio steroids of intermediate duration of action, such as vecuronium, rocuronium, and rapacuronium (*see* Table 9–1), are more rapidly cleared by the liver than are pancuronium and pipecuronium. The more rapid offset of neuromuscular blockade with compounds of intermediate duration argues for sequential dosing of these agents, rather than administering a single dose of a long-duration neuromuscular blocking agent (Savarese *et al.*, 2000).

Atracurium is converted to less-active metabolites by plasma esterases and spontaneous degradation. These alternative routes of metabolism are responsible for atracurium not exhibiting an increase in half-life in patients with compromised renal function. Hence, it becomes the agent of choice under these conditions (Hunter, 1994). Mivacurium shows an even greater susceptibility to butyryl-

cholinesterase catalysis, thus conferring to it the shortest duration among the nondepolarizing blockers.

The extremely brief duration of action of succinylcholine also is due largely to its rapid hydrolysis by the butyrylcholinesterase of liver and plasma. Among the occasional patients who exhibit prolonged apnea following the administration of succinylcholine or mivacurium, most have an atypical plasma cholinesterase or a deficiency of the enzyme, due to allelic variations (Pantuck, 1993; Primo-Parmo *et al.*, 1996), hepatic or renal disease, or a nutritional disturbance; however, in some the enzymatic activity in plasma is normal (Whittaker, 1986).

Therapeutic Uses

The main clinical use of the neuromuscular blocking agents is as an adjuvant in surgical anesthesia to obtain relaxation of skeletal muscle, particularly of the abdominal wall, so that operative manipulations are facilitated. With muscle relaxation no longer dependent upon the depth of general anesthesia, a much lighter level of anesthesia suffices. This situation is of obvious advantage, since the risk of respiratory and cardiovascular depression is minimized. Moreover, the postanesthetic recovery period is shortened.

These considerations notwithstanding, neuromuscular blocking agents cannot be used to substitute for inadequate depth of anesthesia in the surgical planes. Otherwise, a risk of reflex responses to painful stimuli and conscious recall may occur. Muscle relaxation is also of value in various orthopedic procedures, such as the correction of dislocations and the alignment of fractures. Neuromuscular blocking agents of short duration often are used to facilitate intubation with an endotracheal tube and have been used to facilitate laryngoscopy, bronchoscopy, and esophagoscopy in combination with a general anesthetic agent.

Neuromuscular blocking agents are administered parenterally and nearly always intravenously. As potentially hazardous drugs, they should be administered to patients only by anesthesiologists and other clinicians who have had extensive training in their use and in a setting where facilities for respiratory and cardiovascular resuscitation are immediately at hand. Detailed information on dosage and monitoring the extent of muscle relaxation can be found in anesthesiology textbooks (Pollard, 1994; Savarese *et al.*, 2000).

Measurement of Neuromuscular Blockade in Human Beings. Assessment of neuromuscular block usually is performed by stimulation of the ulnar nerve. Responses are monitored from compound action potentials or muscle tension developed in the adductor pollicis (thumb) muscle. Responses to repetitive or tetanic stimuli are most useful for evaluation of blockade of transmission, since individual measurements of twitch tension must be related to control values obtained prior to the administration of drugs. Thus, stimulus schedules such as the "train of four" and the "double burst" or responses to tetanic stimulation are preferred procedures (Waud and Waud, 1972; Drenck *et al.,* 1989). Rates of onset of blockade and recovery are more rapid in the airway musculature (jaw, larynx, and diaphragm) than in the thumb. Hence, tracheal intubation can be performed before onset of complete block at the adductor pollicis, while partial recovery of function of this muscle allows sufficient recovery of respiration for extubation (Savarese *et al.,* 2000). Differences in rates of onset of blockade, recovery from blockade, and intrinsic sensitivity between the stimulated muscle and those of the larynx, abdomen, and diaphragm should be considered.

Use to Prevent Trauma during Electroshock Therapy. Electroconvulsive therapy of psychiatric disorders occasionally is complicated by trauma to the patient; the seizures induced may cause dislocations or fractures. Inasmuch as the muscular component of the convulsion is not essential for benefit from the procedure, neuromuscular blocking agents and thiopental are employed. The combination of the blocking drug, the anesthetic agent, and postictal depression usually results in respiratory depression or temporary apnea. An endotracheal tube and oxygen always should be available. An oropharyngeal airway should be inserted as soon as the jaw muscles relax (after the seizure) and provision made to prevent aspiration of mucus and saliva. Succinylcholine or mivacurium is most often used because of the brevity of relaxation. A cuff may be applied to one extremity to prevent the effects of the drug in that limb; evidence of an effective electroshock is provided by contraction of the group of protected muscles.

Control of Muscle Spasms. Several agents, many of which have rather limited efficacy, have been used to treat spasticity involving the α-motor neuron with the objective of increasing functional capacity and relieving discomfort. Some agents that act in the CNS at either higher centers or the spinal cord are considered in Chapter 22. These include baclofen, the benzodiazepines, and tizandine. Botulinum toxin and dantrolene act peripherally.

The anaerobic bacterium *Clostridium botulinum* produces a family of toxins targeted to presynaptic proteins and that block the release of acetylcholine (ACh) (*see* Chapter 6). Botulinum toxin–A (BOTOX), in blocking ACh release, produces flaccid paralysis of skeletal muscle and diminished activity of parasympathetic and sympathetic cholinergic synapses. Inhibition lasts from several weeks to 3 to 4 months, and restoration of function requires nerve sprouting. Immunoresistance may develop with continued use (Davis and Barnes, 2000).

Originally approved for the treatment of the ocular conditions of strabismus and blepharospasm and for hemifacial spasms, botulinum toxin has received wider use in the treatment of spasms and dystonias such as adductor spasmodic dysphonia, oromandibular dystonia, cervical dystonia, and spasms associated with the lower esophageal sphincter and anal fissures. Its dermatological uses include treatment of hyperhidrosis of the palms and axillae that is resistant to topical and iontophoretic remedies and removal of facial lines associated with excessive nerve stimulation and muscle activity. Treatment involves local intramuscular or intradermal injections (Boni *et al.,* 2000).

In addition to its use in managing an acute attack of malignant hyperthermia (*see* above), dantrolene also has been explored in the treatment of spasticity and hyperreflexia. With its peripheral action, it causes a generalized weakness. As such, its use should be reserved to nonambulatory patients with severe spasticity. Hepatotoxicity has been reported with continued use, requiring liver function tests (Kita and Goodkin, 2000).

GANGLIONIC NEUROTRANSMISSION

Neurotransmission in autonomic ganglia has long been recognized to be a far more complex process than that described by a single neurotransmitter–receptor system; intracellular recordings reveal at least four different changes in potential that can be elicited by stimulation of the preganglionic nerve (Eccles and Libet, 1961; Weight *et al.,* 1979) (Figure 9–4). The primary event involves a rapid depolarization of postsynaptic sites by ACh. The receptors are nicotinic, and the pathway is sensitive to classical blocking agents such as hexamethonium and trimethaphan. Activation of this primary pathway gives rise to an initial excitatory postsynaptic potential (EPSP). This rapid depolarization is due primarily to an inward Na^+ and perhaps Ca^{2+} current through a neuronal type of nicotinic receptor channel. Multiple nicotinic receptor subunits or their mRNAs ($\alpha3$, $\alpha5$, $\alpha7$, $\beta2$, $\beta4$) have been identified in ganglia with $\alpha3$ and $\beta2$ being in abundance.

An action potential is generated in the postganglionic neuron when the initial EPSP attains a critical amplitude. In mammalian sympathetic ganglia *in vivo,* it may be necessary for multiple synapses to be activated before transmission is effective. Discrete end plates with focal localization of receptors do not exist in ganglia; rather, the dendrites and nerve cell bodies contain the receptors.

Iontophoretic application of ACh to the ganglion results in a depolarization with a latency of less than 1 millisecond; this decays over a period of 10 to 50 milliseconds (Ascher *et al.,* 1979). Measurements of single-channel conductances indicate that the characteristics of nicotinic receptor channels of the ganglia and the neuromuscular junction are quite similar.

The secondary events that follow the initial depolarization are insensitive to hexamethonium or other nicotinic antagonists.

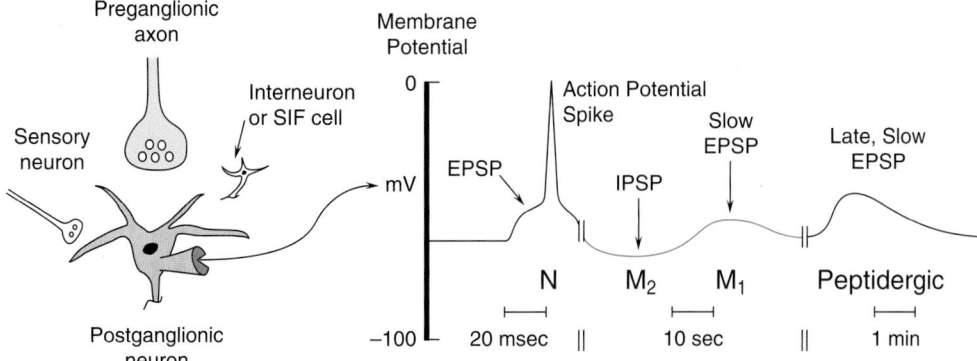

Figure 9–4. Representation of autonomic ganglion cells and the excitatory and inhibitory postsynaptic potentials (EPSP and IPSP) recorded from the postganglionic nerve cell body after stimulation of the preganglionic nerve fiber.

The initial EPSP, if of sufficient magnitude, triggers an action potential spike, which is followed by a slow IPSP, a slow EPSP, and a late, slow EPSP. The slow IPSP and slow EPSP are not seen in all ganglia. The subsequent electrical events are thought not to trigger spikes directly but rather to increase or decrease the probability of a subsequent EPSP reaching a threshold to trigger a spike. Other interneurons, such as catecholamine-containing, small, intensely fluorescent cells, and axon terminals from sensory, afferent neurons also release transmitters and are thought to influence the slow potentials of the postganglionic neuron. A variety of cholinergic, peptidergic, adrenergic, and amino acid receptors are found on the dendrites and soma of the postganglionic neuron and the interneurons. The preganglionic terminal releases acetylcholine and peptides; the interneurons store and release catecholamines, amino acids, and peptides; and the sensory afferent nerve terminals release peptides. The initial EPSP is mediated through nicotinic (N) receptors, the slow IPSP and EPSP through M_2 and M_1 muscarinic receptors, and the late, slow EPSP through several types of peptidergic receptors, as detailed in the text. (After; Weight *et al.,* 1979; Jan and Jan, 1983; Elfvin *et al.,* 1993.)

They include the slow EPSP, the late slow EPSP, and an inhibitory postsynaptic potential (IPSP). The slow EPSP is generated by ACh acting on muscarinic receptors, and it is blocked by atropine or antagonists that are selective for M_1 muscarinic receptors (*see* Chapter 7). The slow EPSP has a longer latency and a duration of 30 to 60 seconds. In contrast, the late slow EPSP lasts for several minutes and is initiated by the action of peptides released from presynaptic nerve endings or interneurons in specific ganglia (Dun, 1983). The peptides and ACh may be released from the same nerve ending, but the enhanced stability of the peptide in the ganglion extends its sphere of influence to postsynaptic sites beyond those in immediate proximity to the nerve ending. The slow EPSPs result from decreased K^+ conductance (Weight *et al.,* 1979). The K^+ conductance has been called an *M current,* and it regulates the sensitivity of the cell to repetitive fast-depolarizing events (Adams *et al.,* 1982).

Like the slow EPSP, the IPSP is unaffected by the classical nicotinic-receptor blocking agents. Substantial electrophysiological and morphological evidence has accumulated to suggest that catecholamines participate in the generation of the IPSP. Dopamine and norepinephrine cause hyperpolarization of ganglia, and both the IPSP and the catecholamine-induced hyperpolarization are blocked by α-adrenergic receptor antagonists. Since the IPSP is sensitive in most systems to blockade by both atropine and α-adrenergic antagonists, ACh that is released at the preganglionic terminal may act on a catecholamine-containing interneuron to stimulate the release of dopamine or

norepinephrine; the catecholamine, in turn, produces hyperpolarization (an IPSP) of the ganglion cell (Eccles and Libet, 1961). At least in some ganglia, a muscarinic link in the IPSP is mediated through M_2 muscarinic receptors (*see* Chapter 7). Histochemical studies indicate that catecholamine-containing cells are present in ganglia. These include the dopamine- or norepinephrine-containing small, intensely fluorescent (SIF) cells and adrenergic nerve terminals. Details of the functional linkage between the SIF cells and the electrogenic mechanism of the IPSP remain to be resolved (Eränkö *et al.,* 1980).

The relative importance of the secondary pathways and even the nature of the modulating transmitters appear to differ among individual ganglia and between parasympathetic and sympathetic ganglia. A variety of peptides, including luteinizing hormone–releasing hormone, substance P, angiotensin, calcitonin gene-related peptide, vasoactive intestinal polypeptide, neuropeptide Y, and enkephalins, have been identified in ganglia by immunofluorescence. They appear localized to particular cell bodies, nerve fibers, or SIF cells; are released upon nerve stimulation; and are presumed to mediate the late slow EPSP (Dun, 1983; Elfvin *et al.,* 1993). Other neurotransmitter substances, such as 5-hydroxytryptamine and gamma-aminobutyric acid, are known to modify ganglionic transmission. Precise details of their modulatory actions are not understood, but they appear to be most closely associated with the late slow EPSP and inhibition of the M current in various ganglia. It should be emphasized that the secondary synaptic events only modulate the initial EPSP. Conventional ganglionic blocking agents can inhibit ganglionic transmission completely; the same cannot be said for muscarinic antagonists or α-adrenergic agonists (*see* Weight *et al.,* 1979; Volle, 1980).

Drugs that stimulate cholinergic receptor sites on autonomic ganglia can be grouped into two major categories. The first group consists of drugs with nicotinic specificity, including nicotine itself. Their excitatory effects on ganglia are rapid in onset, are blocked by ganglionic nicotinic-receptor antagonists, and mimic the initial EPSP. The second group is composed of agents such as *muscarine, McN-A-343,* and *methacholine.* Their excitatory effects on ganglia are delayed in onset, blocked by atropine-like drugs, and mimic the slow EPSP.

Ganglionic blocking agents acting on the nicotinic receptor may be classified into two groups. The first group includes those drugs that initially stimulate the ganglia by an ACh-like action and then block them because of a persistent depolarization (*e.g., nicotine*); prolonged application of nicotine results in desensitization of the cholinergic receptor site and continued blockade. (*See* review by Volle, 1980.) The blockade of autonomic ganglia produced by the second group of blocking drugs, of which *hexamethonium* and *trimethaphan* can be regarded as prototypes, does not involve prior ganglionic stimulation or changes in ganglionic potentials. These agents impair transmission either by competing with ACh for ganglionic nicotinic receptor sites or by blocking the channel when it is open. Trimethaphan acts by competition with ACh, analogous to the mechanism of action of curare at the neuromuscular junction. Hexamethonium appears to block the channel after it opens. This action shortens the duration of current flow, since the open channel either becomes occluded or closes (Gurney and Rang, 1984). Regardless of the mechanism, the initial EPSP is blocked and ganglionic transmission is inhibited.

GANGLIONIC STIMULATING DRUGS

History. Two natural alkaloids, nicotine and lobeline, exhibit peripheral actions by stimulating autonomic ganglia. Nicotine (*see* Figure 9–5) was first isolated from leaves of tobacco, *Nicotiana tabacum,* by Posselt and Reiman in 1828, and Orfila initiated the first pharmacological studies of the alkaloid in 1843. Langley and Dickinson (1889) painted the superior cervical ganglion of rabbits with nicotine and demonstrated that its site of action was the ganglion, rather than the preganglionic or postganglionic nerve fiber. Lobeline, from *Lobelia inflata,* has many of the same actions as nicotine but is less potent.

A number of synthetic compounds also have prominent actions at ganglionic receptor sites. The actions of the "onium" compounds, of which tetramethylammonium (TMA) is the simplest prototype, were explored in considerable detail in the last half of the nineteenth century and in the early twentieth century.

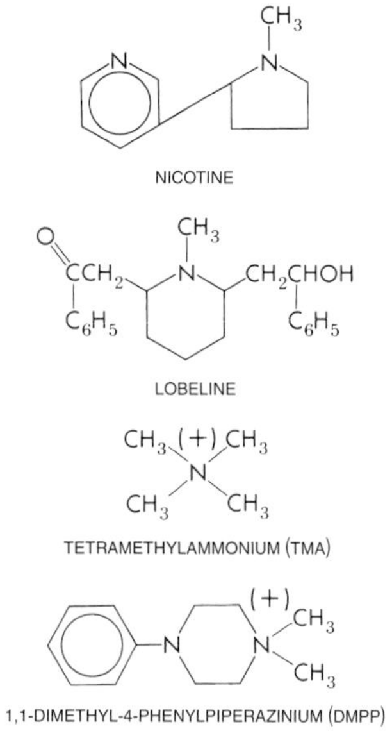

Figure 9–5. Ganglionic stimulants.

Nicotine

Nicotine is of considerable medical significance because of its toxicity, presence in tobacco, and propensity for conferring a dependence on its users. The chronic effects of nicotine and the untoward effects of the chronic use of tobacco are considered in Chapter 24.

Nicotine is one of the few natural liquid alkaloids. It is a colorless, volatile base ($pK_a = 8.5$) that turns brown and acquires the odor of tobacco on exposure to air.

Pharmacological Actions. The complex and often unpredictable changes that occur in the body after administration of nicotine are due not only to its actions on a variety of neuroeffector and chemosensitive sites but also to the fact that the alkaloid can stimulate and desensitize receptors. The ultimate response of any one system represents the summation of stimulatory and inhibitory effects of nicotine. For example, the drug can increase heart rate by excitation of sympathetic or paralysis of parasympathetic cardiac ganglia, and it can slow heart rate by paralysis of sympathetic or stimulation of parasympathetic cardiac ganglia. In addition, the effects of the drug on the chemoreceptors of the carotid and aortic bodies and on brain centers influence heart rate, as do also the cardiovascular compensatory reflexes resulting from changes in blood pressure caused by nicotine. Finally, nicotine elicits a discharge of epinephrine from the adrenal medulla, and this hormone accelerates cardiac rate and raises blood pressure.

Peripheral Nervous System. The major action of nicotine consists initially of transient stimulation and subsequently of a more persistent depression of all autonomic ganglia. Small doses of nicotine stimulate the ganglion cells directly and may facilitate the transmission of impulses. When larger doses of the drug are applied, the initial stimulation is followed very quickly by a blockade of transmission. Whereas stimulation of the ganglion cells coincides with their depolarization, depression of transmission by adequate doses of nicotine occurs both during the depolarization and after it has subsided. Nicotine also possesses a biphasic action on the adrenal medulla; small doses evoke the discharge of catecholamines, and larger doses prevent their release in response to splanchnic nerve stimulation.

The effects of nicotine on the neuromuscular junction are similar to those on ganglia. However, with the exception of avian and denervated mammalian muscle, the stimulant phase is largely obscured by the rapidly developing paralysis. In the latter stage, nicotine also produces neuromuscular blockade by receptor desensitization.

Nicotine, like ACh, is known to stimulate a number of sensory receptors. These include mechanoreceptors that respond to stretch or pressure of the skin, mesentery, tongue, lung, and stomach; chemoreceptors of the carotid body; thermal receptors of the skin and tongue; and pain receptors. Prior administration of hexamethonium prevents the stimulation of the sensory receptors by nicotine but has little, if any, effect on the activation of the sensory receptors by physiological stimuli.

Central Nervous System.   Nicotine markedly stimulates the CNS. Low doses produce weak analgesia; with higher doses, tremors leading to convulsions at toxic doses are evident. The excitation of respiration is a prominent action of nicotine; although large doses act directly on the medulla oblongata, smaller doses augment respiration reflexly by excitation of the chemoreceptors of the carotid and aortic bodies. Stimulation of the CNS with large doses is followed by depression, and death results from failure of respiration due to both central paralysis and peripheral blockade of muscles of respiration.

Nicotine induces vomiting by both central and peripheral actions. The central component of the vomiting response is due to stimulation of the emetic chemoreceptor trigger zone in the area postrema of the medulla oblongata. In addition, nicotine activates vagal and spinal afferent nerves that form the sensory input of the reflex pathways involved in the act of vomiting. Studies in isolated higher centers of the brain and spinal cord reveal that the primary sites of action of nicotine in the CNS are prejunctional, causing the release of other transmitters. Accordingly, the stimulatory and pleasure-reward actions of nicotine appear to result from release of excitatory amino acids, dopamine, and other biogenic amines from various CNS centers (MacDermott *et al.,* 1999).

Chronic exposure to nicotine in several systems causes an increase in the density or number of nicotinic receptors (*see* Di Chiara *et al.,* 2000; Stitzel *et al.,* 2000). While the details of the mechanism are not yet understood, the response may be compensatory to the desensitization of receptor function by nicotine.

Cardiovascular System.   When administered intravenously to dogs, nicotine characteristically produces an increase in heart rate and blood pressure. The latter is usually a more sustained response. In general, the cardiovascular responses to nicotine are due to stimulation of sympathetic ganglia and the adrenal medulla, together with the discharge of catecholamines from sympathetic nerve endings. Also contributing to the sympathomimetic response to nicotine is the activation of chemoreceptors of the aortic and carotid bodies, which reflexly results in vasoconstriction, tachycardia, and elevated blood pressure.

Gastrointestinal Tract.   The combined activation of parasympathetic ganglia and cholinergic nerve endings by nicotine results in increased tone and motor activity of the bowel. Nausea, vomiting, and occasionally diarrhea are observed following systemic absorption of nicotine in an individual who has not been exposed to nicotine previously.

Exocrine Glands.   Nicotine causes an initial stimulation of salivary and bronchial secretions that is followed by inhibition.

Absorption, Fate, and Excretion.   Nicotine is readily absorbed from the respiratory tract, buccal membranes, and skin. Severe poisoning has resulted from percutaneous absorption. Being a relatively strong base, its absorption from the stomach is limited, and intestinal absorption is far more efficient. Nicotine in chewing tobacco, because it is more slowly absorbed than inhaled nicotine, has a longer duration of effect. The average cigarette contains 6 to 11 mg of nicotine and delivers about 1 to 3 mg of nicotine systemically to the smoker; bioavailability can increase as much as threefold with intensity of puffing and technique of the smoker (Henningfield, 1995; Benowitz, 1998). Nicotine is available in several dosage forms to help achieve abstinence from tobacco use. Efficacy primarily results from preventing a withdrawal or abstinence syndrome. Nicotine may be administered orally as a gum (nicotine polacrilex; NICORETTE), transdermal patch (NICODERM, HABITROL, others), a nasal spray (NICOTROL NS), and vapor inhaler (NICOTROL INHALER). The first two are most widely used, and the objective is to obtain a sustained plasma nicotine concentration lower than venous blood concentrations after smoking. Arterial blood concentrations immediately following inhalation can be as much as tenfold higher than venous concentrations. The efficacy of the above dosage forms in producing abstinence from smoking is enhanced when linked to counseling and motivational therapy (Henningfield, 1995; Fant *et al.,* 1999; Benowitz, 1999; *see also* Chapter 24).

Approximately 80% to 90% of nicotine is altered in the body, mainly in the liver but also in the kidney and lung. Cotinine is the major metabolite, with nicotine-1'-*N*-oxide and 3-hydroxycotinine and conjugated metabolites found in lesser quantities (Benowitz, 1998). The profile of metabolites and the rate of metabolism appear to be similar in the smoker and nonsmoker. The half-life of nicotine following inhalation or parenteral administration is about 2 hours. Both nicotine and its metabolites are eliminated rapidly by the kidney. The rate of urinary excretion of nicotine is dependent upon the pH of the urine; excretion diminishes when the urine is alkaline. Nicotine also is excreted in the milk of lactating women who smoke; the milk of heavy smokers may contain 0.5 mg per liter.

Acute Nicotine Poisoning.   Poisoning from nicotine may occur from accidental ingestion of nicotine-containing insecticide sprays or in children from ingestion of tobacco products. The acutely fatal dose of nicotine for an adult is probably about 60 mg of the base. Smoking tobacco usually contains 1% to 2% nicotine. Apparently, the gastric absorption of nicotine from tobacco taken by mouth is delayed because of slowed gastric emptying, so that vomiting caused by the central effect of the initially absorbed fraction may remove much of the tobacco remaining in the gastrointestinal tract.

The onset of symptoms of acute, severe nicotine poisoning is rapid; they include nausea, salivation, abdominal pain, vomiting, diarrhea, cold sweat, headache, dizziness, disturbed hearing and vision, mental confusion, and marked weakness. Faintness and prostration ensue; the blood pressure falls; breathing is difficult; the pulse is weak, rapid, and irregular; and collapse may be followed by terminal convulsions. Death may result within a few minutes from respiratory failure.

Therapy. Vomiting should be induced with syrup of ipecac or gastric lavage should be performed. Alkaline solutions should be avoided. A slurry of activated charcoal is then passed through the tube and left in the stomach. Respiratory assistance and treatment of shock may be necessary.

Other Ganglionic Stimulants

Stimulation of ganglia by tetramethylammonium (TMA) or 1,1-dimethyl-4-phenylpiperazinium iodide (DMPP) differs from that produced by nicotine in that the initial stimulation is not followed by a dominant blocking action. DMPP is about three times more potent and slightly more ganglion-selective than nicotine. Although parasympathomimetic drugs stimulate ganglia, their effects usually are obscured by stimulation of other neuroeffector sites. McN-A-343 represents an exception to this; in certain tissues its primary action appears to occur at muscarinic M_1 receptors in ganglia.

GANGLIONIC BLOCKING DRUGS

The chemical diversity of compounds that block autonomic ganglia without causing prior stimulation is shown in Figure 9–6.

History and Structure–Activity Relationship. Although Marshall (1913) first described the "nicotine paralyzing" action of tetraethylammonium (TEA) on ganglia, TEA was largely overlooked until Acheson and Moe (1946) published their definitive analyses of the effects of the ion on the cardiovascular system and autonomic ganglia. The *bis*-quaternary ammonium salts were developed and studied independently by Barlow and Ing (1948) and Paton and Zaimis (1952). The prototypical ganglionic blocking drug in this series, *hexamethonium* (C6), has a bridge of six methylene groups between the two quaternary

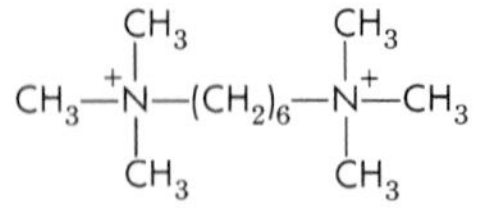

HEXAMETHONIUM (C6)

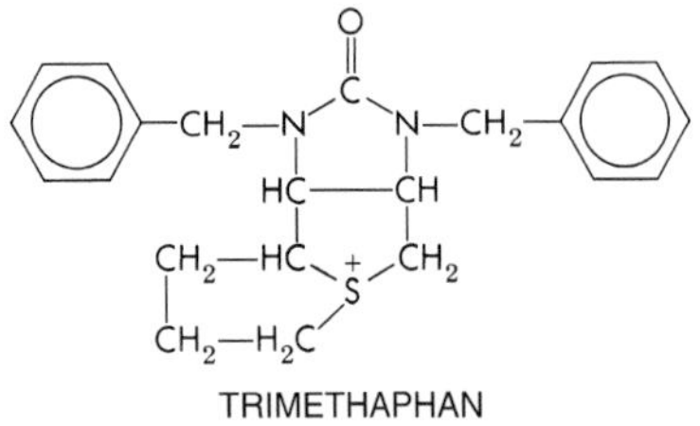

TRIMETHAPHAN

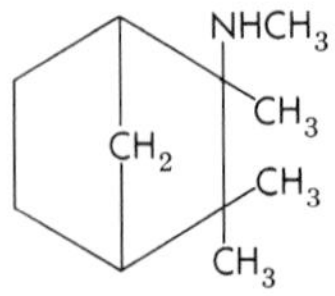

MECAMYLAMINE

Figure 9–6. Ganglionic blocking agents.

nitrogen atoms (*see* Figure 9–6). It has minimal neuromuscular and muscarinic blocking activities.

Triethylsulfoniums, like the quaternary and *bis*-quaternary ammonium ions, possess ganglionic blocking actions. This knowledge led to the development of sulfonium ganglionic blocking agents such as *trimethaphan* (*see* Figure 9–6). *Mecamylamine,* a secondary amine, was introduced into therapy for hypertension in the mid-1950s.

Pharmacological Properties. Nearly all of the physiological alterations observed after the administration of ganglionic blocking agents can be anticipated with reasonable accuracy by a careful inspection of Figure 6–1 and by knowing which division of the autonomic nervous system exercises dominant control of various organs (Table 9–4). For example, blockade of sympathetic ganglia interrupts adrenergic control of arterioles and results in vasodilation, improved peripheral blood flow in some vascular beds, and a fall in blood pressure.

Generalized ganglionic blockade may result also in atony of the bladder and gastrointestinal tract, cycloplegia, xerostomia, diminished perspiration, and, by abolishing circulatory reflex pathways, postural hypotension. These changes represent the generally undesirable features of ganglionic blockade, which severely limit the therapeutic efficacy of ganglionic blocking agents.

Cardiovascular System. The importance of existing sympathetic tone in determining the degree to which blood pressure is lowered by ganglionic blockade is illustrated by the fact that blood pressure may be decreased only minimally in recumbent normotensive subjects but may fall markedly in sitting or standing subjects. Postural hypotension is a major problem in ambulatory patients receiving ganglionic blocking drugs; it is relieved to some extent by muscular activity and completely by recumbency.

Changes in cardiac rate following ganglionic blockade depend largely on existing vagal tone. In human beings, mild tachycardia usually accompanies the hypotension, a sign that indicates fairly complete ganglionic blockade. However, a decrease may occur if the heart rate is initially high.

Cardiac output often is reduced by ganglionic blocking drugs in patients with normal cardiac function as a consequence of diminished venous return resulting from venous dilation and peripheral pooling of blood. In patients with cardiac failure, ganglionic blockade frequently results in increased cardiac output due to a reduction in peripheral resistance. In hypertensive subjects, cardiac output, stroke volume, and left ventricular work are diminished.

Although total systemic vascular resistance is decreased in patients who receive ganglionic blocking agents, changes in blood flow and vascular resistance of individual vascular beds are variable. Reduction of cerebral blood flow is small unless mean systemic blood pressure falls below 50 to 60 mm Hg. Skeletal muscle blood flow is unaltered, but splanchnic and renal blood flow decrease following the administration of a ganglionic blocking agent.

Absorption, Fate, and Excretion. The absorption of quaternary ammonium and sulfonium compounds from the enteric tract is incomplete and unpredictable. This is due both to the

Table 9–4
Usual Predominance of Sympathetic (Adrenergic) or Parasympathetic (Cholinergic) Tone at Various Effector Sites, with Consequent Effects of Autonomic Ganglionic Blockade

SITE	PREDOMINANT TONE	EFFECT OF GANGLIONIC BLOCKADE
Arterioles	Sympathetic (adrenergic)	Vasodilation; increased peripheral blood flow; hypotension
Veins	Sympathetic (adrenergic)	Dilation: peripheral pooling of blood; decreased venous return; decreased cardiac output
Heart	Parasympathetic (cholinergic)	Tachycardia
Iris	Parasympathetic (cholinergic)	Mydriasis
Ciliary muscle	Parasympathetic (cholinergic)	Cycloplegia—focus to far vision
Gastrointestinal tract	Parasympathetic (cholinergic)	Reduced tone and motility; constipation; decreased gastric and pancreatic secretions
Urinary bladder	Parasympathetic (cholinergic)	Urinary retention
Salivary glands	Parasympathetic (cholinergic)	Xerostomia
Sweat glands	Sympathetic (cholinergic)	Anhidrosis
Genital tract	Sympathetic and parasympathetic	Decreased stimulation

limited ability of these ionized substances to penetrate cell membranes and to the depression of propulsive movements of the small intestine and gastric emptying. Although the absorption of mecamylamine is less erratic, a danger exists of reduced bowel activity leading to frank paralytic ileus.

After absorption, the quaternary ammonium and sulfonium blocking agents are confined primarily to the extracellular space and are excreted mostly unchanged by the kidney. Mecamylamine concentrates in the liver and kidney and is slowly excreted in an unchanged form.

Untoward Responses and Severe Reactions. Among the milder untoward responses observed are visual disturbances, dry mouth, conjunctival suffusion, urinary hesitancy, decreased potentia, subjective chilliness, moderate constipation, occasional diarrhea, abdominal discomfort, anorexia, heartburn, nausea, eructation and bitter taste, and the signs and symptoms of syncope caused by postural hypotension. More severe reactions include marked hypotension, constipation, syncope, paralytic ileus, urinary retention, and cycloplegia.

Therapeutic Uses. Of the ganglionic blocking agents that have appeared on the therapeutic scene, only *mecamylamine* (INVERSINE) and *trimethaphan* (ARFONAD) currently are utilized in the United States.

Ganglionic blocking agents have been supplanted by superior agents for the treatment of chronic hypertension (*see* Chapter 33). Alternative agents also are available for management of acute hypertensive crises (Murphy, 1995; *see* Chapter 33). A remaining use of ganglionic blockers in a hypertensive crisis is for the initial control of blood pressure in

patients with acute dissecting aortic aneurysm, particularly when preexisting conditions make β-adrenergic receptor antagonists a relative contraindication (Varon and Marik, 2000). Ganglionic blocking agents are well suited for this condition because they not only reduce blood pressure but also inhibit sympathetic reflexes and thereby reduce the rate of rise of pressure at the site of the tear. In such situations, trimethaphan is infused intravenously at a rate of 0.5 to 3 mg per minute with frequent monitoring of blood pressure. In the absence of symptoms or signs of renal, cerebral, or myocardial ischemia, the dose is increased until the pressure is in the low-normal range. Disappearance of pain is a sign that the dissection has stopped. A disadvantage of trimethaphan is the development of tolerance over the first 48 hours of therapy; this is in part related to fluid retention.

An additional therapeutic use of the ganglionic blocking agents is in the production of controlled hypotension; a reduction in blood pressure during surgery may be sought deliberately to minimize hemorrhage in the operative field, to reduce blood loss in various orthopedic procedures, and to facilitate surgery on blood vessels (Fukusaki *et al.*, 1999). Trimethaphan, as an infusion, may be used as an alternative to or in combination with sodium nitroprusside, since some patients are resistant to the latter drug. Trimethaphan blunts the sympathoadrenal stimulation caused by nitroprusside and reduces the required dosage (Fahmy, 1985).

Trimethaphan can be used in the management of autonomic hyperreflexia or reflex sympathetic dystrophy. This syndrome typically is seen in patients with injuries of the upper spinal cord and results from a massive sympathetic discharge. Since normal central inhibition of the reflex is lacking in such patients, the spinal reflex is dominant.

BIBLIOGRAPHY

Acheson, G.H., and Moe, G.K. The action of tetraethylammonium ion on the mammalian circulation. *J. Pharmacol. Exp. Ther.,* **1946,** *87:*220–236.

Adams, P.R., Brown, D.A., and Constanti, A. Pharmacological inhibition of the M-current. *J. Physiol.,* **1982,** *332:*223–262.

Adams, P.R., and Sakmann, B. Decamethonium both opens and blocks endplate channels. *Proc. Natl. Acad. Sci. U.S.A.,* **1978,** *75:*2994–2998.

Ascher, P., Large, W.A., and Rang, H.P. Studies on the mechanism of action of acetylcholine antagonists on rat parasympathetic ganglion cells. *J. Physiol.,* **1979,** *295:*139–170.

Barlow, R.B., and Ing, H.R. Curare-like action of polymethylene *bis*-quaternary ammonium salts. *Br. J. Pharmacol. Chemother.,* **1948,** *3:*298–304.

Chang, C.C., and Lee, C.Y. Isolation of neurotoxins from the venom of *Bungarus multicinctus* and their modes of neuromuscular blocking action. *Arch. Int. Pharmacodyn. Ther.,* **1963,** *144:*241–257.

Colquhoun, D., Dreyer, F., and Sheridan, R.E. The actions of tubocurarine at the frog neuromuscular junction. *J. Physiol.,* **1979,** *293:*247–284.

Drenck, N.E., Ueda, N., Olsen, N.V., Engbaek, J., Jensen, E., Skovgaard, L.T., and Viby-Mogensen, J. Manual evaluation of residual curarization using double-burst stimulation: a comparison with train-of-four. *Anesthesiology,* **1989,** *70:*578–581.

Eccles, R.M., and Libet, B. Origin and blockade of the synaptic responses of curarized sympathetic ganglia. *J. Physiol.,* **1961,** *157:*484–503.

Fahmy, N.R. Nitroprusside vs. a nitroprusside-trimethaphan mixture for induced hypotension: hemodynamic effects and cyanide release. *Clin. Pharmacol. Ther.,* **1985,** *37:*264–270.

Fogdall, R.P., and Miller, R.D. Neuromuscular effects of enflurane, alone and combined with *d*-tubocurarine, pancuronium, and succinylcholine, in man. *Anesthesiology,* **1975,** *42:*173–178.

Fruen, B.R., Mickelson, J.R., and Louis, C.F. Dantrolene inhibition of sarcoplasmic reticulum Ca^{2+} release by direct and specific action at skeletal muscle ryanodine receptors. *J. Biol. Chem.,* **1997,** *272:*26965–26971.

Fukusaki, M., Miyako, M., Hara, T., Maekawa, T., Yamaguchi, K., and Sumikawa, K. Effects of controlled hypotension with sevoflurane anesthesia on hepatic function of surgical patients. *Eur. J. Anaesthesiol.,* **1999,** *16:*111–116.

Griffith, H.R., and Johnson, G.E. The use of curare in general anesthesia. *Anesthesiology,* **1942,** *3:*418–420.

Gurney, A.M., and Rang, H.P. The channel-blocking action of methonium compounds on rat submandibular ganglion cells. *Br. J. Pharmacol.,* **1984,** *82:*623–642.

Jan, Y.N., and Jan, L.Y. A LHRH-like peptidergic neurotransmitter capable of action at a distance in autonomic ganglia. *Trends Neurosci.,* **1983,** *6:*320–325.

Katz, B., and Miledi, R. A re-examination of curare action at the motor end plate. *Proc. R. Soc. Lond. [Biol.],* **1978,** *203:*119–133.

Katz, B., and Thesleff, S. A study of the "desensitization" produced by acetylcholine at the motor end-plate. *J. Physiol. (Lond.),* **1957,** *138:*63–80.

Langley, J.N., and Dickinson, W.L. On the local paralysis of peripheral ganglia, and on the connexion of different classes of nerve fibers with them. *Proc. R. Soc. Lond. [Biol.],* **1889,** *46:*423–431.

Marshall, C.R. Studies on the pharmaceutical action of tetra-alkyl-ammonium compounds. *Trans. R. Soc. Edinb.,* **1913,** *1:*17–40.

Miyazawa, A., Fujiyoshi, Y., Stowell, M., and Unwin, N. Nicotinic acetylcholine receptor at 4.6 Å resolution: transverse tunnels in the channel wall. *J. Mol. Biol.,* **1999,** *288:*765–786.

Pantuck, E.J. Plasma cholinesterase: gene and variations. *Anesth. Analg.,* **1993,** *77:*380–386.

Primo-Parmo, S.L., Bartels, C.F., Wiersema, B., van deer Spek, A.F., Innis, J.W., and La Du, B.N. Characterization of 12 silent alleles of the human butyrylcholinesterase (BCHE) gene. *Am. J. Hum. Genet.,* **1996,** *58:*52–64.

Sine, S.M., and Claudio, T. γ- and δ-subunits regulate the affinity and cooperativity of ligand binding to the acetylcholine receptor. *J. Biol. Chem.* **1991,** *266:*19369–19377.

Smith, S.M., Brown, H.O., Toman, J.E.P., and Goodman, L.S. The lack of cerebral effects of *d*-tubocurarine. *Anesthesiology,* **1947,** *8:*1–14.

Unwin, N. Nicotinic acetylcholine receptor at 9 Å resolution. *J. Mol. Biol.,* **1993,** *229:*1101–1124.

Vita, G.M., Olckers, A., Jedlicka, A.E., George, A.L., Heiman-Patterson, T., Rosenberg, H., Fletcher, J.E., and Levitt, R.C. Masseter muscle rigidity associated with glycine1306-to-alanine mutation in the adult muscle sodium channel α-subunit gene. *Anesthesiology,* **1995,** *82:*1097–1103.

Waud, B.E., and Waud, D.R. The relation between the response to "train-of-four" stimulation and receptor occlusion during competitive neuromuscular block. *Anesthesiology,* **1972,** *37:*413–416.

MONOGRAPHS AND REVIEWS

Basta, S.J. Modulation of histamine release by neuromolecular blocking drugs. *Curr. Opin. Anaesthesiol.,* **1992,** *5:*512–566.

Benowitz, N.L. In, *Nicotine Safety and Toxicity.* (Benowitz, N.L., ed.) Oxford University Press, New York, **1998,** pp. 3–28.

Benowitz, N.L. Nicotine addiction. *Prim. Care,* **1999,** *26:*611–653.

Bernard, C. Analyse physiologique des propriétés des systèmes musculaires et nerveux au moyen du curare. *C. R. Acad. Sci.,* **1856,** *43:*825–829.

Bevan, D.R. Newer neuromuscular blocking agents. *Pharmacol. Toxicol.,* **1994,** *74:*3–9.

Boni, R., Kryden, O.P., and Burg, G. Revival of the use of botulinum toxin: application in dermatology. *Dermatology,* **2000,** *200:*287–291.

Bovet, D. Synthetic inhibitors of neuromuscular transmission, chemical structures and structure-activity relationships. In, *Neuromuscular Blocking and Stimulating Agents.* Vol. 1. *International Encyclopedia of Pharmacology and Therapeutics,* Sect. 14. (Cheymol, J., ed.) Pergamon Press, Oxford, **1972,** pp. 243–294.

Bowman, W.C., Prior, C., and Marshall, I.G. Presynaptic receptors in the neuromuscular junction. *Ann. N.Y. Acad. Sci.,* **1990,** *604:*69–81.

Changeux, J.P., and Edelstein, S.J. Allosteric receptors after 30 years. *Neuron,* **1998,** *21:*959–980.

Davis, E., and Barnes, M.P. Botulinum toxin and spasticity. *J. Neurol. Neurosurg. Psychiatry,* **2000,** *68:*141–147.

Di Chiara, G. Behavioral pharmacology and neurobiology of nicotine reward and dependence. In, *Neuronal Nicotinic Receptors.* (Clementi, F., Fornasari, D., and Gotti, C., eds.) Springer-Verlag, Berlin, **2000,** pp. 603–750.

Dorkins, H.R. Suxamethonium—the development of a modern drug from 1906 to the present day. *Med. Hist.,* **1982,** *26:*145–168.

Dripps, R.D. The clinician looks at neuromuscular blocking drugs. In, *Neuromuscular Junction.* (Zaimis, E., ed.) Springer-Verlag, Berlin, **1976,** pp. 583–592.

Dun, N.J. Peptide hormones and transmissions in sympathetic ganglia. In, *Autonomic Ganglia.* (Elfvin, L.G. ed.) Wiley, New York, **1983,** pp. 345–666.

Durant, N.N., and Katz, R.L. Suxamethonium. *Br. J. Anaesth.,* **1982,** *54:*195–208.

Elfvin, L.G., Lindh, B., and Hokfelt, T. The chemical neuroanatomy of sympathetic ganglia. *Annu. Rev. Neurosci.,* **1993,** *16:*471–507.

Engel, A.G., Ohno, K., Milone, M., and Sine, S.M. Congenital myasthenic syndromes. New insights from molecular genetic and patch–clamp studies. *Ann. N.Y. Acad. Sci.,* **1998,** *841:*140–156.

Eränkö, O., Sonila, S., and Päivärinta, H., eds. *Histochemistry and Cell Biology of Autonomic Neurons, SIF Cells, and Paraneurons.* Raven Press, New York, **1980.**

Fant, R.V., Owen, L.L., and Henningfield, J.E. Nicotine replacement therapy. *Primary Care,* **1999,** *26:*633–652.

Feldman, S.A., and Fauvel, N. Onset of neuromuscular block. In, *Applied Neuromuscular Pharmacology.* (Pollard, B.J., ed.) Oxford University Press, Oxford, **1994,** pp. 69–84.

Gill, R.C. *White Waters and Black Magic.* Holt, New York, **1940.**

Harper, N.J.N. Neuromuscular blockage: measurement and monitoring. In, *Applied Neuromuscular Pharmacology.* (Pollard, B.J., ed.) Oxford University Press, Oxford, **1994,** pp. 319–344.

Henningfield, J.E. Nicotine medications for smoking cessation. *N. Engl. J. Med.,* **1995,** *333:*1196–1203.

Hopkins, P.M. Malignant hyperthermia: advances in clinical management and diagnosis. *Br. J. Anaesth.,* **2000,** *85:*118–128.

Hunter, J.M. Muscle relaxants in renal disease. *Acta Anaesthesiol. Scand. Suppl.,* **1994,** *102:*2–5.

Jurkat-Rott, K., McCarthy, T., and Lehmann-Horn, F. Genetics and pathogenesis of malignant hyperthermia. *Muscle Nerve,* **2000,** *23:*4–17.

Karlin, A., and Akabas, M.H. Toward a structural basis for the function of nicotinic acetylcholine receptors and their cousins. *Neuron,* **1995,** *15:*1231–1244.

Kita, M., and Goodkin, D.E. Drugs used to treat spasticity. *Drugs,* **2000,** *59:*487–495.

Lehmann-Horn, F., and Jurkat-Rott, K. Voltage-gated ion channels and hereditary disease. *Physiol. Rev.,* **1999,** *79:*1317–1372.

Lindstrom, J.M. The structures of neuronal nicotinic receptors. *Neuronal Nicotinic Receptors.* (Clementi, F., Fornasari, D., Gotti, C., eds.) Springer-Verlag, Berlin, **2000,** pp. 101–162.

MacDermott, A.B., Role, L.W., and Siegelbaum, S.A. Presynaptic ionotropic receptors and the control of transmitter release. *Annu. Rev. Neurosci.,* **1999,** *22:*443–485.

McIntyre, A.R. *Curare: Its History, Nature and Clinical Use.* University of Chicago Press, Chicago, **1947.**

Murphy, C. Hypertensive emergencies. *Emerg. Med. Clin. North Am.,* **1995,** *13:*973–1007.

Numa, S., Noda, M., Takahashi, H., Tanabe, T., Toyosato, M., Furutani, Y., and Kikyotani, S. Molecular structure of the nicotinic acetylcholine receptor. *Cold Spring Harbor Symp. Quant. Biol.,* **1983,** *48(Pt. 1):*57–69.

Paterson, D., and Nordberg, A. Neuronal nicotinic receptors in the human brain. *Prog. Neurobiol.,* **2000,** *61:*75–111.

Paton, W.D.M., and Zaimis, E.J. The methonium compounds. *Pharmacol. Rev.,* **1952,** *4:*219–253.

Pollard, B.J. Interactions involving relaxants. In, *Applied Neuromuscular Pharmacology.* (Pollard, B.J., ed.) Oxford University Press, Oxford, **1994,** pp. 202–248.

Sakmann, B. Elementary steps in synaptic transmission revealed by currents through single ion channels. *Science,* **1992,** *256:*503–512.

Savarese, J.J., Caldwell, J.E., Lein, C.A., and Miller, R.D. Pharmacology of muscle relaxants and their antagonists. In, *Anesthesia,* 5th ed. (Miller, R.D., ed.) Churchill Livingstone, Philadelphia, **2000,** pp. 412–490.

Stitzel, J.A., Leonard, S.S., and Collins, A.C. Genetic regulation of nicotine-related behaviors and brain nicotinic receptors. In, *Neuronal Nicotinic Receptors.* (Clementi, F., Fornasari, D., and Gotti, C., eds.) Springer-Verlag, Berlin, **2000,** pp. 563–586.

Taylor, P., Brown, R.D., and Johnson, D.A. The linkage between ligand occupation and response of the nicotinic acetylcholine receptor. In, *Current Topics in Membranes and Transport.* Vol. 18. (Kleinzeller, A., and Martin, B.R., eds.) Academic Press, New York, **1983,** pp. 407–444.

Taylor, P., Osaka, H., Molles, B., Keller, S.H., and Malany, S. Contributions of studies of the nicotinic receptor from muscle to defining structural and functional properties of ligand-gated ion channels. In, *Neuronal Nicotinic Receptors.* (Clementi, F., Fornasari, D., and Gotti, C., eds.) Springer-Verlag, Berlin, **2000,** pp. 79–100.

Van der Kloot, W., and Molgo, J. Quantal acetylcholine release at the vertebrate neuromuscular junction. *Physiol. Rev.,* **1994,** *74:*899–991.

Varon, J., and Marik, P.E. The diagnosis and management of hypertensive crises. *Chest,* **2000,** *118:*214–227.

Volle, R.L. Nicotinic ganglion-stimulating agents. In, *Pharmacology of Ganglionic Transmission.* (Kharkevich, D.A., ed.) Springer-Verlag, Berlin, **1980,** pp. 281–312.

Watkins, J. Adverse reaction to neuromuscular blockers: frequency, investigation, and epidemiology. *Acta Anaesthesiol. Scand. Suppl.,* **1994,** *102:*6–10.

Weight, F.F., Schulman, J.A., Smith, P.A., and Busis, N.A., Long-lasting synaptic potentials and the modulation of synaptic transmission. *Fed. Proc.,* **1979,** *38:*2084–2094.

Whittaker, M. Cholinesterase. In, *Monographs in Human Genetics.* Vol. 11. (Beckman, L., ed.) S. Karger, Basel, **1986,** p. 231.

Zaimis, E. The neuromuscular junction: area of uncertainty. In, *Neuromuscular Junction.* (Zaimis, E., ed.) Springer-Verlag, Berlin, **1976,** pp. 1–18.

CATECHOLAMINES, SYMPATHOMIMETIC DRUGS, AND ADRENERGIC RECEPTOR ANTAGONISTS

Brian B. Hoffman

Catecholamines released by the sympathetic nervous system and adrenal medulla are involved in regulating a host of physiological functions, particularly in integrating responses to a range of stresses that would otherwise threaten homeostatic mechanisms. Norepinephrine is the major neurotransmitter in the peripheral sympathetic nervous system, whereas epinephrine is the primary hormone secreted by the adrenal medulla in mammals. Activation of the sympathetic nervous system occurs in response to diverse stimuli, including physical activity, psychological stress, blood loss, and many other normal or disease-related provocations. Because the functions mediated or modified by the sympathetic nervous system are diverse, drugs that mimic, alter, or antagonize its activity are useful in the treatment of many clinical disorders, including hypertension, cardiovascular shock, arrhythmias, asthma, and anaphylactic reactions. Some of these indications are discussed elsewhere (see Chapters 28, 32, 33, 34, and 35).

The physiological and metabolic responses that follow stimulation of sympathetic nerves in mammals usually are mediated by the neurotransmitter norepinephrine, although cotransmitters such as peptides potentially may contribute to sympathetic effects. As part of the response to stress, the adrenal medulla also is stimulated, resulting in elevation of the concentration of epinephrine in the circulation; epinephrine functions as a hormone, acting at distant sites in the circulation. The actions of these two catecholamines are very similar at some sites but differ significantly at others. For example, both compounds stimulate the myocardium; however, epinephrine dilates blood vessels to skeletal muscle, whereas norepinephrine causes constriction of blood vessels in skin, mucosa, and kidney.

Dopamine is a third naturally occurring catecholamine. Although it is found predominantly in the basal ganglia of the central nervous system (CNS), dopaminergic nerve endings and specific receptors for this catecholamine have been identified elsewhere in the CNS and in the periphery. The role of catecholamines in the CNS is detailed in Chapter 12 and elsewhere. As might be expected, sympathomimetic amines—naturally occurring catecholamines and drugs that mimic their actions—and adrenergic receptor antagonists—drugs that block the effects of sympathetic stimulation—constitute two of the more extensively studied groups of pharmacological agents.

Many of the actions of agonists or antagonists that activate or inhibit adrenergic receptors are understandable in terms of the known physiological effects of catecholamines. Whereas endogenous catecholamines such as epinephrine are sometimes used as drugs, most of the available agonists are structural analogs of epinephrine or norepinephrine. These synthetic compounds have a variety of advantages as therapeutic agents—such as oral bioavailability, prolonged duration of action, and specificity for particular subtypes of adrenergic receptors—which serve to enhance their therapeutic actions and to diminish potential adverse effects. The structure, cellular function, and physiological effects of adrenergic agonists and antagonists are outlined in this chapter.

I. CATECHOLAMINES AND SYMPATHOMIMETIC DRUGS

Most of the actions of catecholamines and sympathomimetic agents can be classified into seven broad types: (1) a peripheral excitatory action on certain types of smooth muscle, such as those in blood vessels supplying skin, kidney, and mucous membranes, and on gland cells, such as those in salivary and sweat glands; (2) a peripheral inhibitory action on certain other types of smooth muscle, such as those in the wall of the gut, in the bronchial tree, and in blood vessels supplying skeletal muscle; (3) a cardiac excitatory action, responsible for an increase in heart rate and force of contraction; (4) metabolic actions, such as an increase in rate of glycogenolysis in liver and muscle and liberation of free fatty acids from adipose tissue; (5) endocrine actions, such as modulation (increasing or decreasing) of the secretion of insulin, renin, and pituitary hormones; (6) central nervous system (CNS) actions, such as respiratory stimulation and, with some of the drugs, an increase in wakefulness and psychomotor activity and a reduction in appetite; and (7) presynaptic actions that result in either inhibition or facilitation of the release of neurotransmitters such as norepinephrine and acetylcholine; physiologically, the inhibitory action is more important than the excitatory action. Many of these actions and the receptors that mediate them are summarized in Tables 6–1 and 6–3. Not all sympathomimetic drugs show each of the above types of action to the same degree. However, many of the differences in their effects are only quantitative, and descriptions of the effects of each compound would be unnecessarily repetitive. Therefore, the pharmacological properties of these drugs as a class are described in detail for the prototypical agent, epinephrine.

Appreciation of the pharmacological properties of the drugs that are described in this chapter is critically dependent on understanding the classification, distribution, and mechanism of action of the various subtypes of adrenergic receptors (α, β) (Figure 10–1). This information is presented in Chapter 6.

History.   The pressor effect of adrenal extracts was first shown by Oliver and Schäfer in 1895. The active principle was named *epinephrine* by Abel in 1899 and synthesized independently by Stolz and Dakin (*see* Hartung, 1931). The development of our knowledge of epinephrine and *norepinephrine* as neurohumoral transmitters is outlined in Chapter 6. Barger and Dale (1910) studied the pharmacological activity of a large series of synthetic amines related to epinephrine and termed their action *sympathomimetic*. This important study determined the basic structural requirements for activity. When it was later found that cocaine or chronic denervation of effector organs reduced the responses to ephedrine and tyramine but enhanced the ef-

fects of epinephrine, it became clear that the differences between sympathomimetic amines were not simply quantitative. It was suggested that epinephrine acted directly on the effector cell, whereas ephedrine and tyramine had an indirect effect by acting on the nerve endings. The discovery that reserpine depletes tissues of norepinephrine (Bertler *et al.,* 1956) was followed by evidence that tyramine and certain other sympathomimetic amines do not act on tissues from animals that have been treated with reserpine; this, too, indicated that they act by releasing endogenous norepinephrine (Burn and Rand, 1958).

Chemistry and Structure-Activity Relationship of Sympathomimetic Amines. β-Phenylethylamine (Table 10–1) can be viewed as the parent compound of the sympathomimetic amines, consisting of a benzene ring and an ethylamine side chain. The structure permits substitutions to be made on the aromatic ring, the α- and β-carbon atoms, and the terminal amino group to yield a variety of compounds with sympathomimetic activity. Norepinephrine, epinephrine, *dopamine, isoproterenol,* and a few other agents have hydroxyl groups substituted at positions 3 and 4 of the benzene ring. Since *o*-dihydroxybenzene also is known as catechol, sympathomimetic amines with these hydroxyl substitutions in the aromatic ring are termed *catecholamines.*

Many directly acting sympathomimetic drugs influence both α and β receptors, but the ratio of activities varies among drugs in a continuous spectrum from predominantly α activity (*phenylephrine*) to predominantly β activity (*isoproterenol*). Despite the multiplicity of the sites of action of sympathomimetic amines, several generalizations can be made (*see* Table 10–1).

Separation of Aromatic Ring and Amino Group.   By far the greatest sympathomimetic activity occurs when two carbon atoms separate the ring from the amino group. This rule applies with few exceptions to all types of action.

Substitution on the Amino Group.   The effects of amino substitution are most readily seen in the actions of catecholamines on α and β receptors. Increase in the size of the alkyl substituent increases β-receptor activity (*e.g.,* isoproterenol). Norepinephrine has, in general, rather feeble β_2 activity; this activity is greatly increased in epinephrine with the addition of a methyl group. A notable exception is phenylephrine, which has an *N*-methyl substituent but is an α-selective agonist. β_2-Selective compounds require a large amino substituent, but depend on other substitutions to define selectivity for β_2 rather than for β_1 receptors. In general, the smaller the substitution on the amino group the greater the selectivity for α activity, although *N*-methylation increases the potency of primary amines. Thus, α activity is maximal in epinephrine, less in norepinephrine, and almost absent in isoproterenol.

Substitution on the Aromatic Nucleus.   Maximal α and β activity depends on the presence of hydroxyl groups on positions 3 and 4. When one or both of these groups are absent, with no other aromatic substitution, the overall potency is reduced. Phenylephrine is thus less potent than epinephrine at both α and β receptors, with β_2 activity almost completely absent. Studies of the β-adrenergic receptor suggest that the hydroxyl groups on serine residues 204 and 207 probably form hydrogen bonds with the catechol hydroxyl groups at positions 3 and 4, respectively (Strader *et al.,* 1989). It also appears that aspartate 113 is a point of electrostatic interaction with the amine group on

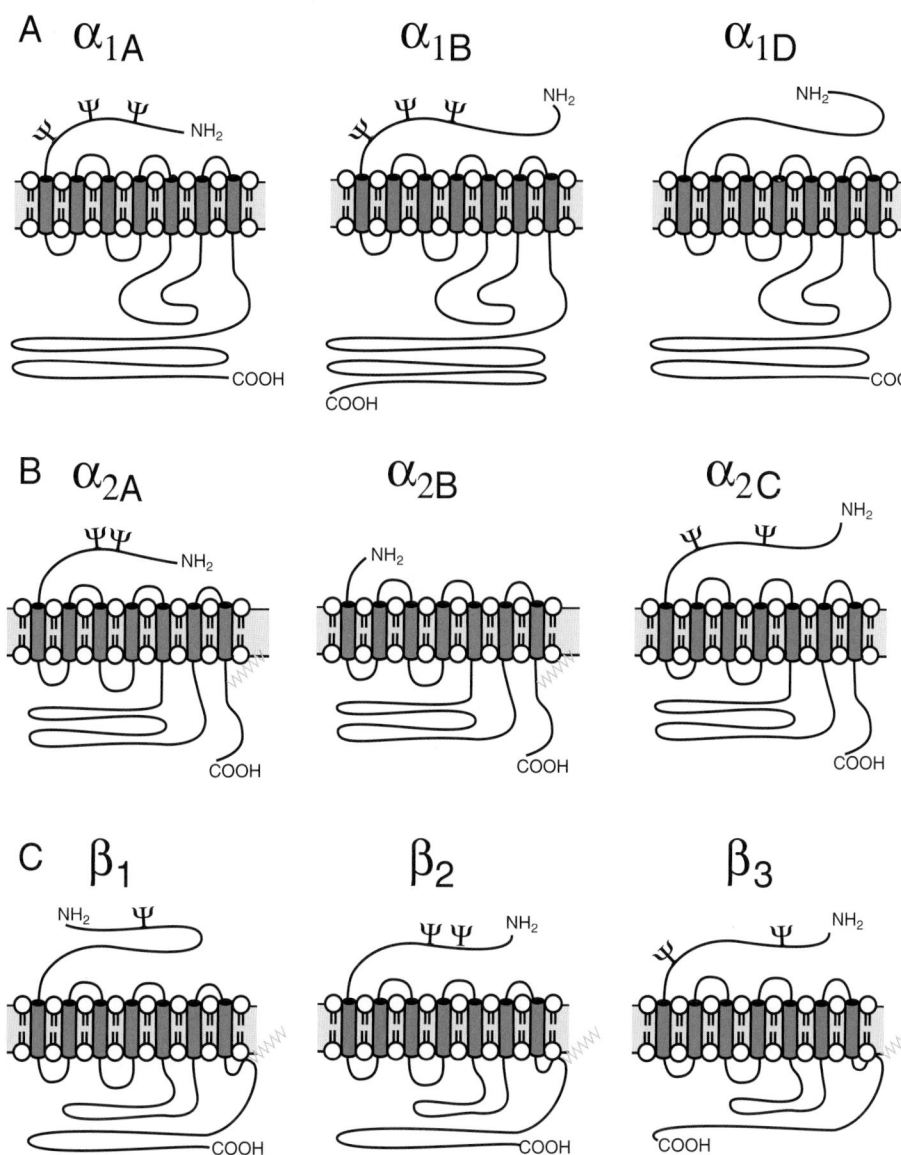

Figure 10–1. Subtypes of adrenergic receptors.

There are three known subtypes of each of the α_1-, α_2-, and β-adrenergic receptor populations. All β-adrenergic receptor subtypes are coupled to stimulation of adenylyl cyclase activity; similarly, all α_2-adrenergic receptor subtypes affect the same effector systems, *i.e.,* inhibition of adenylyl cyclase, activation of receptor-operated K^+ channels, and inhibition of voltage-sensitive Ca^{2+} channels. In contrast, there is evidence that different α_1-adrenergic receptor subpopulations couple to different effector systems. Ψ indicates a site for *N*-glycosylation; wwww indicates a site for thio-acylation.

the ligand. Since the serines are in the fifth membrane-spanning region and the aspartate is in the third (*see* Chapter 6), it is likely that catecholamines bind parallel to the plane of the membrane, forming a bridge between the two membrane spans. However, models involving dopamine receptors suggest alternative possibilities (Hutchins, 1994).

Hydroxyl groups in positions 3 and 5 confer β_2-receptor selectivity on compounds with large amino substituents. Thus, metaproterenol, terbutaline, and other similar compounds relax the bronchial musculature in patients with asthma but cause less direct cardiac stimulation than do the nonselective drugs. The response to noncatecholamines is in part determined by their capacity to release norepinephrine from storage sites. These agents thus cause effects that are mostly mediated by α and β_1 receptors, since norepinephrine is a weak β_2 agonist. Phenylethyl-

amines that lack hydroxyl groups on the ring and the β-hydroxyl group on the side chain act almost exclusively by causing the release of norepinephrine from adrenergic nerve terminals.

Since substitution of polar groups on the phenylethylamine structure makes the resultant compounds less lipophilic, unsubstituted or alkyl-substituted compounds cross the blood–brain barrier more readily and have more central activity. Thus, *ephedrine, amphetamine,* and *methamphetamine* exhibit considerable CNS activity. In addition, as noted above, the absence of polar hydroxyl groups results in a loss of direct sympathomimetic activity.

Catecholamines have only a brief duration of action and are ineffective when administered orally, because they are rapidly inactivated in the intestinal mucosa and in the liver before

Table 10–1
Chemical Structures and Main Clinical Uses of Important Sympathomimetic Drugs†

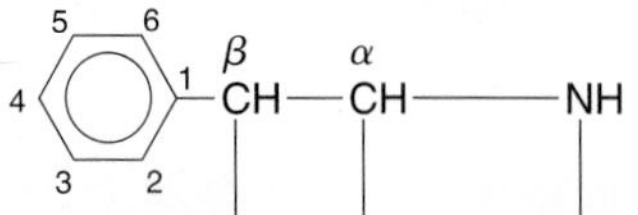

Prototypical formula: positions 4,5,6 / 3,2 on the phenyl ring; side chain βCH—αCH—NH.

Drug	Ring substituent	β	α	NH	α Receptor A N P V	β Receptor B C U	CNS, 0
Phenylethylamine		H	H	H			
Epinephrine	3-OH,4-OH	OH	H	CH₃	A, P, V	B,C	
Norepinephrine	3-OH,4-OH	OH	H	H	P		
Dopamine	3-OH,4-OH	H	H	H	P		
Dobutamine	3-OH,4-OH	H	H	1 *		C	
Colterol	3-OH,4-OH	OH	H	C(CH₃)₃		B	
Ethylnorepinephrine	3-OH,4-OH	OH	CH₂CH₃	H		B	
Isoproterenol	3-OH,4-OH	OH	H	CH(CH₃)₂		B,C	
Isoetharine	3-OH,4-OH	OH	CH₂CH₃	CH(CH₃)₂		B	
Metaproterenol	3-OH,5-OH	OH	H	CH(CH₃)₂		B	
Terbutaline	3-OH,5-OH	OH	H	C(CH₃)₃		B, U	
Metaraminol	3-OH	OH	CH₃	H	P		
Phenylephrine	3-OH	OH	H	CH₃	N, P		
Tyramine	4-OH	H	H	H			
Hydroxyamphetamine	4-OH	H	CH₃	H			
Ritodrine	4-OH	OH	CH₃	2 *		U	
Prenalterol	4-OH	OH ‡	H	–CH(CH₃)₂		C	
Methoxamine	2-OCH₃,5-OCH₃	OH	CH₃	H	P		
Albuterol	3-CH₂OH,4-OH	OH	H	C(CH₃)₃		B, U	
Amphetamine		H	CH₃	H			CNS, 0
Methamphetamine		H	CH₃	CH₃			CNS, 0
Benzphetamine		H	CH₃	3 *			0
Ephedrine		OH	CH₃	CH₃	N,P	B,C	
Phenylpropanolamine		OH	CH₃	H	N		0
Mephentermine		H	4 *	CH₃	N,P		
Phentermine		H	4 *	H			0
Propylhexedrine	5 *	H	CH₃	CH₃	N		
Diethylpropion		6 *					0
Phenmetrazine		7 *					0
Phendimetrazine		8 *					0

Substituent structures:

1. —CH—(CH₂)₂—⟨C₆H₄⟩—OH, with CH₃ on the CH
2. —CH₂—CH₂—⟨C₆H₄⟩—OH
3. —N(CH₃)(CH₂—C₆H₅)
4. —C(CH₃)₃ (C with CH₃, CH₃, CH₃)
5. cyclohexane ring
6. —C(=O)—CH(CH₃)—N(C₂H₅)(C₂H₅)
7. morpholine ring: O—CH₂, CH₂, CH—NH, CH—CH₃
8. morpholine ring: O—CH₂, CH₂, CH—N—CH₃, CH—CH₃

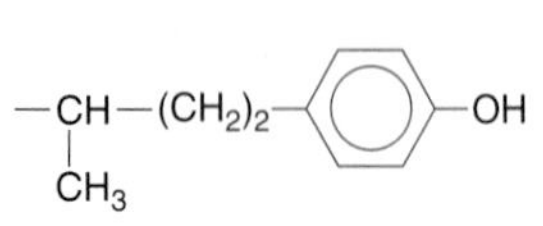

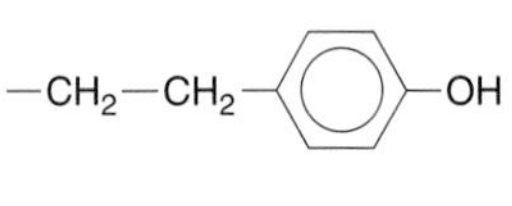

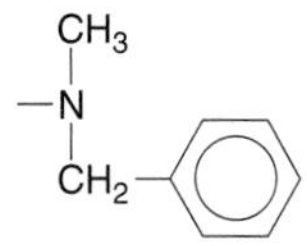

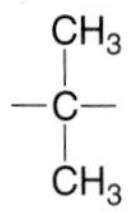

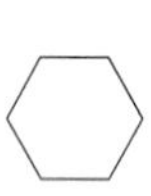

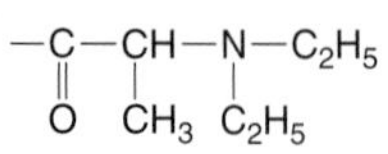

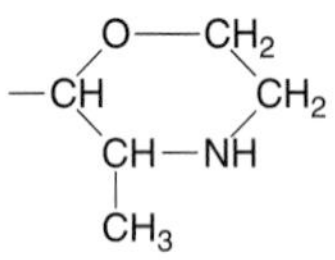

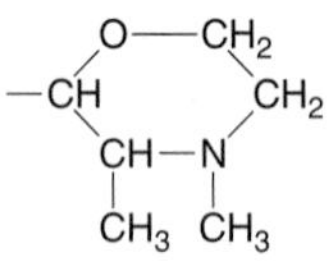

α Activity
A = Allergic reactions (includes β action)
N = Nasal decongestion
P = Pressor (may include β action)
V = Other local vasoconstriction
   (e.g., in local anesthesia)

β Activity
B = Bronchodilator
C = Cardiac
U = Uterus

CNS = Central nervous system
0 = Anorectic

*Numbers bearing an asterisk refer to the substituents numbered in the bottom rows of the table; substituent 3 replaces the N atom, substituent 5 replaces the phenyl ring, and 6, 7, and 8 are attached directly to the phenyl ring, replacing the ethylamine side chain.

†The α and β in the prototypical formula refer to positions of the C atoms in the ethylamine side chain.

‡Prenalterol has —OCH₂— between the aromatic ring and the carbon atom designated as β in the prototypical formula.

reaching the systemic circulation (*see* Chapter 6). Compounds without one or both hydroxyl substituents are not acted upon by catechol-*O*-methyltransferase (COMT), and their oral effectiveness and duration of action are enhanced.

Groups other than hydroxyls have been substituted on the aromatic ring. In general, potency at α receptors is reduced and β-receptor activity is minimal; the compounds may even block β receptors. For example, *methoxamine*, with methoxy substituents at positions 2 and 5, has highly selective α-stimulating activity and, in large doses, blocks β receptors. *Albuterol*, a β_2-selective agonist, has a substituent at position 3 and is an important exception to the general rule of low β-receptor activity. The structure of albuterol is as follows:

$$CH_2OH$$

$$HO-\bigcirc-CHOHCH_2NHC(CH_3)_3$$

ALBUTEROL

Substitution on the α-Carbon Atom. This substitution blocks oxidation by monoamine oxidase (MAO), greatly prolonging the duration of action of noncatecholamines because their degradation depends largely on the action of MAO. The duration of action of drugs such as ephedrine or amphetamine is thus measured in hours rather than in minutes. Similarly, compounds with an α-methyl substituent persist in the nerve terminal and are more likely to release norepinephrine from storage sites. Agents such as *metaraminol* exhibit a greater degree of indirect sympathomimetic activity.

Substitution on the β Carbon. Substitution of a hydroxyl group on the β carbon generally decreases actions within the CNS, largely because of the lower lipid solubility of such compounds. However, such substitution greatly enhances agonist activity at both α and β receptors. Although ephedrine is less potent than methamphetamine as a central stimulant, it is more powerful in dilating bronchioles and increasing blood pressure and heart rate.

Optical Isomerism. Substitution on either α or β carbon yields optical isomers. Levorotatory substitution on the β carbon confers the greater peripheral activity, so that the naturally occurring *l*-epinephrine and *l*-norepinephrine are at least ten times as potent as their unnatural *d*-isomers. Dextrorotatory substitution on the α carbon generally results in a more potent compound. *d*-Amphetamine is more potent than *l*-amphetamine in central but not peripheral activity.

Physiological Basis of Adrenergic Receptor Function.

An important factor in the response of any cell or organ to sympathomimetic amines is the density and proportion of α- and β-adrenergic receptors. For example, norepinephrine has relatively little capacity to increase bronchial airflow, since the receptors in bronchial smooth muscle are largely of the β_2 subtype. In contrast, isoproterenol and epinephrine are potent bronchodilators. Cutaneous blood vessels physiologically express almost exclusively α receptors; thus, norepinephrine and epinephrine cause constriction of such vessels, whereas isoproterenol

has little effect. The smooth muscle of blood vessels that supply skeletal muscles has both β_2 and α receptors; activation of β_2 receptors causes vasodilation, and stimulation of α receptors constricts these vessels. In such vessels, the threshold concentration for activation of β_2 receptors by epinephrine is lower than that for α receptors, but when both types of receptors are activated at high concentrations of epinephrine, the response to α receptors predominates. Physiological concentrations of epinephrine cause primarily vasodilation.

The ultimate response of a target organ to sympathomimetic amines is dictated not only by the direct effects of the agents but also by the reflex homeostatic adjustments of the organism. One of the most striking effects of many sympathomimetic amines is a rise in arterial blood pressure caused by stimulation of vascular α receptors. This stimulation elicits compensatory reflexes which are mediated by the carotid aortic baroreceptor system. As a result, sympathetic tone is diminished and vagal tone is enhanced; each of these responses leads to slowing of the heart rate. This reflex effect is of special importance for drugs that have little capacity to activate β-adrenergic receptors directly. With diseases such as atherosclerosis, which may impair baroreceptor mechanisms, the effects of sympathomimetic drugs may be magnified (Chapleau *et al.,* 1995).

Indirectly Acting Sympathomimetic Drugs.

For many years, it was presumed that sympathomimetic amines produced their effects by acting directly on adrenergic receptors. However, this notion was dispelled by the finding that the effects of tyramine and many other noncatecholamines were reduced or abolished after chronic postganglionic denervation or treatment with cocaine or reserpine. Under these circumstances, the effects of exogenously administered epinephrine, and especially norepinephrine, often were enhanced. These observations led to the proposal that tyramine and related amines act indirectly, following uptake into the adrenergic nerve terminal, by displacing norepinephrine from storage sites in the synaptic vesicles or from extravesicular binding sites. Norepinephrine could then exit from the adrenergic nerve terminal and interact with receptors to produce sympathomimetic effects. The depletion of tissue stores of catecholamines that follows treatment with reserpine or degeneration of adrenergic nerve terminals would explain the lack of effect of tyramine under these conditions. In the presence of cocaine, the high-affinity neuronal transport system for catecholamines and certain congeners is inhibited, and tyramine and related amines are unable to enter the adrenergic nerve terminal. In this manner, cocaine inhibits the actions of indirectly acting sympathomimetic amines while potentiating the effects of directly acting agents that are normally removed from the synaptic cleft by this transport system (*see* Chapter 6).

In assessing the proportion of direct and indirect actions of a sympathomimetic amine, the most common experimental procedure is to compare the dose-response curves for the agent on a particular target tissue before and after treatment with reserpine (Trendelenburg, 1972). Those drugs whose actions are essentially unaltered after treatment with reserpine are classified as *directly acting* sympathomimetic amines (*e.g.,* norepinephrine, phenylephrine), whereas those whose actions are abolished are termed *indirectly acting* (*e.g.,* tyramine). Many agents exhibit some degree of residual sympathomimetic activity after the administration of reserpine, but higher doses of these amines are required to produce comparable effects. These are classified as mixed-acting sympathomimetic amines; that is, they have both direct and indirect actions. The proportion of direct and indirect actions can vary considerably among different tissues and species. In some cases, relatively little is known about these properties in human beings.

Since the actions of norepinephrine are more marked on α and β_1 receptors than on β_2 receptors, many noncatecholamines that release norepinephrine have predominantly α-receptor–mediated and cardiac effects. However, certain noncatecholamines with both direct and indirect effects on adrenergic receptors show significant β_2 activity and are used clinically for these effects. Thus, ephedrine, although dependent on release of norepinephrine for some of its effects, relieves bronchospasm by its action on β_2 receptors in bronchial muscle, an effect not seen with norepinephrine. It also must be recalled that some noncatecholamines—phenylephrine, for example—act primarily and directly on effector cells. It is therefore impossible to predict precisely the characteristic effects of noncatecholamines simply on the basis that they may provoke the release of at least some norepinephrine.

False-Transmitter Concept. As indicated above, indirectly acting amines are taken up into adrenergic nerve terminals and storage vesicles, where they replace norepinephrine in the storage complex. Phenylethylamines that lack a β-hydroxyl group are retained there poorly, but β-hydroxylated phenylethylamines and compounds that subsequently become hydroxylated in the synaptic vesicle by dopamine β-hydroxylase are retained in the synaptic vesicle for relatively long periods of time. Such substances can produce a persistent diminution in the content of norepinephrine at functionally critical sites. When the nerve is stimulated, the contents of a relatively constant number of synaptic vesicles are apparently released by exocytosis. If these vesicles contain phenylethylamines that are much less potent

than norepinephrine, activation of postsynaptic adrenergic receptors will be diminished.

This hypothesis, known as the *false-transmitter concept,* is a possible explanation for some of the effects of inhibitors of MAO. Phenylethylamines normally are synthesized in the gastrointestinal tract as a result of the action of bacterial tyrosine decarboxylase. The tyramine formed in this fashion usually is oxidatively deaminated in the gastrointestinal tract and the liver, and the amine does not reach the systemic circulation in significant concentrations. However, when a MAO inhibitor is administered, tyramine may be absorbed systemically and is transported into adrenergic nerve terminals, where its catabolism is again prevented because of the inhibition of MAO at this site; it is then β-hydroxylated to octopamine and stored in the vesicles in this form. As a consequence, norepinephrine gradually is displaced, and stimulation of the nerve terminal results in the release of a relatively small amount of norepinephrine along with a fraction of octopamine. The latter amine has relatively little ability to activate either α- or β-adrenergic receptors. Thus, a functional impairment of sympathetic transmission parallels long-term administration of MAO inhibitors.

Despite such functional impairment, patients who have received MAO inhibitors may experience severe hypertensive crises if they ingest cheese, beer, or red wine. These and related foods, which are produced by fermentation, contain a large quantity of tyramine and, to a lesser degree, other phenylethylamines. When gastrointestinal and hepatic MAO are inhibited, the large quantity of tyramine that is ingested is absorbed rapidly and reaches the systemic circulation in high concentration. A massive and precipitous release of norepinephrine can result, with consequent hypertension that can be severe enough to cause myocardial infarction or a stroke. The properties of various MAO inhibitors (reversible or irreversible; selective or nonselective at MAO-A and MAO-B) are discussed in Chapter 19.

ENDOGENOUS CATECHOLAMINES

Epinephrine

Epinephrine (adrenaline) is a potent stimulant of both α- and β-adrenergic receptors, and its effects on target organs are thus complex. Most of the responses listed in Table 6–1 are seen after injection of epinephrine, although the occurrence of sweating, piloerection, and mydriasis depends on the physiological state of the subject. Particularly prominent are the actions on the heart and on vascular and other smooth muscle.

Blood Pressure. Epinephrine is one of the most potent vasopressor drugs known. If a pharmacological dose is given rapidly by an intravenous route, it evokes a characteristic effect on blood pressure, which rises rapidly to a peak that is proportional to the dose. The increase in systolic pressure is greater than the increase in diastolic pressure, so that the pulse pressure increases. As the response wanes, the mean pressure may fall below normal before returning to control levels.

The mechanism of the rise in blood pressure due to epinephrine is threefold: (1) a direct myocardial stimulation that increases the strength of ventricular contraction (positive inotropic action); (2) an increased heart rate (positive chronotropic action); and (3) vasoconstriction in many vascular beds—especially in the precapillary resistance vessels of skin, mucosa, and kidney—along with marked constriction of the veins. The pulse rate, at first accelerated, may be slowed markedly at the height of the rise of blood pressure by compensatory vagal discharge. Small doses of epinephrine (0.1 μg/kg) may cause the blood pressure to fall. The depressor effect of small doses and the biphasic response to larger doses are due to greater sensitivity to epinephrine of vasodilator β_2 receptors than of constrictor α receptors.

The effects are somewhat different when the drug is given by slow intravenous infusion or by subcutaneous injection. Absorption of epinephrine after subcutaneous injection is slow due to local vasoconstrictor action; the effects of doses as large as 0.5 to 1.5 mg can be duplicated by intravenous infusion at a rate of 10 to 30 μg per minute. There is a moderate increase in systolic pressure due to increased cardiac contractile force and a rise in cardiac output (Figure 10–2). Peripheral resistance decreases, owing to a dominant action on β_2 receptors of vessels in skeletal muscle, where blood flow is enhanced; as a consequence, diastolic pressure usually falls. Since the mean blood pressure is not, as a rule, greatly elevated, compensatory baroreceptor reflexes do not appreciably antagonize the direct cardiac actions. Heart rate, cardiac output, stroke volume, and left ventricular work per beat are increased as a result of direct cardiac stimulation and increased venous return to the heart, which is reflected by an increase in right atrial pressure. At slightly higher rates of infusion, there may be no change or a slight rise in peripheral resistance and diastolic pressure, depending on the dose and the resultant ratio of α to β responses in the various vascular beds; compensatory reflexes also may come into play. The details of the effects of intravenous infusion of epinephrine, norepinephrine, and isoproterenol in human beings are compared in Table 10–2 and Figure 10–2.

Vascular Effects.   The chief vascular action of epinephrine is exerted on the smaller arterioles and precapillary sphincters, although veins and large arteries also respond to the drug. Various vascular beds react differently, which results in a substantial redistribution of blood flow.

Injected epinephrine markedly decreases cutaneous blood flow, constricting precapillary vessels and small venules. Cutaneous vasoconstriction accounts for a marked decrease in blood flow in the hands and feet. The "after-congestion" of mucosae following the vasoconstriction from locally applied epinephrine probably is due to changes in vascular reactivity as a result of tissue hypoxia rather than to β-receptor activity of the drug on mucosal vessels.

Blood flow to skeletal muscles is increased by therapeutic doses in human beings. This is due in part to a powerful β_2-receptor vasodilator action that is only partially counterbalanced by a vasoconstrictor action on the α receptors that also are present in the vascular bed. If an α-adrenergic receptor antagonist is given, the vasodilation in muscle is more pronounced, the total peripheral resistance is decreased, and the mean blood pressure falls

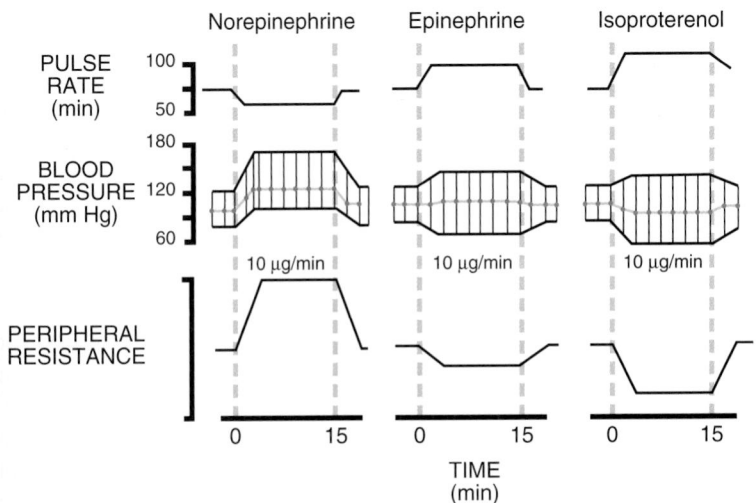

Figure 10–2. Effects of intravenous infusion of norepinephrine, epinephrine, or isoproterenol in human beings. (Modified from Allwood et al., 1963, with permission.)

Table 10–2

Comparison of the Effects of Intravenous Infusion of Epinephrine and Norepinephrine in Human Beings*

EFFECT	EPINEPH-RINE	NOREPINEPH-RINE
Cardiac		
Heart rate	+	$-$†
Stroke volume	++	++
Cardiac output	+++	0,$-$
Arrhythmias	++++	++++
Coronary blood flow	++	++
Blood pressure		
Systolic arterial	+++	+++
Mean arterial	+	++
Diastolic arterial	+,0,$-$	++
Mean pulmonary	++	++
Peripheral circulation		
Total peripheral resistance	$-$	++
Cerebral blood flow	+	0,$-$
Muscle blood flow	+++	0,$-$
Cutaneous blood flow	$--$	$--$
Renal blood flow	$-$	$-$
Splanchnic blood flow	+++	0,+
Metabolic effects		
Oxygen consumption	++	0,+
Blood glucose	+++	0,+
Blood lactic acid	+++	0,+
Eosinopenic response	+	0
Central nervous system		
Respiration	+	+
Subjective sensations	+	+

*0.1 to 0.4 μg/kg per minute.

Abbreviations: + = increase; 0 = no change; $-$ = decrease; † = after atropine, +

SOURCE: After Goldenberg *et al.,* 1950. Courtesy of *Archives of Internal Medicine.*

(epinephrine reversal). After the administration of a non-selective β-adrenergic receptor antagonist, only vasoconstriction occurs, and the administration of epinephrine is associated with a considerable pressor effect.

The effect of epinephrine on cerebral circulation is related to systemic blood pressure. In usual therapeutic doses, the drug has relatively little constrictor action on cerebral arterioles. It is physiologically advantageous that the cerebral circulation does not constrict in response to activation of the sympathetic nervous system by stressful stimuli. Indeed, autoregulatory mechanisms tend to limit the increase in cerebral blood flow caused by increased blood pressure.

Doses of epinephrine that have little effect on mean arterial pressure consistently increase renal vascular resistance and reduce renal blood flow by as much as 40%. All segments of the renal vascular bed contribute to the increased resistance. Since the glomerular filtration rate is only slightly and variably altered, the filtration fraction is consistently increased. Excretion of Na^+, K^+, and Cl^- is decreased; urine volume may be increased, decreased, or unchanged. Maximal tubular reabsorptive and excretory capacities are unchanged. The secretion of renin is increased as a consequence of a direct action of epinephrine on β_1 receptors in the juxtaglomerular apparatus.

Arterial and venous pulmonary pressures are raised. Although direct pulmonary vasoconstriction occurs, redistribution of blood from the systemic to the pulmonary circulation, due to constriction of the more powerful musculature in the systemic great veins, doubtless plays an important part in the increase in pulmonary pressure. Very high concentrations of epinephrine may cause pulmonary edema precipitated by elevated pulmonary capillary filtration pressure and possibly by "leaky" capillaries.

Coronary blood flow is enhanced by epinephrine or by cardiac sympathetic stimulation under physiological conditions. The increased flow occurs even with doses that do not increase the aortic blood pressure and is the result of two factors. The first is the increased relative duration of diastole at higher heart rates (*see* below); this is partially offset by decreased blood flow during systole because of more forceful contraction of the surrounding myocardium and an increase in mechanical compression of the coronary vessels. The increased flow during diastole is further enhanced if aortic blood pressure is elevated by epinephrine, and, as a consequence, total coronary flow may be increased. The second factor is a metabolic dilator effect that results from the increased strength of contraction and myocardial oxygen consumption due to the direct effects of epinephrine on cardiac myocytes. This vasodilation is mediated in part by adenosine released from cardiac myocytes, which tends to override a direct vasoconstrictor effect of epinephrine that results from activation of α receptors in coronary vessels.

Cardiac Effects. Epinephrine is a powerful cardiac stimulant. It acts directly on the predominant β_1 receptors of the myocardium and of the cells of the pacemaker and conducting tissues; β_2 and α receptors also are present in the heart, although there are considerable species differences. Considerable recent interest has focused on the role of β_1 and β_2 receptors in the human heart, especially in heart failure. The heart rate increases, and the rhythm often is altered. Cardiac systole is shorter and more powerful, cardiac output is enhanced, and the work of the heart and its oxygen consumption are markedly increased. Cardiac efficiency (work done relative to oxygen consumption) is lessened. Direct responses to epinephrine include increases in contractile force, accelerated rate of rise of isometric tension, enhanced rate of relaxation, decreased time to peak tension, increased excitability, acceleration of the rate of spontaneous beating, and induction of automaticity in specialized regions of the heart.

In accelerating the heart, epinephrine preferentially shortens systole so that the duration of diastole usually is not reduced. Indeed, activation of β receptors increases the rate of relaxation of ventricular muscle. Epinephrine speeds the heart by accelerating the slow depolarization of sinoatrial (SA) nodal cells that takes place during diastole, *i.e.,* during phase 4 of the action potential (*see* Chapter 35). Consequently, the transmembrane potential of the pacemaker cells rises more rapidly to the threshold level at which the action potential is initiated. The amplitude of the action potential and the maximal rate of depolarization (phase 0) also are increased. A shift in the location of the pacemaker within the SA node often occurs, owing to activation of latent pacemaker cells. In Purkinje fibers, epinephrine also accelerates diastolic depolarization and may cause activation of latent pacemaker cells. These changes do not occur in atrial and ventricular muscle fibers, where epinephrine has little effect on the stable, phase 4 membrane potential after repolarization. If large doses of epinephrine are given, premature ventricular systoles occur and may herald more serious ventricular arrhythmias. This rarely is seen with conventional doses in human beings, but ventricular extrasystoles, tachycardia, or even fibrillation may be precipitated by release of endogenous epinephrine when the heart has been sensitized to this action of epinephrine by certain anesthetics or in cases of myocardial infarction. The mechanism of induction of these cardiac arrhythmias is not clear.

Some effects of epinephrine on cardiac tissues are largely secondary to the increase in heart rate, and are small or inconsistent when the heart rate is kept constant. For example, the effect of epinephrine on repolarization of atrial muscle, Purkinje fibers, or ventricular muscle is small if the heart rate is unchanged. When the heart rate is increased, the duration of the action potential is consistently shortened, and the refractory period is correspondingly decreased.

Conduction through the Purkinje system depends on the level of membrane potential at the time of excitation. Excessive reduction of this potential results in conduction disturbances, ranging from slowed conduction to complete block. Epinephrine often increases the membrane potential and improves conduction in Purkinje fibers that have been excessively depolarized.

Epinephrine normally shortens the refractory period of the human atrioventricular (AV) node by direct effects on the heart, although doses of epinephrine that slow the heart through reflex vagal discharge may indirectly tend to prolong it. Epinephrine also decreases the grade of AV block that occurs as a result of disease, drugs, or vagal stimulation. Supraventricular arrhythmias are apt to occur from the combination of epinephrine and cholinergic stimulation. Depression of sinus rate and AV conduction by vagal discharge probably plays a part in epinephrine-induced ventricular arrhythmias, since various drugs that block the vagal effect confer some protection. The action of epinephrine in enhancing cardiac automaticity and its action in causing arrhythmias are effectively antagonized by β-adrenergic receptor antagonists such as propranolol. However, α_1 receptors exist in most regions of the heart, and their activation prolongs the refractory period and strengthens myocardial contractions.

Cardiac arrhythmias have been seen in patients after inadvertent intravenous administration of conventional subcutaneous doses of epinephrine. Ventricular premature systoles can appear, which may be followed by multifocal ventricular tachycardia or ventricular fibrillation. Pulmonary edema also may occur.

Epinephrine decreases the amplitude of the T wave of the electrocardiogram (ECG) in normal persons. In animals given relatively larger doses, additional effects are seen on the T wave and the ST segment. After decreasing in amplitude, the T wave may become biphasic, and the ST segment can deviate either above or below the isoelectric line. Such ST-segment changes are similar to those seen in patients with angina pectoris during spontaneous or epinephrine-induced attacks of pain. These electrical changes therefore have been attributed to myocardial ischemia. Also, epinephrine as well as other catecholamines may cause myocardial cell death, particularly after intravenous infusions. Acute toxicity is associated with contraction band necrosis and other pathological changes. Recent interest has focused on the possiblilty that prolonged sympathetic stimulation of the heart, such as in congestive cardiomyopathy, may promote apoptosis of cardiomyocytes.

Effects on Smooth Muscles. The effects of epinephrine on the smooth muscles of different organs and systems depend on the type of adrenergic receptor in the muscle (*see* Table 6–1). The effects on vascular smooth muscle are of major physiological importance, whereas those on gastrointestinal smooth muscle are relatively minor. Gastrointestinal smooth muscle is, in general, relaxed by epinephrine. This effect is due to activation of both α- and β-adrenergic receptors. Intestinal tone and the frequency and amplitude of spontaneous contractions are reduced. The stomach usually is relaxed and the pyloric and ileocecal sphincters are contracted, but these effects depend on the preexisting tone of the muscle. If tone already is high, epinephrine causes relaxation; if low, contraction.

The responses of uterine muscle to epinephrine vary with species, phase of the sexual cycle, state of gestation, and dose given. Epinephrine contracts strips of pregnant or nonpregnant human uterus *in vitro* by interaction with α receptors. The effects of epinephrine on the human uterus *in situ,* however, differ. During the last month of pregnancy and at parturition, epinephrine inhibits uterine tone and contractions. β_2-Selective agonists, such as ritodrine or terbutaline, have been used to delay premature labor, although their efficacy is limited. Effects of these and other drugs on the uterus are discussed later in this chapter.

Epinephrine relaxes the detrusor muscle of the bladder as a result of activation of β receptors and contracts the trigone and sphincter muscles owing to its α-agonist activity. This can result in hesitancy in urination and may contribute to retention of urine in the bladder. Activation of smooth muscle contraction in the prostate promotes urinary retention.

Respiratory Effects. Epinephrine affects respiration primarily by relaxing bronchial muscle. It has a powerful bronchodilator action, most evident when bronchial muscle is contracted because of disease, as in bronchial asthma, or in response to drugs or various autacoids. In such situations, epinephrine has a striking therapeutic effect as a physiological antagonist to substances that cause bronchoconstriction.

The beneficial effects of epinephrine in asthma also may arise from inhibition of antigen-induced release of inflammatory mediators from mast cells, and to a lesser extent from diminution of bronchial secretions and congestion within the mucosa. Inhibition of mast cell secretion is mediated by β_2-adrenergic receptors, while the effects on the mucosa are mediated by α receptors; however, other drugs, such as glucocorticoids and leukotriene antagonists, have much more profound antiinflammatory effects in asthma (see Chapter 28).

Effects on the Central Nervous System. Because of the inability of this rather polar compound to enter the CNS, epinephrine in conventional therapeutic doses is not a powerful CNS stimulant. While the drug may cause restlessness, apprehension, headache, and tremor in many persons, these effects in part may be secondary to the effects of epinephrine on the cardiovascular system, skeletal muscles, and intermediary metabolism; that is, they may be the result of somatic manifestations of anxiety. Some other sympathomimetic drugs more readily cross the blood–brain barrier.

Metabolic Effects. Epinephrine has a number of important influences on metabolic processes. It elevates the concentrations of glucose and lactate in blood by mechanisms described in Chapter 6. Insulin secretion is inhibited through an interaction with α_2 receptors and is enhanced by activation of β_2 receptors; the predominant effect seen with epinephrine is inhibition. Glucagon secretion is enhanced by an action on the β receptors of the α cells of pancreatic islets. Epinephrine also decreases the uptake of glucose by peripheral tissues, at least in part because of its effects on the secretion of insulin, but also possibly due to direct effects on skeletal muscle. Glycosuria rarely occurs. The effect of epinephrine to stimulate glycogenolysis in most tissues and in most species involves β receptors (see Chapter 6).

Epinephrine raises the concentration of free fatty acids in blood by stimulating β receptors in adipocytes. The result is activation of triglyceride lipase, which accelerates the breakdown of triglycerides to form free fatty acids and glycerol. The calorigenic action of epinephrine (increase in metabolism) is reflected in human beings by an increase of 20% to 30% in oxygen consumption after conventional doses. This effect is mainly due to enhanced breakdown of triglycerides in brown adipose tissue, providing an increase in oxidizable substrate (see Chapter 6).

Miscellaneous Effects. Epinephrine reduces circulating plasma volume by loss of protein-free fluid to the extracellular space, thereby increasing erythrocyte and plasma protein concentrations. However, conventional doses of epinephrine do not significantly alter plasma volume or packed red-cell volume under normal conditions, although such doses are reported to have variable effects in the presence of shock, hemorrhage, hypotension, and anesthesia. Epinephrine rapidly increases the number of circulating polymorphonuclear leukocytes, likely due to β-receptor–mediated demargination of these cells. Epinephrine accelerates blood coagulation in laboratory animals and human beings and promotes fibrinolysis.

The effects of epinephrine on secretory glands are not marked; in most glands secretion usually is inhibited, partly owing to the reduced blood flow caused by vasoconstriction. Epinephrine stimulates lacrimation and a scanty mucous secretion from salivary glands. Sweating and pilomotor activity are minimal after systemic administration of epinephrine, but occur after intradermal injection of very dilute solutions of either epinephrine or norepinephrine. Such effects are inhibited by α-receptor antagonists.

Mydriasis is readily seen during physiological sympathetic stimulation but not when epinephrine is instilled into the conjunctival sac of normal eyes. However, epinephrine usually lowers intraocular pressure from normal levels and in wide-angle glaucoma; the mechanism of this effect is not clear, but both reduced production of aqueous humor due to vasoconstriction and enhanced outflow probably occur (see Chapter 66).

Although epinephrine does not directly excite skeletal muscle, it facilitates neuromuscular transmission, particularly that following prolonged rapid stimulation of motor nerves. In apparent contrast to the effects of α-receptor activation at presynaptic nerve terminals in the autonomic nervous system (α_2 receptors), stimulation of α receptors causes a more rapid increase in transmitter release from the somatic motor neuron, perhaps as a result of enhanced influx of Ca^{2+}. These responses likely are mediated by α_1 receptors. These actions may explain in part the ability of epinephrine (given intraarterially) to cause a brief increase in motor power of the injected limb of patients with myasthenia gravis. Epinephrine also acts directly on white, fast-contracting muscle fibers to prolong the active state, thereby increasing peak tension. Of greater physiological and clinical importance is the capacity of epinephrine and selective β_2-agonists to increase physiological tremor, at least in part due to β-receptor–mediated enhancement of discharge of muscle spindles.

Epinephrine promotes a fall in plasma K^+ largely due to stimulation of K^+ uptake into cells, particularly skeletal muscle, due to activation of β_2 receptors. This is associated with decreased renal K^+ excretion. These receptors have been exploited in the management of hyperkalemic familial periodic paralysis, which is characterized by episodic flaccid paralysis, hyperkalemia, and depolarization of skeletal muscle. The β_2-selective agonist albuterol apparently is able to ameliorate the impairment in the ability of the muscle to accumulate and retain K^+.

Large or repeated doses of epinephrine or other sympathomimetic amines given to experimental animals lead to damage to arterial walls and myocardium, which is so severe as to cause the appearance of necrotic areas in the heart indistinguishable from myocardial infarcts. The mechanism of this injury is not yet clear, but α- and β-receptor antagonists and Ca^{2+} channel blockers may afford substantial protection against the damage.

Similar lesions occur in many patients with pheochromocytoma or after prolonged infusions of norepinephrine.

Absorption, Fate, and Excretion. As indicated above, epinephrine is not effective after oral administration, because it is rapidly conjugated and oxidized in the gastrointestinal mucosa and liver. Absorption from subcutaneous tissues occurs relatively slowly because of local vasoconstriction and the rate may be further decreased by systemic hypotension, for example in a patient with shock. Absorption is more rapid after intramuscular injection. In emergencies, it may be necessary in some cases to administer epinephrine intravenously. When relatively concentrated solutions (1%) are nebulized and inhaled, the actions of the drug largely are restricted to the respiratory tract; however, systemic reactions such as arrhythmias may occur, particularly if larger amounts are used.

Epinephrine is rapidly inactivated in the body. The liver, which is rich in both of the enzymes responsible for destroying circulating epinephrine (COMT and MAO), is particularly important in this regard (*see* Figure 6–5). Although only small amounts appear in the urine of normal persons, the urine of patients with pheochromocytoma may contain relatively large amounts of epinephrine, norepinephrine, and their metabolites.

Epinephrine is available in a variety of formulations geared for different clinical indications and routes of administration, such as by injection (usually subcutaneously but sometimes intravenously), by inhalation, or topically. Several practical points are worth noting. First, epinephrine is unstable in alkaline solution; when exposed to air or light, it turns pink from oxidation to adrenochrome and then brown from formation of polymers. *Epinephrine injection* is available in 1:1,000, 1:10,000, and 1:100,000 solutions. The usual adult dose given subcutaneously ranges from 0.3 mg to 0.5 mg. The intravenous route is used cautiously if an immediate and reliable effect is mandatory. If the solution is given by vein, it must be adequately diluted and injected very slowly. The dose is seldom as much as 0.25 mg, except for cardiac arrest, when larger doses may be required. Epinephrine suspensions (*e.g.,* SUS-PHRINE) are used to slow subcutaneous absorption and must never be injected intravenously. *Also, a 1% (1:100) formulation is available for administration* via *inhalation; every precaution must be taken not to confuse this 1:100 solution with the 1:1000 solution designed for parenteral administration, because inadvertent injection of the 1:100 solution can be fatal.*

Toxicity, Adverse Effects, and Contraindications. Epinephrine may cause disturbing reactions, such as rest-

lessness, throbbing headache, tremor, and palpitations. The effects rapidly subside with rest, quiet, recumbency, and reassurance.

More serious reactions include cerebral hemorrhage and cardiac arrhythmias. The use of large doses or the accidental, rapid intravenous injection of epinephrine may result in cerebral hemorrhage from the sharp rise in blood pressure. Ventricular arrhythmias may follow the administration of epinephrine. Angina may be induced by epinephrine in patients with coronary artery disease.

The use of epinephrine generally is contraindicated in patients who are receiving nonselective β-adrenergic receptor blocking drugs, since its unopposed actions on vascular α_1-adrenergic receptors may lead to severe hypertension and cerebral hemorrhage.

Therapeutic Uses. Epinephrine has limited clinical uses. In general, these are based on the actions of the drug on blood vessels, heart, and bronchial muscle. In the past, the most common use of epinephrine was to relieve respiratory distress due to bronchospasm; however, β_2-selective agonists now are preferred. A major use is to provide rapid relief of hypersensitivity reactions, including anaphylaxis, to drugs and other allergens. Also, epinephrine may be used to prolong the action of local anesthetics, presumably by decreasing local blood flow. Its cardiac effects may be of use in restoring cardiac rhythm in patients with cardiac arrest due to various causes. It also is used as a topical hemostatic agent on bleeding surfaces such as in the mouth or in bleeding peptic ulcers during endoscopy of the stomach/duodenum. Systemic absorption of the drug can occur with dental application. In addition, inhalation of epinephrine may be useful in the treatment of postintubation and infectious croup. The therapeutic uses of epinephrine are discussed later in this chapter, in relation to other sympathomimetic drugs.

Norepinephrine

Norepinephrine (levarterenol, *l*-noradrenaline, *l*-β-[3,4-dihydroxyphenyl]-α-aminoethanol) is the major chemical mediator liberated by mammalian postganglionic adrenergic nerves. It differs from epinephrine only by lacking the methyl substitution in the amino group (*see* Table 10–1). Norepinephrine constitutes 10% to 20% of the catecholamine content of human adrenal medulla and as much as 97% in some pheochromocytomas, which may not express the enzyme phenylethanolamine-*N*-methyltransferase. The history of its discovery and its role as a neurohumoral mediator are discussed in Chapter 6.

Pharmacological Properties. The pharmacological actions of norepinephrine and epinephrine have been extensively compared *in vivo* and *in vitro* (*see* Table 10–2). Both drugs are direct agonists on effector cells, and their actions differ mainly in the ratio of their effectiveness in stimulating α and β_2 receptors. They are approximately equipotent in stimulating β_1 receptors. Norepinephrine is a potent agonist at α receptors and has relatively little action on β_2 receptors; however, it is somewhat less potent than epinephrine on the α receptors of most organs.

Cardiovascular Effects. The cardiovascular effects of an intravenous infusion of 10 μg of norepinephrine per minute in human beings are shown in Figure 10–2. Systolic and diastolic pressures and, usually, pulse pressure are increased. Cardiac output is unchanged or decreased, and total peripheral resistance is raised. Compensatory vagal reflex activity slows the heart, overcoming a direct cardioaccelerator action, and stroke volume is increased. The peripheral vascular resistance increases in most vascular beds, and blood flow is reduced to the kidneys. Norepinephrine constricts mesenteric vessels and reduces splanchnic and hepatic blood flow. Coronary flow usually is increased, probably owing both to indirectly induced coronary dilation, as with epinephrine, and to elevated blood pressure. However, patients with Prinzmetal's variant angina may be supersensitive to the α-adrenergic vasoconstrictor effects of norepinephrine (*see* Chapter 32).

Unlike epinephrine, small doses of norepinephrine do not cause vasodilation or lower blood pressure, since the blood vessels of skeletal muscle constrict rather than dilate; α-adrenergic receptor blocking agents therefore abolish the pressor effects but do not cause significant reversal, *i.e.*, hypotension.

Other Effects. Other responses to norepinephrine are not prominent in human beings. The drug causes hyperglycemia and other metabolic effects similar to those produced by epinephrine, but these are observed only when large doses are given; that is, norepinephrine is not as effective a "hormone" as epinephrine. Intradermal injection of suitable doses causes sweating that is not blocked by atropine.

Absorption, Fate, and Excretion. Norepinephrine, like epinephrine, is ineffective when given orally and is absorbed poorly from sites of subcutaneous injection. It is rapidly inactivated in the body by the same enzymes that methylate and oxidatively deaminate epinephrine (*see* above). Small amounts normally are found in the urine. The excretion rate may be greatly increased in patients with pheochromocytoma.

Toxicity, Adverse Effects, and Precautions. The untoward effects of norepinephrine are similar to those of epinephrine, although there is typically greater elevation of blood pressure with norepinephrine. Excessive doses can cause severe hypertension, so careful blood pressure monitoring generally is indicated during systemic administration of this agent.

Care must be taken that necrosis and sloughing do not occur at the site of intravenous injection owing to extravasation of the drug. The infusion should be made high in the limb, preferably through a long plastic cannula extending centrally. Impaired circulation at injection sites, with or without extravasation of norepinephrine, may be relieved by infiltrating the area with phentolamine, an α-receptor antagonist. Blood pressure must be determined frequently during the infusion and particularly during adjustment of the rate of the infusion. Reduced blood flow to organs such as kidney and intestines is a constant danger with the use of norepinephrine.

Therapeutic Uses and Status. Norepinephrine (*norepinephrine bitartrate*, LEVOPHED) has only limited therapeutic value. The use of it and other sympathomimetic amines in shock is discussed later in this chapter. In the treatment of low blood pressure, the dose is titrated to the desired pressor response.

Dopamine

Dopamine (3,4-dihydroxyphenylethylamine) (*see* Table 10–1) is the immediate metabolic precursor of norepinephrine and epinephrine; it is a central neurotransmitter particularly important in the regulation of movement (Chapters 12, 20, and 22) and possesses important intrinsic pharmacological properties. Dopamine is a substrate for both MAO and COMT and thus is ineffective when administered orally. Classification of dopamine receptors is described in Chapter 22.

Pharmacological Properties. ***Cardiovascular Effects.*** The cardiovascular effects of dopamine are mediated by several distinct types of receptors that vary in their affinity for dopamine (Goldberg and Rajfer, 1985). At low concentrations, the primary interaction of dopamine is with vascular D_1-dopaminergic receptors, especially in the renal, mesenteric, and coronary beds. By activating adenylyl cyclase and raising intracellular concentrations of cyclic AMP, D_1-receptor stimulation leads to vasodilation (Missale *et al.*, 1998). Infusion of low doses of dopamine causes an increase in glomerular filtration rate, renal blood flow, and Na^+ excretion. As a consequence, dopamine has pharmacologically appropriate effects in the management of states of low cardiac output associated with compromised renal function, such as severe congestive heart failure.

At somewhat higher concentrations, dopamine exerts a positive inotropic effect on the myocardium, acting on β_1-adrenergic receptors. Dopamine also causes the release of norepinephrine from nerve terminals, which contributes to its effects on the heart. Tachycardia is less prominent during infusion of dopamine than of isoproterenol (*see* below). Dopamine usually increases systolic blood pressure and pulse pressure and either has no effect on diastolic blood pressure or increases it slightly. Total peripheral resistance usually is unchanged when low or intermediate doses of dopamine are given, probably because of the ability of dopamine to reduce regional arterial resistance in some vascular beds, such as mesenteric and renal, while causing only minor increases in other vascular beds. At high concentrations, dopamine activates vascular α_1-adrenergic receptors, leading to more general vasoconstriction.

Other Effects. Although there are specific dopamine receptors in the CNS, injected dopamine usually has no central effects because it does not readily cross the blood–brain barrier.

Precautions, Adverse Reactions, and Contraindications.
Before dopamine is administered to patients in shock, hypovolemia should be corrected by transfusion of whole blood, plasma, or other appropriate fluid. Untoward effects due to overdosage generally are attributable to excessive sympathomimetic activity (although this also may be the response to worsening shock). Nausea, vomiting, tachycardia, anginal pain, arrhythmias, headache, hypertension, and peripheral vasoconstriction may be encountered during an infusion of dopamine. Extravasation of large amounts of dopamine during infusion may cause ischemic necrosis and sloughing. Rarely, gangrene of the fingers or toes has followed the prolonged infusion of the drug.

Dopamine should be avoided or used at a much reduced dosage (one-tenth or less) if the patient has received a MAO inhibitor. Careful adjustment of dosage also is necessary for the patient who is taking tricyclic antidepressants, as responses may be particularly variable.

Therapeutic Uses.
Dopamine (*dopamine hydrochloride;* INTROPIN) is used in the treatment of severe congestive failure, particularly in patients with oliguria and with low or normal peripheral vascular resistance. The drug also may improve physiological parameters in the treatment of cardiogenic and septic shock. While dopamine may acutely improve cardiac and renal function in severely ill patients with chronic heart disease or renal failure, there is relatively little evidence supporting long-term changes in clinical outcome (Marik and Iglesias, 1999). The management of shock is discussed later in this chapter.

Dopamine hydrochloride is used only intravenously. The drug is initially administered at a rate of 2 to 5 μg/kg per minute; this rate may be increased gradually up to 20 to 50 μg/kg per minute or more as the clinical situation dictates. During the infusion, patients require clinical assessment of myocardial function, perfusion of vital organs such as the brain, and the production of urine. Most patients should receive intensive care, with monitoring of arterial and venous pressures and the ECG. Reduction in urine flow, tachycardia, and the development of arrhythmias may be indications to slow or terminate the infusion. The duration of action of dopamine is brief, and hence the rate of administration can be used to control the intensity of effect.

Related drugs include *fenoldopam* and *dopexamine*. Fenoldopam (CORLOPAM) is a D_1-receptor-selective agonist, which lowers blood pressure in severe hypertension (Elliott *et al.,* 1990; Nichols *et al.,* 1990). Fenoldopam does not appear to activate α- or β-adrenergic receptors. Intravenous infusions of fenoldopam dilate a variety of blood vessels including coronary, renal (both afferent and efferent arterioles), and mesenteric arteries (Brogden and Markham, 1997). The drug is indicated for short-term management of severe hypertension where rapid reduction of blood pressure is clinically indicated. Dopexamine (DOPACARD) is a synthetic analog related to dopamine with intrinsic activity at dopamine receptors as well as at β_2-adrenergic receptors; it may have other effects such as inhibition of catecholamine uptake (Fitton and Benfield, 1990). It appears to have favorable hemodynamic actions in patients with severe congestive heart failure, sepsis, and shock. Dopexamine is not available in the United States.

β-ADRENERGIC AGONISTS

β-Adrenergic receptor agonists have been utilized in many clinical settings but now play a major role only in the treatment of bronchoconstriction in patients with asthma (reversible airway obstruction) or chronic obstructive pulmonary disease.

Epinephrine was first used as a bronchodilator at the beginning of this century, and ephedrine was introduced into western medicine in 1924, although it had been used in China for thousands of years (Chen and Schmidt, 1930). The next major advance was the development in the 1940s of isoproterenol, a β-receptor-selective agonist; this provided a drug for asthma that lacked α-adrenergic activity. The recent development of β_2-selective agonists has resulted in drugs with even more valuable characteristics, including adequate oral bioavailability, lack of α-adrenergic activity, and diminished likelihood of adverse cardiovascular effects.

β-Adrenergic agonists may be used to stimulate the rate and force of cardiac contraction. The chronotropic effect is useful in the emergency treatment of arrhythmias such as *torsades de pointes,* bradycardia, or heart block (Chapter 35), whereas the inotropic effect is useful when it is desirable to augment myocardial contractility. The various therapeutic uses of β-adrenergic agonists are discussed later in the chapter.

Isoproterenol

Isoproterenol (isopropylarterenol, isopropylnorepinephrine, isoprenaline, isopropylnoradrenaline, d,l-β-[3,4-dihydroxyphenyl]-α-isopropylaminoethanol) (*see* Table 10–1) is a potent, nonselective β-adrenergic agonist with very low affinity for α-adrenergic receptors. Consequently, isoproterenol has powerful effects on all β receptors and almost no action at α receptors.

Pharmacological Actions. The major cardiovascular effects of isoproterenol (compared with epinephrine and norepinephrine) are illustrated in Figure 10–2. Intravenous infusion of isoproterenol lowers peripheral vascular resistance, primarily in skeletal muscle but also in renal and mesenteric vascular beds. Diastolic pressure falls. Systolic blood pressure may remain unchanged or rise, although mean arterial pressure typically falls. Cardiac output is increased because of the positive inotropic and chronotropic effects of the drug in the face of diminished peripheral vascular resistance. The cardiac effects of isoproterenol may lead to palpitations, sinus tachycardia, and more serious arrhythmias; large doses of isoproterenol may cause myocardial necrosis in animals.

Isoproterenol relaxes almost all varieties of smooth muscle when the tone is high, but this action is most pronounced on bronchial and gastrointestinal smooth muscle. It prevents or relieves bronchoconstriction. Its effect in asthma may be due in part to an additional action to inhibit antigen-induced release of histamine and other mediators of inflammation; this action is shared by β_2-receptor–selective stimulants.

Absorption, Fate, and Excretion. Isoproterenol is readily absorbed when given parenterally or as an aerosol. It is metabolized primarily in the liver and other tissues by COMT. Isoproterenol is a relatively poor substrate for MAO and is not taken up by sympathetic neurons to the same extent as are epinephrine and norepinephrine. The duration of action of isoproterenol therefore may be longer than that of epinephrine, but it still is brief.

Toxicity and Adverse Effects. Palpitations, tachycardia, headache, and flushed skin are common. Cardiac ischemia and arrhythmias may occur, particularly in patients with underlying coronary artery disease.

Therapeutic Uses. Isoproterenol (*isoproterenol hydrochloride;* ISUPREL) may be used in emergencies to stimulate heart rate in patients with bradycardia or heart block, particularly in anticipation of inserting an artificial cardiac pacemaker or in patients with the ventricular arrhythmia *torsades de pointes.* In disorders such as asthma and shock, isoproterenol largely has been replaced by other sympathomimetic drugs (*see* below and Chapter 28).

Dobutamine

Dobutamine resembles dopamine structurally but possesses a bulky aromatic substituent on the amino group (*see* Table 10–1). The pharmacological effects of dobutamine are due to direct interactions with α- and β-adrenergic receptors; its actions do not appear to be a result of release of norepinephrine from sympathetic nerve endings, nor are they exerted *via* dopaminergic receptors. Although dobutamine originally was thought to be a relatively selective β_1-adrenergic agonist, it is now clear that its pharmacological effects are complex. Dobutamine possesses a center of asymmetry; the two enantiomeric forms are present in the racemic mixture that is used clinically (Ruffolo *et al.,* 1981). The ($-$) isomer of dobutamine is a potent agonist at α_1 receptors and is capable of causing marked pressor responses (Ruffolo and Yaden, 1983). In contrast, ($+$)-dobutamine is a potent α_1-adrenergic receptor antagonist, which can block the effects of ($-$)-dobutamine. The effects of these two isomers are mediated *via* β-adrenergic receptors. The ($+$) isomer is about ten times more potent as a β-adrenergic receptor agonist than is the ($-$) isomer. Both isomers appear to be full agonists.

Cardiovascular Effects. The cardiovascular effects of racemic dobutamine represent a composite of the distinct pharmacological properties of the ($-$) and ($+$) stereoisomers. Dobutamine has relatively more prominent inotropic than chronotropic effects on the heart compared to isoproterenol. The explanation for this useful selectivity is not clear. It may be due in part to the fact that peripheral resistance is relatively unchanged. Alternatively, cardiac α_1 receptors may contribute to the inotropic effect. At equivalent inotropic doses, dobutamine enhances automaticity of the sinus node to a lesser extent than does isoproterenol; however, enhancement of atrioventricular and intraventricular conduction is similar for the two drugs.

In animals, administration of dobutamine at a rate of 2.5 to 15 μg/kg per minute increases cardiac contractility and cardiac output. Total peripheral resistance is not greatly affected. The relative constancy of peripheral resistance presumably reflects counterbalancing of α_1-adrenergic receptor–mediated vasoconstriction and β_2-receptor–mediated vasodilation (Ruffolo, 1987). The heart rate increases only modestly when the rate of administration of dobutamine is maintained at less than 20 μg/kg per minute. After administration of β-adrenergic blocking agents, infusion of dobutamine fails to increase cardiac output, but total peripheral resistance increases, confirming that dobutamine does have modest direct effects on α receptors in the vasculature.

Adverse Effects. In some patients, blood pressure and heart rate may increase significantly during administration of dobutamine; this may require reduction of the rate of infusion. Patients with a history of hypertension may be at greater risk of developing an exaggerated pressor response. Since dobutamine facilitates atrioventricular conduction, patients with atrial fibrillation are at risk of marked increases in ventricular response rates; digoxin or other measures may be required to prevent this from occurring. Some patients may develop ventricular ectopic activity. As with any inotropic agent, dobutamine potentially may increase the size of a myocardial infarct by increasing myocardial oxygen demand. This risk must be balanced against the patient's overall clinical status. The efficacy of dobutamine over a period of more than a few days is uncertain; there is evidence for the development of tolerance (Unverferth *et al.*, 1980).

Therapeutic Uses. Dobutamine (*dobutamine hydrochloride;* DOBUTREX) is indicated for the short-term treatment of cardiac decompensation that may occur after cardiac surgery or in patients with congestive heart failure or acute myocardial infarction. Dobutamine increases cardiac output and stroke volume in such patients, usually without a marked increase in heart rate. Alterations in blood pressure or peripheral resistance usually are minor, although some patients may have marked increases in blood pressure or heart rate. Clinical evidence of longer-term efficacy remains uncertain. Interestingly, an infusion of dobutamine in combination with echocardiography is useful in the noninvasive assessment of patients with coronary artery disease (Madu *et al.*, 1994). Stressing of the heart with dobutamine may reveal cardiac abnormalities in carefully selected patients.

Dobutamine has a half-life of about 2 minutes; the major metabolites are conjugates of dobutamine and 3-*O*-methyldobutamine. The onset of effect is rapid. Consequently, a loading dose is not required, and steady-state concentrations generally are achieved within 10 minutes of initiation of an infusion. The rate of infusion required to increase cardiac output is typically between 2.5 and 10 μg/kg per minute, although higher infusion rates occasionally are required. The rate and duration of the infusion are determined by the clinical and hemodynamic responses of the patient.

β_2-Selective Adrenergic Agonists

Some of the major adverse effects of β-adrenergic agonists in the treatment of asthma are caused by stimulation of β_1-adrenergic receptors in the heart. Accordingly, drugs with preferential affinity for β_2 receptors compared with β_1 receptors have been developed. However, this selectivity is not absolute, and it is lost at sufficiently high concentrations of these drugs.

A second strategy that has increased the usefulness of several β_2-selective agonists in the treatment of asthma has been structural modification that results in lower rates of metabolism and enhanced oral bioavailability (compared with catecholamines). Modifications have included placing the hydroxyl groups at positions 3 and 5 of the phenyl ring or substituting another moiety for the hydroxyl group at position 3. This has yielded drugs such as *metaproterenol, terbutaline,* and *albuterol,* which are not substrates for COMT. Bulky substituents on the amino group of catecholamines contribute to potency at β-adrenergic receptors with decreased activity at α-adrenergic receptors and decreased metabolism by MAO (Nelson, 1982).

A final strategy to enhance preferential activation of pulmonary β_2 receptors is the administration by inhalation of small doses of the drug in aerosol form. This approach typically leads to effective activation of β_2 receptors in the bronchi but very low systemic drug concentrations (Newhouse and Dolovich, 1986). Consequently, there is less potential to activate cardiac β_1 receptors or to stimulate β_2 receptors in skeletal muscle, which can cause tremor and thereby limit oral therapy.

Administration of β-adrenergic agonists by aerosol (*see* Chapter 28) typically leads to a very rapid therapeutic response, generally within minutes, although some agonists such as salmeterol have a delayed onset of action. While subcutaneous injection also causes prompt bronchodilation, the peak effect of a drug given orally may be delayed for several hours. Aerosol therapy depends on the delivery of drug to the distal airways. This, in turn, depends on the size of the particles in the aerosol and respiratory parameters such as inspiratory flow rate, tidal volume, breath-holding time, and airway diameter (Newhouse and Dolovich, 1986). Only about 10% of an inhaled dose actually enters the lungs; much of the remainder is swallowed and ultimately may be absorbed. Successful aerosol therapy requires that each patient master the technique of drug administration. Many patients, particularly children and the elderly, do not use optimal techniques, often because of inadequate instructions (Kelly, 1985; Newhouse and Dolovich, 1986). In these patients, spacer devices may enhance the efficacy of inhalation therapy (*see* Chapter 28).

In the treatment of asthma, β-adrenergic agonists are used to activate pulmonary receptors that relax bronchial smooth muscle and decrease airway resistance. Although this action appears to be a major therapeutic effect of these drugs in patients with asthma, evidence suggests that β-adrenergic agonists also may suppress the release of leukotrienes and histamine from mast cells in lung tissue (Hughes *et al.,* 1983), enhance mucociliary function, decrease microvascular permeability, and possibly inhibit phospholipase A_2 (Seale, 1988). The relative importance of these actions in the treatment of human asthma remains to be determined. However, it is becoming increasingly clear that airway inflammation is directly involved in airway hyperresponsiveness (*see* Chapter 28); consequently, the use of antiinflammatory drugs such as inhaled steroids may have primary importance. The use of β-adrenergic agonists for the treatment of asthma is discussed in Chapter 28.

Metaproterenol. *Metaproterenol* (called *orciprenaline* in Europe), along with terbutaline and fenoterol, belongs to the structural class of resorcinol bronchodilators that have hydroxyl groups at positions 3 and 5 of the phenyl ring (rather than at positions 3 and 4 as in catechols) (*see* Table 10–1). Consequently, metaproterenol is resistant to methylation by COMT, and a substantial fraction (40%) is absorbed in active form after oral administration. It is excreted primarily as glucuronic acid conjugates. Metaproterenol is considered to be β_2-selective, although it probably is less selective than albuterol or terbutaline. Effects occur within minutes of inhalation and persist for several hours. After oral administration, onset of action is slower, but effects last 3 to 4 hours. Metaproterenol (*metaproterenol sulfate;* ALUPENT) is used for the long-term treatment of obstructive airway diseases and for treatments of acute bronchospasm (*see* Chapter 28).

Terbutaline. *Terbutaline* is a β_2-selective bronchodilator. It contains a resorcinol ring and thus is not a substrate for methylation by COMT. It is effective when taken orally, subcutaneously, or by inhalation. Effects are observed rapidly after inhalation or parenteral administration; after inhalation its action may persist for 3 to 6 hours. With oral administration, the onset of effect may be delayed for 1 to 2 hours. Terbutaline (*terbutaline sulfate;*

BRETHINE, others) is used for the long-term treatment of obstructive airway diseases and for treatment of acute bronchospasm; furthermore, it is available for parenteral use for the emergency treatment of status asthmaticus (*see* Chapter 28).

Albuterol. *Albuterol* (salbutamol; VENTOLIN, PROVENTIL, others) is a selective β_2-adrenergic agonist with pharmacological properties and therapeutic indications similar to those of terbutaline. It is administered either by inhalation or orally for the symptomatic relief of bronchospasm. When administered by inhalation, it produces significant bronchodilation within 15 minutes, and effects are demonstrable for 3 to 4 hours. The cardiovascular effects of albuterol are considerably weaker than those of isoproterenol when doses that produce comparable bronchodilatation are administered by inhalation.

Isoetharine. *Isoetharine* was the first drug with β_2 selectivity widely used for the treatment of airway obstruction. However, its degree of selectivity for β_2-adrenergic receptors may not approach that of some of the other agents. Although resistant to metabolism by MAO, it is a catecholamine and thus is a good substrate for COMT (*see* Table 10–1). Consequently, it is used only by inhalation for the treatment of acute episodes of bronchoconstriction.

Pirbuterol. *Pirbuterol* is a relatively selective β_2 agonist. It is structurally identical to albuterol except for the substitution of a pyridine ring for the benzene ring (Richards and Brogden, 1985). Pirbuterol acetate (MAXAIR) is available for inhalation therapy; dosing is typically every 4 to 6 hours.

Bitolterol. *Bitolterol* (*bitolterol mesylate;* TORNALATE) is a novel β_2 agonist in which the hydroxyl groups in the catechol moiety are protected by esterification with 4-methylbenzoate. Esterases in the lung and other tissues hydrolyze this prodrug to the active form, colterol, or terbutylnorepinephrine (*see* Table 10–1). Results of animal studies have suggested that these esterases are present in higher concentration in lung than in tissues such as the heart (Nelson, 1986; Friedel and Brogden, 1988). The duration of effect of bitolterol after inhalation ranges from 3 to 6 hours.

Fenoterol. *Fenoterol* (BEROTEC) is a β_2-selective adrenergic receptor agonist. After inhalation, it has a prompt onset of action, and its effect typically is sustained for 4 to 6 hours. Fenoterol is not available in the United States. The possible association of fenoterol use with increased deaths from asthma in New Zealand is controversial (Pearce *et al.,* 1995; Suissa and Ernst, 1997).

Formoterol. *Formoterol* (FORADIL) is a long-acting β_2-selective adrenergic receptor agonist. Significant bronchodilation occurs within minutes of inhalation of a therapeutic dose, and this action may persist for up to 12 hours (Faulds *et al.,* 1991). Its major advantage over many other β_2-selective agonists is this prolonged duration of action, which may be particularly advantageous in settings such as nocturnal asthma. Formoterol is not available in the United States.

Procaterol. *Procaterol* (MASCACIN, others) is a β_2-selective adrenergic receptor agonist. After inhalation, it has a prompt onset of action, and action is sustained for about 5 hours. Procaterol is not available in the United States.

Salmeterol. *Salmeterol* (SEREVENT) is a β_2-selective adrenergic receptor agonist with a prolonged duration of action, about 12 hours. However, it has a relatively slow onset of action after inhalation, so is not suitable alone for prompt relief of breakthrough attacks of bronchospasm (Lötvall and Svedmyr, 1993; Brogden and Faulds, 1991).

Ritodrine. *Ritodrine* is a selective β_2-adrenergic agonist that was developed specifically for use as a uterine relaxant. Nevertheless, its pharmacological properties closely resemble those of the other agents in this group. Ritodrine is rapidly but incompletely (30%) absorbed following oral administration, and 90% of the drug is excreted in the urine as inactive conjugates; about 50% of ritodrine is excreted unchanged after intravenous administration. The pharmacokinetic properties of ritodrine are complex and incompletely defined, especially in pregnant women.

Therapeutic Uses. Ritodrine may be administered intravenously to selected patients to arrest premature labor. Ritodrine and related drugs can prolong pregnancy (King *et al.,* 1988). However, β_2-selective agonists may not have clinically significant benefits on perinatal mortality and may actually increase maternal morbidity (The Canadian Preterm Labor Investigators Group, 1992; Higby *et al.,* 1993; Johnson, 1993). Given modern improvements in the care of premature babies, it is possible that existing clinical trials may not have had sufficient statistical power to demonstrate subtle, but potentially important, clinical effects. Many other drugs are used to delay labor (Bossmar, 1998; Norwitz *et al.,* 1999). Magnesium therapy may prolong labor in preterm women. There is some evidence suggesting that indomethacin may prolong preterm labor, but a favorable risk-to-benefit ratio has not been established (Panter *et al.,* 1999). Also, while calcium channel blockers prolong preterm labor, their long-term benefits are unclear (*see* Chapter 32; Carr *et al.,* 1999).

Adverse Effects of β_2-Selective Agonists. The major adverse effects of β-adrenergic agonists occur as a result of excessive activation of β-adrenergic receptors. Patients with underlying cardiovascular disease are particularly at risk for significant reactions. However, the likelihood of adverse effects can be greatly decreased in patients with lung disease by administering the drug by inhalation rather than orally or parenterally.

Skeletal muscle tremor is a relatively common adverse effect of the β_2-selective adrenergic agonists. Tolerance generally develops to this effect; it is not clear whether tolerance reflects desensitization of the β_2 receptors of skeletal muscle or adaptation within the CNS. This adverse effect can be minimized by starting oral therapy with a low dose of drug and progressively increasing the dose as tolerance to the tremor develops. Feelings of restlessness, apprehension, and anxiety may limit therapy with these drugs, particularly after oral or parenteral treatment.

Tachycardia is a common adverse effect of systemically administered β-adrenergic agonists. Stimulation of heart rate occurs primarily *via* β_1 receptors. It is uncertain to what extent the increase in heart rate also is due to activation of cardiac β_2 receptors or to reflex effects that stem from β_2-receptor–mediated peripheral vasodilation. However, during a severe asthmatic attack, heart rate may actually decrease during therapy with a β-adrenergic agonist, presumably because of improvement in pulmonary function with consequent reduction in endogenous cardiac sympathetic stimulation. In patients without cardiac disease, β agonists rarely cause significant arrhythmias or myocardial ischemia; however, patients with underlying coronary artery disease or preexisting arrhythmias are at greater risk. The risk of adverse cardiovascular effects also is increased in patients who are receiving MAO inhibitors.

Arterial oxygen tension may fall when treatment of patients with an acute exacerbation of asthma is begun; this may be due to drug-induced pulmonary vascular dilation, which leads to increased mismatching of ventilation and perfusion. This effect usually is small and transient. Supplemental oxygen should be given if necessary. Severe pulmonary edema has been reported in women receiving ritodrine or terbutaline for premature labor.

The results of a number of epidemiologic studies have suggested a possible adverse connection between prolonged use of β-adrenergic agonists and death or near-death from asthma (Suissa *et al.,* 1994). While exact interpretation of these results is difficult, these studies have raised questions about the role of β-adrenergic agonists in the treatment of chronic asthma. Tolerance to effects of β-adrenergic agonists has been studied extensively, both *in vitro* and *in vivo* (*see* Chapter 6). Long-term systemic administration of β-adrenergic agonists leads to down-regulation of β receptors in some tissues and decreased pharmacological responses. However, it appears likely that tolerance to the pulmonary effects of these drugs is not a major clinical problem for the majority of asthmatics who do not exceed recommended dosages of β-adrenergic agonists over prolonged periods (Jenne, 1982; Tattersfield, 1985).

There is some evidence suggesting that regular use of β_2-selective agonists may cause increased bronchial hyperreactivity and deterioration in disease control (Lipworth and McDevitt, 1992; Hancox *et al.*, 1999). To what extent this potential adverse association may be even more unfavorable for very long-acting β agonists or excess doses of medication is not yet known (Beasley *et al.*, 1999). However, for patients requiring regular use of these drugs over prolonged periods, strong consideration should be given to additional or alternative therapy, such as the use of inhaled corticosteroids.

Large doses of β-adrenergic agonists cause myocardial necrosis in laboratory animals. When given parenterally, these drugs also may increase the concentrations of glucose, lactate, and free fatty acids in plasma and decrease the concentration of K^+. The decrease in K^+ concentration may be especially important in patients with cardiac disease, particularly those taking cardiac glycosides and diuretics. In some diabetic patients, hyperglycemia may be worsened by these drugs, and higher doses of insulin may be required. All these adverse effects are far less likely with inhalation therapy than with parenteral or oral therapy.

α_1-SELECTIVE ADRENERGIC AGONISTS

The major clinical effects of a number of sympathomimetic drugs are due to activation of α-adrenergic receptors in vascular smooth muscle. As a result, peripheral vascular resistance is increased and blood pressure is maintained or elevated. Although the clinical utility of these drugs is limited, they may be useful in the treatment of some patients with hypotension or shock. *Phenylephrine* and *methoxamine* are direct-acting vasoconstrictors and are selective activators of α_1 receptors. *Mephentermine* and *metaraminol* act both directly and indirectly; *i.e.,* a portion of their effects is mediated through the release of endogenous norepinephrine.

Methoxamine

Methoxamine (*methoxamine hydrochloride;* VASOXYL; *see* Table 10–1) is a relatively specific α_1-receptor–selective adrenergic agonist; as such, it causes a dose-related increase in peripheral vascular resistance. The drug may have different intrinsic activities at α_1 receptors in different tissues (Garcia-Sainz *et al.,* 1985). Methoxamine does not activate β-adrenergic receptors, nor does it cause stimulation of the CNS. However, at high concentrations, methoxamine has some capacity to block β receptors. The

major cardiovascular response to the drug is a rise in blood pressure, which is associated with sinus bradycardia because of activation of vagal reflexes; the slowing of the heart rate is largely blocked by atropine. Methoxamine may be used intravenously in the treatment of hypotensive states.

Phenylephrine

Phenylephrine is an α_1-selective agonist; it activates β-adrenergic receptors only at much higher concentrations. Chemically, phenylephrine differs from epinephrine only in lacking a hydroxyl group at position 4 on the benzene ring (*see* Table 10–1). The pharmacological effects of phenylephrine are similar to those of methoxamine. The drug causes marked arterial vasoconstriction during intravenous infusion. Phenylephrine (*phenylephrine hydrochloride;* NEOSYNEPHRINE, others) also is used as a nasal decongestant and as a mydriatic in various nasal and ophthalmic formulations (*see* Chapter 66 for ophthalmic uses).

Mephentermine

Mephentermine (*see* Table 10–1) is a sympathomimetic drug that acts both directly and indirectly; it has many similarities to ephedrine (*see* below). After an intramuscular injection, the onset of action is prompt (within 5 to 15 minutes), and effects may last for several hours. Since the drug releases norepinephrine, cardiac contraction is enhanced, and cardiac output and systolic and diastolic pressures usually are increased. The change in heart rate is variable, depending on the degree of vagal tone. Adverse effects are related to CNS stimulation, excessive rises in blood pressure, and arrhythmias. Mephentermine (*mephentermine sulfate;* WYAMINE SULFATE) is used to prevent hypotension, which frequently accompanies spinal anesthesia.

Metaraminol

Metaraminol (*metaraminol bitartrate;* ARAMINE) (*see* Table 10–1) is a sympathomimetic drug with prominent direct effects on vascular α-adrenergic receptors. Metaraminol also is an indirectly acting agent that stimulates the release of norepinephrine. The drug has been used in the treatment of hypotensive states or to relieve attacks of paroxysmal atrial tachycardia, particularly those associated with hypotension (*see* Chapter 35 for preferable treatments of this arrhythmia).

Midodrine

Midodrine (PROAMATINE) is an orally effective, α_1-adrenergic agonist (Fouad-Tarazi *et al.*, 1995). It is a prodrug; its activity is due to its conversion to an active metabolite, desglymidodrine, which achieves peak concentrations about 1 hour after a dose of midodrine. The half-life of desglymidodrine is about 3 hours. Consequently, the duration of action is about 4 to 6 hours. Midodrine-induced rises in blood pressure are associated with both arterial and venous smooth muscle contraction. This is advantageous in the treatment of patients with autonomic insufficiency and postural hypotension (McClellan *et al.,* 1998). A frequent complication in these patients is supine hypertension. This can be minimized by avoiding dosing prior to bedtime and elevating the head of the bed. Very cautious use of a short-acting antihypertensive drug at bedtime may be useful in some patients. Typical dosing, achieved by careful titration of blood pressure responses, varies between 2.5 and 10 mg three times daily, at 4-hour intervals.

α_2-SELECTIVE ADRENERGIC AGONISTS

α_2-Receptor-selective adrenergic agonists are used primarily for the treatment of systemic hypertension. Their efficacy as antihypertensive agents is somewhat surprising, since many blood vessels contain postsynaptic α_2 receptors that promote vasoconstriction (*see* Chapter 6). Indeed, clonidine was initially developed as a vasoconstricting nasal decongestant. Its capacity to lower blood pressure results from activation of α_2-adrenergic receptors in the cardiovascular control centers of the CNS; such activation suppresses the outflow of sympathetic nervous system activity from the brain.

Clonidine

Clonidine, an imidazoline, was synthesized in the early 1960s and found to produce vasoconstriction that was mediated by α-adrenergic receptors. During clinical testing of the drug as a topical nasal decongestant, clonidine was found to cause hypotension, sedation, and bradycardia. The structural formula of clonidine is as follows:

CLONIDINE

Pharmacological Effects. The major pharmacological effects of clonidine involve changes in blood pressure and heart rate, although the drug has a variety of other important actions. Intravenous infusion of clonidine causes an acute rise in blood pressure, apparently because of activation of postsynaptic α_2 receptors in vascular smooth muscle (Kobinger, 1978). The affinity of clonidine for these receptors is high, although the drug is a partial agonist with relatively low efficacy at these sites. The hypertensive response that follows parenteral administration of clonidine generally is not seen when the drug is given orally. However, even after intravenous administration, the transient vasoconstriction is followed by a more prolonged

hypotensive response which results from decreased central outflow of impulses in the sympathetic nervous system. The exact mechanism by which clonidine lowers blood pressure is not completely understood. The effect appears to result, at least in part, from activation of α_2 receptors in the lower brainstem region. This central action has been demonstrated by infusing small amounts of the drug into the vertebral arteries or by injecting it directly into the cisterna magna.

Data obtained using [^{3}H]clonidine as a radioligand in receptor-binding assays suggest that noradrenergic imidazoline-preferring binding sites exist in the brain. These sites, however, do not bind catecholamines and thus cannot mediate the centrally mediated hypotensive effects of norepinephrine. There is increasing evidence that these imidazoline-preferring sites may represent a new family of receptors through which clonidine and other imidazolines may elicit hypotensive effects (van Zwieten, 1999). However, the lack of an antihypertensive effect of clonidine and other imidazoline-site ligands in genetically engineered mice lacking functional α_{2A}-adrenergic receptors affirms the importance of this receptor subtype in mediating the effects of clonidine and currently available imidazoline-site ligands, such as moxonidine and rilmenidine (MacMillan *et al.,* 1996; Zhu *et al.,* 1999).

Clonidine decreases discharges in sympathetic preganglionic fibers in the splanchnic nerve as well as in postganglionic fibers of cardiac nerves (Langer *et al.,* 1980). These effects are blocked by α_2-selective antagonists such as yohimbine. Clonidine also stimulates parasympathetic outflow, and this may contribute to the slowing of heart rate as a consequence of increased vagal tone as well as diminished sympathetic drive. In addition, some of the antihypertensive effects of clonidine may be mediated by activation of presynaptic α_2 receptors that suppress the release of norepinephrine from peripheral nerve endings. Clonidine decreases the plasma concentration of norepinephrine and reduces its excretion in the urine.

Absorption, Fate, and Excretion. Clonidine is well absorbed after oral administration, and bioavailability is nearly 100%. The peak concentration in plasma and the maximal hypotensive effect are observed 1 to 3 hours after an oral dose. The elimination half-life of the drug ranges from 6 to 24 hours, with a mean of about 12 hours (Lowenthal *et al.,* 1988). About half of an administered dose can be recovered unchanged in the urine, and the half-life of the drug may increase with renal failure. There is good correlation between plasma concentrations of clonidine and its pharmacological effects. A transdermal delivery patch permits continuous administration of clonidine as an alternative to oral therapy. The drug is released at an approximately constant rate for a week; 3 or 4 days are required to reach steady-state concentrations in plasma. When the patch is removed, plasma concentrations remain stable for about 8 hours and then decline gradually over a period of several days; this decrease is associated with a rise in blood pressure (Langley and Heel, 1988; Lowenthal *et al.*, 1988).

Adverse Effects.   The major adverse effects of clonidine are dry mouth and sedation. These responses occur in at least 50% of patients and may require discontinuation of drug administration. However, they may diminish in intensity after several weeks of therapy. Sexual dysfunction also may occur. Marked bradycardia is observed in some patients. These and some of the other adverse effects of clonidine are frequently related to dose, and their incidence may be lower with transdermal administration of clonidine, since antihypertensive efficacy may be achieved while avoiding the relatively high peak concentrations that occur after oral administration of the drug; however, this possibility requires further evaluation (Langley and Heel, 1988). About 15% to 20% of patients develop contact dermatitis when using clonidine in the transdermal system. Withdrawal reactions follow abrupt discontinuation of long-term therapy with clonidine in some hypertensive patients (Parker and Atkinson, 1982; *see* also Chapter 33).

Therapeutic Uses.   The major therapeutic use of clonidine (*clonidine hydrochloride;* CATAPRES) is in the treatment of hypertension (*see* Chapter 33). Clonidine also has apparent efficacy in the treatment of a range of other disorders. Stimulation of α_2-adrenergic receptors in the gastrointestinal tract may increase absorption of sodium chloride and fluid and inhibit secretion of bicarbonate (Chang *et al.*, 1986). This may explain why clonidine has been found to improve diarrhea in some diabetic patients with autonomic neuropathy (Fedorak *et al.*, 1985). Clonidine also is useful in treating and preparing addicted subjects for withdrawal from narcotics (Gold *et al.*, 1978), alcohol (Bond, 1986), and tobacco (Glassman *et al.*, 1988) (*see* Chapter 24). Clonidine may help ameliorate some of the adverse sympathetic nervous activity associated with withdrawal from these agents, as well as decrease craving for the drug. The long-term benefits of clonidine in these settings and in neuropsychiatric disorders remain to be determined (Bond, 1986). Clonidine may be useful in selected patients receiving anesthesia because it may decrease the requirement for anesthetic and increase hemodynamic stability (Flacke *et al.*, 1987; Hayashi and Maze, 1993; *see* also Chapter 14). Other potential benefits of clonidine and related drugs such as *dexmedetomidine* in anesthesia include preoperative sedation and anxiolysis, drying of secretions, and analgesia. Transdermal administration of clonidine (CATAPRES-TTS) may be useful in reducing the incidence of menopausal hot flashes (Nagamani *et al.*, 1987).

Acute administration of clonidine has been used in the differential diagnosis of patients with hypertension and suspected pheochromocytoma. In patients with primary hypertension, plasma concentrations of norepinephrine are markedly suppressed after a single dose of clonidine; this response is not observed in many patients with pheochromocytoma (Bravo *et al.*, 1981). The capacity of clonidine to activate postsynaptic α_2 receptors in vascular smooth muscle has been exploited in a limited

number of patients whose autonomic failure is so severe that reflex sympathetic responses on standing are absent; postural hypotension is thus marked. Since the central effect of clonidine on blood pressure is unimportant in these patients, the drug can elevate blood pressure and improve the symptoms of postural hypotension (Robertson *et al.*, 1983a).

Apraclonidine

Apraclonidine (IOPIDINE) is a relatively selective α_2-adrenergic agonist used locally to reduce intraocular pressure. While the mechanism is unclear, it may relate to reduction in formation of aqueous humor (*see* Chapter 66).

Guanfacine

Guanfacine is a phenylacetylguanidine derivative. Its structural formula is as follows:

GUANFACINE

Guanfacine (*guanfacine hydrochloride;* TENEX) is an α_2-adrenergic agonist that is more selective for α_2 receptors than is clonidine. Like clonidine, guanfacine lowers blood pressure by activation of brain stem receptors with resultant suppression of sympathetic nervous system activity (Sorkin and Heel, 1986). The drug is well absorbed after oral administration and has a large volume of distribution (4 to 6 liters/kg). About 50% of guanfacine appears unchanged in the urine; the rest is metabolized. The half-time for elimination ranges from 12 to 24 hours. Guanfacine and clonidine appear to have similar efficacy for the treatment of hypertension. The pattern of adverse effects also is similar for the two drugs, although it has been suggested that some of these effects may be milder and occur less frequently with guanfacine (Sorkin and Heel, 1986). A withdrawal syndrome may occur after the abrupt discontinuation of guanfacine, but it appears to be less frequent and milder than the syndrome that follows withdrawal of clonidine. Part of this difference may relate to the longer half-life of guanfacine.

Guanabenz

Guanabenz and guanfacine are closely related chemically and pharmacologically. The structural formula of guanabenz is as follows:

GUANABENZ

Guanabenz (*guanabenz acetate;* WYTENSIN) is a centrally acting α_2 agonist that decreases blood pressure by a mechanism similar to those of clonidine and guanfacine (Holmes *et al.*,

1983). Guanabenz has a half-life of 4 to 6 hours and is extensively metabolized by the liver. Dosage adjustment may be necessary in patients with hepatic cirrhosis. The adverse effects caused by guanabenz (*e.g.,* dry mouth and sedation) are similar to those seen with clonidine.

Methyldopa

Methyldopa (α-methyl-3,4-dihydroxyphenylalanine) is a centrally acting antihypertensive agent. It is metabolized to α-methylnorepinephrine in the brain, and this compound is thought to activate central α_2-adrenergic receptors and lower blood pressure in a manner similar to that of clonidine. Methyldopa is discussed in more detail in Chapter 33.

Tizanidine

Tizanidine (ZANAFLEX) is a muscle relaxant drug used for the treatment of spasticity associated with cerebral and spinal disorders. It also is an α_2-receptor agonist with some properties similar to those of clonidine (Wagstaff and Bryson, 1997).

Brimonidine

Brimonidine tartrate (ALPHAGAN) is an α_2-adrenergic receptor agonist administered ocularly to lower intraocular pressure in patients with ocular hypertension or open-angle glaucoma (*see* Chapter 66).

MISCELLANEOUS ADRENERGIC AGONISTS

Amphetamine

Amphetamine, racemic β-phenylisopropylamine (*see* Table 10–1), has powerful CNS stimulant actions in addition to the peripheral α and β actions common to indirect-acting sympathomimetic drugs. Unlike epinephrine, it is effective after oral administration and its effects last for several hours.

Cardiovascular Responses. Amphetamine given orally raises both systolic and diastolic blood pressure. Heart rate is often reflexly slowed; with large doses, cardiac arrhythmias may occur. Cardiac output is not enhanced by therapeutic doses, and cerebral blood flow does not change much. The *l* isomer is slightly more potent than the *d* isomer in its cardiovascular actions.

Other Smooth Muscles. In general, smooth muscles respond to amphetamine as they do to other sympathomimetic amines. The contractile effect on the sphincter of the urinary bladder is particularly marked, and for this reason amphetamine has been used in treating enuresis and incontinence. Pain and difficulty in micturition occasionally occur. The gastrointestinal effects of amphetamine are unpredictable. If enteric activity is pronounced, amphetamine may cause relaxation and delay the movement of intestinal contents; if the gut already is relaxed, the opposite effect may occur. The response of the human uterus varies, but there usually is an increase in tone.

Central Nervous System. Amphetamine is one of the most potent sympathomimetic amines in stimulating the CNS. It stimulates the medullary respiratory center, lessens the degree of central depression caused by various drugs, and produces other signs of stimulation of the CNS. These effects are thought to be due to cortical stimulation and possibly to stimulation of the reticular activating system. In contrast, the drug can obtund the maximal electroshock seizure discharge and prolong the ensuing period of depression. In elicitation of CNS excitatory effects, the *d* isomer (dextroamphetamine) is three to four times as potent as the *l* isomer.

The psychic effects depend on the dose and the mental state and personality of the individual. The main results of an oral dose of 10 to 30 mg include wakefulness, alertness, and a decreased sense of fatigue; elevation of mood, with increased initiative, self-confidence, and ability to concentrate; often, elation and euphoria; and increase in motor and speech activities. Performance of simple mental tasks is improved, but, although more work may be accomplished, the number of errors may increase. Physical performance—in athletes, for example—is improved, and the drug often is abused for this purpose. These effects are not invariable, and may be reversed by overdosage or repeated usage. Prolonged use or large doses are nearly always followed by depression and fatigue. Many individuals given amphetamine experience headache, palpitation, dizziness, vasomotor disturbances, agitation, confusion, dysphoria, apprehension, delirium, or fatigue (*see* Chapter 24).

Fatigue and Sleep. Prevention and reversal of fatigue by amphetamine have been studied extensively in the laboratory, in military field studies, and in athletics. In general, the duration of adequate performance is prolonged before fatigue appears, and the effects of fatigue are at least partly reversed. The most striking improvement appears to occur when performance has been reduced by fatigue and lack of sleep. Such improvement may be partly due to alteration of unfavorable attitudes toward the task. However, amphetamine reduces the frequency of attention lapses that impair performance after prolonged sleep deprivation and thus improves execution of tasks requiring sustained attention. The need for sleep may be postponed, but it cannot be avoided indefinitely. When the drug is discontinued after long use, the pattern of sleep may take as long as two months to return to normal.

Analgesia. Amphetamine and some other sympathomimetic amines have a small analgesic effect, but it is not sufficiently pronounced to be therapeutically useful. However, amphetamine can enhance the analgesia produced by morphine-like drugs.

Respiration. Amphetamine stimulates the respiratory center, increasing the rate and depth of respiration. In normal human beings, usual doses of the drug do not appreciably increase respiratory rate or minute volume. Nevertheless, when respiration is depressed by centrally acting drugs, amphetamine may stimulate respiration.

Depression of Appetite. Amphetamine and similar drugs have been used for the treatment of obesity, although the wisdom of this use is at best questionable. Weight loss in obese human beings treated with amphetamine is almost entirely due to reduced food intake and only in small measure to increased metabolism. The site of action is probably in the lateral hypothalamic feeding center; injection of amphetamine into this area, but not into the ventromedial satiety center, suppresses food intake. Neurochemical mechanisms of action are unclear but may involve increased release of norepinephrine and/or dopamine (Samanin and Garattini, 1993). In human beings, tolerance to the appetite suppression develops rapidly. Hence, continuous weight reduction usually is not observed in obese individuals without dietary restriction (Silverstone, 1992; Bray, 1993).

Mechanisms of Action in the CNS. Amphetamine appears to exert most or all of its effects in the CNS by releasing biogenic amines from their storage sites in nerve terminals. The alerting effect of amphetamine, its anorectic effect, and at least a component of its locomotor-stimulating action are presumably mediated by release of norepinephrine from central noradrenergic neurons. These effects can be prevented in experimental animals by treatment with α-methyltyrosine, an inhibitor of tyrosine hydroxylase and, therefore, of catecholamine synthesis. Some aspects of locomotor activity and the stereotyped behavior induced by amphetamine probably are a consequence of the release of dopamine from dopaminergic nerve terminals, particularly in the neostriatum. Higher doses are required to produce these behavioral effects, and this correlates with the higher concentrations of amphetamine required to release dopamine from brain slices or synaptosomes *in vitro*. With still higher doses of amphetamine, disturbances of perception and overt psychotic behavior occur. These effects may be due to release of 5-hydroxytryptamine (serotonin, 5-HT) from tryptaminergic neurons and of dopamine in the mesolimbic system. In addition, amphetamine may exert direct effects on central receptors for 5-HT (*see* Chapter 11).

Toxicity and Adverse Effects. The acute toxic effects of amphetamine usually are extensions of its therapeutic actions and, as a rule, result from overdosage. The central effects commonly include restlessness, dizziness, tremor, hyperactive reflexes, talkativeness, tenseness, irritability, weakness, insomnia, fever, and sometimes euphoria. Confusion, aggressiveness, changes in libido, anxiety, delirium, paranoid hallucinations, panic states, and suicidal or homicidal tendencies occur, especially in mentally ill patients. However, these psychotic effects can be elicited in any individual if sufficient quantities of amphetamine are ingested for a prolonged period. Fatigue and depression usually follow central stimulation. Cardiovascular effects are common and include headache, chilliness, pallor or flushing, palpitation, cardiac arrhythmias, anginal pain, hypertension or hypotension, and circulatory collapse. Excessive sweating occurs. Symptoms referable to the gastrointestinal system include dry mouth, metallic taste, anorexia, nausea, vomiting, diarrhea, and abdominal cramps. Fatal poisoning usually terminates in convulsions and coma, and cerebral hemorrhages are the main pathological findings.

The toxic dose of amphetamine varies widely. Toxic manifestations occasionally occur as an idiosyncrasy after as little as 2 mg, but are rare with doses of less than 15 mg. Severe reactions have occurred with 30 mg, yet doses of 400 to 500 mg are not uniformly fatal. Larger doses can be tolerated after chronic use of the drug.

Treatment of acute amphetamine intoxication may include acidification of the urine by administration of ammonium chloride; this enhances the rate of elimination. Sedatives may be required for the CNS symptoms. Severe hypertension may require administration of sodium nitroprusside or an α-adrenergic antagonist.

Chronic intoxication with amphetamine causes symptoms similar to those of acute overdosage, but abnormal mental conditions are more common. Weight loss may be marked. A psychotic reaction with vivid hallucinations and paranoid delusions, often mistaken for schizophrenia, is the most common serious effect. Recovery usually is rapid after withdrawal of the drug, but occasionally the condition becomes chronic. In these persons, amphetamine may act as a precipitating factor hastening the onset of an incipient schizophrenia.

The abuse of amphetamine as a means of overcoming sleepiness and of increasing energy and alertness should be discouraged. The drug should be used only under medical supervision. The amphetamines are schedule II drugs under federal regulations (*see* Appendix I). The additional contraindications and precautions for the use of amphetamine generally are similar to those described above for epinephrine. Its use is inadvisable in patients with anorexia, insomnia, asthenia, psychopathic personality, or a history of homicidal or suicidal tendencies.

Dependence and Tolerance. Psychological dependence often occurs when amphetamine or dextroamphetamine is used chronically, as discussed in Chapter 24. Tolerance almost invariably develops to the anorexigenic effect of amphetamines, and is often seen also in the need for increasing doses to maintain improvement of mood in psychiatric patients. Tolerance is striking in individuals who are dependent on the drug, and a daily intake of 1.7 g without apparent ill effects has been reported. Development of tolerance is not invariable, and cases of narcolepsy have been treated for years without requiring an increase in the initially effective dose.

Therapeutic Uses.   Amphetamine and dextroamphetamine are used chiefly for their CNS effects. Dextroamphetamine (*dextroamphetamine sulfate;* DEXEDRINE), with greater CNS action and less peripheral action, generally is preferred to amphetamine; it is used in obesity, narcolepsy, and attention-deficit hyperactivity disorder. These uses are discussed later in this chapter.

Methamphetamine

Methamphetamine (*methamphetamine hydrochloride;* DESOXYN) is closely related chemically to amphetamine and ephedrine (*see* Table 10–1). Small doses have prominent central stimulant effects without significant peripheral actions; somewhat larger doses produce a sustained rise in systolic and diastolic blood pressures, due mainly to cardiac stimulation. Cardiac output is increased, although the heart rate may be reflexly slowed. Venous constriction causes peripheral venous pressure to increase. These factors tend to increase the venous return and, therefore, the cardiac output. Pulmonary arterial pressure is raised, probably owing to increased cardiac output. Methamphetamine is a schedule II drug under federal regulations and has high potential for abuse (*see* Chapter 24 and Appendix I). It is used principally for its central effects, which are more pronounced than those of amphetamine and are accompanied by less prominent peripheral actions. These uses are discussed below in the section of this chapter on therapeutic uses.

Methylphenidate

Methylphenidate is a piperidine derivative that is structurally related to amphetamine and has the following formula:

METHYLPHENIDATE

Methylphenidate (*methylphenidate hydrochloride;* RITALIN) is a mild CNS stimulant with more prominent effects on mental than on motor activities. However, large doses produce signs of generalized CNS stimulation that may lead to convulsions. Its pharmacological properties are essentially the same as those of the amphetamines. Methylphenidate also shares the abuse potential of the amphetamines. Methylphenidate is effective in the treatment of narcolepsy and attention-deficit hyperactivity disorder, as described below.

Methylphenidate is readily absorbed after oral administration and reaches peak concentrations in plasma in about 2 hours. Methylphenidate is a racemate; its more potent (+) enantiomer has a half-life of about 6 hours, and the less potent (−) enantiomer has a half-life of about 4 hours. Concentrations in the brain exceed those in plasma. The main urinary metabolite is a deesterified product, ritalinic acid, which accounts for 80% of the dose. The use of methylphenidate is contraindicated in patients with glaucoma.

Pemoline

Pemoline (CYLERT) is structurally dissimilar to methylphenidate but elicits similar changes in CNS function with minimal effects on the cardiovascular system. It is employed in treating attention-deficit hyperactivity disorder and can be given once daily because of its long half-life. Clinical improvement may require treatment for 3 to 4 weeks. Its use has been associated with severe hepatic failure.

Ephedrine

Ephedrine (*ephedrine sulfate*) is both an α- and a β-adrenergic agonist; in addition, it enhances release of norepinephrine from sympathetic neurons. Ephedrine contains two asymmetrical carbon atoms (*see* Table 10–1); only *l*-ephedrine and racemic ephedrine are used clinically.

Pharmacological Actions.   Ephedrine does not contain a catechol moiety, and it is effective after oral administration. The drug stimulates heart rate and cardiac output and variably increases peripheral resistance; as a result, ephedrine usually increases blood pressure. Stimulation of the α-adrenergic receptors of smooth muscle cells in the bladder base may increase the resistance to the outflow of urine. Activation of β-adrenergic receptors in the lungs promotes bronchodilation. Ephedrine is a potent CNS stimulant. After oral administration, effects of the drug may persist for several hours. Ephedrine is eliminated in the urine largely as unchanged drug, with a half-life of about 3 to 6 hours.

Therapeutic Uses and Toxicity.   In the past, ephedrine was used to treat Stokes-Adams attacks with complete heart block and as a CNS stimulant in narcolepsy and depressive states. It has been replaced by alternative modes of treatment in each of these disorders. In addition, its use as a bronchodilator in patients with asthma has become much less extensive with the development of β_2-selective agonists. Ephedrine has been used to promote urinary continence, although its efficacy is not clear. Indeed, the drug may cause urinary retention, particularly in men with benign prostatic hyperplasia. Ephedrine also has been used to treat the hypotension that may occur with spinal anesthesia.

Untoward effects of ephedrine include the risk of hypertension, particularly after parenteral administration or with higher than recommended oral dosing. Insomnia is a common CNS

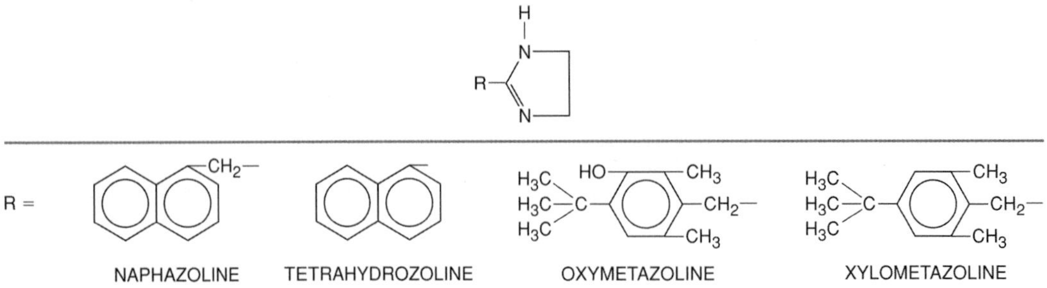

Figure 10–3. Chemical structures of imidazoline derivatives.

adverse effect. Tachyphylaxis may occur with repetitive dosing. Concerns have been raised about the safety of ephedrine. Usual or higher than recommended doses may cause important adverse effects in susceptible individuals and be especially of concern in patients with underlying cardiovascular disease that might be unrecognized. Of potentially greater cause for concern, large amounts of herbal preparations containing ephedrine (ma huang, *Ephedra*) are utilized around the world. There can be considerable variability in the content of ephedrine in these preparations, which may lead to inadvertent consumption of higher than usual does of ephedrine and its isomers.

Other Sympathomimetic Agents

Several sympathomimetic drugs are used primarily as vasoconstrictors for local application to the nasal mucous membrane or the eye. The structures of *propylhexedrine* (BENZEDREX), *naphazoline hydrochloride* (PRIVINE, NAPHCON, others), *tetrahydrozoline hydrochloride* (TYZINE, VISINE ORIGINAL, others), *oxymetazoline hydrochloride* (AFRIN, OCUCLEAR, others), and *xylometazoline hydrochloride* (OTRIVIN) are depicted in Table 10–1 and Figure 10–3. *Ethylnorepinephrine hydrochloride* (BRONKEPHRINE) (*see* Table 10–1) is a β-adrenergic agonist that is used as a bronchodilator. The drug also has α-adrenergic agonist activity; this effect may cause local vasoconstriction and thereby reduce bronchial congestion.

Phenylephrine (*see* above), *pseudoephedrine* (SUDAFED, others) (a stereoisomer of ephedrine), and *phenylpropanolamine* (PROPAGEST, others) are the sympathomimetic drugs that have been used most commonly in oral preparations for the relief of nasal congestion. Pseudoephedrine hydrochloride is available without a prescription in a variety of solid and liquid dosage forms. Phenylpropanolamine hydrochloride shares the pharmacological properties of ephedrine and is approximately equal in potency except that it causes less CNS stimulation. The drug has been available without prescription in tablets and capsules. In addition, numerous proprietary mixtures marketed for the oral treatment of nasal and sinus congestion contain one of these sympathomimetic amines, usually in combination with an H_1-histamine receptor antagonist. Also, phenylpropanolamine suppresses appetite by mechanisms possibly different from those of amphetamines (Wellman, 1992). Concern about the possibility that phenylpropanolamine increases the risk of hemorrhagic stroke in young women led the United States Food and Drug Administration (FDA) recently to consider banning the sale of the drug. The FDA has issued a public warning about the risk

and has asked manufacturers of over-the-counter products containing phenylpropanolamine to stop marketing them; several manufacturers have complied with the request.

THERAPEUTIC USES OF SYMPATHOMIMETIC DRUGS

The success that has attended efforts to develop therapeutic agents that can influence adrenergic receptors selectively and the variety of vital functions that are regulated by the sympathetic nervous system have resulted in a class of drugs with a large number of important therapeutic uses.

Shock. Shock is a clinical syndrome characterized by inadequate perfusion of tissues; it usually is associated with hypotension and ultimately with the failure of organ systems (Hollenberg *et al.,* 1999). Shock is an immediately life-threatening impairment of delivery of oxygen and nutrients to the organs of the body. Causes of shock include hypovolemia (due to dehydration or blood loss), cardiac failure (extensive myocardial infarction, severe arrhythmia, or cardiac mechanical defects such as ventricular septal defect), obstruction to cardiac output (due to pulmonary embolism, pericardial tamponade, or aortic dissection), and peripheral circulatory dysfunction (sepsis or anaphylaxis). The treatment of shock consists of specific efforts to reverse the underlying pathogenesis as well as nonspecific measures aimed at correcting hemodynamic abnormalities. Regardless of the etiology, the accompanying fall in blood pressure generally leads to marked activation of the sympathetic nervous system. This, in turn, causes peripheral vasoconstriction and an increase in the rate and force of cardiac contraction. In the initial stages of shock these mechanisms may maintain blood pressure and cerebral blood flow, although blood flow to the kidneys, skin, and other organs may be decreased, leading to impaired production of urine and metabolic acidosis (Ruffolo, 1992).

The initial therapy of shock involves basic life-support measures. It is essential to maintain blood volume, which often requires monitoring of hemodynamic parameters. Specific therapy (*e.g.,* antibiotics for patients in septic shock) should be initiated immediately. If these measures do not lead to an adequate therapeutic response, it may be necessary to use vasoactive drugs in an effort to improve abnormalities in blood pressure and flow. This therapy is generally empirically based on response to hemodynamic measurements. Many of these pharmacological approaches, while apparently clinically reasonable, are of uncertain efficacy. Adrenergic agonists may be used in an attempt to increase myocardial contractility or to modify peripheral vascular resistance. In general terms, β-adrenergic agonists increase heart rate and force of contraction, α-adrenergic agonists increase peripheral vascular resistance, and dopamine promotes dilation of renal and splanchnic vascular beds, in addition to activating β- and α-adrenergic receptors (Breslow and Ligier, 1991).

Cardiogenic shock due to myocardial infarction has a poor prognosis; therapy is aimed at improving peripheral blood flow. Definitive therapy, such as emergency cardiac catheterization following surgical revascularization or angioplasty, may be very important. Mechanical left ventricular assist devices also may be important in maintaining cardiac output and coronary perfusion in critically ill patients. In the setting of severely impaired cardiac output, falling blood pressure leads to intense sympathetic outflow and vasoconstriction. This may further decrease cardiac output as the damaged heart pumps against a higher peripheral resistance. Medical intervention is designed to optimize cardiac filling pressure (preload), myocardial contractility, and peripheral resistance (afterload). Preload may be increased by administration of intravenous fluids or reduced with drugs such as diuretics and nitrates. A number of sympathomimetic amines have been used to increase the force of contraction of the heart. Some of these drugs have disadvantages: isoproterenol is a powerful chronotropic agent and can greatly increase myocardial oxygen demand; norepinephrine intensifies peripheral vasoconstriction; and epinephrine increases heart rate and may predispose the heart to dangerous arrhythmias. Dopamine is an effective inotropic agent that causes less increase in heart rate than does isoproterenol. It also promotes renal arterial dilation; this may be useful in preserving renal function. When given in high doses (greater than 10 to 20 μg/kg per minute), dopamine activates α-adrenergic receptors, causing peripheral and renal vasoconstriction. Dobutamine has complex pharmacological actions that are mediated by its stereoisomers; the clinical effects of the drug are to increase myocardial contractility with little increase in heart rate or peripheral resistance.

In some patients in shock, hypotension is so severe that vasoconstricting drugs are required to maintain a blood pressure that is adequate for perfusion of the CNS (Kulka and Tryba, 1993). α-Adrenergic agonists such as norepinephrine, phenylephrine, metaraminol, mephentermine, and methoxamine have been used for this purpose. This approach may be advantageous in patients with hypotension due to failure of the sympathetic nervous system (*e.g.,* after spinal anesthesia or injury). However, in patients with other forms of shock, such as cardiogenic shock, reflex vasoconstriction is generally intense, and α-adrenergic agonists may further compromise blood flow to organs such as the kidneys and gut as well as adversely increase the work of the heart. Indeed, vasodilating drugs such as nitroprusside are more likely to improve blood flow and decrease cardiac work in such patients by decreasing afterload if a minimally adequate blood pressure can be maintained.

The hemodynamic abnormalities in septic shock are complex and are not well understood. Most patients with septic shock initially have low or barely normal peripheral vascular resistance, possibly owing to excessive effects of endogenously produced nitric oxide as well as normal or increased cardiac output. If the syndrome progresses, myocardial depression, increased peripheral resistance, and impaired tissue oxygenation occur. The primary treatment of septic shock is antibiotics. Data on the comparative value of various adrenergic agents in the treatment of septic shock are limited (Chernow and Roth, 1986). Therapy with drugs such as dopamine or dobutamine is guided by hemodynamic monitoring, with individualization of therapy depending on the patient's overall clinical condition.

Hypotension. Drugs with predominantly α-adrenergic activity can be used to raise blood pressure in patients with decreased peripheral resistance in conditions such as spinal anesthesia or intoxication with antihypertensive medications. However, hypotension *per se* is not an indication for treatment with these agents unless there is inadequate perfusion of organs such as the brain, heart, or kidneys. Furthermore, adequate replacement of fluid or blood may be more appropriate than drug therapy for many patients with hypotension. In patients with spinal anesthesia that interrupts sympathetic activation of the heart, injections of ephedrine increase heart rate as well as peripheral vascular resistance; tachyphylaxis may occur with repetitive injections, necessitating the use of a directly acting drug.

Patients with orthostatic hypotension (excessive fall in blood pressure with standing) represent a pharmacological challenge in many cases. There are diverse causes for this disorder, including the Shy–Drager syndrome and idiopathic autonomic failure. There are several therapeutic approaches including physical maneuvers and a variety of drugs (fludrocortisone, prostaglandin synthesis inhibitors, somatostatin analogs, caffeine, vasopressin analogs, and dopamine antagonists). A number of sympathomimetic drugs have been used in treating this disorder. The ideal agents would enhance venous constriction prominently and produce relatively little arterial constriction so as to avoid supine hypertension. No such agent currently is available. Drugs used in this disorder to activate α_1 receptors include both direct- and indirect-acting agents. Midodrine shows promise in treating this challenging disorder.

Hypertension. Centrally acting α_2-adrenergic agonists such as clonidine are useful in the treatment of hypertension. Drug therapy of hypertension is discussed in Chapter 33.

Cardiac Arrhythmias. Cardiopulmonary resuscitation in patients with cardiac arrest due to ventricular fibrillation, electromechanical dissociation, or asystole may be facilitated by drug treatment. Epinephrine is an important therapeutic agent in patients with cardiac arrest; epinephrine and other α-adrenergic agonists increase diastolic pressure and improve coronary blood flow (Raehl, 1987). α-Adrenergic agonists also help to preserve cerebral blood flow during resuscitation. Cerebral blood vessels are relatively insensitive to the vasoconstricting effects of catecholamines, and perfusion pressure is increased. Consequently, during external cardiac massage, epinephrine facilitates distribution of the limited cardiac output to the cerebral and coronary circulations. Although it had been thought that the β-adrenergic effects of epinephrine on the heart made ventricular fibrillation more susceptible to conversion with electrical countershock, tests in animal models have not confirmed this hypothesis (Raehl, 1987). The optimal dose of epinephrine in patients with cardiac arrest is unclear. Once a cardiac rhythm has been restored, it may be necessary to treat arrhythmias, hypotension, or shock.

In patients with paroxysmal supraventricular tachycardias, particularly those associated with mild hypotension, careful infusion of an α-adrenergic agonist such as phenylephrine or methoxamine to raise blood pressure to about 160 mm Hg may end the arrhythmia by increasing vagal tone. However, this method of treatment has been replaced largely by drugs such as Ca^{2+} channel blockers with clinically significant effects on the AV node, β-adrenergic antagonists, and adenosine, and by electrical cardioversion (see Chapter 35). β-Adrenergic agonists such as isoproterenol may be used as adjunctive or temporizing therapy with atropine in patients with marked bradycardia who are compromised hemodynamically; if long-term therapy is required, a cardiac pacemaker usually is the treatment of choice.

Congestive Heart Failure. Sympathetic stimulation of β-adrenergic receptors in the heart is a very important compensatory mechanism for maintenance of cardiac function in patients with congestive heart failure (Francis and Cohn, 1986). Evidence indicates that responses mediated by β-adrenergic receptors are blunted in the failing human heart (Bristow et al., 1985). While β-adrenergic agonists may increase cardiac output in acute emergency settings such as shock, long-term therapy with β-adrenergic agonists as inotropic agents is not efficacious. Indeed, interest has grown in the use of β-adrenergic receptor antagonists in the treatment of patients with congestive heart failure (see Chapter 34).

Local Vascular Effects of α-Adrenergic Agonists. Epinephrine is used in many surgical procedures in the nose, throat, and larynx to shrink the mucosa and improve visualization by limiting hemorrhage. Simultaneous injection of epinephrine with local anesthetics retards the absorption of the anesthetic and increases the duration of anesthesia (see Chapter 15). Injection of α-adrenergic agonists into the penis may be useful in reversing priapism, which may complicate the use of α-adrenergic antagonists in the treatment of erectile dysfunction. Both phenylephrine and oxymetazoline are efficacious vasoconstrictors when applied locally during sinus surgery (Riegle et al., 1992).

Nasal Decongestion. α-Adrenergic agonists are used extensively as nasal decongestants in patients with allergic or vasomotor rhinitis and in acute rhinitis in patients with upper respiratory infections (Empey and Medder, 1981). These drugs probably decrease resistance to airflow by decreasing the volume of the nasal mucosa; this may occur by activation of α-adrenergic receptors in venous capacitance vessels in nasal tissues that have erectile characteristics (Cole et al., 1983). The receptors that mediate this effect appear to be α_1-adrenergic receptors. Interestingly, α_2 receptors may mediate contraction of arterioles that supply nutrition to the nasal mucosa (Andersson and Bende, 1984). Intense constriction of these vessels may cause structural damage of the mucosa (DeBernardis et al., 1987). A major limitation of therapy with nasal decongestants is that loss of efficacy and "rebound" hyperemia and worsening of symptoms often occur with chronic use or when the drug is stopped. Although mechanisms are uncertain, possibilities include receptor desensitization and damage to the mucosa. Agonists that are selective for α_1 receptors may be less likely to induce mucosal damage (DeBernardis et al., 1987).

For decongestion, α-adrenergic agonists may be administered either orally or topically. Oral ephedrine often causes CNS adverse effects. Pseudoephedrine is a stereoisomer of ephedrine that is less potent than ephedrine in producing tachycardia, increased blood pressure, and CNS stimulation (Empey and Medder, 1981). Sympathomimetic decongestants should be used with great caution in patients with hypertension and in men with prostatic enlargement, and they are contraindicated in patients who are taking an MAO inhibitor. A variety of compounds (see above) are available for topical use in patients with rhinitis. Topical decongestants are particularly useful in acute rhinitis because of their more selective site of action, but they are apt to be used excessively by patients, leading to rebound congestion. Oral decongestants are much less likely to cause rebound congestion but carry a greater risk of inducing adverse systemic effects. Indeed, patients with uncontrolled hypertension or ischemic heart disease generally should carefully avoid the oral consumption of over-the-counter products or herbal preparations containing sympathomimetic drugs.

Asthma. Use of adrenergic agents in the treatment of asthma is discussed in Chapter 28.

Allergic Reactions. Epinephrine is the drug of choice to reverse the manifestations of serious, acute hypersensitivity reactions (e.g., from a food, bee sting, or drug allergy). A subcutaneous injection of epinephrine rapidly relieves itching, hives, and swelling of lips, eyelids, and tongue. In some patients, careful intravenous infusion of epinephrine may be required to ensure prompt pharmacological effects. This treatment may be lifesaving when edema of the glottis threatens patency of the airway or when there is hypotension or shock in patients with anaphylaxis. In addition to its cardiovascular effects, epinephrine is thought to activate β-adrenergic receptors that suppress the release from mast cells of mediators such as histamine or leukotrienes. Although glucocorticoids and antihistamines frequently are administered to patients with severe hypersensitivity reactions, epinephrine remains the mainstay of treatment.

Ophthalmic Uses. Application of various sympathomimetic amines for diagnostic and therapeutic ophthalmic use is discussed in Chapter 66.

Narcolepsy. Narcolepsy is characterized by hypersomnia, including attacks of sleep that may occur suddenly under conditions that are not normally conducive to sleep. Some patients respond to treatment with tricyclic antidepressants or MAO inhibitors. Alternatively, CNS stimulants such as amphetamine, dextroamphetamine, or methamphetamine may be useful (Mitler et al., 1993). *Modafinil* (PROVIGIL), a CNS stimulant, may have benefit in narcolepsy (Fry, 1998). In the United States, it is a controlled substance (schedule IV; see Appendix I). Its mechanism of action in narcolepsy is unclear and may not involve adrenergic receptors. Therapy with amphetamines is complicated by the risk of abuse and the likelihood of the development of tolerance. Depression, irritability, and paranoia also may occur. Amphetamines may disturb nocturnal sleep, which increases the difficulty of avoiding daytime attacks of sleep in these patients.

Weight Reduction. Obesity arises as a consequence of positive caloric balance. Optimally, weight loss is achieved by a gradual increase in energy expenditure from exercise combined with dieting to decrease the caloric intake. However, this obvious approach has a relatively low success rate. Consequently, alternative forms of treatment, including surgery or medications, have been developed in an effort to increase the likelihood of achieving and maintaining weight loss. Amphetamine was found to produce weight loss in early studies of patients with narcolepsy and was subsequently used in the treatment of obesity (Silverstone, 1986). The drug promotes weight loss by suppressing appetite rather than by increasing energy expenditure. Other anorexiant drugs include methamphetamine, dextroamphetamine, phentermine, benzphetamine, phendimetrazine, phenmetrazine, diethylpropion, mazindol, and phenylpropanolamine. In short-term (up to 20 weeks), double-blind, controlled studies, amphetamine-like drugs have been shown to be more effective than placebo in promoting weight loss; the rate of weight loss is typically increased by about 0.5 pound per week with these drugs. There is little to choose among these drugs in terms of efficacy. However, long-term weight loss has not been demonstrated unless these drugs are taken continuously (Bray, 1993). In addition, other important issues have not yet been resolved; these include the selection of patients who might be benefited by these drugs, whether the drugs should be administered continuously or intermittently, and the duration of treatment (Silverstone, 1986). Adverse effects of treatment include the potential for drug abuse and habituation, serious worsening of hypertension (although in some patients blood pressure may actually fall, presumably as a consequence of weight loss), sleep disturbances, palpitations, and dry mouth. These agents may be effective as adjuncts in the treatment of obese patients. However, available evidence does not support the isolated use of these drugs in the absence of a more comprehensive program that stresses exercise and modification of diet.

Attention-Deficit Hyperactivity Disorder (ADHD). This syndrome, usually first evident in childhood, is characterized by excessive motor activity, difficulty in sustaining attention, and impulsiveness. Children with this disorder frequently are troubled by difficulties in school, impaired interpersonal relationships, and excitability. Academic underachievement is an important characteristic. A substantial number of children with this syndrome have characteristics that persist into adulthood, although in modified form (American Psychiatric Association, 1987). Behavioral therapy may be helpful in some patients.

Catecholamines may be involved in the control of attention at the level of the cerebral cortex. A variety of stimulant drugs have been utilized in the treatment of ADHD, and they are particularly indicated in moderate-to-severe cases. Dextroamphetamine has been demonstrated to be more effective than placebo (Klein et al., 1980); methylphenidate also is effective in children with ADHD, although information about the long-term efficacy of both drugs is limited. Treatment may start with a dose of 5 mg of methylphenidate in the morning and at lunch; the dose is increased gradually over a period of weeks depending on the response as judged by parents, teachers, and the physician. The total daily dose generally should not exceed 60 mg; because of its short duration of action, most children require two or three doses of methylphenidate each day. The timing of doses is adjusted individually in accordance with rapidity of onset of effect and duration of action. Some children may not respond, and the drug should be discontinued after one month of dosage adjustment. Methylphenidate and dextroamphetamine probably have similar efficacy in ADHD and are the preferred drugs for this disorder (Elia et al., 1999). Pemoline appears to be less effective, although it may be used once daily in some children (Klein et al., 1980). Potential adverse effects of these medications in children include insomnia, abdominal pain, anorexia, and weight loss that may be associated with suppression of growth. Minor symptoms may be transient or may respond to adjustment of dosage or administration of the drug with meals. Other drugs that have been utilized include tricyclic antidepressants, antipsychotic agents, and clonidine (Fox and Rieder, 1993). There is evidence that stimulant medications are effective in adults with similar disorders (Chiarello and Cole, 1987).

II. ADRENERGIC RECEPTOR ANTAGONISTS

Many types of drugs interfere with the function of the sympathetic nervous system and thus have profound effects on the physiology of sympathetically innervated organs. Several of these drugs are important in clinical medicine, particularly for the treatment of cardiovascular diseases. Drugs that decrease the amount of norepinephrine released as a consequence of sympathetic nerve stimulation as well as drugs that inhibit sympathetic nervous activity by suppressing sympathetic outflow from the brain are discussed in Chapter 33.

The remainder of this chapter focuses on drugs termed *adrenergic receptor antagonists,* which inhibit the interaction of norepinephrine, epinephrine, and other sympathomimetic drugs with adrenergic receptors. Almost all of these agents are competitive antagonists in their interactions with either α- or β-adrenergic receptors; one exception is phenoxybenzamine, an irreversible antagonist that binds covalently to α-adrenergic receptors. There are important structural differences among the various types of adrenergic receptors (*see* also Chapter 6). Since compounds have been developed that have different affinities for the various receptors, it is possible to interfere selectively with responses that result from stimulation of the sympathetic nervous system. For example, selective antagonists of β_1-adrenergic receptors block most actions of epinephrine and norepinephrine on the heart, while having less effect on β_2-adrenergic receptors in bronchial smooth muscle and no effect on responses mediated by α_1- or α_2-adrenergic receptors. Detailed knowledge of the autonomic nervous system and the sites of action of drugs that act on adrenergic receptors is essential for understanding the pharmacological properties and therapeutic uses of this important class of drugs. Additional background material is presented in Chapter 6. Because of their unique activity in the CNS, drugs that block dopamine receptors are considered in Chapter 20.

α-ADRENERGIC RECEPTOR ANTAGONISTS

α-Adrenergic receptors mediate many of the important actions of endogenous catecholamines. Responses of particular clinical relevance include α_1-receptor-mediated contraction of arterial and venous smooth muscle. α_2-Adrenergic receptors are involved in suppressing sympathetic output, increasing vagal tone, facilitating platelet aggregation, inhibiting the release of norepinephrine and acetylcholine from nerve endings, and regulating metabolic effects. These effects include suppression of insulin secretion and inhibition of lipolysis. α_2-Receptors also mediate contraction of some arteries and veins.

α-Adrenergic receptor antagonists have a wide spectrum of pharmacological specificities and are chemically heterogeneous. Some of these drugs have markedly different affinities for α_1 and α_2 receptors. For example, prazosin is much more potent in blocking α_1 than α_2 receptors (and is termed α_1-selective), whereas yohimbine is α_2-selective; phentolamine has similar affinities for both of these receptor subtypes. More recently, agents that discriminate among the various subtypes of a particular receptor have become available; for example *tamsulosin* has higher potency at α_{1A} than at α_{1B} receptors.

Chemistry.   The structural formulas of a number of α-adrenergic antagonists are shown in Figure 10–4. These structurally diverse drugs can be divided into a number of major groups including β-haloethylamine alkylating agents, imidazoline analogs, piperazinyl quinazolines, and indole derivatives.

Pharmacological Properties

Cardiovascular System.   The most important effects of α-adrenergic antagonists observed clinically are on the cardiovascular system. Actions in both the CNS and the periphery are involved, and the outcome depends on the cardiovascular status of the patient at the time of drug administration and the relative selectivity of the agent for α_1 or α_2 receptors.

α_1-Adrenergic Antagonists.   Blockade of α_1-adrenergic receptors inhibits vasoconstriction induced by endogenous catecholamines; vasodilation may occur in both arteriolar resistance vessels and veins. The result is a fall in blood pressure because of decreased peripheral resistance. The magnitude of such effects depends on the activity of the sympathetic nervous system at the time the antagonist is administered and thus is less in supine than in upright subjects and is particularly marked if there is hypovolemia. For most α-adrenergic antagonists, the fall in blood pressure is opposed by baroreceptor reflexes that cause increases in heart rate and cardiac output, as well as fluid retention. These reflexes are exaggerated if the antagonist also blocks α_2 receptors on peripheral sympathetic nerve endings, leading to enhanced release of norepinephrine and increased stimulation of postsynaptic β_1 receptors in the heart and on juxtaglomerular cells (Langer, 1981; Starke *et al.*, 1989; *see* also Chapter 6). Although stimulation of α_1-adrenergic receptors in the heart may cause an increased force of contraction, the importance of blockade at this site in human beings is uncertain.

Blockade of α_1-adrenergic receptors also inhibits vasoconstriction and the increase in blood pressure produced by the administration of a sympathomimetic amine. The pattern of effects depends on the adrenergic agonist that is administered: pressor responses to phenylephrine can be completely suppressed; those to norepinephrine are only incompletely blocked because of residual stimulation of cardiac β_1 receptors; and pressor responses to epinephrine may be transformed to vasodepressor effects (epinephrine "reversal") because of residual stimulation of β_2 receptors in the vasculature with resultant vasodilation.

α_2-Adrenergic Antagonists. α_2-Adrenergic receptors have an important role in regulation of the activity of the sympathetic nervous system, both peripherally and centrally. As mentioned above, activation of presynaptic α_2 receptors inhibits the release of norepinephrine from peripheral sympathetic nerve endings. Activation of α_2 receptors in the pontomedullary region of the CNS inhibits sympathetic nervous system activity and leads to a fall in blood pressure; these receptors are a site of action of drugs such as clonidine. Blockade of α_2-adrenergic receptors with selective antagonists such as yohimbine can thus increase sympathetic outflow and potentiate the release of norepinephrine from nerve endings, leading to activation of α_1 and β_1 receptors in the heart and peripheral vasculature with a consequent rise in blood pressure (Goldberg and Robertson, 1983). Antagonists that also block α_1 receptors give rise to similar effects on sympathetic outflow and release of norepinephrine, but the net increase in blood pressure is prevented by inhibition of vasoconstriction.

Although certain vascular beds contain α_2-adrenergic receptors that promote contraction of smooth muscle, it is thought that these receptors are preferentially stimulated by circulating catecholamines, whereas α_1 receptors are activated by norepinephrine released from sympathetic

Alkylating agent

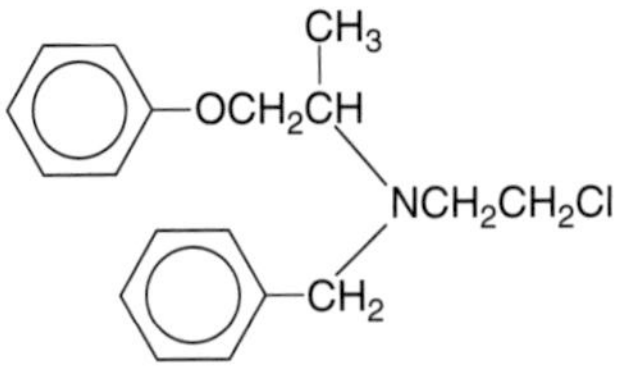

Benzenesulfonamide

PHENOXYBENZAMINE

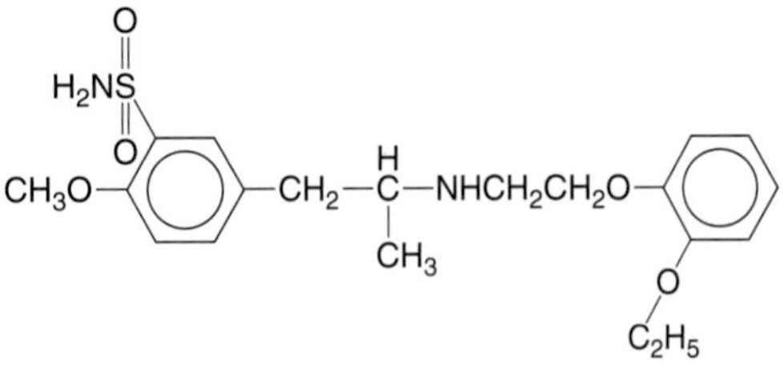

TAMSULOSIN

Imidazolines

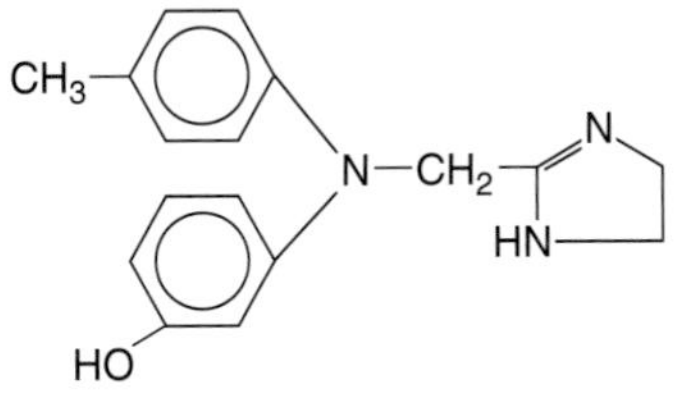

PHENTOLAMINE

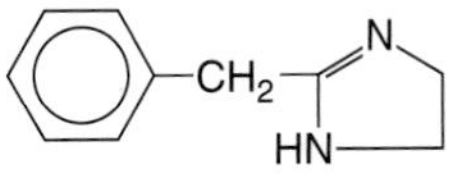

TOLAZOLINE

Piperazinyl quinazolines

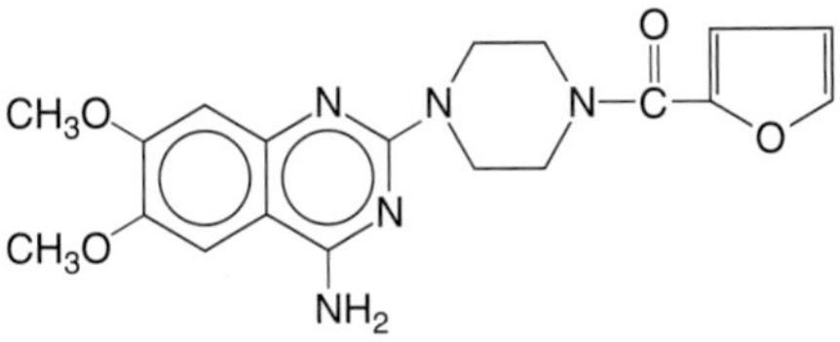

PRAZOSIN

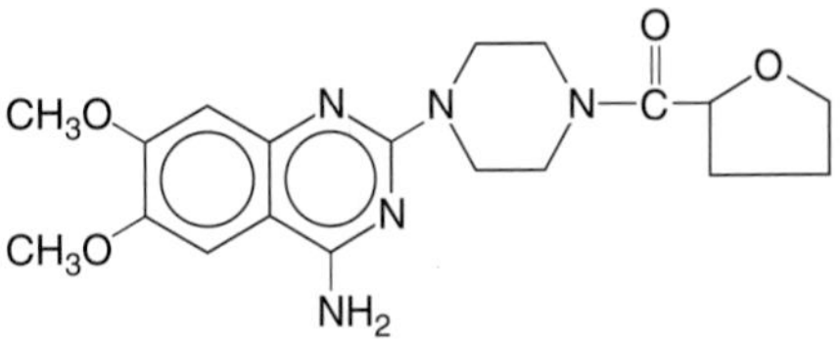

TERAZOSIN

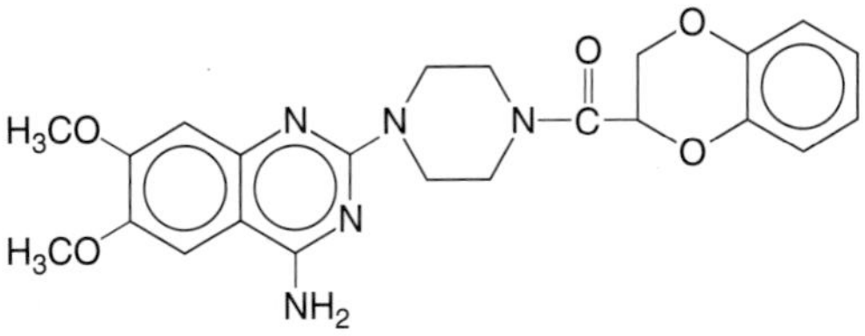

DOXAZOSIN

Indoles

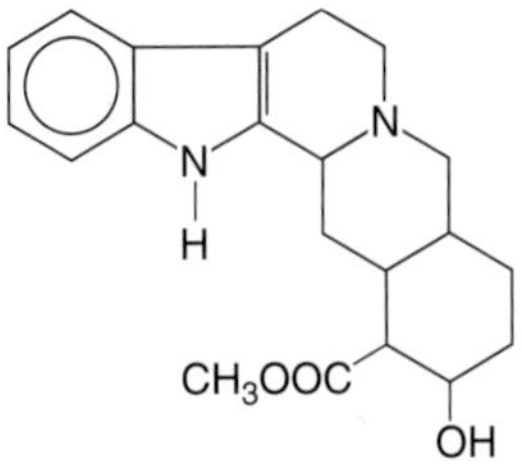

YOHIMBINE

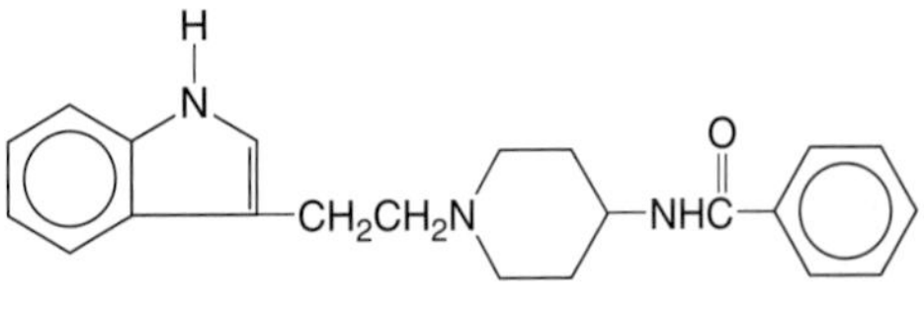

INDORAMIN

Figure 10–4. Structural formulas of some α-adrenergic receptor antagonists.

nerve fibers (Davey, 1987; van Zwieten, 1988). In other vascular beds, α_2 receptors promote vasodilation by stimulating the release of endothelium-derived relaxing factor (nitric oxide). The physiological role of vascular α_2-adrenergic receptors in the regulation of blood flow within various vascular beds is uncertain (Cubeddu, 1988). α_2-Adrenergic receptors contribute to smooth muscle contraction in human saphenous vein, whereas α_1 receptors are more prominent in dorsal hand veins (Haefeli et al., 1993; Gavin et al., 1997). The effects of α_2-adrenergic antagonists on the cardiovascular system are dominated by actions in the CNS and on sympathetic nerve endings.

Other Actions of α-Adrenergic Antagonists. α-Adrenergic antagonists can block α receptors that mediate contraction of nonvascular smooth muscle. For example, contraction of the trigone and sphincter muscles in the base of the urinary bladder and in the prostate may be inhibited by α_1-receptor antagonists, leading to decreased resistance to urinary outflow. Recent evidence suggests that α_{1A} receptors are important in mediating catecholamine-induced prostate smooth muscle contraction (Ruffolo and Hieble, 1999). Although α receptors may promote contraction of bronchial smooth muscle, the importance of this effect is minimal. Catecholamines increase the output of glucose from the liver; in human beings, this effect is mediated predominantly by β-adrenergic receptors, although α receptors may contribute (Rosen et al., 1983). α_2-Adrenergic receptors of the α_{2A} subtype facilitate platelet aggregation; the effect of blockade of platelet α_2 receptors in vivo is not clear. Activation of α_2 receptors in the pancreatic islets greatly suppresses insulin secretion; blockade of pancreatic α_2 receptors may facilitate insulin release (Kashiwagi et al., 1986).

Phenoxybenzamine and Related Haloalkylamines

Phenoxybenzamine is a haloalkylamine that blocks α_1- and α_2-adrenergic receptors irreversibly. Although phenoxybenzamine may have slight selectivity for α_1 receptors, it is not clear whether or not this has any significance in human beings.

Chemistry. The haloalkylamine adrenergic blocking drugs are closely related chemically to the nitrogen mustards; as in the latter, the tertiary amine cyclizes with the loss of chlorine to form a reactive ethyleniminium or aziridinium ion (see Chapter 52). The molecular configuration directly responsible for blockade is probably a highly reactive carbonium ion formed upon cleavage of the three-membered ring. It is presumed that the arylalkyl

amine moiety of the molecule is responsible for the relative specificity of action of these agents, since the reactive intermediate probably reacts with sulfhydryl, amino, and carboxyl groups in many proteins. Because of these chemical reactions, phenoxybenzamine is covalently conjugated with α-adrenergic receptors. Consequently, receptor blockade is irreversible, and restoration of cellular responsiveness to α-adrenergic agonists probably requires the synthesis of new receptors.

Pharmacological Properties. The major effects of phenoxybenzamine result from blockade of α-adrenergic receptors in smooth muscle. Phenoxybenzamine causes a progressive decrease in peripheral resistance and an increase in cardiac output that is due, in part, to reflex sympathetic nerve stimulation. Tachycardia may be accentuated by enhanced release of norepinephrine (because of α_2 blockade) and decreased inactivation of the amine because of inhibition of neuronal and extraneuronal uptake mechanisms (see below; see also Chapter 6). Pressor responses to exogenously administered catecholamines are impaired. Indeed, hypotensive responses to epinephrine occur because of unopposed β-adrenergic receptor–mediated vasodilation. Although phenoxybenzamine has relatively little effect on supine blood pressure in normotensive subjects, there is a marked fall in blood pressure on standing because of antagonism of compensatory vasoconstriction. In addition, the ability to respond to hypovolemia and anesthetic-induced vasodilation is impaired.

Phenoxybenzamine inhibits the uptake of catecholamines into both adrenergic nerve terminals and extraneuronal tissues. In addition to blockade of α-adrenergic receptors, substituted β-haloalkylamines irreversibly inhibit responses to 5-HT, histamine, and acetylcholine. However, somewhat higher doses of phenoxybenzamine are required to produce these effects than to produce blockade of α-adrenergic receptors. The general pharmacology of the haloalkylamines has been reviewed by Nickerson and Hollenberg (1967) and Furchgott (1972); also, more detailed discussion can be found in earlier editions of this textbook.

The pharmacokinetic properties of phenoxybenzamine are not well understood. The half-life of phenoxybenzamine is probably less than 24 hours. However, since the drug inactivates α-adrenergic receptors irreversibly, the duration of its effect is dependent not only on the presence of the drug but also on the rate of synthesis of α-adrenergic receptors. Many days may be required before the number of functional α-adrenergic receptors on the surface of target cells returns to normal (Hamilton et al., 1982). Blunted maximal responses to catecholamines may not be as persistent, since there are so-called spare α_1 receptors in vascular smooth muscle (Hamilton et al., 1983).

Therapeutic Uses. A major use of phenoxybenzamine (*phenoxybenzamine hydrochloride;* DIBENZYLINE) is in the treatment of pheochromocytoma. Pheochromocytomas are tumors of the adrenal medulla and sympathetic neurons that secrete enormous quantities of catecholamines into the circulation. The usual result is hypertension, which may be episodic and severe. The vast majority of pheochromocytomas are treated surgically; however, phenoxybenzamine is frequently used to treat the patient in preparation for surgery. The drug controls episodes of severe hypertension and minimizes other adverse effects of catecholamines, such as contraction of plasma volume and injury of the myocardium. A conservative approach is to initiate treatment with phenoxybenzamine (at a dosage of 10 mg twice daily) 1 to 3 weeks before the operation. The dose is increased every other day until the desired effect on blood pressure is achieved. Therapy may be limited by postural hypotension; nasal stuffiness is another frequent adverse effect. The usual total daily dose of phenoxybenzamine in patients with pheochromocytoma is 40 to 120 mg given in two or three divided portions. Some physicians do not use phenoxylenzamine preoperatively in patients with pheochromocytoma (Boutros *et al.,* 1990). Prolonged treatment with phenoxybenzamine may be necessary in patients with inoperable or malignant pheochromocytoma. In some patients, particularly those with malignant disease, administration of metyrosine may be a useful adjuvant (Brogden *et al.,* 1981; Perry *et al.,* 1990). Metyrosine is a competitive inhibitor of tyrosine hydroxylase, the rate-limiting enzyme in the synthesis of catecholamines (*see* Chapter 6). β-Adrenergic receptor antagonists also are used to treat pheochromocytoma, but only after the administration of an α-receptor antagonist (*see* below).

Phenoxybenzamine was the first α-receptor antagonist used in the medical therapy of benign prostatic hyperplasia (BPH); blockade of α receptors in smooth muscle of the prostate and bladder base may decrease both obstructive symptoms and the need to urinate at night (Caine *et al.,* 1981). However, *terazosin* and related drugs are safer and preferable α-adrenergic antagonists for this disorder (*see* below). Phenoxybenzamine has been used to control the manifestations of autonomic hyperreflexia in patients with spinal cord transection (Braddom and Rocco, 1991).

Toxicity and Adverse Effects.

The major adverse effect of phenoxybenzamine is postural hypotension. This is often accompanied by reflex tachycardia and other arrhythmias. Hypotension can be particularly severe in hypovolemic patients or under conditions that promote vasodilation (administration of vasodilator drugs, exercise, ingestion of alcohol or large quantities of food). Reversible inhibition of ejaculation and aspermia after orgasm may occur because of impaired smooth muscle contraction in the vas deferens and ejaculatory ducts. Phenoxybenzamine has mutagenic activity in the Ames test, and repeated administration of this drug to experimental animals causes peritoneal sarcomas and lung tumors (IARC, 1980). The clinical significance of these findings is not known.

Phentolamine and Tolazoline

Phentolamine, an imidazoline, is a competitive α-adrenergic antagonist that has similar affinities for α_1 and α_2 receptors. Its effects on the cardiovascular system are very similar to those of phenoxybenzamine. Phentolamine also can block receptors for 5-HT, and it causes release of histamine from mast cells. In addition, phentolamine has been found to block K^+ channels (McPherson, 1993). Tolazoline is a related but somewhat less potent compound. Tolazoline and phentolamine stimulate gastrointestinal smooth muscle, an effect that is antagonized by atropine, and they also enhance gastric acid secretion. Tolazoline stimulates secretion by salivary, lacrimal, and sweat glands as well.

The pharmacokinetic properties of phentolamine are not known, although the drug is extensively metabolized. Tolazoline is well absorbed after oral administration and is excreted in the urine.

Therapeutic Uses. Phentolamine (*phentolamine mesylate;* REGITINE) can be used in the short term to control hypertension in patients with pheochromocytoma. Rapid infusions of phentolamine may cause severe hypotension, and the drug should be administered cautiously. Phentolamine also may be useful to relieve pseudoobstruction of the bowel in patients with pheochromocytoma; this condition may result from the inhibitory effects of catecholamines on intestinal smooth muscle. Phentolamine has been used locally to prevent dermal necrosis after the inadvertent extravasation of an α-adrenergic agonist. The drug also may be useful for the treatment of hypertensive crises that follow the abrupt withdrawal of clonidine or that may result from the ingestion of tyramine-containing foods during the use of nonselective inhibitors of monoamine oxidase. Although excessive activation of α-adrenergic receptors is important in the development of severe hypertension in these settings, there is little information about the safety and efficacy of phentolamine compared with those of other antihypertensive agents in the treatment of such patients. Direct intracavernous injection of phentolamine (in combination with papaverine) has been proposed as a treatment for male sexual dysfunction (Sidi, 1988; Zentgraf *et al.,* 1988). The long-term efficacy of this treatment is not known. Intracavernous injection of phentolamine may cause orthostatic hypotension and priapism; pharmacological reversal of drug-induced erections can be achieved with an α-adrenergic agonist such as phenylephrine. Repetitive intrapenile injections may cause fibrotic reactions (Sidi, 1988). Interestingly, there is preliminary evidence suggesting that buccally or orally administered phentolamine may have efficacy in some men with sexual dysfunction (Zorgniotti, 1994; Becker *et al.,* 1998).

Tolazoline (*tolazoline hydrochloride;* PRISCOLINE) has been used in the treatment of persistent pulmonary hypertension of the newborn and as an aid in visualizing distal peripheral vessels during arteriography (Gouyon and Francoise, 1992; Wilms *et al.,* 1993). The use of tolazoline in the newborn may be replaced by the use of prostaglandins or nitric oxide (Gouyon and Francoise, 1992).

Toxicity and Adverse Effects. Hypotension is the major adverse effect of phentolamine. In addition, reflex cardiac stimulation may cause alarming tachycardia, cardiac arrhythmias, and ischemic cardiac events, including myocardial infarction. Gastrointestinal stimulation may result in abdominal pain, nausea, and exacerbation of peptic ulcer. Phentolamine should be used with particular caution in patients with coronary artery disease or a history of peptic ulcer.

Prazosin and Related Drugs

Prazosin, the prototype of a family of agents that contain a piperazinyl quinazoline nucleus, is a very potent and selective α_1-adrenergic antagonist. Its affinity for α_1 receptors is about 1000-fold greater than that for α_2 receptors. Prazosin has similar potencies at α_{1A}, α_{1B}, and α_{1D} receptor subtypes. Interestingly, the drug also is a relatively potent inhibitor of cyclic nucleotide phosphodiesterases, and it was originally synthesized for this purpose (Hess, 1975). The pharmacological properties of prazosin have been characterized extensively, and the drug is used frequently for the treatment of hypertension (*see* Chapter 33).

Pharmacological Properties. *Prazosin.* The major effects of prazosin are a result of its blockade of α_1-adrenergic receptors in arterioles and veins. This leads to a fall in peripheral vascular resistance and in venous return to the heart. Administration of prazosin usually does not increase heart rate, a response that occurs frequently with other vasodilating drugs. Since prazosin has little or no α_2-receptor–blocking effect at concentrations achieved clinically, it probably does not promote the release of norepinephrine from sympathetic nerve endings in the heart. In addition, prazosin decreases cardiac preload and thus has little tendency to increase cardiac output and rate, in contrast to vasodilators such as hydralazine that have minimal dilatory effects on veins. Although the combination of reduced preload and selective α_1-receptor blockade might be sufficient to account for the relative absence of reflex tachycardia, prazosin also may act in the CNS to suppress sympathetic outflow (*see* Cubeddu, 1988). Prazosin appears to depress baroreflex function in hypertensive patients (Sasso and O'Connor, 1982). Prazosin and related drugs in this class tend to have small but favorable effects on serum lipids in human beings, decreasing low-density lipoproteins (LDL) and triglycerides while increasing concentrations of high-density lipoproteins (HDL). The clinical significance of these changes is not known. Prazosin and related drugs may have effects on cell growth unrelated to antagonism of α_1 receptors (Yang *et al.,* 1997; Hu *et al.,* 1998).

Prazosin (*prazosin hydrochloride;* MINIPRESS) is well absorbed after oral administration, and bioavailability is about 50% to 70%. Peak concentrations of prazosin in plasma are generally reached 1 to 3 hours after an oral dose. The drug is tightly bound to plasma proteins (primarily α_1-acid glycoprotein), and only 5% of the drug is free in the circulation; diseases that modify the concentration of this protein (*e.g.,* inflammatory processes)

may change the free fraction (Rubin and Blaschke, 1980). Prazosin is extensively metabolized in the liver, and little unchanged drug is excreted by the kidneys. The plasma half-life is approximately 2 to 3 hours (this may be prolonged to 6 to 8 hours in congestive heart failure). The duration of action of the drug is typically 7 to 10 hours in the treatment of hypertension.

The initial dose should be 1 mg, usually given at bedtime, so that the patient will remain recumbent for at least several hours to reduce the risk of syncopal reactions that may follow the first dose of prazosin. Therapy is begun with 1 mg given two or three times daily, and the dose is titrated upward depending on the blood pressure. A maximal effect generally is observed with a total daily dose of 20 mg in patients with hypertension. In the treatment of benign prostatic hyperplasia (BPH), doses from 1 to 5 mg twice daily typically are used. The twice-daily dosing requirement for prazosin is a disadvantage compared with newer α_1-receptor antagonists.

Terazosin. Terazosin (*terazosin hydrochloride;* HYTRIN) is a close structural analog of prazosin (Kyncl, 1993; Wilde *et al.,* 1993). It is less potent than prazosin but retains high specificity for α_1 receptors; terazosin does not discriminate among α_{1A}, α_{1B}, and α_{1D} receptors. The major distinction between the two drugs is in their pharmacokinetic properties. Terazosin is more soluble in water than is prazosin, and its bioavailability is high ($>90\%$) (Cubeddu, 1988; Frishman *et al.,* 1988); this may facilitate titration of dosage. The half-time of elimination of terazosin is approximately 12 hours, and its duration of action usually extends beyond 18 hours. Consequently, the drug may be taken once daily to treat hypertension and BPH in most patients. Terazosin has been found more effective that *finasteride* in treatment of BPH (Lepor *et al.,* 1996). Only about 10% of terazosin is excreted unchanged in the urine. An initial first dose of 1 mg is recommended. Doses are titrated upward depending on the therapeutic response. Doses of 10 mg/day may be required for maximal effect in BPH.

Doxazosin. Doxazosin (CARDURA) is another structural analog of prazosin. It, too, is a highly selective antagonist at α_1-adrenergic receptors, although nonselective among α_1-receptor subtypes, but it differs in its pharmacokinetic profile (Babamoto and Hirokawa, 1992). The half-life of doxazosin is approximately 20 hours, and its duration of action may extend to 36 hours (Cubeddu, 1988). The bioavailability and extent of metabolism of doxazosin and prazosin are similar. Most doxazosin metabolites are eliminated in the feces. The hemodynamic effects of doxazosin appear to be similar to those of prazosin. Doxazosin should be given initially as a one-mg dose in the treatment of hypertension or BPH. The role of doxazosin in the monotherapy of hypertension recently has been questioned by the results of a clinical trial. A slow-release formulation of doxazosin is under investigation; preliminary evidence suggests that this might ease dose titration (Os and Stokke, 1999).

Alfuzosin. *Alfuzosin* is a quinozoline-based α_1-receptor antagonist with similar affinity at all of the α_1-receptor subtypes (Foglar *et al.*, 1995; Kenny *et al.*, 1996). It has been used extensively in treating BPH. Its bioavailability is about 64%; it has a half-life of 3 to 5 hours. Alfuzosin is not currently available in the United States.

Tamsulosin. *Tamsulosin* (FLOMAX), a benzenesulfonamide, is an α_1 receptor antagonist with some selectivity for α_{1A} (and α_{1D}) receptor subtypes compared to α_{1B} receptor subtype (Kenny *et al.*, 1996). This selectivity may favor blockade of α_{1A} receptors in prostate compared to α_{1B} receptors, which are important in vascular smooth muscle. Tamsulosin is efficacious in the treatment of BPH with little effect on blood pressure (Wilde and McTavish, 1996; Beduschi *et al.*, 1998). Tamsulosin is well absorbed and has a half-life of 5 to 10 hours. It is extensively metabolized by the cytochrome P450 system. Tamsulosin may be administered at a 0.4-mg starting dose; a dose of 0.8 mg ultimately will be more efficacious in some patients. Abnormal ejaculation is an adverse effect of tamsulosin.

Adverse Effects. A major potential adverse effect of prazosin and its congeners is the so-called first-dose phenomenon; marked postural hypotension and syncope are sometimes seen 30 to 90 minutes after a patient takes an initial dose. Occasionally, syncopal episodes also have occurred with a rapid increase in dosage or with the addition of a second antihypertensive drug to the regimen of a patient who is already taking a large dose of prazosin. The mechanisms responsible for such exaggerated hypotensive responses or for the development of tolerance to these effects are not clear. An action in the CNS to reduce sympathetic outflow may contribute (*see* above). The risk of the first-dose phenomenon is minimized by limiting the initial dose to 1 mg at bedtime, by increasing the dosage slowly, and by introducing additional antihypertensive drugs cautiously. Since orthostatic hypotension may be a problem during long-term treatment with prazosin or its congeners, it is essential to check standing as well as recumbent blood pressure. Nonspecific adverse effects such as headache, "dizziness," and asthenia do not often limit treatment with prazosin. The nonspecific complaint of "dizziness" is generally not due to orthostatic hypotension. Although not extensively documented, the adverse effects of the structural analogs of prazosin appear to be similar to those of the parent compound. For tamsulosin,

at a dose of 0.4 mg daily, effects on blood pressure are not expected, although impaired ejaculation may occur.

Therapeutic Uses. Prazosin and its congeners have been used successfully in the treatment of primary systemic hypertension (*see* Chapter 33). The most important distinction among these drugs relates to their duration of action and thus the required dosing interval. Considerable recent interest has focused on the use of α_1-adrenergic antagonists in the treatment of hypertension in view of the tendency of these drugs to improve rather than worsen lipid profiles and glucose-insulin metabolism in patients with hypertension who are at risk for atherosclerotic disease (Grimm, 1991). Also, catecholamines are powerful stimulators of vascular smooth muscle hypertrophy, acting *via* α_1 receptors (Majesky *et al.*, 1990; Okazaki *et al.*, 1994). To what extent these effects of α_1 antagonists have clinical significance in diminishing risk of atherosclerosis is not known.

Congestive Heart Failure. α-Adrenergic antagonists have been used in the treatment of congestive heart failure, as have other vasodilating drugs. The short-term effects of prazosin in these patients are due to dilation of both arteries and veins, resulting in a reduction of preload and afterload, which increases cardiac output and reduces pulmonary congestion (Colucci, 1982). In contrast to results obtained with inhibitors of angiotensin converting enzyme or a combination of hydralazine and an organic nitrate, prazosin has not been found to prolong life in patients with congestive heart failure (Cohn *et al.*, 1986).

Benign Prostatic Hyperplasia. α_1-Adrenergic receptors in the trigone muscle of the bladder and urethra contribute to the resistance to outflow of urine. Prazosin reduces this resistance in some patients with impaired bladder emptying caused by prostatic obstruction or parasympathetic decentralization from spinal injury (Kirby *et al.*, 1987; Andersson, 1988). The efficacy and importance of α_1-adrenergic-receptor antagonists in the medical treatment of benign prostatic hyperplasia have been demonstrated in multiple controlled clinical trials. Transurethral resection of the prostate has been the accepted surgical treatment for symptoms of urinary obstruction in men with BPH; however, there are some serious potential complications, and improvement may not be permanent. Other, less invasive procedures also are available. Medical therapy has utilized α-adrenergic antagonists for many years. Finasteride, a drug that inhibits conversion of testosterone to dihydrotestosterone (*see* Chapter 59), and can reduce prostate volume in some patients, has been approved for this indication. However, its overall efficacy appears less than that observed with α_1 receptor antagonists (Lepor *et al.*, 1996). α_1-Selective adrenergic antagonists have efficacy in benign prostatic hyperplasia owing to relaxation of smooth muscle in the bladder neck, prostate capsule, and prostatic urethra. These drugs rapidly improve urinary flow, whereas the actions of finasteride are typically delayed for months. Phenoxybenzamine was the first adrenergic antagonist used extensively for benign prostatic hyperplasia; however, the relative lack of extensive safety information about this drug has led to its replacement by newer, reversible antagonists for this indication. Prazosin, terazosin, doxazosin, tamsulosin, and alfuzosin have been studied extensively and used widely in patients with benign prostatic hyperplasia (Cooper *et al.*, 1999). With the exception on tamsulosin, the comparative efficacies of each of these drugs, especially in comparison with relative adverse effects such as postural hypotension, appear similar, although direct comparisons are limited. Tamsulosin at the recommended dose of 0.4 mg daily is less likely to cause orthostatic hypotension than are the other drugs; its relative efficacy in BPH requires further study. Animal models have some utility in comparing potencies of adrenergic antagonists but may not adequately reflect the human prostate or predict clinical efficacy (Breslin *et al.*, 1993). The nature of the subtype(s) of α_1 receptors contributing to contraction in human prostate is unclear. However, there is growing evidence that the predominant α_1-receptor subtype expressed in the prostate is the α_{1A} receptor (Price *et al.*, 1993; Faure *et al.*, 1994; Forray *et al.*, 1994). Indeed, studies of receptor binding and smooth muscle contraction in the human prostate also suggest the importance of the cloned α_{1A} receptor (Forray *et al.*, 1994). Developments in this area will provide the basis for the selection of α-adrenergic antagonists with specificity for the relevant subtype of α_1 receptor in human prostate. However, the possibility remains that some of the symptoms of BPH are due to α_1 receptors in other sites, such as bladder, spinal cord, or brain.

Other Disorders.   Although anecdotal evidence suggested that prazosin might be useful in the treatment of patients with variant angina (Prinzmetal's angina) due to coronary vasospasm, several small controlled trials have failed to demonstrate a clear benefit (Robertson *et al.*, 1983b; Winniford *et al.*, 1983). Some studies have indicated that prazosin can decrease the incidence of digital vasospasm in patients with Raynaud's disease; however, its relative efficacy as compared with other vasodilators (*e.g.*, Ca^{2+} channel blockers) is not known (Surwit *et al.*, 1984; Wollersheim *et al.*, 1986). Prazosin may have some benefit in patients with other vasospastic disorders (Spittell and Spittell, 1992). Prazosin decreases ventricular arrhythmias induced by coronary artery ligation or reperfusion in laboratory animals; the therapeutic potential for this use in human beings is not known (Davey, 1986). Prazosin also might be useful for the treatment of patients with mitral or aortic valvular insufficiency, presumably because of reduction of afterload; additional data are needed (Jebavy *et al.*, 1983; Stanaszek *et al.*, 1983).

Ergot Alkaloids

The ergot alkaloids were the first adrenergic blocking agents to be discovered, and most aspects of their general pharmacology were disclosed in the classic studies of Dale (1906). Ergot alkaloids exhibit a complex variety of pharmacological properties. To varying degrees, these agents act as partial agonists or antagonists at α-adrenergic, 5-HT, and dopamine receptors.

Chemistry.   Details of the chemistry of the ergot alkaloids are presented in Chapter 11. In general, compounds of the ergonovine type, which lack a peptide side chain, have no adrenergic blocking activity. Of the natural ergot preparations, "ergotoxine" has the greatest α-adrenergic blocking potency. It is a mixture of three alkaloids—ergocornine, ergocristine, and ergocryptine. Dihydrogenation of the lysergic acid nucleus increases α-adrenergic blocking activity and decreases, but does not eliminate, the ability to stimulate smooth muscle by an action on tryptaminergic receptors.

Pharmacological Properties.   Both the natural and the dihydrogenated peptide alkaloids produce α-adrenergic blockade.

This is relatively persistent for a competitive antagonist, but it is of much shorter duration than that produced by phenoxybenzamine. These drugs also are effective antagonists of 5-HT. Although the hydrogenated ergot alkaloids are among the most potent α-adrenergic blocking agents known, a plethora of adverse effects prevents the administration of doses that could produce more than minimal blockade in human beings.

The most important effects of the ergot alkaloids are due to actions on the CNS and direct stimulation of smooth muscle. The latter occurs in many different organs (*see* Chapter 11), and even *dihydroergotoxine* (ergoloid mesylate) has been observed to produce spastic contractions of the intestine.

The peptide ergot alkaloids can reverse the pressor response to epinephrine to a depressor action. However, all the natural ergot alkaloids cause a significant rise in blood pressure as a result of peripheral vasoconstriction, which is more pronounced in postcapillary than in precapillary vessels. Although hydrogenation reduces this action, dihydroergotamine still is an effective vasoconstrictor; a residual constrictor action of dihydroergotoxine also is demonstrable. *Ergotamine, ergonovine,* and other ergot alkaloids can produce coronary vasoconstriction, often with associated ischemic changes and anginal pain in patients with coronary artery disease. The ergot alkaloids usually induce bradycardia even when the blood pressure is not increased. This is predominantly due to increased vagal activity, but a central reduction in sympathetic tone and direct myocardial depression also may be involved.

Toxicity and Adverse Effects.   The dose of dihydroergotoxine in human beings is limited by the occurrence of nausea and vomiting. Prolonged or excessive administration of any of the natural peptide ergot alkaloids can cause vascular insufficiency, including myocardial ischemia and gangrene of the extremities due to marked arterial constriction (Galer *et al.*, 1991). This is particularly likely to occur in the presence of preexisting vascular pathological processes. In severe cases, prompt vasodilation is essential. There have been no comparative studies on the treatment of this sporadic condition, but a directly acting drug such as nitroprusside appears to be most effective (Carliner *et al.*, 1974). Toxic effects of the ergot alkaloids are described in more detail in Chapter 11.

Therapeutic Uses.   The primary uses of ergot alkaloids are to stimulate contraction of the uterus postpartum and to relieve the pain of migraine (Mitchell and Elbourne, 1993; Saxena and De Deyn, 1992; *see* Chapter 11). However, newer alternatives, such as sumatriptan and other 5-HT$_1$-receptor agonists, may have better efficacy and safety in migraine (Dechant and Clissold, 1992; *see* also Chapter 11). Ergonovine and *methylergonovine* are useful in preventing and treating postpartum hemorrhage due to uterine atonia, probably by stimulating uterine contraction, which compresses bleeding blood vessels. Synthetic preparations of the posterior pituitary hormone *oxytocin* also are used to enhance uterine contractions (*see* Chapter 56); this may have the benefit not only of preventing or treating uterine hemorrhage but also of inducing or augmenting labor. *Dinoprostone* (prostaglandin E$_2$) also inhibits postpartum bleeding and may be efficacious if there is an inadequate response to ergot alkaloids or oxytocin (Winkler and Rath, 1999). Ergot alkaloids have been used clinically in many settings: diagnostically to stimulate coronary artery contraction; as putative cognition enhancers

(Wadworth and Chrisp, 1992); and in the management of orthostatic hypotension (Stumpf and Mitrzyk, 1994). The effect of bromocriptine on the secretion of prolactin is described in Chapter 56.

Additional α-Adrenergic Antagonists

Indoramin. *Indoramin* is a selective, competitive α_1-receptor antagonist that has been used for the treatment of hypertension. Competitive antagonism of histamine H_1 and 5-HT receptors also is evident (Cubeddu, 1988). As an α_1-selective antagonist, indoramin lowers blood pressure with minimal tachycardia. The drug also decreases the incidence of attacks of Raynaud's phenomenon (Holmes and Sorkin, 1986).

The bioavailability of indoramin is generally less than 30% (with considerable variability), and it undergoes extensive first-pass metabolism (Holmes and Sorkin, 1986; Pierce, 1990). Little unchanged drug is excreted in the urine, and some of the metabolites may be biologically active. The elimination half-life is about 5 hours. Some of the adverse effects of indoramin include sedation, dry mouth, and failure of ejaculation. Although indoramin is an effective antihypertensive agent, it has complex pharmacokinetics and lacks a well-defined place in current therapy. Indoramin currently is not available in the United States.

Labetalol. *Labetalol,* a potent β-adrenergic receptor antagonist, competitively blocks α_1 receptors as well (*see* below).

Ketanserin. Although developed as a 5-HT-receptor antagonist, *ketanserin* also blocks α_1-adrenergic receptors. Ketanserin is discussed in Chapter 11.

Urapidil. *Urapidil* is a novel, selective α_1-adrenergic antagonist that has a chemical structure distinct from those of prazosin and related compounds. Blockade of peripheral α_1 receptors appears to be primarily responsible for the hypotension produced by urapidil, although it has actions in the CNS as well (Cubeddu, 1988; van Zwieten, 1988). The drug is extensively metabolized and has a half-life of 3 hours. The role of urapidil in the treatment of hypertension remains to be determined. Urapidil is not currently available for clinical use in the United States.

Bunazosin. *Bunazosin* is an α_1-selective antagonist of the quinazoline class of compounds. Bunazosin has been shown to lower blood pressure in patients with hypertension (Harder and Thurmann, 1994). Bunazosin is not currently available in the United States.

Yohimbine. *Yohimbine* (YOCON) is a competitive antagonist that is selective for α_2-adrenergic receptors. The compound is an indolealkylamine alkaloid and is found in the bark of the tree *Pausinystalia yohimbe* and in *Rauwolfia* root; its structure resembles that of reserpine. Yohimbine readily enters the CNS, where it acts to increase blood pressure and heart rate; it also enhances motor activity and produces tremors. These actions are opposite to those of clonidine, an α_2 agonist (*see* Goldberg and Robertson, 1983; Grossman *et al.,* 1993). Yohimbine also is an antagonist of 5-HT. In the past, it has been used extensively to treat male sexual dysfunction. Although efficacy was never clearly demonstrated, there is renewed interest in the use of yohimbine in the treatment of male sexual dysfunction.

The drug enhances sexual activity in male rats (Clark *et al.,* 1984), and it may benefit some patients with psychogenic erectile dysfunction (Reid *et al.,* 1987). However, the efficacies of sildenafil and apomorphine have been much more conclusively demonstrated in oral treatment of erectile dysfunction. Several small studies suggest that yohimbine also may be useful for diabetic neuropathy and in the treatment of postural hypotension.

Neuroleptic Agents. Natural and synthetic compounds of several other chemical classes developed primarily because they are antagonists of D_2 dopamine receptors also exhibit α-adrenergic blocking activity. Chlorpromazine, haloperidol, and other neuroleptic drugs of the phenothiazine and butyrophenone types produce significant α-receptor blockade in both laboratory animals and human beings.

β-ADRENERGIC RECEPTOR ANTAGONISTS

β-Adrenergic receptor antagonists (β blockers) have received enormous clinical attention because of their efficacy in the treatment of hypertension, ischemic heart disease, congestive heart failure, and certain arrhythmias.

History. Ahlquist's hypothesis that the effects of catecholamines were mediated by activation of distinct α- and β-adrenergic receptors provided the initial impetus for the synthesis and pharmacological evaluation of β-adrenergic blocking agents (*see* Chapter 6). The first such selective agent was dichloroisoproterenol (Powell and Slater, 1958). However, this compound is a partial agonist, and this property was thought to preclude its safe clinical use. Sir James Black and his colleagues initiated a program in the late 1950s to develop additional agents of this type. Although the usefulness of their first antagonist, pronethalol, was limited by the production of thymic tumors in mice, *propranolol* soon followed (Black and Stephenson, 1962; Black and Prichard, 1973). Propranolol is a competitive β-adrenergic receptor antagonist and remains the prototype to which other β-adrenergic antagonists are compared. Subsequent efforts to generate additional antagonists have resulted in compounds that can be distinguished by the following properties: relative affinity for β_1 and β_2 receptors, intrinsic sympathomimetic activity, blockade of α-adrenergic receptors, differences in lipid solubility, capacity to induce vasodilation, and general pharmacokinetic properties. Some of these distinguishing characteristics have clinical significance, and they help guide the appropriate choice of a β-adrenergic antagonist for an individual patient.

Propranolol has equal affinity for β_1 and β_2 receptors; thus, it is a nonselective β-adrenergic antagonist. Agents such as metoprolol and atenolol have somewhat greater affinity for β_1 than for β_2 receptors; these are examples of selective β_1 antagonists, even though the selectivity is not absolute. Propranolol is a pure antagonist, and it has no capacity to activate β-adrenergic receptors. Several β blockers (*e.g.,* pindolol and acebutolol) activate

β receptors partially in the absence of catecholamines; however, the intrinsic activities of these drugs are less than that of a full agonist such as isoproterenol. These partial agonists are said to have intrinsic sympathomimetic activity. Substantial sympathomimetic activity would be counterproductive to the response desired from a β-adrenergic antagonist; however, slight residual activity may, for example, prevent profound bradycardia or negative inotropy in a resting heart. The potential clinical advantage of this property, however, is unclear and may be a disadvantage in the context of secondary prevention of myocardial infarction (see below). In addition, other β-receptor antagonists have been found to have the property of so-called inverse agonism (see Chapter 2). These drugs can decrease basal activation of β-receptor signaling by shifting the equilibrium of spontaneously active receptors toward the inactive state (Chidiac et al., 1994). The clinical significance of this property is unknown. Although most β-adrenergic antagonists do not block α-adrenergic receptors, *labetalol* and *carvedilol* are examples of agents that block both α_1 and β receptors. *Celiprolol* is an example of a drug that is a β_1-selective antagonist and a β_2-selective agonist and that promotes vasodilation.

Chemistry. The structural formulas of some β-adrenergic antagonists in general use are shown in Figure 10–5. The structural similarities between agonists and antagonists that act on β receptors are closer than those between α-receptor agonists and antagonists. Substitution of an isopropyl group or other bulky substituent on the amino nitrogen favors interaction with β-adrenergic receptors. There is a rather wide tolerance for the nature of the aromatic moiety in the nonselective β-receptor antagonists; however, the structural tolerance for β_1-selective antagonists is far more constrained. The β-adrenergic receptor, as shown in Figure 10–1 and discussed in Chapter 6, is a member of the G protein–coupled receptor family with seven membrane-spanning domains.

Pharmacological Properties

As in the case of α-adrenergic blocking agents, the pharmacological properties of β-adrenergic antagonists can be explained largely from knowledge of the responses elicited by the receptors in the various tissues and the activity of the sympathetic nerves that innervate these tissues (see Table 6–1). For example, β-receptor blockade has relatively little effect on the normal heart of an individual at rest but has profound effects when sympathetic control of the heart is dominant, as during exercise or stress.

Cardiovascular System. The major therapeutic effects of β-adrenergic antagonists are on the cardiovascular system. It is important to distinguish these effects in normal

subjects from those in subjects with cardiovascular disease such as hypertension or myocardial ischemia.

Since catecholamines have positive chronotropic and inotropic actions, β-adrenergic antagonists slow the heart rate and decrease myocardial contractility. When tonic stimulation of β receptors is low, this effect is correspondingly modest. However, when the sympathetic nervous system is activated, as during exercise or stress, β-adrenergic antagonists attenuate the expected rise in heart rate. Short-term administration of β-adrenergic antagonists such as propranolol decreases cardiac output; peripheral resistance increases in proportion to maintain blood pressure as a result of blockade of vascular β_2 receptors and compensatory reflexes, such as increased sympathetic nervous system activity, leading to activation of vascular α-adrenergic receptors. However, with long-term use of β-adrenergic antagonists, total peripheral resistance returns to initial values (Mimran and Ducailar, 1988) or decreases in patients with hypertension (Man in't Veld et al., 1988). With β-receptor antagonists that also are α_1-receptor antagonists, such as labetalol and carvedilol, cardiac output is maintained with a greater fall in peripheral resistance.

β-Adrenergic receptor antagonists have significant effects on cardiac rhythm and automaticity. Although it had been thought that these effects were due exclusively to blockade of β_1 receptors, β_2-adrenergic receptors likely also are involved in regulating heart rate in human beings (Brodde, 1988). β-Adrenergic antagonists reduce sinus rate, decrease the spontaneous rate of depolarization of ectopic pacemakers, slow conduction in the atria and in the AV node, and increase the functional refractory period of the AV node.

Although high concentrations of many β blockers produce quinidine-like effects ("membrane-stabilizing activity"), it is doubtful that this is significant at usual doses of these agents. However, this effect may be important when there is overdosage. Interestingly, there is some evidence suggesting that d-propranolol may suppress ventricular arrhythmias independently of β-receptor blockade (Murray et al., 1990).

The cardiovascular effects of β-adrenergic antagonists are most evident during dynamic exercise. In the presence of β-receptor blockade, the exercise-induced increases in heart rate and myocardial contractility are attenuated. However, the exercise-induced increase in cardiac output is less affected because of an increase in stroke volume (Shephard, 1982; Tesch, 1985; Van Baak, 1988). The effects of β-adrenergic antagonists on exercise are somewhat analogous to the changes that occur with normal aging. In healthy elderly persons, catecholamine-induced increases in heart rate are smaller than in younger individuals; however, the increase in cardiac output in older people may be preserved because of an increase in stroke volume during exercise. β Blockers tend to decrease work

Nonselective antagonists

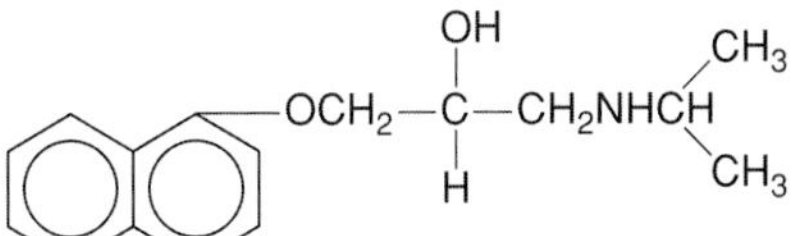

PROPRANOLOL

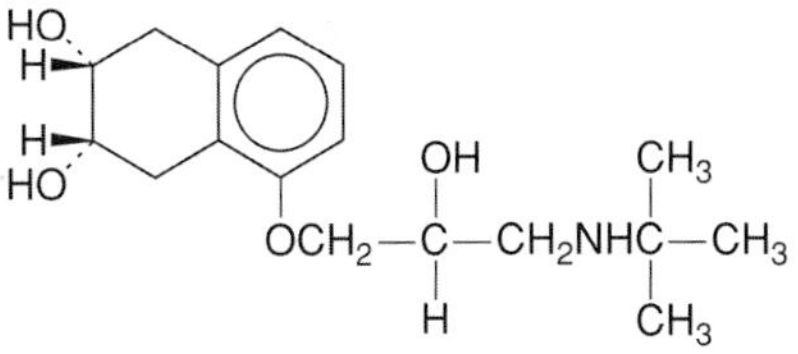

NADOLOL

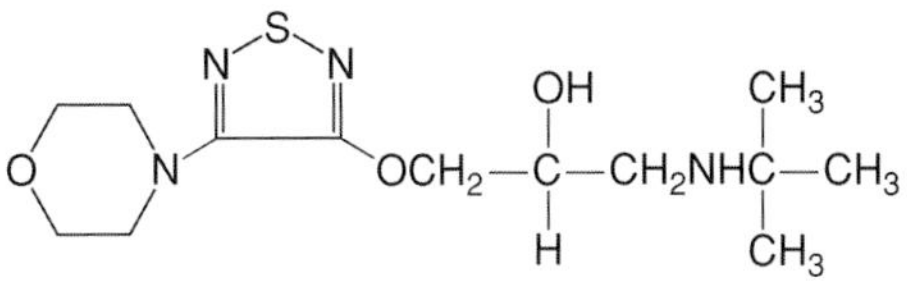

TIMOLOL

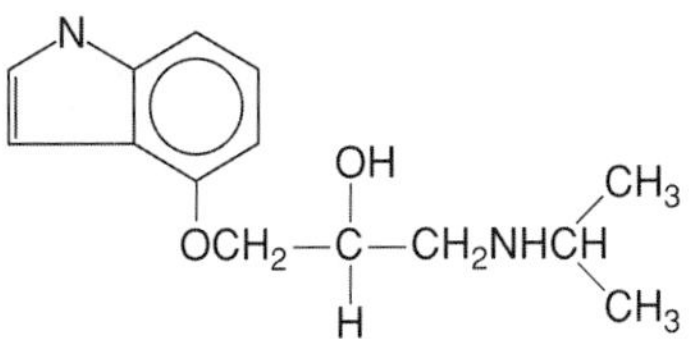

PINDOLOL

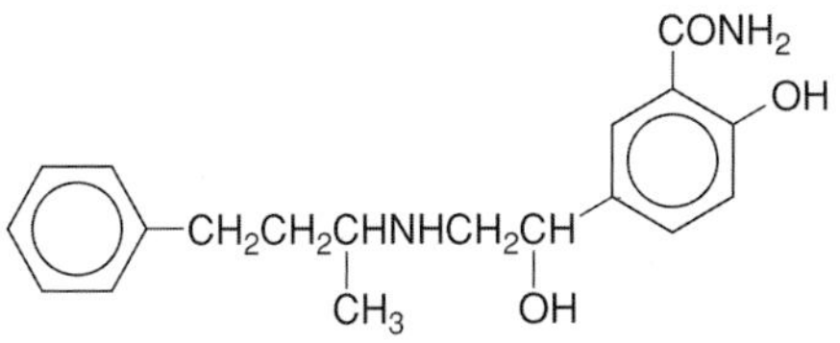

LABETALOL

β_1-selective antagonists

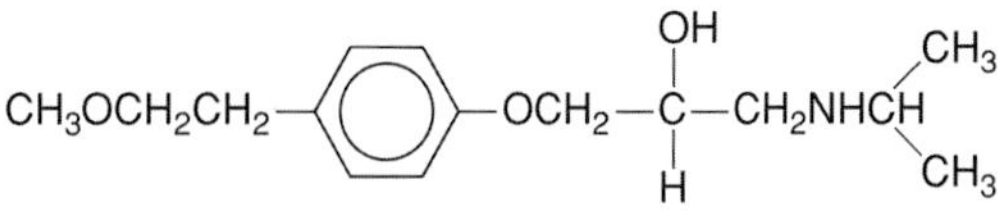

METOPROLOL

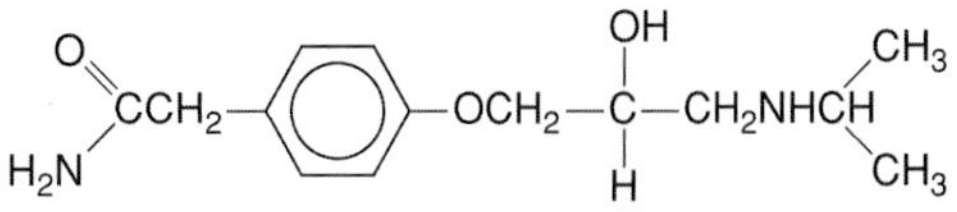

ATENOLOL

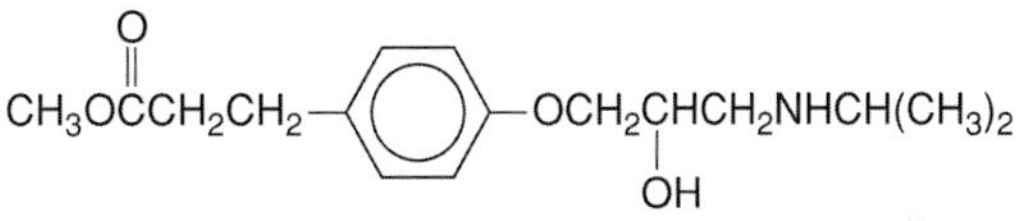

ESMOLOL

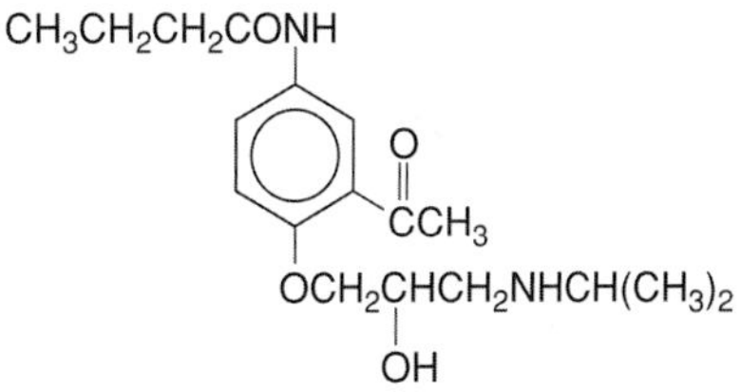

ACEBUTOLOL

Figure 10–5. Structural formulas of some β-adrenergic receptor antagonists.

capacity, as assessed by their effects on intense short-term or more prolonged steady-state exertion (Kaiser *et al.,* 1986). Exercise performance may be impaired to a lesser extent by β_1-selective agents than by nonselective antagonists (Tesch, 1985). Blockade of β_2 receptors tends to blunt the increase in blood flow to active skeletal muscle during submaximal exercise (Van Baak, 1988). Blockade of β receptors also may attenuate catecholamine-induced activation of glucose metabolism and lipolysis.

Coronary arterial blood flow increases during exercise or stress to meet the metabolic demands of the heart. By increasing heart rate, contractility, and systolic pressure, catecholamines increase myocardial oxygen demand. However, in patients with coronary artery disease, fixed narrowing of these vessels attenuates the expected increase in flow, leading to myocardial ischemia. β-Adrenergic antagonists decrease the effects of catecholamines on the determinants of myocardial oxygen consumption. However, these agents may tend to increase the requirement for oxygen by increasing end-diastolic pressure and systolic ejection period. Usually, the net effect is to improve the relationship between cardiac oxygen supply and demand; exercise tolerance generally is improved in patients with angina, whose capacity to exercise is limited by the development of chest pain (*see* Chapter 32).

Activity as Antihypertensive Agents. β-Adrenergic antagonists generally do not cause a reduction in blood pressure in patients with normal blood pressure. However, these drugs do lower blood pressure in patients with hypertension. Despite their widespread use, the mechanisms responsible for this important clinical effect are not well understood. The release of renin from the juxtaglomerular apparatus is stimulated by the sympathetic nervous system, and this effect is blocked by β-adrenergic antagonists (*see* Chapter 31). However, the relationship between this phenomenon and the fall in blood pressure is not clear. Some investigators have found that the antihypertensive effect of propranolol is most marked in patients with elevated concentrations of plasma renin, as compared with patients with low or normal concentrations of renin. However, β-receptor antagonists are effective even in patients with low plasma renin, and pindolol is an effective antihypertensive agent that has little or no effect on plasma renin activity (Frishman, 1983).

Presynaptic β-adrenergic receptors enhance the release of norepinephrine from sympathetic neurons, but the importance of diminished release of norepinephrine to the antihypertensive effects of β-adrenergic antagonists is unclear. Although β blockers would not be expected to decrease the contractility of vascular smooth muscle, long-term administration of these drugs to hypertensive patients ultimately leads to a fall in peripheral vascular resistance (Man in't Veld *et al.*, 1988). The mechanism for this important effect is not known, but this delayed fall in peripheral vascular resistance in the face of a persistent reduction of cardiac output appears to account for much of the antihypertensive effect of these drugs. Although it has been hypothesized that central actions of β blockers also may contribute to their antihypertensive effects, there is relatively little evidence to support this possibility.

As indicated above, some β-adrenergic receptor antagonists have additional effects that may contribute to their ability to lower blood pressure. Three properties of some β-receptor antagonists have been suggested to contribute to peripheral vasodilation: α-adrenergic receptor blockade; β-adrenergic receptor agonism; and mechanism(s) independent of adrenergic receptors. For example, drugs such as labetalol and carvedilol, which block α_1-adrenergic receptors directly, decrease peripheral resistance. Celiprolol appears to be a partial β_2-receptor agonist and additionally to have nonadrenergic-receptor–mediated vasodilating properties, which contribute to decreasing peripheral resistance (Shanks, 1991; Milne and Buckley, 1991). The clinical significance in human beings of some of these relatively subtle differences in pharmacological properties is unclear (Fitzgerald, 1991). Particular interest has focused on patients with congestive heart failure or peripheral arterial occlusive disease.

Propranolol and other nonselective β-adrenergic antagonists inhibit the vasodilation caused by isoproterenol and augment the pressor response to epinephrine. This is particularly significant in patients with a pheochromocytoma, in whom β-adrenergic antagonists should be used only after adequate α-adrenergic blockade has been established. This avoids uncompensated α-receptor-mediated vasoconstriction caused by epinephrine secreted from the tumor.

Pulmonary System.   Nonselective β-adrenergic antagonists such as propranolol block β_2-adrenergic receptors in bronchial smooth muscle. This usually has little effect on pulmonary function in normal individuals. However, in patients with asthma or chronic obstructive pulmonary disease, such blockade can lead to life-threatening bronchoconstriction. Although β_1-selective antagonists or antagonists with intrinsic sympathomimetic activity are less likely than propranolol to increase airway resistance in patients with asthma, these drugs should be used only with great caution, if at all, in patients with bronchospastic diseases. Drugs such as celiprolol, with β_1-receptor selectivity and β_2-receptor partial agonism, are of potential promise, although clinical experience is limited (Pujet *et al.*, 1992).

Metabolic Effects. β-Adrenergic antagonists modify the metabolism of carbohydrates and lipids. Catecholamines promote glycogenolysis and mobilize glucose in response to hypoglycemia. Nonselective β blockers may adversely affect recovery from hypoglycemia in insulin-dependent diabetics. β-Adrenergic antagonists should be used with great caution in patients with labile diabetes and frequent hypoglycemic reactions. If such a drug is strongly indicated, a β_1-selective compound is preferable, since these drugs are less likely to delay recovery from hypoglycemia. All β blockers mask the tachycardia that is typically seen with hypoglycemia, denying the patient an important warning sign. Although insulin secretion is enhanced by

β-adrenergic agonists, β blockade only rarely impairs insulin release.

β-Adrenergic receptors mediate activation of hormone-sensitive lipase in fat cells, leading to the release of free fatty acids into the circulation. The potential role of β_3 receptors in mediating this response in human beings is discussed in Chapter 6. This increased flux of fatty acids is an important energy source for exercising muscle. β-Adrenergic antagonists can attenuate the release of free fatty acids from adipose tissue. Nonetheless, in some patients, nonselective β blockers modestly elevate plasma concentrations of triglycerides and decrease those of high-density lipoproteins. Concentrations of LDLs usually do not change (Miller, 1987). Although the significance of these changes is not known, there is concern that they may be undesirable effects, particularly in patients with hypertension (Reaven and Hoffman, 1987; Rabkin, 1993). β_1-Selective antagonists and those with intrinsic sympathomimetic activity may cause less of an effect on lipid metabolism than do nonselective antagonists. The mechanism of these effects is not clear.

β-Adrenergic agonists decrease the plasma concentration of K^+ by promoting the uptake of the ion, predominantly into skeletal muscle. At rest, an infusion of epinephrine causes a decrease in the plasma concentration of K^+ (Brown *et al.*, 1983). The marked increase in the concentration of epinephrine that occurs with stress (such as myocardial infarction) may cause hypokalemia, which could predispose to cardiac arrhythmias (Struthers and Reid, 1984). The hypokalemic effect of epinephrine is blocked by an experimental antagonist, ICI 118551, which has a high affinity for β_2- and β_3-adrenergic receptors (Brown *et al.*, 1983; Emorine *et al.*, 1989). Exercise causes an increase in the efflux of K^+ from skeletal muscle. Catecholamines tend to buffer the rise in K^+ by increasing its influx into muscle. β-blocking agents negate this buffering effect (Brown, 1985).

Other Effects. β-Adrenergic antagonists block catecholamine-induced tremor. They also block inhibition of mast-cell degranulation by catecholamines (*see* Chapter 25).

NON-SUBTYPE-SELECTIVE β-ADRENERGIC ANTAGONISTS

Propranolol

In view of the extensive experience with propranolol (*propranolol hydrochloride;* INDERAL), it is useful as a prototype (*see* Table 10–3). Propranolol interacts with β_1 and β_2 receptors with equal affinity, lacks intrinsic sympathomimetic activity, and does not block α-adrenergic receptors.

Absorption, Fate, and Excretion. Propranolol is highly lipophilic and is almost completely absorbed after oral administration. However, much of the drug is metabolized by the liver during its first passage through the portal circulation; on average, only about 25% reaches the systemic circulation. In addition, there is great interindividual variation in the presystemic clearance of propranolol by the liver; this contributes to enormous variability in plasma concentrations (approximately 20-fold) after oral administration of the drug and contributes to the wide range of

Table 10–3
Pharmacological Characteristics of β-Adrenergic Antagonists

COMPOUND	INTRINSIC SYM-PATHOMIMETIC ACTIVITY	MEMBRANE-STABILIZING ACTIVITY	LIPID SOLUBILITY, LOG Kp*	ORAL BIO-AVAILABILITY, %	HALF-LIFE IN PLASMA, HOURS†
I. Nonselective β-(β_1+β_2) Adrenergic Antagonists					
Propranolol	0	++	3.65	~25	3–5
Nadolol	0	0	0.7	~35	10–20
Timolol	0	0	2.1	~50	3–5
Pindolol	++	±	1.75	~75	3–4
Labetalol‡	−‡	±	—	~20	4–6
II. Selective β_1-Adrenergic Antagonists					
Metoprolol	0	±	2.15	~40	3–4
Atenolol	0	0	0.23	~50	5–8
Esmolol	0	0	—	—	0.13
Acebutolol	+	+	1.9	~40	2–4

*Kp refers to the octanol: water partition coefficient; propranolol and atenolol are at the lipophilic and hydrophilic extremes, respectively.
†The duration of effect, in general, is longer than might be expected from the plasma $t_{1/2}$.
‡Labetalol is also a potent α_1-adrenergic antagonist. *See* text for a description of the activities of the individual isomers of labetalol.
SOURCE: Based on data in Drayer (1987), McDevitt (1987), and other references cited in the text.

doses in terms of clinical efficacy. In other words, a clinical disadvantage of propranolol is that multiple, increasing steps in drug dose may be required over time. The degree of hepatic extraction of propranolol declines as the dose is increased. The bioavailability of propranolol may be increased by the concomitant ingestion of food and during long-term administration of the drug.

Propranolol has a large volume of distribution (4 liters/kg) and readily enters the CNS. Approximately 90% of the drug in the circulation is bound to plasma proteins. It is extensively metabolized, with most metabolites appearing in the urine. One product of hepatic metabolism is 4-hydroxypropranolol, which has some β-adrenergic-antagonist activity.

Analysis of the distribution of propranolol, its clearance by the liver, and its activity is complicated by the stereospecificity of these processes (Walle *et al.,* 1988). The (−)-enantiomers of propranolol and other β blockers are the active forms of the drug. This enantiomer of propranolol appears to be cleared more slowly from the body than is the inactive enantiomer. The clearance of propranolol may vary with hepatic blood flow and liver disease, and it also may change during the administration of other drugs that affect hepatic metabolism. Monitoring of plasma concentrations of propranolol has found little application, since the clinical end-points (reduction of blood pressure and heart rate) are readily determined. The relationships between the plasma concentrations of propranolol and its pharmacodynamic effects are complex; for example, despite its short half-life in plasma (about 4 hours), its antihypertensive effect is sufficiently long-lived to permit administration twice daily. Some of the (−)-enantiomer of propranolol and other β blockers is taken up into sympathetic nerve endings and is released upon sympathetic nerve stimulation (Walle *et al.,* 1988).

A sustained-release formulation of propranolol (INDERAL LA) has been developed to maintain therapeutic concentrations of propranolol in plasma throughout a 24-hour period (Nace and Wood, 1987). Suppression of exercise-induced tachycardia is maintained throughout the dosing interval, and patient compliance may be improved.

Therapeutic Uses. For the treatment of hypertension and angina, the initial oral dose of propranolol is generally 40 to 80 mg per day. The dose may then be titrated upward until the optimal response is obtained. For the treatment of angina, the dose may be increased at intervals of less than one week, as indicated clinically. In hypertension, the full blood-pressure response may not develop for several weeks. Typically, doses are less than 320 mg per day. If propranolol is taken twice daily for hypertension, blood pressure should be measured just prior to a dose to ensure that the duration of effect is sufficiently prolonged. Adequacy of β-adrenergic blockade can be assessed by measuring suppression of exercise-induced tachy-

cardia. Propranolol may be administered intravenously for the management of life-threatening arrhythmias or to patients under anesthesia. Under these circumstances, the usual dose is 1 to 3 mg, administered slowly (less than 1 mg per minute) with careful and frequent monitoring of blood pressure, ECG, and cardiac function. If an adequate response is not obtained, a second dose may be given after several minutes. If bradycardia is excessive, atropine should be administered to increase heart rate. Change to oral therapy should be initiated as soon as possible.

Nadolol

Nadolol (CORGARD) is a long-acting antagonist with equal affinity for β_1- and β_2-adrenergic receptors. It is devoid of both membrane-stabilizing and intrinsic sympathomimetic activity. A distinguishing characteristic of nadolol is its relatively long half-life.

Absorption, Fate, and Excretion. Nadolol is very soluble in water and is incompletely absorbed from the gut; its bioavailability is about 35% (Frishman, 1981). Interindividual variability is less than with propranolol. The low solubility of nadolol in fat may result in lower concentrations of the drug in the brain as compared with more lipid-soluble β-adrenergic antagonists. Although it frequently has been suggested that the incidence of CNS adverse effects is lower with hydrophilic β-adrenergic antagonists, data from controlled trials to support this contention are limited. Nadolol is not extensively metabolized and is largely excreted intact in the urine. The half-life of the drug in plasma is approximately 20 hours; consequently, it generally is administered once daily. Nadolol may accumulate in patients with renal failure, and dosage should be reduced in such individuals.

Timolol

Timolol (*timolol maleate;* BLOCADREN) is a potent, non-subtype-selective β-adrenergic antagonist. It has no intrinsic sympathomimetic activity and no membrane-stabilizing activity.

Absorption, Fate, and Excretion. Timolol is well absorbed from the gastrointestinal tract and is subject to moderate first-pass metabolism. It is metabolized extensively by the liver, and only a small amount of unchanged drug appears in the urine. The half-life in plasma is about 4 hours. Interestingly, the ocular formulation of timolol (TIMOPTIC), used for the treatment of glaucoma, may be extensively absorbed systemically (*see* Chapter 66); adverse effects can occur in susceptible patients, such as those with asthma or congestive heart failure.

Pindolol

Pindolol (VISKEN) is a non-subtype-selective β-adrenergic antagonist with intrinsic sympathomimetic activity. It has low membrane-stabilizing activity and is moderately soluble in lipid.

Although only limited data are available, β blockers with slight partial agonist activity may produce smaller reductions in resting heart rate and blood pressure. Hence, such drugs may be preferred as antihypertensive agents in individuals with diminished cardiac reserve or a propensity for bradycardia. Nonetheless, the clinical significance of partial agonism has not been substantially demonstrated in controlled trials but may be of importance in individual patients (Fitzgerald, 1993). Agents like pindolol do block exercise-induced increases in heart rate and cardiac output.

Absorption, Fate, and Excretion. Pindolol is almost completely absorbed after oral administration and has moderately high bioavailability. These properties tend to minimize interindividual variation in the plasma concentrations of the drug that are achieved after its oral administration. Approximately 50% of pindolol ultimately is metabolized in the liver. The principal metabolites are hydroxylated derivatives that subsequently are conjugated with either glucuronide or sulfate before renal excretion. The remainder of the drug is excreted unchanged in the urine. The plasma half-life of pindolol is about 4 hours; clearance is reduced in patients with renal failure.

Labetalol

Labetalol (*labetalol hydrochloride;* NORMODYNE, TRANDATE) is representative of a class of drugs that act as competitive antagonists at both α_1- and β-adrenergic receptors. Labetalol has two optical centers, and the formulation used clinically contains equal amounts of the four diastereomers (Gold *et al.*, 1982). The pharmacological properties of the drug are complex, because each isomer displays different relative activities. The properties of the mixture include selective blockade of α_1-adrenergic receptors (as compared with the α_2 subtype), blockade of β_1 and β_2 receptors, partial agonist activity at β_2 receptors, and inhibition of neuronal uptake of norepinephrine (cocaine-like effect) (*see* Chapter 6). The potency of the mixture for β-adrenergic blockade is fivefold to tenfold that for α-adrenergic blockade.

The pharmacological effects of labetalol have become clearer since the four isomers were separated and tested individually. The R,R isomer is about four times more potent as a β-adrenergic antagonist than is racemic labetalol, and it accounts for much of the β-blockade produced by the mixture of isomers, although it is no longer in development as a separate drug (*dilevalol*). As an α_1 antagonist, this isomer is less than 20% as potent as the racemic mixture (Sybertz *et al.*, 1981; Gold *et al.*, 1982). The R,S isomer is almost devoid of both α- and β-adrenergic blocking effects. The S,R isomer has almost no β-adrenergic-blocking activity, yet is about five times more potent as an α_1 blocker than is racemic labetalol. The S,S isomer is devoid of β-blocking activity and has a potency similar to that of racemic labetalol as an α_1-receptor antagonist (Gold *et al.*, 1982). The R,R isomer has some intrinsic sympathomimetic activity at β_2 receptors; this may contribute to vasodilation (Baum *et al.*, 1981). Labetalol also may have some direct vasodilating capacity.

The actions of labetalol on both α_1- and β-adrenergic receptors contribute to the fall in blood pressure observed in patients with hypertension. α_1-Receptor blockade leads to relaxation of arterial smooth muscle and vasodilation, particularly in the upright position. The β_1 blockade also contributes to a fall in blood pressure, in part by blocking reflex sympathetic stimula-

tion of the heart. In addition, the intrinsic sympathomimetic activity of labetalol at β_2 receptors may contribute to vasodilation.

Labetalol is available in oral form for therapy of chronic hypertension and as an intravenous formulation for use in hypertensive emergencies. Labetalol has been associated with hepatic injury in a limited number of patients (Clark *et al.*, 1990).

Absorption, Fate, and Excretion. Although labetalol is completely absorbed from the gut, there is extensive first-pass clearance; bioavailability is only about 20% to 40% and is highly variable (McNeil and Louis, 1984). Bioavailability may be increased by food intake. The drug is rapidly and extensively metabolized in the liver by oxidative biotransformation and glucuronidation; very little unchanged drug is found in the urine. The rate of metabolism of labetalol is sensitive to changes in hepatic blood flow. The elimination half-life of the drug is about 8 hours. The half-life of the R,R isomer of labetalol (dilevalol) is about 15 hours. Labetalol provides an interesting and challenging example of pharmacokinetic-pharmacodynamic modeling applied to a drug that is a racemic mixture of isomers with different kinetics and pharmacological actions (Donnelly and Macphee, 1991).

Carvedilol

Carvedilol (COREG) is a non-subtype-selective β-receptor antagonist that also is an antagonist of α_1 receptors (McTavish *et al.*, 1993; Dunn *et al.*, 1997; Frishman, 1998). Interestingly, carvedilol also has antioxidant activity (Yue *et al.*, 1995; Tadolini and Franconi, 1998). The clinical significance of this action, especially in patients with congestive heart failure, is not clear.

Absorption, Fate, and Excretion. Carvedilol has a bioavailability of about 25% to 35% because of extensive first-pass metabolism. Carvedilol is eliminated by hepatic metabolism and has a terminal half-life of 7 to 10 hours, but most of the drug is eliminated with a half-life of about 2 hours.

Therapeutic Uses. In the treatment of hypertension, the usual starting dose is 6.25 mg twice daily; if an adequate therapeutic response is not achieved, the dose may be increased progressively over time, typically to a maximum of 25 mg twice daily. In the treatment of congestive heart failure, dosing is much more cautious due to possibility of acutely worsening heart failure. Dosing often starts at 3.125 mg twice per day with cautious increases over time.

β_1-SELECTIVE ADRENERGIC ANTAGONISTS

Metoprolol

Metoprolol (*metoprolol tartrate;* LOPRESSOR) is a β_1-selective adrenergic antagonist that is devoid of intrinsic sympathomimetic activity.

Absorption, Fate, and Excretion. Metoprolol is almost completely absorbed after oral administration, but bioavailability is relatively low (about 40%) because of first-pass metabolism. Plasma concentrations of the drug vary widely (up to 17-fold), perhaps because of genetically determined differences in the rate of metabolism (Benfield *et al.*, 1986). Metoprolol is extensively metabolized by the hepatic monooxygenase system, and only 10% of the administered drug is recovered unchanged in the urine. The half-life of metoprolol is 3 to 4 hours. An extended-release formulation (TOPROL XL) is available for once-daily administration (Plosker and Clissold, 1992).

Therapeutic Uses. For the treatment of hypertension, the usual initial dose is 100 mg per day. The drug is sometimes effective when given once daily, although it is frequently used in two divided doses. Dosage may be increased at weekly intervals until optimal reduction of blood pressure is achieved. If the drug is taken only once daily, it is important to confirm that blood pressure is controlled for the entire 24-hour period. Metoprolol is generally used in two divided doses for the treatment of stable angina. Conventional dosage forms of metoprolol have been extensively established for indications in hypertension and ischemic heart disease. The extended-release formulation, which provides relatively constant rates of drug delivery over 24-hour periods, may be given once daily. For the initial treatment of patients with acute myocardial infarction, an intravenous formulation of metoprolol tartrate is available. Oral dosing is initiated as soon as the clinical situation permits. Metoprolol generally is contraindicated for the treatment of acute myocardial infarction in patients with heart rates of less than 45 beats per minute, heart block greater than first degree (PR interval greater than or equal to 0.24 second), systolic blood pressure less than 100 mm Hg, or moderate-to-severe heart failure.

Atenolol

Atenolol (TENORMIN) is a β_1-selective antagonist that is devoid of intrinsic sympathomimetic activity (Wadworth *et al.*, 1991). Atenolol is very hydrophilic and appears to penetrate the brain only to a limited extent. Its half-life is somewhat longer than that of metoprolol.

Absorption, Fate, and Excretion. Atenolol is incompletely absorbed (about 50%), but most of the absorbed dose reaches the systemic circulation. There is relatively little interindividual variation in the plasma concentrations of atenolol; peak concentrations in different patients vary over only a fourfold range (Cruickshank, 1980). The drug is excreted largely unchanged in the urine, and the elimination half-life is about 5 to 8 hours. The drug accumulates in patients with renal failure, and dosage should be adjusted for patients whose creatinine clearance is less than 35 ml/minute.

Therapeutic Uses. The initial dose of atenolol for the treatment of hypertension usually is 50 mg per day, given once daily. If an adequate therapeutic response is not evident within several weeks, the daily dose may be increased to 100 mg; higher doses are unlikely to provide any greater antihypertensive effect. Atenolol has been shown to be efficacious, in combina-

tion with a diuretic, in elderly patients with isolated systolic hypertension.

Esmolol

Esmolol (*esmolol hydrochloride;* BREVIBLOC) is a β_1-selective antagonist with a very short duration of action. It has little if any intrinsic sympathomimetic activity, and it lacks membrane-stabilizing actions. Esmolol is administered intravenously and is used when β blockade of short duration is desired or in critically ill patients in whom adverse effects of bradycardia, heart failure, or hypotension may necessitate rapid withdrawal of the drug.

Absorption, Fate, and Excretion. Esmolol has a half-life of about 8 minutes and an apparent volume of distribution of approximately 2 liters/kg. The drug contains an ester linkage, and it is hydrolyzed rapidly by esterases in erythrocytes. The half-life of the carboxylic acid metabolite of esmolol is far longer (4 hours), and it accumulates during prolonged infusion of esmolol (*see* Benfield and Sorkin, 1987). However, this metabolite has very low potency as a β-adrenergic antagonist (1/500 of the potency of esmolol; Reynolds *et al.*, 1986); it is excreted in the urine.

The onset and cessation of β-adrenergic blockade with esmolol are rapid; peak hemodynamic effects occur within 6 to 10 minutes of administration of a loading dose, and there is substantial attenuation of β blockade within 20 minutes of stopping an infusion. Esmolol may have striking hypotensive effects in normal subjects, although the mechanism of this effect is unclear (Reilly *et al.*, 1985).

Since esmolol is used in urgent settings where immediate onset of β-adrenergic receptor blockade is warranted, a partial loading dose typically is administered, followed by a continuous infusion of the drug. If an adequate therapeutic effect is not observed within 5 minutes, the same loading dose is repeated, followed by a maintenance infusion at a higher rate. This process, including progressively greater infusion rates, may need to be repeated until the desired end point (*e.g.*, lowered heart rate or blood pressure) is approached.

Acebutolol

Acebutolol (*acebutolol hydrochloride;* SECTRAL) is a selective β_1-adrenergic antagonist with some intrinsic sympathomimetic activity.

Absorption, Fate, and Excretion. Acebutolol is well absorbed, but it is extensively metabolized to an active metabolite, diacetolol, which accounts for most of the drug's activity (Singh *et al.*, 1985). The elimination half-life of acebutolol is typically about 3 hours, but the half-life of diacetolol is 8 to 12 hours; it is excreted in the urine.

Therapeutic Uses. The initial dose of acebutolol in hypertension is usually 400 mg per day; it may be given as a single dose, but two divided doses may be required for adequate control of blood pressure. Optimal responses usually occur with doses of 400 to 800 mg per day (range 200 to 1200 mg). For treatment of ventricular arrhythmias, the drug should be given twice daily.

OTHER β-ADRENERGIC ANTAGONISTS

A plethora of other β-adrenergic antagonists also have been synthesized and evaluated to varying extents. *Bopindolol* (SANDONORM, others; not available in the United States), *carteolol* (CARTROL, OCUPRESS), *oxprenolol,* and *penbutolol* (LEVATOL) are non-subtype-selective β blockers with intrinsic sympathomimetic activity. *Medroxalol* and *bucindolol* are nonselective β-adrenergic blockers with α_1-receptor-blocking activity (Rosendorff, 1993). *Levobunolol* (BETAGAN LIQUIFILM, others) and *metipranolol* (OPTIPRANOLOL) are non-subtype-selective β antagonists used as topical agents in the treatment of glaucoma (Brooks and Gillies, 1992). *Bisoprolol* (ZEBETA) and *nebivolol* are β_1-selective antagonists without partial agonist activity (Jamin *et al.,* 1994; Van de Water *et al.,* 1988). *Betaxolol* (BETOPTIC), a β_1-selective antagonist, is available as an ophthalmic preparation for glaucoma and an oral formulation for systemic hypertension. Betaxolol may be less likely to induce bronchospasm than are the ophthalmic preparations of the nonselective β blockers timolol and levobunolol. Similarly, there have been suggestions that ocular administration of carteolol may be less likely than timolol to have systemic effects, possibly because of its intrinsic sympathomimetic activity; cautious monitoring is required, nonetheless (Chrisp and Sorkin, 1992). *Celiprolol* (SELECTOR) is a β_1-selective adrenergic receptor antagonist with mild β_2-selective agonism as well as additional weak vasodilator properties of uncertain mechanism (Milne and Buckely, 1991). *Sotalol* (BETAPACE) is a nonselective β antagonist that is devoid of membrane-stabilizing actions. However, it has antiarrhythmic actions independent of its ability to block β-adrenergic receptors (Fitton and Sorkin, 1993; *see* Chapter 35). *Propafenone* (RYTHMOL) is a Na^+-channel blocking drug that also is a β-adrenergic receptor antagonist (Bryson *et al.,* 1993).

ADVERSE EFFECTS AND PRECAUTIONS

The most common adverse effects of β-adrenergic antagonists arise as pharmacological consequences of blockade of β receptors; serious adverse effects unrelated to β-receptor blockade are rare.

Cardiovascular System. β-Adrenergic antagonists may induce congestive heart failure in susceptible patients, since the sympathetic nervous system provides critical support for cardiac performance in many individuals with impaired myocardial function. Thus, β-adrenergic blockade may cause or exacerbate heart failure in patients with compensated heart failure, acute myocardial infarction, or cardiomegaly. It is not known whether β-adrenergic antagonists that possess intrinsic sympathomimetic activity or peripheral vasodilating properties are safer in these settings. Nonetheless, there now is convincing evidence that chronic administration of β-adrenergic antagonists is efficacious in prolonging life in the therapy of heart failure in selected patients (*see* below; *see also* Chapter 34).

Bradycardia is a normal response to β-adrenergic blockade; however, in patients with partial or complete atrioventricular conduction defects, β-adrenergic antagonists may cause life-threatening bradyarrhythmias. Particular caution is indicated in patients who are taking other drugs, such as verapamil or various antiarrhythmic agents, which may impair sinus-node function or AV conduction.

Some patients complain of cold extremities while taking β-adrenergic antagonists. Symptoms of peripheral vascular disease may worsen, although this is uncommon (Lepäntalo, 1985), or Raynaud's phenomenon may develop. The risk of worsening intermittent claudication is probably very small with this class of drugs, and the clinical benefits of β-adrenergic antagonists in patients with peripheral vascular disease and coexisting coronary artery disease may be very important.

Abrupt discontinuation of β-adrenergic antagonists after long-term treatment can exacerbate angina and may increase the risk of sudden death. The underlying mechanism is unclear, but it is well established that there is enhanced sensitivity to β-adrenergic agonists in patients who have undergone long-term treatment with certain β-adrenergic antagonists after the blocker is withdrawn abruptly. For example, chronotropic responses to isoproterenol are blunted in patients who are receiving β-adrenergic antagonists; however, abrupt discontinuation of propranolol leads to greater-than-normal sensitivity to isoproterenol. This increased sensitivity is evident several days after stopping propranolol and may persist for at least one week (Nattel *et al.,* 1979). Such enhanced sensitivity can be attenuated by tapering the dose of the β blocker for several weeks before discontinuation (Rangno *et al.,* 1982). Supersensitivity to isoproterenol also has been observed after abrupt discontinuation of metoprolol, but not of pindolol (Rangno and Langlois, 1982). The concentration of β-adrenergic receptors on circulating lymphocytes is increased in subjects who have received propranolol for long periods; pindolol has the opposite effect (Hedberg *et al.,* 1986). Optimal strategies for discontinuation of β blockers are not known, but it is prudent to decrease the dose gradually and to restrict exercise during this period.

Pulmonary Function. A major adverse effect of β-adrenergic antagonists is caused by blockade of β_2

receptors in bronchial smooth muscle. These receptors are particularly important for promoting bronchodilation in patients with bronchospastic disease, and β blockers may cause a life-threatening increase in airway resistance in such patients. Drugs with selectivity for β_1 receptors or those with intrinsic sympathomimetic activity at β_2 receptors may be somewhat less likely to induce bronchospasm. Since the selectivity of current β blockers for β_1-adrenergic receptors is modest, these drugs should be avoided if at all possible in patients with asthma. However, in some patients with chronic obstructive pulmonary disease, the potential advantage of using β-receptor antagonists after myocardial infarction may outweigh the risk of worsening pulmonary function (Gottlieb *et al.,* 1998).

Central Nervous System. The adverse effects of β-adrenergic antagonists that are referable to the CNS may include fatigue, sleep disturbances (including insomnia and nightmares), and depression. The previously ascribed association between these drugs and depression (Thiessen *et al.,* 1990) may not be substantiated by more recent clinical studies (Gerstman *et al.,* 1996; Ried *et al.,* 1998). Interest has focused on the relationship between the incidence of the adverse effects of β-adrenergic-receptor antagonists and their lipophilicity; however, no clear correlation has emerged (Drayer, 1987; Gengo *et al.,* 1987).

Metabolism. As described above, β-adrenergic blockade may blunt recognition of hypoglycemia by patients; it also may delay recovery from insulin-induced hypoglycemia. β-Adrenergic antagonists should be used with great caution in patients with diabetes who are prone to hypoglycemic reactions; β_1-selective agents may be preferable for these patients. The benefits of β-receptor antagonists in type I diabetes with myocardial infarction may outweigh the risk in selected patients (Gottlieb *et al.,* 1998).

Miscellaneous. The incidence of sexual dysfunction in men with hypertension who are treated with β-adrenergic antagonists is not clearly defined. Although experience with the use of β-adrenergic antagonists in pregnancy is increasing, information about the safety of these drugs during pregnancy is still limited (*see* Widerhorn *et al.,* 1987).

Overdosage. The manifestations of poisoning with β-adrenergic antagonists depend on the pharmacological properties of the ingested drug, particularly its β_1 selectivity, intrinsic sympathomimetic activity, and membrane-stabilizing properties (*see* Frishman *et al.,* 1984). Hypotension, bradycardia, prolonged AV conduction times, and widened QRS complexes are common manifestations of overdosage. Seizures and/or depression

may occur. Hypoglycemia is rare, and bronchospasm is uncommon in the absence of pulmonary disease. Significant bradycardia should be treated initially with atropine, but a cardiac pacemaker often is required. Large doses of isoproterenol or an α-adrenergic agonist may be necessary to treat hypotension. Glucagon has positive chronotropic and inotropic effects on the heart that are independent of interactions with β-adrenergic receptors, and the drug has been useful in some patients.

Drug Interactions. Both pharmacokinetic and pharmacodynamic interactions have been noted between β-adrenergic-blocking agents and other drugs. Aluminum salts, cholestyramine, and colestipol may decrease the absorption of β blockers. Drugs such as phenytoin, rifampin, and phenobarbital, as well as smoking, induce hepatic biotransformation enzymes and may decrease plasma concentrations of β-adrenergic antagonists that are metabolized extensively (*e.g.,* propranolol). Cimetidine and hydralazine may increase the bioavailability of agents such as propranolol and metoprolol by affecting hepatic blood flow. β-Adrenergic antagonists can impair the clearance of lidocaine.

Other drug interactions have pharmacodynamic explanations. For example, β-adrenergic antagonists and Ca^{2+} channel blockers have additive effects on the cardiac conducting system. Additive effects on blood pressure between β blockers and other antihypertensive agents often are sought. However, the antihypertensive effects of β-adrenergic antagonists can be opposed by indomethacin and other nonsteroidal antiinflammatory drugs (*see* Chapter 27).

THERAPEUTIC USES

Cardiovascular Diseases

β-Adrenergic antagonists are used extensively in the treatment of hypertension (*see* Chapter 33), angina and acute coronary syndromes (*see* Chapter 32), and congestive heart failure (*see* Chapter 34). These drugs also are used frequently in the treatment of supraventricular and ventricular arrhythmias (*see* Chapter 35).

Myocardial Infarction. A great deal of interest has focused on the use of β-adrenergic antagonists in the treatment of acute myocardial infarction and in the prevention of recurrences for those who have survived an initial attack. Numerous trials have shown that β-adrenergic antagonists administered during the early phases of acute myocardial infarction and continued long-term may decrease mortality by about 25% (Freemantle *et al.,* 1999). The precise mechanism is not known, but the favorable effects of β-adrenergic antagonists may stem from decreased myocardial oxygen demand, redistribution of myocardial blood flow, and antiarrhythmic actions. There is likely much less benefit if β-receptor antagonists are administered for only a short time. In studies of secondary prevention, the most extensive, favorable clinical trial data are available for propranolol, metoprolol, and timolol. In spite of these benefits, many patients with myocardial infarction do not receive a β-receptor antagonist.

Congestive Heart Failure. It is a common clinical observation that acute administration of β-adrenergic antagonists can worsen markedly or even precipitate congestive heart failure in compensated patients with multiple forms of heart disease, such as ischemic or congestive cardiomyopathy. Consequently, the hypothesis that β-adrenergic antagonists might be efficacious in the long-term treatment of heart failure originally seemed counterintuitive to many physicians. Nonetheless, after the completion of a number of well-designed, randomized control clinical trials, it is clear that some of these drugs are beneficial in patients with mild to moderate heart failure (Packer, 1998; Krum, 1999; and Teerlink and Massie, 1999; see also Chapter 34). From the point of view of the history of therapeutic advances in the treatment of congestive heart failure, it is interesting to note how a drug class has moved from being completely contraindicated to being almost the standard of modern care in many settings.

Alterations in cardiac responsiveness to catecholamines have been found in heart failure. A consistent observation is that sympathetic nervous system activity is increased in patients with congestive heart failure (Bristow, 1993). Infusions of β-adrenergic agonists have been found toxic to the heart in several animal models. Also, overexpression of β-adrenergic receptors in mice leads to a dilated cardiomyopathy (Engelhardt et al., 1999). A number of changes in β-adrenergic receptor signaling occur in the myocardium from patients with heart failure as well as in a variety of animal models (Post et al., 1999). Decreased numbers and functioning of β_1-adrenergic receptors consistently have been found in heart failure, leading to attenuation of β-adrenergic receptor–mediated stimulation of positive inotropic responses in the failing heart. These changes may be due in part to increased expression of β-adrenergic receptor kinase-1 (βARK-1, GRK2) (Lefkowitz et al., 2000; see also Chapter 6).

It is of potential interest that β_2-receptor expression is relatively maintained in these settings of heart failure. While both β_1 and β_2 receptors activate adenylyl cyclase via G_s, there is evidence suggesting that β_2-adrenergic receptors also stimulate G_i; this capacity to activate G_i may attenuate contractile responses to activation of β_2 receptors as well as lead to activation of other effector pathways downstream of G_i (Lefkowitz et al., 2000). Overexpression of β_2 receptors in mouse heart may be associated with increased cardiac force without the development of cardiomyopathy (Liggett et al., 2000).

The mechanism(s) utilized by β-adrenergic receptor antagonists in decreasing mortality in patients with congestive heart failure is unclear. Perhaps this is not surprising, given that the mechanism by which this class of drugs lowers blood pressure in patients with hypertension, in spite of years of investigation, remains elusive (see Chapter 33). At the moment there are sev-

eral hypotheses, all of which require further experimental testing. This is much more than an academic undertaking; a deeper understanding of involved pathways could lead to selection of the most appropriate available drugs as well as the development of novel compounds with especially desirable properties. The potential differences between β_1- and β_2-receptor function in heart failure is one example of the complexity of adrenergic pharmacology of this syndrome.

A number of mechanisms have been proposed to play a role in the beneficial effects of β-adrenergic receptor antagonists in heart failure. Since excess effects of catecholamines may be toxic to the heart, especially via activation of β_1 receptors, inhibition of the pathway may help preserve myocardial function. Also, antagonism of β receptors in the heart may attenuate cardiac remodeling, which ordinarily might have deleterious effects on cardiac function. Interestingly, activation of β receptors may promote myocardial cell death via apoptosis (Singh et al., 2000). In addition, properties of certain β-receptor antagonists that are due to other, unrelated properties of these drugs may be potentially important. For example, afterload reductions mediated by α_1-adrenergic antagonism by drugs such as carvedilol may be relevant. The potential importance of the role of the antioxidant properties of carvedilol in its beneficial effects in patients with heart failure is not clear (Ma et al., 1996).

Studies involving numerous patients have demonstrated that certain β-receptor antagonists may improve myocardial function and prolong life in patients with mild to moderate congestive heart failure. Data from randomized trials are available for several drugs in this class. It is important to emphasize that beneficial effects in congestive heart failure may not be true of all β-receptor antagonists. Extensive favorable experience is available for metoprolol. The β_1-subtype selective receptor antagonist bisoprolol also has been demonstrated to prolong life in patients with moderate heart failure (Teerlink and Massie, 1999). Carvedilol has favorable effects in patients with congestive heart failure. *Bucindolol* likely improves cardiac function in patients with heart failure; the results of a study [Beta-blocker Estimation of Survival Trial (BEST)] of its potential effects on mortality are not yet available.

Because of the real possibility of acutely worsening cardiac function in patients with congestive heart failure, particular caution and the involvement of an experienced physician are required in initiating therapy with a β-receptor antagonist in these patients. As might be anticipated, starting with very low doses of drug and advancing doses slowly over time, depending on each patient's response, are critical for the safe use of these drugs in patients with congestive heart failure.

Other Cardiovascular Diseases. β-Adrenergic antagonists, particularly propranolol, are used in the treatment of hypertrophic obstructive cardiomyopathy. Propranolol is useful for relieving angina, palpitations, and syncope in patients with this disorder. Efficacy probably is related to partial relief of the pressure gradient along the outflow tract. β blockers also may attenuate catecholamine-induced cardiomyopathy in pheochromocytoma (Rosenbaum *et al.*, 1987).

β-Adrenergic antagonists are used to treat arrhythmias in patients with mitral valve prolapse and to combat arrhythmias in patients with pheochromocytoma (*see also* Chapter 35). However, it is very important to initiate treatment with an α-receptor antagonist before a β-receptor antagonist is administered. Otherwise, hypertension may be exacerbated because of the loss of β_2-receptor–mediated vasodilation.

β blockers are used frequently in the medical management of acute dissecting aortic aneurysm; their usefulness comes from reduction in the force of myocardial contraction and the rate of development of such force. Nitroprusside is an alternative, but when given in the absence of β-adrenergic blockade, it causes an undesirable tachycardia. Patients with Marfan's syndrome may progressively develop dilation of the aorta, which may lead to aortic dissection and regurgitation, a major cause of shortened life expectancy in these patients. There is evidence suggesting that chronic treatment with propranolol may be efficacious in slowing the progression of aortic dilation and its complications in patients with Marfan's syndrome (Shores *et al.*, 1994).

Other Uses

Many of the signs and symptoms of hyperthyroidism are reminiscent of the manifestations of increased sympathetic nervous system activity. Indeed, excess thyroid hormone increases the expression of β-adrenergic receptors in some types of cells. β-Adrenergic antagonists control many of the cardiovascular signs and symptoms of hyperthyroidism and are useful adjuvants to more definitive therapy (Geffner and Hershman, 1992). In addition, propranolol inhibits the peripheral conversion of thyroxine to triiodothyronine, an effect that may be independent of β-receptor blockade. However, caution is advised in treating patients with cardiac enlargement, since the use of β-adrenergic blockers may precipitate congestive heart failure (*see* Chapter 57 for further discussion of the treatment of hyperthyroidism).

Propranolol, timolol, and metoprolol are effective for the prophylaxis of migraine (Tfelt-Hansen, 1986); the mechanism of this effect is not known, and these drugs are not useful for treatment of acute attacks of migraine.

Propranolol and other β blockers are effective in controlling acute panic symptoms in individuals who are required to perform in public or in other anxiety-provoking situations (Lader, 1988). Thus, public speakers may be calmed by the prophylactic administration of the drug, and the performance of musicians may be improved (Brantigan *et al.*, 1982). Tachycardia, muscle tremors, and other evidence of increased sympathetic activity are reduced. Propranolol also may be useful in the treatment of essential tremor.

β-Adrenergic antagonists decrease intraocular pressure, probably by decreasing the rate of production of aqueous humor by the ciliary body. The use of topically administered β blockers for the treatment of glaucoma is discussed in Chapter 66. Topically administered β blockers usually are well tolerated; however, they are systemically absorbed, which can lead to adverse cardiovascular and pulmonary effects in susceptible patients. The agents therefore should be used with great caution in glaucoma patients at risk for adverse systemic effects of

β-receptor antagonists. Use of a β_1-receptor–selective drug, such as betaxolol, may be preferable in these cases.

β blockers may be of some value in the treatment of patients undergoing withdrawal from alcohol or those with akathisia. Propranolol and nadolol are efficacious in the primary prevention of variceal bleeding in patients with portal hypertension, caused by cirrhosis of the liver (Villanueva *et al.*, 1996; Bosch, 1998). Isosorbide mononitrate may augment the fall in portal pressure seen in some patients treated with β-receptor antagonists. These drugs also may be beneficial in reducing the risk of recurrent variceal bleeding.

Selection of a β-Adrenergic Antagonist

The various β-adrenergic antagonists that are used for the treatment of hypertension and angina appear to have similar efficacies. Selection of the most appropriate drug for an individual patient should be based on pharmacokinetic and pharmacodynamic differences among the drugs, cost, and whether or not there are associated medical problems. For some diseases (*e.g.,* myocardial infarction, migraine, cirrhosis with varices, congestive heart failure), it should not be assumed that all members of this class of drugs are interchangeable; the appropriate drug should be selected from those that have documented efficacy for the disease. β_1-Selective antagonists are preferable in patients with bronchospasm, diabetes, peripheral vascular disease, or Raynaud's phenomenon. Although no clinical advantage of β-adrenergic antagonists with intrinsic sympathomimetic activity has been established clearly, such drugs might be preferable in patients with bradycardia. In addition, β-adrenergic antagonists that dilate the peripheral vasculature, *via* α_1-adrenergic blockade, selective β_2-receptor partial agonism, or some other mechanism, may be potentially advantageous in patients with hypertension, occlusive peripheral arterial disease or congestive heart failure.

PROSPECTUS

Despite the large number of available drugs that modify sympathetic responses and their application in many areas of therapeutics, there remains considerable interest in developing novel compounds for both experimental and clinical applications. Information about the physiological roles in different organ systems of the various subtypes of the major classes of adrenergic receptors has not kept pace with knowledge of the expression of these subtypes gained from molecular biological techniques. Consequently, the rigorous demonstration of the existence of these subtypes as distinct gene products affords the tantalizing possibility for medicinal chemists to develop novel drugs that will act on particular subtypes of receptors in particular organs or regions of the CNS. Such increased specificity could make possible novel therapeutic actions and improve safety profiles. The pharmaceutical industry has discovered and developed, at an unrelenting pace, a wide range of drugs that activate or inhibit adrenergic receptors. It remains a major challenge to characterize the potential clinical significance of pharmacological differences among the many drugs already available. In addition, discoveries relating to heterogeneity of receptor subtypes at the molecular level afford numerous opportunities for the explicit development of novel compounds with specificity for a particular subtype. Moreover, recent discoveries of polymorphisms in some adrenergic receptors, for example the β_2 receptor, could lead to predictions about the potential responsiveness of patients, such as those with asthma, to different therapeutic approaches.

Considerable interest has focused on the possibility that novel β_3-adrenergic receptor agonists might have utility in mobilizing fat or increasing energy expenditure (Weyer *et al.*, 1999) in obese human beings. The pharmacological and clinical implications of this approach have not yet been demonstrated. However, there is increasing evidence suggesting that polymorphisms involving the β_3 receptor gene may contribute to obesity or type II diabetes (Arner, 1995).

A plethora of β-adrenergic antagonists exist, with a range of selectivities for β_1 receptors, lipophilicity, duration of action, partial agonism at β_1 or β_2 receptors, and capacity to block α_1-adrenergic receptors, as well as with vasodilating activity independent of adrenergic receptors. How these drugs compare clinically in terms of adverse effects and efficacy is not generally clear. This issue may be of particular importance in the therapy of congestive heart failure. Also, these multiple actions of a single drug should not be presumed necessarily to enhance clinical efficacy, as there may be considerable interperson variability in the actions of such drugs. While there still may be possibilities for developing additional β-adrenergic antagonists with novel properties, there is a considerable need for rigorous clinical investigation to sort out the advan-

tages (if any) of some of these recently developed drugs in various clinical settings, such as coronary artery disease, myocardial infarction, hypertension, and congestive heart failure. For example, carvedilol, a vasodilating β-receptor antagonist with antioxidant activity, decreases mortality in patients receiving standard therapy for congestive heart failure. An understanding of the mechanisms responsible for decreases in mortality in patients with congestive heart failure when treated with β-adrenergic receptor antagonists could lead to the development of novel compounds with especially desirable properties.

α_1-Adrenergic antagonists are growing in popularity in the treatment of BPH; how the efficacy and adverse effects of various available drugs compare needs to be carefully examined. This situation is particularly complex, since α_1 receptors outside the prostate, possibly in neurons, may be involved in mediating the unpleasant symptoms of BPH. The reality of the theoretical advantages of α_1-adrenergic antagonists in hypertension in terms of favorable effects on plasma lipids and glucose tolerance requires testing with clinically significant end points, such as myocardial infarction or stroke. The recent observation that congestive heart failure may develop more commonly with doxazosin than with a diuretic in treatment of hypertension with a single drug complicates this issue. The recent appreciation of various subtypes of α_1 receptors affords an opportunity to develop novel compounds with potential specificity for α-adrenergic receptors expressed in vascular or prostatic smooth muscle, for example. The potential clinical significance of inverse agonists at the α_1-receptor subtypes is unknown but potentially of importance (Rossier *et al.*, 1999).

α_2-Adrenergic agonists such as clonidine have been used mainly for treatment of hypertension. However, the increasing recognition of the physiological roles of particular α_2-receptor subtypes holds promise for the development of increasingly selective α_2 agonists (Link *et al.*, 1996), such as dexmedetomidine, which could lead to improved safety and efficacy profiles for indications in anesthesia and pain control (*see also* Chapter 14). Also, α_2 agonists have shown promise in experimental treatment of cerebral and myocardial ischemia.

BIBLIOGRAPHY

Allwood, M.J., Cobbold, A.F., and Ginsberg, J. Peripheral vascular effects of noradrenaline, isopropylnoradrenaline, and dopamine. *Br. Med. Bull.*, **1963**, *19*:132–136.

Andersson, K.E., and Bende, M. Adrenoceptors in the control of human nasal mucosal blood flow. *Ann. Otol. Rhinol. Laryngol.*, **1984**, *93*:179–182.

Barger, G., and Dale, H.H. Chemical structure and sympathomimetic action of amines. *J. Physiol. (Lond.),* **1910,** *41:*19–59.

Baum, T., Watkins, R.W., Sybertz, E.J., Vemulapalli, S., Pula, K.K., Eynon, E., Nelson, S., Vliet, G.V., Glennon, J., and Moran, R.M. Antihypertensive and hemodynamic actions of SCH 19927, the *R,R-*isomer and labetalol. *J. Pharmacol. Exp. Ther.,* **1981,** *218:*444–452.

Becker, A.J., Stief, C.G., Machtens, S., Schultheiss, D., Hartmann, U., Truss, M.C., and Jonas, U. Oral phentolamine as treatment for erectile dysfunction. *J. Urol.,* **1998,** *159:*1214–1216.

Bertler, A., Carlsson, A., and Rosengren, E. Release by reserpine of catecholamines from rabbit hearts. *Naturwissenschaften,* **1956,** *43:*521.

Black, J.W., and Stephenson, J.S. Pharmacology of a new adrenergic beta-receptor blocking compound. *Lancet,* **1962,** *2:*311–314.

Boutros, A.R., Bravo, E.L., Zanettin, G., and Straffon, R.A. Perioperative management of 63 patients with pheochromocytoma. *Clev. Clin. J. Med.,* **1990,** *57:*613–617.

Brantigan, C.O., Brantigan, T.A., and Joseph, N. Effect of beta blockade and beta stimulation on stage fright. *Am. J. Med.,* **1982,** *72:*88–94.

Bravo, E.L., Tarazi, R.C., Fouad, R.M., Vidt, D.G., and Gifford, R.W., Jr. Clonidine-suppression test: a useful aid in the diagnosis of pheochromocytoma. *N. Engl. J. Med.,* **1981,** *305:*623–626.

Breslin, D., Fields, D.W., Chou, T.C., Marion, D.N., Kane, M., Vaughan, E.D., Jr., and Felsen, D. Medical management of benign prostatic hyperplasia: a canine model comparing the in vivo efficacy of alpha-1 adrenergic antagonists in the prostate. *J. Urol.,* **1993,** *149:*395–399.

Brown, M.J., Brown, D.C., and Murphy, M.B. Hypokalemia from β_2-receptor stimulation by circulating epinephrine. *N. Engl. J. Med.,* **1983,** *309:*1414–1419.

Burn, J.H., and Rand, M.J. The action of sympathomimetic amines in animals treated with reserpine. *J. Physiol. (Lond.),* **1958,** *144:*314–336.

Caine, M., Perlberg, S., and Shapiro, A. Phenoxybenzamine for benign prostatic obstruction: review of 200 cases. *Urology,* **1981,** *17:*542–546.

The Canadian Preterm Labor Investigators Group. Treatment of preterm labor with the beta-adrenergic agonist ritodrine. *N. Engl. J. Med.,* **1992,** *327:*308–312.

Carliner, N.H., Denune, D.P., Finch, C.S., Jr., and Goldberg, L.I. Sodium nitroprusside treatment of ergotamine-induced peripheral ischemia. *JAMA,* **1974,** *227:*308–309.

Carr, D.B., Clark, A.L., Kernek, K., and Spinnato, J.A. Maintenance oral nifedipine for preterm labor: a randomized clinical trial. *Am. J. Obstet. Gynecol.,* **1999,** *181:*822–827.

Chang, E.B., Fedorak, R.N., and Field, M. Experimental diabetic diarrhea in rats. Intestinal mucosal denervation hypersensitivity and treatment with clonidine. *Gastroenterology,* **1986,** *91:*564–569.

Chapleau, M.W., Cunningham, J.T., Sullivan, M.J., Wachtel, R.E., and Abboud, F.M. Structural versus functional modulation of the arterial baroreflex. *Hypertension,* **1995,** *26:*341–347.

Chidiac, P., Hebert, T.E., Valiquette, M., Dennis, M., and Bouvier, M. Inverse agonist activity of beta-adrenergic antagonists. *Mol. Pharmacol.,* **1994,** *45:*490–499.

Clark, J.A., Zimmerman, H.J., and Tanner, L.A. Labetalol hepatotoxicity. *Ann. Intern. Med.,* **1990,** *113:*210–213.

Clark, J.T., Smith, E.R., and Davidson, J.M. Enhancement of sexual motivation in male rats by yohimbine. *Science,* **1984,** *225:*847–849.

Cohn, J.N., Archibald, D.G., Ziesche, S., Franciosa, J.A., Harston, W.E., Tristani, F.E., Dunkman, W.B., Jacobs, W., Francis, G.S., Flohr, K.H., Goldman, S., Cobb, F.R., Shah, P.M., Saunders, R.,

Fletcher, R.D., Loeb, H.S., Hughes, V.C., and Baker, B. Effect of vasodilator therapy on mortality in chronic congestive heart failure. Results of a Veterans Administration Cooperative Study. *N. Engl. J. Med.,* **1986,** *314:*1547–1552.

Cole, P., Haight, J.S., Cooper, P.W., and Kassel, E.E. A computed tomographic study of nasal mucosa: effects of vasoactive substances. *J. Otolaryngol.,* **1983,** *12:*58–60.

DeBernardis, J.F., Winn, M., Kerkman, D.J., Kyncl, J.J., Buckner, S., and Horrom, B. A new nasal decongestant, A-57219: a comparison with oxymetazoline. *J. Pharm. Pharmacol.,* **1987,** *39:*760–763.

Emorine, L.J., Marullo, S., Briend-Sutren, M.M., Patey, G., Tate, K., Delavier-Klutchko, C., and Strosberg, D. Molecular characterization of the human β_3-adrenergic receptor. *Science,* **1989,** *245:*1118–1121.

Engelhardt, S., Hein, L., Wiesmann, F., and Lohse, M.J. Progressive hypertrophy and heart failure in beta₁-adrenergic receptor transgenic mice. *Proc. Natl. Acad. Sci. U.S.A.,* **1999,** *96:*7059–7064.

Faure, C., Pimoule, C., Vallancien, G., Langer, S.Z., and Graham, D. Identification of α_1-adrenoceptor subtypes in the human prostate. *Life Sci.,* **1994,** *54:*1595–1605.

Fedorak, R.N., Field, M., and Chang, E.B. Treatment of diabetic diarrhea with clonidine. *Ann. Intern. Med.,* **1985,** *102:*197–199.

Flacke, J.W., Bloor, B.C., Flacke, W.E., Wong, D., Dazza, S., Stead, S.W., and Laks, H. Reduced narcotic requirement by clonidine with improved hemodynamic and adrenergic stability in patients undergoing coronary bypass surgery. *Anesthesiology,* **1987,** *67:*11–19.

Foglar, R., Shibata, K., Horie, K., Hirasawa, A., and Tsujimoto, G. Use of recombinant alpha₁-adrenoceptors to characterize subtype selectivity of drugs for the treatment of prostatic hypertrophy. *Eur. J. Pharmacol.,* **1995,** *288:*201–207.

Forray, C., Bard, J.A., Wetzel, J.M., Chiu, G., Shapiro, E., Tang, R., Lepor, H., Hartig, P.R., Weinshank, R.L., Branchek, T.A., and Gluchowski, C. The α_1-adrenergic receptor that mediates smooth muscle contraction in human prostate has the pharmacological properties of the cloned human alpha 1c subtype. *Mol. Pharmacol.,* **1994,** *45:*703–708.

Fouad-Tarazi, F.M., Okabe, M., and Goren, H. Alpha sympathomimetic treatment of autonomic insufficiency with orthostatic hypotension. *Am. J. Med.,* **1995,** *99:*604–610.

Garcia-Sainz, J.A., Villalobos-Molina, R., Corvera, S., Huerta-Bahena, J., Tsujimoto, G., and Hoffman, B.B. Differential effects of adrenergic agonists and phorbol esters on the α_1-adrenoceptors of hepatocytes and aorta. *Eur. J. Pharmacol.,* **1985,** *112:*393–397.

Gavin, K.T., Colgan, M.P., Moore, D., Shanik, G., and Docherty, J.R. Alpha 2C-adrenoceptors mediate contractile responses to noradrenaline in the human saphenous vein. *Naunyn Schmiedebergs Arch. Pharmacol.,* **1997,** *355:*406–411.

Gengo, F.M., Huntoon, L., and McHugh, W.B. Lipid-soluble and water-soluble beta-blockers. Comparison of the central nervous system depressant effect. *Arch. Intern. Med.,* **1987,** *147:*39–43.

Glassman, A.H., Stetner, F., Walsh, B.T., Raizman, P.S., Fleiss, J.L., Cooper, T.B., and Covey, L.S. Heavy smokers, smoking cessation, and clonidine. Results of a double-blind, randomized trial. *JAMA,* **1988,** *259:*2863–2866.

Gold, E.H., Chang, W., Cohen, M., Baum, T., Ehrreich, S., Johnson, G., Prioli, N., and Sybertz, E.J. Synthesis and comparison of some cardiovascular properties of the stereoisomers of labetalol. *J. Med. Chem.,* **1982,** *25:*1363–1370.

Gold, M.S., Redmond, D.E. Jr., and Kleber, H.D. Clonidine blocks acute opiate-withdrawal symptoms. *Lancet,* **1978,** *2:*599–602.

Goldberg, L.I., and Rajfer, S.I. Dopamine receptors: applications in clinical cardiology. *Circulation,* **1985,** 72:245–248.

Goldenberg, M., Aranow, H., Jr., Smith, A.A., and Faber, M. Pheochromocytoma and essential hypertensive vascular disease. *Arch. Intern. Med.,* **1950,** 86:823–836.

Gottlieb, S.S., McCarter, R.J., and Vogel, R.A. Effect of beta-blockade on mortality among high-risk and low-risk patients after myocardial infarction. *N. Engl. J. Med.,* **1998,** 339:489–497.

Grossman, E., Rosenthal, T., Peleg, E., Holmes, C., and Goldstein, D.S. Oral yohimbine increases blood pressure and sympathetic nervous outflow in hypertensive patients. *J. Cardiovasc. Pharmacol.,* **1993,** 22:22–26.

Haefeli, W.E., Srivastava, N., Kongpatanakul, S., Blaschke, T.F., and Hoffman, B.B. Lack of role of endothelium-derived relaxing factor in effects of alpha-adrenergic agonists in cutaneous veins in humans. *Am. J. Physiol.,* **1993,** 264:H364–H369.

Hamilton, C., Dalrymple, H., and Reid, J. Recovery in vivo and in vitro of α-adrenoceptor responses and radioligand binding after phenoxybenzamine. *J. Cardiovasc. Pharmacol.,* **1982,** 4(suppl 1):S125–S128.

Hamilton, C.A., Reid, J.L., and Sumner, D.J. Acute effects of phenoxybenzamine on α-adrenoceptor responses in vivo and in vitro: relation of in vivo pressor responses to the number of specific adrenoceptor binding sites. *J. Cardiovasc. Pharmacol.,* **1983,** 5:868–873.

Hancox, R.J., Aldridge, R.E., Cowan, J.O., Flannery, E.M., Herbison, G.P., McLachlan, C.R., Town, G.I., and Taylor, D.R. Tolerance to beta-agonists during acute bronchoconstriction. *Eur. Respir. J.,* **1999,** 14:283–287.

Harder, S., and Thurmann, P. Concentration/effect relationship of bunazosin, a selective α₁-adrenoceptor antagonist in hypertensive patients after single and multiple oral doses. *Int. J. Clin. Pharmacol. Ther.,* **1994,** 32:38–43.

Hartung, W.H. Epinephrine and related compounds: influence of structure on physiologic activity. *Chem. Rev.,* **1931,** 9:389–465.

Hedberg, A., Gerber, J.G., Nies, A.S., Wolfe, B.B., and Molinoff, P.B. Effects of pindolol and propranolol on beta adrenergic receptors on human lymphocytes. *J. Pharmacol. Exp. Ther.,* **1986,** 239:117–123.

Holmes, B., Brogden, R.N., Heel, R.C., Speight, T.M., and Avery, G.S. Guanabenz. A review of its pharmacodynamic properties and therapeutic efficacy in hypertension. *Drugs,* **1983,** 26:212–229.

Hu, Z.W., Shi, X.Y., and Hoffman, B.B. Doxazosin inhibits proliferation and migration of human vascular smooth-muscle cells independent of alpha₁-adrenergic receptor antagonism. *J. Cardiovasc. Pharmacol.,* **1998,** 31:833–839.

Hughes, J.M., Seale, J.P., and Temple, D.M. Effect of fenoterol on immunological release of leukotrienes and histamine from human lung in vitro: selective antagonism by β-adrenoceptor antagonists. *Eur. J. Pharmacol.,* **1983,** 95:239–245.

Jebavy, P., Koudelkova, E., and Henzlova, M. Unloading effects of prazosin in patients with chronic aortic regurgitation. *Am. Heart J.,* **1983,** 105:567–574.

Kaiser, P., Tesch, P.A., Frisk-Holmberg, M., Juhlin-Dannfelt, A., and Kaijser, L. Effect of beta₁-selective and nonselective beta-blockade on work capacity and muscle metabolism. *Clin. Physiol.,* **1986,** 6:197–207.

Kashiwagi, A., Harano, Y., Suzuki, M., Kojima, H., Harada, M., Nishio, Y., and Shigeta, Y. New α₂-adrenergic blocker (DG-5128) improves insulin secretion and in vivo glucose disposal in NIDDM patients. *Diabetes,* **1986,** 35:1085–1089.

Kelly, H.W. New β₂-adrenergic agonist aerosols. *Clin. Pharm.,* **1985,** 4:393–403.

Kenny, B.A., Miller, A.M., Williamson, I.J., O'Connell, J., Chalmers, D.H., and Naylor, A.M. Evaluation of the pharmacological selectivity profile of alpha₁ adrenoceptor antagonists at prostatic alpha₁ adrenoceptors: binding, functional and in vivo studies. *Br. J. Pharmacol.,* **1996,** 118:871–878.

Kirby, R.S., Coppinger, S.W., Corcoran, M.O., Chapple, C.R., Flannigan, M., and Milroy, E.J. Prazosin in the treatment of prostatic obstruction. A placebo-controlled study. *Br. J. Urol.,* **1987,** 60:136–142.

Lepäntalo, M. Chronic effects of labetalol, pindolol, and propranolol on calf blood flow in intermittent claudication. *Clin. Pharmacol. Ther.,* **1985,** 37:7–12.

Lepor, H., Williford, W.O., Barry, M.J., Brawer, M.K., Dixon, C.M., Gormley, G., Haakenson, C., Machi, M., Narayan, P., and Padley, R.J. The efficacy of terazosin, finasteride, or both in benign prostatic hyperplasia. Veterans Affairs Cooperative Studies Benign Prostatic Hyperplasia Study Group. *N. Engl. J. Med.,* **1996,** 335:533–539.

Liggett, S.B., Tepe, N.M., Lorenz, J.N., Canning, A.M., Jantz, T.D., Mitarai, S., Yatani, A., and Dorn, G.W. II. Early and delayed consequences of beta(2)-adrenergic receptor overexpression in mouse hearts: critical role for expression level. *Circulation,* **2000,** 101:1707–1714.

Link, R.E., Desai, K., Hein, L., Stevens, M.E., Chruscinski, A., Bernstein, D., Barsh, G.S., and Kobilka, B.K. Cardiovascular regulation in mice lacking alpha₂ adrenergic receptor subtypes b and c. *Science,* **1996,** 273:803–805.

Ma, X.L., Yue, T.L., Lopez, B.L., Barone, F.C., Christopher, T.A., Ruffolo, R.R., Jr., and Feuerstein, G.Z. Carvedilol, a new beta adrenoreceptor blocker and free radical scavenger, attenuates myocardial ischemia–reperfusion injury in hypercholesterolemic rabbits. *J. Pharmacol. Exp. Ther.,* **1996,** 277:128–136.

MacMillan, L.B., Hein, L., Smith, M.S., Piascik, M.T., and Limbird, L.E. Central hypotensive effects of the alpha₂ₐ adrenergic receptor subtype. *Science,* **1996,** 273:801–803.

Majesky, M.W., Daemen, M.J., and Schwartz, S.M. α₁-Adrenergic stimulation of platelet-derived growth factor A-chain gene expression in rat aorta. *J. Biol. Chem.,* **1990,** 265:1082–1088.

Marik, P.E., and Iglesias, J. Low-dose dopamine does not prevent acute renal failure in patients with septic shock and oliguria. NORASEPT II Study Investigators. *Am. J. Med.,* **1999,** 107:387–390.

Mitchell, G.G., and Elbourne, D.R. The Salford Third Stage Trial. Oxytocin plus ergometrine versus oxytocin alone in the active management of the third stage of labor. *Online J. Curr. Clin. Trials,* **1993,** Doc. No. 83.

Murray, K.T., Reilly, C, Koshakji, R.P., Roden, D.M., Lineberry, M.D., Wood, A.J., Siddoway, L.A., Barbey, J.T., and Woosley, R.L. Suppression of ventricular arrhythmias in man by d-propranolol independent of beta-adrenergic receptor blockade. *J. Clin. Invest.,* **1990,** 85:836–842.

Nagamani, M., Kelver, M.E., and Smith, E.R. Treatment of menopausal hot flashes with transdermal administration of clonidine. *Am. J. Obstet. Gynecol.,* **1987,** 156:561–565.

Nattel, S., Rangno, R.E., and Van Loon, G. Mechanism of propranolol withdrawal phenomena. *Circulation,* **1979,** 59:1158–1164.

Okazaki, M., Hu, Z.-W., Fujinaga, M., and Hoffman, B.B. Alpha₁ adrenergic receptor-induced c-*fos* gene expression in rat aorta and cultured vascular smooth muscle cells. *J. Clin. Invest.,* **1994,** 94:210–218.

Oliver, G., and Schäfer, E.A. The physiological action of extract of the suprarenal capsules. *J. Physiol. (Lond.),* **1895,** 18:230–276.

Os, I., and Stokke, H.P. Effects of doxazosin in the gastrointestinal therapeutic system formulation versus doxazosin standard and placebo in mild-to-moderate hypertension. Doxazosin Investigators' Study Group. *J. Cardiovasc. Pharmacol.*, **1999**, *33*:791–797.

Panter, K.R., Hannah, M.E., Amankwah, K.S., Ohlsson, A., Jefferies, A.L., and Farine, D. The effect of indomethacin tocolysis in preterm labour on perinatal outcome: a randomised placebo-controlled trial. *Br. J. Obstet. Gynaecol.*, **1999**, *106*:467–473.

Pearce, N., Beasley, R., Crane, J., Burgess, C., and Jackson, R. End of the New Zealand asthma mortality epidemic. *Lancet,* **1995**, *345*: 41–44.

Perry, R.R., Keiser, H.R., Norton, J.A., Wall, R.T., Robertson, C.N., Travis, W., Pass, H.I., Walther, M.M, and Linehan, W.M. Surgical management of pheochromocytoma with the use of metyrosine. *Ann. Surg.,* **1990**, *212*:621–628.

Powell, C.E., and Slater, I.H. Blocking of inhibitory adrenergic receptors by a dichloro analog of isoproterenol. *J. Pharmacol. Exp. Ther.,* **1958**, *122*:480–488.

Price, D.T., Schwinn, D.A., Lomasney, J.W., Allen, L.F., Caron, M.G., and Lefkowitz, R.J. Identification, quantification, and localization of mRNA for three distinct α_1 adrenergic receptor subtypes in human prostate. *J. Urol.,* **1993**, *150*:546–551.

Pujet, J.C., Dubreuil, C., Fleury, B., Provendier, O., and Abella, M.L. Effects of celiprolol, a cardioselective beta-blocker, on respiratory function in asthmatic patients. *Eur. Respir. J.,* **1992**, *5*:196–200.

Rangno, R.E., and Langlois, S. Comparison of withdrawal phenomena after propranolol, metoprolol, and pindolol. *Am. Heart J.,* **1982**, *104*: 473–478.

Rangno, R.E., Nattel, S., and Lutterodt, A. Prevention of propranolol withdrawal mechanism by prolonged small dose propranolol schedule. *Am. J. Cardiol.,* **1982**, *49*:828–833.

Reid, D., Surridge, D.H., Morales, A., Condra, M., Harris, C., Owen, J., and Fenemore, J. Double-blind trial of yohimbine in treatment of psychogenic impotence. *Lancet,* **1987**, *2*:421–423.

Reilly, C.S., Wood, M., Koshakji, R.P., and Wood, A.J. Ultra-short-acting beta-blockade: a comparison with conventional beta-blockade. *Clin. Pharmacol. Ther.,* **1985**, *38*:579–585.

Riegle, E.V., Gunter, J.B., Lusk, R.P., Muntz, H.R., and Weiss, K.L. Comparison of vasoconstrictors for functional endoscopic sinus surgery in children. *Laryngoscope,* **1992**, *102*:820–823.

Robertson, D., Goldberg, M.R., Hollister, A.S., Wade, D., and Robertson, R.M. Clonidine raises blood pressure in severe idiopathic orthostatic hypotension. *Am J. Med.,* **1983a**, *74*:193–200.

Robertson, R.M., Bernard, Y.D., Carr, R.K., and Robertson, D. Alpha-adrenergic blockade in vasotonic angina: lack of efficacy of specific α_1-receptor blockade with prazosin. *J. Am. Coll. Cardiol.,* **1983b**, *2*:1146–1150.

Rosen, S.G., Clutter, W.E., Shah, S.D., Miller, J.P., Bier, D.M., and Cryer, P.E. Direct α-adrenergic stimulation of hepatic glucose production in human subjects. *Am. J. Physiol.,* **1983**, *245*:E616–E626.

Rosenbaum, J.S., Ginsburg, R., Billingham, M.E., and Hoffman, B.B. Effects of adrenergic receptor antagonists on cardiac morphological and functional alterations in rats harboring pheochromocytoma. *J. Pharmacol. Exp. Ther.,* **1987**, *241*:354–360.

Rossier, O., Abuin, L., Fanelli, F., Leonardi, A., and Cotecchia, S. Inverse agonism and neutral antagonism at alpha(1a)- and alpha(1b)-adrenergic receptor subtypes. *Mol. Pharmacol.,* **1999**, *56*:858–866.

Ruffolo, R.R., Jr., and Yaden, E.L. Vascular effects of the stereoisomers of dobutamine. *J. Pharmacol. Exp. Ther.,* **1983**, *224*:46–50.

Ruffolo, R.R., Jr., Spradlin, T.A., Pollock, G.D., Waddell, J.E., and Murphy, P.J. Alpha and beta adrenergic effects of the stereoisomers of dobutamine. *J. Pharmacol. Exp. Ther.,* **1981**, *219*:447–452.

Sasso, E.H., and O'Connor, D.T. Prazosin depression of baroreflex function in hypertensive man. *Eur. J. Clin. Pharmacol.,* **1982**, *22*:7–14.

Shores, J., Berger, K.R., Murphy, E.A., and Pyeritz, R.E. Progression of aortic dilatation and the benefit of long-term β-adrenergic blockade in Marfan's syndrome. *N. Engl. J. Med.,* **1994**, *330*:1335–1341.

Spittell, J.A. Jr., and Spittell, P.C. Chronic pernio: another cause of blue toes. *Int. Angiol.,* **1992**, *11*:46–50.

Strader, C.D., Candelore, M.R., Hill, W.S., Sigal, I.S., and Dixon, R.A. Identification of two serine residues involved in agonist activation of the β-adrenergic receptor. *J. Biol. Chem.,* **1989**, *264*:13572–13578.

Suissa, S., and Ernst, P. Optical illusions from visual data analysis: example of the New Zealand asthma mortality epidemic. *J. Clin. Epidemiol.,* **1997**, *50*:1079–1088.

Suissa, S., Ernst, P., Boivin, J.F., Horwitz, R.I., Habbick, B., Cockroft, D., Blais, L., McNutt, M., Buist, A.S., and Spitzer, W.O. A cohort analysis of excess mortality in asthma and the use of inhaled beta-agonists. *Am. J. Respir. Crit. Care. Med.,* **1994**, *149*:604–610.

Surwit, R.S., Gilgor, R.S., Allen, L.M., and Duvic, M. A double-blind study of prazosin in the treatment of Raynaud's phenomenon in scleroderma. *Arch. Dermatol.,* **1984**, *120*:329–331.

Sybertz, E.J., Sabin, C.S., Pula, K.K., Vliet, G.V., Glennon, J., Gold, E.H., and Baum, T. Alpha and beta adrenoceptor blocking properties of labetalol and its *R,R*-isomer, SCH 19927. *J. Pharmacol. Exp. Ther.,* **1981**, *218*:435–443.

Tadolini, B., and Franconi, F. Carvedilol inhibition of lipid peroxidation. A new antioxidative mechanism. *Free Radic. Res.,* **1998**, *29*:377–387.

Thiessen, B.Q., Wallace, S.M., Blackburn, J.L., Wilson, T.W., and Bergman, U. Increased prescribing of antidepressants subsequent to beta-blocker therapy. *Arch. Intern. Med.,* **1990**, *150*:2286–2290.

Unverferth, D.A., Blanford, M., Kates, R.E., and Leier, C.V. Tolerance to dobutamine after a 72 hour continuous infusion. *Am. J. Med.,* **1980**, *69*:262–266.

Villanueva, C., Balanzo, J., Novella, M.T., Soriano, G., Sainz, S., Torras, X., Cusso, X., Guarner, C., and Vilardell, F. Nadolol plus isosorbide mononitrate compared with sclerotherapy for the prevention of variceal rebleeding. *N. Engl. J. Med.,* **1996**, *334*:1624–1629.

Wilms, G., Stockx, L., and Baert, A.L. Optimization of distal artery opacification in peripheral arteriography: comparison between nitroglycerin, tolazoline and buflomedyl. *J. Belge Radiol.,* **1993**, *76*:311–313.

Winniford, M.D., Filipchuk, N., and Hillis, L.D. Alpha-adrenergic blockade for variant angina: a long-term, double-blind, randomized trial. *Circulation,* **1983**, *67*:1185–1188.

Wollersheim, H., Thien, T., Fennis, J., van Elteren, P., and van't Laar, A. Double-blind, placebo-controlled study of prazosin in Raynaud's phenomenon. *Clin. Pharmacol. Ther.,* **1986**, *40*:219–225.

Yang, G., Timme, T.L., Park, S.H., Wu, X., Wyllie, M.G., and Thompson, T.C. Transforming growth factor beta 1 transduced mouse prostate reconstitutions: II. Induction of apoptosis by doxazosin. *Prostate,* **1997**, *33*:157–163.

Yue, T.L., Wang, X., Gu, J.L., Ruffolo, R.R., Jr., and Feuerstein, G.Z. Carvedilol, a new vasodilating beta-adrenoceptor blocker, inhibits oxidation of low-density lipoproteins by vascular smooth muscle cells and prevents leukocyte adhesion to smooth muscle cells. *J. Pharmacol. Exp. Ther.,* **1995**, *273*:1442–1449.

Zhu, Q.-M., Lesnick, J.D., Jasper, J.R., MacLennan, S.J., Dillon, M.P., Eglen, R.M., and Blue, D.R., Jr. Cardiovascular effects of rilmedidine, moxonidine and clonidine in conscious wild-type and D79N α_{2A}-adrenoreceptor transgenic mice. *Br. J. Pharmacol.,* **1999**, *126*:1522–1530.

Zorgniotti, A.W. Experience with buccal phentolamine mesylate for impotence. *Int. J. Impot. Res.,* **1994**, *6*:37–41.

MONOGRAPHS AND REVIEWS

American Psychiatric Association. Attention-deficit hyperactivity disorder. In, *Diagnostic and Statistical Manual of Mental Disorders: DSM-III-R.* American Psychiatric Association, Washington, D.C., **1987**, pp. 50–53.

Andersson, K.E. Current concepts in the treatment of disorders of micturition. *Drugs,* **1988,** *35*:477–494.

Arner, P. The β_3-adrenergic receptor—a cause and cure of obesity? *N. Engl. J. Med.,* **1995,** *333*:382–383.

Babamoto, K.S., and Hirokawa, W.T. Doxazosin: a new α_1-adrenergic antagonist. *Clin. Pharm.,* **1992,** *11*:415–427.

Beasley, R., Pearce, N., Crane, J., and Burgess, C. Beta-agonists: what is the evidence that their use increases the risk of asthma morbidity and mortality? *J. Allergy Clin. Immunol.,* **1999,** *104*:S18–S30.

Beduschi, M.C., Beduschi, R., and Oesterling, J.E. Alpha-blockade therapy for benign prostatic hyperplasia: from a nonselective to a more selective alpha1A-adrenergic antagonist. *Urology,* **1998,** *51*:861–872.

Benfield, P., and Sorkin, E.M. Esmolol. A preliminary review of its pharmacodynamic and pharmacokinetic properties, and therapeutic efficacy. *Drugs,* **1987,** *33*:392–412.

Benfield, P., Clissold, S.P., and Brogden, R.N. Metoprolol. An updated review of its pharmacodynamic and pharmacokinetic properties, and therapeutic efficacy, in hypertension, ischemic heart disease and related cardiovascular disorders. *Drugs,* **1986,** *31*:376–429.

Black, J.W., and Prichard, B.N. Activation and blockade of β adrenoceptors in common cardiac disorders. *Br. Med. Bull.,* **1973,** *29*:163–167.

Bond, W.S. Psychiatric indications for clonidine: the neuropharmacologic and clinical basis. *J. Clin. Psychopharmacol.,* **1986,** *6*:81–87.

Bosch, J. Medical treatment of portal hypertension. *Digestion,* **1998,** *59*:547–555.

Bossmar, T. Treatment of preterm labor with the oxytocin and vasopressin antagonist Atosiban. *J. Perinat. Med.,* **1998,** *26*:458–465.

Braddom, R.L., and Rocco, J.F. Autonomic dysreflexia. A survey of current treatment. *Am. J. Phys. Med. Rehabil.,* **1991,** *70*:234–241.

Bray, G.A. Use and abuse of appetite-suppressant drugs in the treatment of obesity. *Ann. Intern. Med.,* **1993,** *119*:707–713.

Breslow, M.J., and Ligier, B. Hyperadrenergic states. *Crit. Care Med.,* **1991,** *19*:1566–1579.

Bristow, M.R. Pathophysiologic and pharmacologic rationales for clinical management of chronic heart failure with beta-blocking agents. *Am. J. Cardiol.,* **1993,** *71*:12C–22C.

Bristow, M.R., Kantrowitz, N.E., Ginsburg, R., and Fowler, M.B. Beta-adrenergic functions in heart muscle disease and heart failure. *J. Mol. Cell Cardiol.,* **1985,** *17*(suppl 2):41–52.

Brodde, O.E. The functional importance of β_1 and β_2 adrenoceptors in the human heart. *Am. J. Cardiol.,* **1988,** *62*:24C–29C.

Brogden, R.N., and Faulds, D. Salmeterol xinafoate. A review of its pharmacological properties and therapeutic potential in reversible obstructive airways disease. *Drugs,* **1991,** *42*:895–912.

Brogden, R.N., Heel, R.C., Speight, T.M., and Avery, G.S. α-Methyl-p-tyrosine: a review of its pharmacology and clinical use. *Drugs,* **1981,** *21*:81–89.

Brogden, R.N., and Markham, A. Fenoldopam: a review of its pharmacodynamic and pharmacokinetic properties and intravenous clinical potential in the management of hypertensive urgencies and emergencies. *Drugs,* **1997,** *54*:634–650.

Brooks, A.M., and Gillies, W.E. Ocular beta-blockers in glaucoma management. Clinical pharmacological aspects. *Drugs Aging,* **1992,** *2*:208–221.

Brown, M.J. Hypokalemia from β_2-receptor stimulation by circulating epinephrine. *Am. J. Cardiol.,* **1985,** *56*:3D–9D.

Bryson, H.M., Palmer K.J., Langtry H.D., and Fitton, A. Propafenone. A reappraisal of its pharmacology, pharmacokinetics and therapeutic use in cardiac arrhythmias. *Drugs,* **1993,** *45*:85–130.

Chen, K.K., and Schmidt, C.F. Ephedrine and related substances. *Medicine (Baltimore),* **1930,** *9*:1–117.

Chernow, B., and Roth, B.L. Pharmacologic manipulation of the peripheral vasculature in shock: clinical and experimental approaches. *Circ. Shock,* **1986,** *18*:141–155.

Chiarello, R.J., and Cole, J.O. The use of psychostimulants in general psychiatry. A reconsideration. *Arch. Gen. Psychiatry,* **1987,** *44*:286–295.

Chrisp, P., and Sorkin, E.M. Ocular carteolol. A review of its pharmacological properties, and therapeutic use in glaucoma and ocular hypertension. *Drugs Aging,* **1992,** *2*:58–77.

Colucci, W.S. Alpha-adrenergic receptor blockade with prazosin. Consideration of hypertension, heart failure, and potential new applications. *Ann. Intern. Med.,* **1982,** *97*:67–77.

Cooper, K.L., McKiernan, J.M., and Kaplan, S.A. Alpha-adrenoceptor antagonists in the treatment of benign prostatic hyperplasia. *Drugs,* **1999,** *57*:9–17.

Cruickshank, J.M. The clinical importance of cardioselectivity and lipophilicity in beta blockers. *Am. Heart J.,* **1980,** *100*:160–178.

Cubeddu, L.X. New α_1-adrenergic receptor antagonists for the treatment of hypertension: role of vascular alpha receptors in the control of peripheral resistance. *Am. Heart J.,* **1988,** *116*:133–162.

Dale, H.H. On some physiological actions of ergot. *J. Physiol. (Lond.),* **1906,** *34*:163–206.

Davey, M.J. Alpha adrenoceptors—an overview. *J. Mol. Cell. Cardiol.,* **1986,** *18*(suppl. 5):1–15.

Davey, M. Mechanism of alpha blockade for blood pressure control. *Am. J. Cardiol.,* **1987,** *59*:18G–28G.

Dechant, K.L., and Clissold, S.P. Sumatriptan. A review of its pharmacodynamic and pharmacokinetic properties, and therapeutic efficacy in the acute treatment of migraine and cluster headache. *Drugs,* **1992,** *43*:776–798.

Donnelly, R., and Macphee, G.J. Clinical pharmacokinetics and kinetic-dynamic relationships of dilevalol and labetalol. *Clin. Pharmacokinet.,* **1991,** *21*:95–109.

Drayer, D.E. Lipophilicity, hydrophilicity, and the central nervous system side effects of beta blockers. *Pharmacotherapy,* **1987,** *7*:87–91.

Dunn, C.J., Lea, A.P., and Wagstaff, A.J. Carvedilol. A reappraisal of its pharmacological properties and therapeutic use in cardiovascular disorders. *Drugs,* **1997,** *54*:161–185.

Elia, J., Ambrosini, P.J., and Rapoport, J.L. Treatment of attention-deficit-hyperactivity disorder. *N. Engl. J. Med.,* **1999,** *340*:780–788.

Elliott, W.J., Weber, R.R., Nelson, K.S., Oliner, C.M., Fumo, M.T., Gretler, D.D., McCray, G.R., and Murphy, M.B. Renal and hemodynamic effects of intravenous fenoldopam versus nitroprusside in severe hypertension. *Circulation,* **1990,** *81*:970–977.

Empey, D.W., and Medder, K.T. Nasal decongestants. *Drugs,* **1981,** *21*:438–443.

Faulds, D., Hollingshead, L.M., and Goa, K.L. Formoterol. A review of its pharmacological properties and therapeutic potential in reversible obstructive airways disease. *Drugs,* **1991,** *42*:115–137.

Fitton, A, and Benfield, P. Dopexamine hydrochloride. A review of its pharmacodynamic and pharmacokinetic properties and therapeutic potential in acute cardiac insufficiency. *Drugs,* **1990,** *39*:308–330.

Fitton, A., and Sorkin, E.M. Sotalol. An updated review of its pharmacological properties and therapeutic use in cardiac arrhythmias. *Drugs,* **1993,** *46*:678–719.

Fitzgerald, J.D. The applied pharmacology of beta-adrenoceptor antagonist (beta blockers) in relation to clinical outcomes. *Cardiovasc. Drugs Ther.,* **1991,** *5*:561–576.

Fitzgerald, J.D. Do partial agonist beta-blockers have improved clinical utility? *Cardiovasc. Drugs Ther.,* **1993,** *7*:303–310.

Fox, A.M., and Rieder, M.J. Risks and benefits of drugs used in the management of the hyperactive child. *Drug Saf.,* **1993,** *9*:38–50.

Francis, G.S., and Cohn, J.N. The autonomic nervous system in congestive heart failure. *Annu. Rev. Med.,* **1986,** *37*:235–247.

Freemantle, N., Cleland, J., Young, P., Mason, J., and Harrison, J. β Blockade after myocardial infarction: systematic review and meta regression analysis. *BMJ,* **1999,** *318*:1730–1737.

Friedel, H.A., and Brogden, R.N. Bitolterol. A preliminary review of its pharmacological properties and therapeutic efficacy in reversible obstructive airways disease. *Drugs,* **1988,** *35*:22–41.

Frishman, W.H. Nadolol: a new β-adrenoceptor antagonist. *N. Engl. J. Med.,* **1981,** *305*:678–682.

Frishman, W.H. Pindolol: a new β-adrenoceptor antagonist with partial agonist activity. *N. Engl. J. Med.,* **1983,** *308*:940–944.

Frishman, W.H. Carvedilol. *N. Engl. J. Med.,* **1998,** *339*:1759–1765.

Frishman, W.H., Eisen, G., and Lapsker, J. Terazosin: a new long-acting α_1-adrenergic antagonist for hypertension. *Med. Clin. North Am.,* **1988,** *72*:441–448.

Frishman, W.H., Jacob, H., Eisenberg, E., and Spivack, C.R. Overdosage with beta-adrenoceptor blocking drugs: Pharmacologic considerations and clinical management. In, *Clinical Pharmacology of the β-Adrenoceptor Blocking Drugs,* 2nd ed. (Frishman, W.H., ed.) Appleton-Century-Crofts, Norwalk, CT, **1984,** pp. 169–203.

Fry, J.M. Treatment modalities for narcolepsy. *Neurology,* **1998,** *50*: S43–S48.

Furchgott, R.F. The classification of adrenoceptors (adrenergic receptors). An evaluation from the standpoint of receptor theory. In, *Catecholamines.* (Blaschko, H., and Muscholl, E., eds.) *Handbuch der Experimentellen Pharmakologie.* Vol. 33. Springer-Verlag, Berlin, **1972,** pp. 283–335.

Galer, B.S., Lipton, R.B., Solomon, S., Newman, L.C., and Spierings, E.L. Myocardial ischemia related to ergot alkaloids: a case report and literature review. *Headache,* **1991,** *31*:446–450.

Geffner, D.L., and Hershman, J.M. Beta-adrenergic blockade for the treatment of hyperthyroidism. *Am. J. Med.,* **1992,** *93*:61–68.

Gerstman, B.B., Jolson, H.M., Bauer, M., Cho, P., Livingston, J.M., and Platt, R. The incidence of depression in new users of beta-blockers and selected antihypertensives. *J. Clin. Epidemiol.,* **1996,** *49*:809–815.

Goldberg, M.R., and Robertson, D. Yohimbine: a pharmacological probe for study of the α_2-adrenoreceptor. *Pharmacol. Rev.,* **1983,** *35*:143–180.

Gouyon, J.B., and Francoise, M. Vasodilators in persistent pulmonary hypertension of the newborn: a need for optimal appraisal of efficacy. *Dev. Pharmacol. Ther.,* **1992,** *19*:62–68.

Grimm, R.H., Jr. Antihypertensive therapy: taking lipids into consideration. *Am. Heart J.,* **1991,** *122*:910–918.

Haspel, T. Beta-blockers and the treatment of aggression. *Harv. Rev. Psychiatry,* **1995,** *2*:274–281.

Hayashi, Y., and Maze, M. Alpha$_2$ adrenoceptor agonists and anaesthesia. *Br. J. Anaesth.,* **1993,** *71*:108–118.

Hess, H.J. Prazosin: biochemistry and structure-activity studies. *Postgrad. Med.,* **1975,** *Spec. No.*:9–17.

Higby, K., Xenakis, E.M., and Pauerstein, C.J. Do tocolytic agents stop preterm labor? A critical and comprehensive review of efficacy and safety. *Am. J. Obstet. Gynecol.,* **1993,** *168*:1247–1256.

Hollenberg, S.M., Kavinsky, C.J., and Parrillo, J.E. Cardiogenic shock. *Ann. Intern. Med.,* **1999,** *131*:47–59.

Holmes, B., and Sorkin, E.M. Indoramin. A review of its pharmacodynamic and pharmacokinetic properties, and therapeutic efficacy in hypertension and related vascular, cardiovascular and airway diseases. *Drugs,* **1986,** *31*:467–499.

Hutchins, C. Three-dimensional models of the D1 and D2 dopamine receptors. *Endocr. J.,* **1994,** *23*:7–23.

IARC. Phenoxybenzamine and phenoxybenzamine hydrochloride. *IARC Monogr. Eval. Carcinog. Risk Chem. Hum.,* **1980,** *24*:185–194.

Jamin, P., LeCoz, F., Funck-Brentano, C., Poirier, J.M., and Jaillon, P. Relationships between acute and chronic beta-blocking effects of bisoprolol in healthy volunteers: a practical approach to predict intensity of beta-blockade. *J. Cardiovasc. Pharmacol.,* **1994,** *23*:658–663.

Jenne, J.W. Whither beta-adrenergic tachyphylaxis? *J. Allergy Clin. Immunol.,* **1982,** *70*:413–416.

Johnson, P. Suppression of preterm labour. Current concepts. *Drugs,* **1993,** *45*:684–692.

King, J.F., Grant, A., Keirse, M.J., and Chalmers, I. Beta-mimetics in preterm labour: an overview of the randomized controlled trials. *Br. J. Obstet. Gynaecol.,* **1988,** *95*:211–222.

Klein, D.F., Gittleman, R., Quitkin, F., and Rifkin, A. Diagnosis and drug treatment of childhood disorders. In, *Diagnosis and Drug Treatment of Psychiatric Disorders: Adults and Children,* 2nd ed. Williams & Wilkins, Baltimore, **1980,** pp. 590–775.

Kobinger, W. Central α-adrenergic systems as targets for hypotensive drugs. *Rev. Physiol. Biochem. Pharmacol.,* **1978,** *81*:39–100.

Krum, H. Beta-blockers in heart failure. The "new wave" of clinical trials. *Drugs,* **1999,** *58*:203–210.

Kulka, P.J., and Tryba, M. Inotropic support of the critically ill patient. A review of the agents. *Drugs,* **1993,** *45*:654–667.

Kyncl, J.J. Pharmacology of terazosin: an α_1-selective blocker. *J. Clin. Pharmacol.,* **1993,** *33*:878–883.

Lader, M. Beta-adrenoceptor antagonists in neuropsychiatry: an update. *J. Clin. Psychiatry,* **1988,** *49*:213–223.

Langer, S.Z. Presynaptic regulation of the release of catecholamines. *Pharmacol. Rev.,* **1981,** *32*:337–362.

Langer, S.Z., Cavero, I., and Massingham, R. Recent developments in noradrenergic neurotransmission and its relevance to the mechanism of action of certain antihypertensive agents. *Hypertension,* **1980,** *2*: 372–382.

Langley, M.S., and Heel, R.C. Transdermal clonidine. A preliminary review of its pharmacodynamic properties and therapeutic efficacy. *Drugs,* **1988,** *35*:123–142.

Lefkowitz, R.J., Rockman, H.A., and Koch, W.J. Catecholamines, cardiac beta-adrenergic receptors, and heart failure. *Circulation,* **2000,** *101*:1634–1637.

Lipworth, B.J., and McDevitt, D.G. Inhaled β_2-adrenoceptor agonists in asthma: help or hindrance? *Br. J. Clin. Pharmacol.,* **1992,** *33*:129–138.

Lötvall, J., and Svedmyr, N. Salmeterol: an inhaled β_2-agonist with prolonged duration of action. *Lung,* **1993,** *171*:249–264.

Lowenthal, D.T., Matzek, K.M., and MacGregor, T.R. Clinical pharmacokinetics of clonidine. *Clin. Pharmacokinet.,* **1988,** *14*:287–310.

Madu, E.C., Ahmar, W., Arthur, J., and Fraker, T.D., Jr. Clinical utility of digital dobutamine stress echocardiography in the noninvasive evaluation of coronary artery disease. *Arch. Intern. Med.,* **1994,** *154*: 1065–1072.

Man in't Veld, A.J., Van den Meiracker, A.H., and Schalekamp, M.A. Do beta blockers really increase peripheral vascular resistance?

Review of the literature and new observations under basal conditions. *Am. J. Hypertens.*, **1988,** *1*:91–96.

McClellan, K.J., Wiseman, L.R., and Wilde, M.I. Midodrine. A review of its therapeutic use in the management of orthostatic hypotension. *Drugs Aging,* **1998,** *12*:76–86.

McDevitt, D.G. Comparison of pharmacokinetic properties of beta-adrenoceptor blocking drugs. *Eur. Heart J.,* **1987,** *8*(suppl M):9–14.

McNeil, J.J., and Louis, W.J. Clinical pharmacokinetics of labetalol. *Clin. Pharmacokinet.,* **1984,** *9*:157–167.

McPherson, G.A. Current trends in the study of potassium channel openers. *Gen. Pharmacol.,* **1993,** *24*:275–281.

McTavish, D., Campoli-Richards, D., and Sorkin, E.M. Carvedilol. A review of its pharmacodynamic and pharmacokinetic properties, and therapeutic efficacy. *Drugs,* **1993,** *45*:232–258.

Miller, N.E. Effects of adrenoceptor-blocking drugs on plasma lipoprotein concentrations. *Am. J. Cardiol.,* **1987,** *60*:17E–23E.

Milne, R.J, and Buckley, M.M. Celiprolol. An updated review of its pharmacodynamic and pharmacokinetic properties, and therapeutic efficacy in cardiovascular disease. *Drugs,* **1991,** *41*:941–969.

Mimran, A., and Ducailar, G. Systemic and regional haemodynamic profile of diuretics and α- and β-blockers. A review comparing acute and chronic effects. *Drugs,* **1988,** *35*(suppl 6):60–69.

Missale, C., Nash, S.R., Robinson, S.W., Jaber, M., and Caron, M.G. Dopamine receptors: from structure to function. *Physiol. Rev.,* **1998,** *78*:189–225.

Mitler, M.M., Erman, M., and Hajdukovic, R. The treatment of excessive somnolence with stimulant drugs. *Sleep,* **1993,** *16*:203–206.

Nace, G.S., and Wood, A.J. Pharmacokinetics of long acting propranolol: implications for therapeutic use. *Clin. Pharmacokinet.,* **1987,** *13*:51–64.

Nelson, H.S. Beta adrenergic agonists. *Chest,* **1982,** *82*:33S–38S.

Nelson, H.S. Adrenergic therapy of bronchial asthma. *J. Allergy Clin. Immunol.,* **1986,** *77*:771–785.

Newhouse, M.T., and Dolovich, M.B. Control of asthma by aerosols. *N. Engl. J. Med.,* **1986,** *315*:870–874.

Nichols, A.J., Ruffolo, R.R., Jr., and Brooks, D.P. The pharmacology of fenoldopam. *Am. J. Hypertens.,* **1990,** *3*:116S–119S.

Nickerson, M., and Hollenberg, N.K. Blockade of α-adrenergic receptors. In, *Physiological Pharmacology: A Comprehensive Treatise.* Vol. 4. (Root, W.S., and Hofmann, F.G., eds.) Academic Press, New York, **1967,** pp. 243–305.

Norwitz, E.R., Robinson, J.N., and Challis, J.R. The control of labor. *N. Engl. J. Med.,* **1999,** *341*:660–666.

Packer, M. Beta-adrenergic blockade in chronic heart failure: principles, progress, and practice. *Prog. Cardiovasc. Dis.,* **1998,** *41*:39–52.

Parker, M., and Atkinson, J. Withdrawal syndromes following cessation of treatment with antihypertensive drugs. *Gen. Pharmacol.,* **1982,** *13*:79–85.

Pierce, D.M. A review of the clinical pharmacokinetics and metabolism of the alpha$_1$-adrenoceptor antagonist indoramin. *Xenobiotica,* **1990,** *20*:1357–1367.

Plosker, G.L., and Clissold, S.P. Controlled release metoprolol formulations. A review of their pharmacodynamic and pharmacokinetic properties, and therapeutic use in hypertension and ischaemic heart disease. *Drugs,* **1992,** *43*:382–414.

Post, S.R., Hammond, H.K., and Insel, P.A. Beta-adrenergic receptors and receptor signaling in heart failure. *Annu. Rev. Pharmacol. Toxicol.,* **1999,** *39*:343–360.

Rabkin, S.W. Mechanisms of action of adrenergic receptor blockers on lipids during antihypertensive drug treatment. *J. Clin. Pharmacol.,* **1993,** *33*:286–291.

Raehl, C.L. Advances in drug therapy of cardiopulmonary arrest. *Clin. Pharm.,* **1987,** *6*:118–139.

Reaven, G.M., and Hoffman, B.B. A role for insulin in the aetiology and course of hypertension? *Lancet,* **1987,** *2*:435–437.

Reynolds, R.D., Gorczynski, R.J., and Quon, C.Y. Pharmacology and pharmacokinetics of esmolol. *J. Clin. Pharmacol.,* **1986,** *26*:A3–A14.

Richards, D.M., and Brogden, R.N. Pirbuterol. A preliminary review of its pharmacological properties and therapeutic efficacy in reversible bronchospastic disease. *Drugs,* **1985,** *30*:6–21.

Ried, L.D., McFarland, B.H., Johnson, R.E., and Brody, K.K. Beta-blockers and depression: the more the murkier? *Ann. Pharmacother.,* **1998,** *32*:699–708.

Rosendorff, C. Beta-blocking agents with vasodilator activity. *J. Hypertens. Suppl.,* **1993,** *11*:S37–S40.

Rubin, P., and Blaschke, T. Prazosin protein binding in health and disease. *Br. J. Clin. Pharmacol.,* **1980,** *9*:177–182.

Ruffolo, R.R., Jr. The pharmacology of dobutamine. *Am. J. Med. Sci.,* **1987,** *294*:244–248.

Ruffolo, R.R., Jr. Fundamentals of receptor theory: basics for shock research. *Circ. Shock,* **1992,** *37*:176–184.

Ruffolo, R.R., Jr., and Hieble, J.P. Adrenoceptor pharmacology: urogenital applications. *Eur. Urol.,* **1999,** *36*(suppl 1):17–22.

Samanin, R., and Garattini, S. Neurochemical mechanisms of action of anorectic drugs. *Pharmacol. Toxicol.,* **1993,** *73*:63–68.

Saxena, V.K., and De Deyn, P.P. Ergotamine: its use in the treatment of migraine and its complications. *Acta Neurol. (Napoli),* **1992,** *14*:140–146.

Seale, J.P. Whither beta-adrenoceptor agonists in the treatment of asthma? *Prog. Clin. Biol. Res.,* **1988,** *263*:367–377.

Shanks, R.G. Clinical pharmacology of vasodilatory beta-blocking drugs. *Am. Heart J.,* **1991,** *121*:1006–1011.

Shephard, R.J. *Physiology and Biochemistry of Exercise.* Praeger, New York, **1982,** pp. 228–229.

Sidi, A.A. Vasoactive intracavernous pharmacotherapy. *Urol. Clin. North Am.,* **1988,** *15*:95–101.

Silverstone, T. Appetite suppressants. A review. *Drugs,* **1992,** *43*:820–836.

Silverstone, T. Clinical use of appetite suppressants. *Drug Alcohol Depend.,* **1986,** *17*:151–167.

Singh, K., Communal, C., Sawyer, D.B., and Colucci, W.S. Adrenergic regulation of myocardial apoptosis. *Cardiovasc. Res.,* **2000,** *45*:713–719.

Singh, B.N., Thoden, W.R., and Ward, A. Acebutolol. A review of its pharmacological properties and therapeutic efficacy in hypertension, angina pectoris, and arrhythmia. *Drugs,* **1985,** *29*:531–569.

Sorkin, E.M., and Heel, R.C. Guanfacine. A review of its pharmacodynamic and pharmacokinetic properties and therapeutic efficacy in the treatment of hypertension. *Drugs,* **1986,** *31*:301–336.

Stanaszek, W.F., Kellerman, D., Brogden, R.N., and Romankiewicz, J.A. Prazosin update. A review of its pharmacological properties and therapeutic use in hypertension and congestive heart failure. *Drugs,* **1983,** *25*:339–384.

Starke, K., Gothert, M., and Kilbinger, H. Modulation of neurotransmitter release by presynaptic autoreceptors. *Physiol. Rev.,* **1989,** *69*:864–989.

Struthers, A.D., and Reid, J.L. The role of adrenal medullary catecholamines in potassium homeostasis. *Clin. Sci.,* **1984,** *66*:377–382.

Stumpf, J.L., and Mitrzyk, B. Management of orthostatic hypotension. *Am. J. Hosp. Pharm.,* **1994,** *51*:648–660.

Tattersfield, A.E. Tolerance to beta-agonists. *Bull. Eur. Physiopathol. Respir.,* **1985,** *21*:1S–5S.

Teerlink, J.R., and Massie, B.M. Beta-adrenergic blocker mortality trials in congestive heart failure. *Am. J. Cardiol.,* **1999,** *84*:94R–102R.

Tesch, P.A. Exercise performance and beta-blockade. *Sports Med.,* **1985,** *2*:389–412.

Tfelt-Hansen, P. Efficacy of beta-blockers in migraine. A critical review. *Cephalalgia.,* **1986,** *6*(suppl 5):15–24.

Trendelenburg, U. Factors influencing the concentration of catecholamines at the receptors. In, *Catecholamines.* (Blaschko, H., and Muscholl E., eds.) *Handbuch der Experimentellen Pharmakologie.* Vol. 33. Springer-Verlag, Berlin, **1972,** pp. 726–761.

Van Baak, M.A. Beta-adrenoceptor blockade and exercise. An update. *Sports Med.,* **1988,** *5*:209–225.

Van de Water, A., Janssens, W., Van Neuten, J., Xhonneux, R., De Cree, J., Verhaegen, H., Reneman, R.S., and Janssen, P.A. Pharmacological and hemodynamic profile of nebivolol, a chemically novel, potent, and selective β_1-adrenergic antagonist. *J. Cardiovasc. Pharmacol.,* **1988,** *11*:552–563.

van Zwieten, P.A. Antihypertensive drugs interacting with α- and β-adrenoceptors. A review of basic pharmacology. *Drugs,* **1988,** *35*(suppl. 6):6–19.

van Zwieten, P.A. The renaissance of centrally acting antihypertensive drugs. *J. Hypertens.,* **1999,** *17*(suppl. *3*):S15–S21.

Wadworth, A.N., and Chrisp, P. Co-dergocrine mesylate. A review of its pharmacodynamic and pharmacokinetic properties and therapeutic use in age-related cognitive decline. *Drugs Aging,* **1992,** *2*:153–173.

Wadworth, A.N., Murdoch, D., and Brogden, R.N. Atenolol. A reappraisal of its pharmacological properties and therapeutic use in cardiovascular disorders. *Drugs,* **1991,** *42*:468–510.

Wagstaff, A.J., and Bryson, H.M. Tizanidine. A review of its pharmacology, clinical efficacy and tolerability in the management of spasticity associated with cerebral and spinal disorders. *Drugs,* **1997,** *53*:435–452.

Walle, T., Webb, J.G., Bagwell, E.E., Walle, U.K., Daniell, H.B., and Gaffney, T.E. Stereoselective delivery and actions of beta receptor antagonists. *Biochem. Pharmacol.,* **1988,** *37*:115–124.

Wellman, P.J. Overview of adrenergic anorectic agents. *Am. J. Clin. Nutr.,* **1992,** *55*:193S–198S.

Weyer, C., Gautier, J.F., and Danforth, E., Jr. Development of beta 3-adrenoceptor agonists for the treatment of obesity and diabetes—an update. *Diabetes Metab.,* **1999,** *25*:11–21.

Widerhorn, J., Rubin, J.N., Frishman, W.H., and Elkayam, U. Cardiovascular drugs in pregnancy. *Cardiol. Clin.,* **1987,** *5*:651–674.

Wilde, M.I., Fitton, A., and Sorkin, E.M. Terazosin. A review of its pharmacodynamic and pharmacokinetic properties, and therapeutic potential in benign prostatic hyperplasia. *Drugs Aging,* **1993,** *3*:258–277.

Wilde, M.I., and McTavish, D. Tamsulosin. A review of its pharmacological properties and therapeutic potential in the management of symptomatic benign prostatic hyperplasia. *Drugs,* **1996,** *52*:883–898.

Winkler, M., and Rath, W. A risk-benefit assessment of oxytocics in obstetric practice. *Drug Saf.,* **1999,** *20*:323–345.

Zentgraf, M., Baccouche, M., and Junemann, K.P. Diagnosis and therapy of erectile dysfunction using papaverine and phentolamine. *Urol. Int.,* **1988,** *43*:65–75.

5-HYDROXYTRYPTAMINE (SEROTONIN): RECEPTOR AGONISTS AND ANTAGONISTS

Elaine Sanders-Bush and Steven E. Mayer

This chapter deals with the diverse physiological roles of 5-hydroxytryptamine (5-HT, serotonin) as a neurotransmitter in the central nervous system, as a regulator of smooth muscle function in the cardiovascular and gastrointestinal systems, and as a regulator of platelet function. Molecular cloning has revealed an unexpected diversity of receptor subtypes, which fall into four structural and functional families. Three subtype families (5-HT$_1$, 5-HT$_2$, and 5-HT$_4$) are coupled via *G proteins to a variety of enzymatic and electrical effector systems; the 5-HT$_3$ receptor, in marked contrast, serves as a 5-HT–gated ion channel. This chapter covers 5-HT-receptor agonists and antagonists including new ones emerging as a result of the use of recombinant receptors as tools to screen for subtype-selective agents. Experimental models used to test for drugs that alter complex behaviors, such as compulsion, aggression, anxiety, depression, and sleep-wake cycles, also are described. New subtype-selective 5-HT-receptor agonists already have demonstrated therapeutic effectiveness in the acute treatment of migraine headaches and in anxiety (see Chapter 19); subtype-selective antagonists have proven to be effective for treatment of various gastrointestinal disorders (see Chapter 38). Serotonin actions* in vivo *also can be regulated by pharmacological agents that control its availability as a neurotransmitter, such as selective inhibitors of neuronal reuptake of serotonin. These agents have proven to be efficacious in depression and anxiety disorders and are discussed in Chapter 19.*

5-Hydroxytryptamine (5-HT, serotonin) has been recognized for more than 50 years as an effector on various types of smooth muscle and, subsequently, as an agent that enhances platelet aggregation and as a neurotransmitter in the central nervous system (CNS). 5-HT is found in high concentrations in enterochromaffin cells throughout the gastrointestinal tract, in platelets, and in specific regions of the CNS. Although implicated in the regulation of a number of physiological processes and their malfunction, the exact sites and modes of action of 5-HT remain ill-defined and elusive. These ambiguities are probably, in large part, the consequence of the large number of 5-HT-receptor subtypes defined initially by pharmacological analyses and confirmed by cDNA cloning. The availability of cloned receptors is allowing the development of subtype-selective drugs and elucidation of the various actions of 5-HT at a molecular level. Furthermore, an increasing number of therapeutic goals can be approached by drugs that target one or more of the subtypes of serotonin receptors.

History. In the 1930s, Erspamer began to study the distribution of enterochromaffin cells, which stained with a reagent for indoles. The highest concentrations were found in gastrointestinal mucosa, followed by platelets and the CNS (Erspamer, 1966). Page and his colleagues at the Cleveland Clinic were the first to isolate and chemically characterize a vasoconstrictor substance released from platelets in clotting blood (Rapport *et al.,* 1948). This substance was called *serotonin* (Page, 1976) and was shown to be identical to the indole isolated by Erspamer. The discovery of biosynthetic and degradative pathways (Udenfriend, 1959) and clinical interest in the pressor effects of 5-HT (Sjoerdsma, 1959) led to the hypothesis that the symptoms of patients with tumors of intestinal enterochromaffin cells (carcinoid syndrome) are the result of abnormally high production of 5-HT. Several hundred milligrams of 5-HT and its metabolites may be excreted within a 24-hour period in patients with carcinoid tumors. The gross effects of 5-HT, produced in excess in malignant carcinoid, give some indication of the actions of 5-HT. For example, these patients may display psychotic behaviors similar to those produced by lysergic acid diethylamide (LSD). Several naturally occurring hallucinogenic tryptamine-like substances were identified from animal and plant sources, suggesting that these substances may be formed *in vivo* and could explain the abnormal behavior of carcinoid patients.

An early explanation of the action of 5-HT was obtained with the parasitic liver fluke, *Fasciola hepatica* (Mansour, 1979). Exposure of the fluke to 5-HT elicited a marked increase in motility and a concomitant increase in cyclic AMP formation. Both effects were blocked by LSD. The increased motility was mediated by regulation of glycolysis at its rate-limiting step, phosphofructokinase, *via* a cyclic AMP–dependent phosphorylation of the enzyme. The 5-HT receptor involved appears to be unrelated to mammalian receptors linked to adenylyl cyclase. Such detailed explanations of the neurohumoral effects of 5-HT have not yet been achieved in mammals.

In the mid-1950s, it was suggested that 5-HT may function as a neurotransmitter in the mammalian brain (*see* Brodie and Shore, 1957). 5-HT appeared early in the evolution of the plant and animal kingdoms. This may explain why there are so many 5-HT-receptor subtypes (Peroutka and Howell, 1994). Recent cloning of 5-HT-receptor subtypes has revealed that some drugs previously considered to be subtype-selective have high affinities for multiple molecularly defined receptors (*see* Table 11–1; *see also* Sjoerdsma and Palfreyman, 1990, for additional details about the discovery and effects of 5-HT).

Source and Chemistry. 5-HT, 3-(β-aminoethyl)-5-hydroxy-indole, is widely distributed in the animal and plant kingdoms (*see* Figure 11–1 for chemical structures). It occurs in vertebrates; in tunicates, mollusks, arthropods, and coelenterates; and in fruits and nuts. It also is present in venoms, including those of the common stinging nettle and of wasps and scorpions. Numerous synthetic or naturally occurring congeners of 5-HT have varying degrees of peripheral and central pharmacological activity. Many of the *N*- and *O*-methylated indoleamines, such as *N,N*-dimethyltryptamine, have hallucinogenic activity. Because these compounds are behaviorally active and might be synthesized *via* known metabolic pathways, they have long been considered candidates for endogenous psychotomimetic substances, potentially responsible for some psychotic behaviors. Another close relative of 5-HT, melatonin (5-methoxy-*N*-acetyltryptamine), is formed by sequential *N*-acetylation and *O*-methylation (Figure 11–2). Melatonin is the principal indoleamine in the pineal gland, where its synthesis is controlled by external factors including environmental light. Melatonin also induces pigment lightening in skin cells and suppresses ovarian functions. It also may serve a role in biological rhythms and shows promise in the treatment of jet lag and other sleep disturbances.

Synthesis and Metabolism. 5-HT is synthesized by a two-step pathway from the essential amino acid tryptophan (*see* Figure 11–2). Tryptophan hydroxylase, a mixed-function oxidase that requires molecular oxygen and a reduced pteridine cofactor for activity, is the rate-limiting enzyme in the pathway. The active uptake of tryptophan is the first step in the synthesis of 5-HT in the brain. Unlike tyrosine hydroxylase, tryptophan hydroxylase is not regulated by end-product inhibition, although regulation by phosphorylation is common to both enzymes. Brain tryptophan hydroxylase is not saturated with substrate; consequently, the amount of tryptophan in the brain influences the synthesis of 5-HT. Tryptophan is actively transported into the brain by a carrier that also transports other large neutral and branch-chain amino acids. The levels of tryptophan in the brain are influenced not only by its plasma concentration but also by the plasma concentrations of other amino acids that compete for the brain uptake carrier.

The enzyme that converts L-5-hydroxytryptophan to 5-HT, aromatic L-amino acid decarboxylase, is widely distributed and has a broad substrate specificity. A longstanding debate about whether or not L-5-hydroxytryptophan decarboxylase and L-dopa decarboxylase are identical enzymes was clarified when cDNA cloning confirmed that a single gene product decarboxylates both amino acids. 5-Hydroxytryptophan is not detected in the brain, because the amino acid is rapidly decarboxylated. Therefore, it is not possible to alter levels of 5-HT in the brain by manipulating the levels of 5-hydroxytryptophan.

The principal route of metabolism of 5-HT involves monoamine oxidase (MAO) forming 5-hydroxyindole acetic acid (5-HIAA) by a two-step process (*see* Figure 11–2). The aldehyde formed by the action of MAO is converted to 5-HIAA by an ubiquitous enzyme, aldehyde dehydrogenase. An alternative route, reduction of the acetaldehyde to an alcohol, 5-hydroxytryptophol, is normally insignificant. 5-HIAA is actively transported out of the brain by a process that is sensitive to the nonspecific transport inhibitor probenecid. Since 5-HIAA accounts for nearly 100% of the metabolism of 5-HT in brain, the turnover rate of brain 5-HT is estimated by measuring the rate of rise of 5-HIAA after administration of probenecid. 5-HIAA from brain and peripheral sites of 5-HT storage and metabolism is excreted in the urine along with small amounts of 5-hydroxytryptophol sulfate or glucuronide conjugates. The usual urinary excretion of 5-HIAA by a normal adult is 2 to 10 mg daily. Larger amounts are excreted by patients with malignant carcinoid, providing a reliable diagnostic test for the disease. The massive amounts of pyridine nucleotides and tryptophan that are required for 5-HT synthesis in patients with malignant carcinoid may produce symptoms of niacin and tryptophan deficiencies. Ingestion of ethyl alcohol results in elevated amounts of NADH, which diverts 5-hydroxyindoleacetaldehyde from the oxidative route to the reductive pathway (*see* Figure 11–2). This tends to increase the excretion of 5-hydroxytryptophol and correspondingly reduces the excretion of 5-HIAA.

Two isoforms of monoamine oxidase (MAO-A and -B) were distinguished initially on the basis of substrate and inhibitor specificities. Both isoforms have been cloned, and the properties of the cloned enzymes are consistent with the pharmacological profiles established previously (Shih, 1991; *see* Chapter 10). MAO-A preferentially metabolizes 5-HT and nor-epinephrine; *clorgyline* is a specific inhibitor of this enzyme. MAO-B prefers β-phenylethylamine and benzylamine as substrates; *selegiline* (ELDEPRYL) is a selective inhibitor. Dopamine and tryptamine are metabolized equally well by both isoforms. Neurons contain both isoforms of MAO, localized primarily in the outer membrane of mitochondria. MAO-B is the principal isoform in platelets, which contain large amounts of 5-HT.

Other minor pathways of metabolism of 5-HT, such as sulfation and *O*- or *N*-methylation, have been suggested. The latter reaction could lead to formation of an endogenous psychotropic substance, 5-hydroxy-*N,N*-dimethyltryptamine (*bufotenine; see* Figure 11–1). However, other methylated indoleamines such as *N,N*-dimethyltryptamine and 5-methoxy-*N,N*-dimethyltryptamine are far more active hallucinogenic agents and are more likely candidates as endogenous psychotomimetics.

Table 11–1

Serotonin Receptor Subtypes

Structural Families

| | | | 5-HT$_1$, 5-HT$_2$, 5-HT$_{4-7}$ | | 5-HT$_3$ | |
| | | | G protein–coupled receptor | | 5-HT–gated ion channel | |

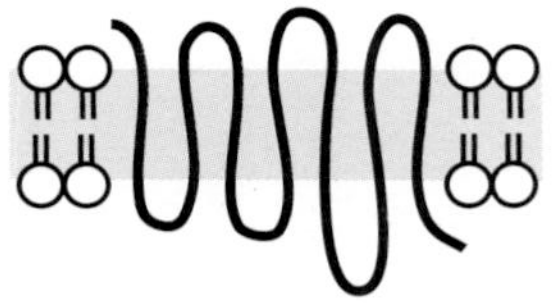

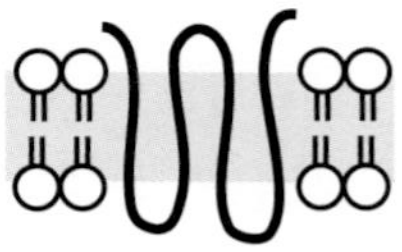

SUBTYPE	GENE STRUCTURE	SIGNAL TRANSDUCTION	LOCALIZATION	FUNCTION	SELECTIVE AGONIST	SELECTIVE ANTAGONIST
5-HT$_{1A}$	Intronless	Inhibition of AC	Raphe nuclei Hippocampus	Autoreceptor	8-OH-DPAT	WAY 100135
5-HT$_{1B}$*	Intronless	Inhibition of AC	Subiculum Substantia nigra	Autoreceptor	—	—
5-HT$_{1D}$	Intronless	Inhibition of AC	Cranial blood vessels	Vasoconstriction	Sumatriptan	—
5-HT$_{1E}$	Intronless	Inhibition of AC	Cortex Striatum	—	—	—
5-HT$_{1F}$†	Intronless	Inhibition of AC	Brain and periphery	—	—	—
5-HT$_{2A}$ (D Receptor)	Introns	Activation of PLC	Platelets Smooth muscle Cerebral cortex	Platelet aggregation Contraction Neuronal excitation	α-Methyl-5-HT, DOI	Ketanserin LY53857 MDL 100,907
5-HT$_{2B}$	Introns	Activation of PLC	Stomach fundus	Contraction	α-Methyl-5-HT, DOI	LY53857
5-HT$_{2C}$	Introns	Activation of PLC	Choroid plexus	—	α-Methyl-5-HT, DOI	LY53857
5-HT$_3$ (M Receptor)	Introns	Ligand-operated ion channel	Peripheral nerves Area postrema	Neuronal excitation	2-Methyl-5-HT	Mesulergine Ondansetron Tropisetron
5-HT$_4$	Introns	Activation of AC	Hippocampus Gastrointestinal tract	Neuronal excitation	Renzapride	GR 113808
5-HT$_{5A}$	Introns	Inhibition of AC	Hippocampus	Unknown	—	—
5-HT$_{5B}$	Introns	Unknown			—	—
5-HT$_6$	Introns	Activation of AC	Striatum	Unknown	—	—
5-HT$_7$	Introns	Activation of AC	Hypothalamus Intestine	Unknown	—	—

*Also referred to as 5-HT$_{1D\beta}$

†Also referred to as 5-HT$_{1E\beta}$

NOTE: AC, adenylyl cyclase; PLC, phospholipase C; 8-OH-DPAT, 8-hydroxy-(2-N,N-dipropylamino)-tetraline; DOI, 1-(2,5-dimethoxy-4-iodophenyl)isopropylamine.

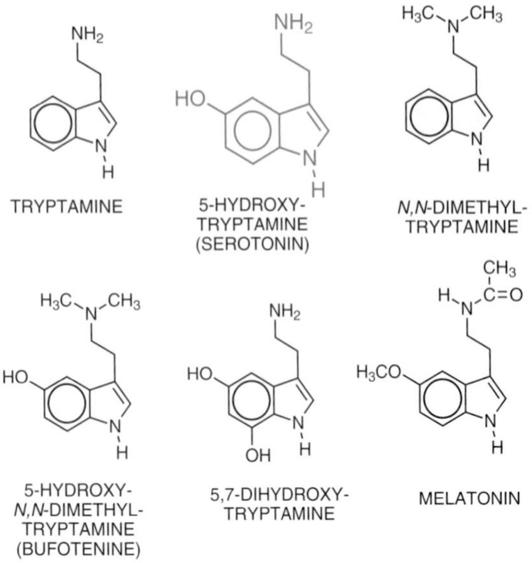

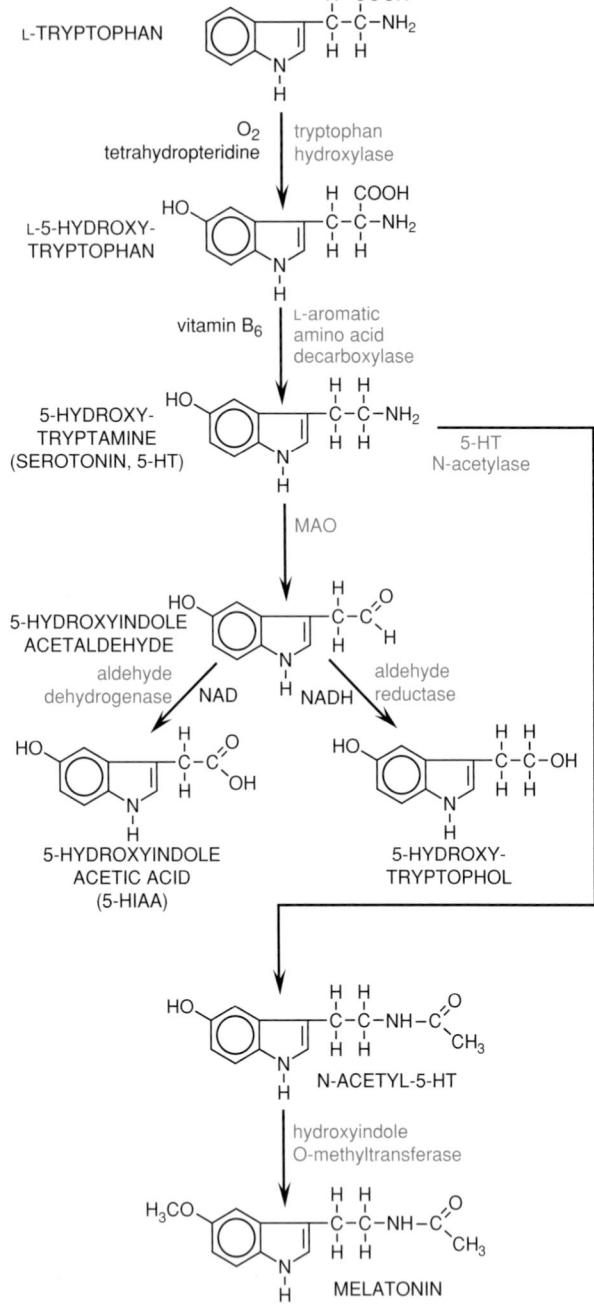

Figure 11–1. Structures of representative indolealkylamines.

In addition to metabolism by MAO, a Na$^+$-dependent, carrier-mediated uptake process exists and is involved in terminating the action of 5-HT. The 5-HT transporter is localized in the outer membrane of serotonergic axon terminals (where it terminates the action of 5-HT in the synapse) and in the outer membrane of platelets (where it takes up 5-HT from the blood). This uptake system is the only way that platelets acquire 5-HT, as they do not have the enzymes required for synthesis of 5-HT. The 5-HT transporter, as well as other monoamine transporters, has been cloned (see Chapter 12). The deduced amino acid sequence and predicted membrane topology place the amine transporters in a family clearly distinct from the transport proteins that concentrate amines in intracellular storage vesicles. Furthermore, the vesicular transporter is a nonspecific amine carrier, while the 5-HT transporter and the other amine transporters are highly specific. Neither pharmacological studies nor cDNA cloning has provided evidence to support the existence of multiple 5-HT transporters. Recent studies have found that the 5-HT transporter is regulated by phosphorylation with subsequent internalization (Ramamoorthy and Blakely, 1999), providing an unexpected mechanism for dynamic regulation of serotonergic transmission.

PHYSIOLOGICAL FUNCTIONS OF SEROTONIN

Multiple 5-HT Receptors

Early studies of peripheral tissues advanced the hypothesis that the multiple actions of 5-HT are explained by an interaction with more than one 5-HT-receptor subtype. Extensive pharmacological characterizations, as well as recent cloning of receptor cDNAs, have provided ample support for this hypothesis. The multiple 5-HT-receptor

Figure 11–2. Synthesis and inactivation of serotonin.

Synthetic enzymes are identified in blue text, and cofactors are shown in black lowercase text.

subtypes cloned to date are the largest of all known neurotransmitter receptor families. The 5-HT-receptor subtypes are expressed in distinct but often overlapping patterns (Palacios *et al.*, 1990) and are coupled to different transmembrane-signaling mechanisms (*see* Table 11–1). Four 5-HT-receptor families with defined functions, 5-HT_1 through 5-HT_4, currently are recognized. The 5-HT_1, 5-HT_2, and 5-HT_{4-7} receptor families are members of the superfamily of G protein–coupled receptors with a predicted membrane topology composed of an extracellular *N*-terminal segment linked to an intracellular C terminus by seven transmembrane-spanning segments (*see* Chapters 2 and 12). The 5-HT_3 receptor, on the other hand, is a ligand-gated ion channel that gates Na^+ and K^+ and has a predicted membrane topology akin to that of the nicotinic cholinergic receptor (*see* Chapter 9).

History of 5-HT Receptor Subtypes. Gaddum and Picarelli (1957) in a pioneering paper proposed the existence of two 5-HT-receptor subtypes, which they termed *M* and *D receptors.* M receptors were believed to be located on parasympathetic nerve endings, controlling the release of acetylcholine, whereas D receptors were thought to be located on smooth muscle. Although results of subsequent studies in both the periphery and brain were consistent with the notion of multiple subtypes of 5-HT receptor, the radioligand-binding studies of Peroutka and Snyder (1979) provided the first definitive evidence for two distinct recognition sites for 5-HT. 5-HT_1 receptors had a high affinity for $[^3\text{H}]$-5-HT, while 5-HT_2 receptors had a low affinity for $[^3\text{H}]$-5-HT and a high affinity for $[^3\text{H}]$-spiperone. Subsequently, high affinity for 5-HT was used as a primary criterion for classifying a receptor subtype as a member of the 5-HT_1 receptor family. This classification strategy proved to be invalid; for example, a receptor expressed in the choroid plexus was named the 5-HT_{1C} receptor because it was the third receptor shown to have a high affinity for 5-HT. However, based on its pharmacological properties, second-messenger function, and deduced amino acid sequence, the 5-HT_{1C} receptor clearly belonged to the 5-HT_2 receptor family and recently has been renamed the 5-HT_{2C} receptor. The current, widely accepted classification scheme (Hoyer *et al.*, 1994) proposes seven subfamilies of 5-HT receptors (*see* Table 11–1). It is likely that further modifications of this scheme will be required. For example, convincing evidence suggests that the $5\text{-HT}_{1D\beta}$ receptor is the human homolog of the 5-HT_{1B} receptor originally characterized and subsequently cloned from rodent brain. The current designation for species homologs of the same receptor protein is confusing and likely will be resolved in the future. Interestingly, although the amino acid sequences of the rat 5-HT_{1B} receptor and the human 5-HT_{1D} receptor show greater than 95% homology, these two receptors have distinct pharmacological properties. The rat 5-HT_{1B} receptor has an affinity for β-adrenergic antagonists, such as pindolol and propranolol, that is two to three orders of magnitude higher than that of the human 5-HT_{1D} receptor. This difference appears to be due to a single amino acid in the seventh transmembrane-spanning region, where the threonine present in the human 5-HT_{1D} receptor is substituted with an asparagine in the rodent 5-HT_{1B} receptor.

5-HT_1 Receptors. All five members of the 5-HT_1-receptor subfamily are negatively coupled to adenylyl cyclase.

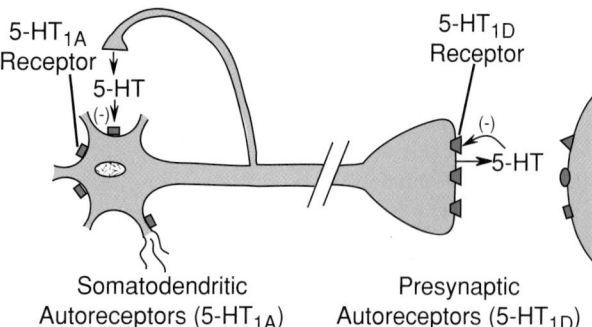

Figure 11–3. Two classes of 5-HT autoreceptors with differential localizations.

Somatodendritic 5-HT_{1A} autoreceptors decrease raphe cell firing when activated by 5-HT released from axon collaterals of the same or adjacent neurons. The receptor subtype of the presynaptic autoreceptor on axon terminals in the forebrain has different pharmacological properties and has been classified as 5-HT_{1D} (in human beings) or 5-HT_{1B} (in rodents). This receptor modulates the release of 5-HT. Postsynaptic 5-HT_1 receptors are also indicated.

At least one 5-HT_1-receptor subtype, the 5-HT_{1A} receptor, also activates a receptor-operated K^+ channel and inhibits a voltage-gated Ca^{2+} channel, a common property of receptors coupled to the pertussis toxin–sensitive G_i/G_o family of G proteins (Limbird, 1988). The 5-HT_{1A} receptor is found in the raphe nuclei of the brainstem, where it functions as an inhibitory, somatodendritic autoreceptor on cell bodies of serotonergic neurons (Figure 11–3). Another subtype, the 5-HT_{1D} receptor (and its rat homolog, 5-HT_{1B}), functions as an autoreceptor on axon terminals, inhibiting 5-HT release. 5-HT_{1D} receptors, abundantly expressed in the substantia nigra and basal ganglia, may regulate the firing rate of dopamine-containing cells and the release of dopamine at axonal terminals.

5-HT_2 Receptors. The three subtypes of 5-HT_2 receptors are linked to phospholipase C with the generation of two second messengers, diacylglycerol (which activates protein kinase C) and inositol trisphosphate (which releases intracellular stores of Ca^{2+}). The 5-HT_2-receptor subtypes couple to pertussis toxin–insensitive G proteins, such as G_q and G_{11}. For the 5-HT_{2A}-receptor subtype, however, coupling to pertussis toxin–sensitive proteins (G_i/G_o) *versus* insensitive proteins (G_q, and perhaps others) varies in different cellular preparations. 5-HT_{2A} receptors are broadly distributed in the CNS, primarily in serotonergic terminal areas. High densities of 5-HT_{2A} receptors are found in prefrontal cortex, claustrum, and platelets. 5-HT_{2A} receptors in the gastrointestinal tract are thought to correspond to the D subtype of 5-HT receptor described by Gaddum and Picarelli (1957). 5-HT_{2B} receptors originally were described in stomach fundus. The expression of 5-HT_{2B} receptor mRNA is highly restricted in the CNS. 5-HT_{2C} receptors have a very high density in the choroid plexus, an epithelial tissue that is the primary site of cerebrospinal fluid production. Despite the high density of 5-HT_{2C} receptors in choroid plexus, the role of these receptors is unknown. The 5-HT_{2C} receptor has been shown to be regulated by RNA editing, a posttranscriptional event that alters expression of the genetic code at the level of RNA (Burns *et al.*, 1997). Multiple receptor isoforms with alterations of as many as three amino acids within the second intracellular loop are predicted, and these edited isoforms have modified G protein–coupling efficiency.

5-HT_3 Receptors. The 5-HT_3 receptor is unique, being the only monoamine neurotransmitter receptor that is known to function as a ligand-operated ion channel. The 5-HT_3 receptor corresponds to Gaddum and Picarelli's M receptor (Richardson *et al.*, 1985). Activation of 5-HT_3 receptors elicits a rapidly desensitizing depolarization mediated by the gating of cations. These receptors are located on parasympathetic terminals in the gastrointestinal tract, including vagal and splanchnic afferents. In the CNS, a high density of 5-HT_3 receptors is found in the nucleus tractus solitarii and in the area postrema. 5-HT_3 receptors in both the gastrointestinal tract and the CNS participate in the emetic response, providing an anatomical basis for the antiemetic property of 5-HT_3-receptor antagonists. Most ligand-operated ion channels are composed of multiple subunits; however, the original, cloned 5-HT_3-receptor subunit is able to form functional channels that gate cations when expressed in *Xenopus* oocytes or in cultured cells (Maricq *et al.*, 1991). Nevertheless, extensive pharmacological and physiological evidence obtained in tissues and in intact animals clearly suggests the existence of multiple components of 5-HT_3 receptors. Recently, splice variants of the 5-HT_3 receptor have been identified, perhaps explaining the observed functional diversity.

5-HT_4 Receptors. 5-HT_4 receptors are widely distributed throughout the body. In the CNS, the receptors are found on neurons of the superior and inferior colliculi and in the hippocampus. In the gastrointestinal tract, 5-HT_4 receptors are located on neurons (*e.g.*, myenteric plexus) as well as on smooth muscle and secretory cells. The 5-HT_4 receptor is thought to evoke secretion in the alimentary tract and to facilitate the peristaltic reflex. 5-HT_4 receptors activate adenylyl cyclase, leading to a rise in intracellular levels of cyclic AMP (Hedge and Eglen, 1996). The latter

effect may explain the utility of prokinetic benzamides in gastrointestinal disorders (*see* Chapter 38).

Additional Cloned 5-HT Receptors. Two other cloned receptors, 5-HT_6 and 5-HT_7 receptors, are linked to activation of adenylyl cyclase. Multiple splice variants of the 5-HT_7 receptor have been found, although functional distinctions are not clear. The absence of selective agonists and antagonists has foiled definitive studies of the role of the 5-HT_6 and 5-HT_7 receptors. Circumstantial evidence suggests that 5-HT_7 receptors play a role in smooth muscle relaxation both in the gut and the vasculature. The atypical antipsychotic drug clozapine has a high affinity for 5-HT_6 and 5-HT_7 receptors. It remains to be determined whether or not this property is related to the broader effectiveness of clozapine compared to conventional antipsychotic drugs. Clozapine appears to be effective in many patients who do not respond to conventional antipsychotic drugs (*see* Chapter 20). Two subtypes of the 5-HT_5 receptor have been cloned; although the 5-HT_{5A} receptor recently has been shown to inhibit adenylyl cyclase, functional coupling of the cloned 5-HT_{2B} receptor has not yet been described.

Sites of 5-HT Action

5-HT has a major role in the regulation of gastrointestinal motility; it is stored and secreted by enterochromaffin cells and by platelets. Although peripheral stores account for most of the 5-HT in the body, this monoamine also acts as a neurotransmitter in the CNS.

Enterochromaffin Cells. Enterochromaffin cells, identified histologically, are located in the gastrointestinal mucosa, with the highest density found in the duodenum. These cells synthesize 5-HT from tryptophan and store 5-HT and other autacoids, such as the vasodilator peptide substance P and other kinins. Basal release of enteric 5-HT is augmented by mechanical stretching, such as that caused by food or the administration of hypertonic saline, and also by efferent vagal stimulation. 5-HT probably has an additional role in stimulating motility *via* the myenteric network of neurons, located between the layers of smooth muscle (Gershon, 1991; *see also* Chapter 38). The greatly enhanced secretion of 5-HT and other autacoids in malignant carcinoid leads to a multitude of cardiovascular, gastrointestinal, and CNS abnormalities. In addition, the synthesis of large amounts of 5-HT by carcinoid tumors may result in tryptophan and niacin deficiencies (pellagra).

Platelets. Platelets differ from other formed elements of blood in expressing mechanisms for uptake, storage, and endocytotic release of 5-HT. 5-HT is not synthesized in platelets but is taken up from the circulation and stored in secretory granules by active transport, similar to the uptake and storage of norepinephrine by sympathetic nerve terminals (*see* Chapters 6 and 12). Thus, Na^+-dependent transport across the surface membrane of platelets is followed by uptake into dense core granules *via* an electrochemical gradient generated by a H^+-translocating ATPase. A gradient of 5-HT as high as 1000:1 with an internal concentration of 0.6 M in the dense core storage vesicles can be maintained by platelets. Measuring the rate

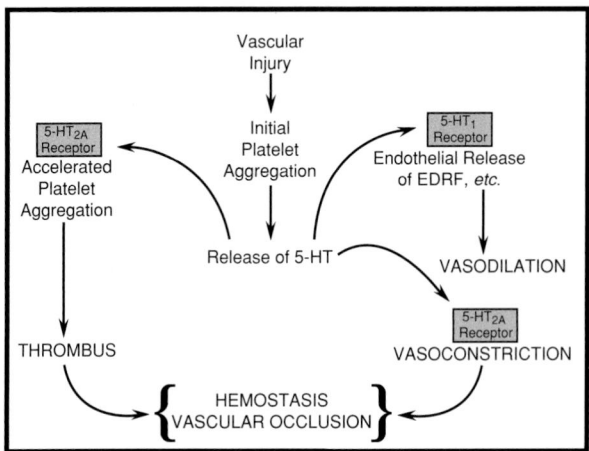

Figure 11–4. Schematic representation of the local influences of platelet 5-HT.

 The release of 5-HT stored in platelets is triggered by aggregation. The local actions of 5-HT include feedback actions on platelets (shape change and accelerated aggregation) mediated by interaction with platelet 5-HT$_{2A}$ receptors, release of endothelium-derived relaxing factor (EDRF) mediated by 5-HT$_1$-like receptors on vascular endothelium, and contraction of vascular smooth muscle mediated by 5-HT$_{2A}$ receptors. These influences act in concert with many other mediators that are not shown to promote thrombus and hemostasis.

of Na$^+$-dependent 5-HT-uptake by platelets provides a sensitive assay for 5-HT-uptake inhibitors.

 The main function of platelets is to plug holes in injured endothelial cells. Conversely, the functional integrity of the endothelium is critical for the action of platelets (Furchgott and Vanhoutte, 1989). The endothelial surface is exposed constantly to platelets, because the shear forces of circulating blood favor centrifugal stratification of platelets (Gibbons and Dzau, 1994). Release of endothelium-derived relaxing factor (EDRF; nitric oxide and perhaps other components) antagonizes the vasoconstrictor action of thromboxane and 5-HT (Furchgott and Vanhoutte, 1989; Figure 11–4). The net effect of platelet aggregation is critically determined by the functional status of the endothelium (Hawiger, 1992; Ware and Heistad, 1993). When platelets make contact with injured endothelium, they release substances that promote platelet adhesion and release of 5-HT, including ADP, thrombin, and thromboxane A$_2$ (*see* Chapters 26 and 55). 5-HT binding to platelet 5-HT$_{2A}$ receptors elicits a weak aggregation response that is markedly enhanced in the presence of collagen. If the damaged blood vessel is injured to a depth where vascular smooth muscle is exposed, 5-HT exerts a direct constrictor effect, thereby promoting hemostasis. Locally released autacoids (thromboxane A$_2$, kinins, and vasoactive peptides) enhance this action. In atherosclerosis, thrombus formation is potentiated by the destruction of endothelium and, therefore, a deficiency of EDRF. An amplification cycle involving 5-HT in thrombus formation is induced. In addition to atherosclerosis, a cycle of this kind may be involved in other vascular diseases including Raynaud's phenomenon and coronary vasospasm.

Cardiovascular System. The classical response of blood vessels to 5-HT is contraction, particularly in the splanchnic, renal, pulmonary, and cerebral vasculatures. This response also occurs in bronchial smooth muscle. 5-HT also induces a variety of responses by the heart that are the result of activation of 5-HT-receptor subtypes, stimulation or inhibition of autonomic activity, or dominance of reflex responses to 5-HT (Saxena and Villalón, 1990). Thus, 5-HT has positive inotropic and chronotropic actions on the heart that may be blunted by simultaneous stimulation of afferent nerves from baroreceptors and chemoreceptors. An effect on vagus nerve endings elicits the Bezold-Jarisch reflex, causing extreme bradycardia and hypotension. The local response of arterial blood vessels to 5-HT also may be inhibitory, the result of the release of EDRF and prostaglandins and blockade of norepinephrine release from sympathetic nerves. On the other hand, 5-HT amplifies the local constrictor action of norepinephrine, angiotensin II, and histamine, which reinforce the hemostatic response to 5-HT (*see* Gershon, 1991).

Gastrointestinal Tract. Enterochromaffin cells in the mucosa appear to be the location of the synthesis and most of the storage of 5-HT in the body and are the source of circulating 5-HT. 5-HT released from these cells enters the portal vein and is subsequently metabolized by MAO-A in the liver (Gillis, 1985). 5-HT that survives oxidation in the liver is rapidly removed by the endothelium of lung capillaries and then inactivated by MAO. 5-HT released by mechanical or vagal stimulation also acts locally to regulate gastrointestinal function. Motility of gastric and intestinal smooth muscle may be either enhanced or inhibited (Dhasmana *et al.*, 1993) *via* at least six subtypes of 5-HT receptors (Table 11–2). The stimulatory response occurs at nerve endings on longitudinal and circular enteric muscle (5-HT$_4$), at postsynaptic cells of the enteric ganglia (5-HT$_3$ and 5-HT$_{1P}$), and by direct effects of 5-HT on the smooth muscle cells (5-HT$_{2A}$ in intestine and 5-HT$_{2B}$ in stomach fundus). In esophagus, 5-HT acting at 5-HT$_4$ receptors causes either relaxation or contraction, depending on the species. Abundant 5-HT$_3$ receptors on vagal and other afferent neurons and on enterochromaffin cells play a pivotal role in emesis (Grunberg and Hesketh, 1993). Serotonergic terminals have been described in the myenteric plexus. Release of enteric 5-HT occurs in response to acetylcholine, noradrenergic nerve stimulation, increases in intraluminal pressure, and lowered pH (Gershon, 1991), triggering peristaltic contraction.

Central Nervous System. A multitude of brain functions are influenced by 5-HT, including sleep, cognition, sensory perception, motor activity, temperature regulation, nociception, appetite, sexual behavior, and hormone secretion. All of the cloned 5-HT receptors are expressed in the brain, often in overlapping areas. Although patterns of 5-HT receptor expression in individual neurons have not been defined, it is likely that multiple 5-HT receptor subtypes with similar or opposing actions are expressed in individual neurons, leading to a tremendous diversity of actions.

 The principal cell bodies of 5-HT neurons are located in raphe nuclei of the brainstem and project throughout the brain and spinal cord (*see* Chapter 12). In addition to being released at discrete synapses, evidence suggests that release of serotonin also occurs at sites of axonal swelling, termed *varicosities,* which do not form distinct synaptic contacts (Descarries *et al.*,

Table 11–2

Some Actions of 5-HT in the Gastrointestinal Tract

SITE	RESPONSE	RECEPTOR
Enterochromaffin cells	Release of 5-HT	$5\text{-}HT_3$
	Inhibition of 5-HT release	$5\text{-}HT_4$
Enteric ganglion cells (presynaptic)	Release of ACh	$5\text{-}HT_4$
	Inhibition of ACh release	$5\text{-}HT_{1P}$, $5\text{-}HT_{1A}$
Enteric ganglion cells (postsynaptic)	Fast depolarization	$5\text{-}HT_3$
	Slow depolarization	$5\text{-}HT_{1P}$
Smooth muscle, intestinal	Contraction	$5\text{-}HT_{2A}$
Smooth muscle, stomach fundus	Contraction	$5\text{-}HT_{2B}$
Smooth muscle, esophagus	Contraction	$5\text{-}HT_4$

NOTE: ACh, acetylcholine.

1990). 5-HT released at nonsynaptic varicosities is thought to diffuse to outlying targets, rather than acting on discrete synaptic targets. Such nonsynaptic release with an ensuing widespread influence of 5-HT is consistent with a longstanding belief that 5-HT acts as a neuromodulator as well as a neurotransmitter (*see* Chapter 12).

Serotonergic nerve terminals contain all of the proteins needed to synthesize 5-HT from L-tryptophan (*see* Figure 11–2). Newly formed 5-HT is rapidly accumulated in synaptic vesicles, where it is protected from MAO. 5-HT released by nerve-impulse flow is reaccumulated into the presynaptic terminal by a Na^+-dependent carrier, the 5-HT transporter. Presynaptic reuptake is a highly efficient mechanism for terminating the action of 5-HT released by nerve-impulse flow. MAO localized in postsynaptic elements and surrounding cells rapidly inactivates 5-HT that escapes reuptake.

Electrophysiology.   The physiological consequences of 5-HT release vary with the brain area and the neuronal element involved, as well as with the population of 5-HT receptor subtype(s) expressed (*see* Aghajanian, 1995). 5-HT has direct excitatory and inhibitory actions (Table 11–3), which may occur in the same preparation but with distinct temporal patterns. For example, in hippocampal neurons, 5-HT elicits hyperpolarization mediated by $5\text{-}HT_{1A}$ receptors followed by a slow depolarization mediated by $5\text{-}HT_4$ receptors.

Table 11–3

Physiological Effects of Serotonin Receptors

SUBTYPE	RESPONSE
$5\text{-}HT_{1A,B}$	Increase K^+ conductance Hyperpolarization
$5\text{-}HT_{2A}$	Decrease K^+ conductance Slow depolarization
$5\text{-}HT_3$	Gating of Na^+, K^+ Fast depolarization
$5\text{-}HT_4$	Decrease K^+ conductance Slow depolarization

$5\text{-}HT_{1A}$ receptor–induced membrane hyperpolarization and reduction in input resistance is the result of an increase in K^+ conductance. These ionic effects, which are blocked by pertussis toxin, are independent of cyclic AMP, suggesting that $5\text{-}HT_{1A}$ receptors couple directly, *via* G_i-like G proteins, to receptor-operated K^+ channels (Andrade *et al.*, 1986). Somatodendritic $5\text{-}HT_{1A}$ receptors on raphe cells also elicit a K^+-dependent hyperpolarization. The G protein involved is pertussis toxin–sensitive, but the K^+ current apparently is different from the current elicited at postsynaptic $5\text{-}HT_{1A}$ receptors in the hippocampus. The precise signaling mechanism involved in inhibition of 5-HT release by the $5\text{-}HT_{1D}$ autoreceptor is not known, although inhibition of voltage-gated calcium channels likely contributes to the mechanism.

Slow depolarization induced by $5\text{-}HT_{2A}$-receptor activation in areas such as the prefrontal cortex, nucleus accumbens, and facial motor nucleus involves a decrease in K^+ conductance (Aghajanian *et al.*, 1987). A second, distinct mechanism involving Ca^{2+}-activated membrane currents enhances neuronal excitability and potentiates the response to excitatory signals such as glutamate. The role of the phosphoinositide hydrolysis signaling cascade in these physiological actions of $5\text{-}HT_{2A}$ receptors has not been clearly defined. It appears that in areas where $5\text{-}HT_1$ and $5\text{-}HT_{2A}$ receptors coexist, the effect of 5-HT reflects a combination of the two opposing responses, with a prominent $5\text{-}HT_1$ receptor–mediated hyperpolarization and an opposing $5\text{-}HT_{2A}$ receptor–mediated depolarization. When $5\text{-}HT_{2A}$ receptors are blocked, hyperpolarization is enhanced. In many cortical areas, $5\text{-}HT_{2A}$ receptors are localized on GABAergic interneurons and on pyramidal cells. Activation of interneurons enhances GABA (gamma-aminobutyric acid) release, which secondarily slows the firing rate of pyramidal cells. Thus, there is the potential for the $5\text{-}HT_{2A}$ receptor to regulate differentially cortical pyramidal cells, depending on the specific target cells (interneurons *versus* pyramidal cells). $5\text{-}HT_{2C}$ receptors have been shown to depress a K^+ current in *Xenopus* oocytes expressing the cloned receptor mRNA; a similar action has not been definitively identified in the brain. The $5\text{-}HT_4$ receptor, which is coupled to activation of adenylyl cyclase, also elicits a slow neuronal depolarization mediated by a decrease in K^+ conductance. It is not clear why two distinct 5-HT receptor families linked to different signaling pathways are capable of eliciting a common neurophysiological action. Yet another receptor, the 5-HT$_{1P}$ receptor, elicits a slow depolarization. This receptor, which couples to activation of adenylyl cyclase, is restricted to the enteric nervous system and has a unique pharmacological profile (Gershon, 1991).

The fast depolarization elicited by 5-HT$_3$ receptors reflects direct gating of an ion channel intrinsic to the receptor structure itself. The 5-HT$_3$ receptor–induced inward current has the characteristics of a cation-selective ligand-operated channel. Membrane depolarization is mediated by simultaneous increases in Na$^+$ and K$^+$ conductance (Higashi and Nishi, 1982). Patch–clamp analyses confirmed that the 5-HT$_3$ receptor functions as a receptor–ion channel complex, comparable to the nicotinic cholinergic receptor. 5-HT$_3$ receptors have been characterized in the CNS and in sympathetic ganglia, primary afferent parasympathetic and sympathetic nerves, enteric neurons, and neuronally derived clonal cell lines, such as NG108-15 cells. The pharmacological properties of 5-HT$_3$ receptors, which are different from those of other 5-HT receptors, suggest that multiple 5-HT$_3$ receptor subtypes may exist and may correspond to different combinations of subunits (see Chapter 12).

Behavior.   The behavioral alterations elicited by drugs that interact with 5-HT receptors are extremely diverse. Many animal behavioral models for initial assessment of agonist and antagonist properties of drugs depend on aberrant motor or reflex responses, such as startle reflexes, hind-limb abduction, head twitches, and other stereotypical behaviors. Operant behavioral paradigms, such as drug discrimination, provide models of specific 5-HT receptor activation and are useful for exploring the action of CNS-active drugs, including agents that interact with 5-HT. For example, investigations of the mechanism of action of hallucinogenic drugs have relied heavily on drug discrimination (as discussed below). The following discussion focuses on animal models that may relate to pathological conditions in human beings and will not attempt to cover the voluminous literature dealing with 5-HT and behavior. *See* Glennon and Lucki, 1988; Zifa and Fillion, 1992; and Koek *et al.,* 1992, for excellent reviews on this topic.

Sleep-Wake Cycle.   Control of the sleep-wake cycle is one of the first behaviors in which a role for 5-HT was identified. Following the pioneering work in cats by Mouret *et al.* (1967), many studies showed that depletion of 5-HT with *p*-chlorophenylalanine elicited insomnia, which was reversed by administration of the 5-HT precursor 5-hydroxytryptophan. Conversely, treatment with L-tryptophan or with nonselective 5-HT agonists accelerated sleep onset and prolonged total sleep time. 5-HT antagonists were reported to both increase and decrease slow-wave sleep, probably reflecting interacting or opposing roles for subtypes of 5-HT receptors (for review, *see* Wasquier and Dugovic, 1990). One relatively consistent finding reported in human beings as well as in laboratory animals is an increase in slow-wave sleep following administration of a selective 5-HT$_{2A/2C}$ receptor antagonist such as ritanserin.

Aggression and Impulsivity.   Results of studies in laboratory animals and in human beings suggest that 5-HT serves a critical role in aggression and impulsivity. Many human studies reveal a correlation between low cerebrospinal fluid 5-HIAA and violent impulsivity and aggression (Brown and Linnoila, 1990). As an example, low 5-HIAA is associated with violent suicide acts but not with suicidal ideation *per se* (Virkkunen *et al.,* 1995). As with so many of the effects of 5-HT, pharma-

cological studies of aggressive behavior in laboratory animals have not been definitive, although a role for 5-HT is suggested. Two genetic studies have reinforced and amplified this notion. The 5-HT$_{1B}$ receptor was the first 5-HT receptor to be investigated using gene targeting *via* homologous recombination to eliminate the gene encoding the 5-HT$_{1B}$ receptor protein in mice (Saudau *et al.,* 1994). These so-called 5-HT$_{1B}$ "knock-out" mice develop extreme aggression, suggesting either a role for 5-HT$_{1B}$ receptors in the development of neuronal pathways important in aggression or a direct role in the mediation of aggressive behavior. A genetic study in human beings identified a point mutation in the gene coding for MAO-A that was associated with extreme aggressiveness and mental retardation (Brunner *et al.,* 1993), and this has been confirmed in mutant mice lacking MAO-A (Cases *et al.,* 1995). These genetic studies add credence to the proposition that abnormalities in 5-HT are correlated with aggressive behaviors.

Anxiety and Depression.   The effects of 5-HT-active drugs, like the selective serotonin-reuptake inhibitors (SSRIs), in anxiety and depressive disorders strongly suggest an effect of 5-HT in the neurochemical mediation of these disorders. However, 5-HT-related drugs with clinical effects in anxiety and depression have varied effects in classical animal models of these disorders, depending on factors such as the experimental paradigm as well as animal species and strain. For example, the effective anxiolytic *buspirone* (BUSPAR, *see* Chapter 19), a 5-HT$_{1A}$-receptor partial agonist, does not reduce anxiety in classical approach-avoidance paradigms that were instrumental in development of anxiolytic benzodiazepines. However, buspirone and other 5-HT$_{1A}$-receptor agonists are effective in other animal behavioral tests used to predict anxiolytic effects (Barrett and Vanover, 1993). Further, recent studies in 5-HT$_{1A}$-receptor "knockout" mice suggest a role for this receptor in anxiety and, possibly, depression (Parks *et al.,* 1998; Ramboz *et al.,* 1998). Agonists of certain 5-HT receptors, including 5-HT$_{2A}$, 5-HT$_{2C}$, and 5-HT$_3$ receptors [*e.g., m*-chlorophenylpiperazine (mCPP)], have been shown to have anxiogenic properties in laboratory-animal and human studies. Similarly, these receptors have been implicated in the animal models of depression, such as learned helplessness.

An impressive finding in human beings with depression is the abrupt reversal of the antidepressant effects of drugs, such as SSRIs, by manipulations that rapidly reduce the amount of 5-HT in brain. These approaches include administration of *p*-chlorophenylalanine or a tryptophan-free drink containing large quantities of neutral amino acids (Delgado *et al.,* 1990). Curiously, this kind of 5-HT depletion has not been shown to worsen depression or induce depression in nondepressed subjects, suggesting that the continued presence of 5-HT is required to maintain the effects of these drugs. This clinical finding adds credence to somewhat less convincing neurochemical findings that suggest a role for 5-HT in the pathogenesis of depression.

Pharmacological Manipulation of the Amount of 5-HT in Tissues

Experimental strategies for evaluating the role of 5-HT depend on techniques that manipulate tissue levels of 5-HT or block 5-HT receptors. Until recently, manipulation of the levels of endogenous 5-HT was the most commonly used strategy, because the actions of 5-HT antagonists were poorly understood.

Tryptophan hydroxylase, the rate-limiting enzyme in 5-HT synthesis, is a vulnerable site. A diet low in tryptophan reduces the concentration of brain 5-HT; conversely, ingestion of a tryptophan load increases levels of 5-HT in the brain. In addition, administration of a tryptophan hydroxylase inhibitor causes a profound depletion of 5-HT. The most widely used selective tryptophan hydroxylase inhibitor is *p*-chlorophenylalanine, which acts irreversibly. *p*-Chlorophenylalanine produces profound, long-lasting depletion of 5-HT levels with no change in levels of catecholamines.

p-Chloroamphetamine and other halogenated amphetamines promote 5-HT release from platelets and neurons. A rapid release of 5-HT is followed by a prolonged and selective depletion of 5-HT in brain. The halogenated amphetamines are valuable experimental tools and two of them, *fenfluramine* and *dexfenfluramine,* were used clinically to reduce appetite. These drugs were withdrawn from the United States market in 1998 after there were reports of cardiac toxicity associated with their use. The mechanism of action of this class of drugs is controversial. A profound reduction in levels of 5-HT in the brain lasts for weeks and is accompanied by an equivalent loss of proteins selectively localized in 5-HT neurons (5-HT transporter and tryptophan hydroxylase), suggesting that the halogenated amphetamines have a neurotoxic action. Despite these long-lasting, biochemical deficits, neuroanatomical signs of neuronal death are not readily apparent. Another class of compounds, ring-substituted tryptamine derivatives such as 5,7-dihydroxytryptamine (*see* structure in Figure 11–1), leads to unequivocal degeneration of 5-HT neurons. In adult animals, 5,7-dihydroxytryptamine selectively destroys serotonergic axon terminals; the remaining intact cell bodies allow eventual regeneration of axon terminals. In newborn animals, degeneration is permanent, because 5,7-dihydroxytryptamine destroys serotonergic cell bodies as well as axon terminals.

Another highly specific mechanism for altering synaptic availability of 5-HT is inhibition of presynaptic reaccumulation of neuronally released 5-HT. SSRIs, such as *fluoxetine* (PROZAC), potentiate the action of 5-HT released by neuronal activity. When coadministered with L-5-hydroxytryptophan, SSRIs elicit a profound activation of serotonergic responses. SSRIs are one of the newest and most widely used treatments for endogenous depression (*see* Chapter 19). *Sibutramine* (MERIDIA), an inhibitor of the reuptake of 5-HT, norepinephrine, and dopamine,

is used as an appetite suppressant in the management of obesity. The drug is converted to two active metabolites that probably account for its therapeutic effects. Which neurotransmitter is primarily responsible for sibutramine's effects in obese patients is unclear.

Nonselective treatments that alter 5-HT levels include MAO inhibitors and reserpine. MAO inhibitors block the principal route of degradation, thereby increasing levels of 5-HT, whereas reserpine treatment releases intraneuronal stores with subsequent depletion of 5-HT. These treatments profoundly alter levels of 5-HT throughout the body. However, because comparable changes occur in the levels of catecholamines, reserpine and MAO inhibitors are of limited utility as research tools. Both, at one time or another, have been useful in the treatment of mental diseases: reserpine as an antipsychotic drug (*see* Chapter 20) and MAO inhibitors as antidepressants (*see* Chapter 19).

5-HT-RECEPTOR AGONISTS AND ANTAGONISTS

5-HT-Receptor Agonists

Direct-acting 5-HT-receptor agonists have widely different chemical structures, as well as diverse pharmacological properties (*see* Table 11–4). This diversity is not surprising in light of the number of 5-HT-receptor subtypes. $5-HT_{1A}$ receptor–selective agonists have helped elucidate the functions of this receptor in the brain and have resulted in a new class of antianxiety drugs including *buspirone, gepirone,* and *ipsaperone* (*see* Chapter 19). $5-HT_{1D}$ receptor–selective agonists, such as *sumatriptan,* have unique properties that result in constriction of intracranial blood vessels. Sumatriptan was first in a series of new serotonin-receptor agonists available for treatment of acute migraine attacks (*see* below). Other such agents now FDA-approved in the United States for the acute treatment of migraine include *zolmitriptan* (ZOMIG), *naratriptan* (AMERGE), and *rizatriptan* (MAXALT), all of which are selective for $5-HT_{1D}$ and $5-HT_{1B}$ receptors. A large series of $5-HT_4$ receptor–selective agonists have been developed or are being developed for the treatment of disorders of the gastrointestinal tract (*see* Chapter 38). These classes of selective 5-HT-receptor agonists are discussed in more detail in the chapters that deal directly with treatment of the relevant pathological conditions.

5-HT-Receptor Agonists and Migraine.   Migraine headache afflicts 10% to 20% of the population, producing a morbidity estimated to be approximately sixty-four million

Table 11–4
Serotonergic Drugs: Primary Actions and Clinical Uses

RECEPTOR	ACTION	DRUG EXAMPLES	CLINICAL DISORDER
5-HT$_{1A}$	Partial agonist	Buspirone, ipsaperone	Anxiety, depression
5-HT$_{1D}$	Agonist	Sumatriptan	Migraine
5-HT$_{2A/2C}$	Antagonist	Methysergide, trazodone, risperidone, ketanserin	Migraine, depression, schizophrenia
5-HT$_3$	Antagonist	Ondansetron	Chemotherapy-induced emesis
5-HT$_4$	Agonist	Cisapride	Gastrointestinal disorders
5-HT transporter	Inhibitor	Fluoxetine, sertraline	Depression, obsessive-compulsive disorder, panic disorder, social phobia, posttraumatic stress disorder

workdays per year in the United States. Although migraine is a specific neurological syndrome, there is a wide variety of manifestations. The principal types are: migraine without aura (common migraine); migraine with aura (classic migraine), which includes subclasses of migraine with typical aura, migraine with prolonged aura, migraine without headache, and migraine with acute-onset aura; and several other rarer types. Auras also may appear without a subsequent headache. Premonitory aura may begin as long as 24 hours before the onset of pain and often is accompanied by photophobia, hyperacusis, polyuria, and diarrhea, and by disturbances of mood and appetite. A migraine attack may last for hours or days and be followed by prolonged pain-free intervals. The frequency of migraine attacks is extremely variable, but usually ranges from one to two a year to one to four per month.

The therapy of headaches classified as migraine is complicated by the variability of the responses among and within individual patients and by the lack of a firm experimental foundation of the pathophysiology of the syndrome. The efficacy of antimigraine drugs varies with the absence or presence of aura, duration of the headache, its severity and intensity, and as yet undefined environmental and genetic factors (Deleu *et al.,* 1998). A rather vague and inconsistent pathophysiological characteristic of migraine is the spreading depression of neural impulses from a focal point of vasoconstriction followed by vasodilation (Olesen *et al.,* 1981). However, it is unlikely that vasoconstriction followed by vasodilation (spreading depression) or vasodilation alone accounts for the local edema and focal tenderness often observed in migraine patients.

Consistent with the hypothesis that 5-HT is a key mediator in the pathogenesis of migraine, 5-HT-receptor agonists have become the mainstay for acute treatment of migraine headaches. This hypothesis is based on evi-

dence obtained in laboratory experiments and on the following evidence obtained in human beings: (1) Plasma and platelet concentrations of 5-HT vary with the different phases of the migraine attack. (2) Urinary concentrations of 5-HT and its metabolites are elevated during most migraine attacks. (3) Migraine may be precipitated by agents such as reserpine and fenfluramine that release biogenic amines, including serotonin, from intracellular storage sites.

5-HT$_1$-Receptor Agonists: The Triptans.   The introduction of *sumatriptan* (IMITREX), *zolmitriptan* (ZOMIG), *naratriptan* (AMERGE), and *rizatriptan* (MAXALT and MAXALT-MLT) in the therapy of migraine has led to significant progress in preclinical and clinical research on migraine. At the scientific level, the selective pharmacological effects of these agents, dubbed the *triptans,* at 5-HT$_1$ receptors have led to new insights into the pathophysiology of migraine. At the clinical level, the drugs are effective, acute antimigraine agents. Their ability to decrease, rather than exacerbate, the nausea and vomiting of migraine is an important advance in the treatment of the condition.

History.   The development of sumatriptan was the first experimentally based approach to identify and develop a novel therapy for migraine. In 1972, Humphrey and colleagues initiated a long-term project aimed at identifying novel therapeutic agents in the treatment of migraine (*see* Humphrey *et al.,* 1990). The goal of this project was to develop selective vasoconstrictors of the extracranial circulation based on the theories of the etiology of migraine prevalent in the early 1970s. Humphrey and his colleagues focused on the identification of 5-HT receptors in the carotid vasculature based on the evidence that the efficacy of traditional antimigraine drugs such as ergotamine derived from their ability to induce vasoconstriction of the carotid arteriovenous anastomoses, presumably *via* their effects on 5-HT receptors (Saxena, 1978). The synthesis of many novel tryptamine analogs was followed by determination of their

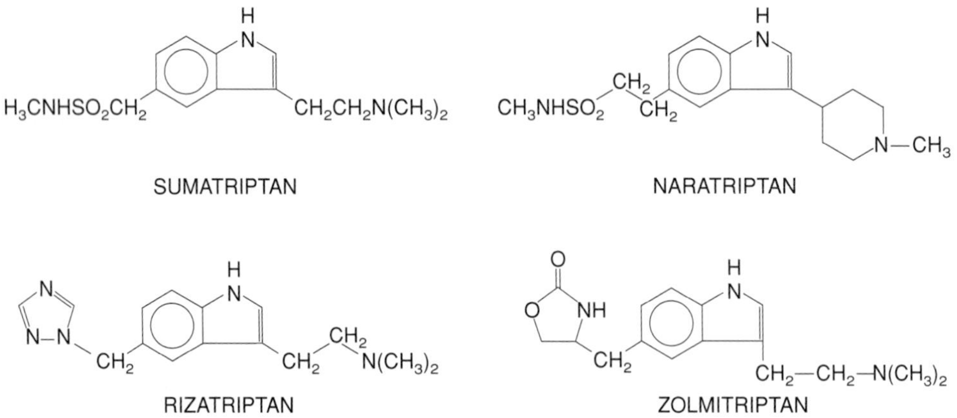

Figure 11–5. Structures of the triptans (selective 5-HT₁-receptor agonists).

actions on *in vitro* vascular preparations and in intact animals. Sumatriptan, first synthesized in 1984, potently contracted the dog isolated saphenous vein (Humphrey *et al.,* 1988), a vessel believed to contain the novel 5-HT receptor located in the carotid circulation. Sumatriptan became available for clinical use in the United States in 1992, and the other three currently available triptans were approved by the Food and Drug Administration in the late 1990s (*see* Limmroth and Diener, 1998).

Chemistry. The triptans are derivatives of indole, with substituents on the 3 and 5 positions. Their structures are given in Figure 11–5.

Pharmacological Properties. In contrast to ergot alkaloids (*see* below), the pharmacological effects of the triptans appear to be limited to the 5-HT₁ family of receptors, providing evidence that this receptor subclass plays an important role in the acute relief of a migraine attack. The triptans are much more selective agents than are ergot alkaloids in that they interact potently with 5-HT₁D and 5-HT₁B receptors and have a low or no affinity for other subtypes of 5-HT receptors. The triptans are essentially inactive at α_1- and α_2-adrenergic, β-adrenergic, dopamine, muscarinic cholinergic, and benzodiazepine receptors. Clinically effective doses of the triptans and ergot alkaloids do not correlate well with their affinity for either 5-HT₁A or 5-HT₁E receptors but do correlate well with their affinities for both 5-HT₁B and 5-HT₁D receptors. Current data are thus consistent with the hypothesis that 5-HT₁B and/or 5-HT₁D receptors are the most likely receptor site(s) involved in the mechanism of action of acute antimigraine drugs.

Mechanism of Action. Two hypotheses have been proposed to explain the efficacy of 5-HT₁B/₁D receptor agonists in migraine. One hypothesis implicates the ability of these receptors to cause constriction of intracranial blood vessels including arteriovenous anastomoses. According to a prominent pathophysiological model of migraine, as yet unknown events lead to the abnormal dilation of carotid arteriovenous anastomoses in the head. As much as 80% of carotid arterial blood flow has been reported to be "shunted" *via* these anastomoses, located mainly in the cranial skin and ears, diverting blood from the capillary beds, thus producing cerebral ischemia and hypoxia. Based on this model, an effective antimigraine agent would close the shunts and restore blood flow to the brain. Indeed, ergotamine, dihydroergotamine, and sumatriptan share the ability to produce this vascular effect with a pharmacological specificity that mirrors the effects of these agents on 5-HT₁B and 5-HT₁D receptor subtypes (den Boer *et al.,* 1991).

An alternative hypothesis concerning the significance of one or more 5-HT₁ receptors in migraine pathophysiology relates to the observation that both 5-HT₁B and 5-HT₁D receptors serve as presynaptic autoreceptors, modulating neurotransmitter release from neuronal terminals (*see* Figure 11–3). 5-HT₁ agonists may block the release of proinflammatory neuropeptides at the level of the nerve terminal in the perivascular space. Indeed, ergotamine, dihydroergotamine, and sumatriptan are able to block the development of neurogenic plasma extravasation in dura mater that follows depolarization of perivascular axons following capsaicin injection or unilateral electrical stimulation of the trigeminal nerve (Moskowitz, 1992). The ability of potent 5-HT₁-receptor agonists to inhibit endogenous neurotransmitter release in the perivascular space could account for their efficacy in the acute treatment of migraine.

Absorption, Fate, and Excretion. When given subcutaneously, sumatriptan reaches its peak plasma concentration in approximately 12 minutes. Following oral administration, peak plasma concentrations occur within 1 to 2 hours. Bioavailability following the subcutaneous route of administration is approximately 97%; after oral administration or nasal spray, bioavailability is only 14% to 17%. The elimination half-life is approximately 1 to 2 hours. Sumatriptan is metabolized predominantly by MAO-A, and its metabolites are excreted in the urine.

Zolmitriptan reaches its peak plasma concentration 1.5 to 2 hours after oral administration. Its bioavailability is about 40% following oral ingestion. Zolmitriptan is converted to an active N-desmethyl metabolite, which has severalfold higher affinity for 5-HT_{1B} and 5-HT_{1D} receptors than does the parent drug. Both the metabolite and the parent drug have half-lives of 2 to 3 hours.

Naratriptan, administered orally, reaches its peak plasma concentration in 2 to 3 hours and has an absolute bioavailability of about 70%. It is the longest acting of the triptans, having a half-life of about 6 hours. Fifty percent of an administered dose of naratriptan is excreted unchanged in the urine, and about 30% is excreted as products of cytochrome P450 oxidation.

Rizatriptan has an oral absolute bioavailability of about 45% and reaches peak plasma levels within 1 to 1.5 hours after oral ingestion of tablets of the drug. An orally disintegrating dosage form has a somewhat slower rate of absorption, yielding peak plasma levels of the drug 1.6 to 2.5 hours after administration. The principal route of metabolism of rizatriptan is *via* oxidative deamination by MAO-A.

Plasma protein-binding of the triptans ranges from about 14% (sumatriptan, rizatriptan) to 30% (naratriptan).

Adverse Effects and Contraindications.   Rare but serious cardiac events have been associated with the administration of 5-HT_1 agonists, including coronary artery vasospasm, transient myocardial ischemia, atrial and ventricular arrhythmias, and myocardial infarction. Most such events have occurred in patients with risk factors for coronary artery disease. In general, however, only minor side effects are seen with the triptans in the acute treatment of migraine. As many as 83% of patients experience at least one side effect after subcutaneous injection of sumatriptan (Simmons and Blakeborough, 1994). After subcutaneous injection, a majority of patients report transient mild pain, stinging, or burning sensations at the site of injection. The most common side effect of sumatriptan nasal spray is a bitter taste. Orally administered triptans can cause paresthesia; asthenia and fatigue; flushing; feelings of pressure, tightness, or pain in the chest, neck, and jaw; drowsiness; dizziness; nausea; and sweating.

The triptans are contraindicated in patients who have a history of ischemic or vasospastic coronary artery disease, cerebrovascular or peripheral vascular disease, or other significant cardiovascular diseases. These drugs also are contraindicated in patients with uncontrolled hypertension. Naratriptan is contraindicated in patients with severe renal or hepatic impairment. Rizatriptan should be used with caution in patients with renal or hepatic disease, but it is not contraindicated in such patients. Sumatriptan, rizatriptan, and zolmitriptan are contraindicated in patients who are taking monoamine oxidase inhibitors.

Use in Treatment of Migraine.   The triptans are effective in the acute treatment of migraine (with or without aura), but are not intended for use in prophylaxis of migraine. Treatment with these agents should begin as soon as possible after onset of a migraine attack. Oral dosage forms of the triptans are the most convenient to use, but they may not be practical in patients experiencing nausea and vomiting with migraine attack. Approximately 70% of individuals report significant headache relief from a 6-mg subcutaneous dose of sumatriptan. This dose may be repeated once within a 24-hour period if the first dose does not relieve the headache. An oral formulation and a nasal spray of sumatriptan also are available. The onset of action is as early as 15 minutes with the nasal spray. The recommended oral dose of sumatriptan is 25 to 100 mg, which may be repeated after 2 hours up to a total dose of 200 mg over a 24-hour period. When administered by nasal spray, from 5 to 20 mg of sumatriptan is recommended. The dose can be repeated after 2 hours up to a maximum dose of 40 mg over a 24-hour period. Zolmitriptan is given orally in a 1.25- to 2.5-mg dose, which can be repeated after 2 hours, up to a maximum dose of 10 mg over 24 hours, if the migraine attack persists. Naratriptan is given orally in a 1 to 2.5-mg dose, which should not be repeated until 4 hours after the previous dose. The maximum dose over a 24-hour period should not exceed 5 mg. The recommended oral dose of rizatriptan is 5 to 10 mg. The dose can be repeated after 2 hours up to a maximum dose of 30 mg over a 24-hour period. The safety of treating more than 3 or 4 headaches over a 30-day period with triptans has not been established. Because triptans may cause an acute, although usually small, increase in blood pressure, they should not be given to individuals with uncontrolled hypertension. Triptans should not be used concurrently with (or within 24 hours of) an ergot derivative (*see* below) nor should more than one triptan be used concurrently or within 24 hours of each other.

Ergot and the Ergot Alkaloids.   The dramatic effect of ergot ingested during pregnancy has been recognized for more than 2000 years. Early in the 20th century, the isolation and chemical identification of the active principles of ergot were accomplished, and detailed study of their biological activity was begun. The elucidation of the constituents of ergot and their complex actions was an important chapter in the evolution of modern pharmacology. The ergot alkaloids are therefore discussed here, even though the very complexity of their actions limits their therapeutic uses (Table 11–5). The pharmacological effects of the ergot alkaloids are varied and complex; however, in general, the effects result from their actions as partial agonists or antagonists at adrenergic, dopaminergic, and

Table 11–5
Pharmacological Actions of Selected Ergot Alkaloids

Compound	INTERACTIONS WITH TRYPTAMINERGIC RECEPTORS	Pharmacological Actions INTERACTIONS WITH DOPAMINERGIC RECEPTORS	INTERACTIONS WITH α-ADRENERGIC RECEPTORS
Ergotamine	Partial agonist in certain blood vessels; nonselective antagonist in various smooth muscles; poor agonist/antagonist in CNS	No notable actions on central or peripheral structures, but high emetic potency after intravenous administration	Partial agonist and antagonist in blood vessels and various smooth muscles; mainly antagonist in peripheral and central nervous systems
Dihydro-ergotamine	Partial agonist and antagonist in a few smooth muscles; may be agonist in lateral geniculate nucleus	Nonselective antagonist in sympathetic ganglia; low emetic potency	Partial agonist in veins; antagonist in blood vessels, various smooth muscles, and peripheral and central nervous systems
Bromocriptine	Only a few weak antagonistic actions reported	Partial agonist and antagonist in various areas of CNS; presumed agonist in inhibiting secretion of prolactin; less emetic potency than ergotamine	No agonistic effects; somewhat less potent antagonist than dihydro-ergotamine in various tissues
Ergonovine and methyl ergonovine	Partial agonists in human umbilical and placental blood vessels; selective and fairly potent antagonists in various smooth muscles; partial agonists and antagonists in some areas of CNS	Weak antagonists in certain blood vessels; partial agonists and antagonists in various areas of CNS; less potent than bromocriptine in producing emesis or inhibiting secretion of prolactin	Partial agonists in blood vessels (less than ergotamine); little antagonistic action
Methysergide	Partial agonist in certain blood vessels and areas of CNS; selective and very potent antagonist in many tissues and areas of CNS	Little evidence for agonistic or antagonistic activity; no emetic activity	Little or no agonistic or antagonistic action

Table 11-6
Natural and Semisynthetic Ergot Alkaloids

	A. AMINE ALKALOIDS AND CONGENERS		B. AMINO ACID ALKALOIDS		

ALKALOID	X	Y	ALKALOID §	R(2′)	R′(5′)
d-Lysergic acid	—COOH	—H	Ergotamine	—CH₃	—CH₂—phenyl
d-Isolysergic acid	—H	—COOH	Ergosine	—CH₃	—CH₂CH(CH₃)₂
d-Lysergic acid diethylamide (LSD)	—C—N(CH₂CH₃)₂ (C=O)	—H	Ergostine	—CH₂CH₃	—CH₂—phenyl
			Ergotoxine group:		
Ergonovine (ergometrine)	—C—NH—CHCH₂OH / CH₃ (C=O)	—H	Ergocornine	—CH(CH₃)₂	—CH(CH₃)₂
			Ergocristine	—CH(CH₃)₂	—CH₂—phenyl
			α-Ergocryptine	—CH(CH₃)₂	—CH₂CH(CH₃)₂
Methylergonovine	—C—NH—CH / CH₂CH₃ CH₂OH (C=O)	—H	β-Ergocryptine	—CH(CH₃)₂	—CHCH₂CH₃ CH₃
Methysergide *	—C—NH—CH / CH₂CH₃ CH₂OH (C=O)	—H	Bromocriptine ¶	—CH(CH₃)₂	—CH₂CH(CH₃)₂
Lisuride	—H	—NH—C—N(CH₂CH₃)₂ (C=O)			
Lysergol	—CH₂OH	—H			
Lergotrile †,‡	—CH₂CN	—H			
Metergoline *,†	—CH₂—NH—C—O—CH₂—phenyl (C=O)	—H			

* Contains methyl substitution at N 1.
† Contains hydrogen atoms at C 9 and C 10.
‡ Contains chlorine atom at C 2.

§ Dihydro derivatives contain hydrogen atoms at C 9 and C 10.
¶ Contains bromine atom at C 2.

serotonergic receptors (*see* also Chapter 10). The spectrum of effects depends on the agent, dosage, species, tissue, physiological and endocrinological state, and experimental conditions.

History. Ergot is the product of a fungus (*Claviceps purpurea*) that grows on rye and other grains. The contamination of an edible grain by a poisonous, parasitic fungus spread death for centuries. As early as 600 B.C., an Assyrian tablet alluded to a "noxious pustule in the ear of grain." Written descriptions of ergot poisoning first appeared in the Middle Ages. Strange epidemics were described in which the characteristic symptom was gangrene of the feet, legs, hands, and arms. In severe cases, the tissue became dry and black and mummified limbs separated off without loss of blood. Limbs were said to be consumed by the holy fire, blackened like charcoal with agonizing burning sensations. The disease was called holy fire or St. Anthony's fire in honor of the saint at whose shrine relief was said to be obtained. The relief that followed migration to the shrine of St. Anthony was probably real, for the sufferers received a diet free of contaminated grain during their sojourn at the shrine. The symptoms of ergot poisoning were not restricted to limbs. A frequent complication of ergot poisoning was abortion. Indeed, ergot was known as an obstetrical herb before it was identified as the cause of St. Anthony's fire.

Chemistry. The ergot alkaloids can all be considered to be derivatives of the tetracyclic compound 6-methylergoline

(Table 11–6). The naturally occurring alkaloids contain a substituent in the beta configurations at position 8 and a double bond in ring D. The natural alkaloids of therapeutic interest are amide derivatives of *d*-lysergic acid. The first pure ergot alkaloid, ergotamine, was obtained in 1920, followed by the isolation of ergonovine in 1932. Numerous semisynthetic derivatives of the ergot alkaloids have been prepared by catalytic hydrogenation of the natural alkaloids, *e.g.,* dihydroergotamine. Another synthetic derivative, *bromocriptine* (2-bromo-α-ergocryptine), is used to control the secretion of prolactin (*see* Chapter 56). However, this property is derived from a dopamine agonist effect of the drug. Other products of this series include lysergic acid diethylamide (LSD), a potent hallucinogenic drug, and methysergide, a serotonin antagonist. These drugs are discussed later in this chapter.

Absorption, Fate, and Excretion. The pharmacokinetic properties of the ergot alkaloids have been reviewed by Perrin (1985). The oral administration of ergotamine by itself results in undetectable systemic drug concentrations, because of extensive first-pass metabolism. Bioavailability after sublingual administration also is poor and often is inadequate for therapeutic purposes. Although the concurrent administration of caffeine is said to improve both the rate and extent of absorption, the bioavailability of ergotamine still is probably less than 1%. The bioavailability after administration of rectal suppositories is greater.

Ergotamine is metabolized in the liver by largely undefined pathways, and 90% of the metabolites are excreted in the bile.

Only traces of unmetabolized drug can be found in urine and feces. Ergotamine produces vasoconstriction that endures for 24 hours or longer, despite a plasma half-life of approximately 2 hours. Dihydroergotamine is much less completely absorbed and is eliminated more rapidly than ergotamine, presumably due to its rapid hepatic clearance.

Ergonovine and methylergonovine are rapidly absorbed after oral administration and reach peak concentrations in plasma within 60 to 90 minutes that are more than tenfold those achieved with an equivalent dose of ergotamine. An uterotonic effect can be observed within 10 minutes after oral administration of 0.2 mg of ergonovine to women postpartum. Judging from the relative duration of action, ergonovine is metabolized and/or eliminated more rapidly than is ergotamine. The half-life of methylergonovine in plasma ranges between 0.5 and 2 hours.

Use in the Treatment of Migraine. Ergot derivatives were first found to be effective antimigraine agents in the 1920s, and they continue to be a class of therapeutic agents used for the acute relief of migraine; however, ergot alkaloids are nonselective pharmacological agents in that they interact with numerous neurotransmitter receptors, including 5-HT$_1$ and 5-HT$_2$ receptors as well as adrenergic and dopaminergic receptors. For example, the ergot alkaloid dihydroergotamine can compete potently for radioligand binding to a variety of receptor subpopulations, including all known 5-HT$_1$ receptors as well as a number of other biogenic amine receptors, such as 5-HT$_{2A}$, 5-HT$_{2B}$, D$_2$ dopamine, and α_1- and α_2-adrenergic receptors. The multiple pharmacological effects of ergot alkaloids have complicated the determination of their precise mechanism of action in the acute treatment of migraine. Based on the mechanism of action of sumatriptan and other 5-HT$_{1B/1D}$-receptor agonists (discussed above), the actions of ergot alkaloids at 5-HT$_{1B/1D}$ receptors likely mediate their *acute* antimigraine effects. The ergot derivative *methysergide,* which acts more commonly as a 5-HT-receptor *antagonist,* has been used for the prophylactic treatment of migraine headaches and is discussed later in the section on 5-HT-receptor antagonists.

The use of ergot alkaloids for migraine should be restricted to patients having frequent, moderate migraine or infrequent, severe migraine attacks. As with other medications used to abort an attack, the patient should be advised to take ergot preparations as soon as possible after the onset of a headache. Gastrointestinal absorption of ergot alkaloids is erratic, perhaps explaining the large variation in patient response to these drugs. Accordingly, currently available preparations in the United States include sublingual tablets of *ergotamine tartrate* (ERGOMAR) and a nasal spray and solution for injection of *dihydroergotamine mesylate* (MIGRANAL and D.H.E. 45, respectively). The recommended dose for ergotamine tartrate is 2 mg sublingually, which can be repeated at 30-minute intervals if necessary up to a total dose of 6 mg in a 24-hour period or 10 mg a week. Dihydroergotamine mesylate injections can be given intravenously, subcutaneously, or intramuscularly. The recommended dose is 1 mg, which can be repeated after 1 hour if necessary up to a total dose of 2 mg (intravenously) or 3 mg (subcutaneously or intramuscularly) in a 24-hour period or 6 mg in a week. The dose of dihydroergotamine mesylate administered as a nasal spray is 0.5 mg (one spray) in each nostril, repeated after 15 minutes for a total dose of 2 mg (4 sprays). The safety of more than 3 mg over 24 hours or 4 mg over 7 days has not been established.

Adverse Effects and Contraindications. Nausea and vomiting, due to a direct effect on CNS emetic centers, occur in approximately 10% of patients after oral administration of ergotamine and in about twice that number after parental administration. This side effect is problematic, since nausea and sometimes vomiting are part of the symptomatology of a migraine headache. Leg weakness is common, and muscle pains, which occasionally are severe, may occur in the extremities. Numbness and tingling of fingers and toes are other reminders of the ergotism that this alkaloid may cause. Precordial distress and pain suggestive of angina pectoris, as well as transient tachycardia or bradycardia, also have been noted, presumably as a result of coronary vasospasm induced by ergotamine. Localized edema and itching may occur in an occasional hypersensitive patient, but usually do not necessitate interruption of ergotamine therapy. In the event of acute or chronic poisoning (ergotism), treatment consists of complete withdrawal of the offending drug and symptomatic measures. The latter include attempts to maintain adequate circulation by agents such as anticoagulants, low-molecular-weight dextran, and potent vasodilator drugs, such as intravenous sodium nitroprusside. Dihydroergotamine has lower potency than does ergotamine as an emetic and as a vasoconstrictor and oxytocic.

Ergot alkaloids are contraindicated in women who are or may become pregnant, because the drugs may cause fetal distress and miscarriage. Ergot alkaloids also are contraindicated in patients with peripheral vascular disease, coronary heart disease, hypertension, impaired hepatic or renal function, and sepsis. Ergot alkaloids should not be taken within 24 hours of the use of the triptans and should not be used concurrently with other drugs that can cause vasocontriction.

Use of Ergot Alkaloids in Postpartum Hemorrhage. All of the natural ergot alkaloids markedly increase the motor activity of the uterus. After small doses, contractions are increased in force or frequency, or both, but are followed by a normal degree of relaxation. As the dose is increased, contractions become more forceful and prolonged, resting tonus is dramatically increased, and sustained contracture can result. Although this characteristic precludes their use for induction or facilitation of labor, it is quite compatible with their use postpartum or after abortion to control bleeding and maintain uterine contraction. The gravid uterus is very sensitive, and small doses of ergot alkaloids can be given immediately postpartum to obtain a marked uterine response, usually without significant side effects. In current obstetric practice, ergot alkaloids are used primarily to prevent postpartum hemorrhage. Although all natural ergot alkaloids have qualitatively the same effect on the uterus, *ergonovine* is the most active and also less toxic than ergotamine. For these reasons ergonovine and its semisynthetic derivative *methylergonovine* have replaced other ergot preparations as uterine-stimulating agents in obstetrics.

D-Lysergic Acid Diethylamide (LSD).

Of the many drugs that are nonselective 5-HT agonists, LSD is the most remarkable. This ergot derivative profoundly alters human behavior, eliciting perception disturbances, such as sensory distortion (especially visual and auditory), and hallucinations at doses as low as 1 μg/kg. The potent, mind-altering effects of LSD explain its abuse by human beings (*see* Chapter 24) as well as the fascination of scientists with the mechanism of action of LSD. The chemical structure of LSD is shown in Table 11–6.

LSD was synthesized in 1943 by Albert Hoffman, who discovered its unique properties when he accidentally ingested the drug. The chemical precursor, lysergic acid, occurs naturally in a fungus that grows on wheat and rye, but it is devoid of hallucinogenic actions. LSD contains an indolealkylamine moiety embedded within its structure, and early investigators postulated that it would interact with 5-HT receptors. Extensive studies have shown that LSD interacts with brain 5-HT receptors as an agonist/partial agonist. LSD mimics 5-HT at 5-HT$_{1A}$ autoreceptors on raphe cell bodies, producing a marked slowing of the firing rate of serotonergic neurons. In the raphe, LSD and 5-HT are equieffective; however, in areas of serotonergic axonal projections (such as visual relay centers), LSD is far less effective than is 5-HT (Aghajanian *et al.*, 1987). This nonuniform action in cell body and target areas may explain the abnormal visual responses that LSD produces. In drug discrimination, an animal behavioral model thought to reflect the subjective effects of abused drugs, the discriminative stimulus effects of LSD and other hallucinogenic drugs appear to be mediated by activation of 5-HT$_{2A}$ receptors (Glennon, 1990). Consistent with these behavioral results, analyses of receptor-linked phosphoinositide hydrolysis show that LSD and other hallucinogenic drugs act as partial or full agonists at 5-HT$_{2A}$ and 5-HT$_{2C}$ receptors. An important unanswered question is whether or not the agonist property of hallucinogenic drugs at 5-HT$_{2C}$ receptors contributes to the behavioral alterations. LSD also interacts potently with many other 5-HT receptors, including recently cloned receptors whose functions have not yet been determined. The hallucinogenic phenethylamine derivatives such as 1-(4-bromo-2,5-dimethoxyphenyl)-2-aminopropane, on the other hand, are selective 5-HT$_{2A/2C}$-receptor agonists. Promising signs of progress in understanding the actions of hallucinogens are the results of clinical investigations of hallucinogens. It is now possible to test in human beings the hypotheses developed in animal models. For example, PET imaging studies (Vollenweider *et al.*, 1997) revealed that administration of the hallucinogen psilocybin mimics the pattern of brain activation found in schizophrenic patients experiencing hallucinations. Consistent with results of animal studies, this action of psilocybin is blocked by pretreatment with 5-HT$_{2A/2C}$ antagonists (Vollenweider *et al.*, 1998).

8-Hydroxy-(2-N,N-Dipropylamino)-Tetraline (8-OH-DPAT). This prototypic selective 5-HT$_{1A}$ receptor agonist is a valuable experimental tool. The structure of 8-OH-DPAT is given below.

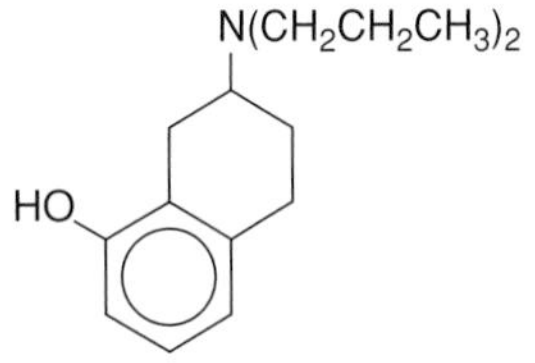

8-OH-DPAT

8-OH-DPAT does not interact with other members of the 5-HT$_1$ receptor subfamily or with 5-HT$_2$, 5-HT$_3$, or 5-HT$_4$ receptors. 8-OH-DPAT reduces the firing rate of raphe cells by activating 5-HT$_{1A}$ autoreceptors and inhibits neuronal firing in terminal fields (*e.g.*, hippocampus) by direct interaction with postsynaptic 5-HT$_{1A}$ receptors. A series of long-chain arylpiper-

azines, such as *buspirone, gepirone,* and *ipsapirone,* are selective partial agonists at 5-HT$_{1A}$ receptors. Other closely related arylpiperazines act as 5-HT$_{1A}$-receptor antagonists. Buspirone, the first clinically available drug in this series, has been effective in the treatment of anxiety (*see* Chapter 19). It has been postulated that the sedative properties of the benzodiazepines, which buspirone does not have, may explain why patients usually prefer the benzodiazepines to relieve anxiety. Other arylpiperazines (gepirone and ipsapirone) are being developed for treatment of depression as well as anxiety.

***m*-Chlorophenylpiperazine (mCPP).** The *in vivo* actions of mCPP primarily reflect activation of 5-HT$_{1B}$ and/or 5-HT$_{2A/2C}$ receptors, although this agent is not subtype-selective in radioligand-binding studies *in vitro*. mCPP (structure below) is an active metabolite of the antidepressant drug *trazodone* (DESYREL).

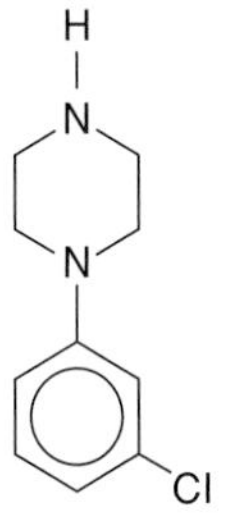

mCPP

mCPP has been extensively employed to probe brain 5-HT function in human beings. The drug alters a number of neuroendocrine parameters and elicits profound behavioral effects, with anxiety as a prominent symptom (Murphy, 1990). mCPP elevates cortisol and prolactin secretion, probably *via* a combination of 5-HT$_1$- and 5-HT$_{2A/2C}$-receptor activation. It also increases growth-hormone secretion, apparently by a 5-HT-independent mechanism. 5-HT$_{2A/2C}$ receptors appear to mediate at least part of the anxiogenic effects of mCPP, as 5-HT$_{2A/2C}$-receptor antagonists attenuate mCPP-induced anxiety. Animal studies suggest a greater involvement of the 5-HT$_{2C}$ receptor in anxiogenic actions of mCPP.

5-HT-Receptor Antagonists

The properties of 5-HT-receptor antagonists also vary widely. Ergot alkaloids and related compounds tend to be nonspecific 5-HT-receptor antagonists; however, a few ergot derivatives such as *metergoline* bind preferentially to members of the 5-HT$_2$-receptor family. A number of selective antagonists for 5-HT$_{2A/2C}$ and 5-HT$_3$ receptors are currently available. Members of these drug classes have widely different chemical structures, with no common structural motif predictably conveying high affinity.

Ketanserin is the prototypic 5-HT$_{2A}$-receptor antagonist (*see* below). A large series of 5-HT$_3$-receptor antagonists are being explored for treatment of various gastrointestinal disturbances (*see* Chapter 38). *Ondansetron* (ZOFRAN), *dolasetron* (ANZEMET), and *granisetron* (KYTRIL), all 5-HT$_3$-receptor antagonists, have proven to be highly efficacious in the treatment of chemotherapy-induced nausea (Grunberg and Hesketh, 1993; *see also* Chapter 38).

Clinical effects of 5-HT-related drugs often exhibit a significant delay in onset. This is particularly the case with drugs used to treat affective disorders such as anxiety and depression (*see* Chapter 19). This delayed onset has generated considerable interest in potential adaptive changes in 5-HT-receptor density and sensitivity after chronic drug treatments. Laboratory studies have documented agonist-promoted receptor subsensitivity and down-regulation of the 5-HT-receptor subtypes, a compensatory response common to many neurotransmitter systems. However, an unusual adaptive process, *antagonist*-induced down-regulation of 5-HT$_{2C}$ receptors, takes place in rats and mice after chronic treatment with receptor antagonists (Sanders-Bush, 1990). The mechanism of this paradoxical regulation of 5-HT$_{2A/2C}$ receptors has generated considerable interest, since many clinically effective drugs, including clozapine, ketanserin, and amitriptyline, exhibit this unusual property. These drugs, as well as several other 5-HT$_{2A/2C}$-receptor antagonists, possess negative intrinsic activity, reducing constitutive (spontaneous) receptor activity in a cell line expressing the 5-HT$_{2C}$-receptor cDNA (Barker *et al.*, 1994). This property of negative intrinsic activity is contrary to classical concepts, where receptor antagonists are thought to block the action of an agonist but have no effect alone. Another group of 5-HT$_{2A/2C}$-receptor antagonists was found to act in the classical manner. It is not known if these differences in the properties of 5-HT$_{2A/2C}$-receptor antagonists are clinically significant.

Ketanserin. *Ketanserin* (SUFREXAL) (structure below) opened a new era in 5-HT-receptor pharmacology. Ketanserin potently blocks 5-HT$_{2A}$ receptors, less potently blocks 5-HT$_{2C}$ receptors, and has no significant effect on 5-HT$_3$ or 5-HT$_4$ receptors or any members of the 5-HT$_1$-receptor family. It is important to note, however, that ketanserin also has high affinity for α-adrenergic receptors and histamine H$_1$ receptors (Janssen, 1983).

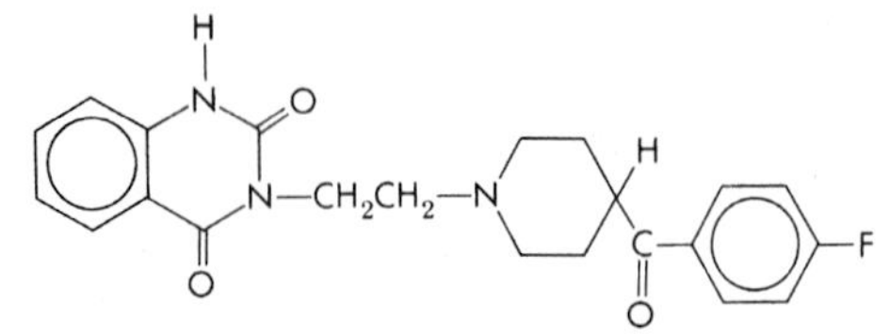

KETANSERIN

Ketanserin lowers blood pressure in patients with hypertension, causing a reduction comparable to that seen with β-adrenergic receptor antagonists or diuretics. The drug appears to reduce the tone of both capacitance and resistance vessels. This effect likely relates to its blockade of α_1-adrenergic receptors, not its blockade of 5-HT$_{2A}$ receptors. Ketanserin inhibits 5-HT–induced platelet aggregation, but it does not greatly reduce the ability of other agents to cause aggregation. Ketanserin is not yet marketed in the United States but is available in other countries, including Italy, the Netherlands, and Switzerland. Severe side effects after treatment with ketanserin have not been reported. Its oral bioavailability is about 50%, and its plasma half-life is about 12 to 25 hours. The primary mechanism of elimination is hepatic metabolism.

Chemical relatives of ketanserin such as *ritanserin* are more selective 5-HT$_{2A}$-receptor antagonists with low affinity for α_1-adrenergic receptors. However, ritanserin, as well as most other 5-HT$_{2A}$-receptor antagonists, also potently antagonize 5-HT$_{2C}$ receptors. The physiological significance of 5-HT$_{2C}$-receptor blockade is unknown. MDL 100,907 is the prototype of a new series of potent 5-HT$_{2A}$-receptor antagonists, with high selectivity for 5-HT$_{2A}$ *versus* 5-HT$_{2C}$ receptors. Early clinical trials of MDL 100,907 in the treatment of schizophrenia have been inconclusive.

Atypical Antipsychotic Drugs. *Clozapine* (CLOZARIL), a 5-HT$_{2A/2C}$-receptor antagonist, represents a new class of atypical antipsychotic drugs with reduced incidence of extrapyramidal side effects, compared to the classical neuroleptics, and a greater efficacy for reducing negative symptoms of schizophrenia (*see* Chapter 20). Clozapine also has a high affinity for subtypes of dopamine receptors.

One of the newest strategies for the design of additional atypical antipsychotic drugs is to combine 5-HT$_{2A/2C}$ and dopamine D$_2$ receptor–blocking actions in the same molecule (Leysen *et al.*, 1993). *Risperidone* (RISPERDAL), for example, is a potent 5-HT$_{2A}$- and D$_2$-receptor antagonist. Low doses of risperidone have been reported to attenuate negative symptoms of schizophrenia with a low incidence of extrapyramidal side effects. Extrapyramidal effects are commonly seen, however, with doses of risperidone in excess of 6 mg/day. Other atypical antipsychotic agents—*quetiapine* (SEROQUEL) and *olanzapine* (ZYPREXA)—act on multiple receptors, but their antipsychotic effects are thought to be due to antagonism of dopamine and serotonin.

Methysergide. *Methysergide* (SANSERT; 1-methyl-*d*-lysergic acid butanolamide) is a congener of methylergonovine (*see* Table 11–6).

Methysergide blocks 5-HT$_{2A}$ and 5-HT$_{2C}$ receptors but appears to have partial agonist activity in some preparations. Methysergide inhibits the vasoconstrictor and pressor effects of 5-HT as well as the actions of 5-HT on various types of extravascular smooth muscle. It has been found to both block and mimic the central effects of 5-HT. Methysergide is not selective (it also interacts with 5-HT$_1$ receptors), but its therapeutic effects appear primarily to reflect blockade of 5-HT$_2$ receptors. Although methysergide is an ergot derivative, it has only weak vasoconstrictor and oxytocic activity.

Methysergide has been used for the prophylactic treatment of migraine and other vascular headaches, including Horton's syndrome. It is without benefit when given during an acute migraine attack. The protective effect takes 1 to 2 days to develop and disappears slowly when treatment is terminated. This might be due to the accumulation of an active metabolite of methysergide, methylergometrine, which is more potent than the parent drug. Methysergide also has been used to combat diarrhea and malabsorption in patients with carcinoid tumors and may be beneficial in the postgastrectomy dumping syndrome. Both of these conditions have a 5-HT–mediated component. However, methysergide is not effective against other substances (*e.g.,* kinins) that also are released by carcinoid tumors. For this reason, the preferred agent to treat malabsorption in carcinoid patients is a somatostatin analog, *octreotide acetate* (SANDOSTATIN), which inhibits the secretion of all the mediators released by the carcinoid tumors.

Side effects of methysergide are usually mild and transient, although drug withdrawal is infrequently required to reverse more severe reactions. Common side effects consist of gastrointestinal disturbances, including heartburn, diarrhea, cramps, nausea, and vomiting, and symptoms related to vasospasm-induced ischemia (numbness and tingling of extremities, pain in the extremities, low back and abdominal pain). Effects attributable to central actions include unsteadiness, drowsiness, weakness, lightheadedness, nervousness, insomnia, confusion, excitement, hallucinations, and even frank psychotic episodes. Reactions suggestive of vascular insufficiency have been observed in a few patients, as well as exacerbation of angina pectoris. A potentially serious complication of prolonged treatment is inflammatory fibrosis, giving rise to various syndromes, including retroperitoneal fibrosis, pleuropulmonary fibrosis, and coronary and endocardial fibrosis. Usually the fibrosis regresses after drug withdrawal, although persistent cardiac valvular damage has been reported. Because of this danger, other drugs are preferred for the prophylactic treatment of migraine. β-Adrenergic receptor antagonists (such as propranolol; *see* Chapter 10), amitriptyline (Chapter 19), and nonsteroidal antiinflammatory drugs (Chapter 27) are alternatives that may be used as prophylactic treatment of migraine headaches. If methysergide is used chronically, treatment should be interrupted for 3 weeks or more every 6 months.

Cyproheptadine. The structure of *cyproheptadine* (PERIACTIN; *see* below) resembles that of the phenothiazine histamine H$_1$-receptor antagonists, and, indeed, it is an effective H$_1$-receptor antagonist. Cyproheptadine also has prominent 5-HT-blocking activity on smooth muscle by virtue of its binding to 5-HT$_{2A}$ receptors. In addition, it has weak anticholinergic activity and possesses mild central depressant properties.

CYPROHEPTADINE

Cyproheptadine shares the properties and uses of other H$_1$-receptor antagonists (*see* Chapter 25). It is effective in controlling skin allergies, particularly the accompanying pruritus, and appears to be useful in cold urticaria. In allergic conditions, the action of cyproheptadine as a 5-HT-receptor antagonist is irrelevant, since 5-HT$_{2A}$ receptors are not involved in human allergic responses. Some physicians recommend cyproheptadine to counteract the sexual side effects of selective 5-HT-reuptake inhibitors such as fluoxetine and sertraline (*see* Chapter 19). The 5-HT-blocking actions of cyproheptadine explain its value in the postgastrectomy dumping syndrome, intestinal hypermotility of carcinoid, and migraine prophylaxis. Cyproheptadine is not, however, a preferred treatment for these conditions.

Side effects of cyproheptadine include those common to other H$_1$-receptor antagonists, such as drowsiness. Weight gain and increased growth in children have been observed and attributed to an interference with regulation of the secretion of growth hormone.

PROSPECTUS

The availability of molecular reagents, such as cDNA clones coding for 5-HT-receptor subtypes and 5-HT-selective neurotransmitter transporters (Chapter 19), as well as genetically altered mice, will enhance the development of more selective therapeutic agents. It is now known that 5-HT-receptor subtypes have varying degrees of constitutive/spontaneous activity. Moreover, 5-HT receptor antagonists exist that either simply block receptor occupancy by agonists (*antagonists*) or stabilize unproductive receptor conformations as well as block agonist occupancy (*inverse agonists*). Even though there is only scant evidence for constitutive activity *in vivo,* drug development has been further refined by focusing on reduction of preexisting constitutive neuronal activity as opposed to blockade of excess neurotransmitter action. Improved experimental models for behavioral dysfunctions of complex origin, such as anxiety, depression, aggression, compulsivity, and others, already have revealed therapeutic outcomes that can be achieved by simultaneously blocking multiple receptor populations. Development of animal models that reflect physiological mechanisms influencing, for example, sleep, sex, appetite, emotions, sensory and pain perception, motor control, and digestion in human beings should permit further elucidation of receptor subpopulations that can be targeted to relieve dysfunctions in these complex processes.

For further discussion of migraines, *see* Chapter 364 in *Harrison's Principles of Internal Medicine,* 14th ed., McGraw-Hill, New York, 1998.

BIBLIOGRAPHY

Andrade, R., Malenka, R.C., and Nicoll, R.A. A G protein couples serotonin and GABA-B receptors to the same channels in hippocampus. *Science,* **1986,** *234:*1261–1265.

Barker, E.L., Westphal, R.S., Schmidt, D., and Sanders-Bush, E. Constitutively active 5HT$_{2C}$ receptors reveal novel inverse agonist activity of receptor ligands. *J. Biol. Chem.,* **1994,** *296:*11687–11690.

Brunner, H.C., Nelen, M., Breakefield, X.O., Ropers, H.H., and van Oost, B.A. Abnormal behavior associated with a point mutation in the structural gene for monoamine oxidase A. *Science,* **1993,** *262:* 578–580.

Burns, C.M., Chu, H., Rueter, S.M., Hutchinson, L.K., Canton, H., Sanders-Bush, E., and Emerson, R.B. Regulation of serotonin-2C receptor G-protein coupling by RNA editing. *Nature,* **1997,** *387:*303–308.

Cases, O., Seif, I., Grimsby, J., Gaspar, P., Chen, K., Pournin, S., Muller, U., Aguet, M., Babinet, C., Shih, J.C., *et al.* Aggressive behavior and altered amounts of brain serotonin and norepinephrine in mice lacking MAOA. *Science,* **1995,** *268:*1763–1766.

Delgado, P.L., Charney, D.S., Price, L.H., Aghajanian, G.K., Landis, H., and Heninger, G.R. Serotonin function and the mechanism of antidepressant action. Reversal of antidepressant-induced remission by rapid depletion of plasma tryptophan. *Arch. Gen. Psychiatry,* **1990,** *47:*411–418.

den Boer, M.O., Villalon, C.M., Heiligers, J.P., Humphrey, P.P., and Saxena, P.R. Role of 5-HT1-like receptors in the reduction of porcine cranial arteriovenous anastomotic shunting by sumatriptan. *Br. J. Pharmacol.,* **1991,** *102:*323–330.

Doenicke, A., Brand, J., and Perrin, V.L. Possible benefit of GR43175, a novel 5-HT1-like receptor agonist, for the acute treatment of severe migraine. *Lancet,* **1988,** *1:*1309–1311.

Gaddum, J.H., and Picarelli, Z.P. Two kinds of tryptamine receptors. *Br. J. Pharmacol.,* **1957,** *12:*323–328.

Higashi, H., and Nishi, S. 5-Hydroxytryptamine receptors of visceral primary afferent neurons on rabbit nodose ganglia. *J. Physiol. (Lond.),* **1982,** *323:*543–567.

Humphrey, P.P., Feniuk, W., Perren, M.J., Connor, H.E., Oxford, A.W., Coates, L.H., and Butina, D. GR43175, a selective agonist for the 5-HT1-like receptor in dog isolated saphenous vein. *Br. J. Pharmacol.,* **1988,** *94:*1123–1132.

Maricq, A.V., Peterson, A.S., Brake, A.J., Myers, R.M., and Julius, D. Primary structure and functional expression of the 5HT3 receptor, a serotonin-gated ion channel. *Science,* **1991,** *254:*432–437.

Mouret, J., Froment, J.L., Bobillier, P., and Jouvet, M. Étude neuropharmacologique et biochemique des insomnies provoquées par la P.-chlorophénylalanine. *J. Physiol. (Paris),* **1967,** *59:*463–464.

Parks, C.L., Robinson, P.S., Sibille, E., Shenk, T., and Toth, M. Increased anxiety of mice lacking the serotonin 1A receptor. *Proc. Natl. Acad. Sci. U.S.A.,* **1998,** *95:*10734–10739.

Peroutka, S.J., and Snyder, S.H. Multiple serotonin receptors: differential binding of [^{3}H]5-hydroxytryptamine, [^{3}H]-lysergic acid diethylamide and [^{3}H]-spiroperidol. *Mol. Pharmacol.,* **1979,** *16:*687–699.

Perrin, V.L. Clinical pharmacokinetics of ergotamine in migraine and cluster headache. *Clin. Pharmacokinet.,* **1985,** *10:*334–352.

Ramamoorthy, S., and Blakely, R.D. Phosphorylation and sequestration of serotonin transporters differentially modulated by psychostimulants. *Science,* **1999,** *285:*763–766.

Ramboz, S., Oosting, R., Amara, D.A., Kung, H.F., Blier, P., Mendelsohn, M., Mann, J.J., Brunner, D., and Hen, R. Serotonin receptor 1A knockout: an animal model of anxiety-related disorder. *Proc. Natl. Acad. Sci. U.S.A.,* **1998,** *95:*14476–14481.

Rapport, M.M., Green, A.A., and Page, I.H. Serum vasoconstrictor (serotonin). IV. Isolation and characterization. *J. Biol. Chem.,* **1948,** *176:*1243–1251.

Richardson, B.P., Engel, G., Donatsch, P., and Stadler, P.A. Identification of serotonin M-receptor subtypes and their specific blockade by a new class of drugs. *Nature,* **1985,** *316:*126–131.

Saudou, F., Amara, D.A., Dierich, A., LeMeur, M., Ramboz, S., Segu, L., Buhot, M.-C., and Hen, R. Enhanced aggressive behavior in mice lacking 5-HT$_{1B}$ receptor. *Science,* **1994,** *265:*1875–1878.

Simmons, V.E., and Blakeborough, P. The safety profile of sumatriptan. *Rev. Contemp. Pharmacother,* **1994,** *5*:319–328.

Vollenweider, F.X., Leenders, K.L., Scharfetter, C., Maguire, P., Stadelmann, O., and Angst, J. Positron emission tomography and fluorodeoxyglucose studies of metabolic hyperfrontality and psychopathology in the psilocybin model of psychosis. *Neuropsychopharmacology,* **1997,** *16*:357–372.

Vollenweider, F.X., Vollenweider-Scherpenhuyzen, M.F., Babler, A., Vogel, H., and Hell, D. Psilocybin induces schizophrenia-like psychosis in humans via a serotonin-2 agonist action. *Neuroreport,* **1998,** *9*:3897–3902.

MONOGRAPHS AND REVIEWS

Aghajanian, G.K. Electrophysiology of serotonin receptor subtypes and signal transduction pathways. In, *Psychopharmacology: The Fourth Generation of Progress.* (Bloom, F.E., and Kupfer, D.J., eds.) Raven Press, New York, **1995,** pp. 451–460.

Aghajanian, G.K., Sprouse, J.S., and Rasmussen, K. Physiology of the midbrain serotonin system. In, *Psychopharmacology: The Third Generation of Progress.* (Meltzer, H., ed.) Raven Press, New York, **1987,** pp. 141–149.

Barrett, J.E., and Vanover, K.E. 5-HT receptors as targets for the development of novel anxiolytic drugs: models, mechanisms and future directions. *Psychopharmacology (Berl.),* **1993,** *112*:1–12.

Brodie, B.B., and Shore, P.A. A concept for a role of serotonin and norepinephrine as chemical mediators in the brain. *Ann. N.Y. Acad. Sci.,* **1957,** *66*:631–642.

Brown, G.L., and Linnoila, M.I. CSF serotonin metabolite (5-HIAA) studies in depression, impulsivity, and violence. *J. Clin. Psychiatry,* **1990,** *51(suppl)*:31–41.

Deleu, D., Hanssens, Y., and Worthing, E.A. Symptomatic and prophylactic treatment of migraine: a critical appraisal. *Clin. Neuropharmacol.,* **1998,** *21*:267–279.

Descarries, L., Audet, M.A., Doucet, G., Garcia, S., Oleskevich, S., Seguela, P., Soghomonian, J.J., and Watkins, K.C. Morphology of central serotonin neurons. Brief review of quantified aspects of their distribution and ultrastructural relationships. *Ann. N.Y. Acad. Sci.,* **1990,** *600*:81–92.

Dhasmana, K.M., Zhu, Y.N., Cruz, S.L., and Villalon, C.M. Gastrointestinal effects of 5-hydroxytryptamine and related drugs. *Life Sci.,* **1993,** *53*:1651–1661.

Erspamer, V. Occurrence of indolealkylamines in nature. In, *5-Hydroxytryptamine and Related Indolealkylamines.* (Erspamer, V., ed.) *[Handbuch der Experimentellen Pharmakologie],* Vol. 19. Springer-Verlag, Berlin, **1966,** pp. 132–181.

Furchgott, R.F., and Vanhoutte, P.M. Endothelium-derived relaxing and contracting factors. *FASEB J.,* **1989,** *3*:2007–2018.

Gershon, M.D. Serotonin, its role and regulation in enteric neurotransmission. In, *Kynurenine and Serotonergic Pathways.* (Schwarcz, R., ed.) *Advances in Experimental Medicine and Biology,* Vol. 294. Plenum Press, New York, **1991,** pp. 221–230.

Gibbons, G.H., and Dzau, V.J. The emerging concept of vascular remodeling. *N. Engl. J. Med.,* **1994,** *330*:1431–1438.

Gillis, C.N. Peripheral metabolism of serotonin In, *Serotonin and the Cardiovascular System.* (Vanhoutte, P.M., ed.) Raven Press, New York, **1985,** pp. 27–42.

Glennon, R.A. Do classical hallucinogens act as 5-HT$_2$ agonists or antagonists? *Neuropsychopharmacology,* **1990,** *3*:509–517.

Glennon, R.A., and Lucki, I. Behavioral models of serotonin receptor

activation. In, *The Serotonin Receptors.* (Sanders-Bush, E., ed.) The Humana Press, Clifton, N.J., **1988,** pp. 253–293.

Grunberg, S.M., and Hesketh, P.J. Control of chemotherapy-induced emesis. *N. Engl. J. Med.,* **1993,** *329*:1790–1796.

Hawiger, J. Repertoire of platelet receptors. In, *Platelets: Receptors, Adhesion, Secretion.* (Hawiger, J., ed.) *Methods in Enzymology,* Vol. 215. Academic Press, San Diego, CA, **1992,** pp. 131–136.

Hegde, S.S., and Eglen, R.M. Peripheral 5-HT4 receptors. *FASEB J.,* **1996,** *10*:1398–1407.

Hoyer, D., Clarke, D.E., Fozard, J.R., Hartig, P.R., Martin, G.R., Mylecharane, E.J., Saxena, P.R., and Humphrey, P.P. International Union of Pharmacology classification of receptors for 5-hydroxytryptamine (serotonin). *Pharmacol. Rev.,* **1994,** *46*:157–203.

Humphrey, P.P., Aperley, E., Feniuk, W., and Perren, M.J. A rational approach to identifying a fundamentally new drug for the treatment of migraine. In, *Cardiovascular Pharmacology of 5-Hydroxytryptamine* (Saxena, P.R., Wallis, D.I., Wouters, W., and Bevan, P., eds.). Kluwer Academic Publishers, Dordrecht, Netherlands, **1990,** pp. 417–431.

Janssen, P.A.J. 5-HT$_2$ receptor blockade to study serotonin-induced pathology. *Trends Pharmacol. Sci.,* **1983,** *4*:198–206.

Koek, W., Jackson, A., and Colpaert, F.C. Behavioral pharmacology of antagonists at 5-HT$_2$/5-HT$_{1C}$ receptors. *Neurosci. Biobehav. Rev.,* **1992,** *16*:95–105.

Leysen, J.E., Janssen, P.M., Schotte, A., Luyten, W.H., and Megens, A.A. Interaction of antipsychotic drugs with neurotransmitter receptor sites *in vitro* and *in vivo* in relation to pharmacological and clinical effects: role of 5-HT$_2$ receptors. *Psychopharmacology (Berl.),* **1993,** *112*:S40–S54.

Limbird, L.E. Receptors linked to inhibition of adenylate cyclase: additional signaling mechanisms. *FASEB J.,* **1988,** *2*:2686–2695.

Limmroth, V., and Diener, H.C. New anti-migraine drugs: present and beyond the millennium. *Int. J. Clin. Pract.,* **1998,** *52*:566–570.

Mansour, T.E. Chemotherapy of parasitic worms: new biochemical strategies. *Science,* **1979,** *205*:462–469.

Moskowitz, M.A. Neurogenic versus vascular mechanisms of sumatriptan and ergot alkaloids in migraine. *Trends Pharmacol. Sci.,* **1992,** *13*:307–311.

Murphy, D.L. Neuropsychiatric disorders and the multiple human brain serotonin receptor subtypes and subsystems. *Neuropsychopharmacology,* **1990,** *3*:457–471.

Olesen, J., Larsen, B., and Lauritzen, M. Focal hyperemia followed by spreading oligemia and impaired activation of rCBF in classic migraine. *Ann. Neurol.,* **1981,** *9*:344–352.

Page, I.H. The discovery of serotonin. *Perspect. Biol. Med.,* **1976,** *20*:1–8.

Palacios, J.M., Waeber, C., Hoyer, D., and Mengod, G. Distribution of serotonin receptors. *Ann. N.Y. Acad. Sci.,* **1990,** *600*:36–52.

Peroutka, S.J., and Howell, T.A. The molecular evolution of G protein-coupled receptors: focus on 5-hydroxytryptamine receptors. *Neuropharmacology,* **1994,** *33*:319–324.

Sanders-Bush, E. Adaptive regulation of central serotonin receptors linked to phosphoinositide hydrolysis. *Neuropsychopharmacology,* **1990,** *3*:411–416.

Saxena, P.R. Arteriovenous shunting and migraine. *Res. Clin. Stud. Headache,* **1978,** *6*:89–102.

Saxena, P.R., and Villalón, C.M. Cardiovascular effects of serotonin agonists and antagonists. *J. Cardiovasc. Pharmacol.,* **1990,** *15 (suppl 7)*:S17–S34.

Shih, J.C. Molecular basis of human MAO A and B. *Neuropsychopharmacology,* **1991,** *4*:1–7.

Sjoerdsma, A. Medical progress—serotonin. *N. Engl. J. Med.,* **1959,** *261*:181–188.

Sjoerdsma, A., and Palfreyman, M.G. History of serotonin and serotonin disorders. *Ann. N.Y. Acad. Sci.,* **1990,** *600*:1–8.

Udenfriend, S. Biochemistry of serotonin and other indoleamines. *Vitam. Horm.,* **1959,** *17*:133–151.

Virkkunen, M., Golman, D., Nielsen, D.A., and Linnoila, M. Low brain serotonin turnover rate (low CSF 5-HIAA) and impulsive violence. *J. Psychiatry Neurosci.,* **1995,** *20*:271–275.

Ware, J.A., and Heistad, D.D. Seminars in medicine of the Beth Israel Hospital, Boston. Platelet-endothelium interactions. *N. Engl. J. Med.,* **1993,** *328*:628–635.

Wauquier, A., and Dugovic, C. Serotonin and sleep-wakefulness. *Ann. N.Y. Acad. Sci.,* **1990,** *600*:447–459.

Zifa, E., and Fillion, G. 5-Hydroxytryptamine receptors. *Pharmacol. Rev.,* **1992,** *44*:401–458.

SECTION III

DRUGS ACTING ON THE CENTRAL NERVOUS SYSTEM

NEUROTRANSMISSION AND THE CENTRAL NERVOUS SYSTEM

Floyd E. Bloom

Drugs that act upon the central nervous system (CNS) influence the lives of everyone, every day. These agents are invaluable therapeutically because they can produce specific physiological and psychological effects. Without general anesthetics, modern surgery would be impossible. Drugs that affect the CNS can selectively relieve pain, reduce fever, suppress disordered movement, induce sleep or arousal, reduce the desire to eat, or allay the tendency to vomit. Selectively acting drugs can be used to treat anxiety, mania, depression, or schizophrenia and do so without altering consciousness (see Chapters 19 and 20).

The nonmedical self-administration of CNS-active drugs is a widespread practice. Socially acceptable stimulants and antianxiety agents produce stability, relief, and even pleasure for many. However, the excessive use of these and other drugs also can affect lives adversely when their uncontrolled, compulsive use leads to physical dependence on the drug or to toxic side effects, which may include lethal overdosage (see Chapter 24).

The unique quality of drugs that affect the nervous system and behavior places investigators who study the CNS in the midst of an extraordinary scientific challenge—the attempt to understand the cellular and molecular basis for the enormously complex and varied functions of the human brain. In this effort, pharmacologists have two major goals: to use drugs to elucidate the mechanisms that operate in the normal CNS and to develop appropriate drugs to correct pathophysiological events in the abnormal CNS.

Approaches to the elucidation of the sites and mechanisms of action of CNS drugs demand an understanding of the cellular and molecular biology of the brain. Although knowledge of the anatomy, physiology, and chemistry of the nervous system is far from complete, the acceleration of interdisciplinary research on the CNS has led to remarkable progress. This chapter introduces guidelines and fundamental principles for the comprehensive analysis of drugs that affect the CNS. Specific therapeutic approaches to neurological and psychiatric disorders are discussed in the chapters that follow in this section (see Chapters 13 through 24).

ORGANIZATIONAL PRINCIPLES OF THE BRAIN

The brain is an assembly of interrelated neural systems that regulate their own and each other's activity in a dynamic, complex fashion.

Macrofunctions of Brain Regions

The large anatomical divisions provide a superficial classification of the distribution of brain functions.

Cerebral Cortex. The two cerebral hemispheres constitute the largest division of the brain. Regions of the cortex are classified in several ways: (1) by the modality of information processed (*e.g.,* sensory, including somatosensory, visual, auditory, and olfactory, as well as motor and associational); (2) by anatomical position (frontal, temporal, parietal, and occipital); and (3) by the geometrical relationship between cell types in the major cortical layers ("cytoarchitectonic" classifications). The cerebral cortex exhibits a relatively uniform laminar appearance within any given local region. Columnar sets of approximately 100 vertically connected neurons are thought to form an elemental processing module. The specialized functions of a cortical region arise from the interplay upon this basic module of connections among other regions of the cortex (corticocortical systems) and noncortical areas of the brain (subcortical systems) (*see* Mountcastle, 1997). Varying numbers of adjacent columnar modules may be functionally, but transiently, linked into larger information-processing ensembles. The pathology of Alzheimer's disease, for example, destroys the integrity of the columnar modules and the corticocortical connections (*see* Morrison and Hof, 1997; *see* also Chapter 22).

These columnar ensembles serve to interconnect nested distributed systems in which sensory associations are rapidly modifiable as information is processed (*see* Mountcastle, 1997; Tononi and Edelman, 1998). Cortical areas termed *association areas* receive and somehow process information from primary cortical sensory regions to produce higher cortical functions such as abstract thought, memory, and consciousness. The cerebral cortices also provide supervisory integration of the autonomic nervous system, and they may integrate somatic and vegetative functions, including those of the cardiovascular and gastrointestinal systems.

Limbic System.   The "limbic system" is an archaic term for an assembly of brain regions (hippocampal formation, amygdaloid complex, septum, olfactory nuclei, basal ganglia, and selected nuclei of the diencephalon) grouped around the subcortical borders of the underlying brain core to which a variety of complex emotional and motivational functions have been attributed. Modern neuroscience avoids this term, because the components of the limbic system neither function consistently as a system nor are the boundaries of such a system precisely defined. Parts of the limbic system also participate individually in functions that are capable of more precise definition. Thus, the basal ganglia or neostriatum (the *caudate nucleus, putamen, globus pallidus,* and *lentiform nucleus*) form an essential regulatory segment of the so-called *extrapyramidal motor system.* This system complements the function of the pyramidal (or voluntary) motor system. Damage to the extrapyramidal system depresses the ability to initiate voluntary movements and causes disorders characterized by involuntary movements, such as the tremors and rigidity of Parkinson's disease or the uncontrollable limb movements of Huntington's chorea (*see* Chapter 22). Similarly, the hippocampus may be crucial to the formation of recent memory, since this function is lost in patients with extensive bilateral damage to the hippocampus. Memory also is disrupted with Alzheimer's disease, which destroys the intrinsic structure of the hippocampus as well as parts of the frontal cortex (*see* also Squire, 1998).

Diencephalon.   The *thalamus* lies in the center of the brain, beneath the cortex and basal ganglia and above the hypothalamus. The neurons of the thalamus are arranged into distinct clusters, or nuclei, which are either paired or midline structures. These nuclei act as relays between the incoming sensory pathways and the cortex, between the discrete regions of the thalamus and the hypothalamus, and between the basal ganglia and the association regions of the cerebral cortex. The thalamic nuclei and the basal ganglia also exert regulatory control over visceral functions; aphagia and adipsia, as well as general sensory neglect, follow damage to the corpus striatum or to selected circuits ending there (*see* Jones, 1998).

The *hypothalamus* is the principal integrating region for the entire autonomic nervous system, and, among other functions, it regulates body temperature, water balance, intermediary metabolism, blood pressure, sexual and circadian cycles, secretion of the adenohypophysis, sleep, and emotion. Recent advances in the cytophysiological and chemical dissection of the hypothalamus have clarified the connections and possible functions of individual hypothalamic nuclei (Swanson, 1999).

Midbrain and Brainstem.   The *mesencephalon, pons,* and *medulla oblongata* connect the cerebral hemispheres and thalamus-hypothalamus to the spinal cord. These "bridge portions" of the CNS contain most of the nuclei of the cranial nerves, as well as the major inflow and outflow tracts from the cortices and spinal cord. These regions contain the reticular activating system, an important but incompletely characterized region of gray matter linking peripheral sensory and motor events with higher levels of nervous integration. The major monoamine-containing neurons of the brain (*see* below) are found here. Together, these regions represent the points of central integration for coordination of essential reflexive acts, such as swallowing and vomiting, and those that involve the cardiovascular and respiratory systems; these areas also include the primary receptive regions for most visceral afferent sensory information. The *reticular activating system* is essential for the regulation of sleep, wakefulness, and level of arousal as well as for coordination of eye movements. The fiber systems projecting from the reticular formation have been called "nonspecific," because the targets to which they project are relatively more diffuse in distribution than those of many other neurons (*e.g.,* specific thalamocortical projection). However, the chemically homogeneous components of the reticular system innervate targets in a coherent, functional manner despite their broad distribution (*see* Foote and Aston-Jones, 1995; Usher *et al.,* 1999).

Cerebellum.   The cerebellum arises from the posterior pons behind the cerebral hemispheres. It is also highly laminated and redundant in its detailed cytological organization. The lobules and folia of the cerebellum project onto specific deep cerebellar nuclei, which in turn make relatively selective projections to the motor cortex (by way of the thalamus) and to the brainstem nuclei concerned with vestibular (position-stabilization) function. In addition to maintaining the proper tone of antigravity musculature and providing continuous feedback during volitional movements of the trunk and extremities, the cerebellum also may regulate visceral function (*e.g.,* heart rate, so as to maintain blood flow despite changes in posture). In addition, the cerebellum has been shown in recent studies to play a significant role in learning and memory (*see* Middleton and Strick, 1998).

Spinal Cord.   The spinal cord extends from the caudal end of the medulla oblongata to the lower lumbar vertebrae. Within this mass of nerve cells and tracts, the sensory information from skin, muscles, joints, and viscera is locally coordinated with motoneurons and with primary sensory relay cells that project to and receive signals from higher levels. The spinal cord is divided into anatomical segments (cervical, thoracic, lumbar, and sacral) that correspond to divisions of the peripheral nerves and spinal column. Ascending and descending tracts of the spinal cord are located within the white matter at the perimeter of the cord, while intersegmental connections and synaptic contacts are concentrated within the H-shaped internal mass of gray matter. Sensory information flows into the dorsal cord, and motor commands exit *via* the ventral portion. The preganglionic neurons of the autonomic nervous system (*see* Chapter 6) are found in the intermediolateral columns of the gray matter. Autonomic reflexes (*e.g.,* changes in skin vasculature with alteration of temperature) easily can be elicited within local segments of the spinal cord, as shown by the maintenance of these reflexes after the cord is severed.

Microanatomy of the Brain

Neurons operate either within layered structures (such as the olfactory bulb, cerebral cortex, hippocampal formation, and cerebellum) or in clustered groupings (the defined collections of central neurons that aggregate into nuclei). The specific connections between neurons within or across the macrodivisions of the brain are essential to the brain's functions. It is through their patterns of neuronal circuitry that individual neurons form functional ensembles to regulate the flow of information within and between the regions of the brain.

Cellular Organization of the Brain. Present understanding of the cellular organization of the CNS can be viewed simplistically according to three main patterns of neuronal connectivity (*see* Shepherd, 1998).

Long-hierarchical neuronal connections typically are found in the primary sensory and motor pathways. Here the transmission of information is highly sequential, and interconnected neurons are related to each other in a hierarchical fashion. Primary receptors (in the retina, inner ear, olfactory epithelium, tongue, or skin) transmit first to primary relay cells, then to secondary relay cells, and finally to the primary sensory fields of the cerebral cortex. For motor output systems, the reverse sequence exists with impulses descending hierarchically from motor cortex to spinal motoneuron. This hierarchical scheme of organization provides a precise flow of information, but such organization suffers the disadvantage that destruction of any link incapacitates the entire system.

Local-circuit neurons establish their connections mainly within their immediate vicinity. Such local-circuit neurons frequently are small and may have very few processes. They are believed to regulate (*i.e.,* expand or constrain) the flow of information through their small spatial domain. Given their short axons, they may function without generating action potentials, which are essential for the long-distance transmission between hierarchically connected neurons. The neurotransmitters for many local-circuit neurons in most brain regions have been inferred through pharmacological tests (*see* below).

Single-source divergent circuitry is utilized by certain neuronal systems of the hypothalamus, pons, and medulla. From their clustered anatomical location, these neurons extend multiple-branched and divergent connections to many target cells, almost all of which lie outside the brain region in which the neurons are located.

Neurons with divergent circuitry can be conceived of as special local-circuit neurons whose spatial domains are one to two orders of magnitude larger than those of the classical intraregional interneurons rather than as sequential elements within any known hierarchical system. For example, neurons of the locus ceruleus project from the pons to the cerebellum, spinal cord, thalamus, and several cortical zones, whose function is only subtly disrupted when the adrenergic fibers are destroyed experimentally. Abundant data suggest that these systems could mediate linkages between regions that may require temporary integration (*see* Foote and Aston-Jones, 1995; Aston-Jones *et al.,* 1999). The neurotransmitters for some of these connections are well known (*see* below), while others remain to be identified.

Cell Biology of Neurons. Neurons are classified in many different ways, according to function (sensory, motor, or interneuron), location, or identity of the transmitter they synthesize and release. Microscopic analysis focuses on their general shape and, in particular, the number of extensions from the cell body. Most neurons have one axon to carry signals to functionally interconnected target cells. Other processes, termed *dendrites,* extend from the nerve cell body to receive synaptic contacts from other neurons; these dendrites may branch in extremely complex patterns. Neurons exhibit the cytological characteristics of highly active secretory cells with large nuclei; large amounts of smooth and rough endoplasmic reticulum; and frequent clusters of specialized smooth endoplasmic reticulum (Golgi apparatus), in which secretory products of the cell are packaged into membrane-bound organelles for transport out of the cell body proper to the axon or dendrites (Figure 12–1). Neurons and their cellular extensions are rich in microtubules—elongated tubules approximately 24 nm in diameter. Their functions may be to support the elongated axons and dendrites and to assist in the reciprocal transport of essential macromolecules and organelles between the cell body and the distant axon or dendrites.

The sites of interneuronal communication in the CNS are termed *synapses* (*see* below). Although synapses are functionally analogous to "junctions" in the somatic motor and autonomic nervous systems, the central junctions are characterized morphologically by various additional forms of paramembranous deposits of specific proteins (essential for transmitter release, response, and catabolism; *see* Liu and Edwards, 1997; Geppert and Südhoff, 1998). These specialized sites are presumed to be the active zone for transmitter release and response. The paramembranous proteins constitute a specialized junctional adherence zone, termed the *synaptolemma* (*see* Bodian, 1972). Like peripheral "junctions," central synapses also are denoted by accumulations of tiny (500 to 1500 Å) organelles, termed *synaptic vesicles.* The proteins of these vesicles have been shown to have specific roles in transmitter storage, vesicle docking onto presynaptic membranes, voltage- and Ca^{2+}-dependent secretion (*see* Chapter 6), and recycling and restorage of released transmitter (*see* Augustine *et al.,* 1999).

Synaptic Relationships. Synaptic arrangements in the CNS fall into a wide variety of morphological and functional forms

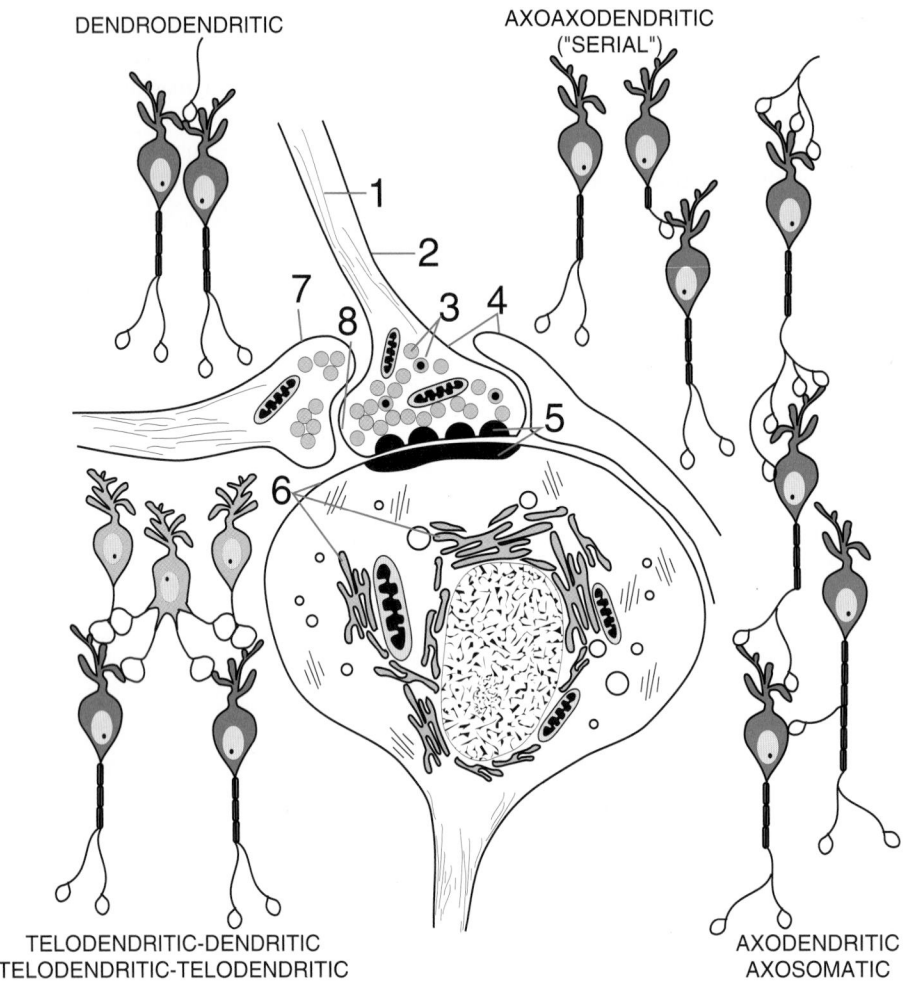

DENDRODENDRITIC

AXOAXODENDRITIC
("SERIAL")

TELODENDRITIC-DENDRITIC
TELODENDRITIC-TELODENDRITIC

AXODENDRITIC
AXOSOMATIC

Figure 12–1. Drug-sensitive sites in synaptic transmission.

Schematic view of the drug-sensitive sites in prototypical synaptic complexes. In the center, a post-synaptic neuron receives a somatic synapse (shown greatly oversized) from an axonic terminal; an axoaxonic terminal is shown in contact with this presynaptic nerve terminal. Drug-sensitive sites include: (1) microtubules responsible for bidirectional transport of macromolecules between the neuronal cell body and distal processes; (2) electrically conductive membranes; (3) sites for the synthesis and storage of transmitters; (4) sites for the active uptake of transmitters by nerve terminals or glia; (5) sites for the release of transmitter; (6) postsynaptic receptors, cytoplasmic organelles, and postsynaptic proteins for expression of synaptic activity and for long-term mediation of altered physiological states; and (7) presynaptic receptors on adjacent presynaptic processes and (8) on nerve terminals (autorecep-tors). Around the central neuron are schematic illustrations of the more common synaptic relationships in the CNS. (Modified from Bodian, 1972, and Cooper *et al.,* 1996, with permission.)

that are specific for the cells involved. Many spatial arrangements are possible within these highly individualized synaptic relationships (*see* Figure 12–1). The most common arrangement, typical of the hierarchical pathways, is the axodendritic or axosomatic synapse in which the axons of the cell of origin make their functional contact with the dendrites or cell body of the target. In other cases, functional contacts may occur more rarely between adjacent cell bodies (somasomatic) or overlapping dendrites (dendrodendritic). Some local-circuit neurons can enter

into synaptic relationships through modified dendrites, *teloden-drites,* that can be either presynaptic or postsynaptic. Within the spinal cord, serial axoaxonic synapses are relatively frequent. Here, the axon of an interneuron ends on the terminal of a long-distance neuron as that terminal contacts a dendrite in the dorsal horn. Many presynaptic axons contain local collections of typical synaptic vesicles with no opposed specialized synap-tolemma (termed *boutons en passant*). Release of transmitter may not occur at such sites.

The bioelectric properties of neurons and junctions in the CNS generally follow the outlines and details already described for the peripheral autonomic nervous system (*see* Chapter 6). However, in the CNS there is found a much more varied range of intracellular mechanisms (Nicoll *et al.,* 1990; Tzounopoulos *et al.,* 1998).

Supportive Cells. Neurons are not the only cells in the CNS. According to most estimates, neurons are outnumbered, perhaps by an order of magnitude, by the various nonneuronal supportive cellular elements (*see* Cherniak, 1990). Nonneuronal cells include the macroglia, microglia, the cells of the vascular elements (including the intracerebral vasculature as well as the cerebrospinal fluid-forming cells of the *choroid plexus* found within the intracerebral ventricular system), and the meninges, which cover the surface of the brain and comprise the cerebrospinal fluid-containing envelope. Macroglia are the most abundant supportive cells; some are categorized as *astrocytes* (nonneuronal cells interposed between the vasculature and the neurons, often surrounding individual compartments of synaptic complexes). Astrocytes play a variety of metabolic support roles including furnishing energy intermediates and supplementary removal of excessive extracellular neurotransmitter secretions (*see* Magistretti *et al.,* 1995). A second prominent category of macroglia are the myelin-producing cells, the *oligodendroglia*. Myelin, made up of multiple layers of their compacted membranes, insulates segments of long axons bioelectrically and accelerates action-potential conduction velocity. Microglia are relatively uncharacterized supportive cells believed to be of mesodermal origin and related to the macrophage/monocyte lineage (*see* Aloisi, 1999; González-Scarano and Baltuch, 1999). Some microglia are resident within the brain, while additional cells of this class may be attracted to the brain during periods of inflammation following either microbial infection or other postinjury inflammatory reactions. The response of the brain to inflammation differs strikingly from that of other tissues (*see* Andersson *et al.,* 1992; Raber *et al.,* 1998; Schnell *et al.,* 1999) and may in part explain its unique reactions to trauma (*see* below).

Blood–Brain Barrier. Apart from the exceptional instances in which drugs are introduced directly into the CNS, the concentration of the agent in the blood after oral or parenteral administration will differ substantially from its concentration in the brain. Although not thoroughly defined anatomically, the *blood–brain barrier* is an important boundary between the periphery and the CNS in the form of a permeability barrier to the passive diffusion of substances from the bloodstream into various regions of the CNS (*see* Park and Cho, 1991; Rubin and Staddon, 1999). Evidence of the barrier is provided by the greatly diminished rate of access of chemicals from plasma to the brain (*see* Chapter 1). This barrier is much less prominent in the hypothalamus and in several small, specialized organs lining the third and fourth ventricles of the brain: the median eminence, area postrema, pineal gland, subfornical organ, and subcommissural organ. In addition, there is little evidence of a barrier between the circulation and the peripheral nervous system (*e.g.,* sensory and autonomic nerves and ganglia). While severe limitations are imposed on the diffusion of macromolecules, selective barriers to permeation also exist for small charged molecules such as neurotransmitters, their precursors and metabolites, and some

drugs. These diffusional barriers are at present best thought of as a combination of the partition of solute across the vasculature (which governs passage by definable properties such as molecular weight, charge, and lipophilicity) and the presence or absence of energy-dependent transport systems. Active transport of certain agents may occur in either direction across the barriers. The diffusional barriers retard the movement of substances from brain to blood as well as from blood to brain. The brain clears metabolites of transmitters into the cerebrospinal fluid by excretion through the acid transport system of the choroid plexus (*see* Cserr and Bundgaard, 1984; Strange, 1993). Substances that rarely gain access to the brain from the bloodstream often can reach the brain after injection directly into the cerebrospinal fluid. Under certain conditions, it may be possible to open the blood–brain barrier, at least transiently, to permit the entry of chemotherapeutic agents (*see* Emerich *et al.,* 1998; Granholm *et al.,* 1998; LeMay *et al.,* 1998, for discussion). Cerebral ischemia and inflammation also modify the blood–brain barrier, resulting in increased access to substances that ordinarily would not affect the brain.

Response to Damage: Repair and Plasticity in the CNS

Because the neurons of the CNS are terminally differentiated cells, they do not undergo proliferative responses to damage, although recent evidence suggests the possibility of neural stem-cell proliferation as a natural means for selected neuronal replacement (*see* Gage, 2000). As a result, neurons have evolved other adaptive mechanisms to provide for maintenance of function following injury. These adaptive mechanisms endow the brain with considerable capacity for structural and functional modification well into adulthood (*see* Yang *et al.,* 1994; Jones *et al.,* 2000), and they may represent some of the mechanisms employed in the phenomena of memory and learning (*see* Kandel and O'Dell, 1992). Recent studies have shown that molecular signaling processes employed during brain development also may be involved in the plasticity seen in the adult brain, relying on specific neurotrophic agents (*see* Bothwell, 1995; Casaccia-Bonnefil *et al.,* 1998; Chao *et al.,* 1998); *see* below).

INTEGRATIVE CHEMICAL COMMUNICATION IN THE CENTRAL NERVOUS SYSTEM

The capacity to integrate information from a variety of external and internal sources epitomizes the cardinal role of the CNS, namely to optimize the needs of the organism within the demands of the individual's environment. These integrative concepts transcend individual transmitter systems and emphasize the means by which neuronal activity is normally coordinated. Only through a detailed understanding of these integrative functions, and their failure in certain pathophysiological conditions, can effective and specific therapeutic approaches be developed for neurological and psychiatric disorders. The identification of molecular and cellular mechanisms of neural integration is productively linked to clinical therapeutics, because untreatable diseases and unexpected nontherapeutic side effects of drugs often reveal ill-defined mechanisms of pathophysiology. Such observations can then drive the search for novel mechanisms of cellular regulation. The capacity to link molecular processes to behavioral operations, both normal and pathological, provides one of the most exciting aspects of modern neuropharmacological research. A central underlying concept of neuropsychopharmacology is that drugs that influence behavior and improve the functional status of patients with neurological or psychiatric diseases act by enhancing or blunting the effectiveness of specific combinations of synaptic transmitter actions.

Four research strategies provide the neuroscientific substrates of neuropsychological phenomena: molecular, cellular, multicellular (or systems), and behavioral. The intensively exploited molecular level has been the traditional focus for characterizing drugs that alter behavior. Molecular discoveries provide biochemical probes for identifying the appropriate neuronal sites and their mediative mechanisms. Such mechanisms include: (1) the ion channels, which provide for changes in excitability induced by neurotransmitters; (2) the neurotransmitter receptors (*see* below); (3) the auxiliary intramembranous and cytoplasmic transductive molecules that couple these receptors to intracellular effectors for short-term changes in excitability and for longer-term regulation *e.g.*, through alterations in gene expression (*see* Neyroz *et al.*, 1993; Gudermann *et al.*, 1997); (4) transporters for the conservation of released transmitter molecules by reaccumulation into nerve terminals, and then into synaptic vesicles (Blakely *et al.*, 1994; Amara and Sonders, 1998; Fairman and Amara, 1999). Transport across vesicle membranes utilizes a transport protein distinct from that involved in reuptake into nerve terminals (Liu and Edwards, 1997).

Research at the molecular level also provides the pharmacological tools to verify the working hypotheses of other molecular, cellular, and behavioral strategies and allows for a means to pursue their genetic basis. Thus, the most basic cellular phenomena of neurons now can be understood in terms of such discrete molecular entities. It has been known for some time that the basic excitability of neurons is achieved through modifications of the ion channels that all neurons express in abundance in their plasma membranes. However, it is now possible to understand precisely how the three major cations, Na^+, K^+, and Ca^{2+}, as well as the Cl^- anion are regulated in their flow through highly discriminative ion channels (*see* Figures 12–2 and 12–3). The voltage-dependent ion channels (Figure 12–2), which are contrasted with the "ligand-gated ion channels" (Figure 12–3), provide for rapid changes in ion permeability. These rapid changes underlie the rapid propagation of signals along axons and dendrites, and for the excitation-secretion coupling that releases neurotransmitters from presynaptic sites (Catterall, 1988, 1993). Cloning, expression, and functional assessment of constrained molecular modifications have defined conceptual chemical similarities among the major

cation channels (*see* Figure 12–2A). The intrinsic membrane-embedded domains of the Na^+ and Ca^{2+} channels are envisioned as four tandem repeats of a putative six-transmembrane domain, while the K^+ channel family contains greater molecular diversity. X-ray crystallography has now confirmed these configurations for the K^+ channel (Doyle *et al.*, 1998). One structural form of voltage-regulated K^+ channels, shown in Figure 12–2C, consists of subunits composed of a single putative six-transmembrane domain. The inward rectifier K^+ channel structure, in contrast, retains the general configuration corresponding to transmembrane spans 5 and 6 with the interposed "pore region" that penetrates only the exofacial surface membrane. These two structural categories of K^+ channels can form heteroligomers, giving rise to multiple possibilities for regulation by voltage, neurotransmitters, assembly with intracellular auxiliary proteins, or posttranslational modifications (Krapivinsky *et al.*, 1995). The structurally defined channel molecules (*see* Jan *et al.*, 1997; Doyle *et al.*, 1998) now can be examined to determine how drugs, toxins, and imposed voltages alter the excitability of a neuron, permitting a cell either to become spontaneously active or to die through prolonged opening of such channels (*see* Adams and Swanson, 1994). Within the CNS, variants of the K^+ channels (the delayed rectifier, the Ca^{2+}-activated K^+ channel, and the afterhyperpolarizing K^+ channel) regulated by intracellular second messengers repeatedly have been shown to underlie complex forms of synaptic modulation (*see* Nicoll, *et al.*, 1990; Malenka and Nicoll, 1999).

Research at the cellular level determines which specific neurons and which of their most proximate synaptic connections may mediate a behavior or the behavioral effects of a given drug. For example, research at the cellular level into the basis of emotion exploits both molecular and behavioral leads to determine the most likely brain sites at which behavioral changes pertinent to emotion can be analyzed. Such research provides clues as to the nature of the interactions in terms of interneuronal communication (*i.e.*, excitation, inhibition, or more complex forms of synaptic interaction; *see* Aston-Jones *et al.*, 1999; Brown *et al.*, 1999).

An understanding at the systems level is required to assemble the descriptive structural and functional properties of specific central transmitter systems, linking the neurons that make and release this transmitter to the possible effects of this release at the behavioral level. While many such transmitter-to-behavior linkages have been postulated, it has proven difficult to validate the essential involvement of specific transmitter-defined neurons in the mediation of specific mammalian behavior.

Research at the behavioral level often can illuminate the integrative phenomena that link populations of neurons (often through operationally or empirically defined ways) into extended specialized circuits, ensembles, or more pervasively distributed systems that integrate the physiological expression of a learned, reflexive, or spontaneously generated behavioral response. The entire concept of animal models of human psychiatric diseases rests on the assumption that scientists can appropriately infer from observations of behavior and physiology (heart rate, respiration, locomotion, *etc.*) that the states experienced by animals are equivalent to the emotional states experienced by human beings expressing similar physiological changes (*see* Kandel, 1998).

Ion Channels

A α_1 Subunits for Ca^{2+}, Na^+ Channels

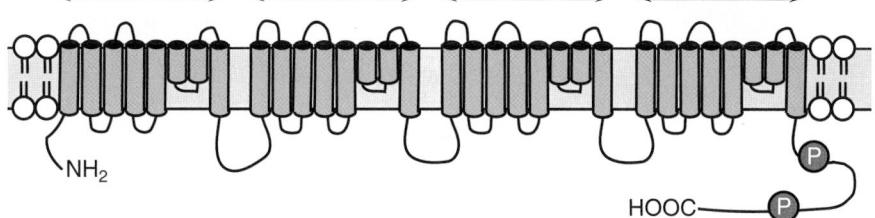

NH₂ HOOC

B   Multi-subunit Assembly for Ca^{2+} Channels

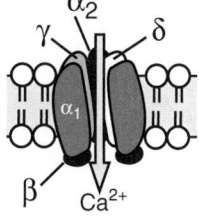 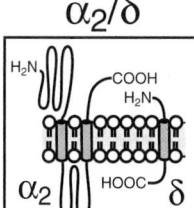 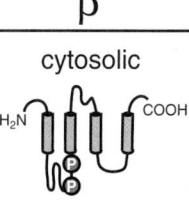 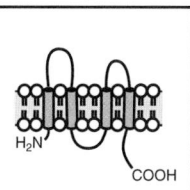

α_2/δ β γ

C   Structural Diversity of K^+ Channels

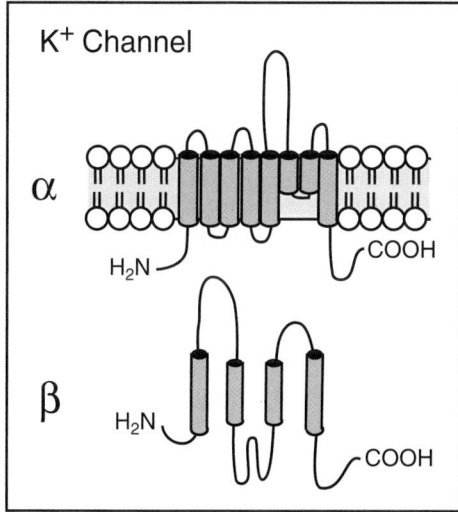 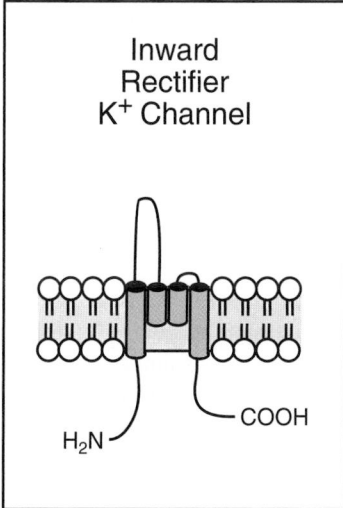

Figure 12–2. The major molecular motifs of ion channels that establish and regulate neuronal excitability in the CNS.

A. The α subunits of the Ca^{2+} and Na^+ channels share a similar presumptive six-transmembrane structure, repeated four times, in which an intramembranous segment separates transmembrane segments 5 and 6. **B.** The Ca^{2+} channel also requires several auxiliary small proteins (α_2, β, γ, and δ). The α_2 and δ subunits are linked by a disulfide bond (*not shown*). Regulatory subunits also exist for Na^+ channels. **C.** Voltage-sensitive K^+ channels (K_v) and the rapidly activating K^+ channel (K_a) share a similar presumptive six-transmembrane domain currently indistinguishable in overall configuration to one repeat unit within the Na^+ and Ca^{2+} channel structure, while the inwardly rectifying K^+ channel protein (K_{ir}) retains the general configuration of just loops 5 and 6. Regulatory β subunits can alter K_v channel functions. Channels of these two overall motifs can form heteromultimers (Krapivinsky *et al.*, 1995).

Identification of Central Transmitters

An essential step in understanding the functional properties of neurotransmitters within the context of the circuitry of the brain is to identify which substances are the transmitters for specific interneuronal connections. The criteria for the rigorous identification of central transmitters require the same data used to establish the transmitters of the autonomic nervous system (*see* Chapter 6).

1. *The transmitter must be shown to be present in the presynaptic terminals of the synapse and in the neurons from which those presynaptic terminals arise.* Extensions of this criterion involve the demonstration

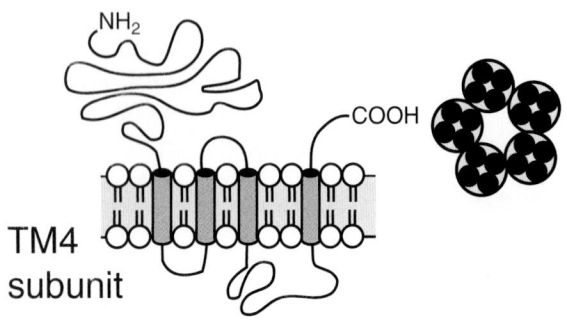

Figure 12–3. Ionophore receptors for neurotransmitters are composed of subunits with four presumptive transmembrane domains and are assembled as tetramers or pentamers (at right).

The predicted motif shown likely describes nicotinic cholinergic receptors for ACh, $GABA_A$ receptors for gamma-aminobutyric acid, $5HT_3$ receptors for serotonin, and receptors for glycine. Ionophore receptors for glutamate, however, probably are not accurately represented by this schematic motif.

that the presynaptic neuron synthesizes the transmitter substance, rather than simply storing it after accumulation from a nonneural source. Microscopic cytochemistry with antibodies or *in situ* hybridization, subcellular fractionation, and biochemical analysis of brain tissue are particularly suited to satisfy this criterion. These techniques often are combined in experimental animals with the production of surgical or chemical lesions of presynaptic neurons or their tracts to demonstrate that the lesion eliminates the proposed transmitter from the target region. Detection of the mRNA for receptors within postsynaptic neurons using molecular biological methods can strengthen the satisfaction of this criterion.

2. *The transmitter must be released from the presynaptic nerve concomitantly with presynaptic nerve activity.* This criterion is best satisfied by electrical stimulation of the nerve pathway *in vivo* and collection of the transmitter in an enriched extracellular fluid within the synaptic target area. Demonstrating release of a transmitter used to require sampling for prolonged intervals, but modern approaches employ minute microdialysis tubing or microvoltametric electrodes capable of sensitive detection of amine and amino acid transmitters within spatially and temporally meaningful dimensions (*see* Parsons and Justice, 1994; Humpel *et al.*, 1996). Release of transmitter also can be studied *in vitro* by ionic or electrical activation of thin brain slices or subcellular fractions that are enriched

in nerve terminals. The release of all transmitter substances so far studied, including presumptive transmitter release from dendrites (Morris *et al.*, 1998), is voltage-dependent and requires the influx of Ca^{2+} into the presynaptic terminal. However, transmitter release is relatively insensitive to extracellular Na^+ or to tetrodotoxin, which blocks transmembrane movement of Na^+.

3. *When applied experimentally to the target cells, the effects of the putative transmitter must be identical to the effects of stimulating the presynaptic pathway.* This criterion can be met loosely by qualitative comparisons (*e.g.*, both the substance and the pathway inhibit or excite the target cell). More convincing is the demonstration that the ionic conductances activated by the pathway are the same as those activated by the candidate transmitter. Alternatively, the criterion can be satisfied less rigorously by demonstration of the pharmacological identity of receptors. In general, pharmacological antagonism of the actions of the pathway and those of the candidate transmitter should be achieved by similar doses of the same drug. To be convincing, the antagonistic drug should not affect responses of the target neurons to other unrelated pathways or to chemically distinct transmitter candidates. Actions that are qualitatively identical to those that follow stimulation of the pathway also should be observed with synthetic agonists that mimic the actions of the transmitter.

Other studies, especially those that have implicated peptides as transmitters in the central and peripheral nervous systems, suggest that many brain and spinal cord synapses contain more than one transmitter substance (*see* Hökfelt *et al.*, 2000). Although rigorous proof is lacking, substances that coexist in a given synapse are presumed to be released together and to act jointly on the postsynaptic membrane (*see* Derrick and Martinez, 1994; Jin and Chavkin, 1999). Clearly, if more than one substance transmits information, no single agonist necessarily would provide faithful mimicry, nor would an antagonist provide total antagonism of activation of a given presynaptic element.

CNS Transmitter Discovery Strategies

The earliest transmitters considered for central roles were acetylcholine and norepinephrine, largely because of their established roles in the somatic motor and autonomic nervous systems. In the 1960s, serotonin, epinephrine, and dopamine also were investigated as potential CNS transmitters. Histochemical as well as biochemical and pharmacological data yielded results consistent with roles as neurotransmitters, but complete satisfaction of all criteria was not achieved. In the early 1970s, the availability of selective and potent antagonists of gamma-aminobutyric acid (GABA), glycine, and glutamate, all known to be enriched in brain, led to their acceptance as transmitter substances in general. Also at this time, a search for hypothalamic-hypophyseal factors led to an improvement in the technology to isolate, purify, sequence, and synthetically replicate a growing family of neuropeptides (*see* Hökfelt, *et al.,* 2000, for an overview). This advance, coupled with the widespread application of immunohistochemistry, strongly supported the view that neuropeptides may act as transmitters. Adaptation of bioassay technology from studies of pituitary secretions to other effectors (such as smooth-muscle contractility and, later, ligand-displacement assays) gave rise to the discovery of endogenous peptide ligands for drugs acting at opiate receptors (*see* Chapter 23). The search for endogenous factors whose receptors constituted the drug-binding sites was extended later to the benzodiazepine receptors (Costa and Guidotti, 1991). A more recent extension of this strategy has identified a series of endogenous lipid amides as the natural ligands for the tetrahydrocannabinoid receptors (*see* Piomelli *et al.,* 1998).

Assessment of Receptor Properties. Until quite recently, central synaptic receptors were characterized either by examination of their ability to bind radiolabeled agonists or antagonists (and on the ability of other unlabeled compounds to compete for such binding sites) or by electrophysiological or biochemical consequences of receptor activation of neurons *in vivo* or *in vitro.* Radioligand-binding assays can quantify binding sites within a region, track their appearance throughout the phylogenetic scale and during brain development, and evaluate how physiological or pharmacological manipulation regulates receptor number or affinity (*see* Dumont *et al.,* 1998; Redrobe *et al.,* 1999, for examples).

The properties of the cellular response to the transmitter can be studied electrophysiologically by the use of microiontophoresis (involving recording from single cells and highly localized drug administration). The patch-clamp technique can be used to study the electrical properties of single ionic channels and their regulation by neurotransmitters. These direct electrophysiological tests of neuronal responsiveness can provide qualitative and quantitative information on the effects of a putative transmitter substance (*see* Jardemark *et al.,* 1998, for recent examples). Receptor properties also can be studied biochemically when the activated receptor is coupled to an enzymatic reaction, such as the synthesis of a second messenger and the ensuing biochemical changes measured.

In the current era, molecular biological techniques have led to identification of mRNAs (or cDNAs) for the receptors for virtually every natural ligand considered as a neurotransmitter. A common practice is to introduce these coding sequences into test cells (frog oocytes or mammalian cells) and to assess the relative effects of ligands and of second-messenger production in such cells. Molecular cloning studies have revealed two major (*see* Figures 12–3 and 12–4) and one minor molecular motif of transmitter receptors. Oligomeric ion-channel receptors composed of multiple subunits usually have four putative

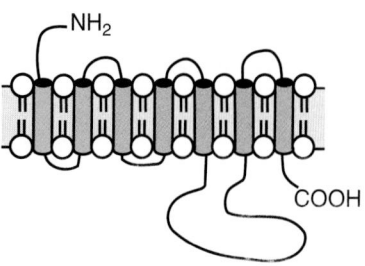

Figure 12–4. G protein–coupled receptors are composed of a single subunit, with seven presumptive transmembrane domains.

For small neurotransmitters, the binding pocket is buried within the bilayer; sequences in the second cytoplasmic loop and projecting out of the bilayer at the base of transmembrane spans 5 and 6 have been implicated in agonist-facilitated G protein coupling (*see* Chapter 2).

"transmembrane domains" consisting of 20 to 25 generally hydrophobic amino acids (*see* Figure 12–3). The ion channel receptors (called *ionotropic receptors*) for neurotransmitters contain sites for reversible phosphorylation by protein kinases and phosphoprotein phosphatases and for voltage-gating. Receptors with this structure include nicotinic cholinergic (or nicotinic acetylcholine) receptors (*see* Chapters 2 and 7); the receptors for the amino acids GABA, glycine, glutamate, and aspartate, and for the 5-HT$_3$ receptor (*see* Chapter 11).

The second major structural motif for transmitter receptors is manifest by G protein–coupled receptors (GPCR), in which a monomeric receptor has seven putative transmembrane domains, with varying intra- and extracytoplasmic loop lengths (*see* Figure 12–4). Multiple mutagenesis strategies have defined how the activated receptors (themselves subject to reversible phosphorylation at one or more functionally distinct sites) can interact with the heterotrimeric GTP-binding protein complex to ultimately activate, inhibit, or otherwise regulate enzymatic effector systems, *e.g.,* adenylyl cyclase or phospholipase C, or ion channels, such as voltage-gated Ca^{2+} channels or receptor-operated K^+ channels (*see* Figure 2–1 and related text in Chapter 2). The GPCR family includes muscarinic cholinergic receptors, GABA$_B$ and metabotropic glutamate receptors, and all other aminergic and peptidergic receptors. By transfecting "null cells" with uncharacterized GPCR mRNAs, novel neuropeptides have been identified (*see* Reinscheid *et al.,* 1995). A third receptor motif is represented by cell-surface receptors whose cytoplasmic domains possess catalytic activities, in particular, guanylyl cyclase (*see* Chapter 2).

An additional molecular motif expressed within the CNS involves the transporters that remove transmitters after secretion by an ion-dependent reuptake process (Figure 12–5). Transporters exhibit a molecular motif with 12 hypothetical transmembrane domains similar to glucose transporters and to mammalian adenylyl cyclase (*see* Tang and Gilman, 1992).

Postsynaptic receptivity of CNS neurons is regulated continuously in terms of the number of receptor sites and the threshold required for generation of a response. Receptor number often is dependent on the concentration of agonist to which the target

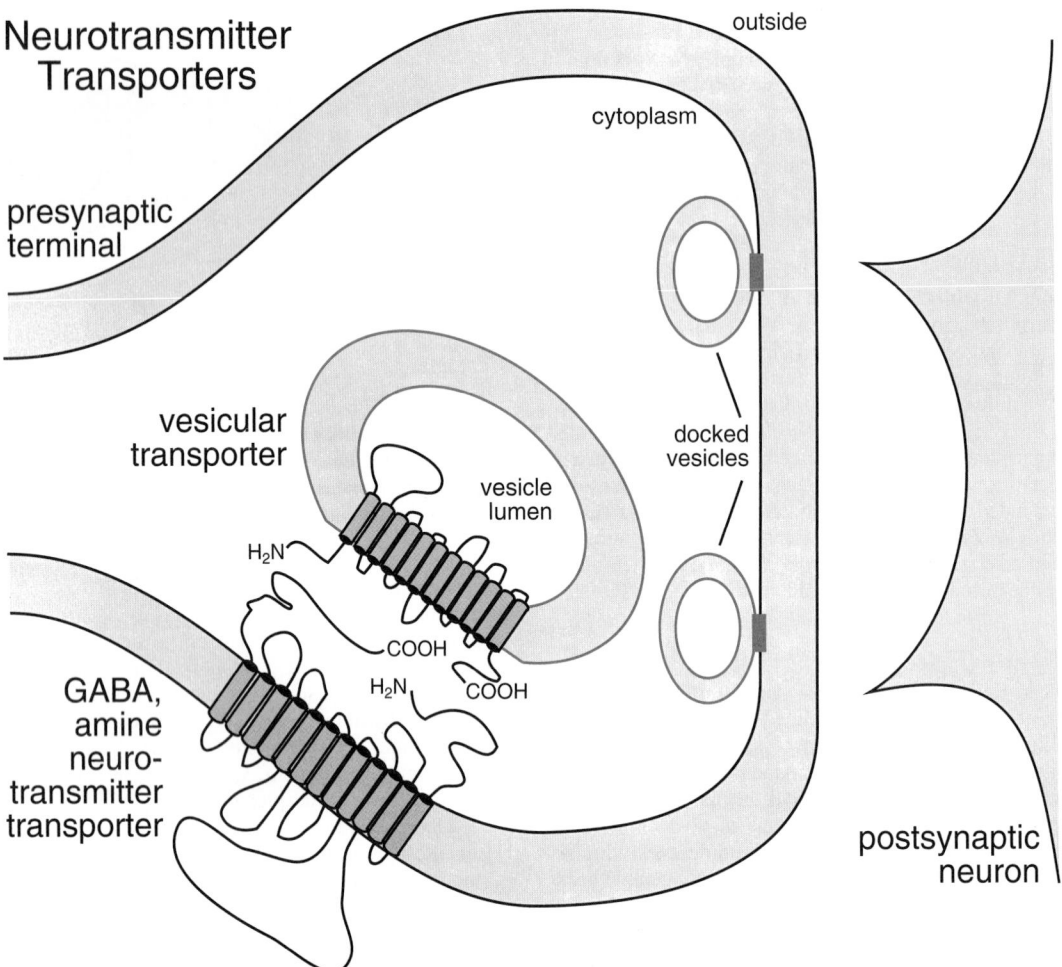

Figure 12–5. Predicted structural motif for neurotransmitter transporters.

Transporters for the conservation of released amino acid or amine transmitters all share a presumptive twelve-transmembrane domain structure, although the exact orientation of the amino terminus is not clear. Transporters for amine transmitters found on synaptic vesicles also share a presumptive twelve-transmembrane domain structure, but one which is distinct from the transporters of the plasma membrane.

cell is exposed. Thus, chronic excess of agonist can lead to a re-duced number of receptors (desensitization or down-regulation) and consequently to subsensitivity or tolerance to the transmit-ter. A deficit of transmitter can lead to increased numbers of receptors and supersensitivity of the system. These adaptive pro-cesses become especially important when drugs are used to treat chronic illness of the CNS. With prolonged periods of exposure to drug, the actual mechanisms underlying the therapeutic effect may differ strikingly from those that operate when the agent is first introduced into the system. Similar adaptive modifications of neuronal systems also can occur at presynaptic sites, such as those concerned with transmitter synthesis, storage, reuptake, and release.

NEUROTRANSMITTERS, NEUROHORMONES, AND NEUROMODULATORS: CONTRASTING PRINCIPLES OF NEURONAL REGULATION

Neurotransmitters. Satisfaction of the experimental cri-teria for identification of synaptic transmitters can lead to the conclusion that a substance contained in a neuron is secreted by that neuron to transmit information to its postsynaptic target. Given a definite effect of neuron A on target cell B, a substance found in or secreted by neuron A and producing the effect of A on B operationally would be the transmitter from A to B. In some cases, transmitters may produce minimal effects on bioelectric properties yet activate or inactivate biochemical mechanisms necessary for responses to other circuits. Alternatively, the action of a transmitter may vary with the context of ongoing synaptic events—enhancing excitation or inhibition, rather than operating to impose direct excitation or inhibition (see Bourne and Nicoll, 1993). Each chemical substance that fits within the broad definition of a transmitter may, therefore, require operational definition within the spatial and temporal domains in which a specific cell-cell circuit is defined. Those same properties may or may not be generalized to other cells that are contacted by the same presynaptic neurons, with the differences in operation related to differences in postsynaptic receptors and the mechanisms by which the activated receptor produces its effect.

Classically, electrophysiological signs of the action of a *bona fide* transmitter fall into two major categories: (1) *excitation,* in which ion channels are opened to permit net influx of positively charged ions, leading to depolarization with a reduction in the electrical resistance of the membrane; and (2) *inhibition,* in which selective ion movements lead to hyperpolarization, also with decreased membrane resistance. More recent work suggests there may be many "nonclassical" transmitter mechanisms operating in the CNS. In some cases, either depolarization or hyperpolarization is accompanied by a *decreased* ionic conductance (increased membrane resistance) as actions of the transmitter lead to the closure of ion channels (so-called leak channels) that normally are open in some resting neurons (Shepherd, 1998). For some transmitters, such as monoamines and certain peptides, a "conditional" action may be involved. That is, a transmitter substance may enhance or suppress the response of the target neuron to classical excitatory or inhibitory transmitters while producing little or no change in membrane potential or ionic conductance when applied alone. Such conditional responses have been termed *modulatory,* and specific categories of modulation have been hypothesized (see Nicoll et al., 1990; Foote and Aston-Jones, 1995). Regardless of the mechanisms that underlie such synaptic operations, their temporal and biophysical characteristics differ substantially from the rapid onset-offset type of effect previously thought to describe all synaptic events. These differences have thus raised the issue of whether or not substances that produce slow synaptic effects should be described with the same term—*neurotransmitter.* Some of the alternative terms and the molecules they describe

deserve brief mention with regard to mechanisms of drug action.

Neurohormones. Peptide-secreting cells of the hypothalamico-hypophyseal circuits originally were described as neurosecretory cells, a form of neuron that was both fish and fowl, receiving synaptic information from other central neurons yet secreting transmitters in a hormone-like fashion into the circulation. The transmitter released from such neurons was termed a *neurohormone—i.e.,* a substance secreted into the blood by a neuron. However, this term has lost most of its original meaning, because these hypothalamic neurons also may form traditional synapses with central neurons (Hökfelt et al., 1995, 2000). Cytochemical evidence indicates that the same substance that is secreted as a hormone from the posterior pituitary (oxytocin, antidiuretic hormone), mediates transmission at these sites. Thus, the designation *hormone* relates to the site of release at the pituitary and does not necessarily describe all of the actions of the peptide.

Neuromodulators. Florey (1967) employed the term *modulator* to describe substances that can influence neuronal activity in a manner different from that of neurotransmitters. In the context of this definition, the distinctive feature of a modulator is that it originates from cellular and nonsynaptic sites, yet influences the excitability of nerve cells. Florey specifically designated substances such as CO_2 and ammonia, arising from active neurons or glia, as potential modulators through nonsynaptic actions. Similarly, circulating steroid hormones, steroids produced in the nervous system (Baulieu, 1998), locally released adenosine and other purines, prostaglandins and other arachidonic acid metabolites, and nitric oxide (NO) (Gally et al., 1990) might all now be regarded as modulators.

Neuromediators. Substances that participate in the elicitation of the postsynaptic response to a transmitter fall under this heading. The clearest examples of such effects are provided by the involvement of adenosine 3',5'-monophosphate (cyclic AMP), guanosine 3',5'-monophosphate (cyclic GMP), and inositol phosphates as second messengers at specific sites of synaptic transmission (see Chapters 6, 7, 10, and 11). However, it is technically difficult to demonstrate in brain that a change in the concentration of cyclic nucleotides occurs prior to the generation of the synaptic potential and that this change in concentration is both necessary and sufficient for its generation. It is possible that changes in the concentration of second messengers can occur and enhance the generation of synaptic potentials. Activation of second messenger-dependent protein phosphorylation reactions can initiate a complex cascade of precise molecular events that regulate the properties of membrane and cytoplasmic proteins that are central to neuronal excitability (Greengard et al., 1999). These possibilities are particularly pertinent to the action of drugs that augment or reduce transmitter effects (see below).

Neurotrophic Factors. Neurotrophic factors are substances produced within the CNS by neurons, astrocytes, microglia, or transiently invading peripheral inflammatory or immune cells that assist neurons in their attempts to repair damage. Seven categories of peptide factors have been recognized to operate in this fashion (see Black, 1999; McKay et al., 1999, for recent reviews): (1) the classic neurotrophins (nerve growth factor, brain-derived neurotrophic factor, and the related neurotrophins); (2) the neuropoietic factors, which have effects both in brain and in myeloid cells [*e.g.*, cholinergic differentiation factor (also called leukemia inhibitory factor), ciliary neurotrophic factor, and some interleukins]; (3) growth factor peptides, such as epidermal growth factor, transforming growth factors α and β, glial-cell line-derived neurotrophic factor, and activin A; (4) the fibroblast growth factors; (5) insulin-like growth factors; (6) platelet-derived growth factors; and (7) axon-guidance molecules, some of which also are capable of affecting cells of the immune system (*see* Song and Poo, 1999; Spriggs, 1999). Drugs designed to elicit the formation and secretion of these products as well as to emulate their actions could provide useful adjuncts to rehabilitative treatments.

CENTRAL NEUROTRANSMITTERS

In examining the effects of drugs on the CNS with reference to the neurotransmitters for specific circuits, attention should be devoted to the general organizational principles of neurons. The view that synapses represent drug-modifiable control points within neuronal networks thus requires explicit delineation of the sites at which given neurotransmitters may operate and the degree of specificity with which such sites may be affected. One principle that underlies the following summaries of individual transmitter substances is the chemical-specificity hypothesis of Dale (1935), which holds that a given neuron releases the same transmitter substance at each of its synaptic terminals. In the face of growing indications that some neurons may contain more than one transmitter substance (Hökfelt, *et al.*, 1995, 2000), Dale's hypothesis has been modified to indicate that a given neuron will secrete the same set of transmitters from all of its terminals. However, even this theory may require revision. For example, it is not clear whether or not a neuron that secretes a given peptide will process the precursor peptide to the same end product at all of its synaptic terminals. Table 12–1 provides an overview of the pharmacological properties of the transmitters in the CNS that have been studied extensively. Neurotransmitters are discussed below in terms of the groups of substances within given chemical categories: amino acids, amines, and neuropeptides. Other substances that may participate in central synaptic transmission include purines (such as adenosine and ATP (*see* Edwards and Robertson, 1999; Moreau and Huber, 1999; Baraldi *et al.*, 2000), nitric oxide (*see* Cork *et al.*, 1998), and arachidonic acid derivatives (*see* Mechoulam *et al.*, 1996; Piomelli, *et al.*, 1998).

Amino Acids. The CNS contains uniquely high concentrations of certain amino acids, notably glutamate and GABA; these amino acids are extremely potent in their ability to alter neuronal discharge. Initially, physiologists were reluctant to accept these simple substances as central neurotransmitters. Their ubiquitous distribution within the brain and the consistent observation that they produced prompt, powerful, and readily reversible but redundant effects on every neuron tested seemed out of keeping with the extreme heterogeneity of distribution and responsivity seen for other putative transmitters. The dicarboxylic amino acids produced near-universal excitation, and the monocarboxylic ω-amino acids (*e.g.*, GABA, glycine, β-alanine, taurine) produced qualitatively similar and consistent inhibitions (Kelly and Beart, 1975). Following the emergence of selective antagonists to the amino acids, identification of selective receptors and receptor subtypes became possible. Together with the development of methods for mapping the ligands and their receptors, there is now strong evidence and widespread acceptance that the amino acids GABA, glycine, and glutamate are central transmitters.

GABA. GABA was identified as a unique chemical constituent of brain in 1950, but its potency as a CNS depressant was not immediately recognized. At the crustacean stretch receptor, GABA was identified as the only inhibitory amino acid found exclusively in crustacean inhibitory nerves and the inhibitory potency of extracts of these nerves was accounted for by their content of GABA. Release of GABA correlated with the frequency of nerve stimulation, and application of GABA and inhibitory nerve stimulation produced identical increases of Cl^- conductance in the muscle, fully satisfying the criteria for identification of GABA as the transmitter for this nerve (for further historical references, *see* Bloom, 1996).

These same physiological and pharmacological properties later were found to be useful models in tests of a role for GABA in the mammalian CNS. Substantial data support the idea that GABA mediates the inhibitory actions of local interneurons in the brain and that GABA also may mediate presynaptic inhibition within the spinal cord. Presumptive GABA-ergic inhibitory synapses have been demonstrated most clearly between cerebellar Purkinje neurons and their targets in Deiter's nucleus; between small interneurons and the major output cells of the cerebellar cortex, olfactory bulb, cuneate nucleus, hippocampus, and lateral septal nucleus; and between the vestibular nucleus and the trochlear motoneurons. GABA also mediates inhibition within the cerebral cortex and between the caudate nucleus and the substantia nigra. GABA-ergic neurons and nerve terminals have been localized with immunocytochemical methods that visualize glutamic acid decarboxylase, the enzyme that catalyzes the synthesis of GABA from glutamic acid, or by *in situ* hybridization of the mRNAs for this protein. GABA-containing neurons frequently have been found to coexpress one or more neuropeptides. The most useful drugs for confirmation of GABA-ergic mediation have been bicuculline and

Table 12–1
Overview of Transmitter Pharmacology in the Central Nervous System

TRANSMITTER	TRANSPORTER BLOCKER*	RECEPTOR SUBTYPE & MOTIF (IR/GPCR)	SELECTIVE AGONISTS	SELECTIVE ANTAGONISTS
GABA	Guvacine Nipecotic acid	$GABA_A$ (IR) $\alpha, \beta, \gamma, \delta, \sigma$ isoforms	Muscimol Isoguvacine THIP	Bicuculline Picrotoxin SR 95531
	(β-Alanine for glia)	$GABA_B$ (GPCR)	Baclofen 3-Aminopropylphosphinic acid	2-hydroxy-s-Saclofen CGP35348 CGP55845 CPG64213
Glycine	? Sarcosine	α and β subunits (IR)	β-Alanine; taurine	Strychnine
Glutamate Aspartate	—	AMPA (IR) GLU 1-4 (IR)	Quisqualate	NBQX, LY215490
		KA (IR) GLU 5-7; KA 1,2 (IR)	Domoic acid	MK801; AP5; LY223053
		NMDA (IR) NMDA $1,2_{A-D}$ (IR)	—	α-Me-4-carboxyphenylglycine
		mGLU 1-7 (GPCR)	—	—
Acetylcholine		Nicotinic (IR) Multiple α and β isoforms	—	α-Bungarotoxin Me-Lycaconitine
	—	Muscarinic M_1-M_4 (GPCR)	—	M_1: Pirenzepine M_2: Methoctramine M_3: Hexahydrosiladifenidol M_4: Tropicamide
Dopamine	Cocaine; mazindol; GBR12-395; nomifensine	D_{1-5} (GPCR)	D_1: SKF38393 D_2: Bromocriptine D_3: 7-OH-DPAT	D_1: SCH23390 D_2: Sulpiride; domperidone
Norepinephrine	Desmethylimipramine; mazindol; cocaine	α_{1A-D} (GPCR)	α_{1A}: NE > EPI	WB4101

Table 12-1
Overview of Transmitter Pharmacology in the Central Nervous System (*Continued*)

TRANSMITTER	TRANSPORTER BLOCKER*	RECEPTOR SUBTYPE & MOTIF (IR/GPCR)	SELECTIVE AGONISTS	SELECTIVE ANTAGONISTS
		α_{2A-C} (GPCR)	α_{2A}: Oxymetazoline, dexmedetomidine	$\alpha_{2A}-\alpha_{2C}$: Yohimbine α_{2B}, α_{2C}: Prazosin
		β_{1-3} (GPCR)	β_1: EPI = NE β_2: EPI $\gg$ NE β_3: NE > EPI	β_1: Atenolol β_2: Butoxamine β_3: BRL 37344
Serotonin	Clomipramine; sertraline; fluoxetine	5-HT$_{1A-F}$ (GPCR)	5-HT$_{1A}$: 8-OH-DPAT 5-HT$_{1B}$: CP93129 5-HT$_{1D}$: LY694247	5-HT$_{1A}$: WAY101135 5-HT$_{1D}$: GR127935
		5-HT$_{2A-C}$ (GPCR)	α-Me-5-HT, DOB	LY53857; ritanserin; mesulergine; ketanserin
		5-HT$_3$ (IR)	2-Me-5-HT; m-CPB	Tropisetron; ondansetron; granisetron
		5-HT$_{4-7}$ (GPCR)	5-HT$_4$: BIMU8; RS67506; ML10302	5-HT$_4$: GR113808; SB204070
Histamine		H$_1$ (GPCR)	2 (m-F-phenylhistamine); 2-methylhistamine	Mepyramine; chlorpheniramine
	—	H$_2$ (GPCR)	Dimaprit; impromadine	Ranitidine; famotidine; cimetidine
	—	H$_3$ (?)	R-α-Me-histamine; imetit	Thioperamide; iodophenpropit
Vasopressin	—	V1$_{A,B}$ (GPCR)	—	V1$_A$: SR 49059
	—	V2 (GPCR)	d[dArg^8]VP	d(CH$_2$)$_5$ [dIle^{2}Ile^4]AVP
Oxytocin	—	(GPCR)	[Thr^4,Gly^7]OT	d(CH$_2$)$_5$ [Tyr(Me)^2, Thr^4, Orn^8]OT$_{1-8}$
Tachykinins	—	NK1 (SP > NKA > NKB) (GPCR)	Substance P Me ester	SR140333 LY303870 CP99994
		NK2 (NKA > NKB > SP) (GPCR)	β–[Ala^8]NKA$_{4-10}$	GR94800 GR159897
		NK3 (NKB > NKA > SP) (GPCR)	GR138676	SR142802 SB223412

CCK	—	CCK$_1$ (GPCR)	CCK8 $\gg$ gastrin = CCK4; A71623	Devazepide; lorglumide
		CCK$_2$ (GPCR)	CCK8 $\geq$ gastrin = CCK4	CI988; L365260; YM022
NPY	—	Y1 (GPCR) Y2 (GPCR) Y4–Y6 (GPCR)	[Pro$_{34}$]NPY NPY$_{13-16}$	GR231118; SR 120107A NPY
		Y2 (GPCR)	NPY$_{13-36}$, NPY$_{18-36}$	
Neurotensin	—	(GPCR)	—	SR48692
Opioid peptides		μ (β-endorphin) (GPCR)	DAMGO, sufentanil, DALDA	CTOP, CTAP, β–FNA
		δ (Met^5-Enk) (GPCR)	DPDPE; DSBULET; SNC–80	Naltrindole, TIPP4, DALCE ICI174864
	—	κ (Dyn A) (GPCR)	U69593; CI977 ICI174864	nor-Binaltorphimine, DIPPA, UPHIT
Somatostatin	—	sst$_1$ (GPCR)	sst des-Ala^{1,2,5}	—
		sst$_2$ (GPCR)	Octreotide, seglitide, BIM23027	Cyanamid 154806
		sst$_{3,4}$ (GPCR)	BIM23052, NNC269100	—
		sst$_5$ (GPCR)	L362855	BIM23056
Purines		P1 (A$_{1,2a,2b,3}$) (GPCR)	A$_1$: N^6-cyclopentyladenosine	8-Cyclopentyltheophylline; DPCPX
			A$_{2a}$: CGS21680, APEC, HENECA	CO66713, SCH58261, ZM241385
		P2X (IR)	α,β–methylene ATP	Suramin (nonselective)
	—	P2Y (GPCR)	ADPβF	Suramin

*In some instances (*e.g.*, acetylcholine, purines), agents that inhibit metabolism of the transmitter(s) have effects that are analogous to those of inhibitors of transport of other transmitters.

Abbreviations: CCK: cholecystokinin; NPY: neuropeptide Y; NK: neurokinin; SP: substance P; GPCR: G protein–coupled receptor; IR: ionophore receptor; 5-HT: 5-hydroxytryptamine (serotonin); NE: norepinephrine; EPI: epinephrine; VP: vasopressin; AVP: arginine vasopressin; OT: Oxytocin; 7-OH-DPAT: 7-hydroxy-2(di-n-propylamino) tetralin; DOB: dobutamine; DAMGO: d-Ala-2, Me-Phe4, Gly (01) 5 enkephalin; DPDPE: [d-Pen2; d-Pen5] enkephalin; DSBULET: Tyr-d-Ser-O-tbutyl-Gly-Phe-Leu-Thr. *See* Chapter 2 for discussion of mechanisms linking receptor occupancy to effector activation.

picrotoxin; however, many convulsants whose actions previously were unexplained (including penicillin and pentylenetetrazol) also may act as relatively selective antagonists of the action of GABA (Macdonald *et al.,* 1992; Macdonald and Olsen, 1994). Useful therapeutic effects have not yet been obtained through the use of agents that mimic GABA (such as muscimol), inhibit its active reuptake (such as 2,4-diaminobutyrate, nipecotic acid, and guvacine), or alter its turnover (such as aminooxyacetic acid).

GABA is the major inhibitory neurotransmitter in the mammalian CNS. Its receptors have been divided into two main types. The more prominent GABA receptor subtype, the GABA$_A$ receptor, is a ligand-gated Cl$^-$ ion channel, an "ionotropic receptor" that is opened after release of GABA from presynaptic neurons. A second receptor, the GABA$_B$ receptor, is a member of the GPCR family, as noted above, and is coupled both to biochemical pathways and to regulation of ion channels, a class of receptor generally referred to as "metabotropic" (Grifa *et al.,* 1998; Billinton *et al.,* 1999; Brauner-Osborne and Krogsgaard-Larsen, 1999).

The GABA$_A$ receptor subunit proteins have been well characterized due to their high abundance and the receptor's role in almost every neuronal circuit. The receptor also has been extensively characterized in its role as the site of action of many neuroactive drugs (*see* Chapter 17). Notable among these are benzodiazepines and barbiturates. It has been suggested recently that direct interactions occur between GABA$_A$ receptors and anesthetic steroids, volatile anesthetics, and alcohol (Macdonald, Twyman *et al.,* 1992).

Based on sequence homology to the first GABA$_A$ subunit cDNAs, more than 15 other subunits have been cloned. In addition to these subunits, which are products of separate genes, mRNA splice variants for several subunits have been described. The GABA$_A$ receptor, by analogy with the classical ionotropic nicotinic cholinergic receptor, may be either a pentameric or tetrameric protein in which the subunits assemble together around a central ion pore, a structural format typical for all ionotropic receptors.

Abundant evidence has shown that there are multiple subtypes of GABA$_A$ receptors in the brain. The existence of subtypes was first suggested by pharmacological differences. It is now known that receptors composed of particular subunits have distinct pharmacological properties (Barnard *et al.,* 1988; Olsen *et al.,* 1990; Seeburg *et al.,* 1990), but the true heterogeneity of GABA$_A$-receptor subtypes has yet to be fully defined. Differences in anatomical distribution of subunits and differences in the time course of development of genes expressing each subunit suggest that there are important functional differences among the subtypes.

The subunit composition of the major form of the GABA$_A$ receptor contains at least three different subunits—α, β, and γ. The stoichiometry of these subunits is not known (De Blas, 1996). To interact with benzodiazepines with the profile expected of the native GABA$_A$ receptor, the receptor must contain each of these subunits. Inclusion of variant α, β, or γ subunits results in receptors with different pharmacological profiles (*see* Chapter 17).

Glycine. Many of the features described for the GABA$_A$ receptor family also are features of the inhibitory glycine receptor that is prominent in the brainstem and spinal cord. Multiple subunits have been cloned, and they can assemble into a variety of glycine-receptor subtypes (Grenningloh *et al.,* 1987; Malosio *et al.,* 1991). These pharmacological subtypes are detected in brain tissue with particular neuroanatomical and neurodevelopmental profiles. However, as with the GABA$_A$ receptor, the complete functional significance of the glycine receptor subtypes is not known.

Glutamate and Aspartate. Glutamate and aspartate are found in very high concentrations in brain, and both amino acids have extremely powerful excitatory effects on neurons in virtually every region of the CNS. Their widespread distribution tended to obscure their roles as transmitters, but there is now broad acceptance of the view that glutamate and possibly aspartate function as the principal fast ("classical") excitatory transmitters throughout the CNS (*see* Seeburg, 1993; Cotman *et al.,* 1995; Herrling, 1997). Furthermore, over the past decade, multiple subtypes of receptors for excitatory amino acids have been characterized pharmacologically, based on the relative potencies of synthetic agonists and the discovery of potent and selective antagonists (*see* Herrling, 1997).

Glutamate receptors, like those for GABA, are classified functionally either as ligand-gated ion channels ("ionotropic" receptors) or as "metabotropic" (G protein–coupled) receptors. Neither the precise number of subunits that assemble to generate a functional glutamate receptor ion channel *in vivo* nor the topography of each subunit has been established unequivocally (Borges and Dingledine, 1998; Dingledine *et al.,* 1999).

The ligand-gated ion channels are further classified according to the identity of agonists that selectively activate each receptor subtype. These receptors include α-amino-3-hydroxy-5-methyl-4-isoxazole propionic acid (AMPA), kainate, and *N*-methyl-D aspartate (NMDA) receptors (Borges and Dingledine, 1998; Dingledine *et al.,* 1999). A number of selective antagonists for these receptors now are available (Herrling, 1997). In the case of NMDA receptors, noncompetitive antagonists acting at various sites on the receptor protein have been described in addition to competitive (glutamate site) antagonists. These include open-channel blockers such as phencyclidine (PCP or angel dust), antagonists such as 5,7-dichlorokynurenic acid that act at an allosteric glycine-binding site, and the novel antagonist ifenprodil, which may act as a closed-channel blocker. In addition, the activity of NMDA receptors is sensitive to pH and also can be modulated by a variety of endogenous modulators including Zn^{2+}, some neurosteroids, arachidonic acid, redox reagents, and polyamines such as spermine (for review, *see* Dingledine *et al.,* 1999).

Multiple cDNAs encoding metabotropic receptors and subunits of NMDA, AMPA, and kainate receptors have been cloned in recent years (Borges and Dingledine, 1998; Dingledine *et al.,* 1999). The diversity of gene expression and, consequently, of the protein structure of glutamate receptors also arises by alternative splicing and in some cases by single-base editing of mRNAs encoding the receptors or receptor subunits. Alternative splicing has been described for metabotropic receptors and for subunits of NMDA, AMPA, and kainate receptors (Hollmann and Heinemann, 1994). A remarkable form of endogenous molecular engineering occurs with some subunits of AMPA and kainate receptors in which the RNA sequence differs from the genomic sequence in a single codon of the receptor subunit and determines the extent of Ca^{2+} permeability of the receptor channel (Traynelis *et al.,* 1995). This RNA-editing process alters the identity of a single amino acid (out of about 900 amino acids) that dictates whether or not the receptor channel gates Ca^{2+}.

The glutamate receptor genes seem to be unique families with only limited similarity to other ligand-gated channels such as the nicotinic acetylcholine receptor or, in the case of metabotropic receptors, to members of the GPCR superfamily.

AMPA and kainate receptors mediate fast depolarization at most glutamatergic synapses in the brain and spinal cord. NMDA receptors also are involved in normal synaptic transmission, but activation of NMDA receptors is more closely associated with the induction of various forms of synaptic plasticity rather than with fast point-to-point signaling in the brain. AMPA or kainate receptors and NMDA receptors may be colocalized at many glutamatergic synapses. A well-characterized phenomenon that involves NMDA receptors is the induction of long-term potentiation (LTP). LTP refers to a prolonged (hours to days) increase in the size of a postsynaptic response to a presynaptic stimulus of given strength. Activation of NMDA receptors is obligatory for the induction of one type of LTP that occurs in the hippocampus (Bliss and Collingridge, 1993). NMDA receptors normally are blocked by Mg^{2+} at resting membrane potentials. Thus, activation of NMDA receptors requires not only binding of synaptically released glutamate but simultaneous depolarization of the postsynaptic membrane. This is achieved by activation of AMPA/kainate receptors at nearby synapses from inputs from different neurons. Thus, NMDA receptors may function as coincidence detectors, being activated only when there is simultaneous firing of two or more neurons. Interestingly, NMDA receptors also can induce long-term depression (LTD; the flip side of LTP) at CNS synapses (Malenka and Nicoll, 1998). It seems that the frequency and pattern of synaptic stimulation is what dictates whether a synapse undergoes LTP or LTD (see Malenka and Nicoll, 1999).

Glutamate Excitotoxicity. The ability of high concentrations of glutamate to produce neuronal cell death has been known for more than three decades (Olney, 1969), but the mechanisms by which glutamate and selective, rigid agonists of its receptors produce this effect only recently have begun to be clarified. The cascade of events leading to neuronal death initially was thought to be triggered exclusively by excessive activation of NMDA or AMPA/kainate receptors, which allow significant influx of Ca^{2+} into the neurons. Such glutamate neurotoxicity was thought to underlie the damage that occurs after ischemia or hypoglycemia in the brain, during which a massive release and impaired reuptake of glutamate in the synapse would lead to excess stimulation of glutamate receptors and subsequent cell death. Although NMDA receptor antagonists can attenuate or block neuronal cell death induced by activation of these receptors (see Herrling, 1997), even the most potent antagonists could not prevent all such damage. More recent studies (see Choi and Koh, 1998; Lee et al., 1999; Zipfel et al., 1999) implicate both local depletion of Na^+ and K^+, as well as small but significant elevations of extracellular Zn^{2+} as factors that can activate both necrotic and proapoptotic cascades (Merry and Korsmeyer, 1997) leading to neuronal death. NMDA receptors also may be involved in the development of susceptibility to epileptic seizures and in the occurrence of seizure activity (Blumcke et al., 1995). Cases of Rasmussen's encephalitis, a childhood disease leading to intractable seizures and dementia, were found to correlate with levels of serum antibodies to a glutamate receptor subunit (Rogers et al., 1994).

Because of the widespread distribution of glutamate receptors in the CNS, it is likely that these receptors ultimately will become the targets for diverse therapeutic interventions. For example, a role for disordered glutamatergic transmission in the etiology of chronic neurodegenerative diseases and in schizophrenia has been postulated (Farber et al., 1998; Olney et al., 1999).

Acetylcholine. After acetylcholine (ACh) was identified as the transmitter at neuromuscular and parasympathetic neuroeffector junctions, as well as at the major synapse of autonomic ganglia (see Chapter 6), the amine began to receive considerable attention as a potential central neurotransmitter. Based on its irregular distribution within the CNS and the observation that peripheral cholinergic drugs could produce marked behavioral effects after central administration, many investigators were willing to consider the possibility that ACh also might be a central neurotransmitter. In the late 1950s, Eccles and colleagues demonstrated that the recurrent excitation of spinal Renshaw neurons was sensitive to nicotinic cholinergic antagonists; these cells also were found to be cholinoceptive. Such observations were consistent with the chemical and functional specificity of Dale's hypothesis that all branches of a neuron released the same transmitter substance and, in this case, produced similar types of postsynaptic action (see Eccles, 1964). Although the ability of ACh to elicit neuronal discharge subsequently has been replicated on scores of CNS cells (see Shepherd, 1998), the spinal Renshaw cell remains the prototype for central nicotinic cholinergic synapses. Nevertheless, the search for selectively acting, central nicotinic drugs continues (Decker et al., 1997; Bannon et al., 1998).

In most regions of the CNS, the effects of ACh, assessed either by iontophoresis or by radioligand receptor–displacement assays, appear to be generated by interaction with a mixture of nicotinic and muscarinic receptors. Several sets of presumptive cholinergic pathways have been proposed in addition to that of the motoneuron-Renshaw cell. By combination of immunocytochemistry of choline acetyltransferase (ChAT; the enzyme that synthesizes ACh) and ligand binding or *in situ* hybridization studies for the detection of neurons expressing subunits of nicotinic and muscarinic receptors, eight major clusters of ACh neurons and their pathways have been characterized (Mesulam, 1995). Four separate groups of cell bodies located in the basal forebrain, between the septum and the nucleus basalis of Meynert, send largely autonomous projections to the neocortex, hippocampal formation, and olfactory bulb. While rodent brains exhibit cholinergic neurons that are intrinsic to the neocortex, these neurons are not found in primate brain. Two collections of cholinergic neurons in the upper pons provide the major cholinergic innervation of thalamus and striatum, while medullary cholinergic neurons provide the cholinergic innervation of midbrain and brainstem regions. The intense cholinergic projections to neocortex and hippocampal formation will atrophy if these neurons are deprived of the trophic growth factors provided to them by retrograde axonal transport from their target neurons (Sofroniew *et al.*, 1993). This occurs in Alzheimer's disease when these target neurons are diseased (*see* Chapter 22) and has driven therapeutic efforts to restore residual cholinergic signaling.

Catecholamines.   The brain contains separate neuronal systems that utilize three different catecholamines—*dopamine, norepinephrine,* and *epinephrine.* Each system is anatomically distinct and serves separate, but similar, functional roles within their fields of innervation. Much of the original mapping was performed in rodent brains (Hökfelt *et al.*, 1976, 1977), but recent studies have extended these maps into primates (Foote, 1997; Lewis, 1997).

Dopamine.   Although dopamine originally was regarded only as a precursor of norepinephrine, assays of distinct regions of the CNS eventually revealed that the distributions of dopamine and norepinephrine are markedly different. In fact, more than half the CNS content of catecholamine is dopamine, and extremely large amounts are found in the basal ganglia (especially the caudate nucleus), the nucleus accumbens, the olfactory tubercle, the central nucleus of the amygdala, the median eminence, and restricted fields of the frontal cortex. The anatomical connections of the dopamine-containing neurons are known with some precision.

Dopaminergic neurons fall into three major morphological classes: (1) ultrashort neurons within the amacrine cells of the retina and periglomerular cells of the olfactory bulb; (2) intermediate-length neurons within the tuberobasal ventral hypothalamus that innervate the median eminence and intermediate lobe of the pituitary, connect the dorsal and posterior hypothalamus with the lateral septal nuclei, and extend caudally to the dorsal motor nucleus of the vagus, the nucleus of the solitary tract, and the periaqueductal gray matter; and (3) long projections between the major dopamine-containing nuclei in the substantia nigra and ventral tegmentum and their targets in the striatum, in the limbic zones of the cerebral cortex, and in other major regions of the limbic system except the hippocampus (*see* Hökfelt, *et al.*, 1976, 1977). At the cellular level, the actions of dopamine depend on receptor subtype expression and the contingent convergent actions of other transmitters to the same target neurons.

Although initial pharmacological studies discriminated between two subtypes of dopamine receptors, D_1 (by which dopamine activates adenylyl cyclase) and D_2 (by which dopamine inhibits adenylyl cyclase), subsequent cloning studies identified at least five genes encoding subtypes of dopamine receptors. Nevertheless, the two major categories, D_1-like or D_2-like, persist. The D_1-like receptors include the D_1 and the D_5 receptors, whereas the D_2-like receptors include the two isoforms of the D_2 receptor, differing in the length of their predicted third cytoplasmic loop, dubbed D_2 *short* (D_{2S}) and D_2 *long* (D_{2L}), the D_3, and the D_4 receptors (*see* Grandy and Civelli, 1992; Gingrich and Caron, 1993; Civelli, 1994). The D_1 and D_5 receptors activate adenylyl cyclase. The D_2 receptors couple to multiple

effector systems, including the inhibition of adenylyl cyclase activity, suppression of Ca^{2+} currents, and activation of K^+ currents. The effector systems to which the D_3 and D_4 receptors couple have not been unequivocally defined (Sokoloff and Schwartz, 1995; Schwartz *et al.*, 1998). D_2 dopamine receptors have been implicated in the pathophysiology of schizophrenia and Parkinson's disease (*see* Chapters 20 and 22).

Norepinephrine.   There are relatively large amounts of norepinephrine within the hypothalamus and in certain zones of the limbic system, such as the central nucleus of the amygdala and the dentate gyrus of the hippocampus. However, this catecholamine also is present in significant, although lower, amounts, in most brain regions. Detailed mapping studies indicate that most noradrenergic neurons arise either in the locus ceruleus of the pons or in neurons of the lateral tegmental portion of the reticular formation. From these neurons, multiple branched axons innervate specific target cells in a large number of cortical, subcortical, and spinomedullary fields (Hökfelt, *et al.*, 1976, 1977; Foote and Aston-Jones, 1995; Foote, 1997).

Although norepinephrine has been firmly established as the transmitter at synapses between presumptive noradrenergic pathways and a wide variety of target neurons, a number of features of the mode of action of this biogenic amine have complicated the acquisition of convincing evidence. In large part, these problems reflect its "nonclassical" electrophysiological synaptic actions, which result in "state-dependent" or "enabling" effects. In some instances, the pharmacological properties of such synapses have been complex, with evidence for mediation by both α- and β-adrenergic receptors. For example, stimulation of the locus ceruleus depresses the spontaneous activity of target neurons in the cerebellum; this is associated with a slowly developing hyperpolarization and a decrease in membrane conductance. However, activation of the locus ceruleus affects the higher firing rates produced by stimulation of excitatory inputs to these neurons to a lesser degree, and excitatory postsynaptic potentials are enhanced. All consequences of activation of the locus ceruleus are emulated by the iontophoretic application of norepinephrine and are effectively blocked by β-adrenergic antagonists. Although the mechanisms underlying these effects are not at all clear, there is convincing evidence for intracellular mediation by cyclic AMP. The afferent projections to locus ceruleus neurons include medullary cholinergic neurons, opioid peptide neurons, raphe (5-HT) neurons, and corticotropin-releasing hormone neurons from the hypothalamus. The latter provides a link to stress reactions for this system (*see* Aston-Jones *et al.*, 1999).

As in the periphery, three families of adrenergic receptors have been described in the CNS (*i.e.*, α_1, α_2, and β). Subtypes of α_1-, α_2-, and β-adrenergic receptors also exist in the CNS. These subtypes can be distinguished in terms of their pharmacological properties and their distribution (*see* Chapter 10). The three subtypes of β-adrenergic receptor are all coupled to stimulation of adenylyl cyclase activity. Even though the proportion varies from region to region, β_1-adrenergic receptors may be associated predominantly with neurons, while β_2-adrenergic receptors may be more characteristic of glial and vascular elements.

The α_1 receptors on noradrenergic target neurons of the neocortex and thalamus respond to norepinephrine with prazosin-sensitive, depolarizing responses due to decreases in K^+ conductances (both voltage-sensitive and voltage-insensitive; *see*

Wang and McCormick, 1993). However, α_1 receptors also can augment the generation of cyclic cAMP by neocortical slices in response to vasoactive intestinal polypeptide (Magistretti *et al.,* 1995). α_1-Adrenergic receptors also are coupled to stimulation of phospholipase C, leading to release of inositol trisphosphate and diacylglycerol (*see* Chapter 2). α_2-Adrenergic receptors are prominent on noradrenergic neurons, where they mediate a hyperpolarizing response due to enhancement of an inwardly rectifying K^+ conductance. The latter type of K^+ conductance also can be regulated by other transmitter systems (*see* Foote and Aston-Jones, 1995; *see* also Figure 12–2). In cortical projection fields, α_2 receptors may help restore functional declines of senescence (Arnsten, 1993). α_2-Adrenergic receptors, like D_2 dopamine receptors, are coupled to inhibition of adenylyl cyclase activity, but their effects in the CNS likely rely more on their ability to activate receptor-operated K^+ channels and to suppress voltage-gated Ca^{2+} channels, both mediated *via* pertussis toxin-sensitive G proteins. Based on ligand-binding patterns and the properties of cloned receptors, three subtypes of α_2-adrenergic receptor have been defined (α_{2A}, α_{2B}, and α_{2C}), but all appear to couple to similar signaling pathways (*see* Bylund, 1992). Functional roles for these receptor subtypes are being defined based on studies on transgenic mice in which these receptors are functionally absent may be revealing (MacDonald *et al.,* 1997).

Epinephrine.   Neurons in the CNS that contain epinephrine were recognized only after the development of sensitive enzymatic assays for phenylethanolamine-*N*-methyltransferase and immunocytochemical staining techniques for the enzyme (*see* Hökfelt *et al.,* 1976 and references therein). Epinephrine-containing neurons are found in the medullary reticular formation and make restricted connections to a few pontine and diencephalic nuclei, eventually coursing as far rostrally as the paraventricular nucleus of the dorsal midline thalamus. Their physiological properties have not been identified.

5-Hydroxytryptamine.

5-Hydroxytryptamine.   Following the chemical determination that a biogenic substance found both in serum ("serotonin") and in gut ("enteramine") was 5-hydroxytryptamine (5-HT), assays for this substance revealed its presence in brain (*see* Chapter 11). Since that time, studies of 5-HT have had a pivotal role in advancing our understanding of the neuropharmacology of the CNS. Various cytochemical methods have been used to trace the central anatomy of 5-HT-containing neurons in several species. Tryptaminergic neurons are found in nine nuclei lying in or adjacent to the midline (raphe) regions of the pons and upper brainstem, corresponding to well-defined nuclear ensembles (Steinbusch and Mulder, 1984).

The rostral raphe nuclei innervate forebrain regions, while the caudal raphe nuclei project within the brainstem and spinal cord with some overlaps. The median raphe nucleus makes a major contribution to the innervation of the limbic system, and the dorsal raphe nucleus makes a similar contribution to cortical regions and the neostriatum. In the mammalian CNS, cells receiving cytochemically demonstrable tryptaminergic input, such as the suprachiasmatic nucleus, ventrolateral genicu-

late body, amygdala, and hippocampus, exhibit a uniform and dense investment of reactive terminals.

Molecular biological approaches have led to identification of 14 distinct mammalian 5-HT-receptor subtypes. These subtypes exhibit characteristic ligand-binding profiles, couple to different intracellular signaling systems, exhibit subtype-specific distributions within the CNS, and mediate distinct behavioral effects of 5-HT. Present terminology has grouped the known 5-HT receptor subtypes into multiple classes: the 5-HT_1 and 5-HT_2 classes of receptor are both G protein–coupled receptors with a seven-transmembrane-spanning-domain motif and include multiple isoforms within each class, while the 5-HT_3 receptor is a ligand-gated ion channel with structural similarity to the α subunit of the nicotinic acetylcholine receptor. The 5-HT_4, 5-HT_5, 5-HT_6, and 5-HT_7 classes of receptor are all apparent GPCRs, but have not yet been well studied electrophysiologically or operationally (Hoyer and Martin, 1996). Structural diversity among these subtypes of receptors indicates that they are representatives of distinct 5-HT receptor classes (*see* Chapter 11 for further discussion of pharmacological properties of 5-HT receptor subtypes). As with all other genetically identified receptors, the new genetic perturbation models are assisting in the specification of function (*see* Murphy *et al.,* 1999).

The 5-HT_1 receptor subset is composed of at least five intronless receptor subtypes (5-HT_{1A}, 5-HT_{1B}, 5-HT_{1D}, 5-HT_{1E}, 5-HT_{1F}) that are linked to inhibition of adenylyl cyclase activity or to regulation of K^+ or Ca^{2+} channels. The 5-HT_{1A} receptors are abundantly expressed on 5-HT neurons of the dorsal raphe nucleus, where they are thought to be involved in temperature regulation. They also are found in regions of the CNS associated with mood and anxiety such as the hippocampus and amygdala. Activation of 5-HT_{1A} receptors leads to opening of an inwardly rectifying K^+ conductance, which leads to hyperpolarization and neuronal inhibition. These receptors can be activated by the drugs buspirone and ipsapirone, which are used to treat anxiety and panic disorders (*see* Aghajanian, 1995). 5-HT_{1D} receptors are potently activated by the drug sumatriptan, which is currently prescribed for acute management of migraine headaches.

Three receptor subtypes constitute the 5-HT_2 receptor class: 5-HT_{2A}, 5-HT_{2B}, and 5-HT_{2C}. In contrast to 5-HT_1 receptors, these 5-HT_2 receptors contain introns and all are linked to activation of phospholipase C. Based on ligand binding and mRNA *in situ* hybridization patterns, 5-HT_{2A} receptors are enriched in forebrain regions such as neocortex and olfactory tubercle, as well as in several nuclei arising from the brainstem. On facial motoneurons, 5-HT enhances excitability by two mechanisms: (1) slow closure of resting K^+ conductances, increasing membrane resistance; and (2) a more potent, ritanserin-antagonizable opening of a voltage-sensitive K^+ conductance that is activated by hyperpolarization (Aghajanian, 1995). In piriform cortex, Aghajanian and colleagues have observed an indirect inhibition of pyramidal neurons through activation of local-circuit, GABA-mediated inhibitory interneurons, an effect that is blocked by ritanserin. In the cerebral cortex, 5-HT_{2A}-receptor agonists (but not 5-HT itself) also produce neuronal inhibition, but other effects reported may be the result of coexpression of multiple 5-HT-receptor subtypes on the same neuron. The 5-HT_{2C} receptor, which is very similar in sequence and pharmacology to the 5-HT_{2A} receptor, is expressed abundantly in the choroid plexus where it regulates transferrin and cerebrospinal fluid production (*see* Chapter 11).

Receptors of the 5-HT$_3$ class first were recognized in the peripheral autonomic system. They also are expressed in brain within the area postrema and nucleus tractus solitarius, where they couple to potent depolarizing responses that show rapid desensitization to continued 5-HT exposure. The 5-HT$_3$ receptor leads to enhanced Na$^+$ and K$^+$ currents but does not seem to affect Ca^{2+} permeability. At the behavioral level, actions of 5-HT at central 5-HT$_3$ receptors can lead to emesis and antinociceptive actions; 5-HT$_3$-receptor antagonists such as ondansetron are beneficial in the management of chemotherapy-induced emesis (see Chapter 38).

The hallucinogen LSD is among the most interesting of the compounds that interact with 5-HT, primarily through 5-HT$_2$ receptors. In iontophoretic tests, LSD and 5-HT are both potent inhibitors of the firing of raphe (5-HT) neurons, whereas LSD and other hallucinogens are far more potent excitants on facial motoneurons that receive innervation from the raphe. The inhibitory effect of LSD on raphe neurons offers a plausible explanation for the drug's hallucinogenic effects, namely, that these effects result from depression of activity in a system that tonically inhibits visual and other sensory inputs. However, typical LSD-induced behavior is still seen in animals with destroyed raphe nuclei or after blockade of the synthesis of 5-HT by p-chlorophenylalanine. Other evidence against this explanation of LSD-induced hallucinations is potentiation of the effects of LSD by administration of the precursor of 5-HT, 5-hydroxytryptophan. More precise definition of the various functional roles of tryptaminergic pathways in the CNS awaits the results of studies using more specific agents, whose number is steadily increasing (see Aghajanian and Marek, 1999).

Histamine.   For many years, histamine and antihistamines that are active in the periphery have been known to produce significant effects on animal behavior. Relatively recently, however, evidence has accumulated to suggest that histamine also might be a central neurotransmitter. Biochemical detection of histamine synthesis by neurons, as well as direct cytochemical localization of these neurons, has established the existence of a histaminergic system in the CNS. Most of these neurons are located in the ventral posterior hypothalamus; they give rise to long ascending and descending tracts to the entire CNS that are typical of the patterns characteristic of other aminergic systems. Based on the presumptive central effects of histamine antagonists, the histaminergic system is thought to function in the regulation of arousal, body temperature, and vascular dynamics.

Three subtypes of histamine receptors have been described. H$_1$ receptors, the most prominent, may be located on glia and vessels as well as on neurons and may act to mobilize Ca^{2+} in receptive cells. H$_2$ receptors are linked to the activation of adenylyl cyclase, perhaps in concert with H$_1$ receptors in certain circumstances. H$_3$ receptors, which have the greatest sensitivity to histamine, are localized much more selectively in basal ganglia and olfactory regions in the rat, but consequences of their activation remain unresolved. Unlike the monoamines and amino acid transmitters, there does not appear to be an active reuptake process for histamine after its release. In addition, no direct evidence has been obtained for release of histamine from neurons either in vivo or in vitro (see Schwartz et al., 1995, for additional recent references).

Peptides.   The discovery during the 1980s of numerous novel peptides in the CNS, each capable of regulating one or another aspect of neural function, produced considerable excitement and an imposing catalog of entities (see Hökfelt et al., 1995; Darlison and Richter, 1999). In addition, certain peptides previously thought to be restricted to the gut or to endocrine glands also have been found in the CNS. Relatively detailed neuronal maps are available that show immunoreactivity to peptide-specific antisera. While some CNS peptides may function on their own, most are now thought to act mainly in concert with coexisting transmitters, both amines and amino acids. Some neurons may contain more than two possible transmitters (see Hökfelt et al., 1995), and they can be independently regulated. At this time at least three approaches appear to have utility in attempting to grasp the continuously enlarging peptidergic systems of neurons.

Organization by Peptide Families.   Because of significant homology in amino acid sequences, families of related molecules can be defined as either *ancestral* or *concurrent*. The ancestral relationship is illustrated by peptides such as the tachykinin/substance P or the vasotocin (vasopressin/oxytocin) family, in which species differences can be correlated with modest variations in peptide structure. The concurrent relationship is best exemplified by the endorphins and by the glucagon-secretin family. In the endorphin "superfamily," three major systems of endorphin peptides (proopiomelanocortin, proenkephalin, and prodynorphin) exist in independent neuronal circuits (see Akil et al., 1998 for recent review). These natural opioid peptides arise from independent, but homologous, genes. The peptides all share some actions at receptors once classed generally as "opioid" but now are undergoing progressive refinement (see Chapter 23). In the glucagon family, multiple and somewhat homologous peptides are found simultaneously in different cells of the same organism but in separate organ systems: glucagon and vasoactive intestinal polypeptide (VIP) in pancreatic islets; secretin in duodenal mucosa; VIP and related peptides in enteric, autonomic, and central neurons (see Magistretti et al., 1998); and growth hormone-releasing factor in central neurons only (Guillemin et al., 1984). The general metabolic effects produced by this family can be viewed as leading to increased blood glucose. To some degree, ancestral and concurrent relationships are not mutually exclusive. For example, multiple members of the tachykinin/substance P family within mammalian brains and intestines may account for the apparent existence of subsets of receptors for these peptides (Vanden Broeck et al., 1999). The mammalian terminus of the vasotocin family shows two concurrent products as well, vasopressin and oxytocin, each having evolved to perform separate functions once executed by single vasotocin-related peptides in lower phyla.

Organization by Anatomic Pattern. Some peptide systems follow rather consistent anatomical organizations. Thus, the hypothalamic peptides oxytocin, vasopressin, proopiomelanocortin, gonadotropin-releasing hormone, and growth hormone–releasing hormone all tend to be synthesized by single large clusters of neurons that give off multibranched axons to several distant targets. Others, such as systems that contain somatostatin, cholecystokinin, and enkephalin, can have many forms, with patterns varying from moderately long, hierarchical connections to short-axon, local-circuit neurons that are widely distributed throughout the brain (*see* Hökfelt *et al.*, 2000).

Organization by Function. Since almost all peptides initially were identified on the basis of bioassays, their names reflect these biologically assayed functions (*e.g.,* thyrotropin-releasing hormone, vasoactive intestinal polypeptide). These names become trivial if more ubiquitous distributions and additional functions are discovered. Some general integrative role might be hypothesized for widely separated neurons (and other cells) that make the same peptide. However, a more parsimonious view would be that each peptide has unique messenger roles at the cellular level and that these are used repeatedly in functionally similar pathways within large systems that differ in their overall functions. The cloning of the major members of the opioid-peptide receptors revealed unexpected and as yet unexplained conservation of sequences with receptors for somatostatin, angiotensin, and other peptides (*see* Uhl *et al.*, 1994).

Comparison with Other Transmitters. Peptides differ in several important respects from the monoamine and amino acid transmitters considered earlier. Synthesis of a peptide is performed in the rough endoplasmic reticulum, where mRNA for the propeptide can be translated into an amino-acid sequence. The propeptide is cleaved (processed) to the form that is secreted as the secretory vesicles are transported from the perinuclear cytoplasm to the nerve terminals. Further, no active reuptake mechanisms for peptides have been described (*but see* Honor *et al.*, 1999, for possible exception). This increases the dependency of peptidergic nerve terminals on distant sites of synthesis. Perhaps most importantly, linear chains of amino acids can assume many conformations at their receptors, making it difficult to define the sequences and their steric relationships that are critical for activity.

Until recently, it has been difficult to develop nonpeptidic, synthetic agonists or antagonists that will interact with specific receptors for peptides. However, such drugs are now being developed (for cholecystokinin CCK_1 and CCK_2 receptors, for neurotensin receptors, and for corticotropin-releasing-hormone receptors), and some (against substance P NK-1 receptors) have entered clinical trials (*see* Rupniak and Kramer, 1999; Hökfelt *et al.*, 2000). Nature also has had limited success in this regard, since only one plant alkaloid, morphine, has been found to act selectively at peptidergic synapses. Fortunately for pharmacologists, morphine was discovered before the endorphins, or rigid molecules capable of acting at peptide receptors might have been deemed impossible to develop.

Other Regulatory Substances.

In addition to these major families of neurotransmitters, other endogenous substances also may participate in the regulated flow of signals between neurons, but in sequences of events that differ somewhat from the conventional concepts of neurotransmitter function. These substances have significant potential importance as regulatory factors and as targets for future drug development.

Purines. In addition to their roles as essential biochemical anabolites, *adenosine monophosphate, adenosine triphosphate,* and free *adenosine* have gained attention as independent, neuronal signaling molecules in their own right (*see* Moreau and Huber, 1999; Williams *et al.*, 1999; Baraldi *et al.*, 2000). Two large families of purinergic receptors have been characterized. Those in the P1 class are GPCRs. These have been further divided into four subtypes (A_1–A_4) based on agonist actions of adenosine; A_1 and A_2 adenosine receptors are antagonized by xanthines, whereas A_3 and A_4 adenosine receptors are not. A_1 adenosine receptors have been associated with inhibition of adenylyl cyclase, activation of K^+ currents, activation of phospholipase C in some circumstances, and ion-channel regulation, while A_2 receptors activate adenylyl cyclase. The P2 class of purine receptors refers to the receptors for ATP and related triphosphate nucleotides such as UTP. The P2X subtype of receptor is a ligand-gated ion channel, while the P2Y subtype is a GPCR. Adenosine can act presynaptically throughout the cortex and hippocampal formation to inhibit the release of amine and amino acid transmitters. ATP-regulated responses have been linked pharmacologically to a variety of supracellular functions including anxiety, stroke, and epilepsy (Williams, 1995).

Diffusible Mediators. Certain potent agents shown to be active under pharmacological conditions and inferred to be physiological regulators in systems throughout the body recently have been examined for their roles within the central nervous system.

Arachidonic acid, normally stored within the cell membrane as a glycerol ester, can be liberated during phospholipid hydrolysis (by pathways involving phospholipases A_2, C, and D). Phospholipases are activated by a variety of receptors. Arachidonic acid can be converted to highly reactive regulators by three major enzymatic pathways (*see* Chapter 26): cyclooxygenases (leading to *prostaglandins* and *thromboxanes*), lipoxygenases (leading to the *leukotrienes* and other transient catabolites of eicosatetraenoic acid), and cytochrome P450 (which is inducible although expressed at low levels in brain). These arachidonic acid metabolites have been implicated as diffusible modulators in the CNS, particularly for long-term potentiation and other forms of plasticity (Mechoulam *et al.*, 1996; Piomelli *et al.*, 1998).

Nitric oxide has been recognized as an important regulator of vascular and inflammatory mediation for more than a decade, but came into focus with respect to roles in the CNS after successful efforts to characterize brain nitric oxide synthases (NOS; *see* Snyder and Dawson, 1995). Molecular cloning studies have now revealed at least four isoforms of this biosynthetic enzyme in the brain, a constitutive form present in some neurons, capillary endothelial cells, and macrophages, as well as inducible forms of the enzyme. The availability of potent activators and inhibitors of NOS has led to reports of the presumptive involvement of nitric oxide in a host of phenomena in the brain including long-term potentiation, guanylyl cyclase activation, neurotransmitter release and reuptake, and enhancement of glutamate (NMDA)-mediated neurotoxicity. Subsequently, rational analysis based on proposed mechanisms of NO action through binding to the iron in the active site of target enzymes led to the idea that carbon monoxide may be a second gaseous, labile, diffusible intercellular regulator, at least in the regulation of guanylyl cyclase in neurons *in vitro*.

Cytokines.   The term *cytokines* encompasses a large and diverse family of polypeptide regulators, produced widely throughout the body by cells of diverse embryological origin. In general, these regulators have multiple functions attributed to effects under controlled conditions *in vitro*. *In vivo*, the effects of cytokines are known to be further regulated by the conditions imposed by other cytokines, interacting as a network with variable effects leading to synergistic, additive, or opposing actions. Within the cytokines, tissue-produced peptidic factors termed *chemokines* serve to attract cells of the immune and inflammatory lines into interstitial spaces. These special cytokines have received much attention as potential regulators in nervous system inflammation (as in early stages of dementia, following infection with human immunodeficiency virus; *see* Asensio *et al.,* 1999; Mennicken *et al.,* 1999) and during recovery from traumatic injury. The more conventional neuronal and glial-derived growth-enhancing and growth-retardant factors were mentioned above. The fact that, under some pathophysiological conditions, neurons and astrocytes may be induced to express cytokines or other growth factors further blurs the dividing line between neurons and glia.

ACTIONS OF DRUGS IN THE CNS

Specificity and Nonspecificity of CNS Drug Actions. The effect of a drug is considered to be specific when it affects an identifiable molecular mechanism unique to target cells that bear receptors for that drug. Conversely, a drug is regarded as nonspecific when it produces effects on many different target cells and acts by diverse molecular mechanisms. This distinction is often a property of the dose-response relationship of the drug and the cell or mechanisms under scrutiny (*see* Chapter 3). Even a drug that is highly specific when tested at a low concentration may exhibit nonspecific actions at substantially higher doses. Conversely, even generally acting drugs may not act equally on all levels of the CNS. For example, sedatives, hypnotics, and general anesthetics would have very limited utility if central neurons that control the respiratory and cardiovascular systems were sensitive to their actions. Drugs with specific actions may produce nonspecific effects if the dose and route of administration produce high tissue concentrations.

Drugs whose mechanisms currently appear to be primarily general or nonspecific are classed according to whether they produce behavioral depression or stimulation. Specifically acting CNS drugs can be classed more definitively according to their locus of action or specific therapeutic usefulness. It must be remembered that the absence of overt behavioral effects does not rule out the existence of important central actions for a given drug.

For example, the impact of muscarinic cholinergic antagonists on the behavior of normal animals may be subtle, but these agents are used extensively in the treatment of movement disorders and motion sickness (*see* Chapter 7).

General (Nonspecific) CNS Depressants.   This category includes the anesthetic gases and vapors, the aliphatic alcohols, and some hypnotic-sedative drugs. These agents share the ability to depress excitable tissue at all levels of the CNS, leading to a decrease in the amount of transmitter released by the nerve impulse, as well as to general depression of postsynaptic responsiveness and ion movement. At subanesthetic concentrations, these agents (*e.g.,* ethanol) can exert relatively specific effects on certain groups of neurons, which may account for differences in their behavioral effects, especially the propensity to produce dependence (Koob and Le Moal, 1997; Koob *et al.,* 1998; *see also* Chapters 14, 17, 18, and 24).

General (Nonspecific) CNS Stimulants.   The drugs in this category include pentylenetetrazol and related agents that are capable of powerful excitation of the CNS and the methylxanthines, which have a much weaker stimulant action. Stimulation may be accomplished by one of two general mechanisms: (1) by blockade of inhibition or (2) by direct neuronal excitation (which may involve increased transmitter release, more prolonged transmitter action, labilization of the postsynaptic membrane, or decreased synaptic recovery time).

Drugs That Selectively Modify CNS Function.   The agents in this group may cause either depression or excitation. In some instances, a drug may produce both effects simultaneously on different systems. Some agents in this category have little effect on the level of excitability in doses that are used therapeutically. The principal classes of these CNS drugs include the following: anticonvulsants, antiparkinsonism drugs, opioid and nonopioid analgesics, appetite suppressants, antiemetics, analgesic-antipyretics, certain stimulants, antidepressants, antimanic agents, antipsychotic agents, sedatives, and hypnotics.

Although selectivity of action may be remarkable, a drug usually affects several CNS functions to varying degrees. When only one constellation of effects is wanted in a therapeutic situation, the remaining effects of the drug are regarded as limitations in selectivity (*i.e.,* unwanted side effects). The specificity of a drug's action frequently is overestimated. This is partly due to the fact that the drug is identified with the effect that is implied by the class name.

General Characteristics of CNS Drugs.   Combinations of centrally acting drugs frequently are administered to therapeutic advantage (*e.g.,* an anticholinergic drug and levodopa for Parkinson's disease). However, other combinations of drugs may be detrimental because of potentially dangerous additive or mutually antagonistic effects.

The effect of a CNS drug is additive with the physiological state and with the effects of other depressant and stimulant drugs. For example, anesthetics are less effective in a hyperexcitable subject than in a normal patient; the converse is true with respect to the effects of stimulants. In general, the depressant effects of drugs from all categories are additive (*e.g.,* the fatal combination of barbiturates or benzodiazepines with ethanol), as are the effects of stimulants. Therefore, respiration depressed by morphine is further impaired by depressant drugs, while stimulant drugs can augment the excitatory effects of morphine to produce vomiting and convulsions.

Antagonism between depressants and stimulants is variable. Some instances of true pharmacological antagonism among CNS drugs are known; for example, opioid antagonists are very selective in blocking the effects of opioid analgesics. However, the antagonism exhibited between two CNS drugs is usually physiological in nature. Thus, an individual who has received one drug cannot be returned entirely to normal by another.

The selective effects of drugs on specific neurotransmitter systems may be additive or competitive. This potential for drug interaction must be considered whenever such drugs are administered concurrently. To minimize such interactions, a drug-free period may be required when modifying therapy. An excitatory effect is commonly observed with low concentrations of certain depressant drugs due either to depression of inhibitory systems or to a transient increase in the release of excitatory transmitters. Examples are the "stage of excitement" during induction of general anesthesia and the "stimulant" effects of alcohol. The excitatory phase occurs only with low concentrations of the depressant; uniform depression ensues with increasing drug concentration. The excitatory effects can be minimized, when appropriate, by pretreatment with a depressant drug that is devoid of such effects (*e.g.,* benzodiazepines in preanesthetic medication). Acute, excessive stimulation of the cerebrospinal axis normally is followed by depression, which is in part a consequence of neuronal fatigue and exhaustion of stores of transmitters. Postictal depression is additive with the effects of depressant drugs. Acute, drug-induced depression is not, as a rule, followed by stimulation. However, chronic drug-induced sedation or depression may be followed by prolonged hyperexcitability upon abrupt withdrawal of the medication (barbiturates, alcohol). This type of hyperexcitability can be controlled effectively by the same or another depressant drug (*see* Chapters 17 and 18).

Organization of CNS–Drug Interactions. The structural and functional properties of neurons provide a means to specify the possible sites at which drugs could interact specifically or generally in the CNS (*see* Figure 12–1). In this scheme, drugs that affect neuronal energy metabolism, membrane integrity, or transmembrane ionic equilibria would be generally acting compounds. Similarly general in action would be drugs that affect the

two-way intracellular transport systems (*e.g.,* colchicine). These general effects still can exhibit different dose-response or time-response relationships based, for example, on such neuronal properties as rate of firing, dependence of discharge on external stimuli or internal pacemakers, resting ionic fluxes, or axon length. In contrast, when drug actions can be related to specific aspects of the metabolism, release, or function of a neurotransmitter, the site, specificity, and mechanism of action of a drug can be defined by systematic studies of dose-response and time-response relationships. From such data the most sensitive, rapid, or persistent neuronal event can be identified.

Transmitter-dependent actions of drugs can be organized conveniently into presynaptic and postsynaptic categories. The presynaptic category includes all of the events in the perikaryon and nerve terminal that regulate transmitter synthesis (including the acquisition of adequate substrates and cofactors), storage, release, reuptake, and catabolism. Transmitter concentrations can be lowered by blockade of synthesis, storage, or both. The amount of transmitter released per impulse is generally stable but also can be regulated. The effective concentration of transmitter may be increased by inhibition of reuptake or by blockade of catabolic enzymes. The transmitter that is released at a synapse also can exert actions on the terminal from which it was released by interacting with receptors at these sites (termed *autoreceptors; see* above). Activation of presynaptic autoreceptors can slow the rate of discharge of transmitter and thereby provide a feedback mechanism that controls the concentration of transmitter in the synaptic cleft.

The postsynaptic category includes all the events that follow release of the transmitter in the vicinity of the postsynaptic receptor in particular, the molecular mechanisms by which occupancy of the receptor by the transmitter results in changes in the properties of the membrane of the postsynaptic cell (shifts in membrane potential) as well as more enduring biochemical actions (changes in intracellular cyclic nucleotides, protein kinase activity, and related substrate proteins). Direct postsynaptic effects of drugs generally require relatively high affinity for the receptors or resistance to metabolic degradation. Each of these presynaptic or postsynaptic actions is potentially highly specific and can be envisioned as being restricted to a single, chemically defined subset of CNS cells.

Convergence, Synergism, and Antagonism Result from Transmitter Interactions. A hallmark of modern neuropharmacology is the capacity to clone receptor or receptor-subunit cDNAs and to determine their properties by expression in cells that do not normally express the receptor or subunit being studied. The simplicity of *in vitro* models of this type may divert one's attention from the fact that, in the intact CNS, a given neurotransmitter may interact simultaneously with all of the various isoforms of its receptor on neurons that are also under the influence of multiple other afferent pathways and their transmitters. Thus, attempts to predict the behavioral or therapeutic consequences of drugs designed to elicit precise and restricted receptor actions may fail due to differences under normal as compared to diseased conditions, and as a consequence of the complexity of the interactions possible.

PROSPECTUS

With the ability to clone, sequence, and express the genes that encode the molecules that underlie every step of neurotransmission, a new era in drug development is approaching. Such studies already have permitted the identification of novel receptor subtypes that were undetected or ambiguously defined by traditional pharmacological approaches. The pace of such discovery undoubtedly will accelerate. Receptor heterogeneity provides an opportunity, in principle, for greater pharmacological selectivity. *In situ* hybridization facilitates unambiguous localization of expression of individual forms of a receptor; immunodetection affords precise receptor localization; and expression of the receptor in cultured cell systems allows characterization of its pharmacological properties. Molecular modeling based on the primary amino acid sequence of a receptor eventually may make it possible to define the precise structure of the ligand-binding site and permit synthesis of novel compounds tailored to these sites, particularly once the X-ray structure of a prototypical neurotransmitter receptor is obtained as a guide. Molecular studies also facilitate development of new methods to evaluate the importance of regulation of receptor number and the precise nature of the protein-protein interactions by which GPCR and ionotropic receptors transduce their effects.

Future efforts to provide explanations for drug-induced neurological changes undoubtedly will continue to focus on synaptic transmitters and their mechanisms. If estimates of the complexity of brain-specific mRNA are any indication, many more transmitter peptides remain to be discovered. As more transmitters, including more nonclassical signaling molecules, are discovered and their neuronal systems are mapped, new target cells will become available for the study of unique or common mechanisms of action. In this regard it may be useful to consider three general properties by which neuronal circuits can be described and to employ them in efforts to correlate the molecular actions of drugs with their resulting neurological and behavioral effects. A spatial domain describes those areas of the brain or of peripheral receptive fields that feed signals to a given cell and those areas to which that cell sends its signals. A temporal domain describes the duration of the effects of a cell on its targets. A functional domain describes the molecular mechanisms by which the cell influences its targets. Within these three domains, neurons can be defined in terms of their transmitters, receptors, and functional location, as well as in the more classical categories of sensory, motor, or interneuronal. All these properties must be borne in mind simultaneously in the attempt to develop comprehensive explanations of the acute and chronic effects of drugs.

Lastly, given the pace of present work, it seems likely that the molecular biological strategies that have already fostered discovery of molecular mechanisms, motifs, and new messenger moieties will now be further exploited for assessment of changes in gene expression with disease and with the development of new therapeutic strategies. The possibility of replacing lost or dysfunctional neurons by CNS transplantation of neuronal or glial stem cells suggests previously unrecognized new opportunities (*see* Brustle *et al.,* 1999; McDonald *et al.,* 1999; McKay, 2000). Ultimately, the goal must be to find ways to diminish genetically transmittable vulnerabilities to the complex disorders of the CNS.

BIBLIOGRAPHY

Aloisi, F. The role of microglia and astrocytes in CNS immune surveillance and immunopathology. *Adv. Exp. Med. Biol.,* **1999,** *468*:123–133.

Andersson, P.-B., Perry, V.H., and Gordon, S. The acute inflammatory response to lipopolysaccharide in CNS parenchyma differs from that in other body tissues. *Neuroscience,* **1992,** *48*:169–186.

Arnsten, A.P. Catecholamine mechanisms in age-related cognitive decline. *Neurobiol. Aging,* **1993,** *14*:639–641.

Asensio, V.C., Kincaid, C., and Campbell, I.L. Chemokines and the inflammatory response to viral infection in the central nervous system with a focus on lymphocytic choriomeningitis virus. *J. Neurovirol.,* **1999,** *5*:65–75.

Aston-Jones, G., Rajkowski, J., and Cohen, J. Role of locus coeruleus in attention and behavioral flexibility. *Biol. Psychiatry,* **1999,** *46*:1309–1320.

Augustine, G.J., Burns, M.E., DeBello, W.M., Hilfiker, S., Morgan, J.R., Schweizer, F.E., Tokumaru, H., and Umayahara, K. Proteins involved in synaptic vesicle trafficking. *J. Physiol.,* **1999,** *520(pt.1)*:33–41.

Bannon, A.W., Decker, M.W., Holladay, M.W., Curzon, P., Donnelly-Roberts, D., Puttfarcken, P.S., Bitner, R.S., Diaz, A., Dickenson, A.H., Porsolt, R.D., Williams, M., and Arneric, S.P. Broad-spectrum, non-opioid analgesic activity by selective modulation of neuronal nicotinic acetylcholine receptors. *Science,* **1998,** *279*:77–81.

Barnard, E.A., Darlison, M.G., Fujita, N., Glencorse, T.A., Levitan, E.S., Reale, V., Schofield, P.R., Seeburg, P.H., Squire, M.D., and Stephenson, F.A. Molecular biology of the GABAA receptor. *Adv. Exp. Med. Biol.,* **1988,** *236*:31–45.

Billinton, A., Upton, N., and Bowery, N.G. GABA(B) receptor isoforms GBR1a and GBR1b, appear to be associated with pre- and post-synaptic elements respectively in rat and human cerebellum. *Br. J. Pharmacol.,* **1999,** *126*:1387–1392.

Blakely, R.D., De Felice, L.J., and Hartzell, H.C. Molecular physiology of norepinephrine and serotonin transporters. *J. Exp. Biol.,* **1994,** *196*:263–281.

Bliss, T.V., and Collingridge, G.L. A synaptic model of memory: long-term potentiation in the hippocampus. *Nature,* **1993,** *361*:31–39.

Blumcke, I., Wolf, H.K., Hof, P.R., Morrison, J.H., and Wiestler, O.D. Regional distribution of the AMPA glutamate receptor subunits GluR2(4) in human hippocampus. *Brain Res.,* **1995,** *682*:239–244.

Brauner-Osborne, H., and Krogsgaard-Larsen, P. Functional pharmacology of cloned heterodimeric GABAB receptors expressed in mammalian cells. *Br. J. Pharmacol.,* **1999,** *128*:1370–1374.

Brown, E.S., Rush, A.J., and McEwen, B.S. Hippocampal remodeling and damage by corticosteroids: implications for mood disorders. *Neuropsychopharmacology,* **1999,** *21*:474–484.

Brustle, O., Jones, K.N., Learish, R.D., Karram, K., Choudhary, K., Wiestler, O.D., Duncan, I.D., and McKay, R.D. Embryonic stem cell-derived glial precursors: a source of myelinating transplants. *Science,* **1999,** *285*:754–756.

Casaccia-Bonnefil, P., Kong, H., and Chao, M.V. Neurotrophins: the biological paradox of survival factors eliciting apoptosis. *Cell Death Differ.,* **1998,** *5*:357–364.

Cork, R.J., Perrone, M.L., Bridges, D., Wandell, J., Scheiner, C.A., and Mize, R.R. A web-accessible digital atlas of the distribution of nitric oxide synthase in the mouse brain. *Prog. Brain Res.,* **1998,** *118*:37–50.

Costa, E., and Guidotti, A. Diazepam binding inhibitor (DBI): a peptide with multiple biological actions. *Life Sci.,* **1991,** *49*:325–344.

Cserr, H.F., and Bundgaard, M. Blood-brain interfaces in vertebrates: a comparative approach. *Am. J. Physiol.,* **1984,** *246*:R277–R288.

De Blas, A.L. Brain GABAA receptors studied with subunit-specific antibodies. *Mol. Neurobiol.,* **1996,** *12*:55–71.

Decker, M.W., Bannon, A.W., Curzon, P., Gunther, K.L., Brioni, J.D., Holladay, M.W., Lin, N.H., Li, Y., Daanen, J.F., Buccafusco, J.J., Prendergast, M.A., Jackson, W.J., and Arneric, S.P. ABT-089 [2-methyl-3-(2-(S)-pyrrolidinylmethoxy)pyridine dihydrochloride]: II. A novel cholinergic channel modulator with effects on cognitive performance in rats and monkeys. *J. Pharmacol. Exp. Ther.,* **1997,** *283*:247–258.

Derrick, B.E., and Martinez, J.L. Jr. Opioid receptor activation is one factor underlying the frequency dependence of mossy fiber LTP induction. *J. Neurosci.,* **1994,** *14*:4359–4367.

Doyle, D.A., Morais Cabral, J., Pfuetzner, R.A., Kuo, A., Gulbis, J.M., Cohen, S.L., Chait, B.T., and MacKinnon, R. The structure of the potassium channel: molecular basis of K+ conduction and selectivity. *Science,* **1998,** *280*:69–77.

Dumont, Y., Jacques, D., Bouchard, P., and Quirion, R. Species differences in the expression and distribution of the neuropeptide Y Y1, Y2, Y4, and Y5 receptors in rodents, guinea pig, and primates brains. *J. Comp. Neurol.,* **1998,** *402*:372–384.

Emerich, D.F., Snodgrass, P., Pink, M., Bloom, F., and Bartus, R.T. Central analgesic actions of loperamide following transient permeation of the blood brain barrier with Cereport (RMP-7). *Brain Res.,* **1998,** *801*:259–266.

Fairman, W.A., and Amara, S.G. Functional diversity of excitatory amino acid transporters: ion channel and transport modes. *Am. J. Physiol.,* **1999,** *277*:F481–F486.

Farber, N.B., Newcomer, J.W., and Olney, J.W. The glutamate synapse in neuropsychiatric disorders. Focus on schizophrenia and Alzheimer's disease. *Prog. Brain Res.,* **1998,** *116*:421–437.

Gally, J.A., Montague, P.R., Reeke, G.N. Jr., and Edelman, G.M. The NO hypothesis: possible effects of a short-lived, rapidly diffusible signal in the development and function of the nervous system. *Proc. Natl. Acad. Sci. U.S.A.,* **1990,** *87*:3547–3551.

Grenningloh, G., Rienitz, A., Schmitt, B., Methfessel, C., Zensen, M., Beyreuther, K., Gundelfinger, E.D., and Betz, H. The strychnine-binding subunit of the glycine receptor shows homology with nicotinic acetylcholine receptors. *Nature,* **1987,** *328*:215–220.

Grifa, A., Totaro, A., Rommens, J.M., Carella, M., Roetto, A., Borgato, L., Zelante, L., and Gasparini, P. GABA (gamma-amino-butyric acid) neurotransmission: identification and fine mapping of the human GABAB receptor gene. *Biochem. Biophys. Res. Commun.,* **1998,** *250*:240–245.

Guillemin, R., Zeytin, F., Ling, N., Bohlen, P., Esch, F., Brazeau, P., Bloch, B., and Wehrenberg, W.B. Growth hormone-releasing factor: chemistry and physiology. *Proc. Soc. Exp. Biol. Med.,* **1984,** *175*:407–413.

Hökfelt, T., Johansson, O., Fuxe, K., Goldstein, M., and Park, D. Immunohistochemical studies on the localization and distribution of monoamine neuron systems in the rat brain. I. Tyrosine hydroxylase in the mesand diencephalon. *Med. Biol.,* **1976,** *54*:427–453.

Hökfelt, T., Johansson, O., Fuxe, K., Goldstein, M., and Park, D. Immunohistochemical studies on the localization and distribution of monoamine neuron systems in the rat brain. II. Tyrosine hydroxylase in the telencephalon. *Med. Biol.,* **1977,** *55*:21–40.

Honor, P., Menning, P.M., Rogers, S.D., Nichols, M.L., Basbaum, A.I., Besson, J.M., and Mantyh, P.W. Spinal substance P receptor expression and internalization in acute, short-term, and long-term inflammatory pain states. *J. Neurosci.,* **1999,** *19*:7670–7678.

Hoyer, D., and Martin, G.R. Classification and nomenclature of 5-HT receptors: a comment on current issues. *Behav. Brain Res.,* **1996,** *73*:263–268.

Humpel, C., Ebendal, T., and Olson, L. Microdialysis: a way to study in vivo release of neurotrophic bioactivity: a critical summary. *J. Mol. Med.,* **1996,** *74*:523–526.

Jardemark, K., Farre, C., Jacobson, I., Zare, R.N., and Orwar, O. Screening of receptor antagonists using agonist-activated patch clamp detection in chemical separations. *Anal. Chem.,* **1998,** *70*:2468–2474.

Jin, W., and Chavkin, C. Mu opioids enhance mossy fiber synaptic transmission indirectly by reducing GABAB receptor activation. *Brain Res.,* **1999,** *821*:286–293.

Jones, E.G. Viewpoint: the core and matrix of thalamic organization. *Neuroscience,* **1998,** *85*:331–345.

Kandel, E.R., and O'Dell, T.J. Are adult learning mechanisms also used for development? *Science,* **1992,** *258*:243–245.

Koob, G.F., Sanna, P.P., and Bloom, F.E. Neuroscience of addiction. *Neuron,* **1998,** *21*:467–476.

Krapivinsky, G., Gordon, E.A., Wickman, K., Velimirovic, B., Krapivinsky, L., and Clapham, D.E. The G-protein–gated atrial K$^+$ channel IKACh is a heteromultimer of two inwardly rectifying K(+)-channel proteins. *Nature,* **1995,** *374*:135–141.

Lee, J.M., Zipfel, G.J., and Choi, D.W. The changing landscape of ischaemic brain injury mechanisms. *Nature,* **1999,** *399*:A7–A14.

LeMay, D.R., Kittaka, M., Gordon, E.M., Gray, B., Stins, M.F., McComb, J.G., Jovanovic, S., Tabrizi, P., Weiss, M.H., Bartus, R., Anderson, W.F., and Zlokovic, B.V. Intravenous RMP-7 increases delivery of ganciclovir into rat brain tumors and enhances the effects of herpes simplex virus thymidine kinase gene therapy. *Hum. Gene Ther.,* **1998,** *9*:989–995.

Magistretti, P.J., Cardinaux, J.R., and Martin, J.L. VIP and PACAP in the CNS: regulators of glial energy metabolism and modulators of glutamatergic signaling. *Ann. N.Y. Acad. Sci.,* **1998,** *865*:213–225.

Malenka, R.C., and Nicoll, R.A. Long-term potentiation—a decade of progress? *Science,* **1999,** *285*:1870–1874.

Malosio, M.L., Marqueze-Pouey, B., Kuhse, J., and Betz, H. Widespread expression of glycine receptor subunit mRNAs in the adult and developing rat brain. *EMBO J.,* **1991,** *10*:2401–2409.

McDonald, J.W., Liu, X.Z., Qu, Y., Liu, S., Mickey, S.K., Turetsky, D., Gottlieb, D.I., and Choi, D.W. Transplanted embryonic stem cells survive, differentiate and promote recovery in injured rat spinal cord. *Nat. Med.,* **1999,** *5*:1410–1412.

McKay, R. Stem cells and the cellular organization of the brain. *J. Neurosci. Res.,* **2000,** *59*:298–300.

Mechoulam, R., Ben Shabat, S., Hanus, L., Fride, E., Vogel, Z., Bayewitch, M., and Sulcova, A.E. Endogenous cannabinoid ligands—chemical and biological studies. *J. Lipid Mediat. Cell Signal.,* **1996,** *14*:45–49.

Neyroz, P., Desdouits, F., Benfenati, F., Knutson, J.R., Greengard, P., and Girault, J.A. Study of the conformation of DARPP-32, a dopamine- and cAMP-regulated phosphoprotein, by fluorescence spectroscopy. *J. Biol. Chem.,* **1993,** *268*:24022–24031.

Olney, J.W. Brain lesions, obesity, and other disturbances in mice treated with monosodium glutamate. *Science,* **1969,** *164*:719–721.

Olney, J.W., Newcomer, J.W., and Farber, N.B. NMDA receptor hypofunction model of schizophrenia. *J. Psychiatr. Res.,* **1999,** *33*:523–533.

Olsen, R.W., McCabe, R.T., and Wamsley, J.K. GABAA receptor subtypes: autoradiographic comparison of GABA, benzodiazepine, and convulsant binding sites in the rat central nervous system. *J. Chem. Neuroanat.,* **1990,** *3*:59–76.

Park, K.H., and Cho, Y.D. Purification of monomeric agmatine iminohydrolase from soybean. *Biochem. Biophys. Res. Commun.,* **1991,** *174*:32–36.

Piomelli, D., Beltramo, M., Giuffrida, A., and Stella, N. Endogenous cannabinoid signaling. *Neurobiol. Dis.,* **1998,** *5*:462–473.

Redrobe, J.P., Dumont, Y., St-Pierre, J.A., and Quirion, R. Multiple receptors for neuropeptide Y in the hippocampus: putative roles in seizures and cognition. *Brain Res.,* **1999,** *848*:153–166.

Reinscheid, R.K., Nothacker, H.P., Bourson, A., Ardati, A., Henningsen, R.A., Bunzow, J.R., Grandy, D.K., Langen, H., Monsma, F.J. Jr., and Civelli, O. Orphanin FQ: a neuropeptide that activates an opioidlike G protein-coupled receptor. *Science,* **1995,** *270*:792–794.

Rogers, S.W., Andrews, P.I., Gahring, L.C., Whisenand, T., Cauley, K., Crain, B., Hughes, T.E., Heinemann, S.F., and McNamara, J.O.

Autoantibodies to glutamate receptor GluR3 in Rasmussen's encephalitis. *Science,* **1994,** *265*:648–651.

Schnell, L., Fearn, S., Klassen, H., Schwab, M.E., and Perry, V.H. Acute inflammatory responses to mechanical lesions in the CNS: differences between brain and spinal cord. *Eur. J. Neurosci.,* **1999,** *11*:3648–3658.

Sofroniew, M.V., Cooper, J.D., Svendsen, C.N., Crossman, P., Ip, N.Y., Lindsay, R.M., Zafra, F., and Lindholm, D. Atrophy but not death of adult septal cholinergic neurons after ablation of target capacity to produce mRNAs for NGF, BDNF, and NT3. *J. Neurosci.,* **1993,** *13*:5263–5276.

Song, H.J., and Poo, M.M. Signal transduction underlying growth cone guidance by diffusible factors. *Curr. Opin. Neurobiol.,* **1999,** *9*:355–363.

Squire, L.R. Memory systems. *C. R. Acad. Sci. III,* **1998,** *321*:153–156.

Strange, K. Maintenance of cell volume in the central nervous system. *Pediatr. Nephrol.,* **1993,** *7*:689–697.

Swanson, L.W. The neuroanatomy revolution of the 1970s and the hypothalamus. *Brain Res. Bull.,* **1999,** *50*:397.

Traynelis, S.F., Hartley, M., and Heinemann, S.F. Control of proton sensitivity of the NMDA receptor by RNA splicing and polyamines. *Science,* **1995,** *268*:873–876.

Tzounopoulos, T., Janz, R., Sudhof, T.C., Nicoll R.A., and Malenka, R.C. A role for cAMP in long-term depression at hippocampal mossy fiber synapses. *Neuron,* **1998,** *21*:837–845.

Usher, M., Cohen, J.D., Servan-Schreiber, D., Rajkowski, J., and Aston-Jones, G. The role of locus coeruleus in the regulation of cognitive performance. *Science,* **1999,** *283*:549–554.

Wang, Z., and McCormick, D.A. Control of firing mode of corticotectal and corticopontine layer V burst-generating neurons by norepinephrine, acetylcholine, and 1S,3R-ACPD. *J. Neurosci.,* **1993,** *13*:2199–2216.

Yang, T.T., Gallen, C., Schwartz, B., Bloom, F.E., Ramachandran, V.S., and Cobb, S. Sensory maps in the human brain. *Nature,* **1994,** *368*:592–593.

Zipfel, G.J., Lee, J.M., and Choi, D.W. Reducing calcium overload in the ischemic brain. *N. Engl. J. Med.,* **1999,** *341*:1543–1544.

MONOGRAPHS AND REVIEWS

Adams, M.E., and Swanson, G. Neurotoxins supplement. *Trends Neurosci.,* **1994,** *17*:1–31.

Aghajanian, G.K. Electrophysiology of serotonin receptor subtypes and signal transduction pathways. *Psychopharmacology: The Fourth Generation of Progress.* (Bloom, F.E., and Kupfer, D.J., eds.) Raven Press, New York, **1995,** pp. 451–460.

Aghajanian, G.K., and Marek, G.J. Serotonin and hallucinogens. *Neuropsychopharmacology,* **1999,** *21*:16S–23S.

Akil, H., Owens, C., Gutstein, H., Taylor, L., Curran, E., and Watson, S. Endogenous opioids: overview and current issues. *Drug Alcohol Depend.,* **1998,** *51*:127–140.

Amara, S.G., and Sonders, M.S. Neurotransmitter transporters as molecular targets for addictive drugs. *Drug Alcohol Depend.,* **1998,** *51*:87–96.

Baraldi, P.G., Cacciari, B., Romagnoli, R., Merighi, S., Varani, K., Borea, P.A., and Spalluto, G. A(3) adenosine receptor ligands: history and perspectives. *Med. Res. Rev.,* **2000,** *20*:103–128.

Baulieu, E.E. Neurosteroids: a novel function of the brain. *Psychoneuroendocrinology,* **1998,** *23*:963–987.

Black, I.B. Trophic regulation of synaptic plasticity. *J. Neurobiol.,* **1999,** *41*:108–118.

Bloom, F.E. Neurotransmission and the central nervous system. In, *Goodman and Gilman's The Pharmacological Basis of Therapeutics,* 9th ed. (Hardman, J.G., and Limbird, L.E., eds.) McGraw-Hill, New York, **1996**, pp. 267–293.

Bodian, D. Neuron junctions: a revolutionary decade. *Anat. Rec.,* **1972,** *174:*73–82.

Borges, K., and Dingledine, R. AMPA receptors: molecular and functional diversity. *Prog. Brain Res.,* **1998,** *116:*153–170.

Bothwell, M. Functional interactions of neurotrophins and neurotrophin receptors. *Annu. Rev. Neurosci.,* **1995,** *18:*223–253.

Bourne, H.R., and Nicoll, R. Molecular machines integrate coincident synaptic signals. *Cell,* **1993,** *72(suppl.):*65–75.

Bylund, D.B. Subtypes of α_1- and α_2-adrenergic receptors. *FASEB J.,* **1992,** *6:*832–839.

Catterall, W.A. Structure and function of voltage-gated ion channels. *Trends Neurosci.,* **1993,** *16:*500–506.

Catterall, W.A. Structure and function of voltage-sensitive ion channels. *Science,* **1988,** *242:*50–61.

Chao, M., Casaccia-Bonnefil, P., Carter, B., Chittka, A., Kong, H., and Yoon, S.O. Neurotrophin receptors: mediators of life and death. *Brain Res. Brain Res. Rev.,* **1998,** *26:*295–301.

Cherniak, C. The bounded brain: toward quantitative neuroanatomy. *J. Cogn. Neurosci.,* **1990,** *2:*58–68.

Choi, D.W., and Koh, J.Y. Zinc and brain injury. *Annu. Rev. Neurosci.,* **1998,** *21:*347–375.

Civelli, O. Molecular biology of the dopamine receptor subtypes. In, *Psychopharmacology: The Fourth Generation of Progress.* (Bloom, F.E., and Kupfer, D.J., eds.) Raven Press, New York, **1995,** pp. 155–162.

Cooper, J.R., Bloom, F.E., and Roth, R.H., eds. *The Biochemical Basis of Neuropharmacology.* Oxford University Press, New York, **1996.**

Cotman, C.W., Kahle, J.S., Miller, S., Ulas, J., and Bridges, R.J. Excitatory amino acid neurotransmission. In, *Psychopharmacology: The Fourth Generation of Progress.* (Bloom, F.E., and Kupfer, D.J., eds.) Raven Press, New York, **1995,** pp. 75–86.

Dale, H.H. Pharmacology and nerve endings. *Proc. R. Soc. Med.,* **1935,** *28:*319–332.

Darlison, M.G., and Richter, D. Multiple genes for neuropeptides and their receptors: co-evolution and physiology. *Trends Neurosci.,* **1999,** *22:*81–88.

Dingledine, R., Borges, K., Bowie, D., and Traynelis, S.F. The glutamate receptor ion channels. *Pharmacol. Rev.,* **1999,** *51:*7–61.

Eccles, J.C. *The Physiology of Synapses.* Academic Press, New York, **1964.**

Edwards, F.A., and Robertson, S.J. The function of A2 adenosine receptors in the mammalian brain: evidence for inhibition vs. enhancement of voltage gated calcium channels and neurotransmitter release. *Prog. Brain Res.,* **1999,** *120:*265–273.

Florey, E. Neurotransmitters and modulators in the animal kingdom. *Fed. Proc.* **1967,** *26:*1164–1176.

Foote, S.L. The primate locus coeruleus: the chemical neuroanatomy of the nucleus, its efferent projections, and its target receptors. In, *Handbook of Chemical Neuroanatomy.* Vol. 13. (Bloom, F.E., Björklund, A., and Hökfelt, T., eds.) Elsevier, Amsterdam, **1997,** pp. 187–215.

Foote, S.L., and Aston-Jones, G. Pharmacology and physiology of central noradrenergic systems. In, *Psychopharmacology: The Fourth Generation of Progress.* (Bloom, F.E., and Kupfer, D.J., eds.) Raven Press, New York, **1995,** pp. 335–346.

Gage, F.H. Mammalian neural stem cells. *Science,* **2000,** *287:*1433–1438.

Geppert, M., and Südhof, T.C. RAB3 and synaptotagmin: The yin and yang of synaptic membrane fusion. *Annu. Rev. Neurosci.,* **1998,** *21:*75–95.

Gingrich, J.A., and Caron, M.G. Recent advances in the molecular biology of dopamine receptors. *Annu. Rev. Neurosci.,* **1993,** *16:*299–321.

González-Scarano, F., and Baltuch, G. Microglia as mediators of inflammatory and degenerative diseases. *Annu. Rev. Neurosci.,* **1999,** *22:*219–240.

Grandy, D.K., and Civelli, O. G-protein-coupled receptors: the new dopamine receptor subtypes. *Curr. Opin. Neurobiol.,* **1992,** *2:*275–281.

Granholm, A.C., Albeck, D., Backman, C., Curtis, M., Ebendal, T., Friden, P., Henry, M., Hoffer, B., Kordower, J., Rose, G.M., Soderstrom, S., and Bartus, R.T. A non-invasive system for delivering neural growth factors across the blood-brain barrier: a review. *Rev. Neurosci.,* **1998,** *9:*31–55.

Greengard, P., Allen, P.B., and Nairn, A.C. Beyond the dopamine receptor: the DARPP-32/protein phophatase-1 cascade. *Neuron,* **1999,** *23:*435–447.

Gudermann, T., Schöneberg, T., and Schultz, G. Functional and structural complexity of signal transduction via G-protein–coupled receptors. *Annu. Rev. Neurosci.,* **1997,** *20:*399–427.

Herrling, P., ed. *Excitatory Amino Acids: Clinical Results with Antagonists.* Academic Press, San Diego, CA, **1997.**

Hökfelt, T., Broberger, C., Xu, D., Sergeyev, V., Ubink, R., and Diez, M. Neuropeptides—an overview. *Neuropharmacology,* **2000,** *39:*1337–1356.

Hökfelt, T., Castel, M.-N., Morino, P., Zhang, X., and Dagerlind, A. General overview of neuropeptides. *Psychopharmacology: The Fourth Generation of Progress.* (Bloom, F.E., and Kupfer, D.J., eds.) Raven Press, New York, **1995.**

Hollmann, M., and Heinemann, S. Cloned glutamate receptors. *Annu. Rev. Neurosci.,* **1994,** *17:*31–108.

Jan, L.Y., Jan, Y.N. Cloned potassium channels from eukaryotes and prokaryotes. *Annu. Rev. Neurosci.,* **1997,** *20:*91–123.

Jones, E.G. Cortical and subcortical contributions to activity-dependent plasticity in primate somatosensory cortex. *Annu. Rev. Neurosci.,* **2000,** *23:*1–37.

Kandel, E.R. A new intellectual framework for psychiatry. *Am. J. Psychiatry,* **1998,** *155:*457–469.

Kelly, J.S., and Beart, P.M. Amino acid receptors in CNS. II. GABA in supraspinal regions. In, *Handbook of Psychopharmacology.* Vol. 4. (Iversen L.L., Iversen, S.D., and Snyder, S.H., eds.) Raven Press, New York, **1975,** pp. 129–209.

Koob, G.F., and Le Moal, M. Drug abuse: hedonic homeostatic dysregulation. *Science,* **1997,** *278:*52–58.

Lewis, D.A. Dopamine systems in the primate brain. In, *Handbook of Chemical Neuroanatomy.* Vol. 13. (Bloom, F.E., Björklund, A., and Hökfelt, T. eds.) Elsevier, Amsterdam, **1997,** pp. 263–375.

Liu, Y., and Edwards, R.H. The role of vesicular transport proteins in synaptic transmission and neural degeneration. *Annu. Rev. Neurosci.,* **1997,** *20:*125–156.

MacDonald, E., Kobilka, B., and Scheinin, M. Gene targeting—homing in on α_2-adrenoceptor-subtype function. *Trends Pharmacol. Sci.,* **1997,** *18:*211–219.

Macdonald, R.L., and Olsen, R.W. GABAA receptor channels. *Annu. Rev. Neurosci.,* **1994,** *17:*569–602.

Macdonald, R.L., Twyman, R.E., Ryan-Jastrow, T., and Angelotti, T.P. Regulation of GABAA receptor channels by anticonvulsant and convulsant drugs and by phosphorylation. *Epilepsy Res. Suppl.,* **1992,** *9:*265–277.

McKay, S.E., Purcell, A.L., and Carew, T.J. Regulation of synaptic function by neurotrophic factors in vertebrates and invertebrates: implications for development and learning. *Learn. Mem.,* **1999,** *6*:193–215.

Magistretti, P.J., Pellerin, L., and Martin, J.-L. Brain energy metabolism: an integrated cellular perspective. In, *Psychopharmacology: The Fourth Generation of Progress.* (Bloom, F.E., and Kupfer, D.J., eds.) Raven Press, New York, **1995.**

Malenka, R.C., and Nicoll, R.A. Long-term depression with a flash. *Nat. Neurosci.,* **1998,** *1*:89–90.

Mennicken, F., Maki, R., de Souza, E.B., and Quirion, R. Chemokines and chemokine receptors in the CNS: a possible role in neuroinflammation and patterning. *Trends Pharmacol. Sci.,* **1999,** *20*:73–78.

Merry, D.E., and Korsmeyer, S.J. Bcl-2 gene family in the nervous system. *Annu. Rev. Neurosci.,* **1997,** *70*:245–267.

Mesulam, M.-M. Structure and function of cholinergic pathways in the cerebral cortex, limbic system, basal ganglia and thalamus of the human brain. In, *Psychopharmacology: The Fourth Generation of Progress.* (Bloom, F.E., and Kupfer, D.J., eds.) Raven Press, New York, **1995,** pp. 135–146.

Middleton, F.A., and Strick, P.L. The cerebellum: an overview. *Trends Neurosci.,* **1998,** *21*:367–369.

Moreau, J.L., and Huber, G. Central adenosine A(2A) receptors: an overview. *Brain Res. Brain Res. Rev.,* **1999,** *31*:65–82.

Morris, J.F., Budd, T.C., Epton, M.J., Ma, D., Pow, D.V., and Wang, H. Functions of the perikaryon and dendrites in magnocellular vasopressin-secreting neurons: new insights from ultrastructural studies. *Prog. Brain Res.,* **1998,** *119*:21–30.

Morrison, J.H., and Hof, P.R. Life and death of neurons in the aging brain. *Science,* **1997,** *278*:412–419.

Mountcastle, V.B. The columnar organization of the neocortex. *Brain,* **1997,** *120*:701–722.

Murphy, D.L., Wichems, C., Li, Q., and Heils, A. Molecular manipulations as tools for enhancing our understanding of 5-HT neurotransmission. *Trends Pharmacol. Sci.,* **1999,** *20*:246–252.

Nelson, T.J., Gusev, P.A., and Alkon, D.L. Identification of ion channel regulating proteins by patch-clamp analysis. *Methods Enzymol.,* **1998,** *293*:194–201.

Nicoll, R.A., Malenka, R.C., and Kauer, J.A. Functional comparison of neurotransmitter receptor subtypes in mammalian central nervous system. *Physiol. Rev.,* **1990,** *70*:513–565.

Parsons, L.H., and Justice, J.B. Jr. Quantitative approaches to in vivo brain microdialysis. *Crit. Rev. Neurobiol.,* **1994,** *8*:189–220.

Raber, J., Sorg, O., Horn, T.F., Yu, N., Koob, G.F., Campbell, I.L., and Bloom, F.E. Inflammatory cytokines: putative regulators of neuronal and neuro-endocrine function. *Brain Res. Brain Res. Rev.,* **1998,** *26*:320–326.

Rubin, L.L., and Staddon, J.M. The cell biology of the blood-brain barrier. *Annu. Rev. Neurosci.,* **1999,** *22*:11–28.

Rupniak, N.M., and Kramer, M.S. Discovery of the antidepressant and anti-emetic efficacy of substance P (NK1) receptor antagonists. *Trends Pharmacol. Sci.,* **1999,** *20*:485–490.

Schwartz, J.C., Diaz, J., Bordet, R., Griffon, N., Perachon, S., Pilon, C., Ridray, S., and Sokoloff, P. Functional implications of multiple dopamine receptor subtypes: the D1/D3 receptor coexistence. *Brain Res. Brain Res. Rev.,* **1998,** *26*:236–242.

Schwartz, J.-C., Arrang, J.-M., Garbarg, M., and Traiffort, E. Histamine. In, *Psychopharmacology: The Fourth Generation of Progress.* (Bloom, F.E., and Kupfer, D.J., eds.) Raven Press, New York, **1995,** pp. 397–406.

Seeburg, P.H. The TINS/TiPS Lecture. The molecular biology of mammalian glutamate receptor channels. *Trends Neurosci.,* **1993,** *16*:359–365.

Seeburg, P.H., Wisden, W., Verdoorn, T.A., Pritchett, D.B., Werner, P., Herb, A., Luddens, H., Sprengel, R., and Sakmann, B. The $GABA_A$ receptor family: molecular and functional diversity. *Cold Spring Harb. Symp. Quant. Biol.,* **1990,** *55*:29–40.

Shepherd, G.M., ed. *The Synaptic Organization of the Brain,* 4th ed. Oxford University Press, New York, **1998.**

Snyder, S.H., and Dawson, T.M. Nitric oxide and related substances as neural messengers. In, *Psychopharmacology: The Fourth Generation of Progress.* (Bloom, F.E., and Kupfer, D.J., eds.) Raven Press, New York, **1995,** pp. 609–618.

Sokoloff, P., and Schwartz, J.C. Novel dopamine receptors half a decade later. *Trends Pharmacol. Sci.,* **1995,** *16*:270–275.

Spriggs, M.K. Shared resources between the neural and immune systems: semaphorins join the ranks. *Curr. Opin. Immunol.,* **1999,** *11*:387–391.

Steinbusch, H., and Mulder, A.H. Serotonin-immunoreactive neurons and their projections in the CNS. In, *Handbook of Chemical Neuroanatomy.* Vol. 3. (Björklund, A., Hökflet, T., and Kuhar, M., eds.) Elsevier, Amsterdam, **1984,** pp. 101–125.

Tang, W.J., and Gilman, A.G. Adenylyl cyclases. *Cell,* **1992,** *70*:869–872.

Tononi, G., and Edelman, G.M. Consciousness and complexity. *Science,* **1998,** *28*:1846–1851.

Uhl, G.R., Childers, S., and Pasternak, G. An opiate receptor gene family reunion. *Trends Neurosci.,* **1994,** *17*:89–93.

Vanden Broeck, J., Torfs, H., Poels, J., Van Poyer, W., Swinnen, E., Ferket, K., and De Loof, A. Tachykinin-like peptides and their receptors. A review. *Ann. N.Y. Acad. Sci.,* **1999,** *897*:374–387.

Williams, M. Purinoceptors in central nervous system function: targets for therapeutic intervention. In, *Psychopharmacology: The Fourth Generation of Progress.* (Bloom, F.E., and Kupfer, D.J., eds.) Raven Press, New York, **1995.**

Williams, M., Kowaluk, E.A., and Arneric, S.P. Emerging molecular approaches to pain therapy. *J. Med. Chem.,* **1999,** *42*:1481–1500.

C H A P T E R   1 3

HISTORY AND PRINCIPLES OF ANESTHESIOLOGY

Charles Beattie

Prior to 1846, attempts to provide comfort during operative procedures were minimally effective and the development of surgery was necessarily limited. William T.G. Morton's public demonstration of ether in that year revolutionized medical care throughout the world. The evolution of anesthesiology as a medical specialty has facilitated the success of modern, complex surgical procedures. Beyond the obtundation of consciousness and creation of a quiescent surgical field, anesthesiology applies principles of physiology, pathophysiology, and pharmacology to assess and reduce surgical risk, maintain homeostasis, attenuate the surgical stress response, and provide analgesia. In this chapter, we explore the salient features of the preoperative, intraoperative, and postoperative periods, highlighting recent discoveries including anesthetic receptor specificity, identification of the neural correlates of consciousness, and new technology to assess levels of awareness.

HISTORY OF SURGICAL ANESTHESIA

Anesthesia before 1846. Surgical procedures were uncommon before 1846. Understanding of the pathophysiology of disease and of the rationale for its treatment by surgery was rudimentary. Aseptic technique and the prevention of wound infection were almost unknown. In addition, the lack of satisfactory anesthesia was a major deterrent. Because of all these factors, few operations were attempted, and mortality was frequent. Typically, surgery was of an emergency nature—for example, amputation of a limb for open fracture or drainage of an abscess. Fine dissection and careful technique were not possible in patients for whom relief of pain was inadequate.

Some means of attempting to relieve surgical pain were available and, in fact, had been used since ancient times. Drugs like alcohol, hashish, and opium derivatives, taken by mouth, provided some consolation. Physical methods for the production of analgesia, such as packing a limb in ice or making it ischemic with a tourniquet, occasionally were used. Unconsciousness induced by a blow to the head or by strangulation did provide relief from pain, although at a high cost. However, the most common method used to achieve a relatively quiet surgical field was simple restraint of the patient by force. It is no wonder that surgery was looked upon as a last resort.

Although the analgesic properties of both nitrous oxide and diethyl ether had been known to a few for years, the agents were not used for medical purposes. Nitrous oxide was synthesized by Priestley in 1776, and both he and Humphry Davy some 20 years later commented upon its anesthetic properties (Faulconer and Keys, 1965). Davy in fact suggested that ". . . it may probably be used with advantage during surgical operations in which no great effusion of blood takes place." Another 20 years passed

before Michael Faraday wrote that the inhalation of diethyl ether produced effects similar to those of nitrous oxide. However, except for their inhalation in carnival exhibitions or to produce "highs" at "ether frolics," these drugs were not used in human beings until the mid–nineteenth century.

Greene (1971) has presented an analysis of the reasons for the introduction of anesthesia in the 1840s. The time was then right, since concern for the well-being of one's fellows, a humanitarian attitude, was more prevalent than it had been in the previous century. "So long as witches were being burned in Salem, anesthesia could not be discovered 20 miles away in Boston." While humanitarian concern extended to the relief of pain, chemistry and medicine had simultaneously advanced to such an extent that a chemically pure drug could be prepared and then used with some degree of safety. There was, too, growth of the inquisitive spirit—a search for improvement of the human condition.

Public Demonstration of Ether Anesthesia. Dentists were instrumental in the introduction of both diethyl ether and nitrous oxide. They, even more than physicians, came into daily contact with persons complaining of pain; often, as a by-product of their work, they produced pain. It was at a stage show that Horace Wells, a dentist, noted that one of the participants, while under the influence of nitrous oxide, injured himself yet felt no pain. The next day Wells, while breathing nitrous oxide, had one of his own teeth extracted, painlessly, by a colleague. Shortly thereafter, in 1845, Wells attempted to demonstrate his discovery at the Massachusetts General Hospital in Boston. Unfortunately the patient cried out during the operation, and the demonstration was deemed a failure.

William T. G. Morton, a Boston dentist (and medical student), was familiar with the use of nitrous oxide from a previous association with Horace Wells. Morton learned of ether's anesthetic effects, thought it more promising, and practiced with it on animals and then on himself. Finally, he asked permission to demonstrate the drug's use, publicly, as a surgical anesthetic.

The story of this classical demonstration in 1846 has been retold countless times. The operating room ("ether dome") at the Massachusetts General Hospital remains as a memorial to the first public demonstration of surgical anesthesia. In the gallery of this room skeptical spectators gathered, for the news had spread that a second-year medical student had developed a method for abolishing surgical pain. The patient, Gilbert Abbott, was brought in and Dr. Warren, the surgeon, waited in formal morning clothes. Operating gowns, masks, gloves, surgical asepsis, and the bacterial origin of infection were entirely unknown at that time. Everyone was ready and waiting, including the strong men to hold down the struggling patient, but Morton did not appear. Fifteen minutes passed, and the surgeon, becoming impatient, took his scalpel and turning to the gallery said, "As Dr. Morton has not arrived, I presume he is otherwise engaged." While the audience smiled and the patient cringed, the surgeon turned to make his incision. Just then Morton entered, his tardiness being due to the necessity for completing an apparatus with which to administer the ether. Warren stepped back, and pointing to the man strapped to the operating table said, "Well, sir, your patient is ready." Surrounded by a silent and unsympathetic audience, Morton went quietly to work. After a few minutes of ether inhalation, the patient was unconscious, whereupon Morton looked up and said, "Dr. Warren, *your* patient is ready." The operation was begun. The patient showed no sign of pain, yet he was alive and breathing. The strong men were not needed. When the operation was completed, Dr. Warren turned to the astonished audience and made the famous statement, "Gentlemen, this is no humbug." Dr. Henry J. Bigelow, an eminent surgeon attending the demonstration, remarked, "I have seen something today that will go around the world."

Following initial disbelief, news of the successful demonstration spread rapidly. Within a month, ether was in use in other cities of the United States and had been given in Great Britain as well. Its use soon was established as legitimate medical therapy.

The lives of those involved in the introduction of surgical anesthesia did not have so salubrious an outcome. Morton initially tried to patent the use of ether to produce anesthesia and, when this failed, patented instead his device for its administration. Considerable wrangling ensued as to who was the legitimate discoverer of anesthesia. Never receiving what he felt to be his due, Morton died an embittered man.

Charles Jackson, Morton's chemistry teacher at Harvard, also claimed priority in the discovery; it was he who had suggested that Morton use pure sulfuric ether. Jackson became insane, a fate that also befell Horace Wells, the man who had failed in the public demonstration of nitrous oxide anesthesia. Crawford Long, a physician in rural Georgia, had used ether anesthesia since 1842 but neglected to publish his experiences. He survived and prospered, but Morton rightfully receives credit for the introduction of surgical anesthesia. A monument erected by the citizens of Boston over the grave of Dr. Morton, in

Mt. Auburn Cemetery near Boston, bears the following inscription, written by Dr. Jacob Bigelow:

WILLIAM T. G. MORTON

Inventor and Revealer of Anaesthetic Inhalation.
Before Whom, in All Time, Surgery Was Agony.
By Whom Pain in Surgery Was Averted and Annulled.
Since Whom Science Has Control of Pain.

Anesthesia after 1846. Although it is rarely used today, ether was the ideal "first" anesthetic. Chemically, it is readily made in pure form. It is relatively easy to administer, since it is a liquid at room temperature but is readily vaporized. Ether is potent, unlike nitrous oxide, and thus a few volumes percent can produce anesthesia without diluting the oxygen in room air to hypoxic levels. It supports both respiration and circulation, crucial properties at a time when human physiology was not understood well enough for assisted respiration and circulation to be possible. And ether is not toxic to vital organs.

The next anesthetic to receive wide use was chloroform. Introduced by the Scottish obstetrician James Simpson in 1847, it became quite popular, perhaps because of its more pleasant odor. Other than this and its nonflammability, there was little to recommend it (Sykes, 1960). The drug is a hepatotoxin and a severe cardiovascular depressant. Despite the relatively high incidence of intraoperative and postoperative death associated with the use of chloroform, it was championed, especially in Great Britain, for nearly 100 years. Because of the danger and difficulty in administering chloroform, distinguished British physicians became interested in anesthetics and their administration, a trend that was not evident in the United States until 100 years later.

The course of anesthesiology in the United States, after the initial burst of enthusiasm, was one of slow change and limited progress. Furthermore, despite the relative comfort that the surgical patient experienced, the amount and scope of surgery increased only slightly during the 1840s and 1850s (Greene, 1979). The incidence of mortality was little changed, for postoperative infection was still a serious problem. Only with the introduction of aseptic techniques 20 years after the discovery of anesthesia did surgery come into its own.

Other Anesthetic Agents. Nitrous oxide fell into disuse after the apparent failure in Boston in 1845. It was reintroduced in 1863 into American dental and surgical practice, largely through the efforts of Gardner Q. Colton, a showman, entrepreneur, and partially trained physician. In 1868, the administration of nitrous oxide with oxygen was described by Edmond Andrews, a Chicago surgeon, and soon thereafter the two gases became available in steel cylinders, greatly increasing their practicality. Nitrous oxide still is used widely today.

The anesthetic properties of cyclopropane were accidentally discovered in 1929, when chemists were analyzing impurities in an isomer, propylene. After extensive clinical trial at the University of Wisconsin, the drug was introduced into practice; cyclopropane was perhaps the most widely used general anesthetic for the next 30 years. However, with the increasing risk of explosion in the operating room brought about by the use of electronic equipment, the need for a safe, nonflammable anesthetic increased, and several groups pursued the search. Efforts by the British Research Council and by chemists at Imperial Chemical

Industries were rewarded by the development of halothane, a nonflammable anesthetic agent that was introduced into clinical practice in 1956; it revolutionized inhalational anesthesia. Most of the newer agents, which are halogenated hydrocarbons and ethers, are modeled after halothane.

The skeletal muscle relaxants (neuromuscular blocking agents) also were discovered and their pharmacological properties demonstrated long before their introduction into clinical practice. Curare, in crude form, had long been used by South American Indians as a poison on their arrow tips (*see* Chapter 9). Its first clinical use was in spastic disorders, where it could decrease muscle tone without compromising respiration excessively. It was then used to modify the violent muscle contractions associated with electroconvulsive therapy of psychiatric disorders. Finally, in the 1940s, anesthesiologists used curare to provide the muscular relaxation that previously could be obtained only with deep levels of general anesthesia. Over the next half-dozen years several synthetic substitutes were used clinically. It is difficult to overemphasize the importance of muscle relaxants in anesthetic practice. Their use permits adequate conditions for surgery with light levels of general anesthesia; cardiovascular depression is thus minimized, and the patient awakens promptly when the anesthetic is discontinued.

Although the desirability of an intravenous anesthetic agent must have been apparent to physicians early in the twentieth century, the drugs at hand were few and unsatisfactory. The situation changed dramatically in 1935, when Lundy demonstrated the clinical usefulness of thiopental, a rapidly acting thiobarbiturate. It was originally considered useful as a sole anesthetic agent, but the doses required resulted in serious depression of the circulatory, respiratory, and nervous systems. Thiopental, however, has been enthusiastically accepted as an agent for the rapid induction of general anesthesia.

Various combinations of intravenous drugs from several classes have been used recently as anesthetic agents, usually together with nitrous oxide. The administration of short-acting opioids by constant intravenous infusion (with little or no potent inhalational agent) is an exciting current development in the practice of anesthesia.

MODERN ANESTHESIOLOGY

What Is Anesthesia? The answer to this question is both more complex and more elusive than generally appreciated. To guide the discussion we may first consider the basic goals of anesthesia, namely *to create a reversible condition of comfort, quiescence, and physiological stability in a patient before, during, and after performance of a procedure that would otherwise be painful, frightening, or hazardous.* This statement embodies concepts that have evolved with modern developments within the specialty of anesthesiology that were not necessarily envisioned by early workers.

After the public demonstration of diethyl ether in 1846, anesthesia was eagerly embraced by the general public and the medical profession even as complications associated with its use were noted with concern (Codman,

1917). For several decades, the dramatic increase in surgical procedures performed was tracked precisely by increases in the deaths and major morbidities attributed to the anesthesia (Sykes, 1960). Foremost among the complications were regurgitation and aspiration of stomach contents and cardiovascular collapse, now thought to be disturbances of heart rhythm resulting from an interaction between direct effects of the agents that were used with the physiological response to surgical stress.

To realize fully the benefits and the promise of anesthesia, laboratory and clinical researchers have investigated the pharmacological and physiological actions of potent new therapeutic agents, guided development of monitoring equipment and drug-delivery devices, and created advanced techniques and principles of practice (Wiklund and Rosenbaum, 1997). Recent refinements have included progressive attention to issues of risk assessment and risk reduction.

Unlike the practice of every other branch of medicine, anesthesia usually is considered to be neither therapeutic nor diagnostic. The notable exceptions to this, including treatments of status asthmaticus with halothane and intractable angina with epidural local anesthetics (and other examples), should not obscure the critical point, which permeates the training and practice of the specialty. Patients present for surgery with an array of medical conditions both known and unknown, while ingesting drugs that alter cardiovascular and other responses. They will then undergo a series of physiological stressors from which they must be protected, including effects of the very agents used to initiate and sustain the anesthetic condition. Reduction of complications may be separated for illustrative purposes into three categories:

1. *Minimizing the potentially deleterious direct and indirect effects of anesthetic agents and techniques,* including perturbations of cardiac rhythm and contractility, alterations of vascular tone, blunting of protective reflexes, and changes in metabolic rate and thermoregulation.
2. *Sustaining homeostasis during surgical procedures* that involve major blood loss, tissue ischemia, reperfusion of ischemic tissue, fluid shifts, exposure to cold environment, and impaired coagulation.
3. *Improving postoperative outcomes* by choosing techniques that block or treat components of the *surgical stress response,* which would otherwise lead to short- or long-term sequalae.

The Surgical Stress Response. The stress of surgery includes (presumably) adaptive responses involving three systems, the hypothalamic-pituitary-adrenal axis, the sympathetic nervous system, and the acute-phase response, all of which may be activated by psychological stress, tissue injury, intravascular volume changes, anesthetic agents, pain, and organ manipulation (Udelsman and Holbrook, 1994). These stimuli trigger a cascade of neurohumeral responses, including increases in cortisol, catecholamines, heat shock proteins, and cytokines which, in turn, provoke tachycardia, hypertension, increased metabolism, hypercoagulability, and decreased immune function (Breslow, 1998). Specific associated morbidities include myocardial ischemia and infarction (Mangano *et al.*, 1996), arrhythmias (Balser *et al.*, 1998), thrombosis, infection, and delayed wound healing. The effects of anesthesia attenuate some components of the surgical stress response.

In addition to promoting stability within the clinical milieu described above, it should be emphasized that the kinetics of anesthetic agents and the techniques used must conform to certain time constraints so that the duration and depth of anesthetic states parallel the tempo of the surgical procedure. Hence the uptake, distribution, and elimination of anesthetic drugs are important matters, and the discovery of agents with rapid onset and elimination has greatly improved this aspect of care.

The rest of this chapter will be organized around discussions of the functionally separable time periods: before (*preoperative*), during (*intraoperative*), and after (*postoperative*) surgery, illustrating within each period the principles of perioperative medical care and the anesthesia-specific issues as they logically appear.

PREOPERATIVE PERIOD

Anesthetic considerations prior to surgery include patient evaluation and the administration of medications that treat chronic or acute disease and that facilitate the impending anesthetic experience.

Preexisting comorbidities are important determinants of perioperative risk. Risk prediction indices or algorithms have been developed (Goldman *et al.*, 1977; Palda and Detsky, 1997) that incorporate several pathophysiological conditions, including known or probable coronary artery disease; electrocardiogram (ECG) changes; signs and symptoms of congestive heart failure; abnormalities indicating pulmonary, renal, or hepatic disease; patient age; and invasiveness of the planned surgical procedure. Each one of these conditions has one or more treatment options that have been developed to neutralize its effect and prevent it from worsening during or after the procedure. This is a major feature of the practice of anesthesiology. Decisions are made with regard to the techniques employed, agents chosen, and monitors used based on the preoperative information (Sweitzer, 2000). Depending on the patient's condition, interventions suggested by

the preoperative evaluation range from preoperative coronary angiography (with balloon angioplasty or coronary artery bypass grafting in appropriate cases) (Eagle *et al.*, 1996), optimization of cardiac loading conditions guided by data from pulmonary artery catheters prior to surgery (Berlauk *et al.*, 1991), simple corrections of electrolyte and hemoglobin abnormalities, and institution of antihypertensive therapy.

Novel proposals for preoperative assessment are emerging from modern techniques of molecular biology. Genetic polymorphisms, the discovery of which has been accelerated as a consequence of the mapping of the human genome, are being linked to medical conditions (hypertension, coagulation disorders, arrhythmias) and variable responses to therapy. The challenge now is to apply these same concepts to the surgical environment. Preoperative evaluation and risk assessment may evolve to include broad screenings for polymorphism associated with morbidity and, thereby, guide risk-reduction therapies.

Preoperative Medication

Chronic Medications. Preoperative medication begins with virtually all of the patient's normal daily morning doses of significant drugs. This includes inotropic, chronotropic, dromotropic, and vasoactive agents, especially antihypertensive agents. Diuretics are controversial, as are metformin and monoamine oxidase inhibitors. The latter agents have serious interactions with meperidine and other drugs used during surgery, but these interactions can be managed. The management of insulin-dependent diabetes and chronic steroid use is addressed formally by protocols. Patients dependent on drugs that are associated with withdrawal symptoms must be given special treatment.

The importance of maintaining cardiovascular medications is illustrated by clinical studies showing that the incidence and severity of myocardial ischemia is associated with elevated heart rates in the postoperative period. This finding led to clinical trials of prophylactic, perioperative administration of β-adrenergic receptor antagonists in high-risk patients. Preoperative and postoperative administration of the β-receptor antagonist atenolol yielded significant reduction of myocardial ischemia and a reduction in mortality (at two years) in the treatment group (Mangano *et al.*, 1996). This has been confirmed in a study of high-risk patients given bisoprolol who had significantly lower rates of myocardial infarction and death than did control patients (Poldermans *et al.*, 1999). Previous studies of prophylactic nitroglycerin and calcium channel blockers had failed to show a benefit.

Other preoperative medications are used to treat conditions directly related to anesthetic issues that may arise before, during, and after surgery.

Anticholinergic Drugs. Though previously widely employed for their vagolytic and membrane-drying properties, anticholinergic agents (*see* Chapter 7) are little used, preoperatively, in adults in modern practice, except in specific situations requiring reduced secretions. Vagotonia may occur intraoperatively from increases in ocular pressure, visceral traction, and other reasons, and it is treated by interrupting the stimulus temporarily while administering anticholinergic drugs.

Drugs That Reduce the Acidity and Volume of Gastric Contents. The induction of general anesthesia eliminates the patient's ability to protect the airway should regurgitation of stomach contents occur. This is why nothing-by-mouth ("npo") status is emphasized so strongly for patients having elective procedures. Decreasing the volume of gastric contents further reduces the likelihood of regurgitation, and increasing the gastric pH above 2.5 reduces damage to the lungs in the event of aspiration. Histamine H_2-receptor antagonists, antacids, and prokinetic agents (*see* Chapters 37 and 38) frequently are administered to achieve these conditions.

Sedative-Hypnotics and Antianxiety Agents. Drugs such as benzodiazepines and butyrophenones (*see* Chapter 17) are useful when administered before surgery both for patient comfort and for facilitation of the anesthetic state. When given in conjunction with opioids, there is reduction of catecholamine release in response to surgical stimuli (Newman and Reves, 1993).

Opioids. Opioids (*see* Chapters 14 and 23) may be used preoperatively in small doses to act synergistically with sedatives in creating a tranquil patient. Only in persons actually having pain or experiencing incipient withdrawal symptoms are they specifically indicated before surgery.

INTRAOPERATIVE PERIOD

Monitoring

Standard monitoring (Pierce, 1989) during anesthesia includes continuous electrocardiography, monitoring of heart rate and body temperature, pulse oximetry, and capnography (the measurement of carbon dioxide concentration in exhaled gas) and frequent noninvasive blood pressure measurement. Additional parameters measured may include urine output, blood loss, and ventilation-related parameters—including inspired oxygen, tidal volume, minute ventilation, peak inspired airway pressure, and all gas flows. Direct measurement of inspired and expired levels of volatile anesthesic agents is desirable. In selected cases, invasive measurements are made of arterial pressure, central venous pressure, pulmonary artery pressure, cardiac output, pulmonary capillary wedge pressure, right ventricular ejection fraction, and pulmonary artery oxygen saturation. Transesophageal echocardiography has proven to be most useful in cardiac surgery and in other special situations.

General Anesthesia

There are two fundamentally different ways of achieving the basic anesthetic conditions required to perform surgical procedures, *general anesthesia* and *regional (or conduction) anesthesia*. The hallmark of general anesthesia is loss of consciousness as represented by the historical vignette and the description "going to sleep," which continues to be used by lay persons and professionals alike. Regional anesthesia is effected by the injection or infiltration of certain amides or esters that block signal conduction (usually voltage-gated sodium channels) near nerves either peripherally or more centrally (*see* Chapter 15). This widely used technique has advantages (including intense attenuation of noxious stimuli) as well as drawbacks, as discussed in a later section of this chapter.

General anesthesia is classically described by four qualities: *hypnosis* (usually meaning sleep or loss of consciousness), *amnesia, analgesia,* and *muscle relaxation.* To these must be added the broader concepts of maintaining physiological stability, attenuation of the surgical stress response, and a host of techniques to lessen the aforementioned categories of risk.

The intraoperative period for general anesthesia is normally broken down into three phases—*induction, maintenance,* and *emergence*—each with its special considerations.

Induction. The "induction" of general anesthesia occurs when a conscious or otherwise responsive being is rendered unconscious by the effects on the nervous system of inhaled or intravenously injected agents.

Loss of Consciousness. Oddly, after 150 years of investigation, researchers still do not know with certainty either the molecular mechanisms whereby general anesthetic agents exert their neurological effect or the brain structures or circuitry involved in the loss of consciousness. It may be disconcerting, but a corollary of this lack of understanding is that assessment of the "depth" of anesthesia must be determined by indirect means (*i.e.,* changes in vital signs) that are only variably reliable.

The variety of structurally diverse molecules that can create the condition we call general anesthesia is astonishing (*see* Chapter 14). The group includes volatile organic agents (halogenated hydrocarbons, diethyl ether, chloroform); inorganic gases such as nitrous oxide and xenon; alcohols; and an array of intravenous agents, including barbiturates, etomidate, propofol, and ketamine. Exactly how and precisely where anesthetic agents produce their remarkable effects have been under investigation for a century (Meyer, 1899, 1901; Overton, 1901).

At the cellular level, fundamental discoveries in the last decade have greatly changed traditional concepts that attributed anesthetic action to nonspecific membrane solubility of anesthetic molecules with resulting perturbed structural and dynamic properties of the lipid membrane.

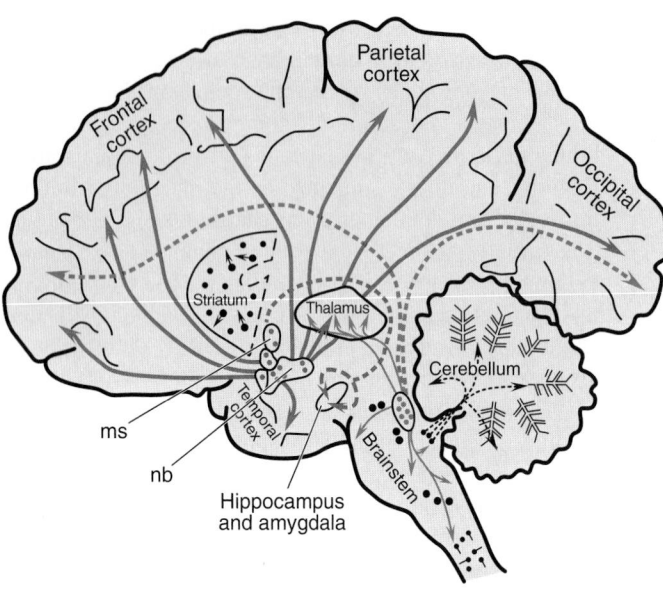

Figure 13–1. Cholinergic systems in the human brain.

Two major pathways project widely to different brain areas: basal-forebrain cholinergic neurons (blue) [including the nucleus basalis (nb) and medial septal nucleus (ms)] and pedunculopontine–lateral dorsal tegmental neurons (gray). Other cholinergic neurons include striatal interneurons, cranial nerve nuclei, vestibular nuclei, and spinal cord preganglionic and motoneurons. (Modified from Perry *et al.,* 1999, with permission.)

Recent work has identified functional targets for a wide range of intravenous and inhalational anesthetic molecules. These primarily include ligand-gated ion channels, such as the gamma-aminobutyric acid type A (GABA$_A$), glycine, 5-HT$_3$ serotonin, nicotinic acetylcholine (ACh), and subtypes of glutamate receptors (NMDA, AMPA, and kainate) (*see* Chapters 12 and 14). GABA$_A$ and glutamate receptors are found throughout the brain, while ACh and serotonin receptors are associated with specific pathways of interconnecting nuclei. Identifying the location of these receptors in the central nervous system (CNS), the function of pathways that incorporate them, and the behavioral and physiological changes induced by their interaction with anesthetic molecules are some of the fundamental challenges to modern research.

Any discussion of loss of consciousness immediately begs the question: What is consciousness? Descriptions include the qualities of perception, attention, volition, self-awareness, and memory. Purposeful movement and response to auditory, tactile, or noxious stimulation classically have suggested consciousness, but the role of spinal cord reflexes complicates this idea. Consciousness has been dubbed a "prescientific" concept (Kulli and Koch, 1991), but it is enjoying a resurgence of attention from a range of investigators from philosophers to molecular biologists (Crick and Koch, 1998; Chalmers, 1996).

Neural Correlates of Consciousness. Two components of conscious awareness have been proposed: "arousal-access-vigilance" and "mental experience-selective attention" (Block, 1996). Crick and Koch (1995) postulate that some identifiable, active neuronal processes in the brain are associated with states of awareness. The quest is to determine what is special, if anything,

about their connections and manner of activation. Such circuitry would be called the "neural correlates of consciousness" (Crick and Koch, 1998), and work is in progress to establish the concept's validity using *in vivo* imaging, single neuronal types, and intracellular components. Several observations suggest that neural pathways mediated by ACh control both the content of conscious awareness and its level of intensity (Perry *et al.,* 1999). Mental disturbances seen with degenerative brain diseases include fluctuating levels of conscious awareness and are associated with deficits in neocortical ACh systems (Perry and Perry, 1995). The cholinergic system is distributed in various nuclei (Figure 13–1), including two major groups—the basal forebrain and pedunculopontine nuclei with extensive bidirectional connections to the cortex and thalamus. These are considered to be essential for controlling selective attention (Bentivoglio and Steriade, 1990). The extent of cholinergic projections from the nucleus basalis to the human cortex suggests a major role in regulatory modulation. Continuous firing during rapid-eye-movement (REM) sleep is sufficient to activate the cortex (Perry *et al.,* 1999). The phenomenon of brain stem activation of cortical processes (accepted as necessary for consciousness as defined in higher animals) has received attention, because the midbrain reticular formation (MRF) has neural projections from brainstem to thalamic nuclei to cortical structures, and the main neurotransmitters (ACh and glutamate) have been described (Steriade, 1996). Note that either ACh receptors or glutamate receptors or both are inhibited by a wide range of anesthetic agents including the volatile agents, barbiturates, and ketamine (Krasowski and Harrison, 1999).

In human beings engaging in tasks that require alertness and attention, there is increased blood flow in the MRF (Kinomura *et al.,* 1996). Stimulation of the MRF in anesthetized animals causes changes in the cortical EEG to resemble the awake state. Finally, Shimoji *et al.* (1984) have shown that the excitatory responses of MRF neurons, evoked by somatosensory stimulation in cats, are suppressed by anesthetic agents from several classes, while inhibitory responses of the MRF neurons are potentiated by barbiturates and ether.

It has been proposed that awareness uses a serial attention mechanism consisting of high-frequency (40-Hz), synchronized oscillations that transiently "bind together" widely distributed cortical neurons related to different aspects of a perceived object (color, size, motion, sound, *etc.*) (Crick and Koch, 1990; Steriade *et al.,* 1996). Direct application of ACh induces just such fast synchronized activity in hippocampal slice preparation (Fisahn *et al.,* 1998). Again, ACh receptors are inhibited by halogenated agents, barbiturates, and ketamine (Perry *et al.,* 1999). It has been suggested that the thalamus is the most likely source of this oscillatory activity because of its extensive bidirectional connections with higher and lower structures. It seems likely that the action of ACh in the cortex and thalamus is central to the normal maintenance of conscious awareness, as are interactions among ACh, GABA, and glutamate, all three of which control the cholinergic neurons in the basal forebrain and pedunculopontine projections.

Other pathway candidates for neural correlates of consciousness include noradrenergic projections from pontine locus ceruleus nuclei, which distribute axons cephalad to the dorsal thalamus, hypothalamus, cerebellum, forebrain, and neocortex. Not only does this system contain 50% of all noradrenergic cells in the brainstem, but changes in concentrations of norepinephrine alter anesthetic dose requirements (Angel, 1993). α_2-Adrenergic receptor agonists increase the depth of anesthesia, whereas α_2-receptor antagonists increase the amount of anesthesia required (Angel *et al.,* 1986). Obviously, these findings support a role for noradrenergic mechanisms contributing to consciousness.

Hemodynamic Effects. The physiological effects of anesthesia induction associated with the majority of both intravenous and inhalational agents include most prominently a decrease in systemic arterial blood pressure. The cause is either direct vasodilation or myocardial depression or both, a blunting of baroreceptor control, and a generalized decrease in central sympathetic tone (Sellgren *et al.,* 1990). Agents vary in the magnitude of their specific effects (*see* Chapter 14), but in all cases the hypotensive response is enhanced in the face of underlying volume depletion, intrinsic depressed myocardial function, and cardiovascular medications. Even anesthetics that show minimal hypotensive tendencies under normal conditions (etomidate, ketamine) must be used with caution in trauma victims, in whom intravascular volume depletion is being compensated by intense sympathetic discharge. Smaller than normal induction dosages are employed in patients presumed to be sensitive to hemodynamic effects of anesthetics (*e.g.,* elderly or debilitated patients, those with systolic and diastolic dysfunction, those taking diuretics or who have had recent dye studies or preparation for bowel surgery). Administration of direct- and indirect-acting sympathomimetics (*see* Chapter 10) will contribute to stability. Also, it is common to administer intravenous fluids liberally prior to and during induction to avoid hypotension. In some cases, fluid is relatively contraindi-

cated, requiring the use of inotropic agents and/or vasoconstrictors to support the circulation.

Airway Maintenance. Airway maintenance is essential following induction. Ventilation must be assisted or controlled for at least some period and perhaps throughout surgery. The gag reflex is lost, and the stimulus to cough is blunted. Lower esophageal sphincter tone is reduced. Both passive and active regurgitation may occur. Endotracheal intubation was introduced in the early 1900s (Kuhn, 1901) and was a major reason for a decline in the number of aspiration deaths.

Muscle relaxation is valuable during the induction of general anesthesia where it facilitates management of the airway including endotracheal intubation. Neuromuscular blocking agents are commonly used to effect such relaxation (*see* Chapter 9).

Endotracheal intubation both prevents aspiration and permits control of ventilation. While the procedure is used broadly, there also are alternative procedures. In patients who have had nothing to eat and are without symptoms of reflux, maintenance of ventilation (usually assisted-spontaneous) with an externally applied mask has been common for certain procedures not requiring muscle relaxation. It is important to note that the combination of direct laryngoscopy and intubation are stimuli fully comparable to an abdominal incision. Instrumentation of the subglottic airway stimulates secretions and exacerbates bronchospastic reactions as well, so when feasible, it might be desirable to avoid the procedure. An instrument called the laryngeal mask airway (Brain, 1983) has been progressively employed. This device consists of a flexible oval fenestrated diaphragm that is inserted blindly into the oropharynx. When seated, the diaphragm covers the laryngeal opening and can be sealed by inflation of a balloon around its circumference. Use of the laryngeal mask is becoming very popular; more than half of the anesthetics administered in Great Britain are thought to involve its use. There is controversy about its employment during controlled ventilation and in patients with symptoms of gastric reflux, since it does not provide complete airway protection.

Stabilizing the Anesthetic State. Following induction, continued management of the patient may be associated with fluctuations in blood pressure under the competing influences of anesthetic-induced depression and surgical stimulation. Part of the art and science of administering anesthetics is learning to manage the process smoothly, matching metabolic demands with appropriate oxygen supply while ensuring unconsciousness in preparation for the impending surgical stimulation, which will continue (not necessarily uniformly) throughout the case. Assessing the patient's level of consciousness, assuring adequate depth of anesthesia, and minimizing recall obviously are central to the goals of general anesthesia.

Signs and Stages of Anesthesia.   Between 1847 and 1858, John Snow described certain signs that helped him determine the depth of anesthesia in patients receiving chloroform or ether. In 1920, Guedel, using these and other signs, outlined four stages of general anesthesia, dividing the third stage—surgical anesthesia—into four planes. The somewhat arbitrary division is as follows: I, stage of analgesia; II, stage of delirium; III, stage of surgical anesthesia; IV, stage of medullary depression.

Although the classical signs and stages of anesthesia are partly recognizable during administration of volatile anesthetics, they are most often obscured by modern anesthetic techniques. Intravenous induction agents (thiopental, etomidate, propofol) produce a deep plane of anesthesia virtually within one circulation time, while certain properties of new inhalational agents—such as low blood solubility (desflurane) and minimal airway irritability (sevoflurane)—allow for such rapid establishment of anesthesia that the transition to unconsciousness is almost immediate. Furthermore, Cullen and coworkers (1972) demonstrated that no single one of the major signs described by Guedel correlated satisfactorily with the measured alveolar concentrations of anesthetic during prolonged, stable states. Thus, only the term *stage two* remains in common use today, signifying a state of delirium in the partially anesthetized patient most frequently seen during *emergence* from anesthesia where volatile inhalational agents have been used.

Maintenance.   The maintenance phase of general anesthesia is associated with changes in intensity of stimulation, fluid shifts (third spacing), blood loss, acid-base disturbances, hypothermia, coagulopathies, and other conditions. Of course, in many cases none of these things occurs, but special measurements, monitors, and precautions are necessary when they do—or in their anticipation. Management of the anesthetic interplays constantly with the general physiology of the patient. Historically, and continuing to the present, the great majority of cases involves the administration of one or more of the anesthetic gases during the maintenance phase. Special factors govern the transport of anesthetic molecules from inspired gas through the lungs to blood and then to the brain, including (1) concentration of the anesthetic agent in inspired gas, (2) pulmonary ventilation delivering the anesthetic to the lungs, (3) transfer of the gas from the alveoli to the

blood flowing through the lungs, and (4) loss of the agent from the arterial blood to all the tissues of the body. Obviously, the concentration in neural tissues is of greatest importance. The details of the uptake and distribution of anesthetic agents are covered in Chapter 14. With full cognizance of the factors related to the delivery of anesthetic gases to the brain, there remains the need to characterize and quantify the relative potencies of volatile anesthetic agents in a practical way.

The Minimum Alveolar Concentration (MAC).   Since 1965, the relative potencies of volatile anesthetic agents (halothane, enflurane, isoflurane, *etc.*) and N_2O and xenon have been described by the concentration (minimum alveolar concentration or MAC) that renders immobile 50% of subjects exposed to a strong noxious stimulation (1.0 MAC) (Eger *et al.*, 1965), such as surgical incision. Lack of movement in response to incision has been assumed to imply unconsciousness and amnesia in an unparalyzed patient.

A major strength of this concept stems from the facts that the concentration of anesthetic gases can be measured and displayed in each breath and that the end-tidal expired partial pressures approximate the brain concentration. The latter assumption fails during periods of rapid change. Also useful is the fact that doses of different agents expressed as MAC equivalents appear to be additive (Cullen *et al.*, 1969; Miller *et al.*, 1969).

In human beings exposed to modern inhalational agents, mild analgesia begins at about 0.3 MAC; amnesia is present at 0.5 MAC, where the patient can respond to command or even speak but does not recall this later (Levy, 1986). Obtundation deepens with 1.0 MAC where (by definition) 50% of patients remain immobile after stimulation. At higher doses (about 1.3 MAC), the sympathetically mediated response to surgery is blunted (Roizen *et al.*, 1981). Doses of inhalational agents higher than 2.0 MAC (equilibrated) are said to be potentially lethal, but in fact, such MAC multiples using balanced combinations of inhalational and intravenous agents are commonly achieved and sustained without untoward effect. Pharmacological support of the circulation may be required.

Obviously, a similar concept exists for intravenous anesthetics (barbiturates, propofol, etomidate) and adjuvants, but there is currently no on-line, real-time measurement of blood drug concentration for these compounds. The clinician must rely on body weight and age-adjusted dose guidelines to approximate the target blood levels, and then adjust the delivery rates according to various physiological responses, notably changes in blood pressure and heart rate.

Knowledge of the MAC fraction or multiple does not necessarily convey all of the necessary information. The anesthesiologist needs to assess both the level of responsiveness that exists at a point in time (with the level of stimulation existing at that moment) and the likelihood that the patient will react to an anticipated increase in the stimulation (such as laryngoscopy, incision, use of a retractor).

As surgery proceeds, continuous adjustments in the delivery rates of both inhalational and intravenous agents are required in an attempt to ensure unconsciousness, amnesia, immobility, and analgesia while simultaneously attending to the drifting physiological conditions.

Limitation of MAC. It is important to note that the concept of MAC leaves 50% of patients who actually move with stimulation and who thereby fail one measure of lack of awareness. While the dose-response curve is steep with 99% of subjects immobile at 1.3 MAC, the possibility of awareness and recall still may exist. Moreover, movement itself is of no use in the large number of patients who receive muscle relaxants. Other indicators of awareness that are independent of muscle relaxation include lacrimation, diaphoresis, and pupillary dilation. These signs are highly suggestive if they are present, but their absence is not definitive.

While the absence of movement does not ensure unconsciousness, neither does its presence necessarily imply consciousness. Elegant experiments with laboratory animals using EEG and MRF recordings that split the circulation between the brain and torso show that 1.0 MAC of isoflurane delivered to both circulations largely suppressed both EEG and MRF responses to noxious stimuli delivered to the torso. However, there were marked effects when the torso concentration was lowered to 0.3 MAC while the brain remained at 1.0 MAC (Antognini *et al.,* 2000). The animals moved with torso stimulation although the brain remained unconscious by EEG criteria. It has been appreciated for some time that spinal cord effects are important in general anesthesia (Kendig, 1993). Indeed, subarachnoid injection of local anesthetics lowers the dose of sedative required to achieve a hypnotic response (Ben-David *et al.,* 1995). These observations explain the long-noted clinical experience that a patient who moves with incision is not necessarily "awake" and one who does not move is not necessarily unconscious or amnesic. The experimental validation of this phenomenon clearly calls into question the applicability of MAC as classically defined and sets the stage for new efforts to better assess brain states during anesthesia.

Amnesia. Memory processes associated with anesthesia and surgery are complex (Bailey and Jones, 1997). Both explicit (free recall) memory and implicit (subconscious) phenomena are described. The latter may be identified by tests such as category generation, free association, and forced choice recognition.

Recent large studies have suggested that the incidence of explicit recall is 0.15% following general anesthesia (0.18% when using muscle relaxants, 0.10% without muscle relaxants) in patients undergoing surgery and anesthesia when interviewed three times following the case (Sandin *et al.,* 2000). Interestingly, the incidence of recall was unaffected by the use of preoperative benzodiazepines. Since many millions of anesthetic procedures are performed each year, thousands of people actually will experience intraoperative awareness. Further, it is well established (Schwender *et al.,* 1998) that delayed neurotic symptoms (posttraumatic stress disorder) can follow awareness during general anesthesia.

Monitoring Consciousness. The search for a monitor of level of consciousness or anesthetic depth obviously has centered on electroencephalography (and evoked potentials). Whereas the processed EEG power spectrum median frequency falls from about 10 Hz in the awake state to 5 Hz or less in both natural sleep and anesthesia in the absence of verbal stimuli, it does so only for some agents, and it can be altered further by hypoxia, hypocarbia, hypothermia, and other common conditions during surgery (Jessop and Jones, 1992). The volatile agents, as previously noted, elicit an excitement phase registered by the EEG as high frequency and high power transiently, as the subject passes through the planes of anesthetic depth. The EEG has been deemed unreliable as a measure of anesthetic dose or as a predictor of awareness or recall (Levy, 1986). Recent developments have changed that impression. Highly processed EEG signals have evolved from first order (signal amplitude mean and variance) to second order (power spectrum) and now to higher order statistics. The latter include the bispectrum and trispectrum (third- and fourth-order statistics, respectively) (Rampil, 1998). Special attention is focused on the bispectrum, which measures the correlation between phase and frequency components. Four derived subparameters have been defined and combined through weighting factors, determined empirically to produce a dimensionless number, called the bispectral index or BIS (Aspect Medical Systems, Inc., Natick, MA), which varies from 0 to 100. The proprietary algorithms, which give rise to the BIS value, have evolved by incorporating data from thousands of patients undergoing anesthesia with agents from different classes. A monitor receives signals from electrodes placed on the forehead and displays the BIS value continuously. Table 13–1 shows the experimentally derived correlation between absolute value and effect.

Figure 13–2 shows the hypnotic level (BIS) *versus* time in a volunteer receiving a propofol infusion demonstrating a direct relationship between blood level of the hypnotic drug and level of consciousness. This technology has become available at a time of growing international concerns regarding intraoperative awareness (Ghoneim, 2000). It must be emphasized that the ability of the device to assure lack of consciousness or recall has not been established, but recall below a reading of 60 apparently has not been reported.

Analgesia. Although inhalational anesthetic agents have an analgesic component in that the response to noxious impulses are blunted, this is mild at low doses and is only

Table 13–1

Relationship among Clinical State, Predominant Electroencephalogram (EEG) Pattern, and Corresponding Bispectral Index (BIS) Ranges Induced by Sedative/Hypnotic Agents

BIS LEVEL	CLINICAL STATE	MAIN EEG FEATURE
100	Awake	
80	Sedated	Synchronized high-frequency activity
60	Moderate hypnotic level (no recall)	Normalized low-frequency activity (proprietary bispectral feature)
40	Deep hypnotic level	High amount of EEG suppression
0		Isoelectric EEG

SOURCE: Modified from Rosow and Manberg, **1998,** with permission.

effective for surgery at higher concentrations (1.3 MAC or greater) where other side effects may be limiting. Most general anesthetics employ some dose of an opioid to provide analgesia.

Opioids. Opioids have been used for centuries for their analgesic properties. The identification of opioid receptors in the spinal cord (Kitahata *et al.,* 1974) and brainstem, and the manufacture of synthetic opioids of great potency (fentanyl, alfentanil, sufentanil) have transformed the practice of anesthesia over the past 30 years. The pharmacology of opioids is covered in Chapters 14 and 23.

Opioids are synergistic with sedative-hypnotic agents and inhalational agents, including nitrous oxide. The ability of opi-

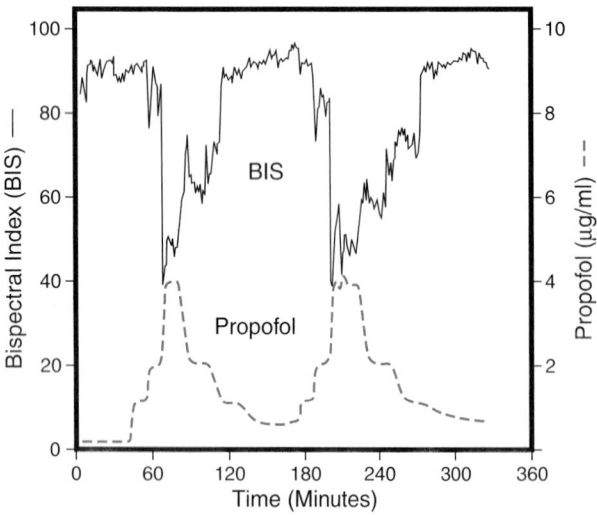

Figure 13–2. Hypnotic state and sedative concentration.

The figure shows a continuous read-out of hypnotic state assessed by bispectral index (BIS) monitoring as propofol blood level is varied. (From Rosow and Manberg, 1998, with permission.)

oids to block painful stimuli, accompanied by intrinsic hemodynamic stability, has led to so called "high-dose" techniques, notably for cardiac surgery (a maximal stimulus). In this approach, opioids are combined only with an amnesic agent such as midazolam (Curran, 1986), since the opioid doses that cause autonomic stability (and lack of movement) will not reliably cause loss of consciousness or amnesia (Ausems *et al.,* 1983). More common is the use of lower doses of opioids administered continuously or intermittently during surgery in conjunction with a volatile general anesthetic, the latter given in fractions of MAC (0.5 to 0.8), and nitrous oxide, where not contraindicated. This combination, called "balanced anesthesia" by some, permits sustaining unconsciousness (presumably) with the volatile anesthetic while supplying analgesia with opiates for the duration of surgery and into the postoperative period. Return to responsiveness at surgery's end can be prompt.

The introduction of remifentanil, an ester opioid metabolized by plasma esterases, has created a new dimension for intensity of analgesia during surgery and for rapid awakening during recovery. This agent is not only intrinsically very potent, but it has a very short half-life, allowing for higher infusion rates during the intense periods of stimulation (Bürkle *et al.,* 1996). ***Contribution of Analgesia to the Hypnotic State.*** To separate the influences of analgesia and hypnosis on anesthetic requirements in conditions of variable stimulation, we consider a study of patients who received an infusion of the hypnotic propofol in a dose predicted to induce marked loss of consciousness (blood level 4 µg/ml) (Guignard *et al.,* 2000). Following equilibration and determination of hypnotic state (by BIS monitoring), the opioid remifentanil was administered in five graded doses to achieve blood levels of 0 (placebo), 2, 4, 8, and 16 ng/ml. At steady state, an intense noxious stimulus (laryngoscopy) was applied. Figure 13–3 shows the level of consciousness at each step in aggregate. Note that (1) propofol alone produced a level of deep hypnosis (BIS = 50); (2) the addition of the opioid did not deepen the hypnotic state; (3) the effect of the stimulus on arousal varied with opioid blood level, with the lowest level (0) leading to a marked rise in the BIS value, while the highest opioid concentration completely removed the tendency to arousal, leaving the hypnotic state unchanged.

The methodology in this study illustrates an alternative technique for managing general anesthesia with only intravenous

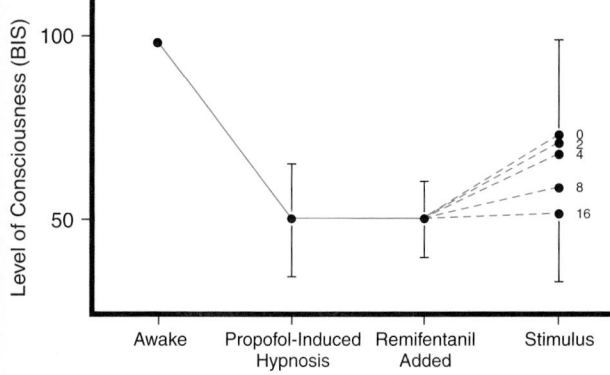

Figure 13–3. Level of consciousness [assessed by bispectral index (BIS) monitoring] following sedation, analgesia, and stimulation.

The numerals on the right side of the figure represent the blood levels of remifentanil (ng/ml) after four different doses or placebo (0). The stimulus was laryngoscopy. *See* text for details. (Adapted from Guignard *et al.,* 2000, with permission.)

agents. Called TIVA, for *total intravenous anesthesia*, it frequently incorporates an amnesic drug such as midazolam to ensure lack of recall (Newman and Reves, 1993) and a muscle relaxant in addition to analgesic and hypnotic agents. The ability to assess levels of consciousness objectively enhances the appeal of TIVA. The technique may increase in popularity, especially if the cost of the newer, shorter-acting agents can be justified.

Muscle Relaxation.   The fourth quality of general anesthesia is muscle relaxation. This, at least, implies that patients should not move with incision—an achievable goal with sufficient doses of inhalational anesthetics, intravenous anesthetics, opioids, or some combination. However, following the need for brief muscle paralysis to achieve intubation, more prolonged relaxation is required for some orthopedic, general abdominal, and otolaryngology surgeries. Muscle relaxants are further discussed in Chapters 9 and 14. Their usual, ready reversal by cholinesterase inhibitors (*e.g.,* neostigmine; *see* Chapter 8), along with development of drugs with a wide range of half-lives, has made use of muscle-relaxant drugs widespread in surgery.

Emergence.   As surgical stimulation begins to lessen during wound closure, delivered doses of anesthetic agents will be reduced in a manner that reflects their specific pharmacokinetics. Both inhaled and intravenous drugs can exhibit delayed dissipation caused by either slow washout (from poorly perfused fat-rich tissue) or by the character

of their distribution and metabolism. The major factors that affect rate of elimination of inhaled anesthetics are the same as those that are important in the uptake phase: pulmonary ventilation, blood flow, and solubility in blood and tissue. Because of the high blood flow to brain, the tension of anesthetic gas in the brain decreases rapidly, accounting for the rapid awakening from anesthesia noted with relatively insoluble agents such as nitrous oxide (*see* Chapter 14).

The physiological changes accompanying emergence from general anesthesia can be profound. Hypertension and tachycardia are common as the sympathetic nervous system regains its tone and is enhanced by pain (Breslow, 1998). Myocardial ischemia can appear or markedly worsen during emergence in patients with coronary artery disease. Emergence excitement occurs in 5% to 30% of patients and is characterized by tachycardia, restlessness, crying, moaning and thrashing, and various neurological signs (Eckenhoff *et al.,* 1961). Postanesthesia shivering occurs frequently because of core hypothermia, which was common before modern realization of its negative effects. A small dose of meperidine (12.5 mg) lowers the shivering trigger temperature and effectively stops the activity. The incidence of all of these emergence phenomena is greatly reduced when opioids are employed as part of the intraoperative regimen.

Hypothermia.   Patients develop hypothermia (body temperature <36°C) during surgery for several reasons, including low ambient temperature (and exposed body cavities), cold intravenous fluids, altered thermoregulatory control, and reduced metabolic rate. General anesthetics lower the core temperature set point, at which thermoregulatory vasoconstriction is activated to defend against heat loss. Further, vasodilation caused by both general and regional anesthesia blocks the normal thermal constriction, thereby redistributing heat in the body mass and leading to a rapid decline in core temperature until the new (lower) set point is reached (Sessler, 2000). Total body oxygen consumption decreases with general anesthesia by about 30%, and thus heat generation is reduced.

Even small drops in body temperatures may lead to an increase in perioperative morbidity, including cardiac complications (Frank *et al.,* 1997), wound infections (Kurz *et al.,* 1996), and blood loss. Prevention of hypothermia has emerged as a major goal of anesthetic care. Modalities to maintain normothermia include using warm intravenous fluids, heat exchangers in the anesthesia circuit, forced-warm-air covers, and new technology involving water-filled garments with microprocessor feedback control to a core temperature set point.

Regional (Local) Anesthesia

Local anesthetics include esters (*e.g.,* cocaine, procaine, tetracaine) and amides (*e.g.,* lidocaine, bupivicaine, ropivicaine) that are injected in the vicinity of nerves to cause temporary, virtually complete interruption of neural traffic (*see* Chapter 15), enabling surgery to proceed in comfort. Upper limb procedures may be facilitated by plexus blockade, while surgery on the thorax, abdomen, and lower extremities may be accomplished by neuraxial blockade (epidural and spinal), either in conjunction with general anesthesia or as the sole modality employed.

Spinal anesthesia, first performed in 1889 (*see* Wulf, 1998) is effected by injection of local anesthetic agents into the lumbar (L3–4, L4–5) subarachnoid cerebrospinal fluid. Since the spinal cord rarely extends below L2, the injection needle harmlessly pushes aside the strands of the cauda equina. Depending on the volume of injectate (usually 1 to 3 ml), specific gravity (may be either hyper-, hypo-, or isobaric, varying with the diluent), manner of injection, and the position of the patient, spinal blockade may extend from T2 down through the sacral roots.

Epidural anesthesia proceeds with injection of a volume (10 to 25 ml) of local anesthetic solution into the epidural "potential" space. Because dural puncture is not intended, the site of entry may be at any vertebral level permitting a band of "segmental" blockade approximately limited to the region of interest. Spinal and epidural anesthesia share many similarities and will be discussed together as "neuraxial" techniques with specific differences highlighted.

The sympathetic nervous system is mediated through spinal segments T1–L2, and neuraxial blockade will most commonly involve several of these. The drop in blood pressure that ensues is anticipated and compensated for, as necessary, with fluid administration and vasopressor agents. In volume-depleted patients, aggressive prophylactic measures are taken. Arterial and venous dilation cause most of the pressure drop, but cardiac sympathetic nerves emerge from T1–T4 and also may be blocked. This blockade of sympathetic nerves going to the heart is used to advantage in the treatment of myocardial ischemia refractory to conventional medical therapy by administering a thoracic epidural injection of a local anesthetic agent (Blomberg *et al.*, 1989). Further, the decrease in afterload seen with all levels of neuraxial blockade can improve cardiac output in patients with congestive heart failure.

To achieve neuraxial blockade over a prolonged period (more than 3 hours), a catheter is placed in either the subarachnoid or epidural space for either bolus injection or continuous infusion. This allows continuance of neural blockade into the postoperative period.

As previously noted, regional anesthesia may have special advantages over general anesthesia, including attenuation of the surgical stress response. Intense block-ade using regional anesthesia can hold intraoperative catecholamines to presurgical values (Breslow *et al.*, 1993). There is evidence that successful blockade of components of the stress response can result in improved outcome. Hypercoagulability, seen postoperatively in patients having lower extremity vascular surgery under general anesthesia, is eliminated when stress ablation is achieved. Unfortunately, stimuli from upper abdominal and thoracic surgery are difficult to block completely with regional techniques. In these cases, direct suppression of sympathetic nervous system by α_2-adrenergic receptor agonists or end-organ blockade (β-adrenergic receptor antagonists) may be required. Other benefits include shorter periods of ileus (Liu *et al.*, 1995).

The discovery of opioid receptors in the dorsal column of the spinal cord suggested the addition of a neuraxial opioid to induce analgesia. This practice is now common, and the combination of opioids and local anesthetic agents is used to advantage, especially in the management of postoperative pain.

Unattenuated surgical stimuli cause sensitization of excitable spinal neurons, a phenomenon called neuroplasticity (King *et al.*, 1988) or "wind-up." This condition produces long-lasting depolarization of posterior horn neurons and heightens the perception of pain. Wind-up can be prevented by intense blockade *prior to the stimulus* (preemptive analgesia) as with epidural or spinal anesthesia, or by adequately performed local infiltration of the proposed incision site.

Complications of regional anesthesia include "high" spinal blockade, hypotension, headache, cardiac and vascular toxicity, neuropathies, and epidural hematoma.

POSTOPERATIVE PERIOD

The postoperative period can be a turbulent experience for patients and health-care providers. In addition to the emergence phenomena listed above, other problems arise involving the airway, lungs, and cardiovascular system.

Airway obstruction may occur because residual anesthesia effects continue partially to obtund consciousness and reflexes (especially seen among patients who normally snore or who have sleep apnea). Strong inspiratory efforts against a closed glottis can lead to negative-pressure pulmonary edema. Pulmonary functional residual capacity is reduced postoperatively following all types of anesthesia and surgery, and hypoxemia may occur. Hypertension can be prodigious and must be treated with α_1-adrenergic receptor antagonists, β-adrenergic receptor antagonists, α_2-adrenergic receptor antagonists, angiotensin converting enzyme inhibitors, calcium channel antagonists, or other intravenous antihypertensive agents.

Pain control can be complicated in the immediate postoperative period, especially if opioids have not been part of a balanced anesthetic. Administration of opioids in the recovery room can be problematic among patients who still have a substantial residual anesthetic effect. Patients can alternate between screaming in apparent agony and being deeply somnolent with airway obstruction, all in a matter of moments. The nonsteroidal antiinflammatory agent ketorolac (30 to 60 mg intravenously) frequently is effective, and the development of cyclooxygenase-2 inhibitors (*see* Chapter 27) holds promise for analgesia without respiratory depression.

Regional anesthetic techniques are an important part of a perioperative "multimodal" approach that employs local anesthetic wound infiltration, epidural, spinal, and plexus blocks, nonsteroidal antiinflammatory drugs, opioids, α_2-adrenergic receptor agonists, and NMDA-receptor antagonists (which prevent neuroplasticity) (Kehlet, 1997).

Patient-controlled administration of intravenous and epidural analgesics makes use of small computerized pumps activated on demand but programmed with safety limits to prevent overdose. The agents used are opioids (frequently morphine) by the intravenous route and opioid, local anesthetic, or both, by the epidural route. These techniques have revolutionized postoperative pain management, which can be continued for hours or days, promoting ambulation and improved bowel function while oral medications are stabilized.

Nausea and Vomiting.   Nausea and vomiting in the postoperative period continue to be a significant problem following general anesthesia and are caused by an action of anesthetics on the chemoreceptor trigger zone and the brainstem vomiting center, which are modulated by serotonin, histamine, ACh muscarinic, and dopamine receptors. The 5-HT$_3$ serotonin receptor antagonist ondansetron (*see* Chapter 38) is very effective in suppressing nausea and vomiting. Common treatment also includes droperidol, metaclopromide, dexamethasone, and avoidance of N$_2$O. The use of propofol as an induction agent and the nonsteroidal antiinflammatory drug ketorolac as a substitute for opioids may decrease the incidence and severity of postoperative nausea and vomiting.

PROSPECTUS

A major goal, and promise, of current research in anesthesia is to elucidate the molecular mechanisms of action of general anesthetics, with the intent to increase efficacy and minimize complications. Historical theories of anesthetic action (Meyer, 1899, 1901; Overton, 1901) were based on the physicochemical characteristics of anesthetic drugs and related to the correlation between the potency of an anesthetic agent and the solubility of the drug in oil, implicating changes in the lipid bilayer as the mechanism of anesthetic action. Current work implicates proteins (or the protein-lipid interface) as the site of action, although still with the premise that anesthetics act in hydrophobic domains. While they are not completely characterized at the molecular level, much is known about mechanisms of action of general anesthetics. The effect of clinically relevant concentrations of anesthetics on both voltage-gated and ligand-gated ion channels has fostered significant research using recombinant chimeric and mutated receptors to identify the sites for allosteric modulation of ligand-gated ion channels (Franks and Lieb, 1994) and thus aid the development of target-specific anesthetic agents (*see* Chapter 18 for discussion of actions of ethanol on ligand-gated channels). The growing knowledge about both receptor-specific anesthetic action and the neural pathways that correlate with consciousness suggests a future for drug design that will increase the desirable characteristics and decrease the behavioral and other unwanted responses of anesthetic action.

BIBLIOGRAPHY

Angel, A., Goldman, P., Halsey, M.J., Kendig, J., and Kajeed, A.B.A. A possible anaesthetic action of clonidine. In Proceedings of the Physiological Society. *J. Physiol.,* **1986,** *378*:10P.

Antognini, J.F., Wang, X.W., and Carstens, E. Isoflurane action in the spinal cord blunts electroencephalographic and thalamic-reticular formation responses to noxious stimulation in goats. *Anesthesiology,* **2000,** *92*:559–566.

Ausems, M.E., Hug, C.C., Jr., and de Lange, S. Variable rate infusion of alfentanil as a supplement to nitrous oxide anesthesia for general surgery. *Anesth. Analg.,* **1983,** *62*:982–986.

Balser, J.R., Martinez, E.A., Winters, B.D., Purdue, P.W., Clarke, A.W., Huang, W., Tomaselli, G.F., Dorman, T., Campbell, K., Lipsett, P., Breslow, M.J., and Rosenfeld, B.A. Beta-adrenergic blockade accelerates conversion of postoperative supraventricular tachyarrhythmias. *Anesthesiology,* **1998,** *89*:1052–1059.

Ben-David, B., Vaida, S., and Gaitini, L. The influence of high spinal anesthesia on sensitivity to midazolam sedation. *Anesth. Analg.,* **1995,** *81*:525–528.

Berlauk, J.F., Abrams, J.H., Gilmour, I.J., O'Connor, S.R., Knighton, D.R., and Cerra, F.B. Preoperative optimization of cardiovascular hemodynamics improves outcome in peripheral vascular surgery. A prospective, randomized clinical trial. *Ann Surg,* **1991,** *214:*289–297.

Block, N. How can we find the neural correlate of consciousness? *Trends Neurosci.,* **1996,** *19:*456–459.

Blomberg, S., Curelaru, I., Emanuelsson, H., Herlitz, J., Ponten, J., and Ricksten, S.E. Thoracic epidural anaesthesia in patients with unstable angina pectoris. *Eur. Heart J.,* **1989,** *10:*437–444.

Brain, A.I. The laryngeal mask–a new concept in airway management. *Br. J. Anaesth.,* **1983,** *55:*801–805.

Breslow, M.J., Parker, S.D., Frank, S.M., Norris, E.J., Yates, H., Raff, H., Rock, P., Christopherson, R., Rosenfeld, B.A., and Beattie, C. Determinants of catecholamine and cortisol responses to lower extremity revascularization. The PIRAT Study Group. *Anesthesiology,* **1993,** *79:*1202–1209.

Bürkle, H., Dunbar, S., and Van Aken, H. Remifentanil: a novel, short-acting, μ-opioid. *Anesth. Analg.,* **1996,** *83:*646–651.

Codman, E.A. *A Study in Hospital Efficiency.* Thomas Todd Co., Boston, **1917.**

Cullen, D.J., Eger, E.I. II, Stevens, W.C., Smith, N.T., Cromwell, T.H., Cullen, B.F., Gregory, G.A., Bahlman, S.H., Dolan, W.M., Stoelting, R.K., and Fourcade, H.E. Clinical signs of anesthesia. *Anesthesiology,* **1972,** *36:*21–36.

Cullen, S.C., Eger, E.I. II, Cullen, B.F., and Gregory, P. Observations on the anesthetic effect of the combination of xenon and halothane. *Anesthesiology,* **1969,** *31:*305–309.

Eagle, K.A., Brundage, B.H., Chaitman, B.R., Ewy, G.A., Fleisher, L.A., Hertzer, N.R., Leppo, J.A., Ryan, T., Schlant, R.C., Spencer, W.H. III, Spittell, J.A., Jr., Twiss, R.D., Ritchie, J.L., Cheitlin, M.D., Gardner, T.J., Garson, A., Jr., Lewis, R.P., Gibbons, R.J., O'Rourke, R.A., and Ryan, T.J. Guidelines for perioperative cardiovascular evaluation for noncardiac surgery. Report of the American College of Cardiology/American Heart Association Task Force on Practice Guidelines (Committee on Perioperative Cardiovascular Evaluation for Noncardiac Surgery). *J. Am. Coll. Cardiol.,* **1996,** *27:*910–948.

Eckenhoff, J.E., Kneale, D.H., and Dripps, R.D. The incidence and etiology of postanesthetic excitement. A clinical survey. *Anesthesiology,* **1961,** *22:*667–673.

Eger, E.I., Saidman, L.J., and Brandstater, B. Minimum alveolar anesthetic concentration, a standard of anesthetic potency. *Anesthesiology,* **1965,** *26:*756–763.

Fisahn, A., Pike, F.G., Buhl, E.H., and Paulsen, O. Cholinergic induction of network oscillations at 40 Hz in the hippocampus in vitro. *Nature,* **1998,** *394:*186–189.

Frank, S.M., Fleisher, L.A., Breslow, M.J., Higgins, M.S., Olson, K.F., Kelly, S., and Beattie, C. Perioperative maintenance of normothermia reduces the incidence of morbid cardiac events. A randomized clinical trial. *JAMA,* **1997,** *277:*1127–1134.

Franks, N.P., and Lieb, W.R. Molecular and cellular mechanisms of general anesthesia. *Nature,* **1994,** *367:*607–614.

Ghoneim, M.M. Awareness during anesthesia. *Anesthesiology,* **2000,** *92:*597–602.

Goldman, L., Caldera, D.L., Nussbaum, S., Southwick, F.S., Krogstad, D., Murray, B., Burke, D.S., O'Malley, T.A., Goroll, A.H., Caplan, C.H., Nolan, J., Carabello, B., and Slater, E.E. Multifactorial index of cardiac risk in noncardiac surgical procedures. *N. Engl. J. Med.,* **1977,** *297:*845–850.

Greene, N.M. A consideration of factors in the discovery of anesthesia and their effects on its development. *Anesthesiology,* **1971,** *35:*515–522.

Guignard, B., Menigaux, C., Dupont, X., Fletcher, D., and Chauvin, M. The effect of remifentanil on the bispectral index change and

hemodynamic responses after orotracheal intubation. *Anesth. Analg.,* **2000,** *90:*161–167.

Jessop, J., and Jones, J.G. Evaluation of the actions of general anaesthetics in the human brain. *Gen. Pharmacol.,* **1992,** *23:*927–935.

Kehlet, H. Multimodal approach to control postoperative pathophysiology and rehabilitation. *Br. J. Anaesth.,* **1997,** *78:*606–617.

Kendig, J.J. Spinal cord as a site of anesthetic action. *Anesthesiology,* **1993,** *79:*1161–1162.

King, A.E., Thompson, S.W., Urban, L., and Woolf, C.J. The responses recorded in vitro of deep dorsal horn neurons to direct and orthodromic stimulation in the young rat spinal cord. *Neuroscience,* **1988,** *27:*231–242.

Kinomura, S., Larsson, J., Gulyas, B., and Roland, P.E. Activation by attention of the human reticular formation and thalamic intralaminar nuclei. *Science,* **1996,** *271:*512.

Kitahata, L.M., Kosaka, Y., Taub, A., Bonikos, K., and Hoffert, M. Lamina-specific suppression of dorsal-horn unit activity by morphine sulfate. *Anesthesiology,* **1974,** *41:*39–48.

Krasowski, M.D., and Harrison, N.L. General anaesthetic actions on ligand-gated ion channels. *Cell Mol. Life Sci.,* **1999,** *55:*1278–1303.

Kuhn, F. Die perorale Intubation (Orotracheal intubation). *Centralblatt Chir,* **1901,** *28:*1281–1285.

Kulli, J., and Koch, C. Does anesthesia cause loss of consciousness? *Trends Neurosci.,* **1991,** *14:*6–10.

Kurz, A., Sessler, D.I., and Lenhardt, R. Perioperative normothemia to reduce the incidence of surgical-wound infection and shorten hospitalization. Study of Wound Infection and Temperature Group. *N. Engl. J. Med.,* **1996,** *334:*1209–1215.

Levy, W.J. Power spectrum correlates of changes in consciousness during anesthetic induction with enflurane. *Anesthesiology,* **1986,** *64:*688–693.

Mangano, D.T., Layug, E.L., Wallace, A., and Tateo, I. Effect of atenolol on mortality and cardiovascular morbidity after noncardiac surgery. Multicenter Study of Perioperative Ischemia Research Group. *N. Engl. J. Med.,* **1996,** *335:*1713–1720.

Meyer, H.H. Zur Theorie de Alkoholnarkose. I. Mitt. Welche Eigenschaft der Anästhetika bedingt ihre narkotische Wirkung? *Arch. Exp. Pathol. Pharmakol.,* **1899,** *42:*109.

Meyer, H.H. Zur Theorie der Alkolnarkose. III. Mitt. Der Einfuss wechselnder Temperatur auf Wirkungsstärke und Teilungskoeffizient der Narkotika. *Arch. Exp. Pathol. Pharmakol.,* **1901,** *46:*338.

Miller, R.D., Wahrenbrock, E.A., Schroeder, C.F., Knipstein, T.W., Eger, E.I. II, and Buechel, D.R. Ethylene-halothane anesthesia: addition or synergism? *Anesthesiology,* **1969,** *31:*301–304.

Newman, M., and Reves, J.G. Pro: midazolam is the sedative of choice to supplement narcotic anesthesia. *J. Cardiothorac. Vasc. Anesth.,* **1993,** *7:*615–619.

Overton, C.E. *Studien über die Narkose: Zugleich ein Beitrag zur allgemeinen Pharmakologie.* G. Fischer, Jena, **1901.**

Palda, V.A., and Detsky, A.S. Guidelines for assessing and managing the perioperative risk from coronary artery disease associated with major noncardiac surgery. *Ann. Intern. Med.,* **1997,** *127:*309.

Perry, E.K., and Perry, R.H. Acetylcholine and hallucinations: disease-related compared to drug-induced alterations in human consciousness. *Brain Cogn.,* **1995,** *28:*240–258.

Pierce, E.C. Jr. Anesthesia: standards of care and liability. *JAMA,* **1989,** *262:*773.

Poldermans, D., Boersma, E., Bax, J.J., Thomson, I.R., van de Ven, L.L., Blankensteijn, J.D., Baars, H.F., Yo, T.I., Trocino, G., Vigna, C., Roelandt, J.R., and van Urk, H. The effect of bisoprolol on perioperative mortality and myocardial infarction in high-risk patients undergoing vascular surgery. Dutch Echocardiographic Cardiac Risk Evaluation Applying Stress Echocardiography Study Group. *N. Engl. J. Med.,* **1999,** *341*:1789–1794.

Roizen, M.F., Horrigan, R.W., and Frazer, B.M. Anesthetic doses blocking adrenergic (stress) and cardiovascular responses to incision—MAC BAR. *Anesthesiology,* **1981,** *54*:390–398.

Rosow, C., and Manberg, P.J. Bispectral index monitoring. *Anesthesiol. Clin. North Am.: Annu. Anesth. Pharmacol.,* **1998,** *2*:89–107.

Sandin, R.H., Enlund, G., Samuelsson, P., and Lennmarken, C. Awareness during anaesthesia: a prospective case study. *Lancet,* **2000,** *355*:707–711.

Schwender, D., Kunze-Kronawitter, H., Dietrich, P., Klasing, S., Forst, H., and Madler, C. Conscious awareness during general anesthesia: patients' perceptions, emotions, cognition and reactions. *Br. J. Anaesth.,* **1998,** *80*:133–139.

Sellgren, J., Ponten, J., and Wallin, G. Percutaneous recording of muscle nerve sympathetic activity during propofol, nitrous oxide, and isoflurane anesthesia in humans. *Anesthesiology,* **1990,** *73*:20–27.

Shimoji, K., Fujioka, H., Fukazawa, T., Hashiba, M., and Maruyama, Y. Anesthetics and excitatory/inhibitory responses of midbrain reticular neurons. *Anesthesiology,* **1984,** *61*:151–155.

Steriade, M. Arousal: revisiting the reticular activating system. *Science,* **1996,** *272*:225–226.

Steriade, M., Amzica, F., and Contreras, D. Synchronization of fast (30–40 Hz) spontaneous cortical rhythms during brain activation. *J. Neurosci.,* **1996,** *16*:392–417.

MONOGRAPHS AND REVIEWS

Angel, A. Central neuronal pathways and the process of anaesthesia. *Br. J. Anaesth.,* **1993,** *71*:148–163.

Bailey, A.R., and Jones, J.G. Patients' memories of events during general anaesthesia. *Anaesthesia,* **1997,** *52*:460–476.

Bentivoglio, M., and Steriade, M. *The Diencephalon and Sleep.* (Mancia, M., Marini, G., eds.) Raven Press, New York, **1990,** pp. 7–29.

Breslow, M.J. Clinical implications of the stress response to surgery. In, *Principles and Practice of Anesthesiology,* 2nd ed. (Longnecker,

D.E., Tinker, J.H., and Morgan, G.E., Jr., eds.) Mosby, St. Louis, **1998,** pp. 117–129.

Chalmers, D.J. *The Conscious Mind: In Search of a Fundamental Theory.* Oxford University Press, New York, **1996.**

Crick, F., and Koch, C. *Semin. Neurosci.,* **1990,** 2:263–275.

Crick, F., and Koch, C. Why neuroscience may be able to explain consciousness. *Sci. Am.,* **1995,** *273*:84–85, as found in: Chalmers, D.J. The puzzle of conscious experience. *Sci. Am.,* **1995,** *273*:80–86.

Crick F., and Koch C. Consciousness and neuroscience. *Cereb. Cortex,* **1998,** *8*:97–107.

Curran, H.V. Tranquillising memories: a review of the effects of benzodiazepines on human memory. *Biol. Psychol.,* **1986,** *23*:179–213.

Faulconer, A. Jr., and Keys, T.E., eds. *Foundations of Anesthesiology.* Charles C. Thomas, Springfield, IL, **1965.**

Greene, N.M. Anesthesia and the development of surgery (1846–1896). *Anesth. Analg.,* **1979,** *58*:5–12.

Liu, S., Carpenter, R.L., and Neal, J.M. Epidural anesthesia and analgesia. Their role in postoperative outcome. *Anesthesiology,* **1995,** *82*:1474–1506.

Perry, E., Walker, M., Grace, J., and Perry, R. Acetylcholine in mind: a neurotransmitter correlate of consciousness? *Trends Neurosci.,* **1999,** *22*:273–280.

Rampil, I.J. A primer for EEG signal processing in anesthesia. *Anesthesiology,* **1998,** *89*:980–1002.

Sessler, D.I. Perioperative heat balance. *Anesthesiology,* **2000,** *92*:578–596.

Sweitzer, B.J. *Handbook of Preoperative Assessment and Management.* Lippincott Williams & Wilkins, Philadelphia, **2000.**

Sykes, W.S. *Essays on the First Hundred Years of Anaesthesia.* E. & S. Livingstone, Edinburgh, **1960.**

Udelsman, R., and Holbrook, N.J. Endocrine and molecular responses to surgical stress. In, *Current Problems in Surgery.* Vol. 31, no. 8. Mosby, St. Louis, **1994,** pp. 653–720.

Wiklund, R.A., and Rosenbaum, S.H. Medical progress review article in two parts. *N. Engl. J. Med.,* **1997,** *337*:1132–1141 (part I) and *337*:1215–1219 (part II).

Wulf, H.F. The centennial of spinal anesthesia. *Anesthesiology,* **1998,** *89*:500–506.

Acknowledgment

The author wishes to acknowledge Sean K. Kennedy and David E. Longnecker, the authors of this chapter in the ninth edition of *Goodman and Gilman's The Pharmacological Basis of Therapeutics,* some of whose text has been retained in this edition.

GENERAL ANESTHETICS

Alex S. Evers and C. Michael Crowder

General anesthetics are a class of drugs used to depress the central nervous system to a sufficient degree to permit the performance of surgery and other noxious or unpleasant procedures. Not surprisingly, general anesthetics have very low therapeutic indices and thus are dangerous drugs that require great care in administration. Indeed, an entire specialty of medicine has grown around the administration of this class of drugs. General anesthetics can be administered by a variety of routes, but intravenous or inhalational administration is preferred because effective doses can be more accurately administered and the time course of action more carefully controlled. While all general anesthetics produce a relatively similar anesthetic state, the drugs are quite dissimilar in their secondary actions (side effects) on other organ systems. The selection of specific drugs and routes of administration to produce general anesthesia is based on their pharmacokinetic properties and on the secondary effects of the various drugs, in the context of the individual patient's age, pathophysiology, and medication use. This chapter will review basic aspects of anesthetic action and then will focus on the specific properties of inhalational and intravenous anesthetics as well as on practical aspects of their use.

INTRODUCTION

Definition of Anesthetic State

General anesthetics are a structurally diverse class of drugs that produce a common end point—a behavioral state referred to as *general anesthesia*. In the broadest sense, general anesthesia can be defined as a global but reversible depression of central nervous system (CNS) function resulting in the loss of response to and perception of all external stimuli. While this definition is appealing in its simplicity, it is not useful for two reasons: First, it is inadequate because anesthesia is not simply a deafferented state; for example, amnesia is an important aspect of the anesthetic state. Second, not all general anesthetics produce identical patterns of deafferentation. Barbiturates, for example, are very effective at producing amnesia and loss of consciousness but are not effective as analgesics.

An alternative way of defining the anesthetic state is to consider it as a collection of "component" changes in behavior or perception. The components of the anesthetic state include *amnesia, immobility* in response to noxious stimulation, *attenuation of autonomic responses* to noxious stimulation, *analgesia,* and *unconsciousness.* It is important to remember that general anesthesia is useful only insofar as it facilitates the performance of surgery or other noxious procedures. The performance of surgery requires an immobilized patient who does not have an excessive autonomic response to surgery (blood pressure, heart rate) and who has amnesia for the procedure. Thus the essential components of the anesthetic state are immobilization, amnesia, and attenuation of autonomic responses to noxious stimulation. Indeed, if an anesthetic produces profound amnesia, it can be difficult, in principle, to determine if it also produces either analgesia or unconsciousness.

Measurement of Anesthetic Potency

Given the essential requirement that a general anesthetic agent provide an immobilized patient who does not move in response to surgical stimulation, the potency of general anesthetic agents usually is measured by determining the concentration of general anesthetic that prevents movement in response to surgical stimulation. As described in Chapter 13, anesthetic potency is measured in MAC units, with 1 MAC defined as the *minimum alveolar concentration* that prevents movement in response to surgical stimulation in 50% of subjects. The strengths of MAC as a measurement are that (1) it can be monitored continuously by measuring end-tidal anesthetic concentration using infrared spectroscopy or mass spectrometry; (2) it provides a direct correlate of the free concentration of the anesthetic at its site(s) of action in the central nervous system; (3) it is a simple-to-measure endpoint that reflects an important clinical goal. End points other than immobilization also can be used to measure anesthetic potency. For example, the ability to respond to verbal commands (MAC$_{awake}$) (Stoelting *et al.*, 1970) and the ability to form memories (Dwyer *et al.*, 1992) also have been correlated with alveolar anesthetic concentration. Interestingly, verbal response and memory formation are both suppressed at a fraction of MAC. Furthermore, the ratio of the anesthetic concentrations required to produce amnesia and immobility vary significantly among different inhalational anesthetic agents (nitrous oxide *vs.* isoflurane, Table 14–1), suggesting that anesthetic agents may produce these behavioral end points *via* different cellular and molecular mechanisms. The potency of intravenous anesthetic agents is somewhat more difficult to measure, because there is not an available method to measure blood or plasma anesthetic concentration continuously and because the free concentration of the drug at its site of action cannot be determined. Generally, the potency of intravenous agents is defined as the free plasma concentration (at equilibrium) that produces loss of response to surgical incision (or other end points) in 50% of subjects (Franks and Lieb, 1994).

Mechanisms of Anesthesia

The molecular mechanisms by which general anesthetics produce their effects have remained one of the great mysteries of pharmacology. For most of the twentieth century, it was theorized that all anesthetics act by a common mechanism (*the unitary theory of anesthesia*) and that anesthesia is produced by perturbation of the physical properties of cell membranes. This thinking was based largely on observations made in the late nineteenth century that the potency of a gas as an anesthetic correlated with its solubility in olive oil. This correlation, referred to as the Meyer-Overton rule, was interpreted as indicating the lipid bilayer as the likely target of anesthetic action. In the past decade, clear exceptions to the Meyer-Overton rule have been noted (Koblin *et al.*, 1994). For example, it has been shown that inhalational and intravenous anesthetics can be enantioselective in their action as anesthetics (etomidate, steroids, isoflurane) (Tomlin *et al.*, 1998; Lysko *et al.*, 1994; Wittmer *et al.*, 1996). The fact that enantiomers have unique actions but identical physical properties indicates that properties other than bulk solubility are important in determining anesthetic action. This realization has focused thinking on identification of specific protein binding sites for anesthetics.

One impediment to understanding the mechanisms of anesthesia has been the difficulty in precisely defining anesthesia. It has now become clear that an anesthetic agent produces different components of the anesthetic state *via* actions at different anatomic loci in the nervous system and may produce these component effects *via* different cellular and/or molecular actions. It also is becoming clear that different anesthetic agents can produce a specific component of anesthesia *via* actions at different molecular targets. Given these insights, the unitary theory of anesthesia has been largely discarded. The ensuing section will focus on the identification of specific anatomic, cellular, and molecular targets of anesthetic action. The complete mechanism(s) of anesthetic action have not been defined. The most difficult issue is mapping the effects of anesthetics on specific molecular targets to the complex component behaviors that compose anesthesia. This is a particularly vexing problem for poorly understood behaviors such as consciousness (*see* Chapter 13).

Anatomic Sites of Anesthetic Action. General anesthetics could, in principle, interrupt nervous system function at myriad levels, including peripheral sensory neurons, the spinal cord, the brain stem, and the cerebral cortex. Delineation of the precise anatomic sites of action is difficult because many anesthetics diffusely inhibit electrical activity in the CNS. For example, isoflurane at 2 MAC can cause electrical silence in the brain (Newberg *et al.*, 1983)! Despite this, *in vitro* studies have shown that specific cortical pathways exhibit markedly different sensitivities to both inhalational and intravenous anesthetics (MacIver and Roth, 1988; Richards and White, 1975; Nicoll, 1972). This suggests that anesthetics may produce specific components of the anesthetic state *via* actions at specific sites in the CNS. Consistent with this possibility, studies by Rampil (1994) and Antognini and Schwartz (1993) have demonstrated that immobilization in response to a surgical incision (the end point used in determining MAC) results from inhalational anesthetic action in the spinal cord. It is unlikely that amnesia or unconsciousness are the result of anesthetic actions in the spinal cord; thus different components of anesthesia are produced at different sites in the CNS. One intravenous anesthetic, dexmedetomidine (an α_2-adrenergic receptor agonist), has been shown to produce unconsciousness *via* actions in the locus coeruleus (Mizobe *et al.*, 1996). While the sites at which other intravenous and inhalational anesthetics produce unconsciousness have not been identified, inhalational anesthetics have been shown recently to depress the excitability of thalamic neurons (Ries and Puil, 1999). This suggests the thalamus as a potential locus for the sedative effects of inhalational anesthetics, since blockade of thalamocortical communication would produce unconsciousness. Finally, both intravenous and inhalational anesthetics depress hippocampal neurotransmission (Kendig *et al.*, 1991). This provides a probable locus for the amnesic effects of anesthetics.

Physiological Mechanisms of Anesthesia. General anesthetics produce two important physiologic effects at the cellular level. First, the inhalational anesthetics can hyperpolarize neurons (Nicoll and Madison, 1982). This may be an important effect on neurons serving a pacemaker role and on pattern-generating circuits. It also may be important in synaptic communication, since reduced excitability in a postsynaptic neuron

Table 14–1

Properties of Inhalational Anesthetic Agents

ANESTHETIC AGENT	MAC,* (%)	MAC-AWAKE,† (%)	EC$_{50}$‡ SUPPRESSION OF MEMORY (%)	VAPOR PRESSURE mm Hg at 20°C	PARTITION COEFFICIENT AT 37°C			RECOVERED AS METABOLITES (%)
					Blood:Gas	Brain:Blood	Fat:Blood	
Halothane	0.75	0.41	—	243	2.3	2.9	51	20.0
Isoflurane	1.2	0.4	0.24	250	1.4	2.6	45	0.2
Enflurane	1.6	0.4	—	175	1.8	1.4	36	2.4
Sevoflurane	2.0	0.6	—	160	0.65	1.7	48	3.0
Desflurane	6.0	2.4	—	664	0.45	1.3	27	0.02
Nitrous oxide	105.0§	60.0	52.5	Gas	0.47	1.1	2.3	0.004
Xenon	71.0	32.6	—	Gas	0.12	—	—	0

*MAC is minimum alveolar concentration.

†MAC-awake is the concentration at which appropriate responses to commands are lost.

‡EC$_{50}$ is the concentration that produces memory suppression in 50% of patients.

§A value of MAC greater than 100% means that hyperbaric conditions would be required to reach 1 MAC.

— Not available.

may reduce the likelihood that an action potential will be initiated in response to neurotransmitter release. Second, both inhalational and intravenous anesthetics have substantial effects on synaptic function. In this regard it is noteworthy that anesthetics appear to have minimal effects on action-potential generation or propagation at concentrations that affect synapses (Larrabee and Posternak, 1952). The inhalational anesthetics have been shown to inhibit excitatory synapses and enhance inhibitory synapses in various preparations. It seems likely that these effects are produced by both pre- and postsynaptic actions of the inhalational anesthetics. There is clear evidence that the inhalational anesthetic isoflurane can inhibit neurotransmitter release (Perouansky et al., 1995; MacIver et al., 1996); this may be mediated via an effect on the neurosecretory machinery (van Swinderen et al., 1999). It also is abundantly clear that inhalational anesthetics can act postsynaptically, altering the response to released neurotransmitter. These actions are thought to be due to specific interactions of anesthetic agents with neurotransmitter receptors.

The intravenous anesthetics produce a narrower range of physiological effects. Their predominant actions are at the synapse, where they have profound but relatively specific effects on the postsynaptic response to released neurotransmitter. Most of the intravenous agents act predominantly by enhancing inhibitory neurotransmission, whereas ketamine predominantly inhibits excitatory neurotransmission at glutamatergic synapses.

Molecular Actions of General Anesthetics.   The electrophysiological effects of general anesthetics at the cellular level suggest several potential molecular targets for anesthetic action. There is strong evidence supporting ligand-gated ion channels as important targets for anesthetic action. Chloride channels gated by the inhibitory neurotransmitter gamma-aminobutyric acid (GABA$_A$ receptors; see Chapter 17) are sensitive to clinical concentrations of a wide variety of anesthetics, including the halogenated inhalational agents and many intravenous agents (propofol, barbiturates, etomidate, and neurosteroids) (Krasowski and Harrison, 1999). At clinical concentrations, general anesthetics increase the sensitivity of the GABA$_A$ receptor to GABA, thus enhancing inhibitory neurotransmission and depressing nervous system activity. It appears likely that action of anesthetics on the GABA$_A$ receptor is mediated by binding of the anesthetics to specific sites on the GABA$_A$-receptor protein, as point mutations on the receptor can eliminate the effects of the anesthetic on ion channel function (Mihic et al., 1997). It also seems likely that there are specific binding sites for at least several classes of anesthetics, as mutations in various regions (and subunits) of the GABA$_A$ receptor selectively affect the actions of various anesthetics (Belelli et al., 1997; Krasowski and Harrison, 1999). It should be noted that none of the general anesthetics competes with GABA for its binding site on the receptor. Which components of anesthesia are mediated by actions of anesthetics on GABA$_A$ receptors remains a subject of conjecture. The fact that GABA mimetics themselves can produce unconsciousness suggests a role for GABA$_A$ receptors in mediating the hypnotic effects of general anesthetics (Cheng and Brunner, 1985).

Closely related to the GABA$_A$ receptors are other ligand-gated ion channels including glycine receptors and neuronal nicotinic acetylcholine receptors. Clinical concentrations of the inhalational anesthetics enhance the ability of glycine to activate glycine-gated chloride channels (glycine receptors), which play an important role in inhibitory neurotransmission in the spinal cord and brain stem. Propofol (Hales and Lambert, 1988), neurosteroids, and barbiturates also potentiate glycine-activated currents, whereas etomidate and ketamine do not (Mascia et al., 1996). Glycine receptors may play a role in mediating inhibition by anesthetics of responses to noxious stimuli. Subanesthetic concentrations of the inhalational anesthetics inhibit some classes of neuronal nicotinic acetylcholine receptors (Violet et al., 1997, Flood et al., 1997). The neuronal nicotinic receptors may play a role in mediating the analgesic effects of inhalational anesthetic agents.

The only general anesthetics that do not have significant effects on GABA$_A$ or glycine receptors are ketamine, nitrous oxide, and xenon. All of these agents have been shown to inhibit a different type of ligand-gated ion channel, the N-methyl-D-aspartate (NMDA) receptor (see Chapter 12). NMDA receptors are glutamate-gated cation channels that are somewhat selective for calcium and are involved in long-term modulation of synaptic responses (long-term potentiation) and glutamate-mediated neurotoxicity. Ketamine inhibits NMDA receptors by binding to the phencyclidine site on the NMDA-receptor protein (Lodge et al., 1982; Anis et al., 1983; Zeilhofer et al., 1992). The NMDA receptor is thought to be the principal molecular target for the anesthetic actions of ketamine. Recent studies also show that nitrous oxide (Mennerick et al., 1998; Jevotvic-Todorovic et al., 1998) and xenon (Franks et al., 1998; de Sousa et al., 2000) are potent and selective inhibitors of NMDA-activated currents, suggesting that these agents also may produce unconsciousness via actions on NMDA receptors.

Inhalational anesthetics have two other identified molecular targets that may be important in some of their actions. Some members of a class of potassium channels known as two-pore domain channels are activated by inhalational anesthetics (Gray et al., 1998; Patel et al., 1999). These channels are important in setting the resting membrane potential of a neuron and may be the molecular locus through which these agents hyperpolarize neurons. A second target is the molecular machinery involved in neurotransmitter release. Recent evidence shows that the action of inhalational anesthetics requires a protein complex (syntaxin, SNAP-25, synaptobrevin) involved in synaptic neurotransmitter release (van Swinderen et al., 1999). These molecular interactions may explain the ability of inhalational anesthetics to cause presynaptic inhibition in the hippocampus, and could contribute to the amnesic effect of inhalational anesthetics.

Summary.   Current evidence supports the view that most of the intravenous general anesthetics act predominantly through GABA$_A$ receptors and perhaps through some interactions with other ligand-gated ion channels. The halogenated inhalational agents have a variety of molecular targets, consistent with their status as complete (all components) anesthetics. Nitrous oxide, ketamine, and xenon constitute a third category of general anesthetics that are likely to produce unconsciousness via inhibition of the NMDA receptor.

PARENTERAL ANESTHETICS

Pharmacokinetic Principles

Parenteral anesthetics are small, hydrophobic, substituted aromatic or heterocyclic compounds (Figure 14–1). Hydrophobicity is the key factor governing the pharmacokinetics of this class of drugs (Bischoff and Dedrick, 1968; Burch and Stanski, 1983; Shafer and Stanski, 1992). After a single intravenous bolus, each of these drugs preferentially partitions into the highly perfused and lipophilic brain and spinal cord tissue where it produces anesthesia within a single circulation time. Subsequently, blood levels fall rapidly, resulting in redistribution of anesthetic out of the central nervous system back into the blood, where it then diffuses into less-well-perfused tissues such as muscle, viscera and, at a slower rate, into the poorly perfused but very hydrophobic adipose tissue. Termination of anesthesia after single boluses of parenteral anesthetics is primarily by redistribution out of the nervous system rather than by metabolism (for example, *see* Figure 14–2). After redistribution, anesthetic blood levels fall according to a complex interaction between the metabolic rate and the amount and lipophilicity of the drug stored in the peripheral compartments (Hughes *et al.,* 1992; Shafer and Stanski, 1992). Thus, parenteral anesthetic half-lives are "context-sensitive," and the degree to which a half-life is contextual varies greatly from drug to drug as might be predicted based on their markedly different hydrophobic-

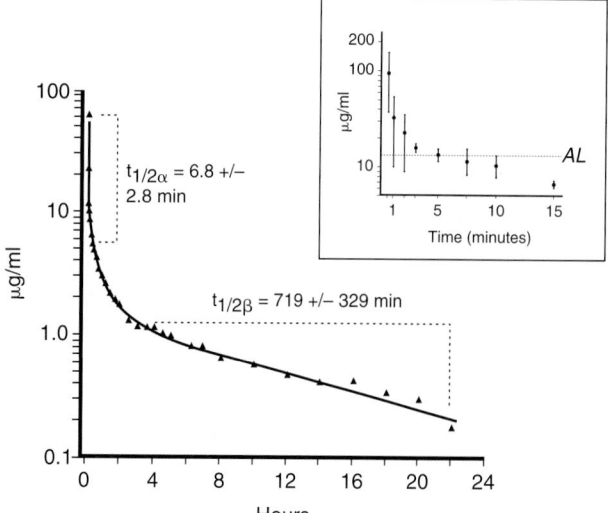

Figure 14–2. Thiopental serum levels after a single intravenous induction dose.

Thiopental serum levels after a bolus can be described by two time constants, $t_{1/2\alpha}$ and $t_{1/2\beta}$. The initial fall is rapid ($t_{1/2\alpha} < 10$ min) and is due to redistribution of drug from the plasma and the highly perfused brain and spinal cord into less well-perfused tissues such as muscle and fat. During this redistribution phase, serum thiopental concentration falls to levels (AL—awakening level) where patients awaken (*see* inset—the average thiopental serum concentration in 12 patients after a 6 mg/kg intravenous bolus of thiopental). Subsequent metabolism and elimination is much slower and is characterized by a half-life ($t_{1/2\beta}$ of more than 10 hours. (Adapted with permission from Burch and Stanski, 1983.)

ities and metabolic clearances (Table 14–2; and Figure 14–3). For example, after a single bolus of thiopental, patients usually emerge from anesthesia within 10 minutes; however, a patient may require more than a day to awaken from a prolonged thiopental infusion. The majority of individual variability in sensitivity to parenteral anesthetics can be accounted for by pharmacokinetic factors (Wada *et al.,* 1997; Wulfsohn and Joshi, 1969). For example, in patients with lower cardiac output, the relative perfusion of and fraction of anesthetic dose delivered to the brain is higher; thus, patients in septic shock and those with cardiomyopathy usually require lower doses of anesthetic. Elderly patients typically require a smaller anesthetic dose, primarily because of a smaller initial volume of distribution (Arden *et al.,* 1986; Homer and Stanski, 1985). As described below, similar principles govern the pharmacokinetics of the hydrophobic inhalational anesthetics with the added complexity of drug uptake by inhalation.

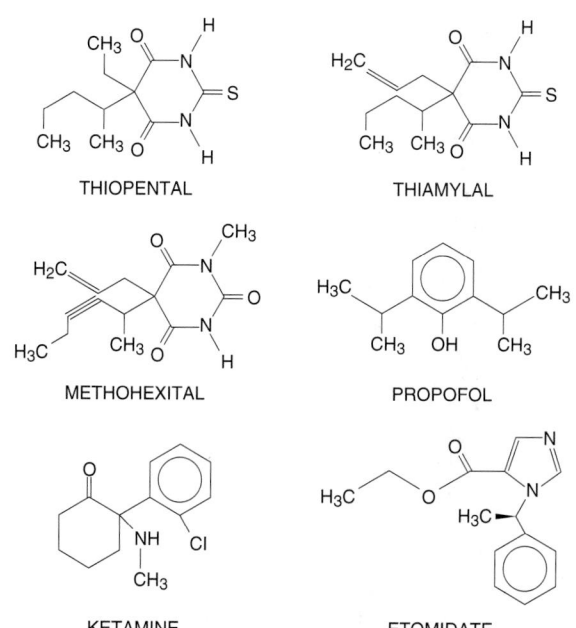

Figure 14–1. Structures of parenteral anesthetics.

Table 14–2
Pharmacological Properties of Parenteral Anesthetics

DRUG	FORMULATION	IV INDUCTION DOSE (mg/kg)	MINIMAL HYPNOTIC LEVEL (μg/ml)	DURATION OF INDUCTION DOSE (min)	$t_{1/2\beta}$* (hours)	CL (ml·min^{-1}·kg^{-1})	PROTEIN BINDING (%)	V_{ss} (l/kg)
Thiopental	25 mg/ml in aqueous solution + 1.5 mg/ml Na$_2$CO$_3$; pH = 10–11	3–5	15.6	5–8	12.1	3.4	85	2.3
Methohexital	10 mg/ml in aqueous solution + 1.5 mg/ml Na$_2$CO$_3$; pH = 10–11	1–2	10	4–7	3.9	10.9	85	2.2
Propofol	10 mg/ml in 10% soybean oil, 2.25% glycerol, 1.2% egg phospholipid, 0.005% EDTA or 0.025% Na metabisulfite; pH = 4.5–7	1.5–2.5	1.1	4–8	1.8	30	98	2.3
Etomidate	2 mg/ml in 35% propylene glycol; pH = 6.9	0.2–0.4	0.3	4–8	2.9	17.9	76	2.5
Ketamine	10, 50, or 100 mg/ml in aqueous solution; pH = 3.5–5.5	0.5–1.5	1	10–15	3.0	19.1	27	3.1

SOURCES: Data for thiopental from Clarke *et al.*, 1968; Burch and Stanski, 1983; Hudson *et al.*, 1983; Hung *et al.*, 1992; for methohexital from Brand *et al.*, 1963; Clarke *et al.*, 1968; Kay and Stephenson, 1981; Hudson *et al.*, 1983; McMurray *et al.*, 1986; for propofol from Kirkpatrick *et al.*, 1988; Langley and Heel, 1988; Shafer *et al.*, 1988; for etomidate from Doenicke, 1974; Meuldermans and Heykants, 1976; Fragen *et al.*, 1983; Hebron *et al.*, 1983; for ketamine from Chang and Glazko, 1974; Clements and Nimmo, 1981; White *et al.*, 1982; Dayton *et al.*, 1983.

*$t_{1/2\beta}$ = β phase half-life; CL = clearance; V_{ss} = volume of distribution at steady state; EDTA = ethylenediaminetetraacetic acid.

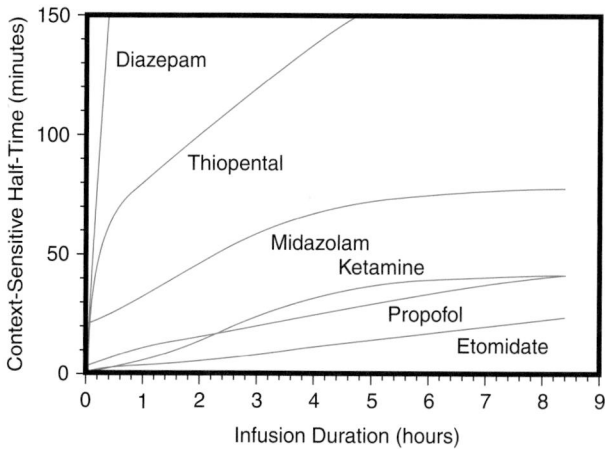

Figure 14–3. Context-sensitive half-time of general anesthetics.

The duration of action of single intravenous doses of anesthetic/hypnotic drugs is similarly short for all and is determined by redistribution of the drugs away from their active sites. However, after prolonged infusions, drug half-lives and durations of action are dependent on a complex interaction between the rate of redistribution of the drug, the amount of drug accumulated in fat, and the drug's metabolic rate. Thus, drug half-lives vary greatly. This phenomenon has been termed the *context-sensitive half-time* (that is, the half-time of a drug can only be estimated if one knows the context—the total dose and over what time it has been given). Note that the half-times of some drugs such as etomidate, propofol, and ketamine increase only modestly with prolonged infusions; others (*e.g.,* diazepam and thiopental) increase dramatically. (Reproduced with permission from Reves *et al.,* 1994.)

Barbiturates

Chemistry and Formulations. Anesthetic barbiturates are derivatives of barbituric acid (2,4,6-trioxohexahydropyrimidine), with either an oxygen or sulfur at the 2-position (Figure 14–1). The three barbiturates used for clinical anesthesia are *sodium thiopental* (PENTOTHAL), *thiamylal* (SURITAL), and *methohexital* (BREVITAL). Sodium thiopental is the most frequently used of the barbiturates for inducing anesthesia. All three barbiturate anesthetics are supplied as racemic mixtures despite enantioselectivity in their anesthetic potency (Andrews and Mark, 1982; Christensen and Lee, 1973; Nguyen *et al.,* 1996). Barbiturates are formulated as the sodium salts with 6% sodium carbonate and reconstituted in water or isotonic saline solution to produce 1% (methohexital), 2% (thiamylal), or 2.5% (thiopental) alkaline solutions with pHs of 10 to 11. Once reconstituted, the thiobarbiturates are stable in solution for up to 1 week and methohexital for up to 6 weeks if refrigerated. Mixing with more acidic drugs commonly used during anesthetic induction can result in precipitation of the barbiturate as the free acid; thus, standard practice is to delay the administration of other drugs until the barbiturate has cleared the intravenous tubing.

Pharmacokinetics. Pharmacokinetic parameters for each drug are given in Table 14–2. As discussed above, the principal mechanism limiting anesthetic duration after single doses is redistribution of these hydrophobic drugs from the brain to other tissues. However, after multiple doses or infusions, the duration of action of the barbiturates varies considerably depending on their clearances. Methohexital differs from the other two barbiturates in its much more rapid clearance; thus, it accumulates less during prolonged infusions (Schwilden and Stoeckel, 1990). Prolonged infusions or very large doses of thiopental and thiamylal can produce unconsciousness lasting several days because of their slow elimination and large volume of distributions (Stanski *et al.,* 1980). Even single induction doses of thiopental and, to a lesser degree, methohexital can produce psychomotor impairment lasting up to 8 hours (Beskow *et al.,* 1995; Korttila *et al.,* 1975). Methohexital had been used frequently for outpatient procedures where rapid return to an alert state is particularly desirable, but this role now has been filled largely by the anesthetic propofol (*see* below). All three drugs are eliminated primarily by hepatic metabolism and renal excretion of inactive metabolites (Broadie *et al.,* 1950); a small fraction of thiopental undergoes a desulfuration reaction to the longer-acting hypnotic pentobarbital (Chan *et al.,* 1985). Each drug is highly protein bound (Table 14–2). Hepatic disease or other conditions that reduce serum protein concentrations will decrease the volume of distribution and thereby increase the initial free concentration and hypnotic effect of an induction dose (Ghoneim and Pandya, 1975).

Clinical Use. Recommended intravenous doses for all three drugs in a healthy young adult are given in Table 14–2. The typical induction dose of thiopental (3 to 5 mg/kg) produces unconsciousness in 10 to 30 seconds with a peak effect in one minute and duration of anesthesia of 5 to 8 minutes (Dundee *et al.,* 1982). Neonates and infants usually require a higher induction dose (5 to 8 mg/kg), whereas elderly and pregnant patients require less (1 to 3 mg/kg) (Gin *et al.,* 1997; Homer and Stanski, 1985; Jonmarker *et al.,* 1987). Dosage calculation based on lean body mass reduces individual variation in dosage requirements. Doses can be reduced 10% to 50% after premedication with benzodiazepines, opioids, and/or α_2-adrenergic receptor agonists because of their additive hypnotic effect (Nishina *et al.,* 1994; Short *et al.,* 1991; Wang *et al.,* 1996). Thiamylal is approximately equipotent with and in all aspects very similar to thiopental (Tovell *et al.,* 1955). Methohexital is three times as potent as but otherwise similar to thiopental in onset and duration of action (Thornton, 1970; Tovell *et al.,* 1955). Thiopental and thiamylal produce little or no pain on injection; methohexital elicits mild pain. Venoirritation can be reduced by injection into larger non-hand veins and by prior intravenous injection of lidocaine (0.5 to 1 mg/kg). Intraarterial injection of thiobarbiturates can induce a severe inflammatory and potentially necrotic reaction and should be avoided

(Dohi and Naito, 1983; Waters, 1966). Thiopental often evokes the taste of garlic just prior to inducing anesthesia (Nor *et al.*, 1996). Methohexital and, to a lesser degree, the other barbiturates can produce excitement phenomena such as muscle tremor, hypertonus, and hiccoughs (Clarke, 1981; Thornton, 1970). For induction of pediatric patients without intravenous access, all three drugs can be given by rectum at approximately 10 times the intravenous dose.

Side Effects. *Nervous System.* Besides producing general anesthesia, barbiturates dose-dependently reduce cerebral metabolic rate as measured by cerebral oxygen utilization (cerebral metabolic rate for oxygen; CMR_{O_2}). Induction doses of thiopental reduce CMR_{O_2} about 25% to 30% with a maximal decrease of 55% occurring at about 2 to 5 times the induction dose (Pierce *et al.*, 1962; Stullken *et al.*, 1977). As a consequence of the decrease in CMR_{O_2}, cerebral blood flow and intracranial pressure are similarly reduced (Pierce *et al.*, 1962; Shapiro *et al.*, 1973). Because it markedly lowers cerebral metabolism, thiopental has been tried as a protective agent against cerebral ischemia. At least one human study suggests that thiopental may be efficacious in ameliorating ischemic damage in the perioperative setting (Nussmeier *et al.*, 1986). Thiopental also reduces intraocular pressure (Joshi and Bruce, 1975). Presumably because of their CNS-depressant activity, barbiturates are effective anticonvulsants (*see* Chapter 21). Thiopental in particular is of proven value in the treatment of status epilepticus (Modica *et al.*, 1990).

Cardiovascular System. The anesthetic barbiturates produce dose-dependent decreases in blood pressure. The effect primarily is caused by vasodilation, particular venodilation, and to a lesser degree by a mild direct decrease in myocardial contractility (Elder *et al.*, 1955; Etsten and Li, 1955; Fieldman *et al.*, 1955). Typically, heart rate increases as a compensatory response to a lower blood pressure, although barbiturates do blunt the baroreceptor reflex (Bristow *et al.*, 1969). Drops in blood pressure can be severe in patients with impaired ability to compensate for venodilation, such as those with hypovolemia, cardiomyopathy, valvular heart disease, coronary artery disease, cardiac tamponade, or β-adrenergic-receptor blockade. Thiopental is not necessarily contraindicated in patients with coronary artery disease, because the ratio of myocardial oxygen supply to demand appears to be adequately maintained within a patient's normal blood pressure range (Reiz *et al.*, 1981). None of the barbiturates has been shown to be arrythmogenic.

Respiratory System. Barbiturates are respiratory depressants. Induction doses of thiopental decrease minute ventilation and tidal volume with a smaller and inconsistent reduction in respiratory rate (Grounds *et al.*, 1987). Reflex responses to hypercarbia and hypoxia are diminished by anesthetic barbiturates (Gross *et al.*, 1983; Hirshman *et al.*, 1975), and apnea can result at higher doses or in the presence of other respiratory depressants such as opioids. With the exception of uncommon anaphylactoid reactions, these drugs have little effect on bronchomotor tone and can be used safely in asthmatic patients (Kingston and Hirshman, 1984).

Other Side Effects. Short-term administration of barbiturates has no clinically significant effects on the hepatic, renal, or endocrine systems. A single induction dose of thiopental does not alter gravid uterine tone but produces mild, transient depression of activity of the newborn (Kosaka *et al.*, 1969). True allergies to barbiturates are rare (Baldo *et al.*, 1991); however, drug-induced histamine release occasionally is seen (Hirshman *et al.*, 1982; Sprung *et al.*, 1997). Barbiturates can induce fatal attacks of porphyria in patients with acute intermittent or variegate porphyria and are contraindicated in such patients (Dundee *et al.*, 1962). Unlike inhalational anesthetics and succinylcholine, barbiturates and all other parenteral anesthetics do not appear to trigger malignant hyperthermia (Rosenberg *et al.*, 1997).

Propofol

Chemistry and Formulations. Along with thiopental, *propofol* (DIPRIVAN) is the most commonly used parenteral anesthetic. Propofol, 2,6-diisopropylphenol, is essentially insoluble in aqueous solutions and is formulated only for intravenous administration as a 1% (10 mg/ml) emulsion in 10% soybean oil, 2.25% glycerol, and 1.2% purified egg phospholipid. In the United States, disodium EDTA (0.05 mg/ml) or sodium metabisulfite (0.25 mg/ml) is added to inhibit bacterial growth. Nevertheless, significant bacterial contamination of open containers still has been reported and associated with serious infection (Bennett *et al.*, 1995); propofol should be administered shortly after removal from sterile packaging or discarded.

Pharmacokinetics. The pharmacokinetics of propofol are governed by the same principles that apply to barbiturates. Onset and duration of anesthesia after a single bolus are similar to those of thiopental (Langley and Heel, 1988). However, recovery after multiple doses or infusion has been shown to be much faster after propofol than after thiopental or even methohexital (Doze *et al.*, 1986; Langley and Heel, 1988). The rapid rate of recovery after infusion of propofol can be explained by its very high clearance coupled with the slow diffusion of drug from the peripheral to the central compartment (Figure 14–3). The rapid clearance of propofol explains its less severe hangover compared to barbiturates and may allow for a more rapid discharge from the recovery room (Bryson *et al.*, 1995). Propofol is metabolized primarily in the liver to less-active metabolites that are renally excreted (Simons *et al.*, 1988); however, its clearance exceeds hepatic blood flow, and extrahepatic metabolism has been demonstrated (Veroli *et al.*, 1992). Propofol is highly protein bound, and its pharmacokinetics, like that of the barbiturates, may be affected by conditions that alter serum protein levels (Kirkpatrick *et al.*, 1988).

Clinical Use. The induction dose of propofol in a healthy adult is 1.5 to 2.5 mg/kg. Propofol has an onset and duration of anesthesia similar to those of thiopental (Table 14–2). As with barbiturates, dosages should be reduced in elderly patients and in the presence of other sedatives and increased in young children (Aun *et al.*, 1992; Dundee *et al.*, 1986). Propofol often is used for maintenance of anesthesia as well as induction. For short procedures, small boluses (10% to 50% of the induction dose) every 5 minutes or as needed are effective. Because they produce more stable drug levels, propofol infusions (100 to 300 μg/kg per minute) are better suited for longer-term anesthetic maintenance. Infusion rates should be tailored to patient response and the levels of other hypnotics. Sedating doses of propofol are 20% to 50% of those required for general anesthesia. However, even at these lower doses, caregivers should be vigilant and prepared for all of the side effects of propofol discussed below, particularly airway obstruction and apnea. Propofol elicits pain on injection, which can be reduced with lidocaine and the use of larger arm and antecubital veins (McCulloch and Lees, 1985; Picard and Tramer, 2000). Excitatory phenomena during induction with propofol occur at about the same frequency as with thiopental but much less frequently than with methohexital (Langley and Heel, 1988).

Side Effects. *Nervous System.* The central nervous system effects of propofol are similar to those of barbiturates. Propofol decreases CMR_{O_2}, cerebral blood flow, and intracranial and intraocular pressures by about the same amount as does thiopental (Langley and Heel, 1988; Ravussin *et al.*, 1988; Vandesteene *et al.*, 1988). Like thiopental, propofol has been used in patients at risk for cerebral ischemia (Ravussin and de Tribolet, 1993); however, no human outcome studies have been performed to determine propofol's efficacy as a neuroprotectant. Results from studies on the anticonvulsant effects of propofol have been mixed, with some data even suggesting that it has proconvulsant activity when combined with other drugs (Modica *et al.*, 1990). Thus, unlike thiopental, propofol is not a proven acute intervention for seizures.

Cardiovascular System. Propofol produces a dose-dependent decrease in blood pressure that is significantly greater than that produced by thiopental (Grounds *et al.*, 1985; Langley and Heel, 1988). The fall in blood pressure can be explained by both vasodilation and mild depression of myocardial contractility (Claeys *et al.*, 1988; Grounds *et al.*, 1985). Propofol appears to blunt the baroreceptor reflex and/or is directly vagotonic, because smaller increases in heart rate are seen for any given drop in blood pressure after doses of propofol (Claeys *et al.*, 1988; Langley

and Heel, 1988). As with thiopental, propofol should be used with caution in patients at risk for or intolerant of decreases in blood pressure.

Respiratory and Other Side Effects. At equianesthetic doses, propofol produces a slightly greater degree of respiratory depression than does thiopental (Blouin *et al.*, 1991; Taylor *et al.*, 1986). Patients given propofol should be monitored to ensure adequate oxygenation and ventilation. Propofol appears to be less likely than barbiturates to provoke bronchospasm (Eames *et al.*, 1996; Pizov *et al.*, 1995). It has no clinically significant effects on hepatic, renal, or endocrine organ systems. Unlike thiopental, propofol appears to have significant antiemetic action and is a good choice for sedation or anesthesia in patients at high risk for nausea and vomiting (Gan *et al.*, 1996; McCollum *et al.*, 1988). Propofol provokes anaphylactoid reactions and histamine release at about the same low frequency as does thiopental (Bryson *et al.*, 1995; Laxenaire *et al.*, 1992). Although propofol does cross placental membranes, it is considered safe for use in pregnant patients and transiently depresses activity of the newborn similarly to thiopental (Abboud *et al.*, 1995).

Etomidate

Chemistry and Formulation. *Etomidate* (AMIDATE) is a substituted imidazole that is supplied as the active D-isomer (Figure 14–1). Etomidate is poorly soluble in water and is formulated as a 2-mg/ml solution in 35% propylene glycol. Unlike thiopental, etomidate does not induce precipitation of neuromuscular blocking agents or other drugs frequently given during anesthetic induction (Hadzija and Lubarsky, 1995).

Pharmacokinetics. An induction dose of etomidate has a rapid onset and redistribution-limited duration of action (Table 14–2). Metabolism of etomidate occurs in the liver, where it is primarily hydrolyzed to inactive compounds (Gooding and Corssen, 1976; Heykants *et al.*, 1975). Elimination is both renal (78%) and biliary (22%). Compared to thiopental, the duration of action of etomidate increases less with repeated doses (Figure 14–3). The plasma-protein binding of etomidate is high but less than that of barbiturates and propofol (Table 14–2).

Clinical Use. Etomidate primarily is used for anesthetic induction of patients at risk for hypotension. Induction doses of etomidate (0.2 to 0.4 mg/kg) have a rapid onset and a short duration of action (Table 14–2); they are accompanied by a high incidence of pain on injection and myoclonic movements (Giese and Stanley, 1983). As with propofol, lidocaine effectively reduces the pain of injection (Galloway *et al.*, 1982). The myoclonic movements can be reduced by premedication with either benzodiazepines or opioids (Zacharias *et al.*, 1979). Etomidate is pharmacokinetically suitable for infusion for anesthetic maintenance (10 μg/kg per minute) or sedation (5 μg/kg per minute) (Fragen et al., 1983); however, long-term infusions are not recommended for reasons discussed below. Etomidate also may be given by rectum (6.5 mg/kg) with an onset of about 5 minutes (Linton and Thornington, 1983).

Side Effects. *Nervous System.* The effects of etomidate on cerebral blood flow, metabolism, and intracranial and intraocular pressures are similar to those of thiopental (Modica and Tempelhoff, 1992; Renou et al., 1978; Thomson et al., 1982). Etomidate has been tried as a protective agent against cerebral ischemia (Batjer, 1993). However, animal studies have failed to show a consistent beneficial effect (Drummond et al., 1995; Guo et al., 1995), and no controlled human trials have been performed. Etomidate has been shown in some studies to be a proconvulsant and is not a proven treatment for seizures (Modica et al., 1990).
Cardiovascular System. Cardiovascular stability after induction is a major advantage of etomidate over either barbiturates or propofol. Induction doses of etomidate typically produce a small increase in heart rate and little to no decrease in blood pressure or cardiac output (Criado et al., 1980; Gooding and Corssen, 1977; Gooding et al., 1979). Etomidate has little effect on coronary perfusion pressure and reduces myocardial oxygen consumption (Kettler et al., 1974). Thus, of all induction agents, etomidate is best suited to maintain cardiovascular stability in patients with coronary artery disease, cardiomyopathy, cerebral vascular disease, and/or hypovolemia.
Respiratory and Other Side Effects. The degree of respiratory depression by etomidate appears to be less than that by thiopental (Colvin et al., 1979; Morgan et al., 1977). Like methohexital, it sometimes induces hiccups but does not significantly stimulate histamine release (Doenicke et al., 1973; Zacharias et al., 1979). Despite minimal cardiac and respiratory effects, etomidate does have two major drawbacks. First, etomidate has been associated with a significant increase in nausea and vomiting (Fragen and Caldwell, 1979). A second problem was discovered when an increase in the mortality of intensive-care-unit patients sedated with etomidate infusions was observed (Ledingham and Watt, 1983). The increased mortality was linked to suppression of the adrenocortical stress response (Ledingham et al., 1983). Indeed, etomidate inhibits certain adrenal biosynthetic enzymes required for the production of cortisol and some other steroids. Even single induction doses of etomidate may mildly and transiently reduce cortisol levels (Allolio et al., 1985; Fragen et al., 1984;

Wagner et al., 1984), but no significant differences in outcome after short-term administration have been found even for variables specifically known to be associated with adrenocortical suppression (Wagner et al., 1984). Thus, while etomidate is not recommended for long-term infusion, it appears to be safe for anesthetic induction and has some unique advantages in patients prone to hemodynamic instability.

Ketamine

Chemistry and Formulation. *Ketamine* (KETALAR) is an aryl-cyclohexylamine, a congener of phencyclidine (Figure 14–1). It is supplied as a racemic mixture, despite the (S)-isomer being more potent and having less side effects than the (R)-isomer (White et al., 1982). Although more lipophilic than thiopental, ketamine is water-soluble and available as 10, 50, and 100 mg/ml in sodium chloride solution plus the preservative benzethonium chloride.

Pharmacokinetics. The onset and duration of an induction dose of ketamine is determined by the same distribution/redistribution mechanism operant for all the other parenteral anesthetics. Ketamine is hepatically metabolized to norketamine, which has reduced CNS activity; norketamine is further metabolized and excreted in the urine and bile (Chang and Glazko, 1974). Ketamine has a large volume of distribution and rapid clearance that makes it suitable for continuous infusion without the drastic lengthening in duration of action seen with thiopental (Table 14–2 and Figure 14–3). Protein binding is much lower with ketamine than with the other parenteral anesthetics (Table 14–2).

Clinical Use. Ketamine has unique properties that make it useful for certain pediatric procedures and for anesthetizing patients at risk for hypotension or bronchospasm. However, it has significant side effects that limit its routine use. Ketamine rapidly produces a hypnotic state distinct from that of other anesthetics. Patients have profound analgesia, unresponsiveness to commands, and amnesia but may have their eyes open, move their limbs involuntarily, and usually have spontaneous respiration. This cataleptic state has been termed *dissociative anesthesia*. Ketamine is typically administered intravenously but also is effective by intramuscular, oral, and rectal routes. The induction doses are 0.5 to 1.5 mg/kg intravenously, 4 to 6 mg/kg intramuscularly, and 8 to 10 mg/kg rectally (White et al., 1982). The onset of action after an intravenous dose is similar to that of the other parenteral anesthetics, but the duration of anesthesia of a single dose is longer (Table 14–2). For anesthetic maintenance, ketamine occasionally is continued as an infusion (25 to 100 μg/kg per minute) (White et al., 1982). Ketamine does not elicit pain on injection or true excitatory behavior as described for methohexital, although involuntary movements produced by ketamine can be mistaken for anesthetic excitement.

Side Effects. *Nervous System.* As mentioned, ketamine has behavioral effects distinct from those of other anesthetics. The ketamine-induced cataleptic state is accompanied by nystagmus with pupillary dilation, salivation and/or lacrimation, and spontaneous limb movements with increased overall muscle tone. Although ketamine does not produce the classic anesthetic state, patients are anesthetized in that they are amnestic and unresponsive to painful stimuli. Indeed, ketamine produces profound analgesia, a distinct advantage over other parenteral anesthetics (White *et al.*, 1982). Unlike other parenteral anesthetics, ketamine increases cerebral blood flow and intracranial pressure with minimal alteration of cerebral metabolism (Gardner *et al.*, 1971; Takeshita *et al.*, 1972; Wyte *et al.*, 1972). These effects can be attenuated by concurrent administration of thiopental and/or benzodiazepines along with hyperventilation (Belopavlovic and Buchthal, 1982; Mayberg *et al.*, 1995). However, given that other anesthetics actually reduce intracranial pressure and cerebral metabolism, ketamine is relatively contraindicated for patients with increased intracranial pressure or those at risk for cerebral ischemia. In some studies, ketamine has been shown to increase intraocular pressure, and its use for induction of patients with open eye injuries is controversial (Whitacre and Ellis, 1984). The effects of ketamine on seizure activity appear to be mixed, with neither strong pro- nor anticonvulsant activity (Modica *et al.*, 1990). Emergence delirium characterized by hallucinations, vivid dreams, and illusions is a frequent complication of ketamine that can result in serious patient dissatisfaction and can complicate postoperative management (White *et al.*, 1982). Delirium symptoms are most frequent in the first hour after emergence and occur less frequently in children (Sussman, 1974). Benzodiazepines reduce the incidence of emergence delirium (Dundee and Lilburn, 1978).

Cardiovascular System. Unlike other anesthetics, induction doses of ketamine typically increase blood pressure, heart rate, and cardiac output (Stanley *et al.*, 1968). The cardiovascular effects are indirect and are most likely mediated by inhibition of both central and peripheral catecholamine reuptake (White *et al.*, 1982). Ketamine has direct negative inotropic and vasodilating activity, but these effects usually are overwhelmed by the indirect sympathomimetic action (Pagel *et al.*, 1992). Thus, ketamine is a useful drug in patients at risk for hypotension during anesthesia. While not arrythmogenic, ketamine increases myocardial oxygen consumption and is not an ideal drug for patients at risk for myocardial ischemia (Reves *et al.*, 1978).

Respiratory System. The respiratory effects of ketamine are perhaps the best indication for its use. Induction doses of ketamine produce small and transient decreases in minute ventilation, but respiratory depression is less severe than with other general anesthetics (White *et al.*, 1982). Ketamine is a potent bronchodilator due to its indirect sympathomimetic activity and perhaps some direct bronchodilating activity (Hirshman *et al.*, 1979; Wanna and Gergis, 1978). Thus, ketamine is particularly well suited for anesthetizing patients at high risk for bronchospasm.

Summary of Parenteral Anesthetics

Parenteral anesthetics are the most commonly used drugs for anesthetic induction of adults. Their lipophilicity coupled with the relatively high perfusion of the brain and spinal cord results in a rapid onset and short duration after a single bolus dose. However, these drugs ultimately accumulate in fatty tissue, prolonging the patient's recovery if multiple doses are given, particularly for drugs with lower rates of clearance. Each anesthetic has its own unique set of properties and side effects (summarized in Table 14–3). Thiopental and propofol are the two most commonly used parenteral agents. Thiopental has a long-established track record of safety. Propofol is advantageous for procedures where rapid return to a preoperative mental status is desirable. Etomidate usually is reserved for patients at risk for hypotension and/or myocardial ischemia. Ketamine is best suited for patients with asthma and/or for children undergoing short, painful procedures.

INHALATIONAL ANESTHETICS

Introduction

A wide variety of gases and volatile liquids can produce anesthesia. The first widely used inhalational anesthetic was diethyl ether (*see* Chapter 13). Subsequently, a variety of structurally unrelated compounds have been used as inhalational anesthetics including cyclopropane, elemental xenon, nitrous oxide, and more recently, short-chain halogenated alkanes and ethers. The structures of the currently used inhalational anesthetics are shown in Figure 14–4. One of the troublesome properties of the inhalational anesthetics is their low safety margin. The inhalational anesthetics have therapeutic indices (LD_{50}/ED_{50}) that range from 2 to 4, making these among the most dangerous drugs in clinical use. The toxicity of these drugs is largely a function of their side effects, and each of the

Table 14–3
Some Pharmacological Effects of Parenteral Anesthetics*

DRUG	CBF	CMR_{O_2}	ICP	MAP	HR	CO	RR	$\dot{V}_E$
Thiopental	– – –	– – –	– – –	–	+	–	–	– –
Etomidate	– – –	– – –	– – –	+/–	+/–	+/–	–	–
Ketamine	+ +	+/–	+ +	+	+ +	+	+/–	+/–
Propofol	– – –	– – –	– – –	– –	+	–	– –	– – –

KEY: CBF, cerebral blood flow; CMR_{O_2}, cerebral metabolic rate for oxygen; ICP, intracranial pressure; MAP,
    mean arterial pressure; HR, heart rate; CO, cardiac output; RR, respiratory rate; $\dot{V}_E$, minute ventilation.
*Typical effects of a single induction dose in human beings; see text for references.
Qualitative scale from – – – to + + + = slight, moderate, or large decrease or increase, respectively;
    +/– indicates no significant change.

inhalational anesthetics has a unique side-effect profile.
Hence, the selection of an inhalational anesthetic often is
based on matching a patient's pathophysiology with drug
side-effect profiles. The specific adverse effects of each of
the inhalational anesthetics are emphasized in the following sections. The inhalational anesthetics also vary widely
in their physical properties. Table 14–1 lists the important
physical properties of the inhalational agents in clinical
use. These properties are important because they govern
the pharmacokinetics of the inhalational agents. Ideally,

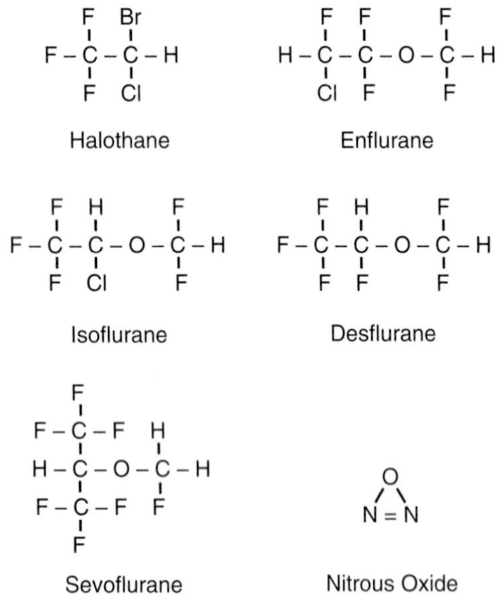

an inhalational agent would produce a rapid induction
of anesthesia and a rapid recovery following discontinuation. The pharmacokinetics of the inhalational agents is
reviewed in the following section.

Pharmacokinetic Principles

The inhalational agents are some of the very few pharmacological agents administered as gases. The fact that these
agents behave as gases rather than as liquids requires that
different pharmacokinetic constructs be used in analyzing
their uptake and distribution. It is essential to understand
that inhalational anesthetics distribute between tissues (or
between blood and gas) such that equilibrium is achieved
when the partial pressure of anesthetic gas is equal in the
two tissues. When a person has breathed an inhalational
anesthetic for a sufficiently long time that all tissues are
equilibrated with the anesthetic, the partial pressure of the
anesthetic in all tissues will be equal to the partial pressure
of the anesthetic in inspired gas. It is important to note that
while the partial pressure of the anesthetic may be equal
in all tissues, the concentration of anesthetic in each tissue
will be different. Indeed, anesthetic partition coefficients
are defined as the ratio of anesthetic concentration in two
tissues when the partial pressures of anesthetic are equal
in the two tissues. Blood:gas, brain:blood, and blood:fat
partition coefficients for the various inhalational agents
are listed in Table 14–1. These partition coefficients show
that inhalational anesthetics are more soluble in some tissues (*e.g.*, fat) than they are in other (*e.g.*, blood), and that
there is significant range in the solubility of the various
inhalational agents in such tissues.

In clinical practice, one can monitor the equilibration
of a patient with anesthetic gas. Equilibrium is achieved
when the partial pressure in inspired gas is equal to the
partial pressure in end-tidal (alveolar) gas. This defines

Figure 14–4. Structures of inhalational general anesthetics.

Note that all inhalational general anesthetic agents except
nitrous oxide and halothane are ethers and that fluorine
progressively replaces other halogens in the development
of the halogenated agents. All structural differences are
associated with important differences in pharmacological
properties.

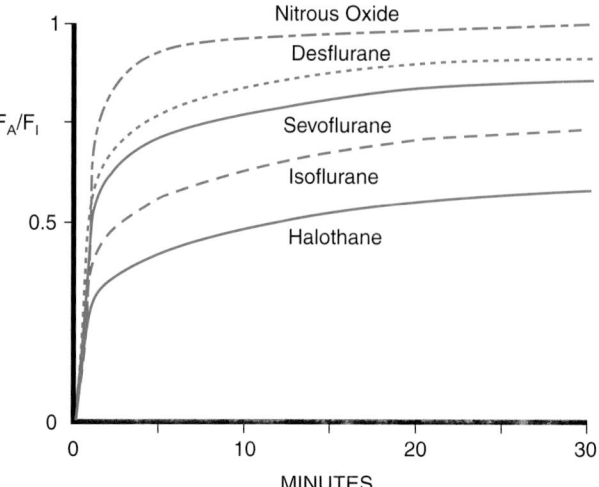

Figure 14–5. Uptake of inhalational general anesthetics.

The rise in alveolar (F_A) anesthetic concentration toward the inspired (F_I) concentration is most rapid with the least soluble anesthetics, nitrous oxide and desflurane, and slowest with the most soluble anesthetic, halothane. All data are from human studies. (Reproduced with permission from Eger, 2000.)

equilibrium, because it is the point when there is no net uptake of anesthetic from the alveoli into the blood. For inhalational agents that are not very soluble in blood or any other tissue, equilibrium is achieved quickly, as illustrated for nitrous oxide in Figure 14–5. If an agent is more soluble in a tissue such as fat, equilibrium may take many hours to reach. This occurs because fat represents a huge reservoir for the anesthetic, which will be filled slowly because of the modest blood flow to fat. This is illustrated by the slow approach of halothane alveolar partial pressure to inspired partial pressure in Figure 14–5.

In considering the pharmacokinetics of anesthetics, one important parameter is the speed of anesthetic induction. Anesthetic induction requires that brain partial pressure be equal to MAC. Because the brain is well perfused, anesthetic partial pressure in brain becomes equal to the partial pressure in alveolar gas (and in blood) over the course of several minutes. Therefore, anesthesia is achieved shortly after alveolar partial pressure reaches MAC. While the rate of rise of alveolar partial pressure will be slower for anesthetics that are highly soluble in blood and other tissues, this limitation on speed of induction can be overcome largely by delivering higher inspired partial pressures of the anesthetic.

Elimination of inhalational anesthetics is largely the reverse process of uptake. For agents with low blood and tissue solubility, recovery from anesthesia should mirror anesthetic induction, regardless of the duration of anesthetic administration. For inhalational agents with high blood and tissue solubility, recovery will be a function of the duration of anesthetic administration. This occurs because the accumulated amounts of anesthetic in the fat reservoir will prevent blood (and therefore alveolar) partial pressures from falling rapidly. Patients will be arousable when alveolar partial pressure reaches MAC_{awake}, a partial pressure somewhat lower than MAC (*see* Table 14–1).

Halothane

Chemistry and Formulation. *Halothane* (FLUOTHANE) is 2-bromo-2-chloro-1,1,1-trifluoroethane (*see* Figure 14–4). Halothane is a volatile liquid at room temperature and must be stored in a sealed container. Because halothane is a light-sensitive compound that also is subject to spontaneous breakdown, it is marketed in amber bottles with thymol added as a preservative. Mixtures of halothane with oxygen or air are neither flammable nor explosive.

Pharmacokinetics. Halothane has a relatively high blood:gas partition coefficient and high blood:fat partition coefficient (*see* Table 14–1). Induction with halothane therefore is relatively slow, and the alveolar halothane concentration remains substantially lower than the inspired halothane concentration for many hours of administration. Because halothane is soluble in fat and other body tissues, it will accumulate during prolonged administration. Therefore, the speed of recovery from halothane is lengthened as a function of duration of administration (Stoelting and Eger, 1969).

Approximately 60% to 80% of halothane taken up by the body is eliminated unchanged *via* the lungs in the first 24 hours after its administration. A substantial amount of the halothane not eliminated in exhaled gas is biotransformed in the liver by cytochrome P450 enzymes. The major metabolite of halothane is trifluoroacetic acid, which is formed by removal of bromine and chlorine ions (Gruenke *et al.*, 1988). Trifluoroacetic acid, bromine, and chlorine all can be detected in the urine. Trifluoroacetylchloride, an intermediate in oxidative metabolism of halothane, can trifluoroacetylate covalently several proteins in the liver. An immune reaction to these altered proteins may be responsible for the rare cases of fulminant halothane-induced hepatic necrosis (Kenna *et al.*, 1988). There also is a minor reductive pathway accounting for approximately 1% of halothane metabolism and generally observed only under hypoxic conditions (Van Dyke *et al.*, 1988).

Clinical Use. Halothane, introduced in 1956, was the first of the modern, halogenated inhalational anesthetics used in clinical practice. It is a potent agent that usually is used for maintenance of anesthesia. It is not pungent and is therefore well tolerated for inhalation induction of anesthesia. This is most commonly done in children, where preoperative placement of an intravenous catheter can be difficult. Anesthesia is produced by halothane at end-tidal concentrations of 0.7% to 1.0% halothane. The end-tidal concentration of halothane required to produce anesthesia is substantially reduced when it is coadministered with nitrous oxide. The use of halothane in the United States has diminished substantially in the past decade because of the introduction of newer inhalational agents with better pharmacokinetic and side-effect profiles. Halothane continues to be extensively used in children because it is well tolerated for inhalation induction and because the serious side effects appear to be diminished in children. Halothane has a low cost and is therefore still widely used in developing countries.

Side Effects. *Cardiovascular System.* The most predictable side effect of halothane is a dose-dependent reduction in arterial blood pressure. Mean arterial pressure decreases about 20% to 25% at MAC concentrations of halothane. This reduction in blood pressure primarily is the result of direct myocardial depression leading to reduced cardiac output (*see* Figure 14–6). Myocardial depression is thought to result from attenuation of depolarization-induced intracellular calcium transients (Lynch, 1997). Halothane-induced hypotension usually is accompanied by either bradycardia or a normal heart rate. This absence of a tachycardic (or contractile) response to reduced blood pressure is thought to be due to an inability of the heart to respond to the effector arm of the baroceptor reflex. Heart rate can be increased during halothane anesthesia by exogenous catecholamine or by sympathoadrenal stimulation. Halothane-induced reductions in blood pressure and heart rate generally disappear after several hours of constant halothane administration. This is thought to occur because of progressive sympathetic stimulation (Eger *et al.*, 1970).

Halothane does not cause a significant change in systemic vascular resistance. Nonetheless, it causes changes in the resistance and autoregulation of specific vascular beds leading to redistribution of blood flow. The vascular beds of the skin and brain are dilated directly by halothane, leading to increased cerebral blood flow and skin perfusion. Conversely, autoregulation of renal, splanchnic, and cerebral blood flow is inhibited by halothane, leading to reduced perfusion of these organs in the face of reduced blood pressure. Coronary autoregulation is largely preserved during halothane anesthesia. Finally, halothane does inhibit hypoxic pulmonary vasoconstriction, which leads to increased perfusion to poorly ventilated regions of the lung and an increased alveolar:arterial oxygen gradient.

Halothane also has significant effects on cardiac rhythm. Sinus bradycardia and atrioventricular rhythms occur frequently during halothane anesthesia but are usu-

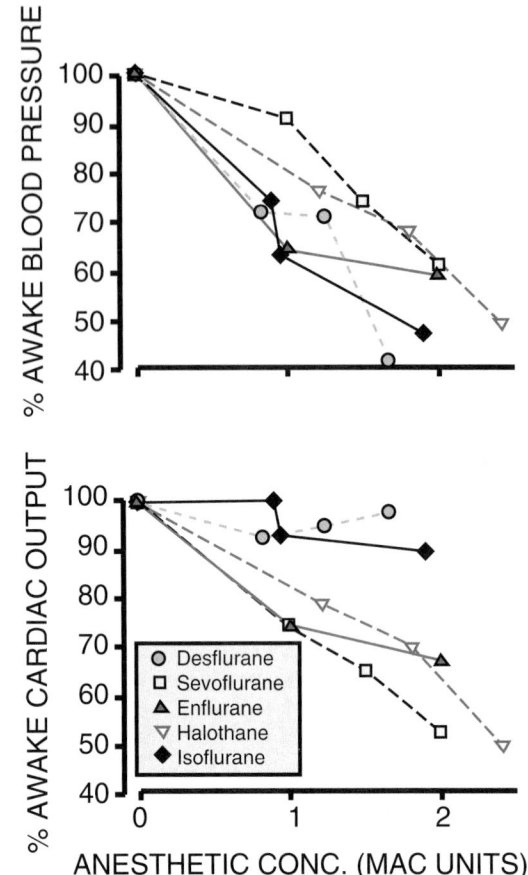

Figure 14–6. Influence of inhalational general anesthetics on the systemic circulation.

While all of the inhalational anesthetics reduce systemic blood pressure in a dose-related manner (top), the lower figure shows that cardiac output is well preserved with isoflurane and desflurane and, therefore, that the causes of hypotension vary with the agent. (Data are from human studies except for sevoflurane, where data are from swine: Bahlman *et al.*, 1972; Cromwell *et al.*, 1971; Weiskopf *et al.*, 1991; Calverley *et al.*, 1978; Stevens *et al.*, 1971; Eger *et al.*, 1970; Weiskopf *et al.*, 1988).

ally benign. These rhythms result mainly from a direct depressive effect of halothane on sinoatrial node discharge. Halothane also can sensitize the myocardium to the arrythmogenic effects of epinephrine (Sumikawa *et al.*, 1983). Premature ventricular contractions and sustained ventricular tachycardia can be observed during halothane anesthesia when exogenous administration or endogenous adrenal production elevates plasma epinephrine levels. Epinephrine-induced arrhythmias during halothane anesthesia are thought to be mediated by a synergistic effect on α_1- and β_1-adrenergic receptors (Hayashi *et al.*, 1988).

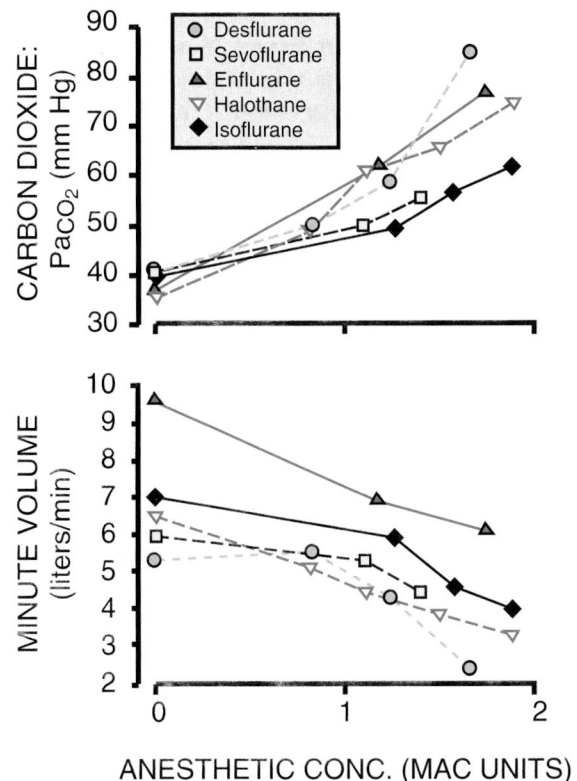

Figure 14–7. Respiratory effects of inhalational anesthetics.

Spontaneous ventilation with all of the halogenated inhalational anesthetics reduces minute volume of ventilation in a dose-dependent manner (lower panel). This results in an increased arterial carbon dioxide tension (top panel). Differences among agents are modest. (Data are from Doi and Ikada, 1987; Lockhart *et al.*, 1991; Munson *et al.*, 1966; Calverley *et al.*, 1978; Fourcade *et al.*, 1971.)

Respiratory System. Spontaneous respiration is rapid and shallow during halothane anesthesia. This produces a decrease in alveolar ventilation resulting in an elevation in arterial carbon dioxide tension from 40 mm Hg to >50 mm Hg at 1 MAC (*see* Figure 14–7). The elevated carbon dioxide does not provoke a compensatory increase in ventilation, because halothane causes a concentration-dependent inhibition of the ventilatory response to carbon dioxide (Knill and Gelb, 1978). This action of halothane is thought to be mediated by depression of central chemoceptor mechanisms. Halothane also inhibits peripheral chemoceptor responses to arterial hypoxemia. Thus, neither hemodynamic (tachycardia, hypertension) nor ventilatory responses to hypoxemia are observed during halothane anesthesia, making it prudent to monitor arterial oxygenation directly. Halothane also is an effective bronchodilator, producing

direct relaxation of bronchial smooth muscle (Yamakage, 1992) and has been effectively used as a treatment of last resort in patients with status asthmaticus (Gold and Helrich, 1970).

Nervous System. Halothane dilates the cerebral vasculature, increasing cerebral blood flow under most conditions. This increase in blood flow can increase intracranial pressure in patients with space-occupying intracranial masses, brain edema, or preexisting intracranial hypertension. For this reason, halothane is relatively contraindicated in patients at risk for elevated intracranial pressure. Halothane also attenuates autoregulation of cerebral blood flow. For this reason, cerebral blood flow can decrease when arterial blood pressure is markedly decreased. Modest decreases in cerebral blood flow generally are well tolerated, because halothane also reduces cerebral metabolic consumption of oxygen.

Muscle. Halothane causes some relaxation of skeletal muscle *via* its central-depressant effects. Halothane also potentiates the actions of nondepolarizing muscle relaxants (curariform drugs; *see* Chapter 9), increasing both their duration of action and the magnitude of their effect. Halothane also is one of the triggering agents for malignant hyperthermia, a syndrome characterized by severe muscle contraction, rapid development of hyperthermia, and a massive increase in metabolic rate in genetically susceptible patients. This syndrome frequently is fatal and is treated by immediate discontinuation of the anesthetic and administration of dantrolene.

Uterine smooth muscle is relaxed by halothane. This is a useful property for manipulation of the fetus (version) in the prenatal period and for delivery of retained placenta postnatally. Halothane, however, does inhibit uterine contractions during parturition, prolonging labor and increasing blood loss. Halothane therefore is not used as an analgesic or anesthetic for labor and vaginal delivery.

Kidney. Patients anesthetized with halothane usually produce a small volume of concentrated urine. This is the consequence of halothane-induced reduction of renal blood flow and glomerular filtration rate; these parameters may be reduced by 40% to 50% at 1 MAC. (Mazze *et al.*, 1963). Halothane-induced changes in renal function are fully reversible and are not associated with long-term nephrotoxicity.

Liver and Gastrointestinal Tract. Halothane reduces splanchnic and hepatic blood flow as a consequence of reduced perfusion pressure, as discussed above. This reduced blood flow has not been shown to produce detrimental effects on hepatic or gastrointestinal function.

Halothane can produce fulminant hepatic necrosis in a small number of patients. This syndrome generally is characterized by fever, anorexia, nausea, and vomiting developing several days after anesthesia and can be accompanied by a rash and peripheral eosinophilia. There is a rapid progression to hepatic failure, with a fatality rate of approximately 50%. This syndrome occurs in about 1 in 10,000 patients receiving halothane and is referred to as *halothane hepatitis* (Subcommittee on the National Halothane Study, 1966). Current thinking is that halothane hepatitis is the result of an immune response to trifluoroacetylated proteins on hepatocytes (*see* "Pharmacokinetics," above).

Isoflurane

Chemistry and Physical Properties. *Isoflurane* (FORANE) is 1-chloro-2,2,2-trifluoroethyl difluoromethyl ether (*see* Figure 14–4). It is a volatile liquid at room temperature and is neither flammable nor explosive in mixtures of air or oxygen.

Pharmacokinetics. Isoflurane has a blood:gas partition coefficient substantially lower than that of halothane or enflurane (*see* Table 14–1). Consequently, induction with isoflurane and recovery from isoflurane are relatively rapid. Changes in anesthetic depth also can be achieved more rapidly with isoflurane than with halothane or enflurane. More than 99% of inhaled isoflurane is excreted unchanged *via* the lungs. Approximately 0.2% of absorbed isoflurane is oxidatively metabolized by cytochrome P450 2E1 (Kharasch *et al.*, 1993). The small amount of isoflurane degradation products produced are insufficient to produce any renal, hepatic, or other organ toxicity. Isoflurane does not appear to be a mutagen, teratogen, or carcinogen (Eger *et al.*, 1978).

Clinical Use. Isoflurane is the most commonly used inhalational anesthetic in the United States. Induction of anesthesia can be achieved in less than 10 minutes with an inhaled concentration of 3% isoflurane in oxygen; this concentration is reduced to 1.5% to 2.5% for maintenance of anesthesia. The use of other drugs such as opioids or nitrous oxide reduces the concentration of isoflurane required for surgical anesthesia.

Side Effects. *Cardiovascular System.* Isoflurane produces a concentration-dependent decrease in arterial blood pressure. Unlike halothane, cardiac output is well maintained with isoflurane, and hypotension is the result of decreased systemic vascular resistance (*see* Figure 14–6). Isoflurane produces vasodilation in most vascular beds, with particularly pronounced effects in skin and muscle. Isoflurane is a potent coronary vasodilator, simultaneously producing increased coronary blood flow and decreased myocardial oxygen consumption. In theory, this makes

isoflurane a particularly safe anesthetic to use for patients with ischemic heart disease. However, concern has been raised that isoflurane may produce myocardial ischemia by inducing "coronary steal" (*i.e.*, the diversion of blood flow from poorly perfused to well-perfused areas) (Buffington *et al.*, 1988). This concern has not been substantiated in subsequent animal and human studies. Patients anesthetized with isoflurane generally have mildly elevated heart rates, and rapid changes in isoflurane concentration can produce transient tachycardia and hypertension. This is the result of direct isoflurane-induced sympathetic stimulation.

Respiratory System. Isoflurane produces concentration-dependent depression of ventilation. Patients spontaneously breathing isoflurane have a normal rate of respiration but a reduced tidal volume, resulting in a marked reduction in alveolar ventilation and an increase in arterial carbon dioxide tension (*see* Figure 14–7). Isoflurane is particularly effective at depressing the ventilatory response to hypercapnia and hypoxia (Hirshman *et al.*, 1977). While isoflurane is an effective bronchodilator, it also is an airway irritant and can stimulate airway reflexes during induction of anesthesia, producing coughing and laryngospasm.

Nervous System. Isoflurane, like halothane, dilates the cerebral vasculature, producing increased cerebral blood flow and the risk of increased intracranial pressure. Isoflurane also reduces cerebral metabolic oxygen consumption. Isoflurane causes less cerebral vasodilation than do either enflurane or halothane, making it a preferred agent for neurosurgical procedures (Drummond *et al.*, 1983). The modest effects of isoflurane on cerebral blood flow can be reversed readily by hyperventilation (McPherson *et al.*, 1989).

Muscle. Isoflurane produces some relaxation of skeletal muscle *via* its central effects. It also enhances the effects of both depolarizing and nondepolarizing muscle relaxants. Isoflurane is more potent than halothane in its potentiation of neuromuscular blocking agents. Isoflurane, like other halogenated inhalational anesthetics, relaxes uterine smooth muscle and is not recommended for analgesia or anesthesia for labor and vaginal delivery.

Kidney. Isoflurane reduces renal blood flow and glomerular filtration rate. This results in a small volume of concentrated urine. Changes in renal function observed during isoflurane anesthesia are rapidly reversed, and there are no long-term renal sequelae or toxicity associated with isoflurane.

Liver and Gastrointestinal Tract. Splanchnic (and hepatic) blood flow is reduced with increasing doses of isoflurane, as systemic arterial pressure decreases. Liver function tests are minimally affected by isoflurane, and there is no described incidence of hepatic toxicity with isoflurane.

Enflurane

Chemical and Physical Properties. *Enflurane* (ETHRANE) is 2-chloro-1,1,2-trifluoroethyl difluoromethyl ether (*see* Figure 14–4). It is a clear colorless liquid at room temperature with a mild, sweet odor. Like other inhalational anesthetics, it is volatile and must be stored in a sealed bottle. It is nonflammable and nonexplosive in mixtures of air or oxygen.

Pharmacokinetics. Because of its relatively high blood:gas partition coefficient, induction of anesthesia and recovery from enflurane are relatively slow (*see* Table 14–1). Enflurane is metabolized to a modest extent, with 2% to 8% of absorbed enflurane undergoing oxidative metabolism in the liver by cytochrome P450 2E1 (Kharasch *et al.,* 1994). Fluoride ions are a by-product of enflurane metabolism, but plasma fluoride levels are low and nontoxic. Patients taking isoniazid exhibit enhanced metabolism of enflurane with significantly elevated serum fluoride concentrations (Mazze *et al.,* 1982).

Clinical Use. Surgical anesthesia can be induced with enflurane in less than 10 minutes with an inhaled concentration of 4% in oxygen. Anesthesia can be maintained with concentrations from 1.5% to 3%. As with other anesthetics, the enflurane concentrations required to produce anesthesia are reduced when it is coadministered with nitrous oxide or opioids. Use of enflurane has decreased substantially in recent years with the introduction of newer inhalational agents with preferable pharmacokinetic and side-effect profiles.

Side Effects. *Cardiovascular System.* Enflurane causes a concentration-dependent decrease in arterial blood pressure. Hypotension is due, in part, to depression of myocardial contractility with some contribution from peripheral vasodilation (*see* Figure 14–6). Enflurane has minimal effects on heart rate and produces neither the bradycardia seen with halothane nor the tachycardia seen with isoflurane.

Respiratory System. The respiratory effects of enflurane are similar to those of halothane. Spontaneous ventilation with enflurane produces a pattern of rapid, shallow breathing. Minute ventilation is markedly decreased, and a Pa_{CO_2} of 60 mm Hg is seen with 1 MAC of enflurane (*see* Figure 14–7). Enflurane produces a greater depression of the ventilatory responses to hypoxia and hypercarbia than do either halothane or isoflurane (Hirshman *et al.,* 1977). Enflurane, like other inhalational anesthetics, is an effective bronchodilator.

Nervous System. Enflurane is a cerebral vasodilator and thus can increase intracranial pressure in some patients. Like other inhalational anesthetics, enflurane reduces cerebral metabolic oxygen consumption. Enflurane has an unusual property of producing electrical seizure activity. High concentrations of enflurane or profound hypocarbia during enflurane anesthesia result in a characteristic high-voltage, high-frequency electroencephalographic (EEG) pattern, which progresses to spike-and-dome complexes. The spike-and-dome pattern can be punctuated by frank seizure activity, which may or may not be accompanied by peripheral motor manifestations of seizure activity. The seizures are self-limited and are not thought to produce permanent damage. Enflurane is not thought to precipitate seizures in epileptic patients. Nonetheless, enflurane is generally not used in patients with seizure disorders.

Muscle. Enflurane produces significant skeletal muscle relaxation in the absence of muscle relaxants. It also significantly enhances the effects of nondepolarizing muscle relaxants. As with other inhalational agents, enflurane relaxes uterine smooth muscle. It thus is not widely used for obstetrical anesthesia.

Kidney. Like other inhalational anesthetics, enflurane reduces renal blood flow, glomerular filtration rate, and urinary output. These effects are rapidly reversed with discontinuation of the drug. Enflurane metabolism produces significant plasma levels of fluoride ions (20 to 40 μM) and can produce transient urinary-concentrating defects following prolonged administration (Mazze *et al.,* 1977). There is scant evidence of long-term nephrotoxicity following enflurane use, and it is safe to use in patients with renal impairment, provided that the depth of enflurane anesthesia and the duration of administration are not excessive.

Liver and Gastrointestinal Tract. Enflurane reduces splanchnic and hepatic blood flow in proportion to reduced arterial blood pressure. Enflurane does not appear to alter liver function or to be hepatotoxic.

Desflurane

Chemistry and Physical Properties. *Desflurane* (SUPRANE) is difluoromethyl 1-fluoro-2,2,2-trifluoromethyl ether (*see* Figure 14–4). It is a highly volatile liquid at room temperature (vapor pressure = 681 mm Hg) and thus must be stored in tightly sealed bottles. Delivery of a precise concentration of desflurane requires the use of a specially heated vaporizer that delivers pure vapor that is then diluted appropriately with other gases (oxygen, air, nitrous oxide). Desflurane is nonflammable and nonexplosive in mixtures of air or oxygen.

Pharmacokinetics. Desflurane has a very low blood:gas partition coefficient (0.42) and also is not very soluble in fat or other peripheral tissues (*see* Table 14–1). For this reason, the alveolar (and blood) concentration rapidly rises to the level of inspired concentration. Indeed, within five minutes of administration, the alveolar concentration reaches 80% of the inspired concentration. This provides for a very rapid induction of anesthesia and for rapid changes in depth of anesthesia following changes in the inspired concentration. Emergence from anesthesia also is very rapid with desflurane. The time to awakening following desflurane is half as long as with halothane or sevoflurane and usually does not exceed 5 to 10 minutes (Smiley *et al.,* 1991).

Desflurane is metabolized to a minimal extent, and more than 99% of absorbed desflurane is eliminated unchanged *via* the lungs. A small amount of absorbed desflurane is oxidatively metabolized by hepatic cytochrome P450 enzymes. Virtually no serum fluoride ions are detectable in serum after desflurane administration, but low concentrations of trifluoroacetic acid are detectable in serum and urine (Koblin *et al.,* 1988).

Clinical Use.   Desflurane is a widely used anesthetic for outpatient surgery because of its rapid onset of action and rapid recovery. Desflurane is irritating to the airway in awake patients and can provoke coughing, salivation, and bronchospasm. Anesthesia therefore usually is induced with an intravenous agent, with desflurane subsequently administered for maintenance of anesthesia. Maintenance of anesthesia usually requires inhaled concentrations of 6% to 8%. Lower concentrations of desflurane are required if it is coadministered with nitrous oxide or opioids.

Side Effects.   *Cardiovascular System.*   Desflurane, like all inhalational anesthetics, causes a concentration-dependent decrease in blood pressure. Desflurane has a very modest negative inotropic effect and produces hypotension primarily by decreasing systemic vascular resistance (Eger, 1994) (*see* Figure 14–6). Cardiac output thus is well preserved during desflurane anesthesia, as is blood flow to the major organ beds (splanchnic, renal, cerebral, coronary). Marked increases in heart rate often are noted during induction of desflurane anesthesia and during abrupt increases in the delivered concentration of desflurane. This tachycardia is transient and is the result of desflurane-induced stimulation of the sympathetic nervous system (Ebert and Muzi, 1993). While the hypotensive effects of some inhalational anesthetics are attenuated as a function of duration of administration, this is not the case with desflurane (Weiskopf *et al.,* 1991).

Respiratory System.   Similar to halothane and enflurane, desflurane causes a concentration-dependent increase in respiratory rate and a decrease in tidal volume. At low concentrations (less than 1 MAC) the net effect is to preserve minute ventilation. At desflurane concentrations greater than 1 MAC, minute ventilation is markedly depressed, resulting in elevated arterial carbon dioxide tension (*see* Figure 14–7) (Lockhart *et al.,* 1991). Patients spontaneously breathing desflurane at concentrations greater than 1.5 MAC will have extreme elevations of arterial carbon dioxide tension and may become apneic. Desflurane, like other

inhalational agents, is a bronchodilator. It is also a strong airway irritant, however, and can cause coughing, breath-holding, laryngospasm, and excessive respiratory secretions. Because of its irritant properties, desflurane is not used for induction of anesthesia.

Nervous System.   Desflurane decreases cerebral vascular resistance and cerebral metabolic oxygen consumption. Under conditions of normocapnia and normotension, desflurane produces an increase in cerebral blood flow and can increase intracranial pressure in patients with poor intracranial compliance. The vasoconstrictive response to hypocapnia is preserved during desflurane anesthesia, and increases in intracranial pressure thus can be prevented by hyperventilation.

Muscle.   Desflurane produces direct skeletal muscle relaxation as well as enhancing the effects of nondepolarizing and depolarizing neuromuscular blocking agents (Caldwell *et al.,* 1991).

Kidney.   Desflurane has no reported nephrotoxicity. This is consistent with its minimal metabolic degradation.

Liver and Gastrointestinal Tract.   Desflurane is not known to affect liver function tests or to cause hepatotoxicity.

Sevoflurane

Chemistry and Physical Properties.   *Sevoflurane* (ULTANE) is fluoromethyl 2,2,2-trifluoro-1-[trifluoromethyl]ethyl ether (*see* Figure 14–4). It is a clear, colorless, volatile liquid at room temperature and must be stored in a sealed bottle. It is nonflammable and nonexplosive in mixtures of air or oxygen.

Pharmacokinetics.   The low solubility of sevoflurane in blood and other tissues provides for rapid induction of anesthesia, rapid changes in anesthetic depth following changes in delivered concentration, and rapid emergence following discontinuation of administration (*see* Table 14–1). Approximately 3% of absorbed sevoflurane is biotransformed. Sevoflurane is metabolized in the liver by cytochrome P450 2E1, with the predominant product being hexafluoroisopropanol (Kharasch *et al.,* 1995). Hepatic metabolism of sevoflurane also produces inorganic fluoride. Serum fluoride concentrations reach a peak shortly after surgery and decline rapidly. Interaction of sevoflurane with soda lime also produces decomposition products. The major product of interest is referred to as compound A and is pentafluoroisopropenyl fluoromethyl ether (*see* "Side Effects"— "Kidney," below) (Hanaki *et al.,* 1987).

Clinical Use.   Sevoflurane has been widely used in Japan for a number of years and is enjoying increasing use in the United States. Sevoflurane is widely used for outpatient anesthesia because of its rapid recovery profile. It also is a useful drug for inhalation induction of anesthesia (particularly in children), because it is not irritating to the airway. Induction of anesthesia is rapidly achieved using inhaled concentrations of 2% to 4% sevoflurane.

Side Effects. *Cardiovascular System.*   Sevoflurane, like all other halogenated inhalational anesthetics, produces a concentration-dependent decrease in arterial blood pressure. This hypotensive effect primarily is due to systemic vasodilation, although sevoflurane also produces a concentration-dependent decrease in cardiac output (*see* Figure 14–6). Unlike isoflurane or desflurane, sevoflurane does not produce tachycardia and thus may be a preferable agent in patients prone to myocardial ischemia.
Respiratory System.   Sevoflurane produces a concentration-dependent reduction in tidal volume and increase in respiratory rate in spontaneously breathing patients. The increased respiratory frequency is not adequate to compensate for reduced tidal volume, with the net effect being a reduction in minute ventilation and an increase in arterial carbon dioxide tension (Doi and Ikeda, 1987) (*see* Figure 14–7). Sevoflurane is not irritating to the airway and is a potent bronchodilator. Because of this combination of properties, sevoflurane is the most effective clinical bronchodilator of the inhalational anesthetics (Rooke *et al.,* 1997).
Nervous System.   Sevoflurane produces effects on cerebral vascular resistance, cerebral metabolic oxygen consumption, and cerebral blood flow that are very similar to those produced by isoflurane and desflurane. While sevoflurane thus can increase intracranial pressure in patients with poor intracranial compliance, the response to hypocapnia is preserved during sevoflurane anesthesia, and increases in intracranial pressure thus can be prevented by hyperventilation.
Muscle.   Sevoflurane produces direct skeletal muscle relaxation as well as enhancing the effects of nondepolarizing and depolarizing neuromuscular blocking agents. Its effects are similar to those of other halogenated inhalational anesthetics.
Kidney.   Controversy has surrounded the potential nephrotoxicity of compound A, the degradation product produced by interaction of sevoflurane with the carbon dioxide absorbant soda lime. There has been a report showing transient biochemical evidence of renal injury in studies with human volunteers but no evidence of permanent renal injury (Eger *et al.,* 1997). Large clinical studies have showed no evidence of increased serum creatinine, blood urea nitrogen, or any other evidence of renal impairment following sevoflurane administration (Mazze *et al.,* 2000). The current recommendation of the U.S. Food and Drug Administration is that sevoflurane be administered with fresh

gas flows of at least 2 liters/minute to minimize accumulation of compound A.

Liver and Gastrointestinal Tract.   Sevoflurane is not known to cause hepatotoxicity or alterations of hepatic function tests.

Nitrous Oxide

Chemical and Physical Properties.   *Nitrous oxide* (dinitrogen monoxide; N_2O) is a colorless, odorless gas at room temperature (*see* Figure 14–4). It is sold in steel cylinders and must be delivered through calibrated flow meters provided on all anesthesia machines. Nitrous oxide is neither flammable nor explosive, but it does support combustion as actively as oxygen does when it is present in proper concentration with a flammable anesthetic or material.

Pharmacokinetics.   Nitrous oxide is very insoluble in blood and other tissues (*see* Table 14–1). This results in rapid equilibration between delivered and alveolar anesthetic concentrations and provides for rapid induction of anesthesia and rapid emergence following discontinuation of administration. The rapid uptake of nitrous oxide from alveolar gas serves to concentrate coadministered halogenated anesthetics; this effect (the "second gas effect") speeds induction of anesthesia. On discontinuation of nitrous oxide administration, nitrous oxide gas can diffuse from blood to the alveoli, diluting oxygen in the lung. This can produce an effect called *diffusional hypoxia.* To avoid hypoxia, 100% oxygen rather than air should be administered when nitrous oxide is discontinued.

Nitrous oxide is almost completely eliminated by the lungs, with some minimal diffusion through the skin. Nitrous oxide is not biotransformed by enzymatic action in human tissue, and 99.9% of absorbed nitrous oxide is eliminated unchanged. Nitrous oxide can be degraded by interaction with vitamin B_{12} in intestinal bacteria. This results in inactivation of methionine synthesis and can produce signs of vitamin B_{12} deficiency (megaloblastic anemia, peripheral neuropathy) following long-term nitrous oxide administration (O'Sullivan *et al.,* 1981). For this reason, nitrous oxide is not used as a chronic analgesic or as a sedative in critical care settings.

Clinical Use.   Nitrous oxide is a weak anesthetic agent and produces reliable surgical anesthesia only under hyperbaric conditions. It does produce significant analgesia at concentrations as low as 20% and usually produces sedation in concentrations between 30% and 80%. It is used frequently in concentrations of approximately 50% to provide analgesia and sedation in outpatient dentistry. Nitrous oxide cannot be used at concentrations above 80%, because this limits the delivery of an adequate amount of oxygen. Because of this limitation, nitrous oxide is used primarily as an adjunct to other inhalational or intravenous anesthetics. Nitrous oxide substantially reduces the requirement for inhalational anesthetics. For example, at 70% nitrous oxide, MAC for other inhalational agents is reduced by about 60%, allowing for lower concentrations of halogenated anesthetics and a lesser degree of side effects.

One major problem with nitrous oxide is that it will exchange with nitrogen in any air-containing cavity in the body. Moreover, nitrous oxide will enter the cavity faster than nitrogen escapes, thereby increasing the volume and/or pressure in this cavity. Examples of air collections that can be expanded by nitrous oxide include a pneumothorax, an obstructed middle ear, an air embolus, an obstructed loop of bowel, an intraocular air bubble, a pulmonary bulla, and intracranial air. Nitrous oxide should be avoided in these clinical settings.

Side Effects. *Cardiovascular System.* Although nitrous oxide produces a negative inotropic effect on heart muscle *in vitro,* depressant effects on cardiac function generally are not observed in patients. This is because of the stimulatory effects of nitrous oxide on the sympathetic nervous system. The cardiovascular effects of nitrous oxide also are heavily influenced by the concomitant administration of other anesthetic agents. When nitrous oxide is coadministered with halogenated inhalational anesthetics, it generally produces an increase in heart rate, arterial blood pressure, and cardiac output. In contrast, when nitrous oxide is coadministered with an opioid, it generally decreases arterial blood pressure and cardiac output. Nitrous oxide also increases venous tone in both the peripheral and pulmonary vasculature. The effects of nitrous oxide on pulmonary vascular resistance can be exaggerated in patients with preexisting pulmonary hypertension (Schulte-Sasse *et al.,* 1982). Nitrous oxide, therefore, is not generally used in patients with pulmonary hypertension.
Respiratory System. Nitrous oxide causes modest increases in respiratory rate and decreases in tidal volume in spontaneously breathing patients. The net effect is that minute ventilation is not significantly changed and arterial carbon dioxide tension remains normal. However, even modest concentrations of nitrous oxide markedly depress the ventilatory response to hypoxia (Yacoub *et al.,* 1975). Thus it is prudent to monitor arterial oxygen saturation directly in patients receiving or recovering from nitrous oxide.
Nervous System. When nitrous oxide is administered alone, it can produce significant increases in cerebral blood flow and intracranial pressure. When nitrous oxide is coadministered with intravenous anesthetic agents, increases in cerebral blood flow are attenuated or abolished. When nitrous oxide is added to a halogenated inhalational anesthetic, its vasodilatory effect on the cerebral vasculature is slightly reduced.

Muscle. Nitrous oxide does not relax skeletal muscle and does not enhance the effects of neuromuscular blocking drugs. Unlike the halogenated anesthetics, nitrous oxide is not a triggering agent for malignant hyperthermia.

Kidney, Liver, and Gastrointestinal Tract. Nitrous oxide is not known to produce any changes in renal or hepatic function and is neither nephrotoxic nor hepatotoxic.

Xenon

Xenon is an inert gas that was first identified as an anesthetic agent in 1951 (Cullen and Gross, 1951). It is not approved for use in the United States and is unlikely to enjoy widespread use, because it is a rare gas that cannot be manufactured and must be extracted from air. This limits the quantities of available xenon gas and renders xenon a very expensive agent. Despite these shortcomings, xenon has properties that make it a virtually ideal anesthetic gas that ultimately may be used in critical situations (Lynch *et al.,* 2000).

Xenon is extremely insoluble in blood and other tissues, providing for rapid induction and emergence from anesthesia (*see* Table 14–1). It is sufficiently potent to produce surgical anesthesia when administered with 30% oxygen. Most importantly, xenon has minimal side effects. It has no effects on cardiac output or cardiac rhythm and is not thought to have a significant effect on systemic vascular resistance. It also does not affect pulmonary function and is not known to have any hepatic or renal toxicity. Finally, xenon is not metabolized at all in the human body. Xenon is an anesthetic that may be available in the future if limitations on its availability and its high cost can be overcome.

ANESTHETIC ADJUNCTS

General anesthetics rarely are given as the sole agent. Rather, anesthetic adjuncts usually are used to augment specific components of anesthesia, permitting lower doses of general anesthetics with fewer side effects. Because they are such an integral part of general anesthetic drug regimens, why and how they are utilized as anesthetic adjuncts will be described briefly here. The detailed pharmacology of each drug is covered in other chapters.

Benzodiazepines

Benzodiazepines (*see* Chapter 17) are commonly used for sedation rather than general anesthesia because of the prolonged amnesia and sedation that may result from anesthetizing doses. As adjuncts, benzodiazepines are used for anxiolysis, amnesia, and sedation prior to induction of anesthesia or for sedation during procedures not requiring general anesthesia. The benzodiazepine most frequently used in the perioperative period is *midazolam* (VERSED) followed distantly by *diazepam* (VALIUM) and *lorazepam*

(ATIVAN). Midazolam is water soluble and is typically administered intravenously but also can be given orally, intramuscularly, or rectally; oral midazolam is particularly useful for sedation of young children. Midazolam produces minimal venous irritation as opposed to diazepam and lorazepam, which are formulated in propylene glycol and are painful on injection, sometimes producing thrombophlebitis. Midazolam has the pharmacokinetic advantage, particularly over lorazepam, of being more rapid in onset and shorter in duration of effect. Sedative doses of midazolam (0.01 to 0.07 mg/kg intravenously) reach peak effect in about 2 minutes and provide sedation for about 30 minutes (Reves *et al.,* 1985). Elderly patients tend to be more sensitive to and have a slower recovery from benzodiazepines (Jacobs *et al.,* 1995); thus, titration of smaller doses in this age group is prudent. Midazolam is hepatically metabolized with a clearance (6 to 11 ml/min per kg) similar to that of methohexital and about 20 and 7 times higher than those of diazepam and lorazepam, respectively (Greenblatt *et al.,* 1981; Reves *et al.,* 1985). Either for prolonged sedation or for general anesthetic maintenance, midazolam is more suitable for infusion than are other benzodiazepines, although its duration of action does significantly increase with prolonged infusions (Figure 14–3). Benzodiazepines reduce both cerebral blood flow and metabolism but at equianesthetic doses are less potent in this respect than are barbiturates. They are effective anticonvulsants and are sometimes given to treat status epilepticus (Modica *et al.,* 1990). Benzodiazepines modestly decrease blood pressure and respiratory drive, occasionally resulting in apnea (Reves *et al.,* 1985). Thus, blood pressure and respiratory rate should be monitored in patients sedated with intravenous benzodiazepines.

Analgesics

With the exception of ketamine, neither parenteral nor currently available inhalational anesthetics are effective analgesics. Thus, analgesics typically are administered with general anesthetics to reduce anesthetic requirement and minimize hemodynamic changes produced by painful stimuli. Nonsteroidal antiinflammatory drugs, including *cyclooxygenase-2 inhibitors* or *acetaminophen,* sometimes provide adequate analgesia for minor surgical procedures. However, because of the rapid and profound analgesia produced, opioids are the primary analgesics used during the perioperative period. *Fentanyl* (SUBLIMAZE), *sufentanil* (SUFENTA), *alfentanil* (ALFENTA), *remifentanil* (ULTIVA), *meperidine* (DEMEROL), and *morphine* are the major parenteral opioids used in the perioperative period. The primary analgesic activity of each of these drugs is produced

by agonist activity at μ-opioid receptors (Pasternak, 1993). Their order of potency (relative to morphine) is: sufentanil ($1000\times$) > remifentanil ($300\times$) > fentanyl ($100\times$) > alfentanil ($15\times$) > morphine ($1\times$) > meperidine ($0.1\times$) (Clotz and Nahata, 1991; Glass *et al.,* 1993; Martin, 1983). Pharmacological properties of these agents are discussed in more detail in Chapter 23.

The choice of a perioperative opioid is based primarily on duration of action, given that, at appropriate doses, all produce similar analgesia and side effects. Remifentanil has an ultra-short duration of action (≈10 min) and minimally accumulates with repeated doses or infusion (Glass *et al.,* 1993); it is particularly well suited for procedures that are briefly painful but for which little analgesia is required postoperatively. Single doses of fentanyl, alfentanil, and sufentanil all have similar intermediate durations of action (30, 20, and 15 minutes, respectively), but as for general anesthetics, recovery after prolonged administration varies considerably (Shafer and Varvel, 1991). Fentanyl's duration of action lengthens most with infusion, sufentanil's much less so, and alfentanil's the least. Except for remifentanil, all of the above-mentioned opioids are metabolized in the liver followed by renal and biliary excretion of the metabolites (Tegeder *et al.,* 1999). Remifentanil is hydrolyzed by tissue and plasma esterases (Westmoreland *et al.,* 1993). After prolonged administration, morphine metabolites have significant analgesic and hypnotic activity (Christrup, 1997).

During the perioperative period, opioids often are given at induction to preempt responses to predictable painful stimuli (*e.g.,* endotracheal intubation and surgical incision). Subsequent doses either by bolus or infusion are titrated to the surgical stimulus and the patient's hemodynamic response. Marked decreases in respiratory rate and heart rate with much smaller reductions in blood pressure are seen to varying degrees with all opioids (Bowdle, 1998). Muscle rigidity that can impair ventilation sometimes accompanies larger doses of opioids. The incidence of sphincter of Oddi spasm is increased with all opioids, although morphine appears to be more potent in this regard (Hahn *et al.,* 1988; Thune *et al.,* 1990). After emergence from anesthesia, the frequency and severity of nausea, vomiting, and pruritus are increased by all opioids to about the same degree (Watcha and White, 1992). A useful side effect of meperidine is its ability to reduce shivering, a common problem during emergence from anesthesia (Pauca *et al.,* 1984); other opioids are not as efficacious against shivering perhaps due to less κ-receptor agonist activity. Opioids sometimes are combined with the neuroleptic *droperidol* (*see* Chapter 20) to produce what is termed *neurolept analgesia/anesthesia* (analgesia accompanied by a quiescent state with or without loss of consciousness); the addition of 70% nitrous oxide usually is enough to produce anesthesia. Neurolept anesthesia currently is not a commonly used technique and is usually reserved for clinical scenarios where inhalational and/or other parenteral anesthetics are relatively contraindicated. Finally, opioids often are administered intrathecally and epidurally for management of acute and chronic pain. Neuraxial opioids with or without local anesthetics can provide profound analgesia for many surgical procedures; however, respiratory depression and pruritus usually limit their use to major operations.

Neuromuscular Blocking Agents

The practical aspects of the use of neuromuscular blockers as anesthetic adjuncts are briefly described here. The detailed pharmacology of this drug class is presented in Chapter 9. Depolarizing (*e.g., succinylcholine*) and nondepolarizing muscle relaxants (*e.g., pancuronium*) often are administered during the induction of anesthesia to relax muscles of the jaw, neck, and airway and thereby facilitate laryngoscopy and endotracheal intubation. As mentioned above, barbiturates will precipitate when mixed with muscle relaxants and should be allowed to clear from the intravenous line prior to injection of a muscle relaxant. Following induction, continued muscle relaxation is desirable for many procedures to aid surgical exposure and/or to provide additional insurance of immobility. Of course, muscle relaxants are not by themselves anesthetics and should not be used in lieu of adequate anesthetic depth. The action of nondepolarizing muscle relaxants is usually antagonized, once muscle paralysis is no longer desired, with an acetylcholine esterase inhibitor such as neostigmine or edrophonium (*see* Chapter 8) combined with a muscarinic receptor antagonist (*see* Chapter 7) (*e.g.,* glycopyrrolate or atropine to offset the muscarinic activation of the esterase inhibitors). Other than histamine release by some agents, nondepolarizing muscle relaxants have little in the way of side effects. However, succinylcholine has multiple serious side effects (bradycardia, hyperkalemia, severe myalgia) including induction of malignant hyperthermia in susceptible individuals (*see* Chapter 9).

PROSPECTUS

Two drug classes, α_2-adrenergic receptor agonists and neurosteroids, appear to hold great promise for providing

new anesthetics. Currently, the α_2-receptor agonist *clonidine* is being used as an anesthetic adjunct for its sedative and analgesic actions, but its role has been limited by cardiovascular side effects that include bradycardia and hypotension (Hayashi and Maze, 1993). Newer α_2-receptor agonists have been under investigation, and recently *dexmedetomidine* (PRECEDEX) has been approved in the United States for sedation in the intensive care unit (ICU). When used alone, dexmedetomidine, like clonidine, does not reliably provide general anesthesia. However, dexmedetomidine can reduce the MAC of inhalational anesthetics by as much as 90%, a property referred to as *anesthetic sparing* (Aho *et al.,* 1992). Thus, α_2-receptor agonists allow a reduction in the amount of anesthetic and opioids needed to maintain the anesthetized state, perhaps resulting in a more rapid recovery with fewer side effects. Moreover unlike other anesthetics, α_2-receptor agonists can be antagonized specifically by agents such as *atipamezole* (Karhuvaara *et al.,* 1991); this offers the possibility of an immediate and predictable emergence from anesthesia. Sedation of intensive-care-unit patients by dexmedotomidine (0.2 to 0.7 mg/kg per hour) has the advantage of causing less respiratory depression than do opioids and benzodiazepines; however, infusions of longer than 24 hours are not recommended because of the potential for rebound hypertension.

For some time, certain steroids have been known to produce sedation and anesthesia. In 1971, the neurosteroid *alphaxalone* (ALTHESIN) was approved in Europe for use as a parenteral anesthetic but was subsequently withdrawn from the market because of several severe anaphylactic reactions to the cremaphor EL formulation (Moneret-Vautrin *et al.,* 1983; Tachon *et al.,* 1983). No neurosteroid has been approved subsequently for general anesthesia. Nevertheless, neurosteroids have several properties that make them potentially useful parenteral anesthetics, and newer agents have been examined in clinical trials (Gray *et al.,* 1992; Powell *et al.,* 1992). *Pregnanolone* is capable of providing general anesthesia when used as the sole anesthetic drug and produces minimal pain on injection. It appears to have somewhat less cardiovascular side effects than do barbiturates or propofol (Van Hemelrijck *et al.,* 1994). However, recovery after induction with pregnanolone is significantly slower than after propofol. Developing new neurosteroid agonists and antagonists and understanding their mechanism of action are active areas of research in the quest for an ideal anesthetic agent (Covey *et al.,* 2000; Wittmer *et al.,* 1996).

BIBLIOGRAPHY

Abboud, T.K., Zhu, J., Richardson, M., Peres Da Silva, E., and Donovan, M. Intravenous propofol vs thiamylal-isoflurane for caesarean section, comparative maternal and neonatal effects. *Acta. Anaesthesiol. Scand.,* **1995,** *39*:205–209.

Aho, M., Erkola, O., Kallio, A., Scheinin, H., and Korttila, K. Dexmedetomidine infusion for maintenance of anesthesia in patients undergoing abdominal hysterectomy. *Anesth. Analg.,* **1992,** *75*:940–946.

Allolio, B., Dorr, H., Stuttmann, R., Knorr, D., Engelhardt, D., and Winkelmann, W. Effect of a single bolus of etomidate upon eight major corticosteroid hormones and plasma ACTH. *Clin. Endocrinol. (Oxf.),* **1985,** *22*:281–286.

Anis, N.A., Berry, S.C., Burton, N.R., and Lodge, D. The dissociative anaesthetics, ketamine and phencyclidine, selectively reduce excitation of central mammalian neurons by *N*-methyl aspartate. *Br. J. Pharmacol.,* **1983,** *79*:565–575.

Antognini, J.F., and Schwartz, K. Exaggerated anesthetic requirements in the preferentially anesthetized brain. *Anesthesiology,* **1993,** *79*:1244–1249.

Arden, J.R., Holley, F.O., and Stanski, D.R. Increased sensitivity to etomidate in the elderly: initial distribution versus altered brain response. *Anesthesiology,* **1986,** *65*:19–27.

Aun, C.S., Short, S.M., Leung, D.H., and Oh, T.E. Induction dose-response of propofol in unpremedicated children. *Br. J. Anaesth.,* **1992,** *68*:64–67.

Bahlman, S.H., Eger, E.I. II, Halsey, M.J., Stevens, W.C., Shakespeare, T.F., Smith, N.T., Cromwell, T.H., and Fourcade, H. The cardiovascular effects of halothane in man during spontaneous ventilation. *Anesthesiology,* **1972,** *36*:494–502.

Belelli, D., Lambert, J.J., Peters, J.A., Wafford, K., and Whiting, P.J. The interaction of the general anesthetic etomidate with the gammaaminobutyric acid type A receptor is influenced by a single amino acid. *Proc. Natl. Acad. Sci. U.S.A.,* **1997,** *94*:11031–11036.

Belopavlovic, M., and Buchthal, A. Modification of ketamine-induced intracranial hypertension in neurosurgical patients by pretreatment with midazolam. *Acta. Anaesthesiol. Scand.,* **1982,** *26*:458–462.

Bennett, S.N., McNeil, M.M., Bland, L.A., Arduino, M.J., Villarino, M.E., Perrotta, D.M., Burwen, D.R., Welbel, S.F., Pegues, D.A., Stroud, L., Zeitz, P.S., and Jarvis, W.R. Postoperative infections traced to contamination of an intravenous anesthetic, propofol. *N. Engl. J. Med.,* **1995,** *333*:147–154.

Beskow, A., Werner, O., and Westrin, P. Faster recovery after anesthesia in infants after intravenous induction with methohexital instead of thiopental. *Anesthesiology,* **1995,** *83*:976–979.

Blouin, R.T., Conard, P.F., and Gross, J.B. Time course of ventilatory depression following induction doses of propofol and thiopental. *Anesthesiology,* **1991,** *75*:940–944.

Brand, L., Mark, L.C., Snell, M.M., Vrindten, P., and Dayton, P.G. Physiologic disposition of methohexital in man. *Anesthesiology,* **1963,** *24*:331–335.

Bristow, J.D., Prys-Roberts, C., Fisher, A., Pickering, T.G., and Sleight, P. Effects of anesthesia on baroreflex control of heart rate in man. *Anesthesiology,* **1969,** *31*:422–428.

Broadie, B.B., Mark, L.C., Papper, E.M., Lief, P.A., Bernstein, E., and Rovenstine, E.A. The fate of thiopental in man and a method for its estimation in biological material. *J. Pharmacol. Exp. Ther.,* **1950,** *98*:85–96.

Buffington, C.W., Davis, K.B., Gillespie, S., and Pettinger, M. The prevalence of steal-prone anatomy in patients with coronary artery disease: an analysis of the Coronary Artery Surgery Studio Registry. *Anesthesiology,* **1988,** *69*:721–727.

Burch, P.G., and Stanski, D.R. The role of metabolism and protein binding in thiopental anesthesia. *Anesthesiology,* **1983,** *58*:146–152.

Caldwell, J.E., Laster, M.J., Magorian, T., Heier, T., Yasuda, N., Lynam, D.P., Eger, E.I. II, and Weiskopf, R.B. The neuromuscular effects of desflurane, alone and combined with pancuronium or succinylcholine in humans. *Anesthesiology,* **1991,** *74*:412–418.

Calverley, R.K., Smith, N.T., Jones, C.W., Prys-Roberts, C., and Eger, E.I. II. Ventilatory and cardiovascular effects of enflurane anesthesia during spontaneous ventilation in man. *Anesth. Analg.,* **1978,** *57*:610–618.

Chan, H.N., Morgan, D.J., Crankshaw, D.P., and Boyd, M.D. Pentobarbitone formation during thiopentone infusion. *Anaesthesia,* **1985,** *40*:1155–1159.

Cheng, S.C., and Brunner, E.A. Inducing anesthesia with a GABA analog, THIP. *Anesthesiology,* **1985,** *63*:147–151.

Christensen, H.D., and Lee, I.S. Anesthetic potency and acute toxicity of optically active disubstituted barbituric acids. *Toxicol. Appl. Pharmacol.,* **1973,** *26*:495–503.

Claeys, M.A., Gepts, E., and Camu, F. Haemodynamic changes during anaesthesia induced and maintained with propofol. *Br. J. Anaesth.,* **1988,** *60*:3–9.

Clarke, R.S., Dundee, J.W., Barron, D.W., and McArdle, L. Clinical studies of induction agents. XVXVI. The relative potencies of thiopentone, methohexitone and propanidid. *Br. J. Anaesth.,* **1968,** *40*:593–601.

Clements, J.A., and Nimmo, W.S. Pharmacokinetics and analgesic effect of ketamine in man. *Br. J. Anaesth.,* **1981,** *53*:27–30.

Colvin, M.P., Savege, T.M., Newland, P.E., Weaver, E.J., Waters, A.F., Brookes, J.M., and Inniss, R. Cardiorespiratory changes following induction of anaesthesia with etomidate in patients with cardiac disease. *Br. J. Anaesth.,* **1979,** *51*:551–556.

Covey, D.F., Nathan, D., Kalkbrenner, M., Nilsson, K.R., Hu, Y., Zorumski, C.F., and Evers, A.S. Enantioselectivity of pregnanolone-induced gamma-aminobutyric acid(A) receptor modulation and anesthesia. *J. Pharmacol. Exp. Ther.,* **2000,** *293*:1009–1016.

Criado, A., Maseda, J., Navarro, E., Escarpa, A., and Avello, F. Induction of anaesthesia with etomidate: haemodynamic study of 36 patients. *Br. J. Anaesth.,* **1980,** *52*:803–806.

Cromwell, T.H., Stevens, W.C., Eger, E.I. II, Shakespeare, T.F., Halsey, M.J., Bahlman, S.H., and Fourcade, H.E. The cardiovascular effects of compound 469 (Forane) during spontaneous ventilation and CO_2 challenge in man. *Anesthesiology,* **1971,** *35*:17–25.

Cullen, S.C., and Gross, E.G. The anesthetic properties of xenon in animals and human beings, with additional observations on krypton. *Science,* **1951,** *113*:580–582.

Dayton, P.G., Stiller, R.L., Cook, D.R., and Perel, J.M. The binding of ketamine to plasma proteins: emphasis on human plasma. *Eur. J. Clin. Pharmacol.,* **1983,** *24*:825–831.

de Sousa, S.L., Dickinson, R., Lieb, W.R., and Franks, N.P. Contrasting synaptic actions of the inhalational general anesthetics isoflurane and xenon. *Anesthesiology,* **2000,** *92*:1055–1066.

Doenicke, A. Etomidate, a new intravenous hypnotic. *Acta. Anaesthesiol. Belg.,* **1974,** *25*:307–315.

Doenicke, A., Lorenz, W., Beigl, R., Bezecny, H., Uhlig, G., Kalmar, L., Praetorius, B., and Mann, G. Histamine release after intravenous application of short-acting hypnotics. A comparison of etomidate, Althesin (CT1341) and propanidid. *Br. J. Anaesth.,* **1973,** *45:*1097–1104.

Dohi, S., and Naito, H. Intraarterial injection of 2.5% thiamylal does cause gangrene. *Anesthesiology,* **1983,** *59:*154.

Doi, M., and Ikeda, K. Respiratory effects of sevoflurane. *Anesth. Analg.,* **1987,** *66:*241–244.

Doze, V.A., Westphal, L.M., and White, P.F. Comparison of propofol with methohexital for outpatient anesthesia. *Anesth. Analg.,* **1986,** *65:*1189–1195.

Drummond, J.C., Todd, M.M., Toutant, S.M., and Shapiro, H.M. Brain surface protrusion during enflurane, halothane, and isoflurane anesthesia in cats. *Anesthesiology,* **1983,** *59:*288–293.

Drummond, J.C., Cole, D.J., Patel, P.M., and Reynolds, L.W. Focal cerebral ischemia during anesthesia with etomidate, isoflurane, or thiopental: a comparison of the extent of cerebral injury. *Neurosurgery,* **1995,** *37:*742–748; discussion 748–749.

Dundee, J.W., Hassard, T.H., McGowan, W.A., and Henshaw, J. The "induction" dose of thiopentone. A method of study and preliminary illustrative results. *Anaesthesia,* **1982,** *37:*1176–1184.

Dundee, J.W., and Lilburn, J.K. Ketamine-lorazepam. Attenuation of psychic sequelae of ketamine by lorazepam. *Anaesthesia,* **1978,** *33:*312–314.

Dundee, J.W., McCleery, W.N., and McLoughlin, G. The hazard of thiopental anaesthesia in porphyria. *Anesth. Analg.,* **1962,** *41:*567–574.

Dundee, J.W., Robinson, F.P., McCollum, J.S., and Patterson, C.C. Sensitivity to propofol in the elderly. *Anaesthesia,* **1986,** *41:*482–485.

Dwyer, R., Bennett, H.L., Eger, E.I. II, and Peterson, N. Isoflurane anesthesia prevents unconscious learning. *Anesth. Analg.,* **1992,** *75:*107–112.

Eames, W.O., Rooke, G.A., Wu, R.S., and Bishop, M.J. Comparison of the effects of etomidate, propofol, and thiopental on respiratory resistance after tracheal intubation. *Anesthesiology,* **1996,** *84:*1307–1311.

Ebert, T.J., and Muzi, M. Sympathetic hyperactivity during desflurane anesthesia in healthy volunteers. A comparison with isoflurane. *Anesthesiology,* **1993,** *79:*444–453.

Eger, E.I. II, Koblin, D.D., Bowland, T., Ionescu, P., Laster, M.J., Fang, Z., Gong, D., Sonner, J., and Weiskopf, R.B. Nephrotoxicity of sevoflurane versus desflurane anesthesia in volunteers. *Anesth. Analg.,* **1997,** *84:*160–168.

Eger, E.I. II, Smith, N.T., Stoelting, R.K., Cullen, D.J., Kadis, L.B., and Whitcher, C.E. Cardiovascular effects of halothane in man. *Anesthesiology,* **1970,** *2:*396–409.

Eger, E.I. II, White, A.E., Brown, C.L., Biava, C.G., Corbett, T.H., and Stevens, W.C. A test of the carcinogenicity of enflurane, isoflurane, halothane, methoxyflurane, and nitrous oxide in mice. *Anesth. Analg.,* **1978,** *57:*678–694.

Elder, J.D., Nagano, S.M., Eastwood, D.W., and Harnagel, D. Circulatory changes associated with thiopental anesthesia in man. *Anesthesiology,* **1955,** *16:*394–400.

Etsten, B., and Li, T.H. Hemodynamic changes during thiopental anesthesia in humans: cardiac output, stroke volume, total peripheral resistance, and intrathoracic blood volume. *J. Clin. Invest.,* **1955,** *34:*500–510.

Fieldman, E.J., Ridley, R.W., and Wood, E.H. Hemodynamic studies during thiopental sodium and nitrous oxide anesthesia in humans. *Anesthesiology,* **1955,** *16:*473–489.

Flood, P., Ramirez-Latorre, J., and Role, L. Alpha 4 beta 2 neuronal nicotinic acetylcholine receptors in the central nervous system are inhibited by isoflurane and propofol, but alpha 7-type nicotinic acetylcholine receptors are unaffected. *Anesthesiology,* **1997,** *86:*859–865.

Fourcade, H.E., Stevens, W.C., Larson, C.P. Jr., Cromwell, T.H., Balman, S.H., Hickey, R.F., Halsey, M.J., and Eger, E.I. II. The ventilatory effects of Forane, a new inhaled anesthetic. *Anesthesiology,* **1971,** *35:*26–31.

Fragen, R.J., and Caldwell, N. Comparison of a new formulation of etomidate with thiopental—side effects and awakening times. *Anesthesiology,* **1979,** *50:*242–244.

Fragen, R.J., Avram, M.J., Henthorn, T.K., and Caldwell, N.J. A pharmacokinetically designed etomidate infusion regimen for hypnosis. *Anesth. Analg.,* **1983,** *62:*654–660.

Fragen, R.J., Shanks, C.A., Molteni, A., and Avram, M.J. Effects of etomidate on hormonal responses to surgical stress. *Anesthesiology,* **1984,** *61:*652–656.

Franks, N.P., Dickinson, R., de Sousa, S.L., Hall, A.C., and Lieb, W.R. How does xenon produce anaesthesia? *Nature,* **1998,** *396:*324.

Galloway, P.A., Nicoll, J.M., and Leiman, B.C. Pain reduction with etomidate injection. *Anaesthesia,* **1982,** *37:*352–353.

Gan, T.J., Ginsberg, B., Grant, A.P., and Glass, P.S. Double-blind, randomized comparison of ondansetron and intraoperative propofol to prevent postoperative nausea and vomiting. *Anesthesiology,* **1996,** *85:*1036–1042.

Gardner, A.E., Olson, B.E., and Lichtiger, M. Cerebrospinal-fluid pressure during dissociative anesthesia with ketamine. *Anesthesiology,* **1971,** *35:*226–228.

Ghoneim, M.M., and Pandya, H. Plasma protein binding of thiopental in patients with impaired renal or hepatic function. *Anesthesiology,* **1975,** *42:*545–549.

Gin, T., Mainland, P., Chan, M.T., and Short, T.G. Decreased thiopental requirements in early pregnancy. *Anesthesiology,* **1997,** *86:*73–78.

Glass, P.S., Hardman, D., Kamiyama, Y., Quill, T.J., Marton, G., Donn, K.H., Grosse, C.M., and Hermann, D. Preliminary pharmacokinetics and pharmacodynamics of an ultra-short-acting opioid: remifentanil (GI87084B). *Anesth. Analg.,* **1993,** *77:*1031–1040.

Gold, M.I., and Helrich, M. Pulmonary mechanics during general anesthesia: V. status asthmaticus. *Anesthesiology,* **1970,** *32:*422–428.

Gooding, J.M., and Corssen, G. Etomidate: an ultrashort-acting nonbarbiturate agent for anesthesia induction. *Anesth. Analg.,* **1976,** *55:*286–289.

Gooding, J.M., and Corssen, G. Effect of etomidate on the cardiovascular system. *Anesth. Analg.,* **1977,** *56:*717–719.

Gooding, J.M., Weng, J.T., Smith, R.A., Berninger, G.T., and Kirby, R.R. Cardiovascular and pulmonary responses following etomidate induction of anesthesia in patients with demonstrated cardiac disease. *Anesth. Analg.,* **1979,** *58:*40–41.

Gray, A.T., Winegar, B.D., Leonoudakis, D.J., Forsayeth, J.R., and Yost, C.S. TOK1 is a volatile anesthetic stimulated K^+ channel. *Anesthesiology,* **1998,** *88:*1076–1084.

Gray, H.S., Holt, B.L., Whitaker, D.K., and Eadsforth, P. Preliminary study of a pregnanolone emulsion (Kabi 2213) for i.v. induction of general anaesthesia. *Br. J. Anaesth.,* **1992,** *68:*272–276.

Gross, J.B., Zebrowski, M.E., Carel, W.D., Gardner, S., and Smith, T.C. Time course of ventilatory depression after thiopental and midazolam in normal subjects and in patients with chronic obstructive pulmonary disease. *Anesthesiology,* **1983,** *58:*540–544.

Grounds, R.M., Twigley, A.J., Carli, F., Whitwam, J.G., and Morgan, M. The haemodynamic effects of intravenous induction. Comparison of the effects of thiopentone and propofol. *Anaesthesia,* **1985,** *40:*735–740.

Grounds, R.M., Maxwell, D.L., Taylor, M.B., Aber, V., and Royston, D. Acute ventilatory changes during i.v. induction of anaesthesia with thiopentone or propofol in man. Studies using inductance plethysmography. *Br. J. Anaesth.,* **1987,** *59:*1098–1102.

Gruenke, L.D., Konopka, K., Koop, D.R., and Waskell, L.A. Characterization of halothane oxidation by hepatic microsomes and purified cytochromes P-450 using a gas chromatographic mass spectrometric assay. *J. Pharmacol. Exp. Ther.,* **1988,** *246:*454–459.

Guo, J., White, J.A., and Batjer, H.H. Limited protective effects of etomidate during brain stem ischemia in dogs. *J. Neurosurg.,* **1995,** *82:*278–283.

Hadzija, B.W., and Lubarsky, D.A. Compatibility of etomidate, thiopental sodium, and propofol injections with drugs commonly administered during induction of anesthesia. *Am. J. Health Syst. Pharm.,* **1995,** *52:*997–999.

Hahn, M., Baker, R., and Sullivan, S. The effect of four narcotics on cholecystokinin octapeptide stimulated gallbladder contraction. *Aliment. Pharmacol. Ther.,* **1988,** *2:*129–134.

Hales, T.G., and Lambert, J.J. Modulation of the $GABA_A$ receptor by propofol. *Br. J. Pharmacol.,* **1988,** *93:*84P.

Hanaki, C., Fujii, K., Morio, M., and Tashima, T. Decomposition of sevoflurane by soda lime. *Hiroshima J. Med. Sci.,* **1987,** *36:*61–67.

Hayashi, Y., Sumikawa, K., Tashiro, C., Yamatodani, A., and Yoshiya, I. Arrhythmogenic threshold of epinephrine during sevoflurane, enflurane, and isoflurane anesthesia in dogs. *Anesthesiology,* **1988,** *69:*145–147.

Hebron, B.S., Edbrooke, D.L., Newby, D.M., and Mather, S.J. Pharmacokinetics of etomidate associated with prolonged i.v. infusion. *Br. J. Anaesth.,* **1983,** *55:*281–287.

Heykants, J.J., Meuldermans, W.E., Michiels, L.J., Lewi, P.J., and Janssen, P.A. Distribution, metabolism and excretion of etomidate, a short-acting hypnotic drug, in the rat. Comparative study of (*R*)-(+)-(−)-Etomidate. *Arch. Int. Pharmacodyn. Ther.,* **1975,** *216:*113–129.

Hirshman, C.A., McCullough, R.E., Cohen, P.J., and Weil, J.V. Hypoxic ventilatory drive in dogs during thiopental, ketamine, or pentobarbital anesthesia. *Anesthesiology,* **1975,** *43:*628–634.

Hirshman, C.A., McCullough, R.E., Cohen, P.J., and Weil, J.V. Depression of hypoxic ventilatory response by halothane, enflurane and isoflurane in dogs. *Br. J. Anaesth.,* **1977,** *49:*957–963.

Hirshman, C.A., Downes, H., Farbood, A., and Bergman, N.A. Ketamine block of bronchospasm in experimental canine asthma. *Br. J. Anaesth.,* **1979,** *51:*713–718.

Hirshman, C.A., Peters, J., and Cartwright-Lee, I. Leukocyte histamine release to thiopental. *Anesthesiology,* **1982,** *56:*64–67.

Homer, T.D., and Stanski, D.R. The effect of increasing age on thiopental disposition and anesthetic requirement. *Anesthesiology,* **1985,** *62:*714–724.

Hudson, R.J., Stanski, D.R., and Burch, P.G. Pharmacokinetics of methohexital and thiopental in surgical patients. *Anesthesiology,* **1983,** *59:*215–219.

Hughes, M.A., Glass, P.S., and Jacobs, J.R. Context-sensitive half-time in multicompartment pharmacokinetic models for intravenous anesthetic drugs. *Anesthesiology,* **1992,** *76:*334–341.

Hung, O.R., Varvel, J.R., Shafer, S.L., and Stanski, D.R. Thiopental pharmacodynamics. II. Quantitation of clinical and electroencephalographic depth of anesthesia. *Anesthesiology,* **1992,** *77:*237–244.

Jacobs, J.R., Reves, J.G., Marty, J., White, W.D., Bai, S.A., and Smith, L.R. Aging increases pharmacodynamic sensitivity to the hypnotic effects of midazolam. *Anesth. Analg.,* **1995,** *80:*143–148.

Jevtovic-Todorovic, V., Todorovic, S.M., Mennerick, S., Powell, S., Dikranian, K., Benshoff, N., Zorumski, C.F., and Olney, J.W. Nitrous oxide (laughing gas) is an NMDA antagonist, neuroprotectant and neurotoxin. *Nat. Med.,* **1998,** *4:*460–463.

Jonmarker, C., Westrin, P., Larsson, S., and Werner, O. Thiopental requirements for induction of anesthesia in children. *Anesthesiology,* **1987,** *67:*104–107.

Joshi, C., and Bruce, D.L. Thiopental and succinylcholine: action on intraocular pressure. *Anesth. Analg.,* **1975,** *54:*471–475.

Karhuvaara, S., Kallio, A., Salonen, M., Tuominen, J., and Scheinin, M. Rapid reversal of alpha 2-adrenoceptor agonist effects by atipamezole in human volunteers. *Br. J. Clin. Pharmacol.,* **1991,** *31:*160–165.

Kay, B., and Stephenson, D.K. Dose-response relationship for disoprofol (ICI 35868; Diprivan). Comparison with methohexitone. *Anaesthesia,* **1981,** *36:*863–867.

Kenna, J.G., Satoh, H., Christ, D.D., and Pohl, L.R. Metabolic basis of a drug hypersensitivity: antibodies in sera from patients with halothane hepatitis recognize liver neoantigens that contain the trifluoroacetyl group derived from halothane. *J. Pharmacol. Exp. Ther.,* **1988,** *2435:*1103–1109.

Kettler, D., Sonntag, H., Donath, U., Regensburger, D., and Schenk, H.D. [Haemodynamics, myocardial mechanics, oxygen requirement and oxygenation of the human heart during induction of anaesthesia with etomidate]. *Anaesthesist,* **1974,** *23:*116–121.

Kharasch, E.D., and Thummel, K.E. Identification of cytochrome P450 2E1 as the predominant enzyme catalyzing human liver microsomal defluorination of sevoflurane, isoflurane, and methoxyflurane. *Anesthesiology,* **1993,** *79:*795–807.

Kharasch, E.D., Thummel, K.E., Mautz, D., and Bosse, S. Clinical enflurane metabolism by cytochrome P450 2E1. *Clin. Pharmacol. Ther.,* **1994,** *55:*434–440.

Kharasch, E.D., Armstrong, A.S., Gunn, K., Artru, A., Cox, K., and Karol, M.D. Clinical sevoflurane metabolism and disposition. II. The role of cytochrome P450 2E1 in fluoride and hexafluoroisopropanol formation. *Anesthesiology,* **1995,** *82:*1379–1388.

Kirkpatrick, T., Cockshott, I.D., Douglas, E.J., and Nimmo, W.S. Pharmacokinetics of propofol (diprivan) in elderly patients. *Br. J. Anaesth.,* **1988,** *60:*146–150.

Knill, R.L., and Gelb, A.W. Ventilatory responses to hypoxia and hypercapnia during halothane sedation and anesthesia in man. *Anesthesiology,* **1978,** *49:*244–251.

Koblin, D.D., Chortkoff, B.S., Laster, M.J., Eger, E.I. II, Halsey, M.J., and Ionescu, P. Polyhalogenated and perfluorinated compounds that disobey the Meyer-Overton hypothesis. *Anesth. Analg.,* **1994,** *79:*1043–1048.

Koblin, D.D., Eger, E.I. II, Johnson, B.H., Konopka, K., and Waskell, L. I-653 resists degradation in rats. *Anesth. Analg.,* **1988,** *67:*534–538.

Korttila, K., Linnoila, M., Ertama, P., and Hakkinen, S. Recovery and simulated driving after intravenous anesthesia with thiopental, methohexital, propanidid, or alphadione. *Anesthesiology,* **1975,** *43:*291–299.

Kosaka, Y., Takahashi, T., and Mark, L.C. Intravenous thiobarbiturate anesthesia for cesarean section. *Anesthesiology,* **1969,** *31:*489–506.

Larrabee, M.G., and Posternak, J.M. Selective action of anesthetics on synapses and axons in mammalian sympathetic ganglia. *J. Neurophysiol.,* **1952,** *15:*91–114.

Laxenaire, M.C., Mata-Bermejo, E., Moneret-Vautrin, D.A., and Gueant, J.L. Life-threatening anaphylactoid reactions to propofol. *Anesthesiology,* **1992,** *77:*275–280.

Ledingham, I.M., Finlay, W.E.I., Watt, I., and McKee, J.I. Etomidate and adrenocortical function. *Lancet*, **1983**, *1*:1434.

Ledingham, I.M., and Watt, I. Influence of sedation on mortality in critically ill multiple trauma patients. *Lancet*, **1983**, *1*:1270.

Linton, D.M., and Thornington, R.E. Etomidate as a rectal induction agent. Part II. A clinical study in children. *S. Afr. Med. J.*, **1983**, *64*:309–310.

Lockhart, S.H., Rampil, I.J., Yasuda, N., Eger, E.I. II, and Weiskopf, R.B. Depression of ventilation by desflurane in humans. *Anesthesiology*, **1991**, *74*:484–488.

Lodge, D., Anis, N.A., and Burton, N.R. Effects of optical isomers of ketamine on excitation of cat and rat spinal neurons by amino acids and acetylcholine. *Neurosci. Lett.*, **1982**, *29*:281–286.

Lysko, G.S., Robinson, J.L., Casto, R., and Ferrone, R.A. The stereospecific effects of isoflurane isomers *in vivo*. *Eur. J. Pharmacol.*, **1994**, *263*:25–29.

MacIver, M.B., and Roth, S.H. Inhalational anaesthetics exhibit pathway-specific and differential actions on hippocampal synaptic responses *in vitro*. *Br. J. Anaesth.*, **1988**, *60*:680–691.

MacIver, M.B., Mikulec, A.A., Amagasu, S.M., and Monroe, F.A. Volatile anesthetics depress glutamate transmission *via* presynaptic actions. *Anesthesiology*, **1996**, *85*:823–834.

Mascia, M.P., Machu, T.K., and Harris, R.A. Enhancement of homomeric glycine receptor function by long-chain alcohols and anaesthetics. *Br. J. Pharmacol.*, **1996**, *119*:1331–1336.

Mayberg, T.S., Lam, A.M., Matta, B.F., Domino, K.B., and Winn, H.R. Ketamine does not increase cerebral blood flow velocity or intracranial pressure during isoflurane/nitrous oxide anesthesia in patients undergoing craniotomy. *Anesth. Analg.*, **1995**, *81*:84–89.

Mazze, R.I., Callan, C.M., Galvez, S.T., Delgado-Herrera, L., and Mayer, D.B. The effects of sevoflurane on serum creatinine and blood urea nitrogen concentrations: a retrospective, twenty-two-center, comparative evaluation of renal function in adult surgical patients. *Anesth. Analg.*, **2000**, *90*:683–688.

Mazze, R.I., Calverley, R.K., and Smith, N.T. Inorganic fluoride nephrotoxicity: prolonged enflurane and halothane anesthesia in volunteers. *Anesthesiology*, **1977**, *46*:265–271.

Mazze, R.I., Woodruff, R.E., and Heerdt, M.E. Isoniazid-induced enflurane defluorination in humans. *Anesthesiology*, **1982**, *57*:5–8.

Mazze, R.I., Schwartz, F.D., Slocum, H.C., and Barry, K.G. Renal function during anesthesia and surgery. I. The effects of halothane anesthesia. *Anesthesiology*, **1963**, *24*:279–284.

McCollum, J.S., Milligan, K.R., and Dundee, J.W. The antiemetic action of propofol. *Anaesthesia*, **1988**, *43*:239–240.

McCulloch, M.J., and Lees, N.W. Assessment and modification of pain on induction with propofol (Diprivan). *Anaesthesia*, **1985**, *40*:1117–1120.

McMurray, T.J., Robinson, F.P., Dundee, J.W., Riddell, J.G., and McClean, E. A method for producing constant plasma concentration of drugs. Application to methohexitone. *Br. J. Anaesth.*, **1986**, *58*:1085–1090.

McPherson, R.W., Briar, J.E., and Traystman, R.J. Cerebrovascular responsiveness to carbon dioxide in dogs with 1.4% and 2.8% isoflurane. *Anesthesiology*, **1989**, *70*:843–850.

Mennerick, S., Jevtovic-Todorovic, V., Todorovic, S.M., Shen, W., Olney, J.W., and Zorumski, C.F. Effect of nitrous oxide on excitatory and inhibitory synaptic transmission in hippocampal cultures. *J. Neurosci.*, **1998**, *18*:9716–9726.

Meuldermans, W.E., and Heykants, J.J. The plasma protein binding and distribution of etomidate in dog, rat and human blood. *Arch. Int. Pharmacodyn. Ther.*, **1976**, *221*:150–162.

Mihic, S.J., Ye, Q., Wick, M.J., Koltchine, V.V., Krasowski, M.D., Finn, S.E., Mascia, M.P., Valenzuela, C.F., Hanson, K.K., Greenblatt, E.P., Harris, R.A., and Harrison, N.L. Sites of alcohol and volatile anaesthetic action on GABA(A) and glycine receptors. *Nature*, **1997**, *389*:385–389.

Mizobe, T., Maghsoudi, K., Sitwala, K., Tianzhi, G., Ou, J., and Maze, M. Antisense technology reveals the alpha$_{2A}$ adrenoceptor to be the subtype mediating the hypnotic response to the highly selective agonist, dexmedetomidine, in the locus coeruleus of the rat. *J. Clin. Invest.*, **1996**, *98*:1076–1080.

Modica, P.A., and Tempelhoff, R. Intracranial pressure during induction of anaesthesia and tracheal intubation with etomidate-induced EEG burst suppression. *Can. J. Anaesth.*, **1992**, *39*:236–241.

Moneret-Vautrin, D.A., Laxenaire, M.C., and Viry-Babel, F. Anaphylaxis caused by anti-cremophor EL IgG STS antibodies in a case of reaction to althesin. *Br. J. Anaesth.*, **1983**, *55*:469–471.

Morgan, M., Lumley, J., and Whitwam, J.G. Respiratory effects of etomidate. *Br. J. Anaesth.*, **1977**, *49*:233–236.

Munson, E.S., Larson, C.P., Jr., Babad, A.A., Regan, M.J., Buechel, D.R., and Eger, E.I. II. The effects of halothane, fluroxene and cyclopropane on ventilation: a comparative study in man. *Anesthesiology*, **1966**, *27*:716–728.

Newberg, L.A., Milde, J.J., and Michenfelder, J.D. The cerebral metabolic effects of isoflurane at and above concentrations that suppress cortical electrical activity. *Anesthesiology*, **1983**, *59*:23–28.

Nguyen, K.T., Stephens, D.P., McLeish, M.J., Crankshaw, D.P., and Morgan, D.J. Pharmacokinetics of thiopental and pentobarbital enantiomers after intravenous administration of racemic thiopental. *Anesth. Analg.*, **1996**, *83*:552–558.

Nicoll, R.A. The effects of anaesthetics on synaptic excitation and inhibition in the olfactory bulb. *J. Physiol.*, **1972**, *223*:803–814.

Nicoll, R.A., and Madison, D.V. General anesthetics hyperpolarize neurons in the vertebrate central nervous system. *Science*, **1982**, *217*:1055–1057.

Nishina, K., Mikawa, K., Maekawa, N., Takao, Y., and Obara, H. Clonidine decreases the dose of thiamylal required to induce anesthesia in children. *Anesth. Analg.*, **1994**, *79*:766–768.

Nor, N.B., Fox, M.A., Metcalfe, I.R., and Russell, W.J. The taste of intravenous thiopentone. *Anaesth. Intens. Care*, **1996**, *24*:483–485.

Nussmeier, N.A., Arlund, C., and Slogoff, S. Neuropsychiatric complications after cardiopulmonary bypass: cerebral protection by a barbiturate. *Anesthesiology*, **1986**, *64*:165–170.

O'Sullivan, H., Jennings, F., Ward, K., McCann, S., Scott, J.M., and Weir, D.G. Human bone marrow biochemical function and megaloblastic hematopoiesis after nitrous oxide anesthesia. *Anesthesiology*, **1981**, *55*:645–649.

Pagel, P.S., Kampine, J.P., Schmeling, W.T., and Warltier, D.C. Ketamine depresses myocardial contractility as evaluated by the preload recruitable stroke work relationship in chronically instrumented dogs with autonomic nervous system blockade. *Anesthesiology*, **1992**, *76*:564–572.

Patel, A.J., Honore, E., Lesage, F., Fink, M., Romey, G., and Lazdunski, M. Inhalational anesthetics activate two-pore-domain background K$^+$ channels. *Nat. Neurosci.*, **1999**, *2*:422–426.

Pauca, A.L., Savage, R.T., Simpson, S., and Roy, R.C. Effect of pethidine, fentanyl and morphine on post-operative shivering in man. *Acta. Anaesthesiol. Scand.*, **1984**, *28*:138–143.

Perouansky, M., Barnaov, D., Salman, M., and Yaari, Y. Effects of halothane on glutamate receptor–mediated excitatory postsynaptic currents. A patch-clamp study in adult mouse hippocampal slices. *Anesthesiology*, **1995**, *83*:109–119.

Pierce, E.C., Lambertsen, C.J., Deutsch, S., Chase, P.E., Linde, H.W., Dripps, R.D., and Price, H.L. Cerebral circulation and metabolism during thiopental anesthesia and hyperventilation in man. *J. Clin. Invest.,* **1962,** *41*:1664–1671.

Pizov, R., Brown, R.H., Weiss, Y.S., Baranov, D., Hennes, H., Baker, S., and Hirshman, C.A. Wheezing during induction of general anesthesia in patients with and without asthma. A randomized, blinded trial. *Anesthesiology,* **1995,** *82*:1111–1116.

Powell, H., Morgan, M., and Sear, J.W. Pregnanolone: a new steroid intravenous anaesthetic. Dose-finding study. *Anaesthesia,* **1992,** *47*:287–290.

Rampil, I.J. Anesthetic potency is not altered after hypothermic spinal cord transection in rats. *Anesthesiology,* **1994,** *80*:606–610.

Ravussin, P., Guinard, J.P., Ralley, F., and Thorin, D. Effect of propofol on cerebrospinal fluid pressure and cerebral perfusion pressure in patients undergoing craniotomy. *Anaesthesia,* **1988,** *43*(suppl):37–41.

Ravussin, P., and de Tribolet, N. Total intravenous anesthesia with propofol for burst suppression in cerebral aneurysm surgery: preliminary report of 42 patients. *Neurosurgery,* **1993,** *32*:236–240.

Reiz, S., Balfors, E., Friedman, A., Haggmark, S., and Peter, T. Effects of thiopentone on cardiac performance, coronary hemodynamics and myocardial oxygen consumption in chronic ischemic heart disease. *Acta. Anaesthesiol. Scand.,* **1981,** *25*:103–110.

Renou, A.M., Vernhiet, J., Macrez, P., Constant, P., Billerey, J., Khadaroo, M.Y., and Caille, J.M. Cerebral blood flow and metabolism during etomidate anaesthesia in man. *Br. J. Anaesth.,* **1978,** *50*:1047–1051.

Reves, J.G., Lell, W.A., McCracken, L.E. Jr., Kravetz, R.A., and Prough, D.S. Comparison of morphine and ketamine anesthetic technics for coronary surgery: a randomized study. *South Med. J.,* **1978,** *71*:33–36.

Richards, C.D., and White, A.N. The actions of volatile anaesthetics on synaptic transmission in the dentate gyrus. *J. Physiol.,* **1975,** *252*:241–257.

Ries, C.R., and Puil, E. Mechanism of anesthesia revealed by shunting actions of isoflurane on thalamocortical neurons. *J. Neurophysiol.,* **1999,** *81*:1795–1801.

Rooke, G.A., Choi, J.H., and Bishop, M.J. The effect of isoflurane, halothane, sevoflurane and thiopental/nitrous oxide on respiratory resistance after tracheal intubation. *Anesthesiology,* **1997,** *86*:1294–1299.

Schulte-Sasse, U., Hess, W., and Tarnow, J. Pulmonary vascular responses to nitrous oxide in patients with normal and high pulmonary vascular resistance. *Anesthesiology,* **1982,** *57*:9–13.

Schwilden, H., and Stoeckel, H. Effective therapeutic infusions produced by closed-loop feedback control of methohexital administration during total intravenous anesthesia with fentanyl. *Anesthesiology,* **1990,** *73*:225–229.

Shafer, A., Doze, V.A., Shafer, S.L., and White, P.F. Pharmacokinetics and pharmacodynamics of propofol infusions during general anesthesia. *Anesthesiology,* **1988,** *69*:348–356.

Shafer, S.L., and Stanski, D.R. Improving the clinical utility of anesthetic drug pharmacokinetics. *Anesthesiology,* **1992,** *76*:327–330.

Shafer, S.L., and Varvel, J.R. Pharmacokinetics, pharmacodynamics, and rational opioid selection. *Anesthesiology,* **1991,** *74*:53–63.

Shapiro, H.M., Galindo, A., Wyte, S.R., and Harris, A.B. Rapid intraoperative reduction of intracranial pressure with thiopentone. *Br. J. Anaesth.,* **1973,** *45*:1057–1062.

Short, T.G., Galletly, D.C., and Plummer, J.L. Hypnotic and anaesthetic action of thiopentone and midazolam alone and in combination. *Br. J. Anaesth.,* **1991,** *66*:13–19.

Simons, P.J., Cockshott, I.D., Douglas, E.J., Gordon, E.A., Hopkins, K., and Rowland, M. Disposition in male volunteers of a subanaesthetic intravenous dose of an oil in water emulsion of 14C-propofol. *Xenobiotica,* **1988,** *18*:429–440.

Smiley, R.M., Ornstein, E., Matteo, R.S., Pantuck, E.J., and Pantuck, C.B. Desflurane and isoflurane in surgical patients: comparison of emergence time. *Anesthesiology,* **1991,** *74*:425–428.

Sprung, J., Schoenwald, P.K., and Schwartz, L.B. Cardiovascular collapse resulting from thiopental-induced histamine release. *Anesthesiology,* **1997,** *86*:1006–1007.

Stanley, V., Hunt, J., Willis, K.W., and Stephen, C.R. Cardiovascular and respiratory function with CI-581. *Anesth. Analg.,* **1968,** *47*:760–768.

Stanski, D.R., Mihm, F.G., Rosenthal, M.H., and Kalman, S.M. Pharmacokinetics of high-dose thiopental used in cerebral resuscitation. *Anesthesiology,* **1980,** *53*:169–171.

Stevens, W.C., Cromwell, T.H., Halsey, M.J., Eger, E.I. II, Shakespeare, T.F., and Bahlman, S.H. The cardiovascular effects of a new inhalation anesthetic, Forane, in human volunteers at constant arterial carbon dioxide tension. *Anesthesiology,* **1971,** *35*:8–16.

Stoelting, R.K., and Eger, E.I. II. The effects of ventilation and anesthetic solubility on recovery from anesthesia: an *in vivo* and analog analysis before and after equilibration. *Anesthesiology,* **1969,** *30*:290–296.

Stoelting, R.K., Longnecker, D.E., and Eger, E.I. II. Minimum alveolar concentration in man on awakening from methoxyflurane, halothane, ether and fluroxene anesthesia: MAC$_{awake}$. *Anesthesiology,* **1970,** *33*:5–9.

Stullken, E.H. Jr., Milde, J.H., Michenfelder, J.D., and Tinker, J.H. The nonlinear responses of cerebral metabolism to low concentrations of halothane, enflurane, isoflurane, and thiopental. *Anesthesiology,* **1977,** *46*:28–34.

Subcommittee on the National Halothane Study of the Committee on Anesthesia, National Academy of Sciences–National Research Council. Summary of the National Halothane Study. Possible association between halothane anesthesia and postoperative hepatic necrosis. *JAMA,* **1966,** *197*:775–788.

Sumikawa, K., Ishizaka, N., and Suzaki, M. Arrhythmogenic plasma levels of epinephrine during halothane, enflurane, and pentobarbital anesthesia in the dog. *Anesthesiology,* **1983,** *58*:322–325.

Sussman, D.R. A comparative evaluation of ketamine anesthesia in children and adults. *Anesthesiology,* **1974,** *40*:459–464.

Tachon, P., Descotes, J., Laschi-Loquerie, A., Guillot, J.P., and Evreux, J.C. Assessment of the allergenic potential of althesin and its constituents. *Br. J. Anaesth.,* **1983,** *55*:715–717.

Takeshita, H., Okuda, Y., and Sari, A. The effects of ketamine on cerebral circulation and metabolism in man. *Anesthesiology,* **1972,** *36*:69–75.

Taylor, M.B., Grounds, R.M., Mulrooney, P.D., and Morgan, M. Ventilatory effects of propofol during induction of anaesthesia. Comparison with thiopentone. *Anaesthesia,* **1986,** *41*:816–820.

Thomson, M.F., Brock-Utne, J.G., Bean, P., Welsh, N., and Downing, J.W. Anaesthesia and intra-ocular pressure: a comparative of total intravenous anaesthesia using etomidate with conventional inhalation anaesthesia. *Anaesthesia,* **1982,** *37*:758–761.

Thune, A., Baker, R.A., Saccone, G.T., Owen, H., and Toouli, J. Differing effects of pethidine and morphine on human sphincter of Oddi motility. *Br. J. Surg.,* **1990,** *77*:992–995.

Tomlin, S.L., Jenkins, A., Lieb, W.R., and Franks, N.P. Stereoselective effects of etomidate optical isomers on gamma-aminobutyric acid type A receptors and animals. *Anesthesiology*, **1998**, *88*:708–717.

Tovell, R.M., Anderson, C.C., Sadove, M.S., Artusio, J.F., Papper, E.M., Coakley, C.S., Hudon, F.H., Smith, S.M., and Thomas, G.J. A comparative clinical and statistical study of thiopental and thiamylal in human anesthesia. *Anesthesiology*, **1955**, *16*:910–926.

Vandesteene, A., Trempont, V., Engelman, E., Deloof, T., Focroul, M., Schoutens, A., and de Rood, M. Effect of propofol on cerebral blood flow and metabolism in man. *Anaesthesia*, **1988**, *43*(suppl):42–43.

Van Dyke, R.A., Baker, M.T., Jansson, I., and Schenkman, J. Reductive metabolism of halothane by purified cytochrome P-450. *Biochem. Pharmacol.*, **1988**, *37*:2357–2361.

Van Hemelrijck, J., Muller, P., Van Aken, H., and White, P.F. Relative potency of eltanolone, propofol, and thiopental for induction of anesthesia. *Anesthesiology*, **1994**, *80*:36–41.

van Swinderen, B., Saifee, O., Shebester, L., Roberson, R., Nonet, M.L., and Crowder, C.M. A neomorphic syntaxin mutation blocks volatile-anesthetic action in *Caenorhabditis elegans*. *Proc. Natl. Acad. Sci. U.S.A.*, **1999**, *96*:2479–2484.

Veroli, P., O'Kelly, B., Bertrand, F., Trouvin, J.H., Farinotti, R., and Ecoffey, C. Extrahepatic metabolism of propofol in man during the anhepatic phase of orthotopic liver transplantation. *Br. J. Anaesth.*, **1992**, *68*:183–186.

Violet, J.M., Downie, D.L., Nakisa, R.C., Lieb, W.R., and Franks, N.P. Differential sensitivities of mammalian neuronal and muscle nicotinic acetylcholine receptors to general anesthetics. *Anesthesiology*, **1997**, *86*:866–874.

Wada, D.R., Bjorkman, S., Ebling, W.F., Harashima, H., Harapat, S.R., and Stanski, D.R. Computer simulation of the effects of alterations in blood flows and body composition on thiopental pharmacokinetics in humans. *Anesthesiology*, **1997**, *87*:884–899.

Wagner, R.L., White, P.F., Kan, P.B., Rosenthal, M.H., and Feldman, D. Inhibition of adrenal steroidogenesis by the anesthetic etomidate. *N. Engl. J. Med.*, **1984**, *310*:1415–1421.

Wang, L.P., Hermann, C., and Westrin, P. Thiopentone requirements in adults after varying pre-induction doses of fentanyl. *Anaesthesia*, **1996**, *51*:831–835.

Wanna, H.T., and Gergis, S.D. Procaine, lidocaine, and ketamine inhibit histamine-induced contracture of guinea pig tracheal muscle *in vitro*. *Anesth. Analg.*, **1978**, *57*:25–27.

Waters, D.J. Intra-arterial thiopentone. A physico-chemical phenomenon. *Anaesthesia*, **1966**, *21*:346–356.

Weiskopf, R.B., Cahalan, M.K., Eger, E.I. II, Yasuda, N., Rampil, I.J., Ionescu, P., Lockhart, S.H., Johnson, B.H., Freire, B., and Kelley, S. Cardiovascular actions of desflurane in normocarbic volunteers. *Anesth. Analg.*, **1991**, *73*:143–156.

Weiskopf, R.B., Holmes, M.A., Eger, E.I. II., Johnson, B.H., Rampil, I.J., and Brown, J.G. Cardiovascular effects of I653 in swine. *Anesthesiology*, **1988**, *69*:303–309.

Westmoreland, C.L., Hoke, J.F., Sebel, P.S., Hug, C.C. Jr., and Muir, K.T. Pharmacokinetics of remifentanil (GI87084B) and its major metabolite (GI90291) in patients undergoing elective inpatient surgery. *Anesthesiology*, **1993**, *79*:893–903.

Whitacre, M.M., and Ellis, P.P. Outpatient sedation for ocular examination. *Surv. Ophthalmol.*, **1984**, *28*:643–652.

Wittmer, L.L., Hu, Y., Kalkbrenner, M., Evers, A.S., Zorumski, C.F., and Covey, D.F. Enantioselectivity of steroid-induced gamma-aminobutyric acidA receptor modulation and anesthesia. *Mol. Pharmacol.*, **1996**, *50*:1581–1586.

Wulfsohn, N.L., and Joshi, C.W. Thiopentone dosage based on lean body ms. *Br. J. Anaesth.*, **1969**, *41*:516–521.

Wyte, S.R., Shapiro, H.M., Turner, P., and Harris, A.B. Ketamine-induced intracranial hypertension. *Anesthesiology*, **1972**, *36*:174–176.

Yacoub, O., Doell, D., Kryger, M.H., and Anthonisen, N.R. Depression of hypoxic ventilatory response by nitrous oxide. *Anesthesiology*, **1975**, *45*:385–389.

Yamakage, M. Direct inhibitory mechanisms of halothane on canine tracheal smooth muscle contraction. *Anesthesiology*, **1992**, *77*:546–553.

Zacharias, M., Dundee, J.W., Clarke, R.S., and Hegarty, J.E. Effect of preanaesthetic medication on etomidate. *Br. J. Anaesth.*, **1979**, *51*:127–133.

Zeilhofer, H.U., Swandulla, D., Geisslinger, G., and Brune, K. Differential effects of ketamine enantiomers on NMDA receptor currents in cultured neurons. *Eur. J. Pharmacol.*, **1992**, *213*:155–158.

MONOGRAPHS AND REVIEWS

Andrews, P.R., and Mark, L.C. Structural specificity of barbiturates and related drugs. *Anesthesiology*, **1982**, *57*:314–320.

Baldo, B.A., Fisher, M.M., and Harle, D.G. Allergy to thiopentone. *Clin. Rev. Allergy*, **1991**, *9*:295–308.

Batjer, H.H. Cerebral protective effects of etomidate: experimental and clinical aspects. *Cerebrovasc. Brain Metab. Rev.*, **1993**, *5*:17–32.

Bischoff, K.B., and Dedrick, R.L. Thiopental pharmacokinetics. *J. Pharm. Sci.*, **1968**, *57*:1346–1351.

Bowdle, T.A. Adverse effects of opioid agonists and agonist-antagonists in anaesthesia. *Drug Saf.*, **1998**, *19*:173–189.

Bryson, H.M., Fulton, B.R., and Faulds, D. Propofol. An update of its use in anaesthesia and conscious sedation. *Drugs*, **1995**, *50*:513–559.

Chang, T., and Glazko, A.J. Biotransformation and disposition of ketamine. *Int. Anesthesiol. Clin.*, **1974**, *12*:157–177.

Christrup, L.L. Morphine metabolites. *Acta. Anaesthesiol. Scand.*, **1997**, *41*:116–122.

Clarke, R.S. Adverse effects of intravenously administered drugs used in anaesthetic practice. *Drugs*, **1981**, *22*:26–41.

Clotz, M.A., and Nahata, M.C. Clinical uses of fentanyl, sufentanil, and alfentanil. *Clin. Pharm.*, **1991**, *10*:581–593.

Eger, E.I. II. New inhaled anesthetics. *Anesthesiology*, **1994**, *80*:906–922.

Eger, E.I. II. Uptake and distribution. In, *Anesthesia*, 5th ed. (Miller, R.D., ed.) Churchill Livingstone, Philadelphia, **2000**, pp. 74–95.

Franks, N.P., and Lieb, W.R. Molecular and cellular mechanisms of general anaesthesia. *Nature*, **1994**, *367*:607–614.

Giese, J.L., and Stanley, T.H. Etomidate: a new intravenous anesthetic induction agent. *Pharmacotherapy*, **1983**, *3*:251–258.

Greenblatt, D.J., Shader, R.I., Divoll, M., and Harmatz, J.S. Benzodiazepines: a summary of pharmacokinetic properties. *Br. J. Clin. Pharmacol.*, **1981**, *11*(suppl 1):11S–16S.

Hayashi, Y., and Maze, M. Alpha 2 adrenoceptor agonists and anaesthesia. *Br. J. Anaesth.*, **1993**, *71*:108–118.

Kendig, J.J., MacIver, M.B., and Roth, S.H. Anesthetic actions in the hippocampal formation. *Ann. N.Y. Acad. Sci.*, **1991**, *625*:37–53.

Kingston, H.G., and Hirshman, C.A. Perioperative management of the patient with asthma. *Anesth. Analg.*, **1984**, *63*:844–855.

Krasowski, M.D., and Harrison, N.L. General anaesthetic actions on ligand-gated ion channels. *Cell. Mol. Life Sci.*, **1999**, *55*:1278–1303.

Langley, M.S., and Heel, R.C. Propofol. A review of its pharmacodynamic and pharmacokinetic properties and use as an intravenous anaesthetic. *Drugs*, **1988**, *35*:334–372.

Lynch, C. III. Myocardial excitation-contraction coupling. In, *Anesthesia: Biologic Foundations.* (Yaksh, T.L., Lynch, C. III, and Zapol, W.M., eds.) Lippincott-Raven, Philadelphia, **1997,** pp. 1047–1079.

Lynch, C. III, Baum, J., and Tenbrinck, R. Xenon anesthesia. *Anesthesiology,* **2000,** *92*:865–868.

Martin, W.R. Pharmacology of opioids. *Pharmacol. Rev.,* **1983,** *35*:283–323.

Modica, P.A., Tempelhoff, R., and White, P.F. Pro- and anticonvulsant effects of anesthetics. *Anesth. Analg.,* **1990,** *70*:433–444.

Pasternak, G.W. Pharmacological mechanisms of opioid analgesics. *Clin. Neuropharmacol.,* **1993,** *16*:1–18.

Picard, P., and Tramer, M.R. Prevention of pain on injection with propofol: a quantitative systematic review. *Anesth. Analg.,* **2000,** *90*:963–969.

Reves, J.G., Fragen, R.J., Vinik, H.R., and Greenblatt, D.J. Midazolam: pharmacology and uses. *Anesthesiology,* **1985,** *62*:310–324.

Reves, J.G., Glass, P.S.A., and Lubarsky, D.A. Nonbarbiturate intravenous anesthetics: In, *Anesthesia,* 4th ed. (Miller, R.D., ed.) Churchill Livingstone, New York, **1994,** pp. 228–272.

Rosenberg, H., Fletcher, J.E., and Seitman, D. Pharmacogenetics, In, *Clinical Anesthesia,* 3rd ed. (Barash, P.G., Cullen, B.F., and Stoelting, R.K., eds.) Lippincott-Raven, Philadelphia, **1997,** pp. 489–517.

Tegeder, I., Lotsch, J., and Geisslinger, G. Pharmacokinetics of opioids in liver disease. *Clin. Pharmacokinet.,* **1999,** *37*:17–40.

Thornton, J.A. Methohexitone and its application in dental anaesthesia. *Br. J. Anaesth.,* **1970,** *42*:255–261.

Watcha, M.F., and White, P.F. Postoperative nausea and vomiting. Its etiology, treatment, and prevention. *Anesthesiology,* **1992,** *77*:162–184.

White, P.F., Way, W.L., and Trevor, A.J. Ketamine—its pharmacology and therapeutic uses. *Anesthesiology,* **1982,** *56*:119–136.

Acknowledgment

The authors wish to acknowledge Drs. Bryan E. Marshall and David E. Longnecker, the authors of this chapter in the ninth edition of *Goodman and Gilman's The Pharmacological Basis of Therapeutics,* some of whose material has been retained in this edition.

CHAPTER 15

LOCAL ANESTHETICS

William Catterall and Kenneth Mackie

Local anesthetics prevent or relieve pain by interrupting nerve conduction. They bind to a specific receptor site within the pore of the Na⁺ channels in nerves and block ion movement through this pore. In general, their action is restricted to the site of application and rapidly reverses upon diffusion from the site of action in the nerve. The chemical and pharmacological properties of each drug determine its clinical use. Local anesthetics can be administered by a variety of routes, including topical, infiltration, field or nerve block, intravenous regional, spinal, or epidural, as dictated by clinical circumstances. This chapter covers the mechanism of action of various local anesthetics, their therapeutic use and routes of administration, and individual side effects. The frequency and voltage-dependence of local anesthetics also are properties of antiarrhythmic agents, discussed in Chapter 35.

INTRODUCTION TO LOCAL ANESTHETICS

When applied locally to nerve tissue in appropriate concentrations, local anesthetics reversibly block the action potentials responsible for nerve conduction. They act on any part of the nervous system and on every type of nerve fiber. Thus, a local anesthetic in contact with a nerve trunk can cause both sensory and motor paralysis in the area innervated. The necessary practical advantage of the local anesthetics is that their action is reversible at clinically relevant concentrations; their use is followed by complete recovery in nerve function with no evidence of damage to nerve fibers or cells.

History. The first local anesthetic, cocaine, was serendipitously discovered to have anesthetic properties in the late nineteenth century. Cocaine occurs in abundance in the leaves of the coca shrub (*Erythroxylon coca*). For centuries, Andean natives have chewed an alkali extract of these leaves for its stimulatory and euphoric actions. Cocaine was first isolated in 1860 by Albert Niemann. He, like many chemists of that era, tasted his newly isolated compound and noted that it caused a numbing of the tongue. Sigmund Freud studied cocaine's physiological actions, and Carl Koller introduced cocaine into clinical practice in 1884 as a topical anesthetic for ophthalmological surgery. Shortly thereafter, Halstead popularized its use in infiltration and conduction block anesthesia. The many local anesthetics used in clinical practice today all stem from these early observations.

Chemistry and Structure–Activity Relationship. Cocaine is an ester of benzoic acid and the complex alcohol 2-carbomethoxy, 3-hydroxy-tropane (Figure 15–1). Because of its toxicity and

addictive properties (*see* Chapter 24), a search for synthetic substitutes for cocaine began in 1892 with the work of Einhorn and his colleagues. In 1905, this resulted in the synthesis of procaine, which became the prototype for local anesthetics for nearly half a century. The most widely used agents today are procaine, lidocaine, bupivacaine, and tetracaine.

Figure 15–1 shows that the structure of typical local anesthetics contains hydrophilic and hydrophobic moieties that are separated by an intermediate ester or amide linkage. A broad range of compounds containing these minimal structural features can satisfy the requirements for action as local anesthetics. The hydrophilic group usually is a tertiary amine, but it also may be a secondary amine; the hydrophobic moiety must be aromatic. The nature of the linking group determines certain of the pharmacological properties of these agents. For example, local anesthetics with an ester link are hydrolyzed readily by plasma esterases.

The structure–activity relationship and the physicochemical properties of local anesthetics have been reviewed by Courtney and Strichartz (1987). In brief, hydrophobicity increases both the potency and the duration of action of the local anesthetics. This arises because association of the drug at hydrophobic sites enhances the partitioning of the drug to its sites of action and decreases the rate of metabolism by plasma esterases and liver enzymes. In addition, the receptor site for these drugs on Na⁺ channels is thought to be hydrophobic (*see* below), so that receptor affinity for anesthetic agents is increased for more hydrophobic drugs. Hydrophobicity also increases toxicity, so that the therapeutic index actually is decreased for more hydrophobic drugs.

Molecular size also influences the rate of dissociation of local anesthetics from their receptor sites (Courtney and Strichartz, 1987). Smaller drug molecules can escape from the receptor site more rapidly. This characteristic is important in rapidly firing tissues, in which local anesthetics bind during action potentials and dissociate during the period of membrane repolarization. Rapid

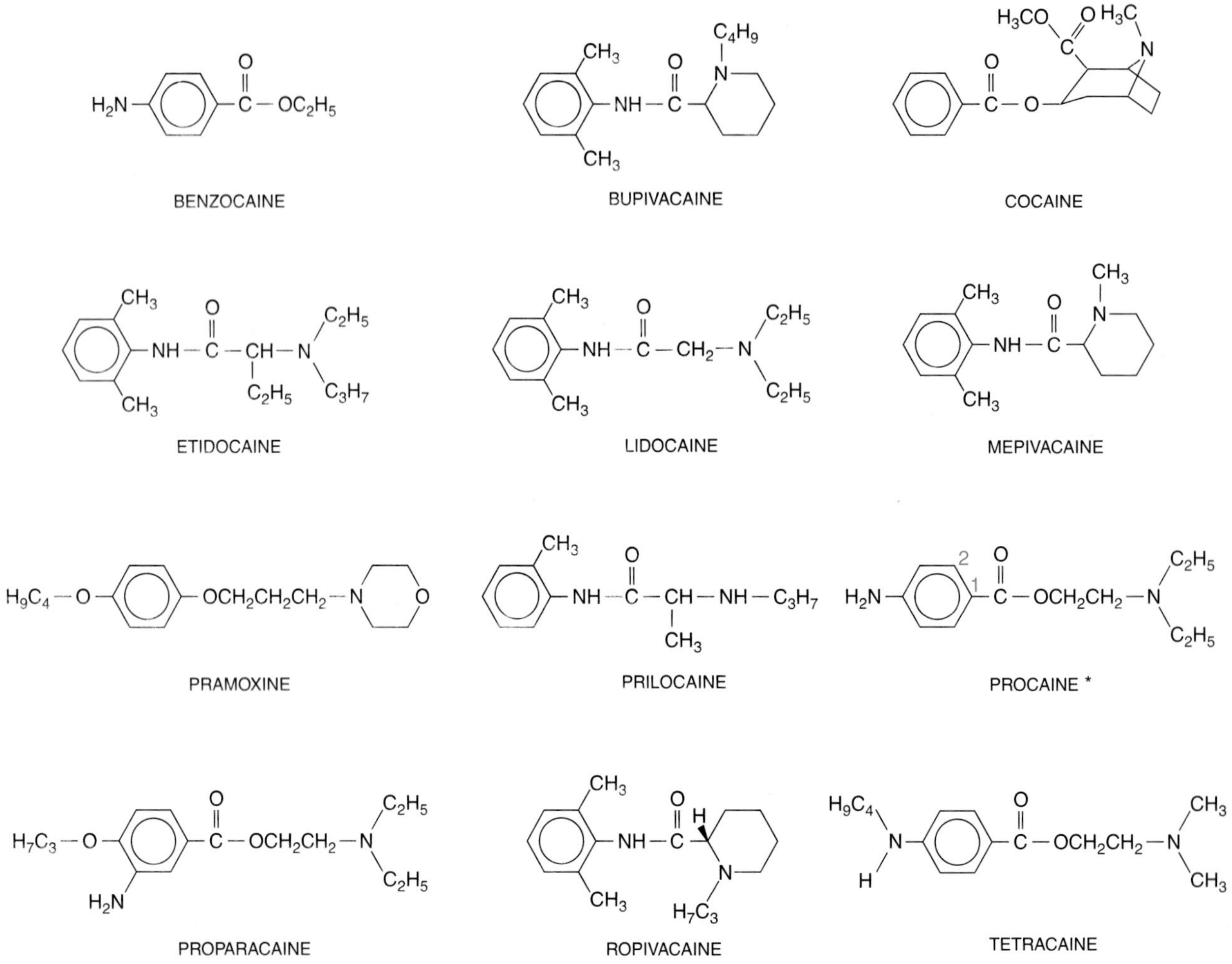

Figure 15–1. Structural formulas of selected local anesthetics.

*Note that chloroprocaine has a chlorine atom in position 2 of the aromatic moiety of procaine.

binding of local anesthetics during action potentials allows the frequency- and voltage-dependence of their action (*see* below).

Mechanism of Action. Local anesthetics prevent the generation and the conduction of the nerve impulse. Their primary site of action is the cell membrane. Conduction block can be demonstrated in squid giant axons from which the axoplasm has been removed.

Local anesthetics block conduction by decreasing or preventing the large transient increase in the permeability of excitable membranes to Na^+ that normally is produced by a slight depolarization of the membrane (*see* Chapter 12 and Strichartz and Ritchie, 1987). This action of local anesthetics is due to their direct interaction with voltage-gated Na^+ channels. As the anesthetic action progressively develops in a nerve, the threshold for electrical excitability

gradually increases, the rate of rise of the action potential declines, impulse conduction slows, and the safety factor for conduction decreases. These factors decrease the probability of propagation of the action potential, and nerve conduction eventually fails.

In addition to Na^+ channels, local anesthetics can bind to other membrane proteins (*see* Butterworth and Strichartz, 1990). In particular, they can block K^+ channels (*see* Strichartz and Ritchie, 1987). However, since the interaction of local anesthetics with K^+ channels requires higher concentrations of drug, blockade of conduction is not accompanied by any large or consistent change in resting membrane potential.

Quaternary analogs of local anesthetics block conduction when applied internally to perfused giant axons of squid, but they are relatively ineffective when applied externally. These observations suggest that the site at which local anesthetics act, at least in their charged form, is accessible only from the inner surface of the membrane (Narahashi and Frazier, 1971; Strichartz and Ritchie, 1987). Therefore, local anesthetics applied externally first must cross the membrane before they can exert a blocking action.

Although a variety of physicochemical models have been proposed to explain how local anesthetics achieve conduction block (*see* Courtney and Strichartz, 1987), it now is generally accepted that the major mechanism of action of these drugs involves their interaction with one or more specific binding sites within the Na^+ channel (*see* Butterworth and Strichartz, 1990). Biochemical, biophysical, and molecular biological investigations during the past two decades have led to a rapid expansion of knowledge about the structure and function of the Na^+ channel and other voltage-gated ion channels (*see* Catterall, 2000, and Chapter 12). The Na^+ channels of the mammalian brain are heterotrimeric complexes of glycosylated proteins with an aggregate molecular size in excess of 300,000 daltons; the individual subunits are designated α (260,000 daltons), β_1 (36,000 daltons), and β_2 (33,000 daltons). The large α subunit of the Na^+ channel contains four homologous domains (I to IV); each domain is thought to consist of six transmembrane segments in α-helical conformation (S1 to S6; *see* Figure 15–2) and an additional, membrane-reentrant pore loop. The Na^+-selective transmembrane pore of the channel is presumed to reside in the center of a nearly symmetrical structure formed by the four homologous domains. The voltage dependence of channel opening is hypothesized to reflect conformational changes that result from the movement of "gating charges" (voltage sensors) in response to changes in the transmembrane potential. The gating charges are located in the S4 transmembrane helix; the S4 helices are both hydrophobic and positively charged, containing lysine or arginine residues at every third position. It is postulated that these residues move perpendicular to the plane of the membrane under the influence of the transmembrane potential, initiating a series of conformational changes in all four domains which leads to the open state of the channel (Catterall, 1988; Figure 15–2).

The transmembrane pore of the Na^+ channel is thought to be surrounded by the S5 and S6 transmembrane helices and the short membrane-associated segments between them, designated SS1 and SS2. Amino acid residues in these short segments are the most critical determinants of the ion conductance and selectivity of the channel.

After it opens, the Na^+ channel inactivates within a few milliseconds due to closure of an inactivation gate. This functional gate is formed by the short intracellular loop of protein that connects homologous domains III and IV (Figure 15–2). The loop folds over the intracellular mouth of the transmembrane pore during the process of inactivation. It may bind to an inactivation gate "receptor" formed by the intracellular mouth of the pore.

Amino acid residues that are important for local anesthetic binding are found in the S6 segment in domain IV (Ragsdale *et al.*, 1994). Hydrophobic amino acid residues near the center and the intracellular end of the S6 segment may interact directly with bound local anesthetics (Figure 15–3). Experimental mutation of a large hydrophobic amino acid residue (isoleucine) to a smaller one (alanine) near the extracellular end of this segment creates a pathway for access of charged local anesthetic drugs from the extracellular solution to the receptor site. These findings place the local anesthetic receptor site within the intracellular half of the transmembrane pore of the Na^+ channel, with part of its structure contributed by amino acids in the S6 segment of domain IV.

Frequency- and Voltage-Dependence of Local Anesthetic Action.   The degree of block produced by a given concentration of local anesthetic depends on how the nerve has been stimulated and on its resting membrane potential. Thus, a resting nerve is much less sensitive to a local anesthetic than one that is repetitively stimulated; higher frequency of stimulation and more positive membrane potential cause a greater degree of anesthetic block. These frequency- and voltage-dependent effects of local anesthetics occur because the local anesthetic molecule in its charged form gains access to its binding site within the pore only when the Na^+ channel is in an open state and because the local anesthetic binds more tightly to and stabilizes the inactivated state of the Na^+ channel (*see* Courtney and Strichartz, 1987; Butterworth and Strichartz, 1990). Local anesthetics exhibit these properties to different extents depending on their pK_a, lipid solubility, and molecular size. In general, the frequency dependence of local anesthetic action depends critically on the rate of dissociation from the receptor site in the pore of the Na^+ channel. A high frequency of stimulation is required for rapidly dissociating drugs so that drug binding during the action potential exceeds drug dissociation between action potentials. Dissociation of smaller and more hydrophobic drugs is more rapid, so a higher frequency of stimulation is required to yield frequency-dependent block. Frequency-dependent block of ion channels is most important for the actions of antiarrhythmic drugs. (*see* Chapter 35).

Differential Sensitivity of Nerve Fibers to Local Anesthetics.   Although there is great individual variation, for

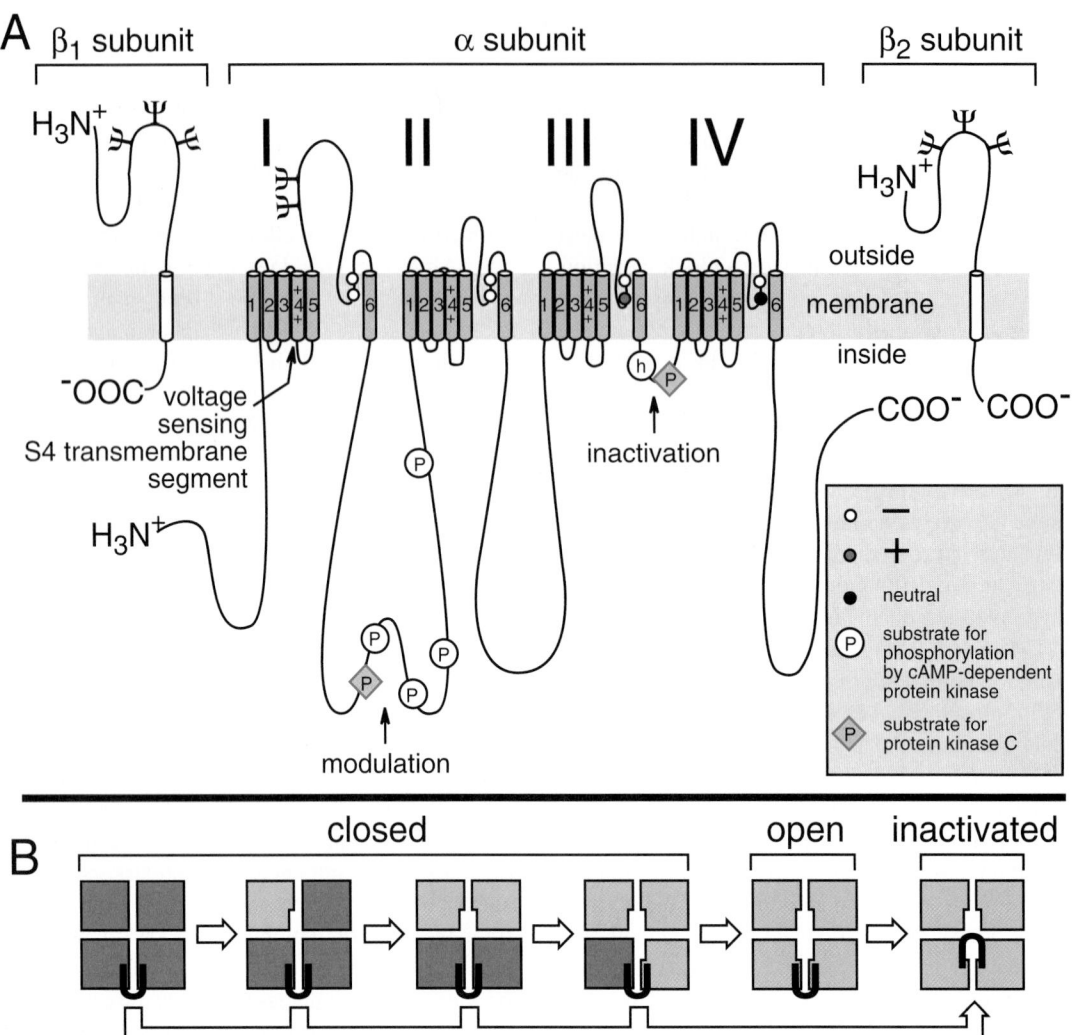

Figure 15–2. Structure and function of voltage-gated Na⁺ channels.

A. A two-dimensional representation of the α (center), β_1 (left), and β_2 (right) subunits of the voltage-gated Na⁺ channel from mammalian brain. The polypeptide chains are represented by continuous lines with length approximately proportional to the actual length of each segment of the channel protein. Cylinders represent regions of transmembrane α helices. Ψ indicates sites of demonstrated N-linked glycosylation. Note the repeated structure of the four homologous domains (I through IV) of the α subunit. **Voltage Sensing.** The S4 transmembrane segments in each homologous domain of the α subunit serve as voltage sensors. (+) represents the positively charged amino acid residues at every third position within these segments. Electrical field (negative inside) exerts a force on these charged amino acid residues, pulling them toward the intracellular side of the membrane. **Pore.** The S5 and S6 transmembrane segments and the short membrane-associated loops between them (segments SS1 and SS2, *see* Figure 15–3) form the walls of the pore in the center of an approximately symmetrical square array of the four homologous domains (*see* Panel B). The amino acid residues indicated by circles in segment SS2 are critical for determining the conductance and ion selectivity of the Na⁺ channel and its ability to bind the extracellular pore blocking toxins tetrodotoxin and saxitoxin. **Inactivation.** The short intracellular loop connecting homologous domains III and IV serves as the inactivation gate of the Na⁺ channel. It is thought to fold into the intracellular mouth of the pore and occlude it within a few milliseconds after the channel opens. Three hydrophobic residues (isoleucine–phenylalanine–methionine, IFM) at the position marked h appear to serve as an inactivation particle, entering the intracellular mouth of the pore and binding to an inactivation gate receptor there. **Modulation.** The gating of the Na⁺ channel can be modulated by protein phosphorylation. Phosphorylation of the inactivation gate between homologous domains III and IV by protein kinase C slows inactivation. Phosphorylation of sites in the intracellular loop between homologous domains I and II by either protein kinase C ⓟ or cyclic AMP-dependent protein kinase Ⓟ reduces Na⁺ channel activation.

B. The four homologous domains of the Na⁺ channel α subunit are illustrated as a square array as viewed looking down on the membrane. The sequence of conformational changes that the Na⁺ channel undergoes during activation and inactivation is diagrammed. Upon depolarization, each of the four homologous domains undergoes a conformational change in sequence to an activated state. After all four domains have activated, the Na⁺ channel can open. Within a few milliseconds after opening, the inactivation gate between domains III and IV closes over the intracellular mouth of the channel and occludes it, preventing further ion conductance. (Adapted from Catterall, 1988, with permission.)

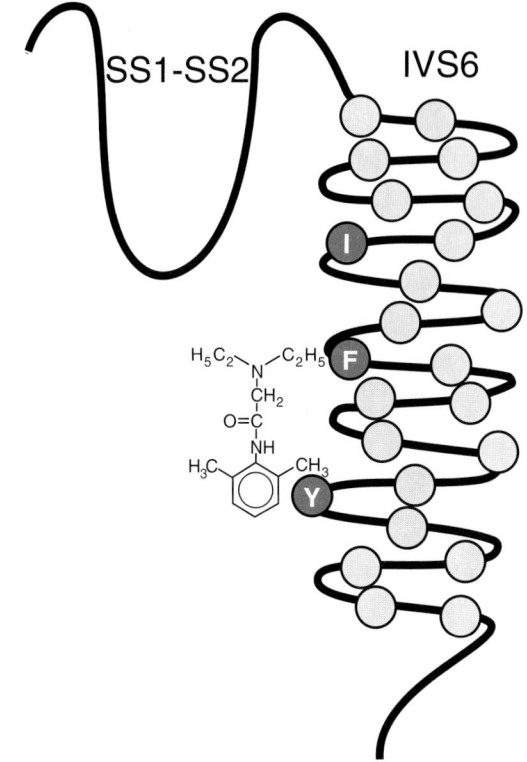

Figure 15–3. The local anesthetic receptor site.

Transmembrane segment S6 in domain IV (IVS6) is illustrated as an α helix along with adjacent short segments SS1 and SS2 that contribute to formation of the extracellular mouth of the pore. Each circle represents an amino acid residue in segment IVS6. The three critical residues for formation of the local anesthetic binding site are shaded blue. The local anesthetic lidocaine is shown docked to two of these residues, which are phenylalanine (F) 1764 and tyrosine (Y) 1771. The third shaded residue is isoleucine (I) 1760. Substitution of a smaller alanine residue at this position by site-directed mutagenesis allows local anesthetics to reach their receptor site from outside the membrane. This residue therefore is assumed to form the outer boundary of the receptor site (*see* Ragsdale *et al.,* 1994).

most patients treatment with local anesthetics causes the sensation of pain to disappear first followed by the sensations of temperature, touch, deep pressure, and finally motor function (Table 15–1). Classical experiments with intact nerves showed that the δ wave in the compound action potential, which represents slowly conducting, small-diameter myelinated fibers, was reduced more rapidly and at lower concentrations of cocaine than was the α wave, which represents rapidly conducting, large-diameter fibers (Gasser and Erlanger, 1929). In general, autonomic fibers,

small unmyelinated C fibers (mediating pain sensations), and small myelinated Aδ fibers (mediating pain and temperature sensations) are blocked before the larger myelinated Aγ, Aβ, and Aα fibers (mediating postural, touch, pressure, and motor information; reviewed in Raymond and Gissen, 1987). The differential rate of block exhibited by fibers mediating different sensations is of considerable practical importance in use of local anesthetics.

The precise mechanisms responsible for this apparent specificity of local anesthetic action on pain fibers are not known, but several factors may contribute. The initial hypothesis from the classical work on intact nerves was that sensitivity to local anesthetic block decreases with increasing fiber size, consistent with high sensitivity for pain sensation mediated by small fibers and low sensitivity for motor function mediated by large fibers (Gasser and Erlanger, 1929). However, when nerve fibers are dissected from nerves to allow direct measurement of action potential generation, no clear correlation of the concentration dependence of local anesthetic block with fiber diameter is observed (Franz and Perry, 1974; Fink and Cairns, 1984; Huang *et al.,* 1997). Therefore, it is unlikely that the fiber size *per se* determines the sensitivity to local anesthetic block under steady-state conditions. However, the spacing of nodes of Ranvier increases with the size of nerve fibers. Because a fixed number of nodes must be blocked to prevent conduction, small fibers with closely spaced nodes of Ranvier may be blocked more rapidly during treatment of intact nerves, because the local anesthetic reaches a critical length of nerve more rapidly (Franz and Perry, 1974). Differences in tissue barriers and location of smaller C fibers and Aδ fibers in nerves also may influence the rate of local anesthetic action.

Effect of pH.   Local anesthetics tend to be only slightly soluble as unprotonated amines. Therefore, they are generally marketed as water-soluble salts, usually hydrochlorides. Inasmuch as the local anesthetics are weak bases (typical pK_a values range from 8 to 9), their hydrochloride salts are mildly acidic. This property increases the stability of the local anesthetic esters and any accompanying vasoconstrictor substance. Under usual conditions of administration, the pH of the local anesthetic solution rapidly equilibrates to that of the extracellular fluids.

Although the unprotonated species of the local anesthetic is necessary for diffusion across cellular membranes, it is the cationic species that interacts preferentially with Na^+ channels. This conclusion has been supported by the results of experiments on anesthetized mammalian

Table 15–1
Susceptibility to Block of Types of Nerve Fibers

CONDUCTION BIOPHYSICAL CLASSIFICATION	ANATOMIC LOCATION	MYELIN	DIAMETER, μm	CONDUCTION VELOCITY, m·sec^{-1}	FUNCTION	SENSITIVITY TO BLOCK
A fibers						
A α	Afferent to and efferent from muscles and joints	Yes	6–22	10–85	Motor and proprioception	+
A β						++
A γ	Efferent to muscle spindles	Yes	3–6	15–35	Muscle tone	++
A δ	Sensory roots and afferent peripheral nerves	Yes	1–4	5–25	Pain, temperature, touch	+++
B fibers	Preganglionic sympathetic	Yes	<3	3–15	Vasomotor, visceromotor, sudomotor, pilomotor	++++
C fibers						
Sympathetic	Postganglionic sympathetic	No	0.3–1.3	0.7–1.3	Vasomotor, visceromotor, sudomotor, pilomotor	++++
Dorsal root	Sensory roots and afferent peripheral nerves	No	0.4–1.2	0.1–2.0	Pain, temperature, touch	++++

SOURCE: Adapted from Carpenter and Mackey, 1992, with permission.

nonmyelinated fibers (Ritchie and Greengard, 1966). In these experiments, conduction could be blocked or unblocked merely by adjusting the pH of the bathing medium to 7.2 or 9.6, respectively, without altering the amount of anesthetic present. The primary role of the cationic form also has been demonstrated clearly by Narahashi and colleagues, who perfused the extracellular and axoplasmic surface of the giant squid axon with tertiary and quaternary amine local anesthetics (Narahashi and Frazier, 1971). However, the unprotonated molecular forms also possess some anesthetic activity (Butterworth and Strichartz, 1990).

Prolongation of Action by Vasoconstrictors. The duration of action of a local anesthetic is proportional to the time during which it is in contact with nerve. Consequently, maneuvers that keep the drug at the nerve prolong the period of anesthesia. Cocaine itself constricts blood vessels by potentiating the action of norepinephrine (*see* Chapters 6 and 10), thereby preventing its own absorption. In clinical practice, preparations of local anesthetics

often contain a vasoconstrictor, usually epinephrine. The vasoconstrictor performs a dual service. By decreasing the rate of absorption, it not only localizes the anesthetic at the desired site but also allows the rate at which it is destroyed in the body to keep pace with the rate at which it is absorbed into the circulation. This reduces its systemic toxicity. It should be noted, however, that epinephrine also dilates skeletal muscle vascular beds through actions at β_2-adrenergic receptors and, therefore, has the potential to increase systemic toxicity of anesthetic deposited in muscle tissue.

Some of the vasoconstrictor agent may be absorbed systemically, occasionally to an extent sufficient to cause untoward reactions (*see* below). There also may be delayed wound healing, tissue edema, or necrosis after local anesthesia. These effects seem to occur partly because sympathomimetic amines increase the oxygen consumption of the tissue; this, together with the vasoconstriction, leads to hypoxia and local tissue damage. The use of vasoconstrictors in local-anesthetic preparations for anatomical regions with limited collateral circulation could produce irreversible hypoxic damage, tissue necrosis, and gangrene and therefore is contraindicated.

Undesired Effects of Local Anesthetics. In addition to blocking conduction in nerve axons in the peripheral nervous system, local anesthetics interfere with the function of all organs in which conduction or transmission of impulses occurs. Thus, they have important effects on the central nervous system (CNS), the autonomic ganglia, the neuromuscular junction, and all forms of muscle (for review *see* Covino, 1987; Garfield and Gugino, 1987; Gintant and Hoffman, 1987). The danger of such adverse reactions is proportional to the concentration of local anesthetic achieved in the circulation.

Central Nervous System. Following absorption, local anesthetics may cause stimulation of the CNS, producing restlessness and tremor that may proceed to clonic convulsions. In general, the more potent the anesthetic, the more readily convulsions may be produced. Alterations of CNS activity are thus predictable from the local anesthetic agent in question and the blood concentration achieved. Central stimulation is followed by depression; death usually is caused by respiratory failure.

The apparent stimulation and subsequent depression produced by applying local anesthetics to the CNS presumably is due solely to depression of neuronal activity; a selective depression of inhibitory neurons is thought to account for the excitatory phase *in vivo*. Rapid systemic administration of local anesthetics may produce death with no or only transient signs of CNS stimulation. Under these conditions, the concentration of the drug probably rises so rapidly that all neurons are depressed simultaneously. Airway control and support of respiration are essential features of treatment in the late stage of intoxication. Benzodiazepines or rapidly acting barbiturates administered intravenously are the drugs of choice for both the prevention and arrest of convulsions (*see* Chapter 17).

Although drowsiness is the most frequent complaint that results from the CNS actions of local anesthetics, lidocaine may produce dysphoria or euphoria and muscle twitching. Moreover, both lidocaine and procaine may produce a loss of consciousness that is preceded only by symptoms of sedation (*see* Covino, 1987). Whereas other local anesthetics also show the effect, cocaine has a particularly prominent effect on mood and behavior. These effects of cocaine and its potential for abuse are discussed in Chapter 24.

Cardiovascular System. Following systemic absorption, local anesthetics act on the cardiovascular system (*see* Covino, 1987). The primary site of action is the myocardium, where decreases in electrical excitability, conduction rate, and force of contraction occur. In addition, most local anesthetics cause arteriolar dilation. Untoward cardiovascular effects usually are seen only after high systemic concentrations are attained and effects on the CNS are produced. However, on rare occasions, lower doses of some local anesthetics will cause cardiovascular collapse and death, probably due to either an action on the pacemaker or the sudden onset of ventricular fibrillation. It should be noted that ventricular tachycardia and fibrillation are relatively uncommon consequences of local anesthetics other than bupivacaine. The effects of local anesthetics such as lidocaine and procainamide, which also are used as antiarrhythmic drugs, are discussed in Chapter 35. Finally, it should be stressed that untoward cardiovascular effects of local anesthetic agents may result from their inadvertent intravascular administration, especially if epinephrine also is present.

Smooth Muscle. The local anesthetics depress contractions in the intact bowel and in strips of isolated intestine (*see* Zipf and Dittmann, 1971). They also relax vascular and bronchial smooth muscle, although low concentrations initially may produce contraction (*see* Covino, 1987). Spinal and epidural anesthesia, as well as instillation of local anesthetics into the peritoneal cavity, cause sympathetic nervous system paralysis, which can result in increased tone of gastrointestinal musculature (*see* below). Local anesthetics may increase the resting tone and decrease the contractions of isolated human uterine muscle; however, uterine contractions seldom are depressed directly during intrapartum regional anesthesia.

Neuromuscular Junction and Ganglionic Synapse. Local anesthetics also affect transmission at the neuromuscular junction. Procaine, for example, can block the response of skeletal muscle to maximal motor-nerve volleys and to acetylcholine at concentrations where the muscle responds normally to direct electrical stimulation. Similar effects occur at autonomic ganglia. These effects are due to block of the ion channel of the acetylcholine receptor by high concentrations of the local anesthetics (Neher and Steinbach, 1978; Charnet *et al.*, 1990).

Hypersensitivity to Local Anesthetics. Rare individuals are hypersensitive to local anesthetics. The reaction may manifest itself as an allergic dermatitis or a typical asthmatic attack (*see* Covino, 1987). It is important to distinguish allergic reactions from toxic side effects and from the effects of coadministered vasoconstrictors. Hypersensitivity seems to occur almost exclusively with local anesthetics of the ester type and frequently extends to chemically related compounds. For example, individuals sensitive to procaine also may react to structurally similar compounds (*e.g.*, tetracaine) through reaction to a common metabolite. Although agents of the amide type are essentially free of this problem, solutions of such agents may contain preservatives such as methylparaben that may provoke an allergic reaction (Covino, 1987). Local anesthetic preparations containing a vasoconstrictor also may elicit allergic responses due to the sulfite contained in them.

Metabolism of Local Anesthetics. The metabolic fate of local anesthetics is of great practical importance, because their toxicity depends largely on the balance between their rates of absorption and elimination. As noted above, the rate of absorption of many anesthetics can be reduced considerably by the incorporation of a vasoconstrictor agent in the anesthetic solution. However, the rate of destruction of local anesthetics varies greatly, and this is a major factor in determining the safety of a particular agent. Since toxicity is related to the free concentration of drug, binding of the anesthetic to proteins in the serum and to tissues reduces the concentration of free drug in the systemic circulation and, consequently, reduces toxicity. For example, in intravenous regional anesthesia of an extremity, about half of the original anesthetic dose is still tissue bound 30 minutes after release of the tourniquet; the lungs also bind large quantities of local anesthetic (Arthur, 1987).

Some of the common local anesthetics (*e.g.,* tetracaine) are esters. They are hydrolyzed and inactivated primarily by a plasma esterase, probably plasma cholinesterase. The liver also participates in hydrolysis of local anesthetics. Since spinal fluid contains little or no esterase, anesthesia produced by the intrathecal injection of an anesthetic agent will persist until the local anesthetic agent has been absorbed into the circulation.

The amide-linked local anesthetics are, in general, degraded by the hepatic endoplasmic reticulum, the initial reactions involving *N*-dealkylation and subsequent hydrolysis (Arthur, 1987). However, with prilocaine, the initial step is hydrolytic, forming *o*-toluidine metabolites that can cause methemoglobinemia. Caution is indicated in the extensive use of amide-linked local anesthetics in patients with severe hepatic disease. The amide-linked local anesthetics are extensively (55% to 95%) bound to plasma proteins, particularly α_1-acid glycoprotein. Many factors increase the concentration of this plasma protein (cancer, surgery, trauma, myocardial infarction, smoking, uremia) or decrease it (oral contraceptive agents). This results in changes in the amount of anesthetic delivered to the liver for metabolism, thus influencing systemic toxicity. Age-related changes in protein binding of local anesthetics also occur. The neonate is relatively deficient in plasma proteins that bind local anesthetics and thereby has greater susceptibility to toxicity. Plasma proteins are not the sole determinant of local anesthetic availability. Uptake by the lung also may play an important role in the distribution of amide-linked local anesthetics in the body (*see* Arthur, 1987).

COCAINE

Chemistry. As outlined in the introduction above, cocaine occurs in abundance in the leaves of the coca shrub and is an ester of benzoic acid and methylecgonine. Egonine is an amino alcohol base closely related to tropine, the amino alcohol in atropine. It has the same fundamental structure as the synthetic local anesthetics (*see* Figure 15–1).

Pharmacological Actions and Preparations. The clinically desired actions of cocaine are the blockade of nerve impulses, as a consequence of its local anesthetic properties, and local vasoconstriction, secondary to inhibition of local norepinephrine reuptake. Toxicity and its potential for abuse have steadily decreased the clinical uses of cocaine. Its high toxicity is due to block of catecholamine uptake in both the central and peripheral nervous systems. Its euphoric properties are due primarily to inhibition of catecholamine uptake, particularly dopamine, at central nervous system synapses. Other local anesthetics do not block the uptake of norepinephrine and do not produce the sensitization to catecholamines, vasoconstriction, or mydriasis characteristic of cocaine. Currently, cocaine is used primarily for topical anesthesia of the upper respiratory tract, where its combined vasoconstrictor and local anesthetic properties provide anesthesia and shrinking of the mucosa with a single agent. Cocaine hydrochloride is used as a 1%, 4%, or 10% solution for topical application. For most applications, the 1% or 4% preparation is preferred to reduce toxicity. Because of its abuse potential, cocaine is listed as a schedule II drug by the United States Drug Enforcement Agency.

LIDOCAINE

Lidocaine (XYLOCAINE, others), introduced in 1948, is now the most widely used local anesthetic. The chemical structure of lidocaine is shown in Figure 15–1.

Pharmacological Actions. The pharmacological actions that lidocaine shares with other local anesthetic drugs have been described. Lidocaine produces faster, more intense, longer-lasting, and more extensive anesthesia than does an equal concentration of procaine. Unlike procaine, it is an aminoethylamide and is the prototypical member of the amide class of local anesthetics. It is an alternative choice for individuals sensitive to ester-type local anesthetics.

Absorption, Fate, and Excretion. Lidocaine is absorbed rapidly after parenteral administration and from the gastrointestinal and respiratory tracts. Although it is effective when used without any vasoconstrictor, in the presence of epinephrine the rate of absorption and the toxicity are decreased, and the duration of action usually is prolonged. In addition to preparations for injection, an iontophoretic, needle-free drug-delivery system for a lidocaine and epinephrine solution (IONTOCAINE) is available. This system generally is used for dermal procedures and provides anesthesia to a depth of up to 10 mm. Lidocaine is dealkylated in the liver by mixed-function oxidases to monoethylglycine xylidide and glycine xylidide, which can be metabolized further to monoethylglycine and xylidide. Both monoethylglycine xylidide and glycine xylidide retain local anesthetic activity. In human beings, about 75% of the xylidide is excreted in the urine as the further metabolite 4-hydroxy-2,6-dimethylaniline (*see* Arthur, 1987).

Toxicity.   The side effects of lidocaine seen with increasing dose include drowsiness, tinnitus, dysgeusia, dizziness, and twitching. As the dose increases, seizures, coma, and respiratory depression and arrest will occur. Clinically significant cardiovascular depression usually occurs at serum lidocaine levels that produce marked CNS effects. The metabolites monoethylglycine xylidide and glycine xylidide may contribute to some of these side effects.

Clinical Uses.   Lidocaine has a wide range of clinical uses as a local anesthetic; it has utility in almost any application where a local anesthetic of intermediate duration is needed. Lidocaine also is used as an antiarrhythmic agent (*see* Chapter 35).

BUPIVACAINE

Pharmacological Actions.   *Bupivacaine* (MARCAINE, SENSORCAINE), introduced in 1963, is a widely used amide local anesthetic; its structure is similar to that of lidocaine except that the amine-containing group is a butyl piperidine (Figure 15–1). It is a potent agent capable of producing prolonged anesthesia. Its long duration of action plus its tendency to provide more sensory than motor block has made it a popular drug for providing prolonged analgesia during labor or the postoperative period. By taking advantage of indwelling catheters and continuous infusions, bupivacaine can be used to provide several days of effective analgesia.

Toxicity.   Bupivacaine (and etidocaine, below) are more cardiotoxic than equieffective doses of lidocaine. Clinically, this is manifested by severe ventricular arrhythmias and myocardial depression after inadvertent intravascular administration of large doses of bupivacaine. The enhanced cardiotoxicity of bupivacaine probably is due to multiple factors. Lidocaine and bupivacaine both rapidly block cardiac Na^+ channels during systole. However, bupivacaine dissociates much more slowly than does lidocaine during diastole, so a significant fraction of Na^+ channels remains blocked at the end of diastole (at physiological heart rates) with bupivacaine (Clarkson and Hondeghem, 1985). Thus the block by bupivacaine is cumulative and substantially more than would be predicted by its local anesthetic potency. At least a portion of the cardiac toxicity of bupivacaine may be mediated centrally, as direct injection of small quantities of bupivacaine into the medulla can produce malignant ventricular arrhythmias (Thomas *et al.*, 1986). Bupivacaine-induced cardiac toxicity can be very difficult to treat, and its severity is enhanced in the presence of acidosis, hypercarbia, and hypoxemia.

OTHER SYNTHETIC LOCAL ANESTHETICS

The number of synthetic local anesthetics is so large that it is impractical to consider them all here. Some local anesthetic agents are too toxic to be given by injection. Their use is restricted to topical application to the eye (*see* Chapter 66), the mucous membranes, or the skin (*see* Chapter 65). Many local anesthetics are suitable, however, for infiltration or injection to produce nerve block; some of them also are useful for topical application. The main categories of local anesthetics are given below; agents are listed alphabetically.

Local Anesthetics Suitable for Injection

Chloroprocaine.   *Chloroprocaine* (NESACAINE), an ester local anesthetic introduced in 1952, is a chlorinated derivative of procaine (Figure 15–1). Its major assets are its rapid onset and short duration of action and its reduced acute toxicity due to its rapid metabolism (plasma half-life approximately 25 seconds). Enthusiasm for its use has been tempered by reports of prolonged sensory and motor block after epidural or subarachnoid administration of large doses. This toxicity appears to have been a consequence of low pH and the use of sodium metabisulfite as a preservative in earlier formulations. There are no reports of neurotoxicity with newer preparations of chloroprocaine, which contain calcium EDTA as the preservative, although these preparations also are not recommended for intrathecal administration. A higher-than-expected incidence of muscular back pain following epidural anesthesia with 2-chloroprocaine also has been reported (Stevens *et al.*, 1993). This back pain is thought to be due to tetany in the paraspinus muscles, which may be a consequence of Ca^{2+} binding by the EDTA included as a preservative; the incidence of back pain appears to be related to the volume of drug injected and its use for skin infiltration.

Etidocaine.   *Etidocaine* (DURANEST), introduced in 1972, is a long-acting amino amide (Figure 15–1). Its onset of action is faster than that of bupivacaine and comparable to that of lidocaine, yet its duration of action is similar to that of bupivacaine. Compared to bupivacaine, etidocaine produces preferential motor blockade. Thus, while it is useful for surgery requiring intense skeletal muscle relaxation, its utility in labor or postoperative analgesia is limited. Its cardiac toxicity is similar to that of bupivacaine (*see* above).

Mepivacaine.   *Mepivacaine* (CARBOCAINE, others), introduced in 1957, is an intermediate-acting amino amide (Figure 15–1). Its pharmacological properties are similar to those of lidocaine. Mepivacaine, however, is more toxic to the neonate and thus is not used in obstetrical anesthesia. The increased toxicity of mepivacaine in the neonate is related to ion trapping of this agent because of the lower pH of neonatal blood and the pK_a of mepivacaine rather than to its slower metabolism in the neonate. It appears to have a slightly higher therapeutic index in adults than does lidocaine. Its onset of action is similar to that of lidocaine and its duration slightly longer (about 20%) than that of lidocaine in the absence of a coadministered vasoconstrictor. Mepivacaine is not effective as a topical anesthetic.

Prilocaine. *Prilocaine* (CITANEST) is an intermediate-acting amino amide (Figure 15–1). It has a pharmacological profile similar to that of lidocaine. The primary differences are that it causes little vasodilation and thus can be used without a vasoconstrictor, if desired, and its increased volume of distribution reduces its CNS toxicity, making it suitable for intravenous regional blocks (below). It is unique among the local anesthetics for its propensity to cause methemoglobinemia. This effect is a consequence of the metabolism of the aromatic ring to *o*-toluidine. Development of methemoglobinemia is dependent on the total dose administered, usually appearing after a dose of 8 mg/kg. In healthy persons, methemoglobinemia usually is not a problem. If necessary, it can be treated by the intravenous administration of methylene blue (1 to 2 mg/kg). Methemoglobinemia following prilocaine has limited its use in obstetrical anesthesia, because it complicates evaluation of the newborn. Also, methemoglobinemia is more common in neonates due to decreased resistance of fetal hemoglobin to oxidant stresses and the immaturity of enzymes in the neonate that convert methemoglobin back to the ferrous state.

Ropivacaine. The cardiac toxicity of bupivacaine stimulated interest in developing a less toxic, long-lasting local anesthetic. The result of that search was the development of a new amino ethylamide, *ropivacaine* (NAROPIN) (Figure 15–1), the *S*-enantiomer of 1-propyl-2′,6′-pipecoloxylidide. The *S*-enantiomer was chosen because, like most local anesthetics with a chiral center, it has a lower toxicity than the *R*-isomer (McClure, 1996). This is presumably due to slower uptake, resulting in lower blood levels for a given dose. Ropivacaine is slightly less potent than bupivacaine in producing anesthesia. In several animal models, it appears to be less cardiotoxic than equieffective doses of bupivacaine. In clinical studies, ropivacaine appears to be suitable for both epidural and regional anesthesia, with a duration of action similar to that of bupivacaine. Interestingly, it seems to be even more motor-sparing than bupivacaine.

Procaine. *Procaine* (NOVOCAIN), introduced in 1905, was the first synthetic local anesthetic and is an amino ester (Figure 15–1). While it formerly was used widely, its use now is confined to infiltration anesthesia and occasionally for diagnostic nerve blocks. This is because of its low potency, slow onset, and short duration of action. While its toxicity is fairly low, it is hydrolyzed *in vivo* to produce paraaminobenzoic acid, which inhibits the action of sulfonamides. Thus, large doses should not be administered to patients taking sulfonamide drugs.

Tetracaine. *Tetracaine* (PONTOCAINE), introduced in 1932, is a long-acting amino ester (Figure 15–1). It is significantly more potent and has a longer duration of action than procaine. Tetracaine may exhibit increased systemic toxicity because it is more slowly metabolized than the other commonly used ester local anesthetics. Currently, it is widely used in spinal anesthesia when a drug of long duration is needed. Tetracaine also is incorporated into several topical anesthesic preparations. With the introduction of bupivacaine, tetracaine is rarely used in peripheral nerve blocks because of the large doses often necessary, its slow onset, and its potential for toxicity.

Local Anesthetics Used Primarily to Anesthetize Mucous Membranes and Skin

Some anesthetics are either too irritating or too ineffective to be applied to the eye. However, they are useful as topical anesthetic agents on the skin and/or mucous membranes. These preparations are effective in the symptomatic relief of anal and genital pruritus, poison ivy rashes, and numerous other acute and chronic dermatoses. They are sometimes combined with a glucocorticoid or antihistamine and are available in a number of proprietary formulations.

Dibucaine (NUPERCAINAL) is a quinoline derivative. Its toxicity resulted in its removal from the United States market as an injectable preparation; however, it retains wide popularity outside the United States as a spinal anesthetic. It currently is available as a cream and an ointment for use on the skin.

Dyclonine hydrochloride (DYCLONE) has a rapid onset of action and a duration of effect comparable to that of procaine. It is absorbed through the skin and mucous membranes. The compound is used as 0.5% or 1.0% solution for topical anesthesia during endoscopy, for oral mucositis pain following radiation or chemotherapy, and for anogenital procedures.

Pramoxine hydrochloride (ANUSOL, TRONOTHANE, others) is a surface anesthetic agent that is not a benzoate ester. Its distinct chemical structure (Figure 15–1) may help minimize the danger of cross-sensitivity reactions in patients allergic to other local anesthetics. Pramoxine produces satisfactory surface anesthesia and is reasonably well tolerated on the skin and mucous membranes. It is too irritating to be used on the eye or in the nose. Various preparations, usually containing 1% pramoxine, are available for topical application.

Anesthetics of Low Solubility

Some local anesthetics are poorly soluble in water and, consequently, too slowly absorbed to be toxic. They can be applied directly to wounds and ulcerated surfaces, where they remain localized for long periods of time, producing a sustained anesthetic action. Chemically, they are esters of paraaminobenzoic acid lacking the terminal amino group possessed by the previously described local anesthetics. The most important member of the series is *benzocaine* (ethyl aminobenzoate; AMERICAINE ANESTHETIC, others). Benzocaine is structurally similar to procaine; the difference is that it lacks the terminal diethylamino group (Figure 15–1). It is incorporated into a large number of topical preparations. Benzocaine has been reported to cause methemoglobinemia (*see* text concerning methemoglobinemia caused by prilocaine, above); consequently, dosing recommendations must be carefully followed.

Local Anesthetics Largely Restricted to Ophthalmological Use

Anesthesia of the cornea and conjunctiva can be obtained readily by topical application of local anesthetics. However, most of the local anesthetics described above are too irritating for ophthalmological use. The first local anesthetic used in ophthalmology, cocaine, has the severe disadvantages of producing mydriasis and corneal sloughing and has fallen out of favor. The two compounds used most frequently today are *proparacaine* (ALCAINE, OPHTHAINE, others) and tetracaine (Figure 15–1). In addition to being less irritating during administration, proparacaine has the added advantage of bearing little antigenic similarity to the other benzoate local anesthetics. Thus, it sometimes can be used in individuals sensitive to the amino ester local anesthetics.

For use in ophthalmology, these local anesthetics are instilled a single drop at a time. If anesthesia is incomplete, successive drops are applied until satisfactory conditions are obtained. The duration of anesthesia is determined chiefly by the vascularity of the tissue; thus it is longest in normal cornea and least in inflamed conjunctiva. In the latter case, repeated instillations are necessary to maintain adequate anesthesia for the duration of the procedure. Long-term administration of topical anesthesia to the eye has been associated with retarded healing, pitting and sloughing of the corneal epithelium, and predisposition of the eye to inadvertent injury. Thus, these drugs should not be prescribed for self-administration. For drug delivery, pharmacokinetic, and toxicity issues unique to drugs for ophthalmic use, *see* Chapter 66.

Tetrodotoxin and Saxitoxin

These toxins are two of the most potent poisons known; the minimal lethal dose of each in the mouse is about 8 μg/kg. Both toxins are responsible for fatal poisoning in human beings. Tetrodotoxin is found in the gonads and other visceral tissues of some fish of the order Tetraodontiformes (to which the Japanese *fugu*, or puffer fish, belongs); it also occurs in the skin of some newts of the family Salamandridae and of the Costa Rican frog *Atelopus*. Saxitoxin, and possibly some related toxins, are elaborated by the dinoflagellates *Gonyaulax catanella* and *Gonyaulax tamerensis* and are retained in the tissues of clams and other shellfish that eat these organisms. Given the right conditions of temperature and light, the *Gonyaulax* may multiply so rapidly as to discolor the ocean—hence the term *red tide*. Shellfish feeding on *Gonyaulax* at this time become extremely toxic to human beings and are responsible for periodic outbreaks of paralytic shellfish poisoning (*see* Kao, 1972; Ritchie, 1980). Although the toxins are chemically different from each other, their mechanism of action is similar (*see* Ritchie, 1980). Both toxins, in nanomolar concentrations, specifically block the outer mouth of the pore of Na$^+$ channels in the membranes of excitable cells. As a result, the action potential is blocked. The receptor site for these toxins is formed by amino acid residues in the SS2 segment of the Na$^+$ channel α subunit (*see* Figure 15–2) in all four domains (Terlau *et al.*, 1991; Catterall, 2000). Not all Na$^+$ channels are equally sensitive to tetrodotoxin; the channels in cardiac myocytes are resistant, and a tetrodotoxin-resistant Na$^+$ channel is expressed when skeletal muscle is denervated. Both toxins cause death by paralysis of the respiratory muscles; therefore, the treatment of severe cases of poisoning requires artificial ventilation. Blockade of vasomotor nerves, together with a relaxation of vascular smooth muscle, seems to be responsible for the hypotension that is characteristic of tetrodotoxin poisoning (Kao, 1972). Early gastric lavage and therapy to support the blood pressure also are indicated. If the patient survives paralytic shellfish poisoning for 24 hours, the prognosis is good (*see* Ogura, 1971; Schantz, 1971).

CLINICAL USES OF LOCAL ANESTHETICS

Local anesthesia is the loss of sensation in a body part without the loss of consciousness or the impairment of central control of vital functions. It offers two major advantages. The first is that the physiological perturbations associated with general anesthesia are avoided; the second is that neurophysiological reponses to pain and stress can be modified beneficially. As discussed above, local anesthetics have the potential to produce deleterious side effects. The choice of a local anesthetic and care in its use are the primary determinants of such toxicity. There is a poor relationship between the amount of local anesthetic injected and peak plasma levels in adults. Furthermore, peak plasma levels vary widely depending on the area of injection. They are highest with interpleural or intercostal block and lowest with subcutaneous infiltration. Thus, recommended maximum doses serve only as general guidelines.

The following discussion concerns the pharmacological and physiological consequences of the use of local anesthetics categorized by method of administration. A more comprehensive discussion of their use and administration is presented in standard anesthesiology texts (*e.g.,* Cousins and Bridenbaugh, 1998).

Topical Anesthesia

Anesthesia of mucous membranes of the nose, mouth, throat, tracheobronchial tree, esophagus, and genitourinary tract can be produced by direct application of aqueous solutions of salts of many local anesthetics or by suspension of the poorly soluble local anesthetics. Tetracaine (2%), lidocaine (2% to 10%), and cocaine (1% to 4%) typically are used. Cocaine is used only in the nose, nasopharynx, mouth, throat, and ear. Cocaine has the unique advantage of producing vasoconstriction as well as anesthesia. The shrinking of mucous membranes decreases operative bleeding while improving surgical visualization. Comparable vasoconstriction can be achieved with other local anesthetics by the addition of a low concentration of a vasoconstrictor such as phenylephrine (0.005%). Epinephrine, topically applied, has no significant local effect and does not prolong the duration of action of local anesthetics applied to mucous membranes because of poor penetration. *Maximal* safe total dosages for topical anesthesia in a healthy 70-kg adult are 300 mg for lidocaine, 150 mg for cocaine, and 50 mg for tetracaine.

Peak anesthetic effect following topical application of cocaine or lidocaine occurs within 2 to 5 minutes (3 to 8 minutes with tetracaine), and anesthesia lasts for 30 to 45 minutes (30 to

60 minutes with tetracaine). Anesthesia is entirely superficial; it does not extend to submucosal structures. This technique does not alleviate joint pain or discomfort from subdermal inflammation or injury.

Local anesthetics are absorbed rapidly into the circulation following topical application to mucous membranes or denuded skin. Thus, it must be kept in mind that topical anesthesia always carries the risk of systemic toxic reactions. Systemic toxicity has occurred even following the use of local anesthetics to control discomfort associated with severe diaper rash in infants. Absorption is particularly rapid when local anesthetics are applied to the tracheobronchial tree. Concentrations in blood after instillation of local anesthetics into the airway are nearly the same as those that follow intravenous injection. Surface anesthetics for the skin and cornea have been described above.

The introduction of an eutectic mixture of lidocaine (2.5%) and prilocaine (2.5%) (EMLA) bridges the gap between topical and infiltration anesthesia. The efficacy of this combination lies in the fact that the mixure of prilocaine and lidocaine has a melting point less than that of either compound alone, existing at room temperature as an oil that can penetrate intact skin. EMLA cream produces anesthesia to a maximum depth of 5 mm and is applied as a cream on intact skin under an occlusive dressing, which must be left in place for at least 1 hour. It is effective for procedures involving skin and superficial subcutaneous structures (e.g., venipuncture and skin graft harvesting). The component local anesthetics will be absorbed into the systemic circulation, potentially producing toxic effects (above). Guidelines are available to calculate the maximum amount of cream that can be applied and area of skin covered. It must not be used on mucous membranes or abraded skin, as rapid absorption across these surfaces may result in systemic toxicity.

Infiltration Anesthesia

Infiltration anesthesia is the injection of local anesthetic directly into tissue without taking into consideration the course of cutaneous nerves. Infiltration anesthesia can be so superficial as to include only the skin. It also can include deeper structures, including intraabdominal organs when these, too, are infiltrated.

The duration of infiltration anesthesia can be approximately doubled by the addition of epinephrine (5 μg/ml) to the injection solution; epinephrine also decreases peak concentrations of local anesthetics in blood. Epinephrine-containing solutions should not, however, be injected into tissues supplied by end arteries—for example, fingers and toes, ears, the nose, and the penis. The intense vasoconstriction produced by epinephrine may result in gangrene. For the same reason, epinephrine should be avoided in solutions injected intracutaneously. Since epinephrine also is absorbed into the circulation, its use should be avoided in those for whom adrenergic stimulation is undesirable.

The local anesthetics most frequently used for infiltration anesthesia are lidocaine (0.5% to 1.0%), procaine (0.5% to 1.0%), and bupivacaine (0.125% to 0.25%). When used without epinephrine, up to 4.5 mg/kg of lidocaine, 7 mg/kg of procaine, or 2 mg/kg of bupivacaine can be employed in adults. When epinephrine is added, these amounts can be increased by one-third.

The advantage of infiltration anesthesia and other regional anesthetic techniques is that it is possible to provide satisfactory anesthesia without disruption of normal bodily functions. The chief disadvantage of infiltration anesthesia is that relatively large amounts of drug must be used to anesthetize relatively small areas. This is no problem with minor surgery. When major surgery is performed, however, the amount of local anesthetic that is required makes systemic toxic reactions likely. The amount of anesthetic required to anesthetize an area can be reduced significantly and the duration of anesthesia increased markedly by specifically blocking the nerves that innervate the area of interest. This can be done at one of several levels: subcutaneously, at major nerves, or at the level of the spinal roots.

Field Block Anesthesia

Field block anesthesia is produced by subcutaneous injection of a solution of local anesthetic in such a manner as to anesthetize the region distal to the injection. For example, subcutaneous infiltration of the proximal portion of the volar surface of the forearm results in an extensive area of cutaneous anesthesia that starts 2 to 3 cm distal to the site of injection. The same principle can be applied with particular benefit to the scalp, the anterior abdominal wall, and the lower extremity.

The drugs used and the concentrations and doses recommended are the same as for infiltration anesthesia. The advantage of field block anesthesia is that less drug can be used to provide a greater area of anesthesia than when infiltration anesthesia is used. Knowledge of the relevant neuroanatomy obviously is essential for successful field block anesthesia.

Nerve Block Anesthesia

Injection of a solution of a local anesthetic into or about individual peripheral nerves or nerve plexuses produces even greater areas of anesthesia than do the techniques described above. Blockade of mixed peripheral nerves and nerve plexuses also usually anesthetizes somatic motor nerves, producing skeletal muscle relaxation, which is essential for some surgical procedures. The areas of sensory and motor block usually start several centimeters distal to the site of injection. Brachial plexus blocks are particularly useful for procedures on the upper extremity and shoulder. Intercostal nerve blocks are effective for anesthesia and relaxation of the anterior abdominal wall. Cervical plexus block is appropriate for surgery of the neck. Sciatic and femoral nerve blocks are useful for surgery distal to the knee. Other useful nerve blocks prior to surgical procedures include blocks of individual nerves at the wrist and at the ankle, blocks of individual nerves such as the median or ulnar at the elbow, and blocks of sensory cranial nerves.

There are four major determinants of the onset of sensory anesthesia following injection near a nerve. These are the proximity of the injection to the nerve, concentration and volume of drug, the degree of ionization of the drug, and time. Local anesthetic is never intentionally injected into the nerve, as this would be painful and could lead to nerve damage. Instead, the anesthetic agent is deposited as close to the nerve as possible. Thus the local anesthetic must diffuse from the site of injection into the nerve, where it acts. The rate of diffusion will be determined chiefly by the concentration of the drug, its degree of ionization (as ionized local anesthetic diffuses more slowly), its hydrophobicity, and the physical characteristics of the tissue surrounding the nerve. Higher concentrations of local anesthetic will result in a more rapid onset of peripheral nerve block. The utility of using higher concentrations, however, is limited by systemic toxicity as well as direct neural toxicity of concentrated local anesthetic solutions. Local anesthetics with lower pK_a values tend to have a more rapid onset of action for a given concentration, because more drug is uncharged at neutral pH. For example, the onset of action of lidocaine occurs in about 3 minutes; 35% of lidocaine is in the basic form at pH 7.4. In contrast, the onset of action of bupivacaine requires about 15 minutes; only 5% to 10% of bupivacaine is in the basic (uncharged) form at this pH. Increased hydrophobicity might be expected to speed onset by increased penetration into nerve tissue. However, it also will increase binding in tissue lipids. Furthermore, the more hydrophobic local anesthetics also are more potent (and toxic) and thus must be used at lower concentrations, decreasing the concentration gradient for diffusion. Tissue factors also play a role in determining the rate of onset of anesthetic effects. The amount of connective tissue that must be penetrated can be significant in a nerve plexus compared to isolated nerves and can serve to slow or even prevent adequate diffusion of local anesthetic to the nerve fibers.

Duration of nerve block anesthesia depends on the physical characteristics of the local anesthetic used and the presence or absence of vasoconstrictors. Especially important physical characteristics are lipid solubility and protein binding. In general, local anesthetics can be divided into three categories: those with a short (20 to 45 minutes) duration of action in mixed peripheral nerves, such as procaine; those with an intermediate (60 to 120 minutes) duration of action, such as lidocaine and mepivacaine; and those with a long (400 to 450 minutes) duration of action, such as bupivacaine, etidocaine, ropivacaine, and tetracaine. Block duration of the intermediate-acting local anesthetics such as lidocaine can be prolonged by the addition of epinephrine (5 μg/ml). The degree of block prolongation in peripheral nerves following the addition of epinephrine appears to be related to the intrinsic vasodilatory properties of the local anesthetic and thus is most pronounced with lidocaine.

The types of nerve fibers that are blocked when a local anesthetic is injected about a mixed peripheral nerve depend on the concentration of drug used, nerve-fiber size, internodal distance, and frequency and pattern of nerve-impulse transmission (*see* above). Anatomical factors are similarly important. A mixed peripheral nerve or nerve trunk consists of individual nerves surrounded by an investing epineurium. The vascular supply is usually centrally located. When a local anesthetic is deposited about a peripheral nerve, it diffuses from the outer surface toward the core along a concentration gradient (DeJong, 1994; Winnie *et al.*, 1977). Consequently, nerves in the outer mantle of the mixed nerve are blocked first. These fibers usually are distributed to more proximal anatomical structures than are those situated near the core of the mixed nerve and are often motor. If the volume and concentration of local anesthetic solution deposited about the nerve are adequate, the local anesthetic eventually will diffuse inwardly in amounts adequate to block even the most centrally located fibers. Lesser amounts of drug will block only nerves in the mantle and the smaller and more sensitive central fibers. Furthermore, since removal of local anesthetics occurs primarily in the core of a mixed nerve or nerve trunk, where the vascular supply is located, the dura-

tion of blockade of centrally located nerves is shorter than that of more peripherally situated fibers.

Choice of local anesthetic, as well as the amount and concentration administered, is determined by the nerves and the types of fibers to be blocked, the duration of anesthesia required, and the size and health of the patient. For blocks of 2 to 4 hours, lidocaine (1.0% to 1.5%) can be used in the amounts recommended above (*see* "Infiltration Anesthesia"). Mepivacaine (up to 7 mg/kg of a 1.0% to 2.0% solution) provides anesthesia that lasts about as long as that from lidocaine. Bupivacaine (2 to 3 mg/kg of a 0.25% to 0.375% solution) can be used when a longer duration of action is required. Addition of 5 μg/ml epinephrine prolongs duration and lowers the plasma concentration of the intermediate-acting local anesthetics.

Peak concentrations of local anesthetics in blood depend on the amount injected, the physical characteristics of the local anesthetic, and whether or not epinephrine is used. They also are determined by the rate of blood flow to the site of injection and the surface area exposed to local anesthetic. This is of particular importance in the safe application of nerve block anesthesia, as the potential for systemic reactions also is related to peak free serum concentrations. For example, peak concentrations of lidocaine in blood following injection of 400 mg without epinephrine for intercostal nerve blocks average 7 μg/ml; the same amount of lidocaine used for block of the brachial plexus results in peak concentrations in blood of approximately 3 μg/ml (Covino and Vassallo, 1976). The amount of local anesthetic that can be injected must, therefore, be adjusted according to the anatomical site of the nerve(s) to be blocked to minimize untoward effects. Addition of epinephrine can decrease peak plasma concentrations by 20% to 30%. Multiple nerve blocks (*e.g.,* intercostal block) or blocks performed in vascular regions require reduction in the amount of anesthetic that can be given safely, because the surface area for absorption or the rate of absorption is increased.

Intravenous Regional Anesthesia (Bier's Block)

This technique relies on using the vasculature to bring the local anesthetic solution to the nerve trunks and endings. In this technique, an extremity is exsanguinated with an Esmarch (elastic) bandage, and a proximally located tourniquet is inflated to 100 to 150 mm Hg above the systolic blood pressure. The Esmarch bandage is removed, and the local anesthetic is injected into a previously cannulated vein. Typically, complete anesthesia of the limb ensues within 5 to 10 minutes. Pain from the tourniquet and the potential for ischemic nerve injury limits tourniquet inflation to 2 hours or less. However, the tourniquet should remain inflated for at least 15 to 30 minutes to prevent toxic amounts of local anesthetic from entering the circulation following deflation. Lidocaine, 40 to 50 ml (0.5 ml/kg in children) of a 0.5% solution, without epinephrine, is the drug of choice for this technique. For intravenous regional anesthesia in adults using a 0.5% solution without epinephrine, the dose administered should not exceed 4 mg/kg. A few clinicians prefer prilocaine (0.5%) over lidocaine because of its higher therapeutic index. The attractiveness of this technique lies in its simplicity. Its primary disadvantages are that it can be used only for a few anatomical regions, sensation (that is, pain) returns quickly after tourniquet deflation, and premature release or failure of the tourniquet can produce toxic levels of local anesthetic (*e.g.,* 50 ml of 0.5% lidocaine contains 250 mg of lidocaine). For the last reason and because their longer durations of action offer no advantages, the more cardiotoxic local anesthetics, bupivacaine and etidocaine, are not recommended for this technique. Intravenous regional anesthesia is used most often for surgery of the forearm and hand but can be adapted for the foot and distal leg.

Spinal Anesthesia

Spinal anesthesia follows the injection of local anesthetic into the cerebrospinal fluid (CSF) in the lumbar space. This technique was first performed in human beings and described by Bier in 1899. For a number of reasons, including the ability to produce anesthesia of a considerable fraction of the body with a dose of local anesthetic that produces negligible plasma levels, it still remains one of the most popular forms of anesthesia. In most adults, the spinal cord terminates above the second lumbar vertebra; between that point and the termination of the thecal sac in the sacrum, the lumbar and sacral roots are bathed in CSF. Thus, in this region, there is a relatively large volume of CSF within which to inject drug, thereby minimizing the potential for direct nerve trauma.

A brief discussion of the physiological effects of spinal anesthesia and those features relating to the pharmacology of the local anesthetics used are presented here. The technical performance and extensive discussion of the physiological consequences of spinal anesthesia are beyond the scope of this text (*see* Greene and Brull, 1993; Cousins and Bridenbaugh, 1998).

Physiological Effects of Spinal Anesthesia.   Most of the physiological side effects of spinal anesthesia are a consequence of the sympathetic blockade produced by local anesthetic block of the sympathetic fibers in the spinal nerve roots. A thorough understanding of these physiological effects is necessary for the safe and successful application of spinal anesthesia. Although some of them may be deleterious and require treatment, others can be beneficial for the patient or can improve operating conditions. Most sympathetic fibers leave the spinal cord between T1 and L2 (Chapter 6, Figure 6–1). Although local anesthetic is injected below these levels in the lumbar portion of the dural sac, cephalad spread of the local anesthetic is seen with all but the smallest volumes injected. This cephalad spread is of considerable importance in the practice of spinal anesthesia and potentially is under the control of numerous variables, of which patient position and baricity (density of the drug relative to the density of the CSF) are the most important (Greene, 1983). The degree of sympathetic block is related to the height of sensory anesthesia; often the level of sympathetic blockade is several spinal segments higher, since the preganglionic sympathetic fibers are more sensitive to block by low concentrations of local anesthetic. The effects of sympathetic blockade involve both the actions (now partially unopposed) of the parasympathetic nervous system as well as the response of the unblocked portion of the sympathetic nervous system. Thus, as the level of sympathetic block ascends, the actions of the parasympathetic nervous system are increasingly dominant, and the compensatory mechanisms of the unblocked sympathetic nervous system are diminished. As most sympathetic nerve fibers leave

the cord at T1 or below, few additional effects of sympathetic blockade are seen with cervical levels of spinal anesthesia. The consequences of sympathetic blockade will vary among patients as a function of age, physical conditioning, and disease state. Interestingly, sympathetic blockade during spinal anesthesia appears to be inconsequential in healthy children.

Clinically, the most important effects of sympathetic blockade during spinal anesthesia are on the cardiovascular system. At all but the lowest levels of spinal blockade, some vasodilation will occur. Vasodilation is more marked on the venous than on the arterial side of the circulation, resulting in a pooling of blood in the venous capacitance vessels. At low levels of spinal anesthesia in healthy patients, this reduction in circulating blood volume is well tolerated. With an increasing level of block, this effect becomes more marked and venous return becomes gravity-dependent. If venous return decreases too much, cardiac output and organ perfusion precipitously decline. Venous return can be increased by modest (10° to 15°) head-down tilt or by elevating the legs. At high levels of spinal blockade, the cardiac accelerator fibers, which exit the spinal cord at T1 to T4, will be blocked. This is detrimental in patients dependent on elevated sympathetic tone to maintain cardiac output (*e.g.,* during congestive heart failure or hypovolemia), and it also removes one of the compensatory mechanisms available to maintain organ perfusion during vasodilation. Thus, as the level of spinal block ascends, the rate of cardiovascular compromise can accelerate if not carefully observed and treated. Sudden asystole also can occur, presumably because of loss of sympathetic innervation in the continued presence of parasympathetic activity at the sinoatrial node (Caplan, *et al.,* 1988). In the usual clinical situation, blood pressure serves as a surrogate marker for cardiac output and organ perfusion. Treatment of hypotension usually is warranted when the blood pressure decreases to about 30% of *resting* values. Therapy is aimed at maintaining brain and cardiac perfusion and oxygenation. To achieve these goals, administration of oxygen, fluid infusion, manipulation of patient position as mentioned above, and the administration of vasoactive drugs are all options. In particular, patients typically are administered a bolus (500 to 1000 ml) of fluid prior to the administration of spinal anesthesia in an attempt to prevent some of the deleterious effects of spinal blockade. As the usual cause of hypotension is decreased venous return, possibly complicated by decreased heart rate, vasoactive drugs with preferential venoconstrictive and chronotropic properties are preferred. For this reason ephedrine, 5 to 10 mg intravenously, often is the drug of choice. In addition to the use of ephedrine to treat deleterious effects of sympathetic blockade, direct-acting α_1-adrenergic receptor agonists such as phenylephrine (*see* Chapter 10) can be administered either by bolus or continuous infusion.

A beneficial effect of spinal anesthesia partially mediated by the sympathetic nervous system is on the intestine. Sympathetic fibers originating from T5 to L1 inhibit peristalsis; thus, their blockade produces a small, contracted intestine. This, together with a flaccid abdominal musculature, produces excellent operating conditions for some types of bowel surgery. The effects of spinal anesthesia on the respiratory system mostly are mediated by effects on the skeletal musculature. Paralysis of the intercostal muscles will reduce a patient's ability to cough and clear secretions, which may be undesirable in a bronchitic or emphysematous patient and may produce dyspnea. It should be noted that respiratory arrest during spinal anesthesia is seldom due to paralysis of the phrenic nerves or to toxic levels of local anesthetic in the CSF of the fourth ventricle. It is much more likely to be due to medullary ischemia secondary to hypotension.

Pharmacology of Spinal Anesthesia.   Currently in the United States, the drugs most commonly used in spinal anesthesia are lidocaine, tetracaine, and bupivacaine. Procaine occasionally is used for diagnostic blocks when a short duration of action is desired. The choice of local anesthetic primarily is determined by the duration of anesthesia desired. General guidelines are to use lidocaine for short procedures, bupivacaine for intermediate to long procedures, and tetracaine for long procedures. As mentioned above, the factors contributing to the distribution of local anesthetics in the CSF have received much attention because of their importance in determining the height of block. The most important pharmacological factors include the amount and, possibly, the volume of drug injected and its baricity. The speed of injection of the local anesthesia solution also may affect the height of the block, just as the position of the patient (*see* below) can influence the rate of distribution of the anesthetic agent and the height of blockade achieved. For a given preparation of local anesthetic, administration of increasing amounts leads to a fairly predictable increase in the level of block attained. For example, 100 mg of lidocaine, 20 mg of bupivacaine, or 12 mg of tetracaine usually will result in a T4 sensory block. More complete tables of these relationships can be found in standard anesthesiology texts. Epinephrine often is added to spinal anesthetics to increase the duration or intensity of block. Epinephrine's effect on duration of block is dependent on the technique used to measure duration. A commonly used measure of block duration is the length of time it takes for the block to recede by two dermatomes from the maximum height of the block, while a second is the duration of block at some specified level, typically L1. In most studies, addition of 200 μg of epinephrine to tetracaine solutions prolongs the duration of block by both measures. However, addition of epinephrine to lidocaine or bupivacaine does not affect the first measure of duration but does prolong the block at lower levels. In different clinical situations, one or the other measure of anesthesia duration may be more relevant, and this must be kept in mind when deciding to add epinephrine to spinal local anesthetics. The mechanism of action of vasoconstrictors in prolonging spinal anesthesia is uncertain. It has been hypothesized that these agents decrease spinal cord blood flow, decreasing clearance of local anesthetic from the CSF, but this has not been convincingly demonstrated. Epinephrine and other α-adrenergic agonists have been shown to decrease nociceptive transmission in the spinal cord, and studies in genetically modified mice suggest that α_{2A}-adrenergic receptors play a principal role in this response (Stone *et al.,* 1997). It is possible that these actions contribute to the effects of epinephrine.

Drug Baricity and Patient Position.   The baricity of the local anesthetic injected will determine the direction of migration within the dural sac. Hyperbaric solutions will tend to settle in the dependent portions of the sac, while hypobaric solutions will tend to migrate in the opposite direction. Isobaric solutions usually will stay in the vicinity where they were injected, diffusing slowly in all directions. Consideration of the patient position during and after the performance of the block and the choice of a local anesthetic of the appropriate baricity is crucial for a successful block during some surgical procedures.

For example, a saddle (perineal) block is best performed with a hyperbaric anesthetic in the sitting position, with the patient remaining in that position until the anesthetic level has become "fixed." On the other hand, for a saddle block in the prone, jackknife position, a hypobaric local anesthetic is appropriate. Lidocaine and bupivacaine are marketed in both isobaric and hyperbaric preparations and, if desired, can be diluted with sterile, preservative-free water to make them hypobaric.

Complications of Spinal Anesthesia.   Persistent neurological deficits following spinal anesthesia are extremely rare. Thorough evaluation of a suspected deficit should be performed in collaboration with a neurologist. Neurological sequelae can be both immediate and late. Possible causes include introduction of foreign substances (such as disinfectants or talc) into the subarachnoid space, infection, hematoma, or direct mechanical trauma. Aside from drainage of an abscess or hematoma, treatment usually is ineffective; thus, avoidance and careful attention to detail while performing spinal anesthesia are necessary. High concentrations of local anesthetic can cause irreversible block. After administration, local anesthetic solutions are diluted rapidly, quickly reaching nontoxic concentrations. However, there are several reports of transient or longer-lasting neurological deficits following lidocaine spinal anesthesia, particularly with 5% lidocaine (*i.e.,* 180 mM) in 7.5% glucose (Hodgson *et al.,* 1999). Spinal anesthesia sometimes is regarded as contraindicated in patients with preexisting disease of the spinal cord. No experimental evidence exists to support this hypothesis. Nonetheless, it is prudent to avoid spinal anesthesia in patients with progressive diseases of the spinal cord. However, spinal anesthesia may be very useful in patients with fixed, chronic spinal cord injury.

A more common sequela following any lumbar puncture, including spinal anesthesia, is a postural headache with classic features. The incidence of headache decreases with increasing age of the patient and decreasing needle diameter. Headache following lumbar puncture must be thoroughly evaluated to exclude serious complications such as meningitis. Treatment usually is conservative, with bed rest and analgesics. If this approach fails, an epidural blood patch can be performed; this procedure usually is successful in alleviating post–dural puncture headaches, although a second blood patch may be necessary. If two epidural blood patches are ineffective in relieving the headache, the diagnosis of post–dural puncture headache should be reconsidered. Intravenous caffeine (500 mg as the benzoate salt administered over 4 hours) also has been advocated for the treatment of post–dural puncture headache. However, the efficacy of caffeine is less than that of a blood patch, and relief usually is transient.

Evaluation of Spinal Anesthesia.   Spinal anesthesia is a safe and effective technique. Its value is greatest during surgery involving the lower abdomen, the lower extremities, and the perineum. It often is combined with intravenous medication to provide sedation and amnesia. The physiological perturbations associated with low spinal anesthesia often have less potential harm than those associated with general anesthesia. The same does not apply for high spinal anesthesia. The sympathetic blockade that accompanies levels of spinal anesthesia adequate for mid- or upper-abdominal surgery, coupled with the difficulty in achieving visceral analgesia, is such that equally satisfactory and safer operating conditions can be realized by combining the spinal anesthetic with a "light" general anesthetic or by the administration of a general anesthetic and a neuromuscular blocking agent.

Epidural Anesthesia

Epidural anesthesia is administered by injecting local anesthetic into the epidural space—the space bounded by the ligamentum flavum posteriorly, the spinal periosteum laterally, and the dura anteriorly. Epidural anesthesia can be performed in the sacral hiatus (caudal anesthesia) or in the lumbar, thoracic, or cervical regions of the spine. Its current popularity arises from the development of catheters that can be placed into the epidural space, allowing either continuous infusions or repeated bolus administration of local anesthetics. The primary site of action of epidurally administered local anesthetics is on the spinal nerve roots. However, epidurally administered local anesthetics also may act on the spinal cord and on the paravertebral nerves.

The selection of drugs available for epidural anesthesia is similar to that for major nerve blocks. As for spinal anesthesia, the choice of drugs to be used during epidural anesthesia is dictated primarily by the duration of anesthesia desired. However, when an epidural catheter is placed, short-acting drugs can be administered repeatedly, providing more control over the duration of block. Bupivacaine, 0.5% to 0.75%, is used when a long duration of surgical block is desired. Due to enhanced cardiotoxicity in pregnant patients, the 0.75% solution is not approved for obstetrical use. Lower concentrations—0.25%, 0.125%, or 0.0625%—of bupivacaine, often with 2 μg/ml of fentanyl added, frequently are used to provide analgesia during labor. They also are useful preparations for providing postoperative analgesia in certain clinical situations. Etidocaine, 1.0% or 1.5%, is useful for providing surgical anesthesia with excellent muscle relaxation of long duration. Lidocaine, 2%, is the most frequently used intermediate-acting epidural local anesthetic. Chloroprocaine, 2% or 3%, provides rapid onset and a very short duration of anesthetic action. However, its use in epidural anesthesia has been clouded by controversy regarding its potential ability to cause neurological complications if the drug is accidentally injected into the subarachnoid space (*see* above). The duration of action of epidurally administered local anesthetics is frequently prolonged, and systemic toxicity decreased, by addition of epinephrine. Addition of epinephrine also makes inadvertent intravascular injection easier to detect and modifies the effect of sympathetic blockade during epidural anesthesia.

For each anesthetic agent, a relationship exists between the volume of local anesthetic injected epidurally and the segmental level of anesthesia achieved. For example, in 20- to 40-year-old, healthy, nonpregnant patients, each 1 to 1.5 ml of 2% lidocaine will give an additional segment of anesthesia. The amount needed will decrease with increasing age and also will be decreased during pregnancy and in children.

The concentration of local anesthetic used determines the type of nerve fibers blocked. The highest concentrations are used when sympathetic, somatic sensory, and somatic motor blockade are required. Intermediate concentrations allow somatic sensory anesthesia without muscle relaxation. Low concentrations will block only preganglionic sympathetic fibers. As an example, with bupivacaine these effects might be achieved with concentrations of 0.5%, 0.25%, and 0.0625%, respectively. The total amounts of drug that can be injected with safety at one

time are approximately those mentioned above under "Nerve Block Anesthesia" and "Infiltration Anesthesia." Performance of epidural anesthesia requires a greater degree of skill than does spinal anesthesia. The technique of epidural anesthesia and the volumes, concentrations, and types of drugs used are described in detail in standard anesthesiology texts (*e.g., see* Cousins and Bridenbaugh, 1998).

A significant difference between epidural and spinal anesthesia is that the dose of local anesthetic used can produce high concentrations in blood following absorption from the epidural space. Peak concentrations of lidocaine in blood following injection of 400 mg (without epinephrine) into the lumbar epidural space average 3 to 4 μg/ml; peak concentrations of bupivacaine in blood average 1.0 μg/ml after the lumbar epidural injection of 150 mg. Addition of epinephrine (5 μg/ml) decreases peak plasma concentrations by about 25%. Peak blood concentrations are a function of the total dose of drug administered rather than the concentration or volume of solution following epidural injection (Covino and Vassallo, 1976). The risk of inadvertent intravascular injection is increased in epidural anesthesia, as the epidural space contains a rich venous plexus.

Another major difference between epidural and spinal anesthesia is that there is no zone of differential sympathetic blockade with epidural anesthesia; thus, the level of sympathetic block is close to the level of sensory block. Because epidural anesthesia does not result in the zone of differential sympathetic blockade that is observed during spinal anesthesia, cardiovascular responses to epidural anesthesia might be expected to be less prominent. In practice, however, this is not the case; this potential advantage of epidural anesthesia is offset by the cardiovascular responses to the high concentration of anesthetic in blood that occurs during epidural anesthesia. This is most apparent when, as is often the case, epinephrine is added to the epidural injection. The resulting concentration of epinephrine in blood is sufficient to produce significant β_2-adrenergic receptor-mediated vasodilation. As a consequence, blood pressure decreases, even though cardiac output increases owing to the positive inotropic and chronotropic effects of epinephrine (*see* Chapter 10). The result is peripheral hyperperfusion and hypotension. Differences in cardiovascular responses to equal levels of spinal and epidural anesthesia also are observed when a local anesthetic such as lidocaine is used without epinephrine. This may be a consequence of the direct effects of high concentrations of lidocaine on vascular smooth muscle and the heart. The magnitude of the differences in responses to equal sensory levels of spinal and epidural anesthesia varies, however, with the local anesthetic used for the epidural injection (assuming no epinephrine is used). For example, local anesthetics such as bupivacaine, which are highly lipid soluble, are distributed less into the circulation than are less lipid-soluble agents such as lidocaine.

High concentrations of local anesthetics in blood during epidural anesthesia are of special importance when this technique is used to control pain during labor and delivery. Local anesthetics cross the placenta, enter the fetal circulation, and at high concentrations may cause depression of the neonate (Scanlon *et al.,* 1974). The extent to which they do so is determined by dosage, acid–base status, the level of protein binding in both maternal and fetal blood (Tucker, *et al.,* 1970), placental blood flow, and solubility of the agent in fetal tissue. These concerns have been lessened by the trend toward using more dilute solutions of bupivacaine for labor analgesia.

Epidural and Intrathecal Opiate Analgesia. Small quantities of opioid injected intrathecally or epidurally produce segmental analgesia (Yaksh and Rudy, 1976). This observation led to the clinical use of spinal and epidural opioids during surgical procedures and for the relief of postoperative and chronic pain (Cousins and Mather, 1984). As with local anesthesia, analgesia is confined to sensory nerves that enter the spinal cord dorsal horn in the vicinity of the injection. Presynaptic opioid receptors inhibit the release of substance P and other neurotransmitters from primary afferents, while postsynaptic opioid receptors decrease the activity of certain dorsal horn neurons in the spinothalamic tracts (Willcockson, *et al.,* 1986; *see* also Chapters 6 and 23). Since conduction in autonomic, sensory, and motor nerves is not affected by the opioids, blood pressure, motor function, and nonnociceptive sensory perception typically are not influenced by spinal opioids. The volume-evoked micturition reflex is inhibited, implicating opioid receptors in this reflex pathway. Clinically, this is manifest by urinary retention. Other side effects include pruritus and nausea and vomiting in susceptible individuals. Delayed respiratory depression and sedation, presumably from cephalad spread of opioid within the CSF, occurs infrequently with the doses of opioids currently used.

Spinally administered opioids by themselves do not provide satisfactory anesthesia for surgical procedures. Thus, opioids have found the greatest use in the treatment of postoperative and chronic pain. In selected patients, spinal or epidural opioids can provide excellent analgesia following thoracic, abdominal, pelvic, or lower extremity surgery without the side effects associated with high doses of systemically administered opioids. For postoperative analgesia, spinally administered morphine, 0.2 to 0.5 mg, usually will provide 8 to 16 hours of analgesia. Placement of an epidural catheter and repeated boluses or an infusion of opioid permits an increased duration of analgesia. Many opioids have been used epidurally. Morphine, 2 to 6 mg, every 6 hours, commonly is used for bolus injections, while fentanyl, 20 to 50 μg/hour, often combined with bupivacaine, 5 to 20 mg/hour, is used for infusions. For cancer pain, repeated doses of epidural opioids can provide analgesia of several months' duration. The dose of epidural morphine, for example, is far less than the dose of systemically administered morphine that would be required to provide similar analgesia. This reduces the complications that usually accompany the administration of high doses of systemic opioids, particularly sedation and constipation. Unfortunately, like systemic opioids, tolerance will develop to the analgesic effects of epidural opioids, but this can usually be managed by increasing the dose.

BIBLIOGRAPHY

Caplan, R.A., Ward, R.J., Posner, K., and Cheney, F.W. Unexpected cardiac arrest during spinal anesthesia: a closed claims analysis of predisposing factors. *Anesthesiology,* **1988,** *68*:5–11.

Catterall, W.A. Structure and function of voltage-sensitive ion channels. *Science,* **1988,** *242*:50–61.

Charnet, P., Labarca, C., Leonard, R.J., Vogelaar, N.J., Czyzyk, L., Gouin, E., Davidson, N., and Lester, H.A. An open-channel blocker interacts with adjacent turns of alpha-helices in the nicotinic acetylcholine receptor. *Neuron,* **1990,** *4*:87–95.

Clarkson, C.W., and Hondeghem, L.M. Mechanism for bupivacaine depression of cardiac conduction: fast block of sodium channels during the action potential with slow recovery from block during diastole. *Anesthesiology,* **1985,** *62*:396–405.

Cousins, M.J., and Mather, L.E. Intrathecal and epidural administration of opioids. *Anesthesiology,* **1984,** *61*:276–310.

Fink, B.R., and Cairns, A.M. Differential slowing and block of conduction by lidocaine in individual afferent myelinated and unmyelinated axons. *Anesthesiology,* **1984,** *60*:111–120.

Franz, D.N., and Perry, R.S. Mechanisms for differential block among single myelinated and nonmyelinated axons by procaine. *J. Physiol.,* **1974,** *236*:193–210.

Gasser, H.S., and Erlanger, J. The role of fiber size in the establishment of a nerve block by pressure or cocaine. *Am. J. Physiol.,* **1929,** *88*:581–591.

Hodgson, P.S., Neal, J.M., Pollock, J.E., and Liu, S.S. The neurotoxicity of drugs given intrathecally. *Anesth. Analg.,* **1999,** *88*:797–809.

Huang, J.H., Thalhammer, J.G., Raymond, S.A., and Strichartz, G.R. Susceptibility to lidocaine of impulses in different somatosensory

fibers of rat sciatic nerve. *J. Pharmacol. Exp. Ther.,* **1997,** *292*:802–811.

Narahashi, T., and Frazier, D.T. Site of action and active form of local anesthetics. *Neurosci. Res. (N.Y.),* **1971,** *4*:65–99.

Neher, E., and Steinbach, J.H. Local anesthetics transiently block currents through single acetylcholine-receptor channels. *J. Physiol.,* **1978,** *277*:153–176.

Ragsdale, D.R., McPhee, J.C., Scheuer, T., and Catterall, W.A. Molecular determinants of state-dependent block of Na$^+$ channels by local anesthetics. *Science,* **1994,** *265*:1724–1728.

Scanlon, J.W., Brown, W.U. Jr., Weiss, J.B., and Alper, M.H. Neurobehavioral responses of newborn infants after maternal epidural anesthesia. *Anesthesiology,* **1974,** *40*:121–128.

Stevens, R.A., Urmey, W.F., Urquhart, B.L., and Kao, T.C. Back pain after epidural anesthesia with chloroprocaine. *Anesthesiology,* **1993,** *78*:492–497.

Stone, L.S., MacMillan, L.B., Kitto, K.F., Limbird, L.E., and Wilcox, G.L. The alpha 2a adrenergic receptor subtype mediates spinal analgesia evoked by alpha 2 agonists and is necessary for spinal adrenergic-opioid synergy. *J. Neurosci.,* **1997,** *37*:1255–1260.

Terlau, H., Heinemann, S.H., Stühmer, W., Pusch, M., Conti, F., Imoto, K., and Numa, S. Mapping the site of block by tetrodotoxin and saxitoxin of sodium channel II. *FEBS Lett.,* **1991,** *293*:93–96.

Thomas, R.D., Behbehani, M.M., Coyle, D.E., and Denson, D.D. Cardiovascular toxicity of local anesthetics: an alternative hypothesis. *Anesth. Analg.,* **1986,** *65*:444–450.

Tucker, G.T., Boyes, R.N., Bridenbaugh, P.O., and Moore, D.C. Binding of anilide-type local anesthetics in human plasma. II. Implications in vivo, with special reference to transplacental distribution. *Anesthesiology,* **1970,** *33:*304–314.

Willcockson, W.S., Kim, J., Shin, H.K., Chung, J.M., and Willis, W.D. Actions of opioid on primate spinothalamic tract neurons. *J. Neurosci.,* **1986,** 6:2509–2520.

Winnie, A.P., Tay, C.H., Patel, K.P., Ramanmurthy, S., and Durrani, Z. Pharmacokinetics of local anesthetics during plexus blocks. *Anesth. Analg.,* **1977,** *56:*852–861.

Yaksh, T.L., and Rudy, T.A. Analgesia mediated by a direct spinal action of narcotics. *Science,* **1976,** *192:*1357–1358.

MONOGRAPHS AND REVIEWS

Arthur, G.R. Pharmacokinetics. In, *Local Anesthetics.* (Strichartz, G.R., ed.) *Handbook of Experimental Pharmacology.* Vol. 81. Springer-Verlag, Berlin, **1987,** pp. 165–186.

Butterworth, J.F. IV, and Strichartz, G.R. Molecular mechanisms of local anesthesia: a review. *Anesthesiology,* **1990,** *72:*711–734.

Carpenter, R.L., and Mackey, D.C. Local anesthetics. In, *Clinical Anesthesia,* 2nd ed. (Barash, P.G., Cullen, B.F., and Stoelting, R.K., eds.) Lippincott, Philadelphia, **1992,** pp. 509–541.

Catterall, W.A. From ionic currents to molecular mechanisms: the structure and function of voltage-gated sodium channels. *Neuron,* **2000,** *26:*13–25.

Courtney, K.R., and Strichartz, G.R. Structural elements which determine local anesthetic activity. In, *Local Anesthetics.* (Strichartz, G.R., ed.) *Handbook of Experimental Pharmacology.* Vol. 81. Springer-Verlag, Berlin, **1987,** pp. 53–94.

Cousins, M.J., and Bridenbaugh, P.O., eds. *Neural Blockade in Clinical Anesthesia and Management of Pain,* 3rd ed. Lippincott-Raven, Philadelphia, **1998.**

Covino, B.G. Toxicity and systemic effects of local anesthetic agents. In, *Local Anesthetics.* (Strichartz, G.R., ed.) *Handbook of Experimental Pharmacology.* Vol. 81. Springer-Verlag, Berlin, **1987,** pp. 187–212.

Covino, B.G., and Vassallo, H.G. *Local Anesthetics: Mechanisms of Action and Clinical Use.* Grune & Stratton, New York, **1976.**

DeJong, R.H. *Local Anesthetics.* Mosby, St. Louis, MO, **1994.**

Garfield, J.M., and Gugino, L. Central effects of local anesthetics. In, *Local Anesthetics.* (Strichartz, G.R., ed.) *Handbook of Experimental Pharmacology.* Vol. 81. Springer-Verlag, Berlin, **1987,** pp. 253–284.

Gintant, G.A., and Hoffman, B.F. The role of local anesthetic effects in the actions of antiarrhythmic drugs. In, *Local Anesthetics.* (Strichartz, G.R., ed.) *Handbook of Experimental Pharmacology.* Vol. 81. Springer-Verlag, Berlin, **1987,** pp. 213–251.

Greene, N.M. Uptake and elimination of local anesthetics during spinal anesthesia. *Anesth. Analg.,* **1983,** *62:*1013–1024.

Greene, N.M., and Brull, S.J. *Physiology of Spinal Anesthesia,* 4th ed. Williams & Wilkins, Baltimore, **1993.**

Kao, C.Y. Pharmacology of tetrodotoxin and saxitoxin. *Fed. Proc.,* **1972,** *31:*1117–1123.

McClure, J.H. Ropivacaine. *Br. J. Anaesth.,* **1996,** *76:*300–307.

Ogura, Y. Fugu (puffer-fish) poisoning and the pharmacology of crystalline tetrodotoxin poisoning. In, *Neuropoisons: Their Pathophysiological Actions.* Vol. 1. *Poisons of Animal Origin.* (Simpson, L.L., ed.) Plenum Press, New York, **1971,** pp. 139–156.

Raymond, S.A., and Gissen, A.J. Mechanism of differential nerve block. In, *Local Anesthetics.* (Strichartz, G.R., ed.) *Handbook of Experimental Pharmacology.* Vol. 81. Springer-Verlag, Berlin, **1987,** pp. 95–164.

Ritchie, J.M. Tetrodotoxin and saxitoxin and the sodium channels of excitable tissues. *Trends Pharmacol. Sci.,* **1980,** *1:*275–279.

Ritchie, J.M., and Greengard, P. On the mode of action of local anesthetics. *Annu. Rev. Pharmacol.,* **1966,** *6:*405–430.

Schantz, E.J. Paralytic shellfish poisoning and saxitoxin. In, *Neuropoisons: Their Pathophysiological Actions.* Vol. 1. *Poisons of Animal Origin.* (Simpson, L.L., ed.) Plenum Press, New York, **1971,** pp. 159–168.

Strichartz, G.R., and Ritchie, J.M. The action of local anesthetics on ion channels of excitable tissues. In, *Local Anesthetics.* (Strichartz, G.R., ed.) *Handbook of Experimental Pharmacology.* Vol. 81. Springer-Verlag, Berlin, **1987,** pp. 21–53.

Zipf, H.F., and Dittmann, E.C. General pharmacological effects of local anesthetics. In, *Local Anesthetics,* Vol. 1. *International Encyclopedia of Pharmacology and Therapeutics,* Sect. 8. (Lechat, P., ed.) Pergamon Press, Ltd., Oxford, **1971,** pp. 191–238.

THERAPEUTIC GASES

Oxygen, Carbon Dioxide, Nitric Oxide, and Helium

Eric J. Moody, Brett A. Simon, and Roger A. Johns

Inhaled nonanesthetic gases, especially oxygen, represent an important therapeutic modality. Normal oxygenation and the physiological consequences of oxygen deprivation and excess are presented together with modes of administration and monitoring. In addition, the therapeutic use and administration of carbon dioxide, nitric oxide, and helium are discussed in this chapter.

OXYGEN

Oxygen is a fundamental requirement for animal existence. Hypoxia is a life-threatening condition in which oxygen delivery is inadequate to meet the metabolic demands of the tissues. Since oxygen delivery is the product of blood flow and oxygen content, hypoxia may result from alterations in tissue perfusion, decreased oxygen tension in the blood, or decreased oxygen carrying capacity. In addition, hypoxia may result from a problem in oxygen transport from the microvasculature to the cells or in utilization within the cell. Irrespective of cause, an inadequate supply of oxygen ultimately results in the cessation of aerobic metabolism and oxidative phosphorylation, depletion of high-energy compounds, cellular dysfunction, and death.

History. Soon after Priestley's discovery of oxygen in 1772 and Lavoisier's elucidation of its role in respiration, oxygen therapy was introduced in England by Beddoes. His publication in 1794, entitled "Considerations on the Medicinal Use and Production of Factitious Airs," can be considered the beginning of inhalational therapy. Beddoes, overcome with enthusiasm for his project, treated all kinds of diseases with oxygen, including such diverse conditions as scrofula, leprosy, and paralysis. Such indiscriminate therapeutic applications naturally led to many failures, and Beddoes died a disconsolate man. Beddoes' assistant Sir Humphrey Davy went on to make significant contributions to our knowledge of the anesthetic gas nitrous oxide. It was as a result of pioneer investigations such as those of Haldane, Hill, Barcroft, Krogh, L. J. Henderson, and Y. Henderson that oxygen therapy achieved a sound physiological basis (Sackner, 1974). Although Paul Bert had studied therapeutic aspects of hyperbaric oxygen in 1870 and identified oxygen toxicity (Bert, 1873), the use of oxygen at pressures above 1 atmosphere for therapeutic purposes did not begin until the 1950s (Lambertsen *et al.*, 1953; Boerema *et al.*, 1960).

Normal Oxygenation

Oxygen makes up 21% of air, which at sea level (1 atmosphere, 101 kPa) represents a partial pressure of 21 kPa (158 mmHg). While the fraction (percentage) of oxygen remains constant regardless of atmospheric pressure and altitude, the partial pressure of oxygen (P_{O_2}) decreases with lower atmospheric pressure. Since it is this partial pressure that drives the diffusion of oxygen, ascent to elevated altitude reduces the uptake and delivery of oxygen to the tissues. Conversely, increases in atmospheric pressure (hyperbaric therapy, or breathing at depth) increase the P_{O_2} in inspired air and result in increased gas uptake. As the air is delivered to the distal airways and alveoli, the P_{O_2} decreases by dilution with carbon dioxide and water vapor and by uptake into the blood. Under ideal conditions, when ventilation and perfusion are uniformly distributed, the alveolar P_{O_2} will be approximately 14.6 kPa (110 mmHg). The corresponding alveolar partial pressures of water and carbon dioxide are 6.2 kPa (47 mmHg) and 5.3 kPa (40 mmHg), respectively. Under normal conditions, there is complete equilibration of alveolar gas and capillary blood, and the P_{O_2} in end capillary blood is typically within a fraction of a kPa of that in the alveoli. Under conditions of disease, when the diffusion barrier for gas transport may be increased, or exercise, when high cardiac output reduces capillary transit time, full equilibration may not occur, and the alveolar–end capillary P_{O_2} gradient may be increased.

The P_{O_2} in arterial blood, however, is further reduced by venous admixture (shunt), the addition of mixed venous blood, which has a P_{O_2} of approximately 5.3 kPa (40 mmHg). Together, the diffusional barrier, inhomogeneities of ventilation and perfusion, and the shunt fraction are the major causes of the alveolar-to-arterial oxygen gradient, which is normally 1.3 to 1.6 kPa (10 to 12 mmHg) when air is breathed and 4.0 to 6.6 kPa (30 to 50 mmHg) when 100% oxygen is breathed (Clark and Lambertsen, 1971).

Oxygen is delivered to the tissue capillary beds by the circulation and again follows a gradient out of the blood and into cells. Tissue extraction of oxygen typically reduces the P_{O_2} of venous blood by an additional 7.3 kPa (55 mmHg). The mean tissue P_{O_2} is much lower than the value in the mixed

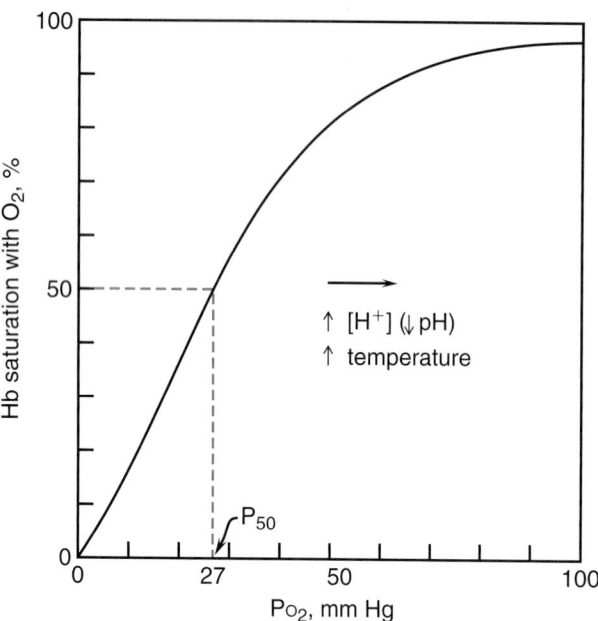

Figure 16–1. Oxyhemoglobin dissociation curve for whole blood.

The relationship between P_{O_2} and hemoglobin (Hb) saturation is shown. The P_{50}, or the P_{O_2} resulting in 50% saturation, is indicated as well. An increase in temperature or a decrease in pH (as in working muscle) shifts this relationship to the right, reducing the hemoglobin saturation at the same P_{O_2} and thus aiding in the delivery of oxygen to the tissues.

venous blood because of substantial diffusional barriers and the consumption of oxygen in the tissues. Although the P_{O_2} at the site of oxygen utilization—the mitochondria—is not known, oxidative phosphorylation can continue at a P_{O_2} of only a few mm Hg (Robiolio *et al.*, 1989).

In the blood, oxygen is carried primarily in chemical combination with hemoglobin and to a small extent dissolved in solution. The quantity of oxygen combined with hemoglobin depends on the P_{O_2}, as illustrated by the sigmoid-shaped oxyhemoglobin dissociation curve (Figure 16–1). Hemoglobin is about 98% saturated with oxygen when air is breathed under normal circumstances, and it binds 1.3 ml of oxygen per gram when fully saturated. The steep slope of this curve with falling P_{O_2} facilitates unloading of oxygen from hemoglobin at the tissue level and reloading when desaturated, mixed venous blood arrives at the lung. Shifting of the curve to the right with increasing temperature, increasing P_{CO_2}, and decreasing pH, as is found in metabolically active tissues, lowers the oxygen saturation for the same P_{O_2} and thus delivers additional oxygen where and when it is most needed. However, the flattening of the curve with higher P_{O_2} indicates that increasing blood P_{O_2} by inspiring oxygen-enriched mixtures only minimally can increase the amount of oxygen carried by hemoglobin. Further increases in blood oxygen content can occur only by increasing the amount of oxygen dissolved in plasma. Because of the low solubility of oxygen (0.226 ml/liter per kPa or 0.03ml/liter

per mm Hg at 37°C), breathing 100% oxygen can increase the amount of oxygen in blood by only 15 ml per liter, less than one third of normal metabolic demands. However, if the inspired P_{O_2} is increased to 3 atmospheres (304 kPa) in a hyperbaric chamber, the amount of dissolved oxygen is sufficient to meet normal metabolic demands even in the absence of hemoglobin (Table 16–1).

Oxygen Deprivation

An understanding of the causes and effects of oxygen deficiency is necessary for the rational therapeutic use of the gas. *Hypoxia* is the term used to denote insufficient oxygenation of the tissues. *Hypoxemia* generally implies a failure of the respiratory system to oxygenate arterial blood.

Pulmonary Mechanisms of Hypoxemia. Classically there are five causes of hypoxemia: low inspired oxygen fraction ($F_{I_{O_2}}$), increased diffusion barrier, hypoventilation, ventilation/perfusion ($\dot{V}/\dot{Q}$) mismatch, and shunt or venous admixture.

Low $F_{I_{O_2}}$ is a cause of hypoxemia only at high altitude or in the event of equipment failure, such as a gas blender malfunction or a mislabeled compressed-gas tank. An increase in the barrier to diffusion of oxygen within the lung is rarely a cause of hypoxemia in a resting subject, except in end-stage parenchymal lung disease. Both of these problems may be alleviated with administration of supplemental oxygen, the former by definition and the latter by increasing the gradient driving diffusion.

Hypoventilation causes hypoxemia by reducing the alveolar P_{O_2} in proportion to the build-up of CO_2 in the alveoli. In essence, during hypoventilation there is decreased delivery of oxygen to the alveoli while its removal by the blood remains the same, causing its alveolar concentration to fall. The opposite occurs with carbon dioxide. This is described by the alveolar gas equation: $P_{A_{O_2}} = P_{I_{O_2}} - (P_{A_{CO_2}}/R)$, where $P_{A_{O_2}}$ and $P_{A_{CO_2}}$ are the alveolar partial pressures of O_2 and CO_2, $P_{I_{O_2}}$ the partial pressure of O_2 in the inspired gas, and R the respiratory quotient. Under normal conditions, breathing room air at sea level (corrected for the partial pressure of water vapor), the $P_{I_{O_2}}$ is about 20 kPa (150 mmHg), the $P_{A_{CO_2}}$ about 5.3 kPa (40 mmHg), R is 0.8, and thus the $P_{A_{O_2}}$ is normally around 13.3 kPa (100 mmHg). It would require substantial hypoventilation, with the $P_{A_{CO_2}}$ rising to over 9.3 kPa (70 mmHg), to cause the $P_{A_{O_2}}$ to fall below 7.8 kPa (60 mmHg). This cause of hypoxemia is readily prevented by administration of even small amounts of supplemental oxygen.

Table 16–1
The Carriage of Oxygen in Blood*

ARTERIAL PO$_2$ kPa (mm Hg)	Arterial O$_2$ Content (ml O$_2$/liter)			MIXED VENOUS PO$_2$ kPa (mm Hg)	Mixed Venous O$_2$ Content (ml O$_2$/liter)			EXAMPLES
	DISSOLVED	BOUND TO HEMOGLOBIN	TOTAL		DISSOLVED	BOUND TO HEMOGLOBIN	TOTAL	
4.0 (30)	1.0	109	110	2.7 (20)	0.6	59	59.6	High altitude or respiratory failure breathing air
12.0 (90)	3.0	192	195	5.4 (41)	1.2	144	145.2	Normal person breathing air
9.0 (300)	9.0	195	204	5.8 (44)	1.2	153	154.2	Normal person breathing 50% O$_2$
79.7 (600)	18	196	214	6.5 (49)	1.4	163	164.2	Normal person breathing 100% O$_2$
239 (1800)	54	196	250	19.9 (150)	4.5	196	200.5	Normal person breathing hyperbaric O$_2$

*This table illustrates the carriage of oxygen in the blood under a variety of circumstances. As arterial oxygen tension increases, the amount of dissolved oxygen increases in direct proportion to the PO$_2$, but the amount of oxygen bound to hemoglobin reaches a maximum of 196 ml O$_2$/liter (100% saturation of hemoglobin at 15 g/dl). Further increases in oxygen content require increases in dissolved oxygen. At 100% inspired oxygen, dissolved oxygen still provides only a small fraction of total demand. Hyperbaric oxygen therapy is required to increase the amount of dissolved oxygen to supply all or a large part of metabolic requirements. Note that, during hyperbaric oxygen therapy, the hemoglobin in the mixed venous blood remains fully saturated with oxygen.

The figures in this table are approximate and are based on the assumptions of 15 g/dl hemoglobin, 50 ml O$_2$/liter whole-body oxygen extraction, and constant cardiac output. When severe anemia is present, arterial PO$_2$ remains the same, but arterial content is lower. Oxygen extraction continues, resulting in lower oxygen content and tension in mixed venous blood. Similarly, as cardiac output falls significantly, the same oxygen extraction occurs from a smaller volume of blood and results in lower mixed venous oxygen content and tension.

Shunt and $\dot{V}/\dot{Q}$ mismatch are related causes of hypoxemia, but with an important distinction in their responses to supplemental oxygen. Optimal gas exchange occurs when blood flow ($\dot{Q}$) and ventilation ($\dot{V}$) are quantitatively matched. However, regional variations in $\dot{V}/\dot{Q}$ matching typically exist within the lung, particularly in the presence of lung disease. As ventilation increases relative to blood flow, the alveolar PO_2 (PA_{O_2}) increases; but because of the flat shape of the oxyhemoglobin dissociation curve at high PO_2 (Figure 16–1), this increased PA_{O_2} does not contribute much to the oxygen content of the blood. In addition, high $\dot{V}/\dot{Q}$ ratio lung regions have a relatively reduced blood flow, eventually becoming pure dead space regions at the extreme—contributing nothing to the oxygenation of the blood while decreasing the efficiency of CO_2 removal. Conversely, as the $\dot{V}/\dot{Q}$ ratio falls and perfusion increases relative to ventilation, the PA_{O_2} of the blood leaving these regions falls relative to regions with better matched ventilation and perfusion. Since the oxyhemoglobin dissociation curve is steep at these lower PO_2 values, the oxygen saturation and content of the pulmonary venous blood falls significantly. At the extreme of low $\dot{V}/\dot{Q}$ ratios, there is no ventilation to a perfused region and pure shunt results, and the blood leaving the region has the same low PO_2 and high PCO_2 as mixed venous blood.

The deleterious effect of $\dot{V}/\dot{Q}$ mismatch on arterial oxygenation is thus a direct result of the asymmetry of the oxyhemoglobin dissociation curve. Adding supplemental oxygen will generally make up for the fall in PA_{O_2} in low $\dot{V}/\dot{Q}$ units and thus improve arterial oxygenation. However, since there is no ventilation to units with pure shunt, supplemental oxygen will not be effective in reversing the hypoxemia from this cause. Because of the steep oxyhemoglobin dissociation curve at low PO_2, even moderate amounts of pure shunt will cause significant hypoxemia despite oxygen therapy (Figure 16–2). For the same reason, factors that decrease mixed venous PO_2, such as decreased cardiac output or increased oxygen consumption, enhance the effects of $\dot{V}/\dot{Q}$ mismatch and shunt in causing hypoxemia.

Nonpulmonary Causes of Hypoxia.   In addition to failure of the respiratory system to adequately oxygenate the blood, there are a number of other factors that can contribute to hypoxia at the tissue level. These may be divided into categories of oxygen delivery and oxygen utilization. Oxygen delivery decreases globally when cardiac output falls or locally when regional blood flow is compromised, as from a vascular occlusion (stenosis, throm-

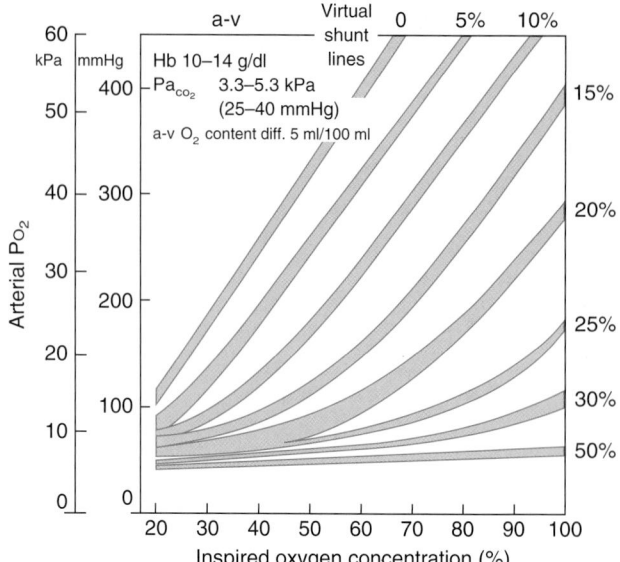

Figure 16–2. Effect of shunt on arterial oxygenation.

The iso-shunt diagram shows the effect of changing inspired oxygen concentration on arterial oxygenation in the presence of different amounts of pure shunt. As shunt fraction increases, even an inspired oxygen fraction (FI_{O_2}) of 1.0 is ineffective at increasing the arterial PO_2. This estimation assumes hemoglobin (Hb) from 10 to 14 g/dl, arterial PCO_2 of 3.3 to 5.3 kPa (25 to 40 mmHg), and an arterial-venous (a-v) O_2 content difference of 5 ml/100 ml. Redrawn from Benatar et al., 1973, with permission.

bosis, microvascular occlusion) or increased downstream pressure to flow (compartment syndrome, venous stasis, or venous hypertension). Decreased oxygen-carrying capacity of the blood will likewise decrease oxygen delivery, as occurs with anemia, carbon monoxide poisoning, or hemoglobinopathy. Finally, hypoxia may occur when transport of oxygen from the capillaries to the tissues is decreased (edema) or utilization of the oxygen by the cells impaired (cyanide toxicity).

Multiple causes of hypoxia often coexist. A victim of smoke inhalation may have an airway obstruction as a result of thermal injury and reduced oxygen carrying capacity because of carbon monoxide poisoning and anemia. An organ with a marginal blood supply because of atherosclerosis may be seriously damaged if the PO_2 of its arterial supply is decreased only slightly.

Effects of Hypoxia.   Regardless of the cause, hypoxia ultimately results in the cessation of aerobic metabolism, exhaustion of high-energy intracellular stores, cellular dysfunction, and death. The time course of cellular demise depends upon the tissue's relative metabolic requirements, oxygen and energy stores, and anaerobic capacity. Survival times (the time from the onset of circulatory arrest to significant organ dysfunction) range from 1 minute in the cerebral cortex to around 5 minutes in the heart and 10 minutes in the kidneys and liver, with the potential for some degree of recovery if reperfused. Revival times (the duration of hypoxia beyond which recovery is no longer possible) are approximately 4 to 5 times longer. Less severe degrees of hypoxia have progressive physiological effects on different organ systems (Nunn, 1993b).

Respiratory System.   Hypoxia stimulates the carotid and aortic baroreceptors to cause increases in both the rate and depth of ventilation. Minute volume almost doubles when normal individuals inspire gas with a PO_2 of 6.6 kPa (50 mm Hg). Dyspnea is not always experienced with simple hypoxia but occurs when the respiratory minute volume approaches half the maximal breathing capacity; this may occur with minimum exertion in patients in whom maximal breathing capacity is reduced by lung disease. In general, little warning precedes the loss of consciousness resulting from hypoxia.

Cardiovascular System.   Hypoxia causes reflex activation of the sympathetic nervous system *via* both autonomic and humoral mechanisms, resulting in tachycardia and increased cardiac output. Peripheral vascular resistance, however, decreases primarily *via* local autoregulatory mechanisms, with the net result that blood pressure is generally maintained unless hypoxia is prolonged or severe. In contrast to the systemic circulation, hypoxia causes pulmonary vasoconstriction and hypertension, an extension of the normal regional vascular response that matches perfusion with ventilation to optimize gas exchange in the lung (hypoxic pulmonary vasoconstriction).

Central Nervous System (CNS).   The CNS is least able to tolerate hypoxia. Hypoxia is manifest initially by decreased intellectual capacity and impaired judgment and psychomotor ability. This state progresses to confusion and restlessness and ultimately to stupor, coma, and death as the arterial PO_2 decreases below 4 to 5.3 kPa (30 to 40 mm Hg). Victims often are unaware of this progression.

Cellular and Metabolic Effects.   When the mitochondrial PO_2 falls below about 0.13 kPa (1 mm Hg), anaerobic metabolism stops, and the less efficient anaerobic pathways of glycolysis become responsible for the production of cellular energy. End-products of anaerobic metabolism, such as lactic acid, may be released into the circulation in measurable quantities. Energy-dependent ion pumps slow and transmembrane ion gradients dissipate. Intracellular concentrations of Na^+, Ca^{2+}, and H^+ increase, finally leading to cell death. The time course of cellular demise depends on the relative metabolic demands, O_2 storage

capacity, and anaerobic capacity of the individual organs. Restoration of perfusion and oxygenation prior to hypoxic cell death paradoxically can result in an accelerated form of cell injury (ischemia-reperfusion syndrome), thought to result from the generation of highly reactive oxygen free radicals (McCord, 1985).

Adaptation to Hypoxia.   Long-term hypoxia results in adaptive physiological changes; these have been studied most thoroughly in persons exposed to high altitude. Adaptations include increased numbers of pulmonary alveoli, increased concentrations of hemoglobin in blood and myoglobin in muscle, and a decreased ventilatory response to hypoxia (Cruz *et al.,* 1980). Short-term exposure to altitude produces similar adaptive changes. In susceptible individuals, however, acute exposure to high altitude may produce "acute mountain sickness," a syndrome characterized by headache, nausea, dyspnea, sleep disturbances, and impaired judgment, progressing to pulmonary and cerebral edema (Johnson and Rock, 1988). Mountain sickness is treated with supplemental oxygen, descent to lower altitude, or an increase in ambient pressure. Diuretics (carbonic anhydrase inhibitors) and steroids also may be helpful. The syndrome usually can be avoided by a slow ascent to altitude, permitting time for adaptation to occur.

It has been noted that certain aspects of fetal and newborn physiology are strongly reminiscent of adaptation mechanisms found in hypoxia-tolerant animals (Mortola, 1999; Singer, 1999), including shifts in the oxyhemoglobin dissociation curve (fetal hemoglobin), reduction in metabolic rate and body temperature (hibernation-like mode), reduction in heart rate and circulatory redistribution (as in diving mammals), and redirection of energy utilization from growth to maintenance metabolism. These adaptations help account for the relative tolerance of the fetus and neonate to both chronic (uterine insufficiency) and short-term hypoxia.

Oxygen Inhalation

Physiological Effects of Oxygen Inhalation.   The primary use for inhalation of oxygen is to reverse or prevent the development of hypoxia; other consequences usually are minor. However, when oxygen is breathed in excessive amounts or for prolonged periods, secondary physiological changes and toxic effects can occur.

Respiratory System.   Inhalation of oxygen at 1 atmosphere or above causes a small degree of respiratory depression in normal subjects, presumably as a result of loss of tonic chemoreceptor activity. However, ventilation typically increases within a few minutes of oxygen inhalation because of a paradoxical increase in the tension of carbon dioxide in tissues. This increase results from the increased concentration of oxyhemoglobin in venous blood, which causes less efficient removal of carbon dioxide from the tissues (Lambertsen *et al.,* 1953; Plewes and Farhi, 1983).

In a small number of patients whose respiratory center is depressed by long-term retention of carbon dioxide, injury, or drugs, ventilation is maintained largely by stimulation of carotid and aortic chemoreceptors, commonly referred to as the hypoxic drive. The provision of too much oxygen can depress this drive, resulting in respiratory acidosis. In these cases, supplemental oxygen should be titrated carefully to ensure adequate arterial saturation. If hypoventilation results, then mechanical ventilatory support with or without tracheal intubation should be provided.

Expansion of poorly ventilated alveoli is maintained in part by the nitrogen content of alveolar gas; nitrogen is poorly soluble and thus remains in the airspaces while oxygen is absorbed. High oxygen concentrations delivered to poorly ventilated lung regions can promote absorption atelectasis, occasionally resulting in an increase in shunt and a paradoxical worsening of hypoxemia after a period of oxygen administration.

Cardiovascular System.   Aside from reversing the effects of hypoxia, the physiological consequences of oxygen inhalation on the cardiovascular system are of little significance. Heart rate and cardiac output are slightly reduced when 100% oxygen is breathed; blood pressure changes little. While pulmonary arterial pressure changes little in normal subjects with oxygen inhalation, elevated pulmonary artery pressures in patients living at altitude who have chronic hypoxic pulmonary hypertension may reverse with oxygen therapy or return to sea level (Grover *et al.,* 1966; Spievogel *et al.,* 1969). In particular, in neonates with congenital heart disease and left-to-right shunting of cardiac output, oxygen supplementation must be carefully regulated because of the risk of further reducing pulmonary vascular resistance and increasing pulmonary blood flow.

Metabolism.   Inhalation of 100% oxygen does not produce detectable changes in oxygen consumption, carbon dioxide production, respiratory quotient, or glucose utilization.

Oxygen Administration

Oxygen is supplied as a compressed gas in steel cylinders, and a purity of 99% is referred to as "medical grade." Most hospitals have oxygen piped from insulated liquid oxygen containers to areas of frequent use. For safety, oxygen cylinders and piping are color-coded (green in the United States), and some form of mechanical indexing of valve connections is used to prevent the connection of other gases to oxygen systems. Oxygen concentrators, which employ molecular sieve, membrane, or electrochemical technologies, are available for low-flow home use. Such

systems produce 30% to 95% oxygen, depending on the flow rate. These devices reduce the resupply problem inherent in the use of compressed or liquid gas systems.

Oxygen is delivered by inhalation except during extracorporeal circulation, when it is dissolved directly into the circulating blood. Only a closed delivery system, with an airtight seal to the patient's airway and complete separation of inspired from expired gases, can precisely control $F_{I_{O_2}}$. In all other systems, the actual delivered $F_{I_{O_2}}$ will depend upon the ventilatory pattern (rate, tidal volume, inspiratory:expiratory time ratio, and inspiratory flow) and delivery system characteristics.

Low-Flow Systems.   Low-flow systems, in which the oxygen flow is lower than the inspiratory flow rate, have a limited ability to raise the $F_{I_{O_2}}$ because they depend upon entrained room air to make up the balance of the inspired gas. The $F_{I_{O_2}}$ of these systems is extremely sensitive to small changes in the ventilatory pattern. Devices such as face tents are used primarily for delivering humidified gases to patients and cannot be relied upon to provide predictable amounts of supplemental oxygen. Nasal cannulae—small, flexible prongs that sit just inside each naris—deliver oxygen at 1 to 6 liters/minute. The nasopharynx acts as a reservoir for storing the oxygen, and patients may breathe through either the mouth or nose as long as the nasal passages remain patent. These devices typically deliver 24% to 28% $F_{I_{O_2}}$ at 2 to 3 liters/minute. Up to 40% $F_{I_{O_2}}$ is possible at higher flow rates, although this is poorly tolerated for more than brief periods because of mucosal drying. The simple facemask, a clear plastic mask with side holes for clearance of expiratory gas and inspiratory air entrainment, is used when higher concentrations of oxygen delivered without tight control are desired. The maximum $F_{I_{O_2}}$ of a facemask can be increased from around 60% at 6 to 15 liters/minute to greater than 85% by adding a 600- to 1000-ml reservoir bag. With this partial rebreathing mask, most of the inspired volume is drawn from the reservoir, avoiding dilution of the $F_{I_{O_2}}$ by entrainment of room air.

High-Flow Systems.   The most commonly used high-flow oxygen delivery device is the Venturi mask, which utilizes a specially designed mask insert to reliably entrain room air in a fixed ratio and thus provides a relatively constant $F_{I_{O_2}}$ at relatively high flow rates. Typically, each insert is designed to operate at a specific oxygen flow rate, and different inserts are required to change the $F_{I_{O_2}}$. Lower delivered $F_{I_{O_2}}$ values use greater entrainment ratios, resulting in higher total (oxygen plus entrained air) flows to the patient, ranging from 80 liters/minute for 24% $F_{I_{O_2}}$ to 40 liters/minute at 50% $F_{I_{O_2}}$. While these flow rates are much higher than those obtained with low-flow devices, they still may be lower than the peak inspiratory flows for patients in respiratory distress, and thus the actual delivered oxygen concentration may be lower than the nominal value. Oxygen nebulizers, another type of Venturi device, provide patients with humidified oxygen at 35% to 100% $F_{I_{O_2}}$ at high flow rates. Finally, oxygen blenders provide high inspired oxygen concentrations at very high flow rates. These devices mix high-pressure, compressed air and oxygen to achieve any concentration of oxygen from 21% to 100% at flow rates up to 100 liters/minute. These same blenders are used to provide control of FI_{O_2} for ventilators, CPAP/BiPAP machines, oxygenators, and other devices with similar requirements. Again, despite the high flows, the delivery of high FI_{O_2} to an individual patient also depends on maintaining a tight-fitting seal to the airway and/or the use of reservoirs to minimize entrainment of diluting room air.

Monitoring of Oxygenation.   Monitoring and titration are required to meet the therapeutic goal of oxygen therapy and to avoid complications and side effects. Although cyanosis is a physical finding of substantial clinical importance, it is not an early, sensitive, or reliable index of oxygenation. Cyanosis appears when about 5 g/dl of deoxyhemoglobin is present in arterial blood (Lundsgaard and Van Slyke, 1923), representing an oxygen saturation of about 67% when a normal amount of hemoglobin (15 g/dl) is present. However, when anemia lowers the hemoglobin to 10 g/dl, then cyanosis does not appear until the arterial blood saturation has decreased to 50%. Invasive approaches for monitoring oxygenation include intermittent laboratory analysis of arterial or mixed venous blood gases and placement of intravascular cannulae capable of continuous measurement of oxygen tension. The latter method, which relies on fiberoptic oximetry, is used frequently for the continuous measurement of mixed venous hemoglobin saturation as an index of tissue extraction of oxygen, usually in critically ill patients.

Noninvasive monitoring of arterial oxygen saturation now is widely available from transcutaneous pulse oximetry, in which oxygen saturation is measured from the differential absorption of light by oxyhemoglobin and deoxyhemoglobin and the arterial saturation determined from the pulsatile component of this signal. Application is simple and calibration not required. Because pulse oximetry measures hemoglobin saturation and not P_{O_2}, it is not sensitive to increases in P_{O_2} that exceed levels required to fully saturate the blood. However, pulse oximetry is very useful for monitoring the adequacy of oxygenation during procedures requiring sedation or anesthesia, rapid evaluation and monitoring of potentially compromised patients, and titrating oxygen therapy in situations where toxicity from oxygen or side effects of excess oxygen are of concern.

Complications of Oxygen Therapy.   Administration of supplemental oxygen is not without potential complications. In addition to the potential to promote absorption atelectasis and depress ventilation, discussed above, high flows of dry oxygen can dry out and irritate mucosal surfaces of the airway and the eyes, as well as decrease mucociliary transport and clearance of secretions. Humidified oxygen thus should be used when therapy of greater than an hour's duration is required. Finally, any oxygen-enriched atmosphere constitutes a fire hazard, and appropriate precautions must be taken both in the operating room and for patients on oxygen at home.

It is important to realize that hypoxemia still can occur despite the administration of supplemental oxygen. Furthermore, when supplemental oxygen is administered, desaturation occurs at a later time after airway obstruction or hypoventilation, potentially delaying the detection of these critical events. Therefore, whether or not oxygen is administered to a patient at risk for these problems, it is essential that both oxygen saturation and adequacy of ventilation be frequently assessed.

Therapeutic Uses of Oxygen

Correction of Hypoxia.   As stated above, the primary therapeutic use of oxygen is to correct hypoxia. However, hypoxia is most commonly a manifestation of an underlying disease, and administration of oxygen thus can be viewed as a symptomatic or temporizing therapy. Only rarely is hypoxia due to a primary deficiency in the inspired gas. Because of the many causes of hypoxia, supplementation of the inspired gas alone will not suffice to correct the problem. Efforts must be directed at correcting the cause of the hypoxia. For example, airway obstruction is unlikely to respond to an increase in inspired oxygen tension without relief of the obstruction. More importantly, while hypoxemia due to hypoventilation after a narcotic overdose can be improved with supplemental oxygen administration, the patient remains at risk for respiratory embarrassment if ventilation is not increased through stimulation, narcotic reversal, or mechanical ventilation. In general, the hypoxia that results from most pulmonary diseases can be alleviated at least partially by administration of oxygen, thereby allowing time for definitive therapy to reverse the primary process. Thus, administration of oxygen is a basic and important treatment to be used in all forms of hypoxia, with the understanding that the response will vary in a way that is generally predictable from knowledge of the underlying pathophysiological processes.

Reduction of Partial Pressure of an Inert Gas.   Since nitrogen constitutes some 79% of ambient air, it also is the predominant gas in most gas-filled spaces in the body. In certain situations, such as bowel distension from obstruction or ileus, intravascular air embolism, or pneumothorax, it is desirable to reduce the volume of these air-filled spaces. Since nitrogen is relatively insoluble, inhalation of high concentrations of oxygen (and thus low concentrations of nitrogen) rapidly lowers total body partial pressure of nitrogen and provides a substantial gradient for the removal of nitrogen from gas spaces. Administration of oxygen for air embolism is additionally beneficial, because it also helps to relieve the localized hypoxia distal to the embolic vascular obstruction. In the case of *decompression sickness* or *bends,* lowering of inert gas tension in blood and tissues by oxygen inhalation prior to or during a barometric decompression can reduce the degree of supersaturation that occurs after decompression so that bubbles do not form. If bubbles do form in either tissues or the vasculature, administration of oxygen is based on the same rationale as that described for gas embolism.

Hyperbaric Oxygen Therapy.   Oxygen is administered at greater than atmospheric pressure for a number of conditions when 100% oxygen at a single atmosphere is insufficient (Buras, 2000; Shank and Muth, 2000; Myers, 2000). To achieve concentrations of greater than 1 atmosphere, a hyperbaric chamber must be used. These chambers range from small, single-person affairs to multiroom establishments, which may include complex medical equipment. Smaller, one-person chambers typically are pressurized with oxygen, while larger ones are filled with air. In the latter case, a patient must wear a mask to receive the oxygen at the increased pressure. The larger chambers are more suitable for critically ill patients who require ventilation, monitoring, and constant attendance. Any chamber must be built to withstand pressures which may range from 200 to 600 kPa (2 to 6 atmospheres), though inhaled oxygen tension that exceeds 300 kPa (3 atmospheres) rarely is used (*see* Oxygen Toxicity, below).

Hyperbaric oxygen therapy has two components: increased hydrostatic pressure and increased oxygen pressure. Both factors are necessary for the treatment of decompression sickness and air embolism. The hydrostatic pressure reduces bubble volume, and the absence of inspired nitrogen increases the gradient for elimination of nitrogen and reduces hypoxia in downstream tissues. Increased oxygen pressure at the tissue level is the primary therapeutic goal for most of the other indications for hyperbaric oxygen. For example, even a small increase in P_{O_2} in previously ischemic areas may enhance the bactericidal activity of leukocytes and increase angiogenesis. Thus, repetitive, brief exposure to hyperbaric oxygen is a useful adjunct in the treatment of chronic refractory osteomyelitis, osteoradionecrosis, or crush injury or for the recovery of compromised skin, tissue grafts, or flaps. Furthermore, increased oxygen tension can itself be bacteriostatic; the spread of infection with *Clostridium perfringens* and production of toxin by the bacteria are slowed when oxygen tensions exceed 33 kPa (250 mm Hg), justifying the early use of hyperbaric oxygen in clostridial myonecrosis (gas gangrene).

Hyperbaric oxygen also is useful in selected instances of generalized hypoxia. In carbon monoxide poisoning, hemoglobin and myoglobin become unavailable for oxygen binding because of the high affinity of CO for these proteins. A high P_{O_2} facilitates competition of oxygen with CO for binding sites, permitting the resumption of normal delivery of oxygen to the tissues. Hyperbaric oxygen decreases the incidence of neurological sequelae after CO intoxication; this effect may be independent of the ability of hyperbaric oxygen to speed the elimination of CO (Thom, 1989). However, a recent randomized study suggests that hyperbaric oxygen is not beneficial in carbon monoxide poisoning and might even be harmful (Scheinkestel *et al.,* 1999). The occasional use of hyperbaric oxygen in cyanide poisoning has a similar rationale. Hyperbaric oxygen also may be useful in severe, short-term anemia, since sufficient oxygen can be dissolved in the plasma at 3 atmospheres to meet metabolic needs. However, such treatment must be limited, because oxygen toxicity is dependent on increased P_{O_2}, not on the oxygen content of the blood.

Hyperbaric oxygen therapy also has been used in such diverse conditions as multiple sclerosis, traumatic spinal cord injury, cerebrovascular accidents, bone grafts and fractures, and leprosy. However, data from well-controlled clinical trials are not sufficient to justify these uses, and the costs of hyperbaric therapy remain very high.

Oxygen Toxicity

Oxygen is used in cellular energy production and is crucial for cellular metabolism. However, oxygen also may have deleterious actions at the cellular level. Oxygen toxicity probably results from increased production of re-

active agents such as superoxide anion, singlet oxygen, hydroxyl radical, and hydrogen peroxide (Turrens *et al.,* 1982). These agents attack and damage biological membranes, and thus eventually result in damage to most cellular components. A variety of factors limit the toxicity of oxygen-derived, reactive agents. These factors include enzymes such as superoxide dismutase, glutathione peroxidase, and catalase, which scavenge toxic byproducts. In addition, there are reducing agents including iron, glutathione, and ascorbate. These factors, however, are insufficient to limit the destructive actions of oxygen when patients are exposed to high concentrations over a period of time. Tissues show differential sensitivity to oxygen toxicity, which is likely the result of differences in both their production of reactive compounds and protective mechanisms. Oxygen toxicity recently was reviewed by Carraway and Piantadosi (1999).

Respiratory Tract.   The pulmonary system is usually the first to exhibit toxicity, a function of its being continuously exposed to the highest oxygen tensions in the body. Subtle changes in pulmonary function can occur after as little as 8 to 12 hours of exposure to 100% oxygen (Sackner *et al.,* 1975). Increases in capillary permeability, which will increase the alveolar/arterial O_2 gradient and ultimately lead to further hypoxemia, and decreased pulmonary function can be seen after only 18 hours of exposure (Davis *et al.,* 1983; Clark, 1988). Serious injury and death, however, require much longer exposures. Pulmonary damage is directly related to the inspired oxygen tension, and concentrations of less than 0.5 atmosphere appear safe over long time periods. The capillary endothelium is the most sensitive tissue of the lung. Endothelial injury results in loss of surface area from interstitial edema and leaks into the alveoli (Crapo *et al.,* 1980).

Decreases of inspired oxygen concentrations remain the cornerstone of therapy for oxygen toxicity. Modest decreases in toxicity have been observed in animals treated with antioxidant enzymes (White *et al.,* 1989). Tolerance also may play a role in protection from oxygen toxicity; animals exposed briefly to high oxygen tension are subsequently more resistant to toxicity (Kravetz *et al.,* 1980; Coursin *et al.,* 1987). Sensitivity in human beings also can be altered by preexposure to both high and low oxygen concentrations (Hendricks *et al.,* 1977; Clark, 1988). These studies strongly suggest that changes in alveolar surfactant and cellular levels of antioxidant enzymes play a role in protection from oxygen toxicity.

Retina.   Retrolental fibroplasia can occur when neonates are exposed to increased oxygen tensions (Betts *et al.,*

1977). These changes can go on to cause blindness and are likely caused by angiogenesis (Kushner *et al.,* 1977; Ashton, 1979). Incidence of this disorder has decreased with an improved appreciation of the issues and avoidance of excessive inspired oxygen concentrations. Adults do not seem to develop the disease.

Central Nervous System.   CNS problems are rare, and toxicity occurs only under hyperbaric conditions where exposure exceeds 200 kPa (2 atmospheres). Symptoms include seizures and visual changes, which resolve when oxygen tensions are returned to normal. These problems are a further reason to replace oxygen with helium under hyperbaric conditions (*see* below).

CARBON DIOXIDE

Transfer and Elimination of Carbon Dioxide

Carbon dioxide is produced by the body's metabolism at approximately the same rate as oxygen consumption. At rest, this value is about 3 ml/kg per minute, but it may increase dramatically with heavy exercise. Carbon dioxide diffuses readily from the cells into the bloodstream, where it is carried partly as bicarbonate ion, partly in chemical combination with hemoglobin and plasma proteins, and partly in solution at a partial pressure of about 6 kPa (46 mmHg) in mixed venous blood. CO_2 is transported to the lung, where it is normally exhaled at the same rate at which it is produced, leaving a partial pressure of about 5.2 kPa (40 mmHg) in the alveoli and in arterial blood. An increase in P_{CO_2} results in a respiratory acidosis and may be due to decreased ventilation or the inhalation of CO_2, while an increase in ventilation results in decreased P_{CO_2} and a respiratory alkalosis. As carbon dioxide is freely diffusible, the changes in blood P_{CO_2} and pH soon are reflected by intracellular changes in P_{CO_2} and pH.

Effects of Carbon Dioxide

Alterations in P_{CO_2} and pH have widespread effects in the body, particularly on respiration, circulation, and the CNS. More complete discussions of these and other effects are found in textbooks of physiology (*see* Nunn, 1993a).

Respiration.   Carbon dioxide is a rapid, potent stimulus to ventilation in direct proportion to the inspired CO_2. Inhalation of 10% carbon dioxide can produce minute volumes of 75 liters per minute in normal individuals. Carbon dioxide acts at multiple sites to stimulate ventilation. Respiratory integration areas in the brainstem are acted upon by impulses from medullary and peripheral arterial chemoreceptors. The mechanism by which carbon dioxide acts on these receptors probably involves changes in pH (Nattie, 1999; Drysdale *et al.,* 1981). Elevated P_{CO_2} causes bronchodilation, whereas hypocarbia causes constriction of airway smooth muscle; these responses may play a role in matching pulmonary ventilation and perfusion (Duane *et al.,* 1979).

Circulation.   The circulatory effects of carbon dioxide result from the combination of its direct local effects and its centrally mediated effects on the autonomic nervous system. The direct effect of carbon dioxide on the heart, diminished contractility, results from pH changes (van den Bos *et al.,* 1979). The direct effect on systemic blood vessels results in vasodilation. Carbon dioxide causes widespread activation of the sympathetic nervous system and an increase in the plasma concentrations of epinephrine, norepinephrine, angiotensin, and other vasoactive peptides (Staszewska-Barczak and Dusting, 1981). The results of sympathetic nervous system activation are, in general, opposite to the local effects of carbon dioxide. The sympathetic effects consist of increases in cardiac contractility, heart rate, and vasoconstriction (*see* Chapter 10).

The balance of opposing local and sympathetic effects, therefore, determines the total circulatory response to carbon dioxide. The net effect of carbon dioxide inhalation is an increase in cardiac output, heart rate, and blood pressure. In blood vessels, however, the direct vasodilating actions of CO_2 appear more important and total peripheral resistance decreases when the P_{CO_2} is increased. Carbon dioxide also is a potent coronary vasodilator (Ely *et al.,* 1982). Cardiac arrhythmias associated with increased P_{CO_2} are due to the release of catecholamines.

Hypocarbia results in opposite effects: decreased blood pressure and vasoconstriction in skin, intestine, brain, kidney, and heart. These actions are exploited clinically in the use of hyperventilation in the presence of intracranial hypertension.

Central Nervous System.   Hypercarbia depresses the excitability of the cerebral cortex and increases the cutaneous pain threshold through a central action. This central depression has therapeutic importance. For example, in patients hypoventilating from narcotics or anesthetics, increasing P_{CO_2} may result in further CNS depression, which in turn may worsen the respiratory depression. This positive feedback cycle can be deadly. The inhalation of high concentrations of carbon dioxide (about 50%) produces marked cortical and subcortical depression of a type similar to that produced by anesthetic agents. Under certain circumstances inspired CO_2 (25% to 30%) can result in subcortical activation and seizures.

Methods of Administration

Carbon dioxide is marketed in gray metal cylinders as the pure gas or as carbon dioxide mixed with oxygen. It usually is administered at a concentration of 5% to 10% in combination with oxygen by means of a facemask. Another method for the temporary administration of carbon dioxide is by rebreathing, for example from an anesthesia breathing circuit when the soda lime canister is bypassed or from something as simple as a paper bag. A potential safety issue exists in that CO_2 tanks containing oxygen are the same color as those that are 100% CO_2. When tanks containing oxygen have been used inadvertently where a fire hazard exists (*e.g.*, in the presence of electrocautery during laparoscopic surgery), explosions and fires have resulted.

Therapeutic Uses

Inhalation of carbon dioxide is used less commonly today than in the past because there are now more effective treatments for most indications. Inhalation of carbon dioxide has been used during anesthesia to increase the speed of induction and emergence from inhalational anesthesia by increasing minute ventilation and cerebral blood flow. However, this technique results in some degree of respiratory acidosis. Hypocarbia with its attendant respiratory alkalosis still has some uses in anesthesia. It constricts cerebral vessels, decreasing brain size slightly, and thus may facilitate the performance of neurosurgical operations. Although carbon dioxide stimulates respiration, it is not useful in situations where respiratory depression has resulted in hypercarbia or acidosis, since further depression results.

A common use of CO_2 is for insufflation during endoscopic procedures (*e.g.*, laparoscopic surgery), because it is highly soluble and does not support combustion. Any inadvertent gas emboli are thus more easily dissolved and eliminated *via* the respiratory system.

Recently CO_2 has been utilized during open cardiac surgery, where it is used to flood the surgical field. Because of its density, CO_2 displaces the air surrounding the open heart so that any gas bubbles trapped in the heart are CO_2 rather than insoluble nitrogen (Nadolny and Svensson, 2000). For the same reasons, CO_2 is used to debubble cardiopulmonary bypass and extracorporeal membrane oxygenation (ECMO) circuits. It also can be used to adjust pH during bypass procedures when a patient is cooled.

NITRIC OXIDE

Nitric oxide (NO), a free radical gas long known as an air pollutant and a potentially toxic agent, particularly when further oxidized (*see* below), recently has been shown to be an endogenous cell-signaling molecule of great physiological importance. As knowledge of the important actions of NO have evolved, the use of NO as a therapeutic agent has grown in interest.

Endogenous NO is produced from the amino acid L-arginine by a family of enzymes called NO synthases. NO is now recognized as a novel cell messenger implicated in a wide range of physiological and pathophysiological events in numerous cell types and processes, including the cardiovascular, immune, and nervous systems. In the vasculature, NO produced by endothelial cells is a primary determinant of resting vascular tone through basal release and causes vasodilation when synthesized in response to shear stress and to a variety of vasodilating agents. It also plays an active role in inhibiting platelet aggregation and adhesion. Impaired NO production has been implicated in disease states such as atherosclerosis, hypertension, cere-

bral and coronary vasospasm, and ischemia-reperfusion injury. In the immune system, NO serves as an important effector of macrophage-induced cytotoxicity, and its overproduction is an important mediator of inflammatory states. In neurons, NO serves multiple functions, acting as a mediator of long-term potentiation, of *N*-methyl-D-aspartate (NMDA)–mediated cytotoxicity, and as the mediator of nonadrenergic noncholingeric neurotransmission; it also has been implicated in mediating central nociceptive pathways. The physiology and pathophysiology of endogenous NO have been extensively reviewed (Moncada and Palmer, 1991; Nathan, 1992; Ignarro *et al.*, 1999).

Therapeutic Use of NO

Inhalation of NO gas has received considerable therapeutic attention due to its ability to dilate selectively the pulmonary vasculature with minimal systemic cardiovascular effects (Steudel *et al.*, 1999). The lack of effect of inhaled NO on the systemic circulation is due to its strong binding and inactivation by oxyhemoglobin upon exposure to the pulmonary circulation. Ventilation-perfusion matching is preserved or improved by NO, because inhaled NO is distributed only to ventilated areas of the lung and dilates only those vessels directly adjacent to the ventilated alveoli. Thus, inhaled NO will decrease elevated pulmonary artery pressure and pulmonary vascular resistance and often improve oxygenation (Steudel *et al.*, 1999; Haddad *et al.*, 2000).

Due to its selective pulmonary vasodilating action, inhaled NO is undergoing intensive study as a potential therapeutic agent for numerous diseases associated with increased pulmonary vascular resistance. Therapeutic trials of inhaled NO in a wide range of such conditions have confirmed its ability to decrease pulmonary vascular resistance and often increase oxygenation, but in all but a few cases these trials have yet to demonstrate long-term improvement in terms of morbidity or mortality (Dellinger, 1999; Cheifetz, 2000). Inhaled NO has been approved by the United States Food and Drug Administration only for use in newborns with persistent pulmonary hypotension. In this disease state, NO inhalation has been shown to reduce significantly the necessity for extracorporeal membrane oxygenation, although overall mortality has been unchanged (Kinsella *et al.*, 1997; Roberts *et al.*, 1997). Notably, numerous trials of inhaled NO in adult and pediatric acute respiratory distress syndrome have failed to demonstrate an impact on outcome (Dellinger, 1999; Cheifetz, 2000). Several small studies and case reports have suggested potential benefits of inhaled NO in a variety of conditions, including weaning from cardiopulmonary bypass in adult and congenital heart disease patients; primary pulmonary hypertension; pulmonary embolism; acute chest syndrome in sickle-cell patients; congenital diaphragmatic hernia; high-altitude pulmonary edema; and lung transplantation (Steudel *et al.,* 1999; Haddad *et al.,* 2000). Larger, prospective, randomized studies, however, have not yet been performed or have failed to confirm any changes in outcome. At the present time, outside of clinical investigation, therapeutic use and benefit of inhaled NO are limited to newborns with persistent pulmonary hypotension.

Diagnostic Uses of NO

Inhaled NO also is used in several diagnostic applications. Inhaled NO can be used during cardiac catheterization to evaluate safely and selectively the pulmonary vasodilating capacity of patients with heart failure and infants with congenital heart disease. Inhaled NO also is used to determine the diffusion capacity (D_L) across the alveolar-capillary unit. NO is more effective than carbon dioxide in this regard because of its greater affinity for hemoglobin and its higher water solubility at body temperature (Steudel *et al.,* 1999; Haddad *et al.,* 2000).

NO is produced from the nasal passages and from the lungs of normal human subjects and can be detected in exhaled gas. The measurement of exhaled NO has been investigated for its utility in assessment of respiratory tract diseases. Measurement of exhaled NO may prove to be useful in diagnosis of asthma and in respiratory tract infections (Haddad *et al.,* 2000).

Toxicity of NO

Administered at low concentrations (0.1 to 50 parts per million), inhaled NO appears to be safe and without significant side effects. Pulmonary toxicity can occur with levels higher than 50 to 100 ppm. In the context of NO as an atmospheric pollutant, the Occupational Safety and Health Administration places the seven-hour exposure limit at 50 ppm. Part of the toxicity of NO may be related to its further oxidation to nitrogen dioxide (NO_2) in the presence of high concentrations of oxygen. Even low concentrations of NO_2 (2 ppm) have been shown to be highly toxic in animal models, with observed changes in lung histopathology, including loss of cilia, hypertrophy, and focal hyperplasia in the epithelium of terminal bronchioles. It is important, therefore, to keep NO_2 formation during NO therapy at a low level. This can be achieved through appropriate filters and scavengers and the use of high-quality gas mixtures. Laboratory studies have suggested potential additional toxic effects of chronic low doses of inhaled NO, including surfactant inactivation and the formation of peroxynitrite by interaction with superoxide. The ability of NO to inhibit or alter the function of a number of iron- and heme-containing proteins—including cyclooxygenase, lipoxygenases, and oxidative cytochromes—as well as its interactions with ADP-ribosylation suggest a need for further investigation of the toxic potential of NO under therapeutic conditions (Steudel *et al.,* 1999; Haddad *et al.,* 2000).

The development of methemoglobinemia is a significant complication of inhaled NO at higher concentrations, and rare deaths have been reported with overdoses of NO. The blood content of methemoglobin, however, generally will not increase to toxic levels with appropriate use of inhaled NO. Methemoglobin concentrations should be intermittently monitored during NO inhalation (Steudel *et al.,* 1999; Haddad *et al.,* 2000).

Inhaled NO can inhibit platelet function and has been shown to increase bleeding time in some clinical studies, although reports of bleeding complications are not apparent in the literature.

In patients with impaired function of the left ventricle, NO has a potential to further impair left ventricular performance by dilating the pulmonary circulation and increasing the blood flow to the left ventricle, thereby increasing left atrial pressure and promoting pulmonary edema formation. Careful monitoring of cardiac output, left atrial pressure or pulmonary capillary wedge pressure is important in this situation (Steudel *et al.,* 1999).

Despite these concerns, there are limited reports of inhaled NO-related toxicity in humans. The most important requirements for safe NO inhalation therapy are outlined by Steudel *et al.* (1999) and include: (1) continuous measurement of NO and NO_2 concentrations using either chemiluminescence or electrochemical analyzers; (2) frequent calibration of monitoring equipment; (3) intermittent analysis of blood methemoglobin levels; (4) the use of certified tanks of NO; and (5) administration of the lowest NO concentration required for therapeutic effect.

Methods of Administration

Courses of treatment of patients with inhaled NO are highly varied, extending from 0.1 to 40 ppm in dose and for periods of a few hours to several weeks in duration. The minimum effective inhaled NO concentration should be determined for each patient to minimize the chance for toxicity. Commercial NO systems are available that will accurately deliver inspired NO concentrations between 0.1 and 80 ppm and simultaneously measure NO and NO_2 concentrations. A constant inspired concentration of NO is obtained by administering NO in nitrogen to the inspiratory limb of the ventilator circuit in either a pulse or continuous mode. While inhaled NO may be administered to spontaneously breathing patients *via* a closely fitting mask, it usually is delivered during mechanical ventilation. Nasal prong administration is being employed in therapeutic trials of home administration for treatment of primary pulmonary hypertension (Steudel *et al.,* 1999; Haddad *et al.,* 2000).

Acute discontinuation of NO inhalation can lead to a rebound pulmonary artery hypertension with an increase in right-to-left intrapulmonary shunting and a decrease in oxygenation. To avoid this phenomenon, a graded decrease of inhaled NO concentration is important in the process of weaning a patient from inhaled NO (Steudel *et al.,* 1999; Haddad *et al.,* 2000).

HELIUM

Helium is an inert gas whose low density, low solubility, and high thermal conductivity provide the basis for its medical and diagnostic use. Helium is produced by separation from liquefied natural gas and supplied in brown cylinders. Helium can be mixed with oxygen and administered by mask or tracheal tube. Under hyperbaric conditions, it can be substituted for the bulk of other gases, resulting in a mixture of much lower density that is easier to breathe.

The primary uses of helium are in pulmonary function testing, the treatment of respiratory obstruction, during laser airway surgery, for diving at depth, and most recently, as a label in imaging studies. The determinations of residual lung volume, functional residual capacity, and related lung volumes require a highly diffusible, nontoxic gas that is insoluble (and thus does not leave the lung *via* the bloodstream), so that, by dilution, the lung volume can be measured. Helium is well suited to these needs and is much cheaper than alternatives. In these tests, a breath of a known concentration of helium is given and the concentration of helium then measured in the mixed expired gas, allowing calculation of the other pulmonary volumes.

Pulmonary gas flow is normally laminar, but with increased flow rate or narrowed flow pathway a component becomes turbulent. Helium can be added to oxygen to treat this turbulence due to airway obstruction. The density of helium is substantially less than that of air, and flow rates under turbulent conditions are increased with lower-density gases. This results in decreased work of breathing with mixtures of helium and oxygen. However, several factors limit the usefulness of this approach. Oxygenation frequently is a principal problem in airway obstruction, and the need for increased inspired oxygen concentration may limit the amount of helium that may be used. Furthermore, the viscosity of helium is higher than that of air, and increased viscosity reduces laminar flow.

Helium has high thermal conductivity, which makes it useful during laser surgery on the airway. This more rapid conduction of heat away from the point of contact of the laser beam reduces the spread of tissue damage and the likelihood that the ignition point of flammable materials in the airway will be reached. Its low density improves the flow through the small endotracheal tubes typically used in such procedures.

Recently, laser-polarized helium has been used as an inhalational contrast agent for pulmonary magnetic resonance imaging. Optical pumping of nonradioactive helium increases the signal from the gas in the lung sufficiently to permit detailed imaging of the airways and inspired airflow patterns (Kauczor *et al.*, 1998).

Hyperbaric Applications. The depth and duration of diving activity are limited by oxygen toxicity, inert gas (nitrogen) narcosis, and nitrogen supersaturation when decompressing. Oxygen toxicity is a problem with prolonged exposure to compressed air at 500 kPa (5 atmospheres) or more. This problem can be minimized by dilution of oxygen with helium, which lacks narcotic potential even at very high pressures and is quite insoluble in body tissues. This low solubility reduces the likelihood of bubble formation after decompression, which can therefore be achieved more rapidly. The low density of helium also reduces the work of breathing in the otherwise dense hyperbaric atmosphere. The lower heat capacity of helium also decreases respiratory heat loss, which can be significant when diving at depth.

BIBLIOGRAPHY

Ashton, N. The pathogenesis of retrolental fibroplasia. *Ophthalmology,* **1979,** *86:*1695–1699.

Benatar, S.R., Hewlett, A.M., and Nunn, J.F. The use of iso-shunt lines for control of oxygen therapy. *Br. J. Anaesth.,* **1973,** *45:*711–718.

Bert, P. Expériencence sur l'empoisonn par l'oxygène. *Gaz. Méd. Paris,* **1873,** *28:*387.

Betts, E.K., Downes, J.J., Schaffer, D.B., and Johns, R. Retrolental fibroplasia and oxygen administration during general anesthesia. *Anesthesiology,* **1977,** *47:*518–520.

Boerema, I., Meyne, N.G., Brummelkamp, W.K., Bouma, S., Mensch, M.H., Kamermans, F., Stern Hanf, M., and van Aalderen, W. Life without blood. *J. Cardiovasc. Surg. (Torino),* **1960,** *1:*133–146.

Cheifetz, I.M. Inhaled nitric oxide: plenty of data, no consensus. *Crit. Care Med.,* **2000,** *28:*902–903.

Clark, J.M. Pulmonary limits of oxygen tolerance in man. *Exp. Lung Res.,* **1988,** *14:*897–910.

Clark, J.M., and Lambertsen, C.J. Alveolar–arterial O_2 differences in man at 0.2, 1.0, 2.0, and at 3.5 Ata inspired P_{O_2}. *J. Appl. Physiol.,* **1971,** *30:*753–763.

Coursin, D.B., Cihla, H.P., Will, J.A., and McCreary, J.L. Adaptation to chronic hyperoxia. Biochemical effects and the response to subsequent lethal hyperoxia. *Am. Rev. Respir. Dis.,* **1987,** *135:*1002–1006.

Crapo, J.D., Barry, B.E., Foscue, H.A., and Shelburne, J. Structural and biochemical changes in rat lungs occurring during exposures to lethal and adaptive doses of oxygen. *Am. Rev. Respir. Dis.,* **1980,** *122:*123–143.

Cruz, J.C., Reeves, J.T., Grover, R.F., Maher, J.T., McCullough, R.E., Cymerman, A., and Denniston, J.C. Ventilatory acclimatization to high altitude is prevented by CO_2 breathing. *Respiration,* **1980,** *39:*121–130.

Davis, W.B., Rennard, S.I., Bitterman, P.B., and Crystal, R.G. Pulmonary oxygen toxicity. Early reversible changes in human alveolar structures induced by hyperoxia. *N. Engl. J. Med.,* **1983,** *309:*878–883.

Dellinger, R.P. Inhaled nitric oxide in acute lung injury and acute respiratory distress syndrome. Inability to translate physiologic benefit to clinical outcome benefit in adult clinical trials. *Intens. Care Med.,* **1999,** *23:*881–883.

Drysdale, D.B., Jensen, J.I., and Cunningham, D.J. The short-latency respiratory response to sudden withdrawal of hypercapnia and hypoxia in man. *Q. J. Exp. Physiol.,* **1981,** *66:*203–210.

Duane, S.F., Weir, E.K., Stewart, R.M., and Niewoehner, D.E. Distal airway responses to changes in oxygen and carbon dioxide tensions. *Respir. Physiol.,* **1979,** *38:*303–311.

Ely, S.W., Sawyer, D.C., and Scott, J.B. Local vasoactivity of oxygen and carbon dioxide in the right coronary circulation of the dog and pig. *J. Physiol. (Lond.),* **1982,** *332:*427–439.

Grover, R.F., Vogel, J.H., Voigt, G.C., and Blount, S.G. Jr. Reversal of high altitude pulmonary hypertension. *Am. J. Cardiol.,* **1966,** *18:*928–932.

Hendricks, P.L., Hall, D.A., Hunter, W.L. Jr., and Haley, P.J. Extension of pulmonary O_2 tolerance in man at 2 ATA by intermittent O_2 exposure. *J. Appl. Physiol.,* **1977,** *42:*593–599.

Johnson, T.S., and Rock, P.B. Current concepts. Acute mountain sickness. *N. Engl. J. Med.,* **1988,** *319*:841–845.

Kauczor, H., Surkau, R., and Roberts, T. MRI using hyperpolarized noble gases. *Eur. Radiol.,* **1998,** 8:820–827.

Kinsella, J.P., Truog, W.E., Walsh, W.F., Goldberg, R.N., Bancalari, E., Mayock, D.E., Redding, G.J., deLemos, R.A., Sardesai, S., McCurnin, D.C., Moreland, S.G., Cutter, G.R., and Abman, S.H. Randomized, multicenter trail of inhaled nitric oxide and high-frequency oscillatory ventilation in severe, persistent pulmonary hypertension of the newborn. *J. Pediatr.,* **1997,** *131*:55–62.

Kravetz, G., Fisher, A.B., and Forman, H.J. The oxygen–adapted rat model: tolerance to oxygen at 1.5 and 2 ATA. *Aviat. Space Environ. Med.,* **1980,** *51*:775–777.

Kushner, B.J., Essner, D., Cohen, I.J., and Flynn, J.T. Retrolental fibroplasia. II. Pathologic correlation. *Arch. Ophthalmol.,* **1977,** *95*:29–38.

Lambertsen, C.J., Kough, R.H., Cooper, D.Y., Emmel, G.L., Loeschcke, H.H., and Schmidt, C.F. Oxygen toxicity. Effects in man of oxygen inhalation at 1 and 3.5 atmospheres upon blood gas transport, cerebral circulation and cerebral metabolism. *J. Appl. Physiol.,* **1953,** *5*:471–486.

McCord, J.M. Oxygen-derived free radicals in postischemic tissue injury. *N. Engl. J. Med.,* **1985,** *312*:159–163.

Mortola, J.P. How newborn mammals cope with hypoxia. *Respir. Physiol.,* **1999,** *116*:95–103.

Nadolny, E.M., and Svensson, L.G. Carbon dioxide field flooding techniques for open heart surgery: monitoring and minimizing potential adverse effects. *Perfusion,* **2000,** *15*:151–153.

Plewes, J.L., and Farhi, L.E. Peripheral circulatory responses to acute hyperoxia. *Undersea Biomed. Res.,* **1983,** *10*:123–129.

Roberts, J.D. Jr., Fineman, J.R., Morin, F.C. III, Shaul, P.W., Rimer, S., Schreiber, M.D., Polin, R.A., Zwass, M.S., Zayek, M.M., Gross, I., Heyman, M.A., and Zapol, W.M. Inhaled nitric oxide and persistent pulmonary hypertension of the newborn. The Inhaled Nitric Oxide Study Group. *N. Engl. J. Med.,* **1997,** *336*:605–610.

Robiolio, M., Rumsey, W.L., and Wilson, D.F. Oxygen diffusion and mitochondrial respiration in neuroblastoma cells. *Am. J. Physiol.,* **1989,** *256*:C1207–C1213.

Sackner, M.A., Landa, J., Hirsch, J., and Zapata, A. Pulmonary effects of oxygen breathing. A 6-hour study in normal men. *Ann. Intern. Med.,* **1975,** *82*:40–43.

Singer, D. Neonatal tolerance to hypoxia: a comparative-physiological approach. *Comp. Biochem. Physiol. A. Mol. Integr. Physiol.,* **1999,** *123*:221–234.

Spievogel, H., Otero-Calderon, L., Calderon, G., Hartmann, R., and Cudkowicz, L. The effects of high altitude on pulmonary hypertension of cardiopathies, at La Paz, Bolivia. *Respiration,* **1969,** *26*:369–386.

Staszewska-Barczak, J., and Dusting, G.J. Importance of circulating angiotensin II for elevation of arterial pressure during acute hypercapnia in anaesthetized dogs. *Clin. Exp. Pharmacol. Physiol.,* **1981,** *8*:189–201.

Turrens, J.F., Freeman, B.A., Levitt, J.G., and Crapo, J.D. The effect of hyperoxia on superoxide production by lung submitochondrial particles. *Arch. Biochem. Biophys.,* **1982,** *217*:401–410.

van den Bos, G.C., Drake, A.J., and Noble, M.I.M. The effect of carbon dioxide upon myocardial contractile performance, blood flow and oxygen consumption. *J. Physiol. (Lond.),* **1979,** *287*:149–161.

White, C.W., Jackson, J.H., Abuchowski, A., Kazo, G.M., Mimmack, R.F., Berger, E.M., Freeman, B.A., McCord, J.M., and Repine, J.E. Polyethylene glycol–attached antioxidant enzymes decrease pulmonary oxygen toxicity in rats. *J. Appl. Physiol.,* **1989,** *66*:584–590.

MONOGRAPHS AND REVIEWS

Buras, J. Basic mechanisms of hyperbaric oxygen in the treatment of ischemia-reperfusion injury. *Int. Anesthesiol. Clin.,* **2000,** *38*:91–109.

Carraway, M.S., and Piantadosi, C.A. Oxygen toxicity. *Respir. Care Clin. North Am.,* **1999,** *5*:265–295.

Haddad, E., Millatt, L.J., and Johns, R.A. Clinical applications of inhaled NO. In, *Lung Physiology.* (P. Kadowitz, ed.) Marcel Dekker, New York, **2000.**

Ignarro, L.J., Cirino, G., Casini, A., and Napoli, C. Nitric oxide as a signaling molecule in the vascular system: an overview. *J. Cardiovasc. Pharmacol.,* **1999,** *34*:879–886.

Lundsgaard, C., and Van Slyke, D.D. Cyanosis. *Medicine (Baltimore),* **1923,** 2:1–76.

Moncada, S., Palmer, R.M., and Higgs, E.A. Nitric oxide: physiology, pathophysiology and pharmacology. *Pharmacol. Rev.,* **1991,** *43*:109–142.

Myers, R.A. Hyperbaric oxygen therapy for trauma: crush injury, compartment syndrome, and other acute traumatic peripheral ischemias. *Int. Anesthesiol. Clin.,* **2000,** *38*:139–151.

Nathan, C. Nitric oxide as a secretory product of mammalian cells. *F.A.S.E.B. J.,* **1992,** *6*:3051–3064.

Nattie, E. CO_2, brainstem chemoreceptors and breathing. *Prog. Neurobiol.,* **1999,** *59*:299–331.

Nunn, J.F. Carbon dioxide. In, *Nunn's Applied Respiratory Physiology,* 4th ed. (Nunn, J.F., ed.) Butterworth-Heineman, Oxford, **1993a,** pp. 219–246.

Nunn, J.F. Hypoxia. In, *Nunn's Applied Respiratory Physiology,* 4th ed. (Nunn, J.F., ed.) Butterworth-Heineman, Oxford, **1993b,** pp. 535–536.

Sackner, M.A. A history of oxygen usage in chronic obstructive pulmonary disease. *Am. Rev. Respir. Dis.,* **1974,** *110*(suppl):25–34.

Scheinkestel, C.D., Bailey, M., Myles, P.S., Jones, K., Cooper, D.J., Millar, I.L., and Tuxen, D.V. Hyperbaric or normobaric oxygen for acute carbon monoxide poisoning: a randomised controlled clinical trial. *Med. J. Aust.,* **1999,** *170*:203–210.

Shank, E.S., and Muth, C.M. Decompression illness, iatrogenic gas embolism, and carbon monoxide poisoning: the role of hyperbaric oxygen therapy. *Int. Anesthesiol. Clin.,* **2000,** *38*:111–138.

Steudel, W., Hurford, W.E., and Zapol, W.M. Inhaled NO: basic biology and clinical applications. *Anesthesiology,* **1999,** *91*:1090–1121.

Thom, S.R. Smoke inhalation. *Emerg. Med. Clin. North Am.,* **1989,** 7:371–387.

Acknowledgment

The authors wish to acknowledge Drs. Roderic G. Eckenhoff and David E. Longnecker, authors of this chapter in the ninth edition of *Goodman and Gilman's The Pharmacological Basis of Therapeutics,* some of whose text we have retained in this edition.

CHAPTER 17

HYPNOTICS AND SEDATIVES

Dennis S. Charney, S. John Mihic, and R. Adron Harris

A wide variety of agents have the capacity to depress the function of the central nervous system (CNS) such that calming or drowsiness (sedation) is produced. Older sedative-hypnotic drugs depress the CNS in a dose-dependent fashion, progressively producing sedation, sleep, unconsciousness, surgical anesthesia, coma, and, ultimately, fatal depression of respiration and cardiovascular regulation. The CNS depressants that are addressed in this chapter include the benzodiazepines and barbiturates as well as sedative-hypnotic agents of diverse chemical structure (e.g., paraldehyde, chloral hydrate). Volatile anesthetics are discussed in Chapter 14.

Benzodiazepines have only a limited capacity to produce profound and potentially fatal CNS depression. Although coma may be produced at very high doses, benzodiazepines cannot induce a state of surgical anesthesia by themselves and virtually are incapable of causing fatal respiratory depression or cardiovascular collapse unless other CNS depressants also are present. Because of this measure of safety, benzodiazepines and their newer analogs have largely replaced older agents for the treatment of insomnia or anxiety.

Sedative-hypnotic drugs, particularly the benzodiazepines, also are used to produce sedation and amnesia before or during diagnostic or operative procedures, and some, notably certain barbiturates, are used at high doses to induce or maintain surgical anesthesia (see Chapter 14). A few barbiturates and benzodiazepines are used as antiepileptic agents (see Chapter 21), and a few benzodiazepines may be used as muscle relaxants (see Chapter 22). The role of the benzodiazepines and other agents in the pharmacotherapy of anxiety will be discussed in Chapter 19.

CNS depressants also include the aliphatic alcohols, particularly ethanol. Ethanol shares many pharmacological properties with the nonbenzodiazepine sedative-hypnotic drugs. However, its usefulness in the treatment of sleep disorders is limited, and often it may be more disruptive than beneficial. The pharmacology of ethanol is discussed in Chapter 18. Abuse of ethanol and other CNS depressants is discussed in Chapter 24.

A *sedative* drug decreases activity, moderates excitement, and calms the recipient, whereas a *hypnotic* drug produces drowsiness and facilitates the onset and maintenance of a state of sleep that resembles natural sleep in its electroencephalographic characteristics and from which the recipient can be aroused easily. The latter effect sometimes is called hypnosis, but the sleep induced by hypnotic drugs does not resemble the artificially induced passive state of suggestibility also called hypnosis.

The nonbenzodiazepine sedative-hypnotic drugs belong to a group of agents that depress the central nervous system (CNS) in a dose-dependent fashion, progressively producing calming or drowsiness (sedation), sleep (pharmacological hypnosis), unconsciousness, coma, surgical anesthesia, and fatal depression of respiration and car-

diovascular regulation. They share these properties with a large number of chemicals, including general anesthetics (*see* Chapter 14) and aliphatic alcohols, most notably ethanol (*see* Chapter 18). Only two landmarks on the continuum of CNS depression produced by increasing concentrations of these agents can be defined with a reasonable degree of precision: surgical anesthesia, a state in which painful stimuli elicit no behavioral or autonomic response (*see* Chapter 13), and death, resulting from sufficient depression of medullary neurons to disrupt coordination of cardiovascular function and respiration. The "end points" at lower concentrations of CNS depressants are defined with less precision—in terms of deficits in cognitive function (including attention to environmental stimuli) or motor skills (*e.g.,* ataxia), or of the intensity of sensory stimuli needed to elicit some reflex or behavioral response. Other important indices of decreased activity of the CNS, such as analgesia and seizure suppression, do not necessarily fall along this continuum; they may not be present at subanesthetic concentrations of a CNS-depressant drug (*e.g.,* a barbiturate), or they may be achieved with minimal sedation or other evidence of CNS depression (*e.g.,* with low doses of opioids, phenytoin, ethosuximide).

Sedation is a side effect of many drugs that are not general CNS depressants (*e.g.,* antihistamines, neuroleptics). Although such agents can intensify the effects of CNS depressants, they usually produce more specific therapeutic effects at concentrations far lower than those causing substantial CNS depression. They cannot, for example, induce surgical anesthesia in the absence of other agents. The benzodiazepine sedative-hypnotics resemble such agents; although coma may occur at very high doses, neither surgical anesthesia nor fatal intoxication is produced by benzodiazepines in the absence of other drugs with CNS-depressant actions. Moreover, certain congeners can specifically antagonize the actions of benzodiazepines without eliciting significant effects in their absence. This constellation of properties sets the benzodiazepines apart from other sedative-hypnotic drugs and imparts a measure of safety that has resulted in benzodiazepines largely displacing older agents for the treatment of insomnia and anxiety.

History. Since antiquity, alcoholic beverages and potions containing laudanum and various herbals have been used to induce sleep. The first agent to be introduced specifically as a sedative and soon thereafter as a hypnotic was bromide, in the middle of the nineteenth century. *Chloral hydrate, paraldehyde, urethane,* and *sulfonal* came into use before the introduction of *barbital* in 1903 and *phenobarbital* in 1912. Their success spawned the synthesis and testing of over 2500 barbiturates, of which approximately 50 were distributed commercially. The barbiturates so dominated the stage that less than a dozen other sedative-hypnotics were successfully marketed before 1960.

The partial separation of sedative-hypnotic-anesthetic from anticonvulsant properties embodied in phenobarbital led to searches for agents with more selective effects on the functions of the CNS. As a result, relatively nonsedative anticonvulsants, notably *phenytoin* and *trimethadione,* were developed in the late 1930s and early 1940s (*see* Chapter 21). The advent of chlorpromazine and meprobamate in the early 1950s, with their taming effects in animals, and the development of increasingly sophisticated methods for evaluating the behavioral effects of drugs set the stage in the 1950s for the synthesis of chlordiazepoxide by Sternbach and the discovery of its unique pattern of actions by Randall (*see* Symposium, 1982). The introduction of *chlordiazepoxide* into clinical medicine in 1961 ushered in the era of benzodiazepines. Most of the benzodiazepines that have reached the marketplace were selected for high anxiolytic potency in relation to their depression of CNS function. However,

all benzodiazepines possess sedative-hypnotic properties to varying degrees; these properties are extensively exploited clinically, especially to facilitate sleep. Mainly because of their remarkably low capacity to produce fatal CNS depression, the benzodiazepines have displaced the barbiturates as sedative-hypnotic agents.

Over the past decade, it has become clear that all benzodiazepines in clinical use have the capacity to promote the binding of the major inhibitory neurotransmitter, gamma-aminobutyric acid (GABA), to the $GABA_A$ subtype of GABA receptors, which exist as multisubunit, ligand-gated chloride channels. Benzodiazepines enhance the GABA-induced ionic currents through these channels. Pharmacological investigations have provided evidence for heterogeneity among sites of binding and action of benzodiazepines, while biochemical and molecular biological investigations have revealed the numerous varieties of subunits that make up the GABA-gated chloride channels expressed in different neurons. Since receptor subunit composition appears to govern the interaction of various allosteric modulators with these channels, there has been a surge in efforts to find agents displaying a different mixture of benzodiazepine-like properties that may reflect selective actions on one or more subtypes of GABA receptors. One result of these efforts has been the introduction of *zolpidem,* one of several imidazopyridine compounds that appear to exert sedative-hypnotic actions by interacting with a subset of benzodiazepine binding sites. *Zaleplon,* a pyrazolopyrimidine, also has specificity for a subset of $GABA_A$ receptors. Investigation of compounds in many other chemical classes is in progress.

BENZODIAZEPINES

Although the benzodiazepines in clinical use exert qualitatively similar effects, important quantitative differences in their pharmacodynamic spectra and pharmacokinetic properties have led to varying patterns of therapeutic application. There is reason to believe that a number of distinct mechanisms of action contribute in varying degrees to the sedative-hypnotic, muscle-relaxant, anxiolytic, and anticonvulsant effects of the benzodiazepines. Recent findings provide evidence that specific subunits of $GABA_A$ receptor are responsible for specific pharmacological properties of benzodiazepines. While only the benzodiazepines used primarily for hypnosis will be discussed in detail, this chapter will describe the general properties of the group and the important differences among individual agents (*see also* Chapters 19 and 21).

Chemistry. The structures of the benzodiazepines in use in the United States are shown in Table 17–1, as are those of a few related compounds, discussed below. The term *benzodiazepine* refers to the portion of the structure composed of a benzene ring (A) fused to a seven-membered diazepine ring (B). However, since all the important benzodiazepines contain a 5-aryl substituent (ring C) and a 1,4-diazepine ring, the term has come to mean the 5-aryl-1,4-benzodiazepines. Various modifications in the structure of the ring systems have yielded compounds

Table 17–1

Benzodiazepines: Names and Structures*

BENZODIAZEPINE	R_1	R_2	R_3	R_7	R_2'
Alprazolam	[Fused triazolo ring][b]	—H	—H	—Cl	—H
Brotizolam†	[Fused triazolo ring][b]	—H	—H	[Thieno ring A][c]	—Cl
Chlordiazepoxide[a]	(—)	—NHCH$_3$	—H	—Cl	—H
Clobazam[a],†	—CH$_3$	=O	—H	—Cl	—H
Clonazepam	—H	=O	—H	—NO$_2$	—Cl
Clorazepate	—H	=O	—COO$^-$	—Cl	—H
Demoxepam[a],†,‡	—H	=O	—H	—Cl	—H
Diazepam	—CH$_3$	=O	—H	—Cl	—H
Estazolam	[Fused triazolo ring][d]	—H	—H	—Cl	—H
Flumazenil[a]	[Fused imidazo ring][e]	—H	—H	—F	[=O at C$_5$][g]
Flurazepam	—CH$_2$CH$_2$N(C$_2$H$_5$)$_2$	=O	—H	—Cl	—F
Halazepam	—CH$_2$CF$_3$	=O	—H	—Cl	—H
Lorazepam	—H	=O	—OH	—Cl	—Cl
Midazolam	[Fused imadazo ring][f]	—H	—H	—Cl	—F
Nitrazepam†	—H	=O	—H	—NO$_2$	—H
Nordazepam†,§	—H	=O	—H	—Cl	—H
Oxazepam	—H	=O	—OH	—Cl	—H
Prazepam†	—CH$_2$—CH⟨CH$_2$/CH$_2$⟩	=O	—H	—Cl	—H
Quazepam	—CH$_2$CF$_3$	=S	—H	—Cl	—F
Temazepam	—CH$_3$	=O	—OH	—Cl	—H
Triazolam	[Fused triazolo ring][b]	—H	—H	—Cl	—Cl

*Alphabetical footnotes refer to alterations of the general formula; symbolic footnotes are used for other comments.

†Not available for clinical use in the United States.

‡Major metabolite of chlordiazepoxide.

§Major metabolite of diazepam and others; also referred to as nordiazepam and desmethyldiazepam.

[a]No substituent at position 4, except for chlordiazepoxide and demoxepam, which are N-oxides; R_4 is —CH$_3$ in flumazenil, in which there is no double bond between positions 4 and 5; R_4 is =O in clobazam, in which position 4 is C and position 5 is N.

[g]No ring C.

with similar activities. These include 1,5-benzodiazepines (*e.g.,* *clobazam*) and the replacement of the fused benzene ring (A) with heteroaromatic systems such as thieno (*e.g., brotizolam*). The chemical nature of substituents at positions 1 to 3 can vary widely and can include triazolo or imidazolo rings fused at positions 1 and 2. Replacement of ring C with a keto function at position 5 and a methyl substituent at position 4 are important structural features of the benzodiazepine antagonist, *flumazenil* (ROMAZICON; Ro 15-1788; *see* Haefely, 1983).

In addition to various benzodiazepine or imidazobenzodiazepine derivatives, a large number of nonbenzodiazepine compounds have been synthesized that compete with classic benzodiazepines or flumazenil for binding at specific sites in the CNS (*see* Gardner *et al.,* 1993). These include representatives from the β-carbolines (containing an indole nucleus fused to a pyridine ring), imidazopyridines (*e.g., zolpidem; see* below), imidazopyrimidines and imidazoquinolones, and cyclopyrrolones (*e.g., zopiclone*).

Pharmacological Properties

Virtually all effects of the benzodiazepines result from actions of these drugs on the CNS. The most prominent of these effects are sedation, hypnosis, decreased anxiety, muscle relaxation, anterograde amnesia, and anticonvulsant activity. Only two effects of these drugs appear to result from actions on peripheral tissues: coronary vasodilation, seen after intravenous administration of therapeutic doses of certain benzodiazepines, and neuromuscular blockade, seen only with very high doses.

A variety of benzodiazepine-like effects have been observed *in vivo* and *in vitro* and have been classified as *full agonistic effects* (*i.e.,* faithfully mimicking agents such as diazepam with relatively low fractional occupancy of binding sites) or *partial agonistic effects* (*i.e.,* producing less intense maximal effects and/or requiring relatively high fractional occupancy compared to agents such as diazepam). Some compounds produce effects opposite to those of diazepam in the absence of benzodiazepine-like agonists and have been termed *inverse agonists; partial inverse agonists* also have been recognized. The vast majority of effects of agonists and inverse agonists can be reversed or prevented by the benzodiazepine antagonist flumazenil, which competes with agonists and inverse agonists for binding to the benzodiazepine receptor. In addition, representatives from various classes of compounds behave like flumazenil and act only to block the effects of agonists or inverse agonists.

Central Nervous System.   While benzodiazepines affect activity at all levels of the neuraxis, some structures are affected to a much greater extent than others. The benzodiazepines are not capable of producing the same degrees of

neuronal depression as do barbiturates and volatile anesthetics. All of the benzodiazepines have very similar pharmacological profiles. Nevertheless, the drugs differ in selectivity, and the clinical usefulness of individual benzodiazepines thus varies considerably.

As the dose of a benzodiazepine is increased, sedation progresses to hypnosis and then to stupor. The clinical literature often refers to the "anesthetic" effects and uses of certain benzodiazepines, but the drugs do not cause a true general anesthesia, since awareness usually persists, and relaxation sufficient to allow surgery cannot be achieved. However, at "preanesthetic" doses, there is amnesia for events subsequent to the administration of the drug; this may create the illusion of previous anesthesia.

The recent discovery of a molecular basis for numerous benzodiazepine receptor subtypes (*see* below) has provided the rationale for attempts to separate the anxiolytic actions of these drugs from their sedative/hypnotic effects. However, distinguishing between these behaviors remains problematic. Measurements of anxiety and sedation are difficult in human beings, and the validity of animal models for anxiety and sedation is uncertain. The existence of multiple benzodiazepine receptors may partially explain the diversity of pharmacological responses in different species.

Animal Models of Anxiety.   In animal models of anxiety, most attention has been focused on the ability of benzodiazepines to increase locomotor, feeding, or drinking behavior that has been suppressed by novel or aversive stimuli. For such tests, animal behaviors that previously had been rewarded by food or water are periodically punished by an electric shock. The time during which shocks are delivered is signaled by some auditory or visual cue, and untreated animals stop performing almost completely when the cue is perceived. The difference in behavioral responses during the punished and unpunished periods is eliminated by benzodiazepine agonists, usually at doses that do not reduce the rate of unpunished responses or produce other signs of impaired motor function. Similarly, rats placed in an unfamiliar environment exhibit markedly reduced exploratory behavior (neophobia), whereas animals treated with benzodiazepines do not. Opioid analgesics and neuroleptic (antipsychotic) drugs do not increase suppressed behaviors, and phenobarbital and meprobamate usually do so only at doses that also reduce spontaneous or unpunished behaviors or produce ataxia.

The difference between the dose required to impair motor function and that necessary to increase punished behavior varies widely among the benzodiazepines and depends on the species and experimental protocol. Although such differences may have encouraged the marketing of some benzodiazepines as selective sedative-hypnotic agents, they have not predicted with any accuracy the magnitude of sedative effects among those benzodiazepines marketed as anxiolytic agents.

Tolerance to Benzodiazepines.   Studies on tolerance in laboratory animals often are cited to support the belief that disinhibitory effects of benzodiazepines are separate from their sedative-ataxic effects. For example, tolerance to the depressant effects on rewarded or neutral behavior occurs after several days of treatment with benzodiazepines; the disinhibitory effects of the drugs on punished behavior are augmented initially and decline after 3 to 4 weeks (*see* File, 1985). Although most patients who chronically ingest benzodiazepines report that drowsiness wanes over a few days, tolerance to the impairment of some measures of psychomotor performance (*e.g.,* visual tracking) usually is not observed. The development of tolerance to the anxiolytic effects of benzodiazepines is a subject of debate (Lader and File, 1987). However, many patients can maintain themselves on a fairly constant dose; increases or decreases in dosage appear to correspond to changes in problems or stresses. Nevertheless, some patients either do not reduce their dosage when stress is relieved or steadily escalate dosage. Such behavior may be associated with the development of drug dependence (*see* Woods *et al.,* 1987; DuPont, 1988).

Some benzodiazepines induce muscle hypotonia without interfering with normal locomotion and can decrease rigidity in patients with cerebral palsy. However, in contrast to effects in animals, there is only a limited degree of selectivity in human beings. Clonazepam in nonsedative doses does cause muscle relaxation in patients, but diazepam and most other benzodiazepines do not. Tolerance occurs to both the muscle relaxant and ataxic effects of these drugs.

Experimentally, benzodiazepines inhibit seizure activity induced by either pentylenetetrazol or picrotoxin, but strychnine- and maximal electroshock-induced seizures are suppressed only with doses that also severely impair locomotor activity. *Clonazepam, nitrazepam,* and *nordazepam* are among those compounds with more selective anticonvulsant activity than most other benzodiazepines. Benzodiazepines also suppress photic seizures in baboons and ethanol-withdrawal seizures in human beings. However, the development of tolerance to the anticonvulsant effects has limited the usefulness of benzodiazepines in the treatment of recurrent seizure disorders in human beings (*see* Chapter 21).

Although analgesic effects of benzodiazepines have been observed in experimental animals, only transient analgesia is apparent in human patients after intravenous administration. Such effects actually may involve the production of amnesia. However, it is clear that benzodiazepines do not cause hyperalgesia, unlike the barbiturates.

Effects on the Electroencephalogram (EEG) and Sleep Stages.
The effects of benzodiazepines on the waking EEG resemble those of other sedative-hypnotic drugs. Alpha activity is decreased, but there is an increase in low-voltage fast activity. Tolerance occurs to these effects.

Most benzodiazepines decrease sleep latency, especially when first used, and diminish the number of awakenings and the time spent in stage 0 (a stage of wakefulness). Time in stage 1 (descending drowsiness) usually is decreased, and there is a prominent decrease in the time spent in slow-wave sleep (stages 3 and 4). Most benzodiazepines increase the time from onset of spindle sleep to the first burst of rapid-eye-movement (REM) sleep, and the time spent in REM sleep usually is shortened. However, the number of cycles of REM sleep usually is increased, mostly late in the sleep time. *Zolpidem* does not suppress REM sleep to the same extent as do benzodiazepines and thus may be superior to benzodiazepines for use as a hypnotic (Dujardin *et al.,* 1998).

Despite the shortening of stage 4 and REM sleep, the net effect of administration of benzodiazepines typically is an increase in total sleep time, largely because of an increase in time spent in stage 2 (which is the major fraction of non-REM sleep). The effect is greatest in subjects with shortest baseline total sleep time. In addition, despite the increase in the number of REM cycles, the number of shifts to lighter sleep stages (1 and 0) and the amount of body movement are diminished. The nocturnal peaks in the concentrations of growth hormone, prolactin, and luteinizing hormone in plasma are not affected. During chronic nocturnal use of benzodiazepines, the effects on the various stages of sleep usually decline within a few nights. When such use is discontinued, the pattern of drug-induced changes in sleep parameters may "rebound," and an increase in the amount and density of REM sleep may be especially prominent. However, if the dosage has not been excessive, patients usually will note only a shortening of sleep time rather than an exacerbation of insomnia.

Although some differences in the patterns of effects exerted by the various benzodiazepines have been noted, their use usually imparts a sense of deep or refreshing sleep. It is uncertain to which effect on sleep parameters this feeling can be attributed. As a result, variations in the pharmacokinetic properties of individual benzodiazepines appear to be much more important determinants of the utility of the available drugs for their effects on sleep than are any potential differences in their pharmacodynamic properties.

Molecular Targets for Benzodiazepine Actions in the CNS.
Benzodiazepines are believed to exert most of their effects by interacting with inhibitory neurotransmitter receptors directly activated by GABA. GABA receptors are membrane-bound proteins that can be divided into two major subtypes: $GABA_A$ and $GABA_B$ receptors. The ionotropic $GABA_A$ receptors are composed of five subunits that coassemble to form an integral chloride channel. $GABA_A$ receptors are responsible for most inhibitory neurotransmission in the CNS. In contrast, the metabotropic $GABA_B$ receptors, made up of single peptides with seven transmembrane domains, are coupled to their signal transduction mechanisms by G proteins. Benzodiazepines act at $GABA_A$ but not $GABA_B$ receptors by binding directly to a specific site that is distinct from that of GABA binding on the receptor/ion channel complex. Unlike barbiturates, benzodiazepines do not directly activate $GABA_A$ receptors but require GABA to express their effects; *i.e.,* they only modulate the effects of GABA. Benzodiazepines and GABA analogs bind to their respective sites on brain membranes with nanomolar affinity. Benzodiazepines modulate GABA binding and GABA alters benzodiazepine binding in an allosteric fashion. Benzodiazepine-receptor ligands can act as agonists, antagonists, or inverse agonists at the benzodiazepine receptor site, depending on the compound. Agonists at the benzodiazepine receptor increase, while inverse agonists decrease, the amount of chloride current

generated by GABA$_A$-receptor activation. Benzodiazepine receptor agonists produce shifts of GABA concentration-response curves to the left, while inverse agonists shift the curves to the right. Both of these effects can be blocked by antagonists at the benzodiazepine-receptor site. In the absence of a benzodiazepine-receptor agonist or inverse agonist, a benzodiazepine-receptor antagonist does not affect GABA$_A$-receptor function. One such antagonist, flumazenil, is used clinically to reverse the effects of high doses of benzodiazepines. The behavioral and electrophysiological effects of benzodiazepines also can be reduced or prevented by prior treatment with antagonists (*e.g.* bicuculline) at the GABA binding site.

The strongest evidence that benzodiazepines act directly on GABA$_A$ receptors comes from molecular cloning of cDNAs encoding subunits of the GABA$_A$ receptor complex (Schofield *et al.*, 1987; Pritchett *et al.*, 1989). When receptors formed of the appropriate subunits (*see* below) are studied in an *in vitro* expression system, high-affinity benzodiazepine binding sites are seen, as are GABA-activated chloride conductances that are enhanced by benzodiazepine-receptor agonists. The properties of the expressed receptors are generally similar to those of GABA$_A$ receptors found in most CNS neurons. Each GABA$_A$ receptor is believed to consist of a pentamer of homologous subunits. Thus far, 16 different subunits have been identified and classified into seven subunit families: six α, three β, three γ, and single δ, ε, π, and θ subunits. Additional complexity arises from RNA splice variants of some of these subunits (*e.g.*, $\gamma2$ and $\alpha6$). The exact subunit structures of native GABA receptors remains unknown, but it is thought that most GABA receptors are composed of α, β, and γ subunits that coassemble with some uncertain stoichiometry. The multiplicity of subunits generates heterogeneity in GABA$_A$ receptors and is responsible, at least in part, for the pharmacological diversity in benzodiazepine receptors detected by behavioral, biochemical, and functional studies. Studies of cloned GABA$_A$ receptors have shown that the coassembly of a γ subunit with α and β subunits confers benzodiazepine sensitivity to GABA$_A$ receptors (Pritchett *et al.*, 1989). Receptors composed solely of α and β subunits produce functional GABA$_A$ receptors that also respond to barbiturates, but they neither bind nor are affected by benzodiazepines. Benzodiazepines are believed to bind at the interface between α and β subunits, and both subunits determine the pharmacology of the benzodiazepine receptor site (McKernan *et al.*, 1995). For example, combinations containing the $\alpha1$ subunit show pharmacology distinct from that of receptors containing $\alpha2$, $\alpha3$, or $\alpha5$ subunits (Pritchett and Seeburg, 1990), reminiscent of the pharmacological heterogeneity detected with radioligand binding studies using brain membranes. Receptors containing the $\alpha6$ subunit do not display high-affinity binding of diazepam and appear to be selective for the benzodiazepine-receptor inverse agonist RO 15-4513, which has been tested as an alcohol antagonist (Lüddens *et al.*, 1990). The subtype of γ subunit present in receptors also determines benzodiazepine pharmacology, with lower affinity binding observed in receptors containing the $\gamma1$ subunit (McKernan *et al.*, 1995). Although theoretically hundreds of thousands of different GABA$_A$ receptors could be assembled from all these different subunits, there are constraints

for the assembly of these receptors that limit their numbers (Sieghart *et al.*, 1999).

Recent work is beginning to show which GABA$_A$-receptor subunits are responsible for particular effects of benzodiazepines *in vivo*. The mutation to arginine of a histidine residue at position 101 of the GABA$_A$ receptor $\alpha1$ subunit renders receptors containing that subunit insensitive to the GABA-enhancing effects of diazepam (Kleingoor *et al.*, 1993). Mice bearing these mutated subunits fail to exhibit the sedative, amnestic, and, in part, the anticonvulsant effects of diazepam, while retaining sensitivity to the anxiolytic, muscle-relaxant, and ethanol-enhancing effects (Rudolph *et al.*, 1999; McKernan *et al.*, 2000). Conversely, mice bearing the equivalent mutation in the $\alpha2$ subunit of the GABA$_A$ receptor display insensitivity to the anxiolytic effects of diazepam (Löw, *et al.*, 2000). The attribution of specific behavioral effects of benzodiazepines to individual receptor subunits will aid in the development of new compounds exhibiting fewer undesired side effects. For example, the experimental compound L838,417 enhances the effects of GABA on receptors composed of $\alpha2$, $\alpha3$, or $\alpha5$ subunits but lacks efficacy on receptors containing the $\alpha1$ subunit; it is thus anxiolytic but not sedating (McKernan *et al.*, 2000).

GABA$_A$-receptor subunits also may play roles in the proper targeting of assembled receptors to their proper locations in synapses. The production of $\gamma2$ subunit knockout mice demonstrated that receptors lacking a $\gamma2$ subunit were not properly localized to synapses, although receptors lacking these subunits were formed and translocated to cell surfaces (Essrich *et al.*, 1998). The synaptic clustering molecule gephyrin also was found to play a role in receptor localization.

GABA$_A$ Receptor-Mediated Electrical Events: In Vivo Properties.
The remarkable safety of the benzodiazepines is likely related to the fact that the production of their effects *in vivo* depends on the presynaptic release of GABA; in the absence of GABA, benzodiazepines have no effects on GABA$_A$-receptor function. Although barbiturates also enhance the effects of GABA at low doses, they directly activate GABA receptors at higher doses, which can lead to profound CNS depression (*see* below). Further, the ability of benzodiazepines to release suppressed behaviors and to produce sedation can be ascribed in part to potentiation of GABA-ergic pathways that serve to regulate the firing of neurons containing various monoamines (*see* Chapter 12). These neurons are known to promote behavioral arousal and are important mediators of the inhibitory effects of fear and punishment on behavior. Finally, inhibitory effects on muscular hypertonia or the spread of seizure activity can be rationalized by potentiation of inhibitory GABA-ergic circuits at various levels of the neuraxis. In most studies conducted *in vivo* or *in situ*, the local or systemic administration of benzodiazepines reduces the spontaneous or evoked electrical activity of major (large) neurons in all regions of the brain and spinal cord. The activity of these neurons is regulated in part by small inhibitory interneurons (predominantly GABA-ergic) arranged in both feedback and feedforward types of circuits. The magnitude of the effects produced by benzodiazepines can vary widely and depends on such factors as the types of inhibitory circuits that are operating, the sources and intensity of excitatory input, and the manner in which experimental manipulations are performed and assessed. For example, feedback circuits often involve powerful inhibitory synapses on the neuronal soma near the axon hillock, which are supplied predominantly by recurrent pathways. The synaptic or exogenous application of GABA to this region increases

chloride conductance and can prevent neuronal discharge by shunting electrical currents that would otherwise depolarize the membrane of the initial segment. Accordingly, benzodiazepines markedly prolong the period following brief activation of recurrent GABA-ergic pathways during which neither spontaneous nor applied excitatory stimuli can evoke neuronal discharge; this effect is reversed by the $GABA_A$-receptor antagonist *bicuculline*.

Molecular Basis for Benzodiazepine Regulation of GABA$_A$ Receptor-Mediated Electrical Events. Electrophysiological studies *in vitro* have shown that the enhancement of GABA-induced chloride currents by benzodiazepines results primarily from an increase in the frequency of bursts of openings of chloride channels produced by submaximal amounts of GABA (Twyman *et al.,* 1989). Inhibitory synaptic transmission measured after stimulation of afferent fibers is potentiated by benzodiazepines at therapeutically relevant concentrations. Prolongation of spontaneous miniature inhibitory postsynaptic currents (IPSCs) by benzodiazepines also has been observed. Although sedative barbiturates also enhance such chloride currents, they do so by prolonging the duration of individual channel-opening events. Macroscopic measurements of $GABA_A$ receptor-mediated currents indicate that benzodiazepines shift the GABA concentration-response curve to the left without increasing the maximum current evoked with GABA. Taken together with the *in vivo* data, these findings are consistent with a model in which benzodiazepines exert their major actions by increasing the gain of inhibitory neurotransmission mediated by $GABA_A$ receptors. As noted above, certain experimental benzodiazepines and other structurally related compounds act as inverse agonists to reduce GABA-induced chloride currents, promote convulsions, and produce other *in vivo* effects opposite to those induced by the benzodiazepines in clinical use (*see* Gardner, 1988; Gardner *et al.,* 1993). A few compounds, most notably flumazenil, can block the effects of both clinically used benzodiazepines and inverse agonists *in vitro* and *in vivo* but have no detectable actions by themselves. The conceptual advances brought about by molecular studies have strengthened the hypothesis that benzodiazepines act mainly at $GABA_A$ receptors. Moreover, molecular diversity helps clarify many previous observations that appeared to conflict with this hypothesis (for reviews, *see* De Lorey and Olsen, 1992; Doble and Martin, 1992; Sieghart, 1992; Ragan *et al.,* 1993; and Symposium, 1992). Nonetheless, some observations are difficult to reconcile with the hypothesis that all effects of benzodiazepines are mediated *via* $GABA_A$ receptors. Low concentrations of benzodiazepines that are not blocked by bicuculline or picrotoxin induce depressant effects on hippocampal neurons (Polc, 1988). The induction of sleep in rats by benzodiazepines also is insensitive to bicuculline or picrotoxin but is prevented by flumazenil (*see* Mendelson, 1992). At higher concentrations, corresponding to those producing hypnosis and amnesia during preanesthetic medication (*see* Chapter 14) or those achieved during the treatment of status epilepticus (*see* Chapter 21), the actions of the benzodiazepines may involve the participation of a number of other mechanisms. These include inhibition of the uptake of adenosine and the resultant potentiation of the actions of this endogenous neuronal depressant (*see* Phillis and O'Regan, 1988), as well as the GABA-independent inhibition of Ca^{2+} currents, Ca^{2+}-dependent release of neurotransmitter, and tetrodotoxin-sensitive Na^+ channels (*see* Macdonald and McLean, 1986).

The macromolecular complex containing GABA-regulated chloride channels also may be a site of action of general anesthetics, ethanol, inhaled drugs of abuse, and certain metabolites of endogenous steroids (Mehta and Ticku, 1999; Beckstead *et al.,* 2000). Among the latter, allopregnanolone (3α hydroxy, 5α-dihydroprogesterone) is of particular interest. This compound, a metabolite of progesterone that can be formed in the brain from precursors in the circulation as well as from those synthesized by glial cells, produces barbiturate-like effects including promotion of GABA-induced chloride currents and enhanced binding of benzodiazepines and GABA-receptor agonists. Like the barbiturates, higher concentrations of the steroid activate chloride currents in the absence of GABA, and its effects do not require the presence of a γ subunit in $GABA_A$ receptors expressed in transfected cells. Unlike the barbiturates, however, the steroid cannot reduce excitatory responses to glutamate (*see* below). These effects are produced very rapidly and apparently are mediated by interactions at sites on the cell surface. A congener of allopregnanolone (alfaxalone) previously was used outside the United States for the induction of anesthesia.

Respiration. Hypnotic doses of benzodiazepines are without effect on respiration in normal subjects, but special care must be taken in the treatment of children (Kriel *et al.,* 2000) and individuals with impaired hepatic function, such as alcoholics (Guglielminotti *et al.,* 1999). At higher doses, such as those used for preanesthetic medication or for endoscopy, benzodiazepines slightly depress alveolar ventilation and cause respiratory acidosis as the result of a decrease in hypoxic rather than hypercapnic drive; these effects are exaggerated in patients with chronic obstructive pulmonary disease (COPD), and alveolar hypoxia and/or CO_2 narcosis may result. These drugs can cause apnea during anesthesia or when given with opioids, and patients severely intoxicated with benzodiazepines usually require respiratory assistance only when they also have ingested another CNS-depressant drug, most commonly alcohol.

By contrast, hypnotic doses of benzodiazepines may worsen sleep-related breathing disorders by adversely affecting the control of the upper airway muscles or by decreasing the ventilatory response to CO_2 (*see* Guilleminault, in Symposium, 1990b). The latter effect may be sufficient to cause hypoventilation and hypoxemia in some patients with severe COPD, although benzodiazepines may improve sleep and sleep structure in some instances. In patients with obstructive sleep apnea (OSA), hypnotic doses of benzodiazepines may decrease muscular tone in the upper airway and exaggerate the impact of apneic episodes on alveolar hypoxia, pulmonary hypertension, and cardiac ventricular load. Many physicians consider the presence of OSA to be a contraindication for the use of alcohol or any sedative-hypnotic agent, including a benzodiazepine; caution also should be exercised in patients who snore regularly, because partial airway obstruction may be converted to OSA under the influence of these drugs. In addition, benzodiazepines may promote the appearance of episodes of apnea during REM sleep (associated with decreases in oxygen saturation) in patients recovering from a myocardial infarction (Guilleminault, in *Symposium*, 1990b); however, the potential impact of these drugs on survival of patients with cardiac disease has not been investigated as yet.

Cardiovascular System.   The cardiovascular effects of benzodiazepines are minor in normal subjects except in severe intoxication; the adverse effects in patients with obstructive sleep disorders or cardiac disease were noted above. In preanesthetic doses, all benzodiazepines decrease blood pressure and increase heart rate. With midazolam, the effects appear to be secondary to a decrease in peripheral resistance, but with diazepam they are secondary to a decrease in left ventricular work and cardiac output. Diazepam increases coronary flow, possibly by an action to increase interstitial concentrations of adenosine, and the accumulation of this cardiodepressant metabolite also may explain the negative inotropic effects of the drug. In large doses, midazolam decreases considerably both cerebral blood flow and oxygen assimilation (Nugent *et al.,* 1982).

Gastrointestinal Tract.   Benzodiazepines are thought by some gastroenterologists to improve a variety of "anxiety-related" gastrointestinal disorders. There is a paucity of evidence for direct actions. Benzodiazepines partially protect against stress ulcers in rats, and diazepam markedly decreases nocturnal gastric secretion in human beings.

Absorption, Fate, and Excretion.   The physicochemical and pharmacokinetic properties of the benzodiazepines greatly affect their clinical utility. They all have high lipid:water distribution coefficients in the nonionized form; nevertheless, lipophilicity varies more than 50-fold according to the polarity and electronegativity of various substituents.

All of the benzodiazepines essentially are completely absorbed, with the exception of clorazepate; this drug is rapidly decarboxylated in gastric juice to *N*-desmethyldiazepam (nordazepam), which subsequently is absorbed completely. Some benzodiazepines (*e.g.,* prazepam and flurazepam) reach the systemic circulation only in the form of active metabolites.

Drugs active at the benzodiazepine receptor may be divided into four categories based on their elimination half-lives: (1) ultra-short-acting benzodiazepines; (2) short-acting agents, with $t_{1/2}$ less than 6 hours, including triazolam, the nonbenzodiazepine zolpidem ($t_{1/2}$ approximately 2 hours), and zopiclone ($t_{1/2}$ 5 to 6 hours); (3) intermediate-

acting agents, with $t_{1/2}$ of 6 to 24 hours, including estazolam and temazepam; and (4) long-acting agents, with $t_{1/2}$ greater than 24 hours, including flurazepam, diazepam, and quazepam.

The benzodiazepines and their active metabolites bind to plasma proteins. The extent of binding correlates strongly with lipid solubility and ranges from about 70% for alprazolam to nearly 99% for diazepam. The concentration in the cerebrospinal fluid (CSF) is approximately equal to the concentration of free drug in plasma. While competition with other protein-bound drugs may occur, no clinically significant examples have been reported.

The plasma concentrations of most benzodiazepines exhibit patterns that are consistent with two-compartment models (*see* Chapter 1), but three-compartment models appear to be more appropriate for the compounds with the highest lipid solubility. Accordingly, there is rapid uptake of benzodiazepines into the brain and other highly perfused organs after intravenous administration (or oral administration of a rapidly absorbed compound); rapid uptake is followed by a phase of redistribution into tissues that are less well perfused, especially muscle and fat. Redistribution is most rapid for drugs with the highest lipid solubility. In the regimens used for nighttime sedation, the rate of redistribution sometimes can have a greater influence than the rate of biotransformation on the duration of CNS effects (Dettli, in *Symposium*, 1986a). The kinetics of redistribution of diazepam and other lipophilic benzodiazepines are complicated by enterohepatic circulation. The volumes of distribution of the benzodiazepines are large, and in many cases are increased in elderly patients (Swift and Stevenson, in *Symposium*, 1983). These drugs cross the placental barrier and are secreted into breast milk.

The benzodiazepines are metabolized extensively by enzymes in the cytochrome P450 family, particularly CYP3A4 and CYP2C19. Some benzodiazepines, such as oxazepam, are conjugated directly and are not metabolized by these enzymes (*see* Tanaka, 1999). Erythromycin, clarithromycin, ritonavir, itraconazole, ketoconazole, nefazodone, and grapefruit juice are inhibitors of CYP3A4 and can affect the metabolism of benzodiazepines (Dresser *et al.,* 2000). Because active metabolites of some benzodiazepines are biotransformed more slowly than are the parent compounds, the duration of action of many benzodiazepines bears little relationship to the half-time of elimination of the drug that has been administered. For example, the half-life of flurazepam in plasma is 2 to 3 hours, but that of a major active metabolite (*N*-desalkylflurazepam) is 50 hours or more. Conversely, the rate of biotransformation of those agents that are inactivated by the initial reaction is an important determinant of their duration of action; these agents include oxazepam, lorazepam,

Table 17–2
Major Metabolic Relationships among Some of the Benzodiazepines*

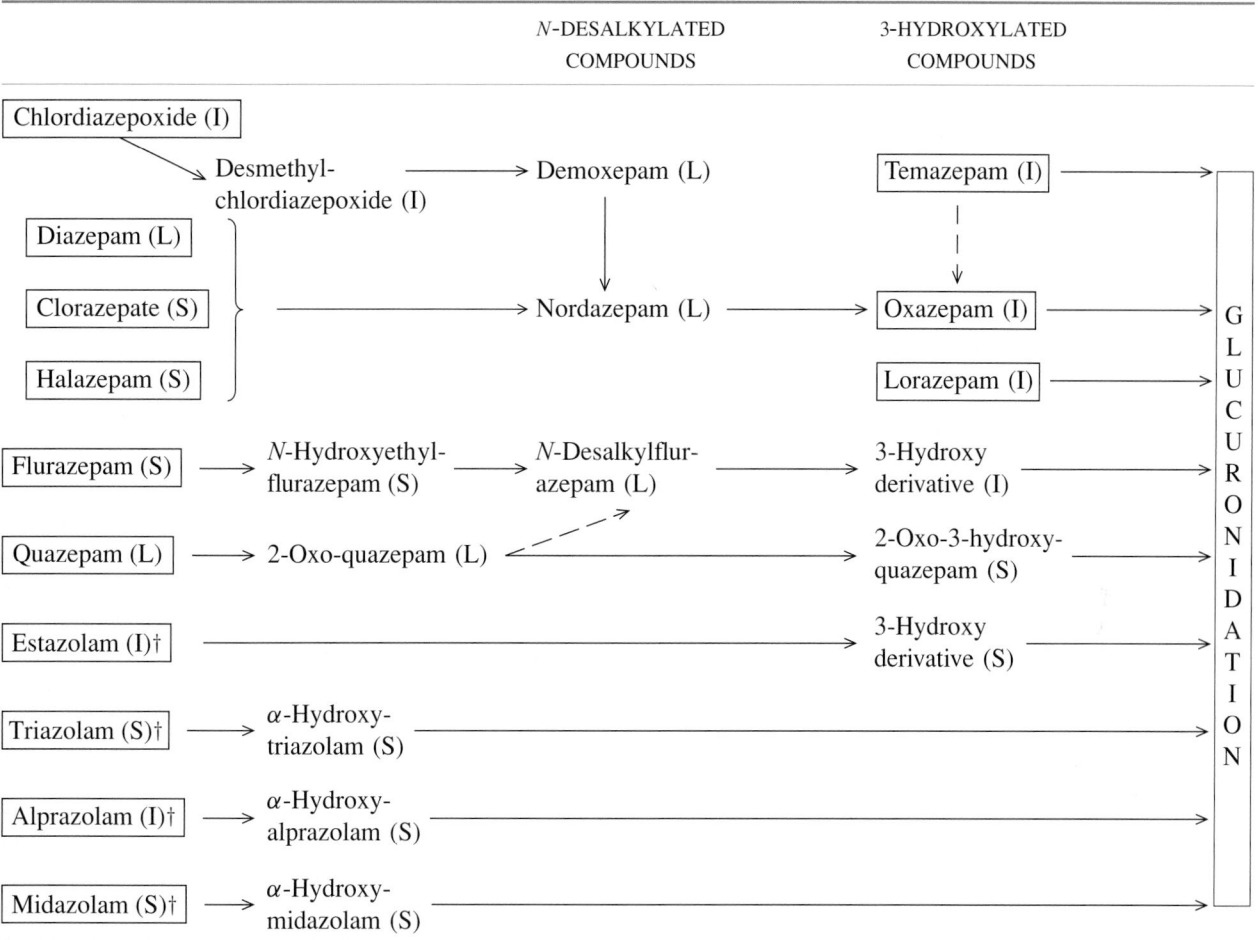

*Compounds enclosed in boxes are marketed in the United States. The approximate half-lives of the various compounds are denoted in parentheses; S (short-acting), $t_{1/2} < 6$ hours; I (intermediate-acting), $t_{1/2} = 6$ to 24 hours; L (long-acting), $t_{1/2} = >24$ hours. All compounds except clorazepate are biologically active; the activity of 3-hydroxydesalkylflurazepam has not been determined. Clonazepam (not shown) is an N-desalkyl compound, and it is metabolized primarily by reduction of the 7-NO_2 group to the corresponding amine (inactive), followed by acetylation; its half-life is 20 to 40 hours.
†*See* text for discussion of other pathways of metabolism.

temazepam, triazolam, and midazolam. Metabolism of the benzodiazepines occurs in three major stages. These and the relationships between the drugs and their metabolites are shown in Table 17–2.

For those benzodiazepines that bear a substituent at position 1 (or 2) of the diazepine ring, the initial and most rapid phase of metabolism involves modification and/or removal of the substituent. With the exception of triazolam, alprazolam, estazolam, and midazolam, which contain either a fused triazolo or imidazolo ring, the eventual products are N-desalkylated compounds; these are all biologically active. One such compound, nordazepam, is a major metabolite common to the biotransformation of diazepam, clorazepate, prazepam, and halazepam; it

also is formed from demoxepam, an important metabolite of chlordiazepoxide.

The second phase of metabolism involves hydroxylation at position 3 and also usually yields an active derivative (*e.g.,* oxazepam from nordazepam). The rates of these reactions are usually very much slower than the first stage (half-times greater than 40 to 50 hours), such that appreciable accumulation of hydroxylated products with intact substituents at position 1 does not occur. There are two significant exceptions to this rule: (1) Small amounts of temazepine accumulate during the chronic administration of diazepam (not shown in Table 17–2) and (2) following the replacement of sulfur with oxygen in quazepam, most of the resultant 2-oxoquazepam is slowly hydroxylated at position 3 without removal of the N-alkyl group. However, only small amounts of the 3-hydroxyl derivative accumulate during the chronic administration of quazepam, because this compound is conjugated at an unusually rapid rate. By contrast, the *N*-desalkylflurazepam that is formed by the "minor" metabolic pathway does accumulate during quazepam administration, and it contributes significantly to the overall clinical effect.

The third major phase of metabolism is the conjugation of the 3-hydroxyl compounds, principally with glucuronic acid; the half-times of these reactions are usually between 6 and 12 hours, and the products are invariably inactive. Conjugation is the only major route of metabolism available for oxazepam and lorazepam, and it is the preferred pathway for temazepam because of the slower conversion of this compound to oxazepam. Triazolam and alprazolam are metabolized principally by initial hydroxylation of the methyl group on the fused triazolo ring; the absence of a chlorine residue in ring C of alprazolam slows this reaction significantly. The products, sometimes referred to as *α-hydroxylated compounds,* are quite active but are metabolized very rapidly, primarily by conjugation with glucuronic acid, such that there is no appreciable accumulation of active metabolites. The fused triazolo ring in estazolam lacks a methyl group, and it is hydroxylated to only a limited extent; the major route of metabolism involves the formation of the 3-hydroxyl derivative. The corresponding hydroxyl derivatives of triazolam and alprazolam also are formed to a significant extent. Compared to compounds without the triazolo ring, the rate of this reaction for all three drugs is unusually swift, and the 3-hydroxyl compounds are rapidly conjugated or oxidized further to benzophenone derivatives before excretion.

Midazolam is metabolized rapidly, primarily by hydroxylation of the methyl group on the fused imidazo ring; only small amounts of 3-hydroxyl compounds are formed. The *α*-hydroxylated compound, which has appreciable biological activity, is eliminated with a half-life of 1 hour after conjugation with glucuronic acid. Variable and sometimes substantial accumulation of this metabolite has been noted during intravenous infusion (Oldenhof *et al.,* 1988).

The aromatic rings (A and C) of the benzodiazepines are hydroxylated to only a small extent. The only important metabolism at these sites is the reduction of the 7-nitro substituents of clonazepam, nitrazepam, and flunitrazepam; the half-lives of these reactions are usually 20 to 40 hours. The resulting amines are inactive and are acetylated to varying degrees before excretion.

Because the benzodiazepines apparently do not significantly induce the synthesis of hepatic microsomal enzymes, their chronic administration usually does not result in the accelerated metabolism of other substances or of the benzodiazepines. Cimetidine and oral contraceptives inhibit *N*-dealkylation and 3-hydroxylation of benzodiazepines. Ethanol, isoniazid, and phenytoin are less effective in this regard. These reactions usually are reduced to a greater extent in elderly patients and in patients with chronic liver disease than are those involving conjugation.

Ideally, a useful hypnotic agent would have a rapid onset of action when taken at bedtime, a sufficiently sustained action to facilitate sleep throughout the night, and no residual action by the following morning. Among those benzodiazepines that are commonly used as hypnotic agents, triazolam theoretically fits this description most

closely. Because of the slow rate of elimination of des-alkylflurazepam, flurazepam (or quazepam) might seem to be unsuitable for this purpose. However, in practice there appear to be some disadvantages to the use of agents that have a relatively rapid rate of disappearance; these disadvantages include the early-morning insomnia that is experienced by some patients and a greater likelihood of rebound insomnia upon discontinuance of use (*see* Gillin *et al.,* 1989; Roehrs *et al.,* in Symposium, 1990b; Roth and Roehrs, 1992). With careful selection of dosage, flurazepam and other benzodiazepines with slower rates of elimination than triazolam can be used effectively (*see* Vogel, 1992). The biotransformation and pharmacokinetic properties of the benzodiazepines have been reviewed by Greenblatt (1991), Greenblatt and Wright (1993), Greenblatt *et al.* (1983a,b, 1991), and Hilbert and Battista (1991).

Untoward Effects.   At the time of peak concentration in plasma, hypnotic doses of benzodiazepines can be expected to cause varying degrees of lightheadedness, lassitude, increased reaction time, motor incoordination, impairment of mental and motor functions, confusion, and anterograde amnesia. Cognition appears to be affected less than motor performance. All of these effects can greatly impair driving and other psychomotor skills. Interaction with ethanol may be especially serious. When the drug is given at the intended time of sleep, the persistence of these effects during the waking hours is adverse. These residual effects are clearly dose-related and can be insidious, since most subjects underestimate the degree of their impairment. Residual daytime sleepiness also may be present as an adverse effect, even though successful drug therapy can reduce the daytime sleepiness resulting from chronic insomnia (*see* Dement, 1991). The intensity and incidence of CNS toxicity generally increase with age; both pharmacokinetic and pharmacodynamic factors are involved (*see* Meyer, 1982; Swift *et al.,* in Symposium, 1983; Monane, 1992).

Other relatively common side effects of benzodiazepines are weakness, headache, blurred vision, vertigo, nausea and vomiting, epigastric distress, and diarrhea; joint pains, chest pains, and incontinence may occur in a few recipients. Anticonvulsant benzodiazepines sometimes actually increase the frequency of seizures in patients with epilepsy.

The possible adverse effects of alterations in the sleep pattern are discussed at the end of this chapter.

Adverse Psychological Effects.   Benzodiazepines may cause paradoxical effects. For example, flurazepam may occasionally increase the incidence of nightmares, especially during the first week of use, and sometimes causes garrulousness, anxiety, irritability, tachycardia, and sweating. Amnesia, euphoria, restlessness, hallucinations, and hypomanic behavior have been reported to occur during use of various benzodiazepines. The release of bizarre uninhibited behavior has been noted in some users, while hostility and rage may occur in others; collectively, these are sometimes referred to as *disinhibition* or *dyscontrol* reactions. Paranoia, depression, and suicidal ideation also occasionally may accompany the use of these agents. The incidence of such paradoxical or disinhibition reactions is rare and appears to be dose-related. Because of reports of an increased incidence of confusion and abnormal behaviors, triazolam has been banned in the United Kingdom. Review by the United States Food and Drug Administration (FDA), however, declared triazolam to be safe and effective in low doses of 0.125 to 0.25 mg. Hindmarch *et al.* (1993) surveyed British family practitioners who had switched their patients from triazolam to a variety of other hypnotics after the ban in the United Kingdom and found that the patients did not have fewer side effects with replacement treatments. This report is consonant with controlled studies that do not support the conclusion that such reactions occur more frequently with any one benzodiazepine than with others (*see* Jonas *et al.,* 1992; Rothschild, 1992).

Chronic benzodiazepine use poses a risk for development of dependence and abuse, but not to the same extent as seem with older sedatives and other recognized drugs of abuse (Ulemhuth *et al.,* 1999). Abuse of benzodiazepines includes the use of *flunitrazepam* (ROHYPNOL) as a "date-rape" drug (Woods and Winger, 1997). Mild dependence may develop in many patients who have taken therapeutic doses of benzodiazepines on a regular basis for prolonged periods. Withdrawal symptoms may include temporary intensification of the problems that originally prompted their use (*e.g.,* insomnia, anxiety). Dysphoria, irritability, sweating, unpleasant dreams, tremors, anorexia, and faintness or dizziness also may occur, especially when withdrawal of the benzodiazepine occurs abruptly (Petursson, 1994). Hence, it is prudent to taper the dosage gradually when therapy is to be discontinued. During conventional treatment regimens, very few individuals increase their intake without instructions to do so, and very few manifest compulsive drug-seeking behavior upon discontinuation of a benzodiazepine. Patients who have histories of drug or alcohol abuse are most apt to use these agents inappropriately, and abuse of benzodiazepines usually occurs as part of a pattern of abuse of multiple drugs. In such individuals, benzodiazepines seldom are preferred to barbiturates or even alcohol, but they often are combined with those drugs to either accentuate their effect (*e.g.,* alcohol, opiates) or reduce their toxicity (*e.g.,* cocaine). The use of high doses of benzodiazepines over prolonged periods can lead to more severe symptoms after discontinuing the drug, including agitation, depression, panic, paranoia, myalgia, muscle twitches, and even convulsions and delirium. Dependence on benzodiazepines and their abuse have been reviewed by Woods *et al.* (1992) and in a report edited by DuPont (1988).

In spite of the adverse effects reviewed above, the benzodiazepines are relatively safe drugs. Even huge doses are rarely fatal unless other drugs are taken concomitantly. Ethanol is a common contributor to deaths involving benzodiazepines, and true coma is uncommon in the absence of another CNS depressant. Although overdosage with a benzodiazepine rarely causes severe cardiovascular or respiratory depression, therapeutic doses can further compromise respiration in patients with COPD or obstructive sleep apnea (*see* discussion of effects on respiration, above).

A wide variety of allergic, hepatotoxic, and hematologic reactions to the benzodiazepines may occur, but the incidence is quite low; these reactions have been associated with the use of flurazepam and triazolam but not with temazepam. Large doses taken just prior to or during labor may cause hypothermia, hypotonia, and mild respiratory depression in the neonate. Abuse by the pregnant mother can result in a withdrawal syndrome in the newborn.

Except for additive effects with other sedative or hypnotic drugs, reports of clinically important, pharmacodynamic interactions between benzodiazepines and other drugs have been infrequent. Ethanol increases both the rate of absorption of benzodiazepines and the associated CNS depression. Valproate and benzodiazepines in combination may cause psychotic episodes. Pharmacokinetic interactions are mentioned above.

Therapeutic Uses

The therapeutic uses and routes of administration of individual benzodiazepines that currently are marketed in the United States are summarized in Table 17–3. It should be emphasized that most benzodiazepines can be used interchangeably. For example, diazepam can be used for alcohol withdrawal, and most benzodiazepines work as hypnotics. In general, the therapeutic uses of a given benzodiazepine depend on its half-life and may not match the marketed indications. Benzodiazepines that are useful as anticonvulsants have a long half-life, and rapid entry into the brain is required for efficacy in treatment of status epilepticus. A short elimination half-life is desirable for hypnotics, although it carries the drawback of increased abuse liability and severity of withdrawal after discontinuation of chronic use. Antianxiety agents, in contrast, should have a long half-life, despite the drawback of the risk of neuropsychological deficits caused by drug accumulation.

The use of the benzodiazepines as hypnotics and sedatives is discussed later in this chapter (*see also* Symposium, 1990b; Teboul and Chouinard, 1991; Vogel, 1992; Dement, 1992; Walsh and Engelhardt, 1992; Maczaj, 1993). The use of benzodiazepines as antianxiety agents and anticonvulsants is discussed in Chapters 19 and 21, respectively, and their roles in preanesthetic medication and anesthesia are described in Chapters 13 and 14. The utility of benzodiazepines as muscle relaxants is discussed in Chapter 22.

Novel Benzodiazepine-Receptor Agonists

Hypnotics in this class include *zolpicone* (not available in the United States), *zolpidem* (AMBIEN), and *zaleplon*

Table 17–3

Trade Names, Routes of Administration, and Therapeutic Uses of Benzodiazepines

COMPOUND (TRADE NAME)	ROUTES OF ADMINISTRATION*	EXAMPLES OF THERAPEUTIC USES†	COMMENTS	$t_{1/2}$, hours‡	USUAL SEDATIVE-HYPNOTIC DOSAGE, mg¶
Alprazolam (XANAX)	Oral	Anxiety disorders, agoraphobia	Withdrawal symptoms may be especially severe	12 ± 2	—
Chlordiazepoxide (LIBRIUM, others)	Oral, I.M., I.V.	Anxiety disorders, management of alcohol withdrawal, anesthetic premedication	Long-acting and self-tapering because of active metabolites	10 ± 3.4	50–100, qd–qid§
Clonazepam (KLONOPIN)	Oral	Seizure disorders, adjunctive treatment in acute mania and certain movement disorders	Tolerance develops to anticonvulsant effects	23 ± 5	—
Clorazepate (TRANXENE, others)	Oral	Anxiety disorders, seizure disorders	Prodrug; activity due to formation of nordazepam during absorption	2.0 ± 0.9	3.75–20, bid–qid§
Diazepam (VALIUM, others)	Oral, I.M., I.V., rectal	Anxiety disorders, status epilepticus, skeletal muscle relaxation, anesthetic premedication	Prototypical benzodiazepine	43 ± 13	5–10, tid–qid§
Estazolam (PROSOM)	Oral	Insomnia	Contains triazolo ring; adverse effects may be similar to those of triazolam	10–24	1–2
Flurazepam (DALMANE)	Oral	Insomnia	Active metabolites accumulate with chronic use	74 ± 24	15–30
Halazepam (PAXIPAM)	Oral	Anxiety disorders	Activity largely due to metabolic conversion to nordazepam	14	—
Lorazepam (ATIVAN)	Oral, I.M., I.V.	Anxiety disorders, preanesthetic medication	Metabolized solely by conjugation	14 ± 5	2–4

(SONATA). Although the chemical structures of these compounds do not resemble those of benzodiazepines, it is assumed that their therapeutic efficacies are due to their agonist effects on the benzodiazepine receptor.

Zaleplon and zolpidem are effective in relieving sleep-onset insomnia. Both drugs have been approved by the FDA for use for up to 7 to 10 days at a time. There is evidence that both zaleplon and zolpidem have sustained hypnotic efficacy, without occurrence of rebound insomnia on abrupt discontinuation (Mitler, 2000; Walsh *et al.,* 2000). Zaleplon and zolpidem have similar degrees of efficacy. Zolpidem has a half-life of about 2 hours, which is sufficient to cover most of a typical 8-hour sleep period, and is presently approved for bedtime use only.

Zaleplon has a shorter half-life, about 1 hour, which offers up the possibility for safe dosing later in the night, within 4 hours of the anticipated rising time. As a result, zaleplon is approved for use immediately at bedtime or when the patient has difficulty falling asleep after bedtime. Because of its short half-life, zaleplon has not been shown to be different from placebo in measures of duration of sleep and number of awakenings. Zaleplon and zolpidem may differ in residual side effects; late-night administration of zolpidem has been associated with morning sedation, delayed reaction time, and anterograde amnesia, whereas zaleplon has had no more side effects than has placebo. The abuse potential of these drugs appears to be similar to that of benzodiazepines.

Table 17–3

Trade Names, Routes of Administration, and Therapeutic Uses of Benzodiazepines (*Continued*)

COMPOUND (TRADE NAME)	ROUTES OF ADMINISTRATION*	EXAMPLES OF THERAPEUTIC USES†	COMMENTS	$t_{1/2}$, hours‡	USUAL SEDATIVE-HYPNOTIC DOSAGE, mg¶
Midazolam (VERSED)	I.V., I.M.	Preanesthetic and intra-operative medication	Most rapidly inactivated benzodiazepine used for anesthetic premedication	1.9 ± 0.6	—#
Oxazepam (SERAX)	Oral	Anxiety disorders	Metabolized solely by conjugation	8.0 ± 2.4	15–30, tid–qid§
Quazepam (DORAL)	Oral	Insomnia	Active metabolites accumulate with chronic use	39	7.5–15
Temazepam (RESTORIL)	Oral	Insomnia	Metabolized mainly by conjugation	11 ± 6	7.5–30
Triazolam (HALCION)	Oral	Insomnia	Most rapidly inactivated benzodiazepine used for insomnia; may cause disturbing daytime side effects	2.9 ± 1.0	0.125–0.25

*I.M., intramuscular injection; I.V., intravenous administration; qd, once a day; bid, twice a day; tid, three times a day; qid, four times a day.

†The therapeutic uses are identified as *examples* to emphasize that most benzodiazepines can be used interchangeably. In general, the therapeutic uses of a given benzodiazepine are related to its half-life and may not match the marketed indications. The issue is addressed more extensively in the text.

‡Half-life of active metabolite may differ. *See* Appendix II for additional information.

¶For additional dosage information, *see* Chapter 14 (anesthesia), Chapter 19 (anxiety), and Chapter 21 (seizure disorders).

§Approved as a sedative-hypnotic only for management of alcohol withdrawal; doses in a nontolerant individual would be smaller.

#Recommended doses vary considerably depending on specific use, condition of patient, and concomitant administration of other drugs.

Zaleplon. Zaleplon (SONATA) is a nonbenzodiazepine and is a member of the pyrazolopyrimidine class of compounds. The structural formula is shown below.

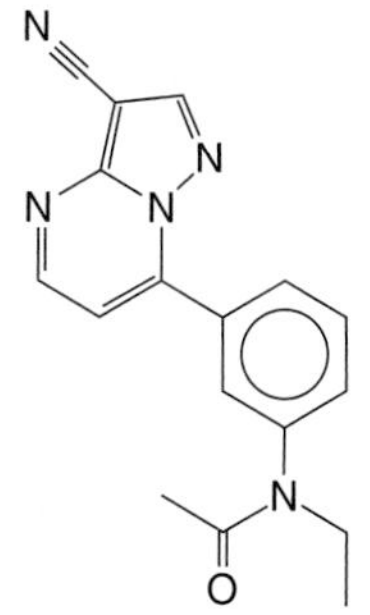

ZALEPLON

Although its chemical structure is unrelated to that of benzodiazepines, zaleplon preferentially binds to the benzodiazepine receptor site on $GABA_A$ receptors containing the $\alpha 1$ subunit of the receptor. Zaleplon is rapidly absorbed and reaches peak plasma concentrations in about one hour. Its half-life is approximately one hour. Its bioavailability is approximately 30% because of presystemic metabolism. Zaleplon has a volume of distribution of approximately 1.4 liters/kg and plasma-protein binding of approximately 60%. Zaleplon is metabolized largely by aldehyde oxidase and to a lesser extent by CYP3A4. Its oxidative metabolites are converted to glucuronides and elimi-

nated in urine. Less than 1% of zaleplon is excreted unchanged in urine. None of zaleplon's metabolites are pharmacologically active.

Zaleplon (usually administered in 5-, 10-, or 20-mg doses) has been studied in clinical trials on patients with chronic or transient insomnia (for a review, *see* Dooley and Plosker, 2000). Studies have focused on its effects in decreasing sleep latency. Zaleplon-treated subjects with either chronic or transient insomnia have experienced shorter periods of sleep latency than have placebo-treated subjects. Tolerance to zaleplon does not appear to occur, nor do rebound insomnia or withdrawal symptoms after stopping treatment.

Zolpidem. Zolpidem (AMBIEN) is a nonbenzodiazepine sedative-hypnotic drug that became available in the United States in 1993 after 5 years of use in Europe. It is classified as an imidazopyridine and has the following chemical structure:

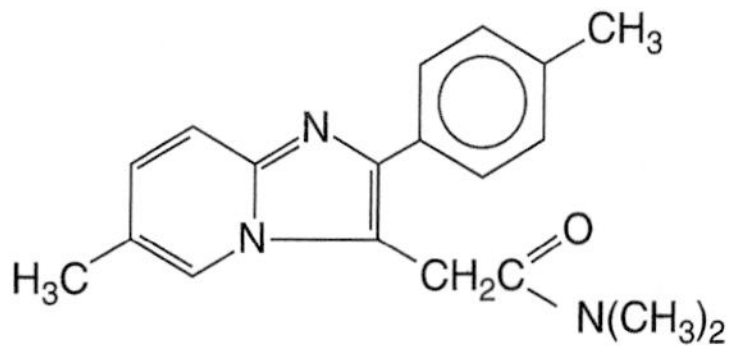

ZOLPIDEM

Although the actions of zolpidem are due to agonist effects on benzodiazepine receptors and generally resemble those of benzodiazepines, it produces only weak anticonvulsant effects in experimental animals, and its relatively strong sedative actions appear to mask anxiolytic effects in various animal models of anxiety (*see* Langtry and Benfield, 1990). Although the chronic administration of zolpidem to rodents produces neither tolerance to its sedative effects nor signs of withdrawal when the drug is discontinued and flumazenil is injected (Perrault *et al.,* 1992), evidence of tolerance and physical dependence has been observed with chronic administration of zolpidem to baboons (Griffiths *et al.,* 1992).

Unlike the benzodiazepines, zolpidem has little effect on the stages of sleep in normal human subjects. The drug is as effective as benzodiazepines in shortening sleep latency and prolonging total sleep time in patients with insomnia. Following discontinuation of zolpidem, the beneficial effects on sleep have been reported to persist for up to one week (Herrmann *et al.,* 1993), but mild rebound insomnia on the first night also has occurred (Anonymous, 1993). The development of tolerance and physical dependence has been seen only very rarely and under unusual circumstances (Cavallaro *et al.,* 1993; Morselli, 1993). Indeed, zolpidem-induced improvement in sleep time of chronic insomniacs was found in one study to be sustained during as much as 6 months of treatment without signs of withdrawal or rebound after stopping the drug (Kummer *et al.,* 1993). Nevertheless, zolpidem currently is approved only for the short-term treatment of insomnia despite the apparently benign consequences of its chronic administration. At therapeutic doses (10 to 20 mg; 5 to 10 mg in elderly patients), zolpidem infrequently produces residual daytime sedation or amnesia, and the incidence of other adverse effects (*e.g.,* gastrointestinal complaints, dizziness) also is low. Like the benzodiazepines, large overdoses of zolpidem do not produce severe respiratory depression unless other agents (*e.g.,* alcohol) also are ingested (Garnier *et al.,* 1994). Hypnotic doses increase the hypoxia and hypercarbia of patients with obstructive sleep apnea.

Zolpidem is absorbed readily from the gastrointestinal tract; first-pass hepatic metabolism results in an oral bioavailability of about 70%, but this value is lower when the drug is ingested with food because of slowed absorption and increased hepatic blood flow. Zolpidem is eliminated almost entirely by conversion to inactive products in the liver, largely through oxidation of the methyl groups on the phenyl and imidazopyridine rings to the corresponding carboxylic acids. Its half-life in plasma is approximately 2 hours in individuals with normal hepatic blood flow or function. This value may be increased twofold or more in those with cirrhosis, and it also tends to be greater in older patients; adjustment of dosage often is necessary in both categories of patients. Although little or no unchanged zolpidem is found in the urine, the elimination of the drug is slower in patients with chronic renal insufficiency, largely owing to an increase in its apparent volume of distribution.

The properties of zolpidem and its therapeutic utility have been reviewed by Langtry and Benfield (1990) and by Hoehns and Perry (1993).

Flumazenil: A Benzodiazepine-Receptor Antagonist

Flumazenil (ROMAZICON) is an imidazobenzodiazepine (*see* Table 17–1) that behaves as a specific benzodiazepine antagonist. It is the first such agent to undergo an extensive clinical trial, and it was released for clinical use in 1991. As noted above, flumazenil binds with high affinity to specific sites, where it competitively antagonizes the binding and allosteric effects of benzodiazepines and other ligands. Both the electrophysiological and behavioral effects of agonist or inverse-agonist benzodiazepines or β-carbolines also are antagonized. In animal studies, the intrinsic pharmacological actions of flumazenil have been subtle; effects resembling those of inverse agonists sometimes have been detected at low doses, while slight benzodiazepine-like effects often have been evident at high doses. The evidence for intrinsic activity in human subjects is even more vague, except for modest anticonvulsant effects at high doses. However, anticonvulsant effects cannot be relied upon for therapeutic utility, as the administration of flumazenil may precipitate seizures under certain circumstances (*see* below).

Flumazenil is available only for intravenous administration. Although it is rapidly absorbed after oral administration, less than 25% of the drug reaches the systemic circulation as a result of extensive first-pass hepatic metabolism; effective oral doses are apt to cause headache and dizziness (Roncari *et al.,* 1993). Upon intravenous administration, flumazenil is eliminated almost entirely by hepatic metabolism to inactive products with a half-life of about 1 hour; the duration of clinical effects is thus brief, and they usually persist for only 30 to 60 minutes.

The primary indications for the use of flumazenil are the management of suspected benzodiazepine overdose and the reversal of sedative effects produced by benzodiazepines administered during either general anesthesia or diagnostic and/or therapeutic procedures.

The administration of a series of small injections is preferred to a single bolus injection. A total of 1 mg of flumazenil given over 1 to 3 minutes usually is sufficient to abolish the effects of therapeutic doses of benzodiazepines; patients with suspected benzodiazepine overdose should respond adequately to a cumulative dose of 1 to 5 mg given over 2 to 10 minutes, and a lack of response to 5 mg of flumazenil strongly suggests that a benzodiazepine is not the major cause of sedation. Additional courses of treatment with flumazenil may be necessary within 20 to 30 minutes should sedation reappear. Flumazenil is not effective in single-drug overdoses with either barbiturates or tricyclic antidepressants. To the contrary, the administration of flumazenil may be associated with the onset of seizures under these circumstances; the risk of seizures is especially high in patients poisoned with tricyclic antidepressants (Spivey, 1992). Seizures or other withdrawal symptoms also may be precipitated in patients who had been taking benzodiazepines for protracted periods and in whom tolerance and/or dependence may have developed. The properties and therapeutic uses of flumazenil have been reviewed by Hoffman and Warren (1993).

BARBITUATES

The barbiturates enjoyed a long period of extensive use as sedative-hypnotic drugs; however, except for a few specialized uses, they have been largely replaced by the much safer benzodiazepines. A more detailed description of the barbiturates can be found in the *fifth edition* of this textbook.

Chemistry. Barbituric acid is 2,4,6-trioxohexahydropyrimidine. This compound lacks central-depressant activity, but the presence of alkyl or aryl groups at position 5 confers sedative-hypnotic and sometimes other activities. The general structural formula for the barbiturates and the structures of selected compounds are included in Table 17–4.

The carbonyl group at position 2 takes on acidic character because of lactam–lactim ("keto"–"enol") tautomerization, which is favored by its location between the two electronegative amido nitrogens. The lactim form is favored in alkaline solution, and salts result. Barbiturates in which the oxygen at C2 is replaced by sulfur are sometimes called thiobarbiturates. These compounds are more lipid-soluble than the corresponding oxybarbiturates. In general, structural changes that increase lipid solubility decrease duration of action, decrease latency to onset of activity, accelerate metabolic degradation, and often increase hypnotic potency.

Pharmacological Properties

The barbiturates reversibly depress the activity of all excitable tissues. The CNS is exquisitely sensitive, and, even when barbiturates are given in anesthetic concentrations, direct effects on peripheral excitable tissues are weak. However, serious deficits in cardiovascular and other peripheral functions occur in acute barbiturate intoxication.

Central Nervous System. The barbiturates can produce all degrees of depression of the CNS, ranging from mild sedation to general anesthesia. The use of barbiturates for general anesthesia is discussed in Chapter 14. Certain barbiturates, particularly those containing a 5-phenyl substituent (phenobarbital, mephobarbital), have selective anticonvulsant activity (see Chapter 20). The antianxiety properties of the barbiturates are not equivalent to those exerted by the benzodiazepines, especially with respect to the degree of sedation that is produced. The barbiturates may have euphoriant effects.

Except for the anticonvulsant activities of phenobarbital and its congeners, the barbiturates possess a low degree of selectivity and therapeutic index. Thus, it is not possible to achieve a desired effect without evidence of general depression of the CNS. Pain perception and reaction are relatively unimpaired until the moment of unconsciousness, and in small doses the barbiturates increase the reaction to painful stimuli. Hence, they cannot be relied upon to produce sedation or sleep in the presence of even moderate pain. In some individuals and in some circumstances, such as in the presence of pain, barbiturates cause overt excitement instead of sedation. The fact that such paradoxical excitement occurs with other CNS depressants suggests that it may result from depression of inhibitory centers.
Effects on Stages of Sleep. Hypnotic doses of barbiturates increase the total sleep time and alter the stages of sleep in a dose-dependent manner. Like the benzodiazepines, these drugs decrease sleep latency, the number of awakenings, and the durations of REM and slow-wave sleep. During repetitive nightly administration, some tolerance to the effects on sleep occurs within a few days, and the effect on total sleep time may be reduced by as much as 50% after 2 weeks of use. Discontinu-

ation leads to rebound increases in all the parameters reported to be decreased by barbiturates.

Tolerance. Both pharmacodynamic (functional) and pharmacokinetic tolerance to barbiturates can occur. The former contributes more to the decreased effect than does the latter. With chronic administration of gradually increasing doses, pharmacodynamic tolerance continues to develop over a period of weeks to months, depending on the dosage schedule, whereas pharmacokinetic tolerance reaches its peak in a few days to a week. Tolerance to the effects on mood, sedation, and hypnosis occurs more readily and is greater than that to the anticonvulsant and lethal effects; thus, as tolerance increases, the therapeutic index decreases. Pharmacodynamic tolerance to barbiturates confers tolerance to all general CNS-depressant drugs, including ethanol.

Abuse and Dependence. Like other CNS-depressant drugs, barbiturates are abused, and some individuals develop a dependence upon them. These topics are discussed in Chapter 24.

Sites and Mechanisms of Action on the CNS. Barbiturates act throughout the CNS; nonanesthetic doses preferentially suppress polysynaptic responses. Facilitation is diminished, and inhibition usually is enhanced. The site of inhibition is either postsynaptic, as at cortical and cerebellar pyramidal cells and in the cuneate nucleus, substantia nigra, and thalamic relay neurons, or presynaptic, as in the spinal cord. Enhancement of inhibition occurs primarily at synapses where neurotransmission is mediated by GABA acting at $GABA_A$ receptors.

The barbiturates exert several distinct effects on excitatory and inhibitory synaptic transmission. For example, (−)-pentobarbital potentiates GABA-induced increases in chloride conductance and depresses voltage-activated Ca^{2+} currents at similar concentrations (below 10 μM) in isolated hippocampal neurons; above 100 μM, chloride conductance is increased in the absence of GABA (ffrench-Mullen et al., 1993). Phenobarbital is less efficacious and much less potent in producing these effects, while (+)-pentobarbital has only weak activity. Thus, the more selective anticonvulsant properties of phenobarbital and its higher therapeutic index may be explained by its lower capacity to produce profound depression of neuronal function as compared with the anesthetic barbiturates.

As noted earlier in this chapter, the mechanisms underlying the actions of barbiturates on $GABA_A$ receptors appear to be distinct from those of either GABA or the benzodiazepines, for reasons that include the following: (1) Although barbiturates also enhance the binding of GABA to $GABA_A$ receptors in a chloride-dependent and picrotoxin-sensitive fashion, they promote (rather than displace) the binding of benzodiazepines. (2) Barbiturates potentiate GABA-induced chloride currents by prolonging periods during which bursts of channel opening occur rather than by increasing the frequency of these bursts, as benzodiazepines do. (3) Only α and β (not γ) subunits are required for barbiturate action. (4) Barbiturate-induced increases in chloride conductance are not affected by the deletion of the tyrosine and threonine residues in the β subunit that govern the sensitivity of $GABA_A$ receptors to activation by agonists (Amin and Weiss, 1993).

Table 17–4

Structures, Trade Names, and Major Pharmacological Properties of Selected Barbiturates

GENERAL FORMULA:

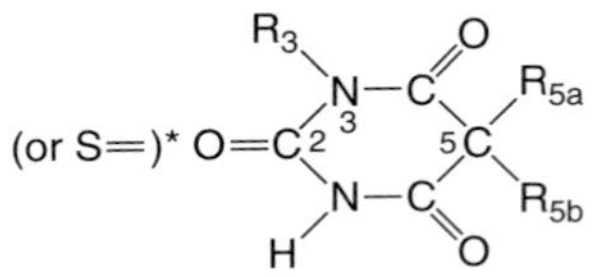

COMPOUND (TRADE NAMES)	R_3	R_{5a}	R_{5b}	ROUTES OF ADMINISTRATION†	HALF-LIFE, HOURS	THERAPEUTIC USES	COMMENTS
Amobarbital (AMYTAL)	—H	—C_2H_5	—$CH_2CH_2CH(CH_3)_2$	Oral, I.M., I.V.	10–40	Insomnia, preoperative sedation, emergency management of seizures	Only sodium salt used for parenteral administration
Aprobarbital (ALURATE)	—H	—$CH_2CH{=}CH_2$	—$CH(CH_3)_2$	Oral	14–34	Insomnia	Largely excreted unchanged in the urine; alkanization of the urine greatly increases excretion
Butabarbital (BUTISOL, others)	—H	—C_2H_5	—$CH(CH_3)CH_2CH_3$	Oral	35–50	Insomnia, preoperative sedation	Redistribution shortens duration of action of single doses to 8 hours
Butalbital	—H	—$CH_2CH{=}CH_2$	$CH_2CH(CH_3)_2$	Oral	35–88	Marketed in combination with analgesic agents	Therapeutic efficacy questionable. Other barbiturates may increase reaction to painful stimuli
Mephobarbital (MEBARAL)	—CH_3	—C_2H_5	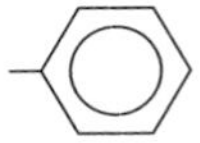 —(phenyl)	Oral	10–70	Seizure disorders, daytime sedation	Second-line anticonvulsant
Methohexital (BREVITAL)	—CH_3	—$CH_2CH{=}CH_2$	—$CH(CH_3)C{\equiv}CCH_2CH_3$	I.V.	3–5‡	Induction and/or maintenance of anesthesia	Only sodium salt is available; single injections provide 5 to 7 minutes of anesthesia‡

(Continued)

Table 17-4
Structures, Trade Names, and Major Pharmacological Properties of Selected Barbiturates (*Continued*)

GENERAL FORMULA:

COMPOUND (TRADE NAMES)	R_3	R_{5a}	R_{5b}	ROUTES OF ADMINISTRATION†	HALF-LIFE, HOURS	THERAPEUTIC USES	COMMENTS
Pentobarbital (NEMBUTAL)	—H	—C_2H_5	—$CH(CH_3)CH_2CH_2CH_3$	Oral, I.M., I.V., rectal	15–50	Insomnia, preoperative sedation, emergency management of seizures	Only sodium salt used for parenteral administration
Phenobarbital (LUMINAL, others)	—H	—C_2H_5	(phenyl group)	Oral, I.M., I.V.	80–120	Seizure disorders, status epilepticus, daytime sedation	First-line anticonvulsant; only sodium salt used for parenteral administration; up to 25% excreted unchanged in the urine
Secobarbital (SECONAL)	—H	—$CH_2CH=CH_2$	—$CH(CH_3)CH_2CH_2CH_3$	Oral, I.M., I.V., rectal	15–40	Insomnia, preoperative sedation, emergency management of seizures	Only sodium salt is available
Thiopental (PENTOTHAL)	—H	—C_2H_5	—$CH(CH_3)CH_2CH_2CH_3$	I.V., rectal	8–10‡	Induction and/or maintenance of anesthesia, preoperative sedation, emergency management of seizures	Only sodium salt is available; single injections provide short periods of anesthesia‡

*O except in thiopental, where it is replaced by S.

†I.M., intramuscular injection; I.V., intravenous administration.

‡Value represents terminal half-life due to metabolism by the liver; redistribution following parenteral administration produces effects lasting only a few minutes.

Subanesthetic concentrations of barbiturates also can reduce glutamate-induced depolarizations (*see* Chapter 12; Macdonald and McLean, 1982); only the AMPA subtypes of glutamate receptors sensitive to kainate or quisqualate appear to be affected (Marszalec and Narahashi, 1993). Recombinant AMPA receptors also are blocked by barbiturates. At higher concentrations that produce anesthesia, pentobarbital suppresses high-frequency, repetitive firing of neurons, apparently as a result of inhibiting the function of voltage-dependent, tetrodotoxin-sensitive Na^+ channels; in this case, however, both stereoisomers are about equally effective (Frenkel *et al.,* 1990). At still higher concentrations, voltage-dependent K^+ conductances are reduced.

Taken together, the findings that barbiturates activate inhibitory $GABA_A$ receptors and inhibit excitatory AMPA receptors can explain the CNS-depressant effects of these agents. The mechanism of action of barbiturates has been reviewed by Saunders and Ho (1990).

Peripheral Nervous Structures. Barbiturates selectively depress transmission in autonomic ganglia and reduce nicotinic excitation by choline esters. This effect may account, at least in part, for the fall in blood pressure produced by intravenous oxybarbiturates and by severe barbiturate intoxication. At skeletal neuromuscular junctions, the blocking effects of both tubocurarine and decamethonium are enhanced during barbiturate anesthesia. These actions probably result from the capacity of barbiturates at hypnotic or anesthetic concentrations to inhibit the passage of current through nicotinic cholinergic receptors. Several distinct mechanisms appear to be involved, and little stereoselectivity is evident (Roth *et al.,* 1989).

Respiration. Barbiturates depress both the respiratory drive and the mechanisms responsible for the rhythmic character of respiration. The neurogenic drive is diminished by hypnotic doses, but usually no more so than during natural sleep. However, neurogenic drive is essentially eliminated by a dose three times greater than that normally used to induce sleep. Such doses also suppress the hypoxic drive and, to a lesser extent, the chemoreceptor drive. At still higher doses, the powerful hypoxic drive also fails. However, the margin between the lighter planes of surgical anesthesia and dangerous respiratory depression is sufficient to permit the ultra-short-acting barbiturates to be used, with suitable precautions, as anesthetic agents.

The barbiturates only slightly depress protective reflexes until the degree of intoxication is sufficient to produce severe respiratory depression. Coughing, sneezing, hiccoughing, and laryngospasm may occur when barbiturates are employed as intravenous anesthetic agents. Indeed, laryngospasm is one of the chief complications of barbiturate anesthesia.

Cardiovascular System. When given orally in sedative or hypnotic doses, the barbiturates do not produce significant overt cardiovascular effects except for a slight decrease in blood pressure and heart rate such as occurs in normal sleep. In general, the effects of thiopental anesthesia on the cardiovascular system are benign in comparison with those of the volatile anesthetic agents; there is usually either no change or a fall in mean arterial pressure. Apparently, a decrease in cardiac output usually is sufficient to offset an increase in total calculated peripheral resistance, which sometimes is accompanied by an increase in heart rate. Cardiovascular reflexes are obtunded by partial inhibition of ganglionic transmission. This is most evident in patients with congestive heart failure or hypovolemic shock whose reflexes already are operating maximally and in whom barbiturates can cause an exaggerated fall in blood pressure. Because barbiturates also impair reflex cardiovascular adjustments to inflation of the lung, positive-pressure respiration should be used cautiously and only when necessary to maintain adequate pulmonary ventilation in patients who are anesthetized or intoxicated with a barbiturate.

Other cardiovascular changes often noted when thiopental and other intravenous thiobarbiturates are administered after conventional preanesthetic medication include a decrease in renal plasma flow and in cerebral blood flow, with a marked fall in CSF pressure. Although cardiac arrhythmias are observed only infrequently, intravenous anesthesia with barbiturates can increase the incidence of ventricular arrhythmias, especially when epinephrine and halothane are also present. Anesthetic concentrations of barbiturates have direct electrophysiological effects in the heart; in addition to depressing Na^+ channels, they reduce the function of at least two types of K^+ channels (Nattel *et al.,* 1990; Pancrazio *et al.,* 1993). However, direct depression of cardiac contractility occurs only when doses several times those required to cause anesthesia are administered, which probably contributes to the cardiovascular depression that accompanies acute barbiturate poisoning.

Gastrointestinal Tract. The oxybarbiturates tend to decrease the tonus of the gastrointestinal musculature and the amplitude of rhythmic contractions. The locus of action is partly peripheral and partly central, depending on the dose. A hypnotic dose does not significantly delay gastric emptying in human beings. The relief of various gastrointestinal symptoms by sedative doses is probably largely due to the central-depressant action.

Liver. The best-known effects of barbiturates on the liver are those on the microsomal drug-metabolizing system (*see* Chapter 1). Acutely, the barbiturates combine with several species of cytochrome P450 and competitively interfere with the biotransformation of a number of other drugs as well as of endogenous substrates, such as steroids; other substrates may reciprocally inhibit barbiturate biotransformations. Drug interactions may result even when the other substances and barbiturates are oxidized by different microsomal enzyme systems.

The chronic administration of barbiturates causes a marked increase in the protein and lipid content of the hepatic smooth endoplasmic reticulum, as well as in the activities of glucuronyl transferase and the oxidases containing cytochrome P450. The inducing effect on these enzymes results in an increased rate of metabolism of a number of drugs and endogenous substances, including steroid hormones, cholesterol, bile salts, and vitamins K and D. An increase in the rate of barbiturate metabolism also results, which accounts for part of the tolerance to barbiturates. Many sedative-hypnotics, various anesthetics, and ethanol also are metabolized by and/or induce the microsomal enzymes, and some degree of cross-tolerance can occur on this basis. Not all microsomal biotransformations of drugs and endogenous substrates are affected to the same degree, but a convenient rule of thumb is that, at maximal induction in human beings, the rates are approximately doubled. The inducing effect is not limited to the microsomal enzymes; for example, there is an increase in δ-aminolevulinic acid (ALA) synthetase, a mitochondrial enzyme, and aldehyde dehydrogenase, a cytoplasmic enzyme. The effect of barbiturates on ALA synthetase can cause dangerous exacerbations of disease in persons with intermittent porphyria.

Kidney. Severe oliguria or anuria may occur in acute barbiturate poisoning, largely as a result of the marked hypotension.

Absorption, Fate, and Excretion. For sedative-hypnotic use, the barbiturates usually are administered orally (*see* Table 17–4). Such doses are rapidly and probably completely absorbed; sodium salts are absorbed more rapidly than the corresponding free acids, especially from liquid formulations. The onset of action varies from 10 to 60 minutes, depending on the agent and the formulation, and is delayed by the presence of food in the stomach. When necessary, intramuscular injections of solutions of the sodium salts should be placed deeply into large muscles in order to avoid the pain and possible necrosis that can result at more superficial sites. With some agents, special preparations are available for rectal administration. The intravenous route is usually reserved for the management of status epilepticus (phenobarbital sodium) or for the induction and/or maintenance of general anesthesia (*e.g.,* thiopental, methohexital).

Barbiturates are distributed widely and readily cross the placenta. The highly lipid-soluble barbiturates, led by those used to induce anesthesia, undergo redistribution after intravenous injection. Uptake into less vascular tissues, especially muscle and fat, leads to a decline in the concentration of barbiturate in the plasma and brain. With thiopental and methohexital, this results in the awakening of patients within 5 to 15 minutes of the injection of the usual anesthetic doses.

With the exception of the less lipid-soluble aprobarbital and phenobarbital, nearly complete metabolism and/or conjugation of barbiturates in the liver precedes their renal excretion. The oxidation of radicals at C5 is the most important biotransformation responsible for termination of biological activity. Oxidation results in the formation of alcohols, ketones, phenols, or carboxylic acids, which may appear in the urine as such or as glucuronic acid conjugates. In some instances (*e.g.,* phenobarbital), *N*-glycosylation is an important metabolic pathway. Other biotransformations include *N*-hydroxylation, desulfuration of thiobarbiturates to oxybarbiturates, opening of the barbituric acid ring, and *N*-dealkylation of *N*-alkylbarbiturates to active metabolites (*e.g.,* mephobarbital to phenobarbital). About 25% of phenobarbital and nearly all of aprobarbital are excreted unchanged in the urine. Their re-

nal excretion can be greatly increased by osmotic diuresis and/or alkalinization of the urine.

The metabolic elimination of barbiturates is more rapid in young people than in the elderly and infants, and half-lives are increased during pregnancy, partly because of the expanded volume of distribution. Chronic liver disease, especially cirrhosis, often increases the half-life of the biotransformable barbiturates. Repeated administration, especially of phenobarbital, shortens the half-life of barbiturates that are metabolized as a result of the induction of microsomal enzymes (*see* above).

The data on half-lives given in Table 17–4 show that none of the barbiturates used for hypnosis in the United States appears to have an elimination half-life that is short enough for elimination to be virtually complete in 24 hours. However, the relationship between duration of action and half-time of elimination is complicated in part by the fact that enantiomers of optically active barbiturates often differ in both biological potencies and rates of biotransformation. Nevertheless, all of these barbiturates will accumulate during repetitive administration unless appropriate adjustments in dosage are made. Furthermore, the persistence of the drug in plasma during the day favors the development of tolerance and abuse.

Untoward Effects. *After Effects.* Drowsiness may last for only a few hours after a hypnotic dose of barbiturate, but residual depression of the CNS sometimes is evident the following day. Even in the absence of overt evidence of residual depression, subtle distortions of mood and impairment of judgment and fine motor skills may be demonstrable. For example, a 200-mg dose of secobarbital has been shown to impair performance of driving or flying skills for 10 to 22 hours. Residual effects also may take the form of vertigo, nausea, vomiting, or diarrhea, or sometimes may be manifested as overt excitement. The user may awaken slightly intoxicated and feel euphoric and energetic; later, as the demands of daytime activities challenge possibly impaired faculties, the user may display irritability and temper.

Paradoxical Excitement. In some persons, barbiturates repeatedly produce excitement rather than depression, and the patient may appear to be inebriated. This type of idiosyncrasy is relatively common among geriatric and debilitated patients and occurs most frequently with phenobarbital and *N*-methylbarbiturates.

Pain. Barbiturates have been prescribed for localized or diffuse myalgic, neuralgic, or arthritic pain but often do not effectively treat these symptoms, especially in psychoneurotic patients with insomnia. Barbiturates may cause restlessness, excitement, and even delirium when given in the presence of pain and may make a patient's perception of pain worse.

Hypersensitivity. Allergic reactions occur especially in persons who tend to have asthma, urticaria, angioedema, and similar conditions. Hypersensitivity reactions in this category include localized swellings, particularly of the eyelids, cheeks, or lips, and erythematous dermatitis. Rarely, exfoliative dermatitis may be caused by phenobarbital and can prove fatal; the skin eruption may be associated with fever, delirium, and marked degenerative changes in the liver and other parenchymatous organs.

Drug Interactions. Barbiturates combine with other CNS depressants to cause severe depression; ethanol is the most frequent offender, and interactions with antihistamines are also common. Isoniazid, methylphenidate, and monoamine oxidase inhibitors also increase the CNS-depressant effects.

Barbiturates competitively inhibit the metabolism of certain other drugs; however, the greatest number of drug interactions results from induction of hepatic microsomal enzymes and the accelerated disappearance of many drugs and endogenous substances. The metabolism of vitamins D and K are accelerated, which may hamper bone mineralization and lower Ca^{2+} absorption in patients taking phenobarbital and may be responsible for the reported instances of coagulation defects in neonates whose mothers had been taking phenobarbital. Hepatic enzyme induction enhances metabolism of endogenous steroid hormones, which may cause endocrine disturbances, as well as of oral contraceptives, which may result in unwanted pregnancy. Barbiturates also induce the hepatic generation of toxic metabolites of chlorocarbon anesthetics and carbon tetrachloride and consequently promote lipid peroxidation, which facilitates the periportal necrosis of the liver caused by these agents.

Other Untoward Effects. Because barbiturates enhance porphyrin synthesis, they are absolutely contraindicated in patients with acute intermittent porphyria or porphyria variegata. In hypnotic doses, the effects of barbiturates on the control of respiration are minor; however, in the presence of pulmonary insufficiency, serious respiratory depression may occur, and the drugs are thus contraindicated. Rapid intravenous injection of a barbiturate may cause cardiovascular collapse before anesthesia ensues, so that the CNS signs of depth of anesthesia may fail to give an adequate warning of impending toxicity. Blood pressure can fall to shock levels; even slow intravenous injection of barbiturates often produces apnea and occasionally laryngospasm, coughing, and other respiratory difficulties.

Barbiturate Poisoning

The incidence of barbiturate poisoning has declined markedly in recent years, largely as a result of the decline in the use of these drugs as sedative-hypnotic agents. Nevertheless, poisoning with barbiturates is a significant clinical problem; death occurs in a few percent of cases. Most of the cases are the result of deliberate attempts at suicide, but some are from accidental poisonings in children or in drug abusers. The lethal dose of barbiturate varies with many factors, but severe poisoning is likely to occur when more than ten times the full hypnotic dose has been ingested at once. If alcohol or other depressant drugs are also present, the concentrations that can cause death are lower.

In severe intoxication, the patient is comatose; respiration is affected early. Breathing may be either slow or else rapid and shallow. Superficial observation of respiration may be misleading with regard to actual minute volume and to the degree of respiratory acidosis and cerebral hypoxia. Eventually, blood pressure falls owing to the effect of the drug and of hypoxia on medullary vasomotor centers; depression of cardiac contractility and sympathetic ganglia also contribute. Pulmonary complications (atelectasis, edema, and bronchopneumonia) and renal failure are likely to be the fatal complications of severe barbiturate poisoning.

The optimal treatment of acute barbiturate intoxication is based on general supportive measures. Hemodialysis or hemoperfusion is only rarely necessary, and the use of CNS stimulants increases the rate of mortality. The present treatment is applicable in most respects to poisoning by any CNS depressant.

Constant attention must be given to the maintenance of a patent airway and adequate ventilation and to the prevention of pneumonia; oxygen should be administered. After precautions to avoid aspiration, gastric lavage should be considered if fewer than 24 hours have elapsed since ingestion, since the barbiturate can reduce gastrointestinal motility. After lavage, the administration of activated charcoal and a cathartic such as sorbitol may shorten the half-life of the less lipid-soluble agents such as phenobarbital. If renal and cardiac function are satisfactory and the patient is hydrated, forced diuresis and alkalinization of the urine will hasten the excretion of aprobarbital and phenobarbital. Measures to prevent or treat atelectasis should be taken, and mechanical ventilation should be initiated when indicated.

In severe acute barbiturate intoxication, circulatory collapse is a major threat. Often the patient is admitted to the hospital with severe hypotension or shock, and dehydration is often severe. Hypovolemia must be corrected, and, if necessary, the blood pressure can be supported with dopamine. Acute renal failure consequent to shock and hypoxia accounts for perhaps one-sixth of the deaths. In the event of renal failure, hemodialysis should be instituted. Intoxication by barbiturates and its management have been reviewed by Gary and Tresznewsky (1983).

Therapeutic Uses

The use of barbiturates as sedative-hypnotic drugs has declined enormously because they lack specificity of effect in the CNS, they have a lower therapeutic index than do the benzodiazepines, tolerance occurs more frequently than with benzodiazepines, the liability for abuse is greater, and the number of drug interactions is considerable. The major uses of individual barbiturates are listed in Table 17–4. Like the benzodiazepines, selection of particular barbiturates for a given therapeutic indication is based primarily on pharmocokinetic considerations.

CNS Uses. Although barbiturates largely have been replaced by benzodiazepines and other compounds for daytime sedation, phenobarbital and butabarbital are still available as "sedatives" in a host of combinations of questionable efficacy for the treatment of functional gastrointestinal disorders and asthma. They also are included in analgesic combinations, possibly counterproductively. Barbiturates, especially butabarbital and phenobarbital, are sometimes used to antagonize unwanted CNS-stimulant effects of various drugs, such as ephedrine, dextroamphetamine, and theophylline, although a preferred approach is adjustment of dosage or substitution of alternative therapy for the primary agents. Phenobarbital still is a widely used, and probably the only effective, treatment for hypnosedative withdrawal (Martin *et al.,* 1979).

Barbiturates are still employed in the emergency treatment of convulsions, such as occur in tetanus, eclampsia, status epilepticus, cerebral hemorrhage, and poisoning by convulsant drugs; however, benzodiazepines generally are superior in these uses. Phenobarbital sodium is most frequently used because of its anticonvulsant efficacy; however, even when administered intravenously, 15 minutes or more may be required for it to attain peak concentrations in the brain. The ultrashort- and short-acting barbiturates have a low ratio of anticonvulsant to hypnotic action, and these drugs or inhalational anesthetic agents are employed only when general anesthesia must be used to control seizures refractory to other measures. Diazepam usually is chosen for the emergency treatment of seizures. The use of barbiturates in the symptomatic therapy of epilepsy is discussed in Chapter 21.

Ultrashort-acting agents such as thiopental or methohexital continue to be employed as intravenous anesthetics (Chapter 14). In children, the rectal administration of methohexital sometimes is used for the induction of anesthesia or for sedation during imaging procedures (Manuli and Davies, 1993). Short- and ultrashort-acting barbiturates occasionally are used as adjuncts to other agents in the production of obstetrical anesthesia. Several studies have failed to affirm gross depression of respiration in full-term infants, but premature infants clearly are more susceptible. Since evaluation of the effects on the fetus and neonate is difficult, it is prudent to avoid the use of barbiturates in obstetrics.

The barbiturates are employed as diagnostic and therapeutic aids in psychiatry; these uses sometimes are referred to as *narcoanalysis* and *narcotherapy,* respectively. In low concentrations, amobarbital has been administered directly into the carotid artery prior to neurosurgery as a means of identifying the dominant cerebral hemisphere for speech. The use of this procedure has been expanded to include a more extensive neuropsychological evaluation of patients with medically intractable seizure disorders who may benefit from surgical therapy (*see* Smith and Riskin, 1991).

Anesthetic doses of barbiturates attenuate cerebral edema resulting from surgery, head injury, or cerebral ischemia, and they may decrease infarct size and increase survival. General anesthetics do not provide protection. The procedure is not without serious danger, however, and the ultimate benefit to the patient has been questioned (*see* Shapiro, 1985; Smith and Riskin, 1991).

Hepatic Metabolic Uses. Because hepatic glucuronyl transferase and the bilirubin-binding Y protein are increased by the barbiturates, phenobarbital has been used successfully to treat hyperbilirubinemia and kernicterus in the neonate. The nondepressant barbiturate phetharbital (*N*-phenylbarbital) works equally well. Phenobarbital may improve the hepatic transport of bilirubin in patients with hemolytic jaundice.

MISCELLANEOUS SEDATIVE-HYPNOTIC DRUGS

Over the years, many drugs with diverse structures have been used for their sedative-hypnotic properties, including *paraldehyde* (introduced before the barbiturates), *chloral hydrate, ethchlorvynol, glutethimide, methyprylon, ethinamate,* and *meprobamate* (introduced just before the benzodiazepines). With the exception of meprobamate, the pharmacological actions of these drugs generally resemble those of the barbiturates: They all are general CNS depressants that can produce profound hypnosis with little or no analgesia; their effects on the stages of sleep are similar to those of the barbiturates; their therapeutic index is limited, and acute intoxication, which produces respiratory depression and hypotension, is managed similarly to barbiturate poisoning; their chronic use can result in tolerance and physical dependence; and the syndrome following chronic use can be severe and life threatening. The properties of meprobamate bear some resemblance to those of the benzodiazepines, but the drug has a distinctly higher potential for abuse and has less selective antianxiety effects. The clinical use of these agents has decreased markedly, and deservedly so. Nevertheless, some of them are useful in certain settings, particularly in hospitalized patients.

The chemical structures and major pharmacological properties of paraldehyde, ethchlorvynol, chloral hydrate, and meprobamate are presented in Table 17–5. Further information

Table 17–5

Structures, Trade Names, and Major Pharmacological Properties of Miscellaneous Sedative-Hypnotic Drugs

COMPOUND (TRADE NAMES)	STRUCTURE	ROUTES OF ADMINISTRATION	HALF-LIFE, HOURS	COMMENTS
Paraldehyde (PARAL)	CH_3 CH O O H_3C—HC CH—CH_3 O	Oral, rectal	4–10	Used to treat delirium tremens in hospitalized patients; eliminated by hepatic metabolism (75%) and exhalation (25%), toxicities include acidosis, hepatitis, and nephrosis
Chloral hydrate	$CCl_3CH(OH)_2$	Oral, rectal	5–10*	Rapidly converted by hepatic alcohol dehydrogenase to trichloroethanol, which is largely responsible for the effects of chloral hydrate; chronic use may cause hepatic damage; withdrawal syndrome is severe
Ethchlorvynol (PLACIDYL)	$C\equiv CH$ CH_3CH_2—C—CH=$CHCl$ OH	Oral	10–20†	Redistribution shortens duration of action of single doses to 4 to 5 hours, which may result in early morning awakening; idiosyncratic responses include marked excitement, especially in the presence of pain
Meprobamate (MILTOWN, others)	O C_3H_7 O H_2N—C—OCH_2—C—CH_2O—C—NH_2 CH_3	Oral	6–17	Approved only for treatment of anxiety disorders, but widely used as a nighttime sedative; overdosage can cause severe hypotension, respiratory depression, and death

*Value is for elimination of trichloroethanol, to which effects can be attributed.

†Value represents terminal half-life due to metabolism by the liver; redistribution shortens duration of action to less than 5 hours.

on glutethimide, methyprylon, and ethinamate can be found in previous editions of this book.

Paraldehyde. Paraldehyde is a polymer of acetaldehyde, but it perhaps is best regarded as a polyether of cyclic structure. It has a strong aromatic odor and a disagreeable taste. Orally, it is irritating to the throat and stomach, and it is not administered parenterally because of its injurious effects on tissues. When given rectally as a retention enema, the drug is diluted with olive oil.

Oral paraldehyde is rapidly absorbed and widely distributed; sleep usually ensues in 10 to 15 minutes after hypnotic doses. About 70% to 80% of a dose is metabolized in the liver, probably by depolymerization to acetaldehyde and subsequent oxidation to acetic acid, which is ultimately converted to carbon dioxide and water; most of the remainder is exhaled, producing a strong, characteristic smell to the breath. Commonly observed consequences of poisoning with the drug include acidosis, bleeding gastritis, and fatty changes in the liver and kidney with toxic hepatitis and nephrosis.

The clinical uses of paraldehyde include the treatment of abstinence phenomena (especially delirium tremens in hospitalized patients) and other psychiatric states characterized by

excitement. Paraldehyde also has been used for the treatments of convulsions (including status epilepticus) in children. Individuals who become addicted to paraldehyde may have become acquainted with the drug during treatment of their alcoholism and then, surprisingly in view of its disagreeable taste and odor, prefer it to alcohol.

Chloral Hydrate. Chloral hydrate is formed by adding one molecule of water to the carbonyl group of chloral (2,2,2-trichloroacetaldehyde). In addition to its hypnotic use, the drug has been employed in the past for the production of sedation in children undergoing diagnostic, dental, or other potentially uncomfortable procedures.

Chloral hydrate is rapidly reduced to the active compound, trichloroethanol (CCl_3CH_2OH), largely by alcohol dehydrogenase in the liver; significant amounts of chloral hydrate are not found in the blood after its oral administration. Therefore, its pharmacological effects probably are caused by trichloroethanol. Indeed, the latter compound can exert barbiturate-like effects on $GABA_A$ receptor channels *in vitro* (Lovinger *et al.*, 1993). Trichloroethanol is mainly conjugated with glucuronic acid, and the product (urochloralic acid) is excreted mostly into the urine.

Chloral hydrate is irritating to the skin and mucous membranes. These irritant actions give rise to an unpleasant taste, epigastric distress, nausea, and occasional vomiting, all of which are particularly likely to occur if the drug is insufficiently diluted or if it is taken on an empty stomach. Undesirable CNS effects include light-headedness, malaise, ataxia, and nightmares. "Hangover" also may occur, although it is less common than with most barbiturates and some benzodiazepines. Rarely, patients exhibit idiosyncratic reactions to chloral hydrate and may be disoriented and incoherent and show paranoid behavior. Acute poisoning by chloral hydrate may cause icterus. Individuals using chloral hydrate chronically may exhibit sudden, acute intoxication, which can be fatal; this situation results either from an overdose or from a failure of the detoxification mechanism owing to hepatic damage; parenchymatous renal injury also may occur. Sudden withdrawal from the habitual use of chloral hydrate may result in delirium and seizures, with a high frequency of death when untreated.

Ethchlorvynol. In addition to pharmacological actions that are very similar to those of barbiturates, ethchlorvynol has anticonvulsant and muscle relaxant properties. Ethchlorvynol is rapidly absorbed and widely distributed following oral administration. Two-compartment kinetics is manifest, with a distribution half-life of about 1 to 3 hours and an elimination half-life of 10 to 20 hours. As a result, the duration of action of the drug is relatively short, and early morning awakening may occur after its administration at bedtime. Approximately 90% of the drug eventually is destroyed in the liver. Ethchlorvynol is used as a short-term hypnotic for the management of insomnia.

The most common side effects caused by ethchlorvynol are mint-like aftertaste, dizziness, nausea, vomiting, hypotension, and facial numbness. Mild "hangover" also is relatively common. An occasional patient responds with profound hypnosis, muscular weakness, and syncope unrelated to marked hypotension. Idiosyncratic responses range from mild stimulation to marked excitement and hysteria. Hypersensitivity reactions include urticaria, rare but sometimes fatal thrombocytopenia, and occasionally cholestatic jaundice. Acute intoxication resembles that produced by barbiturates, except for more severe respiratory depression and a relative bradycardia. Ethchlorvynol may enhance the hepatic metabolism of other drugs such as oral anticoagulants, and it is contraindicated in patients with intermittent porphyria.

Meprobamate. Meprobamate is a *bis*-carbamate ester; it was introduced as an antianxiety agent in 1955, and this remains its only approved use in the United States. However, it also became popular as a sedative-hypnotic drug, and it is discussed here mainly because of the continuing practice of using this drug for such purposes. The question of whether or not the sedative and antianxiety actions of meprobamate differ remains unanswered, and clinical proof for the efficacy of meprobamate as a selective antianxiety agent in human beings is lacking.

The pharmacological properties of meprobamate resemble those of the benzodiazepines in a number of ways. Like the benzodiazepines, meprobamate can release suppressed behaviors in experimental animals at doses that cause little impairment of locomotor activity, and, although it can cause widespread depression of the CNS, it cannot produce anesthesia. Unlike the benzodiazepines, ingestion of large doses of meprobamate alone

may cause severe or even fatal respiratory depression, hypotension, shock, and heart failure. Meprobamate appears to have a mild analgesic effect in patients with musculoskeletal pain, and it enhances the analgesic effects of other drugs.

Meprobamate is well absorbed when administered orally. Nevertheless, an important aspect of intoxication with meprobamate is the formation of gastric bezoars consisting of undissolved meprobamate tablets; hence, treatment may require endoscopy, with mechanical removal of the bezoar. Most of the drug is metabolized in the liver, mainly to a side-chain hydroxy derivative and a glucuronide; the kinetics of elimination may be dependent on the dose. The half-life of meprobamate may be prolonged during its chronic administration, even though the drug can induce some hepatic microsomal enzymes.

The major unwanted effects of the usual sedative doses of meprobamate are drowsiness and ataxia; larger doses produce considerable impairment of learning and motor coordination and prolongation of reaction time. Like the benzodiazepines, meprobamate enhances the CNS depression produced by other drugs.

The abuse of meprobamate has continued despite a substantial decrease in the clinical use of the drug. *Carisoprodol* (SOMA), a skeletal muscle relaxant whose active metabolite is meprobamate, also has abuse potential and has become a popular "street drug" (Reeves *et al.,* 1999). Meprobamate is preferred to the benzodiazepines by subjects with a history of drug abuse. After long-term medication, abrupt discontinuation evokes a withdrawal syndrome usually characterized by anxiety, insomnia, tremors, and, frequently, hallucinations; generalized seizures occur in about 10% of cases. The intensity of symptoms depends on the dosage ingested.

Others. *Etomidate* (AMIDATE) is used in the United States and other countries as an intravenous anesthetic, often in combination with fentanyl. It is advantageous because it lacks pulmonary and vascular depressant activity, although it has a negative inotropic effect on the heart. Its pharmacology and anesthetic uses are described in Chapter 14. It also is used abroad as a sedative-hypnotic drug in intensive care units, during intermittent positive-pressure breathing, in epidural anesthesia, and in other situations. Because it is administered only intravenously, its use is limited to hospital settings. The myoclonus commonly seen after anesthetic doses is not seen after sedative-hypnotic doses.

Clomethiazole has sedative, muscle relaxant, and anticonvulsant properties. It is used outside the United States for hypnosis in elderly and institutionalized patients, for preanesthetic sedation, and especially in the management of withdrawal from ethanol (*see* Symposium, 1986b). Given alone, its effects on respiration are slight, and the therapeutic index is high. However, deaths from adverse interactions with ethanol are relatively frequent.

Nonprescription Hypnotic Drugs. An advisory review panel of the FDA has recommended that, except for certain antihistamines (doxylamine, diphenhydramine, and pyrilamine), all putative active ingredients be eliminated from nonprescription sleep aids. Despite the prominent sedative side effects encountered during their use in the treatment of allergic diseases (*see* Chapter 25), these antihistamines are not consistently effective in the treatment of sleep disorders. Contributing factors may include the rapid development of tolerance, paradoxical stimulation, and the inadequacy of the doses that currently are approved. Nevertheless, these doses sometimes produce prominent residual daytime CNS depression. For example, the elimination half-lives of doxylamine and diphenhydramine are about 9 hours.

MANAGEMENT OF INSOMNIA

Insomnia is one of the most common complaints in general medical practice and its treatment is predicated upon proper diagnosis. A variety of pharmacological agents are available for the treatment of insomnia. The "perfect" hypnotic would allow sleep to occur, with normal sleep architecture, rather than produce a pharmacologically altered sleep pattern. It would not cause next-day effects, either of rebound anxiety or continued sedation. It would not interact with other medications. It could be used chronically without causing dependence or rebound insomnia on discontinuation. Regular moderate exercise meets these criteria, but often is not effective by itself, and patients with significant cardiorespiratory disease may not be able to exercise. However, even small amounts of exercise often are effective in promoting sleep. Although the precise function of sleep is not known, adequate sleep improves the quality of daytime wakefulness, and hypnotics should be used judiciously to avoid its impairment.

Controversy in the management of insomnia revolves around two issues: pharmacological *versus* nonpharmacological treatment and the use of short-acting *versus* long-acting hypnotics. Benzodiazepine hypnotics have been prescribed less commonly over the past decade. The British tend to take a conservative attitude toward prescribing benzodiazepines, for either anxiety or insomnia (Livingston, 1994). However, Walsh and Engelhardt (1992) think that this reduction in benzodiazepine prescribing may have more to do with media coverage of benzodiazepine side effects than with scientific data and that some patients may be undertreated with hypnotics. Perhaps related to this controversy, Yeo *et al.* (1994) found that physician self-rating of benzodiazepine prescribing generally greatly underestimated actual prescribing patterns. The side effects of hypnotic medications must be weighed against the sequelae of chronic insomnia, which include a fourfold increase in serious accidents (Balter, 1992).

Two aspects of the management of insomnia traditionally have been underappreciated. They are a search for specific medical causes and the use of nonpharmacological treatments. In addition to appropriate pharmacological treatment, the management of insomnia should correct identifiable causes, address inadequate sleep hygiene, eliminate performance anxiety related to falling asleep,

provide entrainment of the biological clock so that maximum sleepiness occurs at the hour of attempted sleep, and suppress the use of alcohol and over-the-counter sleep medications (Nino-Murcia, 1992).

Categories of Insomnia.   The National Institute of Mental Health Consensus Development Conference (1984) divided insomnia into three categories:

1. *Transient insomnia* lasts less than three days and usually is caused by a brief environmental or situational stressor. It may respond to attention to sleep hygiene rules. If hypnotics are prescribed, they should be used at the lowest dose and for only two to three nights. However, benzodiazepines given acutely prior to important life events, such as examinations, may result in impaired performance (James and Savage, 1984).
2. *Short-term insomnia* lasts from 3 days to 3 weeks and usually is caused by a personal stressor such as illness, grief, or job problems. Again, sleep hygiene education is the first step. Hypnotics may be used adjunctively for 7 to 10 nights. Hypnotics are best used intermittently during this time, with the patient skipping a dose after one to two nights of good sleep.
3. *Long-term insomnia* is insomnia that has lasted for more than 3 weeks; no specific stressor may be identifiable. A more complete medical evaluation is necessary in these patients, but most do not need an all-night sleep study.

Insomnia Accompanying Major Psychiatric Illnesses.   The insomnia caused by major psychiatric illnesses often responds to specific pharmacological treatment for that illness. For example, in major depressive episodes with insomnia, even such medications as the selective serotonin-reuptake inhibitors, which may cause insomnia as a side effect, usually will result in *improved* sleep as they treat the depressive syndrome. In patients whose depression is responding to the serotonin-reuptake inhibitor but who have persistent insomnia as a side effect of the medication, judicious use of evening trazodone may improve sleep (Nierenberg *et al.*, 1994) as well as augment the antidepressant effect of the reuptake inhibitor. However, the patient should be monitored for priapism, orthostatic hypotension, and arrhythmias.

Adequate control of anxiety in patients with anxiety disorders often produces adequate resolution of the accompanying insomnia. Sedative use in the anxiety disorders is decreasing because of a growing appreciation of the effectiveness of other agents, such as β-adrenergic receptor antagonists (*see* Chapter 10) for performance anxiety and serotonin-reuptake inhibitors for obsessive-compulsive disorder and perhaps generalized anxiety disorder. The profound insomnia of patients with acute psychosis due to schizophrenia or mania usually responds to dopamine-receptor antagonists. Benzodiazepines often are used adjunctively in this situation to reduce agitation; their use also will result in improved sleep.

Insomnia Accompanying Other Medical Illnesses. For long-term insomnia due to other medical illnesses, adequate treatment of the underlying disorder, such as congestive heart failure, asthma, or chronic obstructive pulmonary disease, may resolve the insomnia.

Adequate pain management in conditions of chronic pain, including terminal cancer pain, will treat both the pain and the insomnia and may make hypnotics unnecessary.

Many patients simply manage their sleep poorly. Adequate attention to sleep hygiene, including reduced caffeine intake, avoidance of alcohol, adequate exercise, and regular sleep and wake times often will reduce the insomnia.

Conditioned (Learned) Insomnia. In those who have no major psychiatric or other medical illness and in whom attention to sleep hygiene is ineffective, attention should be directed to conditioned (learned) insomnia. These patients have associated the bedroom with activities consistent with wakefulness rather than sleep. In such patients, the bed should be used only for sex and sleep. All other activities associated with waking, even such quiescent activities as reading and watching television, should be done outside of the bedroom.

Sleep State Misperception. Some patients complain of poor sleep but have been shown to have no objective polysomnographic evidence of insomnia. They are difficult to treat.

Some patients are simply consitutional short sleepers, who do not need the typical seven to eight hours of sleep per day to function. If daytime wakefulness, mood, and functioning are unimpaired, no treatment is necessary.

Some patients with sleep apnea may ask for sleeping pills because they do not feel rested in the morning. Hypnotic agents usually are contraindicated in such patients. These individuals benefit from all-night sleep studies for proper evaluation and recommendations for appropriate treatment.

Long-Term Insomnia. Nonpharmacological treatments are important for all patients with long-term insomnia. These include education about sleep hygiene, adequate exercise (where possible), relaxation training, and behavioral modification approaches, such as sleep restriction and stimulus control therapy. In sleep restriction therapy, the patient keeps a diary of the amount of time spent in bed and then chooses a time in bed of 30 to 60 minutes less than this time. This induces a mild sleep debt, which aids sleep onset. In stimulus control therapy, the patient is instructed to go to bed only when sleepy, to use the bedroom only for sleep and sex, to get up and leave the bedroom if sleep does not occur within 15 to 20 minutes, to return to bed again only when sleepy, to arise at the same time each morning regardless of sleep quality the preceding night, and to avoid daytime naps. Nonpharmacological treatments for insomnia have been found to be particularly effective in reducing sleep-onset latency and time awake after sleep onset (Morin *et al.,* 1994).

Side effects of hypnotic agents may limit their usefulness for insomnia management. The use of hypnotics for long-term insomnia is problematic for many reasons. Long-term hypnotic use leads to a decrease in effectiveness and may produce rebound insomnia upon discontinuance. Almost all hypnotics change sleep architecture. The barbiturates reduce REM sleep; the benzodiazepines reduce slow-wave non-REM sleep and, to a lesser extent, REM sleep. While the significance of these findings is still unclear, there is an emerging consensus that slow-wave sleep is particularly important for physical restorative processes. REM sleep may aid in the consolidation of learning. The blockade of slow-wave sleep by benzodiazepines may help to account for their diminishing effectiveness over the long term, and it also may explain their effectiveness in blocking sleep terrors, a disorder of arousal from slow-wave sleep.

Benzodiazepines produce cognitive changes. Long-acting agents can cause next-day confusion, with a concomitant increase in falls, while shorter-acting agents can produce rebound next-day anxiety. Paradoxically, the acute amnestic effects of benzodiazepines may be responsible for the patient's subsequent report of restful sleep. Triazolam has been postulated to induce cognitive changes that blur the subjective distinction between waking and sleeping (Mendelson, 1993). Anterograde amnesia may be more common with triazolam. While the performance-disruptive effects of alcohol and diphenhydramine are reduced after napping, those of triazolam are not (Roehrs *et al.,* 1993).

Benzodiazepines may worsen sleep apnea. Some hypersomnia patients do not feel refreshed after a night's sleep and so may ask for sleeping pills to improve the quality of their sleep. The consensus is that hypnotics should not be given to the patients with sleep apnea, especially of the obstructive type, because these agents decrease upper airway muscle tone while also decreasing the arousal response to hypoxia (Robinson and Zwillich, 1989).

Insomnia in Older Patients. The elderly, like the very young, tend to sleep in a *polyphasic* (multiple sleep episodes per day) pattern, rather than the *monophasic* pattern characteristic of younger adults. They may have single or multiple daytime naps in addition to nighttime sleep. This pattern makes assessment of adequate sleep time difficult. Anyone who naps regularly will have shortened nighttime sleep without evidence of impaired daytime wakefulness, regardless of age. This pattern is exemplified in "siesta" cultures and probably is adaptive.

Changes in the pharmacokinetic profiles of hypnotic agents occur in the elderly because of reduced body water, reduced renal function, and increased body fat, leading to a longer half-life for benzodiazepines. A dose that produces pleasant sleep and adequate daytime wakefulness during week 1 of administration may produce daytime confusion and amnesia by week 3 as the level continues to rise, particularly with long-acting hypnotics. For example, the benzodiazepine diazepam is highly lipid soluble and is excreted by the kidney. Because of the increase in body fat and the decrease in renal excretion that typically occurs from age 20 to 80, the half-life of the drug may increase fourfold over this span.

Elderly people who are living full lives with relatively unimpaired daytime wakefulness may complain of insomnia because they are not sleeping as long as they did when they were younger. Injudicious use of hypnotics in these individuals can produce daytime cognitive impairment and so impair overall quality of life.

Once an older patient has been taking benzodiazepines for an extended period, whether for daytime anxiety or nighttime sedation, terminating administration of the drug can be a long, involved process. It may be warranted to leave the patient on the medication, with adequate attention to daytime side effects.

Management of Patients Following Long-Term Treatment with Hypnotic Agents. Patients who have been taking hypnotics for many months or even years represent a special problem group (Fleming, 1993). If a benzodiazepine has been used regularly for more than 2 weeks, it should be tapered rather than discontinued abruptly. In some patients on hypnotics with a short half-life, it is easier to switch first to a hypnotic with a long half-life and then taper. In a study of nine patients in whom the nonbenzodiazepine agent zopiclone was abruptly substituted for a benzodiazepine agent for 1 month and then itself abruptly terminated, improved sleep was reported during the zopiclone treatment, and withdrawal effects were absent on discontinuation of zopiclone (Shapiro *et al.,* 1993).

The onset of withdrawal symptoms from medications with a long half-life may be delayed. Consequently, the patient should be warned about the symptoms associated with withdrawal effects.

Prescribing Guidelines for the Management of Insomnia. Hypnotics that act at benzodiazepine receptors, including the benzodiazepine hypnotics as well as the newer agents zolpidem, zopiclone, and zaleplon are preferred to barbiturates because they have a greater therapeutic index, are less toxic in overdose, have smaller effects on sleep architecture, and have less abuse potential. Compounds with a shorter half-life are favored in patients with sleep-onset insomnia but without significant daytime anxiety who need to function at full effectiveness all day.

These compounds also are appropriate for the elderly, because of a decreased risk of falls and respiratory depression. However, the patient and physician should be aware that early morning awakening, rebound daytime anxiety, and amnestic episodes also may occur. These undesirable side effects are more common at higher doses of the benzodiazepines.

Benzodiazepines with a longer half-life are favored for patients who have significant daytime anxiety and who may be able to tolerate next-day sedation but would be impaired further by rebound daytime anxiety. These benzodiazepines also are appropriate for patients receiving treatment for major depressive episodes, because the short-acting agents can worsen early morning awakening. However, longer-acting benzodiazepines can be associated with next-day cognitive impairment or delayed daytime cognitive impairment (after 2 to 4 weeks of treatment) as a result of drug accumulation with repeated administration.

Older agents such as barbiturates, glutethimide, and meprobamate should be avoided for the management of insomnia. They have high abuse potential and are dangerous in overdose.

PROSPECTUS

The emerging molecular understandings of the multisubunit structures that assemble to form the excitatory glutamate receptors and the inhibitory GABA receptors promise the availability of cell-based screens to identify and develop subtype-selective agents with improved therapeutic specificity and minimized side effects. Improvement in the management of insomnia will rely not only on the future availability of hypnotic agents with refined pharmacokinetic and pharmacodynamic properties but also on informed implementations of nonpharmacological strategies, such as behavioral modification, improved sleep hygiene, and judicious reliance on exercise.

For further discussion of sleep disorders, *see* Chapter 27 in *Harrison's Principles of Internal Medicine,* 14th ed., McGraw-Hill, 1998.

BIBLIOGRAPHY

Amin, J., and Weiss, D.S. GABA$_A$ receptor needs two homologous domains of the β-subunit for activation by GABA but not by pentobarbital. *Nature,* **1993,** *366*:565–569.

Balter, M.B., and Uhlenhuth, E.H. New epidemiologic findings about insomnia and its treatment. *J. Clin. Psychiatry,* **1992,** *53*(suppl): 34–39.

Beckstead, M.J., Weiner, J.L., Eger, E.I. II, Gong, D.H., and Mihic, S.J. Glycine and gamma-aminobutyric acid(A) receptor function is enhanced by inhaled drugs of abuse. *Mol. Pharmacol.,* **2000,** *57*:1199–1205.

Cavallaro, R., Regazzetti, M.G., Covelli, G., and Smeraldi, E. Tolerance and withdrawal with zoldipem. *Lancet,* **1993,** *342*:374–375.

DeLorey, T.M., and Olsen, R.W. γ-Aminobutyric acid$_A$ receptor structure and function. *J. Biol. Chem,* **1992,** *267*:16747–16750.

Dresser, G.K., Spence, J.D., and Bailey, D.G. Pharmacokinetic-pharmacodynamic consequences and clinical relevance of cytochrome P450 3A4 inhibition. *Clin. Pharmacokinet.,* **2000,** *38*:41–57.

Dujardin, K., Guieu, J.D., Leconte-Lambert, C., Leconte, P., Borderies, P., and de La Giclais, B. Comparison of the effects of zolpidem and flunitrazepam on sleep structure and daytime cognitive functions. A study of untreated insomniacs. *Pharmacopsychiatry,* **1998,** *31*:14–18.

Fleming, J.A. The difficult to treat insomniac patient. *J. Psychosom. Res.,* **1993,** *37*(suppl 1):45–54.

ffrench-Mullen, J.M., Barker, J.L., and Rogawski, M.A. Calcium current block by (−)-pentobarbital, phenobarbital, and CHEB but not (+)-pentobarbital in acutely isolated hippocampal CA1 neurons: comparison with effects on GABA-activated Cl⁻ current. *J. Neurosci.,* **1993,** *13*:3211–3221.

Frenkel, C., Duch, D.S., and Urban, B.W. Molecular actions of pentobarbital isomers on sodium channels from human brain cortex. *Anesthesiology,* **1990,** *72*:640–649.

Griffiths, R.R., Sannerud, C.A., Ator, N.A., and Brady, J.V. Zolpidem behavioral pharmacology in baboons: self-injection, discrimination, tolerance and withdrawal. *J. Pharmacol. Exp. Ther.,* **1992,** *260*:1199–1208.

Guglielminotti, J., Maury, E., Alzieu, M., Delhotal Landes, B., Becquemont, L., Guidet, B., and Offenstadt, G. Prolonged sedation requiring mechanical ventilation and continuous flumazenil infusion after routine doses of clorazepam for alcohol withdrawal syndrome. *Intens. Care Med.,* **1999,** *25*:1435–1436.

Haefely, W. Antagonists of benzodiazepines: functional aspects. *Adv. Biochem. Psychopharmacol.,* **1983,** *38*:73–93.

Hamburger, L.P. Some minor ailments: their importance in the medical curriculum. *Yale J. Biol. Med.,* **1936,** *8*:365–386.

Herrmann, W.M., Kubicki, S.T., Boden, S., Eich, F.X., Attali, P., and Coquelin, J.P. Pilot controlled double-blind study of the hypnotic effects of zolpidem in patients with chronic "learned" insomnia: psychometric and polysomnographic evaluation. *J. Int. Med. Res.,* **1993,** *21*:306–322.

Hindmarch, I., Fairweather, D.B., and Rombaut, N. Adverse events after triazolam substitution. *Lancet,* **1993,** *341*:55.

James, I., and Savage, I. Beneficial effect of nadolol on anxiety-induced disturbances of performance in musicians: a comparison with diazepam and placebo. *Am. Heart J.,* **1984,** *108*:1150–1155.

Kriel, R.L., Cloyd, J.C., and Pellock, J.M. Respiratory depression in children receiving diazepam for acute seizures: a prospective study. *Dev. Med. Child Neurol.,* **2000,** *42*:429–430.

Kummer, J., Guendel, L., Linden, J., Eich, F.X., Attali, P., Coquelin, J.P., and Kyrein, H.J. Long-term polysomnographic study of the efficacy and safety of zolpidem in elderly psychiatric in-patients with insomnia. *J. Int. Med. Res.,* **1993,** *21*:171–184.

Lader, M., and File, S. The biological basis of benzodiazepine dependence. *Psychol. Med.,* **1987,** *17*:539–547.

Lovinger, D.M., Zimmerman, S.A., Levitin, M., Jones, M.V., and Harrison, N.L. Trichloroethanol potentiates synaptic transmission mediated by γ-aminobutyric acid$_A$ receptors in hippocampal neurons. *J. Pharmacol. Exp. Ther.,* **1993,** *264*:1097–1103.

Löw, K., Crestani, F., Keist, R., Benke, D., Brunig, I., Benson, J.A., Fritschy, J.M., Rülicke, T., Bluethmann, H., Möhler, H., and Rudolph, U. Molecular and neuronal substrate for the selective attenuation of anxiety. *Science,* **2000,** *290*:131–134.

Lüddens, H., Pritchett, D.B., Köhler, M., Killisch, I., Keinänen, K., Monyer, H., Sprengel, R., and Seeburg, P.H. Cerebellar GABA$_A$

receptor selective for a behavioural alcohol antagonist. *Nature,* **1990,** *346*:648–651.

Macdonald, R.L., and McLean, M.J. Cellular bases of barbiturate and phenytoin anticonvulsant drug action. *Epilepsia,* **1982,** *23*(suppl 1): S7–S18.

Manuli, M.A., and Davies, L. Rectal methohexital for sedation of children during imaging procedures. *AJR Am. J. Roentgenol.,* **1993,** *160*:577–580.

Marszalec, W., and Narahashi, T. Use-dependent pentobarbital block of kainate and quisqualate currents. *Brain Res.,* **1993,** *608*:7–15.

Martin, P.R., Bhushan, C.M., Kapur, B.M., Whiteside, E.A., and Sellers, E.M. Intravenous phenobarbital therapy in barbiturate and other hypnosedative withdrawal reactions: a kinetic approach. *Clin. Pharmacol. Ther.* **1979,** *26*:256–264.

Mendelson, W.B. Pharmacologic alteration of the perception of being awake or asleep. *Sleep,* **1993,** *16*:641–646.

Meyer, B.R. Benzodiazepines in the elderly. *Med. Clin. North Am.,* **1982,** *66*:1017–1035.

Monane, M. Insomnia in the elderly. *J. Clin. Psychiatry,* **1992,** *53*(suppl):23–28.

Morin, C.M., Culbert, J.P., and Schwartz, S.M. Nonpharmacological interventions for insomnia: a meta-analysis of treatment efficacy. *Am. J. Psychiatry,* **1994,** *151*:1172–1180.

Morselli, P.L. Zolpidem side-effects. *Lancet,* **1993,** *342*:868–869.

Nattel, S., Wang, Z.G., and Matthews, C. Direct electrophysiological actions of pentobarbital at concentrations achieved during general anesthesia. *Am. J. Physiol.,* **1990,** *259*:H1743–H1751.

Nierenberg, A.A., Adler, L.A., Peselow, E., Zornberg, G., and Rosenthal, M. Trazodone for antidepressant-associated insomnia. *Am. J. Psychiatry,* **1994,** *151*:1069–1072.

Nugent, M., Artru, A.A., and Michenfelder, J.D. Cerebral metabolic, vascular and protective effects of midazolam maleate: comparison to diazepam. *Anesthesiology,* **1982,** *56*:172–176.

Oldenhof, H., de Jong, M., Steenhoek, A., and Janknegt, R. Clinical pharmacokinetics of midazolam in intensive care patients, a wide interpatient variability? *Clin. Pharmacol. Ther.,* **1988,** *43*:263–269.

Pancrazio, J.J., Frazer, M.J., and Lynch, C. III. Barbiturate anesthetics depress the resting K⁺ conductance of myocardium. *J. Pharmacol. Exp. Ther.,* **1993,** *265*:358–365.

Perrault, G., Morel, E., Sanger, D.J., and Zivkovic, B. Lack of tolerance and physical dependence upon repeated treatment with the novel hypnotic zolpidem. *J. Pharmacol. Exp. Ther.,* **1992,** *263*:298–303.

Polc, P. Electrophysiology of benzodiazepine receptor ligands: multiple mechanisms and sites of action. *Prog. Neurobiol.,* **1988,** *31*:349–423.

Pritchett, D.B., Sontheimer, H., Shivers, B.D., Ymer, S., Kettenmann, H., Schofield, P.R., and Seeburg, P.H. Importance of a novel GABA$_A$ receptor subunit for benzodiazepine pharmacology. *Nature,* **1989,** *338*:582–585.

Reeves, R.R., Carter, O.S., Pinkofsky, H.B., Struve, F.A., and Bennett, D.M. Carisoprodol (SOMA): abuse potential and physician unawareness. *J. Addict. Dis.,* **1999,** *18*:51–56.

Roehrs, T., Claiborue, D., Knox, M., and Roth, T. Effects of ethanol, diphenhydramine, and triazolam after a nap. *Neuropsychopharmacology,* **1993,** *9*:239–245.

Roncari, G., Timm, U., Zell, M., Zumbrunnen, R., and Weber, W. Flumazenil kinetics in the elderly. *Eur. J. Clin. Pharmacol.,* **1993,** *45*:585–587.

Roth, S.H., Forman, S.A., Braswell, L.M., and Miller, K.W. Actions of pentobarbital enantiomers on nicotinic cholinergic receptors. *Mol. Pharmacol.,* **1989,** *36*:874–880.

Roth, T., and Roehrs, T.A. Issues in the use of benzodiazepine therapy. *J. Clin. Psychiatry,* **1992,** *53*(suppl):14–18.

Schofield, P.R., Darlison, M.G., Fujita, N., Burt, D.R., Stephenson, F.A., Rodriguez, H., Rhee, L.M., Ramachandran, J., Reale, V., Glencourse, T.A., Seeburg, P.H., and Barnard, E.A. Sequence and functional expression of the GABA$_A$ receptor shows a ligand-gated receptor super-family. *Nature,* **1987,** *328:*221–227.

Shapiro, C.M., MacFarlane, J.G., and MacLean, A.W. Alleviating sleep-related discontinuance symptoms associated with benzodiazepine withdrawal: a new approach. *J. Psychosom. Res.,* **1993,** *37*(suppl 1): 55–57.

Spivey, W.H. Flumazenil and seizures: an analysis of 43 cases. *Clin. Ther.,* **1992,** *14:*292–305.

Twyman, R.E., Rogers, C.J., and Macdonald, R.L. Differential regulation of γ-aminobutyric acid receptor channels by diazepam and phenobarbital. *Ann. Neurol.,* **1989,** *25:*213–220.

Uhlenhuth, E.H., Balter, M.B., Ban, T.A., and Yang, K. International study of expert judgment on therapeutic use of benzodiazepines and other psychotherapeutic medications: IV Therapeutic dose dependence and abuse liability of benzodiazepines in the long-term treatment of anxiety disorders. *J. Clin Psychopharmacol.,* **1999,** *19* (6 suppl 2):23S–29S.

Vogel, G. Clinical uses and advantages of low doses of benzodiazepine hypnotics. *J. Clin. Psychiatry,* **1992,** *53*(suppl):19–22.

Walsh, J.K., Vogel, G.W., Schart, M., Erman, M., Erwin, C.W., Schweitzer, P.K, Mangano, R.M., and Roth, T. A five week, polysomnographic assessment of zaleplon 10 mg for the treatment of primary insomnia. *Sleep Med.,* **2000,** *1:*41–49.

Yeo, G.T., de Burgh, S.P., Letton, T., Shaw, J., Donnelly, N., Swinburn, M.E., Phillips, S., Bridges-Webb, C., and Mant, A. Educational visiting and hypnosedative prescribing in general practice. *Fam. Pract.,* **1994,** *11:*57–61.

MONOGRAPHS AND REVIEWS

Anonymous. Zolpidem for insomnia. *Med. Lett. Drugs Ther.,* **1993,** *35:*35–36.

Dement, W.C. Objective measurements of daytime sleepiness and performance comparing quazepam with flurazepam in two adult populations using the Multiple Sleep Latency Test. *J. Clin. Psychiatry,* **1991,** *52*(suppl):31–37.

Dement, W.C. The proper use of sleeping pills in the primary-care setting. *J. Clin. Psychiatry,* **1992,** *53*(suppl):50–56.

Diamond, I., Nagy, L., Mochly-Rosen, D., and Gordon, A. The role of adenosine and adenosine transport in ethanol-induced cellular tolerance and dependence. Possible biologic and genetic markers of alcoholism. *Ann. N.Y. Acad. Sci.,* **1991,** *625:*473–487.

Doble, A., and Martin, I.L. Multiple benzodiazepine receptors: no reason for anxiety. *Trends Pharmacol. Sci.,* **1992,** *13:*76–81.

Dooley, M., and Plosker, G.L. Zaleplon: a review of its use in the treatment of insomnia. *Drugs,* **2000,** *60:*413–445.

DuPont, R.L. (ed.). Abuse of benzodiazepines: the problems and the solutions. A report of a committee of the Institute for Behavior and Health, Inc. *Am. J. Drug Alcohol Abuse,* **1988,** *14*(suppl 1): 1–69.

Essrich, C., Lorez, M., Benson, J.A., Fritschy, J.M., and Luscher, B. Postsynaptic clustering of major GABA$_A$ receptor subtypes requires the γ2 subunit and gephyrin. *Nat. Neurosci.,* **1998,** *1:*563–571.

File, S.E. Tolerance to the behavioral actions of benzodiazepines. *Neurosci. Biobehav. Rev.,* **1985,** *9:*113–121.

Fisher, S.E., and Karl, P.I. Maternal ethanol use and selective fetal malnutrition. *Recent Dev. Alcohol.,* **1988,** *6:*277–289.

Gardner, C.R. Functional *in vivo* correlates of the benzodiazepine agonist-inverse agonist continuum. *Prog. Neurobiol.,* **1988,** *31:*425–476.

Gardner, C.R., Tully, W.R., and Hedgecock, C.J. The rapidly expanding range of neuronal benzodiazepine receptor ligands. *Prog. Neurobiol.,* **1993,** *40:*1–61.

Garnier, R., Guerault, E., Muzard, D., Azoyan, P., Chaumet-Riffaud, A.E., and Efthymiou, M.L. Acute zolpidem poisoning—analysis of 344 cases. *J. Toxicol. Clin. Toxicol.,* **1994,** *32:*391–404.

Gary, N.E., and Tresznewsky, O. Clinical aspects of drug intoxication: barbiturates and a potpourri of other sedatives, hypnotics, and tranquilizers. *Heart Lung,* **1983,** *12:*122–127.

Gillin, J.C., Spinweber, C.L., and Johnson, L.C. Rebound insomnia: a critical review. *J. Clin. Psychopharmacol.,* **1989,** *9:*161–172.

Greenblatt, D.J., Divoll, M., Abernethy, D.R., Ochs, H.R., and Shader, R.I. Benzodiazepine kinetics: implications for therapeutics and pharmacogeriatrics. *Drug Metab. Rev.,* **1983a,** *14:*251–292.

Greenblatt, D.J., Divoll, M., Abernethy, D.R., Ochs, H.R., and Shader, R.I. Clinical pharmacokinetics of the newer benzodiazepines. *Clin. Pharmacokinet.,* **1983b,** *8:*233–252.

Greenblatt, D.J., Harmatz, J.S., and Shader, R.I. Clinical pharmacokinetics of anxiolytics and hypnotics in the elderly. Therapeutic considerations (Part I). *Clin. Pharmacokinet.,* **1991,** *21:*165–177.

Greenblatt, D.J. Benzodiazepine hypnotics: sorting the pharmacokinetic facts. *J. Clin. Psychiatry,* **1991,** *52*(suppl):4–10.

Greenblatt, D.J., and Wright, C.E. Clinical pharmacokinetics of alprazolam. Therapeutic implications. *Clin. Pharmacokinet.,* **1993,** *24:*453–471.

Hilbert, J.M., and Battista, D. Quazepam and flurazepam: differential pharmacokinetic and pharmacodynamic characteristics. *J. Clin. Psychiatry,* **1991,** *52*(suppl):21–26.

Hoehns, J.D., and Perry, P.J. Zolpidem: a nonbenzodiazepine hypnotic for treatment of insomnia. *Clin. Pharm.,* **1993,** *12:*814–828.

Hoffman, E.J., and Warren, E.W. Flumazenil: a benzodiazepine antagonist. *Clin. Pharm.,* **1993,** *12:*641–656.

Jonas, J.M., Coleman, B.S., Sheridan, A.Q., and Kalinske, R.W. Comparative clinical profiles of triazolam versus other shorter-acting hypnotics. *J. Clin. Psychiatry,* **1992,** *53*(suppl):19–31.

Kleingoor, C., Wieland, H.A., Korpi, E.R., Seeburg, P.H., and Kettenmann, H. Current potentiation by diazepam but not GABA sensitivity is determined by a single histidine residue. *Neuroreport,* **1993,** *4:*187–190.

Langtry, H.D., and Benfield, P. Zolpidem. A review of its pharmacodynamic and pharmacokinetic properties and therapeutic potential. *Drugs,* **1990,** *40:*291–313.

Livingston, M.G. Benzodiazepine dependence. *Br. J. Hosp. Med.,* **1994,** *51:*281–286.

Macdonald, R.L., and McLean, M.J. Anticonvulsant drugs: mechanisms of action. *Adv. Neurol.,* **1986,** *44:*713–736.

Maczaj, M. Pharmacological treatment of insomnia. *Drugs,* **1993,** *45:* 44–55.

McKernan, R.M., Rosahl, T.W., Reynolds, D.S., Sur, C., Wafford, K.A., Atack, J.R., Farrar, S., Myers, J., Cook, G., Ferris, P., Garrett, L., Bristow, L., Marshall, G., Macaulay, A., Brown, N., Howell, O., Moore, K.W., Carling, R.W., Street, L.J., Castro, J.L., Ragan, C.I., Dawson, G.R., and Whiting, P.J. Sedative but not anxiolytic properties of benzodiazepines are mediated by the GABA$_A$ receptor α1 subtype. *Nat. Neurosci.,* **2000,** *3:*587–592.

McKernan, R.M., Wafford, K., Quirk, K., Hadingham, K.L., Harley, E.A., Ragan, C.I., and Whiting, P.J. The pharmacology of the benzodiazepine site of the GABA-A receptor is dependent on the type of γ-subunit present. *J. Recept. Signal Transduct. Res.,* **1995,** *15:* 173–183.

Maczaj, M. Pharmacological treatment of insomnia. *Drugs,* **1993,** *45:* 44–55.

Mehta, A.K., and Ticku, M.K. An update on GABA$_A$ receptors. *Brain Res. Brain Res. Rev.,* **1999,** *29:*196–217.

Mendelson, W.B. Neuropharmacology of sleep induction by benzodiazepines. *Crit. Rev. Neurobiol.,* **1992,** *6:*221–232.

Mitler, M.M. Nonselective and selective benzodiazepine receptor agonists—where are we today? *Sleep,* **2000,** *23*(suppl 1):S39–S47.

National Institute of Mental Health Consensus Development Conference. Drugs and insomnia. The use of medications to promote sleep. *JAMA,* **1984,** *251:*2410–2414.

Nino-Murcia, G. Diagnosis and treatment of insomnia and risks associated with lack of treatment. *J. Clin. Psychiatry,* **1992,** *53*(suppl):43–47.

Petursson, H. The benzodiazepine withdrawal syndrome. *Addiction,* **1994,** *89:*1455–1459.

Phillis, J.W., and O'Regan, M.H. The role of adenosine in the central actions of the benzodiazepines. *Prog. Neuropsychopharmacol. Biol. Psychiatry,* **1988,** *12:*389–404.

Pritchett, D.B, and Seeburg, P.H. Gamma-aminobutyric acidA receptor alpha 5-subunit creates novel type II benzodiazepine receptor pharmacology. *J Neurochem.,* **1990,** *54:*1802–1804.

Ragan, C.I., McKernan, R.M., Wafford, K., and Whiting, P.J. γ-Aminobutyric acid-A (GABA-A) receptor/ion channel complex. *Biochem. Soc. Trans.,* **1993,** *21:*622–626.

Robinson, R.W., and Zwillich, C.W. The effect of drugs on breathing during sleep. In, *Principles and Practice of Sleep Medicine.* (Kryger, M.H., Roth, T., and Dement, W.C., eds.) Saunders, Philadelphia, **1989.**

Rothschild, A.J. Disinhibition, amnestic reactions, and other adverse reactions secondary to triazolam: a review of the literature. *J. Clin. Psychiatry,* **1992,** *53*(suppl):69–79.

Rudolph, U., Crestani, F., Benke, D., Brunig, I., Benson, J.A., Fritschy, J.M., Martin, J.R., Bluethmann, H., and Mohler, H. Benzodiazepine actions mediated by specific gamma-aminobutyric acid(A) receptor subtypes. *Nature,* **1999,** *401:*796–800.

Saunders, P.A., and Ho, I.K. Barbiturates and the GABA$_A$ receptor complex. *Prog. Drug Res.,* **1990,** *34:*261–286.

Shapiro, H.M. Barbiturates in brain ischaemia. *Br. J. Anaesth.,* **1985,** *57:*82–95.

Sieghart, W. GABA$_A$ receptors: ligand-gated Cl$^-$ ion channels modulated by multiple drug-binding sites. *Trends Pharmacol. Sci.,* **1992,** *13:*446–450.

Sieghart, W., Fuchs, K., Tretter, V., Ebert, V., Jechlinger, M., Hoger, H., and Adamiker, D. Structure and subunit composition of GABA(A) receptors. *Neurochem Int.,* **1999,** *34:*379–385.

Smith, M.C., and Riskin, B.J. The clinical use of barbiturates in neurological disorders. *Drugs,* **1991,** *42:*365–378.

Symposium (various authors). *Pharmacology of Benzodiazepines.* (Usdin, E., Skolnick, P., Tallman, J.F., Greenblatt, O., and Paul, S.M., eds.) Macmillan Press, London, **1982.**

Symposium (various authors). *The Benzodiazepines: From Molecular Biology to Clinical Practice.* (Costa, E., ed.) Raven Press, New York, **1983.**

Symposium (various authors). Modern hypnotics and performance. (Nicholson, A., Hippius, H., Rüther, E., and Dunbar, G., eds.) *Acta Psychiatr. Scand. Suppl.,* **1986a,** *332:*3–174.

Symposium (various authors). Chlormethiazole 25 years: recent developments and historical perspectives. (Evans, J.G., Feuerlein, W., Glatt, M.M., Kanowski, S., and Scott, D.B., eds.) *Acta Psychiatr. Scand. Suppl.,* **1986b,** *329:*1–198.

Symposium (various authors). GABA and benzodiazepine receptor subtypes. Molecular biology, pharmacology, and clinical aspects. (Biggio, G., and Costa, E., ed.) *Adv. Biochem. Psychopharmacol.,* **1990a,** *46:*1–239.

Symposium (various authors). Critical issues in the management of insomnia: investigators report on estazolam. (Roth. T., ed.) *Am. J. Med.,* **1990b,** *88*(suppl):IS–48S.

Symposium (various authors). GABAergic synaptic transmission: molecular, pharmacological, and clinical aspects. (Biggio, G., Concas, A., and Costa, E., eds.) *Adv. Biochem. Psychopharmacol.,* **1992,** *47:*1–460.

Tanaka, E. Clinically significant pharmacokinetic drug interactions with benzodiazepines. *J. Clin. Pharm. Ther.,* **1999,** *24:*347–355.

Teboul, E, and Chouinard, G. A guide to benzodiazepine selection. Part II: Clinical aspects. *Can. J. Psychiatry,* **1991,** *36:*62–73.

Walsh, J.K., and Engelhardt, C.L. Trends in the pharmacologic treatment of insomnia. *J. Clin. Psychiatry,* **1992,** *53*(suppl):10–17.

Woods, J.H., Katz, J.L., and Winger, G. Abuse liability of benzodiazepines. *Pharmacol. Rev.,* **1987,** *39:*1–413.

Woods, J.H., Katz, J.L., and Winger, G. Benzodiazepines: use, abuse, and consequences. *Pharmacol. Rev.,* **1992,** *44:*151–347.

Woods, J.H., and Winger, G. Abuse liability of flunitrazepam. *J. Clin. Psychopharmacol.,* **1997,** *17:*1S–57S.

Acknowledgment

The authors wish to acknowledge William R. Hobbs, Theodore W. Rall, and Todd A. Verdoorn, authors of this chapter in the ninth edition of *Goodman & Gilman's The Pharmacological Basis of Therapeutics,* much of whose text we have retained in this edition.

C H A P T E R   1 8

ETHANOL

Michael Fleming, S. John Mihic, and R. Adron Harris

Ethanol is one of a wide variety of structurally dissimilar agents that depress the functioning of the central nervous system (CNS). Ethanol differs from most other CNS depressants in that it is widely available to adults, and its use is legal and accepted in many societies. Associated with this widespread availability of ethanol are the enormous personal and societal costs of its abuse, with millions of individuals becoming alcohol abusers, or alcoholics. This chapter describes the pharmacological properties of ethanol in terms of its effects on a variety of organ systems—including the gastrointestinal, cardiovascular, and central nervous systems—and how ethanol affects disease processes. Effects of ethanol on the developing embryo and fetus are reviewed, as well as the long-term consequences of prenatal exposure to ethanol. Ethanol disturbs the fine balance that exists between excitatory and inhibitory influences in the brain, producing the disinhibition, ataxia, and sedation that follow its consumption. Tolerance to ethanol develops after chronic use, and physical dependence is demonstrated upon alcohol withdrawal. Existing and emerging pharmacotherapies for alcohol dependence are discussed, as well as recent research into the cellular and molecular mechanisms of ethanol actions in vivo, *which should aid in the development of rational therapies for alcohol abuse and alcoholism.*

HISTORY AND OVERVIEW

Alcoholic beverages are so strongly associated with human society that fermentation is said to have developed in parallel with civilization. Until recently, alcoholic beverages contained relatively low concentrations of ethanol (the terms *ethanol* and *alcohol* are used interchangeably in this chapter), and there is speculation that human alcohol use is linked evolutionarily to a preference for fermenting fruit, where the presence of ethanol signals that the fruit is ripe but not yet rotten (Dudley, 2000).

The Arabs developed distillation about A.D. 800, and the word *alcohol* is derived from the Arabic for "something subtle." Alchemists of the Middle Ages were captivated by the invisible "spirit" that was distilled from wine and thought it to be a remedy for practically all diseases. The term *whiskey* is derived from *usquebaugh,* Gaelic for "water of life," and alcohol became the major ingredient of widely marketed "tonics" and "elixirs."

Although alcohol abuse and alcoholism are major health problems in many countries, the medical and social impacts of alcohol abuse have not always been appreciated. The economic burden to the United States economy is about $170 billion each year, and alcohol is responsible for more than 100,000 deaths annually. At least 14 million Americans meet the criteria for alcohol abuse or alcoholism, but medical diagnosis and treatment often are delayed until the disease is advanced and complicated by multiple social and health problems, making treatment difficult. Biological and genetic studies clearly place alcoholism among other diseases with both genetic and environmental influences, but persistent stigmas and attribution to moral failure have impeded recognition and treatment of alcohol problems. A major challenge for physicians and researchers is to devise diagnostic and therapeutic approaches aimed at this major health problem.

Compared with other drugs, surprisingly large amounts of alcohol are required for physiological effects, resulting in its consumption more like a food than a drug. The alcohol content of beverages ranges from 4% to 6% (volume/volume) for beer, 10% to 15% for wine, and 40% and higher for distilled spirits. The "proof" of an alcohol-containing beverage is twice its percent alcohol (*e.g.,* 40% alcohol is 80 proof). Remarkably, and contrary to public impressions, the serving size for alcoholic beverages is adjusted so that about 14 grams of alcohol is contained in a glass of beer or wine or a shot of spirits. Thus, alcohol is consumed in gram quantities, whereas most other drugs are taken in milligram or microgram doses. Blood alcohol levels (BALs) in human beings can be estimated readily by the measurement of alcohol levels in expired air; the partition coefficient for ethanol between blood and alveolar air is approximately 2000:1. Because of the causal relationship between excessive alcohol consumption and vehicular accidents, there has been a near universal adoption of laws attempting to limit the operation of vehicles while under the influence of alcohol. Legally allowed BALs typically are set at or below 100 mg% (100 mg of ethanol per deciliter of blood; 0.1% w/v), which is equivalent to a concentration of 22 mM ethanol in blood. A 12-ounce bottle of beer, a 5-ounce glass of wine, and a 1.5-ounce shot of 40% liquor all contain roughly 14 grams of ethanol, and the consumption of one of those beverages by a 70-kg person would produce a BAL of approximately 30 mg%. However, it is important to note that this is approximate, because the blood alcohol level is determined by a number of factors, including the rate of drinking, gender, body weight and water percentage, and the rates of metabolism and stomach emptying (*see* section on "Acute Alcohol Intoxication").

PHARMACOLOGICAL PROPERTIES

Absorption, Distribution, and Metabolism

After oral administration, ethanol is rapidly absorbed into the bloodstream from the stomach and small intestine and distributes into total body water. Because absorption occurs more rapidly from the small intestine than from the stomach, delays in gastric emptying (due, for example, to the presence of food) slow ethanol absorption. After it enters the bloodstream, alcohol first travels to the liver before it quickly distributes into all body fluids. After oral consumption of alcohol, first-pass metabolism by gastric and liver alcohol dehydrogenase (ADH) enzymes leads to lower blood alcohol levels than would be obtained if the same dose were administered intravenously. Less gastric metabolism of ethanol occurs in women than in men, which may explain in part the greater susceptibility of women to ethanol (Lieber, 2000). Aspirin increases ethanol bioavailability by inhibiting gastric ADH. Although a small amount of ethanol is excreted unchanged in urine, sweat, and breath, most of it (90% to 98%) is metabolized to acetaldehyde and then to acetate, primarily in the liver. ADH, catalase, and a microsomal cytochrome P450 ethanol-oxidizing system all catalyze the oxidation of ethanol to acetaldehyde, with ADH playing the predominant role in the liver. This first step in alcohol metabolism also is the rate-limiting step in determining how quickly ethanol is cleared from the body. The oxidation of ethanol differs from that of most substances, in that it is relatively independent of concentration in blood and is constant with

time (zero-order kinetics). On average, about 10 ml of ethanol are oxidized by a 70-kg person each hour (or about 120 mg/kg per hour). Acetaldehyde is rapidly metabolized to acetate by cytosolic and mitochondrial aldehyde dehydrogenase in the liver.

Although the cytochrome P450 system is not usually a major factor in the metabolism of ethanol, it can be an important site of interactions of ethanol with other drugs. The enzyme system is induced by chronic consumption of ethanol, leading to increased clearance of drugs that are substrates for it. There can be decreased clearance of the same drugs, however, after acute consumption of ethanol, as ethanol competes with them for oxidation by the enzyme system (*e.g.,* phenytoin, warfarin).

Central Nervous System

The public often views alcoholic drinks as stimulating, but ethanol is primarily a central nervous system (CNS) depressant. Ingestion of moderate amounts of ethanol, like that of other depressants such as barbiturates and benzodiazepines, can have antianxiety actions and produce behavioral disinhibition with a wide range of doses. Individual signs of intoxication vary from expansive and vivacious affect to uncontrolled mood swings and emotional outbursts that may have violent components. With more severe intoxication, a general impairment of CNS function occurs, and a condition of general anesthesia ultimately prevails. However, there is little margin between the anesthetic actions and lethal effects (usually due to respiratory depression).

About 10% of alcohol drinkers progress to levels of consumption that are physically and socially detrimental. Chronic abuse is accompanied by tolerance, dependence, and craving for the drug (*see* below for a discussion of neuronal mechanisms; *see* also Chapter 24). Alcoholism is characterized by compulsive use despite clearly deleterious social and medical consequences. Alcoholism is a progressive illness, and brain damage from chronic alcohol abuse contributes to the deficits in cognitive functioning and judgment seen in alcoholics. Alcoholism is a leading cause of dementia in the United States (Oslin *et al.,* 1998). Chronic alcohol abuse results in shrinkage of the brain due to loss of both white and gray matter (Kril and Halliday, 1999). The frontal lobes are particularly sensitive to damage by alcohol, and the extent of damage is determined by the amount and duration of alcohol consumption, with older alcoholics being more vulnerable than younger ones (Pfefferbaum *et al.,* 1998). It is important to note that ethanol itself is neurotoxic and, although malnutrition or vitamin deficiencies probably play roles in complications of alcoholism such as Wernicke's encephalopathy and Korsakoff's psychosis, in western countries most of the brain damage in these disorders is due to alcohol *per se.* In addition to loss of brain tissue, alcohol abuse also reduces brain metabolism (as determined by positron emission tomography), and this hypometabolic state rebounds to a level of increased metabolism during detoxification. The magnitude of decrease in metabolic state is determined by the number of years of alcohol use and the age of the patients (Volkow *et al.*, 1994; *see* "Mechanisms of CNS Actions," below).

Cardiovascular System

Serum Lipoproteins and Cardiovascular Effects. In most countries, the risk of mortality due to coronary heart disease (CHD) is correlated with a high dietary intake of saturated fat and elevated serum cholesterol levels. France is an exception to this rule, with relatively low mortality from CHD despite the consumption of high quantities of saturated fats by the French (the "French paradox"). Epidemiological studies suggest that widespread wine consumption by the French (20 to 30 g of ethanol per day) is one of the factors conferring a cardioprotective effect, with 1 to 3 drinks per day resulting in a 10% to 40% decreased risk of coronary heart disease, compared to abstainers. In contrast, daily consumption of greater amounts of alcohol leads to an increased incidence of noncoronary causes of cardiovascular failure, such as arrhythmias, cardiomyopathy, and hemorrhagic stroke, offsetting the beneficial effects of alcohol on coronary arteries; *i.e.*, alcohol has a "J-shaped" dose-mortality curve. Reduced risks for CHD are seen at intakes as low as one-half drink per day (Maclure, 1993). Young women and others at low risk for heart disease derive little benefit from light to moderate alcohol intake, while those of both sexes who are at high risk and who may have had a myocardial infarction clearly benefit. Data based on a number of prospective, cohort, cross-cultural, and case-control studies in diverse populations consistently reveal lower rates of angina pectoris, myocardial infarction, and peripheral artery disease in those consuming light (1 to 20 g/day) to moderate (21 to 40 g/day) amounts of alcohol.

One possible mechanism by which alcohol could reduce the risk of CHD is through its effects on blood lipids. Changes in plasma lipoprotein levels, particularly increases in high-density lipoprotein (HDL; *see* Chapter 36), have been associated with the protective effects of ethanol. HDL binds cholesterol and returns it to the liver for elimination or reprocessing, decreasing tissue cholesterol levels. Ethanol-induced increases in HDL-cholesterol could thus be expected to antagonize cholesterol buildup on arterial walls, lessening the risk of infarction. Approximately half of the risk reduction associated with ethanol consumption is explained by changes in total HDL levels (Langer *et al.*, 1992). HDL is found as two subfractions, named HDL_2 and HDL_3. Increased levels of HDL_2 (and possibly also HDL_3) are associated with reduced risk of myocardial infarction. Levels of both subfractions are increased following alcohol consump-

tion (Gaziano *et al.*, 1993) and decrease when alcohol consumption ceases. Apolipoproteins A-I and A-II are constituents of HDL, with some HDL particles containing only the former, while others are composed of both. Increased levels of both apolipoproteins A-I and A-II are seen in individuals regularly consuming alcohol. In contrast, there are reports of decreased serum apolipoprotein(a) levels following periods of alcohol consumption. Elevated apolipoprotein(a) levels have been associated with an increased risk for the development of atherosclerosis.

Although the cardioprotective effects of ethanol initially were noted in wine drinkers, all forms of alcoholic beverages confer cardioprotection. A variety of alcoholic beverages increase HDL levels while decreasing the risk of myocardial infarction. The flavonoids found in red wine (and purple grape juice) may play an extra role in protecting LDL from oxidative damage. Oxidized LDL has been implicated in several steps of atherogenesis. The antiatherogenic effects of alcohol could be mediated by changes in LDL oxidation and elevated estrogen levels (Hillbom *et al.*, 1998). Flavonoids also induce endothelium-dependent vasodilation (Stein *et al.*, 1999). Another way in which alcohol consumption conceivably could play a cardioprotective role is by altering factors involved in blood clotting. The formation of clots is an important step in the genesis of myocardial infarctions, and a number of factors maintain a balance between bleeding and clot dissolution. Alcohol consumption elevates the levels of tissue plasminogen activator, a clot-dissolving enzyme (Ridker *et al.*, 1994; *see* Chapter 55), decreasing the likelihood of clot formation. Decreased fibrinogen concentrations seen following ethanol consumption also could have cardioprotective effects (Rimm *et al.*, 1999), and epidemiological studies have linked the moderate consumption of ethanol to an inhibition of platelet activation (Rubin, 1999).

A question worth addressing is whether or not abstainers from alcohol should be advised to begin the consumption of moderate amounts of ethanol. The answer is *no*. It is important to note that there have been no randomized clinical trials to test the efficacy of daily alcohol use in reducing rates of coronary heart disease and mortality, and it is not appropriate for physicians to advocate the ingestion of alcohol solely to prevent heart disease. Many abstainers avoid alcohol because of a family history of alcoholism or for other health reasons, and it is not prudent to suggest that they begin drinking. Other lifestyle changes or medical treatments should be encouraged if patients are at risk for the development of CHD.

Hypertension. Heavy alcohol use can raise diastolic and systolic blood pressure (Klatsky, 1996). Studies indicate a positive, nonlinear association between alcohol use and hypertension, unrelated to age, education, smoking status, or the use of birth control medication. Consumption above 30 grams of alcohol per day (more than two standard drinks) is associated with a 1.5- to 2.3-mm Hg rise in diastolic and systolic blood pressure. A time effect also has been demonstrated, with diastolic and systolic blood pressure elevation being greatest for persons who consumed alcohol within 24 hours of examination (Moreira et al., 1998). Women may be at greater risk than men (Seppa et al., 1996).

A number of hypotheses have been proposed to explain the cause of alcohol-induced hypertension. One is that some hypertensive alcoholic patients abstain before a physician visit (Iwase et al., 1995). As blood alcohol levels fall, acute withdrawal causes an elevation in blood pressure that is reflected in elevated blood pressure readings in the physician's office. Another hypothesis holds that there is a direct pressor effect of alcohol caused by an unknown mechanism. Studies that have examined levels of renin, angiotensin, norepinephrine, antidiuretic hormone, cortisol, and other pressor mediators have been inconclusive. Newer hypotheses include increased intracellular Ca^{2+} levels with a subsequent increase in vascular reactivity, stimulation of the endothelium to release endothelin, and inhibition of endothelium-dependent nitric oxide production (Grogan and Kochar, 1994).

The prevalence of hypertension attributable to excess alcohol consumption is not known, but studies suggest a range of 5% to 11%. The prevalence probably is higher for men than for women because of higher alcohol consumption by men. A reduction or cessation of alcohol use in heavy drinkers may reduce the need for antihypertensive medication or reduce the blood pressure to the normal range. A safe amount of alcohol consumption for hypertensive patients who are light drinkers (one to two drinks per occasion, and less than 14 per week) has not been determined. Factors to consider are a personal history of ischemic heart disease, a history of binge drinking, or a family history of alcoholism or of cerebrovascular accident. Hypertensive patients with any of these risk factors should abstain from alcohol use.

Cardiac Arrhythmias. Alcohol has a number of pharmacological effects on cardiac conduction, including prolongation of the QT interval, prolongation of ventricular repolarization, and sympathetic stimulation (Rossinen et al., 1999; Kupari and Koskinen, 1998). Atrial arrhythmias associated with chronic alcohol use include supraventricular tachycardia, atrial fibrillation, and atrial flutter. Some 15% to 20% of idiopathic cases of atrial fibrillation may be induced by chronic ethanol use (Braunwald, 1997). Ventricular tachycardia may be responsible for the increased risk of unexplained sudden death that has been observed in persons who are alcohol-dependent (Kupari and Koskinen, 1998). During continued alcohol use, treatment of these arrhythmias may be more resistant to cardioversion, digitalis, or Ca^{2+} channel–blocking agents (see Chapter 35). Patients with recurrent or refractory atrial arrhythmias should be questioned carefully about alcohol use.

Cardiomyopathy. Ethanol is known to have dose-related toxic effects on both skeletal and cardiac muscle (Preedy

et al., 1994). Numerous studies have shown that alcohol can depress cardiac contractility and lead to cardiomyopathy (Thomas et al., 1994). Echocardiography demonstrates global hypokinesis. Fatty acid ethyl esters (formed from the enzymatic reaction of ethanol with free fatty acids) appear to play a role in the development of this disorder (Beckemeier and Bora, 1998). Approximately half of all patients with idiopathic cardiomyopathy are alcohol-dependent. Although the clinical signs and symptoms of idiopathic- and alcohol-induced cardiomyopathy are similar, alcohol-induced cardiomyopathy has a better prognosis if patients are able to stop drinking. Women are at greater risk than are men (Urbano-Marquez et al., 1995). As 40% to 50% of persons with alcohol-induced cardiomyopathy who continue to drink die within 3 to 5 years, abstinence remains the primary treatment. Some patients respond to diuretics, angiotensin converting enzyme inhibitors, and vasodilators.

Stroke. Clinical studies indicate a higher than normal incidence of hemorrhagic and ischemic stroke in persons who drink more than 40 to 60 grams of alcohol per day (Hansagi et al., 1995). Many cases of stroke follow prolonged binge drinking, especially when stroke occurs in younger patients. Proposed etiological factors include alcohol-induced (1) cardiac arrhythmias and associated thrombus formation; (2) high blood pressure and subsequent cerebral artery degeneration; (3) acute increases in systolic blood pressure and alteration in cerebral artery tone; and (4) head trauma. The effects on hemostasis, fibrinolysis, and blood clotting are variable and could prevent or precipitate acute stroke (Numminen et al., 1996). The effects of alcohol on the formation of intracranial aneurysms are controversial, but the statistical association disappears when one controls for tobacco use and gender (Qureshi et al., 1998).

Skeletal Muscle

Alcohol has a number of effects on skeletal muscle (Panzak et al., 1998). Chronic, heavy, daily alcohol consumption is associated with decreased muscle strength even when studies are controlled for other factors such as age, nicotine use, or chronic illness (Clarkson and Reichsman, 1990). Heavy doses of alcohol also cause irreversible damage to muscle, reflected by a marked increase in the activity of creatine phosphokinase in plasma. Muscle biopsies from heavy drinkers also reveal decreased levels of glycogen stores and pyruvate kinase activity (Vernet et al., 1995). Approximately 50% of chronic heavy drinkers have evidence of type II fiber atrophy. These changes correlate with reductions in muscle protein synthesis and serum carnosinase activities (Wassif *et al.*, 1993). Most patients with chronic alcoholism show electromyographical changes, and many show evidence of a skeletal myopathy similar to alcoholic cardiomyopathy (Fernandez-Sola *et al.*, 1994).

Body Temperature

Ingestion of ethanol causes a feeling of warmth, because alcohol enhances cutaneous and gastric blood flow. Increased sweating also may occur. Heat, therefore, is lost more rapidly and the internal temperature falls. After consumption of large amounts of ethanol, the central temperature-regulating mechanism itself becomes depressed, and the fall in body temperature may become pronounced. The action of alcohol in lowering body temperature is greater and more dangerous when the ambient environmental temperature is low. Studies of hypothermia deaths suggest that alcohol is a major risk factor in these events (Kortelainen, 1991). Patients with ischemic limbs secondary to peripheral vascular disease are particularly susceptible to cold damage (Proano and Perbeck, 1994).

Diuresis

Alcohol inhibits the release of vasopressin (antidiuretic hormone; *see* Chapter 30) from the posterior pituitary gland, resulting in enhanced diuresis (Leppaluoto *et al.*, 1992). This may be complemented by ethanol-induced increases in plasma levels of atrial natriuretic peptide (Colantonio *et al.*, 1991). Alcoholics have less urine output than do control subjects in response to a challenge dose with ethanol, suggesting that tolerance develops to the diuretic effects of ethanol (Collins *et al.*, 1992). Alcoholics withdrawing from alcohol exhibit increased vasopressin release and a consequent retention of water, as well as dilutional hyponatremia.

Gastrointestinal System

Esophagus. Alcohol frequently is either the primary etiologic factor or one of multiple causal factors associated with esophageal dysfunction. Ethanol also is associated with the development of esophageal reflux, Barrett's esophagus, traumatic rupture of the esophagus, Mallory-Weiss tears, and esophageal cancer. When compared to nonalcoholic nonsmokers, alcohol-dependent patients who smoke have a tenfold increased risk of developing cancer of the esophagus. There is little change in esophageal function at low blood alcohol concentrations, but at higher blood alcohol concentrations, a decrease in peristalsis and decreased lower esophageal sphincter pressure occur. Patients with chronic reflux esophagitis may respond to proton pump inhibitors (*see* Chapter 37).

Stomach. Heavy alcohol use can disrupt the gastric mucosal barrier and cause acute and chronic gastritis. Ethanol appears to stimulate gastric secretions by exciting sensory nerves in the buccal and gastric mucosa and promoting the release of gastrin and histamine. Beverages containing more than 40% alcohol also have a direct toxic effect on gastric mucosa. While these effects are seen most often in chronic heavy drinkers, they can occur after moderate and/or short-term alcohol use. Clinical symptoms include acute epigastric pain that is relieved with antacids or histamine H_2-receptor blockers (*see* Chapter 37). The diagnosis may not be clear, because many patients have normal endoscopic examinations and upper gastrointestinal radiographs.

Alcohol is not thought to play a role in the pathogenesis of peptic ulcer disease. Unlike acute and chronic gastritis, peptic ulcer disease is not more common in alcoholics. Nevertheless, alcohol exacerbates the clinical course and severity of ulcer symptoms. It appears to act synergistically with *Helicobacter pylori* to delay healing (Lieber, 1997a). Acute bleeding from the gastric mucosa, while uncommon, can be a life-threatening emergency. Upper gastrointestinal bleeding more commonly is associated with esophageal varices, traumatic rupture of the esophagus, and clotting abnormalities.

Intestines. Many alcoholics have chronic diarrhea as a result of malabsorption in the small intestine (Addolorato *et al.*, 1997). The major symptom is frequent loose stools. The rectal fissures and pruritis ani that are frequently associated with heavy drinking probably are related to chronic diarrhea. The diarrhea is caused by structural and functional changes in the small intestine (Papa *et al.*, 1998); the intestinal mucosa has flattened villi, and digestive enzyme levels are often decreased. These changes frequently are reversible after a period of abstinence. Treatment is based on replacing essential vitamins and electrolytes, slowing transit time with an agent such as loperamide (*see* Chapter 39), and abstaining from all alcoholic beverages. Patients with severe magnesium deficiencies (serum magnesium less than 1.0 mEq/liter) or symptomatic patients (a positive Chvostek's sign or asterixis) should have replacement with 1 gram of magnesium sulfate intravenously or intramuscularly every four hours until the serum magnesium is greater than 1.0 mEq/liter (Sikkink and Fleming, 1992).

Pancreas.   Heavy alcohol use is the most common cause of both acute and chronic pancreatitis in the United States. While pancreatitis has been known to occur after a single episode of heavy alcohol use, prolonged heavy drinking is common in most cases. Acute alcoholic pancreatitis is characterized by the abrupt onset of abdominal pain, nausea, vomiting, and increased levels of serum or urine pancreatic enzymes. Computed tomography is being used increasingly for diagnostic testing. While most attacks are not fatal, hemorrhagic pancreatitis can develop and lead to shock, renal failure, respiratory failure, and death. Management usually involves intravenous fluid replacement—often with nasogastric suction—and opioid pain medication. The etiology of acute pancreatitis probably is related to a direct toxic-metabolic effect of alcohol on pancreatic acinar cells. Fatty acid esters and cytokines appear to play a major role (Schenker and Montalvo, 1998).

Two-thirds of patients with recurrent alcoholic pancreatitis will develop chronic pancreatitis. Chronic pancreatitis is treated by replacing the endocrine and exocrine deficiencies that result from pancreatic insufficiency. The development of hyperglycemia often requires insulin for control of blood-sugar levels. Pancreatic enzyme capsules containing lipase, amylase, and proteases may be necessary to treat malabsorption. The average lipase dose is 4000 units to 24,000 units with each meal and snack. Many patients with chronic pancreatitis develop a chronic pain syndrome. While opioids may be helpful, nonnarcotic methods for pain relief such as antiinflammatory drugs, tricyclic antidepressants, exercise, relaxation techniques, and self-hypnosis are preferred treatments for this population, since cross-dependence to other drugs is not uncommon among alcoholics. Treatment contracts and frequent assessments for signs of addiction are important for patients receiving chronic opioid therapy for chronic pancreatitis since alcohol-dependent patients receiving chronic opioid therapy are at greater risk for narcotic addiction than are nonalcoholic patients.

Liver.   Ethanol produces a constellation of dose-related deleterious effects in the liver (Fickert and Zatloukal, 2000). The primary effects are fatty infiltration of the liver, hepatitis, and cirrhosis. Because of its intrinsic toxicity, alcohol can injure the liver in the absence of dietary deficiencies (Lieber, 1994). The accumulation of fat in the liver is an early event and can occur in normal individuals after the ingestion of relatively small amounts of ethanol. This accumulation results from inhibition of both the tricarboxylic acid cycle and the oxidation of fat, in part owing to the generation of excess NADH produced by the actions of alcohol dehydrogenase and aldehyde dehydrogenase.

Fibrosis, resulting from tissue necrosis and chronic inflammation, is the underlying cause of alcoholic cirrhosis. Normal liver tissue is replaced by fibrous tissue.

Alcohol can affect directly stellate cells in the liver, causing deposition of collagen around terminal hepatic venules (Worner and Lieber, 1985). Chronic alcohol use is associated with transformation of stellate cells into collagen-producing, myofibroblast-like cells (Lieber, 1998). The histologic hallmark of alcoholic cirrhosis is the formation of Mallory bodies, which are thought to be related to an altered cytokeratin intermediate cytoskeleton (Denk et al., 2000). A number of underlying molecular mechanisms have been proposed.

Phospholipids are a primary target of peroxidation and can be altered by alcohol in nonhuman primate models. Phosphatidylcholine levels are decreased in hepatic mitochondria and are associated with decreased oxidase activity and oxygen consumption (Lieber et al., 1994a,b). Cytokines, such as transforming-growth factor β and tumor-necrosis factor α, can increase rates of fibrinogenesis and fibrosis within the liver (McClain et al., 1993). Acetaldehyde is thought to have a number of adverse effects including depletion of glutathione (Lieber, 2000), depletion of vitamins and trace metals, and decreased transport and secretion of proteins owing to inhibition of tubulin polymerization (Lieber, 1997b). Acetaminophen-induced hepatic toxicity (see Chapter 27) has been associated with alcoholic cirrhosis as a result of alcohol-induced increases in microsomal production of toxic acetaminophen metabolites (Whitcomb and Block, 1994; Seeff et al., 1986). Persons who are alcohol dependent may take large amounts of acetaminophen because of chronic pain. Alcohol also appears to increase intracellular free hydroxy-ethyl radical formation (Mantle and Preedy, 1999), and there is evidence that endotoxins may play a role in the initiation and exacerbation of alcohol-induced liver disease (Bode et al., 1987). Hepatitis C appears to be an important cofactor in the development of end-stage alcoholic liver disease (Regev and Jeffers, 1999).

Several strategies to treat alcoholic liver disease have been evaluated. Prednisolone may improve survival in patients with hepatic encephalopathy (Lieber, 1998). Nutrients such as S-adenosylmethionine and polyunsaturated lecithin have been found to have beneficial effects in nonhuman primates and are undergoing clinical trials. Other medications that have been tested include *oxandrolone, propythiouracil* (Orrego et al., 1987), and *colchicine* (Leiber, 1997b). At present, however, none of these drugs is approved by the United States Food and Drug Administration (FDA) for the treatment of alcoholic liver disease. The current primary treatment for liver failure, including alcoholic liver disease, is transplantation. Long-term outcome studies suggest that patients who are alcohol dependent have survival rates similar to those of patients with other types of liver disease. Alcoholics with hepatitis C may respond to interferon (McCullough and O'Connor, 1998).

Vitamins and Minerals

The almost complete lack of protein, vitamins, and most other nutrients in alcoholic beverages predisposes those who consume large quantities of alcohol to nutritional deficiencies. Alcoholics often present with these deficiencies due to decreased intake, decreased absorption, or impaired utilization of nutrients. The peripheral neuropathy, Korsakoff's psychosis, and Wernicke's encephalopathy seen in alcoholics probably are caused by deficiencies of the B-complex of vitamins (particularly thiamine), although direct toxicity produced by alcohol itself has not been ruled out (Harper, 1998). Liver failure secondary to cirrhosis, resulting in impaired clearance of toxins, also may result in alcohol-induced brain damage. Chronic alcohol abuse decreases the dietary intake of retinoids and carotenoids and enhances the metabolism of retinol by the induction of degradative enzymes (Leo and Lieber, 1999). Retinol and ethanol compete for metabolism by alcohol dehydrogenases; vitamin A supplementation therefore should be monitored carefully in alcoholics when they are consuming alcohol to avoid retinol-induced hepatotoxicity. The chronic consumption of alcohol inflicts an oxidative stress on the liver due to generation of free radicals, contributing to ethanol-induced liver injury. The antioxidant effects of α-tocopherol (vitamin E) may ameliorate some of this ethanol-induced toxicity in the liver (Nordmann, 1994). Plasma levels of α-tocopherol often are reduced in myopathic alcoholics compared to alcoholic patients without myopathy.

Chronic alcohol consumption has been implicated in osteoporosis. The reasons for this decreased bone mass remain unclear, although impaired osteoblastic activity has been implicated. Acute administration of ethanol produces an initial reduction in serum parathyroid hormone (PTH) and Ca^{2+} levels, followed by a rebound increase in PTH that does not restore Ca^{2+} levels to normal. The hypocalcemia observed after chronic alcohol intake also appears to be unrelated to effects of alcohol on PTH levels, and alcohol likely inhibits bone remodeling by a mechanism independent of Ca^{2+}-regulating hormones (Sampson, 1997). Vitamin D also may play a role. Since vitamin D requires hydroxylation in the liver for activation, alcohol-induced liver damage can indirectly affect the role of vitamin D in the intestinal and renal absorption of Ca^{2+}.

Alcoholics tend to have lowered serum and brain levels of magnesium, which may contribute to their predispositions to brain injuries such as stroke (Altura and Altura, 1999). Deficits in intracellular magnesium levels may disturb cytoplasmic and mitochondrial bioenergetic pathways, potentially leading to calcium overload and ischemia. Although there is general agreement that total magnesium levels are decreased in alcoholics, it is less clear that this also applies to ionized magnesium, the phys-

iologically active form (Hristova *et al.*, 1997). Magnesium sulfate is sometimes used in the treatment of alcohol withdrawal, but its efficacy has been questioned (Erstad and Cotugno, 1995).

Sexual Function

Despite the widespread belief that alcohol can enhance sexual activities, the opposite effect is noted more often. Many drugs of abuse, including alcohol, have disinhibiting effects that may lead initially to increased libido. With excessive, long-term use, however, alcohol often leads to a deterioration of sexual function. While alcohol cessation may reverse many sexual problems, patients with significant gonadal atrophy are less likely to respond to discontinuation of alcohol consumption (Sikkink and Fleming, 1992).

Alcohol can lead to impotence in men with both acute and chronic use. Increased blood alcohol concentrations lead to decreased sexual arousal, increased ejaculatory latency, and decreased orgasmic pleasure. The incidence of impotence may be as high as 50% in patients with chronic alcoholism. Additionally, many chronic alcoholics will develop testicular atrophy and decreased fertility. The mechanism involved in this is complex and likely involves altered hypothalamic function and a direct toxic effect of alcohol on Leydig cells. Testosterone levels may be depressed, but many men who are alcohol dependent have normal testosterone and estrogen levels. Gynecomastia is associated with alcoholic liver disease and is related to increased cellular response to estrogen and to accelerated metabolism of testosterone.

Sexual function in alcohol-dependent women is less clearly understood. Many female alcoholics complain of decreased libido, decreased vaginal lubrication, and menstrual cycle abnormalities. Their ovaries often are small and without follicular development. Some data suggest that fertility rates are lower for alcoholic women. The presence of comorbid disorders such as anorexia nervosa or bulimia is likely to aggravate the problem. The prognosis for men and women who become abstinent is favorable in the absence of significant hepatic or gonadal failure (O'Farrell *et al.*, 1997).

Hematological and Immunological Effects

Chronic alcohol use is associated with a number of anemias. Microcytic anemia can occur because of chronic blood loss and iron deficiency. Macrocytic anemias and increases in mean corpuscular volume are common and may occur in the absence of vitamin deficiencies. Normochromic anemias also can occur due to effects of chronic illness on hematopoiesis. In the presence of severe liver disease, morphological changes can include the development of burr cells, schistocytes, and ring sideroblasts. Alcohol-induced sideroblastic anemia may respond to vitamin B_6 replacement (Wartenberg, 1998). Alcohol use also is associated with reversible thrombocytopenia. Platelet counts under 20,000 are rare. Bleeding is uncommon unless there is an alteration in vitamin K_1-dependent clotting factors. Proposed mechanisms focus on platelet trapping in the spleen and marrow.

Alcohol also affects granulocytes and lymphocytes (Schirmer et al., 2000). Effects include leukopenia, alteration of lymphocyte subsets, decreased T-cell mitogenesis, and changes in immunoglobulin production. These disorders may play a role in alcohol-related liver disease. In some patients, a depression of leukocyte migration into inflamed areas may account in part for the poor resistance of alcoholics to some types of infection (i.e., Klebsiella pneumonia, listeriosis, tuberculosis). Alcohol consumption also may alter the distribution and function of lymphoid cells by disrupting cytokine regulation, in particular that involving interleukin-2 (IL-2). Alcohol appears to play a role in the development of HIV infection. In vitro studies with human lymphocytes suggest that alcohol can suppress CD4 T-lymphocyte function and concanavalin-A–stimulated IL-2 production and enhance in vitro replication of HIV. Moreover, persons who abuse alcohol have higher rates of high-risk sexual behavior.

Teratogenic Effects: Fetal Alcohol Syndrome

Although long suspected to be true, the possibility that alcohol consumption during pregnancy has deleterious consequences for the offspring has been examined rigorously only in the latter half of the twentieth century. In 1968, French researchers first noted that children born to alcoholic mothers displayed a common pattern of distinct dysmorphology that later came to be known as fetal alcohol syndrome (FAS) (Lemoine et al., 1968; Jones and Smith, 1973). The diagnosis of FAS typically is based on the observance of a triad of abnormalities in the newborn, including (1) a cluster of craniofacial abnormalities, (2) CNS dysfunction, and (3) pre- and/or postnatal stunting of growth. Hearing, language, and speech disorders also may become evident as the child ages (Church and Kaltenbach, 1997). Children who do not meet all the criteria for a diagnosis of FAS still may show physical and/or mental deficits consistent with a partial phenotype, termed fetal alcohol effects (FAEs) or alcohol-related neurodevelopmental disorders (ARNDs). The incidence of FAS is

believed to be in the range of 0.5 to 1 per thousand live births in the general population, with rates as high as 2 to 3 per thousand in African-American and Native-American populations. A lower socioeconomic status of the mother, rather than racial background per se, appears to be primarily responsible for the higher incidence of FAS observed in those groups (Abel, 1995). The incidence of FAE is likely higher than that of FAS, making alcohol consumption during pregnancy a major public health problem.

Craniofacial abnormalities commonly observed in the diagnosis of FAS consist of a pattern of microcephaly, a long and smooth philtrum, shortened palpebral fissures, a flat midface, and epicanthal folds. Magnetic resonance imaging studies demonstrate decreased volumes in the basal ganglia, corpus callosum, cerebrum, and cerebellum (Mattson et al., 1992). The severity of alcohol effects can vary greatly and depends on the drinking patterns and amount of alcohol consumed by the mother. Maternal drinking in the first trimester has been associated with craniofacial abnormalities; facial dysmorphology also is seen in mice exposed to ethanol at the equivalent time in gestation.

CNS dysfunction following in utero exposure to alcohol manifests itself in the form of hyperactivity, attention deficits, mental retardation, and/or learning disabilities. FAS is the most common cause of preventable mental retardation in the western world (Abel and Sokol, 1987), with afflicted children consistently scoring lower than their peers on a variety of IQ tests. It is now clear that FAS represents the severe end of a spectrum of alcohol effects. A number of studies have documented intellectual deficits, including mental retardation, in children not displaying the craniofacial deformities or retarded growth seen in FAS. Although cognitive improvements are seen with time, decreased IQ scores of FAS children tend to persist as they mature, indicating that the deleterious prenatal effects of alcohol are irreversible. Although a correlation exists between the amount of alcohol consumed by the mother and infant scores on mental and motor performance tests, there is considerable diversity in performance on such tests among children of mothers consuming similar quantities of alcohol. It appears that the peak blood-alcohol concentration reached may be a critical factor in determining the severity of deficits seen in the offspring. Although the evidence is not conclusive, there is a suggestion that even moderate alcohol consumption (two drinks per day) in the second trimester of pregnancy is correlated with impaired academic performance of offspring at age 6 (Goldschmidt et al., 1996). Maternal age also may be a factor. Pregnant women over the age of 30 who drink alcohol create greater risks to their children than do younger women who consume similar amounts of alcohol (Jacobson et al., 1996).

Children prenatally exposed to alcohol most frequently present with attentional deficits and hyperactivity, even in the absence of intellectual deficits or craniofacial abnormalities. Furthermore, attentional problems have been observed in the absence of hyperactivity, suggesting that the two phenomena are not necessarily related. Fetal alcohol exposure also has been identified as a risk factor for alcohol abuse by adolescents (Baer et al., 1998). Apart from the risk of FAS or FAE to the child, the intake of high amounts of alcohol by a pregnant woman, particularly during the first trimester, greatly increases the chances of spontaneous abortion.

Studies with laboratory animals have demonstrated many of the consequences of *in utero* exposure to ethanol observed in human beings, including hyperactivity, motor dysfunction, and learning deficits. In animals, *in utero* exposure to ethanol alters the expression patterns of a wide variety of proteins, changes neuronal migration patterns, and results in brain region–specific and cell type–specific alterations in neuronal numbers. Indeed, specific periods of vulnerability may exist for the various neuronal populations in the brain. Genetics also may play a role in determining vulnerability to ethanol; there are differences among strains of rats in susceptibility to the prenatal effects of ethanol. Finally, multidrug abuse, such as the concomitant administration of cocaine with ethanol, enhances fetal damage and mortality.

ACUTE ETHANOL INTOXICATION

An increased reaction time, diminished fine motor control, impulsivity, and impaired judgment become evident when the concentration of ethanol in the blood is 20 to 30 mg/dl. More than 50% of persons are grossly intoxicated by a concentration of 150 mg/dl. In fatal cases, the average concentration is about 400 mg/dl, although alcohol-tolerant individuals often can withstand these blood alcohol levels. The definition of intoxication varies by state and country. In the United States, most states set the ethanol level defined as intoxication at 80 to 100 mg/dl. There is increasing evidence that lowering the limit to 50 to 80 mg/dl can reduce motor vehicle injuries and fatalities significantly. While alcohol can be measured in saliva, urine, sweat, and blood, measurement of levels in exhaled air remain the primary method of assessing the level of intoxication.

Many factors, such as body weight and composition and the rate of absorption from the gastrointestinal tract, determine the concentration of ethanol in the blood after ingestion of a given amount of ethanol. On average, the ingestion of three standard drinks (42 grams of alcohol) on an empty stomach results in a maximum blood concentration of 67 to 92 mg/dl in men. After a mixed meal, the maximal blood concentration from three drinks is 30 to 53 mg/dl in men. Concentrations of alcohol in blood will be higher in women than in men consuming the same amount of alcohol because, on average, women are smaller than men, have less body water per unit of weight into which ethanol can distribute, and have less gastric alcohol dehydrogenase activity than men. For individuals with normal hepatic function, ethanol is metabolized at a rate of one standard drink every 60 to 90 minutes.

The characteristic signs and symptoms of alcohol intoxication are well known. Nevertheless, an erroneous diagnosis of drunkenness may occur with patients who appear inebriated but who have not ingested ethanol. Diabetic coma, for example, may be mistaken for severe alcoholic intoxication. Drug intoxication, cardiovascular accidents, and skull fractures also may be confused with alcohol intoxication. The odor of the breath of a person who has consumed ethanol is due not to ethanol vapor but to impurities in alcoholic beverages. Breath odor in a case of suspected intoxication can be misleading, as there can be other causes of breath odor similar to that after alcohol consumption. Blood alcohol levels are necessary to confirm the presence or absence of alcohol intoxication (Schuckit, 1995).

The treatment of acute alcohol intoxication is based on the severity of respiratory and CNS depression. Acute alcohol intoxication can be a medical emergency, and a number of young people die every year from this disorder. Patients who are comatose and who exhibit evidence of respiratory depression should be intubated to protect the airway and to provide ventilatory assistance. The stomach may be lavaged, but care must be taken to prevent pulmonary aspiration of the return flow. Since ethanol is freely miscible with water, ethanol can be removed from blood by hemodialysis (Schuckit, 1995).

Acute alcohol intoxication is not always associated with coma, and careful observation is the primary treatment. Usual care involves observing the patient in the emergency room for 4 to 6 hours while the patient's tissues metabolize the ingested ethanol. Blood alcohol levels will be reduced at a rate of about 15 mg/dl per hour. During this period, some individuals may display extremely violent behavior. Sedatives and antipsychotic agents have been employed to quiet such patients. Great care must be taken, however, when using sedatives to treat patients who have ingested an excessive amount of another CNS depressant, *i.e.,* ethanol.

CLINICAL USES OF ETHANOL

Dehydrated alcohol may be injected in the close proximity of nerves or sympathetic ganglia to relieve the long-lasting pain related to trigeminal neuralgia, inoperable carcinoma, and other conditions. Epidural, subarachnoid, and lumbar paravertebral injections of ethanol also have been employed for inoperable pain. For example, lumbar paravertebral injections of ethanol may destroy sympathetic ganglia and thereby produce vasodilation, relieve pain, and promote healing of lesions in patients with vascular disease of the lower extremities.

Systemically administered ethanol is confined to the treatment of poisoning by methyl alcohol and ethylene glycol (*see* Chapter 68). The accidental or intentional consumption of methanol leads to retinal and optic nerve damage, potentially resulting in blindness. Formic acid, a metabolite of methanol, is responsible for the toxicity. Treatment consists of sodium bicarbonate to combat acidosis, hemodialysis, and the administration of ethanol, which competes with methanol for metabolism by alcohol dehydrogenase.

The use of alcohol to treat patients in alcohol withdrawal or obstetrical patients with premature contractions is no longer recommended. Some medical centers continue to use alcohol to prevent or reduce the risk of alcohol withdrawal in postoperative patients, but administering a combination of a benzodiazepine with haloperidol or clonidine may be more appropriate (Spies and Rommelspacher, 1999).

MECHANISMS OF CNS EFFECTS OF ETHANOL

Acute Intoxication

Alcohol disturbs the fine balance that exists between excitatory and inhibitory influences in the brain, resulting in the anxiolysis, ataxia, and sedation that follow alcohol consumption. This is accomplished by either enhancing inhibitory or antagonizing excitatory neurotransmission. Although ethanol was long thought to act nonspecifically by disordering lipids in cell membranes, it is now believed that proteins constitute the primary molecular sites of action for ethanol. A number of putative sites at which ethanol may act have been identified, and ethanol likely produces its effects by simultaneously altering the functioning of a number of proteins that can affect neuronal excitability. A key issue has been to identify those proteins that determine neuronal excitability and are sensitive to ethanol at the low concentrations (5 to 20 mM) that produce behavioral effects.

Ion Channels. A number of different types of ion channels in the CNS are sensitive to ethanol, including representatives of the ligand-gated and G protein–regulated channel families and voltage-gated ion channels. The primary mediators of inhibitory neurotransmission in the brain are the ligand-gated $GABA_A$ receptors (*see* Chapter 12), whose function is markedly enhanced by a number of classes of sedative, hypnotic, and anesthetic agents including barbiturates, benzodiazepines, and volatile anesthetics (Mehta and Ticku, 1999). Substantial biochemical, electrophysiological, and behavioral data implicate the $GABA_A$ receptor as an important target for the *in vivo* actions of ethanol. The $GABA_A$-receptor antagonist bicuculline as well as antagonists at the benzodiazepine binding site on $GABA_A$ receptors decrease alcohol consumption in animal models (Harris *et al.*, 1998). Furthermore, administration of the $GABA_A$-receptor agonist muscimol into specific regions of the limbic system in rats can substitute for ethanol in discrimination studies (Mihic, 1999). Phosphorylation, particularly by protein kinase C (PKC), appears to play a major role in determining the $GABA_A$ receptor's sensitivity to ethanol.

Neuronal nicotinic acetylcholine receptors (*see* Chapter 9) also may be prominent molecular targets of alcohol action (Narahashi *et al.*, 1999). Both enhancement and inhibition of

nicotinic acetylcholine receptor function have been reported, depending on receptor subunit concentration and the concentrations of ethanol tested. Effects of ethanol on these receptors may be particularly important, as there is an observed association between smoking and alcohol consumption in human beings (Collins, 1990). Furthermore, several studies indicate that nicotine increases alcohol consumption in animal models (Smith *et al.*, 1999). Another member of the cation-selective ion-channel superfamily of receptors is the serotonin 5-HT_3 receptor (*see* Chapter 11). Electrophysiological studies demonstrate enhancement by ethanol of 5-HT_3-receptor function (Lovinger, 1999).

Excitatory ionotropic glutamate receptors are divided into the NMDA and nonNMDA receptor classes, with the latter being composed of kainate- and AMPA-receptor subtypes (*see* Chapter 12). Ethanol inhibits the function of the NMDA- and kainate-receptor subtypes, whereas AMPA receptors are largely resistant to alcohol (Weiner *et al.*, 1999). As with the $GABA_A$ receptors, phosphorylation of the glutamate receptor can determine sensitivity to ethanol. The nonreceptor tyrosine kinase *Fyn* phosphorylates NMDA receptors, rendering them less sensitive to inhibition by ethanol (Anders *et al.*, 1999) and perhaps explaining why null mutant mice lacking *Fyn* display significantly greater sensitivity to the hypnotic effects of ethanol. NMDA receptors play a crucial role in the development of long-term potentiation (LTP), a form of neuronal plasticity that may constitute a cellular substrate for memory. Ethanol inhibits LTP, although this does not appear to be accomplished solely through inhibition of NMDA receptors (Schummers *et al.*, 1997).

Although considerable research effort has been expended on the ligand-gated ion channels, a number of other types of channels recently have been found to be sensitive to alcohol at concentrations routinely achieved *in vivo*. Ethanol enhances the activity of large conductance, calcium-activated potassium channels in neurohypophyseal terminals (Dopico *et al.*, 1999), perhaps contributing to the reduced release of oxytocin and vasopressin after ethanol consumption. Ethanol also inhibits N- and P/Q-type Ca^{2+} channels in a manner that can be antagonized by channel phosphorylation by protein kinase A (PKA) (Solem *et al.*, 1997). Finally, G protein–coupled, inwardly rectifying potassium channels, which regulate synaptic transmission and neuronal firing rates, exhibit enhanced function in the presence of low concentrations of ethanol (Lewohl *et al.*, 1999; Kobayashi *et al.*, 1999).

Kinases and Signaling Enzymes. As mentioned above, phosphorylation by a number of protein kinases can affect the functioning of many receptors. The behavioral consequences of this were illustrated in null mutant mice lacking the γ isoform of PKC; these mice display reduced effects of ethanol measured behaviorally and a loss of enhancement by ethanol of GABA's effects measured *in vitro* (Harris *et al.*, 1995). There is some uncertainty as to whether or not ethanol directly interacts with PKC. Some investigators have reported inhibition of function, while others have seen no effect (Stubbs and Slater, 1999), perhaps due to differential sensitivity to ethanol of specific PKC isoforms. Intracellular signal transduction cascades, such as those involving MAP and tyrosine kinases and neurotrophic factor receptors, also are thought to be affected by ethanol (Valenzuela and Harris, 1997). Translocation of PKC and PKA between subcellular compartments also is sensitive to alcohol (Constantinescu *et al.*, 1999).

Ethanol enhances the activities of some of the nine isoforms of adenylyl cyclase, with the type VII isoform being the most sensitive (Tabakoff and Hoffman, 1998). This promotes increased production of cyclic AMP and thus increased activity of PKA. Ethanol's actions appear to be mediated by activation of the stimulatory G protein G_s as well as by promotion of the interaction between the G protein and the catalytic moiety of adenylyl cyclase. Decreased adenylyl cyclase activities have been reported in alcoholics (Parsian et al., 1996) and even in nondrinkers with family histories of alcoholism, suggesting that lowered adenylyl cyclase activity may be a trait marker for alcoholism (Menninger et al., 1998).

Tolerance and Dependence

Tolerance is defined as a reduced behavioral or physiological response to the same dose of ethanol (*see* Chapter 24). There is a marked acute tolerance that is detectable soon after administration of ethanol. Acute tolerance can be demonstrated by measuring behavioral impairment at the same BALs on the ascending limb of the absorption phase of the BAL-time curve (minutes after ingestion of ethanol) and on the descending limb of the curve as BALs are lowered by metabolism (one or more hours after ingestion). Behavioral impairment and subjective feelings of intoxication are much greater at a given BAL on the ascending than on the descending limb. There also is a chronic tolerance that develops in the long-term heavy drinker. In contrast to acute tolerance, chronic tolerance often has a metabolic component due to induction of alcohol-metabolizing enzymes.

Physical dependence is demonstrated by the elicitation of a withdrawal syndrome when alcohol consumption is terminated. The symptoms and severity are determined by the amount and duration of alcohol consumption and include sleep disruption, autonomic nervous system (sympathetic) activation, sleeplessness, tremors, and, in severe cases, seizures. In addition, two or more days after withdrawal, some individuals experience *delirium tremens*, characterized by hallucinations, delirium, fever, and tachycardia. This is sometimes fatal. Another aspect of dependence is craving and drug-seeking behavior, often termed *psychological dependence*.

Ethanol tolerance and physical dependence are readily studied in animal models. Lines of mice with genetic differences in tolerance and dependence have been characterized, and a search for the relevant genes is under way (Crabbe et al., 1999). Neurobiological mechanisms of tolerance and dependence are not understood completely, but chronic alcohol consumption results in changes in synaptic and intracellular signaling, likely due to changes in gene expression. Most of the systems that are acutely affected by ethanol also are affected by chronic exposure, resulting in an adaptive or maladaptive response that

can cause tolerance and dependence. In particular, chronic actions of ethanol likely require changes in signaling by glutamate and GABA receptors and intracellular systems such as PKC (Diamond and Gordon, 1997). There is an increase in NMDA receptor function after chronic alcohol ingestion, which may contribute to the CNS hyperexcitability and neurotoxicity seen during ethanol withdrawal (Tabakoff and Hoffman, 1996; Chandler et al., 1998). Arginine vasopressin, acting on V_1 receptors, maintains tolerance to ethanol in laboratory animals even after chronic ethanol administration has ceased (Hoffman et al., 1990).

The neurobiological basis of the switch from controlled, volitional alcohol use to compulsive and uncontrolled addiction remains obscure. Impairment of the dopaminergic reward system and the resultant increase in alcohol consumption in an attempt to regain activation of the system is a possibility. In addition, the prefrontal cortex is particularly sensitive to damage from alcohol abuse and influences decision making and emotion, processes clearly compromised in the alcoholic (Pfefferbaum et al., 1998). Thus, impairment of executive function in cortical regions by chronic alcohol consumption may be responsible for some of the lack of judgment and control that is expressed as obsessive alcohol consumption. It should be reiterated that the loss of brain volume and impairment of function seen in the chronic alcoholic is at least partially reversible by abstinence but will worsen with continued drinking (Pfefferbaum et al., 1998). Obviously, early diagnosis and treatment of alcoholism is important, as it can limit the brain damage that promotes the spiraling descent into progressively severe addiction.

Genetic Influences

The concept of alcoholism as a disease was first articulated by Jellinek in 1960; the subsequent acceptance of alcoholism and addiction as "brain diseases" led to a search for biological causes. Studies of rats and mice carried out in Chile, Finland, and the United States showed significant heritabilities (roughly 60%) for many behavioral actions of alcohol, including sedation, ataxia, and, most notably, consumption (Crabbe and Harris, 1991). It has long been appreciated that alcoholism "runs in families," and definitive studies of genetics and human alcoholism appeared about 30 years ago. A series of adoption (cross-fostering) and twin studies showed that human alcohol dependence has a genetic component. It is important to note that, although the genetic contribution has varied among studies, it is generally in the range of 40% to 60%, which means that environmental variables also are critical for individual susceptibility to alcoholism (Begleiter and Kissin, 1995).

The search for the genes and alleles responsible for alcoholism is complicated by the polygenetic nature of the disease and the general difficulty in defining the multiple genes responsible for complex diseases. One area of research that has been fruitful has been the study of why some populations (mainly Asian) are protected from alcoholism. This has been found to be caused by genetic differences in alcohol- and aldehyde-metabolizing enzymes. Specifically, genetic variants of alcohol dehydrogenase that exhibit high activity and variants of aldehyde dehydrogenase that exhibit low activity protect against heavy drinking. This is because alcohol consumption by individuals who have these variants results in accumulation of acetaldehyde, which produces a variety of unpleasant effects (Li, 2000). These effects are similar to those of disulfiram therapy (*see* below), but the prophylactic, genetic form of inhibition of alcohol consumption is more effective than the pharmacotherapeutic approach, which is applied after alcoholism has developed.

In contrast to these protective genetic variants, there is little information about genes responsible for increased risk for alcoholism. The recent history of psychiatric genetics is that genes identified in one study are not consistently found in other populations. This also is true for alcoholism. Sequence differences in several candidate genes from alcoholics, including genes for a dopamine receptor (D_2) and for serotonin-related transporters and enzymes, are not consistently different from the sequences of those genes from nonalcoholic subjects. Several large-scale genetic studies of alcoholism currently are in progress, and these efforts, together with genetic studies in laboratory animals, should lead to identification of alcoholism susceptibility genes. It is possible that these studies also will allow genetic classification of subtypes of alcoholism and thereby resolve some of the inconsistencies among study populations. For example, antisocial alcoholism is linked with a polymorphism in a serotonin receptor ($5HT_{1B}$), but there is no association of this gene with nonantisocial alcoholism (Lappalainen *et al.*, 1998).

Another approach to understanding the inherited biology of alcoholism is to ask what behavioral or functional differences exist between individuals with high and low genetic risks for alcoholism. This may be accomplished by studying young social drinkers with many or few alcoholic relatives [family history positive (FHP) and family history negative (FHN)]. Brain imaging by positron emission tomography has been used in this context. A family history of alcoholism is linked to lower cerebellar metabolism and a blunted effect of a benzodiazepine (lorazepam) on cerebellar metabolism (Volkow *et al.*, 1995). Because $GABA_A$ receptors are the molecular site of benzodiazepine action, these results suggest that a genetic predisposition to alcoholism may be reflected in abnormal function of $GABA_A$ receptors.

Schuckit and colleagues have studied actions of alcohol in FHP college students and have followed the study subjects for almost 20 years to determine which ones will develop alcoholism or alcohol abuse. It is remarkable that a blunted behavioral and physiological response to alcohol in the original test is associated with a significantly greater risk for later development of alcohol-related problems (Schuckit, 1994). The genes that control initial sensitivity to ethanol are not known, but they may be important for risk for alcohol abuse. At present, there is little evidence that the genes important for alcoholism also are important for other addictions and diseases with the exception of tobacco use. Studies with twins indicate a common genetic vulnerability for alcohol and nicotine dependence (True *et al.*, 1999), which is consistent with the high rate of smoking among alcoholics.

PHARMACOTHERAPY OF ALCOHOLISM

Currently, only two drugs are approved in the United States for treatment of alcoholism: *disulfiram* (ANTABUSE) and *naltrexone* (REVIA). Disulfiram has a long history of use but has fallen out of favor because of its side effects and compliance problems. Naltrexone was introduced more recently. The goal of both of these medications is to assist the patient in maintaining abstinence.

Naltrexone

Naltrexone was approved by the FDA for treatment of alcoholism in 1994. It is chemically related to the highly selective opioid-receptor antagonist *naloxone* (NARCAN), but it has higher oral bioavailability and a longer duration of action than does naloxone. Neither drug has appreciable opioid-receptor agonist effects. These drugs were used initially in the treatment of opioid overdose and dependence because of their ability to antagonize all of the actions of opioids (*see* Chapters 23 and 24). There were suggestions from both animal research and clinical experience that naltrexone might reduce alcohol consumption and craving, and this was confirmed in clinical trials in the early 1990s (*see* O'Malley *et al.*, 2000; Johnson and Ait-Daoud, 2000). There is evidence that naltrexone blocks activation by alcohol of dopaminergic pathways in the brain that are thought to be critical to reward.

Naltrexone helps to maintain abstinence by reducing the urge to drink and increasing control when a "slip" occurs. It is not a "cure" for alcoholism and does not prevent relapse in all patients. Naltrexone works best when used in conjunction with some form of psychosocial therapy, such as cognitive behavioral therapy (Anton *et al.*, 1999). It is typically administered after detoxification and given at a dose of 50 mg per day for several months. Good compliance is important to ensure the therapeutic value of naltrexone and has proven to be a problem for some patients (Johnson and Ait-Daoud, 2000). The most common side effect of naltrexone is nausea, which is more common in women than in men and subsides if the patients remain abstinent (O'Malley *et al.*, 2000). When given in excessive doses, naltrexone can cause liver damage. It is contraindicated in patients with liver failure or acute hepatitis and should be used only after careful consideration in patients with active liver disease.

Nalmefene (REVEX) is another opioid antagonist that appears promising in preliminary clinical tests. It has a number of advantages over naltrexone, including greater oral bioavailability, longer duration of action, and lack of dose-dependent problems with liver toxicity.

Disulfiram

Disulfiram (tetraethylthiuram disulfide; ANTABUSE) was taken in the course of an investigation of its potential anthelminthic usefulness by two Danish physicians, who became ill at a cocktail party and were quick to realize that the compound had altered their responses to alcohol. They initiated a series of pharmacological and clinical studies that provided the basis for the use of disulfiram as an adjunct in the treatment of chronic alcoholism. Similar responses to alcohol ingestion are produced by various congeners of disulfiram, cyanamide, the fungus *Coprinus atramentarius,* the hypoglycemic sulfonylureas, metronidazole, certain cephalosporins, and the ingestion of animal charcoal.

Disulfiram, given alone, is a relatively nontoxic substance, but it alters the metabolism of alcohol and causes the blood acetaldehyde concentration to rise to five to ten times above the level achieved when ethanol is given to an individual not pretreated with disulfiram. Acetaldehyde, produced as a result of the oxidation of ethanol by alcohol dehydrogenase, ordinarily does not accumulate in the body, because it is further oxidized almost as soon as it is formed, primarily by aldehyde dehydrogenase. Following the administration of disulfiram, both cytosolic and mitochondrial forms of this enzyme are irreversibly inactivated to varying degrees, and the concentration of acetaldehyde rises. It is unlikely that disulfiram itself is responsible for the enzyme inactivation *in vivo;* several active metabolites of the drug, especially diethylthiomethylcarbamate, behave as suicide-substrate inhibitors of aldehyde dehydrogenase *in vitro.* These metabolites reach significant concentrations in plasma following the administration of disulfiram (Johansson, 1992).

The ingestion of alcohol by individuals previously treated with disulfiram gives rise to marked signs and symptoms. Within about 5 to 10 minutes, the face feels hot, and soon afterwards it is flushed and scarlet in appearance. As the vasodilation spreads over the whole body, intense throbbing is felt in the head and neck, and a pulsating headache may develop. Respiratory difficulties, nausea, copious vomiting, sweating, thirst, chest pain, considerable hypotension, orthostatic syncope, marked uneasiness, weakness, vertigo, blurred vision, and confusion are observed. The facial flush is replaced by pallor, and the blood pressure may fall to shock levels. Disulfiram and/or its metabolites can inhibit many enzymes with crucial sulfhydryl groups, and it thus has a wide spectrum of biological effects. It inhibits hepatic microsomal drug–metabolizing enzymes and thereby interferes with the metabolism of phenytoin, chlordiazepoxide, barbiturates, and other drugs.

Disulfiram by itself is usually innocuous, but it may cause acneform eruptions, urticaria, lassitude, tremor, restlessness, headache, dizziness, a garlic-like or metallic taste, and mild gastrointestinal disturbances. Peripheral neuropathies, psychosis, and acetonemia also have been reported. Alarming reactions may result from the ingestion of even small amounts of alcohol in persons being treated with disulfiram. The use of disulfiram as a therapeutic agent thus is not without danger, and it should be attempted only under careful medical and nursing supervision. Patients must be warned that as long as they are taking disulfiram, the ingestion of alcohol in any form will make them sick and may endanger their lives. Patients must learn to avoid disguised forms of alcohol, as in sauces, fermented vinegar, cough syrups, and even after-shave lotions and back rubs.

The drug never should be administered until the patient has abstained from alcohol for at least 12 hours. In the initial phase of treatment, a maximal daily dose of 500 mg is given for 1 to 2 weeks. Maintenance dosage then ranges from 125 to 500 mg daily, depending on tolerance to side effects. Unless sedation is prominent, the daily dose should be taken in the morning, the time when the resolve not to drink may be strongest. Sensitization to alcohol may last as long as 14 days after the last ingestion of disulfiram because of the slow rate of restoration of aldehyde dehydrogenase (Johansson, 1992).

Acamprosate

Acamprosate (*N*-acetylhomotaurine, calcium salt), an analog of GABA widely used in Europe for the treatment of alcoholism, is not yet approved for use in the United States. A number of double-blind, placebo-controlled studies have demonstrated that acamprosate decreases drinking frequency and reduces relapse drinking in abstinent alcoholics. It acts in a dose-dependent manner (1.3 to 2 g/day; Paille *et al.,* 1995) and appears to have efficacy similar to that of naltrexone. Studies in laboratory animals have shown that acamprosate decreases alcohol intake without affecting food or water consumption. Acamprosate generally is well tolerated by patients, with diarrhea being the main side effect (Garbutt *et al.,* 1999). No abuse liability has been noted. The drug undergoes minimal metabolism in the liver, is primarily excreted by the kidneys, and has an elimination half-life of 18 hours after oral administration (Wilde and Wagstaff, 1997). Concomitant use of disulfiram appears to increase the effectiveness of acamprosate, without any adverse drug interactions being noted (Besson *et al.,* 1998). The mechanism of action of acamprosate is obscure, although there is some evidence that it affects the function of the NMDA subtype of ionotropic glutamate receptors in brain. Whether or not this modulation of NMDA receptor function is responsible for the drug's therapeutic effects is unknown (Johnson and Ait-Daoud, 2000).

Other Agents

Ondansetron, a 5-HT$_3$-receptor antagonist and antiemetic drug (*see* Chapters 11 and 38), reduces alcohol consumption in laboratory animals and currently is being tested in alcoholic subjects. Preliminary findings suggest that ondansetron is effective in the treatment of early-onset alcoholics, who respond poorly to psychosocial treatment alone, although the drug does not appear to work well in other types of alcoholics (Johnson and Ait-Daoud, 2000). Ondansetron administration lowers the amount of alcohol consumed, particularly by drinkers who consume fewer than ten drinks per day (Sellers *et al.,* 1994). It also decreases the subjective effects of ethanol on 6 of 10 scales measured, including the desire to drink (Johnson *et al.,* 1993a), while at the same time not having any effect on the pharmacokinetics of ethanol (Johnson *et al.*, 1993b).

Initial studies suggested that lithium or selective serotonin-reuptake inhibitors (SSRIs) might be useful in reducing alcohol consumption, but subsequent clinical trials have not provided evidence for beneficial effects (*see* Garbutt *et al.*, 1999). There have been limited clinical tests of several dopaminergic agonists and antagonists, serotonergic agonists, and calcium channel antagonists in reducing ethanol consumption, but the results with these agents generally have not been encouraging (Johnson and Ait-Daoud, 2000). An emerging approach is treatment with a combination of two or more drugs, particularly combining drugs with different mechanisms of action (*e.g.*, naltrexone plus ondansetron or acamprosate); this approach may be useful if a limited therapeutic response is obtained with a single agent.

PROSPECTUS

Alcoholism and alcohol abuse are major health problems and yet have not received the attention fitting their social and economic impacts. Many cases remain undetected, undiagnosed, and untreated until they have progressed to the points of advanced or fatal organ damage. As with many other diseases, progress will require effective prevention measures, early diagnosis, and effective treatments. At present, these modalities are in the early stages of development and are inadequate. In particular, detection and diagnosis would be facilitated by biomarkers with high selectivity and specificity for alcoholism (rather than for liver damage); such markers also might allow biological classification of subtypes of alcoholism. The pharmacotherapy of alcoholism also is in its infancy, and more effective treatments are essential to limiting the progression of the disease. It is reasonable to ask why such an important health problem still receives so little attention; part of the answer must be that alcoholism still retains the stigma of a moral failing rather than a biological disease. Physicians have an opportunity and an obligation to change this perception.

For further discussion of alcoholism and alcoholic liver disease, *see* Chapters 298 and 386 in *Harrison's Principles of Internal Medicine,* 14th ed., McGraw-Hill, New York, 1998.

BIBLIOGRAPHY

Addolorato, G., Montalto, M., Capristo, E., Certo, M., Fedeli, G., Gentiloni, N., Stefanini, G.F., and Gasbarrini, G. Influence of alcohol on gastrointestinal motility: lactulose breath hydrogen testing in orocecal transit time in chronic alcoholics, social drinkers, and teetotaler subjects. *Hepatogastroenterology,* 1997, *44*:1076–1081.

Anders, D.L., Blevins, T., Sutton, G., Swope, S., Chandler, L.J., and Woodward, J.J. Fyn tyrosine kinase reduces the ethanol inhibition of recombinant NR1/NR2A but not NR1/NR2B NMDA receptors expressed in HEK 293 cells. *J. Neurochem.,* 1999, *72*:1389–1393.

Anton, R.F., Moak, D.H., Waid, L.R., Latham, P.K., Malcolm, R.J., and Dias, J.K. Naltrexone and cognitive behavioral therapy for the treatment of outpatient alcoholics: results of a placebo-controlled trial. *Am. J. Psychiatry,* 1999, *156*:1758–1764.

Baer, J.S., Barr, H.M., Bookstein, F.L., Sampson, P.D., and Streissguth, A.P. Prenatal alcohol exposure and family history of alcoholism in the etiology of adolescent alcohol problems. *J. Stud. Alcohol.,* 1998, *59*:533–543.

Beckemeier, M.E., and Bora, P.S. Fatty acid ethyl esters: potentially toxic products of myocardial ethanol metabolism. *J. Mol. Cell. Cardiol.,* 1998, *30*:2487–2494.

Besson, J., Aeby, F., Kasas, A., Lehert, P., and Potgieter, A. Combined efficacy of acamprosate and disulfiram in the treatment of alcoholism: a controlled study. *Alcohol. Clin. Exp. Res.,* 1998, *22*:573–579.

Bode, C., Kugler, V., and Bode, J.C. Endotoxemia in patients with alcoholic and non-alcoholic cirrhosis and in subjects with no evidence of chronic liver disease following acute alcohol excess. *J. Hepatol.,* 1987, *4*:8–14.

Clarkson, P.M., and Reichsman, F. The effect of ethanol on exercise-induced muscle damage. *J. Stud. Alcohol,* 1990, *51*:19–23.

Colantonio, D., Casale, R., Desiati, P., De Michele, G., Mammarella, M., and Pasqualetti, P. A possible role of atrial natriuretic peptide in ethanol-induced acute diuresis. *Life Sci.,* 1991, *48*:635–642.

Collins, G.B., Brosnihan, K.B., Zuti, R.A., Messina, M., and Gupta, M.K. Neuroendocrine, fluid balance, and thirst responses to alcohol in alcoholics. *Alcohol. Clin. Exp. Res.,* 1992, *16*:228–233.

Constantinescu, A., Diamond, I., and Gordon, A.S. Ethanol-induced translocation of cAMP-dependent protein kinase to the nucleus. Mechanism and functional consequences. *J. Biol. Chem.,* 1999, *274*: 26985–26991.

Denk, H., Stumptner, C., and Zatloukal, K. Mallory bodies revisited. *J. Hepatol.,* 2000, *32*:689–702.

Fernandez-Sola, J., Estruch, R., Grau, J.M., Pare, J.C., Rubin, E., and Urbano-Marquez, A. The relation of alcoholic myopathy to cardiomyopathy. *Ann. Intern. Med.,* 1994, *120*:529–536.

Gaziano, J.M., Buring, J.E., Breslow, J.L., Goldhaber, S.Z., Rosner, B., VanDenburgh, M., Willett, W., and Hennekens, C.H. Moderate alcohol intake, increased levels of high-density lipoprotein and its subfractions, and decreased risk of myocardial infarction. *N. Engl. J. Med.,* 1993, *329*:1829–1834.

Goldschmidt, L., Richardson, G.A., Stoffer, D.S., Geva, D., and Day, N.L. Prenatal alcohol exposure and academic achievement at age six: a nonlinear fit. *Alcohol. Clin. Exp. Res.,* 1996, *20*:763–770.

Hansagi, H., Romelsjo, A., Gerhardsson de Verdier, M., Andreasson, S., and Leifman, A. Alcohol consumption and stroke mortality.

20-year follow-up of 15,077 men and women. *Stroke,* **1995,** *26*:1768–1773.

Harris, R.A., McQuilkin, S.J., Paylor, R., Abeliovich, A., Tonegawa, S., and Wehner, J.M. Mutant mice lacking the γ isoform of protein kinase C show decreased behavioral actions of ethanol and altered function of γ-aminobutyrate type A receptors. *Proc. Natl. Acad. Sci. U.S.A.,* **1995,** *92*:3658–3662.

Hristova, E.N., Rehak, N.N., Cecco, S., Ruddel, M., Herion, D., Eckardt, M., Linnoila, M., and Elim, R.J. Serum ionized magnesium in chronic alcoholism: is it really decreased? *Clin. Chem.,* **1997,** *43*:394–399.

Iwase, S., Matsukawa, T., Ishihara, S., Tanaka, A., Tanabe, K., Danbara, A., Matsuo, M., Sugiyama, Y., and Mano, T. Effect of oral ethanol intake on muscle sympathetic nerve activity and cardiovascular functions in humans. *J. Auton. Nerv. Syst.,* **1995,** *54*:206–214.

Jacobson, J.L., Jacobson, S.W., and Sokol, R.J. Increased vulnerability to alcohol-related birth defects in the offspring of mothers over 30. *Alcohol. Clin. Exp. Res.,* **1996,** *20*:359–363.

Johnson, B.A., and Ait-Daoud, N. Neuropharmacological treatments for alcoholism: scientific basis and clinical findings. *Psychopharmacology (Berl.),* **2000,** *149*:327–344.

Johnson, B.A., Campling, G.M., Griffiths, P., and Cowen, P.J. Attenuation of some alcohol-induced mood changes and the desire to drink by 5-HT$_3$ receptor blockade: a preliminary study in healthy male volunteers. *Psychopharmacology (Berl.),* **1993a,** *112*:142–144.

Johnson, B.A., Rue, J., and Cowen, P.J. Ondansetron and alcohol pharmacokinetics. *Psychopharmacology (Berl.),* **1993b,** *112*:145.

Jones, K.L., and Smith, D.W. Recognition of the fetal alcohol syndrome in early infancy. *Lancet,* **1973,** *2*:999–1001.

Kobayashi, T., Ikeda, K., Kojima, H., Niki, H., Yano, R., Yoshioka, T., and Kumanishi, T. Ethanol opens G-protein-activated inwardly rectifying K$^+$ channels. *Nat. Neurosci.,* **1999,** *2*:1091–1097.

Kortelainen, M.L. Hyperthermia deaths in Finland in 1970–86. *Am. J. Forensic Med. Pathol.,* **1991,** *12*:115–118.

Langer, R.D., Criqui, M.H., and Reed, D.M. Lipoproteins and blood pressure as biological pathways for effect of moderate alcohol consumption on coronary heart disease. *Circulation,* **1992,** *85*:910–915.

Lappalainen, J., Long, J.C., Eggert, M., Ozaki, N., Robin, R.W., Brown, G.L., Naukkarinen, H., Virkkunen, M., Linnoila, M., and Goldman, D. Linkage of antisocial alcoholism to the serotonin 5-HT1B receptor gene in 2 populations. *Arch. Gen. Psychiatry,* **1998,** *55*:989–994.

Lemoine, P., Harousseau, H., Borteyru, J.-P., and Menuet, J.-C. Les enfants de perents alcooliques: anomalies observees. A propos de 127 cas. *Quest Medicale,* **1968,** *25*:476–482.

Leppaluoto, J., Vuolteenaho, O., Arjamaa, O., and Ruskoaho, H. Plasma immunoreactive atrial natriuretic peptide and vasopressin after ethanol intake in man. *Acta. Physiol. Scand.,* **1992,** *144*:121–127.

Lewohl, J.M., Wilson, W.R., Mayfield, R.D., Brozowski, S.J., Morrisett, R.A., and Harris, R.A. G-protein–coupled inwardly rectifying potassium channels are targets of alcohol action. *Nat. Neurosci.,* **1999,** *2*:1084–1090.

Lieber, C.S., Robins, S.J., and Leo, M.A. Hepatic phosphatidylethanolamine methyltransferase activity is decreased by ethanol and increased by phosphatidylcholine. *Alcohol. Clin. Exp. Res.,* **1994b,** *18*:592–595.

Lieber, C.S., Robins, S.J., Li, J., DeCarli, L.M., Max, K.M., Fasulo, J.M., and Leo, M.A. Phosphatidylcholine protects against fibrosis and cirrhosis in the baboon. *Gastroenterology,* **1994a,** *106*:152–159.

Mattson, S.N., Riley, E.P., Jernigan, T.L., Ehlers, C.L., Delis, D.C., Jones, K.L., Stern, C., Johnson, K.A., Hesselink, J.R., and Bellugi, U. Fetal alcohol syndrome: a case report of neuropsychological, MRI, and EEG assessment of two children. *Alcohol. Clin. Exp. Res.,* **1992,** *16*:1001–1003.

McCullough, A.J., and O'Connor, J.F. Alcoholic liver disease: proposed recommendations for the American College of Gastroenterology. *Am. J. Gastroenterol.,* **1998,** *93*:2022–2036.

Menninger, J.A., Baron, A.E., and Tabakoff, B. Effects of abstinence and family history for alcoholism on platelet adenylyl cyclase activity. *Alcohol. Clin. Exp. Res.,* **1998,** *22*:1955–1961.

Moreira, L.B., Fuchs, F.D., Moraes, R.S., Bredemeier, M., and Duncan, B.B. Alcohol intake and blood pressure: the importance of time elapsed since last drink. *J. Hypertens.,* **1998,** *16*:175–180.

Numminen, H., Hillbom, M., and Juvela, S. Platelets, alcohol consumption, and onset of brain infarction. *J. Neurol. Neurosurg. Psychiatry,* **1996,** *61*:376–380.

O'Farrell, T.J., Choquette, K.A., Cutter, H.S., and Birchler, G.R. Sexual satisfaction and dysfunction in marriages of male alcoholics: comparison with nonalcoholic maritally conflicted and nonconflicted couples. *J. Stud. Alcohol.,* **1997,** *58*:91–99.

O'Malley, S.S., Krishnan-Sarin, S., Farren, C., and O'Connor, P.G. Naltrexone-induced nausea in patients treated for alcohol dependence: clinical predictors and evidence for opioid-mediated effects. *J. Clin. Psychopharmacol.,* **2000,** *20*:69–76.

Orrego, H., Blake, J.E., Blendis, L.M., Comptom, K.V., and Israel, Y. Long-term treatment of alcoholic liver disease with propylthiouracil. *N. Engl. J. Med.,* **1987,** *317*:1421–1427.

Paille, F.M., Guelfi, J.D., Perkins, A.C., Royer, R.J., Steru, L., and Parot, P. Double-blind randomized multicentre trial of acamprosate in maintaining abstinence from alcohol. *Alcohol Alcohol.,* **1995,** *30*:239–247.

Panzak, G., Tarter, R., Murali, S., Switala, J., Lu, S., Maher, B., and Van Thiel, D.H. Isometric muscle strength in alcoholic and nonalcoholic liver-transplantation candidates. *Am. J. Drug Alcohol Abuse,* **1998,** *24*:449–512.

Papa, A., Tursi, A., Cammarota, G., Certo, M., Cuoco, L., Montalto, M., Cianci, R., Papa, V., Fedeli, P., Fedeli, G., and Gasbarrini, G. Effect of moderate and heavy alcohol consumption on intestinal transit time. *Panminerva Med.,* **1998,** *40*:183–185.

Parsian, A., Todd, R.D., Cloninger, C.R., Hoffman, P.L., Ovchinnikova, L., Ikeda, H., and Tabakoff, B. Platelet adenylyl cyclase activity in alcoholics and subtypes of alcoholics. WHO/ISBRA Study Clinical Centers. *Alcohol. Clin. Exp. Res.,* **1996,** *20*:745–751.

Pfefferbaum, A., Sullivan, E.V., Rosenbloom, M.J., Mathalon, D.H., and Lim, K.O. A controlled study of cortical gray matter and ventricular changes in alcoholic men over a 5-year interval. *Arch. Gen. Psychiatry,* **1998,** *55*:905–912.

Proano, E., and Perbeck, L. Effect of exposure to heat and intake of ethanol on the skin circulation and temperature in ischaemic limbs. *Clin. Physiol.,* **1994,** *14*:305–310.

Qureshi, A.I., Suarez, J.I., Parekh, P.D., Sung, G., Geocadin, R., Bhardwaj, A., Tamargo, R.J., and Ulatowski, J.A. Risk factors for multiple intracranial aneurysms. *Neurosurgery,* **1998,** *43*:22–26.

Ridker, P.M., Vaughan, D.E., Stampfer, M.J., Glynn, R.J., and Hennekens, C.H. Association of moderate alcohol consumption and plasma concentration of endogenous tissue-type plasminogen activator. *JAMA,* **1994,** *272*:929–933.

Rimm, E.B., Williams, P., Fosher, K., Criqui, M., and Stampfer, M.J. Moderate alcohol intake and lower risk of coronary heart disease:

meta-analysis of effects on lipids and haemostatic factors. *BMJ,* **1999,** *319:*1523–1528.

Rossinen, J., Sinisalo, J., Partanen, J., Nieminen, M.S., and Viitasalo, M. Effects of acute alcohol infusion on duration and dispersion of QT interval in male patients with coronary artery disease and in healthy controls. *Clin. Cardiol.,* **1999,** *22:*591–594.

Schuckit, M.A. Low level of response to alcohol as a predictor of future alcoholism. *Am. J. Psychiatry,* **1994,** *151:*184–189.

Schummers, J., Bentz, S., and Browning, M.D. Ethanol's inhibition of LTP may not be mediated solely via direct effects on the NMDA receptor. *Alcohol. Clin. Exp. Res.,* **1997,** *21:*404–408.

Sellers, E.M., Toneatto, T., Romach, M.K., Somer, G.R., Sobell, L.C., and Sobell, M.B. Clinical efficacy of the 5-HT$_3$ antagonist ondansetron in alcohol abuse and dependence. *Alcohol. Clin. Exp. Res.,* **1994,** *18:*879–885.

Seppa, K., Laippala, P., and Sillanaukee, P. High diastolic blood pressure: common among women who are heavy drinkers. *Alcohol. Clin. Exp. Res.,* **1996,** *20:*47–51.

Smith, B.R., Horan, J.T., Gaskin, S., and Amit, Z. Exposure to nicotine enhances acquisition of ethanol drinking by laboratory rats in a limited access paradigm. *Psychopharmacology (Berl.),* **1999,** *142:*408–412.

Solem, M., McMahon, T., and Messing, R.O. Protein kinase A regulates inhibition of N- and P/Q-type calcium channels by ethanol in PC12 cells. *J. Pharmacol. Exp. Ther.,* **1997,** *282:*1487–1495.

Stein, J.H., Keevil, J.G., Wiebe, D.A., Aeschlimann, S., and Folts, J.D. Purple grape juice improves endothelial function and reduces the susceptibility of LDL cholesterol to oxidation in patients with coronary artery disease. *Circulation,* **1999,** *100:*1050–1055.

True, W.R., Xian, H., Scherrer, J.F., Madden, P.A., Bucholz, K.K., Heath, A.C., Eisen, S.A., Lyons, M.J., Goldberg, J., and Tsuang, M. Common genetic vulnerability for nicotine and alcohol dependence in men. *Arch. Gen. Psychiatry,* **1999,** *56:*655–661.

Urbano-Marquez, A., Estruch, R., Fernandez-Sola, J., Nicolas, J.M., Pare, J.C., and Rubin, E. The greater risk of alcoholic cardiomyopathy and myopathy in women compared with men. *JAMA,* **1995,** *274:*149–154.

Vernet, M., Cadefau, J.A., Balaque, A., Grau, J.M., Urbano-Marquez, A.U., and Cusso, R. Effect of chronic alcoholism on human muscle glycogen and glucose metabolism. *Alcohol. Clin. Exp. Res.,* **1995,** *19:*1295–1299.

Volkow, N.D., Wang, G.J., Begleiter, H., Hitzemann, R., Pappas, N., Burr, G., Pascani, K., Wong, C., Fowler, J.S., and Wolf, A.P. Regional brain metabolic response to lorazepam in subjects at risk for alcoholism. *Alcohol. Clin. Exp. Res.,* **1995,** *19:*510–516.

Volkow, N.D., Wang, G.J., Hitzemann, R., Fowler, J.S., Overall, J.E., Burr, G., and Wolf, A.P. Recovery of brain glucose metabolism in detoxified alcoholics. *Am. J. Psychiatry,* **1994,** *151:*178–183.

Wassif, W.S., Preedy, V.R., Summers, B., Duane, P., Leigh, N., and Peters, T.J. The relationship between muscle fibre atrophy factor, plasma carnosinase activities, and muscle RNA and protein composition in chronic alcoholic myopathy. *Alcohol Alcohol.,* **1993,** *28:*325–331.

Weiner, J.L., Dunwiddie, T.V., and Valenzuela, C.F. Ethanol inhibition of synaptically evoked kainate responses in rat hippocampal CA3 pyramidal neurons. *Mol. Pharmacol.,* **1999,** *56:*85–90.

Whitcomb, D.C., and Block, G.D. Association of acetaminophen hepatotoxicity with fasting and ethanol use. *JAMA,* **1994,** *272:*1845–1850.

Worner, T.M., and Lieber, C.S. Perivenular fibrosis as precursor lesion of cirrhosis. *JAMA,* **1985,** *254:*627–630.

MONOGRAPHS AND REVIEWS

Abel, E.L. An update on incidence of FAS: FAS is not an equal opportunity birth defect. *Neurotoxicol. Teratol.,* **1995,** *17:*437–443.

Abel, E.L., and Sokol, R.J. Incidence of fetal alcohol syndrome and economic impact of FAS-related anomalies. *Drug Alcohol Depend.,* **1987,** *19:*51–70.

Altura, B.M., and Altura, B.T. Association of alcohol in brain injury, headaches, and stroke with braintissue and serum levels of ionized magnesium: a review of recent findings and mechanisms of action. *Alcohol,* **1999,** *19:*119–130.

Begleiter, H., and Kissin, B. eds. *The Genetics of Alcoholism.* Oxford University Press, New York, **1995.**

Braunwald, E., ed. *Heart Disease: A Textbook of Cardiovascular Medicine.* Saunders, Philadelphia, **1997.**

Chandler, L.J., Harris, R.A., and Crews, F.T. Ethanol tolerance and synaptic plasticity. *Trends Pharmacol. Sci.,* **1998,** *19:*491–495.

Church, M.W., and Kaltenbach, J.A. Hearing, speech, language, and vestibular disorders in the fetal alcohol syndrome: a literature review. *Alcohol. Clin. Exp. Res.,* **1997,** *21:*495–512.

Collins, A.C. Interactions of ethanol and nicotine at the receptor level. *Recent Dev. Alcohol.,* **1990,** *8:*221–231.

Crabbe, J.C., and Harris, R.A., eds. *The Genetic Basis of Alcohol and Drug Actions.* Plenum Press, New York, **1991.**

Crabbe, J.C., Phillips, T.J., Buck, K.J., Cunningham, C.L., and Belknap, J.K. Identifying genes for alcohol and drug sensitivity: recent progress and future directions. *Trends Neurosci.,* **1999,** *22:*173–179.

Diamond, I., and Gordon, A.S. Cellular and molecular neuroscience of alcoholism. *Physiol. Rev.,* **1997,** *77:*1–20.

Dopico, A.M., Chu, B., Lemos, J.R., and Treistman, S.N. Alcohol modulation of calcium-activated potassium channels. *Neurochem. Int.,* **1999,** *35:*103–106.

Dudley, R. Evolutionary origins of human alcoholism in primate frugivory. *Q. Rev. Biol.,* **2000,** *75:*3–15.

Erstad, B.L., and Cotugno, C.L. Management of alcohol withdrawal. *Am. J. Health Syst. Pharm.,* **1995,** *52:*697–709.

Fickert, P., and Zatloukal, K. Pathogenesis of alcoholic liver disease. In, *Handbook of Alcoholism* (Zernig, G., Saria, A., Kurz, M., and O'Malley, S., eds.) CRC Press, Boca Raton, FL., **2000,** pp. 317–323.

Garbutt, J.C., West, S.L., Carey, T.S., Lohr, K.N., and Crews, F.T. Pharmacological treatment of alcohol dependence: a review of the evidence. *JAMA,* **1999,** *281:*1318–1325.

Grogan, J.R., and Kochar, M.S. Alcohol and hypertension. *Arch. Fam. Med.,* **1994,** *3:*150–154.

Harper, C. The neuropathology of alcohol-specific brain damage, or does alcohol damage the brain? *J. Neuropathol. Exp. Neurol.,* **1998,** *57:*101–110.

Harris, R.A., Mihic, S.J., and Valenzuela, C.F. Alcohol and benzodiazepines: recent mechanistic studies. *Drug Alcohol Depend.,* **1998,** *51:*155–164.

Hillbom, M., Juvela, S., and Karttunen, V. Mechanisms of alcohol-related strokes, In, *Alcohol and Cardiovascular Diseases.* (Goode, J., ed.) John Wiley & Sons, Chichester, England, **1998,** p. 193.

Hoffman, P.L., Ishizawa, H., Giri, P.R., Dave, J.R., Grant, K.A., Liu, L.I., Gulya, K., and Tabakoff, B. The role of arginine vasopressin in alcohol tolerance. *Ann. Med.,* **1990,** *22:*269–274.

Johansson, B. A review of the pharmacokinetics and pharmacodynamics of disulfiram and its metabolites. *Acta Psychiatr. Scand. Suppl.,* **1992,** *369:*15–26.

Klatsky, A.L. Alcohol, coronary disease, and hypertension. *Annu. Rev. Med.,* **1996,** *47*:149–160.

Kril, J.J., and Halliday, G.M. Brain shrinkage in alcoholics: a decade on and what have we learned? *Prog. Neurobiol.,* **1999,** *58*:381–387.

Kupari, M., and Koskinen, P. Alcohol, cardiac arrhythmias, and sudden death. In, *Alcohol and Cardiovascular Diseases.* (Goode, J., ed.) John Wiley & Sons, Chichester, England, **1998,** p. 68.

Leo, M.A., and Lieber, C.S. Alcohol, vitamin A, and beta-carotene: adverse interactions, including hepatotoxicity and carcinogenicity. *Am. J. Clin. Nutr.,* **1999,** *69*:1071–1085.

Li, T.K. Pharmacogenetics of responses to alcohol and genes that influence alcohol drinking. *J. Stud. Alcohol.,* **2000,** *61*:5–12.

Lieber, C.S. Alcohol and the liver: metabolism of alcohol and its role in hepatic and extrahepatic diseases. *Mt. Sinai J. Med.,* **2000,** *67*:84–94.

Lieber, C.S. Alcohol and the liver: 1994 update. *Gastroenterology,* **1994,** *106*:1085–1105.

Lieber, C.S. Gastric ethanol metabolism and gastritis: interactions with other drugs, *Helicobacter pylori,* and antibiotic therapy (1957–1997)—a review. *Alcohol. Clin. Exp. Res.,* **1997a,** *21*:1360–1366.

Lieber, C.S. Hepatic and other medical disorders of alcoholism: from pathogenesis to treatment. *J. Stud. Alcohol.,* **1998,** *59*:9–25.

Lieber, C.S. Pathogenesis and treatment of liver fibrosis in alcoholics: 1996 update. *Dig. Dis.,* **1997b,** *15*:42–66.

Lovinger, D.M. 5-HT$_3$ receptors and the neural actions of alcohols: an increasingly exciting topic. *Neurochem. Int.,* **1999,** *35*:125–130.

Maclure, M. Demonstration of deductive meta-analysis: ethanol intake and risk of myocardial infarction. *Epidemiol Rev.,* **1993,** *15*:328–351.

Mantle, D., and Preedy, V.R. Free radicals as mediators of alcohol toxicity. *Adverse Drug React. Toxicol. Rev.,* **1999,** *18*:235–252.

McClain, C., Hill, D., Schmidt, J., and Diehl, A.M. Cytokines and alcoholic liver disease. *Semin. Liver Dis.,* **1993,** *13*:170–182.

Mehta, A.K., and Ticku, M.K. An update on GABA$_A$ receptors. *Brain Res. Brain Res. Rev.,* **1999,** *29*:196–217.

Mihic, S.J. Acute effects of ethanol on GABA$_A$ and glycine receptor function. *Neurochem. Int.,* **1999,** *35*:115–123.

Narahashi, T., Aistrup, G.L., Marszalec, W., and Nagata, K. Neuronal nicotinic acetylcholine receptors: a new target site of ethanol. *Neurochem. Int.,* **1999,** *35*:131–141.

Nordmann, R. Alcohol and antioxidant systems. *Alcohol Alcohol.,* **1994,** *29*:513–522.

Oslin, D., Atkinson, R.M., Smith, D.M., and Hendrie, H. Alcohol related dementia: proposed clinical criteria. *Int. J. Geriatr. Psychiatry,* **1998,** *13*:203–212.

Preedy, V.R., Siddiq, T., Why, H., and Richardson, P.J. The deleterious effects of alcohol on the heart: involvement of protein turnover. *Alcohol Alcohol.,* **1994,** *29*:141–147.

Regev, A., and Jeffers, L.J. Hepatitis C and alcohol. *Alcohol. Clin. Exp. Res.,* **1999,** *23*:1543–1551.

Rubin, R. Effect of ethanol on platelet function. *Alcohol. Clin. Exp. Res.,* **1999,** *23*:1114–1118.

Sampson, H.W. Alcohol, osteoporosis, and bone regulating hormones. *Alcohol. Clin. Exp. Res.,* **1997,** *21*:400–403.

Schenker, S., and Montalvo, R. Alcohol and the pancreas. *Recent Dev. Alcohol.,* **1998,** *14*:41–65.

Schirmer, M., Widerman, C., and Konwalinka, G. Immune system. In, *Handbook of Alcoholism* (Zernig, G., Saria, A., Kurz, M., and O'Malley, S., eds.) CRC Press, Boca Raton, FL, **2000,** pp. 225–230.

Schuckit, M.A. *Drug and Alcohol Abuse: Clinical Guide to Diagnosis and Treatment,* 4th ed. Plenum Publishing, New York, **1995.**

Seeff, L.B., Cuccherini, B.A., Zimmerman, H.J., Adler, E., and Benjamin, S.B. Acetaminophen hepatotoxicity in alcoholics. A therapeutic misadventure. *Ann. Intern. Med.,* **1986,** *104*:399–404.

Sikkink, J., and Fleming, M. Health effects of alcohol. In, *Addictive Disorders.* (Fleming, M.F., and Barry, K.L., eds.) Mosby–Year Book, St. Louis, **1992,** pp. 172–203.

Spies, C.D., and Rommelspacher, H. Alcohol withdrawal in the surgical patient: prevention and treatment. *Anesth. Analg.,* **1999,** *88*:946–954.

Stubbs, C.D., and Slater, S.J. Ethanol and protein kinase C. *Alcohol. Clin. Exp. Res.,* **1999,** *23*:1552–1560.

Tabakoff, B., and Hoffman, P.L. Adenylyl cyclases and alcohol. *Adv. Second Messenger Phosphoprotein Res.,* **1998,** *32*:173–193.

Tabakoff, B., and Hoffman, P.L. Alcohol addiction: an enigma among us. *Neuron,* **1996,** *16*:909–912.

Thomas, A.P., Rozanski, D.J., Renard, D.C., and Rubin, E. Effects of ethanol on the contractile function of the heart: a review. *Alcohol. Clin. Exp. Res.,* **1994,** *18*:121–131.

Valenzuela, C.F., and Harris, R.A. Alcohol: Neurobiology. In, *Substance Abuse: A Comprehensive Textbook.* (Lowinson, J.H., Ruiz, P., Millman, R.B., Langrod, J.B., eds.) Williams & Wilkins, Baltimore, **1997,** pp. 119–142.

Wartenberg, A.A. Management of common medical problems. In, *Principles of Addiction Medicine,* 2nd ed. (Graham, A.W. and Shultz, T.K., eds.) American Society of Addiction Medicine, Chevy Chase, MD, **1998,** pp. 731–740.

Wilde, M.I., and Wagstaff, A.J. Acamprosate. A review of its pharmacology and clinical potential in the management of alcohol dependence after detoxification. *Drugs,* **1997,** *53*:1038–1053.

DRUGS AND THE TREATMENT OF PSYCHIATRIC DISORDERS

Depression and Anxiety Disorders

Ross J. Baldessarini

Drugs with demonstrated efficacy in a broad range of severe psychiatric disorders have been developed since the 1950s, leading to development of the subspecialty of psychopharmacology. Knowledge of the actions of such agents has greatly stimulated research in biological psychiatry aimed at defining pathophysiological changes. This chapter reviews current knowledge of the pharmacology of antidepressants and the treatment of depression and anxiety disorders. Chapter 20 covers antipsychotic and antimanic agents and the treatment of psychotic and manic-depressive illness.

The treatment of depression relies on a varied group of antidepressant therapeutic agents, in part because clinical depression is a complex syndrome of widely varying severity. The first agents used successfully were tricyclic antidepressants, which elicit a wide range of neuropharmacological effects in addition to their presumed primary action of inhibiting norepinephrine and, variably, serotonin transport into nerve endings, thus leading to sustained facilitation of noradrenergic and perhaps serotonergic function in the brain. Inhibitors of monoamine oxidase, which increase the brain concentrations of many amines, also have been used. Currently, a series of innovative agents—most notably the selective serotonin-reuptake inhibitors (see Chapter 11)—dominate the treatment of depressive disorders and are widely used to treat severe anxiety disorders.

In addition to the widespread use of antidepressants, the pharmacological treatment of anxiety disorders commonly employs benzodiazepine sedative–antianxiety agents, which facilitate neuronal hyperpolarization through the gamma-aminobutyric acid (GABA)-receptor–Cl^--channel macromolecular complex. Potent benzodiazepines are effective in panic disorder as well as in generalized anxiety disorder. Their long-term risk:benefit ratio remains controversial. Serotonin 5-HT_{1A}–receptor partial agonists such as buspirone also have useful anxiolytic and other psychotropic activity and less likelihood of inducing sedation or dependence. Specialized uses of antidepressants discussed in this chapter include the treatment of anxiety disorders, including obsessive-compulsive disorder, panic-agoraphobia, and social phobias.

INTRODUCTION: PSYCHOPHARMACOLOGY

The use of drugs with demonstrated efficacy in psychiatric disorders has become widespread since the mid-1950s. Today, about 10% to 15% of prescriptions written in the United States are for medications intended to affect mental processes: to sedate, stimulate, or otherwise change mood, thinking, or behavior. This practice reflects both the high frequency of primary psychiatric disorders and the nearly inevitable emotional reactions of persons with medical ill-nesses. In addition, many drugs used for other purposes also modify emotions and cognition, either as part of their usual actions or as toxic effects of overdosage (*see* especially Chapter 24). This and the following chapter discuss psychotropic agents used primarily for the treatment of psychiatric disorders. The study of the chemistry, disposition, actions, and clinical pharmacology of such drugs has led to development of the specialty *psychopharmacology*.

Psychotropic agents can be placed into four major categories. *Antianxiety-sedative* agents, particularly the benzodiazepines, are those used for the drug therapy of anxiety disorders; their pharmacology is reviewed in Chapter 17. *Antidepressants* (mood-elevating agents) and antimanic or *mood-stabilizing* drugs (notably, lithium salts and certain anticonvulsants; *see* Chapter 20) are those used to treat affective or mood disorders and related conditions. *Antipsychotic* or *neuroleptic* drugs (*see* Chapter 20) are those used to treat very severe psychiatric illnesses—the psychoses and mania; they have beneficial effects on mood and thought, but many standard neuroleptic agents carry the risk of producing characteristic side effects that mimic neurological diseases, whereas modern antipsychotics are associated with weight gain and adverse metabolic effects such as diabetes.

The use of drugs in the treatment of psychiatric disorders is becoming more precise as psychiatric diagnoses continue to gain objectivity, coherence, and reliability. Searches for biological bases of psychiatric illnesses have been stimulated by knowledge of the mechanisms of action of psychotropic agents and the emergence of a medical discipline commonly known as *biological psychiatry* (Baldessarini, 2000). The diagnostic terminology and criteria for psychiatric disorders currently employed in the United States are well described in the *Diagnostic and Statistical Manual of Mental Disorders* of the American Psychiatric Association (2000), and updated reviews of psychiatric science are provided in Sadock and Sadock (2000).

History. Modification of behavior, mood, and emotion by drugs always has been a favorite practice of human beings. The use of psychoactive drugs evolved along two related paths: the use of substances to modify normal behavior and to produce altered states of feeling for religious, ceremonial, or recreational purposes, and their use to alleviate mental ailments. Fascinating accounts of the early history and characteristics of many psychoactive compounds, particularly those derived from natural products, are presented by Lewin (1931) and Efron and associates (1967) (*see* Ayd and Blackwell, 1970; Baldessarini, 1985; Caldwell, 1978). In 1845, Moreau proposed that hashish intoxication provided a model psychosis useful in the study of insanity. Three decades later, Freud presented his study of cocaine and suggested its potential uses in pharmacotherapy. Soon thereafter, Kraepelin founded the first laboratory of clinical psychopharmacology in Germany and evaluated psychological effects of drugs in human beings. In 1931, Sen and Bose published the first report of the use of *Rauwolfia serpentina* in the treatment of insanity. Insulin shock, pentylenetetrazole-induced convulsions, and electroconvulsive therapy (ECT) followed in 1933, 1934, and 1937, respectively. Treatments for both severe depression and schizophrenia thus became available. *Amphetamine* (a congener of ephedrine, an active component of the Chinese herbal agent *ma huang*) was the first synthetic drug to provide a model psychosis. In 1943, Hofmann ingested a minute amount of the ergot derivative *lysergic acid diethylamide* (LSD) and experienced its hallucinogenic effects. His report of

the high potency of LSD popularized the concept that a toxic substance or product of metabolism might be a cause of mental illness.

The first modern report on the treatment of psychotic excitement or mania with *lithium* salts was that of Cade in 1949 (*see* Chapter 20). Because of concerns about the toxicity of lithium, this discovery was slow in gaining general acceptance by the medical community. In 1950, *chlorpromazine* was synthesized in France. Recognition of the unique effects of chlorpromazine by Laborit and colleagues and its use in psychiatric patients in 1952 by Delay and Deniker marked the beginnings of modern psychopharmacology (*see* Ayd and Blackwell, 1970; Chapter 20).

A report on *meprobamate* by Berger (1954) marked the beginning of investigations of modern sedatives with useful antianxiety properties. An antitubercular drug, *iproniazid,* was introduced in the early 1950s and soon recognized as a monoamine oxidase inhibitor and antidepressant (Kline, 1958); in 1958, Kuhn recognized the antidepressant effect of *imipramine.* The first of the antianxiety benzodiazepines, *chlordiazepoxide,* was developed by Sternbach in 1957 (*see* Chapter 17). In the following year, Janssen discovered the antipsychotic properties of *haloperidol,* a butyrophenone (*see* Chapter 20), and thus still another class of antipsychotic agents became available. During the 1960s, the expansion of psychopharmacological research was rapid, and many new theories of psychoactive drug effects were introduced. The clinical efficacy of many of these agents was firmly established during that decade.

For many years, the role of biogenic amines and their receptors in the central nervous system (CNS) in mediating effects of psychotropic drugs has been emphasized and has stimulated searches for the causes of mental illness (*see* Baldessarini, 2000). In addition, increasing attention has been paid to the liabilities of treatment with psychotherapeutic drugs, especially their limited efficacy in severe or chronic mental illnesses, their risk of sometimes serious adverse effects, and the limitations, conservatism, and basic circularity of screening and testing methods used to develop new agents (*see* Baldessarini, 2000). The antipsychotic, mood-stabilizing, and antidepressant agents used to treat the most severe mental illnesses have had a remarkable impact on psychiatric practice and theory—an impact that legitimately can be called revolutionary and one that is experiencing continued innovation.

Nosology. The different classes of psychotropic agents are selective in their ability to modify symptoms of mental illnesses. The optimal use of such drugs thus requires familiarity with the differential diagnosis of psychiatric conditions (*see* Sadock and Sadock, 2000; American Psychiatric Association, 2000). A few salient aspects of psychiatric classification are summarized briefly here, and additional information is provided in the discussion of specific classes of drugs.

Basic distinctions are made among the cognitive disorders, psychotic disorders, mood disorders, anxiety disorders, and disorders of personality. The cognitive disorder syndromes of *delirium* and *dementia* commonly are associated with definable neuropathological, metabolic, or toxic (including drug-induced) changes and are characterized by confusion, disorientation, and memory disturbances as well as behavioral disorganization. In general, the effectiveness of pharmacological treatment of the core cognitive impairment in the dementias remains limited, despite extensive efforts to develop effective treatments. These have included use of stimulants, so-called noötropics (*e.g.*, periacetam), cholinesterase inhibitors, putative cerebral vasodilators (*e.g.*, ergot alkaloids, papaverine, isoxuprine), and the calcium channel blockers, such as nimodipine (*see* Chapters 32 and 33; Knapp *et al.*, 1994; Marin and Davis, 1998). This topic is not specifically covered in this chapter.

The psychoses are among the most severe psychiatric disorders, in which there is not only marked impairment of behavior but also a serious inability to think coherently, to comprehend reality, or to gain insight into the presence of these abnormalities. These common disorders (affecting perhaps 0.5% to 1.0% of the population at some age) typically include symptoms of false beliefs (*delusions*) and abnormal sensations (*hallucinations*). The psychotic disorders are suspected of having a neurobiological basis but usually are distinguished from the cognitive disorders. The etiological basis of the psychotic disorders remains unknown, although genetic and neurodevelopmental as well as environmental causative factors have been proposed. Representative syndromes in this category include schizophrenia, brief psychoses, and delusional disorders, although psychotic features also are not uncommon in the major mood disorders, particularly mania and severe melancholic depression. Psychotic illnesses are characterized by disorders of thinking processes, as inferred from illogical or highly idiosyncratic communications, with disorganized or irrational behavior and varying degrees of altered mood that can range from excited agitation to severe emotional withdrawal. Idiopathic psychoses characterized mainly by chronically disordered thinking and emotional withdrawal and often associated with delusions and auditory hallucinations are called *schizophrenia*. Acute or recurrent idiopathic psychoses also occur that bear an uncertain relationship to schizophrenia or the major affective disorders. In addition, more or less isolated delusions can arise in *delusional disorder* or *paranoia*.

Antipsychotic drugs exert beneficial effects in many types of psychotic illness and are *not* selective for schizophrenia. Their beneficial actions are found in disorders ranging from postsurgical delirium and amphetamine intoxication to paranoia, mania, and psychotic depression, and they can be beneficial against the agitation of Alzheimer's dementia. They are especially beneficial in severe depression and possibly other conditions marked by severe turmoil or agitation. This class of agents is discussed in Chapter 20.

The major disorders of mood or affect include the syndromes of *major depression* (formerly including melancholia) and *bipolar disorder* (formerly manic-depressive disorder). These disorders are quite prevalent, affecting several percent of the population at some time. They commonly include disordered autonomic functioning (*e.g.*, altered activity rhythms, sleep, and appetite) and behavior, as well as persistent abnormalities of mood. These disorders parallel an increased risk of self-harm or suicide as well as increased mortality from stress-related general medical conditions, medical complications of commonly comorbid abuse of alcohol or drugs, or from accidents. Bipolar disorder is marked by a high likelihood of recurrences of severe depression and manic excitement, often with psychotic features.

Major depression is usually treated with a variety of agents generally considered to be *antidepressants*, which have beneficial effects on the symptoms of major depression as well as on those of anxiety disorders. They are discussed further in this chapter. Bipolar disorder usually is treated primarily with lithium, certain anticonvulsants, or other agents with mood-stabilizing effects, as discussed in Chapter 20.

The less pervasive psychiatric disorders include conditions formerly termed *psychoneuroses,* which currently are viewed as anxiety-associated disorders. Whereas the ability to comprehend reality is retained, suffering and disability sometimes are severe. Anxiety disorders may be acute and transient or, commonly, recurrent or persistent. Their symptoms may include mood changes (fear, panic, dysphoria) or limited abnormalities of thought (obsessions, irrational fears or phobias) or of behavior (avoidance, rituals or compulsions, pseudoneurological or "hysterical" conversion signs, or fixation on imagined or exaggerated physical symptoms). In such disorders, drugs may have some beneficial effects, particularly by modifying associated anxiety and depression and so facilitating a more comprehensive program of treatment and rehabilitation. Currently, antidepressants as well as sedative-antianxiety agents commonly are used to treat anxiety disorders, which are considered later in this chapter.

Other typically lifelong conditions—including the personality disorders, substance-use disorders, and hypochondriasis—may or may not respond appreciably to pharmacological intervention. Personality disorders have prominent avoidant, antisocial, paranoid, withdrawn, dependent, or unstable characteristics. Other disorders involve patterns of behavior (*e.g.*, abuse of alcohol or other substances, deviant eating, exaggerated somatic preoccupations, or other abnormal behaviors). Typically, psychotropic drugs alone are not effective in such long-term conditions except when anxiety or depression occur. Pharmacological treatment also is an important component of the medical management of withdrawal from addicting substances and in supporting their avoidance (*see* Chapter 24; Cornish *et al.*, 1998).

Biological Hypotheses in Mental Illness. The introduction in the 1950s of relatively effective and selective drugs for the management of schizophrenic and manic-depressive patients encouraged formulation of biological concepts of the pathogenesis of these major mental illnesses. In addition, other agents were discovered that mimic some of the symptoms of severe mental illnesses. These include LSD, which induces hallucinations and altered emotional states; antihypertensive agents such as reserpine, which can induce depression; and stimulants that can induce manic or psychotic states when taken in excess. A leading hypothesis that arose from such considerations was based on observations indicating that antidepressants enhance the biological activity of monoamine neurotransmitters in the CNS and that antiadrenergic compounds may induce depression. These observations led to speculation that a deficiency of aminergic transmission in the CNS might be causative of depression or that an excess could result in mania. Further, since antipsychotic agents antagonize the actions of dopamine as a neurotransmitter in the forebrain, it was proposed that there may be a state of functional overactivity of dopamine in the limbic system or cerebral cortex in schizophrenia or mania. Alternatively, an endogenous psychotomimetic compound might be produced either uniquely or in excessive quantities in psychotic patients.

This "pharmacocentric" approach to the construction of hypotheses was appealing and gained strong encouragement from studies of the actions of antipsychotic and antidepressant drugs while also encouraging further development of similar agents. In turn, the plausibility of such biological hypotheses has encouraged interest in genetic studies as well as in clinical biochemical studies. Despite extensive efforts, attempts to document metabolic changes in human subjects predicted by these hypotheses have not, on balance, provided consistent or compelling corroboration (Baldessarini, 2000; Bloom and Kupfer, 1995; Musselman *et al.*, 1998). Moreover, results of genetic studies have provided evidence that inheritance can account for only a portion of the causation of mental illnesses, leaving room for environmental and psychological hypotheses.

The antipsychotic, antianxiety, antimanic, and antidepressant drugs have effects on cortical, limbic, hypothalamic, and brainstem mechanisms that are of fundamental importance in the regulation of arousal, consciousness, affect, and autonomic functions. It is quite possible that physiological and pharmacological modification of these brain regions have important behavioral consequences and useful clinical effects regardless of the fundamental nature or cause of the mental disorder in question. The lack of symptomatic or even syndromal specificity of most psychotropic drugs tends to reduce the chances of finding a discrete metabolic correlate for a specific disease conceived simply on the actions of therapeutic agents. Finally, the technical problems associated with attempts to study changes in the *in vivo* metabolism or the postmortem chemistry of the human brain are formidable. Among these are artifacts introduced by drug treatment itself.

In summary, the available information does not permit a conclusion as to whether or not discrete biological lesions are the crucial basis of the most severe mental illnesses (other than the deliria and dementias). Moreover, it is not necessary to presume that such a basis is operative to provide effective medical treatment for psychiatric patients. Furthermore, it would be clinical folly to underestimate the importance of psychological and social factors in the manifestations of mental illnesses or to overlook psychological aspects of the conduct of biological therapies (Baldessarini, 2000).

Identification and Evaluation of Psychotropic Drugs. Although rational, predictive development and assessment of the efficacy of any drug is problematic, the difficulties in evaluating psychoactive drugs are particularly challenging. The essential characteristics of human mental disorders cannot be reproduced in animals. Cognition, communication, and social relationships in animals are difficult to compare with human conditions. Thus, screening procedures in animals are of limited utility for the discovery of unique therapeutic agents. Contemporary pharmacology has provided many techniques for characterizing the actions of known psychotropic and other CNS agents at the cellular and molecular levels. Characteristics such as affinity for specific receptors or transporters can lead to the identification of new agents. Further innovation has been emerging slowly from the rapid recent progress in identifying novel subtypes of classical neurotransmitter receptors, effectors, and many other macromolecular target sites in brain tissue for potential new drugs (Baldessarini, 2000). In addition, clinical evaluation of new drugs is hampered by the lack of homogeneity within diagnostic groups and difficulty in application of valid, sensitive measurements of the effects of therapy. As a consequence, the results of clinical trials of psychotropic agents sometimes seem equivocal or inconsistent.

TREATMENT OF DEPRESSIVE AND ANXIETY DISORDERS

Major depression is characterized by clinically significant depression of mood and impairment of functioning as its primary clinical manifestations. Its clinical manifestations and current treatment overlap the anxiety disorders, including *panic-agoraphobia* syndrome, severe *phobias, generalized anxiety disorder, social anxiety disorder, posttraumatic stress disorder,* and *obsessive-compulsive disorder.* Extremes of mood may be associated with psychosis, manifested as disordered or delusional thinking and perceptions, often congruent with the predominant mood. Conversely, psychotic disorders may have associated or secondary changes in mood. This overlap of disorders may lead to errors in diagnosis and clinical management (American Psychiatric Association, 2000). Each with a lifetime morbid risk of perhaps 10% in the general population, major mood and anxiety disorders are the most common mental illnesses (Kessler *et al.,* 1994). Clinical depression is distinguished from normal grief, sadness, disappointment, and the dysphoria or demoralization often associated with medical illness. The condition is underdiagnosed and frequently undertreated (McCombs *et al.,* 1990; Suominen *et al.,* 1998). Major depression is characterized by feelings of intense sadness and despair, mental slowing and loss of concentration, pessimistic worry, lack of pleasure, self-deprecation, and variable agitation. Physical changes also occur, particularly in severe, vital, or "melancholic" depression. These include insomnia or hypersomnia; altered eating patterns, with anorexia and weight loss or sometimes overeating; decreased energy and libido; and disruption of the normal circadian and ultradian rhythms of activity, body temperature, and many endocrine functions. As many as 10% to 15% of individuals with this disorder, and up to 25% of those with bipolar disorder, display suicidal behavior during their lifetime (Baldessarini and Jamison, 1999). Depressed patients usually respond to antidepressant drugs or, in severe or treatment-resistant cases, to ECT (*see* Rudorfer *et al.,* 1997). The decision to treat with an antidepressant is guided by the presenting clinical syndrome and its severity and by the patient's personal and family history. Most antidepressants exert important actions on the metabolism of monoamine neurotransmitters and their receptors, particularly norepinephrine and serotonin (Buckley and Waddington, 2000; Owens *et al.,* 1997). Their therapeutic effectiveness and actions, together with strong evidence for genetic predisposition, have led to speculation that the biological basis of major mood disorders may include abnormal function of monoamine neurotransmission.

However, the direct evidence for this view is limited and inconsistent (*see* Baldessarini, 2000; Bloom and Kupfer, 1995; Heninger and Charney, 1987; Musselman *et al.,* 1998).

Diagnosis and treatment of the severe anxiety disorders has advanced recently, stimulated by the discovery that selective serotonin-reuptake inhibitors, which are effective antidepressants, also are powerful antianxiety agents. Disorders including panic-agoraphobia, social and other phobias, generalized anxiety, and obsessive-compulsive disorder as well as apparently related disorders of impulse control all appear to be responsive to treatment with serotonin-reuptake inhibitors (Taylor, 1998). Benzodiazepines, azapirones, and other sedative-anxiolytic drugs also are employed in anxiety disorders. Their pharmacology is discussed in Chapter 17.

Mania and the alternation or admixture of mania and depression (bipolar disorder) are less common than nonbipolar major depression. Mania and its milder form (hypomania) are treated with antipsychotic drugs, anticonvulsants, or lithium salts, sometimes supplemented with a potent sedative in the short term and lithium salts or certain anticonvulsants with mood-stabilizing properties (*see* Chapters 17 and 20) for longer-term prevention of recurrences. Mania is characterized by excessive elation, typically tinged with dysphoria or marked by irritability, severe insomnia, hyperactivity, uncontrollable speech and activity, impaired judgment, and risky behaviors, and sometimes by psychotic features. The selection and administration of appropriate treatment for depression and anxiety disorders are discussed below.

Antidepressants

Imipramine, amitriptyline, their *N*-demethyl derivatives, and other similar compounds were the first successful antidepressants and, since the early 1960s, have been widely used for the treatment of major depression. Because of their structures (*see* Table 19–1), these agents often are referred to as the "tricyclic" antidepressants (Frazer, 1997). Their efficacy in alleviating major depression is well established, and they also have proved useful in a number of other psychiatric disorders. Just prior to the discovery of the antidepressant properties of imipramine in the late 1950s, the ability of monoamine oxidase (MAO) inhibitors to cause mania was noted, and during the early 1960s, both types of agents were studied intensively in the treatment of clinical depression. Early MAO inhibitors appeared to be limited in efficacy at the doses used and presented both toxic risks and potentially dangerous inter-

actions with other agents, thus limiting their acceptance in favor of the tricyclic agents.

After decades of limited progress, a series of innovative antidepressants has emerged. Most—like *citalopram, fluoxetine, fluvoxamine, paroxetine, sertraline,* and *venlafaxine*—are inhibitors of the active reuptake (transport) of serotonin (5-hydroxytryptamine, 5-HT) into nerve terminals (*see* Chapter 11). Others—including *bupropion, nefazodone,* and *mirtazapine*—have a less well defined neuropharmacology and can be considered "atypical." Whereas the efficacy of the newer agents is not superior to that of the older agents, their relative safety and tolerability has led to their rapid acceptance as the most commonly prescribed antidepressants.

History. *Monoamine Oxidase Inhibitors.* In 1951, *isoniazid* and its isopropyl derivative, *iproniazid,* were developed for the treatment of tuberculosis. Iproniazid had mood-elevating effects in tuberculosis patients. In 1952, Zeller and coworkers found that iproniazid, in contrast to isoniazid, was capable of inhibiting the enzyme MAO. Following investigations by Kline and by Crane in the mid-1950s, iproniazid was used for the treatment of depressed patients; historically, it is the first clinically successful modern antidepressant (Healy, 1997).

Tricyclic Antidepressants. Häfliger and Schindler in the late 1940s synthesized a series of more than 40 iminodibenzyl derivatives for possible use as antihistamines, sedatives, analgesics, and antiparkinsonism drugs. One of these was *imipramine,* a dibenzazepine compound, which differs from the phenothiazines only by replacement of the sulfur with an ethylene bridge to produce a seven-membered central ring analogous to the benzazepine antipsychotic agents (*see* Chapter 20). Following screening in animals, a few compounds, including imipramine, were selected on the basis of sedative or hypnotic properties for therapeutic trial. During clinical investigation of these putative phenothiazine analogs, Kuhn (1958) fortuitously found that, unlike the phenothiazines, imipramine was relatively ineffective in quieting agitated psychotic patients, but it had a remarkable effect on depressed patients; indisputable evidence of its effectiveness in these patients has accumulated (*see* Baldessarini, 1989; Hollister, 1978; Potter *et al.,* 1998; Thase and Nolen, 2000).

Older tricyclic antidepressants with a tertiary-amine side chain (including amitriptyline, doxepin, and imipramine) block neuronal uptake of both serotonin and norepinephrine, and clomipramine is relatively selective against serotonin (*see* Table 19–2). Following this lead, even more selective serotonin-reuptake inhibitors were developed in the early 1970s, arising from observations by Carlsson that antihistamines including chlorpheniramine and diphenhydramine inhibited the transport of serotonin or norepinephrine. Chemical modifications led to the earliest selective serotonin-reuptake inhibitor, *zimelidine,* soon followed by development of *fluoxetine* and *fluvoxamine* (Carlsson and Wong, 1997; Fuller, 1992; Masand and Gupta, 1999; Tollefson and Rosenbaum, 1998; Wong and Bymaster, 1995). Zimelidine was first in clinical use, but withdrawn due to association with febrile illnesses and cases of Guillain-Barré ascending paralysis, leaving fluoxetine and fluvoxamine as the first widely used

Table 19–1
Antidepressants: Chemical Structures, Dose and Dosage Forms, and Side Effects

NONPROPRIETARY NAME (TRADE NAME)	Usual Dose, mg/day	Extreme Dose, mg/day	Dosage Form	AMINE EFFECTS	Agitation	Seizures	Sedation	Hypo-tension	Anti-cholinergic Effects	Gastro-intestinal Effects	Weight Gain	Sexual Effects	Cardiac Effects
Norepinephrine-Reuptake Inhibitors: **Tertiary Amine Tricyclics**													
Amitriptyline (ELAVIL and others) C H C=CH(CH₂)₂N(CH₃)₂	100–200	25–300	O, I	NE, 5-HT	0	2+	3+	3+	3+	0/+	2+	2+	3+
Clomipramine (ANAFRANIL) C Cl N—(CH₂)₃N(CH₃)₂	100–200	25–250	O	NE, 5-HT	0	3+	2+	2+	3+	+	2+	3+	3+
Doxepin (ADAPIN, SINEQUAN) O H C=CH(CH₂)₂N(CH₃)₂	100–200	25–300	O	NE, 5-HT	0	2+	3+	2+	2+	0/+	2+	2+	3+
Imipramine (TOFRANIL and others) C H N—(CH₂)₃N(CH₃)₂	100–200	25–300	O, I	NE, 5-HT	0/+	2+	2+	2+	2+	0/+	2+	2+	3+
(+)-Trimipramine (SURMONTIL) C H N—CH₂CHCH₂N(CH₃)₂ (CH₃)	75–200	25–300	O	NE, 5-HT	0	2+	3+	2+	3+	0/+	2+	2+	3+
Norepinephrine-Reuptake Inhibitors: **Secondary Amine Tricyclics**													
Amoxapine (ASENDIN) 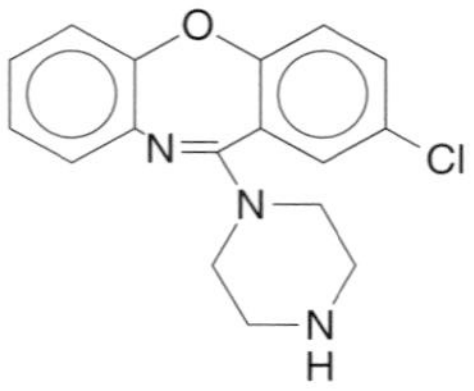	200–300	50–600	O	NE, DA	0	2+	+	2+	+	0/+	+	2+	2+
Desipramine (NORPRAMIN) 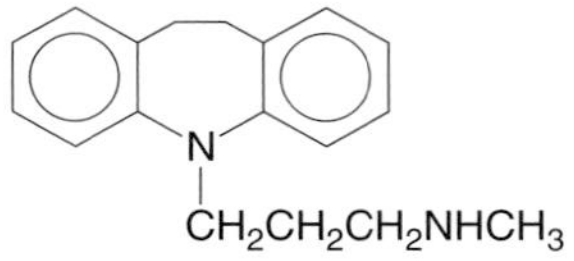	100–200	25–300	O	NE	+	+	0/+	+	+	0/+	+	2+	2+

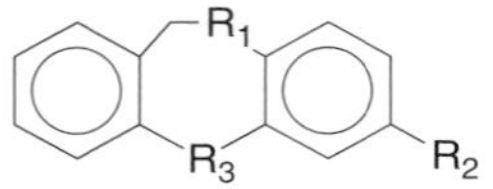

R_1 R_2 / R_3

CH₂CH₂CH₂NHCH₃

Table 19-1
Antidepressants: Chemical Structures, Dose and Dosage Forms, and Side Effects (Continued)

NONPROPRIETARY NAME (TRADE NAME)	Usual Dose, mg/day	Extreme Dose, mg/day	Dosage Form	AMINE EFFECTS	Agitation	Seizures	Sedation	Hypotension	Anticholinergic Effects	Gastrointestinal Effects	Weight Gain	Sexual Effects	Cardiac Effects
Secondary Amine Tricyclics (*cont.*)													
Maprotiline (LUDIOMIL)	100–150	25–225	O	NE	0/+	3+	2+	2+	2+	0/+	+	2+	2+
Nortriptyline (PAMELOR)	75–150	25–250	O	NE	0	+	+	+	+	0/+	+	2+	2+
Protriptyline (VIVACTIL)	15–40	10–60	O	NE	2+	2+	0/+	+	2+	0/+	+	2+	3+
Selective Serotonin-Reuptake Inhibitors													
(±)-Citalopram (CELEXA)	20–40	10–60	O	5-HT	0/+	0	0/+	0	0	3+	0	3+	0
(±)-Fluoxetine (PROZAC)	20–40	5–80	O	5-HT	+	0/+	0/+	0	0	3+	0/+	3+	0/+
Fluvoxamine (LUVOX)	100–200	50–300	O	5-HT	0	0	0/+	0	0	3+	0	3+	0

453

Table 19-1

Antidepressants: Chemical Structures, Dose and Dosage Forms, and Side Effects (*Continued*)

NONPROPRIETARY NAME (TRADE NAME)	DOSE AND DOSAGE FORMS			AMINE EFFECTS	SIDE EFFECTS								
	Usual Dose, mg/day	Extreme Dose, mg/day	Dosage Form		Agitation	Seizures	Sedation	Hypotension	Anticholinergic Effects	Gastrointestinal Effects	Weight Gain	Sexual Effects	Cardiac Effects
Selective Serotonin-Reuptake Inhibitors (*cont.*)													
(−)-Paroxetine (PAXIL)	20–40	10–50	O	5-HT	+	0	0/+	0	0/+	3+	0	3+	0
(+)-Sertraline (ZOLOFT)	100–150	50–200	O	5-HT	+	0	0/+	0	0	3+	0	3+	0
(±)-Venlafaxine (EFFEXOR)	75–225	25–375	O	5-HT, NE	0/+	0	0	0	0	3+	0	3+	0/+
Atypical Antidepressants Bupropion (WELLBUTRIN)	200–300	100–450	O	DA, ?NE	3+	4+	0	0	0	2+	0	0	0
(±)-Mirtazapine (REMERON)	15–45	7.5–45	O	5-HT, NE	0	0	4+	0/+	0	0/+	0/+	0	0

Table 19-1

Antidepressants: Chemical Structures, Dose and Dosage Forms, and Side Effects *(Continued)*

NONPROPRIETARY NAME (TRADE NAME)	Usual Dose, mg/day	Extreme Dose, mg/day	Dosage Form	AMINE EFFECTS	Agitation	Seizures	Sedation	Hypotension	Anticholinergic Effects	Gastrointestinal Effects	Weight Gain	Sexual Effects	Cardiac Effects
Atypical Antidepressants *(cont.)*													
Nefazodone* (SERZONE)	200–400	100–600	O	5-HT	0	0	3+	0	0	2+	0/+	0/+	0/+
Trazodone† (DESYREL)	150–200	50–600	O	5-HT	0	0	3+	0	0	2+	+	+	0/+
Monoamine Oxidase Inhibitors													
Phenelzine (NARDIL)	30–60	15–90	O	NE, 5-HT, DA	0/+	0	+	+	0	0/+	+	3+	0
Tranylcypromine (PARNATE)	20–30	10–60	O	NE, 5-HT, DA	2+	0	0	+	0	0/+	+	2+	0
(−)-Selegiline (ELDEPRYL)	10	5–20	O	DA, ?NE, ?5-HT	0	0	0	0	0	0	0	+	0

Note: Most of the drugs are hydrochloride salts, but SURMONTIL and LUVOX are maleates; CELEXA is a hydrobromide, and REMERON is a free-base. Selegiline is approved for early Parkinson's disease, but may have antidepressant effects, especially at daily doses ≥20 mg, and is under investigation for administration by transdermal patch.

Abbreviations: O, oral tablet or capsule; I, injectable; NE, norepinephrine; DA, dopamine; 5-HT, 5-hydroxytryptamine, serotonin; 0, negligible; 0/+, minimal; +, mild; 2+, moderate; 3+, moderately severe; 4+, severe.

*Nefazodone: additional side effect of impotence (+).

†Trazodone: additional side effect of priapism (+).

Table 19–2
Potencies of Antidepressants at Human Transporters for Monoamine Neurotransmitters

DRUG	NE-T	5-HT-T	DA-T	SELECTIVITY FOR NE OR 5-HT
NE-selective agents				
Desipramine	0.83	17.5	3200	21.1
Protriptyline	1.40	19.6	2130	14.0
Tomoxetine	2.04	9.10	1090	4.46
Norclomipramine	2.50	41.0	—	16.4
Nortriptyline	4.35	18.5	1140	4.25
Oxaprotiline	5.00	4000	4350	800
Lofepramine	5.30	71.4	18,500	13.5
Reboxetine	7.14	58.8	11,500	8.24
Maprotiline	11.1	5900	1000	532
Nomifensine	15.6	1000	55.6	64.1
Amoxapine	16.1	58.5	4350	3.63
Doxepin	29.4	66.7	12,200	2.27
Mianserin	71.4	4000	9100	56.0
Viloxazine	156	17,000	100,000	109
Mirtazapine	4760	100,000	100,000	21.0
5-HT–selective agents				
Paroxetine	40.0	0.125	500	320
Clomipramine	37.0	0.280	2200	132
Sertraline	417	0.293	25.0	1423
Fluoxetine	244	0.810	3600	301
Citalopram	4000	1.16	28,000	3448
Imipramine	37.0	1.41	8300	26.2
Fluvoxamine	1300	2.22	9100	586
Amitriptyline	34.5	4.33	3200	7.97
Nor$_1$-citalopram	780	7.40	—	105
Dothiepin	45.5	8.33	5300	5.46
Venlafaxine	1060	9.10	9100	116
Milnacipran	83.3	9.10	71,400	9.15
Nor$_2$-citalopram	1500	24.0	—	62.5
Norfluoxetine	410	25.0	1100	16.4
Norsertraline	420	76	440	55.0
Trimipramine	2400	1500	10,000	264
Zimelidine	9100	152	12,000	59.9
Trazodone	8300	160	7140	51.9
Nefazodone	60	200	360	1.80
Bupropion	52,600	9100	526	5.78

Note: Potency is expressed as inhibition constant (Ki) in nM, based on radiotransporter competition assays with membranes from cell lines transfected with human genes for specific transporter proteins (T). Selectivity is based on the ratio of Ki values. Some drugs listed are not available for clinical use in the United States. Note that the most potent norepinephrine-transporter (NE-T)–selective agent is desipramine; the least is mirtazapine, and the most selective for NE-T over the serotonin transporter (5-HT-T) are oxaprotiline and its congener maprotiline. For 5-HT-T, the most potent agents are paroxetine and clomipramine; least is bupropion, and citalopram is the most selective over NE-T. Bupropion is the only agent with some selectivity for DA-T over both other transporters.
SOURCES: Data adapted from Frazer, 1997; Owens *et al.*, 1997; and Leonard and Richelson, 2000.

selective serotonin-reuptake inhibitors (dubbed SSRIs). The development of these agents was paralleled by identification of compounds with selectivity for norepinephrine reuptake and others effective against both serotonin and norepinephrine reuptake (*see* "Prospectus," below).

Chemistry and Structure-Activity Relationships. *Tricyclic Antidepressants.*

The search for compounds related chemically to imipramine yielded multiple analogs. In addition to the dibenzazepines, imipramine and its secondary-amine congener (and major metabolite) *desipramine,* as well as its 3-chloro derivative *clomipramine,* there are *amitriptyline* and its *N*-demethylated metabolite *nortriptyline* (dibenzocycloheptadienes), as well as *doxepin* (a dibenzoxepine) and *protriptyline* (a dibenzocycloheptatriene). Other structurally related agents are *trimipramine* (a dibenzazepine, with only weak effects on amine transport); *maprotiline* (containing an additional ethylene bridge across the central six-carbon ring); and *amoxapine* (a piperazinyldibenzoxazepine with mixed antidepressant and neuroleptic properties). Since these agents all have a three-ring molecular core and most share pharmacological (norepinephrine-reuptake inhibition) and clinical (antidepressant, anxiolytic) properties, the trivial name "tricyclic antidepressants" can be used for this group. Structures and other features of antidepressant compounds are given in Table 19–1.

Selective Serotonin-Reuptake Inhibitors.

Most are aryl or aryloxyalkylamines. Several (including citalopram, fluoxetine, and zimelidine) are racemates; sertraline and paroxetine are separate enantiomers. The (*S*)-enantiomers of citalopram and of fluoxetine and its major metabolite norfluoxetine are highly active against serotonin transport and also may have antimigraine effects not found with the (*R*)-enantiomer of fluoxetine. The (*R*)-enantiomer of fluoxetine also is active against serotonin transport and is shorter-acting than the (*S*)-enantiomer. (*R*)-Norfluoxetine is virtually inactive (Wong *et al.,* 1993). Structure-activity relationships are not well established for serotonin-reuptake inhibitors. However, it is known that the *para*-location of the CF_3 substituent of fluoxetine (*see* Table 19–1) is critical for serotonin transporter potency. Its removal and substitution at the *ortho*-position of a methoxy group yields *nisoxetine,* a highly selective norepinephrine-uptake inhibitor.

Monoamine Oxidase Inhibitors.

The first MAO inhibitors to be used in the treatment of depression were derivatives of hydrazine, a highly hepatotoxic substance. *Phenelzine* is the hydrazine analog of phenethylamine, a substrate for MAO; *isocarboxazide* is a hydrazide derivative that probably is converted to the corresponding hydrazine to produce long-lasting inhibition of MAO. Subsequently, compounds unrelated to hydrazine were found to be potent MAO inhibitors. Several of these agents were structurally related to amphetamine and were synthesized in an attempt to enhance central stimulant properties. Cyclization of the side chain of amphetamine resulted in *tranylcypromine,* which also produces long-acting inhibition of MAO without covalent bonding. *Selegiline* and several experimental MAO inhibitors are propargylamines containing a reactive acetylenic bond that interacts irreversibly with the flavin cofactor of MAO (Cesura and Pletscher, 1992). Short-acting, reversible MAO inhibitors include *brofaromine* (a piperidylbenzofuran), *moclobemide* (a morpholinobenzamide), and *toloxatone* (an oxazolidinone). Moclobemide has at least moderate antidepressant activity (Lotufo-Neto *et al.,* 1999).

Pharmacological Properties: Central Nervous System. *Tricyclic Antidepressants and Other Norepinephrine-Reuptake Inhibitors.*

Knowledge of the pharmacological properties of antidepressant drugs remains incomplete, and its coherent interpretation is limited by a lack of a compelling psychobiological theory of mood disorders. The actions of imipramine-like tricyclic antidepressants include a range of complex, secondary adaptations to their initial actions as inhibitors of neuronal transport (reuptake) of norepinephrine and variable blockade of serotonin transport (*see* Table 19–2; Barker and Blakely, 1995; Beasley *et al.,* 1992; Heninger and Charney, 1987; Leonard and Richelson, 2000; Potter *et al.,* 1998; Wamsley *et al.,* 1987). Tricyclic type antidepressants with secondary amine side chains or the *N*-demethylated (*nor*) metabolites of agents with tertiary-amine moieties (*e.g., amoxapine, desipramine, maprotiline, norclomipramine, nordoxepin, nortriptyline*) are relatively selective inhibitors of norepinephrine transport. Most tertiary-amine tricyclic antidepressants also inhibit the uptake-inactivation of serotonin. The amine transport–inhibiting effects of antidepressants occur immediately and are sustained indefinitely.

It is likely that selective inhibitors of norepinephrine reuptake, including *reboxetine,* share many of the actions of older norepinephrine-transport inhibitors like desipramine (Delgado and Michaels, 1999). Among the tricyclic antidepressants, trimipramine is exceptional in that it lacks prominent inhibitory effects at monoamine transport (*see* Table 19–2), and its actions remain unexplained.

The tricyclic and other norepinephrine-active antidepressants do not block dopamine transport (*see* Table 19–2) and in that way differ from CNS stimulants, including cocaine, methylphenidate, and the amphetamines (*see* Chapter 10). Nevertheless, they may have indirect dopamine-facilitating effects through interactions of increased perisynaptic abundance of norepinephrine, particularly in cerebral cortex, where adrenergic terminals exceed those releasing dopamine. Tricyclic antidepressants also can desensitize D_2 dopamine autoreceptors, perhaps indirectly enhancing forebrain dopaminergic mechanisms, and so contribute to elevation of mood and behavioral activity (Potter *et al.,* 1998).

In addition to their transport-inhibiting effects, tricyclic antidepressants have variable interactions with adrenergic receptors (*see* Table 19–3). The presence or absence of such receptor interactions appears to be critical for subsequent responses to increased availability of extracellular norepinephrine in or near synapses. Most tricyclic antidepressants have at least moderate and selective affinity for α_1-adrenergic receptors, much less for α_2, and virtually none for β receptors. The α_2 receptors include presynaptic

Table 19–3

Potencies of Selected Antidepressants at Three Neurotransmitter Receptors

DRUG	MUSCARINIC CHOLINERGIC RECEPTOR[*]	HISTAMINE H_1 RECEPTOR	ADRENERGIC α_1 RECEPTOR
Amitriptyline	17.9	1.10	27.0
Amoxapine	1000	25.0	50.0
Bupropion	40,000	6700	4550
Citalopram	2200	476	1890
Clomipramine	37.0	31.2	38.5
Desipramine	196	110	130
Doxepin	83.3	0.24	23.8
Fluoxetine	2000	6250	5900
Fluvoxamine	24,000	>100,000	7700
Imipramine	90.9	11.0	90.9
Maprotiline	560	2.00	90.9
Mirtazapine	670	0.14	500
Nefazodone	11,000	21.3	25.6
Nortriptyline	149	10.0	58.8
Paroxetine	108	22,000	>100,000
Protriptyline	25.0	25.0	130
Reboxetine	6700	312	11,900
Sertraline	625	24,000	370
Trazodone	>100,000	345	35.7
Trimipramine	58.8	0.27	23.8
Venlafaxine	>100,000	>100,000	>100,000

Note: Data (*Ki* values in nM) are adapted from Leonard and Richelson, 2000, and reflect the ability of the antidepressant drug to compete with radioligands selective for the three receptors. Note that anticholinergic potency is particularly high with amitriptyline, protriptyline, clomipramine, trimipramine, doxepin, and imipramine; relatively high with paroxetine among selective serotonin-reuptake inhibitors; and lowest with venlafaxine, trazodone, bupropion, fluvoxamine, and nefazodone. This effect contributes to many diverse autonomic effects. Antihistaminic potency is highest with the relatively sedating agents mirtazapine, doxepin, trimipramine, and amitriptyline, and lowest with venlafaxine, fluvoxamine, sertraline, and paroxetine. Anti-α_1–adrenergic potency is highest with doxepin, trimipramine, nefazodone, amitriptyline, trazodone, clomipramine, amoxapine, nortriptyline, imipramine, and maptrotiline and particularly low with paroxetine, venlafaxine, reboxetine, fluvoxamine and fluoxetine.

[*]Data were obtained with a radioligand that is nonselective for muscarinic receptor subtypes.

autoreceptors that limit the neurophysiological activity of noradrenergic neurons ascending from the locus ceruleus in brainstem to supply mid- and forebrain projections, as well as descending projections to the spinal cord cholinergic preganglionic efferents to the peripheral autonomic ganglia (*see* Chapters 6 and 10). Autoreceptor mechanisms also reduce the synthesis of norepinephrine through the rate-limiting step at tyrosine hydroxylase, presumably through α_2-adrenergic receptor attenuation of cyclic AMP–mediated phosphorylation. Activation of these receptors inhibits transmitter release by incompletely defined molecular and cellular actions, but likely including suppression of voltage-gated Ca^{2+} currents and activa-

tion of G protein–coupled, receptor-operated K^+ currents (Foote and Aston-Jones, 1995).

The α_2-receptor–mediated negative-feedback mechanisms are rapidly activated on administration of tricyclic antidepressants. By limiting synaptic availability of norepinephrine, tricyclic antidepressants tend to maintain functional homeostasis. However, with repeated drug exposure, α_2-receptor responses are eventually diminished. This loss may result from desensitization secondary to increased exposure to the endogenous agonist ligand norepinephrine or, alternatively, from prolonged occupation of the norepinephrine transporter itself *via* an allosteric effect, as suggested for inhibitors of serotonin transporters on serotonergic neurons (Chaput *et al.*, 1991). Over a period of days to weeks, this adaptation allows the presynaptic production and release of norepinephrine to return to, or even exceed, baseline levels (Baldessarini, 1989; Heninger and Charney, 1987; Foote and Aston-Jones, 1995; Potter *et al.*, 1998). However, long-term treatment eventually can reduce the expression of tyrosine hydroxylase (Nestler *et al.*, 1990).

Postsynaptic β-adrenergic receptors also gradually down-regulate in functional receptor density over several weeks. This adaptive response accompanies repeated treatment with various types of antidepressants, including tricyclics, some serotonin-reuptake inhibitors, MAO inhibitors, and electroshock treatment in animals (Sulser and Mobley, 1980). Combinations of a serotonin transport inhibitor with a tricyclic antidepressant may have a more rapid β-adrenergic receptor–desensitizing effect. The pharmacodynamic or pharmacokinetic basis of this interaction is not clear, nor are its contributions to superior clinical efficacy proven (Nelson *et al.*, 1991). It is unlikely that loss of β-receptor functioning contributes directly to the mood-elevating effects of antidepressant treatment, since β blockers tend to induce or worsen depression in vulnerable persons. Nevertheless, loss of inhibitory β-adrenergic influences on serotonergic neurons may enhance release of serotonin and thus contribute indirectly to antidepressant effects (Leonard and Richelson, 2000; Wamsley *et al.*, 1987; *see* Chapter 10).

Postsynaptic α_1-adrenergic receptors may be partially blocked initially, probably contributing to early hypotensive effects of many tricyclic antidepressants. Over weeks of treatment they remain available and may even become more sensitive to norepinephrine, as mood-elevating effects gradually emerge clinically. At the time of clinical efficacy, therefore, inactivation of transmitter reuptake continues to be blocked; presynaptic production and release of norepinephrine has returned to or may exceed baseline levels; and a postsynaptic α_1-adrenergic mechanism is in place to provide a functional output believed to contribute to antidepressant activity (Baldessarini, 1989).

Additional neuropharmacological changes that may contribute to the clinical effects of tricyclic antidepressants include indirect facilitation of serotonin and perhaps dopamine neurotransmission through excitatory α_1 receptors on other monoaminergic neurons, or desensitized, inhibitory α_2 receptors, as well as D_2 dopamine autoreceptors. Activated release of serotonin and dopamine may, in turn, lead to secondary down-regulation of serotonin 5-HT$_1$ autoreceptors, postsynaptic 5-HT$_2$ receptors, and perhaps dopamine D_2 autoreceptors and postsynaptic D_2 receptors (Leonard and Richelson, 2000).

Other adaptive changes have been observed in response to long-term treatment with tricyclic antidepressants. These include altered sensitivity of muscarinic acetylcholine receptors as well as decreases of GABA$_B$ gamma-aminobutyric acid receptors and possibly also NMDA glutamate receptors (Kitamura *et al.*, 1991; Leonard and Richelson, 2000). In addition, there is a net gain in cyclic AMP production and altered activity of protein kinases in some cells, including those acting on cytoskeletal and other structural proteins that may alter neuronal growth and sprouting (Racagni *et al.*, 1991; Wong *et al.*, 1991). Nuclear genetic-regulatory factors also are affected, including the cyclic AMP–response-element binding protein (CREB) and brain-derived neurotrophic factor (BDNF) (Duman *et al.*, 1997; Siuciak *et al.*, 1997). Additional changes may be indirect effects of antidepressant treatment or may reflect recovery from depressive illness. These include normalization of corticosteroid release and the sensitivity of corticosteroid receptors, as well as shifts in the production of prostaglandins and cytokines and in lymphocyte functions (Kitayama *et al.*, 1988; Leonard and Richelson, 2000).

Understanding of the physiological and psychobiological implications of these many molecular and cellular changes during repeated antidepressant treatment remains incomplete. Nevertheless, their occurrence underscores the important concept that repeated administration of neuroactive or psychotropic agents sets off a complex series of adaptive processes. Specifically regarding the tricyclic antidepressants, their neuropharmacology is not accounted for simply by blocking the transport-mediated removal of norepinephrine, even though this effect is no doubt a crucial initiating event leading to a cascade of important secondary adaptations (Duman *et al.*, 1997; Hyman and Nestler, 1996; Leonard and Richelson, 2000). Interactions of antidepressants with monoaminergic synaptic transmission are illustrated in Figure 19–1.

Selective Serotonin-Reuptake Inhibitors (SSRIs). Understanding of the late and indirect actions of this very commonly used class of antidepressant and antianxiety agents remains much less well developed than does that of the actions of tricyclic antidepressants. However, there are striking parallels between responses in the noradrenergic and serotonergic systems. Like tricyclic antidepressants, which block norepinephrine reuptake, the serotonin-reuptake inhibitors block neuronal transport of serotonin immediately, and apparently indefinitely, leading to complex secondary responses (*see* Table 19–2).

Increased synaptic availability of serotonin stimulates a large number of postsynaptic 5-HT receptor types (Azmitia and Whitaker-Azmitia, 1995; *see* Chapter 11).

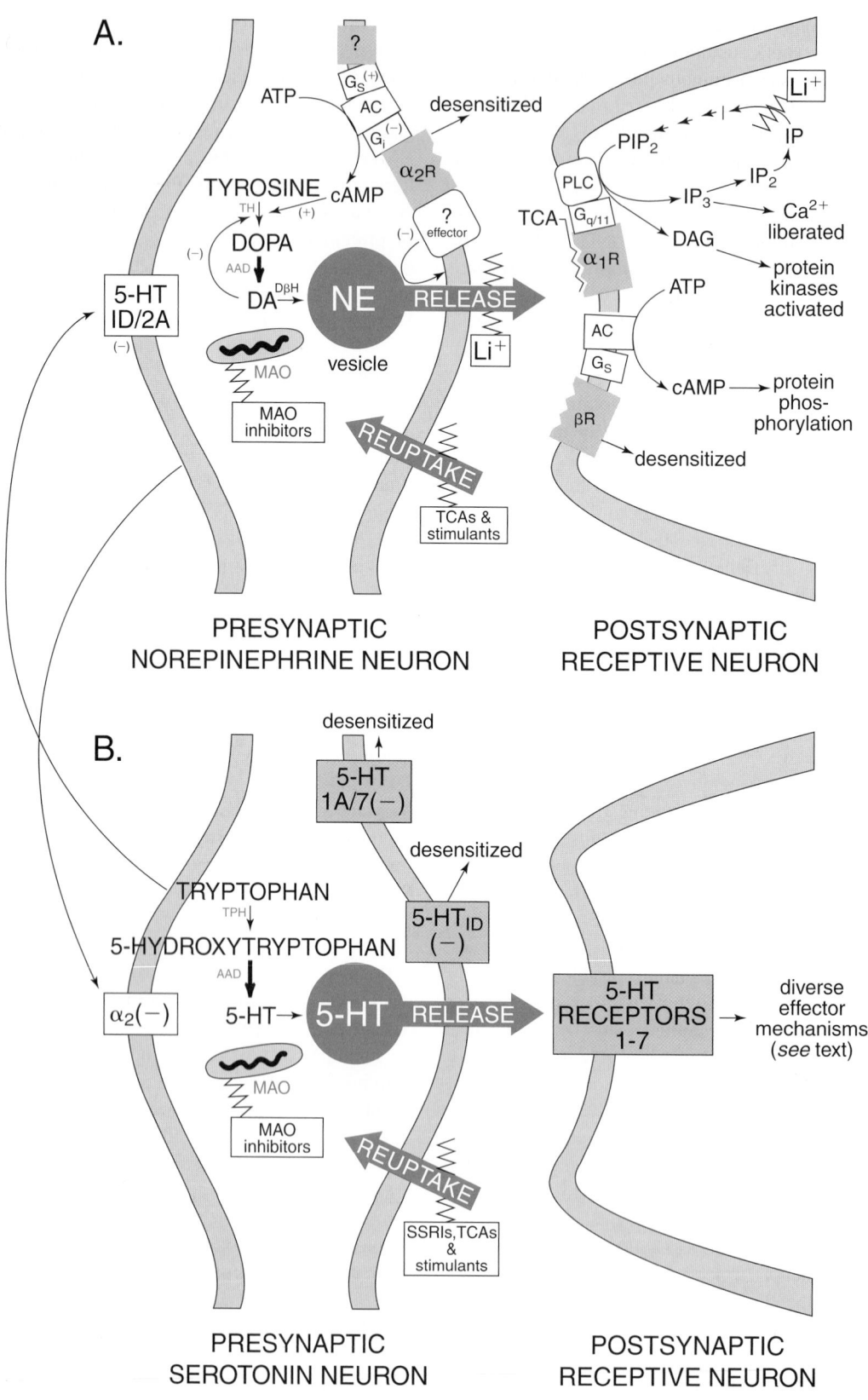

A.

PRESYNAPTIC
NOREPINEPHRINE NEURON

POSTSYNAPTIC
RECEPTIVE NEURON

B.

PRESYNAPTIC
SEROTONIN NEURON

POSTSYNAPTIC
RECEPTIVE NEURON

Stimulation of 5-HT$_3$ receptors is suspected to contribute to common adverse effects characteristic of this class of drugs, including gastrointestinal (nausea, vomiting) and sexual effects (delayed or impaired orgasm). In addition, stimulation of 5-HT$_{2C}$ receptors may contribute to risk of agitation or restlessness sometimes induced by serotonin-reuptake inhibitors.

An important parallel in responses of serotonin and norepinephrine neurons is that negative feedback mechanisms rapidly emerge to restore homeostasis (Azmitia and Whitaker-Azmitia, 1995). In the serotonin system, 5-HT$_1$ subtype autoreceptors (types 1A and 7 at raphe cell bodies and dendrites, type 1D at terminals) suppress serotonin neurons in the raphe nuclei of the brainstem, including inhibition of tryptophan hydroxylase (again, probably through reduced phosphorylation-activation) and neuronal release of serotonin. Repeated treatment leads to gradual downregulation and desensitization of autoreceptor mechanisms over several weeks (particularly of 5-HT$_{1D}$ receptors at nerve terminals), with a return or increase of presynaptic activity, production, and release of serotonin (Blier et al., 1990; Chaput et al., 1991; Tome et al., 1997). Additional secondary changes include gradual down-regulation of postsynaptic 5-HT$_{2A}$ receptors that may contribute to antidepressant effects, as well as influencing the function of other neurons via serotonergic "heteroceptors."

Many other postsynaptic 5-HT receptors presumably remain available to mediate increased serotonergic transmission and contribute to the mood-elevating and anxiolytic effects of this class of drugs.

As in responses to norepinephrine-transport inhibitors, complex late adaptations to repeated treatment with serotonin-reuptake inhibitors occur. These may include indirect enhancement of norepinephrine output by reduction of tonic inhibitory effects of 5-HT$_{2A}$ heteroceptors. Finally, similar nuclear and cellular adaptations occur as with the tricyclic antidepressants, including a net gain of intraneuronal cyclic AMP and of nuclear regulatory factors including CREB and BDNF (Azmitia and Whitaker-Azmitia, 1995; Hyman and Nestler, 1996).

Atypical Antidepressants. Several antidepressants have effects on both noradrenergic and serotonergic neurotransmission. These include the older tricyclic antidepressants, particularly the tertiary amines including amitriptyline, clomipramine, doxepin, and imipramine (*see* Table 19–2). However, even relatively potent serotonin-transport inhibitors like clomipramine and amitriptyline produce *N*-dealkylated metabolites with potent norepinephrine-uptake–inhibiting effects. Venlafaxine also has some effect on norepinephrine transport, and a series of novel agents with mixed effects on both transport systems is emerging (*e.g., duloxetine* and *milnacipran*).

Drugs with significant dopamine-uptake–inhibiting actions include the older psychostimulants (*see* Chapter 10; Fawcett

---

Figure 19–1. Sites of action of antidepressants.

A. In varicosities ("terminals") along terminal arborizations of norepinephrine (NE) neurons projecting from brainstem to forebrain, tyrosine is oxidized to dihydroxyphenylalanine (DOPA) by tyrosine hydroxylase (TH), then decarboxylated to dopamine by aromatic L-amino acid decarboxylase (AAD) and stored in vesicles, where side-chain oxidation by dopamine β-hydroxylase (DβH) converts DA to NE. Following exocytotic release by depolarization in the presence of Ca^{2+} (inhibited by lithium), NE interacts with postsynaptic α- and β-adrenergic receptor (R) subtypes as well as presynaptic α_2 autoreceptors. Regulation of NE release by α_2 receptors is principally through attenuation of Ca^{2+} currents and activation of K$^+$ currents. Inactivation of transsynaptic communication occurs primarily by active transport ("reuptake") into presynaptic terminals [inhibited by most tricyclic antidepressants (TCAs) and stimulants], with secondary deamination [by mitochondrial monoamine oxidase (MAO), blocked by MAO inhibitors]. Blockade of inactivation of NE by TCAs initially leads to α_2-receptor–mediated inhibition of firing rates, metabolic activity, and transmitter release from NE neurons; gradually, however, α_2-autoreceptor response diminishes and presynaptic activity returns. Postsynaptically, β-adrenergic receptors activate adenylyl cyclase (AC) through G$_s$ proteins to convert adenosine triphosphate (ATP) to cyclic AMP (cAMP). Adrenergic α_1 (and other) receptors activate phospholipase C (PLC) *via* additional G proteins, converting phosphatidylinositol bisphosphate (PIP$_2$) to inositol trisphosphate (IP$_3$) and diacylglycerol (DAG), with secondary modulation of intracellular Ca^{2+} and protein kinases. Postsynaptic β receptors also desensitize, but α_1 receptors do not. ***B.*** Selective serotonin-reuptake inhibitors (SSRIs) have analogous actions to TCAs at serotonin-containing neurons, and TCAs can interact with serotonergic neurons and receptors (*see also* text and Chapters 11 and 12). Serotonin is synthesized from L-tryptophan by a relatively rate-limiting hydroxylase (TPH), and the resulting 5-hydroxytryptophan is deaminated by AAD to 5-hydroxytryptamine (5-HT, serotonin). Following release, 5-HT interacts with a large number of post-synaptic receptors in major groups 1–7, which exert their effects through a variety of phospholipase- and cyclase-mediated mechanisms. Inhibitory autoreceptors include types 5-HT$_{1A}$ and perhaps 5-HT$_7$ subtypes at serotonin cell bodies and dendrites, as well as 5-HT$_{1D}$ receptors at the nerve terminals; these receptors probably become desensitized following prolonged treatment with a SSRI antidepressant that blocks 5-HT transporters. The adrenergic and serotonergic systems also influence each other, in part through complementary heteroceptor mechanisms (inhibitory α_2 receptors on 5-HT neurons, and inhibitory 5-HT$_{1D}$ and 5-HT$_{2A}$ receptors on noradrenergic neurons).

and Busch, 1998). These agents provide only limited benefits in major depression and may worsen agitation, psychosis, insomnia, and anorexia associated with severe depressive illness. *Nomifensine* is an effective antidepressant that inhibits the uptake of both norepinephrine and dopamine (*see* Table 19–2). The aromatic aminoketone *bupropion* (*amfebutamone*) and its amphetamine-like active metabolites also affect dopamine and norepinephrine transport (Ascher *et al.*, 1995). The MAO inhibitor tranylcypromine is amphetamine-like in structure but interacts only weakly at dopamine transporters.

The phenylpiperazine *nefazodone* and, to a lesser extent, the structurally related *trazodone* have at least weak inhibitory actions on serotonin transport, and nefazodone also may have a minor effect on norepinephrine transport. This agent also has a prominent direct antagonistic effect at 5-HT$_{2A}$ receptors that may contribute to antidepressant and anxiolytic activity. Both drugs also may inhibit presynaptic 5-HT$_1$ subtype autoreceptors to enhance neuronal release of serotonin, though they probably also exert at least partial agonist effects on postsynaptic 5-HT$_1$ receptors (*see* Table 19–3; Golden *et al.*, 1998). Trazodone also blocks cerebral α_1-adrenergic and H$_1$-histamine receptors, possibly contributing to its tendency to induce priapism and sedation, respectively.

Finally, the structurally similar atypical antidepressants *mirtazapine* and *mianserin* have potent antagonistic effects at several postsynaptic serotonin receptor types (including 5-HT$_{2A}$, 5-HT$_{2C}$, and 5-HT$_3$ receptors) and can produce gradual downregulation of 5-HT$_{2A}$ receptors (Golden *et al.*, 1998). Mirtazapine also limits the effectiveness of inhibitory α_2-adrenergic heteroceptors on serotonergic neurons as well as inhibitory α_2 autoreceptors and 5-HT$_{2A}$ heteroceptors on noradrenergic neurons. These effects may enhance release of both amines, and these several actions probably contribute to the antidepressant effects of these drugs. Mirtazapine also is a potent histamine H$_1$-receptor antagonist, and, correspondingly, relatively sedating.

Monoamine Oxidase Inhibitors. MAO is a flavin-containing enzyme localized in mitochondrial membranes found in nerve terminals, the liver, intestinal mucosa, and other organs (Cesura and Pletscher, 1992). MAO differs biochemically from nonspecific amine oxidases in plasma. It is closely linked functionally with an aldehyde reductase and an aldehyde dehydrogenase. The products of these reactions can be carboxylic acids or alcohols, depending on the substrate and the tissue. MAO regulates the metabolic degradation of catecholamines and serotonin in the CNS or peripheral tissues. Hepatic MAO has a crucial defensive role in inactivating circulating monoamines or those, such as tyramine, that are ingested or originate in the gut and are absorbed into the portal circulation. Of the two major molecular species of MAO, type A is selectively inhibited by *clorgyline* and prefers serotonin as a substrate; type B is inhibited by *selegiline* ([–]-deprenyl) and prefers phenethylamine as a substrate. Both types are found in liver and brain of most species. Serotonin and norepinephrine nerve terminals contain mainly MAO-A; human gut, MAO-A; and blood platelets, MAO-B. Except for selegiline (in low doses), clinically employed MAO inhibitors (phenelzine and tranylcypromine) inhibit both MAO-A and -B.

Selective inhibitors of MAO-A usually are more effective in treating major depression than are type B inhibitors (Murphy *et al.*, 1987, 1995; Krishnan, 1998). The MAO-B inhibitor selegiline is approved for treatment of early Parkinson's disease

and acts by potentiating remaining dopamine in degenerating nigrostriatal neurons and possibly reducing neuronal damage due to reactive products of the oxidative metabolism of dopamine or other potential neurotoxins (*see* Chapter 22). Selegiline also may have antidepressant effects, particularly at higher doses that also may inhibit MAO-A or yield amphetaminelike metabolites (Murphy *et al.*, 1987). Several short-acting selective inhibitors of MAO-A [*e.g.*, brofaromine, moclobemide (MANERIX, in Canada)] have at least moderate antidepressant effects and are much less likely to potentiate the pressor actions of tyramine and other indirectly acting sympathomimetic amines than do the nonselective, irreversible MAO inhibitors (Delini-Stula *et al.*, 1988; Lotufo-Neto *et al.*, 1999).

MAO inhibitors in clinical use are site-directed and irreversible, as reactive hydrazines (*phenelzine, isocarboxazide*) or acetylenic agents (*pargyline, clorgyline, selegiline*) that attack and inactivate the flavin prosthetic group following their oxidation to reactive intermediates by MAO (Krishnan, 1998). Inhibition by the cyclopropylamine tranylcypromine may involve the reaction of a sulfhydryl group in the active center of MAO following formation of a reactive imine intermediate by the action of MAO. In the clinical setting, maximal inhibition usually is achieved within a few days, although the antidepressant effect of these drugs may be delayed for several weeks, as with most antidepressants. Evaluation of MAO activity in human subjects taking these drugs has led to the impression that favorable clinical responses are likely to occur when human platelet MAO-B is inhibited by at least 85% (Robinson *et al.*, 1978). This relationship is best established for phenelzine, but it suggests the need to use aggressive dosages of MAO inhibitors to achieve their maximal therapeutic potential.

Due to the irreversible actions of clinically used MAO inhibitors (other than *moclobemide*), up to 2 weeks may be required to regenerate fresh MAO enzyme and restore amine metabolism to normal after discontinuation of the drugs (Singer *et al.*, 1979). Nevertheless, optimal therapeutic benefit appears to require daily dosing. The capacity of MAO inhibitors to act as antidepressants usually is assumed to reflect increased availability of monoamine neurotransmitters in the CNS or sympathetic nervous system, but this assumption is difficult to prove. MAO inhibition occurs rapidly, but clinical benefits are usually delayed for several weeks. This delay of therapeutic effects remains unexplained. The delay may reflect secondary adaptations already described for tricyclic and serotonin-reuptake–inhibitor antidepressants, including downregulation of α_2- and β-adrenergic receptors (Murphy *et al.*, 1987).

Pharmacological Screening for Novel Antidepressants. Despite their clinical mood-elevating effects, most antidepressants lack the behavioral-arousal inducing actions of stimulant drugs (*see* Chapter 10; Fawcett and Busch, 1998). Nevertheless, several behavioral models have been widely employed in laboratory screening for potential antidepressants. Most are based on the ability of antidepressants to support animal behavior in stressful situations that ordinarily lead to diminished behavioral responsiveness ("learned helplessness"), such as repeated noxious shocks, forced swimming, or separation from other animals; other models involve increasing aggression toward an intruder or shifting dominance hierarchies in animal social settings (*see* Henn and McKinney, 1987; Weiss and Kilts, 1998). Such testing can detect both norepinephrine- and serotonin-reuptake inhibitors (Page *et al.*, 1999). Behavioral models sometimes are used following initial biochemical screening of novel agents with potential antidepressant activity. Such initial screening has relied increasingly on molecular techniques that include assessing potency for cellular transport of radiolabeled monoamines or the binding of selective radioligands to specific monoamine transporter proteins in animal brain tissue or to human transporters encoded by cDNAs expressed in transfected cell lines.

Absorption, Distribution, Fate, and Excretion. Most antidepressants are fairly well absorbed after oral administration. Although they usually are used initially in divided doses, their relatively long half-lives and rather wide range of tolerated concentrations permit a gradual transition toward a single daily dose given at bedtime. With the tricyclic antidepressants, dosing is most safely done with single doses up to the equivalent of 150 mg of imipramine. High doses of the strongly anticholinergic tricyclic agents can slow gastrointestinal activity and gastric emptying time, resulting in slower or erratic drug absorption and complicating management of acute overdosages. Serum concentrations of most tricyclic antidepressants peak within several hours. Intramuscular administration of some tricyclic antidepressants (notably amitriptyline and clomipramine) can be performed under special circumstances, particularly with severely depressed, anorexic patients who may refuse oral medication or ECT, but most antidepressants are available only in oral form (*see* Table 19–1; DeBattista and Schatzberg, 1999).

Once absorbed, tricyclic antidepressants, relatively lipophilic drugs, are widely distributed. They are strongly bound to plasma protein and to constituents of tissues, leading to large apparent volumes of distribution, which can be as high as 10 to 50 liters per kilogram with some antidepressants. The tendency of tricyclic antidepressants and their relatively cardiotoxic, ring-hydroxy metabolites to accumulate in cardiac tissue add to their cardiotoxic risks (Pollock and Perel, 1989; Prouty and Anderson, 1990; Wilens *et al.*, 1992). Serum concentrations of antidepressants that correlate meaningfully with clinical effects are not securely established except for a few tricyclic antidepressants (particularly amitriptyline, desipramine, imipramine, and nortriptyline), typically at concentrations of approximately 100 to 250 ng/ml (Perry *et al.*, 1994; *see* Table 19–4). Toxic effects of tricyclic antidepressants can be expected at serum concentrations above 500 ng/ml, and levels above 1 μg/ml can be fatal (Baldessarini, 1989; Burke and Preskorn, 1995; Catterson *et al.*, 1997; Preskorn, 1997; van Harten, 1993).

The utility of therapeutic drug monitoring in the routine clinical use of antidepressants is limited, and the relative safety of modern antidepressants has led to a diminished interest in this approach to guiding clinical

dosing. Individual variance in tricyclic antidepressant levels in response to a given dose is as high as 10- to 30-fold and is due largely to genetic control of hepatic microsomal oxidative enzymes (DeVane and Nemeroff, 2000). Predictable relationships between initial disposition of a relatively small test dose of nortriptyline or desipramine and doses required to achieve theoretically optimal serum concentrations have been proposed as a guide to clinical dosing of individual patients (Nelson *et al.*, 1987). Serum concentrations of antidepressants, by themselves, are not reliable predictors of the course and outcome of toxic overdoses, and they can be misleading when obtained postmortem for forensic purposes (Prouty and Anderson, 1990).

Tricyclic antidepressants are oxidized by hepatic microsomal enzymes, followed by conjugation with glucuronic acid. The major route of metabolism of imipramine is to the active product desipramine; biotransformation of either compound occurs largely by oxidation to 2-hydroxy metabolites, which retain some ability to block the uptake of amines and may have particularly prominent cardiac depressant actions. In contrast, amitriptyline and its major demethylated by-product, nortriptyline, undergo preferential oxidation at the 10 position; the 10-hydroxy metabolites may have some biological activity, but they may be less cardiotoxic than the 2-hydroxy metabolites of imipramine or desipramine (Pollock and Perel, 1989). The conjugation of ring-hydroxylated metabolites with glucuronic acid extinguishes any remaining biological activity. Although the demethylated metabolites of several tricyclic antidepressants are pharmacologically active and may accumulate in concentrations approaching or exceeding those of the parent drug, it is not known to what extent they account for the activity of the parent drugs.

Amoxapine is oxidized predominantly to the 8-hydroxy metabolite, with some production of the 7-hydroxy metabolite; the former is pharmacologically active, probably including antagonistic interactions with D_2 dopamine receptors. There is some risk of extrapyramidal side effects, including tardive dyskinesia, reminiscent of those of the *N*-methylated congener loxapine, a typical neuroleptic (*see* Chapter 20).

Mirtazapine is also *N*-demethylated and undergoes aromatic hydroxylation. Trazodone and nefazodone are both *N*-dealkylated and yield *meta*-chlorophenylpiperazine (mCPP), an active metabolite with serotonergic activity. Bupropion yields active metabolites that include amphetamine-like compounds. The serotonin-reuptake inhibitors clomipramine, fluoxetine, sertraline, and venlafaxine all are *N*-demethylated to norclomipramine, norfluoxetine, norsertraline, and desmethylvenlafaxine, respectively

Table 19–4
Disposition of Antidepressants

DRUG	ELIMINATION HALF-LIFE,* hours parent, (metabolite)	TYPICAL SERUM CONCENTRATIONS, ng/ml
Tertiary-amine tricyclic antidepressants		
Amitriptyline	16 (30)	100–250
Clomipramine	32 (70)	150–500
Doxepin	16 (30)	150–250
Imipramine	12 (30)	200–300
Trimipramine	16 (30)	100–300
Secondary-amine tricyclic antidepressants		
Amoxapine	8 (30)	200–500
Desipramine	30	125–300
Maprotiline	48	200–400
Nortriptyline	30	60–150
Protriptyline	80	100–250
Serotonin reuptake inhibitors		
Citalopram	36	75–150
Fluoxetine	50 (240)	100–500
Fluvoxamine	15–20	100–200
Paroxetine	22	30–100
Sertraline	24 (65)	25–50
Venlafaxine†	5 (11)	—
Atypical agents		
Bupropion†	14	75–100
Mirtazapine	16–30	—
Nefazodone	3	—
Reboxetine	12	—
Trazodone	6	800–1600

*Half-life is the approximate elimination (β) half-life (limited data for mirtazapine and nefazodone). Half-life values given in parentheses are those of active metabolites (commonly N-demethylated) that contribute to overall duration of action.

†Agents available in slow-release forms that delay absorption but not elimination half-life.

Serum concentrations are levels encountered at typical clinical doses and not intended as guidelines to optimal dosing. Information was obtained from manufacturers' product information summaries.

(DeVane and Nemeroff, 2000; van Harten, 1993). As occurs with the tertiary-amine tricyclic antidepressants, the N-demethylated serotonin-reuptake inhibitor metabolites also are eliminated more slowly, and some are pharmacologically active. Norclomipramine contributes noradrenergic activity. Norfluoxetine is a very long-acting (elimination half-life approximately 10 days; see Table 19–4) inhibitor of serotonin transport, particularly the (S)-enantiomer (Wong et al., 1993). Norfluoxetine also competes with other agents for hepatic oxidases to elevate circulating concentrations of other agents, including tricyclic antidepressants, days after administration of the parent drug has been stopped. Norsertraline, though also eliminated relatively slowly (half-life of 60 to 70 hours), appears to contribute limited pharmacological activity or risk of drug interactions. Nornefazodone contributes little to the biological activity or duration of action of nefazodone.

Inactivation and elimination of most antidepressants occurs over a period of several days, but there are some notable exceptions. Generally, secondary-amine tricyclic antidepressants and the *N*-demethylated derivatives of serotonin-reuptake inhibitors have elimination half-lives about twice those of the parent drugs (van Harten, 1993). Nevertheless, most tricyclics are almost completely eliminated within 7 to 10 days. An exceptionally long-acting tricyclic antidepressant is protriptyline (half-life of about 80 hours). Whereas the half-life of fluoxetine is about 50 hours, its *N*-demethylated by-product may require several weeks for elimination. Also, most MAO inhibitors are long acting, and recovery from their effects requires the synthesis of new enzyme over a period of 1 to 2 weeks; several experimental inhibitors of MAO-A (*e.g.,* brofaromine, moclobemide) are reversible and short acting (Danish University Antidepressant Group, 1993; Delini-Stula *et al.,* 1988; Murphy *et al.,* 1987).

At the other extreme, trazodone, nefazodone, and venlafaxine have short half-lives (about 3 to 6 hours), as does the active 4-hydroxy metabolite of venlafaxine (half-life of about 11 hours). The half-life of bupropion is about 14 hours. The bioavailability of nefazodone is only about 20%, and its half-life is very short (about 3 hours), owing to rapid aromatic hydroxylation. The shorter duration of action of these agents usually implies the need for multiple daily doses. Some short-acting antidepressants have been prepared in slow-release preparations (notably bupropion and venlafaxine), to extend absorption time, but without an effect on elimination half-life.

As with many other drugs, antidepressants are metabolized more rapidly by children and more slowly by patients over 60 years of age as compared with young adults (*see* Baldessarini 1985; Wilens *et al.,* 1992), and dosages are adjusted accordingly, sometimes to mg/kg daily doses that far exceed those typically given to adults (*see* Wilens *et al.,* 1992).

The MAO inhibitors are absorbed readily when given by mouth and produce maximal inhibition of MAO within 5 to 10 days (Murphy *et al.,* 1987). Little information is available on their pharmacokinetics. Although their biological activity is prolonged because of the characteristics of their interaction with the enzyme, their clinical efficacy appears to be reduced when the drug is given less frequently than once daily. The hydrazide MAO inhibitors are thought to be cleaved, with resultant liberation of active products (*e.g.,* hydrazines). They are inactivated primarily by acetylation. About one-half the population of the United States and Europe (and more in certain Asian countries) are "slow acetylators" of hydrazine-type drugs, including phenelzine, and this may contribute to the exaggerated effects observed in some patients given standard doses of phenelzine (*see* Chapters 1 and 4).

The metabolism of most antidepressants is greatly dependent on the activity of isozymes of the hepatic microsomal cytochrome P450 (CYP) system (*see* Chapter 1). Most tricyclic antidepressants are extensively oxidized by the CYP1A2 isozyme; citalopram, imipramine, the *m*-chlorophenylpiperidine metabolite of trazodone and nefazodone are substrates for CYP2C19; mirtazapine, paroxetine, trazodone, and some tricyclics are substrates for CYP2D6; and nefazodone as well as some tricyclic and serotonin-reuptake–inhibitor antidepressants are oxidized by CYP3A3/4 (DeVane and Nemeroff, 2000; van Harten, 1993). In general, CYP enzymes 1A2 and 2D6 mediate aromatic hydroxylation, and 3A3/4 mediate *N*-dealkylation and *N*-oxidation reactions in the metabolism of antidepressants. Glucuronidation is effected by a non-CYP system.

Some antidepressants not only are substrates for metabolism by the CYP system but also can inhibit the metabolic clearance of other drugs, sometimes producing clinically significant drug-drug interactions (*see* below, "Interactions with Other Drugs"). Notable inhibitory interactions include fluvoxamine with CYP1A2; fluoxetine and fluvoxamine with CYP2C9, and fluvoxamine with CYP2C19; paroxetine, fluoxetine and, less actively, sertraline with CYP2D6; and fluvoxamine and nefazodone with CYP3A3/4 (*see* DeVane and Nemeroff, 2000; Hansten and Horn, 2000; Preskorn, 1997; Weber, 1999).

Potentially clinically significant interactions include the tendency for fluvoxamine to increase circulating concentrations of oxidatively metabolized benzodiazepines, clozapine, theophylline, and warfarin. Fluoxetine and nefazodone also can increase levels of terfenadine and astemizole, and sertraline and fluoxetine can increase levels of warfarin, benzodiazepines, and clozapine. Paroxetine increases levels of theophylline and warfarin. Fluoxetine also potentiates tricyclic antidepressants and some class IC antiarrhythmics with a narrow therapeutic index (including flecainide, encainide, and propafenone; *see* Chapter 35). Nefazodone potentiates benzodiazepines other than lorazepam and oxazepam (glucuronidated).

Tolerance and Physical Dependence.   Some tolerance to sedative and autonomic effects tends to develop with continued use of tricyclic antidepressants and to the initial nausea commonly associated with serotonin-reuptake inhibitors. However, it is important to emphasize that various types of antidepressants have been used for months or years by patients with severe recurring depression with limited risk of loss of their desirable effects, though perhaps more often with serotonin-reuptake inhibitors than with older agents (*see* Cohen and Baldessarini, 1985; Frank *et al.,* 1990; Viguera *et al.,* 1998). Occasionally, patients show physical dependence on the tricyclic antidepressants, with malaise, chills, coryza, muscle aches, and sleep disturbance following abrupt discontinuation, particularly of high doses (Shatan, 1966). Similar reactions, along with gastrointestinal and sensory symptoms (paresthesias) and irritability, also occur with abrupt discontinuation of serotonin-reuptake inhibitors, particularly short-acting agents including paroxetine and venlafaxine (Schatzberg *et al.*, 1997; Tollefson and Rosenbaum, 1998). Some of these effects may reflect increased cholinergic activity following its inhibition by such agents as amitriptyline, imipramine, and paroxetine, but serotonergic mechanisms may contribute to the effects of discontinuing serotonin-reuptake inhibitors. Some of these reactions can be confused with clinical worsening of depressive symptoms. Emergence of agitated or manic reactions also has been observed after abrupt discontinuation of tricyclics (Mirin *et al.*, 1981). Such physiological reactions to antidepressant discontinuation indicate that it is wise to discontinue antidepressants gradually over at least a week, or longer when feasible.

Another type of reaction to treatment discontinuation is suspected with several psychotropic agents, involving a period of risk of recurrence of morbidity that is greater than would be predicted by the natural history of untreated illness, particularly if long-term maintenance medication is withdrawn rapidly (Baldessarini *et al.*, 1999; Viguera *et al.*, 1998). This risk probably extends over several months. Evidence for the occurrence of this phenomenon is particularly strong for lithium in bipolar disorder, but it also may occur with antidepressants (Viguera *et al.*, 1998). Such risk may be reduced by gradual discontinuation of long-term medication over at least several weeks (*see* Chapter 20).

Toxic Reactions and Side Effects. Significant side effects of antidepressants are common. Tricyclic antidepressants routinely produce adverse autonomic effects, in part related to their relatively potent antimuscarinic effects. These include dry mouth and a sour or metallic taste, epigastric distress, constipation, dizziness, tachycardia, palpitations, blurred vision (poor accommodation, with increased risk of glaucoma), and urinary retention. In addition, cardiovascular effects include orthostatic hypotension, sinus tachycardia, and variable prolongation of cardiac conduction times, with the potential of arrhythmias, particularly with overdoses.

In the absence of cardiac disease, the principal problem associated with imipramine-like agents is postural hypotension, probably related to anti-α_1-adrenergic actions. Hypotension can be severe, with falls and injuries (*see*

Ray *et al.*, 1987; Roose, 1992). Among tricyclics, nortriptyline may have a relatively low risk of inducing postural blood pressure changes. Most modern antidepressants, notably the serotonin-reuptake inhibitors, have much less risk. Tricyclic antidepressants are avoided following an acute myocardial infarction, in the presence of defects in bundle-branch conduction, or when other cardiac depressants are being administered. They have direct cardiac-depressing actions like those of class I antiarrhythmics, related to actions at fast Na^+ channels (*see* Chapter 35). Mild congestive heart failure and the presence of some cardiac arrhythmias are not necessarily contraindications to the short-term use of an antidepressant when depression and its associated medical risks are severe and appropriate medical care is provided (*see* Glassman *et al.*, 1993). ECT also can be an option.

Weakness and fatigue are attributable to central effects of tricyclic antidepressants, particularly tertiary amines, and mirtazapine, which have potent central antihistaminic effects. Trazodone and nefazodone also are relatively sedating. Other CNS effects include variable risk of confusion or delirium, in large part owing to atropine-like effects of tricyclic antidepressants. Epileptic seizures also occur; this is especially likely with doses of bupropion above 500 mg, maprotiline above 250 mg per day, or acute overdoses of amoxapine or tricyclics (Johnston *et al.*, 1991). Risk of cerebral or cardiac intoxication can increase if such agents are given in relatively high doses, with some serotonin-reuptake inhibitors capable of inhibiting their metabolism (*see* Table 19–4). MAO inhibitors can induce sedation or behavioral excitation and have a high risk of inducing postural hypotension, sometimes with sustained, mild elevations of diastolic blood pressure.

Miscellaneous toxic effects of tricyclic antidepressants include jaundice, leukopenia, and rashes, but these are very infrequent. Weight gain is a common side effect of most antidepressants, less likely with the serotonin-reuptake inhibitors, and rare with bupropion (*see* Table 19–1). Excessive sweating also is common, but its pathophysiology is not known.

Newer antidepressants generally present fewer or different side effects and toxic risks than older tricyclics and MAO inhibitors. The selective serotonin-reuptake inhibitors, as a group, have a high risk of nausea and vomiting, headache, and sexual dysfunction, including inhibited ejaculation in men and impaired orgasm in women. Adverse sexual effects also occur with tricyclic antidepressants but are much less common with bupropion, nefazodone, and mirtazapine. Trazodone can produce priapism in men, presumably due to antiadrenergic actions. Some serotonin-reuptake inhibitors, and perhaps fluoxetine in particular, have been associated with agitation and restlessness that resembles akathisia (*see* Chapter 20; Hamilton and Opler, 1992). Bupropion can act as a stimulant, with agitation, anorexia, and insomnia. Serotonin-reuptake inhibitors, while generally less likely to produce adverse cardiovascular effects than older antidepressants, can elicit electrophysiological changes in cardiac tissue, including interference with Na^+ and Ca^{2+} channels (Pacher *et al.*, 1999).

Another risk of antidepressants in vulnerable patients (particularly those with unrecognized bipolar depression) is switching, sometimes suddenly, from depression to hypomanic or manic excitement or mixed, dysphoric-agitated, manic-depressive states. To some extent, this effect is dose-related, and it seems to be somewhat more likely with tricyclic antidepressants than with serotonin-reuptake inhibitors or bupropion and perhaps MAO inhibitors. Risk of mania with newer sedating antidepressants, including nefazodone and mirtazapine, also may be relatively low, but some risk of inducing mania can be expected with any treatment that elevates mood (Sachs *et al.*, 1994).

Safety through the Life Cycle. Most antidepressants appear to be generally safe during pregnancy, in that proposed teratogenic associations in newborns exposed to several tricyclic antidepressants and some newer antidepressants (particularly fluoxetine) are not convincing (McGrath *et al.*, 1999; Wisner *et al.*, 1999). Most antidepressants and lithium are secreted in breast milk, at least in small quantities, and their safety in nursing infants is neither established nor safely assumed (Birnbaum *et al.*, 1999). For severe depression during pregnancy and lactation, ECT may be a relatively safe and effective alternative.

Children are vulnerable to cardiotoxic and seizure-inducing effects of high doses of tricyclic compounds (Kutcher, 1997). Deaths have occurred in children after accidental or deliberate overdosage with only a few hundred milligrams of drug, and several cases of unexplained sudden death have been reported in children treated with desipramine (Biederman *et al.*, 1995). Children are relatively protected by vigorous hepatic metabolic clearing mechanisms that eliminate many drugs rapidly. Indeed, attaining serum concentrations of desipramine in children like those encountered in adults (*see* Table 19–4) may require doses of 5 mg/kg of body weight or more in some school-age children compared to only 2 to 3 mg/kg in adults (Wilens *et al.*, 1992). Risk/benefit considerations of antidepressants in pediatric populations remain uncertain, particularly since many trials of antidepressants in children have failed to show substantial superiority to a placebo (Kutcher, 1997).

Among geriatric patients, dizziness, postural hypotension, constipation, delayed micturition, edema, and tremor are found commonly with tricyclic antidepressants; these patients are much more likely to tolerate serotonin-reuptake inhibitors and other modern antidepressants (Catterson *et al.*, 1997; Flint, 1998; Newman and Hassan, 1999; Oshima and Higuchi, 1999; Small, 1998). Their risks are increased due to less-efficient metabolic clearance of antidepressants and less ability to tolerate them.

Acute Overdoses. Acute poisoning with tricyclic antidepressants or MAO inhibitors is potentially life threatening. Such fatalities are much less common since modern antidepressants have widely replaced these drugs, but suicide rates probably have not declined (Baldessarini and Jamison, 1999). Deaths have been reported with doses of approximately 2 g of imipramine, and severe intoxication can be expected at doses above 1 g, or about a week's supply. If a patient is severely depressed, potentially suicidal, impulsive, or has a history of substance abuse, prescribing a relatively safe antidepressant agent with close clinical follow-up is an appropriate step. If a potentially lethal agent is prescribed, it is best dispensed in small, sublethal quantities, with a risk that sustained adherence to recommended treatment may be compromised.

Acute poisoning with a tricyclic antidepressant often is clinically complex (Nicotra *et al.*, 1981). A typical pattern is brief excitement and restlessness, sometimes with myoclonus, tonic-clonic seizures, or dystonia, followed by rapid development of coma, often with depressed respiration, hypoxia, depressed reflexes, hypothermia, and hypotension. Antidepressants that have relatively strong antimuscarinic potency commonly induce mydriasis, flushed dry skin and dry mucosae, absent bowel sounds, urinary retention, and tachycardia or other cardiac arrhythmias. A tricyclic antidepressant–intoxicated patient must be treated early in an intensive care unit. Gastric lavage with activated charcoal sometimes is useful, but dialysis and diuresis are ineffective. Coma abates gradually over 1 to 3 days. Excitement and delirium are then typical. Risk of life-threatening cardiac arrhythmias continues for at least several days, requiring close medical supervision (Boehnert and Lovejoy, 1985).

Cardiac toxicity and hypotension in such poisonings can be especially difficult to manage. The heart is usually hyperactive, with supraventricular tachycardia and a high output, and with electrocardiographic conduction times reduced (prolonged QT interval). Cardiac glycosides and antiarrhythmic drugs such as quinidine or procainamide are contraindicated, but phenytoin has been given safely and also can suppress seizure risk, as can diazepam. In addition, β-adrenergic receptor antagonists and lidocaine have been recommended. Effects of α-adrenergic agonists, used as pressor agents, may be unpredictable, and intravascular volume may be difficult to maintain. Hypoxia, hypertension or hypotension, and metabolic acidosis may occur.

Toxic reactions from overdosage of an MAO inhibitor may occur in a matter of hours despite the long delay in onset of a therapeutic response. Effects of overdosage include agitation, hallucinations, hyperreflexia, hyperpyrexia, and convulsions. Both hypotension and hypertension also occur. Treatment of such intoxication is problematic, but conservative treatment is often successful.

Interactions with Other Drugs.   Antidepressants are involved in several clinically important drug interactions (*see* Hansten and Horn, 2000; Leipzig and Mendelowitz, 1992). Binding of tricyclic antidepressants to plasma albumin can be reduced by competition with a number of drugs including phenytoin, phenylbutazone, aspirin, aminopyrine, scopolamine, and phenothiazines. Other interactions that also may potentiate the effects of tricyclic antidepressants can result from interference with their metabolism in the liver. Barbiturates and many anticonvulsant agents (particularly carbamazepine), as well as cigarette smoking, can increase the hepatic metabolism of the antidepressants by inducing microsomal CYP enzymes.

Conversely, the tendency for several serotonin-reuptake inhibitors to compete for the metabolism of other drugs can lead to significant and potentially dangerous drug-drug interactions. For example, when using combinations of such agents with tricyclic antidepressants, as is sometimes done to attempt to achieve more rapid therapeutic effect or to manage otherwise treatment-resistant depressed patients, serum concentrations of the tricyclic drug may rise to toxic levels, and these may persist for days after discontinuing fluoxetine, due to the prolonged elimination of norfluoxetine (Nelson *et al.*, 1991). Several serotonin-reuptake inhibitors are potent inhibitors of human hepatic CYP microsomal oxidases *in vitro* (Crewe *et al.*, 1992), as was discussed above regarding antidepressant drug metabolism. Venlafaxine, citalopram, and sertraline appear to have relatively low risk of such interactions (Caccia, 1998; Ereshevsky *et al.*, 1996; Preskorn, 1997, 1998). Significant interactions may be most likely in persons who are relatively rapid metabolizers through the microsomal oxidase system, perhaps including children (DeVane and Nemeroff, 2000; Preskorn, 1997, 1998).

Examples of drug interactions with serotonin-reuptake inhibitors include potentiation of agents metabolized prominently by CYP1A2 (*e.g.,* β-adrenergic receptor antagonists, caffeine, several antipsychotic agents, and most tricyclic antidepressants); CYP2C9 (carbamazepine); CYP2C19 (barbiturates, imipramine, propranolol, phenytoin); CYP2D6 (β-adrenergic receptor antagonists, some antipsychotics, many antidepressants); CYP3A3/4 (benzodiazepines, carbamazepine, many antidepressants, and several antibiotics). This specialized topic is reviewed elsewhere (DeVane and Nemeroff, 2000; Hansten and Horn, 2000; Preskorn 1997; Weber, 1999; *see* Chapter 1).

Antidepressants potentiate the effects of alcohol and probably other sedatives. The anticholinergic activity of tricyclic antidepressants can add to that of antiparkinsonism agents, antipsychotic drugs of low potency (especially clozapine and thioridazine), or other compounds with antimuscarinic activity to produce toxic effects. Tricyclic antidepressants have prominent and potentially dangerous interactions with biogenic amines, such as norepinephrine, which normally are removed from their site of action by neuronal uptake. However, drugs that inhibit norepinephrine transport also block the effects of indirectly acting amines, such as tyramine, which must be taken up by sympathetic neurons to release norepinephrine. Presumably by a similar mechanism, tricyclic antidepressants prevent the antihypertensive action of adrenergic neuron blocking agents such as guanadrel. Tricyclic agents and trazodone also can block the centrally mediated antihypertensive action of clonidine.

Serotonin-reuptake inhibitors and virtually any agent with serotonin-potentiating activity can interact dangerously or even fatally with MAO inhibitors (particularly long-acting MAO inhibitors). Other agents also have been implicated in dangerous interactions with MAO inhibitors (notably meperidine and perhaps other phenylpiperidine analgesics, as well as pentazocine, dextromethorphan, fenfluramine, and infrequently, tricyclic antidepressants) (*see* White and Simpson, 1981). The resulting reactions have been referred to as a "serotonin syndrome." This syndrome typically includes akathisia-like restlessness, muscle twitches and myoclonus, hyperreflexia, sweating, penile erection, shivering, and tremor as a prelude to more severe intoxication, with seizures and coma (Sternbach, 1991). The reaction often is self-limiting if the diagnosis is made quickly and the offending agents are discontinued. The precise pathophysiological mechanisms underlying these toxic syndromes remain ill-defined. Newer MAO inhibitors (*e.g.,* selegiline, moclobemide) also should be considered to have some risk of such interactions (Sternbach, 1991). MAO inhibitors also can potentiate effects of bupropion (*see* Weber, 1999; Hansten and Horn, 2000). These reactions are distinguished from the hypertensive interaction of MAO inhibitors with indirectly acting pressor phenethylamines such as tyramine. This reaction requires scrupulous avoidance of many potentially interacting agents, including over-the-counter cold remedies containing indirectly acting sympathomimetic agents (*see* Ayd and Blackwell, 1970; Gardner *et al.*, 1996; Healy, 1997; Leipzig and Mendelowitz, 1992). Sometimes fatal intracranial bleeding has occurred in such hypertensive reactions. Headache is a common symptom, and fever frequently accompanies the hypertensive episode. Meperidine should never be used for such headaches, and blood pressure should be evaluated immediately when a patient taking an MAO inhibitor reports a severe throbbing headache or a feeling of pressure in the head.

Therapeutic Uses.   The clinical use of antidepressants in depressed patients is discussed below. In addition to their use in adult major depression syndrome, the various antidepressant agents have found broad utility in other psychiatric disorders that may or may not be related psychobiologically to the mood disorders. Encouragement to find new indications has increased with the advent of newer agents that are less toxic, simpler to use, and often better accepted by both physicians and patients (Edwards, 1995; Edwards *et al.,* 1997; Tollefson and Rosenbaum, 1998). Current applications include rapid but temporary suppression of enuresis in children and in geriatric patients by uncertain mechanisms; prebedtime doses as low as 25 mg of imipramine or nortriptyline have been found to be safe and effective. Major affective disorders are being recognized more often in children, and antidepressants are being used increasingly in that age group, despite an inexplicable lack of demonstrable efficacy of tricyclic antidepressants in pediatric depression *per se,* even at sufficiently high doses (up to 5 mg/kg) to provide plasma concentrations accepted as therapeutic in adults (Hazel, 1996). Serotonin-reuptake inhibitors also have limited evidence of efficacy in depressed children, and other antidepressants have received little assessment in juveniles with various disorders (Emslie *et al.,* 1999; Kutcher, 1997; Steingard *et al.,* 1995).

Antidepressants have a growing role in other disorders, including *attention deficit–hyperactivity disorder* in children and adults, for which imipramine, desipramine, and nortriptyline appear to be effective, even in patients responding poorly to or intolerant of the stimulants (*e.g.,* methylphenidate) that have been the standard agents for this disorder. Newer norepinephrine-selective-uptake inhibitors also may be useful in this disorder. Utility of serotonin-reuptake inhibitors in this syndrome is not established, and bupropion, despite its similarity to stimulants, appears to have limited efficacy (Kutcher, 1997; Spencer *et al.,* 1993; Wilens *et al.,* 1992). Antidepressants tend to provide a more sustained and continuous improvement of the symptoms of attention deficit–hyperactivity disorder than do the stimulants, and they do not induce tics or other abnormal movements sometimes associated with the use of stimulants. Indeed, desipramine and nortriptyline even may effectively treat tic disorder, either in association with the use of stimulants, or arising in patients with both attention disorder and Tourette's syndrome (Spencer *et al.,* 1993). The future of tricyclic antidepressant use in children is uncertain due to the difficulty of demonstrating the efficacy of these agents in pediatric major depression (Hazell, 1996) and because of reports of several cases of unexplained sudden death during use of desipramine in preadolescent children (Biederman *et al.,* 1995).

Antidepressants also are leading choices in the treatment of severe anxiety disorders, including *panic-agoraphobia syndrome, generalized anxiety disorder, social phobia,* and *obsessive-compulsive disorder* (Bennett *et al.,* 1998; Feighner, 1999; Masand and Gupta, 1999; Pigott and Seay, 1999; Roerig, 1999; Uhlenhuth *et al.,* 1998), including the common comorbidity of anxiety in depressive illness (Boerner and Moller, 1999; Hoehn-Saric *et al.,*

2000). Antidepressants, especially serotonin-reuptake inhibitors, also are employed in the management *of post-traumatic stress disorder,* marked by anxiety, startle, painful recollection of the traumatic events, and disturbed sleep (*see* American Psychiatric Association, 1994; Roerig, 1999). Nonsedating antidepressants often are poorly tolerated initially by anxious patients, requiring slowly increased doses. Their beneficial actions typically are delayed for several weeks in anxiety disorders as in major depression.

For panic disorder, tricyclic antidepressants and MAO inhibitors, as well as high-potency benzodiazepines (notably alprazolam, clonazepam, and lorazepam; *see* Chapter 17) are effective in blocking the autonomic expression of panic itself, thus facilitating a comprehensive rehabilitation program (Argyropoulos and Nutt, 1999; Bennett *et al.,* 1998; Nagy *et al.,* 1993; Uhlenhuth *et al.,* 1998). Imipramine and phenelzine are well-studied antidepressants for panic disorder. The serotonin-reuptake inhibitors also may be effective, but β-adrenergic receptor antagonists, buspirone, and low-potency benzodiazepines usually are not, and bupropion can worsen anxiety (Taylor, 1998).

The serotonin-reuptake inhibitors are agents of choice in obsessive-compulsive disorder, as well as in possibly related syndromes of impulse dyscontrol or obsessive preoccupations, including compulsive habits, bulimia (but usually not anorexia) nervosa, and body dysmorphic disorder (Agras, 1998; Geller *et al.,* 1998; Hoehn-Saric *et al.,* 2000; Pigott and Seay, 1999; *see* Sadock and Sadock, 2000). While their benefits may be limited, serotonin-reuptake inhibitors offer an important advance in the medical treatment of these often chronic and sometimes incapacitating disorders for which no other medical treatment, by itself, has been consistently effective. The effectiveness of pharmacological treatment for these commonly treatment-resistant disorders is greatly enhanced by use of behavioral treatments (Miguel *et al.,* 1997).

In addition to the wide use of modern antidepressants to treat depression commonly associated with general medical illnesses (Schwartz *et al.,* 1989), several psychosomatic disorders may respond at least partly to treatment with antidepressants of the tricyclic, MAO inhibitor, or serotonin–reuptake inhibitor types. These include chronic pain disorders, including diabetic and other peripheral neuropathic syndromes (for which tertiaryamine tricyclics are probably superior to fluoxetine); fibromyalgia; peptic ulcer and irritable bowel syndrome; chronic fatigue; cataplexy; tics; migraine; and sleep apnea (Baldessarini, 1989; Gruber *et al.,* 1996; Masand and Gupta, 1999; Max *et al.,* 1992; Spencer *et al.,* 1993). These disorders may have some psychobiological relationship to mood or anxiety disorders (Hudson and Pope, 1990).

Drug Treatment of Mood Disorders

Disorders of mood (*affective disorders*) are extremely common in general medical practice as well as in psychiatry. The severity of these conditions covers an extraordinarily broad range, from normal grief reactions and dysthymia to severe, incapacitating illnesses that may result in death. The lifetime risk of suicide in severe forms of major affective disorders is 10% to 15%, but this statistic does not begin to represent the morbidity and cost of this group of notoriously underdiagnosed and undertreated illnesses. Perhaps one-fourth to one-third of these cases are diagnosed, and a similar proportion of these are adequately treated (Isaacson *et al.,* 1992; Katon *et al.,* 1992; Kind and Sorensen, 1993; McCombs *et al.,* 1990; Suominen *et al.,* 1998). Clearly, not all types of human grief, misery, and disappointment are indications for medical treatment, and even severe affective disorders have a high rate of spontaneous remission provided that sufficient time (often a matter of months) passes. The antidepressant agents thus generally are reserved for the more severe and otherwise incapacitating depressive disorders, and the most satisfactory results tend to occur in patients who have moderately severe illnesses with "endogenous" or "melancholic" characteristics without psychotic features (*see* American Psychiatric Association, 1994; Baldessarini, 1989; Montgomery, 1995; Peselow *et al.,* 1992; *see* Sadock and Sadock, 2000). The data from clinical research in support of the efficacy of antidepressant agents are convincing (*see* Baldessarini, 1989; Burke and Preskorn, 1995; Keller *et al.,* 1998; Kasper *et al.,* 1994; Montgomery and Roberts, 1994; Workman and Short, 1993), and there is no compelling scientific basis to support the view that newer agents may be less effective than tricyclic antidepressants (Roose *et al.,* 1994). Nevertheless, a number of shortcomings continue to be associated with all drugs used to treat affective disorders.

A somewhat surprising fact is that clinically employed antidepressants, as a group, have outperformed inactive placebos in only about two-thirds to three-fourths of controlled comparisons (*see* Baldessarini, 1989; Healy, 1997), with a similar proportion of depressed adult subjects rated as showing clinically significant responses. Moreover, assessment-based changes in clinical ratings of depressive symptoms, rather than categorization as "treatment-responsive," often yield surprisingly small average differences between active antidepressants and placebo in contemporary outpatient trials involving patients with depressive illness of only moderate severity (Healy, 1997; Kahn *et al.,* 2000). With pediatric and geriatric depression, results are typically even less clear. Pediatric studies often have failed to show superiority of drug over a placebo (Hazell, 1996). Geriatric depression includes an excess of chronic and psychotic illnesses, which tend to respond less well to antidepressant treatment alone but may do better with ECT or when an antipsychotic agent is added, or with *amoxapine,* a mixed antidepressant-neuroleptic (Schatzberg and Rothschild, 1992). Despite their potential for less favorable responses to simple antidepressant therapy, patients with severe, prolonged, disabling, psychotic, suicidal, or bipolar depression require vigorous and prompt medical intervention. Underdiagnosis arises, in part, from the sometimes misleading presentation to physicians of many depressed patients with nonspecific somatic complaints, anxiety, or insomnia. Undertreatment, in part, has arisen in the past from the reluctance of many physicians to prescribe potentially toxic or pharmacologically complicated tricyclic or MAO inhibitor antidepressants, especially to medically ill patients. This pattern is changing with the availability of less-toxic and better-accepted antidepressants among the serotonin-reuptake inhibitors and atypical agents (Olfson and Klerman, 1993).

Another major problem with antidepressant agents is that, because placebo response rates tend to be as high as 30% to 40% in research subjects diagnosed with major depression and possibly even higher in some anxiety disorders, statistical and clinical distinctions between active drug and placebo are difficult to prove (Fairchild *et al.,* 1986; Kahn *et al.,* 2000). Separation of response rates to active antidepressants from placebo improves when patients are selected for moderate severity, presence and persistence of classic melancholic or endogenous symptoms, and absence of psychotic features or of mixed bipolar states. The incorporation of various metabolic, endocrinological, or other physiological testing procedures to predict antidepressant treatment responses has been found to have only marginal predictive power and clinical utility (Arana *et al.,* 1985; Baldessarini, 2000). This situation stresses the importance of continued reliance on placebo-controlled studies in the development of new agents, since comparisons of a new *versus* a standard agent can risk an erroneous inference of equal efficacy. In addition, information on special depressed populations (particularly, pediatric, geriatric, medically ill, hospitalized, and recurrently or chronically ill patients, as well as bipolar depressed patients) continues to be limited, despite the medical need for such information. Moreover, evidence concerning clinical dose-response and dose-risk relationships is especially limited with this class of drugs.

Based on the limited information available, it is evident that increasing doses of a standard agent, such as imipramine, to 200 mg daily or more, with plasma concentrations above 200 ng/ml, yields antidepressant benefit superior to that of lower doses and levels in both short- and long-term treatment; however, tolerance may be limited, and rates of treatment refusal are high (*see* DeBattista and Schatzberg, 1999; Mavissakalian and Perel, 1989). Accordingly, the selection of a dose is based on the attempt to exceed a lower limit of perhaps 150 mg of imipramine or its daily equivalent in an otherwise healthy adult depressed patient. Typically this is done by gradually increasing the dose over several days, with an attempt to attain higher doses, as tolerated, if little progress has been made within several weeks of treatment. Although 4 to 8 weeks are required to determine whether an antidepressant trial is successful or not, some indications of improvement should be evident within the first 2 weeks.

From 1960 to 1990, the imipramine-like tricyclics were the standard antidepressants on which most of the research and clinical practice in the field have been based. However, the newer, less toxic serotonin-reuptake inhibitors and other atypical agents now are accepted broadly as agents of first choice, particularly for medically ill or potentially suicidal patients and in the elderly (Brown and Khan, 1994; Flint, 1998; Oshima and Higuchi, 1999; Small, 1998). MAO inhibitors commonly are reserved for patients who fail to respond to vigorous trials of at least one of the newer agents and a standard tricyclic antidepressant, administered alone or with lithium (lithium is covered in Chapter 20), in an attempt to potentiate the antidepressant response, or with a low dose of triiodothyronine, also in an effort to enhance overall therapeutic effectiveness (*see* Austin *et al.*, 1991; Bauer and Döpfmer, 1999; Lasser and Baldessarini, 1997). Even before the wide acceptance of the newer antidepressants, the somewhat less anticholinergic secondary-amine tricyclics, particularly nortriptyline and desipramine, had come to be preferred, particularly for elderly or medically ill patients; they still can be considered as an alternative or a second choice, particularly if administered in moderate, divided doses (*see* Table 19–1). Despite the general safety of newer agents, they are not without limitations, side effects, and interactions with other agents (*see* above). They also are relatively expensive, and prices for a day's supply of antidepressants can vary by more than tenfold among agents (*see* Baldessarini, 1985, 1989). Moreover, their relative efficacy in the most severely depressed patients, those with psychotic features, and the elderly remains to be further evaluated.

The natural history of major depression is that individual episodes tend to remit spontaneously over 6 to 12 months; however, there is a high risk of relapse of depression for at least several months following discontinuation of a successful trial of antidepressant treatment. This risk is estimated at 50% within 6 months and 65% to 70% at one year of follow-up, rising to 85% by 3 years (*see* Baldessarini and Tohen, 1988; Viguera *et al.*, 1988). To minimize this risk, it is best to continue antidepressant medication for not less than 6 months following apparent full clinical recovery. Continued use of initially therapeutic doses is recommended, although tolerability and acceptance by patients may require flexibility in this regard.

Many depressed patients follow a recurring course of episodic illness, often with lesser levels of symptoms and disability between major episodes, and so require consideration of long-term maintenance medication to reduce the risk of recurrence, particularly in patients with more than three relatively severe episodes or chronic depressive or dysthymic disorders (*see* Keller *et al.*, 1998; Viguera *et al.*, 1998). Such treatment has been tested for as long as 5 years, using relatively high doses of imipramine, with evidence that early dose reduction led to a higher risk of relapse (Frank *et al.*, 1990, 1993; Kupfer *et al.*, 1992). Long-term supplementation of an antidepressant with lithium may enhance the result (*see* Baldessarini and Tohen, 1988). Prolonged maintenance treatment of patients with recurring major depression for more than a year has not been well evaluated with any antidepressant drug other than imipramine, and dose-response data are very limited (Frank *et al.*, 1993; Keller *et al.*, 1998). The decision to recommend indefinitely prolonged maintenance treatment with an antidepressant is guided by the past history of multiple, and especially severe or life-threatening, recurrences and the impression that recurrence risk is greater in older patients. Due to evidence that rapid discontinuation of antidepressants and lithium may contribute to excess early recurrence of illness, very gradual reduction and close clinical follow-up over many weeks are recommended when maintenance treatment is to be discontinued and, ideally, even when stopping continuation therapy within the months following recovery from an acute episode of depression (*see* Greden, 1998; Viguera *et al.*, 1998).

The medical literature contains case reports of possible "tolerance" to the therapeutic effects of antidepressants after prolonged use. Sometimes this loss of benefit may be overcome by increasing the dose of antidepressant, by temporary addition of lithium or perhaps a small dose of an antipsychotic agent, or by changing to an antidepressant in a different class (Cohen and Baldessarini, 1985).

Other forms of biological treatment of depression have not been well established or are no longer regularly employed with the important exception of ECT. This remains the most rapid and effective treatment for severe acute depression and is sometimes lifesaving for acutely suicidal patients (*see* Rudorfer *et al.*, 1997).

The MAO inhibitors generally are considered drugs of late choice for the treatment of severe depression, even though the evidence for efficacy of adequate doses of *tranylcypromine* or *phenelzine* is convincing. Despite the favorable results obtained with tranylcypromine and with doses of phenelzine above 45 mg per day (Davis *et al.*, 1987; Krishnan, 1998), the possibility of unwanted reactions has limited their acceptance by many clinicians and patients. Nevertheless, MAO inhibitors sometimes are used when a vigorous trial of one or more standard antidepressants has been unsatisfactory and when ECT is refused. In addition, MAO inhibitors may have selective benefits for conditions other than typical major depression, including illnesses marked by phobias and anxiety or panic as well as dysphoria (Liebowitz, 1993). Similar benefits, however, may be found with imipramine-like agents or serotonin-reuptake inhibitors; thus, indications for the MAO inhibitors are limited and must be weighed against their potential toxicity and their complex interactions with many other drugs.

Innovative MAO inhibitors selective for types MAO-A and MAO-B enzyme now are available. *Selegiline* [(R)-(–)-deprenyl], an MAO-B-selective inhibitor, was introduced for the treatment of Parkinson's disease, but it also may have some antidepressant or other useful psychotropic effects, and its convenience and possibly its safety have been enhanced by recent development of an experimental transdermal preparation (*see* Table 19–1; Mann *et al.*, 1989; Kuhn and Muller, 1996). For consistent beneficial effects, however, daily doses above 10 mg probably are required, which may compromise MAO-B selectivity, especially following repeated use; also, selegiline may be converted *in vivo* to by-products with amphetamine-like structure and neuropharmacology. The MAO-A–selective inhibitor *clorgyline* is an effective antidepressant (*see* Murphy *et al.*, 1987). Other short-acting, reversible inhibitors of MAO-A (*e.g.*, brofaromine, moclobemide) appear to be moderately effective antidepressants with reduced risk of inducing hypertension when combined with indirectly acting sympathomimetic pressor amines (*see* Chapter 10).

Stimulants, with or without added sedatives, are an outmoded and ineffective treatment for severe depression. However, some clinicians continue to find utility and safety in the short-term treatment of selected patients with a stimulant such as methylphenidate or amphetamine (Fawcett and Busch, 1998). These include patients with mild dysphoria, temporary demoralization, or lack of energy associated with medical illnesses as well as some geriatric patients; however, none of these possible indications has been investigated systematically (Chiarello and Cole, 1987).

A particularly difficult clinical challenge is the safe and effective treatment of bipolar depression (*see* Chapter 20). This condition sometimes is misdiagnosed in states of mixed, dysphoric-agitated moods in patients with bipolar disorder and then inappropriately treated with an antidepressant without a mood-stabilizing agent for protection from worsening agitation or mania (Kukopulos *et al.*, 1983; Wehr and Goodwin, 1987). For this reason, the management of manic, mixed, and depressive mood states in bipolar disorder best relies on lithium or other putative mood-stabilizing agents as the primary treatment (*see* Chapter 20).

An antidepressant can be added cautiously and temporarily to treat depression, but the additional benefit and safety of sustained combinations of an antidepressant with a mood stabilizer have not been proven (Prien and Kocsis, 1995).

The choice of antidepressant in bipolar depression remains uncertain. Moderate doses of desipramine or nortriptyline have been used in the past; currently, the short-acting serotonin-reuptake inhibitors, bupropion, nefazodone, or mirtazapine often are employed despite a lack of formal research support for a rational choice of agent, dose, or timing (*see* Zornberg and Pope, 1993). Some of the newer antidepressants like bupropion may have a reduced tendency to induce cycling.

Drugs Used in the Treatment of Anxiety

Anxiety is a cardinal symptom of many psychiatric disorders and an almost-inevitable component of many medical and surgical conditions. Indeed, it is a universal human emotion, closely allied with appropriate fear and often serving psychobiologically adaptive purposes. A most important clinical generalization is that anxiety is rather infrequently a "disease" in itself. Anxiety that is typically associated with the former "psychoneurotic" disorders is not readily explained in biological or psychological terms; contemporary hypotheses implicate overactivity of adrenergic systems or dysregulation of serotonergic systems in the CNS (Stein and Uhde, 1998). In addition, symptoms of anxiety commonly are associated with depression and especially with dysthymic disorder (chronic depression of moderate severity), panic disorder, agoraphobia and other specific phobias, obsessive-compulsive disorder, eating disorders, and many personality disorders (Boerner and Moller, 1999; Liebowitz, 1993). Sometimes, despite a thoughtful evaluation of a patient, no treatable primary illness is found, or, if one is found and treated, it may be desirable to deal directly with the anxiety at the same time. In such situations, antianxiety medications are frequently and appropriately used (Taylor, 1998).

Currently, the serotonin-reuptake inhibitors discussed above and the benzodiazepines (*see* Chapter 17) are the most commonly employed medicinal treatments for the common clinical anxiety disorders. Some high-potency benzodiazepines (*alprazolam, clonazepam,* and *lorazepam*) are effective in severe anxiety with strong autonomic overactivity (panic disorder), as are several antidepressant agents, as discussed above. For generalized or nonspecific anxiety, the benzodiazepine selected seems to make little difference (Roerig, 1999). In the elderly or in patients with impaired hepatic function, *oxazepam* in small, divided doses is sometimes favored due to its brief action and direct conjugation and elimination. The latter property is shared by lorazepam, but not by alprazolam (*see* Chapter 17). Benzodiazepines sometimes are given to outpatients presenting with anxiety mixed with symptoms of depression, although the efficacy of these agents in altering the core features of severe major depression has not been demonstrated (Argyropoulos and Nutt, 1999; Boerner and Moller, 1999; Liebowitz, 1993). Potent benzodiazepines also commonly are employed adjunctively in the short-term management of acutely psychotic or manic patients (*see* Chapter 20).

The most favorable responses to the benzodiazepines are obtained in situations that involve relatively acute anxiety reactions in medical or psychiatric patients who have either modifiable primary illnesses or primary anxiety disorders. However, this group of anxious patients also has a high response rate to placebo and is likely to undergo spontaneous improvement. Antianxiety drugs also are used in the management of more persistent or recurrent primary anxiety disorders; guidelines for their appropriate use are less clear in these situations (Hollister *et al.*, 1993; Uhlenhuth *et al.*, 1998).

Although there has been concern about the potential for habituation and abuse of sedatives, some studies suggest that physicians tend to be conservative and may even undertreat patients with anxiety. They may either withhold drug unless symptoms or dysfunction are severe or cease treatment within a few weeks, with a high proportion of relapses. Patients with personality disorders or a past history of abuse of sedatives or alcohol may be particularly at risk of dose escalation and dependence on benzodiazepines. Benzodiazepines carry some risk of producing impairment of cognition and skilled motor functions, particularly in the elderly, in whom they are a common cause of confusion, delirium (sometimes mistaken for primary dementia), and falls with fractures (Ray *et al.*, 1987). Risk of fatality on acute overdose of benzodiazepines is limited in the absence of other cerebrotoxins or alcohol; risk of suicide with buspirone is very low. A particularly controversial aspect of the use of benzodiazepines, especially those of high potency, is in long-term management of patients with sustained or recurring symptoms of anxiety (Argyropoulos and Nutt, 1999; Hollister *et al.*, 1993; Uhlenhuth *et al.*, 1998). Clinical benefit has been found for at least several months in such cases, but it is unclear to what extent the long-term benefits can be distinguished from nonspecific ("placebo") effects following development of tolerance, on the one hand, or prevention of related withdrawal-emergent anxiety on the other.

Many other classes of drugs that act on the CNS have been used for daytime sedation and the treatment of anxiety, but their use for these conditions is now virtually obsolete. Such drugs include the *propanediol carbamates* (notably, *meprobamate* and *tybamate*), the barbiturates (*see* Chapter 17), and many other pharmacologically similar nonbarbiturates.

The demise of older sedative agents in modern psychiatric practice is due primarily to their tendency to cause unwanted degrees of sedation or frank intoxication at doses required to alleviate anxiety; meprobamate and the barbiturates are likely to produce tolerance, physical dependence, severe withdrawal reactions, and life-threatening toxicity with overdosage.

Other drugs that have been used in the treatment of anxiety include certain anticholinergic agents and antihistamines. Among these is *hydroxyzine,* an antihistamine that is not an effective antianxiety agent unless given in doses (400 mg per day) that produce marked sedation (*see* Chapter 25). *Propranolol* and other β-adrenergic receptor antagonists can reduce the autonomic symptoms associated with specific situational or social phobias but do not appear to be effective in generalized anxiety or panic disorder; similarly, other antiadrenergic agents including clonidine may modify autonomic expression of anxiety but have not been demonstrated convincingly to be clinically useful in the treatment of severe anxiety disorders (*see* Chapters 10 and 33).

Another class of agents with beneficial effects in disorders marked by anxiety or dysphoria of moderate intensity are the *azapirones* (azaspirodecanediones), currently represented clinically by *buspirone* (BUSPAR; Ninan *et al.*, 1998). Originally developed as a potential antipsychotic agent with weak antidopaminergic activity, buspirone has pharmacological properties distinct from those of both neuroleptics and sedatives including the benzodiazepines. The antidopaminergic actions of azapirones are limited *in vivo,* and they do not induce clinical extrapyramidal side effects. Also, they do not interact with binding sites for benzodiazepines or facilitate the action of GABA, are not anticonvulsant (and may even lower seizure threshold weakly), do not appear to cause tolerance or withdrawal reactions, and do not show cross-tolerance with benzodiazepines or other sedatives. Buspirone and several experimental congeners (*e.g., gepirone, ipsapirone, tiospirone*) have selective affinity for serotonin receptors of the 5-HT$_{1A}$ type, for which they appear to be partial agonists (*see* Chapter 11).

Buspirone has beneficial actions in anxious patients, particularly those with generalized anxiety of mild or moderate severity (Ninan *et al.*, 1998; Taylor, 1998). Unlike potent benzodiazepines and antidepressants, buspirone lacks beneficial actions in severe anxiety with panic attacks. It also does not share with serotonin-reuptake inhibitors their efficacy as a monotherapy in obsessive-compulsive disorder, although it may have useful antiobsessional activity when added to serotonin-active antidepressants. A lack of cross-tolerance is consistent with a lack of clinical protection against withdrawal-emergent anxiety when changing abruptly from treatment with a benzodiazepine to buspirone; a gradual transition between these classes of antianxiety agents is more likely to be tolerated (Lader, 1987).

PROSPECTUS

Major affective and anxiety disorders continue to represent the most common psychiatric illnesses; they include the most prevalent disorders of unknown cause with psychotic features and represent enormous costs to society in morbidity, disability, and premature mortality (Kessler *et al.,* 1994). Rates of diagnosis and appropriate treatment of major mood disorders have improved somewhat in recent years with the advent of better accepted modern mood-altering medicines. Nevertheless, the majority of patients with depression and bipolar disorder are diagnosed after years of delay, if at all, and many remain inadequately treated (McCombs *et al.,* 1990; Newman and Hassan, 1999). Given these unmet needs, the clinical needs and economic incentives for developing additional, improved mood-altering medicines are clear.

Several groups of depressed patients continue to be particularly inadequately treated or studied. They include children and the elderly, those with bipolar depression, and those with severe, chronic, or psychotic forms of depression (*see* Shulman *et al.,* 1996; Kutcher, 1997). Whereas ambulatory depressed patients are much greater in number, have the highest likelihood of improvement and recovery, and represent the largest potential market, they also are most likely to respond to a placebo or other nonspecific treatment and thus represent a special challenge for the development of clinically useful and cost-effective treatments.

A major limitation of efforts to develop new mood-altering agents is the lack of compelling rationales other than imitation or modification of successful precedents. The fundamental problem is the continued lack of a coherent pathophysiology, let alone an etiology, of major depression, bipolar disorder and the common anxiety disorders despite decades of important and useful contributions to the description of the syndromes. Major depression may well represent a spectrum of disorders, varying in severity from relatively mild and self-limited disorders that approach everyday human distress to extraordinarily severe, psychotic, incapacitating, and deadly illnesses. It remains difficult to conceive of a mood-altering agent that does not affect central monoaminergic synaptic neurotransmission, particularly that mediated by either norepinephrine or serotonin, which limits the identification of novel therapeutic targets for these disorders (Murphy *et al.,* 1995; Bloom and Kupfer, 1995; Healy, 1997).

Novel Treatments for Major Depression and Anxiety Disorders

Many of the large number of potential antidepressants in development continue to exploit interactions with either noradrenergic or serotonergic systems in proven ways (Evrard and Harrison, 1999; Kent, 2000). These agents conceptually are remarkably similar to the tricyclic-type antidepressants and include several relatively selective inhibitors of the neuronal transport of norepinephrine (*e.g., oxaprotiline, levoprotiline, lofepramine, nisoxetine, reboxetine, (R)-thionisoxetine, tomoxetine,* and *viloxazine*) that are less cardiotoxic or lethal on overdose than traditional tricyclic antidepressants.

Development of additional serotonin-reuptake inhibitors has slowed, although their range of approved indications continues to expand, particularly into the anxiety, impulsive or compulsive, and eating disorders. However, several novel serotonin-reuptake inhibitors including *Ro-15-8081* and *aryl-* or *naphthylpiperidines* and *thiodiphenyls* have been developed; *tianeptine* has complex effects on the storage and release of serotonin and may facilitate its uptake *in vivo*. Also, some substituted phenyltropane analogs of cocaine are serotonin transporter–selective and much less potent at dopamine transporters than are cocaine and older phenyltropanes (Robertson, 1999). Some of these agents have been evaluated as potential antidepressants in clinical trials (*see* Leonard, 1994; Murphy *et al.,* 1995).

The clinical efficacy of the mixed serotonin/norepinephrine transport antagonist, *venlafaxine,* and the interesting beneficial properties of an older, similar agent, *clomipramine* (*see* above) have encouraged further exploration of the principle of mixed aminergic potentiation (Kent, 2000). This strategy has led to such drugs as *duloxetine* (*LY-248686*), *milnacipran,* and analogs of bupropion. These developments arose conceptually from pursuing the transport-blocking activities of the original tricyclic antidepressants, with efforts to avoid their familiar toxic properties (including potent antimuscarinic and cardiac depressant activities).

Surprisingly underexplored are agents with dopamine-potentiating activity (Murphy *et al.,* 1995). *Nomifensine* is a mixed antagonist of norepinephrine and dopamine transporters (*see* Table 19–2; Zahniser *et al.,* 1999). An effective antidepressant, it was withdrawn from clinical use due to association with febrile illnesses and ascending paralysis of the Guillain-Barré type. The stimulant-antidepressant bupropion also has mixed antagonistic effects on the same amine transporters. Other dopamine-receptor agonists also may have antidepressant effects (Murphy *et al.,* 1995; Mattox *et al.,* 1986; Wells and Marken, 1989; D'Acquila *et al.,* 1994). Additional agents whose actions include inhibition of dopamine transport are the tricyclic-like agent *amineptine, medifoxamine,* and a series of potent piperazine derivatives (*GBR-12909* and others). Antiparkinsonism, directly acting dopamine-receptor agonists—including *bromocriptine, pramipexole, lisuride,* and *roxindole* (the latter two also serotonergic)—also have been reported to have mood-elevating properties (Murphy *et al.*, 1995; *see* Chapter 22).

Novel approaches to enhancing central adrenergic function include the use of α_2-adrenergic–receptor antagonists. This is one of several activities of the complex atypical antidepressants *mianserin* and *mirtazapine*. The α_2-receptor antagonist *yohimbine* is stimulant-like, whereas other selective α_2 antagonists including *idazoxan, fluparoxan, R-47,243,* and *setiptiline* have questionable or untested antidepressant activity. Centrally acting β-adrenergic receptor agonists including *clenbuterol, albuterol,* and *SR-58611A* have not been clinically useful antidepressants, and direct-acting α_1-adrenergic receptor agonists (including *adrafinil* and *modafinil*) have had inconsistent effects on depression and may even have deleterious cognitive actions (*see* Leonard, 1994; Murphy *et al.*, 1995; Arnsten *et al.*, 1999). Phosphodiesterase inhibitors including *rolipram* have been considered as potential antidepressants but have dubious clinical effects and an uncertain neuropharmacology aside from the ability to prevent hydrolysis of cyclic AMP (Murphy *et al.*, 1995).

Interest in MAO inhibitors has continued despite their risks of dangerous interactions with other substances. Selective irreversible propargyl inhibitors of MAO-A (*e.g.*, clorgyline) with mood-elevating activity, as well as inhibitors of MAO-B (*e.g.*, selegiline) with dopamine-sparing, antiparkinsonism, and antidepressant activities (at least, at high doses probably not selective for MAO-B), represent potentially important leads to novel psychotropic or neurotropic agents. In addition, several short-acting reversible inhibitors of MAO-A have at least moderate antidepressant activity and limit the risk of inducing acute hypertension by potentiating pressor amines. Such short-acting MAO-A inhibitors include *brofaromine, moclobemide* (MANERIX), *pirlindole,* and *toloxatone* (*see* Danish University Antidepressant Group, 1993; Leonard, 1994; Murphy *et al.*, 1995). At least one short-acting inhibitor of MAO-B (*Ro-19-6327*) also has been described. *Minaprine* is an experimental antidepressant that appears to enhance dopamine and serotonin neurotransmission, possibly through weak anti-MAO-A actions (Murphy *et al.*, 1995). Another approach has been to develop CNS-selective MAO inhibitors in order to avoid blocking hepatic MAO or potentiating peripheral sympathetic function. A lead compound for a CNS-selective MAO inhibitor is *MDL-72394*, a prodrug that evidently is converted by cerebral decarboxylation into an irreversible, central MAO inhibitor (Oxenkrug *et al.*, 1999).

The large number of serotonin receptor subtypes provides many opportunities for developing novel agonists, partial agonists, antagonists, and negative antagonists (or inverse agonists), some of which may alter mood or treat anxiety disorders. *Pindolol,* a mixed β-adrenergic, serotonin 5-HT$_{1A}$–somatodendritic-autoreceptor antagonist, has been reported to accelerate or potentiate some serotonin-reuptake inhibitor antidepressants. These observations have stimulated efforts to develop agents with mixed antiserotonin transport and anti-5-HT$_{1A}$–receptor activity in the same molecule. Several such agents are known, including derivatives of pindolol and the naphthylpyrrolidine *EMD-95750*.

An opposite strategy is to evaluate 5-HT$_{1A}$–receptor agonists as possible mood-altering or antianxiety agents. Such agents may act in part by enhancing release of norepinephrine (Cohen *et al.*, 1999). An example of a 5-HT$_{1A}$ partial agonist with anxiolytic effects is *flesinoxan* (Albert *et al.*, 1999). Several partial agonists of 5-HT$_{1A}$ receptors have been explored for potential utility both in anxiety disorders and in milder cases of mixed anxiety-depression (Dubovsky and Buzan, 1995; Murphy *et al.*, 1995). Some 5-HT$_{1A}$–receptor partial agonists that may have antidepressant activity (*e.g., gepirone, ipsapirone,* and *zalospirone*) are azapirones related chemically to buspirone. An additional opportunity for modifying serotonin function is to antagonize the 5-HT$_{1A}$ receptor subtypes that serve as autoreceptors; several such antagonists are known, including *GR-127935* (Robertson, 1999).

Some recently developed antidepressants, notably *nefazodone*, combine activity as serotonin reuptake inhibitors and 5-HT$_{2A}$ antagonists. Several innovative agents, including *YM-35992*, have followed this precedent.

The 5-HT$_{2C}$ serotonin receptor is prominent in limbic forebrain and cerebral cortex. This receptor subtype has been postulated to be a reasonable therapeutic target for depression or anxiety (Murphy *et al.*, 1995). Nefazodone and the trazodone metabolite m-*chlorophenylpiperazine* (*mCPP*), as well as *Ro-60-0175, Ro-60-0332, Org-12962,* and *Org-8484* all have 5-HT$_{2C}$ agonist or partial-agonist properties. *Norfluoxetine* also interacts potently with 5-HT$_{2C}$ receptors.

There also are selective ligands for the 5-HT$_6$ receptor (*Ro-63-0563, SB-171046*) and emerging compounds for 5-HT$_7$ receptors (Robertson, 1999). However, the potential psychotropic properties of such agents remain obscure, requiring substantial investment in preclinical and exploratory investigations to evaluate their clinical utility in treatment of depression or anxiety.

Agents acting at amino-acid neurotransmission systems also provide leads to potential psychotropic drugs. For example, certain analogs of progesterone interact with a distinct allosteric regulatory site in the GABA$_A$-receptor complex to activate hyperpolarizing chloride channels, and so may have anxiolytic properties (Robertson, 1999; Nabeshima and Muraoka, 1999). Agents that interact with *N*-methyl-D-aspartate (NMDA) glutamate receptors have antidepressantlike activity in some animal behavioral models. They include the NMDA antagonist *dizolcipine* (*MK-801*) and NMDA-receptor partial agonist *AP-7* (Murphy *et al.,* 1995).

Receptors for cerebral peptides also provide targets for psychotropic drug development. Opioids may have mood-elevating effects, but exploration of drugs acting at opioid receptors as potential antidepressants has been limited (Tejedor-Real *et al.,* 1995). Cerebral sigma receptors (σ_1, σ_2) were identified initially as opioid receptors; their role remains obscure, but they may regulate release of norepinephrine, mediating the action of at least one agent, *igmesine* (*JO-1784*). Such agents might lead to novel antidepressants (Maurice *et al.,* 1996). Neurokinin-1 (NK_1, substance P) antagonists also may have antidepressant effects (Swain and Rupniak, 1999). A series of more potent successors of lead agent *MK-869* are under development (Nutt, 1998; Saria, 1999). Some neuroactive steroids that may have antidepressant or anxiolytic activity include agents that appear to act at NK_1 receptors (Maurice *et al.,* 1999).

Another neuropeptide-based strategy for developing antidepressant or antianxiety drugs derives from pronounced behavioral effects of intracerebral administration of the large corticotrophin (ACTH)-releasing peptide (CRF). Observed responses include suggestions of fear or anxiety, increased startle response, loss of interest in food or sex, altered sleep, and eventually epileptic seizures. Small-molecule antagonists of receptors for CRF and related peptides can penetrate the blood-brain barrier and reverse these effects. A growing list of CRF_1 receptor-selective antagonists includes *antialarmin, CP-154,526, SP-904, NBI-30545, DNP-606, DNP-695, CRA-1000,* and *SC-241*. Some of these agents also interact with CRF_2 receptors, but no highly selective CRF_2 antagonists have been identified. The precise cerebral localization and function of the two CRF receptors should yield to exploration with site-selective ligands. Some CRF_1 antagonists are in clinical testing (Mansbach *et al.,* 1997; McCarthy *et al.,* 1999; Steckler and Holsboer, 1999).

There also is a search for natural products for the treatment of depression and anxiety disorders (Wong *et al.,* 1998). *Hypericum* or *St. John's wort* extracts have shown at least moderate antidepressant activity in some controlled trials (Philipp *et al.,* 1999) but not in others (Shelton *et al.,* 2001). At least 10 active agents are found in hyper-

icum; among these, *hypericin* and *hyperforin* have some activity as inhibitors of amine transport *in vitro* (Neary and Bu, 1999). An active constituent of psychoactive South African *Sceletium* plants, *mesembrine,* also may have clinically useful properties (Smith *et al.,* 1996). Another natural product is the autacoid metabolic product of L-methionine and ATP, S-*adenosyl*-L-*methionine,* or active *methionine,* a ubiquitous methyl donor. It, too, has shown mood-elevating effects in human subjects and is sold as a "nutriceutical" product (Baldessarini, 1987). Finally, there may be some evidence of beneficial effects of *Ginkgo biloba* extract in mild dementia, but the extract probably is ineffective in depressive illness (Lingaerde *et al.,* 1999; Wong *et al.,* 1998). Some of these agents can produce adverse interactions with other drugs and should not be considered innocuous (Fugh-Berman, 2000).

New Treatments for Anxiety Disorders

Innovative prospects for the treatment of anxiety disorders include extensions of the pharmacology of benzodiazepines (*see* Chapter 17). Advances in a molecular understanding of the $GABA_A$ receptor–benzodiazepine receptor-Cl^- channel complex indicate that this ring-shaped collection of transmembrane proteins includes representatives of at least 16 subunit proteins in five groups (α, β, γ, δ, ρ (*see,* Chapter 17)); benzodiazepines are believed to bind to α subunits and GABA to β subunits. Various combinations of the subunits occur in different cell populations. This complexity may provide leads to receptor subtype–selective or even regionally selective agents with improved pharmacological properties. Ligands for specific benzodiazepine-receptor types include some nonbenzodiazepines. One, *alpidem,* an imidazole pyridine, has useful anxiolytic activity in human beings, but hepatic toxicity prompted its discontinuation. Alternatively, some benzodiazepine derivatives have been found to have central anticholecystokinin activity; *cholecystokinin* has been implicated as a biological substrate for anxiety, and antagonists have been proposed as potential antianxiety agents (Browne and Shaw, 1991).

A particularly encouraging approach is the development and clinical testing of benzodiazepine-receptor ligands with agonist activity intermediate between a full agonist, such as diazepam, and an antagonist, such as flumazenil (*see* Chapter 17; Browne and Shaw, 1991; Potokar and Nutt, 1994). Benzodiazepines and β-carbolines can have various agonist, partial-agonist, inverse-agonist (reduce GABA effects on Cl^- influx), and antagonist (block full, partial, and inverse agonists) actions. Some with partial-agonist activity appear to have useful antianxiety effects with low risks of excessive sedation and cognitive impairment or tolerance and dependence. Alpidem is a partial agonist; other examples of benzodiazepine partial agonists include the imidazole benzodiazepines *bretazenil* and *imidazenil*. Bretazenil reportedly shows antipanic activity even when taken intermittently, with low abuse potential or risk of dependence. Other partial agonists that are not benzodiazepine derivatives include the β-carboline *abecarnil* and the heterocyclic *pazinaclone*. Abecarnil also is selective for particular benzodiazepine-receptor subtypes.

Elucidation of a growing number of serotonin-receptor subtypes and agents that interact with them has strongly encouraged development of additional psychotropic agents acting on the serotonin system. One approach includes further development of azapirone analogs as 5-HT$_{1A}$ receptor ligands. Another is the use of 5-HT$_3$ receptor antagonists; some of these modulate dopamine synthesis and release, and others have shown properties in animal tests that suggest antianxiety activity. Agents with anti-5-HT$_3$–selective activity include the short-term antiemetic compound *on-*

dansetron and the benzamide *zacopride*; many others are known but have been subjected to only limited clinical testing in psychiatric disorders including psychosis and anxiety.

Other approaches to the pharmacotherapy of anxiety disorders have included the use of antiadrenergic compounds usually employed for hypertension or other cardiovascular indications, including the β-adrenergic receptor antagonists *propranolol* and *atenolol* and the α$_2$-receptor agonist *clonidine* (Cooper *et al.,* 1990; *see* Chapters 10 and 33). Such compounds have not proven to be effective in severe anxiety disorders, but they may modify autonomic expression of situational phobias such as performance anxiety (Rosenbaum and Pollock, 1994). A new technical aspect of the study of antianxiety agents has been the introduction of various laboratory procedures that can induce panic-like symptoms in a controlled setting as a basis for testing new antipanic treatments (Sullivan *et al.,* 1999).

It is reasonable to anticipate that the expansion of novel macromolecular target sites for CNS-active drug development may lead to innovative principles and agents for treating depressive and anxiety disorders in the future.

For further discussion of psychiatric disorders, *see* Chapter 385 in *Harrison's Principles of Internal Medicine,* 14th ed., McGraw-Hill, New York, 1998.

BIBLIOGRAPHY

Albert, P.R., Sajedi, N., Lemonde, S., and Ghahremani, M.H. Constitutive G(i2)-dependent activation of adenylyl cyclase type II by the 5-HT$_{1A}$ receptor. Inhibition by anxiolytic partial agonists. *J. Biol. Chem.,* 1999, *274*:35469–35474.

Arana, G.W., Baldessarini, R.J., and Ornsteen, M. The dexamethasone suppression test for diagnosis and prognosis in psychiatry. *Arch. Gen. Psychiatry,* 1985, *42*:1193–1204.

Argyropoulos, S.V., and Nutt, D.J. The use of benzodiazepines in anxiety and other disorders. *Eur. Neuropsychopharmacol.,* 1999, *9*(suppl. 6):S407–S412.

Arnsten, A.F., Mathew, R., Ubriani, R., Taylor, J.R., and Li, B.M. Alpha-1 noradrenergic receptor stimulation impairs prefrontal cortical cognitive function. *Biol. Psychiatry,* 1999, *45*:26–31.

Ascher, J.A., Cole, J.O., Colin, J.N., Feighner, J.P., Ferris, R.M., Fibiger, H.C., Golden, R.N., Martin, P., Potter, W.Z., Richelson, E., and Sulser, F. Bupropion: a review of its mechanism of antidepressant activity. *J. Clin. Psychiatry,* 1995, *56*:395–401.

Austin, M.P., Souza, F.G., and Goodwin, G.M. Lithium augmentation in antidepressant-resistant patients. A quantitative analysis. *Br. J. Psychiatry,* 1991, *159*:510–514.

Azmitia, E.C., and Whitaker-Azmitia, P.M. Anatomy, cell biology, and plasticity of the seronergic system. In, *Psychopharmacology: The*

Fourth Generation of Progress. (Bloom, F.E., and Kupfer, D.L., eds.) Raven Press, New York, 1995, pp. 443–449.

Baldessarini, R.J. Neuropharmacology of S-adenosyl-L-methionine. *Am. J. Med.,* 1987, *83*:95–103.

Baldessarini, R.J., and Jamison, J.R. Effects of medical interventions on suicidal behavior. Summary and conclusions. *J. Clin. Psychiatry,* 1999, *60*(suppl. 2):117–122.

Baldessarini, R.J., and Tohen, M. Is there a long-term protective effect of mood-altering agents in unipolar depressive disorder? In, *Psychopharmacology: Current Trends.* (Casey, D.E., and Christensen, A.V., eds.) Springer-Verlag, Berlin, 1988, pp. 130–139.

Barker, E.L., and Blakely, R.D. Norepinephrine and serotonin transporters: molecular targets of antidepressant drugs. In, *Psychopharmacology: The Fourth Generation of Progress.* (Bloom, F.E., and Kupfer, D.L., eds.) Raven Press, New York, 1995, pp. 321–333.

Bauer, M., and Döpfmer, S. Lithium augmentation in treatment-resistant depression: meta-analysis of placebo-controlled studies. *J. Clin. Psychopharmacol.,* 1999, *19*:427–434.

Beasley, C.M., Masica, D.N., and Potvin, J.H. Fluoxetine: a review of receptor and functional effects and their clinical implications. *Psychopharmacology (Berl.),* 1992, *107*:1–10.

Bennett, J.A., Moioffer, M., Stanton, S.P., Dwight, M., and Keck, P.E. Jr. A risk-benefit assessment of pharmacological treatments for panic disorder. *Drug Saf.*, **1998**, *18*:419–430.

Berger, F.M. The pharmacological properties of 2-methyl-2-n-propyl-1,3 propanediol dicarbamate (MILTOWN), a new interneuronal blocking agent. *J. Pharmacol. Exp. Ther.*, **1954**, *112*:413–423.

Biederman, J., Thisted, R.A., Greenhill, L.L., and Ryan, N.D. Estimation of the association between desipramine and the risk for sudden death in 5- to 14-year-old children. *J. Clin. Psychiatry*, **1995**, *56*:87–93.

Birnbaum, C.S., Cohen, L.S., Bailey, J.W., Crush, L.P., Robertson, L.M., and Stowe, Z.N. Serum concentrations of antidepressants and benzodiazepines in nursing infants: a case series. *Pediatrics*, **1999**, *104*:1–11.

Blier, P., de Montigny C., and Chaput, Y. A role for the serotonin system in the mechanism of action of antidepressant treatments: preclinical evidence. *J. Clin. Psychiatry*, **1990**, *51*(suppl.):14–20.

Boehnert, M.T., and Lovejoy, F.H. Jr. Value of the QRS duration versus the serum drug level in predicting seizures and ventricular arrhythmias after an acute overdose of tricyclic antidepressants. *N. Engl. J. Med.*, **1985**, *313*:474–479.

Boerner, R.J., and Moller, H.J. The importance of new antidepressants in the treatment of anxiety/depressive disorders. *Pharmacopsychiatry*, **1999**, *32*:119–126.

Brown, W.A., and Khan, A. Which depressed patients should receive antidepressants? *CNS Drugs*, **1994**, *1*:341–347.

Burke, M.J., and Preskorn, S.H. Short-term treatment of mood disorders with standard antidepressants. In, *Psychopharmacology: The Fourth Generation of Progress.* (Bloom, F.E., and Kupfer, D.L., eds.) Raven Press, New York, **1995**, pp. 1053–1065.

Caccia, S. Metabolism of the newer antidepressants. An overview of the pharmacological and pharmacokinetic implications. *Clin. Pharmacokinet.*, **1998**, *34*:281–302.

Carlsson A., and Wong, D.T. Correction: a note on the discovery of selective serotonin reuptake inhibitors. *Life Sci.*, **1997**, *61*:1203.

Catterson, M.L., Preskorn, S.H., and Martin, R.L. Pharmacodynamic and pharmacokinetic considerations in geriatric psychopharmacology. *Psychiatr. Clin. North Am.*, **1997**, *20*:205–218.

Cesura, A.M., and Pletscher, A. The new generation of monoamine oxidase inhibitors. *Prog. Drug Res.*, **1992**, *38*:171–297.

Chaput, Y., de Montigny, C., and Blier, P. Presynaptic and postsynaptic modifications of the serotonin system by long-term administration of antidepressant treatments. An *in vivo* electrophysiologic study in the rat. *Neuropsychopharmacology*, **1991**, *5*:219–229.

Chiarello, R.J., and Cole, J.O. The use of psychostimulants in general psychiatry. A reconsideration. *Arch. Gen. Psychiatry*, **1987**, *44*:286–295.

Cohen, B.M., and Baldessarini, R.J. Tolerance to therapeutic effects of antidepressants. *Am. J. Psychiatry*, **1985**, *142*:489–490.

Cohen, M.L., Schenck, K.W., and Hemrick-Leucke, S.H. 5-Hydroxytryptamine(1A) receptor activation enhances norepinephrine release from nerves in the rabbit saphenous vein. *J. Pharmacol. Exp. Ther.*, **1999**, *290*:1195–1201.

Cooper, S.J., Kelly, C.B., McGilloway, S., and Gilliland, A. Beta$_2$-adrenoreceptor antagonism in anxiety. *Eur. Neuropsychopharmacol.*, **1990**, *1*:75–77.

Crewe, H.K., Lennard, M.S., Tucker, G.T., Woods, F.R., and Haddock, R.E. The effect of selective serotonin reuptake inhibitors on cytochrome P450 2D6 (CYP2D6) activity in human liver microsomes. *Br. J. Clin. Pharmacol.*, **1992**, *34*:262–265.

D'Acquila, P.S., Collu, M., Pani, L., Gessa, G.L., and Serra, G. Antidepressant-like effect of selective dopamine D$_1$ receptor agonists in the behavioural despair animal model of depression. *Eur. J. Pharmacol.*, **1994**, *262*:107–111.

Danish University Antidepressant Group. Moclobemide: a reversible MAO-A inhibitor showing weaker antidepressant effect than clomipramine in a controlled multicenter study. *J. Affect. Disord.*, **1993**, *28*:105–116.

Davis, J.M., Janicak, P.G., and Bruninga, K. The efficacy of MAO inhibitors in depression; a meta-analysis. *Psychiatric Ann.*, **1987**, *17*:825–831.

Delgado, P.L., and Michaels, T. Reboxetine. *Drugs Today*, **1999**, *35*:725–737.

Delini-Stula, A., Radeke, E., and Waldmeier, P.S. Basic and clinical aspects of the new monoamine oxidase inhibitors. In, *Psychopharmacology: Current Trends.* (Casey, D.E., and Christensen, A.V., eds.) Springer-Verlag, Berlin, **1988**, pp. 147–158.

Dubovsky, S.L., and Buzan, R. The role of calcium channel blockers in the treatment of psychiatric disorders. *CNS Drugs*, **1995**, *4*:47–57.

Duman, R.S., Heninger, G.R., and Nestler, E.J. A molecular and cellular theory of depression. *Arch. Gen. Psychiatry*, **1997**, *54*:597–606.

Edwards, J.G. Drug choice in depression: selective serotonin reuptake inhibitors or tricyclic antidepressants? *CNS Drugs*, **1995**, *4*:141–159.

Edwards, J.G., Inman, W.H.W., Wilton, L., Pearce, G.L., and Kubota, K. Drug safety monitoring of 12,692 patients treated with fluoxetine. *Hum. Psychopharmacol. Clin. Exp.*, **1997**, *12*:127–137.

Emslie, G.J., Walkup, J.T., Pliszka, S.R., and Ernst, M. Nontricyclic antidepressants: current trends in children and adolescents. *J. Am. Acad. Child Adolesc. Psychiatry*, **1999**, *38*:517–528.

Ereshevsky, L., Riesenman, C., and Lam, Y.W. Serotonin selective reuptake inhibitor drug interactions and the cytochrome P450 system. *J. Clin. Psychiatry*, **1996**, *57*(suppl. 8):17–24.

Evrard, D.A., and Harrison, B.L. Recent approaches to novel antidepressant therapy. *Ann. Rep. Med. Chem.*, **1999**, *34*:1–10.

Fairchild, C.J., Rush, A.J., Vasavada, N., Giles, D.E., and Khatami, M. Which depressions respond to placebo? *Psychiatry Res.*, **1986**, *18*:217–226.

Flint, A.J. Choosing appropriate antidepressant therapy in the elderly. A risk-benefit assessment of available agents. *Drugs Aging*, **1998**, *13*:269–280.

Foote, S.L., and Aston-Jones, G.S. Pharmacology and physiology of central noradrenergic systems. In, *Psychopharmacology: The Fourth Generation of Progress.* (Bloom, F.E., and Kupfer, D.L., eds.) Raven Press, New York, **1995**, pp. 335–345.

Frank, E., Kupfer, D.J., Perel, J.M., Cornes, C., Jarrett, D.B., Mallinger, A.G., Thase, M.E., McEachran, A.B., and Grochocinski, V.J. Three-year outcomes for maintenance therapies in recurrent depression. *Arch. Gen. Psychiatry*, **1990**, *47*:1093–1099.

Frank, E., Kupfer, D.J., Perel, J.M., Cornes, C., Mallinger, A.G., Thase, M.E., McEachran, A.B., and Grochocinski, V.J. Comparison of full-dose versus half-dose pharmacotherapy in the maintenance treatment of recurrent depression. *J. Affect. Disord.*, **1993**, *27*:139–145.

Fugh-Berman, A. Herb-drug interactions. *Lancet*, **2000**, *355*:134–138.

Gardner, D.M., Shulman, K.I., Walker, S.E., and Tailor, S.A. The making of a user-friendly MAOI diet. *J. Clin. Psychiatry*, **1996**, *57*:99–104.

Glassman, A.H., Roose, S.P., and Bigger, J.T. Jr. The safety of tricyclic antidepressants in cardiac patients. Risk-benefit reconsidered. *JAMA*, **1993**, *269*:2673–2675.

Greden, J.F. Do long-term treatments alter lifetime course? *J. Psychiatr. Res.*, **1998**, *32*:197–199.

Gruber, A.J., Hudson, J.I., and Pope, H.G. Jr. The management of treatment-resistant depression in disorders on the interface of psychiatry and medicine. Fibromyalgia, chronic fatigue syndrome, migraine, irritable bowel syndrome, atypical facial pain, and premenstrual dysphoric disorder. *Psychiatr. Clin. North Am.,* **1996,** *19*:351–369.

Hamilton, M.S., and Opler, L.A. Akathisia, suicidality, and fluoxetine. *J. Clin. Psychiatry,* **1992,** *53*:401–406.

Hazell, P. Tricyclic antidepressants in children: is there a rationale for use? *CNS Drugs,* **1996,** *5*:233–239.

Heninger, G.R., and Charney, D.S. Mechanisms of action of antidepressant treatments: implications for the etiology and treatment of depressive disorders. In, *Psychopharmacology: The Third Generation of Progress.* (Meltzer, H.Y., ed.) New York, Raven Press, **1987,** pp. 535–544.

Henn, F.A., and McKinney, W.T. Animal models in psychiatry. In, *Psychopharmacology: The Third Generation of Progress.* (Meltzer, H.Y., ed.) New York, Raven Press, **1987,** pp. 687–695.

Hoehn-Saric, R., Ninan, P., Black, D.W., Stahl, S., Greist, J.H., Lydiard, B., McElroy, S., Zajecka, J., Chapman, D., Clary C., and Harrison, W. Multicenter double-blind comparison of sertraline and desipramine for concurrent obsessive-compulsive and major depressive disorders. *Arch. Gen. Psychiatry,* **2000,** *57*:76–82.

Hollister, L.E. Tricyclic antidepressants. *N. Engl. J. Med.,* **1978,** *299*:1106–1109, 1168–1172.

Hudson, J.I., and Pope, H.G. Jr. Affective spectrum disorder: does antidepressant response identify a family of disorders with a common pathophysiology? *Am. J. Psychiatry,* **1990,** *147*:552–564.

Hyman, S.E., and Nestler, E.J. Initiation and adaptation: a paradigm for understanding psychotropic drug action. *Am. J. Psychiatry,* **1996,** *153*:151–162.

Isaacsson, G., Boëthius, G., and Bergman, U. Low level of antidepressant prescription for people who later commit suicide: 15 years of experience from a population-based drug database in Sweden. *Acta Psychiatr. Scand.,* **1992,** *85*:444–448.

Johnston, J.A., Lineberry, C.G., Ascher, J.A., Davidson, J., Khayrallah, M.A., Feighner, J.P., and Stark, P. A 102-center prospective study of seizure in association with bupropion. *J. Clin. Psychiatry,* **1991,** *52*:450–456.

Kahn, A., Warner, H.A., and Brown, W.A. Symptom reduction and suicide risk in patients treated with placebo in antidepressant clinical trials: an analysis of the Food and Drug Administration database. *Arch. Gen. Psychiatry,* **2000,** *57*:311–317.

Kasper, S., Höflich, G., Scholl, H.-P., and Möller, H.-J. Safety and antidepressant efficacy of selective serotonin re-uptake inhibitors. *Hum. Psychopharmacol.,* **1994,** *9*:1–12.

Katon, W., von Korff M., Lin, E., Bush, T., and Ormel, J. Adequacy and duration of antidepressant treatment in primary care. *Med. Care,* **1992,** *30*:67–76.

Keller, M.B., Kocsis, J.K., Thase, M.E., Gelenberg, A.J., Rush, A.J., Koran, L., Schatzberg, A., Russel, J., Hirshfeld, R., Klein, D., McCullough, J.P., Fawcett, J.A., Kornstein, S., La Vange, L., and Harrison, W. Maintenance phase efficacy of sertraline for chronic depression: a randomized controlled trial. *JAMA,* **1998,** *280*:1665–1672.

Kessler, R.C., McGonagle, K.A., Zhao, S., Nelson, C.B., Hughes, M., Eshleman, S., Wittchen, H.U., and Kendler, K.S. Lifetime and 12-month prevalence of DSM-III-R psychiatric disorders in the United States. Results from the National Comorbidity Study. *Arch. Gen. Psychiatry,* **1994,** *51*:8–19.

Kind, P., and Sorensen, J. The costs of depression. *Int. Clin. Psychopharmacol.,* **1993,** *7*:191–195.

Kitamura, Y., Zhao, X.H., Takei, M., and Nomura, Y. Effects of antidepressants on the glutamatergic system in mouse brain. *Neurochem. Int.,* **1991,** *19*:247–253.

Kitayama, I., Janson, A.M., Cintra, A., Fuxe, K., Agnati, L.F., Ogren, S.O., Harfstrand, A., Eneroth, P., and Gustafsson, J.A. Effects of chronic imipramine treatment on glucocorticoid receptor immunoreactivity in various regions of the rat brain. Evidence for selective increases of glucocorticoid receptor immunoreactivity in the locus coeruleus and 5-hydroxytryptamine nerve cell groups of the rostral ventromedial medulla. *J. Neural Transm.,* **1988,** *73*:191–203.

Kline, N.S. Clinical experience with iproniazid (Marsilid). *J. Clin. Exp. Psychopathol.,* **1958,** *19*(suppl.):72–78.

Knapp, M.J., Knopman, D.S., Solomon, P.R., Pendlebury, W.W., Davis, C.S., and Gracon, S.I. A 30-week randomized controlled trial of high-dose tacrine in patients with Alzheimer's disease. The Tacrine Study Group. *JAMA,* **1994,** *271*:985–991.

Kuhn, R. The treatment of depressive states with G22355 (imipramine hydrochloride). *Am. J. Psychiatry,* **1958,** *115*:459–464.

Kuhn, W., and Muller, T. The clinical potential of deprenyl in neurologic and psychiatric disorders. *J. Neural Transm. Suppl.,* **1996,** *48*:85–93.

Kukopulos, A., Caliari, B., Tundo, A., Minnai, G., Floris, G., Reginaldi, G., and Tondo, L. Rapid cyclers, temperament, and antidepressants. *Compr. Psychiatry,* **1983,** *24*:249–258.

Kupfer, D.J., Frank, E., Perel, J.M., Cornes, C., Mallinger, A.G., Thase, M.E., McEachran, A.B., and Grochocinski, V.J. Five-year outcome for maintenance therapies in recurrent depression. *Arch. Gen. Psychiatry,* **1992,** *49*:769–773.

Lader, M. Long-term anxiolytic therapy: the issue of drug withdrawal. *J. Clin. Psychiatry,* **1987,** *48*(suppl. *12*):12–16.

Lasser, R.A., and Baldessarini, R.J. Thyroid hormones in depressive disorders: a reappraisal of clinical utility. *Harv. Rev. Psychiatry,* **1997,** *4*:291–305.

Leonard, B.E. Biochemical strategies for the development of antidepressants. *CNS Drugs,* **1994,** *1*:285–304.

Liebowitz, M.R. Depression with anxiety and atypical depression. *J. Clin. Psychiatry,* **1993,** *54*(suppl.):10–14.

Lingaerde, O., Foreland, A.R., and Magnusson, A. Can winter depression be prevented by Ginkgo biloba extract? A placebo-controlled trial. *Acta Psychiatr. Scand.,* **1999,** *100*:62–66.

Lotufo-Neto, F., Trivedi, M., and Thase, M.E. Meta-analysis of the reversible inhibitors of monoamine oxidase type A moclobemide and brofaromine in the treatment of depression. *Neuropsychopharmacology,* **1999,** *20*:226–247.

Mann, J.J., Aarons, S.F., Wilner, P.J., Keilp, J.G., Sweeney, J.A., Pearlstein, T., Frances, A.J., Kocsis, J.H., and Brown, R.P. A controlled study of the antidepressant efficacy and side effects of (–)-deprenyl. A selective monoamine oxidase inhibitor. *Arch. Gen. Psychiatry,* **1989,** *46*:45–50.

Mansbach, R.S., Brooks, E.N., and Chen, Y.L. Antidepressant-like effects of CP-154,526, a selective $CFRF_1$-receptor antagonist. *Eur. J. Pharmacol.,* **1997,** *323*:21–26.

Mattox, J.H., Buckman, M.T., Bernstein, J., Pathak, D., and Kellner, R. Dopamine agonists for reducing depression associated with hyperprolactinemia. *J. Reprod. Med.* **1986,** *31*:694–698.

Maurice, T., Phan, V.L., Urani, A., Kamei, H., Noda, Y., and Nabeshima, T. Neuroactive neurosteroids as endogenous effectors for the sigma (σ_1) receptor: pharmacological evidence and therapeutic opportunities. *Jpn. J. Pharmacol.,* **1999,** *81*:125–155.

Maurice, T., Roman, F.J., Su, T.P., and Privat, A. Beneficial effects of sigma agonists on the age-related learning impairment in the senescence-accelerated mouse (SAM). *Brain Res.,* **1996,** *733*:219–230.

Mavissakalian, M.R., and Perel, J.M. Imipramine dose-response relationship in panic disorder with agoraphobia. Preliminary findings. *Arch. Gen. Psychiatry,* **1989,** *46*:127–131.

Max, M.B., Lynch, S.A., Muir, J., Shoaf, S.E., Smoller, B., and Dubner, R. Effects of desipramine, amitriptyline, and fluoxetine on pain in diabetic neuropathy. *N. Engl. J. Med.,* **1992,** *326*:1250–1256.

McCarthy, J.R., Heinrichs, S.C., and Grigoriadis, D.E. Recent progress in corticotrophin-releasing factor receptor agents. *Ann. Rep. Med. Chem.,* **1999,** *34*:11–20.

McCombs, J.S., Nichol, M.B., Stimmel, G.L., Sclar, D.A., Beasley, C.M. Jr., and Gross, L.S. The cost of antidepressant drug therapy failure: a study of antidepressant use patterns in a Medicaid population. *J. Clin. Psychiatry,* **1990,** *51*(*suppl.*):60–69.

McGrath, C., Buist, A., and Norman, T.R. Treatment of anxiety during pregnancy: effects of psychotropic drug treatment on the developing fetus. *Drug Saf.,* **1999,** *20*:171–186.

Miguel, E.C., Rauch, S.L., and Jenicke, M.A. Obsessive-compulsive disorder. *Psychiatr. Clin. North Am.,* **1997,** *20*:863–883.

Mirin, S.M., Schatzberg, A.F., and Creasey, D.E. Hypomania and mania after withdrawal of tricyclic antidepressants. *Am. J. Psychiatry,* **1981,** *138*:87–89.

Montgomery, S.A. Selective serotonin reuptake inhibitors in the acute treatment of depression. In, *Psychopharmacology: The Fourth Generation of Progress.* (Bloom, F.E., and Kupfer, D.L., eds.) Raven Press, New York, **1995,** pp. 1043–1051.

Montgomery, S.A., and Roberts, A. SSRIs: well tolerated treatment for depression. *Hum. Psychopharmacol.,* **1994,** *9*(*suppl. 1*):S7–S10.

Murphy, D.L., Aulakh, C.S., Garrick, N.A., and Sunderland, T. Monoamine oxidase inhibitors as antidepressants. In, *Psychopharmacology: The Third Generation of Progress.* (Meltzer, H.Y., ed.) New York, Raven Press, **1987,** pp. 545–552.

Nabeshima, T., and Muraoka, I. [Development of sigma-receptor ligands and clinical trials.] *Nippon Yakurigaku Zasshi,* **1999,** *114*:3–11.

Nagy, L.M., Krystal, J.H., Charney, D.S., Merikangas, K.R., and Woods, S.W. Long-term outcome of panic disorder after short-term imipramine and behavioral group treatment: 2.9-year naturalistic follow-up study. *J. Clin. Psychopharmacol.,* **1993,** *13*:16–24.

Neary, J.T., and Bu, Y. Hypericum LI 160 inhibits uptake of serotonin and norepinephrine in astrocytes. *Brain Res.,* **1999,** *816*:358–363.

Nelson, J.C., Jatlow, P.I., and Mazure, C. Rapid desipramine dose adjustment using 24-hour levels. *J. Clin. Psychopharmacol.,* **1987,** *7*:72–77.

Nelson, J.C., Mazure, C.M., Bowers, M.B. Jr., and Jatlow, P.I. A preliminary, open study of the combination of fluoxetine and desipramine for rapid treatment of major depression. *Arch. Gen. Psychiatry,* **1991,** *48*:303–307.

Nestler, E.J., McMahohn, A., Sabban, E.L., Tallman, J.F., and Duman, R.S. Chronic antidepressant administration decreases the expression of tyrosine hydroxylase in the rat locus coeruleus. *Proc. Natl. Acad. Sci. U.S.A.,* **1990,** *87*:7522–7526.

Newman, S.C., and Hassan, A.I. Antidepressant use in the elderly population in Canada: results from a national survey. *J. Gerontol. A. Biol. Sci. Med. Sci.,* **1999,** *54*:M527–M530.

Nicotra, M.B., Rivera, M., Pool, J.L., and Noall, M.W. Tricyclic antidepressant overdose: clinical and pharmacologic observations. *Clin. Toxicol.,* **1981,** *18*:599–613.

Nutt, D. Substance-P antagonists: a new treatment for depression? *Lancet,* **1998,** *352*:1644–1646.

Olfson, M., and Klerman, G.L. Trends in the prescription of antidepressants by office-based psychiatrists. *Am. J. Psychiatry,* **1993,** *150*:571–577.

Oshima, A., and Higuchi, T. Treatment guidelines for geriatric mood disorders. *Psychiatry Clin. Neurosci.,* **1999,** *53*(*suppl.*):S55–S59.

Owens, M.J., Morgan, W.N., Plott, S.J., and Nemeroff, C.B. Neurotransmitter receptor and transporter binding profile of antidepressants and their metabolites. *J. Pharmacol. Exp. Ther.,* **1997,** *283*:1305–1322.

Oxenkrug, G.F., Requintina, P.J., Yuwiler, A., and Palfereyman, M.G. The acute effect of the bioprecursor of the selective brain MAO-A inhibitor, MDL 72392, on rat pineal melatonin biosynthesis. *J. Neural Transm. Suppl.,* **1999,** *41*:377–379.

Pacher, P., Ungvari, Z., Nanasi, P.P., Furst, S., and Kecskemeti, V. Speculations on difference between tricyclic and selective serotonin reuptake inhibitor antidepressants on their cardiac effects. Is there any? *Curr. Med. Chem.,* **1999,** *6*:469–480.

Page, M.E., Detke, M.J., Dalvi, A., Kirby, L.G., and Lucki, I. Serotonergic mediation of the effects of fluoxetine, but not desiptamine, in the rat forced swimming test. *Psychopharmacology (Berl.),* **1999,** *147*:162–167.

Perry, P.J., Zeilman, C., and Arndt, S. Tricyclic antidepressant concentrations in plasma: an estimate of their sensitivity and specificity as a predictor of response. *J. Clin. Psychopharmacol.,* **1994,** *14*:230–240.

Peselow, E.D., Sanfilipo, M.P., Difiglia, C., and Fieve, R.R. Melancholic/endogenous depression and response to somatic treatment and placebo. *Am. J. Psychiatry,* **1992,** *149*:1324–1334.

Philipp, M., Kohnen, R., and Hiller, K.O. Hypericum extract versus imipramine or placebo in patients with moderate depression: randomised multicentre study of treatment for eight weeks. *BMJ,* **1999,** *319*:1534–1538.

Pigott, T.A., and Seay, S.M. A review of the efficacy of selective serotonin reuptake inhibitors in obsessive-compulsive disorder. *J. Clin. Psychiatry,* **1999,** *60*:101–106.

Pollock, B.G., and Perel, J.M. Hydroxy metabolites of tricyclic antidepressants: evaluation of relative cardiotoxicity. In, *Clinical Pharmacology in Psychiatry: From Molecular Studies to Clinical Reality.* (Dahl, S.G., and Gram, L.F., eds.) Springer-Verlag, Berlin, **1989,** pp. 232–236.

Potokar, J., and Nutt, D.J. Anxiolytic potential of benzodiazepine receptor partial agonists. *CNS Drugs,* **1994,** *1*:305–315.

Preskorn, S.H. Debate resolved: there are differential effects of serotonin selective reuptake inhibitors on cytochrome P450 enzymes. *J. Psychopharmacol.,* **1998,** *12*:S89–S97.

Prouty, R.W., and Anderson, W.H. The forensic science implications of site and temporal influences on postmortem blood-drug concentrations. *J. Forensic Sci.,* **1990,** *35*:243–270.

Racagni, G., Tinelli, D., and Bianchi, E. cAMP-dependent binding proteins and endogenous phosphorylation after antidepressant treatment. In, *5-Hydroxytryptamine in Psychiatry: A Spectrum of Ideas.* (Sandler, M., Coppen, A., and Hartnet, S., eds.) Oxford University Press, New York, **1991,** pp. 116–123.

Ray, W.A., Griffin, M.R., Schaffner, W., Baugh, D.K., and Melton, L.J. III. Psychotropic drug use and the risk of hip fracture. *N. Engl. J. Med.,* **1987,** *316*:363–369.

Robinson, D.S., Nies, A., Ravaris, C.L., Ives, J.O., and Bartlett, D. Clinical pharmacology of phenelzine. *Arch. Gen. Psychiatry,* **1978,** *35*:629–635.

Roerig, J.L. Diagnosis and management of generalized anxiety disorder. *J. Am. Pharm. Assoc. (Wash.),* **1999,** *39*:811–821.

Roose, S.P. Modern cardiovascular standards for psychotropic drugs. *Psychopharmacol. Bull.,* **1992,** *28*:35–43.

Roose, S.P., Glassman, A.H., Attia, E., and Woodring, S. Comparative efficacy of selective serotonin reuptake inhibitors and tricyclics in the treatment of melancholia. *Am. J. Psychiatry,* **1994,** *151*:1735–1739.

Rosenbaum, J.F., and Pollock, R.A. The psychopharmacology of social phobia and comorbid disorders. *Bull. Menninger Clin.,* **1994,** *58*:A67–A83.

Sachs, G.S., Lafer, B., Stoll, A.L., Banov, M., Thibault, A.B., Tohen, M., and Rosenbaum, J.F. A double-blind trial of bupropion versus desipramine for bipolar depression. *J. Clin. Psychiatry,* **1994,** 55:391–393.

Saria, A. The tachykinin NK-1 receptor in the brain: pharmacology and putative functions. *Eur. J. Pharmacol.,* **1999,** *375*:51–60.

Schatzberg, A.F., and Rothschild, A.J. Psychotic (delusional) major depression: should it be included as a distinct syndrome in DSM-IV? *Am. J. Psychiatry,* **1992,** *149*:733–745.

Schatzberg, A.F., Haddad, P., Kaplan, E.M., Lejoyeux M., Rosenbaum, J.F., Young, A.H., and Zajecka, J. Serotonin reuptake discontinuation syndrome: a hypothetical definition. Discontinuation Consensus panel. *J. Clin. Psychiatry,* **1997,** *58(suppl. 7)*:5–10.

Schwartz, J.A., Speed, N., and Bereford, T.P. Antidepressants in the medically ill: prediction of benefits. *Int. J. Psychiatry Med.,* **1989,** *19*:363–369.

Shatan, C. Withdrawal symptoms after abrupt termination of imipramine. *Can. Psychiatr. Assoc. J.,* **1966,** *11(suppl.)*:150–158.

Shelton, R.C., Keller, M.B., Gelenberg, A., Dunner, D.L., Hirschfeld, R., Thase, M.E., Russell, J., Lydiard, R.B., Crits-Cristoph, P., Gollop, R., Todd, L., Hellerstein, D., Goodnick, P., Keitner, G., Stahl, S.M., and Halbreich, U. Effectiveness of St. John's wort in major depression: a randomized controlled trial. *JAMA,* **2001,** *285*:1978–1986.

Siuciak, J.A., Lewis, D.R., Wiegand, S.J., and Lindsay, R.M. Antidepressant-like effect of brain-derived neurotrophic factor (BDNF). *Pharmacol. Biochem. Behav.,* **1997,** *56*:131–137.

Small, G.W. Treatment of geriatric depression. *Depression Anxiety,* **1998,** 8*(suppl. 1)*:32–42.

Smith, M.T., Crouch, N.R., Gericke, N., and Hirst, M. Psychoactive constituents of the genus *Sceletium* N.E.Br. and other Mesembryanthemaceae: a review. *J. Ethnopharmacol.,* **1996,** *50*:119–130.

Spencer, T., Biederman, J., Wilens, T., Steingard, R., and Geist, D. Nortriptyline treatment of children with attention-deficit hyperactivity disorder and tic disorder or Tourette's syndrome. *J. Am. Acad. Child Adolesc. Psychiatry,* **1993,** *32*:205–210.

Steckler, T., and Holsboer, F. Corticotrophin-releasing hormone receptor subtypes and emotion. *Biol. Psychiatry,* **1999,** *46*:1480–1508.

Steingard, R.J., DeMaso, D.R., Goldman, S.J., Shorrock, K.L., and Bucci, J.P. Current perspectives on the pharmacotherapy of depressive disorders in children and adolescents. *Harv. Rev. Psychiatry,* **1995,** 2:313–326.

Sternbach, H. The serotonin syndrome. *Am. J. Psychiatry,* **1991,** *148*:705–713.

Stoll, A.L., Mayer, P.V., Kolbrener, M., Goldstein, E., Suplit, B., Lucier, J., Cohen, B.M., and Tohen, M. Antidepressant-associated mania: a controlled comparison with spontaneous mania. *Am. J. Psychiatry,* **1994,** *11*:1642–1645.

Sullivan, G.M., Coplan, J.D., Kent, J.M., and Gorman, J.M. The noradrenergic system in pathological anxiety: a focus on panic with relevance to generalized anxiety and phobias. *Biol. Psychiatry,* **1999,** *46*:1205–1218.

Suominen K.H., Isometsä, E.T., Hendriksson, M.M., Ostamo, A.I., and Lönnqvist, J.K. Inadequate treatment for major depression both before and after attempted suicide. *Am. J. Psychiatry,* **1998,** *155*:1778–1780.

Swain, C., and Rupniak, N.M.J. Progress in the development of neurokinin antagonists. *Ann. Rep. Med. Chem.,* **1999,** *34*:51–60.

Tejedor-Real, P., Mico, J.A., Maldonado, R., Roques, B.P., and Gibert-Rahola, J. Implication of endogenous opioid system in the learned helplessness model of depression. *Pharmacol. Biochem. Behav.,* **1995,** *52*:145–152.

Thase, M.E., and Nolen, W. Tricyclic antidepressants and classical monoamine oxidase inhibitors: contemporary clinical use. In, *Schizophrenia and Mood Disorders: The New Drug Therapies in Clinical Practice.* (Buckley, P.F., and Waddington, J.L., eds.) Butterworth-Heinemann, Boston, **2000,** pp. 85–99.

Tome, M.B., Isaac, M.T., Harte, R., and Holland, C. Paroxetine and pindolol: a randomized trial of serotonergic autoreceptor blockade in the reduction of antidepressant latency. *Int. Clin. Psychopharmacol.,* **1997,** *12*:81–89.

Uhlenhuth, E.H., Balter, M.B., Ban, T.A., and Yang, K. International study of expert judgment on therapeutic use of benzodiazepines and other psychotherapeutic medications: treatment strategies in panic disorder, 1992–1997. *J. Clin. Psychopharmacol.,* **1998,** *18*:27S–31S.

van Harten, J. Clinical pharmacokinetics of selective serotonin reuptake inhibitors. *Clin. Pharmacokinet.,* **1993,** *24*:203–220.

Viguera, A.C., Baldessarini, R.J., and Friedberg, J. Discontinuing antidepressant treatment in major depression. *Harv. Rev. Psychiatry,* **1998,** *5*:293–306.

Wamsley, J.K., Byerley, W.F., McCabe, R.T., McConnell, E.J., Dawson, T.M., and Grosser, B.I. Receptor alterations associated with serotonergic agents: an autoradiographic analysis. *J. Clin. Psychiatry,* **1987,** *48(suppl.)*:19–25.

Wehr, T.A., and Goodwin, F.K. Can antidepressants cause mania and worsen the course of affective illness? *Am. J. Psychiatry,* **1987,** *144*:1403–1411.

Wells, B.G., and Marken, P.A. Bromocriptine in treatment of depression. *Drug Intell. Clin. Pharm.,* **1989,** *23*:600–602.

White, K., and Simpson, G. Combined MAOI-tricyclic antidepressant treatment: a reevaluation. *J. Clin. Psychopharmacol.,* **1981,** *1*:264–282.

Wilens, T.E., Biederman, J., Baldessarini, R.J., Puopolo, P.R., and Flood, J.G. Developmental changes in serum concentrations of desipramine and 2-hydroxydesipramine during treatment with desipramine. *J. Am. Acad. Child Adolesc. Psychiatry,* **1992,** *31*:691–698.

Wisner, K.L., Gelenberg, A.J., Leonard, H., Zarin, D., and Frank, E. Pharmacologic treatment of depression during pregnancy. *JAMA,* **1999,** *282*:1264–1269.

Wong, A.H., Smith, M., and Boon, H.S. Herbal remedies in psychiatric practice. *Arch. Gen. Psychiatry,* **1998,** *55*:1033–1044.

Wong, D.T., and Bymaster, F.P. Development of antidepressant drugs. Fluoxetine (PROZAC) and other selective serotonin reuptake inhibitors. *Adv. Exp. Med. Biol.,* **1995,** *363*:77–95.

Wong, D.T., Bymaster, F.P., Reid, L.R., Mayle, D.A., Krushinski, J.H., and Robertson, D.W. Norfluoxetine enantiomers as inhibitors of serotonin uptake in rat brain. *Neuropsychopharmacology,* **1993,** *8*:337–344.

Wong, K.L., Bruch, R.C., and Farbman, A.I. Amitriptyline-mediated inhibition of neurite outgrowth from chick embryonic cerebral explants involves a reduction in adenylate cyclase activity. *J. Neurochem.,* **1991,** *57*:1223–1230.

Workman, E.A., and Short, D.D. Atypical antidepressants versus imipramine in the treatment of major depression: a meta-analysis. *J. Clin. Psychiatry,* **1993,** *54*:5–12.

Zahniser, N.R., Larson, G.A., and Gerhardt, G.A. *In vivo* dopamine clearance rate in rat striatum: regulation by extracellular dopamine concentration and dopamine transporter inhibitors. *J. Pharmacol. Exp. Ther.,* **1999,** 289:266–277.

Zornberg, G.L., and Pope, H.G. Jr. Treatment of depression in bipolar disorder: new directions for research. *J. Clin. Psychopharmacol.,* **1993,** 13:397–408.

MONOGRAPHS AND REVIEWS

Agras, W.S. Treatment of eating disorders. In, *The American Psychiatric Press Textbook of Psychopharmacology,* 2nd ed. (Schatzberg, A.F., and Nemeroff, C.B., eds.) American Psychiatric Press, Washington, D.C., **1998,** pp. 869–879.

American Psychiatric Association. *Diagnostic and Statistical Manual of Mental Disorders: DSM-IV,* 4th ed., text revision. APA Press, Washington, D.C., **2000.**

Ayd, F.J. Jr., and Blackwell, B., eds. *Discoveries in Biological Psychiatry.* Lippincott, Philadelphia, **1970.**

Baldessarini, R.J. *Chemotherapy in Psychiatry: Principles and Practice,* 2nd ed. Harvard University Press, Cambridge, MA, **1985.**

Baldessarini, R.J. Current status of antidepressants: clinical pharmacology and therapy. *J. Clin. Psychiatry,* **1989,** 50:117–126.

Baldessarini, R.J. Fifty years of biomedical psychiatry and psychopharmacology in America. In, *American Psychiatry After World War II: (1944–1994).* (Menninger R., and Nemiah, J., eds.) American Psychiatric Press, Washington, D.C., **2000,** pp. 369–410.

Bloom, F.E., and Kupfer, D.J., eds. *Psychopharmacology: The Fourth Generation of Progress.* Raven Press, New York, **1995.**

Browne, L.J., and Shaw, K.J. New anxiolytics. *Ann. Rep. Med. Chem.* **1991,** 26:1–10.

Buckley, P.F., and Waddington, J.L., eds. *Schizophrenia and Mood Disorders: The New Drug Therapies in Clinical Practice.* Butterworth-Heinemann, Boston, **2000.**

Caldwell, A.E. History of psychopharmacology. In, *Principles of Psychopharmacology,* 2nd ed. (Clark, W.G., and del Giudice, J., eds.) Academic Press, New York, **1978,** pp. 9–40.

Cornish, J.W., McNicholas, L.F., and O'Brien, C.P. Treatment of substance-related disorders. In, *The American Psychiatric Press Textbook of Psychopharmacology,* 2nd ed. (Schatzberg, A.F., and Nemeroff, C.B., eds.) American Psychiatric Press, Washington, D.C., **1998,** pp. 851–867.

DeBattista, C., and Schatzberg, A.F. Universal psychotropic dosing and monitoring guidelines. *The Economics of Neuroscience (TEN),* **1999,** 1:75–84.

DeVane, C.L., and Nemeroff, C.B. Psychotropic drug interactions. *The Economics of Neuroscience (TEN),* **2000,** 2:55–75.

Efron, D.H., Holmstedt, B., and Kline, N.S., eds. *Ethnopharmacologic Search for Psychoactive Drugs.* Public Health Service Publication No. 67–1645. U.S. Government Printing Office, Washington, D.C., **1967.**

Fawcett, J., and Busch, K.A. Stimulants in psychiatry. In, *The American Psychiatric Press Textbook of Psychopharmacology,* 2nd ed. (Schatzberg, A.F., and Nemeroff, C.B., eds.) American Psychiatric Press, Washington, D.C., **1998,** pp. 503–522.

Feighner, J.P. Overview of antidepressants currently used to treat anxiety disorders. *J. Clin. Psychiatry,* **1999,** 60(suppl. 22):18–22.

Frazer, A. Antidepressants. *J. Clin. Psychiatry,* **1997,** 58(suppl. 6):9–25.

Fuller, R.W. Basic advances in serotonin pharmacology. *J. Clin. Psychiatry,* **1992,** 53(suppl.):36–45.

Geller, D.A., Biederman, J., Jones, J., Shaprio, S., Schwartz, S., and Park, K.S. Obsessive-compulsive disorder in children and adolescents: a review. *Harv. Rev. Psychiatry,* **1998,** 5:260–273.

Golden, R.N., Dawkins, K., Nicholas, L., and Bebchuk, J.M. Trazodone, nefazodone, bupropion, and mirtazapine. In, *The American Psychiatric Press Textbook of Psychopharmacology,* 2nd ed. (Schatzberg, A.F., and Nemeroff, C.B., eds.) American Psychiatric Press, Washington, D.C., **1998,** pp. 251–269.

Goodwin, F.K., and Jamison, K.R. *Manic-Depressive Illness.* Oxford University Press, New York, **1990.**

Hansten, P.D., and Horn, J.R. *Drug Interactions Analysis and Management Quarterly.* Vancouver, WA, Applied Therapeutics, **2000.**

Healy, D. *The Antidepressant Era.* Harvard University Press, Cambridge, MA, **1997.**

Hollister, L.E., Müller-Oerlinghausen, B., Rickels, K., and Shader, R.I. Clinical uses of benzodiazepines. *J. Clin. Psychopharmacol,* **1993,** 13:1S–169S.

Kent, J.M. SNaRIs, NaSSAs, and NaRIs: new agents for the treatment of depression. *Lancet,* **2000,** 355:911–918.

Krishnan, K.R.R. Monoamine oxidase inhibitors. In, *The American Psychiatric Press Textbook of Psychopharmacology,* 2nd ed. (Schatzberg, A.F., and Nemeroff, C.B., eds.) American Psychiatric Press, Washington, D.C., **1998,** pp. 239–249.

Kutcher, S.P. *Child & Adolescent Psychopharmacology.* Saunders, Philadelphia, **1997.**

Leipzig, R.M., and Mendelowitz, A. Adverse psychotropic drug interactions. In, *Adverse Effects of Psychotropic Drugs.* (Kane, J.M., and Lieberman, J.A., eds.) Guilford Press, New York, **1992,** pp. 13–76.

Leonard, B.E., and Richelson, E. Synaptic effects of antidepressants. In, *Schizophrenia and Mood Disorders: The New Drug Therapies in Clinical Practice.* (Buckley, P.F., and Waddington, J.L., eds.) Butterworth-Heinemann, Boston, **2000,** pp. 67–84.

Lewin, L. *Phantastica, Narcotic, and Stimulating Drugs: Their Use and Abuse.* Dutton, New York, **1931.**

Marin, D.B., and Davis, K.L. Cognitive enhancers. In, *The American Psychiatric Press Textbook of Psychopharmacology,* 2nd ed. (Schatzberg, A.F., and Nemeroff, C.B., eds.) American Psychiatric Press, Washington, D.C., **1998,** pp. 473–486.

Masand, P.S., and Gupta, S. Selective serotonin-reuptake inhibitors: an update. *Harv. Rev. Psychiatry,* **1999,** 7:69–84.

Murphy, D.L., Mitchell, P.B., and Potter, W.Z. Novel pharmacological approaches to the treatment of depression. In, *Psychopharmacology: The Fourth Generation of Progress.* (Bloom, F.E., and Kupfer, D.L., eds.) Raven Press, New York, **1995,** pp. 1143–1153.

Musselman, D.L., DeBattista, C., Nathan, K.I., Kilts, C.D., Schatzberg, A.F., and Nemeroff, C.B. Biology of mood disorders. In, *The American Psychiatric Press Textbook of Psychopharmacology,* 2nd ed. (Schatzberg, A.F., and Nemeroff, C.B., eds.) American Psychiatric Press, Washington, D.C., **1998,** pp. 549–588.

Ninan, P.T., Cole, J.O., and Yonkers, K.A. Nonbenzodiazepine anxiolytics. In, *The American Psychiatric Press Textbook of Psychopharmacology,* 2nd ed. (Schatzberg, A.F., and Nemeroff, C.B., eds.) American Psychiatric Press, Washington, D.C., **1998,** pp. 287–300.

Potter, W.Z., Manji, H.K., and Rudorfer, M.V. Tricyclics and tetracyclics. In, *The American Psychiatric Press Textbook of Psychopharmacology,* 2nd ed. (Schatzberg, A.F., and Nemeroff, C.B., eds.) American Psychiatric Press, Washington, D.C., **1998,** pp. 199–218.

Preskorn, S.H. Clinically relevant pharmacology of selective serotonin reuptake inhibitors: an overview with emphasis on pharmacokinetics and effects on oxidative drug metabolism. *Clin. Pharmacokinet.,* **1997,** 32(suppl. 1):1–21.

Prien, R.F., and Kocsis, J.H. Long-term treatment of mood disorders. In, *Psychopharmacology: The Fourth Generation of Progress.*

(Bloom, F.E., and Kupfer, D.L., eds.) Raven Press, New York, **1995,** pp. 1067–1079.

Robertson, D.W., ed. CNS agents. *Ann. Rep. Med. Chem.* **1999,** *34*:1–20.

Rudorfer, M.V., Henry, M.E., and Sackein, H.A. Electroconvulsive therapy. In, *Psychiatry.* Vol. 1. (Tasman, A., Kay, J., and Lieberman, J.A., eds.) Saunders, Philadelphia, **1997,** pp. 1535–1551.

Sadock, B.J., and Sadock, V.A., eds. *Kaplan & Sadock's Comprehensive Textbook of Psychiatry,* 7th ed. Lippincott Williams & Wilkins, Philadelphia, **2000.**

Shulman, K.I., Tohen, M., and Kutcher, S.P., eds. *Mood Disorders Across the Life Span.* Wiley-Liss, New York, **1996.**

Singer, T.P., Von Korff, R.W., and Murphy, D., eds. *Monoamine Oxidase: Structure, Function, and Altered Functions.* Academic Press, New York, **1979.**

Stein, M.B., and Uhde, T.W. Biology of anxiety disorders. In, *The American Psychiatric Press Textbook of Psychopharmacology,* 2nd ed. (Schatzberg, A.F., and Nemeroff, C.B., eds.) American Psychiatric Press, Washington, D.C., **1998,** pp. 609–628.

Sulser, F., and Mobley, P.L. Biochemical effects of antidepressants in animals. In, *Psychotropic Agents. Handbook of Experimental Pharmacology.* Vol. 55, pt. I. (Hoffmeister, F. and Stille, G., eds.) Springer-Verlag, Berlin, **1980,** pp. 471–490.

Taylor, C.B. Treatment of anxiety disorders. In, *The American Psychiatric Press Textbook of Psychopharmacology,* 2nd ed. (Schatzberg, A.F., and Nemeroff, C.B., eds.) American Psychiatric Press, Washington, D.C., **1998,** pp. 775–789.

Tollefson, G.D., and Rosenbaum, J.F. Selective serotonin-reuptake inhibitors. In, *The American Psychiatric Press Textbook of Psychopharmacology,* 2nd ed. (Schatzberg, A.F., and Nemeroff, C.B., eds.) American Psychiatric Press, Washington, D.C., **1998,** pp. 219–237.

Weber, S.S. Drug interactions with antidepressants. *CNS Special Edition,* **1999,** *1*:47–55.

Weiss, J.M., and Kilts, C.D. Animal models of depression and schizophrenia. In, *The American Psychiatric Press Textbook of Psychopharmacology,* 2nd ed. (Schatzberg, A.F., and Nemeroff, C.B., eds.) American Psychiatric Press, Washington, D.C., **1998,** pp. 89–131.

DRUGS AND THE TREATMENT OF PSYCHIATRIC DISORDERS
Psychosis and Mania

Ross J. Baldessarini and Frank I. Tarazi

Clinically effective antipsychotic agents include tricyclic phenothiazines, thioxanthenes, and dibenzepines, as well as butyrophenones and congeners, other heterocyclics, and experimental benzamides. Virtually all of these drugs block D_2-dopamine receptors and reduce dopamine neurotransmission in forebrain; some also interact with D_1- and D_4-dopaminergic, 5-HT_{2A}- and 5-HT_{2C}-serotonergic, and α-adrenergic receptors. Antipsychotic drugs are relatively lipophilic, metabolized mainly by hepatic oxidative mechanisms, and some have complex elimination kinetics.

These drugs offer effective palliative treatment of both organic and idiopathic psychotic disorders with acceptable safety and practicality. Antipsychotic agents of high potency tend to have more adverse extrapyramidal neurological effects, and low-potency agents induce more sedative, hypotensive, and autonomic side effects. Characteristic neurological side effects of typical or "neuroleptic" antipsychotic agents include dystonia, akathisia, bradykinesia, and acute or late dyskinesias. Several antipsychotic agents, including clozapine, olanzapine, quetiapine, and low doses of risperidone, have limited extrapyramidal side effects and so are considered "atypical."

Treatment of acute psychotic illness typically involves daily doses up to the equivalent of 10 to 20 mg of fluphenazine or haloperidol (at serum concentrations of about 5 to 20 ng/ml) or 300 to 600 mg of chlorpromazine; higher doses usually are not more effective but increase risks of adverse effects. Long-term maintenance treatment usually requires lower doses, and tolerance virtually is unknown.

The treatment of mania and recurrences of mania and depression in bipolar disorder for several decades had been based mainly on the use of lithium carbonate or citrate. The therapeutic index of lithium is low, and close control of serum concentrations is required for its safe clinical application. Antipsychotic agents commonly are used to control acute or psychotic mania, and potent sedative-anticonvulsant benzodiazepines (see Chapter 17) also are used adjunctively in acute mania. Additional commonly used alternative or adjunctive treatments for mania include the anticonvulsants sodium divalproex and carbamazepine and other experimental agents (see Chapter 21).

I. DRUGS USED IN THE TREATMENT OF PSYCHOSES

Several classes of drugs are effective in the symptomatic treatment of psychiatric disorders. They are most appropriately used in the therapy of schizophrenia, the manic phase of bipolar (manic-depressive) illness, and other acute idiopathic psychotic illnesses or conditions marked by severe agitation. They also are used as an alternative to electroconvulsive therapy (ECT) in severe depression with psychotic features and sometimes in the management of patients with organic psychotic disorders.

Effective antipsychotic agents include *phenothiazines,* structurally similar *thioxanthenes,* and *benzepines; butyrophenones* (phenylbutylpiperidines) and *diphenylbutylpiperidines;* and *indolones* and other heterocyclic compounds. Since these chemically dissimilar drugs share many properties, information about their pharmacology and clinical uses is presented for the group as a whole. Particular attention is paid to chlorpromazine, the oldest representative of the phenothiazine–thioxanthene group of antipsychotic agents, and haloperidol, the original butyrophenone and representative of several related classes of aromatic butylpiperidine derivatives.

Many patients have been treated with the antipsychotic agents since their introduction in the 1950s. Although they have had a revolutionary, beneficial impact on medical and psychiatric practice, their liabilities, especially the almost relentless association of older, typical or "neuroleptic" agents with extrapyramidal neurological effects, also must be emphasized. Newer antipsychotics are atypical in having less risk of extrapyramidal side effects, but some of them produce hypotension, seizures, weight gain, diabetes, hyperprolactinemia, and other adverse effects.

TRICYCLIC ANTIPSYCHOTIC AGENTS

Antipsychotic agents are used primarily in the management of patients with psychotic or other serious psychiatric illnesses marked by agitation and impaired reasoning. Several dozen antipsychotic drugs are used in psychiatric conditions worldwide; still others are marketed primarily for other uses, including antiemetic and antihistaminic effects. The term *neuroleptic* has taken on connotations, at least in the United States, of relatively prominent experimental and clinical antagonism of D_2-dopamine receptor activity, with substantial risk of extrapyramidal side effects. The term *atypical antipsychotic* has been used to describe agents that are associated with substantially lower risks of adverse extrapyramidal effects. Representative examples include *clozapine, olanzapine, quetiapine,* and low doses of *risperidone* (Blin, 1999; Markowitz *et al.,* 1999).

History. The history of the antipsychotic agents is well summarized by Swazey (1974) and Caldwell (1978). In the early 1950s, some antipsychotic effects were obtained with extracts of the *Rauwolfia* plant and then with large doses of the purified active alkaloid *reserpine,* which was later chemically synthesized by Woodward. Although reserpine and related compounds that share its ability to deplete monoamines from their vesicular storage sites in neurons exert antipsychotic effects, these are relatively weak and are typically associated with severe side effects, including sedation, hypotension, diarrhea, anergy, and depressed mood. Thus, the clinical utility of reserpine primarily has been as an antihypertensive agent (*see* Chapter 33).

Phenothiazine compounds were synthesized in Europe in the late nineteenth century as part of the development of aniline dyes such as methylene blue. In the late 1930s, a phenothiazine derivative, *promethazine,* was found to have antihistaminic and sedative effects. Attempts to treat agitation in

psychiatric patients with promethazine and other antihistamines followed in the 1940s, but with little success.

Meanwhile, the ability of promethazine to prolong barbiturate sleeping time in rodents was discovered, and the drug was introduced into clinical anesthesia as a potentiating and autonomic stabilizing agent (Laborit *et al.,* 1952). This work prompted a search for other phenothiazine derivatives with anesthesia-potentiating actions, and in 1949–1950 Charpentier synthesized *chlorpromazine.* Soon thereafter, Laborit and his colleagues described the ability of this compound to potentiate anesthetics and produce "artificial hibernation." Chlorpromazine by itself did not cause a loss of consciousness but diminished arousal and motility, with some tendency to promote sleep. These central actions became known as *ataractic* or *neuroleptic* soon thereafter.

The first attempts to treat mental illness with chlorpromazine were made in Paris in 1951 and early 1952 by Paraire and Sigwald (*see* Swazey 1974). In 1952, Delay and Deniker became convinced that chlorpromazine achieved more than symptomatic relief of agitation or anxiety and that it had an ameliorative effect upon psychotic processes in diverse disorders. In 1954, Lehmann and Hanrahan in Montreal, followed by Winkelman in Philadelphia, reported the initial use of chlorpromazine in North America for the treatment of psychomotor excitement and manic states as well as schizophrenia (*see* Swazey, 1974). Clinical studies soon revealed that chlorpromazine was effective in the treatment of psychotic disorders of various types.

Chemistry and Structure–Activity Relationships. This topic is reviewed in detail elsewhere (Baldessarini, 1985; Neumeyer and Booth, 2001). Phenothiazines have a three-ring structure in which two benzene rings are linked by a sulfur and a nitrogen atom (*see* Table 20–1). If the nitrogen at position 10 is replaced by a carbon atom with a double bond to the side chain, the compound is a thioxanthene.

Substitution of an electron-withdrawing group at position 2 increases the efficacy of phenothiazines and other tricyclic congeners (*e.g.,* chlorpromazine *vs.* promazine). The nature of the substituent at position 10 also influences pharmacological activity. As can be seen in Table 20–1, the phenothiazines and thioxanthenes can be divided into three groups on the basis of substitution at this site. Those with an *aliphatic* side chain include *chlorpromazine* and *triflupromazine* among the phenothiazines; these compounds are relatively low in potency (but not in clinical efficacy). Those with a *piperidine* ring in the side chain include *thioridazine* and *mesoridazine.* There is a somewhat lower incidence of extrapyramidal side effects with this substitution, possibly due to increased central antimuscarinic activity. Several potent phenothiazine antipsychotic compounds have a *piperazine* group in the side chain; *fluphenazine* and *trifluoperazine* are examples. Use of these potent compounds, most of which have relatively weak anticholinergic activity, entails a greater risk of inducing extrapyramidal side effects but less tendency to produce sedation or autonomic side effects, such as hypotension, unless unusually large doses are employed. Several piperazine phenothiazines have been esterified at a free hydroxyl group with long-chain fatty acids to produce slowly absorbed and hydrolyzed, long-acting, highly lipophilic prodrugs. *The decanoates* of fluphenazine and haloperidol and enanthate of fluphenazine are used commonly in the United States, and several others are available internationally.

Table 20–1

Selected Antipsychotic Drugs: Chemical Structures, Doses and Dosage Forms, and Side Effects*

NONPROPRIETARY NAME / TRADE NAME		DOSE AND DOSAGE FORMS†			SIDE EFFECTS		
Phenothiazines		*Adult Antipsychotic Oral Dose Range— Daily Dosage*		*Single Intramuscular Dose‡*	*Sedative Effects*	*Extra-pyramidal Effects*	*Hypotensive Effects*
R_1	R_2	Usual, mg	Extreme,§ mg	Usual, mg			
Chlorpromazine hydrochloride —$(CH_2)_3$—$N(CH_3)_2$ THORAZINE	—Cl	200–800 O, SR, L, I, S	30–2000	25–50	+++	++	IM +++ Oral ++
Mesoridazine besylate SERENTIL	—SCH_3 ‖ O	75–300 O, L, I	30–400	25	+++	+	++
Thioridazine hydrochloride MELLARIL	—SCH_3	150–600 O, L	20–800		+++	+	+++
Fluphenazine hydrochloride Fluphenazine enanthate Fluphenazine decanoate PERMITIL and PROLIXIN (HYDROCHLORIDES) PROLIXIN (ENANTHATE and DECANOATE) O, L, I	—CF_3	2–20	0.5–30	1.25–2.5 (decanoate or enanthate: 12.5–50 every 1–4 weeks)	+	++++	+
Perphenazine TRILAFON	—Cl	8–32 O, L, I	4–64	5–10	++	++	+
Trifluoperazine hydrochloride STELAZINE	—CF_3	5–20 O, L, I	2–30	1–2	+	+++	+

Table 20–1

Selected Antipsychotic Drugs: Chemical Structures, Doses and Dosage Forms, and Side Effects* (*Continued*)

NONPROPRIETARY NAME	TRADE NAME	DOSE AND DOSAGE FORMS†			SIDE EFFECTS		
Thioxanthenes		*Adult Antipsychotic Oral Dose Range— Daily Dosage*		*Single Intramuscular Dose‡*	*Sedative Effects*	*Extra-pyramidal Effects*	*Hypotensive Effects*
R₁	R₂	Usual, mg	Extreme,§ mg	Usual, mg			
Chlorprothixene CH—(CH₂)₂—N(CH₃)₂ TARACTAN	—Cl	50–400 O, L, I	30–600	25–50	+++	++	++
Thiothixene hydrochloride CH(CH₂)₂—N N—CH₃ NAVANE	—SO₂ N(CH₃)₂	5–30 O, L, I	2–30	2–4	+ to ++	+++	++
Other Heterocyclic Compounds							
Clozapine CLOZARIL		150–450 O	12.5–900		+++	0	+++
Haloperidol and haloperidol decanoate HALDOL		2–20 O, L, I	1–100	2–5 (haloperidol decanoate: 25–250 every 2–4 weeks)	+	++++	+
Loxapine succinate LOXITANE		60–100 O, L, I	20–250	12.5–50	+	++	+
Molindone hydrochloride MOBAN		50–225 O, L	15–225		++	++	+

Table 20–1

Selected Antipsychotic Drugs: Chemical Structures, Doses and Dosage Forms, and Side Effects* (*Continued*)

NONPROPRIETARY NAME	TRADE NAME	DOSE AND DOSAGE FORMS†		SIDE EFFECTS		
Other Heterocyclic Compounds (cont.)						
Olanzapine	ZYPREXA	5–10	2.5–20 O	+	+	++
Pimozide	ORAP	2–6	1–10 O	+	+++	+
Quetiapine fumarate	SEROQUEL	300–500	50–750 O	+++	0	++
Risperidone	RISPERDAL	2–8	0.25–16 O	++	++	+++

*Antipsychotic agents for use in children under age 12 years include chlorpromazine, chlorprothixene (>6 years), thioridazine, and triflupromazine (among agents of low potency); and prochlorperazine and trifluoperazine (>6 years) (among agents of high potency). Haloperidol (orally) has also been used extensively in children.

†Dosage forms are indicated as follows: I, regular or long-acting injection; L, oral liquid or oral liquid concentrate; O, oral solid; S, suppository; SR, oral, sustained release.

‡Except for the enanthate and decanoate forms of fluphenazine and haloperidol decanoate, dosage can be given intramuscularly up to every 6 hours for agitated patients. Haloperidol lactate has been given intravenously; this is experimental.

§Extreme dosage ranges are occasionally exceeded cautiously and only when other appropriate measures have failed.

Side effects: 0, absent; +, low; ++, moderate; +++, moderately high; ++++, high.

The indicated salts are not shown in the formulas but are commercially available forms of the drugs.

Thioxanthenes also have aliphatic or piperazine side-chain substituents. The analog of chlorpromazine among the thioxanthenes is *chlorprothixene.* Piperazine-substituted thioxanthenes include *clopenthixol, flupentixol, piflutixol,* and *thiothixene;* they are all potent and effective antipsychotic agents, although only thiothixene is available in the United States. Since thioxanthenes have an olefinic double bond between the central-ring carbon atom at position 10 and the side chain, geometric isomers exist; the *cis* (or α) isomers are the more active.

The antipsychotic phenothiazines and thioxanthenes have three carbon atoms interposed between position 10 of the central ring and the first amino nitrogen atom of the side chain at this position; the amine is always tertiary. Antihistaminic phenothiazines (*e.g., promethazine*) or strongly anticholinergic phenothiazines (*e.g., ethopropazine, diethazine*) have only two carbon atoms separating the amino group from position 10 of the central ring. Metabolic *N*-dealkylation of the side chain or increasing the size of amino *N*-alkyl substituents reduces antipsychotic activity.

Additional tricyclic antipsychotic agents are the *benzepines,* containing a seven-member central ring, of which *loxapine* (a dibenzoxazepine; *see* Table 20–1) and *clozapine* (a dibenzodiazepine) are available in the United States. *Loxapine*-like agents include potent and typical neuroleptics with prominent antidopaminergic activity (*e.g., clothiapine, metiapine, loxapine, zotepine,* and others). They have an electron-withdrawing moiety at position 2, relatively close to the side-chain nitrogen atoms.

Clozapine-like agents either lack a ring substituent (*e.g., quetiapine,* a dibenzothiazepine), have an analogous methyl substituent (notably *olanzapine,* a thienobenzodiazepine; *see* Table 20–1), or have an electronegative substituent at position 8, away from the side-chain nitrogen atoms (*e.g.,* clozapine, *fluperlapine,* and others). In addition to dopamine receptors, clozapine-like agents interact at several other classes of receptors with varying affinities ($α_1$- and $α_2$-adrenergic, serotonin 5-HT_{2A} and 5-HT_{2C}, muscarinic cholinergic, histamine H_1, and others). Some are highly effective antipsychotic agents, and clozapine, in particular, has proved effective even in chronically ill patients who respond poorly to standard neuroleptics. The basic and clinical pharmacology of clozapine is reviewed elsewhere (Baldessarini and Frankenburg, 1991; Wagstaff and Bryson, 1995; Worrell *et al.,* 2000).

Clozapine strongly stimulated searches for additional, safer agents with antipsychotic activity and an atypically low risk of extrapyramidal neurological side effects. This search led to a series of atypical antipsychotic agents with some pharmacological similarities to clozapine. These include the structurally similar olanzapine and quetiapine, and the mixed antidopaminergic-antiserotonergic agent *risperidone* (a benzisoxazole; *see* Table 20–1; Owens and Risch, 1998; Waddington and Casey, 2000).

The *butyrophenone* (phenylbutylpiperidine) neuroleptics include *haloperidol* (Janssen, 1974). Other experimental heterocyclic-substituted phenylbutylpiperidines include the spiperones. An analogous compound, *droperidol,* is a very short-acting, highly sedative neuroleptic that is used almost exclusively in anesthesia (*see* Chapter 14) but sometimes also in psychiatric emergencies. Additional analogs in the *diphenylbutylpiperidine* series include *fluspirilene, penfluridol,* and *pimozide* (*see* Table 20–1 and Neumeyer and Booth, 2001). These are potent neuroleptics with prolonged action. In the United States, pimozide

is indicated for the treatment of Tourette's syndrome of severe tics and involuntary vocalizations, although it also is an effective antipsychotic.

Several other classes of heterocyclic compounds have antipsychotic effects, but too few are available or sufficiently well characterized to permit conclusions regarding structure–activity relationships (*see* Neumeyer and Booth, 2001). These include several indole compounds [notably, *molindone* (*see* Table 20–1) and *oxypertine*]. Another experimental compound, *butaclamol,* is a potent antidopaminergic agent that has a pentacyclic structure with a dibenzepine core and structural and pharmacological similarity to loxapine-like rather than clozapine-like dibenzepines. Its active (dextrorotatory) and inactive enantiomeric forms have been useful in characterizing the stereochemistry of sites of action of neuroleptics at dopamine receptors.

Risperidone (*see* Table 20–1) has prominent antiserotonergic (5-HT_2) as well as antidopaminergic (D_2) and antihistaminic (H_1) activity. Although risperidone and clozapine share those receptor affinities, risperidone is a much more potent antidopaminergic agent and, unlike clozapine, can induce extrapyramidal symptoms as well as prominent hyperprolactinemia. Nevertheless, risperidone can be considered a "quantitatively atypical" antipsychotic agent in that its extrapyramidal neurological side effects are limited at low daily doses (6 mg or less).

A growing series of heterocyclic antipsychotic agents are the enantiomeric, substituted *benzamides.* These include the gastroenterologic agents *metoclopramide* and *cisapride,* which have antiserotonergic as well as anti–D_2-dopaminergic actions. In addition, several benzamides, like the butyrophenones and their congeners, are relatively selective antagonists at central D_2 dopamine receptors, and many have neuroleptic-antipsychotic activity. Experimental examples include *epidepride, eticlopride, nemonapride, raclopride, remoxipride,* and *sultopride; sulpiride* is employed clinically in other countries, mainly as a sedative.

Pharmacological Properties

Antipsychotic drugs share many pharmacological effects and therapeutic applications (*see* Baldessarini, 1985; Marder, 1998; Owens and Risch, 1998). Chlorpromazine and haloperidol are commonly taken as prototypes for the older, standard neuroleptic-type agents; newer agents can be compared and contrasted to them. Many antipsychotic drugs, especially chlorpromazine and other agents of low potency, have a prominent sedative effect. This is particularly conspicuous early in treatment, although tolerance to this effect is typical; sedation may not be noticeable when very agitated psychotic patients are treated. Despite their sedative effects, neuroleptic drugs generally are not used to treat anxiety disorders, largely because of their autonomic and neurological side effects, which paradoxically can include severe anxiety and restlessness (akathisia). The risk of developing extrapyramidal side effects including tardive dyskinesia following long-term administration of neuroleptic drugs makes these agents less desirable than others for the treatment of anxiety.

The term *neuroleptic* was introduced to denote the effects of chlorpromazine and reserpine on the behavior of laboratory animals and in psychiatric patients and was intended to contrast their effects to those of sedatives and other CNS depressants. The neuroleptic syndrome involves suppression of spontaneous movements and complex behaviors, while spinal reflexes and unconditioned nociceptive-avoidance behaviors remain intact. In human beings, neuroleptic drugs reduce initiative and interest in the environment as well as manifestations of emotion or affect. Such effects led to their being considered "tranquilizers" before their unique antipsychotic effects were well established. In their clinical use, there may be some initial slowness in response to external stimuli and drowsiness. However, subjects are easily aroused, can answer questions, and retain intact cognition. Ataxia, incoordination, or dysarthria do not occur at ordinary doses. Typically, psychotic patients soon become less agitated, and withdrawn or autistic patients sometimes become more responsive and communicative. Aggressive and impulsive behavior diminishes. Gradually (usually over a period of days), psychotic symptoms of hallucinations, delusions, and disorganized or incoherent thinking tend to disappear. Neuroleptic agents also exert characteristic neurological effects—including bradykinesia, mild rigidity, some tremor, and subjective restlessness (akathisia)—that resemble the signs of Parkinson's disease.

Although early use of the term *neuroleptic* appears to have encompassed the whole unique syndrome just described and *neuroleptic* still is used as a synonym for *antipsychotic,* there now is a tendency to use the term *neuroleptic* to emphasize the more neurological aspects of the syndrome (*i.e.,* the parkinsonian and other extrapyramidal effects). Except for clozapine and perhaps olanzapine and quetiapine, all antipsychotic drugs available in the United States also have effects on movement and posture and can thus be called neuroleptic. However, the more general term *antipsychotic* is preferable. Introduction of atypical drugs such as clozapine, olanzapine, and quetiapine that are antipsychotic and have little extrapyramidal action has reinforced this trend.

General Psychophysiological and Behavioral Effects. In laboratory animals and in human beings, the most prominent observable effects of many antipsychotic agents are strikingly similar (Fielding and Lal, 1978). In low doses, operant behavior is reduced but spinal reflexes are unchanged. In laboratory animals, exploratory behavior is diminished, and responses to a variety of stimuli are fewer, slower, and smaller in magnitude, although the ability to discriminate stimuli is retained. Conditioned avoidance

behaviors are selectively inhibited, whereas unconditioned escape or avoidance responses are not. Highly reinforcing self-stimulation of the animal brain (commonly induced with electrodes placed in the monoamine-rich medial forebrain bundle) is blocked, although capacity to press the stimulation-inducing lever is not lost. Behavioral activation, stimulated environmentally or pharmacologically (particularly by stimulants and dopaminergic agonists), is blocked. Feeding is inhibited. Most neuroleptics block the emesis, hyperactivity, and aggression induced by apomorphine and other dopaminergic agonists. In high doses, most neuroleptics induce characteristic cataleptic immobility that allows an animal to be placed in abnormal postures that persist. Muscle tone is increased, and ptosis is typical. The animal appears to be indifferent to most stimuli, although it continues to withdraw from those that are noxious or painful. Many learned tasks still can be performed if sufficient stimulation and motivation are provided. Even very high doses of most neuroleptics do not induce coma, and the lethal dose is extraordinarily high.

Effects on Motor Activity. Nearly all antipsychotic agents diminish spontaneous motor activity in laboratory animals and in human beings. However, one of the more disturbing clinical side effects of these agents is akathisia, which is manifest by an increase in restless activity that is not readily mimicked by animal behavior. The cataleptic immobility of animals treated with neuroleptics resembles the catatonia seen in some psychotic patients as well as in association with a variety of metabolic and neurological disorders affecting the central nervous system (CNS). In patients, catatonic signs, along with other features of psychotic illnesses, are sometimes relieved by antipsychotic agents. However, rigidity and bradykinesia, which mimic catatonia, can be induced in patients, especially by large doses of potent neuroleptics, and reversed by removal of the offending drug or the addition of an antiparkinsonian agent (*see* Fielding and Lal, 1978; Janssen and Van Bever, 1978). Theories concerning the mechanisms underlying these extrapyramidal reactions, as well as descriptions of their clinical presentations and management, are given below.

Effects on Sleep. Antipsychotic drugs have inconsistent effects on sleep patterns, but tend to normalize sleep disturbances characteristic of many psychoses and mania. Ability to prolong and enhance the effect of opioid and hypnotic drugs appears to parallel the sedative rather than the neuroleptic potency of a particular agent. Thus, the more potent neuroleptic agents that do not cause drowsiness also do not enhance hypnosis produced by other drugs.

Effects on Conditioned Responses.   Chlorpromazine and other neuroleptics impair the ability of animals to make a conditioned avoidance response to a learned sensory cue that signals the onset of punishing shock avoidable by moving to a safe place in an experimental chamber. Under the influence of small doses of these drugs, animals ignore the warning signal but still attempt to escape once the shock is applied. General CNS depressants affect both avoidance (the conditioned response) and escape (the unconditioned response) to approximately the same extent, but suppression of unconditioned escape occurs only with doses of neuroleptics that produce ataxia or hypnosis. Passive avoidance behavior, requiring immobility, also is suppressed by neuroleptic drugs, in contrast to what might be expected of drugs that suppress locomotion.

Since correlations between antipsychotic effectiveness and conditioned avoidance tests are good for many types of neuroleptic agents, they have been important in pharmaceutical screening procedures. However, despite their empirical utility and quantitative characteristics, effects on conditioned avoidance have not provided important insights into the basis of clinical antipsychotic effects. For example, the effects of neuroleptic drugs on conditioned avoidance, but not their clinical antipsychotic actions, are subject to tolerance and are blocked by anticholinergic agents. Moreover, the extraordinarily close correlation between the potencies of drugs in conditioned avoidance tests and their ability to block the behavioral effects of dopaminergic agonists such as amphetamine or apomorphine suggests that such avoidance tests may be selective for drugs with extrapyramidal and other neurological effects. The ability of the atypical antipsychotic drugs, such as clozapine and olanzapine, to antagonize dopamine agonists and to block conditioned avoidance responses in animal behavioral tests also supports this interpretation (*see* Fielding and Lal, 1978; Janssen and Van Bever, 1978; Arnt and Skarsfeldt, 1998).

Effects on Complex Behavior.   Antipsychotic drugs can impair vigilance or motor responses in human subjects performing a variety of tasks, such as continuous rotor-pursuit and tapping-speed tests. The drugs produce relatively little impairment of digit–symbol substitution, a test of intellectual functioning. In contrast, barbiturates cause greater impairment in performance in digit–symbol substitution than in continuous performance and other vigilance tests. Moreover, most antipsychotic agents can improve cognitive functioning in psychotic patients with symptomatic improvement.

Effects on Specific Areas of the Nervous System.   Effects of antipsychotic drugs are apparent at all levels in the nervous system. Although knowledge of the actions underlying the antipsychotic and many of the neurological effects of neuroleptic drugs remains incomplete, theories based on their ability to antagonize the actions of dopamine as a neurotransmitter in the basal ganglia and limbic portions of the forebrain have become most prominent and are supported by a large body of data.

Cerebral Cortex.   Since psychosis involves a disorder of higher functions and thought processes, cortical effects of antipsychotic drugs are of great interest. Antipsychotic

drugs interact with dopaminergic projections to the prefrontal and deep-temporal (limbic) regions of the cerebral cortex with relative sparing of these areas from adaptive changes in dopamine metabolism that would suggest tolerance to the actions of neuroleptics (Bunney *et al.*, 1987).

Seizure Threshold.   Many neuroleptic drugs can lower the seizure threshold and induce discharge patterns in the electroencephalogram (EEG) that are associated with epileptic seizure disorders. Clozapine as well as aliphatic phenothiazines with low potency (such as chlorpromazine) seem particularly able to do this, while the more potent piperazine phenothiazines and thioxanthenes (notably fluphenazine and thiothixene), as well as risperidone, seem much less likely to have this effect (Itil, 1978; Baldessarini and Frankenburg, 1991). The butyrophenones have variable and unpredictable effects that cause seizure activity; molindone may have the least activity of this type. Clozapine has a clearly dose-related risk of inducing seizures in nonepileptic patients (Baldessarini and Frankenburg, 1991), and clozapine and olanzapine are associated with more EEG abnormalities than are many high-potency neuroleptics, including risperidone (Centorrino *et al.*, 2001). Antipsychotic agents, especially clozapine and low-potency phenothiazines and thioxanthenes, should be used with *extreme caution,* if at all, in untreated epileptic patients and in patients undergoing withdrawal from central depressants such as alcohol, barbiturates, or benzodiazepines. Most antipsychotic drugs, especially the piperazines, as well as the novel atypical agents quetiapine and risperidone, can be used safely in epileptic patients if moderate doses are attained gradually and if concomitant anticonvulsant drug therapy is maintained (*see* Chapter 21).

Basal Ganglia.   Because the extrapyramidal effects of most clinically used antipsychotic drugs are prominent, a great deal of interest has centered on the actions of these drugs in the basal ganglia, notably the caudate nucleus, putamen, globus pallidus, and allied nuclei, which play a crucial role in the control of posture and the extrapyramidal aspects of movement. The critical role of a deficiency of dopamine in this region in the pathogenesis of Parkinson's disease, the potent activity of neuroleptics as antagonists of dopamine receptors, and the striking resemblance between clinical manifestations of Parkinson's disease and the neurological effects of neuroleptic drugs all have focused attention on the role of a deficiency of dopaminergic activity in some of the neuroleptic-induced extrapyramidal effects (Carlsson, 1990).

The hypothesis that interference with the transmitter function of dopamine in the mammalian forebrain might contribute to the neurological and possibly also the antipsychotic effects of the neuroleptic drugs arose from the observation that neuroleptic drugs consistently increased the concentrations of the metabolites of dopamine but had variable effects on the metabolism of other neurotransmitters. The importance of dopamine also was supported by histochemical studies, which indicated a preferential distribution of dopamine-containing fibers between midbrain and the basal ganglia (notably, the nigrostriatal tract), and within the hypothalamus (see Chapter 12). Other dopamine-containing neurons project from midbrain tegmental nuclei to forebrain regions associated with the limbic system as well as to temporal and prefrontal cerebral cortical areas closely related to the limbic system. A simplistic but attractive concept arose: many extrapyramidal neurological effects of the antipsychotic drugs might be mediated by antidopaminergic effects in the basal ganglia. Their antipsychotic effects might be mediated by modification of dopaminergic neurotransmission in the limbic, mesocortical, and hypothalamic systems.

Antagonism of dopamine-mediated synaptic neurotransmission is an important action of neuroleptic drugs (Carlsson, 1990). Thus, drugs with neuroleptic actions, but not their inactive congeners, initially increase the rate of production of dopamine metabolites, the rate of conversion of the precursor amino acid tyrosine to dihydroxyphenylalanine (DOPA) and its metabolites, and the rate of firing of dopamine-containing cells in the midbrain. These effects usually have been interpreted to represent adaptive responses of neuronal systems that tend to reduce the impact of interrupting synaptic transmission at dopaminergic terminals in the forebrain.

Supporting evidence for such an interpretation includes the observation that small doses of neuroleptic drugs block behavioral or neuroendocrine effects of systemically administered or intracerebrally injected dopaminergic agonists. An example is stereotyped gnawing behavior in the rat induced by apomorphine. Many neuroleptic drugs (except the butyrophenones, their congeners, and the benzamides) also block the effects of agonists on dopamine-sensitive adenylyl cyclase associated with D_1-dopamine receptors in forebrain tissue (Figure 20–1). Atypical antipsychotic drugs such as clozapine and quetiapine are characterized by their low affinity or weak actions in such tests (Campbell et al., 1991). Whereas the initial effect of neuroleptics is to block D_2 receptors and stimulate increased firing and metabolic activity in dopamine neurons, these responses eventually are replaced by diminished activity ("depolarization inactivation"), particularly in the extrapyramidal basal ganglia (Bunney et al., 1987). The timing of these adaptive changes correlates well with the gradual evolution of parkinsonian bradykinesia over days in the clinical application of neuroleptics (Tarsy et al., 2001).

Radioligand-binding assays for dopamine receptor subtypes have been used to define more precisely the mechanism of action of neuroleptic agents (see Civelli et al., 1993; Baldessarini and Tarazi, 1996; Neve and Neve, 1997; see Table 20–2 and Figure 20–1). Estimates of the clinical potency of most types of antipsychotic drugs correlate well with their relative potency in vitro to inhibit binding of these ligands to D_2-dopamine receptors (see Chapter 12). This correlation is obscured to some extent by the tendency of neuroleptics to accumulate in brain tissue to different degrees (Tsuneizumi et al., 1992; Cohen et al., 1992). Nevertheless, almost all clinically effective antipsychotic agents (with the notable exception of clozapine and quetiapine) have characteristically high affinity for D_2 receptors. Although some antipsychotics (especially thioxanthenes, phenothiazines, and clozapine) bind with relatively high affinity to D_1 receptors, they also block D_2 receptors and other D_2-like receptors including the D_3- and D_4-receptor subtypes (Sokoloff et al., 1990; Van Tol et al., 1991; Baldessarini and Tarazi, 1996; Tarazi

and Baldessarini, 1999). Butyrophenones and congeners (e.g., haloperidol, pimozide, N-methylspiperone) as well as experimental benzamide neuroleptics (e.g., eticlopride, nemonapride, raclopride, remoxipride) have relatively high selectivity as antagonists at D_2 and D_3 dopamine receptors, with variable D_4 affinity. The physiological and clinical consequences of selectively blocking D_1 or D_5 receptors remain obscure, although experimental benzazepines (e.g., SCH-23390 and SCH-39166 or ecopipam) with such properties, but apparently weak antipsychotic effects, are known (Daly and Waddington, 1992; Kebabian et al., 1997).

Atypical antipsychotic agents with a low risk of extrapyramidal side effects, such as clozapine and other benzepines, have low affinity for D_2-dopamine receptors and little propensity to produce extrapyramidal side effects. They are, however, active α_1-adrenergic antagonists, as are many other antipsychotic agents (Baldessarini et al., 1992). This action may contribute to sedative and hypotensive side effects or might underlie useful psychotropic effects, although assessment of the psychotropic potential of centrally active antiadrenergic agents is limited. Many antipsychotic agents also have some affinity for 5-HT$_{2A}$-serotonin receptors, and this is particularly prominent in the case of clozapine, olanzapine, quetiapine, risperidone, and other investigational D_2/5-HT$_{2A}$ antagonists (Chouinard et al., 1993; Leysen et al., 1994; see also Chapter 11). This admixture of moderate affinities for several CNS receptor types (including also muscarinic acetylcholine and H_1-histamine receptors) may contribute to the virtually unique pharmacological profile of the atypical antipsychotic agent clozapine (Baldessarini and Frankenburg, 1991). Clozapine also has modest selectivity for dopamine D_4 receptors over other dopamine-receptor types. D_4 receptors, preferentially localized in cortical and limbic brain regions, are upregulated after repeated administration of clozapine and other typical and atypical antipsychotic drugs. These receptors may contribute to the clinical actions of antipsychotic drugs, although agents that are selective D_4 or mixed D_4/5-HT$_{2A}$ antagonists have not proved effective in the treatment of psychotic patients (Baldessarini, 1997; Kramer et al., 1997; Tarazi and Baldessarini, 1999; Truffinet et al., 1999; see "Prospectus," below).

Limbic System. Dopaminergic projections from the midbrain terminate on septal nuclei, the olfactory tubercle, the amygdala, and other structures within the temporal and prefrontal lobes of the cerebrum. Because of the dopamine hypothesis just reviewed, much attention also has been given to the mesolimbic and mesocortical systems as possible sites of mediation of some of the antipsychotic effects of these agents. Speculations about the pathophysiology of the idiopathic psychoses, such as schizophrenia, have for many years centered on the limbic system. Such speculation has been given indirect encouragement by repeated "natural experiments" that have associated psychotic mental phenomena with lesions of the temporal lobe and other portions of the limbic system.

The finding that D_3 and D_4 receptors are preferentially expressed in limbic areas of the CNS has led to

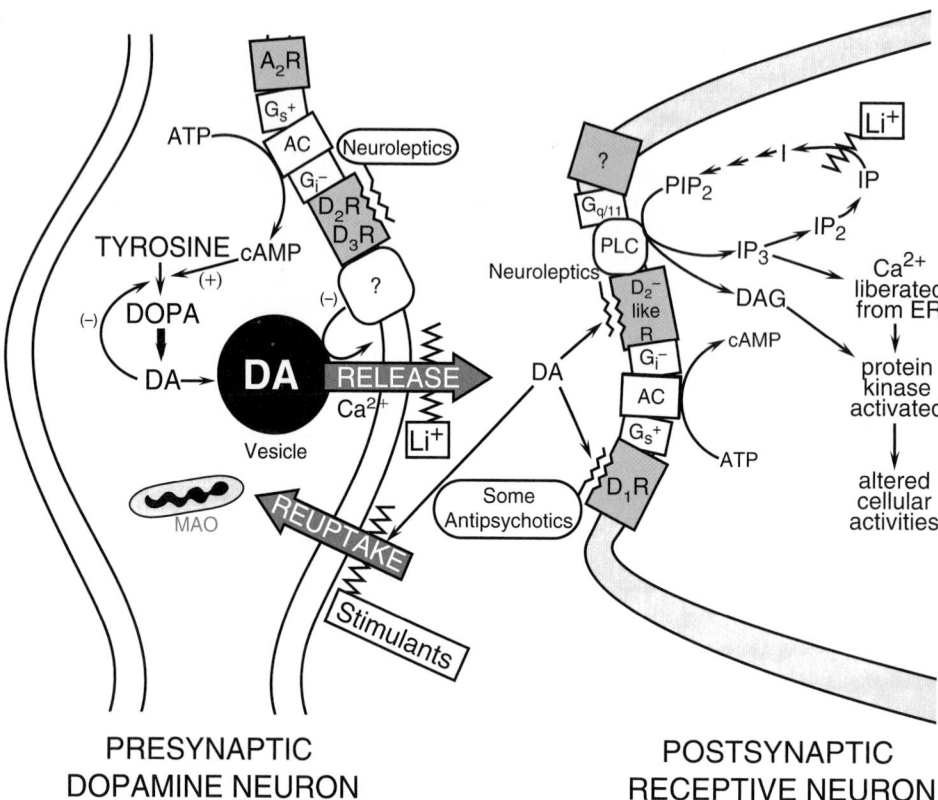

Figure 20–1. Sites of action of neuroleptics and lithium.

In varicosities ("terminals") along terminal arborizations of dopamine (DA) neurons projecting from midbrain to forebrain, tyrosine is oxidized to dihydroxyphenylalanine (DOPA) by tyrosine hydroxylase (TH), the rate-limiting step in catecholamine biosynthesis, then decarboxylated to DA by aromatic L-amino acid decarboxylase (AAD) and stored in vesicles. Following exocytotic release (inhibited by lithium) by depolarization in the presence of Ca^{2+}, DA interacts with postsynaptic receptors (R) of D_1 and D_2 types (and structurally similar but less prevalent D_1-like and D_2-like receptors), as well as with presynaptic D_2 and D_3 autoreceptors. Inactivation of transsynaptic communication occurs primarily by active transport ("reuptake") of DA into presynaptic terminals (inhibited by many stimulants), with secondary deamination by mitochondrial monoamine oxidase (MAO). Postsynaptic D_1 receptors, through G_s-type G proteins, activate adenylyl cyclase (AC) to convert ATP to cyclic AMP (cAMP), whereas D_2 receptors inhibit AC through G_i proteins. D_2 receptors also activate receptor-operated K^+ channels, suppress voltage-gated Ca^{2+} currents, and stimulate phospholipase-C (PLC), perhaps *via* the $\beta\gamma$ subunits liberated from activated G_i (*see* Chapter 2), to convert phosphatidylinositol bisphosphate (PIP_2) to inositol trisphosphate (IP_3) and diacylglycerol (DAG), with secondary modulation of Ca^{2+} and protein kinases. Lithium inhibits the phosphatase that liberates inositol (I) from inositol phosphate (IP). Both Li^+ and valproate can modify the abundance or function of G proteins and effectors, as well as protein kinases and several cell and nuclear regulatory factors. D_2-like autoreceptors suppress synthesis of DA by diminishing phosphorylation of rate-limiting TH, as well as limiting DA release (possibly through modulation of Ca^{2+} or K^+ currents). In contrast, presynaptic A_2 adenosine receptors (A_2R) activate AC and, *via* cyclic AMP production, TH activity. Nearly all antipsychotic agents block D_2 receptors and autoreceptors; some also block D_1 receptors (*see* Table 20–2). Initially in antipsychotic treatment, DA neurons activate and release more DA but, following repeated treatment, they enter a state of physiological depolarization inactivation, with diminished production and release of DA, in addition to continued receptor blockade.

Table 20–2
Potencies of Standard and Experimental Antipsychotic Agents at Neurotransmitter Receptors*†‡

RECEPTOR	DOPAMINE D$_2$	SEROTONIN 5HT$_2$	5HT$_{2A}$/D$_2$ RATIO	DOPAMINE D$_1$	DOPAMINE D$_4$	MUSCARINIC CHOLINERGIC	ADRENERGIC α$_1$	ADRENERGIC α$_2$	HISTAMINE H$_1$
Drugs									
cis-Thiothixene	0.45	130	289	340	77.0	2500	11.0	200	6.00
Sertindole	0.45	0.38	0.84	28.0	21.0	≥10,000	0.77	1700	500
Fluphenazine	0.80	19.0	23.8	15.0	9.30	2000	9.00	1600	20.8
Zotepine	1.00	0.63	0.63	84.0	5.80	550	3.40	960	3.40
Perphenazine	1.40	5.60	4.00	—	—	1500	10.0	510	—
Thioridazine	2.30	41.0	17.8	22.0	12.0	10.0	1.10	—	—
Pimozide	2.50	13.0	5.20	—	30.0	—	—	—	—
Risperidone	3.30	0.16	0.05	750	16.6	>10,000	2.00	55.6	58.8
Haloperidol	4.00	36.0	9.00	45.0	10.3	>20,000	6.20	3800	1890
Ziprasidone	4.79	0.42	0.09	339	39.0	≥10,000	10.5	—	46.8
Mesoridazine	5.00	6.30	1.26	—	13.4	—	—	—	—
Sulpiride	7.40	≥1000	135	≥1000	52.0	≥1000	≥1000	—	—
Olanzapine	11.0	4.00	0.36	31.0	9.60	1.89	19.0	230	7.14
Chlorpromazine	19.0	1.40	0.07	56.0	12.3	60.0	0.60	750	9.10
Loxapine	71.4	1.69	0.02	—	12.0	62.5	27.8	2400	5.00
Pipamperone	93.0	1.20	0.01	2450	—	≥5000	66.0	680	≥5000
Molindone	125	5000	40.0	—	—	—	2500	625	>10,000
Amperozide	140	20.0	0.14	260	1164	1700	130	590	730
Quetiapine	160	294	1.84	455	9.6	120	62.5	2500	11.0
Clozapine	180	1.60	0.01	38.0	9.6	7.50	9.00	160	2.75
Melperone	199	32.0	0.16	—	230	—	—	—	—
Remoxipride	275	≥10,000	36.4	≥10,000	3690	≥10,000	≥10,000	2900	≥10,000

*Data are Ki values (nM) determined by competition with radioligands for binding to the indicated receptors.

†Compounds are in rank-order of dopamine D$_2$-receptor affinity; 5-HT$_{2A}$/D$_2$ ratio indicates relative preference for D$_2$ vs. serotonin 5HT$_{2A}$ receptors. Compounds include clinically used and experimental agents.

‡Muscarinic-cholinergic-receptor Ki values are pooled results obtained with radioligands that are nonselective for muscarinic-receptor subtypes or that are selective for the M$_1$ subtype.

SOURCES: Data are averaged from Roth *et al.* (1995); Seeger *et al.* (1995); Schotte *et al.* (1996); Richelson (1999); and a personal written communication from Dr. E. Richelson (1/26/00).

increased efforts to identify agents selective for these receptors that might have antipsychotic efficacy with a reduced tendency to cause extrapyramidal side effects, so far without success (Kebabian *et al.*, 1997; Kramer *et al.*, 1997; Lahti *et al.*, 1998; Tarazi and Baldessarini, 1999). Moreover, long-term administration of typical and atypical antipsychotic drugs does not alter D_3 receptor levels in rat forebrain regions while increasing expression of D_2 and D_4 receptors (Tarazi *et al.*, 1997). These findings suggest that D_3 receptors are unlikely to play a pivotal role in antipsychotic drug actions, perhaps due to their avid affinity for endogenous dopamine, which may prevent their interaction with antipsychotics (Levant, 1997).

Many of the behavioral, neurophysiological, biochemical, and pharmacological findings with regard to the properties of the dopaminergic system of the basal ganglia have been extended to mesolimbic and mesocortical tissue. Certain important effects of antipsychotic drugs are similar in extrapyramidal and limbic regions, including those on ligand-binding assays for dopaminergic receptors. However, the extrapyramidal and antipsychotic actions of antipsychotic agents differ in several ways. For example, while some acute extrapyramidal effects of neuroleptics tend to diminish or to disappear with time or when anticholinergic drugs are administered concurrently, this is not characteristic of the antipsychotic effects. Dopaminergic subsystems in the forebrain differ functionally and in the physiological regulation of their responses to drugs (*see* Bunney *et al.*, 1987; Moore, 1987; Sulser and Robinson, 1978; Wolf and Roth, 1987). For example, anticholinergic agents block the increase in turnover of dopamine in the basal ganglia induced by neuroleptic agents but not in limbic areas containing dopaminergic terminals. Further, development of tolerance to enhancement of the metabolic turnover of dopamine by antipsychotics is much less prominent in limbic than in extrapyramidal areas (*see* Carlsson, 1990).

In Vivo *Occupation of Cerebral Neurotransmitter Receptors.*
Levels of occupation of dopamine receptors and other receptors in human brain can be estimated with positron emission tomography (PET) in patients treated with antipsychotic drugs. Such analyses not only support conclusions arising from laboratory studies of receptor occupancy (*see* Table 20–2) but also assist in predicting clinical efficacy and extrapyramidal side effects as well as clinical dosing, even in advance of controlled clinical trials (Farde *et al.*, 1995; Waddington and Casey, 2000).

For example, occupation of more than 75% of D_2-like receptors in the basal ganglia is associated with risk of acute extrapyramidal side effects and is commonly found with clinical doses of typical neuroleptics (Farde *et al.*, 1995). In contrast, therapeutic doses of clozapine usually are associated with lower levels of occupation of D_2 receptors (averaging 40% to 50%), but higher (70% to 90%) levels of occupation of cortical 5-HT$_2$ receptors (Kapur *et al.*, 1999; Nordstrom *et al.*, 1995).

Of the novel atypical antipsychotics, only quetiapine has a clozapine-like *in vivo* receptor-occupancy profile, resembling clozapine's levels of occupation of both D_2 (40% to 50%) and 5-HT$_2$ receptors (50% to 70%) (Gefvert *et al.*, 1998). Olanzapine and risperidone also block cortical 5-HT$_2$ receptors at high levels (80% to 100%), with greater effects at D_2 sites (typically,

50% to 90%) than have clozapine or quetiapine (Farde *et al.*, 1995; Nordstrom *et al.*, 1998; Kapur *et al.*, 1999). In addition to its relatively high levels of D_2-receptor occupation, olanzapine is more antimuscarinic than is risperidone, perhaps accounting for its lower risk of acute extrapyramidal effects (*see* Tables 20–1 and 20–2).

Hypothalamus and Endocrine Systems. In addition to neurological and antipsychotic effects that appear to be mediated in part by antidopaminergic actions of neuroleptic drugs, endocrine changes occur as a result of their effects on the hypothalamus or pituitary that also may involve dopamine. Prominent among these is the ability of most antipsychotic drugs to increase the secretion of prolactin.

This effect on prolactin secretion probably is due to a blockade of the pituitary actions of the tuberoinfundibular dopaminergic system that projects from the arcuate nucleus of the hypothalamus to the median eminence. D_2-dopaminergic receptors on mammotrophic cells in the anterior pituitary mediate the prolactin-inhibiting action of dopamine secreted at the median eminence into the hypophyseal portal system (*see* Ben-Jonathan, 1985; *see also* Chapter 56).

Correlations between the potencies of antipsychotic drugs in stimulating prolactin secretion and causing behavioral effects are excellent for many types of agents (Sachar, 1978). Clozapine and quetiapine are exceptional in having minimal effects on prolactin (Arvanitis *et al.*, 1997; Sachar, 1978), and olanzapine produces only minor, transient increases in prolactin levels (Tollefson and Kuntz, 1999), whereas risperidone has an unusually potent prolactin-elevating effect (Grant and Fitton, 1994). The effects of neuroleptics on prolactin secretion tend to occur, however, at lower doses than do their antipsychotic effects; this may reflect their action outside the blood–brain barrier in the adenohypophysis. Little tolerance develops to the effect of antipsychotic drugs on prolactin, even after years of treatment. However, the effect is rapidly reversible when the drugs are discontinued (Bitton and Schnieder, 1992). This effect of antipsychotic agents is presumed to be responsible for the breast engorgement and galactorrhea that occasionally are associated with their use, sometimes even in male patients given high doses of neuroleptic agents. Because antipsychotic drugs are used chronically and thus cause prolonged hyperprolactinemia, there has been concern about their possible contribution to risk of carcinoma of the breast, although clinical evidence has not supported this concern (Dickson and Glazer, 1999; Mortensen, 1994). Nevertheless, neuroleptic and other agents that stimulate secretion of prolactin should be avoided in patients with established carcinoma of the breast, particularly with metastases. Some antipsychotic drugs reduce secretion of gonadotropins, estrogens, and progestins, possibly contributing to amenorrhea.

The effects of neuroleptics on other hypothalamic neuroendocrine functions are much less well characterized, although neuroleptics inhibit the release of growth hormone and may reduce the secretion of corticotropin-releasing hormone (CRH) that occurs in response to stress. Neuroleptics also interfere with secretion of pituitary growth hormone. Nevertheless, neuroleptics are poor therapy for acromegaly, and there is no evidence that they retard growth or development of children. In addition, chlorpromazine can decrease secretion of neurohypophyseal hormones. Weight gain and increased appetite occur with most neuroleptics, particularly clozapine, others of low potency, and olanzapine. Chlorpromazine also may impair glucose tolerance and insulin release to a clinically appreciable degree in some patients (Erle *et al.*, 1977). In addition, several atypical antipsychotic agents (notably clozapine, olanzapine, and quetiapine) have been associated with risk of new-onset type 2 diabetes that may not be accounted for entirely by weight gain (Wirshing *et al.*, 1998).

In addition to neuroendocrine effects, it is likely that other autonomic effects of antipsychotic drugs may be mediated by the hypothalamus. An important example is the poikilothermic effect of chlorpromazine and other neuroleptic agents, which impairs the body's ability to regulate temperature such that hypo- or hyperthermia may result, depending on the ambient temperature. Clozapine can induce elevations of body temperature.

Brainstem. Clinical doses of the antipsychotic agents usually have little effect on respiration. However, vasomotor reflexes mediated by either the hypothalamus or the brainstem are depressed by relatively low doses of chlorpromazine. This effect might occur at many points in the reflex pathway, and the net result is a centrally mediated fall in blood pressure. Even in cases of acute overdosage with suicidal intent, the antipsychotic drugs usually do not cause life-threatening coma or suppression of vital functions; this contributes importantly to their safety. In addition, haloperidol has been administered safely in doses exceeding 500 mg/24 hours intravenously to control agitation in delirious patients (Tesar *et al.*, 1985).

Chemoreceptor Trigger Zone (CTZ). Most neuroleptics protect against the nausea- and emesis-inducing effects of apomorphine and certain ergot alkaloids, all of which can interact with central dopaminergic receptors in the CTZ of the medulla. The antiemetic effect of most neuroleptics occurs with low doses. Drugs or other stimuli that cause emesis by an action on the nodose ganglion or locally on the gastrointestinal tract are not antagonized by antipsychotic drugs, but potent piperazines and butyrophenones are sometimes effective against nausea caused by vestibular stimulation.

Autonomic Nervous System. Since various antipsychotic agents have antagonistic interactions at peripheral, α-adrenergic, serotonin (5-HT$_{2A}$), and histamine (H$_1$) receptors, their effects on the autonomic nervous system are complex and unpredictable. Chlorpromazine, clozapine, and thioridazine have particularly significant α-adrenergic antagonistic activity. The potent piperazine tricyclic neuroleptics (*e.g.,* fluphenazine, trifluoperazine), as well as haloperidol and risperidone, have antipsychotic effects even when used in low doses and show little antiadrenergic activity in patients.

The muscarinic-cholinergic blocking effects of antipsychotic drugs are relatively weak, but the blurring of vision commonly experienced with chlorpromazine may be due to an anticholinergic action on the ciliary muscle. Chlorpromazine regularly produces miosis, which can be due to α-adrenergic blockade. Other phenothiazines can cause mydriasis; this is especially likely to occur with clozapine or thioridazine, which are potent muscarinic antagonists. Chlorpromazine can cause constipation and decreased gastric secretion and motility, and clozapine can decrease the efficiency of clearing saliva and induce severe impairment of intestinal motility (Rabinowitz *et al.*, 1996; Theret *et al.*, 1995). Decreased sweating and salivation are additional manifestations of the anticholinergic effects of such drugs. Acute urinary retention is uncommon but can occur in males with prostatism. Anticholinergic effects are least frequently caused by the potent neuroleptics, including haloperidol and risperidone. The phenothiazines inhibit ejaculation without interfering with erection. Thioridazine produces this effect with some regularity, sometimes limiting its acceptance by male patients. Attribution of this effect to adrenergic blockade is logical but unsubstantiated, inasmuch as thioridazine is less potent than chlorpromazine in its antiadrenergic effects.

Kidney and Electrolyte Balance. Chlorpromazine may have weak diuretic effects in animals and human beings because of a depressant action on the secretion of antidiuretic hormone (ADH), inhibition of reabsorption of water and electrolytes by a direct action on the renal tubule, or both. The slight fall in blood pressure that occurs with chlorpromazine is not associated with a significant change in glomerular filtration rate; indeed, renal blood flow tends to increase. The syndrome of idiopathic polydipsia with potential hyponatremia has been improved with clozapine, presumably through CNS mechanisms (Siegel *et al.*, 1998).

Cardiovascular System. The actions of chlorpromazine on the cardiovascular system are complex because the drug produces direct effects on the heart and blood vessels and also indirect actions through CNS and autonomic reflexes. Chlorpromazine and other low-potency or atypical antipsychotic agents can cause orthostatic hypotension, systolic blood pressure being affected more than diastolic. Tolerance usually develops to the hypotensive effect over several weeks. However, some degree of orthostatic hypotension may persist indefinitely, especially in elderly patients (Ray *et al.*, 1987).

Chlorpromazine and other phenothiazines with low potency can have a direct negative inotropic action and a quinidine-like antiarrhythmic effect on the heart. Electrocardiographic (ECG) changes include prolongation of the QT and PR intervals, blunting of T waves, and depression of the ST segment. Thioridazine, in particular, causes a high incidence of QT- and T-wave changes and may very rarely produce ventricular arrhythmias and sudden death. These effects are uncommon when potent antipsychotic agents are administered. Clozapine has been associated with rare cases of early carditis and later-appearing cardiomyopathy (Killian *et al.*, 1999).

Miscellaneous Pharmacological Effects.   Interactions of antipsychotic drugs with central neurohumors other than dopamine may contribute to their antipsychotic effects or other actions. For example, many antipsychotics enhance the turnover of acetylcholine, especially in the basal ganglia, perhaps secondary to the blockade of inhibitory dopamine heteroceptors on cholinergic neurons. In addition, as discussed above, there is an inverse relationship between antimuscarinic potency of antipsychotic drugs in the brain and the likelihood of extrapyramidal effects (Snyder and Yamamura, 1977). Chlorpromazine and low-potency antipsychotic agents including clozapine have antagonistic actions at histamine receptors that probably contribute to their sedative effects. Antagonistic interactions also occur at serotonin-5-HT$_{2A}$ receptors in the forebrain. The significance of this effect is not certain, but several antipsychotic agents—notably risperidone, olanzapine, quetiapine, sertindole, and ziprasidone—were developed in part to mimic the relatively potent and selective antagonistic activity of clozapine at serotonin-5-HT$_{2A}$ receptors (Ichikawa and Meltzer, 1999; Meltzer and Nash, 1991).

Absorption, Distribution, Fate, and Excretion.   Some antipsychotic drugs tend to have erratic and unpredictable patterns of absorption, particularly after oral administration and even when liquid preparations are used. Parenteral (intramuscular) administration increases the bioavailability of active drug by four to ten times. The drugs are highly lipophilic, highly membrane- or protein-bound, and accumulate in the brain, lung, and other tissues with a high blood supply; they also enter the fetal circulation and breast milk. It is virtually impossible (and usually not necessary) to remove these agents by dialysis.

The usually stated elimination half-lives with respect to total concentrations in plasma are typically 20 to 40 hours, but complex patterns of delayed elimination may occur with some agents, particularly the butyrophenones and their congeners (Cohen *et al.*, 1992). The biological effects of single doses of most neuroleptics usually persist for at least 24 hours; this encourages the common practice of giving the entire daily dose at one time, once the patient has accommodated to the initial side effects of the drug. Elimination from the plasma may be more rapid than from sites of high lipid content and binding, notably in the CNS, but direct pharmacokinetic studies on this issue are few and inconclusive (Sedvall, 1992). Metabolites of some agents have been detected in the urine for as long as several months after administration of the drug has been discontinued. Slow removal of drug may contribute to the typically slow rate of exacerbation of psychosis after stopping drug treatment. Repository ("depot") preparations of

esters of neuroleptic drugs are absorbed and eliminated much more slowly than are oral preparations. For example, whereas half of an oral dose of fluphenazine hydrochloride is eliminated in about 20 hours, the elimination of the decanoate ester following a depot intramuscular injection has a nominal half-life of 7 to 10 days, although the overall clearance of fluphenazine decanoate and normalization of hyperprolactinemia following repeated dosing can require 6 to 8 months (Sampath *et al.*, 1992).

The main routes of metabolism of the antipsychotic drugs are oxidative processes mediated largely by genetically controlled hepatic cytochrome-P450 (CYP) microsomal oxidases and by conjugation processes. Hydrophilic metabolites of these drugs are excreted in the urine and, to some extent, in the bile. Most oxidized metabolites of antipsychotic drugs are biologically inactive, but a few are not (notably, 7-hydroxychlorpromazine, mesoridazine, and several *N*-demethylated metabolites of phenothiazines as well as 9-hydroxyrisperidone) and may contribute to the biological activity of the parent substance as well as complicate the problem of correlating assays of drug in blood with clinical effects. The less potent antipsychotic drugs may weakly induce their own hepatic metabolism, since concentrations of chlorpromazine and other phenothiazines in blood are lower after several weeks of treatment with the same dosage; it also is possible that alterations of gastrointestinal motility are partially responsible. The fetus, the infant, and the elderly have diminished capacity to metabolize and eliminate antipsychotic agents, but children tend to metabolize these drugs more rapidly than do adults (Kutcher, 1997).

Bioavailability of several antipsychotic agents is somewhat increased by the use of liquid concentrates. Peak serum concentrations of chlorpromazine and other phenothiazines are attained within 2 to 4 hours. Their intramuscular administration avoids much of the first-pass metabolism in the liver (and possibly also the gut) and provides measurable concentrations in plasma within 15 to 30 minutes. Bioavailability of chlorpromazine may be increased up to tenfold with injections, but the clinical dose usually is decreased by three- to fourfold. Gastrointestinal absorption of chlorpromazine is modified unpredictably by food and probably is decreased by antacids. Concurrent administration of anticholinergic antiparkinsonian agents probably does not appreciably diminish the intestinal absorption of neuroleptic agents (Simpson *et al.*, 1980). Chlorpromazine and other antipsychotic agents bind significantly to membranes and to plasma proteins. Typically, more than 85% of the drug in plasma is bound to albumin. Concentrations of some neuroleptics (*e.g.*, haloperidol) in brain can be more than ten times those in the blood (Tsuneizumi *et al.*, 1992), and their apparent volume of distribution may be as high as 20 liters per kilogram.

Disappearance of chlorpromazine from plasma includes a rapid distribution phase (half-life about 2 hours) and a slower

Table 20–3
Elimination Half-Lives of Antipsychotic Drugs

DRUG	HALF-LIFE (HOURS)[*]
Chlorpromazine	24 (8–35)
Clozapine	12 (4–66)
Fluphenazine	18 (14–24)
Haloperidol	24 (12–36)[†]
Loxapine	8 (3–12)
Mesoridazine	30 (24–48)
Molindone	12 (6–24)
Olanzapine	30 (20–54)
Perphenazine	12 (8–21)
Pimozide	55 (29–111)[†]
Quetiapine	6
Risperidone	20–24[‡]
Thioridazine	24 (6–40)
Thiothixene	34
Trifluoperazine	18 (14–24)[§]

[*]Average and range.
[†]May have multiphasic elimination with much longer terminal half-life.
[‡]Half-life of the main active metabolite (parent drug half-life ca. 3–4 hours).
[§]Estimated, assuming similarity to fluphenazine.
SOURCES: Data from Ereshefsky (1996) and United States Pharmacopoeia (2000).

elimination phase (half-life about 30 hours), but markedly variable values have been reported; the half-life of elimination from human brain is not known but may be determined using modern brain-scanning technologies (Sedvall, 1992). Approximate elimination half-life of commonly clinically employed antipsychotic agents is provided in Table 20–3.

Attempts to correlate plasma concentrations of chlorpromazine or its metabolites with clinical responses have not been successful (*see* Baldessarini *et al.,* 1988; Cooper *et al.,* 1976). Studies have revealed wide variations (at least tenfold) in plasma concentrations among individuals. Although it appears that plasma concentrations of chlorpromazine below 30 ng/ml are not likely to produce an adequate antipsychotic response and that levels above 750 ng/ml are likely to be associated with unacceptable toxicity (*see* Rivera-Calimlim and Hershey, 1984), it is not yet possible to state with confidence the concentrations in plasma that are associated with optimal clinical responses.

At least 10 or 12 metabolites of chlorpromazine occur in human beings in appreciable quantities (Morselli, 1977). Quantitatively, the most important of these are nor$_2$-chlorpromazine (doubly demethylated), chlorophenothiazine (removal of the entire side chain), methoxy and hydroxy products, and glucuronide conjugates of the hydroxylated compounds. In the urine, 7-hydroxylated and N-dealkylated (nor$_2$) metabolites and their conjugates predominate. Chlorpromazine and other phenothiazines are metabolized extensively through CYP2D6.

The pharmacokinetics and metabolism of thioridazine and fluphenazine are similar to those of chlorpromazine, but the strong anticholinergic action of thioridazine on the gut may modify its own absorption. Major metabolites of thioridazine and fluphenazine include N-demethylated, ring-hydroxylated, and S-oxidized products (Neumeyer and Booth, 2001). Concentrations of thioridazine in plasma are relatively high (hundreds of nanograms per milliliter), possibly because of its relative hydrophilicity. Thioridazine is prominently converted to the active product mesoridazine, a drug in its own right, and probably an important contributor to the neuroleptic activity of thioridazine.

The biotransformation of the thioxanthenes is similar to that of the phenothiazines except that metabolism to sulfoxides is common and ring-hydroxylated products are uncommon. Piperazine derivatives of the phenothiazines and thioxanthenes also are handled much like chlorpromazine, although metabolism of the piperidine ring itself occurs.

Elimination of haloperidol and chemically related agents from human plasma is not a log-linear function, and the apparent half-life increases with time, with a very prolonged terminal half-life of approximately 1 week (Cohen *et al.,* 1992). Haloperidol and other butyrophenones are metabolized primarily by an N-dealkylation reaction; the resultant inactive fragments can be conjugated with glucuronic acid. The metabolites of haloperidol are inactive, with the possible exception of a hydroxylated product formed by reduction of the keto moiety that may be reoxidized to haloperidol (Korpi *et al.,* 1983). A potentially neurotoxic derivative of haloperidol, a substituted phenylpiperidine, analogous to the parkinsonism-inducing agent methylphenyltetrahydropyridine (MPTP), has been described and found in nanomolar quantities in postmortem brain tissue of persons who had been treated with haloperidol (Eyles *et al.,* 1997; Castagnoli *et al.,* 1999). Typical plasma concentrations of haloperidol encountered clinically are about 5 to 20 ng/ml, and these correspond to 80% to 90% occupancy of D$_2$-dopamine receptors in human basal ganglia, as demonstrated by PET brain scanning (Baldessarini *et al.,* 1988; Wolkin *et al.,* 1989).

Typical peak serum concentrations of clozapine after a single oral dose of 200 mg (100 to 770 ng/ml) are reached at 2.5 hours after administration, and typical serum levels during treatment are about 300 to 500 nanograms per milliliter. Clozapine is metabolized preferentially by CYP3A4 into pharmacologically inactive demethylated, hydroxylated, and N-oxide derivatives before excretion in urine and feces. The elimination half-life of clozapine varies with dose and dosing frequency, but average about 12 hours (*see* Table 20–3).

Risperidone is well absorbed, and it is metabolized in the liver preferentially by isozyme CYP2D6 to a major and active circulating metabolite, 9-hydroxyrisperidone. Since this metabolite and risperidone are nearly equipotent, the clinical efficacy of the drug reflects both compounds. Following oral administration of risperidone, peak plasma concentrations of risperidone and of its 9-hydroxy metabolite occur at 1 and 3 hours, respectively. The mean half-life of both compounds is about 22 hours (Table 20–3).

Olanzapine is also well absorbed, but about 40% of an oral dose is metabolized before reaching the systemic circulation. Plasma concentrations of olanzapine peak at about 6 hours after oral administration, and its elimination half-life ranges from 20 to 54 hours (Table 20–3). The major, readily excreted metabolites of olanzapine are the inactive 10-N-glucuronide and 4′-nor derivatives, formed mainly by the action of CYP1A2 with CYP2D6 as a minor alternative pathway (United States Pharmacopoeia, 2000).

Quetiapine fumarate is readily absorbed after oral administration and reaches peak plasma levels after 1.5 hours, with a mean half-life of 6 hours (Table 20–3). It is highly metabolized by hepatic CYP3A4 to inactive and readily excreted sulfoxide and acidic derivatives (United States Pharmacopoeia, 2000).

Tolerance and Physical Dependence. The antipsychotic drugs are not addicting, as the term is defined in Chapter 24. However, some degree of physical dependence may occur, with malaise and difficulty in sleeping developing several days after their abrupt discontinuation.

Tolerance usually develops to the sedative effects of neuroleptics over a period of days or weeks. Tolerance to antipsychotic drugs and cross-tolerance among the agents also are demonstrable in behavioral and biochemical experiments in animals, particularly those directed toward evaluation of the blockade of dopaminergic receptors in the basal ganglia (*see* Baldessarini and Tarsy, 1979). This form of tolerance may be less prominent in limbic and cortical areas of the forebrain. One correlate of tolerance in forebrain dopaminergic systems is the development of disuse supersensitivity of those systems, probably mediated by changes in the receptors for the neurotransmitter. This mechanism may underlie the clinical phenomenon of withdrawal-emergent dyskinesias (choreoathetosis on abrupt discontinuation of antipsychotic agents, especially following prolonged use of high doses of potent agents) (Baldessarini *et al.*, 1980).

Although cross-tolerance for some effects may occur among neuroleptic drugs, clinical problems occur in making rapid changes from high doses of one type of agent to another; sedation, hypotension, and other autonomic effects or acute extrapyramidal reactions can result. Worsening of the clinical condition that routinely follows discontinuation of maintenance treatment with antipsychotic agents appears to be dependent on the rate of drug discontinuation (Viguera *et al.*, 1997). Clinical worsening of psychotic symptoms is particularly likely after rapid discontinuation of clozapine, and it is difficult to control with alternative antipsychotics (Baldessarini *et al.*, 1997).

Preparations and Dosage. The number of agents with known neuroleptic or antipsychotic effects is large. Table 20–1 summarizes only those that are currently marketed in the United States for the treatment of psychotic disorders.

Several available agents are excluded, such as *promazine hydrochloride* (SPARINE) and reserpine and other rauwolfia alkaloids that have inferior antipsychotic effects or that are no longer commonly used for psychiatric patients. *Prochlorperazine* (COMPAZINE) has questionable utility as an antipsychotic agent and frequently produces acute extrapyramidal reactions; it is thus not commonly employed in psychiatry, although it is used as an antiemetic. *Thiethylperazine* (TORECAN), marketed only as an antiemetic, is a potent dopaminergic antagonist with many neuroleptic-like properties; at high doses it may be an efficacious antipsychotic agent (Rotrosen *et al.*, 1978). Several other thioxanthenes, butyrophenones, diphenylbutylpiperidines, benzamides, and long-acting repository preparations of neuroleptic agents are available in other countries.

Toxic Reactions and Side Effects. Antipsychotic drugs have a high therapeutic index and generally are safe agents. Furthermore, most phenothiazines and haloperidol have a relatively flat dose–response curve and can be used over a wide range of dosages. Although occasional deaths from overdosage have been reported, this is rare if the patient is given medical care and if an overdosage is not complicated by the concurrent ingestion of alcohol or other drugs. Based on animal data, the therapeutic index is lower for thioridazine and chlorpromazine than for the more potent agents (Janssen and Van Bever, 1978). Adult patients have survived doses of chlorpromazine up to 10 grams, and deaths from an overdose of haloperidol alone appear to be unknown, although the neuroleptic malignant syndrome and dystonic reactions that compromise respiration can be lethal.

Side effects often are extensions of the many pharmacological actions of these drugs. The most important are those on the cardiovascular system, central and autonomic nervous systems, and on endocrine functions. Other dangerous effects are seizures, agranulocytosis, cardiac toxicity, and pigmentary degeneration of the retina, all of which are rare (*see* below).

Therapeutic doses of phenothiazines may cause faintness, palpitation, and anticholinergic effects including nasal stuffiness, dry mouth, blurred vision, constipation, and, in males with prostatism, urinary retention. The most common troublesome cardiovascular side effect is orthostatic hypotension, which may result in syncope and falls. A fall in blood pressure is most likely to occur from administration of the phenothiazines with aliphatic side chains and of the atypical antipsychotics. Potent neuroleptic agents generally produce less hypotension.

Neurological Side Effects. A variety of neurological syndromes, involving particularly the extrapyramidal motor system, occur following the use of almost all antipsychotic drugs. These reactions are particularly prominent during treatment with the high-potency agents (tricyclic piperazines and butyrophenones). There is less likelihood of acute extrapyramidal side effects with clozapine, quetiapine, olanzapine, thioridazine, or low doses of risperidone. The neurological effects associated with antipsychotic drugs have been reviewed in detail (Baldessarini and Tarsy, 1979; Baldessarini *et al.*, 1980; Baldessarini, 1984; Baldessarini *et al.*, 1990; Kane *et al.*, 1992; Tarsy *et al.*, 2001).

Six varieties of neurological syndromes are characteristic of antipsychotic drugs. Four of these (acute dystonia, akathisia, parkinsonism, and the rare neuroleptic malignant syndrome) usually appear soon after administration of the drug, and two (rare perioral tremor and

Table 20–4
Neurological Side Effects of Neuroleptic Drugs

REACTION	FEATURES	TIME OF MAXIMAL RISK	PROPOSED MECHANISM	TREATMENT
Acute dystonia	Spasm of muscles of tongue, face, neck, back; may mimic seizures; *not* hysteria	1 to 5 days	Unknown	Antiparkinsonian agents are diagnostic and curative*
Akathisia	Motor restlessness; *not* anxiety or "agitation"	5 to 60 days	Unknown	Reduce dose or change drug; antiparkinsonian agents†, benzodiazepines or propranolol‡ may help
Parkinsonism	Bradykinesia, rigidity, variable tremor, mask facies, shuffling gait	5 to 30 days; can recur even after a single dose	Antagonism of dopamine	Antiparkinsonian agents helpful†
Neuroleptic malignant syndrome	Catatonia, stupor, fever, unstable blood pressure, myoglobinemia; can be fatal	Weeks; can persist for days after stopping neuroleptic	Antagonism of dopamine may contribute	Stop neuroleptic immediately: dantrolene or bromocriptine§ may help; antiparkinsonian agents not effective
Perioral tremor ("rabbit syndrome")	Perioral tremor (may be a late variant of parkinsonism)	After months or years of treatment	Unknown	Antiparkinsonian agents often help†
Tardive dyskinesia	Oral-facial dyskinesia; widespread choreoathetosis or dystonia	After months or years of treatment (worse on withdrawal)	Excess function of dopamine hypothesized	Prevention crucial; treatment unsatisfactory

*Many drugs have been claimed to be helpful for acute dystonia. Among the most commonly employed treatments are diphenhydramine hydrochloride, 25 or 50 mg intramuscularly, or benztropine mesylate, 1 or 2 mg intramuscularly or slowly intravenously, followed by oral medication with the same agent for a period of days to perhaps several weeks thereafter.
†For details regarding the use of oral antiparkinsonian agents, *see* the text and Chapter 22.
‡Propranolol often is effective in relatively low doses (20–80 mg per day). Selective β_1-adrenergic receptor antagonists are less effective.
§Despite the response to dantrolene, there is no evidence of an abnormality of Ca^{2+} transport in skeletal muscle; with lingering neuroleptic effects, bromocriptine may be tolerated in large doses (10–40 mg per day).

tardive dyskinesias or dystonias) are late-appearing syndromes that evolve during prolonged treatment. The clinical features of these syndromes and guidelines for their management are summarized in Table 20–4.

Acute dystonic reactions commonly occur with the initiation of antipsychotic drug therapy, particularly with agents of high potency, and may present as facial grimacing, torticollis, or oculogyric crisis. These syndromes may be mistaken for hysterical reactions or seizures, but they respond dramatically to parenteral administration of anti-cholinergic antiparkinsonian drugs. Oral administration of anticholinergic agents also can prevent dystonia, particularly in young male patients who have been given a high-potency neuroleptic drug (Arana *et al.,* 1988). Although treated readily, acute dystonic reactions are terrifying to patients; sudden death has occurred in rare instances, perhaps due to the impaired respiration caused by dystonia of pharyngeal, laryngeal, and other muscles.

Akathisia refers to strong subjective feelings of distress or discomfort, often referred to the legs, as well as to a compelling need to be in constant movement rather than to follow any specific movement pattern. Patients feel that they must get up and walk or continuously move about and may be unable to keep this tendency under control. Akathisia often is mistaken for agitation in psychotic patients; the distinction is critical, since agitation might be treated with an increase in dosage. Because the response of akathisia to antiparkinsonian drugs frequently is unsatisfactory, treatment typically requires reduction of antipsychotic drug dosage or a change of drug. Antianxiety agents or moderate doses of propranolol may be beneficial (Lipinski *et al.*, 1984). This common syndrome often interferes with the acceptance of neuroleptic treatment but frequently is not diagnosed.

A *parkinsonian syndrome* that may be indistinguishable from idiopathic parkinsonism commonly develops gradually during administration of antipsychotic drugs. Its incidence varies with different agents (*see* Tables 20–1 and 20–4). Clinically, there is a generalized slowing of volitional movement (akinesia) with mask facies and a reduction in arm movements. The syndrome characteristically evolves gradually over days to weeks. The most noticeable signs are slowing of movements, sometimes rigidity and variable tremor at rest, especially involving the upper extremities. "Pill-rolling" movements may be seen, although they are not as prominent in neuroleptic-induced as in idiopathic parkinsonism. Parkinsonian side effects may be mistaken for depression, since the flat facial expression and retarded movements may resemble signs of depression. This reaction usually is managed by use of either antiparkinsonian agents with anticholinergic properties or amantadine (*see* Chapter 22); the use of levodopa or a directly acting dopamine agonist incurs the risk of inducing agitation and worsening the psychotic illness. Antipsychotic agents sometimes are required in the clinical management of patients with idiopathic Parkinson's disease with spontaneous psychotic illness or psychotic reactions to dopaminergic therapy (*see* Chapter 22); clozapine and perhaps quetiapine are least likely to worsen the neurological disorder itself (Menza *et al.*, 1999; Parkinson Study Group, 1999).

A rare disorder, *neuroleptic malignant syndrome,* resembles a very severe form of parkinsonism with coarse tremor and catatonia, fluctuating in intensity, as well as signs of autonomic instability (labile pulse and blood pressure, hyperthermia), stupor, elevation of creatine kinase in serum, and sometimes myoglobinemia. In its most severe form, this syndrome may persist for more than a week after stopping the offending agent. Because mortality is high (more than 10%), immediate medical attention is required. This reaction has been associated with various types of neuroleptics, but its prevalence may be greater when relatively high doses of the more potent agents are used, especially when they are administered parenterally. Aside from immediate cessation of neuroleptic treatment and provision of supportive care, specific treatment is unsatisfactory; administration of *dantrolene* or the dopaminergic agonist *bromocriptine* may be helpful (Addonizio *et al.*, 1987; Pearlman, 1986). Although dantrolene also is used to manage the syndrome of malignant hyperthermia induced by general anesthetics, the neuroleptic-induced form of catatonia and hyperthermia probably is not associated with a defect in Ca^{2+} metabolism in skeletal muscle.

A rare movement disorder that can appear late in the treatment of chronically ill patients with antipsychotic agents is *perioral tremor,* often referred to as the "rabbit syndrome" (Jus *et al.*, 1974) because of the peculiar movements that characterize this condition. While sometimes categorized with other tardive (late or slowly evolving) dyskinesias, this term usually is reserved for choreoathetotic or dystonic reactions that develop after prolonged therapy. The rabbit syndrome, in fact, shares many features with parkinsonism, because the tremor has a frequency of about 5 to 7 Hz and there is a favorable response to anticholinergic agents and to the removal of the offending agent.

Tardive dyskinesia is a late-appearing neurological syndrome (or syndromes) associated with the use of neuroleptic drugs. It occurs more frequently in older patients, and risk may be greater in patients with mood disorders than in those with schizophrenia. Prevalence averages 15% to 25% in chronically psychotic young adults, with an annual incidence of 3% to 5% and a somewhat smaller annual rate of spontaneous remission, even with continued neuroleptic treatment. The risk is much lower with clozapine, but that of other recently developed atypical antipsychotic agents is not established (Tarsy *et al.*, 2001). Tardive dyskinesia is characterized by stereotyped, repetitive, painless, involuntary, quick choreiform (tic-like) movements of the face, eyelids (blinks or spasm), mouth (grimaces), tongue, extremities, or trunk. There are varying degrees of slower athetosis (twisting movements) and sustained dystonic postures, which are more common in young men and may be disabling. Late (tardive) emergence of possibly related disorders marked mainly by dystonia or akathisia (restlessness) also are seen. These movements all disappear in sleep (as in many other extrapyramidal syndromes), vary in intensity over time, and are dependent on the level of arousal or emotional distress.

Tardive dyskinetic movements can be suppressed partially by use of a potent neuroleptic, and perhaps with a dopamine-depleting agent such as reserpine or tetrabenazine, but such interventions are reserved for compellingly severe dyskinesia, particularly with continuing psychosis. Some dyskinetic patients, typically those with dystonic features, may benefit from use of clozapine, with which the risk of tardive dyskinesia is very low. Symptoms sometimes persist indefinitely after discontinuation of neuroleptic medication; more often, they diminish or disappear gradually over months of follow-up and are most likely to resolve spontaneously in younger patients (Gardos *et al.*, 1994; Morgenstern and Glazer, 1993; Smith and Baldessarini, 1980). Antiparkinsonism agents typically have little effect on, or may exacerbate, tardive dyskinesia and other forms of choreoathetosis, such as in Huntington's disease; no adequate treatment of these conditions has yet been established (Adler *et al.*, 1999; Soares and McGrath, 1999).

There is no established neuropathology in tardive dyskinesia, and its pathophysiological basis remains obscure. It has been hypothesized that compensatory increases in the function of dopamine as a neurotransmitter in the basal ganglia may be involved, including increased abundance and sensitivity of dopamine D_2-like receptors resulting from long-term administration of neuroleptic drugs (Baldessarini and Tarsy, 1979; Tarazi *et al.*, 1997). This idea is supported by the dissimilarities of therapeutic responses in patients with Parkinson's disease and those with tardive dyskinesia and by the similarities in responses of patients with other choreoathetotic dyskinesias such as Huntington's disease (*see* Chapter 22). Thus, antidopaminergic drugs tend to suppress the manifestations of tardive dyskinesia or Huntington's disease, while dopaminergic agonists worsen these conditions; in contrast to parkinsonism, antimuscarinic agents tend to worsen tardive dyskinesia, but cholinergic agents usually are ineffective. Because supersensitivity to dopaminergic agonists tends not to persist for more than a few weeks after stopping exposure to antagonists of the transmitter, this phenomenon is most likely to play a role in variants of tardive dyskinesia that resolve rapidly; these usually are referred to as *withdrawal-emergent dyskinesias*. The theoretical and clinical aspects of this problem have been reviewed in detail elsewhere (Baldessarini and Tarsy, 1979; Baldessarini *et al.*, 1980; Kane *et al.*, 1992).

It is important to prevent the neurological syndromes that complicate the use of antipsychotic drugs. Certain therapeutic guidelines should be followed. Routine use of antiparkinsonian agents in an attempt to avoid early extrapyramidal reactions usually is unnecessary and adds complexity, side effects, and expense to the treatment regimen. Antiparkinsonian agents are best reserved for cases of overt extrapyramidal reactions that respond favorably to such intervention. The need for such agents for the treatment of acute dystonic reactions ordinarily diminishes with time, but parkinsonism and akathisia tend to persist. The thoughtful and conservative use of antipsy-

chotic drugs in patients with chronic or frequently recurrent psychotic disorders almost certainly can reduce the risk of tardive dyskinesia. Although reduction of the dose of an antipsychotic agent is the best way to minimize its neurological side effects, this may not be practical in a patient with uncontrollable psychotic illness. The best preventive practice is to use the minimum effective dose of an antipsychotic drug for long-term therapy and to discontinue treatment as soon as it seems reasonable to do so or if a satisfactory response cannot be obtained. The use of clozapine, quetiapine, and other novel antipsychotic agents with a low risk of inducing extrapyramidal side effects represents an alternative for some patients, particularly those with continuing psychotic symptoms plus dyskinesia (Baldessarini and Frankenburg, 1991).

Jaundice. Jaundice was observed in patients shortly after the introduction of chlorpromazine. Commonly occurring during the second to fourth week of therapy, the jaundice generally is mild, and pruritus is rare. The reaction is probably a manifestation of hypersensitivity, because eosinophilic infiltration of the liver as well as eosinophilia occur, and there is no correlation with dose. Desensitization to chlorpromazine may occur with repeated administration, and jaundice may or may not recur if the same neuroleptic agent is given again. When the psychiatric disorder calls for uninterrupted drug therapy for a patient with neuroleptic-induced jaundice, it probably is safest to use low doses of a potent, dissimilar agent.

Blood Dyscrasias. Mild leukocytosis, leukopenia, and eosinophilia occasionally occur with antipsychotic medications, particularly with clozapine and less often with low-potency phenothiazines. It is difficult to determine whether a leukopenia occurring during the administration of a phenothiazine is a forewarning of impending agranulocytosis. This serious but rare complication occurs in not more than 1 in 10,000 patients receiving chlorpromazine or other low-potency agents other than clozapine; it usually appears within the first 8 to 12 weeks of treatment (Alvir *et al.*, 1993).

Suppression of the bone marrow or, less commonly, agranulocytosis has been associated particularly with the use of clozapine; the incidence approaches 1% within several months of treatment, independent of dose, and close monitoring of the patient is required for its safe use. Because the onset of blood dyscrasia may be sudden, the appearance of fever, malaise, or apparent respiratory infection in a patient being treated with an antipsychotic drug should be followed immediately by a complete blood count. Risk of agranulocytosis has been greatly reduced, though not eliminated, by frequent white blood cell counts in patients being treated with clozapine.

Other Metabolic Effects. Weight gain and its common long-term complications commonly are associated with long-term treatment with most antipsychotic and antimanic drugs. Among newer antipsychotic agents, weight gain is especially prominent with clozapine and olanzapine and less so with risperidone and quetiapine (Allison *et al.,* 1999). Associated adverse responses include new-onset or worsening of type 2 diabetes mellitus, hypertension, and hyperlipidemia. The anticipated long-term public health impact of these emerging problems is not yet well defined (Gaulin *et al.,* 1999; Wirshing *et al.,* 1998). In some patients with morbid increases in weight, the airway may be compromised, especially during sleep.

Skin Reactions. Dermatological reactions to the phenothiazines are common. Urticaria or dermatitis occurs in about 5% of patients receiving chlorpromazine. Several types of skin disorders may occur. Hypersensitivity reactions that may be urticarial, maculopapular, petechial, or edematous usually occur between the first and eighth weeks of treatment. The skin clears after discontinuation of the drug and may remain so even if drug therapy is reinstituted. Contact dermatitis may occur in personnel who handle chlorpromazine, and there may be a degree of cross-sensitivity to the other phenothiazines. Photosensitivity occurs that resembles severe sunburn. An effective sunscreen preparation should be prescribed for outpatients being treated with phenothiazines during the summer. Gray-blue pigmentation induced by long-term administration of low-potency phenothiazines in high doses is rare with current practices.

Epithelial keratopathy often is observed in patients on long-term therapy with chlorpromazine, and opacities in the cornea and in the lens of the eye also have been noted. The deposits tend to disappear spontaneously, although slowly, following discontinuation of drug administration. Pigmentary retinopathy has been reported, particularly following doses of thioridazine in excess of 1000 mg per day; a maximum daily dose of 800 mg currently is recommended.

Interactions with Other Drugs. The phenothiazines and thioxanthenes, especially those of low potency, affect the actions of a number of other drugs, sometimes with important clinical consequences (*see* DeVane and Nemeroff, 2000; Goff and Baldessarini, 1993). Chlorpromazine originally was introduced to potentiate central depressants in anesthesiology. Antipsychotic drugs can strongly potentiate sedatives and analgesics prescribed for medical purposes, as well as alcohol, nonprescription sedatives and hypnotics, antihistamines, and cold remedies. Chlorpromazine increases the miotic and sedative effects of morphine and may increase its analgesic actions. Furthermore, the drug markedly increases the respiratory depression produced by meperidine and can be expected to have similar effects when administered concurrently with other opioids. Obviously, neuroleptic drugs inhibit the actions of dopaminergic agonists and of levodopa.

Other interactive effects can be manifest on the cardiovascular system. Chlorpromazine and some other antipsychotic drugs, as well as their *N*-demethylated metabolites, may block the antihypertensive effects of guanethidine, probably by blocking its uptake into sympathetic nerves. The more potent antipsychotic agents, as well as molindone, are less likely to cause this effect. Low-potency phenothiazines can promote postural hypotension, possibly due to their α-adrenergic blocking properties. Thus, the interaction between phenothiazines and antihypertensive agents can be unpredictable.

Thioridazine, pimozide, and the experimental agents sertindole and ziprasidone can exert quinidine-like cardiac depressant effects, which can cause myocardial depression, decreased efficiency of repolarization, and increased risk of tachyarrhythmias. These effects may partially nullify the inotropic effect of digitalis. The antimuscarinic action of clozapine and thioridazine can cause tachycardia and enhance the peripheral and central effects (confusion, delirium) of other anticholinergic agents, such as the tricyclic antidepressants and antiparkinsonian agents.

Sedatives or anticonvulsants (*e.g.,* carbamazepine, phenobarbital, and phenytoin but not valproate) that induce microsomal drug-metabolizing enzymes can enhance the metabolism of antipsychotic agents, sometimes with significant clinical consequences. Conversely, serotonin-reuptake inhibitors including fluoxetine (*see* Chapter 19) compete for hepatic oxidases and can elevate circulating levels of neuroleptics (Goff and Baldessarini, 1993).

DRUG TREATMENT OF PSYCHOSES

The antipsychotic drugs are not specific for the type of psychosis to be treated. They are clearly effective in acute psychoses of unknown etiology, including mania, acute idiopathic psychoses, and acute exacerbations of schizophrenia; the greatest amount of controlled clinical data exists for the acute and chronic phases of schizophrenia and in acute mania. In addition, antipsychotic drugs are used empirically in many other neuromedical and idiopathic disorders in which psychotic symptoms and severe agitation are prominent.

The fact that neuroleptic agents are indeed antipsychotic was slow to gain acceptance. However, many clinical trials and five decades of clinical experience have established that these agents are effective and superior to sedatives such as the barbiturates and benzodiazepines, or alternatives such as electroconvulsive shock or other medical or psychological therapies (*see* Baldessarini, 1984, 1985). The "target" symptoms for which antipsychotic agents seem to be especially effective include agitation, combativeness, hostility, hallucinations, acute delusions, insomnia, anorexia, poor self-care, negativism, and sometimes withdrawal and seclusiveness; more variable or delayed are improvements in motivation and cognitive functions including insight, judgment, memory, and orientation. The most favorable prognosis is for patients with acute illnesses of brief duration who had functioned relatively well prior to the illness.

Despite the great success of the antipsychotic drugs, their use alone does not constitute optimal care of psychotic patients. The acute care, protection, and support of acutely psychotic patients, as well as mastery of techniques employed in their long-term care and rehabilitation, also are of critical importance. Detailed reviews of the clinical use of antipsychotic drugs are available (Baldessarini, 1984; Marder, 1998).

No one drug or combination of drugs has a selective effect on a particular symptom complex in groups of psychotic patients; although individual patients may appear to do better with one agent than another, this can be determined only by trial and error. Certain agents (particularly newer antipsychotic drugs) have been claimed to be specifically effective against "negative" symptoms in psychotic disorders (abulia, social withdrawal, lack of motivation), but evidence supporting this proposal remains inconsistent, and such benefits usually are limited (Moller, 1999). Generally, "positive" (irrational thinking, delusions, agitated turmoil, hallucinations) and negative symptoms tend to respond or not respond together. This trend is well documented with typical neuroleptics as well as modern atypical antipsychotic agents. It is clear that clozapine and other modern atypical antipsychotics induce less bradykinesia and other parkinsonian effects than do typical neuroleptics. Minimizing such side effects is sometimes interpreted clinically as a beneficial effect on impoverished affective responsiveness.

It is important to simplify the treatment regimen and to ensure that the patient is receiving the drug. In cases of suspected severe and dangerous noncompliance or with failure of oral treatment, the patient can be treated with injections of fluphenazine decanoate, haloperidol decanoate, or other long-acting preparations. Injectable and long-acting preparations of modern atypical antipsychotics currently are unavailable, but some are in development.

Because the choice of an antipsychotic drug cannot be made reliably on the basis of anticipated therapeutic effect, drug selection often depends on side effects or on a previous favorable response. If the patient has a history of cardiovascular disease or stroke and the threat from hypotension is serious, a potent neuroleptic should be used in the smallest dose that is effective (see Table 20–1; DeBattista and Schatzberg, 1999). If it seems important to minimize the risk of acute extrapyramidal symptoms, quetiapine, a low dose of olanzapine or risperidone, or clozapine should be considered. If the patient would be seriously discomforted by interference with ejaculation or if there are serious risks of cardiovascular or other autonomic toxicity, low doses of a potent neuroleptic might be preferred. If sedative effects are undesirable, a potent agent is preferable. Small doses of antipsychotic drugs of high or moderate potency may be safest in the elderly. If the patient has compromised hepatic function or if there is a potential threat of jaundice, low doses of a high-potency agent may be used. The physician's experience with a particular drug may outweigh other considerations. Skill in the use of antipsychotic drugs depends on selection of an adequate but not excessive dose, knowledge of what to

expect, and judgment as to when to stop therapy or change drugs.

Some patients do not respond satisfactorily to antipsychotic drug treatment, and many chronically ill schizophrenic patients, while helped during periods of acute exacerbation of their disease, may show unsatisfactory responses between the more acute phases of illness. Individual nonresponders cannot be identified beforehand with certainty, and a minority of patients do poorly or sometimes even become worse on medication. If a patient does not improve after a course of seemingly adequate treatment and fails to respond to another drug given in adequate dosage, the diagnosis should be reevaluated.

Usually 2 to 3 weeks or more are required to demonstrate obvious positive effects in schizophrenic patients. Maximum benefit in chronically ill patients may require several months. In contrast, improvement of some acutely psychotic patients can be seen within 48 hours. Aggressive dosing or parenteral administration of an antipsychotic drug at the start of an acute psychosis has not been found to increase the magnitude or the rate of appearance of therapeutic responses (Baldessarini et al., 1988). Sedatives, such as the potent benzodiazepines, can be used for brief periods during the initiation of antipsychotic therapy but are not effective in the long-term treatment of chronically psychotic and, especially, schizophrenic patients. After the initial response, drugs usually are used in conjunction with psychological, supportive, and rehabilitative treatments.

There is no convincing evidence that combinations of antipsychotic drugs offer consistent advantages. A combination of an antipsychotic drug and an antidepressant may be useful in some cases, especially in depressed psychotic patients or in cases of agitated major depression with psychotic features. However, antidepressants and stimulants are unlikely to reduce apathy and withdrawal in schizophrenia, and they may induce clinical worsening in some cases.

Optimal dosage of antipsychotic drugs requires individualization to determine doses that are effective, well tolerated, and accepted by the patient. Dose–response relationships for antipsychotic and side effects overlap, and an end point of a desired therapeutic response can be difficult to determine (DeBattista and Schatzberg, 1999). Typical effective doses are approximately 300 to 500 mg of chlorpromazine, 5 to 15 mg of haloperidol, or their equivalent, daily. Doses of as little as 50 to 200 mg of chlorpromazine per day (or 2 to 6 mg of haloperidol or fluphenazine per day) may be effective and be better tolerated by many patients, especially after the initial improvement of acute symptoms (Baldessarini et al., 1988). Careful observation of the patient's changing response is the best guide to dosage.

In the treatment of acute psychoses, the dose of antipsychotic drug is increased during the first few days to achieve control of symptoms. The dose is then adjusted during the next several weeks as the patient's condition warrants. Parenteral medication sometimes is indicated for acutely agitated patients; 5 mg of haloperidol or fluphenazine or a comparable dose of another agent is given intramuscularly. The desired response usually can be obtained by administering additional doses at intervals of 4 to 8 hours for the first 24 to 72 hours, because the appearance of effects may be delayed for several hours. Rarely is it necessary to administer more than 20 to 30 mg of fluphenazine or haloperidol (or an equivalent amount of another agent) per 24 hours. Severe and otherwise poorly controlled agitation usually can be managed safely by use of adjunctive sedation (*e.g.,* with a benzodiazepine such as lorazepam) and close supervision in a secure setting.

One must remain alert for acute dystonic reactions, which are especially likely early in the aggressive use of potent neuroleptics. Hypotension is most likely to occur if an agent of low potency, such as chlorpromazine, is given in a high dose or by injection and may occur with atypical antipsychotic agents early in treatment. Some antipsychotic drugs, including fluphenazine, other piperazines, and haloperidol, have been given in doses of several hundred milligrams a day without disaster, although such high doses of potent agents do not yield significantly or consistently superior results in the treatment of acute or chronic psychosis, and they may yield inferior antipsychotic effects as well as increasing risks of neurological and other side effects (Baldessarini *et al.*, 1988). After an initial period of stabilization, regimens based on a single daily dose (typically 5 to 10 mg per day of haloperidol or fluphenazine, 2 to 4 mg of risperidone, 5 to 15 mg of olanzapine, or their equivalent) often are effective and safe; such dosing may allow some degree of selection of the time at which unwanted effects occur so as to minimize the patient's discomfort.

Table 20–1 gives the usual and extreme ranges of dosage for antipsychotic drugs used in the United States (*see also* DeBattista and Schatzberg, 1999). The ranges have been established for the most part in the treatment of schizophrenic or manic patients. Although acutely disturbed inpatients often require higher doses of an antipsychotic drug than do more stable outpatients, the concept that a low or flexible maintenance dose will suffice during follow-up care of a partially recovered or chronic psychotic patient is supported by several appropriately controlled trials (Baldessarini *et al.*, 1988; Herz *et al.*, 1991).

In reviews of nearly 30 controlled prospective studies involving several thousand schizophrenic patients, the mean overall relapse rate was 58% for those patients who were withdrawn from antipsychotic drugs and given a placebo, compared with only 16% of those who continued on drug therapy (Baldessarini *et al.*, 1990; Gilbert *et al.*, 1995; Viguera *et al.*, 1997). Dosage in chronic cases often can be lowered to 50 to 200 mg of chlorpromazine (or its equivalent) per day without signs of relapse (Baldessarini *et al.*, 1988), but rapid dose reduction or discontinuation appears to increase risk of exacerbation or relapse (Viguera *et al.*, 1997). Flexible therapy in which dosage is adjusted to changing current requirements can be useful and can reduce the incidence of side effects. Maintenance with injections of the decanoate ester of fluphenazine or haloperidol every 2 to 4 weeks can be very effective (Kane *et al.*, 1983).

The treatment of delirium or dementia is another accepted use of the antipsychotic drugs. They may be administered temporarily while a specific and correctable structural, infectious, metabolic, or toxic cause is vigorously sought. They sometimes are used for prolonged periods when no correctable cause can be found. Once again, there are no drugs of choice or clearly established dosage guidelines for such indications, although agents of high potency are preferred (*see* Prien, 1973). In patients with acute "brain syndromes" without likelihood of seizures, frequent small doses (*e.g.,* 2 to 6 mg) of haloperidol or another potent antipsychotic may be effective in controlling agitation. Agents with low potency should be avoided because of their greater tendency to produce sedation, hypotension, and seizures, and those with central anticholinergic effects may worsen confusion and agitation.

Most antipsychotics are effective in the treatment of mania and often are used concomitantly with the institution of lithium or anticonvulsant therapy (*see* below). In fact, it often is impractical to attempt to manage a manic patient with lithium alone during the first week of illness, when antipsychotic or sedative drugs usually are required. Adequate studies of possible long-term preventive effects of antipsychotic drugs in manic-depressive illness have not been conducted. Antipsychotic drugs also may have a limited role in the treatment of severe depression. Controlled studies have demonstrated the efficacy of several antipsychotic drugs in some depressed patients, especially those with striking agitation or psychotic delusions, and addition of an antipsychotic to an antidepressant in psychotic depression may yield results approaching those obtained with ECT (Brotman *et al.*, 1987; Chan *et al.*, 1987). Antipsychotic agents ordinarily are not used for the treatment of anxiety disorders.

The status of the drug treatment of childhood psychosis and other behavioral disorders of children is confused by diagnostic inconsistencies and a paucity of controlled studies. Antipsychotics can benefit children with disorders characterized by features that occur in adult psychoses or mania as well as those with Tourette's syndrome. Low doses of the more potent agents usually are preferred in an attempt to avoid interference with daytime activities or performance in school (Kutcher, 1997; Findling *et al.*, 1998). Attention disorder, with or without hyperactivity, responds poorly to antipsychotic agents but often very well to stimulants and some antidepressants (Kutcher, 1997). Information on dosages of antipsychotic drugs for children is limited, as is the number of drugs currently approved in the United States for use in preadolescents. The recommended doses of antipsychotic agents for school-aged children with moderate degrees of agitation are lower than those for acutely psychotic children, who may require daily doses similar to those used in adults (Kutcher, 1997; *see also* Table 20–1).

Most relevant experience is with chlorpromazine, for which the recommended single dose is approximately 0.5 mg/kg of body weight given at intervals of 4 to 6 hours orally or 6 to 8 hours intramuscularly. Suggested dosage limits are 200 mg per day (orally) for preadolescents, 75 mg per day (intramuscularly) for children aged 5 to 12 years or weighing 23 to 45 kg, and 40 mg per day (intramuscularly) for children under 5 years of age or weighing less than 23 kg. Usual single doses for other agents of relatively low potency are thioridazine, 0.25 to 0.5 mg/kg, and chlorprothixene, 0.5 to 1.0 mg/kg, to a total of 100 mg/day (over the age of 6). For neuroleptics of high potency, daily doses are trifluoperazine, 1 to 15 mg (6 to 12 years of age) and 1 to 30 mg (over 12 years of age); fluphenazine, 0.05 to 0.10 mg/kg, up to 10 mg (over 5 years of age); and perphenazine, 0.05 to 0.10 mg/kg, up to 6 mg (over 1 year of age). Haloperidol and pimozide have been used in children, especially for Tourette's syndrome; haloperidol is recommended for use in a dosage of 2 to 16 mg per day in children over 12 years of age.

Poor tolerance of the side effects of the antipsychotic drugs often limits the dosage that can be given to elderly patients. One should proceed cautiously, using small, divided doses of agents with moderate or high potency, with the expectation that elderly patients will require doses that are one-half or less of those needed for young adults

MISCELLANEOUS MEDICAL USES FOR ANTIPSYCHOTIC DRUGS

Antipsychotic drugs have a variety of uses in addition to the treatment of psychiatric patients. Predominant among these are the treatment of nausea and vomiting, alcoholic hallucinosis, certain neuropsychiatric diseases marked by movement disorders (notably, Tourette's syndrome and Huntington's disease), and occasionally pruritus (for which trimeprazine is recommended) and intractable hiccough.

Nausea and Vomiting. Many antipsychotic agents can prevent vomiting due to specific etiologies when given in relatively low, nonsedative doses. This use is discussed in Chapter 38.

Other Neuropsychiatric Disorders. Antipsychotic drugs are useful in the management of several syndromes with psychiatric features that also are characterized by movement disorders. These include, in particular, *Tourette's syndrome* (marked by tics, other involuntary movements, aggressive outbursts, grunts, and vocalizations that frequently are obscene) and *Huntington's disease* (marked by severe and progressive choreoathetosis, psychiatric symptoms, and dementia, with a clear genetic basis). Haloperidol currently is regarded as a drug of choice for these conditions, although it probably is not unique in its antidyskinetic actions. Pimozide, a diphenylbutylpiperidine, also is used (typically in daily doses of 2 to 10 mg). Pimozide carries some risk of impairing cardiac repolarization, and it should be discontinued if the QT interval exceeds 470 msec, especially in a child. Clonidine and certain antidepressants also may be effective in Tourette's syndrome (Spencer *et al.,* 1993). Clozapine and quetiapine are relatively well tolerated in psychosis arising with dopamine-receptor agonist treatment in Parkinson's disease (Tarsy *et al.,* 2001).

Withdrawal Syndromes. Antipsychotic drugs are *not* useful in the management of withdrawal from opioids, and their use in the management of withdrawal from barbiturates and other sedatives or alcohol is contraindicated because of the high risk of seizures. They can be used safely and effectively in psychoses associated with chronic alcoholism—especially the syndrome known as *alcoholic hallucinosis* (*see* Sadock and Sadock, 2000).

II. TREATMENT OF MANIA

ANTIMANIC MOOD-STABILIZING AGENTS: LITHIUM

Lithium carbonate was introduced into psychiatry in 1949 for the treatment of mania (Cade, 1949; *see* Mitchell *et al.,* 1999). However, it was not used for this purpose in the United States until 1970, in part due to concerns of American physicians about the safety of this treatment following reports of severe intoxication with lithium chloride from its uncontrolled use as a substitute for sodium chloride in patients with cardiac disease. Evidence for both the safety and the efficacy of lithium salts in the treatment of mania and the prevention of recurrent attacks of manic-depressive illness is both abundant and convincing (Davis *et al.,* 1999; Mitchell *et al.,* 1999). In recent years, the limitations and side effects of lithium salts have become increasingly well appreciated, and efforts to find alternative antimanic or mood-stabilizing agents have intensified (*see* Davis *et al.,* 1999; Goodwin and Jamison, 1990). The most successful alternatives or adjuncts to lithium to date are the anticonvulsants carbamazepine and valproic acid (Post, 2000).

History. Lithium urate is soluble, and lithium salts were used in the nineteenth century as a treatment of gout. Lithium bromide was employed in that era as a sedative (including its use in manic patients) and as a putative anticonvulsant. Thereafter, lithium salts were little used until the late 1940s, when lithium chloride was employed as a salt substitute for cardiac and other chronically ill patients. This ill-advised use led to several reports of severe intoxication and death and to considerable notoriety concerning lithium salts within the medical profession. Cade, in Australia, while looking for toxic nitrogenous substances in the urine of mental patients for testing in guinea pigs, administered lithium salts to the animals in an attempt to increase the solubility of urates. Lithium carbonate made the animals lethargic, and, in an inductive leap, Cade gave lithium carbonate to several agitated or manic psychiatric patients as early as 1948 (*see* Mitchell *et al.,* 1999). In 1949, he reported that this treatment seemed to have a specific effect in mania (Cade, 1949).

Chemistry. Lithium is the lightest of the alkali metals (group Ia); the salts of this monovalent cation share some characteristics with those of Na^+ and K^+. Li^+ is readily assayed in biological fluids by flame-photometric and atomic-absorption spectrophotometric methods, and it can be detected in brain tissue by magnetic resonance spectroscopy (Riedl *et al.,* 1997). Traces of the ion occur normally in animal tissues, but it has no known physiological role. Lithium carbonate and lithium citrate currently are in therapeutic use in the United States.

Pharmacological Properties

Therapeutic concentrations of lithium ion (Li^+) have almost no discernible psychotropic effects in normal individuals. It is not a sedative, depressant, or euphoriant, and this characteristic differentiates Li^+ from other psychotropic agents. The general biology and pharmacology of Li^+ have been reviewed in detail elsewhere (Jefferson *et al.,* 1983). The precise mechanism of action of Li^+ as a mood-stabilizing agent remains unknown, although many cellular actions of Li^+ have been characterized (Manji *et al.,* 1999b).

(Eastham and Jeste, 1997; Jeste *et al.,* 1999a,b; Zubenko and Sunderland, 2000).

An important characteristic of Li$^+$ is that it has a relatively small gradient of distribution across biological membranes, unlike Na$^+$ and K$^+$; although it can replace Na$^+$ in supporting a single action potential in a nerve cell, it is not an adequate "substrate" for the Na$^+$ pump and it cannot, therefore, maintain membrane potentials. It is uncertain whether or not important interactions occur between Li$^+$ (at therapeutic concentrations of about 1 mEq per liter) and the transport of other monovalent or divalent cations by nerve cells.

Central Nervous System. In addition to the possibility of altered distribution of cations in the CNS, much attention has centered on the effects of low concentrations of Li$^+$ on the metabolism of the biogenic monoamines that have been implicated in the pathophysiology of mood disorders as well as on second-messenger and other intracellular molecular mechanisms involved in signal transduction and in cell and gene regulation (Jope, 1999; Lenox and Manji, 1998; Manji *et al.,* 1999a,b).

In animal brain tissue, Li$^+$ at concentrations of 1 to 10 mEq per liter inhibits the depolarization-provoked and Ca^{2+}-dependent release of norepinephrine and dopamine, but *not* serotonin, from nerve terminals (Baldessarini and Vogt, 1988). Li$^+$ may even enhance the release of serotonin, especially in the limbic system, at least transiently (Treiser *et al.,* 1981; Manji *et al.,* 1999a,b; Wang and Friedman, 1989). The ion has limited effects on catecholamine-sensitive adenylyl cyclase activity or on the binding of ligands to monoamine receptors in brain tissue (Manji *et al.,* 1999b; Turkka *et al.,* 1992), although there is some evidence that Li$^+$ can inhibit the effects of receptor-blocking agents that cause supersensitivity in such systems (Bloom *et al.,* 1983). Li$^+$ can modify some hormonal responses mediated by adenylyl cyclase or phospholipase C in other tissues, including the actions of antidiuretic and thyroid-stimulating hormones on their peripheral target tissues (*see* Manji *et al.,* 1999b; Urabe *et al.,* 1991). In part, the actions of Li$^+$ may reflect its ability to interfere with the activity of both stimulatory and inhibitory GTP-binding proteins (G$_s$ and G$_i$) by keeping them in their less active $\alpha\beta\gamma$ trimer state (Jope, 1999; Manji *et al.,* 1999b).

A consistently reported, selective action of Li$^+$ is to inhibit inositol monophosphatase (Berridge *et al.,* 1989) and thus interfere with the phosphatidylinositol pathway (*see* Figure 20–1). This effect can lead to decreases in cerebral inositol concentrations, which can be detected with magnetic resonance spectroscopy in human brain tissue (Manji *et al.,* 1999a,b). However, the physiological consequences of this effect remain uncertain, including interference with neurotransmission mechanisms that are mediated by the phosphatidylinositol pathway (Lenox and Manji, 1998; Manji *et al.,* 1999b).

Lithium treatment also leads to consistent decreases in the functioning of protein kinases in brain tissue, including calcium-activated, phospholipid-dependent protein kinase C (PKC) (Jope, 1999; Lenox and Manji, 1998), particularly subtypes α and ε (Manji *et al.,* 1999b). This effect also is shared with valproic acid (particularly for PKC$_\alpha$) but not carbamazepine, among other proposed antimanic or mood-stabilizing agents (Manji *et al.,* 1993). In turn, these effects may alter the release of amine neurotransmitters and hormones (Wang and Friedman, 1989; Zatz and Reisine, 1985) as well as the activity of tyrosine hydroxylase (Chen *et al.,* 1998). A major substrate for cerebral PKC is the myristolated alanine-rich PKC-kinase substrate protein MARCKS, which has been implicated in synaptic and neuronal plasticity. Its expression is reduced by treatment with both Li$^+$ and valproate, but not by carbamazepine or by antipsychotic, antidepressant, or sedative drugs (Watson and Lenox, 1996; Watson *et al.,* 1998). Another important protein kinase that is inhibited by both Li$^+$ and valproate treatment is glycogen synthase kinase-3β (GSK-3β), which is involved in neuronal and nuclear regulatory processes, including limiting expression of the regulatory protein β-catenin (Chen *et al.,* 1999b; Manji *et al.,* 1999b).

Li$^+$ and valproic acid both interact with nuclear regulatory factors that affect gene expression. Such effects include increasing DNA binding of transcription-regulatory-factor-activator protein-1 (AP-1) as well as altered expression of other transcription regulatory factors, including AMI-1β or PEBP-2β (Chen *et al.,* 1999a,c).

Finally, treatment with both Li$^+$ and valproate has been associated with increased expression of the regulatory protein B-cell lymphocyte protein-2 (bcl-2), which is associated with protection against neuronal degeneration (Chen *et al.,* 1999c, Manji *et al.,* 1999c). The significance of these several interactions of mood-stabilizing agents with cell-regulatory factors remains to be clarified.

Absorption, Distribution, and Excretion. Li$^+$ is absorbed readily and almost completely from the gastrointestinal tract. Complete absorption occurs in about 8 hours, with peak concentrations in plasma occurring 2 to 4 hours after an oral dose. Slow-release preparations of lithium carbonate provide a slower rate of absorption and thereby minimize early peaks in plasma concentrations of the ion. However, absorption can be variable, and the incidence of lower intestinal tract symptoms may be increased. Li$^+$ initially is distributed in the extracellular fluid and then gradually accumulates in various tissues. The concentration gradient across plasma membranes is much smaller than those for Na$^+$ and K$^+$. The final volume of distribution (0.7 to 0.9 liter per kilogram) approaches that of total body water and is much lower than that of most other psychotropic agents, which are lipophilic and protein bound. Passage through the blood–brain barrier is slow, and when a steady state is achieved, the concentration of Li$^+$ in the cerebrospinal fluid is about 40% to 50% of the concentration in plasma. The ion does not bind appreciably to plasma proteins. The kinetics of Li$^+$ can be monitored in human brain with magnetic resonance spectroscopy (Plenge *et al.,* 1994).

Approximately 95% of a single dose of Li$^+$ is eliminated in the urine. From one- to two-thirds of an acute dose is excreted during a 6- to 12-hour initial phase of excretion, followed by slow excretion over the next 10 to

14 days. The elimination half-life averages 20 to 24 hours. With repeated administration, Li^+ excretion increases during the first 5 to 6 days until a steady state is reached between ingestion and excretion. When therapy with Li^+ is stopped, there is a rapid phase of renal excretion followed by a slow 10- to 14-day phase. Since 80% of the filtered Li^+ is reabsorbed by the proximal renal tubules, clearance of Li^+ by the kidney is about 20% of that for creatinine, ranging between 15 and 30 ml per minute. This is somewhat lower in elderly patients (10 to 15 ml per minute). Loading with Na^+ produces a small enhancement of Li^+ excretion, but Na^+ depletion promotes a clinically important degree of retention of Li^+.

Because of the low therapeutic index for Li^+ (as low as 2 or 3), concentrations in plasma or serum are determined to assure safe use of the drug. In the treatment of acutely manic patients, one can postpone treatment with Li^+ until some degree of behavioral control and metabolic stability has been attained with antipsychotics, sedatives, or anticonvulsants. The concentration of Li^+ in blood usually is measured at a trough of the oscillations that result from repetitive administration, but the peaks can be two or three times higher at steady state. When the peaks are reached, intoxication may result, even when concentrations in morning samples of plasma are in the acceptable range of around 1 mEq per liter. Single daily doses, with relatively large oscillations of the plasma concentration of Li^+, may reduce the polyuria sometimes associated with this treatment, but the average reduction is quite small (Baldessarini *et al.*, 1996b; Hetmar *et al.*, 1991). Nevertheless, because of the low margin of safety of Li^+ and because of its short half-life during initial distribution, divided daily doses often are used, and even slow-release formulations usually are given twice daily. Nonetheless, some physicians administer Li^+ once per day and achieve good therapeutic responses safely.

Although the pharmacokinetics of Li^+ vary considerably among subjects, the volume of distribution and clearance are relatively stable in an individual patient. However, a well-established regimen can be complicated by occasional periods of Na^+ loss, as may occur with an intercurrent medical illness or with losses or restrictions of fluids and electrolytes; heavy sweating may be an exception due to a preferential secretion of Li^+ over Na^+ in sweat (Jefferson *et al.*, 1982). Hence, patients taking Li^+ should have plasma concentrations checked at least occasionally. Most of the renal tubular reabsorption of Li^+ seems to occur in the proximal tubule. Nevertheless, Li^+ retention can be increased by any diuretic that leads to depletion of Na^+, particularly the thiazides (Siegel *et al.*, 1998). Renal excretion can be increased by administration of osmotic diuretics, acetazolamide, or aminophylline, although this is of little help in the management of Li^+ intoxication. Triamterene may increase excretion of Li^+, suggesting that some reabsorption of the ion

may occur in the distal nephron; however, spironolactone does not increase the excretion of Li^+. Some nonsteroidal antiinflammatory agents can facilitate renal proximal tubular resorption of Li^+ and thereby increase concentrations in plasma to toxic levels; this interaction appears to be particularly strong with indomethacin; it may occur with ibuprofen and naproxen, and possibly less so with sulindac and aspirin (*see* Siegel *et al.*, 1998). Also a potential drug–drug interaction can occur between Li^+ and angiotensin converting enzyme inhibitors (*see* Chapter 31).

Less than 1% of ingested Li^+ leaves the human body in the feces, and 4% to 5% is secreted in sweat. Li^+ is secreted in saliva in concentrations about twice those in plasma, while its concentration in tears is about equal to that in plasma. Since the ion also is secreted in human milk, women receiving Li^+ should not breast-feed infants.

Toxic Reactions and Side Effects. The occurrence of toxicity is related to the serum concentration of Li^+ and its rate of rise following administration. Acute intoxication is characterized by vomiting, profuse diarrhea, coarse tremor, ataxia, coma, and convulsions. Symptoms of milder toxicity are most likely to occur at the absorptive peak of Li^+ and include nausea, vomiting, abdominal pain, diarrhea, sedation, and fine tremor. The more serious effects involve the nervous system and include mental confusion, hyperreflexia, gross tremor, dysarthria, seizures, and cranial-nerve and focal neurological signs, progressing to coma and death; sometimes, neurological damage may be irreversible. Other toxic effects are cardiac arrhythmias, hypotension, and albuminuria. Side effects including nausea, diarrhea, daytime drowsiness, polyuria, polydipsia, weight gain, fine hand tremor, and dermatological reactions including acne are common even in therapeutic dose ranges (Baldessarini *et al.*, 1996b).

Therapy with Li^+ is associated initially with a transient increase in the excretion of 17-hydroxycorticosteroids, Na^+, K^+, and water. This effect usually is not sustained beyond 24 hours. In the subsequent 4 to 5 days, the excretion of K^+ becomes normal, Na^+ is retained, and in some cases pretibial edema forms. Na^+ retention has been associated with increased aldosterone secretion and responds to administration of spironolactone; however, this maneuver incurs the risk of promoting the retention of Li^+ and increasing its concentration in plasma. Edema and Na^+ retention frequently disappear spontaneously after several days.

A small number of patients treated with Li^+ develop a benign, diffuse, nontender thyroid enlargement suggestive of compromised thyroid function. This effect may be associated with previous thyroiditis, particularly in middle-aged women. In patients treated with Li^+, thyroid uptake of ^{131}I is increased, plasma protein–bound iodine and free thyroxine tend to be slightly low, and thyroid-stimulating hormone (TSH) secretion may be moderately elevated. These effects appear to result from interference with the iodination of tyrosine and, therefore, the synthesis of thyroxine. However, patients usually remain euthyroid, and obvious hypothyroidism is rare. In patients who do develop goiter, discontinuation of Li^+ or treatment with thyroid hormone results in shrinkage of the gland. Adding supplemental triiodothyronine (T_3) to bipolar disorder patients with low-normal thyroid hormone levels and continued depression or anergy may be useful clinically, but proposed use of high doses of thyroxin (T_4) to control rapid-cycling bipolar disorder is not established as a safe practice (Bauer and Whybrow, 1990; Baumgartner et al., 1994; Lasser and Baldessarini, 1997).

Polydipsia and polyuria occur in patients treated with Li^+, occasionally to a disturbing degree. Acquired nephrogenic diabetes insipidus can occur in patients maintained at therapeutic plasma concentrations of the ion (Siegel et al., 1998). Typically, mild polyuria appears early in treatment and then disappears. Late-developing polyuria is an indication to evaluate renal function, lower the dose of Li^+, or consider addition of a thiazide diuretic or a K^+-sparing agent such as amiloride to counteract the polyuria (Batlle et al., 1985; Kosten and Forrest, 1986). The polyuria disappears with termination of Li^+ therapy. The mechanism of this effect may involve inhibition of the action of antidiuretic hormone (ADH) on renal adenylyl cyclase as reflected in elevated circulating ADH and lack of responsiveness to exogenous antidiuretic peptides (Boton et al., 1987; Siegel et al., 1998). The result is decreased ADH stimulation of renal reabsorption of water. However, Li^+ also may act at steps beyond cyclic AMP synthesis to alter renal function. The effect of Li^+ on water metabolism is not sufficiently predictable to be therapeutically useful in treatment of the syndrome of inappropriate secretion of ADH. Evidence of chronic inflammatory changes in biopsied renal tissue has been found in a minority of patients given Li^+ for prolonged periods. Since progressive, clinically significant impairment of renal function is rare, these are considered incidental findings by most experts; nevertheless, plasma creatinine and urine volume should be monitored during long-term use of Li^+ (Boton et al., 1987; Hetmar et al., 1991).

Li^+ also has a weak action on carbohydrate metabolism that resembles that of insulin. In rats, Li^+ causes an increase in skeletal muscle glycogen accompanied by severe depletion of glycogen from the liver.

The prolonged use of Li^+ causes a benign and reversible depression of the T wave of the ECG, an effect not related to depletion of Na^+ or K^+.

Li^+ routinely causes EEG changes characterized by diffuse slowing, widened frequency spectrum, and potentiation with disorganization of background rhythm. Seizures have been reported in nonepileptic patients with plasma concentrations of Li^+ in the therapeutic range. Myasthenia gravis may worsen during treatment with Li^+ (Neil et al., 1976).

A benign, sustained increase in circulating polymorphonuclear leukocytes occurs during the chronic use of Li^+ and is reversed within a week after termination of treatment.

Allergic reactions such as dermatitis and vasculitis can occur with Li^+ administration. Worsening of acne vulgaris is a common problem, and some patients may experience mild alopecia.

In pregnancy, concomitant use of natriuretics and low-Na^+ diets can contribute to maternal and neonatal Li^+ intoxication, and during postpartum diuresis one can anticipate potentially toxic retention of Li^+ by the mother. The use of Li^+ in preg-

nancy has been associated with neonatal goiter, CNS depression, hypotonia, and cardiac murmur. All of these conditions reverse with time. The use of Li^+ in early pregnancy may be associated with an increase in the incidence of cardiovascular anomalies of the newborn, especially Ebstein's malformation (Cohen et al., 1994). The basal risk of Ebstein's anomaly (malformed tricuspid valve, usually with a septal defect) of about 1 per 20,000 live births may rise severalfold, but probably not above 1 per 5000. Moreover, the defect typically is detectable in utero by ultrasonography and often is surgically correctable after birth. In contrast, the antimanic anticonvulsants valproic acid and perhaps carbamazepine have an associated risk of irreversible spina bifida that may exceed 1 per 100 and so do not represent a rational alternative (Viguera et al., 2000). In balancing the risk vs. benefit of using Li^+ in pregnancy, it is important to evaluate the risk of untreated manic-depressive disorder and to consider conservative measures, such as deferring intervention until symptoms arise or using a safer treatment, such as a neuroleptic or ECT (see Cohen et al., 1994; Viguera et al., 2000).

Treatment of Lithium Intoxication.   There is no specific antidote for Li^+ intoxication, and treatment is supportive. Vomiting induced by rapidly rising plasma Li^+ may tend to limit absorption, but fatalities have occurred. Care must be taken to assure that the patient is not Na^+- and water-depleted. Dialysis is the most effective means of removing the ion from the body and should be considered in severe poisonings, i.e., in patients exhibiting symptoms of toxicity or patients with serum Li^+ concentrations greater than 4.0 mEq/l in acute overdoses or greater than 1.5 mEq/l in chronic overdoses.

Interactions with Other Drugs.   Interactions between Li^+ and diuretics and nonsteroidal antiinflammatory agents have been discussed above (see Siegel et al., 1998). Thiazide diuretics as well as amiloride may correct the nephrogenic diabetes insipidus caused by Li^+ (Boton et al., 1987). Retention of Li^+ may be limited during administration of the weakly natriuretic agent amiloride as well as the loop diuretic furosemide, which also reduce the risk of toxic effects of hypokalemia with excessive circulating levels of Li^+. Furosemide also may have lesser interactions with Li^+ than do the thiazides. Amiloride and other diuretic agents (sometimes with reduced doses of Li^+) have been used safely to reverse the syndrome of diabetes insipidus occasionally associated with Li^+ therapy (Batlle et al., 1985; Boton et al., 1987; see Chapter 29). Li^+ often is used in conjunction with antipsychotic, sedative, antidepressant, and anticonvulsant drugs. A few case reports have suggested a risk of increased CNS toxicity with Li^+ when it is combined with haloperidol; however, this finding is at variance with many years of experience with this combination. Antipsychotic drugs may prevent nausea, which can be a sign of Li^+ toxicity. There is, however, no absolute contraindication to the concurrent use of Li^+ and psychotropic drugs. Finally, anticholinergic and other agents that alter gastrointestinal motility also may alter Li^+ concentrations in blood over time.

Therapeutic Uses. The use of Li$^+$ in *bipolar disorder* (manic-depressive illness) is discussed below. Treatment with Li$^+$ is conducted ideally in cooperative patients with normal Na$^+$ intake and with normal cardiac and renal function. Occasionally, patients with severe systemic illnesses can be treated with Li$^+$, provided that the indications are sufficiently compelling. Treatment of acute mania and the prevention of recurrences of mania in otherwise-healthy adults or adolescents currently are the only uses approved by the United States Food and Drug Administration (FDA), even though the primary indication for Li$^+$ treatment is for long-term prevention of recurrences of major affective illness, particularly both mania and depression in bipolar I or II disorders (*see* Baldessarini *et al.*, 1996b; Goodwin and Jamison, 1990; Shulman *et al.*, 1996; Tondo *et al.*, 1998a). In addition, on the basis of compelling evidence of efficacy, Li$^+$ sometimes also is used as an alternative or adjunct to antidepressants in severe recurrent depression, as a supplement to antidepressant treatment in acute major depression, or as an adjunct when later response to an antidepressant alone is unsatisfactory (*see* Austin *et al.*, 1991; Bauer and Döpfmer, 1999).

These beneficial effects in major depression may be associated with the presence of clinical or biological features also found in bipolar affective disorder (*see* Goodwin and Jamison, 1990; Baldessarini *et al.*, 1996b). Growing clinical experience also suggests the utility of Li$^+$ in the management of childhood disorders that are marked by adultlike manic-depression or by severe changes in mood and behavior, which are probable precursors to better-known bipolar disorder in adults (*see* Baldessarini *et al.*, 1996b; Faedda *et al.*, 1995).

Most preparations currently used in the United States are tablets or capsules of lithium carbonate. Slow-release preparations of lithium carbonate also are available, as is a liquid preparation of lithium citrate (with 8 mEq of Li$^+$, equivalent to 300 mg of carbonate salt, per 5 ml or 1 teaspoonful of citrate liquid). Salts other than the carbonate have been used, but the carbonate salt is favored for tablets and capsules because it is relatively less hygroscopic and less irritating to the gut than other salts, especially the chloride salt.

Li$^+$ is not prescribed merely by dose; instead, because of its low therapeutic index, determination of the concentration of the ion in blood is crucial. Li$^+$ cannot be used with adequate safety in patients who cannot be tested regularly. Concentrations considered to be effective and acceptably safe are between 0.60 and 1.25 mEq per liter; the range of 0.9 to 1.1 mEq per liter is favored for treatment of acutely manic or hypomanic patients. Somewhat lower values (0.6 to 0.75 mEq per liter) are considered adequate and are safer for long-term use for prevention of recurrent manic-depressive illness; some patients may not relapse at concentrations as low as 0.5 to 0.6 mEq per liter,

and lower levels usually are better tolerated (Maj *et al.*, 1986; Tondo *et al.*, 1998a). These concentrations refer to serum or plasma samples obtained at 10 to 12 hours after the last oral dose of the day. The recommended concentration usually is attained by doses of 900 to 1500 mg of lithium carbonate per day in outpatients and 1200 to 2400 mg per day in hospitalized manic patients; the optimal dose tends to be larger in younger and heavier individuals. Serum concentrations of Li$^+$ have been found to follow a clear dose-effect relationship between 0.4 and 0.9 mEq per liter, with a corresponding dose-dependent rise in polyuria and tremor as indices of adverse effects, and little gain in benefit at levels above 0.75 mEq per liter (Maj *et al.*, 1986). This pattern indicates the need for individualization of serum levels to obtain a favorable risk/benefit relationship.

Li$^+$ has been evaluated in many additional disorders marked by an episodic course, including premenstrual dysphoria, episodic alcohol abuse, and episodic violence (*see* Baldessarini *et al.*, 1996b). Evidence of efficacy in most of these conditions has been unconvincing. The side effects of the Li$^+$ ion have been exploited in the management of hyperthyroidism and the syndrome of inappropriate ADH secretion, as well as in the reversal of spontaneous or drug-induced leukopenias, but usually with limited benefit.

DRUG TREATMENT OF MANIA

The modern treatment of the manic, depressive, and mixed-mood phases of bipolar disorder was revolutionized by the introduction of lithium in 1949, its gradual acceptance worldwide by the 1960s, and late official acceptance in the United States in 1970 for acute mania only and now primarily for prevention of recurrences of mania. Lithium is effective in acute mania but is now not often employed as a sole treatment due to its slow onset of action and potential difficulty in safe management in a highly agitated and uncooperative manic patient. Initially, an antipsychotic or potent sedative benzodiazepine (such as lorazepam or clonazepam) commonly is used to attain a degree of control of acute agitation (Licht, 1998; Tohen and Zarate, 1998). Alternatively, sodium valproate can bring about rapid antimanic effects (Pope *et al.*, 1991; Bowden *et al.*, 1994), particularly with doses as high as 30 mg/kg and later 20 mg/kg daily, with serum concentrations of 90 to 120 μg/ml (Grunze *et al.*, 1999; Hirschfeld *et al.*, 1999).

Li$^+$ then can be introduced more safely for longer-term mood stabilization, or the anticonvulsant may be continued alone. Li$^+$ or an alternative antimanic agent usually is continued for at least several months after full recovery from a manic episode due to a high risk of relapse or of cycling into depression within 12 months (*see* Goodwin and Jamison, 1990). The clinical decision to recommend more prolonged maintenance treatment is based on balancing the frequency and severity of past episodes of manic-depressive illness, the age and estimated reliability of the patient, and the risk of side effects (*see* Baldessarini *et al.,* 1996b; Zarin and Pass, 1987). Li$^+$ remains by far the most securely established long-term treatment to prevent recurrences of mania and bipolar depression (Baldessarini and Tondo, 2000; Davis *et al.,* 1999; Goodwin and Jamison, 1990). There also is compelling evidence of Li$^+$ lowering risk of suicide substantially (Tondo and Baldessarini, 2000). The potential clinical utility of Li$^+$ in conditions other than recurrences of mania or depression in bipolar I disorder was considered above. Applications include adjunctive use in patients who present clinically with major depression and have only mild mood elevations or hypomania (bipolar II disorder) and adjunctive use in severe, especially melancholic, apparently nonbipolar recurrent major depression.

Owing to the limited tolerability of Li$^+$ and its imperfect protection from recurrences of bipolar illness, antimanic anticonvulsants, particularly carbamazepine and valproic acid or its sodium salt, also are increasingly employed prophylactically in bipolar disorder on an empirical basis. However, their long-term research support remains limited and inconclusive (Calabrese *et al.,* 1992, 1995; Davis *et al.,* 1999; Bowden *et al.,* 2000; Davis *et al.,* 2000). There is even growing evidence for the inferiority of carbamazepine to lithium (Dardennes *et al.,* 1995; Davis *et al.,* 1999; Denicoff *et al.,* 1997; Greil *et al.,* 1997; Post *et al.,* 1998; Post, 2000). The relevant pharmacology and dosing guidelines for these agents in the treatment of epilepsy are provided in Chapter 21. Doses established for their anticonvulsant effects are assumed to be appropriate for the treatment of manic-depressive patients, although formal dose–response studies in psychiatric patients are lacking. Thus, dosing usually is adjusted to provide plasma concentrations of 6 to 12 μg/ml for carbamazepine and 60 to 120 μg/ml for valproic acid. It also is common to combine Li$^+$ with an anticonvulsant, particularly valproate, when patients fail to be fully protected from recurrences of bipolar illness by monotherapy (Freeman and Stoll, 1998).

Antipsychotic drugs commonly are employed empirically to manage psychotic features or failures of prophylaxis against mania in manic-depressive illness (Sernyak *et al.,* 1994), and they have short-term antimanic effects (Segal *et al.,* 1998; Tohen and Zarate, 1998; Tohen *et al.,* 1999). However, there is no credible scientific support for the long-term efficacy of these agents in mood disorders, and the risk of tardive dyskinesia in these syndromes may be even higher than in schizophrenia (Kane, 1999). The empirical use of antimanic-antipsychotic agents in bipolar disorder (particularly in mania and psychosis) is widespread, despite a lack of research demonstrating their

long-term benefits. However, the recent availability of atypical antipsychotic agents with a lower risk of tardive dyskinesia and other neurological side effects, clinical experience suggesting a mood-stabilizing action of clozapine, and evidence of antimanic actions of risperidone and olanzapine all suggest that better-tolerated and safer antipsychotic agents now in development should be considered for treatment of bipolar disorder (Tohen *et al.,* 1999; Keck and Licht, 2000). Other alternatives to lithium and the anticonvulsants have been less well evaluated.

Discontinuation of maintenance treatment with Li$^+$ carries a high risk of early recurrences and of suicidal behavior over a period of several months, even if the treatment has been successful for several years; recurrence is much more rapid than is predicted by the natural history of untreated bipolar disorder, in which cycle lengths average about one year (Baldessarini *et al.,* 1996b, 1999; Tondo *et al.,* 1998b). This risk probably can be moderated by slowing the gradual removal of Li$^+$ when that is medically feasible (Faedda *et al.,* 1993). Significant risk also is suspected after the rapid discontinuation or even sharp dosage reduction during maintenance treatment with other agents, including antipsychotic, antidepressant, and antianxiety drugs at least (*see* Baldessarini *et al.,* 1996b, 1999). This phenomenon affects the design and interpretation of many studies in experimental therapeutics in which an ongoing maintenance treatment is interrupted to compare higher *vs.* lower doses, an alternative agent, or a placebo.

PROSPECTUS

Novel Treatments for Psychotic Disorders

Acceptance of clozapine for general use stimulated renewed interest in discovering other antipsychotic agents with a low risk of extrapyramidal neurological side effects and high efficacy and without the several potentially serious adverse effects of clozapine discussed above (Baldessarini and Frankenburg, 1991). Several benzepine analogs have been introduced and approved by the FDA for clinical use, including olanzapine and quetiapine. These compounds do not induce seizures and lack the hematological toxicity of clozapine, although olanzapine has a higher incidence of motor side effects than does clozapine, as well as a high risk of weight gain and associated metabolic adverse effects. Other compounds currently in development include several substituted-benzamide analogs of sulpiride, the indole derivatives *sertindole* and *ziprasidone,* and the dibenzothiepine analog of clozapine, *zotepine* (Daniel *et al.,* 1999; Waddington and

Casey, 2000). Most of these agents have a complex neuropharmacology resembling that of clozapine, with interactions at several classes of cerebral neurotransmitter receptors.

A specific approach stimulated by clozapine is to test agents with antidopaminergic plus other actions, particularly antagonism of central 5-HT$_{2A}$-serotonin receptors. A lead compound of this type is the benzisoxazole *risperidone*, discussed above. Other compounds that have a risperidone-like binding profile and potential antipsychotic efficacy include ziprasidone (Daniel *et al.*, 1999), sertindole (recently removed from clinical trials due to cardiac depressant actions; *see* Waddington and Casey, 2000), *iloperidone* (Sainati *et al.*, 1995), and *ORG-5222* (Andree *et al.*, 1997).

Compounds selective for dopamine receptors other than the D$_2$ subtype have been considered, but so far have shown little evidence of antipsychotic activity. Substituted enantiomeric R(+)-benzazepines show high selectivity for D$_1$-dopamine receptors; these include the experimental compounds SKF-83566 and SCH-23390 (Kebabian *et al.*, 1997). A modified, longer-acting tetracyclic analog, *ecopipam* (SCH-39166), reached clinical trials as a potential atypical antipsychotic agent, but lacked evidence of efficacy (Karlsson *et al.*, 1995).

Discovery of several gene products that appear to represent new dopamine receptor subtypes also has encouraged a search for agents selective for them. Agents partially selective for the D$_3$-dopamine receptor include several hydroxyaminotetralins [particularly R(+)-7-hydroxy-*N,N*-dipropylaminotetralin, and the tricyclic analog *PD-128,907*], hexahydrobenzophenanthridines, *nafadotride* and *BP-897*, and others in development (Baldessarini *et al.*, 1993; Watts *et al.*, 1993; Sautel *et al.*, 1995; Kebabian *et al.*, 1997; Pilla *et al.*, 1999). The subtle and atypical functional activities of cerebral D$_3$ receptors suggest that D$_3$ agonists rather than antagonists may have useful psychotropic effects (Shafer and Levant, 1998; Pilla *et al.*, 1999).

D$_4$-dopamine receptors also are of interest because of their very low prevalence in the extrapyramidal basal ganglia and their moderate selectivity for clozapine (Van Tol *et al.*, 1991). Selective D$_4$ antagonists or mixed D$_4$/5HT$_2$ antagonists, so far, have proved ineffective in treating the psychotic symptoms of schizophrenia (Kramer *et al.*, 1997; Truffinet *et al.*, 1999). However, D$_4$-selective compounds may emerge as clinically innovative treatments for other neuropsychiatric disorders genetically associated with dopamine D$_4$ receptors, including attention deficit–hyperactivity disorder (Tarazi and Baldessarini, 1999).

In general, the rate of development of novel antipsychotic agents has again slowed following a burst of innovation that led to several new drugs currently in clinical use or advanced clinical trials. Novel principles are needed, particularly involving targets other than dopamine receptors, which have dominated antipsychotic drug development for a half-century.

Novel Treatments for Bipolar Disorder

The clinical success of valproate and carbamazepine as antimanic agents has strongly encouraged further exploration of other anticonvulsant agents, including older agents such as primidone and those that may act by enhancing the function of GABA as a key central inhibitory transmitter (Keck and McElroy, 1998; Manji *et al.*, 2000; Post *et al.*, 1998; Post, 2000). A growing number of such compounds are being introduced into neurological practice (*see* Chapter 21). Several also are in postmarketing evaluation for potential psychiatric applications, including *gabapentin, lamotrigine, oxcarbazepine, tiagabine,* and *topiramate* (*see* Ferrier and Calabrese, 2000; Post, 2000). For bipolar disorder, a critical challenge is to develop effective antidepressants that do not induce mania as well as mood-stabilizing agents that consistently outperform lithium and with greater safety (*see* Baldessarini *et al.*, 1996b; Stoll *et al.*, 1994). Lamotrigine has been found effective in bipolar depression with minimal risk of inducing mania (Calabrese *et al.*, 1999).

Because the sedative-anticonvulsant benzodiazepine clonazepam has useful short-term antimanic or sedative effects, it and lorazepam commonly are used adjunctively in the immediate control of manic excitement (Baldessarini *et al.*, 1996b). Whether or not the anticonvulsant properties of clonazepam actually are greater than those of other potent benzodiazepines and whether or not such agents have a potential for providing a long-term mood-stabilizing action remain uncertain (*see* Chapter 21; Bradwejn *et al.*, 1990).

Despite their theoretical plausibility, central anti-adrenergic drugs have not been considered seriously for the treatment of mania, perhaps due to expectations of excessive sedation or hypotension. In addition to agents acting on central adrenergic receptors, other antihypertensive agents—notably certain lipophilic, highly centrally active L-type Ca^{2+}-channel blockers including nimodipine and other dihydropyridines—deserve further exploration as mood-stabilizing agents (*see* Dubovsky, 1998; Pazzaglia *et al.*, 1998).

Given the several shared actions of lithium and valproate, it may be possible to develop novel antimanic agents that act directly on effector mechanisms that mediate the actions of adrenergic and other neurotransmitter receptors (Manji *et al.*, 1999b). These include drugs that affect protein kinase C, such as the antiestrogen *tamoxifen* (Bebchuk *et al.,* 2000) as well as other novel kinase-inhibiting agents that are under experimental development.

Finally, among natural products, long-chain, unsaturated, omega-3 fatty acids (including docosohexaenoic and linoleic acids) found in seed oils and particularly concentrated in fish flesh oils may have at least moderate mood-stabilizing effects and seem to be particularly helpful in bipolar depression. At least one controlled trial supports this approach (Stoll *et al.,* 1999).

For further discussion of psychiatric disorders, *see* Chapter 385 in *Harrison's Principles of Internal Medicine,* 14th ed., McGraw-Hill, New York, 1998.

BIBLIOGRAPHY

Addonizio, G., Susman, V.L., and Roth, S.D. Neuroleptic malignant syndrome: review and analysis of 115 cases. *Biol. Psychiatry,* **1987,** *22*:1004–1020.

Adler, L.A., Rotrosen, J., Edson, R., Lavori, P., Lohr, J., Hitzemann, R., Raisch, D., Caligiuri, M., and Tracy, K. Vitamin E treatment for tardive dyskinesia. *Arch. Gen. Psychiatry,* **1999,** 56:836–841.

Allison, D.B., Mentore, J.L., Heo, M., Chandler, L.P., Cappelleri, J.C., Infante, M.C., and Weiden, P.J. Antipsychotic-induced weight gain: a comprehensive research synthesis. *Am. J. Psychiatry,* **1999,** *156*:1686–1696.

Alvir, J.M., Lieberman, J.A., Safferman, A.Z., Schwimmer, J.L., and Schaaf, J.A. Clozapine-induced agranulocytosis. Incidence and risk factors in the United States. *N. Engl. J. Med.,* **1993,** *329*:162–167.

Andree, B., Halldin, C., Vrijmoed-de Vries, M., and Farde, L. Central 5-HT$_{2A}$ and D$_2$ dopamine receptor occupancy after sublingual administration of ORG-5222 in healthy men. *Psychopharmacology (Berl.),* **1997,** *131*:339–345.

Arana, G.W., Goff, D.C., Baldessarini, R.J., and Keepers, G.A. Efficacy for anticholinergic prophylaxis of neuroleptic-induced acute dystonia. *Am. J. Psychiatry,* **1988,** *145*:993–996.

Arnt, J., and Skarsfeldt, T. Do novel antipsychotics have similar pharmacological characteristics? A review of the evidence. *Neuropsychopharmacology,* **1998,** *18*:63–101.

Arvanitis, L.A., and Miller, B.G. Multiple fixed doses of "Seroquel" (quetiapine) in patients with acute exacerbation of schizophrenia: a comparison with haloperidol and placebo. The Seroquel Trial 13 Study Group. *Biol. Psychiatry,* **1997,** *42*:233–246.

Austin, M.-P., Souza, F.G., and Goodwin, G.M. Lithium augmentation in andepressant-resistant patients. A quantitative analysis. *Br. J. Psychiatry,* **1991,** *159*:510–514.

Baldessarini, R.J., Cohen, B.M., and Teicher, M.H. Significance of neuroleptic dose and plasma level in the pharmacological treatment of psychoses. *Arch. Gen. Psychiatry,* **1988,** *45*:79–91.

Baldessarini, R.J., Huston-Lyons, D., Campbell, A., Marsh, E., and Cohen, B.M. Do central antiadrenergic actions contribute to the atypical properties of clozapine? *Br. J. Psychiatry Suppl.,* **1992,** 12–16.

Baldessarini, R.J., Kula, N.S., McGrath, C.R., Bakthavachalam, V., Kebabian, J.W., and Neumeyer, J.L. Isomeric selectivity at dopamine D$_3$ receptors. *Eur. J. Pharmacol.,* **1993,** *239*:269–270.

Baldessarini, R.J., Suppes, T., and Tondo, L. Lithium withdrawal in bipolar disorder: implications for clinical practice and experimental therapeutics research. *Am. J. Therapeutics,* **1996a,** *3*:492–496.

Baldessarini, R.J., Tarazi, F.I., Kula, N.S., and Gardner, D.M. Clozapine withdrawal: serotonergic or dopaminergic mechanisms? *Arch. Gen. Psychiatry,* **1997,** *45*:761–762.

Baldessarini, R.J., and Tondo, L. Does lithium treatment still work? Evidence of stable responses over three decades. *Arch. Gen. Psychiatry,* **2000,** *57*:187–190.

Baldessarini, R.J., Tondo, L., and Viguera, A.C. Effects of discontinuing lithium maintenance treatment. *Bipolar Disorders,* **1999,** *1*:17–24.

Baldessarini, R.J., and Vogt, M. Release of [^{3}H]dopamine and analogous monoamines from rat striatal tissue. *Cell. Mol. Neurobiol.,* **1988,** 8:205–216.

Batlle, D.C., von Riotte, A.B., Gaviria, M., and Grupp, M. Amelioration of polyuria by amiloride in patients receiving long-term lithium therapy. *N. Engl. J. Med.,* **1985,** *312*:408–414.

Bauer, M., and Döpfmer, S. Lithium augmentation in treatment-resistant depression: meta-analysis of placebo-controlled studies. *J. Clin. Psychopharmacol.,* **1999,** *19*:427–434.

Bauer, M.E., and Whybrow, P.C. Rapid cycling bipolar affective disorder. II. Treatment of refractory rapid cycling with high-dose levothyroxine: a preliminary study. *Arch. Gen. Psychiatry,* **1990,** *47*:435–440.

Baumgartner, A., Bauer, M., and Hellweg, R. Treatment of intractable non–rapid cycling bipolar affective disorder with high-dose thyroxine: an open clinical trial. *Neuropsychopharmacology,* **1994,** *10*:183–189.

Bebchuk, J.M., Arfken, C.L., Dolan-Manji, S., Murphy, J., Hasant, K., and Manji, H.K. A preliminary investigation of a protein kinase C inhibitor in the treatment of acute mania. *Arch. Gen. Psychiatry,* **2000,** *57*:95–97.

Berridge, M.J., Downes, C.P., and Hanley, M.R. Neural and developmental actions of lithium: a unifying hypothesis. *Cell,* **1989,** *59*:411–419.

Bitton, R., and Schneider, B. Endocrine, metabolic, and nutritional effects of psychotropic drugs. In, *Adverse Effects of Psychotropic Drugs.* (Kane, J.M., and Leiberman, J.A., eds.) Guilford Press, New York, **1992,** pp. 341–355.

Blin, O. A comparative review of new antipsychotics. *Can. J. Psychiatry,* **1999,** *44*:235–244.

Bloom, F.E., Baetge, G., Deyo, S., Ettenberg, A., Koda, L., Magistretti, P.J., Shoemaker, W.J., and Staunton, D.A. Chemical and physiological aspects of the actions of lithium and antidepressant drugs. *Neuropharmacology,* **1983,** *22*(3 Spec. No.):359–365.

Boton, R., Gaviria, M., and Batlle, D.C. Prevalence, pathogenesis, and treatment of renal dysfunction associated with chronic lithium therapy. *Am. J. Kidney Dis.,* **1987,** *10*:329–345.

Bowden, C.L., Brugger, A.M., Swann, A.C., Calabrese, J.R., Janicak, P.G., Petty, F., Dilsaver, S.C., Davis, J.M., Rush, A.J., Small, J.G., Garza-Treviño, E.S., Risch, C., Goodnick, P.J., and Morris, D.D.

Efficacy of divalproex vs. lithium and placebo in the treatment of mania. The Depakote Mania Study Group. *JAMA, 1994, 271*:918–924.

Bowden, C.L., Calebrese, J.R., McElroy, S.L., Gyulai, L., Wassef, A., Petty, F., Pope, H.G. Jr., Chou, J.C., Keck, P.E. Jr., Rhodes, L.J., Swann, A.C., Hirshfeld, R.M., and Wozniak, P.J. A randomized, placebo-controlled 12-month trial of divalproex and lithium in the treatment of outpatients with bipolar I disorder. Divalproex Bipolar Study Group. *Arch. Gen. Psychiatry, 2000, 57*:481–489.

Bradwejn, J., Shriqui, C., Koszycki, D., and Meterissian, G. Double-blind comparison of the effects of clonazepam and lorazepam in acute mania. *J. Clin. Psychopharmacol., 1990, 10*:403–408.

Brotman, A.W., Falk, W.E., and Gelenberg, A.J. Pharmacologic treatment of acute depressive subtypes. In, *Psychopharmacology: The Third Generation of Progress.* (Meltzer, H.Y., ed.) Raven Press, New York, 1987, pp. 1031–1040.

Bunney, B.S., Sesack, S.R., and Silva, N.L. Midbrain dopaminergic systems: neurophysiology and electrophysiological pharmacology. In, *Psychopharmacology: The Third Generation of Progress.* (Meltzer, H.Y., ed.) Raven Press, New York, 1987, pp. 113–126.

Cade, J.F.J. Lithium salts in the treatment of psychotic excitement. *Med. J. Aust., 1949, 2*:349–352.

Calabrese, J.R., Bowden, C.L., Sachs, G.S., Ascher, J.A., Monaghan, E., and Rudd, G.D. A double-blind placebo-controlled study of lamotrigine monotherapy in outpatients with bipolar I depression. Lamictal 602 Study Group. *J. Clin. Psychiatry, 1999, 60*:79–88.

Calabrese, J.R., Markovitz, P.J., Kimmel, S.E., and Wagner, S.C. Spectrum of efficacy of valproate in 78 rapid-cycling bipolar patients. *J. Clin. Psychopharmacol., 1992, 12*:53S–56S.

Campbell, A., Yeghiayan, S., Baldessarini, R.J., and Neumeyer, J.L. Selective antidopaminergic effects of S(+)N-*n*-propylnoraporphines in limbic versus extrapyramidal sites in rat brain: comparisons with typical and atypical antipsychotic agents. *Psychopharmacology, 1991, 103*:323–329.

Castagnoli, N. Jr., Castagnoli, K.P., Van der Schyf, C.J., Usuki, E., Igarashi, K., Steyn, S.J., and Riker, R.R. Enzyme-catalyzed bioactivation of cyclic tertiary amines to form potential neurotoxins. *Pol. J. Pharmacol., 1999, 51*:31–38.

Centorrino, F., Tuttle, M., Bahk, W.-M., Albert, M., Price, B., and Baldessarini, R.J. Effects of typical and atypical antipsychotic drug treatment on the electroencephalogram. *Biol. Psychiatry, 2001,* submitted.

Chan, C.H., Janicak, P.G., Davis, J.M., Altman, E., Andriukaitis, S., and Hedeker, D. Response of psychotic and nonpsychotic depressed patients to tricyclic antidepressants. *J. Clin. Psychiatry, 1987, 48*:197–200.

Chen, G., Yuan, P.X., Jiang, Y.M., Huang, L.D., and Manji, H.K. Lithium increases tyrosine hydroxylase levels both *in vivo* and *in vitro. J. Neurochem., 1998, 70*:1768–1771.

Chen, G., Yuan, P.X., Jiang, Y.M., Huang, L.D., and Manji, H.K. Valproate robustly enhances AP-1 mediated gene expression. *Brain Res. Mol. Brain Res., 1999a, 64*:52–58.

Chen, G., Huang, L.D., Jiang, Y.M., and Manji, H.K. The mood-stabilizing agent valproate inhibits the activity of glycogen synthase kinase-3. *J. Neurochem., 1999b, 72*:1327–1330.

Chen, G., Zeng, W.Z., Yuan, P.X., Huang, L.D., Jiang, Y.M., Zhao, Z.H., and Manji, H.K. The mood-stabilizing agents lithium and valproate robustly increase the levels of the neuroprotective protein bcl-2 in the CNS. *J. Neurochem., 1999c, 72*:879–882.

Chouinard, G., Jones, B., Remington, G., Bloom, D., Addington, D., MacEwan, G.W., Labelle, A., Beauclair, L., and Arnott, W. A Canadian multicenter placebo-controlled study of fixed doses of risperidone and haloperidol in the treatment of chronic schizophrenic patients. *J. Clin. Psychopharmacol., 1993, 13*:25–40.

Cohen, L.S., Friedman, J.M., Jefferson, J.W., Johnson, E.M., and Weiner, M.L. A reevaluation of risk of *in utero* exposure to lithium. *JAMA, 1994, 271*:146–150.

Cohen, B.M., Tsuneizumi, T., Baldessarini, R.J., Campbell, A., and Babb, S.M. Differences between antipsychotic drugs in persistence of brain levels and behavioral effects. *Psychopharmacology (Berl.), 1992, 108*:338–344.

Daly, S.A., and Waddington, J.L. Two directions of dopamine D1/D2 receptor interaction in studies of behavioural regulation: a finding generic to four new, selective dopamine D1 receptor antagonists. *Eur. J. Pharmacol., 1992, 213*:251–258.

Daniel, D.G., Zimbroff, D.L., Potkin, S.G., Reeves, K.R., Harrigan, E.P., and Lakshminarayanan, M. Ziprasidone 80 mg/day and 160 mg/day in the acute exacerbation of schizophrenia and schizoaffective disorder: a 6-week placebo-controlled trial. Ziprasidone Study Group. *Neuropsychopharmacology, 1999, 20*:491–505.

Dardennes, R., Even, C., Bange, F., and Heim, A. Comparison of carbamazepine and lithium in the prophylaxis of bipolar disorders. A meta-analysis. *Br. J. Psychiatry, 1995, 166*:378–381.

Davis, J.M., Janicak, P.G., and Hogan, D.M. Mood stabilizers in the prevention of recurrent affective disorders: a meta-analysis. *Acta Psychiatr. Scand., 1999, 100*:406–417.

Delay, J., and Deniker, P. Trente-huit cas de psychoses traitées par la cure prolongée et continue de 4560 RP. Le Congrès des Al. et Neurol. de Langue Fr. In, *Compte rendu du Congrès.* Masson et Cie, Paris, 1952.

Denicoff, K.D., Smith-Jackson, E.E., Bryan, A.L., Ali, S.O., and Post, R.M. Valproate prophylaxis in a prospective clinical trial of refractory bipolar disorder. *Am. J. Psychiatry, 1997, 154*:1456–1458.

Denicoff, K.D., Smith-Jackson, E.E., Disney, E.R., Ali, S.O., Leverich, G.S., and Post, R.M. Comparative prophylactic efficacy of lithium, carbamazepine, and the combination in bipolar disorder. *J. Clin. Psychiatry, 1997, 58*:470–478.

Dickson, R.A., and Glazer, W.M. Neuroleptic-induced hyperprolactinemia. *Schizophr. Res., 1999, 35*(Suppl.):S75–S86.

Eastham, J.H., and Jeste, D.V. Treatment of schizophrenia and delusional disorder in the elderly. *Eur. Arch. Psychiatry Clin. Neurosci., 1997, 247*:209–218.

Ereshefsky, L. Pharmaocokinetics and drug interactions: update for new antipsychotics. *J. Clin. Psychiatry, 1996, 57*(Suppl. 11):12–25.

Erle, G., Basso, M., Federspil, G., Sicolo, N., and Scandellari, C. Effect of chlorpromazine on blood glucose and plasma insulin in man. *Eur. J. Clin. Pharmacol., 1977, 11*:15–18.

Eyles, D.W., Avent, K.M., Stedman, T.J., and Pond, S.M. Two pyridinium metabolites of haloperidol are present in the brain of patients at post-mortem. *Life Sci., 1997, 60*:529–534.

Faedda, G.L., Baldessarini, R.J., Suppes, T., Tondo, L., Becker, I., and Lipschitz, D.S. Pediatric-onset bipolar disorder: a neglected clinical and public health problem. *Harv. Rev. Psychiatry, 1995, 3*:171–195.

Faedda, G.L., Tondo, L., Baldessarini, R.J., Suppes, T., and Tohen, M. Outcome after rapid vs. gradual discontinuation of lithium treatment in bipolar disorders. *Arch. Gen. Psychiatry, 1993, 50*:448–455.

Farde, L., Nyberg, S., Oxenstierna, G., Nakashima, Y., Halldin, C., and Ericsson, B. Positron emission tomography studies on D_2 and $5HT_2$ receptor binding in risperidone-treated schizophrenic patients. *J. Clin. Psychopharmacol., 1995, 15*:19S–23S.

Freeman, M.P., and Stoll, A.L. Mood stabilizer combinations: a review of safety and efficacy. *Am. J. Psychiatry, 1998, 155*:12–21.

Gardos, G., Casey, D.E., Cole, J.O., Perenyi, A., Kocsis, E., Arato, M., Samson, J.A., and Conley, C. Ten-year outcome of tardive dyskinesia. *Am. J. Psychiatry,* **1994,** *151:*836–841.

Gaulin, B.D., Markowitz, J.S., Caley, C.F., Nesbitt, L.A., and Dufresne, R.L. Clozapine-associated elevation of serum triglycerides. *Am. J. Psychiatry,* **1999,** *156:*1270–1272.

Gefvert, O., Bergstrom, M., Langstrom, B., Lundberg, T., Lindstrom, L., and Yates, R. Time course of central nervous dopamine-D_2 and 5-HT_2 receptor blockade and plasma drug concentrations after discontinuation of quetiapine seroquel in patients with schizophrenia. *Psychopharmacology (Berl.),* **1998,** *135:*119–126.

Gilbert, P.L., Harris, M.J., McAdams, L.A., and Jeste, D.V. Neuroleptic withdrawal in schizophrenic patients. A review of the literature. *Arch. Gen. Psychiatry,* **1995,** *52:*173–188.

Goff, D.C., and Baldessarini, R.J. Drug interactions with antipsychotic agents. *J. Clin. Psychopharmacol.,* **1993,** *13:*57–67.

Grant, S., and Fitton, A. Risperidone. A review of its pharmacology and therapeutic potential in the treatment of schizophrenia. *Drugs,* **1994,** *48:*253–273.

Greil, W., Ludwig-Mayerhofer, W., Erazo, N., Schöchlin, C., Schmidt, S., Engel, R.R., Czernik, A., Giedke, H., Müller-Oerlinghausen, B., Osterheider, M., Rudolf, G.A., Sauer, H., Tegeler, J., and Wetterling, T. Lithium versus carbamazepine in the maintenance treatment of bipolar disorders—a randomised study. *J. Affect. Disord.,* **1997,** *43:*151–161.

Grunze, H., Erfurth, A., Amann, B., Giupponi, G., Kammerer, C., and Walden, J. Intravenous valproate loading in acutely manic and depressed bipolar I patients. *J. Clin. Psychopharmacol.,* **1999,** *19:*303–309.

Herz, M.I., Glazer, W.M., Mostert, M.A., Sheard, M.A., Szymanski, H.V., Hafez, H., Mirza, M., and Vana, J. Intermittent vs. maintenance medication in schizophrenia. Two-year results. *Arch. Gen. Psychiatry,* **1991,** *48:*333–339.

Hetmar, O., Povlsen, U.J., Ladefoged, J., and Bolwig, T.G. Lithium: long-term effects on the kidney. A prospective follow-up study ten years after kidney biopsy. *Br. J. Psychiatry,* **1991,** *158:*53–58.

Hirschfeld, R.M., Allen, M.H., McEvoy, J.P., Keck, P.E. Jr., and Russell, J.M. Safety and tolerability of oral loading divalproex sodium in acutely manic bipolar patients. *J. Clin. Psychiatry,* **1999,** *60:*815–818.

Ichikawa, J., and Meltzer, H.Y. Relationship between dopaminergic and serotonergic neuronal activity in the frontal cortex and the action of typical and atypical antipsychotic drugs. *Eur. Arch. Psychiatry Clin. Neurosci.,* **1999,** *249*(Suppl. 4):90–98.

Jefferson, J.W., Greist, J.H., Clagnaz, P.J., Eischens, R.R., Marten, W.C., and Evenson, M.A. Effect of strenuous exercise on serum lithium level in man. *Am. J. Psychiatry,* **1982,** *139:*1593–1595.

Jeste, D.V., Lacro, J.P., Bailey, A., Rockwell, E., Harris, M.J., and Caligiuri, M.P. Lower incidence of tardive dyskinesia with risperidone compared with haloperidol in older patients. *J. Am. Geriatr. Soc.,* **1999a,** *47:*716–719.

Jeste, D.V., Rockwell, E., Harris, M.J., Lohr, J.B., and Lacro, J. Conventional vs. newer antipsychotics in elderly patients. *Am. J. Geriatr. Psychiatry,* **1999b,** *7:*70–76.

Jope, R.S. A bimodal model of the mechanism of action of lithium. *Mol. Psychiatry,* **1999,** *4:*21–25.

Jus, K., Jus, A., Gautier, J., Villeneuve, A., Pires, P., Pineau, R., and Villeneuve, R. Studies on the action of certain pharmacological agents on tardive dyskinesia and on the rabbit syndrome. *Int. J. Clin. Pharmacol.,* **1974,** *9:*138–145.

Kane, J.M. Tardive dyskinesia in affective disorders. *J. Clin. Psychiatry,* **1999,** *60*(Suppl. 5):43–47.

Kane, J.M., Rifkin, A., Woerner, M., Reardon, G., Sarantakos, S., Schiebel, D., and Ramos-Lorenzi, J. Low-dose neuroleptic treatment of outpatient schizophrenics. I. Preliminary results for relapse rates. *Arch. Gen. Psychiatry,* **1983,** *40:*893–896.

Kapur, S., Zipursky, R.B., and Remington, G. Clinical and theoretical implications of 5-HT_2 and D_2 receptor occupancy of clozapine, risperidone, and olanzapine in schizophrenia. *Am. J. Psychiatry,* **1999,** *156:*286–293.

Karlsson, P., Smith, L., Farde, L., Harnryd, C., Sedvall, G., and Wiesel, F.A. Lack of apparent antipsychotic effect of the D_1-dopamine receptor antagonist SCH-39166 in acutely ill schizophrenic patients. *Psychopharmacology (Berl.),* **1995,** *121:*309–316.

Killian, J.G., Kerr, K., Lawrence, C., and Celermajer, D.S. Myocarditis and cardiomyopathy associated with clozapine. *Lancet,* **1999,** *354:*1841–1845.

Korpi, E.R., Phelps, B.H., Granger, H., Chang, W.-H., Linnoila, M., Meek, J.L., and Wyatt, R.J. Simultaneous determination of haloperidol and its reduced metabolite in serum and plasma by isocratic liquid chromatography with electrochemical detection. *Clin. Chem.,* **1983,** *29:*624–628.

Kosten, T.R., and Forrest, J.N. Treatment of severe lithium-induced polyuria with amiloride. *Am. J. Psychiatry,* **1986,** *143:*1563–1568.

Kramer, M.S., Last, B., Getson, A., and Reines, S.A. The effects of a selective D_4 dopamine receptor antagonist (L-745,870) in acutely psychotic inpatients with schizophrenia. D_4 Dopamine Antagonist Group. *Arch. Gen. Psychiatry,* **1997,** *54:*567–572.

Laborit, H., Huguenard, P., and Alluaume, R. Un nouveau stabilisateur végétatif (LE 4560 RP). *Presse Méd.,* **1952,** *60:*206–208.

Lahti, A.C., Weiler, M., Carlsson, A., and Tamminga, C.A. Effects of the D_3 and autoreceptor-preferring dopamine antagonist (+)-UH232 in schizophrenia. *J. Neural Transm.,* **1998,** *105:*719–734.

Lasser, R.A., and Baldessarini, R.J. Thyroid hormones in depressive disorders: a reappraisal of clinical utility. *Harv. Rev. Psychiatry,* **1997,** *4:*291–305.

Leysen, J.E., Janssen, P.M., Megens, A.A., and Schotte, A. Risperidone: a novel antipsychotic with balanced serotonin-dopamine antagonism, receptor occupancy profile, and pharmacologic activity. *J. Clin. Psychiatry,* **1994,** *55*(Suppl.):5–12.

Licht, R.W. Drug treatment of mania: a critical review. *Acta Psychiatr. Scand.,* **1998,** *97:*387–397.

Lipinski, J.F. Jr., Zubenko, G.S., Cohen, B.M., and Barreira, P.J. Propranolol in the treatment of neuroleptic-induced akathisia. *Am. J. Psychiatry,* **1984,** *141:*412–415.

Maj, M., Starace, F., Nolfe, G., and Kemali, D. Minimum plasma lithium levels required for effective prophylaxis in DSM III bipolar disorder: a prospective study. *Pharmacopsychiatry,* **1986,** *19:*420–423.

Manji, H.K., Etcheberrigaray, G., Chen, R., and Olds, J.L. Lithium decreases membrane-associated protein kinase C in hippocampus: selectivity for the alpha isozyme. *J. Neurochem.,* **1993,** *61:*2303–2310.

Markowitz, J.S., Brown, C.S., and Moore, T.R. Atypical antipsychotics. Part I: Pharmacology, pharmacokinetics, and efficacy. *Ann. Pharmacother.,* **1999,** *33:*73–85.

Meltzer, H.Y., and Nash, J.F. Effects of antipsychotic drugs on serotonin receptors. *Pharmacol. Rev.,* **1991,** *43:*587–604.

Menza, M.M., Palermo, B., and Mark, M. Quetiapine as an alternative to clozapine in the treatment of dopamimetic psychosis in patients with Parkinson's disease. *Ann. Clin. Psychiatry,* **1999,** *11:*141–144.

Moller, H.J. Atypical neuroleptics: a new approach in the treatment of negative symptoms. *Eur. Arch. Psychiatry Clin. Neurosci.,* **1999,** *249*(Suppl. 4):99–107.

Moore, K.E. Hypothalamic dopaminergic neuronal systems. In, *Psychopharmacology: The Third Generation of Progress.* (Meltzer, H.Y., ed.) Raven Press, New York, **1987,** pp. 127–139.

Morgenstern, H., and Glazer, W.M. Identifying risk factors for tardive dyskinesia among long-term outpatients maintained with neuroleptic medications. Results of the Yale Tardive Dyskinesia Study. *Arch. Gen. Psychiatry,* **1993,** *50:*723–733.

Mortensen, P.B. The occurrence of cancer in first admitted schizophrenic patients. *Schizophr. Res.,* **1994,** *12:*185–194.

Neil, J.F., Himmelhoch, J.M., and Licata, S.M. Emergence of myasthenia gravis during treatment with lithium carbonate. *Arch. Gen. Psychiatry,* **1976,** *33:*1090–1092.

Nordstrom, A.-L., Farde, L., Nyberg, S., Karlsson, P., Halldin, C., and Sedvall, G. D_1, D_2, and $5\text{-}HT_2$ receptor occupancy in relation to clozapine serum concentration: a PET study of schizophrenic patients. *Am. J. Psychiatry,* **1995,** *152:*1444–1449.

Nordstrom, A.-L., Nyberg, S., Olsson, H., and Farde, L. Positron emission tomography finding of a high striatal D_2 receptor occupancy in olanzapine-treated patients. *Arch. Gen. Psychiatry,* **1998,** *55:*283–284.

Parkinson Study Group. Low-dose clozapine for the treatment of drug-induced psychosis in Parkinson's disease. *N. Engl. J. Med.,* **1999,** *340:*757–763.

Pazzaglia, P.J., Post, R.M., Ketter, T.A., Callahan, A.M., Marangell, L.B., Frye, M.A., George, M.S., Kimbrell, T.A., Leverich, G.S., Cora-Locatelli, G., and Luckenbaugh, D. Nimodipine monotherapy and carbamazepine augmentation in patients with refractory recurrent affective illness. *J. Clin. Psychopharmacol.,* **1998,** *18:*404–413.

Pearlman, C.A. Neuroleptic malignant syndrome: a review of the literature. *J. Clin. Psychopharmacology,* **1986,** *6:*257–273.

Pilla, M., Perachon, S., Sautel, F., Garrido, F., Mann, A., Wermuth, C.G., Schwartz, J-C., Everitt, B.J., and Sokoloff, P. Selective inhibition of cocaine-seeking behaviour by a partial D_3 receptor agonist. *Nature,* **1999,** *400:*371–375.

Plenge, P., Stensgaard, A., Jensen, H.V., Thomsen, C., Mellerup, E.T., and Henricksen, O. 24-hour lithium concentration in human brain studied by ^7Li magnetic resonance spectroscopy. *Biol. Psychiatry,* **1994,** *36:*511–516.

Pope, H.G. Jr., McElroy, S.L., Keck, P.E. Jr., and Hudson, J.I. Valproate in the treatment of acute mania. A placebo-controlled study. *Arch. Gen. Psychiatry,* **1991,** *48:*62–68.

Post, R.M., Denicoff, K.D., Frye, M.A., Dunn, R.T., Leverich, G.S., Osuch, E., and Speer, A. A history of the use of anticonvulsants as mood stabilizers in the last two decades of the 20th century. *Neuropsychobiology,* **1998,** *38:*152–166.

Rabinowitz, T., Frankenburg, F.R., Centorrino, F., and Kando, J. The effect of clozapine on saliva flow rate: a pilot study. *Biol. Psychiatry,* **1996,** *40:*1132–1134.

Ray, W.A., Griffin, M.R., Schaffner, W., Baugh, D.K., and Milton, L.J. III. Psychotropic drug use and the risk of hip fracture. *N. Engl. J. Med.,* **1987,** *316:*363–369.

Richelson, E. Receptor pharmacology of neuroleptics: relation to clinical effects. *J. Clin. Psychiatry,* **1999,** *60*(Suppl. 10):5–14.

Riedl, U., Barocka, A., Kolem, H., Demling, J., Kaschka, W.P., Schelp, R., Stemmler, M., and Ebert, D. Duration of lithium treatment and brain lithium concentration in patients with unipolar and schizoaffective disorder—a study with magnetic resonance spectroscopy. *Biol. Psychiatry,* **1997,** *41:*844–850.

Roth, B.L., Tandra, S., Burgess, L.H., Sibley, D.R., and Meltzer, H.Y. D_4 dopamine receptor affinity does not distinguish between typical and atypical antipsychotic drugs. *Psychopharmacology (Berl.),* **1995,** *120:*365–368.

Rotrosen, J., Angrist, B.M., Gershon, S., Aronson, M., Gruen, P., Sachar, E.J., Denning, R.K., Matthysse, S., Stanley, M., and Wilk, S. Thiethylperazine: clinical antipsychotic efficacy and correlation with potency in predictive systems. *Arch. Gen. Psychiatry,* **1978,** *35:*1112–1118.

Sainati, S.M., Hubbard, J.W., Chi, E., Grasing, K., and Brecher, M.B. Safety, tolerability, and effect of food on the pharmacokinetics of iloperidone (HP 873), a potential atypical antipsychotic. *J. Clin. Pharmacol.,* **1995,** *35:*713–720.

Sampath, G., Shah, A., Krska, J., and Soni, S.D. Neuroleptic discontinuation in the very stable schizophrenic patient: relapse rates and serum neuroleptic levels. *Hum. Psychopharmacol.,* **1992,** *7:*255–264.

Sautel, F., Griffon, N., Sokoloff, P., Schwartz, J-C., Launay, C., Simon, P., Costentin, J., Schoenfelder, A., Garrido, F., Mann, A., and Wermuth, C.G. Nafadotide, a potent preferential dopamine D_3 receptor antagonist, activates locomotion in rodents. *J. Pharmacol. Exp. Ther.,* **1995,** *275:*1239–1246.

Schotte, A., Janssen, P.F., Gommeren, W., Luyten, W.H., Van Gompel, P., Lesage, A.S., De Loore, K., and Leysen, J.E. Risperidone compared with new and reference antipsychotic drugs: *in vitro* and *in vivo* receptor binding. *Psychopharmacology (Berl.),* **1996,** *124:*57–73.

Sedvall, G. The current status of PET scanning with respect to schizophrenia. *Neuropsychopharmacology,* **1992,** *7:*41–54.

Seeger, T.F., Seymour, P.A., Schmidt, A.W., Zorn, S.H., Schulz, D.W., Lebel, L.A., McLean, S., Guanowsky, V., Howard, H.R., Lowe, J.A. III, and Heym, J. Ziprasidone (CP-88,059): a new antipsychotic with combined dopamine and serotonin receptor antagonists activity. *J. Pharmacol. Exp. Ther.,* **1995,** *275:*101–113.

Segal, J., Berk, M., and Brook, S. Risperidone compared with both lithium and haloperidol in mania: a double-blind ranomized controlled trial. *Clin. Neuropharmacol.,* **1998,** *21:*176–180.

Sernyak, M.J., Griffin, R.A., Johnson, R.M., Pearsall, H.R., Wexler, B.E., and Woods, S.W. Neuroleptic exposure following inpatient treatment of acute mania with lithium and neuroleptic. *Am. J. Psychiatry,* **1994,** *151:*133–135.

Shafer, R.A., and Levant, B. The D_3 dopamine receptor in cellular and organismal function. *Psychopharmacology (Berl.),* **1998,** *135:*1–16.

Siegel, A.J., Baldessarini, R.J., Klepser, M.B., and McDonald, J.C. Primary and drug-induced disorders of water homeostasis in psychiatric patients: principles of diagnosis and management. *Harv. Rev. Psychiatry,* **1998,** *6:*190–200.

Simpson, G.M., Cooper, T.B., Bark, N., Sud, I., and Lee, J.H. Effect of antiparkinsonian medication on plasma levels of chlorpromazine. *Arch. Gen. Psychiatry,* **1980,** *37:*205–208.

Smith, J.M., and Baldessarini, R.J. Changes in prevalence, severity, and recovery in tardive dyskinesia with age. *Arch. Gen. Psychiatry,* **1980,** *37:*1368–1373.

Snyder, S.H., and Yamamura, H.I. Antidepressants and the muscarinic acetylcholine receptor. *Arch. Gen. Psychiatry,* **1977,** *34:*236–239.

Soares, K.V., and McGrath, J.J. The treatment of tardive dyskinesia—a systematic review and meta-analysis. *Schizophr. Res.,* **1999,** *39:*1–16.

Sokoloff, P., Giros, B., Martres, M.P., Bouthenet, M.L., and Schwartz, J.C. Molecular cloning and characterization of a novel dopamine receptor (D_3) as a target for neuroleptics. *Nature,* **1990,** *347:*146–151.

Spencer, T., Biederman, J., Wilens, T., Steingard, R., and Geist, D. Nortriptyline treatment of children with attention-deficit hyperactivity disorder and tic disorder or Tourette's syndrome. *J. Am. Acad. Child Adolesc. Psychiatry,* **1993,** *32:*205–210.

Stoll, A.L., Severus, W.E., Freeman, M.P., Reuter, S., Zboyan, H.A., Diamond, E., Cress, K.K., and Marangell, L.B. Omega 3 fatty acids in bipolar disorder: a preliminary double-blind, placebo-controlled trial. *Arch. Gen. Psychiatry,* **1999,** *56:*407–412.

Stoll, A.L., Mayer, P.V., Kolbrener, M., Goldstein, E., Suplit, B., Lucier, J., Cohen, B.M., and Tohen, M. Antidepressant-associated mania: a controlled comparison with spontaneous mania. *Am. J. Psychiatry,* **1994,** *151:*1642–1645.

Sulser, F., and Robinson, S.E. Clinical implications of pharmacological differences among antipsychotic drugs (with particular emphasis on biochemical central synaptic adrenergic mechanisms). In, *Psychopharmacology: A Generation of Progress.* (Lipton, M.A., DiMascio, A., and Killam, K.F., eds.,) Raven Press, New York, **1978,** pp. 943–954.

Tarazi, F.I., Yeghiayan, S.K., Baldessarini, R.J., Kula, N.S., and Neumeyer, J.L. Long-term effects of S(+)N-*n*-propylnorapomorphine compared with typical and atypical antipsychotics: differential increases of cerebrocortical D_2-like and striatolimbic D_4-like dopamine receptors. *Neuropsychopharmacology,* **1997,** *17:*186–196.

Tesar, G.E., Murray, G.B., and Cassem, N.H. Use of high-dose intravenous haloperidol in the treatment of agitated cardiac patients. *J. Clin. Psychopharmacol.,* **1985,** *5:*344–347.

Theret, L., Germain, M.L., and Burde, A. Current aspects of the use of clozapine in the Chalons-sur-Marne Psychiatric Hospital: intestinal occlusion with clozapine. *Ann. Med. Psychol. (Paris),* **1995,** *153:*474–477.

Tohen, M., Sanger, T.M., McElroy, S.L., Tollefson, G.D., Chengappa, K.N., Daniel, D.G., Petty, F., Centorrino, F., Wang, R., Gundy, S.L., Greaney, M.G., Jacobs, T.G., David, S.R., and Toma, V. Olanzapine versus placebo in the treatment of acute mania. Olanzapine Study Group. *Am. J. Psychiatry,* **1999,** *156:*702–709.

Tohen, M., and Zarate, C.A. Jr. Antipsychotic agents and bipolar disorder. *J. Clin. Psychiatry,* **1998,** *59*(Suppl. 1):38–48.

Tollefson, G.D., and Kuntz, A.J. Review of recent clinical studies with olanzapine. *Br. J. Psychiatry Suppl.,* **1999,** 30–35.

Tondo, L., and Baldessarini, R.J. Reduced suicide risk during lithium maintenance treatment. *J. Clin. Psychiatry,* **2000,** *61*(Suppl. 9):97–104.

Tondo, L., Baldessarini, R.J., Hennen, J., and Floris, G. Lithium maintenance treatment of depression and mania in bipolar I and II bipolar disorders. *Am. J. Psychiatry,* **1998a,** *155:*638–645.

Tondo, L., Baldessarini, R.J., Hennen, J., Floris, G., Silvetti, F., and Tohen, M. Lithium treatment and risk of suicidal behavior in bipolar disorder patients. *J. Clin. Psychiatry,* **1998b,** *59:*405–414.

Turkka, J., Bitram, J.A., Manji, H.K., Linnoilia, M., and Potter, W.Z. Effects of chronic lithium on agonist and antagonist binding to β-adrenergic receptors of rat brain. *Lithium,* **1992,** *3:*43–47.

Treiser, S.L., Cascio, C.S., O'Donohue, T.L., Thoa, N.B., Jacobowitz, D.M., and Kellar, K.J. Lithium increases serotonin release and decreases serotonin receptors in the hippocampus. *Science,* **1981,** *213:*1529–1531.

Truffinet, P., Tamminga, C.A., Fabre, L.F., Meltzer, H.Y., Riviere, M-E., and Papillon-Downey, C. Placebo-controlled study of the D_4/5-HT_{2A} antagonist fanaserin in the treatment of schizophrenia. *Am. J. Psychiatry,* **1999,** *156:*419–425.

Tsuneizumi, T., Babb, S.M., and Cohen, B.M. Drug distribution between blood and brain as a determinant of antipsychotic drug effects. *Biol. Psychiatry,* **1992,** *32:*817–824.

Urabe, M., Hershmann, J.M., Pang, X.P., Murakami, S., and Sugawara, M. Effect of lithium on function and growth of thyroid cells in vitro. *Endocrinology,* **1991,** *129:*807–814.

Van Tol, H.H., Bunzow, J.R., Guan, H.C., Sunahara, R.K., Seeman,

P., Niznik, H.B., and Civelli, O. Cloning of the gene for a human dopamine D_4 receptor with high affinity for the antipsychotic clozapine. *Nature,* **1991,** *350:*610–614.

Viguera, A.C., Baldessarini, R.J., Hegarty, J.M., van Kammen, D.D., and Tohen, M. Clinical risk following abrupt and gradual withdrawal of maintenance neuroleptic treatment. *Arch. Gen. Psychiatry,* **1997,** *54:*49–55.

Viguera, A.C., Nonacs, R., Cohen, L.S., Tondo, L., Murray, A., and Baldessarini, R.J. Risk of recurrence of bipolar disorder in pregnant and nonpregnant women after discontinuing lithium maintenance. *Am. J. Psychiatry,* **2000,** *157:*179–184.

Wang, H.Y., and Friedman, E. Lithium inhibition of protein kinase C activation–induced serotonin release. *Psychopharmacology (Berl.),* **1989,** *99:*213–218.

Watson, D.G., and Lenox, R.H. Chronic lithium-induced down-regulation of MARCKS in immortalized hippocampal cells: potentiation by muscarinic receptor activation. *J. Neurochem.,* **1996,** *67:*767–777.

Watson, D.G., Watterson, J.M., and Lenox, R.H. Sodium valproate down-regulates the myristoylated alanine-rich C kinase substrate (MARCKS) in immortalized hippocampal cells: a property of protein kinase C–mediated mood stabilizers. *J. Pharmacol. Exp. Ther.,* **1998,** *285:*307–316.

Watts, V.J., Lawler, C.P., Knoerzer, T., Mayleben, M.A., Neve, K.A., Nichols, D.E., and Mailman, R.B. Hexahydrobenzo[a]phenanthridines: novel dopamine D_3 receptor ligands. *Eur. J. Pharmacol.,* **1993,** *239:*271–273.

Wirshing, D.A., Spellberg, B.J., Erhard, S.M., Marder, S.R., and Wirshing, W.C. Novel antipsychotics and new onset diabetes. *Biol. Psychiatry,* **1998,** *44:*778–783.

Wolkin, A., Brodie, J.D., Barouche, F., Rotrosen, J., Wolf, A.P., Smith, M., Fowler, J., and Cooper, T.B. Dopamine receptor occupancy and plasma haloperidol levels. *Arch. Gen. Psychiatry,* **1989,** *46:*482–484.

Zarin, D.A., and Pass, T.M. Lithium and the single episode. When to begin long-term prophylaxis for bipolar disorder. *Med. Care,* **1987,** *25:*S76–S84.

Zatz, M., and Reisine, T.D. Lithium induces corticotropin secretion and desensitization in cultured anterior pituitary cells. *Proc. Natl. Acad. Sci. U.S.A.,* **1985,** *82:*1286–1290.

Zubenko, G.S., and Sunderland, T. Geriatric psychopharmacology: why does age matter? *Harv. Rev. Psychiatry,* **2000,** *7:*311–333.

MONOGRAPHS AND REVIEWS

Baldessarini, R.J. Antipsychotic agents. In, *The Psychiatric Therapies.* (Karasu, T.B., ed.) American Psychiatric Association, Washington, D.C., **1984,** pp. 119–170.

Baldessarini, R.J. *Chemotherapy in Psychiatry: Principles and Practice,* 2nd ed. Harvard University Press, Cambridge, MA, **1985.**

Baldessarini, R.J. Dopamine receptors and clinical medicine. In, *The Dopamine Receptors.* (Neve, K.A., and Neve, R.L., eds.) Humana Press, Totowa, NJ, **1997,** pp. 457–498.

Baldessarini, R.J., Cohen, B.M., and Teicher, M.H. Pharmacological treatment. In, *Schizophrenia: Treatment of Acute Psychotic Episodes.* (Levy, S.T., and Ninan, P.T., eds.) American Psychiatric Press, Washington, D.C., **1990,** pp. 61–118.

Baldessarini, R.J., Cole, J.O., Davis, J.M., Gardos, G., Simpson, G., and Tarsy, D. *Tardive Dyskinesia: A Task Force Report of the American Psychiatric Association.* Task Force Report No. 18. American Psychiatric Association, Washington, D.C., **1980.**

Baldessarini, R.J., Faedda, G.L., and Suppes, T. Treatment response in pediatric, adult, and geriatric bipolar disorder patients. In, *Mood Disorders Across the Life Span.* (Shulman, K., Tohen, M., and Kutcher, S.P., eds.) Wiley-Liss, New York, **1996b,** pp. 299–338.

Baldessarini, R.J., and Frankenburg, F.R. Clozapine. A novel antipsychotic agent. *N. Engl. J. Med.,* **1991,** *324*:746–754.

Baldessarini, R.J., and Tarazi, F.I. Brain dopamine receptors: a primer on their current status, basic and clinical. *Harv. Rev. Psychiatry,* **1996,** *3*:301–325.

Baldessarini, R.J., and Tarsy, D. Relationship of the actions of neuroleptic drugs to the pathophysiology of tardive dyskinesia. *Int. Rev. Neurobiol.,* **1979,** *21*:1–45.

Ben-Jonathan, N. Dopamine: a prolactin-inhibiting hormone. *Endocr. Rev.,* **1985,** *6*:564–589.

Calabrese, J.R., Bowden, C.L., and Woyshville, M.J. Lithium and the anticonvulsants in the treatment of bipolar disorder. In, *Psychopharmacology: The Fourth Generation of Progress.* (Bloom, F.E., and Kupfer, D.L., eds.) Raven Press, New York, **1995,** pp. 1099–1111.

Caldwell, A.E. History of psychopharmacology. In, *Principles of Psychopharmacology,* 2nd ed (Clark, W.G., and del Giudice, J., eds.) Academic Press, New York, **1978,** pp. 9–40.

Carlsson, A. Fifteen years of continued research in psychopharmacology. *Pharmacopsychiatry,* **1992,** *25*:22–24.

Civelli, O., Bunzow, J.R., and Grandy, D.K. Molecular diversity of the dopamine receptors. *Annu. Rev. Pharmacol. Toxicol.,* **1993,** *33*:281–307.

Cooper, T.B., Simpson, G.M., and Lee, J.H. Thymoleptic and neuroleptic drug plasma levels in psychiatry: current status. *Int. Rev. Neurobiol.,* **1976,** *19*:269–309.

Davis, J.M., Janicak, P.G., and Hogan, D.M. Mood stabilizers in the prevention of recurrent affective disorders: a meta-analysis. *Acta Psychiatr. Scand.,* **1999,** *100*:406–417.

Davis, L.L., Ryan, W., Adinoff, B., and Petty, F. Comprehensive review of the psychiatric uses of valproate. *J. Clin. Psychopharmacol.,* **2000,** *20*:1S–17S.

DeBattista, C., and Schatzberg, A.F. Universal psychotropic dosing and monitoring guidelines. *The Economics of Neuroscience (TEN),* **1999,** *1*:75–84.

DeVane, C.L., and Nemeroff, C.B. Psychotropic drug interactions. *The Economics of Neuroscience (TEN),* **2000,** *2*:55–75.

Dubovsky, S.L. Calcium channel antagonists as novel agents for the treatment of bipolar disorder. In, *Textbook of Psychopharmacology* (Schatzberg, A.F., and Nemeroff, C.B., eds.) American Psychiatric Press, Washington, D.C., **1998,** pp. 455–469.

Ferrier, N., and Calabrese, J. Lamotrigine, gabapentin, and the new anticonvulsants: efficacy in mood disorders. In, *Schizophrenia and Mood Disorders: The New Drug Therapies in Clinical Practice.* (Buckley, P.F., and Waddington, J.L., eds.) Butterworth-Heinemann, Boston, **2000,** pp. 190–198.

Fielding, S., and Lal, H. Behavioral actions of neuroleptics. In, *Handbook of Psychopharmacology.* Vol. 10. (Iversen, L.L., Iversen, S.D., and Snyder, S.H., eds.) Plenum Press, New York, **1978,** pp. 91–128.

Findling, R.L., Schulz, S.C., Reed, M.D., and Blumer, J.L. The antipsychotics. A pediatric perspective. *Pediatr. Clin. North Am.,* **1998,** *45*:1205–1232.

Goodwin, F.K., and Jamison, K.R. *Manic-Depressive Illness.* Oxford University Press, New York, **1990.**

Itil, T.M. Effects of psychotropic drugs on qualitatively and quantitatively analyzed human EEG. In, *Principles of Psychopharmacology,*

2nd ed. (Clark, W.G., and del Giudice, J., eds.) Academic Press, New York, **1978,** pp. 261–277.

Janssen, P.A.J. Butyrophenones and diphenylbutylpiperidines. In, *Psychopharmacological Agents.* Vol. 3. (Gordon, M., ed.) Academic Press, New York, **1974,** pp. 128–158.

Janssen, P.A.J., and Van Bever, W.F. Preclinical psychopharmacology of neuroleptics. In, *Principles of Psychopharmacology,* 2nd ed. (Clark, W.G., and del Giudice, J., eds.) Academic Press, New York, **1978,** pp. 279–295.

Jefferson, J.W., Greist, J.H., and Ackerman, D.L. *Lithium Encyclopedia for Clinical Practice.* American Psychiatric Press, Washington, D.C., **1983.**

Kane, J.M., Jeste, D.V., Barnes, T.R.E., Casey, D.E., Cole, J.O., Davis, J.M., Gualtieri, C.T., Schooler, N.R., Sprague, R.L., and Wettstein, R.M. *Tardive Dyskinesia: A Task Force Report of the American Psychiatric Association.* American Psychiatric Association, Washington, D.C., **1992.**

Kebabian, J.W., Tarazi, F.I., Kula, N.S and Baldessarini, R.J. Compounds selective for dopamine receptor subtypes. *Drug Discov. Today,* **1997,** *2*:333–340.

Keck, P., and Licht, R. Antipsychotic medications in the treatment of mood disorders. In, *Schizophrenia and Mood Disorders: The New Drug Therapies in Clinical Practice* (Buckley, P.F., and Waddington, J.L., eds.) Butterworth-Heinemann, Boston, **2000,** pp. 199–211.

Keck, P., and McElroy, S.L. Antiepileptic drugs. In, *The American Psychiatric Press Textbook of Psychopharmacology.* (Schatzberg, A.F., and Nemeroff, C.B., eds.) American Psychiatric Press, Washington, D.C., **1998,** pp. 431–454.

Kutcher, S.P. *Child & Adolescent Psychopharmacology.* Saunders, Philadelphia, **1997.**

Lenox, R.H., and Manji, H.K. In, *The American Psychiatric Press Textbook of Psychopharmacology.* (Schatzberg, A.F., and Nemeroff, C.B., eds.) American Psychiatric Press, Washington, D.C., **1998,** pp. 379–429.

Levant, B. The D$_3$ dopamine receptor: neurobiology and potential clinical relevance. *Pharmacol. Rev.,* **1997,** *49*:231–252.

Manji, H.K., Bebchuck, J.M., Moore, G.J., Glitz, D., Hasanat, K.A., and Chen, G. Modulation of CNS signal transduction pathways and gene expression by mood-stabilizing agents: therapeutic implications. *J. Clin. Psychiatry,* **1999a,** *60*(Suppl. 2):27–39.

Manji, H.K., Bowden, C.L., and Belmaker, R.H., eds. *Bipolar Medications: Mechanisms of Action.* American Psychiatric Press, Washington, D.C., **2000.**

Manji, H.K., McNamara, R., Chen, G., and Lenox, R.H. Signalling pathways in the brain: cellular transduction of mood stabilization in the treatment of manic-depressive illness. *Aust. N.Z. J. Psychiatry,* **1999b,** *33*(Suppl.):S65–S83.

Manji, H.K., Moore, G.J., and Chen, G. Lithium at 50: have the neuroprotective effects of this unique cation been overlooked? *Biol. Psychiatry,* **1999c,** *46*:929–940.

Marder, S.R. Antipsychotic medications. In, *The American Psychiatric Press Textbook of Psychopharmacology.* (Schatzberg, A.F., and Nemeroff, C.B., eds.) American Psychiatric Press, Washington, D.C., **1998,** pp. 309–321.

Mitchell, P.B., Hadzi-Pavlovic, D., and Manji, H.K., eds. Fifty years of treatment for bipolar disorder: a celebration of John Cade's discovery. *Aust. N.Z. J. Psychiatry,* **1999,** *33*(Suppl.):S1–S122.

Morselli, P.L. Psychotropic drugs. In, *Drug Disposition During Development.* (Morselli, P.L., ed.) Halsted Press, New York, **1977,** pp. 431–474.

Neumeyer, J.L., and Booth, R.G. Neuroleptics and anxiolytic agents. In, *Principles of Medicinal Chemistry,* 4th ed. (Foye, W.O., Williams, D.A., and Lemke, T.L., eds.) Williams & Wilkins, Baltimore, **2001,** in press.

Neve, K.A., and Neve, R.L. eds. *The Dopamine Receptors.* Humana Press, Totowa, NJ, **1997.**

Owens, M.J., and Risch, S.C. Atypical antipsychotics. In, *The American Psychiatric Press Textbook of Psychopharmacology* (Schatzberg, A.F., and Nemeroff, C.B., eds.) American Psychiatric Press, Washington, D.C., **1998,** pp. 323–348.

Post, R.M. Psychopharmacology of mood-stabilizers. In, *Schizophrenia and Mood Disorders: The New Drug Therapies in Clinical Practice.* (Buckley, P.F., and Waddington, J.L., eds.) Butterworth-Heinemann, Boston, **2000,** pp. 127–154.

Prien, R.F. Chemotherapy in chronic organic brain syndrome—a review of the literature. *Psychopharmacol. Bull.,* **1973,** *9*:5–20.

Rivera-Calimlim, L., and Hershey, L. Neuroleptic concentrations and clinical response. *Annu. Rev. Pharmacol. Toxicol.,* **1984,** *24*:361–386.

Sachar, E.J. Neuroendocrine responses to psychotropic drugs. In, *Psychopharmacology: A Generation of Progress.* (Lipton, M.A., DiMascio, A., and Killam, K.F., eds.) Raven Press, New York, **1978,** pp. 499–507.

Sadock, B.J., and Sadock, V.A., eds. *Kaplan and Sadock's Comprehensive Textbook of Psychiatry,* 7th ed. Lippincott Williams & Wilkins, Philadelphia, **2000.**

Shulman, K., Tohen, M., and Kutcher, S.P., eds. *Mood Disorders Across the Life Span.* John Wiley & Sons, New York, **1996.**

Swazey, J.P. *Chlorpromazine in Psychiatry—A Study in Therapeutic Innovation.* M.I.T. Press, Cambridge, MA, **1974.**

Tarazi, F.I., and Baldessarini, R.J. Dopamine D$_4$ receptors: significance for molecular psychiatry at the millennium. *Int. J. Neuropsychopharmacol.,* **1999,** *2*:41–58.

Tarsy, D., Tarazi, F.I., and Baldessarini, R.J. Extrapyramidal dysfunction associated with modern antipsychotic drugs. *CNS Drugs,* **2001,** in press.

United States Pharmacopoeia. *USP DI. Drug Information for the Health Care Provider.* Micromedex, Englewood, CO, **2000.**

Waddington, J., and Casey, D. Comparative pharmacology of classical and novel (second-generation) antipsychotics. In, *Schizophrenia and Mood Disorders: The New Drug Therapies in Clinical Practice.* (Buckley, P.F., and Waddington, J.L., eds.) Butterworth-Heinemann, Boston, **2000,** pp. 1–13.

Wagstaff, A.J., and Bryson, H.M. Clozapine: a review of its pharmacological properties and therapeutic use. *CNS Drugs,* **1995,** *4*:370–400.

Wolf, M.E., and Roth, R.H. Dopamine autoreceptors. In, *Dopamine Receptors.* (Creese, I., and Fraser, C.M., eds.) A.R. Liss, New York, **1987,** pp. 45–96.

Worrel, J.A., Marken, P.A., Beckman, S.E., and Ruehter, V.L. The atypical antipsychotic agents: a critical review. *Am. J. Health Syst. Pharm.,* **2000,** *57*:238–255.

C H A P T E R   2 1

DRUGS EFFECTIVE IN THE THERAPY OF THE EPILEPSIES

James O. McNamara

The epilepsies are common and frequently devastating disorders, affecting approximately 2.5 million people in the United States alone. More than 40 distinct forms of epilepsy have been identified. Epileptic seizures often cause transient impairment of consciousness, leaving the individual at risk of bodily harm and often interfering with education and employment. Therapy is symptomatic in that available drugs inhibit seizures, but neither effective prophylaxis nor cure is available. Compliance with medication is a major problem because of the need for long-term therapy together with unwanted effects of many drugs.

The mechanisms of action of antiseizure drugs fall into three major categories. Drugs effective against the most common forms of epileptic seizures, partial and secondarily generalized tonic-clonic seizures, appear to work by one of two mechanisms. One is to limit the sustained, repetitive firing of a neuron, an effect mediated by promoting the inactivated state of voltage-activated Na^+ channels. A second mechanism appears to involve enhanced gamma-aminobutyric acid (GABA)–mediated synaptic inhibition, an effect mediated by an action presynaptically for some drugs and postsynaptically for others. Drugs effective against a less common form of epileptic seizure, absence seizure, limit activation of a particular voltage-activated Ca^{2+} channel known as the T current.

Although many treatments are available, much effort is being devoted to novel approaches. Many of these approaches center on elucidating the genetic, cellular, and molecular mechanisms of the hyperexcitability, insights that promise to provide specific targets for novel therapies.

TERMINOLOGY AND EPILEPTIC SEIZURE CLASSIFICATION

The term *seizure* refers to a transient alteration of behavior due to the disordered, synchronous, and rhythmic firing of populations of brain neurons. The term *epilepsy* refers to a disorder of brain function characterized by the periodic and unpredictable occurrence of seizures. Seizures can be "nonepileptic" when evoked in a normal brain by treatments such as electroshock or chemical convulsants or "epileptic" when occurring without evident provocation. Pharmacological agents in current clinical use inhibit seizures, and thus are referred to as antiseizure drugs. Whether any of these agents has prophylactic value in preventing development of epilepsy (epileptogenesis) is uncertain.

Seizures are thought to arise from the cerebral cortex, and not from other central nervous system (CNS) structures such as thalamus, brainstem, or cerebellum. Epileptic seizures have been classified into *partial* seizures, those beginning focally in a cortical site, and *generalized* seizures, those that involve both hemispheres widely from the outset (Commission, 1981). The behavioral manifestations of a seizure are determined by the functions normally served by the cortical site at which the seizure arises. For example, a seizure involving motor cortex is associated with clonic jerking of the body part controlled by this region of cortex. A *simple* partial seizure is associated with preservation of consciousness. A *complex* partial seizure is associated with impairment of consciousness. The majority of complex partial seizures originate from the temporal lobe. Examples of *generalized* seizures include absence, myoclonic, and tonic-clonic. The type of epileptic seizure determines the drug selected for therapy. More detailed information is presented in Table 21–1.

Apart from this epileptic seizure classification, an additional classification specifies *epileptic syndromes*, which refer to a cluster of symptoms frequently occurring together

Table 21–1
Classification of Epileptic Seizures

SEIZURE TYPE	FEATURES	CONVENTIONAL ANTISEIZURE DRUGS	RECENTLY DEVELOPED ANTISEIZURE DRUGS
PARTIAL SEIZURES:			
Simple partial	Diverse manifestations determined by the region of cortex activated by seizure (*e.g.,* if motor cortex representing left thumb, clonic jerking of left thumb results; if somatosensory cortex representing left thumb, paresthesia of left thumb results), lasting approximating 20 to 60 seconds. **Key feature is preservation of consciousness.**	Carbamazepine, phenytoin, valproate	Gabapentin, lamotrigine, levetiracetam, tiagabine, topiramate, zonisamide
Complex partial	Impaired consciousness lasting 30 seconds to two minutes, often associated with purposeless movements such as lip smacking or hand wringing.	Carbamazepine, phenytoin, valproate	Gabapentin, lamotrigine, levetiracetam, tiagabine, topiramate, zonisamide
Partial with secondarily generalized tonic-clonic seizure	Simple or complex partial seizure evolves into a tonic-clonic seizure with loss of consciousness and sustained contractions (tonic) of muscles throughout the body followed by periods of muscle contraction alternating with periods of relaxation (clonic), typically lasting 1 to 2 minutes.	Carbamazepine, phenobarbital, phenytoin, primidone, valproate	Gabapentin, lamotrigine, levetiracetam, tiagabine, topiramate, zonisamide
GENERALIZED SEIZURES:			
Absence seizure	Abrupt onset of impaired consciousness associated with staring and cessation of ongoing activities typically lasting less than 30 seconds.	Ethosuximide, valproate	Lamotrigine
Myoclonic seizure	A brief (perhaps a second), shocklike contraction of muscles which may be restricted to part of one extremity or may be generalized.	Valproate	Lamotrigine, topiramate
Tonic-clonic seizure	As described above for partial with secondarily generalized tonic-clonic seizures except that it is not preceded by a partial seizure.	Carbamazepine, phenobarbital, phenytoin, primidone, valproate	Lamotrigine, topiramate

and include seizure types, etiology, age of onset, and other factors (Commission, 1989). More than 40 distinct epileptic syndromes have been identified. The epileptic syndromes have been categorized into partial *versus* generalized epilepsies. The partial epilepsies may consist of any of the partial seizure types (Table 21–1) and account for roughly 60% of all epilepsies. The etiology commonly consists of a lesion in some part of the cortex, such as a tumor, developmental malformation, damage due to trauma or stroke, etc. Such lesions often are evident on brain imaging studies such as magnetic resonance imaging. Alternatively, the etiology may be genetic. The generalized epilepsies are characterized most commonly by one or more of the generalized seizure types listed in Table 21–1 and account for approximately 40% of all epilepsies. The etiology is usually genetic. The most common generalized epilepsy is referred to as juvenile myoclonic epilepsy, accounting for approximately 10% of all epileptic syndromes. The age of onset is in the early teens, and the condition is characterized typically by myoclonic and tonic-clonic and often absence seizures. Like most of the generalized-onset epilepsies, juvenile myoclonic epilepsy is a complex genetic disorder that is probably due to inheritance of multiple susceptibility genes; there is a familial clustering of cases, but the pattern of inheritance is not mendelian. To date, the classification of epileptic syndromes has had more of an impact on guiding clinical assessment and management than on selection of antiseizure drugs.

NATURE AND MECHANISMS OF SEIZURES AND ANTISEIZURE DRUGS

Partial Epilepsies. More than a century ago, John Hughlings Jackson, the father of modern concepts of epilepsy, proposed that seizures were caused by "occasional, sudden, excessive, rapid and local discharges of gray matter," and that a generalized convulsion resulted when normal brain tissue was invaded by the seizure activity initiated in the abnormal focus. This insightful proposal provided a valuable framework for thinking about mechanisms of partial epilepsy. The advent of the electroencephalogram (EEG) in the 1930s permitted the recording of electrical activity from the scalp of human beings with epilepsy and demonstrated that the epilepsies are disorders of neuronal excitability.

The pivotal role of synapses in mediating communication among neurons in the mammalian brain suggested that defective synaptic function might lead to a seizure. That is, a reduction of inhibitory synaptic activity or enhancement of excitatory synaptic activity might be expected to trigger a seizure; pharmacological studies of seizures supported this notion. The neurotransmitters mediating the bulk of synaptic transmission in the mammalian brain are amino acids, gamma-aminobutyric acid (GABA) and glutamate being the principal inhibitory and excitatory neurotransmitters, respectively (*see* Chapter 12). Pharmacological studies disclosed that microinjection of *antagonists* of the GABA$_A$ receptor or of *agonists* of different glutamate-receptor subtypes (NMDA, AMPA, or kainic acid; *see* Chapter 12) triggers seizures in experimental animals *in vivo*. Pharmacological agents that enhance GABA-mediated synaptic inhibition inhibit seizures in diverse models. Glutamate-receptor antagonists also inhibit seizures in diverse models, including seizures evoked by electroshock and chemical convulsants such as pentylenetetrazol.

Such studies support the idea that pharmacological regulation of synaptic function can regulate the propensity for seizures, and they provide a framework for electrophysiological analyses aimed at elucidating the role of both synaptic and nonsynaptic mechanisms in expression of seizures and epilepsy. Progress in techniques of electrophysiology has fostered the progressive refinement of the level of analysis of seizure mechanisms from the EEG to populations of neurons (field potentials) to individual neurons to individual synapses and individual ion channels on individual neurons. Cellular electrophysiological studies of epilepsy over roughly two decades beginning in the mid-1960s were focused on elucidating the mechanisms underlying the *depolarization shift* (DS), the intracellular correlate of the "interictal spike" (Figure 21–1). The interictal (or between-seizures) spike is a sharp waveform recorded in the EEG of patients with epilepsy; it is asymptomatic in that it is accompanied by no detectable change in the patient's behavior. The location of the interictal spike helps localize the brain region from which seizures originate in a given patient. The DS consists of a large depolarization of the neuronal membrane associated with a burst of action potentials. In most cortical neurons, the DS is generated by a large excitatory synaptic current that can be enhanced by activation of voltage-regulated intrinsic membrane currents (for review *see* Dichter and Ayala, 1987). Although the mechanisms generating the DS are increasingly understood, it remains unclear whether the interictal spike triggers a seizure, inhibits a seizure, or is an epiphenomenon with respect to seizure occurrence in an epileptic brain. While these questions remain unanswered, study of the mechanisms of DS generation set the stage for inquiry into the cellular mechanisms of a seizure.

During the 1980s, a diversity of *in vitro* models of seizures were developed in isolated brain slice preparations, in which many synaptic connections are preserved. Electrographic events with features similar to those recorded during seizures *in vivo* have been produced in hippocampal slices by multiple methods, including altering ionic constituents of media bathing brain slices (for review *see* McNamara, 1994) such as low Ca^{2+}, zero Mg^{2+}, or elevated K^+. The accessibility and experimental control provided by these preparations has permitted mechanistic investigations. Analyses of multiple *in vitro* models confirmed the importance of synaptic function in initiation of a seizure, demonstrating that subtle (*e.g.,* 20%) reductions of inhibitory synaptic function could lead to epileptiform activity and that activation of excitatory synapses could be pivotal in initiation of a seizure. Many other important factors were identified, including the volume of the extracellular space as well as intrinsic

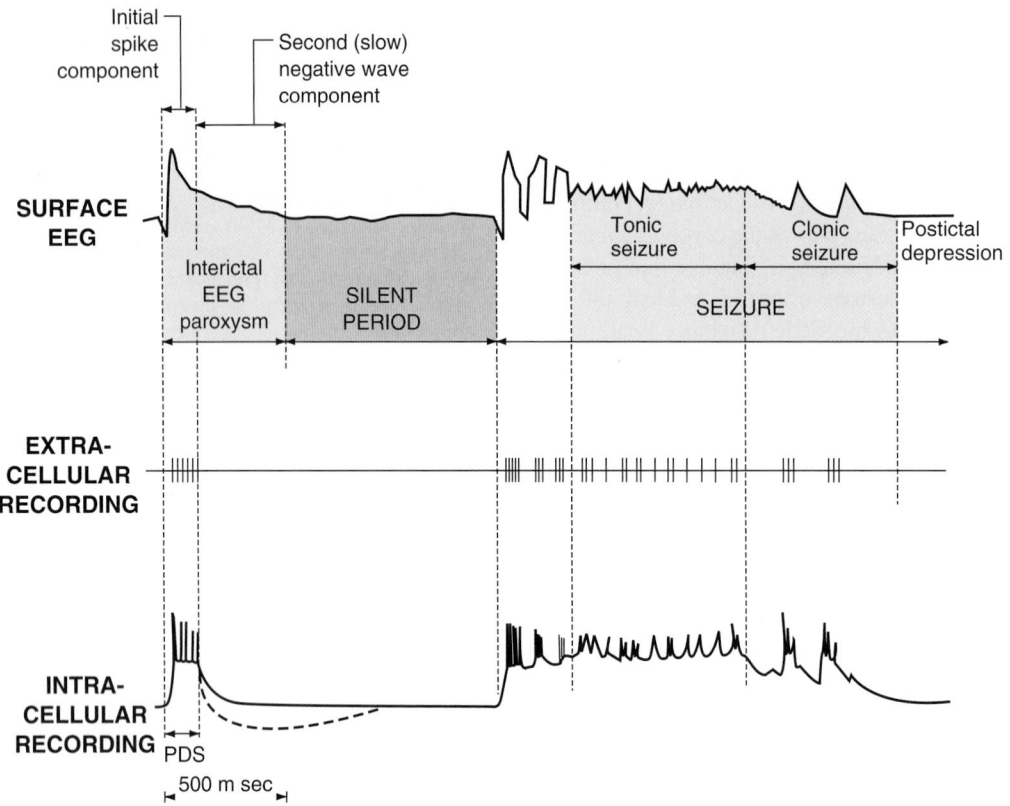

Figure 21–1. Relations among cortical EEG, extracellular, and intracellular recordings in a seizure focus induced by local application of a convulsant agent to mammalian cortex.

The extracellular recording was made through a high-pass filter. Note the high-frequency firing of the neuron evident in both extracellular and intracellular recording during the paroxysmal depolarization shift (PDS). (Modified from Ayala *et al.,* 1973, with permission.)

properties of a neuron such as voltage-regulated ion channels including those gating K^+, Na^+, and Ca^{2+} ions (*see* Traynelis and Dingledine, 1988). Identification of these diverse synaptic and nonsynaptic factors controlling seizures *in vitro* provides potentially valuable pharmacological targets for regulating seizure susceptibility *in vivo*.

An additional line of investigation has centered on understanding the mechanisms by which a normal brain is transformed into an epileptic brain. Some common forms of partial epilepsy arise months to years after injury of cortex sustained as a consequence of stroke, trauma, or other factors. An effective prophylaxis administered to patients at high risk would be highly desirable. The drugs described in this chapter provide symptomatic therapy; that is, the drugs inhibit seizures in patients with epilepsy. No effective antiepileptogenic agent has been identified.

Understanding the mechanisms of epileptogenesis in cellular and molecular terms would provide a framework for development of novel therapeutic approaches. The availability of animal models provides an opportunity to investigate the underlying mechanisms. One model, termed "kindling," is induced by periodic administration of brief, low-intensity electrical stimulation

of the amygdala or other limbic structures. Initial stimulations evoke a brief electrical seizure recorded on the EEG without behavioral change, but repeated (*e.g.,* 10 to 20) stimulations result in progressive intensification of seizures, culminating in tonic-clonic seizures (Goddard *et al.,* 1969). Once established, the enhanced sensitivity to electrical stimulation persists for the life of the animal. Despite the exquisite propensity to intense seizures, spontaneous seizures or a truly epileptic condition do not occur until 100 to 200 stimulations have been administered. The ease of control of kindling induction (*i.e.,* stimulations administered at the investigator's convenience), its graded onset, and the ease of quantitating epileptogenesis (number of stimulations required to evoke tonic-clonic seizures) simplify experimental study. Pharmacological studies have demonstrated that interventions limiting activation of the NMDA subtype of glutamate receptor or the trkB-subtype of neurotrophin receptor inhibit epileptogenesis in this model. These pharmacological data provide valuable clues to the cellular and molecular mechanisms underlying epileptogenesis in this model.

Two additional models are produced by administration of a convulsive chemical, kainic acid or pilocarpine, resulting in an intense limbic and tonic-clonic status epilepticus lasting hours.

In both models, the fleeting episode of status epilepticus is followed weeks later by the onset of spontaneous seizures (Lemos and Cavalheiro, 1995; Longo and Mello, 1998), an intriguing parallel to the scenario of complicated febrile seizures in young children followed by the emergence of spontaneous seizures years later. In contrast to the limited or no neuronal loss characteristic of the kindling model, overt destruction of hippocampal neurons occurs in both the pilocarpine and kainate models, reflecting aspects of hippocampal sclerosis observed in human beings with severe limbic seizures. Indeed, the recent discovery that complicated febrile seizures can cause hippocampal sclerosis in young children (Vanlandingham *et al.*, 1998) establishes yet another commonality between these models and the human condition.

Several questions arise with respect to these models. What transpires during the latent period between status epilepticus induced by pilocarpine or kainate and emergence of spontaneous seizures that causes the epilepsy? Might similar mechanisms be operative in kindling development and during the latent period following status epilepticus? Might an antiepileptogenic agent that was effective in one of these models be effective in the other models?

Important insights into the mechanisms of action of drugs that are effective against partial seizures have emerged in the past two decades (Macdonald and Greenfield, 1997). These insights have emerged in large part from electrophysiological studies of relatively simple *in vitro* models, such as neurons isolated from the mammalian CNS and maintained in primary culture. The experimental control and accessibility provided by these models together with careful attention to clinically relevant concentrations of the drugs led to clarification of the mechanisms. Although it is difficult to prove unequivocally that a given drug effect observed *in vitro* is both necessary and sufficient to inhibit a seizure in an animal or human being *in vivo*, there is an excellent likelihood that the putative mechanisms identified do in fact underlie the clinically relevant antiseizure effects.

Electrophysiological analyses of individual neurons during a partial seizure demonstrate that the neurons undergo depolarization and fire action potentials at high frequencies (Figure 21–1). This pattern of neuronal firing is characteristic of a seizure and is uncommon during physiological neuronal activity. Thus, selective inhibition of this pattern of firing would be expected to reduce seizures with minimal unwanted effects. Carbamazepine, lamotrigine, phenytoin, and valproic acid inhibit high-frequency firing at concentrations known to be effective at limiting seizures in human beings (Macdonald and Greenfield, 1997). Inhibition of the high-frequency firing is thought to be mediated by reducing the ability of Na$^+$ channels to recover from inactivation (Figure 21–2). That is, depolarization-triggered opening of the Na$^+$ channels in the axonal membrane of a neuron is required for an action potential; after opening, the channels spontaneously close, a process termed *inactivation*. This inactivation is thought to cause the refractory period, a short time after an action potential during which it is not possible to evoke another action potential. Upon recovery from inactivation, the Na$^+$ channels are again poised to participate in another action potential. Because firing at a slow rate permits sufficient time for Na$^+$ channels to recover from inactivation, inactivation has little or no effect on low-frequency firing. However, reducing the rate of recovery of Na$^+$ channels from inactivation would limit the ability of a neuron to fire at high

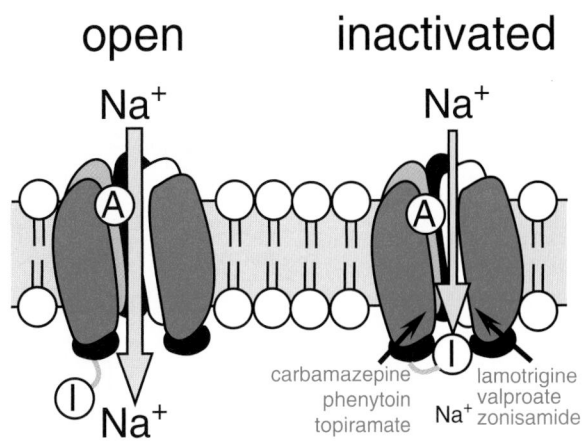

Figure 21–2. Antiseizure drug–enhanced Na$^+$ channel inactivation.

Some antiseizure drugs (shown in blue text) prolong the inactivation of the Na$^+$ channels, thereby reducing the ability of neurons to fire at high frequencies. Note that the inactivated channel itself appears to remain open, but is blocked by the inactivation gate (I). A, activation gate.

frequencies, an effect that likely underlies the effects of carbamazepine, lamotrigine, phenytoin, topiramate, valproic acid, and zonisamide against partial seizures.

Insights into mechanisms of seizures suggest that enhancing GABA-mediated synaptic inhibition would reduce neuronal excitability and raise the seizure threshold. Several drugs are thought to inhibit seizures by regulating GABA-mediated synaptic inhibition through an action at distinct sites of the synapse (Macdonald and Greenfield, 1997). The principal postsynaptic receptor of synaptically released GABA is termed the GABA$_A$ receptor. Activation of the GABA$_A$ receptor effects inhibition of the postsynaptic cell by increasing the flow of Cl$^-$ ions into the cell, which tends to hyperpolarize the neuron. Clinically relevant concentrations of both benzodiazepines and barbiturates can enhance GABA$_A$ receptor-mediated inhibition through distinct actions on the GABA$_A$ receptor (Figure 21–3). This mechanism probably underlies the effectiveness of these compounds against partial and tonic-clonic seizures in human beings. At higher concentrations, such as might be used for status epilepticus, these drugs also can inhibit high-frequency firing of action potentials. γ-Vinyl GABA (vigabatrin) is thought to exert its antiseizure action by irreversibly inhibiting an enzyme that degrades GABA, GABA transaminase; this probably leads to increased amounts of GABA available for synaptic release. A third mechanism of enhancing GABA-mediated synaptic inhibition is thought to underlie the antiseizure mechanism of tiagabine; tiagabine inhibits the GABA transporter, GAT-1, and reduces neuronal and glial uptake of GABA (Suzdak and Jansen, 1995) (Figure 21–3).

Generalized-Onset Epilepsies: Absence Seizures. In contrast to partial seizures, which arise from localized regions of the cerebral cortex, generalized-onset seizures arise from the reciprocal firing of the thalamus and cerebral

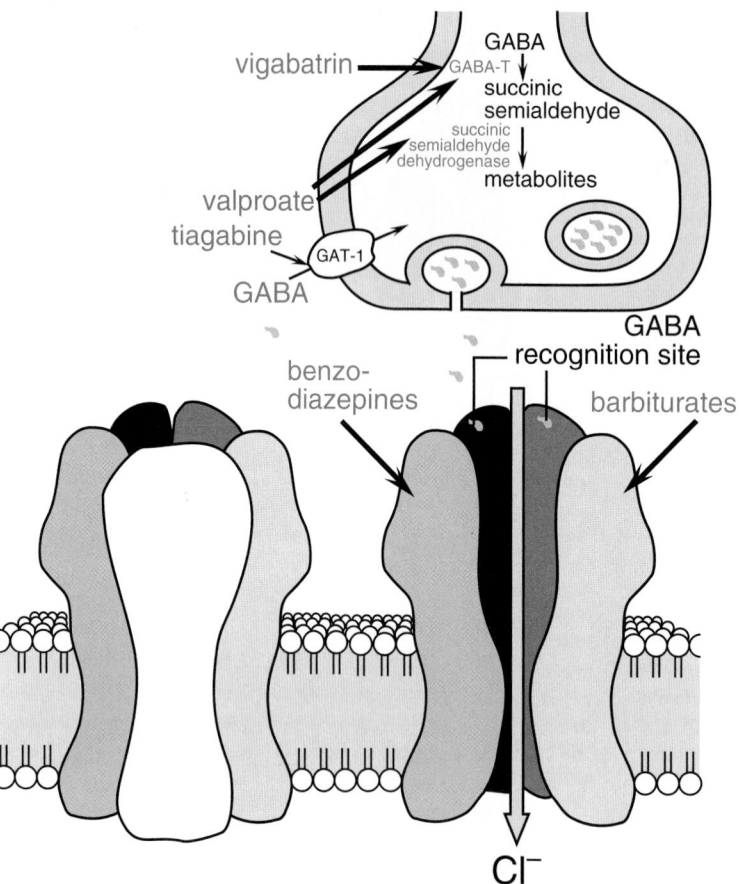

Figure 21–3. Enhanced GABA synaptic transmission.

In the presence of GABA, the $GABA_A$ receptor (structure on left) is opened, allowing an influx of Cl^-, which in turn, increases membrane polarization (*see also* Chapter 17). Some antiseizure drugs (shown in larger blue text) act by reducing the metabolism of GABA. Others act at the $GABA_A$ receptor, enhancing Cl^- influx in response to GABA. As outlined in the text, gabapentin acts presynaptically to promote GABA release; its molecular target is currently under investigation. GABA-T, GABA transaminase. GAT-1, GABA transporter.

cortex (*see* Coulter, 1998, for review). Among the diverse forms of generalized seizures, absence seizures have been most intensively studied. The striking synchrony in appearance of generalized seizure discharges in widespread areas of neocortex led to the idea that a structure in the thalamus and/or brainstem (the "centrencephalon") synchronized these seizure discharges (Penfield and Jasper, 1947). Attention on the thalamus in particular emerged from the demonstration that low-frequency stimulation of midline thalamic structures triggered EEG rhythms in the cortex similar to spike-wave discharges characteristic of absence seizures (Jasper and Droogleever-Fortuyn, 1947). Intracerebral electrode recordings from human beings subsequently demonstrated the presence of thalamic and neocortical involvement in the spike-and-wave discharge of absence seizures.

Many of the structural and functional properties of thalamus and neocortex that lead to the generalized spike-and-wave discharges have been elucidated in the past decade (Coulter, 1998). The EEG hallmark of an absence seizure is generalized spike-and-wave discharges at a frequency of 3 per second. These bilaterally synchronous spike-and-wave discharges,

recorded locally from electrodes in both the thalamus and the neocortex, represent oscillations between thalamus and neocortex. A comparison of EEG and intracellular recordings reveals that the EEG spikes are associated with the firing of action potentials and the following slow wave with prolonged inhibition. These reverberatory, low-frequency rhythms are made possible by a combination of factors, including reciprocal excitatory synaptic connections between neocortex and thalamus as well as intrinsic properties of neurons in the thalamus (*see* Coulter, 1998, for review). One intrinsic property of thalamic neurons that is pivotally involved in the generation of the 3-per-second spike and wave is a particular form of voltage-regulated Ca^{2+} current, the low threshold ("T") current. In contrast to its small size in most neurons, the T current in many neurons throughout the thalamus has a large amplitude. Indeed bursts of action potentials in thalamic neurons are mediated by activation of the T current. The T current plays an amplifying role in thalamic oscillations, one oscillation being the 3-per-second spike and wave of the absence seizure. Importantly, the principal mechanism by which most anti–absence-seizure drugs (ethosuximide, trimethadione, valproic acid) are thought to act is by inhibition of the T current (Figure 21–4; Macdonald and Kelly, 1993). Thus, inhibiting voltage-regulated ion channels is a common mechanism of action of antiseizure drugs, anti–partial-seizure drugs inhibiting voltage-activated Na^+ channels and anti–absence-seizure drugs inhibiting voltage-activated Ca^{2+} channels.

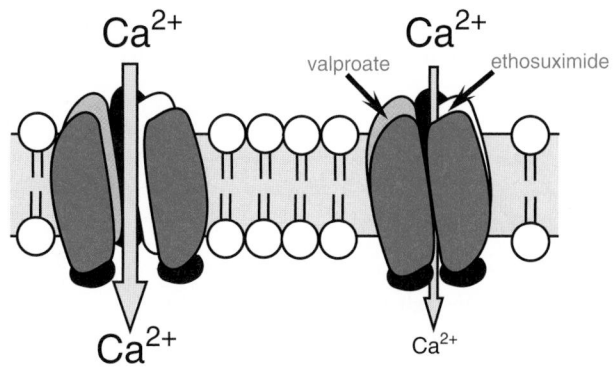

Figure 21–4. Antiseizure drug-induced reduction of current through T-type Ca²⁺ channels.

Some antiepileptic drugs (shown in blue text) reduce the flow of Ca²⁺ through T-type Ca²⁺ channels (*see also* Chapter 12), thus reducing the pacemaker current that underlies the thalamic rhythm in spikes and waves seen in generalized absence seizures.

Genetic Approaches to the Epilepsies. Genetic causes contribute to a wide diversity of human epilepsies. Genetic causes are solely responsible for some rare forms inherited in a mendelian pattern—for example, autosomal dominant or autosomal recessive. Genetic causes also are mainly responsible for some common forms such as juvenile myoclonic epilepsy (JME) or childhood absence epilepsy (CAE), disorders likely due to inheritance of two or more susceptibility genes. Genetic determinants also may contribute some degree of risk to epilepsies caused by injury of the cerebral cortex (Berkovic, 1998).

Enormous progress has been made in understanding the genetics of mammalian epilepsy in the past several years. Whereas prior to 1994, a specific gene defect had been identified in only a single mouse with a phenotype of cortical epilepsy, more than 33 single gene mutations now have been linked to an epileptic phenotype (Puranam and McNamara, 1999). This progress has been paralleled by the genetics of human epilepsy. Prior to 1990, not a single gene causing a form of human epilepsy had been identified; mutations of more than a dozen such genes now have been identified.

Most of the human epilepsies for which mutant genes have been identified are symptomatic epilepsies, in which the epilepsy seems to be a manifestation of some profound neurodegenerative disease. However, most patients with epilepsy are neurologically normal. It is not clear the extent to which the mechanisms underlying the hyperexcitability in a neurologically devastating disease inform mechanisms operative in epilepsies in which the patient is otherwise normal (idiopathic epilepsies). The mutant

genes have been identified in four distinct forms of idiopathic human epilepsy. Remarkably, each of the mutant genes encodes an ion channel gated by voltage or a neurotransmitter; this is of particular interest because several other episodic disorders involving other organs also are caused by mutations of genes encoding ion channels. That is, episodic disorders of the heart (cardiac arrhythmias), skeletal muscle (periodic paralyses), cerebellum (episodic ataxia), vasculature (familial hemiplegic migraine), and other organs all have been linked to mutant genes encoding a component of a voltage-gated ion channel (Ptacek, 1997).

The four idiopathic human epilepsies for which the mutant genes have been identified are the following. Generalized epilepsy with febrile seizures (GEFS+) is caused by a point mutation in the β subunit of a voltage-gated Na⁺ channel (*SCN1B*). Interestingly, several antiseizure drugs act on Na⁺ channels to promote their inactivation; the phenotype of the mutant Na⁺ channel appears to involve defective inactivation (Wallace *et al.,* 1998). Two forms of benign familial neonatal convulsions have been shown to be caused by mutations of two distinct but related novel K⁺-channel genes, *KCNQ2* and *KCNQ3* (Biervert *et al.,* 1998; Singh *et al.,* 1998; Charlier *et al.,* 1998). Autosomal dominant, nocturnal, frontal-lobe epilepsy is a fourth form of idiopathic epilepsy for which a mutant gene has been identified, the mutant gene encoding the α4 subunit of the nicotinic cholinergic receptor (*CHRNA4*) (Steinlein *et al.,*1995). Each of these is a rare syndrome, and together, these four forms likely account for well less than 1% of all of the human epilepsies. In no instance is it yet clear how the genotype leads to the phenotype of epilepsy. Identification of the genes will lead to generation of mutant mice expressing the phenotype; the mutant animals should provide powerful tools with which to elucidate how the genotype produces the phenotype. Importantly, the mutant channels suggest some intriguing molecular targets for development of antiseizure drugs acting by novel mechanisms. These initial successes suggest that many additional epilepsy genes will be identified in the next several years.

ANTISEIZURE DRUGS: GENERAL CONSIDERATIONS

History. Phenobarbital was the first synthetic organic agent recognized as having antiseizure activity (Hauptmann, 1912); its sedative properties led investigators to test and demonstrate its effectiveness for suppressing seizures. In a landmark discovery, Merritt and Putnam (1938a) developed the electroshock seizure test in experimental animals to screen chemical agents for antiseizure effectiveness; in the course of screening a variety of drugs, they discovered that phenytoin suppressed seizures in the absence of sedative effects. The electroshock seizure test is extremely valuable, because drugs that are effective against tonic hindlimb extension induced by electroshock generally have proven to be effective against partial and tonic-clonic seizures in human beings. Another screening test, seizures induced by the chemoconvulsant pentylenetetrazol, is useful in identifying drugs that are effective against absence seizures in human beings. These screening tests remain useful even now. The chemical structures of most of the drugs introduced before 1965 were closely related to phenobarbital. These include the hydantoins, the oxazolidinediones, and the succinimides. The agents introduced after 1965 exhibit a diversity of chemical structures. These include benzodiazepines (clonazepam and clorazepate), an iminostilbene (carbamazepine), a branched-chain carboxylic acid (valproic acid), a phenyltriazine (lamotrigine), a cyclic analog of GABA (gabapentin), a sulfamate-substituted monosaccharide (topiramate), a nipecotic acid derivative (tiagabine), and a pyrrolidine derivative (levetiracetam).

Therapeutic Aspects. The ideal antiseizure drug would suppress all seizures without causing any unwanted effects. Unfortunately, the drugs used currently not only fail to control seizure activity in some patients, but they frequently cause unwanted effects that range in severity from minimal impairment of the CNS to death from aplastic anemia or hepatic failure. The physician who treats patients with epilepsy is thus faced with the task of selecting the appropriate drug or combination of drugs that best controls seizures in an individual patient at an acceptable level of untoward effects. It is generally held that complete control of seizures can be achieved in up to 50% of patients and that another 25% can be improved significantly. The degree of success varies as a function of seizure type, cause, and other factors.

To minimize toxicity, treatment with a single drug should be sought. If seizures are not controlled at adequate plasma concentrations of the initial agent, substitution of a second drug is preferred to the concurrent administration of another agent. However, multiple-drug therapy may be required, especially when two or more types of seizure occur in the same patient.

Measurement of drug concentrations in plasma facilitates optimizing antiseizure medication, especially when therapy is initiated, after dosage adjustments, in the event of therapeutic failure, when toxic effects appear, or when multiple-drug therapy is instituted. However, clinical effects of some drugs do not correlate well with their concentrations in plasma, and recommended concentrations are only guidelines for therapy. The ultimate therapeutic regimen must be determined by clinical assessment of effect and toxicity.

The general principles of the drug therapy of the epilepsies are summarized below, following discussion of the individual agents. Details of diagnosis and therapy can be found in the monographs and reviews listed at the end of the chapter.

HYDANTOINS

Phenytoin

Phenytoin (diphenylhydantoin; DILANTIN; DIPHENYLAN) is effective against all types of partial and tonic-clonic seizures but not absence seizures. Properties of other hydantoins (mephenytoin, ethotoin) are described in earlier editions of this book.

History. Phenytoin was first synthesized in 1908 by Biltz, but its anticonvulsant activity was not discovered until 1938 (Merritt and Putnam, 1938a,b). In contrast to the earlier accidental discovery of the antiseizure properties of bromide and phenobarbital, phenytoin was the product of a search among nonsedative structural relatives of phenobarbital for agents capable of suppressing electroshock convulsions in laboratory animals. It was introduced for the treatment of epilepsy in the same year. The discovery of phenytoin was a signal advance. Since this agent is not a sedative in ordinary doses, it established that antiseizure drugs need not induce drowsiness and encouraged the search for drugs with selective antiseizure action.

Structure-Activity Relationship. Phenytoin has the following structural formula:

PHENYTOIN

A 5-phenyl or other aromatic substituent appears essential for activity against generalized tonic-clonic seizures. Alkyl substituents in position 5 contribute to sedation, a property absent in phenytoin. The position 5 carbon permits asymmetry, but there appears to be little difference in activity between isomers.

Pharmacological Effects. *Central Nervous System.* Phenytoin exerts antiseizure activity without causing general depression of the CNS. In toxic doses it may produce excitatory signs and at lethal levels a type of decerebrate rigidity.

The most significant effect of phenytoin is its ability to modify the pattern of maximal electroshock seizures. The characteristic tonic phase can be abolished completely, but the residual clonic seizure may be exaggerated and prolonged. This seizure-modifying action is observed with many other antiseizure drugs that are effective against generalized tonic-clonic seizures. By contrast, phenytoin does not inhibit clonic seizures evoked by pentylenetetrazol.

Mechanism of Action.   Phenytoin limits the repetitive firing of action potentials evoked by a sustained depolarization of mouse spinal cord neurons maintained *in vitro* (McLean and Macdonald, 1983). This effect is mediated by a slowing of the rate of recovery of voltage-activated Na^+ channels from inactivation, an action that is both voltage- (greater effect if membrane is depolarized) and use-dependent. These effects of phenytoin are evident at concentrations in the range of therapeutic drug levels in cerebrospinal fluid (CSF) in human beings, concentrations that correlate with the free (or unbound) concentration of phenytoin in the serum. At these concentrations, the effects on Na^+ channels are selective, in that no changes of spontaneous activity or responses to iontophoretically-applied GABA or glutamate are detected. At concentrations 5- to 10-fold higher, multiple effects of phenytoin are evident, including reduction of spontaneous activity, enhancement of responses to GABA, and others; these effects may underlie some of the unwanted toxicity associated with high levels of phenytoin.

Pharmacokinetic Properties.   The pharmacokinetic characteristics of phenytoin are influenced markedly by its binding to serum proteins, by the nonlinearity of its elimination kinetics, and by its metabolism by the cytochrome P450 enzyme system. Phenytoin is extensively bound (about 90%) to serum proteins, mainly albumin. Small variations in the percentage of phenytoin that is bound dramatically affect the absolute amount of free (active) drug; increased proportions of free drug are evident in the neonate, in patients with hypoalbuminemia, and in uremic patients. Some agents, such as valproate, can compete with phenytoin for binding sites on plasma proteins; when combined with valproate-mediated inhibition of phenytoin metabolism, marked increases in free phenytoin can result. Measurement of free rather than total phenytoin permits direct assessment of this potential problem in patient management.

Phenytoin is one of the few drugs for which the rate of elimination varies as a function of its concentration (*i.e.,* the rate is nonlinear). The plasma half-life of phenytoin ranges between 6 and 24 hours at plasma concentrations below 10 μg/ml but increases with higher concentrations; as a result, plasma drug concentration increases disproportionately as dosage is increased, even with small adjustments for levels near the therapeutic range.

The majority (95%) of phenytoin is metabolized principally in the hepatic endoplasmic reticulum and mainly by the cytochrome P450 isoform CYP2C9/10 and to a lesser extent CYP2C19 (Table 21–2). The principal metabolite, a parahydroxyphenyl derivative, is inactive. Because its metabolism is saturable, other drugs that are

Table 21–2
Interactions of Antiseizure Drugs with Hepatic Microsomal Enzymes*

DRUG	INDUCES CYP	INDUCES UGT	INHIBITS CYP	INHIBITS UGT	METABOLIZED BY CYP	METABOLIZED BY UGT
Carbamazepine	2C9;3A families	Yes			1A2;2C8;2C9;3A4	No
Ethosuximide	No	No	No	No	Uncertain	Uncertain
Gabapentin	No	No	No	No	No	No
Lamotrigine	No	Yes	No	No	No	Yes
Levetiracetam	No	No	No	No	No	No
Oxcarbazepine	3A4/5	Yes	2C19	Weak	No	Yes
Phenobarbital	2C;3A families	Yes	Yes	No	2C9;2C19	No
Phenytoin	2C;3A families	Yes	Yes	No	2C9;2C19	No
Primidone	2C;3A families	Yes	Yes	No	C9;2C19	No
Tiagabine	No	No	No	No	3A4	No
Topiramate	No	No	2C19	No		
Valproate	No	No	2C9	Yes	2C9;2C19	Yes
Zonisamide	No	No	No	No	3A4	Yes

*CYP, cytochrome P450; UGT, UDP-glucuronosyltransferase.
SOURCE: Based on Anderson, 1998.

metabolized by these enzymes can inhibit phenytoin's metabolism and produce a rise in phenytoin concentration. Conversely, the degradation rate of other drugs that are substrates for these enzymes can be inhibited by phenytoin; one such drug is warfarin, and addition of phenytoin to a patient receiving warfarin can lead to hypoprothrombinemia. An alternative mechanism of drug interactions arises from phenytoin's ability to induce diverse cytochrome P450 enzymes; coadministration of phenytoin and medications metabolized by these enzymes can lead to an increased degradation of such medications. Of particular note in this regard are oral contraceptives, which are metabolized by the CYP3A4; treatment with phenytoin could enhance the metabolism of oral contraceptives and lead to unplanned pregnancy. The potential teratogenic effects of phenytoin underscore the importance of attention to this interaction. Carbamazepine, oxcarbazepine, phenobarbital, and primidone also can induce CYP3A4 and likewise might increase degradation of oral contraceptives.

The low aqueous solubility of phenytoin resulted in diverse problems for intravenous use and led to production of *fosphenytoin,* a water-soluble prodrug. Fosphenytoin (CEREBYX) is converted into phenytoin by phosphatases in liver and red blood cells with a half-life of 8 to 15 minutes. Fosphenytoin is useful for adults with partial or generalized seizures when parenteral administration is indicated.

Toxicity. The toxic effects of phenytoin depend upon the route of administration, the duration of exposure, and the dosage. When fosphenytoin, the water-soluble prodrug, is administered intravenously at an excessive rate in the emergency treatment of status epilepticus, the most notable toxic signs are cardiac arrhythmias, with or without hypotension, and/or CNS depression. Although cardiac toxicity occurs more frequently in older patients and in those with known cardiac disease, it also can develop in young, healthy patients. These complications can be minimized by administering fosphenytoin at a rate of less than 150 mg of phenytoin sodium equivalents per minute. Acute oral overdosage results primarily in signs referable to the cerebellum and vestibular system; high doses have been associated with marked cerebellar atrophy. Toxic effects associated with chronic medication also are primarily dose-related cerebellar-vestibular effects but include other CNS effects, behavioral changes, increased frequency of seizures, gastrointestinal symptoms, gingival hyperplasia, osteomalacia, and megaloblastic anemia. Hirsutism is an annoying untoward effect in young females. Usually, these phenomena can be made bearable by proper adjustment of dosage. Serious adverse effects, including those on the

skin, bone marrow, and liver, probably are manifestations of drug allergy. Although rare, they necessitate withdrawal of the drug. Moderate elevation of the concentrations in plasma of enzymes that are used to assess hepatic function sometimes are observed; since these changes are transient and may result in part from induced synthesis of the enzymes, they do not necessitate withdrawal of the drug.

Electrophysiological evidence of peripheral neuropathy can occur in up to 30% of patients receiving phenytoin, but this phenomenon usually is not clinically significant. Gingival hyperplasia occurs in about 20% of all patients during chronic therapy and is probably the most common manifestation of phenytoin toxicity in children and young adolescents. It may be more frequent in those individuals who also develop coarsened facial features. The overgrowth of tissue appears to involve altered collagen metabolism. Toothless portions of the gums are not affected. The condition does not necessarily require withdrawal of medication, and it can be minimized by good oral hygiene.

A variety of endocrine effects have been reported. Inhibition of release of antidiuretic hormone (ADH) has been observed in patients with inappropriate ADH secretion. Hyperglycemia and glycosuria appear to be due to inhibition of insulin secretion. Osteomalacia, with hypocalcemia and elevated alkaline phosphatase activity, has been attributed to both altered metabolism of vitamin D and inhibition of intestinal absorption of Ca^{2+}. Phenytoin also increases the metabolism of vitamin K and reduces the concentration of vitamin K–dependent proteins that are important for normal Ca^{2+} metabolism in bone. This may explain why the osteomalacia is not always ameliorated by the administration of vitamin D.

Hypersensitivity reactions include morbilliform rash in 2% to 5% of patients and occasionally more serious skin reactions, including Stevens-Johnson syndrome. Systemic lupus erythematosus and potentially fatal hepatic necrosis have been reported rarely. Hematological reactions include neutropenia and leukopenia. A few instances of red-cell aplasia, agranulocytosis, and mild thrombocytopenia also have been reported. Lymphadenopathy, resembling Hodgkin's disease and malignant lymphoma, is associated with reduced immunoglobulin A (IgA) production. Hypoprothrombinemia and hemorrhage have occurred in the newborns of mothers who received phenytoin during pregnancy; vitamin K is effective treatment or prophylaxis.

Plasma Drug Concentrations. A good correlation usually is observed between the total concentration of phenytoin in plasma and the clinical effect. Thus, control of seizures generally is obtained with concentrations above 10 μg/ml, while toxic effects such as nystagmus develop at concentrations around 20 μg/ml.

Drug Interactions. Concurrent administration of any drug metabolized by the 2C9/10 isoform of cytochrome P450 can increase the plasma concentration of phenytoin by decreasing its rate of metabolism. Carbamazepine, which may enhance the metabolism of phenytoin, causes a well-documented *decrease* in phenytoin concentration. Conversely, phenytoin reduces the concentration of carbamazepine. Interaction between phenytoin and phenobarbital is variable.

Therapeutic Uses. *Epilepsy.* Phenytoin is one of the more widely used antiseizure agents, and it is effective against partial and tonic-clonic but not absence seizures. The use of phenytoin and other agents in the therapy of epilepsies is discussed further at the end of this chapter. Various preparations of phenytoin differ significantly in both bioavailability and rate of absorption, and patients should thus be treated with the drug product of a single manufacturer.

Other Uses. Some cases of trigeminal and related neuralgias appear to respond to phenytoin, but carbamazepine may be preferable. The use of phenytoin in the treatment of cardiac arrhythmias is discussed in Chapter 35.

ANTISEIZURE BARBITURATES

The pharmacology of the barbiturates as a class is considered in Chapter 17; discussion in this chapter is limited to the two barbiturates used for therapy of the epilepsies. Although still marketed, a third barbiturate (metharbital) has virtually disappeared from therapeutic use.

Phenobarbital

Phenobarbital (LUMINAL, others) was the first effective organic antiseizure agent (Hauptmann, 1912). It has relatively low toxicity, is inexpensive, and is still one of the more effective and widely used drugs for this purpose.

Structure-Activity Relationship. The structural formula of phenobarbital (5-phenyl-5-ethylbarbituric acid) is shown in Chapter 17. The structure-activity relationship of the barbiturates has been studied extensively. Maximal antiseizure activity is obtained when one substituent at position 5 is a phenyl group. The 5,5-diphenyl derivative has less antiseizure potency than does phenobarbital, but it is virtually devoid of hypnotic activity. By contrast, 5,5-dibenzyl barbituric acid causes convulsions.

Antiseizure Properties. Most barbiturates have antiseizure properties. However, the capacity of some of these agents, such as phenobarbital, to exert maximal antiseizure action at doses below those required for hypnosis determines their clinical utility as antiseizure agents. Phenobarbital is active in most antiseizure tests in animals but is relatively nonselective. It inhibits tonic hindlimb extension in the maximal electroshock model, clonic seizures evoked by pentylenetetrazol, and kindled seizures.

Mechanism of Action. The mechanism by which phenobarbital inhibits seizures likely involves potentiation of synaptic inhibition through an action on the GABA$_A$ receptor. Intracellular recordings of mouse cortical or spinal cord neurons demonstrated that phenobarbital enhances responses to iontophoretically applied GABA (Macdonald and Barker, 1979). These effects have been observed at therapeutically relevant concentrations of phenobarbital. Analyses of single channels in outside-out patches isolated from mouse spinal cord neurons demonstrated that phenobarbital increased the GABA receptor–mediated current by increasing the duration of bursts of GABA receptor–mediated currents without changing the frequency of bursts (Twyman *et al.,* 1989). At levels exceeding therapeutic concentrations, phenobarbital also limits sustained repetitive firing; this may underlie some of the antiseizure effects of higher concentrations of phenobarbital achieved during therapy of status epilepticus.

The mechanisms underlying the antiseizure as opposed to the sedative effects of the barbiturates have been enigmatic. That is, pentobarbital inhibits seizures, but at doses that produce marked sedation; by contrast, phenobarbital inhibits seizures at doses that cause minimal sedative effects. Both pentobarbital and phenobarbital enhance GABA$_A$ receptor–mediated currents. Distinctive effects of pentobarbital and phenobarbital on GABA responses and voltage-activated Ca^{2+} channels may explain this enigma (ffrench-Mullen *et al.,* 1993). The maximal effect of phenobarbital in enhancing GABA responses is only 40% of that of the active isomer of pentobarbital. Moreover, pentobarbital inhibits voltage-activated Ca^{2+} channels with greater potency than does phenobarbital (ffrench-Mullen *et al.,* 1993); one consequence of inhibition of these Ca^{2+} channels could be blockade of Ca^{2+} entry into presynaptic nerve terminals and inhibition of release of neurotransmitters such as glutamate, resulting in net reduction of excitatory synaptic transmission. Thus the powerful sedative actions of pentobarbital could be due to greater maximal enhancement of GABA responses in conjunction with strong inhibition of Ca^{2+} current.

Pharmacokinetic Properties. Oral absorption of phenobarbital is complete but somewhat slow; peak concentrations in plasma occur several hours after a single dose. It is 40% to 60% bound to plasma proteins and bound to a similar extent in tissues, including brain. Up to 25% of a dose is eliminated by pH-dependent renal excretion of the unchanged drug; the remainder is inactivated by hepatic microsomal enzymes. The principal cytochrome P450 responsible is CYP2C9, with minor metabolism by CYP2C19 and 2E1. Phenobarbital induces uridine diphosphate glucuronosyl transferase (UGT) enzymes as well as CYP2C and 3A subfamilies of cytochrome P450. Drugs metabolized by these enzymes can be more rapidly degraded when coadministered with phenobarbital; importantly, oral contraceptives are metabolized by CYP3A4.

Toxicity. Sedation, the most frequent undesired effect of phenobarbital, is apparent to some extent in all patients upon initiation of therapy, but tolerance develops during chronic medication. Nystagmus and ataxia occur at excessive dosage. Phenobarbital sometimes produces irritability and hyperactivity in children, and agitation and confusion in the elderly.

Scarlatiniform or morbilliform rash, possibly with other manifestations of drug allergy, occurs in 1% to 2% of patients. Exfoliative dermatitis is rare. Hypoprothrombinemia with hemorrhage has been observed in the newborn of mothers who have received phenobarbital during pregnancy; vitamin K is effective for treatment or prophylaxis. Megaloblastic anemia that responds to folate and osteomalacia that responds to high doses of vitamin D occur during chronic phenobarbital therapy of epilepsy, as they do during phenytoin medication. Other adverse effects of phenobarbital are discussed in Chapter 17.

Plasma Drug Concentrations. During long-term therapy in adults, the plasma concentration of phenobarbital averages 10 μg/ml per daily dose of 1 mg/kg; in children, the value is 5 to 7 μg/ml per 1 mg/kg. Although a precise relationship between therapeutic results and concentration of drug in plasma does not exist, plasma concentrations of 10 to 35 μg/ml are usually recommended for control of seizures; 15 μg/ml is the minimum for prophylaxis against febrile convulsions.

The relationship between plasma concentration of phenobarbital and adverse effects varies with the development of tolerance. Sedation, nystagmus, and ataxia usually are absent at concentrations below 30 μg/ml during long-term therapy, but adverse effects may be apparent for several days at lower concentrations when therapy is initiated or whenever the dosage is increased. Concentrations greater than 60 μg/ml may be associated with marked intoxication in the nontolerant individual.

Since significant behavioral toxicity may be present despite the absence of overt signs of toxicity, the tendency to maintain patients, particularly children, on excessively high doses of phenobarbital should be resisted. The plasma phenobarbital concentration should be increased above 30 to 40 μg/ml only if the increment is adequately tolerated and only if it contributes significantly to control of seizures.

Drug Interactions. Interactions between phenobarbital and other drugs usually involve induction of the hepatic microsomal enzyme system by phenobarbital (*see* Chapters 1 and 17). The variable interaction with phenytoin has been discussed above. Concentrations of phenobarbital in plasma may be elevated by as much as 40% during concurrent administration of valproic acid (*see* below).

Therapeutic Uses. Phenobarbital is an effective agent for generalized tonic-clonic and partial seizures. Its efficacy, low toxicity, and low cost make it an important agent for these types of epilepsy. However, its sedative effects and its tendency to disturb behavior in children have reduced its use as a primary agent.

Mephobarbital (MEBARAL) is *N*-methylphenobarbital. It is *N*-demethylated in the hepatic endoplasmic reticulum, and most of its activity during long-term therapy can be attributed to the accumulation of phenobarbital. Consequently, the pharmacological properties, toxicity, and clin-

ical uses of mephobarbital are the same as those for phenobarbital.

DEOXYBARBITURATES

Primidone

Primidone (MYSOLINE) is effective against partial and tonic-clonic seizures.

Chemistry. Primidone may be viewed as a congener of phenobarbital in which the carbonyl oxygen of the urea moiety is replaced by two hydrogen atoms:

PRIMIDONE

Antiseizure Properties. Primidone resembles phenobarbital in many laboratory antiseizure effects, but it is much less potent than phenobarbital in antagonizing seizures induced by pentylenetetrazol. The antiseizure effects of primidone are attributed to both the drug and its active metabolites, principally phenobarbital.

Pharmacokinetic Properties. Primidone is rapidly and almost completely absorbed after oral administration, although individual variability can be great. Peak concentrations in plasma usually are observed approximately 3 hours after ingestion. The plasma half-life of primidone is variable; mean values ranging from 5 to 15 hours have been reported.

Primidone is converted to two active metabolites, phenobarbital and phenylethylmalonamide (PEMA). Primidone and PEMA are bound to plasma proteins to only a small extent, whereas about half of phenobarbital is so bound. The half-life of PEMA in plasma is 16 hours; both it and phenobarbital accumulate during long-term therapy. The appearance of phenobarbital in plasma may be delayed several days upon initiation of therapy with primidone. Approximately 40% of the drug is excreted unchanged in the urine; unconjugated PEMA and, to a lesser extent, phenobarbital and its metabolites constitute the remainder.

Toxicity. The more common complaints are sedation, vertigo, dizziness, nausea, vomiting, ataxia, diplopia, and nystagmus. Patients also may experience an acute feeling of intoxication immediately following administration of primidone. This occurs before there is any significant metabolism of the drug. The relationship of adverse effects to dosage is complex, since they result from both the parent drug and its two active metabolites and since tolerance develops during long-term therapy. Side effects are occasionally quite severe when therapy is initiated.

Serious adverse effects are relatively uncommon, but maculopapular and morbilliform rash, leukopenia, thrombocytopenia, systemic lupus erythematosus, and lymphadenopathy have been reported. Acute psychotic reactions also have occurred. Hemorrhagic disease in the neonate, megaloblastic anemia, and osteomalacia similar to those discussed previously in connection with phenytoin and phenobarbital also have been described.

Plasma Drug Concentrations. The relationship between the dose of primidone and the concentration of the drug and its active metabolites in plasma shows marked individual variability. During long-term therapy, the plasma concentrations of primidone and phenobarbital average 1 μg/ml and 2 μg/ml, respectively, per daily dose of 1 mg/kg of primidone. The plasma concentration of PEMA usually is intermediate between those of primidone and phenobarbital. There is no clear relationship between the concentrations of primidone or its metabolites in plasma and therapeutic effect. As an initial guide, the dosage of primidone may be adjusted primarily with reference to the concentration of phenobarbital, as outlined previously for administered phenobarbital, and secondarily with reference to the concentration of the parent drug. Concentrations of primidone greater than 10 μg/ml usually are associated with significant toxic side effects.

Drug Interactions. Phenytoin has been reported to increase the conversion of primidone to phenobarbital. Other drug interactions to be anticipated are those for phenobarbital.

Therapeutic Uses. Primidone is useful against generalized tonic-clonic and both simple and complex partial seizures. Its use in combination with phenobarbital is illogical. Primidone is ineffective against absence seizures but is sometimes useful against myoclonic seizures in young children.

IMINOSTILBENES

Carbamazepine

Carbamazepine (TEGRETOL, CARBATROL, others) was initially approved in the United States for use as an antiseizure agent in 1974. It has been employed since the 1960s for the treatment of trigeminal neuralgia. It is now considered to be a primary drug for the treatment of partial and tonic-clonic seizures.

Chemistry. Carbamazepine is related chemically to the tricyclic antidepressants. It is a derivative of iminostilbene with a carbamyl group at the 5 position; this moiety is essential for potent antiseizure activity. The structural formula of carbamazepine is as follows:

CARBAMAZEPINE

Pharmacological Effects. Although the effects of carbamazepine in animals and human beings resemble those of phenytoin in many ways, the two drugs differ in a number of potentially important ways. Carbamazepine has been found to produce therapeutic responses in manic-depressive patients, including some in whom lithium carbonate is not effective. Further, carbamazepine has antidiuretic effects that are sometimes associated with reduced concentrations of antidiuretic hormone (ADH) in plasma. The mechanisms responsible for these effects of carbamazepine are not clearly understood.

Mechanism of Action. Like phenytoin, carbamazepine limits the repetitive firing of action potentials evoked by a sustained depolarization of mouse spinal cord or cortical neurons maintained *in vitro* (McLean and Macdonald, 1986b). This appears to be mediated by a slowing of the rate of recovery of voltage-activated Na^+ channels from inactivation. These effects of carbamazepine are evident at concentrations in the range of therapeutic drug levels in CSF in human beings. The effects of carbamazepine are selective at these concentrations, in that there are no effects on spontaneous activity or on responses to iontophoretically applied GABA or glutamate. The carbamazepine metabolite, 10,11-epoxycarbamazepine, also limits sustained repetitive firing at therapeutically relevant concentrations, suggesting that this metabolite may contribute to the antiseizure efficacy of carbamazepine.

Pharmacokinetic Properties. The pharmacokinetic characteristics of carbamazepine are complex. They are influenced by its limited aqueous solubility and by the ability of many antiseizure drugs, including carbamazepine itself, to increase their conversion to active metabolites by hepatic oxidative enzymes.

Carbamazepine is absorbed slowly and erratically after oral administration. Peak concentrations in plasma usually are observed 4 to 8 hours after oral ingestion, but may be delayed by as much as 24 hours, especially following the administration of a large dose. The drug distributes rapidly into all tissues. Binding to plasma proteins occurs to the extent of about 75%, and concentrations in the CSF appear to correspond to the concentration of free drug in plasma.

The predominant pathway of metabolism in human beings involves conversion to the 10,11-epoxide. This metabolite is as active as the parent compound in various animals, and its concentrations in plasma and brain may reach 50% of those of carbamazepine, especially during the concurrent administration of phenytoin or phenobarbital. The 10,11-epoxide is metabolized further to inactive compounds, which are excreted in the urine principally as glucuronides. Carbamazepine also is inactivated by conjugation and hydroxylation. The hepatic cytochrome P450 isoform primarily responsible for biotransformation of carbamazepine is CYP3A4. Carbamazepine induces CYP2C and CYP3A and also UDP-glucuronosyltransferase, thus enhancing the metabolism of drugs degraded by these enzymes. Of particular importance in this regard are oral contraceptives, which are metabolized by CYP3A4.

Toxicity. Acute intoxication with carbamazepine can result in stupor or coma, hyperirritability, convulsions, and respiratory depression. During long-term therapy, the more frequent untoward effects of the drug include drowsiness, vertigo, ataxia, diplopia, and blurred vision. The frequency of seizures may increase, especially with overdosage. Other adverse effects include nausea, vomiting, serious hematological toxicity (aplastic anemia, agranulocytosis), and hypersensitivity reactions (dermatitis, eosinophilia, lymphadenopathy, splenomegaly). A late complication of therapy with carbamazepine is retention of water, with decreased osmolality and concentration of Na^+ in plasma, especially in elderly patients with cardiac disease.

Some tolerance develops to the neurotoxic effects of carbamazepine, and they can be minimized by gradual increase in dosage or adjustment of maintenance dosage. Various hepatic or pancreatic abnormalities have been reported during therapy with carbamazepine, most commonly a transient elevation of hepatic enzymes in plasma in 5% to 10% of patients. A transient, mild leukopenia occurs in about 10% of patients during initiation of therapy and usually resolves within the first 4 months of continued treatment; transient thrombocytopenia also has been noted. In about 2% of patients, a persistent leukopenia may develop that requires withdrawal of the drug. The initial concern that aplastic anemia might be a frequent complication of long-term therapy with carbamazepine has not materialized. In the majority of cases, the administration of multiple drugs or the presence of another underlying disease has made it difficult to establish a causal relationship. In any event, the prevalence of aplastic anemia appears to be about 1 in 200,000 patients who are treated with the drug. It is not clear whether or not monitoring of hematological function can avert the development

of irreversible aplastic anemia. Although carbamazepine is carcinogenic in rats, it is not known to be carcinogenic in human beings. The induction of fetal malformations during the treatment of pregnant women is discussed below.

Plasma Drug Concentrations. There is no simple relationship between the dose of carbamazepine and concentrations of the drug in plasma. Therapeutic concentrations are reported to be 6 to 12 μg/ml, although considerable variation occurs. Side effects referable to the CNS are frequent at concentrations above 9 μg/ml.

Drug Interactions. Phenobarbital, phenytoin, and valproate may increase the metabolism of carbamazepine by inducing CYP3A4; carbamazepine may enhance the biotransformation of phenytoin as well as the conversion of primidone to phenobarbital. Administration of carbamazepine may lower concentrations of valproate, lamotrigine, tiagabine, and topiramate given concurrently. Carbamazepine reduces both the plasma concentration and therapeutic effect of haloperidol. The metabolism of carbamazepine may be inhibited by propoxyphene, erythromycin, cimetidine, fluoxetine, and isoniazid.

Therapeutic Uses. Carbamazepine is useful in patients with generalized tonic-clonic and both simple and complex partial seizures. When it is used, renal and hepatic function and hematological parameters should be monitored. The therapeutic use of carbamazepine is discussed further at the end of this chapter.

Carbamazepine was introduced by Blom in the early 1960s and is now the primary agent for treatment of trigeminal and glossopharyngeal neuralgias. It is also effective for lightning tabetic pain. Most patients with neuralgia are benefited initially, but only 70% obtain continuing relief. Adverse effects have required discontinuation of medication in 5% to 20% of patients. The therapeutic range of plasma concentrations for antiseizure therapy serves as a guideline for its use in neuralgia. Carbamazepine also has found use in the treatment of bipolar affective disorders, a use that is discussed further in Chapter 20.

Oxcarbazepine

Oxcarbazepine (TRILEPTAL) (10,11-dihydro-10-oxocarbamazepine) is a keto analog of carbamazepine. In human beings, oxcarbazepine functions as a prodrug, in that it is almost immediately converted to its main active metabolite, a 10-monohydroxy derivative which is inactivated by glucuronide conjugation and eliminated by renal excretion. Its mechanism of action is similar to that of carbamazepine. Oxcarbazepine is a less potent enzyme inducer than is carbamazepine, and substitution of oxcarbazepine for carbamazepine is associated with increased levels of phenytoin and valproic acid, presumably because of reduced induction of hepatic enzymes. There is no induction by oxcarbazepine of hepatic enzymes involved in its degradation. Although oxcarbazepine does not appear to reduce the anticoagulant effect of warfarin, it does induce CYP3A and thus reduces plasma levels of steroid oral contraceptives. It has been approved for monotherapy or adjunct therapy for partial seizures in adults and as adjunctive therapy for partial seizures in children ages 4 to 16.

SUCCINIMIDES

Ethosuximide

The succinimides evolved from a systematic search for effective agents less toxic than the oxazolidinediones for the treatment of absence seizures. *Ethosuximide* (ZARONTIN) is a primary agent for this type of epilepsy.

Structure-Activity Relationship. Ethosuximide has the following structural formula:

ETHOSUXIMIDE

The structure-activity relationship of the succinimides is in accord with that for other antiseizure classes. Methsuximide (CELONTIN) and phensuximide (MILONTIN) have phenyl substituents and are more active against maximal electroshock seizures. Neither of these is now in common use. Discussion of their properties can be found in older editions of this book. Ethosuximide, with alkyl substituents, is the most active of the succinimides against seizures induced by pentylenetetrazol and is the most selective for absence seizures.

Pharmacological Effects. The most prominent characteristic of ethosuximide at nontoxic doses is protection against clonic motor seizures induced by pentylenetetrazol. By contrast, at nontoxic doses, ethosuximide does not inhibit tonic hindlimb extension of electroshock seizures or kindled seizures. This profile correlates with efficacy against absence seizures in human beings.
Mechanism of Action. Ethosuximide reduces low-threshold Ca^{2+} currents (T currents) in thalamic neurons (Coulter *et al.*, 1989). The thalamus plays an important role in generation of 3-Hz spike-wave rhythms typical of absence seizures (Coulter, 1998). Neurons in the thalamus exhibit a large amplitude T-current spike that under-

lies bursts of action potentials and likely plays an important role in thalamic oscillatory activity such as 3-Hz spike-and-wave activity. At clinically relevant concentrations, ethosuximide inhibits the T current, as evident in voltage-clamp recordings of acutely isolated, ventrobasal thalamic neurons from rats and guinea pigs. Ethosuximide reduces this current without modifying the voltage dependence of steady-state inactivation or the time course of recovery from inactivation. By contrast, succinimide derivatives with convulsant properties do not inhibit this current. Ethosuximide does not inhibit sustained repetitive firing or enhance GABA responses at clinically relevant concentrations. Current data are consistent with the idea that inhibition of T currents is the mechanism by which ethosuximide inhibits absence seizures.

Pharmacokinetic Properties. Absorption of ethosuximide appears to be complete, and peak concentrations occur in plasma within about 3 hours after a single oral dose. Ethosuximide is not significantly bound to plasma proteins; during long-term therapy, the concentration in the CSF is similar to that in plasma. The apparent volume of distribution averages 0.7 liter/kg.

In human beings, 25% of the drug is excreted unchanged in the urine. The remainder is metabolized by hepatic microsomal enzymes, but whether or not cytochrome P450 enzymes are responsible is unknown. The major metabolite, the hydroxyethyl derivative, accounts for about 40% of administered drug, is inactive, and is excreted as such and as the glucuronide in the urine. The plasma half-life of ethosuximide averages between 40 and 50 hours in adults and approximately 30 hours in children.

Toxicity. The most common dose-related side effects are gastrointestinal complaints (nausea, vomiting and anorexia) and CNS effects (drowsiness, lethargy, euphoria, dizziness, headache, and hiccough). Some tolerance to these effects develops. Parkinson-like symptoms and photophobia also have been reported. Restlessness, agitation, anxiety, aggressiveness, inability to concentrate, and other behavioral effects have occurred primarily in patients with a prior history of psychiatric disturbance.

Urticaria and other skin reactions, including Stevens-Johnson syndrome—as well as systemic lupus erythematosus, eosinophilia, leukopenia, thrombocytopenia, pancytopenia, and aplastic anemia—also have been attributed to the drug. The leukopenia may be transient despite continuation of the drug, but several deaths have resulted from bone-marrow depression. Renal or hepatic toxicity has not been reported.

Plasma Drug Concentrations. During long-term therapy, the plasma concentration of ethosuximide averages about 2 μg/ml per daily dose of 1 mg/kg. A plasma concentration of 40 to 100 μg/ml is required for satisfactory control of absence seizures in most patients.

Therapeutic Uses. Ethosuximide is effective against absence seizures but not tonic-clonic seizures and has a lower risk of adverse effects than does trimethadione, a drug formerly used to treat absence seizures (its properties are discussed in earlier editions of this book). It is an important therapeutic agent for this type of epilepsy.

An initial daily dose of 250 mg in children (3 to 6 years old) and 500 mg in older children and adults is increased by 250-mg increments at weekly intervals until seizures are adequately controlled or toxicity intervenes. Divided dosage is required occasionally to prevent nausea or drowsiness associated with single daily dosage. The usual maintenance dose is 20 mg/kg per day. Increased caution is required if the daily dose exceeds 1500 mg in adults or 750 to 1000 mg in children. The use of ethosuximide and the other antiseizure agents is discussed further at the end of the chapter.

VALPROIC ACID

Valproic acid (DEPAKENE, others) was approved for use in the United States in 1978. The antiseizure properties of valproate were discovered serendipitously when it was employed as a vehicle for other compounds that were being screened for antiseizure activity.

Chemistry. Valproic acid (*n*-dipropylacetic acid) is a simple branched-chain carboxylic acid; its structural formula is as follows:

$$CH_3CH_2CH_2 \diagdown \atop CH_3CH_2CH_2 \diagup CHCOOH$$

VALPROIC ACID

Certain other branched-chain carboxylic acids have potencies similar to that of valproic acid in antagonizing pentylenetetrazol-induced convulsions. However, increasing the number of carbon atoms to nine introduces marked sedative properties. Straight-chain acids have little or no activity. The primary amide of valproic acid is about twice as potent as the parent compound.

Pharmacological Effects. Valproic acid is strikingly different from phenytoin or ethosuximide in that it is effective in inhibiting seizures in a variety of models. Like phenytoin and carbamazepine, valproate inhibits tonic hindlimb extension in maximal electroshock seizures and kindled seizures at doses without toxicity. Like ethosuximide, valproic acid inhibits clonic motor seizures induced by pentylenetetrazol at subtoxic doses. Its efficacy in diverse models parallels its efficacy against absence as well as partial and generalized tonic-clonic seizures in human beings.

Mechanism of Action. Valproic acid produces effects on isolated neurons similar to those of both phenytoin and ethosuximide. At therapeutically relevant concentrations, valproate inhibits sustained repetitive firing induced by depolarization of mouse cortical or spinal cord neurons (McLean and Macdonald, 1986a). The action is similar to that of both phenytoin and carbamazepine and appears to be mediated by a prolonged recovery of voltage-activated Na^+ channels from inactivation. Valproic acid does not modify neuronal responses to iontophoretically applied GABA. In neurons isolated from a distinct region, the nodose ganglion, valproate also produces small reductions of the low-threshold (T) Ca^{2+} current (Kelly *et al.*, 1990) at clinically relevant but slightly higher concentrations than limit sustained repetitive firing; this effect on T currents is similar to that of ethosuximide in thalamic neurons (Coulter *et al.*, 1989). Together, these actions of limiting sustained repetitive firing and reducing T currents may contribute to the effectiveness of valproic acid against partial and tonic-clonic seizures and absence seizures, respectively.

Another potential mechanism that may contribute to valproate's antiseizure actions involves metabolism of GABA. Although valproate has no effect on responses to GABA, it does increase the amount of GABA that can be recovered from the brain after the drug is administered to animals. *In vitro*, valproate can stimulate the activity of the GABA synthetic enzyme, glutamic acid decarboxylase (Phillips and Fowler, 1982), and inhibit GABA degradative enzymes, GABA transaminase and succinic semialdehyde dehydrogenase (Chapman *et al.*, 1982). Thus far it has been difficult to relate the increased GABA levels to the antiseizure activity of valproate.

Pharmacokinetic Properties. Valproic acid is absorbed rapidly and completely after oral administration. Peak concentration in plasma is observed in 1 to 4 hours, although this can be delayed for several hours if the drug is administered in enteric-coated tablets or is ingested with meals. The apparent volume of distribution for valproate is about 0.2 liter/kg. Its extent of binding to plasma proteins is usually about 90%, but the fraction bound is reduced as the total concentration of valproate is increased through the therapeutic range. Although concentrations of valproate in CSF suggest equilibration with free drug in the blood, there is evidence for carrier-mediated transport of valproate both into and out of the CSF.

The vast majority of valproate (95%) undergoes hepatic metabolism, with less than 5% excreted unchanged. Its hepatic metabolism occurs mainly by UGT enzymes and β-oxidation. Valproate is a substrate for CYP2C9 and CYP2C19, but metabolism by these enzymes accounts for a relatively minor portion of its elimination. Some of the drug's metabolites, notably 2-propyl-2-pentenoic acid and 2-propyl-4-pentenoic acid, are nearly as potent antiseizure agents as the parent compound; however, only the former

(2-en-valproic acid) accumulates in plasma and brain to a potentially significant extent (*see* above). The half-life of valproate is approximately 15 hours but is reduced in patients taking other antiepileptic drugs.

Toxicity. The most common side effects are transient gastrointestinal symptoms, including anorexia, nausea, and vomiting in about 16% of patients. Effects on the CNS include sedation, ataxia, and tremor; these symptoms occur infrequently and usually respond to a decrease in dosage. Rash, alopecia, and stimulation of appetite have been observed occasionally. Valproic acid has several effects on hepatic function. Elevation of hepatic enzymes in plasma is observed in up to 40% of patients and often occurs asymptomatically during the first several months of therapy. A rare complication is a fulminant hepatitis that is frequently fatal (*see* Dreifuss *et al.,* 1989). Pathological examination reveals a microvesicular steatosis without evidence of inflammation or hypersensitivity reaction. Children below 2 years of age with other medical conditions who were given multiple antiseizure agents were especially likely to suffer fatal hepatic injury. At the other extreme, there were no deaths reported for patients over the age of 10 years who received only valproate. Acute pancreatitis and hyperammonemia also have been frequently associated with the use of valproic acid.

Plasma Drug Concentrations.   The concentration of valproate in plasma that is associated with therapeutic effects is approximately 30 to 100 μg/ml. However, the correlation between this concentration and efficacy is poor. There appears to be a threshold at about 30 to 50 μg/ml; this is the concentration at which binding sites on plasma albumin begin to become saturated.

Drug Interactions.   Valproate primarily inhibits drugs metabolized by CYP2C9 including phenytoin and phenobarbital. Valproate also inhibits UGT and thus inhibits the metabolism of lamotrigine and lorazepam. A high proportion of valproate is bound to albumin, and the high molar concentrations of valproate in the clinical setting result in valproate's displacing phenytoin and other drugs from albumin. With respect to phenytoin in particular, valproate's inhibition of the drug's metabolism is countered by displacement of phenytoin from albumin. The concurrent administration of valproate and clonazepam has been associated with the development of absence status epilepticus; however, this complication appears to be rare.

Therapeutic Uses.   Valproate is effective in the treatment of absence, myoclonic, partial, and tonic-clonic seizures. The initial daily dose usually is 15 mg/kg, and this is increased at weekly intervals by 5 to 10 mg/kg per day to a maximum daily dose of 60 mg/kg. Divided doses should be given when the total daily dose exceeds 250 mg. The therapeutic uses of valproate in epilepsy are discussed further at the end of this chapter.

BENZODIAZEPINES

The benzodiazepines are employed clinically primarily as sedative-antianxiety drugs; their pharmacology is presented in detail in Chapters 17 and 19. Discussion in this chapter is limited to consideration of their usefulness in the therapy of the epilepsies. A large number of benzodiazepines have broad antiseizure properties, but only *clonazepam* (KLONOPIN) and *clorazepate* (TRANXENE-SD; others) have been approved in the United States for the long-term treatment of certain types of seizures. *Diazepam* (VALIUM, DIASTAT; others) and *lorazepam* (ATIVAN) have well-defined roles in the management of status epilepticus. The structures of the benzodiazepines are shown in Chapter 17.

Antiseizure Properties. In animals, prevention of pentylenetetrazol-induced seizures by the benzodiazepines is much more prominent than is their modification of the maximal electroshock seizure pattern. Clonazepam is unusually potent in antagonizing the effects of pentylenetetrazol, but it is almost without action on seizures induced by maximal electroshock. Benzodiazepines, including clonazepam, suppress the spread of kindled seizures and generalized convulsions produced by stimulation of the amygdala, but do not abolish the abnormal discharge at the site of stimulation.

Mechanism of Action.   The antiseizure actions of the benzodiazepines, as well as other effects that occur at nonsedating doses, result in large part from their ability to enhance GABA-mediated synaptic inhibition. Molecular cloning and study of recombinant receptors have demonstrated that the benzodiazepine receptor is an integral part of the GABA$_A$ receptor (*see* Chapter 17). At therapeutically relevant concentrations, benzodiazepines act at subsets of GABA$_A$ receptors and increase the frequency, but not duration, of openings at GABA-activated chloride channels (Twyman *et al.,* 1989). At higher concentrations, diazepam and many other benzodiazepines can reduce sustained high-frequency firing of neurons, similar to the effects of phenytoin, carbamazepine, and valproate. Although these concentrations correspond to those achieved in patients during treatment of status epilepticus with diazepam, they are considerably higher than those associated with antiseizure or anxiolytic effects in ambulatory patients.

Pharmacokinetic Properties.   Benzodiazepines are well absorbed after oral administration, and concentrations in plasma are usually maximal within 1 to 4 hours. After intravenous administration, they are redistributed in a manner typical of that for highly lipid-soluble agents (*see* Chapter 1). Central effects develop promptly, but wane rapidly as the drugs move to other tissues. Diazepam is redistributed especially rapidly, with a half-life of redistribution of about 1 hour. The extent of binding of benzodiazepines to plasma proteins correlates with lipid solubility, ranging from approximately 99% for diazepam to about 85% for clonazepam (*see* Appendix II).

The major metabolite of diazepam, *N*-desmethyl-diazepam, is somewhat less active than the parent drug and may behave as a partial agonist. This metabolite also is produced by the rapid decarboxylation of clorazepate following its ingestion. Both diazepam and *N*-desmethyl-diazepam are slowly hydroxylated to other active metabolites, such as oxazepam. The half-life of diazepam in plasma is between 1 and 2 days, while that of *N*-desmethyl-diazepam is about 60 hours. Clonazepam is metabolized principally by reduction of the nitro group to produce inactive 7-amino derivatives. Less than 1% of the drug is recovered unchanged in the urine. The half-life of clonazepam in plasma is about 1 day. Lorazepam is metabolized chiefly by conjugation with glucuronic acid; its half-life in plasma is about 14 hours.

Toxicity.   The principal side effects of long-term oral therapy with clonazepam are drowsiness and lethargy. These occur in about 50% of patients initially, but tolerance often develops with continued administration. Muscular incoordination and ataxia are less frequent. Although these symptoms usually can be kept to tolerable levels by reducing the dosage or the rate at which it is increased, they sometimes force discontinuation of the drug. Other side effects include hypotonia, dysarthria, and dizziness. Behavioral disturbances, especially in children, can be very troublesome; these include aggression, hyperactivity, irritability, and difficulty in concentration. Both anorexia and hyperphagia have been reported. Increased salivary and bronchial secretions may cause difficulties in children. Seizures are sometimes exacerbated, and status epilepticus may be precipitated if the drug is discontinued abruptly. Other aspects of the toxicity of the benzodiazepines are discussed in Chapter 17. Cardiovascular and respiratory depression may occur after the intravenous administration of diazepam, clonazepam, or lorazepam, particularly if other antiseizure agents or central depressants have been administered previously.

Plasma Drug Concentrations.   Because tolerance affects the relationship between drug concentration and drug antiseizure effect, plasma concentrations of benzodiazepines are of limited value.

Therapeutic Uses.   Clonazepam is useful in the therapy of absence seizures as well as myoclonic seizures in children. However, tolerance to its antiseizure effects usually develops after 1 to 6 months of administration, after which some patients no longer will respond to clonazepam at

any dosage. The initial dose of clonazepam for adults should not exceed 1.5 mg per day and for children is 0.01 to 0.03 mg/kg per day. The dose-dependent side effects are reduced if two or three divided doses are given each day. The dose may be increased every 3 days in amounts of 0.25 to 0.5 mg per day in children and 0.5 to 1 mg per day in adults. The maximal recommended dose is 20 mg per day for adults and 0.2 mg/kg per day for children.

While diazepam is an effective agent for treatment of status epilepticus, its short duration of action is a disadvantage, leading to the frequent use of intravenous phenytoin in combination with diazepam. Diazepam is administered intravenously and at a rate of no more than 5 mg per minute. The usual dose for adults is 5 to 10 mg, as required; this may be repeated at intervals of 10 to 15 minutes, up to a maximal dose of 30 mg. If necessary, this regimen can be repeated in 2 to 4 hours, but no more than 100 mg should be administered in a 24-hour period.

Although diazepam is not useful as an oral agent for the treatment of seizure disorders, clorazepate is effective in combination with certain other drugs in the treatment of partial seizures. The maximal inital dose of clorazepate is 22.5 mg per day in three portions for adults and 15 mg per day in two doses in children. Clorazepate is not recommended for children under the age of 9.

OTHER ANTISEIZURE AGENTS

Gabapentin

Gabapentin (NEURONTIN) is an antiseizure drug that was approved by the United States Food and Drug Administration in 1993. The chemical structure of gabapentin is a GABA molecule covalently bound to a lipophilic cyclohexane ring. Gabapentin was designed to be a centrally active GABA agonist, its high lipid solubility aimed at facilitating its transfer across the blood-brain barrier. The structure of gabapentin is shown below:

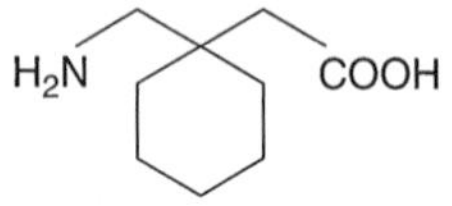

$$H_2N \qquad COOH$$

GABAPENTIN

Pharmacological Effects and Mechanisms of Action.
Gabapentin inhibits tonic hindlimb extension in the electroshock seizure model. Interestingly, gabapentin also inhibits clonic seizures induced by pentylenetetrazol. Its efficacy in both these tests parallels that of valproic acid and distinguishes it from phenytoin and carbamazepine. The

anticonvulsant mechanism of action of gabapentin is unknown. Despite its design as a GABA agonist, gabapentin does not mimic GABA when iontophoretically applied to neurons in primary culture. Gabapentin may promote nonvesicular release of GABA through a poorly understood mechanism (Honmou *et al.*, 1995). Gabapentin does bind a protein in cortical membranes with an amino acid sequence identical to that of the $\alpha 2\delta$ subunit of the L type of voltage-sensitive Ca^{2+} channel. Yet, gabapentin does not affect Ca^{2+} currents of the T, N, or L types of Ca^{2+} channels in dorsal root ganglion cells (Macdonald and Greenfield, 1997). Gabapentin has not been found consistently to reduce sustained repetitive firing of action potentials (Macdonald and Kelly, 1993).

Pharmacokinetics. Gabapentin is absorbed after oral administration and is not metabolized in human beings. It is excreted unchanged, mainly in the urine. Its half-life, when it is used as monotherapy, is 5 to 9 hours. Concurrent administration of gabapentin does not affect the plasma concentrations of phenytoin, carbamazepine, phenobarbital, or valproate.

Therapeutic Uses. Gabapentin is approved by the FDA for treating partial seizures, with and without secondary generalization, in adults when used in addition to other antiseizure drugs. Double-blind, placebo-controlled trials of patients with refractory partial seizures demonstrated that addition of gabapentin to other antiseizure drugs was superior to placebo. The median seizure decrease induced by gabapentin was approximately 27% compared with 12% for placebo. A double-blind study of gabapentin (900 or 1800 mg/day) monotherapy disclosed that gabapentin was similar in efficacy to carbamazepine (600 mg/day). Gabapentin also is being used for migraine, chronic pain, and bipolar disorder.

Gabapentin usually is effective in doses of 900 to 1800 mg daily in three doses. Therapy usually is begun with a low dose (300 mg once on the first day), and the dose is increased in daily increments of 300 mg until an effective dose is reached.

Toxicity. The most common adverse effects of gabapentin are somnolence, dizziness, ataxia, and fatigue. These effects usually are mild to moderate in severity but resolve within two weeks of onset during continued treatment. Overall, gabapentin is well tolerated.

Lamotrigine

Lamotrigine (LAMICTAL) is a phenyltriazine derivative initially developed as an antifolate agent based upon the

incorrect idea that reducing folate would effectively combat seizures. Structure-activity studies indicate that its effectiveness as an antiseizure drug is unrelated to its antifolate properties (Macdonald and Greenfield, 1997). It was approved by the Food and Drug Administration in 1994. Its chemical structure is:

LAMOTRIGINE

Pharmacological Effects and Mechanisms of Action. Lamotrigine suppresses tonic hindlimb extension in the maximal electroshock model and partial and secondarily generalized seizures in the kindling model but does not inhibit clonic motor seizures induced by pentylenetetrazol. Lamotrigine blocks sustained repetitive firing of mouse spinal cord neurons and delays the recovery from inactivation of recombinant Na^+ channels, mechanisms similar to those of phenytoin and carbamazepine (Xie *et al.*, 1995). This may well explain lamotrigine's actions on partial and secondarily generalized seizures. However, as mentioned below, lamotrigine is effective against a broader spectrum of seizures than phenytoin and carbamazepine, suggesting that lamotrigine may have actions in addition to regulating recovery from inactivation of Na^+ channels. The mechanisms underlying its broad spectrum of actions are incompletely understood. One possibility involves lamotrigine's inhibition of glutamate release in rat cortical slices treated with veratridine, a Na^+ channel activator, raising the possibility that lamotrigine inhibits synaptic release of glutamate by acting at Na^+ channels themselves.

Pharmacokinetics. Lamotrigine is completely absorbed from the gastrointestinal tract and is metabolized primarily by glucuronidation. The plasma half-life of a single dose is 24 to 35 hours. Administration of phenytoin, carbamazepine, phenobarbital, or primidone reduces the half-life of lamotrigine to approximately 15 hours and reduces plasma concentrations of lamotrigine. Conversely, addition of valproate markedly increases plasma concentrations of lamotrigine, likely by inhibiting glucuronidation. Addition of lamotrigine to valproic acid produces a reduction of valproate concentrations by approximately 25% over a few weeks. Concurrent use of lamotrigine and carbamazepine is associated with increases of the 10,11-epoxide of carbamazepine and clinical toxicity in some patients.

Therapeutic Use. Lamotrigine is useful for monotherapy and add-on therapy of partial and secondarily generalized tonic-clonic seizures in adults and Lennox-Gastaut syndrome in both children and adults. A double-blind comparison of lamotrigine and carbamazepine monotherapy in newly diagnosed partial or generalized tonic-clonic seizures disclosed similar efficacy for the two drugs, but lamotrigine was better tolerated (Brodie *et al.*, 1995). A double-blind, placebo-controlled trial of addition of lamotrigine to existing antiseizure drugs demonstrated effectiveness of lamotrigine against tonic-clonic seizures and drop attacks in children with the Lennox-Gastaut syndrome (Motte *et al.*, 1997). Lennox-Gastaut syndrome is a disorder of childhood characterized by multiple seizure types, mental retardation, and refractoriness to antiseizure medication. There also is emerging evidence that lamotrigine is effective against juvenile myoclonic epilepsy and absence epilepsy. Patients who already are taking a hepatic enzyme-inducing antiseizure drug (such as carbamazepine, phenytoin, phenobarbital, or primidone, but not valproate) should be given lamotrigine initially at 50 mg per day for 2 weeks. The dose is increased to 50 mg twice per day for 2 weeks and then increased in increments of 100 mg/day each week up to a maintenance dose of 300 to 500 mg/day divided into two doses. For patients taking valproate in addition to an enzyme-inducing antiseizure drug, the initial dose should be 25 mg every other day for 2 weeks, followed by an increase to 25 mg/day for 2 weeks; the dose then can be increased by 25 to 50 mg/day every 1 to 2 weeks up to a maintenance dose of 100 to 150 mg/day divided into two doses.

Toxicity. The most common adverse effects are dizziness, ataxia, blurred or double vision, nausea, vomiting, and rash when lamotrigine was added to another antiseizure drug. A few cases of Stevens-Johnson syndrome and disseminated intravascular coagulation have been reported.

Acetazolamide

Acetazolamide, the prototype for the carbonic anhydrase inhibitors, is discussed in Chapter 29. Its antiseizure actions are discussed in previous editions of this textbook. Although it is sometimes effective against absence seizures, its usefulness is limited by the rapid development of tolerance. Adverse effects are minimal when it is used in moderate dosage for limited periods.

Felbamate

Felbamate (FELBATOL) is a dicarbamate which was approved by the Food and Drug Administration for partial seizures in 1993.

An association between felbamate and aplastic anemia in at least ten cases resulted in a recommendation by the Food and Drug Administration and the manufacturer for the immediate withdrawal of most patients from treatment with this drug. The structure of felbamate is shown below:

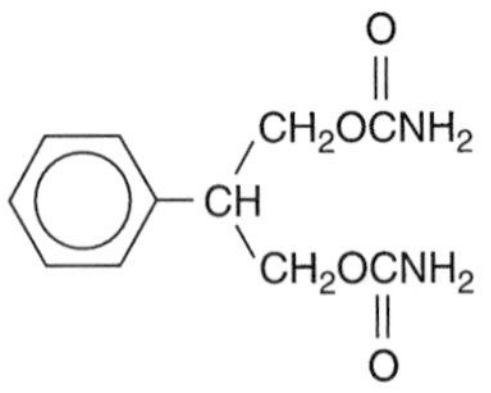

FELBAMATE

Felbamate is effective in both the maximal electroshock and pentylenetetrazol seizure models. Clinically relevant concentrations of felbamate inhibit NMDA-evoked responses and potentiate GABA-evoked responses in whole-cell, voltage-clamp recordings of cultured rat hippocampal neurons (Rho *et al.*, 1994). This dual action on excitatory and inhibitory transmitter responses may contribute to the wide spectrum of action of the drug in seizure models.

An active control, randomized, double-blind protocol demonstrated the efficacy of felbamate in patients with poorly controlled partial and secondarily generalized seizures (Sachdeo *et al.*, 1992). Felbamate also was found to be efficacious against seizures in patients with Lennox-Gastaut syndrome (The Felbamate Study Group in Lennox-Gastaut Syndrome, 1993). The clinical efficacy of this compound, which inhibited responses to NMDA and potentiated those to GABA, underscores the potential value of additional antiseizure agents with similar mechanisms of action.

Levetiracetam

Levetiracetam (KEPPRA) is a pyrrolidine, the racemically pure *S*-enantiomer of α-ethyl-2-oxo-1-pyrrolidineacetamide, which was approved by the Food and Drug Administration in 1999 for treating partial seizures in adults when used in addition to other drugs. Its structure is:

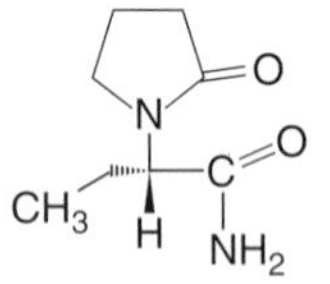

LEVETIRACETAM

Pharmacological Effects and Mechanism of Action. Levetiracetam exhibits a novel pharmacological profile insofar as it inhibits partial and secondarily generalized tonic-clonic seizures in the kindling model yet is ineffective against maximum electroshock- and pentylenetetrazol-induced seizures, findings consistent with effectiveness against partial and secondarily generalized tonic-clonic seizures clinically. The mechanism by which levetiracetam exerts these antiseizure effects is unknown. No evidence for an action on voltage-gated Na^+ channels or either GABA- or glutamate-mediated synaptic transmission has emerged. A stereoselective binding site has been identified in rat brain membranes, but the molecular identity of this site remains obscure.

Pharmacokinetics. Levetiracetam is rapidly and almost completely absorbed after oral administration. Ninety-five percent of the drug and its metabolite are excreted in the urine, 65% of which is unchanged drug; 24% of the drug is metabolized by hydrolysis of the acetamide group. It neither induces nor is a high-affinity substrate for cytochrome P450 isoforms or glucuronidation enzymes and thus is devoid of known interactions with other antiseizure drugs, oral contraceptives, or anticoagulants.

Therapeutic Use. A double-blind, placebo-controlled trial of adults with refractory partial seizures demonstrated that addition of levetiracetam to other antiseizure medications was superior to placebo. Its efficacy for monotherapy is being investigated.

Toxicity. The drug is well tolerated. The most frequently reported adverse effects are somnolence, asthenia, and dizziness.

Tiagabine

Tiagabine (GABITRIL) is a derivative of nipecotic acid that was approved by the Food and Drug Administration in 1998 for treating partial seizures in adults when used in addition to other drugs. Its structure is as follows:

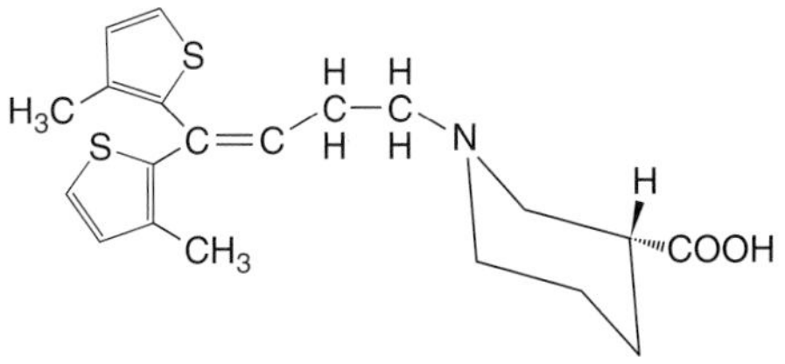

TIAGABINE

Pharmacological Effects and Mechanism of Action. Tiagabine inhibits the GABA transporter, GAT-1, and thereby reduces GABA uptake into neurons and glia. In CA1 neurons of the hippocampus, tiagabine increases the duration of inhibitory synaptic currents, findings consistent with prolonging the effect of GABA at inhibitory synapses through reducing its reuptake by GAT-1. Tiaga-

bine inhibits maximum electroshock seizures and both limbic and secondarily generalized tonic-clonic seizures in the kindling model, results suggestive of efficacy against partial and tonic-clonic seizures clinically.

Pharmacokinetics. Tiagabine is rapidly absorbed after oral administration, extensively bound to proteins, and metabolized mainly in the liver and predominantly by CYP3A. Its half-life is about 8 hours but is shortened by 2 to 3 hours when coadministered with hepatic enzyme-inducing drugs such as phenobarbital, phenytoin, or carbamazepine.

Therapeutic Use. Double-blind, placebo-controlled trials have established tiagabine's efficacy as add-on therapy of refractory partial seizures with or without secondary generalization. Its efficacy for monotherapy for this indication has not yet been established.

Toxicity. The principal adverse effects include dizziness, somnolence, and tremor; they appear to be mild to moderate in severity, and appear shortly after drug initiation. The fact that tiagabine and other drugs thought to enhance effects of synaptically released GABA can facilitate spike-and-wave discharges in animal models of absence seizures raises the possibility that tiagabine may be contraindicated in patients with generalized absence epilepsy.

Topiramate

Topiramate (TOPAMAX) is a sulfamate-substituted monosaccharide that was approved by the Food and Drug Administration in 1996 for partial seizures in adults when used in addition to other drugs. Its structure is as follows:

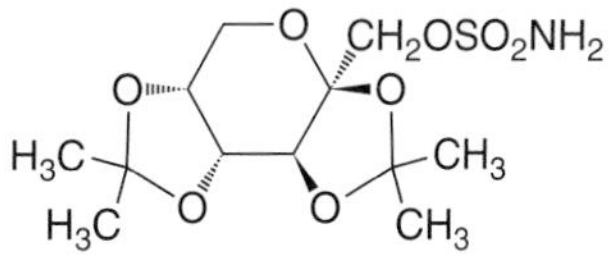

TOPIRAMATE

Pharmacological Effects and Mechanisms of Action. Topiramate reduces voltage-gated Na^+ currents in cerebellar granule cells and may act on the inactivated state of the channel in a manner similar to that of phenytoin. In addition, topiramate enhances postsynaptic $GABA_A$-receptor currents and also limits activation of the AMPA-kainate-subtype(s) of glutamate receptor. Topiramate also is a weak carbonic anhydrase inhibitor. Topiramate inhibits maximal electroshock and pentylenetetrazol-induced seizures as well as partial and secondarily generalized tonic-clonic seizures in the kindling model, findings predictive of a broad spectrum of antiseizure actions clinically.

Pharmacokinetics. Topiramate is rapidly absorbed after oral administration and is mainly excreted unchanged in the urine. The remainder undergoes metabolism by hydroxylation, hydrolysis, and glucuronidation with no one metabolite accounting for more than 5% of an oral dose. Its half-life is about a day. Reduced estradiol plasma concentrations occur with concurrent topiramate, suggesting the need for higher doses of oral contraceptives when coadministered with topiramate.

Therapeutic Use. Double-blind, placebo-controlled studies established the efficacy of topiramate in both adults and children with refractory partial seizures with or without secondary generalized tonic-clonic seizures. Topiramate also was found to be significantly more effective than placebo against both drop attacks and tonic-clonic seizures in patients with Lennox-Gastaut syndrome and against tonic-clonic and myoclonic seizures in adults and children with primary generalized epilepsy. A pilot study suggests that topiramate may be effective against infantile spasms.

Toxicity. Topiramate is well tolerated. The most common adverse effects are somnolence, fatigue, weight loss, and nervousness.

Zonisamide

Zonisamide (ZONEGRAN) is a sulfonamide derivative that was approved by the Food and Drug Administration in 2000 for partial seizures in adults when used in addition to other drugs. Its structure is as follows:

ZONISAMIDE

Pharmacological Effects and Mechanism of Action. Zonisamide inhibits the T-type Ca^{2+} currents. In addition, zonisamide inhibits the sustained, repetitive firing of spinal cord neurons, presumably by prolonging the inactivated state of voltage-gated Na^+ channels in a manner similar to actions of phenytoin and carbamazepine. Zonisamide inhibits tonic hindlimb extension evoked by maximal electroshock and inhibits both partial and secondarily

generalized seizures in the kindling model, results predictive of clinical effectiveness against partial and secondarily generalized tonic-clonic seizures. Zonisamide does not inhibit minimal clonic seizures induced by pentylenetetrazol, suggesting that the drug will not be effective clinically against myoclonic seizures. Zonisamide's inhibition of T-type Ca^{2+} currents suggests that it may be effective against absence seizures, yet its effects in absence models such as the lethargic mouse or the absence epileptic rat of Strasbourg have not been reported.

Pharmacokinetics. Zonisamide is almost completely absorbed after oral administration, has a long half-life (about 63 hours), and is about 40% bound to plasma protein. Approximately 85% of an oral dose is excreted in the urine, principally as unmetabolized zonisamide and a glucuronide of sulfamoylacetyl phenol, which is a product of metabolism by CYP3A4. Phenobarbital, phenytoin, and carbamazepine decrease the plasma concentration/dose ratio of zonisamide, whereas lamotrigine increases this ratio. Conversely, zonisamide has little effect on the plasma concentrations of other antiseizure drugs.

Therapeutic Use. Double-blind, placebo-controlled studies of patients with refractory partial seizures demonstrated that addition of zonisamide to other drugs was superior to placebo. Additional studies of zonisamide have been initiated in absence seizures, infantile spasms, and Lennox-Gastaut syndrome, but only largely anecdotal data are currently available.

Toxicity. Overall, zonisamide is well tolerated. The most common adverse effects include somnolence, ataxia, anorexia, nervousness, and fatigue. Approximately 1% of individuals develop renal calculi during treatment with zonisamide; the mechanism of this effect is obscure.

GENERAL PRINCIPLES AND CHOICE OF DRUGS FOR THE THERAPY OF THE EPILEPSIES

Early diagnosis and treatment of seizure disorders with a single appropriate agent offers the best prospect of achieving prolonged seizure-free periods with the lowest risk of toxicity. An attempt should be made to determine the cause of the epilepsy with the hope of discovering a correctable lesion, either structural or metabolic. The efficacy of antiseizure drugs has been assessed in clinical trials on the basis of seizure type, not epilepsy syndrome type, and thus seizure type determines drug selection. The drugs commonly used for distinct seizure types are listed in Table 21–1. The efficacy combined with the unwanted effects of a given drug determine which particular drug is optimal for a given patient.

The first issue that arises is whether or not and when to initiate treatment. For example, it may not be necessary to initiate antiseizure therapy after an isolated tonic-clonic seizure in a healthy young adult who lacks a family history of epilepsy and who has a normal neurological exam, a normal EEG, and a normal brain magnetic resonance imaging (MRI) scan. That is, the odds of seizure recurrence in the next year (15%) approximate the risk of a drug reaction sufficiently severe to warrant discontinuation of medication (Bazil and Pedley, 1998). Alternatively, a similar seizure occurring in an individual with a positive family history of epilepsy, an abnormal neurological exam, an abnormal EEG, and an abnormal MRI carries a risk of recurrence approximating 60%, odds that favor initiation of therapy.

Unless extenuating circumstances such as status epilepticus exist, medication should be initiated with a single drug. Initial dosage usually is that expected to provide a plasma drug concentration during the plateau state at least in the lower portion of the range associated with clinical efficacy. To minimize dose-related adverse effects, therapy with many drugs is initiated at reduced dosage. Dosage is increased at appropriate intervals, as required for control of seizures or as limited by toxicity, and such adjustment is preferably assisted by monitoring of drug concentrations in plasma. Compliance with a properly selected, single drug in maximal tolerated dosage results in complete control of seizures in approximately 50% of patients. If a seizure occurs despite optimal drug levels, the physician should assess the presence of potential precipitating factors such as sleep deprivation, a concurrent febrile illness, or drugs; drugs might consist of large amounts of caffeine or even over-the-counter medications, which can include drugs that can lower the seizure threshold.

If compliance has been confirmed yet seizures persist, another drug should be substituted. Unless serious adverse effects of the drug dictate otherwise, dosage always should be reduced gradually when a drug is being discontinued to minimize risk of seizure recurrence. In the case of partial seizures in adults, the diversity of available drugs permits selection of a second drug that acts by a distinct mechanism. Smith *et al.* (1987) found that 55% of such patients could be managed satisfactorily on a second single drug, yet others report that only 9% to 11% of patients with complex partial seizures failing an initial drug achieve complete seizure control with a second single drug (Schmidt and Richter, 1986; Dasheiff *et al.,* 1986).

In the event that therapy with a second single drug also is inadequate, many physicians resort to treatment with two drugs simultaneously. This decision should not be taken lightly, because most patients obtain optimal seizure control with fewest unwanted effects when taking a single drug. Nonetheless, some patients will not be controlled adequately without the use of two or more antiseizure agents simultaneously. No properly controlled studies have compared systematically one particular drug combination with another. It seems wise to select two drugs that act by distinct mechanisms (*e.g.*, one that promotes Na^+ channel inactivation and another that enhances GABA-mediated synaptic inhibition). Additional issues that warrant careful consideration are the unwanted effects of each drug and the potential drug interactions. As specified in Table 21–2, many of these drugs induce expression of cytochrome P450 enzymes and thereby impact the metabolism of themselves and/or other drugs. Overall, the more recently developed antiseizure drugs present fewer problems with respect to drug interactions. If a patient fails two drugs in monotherapy, the odds that polytherapy will provide complete control are small. Alternative measures such as epilepsy surgery should be considered.

Essential to optimal management of epilepsy is the filling out of a seizure chart by the patient or a relative. Frequent visits to the physician or seizure clinic may be necessary early in the period of treatment, since hematological and other possible side effects may require consideration of a change in medication. Long-term follow-up with neurological examinations and possibly EEG and neuroimaging studies is appropriate. Most crucial for successful management is regularity of medication, since faulty compliance is the most frequent cause for failure of therapy with antiseizure drugs.

Measurement of plasma drug concentration at appropriate intervals greatly facilitates the initial adjustment of dosage for individual differences in drug elimination and the subsequent adjustment of dosage to minimize dose-related adverse effects without sacrifice of seizure control. Periodic monitoring during maintenance therapy can detect failure of the patient to take the medication as prescribed. Knowledge of plasma drug concentration can be especially helpful during multiple-drug therapy. If toxicity occurs, monitoring helps to identify the particular drug(s) responsible, and if pharmacokinetic drug interaction occurs, monitoring can guide readjustment of dosage.

Duration of Therapy. In an attempt to provide guidelines for withdrawal of antiseizure drugs, Shinnar *et al.* (1994) prospectively studied 264 children in whom antiseizure drugs were discontinued after a mean seizure-free interval of 2.9 years. Children were followed for a mean of 58 months to assess seizure recurrence. Seizures recurred in 36% of children. Factors associated with an increased risk of recurrence included a positive family history of epilepsy, presence of slowing on EEG prior to withdrawal, onset of epilepsy after age 12 (compared with younger ages), atypical febrile seizures, and certain epileptic syndromes such as juvenile myoclonic epilepsy.

In a prospective study, the treatment of patients with generalized or partial seizures was stopped after 2 seizure-free years; only patients who had been treated with a single drug (phenytoin, carbamazepine, or valproate) were included (Callaghan *et al.*, 1988). The overall rate of relapse (within 3 years) was approximately 33% in both children and adults. Although only 92 patients were studied, the risk of relapse was apparently greatest for patients with complex partial seizures or those who had a persistently abnormal EEG.

Although these and other results are encouraging, it is not yet possible to provide clear guidelines for the selection of patients for withdrawal from therapy. Such decisions must be made on an individual basis, weighing both the medical and psychosocial consequences of recurrence of seizures against the potential toxicity associated with prolonged therapy.

If a decision to withdraw antiseizure drugs is made, such withdrawal should be done gradually over a period of months. The risk of status epilepticus is increased with abrupt cessation of therapy.

Simple and Complex Partial and Secondarily Generalized Tonic-Clonic Seizures. The efficacy and toxicity of carbamazepine, phenobarbital, phenytoin, and primidone for treatment of partial and secondarily generalized tonic-clonic seizures in adults have been examined in a double-blind prospective study (Mattson *et al.*, 1985). A subsequent double-blind prospective study compared carbamazepine with valproate (Mattson *et al.*, 1992). Carbamazepine and phenytoin were the most effective overall for single-drug therapy of partial or generalized tonic-clonic seizures. The choice between carbamazepine and phenytoin required assessment of toxic effects of drugs. Primidone was associated with greater incidence of toxicity early in the course of therapy, including nausea, dizziness, ataxia, and somnolence. Decreased libido and impotence were associated with all four drugs (carbamazepine 13%, phenobarbital 16%, phenytoin 11%, and primidone 22%), but significantly more commonly with primidone. The study comparing carbamazepine with valproate revealed that carbamazepine provided superior control of complex partial seizures. With respect to adverse effects, carbamazepine was more commonly associated with skin rash, but valproate was more commonly associated with tremor and weight gain. Overall, the data demonstrated that carbamazepine and phenytoin are preferable for treatment of partial seizures, but phenobarbital, valproic acid, and primidone are efficacious. A double-blind comparison of lamotrigine and carbamazepine disclosed similar efficacy of the two drugs, but lamotrigine was better tolerated (Brodie *et al.*, 1995). Lamotrigine is used for monotherapy of partial and secondarily generalized tonic-clonic seizures. Multiple drugs recently were approved for add-on therapy of these seizures, including gabapentin, levetiracetam, tiagabine, topiramate, and zonisamide.

Control of secondarily generalized tonic-clonic seizures did not differ significantly with carbamazepine, phenobarbital, phenytoin, or primidone (Mattson *et al.*, 1985). Valproate was as effective as carbamazepine for control of secondarily generalized tonic-clonic seizures (Mattson *et al.*, 1992). Since secondarily generalized tonic-clonic seizures usually coexist with partial seizures, carbamazepine, phenytoin, and lamotrigine are the first-line drugs for these conditions.

Absence Seizures. The best current data indicate that ethosuximide and valproate are equally effective in the treatment of absence seizures (*see* Mikati and Browne, 1988). Between 50% and 75% of newly diagnosed patients can be rendered free of seizures. In the event that tonic-clonic seizures are present or emerge during therapy, valproate is the agent of first choice. Emerging evidence suggests that lamotrigine is effective for absence seizures (Bazil and Pedley, 1998).

Myoclonic Seizures. Valproic acid is the drug of choice for myoclonic seizures in the syndrome of juvenile myoclonic epilepsy, in which myoclonic seizures often coexist with tonic-clonic and also absence seizures. Monotherapy with lamotrigine may be effective in some patients with juvenile myoclonic epilepsy in whom valproic acid proves unsatisfactory (Bazil and Pedley, 1998).

Febrile Convulsions. Two percent to 4% of children experience a convulsion associated with a febrile illness. From 25% to 33% of these children will have another febrile convulsion. Only 2% to 3% become epileptic in later years. This is a sixfold increase in risk compared with the general population. Several factors are associated with an increased risk of developing epilepsy: preexisting neurological disorder or developmental delay, a family history of epilepsy, or a complicated febrile seizure (*i.e.*, the febrile seizure lasted more than 15 minutes, was one-sided, or was followed by a second seizure in the same day). If all of these risk factors are present, the risk of developing epilepsy is only 10%.

Concern regarding the increased risk of developing epilepsy or other neurological sequelae led many physicians to prescribe antiseizure drugs prophylactically after a febrile seizure. Uncertainties regarding the efficacy of prophylaxis for reducing epilepsy combined with substantial side effects of phenobarbital prophylaxis (Farwell *et al.*, 1990) argue against the use of chronic therapy for prophylactic purposes (Freeman, 1992). For children at high risk of developing recurrent febrile seizures and epilepsy, rectally administered diazepam at the time of fever may prevent recurrent seizures and avoid side effects of chronic therapy.

Seizures in Infants and Young Children. Infantile spasms with hypsarrhythmia are refractory to the usual antiseizure agents; corticotropin or the adrenocorticosteroids are commonly used. A randomized study found *vigabatrin* (γ-vinyl GABA) to be efficacious in comparison to placebo (Appleton *et al.*, 1999). Constriction of visual fields has been reported in some adults treated with vigabatrin (Miller *et al.*, 1999). The drug has not been approved by the U.S. Food and Drug Administration but is available in other countries.

The Lennox-Gastaut syndrome is a severe form of epilepsy which usually begins in childhood and is characterized by cognitive impairments and multiple types of seizures including tonic-clonic, tonic, atonic, myoclonic, and atypical absence seizures. Addition of lamotrigine to other antiseizure drugs resulted in improved seizure control in comparison to placebo in a double-blind trial (Motte *et al.*, 1997), demonstrating lamotrigine to be an effective and well-tolerated drug for this treatment-resistant form of epilepsy. Felbamate also was found to be effective for seizures in this syndrome, but the occasional occurrence of aplastic anemia has limited its use.

Status Epilepticus and Other Convulsive Emergencies. Status epilepticus is a neurological emergency. Mortality for adults approximates 20% (Lowenstein and Alldredge, 1998). The goal of treatment is rapid termination of behavioral and electrical seizure activity; the longer the episode of status epilepticus is untreated, the more difficult it is to control and the risk of permanent brain damage increases. Critical to the management is a clear plan, prompt treatment with effective drugs in adequate doses, and attention to hypoventilation and hypotension. Since hypoventilation may result from high doses of drugs used for treatment, it may be necessary to assist respiration temporarily. Drugs should be administered by intravenous route only. Because of slow and unreliable absorption, the intramuscular route has no place in treatment of status epilepticus. To assess the optimal initial drug regimen, a double-blind, multicenter trial compared four intravenous treatments: diazepam followed by phenytoin; lorazepam; phenobarbital; and phenytoin alone (Treiman *et al.*, 1998). The treatments were shown to have similar efficacies, in that success rates ranged from 44% to 65%, but lorazepam alone was significantly better than phenytoin alone. No significant differences were found with respect to recurrences or adverse reactions.

Antiseizure Therapy and Pregnancy. Use of antiseizure drugs has diverse implications of great importance for the health of women, issues considered in guidelines articulated by the American Academy of Neurology (Morrell, 1998). These issues include interactions with oral contraceptives, potential teratogenic effects, and effects on vitamin K metabolism in pregnant women.

The effectiveness of oral contraceptives appears to be reduced by concomitant use of antiseizure drugs. The failure rate of oral contraceptives is 3.1/100 years in women receiving antiseizure drugs compared to a rate of 0.7/100 years in nonepileptic women. One attractive explanation of the increased failure rate is the increased rate of oral contraceptive metabolism caused by antiseizure drugs that induce hepatic enzymes (*see* Table 21–2); particular caution is needed with any antiseizure drug that induces CYP3A4. The apparent teratogenic effects of antiseizure drugs add to the deleterious consequences of oral contraceptive failure.

Epidemiological evidence suggests that antiseizure drugs have teratogenic effects. Infants of epileptic mothers are at twofold greater risk of major congenital malformations than offspring of nonepileptic mothers (4% to

8% compared to 2% to 4%). These malformations include congenital heart defects, neural tube defects, and others. Inferring causality from the associations found in large epidemiological studies with many uncontrolled variables can be hazardous, but a causal role for antiseizure drugs is suggested by association of congenital defects with higher concentrations of a drug or with polytherapy compared to monotherapy. Phenytoin, carbamazepine, valproate, and phenobarbital all have been associated with teratogenic effects. Whether or not the recently developed antiseizure drugs also will be associated with teratogenic effects awaits clinical experience with these agents. One consideration for a woman with epilepsy who wishes to become pregnant is a trial free of antiseizure drug; monotherapy with careful attention to drug levels is another alternative. Polytherapy with toxic levels should be avoided. Folate supplementation (0.4 mg/day) has been recommended by the United States Public Health Service for all women of childbearing age to reduce the likelihood of neural tube defects, and this is appropriate for epileptic women as well.

Antiseizure drugs that induce cytochrome P450 enzymes have been associated with vitamin K deficiency in the newborn, which can result in a coagulopathy and intracerebral hemorrhage in the neonate. Treatment with vitamin K_1, 10 mg/day during the last month of gestation, has been recommended for prophylaxis.

PROSPECTUS

Improved therapies for epilepsy are likely to emerge from several lines of investigation over the next decade: (1) Clinical experience and additional clinical trials with the recently approved antiseizure drugs should optimize their utilization for diverse forms of epilepsy. (2) Increased insight into genetic, cellular, and molecular mechanisms of epilepsy emerging from basic investigations should lead to the development of drugs acting by mechanisms distinct from currently available medications. (3) Insight into cellular and molecular mechanisms of epileptogenesis emerging from studies of animal models should lead to pharmacological prophylaxis of individuals at high risk of developing epilepsy. (4) Pharmacogenomic investigations should optimize selection of antiseizure drugs efficacious in a given individual and permit identification of individuals at high risk for devastating, idiosyncratic drug effects.

For further discussion of the epilepsies and convulsive disorders, *see* Chapter 365 in *Harrison's Principles of Internal Medicine,* 14th ed., McGraw-Hill, New York, 1998.

BIBLIOGRAPHY

Anderson, G.D. A mechanistic approach to antiepileptic drug interactions. *Ann. Pharmacother.,* **1998,** *32*:554–563.

Appleton, R.E., Peters, A.C., Mumford, J.P., and Shaw, D.E. Randomised, placebo-controlled study of vigabatrin as first-line treatment of infantile spasms. *Epilepsia,* **1999,** *40*:1627–1633.

Ayala, G.F., Dichter, M., Gumnit, R.J., Matsumoto, H., and Spencer, W.A. Genesis of epileptic interictal spikes. New knowledge of cortical feedback systems suggests a neurophysiological explanation of brief paroxysms. *Brain Res.,* **1973,** *52*:1–17.

Bievert, C., Schroeder, B.C., Kubisch, C., Berkovic, S.F., Propping, P., Jentsch, T.J., and Steinlein, O.K. A potassium channel mutation in neonatal human epilepsy. *Science,* **1998,** *279*:403–406.

Brodie, M.J., Richens, A., and Yuen, A.W. Double-blind comparison of lamotrigine and carbamazepine in newly diagnosed epilepsy. UK Lamotrigine/Carbamazepine Monotherapy Trial Group. *Lancet,* **1995,** *345*:476–479.

Callaghan, N., Garrett, A., and Goggin, T. Withdrawal of anticonvulsant drugs in patients free of seizures for two years. A prospective study. *N. Engl. J. Med.,* **1988,** *318*:942–946.

Chapman, A., Keane, P.E., Meldrum, B.S., Simiand, J., and Vernieres, J.C. Mechanism of anticonvulsant action of valproate. *Prog. Neurobiol.,* **1982,** *19*:315–359.

Charlier, C., Singh, N.A., Ryan, S.G., Lewis, T.B., Reus, B.E., Leach, R.J., and Leppert, M. A pore mutation in a novel KQT-like potassium channel gene in an idiopathic epilepsy family. *Nat. Genet.,* **1998,** *18*:53–55.

Commission on Classification and Terminology of the International League Against Epilepsy. Proposal for revised clinical and electroencephalographic classification of epileptic seizures. *Epilepsia,* **1981,** *22*:489–501.

Commission on Classification and Terminology of the International League Against Epilepsy. Proposal for revised classification of epilepsies and epileptic syndromes. *Epilepsia,* **1989,** *30*:389–399.

Coulter, D.A., Huguenard, J.R., and Prince, D.A. Characterization of ethosuximide reduction of low-threshold calcium current in thalamic neurons. *Ann. Neurol.,* **1989,** *25*:582–593.

Dasheiff, R.M., McNamara, D., and Dickinson, L. Efficacy of second-line antiepileptic drugs in the treatment of patients with medically refractive complex partial seizures. *Epilepsia,* **1986,** *27*:124–127.

Dreifuss, F.E., Langer, D.H., Moline, K.A., and Maxwell, J.E. Valproic acid hepatic fatalities. II. U.S. experience since 1984. *Neurology,* **1989,** *39*:201–207.

Farwell, J.R., Lee, Y.J., Hirtz, D.G., Sulzbacher, S.I., Ellenberg, J.H., and Nelson, K.B. Phenobarbital for febrile seizures—effects on intelligence and on seizure recurrence. *N. Engl. J. Med.,* **1990,** *322*:364–369.

The Felbamate Study Group in Lennox-Gastaut Syndrome. Efficacy of felbamate in childhood epileptic encephalopathy (Lennox-Gastaut syndrome). *N. Engl. J. Med.,* **1993,** *328*: 29–33.

ffrench-Mullen, J.M., Barker, J.L., and Rogawski, M.A. Calcium current block by (−)-pentobarbital, phenobarbital, and CHEB but not (+)-pentobarbital in acutely isolated hippocampal CA1 neurons: comparison with effects on GABA-activated Cl⁻ current. *J. Neurosci.,* **1993,** *13*:3211–3221.

Goddard, G.V., McIntyre, D.C., and Leech, C.K. A permanent change in brain function resulting from daily electrical stimulation. *Exp. Neurol.,* **1969,** *25*:295–330.

Hauptmann, A. Luminal bei Epilepsie Munch. *Med. Wochenschr.,* **1912,** *59*:1907–1909.

Honmou, O., Kocsis, J.D., and Richerson, G.B. Gabapentin potentiates the conductance increase induced by nipecotic acid in CA1 pyramidal neurons *in vitro. Epilepsy Res.,* **1995,** *20*:193–202.

Jasper, H.H., and Droogleever-Fortuyn, J. Experimental studies of the functional anatomy of petit mal epilepsy. *Assoc. Res. Nerv. Ment. Dis. Proc.,* **1947,** *26*:272–298.

Kelly, K.M., Gross, R.A., and Macdonald, R.L. Valproic acid selectively reduces the low-threshold (T) calcium current in rat nodose neurons. *Neurosci. Lett.,* **1990,** *116*:233–238.

Lemos, T., and Cavalheiro, E.A. Suppression of pilocarpine-induced status epilepticus and the late development of epilepsy in rats. *Exp. Brain Res.,* **1995,** *102*:423–428.

Longo, B.M., and Mello, L.E. Supragranular mossy fiber sprouting is not necessary for spontaneous seizures in the intrahippocampal kainate model of epilepsy in the rat. *Epilepsy Res.,* **1998,** *32*:172–182.

Macdonald, R.L., and Barker, J.L. Anticonvulsant and anesthetic barbiturates: different postsynaptic actions in cultured mammalian neurons. *Neurology,* **1979,** *29*:432–447.

Mattson, R.H., Cramer, J.A., Collins, J.F., Smith, D.B., Delgado-Escueta, A.V., Browne, T.R., Williamson, P.D., Treiman, D.M., McNamara, J.O., McCutchen, C.B., Homan, R.W., Crill, W.E., Lubozynski, M.F., Rosenthal, N.P., and Mayersdorf, A. Comparison of carbamazepine, phenobarbital, phenytoin, and primidone in partial and secondarily generalized tonic-clonic seizures. *N. Engl. J. Med.,* **1985,** *313*:145–151.

Mattson, R.H., Cramer, J.A., and Collins, J.F. A comparison of valproate with carbamazepine for the treatment of complex partial seizures and secondarily generalized tonic-clonic seizures in adults. The Department of Veterans Affairs Epilepsy Cooperative Study No. 264 Group. *N. Engl. J. Med.,* **1992,** *327*:765–771.

McLean, M.J., and Macdonald, R.L. Multiple actions of phenytoin on mouse spinal cord neurons in cell culture. *J. Pharmacol. Exp. Ther.,* **1983,** *227*:779–789.

McLean, M.J., and Macdonald, R.L. Sodium valproate, but not ethosuximide, produces use- and voltage-dependent limitation of high-frequency repetitive firing of action potentials of mouse central neurons in cell culture. *J. Pharmacol. Exp. Ther.,* **1986a,** *237*:1001–1011.

McLean, M.J., and Macdonald, R.L. Carbamazepine and 10,11-epoxycarbamazepine produce use- and voltage-dependent limitation of rapidly firing action potentials of mouse central neurons in cell culture. *J. Pharmacol. Exp. Ther.,* **1986b,** *238*:727–738.

McNamara, J.O. Emerging insights into the genesis of epilepsy. *Nature,* **1999,** *399*:A15–A22.

Merritt, H.H., and Putnam, T.J. A new series of anticonvulsant drugs tested by experiments on animals. *Arch. Neurol. Psychiatry,* **1938a,** *39*:1003–1015.

Merritt, H.H., and Putnam, T.J. Sodium diphenyl hydantoinate in treatment of convulsive disorders. *JAMA,* **1938b,** *111*:1068–1073.

Miller, N.R., Johnson, M.A., Paul, S.R., Girkin, C.A., Perry, J.D., Endres, M., and Krauss, G.L. Visual dysfunction in patients receiving vigabatrin: clinical and electrophysiologic findings. *Neurology,* **1999,** *53*:2082–2087.

Morrell, M.J. Guidelines for the care of women with epilepsy. *Neurology,* **1998,** *51*:S21–S27.

Motte, J., Trevathan, E., Arvidsson, J.F., Barrera, M.N., Mullens, E.L., and Manasco, P. Lamotrigine for generalized seizures associated with the Lennox-Gastaut syndrome. Lamictal Lennox-Gastaut Study Group. *N. Engl. J. Med.,* **1997,** *337*:1807–1812.

Penfield, W.G., and Jasper, H.H. Highest level seizures. *Assoc. Res. Nerv. Ment. Dis. Proc.,* **1947,** *26*:252–271.

Phillips, N.I., and Fowler, L.J. The effects of sodium valproate on gamma-aminobutyrate metabolism and behaviour in naive and ethanolamine-0-sulphate pretreated rats and mice. *Biochem. Pharmacol.,* **1982,** *31*:2257–2261.

Ptacek, L.J. Channelopathies: ion channel disorders of muscle as a paradigm for paroxysmal disorders of the nervous system. *Neuromuscul. Disord.,* **1997,** *7*:250–255.

Puranam, R.S., and McNamara, J.O. Seizure disorders in mutant mice: relevance to human epilepsies. *Curr. Opin. Neurobiol.,* **1999,** *9*:281–287.

Rho, J.M., Donevan, S.D., and Rogawski, M.A. Mechanism of action of the anticonvulsant felbamate: opposing effects on *N*-methyl-D-aspartate and GABA$_A$ receptors, *Ann. Neurol.,* **1994,** *35*:229–234.

Sachdeo R., Kramer, L.D., Rosenberg, A., and Sachdeo, S. Felbamate monotherapy: controlled trial in patients with partial onset seizures. *Ann. Neurol.,* **1992,** *32*:386–392.

Schmidt, D., and Richter, K. Alternative single anticonvulsant drug therapy for refractory epilepsy. *Ann. Neurol.,* **1986,** *19*:85–87.

Shinnar, S., Berg, A.T., Moshe, S.L., Kang, H., O'Dell, C., Alemany, M., Goldensohn, E.S., and Hauser, W.A. Discontinuing antiepileptic drugs in children with epilepsy: a prospective study. *Ann. Neurol.,* **1994,** *35*:534–545.

Singh, N.A., Charlier, C., Stauffer, D., DuPont, B.R., Leach, R.J., Melis, R., Ronen, G.M., Bjerre, I., Quattlebaum, T., Murphy, J.V., McHarg, M.L., Gagnon, D., Rosales, T.O., Peiffer, A., Anderson, V.E., and Leppert, M. A novel potassium channel gene, *KCNQ2,* is mutated in an inherited epilepsy of newborns. *Nat. Genet.,* **1998,** *18*:25–29.

Smith, D.B., Mattson, R.H., Cramer, J.A., Collins, J.F., Novelly, R.A., and Craft, B. Results of a nationwide Veterans Administration cooperative study comparing the efficacy and toxicity of carbamazepine, phenobarbital, phenytoin, and primidone. *Epilepsia,* **1987,** *28(suppl 3)*: S50–S58.

Steinlein, O.K., Mulley, J.C., Propping, P., Wallace, R.H., Phillips, H.A., Sutherland, G.R., Scheffer, I.E., and Berkovic, S.F. A missense mutation in the neuronal nicotinic acetylcholine receptor α_4 subunit is associated with autosomal dominant nocturnal frontal lobe epilepsy. *Nat. Genet.,* **1995,** *11*:201–203.

Suzdak, P.D., and Jansen, J.A. A review of the preclinical pharmacology of tiagabine: a potent and selective anticonvulsant GABA uptake inhibitor. *Epilepsia,* **1995,** *36*:612–626.

Traynelis, S.F., and Dingledine, R. Potassium-induced spontaneous electrographic seizures in the rat hippocampal slice. *J. Neurophysiol.,* **1988,** *59*:259–276.

Treiman, D.M., Meyers, P.D., Walton, N.Y., Collins, J.F., Colling, C., Rowan, A.J., Handforth, A., Faught, E., Calabrese, V.P., Uthman,

B.M., Ramsay, R.E., and Mamdani, M.B. A comparison of four treatments for generalized convulsive status epilepticus. Veterans Affairs Status Epilepticus Cooperative Study Group. *N. Engl. J. Med.,* **1998,** *339*:792–798.

Twyman, R.E., Rogers, C.J., and Macdonald, R.L. Differential regulation of γ-aminobutyric acid receptor channels by diazepam and phenobarbital. *Ann. Neurol.,* **1989,** *25*:213–220.

VanLandingham, K.E., Heinz, E.R., Cavazos, J.E., and Lewis, D.V. Magnetic resonance imaging evidence of hippocampal injury after prolonged febrile convulsions. *Ann. Neurol.,* **1998,** *43*:413–426.

Wallace, R.H., Wang, D.W., Singh, R., Scheffer, I.E., George, A.L. Jr., Phillips, H.A., Saar, K., Reis, A., Johnson, E.W., Sutherland, G.R., Berkovic, S.F., and Mulley, J.C. Febrile seizures and generalized epilepsy associated with a mutation in the Na$^+$-channel β1 subunit gene *SCN1B. Nat. Genet.,* **1998,** *19*:366–370.

Xie, X., Lancaster, B., Peakman, T., and Garthwaite, J. Interaction of the antiepileptic drug lamotrigine with recombinant rat brain type IIA Na$^+$ channels and with native Na$^+$ channels in rat hippocampal neurones. *Pflugers Arch.,* **1995,** *430*:437–446.

MONOGRAPHS AND REVIEWS

Bazil, C.W., and Pedley, T.A. Advances in the medical treatment of epilepsy. *Annu. Rev. Med.,* **1998,** *49*:136–162.

Berkovic, S. In, *Epilepsy: A Comprehensive Textbook.* (Engel, J. Jr., and Pedley, T.A., eds.), Lippincott-Raven, Philadelphia, **1998,** pp. 217–224.

Coulter, D.A. Thalamocortical anatomy and physiology. In, *Epilepsy: A Comprehensive Textbook.* Vol. 1. (Engel, J. Jr., and Pedley, T.A., eds.) Lippincott-Raven, Philadelphia, **1998,** pp. 341–353.

Dichter, M.A., and Ayala, G.F. Cellular mechanisms of epilepsy: a status report. *Science,* **1987,** *237*:157–164.

Freeman, J.M. The best medicine for febrile seizures. *N. Engl. J. Med.,* **1992,** *327*:1161–1163.

Lowenstein, D.H., and Alldredge, B.K. Status epilepticus. *N. Engl. J. Med.,* **1998,** *338*:970–976.

Macdonald, R.L., and Greenfield, L.J. Jr. Mechanisms of action of new antiepileptic drugs. *Curr. Opin. Neurol.,* **1997,** *10*:121–128.

Macdonald, R.L., and Kelly, K.M. Antiepileptive drug mechanisms of action. *Epilepsia,* **1993,** *34(suppl 5)*:51–58.

McNamara, J.O. Development of new pharmacological agents for epilepsy: lessons from the kindling model. *Epilepsia,* **1989,** *30(suppl 1)*: S13–S18.

McNamara, J.O. Cellular and molecular basis of epilepsy. *J. Neurosci.,* **1994,** *14*:3413–3425.

Mikati, M.A. and Browne, T.R. Comparative efficacy of antiepileptic drugs. *Clin. Neuropharmacol.,* **1988,** *11*:130–140.

TREATMENT OF CENTRAL NERVOUS SYSTEM DEGENERATIVE DISORDERS

David G. Standaert and Anne B. Young

The neurodegenerative diseases include common and debilitating disorders such as Parkinson's disease, Alzheimer's disease, Huntington's disease, and amyotrophic lateral sclerosis (ALS). Although the clinical and neuropathological aspects of these disorders are distinct, their unifying feature is that each disorder has a characteristic pattern of neuronal degeneration in anatomically or functionally related regions.

Presently available pharmacological treatments for the neurodegenerative disorders are symptomatic and do not alter the course or progression of the underlying disease. The most effective symptomatic therapies are those for Parkinson's disease; a large number of agents from several different pharmacological classes can be used, and, when skillfully applied, these can have a dramatic impact on life span and functional ability. The treatments available for Alzheimer's disease, Huntington's disease, and ALS are less satisfactory but still can make an important contribution to patient welfare.

This chapter reviews current therapeutic agents for treatment of the symptoms of neurodegenerative diseases and introduces the reader to research aimed at developing therapeutic agents that alter the course of neurodegenerative diseases by preventing neuronal death or stimulating neuronal recovery. Related material concerning the serotonergic effects of some of the therapeutic agents employed for Parkinson's disease can be found in Chapter 11, and additional information concerning cholinergic agents that are used in treatment of Alzheimer's disease can be found in Chapters 7 and 8.

Neurodegenerative disorders are characterized by progressive and irreversible loss of neurons from specific regions of the brain. Prototypical neurodegenerative disorders include Parkinson's disease (PD) and Huntington's disease (HD), where loss of neurons from structures of the basal ganglia results in abnormalities in the control of movement; Alzheimer's disease (AD), where the loss of hippocampal and cortical neurons leads to impairment of memory and cognitive ability; and amyotrophic lateral sclerosis (ALS), where muscular weakness results from the degeneration of spinal, bulbar, and cortical motor neurons. As a group, these disorders are relatively common and represent a substantial medical and societal problem. They are primarily disorders of later life, developing in individuals who are neurologically normal, although childhood-onset forms of each of the disorders are recognized. PD is observed in more than 1% of individuals over the age of 65 (Tanner, 1992), whereas AD affects as many as 10% of the same population (Evans *et al.,* 1989). HD, which is a genetically determined autosomal dominant disorder, is less frequent in the population as a whole but affects 50% of each generation in families carrying the gene. ALS also is relatively rare but often leads rapidly to disability and death (Kurtzke, 1982).

At present, the pharmacological therapy of neurodegenerative disorders is limited to symptomatic treatments that do not alter the course of the underlying disease. Symptomatic treatment for PD, where the neurochemical deficit produced by the disease is well defined, is in general relatively successful, and a number of effective agents are available (Lang and Lozano, 1998; Standaert and Stern, 1993). The available treatments for AD, HD, and ALS are much more limited in effectiveness, and the need for new strategies is particularly acute.

SELECTIVE VULNERABILITY AND NEUROPROTECTIVE STRATEGIES

Selective Vulnerability.   The most striking feature of this group of disorders is the exquisite specificity of the disease processes for particular types of neurons. For example, in PD there is extensive destruction of the dopaminergic neurons of the substantia nigra, while neurons in the cortex and many other areas of the brain are unaffected (Gibb, 1992; Fearnley and Lees, 1994). In contrast, neural injury in AD is most severe in the hippocampus and neocortex, and even within the cortex, the loss of neurons is not uniform but varies dramatically in different functional regions (Arnold *et al.,* 1991). Even more striking is the observation that, in HD, the mutant gene responsible for the disorder is expressed throughout the brain and in many other organs, yet the pathological changes are largely restricted to the neostriatum (Vonsattel *et al.,* 1985; Landwehrmeyer *et al.,* 1995). In ALS, there is loss of spinal motor neurons and the cortical neurons that provide their descending input (Tandan and Bradley, 1985). The diversity of these patterns of neural degeneration has led to the proposal that the process of neural injury must be viewed as the interaction of genetic and environmental influences with the intrinsic physiological characteristics of the affected populations of neurons. These intrinsic factors may include susceptibility to excitotoxic injury, regional variation in capacity for oxidative metabolism, and the production of toxic free radicals as products of cellular metabolism (Figure 22–1). The factors that convey selective vulnerability may prove to be important targets for neuroprotective agents to slow the progression of neurodegenerative disorders.

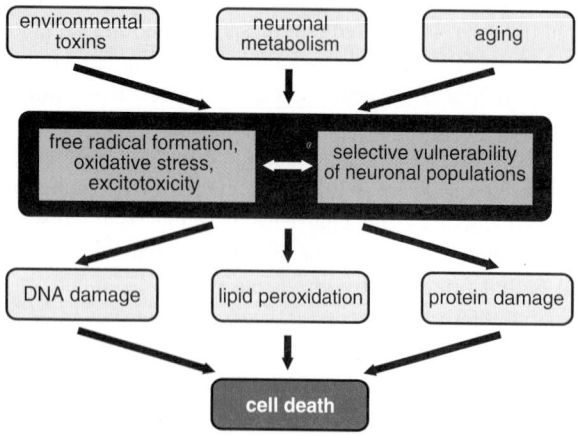

Figure 22–1. Mechanisms of selective neuronal vulnerability in neurodegenerative diseases.

Genetics.   It has been long suspected that genetics plays an important role in the etiology of neurodegenerative disorders, and recent discoveries have begun to shed light on some mechanisms responsible. HD is transmitted by autosomal dominant inheritance, and the molecular nature of the genetic defect has been identified (*discussed below*). Most cases of PD, AD, or ALS are sporadic, but families with a high incidence of each of these diseases have been identified, and these studies have begun to yield important clues to the pathogenesis of the disorders. In the case of PD, mutations in three different proteins can lead to autosomal dominant forms of the disease: alpha-synuclein, an abundant synaptic protein; parkin, a ubiquitin hydrolase; and UCHL1, which also participates in ubiquitin-mediated degradation of proteins in the brain (Duvoisin, 1998; Golbe, 1999; Kitada *et al.,* 1998). In AD, mutations in the genes coding for the amyloid precursor protein (APP) and proteins known as the presenilins (which may be involved in APP processing) lead to inherited forms of the disease (Selkoe, 1998). Mutations in the gene coding for copper-zinc superoxide dismutase (SOD1) account for about 2% of the cases of adult-onset ALS (Cudkowicz and Brown, 1996). Although these mutations are rare, their importance extends beyond the families that carry them, because they point to pathways and mechanisms that also may underlie the more common, sporadic cases of these diseases.

Genetically determined cases of PD, AD, and ALS are infrequent, but it is likely that an individual's genetic background has an important role in determining the probability of acquiring these diseases. Recent studies of AD have revealed the first of what are likely to be many genetic risk factors for neurodegenerative disorders, in the form of apolipoprotein E (apo E). This protein, well known to be involved in transport of cholesterol and lipids in blood, is found in four distinct isoforms. Although all of the isoforms carry out their primary role in lipid metabolism equally well, individuals who are homozygous for the apo E 4 allele ("4/4") have a much higher lifetime risk of AD than do those homozygous for the apo E 2 allele ("2/2"). The mechanism by which the apo E 4 protein increases the risk of AD is not known, but a secondary function of the protein in metabolism of APP has been suggested (Roses, 1997).

Environmental Triggers.   Infectious agents, environmental toxins, and acquired brain injury have been proposed to have a role in the etiology of neurodegenerative disorders. The role of infection is best documented in the numerous cases of PD that developed following the epidemic of encephalitis lethargica (Von Economo's encephalitis) in the early part of the twentieth century. Most contemporary cases of PD are not preceded by encephalitis, and there is no convincing evidence for an infectious contribution to HD, AD, or ALS. Traumatic brain injury has been suggested as a trigger for neurodegenerative disorders, and in the case of AD there is some evidence to support this view (Cummings *et al.,* 1998). At least one toxin, *N*-methyl-4-phenyl-1,2,3,6-tetrahydropyridine (MPTP; *discussed below*), can induce a condition closely resembling PD, but evidence for the widespread occurrence of this or a similar toxin in the environment is lacking (Tanner and Langston, 1990).

Excitotoxicity. The term *excitotoxicity* was coined by Olney (1969) to describe the neural injury that results from the presence of excess glutamate in the brain. Glutamate is used as a neurotransmitter by many different neural systems and is believed to mediate most excitatory synaptic transmission in the mammalian brain (*see* Chapter 12). Although glutamate is required for normal brain function, the presence of excessive amounts of glutamate can lead to excitotoxic cell death (Lipton and Rosenberg, 1994). The destructive effects of glutamate are mediated by glutamate receptors, particularly those of the *N*-methyl-D-aspartate (NMDA) type. Unlike other glutamate-gated ion channels, which primarily regulate the flow of Na^+, activated NMDA receptor-channels allow an influx of Ca^{2+}, which in excess can activate a variety of potentially destructive processes. The activity of NMDA receptor-channels is regulated not only by the concentration of glutamate in the synaptic space but also by a voltage-dependent blockade of the channel by Mg^{2+}; thus, entry of Ca^{2+} into neurons through NMDA receptor-channels requires binding of glutamate to NMDA receptors as well as depolarization of the neuron (*e.g.,* by the activity of glutamate at non-NMDA receptors), which relieves the blockade of NMDA channels by extracellular Mg^{2+}. Excitotoxic injury is thought to make an important contribution to the neural death that occurs in acute processes such as stroke and head trauma (Choi and Rothman, 1990). In the chronic neurodegenerative disorders, the role of excitotoxicity is less certain, but it is thought that regional and cellular differences in susceptibility to excitotoxic injury—conveyed, for example, by differences in types of glutamate receptors—may contribute to selective vulnerability (Young, 1993).

Energy, Metabolism, and Aging. The excitotoxic hypothesis provides a link between selective patterns of neuronal injury, the effects of aging, and observations on the metabolic capacities of neurons (Beal *et al.,* 1993). Since the ability of Mg^{2+} to block the NMDA receptor-channel

is dependent on the membrane potential, disturbances that impair the metabolic capacity of neurons will tend to relieve Mg^{2+} blockade and predispose to excitotoxic injury. The capacity of neurons for oxidative metabolism declines progressively with age, perhaps in part because of a progressive accumulation of mutations in the mitochondrial genome (Wallace, 1992). Patients with PD exhibit several defects in energy metabolism that are even greater than expected for their age, most notably a reduction in the function of complex I of the mitochondrial electron transport chain (Schapira *et al.,* 1990). Additional evidence for the role of metabolic defects in the etiology of neural degeneration comes from the study of patients who inadvertently self-administered MPTP, a "designer drug" that resulted in symptoms of severe and irreversible parkinsonism (Ballard *et al.,* 1985). Subsequent studies have shown that a metabolite of MPTP induces degeneration of neurons similar to that observed in idiopathic PD and that its mechanism of action appears to be related to an ability to impair mitochondrial energy metabolism in dopaminergic neurons (Przedborski and Jackson-Lewis, 1998). In rodents, neural degeneration similar to that observed in HD can be produced either by direct administration of large doses of NMDA receptor agonists or by more chronic administration of inhibitors of mitochondrial oxidative metabolism, suggesting that disturbances of energy metabolism may underlie the selective pathology of HD as well (Beal *et al.,* 1986, 1993).

Oxidative Stress. Although neurons depend on oxidative metabolism for survival, a consequence of this process is the production of reactive compounds such as hydrogen peroxide and oxyradicals (Cohen and Werner, 1994). Unchecked, these reactive species can lead to DNA damage, peroxidation of membrane lipids, and neuronal death. Several mechanisms serve to limit this *oxidative stress,* including the presence of reducing compounds such as ascorbate and glutathione and enzymatic mechanisms such as superoxide dismutase, which catalyzes the reduction of superoxide radicals. Oxidative stress also may be relieved by aminosteroid agents that serve as free radical scavengers. In PD, attention has been focused on the possibility that oxidative stress induced by the metabolism of dopamine may underlie the selective vulnerability of dopaminergic neurons (Jenner, 1998). The primary catabolic pathway of dopamine to 3,4-dihydroxyphenylacetic acid (DOPAC) is catalyzed by monoamine oxidase (MAO) and generates hydrogen peroxide. Hydrogen peroxide, in the presence of ferrous ion, which is relatively abundant in the basal ganglia, may generate hydroxyl free radicals (the

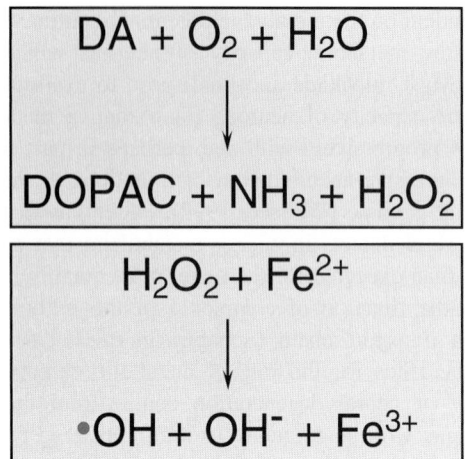

$$DA + O_2 + H_2O$$
$$\downarrow$$
$$DOPAC + NH_3 + H_2O_2$$

$$H_2O_2 + Fe^{2+}$$
$$\downarrow$$
$$\bullet OH + OH^- + Fe^{3+}$$

Figure 22–2. Production of free radicals by the metabolism of dopamine (DA).

DA is converted by monamine oxidase (MAO) and aldehyde dehydrogenase to 3,4-dihydroxyphenylacetic acid (DOPAC), producing hydrogen peroxide (H_2O_2). In the presence of ferrous iron, H_2O_2 undergoes spontaneous conversion, forming a hydroxyl free radical (the Fenton reaction).

Fenton reaction, Figure 22–2; Olanow, 1990). If the protective mechanisms are inadequate because of inherited or acquired deficiency, the oxyradicals could cause degeneration of dopaminergic neurons. This hypothesis has led to several proposals for therapeutic agents to retard neuronal loss in PD. Two candidates, the free radical scavenger *tocopherol* (vitamin E) and the MAO inhibitor *selegiline* (*discussed below*), have been tested in a large-scale clinical trial, but neither was shown to have a substantial neuroprotective effect (The Parkinson Study Group, 1993).

PARKINSON'S DISEASE

Clinical Overview. Parkinsonism is a clinical syndrome comprising four cardinal features: bradykinesia (slowness and poverty of movement), muscular rigidity, resting tremor (which usually abates during voluntary movement), and an impairment of postural balance leading to disturbances of gait and falling. The most common cause of parkinsonism is idiopathic PD, first described by James Parkinson in 1817 as *paralysis agitans,* or the "shaking palsy." The pathological hallmark of PD is a loss of the pigmented, dopaminergic neurons of the substantia nigra pars compacta, with the appearance of intracellular inclusions known as Lewy bodies (Gibb, 1992; Fearnley and Lees, 1994). Progressive loss of dopamine neurons is a feature

of normal aging; however, most people do not lose the 70% to 80% of dopaminergic neurons required to cause symptomatic PD. Without treatment, PD progresses over 5 to 10 years to a rigid, akinetic state in which patients are incapable of caring for themselves. Death frequently results from complications of immobility, including aspiration pneumonia or pulmonary embolism. The availability of effective pharmacological treatment has altered radically the prognosis of PD; in most cases, good functional mobility can be maintained for many years, and the life expectancy of adequately treated patients is substantially increased (Diamond *et al.,* 1987). It is important to recognize that several disorders other than PD also may produce parkinsonism, including some relatively rare neurodegenerative disorders, stroke, and intoxication with dopamine receptor–blocking drugs. Drugs in common clinical use that may cause parkinsonism include antipsychotics such as *haloperidol* and *thorazine* (*see* Chapter 20) and antiemetics such as *prochlorperazine* and *metoclopramide* (*see* Chapter 38). Although a complete discussion of the clinical diagnostic approach to parkinsonism exceeds the scope of this chapter, the distinction between PD and other causes of parkinsonism is important, because parkinsonism arising from other causes usually is refractory to all forms of treatment.

Parkinson's Disease: Pathophysiology. The primary deficit in PD is a loss of the neurons in the substantia nigra pars compacta that provide dopaminergic innervation to the striatum (caudate and putamen). The current understanding of the pathophysiology of PD can be traced to the classical neurochemical investigations in the 1950s and 1960s, in which a more than 80% reduction in the striatal dopamine content was demonstrated. This parallelled the loss of neurons from the substantia nigra, suggesting that replacement of dopamine could restore function (Cotzias *et al.,* 1969; Hornykiewicz, 1973). These fundamental observations led to an extensive investigative effort to understand the metabolism and actions of dopamine and to learn how a deficit in dopamine gives rise to the clinical features of PD. This effort led to a current model of the function of the basal ganglia that admittedly is incomplete but is still useful.

Biosynthesis of Dopamine. Dopamine, a catecholamine, is synthesized in the terminals of dopaminergic neurons from tyrosine, which is transported across the blood–brain barrier by an active process (Figures 22–3 and 22–4). The rate-limiting step in the synthesis of dopamine is the conversion of L-tyrosine to L-dihydroxyphenylalanine (L-DOPA), catalyzed by the enzyme tyrosine hydroxylase which is present within catecholaminergic neurons. L-DOPA is converted rapidly to dopamine by aromatic

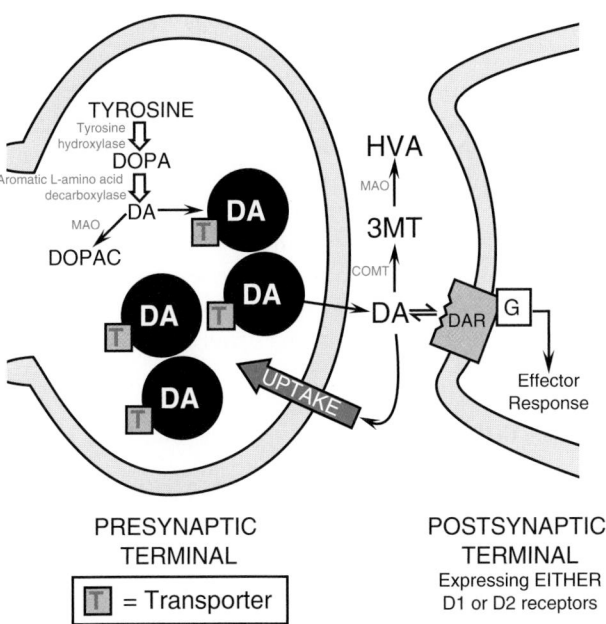

Figure 22–3. Dopaminergic terminal.

Dopamine (DA) is synthesized within neuronal terminals from the precursor tyrosine by the sequential actions of the enzymes tyrosine hydroxylase, producing the intermediary L-dihydroxyphenylalanine (DOPA), and aromatic L-amino acid decarboxylase. In the terminal, dopamine is transported into storage vesicles by a transporter protein (T) associated with the vesicular membrane. Release, triggered by depolarization and entry of Ca^{2+}, allows dopamine to act on postsynaptic dopamine receptors (DAR); as discussed in the text, several distinct types of dopamine receptors are present in the brain, and the differential actions of dopamine on postsynaptic targets bearing different types of dopamine receptors have important implications for the function of neural circuits. The actions of dopamine are terminated by the sequential actions of the enzymes catechol-O-methyltransferase (COMT) and monoamine oxidase (MAO), or by reuptake of dopamine into the terminal.

L-amino acid decarboxylase. In dopaminergic nerve terminals, dopamine is taken up into vesicles by a transporter protein; this process is blocked by reserpine, which leads to depletion of dopamine. Release of dopamine from nerve terminals occurs through exocytosis of presynaptic vesicles, a process that is triggered by depolarization leading to entry of Ca^{2+}. Once dopamine is in the synaptic cleft, its actions may be terminated by reuptake through a membrane carrier protein, a process antagonized by drugs such as cocaine. Alternatively, dopamine can be degraded by the sequential actions of MAO and catechol-O-methyltransferase (COMT) to yield two metabolic products, 3,4-dihydroxyphenylacetic acid (DOPAC) and 3-methoxy-4-hydroxyphenylacetic acid (HVA). In human beings, HVA is the primary product of the metabolism of dopamine (Cooper *et al.*, 1996).

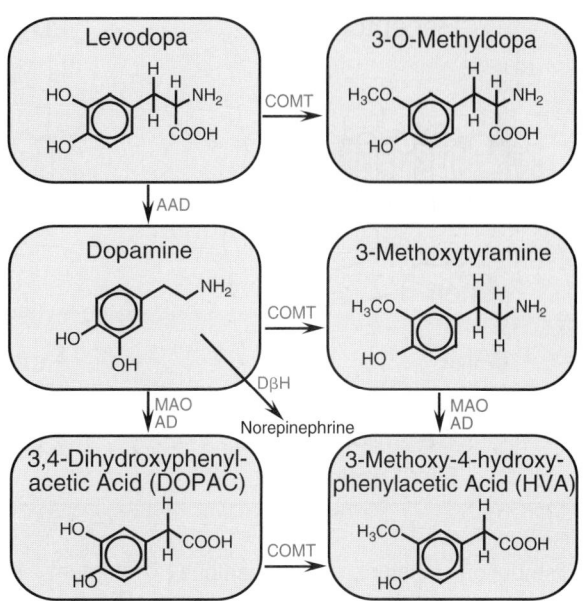

Figure 22–4. Metabolism of levodopa (L-DOPA).

AD, aldehyde dehydrogenase; COMT, catechol-O-methyltransferase; DβH, dopamine β-hydroxylase; AAD, aromatic L-amino acid decarboxylase; MAO, monoamine oxidase.

Dopamine Receptors. The actions of dopamine in the brain are mediated by a family of dopamine receptor proteins (Figure 22–5). Two types of dopamine receptors were identified in the mammalian brain using pharmacological techniques: D_1 receptors, which stimulate the synthesis of the intracellular second messenger cyclic AMP, and D_2 receptors, which inhibit cyclic AMP synthesis as well as suppress Ca^{2+} currents and activate receptor-operated K^+ currents. Application of molecular genetics to the study of dopamine receptors has revealed a more complex receptor situation than originally envisioned. At present, five distinct dopamine receptors are known to exist (*see* Jarvie and Caron, 1993, and Chapter 12). The dopamine receptors share several structural features, including the presence of seven α-helical segments capable of spanning the cell membrane. This structure identifies the dopamine receptors as members of the larger superfamily of seven-transmembrane-region receptor proteins, which includes other important neural receptors such as β-adrenergic receptors, olfactory receptors, and the visual pigment rhodopsin. All members of this superfamily act through guanine nucleotide-binding proteins (G proteins; *see* Chapter 2).

The five dopamine receptors can be divided into two groups on the basis of their pharmacological and structural properties (Figure 22–5). The D_1 and D_5 proteins have a long intracellular carboxy-terminal tail and are members of the pharmacologically defined D_1 class; they stimulate the formation of cyclic AMP and phosphatidyl inositol hydrolysis. The D_2, D_3, and D_4 receptors share a large third intracellular loop and are of the D_2 class. They decrease cyclic AMP formation and modulate K^+ and Ca^{2+} currents. Each of the five dopamine receptor proteins has a distinct anatomical pattern of expression in the

D₁ Receptor Family

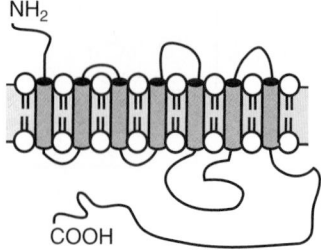

⬆ cAMP
⬆ PIP₂ hydrolysis
  · Ca²⁺ mobilization
  · PKC activation

	D₁	D₅
Distribution	· striatum	· hippocampus
	· neocortex	· hypothalamus

D₂ Receptor Family

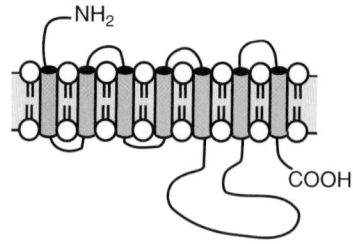

⬇ cAMP
⬆ K⁺ currents
⬇ ψ-gated Ca²⁺ currents

	D₂	D₃	D₄
	· striatum	· olf. tubercle	· frontal cortex
	· SNpc	· n. accumbens	· medulla
	· pituitary	· hypothalamus	· midbrain

Figure 22–5. Distribution and characteristics of dopamine receptors.

SNpc, substantia nigra pars compacta; cAMP, cyclic AMP; Ψ, voltage.

brain. The D₁ and D₂ proteins are abundant in the striatum and are the most important receptor sites with regard to the causes and treatment of PD. The D₄ and D₅ proteins are largely extrastriatal, while D₃ expression is low in the caudate and putamen but more abundant in the nucleus accumbens and olfactory tubercle.

Neural Mechanism of Parkinsonism.   Considerable effort has been devoted to understanding how the loss of dopaminergic input to the neurons of the neostriatum gives rise to the clinical features of PD (for review *see* Albin *et al.,* 1989; Mink and Thach, 1993; and Wichmann and DeLong, 1993). The basal ganglia can be viewed as a modulatory side loop that regulates the flow of information from the cerebral cortex to the motor neurons of the spinal cord (Figure 22–6). The neostriatum is the principal input structure of the basal ganglia and receives excitatory glutamatergic input from many areas of the cortex. The majority of neurons within the striatum are projection neurons that innervate other basal ganglia structures. A small but important subgroup of striatal neurons are interneurons that interconnect neurons within the striatum but do not project beyond its borders. Acetylcholine as well as neuropeptides are used as transmitters by the striatal interneurons. The outflow of the striatum proceeds along two distinct routes, identified as the direct and indirect pathways. The direct pathway is formed by neurons in the striatum that project directly to the output stages of the basal ganglia, the substantia nigra pars reticulata (SNpr) and the medial globus pallidus (MGP); these in turn relay to the ventroanterior and ventrolateral thalamus, which provides excitatory input to the cortex. The neurotransmitter of both links of the direct pathway is gamma-aminobutyric acid (GABA), which is inhibitory, so that the net effect of stimulation of the direct pathway at the level of the striatum is to increase the excitatory outflow from the thalamus to the cortex. The indi-

rect pathway is composed of striatal neurons that project to the lateral globus pallidus (LGP). This structure in turn innervates the subthalamic nucleus (STN), which provides outflow to the SNpr and MGP output stage. As in the direct pathway, the first two links—the projections from striatum to LGP and LGP to STN—use the inhibitory transmitter GABA; however, the final link—the projection from STN to SNpr and MGP—is an excitatory glutamatergic pathway. Thus the net effect of stimulating the indirect pathway at the level of the striatum is to reduce the excitatory outflow from the thalamus to the cerebral cortex.

The key feature of this model of basal ganglia function, which accounts for the symptoms observed in PD as a result of loss of dopaminergic neurons, is the differential effect of dopamine on the direct and indirect pathways (Figure 22–7). The dopaminergic neurons of the substantia nigra pars compacta (SNpc) innervate all parts of the striatum; however, the target striatal neurons express distinct types of dopamine receptors. The striatal neurons giving rise to the direct pathway express primarily the *excitatory* D₁ dopamine receptor protein, while the striatal neurons forming the indirect pathway express primarily the *inhibitory* D₂ type. Thus, dopamine released in the striatum tends to increase the activity of the direct pathway and reduce the activity of the indirect pathway, whereas the depletion that occurs in PD has the opposite effect. The net effect of the reduced dopaminergic input in PD is to increase markedly the inhibitory outflow from the SNpr and MGP to the thalamus and reduce excitation of the motor cortex.

This model of basal ganglia function has important implications for the rational design and use of pharmacological agents in PD. First, it suggests that, to restore the balance of the system through stimulation of dopamine receptors, the complementary effect of actions at both D₁ and D₂ receptors, as well as the possibility of adverse effects that may be mediated by

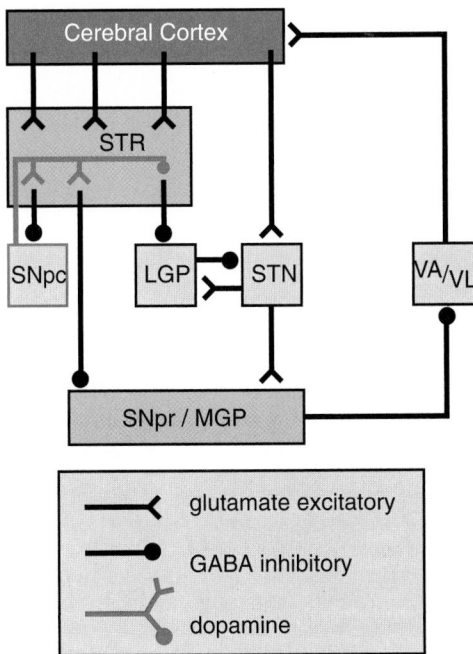

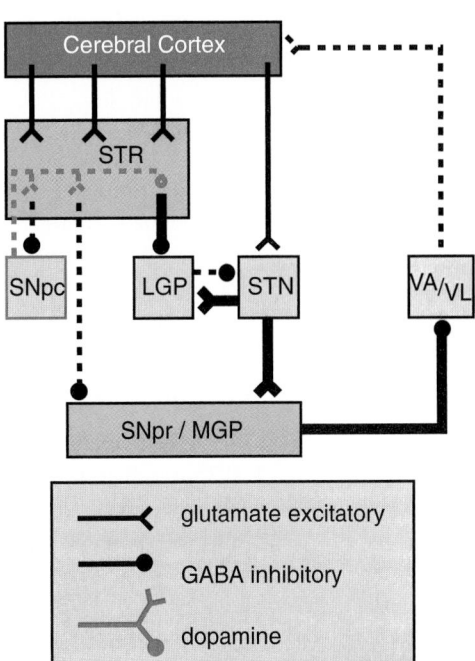

Figure 22–6. Schematic wiring diagram of the basal ganglia.

The neostriatum (STR) is the principal input structure of the basal ganglia and receives excitatory, glutamatergic input from many areas of cerebral cortex. Outflow from the STR proceeds along two routes. The direct pathway, from the STR to the substantia nigra pars reticulata (SNpr) and medial globus pallidus (MGP), uses the inhibitory transmitter GABA. The indirect pathway, from the STR through the lateral globus pallidus (LGP) and the subthalamic nucleus (STN) to the SNpr and MGP consists of two inhibitory, GABAergic links and one excitatory, glutamatergic projection. The substantia nigra pars compacta (SNpc) provides dopaminergic innervation to the striatal neurons giving rise to both the direct and indirect pathways, and regulates the relative activity of these two paths. The SNpr and MGP are the output structures of the basal ganglia, and provide feedback to the cerebral cortex through the ventroanterior and ventrolateral nuclei of the thalamus (VA/VL).

Figure 22–7. The basal ganglia in Parkinson's disease (PD).

The primary defect is destruction of the dopaminergic neurons of the SNpc. The striatal neurons that form the direct pathway from the STR to the SNpr and MGP express primarily the *excitatory* D1 dopamine receptor, while the striatal neurons that project to the LGP and form the indirect pathway express the *inhibitory* D_2 dopamine receptor. Thus, loss of the dopaminergic input to the striatum has a differential effect on the two outflow pathways; the direct pathway to the SNpr and MGP is less active, while the activity in the indirect pathway is increased. The net effect is that neurons in the SNpr and MGP become more active. This leads to increased inhibition of the VA/VL thalamus and reduced excitatory input to the cortex. Thin line, normal pathway activity; thick line, increased pathway activity in PD; dashed line, reduced pathway activity in PD. (*See* legend to Figure 22–6 for definitions of anatomical abbreviations.)

D_3, D_4, or D_5 receptors, must be considered. Second, it explains why replacement of dopamine is not the only approach to the treatment of PD. Drugs that inhibit cholinergic receptors long have been used for treatment of parkinsonism. Although their mechanisms of action are not completely understood, it seems likely that their effect is mediated at the level of the striatal projection neurons which normally receive cholinergic input from striatal cholinergic interneurons. No clinically useful drugs for parkinsonism are presently available based on actions through GABA and glutamate receptors, even though both have crucial roles in the circuitry of the basal ganglia. However, they represent a promising avenue for drug development (Greenamyre and O'Brien, 1991).

Treatment of Parkinson's Disease

Commonly used medications for the treatment of PD are summarized in Table 22–1.

Levodopa.   *Levodopa* (L-DOPA, LARODOPA, DOPAR, L-3,4-dihydroxyphenylalanine), the metabolic precursor of dopamine, is the single most effective agent in the treatment of PD. Levodopa is itself largely inert; its therapeutic as well as adverse effects result from the decarboxylation of levodopa to dopamine. When administered orally, levodopa is rapidly absorbed from the small bowel by an active transport system for aromatic amino acids. Concentrations

Table 22–1
Commonly Used Medications for the Treatment of Parkinson's Disease

AGENT	TYPICAL INITIAL DOSE	TOTAL DAILY DOSE—USEFUL RANGE	COMMENTS
Carbidopa/levodopa	25 mg carbidopa + 100 mg levodopa ("25/100" tablet), twice or three times a day	200–1200 mg levodopa	
Carbidopa/levodopa sustained release	50 mg carbidopa + 200 mg levodopa ("50/200 sustained release" tablet) twice a day	200–1200 mg levodopa	Bioavailability 75% of immediate release form
Bromocriptine	1.25 mg twice a day	3.75–40 mg	Titrate slowly
Pergolide	0.05 mg once a day	0.75–5 mg	Titrate slowly
Ropinirole	0.25 mg three times a day	1.5–24 mg	
Pramipexole	0.125 mg three times a day	1.5–4.5 mg	
Entacapone	200 mg with each dose of levodopa/carbidopa	600–2000 mg	
Tolcapone	100 mg twice a day or three times a day	200–600 mg	May be hepatotoxic; requires monitoring of liver enzymes
Selegiline	5 mg twice a day	2.5–10 mg	
Amantadine	100 mg twice a day	100–200 mg	
Trihexyphenidyl HCl	1 mg twice a day	2–15 mg	

of the drug in plasma usually peak between 0.5 and 2 hours after an oral dose. The half-life in plasma is short (1 to 3 hours). The rate and extent of absorption of levodopa is dependent upon the rate of gastric emptying, the pH of gastric juice, and the length of time the drug is exposed to the degradative enzymes of the gastric and intestinal mucosa. Competition for absorption sites in the small bowel from dietary amino acids also may have a marked effect on the absorption of levodopa; administration of levodopa with meals delays absorption and reduces peak plasma concentrations. Entry of the drug into the central nervous system (CNS) across the blood–brain barrier also is an active process mediated by a carrier of aromatic amino acids, and competition between dietary protein and levodopa may occur at this level. In the brain, levodopa is converted to dopamine by decarboxylation, primarily within the presynaptic terminals of dopaminergic neurons in the striatum. The dopamine produced is responsible for the therapeutic effectiveness of the drug in PD; after release, it is either transported back into dopaminergic terminals by the presynaptic uptake mechanism or metabolized by the actions of MAO and COMT (Mouradian and Chase, 1994).

In modern practice, levodopa is almost always administered in combination with a peripherally acting inhibitor of aromatic L-amino acid decarboxylase, such as *carbidopa* or *benserazide*. If levodopa is administered alone, the drug is largely decarboxylated by enzymes in the intestinal mucosa and other peripheral sites, so that relatively little unchanged drug reaches the cerebral circulation and probably less than 1% penetrates the CNS. In addition, dopamine released into the circulation by peripheral conversion of levodopa produces undesirable effects, particularly nausea. Inhibition of peripheral decarboxylase markedly increases the fraction of administered levodopa that remains unmetabolized and available to cross the blood–brain barrier and reduces the incidence of gastrointestinal side effects. In most individuals, a daily dose of 75 mg of carbidopa is sufficient to prevent the development of nausea. For this reason, the most commonly prescribed form of carbidopa/levodopa (SINEMET, ATAMET) is the *25/100* form, containing 25 mg of carbidopa and 100 mg of levodopa. With this formulation, dosage schedules of three or more tablets daily provide acceptable inhibition of decarboxylase in most individuals. Occasionally, individuals will require larger doses of carbidopa to minimize gastrointestinal side effects, and administration of supplemental carbidopa (LODOSYN) alone may be beneficial.

Levodopa therapy can have a dramatic effect on all the signs and symptoms of PD. Early in the course of the disease, the degree of improvement in tremor, rigidity, and bradykinesia may be nearly complete. In early PD, the duration of the beneficial effects of levodopa may exceed the plasma lifetime of the drug, suggesting that the nigrostriatal dopamine system retains some capacity to store and release dopamine. A principal limitation of the long-term use of levodopa therapy is that, with time, this apparent "buffering" capacity is lost, and the patient's motor state may fluctuate dramatically with each dose of levodopa. A common problem is the development of the "wearing off" phenomenon; each dose of levodopa effectively improves mobility for a period of time, perhaps 1 to 2 hours, but rigidity and akinesia rapidly return at the end of the dosing interval. Increasing the dose and frequency of administration can improve this situation, but this often is limited by development of dyskinesias, excessive and abnormal involuntary movements. Dyskinesias are observed most often when the plasma levodopa concentration is high, although, in some individuals, dyskinesias or dystonia may be triggered when the level is rising or falling. These movements can be as uncomfortable and disabling as the rigidity and akinesia of PD. In the later stages of PD, patients may fluctuate rapidly between being "off," having no beneficial effects from their medications, and being "on" but with disabling dyskinesias, a situation called the "on/off phenomenon."

Recent evidence has indicated that the induction of on/off phenomena and dyskinesias may be the result of an active process of adaptation to variations in brain and plasma levodopa levels. This process of adaptation is apparently complex, involving not only alterations in the expression of dopamine receptor proteins but also downstream changes in the postsynaptic striatal neurons, including modification of NMDA glutamate receptors (Mouradian and Chase, 1994; Chase, 1998). When levodopa levels are maintained at a constant level by intravenous infusion, dyskinesias and fluctuations are greatly reduced, and the clinical improvement is maintained for up to several days after returning to oral levodopa dosing (Mouradian *et al.,* 1990; Chase *et al.,* 1994). A sustained-release formulation consisting of carbidopa/levodopa in an erodable wax matrix (SINEMET CR) has been marketed in an attempt to produce more stable plasma levodopa levels than can be obtained with oral administration of standard carbidopa/levodopa formulations. This formulation is helpful in some cases, but the absorption of the sustained-release formulation is not entirely predictable. Another technique used to overcome the on/off phenomenon is to sum the total daily dose of carbidopa/levodopa and give equal amounts every 2 hours rather than every 4 or 6 hours.

An important unanswered question regarding the use of levodopa in PD is whether this medication alters the course of the underlying disease or merely modifies the symptoms (Agid *et al.,* 1998). Two aspects of levodopa treatment and the outcome of PD are of concern. First, it has been suggested that, if the production of free radicals as a result of dopamine metabolism contributes to the death of nigrostriatal neurons, the addition of levodopa might actually accelerate the process (Olanow, 1990), although no convincing evidence for such an effect has yet been obtained. Second, it is well established that the undesirable on/off fluctuations and wearing off phenomena are observed almost exclusively in patients treated with levodopa, but it is not known if delaying treatment with levodopa will delay the appearance of these effects (Fahn, 1999). In view of these uncertainties, most practitioners have adopted a pragmatic approach, using levodopa only when the symptoms of PD cause functional impairment.

In addition to motor fluctuations and nausea, several other adverse effects may be observed with levodopa treatment. A common and troubling adverse effect is the induction of hallucinations and confusion; these effects are particularly common in the elderly and in those with preexisting cognitive dysfunction and often limit the ability to treat parkinsonian symptoms adequately. Conventional antipsychotic agents, such as the phenothiazines, are effective against levodopa-induced psychosis but may cause marked worsening of parkinsonism, probably through actions at the D_2 dopamine receptor. A recent approach has been to use the "atypical" antipsychotic agents, which are effective in the treatment of psychosis but do not cause or worsen parkinsonism (*see* Chapter 20). The most effective of these are *clozapine* and *quetiapine* (Friedman and Factor, 2000).

Peripheral decarboxylation of levodopa and release of dopamine into the circulation may activate vascular dopamine receptors and produce orthostatic hypotension. The actions of dopamine at α- and β-adrenergic receptors may induce cardiac arrhythmias, especially in patients with preexisting conduction disturbances. Administration of levodopa with nonspecific inhibitors of MAO, such as *phenelzine* and *tranylcypromine,* markedly accentuates the actions of levodopa and may precipitate life-threatening hypertensive crisis and hyperpyrexia; nonspecific MAO inhibitors always should be discontinued at least 14 days before levodopa is administered (note that this prohibition does not include the MAO-B subtype-specific inhibitor *selegiline,* which, as discussed below, often is administered safely in combination with levodopa). Abrupt withdrawal of levodopa or other dopaminergic medications may precipitate the *neuroleptic malignant syndrome* more commonly observed after treatment with dopamine antagonists (Keyser and Rodnitzky, 1991).

Dopamine-Receptor Agonists. An alternative to levodopa is the use of drugs that are direct agonists of striatal dopamine receptors, an approach that offers several potential advantages. Since enzymatic conversion of these drugs is not required for activity, they do not depend on the functional capacities of the nigrostriatal neurons and thus might be more effective than levodopa in late PD. In addition, dopamine-receptor agonists potentially are more selective in their actions; unlike levodopa, which leads to activation of all dopamine receptor types throughout the brain, agonists may exhibit relative selectivity for different subtypes of dopamine receptors. Most of the dopamine-receptor agonists in current clinical use have durations of action substantially longer than that of levodopa and often are useful in the management of dose-related fluctuations in motor state. Finally, if the hypothesis that free radical formation as a result of dopamine metabolism contributes to neuronal death is correct, then dopamine-receptor agonists have the potential to modify the course of the disease by reducing endogenous release of dopamine as well as the need for exogenous levodopa (Goetz, 1990).

Four dopamine-receptor agonists are available for treatment of PD: two older agents *bromocriptine* (PARLODEL) and *pergolide* (PERMAX); and two newer, more selective compounds, *ropinirole* (REQUIP) and *pramipexole* (MIRAPEX). Bromocriptine and pergolide are both ergot derivatives and share a similar spectrum of therapeutic actions and adverse effects. Bromocriptine is a strong agonist of the D_2 class of dopamine receptors and a partial antagonist of the D_1 receptors, while pergolide is an agonist of both classes. Ropinirole and pramipexole (Figure 22–8) have selective activity at D_2 class sites (specifically, at the D_2 and D_3 receptor proteins) and little or no activity at D_1 class sites. All four of the drugs are well absorbed orally, and have similar therapeutic actions. Like levodopa, they can relieve the clinical symptoms of PD. The duration of action of the dopamine agonists often is longer than that of levodopa, and they are particularly effective in the treatment of patients who have developed on/off phenomena. All four also may produce hallucinosis or confusion, similar to that observed with levodopa, and may worsen orthostatic hypotension.

The principal distinction between the newer, more selective agents and the older ergot derivatives is in their tolerability and speed of titration. Initial treatment with

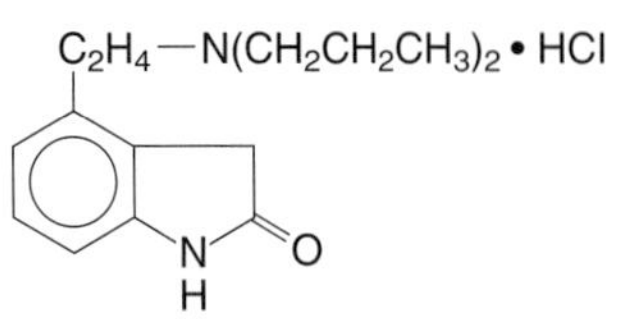

ROPINIROLE HYDROCHLORIDE

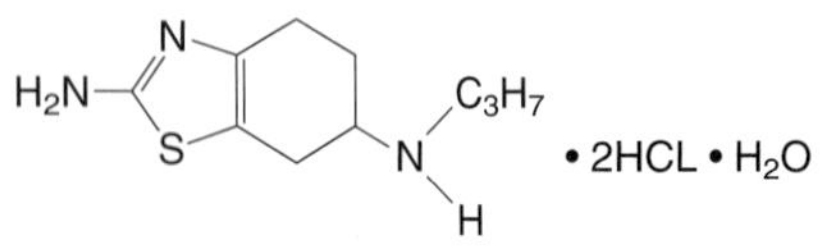

PRAMIPEXOLE DIHYDROCHLORIDE

Figure 22–8. Structures of selective dopamine D_2-receptor agonists.

bromocriptine or pergolide may cause profound hypertension, so they should be initiated at low dosage. The ergot derivatives also often induce nausea and fatigue with initial treatment. Symptoms usually are transient, but they require slow upward adjustment of the dose, over a period of weeks to months. Ropinirole and pramipexole can be initiated more quickly, achieving therapeutically useful doses in a week or less. They generally cause less gastrointestinal disturbance than do the ergot derivatives, but they can produce nausea and fatigue. Although these properties already have led to widespread adoption of the newer drugs in the United States, there are as yet few data on the effects of long-term treatment. One curious adverse effect of pramipexole and ropinirole reported to date is that some individuals treated with these drugs develop a troubling sleep disorder, with sudden attacks of sleep during ordinary daytime activities (Frucht *et al.*, 1999). This effect seems to be uncommon, but it is prudent to advise patients of this possibility and switch to another treatment if these symptoms occur.

The introduction of pramipexole and ropinirole has led to a substantial change in the clinical use of dopamine agonists in PD. Because these selective agonists are well tolerated, they are increasingly used as initial treatment for PD rather than as adjuncts to levodopa. This change has been driven by two factors: (1) the belief that because of their longer duration of action, dopamine agonists may be less likely than levodopa to induce on/off effects and dyskinesias, and (2) the concern that levodopa may contribute to oxidative stress, thereby accelerating loss of dopaminergic neurons. It is important to recognize that, while these concerns are well founded in laboratory experiments, there is at present only limited direct evidence for either of these effects on patients. Two large, controlled clinical trials comparing levodopa to pramipexole or ropinirole as initial treatment of PD recently have revealed a reduced rate of motor fluctuation in patients treated with these agonists, and if confirmed by additional studies, these findings are likely to greatly influence the clinical use of these drugs (Parkinson Study Group, 2000; Rascol *et al.*, 2000).

COMT Inhibitors. A recently developed class of drugs for the treatment of PD are inhibitors of the enzyme catechol-*O*-methyltransferase (COMT). COMT and MAO are responsible for the catabolism of levodopa as well as dopamine. COMT transfers a methyl group from the donor *S*-adenosyl-L-methionine, producing the pharmacologically inactive compounds 3-*O*-methyl DOPA (from levodopa) and 3-methoxytyramine (from dopamine) (Figure 22–9). When levodopa is administered orally, nearly 99%

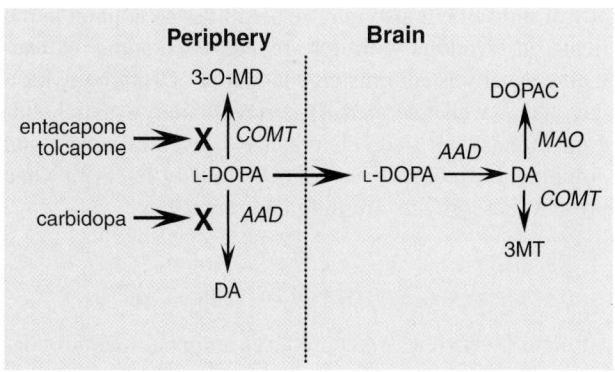

Figure 22–9. Catechol-O-methyltransferase inhibition.

The principal site of action of inhibitors of catechol-*O*-methyltransferase (COMT) (such as tolcapone and entacapone) is in the peripheral circulation. They block the methylation of levodopa (L-DOPA) and increase the fraction of the drug available for delivery to the brain. AAD, aromatic L-amino acid decarboxylase; DA, dopamine; DOPAC, 3,4-dihydroxyphenylacetic acid; MAO, monoamine oxidase; 3MT, 3-methoxytyramine; 3-O-MD, 3-*O*-methylDOPA.

of the drug is catabolized and does not reach the brain. The majority is converted by aromatic L-amino acid decarboxylase (AAD) to dopamine, which causes nausea and hypotension. Addition of an AAD inhibitor, such as carbidopa, reduces the formation of dopamine, but increases the fraction of levodopa that is methylated by COMT. The principal therapeutic action of the COMT inhibitors is to block this peripheral conversion of levodopa to 3-*O*-methyl DOPA, increasing both the plasma half-life of levodopa as well as the fraction of each dose that reaches the central nervous system (Goetz, 1998).

Two COMT inhibitors presently are available for use in the United States, *tolcapone* (TASMAR) and *entacapone* (COMTAN). Both of these agents have been shown in double-blind trials to reduce the clinical symptoms of "wearing-off" in patients treated with levodopa/carbidopa (Parkinson Study Group, 1997; Kurth *et al.,* 1997). Although the magnitude of their clinical effects and mechanisms of action are similar, they differ with respect to pharmacokinetic properties and adverse effects. Tolcapone has a relatively long duration of action, allowing for administration two to three times a day, and appears to act both by central and peripheral inhibition of COMT. The duration of action of entacapone is short, around 2 hours, so it is usually administered simultaneously with each dose of levodopa/carbidopa. The action of entacapone is attributable principally to peripheral inhibition of COMT. The common adverse effects of these agents are similar to those observed in patients treated with levodopa/carbidopa alone,

and include nausea, orthostatic hypotension, vivid dreams, confusion, and hallucinations. An important adverse effect associated with tolcapone is hepatotoxicity. In clinical trials, up to 2% of the patients treated were noted to have an increase in serum alanine aminotransferase and aspartate transaminase; after marketing, three fatal cases of fulminant hepatic failure in patients taking tolcapone were observed. At present, tolcapone should be used only in patients who have not responded to other therapies and with appropriate monitoring for hepatic injury. Entacapone has not been associated with hepatotoxicity and requires no special monitoring.

Selegiline. Two isoenzymes of MAO oxidize monoamines. While both isoenzymes (MAO-A and MAO-B) are present in the periphery and inactivate monoamines of intestinal origin, the isoenzyme MAO-B is the predominant form in the striatum and is responsible for the majority of oxidative metabolism of dopamine in the striatum. At low-to-moderate doses (10 mg/day or less), *selegiline* (ELDEPRYL) is a selective inhibitor of MAO-B, leading to irreversible inhibition of the enzyme (Olanow, 1993). Unlike nonspecific inhibitors of MAO (such as phenelzine, tranylcypromine, and isocarboxazid), selegiline does not inhibit peripheral metabolism of catecholamines; thus, it can be taken safely with levodopa. Selegiline also does not cause the lethal potentiation of catecholamine action observed when patients taking nonspecific MAO inhibitors ingest indirectly acting sympathomimetic amines such as the tyramine found in certain cheeses and wine. Doses of selegiline higher than 10 mg daily can produce inhibition of MAO-A and should be avoided.

Selegiline has been used for several years as a symptomatic treatment for PD, although its benefit is fairly modest. The basis of the efficacy of selegiline is presumed to be its ability to retard the breakdown of dopamine in the striatum. With the recent emergence of interest in the potential role of free radicals and oxidative stress in the pathogenesis of PD, it has been proposed that the ability of selegiline to retard the metabolism of dopamine might confer neuroprotective properties. In support of this idea, it was observed that selegiline could protect animals from MPTP-induced parkinsonism by blocking the conversion of MPTP to its toxic metabolite (1-methyl-4-phenylpyridium ion), a transformation mediated by MAO-B. The potential protective role of selegiline in idiopathic PD was evaluated in multicenter randomized trials; these studies showed a symptomatic effect of selegiline in PD, but longer follow-up failed to provide any definite evidence of ability to retard the loss of dopaminergic neurons (Parkinson Study Group, 1993).

Selegiline is generally well tolerated in patients with early or mild PD. In patients with more advanced PD or underlying cognitive impairment, selegiline may accentuate the adverse motor and cognitive effects of levodopa therapy. Metabolites of selegiline include amphetamine and methamphetamine, which may cause anxiety, insomnia, and other adverse symptoms. Interestingly, it has been observed that selegiline, like the non-specific MAO inhibitors, can lead to the development of stupor, rigidity, agitation, and hyperthermia after administration of the analgesic meperidine; the basis of this interaction is uncertain. There also have been reports of adverse effects resulting from interactions between selegiline and tricyclic antidepressants and between selegiline and serotonin-reuptake inhibitors.

Muscarinic Receptor Antagonists. Antagonists of muscarinic acetylcholine receptors were widely used for the treatment of PD before the discovery of levodopa. The biological basis for the therapeutic actions of anticholinergics is not completely understood. It seems likely that they act within the neostriatum, through the receptors that normally mediate the response to the intrinsic cholinergic innervation of this structure, which arises primarily from cholinergic striatal interneurons. Several muscarinic cholinergic receptors have been cloned (*see* Chapters 7 and 12); like the dopamine receptors, these are proteins with seven transmembrane domains that are linked to second-messenger systems by G proteins. Five subtypes of muscarinic receptors have been identified; at least four and probably all five subtypes are present in the striatum, although each has a distinct distribution (Hersch *et al.,* 1994). Several drugs with anticholinergic properties are currently used in the treatment of PD, including *trihexyphenidyl* (ARTANE, 2 to 4 mg, three times per day), *benztropine mesylate* (COGENTIN, 1 to 4 mg, two times per day), and *diphenhydramine hydrochloride* (BENADRYL, 25 to 50 mg, 3 to 4 times per day). All have a modest antiparkinsonian action, which is useful in the treatment of early PD or as an adjunct to dopamimetic therapy. The adverse effects of these drugs are a result of their anticholinergic properties. Most troublesome is sedation and mental confusion, frequently seen in the elderly. They also may produce constipation, urinary retention, and blurred vision through cycloplegia; they must be used with caution in patients with narrow-angle glaucoma.

Amantadine. *Amantadine* (SYMMETREL), an antiviral agent used for the prophylaxis and treatment of influenza A (*see* Chapter 50), has antiparkinsonian actions. The mechanism of action of amantadine is not clear. It has been suggested that it might alter dopamine release or reuptake; anticholinergic properties also may contribute to its therapeutic actions. Amantadine and the closely related compound *memantadine* have activity at NMDA glutamate receptors, which may contribute to their antiparkinsonian actions (Stoof *et al.,* 1992). In any case, the effects of amantadine in PD are modest. It is used as initial ther-

apy of mild PD. It also may be helpful as an adjunct in patients on levodopa with dose-related fluctuations. Amantadine usually is administered in a dose of 100 mg twice a day and is well tolerated. Dizziness, lethargy, anticholinergic effects, and sleep disturbance, as well as nausea and vomiting, have been observed occasionally, but even when present these effects are mild and reversible.

ALZHEIMER'S DISEASE

Clinical Overview. AD produces an impairment of cognitive abilities that is gradual in onset but relentless in progression. Impairment of short-term memory usually is the first clinical feature, while retrieval of distant memories is preserved relatively well into the course of the disease. As the condition progresses, additional cognitive abilities are impaired, among them the ability to calculate, exercise visuospatial skills, and use common objects and tools (ideomotor apraxia). The level of arousal or alertness of the patient is not affected until the condition is very advanced, nor is there motor weakness, although muscular contractures are an almost universal feature of advanced stages of the disease. Death, most often from a complication of immobility such as pneumonia or pulmonary embolism, usually ensues within 6 to 12 years after onset. The diagnosis of AD is based on careful clinical assessment of the patient and appropriate laboratory tests to exclude other disorders that may mimic AD; at present, no direct antemortem confirmatory test exists.

Pathophysiology. AD is characterized by marked atrophy of the cerebral cortex and loss of cortical and subcortical neurons. The pathological hallmarks of AD are senile plaques, which are spherical accumulations of the protein β-amyloid accompanied by degenerating neuronal processes, and neurofibrillary tangles, composed of paired helical filaments and other proteins (Arnold *et al.,* 1991; Arriagada *et al.,* 1992; Braak and Braak, 1994). Although small numbers of senile plaques and neurofibrillary tangles can be observed in intellectually normal individuals, they are far more abundant in AD, and the abundance of tangles is roughly proportional to the severity of cognitive impairment. In advanced AD, senile plaques and neurofibrillary tangles are numerous. They are most abundant in the hippocampus and associative regions of the cortex, whereas areas such as the visual and motor cortices are relatively spared. This corresponds to the clinical features of marked impairment of memory and abstract reasoning, with preservation of vision and movement. The factors underlying the selective vulnerability of particular cortical neurons to the pathological effects of AD are not known.

Neurochemistry. The neurochemical disturbances that arise in AD have been studied intensively (Johnston, 1992). Direct analysis of neurotransmitter content in the cerebral cortex shows a reduction of many transmitter substances that parallels neuronal loss; there is a striking and disproportionate deficiency of acetylcholine. The anatomical basis of the cholinergic deficit is the atrophy and degeneration of subcortical cholinergic neurons, particularly those in the basal forebrain (nucleus basalis of Meynert), that provide cholinergic innervation to the whole cerebral cortex. The selective deficiency of acetylcholine in AD, as well as the observation that central cholinergic antagonists such as atropine can induce a confusional state that bears some resemblance to the dementia of AD, has given rise to the "cholinergic hypothesis," which proposes that a deficiency of acetylcholine is critical in the genesis of the symptoms of AD (Perry, 1986). Although the conceptualization of AD as a "cholinergic deficiency syndrome" in parallel with the "dopaminergic deficiency syndrome" of PD provides a useful framework, it is important to note that the deficit in AD is far more complex, involving multiple neurotransmitter systems, including serotonin, glutamate, and neuropeptides, and that in AD there is destruction of not only cholinergic neurons but also the cortical and hippocampal targets that receive cholinergic input.

Role of β-Amyloid.   The presence of aggregates of β-amyloid is a constant feature of AD. Until recently, it was not clear whether the amyloid protein was causally linked to the disease process or merely a by-product of neuronal death. The application of molecular genetics has shed considerable light on this question. β-Amyloid was isolated from affected brains and found to be a short polypeptide of 42 to 43 amino acids. This information led to cloning of amyloid precursor protein (APP), a much larger protein of more than 700 amino acids, which is widely expressed by neurons throughout the brain in normal individuals as well as in those with AD. The function of APP is unknown, although the structural features of the protein suggest that it may serve as a cell surface receptor for an as-yet-unidentified ligand. The production of β-amyloid from APP appears to result from abnormal proteolytic cleavage of APP by the recently isolated enzyme BACE (β-site APP-cleaving enzyme). This may be an important target of future therapies (Vassar *et al.,* 1999).

Analysis of APP gene structure in pedigrees exhibiting autosomal dominant inheritance of AD has shown that, in some families, mutations of the β-amyloid–forming region of APP are present, while in others, mutations of proteins involved in the processing of APP have been implicated (Selkoe, 1998). These results demonstrate that it is possible for abnormalities in APP or its processing to cause AD. The vast majority of cases of AD, however, are not familial, and structural abnormality of APP or related proteins has not been observed consistently in these sporadic cases of AD. As noted above, common alleles of the apo E protein have been found to influence the probability of developing AD. This suggests that modifying the metabolism of APP might alter the course of AD in both familial and sporadic cases (Whyte *et al.,* 1994), but no clinically practical strategies have been developed yet.

Treatment of Alzheimer's Disease.   A major approach to the treatment of AD has involved attempts to augment the cholinergic function of the brain (Johnston, 1992). An early approach was the use of precursors of acetylcholine synthesis, such as *choline chloride* and *phosphatidyl choline (lecithin).* Although these supplements generally are well tolerated, randomized trials have failed to demonstrate any clinically significant efficacy. Direct intracerebroventricular injection of cholinergic agonists such as bethanacol appears to have some beneficial effects, although this requires surgical implantation of a reservoir connecting to the subarachnoid space and is too cumbersome and intrusive for practical use. A somewhat more successful strategy has been the use of inhibitors of acetylcholinesterase (AChE), the catabolic enzyme for acetylcholine (*see* Chapter 8). *Physostigmine,* a rapidly acting, reversible AChE inhibitor, produces improved responses in animal models of learning, and some studies have demonstrated mild transitory improvement in memory following physostigmine treatment in patients with AD. The use of physostigmine has been limited because of its short half-life and tendency to produce symptoms of systemic cholinergic excess at therapeutic doses.

Four inhibitors of AChE currently are approved by the United States Food and Drug Administration for treatment of Alzheimer's disease: *tacrine* (1,2,3,4-tetrahydro-9-aminoacridine; COGNEX), *donepezil* (ARICEPT) (Mayeux and Sano, 1999), *rivastigmine* (EXCELON), and *galantamine* (REMINYL). Tacrine is a potent, centrally acting inhibitor of AChE (Freeman and Dawson, 1991). Studies of oral tacrine in combination with lecithin have confirmed that there is indeed an effect of tacrine on some measures of memory performance, but the magnitude of improvement observed with the combination of lecithin and tacrine is modest at best (Chatellier and Lacomblez, 1990). The side effects of tacrine often are significant and dose-limiting; abdominal cramping, anorexia, nausea, vomiting, and diarrhea are observed in up to one-third of patients receiving therapeutic doses, and elevations of serum transaminases are observed in up to 50% of those treated. Because of the significant side-effect profile, tacrine is not widely used in clinical practice. Donepezil is a selective inhibitor of AChE in the CNS with little effect on AChE in peripheral tissues. It produces modest improvements in cognitive scores in Alzheimer's disease patients (Rogers and Friedhoff, 1988) and has a long half-life (*see* Appendix II), allowing once-daily dosing. Rivastigmine and galantamine are dosed twice daily and produce a similar degree of cognitive improvement. Adverse effects associated with donepezil, rivastigmine, and galantamine are similar in character but generally less frequent and less severe than those observed with tacrine; they include nausea, diarrhea, vomiting, and insomnia. Donepezil, rivastigmine, and galantamine are not associated with the hepatotoxicity that limits the use of tacrine.

Drugs currently under development for treatment of Alzheimer's disease include additional anticholinesterase agents as well as agents representing other pharmacological approaches. *Memantine,* an NMDA-receptor antagonist, has shown promise in clinical trials of slowing the progression of AD in patients with moderately severe disease. Antioxidants, antiinflammatory agents, and estrogens have been studied, but none of these has established efficacy. The identification of APP and the enzymes involved in the processing of this protein has opened the door to the development of antiaggregants, a β-amyloid vaccine, and modifiers of APP processing, which may represent the next generation of Alzheimer's therapy.

HUNTINGTON'S DISEASE

Clinical Features. HD is a dominantly inherited disorder characterized by the gradual onset of motor incoordination and cognitive decline in midlife. Symptoms develop insidiously, either as a movement disorder manifest by brief jerk-like movements of the extremities, trunk, face, and neck (chorea) or by personality changes, or both. Fine motor incoordination and impairment of rapid eye movements are early features. Occasionally, especially when the onset of symptoms occurs before the age of 20, choreic movements are less prominent; instead, bradykinesia and dystonia predominate. As the disorder progresses, the involuntary movements become more severe, dysarthria and dysphagia develop, and balance is impaired. The cognitive disorder manifests itself first by slowness of mental processing and difficulty in organizing complex tasks. Memory is affected, but affected persons rarely lose their memory of family, friends, and the immediate situation. Such persons often become irritable, anxious, and depressed. Less frequently, paranoia and delusional states are manifest. The outcome of HD is invariably fatal; over a course of 15 to 30 years, the affected person becomes totally disabled and unable to communicate, requiring full-time care; death ensues from the complications of immobility (Hayden, 1981; Harper, 1991, 1992).

Pathology and Pathophysiology. HD is characterized by prominent neuronal loss in the caudate/putamen of the brain (Vonsattel *et al.,* 1985). Atrophy of these structures proceeds in an orderly fashion, first affecting the tail of the caudate nucleus and then proceeding anteriorly, from medial–dorsal to lateral–ventral. Other areas of the brain also are affected, although much less severely; morphometric analyses indicate that there are fewer neurons in cerebral cortex, hypothalamus, and thalamus. Even within the striatum, the neuronal degeneration of HD is selective. Interneurons and afferent terminals are largely spared, while the striatal projection neurons (the medium spiny neurons) are severely affected. This leads to large decreases in striatal GABA concentrations, whereas somatostatin and dopamine concentrations are relatively preserved (Ferrante *et al.,* 1987; Reiner *et al.,* 1988).

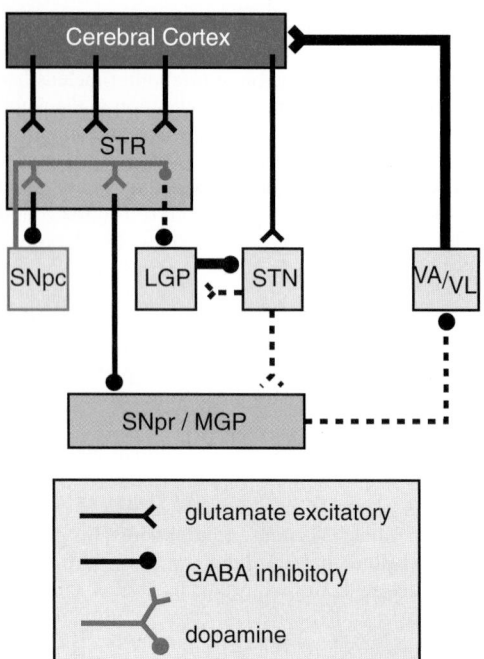

Figure 22–10. The basal ganglia in Huntington's disease (HD).

HD is characterized by loss of neurons from the STR. The neurons that project to the LGP and form the indirect pathway are affected earlier in the course of the disease than those that project to the MGP. This leads to a loss of inhibition of the LGP. The increased activity in this structure in turn inhibits the STN, SNpr, and MGP, resulting in a loss of inhibition to the VA/VL thalamus and increased thalamocortical excitatory drive. Thin line, normal pathway activity; thick line, increased pathway activity in HD; dashed line, reduced pathway activity in HD. (*See* legend to Figure 22–6 for definitions of anatomical abbreviations.)

Selective vulnerability also appears to underlie the most conspicuous clinical feature of HD, the development of chorea. In most adult-onset cases, the medium spiny neurons that project to LGP and SNpr (the indirect pathway) appear to be affected earlier than those projecting to the MGP (the direct pathway; Albin *et al.,* 1990, 1992). The disproportionate impairment of the indirect pathway increases excitatory drive to the neocortex, producing involuntary choreiform movements (Figure 22–10). In some individuals, rigidity rather than chorea is the predominant clinical feature; this is especially common in juvenile-onset cases. In these cases the striatal neurons giving rise to both the direct and indirect pathways are impaired to a comparable degree.

Genetics. HD is an autosomal dominant disorder with nearly complete penetrance. The average age of onset is between 35 and 45 years, but the range varies from as early as age two to as late as the mid-eighties. Although the disease is inherited equally from mother and father, more than 80% of those developing symptoms before the age of 20 inherit the defect from the father. This is an example of *anticipation,* or the tendency for the age of onset of a disease to decline with each succeeding generation, which also is observed in other neurodegenerative diseases with similar genetic mechanisms. Known homozygotes for HD show clinical characteristics identical to the typical HD heterozygote, indicating that the unaffected chromosome does not attenuate the disease symptomatology. Until the discovery of the genetic defect responsible for HD, *de novo* mutations causing HD were thought to be unusual; but it is clear now that the disease can arise from unaffected parents, especially when one carries an "intermediate allele," as described below.

The discovery of the genetic mutation responsible for Huntington's disease was the product of an arduous, ten-year, multi-investigator, collaborative effort. In 1993 a region near the telomere of chromosome 4 was found to contain a polymorphic $(CAG)_n$ trinucleotide repeat that was significantly expanded in all individuals with HD (Huntington's Disease Collaborative Research Group, 1993). The expansion of this trinucleotide repeat is the genetic alteration responsible for HD. The range of CAG repeat length in normal individuals is between 9 and 34 triplets, with a median repeat length on normal chromosomes of 19. The repeat length in HD varies from 40 to over 100. Repeat lengths of 35 to 39 represent intermediate alleles; some of these individuals develop HD late in life, while others are not affected. Repeat length is correlated inversely with age of onset. The younger the age of onset, the higher the probability of a large repeat number. This correlation is most powerful in individuals with onset before the age of 30; with onset above the age of 30, the correlation is weaker. Thus, repeat length cannot serve as an adequate predictor of age of onset in most individuals. Subsequent work has shown that several other neurodegenerative diseases also arise through expansion of a CAG repeat, including hereditary spinocerebellar ataxias and Kennedy's disease, a rare inherited disorder of motor neurons (Paulson and Fischbeck, 1996).

Selective Vulnerability. The mechanism by which the expanded trinucleotide repeat leads to the clinical and pathological features of HD is unknown. The HD mutation lies within a gene designated *IT15*. The *IT15* gene itself is very large (10 kilobases) and encodes a protein of approximately 348,000 daltons or 3144 amino acids. The trinucleotide repeat, which encodes the amino acid glutamine, occurs at the 5'-end of *IT15* and is followed directly by a second, shorter repeat of $(CCG)_n$, which encodes the amino acid proline. The protein, named *huntingtin,* does not resemble any other known protein, and the normal function of the protein has not been identified. Mice with a genetic "knockout" of huntingtin die early in embryonic life, so it must have an essential cellular function. It is thought that the mutation results in a *gain of function;* that is, the mutant protein acquires a new function or property not found in the normal protein.

The HD gene is expressed widely throughout the body. High levels of expression are present in brain, pancreas, intestine, muscle, liver, adrenals, and testes. In brain, expression of *IT15* does not appear to be correlated with neuron vulnerability; although the striatum is most severely affected, neurons in all regions of the brain express similar levels of *IT15* mRNA (Landwehrmeyer *et al.,* 1995). The ability of the HD mutation to produce selective neural degeneration despite nearly universal expression of the gene among neurons may be related

to metabolic or excitotoxic mechanisms. For many years, it has been noted that HD patients are thin, suggesting the presence of a systemic disturbance of energy metabolism. In animal models, agonists for the NMDA subtype of excitatory amino acid receptor can cause pathology similar to that seen in HD when they are injected into the striatum (Beal *et al.,* 1986). More interesting, however, is the fact that inhibitors of complex II of the mitochondrial respiratory chain also can produce HD-like striatal lesions—even when given systemically (Beal *et al.,* 1993). Furthermore, this pathology can be diminished by NMDA-receptor antagonists, suggesting that this is an example of a metabolic impairment giving rise to excitotoxic neuronal injury. Studies employing magnetic resonance imaging (MRI) spectroscopy have provided direct evidence of an alteration in energy metabolism in HD *in vivo* (Jenkins *et al.,* 1993). Thus, the link between the widespread expression of the gene for the abnormal *IT15* protein in HD and the selective vulnerability of neurons in the disease may arise from the interaction of a widespread defect in energy metabolism with the intrinsic properties of striatal neurons, including their capacity and need for oxidative metabolism as well as the types of glutamate receptors present. This hypothesis has a number of potentially important therapeutic implications. It is unlikely that it will be possible in the near future to correct the genetic defect in the brains of individuals with HD, but it may be possible to develop agents that alter metabolic function or protect against excitotoxic injury and thereby arrest or modify the course of the disease.

Symptomatic Treatment of Huntington's Disease. Practical treatment for symptomatic HD emphasizes the selective use of medications (Shoulson, 1992). No current medication slows the progression of the disease, and many medications can impair function because of side effects. Treatment is needed for patients who are depressed, irritable, paranoid, excessively anxious, or psychotic. Depression can be treated effectively with standard antidepressant drugs with the caveat that those drugs with substantial anticholinergic profiles can exacerbate chorea. *Fluoxetine* (Chapter 19) is effective treatment for both the depression and the irritability manifest in symptomatic HD. *Carbamazepine* (Chapter 21) also has been found to be effective for depression. Paranoia, delusional states, and psychosis usually require treatment with antipsychotic drugs, but the doses required often are lower than those usually used in primary psychiatric disorders. These agents also reduce cognitive function and impair mobility and thus should be used in the lowest doses possible and be discontinued when the psychiatric symptoms are resolved. In individuals with predominantly rigid HD, *clozapine* (Chapter 20) or carbamazepine may be more effective for treatment of paranoia and psychosis.

The movement disorder of HD *per se* only rarely justifies pharmacological therapy. For those with large-amplitude chorea causing frequent falls and injury, dopamine-depleting agents such as *tetrabenazine* or *reserpine* (Chapter 33) can be tried, although patients must be monitored for hypotension and depression. Antipsychotic agents also can be used, but these often do not improve overall function because they decrease fine motor coordination and increase rigidity. Many HD patients exhibit worsening of involuntary movements as a result of anxiety or stress. In these situations, judicious use of sedative or anxiolytic benzodiazepines can be very helpful. In juvenile-onset cases where rigidity rather than chorea predominates, dopamine agonists have had variable success in the improvement of rigidity. These individuals also occasionally develop myoclonus and seizures that can be responsive to *clonazepam, valproic acid,* or other anticonvulsants.

AMYOTROPHIC LATERAL SCLEROSIS

Clinical Features and Pathology.   ALS is a disorder of the motor neurons of the ventral horn of the spinal cord and the cortical neurons that provide their afferent input. The ratio of males to females affected is approximately 1.5:1 (Kurtzke, 1982). The disorder is characterized by rapidly progressive weakness, muscle atrophy and fasciculations, spasticity, dysarthria, dysphagia, and respiratory compromise. Sensory function generally is spared, as is cognitive, autonomic, and oculomotor activity. ALS usually is progressive and fatal, with most affected patients dying of respiratory compromise and pneumonia after 2 to 3 years, although occasional individuals have a more indolent course and survive for many years. The pathology of ALS corresponds closely to the clinical features: There is prominent loss of the spinal and brainstem motor neurons that project to striated muscles (although the oculomotor neurons are spared) as well as loss of the large pyramidal motor neurons in layer V of motor cortex, which are the origin of the descending corticospinal tracts. In familial cases, Clarke's column and the dorsal horns sometimes are affected (Caroscio *et al.,* 1987; Rowland, 1994).

Etiology.   About 10% of cases of ALS are familial (FALS), usually with an autosomal dominant pattern of inheritance (Jackson and Bryan, 1998). Most of the mutations responsible have not been identified, but an important subset of FALS patients are families with a mutation in the gene for the enzyme superoxide dismutase (SOD1) (Rosen *et al.,* 1993). Mutations in this protein account for about 20% of cases of FALS. Most of the mutations are alterations of single amino acids, but more than 30 different alleles have been found in different kindreds. Transgenic mice expressing mutant human SOD1 develop a progressive degeneration of motor neurons that closely mimics the

human disease, providing an important animal model for research and pharmaceutical trials. Interestingly, many of the mutations of SOD1 that can cause disease do not reduce the capacity of the enzyme to perform its primary function, the catabolism of potentially toxic superoxide radicals. Thus, as may be the case in HD, mutations in SOD1 may confer a toxic "gain of function," the precise nature of which is unclear.

More than 90% of ALS cases are sporadic and are not associated with abnormalities of SOD1 or any other known gene. The cause of the motor neuron loss in sporadic ALS is unknown, but theories include autoimmunity, excitotoxicity, free radical toxicity, and viral infection (Rowland, 1994; Cleveland, 1999). Most of these ideas are not well supported by available data, but there is evidence that glutamate reuptake may be abnormal in the disease, leading to accumulation of glutamate and excitotoxic injury (Rothstein *et al.,* 1992). The only currently approved therapy for ALS, *riluzole,* is based on these observations.

Spasticity and the Spinal Reflex.   Spasticity is an important component of the clinical features of ALS, in that the presence of spasticity often leads to considerable pain and discomfort and reduces mobility, which already is compromised by weakness. Furthermore, spasticity is the feature of ALS that is most amenable to present forms of treatment. *Spasticity* is defined as an increase in muscle tone characterized by an initial resistance to passive displacement of a limb at a joint, followed by a sudden relaxation (the so-called clasped-knife phenomenon). Spasticity is the result of the loss of descending inputs to the spinal motor neurons, and the character of the spasticity depends on which nervous system pathways are affected (Davidoff, 1990). Whole repertoires of movement can be generated directly at the spinal cord level; it is beyond the scope of this chapter to describe these in detail. The monosynaptic tendon-stretch reflex is the simplest of the spinal mechanisms contributing to spasticity. Primary Ia afferents from muscle spindles, activated when the muscle is rapidly stretched, synapse directly on motor neurons going to the stretched muscle, causing it to contract and resist the movement. A collateral of the primary Ia afferent synapses on an "Ia-coupled interneuron" that inhibits the motor neurons innervating the antagonist of the stretched muscle, allowing the contraction of the muscle to be unopposed. Upper motor neurons from the cerebral cortex (the pyramidal neurons) suppress spinal reflexes and the lower motor neurons indirectly by activating the spinal cord inhibitory interneuron pools. The pyramidal neurons use glutamate as a neurotransmitter. When the pyramidal influences are removed, the reflexes are released from inhibition and become more active, leading to hyperreflexia. Other descending pathways from brainstem—including the rubro-, reticulo-, and vestibulospinal pathways and the descending catecholamine pathways—also influence spinal reflex activity. When just the pyramidal pathway is affected, extensor tone in the legs and flexor tone in the arms are increased. When the vestibulospinal and catecholamine pathways are impaired, increased flexion of all extremities is observed and light cutaneous stimulation can lead to disabling whole-body spasms. In ALS, pyramidal pathways are impaired with relative preservation of the other descending pathways, resulting in hyperactive deep-tendon reflexes, impaired fine motor coordination, increased extensor tone in the legs, and increased flexor tone in the arms. The gag reflex often is overactive as well.

Treatment of ALS with Riluzole. *Riluzole* (2-amino-6-[trifluoromethoxy]benzothiazole; RILUTEK) is an agent with complex actions in the nervous system (Bryson *et al.*, 1996; Wagner and Landis, 1997). Its structure is as follows:

RILUZOLE

Riluzole is orally absorbed and highly protein bound. It undergoes extensive metabolism in the liver by both cytochrome P450-mediated hydroxylation and by glucuronidation. Its half-life is about 12 hours. *In vitro* studies have shown that riluzole has both presynaptic and postsynaptic effects. It inhibits glutamate release, but it also blocks postsynaptic NMDA- and kainate-type glutamate receptors and inhibits voltage-dependent sodium channels. Some of the effects of riluzole *in vitro* are blocked by pertussis toxin, implicating the drug's interaction with an as-yet unidentified G protein–coupled receptor. In clinical trials, riluzole has modest but genuine effects on the survival of patients with ALS. In the largest trial conducted to date, with nearly 1000 patients, the median duration of survival was extended by about 60 days (Lacomblez *et al.*, 1996). The recommended dose is 50 mg every 12 hours, taken 1 hour before or 2 hours after a meal. Riluzole usually is well tolerated, although nausea or diarrhea may occur. Rarely, riluzole may produce hepatic injury with elevations of serum transaminases, and periodic monitoring of these is recommended. Although the magnitude of the effect of riluzole on ALS is small, it represents a significant therapeutic milestone in the treatment of a disease refractory to all previous treatments.

Symptomatic Therapy of Spasticity. The most useful agent for the symptomatic treatment of spasticity in ALS is *baclofen* (LIORESAL), a GABA$_B$ agonist. Initial doses of 5 to 10 mg a day are recommended, but the dose can be increased to as much as 200 mg a day if necessary. If weakness occurs, the dose should be lowered. In addition to oral administration, baclofen also can be delivered directly into the space around the spinal cord by use of a surgically implanted pump and an intrathecal catheter. This approach minimizes the adverse effects of the drug, especially sedation, but it carries the risk of potentially life-threatening CNS depression and should be used only by physicians trained in delivering chronic intrathecal therapy. *Tizanidine* (ZANFLEX) is an agonist of α_2-adrenergic receptors in the central nervous system. It reduces muscle spasticity and is assumed to act by increasing presynap-

tic inhibition of motor neurons. Tizanidine is most widely used in the treatment of spasticity in multiple sclerosis or after stroke, but it also may be effective in patients with ALS. Treatment should be initiated at a low dose of 2 to 4 mg at bedtime, and titrated upwards gradually. Drowsiness, asthenia, and dizziness may limit the dose that can be administered. *Benzodiazepines* (*see* Chapter 17), such as *clonazepam* (KLONIPIN) are effective antispasmodics, but they may contribute to respiratory depression in patients with advanced ALS. *Dantrolene* (DANTRIUM) also is approved in the United States for the treatment of muscle spasm. In contrast to other agents discussed, dantrolene acts directly on skeletal muscle fibers, impairing calcium ion flux across the sarcoplasmic reticulum. Because it can exacerbate muscular weakness, it is not used in ALS, but is effective in treating spasticity associated with stroke or spinal cord injury and in treating malignant hyperthermia. Dantrolene may cause hepatotoxicity, so it is important to perform liver function tests before and during therapy with the drug.

PROSPECTUS

Although advances in the symptomatic therapy of the neurodegenerative disorders, particularly PD, have improved the lives of many patients, the goal of current research is to develop treatments that can prevent, retard, or reverse neuronal cell death. Promising areas for drug development are the mechanisms implicated in several of the disorders: excitotoxicity, defects in energy metabolism, and oxidative stress. Glutamate antagonists have great potential, but their use is limited by the relatively nonselective activity of the available agents. Increased knowledge of the structure and function of glutamate receptor subtypes should make more selective and useful agents available. Pharmacological reduction of oxidative stress also is feasible, despite the disappointing results of initial clinical trials with tocopherol and selegiline. Neural growth factors are another important area for drug development. Several factors that promote the differentiation of neurons and the establishment of neural connections during development have been identified, and these may eventually prove useful in retarding or reversing neuronal death. A more direct and currently accessible approach to reversing neuronal loss is surgical transplantation of neurons; this has been accomplished in PD with a moderate degree of success and has been proposed as a treatment for other conditions such as AD. In addition to these general approaches to neurodegeneration, more specific treatments for the various diseases should become feasible with advances in knowledge of their etiology. For example, discovery of the role of β-amyloid in AD has sparked the study of agents that alter its synthesis or prevent its accumulation; similarly, discovery of the HD gene is likely to lead to novel treatment strategies for that disorder.

For further information regarding neurodegenerative diseases for which the drugs discussed in this chapter are useful, the reader is referred to the following chapters in *Harrison's Principles of Internal Medicine,* 14th ed., McGraw-Hill, New York, 1998: Parkinson's disease, Chapter 368; Alzheimer's disease and Huntington's disease, Chapter 367; and amyotrophic lateral sclerosis, Chapter 370.

BIBLIOGRAPHY

Agid, Y., Chase, T., and Marsden, D. Adverse reactions to levodopa: drug toxicity or progression of disease? *Lancet,* **1998,** *351*:851–852.

Albin, R.L., Reiner, A., Anderson, K.D., Dure, L.S. IV, Handelin, B., Balfour, R., Whetsell, W.O., Jr., Penney, J.B., and Young, A.B. Preferential loss of striato-external pallidal projection neurons in presymptomatic Huntington's disease. *Ann. Neurol.,* **1992,** *31*:425–430.

Albin, R.L., Reiner, A., Anderson, K.D., Penney, J.B., and Young, A.B. Striatal and nigral neuron subpopulations in rigid Huntington's disease: implications for the functional anatomy of chorea and rigidity-akinesia. *Ann. Neurol.,* **1990,** *27*:357–365.

Arnold, S.E., Hyman, B.T., Flory, J., Damasio, A.R., and Van Hoesen, G.W. The topographical and neuroanatomical distribution of neurofibrillary tangles and neuritic plaques in the cerebral cortex of patients with Alzheimer's disease. *Cereb. Cortex,* **1991,** *1*:103–116.

Arriagada, P.V., Growdon, J.H., Hedley-White, E.T., and Hyman, B.T. Neurofibrillary tangles but not senile plaques parallel duration and severity of Alzheimer's disease. *Neurology,* **1992,** *42*:631–639.

Ballard, P.A., Tetrud, J.W., and Lanston, J.W. Permanent human parkinsonism due to N-methyl-4-phenyl-1,2,3,6-tetrahydropyridine (MPTP): seven cases. *Neurology,* **1985,** *35*:949–956.

Beal, M.F., Kowall, N.W., Ellison, D.W., Mazurek, M.F., Swartz, K.J., and Martin, J.B. Replication of the neurochemical characteristics of Huntington's disease by quinolinic acid. *Nature,* **1986,** *321*:168–172.

Caroscio, J.T., Mulvill, M.N., Sterling, R., and Abrams, B. Amyotrophic lateral sclerosis. Its natural history. *Neurol. Clin.,* **1987,** *5*:1–8.

Chase, T.N. Levodopa therapy: consequences of nonphysiologic replacement of dopamine. *Neurology,* **1998,** *50*:S17–S25.

Chase, T.N., Engber, T.M., and Mouradian, M.M. Palliative and prophylactic benefits of continuously administered dopaminomimetics in Parkinson's disease. *Neurology,* **1994,** *44*:S15–S18.

Chatellier, G., and Lacomblez, L. Tacrine (tetrahydroaminoacridine; THA) and lecithin in senile dementia of the Alzheimer type: a multicentre trial. Groupe Français d'Etude de la Tetrahydroaminoacridine. *BMJ,* **1990,** *300*:495–499.

Cohen, G., and Werner, P. Free radicals, oxidative stress and neurodegeneration. In, *Neurodegenerative Diseases.* (Calne, D.B., ed.) Saunders, Philadelphia, **1994,** pp. 139–161.

Cotzias, G.C., Papavasiliou, P.S., and Gellene, R. Modification of Parkinsonism—chronic treatment with L-DOPA. *N. Engl. J. Med.,* **1969,** *280*:337–345.

Cudkowicz, M.E., and Brown, R.H. Jr. An update on superoxide dismutase 1 in familial amyotrophic lateral sclerosis. *J. Neurol. Sci.,* **1996,** *139*(suppl.):10–15.

Diamond, S.G., Markham, C.H., Hoehn, M.M., McDowell, F.H., and Muenter, M.D. Multi-center study of Parkinson mortality with early versus later dopa treatment. *Ann. Neurol.,* **1987,** *22*:8–12.

Duvoisin, R.C. Role of genetics in the cause of Parkinson's disease. *Mov. Disord.,* **1998,** *13*(suppl. 1):7–12.

Evans, D.A., Funkenstein, H.H., Albert, M.S., Scherr, P.A., Cook, N.R., Chown, M.J., Hebert, L.E., Hennekens, C.H., and Taylor, C.O. Prevalence of Alzheimer's disease in a community population of older persons. Higher than previously reported. *JAMA,* **1989,** *262*:2551–2556.

Fahn, S. Parkinson disease, the effect of levodopa, and the ELLDOPA trial. Earlier vs. later L-DOPA. *Arch. Neurol.,* **1999,** *56*:529–535.

Ferrante, R.J., Kowall, N.W., Beal, M.F., Martin, J.B., Bird, E.D., and Richardson, E.P., Jr. Morphologic and histochemical characteristics of a spared subset of striatal neurons in Huntington's disease. *J. Neuropathol. Exp. Neurol.,* **1987,** *46*:12–27.

Friedman, J.H., and Factor, S.A. Atypical antipsychotics in the treatment of drug-induced psychosis in Parkinson's disease. *Mov. Disord.,* **2000,** *15*:201–211.

Frucht, S., Rogers, J.G., Greene, P.E., Gordon, M.F., and Fahn, S. Falling asleep at the wheel: motor vehicle mishaps in persons taking pramipexole and ropinirole. *Neurology,* **1999,** *52*:1908–1910.

Gibb, W.R. Neuropathology of Parkinson's disease and related syndromes. *Neurol. Clin.,* **1992,** *10*:361–376.

Goetz, C.G. Dopaminergic agonists in the treatment of Parkinson's disease. *Neurology,* **1990,** *40*(suppl.):50–54.

Goetz, C.G. Influence of COMT inhibition on levodopa pharmacology and therapy. *Neurology,* **1998,** *50*:S26–S30.

Golbe, L.I. Alpha-synuclein and Parkinson's disease. *Mov. Disord.,* **1999,** *14*:6–9.

Greenamyre, J.T., and O'Brien, C.F. N-methyl-D-aspartate antagonists in the treatment of Parkinson's disease. *Arch. Neurol.,* **1991,** *48*:977–981.

Harper, P.S. The epidemiology of Huntington's disease. *Hum. Genet.,* **1992,** *89*:365–376.

Hersch, S.M., Gutekunst, C.A., Rees, H.D., Heilman, C.J., and Levey, A.I. Distribution of m1-m4 muscarinic receptor proteins in the rat striatum: light and electron microscopic immunocytochemistry using subtype-specific antibodies. *J. Neurosci.,* **1994,** *14*:3351–3363.

Hornykiewicz, O. Dopamine in the basal ganglia. Its role and therapeutic indications (including the clinical use of L-DOPA). *Br. Med. Bull.,* **1973,** *29*:172–178.

Huntington's Disease Collaborative Research Group. A novel gene containing a trinucleotide repeat that is expanded and unstable on Huntington's disease chromosomes. *Cell,* **1993,** *72*:971–983.

Jenkins, B.G., Koroshetz, W.J., Beal, M.F., and Rosen, B.R. Evidence for impairment of energy metabolism *in vivo* in Huntington's disease using localized 1H NMR spectroscopy. *Neurology,* **1993,** *43*:2689–2695.

Jenner, P. Oxidative mechanisms in nigral cell death in Parkinson's disease. *Mov. Disord.,* **1998,** *13(suppl. 1)*:24–34.

Keyser, D.L., and Rodnitzky, R.L. Neuroleptic malignant syndrome in Parkinson's disease after withdrawal or alteration of dopaminergic therapy. *Arch. Intern. Med.,* **1991,** *151*:794–796.

Kitada, T., Asakawa, S., Hattori, N., Matsumine, H., Yamamura, Y., Minoshima, S., Yokochi, M., Mizuno, Y., and Shimizu, N. Mutations in the parkin gene cause autosomal recessive juvenile parkinsonism. *Nature,* **1998,** *392*:605–608.

Kurth, M.C., Adler, C.H., Hilaire, M.S., Singer, C., Waters, C., LeWitt, P., Chernik, D.A., Dorflinger, E.E., and Yoo, K. Tolcapone improves motor function and reduces levodopa requirement in patients with Parkinson's disease experiencing motor fluctuations: a multicenter, double-blind, randomized, placebo-controlled trial. Tolcapone Fluctuator Study Group I. *Neurology,* **1997,** *48*:81–87.

Lacomblez, L., Bensimon, G., Leigh, P.N., Guillet, P., and Meininger, V. Dose-ranging study of riluzole in amyotrophic lateral sclerosis. *Lancet,* **1996,** *347*:1425–1431.

Landwehrmeyer, G.B., McNeil, S.M., Dure, L.S. IV, Ge, P., Aizawa, H., Huang, Q., Ambrose, C.M., Duyao, M.P., Bird, E.D., Bonilla, E., de Young, M., Avila-Gonzales, A.J., Wexler, N.S., DiFiglia, M., Gusella, J.F., MacDonald, M.E., Penney, J.B., Young, A.B., and Vonsattel, J.P. Huntington's disease gene: regional and cellular expression in brain of normal and affected individuals. *Ann. Neurol.,* **1995,** *37*:218–230.

Lipton, S.A., and Rosenberg, P.A. Excitatory amino acids as a final common pathway for neurologic disorders. *N. Engl. J. Med.,* **1994,** *330*:613–622.

Mouradian, M.M., Heuser, I.J., Baronti, F., and Chase, T.N. Modification of central dopaminergic mechanisms by continuous levodopa therapy for advanced Parkinson's disease. *Ann. Neurol.,* **1990,** *27*:18–23.

Olanow, C.W. MAO-B inhibitors in Parkinson's disease. *Adv. Neurol.,* **1993,** *60*:666–671.

Olanow, C.W. Oxidation reactions in Parkinson's disease. *Neurology,* **1990,** *40(suppl.)*:32–37.

Olney, J.W. Brain lesions, obesity, and other disturbances in mice treated with monosodium glutamate. *Science,* **1969,** *164*:719–721.

Parkinson Study Group. Effects of tocopherol and deprenyl on the progression of disability in early Parkinson's disease. *N. Engl. J. Med.,* **1993,** *328*:176–183.

Parkinson Study Group. Entacapone improves motor fluctuations in levodopa-treated Parkinson's disease patients. *Ann. Neurol.,* **1997,** *42*:747–755. [Published erratum appears in *Ann. Neurol.,* **1998,** *44*:292.]

Parkinson Study Group. Pramipexole vs. levodopa as initial treatment for Parkinson's disease: a randomized controlled trial. *JAMA,* **2000,** *284*:1931–1938.

Paulson, H.L., and Fischbeck, K.H. Trinucleotide repeats in neurogenetic disorders. *Annu. Rev. Neurosci.,* **1996,** *19*:79–107.

Przedborski, S., and Jackson-Lewis, V. Mechanisms of MPTP toxicity. *Mov. Disord.,* **1998,** *13(suppl. 1)*:35–38.

Rascol, O., Brooks, D.J., Korczyn, A.D., De Deyn, P.P., Clarke, C.E., and Lang, A.E. A five-year study of the incidence of dyskinesia in patients with early Parkinson's disease who were treated with ropinirole or levodopa. 056 Study Group. *N. Engl. J. Med.,* **2000,** *342*:1484–1491.

Reiner, A., Albin, R.L., Anderson, K.D., D'Amato, C.J., Penney, J.B., and Young, A.B. Differential loss of striatal projection neurons in Huntington disease. *Proc. Natl. Acad. Sci. U.S.A.,* **1988,** *85*:5733–5737.

Rogers, S.L., and Friedhoff, L.T. Long-term efficacy and safety of donepezil in the treatment of Alzheimer's disease: an interim analysis of the results of a US multicentre open label extension study. *Eur. Neuropsychopharmacol.,* **1998,** *8*:67–75.

Rosen, D.R., Siddique, T., Patterson, D., Figlewicz, D.A., Sapp, P., Hentati, A., Donaldson, D., Goto, J., O'Regan, J.P., Deng, H.X., Zohra, R., Krizus, A., McKenna-Yasik, D., Cayabyab, A., Gaston, S.M., Berger, R., Tanzi, R.E., Haperin, J.J., Hertzfeld, B., Van den Bergh, R., Hung, W.Y., Bird, T., Deng, G., Mulder, D.W., Smyth, C., Laing, N.G., Soriano, E., Pericak-Vance, M.A., Haines, J., Rouleau, G.A., Gusella, J.F., Horvitz, H.R., and Brown, R.H. Mutations in Cu/Zn superoxide dismutase gene are associated with familial amyotrophic lateral sclerosis. *Nature,* **1993,** *362*:59–62. [Published erratum appears in *Nature,* **1993,** *364*:362.]

Roses, A.D. Apolipoprotein E, a gene with complex biological interactions in the aging brain. *Neurobiol. Dis.,* **1997,** *4*:170–185.

Rothstein, J.D., Marin, L.J., and Kuncl, R.W. Decreased glutamate transport by the brain and spinal cord in amyotrophic lateral sclerosis. *N. Engl. J. Med.,* **1992,** *326*:1464–1468.

Schapira, A.H., Mann, V.M., Cooper, J.M., Dexter, D., Daniel, S.E., Jenner, P., Clark, J.B., and Marsden, C.D. Anatomic and disease specificity of NADH CoQ1 reductase (complex I) deficiency in Parkinson's disease. *J. Neurochem.,* **1990,** *55*:2142–2145.

Selkoe, D.J. The cell biology of beta-amyloid precursor protein and presenilin in Alzheimer's disease. *Trends Cell Biol.,* **1998,** *8*:447–453.

Standaert, D.G., and Stern, M.B. Update on the management of Parkinson's disease. *Med. Clin. North Am.,* **1993,** *77*:169–183.

Stoof, J.C., Booij, J., and Drukarch, B. Amantadine as *N*-methyl-D-aspartic acid receptor antagonist: new possibilities for therapeutic applications? *Clin. Neurol. Neurosurg.,* **1992,** *94(suppl.)*:S4–S6.

Tandan, R., and Bradley, W.G. Amyotrophic lateral sclerosis: Part 2. Etiopathogenesis. *Ann. Neurol.,* **1985,** *18*:419–431.

Tanner, C.M., and Langston, J.W. Do environmental toxins cause Parkinson's disease? A critical review. *Neurology,* **1990,** *40*(suppl): 17–30.

Vassar, R., Bennett, B.D., Babu-Kahn, S., Kahn, S., Mendiaz, E.A., Denis, P., Teplow, D.B., Ross, S., Amarante, P., Loeloff, R., Luo, Y., Fisher, S., Fuller, J., Edenson, S., Lile, J., Jarosinski, M.A., Biere, A.L., Curran, E., Burgess, T., Louis, J.C., Collins, F., Treanor, J., Rogers, G., and Citron, M. Beta-secretase cleavage of Alzheimer's amyloid precursor protein by the transmembrane aspartic protease BACE. *Science,* **1999,** *286*:735–741.

Vonsattel, J.P., Myers, R.H., Stevens, T.J., Ferrante, R.J., Bird, E.D., and Richardson, E.P., Jr. Neuropathological classification of Huntington's disease. *J. Neuropathol. Exp. Neurol.,* **1985,** *44*:559–577.

Wagner, M.L., and Landis, B.E. Riluzole: a new agent for amyotrophic lateral sclerosis. *Ann. Pharmacother.,* **1997,** *31*:738–744.

Wallace, D.C. Mitochondrial genetics: a paradigm of aging and degenerative diseases? *Science,* **1992,** *256*:628–632.

MONOGRAPHS AND REVIEWS

Albin, R.L., Young, A.B., and Penney, J.B. The functional anatomy of basal ganglia disorders. *Trends Neurosci.,* **1989,** *12*:366–375.

Beal, M.F., Hyman, B.T., and Koroshetz, W. Do defects in mitochondrial energy metabolism underlie the pathology of neurodegenerative diseases? *Trends Neurosci.,* **1993,** *16*:125–131.

Braak, H., and Braak, E. Pathology of Alzheimer's disease. In, *Neurodegenerative Diseases.* (Calne, D.B., ed.) Saunders, Philadelphia, **1994,** pp. 585–614.

Bryson, H.M., Fulton, B., and Benfield, P. Riluzole. A review of its pharmacodynamic and pharmacokinetic properties and therapeutic potential in amyotrophic lateral sclerosis. *Drugs,* **1996,** *52*:549–563.

Choi, D.W., and Rothman, S.M. The role of glutamate neurotoxicity in hypoxic-ischemic neuronal death. *Annu. Rev. Neurosci.,* **1990,** *13*: 171–182.

Cleveland, D.W. From Charcot to SOD1: mechanisms of selective motor neuron death in ALS. *Neuron,* **1999,** *24*:515–520.

Cooper, J.R., Bloom, F.E., and Roth, H.R., eds. *The Biochemical Basis of Neuropharmacology,* 7th ed. Oxford University Press, New York, **1996.**

Cummings, J.L., Vinters, H.V., Cole, G.M., and Khachaturian, Z.S. Alzheimer's disease: etiologies, pathophysiology, cognitive reserve, and treatment opportunities. *Neurology,* **1998,** *51*:S2–S17.

Davidoff, R.A. Spinal neurotransmitters and the mode of action of antispasticity drugs. In, *The Origin and Treatment of Spasticity.* (Benecke, R., Emre, M., and Davidoff, R.A., eds.) Parthenon Publishing Group, Carnforth, England, **1990,** pp. 63–92.

Fearnley, J., and Lees, A. Pathology of Parkinson's disease. In, *Neurodegenerative Diseases.* (Calne, D.B., ed.) Saunders, Philadelphia, **1994,** pp. 545–554.

Freeman, S.E., and Dawson, R.M. Tacrine: a pharmacological review. *Prog. Neurobiol.,* **1991,** *36*:257–277.

Harper, P.S., ed. *Huntington's Disease.* Saunders, London, **1991.**

Hayden, M.R. *Huntington's Chorea.* Springer-Verlag, Berlin, **1981.**

Jackson, C.E., and Bryan, W.W. Amyotrophic lateral sclerosis. *Semin. Neurol.,* **1998,** *18*:27–39.

Jarvie, K.R., and Caron, M.G. Heterogeneity of dopamine receptors. *Adv. Neurol.,* **1993,** *60*:325–333.

Johnston, M.V. Cognitive disorders. In, *Principles of Drug Therapy in Neurology.* (Johnston, M.V., MacDonald, R.L., and Young, A.B., eds.) Davis, Philadelphia, **1992,** pp. 226–267.

Kurtzke, J.F. Epidemiology of amyotrophic lateral sclerosis. In, *Human Motor Neuron Diseases.* (Rowland, L.P., ed.) *Advances in Neurology.* Vol. 36. Raven Press, New York, **1982,** pp. 281–302.

Lang, A.E., and Lozano, A.M. Parkinson's disease. First of two parts. *N. Engl. J. Med.,* **1998,** *339*:1044–1053.

Mayeux, R., and Sano, M. Treatment of Alzheimer's disease. *N. Engl. J. Med.,* **1999,** *341*:1670–1679.

Mink, J.W., and Thach, W.T. Basal ganglia intrinsic circuits and their role in behavior. *Curr. Opin. Neurobiol.,* **1993,** *3*:950–957.

Mouradian, M.M., and Chase, T.N. Improved dopaminergic therapy of Parkinson's disease. In, *Movement Disorders 3.* (Marsden, C.D., and Fahn, S., eds.) Butterworth-Heinemann, Oxford, **1994,** pp. 181–199.

Perry, E.K. The cholinergic hypothesis—ten years on. *Br. Med. Bull.,* **1986,** *42*:63–69.

Rowland, L.P. Amyotrophic lateral sclerosis: theories and therapies. *Ann. Neurol.,* **1994,** *35*:129–130.

Shoulson, I. Huntington's disease. In, *Diseases of the Nervous System: Clinical Neurobiology.* (Asbury, A.K., McKhann, G.M., and McDonald, W.I., eds.) Saunders, Philadelphia, **1992,** pp. 1159–1168.

Tanner, C.M. Epidemiology of Parkinson's disease. *Neurol. Clin.,* **1992,** *10*:317–329.

Whyte, S., Beyreuther, K., and Masters, C.L. Rational therapeutic strategies for Alzheimer's disease. In, *Neurodegenerative Diseases.* (Calne, D.B., ed.) Saunders, Philadelphia, **1994,** pp. 647–664.

Wichmann, T., and DeLong, M.R. Pathophysiology of parkinsonian motor abnormalities. *Adv. Neurol.,* **1993,** *60*:53–61.

Young, A.B. Role of excitotoxins in heredito-degenerative neurologic diseases. *Res. Publ. Assoc. Res. Nerv. Ment. Dis.,* **1993,** *71*:175–189.

OPIOID ANALGESICS

Howard B. Gutstein and Huda Akil

Opioids have been the mainstay of pain treatment for thousands of years, and remain so today. Opioids exert their therapeutic effects by mimicking the action of endogenous opioid peptides at opioid receptors. Effects on both local neurons and intrinsic pain-modulating circuitry lead to analgesia, other therapeutic effects, and also to undesirable side effects. This chapter will provide the background necessary to understand the mechanisms of action and important pharmacological properties of clinically used opioids. First, the endogenous opioid system is discussed with a focus on the receptors and circuitry utilized by the opioids. A discussion of clinically used compounds follows, describing in detail their pharmacological properties and therapeutic uses. Routes of administration, pain treatment strategies, and current therapeutic guidelines also are presented. This information should provide a rational basis for understanding opioid actions, thereby reducing fear of opioid use and encouraging effective treatment of pain.

OVERVIEW

It is now well known that opioids such as heroin and morphine exert their effects by mimicking naturally occurring substances, termed *endogenous opioid peptides* or *endorphins*. Much now is known about the basic biology of the endogenous opioid system and its molecular and biochemical complexity, widespread anatomy, and diversity. The diverse functions of this system include the best-known sensory role, prominent in inhibiting responses to painful stimuli; a modulatory role in gastrointestinal, endocrine, and autonomic functions; an emotional role, evident in the powerful rewarding and addicting properties of opioids; and a cognitive role in the modulation of learning and memory. The endogenous opioid system is complex and subtle, with a great diversity in endogenous ligands (over a dozen), yet with only four major receptor types. This chapter presents key facts about the biochemical and functional nature of the opioid system. This information then is used to establish a basis for understanding the actions of clinically used opioid drugs and current strategies for pain treatment.

Terminology. The term *opioid* refers broadly to all compounds related to opium. The word *opium* is derived from *opos*, the Greek word for juice, the drug being derived from the juice of the opium poppy, *Papaver somniferum*. *Opiates* are drugs derived from opium, and include the natural products morphine, codeine, thebaine, and many semisynthetic congeners derived from them. *Endogenous opioid peptides* are the naturally occurring ligands for opioid receptors. The term *endorphin* is used synonymously with endogenous opioid peptides, but also refers to a specific endogenous opioid, β-endorphin. The term *narcotic* was derived from the Greek word for stupor. At one time, the term referred to any drug that induced sleep, but then it became associated with opioids. It often is used in a legal context to refer to a variety of substances with abuse or addictive potential.

History. The first undisputed reference to opium is found in the writings of Theophrastus in the third century B.C. Arabian physicians were well versed in the uses of opium; Arabian traders introduced the drug to the Orient, where it was employed mainly for the control of dysenteries. During the Middle Ages, many of the uses of opium were appreciated. In 1680, Sydenham wrote: "Among the remedies which it has pleased Almighty God to give to man to relieve his sufferings, none is so universal and so efficacious as opium."

Opium contains more than 20 distinct alkaloids. In 1806, Sertürner reported the isolation of a pure substance in opium that he named morphine, after Morpheus, the Greek god of dreams. The discovery of other alkaloids in opium quickly followed—codeine by Robiquet in 1832, and papaverine by Merck in 1848. By the middle of the nineteenth century, the use of pure alkaloids rather than crude opium preparations began to spread throughout the medical world.

In addition to the remarkable beneficial effects of opioids, the toxic side effects and addictive potential of these drugs also have been known for centuries. These problems stimulated a search for potent, synthetic opioid analgesics free of addictive potential and other side effects. Unfortunately, all of the synthetic compounds that have been introduced into clinical use share the liabilities of classical opioids. However, the search for new opioid agonists led to the synthesis of opioid antagonists and compounds with mixed agonist/antagonist properties, which expanded therapeutic options and provided important tools for exploring mechanisms of opioid actions.

Until the early 1970s, the endogenous opioid system was totally unknown. The actions of morphine, heroin, and other opioids as antinociceptive and addictive agents, while well described, often were studied in the context of interactions with other neurotransmitter systems, such as monoaminergic and cholinergic. Some investigators suggested the existence of a specific opioid receptor because of the unique structural requirements of opiate ligands (Beckett and Casy, 1954), but the presence of an opiate-like system in the brain remained unproven. A particularly misleading observation was that the administration of the opioid antagonist naloxone to a normal animal produced little effect, although the drug was effective in reversing or preventing the effects of exogenous opiates. The first physiological evidence suggesting an endogenous opioid system was the demonstration that analgesia produced by electrical stimulation of certain brain regions was reversed by naloxone (Akil *et al.,* 1972; Akil *et al.,* 1976). Pharmacological evidence for an opiate receptor also was building. In 1973, investigators in three laboratories demonstrated opiate binding sites in the brain (Pert and Snyder, 1973; Simon *et al.,* 1973; Terenius, 1973). This was the first use of radioligand binding assays to demonstrate the presence of membrane-associated neurotransmitter receptors in the brain.

Stimulation-produced analgesia, its naloxone reversibility, and the discovery of opioid receptors strongly pointed to the existence of endogenous opioids. In 1975, Hughes and associates identified an endogenous, opiate-like factor that they called *enkephalin* (from the head) (Hughes *et al.,* 1975). Soon after, two more classes of endogenous opioid peptides were isolated, the *dynorphins* and *endorphins*. Details of these discoveries and the unique properties of the opioid peptides have been reviewed previously (Akil *et al.,* 1984).

Given the large number of endogenous ligands being discovered, it was not surprising that multiple classes of opioid receptors also were found. The concept of opioid-receptor multiplicity arose shortly after the initial demonstration of opiate binding sites. Based on results of *in vivo* studies in dogs, Martin and colleagues postulated the existence of multiple types of opiate receptors (Martin *et al.,* 1976). Receptor-binding studies and subsequent cloning confirmed the existence of three main receptor types, μ, δ, and κ. A fourth member of the opioid peptide receptor family, the *nociceptin/orphanin FQ* (N/OFQ) receptor, was cloned in 1994 (Bunzow *et al.,* 1994; Mollereau *et al.,* 1994). In addition to these four major classes, a number of subtypes have been proposed, such as *epsilon,* often based on bioassays from different species (Schulz *et al.,* 1979); *iota* (Oka, 1980); *lambda* (Grevel and Sadee, 1983); and *zeta* (Zagon *et al.,* 1989). In 2000, the Committee on Receptor Nomenclature and Drug Classification of the International Union of Pharmacology adopted the terms MOP, DOP, and KOP to indicate μ-, δ-, and κ-opioid peptide receptors, respectively. The original Greek letter designation is used in this and other chapters. The Committee also recommended the term NOP for the N/OFQ receptor.

ENDOGENOUS OPIOID PEPTIDES

Three distinct families of classical opioid peptides have been identified: the *enkephalins, endorphins,* and *dynorphins*. Each family is derived from a distinct precursor polypeptide and has a characteristic anatomical distribution. These precursors, preproopiomelanocortin, preproenkephalin, and preprodynorphin, are encoded by three corresponding genes. Each precursor is subject to complex cleavages and posttranslational modifications resulting in the synthesis of multiple active peptides. The opioid peptides share the common amino-terminal sequence of Tyr-Gly-Gly-Phe- (Met or Leu), which has been called the "opioid motif." This motif is followed by various C-terminal extensions yielding peptides ranging from 5 to 31 residues (Table 23–1).

The major opioid peptide derived from proopiomelanocortin (POMC) is β-endorphin. Although β-endorphin contains the sequence for met-enkephalin at its amino terminus, it is not converted to this peptide; met-enkephalin is derived from the processing of preproenkephalin. In addition to β-endorphin, the POMC precursor also is processed into the nonopioid peptides adrenocorticotropic hormone (ACTH), melanocyte-stimulating hormone (α-MSH), and β-lipotropin (β-LPH). Previous biochemical work (Mains *et al.,* 1977) had suggested a common precursor for the stress hormone ACTH and the opioid peptide β-endorphin. This association implied a close physiological linkage between the stress axis and opioid systems, which was validated by many studies of the phenomenon of stress-induced analgesia (Akil *et al.,* 1986). Proenkephalin contains multiple copies of met-enkephalin as well as a single copy of leu-enkephalin. Prodynorphin contains three peptides of differing lengths that all begin with the leu-enkephalin sequence: dynorphin A, dynorphin B, and neoendorphin (Figure 23–1). The anatomical distribution of these peptides in the central nervous system (CNS) has been reviewed thoroughly by Mansour *et al.* (1988).

A novel endogenous opioid peptide was cloned in 1995 (Meunier *et al.,* 1995; Reinscheid *et al.,* 1995). This peptide has a significant sequence homology to dynorphin A, with an identical length of 17 amino acids, identical carboxy-terminal residues, and a slight modification of the amino-terminal opioid core (Phe-Gly-Gly-Phe instead of Tyr-Gly-Gly-Phe; *see* Table 23–1). The removal of this single hydroxyl group is sufficient to abolish interactions with the three classical opioid-peptide receptors. This peptide was called *orphanin FQ* (OFQ) by one group of investigators and *nociceptin* (N) by another, because it lowered pain threshold under certain conditions. The structure of the N/OFQ precursor (Figure 23–2) suggests that it may encode other biologically active peptides (Nothacker *et al.,* 1996; Pan *et al.,* 1996). Immediately downstream of N/OFQ is a 17-amino-acid peptide (orphanin-2), which also starts with phenylalanine and ends with glutamine but is otherwise distinct from N/OFQ, as well as a putative peptide upstream from N/OFQ, which may be liberated

Table 23–1

Endogenous and Synthetic Opioid Peptides

Selected Endogenous Opioid Peptides

[Leu^5]enkephalin	**Tyr-Gly-Gly-Phe-Leu**
[Met^5]enkephalin	**Tyr-Gly-Gly-Phe-Met**
Dynorphin A	**Tyr-Gly-Gly-Phe-Leu-**Arg-Arg-IIe-Arg-Pro-Lys-Leu-Lys-Trp-Asp-Asn-Gln
Dynorphin B	**Tyr-Gly-Gly-Phe-Leu-**Arg-Arg-Gln-Phe-Lys-Val-Val-Thr
α-Neoendorphin	**Tyr-Gly-Gly-Phe-Leu-**Arg-Lys-Tyr-Pro-Lys
β-Neoendorphin	**Tyr-Gly-Gly-Phe-Leu-**Arg-Lys-Tyr-Pro
β_h-Endorphin	**Tyr-Gly-Gly-Phe-Met-**Thr-Ser-Glu-Lys-Ser-Gln-Thr-Pro-Leu-Val-Thr-Leu-Phe-Lys-Asn-Ala-Ile-Ile-Lys-Asn-Ala-Tyr-Lys-Lys-Gly-Glu

Novel Endogenous Opioid-Related Peptides

Orphanin FQ/Nociceptin	Phe-**Gly-Gly-Phe-**Thr-Gly-Ala-Arg-Lys-Ser-Ala-Arg-Lys-Leu-Ala-Asn-Gln
Endomorphin-1	Tyr-Pro-Trp-Phe
Endomorphin-2	Tyr-Pro-Phe-Phe

Selected Synthetic Opioid Peptides

DAMGO	[D-Ala^2,MePhe^4,Gly(ol)^5]enkephalin
DPDPE	[D-Pen^2,D-Pen^5]enkephalin
DSLET	[D-Ser^2,Leu^5]enkephalin-Thr^6
DADL	[D-Ala^2,D-Leu^5]enkephalin
CTOP	D-Phe-Cys-Tyr-D-Trp-Orn-Thr-Pen-Thr-NH$_2$
FK-33824	[D-Ala^2,N-MePhe^4,Met(O)^5-ol]enkephalin
[D-Ala^2]Deltorphin I	Tyr-D-Ala-Phe-Asp-Val-Val-Gly-NH$_2$
[D-Ala^2,Glu^4]Deltorphin (Deltorphin II)	Tyr-D-Ala-Phe-Glu-Val-Val-Gly-NH$_2$
Morphiceptin	Tyr-Pro-Phe-Pro-NH$_2$
PL-017	Tyr-Pro-MePhe-D-Pro-NH$_2$
DALCE	[D-Ala^2,Leu^5,Cys^6]enkephalin

upon posttranslational processing (*nocistatin*). The N/OFQ system represents a new neuropeptide system with a high degree of sequence identity to the opioid peptides. However, the slight change in structure results in a profound alteration in function. N/OFQ has behavioral and pain modulatory properties distinct from those of the three classical opioid peptides (*see* below).

The anatomical distribution of POMC-producing cells is relatively limited within the CNS, occurring mainly in the arcuate nucleus and nucleus tractus solitarius. These neurons project widely to limbic and brainstem areas and to the spinal cord (Lewis *et al.,* 1987). There also is evidence of POMC production in the spinal cord (Gutstein *et al.,* 1992). The distribution of POMC corresponds to areas of the human brain where electrical stimulation can relieve pain (Pilcher *et al.,* 1988). Peptides from POMC occur in both the pars intermedia and the pars distalis of the pituitary and also are contained in pancreatic islet cells. The peptides from prodynorphin and proenkephalin

are distributed widely throughout the CNS and frequently are found together. Although each family of peptides usually is located in different groups of neurons, occasionally more than one family is expressed within the same neuron (Weihe *et al.,* 1988). Of particular note, proenkephalin peptides are present in areas of the CNS that are presumed to be related to the perception of pain (*e.g.,* laminae I and II of the spinal cord, the spinal trigeminal nucleus, and the periaqueductal gray), to the modulation of affective behavior (*e.g.,* amygdala, hippocampus, locus ceruleus, and the cerebral cortex), to the modulation of motor control (caudate nucleus and globus pallidus), and the regulation of the autonomic nervous system (medulla oblongata) and neuroendocrinological functions (median eminence). Although there are a few long enkephalinergic fiber tracts, these peptides are contained primarily in interneurons with short axons. The peptides from proenkephalin also are found in the adrenal medulla and in nerve plexuses and exocrine glands of the stomach and intestine.

The N/OFQ precursor has a unique anatomical distribution (Neal *et al.,* 1999b). The distribution of this system suggests

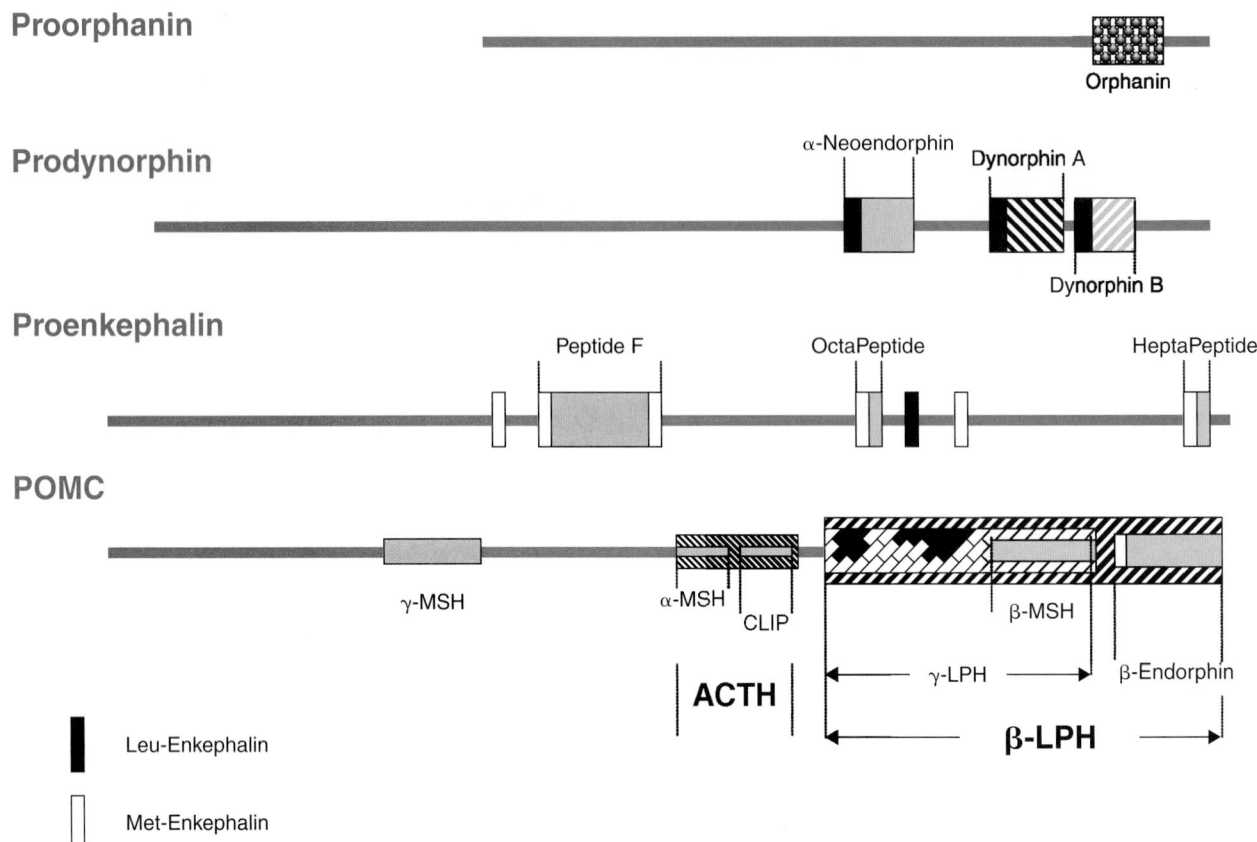

Proorphanin

Prodynorphin

α-Neoendorphin

Dynorphin A

Dynorphin B

Proenkephalin

Peptide F   OctaPeptide   HeptaPeptide

POMC

γ-MSH

α-MSH

CLIP

β-MSH

ACTH

γ-LPH

β-Endorphin

β-LPH

Leu-Enkephalin

Met-Enkephalin

Orphanin

Figure 23–1. Peptide precursors. (From Akil et al., 1998.)
POMC, proopiomelanocortin; ACTH, adrenocorticotropic hormone; β-LPH, β-lipotropin.

important roles in hippocampus, cortex, and numerous sensory sites. N/OFQ produces a complex behavioral profile, including effects on drug reward and reinforcement (Bertorelli *et al.*, 2000; Devine *et al.*, 1996a; Devine *et al.*, 1996b), stress responsiveness (Devine *et al.*, 2001; Koster *et al.*, 1999), and learning and memory processes (Koster *et al.*, 1999; Manabe *et al.*, 1998). Studies of the effect of N/OFQ on pain sensitivity have produced conflicting results, which may be reconciled by data suggesting that the effects of N/OFQ on pain sensitivity depend on the

Orphanin

Nocistatin   Orphanin-2

110-127 Nocistatin   MPRVRSLFQEQEEPEPGMEEAGEMEQKQLQ

130-146 Orphanin   FQFGGFTGARKSARKLANQ

149-165 Orphanin-2   FSEFMRQYLVLSMQSSQ

Figure 23–2. Human proorphanin-derived peptides.

underlying behavioral state of the animal (Pan *et al.*, 2000) (*see below*). Analogous mechanisms also could explain some of the conflicting results with other physiological processes. However, more studies are needed before a general role can be ascribed to the N/OFQ system, including the investigation of other active peptides that may be derived from the N/OFQ precursor (Figure 23–2). Nocistatin has been tested behaviorally and found to produce effects opposite to those of N/OFQ (Okuda-Ashitaka *et al.*, 1998). In sum, these findings, coupled with the extensive anatomy of the system, suggest that the N/OFQ precursor plays a complex role in the brain that is yet to be fully appreciated.

Not all cells that make a given precursor polypeptide store and release the same mixture of active opioid peptides, because of differential processing secondary to variations in the cellular complement of peptidases that produce and degrade the active opioid fragments (Akil *et al.*, 1984). In addition, processing of these peptides is altered by physiological demands, leading to a different mix of peptides being released by the same cell under different conditions. For example, chronic morphine treatment (Bronstein *et al.*, 1990) or stress (Akil *et al.*, 1985) can alter the forms of β-endorphin released by cells, which could possibly underlie some observed physiological adaptations. Although the endogenous opioid peptides appear to function as neurotransmitters, modulators of neurotransmission, or neurohormones, the full extent of their physiological role is not completely understood (Akil *et al.*, 1988). The elucidation of the physiological roles of the opioid peptides has been made more difficult by their frequent coexistence with other putative neurotransmitters within a given neuron.

OPIOID RECEPTORS

Three classical opioid receptor types, μ, δ, and κ, have been studied extensively. The more recently discovered N/OFQ receptor, initially called the opioid-receptor-like 1 (ORL-1) receptor or "orphan" opioid receptor has added a new dimension to the study of opioids. Highly selective ligands that allowed for type-specific labeling of the three classical opioid receptors (*e.g.,* DAMGO for μ, DPDPE for δ, and U-50,488 and U-69,593 for κ) (Handa *et al.,* 1981; Mosberg *et al.,* 1983; Voightlander *et al.,* 1983) became available in the early 1980s. These tools made possible the definition of ligand-binding characteristics of each of the receptor types and the determination of anatomical distribution of the receptors using autoradiographic techniques. Each major opioid receptor has a unique anatomical distribution in brain, spinal cord, and the periphery

(Mansour *et al.,* 1988; Neal *et al.,* 1999b). These distinctive patterns of localization suggested possible functions that subsequently have been investigated in pharmacological and behavioral studies.

The study of the biological functions of opioid receptors *in vivo* was aided by the synthesis of selective antagonists and agonists. Among the most commonly used antagonists are cyclic analogs of somatostatin such as CTOP as μ-receptor antagonists, a derivative of naloxone called naltrindole as a δ-receptor antagonist, and a bivalent derivative of naltrexone called binaltorphimine (nor-BNI) as a κ-receptor antagonist (Gulya *et al.,* 1986; Portoghese *et al.,* 1987; Portoghese *et al.,* 1988). In general, functional studies using selective agonists and antagonists have revealed substantial parallels between μ and δ receptors and dramatic contrasts between μ/δ and κ receptors. *In vivo* infusions of selective antagonists and agonists also were used to establish the receptor types involved in mediating various opioid effects (Table 23–2).

Most of the clinically used opioids are relatively selective for μ receptors, reflecting their similarity to morphine

Table 23–2
Classification of Opioid Receptor Subtypes and Actions from Animal Models

	RECEPTOR SUBTYPE	ACTIONS OF:	
		AGONISTS	ANTAGONISTS
Analgesia			
Supraspinal	μ, κ, δ	Analgesic	No effect
Spinal	μ, κ, δ	Analgesic	No effect
Respiratory function	μ	Decrease	No effect
Gastrointestinal tract	μ, κ	Decrease transit	No effect
Psychotomimesis	κ	Increase	No effect
Feeding	μ, κ, δ	Increase feeding	Decrease feeding
Sedation	μ, κ	Increase	No effect
Diuresis	κ	Increase	
Hormone regulation			
Prolactin	μ	Increase release	Decrease release
Growth hormone	μ and/or δ	Increase release	Decrease release
Neurotransmitter release			
Acetylcholine	μ	Inhibit	
Dopamine	μ, δ	Inhibit	
Isolated organ bioassays			
Guinea pig ileum	μ	Decrease contraction	No effect
Mouse vas deferens	δ	Decrease contraction	No effect

The actions listed for antagonists are seen with the antagonist alone. All the correlations in this table are based on studies in rats and mice, which occasionally show species differences. Thus, any extensions of these associations to human beings are tentative. Clinical studies do indicate that μ receptors elicit analgesia both spinally and supraspinally. Preliminary work with a synthetic opioid peptide, [D-Ala^2,D-Leu^5]enkephalin, suggests that intrathecal δ agonists are analgesic in human beings.

SOURCE: Modified from Pasternak (1993).

Table 23–3

Actions and Selectivities of Some Opioids at the Various Opioid Receptor Classes

	RECEPTOR TYPES		
	μ	δ	κ
Drugs			
Morphine	+++		+
Methadone	+++		
Etorphine	+++	+++	+++
Levorphanol	+++		
Fentanyl	+++		
Sufentanil	+++	+	+
DAMGO	+++		
Butorphanol	P		+++
Buprenorphine	P		−−
Naloxone	−−−	−	−−
Naltrexone	−−−	−	−−−
CTOP	−−−		
Diprenorphine	−−−	−−	−−−
β-Funaltrexamine	−−−	−	++
Naloxonazine	−−−	−	−
Nalorphine	−−−		+
Pentazocine	P		++
Nalbuphine	−−		++
Naloxone benzoylhydrazone	−−−	−	−
Bremazocine	+++	++	+++
Ethylketocyclazocine	P	+	+++
U50,488			+++
U69,593			+++
Spiradoline	+		+++
nor-Binaltorphimine	−	−	−−−
Naltrindole	−	−−−	−
DPDPE		++	
[D-Ala^2,Glu^4]deltorphin		++	
DSLET	+	++	
Endogenous Peptides			
Met-enkephalin	++	+++	
Leu-enkephalin	++	+++	
β-Endorphin	+++	+++	
Dynorphin A	++		+++
Dynorphin B	+	+	+++
α-Neoendorphin	+	+	+++

Activities of drugs are given at the receptors for which the agent has reasonable affinity. +, agonist: −, antagonist: P, partial agonist: DAMGO, CTOP, DPDPE, DSLET, *see* Table 23–1. The number of symbols is an indication of potency: the ratio for a given drug denotes selectivity. These values were obtained primarily from animal studies and should be extrapolated to human beings with caution. Both β-funaltrexamine and naloxonazine are irreversible μ antagonists, but β-funaltrexamine also has reversible κ agonist activity.

Table 23–4

Properties of the Cloned Opioid Receptors

| RECEPTOR SUBTYPE | SELECTIVE LIGANDS | | NONSELECTIVE LIGANDS | | PUTATIVE ENDOGENOUS LIGANDS |
	Agonists	Antagonists	Agonists	Antagonists	
μ	DAMGO Morphine Methadone Fentanyl Dermorphin	CTOP	Levorphanol Etorphine	Naloxone Naltrexone β-Funaltrexamine	Enkephalin Endorphin
κ	Spiradoline U50,488 Dynorphin A	Nor-BNI	Levorphanol Etorphine EKC	Naloxone Naltrexone	Dynorphin A
δ	DPDPE Deltorphin DSLET	Naltrindole NTB BNTX	Levorphanol Etorphine	Naloxone Naltrexone	Enkephalin

ABBREVIATIONS: BNTX, 7 benzylidenenaltroxone; EKC, ethylketocyclazosine NTB, benzofuran analog of naltrindole; nor-BNI, nor-binaltorphimine. DAMGO, CTOR, DPDPE, DSLET, *see* Table 23–1.

SOURCE: Modified from Raynor *et al.* (1994).

(Tables 23–3 and 23–4). However, it is important to note that drugs that are relatively selective at standard doses will interact with additional receptor subtypes when given at sufficiently high doses, leading to possible changes in their pharmacological profile. This is especially true as doses are escalated to overcome tolerance. Some drugs, particularly mixed agonist-antagonist agents, interact with more than one receptor class at usual clinical doses. The actions of these drugs are particularly interesting, since they may act as an agonist at one receptor and an antagonist at another.

There is little agreement regarding the exact classification of opioid receptor subtypes. Pharmacological studies have suggested the existence of multiple subtypes of each receptor. The complex literature on κ opioid-receptor subtypes (*see* Akil and Watson, 1994) strongly suggests the presence of at least one additional subtype with good affinity for the benzomorphan class of opiate alkaloids. The data for δ-opioid receptor subtypes is intriguing. While early support for the possibility of multiple δ receptors came from radioligand-binding studies (Negri *et al.,* 1991), the strongest evidence derives from behavioral studies (Jiang *et al.,* 1991; Sofuoglu *et al.,* 1991), which led to the proposal that two δ-receptor sites exist, δ_1 and δ_2. In the case of the μ receptor, behavioral and pharmacological studies led to the proposal of μ_1 and μ_2 subtypes (Pasternak, 1986). The μ_1 site is proposed to be a very high affinity receptor with little discrimination between μ and δ ligands. A parallel hypothesis (Rothman *et al.,* 1988) holds that there is a high affinity μ/δ complex rather than a distinct μ site. Although molecular cloning studies have not readily supported the existence

of these subtypes as distinct molecules, recent findings (*see* below) regarding modified specificity for opioid ligands due to heterodimerization of receptors may provide an explanation for observed pharmacological diversity (Jordan and Devi, 1999).

Molecular Studies of Opioid Receptors and Their Ligands

For many years, the study of multiple opioid receptors greatly profited from the availability of a rich array of natural and synthetic ligands but was limited by the absence of opioid receptor clones. In 1992, the mouse δ receptor was cloned from the NG-108 cell line (Evans *et al.,* 1992; Kieffer *et al.,* 1992). Subsequently, the other two major types of classical opioid receptors were cloned from various rodent species (Chen *et al.,* 1993; Kong *et al.,* 1994; Meng *et al.,* 1993; Minami *et al.,* 1993; Thompson *et al.,* 1993; Wang *et al.,* 1993; Yasuda *et al.,* 1993). The N/OFQ receptor was cloned as a result of searches for novel types or subtypes of opioid receptors. The coding regions for the opioid-peptide receptors subsequently were isolated and chromosomally assigned (Befort *et al.,* 1994; Yasuda *et al.,* 1994; Wang *et al.,* 1994). In the case of μ, the cloned sequence is the classical morphine-like receptor, rather than the proposed μ_1. With δ, no differentiation between the two proposed types by binding appears possible, and the cloned receptor recognizes all δ-selective ligands regardless of their behavioral assignment as δ_1 or δ_2. For κ, the cloned receptor is the classical receptor, rather than the proposed benzomorphan binding site. All four opioid receptors belong to the G protein-coupled receptor (GPCR) family (*see* Chapter 2) and share extensive sequence homologies (Figure 23–3). The N/OFQ receptor has high structural homology with the classical opioid receptors, but it has very low or no affinity for binding conventional opioid ligands (Bunzow *et al.,* 1994; Chen *et al.,* 1994; Mollereau *et al.,* 1994).

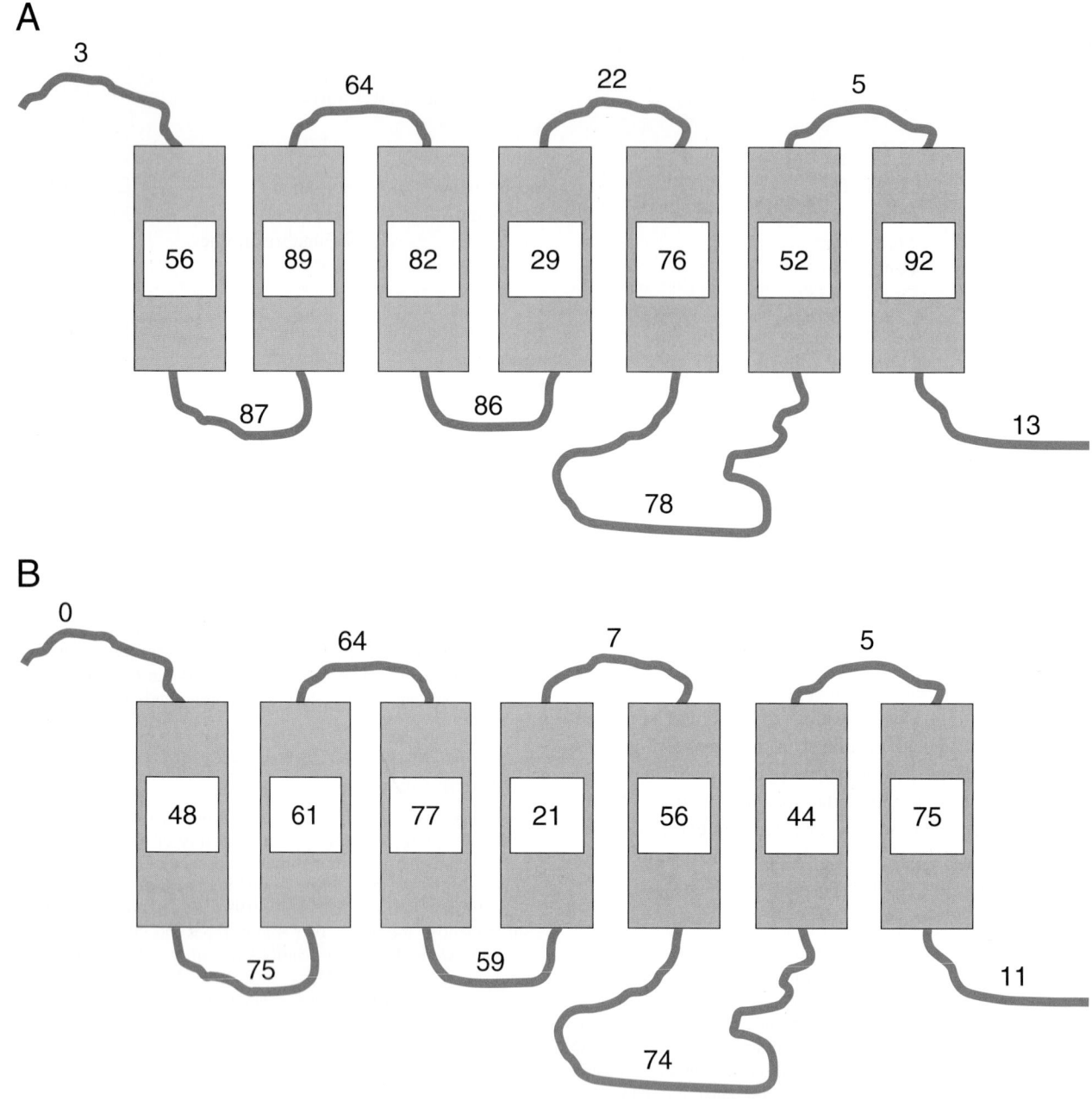

Figure 23–3. A. Structural homology among the three opioid receptors. B. Structural homology among the three opioid receptors and the N/OFQ receptor. (*From Akil* et al., *1998, with permission.*)
Numbers indicate the percent of identical amino acids in the segment.

The structural similarities of the N/OFQ receptor and the three classical opioid receptors are highest in the transmembrane regions and cytoplasmic domains and lowest in the extracellular domains critical for ligand selectivity (Figure 23–3B).

It is possible that further cloning experiments may identify unique genes encoding opioid receptor subtypes. However, it has been suggested that, if multiple opioid receptor subtypes exist,

they could be derived from a single gene, and multiple mechanisms might exist to achieve distinct pharmacological profiles. Two potential pathways to opioid receptor diversity are alternative splicing of receptor RNA and dimerization of receptor proteins.

Alternative splicing of receptor heteronuclear RNA (*e.g.*, exon skipping and intron retention) is thought to play an important role in producing *in vivo* diversity within many members of the GPCR superfamily (Kilpatrick *et al.*, 1999). Splice variants may exist within each of the three opioid receptor families, and this alternative splicing of receptor transcripts may be critical for the diversity of opioid receptors. A technique widely used to identify potential sites of alternative splicing is antisense oligodeoxynucleotide (ODN) mapping. The ability of antisense ODNs to target specific regions of cDNA permits the systematic evaluation of the contribution of individual exons to observed receptor properties. Antisense ODN-targeting of exon 1 of the rat and mouse μ opioid receptors blocks morphine analgesia in these species (Rossi *et al.*, 1995; Rossi *et al.*, 1996a; Rossi *et al.*, 1997). By contrast, administration of antisense ODNs targeting exon 2 does not block morphine analgesia but prevents the analgesia produced by heroin, fentanyl, and the morphine metabolite morphine-6-glucuronide (Rossi *et al.*, 1995; Rossi *et al.*, 1996a; Rossi *et al.*, 1997). An analogous disruption of morphine-6-glucuronide–induced but not morphine-induced analgesia is observed following administration of antisense ODNs targeting exon 3 (Rossi *et al.*, 1997). These results imply that unique μ receptor mechanisms mediate the analgesic effects of a variety of opioids and are consistent with the claim that these unique receptor mechanisms could be achieved *via* alternative splicing. The use of antisense ODNs also has led to the identification of potential sites for splice variation in the κ- and δ-opioid receptors (Pasternak and Standifer, 1995). Central to the claim that these results reflect the existence of splice variants is the *in vivo* isolation of such variants. A μ-opioid receptor splice variant has been identified that differs considerably from the native receptor within its C-terminus (Zimprich *et al.*, 1995). As might be expected on the basis of the splicing location, this variant exhibits a binding profile similar to that of the cloned μ-opioid receptor but does not readily undergo the desensitization frequently observed following exposure to agonist. Thus, the existence of this splice variant cannot explain the differential analgesic sensitivities described above. However, just such a variant was detected in mice with a targeted disruption of exon 1 (Schuller *et al.*, 1999). Transcripts of the μ-opioid receptor that contained exons 2 and 3 were identified in these mice. Moreover, whereas morphine-induced analgesia was abolished, heroin- and M6G-induced analgesia were unaffected.

The interaction of two receptors to form a unique structure (dimerization) also has been accorded an important role in regulating receptor function. For example, dimerization of $GABA_{BR1}$ and $GABA_{BR2}$ subunits is required to form a functional $GABA_B$ receptor for gamma-aminobutyric acid (*e.g.*, Jones *et al.*, 1998). Both cloned κ- and δ-opioid receptors have been shown to exist *in vitro* as homodimers (Cvejic and Devi, 1997). However, the most interesting findings have been generated by studies showing dimerization between different opioid receptor types. Jordan and Devi (1999) showed that κ- and δ-opioid receptors can exist as heterodimers both in heterologous expression systems and in brain, based on coimmunoprecipitation studies. The dimerization of these receptors profoundly alters their pharmacological properties. The affinity of the heterodimers for highly selective agonists and antagonists is greatly reduced. Instead, the heterodimers show greatest affinity for partially selective agonists such as bremazocine, suggesting that receptor hetero dimerization may explain at least part of the discrepancy between molecular and pharmacological properties of opioid receptors.

Given the existence of four families of endogenous ligands and cloned receptors, it seems reasonable to ask if there is a one-to-one correspondence between them. Previous studies using brain homogenates demonstrated that an orderly pattern of association between a set of opioid gene products and a given receptor does not exist. Although proenkephalin products generally are associated with δ and prodynorphin products with κ receptors, much "cross-talk" is present (Mansour *et al.*, 1995). The cloning of the opioid receptors allowed this question to be addressed more systematically, since each receptor could be expressed separately and then compared side by side under identical conditions (Mansour *et al.*, 1997). The κ receptor exhibits the most selectivity across endogenous ligands, with affinities ranging from 0.1 nM for dynorphin A to approximately 100 nM for leu-enkephalin. In contrast, μ and δ receptors show only a 10-fold difference between the most- and least-preferred ligand, with a majority of endogenous ligands exhibiting greater affinity for δ than for μ receptors. The limited selectivity of μ and δ receptors suggests that the μ and δ receptor recognize principally the Tyr-Gly-Gly-Phe core of the endogenous peptide, whereas the κ receptor requires this core *and* the arginine in position 6 of dynorphin A and other prodynorphin products (*see* Table 23–1). Interestingly, proenkephalin products with arginine in position 6 (*i.e.*, met-enkephalin-Arg-Phe and met-enkephalin-Arg-Gly-Leu) are equally good κ-receptor ligands, arguing against the idea of a unique association between a given receptor and a given opioid precursor family. In sum, high affinity interactions are possible between each of the peptide precursor families and each of the three receptor types, the only exception being the lack of high-affinity interaction between POMC-derived peptides and κ receptors. Otherwise, at least one peptide product from each of the families exhibits high affinity (low nanomolar or subnanomolar) for each receptor. The relatively unimpressive affinity of the μ receptor toward all known endogenous ligands suggests that its most avid and selective ligand has not been identified, a notion being put to test (*see* below).

Endomorphins. The search for a high affinity/high selectivity endogenous ligand for the μ receptor led to the discovery of a class of novel endogenous opioids termed *endomorphins* (Zadina *et al.*, 1997). Endomorphin-1 and endomorphin-2 are tetrapeptides with the sequences Tyr-Pro-Trp-Phe and Tyr-Pro-Phe-Phe, respectively (Table 23–1). These novel peptides do not contain the canonical opioid core (Tyr-Gly-Gly-Phe) but nevertheless bind the μ receptor with very high affinity and selectivity. However, an endomorphin gene has yet to be cloned, and much remains to be learned about the endomorphins' anatomical distribution, mode of interaction with the opioid receptors, function *in vivo,* and the potential existence of other related peptides that are highly selective for each of the opioid receptors.

Molecular Basis for Opioid Receptor Selectivity and Affinity. Previous studies of other peptide receptors suggested that peptides and small molecules may bind to GPCRs differently. Mutagenesis studies of small ligand receptors (*e.g.*, adrenergic and dopamine receptors) showed that charged amino acid residues in the transmembrane domains were important in receptor binding and activation (Strader *et al.*, 1988; Mansour *et al.*, 1992). This observation places the bound ligands within the receptor core formed by the transmembrane helices. On the other hand, studies with peptidergic receptors have demonstrated a critical role for extracellular loops in ligand recognition (Xie *et al.,* 1990). All three classical opioid receptors appear to combine both properties: Charged residues located in transmembrane domains have been implicated in the high affinity binding of most opioid ligands, whether alkaloid or peptide (Surratt *et al.,* 1994; Mansour *et al.,* 1997). However, critical interactions of opioid peptides with the extracellular domains also have been shown.

The opioid peptide Tyr-Gly-Gly-Phe core, sometimes termed the "message," appears to be necessary for interaction with the receptor-binding pocket; however, peptide *selectivity* resides in the carboxy-terminal extension beyond the tetrapeptide core, providing the "address" (Schwyzer, 1986). When the carboxy-terminal domain is long, it may interact with extracellular loops of the receptors, contributing to selectivity in a way that cannot be achieved by the much smaller alkaloids. Indeed, dynorphin A selectivity is dependent on the second extracellular loop of the κ receptor (Kong *et al.,* 1994; Xue *et al.,* 1994; Meng *et al.,* 1995), whereas δ- and μ-selective ligands have more complex mechanisms of selectivity that depend on multiple extracellular loops. These findings have led to the proposal that high selectivity is achieved by both attraction to the most-favored receptor and repulsion by the less-favored receptor (Watson *et al.,* 1995; Meng *et al.,* 1995). For example, the N/OFQ receptor does not bind any of the classical endogenous opioid peptides. However, mutating as few as four amino acids endows the N/OFQ receptor with the ability to recognize prodynorphin-derived peptides while retaining recognition of N/OFQ (Meng *et al.,* 1996), suggesting that unique mechanisms have evolved to ensure selectivity of the N/OFQ receptor for N/OFQ and against classical opioid peptides. Mechanisms involved in selectivity can be difficult to separate from mechanisms involved in affinity, because the extracellular domains may not only allow interactions with the peptide ligands but also may be important in stabilizing these interactions.

Results of the research discussed above imply that the alkaloids are small enough to fit completely inside or near the mouth of the receptor core, while peptides bind to the extracellular loops and simultaneously extend to the receptor core to activate the common binding site. That one can truly separate the binding of peptides and alkaloids is demonstrated most clearly by a genetically engineered κ receptor (Coward *et al.,* 1998), which does not recognize endogenous peptide ligands, yet retains full affinity and efficacy for small synthetic κ-receptor ligands, such as spiradoline. Given these differences in binding interactions with the receptor, it is possible that unique classes of ligands may activate the opioid receptor differently, leading to conformational changes of distinct quality or duration that may result in varying magnitudes and possibly different second-messenger events. This hypothesis currently is being tested and, if validated, may lead to novel strategies for differentially altering the interactions between the opioid receptors and signal transduction cascades. With the potential presence of receptor heterodimers and the likelihood that they have unique profiles and signaling properties (Jordan and Devi, 1999), there now are a number of new directions for discovery of drugs that may target receptors in particular states.

Opioid Receptor Signaling and Consequent Intracellular Events

Coupling of Opioid Receptors to Second Messengers. The μ, δ, and κ receptors in endogenous neuronal settings are coupled, *via* pertussis toxin-sensitive GTP-binding proteins, to inhibition of adenylyl cyclase activity (Herz, 1993), activation of receptor-operated K^+ currents, and suppression of voltage-gated Ca^{2+} currents (Duggan and North, 1983). The hyperpolarization of the membrane potential by K^+-current activation and the limiting of Ca^{2+} entry by suppression of Ca^{2+} currents are tenable but unproven mechanisms for explaining blockade by opioids of neurotransmitter release and pain transmission in varying neuronal pathways. Studies with cloned receptors have shown that opioid receptors may couple to an array of other second messenger systems, including activation of the MAP kinases and the phospholipase C (PLC)-mediated cascade leading to the formation of inositol trisphosphate and diacylglycerol (*see* Akil *et al.,* 1997, for review). Prolonged exposure to opioids results in adaptations at multiple levels within these signaling cascades. The significance of these cellular-level adaptations lies in the causal relationship that may exist between them and adaptations seen at the organismic level such as tolerance, sensitization, and withdrawal.

Receptor Desensitization, Internalization, and Sequestration Following Chronic Exposure to Opioids. Transient administration of opioids leads to a phenomenon termed *acute tolerance,* whereas sustained administration leads to the development of "classical" or *chronic tolerance. Tolerance* simply refers to a decrease in effectiveness of a drug with its repeated administration. Recent studies have focused on cellular mechanisms of acute tolerance. Several investigators have shown that short-term desensitization probably involves phosphorylation of the μ and δ receptors *via* protein kinase C (Mestek *et al.,* 1995; Narita *et al.,* 1995; Ueda *et al.,* 1995). A number of other kinases also have been implicated, including protein kinase A and β-adrenergic receptor kinase, βARK (Pei *et al.,* 1995; Wang *et al.,* 1994; also, *see* below).

Like other GPCRs, both μ and δ receptors can undergo rapid agonist-mediated internalization *via* a classic endocytic pathway (Trapaidze *et al.,* 1996; Gaudriault *et al.,* 1997), whereas κ receptors do not internalize following prolonged agonist exposure (Chu *et al.,* 1997). Interestingly, it seems that internalization occurs *via* partially distinct endocytic pathways for the μ and δ receptors, suggesting *receptor*-specific interactions with different mediators of intracellular trafficking (Gaudriault *et al.,* 1997). It also is intriguing that these processes may be induced differentially as a function of the structure of the *ligand.* For example, certain agonists, such as etorphine and enkephalins, cause rapid internalization of the μ receptor, while morphine, although it decreases adenylyl cyclase activity equally well, does not cause μ receptor internalization (Keith *et al.,* 1996). In addition, a truncated μ receptor with normal G protein coupling was shown to recycle constitutively from the membrane to cytosol (Segredo *et al.,* 1997), further indicating that activation of signal transduction and internalization are controlled by distinct molecular mechanisms. These studies also support the hypothesis that different ligands induce different conformational changes in the receptor that result in divergent intracellular events, and they may provide an explanation for differences in the efficacy and abuse potential of various opioids. One of the most interesting studies to evaluate the relevance of these alterations in signaling to the adaptations seen in response to opioid exposure *in vivo* was the demonstration that acute morphine-induced analgesia was enhanced in mice lacking β-arrestin 2 (Bohn *et al.,* 1999). Opioid-receptor internalization is mediated, at least partially, by the actions of GPCR kinases (GRKs). GRKs selectively phosphorylate agonist-bound receptors, thereby promoting interactions with β-arrestins, which interfere with G protein coupling and promote receptor internalization (Bohn *et al.,* 1999). Enhanced analgesia in mice lacking β-arrestin 2 is consistent with a role for the GRKs and arrestins in regulating responsivity to opioids *in vivo.* This result is even more intriguing given the inability of morphine to support arrestin translocation and receptor internalization *in vitro* (Whistler and von Zastrow, 1998).

Traditionally, long-term tolerance has been thought to be associated with increases in adenylyl cyclase activity—a counter-regulation to the decrease in cyclic AMP levels seen after acute opioid administration (Sharma *et al.,* 1977). Chronic treatment with μ-receptor opioids causes superactivation of adenylyl cyclase (Avidor-Reiss *et al.,* 1996). This effect is prevented by pretreatment with pertussis toxin, demonstrating involvement of $G_{i/o}$ proteins, and also by cotransfection with scavengers of G protein-$\beta\gamma$ dimers, indicating a role for this complex in superactivation. Alterations in levels of cyclic AMP clearly bring about numerous secondary changes (*see* Nestler and Aghajanian, 1997).

An "Apparent Paradox." A paradox in evaluating the function of endogenous opioid systems is that a host of endogenous ligands activate a small number of opioid receptors. This pattern is different from that of many other neurotransmitter systems, where a single ligand interacts with a large number of receptors having different structures and second messengers. Is this richness and complexity at the presynaptic level lost as multiple opioid ligands derived from different genes converge on only three receptors, or is this richness preserved through means yet to be discovered? One possibility is that all opioid receptors have not been revealed by molecular cloning. Other options include splice variants, dimerization, and posttranslational modification, as discussed previously. Even assuming that other receptors and variants will be found, the binding of many endogenous ligands to the three cloned classical receptors suggests a great deal of convergence. However, this convergence may be only apparent, since multiple mechanisms for achieving distinctive responses in the context of the biology described above may exist. Some issues to consider are as follows:

1. The *duration of action* of endogenous ligands may be a critical variable that has been overlooked and that may have clinical relevance.
2. The *pattern or profile of activation of multiple receptors by a ligand,* rather than activation of a single receptor, may be a critical determinant of effect.
3. *Opioid genes may give rise to multiple active peptides with unique profiles of activity.* This patterning may be very complex and regulatable by various stimuli.

4. *Patterns and/or efficacy of intracellular signaling* produced by endogenous ligands at opioid receptors are under investigation (Emmerson *et al.,* 1996). This issue may be particularly relevant for understanding physiological alterations following chronic administration of exogenous opioids.
5. *Intracellular trafficking of the receptors* may vary both as a function of the receptor and the ligand. This could have interesting implications for long-term adaptations during sustained treatment with opioids and following their withdrawal.

Understanding the complexity of endogenous opioid peptides and their patterns of interaction with multiple opioid receptors may help define the similarities and differences between the endogenous modulation of these systems and their activation by drugs. These insights could be important in devising treatment strategies that maximize beneficial properties of opioids (*e.g.,* pain relief) while limiting their undesirable side effects such as tolerance, dependence, and addiction.

EFFECTS OF CLINICALLY USED OPIOIDS

Morphine and most other clinically used opioid agonists exert their effects through μ opioid receptors. These drugs affect a wide range of physiological systems. They produce analgesia, affect mood and rewarding behavior (*see also* Chapter 24), and alter respiratory, cardiovascular, gastrointestinal, and neuroendocrine function. δ-Opioid receptor agonists also are potent analgesics in animals, and in isolated cases have proved useful in human beings (Coombs *et al.,* 1985). The main barrier to the clinical use of δ agonists is that most of the available agents are peptides and do not cross the blood–brain barrier, thus requiring intraspinal administration. However, much effort currently is being devoted to the development of clinically useful δ agonists. κ-Selective agonists produce analgesia that has been shown in animals to be mediated primarily at spinal sites. Respiratory depression and miosis may be less severe with κ agonists. Instead of euphoria, κ-receptor agonists produce dysphoric and psychotomimetic effects (Pfeiffer *et al.,* 1986). In neural circuitry mediating both reward and analgesia, μ and κ agonists have been shown to have antagonistic effects (*see* below).

Mixed agonist-antagonist compounds were developed for clinical use with the hope that they would have less addictive potential and less respiratory depression than morphine and related drugs. In practice, however, it has turned out that for the same degree of analgesia, the same intensity of side effects will occur. (American Pain Society, 1999). A "ceiling effect," limiting the amount of analgesia attainable, often is seen with these drugs. Some mixed agonist-antagonist drugs, such as *pentazocine* and *nalorphine,* can produce severe psychotomimetic effects that are not reversible with naloxone (suggesting that these undesirable side effects are not mediated through classical opioid receptors). Also, pentazocine and nalorphine can precipitate withdrawal in opioid-tolerant patients. For these reasons, the clinical use of these mixed agonist-antagonist drugs is limited.

Analgesia

In human beings, morphine-like drugs produce analgesia, drowsiness, changes in mood, and mental clouding. A significant feature of the analgesia is that it occurs without loss of consciousness. When therapeutic doses of morphine are given to patients with pain, they report that the pain is less intense, less discomforting, or entirely gone; drowsiness commonly occurs. In addition to relief of distress, some patients experience euphoria.

When morphine in the same dose is given to a normal, pain-free individual, the experience may be unpleasant. Nausea is common, and vomiting also may occur. There may be feelings of drowsiness, difficulty in mentation, apathy, and lessened physical activity. As the dose is increased, the subjective, analgesic, and toxic effects, including respiratory depression, become more pronounced. Morphine does not have anticonvulsant activity and usually does not cause slurred speech, emotional lability, or significant motor incoordination.

The relief of pain by morphine-like opioids is relatively selective, in that other sensory modalities are not affected. Patients frequently report that the pain is still present, but that they feel more comfortable (*see* section on Therapeutic Uses of Opioid Analgesics). Continuous, dull pain is relieved more effectively than sharp, intermittent pain, but with sufficient amounts of opioid it is possible to relieve even the severe pain associated with renal or biliary colic.

Any meaningful discussion of the action of analgesic agents must include some distinction between *pain as a specific sensation,* subserved by distinct neurophysiological structures, and *pain as suffering* (the original sensation plus the reactions evoked by the sensation). It is generally agreed that all types of painful experiences, whether produced experimentally or occurring clinically as a result of pathology, include both the original sensation and the reaction to that sensation. It also is important to distinguish between pain caused by stimulation of nociceptive receptors and transmitted over intact neural pathways (*nociceptive* pain) and pain that is caused by damage to neural structures, often involving neural supersensitivity (*neuropathic* pain). Although nociceptive pain usually is responsive to opioid analgesics, neuropathic pain typically responds poorly to opi-

oid analgesics and may require higher doses of drug (McQuay, 1988).

In clinical situations, pain cannot be terminated at will, and the meaning of the sensation and the distress it engenders are markedly affected by the individual's previous experiences and current expectations. In experimentally produced pain, measurements of the effects of morphine on pain threshold have not always been consistent; some workers find that opioids reliably elevate the threshold, while many others do not obtain consistent changes. In contrast, moderate doses of morphine-like analgesics are effective in relieving clinical pain and increasing the capacity to tolerate experimentally induced pain. Not only is the sensation of pain altered by opioid analgesics, but the affective response is changed as well. This latter effect is best assessed by asking patients with clinical pain about the degree of relief produced by the drug administered. When pain does not evoke its usual responses (anxiety, fear, panic, and suffering), a patient's ability to tolerate the pain may be markedly increased even when the capacity to perceive the sensation is relatively unaltered. It is clear, however, that alteration of the emotional reaction to painful stimuli is not the sole mechanism of analgesia. Intrathecal administration of opioids can produce profound segmental analgesia without causing significant alteration of motor or sensory function or subjective effects (Yaksh, 1988).

Mechanisms and Sites of Opioid-Induced Analgesia. While cellular and molecular studies of opioid receptors are invaluable in understanding their function, it is critical to place them in their anatomical and physiological context to fully understand the opioid system. Pain control by opioids needs to be considered in the context of brain circuits modulating analgesia and the functions of the various receptor types in these circuits. Excellent reviews of this topic are available (Fields *et al.,* 1991; Harris, 1996).

It has been well established that the analgesic effects of opioids arise from their ability to inhibit directly the ascending transmission of nociceptive information from the spinal cord dorsal horn and to activate pain control circuits that descend from the midbrain, *via* the rostral ventromedial medulla, to the spinal cord dorsal horn. Opioid peptides and their receptors are found throughout these descending pain control circuits (Mansour *et al.,* 1995; Gutstein *et al.,* 1998). μ-Opioid receptor mRNA and/or ligand binding is seen throughout the periaqueductal grey (PAG), pontine reticular formation, median raphe, nucleus raphe magnus, and adjacent gigantocellular reticular nucleus in the rostral ventromedial medulla (RVM) and spinal cord. Evaluation of discrepancies between levels of ligand binding and mRNA expression provides important insights into the mechanisms of μ-opioid receptor-mediated analgesia. For instance, the presence of significant μ-opioid receptor ligand binding in the superficial dorsal horn but scarcity of mRNA expression (Mansour *et al.,* 1995) suggests that the majority of these spinal μ-receptor ligand binding sites are located presynaptically on the terminals of primary afferent nociceptors. This conclusion is consistent with the high levels of μ-opioid receptor mRNA observed in dorsal root ganglia (DRG). A similar mismatch between μ-receptor ligand binding and mRNA expression is seen in the dorsolateral PAG (a high level of binding and sparse mRNA) (Gutstein *et al.,* 1998). δ-Opioid receptor mRNA and ligand binding have been demonstrated in the ventral and ventrolateral quadrants of the PAG, the pontine reticular formation, and the gigantocellular reticular nucleus, but only low levels are seen in the median raphe and nucleus raphe magnus. As with the μ-opioid receptor, there are significant numbers of δ-opioid receptor binding sites in the dorsal horn but no detectable mRNA expression, suggesting an important role for presynaptic actions of the δ-opioid receptor in spinal analgesia. κ-Opioid receptor mRNA and ligand binding are widespread throughout the PAG, pontine reticular formation, median raphe, nucleus raphe magnus and adjacent gigantocellular reticular nucleus. Again, κ-receptor ligand binding but minimal mRNA have been found in the dorsal horn. Although all three receptor mRNAs are found in the DRG, they are localized on different types of primary afferent cells. μ-Opioid receptor mRNA is present in medium and large diameter DRG cells, δ-opioid receptor mRNA in large diameter cells, and κ-opioid receptor mRNA in small and medium diameter cells (Mansour et al., 1995). This differential localization might be linked to functional differences in pain modulation.

The distribution of opioid receptors in descending pain control circuits indicates substantial overlap between μ and κ receptors. μ Receptors and κ receptors are most anatomically distinct from the δ-opioid receptor in the PAG, median raphe, and nucleus raphe magnus (Gutstein et al., 1998). A similar differentiation of μ and κ receptors from δ is seen in the thalamus, suggesting that interactions between the κ receptor and the μ receptor may be important for modulating nociceptive transmission from higher nociceptive centers as well as in the spinal cord dorsal horn. The actions of μ-receptor agonists are invariably analgesic, whereas those of κ-receptor agonists can be either analgesic or antianalgesic. Consistent with the anatomical overlap between the μ and κ receptors, the antianalgesic actions of the κ-receptor agonists appear to be mediated by functional antagonism of the actions of μ-receptor agonists. The μ receptor produces analgesia within descending pain control circuits, at least in part, by the removal of GABAergic inhibition of RVM-projecting neurons in the PAG and spinally projecting neurons in the RVM (Fields et al., 1991). The pain-modulating effects of the κ-receptor agonists in the brainstem appear to oppose those of μ-receptor agonists. Application of a κ-opioid agonist hyperpolarizes the same RVM neurons that are depolarized by a μ-opioid agonist, and microinjections of a κ-receptor agonist into the RVM antagonize the analgesia produced by microinjections of μ agonists into this region (Pan et al., 1997). This is the strongest evidence to date demonstrating that opioids can have antianalgesic as well as analgesic effects. This finding may explain behavioral evidence for a reduction in hyperalgesia that follows injections of naloxone under certain circumstances.

As mentioned above, there is significant opioid-receptor ligand binding, and little detectable receptor mRNA expression in the spinal cord dorsal horn, but high levels of opioid-receptor mRNA in DRG. This distribution might suggest that the actions of opioid-receptor agonists relevant to analgesia at the spinal level are predominantly presynaptic. At least one presynaptic mechanism with potential clinical significance is inhibition of spinal tachykinin signaling. It is well known that opioids decrease the pain-evoked release of tachykinins from primary afferent nociceptors (Jessell and Iversen, 1977; Yaksh et al., 1980). Recently, the significance of this effect has been questioned. Trafton et al. (1999) have demonstrated that at least 80% of tachykinin signaling in response to noxious stimulation remains intact after the intrathecal administration of large doses of

opioids. These results suggest that, while opioid administration may reduce tachykinin release from primary afferent nociceptors, this reduction has little functional impact on the actions of tachykinins on postsynaptic pain-transmitting neurons. This implies that either tachykinins are not central to pain signaling and/or opioid-induced analgesia at the spinal level or that, contrary to the conclusions suggested by anatomical studies, presynaptic opioid actions may be of little analgesic significance.

Just as important insights have been made into mechanisms of opioid-induced analgesia at the brainstem and spinal levels, progress also has been made in understanding forebrain mechanisms. It is well known that the actions of opioids in bulbospinal pathways are critical to their analgesic efficacy. The precise role of forebrain actions of opioids and whether or not these actions are independent of those in bulbospinal pathways are less well defined. It is clear that opioid actions in the forebrain contribute to analgesia, because decerebration prevents analgesia when rats are tested for pain sensitivity using the formalin test (Matthies and Franklin, 1992), and microinjection of opioids into several forebrain regions are analgesic in this test (Manning et al., 1994). However, because these manipulations frequently do not change the analgesic efficacy of opioids in measures of acute phasic nociception, such as the tailflick test, a distinction has been made between forebrain-dependent mechanisms for morphine-induced analgesia in the presence of tissue injury and bulbospinal mechanisms for this analgesia in the absence of tissue injury. In an important series of experiments, Manning and Mayer (1995a; 1995b) have shown that this distinction is not absolute. Analgesia induced by systemic administration of morphine in both the tailflick and formalin tests was disrupted either by lesioning or reversibly inactivating the central nucleus of the amygdala, demonstrating that opioid actions in the forebrain contribute to analgesia in measures of tissue damage as well as acute, phasic nociception. The involvement of the amygdala in analgesia is intriguing, as the amygdala has been implicated in the environmental activation of pain control circuits, and it projects extensively to brainstem regions involved in descending pain control (Manning and Mayer, 1995a; 1995b).

Simultaneous administration of morphine at both spinal and supraspinal sites results in synergy in analgesic response, with a tenfold reduction in the total dose of morphine necessary to produce equivalent analgesia at either site alone. The mechanisms responsible for spinal/supraspinal synergy are readily distinguished from those involved with supraspinal analgesia (Pick et al., 1992a). In addition to the well-described spinal/supraspinal synergy, synergistic μ/μ- and μ/δ-agonist interactions also have been observed within the brainstem between the periaqueductal gray, locus coeruleus, and nucleus raphe magnus (Rossi et al., 1993).

Opioids also can produce analgesia when administered peripherally. Opioid receptors are present on peripheral nerves (Fields et al., 1980) and will respond to peripherally applied opioids and locally released endogenous opioid compounds when "up-regulated" during inflammatory pain states (Stein et al., 1991; Stein, 1993). During inflammation, immune cells capable of releasing endogenous opioids are present near sensory nerves, and a perineural defect allows opioids access to the nerves (Stein, 1993; Stein, 1995). It appears that this also may occur in neuropathic pain models (Kayser et al., 1995), perhaps because of the presence of immune cells near damaged nerves (Monaco et al., 1992) and perineural defects extant in these conditions.

The Role of N/OFQ and Its Receptor in Pain Modulation.
N/OFQ mRNA and peptide are present throughout descending pain control circuits. For instance, N/OFQ-containing neurons are present in the PAG, the median raphe, throughout the RVM, and in the superficial dorsal horn (Neal *et al.,* 1999b). This distribution overlaps with that of opioid peptides, but the extent of colocalization remains unclear. N/OFQ-receptor ligand binding and mRNA are seen in the PAG, median raphe, and RVM (Neal *et al.,* 1999a). Spinally, there is stronger N/OFQ-receptor mRNA expression in the ventral horn than in the dorsal horn, but higher levels of ligand binding in the dorsal horn. There also are high N/OFQ-receptor mRNA levels in the DRG.

Despite clear anatomical evidence for a role of the N/OFQ system in pain modulation, its function remains unclear. Targeted disruption of the N/OFQ receptor in mice had little effect on basal pain sensitivity in several measures, whereas targeted disruption of the N/OFQ precursor consistently elevated basal responses in the tailflick test, suggesting an important role for N/OFQ in regulating basal pain sensitivity (Nishi *et al.,* 1997; Koster *et al.,* 1999). Intrathecal injections of N/OFQ have been shown to be analgesic (Yamamoto *et al.,* 1997; Xu *et al.,* 1996); however, supraspinal administration has produced either hyperalgesia, antiopioid effects, or a biphasic hyperalgesic/analgesic response (Rossi *et al.,* 1996b, Rossi *et al.,* 1997; Grisel *et al.,* 1996). These conflicting findings may be explained in part by a study in which it was shown that N/OFQ inhibits both pain-facilitating and analgesia-facilitating neurons in the RVM (Pan *et al.,* 2000). Activation of endogenous analgesic circuitry was blocked by administration of N/OFQ. If the animal was hyperalgesic, the enhanced pain sensitivity also was blocked by N/OFQ. Thus, the effects of N/OFQ on pain responses appear to depend on the preexisting state of pain in the animal.

Mood Alterations and Rewarding Properties

The mechanisms by which opioids produce euphoria, tranquility, and other alterations of mood (including rewarding properties) are not entirely clear. However, the neural systems that mediate opioid reinforcement are distinct from those involved in physical dependence and analgesia (Koob and Bloom, 1988). Behavioral and pharmacological evidence points to the role of dopaminergic pathways, particularly involving the nucleus accumbens (NAcc), in drug-induced reward. There is ample evidence for interactions between opioids and dopamine in mediating opioid-induced reward.

A full appreciation of mechanisms of drug-induced reward requires a more complete understanding of the NAcc and related structures at the anatomical level as well as a careful examination of the interface between the opioid system and dopamine receptors. The NAcc, portions of the olfactory tubercle, and the ventral and medial portions of the caudate-putamen constitute an area referred to as the ventral striatum (Heimer *et al.,* 1982). The ventral striatum is implicated in motivation and affect (limbic functions), while the dorsal striatum is involved in sensorimotor and cognitive functions (Willner *et al.,* 1991). Both the dorsal and ventral striatum are heterogeneous structures that can be subdivided into distinct compartments. In the middle and caudal third of the NAcc, the characteristic distribution of neuroactive substances results in two unique compartments termed the core and the shell (Zahm and Heimer, 1988; Heimer *et al.,* 1991). It is important to note that other reward-relevant brain regions (*e.g.,* the lateral hypothalamus and medial prefrontal cortex) implicated with a variety of abused drugs are connected reciprocally to the shell of the NAcc. Thus, the *shell of the NAcc* is the site that may be involved directly in the emotional and motivational aspects of drug-induced reward.

Prodynorphin- and proenkephalin-derived opioid peptides are expressed primarily in *output neurons* of the striatum and NAcc. All three opioid receptor types are present in the NAcc (Mansour *et al.,* 1988) and are thought to mediate, at least in part, the motivational effects of opiate drugs. Selective μ- and δ-receptor agonists are rewarding when defined by place preference (Shippenberg *et al.,* 1992) and intracranial self-administration (Devine and Wise, 1994) paradigms. Conversely, selective κ-receptor agonists produce aversive effects (Cooper, 1991; Shippenberg *et al.,* 1992). Naloxone and selective μ antagonists also produce aversive effects (Cooper, 1991). Positive motivational effects of opioids are partially mediated by dopamine release at the level of the NAcc. Thus, κ-receptor activation in these circuits inhibits dopamine release (Mulder *et al.,* 1991; Mulder and Schoffelmeer, 1993), while μ- and δ-receptor activation increases dopamine release (Chesselet *et al.,* 1983; Devine *et al.,* 1993). Distinctive cell clusters in the shell of the accumbens contain proenkephalin, prodynorphin, μ receptors, and κ receptors as well as dopamine receptors. These clusters possibly could be a region where the motivational properties of dopaminergic and opioid drugs are processed. The potential role of these structures and the neural circuits in which they are embedded in the rewarding effects of opioids will be of great interest.

The locus ceruleus (LC) contains both noradrenergic neurons and high concentrations of opioid receptors and is postulated to play a critical role in feelings of alarm, panic, fear, and anxiety. Neural activity in the LC is inhibited by both exogenous opioids and endogenous opioid-like peptides.

Other CNS Effects

While opioids are used clinically primarily for their pain-relieving properties, they produce a host of other effects. This is not surprising in view of the wide distribution of opioids and their receptors, both in the brain and in the periphery. A brief summary of some of these effects is presented below. High doses of opioids can produce muscular rigidity in human beings. Chest wall rigidity severe enough to compromise respiration is not uncommon during anesthesia with fentanyl, alfentanil, remifentanil, and sufentanil (*see* Monk *et al.,* 1988). Opioids and endogenous peptides cause catalepsy, circling, and stereotypical behavior in rats and other animals.

Effects on the Hypothalamus. Opioids alter the equilibrium point of the hypothalamic heat-regulatory mechanisms, such that body temperature usually falls slightly. However, chronic high dosage may increase body temperature (*see* Martin, 1983).

Neuroendocrine Effects.   Morphine acts in the hypothalamus to inhibit the release of gonadotropin-releasing hormone (GnRH) and corticotropin-releasing factor (CRF), thus decreasing circulating concentrations of luteinizing hormone (LH), follicle-stimulating hormone (FSH), ACTH, and β-endorphin; the last two peptides usually are released simultaneously from corticotropes in the pituitary. As a result of the decreased concentrations of pituitary trophic hormones, the concentrations of testosterone and cortisol in plasma decline. Secretion of thyrotropin is relatively unaffected.

The administration of μ agonists increases the concentration of prolactin in plasma, probably by reducing the dopaminergic inhibition of its secretion. Although some opioids enhance the secretion of growth hormone, the administration of morphine or β-endorphin has little effect on the concentration of the hormone in plasma. With chronic administration, tolerance develops to the effects of morphine on hypothalamic releasing factors. Observations in patients maintained on methadone reflect this phenomenon; in women, menstrual cycles that had been disrupted by intermittent use of heroin return to normal; in men, circulating concentrations of LH and testosterone are usually within the normal range.

Although κ-receptor agonists inhibit the release of antidiuretic hormone and cause diuresis, the administration of μ-opioid agonists tends to produce antidiuretic effects in human beings. The effects of opioids on neuroendocrine function have been reviewed by (Howlett and Rees, 1986) and by (Grossman, 1988).

Miosis.   Morphine and most μ and κ agonists cause constriction of the pupil by an excitatory action on the parasympathetic nerve innervating the pupil. Following toxic doses of μ agonists, *the miosis is marked and pinpoint pupils are pathognomonic;* however, marked mydriasis occurs when asphyxia intervenes. Some tolerance to the miotic effect develops, but addicts with high circulating concentrations of opioids continue to have constricted pupils. Therapeutic doses of morphine increase accommodative power and lower intraocular tension in both normal and glaucomatous eyes.

Convulsions.   In animals, high doses of morphine and related opioids produce convulsions. Several mechanisms appear to be involved, and different types of opioids produce seizures with different characteristics. Morphine-like drugs excite certain groups of neurons, especially hippocampal pyramidal cells; these excitatory effects probably result from inhibition of the release of GABA by interneurons (*see* McGinty and Friedman, 1988). Selective δ agonists produce similar effects. These actions may contribute to the seizures that are produced by some agents at doses only moderately higher than those required for analgesia, especially in children. However, with most opioids, convulsions occur only at doses far in excess of those required to produce profound analgesia, and seizures are not seen when potent μ agonists are used to produce anesthesia. Naloxone is more potent in antagonizing convulsions produced by some opioids (*e.g.,* morphine, methadone, and propoxyphene) than those produced by others (*e.g.,* meperidine). The production of convulsant metabolites of the latter agent may be partially responsible (*see* below). Anticonvulsant agents may not always be effective in suppressing opioid-induced seizures.

Respiration.   Morphine-like opioids depress respiration, at least in part by virtue of a direct effect on the brainstem respiratory centers. The respiratory depression is discernible even with doses too small to disturb consciousness and increases progressively as the dose is increased. In human beings, death from morphine poisoning is nearly always due to respiratory arrest. Therapeutic doses of morphine in human beings depress all phases of respiratory activity (rate, minute volume, and tidal exchange) and also may produce irregular and periodic breathing. The diminished respiratory volume is due primarily to a slower rate of breathing, and with toxic amounts the rate may fall to 3 or 4 breaths per minute. Although effects on respiration are readily demonstrated, clinically significant respiratory depression rarely occurs with standard morphine doses in the absence of underlying pulmonary dysfunction. However, the combination of opioids with other medications, such as general anesthetics, tranquilizers, alcohol, or sedative-hypnotics, may present a greater risk of respiratory depression. Maximal respiratory depression occurs within 5 to 10 minutes after intravenous administration of morphine or within 30 or 90 minutes following intramuscular or subcutaneous administration, respectively.

Maximal respiratory depressant effects occur more rapidly with more lipid-soluble agents. Following therapeutic doses, respiratory minute volume may be reduced for as long as 4 to 5 hours. The primary mechanism of respiratory depression by opioids involves a reduction in the responsiveness of the brainstem respiratory centers to carbon dioxide. Opioids also depress the pontine and medullary centers involved in regulating respiratory rhythmicity and the responsiveness of medullary respiratory centers to electrical stimulation (*see* Martin, 1983).

Hypoxic stimulation of the chemoreceptors still may be effective when opioids have decreased the responsiveness to CO_2, and the inhalation of O_2 may thus produce apnea. After large doses of morphine or other μ agonists, patients will breathe if instructed to do so, but without such instruction they may remain relatively apneic.

Because of the accumulation of CO_2, respiratory rate and sometimes even minute volume can be unreliable indicators of the degree of respiratory depression that has been produced by morphine. Natural sleep also produces a decrease in the sensitivity of the medullary center to CO_2, and the effects of morphine and sleep are additive.

Numerous studies have compared morphine and morphine-like opioids with respect to their ratios of analgesic to respiratory-depressant activities. Most studies have found that, when equianalgesic doses are used, the degree of respiratory depression observed with morphine-like opioids is not significantly different from that seen with morphine. Severe respiratory depression is less likely after the administration of large doses of selective κ agonists. High concentrations of opioid receptors and of endogenous peptides are found in the medullary areas believed to be important in ventilatory control.

Cough.   Morphine and related opioids also depress the cough reflex, at least in part by a direct effect on a cough center in the medulla. There is, however, no obligatory relationship between depression of respiration and depression of coughing, and effective antitussive agents are available that do not depress respiration (*see* below). Suppression of cough by such agents appears to involve receptors in the medulla that are less sensitive to naloxone than are those responsible for analgesia.

Nauseant and Emetic Effects.   Nausea and vomiting produced by morphine-like drugs are unpleasant side effects caused by direct stimulation of the chemoreceptor trigger zone for emesis, in the area postrema of the medulla. Certain individuals never vomit after morphine, whereas others do so each time the drug is administered.

Nausea and vomiting are relatively uncommon in recumbent patients given therapeutic doses of morphine, but nausea occurs in approximately 40% and vomiting in 15% of ambulatory patients given 15 mg of the drug subcutaneously. This suggests that a vestibular component also is operative. Indeed, the nauseant and emetic effects of morphine are markedly enhanced by vestibular stimulation, and morphine and related synthetic analgesics produce an increase in vestibular sensitivity. All clinically useful μ agonists produce some degree of nausea and vomiting. Careful, controlled clinical studies usually demonstrate that, in equianalgesic dosage, the incidence of such side effects is not significantly lower than that seen with morphine. Drugs that are useful in motion sickness are sometimes helpful in reducing opioid-induced nausea in ambulatory patients; phenothiazines are also useful (*see* Chapter 20).

Cardiovascular System

In the supine patient, therapeutic doses of morphine-like opioids have no major effect on blood pressure or cardiac rate and rhythm. Such doses do produce peripheral vasodilation, reduced peripheral resistance, and an inhibition of baroreceptor reflexes. Therefore, when supine patients assume the head-up position, orthostatic hypotension and fainting may occur. The peripheral arteriolar and venous dilation produced by morphine involves several mechanisms. Morphine and some other opioids provoke release of histamine, which sometimes plays a large role in the hypotension. However, vasodilation is usually only partially blocked by H_1 antagonists, but it is effectively reversed by naloxone. Morphine also blunts the reflex vasoconstriction caused by increased P_{CO_2}.

Effects on the myocardium are not significant in normal individuals. In patients with coronary artery disease but no acute medical problems, 8 to 15 mg of morphine administered intravenously produces a decrease in oxygen consumption, left ventricular end-diastolic pressure, and cardiac work; effects on cardiac index are usually slight (Sethna *et al.*, 1982). In patients with acute myocardial infarction, the cardiovascular responses to morphine may be more variable than in normal subjects, and the magnitude of changes (*e.g.*, the decrease in blood pressure) may be more pronounced (*see* Roth *et al.*, 1988).

Morphine may exert its well-known therapeutic effect in the treatment of angina pectoris and acute myocardial infarction by decreasing preload, inotropy, and chronotropy, thus favorably altering determinants of myocardial oxygen consumption and helping to relieve ischemia. It is not clear whether the analgesic properties of morphine in this situation are due to the reversal of acidosis that may stimulate local acid-sensing ion channels (Benson *et al.*, 1999; McCleskey and Gold, 1999) or to a direct analgesic effect on nociceptive afferents from the heart.

When administered prior to experimental ischemia, morphine has been shown to produce cardioprotective effects. Morphine can mimic the phenomenon of ischemic preconditioning, where a short ischemic episode paradoxically protects the heart against further ischemia. This effect appears to be mediated through δ receptors signaling through a mitochondrial ATP-sensitive potassium channel in cardiac myocytes; the effect also is produced by other G protein-coupled receptors signaling through G_i subunits (Fryer *et al.*, 2000; Liang and Gross, 1999; Schultz *et al.*, 1996). It also has been suggested recently that δ opioids can be antiarrhythmic and antifibrillatory during and after periods of ischemia (Fryer *et al.*, 2000). Other data, however, suggest that δ opioids can be arrythmogenic (McIntosh *et al.*, 1992).

Very large doses of morphine can be used to produce anesthesia; however, decreased peripheral resistance and blood pressure are troublesome. Fentanyl and sufentanil, which are potent and selective μ agonists, are less likely to cause hemodynamic instability during surgery, in part because they do not cause the release of histamine (Monk *et al.*, 1988).

Morphine-like opioids should be used with caution in patients who have a decreased blood volume, since these agents can aggravate hypovolemic shock. Morphine should be used with great care in patients with cor pulmonale, since deaths following ordinary therapeutic doses have been reported. The concurrent use of certain phenothiazines may increase the risk of morphine-induced hypotension.

Cerebral circulation is not directly affected by therapeutic doses of morphine. However, opioid-induced respiratory depression and CO_2 retention can result in cerebral vasodilation and an increase in cerebrospinal fluid pressure; the pressure increase does not occur when PCO_2 is maintained at normal levels by artificial ventilation.

Gastrointestinal Tract

Stomach. Morphine and other μ agonists usually decrease the secretion of hydrochloric acid, although stimulation is sometimes evident. Activation of opioid receptors on parietal cells enhances secretion, but indirect effects, including increased secretion of somatostatin from the pancreas and reduced release of acetylcholine, appear to be dominant in most circumstances (*see* Kromer, 1988). Relatively low doses of morphine decrease gastric motility, thereby prolonging gastric emptying time; this can increase the likelihood of esophageal reflux (*see* Duthie and Nimmo, 1987). The tone of the antral portion of the stomach and of the first part of the duodenum is increased, which often makes therapeutic intubation of the duodenum more difficult. Passage of the gastric contents through the duodenum may be delayed by as much as 12 hours, and the absorption of orally administered drugs is retarded.

Small Intestine. Morphine diminishes biliary, pancreatic, and intestinal secretions (Dooley *et al.,* 1988) and delays digestion of food in the small intestine. Resting tone is increased, and periodic spasms are observed. The amplitude of the nonpropulsive type of rhythmic, segmental contractions usually is enhanced, but propulsive contractions are markedly decreased. The upper part of the small intestine, particularly the duodenum, is affected more than the ileum. A period of relative atony may follow the hypertonicity. Water is absorbed more completely because of the delayed passage of bowel contents, and intestinal secretion is decreased; this increases the viscosity of the bowel contents.

In the presence of intestinal hypersecretion that may be associated with diarrhea, morphine-like drugs inhibit the transfer of fluid and electrolytes into the lumen by naloxone-sensitive actions on the intestinal mucosa and within the CNS. Enterocytes may possess opioid receptors, but this hypothesis is controversial. However, it is clear that opioids exert important effects on the submucosal plexus that lead to a decrease in the basal secretion by enterocytes and inhibition of the stimulatory effects of acetylcholine, prostaglandin E_2, and vasoactive intestinal peptide. The effects of opioids initiated either in the CNS or the submucosal plexus may be mediated in large part by the release of norepinephrine and stimulation of α_2-adrenergic receptors on enterocytes (*see* Coupar, 1987). The actions of opioids on intestinal secretion have been reviewed by Manara and Bianchetti (1985) and Kromer (1988).

Large Intestine. Propulsive peristaltic waves in the colon are diminished or abolished after administration of morphine, and tone is increased to the point of spasm. The resulting delay in the passage of bowel contents causes considerable desiccation of the feces, which, in turn, retards their advance through the colon. The amplitude of the nonpropulsive type of rhythmic contractions of the colon usually is enhanced. The tone of the anal sphincter is greatly augmented, and reflex relaxation in response to rectal distension is reduced. These actions, combined with inattention to the normal sensory stimuli for defecation reflex due to the central actions of the drug, contribute to morphine-induced constipation.

Mechanism of Action on the Bowel. The usual gastrointestinal effects of morphine primarily are mediated by μ- and δ-opioid receptors in the bowel. However, injection of opioids into the cerebral ventricles or in the vicinity of the spinal cord can inhibit gastrointestinal propulsive activity as long as the extrinsic innervation to the bowel is intact. The relatively poor penetration of morphine into the CNS may explain how preparations such as paregoric can produce constipation at less than analgesic doses and may account for troublesome gastrointestinal side effects during the use of oral morphine for the treatment of cancer pain (*see* Manara and Bianchetti, 1985). Although some tolerance develops to the effects of opioids on gastrointestinal motility, patients who take opioids chronically remain constipated.

Biliary Tract. After the subcutaneous injection of 10 mg of morphine sulfate, the sphincter of Oddi constricts and the pressure in the common bile duct may rise more than tenfold within 15 minutes; this effect may persist for 2 hours or more. Fluid pressure also may increase in the gallbladder and produce symptoms that may vary from epigastric distress to typical biliary colic.

Some patients with biliary colic may experience exacerbation rather than relief of pain when given these drugs. Spasm of the sphincter of Oddi is probably responsible for elevations of plasma amylase and lipase that are sometimes found after patients are given morphine. Atropine only partially prevents morphine-induced biliary spasm, but opioid antagonists prevent or relieve it. Nitroglycerin (0.6 to 1.2 mg) administered sublingually also decreases the elevated intrabiliary pressure (*see* Staritz, 1988).

Other Smooth Muscle

Ureter and Urinary Bladder. Therapeutic doses of morphine may increase the tone and amplitude of contractions of the ureter, although the response is variable. When the antidiuretic effects of the drug are prominent and urine flow decreases, the ureter may become quiescent.

Morphine inhibits the urinary voiding reflex, and both the tone of the external sphincter and the volume of the bladder are increased; catheterization is sometimes required following therapeutic doses of morphine. Stimulation of either μ or δ

receptors in the brain or in the spinal cord exerts similar actions on bladder motility (*see* Dray and Nunan, 1987). Tolerance develops to these effects of opioids on the bladder.

Uterus. If the uterus has been made hyperactive by oxytocics, morphine tends to restore tone, frequency, and the amplitude of contractions to normal. Parenteral administration of opioids within 2 to 4 hours of delivery may lead to transient respiratory depression in the neonate due to transplacental passage of opioids. This may be treated readily with naloxone.

Skin

Therapeutic doses of morphine cause dilation of cutaneous blood vessels. The skin of the face, neck, and upper thorax frequently becomes flushed. These changes may be due in part to the release of histamine and may be responsible for the sweating and some of the pruritus that occasionally follow the systemic administration of morphine (*see* below). Histamine release probably accounts for the urticaria commonly seen at the site of injection; this is not mediated by opioid receptors and is not blocked by naloxone. It is seen with morphine and meperidine, but not with oxymorphone, methadone, fentanyl, or sufentanil (*see* Duthie and Nimmo, 1987).

Pruritus is a common and potentially disabling complication of opioid use. It can be caused by intraspinal and systemic injections of opioids, but it appears to be more intense after intraspinal administration (Ballantyne *et al.*, 1988). The effect appears to be mediated in large part by dorsal horn neurons and is reversible by naloxone (Thomas *et al.*, 1992). An intriguing report suggested that systemic morphine could partially inhibit pruritus caused by intraspinal administration of morphine, implying the existence of an opioid-mediated, itch-inhibition system, possibly supraspinal in origin (Thomas *et al.*, 1993).

Immune System

The effects of opioids on the immune system are complex. Opioids have been shown to modulate immune function by direct effects on cells of the immune system and indirectly *via* centrally mediated neuronal mechanisms (Sharp and Yaksh, 1997). It appears that acute, central immunomodulatory effects of opioids may be mediated by activation of the sympathetic nervous system, whereas the chronic effects of opioids may involve modulation of hypothalamic-pituitary-adrenal (HPA) axis function (Mellon and Bayer, 1998). Direct effects on immune cells may involve unique and as yet incompletely characterized variants of the classical neuronal opioid receptors, with δ-receptor variants being more prominent (Sharp and Yaksh, 1997). Atypical receptors could account for the fact that it has been very difficult to demonstrate significant opioid binding on immune cells in spite of the observance of robust functional effects. In contrast, morphine-induced immune suppression is largely abolished in mice lacking the μ-receptor gene, suggesting that the μ receptor is a major target of morphine's actions on the immune system (Gaveriaux-Ruff *et al.*, 1998). A potential mechanism for the immune suppressive effects of morphine on neutrophils was proposed recently by Welters *et al.* (2000), who demonstrated that NF-κB activation induced by an inflammatory stimulus was inhibited by morphine in a nitric oxide-dependent manner. Another group of investigators has proposed that the induction and activation of MAP kinase also may play a role (Chuang *et al.*, 1997).

The overall effects of opioids on immune function appear to be suppressive; increased susceptibility to infection and tumor spread have been observed in experimental settings. Infusion of the μ-receptor antagonist naloxone has been shown to improve survival after experimentally induced sepsis (Risdahl *et al.*, 1998). Such effects have been inconsistent in clinical situations, possibly because of the use of confounding therapies and necessary opioid analgesics. In some situations, effects on immune function appear more prominent with acute administration than with chronic administration, which could have important implications for the care of the critically ill (Sharp and Yaksh, 1997). In contrast, opioids have been shown to reverse pain-induced immunosuppression and increased tumor metastatic potential in animal models (Page and Ben-Eliyahu, 1997). Therefore, opioids may either inhibit or augment immune function depending on the context in which they are used. These studies also indicate that withholding opioids in the presence of pain in immunocompromised patients could actually worsen immune function. An intriguing recent paper indicated that the partial μ-receptor agonist buprenorphine (*see* below) did not alter immune function when injected centrally into the mesencephalic periaqueductal gray matter, while morphine did (Gomez-Flores and Weber, 2000). Taken together, these studies indicate that opioid-induced immune suppression may be clinically relevant to both the treatment of severe pain and in the susceptibility of opioid addicts to infection (*e.g.*, HIV, tuberculosis). Different opioid agonists also may have unique immunomodulatory properties. Better understanding of these properties eventually should help guide rational use of opioids in patients with cancer or at risk for infection or immune compromise.

Tolerance and Physical Dependence

The development of tolerance and physical dependence with repeated use is a characteristic feature of all the opioid drugs. *Tolerance* to the effect of opioids or other drugs simply means that, over time, the drug loses its effectiveness and an increased dose is required to produce the same physiological response. *Dependence* refers to a complex and poorly understood set of changes in the homeostasis of an organism that cause a disturbance of the homeostatic set point of the organism if the drug is stopped. This disturbance often is revealed when administration of an opioid is abruptly stopped, resulting in *withdrawal*. *Addiction* is a behavioral pattern characterized by compulsive use of a drug and overwhelming involvement with its procurement and use. Tolerance and dependence are physiological responses seen in all patients and are not predictors of addiction (*see* Chapter 24). These processes appear to be quite distinct. For example, cancer pain often requires prolonged treatment with high doses of opioids, leading to tolerance and dependence. Yet, abuse in this setting is very unusual (Foley, 1993). Neither the presence of tolerance and dependence nor the fear that they may develop should *ever* interfere with the appropriate use of opioids. Opioids can be discontinued in dependent patients once the need for analgesics is gone without subjecting them to withdrawal (*see* Chapter 24). Clinically, the dose can be decreased by 10% to 20% every other day and eventually stopped without signs and symptoms of withdrawal.

In vivo studies in animal models demonstrate the importance of other neurotransmitters and their interactions with opioid pathways in the development of tolerance to morphine. Blockade of glutamate actions by NMDA (*N*-methyl-D-aspartate)-receptor antagonists blocks morphine tolerance (Trujillo and Akil, 1997). Since NMDA antagonists have no effect on the potency of morphine in naive animals, their effect cannot be attributed to potentiation of opioid actions. Interestingly, the clinically used antitussive dextromethorphan (*see* below) has been shown to function as an NMDA antagonist. In animals, it can attenuate opioid tolerance development and reverse established tolerance (Elliott *et al.*, 1994). Nitric oxide production, possibly induced by NMDA-receptor activation, also has been implicated in tolerance, as inhibition of nitric oxide synthase (NOS) also blocks morphine tolerance development (Kolesnikov *et al.*, 1993). Administering NOS inhibitors to morphine-tolerant animals also may reverse tolerance in certain circumstances. Although the NMDA antagonists and nitric oxide synthase inhibitors are effective against tolerance to morphine and δ agonists such as DPDPE, they have little effect against tolerance to the κ agonists. Dependence seems to be closely related to tolerance, since the same treatments that block tolerance to morphine also block dependence. Other related signaling systems also are being investigated as mediators of opioid tolerance and dependence. The selective actions of drugs on tolerance and dependence demonstrate that specific mechanisms can be targeted to minimize these two unwanted actions.

MORPHINE AND RELATED OPIOID AGONISTS

There are now many compounds with pharmacological properties similar to those of morphine, yet morphine remains the standard against which new analgesics are measured. However, responses of an individual patient may vary dramatically with different μ-opioid receptor agonists. For example, some patients unable to tolerate morphine may have no problems with an equianalgesic dose of methadone, whereas others can take morphine and not methadone. If problems are encountered with one drug, another should be tried. Mechanisms underlying variations in individual responses to morphine-like agonists are not yet well understood.

Source and Composition of Opium.   Because the laboratory synthesis of morphine is difficult, the drug is still obtained from opium or extracted from poppy straw. Opium is obtained from the unripe seed capsules of the poppy plant, *Papaver somniferum*. The milky juice is dried and powdered to make powdered opium, which contains a number of alkaloids. Only a few—morphine, codeine, and papaverine—have clinical usefulness. These alkaloids can be divided into two distinct chemical classes, *phenanthrenes* and *benzylisoquinolines*. The principal phenanthrenes are *morphine* (10% of opium), *codeine* (0.5%), and *thebaine* (0.2%). The principal benzylisoquinolines are *papaverine* (1.0%), which is a smooth muscle relaxant (*see* the seventh and earlier editions of this book), and *noscapine* (6.0%).

Chemistry of Morphine and Related Opioids.   The structure of morphine is shown in Table 23–5. Many semisynthetic derivatives are made by relatively simple modifications of morphine or thebaine. Codeine is methylmorphine, the methyl substitution being on the phenolic hydroxyl group. Thebaine differs from morphine only in that both hydroxyl groups are methylated and that the ring has two double bonds ($\Delta^{6,7}$, $\Delta^{8,14}$). Thebaine has little analgesic action but is a precursor of several important 14-OH compounds, such as oxycodone and naloxone. Certain derivatives of thebaine are more than 1000 times as potent as morphine (*e.g.*, etorphine). Diacetylmorphine, or heroin, is made from morphine by acetylation at the 3 and 6 positions. Apomorphine, which also can be prepared from morphine, is a potent emetic and dopaminergic agonist. Hydromorphone, oxymorphone, hydrocodone, and oxycodone also are made by modifying the morphine molecule. The structural relationships between morphine and some of its surrogates and antagonists are shown in Table 23–5.

Structure-Activity Relationship of the Morphine-Like Opioids.   In addition to morphine, codeine, and the semisynthetic derivatives of the natural opium alkaloids, a number of other structurally distinct chemical classes of drugs have pharmacological actions similar to those of morphine. Clinically useful compounds include the morphinans, benzomorphans, methadones, phenylpiperidines, and propionanilides. Although the two-dimensional representations of these chemically diverse compounds appear to be quite different, molecular models show certain common characteristics; these are indicated by the heavy lines in the structure of morphine shown in Table 23–5. Among the important properties of the opioids that can be altered by structural modification are their affinities for various species of opioid receptors, their activities as agonists *versus* antagonists, their lipid solubilities, and their resistance to metabolic breakdown. For example, blockade of the phenolic hydroxyl at position 3, as in codeine and heroin, drastically reduces binding to μ receptors; these compounds are converted to the potent analgesics morphine and 6-acetyl morphine, respectively, *in vivo*.

Absorption, Distribution, Fate, and Excretion.   *Absorption.*   In general, the opioids are readily absorbed from the gastrointestinal tract; absorption through the rectal mucosa is adequate, and a few agents (*e.g.*, morphine, hydromorphone) are available in suppositories. The more lipophilic opioids also are readily absorbed through the nasal or buccal mucosa (Weinberg *et al.*, 1988). Those with the greatest lipid solubility also can be absorbed transdermally (Portenoy *et al.*, 1993). Opioids are absorbed

Table 23–5

Structures of Opioids and Opioid Antagonists Chemically Related to Morphine

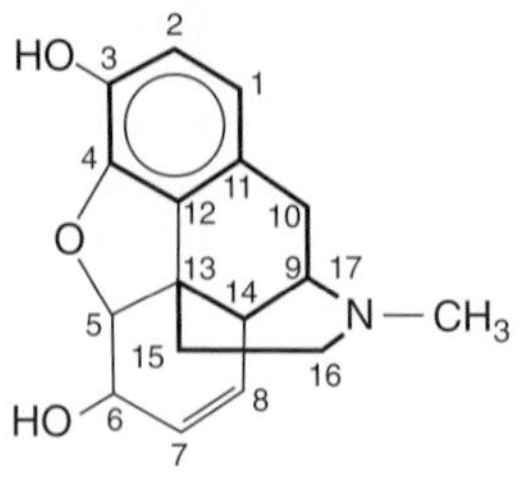

MORPHINE

NONPROPRIETARY NAME	CHEMICAL RADICALS AND POSITION*			OTHER CHANGES†
	3	*6*	*17*	
Morphine	—OH	—OH	—CH$_3$	—
Heroin	—OCOCH$_3$	—OCOCH$_3$	—CH$_3$	—
Hydromorphone	—OH	=O	—CH$_3$	(1)
Oxymorphone	—OH	=O	—CH$_3$	(1), (2)
Levorphanol	—OH	—H	—CH$_3$	(1), (3)
Levallorphan	—OH	—H	—CH$_2$CH=CH$_2$	(1), (3)
Codeine	—OCH$_3$	—OH	—CH$_3$	—
Hydrocodone	—OCH$_3$	=O	—CH$_3$	(1)
Oxycodone	—OCH$_3$	=O	—CH$_3$	(1), (2)
Nalmefene	—OH	=CH$_2$	—CH$_2$—◁ 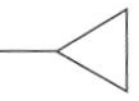	(1), (2)
Nalorphine	—OH	—OH	—CH$_2$CH=CH$_2$	—
Naloxone	—OH	=O	—CH$_2$CH=CH$_2$	(1), (2)
Naltrexone	—OH	=O	—CH$_2$—◁ 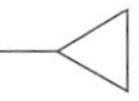	(1), (2)
Buprenorphine	—OH	—OCH$_3$	—CH$_2$—◁ 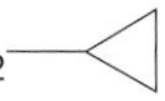	(1), (4)
Butorphanol	—OH	—H	—CH$_2$—◇ 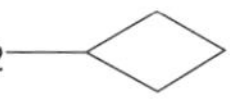	(1), (2), (3)
Nalbuphine	—OH	—OH	—CH$_2$—◇ 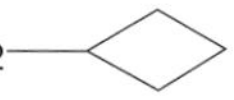	(1), (2)

*The numbers 3, 6, and 17 refer to positions in the morphine molecule, as shown above.
†Other changes in the morphine molecule are as follows:
  (1) Single instead of double bond between C7 and C8.
  (2) OH added to C14.
  (3) No oxygen between C4 and C5.
  (4) *Endo*etheno bridge between C6 and C14; 1-hydroxy-1,2,2-trimethylpropyl substitution on C7.

readily after subcutaneous or intramuscular injection and can adequately penetrate the spinal cord following epidural or intrathecal administration (*also see* section on alternative routes of administration). Small amounts of morphine introduced epidurally or intrathecally into the spinal canal can produce profound analgesia that may last 12 to 24 hours. However, due to the hydrophilic nature of morphine, there is rostral spread of the drug in spinal fluid, and side effects, especially respiratory depression, can emerge up to 24 hours later as the opioid reaches supraspinal respiratory control centers. With highly lipophilic agents such as hydromorphone or fentanyl, rapid absorption by spinal neural tissues produces very localized effects and segmental analgesia. The duration of action is shorter because of distribution of the drug in the systemic circulation, and the severity of respiratory depression may be more directly proportional to its concentration in plasma, due to a lesser degree of rostral spread (Gustafsson and Wiesenfeld-Hallin, 1988). However, patients receiving epidural or intrathecal fentanyl still should be monitored for respiratory depression.

With most opioids, including morphine, the effect of a given dose is less after oral than after parenteral administration, due to variable but significant first-pass metabolism in the liver. For example, the bioavailability of oral preparations of morphine is only about 25%. The shape of the time-effect curve also varies with the route of administration, so that the duration of action is often somewhat longer with the oral route. If adjustment is made for variability of first-pass metabolism and clearance, it is possible to achieve adequate relief of pain by the oral administration of morphine. Satisfactory analgesia in cancer patients has been associated with a very broad range of steady-state concentrations of morphine in plasma (16 to 364 ng/ml; Neumann et al., 1982).

When morphine and most opioids are given intravenously, they act promptly. However, the more lipid-soluble compounds act more rapidly than morphine after subcutaneous administration because of differences in the rates of absorption and entry into the CNS. Compared with other more lipid-soluble opioids such as codeine, heroin, and methadone, morphine crosses the blood–brain barrier at a considerably lower rate.

Distribution and Fate. When therapeutic concentrations of morphine are present in plasma, about one-third of the drug is protein bound. Morphine itself does not persist in tissues, and 24 hours after the last dose tissue concentrations are low.

The major pathway for the metabolism of morphine is conjugation with glucuronic acid. The two major metabolites formed are *morphine-6-glucuronide* and *morphine-3-glucuronide*. Small amounts of morphine 3,6, diglucuronide also may be formed. Although the 3- and 6-glucuronides are quite polar, both can cross the blood–brain barrier to exert significant clinical effects (Christup, 1997). Morphine-6-glucuronide has pharmacological actions indistinguishable from those of morphine. Morphine-6-glucuronide given systemically is approximately twice as potent as morphine in animal models (Paul et al., 1989) and in human beings (Osborne et al., 1988). With chronic administration, it accounts for a significant portion of morphine's analgesic actions (Osborne et al., 1988; Osborne et al., 1990; Portenoy et al., 1991; Portenoy et al., 1992). Indeed, with chronic oral dosing, the blood levels of morphine-6-glucuronide typically exceed those of mor-

phine. Given its greater potency as well as its higher concentrations, morphine-6-glucuronide may be responsible for most of morphine's analgesic activity in patients receiving chronic oral morphine. Morphine-6-glucuronide is excreted by the kidney. In renal failure, the levels of morphine-6-glucuronide can accumulate, perhaps explaining morphine's potency and long duration in patients with compromised renal function. In young adults, the half-life of morphine is about 2 hours; the half-life of morphine-6-glucuronide is somewhat longer. Children achieve adult renal function values by 6 months of age. In elderly patients, lower morphine doses are recommended, based on its smaller volume of distribution (Owen et al., 1983) and the general decline in renal function in the elderly. The 3-glucuronide, also an important metabolite of morphine (Milne et al., 1996), has little affinity for opioid receptors but may contribute to excitatory effects of morphine (Smith, 2000). Some investigators also have shown that morphine-3-glucuronide can antagonize morphine-induced analgesia (Smith et al., 1990), but this finding is not universal (Christup, 1997). Morphine also is metabolized by other pathways. *N*-demethylation to normorphine is a minor metabolic pathway in human beings but is more prominent in rodents (Yeh et al., 1977). *N*-dealkylation is important in the metabolism of some congeners of morphine.

Excretion. Very little morphine is excreted unchanged. It is eliminated by glomerular filtration, primarily as morphine-3-glucuronide; 90% of the total excretion takes place during the first day. Enterohepatic circulation of morphine and its glucuronides occurs, which accounts for the presence of small amounts of morphine in the feces and in the urine for several days after the last dose.

Codeine. In contrast to morphine, codeine is approximately 60% as effective orally as parenterally, both as an analgesic and as a respiratory depressant. Codeine, like levorphanol, oxycodone, and methadone, has a high oral to parenteral potency ratio. The greater oral efficacy of these drugs is due to less first-pass metabolism in the liver. Once absorbed, codeine is metabolized by the liver, and its metabolites are excreted chiefly in the urine, largely in inactive forms. A small fraction (approximately 10%) of administered codeine is *O*-demethylated to form morphine, and both free and conjugated morphine can be found in the urine after therapeutic doses of codeine. Codeine has an exceptionally low affinity for opioid receptors, and the analgesic effect of codeine is due to its conversion to morphine. However, its antitussive actions may involve distinct receptors that bind codeine itself. The half-life of codeine in plasma is 2 to 4 hours.

The conversion of codeine to morphine is effected by the cytochrome P450 enzyme CYP2D6. Well-characterized genetic polymorphisms in CYP2D6 lead to the inability to convert codeine to morphine, thus making codeine ineffective as an analgesic for about 10% of the Caucasian population (Eichelbaum and Evert, 1996). Other polymorphisms can lead to enhanced metabolism and thus increased sensitivity to codeine's effects (Eichelbaum and Evert, 1996). Interestingly, there appears to be variation in metabolic efficiency among different ethnic groups. For example, Chinese produce less morphine from codeine than do Caucasians and also are less sensitive to morphine's effects than are Caucasians (Caraco *et al.*, 1999). The reduced sensitivity to morphine may be due to decreased production of morphine-6-glucuronide (Caraco *et al.*, 1999). Thus, it is important to consider the possibility of metabolic enzyme polymorphism in any patient who does not receive adequate analgesia from codeine or an adequate response to other administered prodrugs.

Tramadol. *Tramadol* (ULTRAM) is a synthetic codeine analog that is a weak μ-opioid receptor agonist. Part of its analgesic effects are produced by inhibition of uptake of norepinephrine and serotonin. Tramadol appears to be as effective as other weak opioids. In the treatment of mild to moderate pain, tramadol is as effective as morphine or meperidine. However, for the treatment of severe or chronic pain, tramadol is less effective. Tramadol is as effective as meperidine in the treatment of labor pain and may cause less neonatal respiratory depression.

Tramadol is 68% bioavailable after a single oral dose and 100% available when administered intramuscularly. Its affinity for the μ opioid receptor is only 1/6000 that of morphine. However, the primary *O*-demethylated metabolite of tramadol is 2- to 4-times as potent as the parent drug and may account for part of the analgesic effect. Tramadol is supplied as a racemic mixture, which is more effective than either enantiomer alone. The (+) enantiomer binds to the μ receptor and inhibits serotonin uptake. The (−) enantiomer inhibits norepinephrine uptake and stimulates α_2-adrenergic receptors (Lewis and Han, 1997). The compound undergoes hepatic metabolism and renal excretion, with an elimination half-life of 6 hours for tramadol and 7.5 hours for its active metabolite. Analgesia begins within an hour of oral dosing, and the effect peaks within 2 to 3 hours. The duration of analgesia is about 6 hours. The maximum recommended daily dose is 400 mg.

Common side effects of tramadol include nausea, vomiting, dizziness, dry mouth, sedation, and headache. Respiratory depression appears to be less than with equi-analgesic doses of morphine, and the degree of constipation is less than that seen after equivalent doses of codeine (Duthie, 1998). Tramadol can cause seizures and possibly exacerbate seizures in patients with predisposing factors. While tramadol-induced analgesia is not entirely reversible by naloxone, tramadol-induced respiratory depression can be reversed by naloxone. However, the use of naloxone increases the risk of seizure. Physical dependence on and abuse of tramadol have been reported. Although its abuse potential is unclear, tramadol probably should be avoided in patients with a history of addiction. Because of its inhibitory effect on serotonin uptake, tramadol should not be used in patients taking monoamine oxidase (MAO) inhibitors (Lewis and Han, 1997; *see also* section on interaction of meperidine with other drugs, below).

Heroin. Heroin (diacetylmorphine) is rapidly hydrolyzed to 6-monoacetylmorphine (6-MAM), which, in turn is hydrolyzed to morphine. Both heroin and 6-MAM are more lipid soluble than morphine and enter the brain more readily. Current evidence suggests that morphine and 6-MAM are responsible for the pharmacological actions of heroin. Heroin is mainly excreted in the urine, largely as free and conjugated morphine.

The absorption, fate, and distribution of heroin and other morphine-like drugs have been reviewed by (Misra, 1978) and by (Chan and Matzke, 1987).

Untoward Effects and Precautions. Morphine and related opioids produce a wide spectrum of unwanted effects, including respiratory depression, nausea, vomiting, dizziness, mental clouding, dysphoria, pruritus, constipation, increased pressure in the biliary tract, urinary retention, and hypotension. The bases of these effects have been described above. Rarely, a patient may develop delirium. Increased sensitivity to pain after the analgesia has worn off also may occur.

A number of factors may alter a patient's sensitivity to opioid analgesics, including the integrity of the blood–brain barrier. For example, when morphine is administered to a newborn infant in weight-appropriate doses extrapolated from adults, unexpectedly profound analgesia and respiratory depression may be observed. This is due to the immaturity of the blood–brain barrier in neonates (Way *et al.*, 1965). As mentioned previously, morphine is hydrophilic, so in the normal situation, proportionately less morphine crosses into the CNS than with more lipophilic opioids. In neonates and in other situations with a compromised blood–brain barrier, lipophilic opioids may give more predictable clinical results than morphine. In adults, the *duration* of the analgesia produced by morphine increases progressively with age; however, the *degree* of analgesia that is obtained with a given dose changes little. Changes in pharmacokinetic parameters only partially explain these observations. The patient with severe pain may tolerate larger doses of morphine. However, as the pain subsides, the patient may exhibit sedation and even respiratory depression as the stimulatory effects of pain are diminished. The reasons for this effect are unclear.

All the opioid analgesics are metabolized by the liver, and the drugs should be used with caution in patients with hepatic disease, since increased bioavailability after oral administration or cumulative effects may occur (*see* Sawe *et al.,* 1981). Renal disease also significantly alters the pharmacokinetics of morphine, codeine, drocode (dihydrocodeine), meperidine, and propoxyphene. Although single doses of morphine are well tolerated, the active metabolite, morphine-6-glucuronide, may accumulate with continued dosing, and symptoms of opioid overdose may result (*see* Chan and Matzke, 1987). This metabolite also may accumulate during repeated administration of codeine to patients with impaired renal function. When repeated doses of meperidine are given to such patients, the accumulation of normeperidine may cause tremor and seizures (Kaiko *et al.,* 1983). Similarly, the repeated administration of propoxyphene may lead to naloxone-insensitive cardiac toxicity caused by the accumulation of norpropoxyphene (*see* Chan and Matzke, 1987).

Morphine and related opioids must be used cautiously in patients with compromised respiratory function, such as those with emphysema, kyphoscoliosis, or severe obesity. In patients with chronic cor pulmonale, death has occurred following therapeutic doses of morphine. Although many patients with such conditions seem to be functioning within normal limits, they are already utilizing compensatory mechanisms, such as increased respiratory rate. Many have chronically elevated levels of plasma CO_2 and may be less sensitive to the stimulating actions of CO_2. The further imposition of the depressant effects of opioids can be disastrous. The respiratory-depressant effects of opioids and the related capacity to elevate intracranial pressure must be considered in the presence of head injury or of an already elevated intracranial pressure. While head injury *per se* does not constitute an absolute contraindication to the use of opioids, the possibility of exaggerated depression of respiration and the potential need to control ventilation of the patient must be considered. Finally, since opioids may produce mental clouding and side effects such as miosis and vomiting, which are im-

portant signs in following the clinical course of patients with head injuries, the advisability of their use must be weighed carefully against these risks.

Morphine causes histamine release, which can cause bronchoconstriction and vasodilation. Morphine has the potential to precipitate or exacerbate asthmatic attacks. The use of morphine should be avoided in patients with a history of asthma. Other μ-receptor agonists that do not release histamine, such as the fentanyl derivatives, may be better choices for such patients.

Patients with reduced blood volume are considerably more susceptible to the vasodilatory effects of morphine and related drugs, and these agents must be used cautiously in patients with hypotension from any cause.

Allergic phenomena occur with opioid analgesics, but they are not common. They usually are manifested as urticaria and other types of skin rashes such as fixed eruptions; contact dermatitis in nurses and pharmaceutical workers also occurs. Wheals at the site of injection of morphine, codeine, and related drugs are probably secondary to the release of histamine. Anaphylactoid reactions have been reported after intravenous administration of codeine and morphine, but such reactions are rare. It has been suggested, but not proven, that such reactions are responsible for some of the sudden deaths, episodes of pulmonary edema, and other complications that occur among addicts who use heroin intravenously (*see* Chapter 24).

Interactions with Other Drugs.   The depressant effects of some opioids may be exaggerated and prolonged by phenothiazines, monoamine oxidase inhibitors, and tricyclic antidepressants; the mechanisms of these supraadditive effects are not fully understood but may involve alterations in the rate of metabolic transformation of the opioid or alterations in neurotransmitters involved in the actions of opioids. Some, but not all, phenothiazines reduce the amount of opioid required to produce a given level of analgesia. However, depending on the specific agent, the respiratory-depressant effects also seem to be enhanced, the degree of sedation is increased, and the hypotensive effects of phenothiazines become an additional complication. Some phenothiazine derivatives enhance the sedative effects, but at the same time seem to be antianalgesic and increase the amount of opioid required to produce satisfactory relief from pain. Small doses of amphetamine substantially increase the analgesic and euphoriant effects of morphine and may decrease its sedative side effects. A number of antihistamines exhibit modest analgesic actions; some (*e.g.,* hydroxyzine) enhance the analgesic effects of low doses of opioids (Rumore and Schlichting, 1986). Antidepressants such as desipramine and amitriptyline are used in the treatment of chronic neuropathic pain but have limited intrinsic analgesic actions in acute pain. However, antidepressants may enhance morphine-induced analgesia (Levine *et al.,* 1986; Pick *et al.,* 1992b). The analgesic synergism between opioids and aspirin-like drugs is discussed below and in Chapter 27.

OTHER μ-RECEPTOR AGONISTS

Levorphanol and Congeners

Levorphanol (LEVO-DROMORAN) is the only commercially available opioid agonist of the morphinan series. The *d*-isomer (dextrorphan) is relatively devoid of analgesic action but may have inhibitory effects at NMDA receptors. The structure of levorphanol is shown in Table 23–5.

The pharmacological effects of levorphanol closely parallel those of morphine. However, clinical reports suggest that it may produce less nausea and vomiting. Although levorphanol is less effective when given orally, its oral–parenteral potency ratio is comparable to that of codeine and oxycodone. The average adult dose (2 mg subcutaneously) produces analgesia for a period of time somewhat longer than that for morphine. Levorphanol is metabolized less rapidly and has a half-life of about 12 to 16 hours; repeated administration at short intervals may thus lead to accumulation of the drug in plasma (Foley, 1985).

Meperidine and Congeners

The structural formulas of *meperidine,* a *phenylpiperidine,* and some of its congeners are shown in Figure 23–4. Meperidine is predominantly a μ-receptor agonist, and it exerts its chief pharmacological action on the CNS and the neural elements in the bowel. The use of meperidine has diminished in recent years due to concerns over metabolite toxicity. For this reason, meperidine is no longer recommended for the treatment of chronic pain and should not be used for longer than 48 hours or in doses greater than 600 mg/24 hrs (Agency for Health Care Policy and Research, 1992).

Pharmacological Properties.   *Central Nervous System.* Meperidine produces a pattern of effects similar but not identical to that described for morphine.

Analgesia.   The analgesic effects of meperidine are detectable about 15 minutes after oral administration, reach a peak in about 1 to 2 hours, and subside gradually. The onset of analgesic effect is faster (within 10 minutes) after subcutaneous or intramuscular administration, and the effect reaches a peak in about 1 hour that corresponds closely to peak concentrations in plasma. In clinical use, the duration of effective analgesia is approximately 1.5 to 3 hours. In general, 75 to 100 mg of *meperidine hydrochloride* (*pethidine,* DEMEROL) given parenterally is approximately equivalent to 10 mg of morphine, and, in equianalgesic doses, meperidine produces as much sedation, respiratory depression, and euphoria as does mor-

phine. In terms of total analgesic effect, meperidine is about one-third as effective when given by mouth as when administered parenterally. A few patients may experience dysphoria.

Other CNS Actions.   Peak respiratory depression is observed within 1 hour after intramuscular administration, and there is a return toward normal starting at about 2 hours. Like other opioids, meperidine causes pupillary constriction, increases the sensitivity of the labyrinthine apparatus, and has effects on the secretion of pituitary hormones similar to those of morphine. Meperidine sometimes causes CNS excitation, characterized by tremors, muscle twitches, and seizures; these effects are due largely to accumulation of a metabolite, normeperidine (*see* below). As with morphine, respiratory depression is responsible for an accumulation of CO_2, which, in turn, leads to cerebrovascular dilation, increase in cerebral blood flow, and elevation of cerebrospinal fluid pressure.

Cardiovascular System.   The effects of meperidine on the cardiovascular system generally resemble those of morphine, including the ability to release histamine upon parenteral administration (Lee *et al.,* 1976). Intramuscular administration of meperidine does not significantly affect heart rate, but intravenous administration frequently produces a marked increase in heart rate.

Smooth Muscle.   Meperidine has effects on certain smooth muscles qualitatively similar to those observed with other opioids. Meperidine does not cause as much constipation as does morphine even when given over prolonged periods of time; this may be related to its greater ability to enter the CNS, thereby producing analgesia at lower systemic concentrations. As with other opioids, clinical doses of meperidine slow gastric emptying sufficiently to delay absorption of other drugs significantly.

The uterus of a nonpregnant woman usually is mildly stimulated by meperidine. Administered prior to an oxytocic, meperidine does not exert any antagonistic effect. Therapeutic doses given during active labor do not delay the birth process; in fact, the frequency, duration, and amplitude of uterine contraction sometimes may be increased (Zimmer *et al.,* 1988). The drug does not interfere with normal postpartum contraction or involution of the uterus, and it does not increase the incidence of postpartum hemorrhage.

Absorption, Fate, and Excretion.   Meperidine is absorbed by all routes of administration, but the rate of absorption may be erratic after intramuscular injection. The peak plasma concentration usually occurs at about 45 minutes, but the range is wide. After oral administration, only about 50% of the drug escapes first-pass metabolism to enter the circulation, and peak concentrations in plasma are usually observed in 1 to 2 hours (Herman *et al.,* 1985).

Meperidine is metabolized chiefly in the liver, with a half-life of about 3 hours. In patients with cirrhosis, the

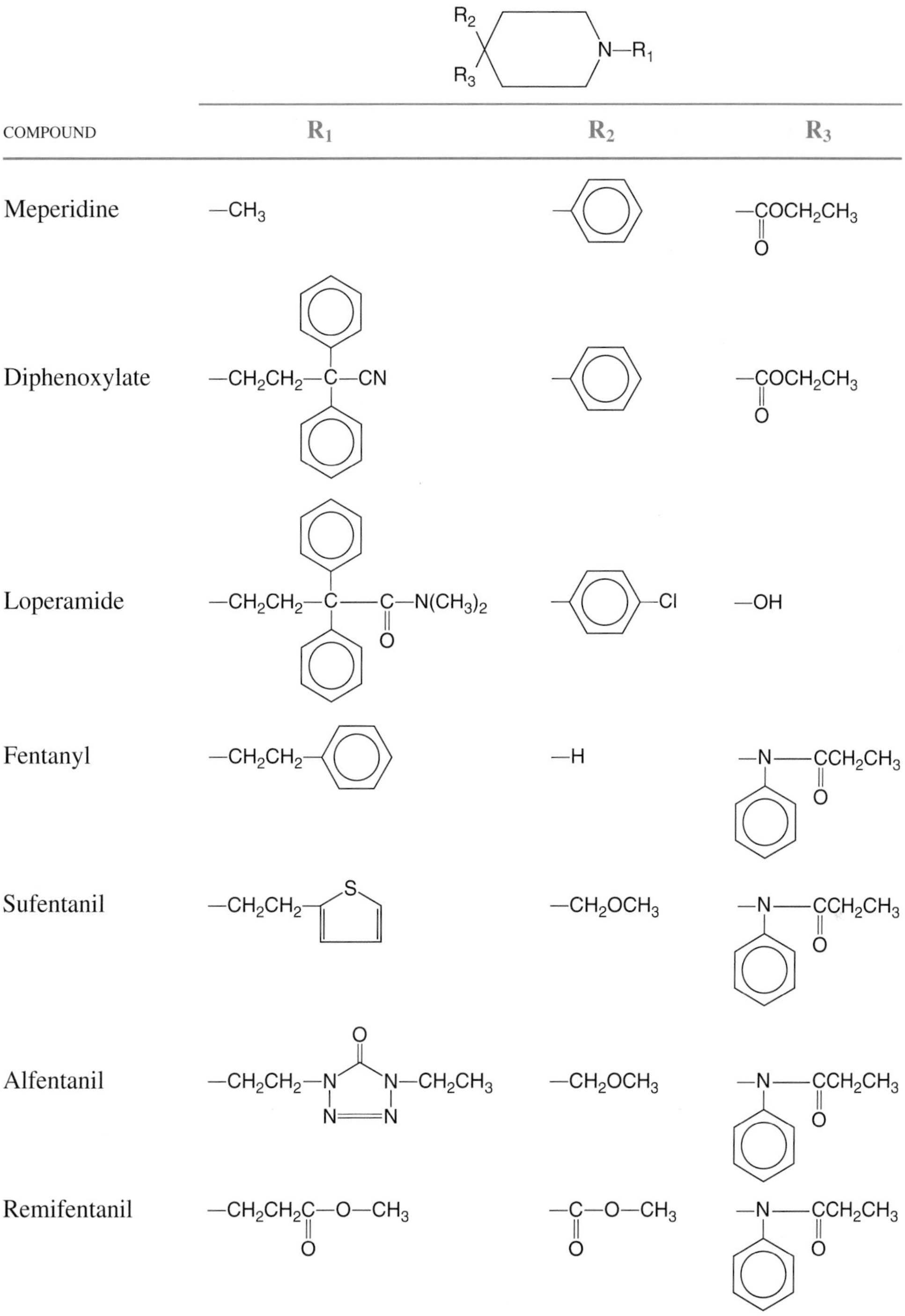

Figure 23–4. Chemical structures of piperidine and phenylpiperidine analgesics.

bioavailability of meperidine is increased to as much as 80%, and the half-lives of both meperidine and normeperidine are prolonged. Approximately 60% of meperidine in plasma is protein bound.

In human beings, meperidine is hydrolyzed to meperidinic acid, which, in turn, is partially conjugated. Meperidine also is N-demethylated to normeperidine, which may then be hydrolyzed to normeperidinic acid and subsequently conjugated. The clinical significance of the formation of normeperidine is discussed further below. Only a small amount of meperidine is excreted unchanged.

Untoward Effects, Precautions, and Contraindications.
The pattern and overall incidence of untoward effects that follow the use of meperidine are similar to those observed after equianalgesic doses of morphine, except that constipation and urinary retention may be less common. Patients who experience nausea and vomiting with morphine may not do so with meperidine; the converse also may be true. As with other opioids, tolerance develops to some of these effects. The contraindications are generally the same as for other opioids. In patients or addicts who are tolerant to the depressant effects of meperidine, large doses repeated at short intervals may produce an excitatory syndrome including hallucinations, tremors, muscle twitches, dilated pupils, hyperactive reflexes, and convulsions. These excitatory symptoms are due to the accumulation of normeperidine, which has a half-life of 15 to 20 hours compared with 3 hours for meperidine. Opioid antagonists can block the convulsant effect of normeperidine in the mouse. Since normeperidine is eliminated by both the kidney and the liver, decreased renal or hepatic function increases the likelihood of such toxicity (Kaiko et al., 1983). Thus, meperidine is not the drug of choice for the treatment of severe or prolonged pain because of its shorter duration of action relative to morphine and the potential for CNS toxicity from normeperidine.

Interaction with Other Drugs. Severe reactions may follow the administration of meperidine to patients being treated with MAO inhibitors. Two basic types of interactions can be observed. The most prominent is an excitatory reaction with delirium, hyperthermia, headache, hyper- or hypotension, rigidity, convulsions, coma, and death. This reaction may be due to the ability of meperidine to block neuronal reuptake of serotonin and the resultant serotonergic overactivity (Stack et al., 1988). Therefore, meperidine and its congeners should not be used in patients taking MAO inhibitors. Dextromethorphan also inhibits neuronal serotonin uptake and should be avoided in these patients. As discussed above, tramadol inhibits uptake of norepinephrine and serotonin and should not be used concomitantly with MAO inhibitors. Similar interactions with other currently used opioids have not been observed clinically. Another type of interaction, a potentiation of opioid effect due to inhibition of hepatic microsomal enzymes, also can be observed in patients taking MAO inhibitors, necessitating a reduction in the doses of opioids.

Chlorpromazine increases the respiratory-depressant effects of meperidine, as do tricyclic antidepressants; this is not true of diazepam. Concurrent administration of drugs such as promethazine or chlorpromazine also may greatly enhance meperidine-induced sedation without slowing clearance of the drug. Treatment with phenobarbital or phenytoin increases systemic

clearance and decreases oral bioavailability of meperidine; this is associated with an elevation of the concentration of normeperidine in plasma (Edwards et al., 1982). As with morphine, concomitant administration of amphetamine has been reported to enhance the analgesic effects of meperidine and its congeners while counteracting sedation.

Therapeutic Uses. The major use of meperidine is for analgesia. Unlike morphine and its congeners, meperidine is not used for the treatment of cough or diarrhea. Single doses of meperidine also appear to be effective in the treatment of postanesthetic shivering.

Meperidine crosses the placental barrier and even in reasonable analgesic doses causes a significant increase in the percentage of babies who show delayed respiration, decreased respiratory minute volume, or decreased oxygen saturation, or who require resuscitation. Both fetal and maternal respiratory depression induced by meperidine can be treated with naloxone. The fraction of drug that is bound to protein is lower in the fetus; concentrations of free drug thus may be considerably higher than in the mother. Nevertheless, meperidine produces less respiratory depression in the newborn than does an equianalgesic dose of morphine or methadone (Fishburne, 1982).

Congeners of Meperidine. *Diphenoxylate.* Diphenoxylate is a meperidine congener that has a definite constipating effect in human beings. Its only approved use is in the treatment of diarrhea. Although single doses in the therapeutic range (see below) produce little or no morphine-like subjective effects, at high doses (40 to 60 mg) the drug shows typical opioid activity, including euphoria, suppression of morphine abstinence, and a morphine-like physical dependence after chronic administration. Diphenoxylate is unusual in that even its salts are virtually insoluble in aqueous solution, thus obviating the possibility of abuse by the parenteral route. *Diphenoxylate hydrochloride* is available only in combination with atropine sulfate (LOMOTIL, others). The recommended daily dosage of diphenoxylate for treatment of diarrhea in adults is 20 mg, in divided doses. *Difenoxin* (difenoxylic acid; MOTOFEN) is one of the metabolites of diphenoxylate; it has actions similar to those of the parent compound.

Loperamide. Loperamide (IMODIUM, others), like diphenoxylate, is a piperidine derivative (see Figure 23–3). It slows gastrointestinal motility by effects on the circular and longitudinal muscles of the intestine, presumably as a result of its interactions with opioid receptors in the intestine. Some part of its antidiarrheal effect may be due to a reduction of gastrointestinal secretion (see above; see also Manara and Bianchetti, 1985; Coupar, 1987; Kromer, 1988). In controlling chronic diarrhea, loperamide is as effective as diphenoxylate. In clinical studies, the most common side effect is abdominal cramps. Little tolerance develops to its constipating effect.

In human volunteers taking large doses of loperamide, concentrations of drug in plasma peak about 4 hours after ingestion; this long latency may be due to inhibition of gastrointestinal motility and to enterohepatic circulation of the drug. The apparent elimination half-life is 7 to 14 hours. Loperamide is not well absorbed after oral administration and, in addition, apparently does not penetrate well into the brain because of exclusion by a P-glycoprotein transporter widely expressed in the blood–brain barrier (Sadeque *et al.,* 2000). Mice with deletions of one of the genes encoding the P-glycoprotein transporter have much higher brain levels and significant central effects after administration of loperamide (Schinkel *et al.,* 1996). Inhibition of P-glycoprotein by many clinically used drugs, such as quinidine, verapamil, and ketoconazole, possibly could lead to enhanced central effects of loperamide.

In general, loperamide is unlikely to be abused parenterally because of its low solubility; large doses of loperamide given to human volunteers do not elicit pleasurable effects typical of opioids. The usual dosage is 4 to 8 mg per day; the daily dose should not exceed 16 mg.

Fentanyl and Congeners

Fentanyl is a synthetic opioid related to the phenylpiperidines (*see* Figure 23–3). It is a μ-receptor agonist and is about 100-times more potent than morphine as an analgesic.

The actions of fentanyl and its congeners, *sufentanil, alfentanil,* and *remifentanil,* are similar to those of other μ-receptor agonists. Fentanyl is a popular drug in anesthetic practice because of its shorter time to peak analgesic effect, rapid termination of effect after small bolus doses, and relative cardiovascular stability (*see* Chapter 14).

Pharmacological Properties. *Analgesia.* The analgesic effects of fentanyl and sufentanil are similar to those of morphine and other μ opioids. Fentanyl is approximately 100-times more potent than morphine, and sufentanil is approximately 1000-times more potent than morphine. These drugs are most commonly administered intravenously, although both also are commonly administered epidurally and intrathecally for acute postoperative and chronic pain management. Fentanyl and sufentanil are far more lipid soluble than morphine; thus the risk of delayed respiratory depression due to rostral spread of intraspinally administered narcotic to respiratory centers is greatly reduced. The time to peak analgesic effect after intravenous administration of fentanyl and sufentanil is less than that for morphine and meperidine, with peak analgesia being reached after about 5 minutes, as opposed to approximately 15 minutes. Recovery from analgesic effects also occurs more quickly. However, with larger doses or prolonged infusions, the effects of these drugs become more long lasting, with durations of action becoming similar to those of longer acting opioids (*see* below).

Other CNS Effects. As with other μ opioids, nausea, vomiting, and itching can be observed with fentanyl. Muscle rigidity, while possible after all narcotics, appears to be more common after administration of bolus doses of fentanyl or its congeners. This effect is felt to be cen-

trally mediated and may be due in part to their increased potency relative to morphine. Rigidity can be mitigated by avoiding bolus dosing, slower administration of boluses, and by pretreatment with a nonopioid anesthetic induction agent. Rigidity can be treated with depolarizing or nondepolarizing neuromuscular blocking agents while controlling the patient's ventilation. Care must be taken to make sure the patient is not aware but unable to move. Respiratory depression is similar to that observed with other μ-receptor agonists, but the onset is more rapid. As with analgesia, respiratory depression after small doses is of shorter duration than with morphine, but of similar duration after large doses or long infusions. As with morphine and meperidine, delayed respiratory depression also can be seen after the use of fentanyl, sufentanil, or alfentanil, possibly due to enterohepatic circulation. High doses of fentanyl can cause neuroexcitation and, rarely, seizure-like activity in human beings (Bailey and Stanley, 1994). Fentanyl has minimal effects on intracranial pressure when ventilation is controlled and the arterial CO_2 concentration is not allowed to rise.

Cardiovascular System. Fentanyl and its derivatives decrease the heart rate and can mildly decrease blood pressure. However, these drugs do not release histamine and in general provide a marked degree of cardiovascular stability. Direct depressant effects on the myocardium are minimal. For this reason, high doses of fentanyl or sufentanil commonly are used as the primary anesthetic for patients undergoing cardiovascular surgery or for patients with poor cardiac function.

Absorption, Fate, and Excretion. These agents are highly lipid soluble and rapidly cross the blood–brain barrier. This is reflected in the half-life for equilibration between the plasma and CSF of approximately 5 minutes for fentanyl and sufentanil. The levels in plasma and CSF rapidly decline due to redistribution of fentanyl from highly perfused tissue groups to other tissues, such as muscle and fat. As saturation of less-well-perfused tissue occurs, the duration of fentanyl's and sufentanil's effects approach the length of their elimination half lives of between 3 and 4 hours (Sanford and Gutstein, 1995). Fentanyl and sufentanil undergo hepatic metabolism and renal excretion. Therefore, with the use of higher doses or prolonged infusions, fentanyl and sufentanil become longer acting.

Therapeutic Uses. *Fentanyl citrate* (SUBLIMAZE) and *sufentanil citrate* (SUFENTA) have gained widespread popularity as anesthetic adjuvants (*see* Chapter 14). They commonly are used either intravenously, epidurally, or intrathecally. A formulation of fentanyl and *droperidol* (INNOVAR) was commonly used for anesthesia. However, dysphoric side effects of droperidol have limited the popularity of this combination. Epidural use of fentanyl and sufentanil for postoperative or labor analgesia has gained increasing popularity. A combination of epidural opioids with local anesthetics permits reduction in the dosage of both components, minimizing the side effects of both local anesthetics (*i.e.,* motor blockade) and opioids (*i.e.,* urinary retention, itching, and delayed respiratory depression in the case of morphine). Intravenous use of fentanyl and sufentanil for postoperative pain has been effective but limited by clinical concerns about muscle rigidity. However, the use of fentanyl and sufentanil in chronic pain treatment has become more widespread. Epidural and intrathecal infusions, both with and without local anesthetic, are used in the management of chronic malignant pain and selected cases of nonmalignant pain. Also, the development of novel, less invasive routes of administration for fentanyl has facilitated the use of these compounds in chronic pain management. Transdermal patches (DURAGESIC) that provide sustained release of fentanyl for 48 hours or more are available. However, factors promoting increased absorption (*e.g.,* fever) can lead to relative overdosage and increased side effects (*see also* the section on alternative routes of administration, below). Also, the FENTANYL ORALET, a formulation that permits rapid absorption of fentanyl through the buccal mucosa (much like a lollipop), was tried as an anesthetic premedicant but did not gain wide acceptance due to undesirable side effects in opioid-naïve patients (nausea, vomiting, pruritus, and respiratory depression). A similar fentanyl product, ACTIQ, is available in higher strengths and is used for relief of breakthrough cancer pain (Ashburn *et al.,* 1989).

Alfentanil and Remifentanil. These compounds were developed in an effort to create analgesics with a more rapid onset and predictable termination of opioid effects. The potency of remifentanil is approximately equal to that of fentanyl and is between 20- and 30-times greater than that of alfentanil. The pharmacological properties of alfentanil and remifentanil are similar to those of fentanyl and sufentanil. They have similar incidences of nausea, vomiting, and dose-dependent muscle rigidity. Nausea, vomiting, itching, and headaches have been reported when remifentanil has been used for conscious analgesia for painful procedures. Intracranial pressure changes are minimal when ventilation is controlled. Seizures after remifentanil administration have not yet been reported.

Absorption, Fate and Excretion. Both alfentanil and remifentanil have a more rapid onset of analgesic action than do fentanyl on sufentanil. Analgesic effects occur within of 1 to 1.5 minutes. After intravenous administration, alfentanil is metabolized in the liver similarly to fentanyl and sufentanil, with an elimination half-life of 1 to 2 hours. The duration of action of alfentanil is dependent on both the dose and length of administration. Remifentanil is unique in that it is metabolized by plasma esterases (Burkle *et al.,* 1996). Elimination is independent of hepatic metabolism or renal excretion, and the elimination half-life is 8 to 20 minutes. There is no prolongation of effect with repeated dosing or prolonged infusion. Age and weight can affect clearance of remifentanil, requiring that dosage be reduced in the elderly and based on lean body mass. However, neither of these conditions causes major changes in duration of effect. After 3- to 5-hour infusions of remifentanil, recovery of respiratory function can be seen within 3 to 5 minutes, while full recovery from all effects of remifentanil is observed within 15 minutes (Glass *et al.,* 1999). The primary metabolite, remifentanil acid, is 2000- to 4000-times less potent than remifentanil and is renally excreted. Peak respiratory depression after bolus doses of remifentanil occurs after 5 minutes (Patel and Spencer, 1996).

Therapeutic Uses. *Alfentanil hydrochloride* (ALFENTA) and *remifentanil hydrochloride* (ULTIVA) are useful for short, painful procedures that require intense analgesia and blunting of stress responses. The titratability of remifentanil and its consistent, rapid offset make it ideally suited for short surgical procedures where rapid recovery is an issue. Remifentanil also has been used successfully for longer neurosurgical procedures, where rapid emergence from anesthesia is important. However, in cases where postprocedural analgesia is required, remifentanil alone is a poor choice. In this situation, either a longer-acting opioid or another analgesic modality should be combined with remifentanil for prolonged analgesia, or another opioid should be used. Alfentanil has been administered intraspinally for pain control. Remifentanil is presently not used intraspinally, as glycine in the drug vehicle can cause temporary motor paralysis. It is generally given by continuous intravenous infusion, as its short duration of action makes bolus administration impractical.

Methadone and Congeners

Methadone is a long-lasting μ-receptor agonist with pharmacological properties qualitatively similar to those of morphine.

Chemistry. Methadone has the following structural formula:

$$CH_3CH_2-\underset{\underset{O}{\|}}{C}-\underset{}{C}-CH_2-CH-N\underset{CH_3}{\overset{CH_3}{<}}$$

METHADONE

The analgesic activity of the racemate is almost entirely the result of its content of *l*-methadone, which is 8- to 50-times more potent than the *d* isomer; *d*-methadone also lacks significant respiratory depressant action and addiction liability, but it does possess antitussive activity.

Pharmacological Actions.

The outstanding properties of methadone are its analgesic activity, its efficacy by the oral route, its extended duration of action in suppressing withdrawal symptoms in physically dependent individuals, and its tendency to show persistent effects with repeated administration. Miotic and respiratory-depressant effects can be detected for more than 24 hours after a single dose and, upon repeated administration, marked sedation is seen in some patients. Effects on cough, bowel motility, biliary tone, and the secretion of pituitary hormones are qualitatively similar to those of morphine.

Absorption, Fate, and Excretion.

Methadone is well absorbed from the gastrointestinal tract and can be detected in plasma within 30 minutes after oral ingestion; it reaches peak concentrations at about 4 hours. After therapeutic doses, about 90% of methadone is bound to plasma proteins. Peak concentrations occur in the brain within 1 or 2 hours after subcutaneous or intramuscular administration, and this correlates well with the intensity and duration of analgesia. Methadone also can be absorbed from the buccal mucosa (Weinberg *et al.,* 1988).

Methadone undergoes extensive biotransformation in the liver. The major metabolites, the results of *N*-demethylation and cyclization to form pyrrolidines and pyrroline, are excreted in the urine and the bile along with small amounts of unchanged drug. The amount of methadone excreted in the urine is increased when the urine is acidified. The half-life of methadone is approximately 15 to 40 hours.

Methadone appears to be firmly bound to protein in various tissues, including brain. After repeated administration there is gradual accumulation in tissues. When administration is discontinued, low concentrations are maintained in plasma by slow release from extravascular

binding sites (*see* Kreek, 1979); this process probably accounts for the relatively mild but protracted withdrawal syndrome.

Side Effects, Toxicity, Drug Interactions, and Precautions. Side effects, toxicity, and conditions that alter sensitivity, as well as the treatment of acute intoxication, are similar to those described for morphine. During long-term administration, there may be excessive sweating, lymphocytosis, and increased concentrations of prolactin, albumin, and globulins in the plasma. Rifampin and phenytoin accelerate the metabolism of methadone and can precipitate withdrawal symptoms (*see* Kreek, 1979).

Tolerance and Physical Dependence. Volunteer postaddicts who receive subcutaneous or oral methadone daily develop partial tolerance to the nauseant, anorectic, miotic sedative, respiratory-depressant, and cardiovascular effects of methadone. Tolerance develops more slowly to methadone than to morphine in some patients, especially with respect to the depressant effects. However, this may be related in part to cumulative effects of the drug or its metabolites. Tolerance to the constipating effect of methadone does not develop as fully as does tolerance to other effects. The behavior of addicts who use methadone parenterally is strikingly similar to that of morphine addicts, but many former heroin users treated with oral methadone show virtually no overt behavioral effects.

Development of physical dependence during the long-term administration of methadone can be demonstrated by drug withdrawal or by administration of an opioid antagonist. Subcutaneous administration of 10 to 20 mg of methadone to former opioid addicts produces definite euphoria equal in duration to that caused by morphine, and its overall abuse potential is comparable to that of morphine.

Therapeutic Uses. The primary uses of *methadone hydrochloride* (DOLOPHINE, others) are relief of chronic pain, treatment of opioid abstinence syndromes, and treatment of heroin users. It is not widely used as an antiperistaltic agent. It should not be used in labor.

Analgesia. The onset of analgesia occurs 10 to 20 minutes following parenteral administration and 30 to 60 minutes after oral medication. The average minimal effective analgesic concentration in blood is about 30 ng/ml (Gourlay *et al.,* 1986). The typical oral dose is 2.5 to 15 mg, depending on the severity of the pain and the response of the patient. The initial parenteral dose is usually 2.5 to 10 mg. Care must be taken when escalating the dosage, because of the prolonged half-life of the drug and its tendency to accumulate over a period of several days with repeated dosing. Despite its longer plasma half-life, the duration of the analgesic action of single doses is essentially the same as that of morphine. With repeated usage, cumulative effects are seen, so that either lower dosage or longer intervals between doses become possible. In contrast to morphine, methadone and many of its congeners retain a considerable degree of their effectiveness when given orally. In terms of total analgesic effects, methadone given orally is about 50% as effective as the same dose administered intramuscularly; however, the oral-parenteral potency ratio is considerably lower when peak analgesic effect is considered. In equianalgesic doses, the pattern and incidence of untoward effects caused by methadone and morphine are similar.

Levomethadyl Acetate.   *Levomethadyl acetate* (*l-α*-acetyl-methadol; ORLAAM) is a congener of methadone that is approved for use in maintenance programs for the treatment of heroin addicts. The drug is thought to act, in part, by its conversion to active metabolites, which explains its slow onset and protracted duration of action. The slow onset of effect can be problematic in the treatment of addicts (*see* Chapter 24). In physically dependent subjects taking levomethadyl acetate, withdrawal symptoms are not perceived for 72 to 96 hours after the last oral dose. Most subjects are comfortable taking a single dose as infrequently as every 72 hours (*see* Ling *et al.,* 1978). The *d* isomer of methadyl acetate is inactive.

Propoxyphene

Propoxyphene is structurally related to methadone (*see* below). Its analgesic effect resides in the dextro isomer, *d*-propoxyphene (dextropropoxyphene). However, levopropoxyphene seems to have some antitussive activity. The structure of propoxyphene is shown below.

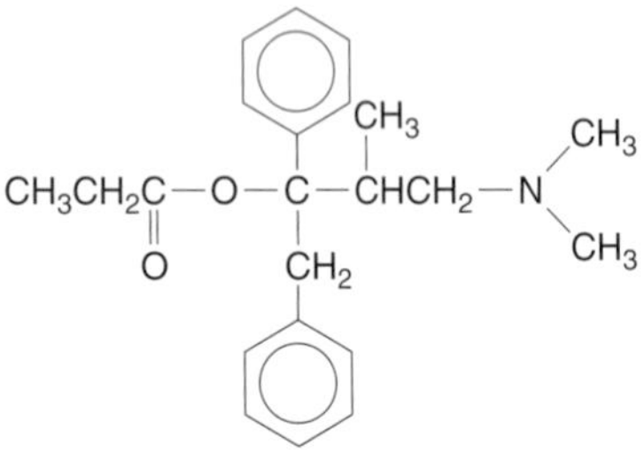

PROPOXYPHENE

Pharmacological Actions.   Although slightly less selective than morphine, propoxyphene binds primarily to μ-opioid receptors and produces analgesia and other CNS effects that are similar to those seen with morphine-like opioids. It is likely that at equianalgesic doses the incidence of side effects such as nausea, anorexia, constipation, abdominal pain, and drowsiness would be similar to those of codeine.

   As an analgesic, propoxyphene is about one-half to two-thirds as potent as codeine given orally. Ninety to 120 mg of propoxyphene hydrochloride administered orally would equal the analgesic effects of 60 mg of codeine, a dose that usually produces about as much analgesia as 600 mg of aspirin. Combinations of propoxyphene and aspirin, like combinations of codeine and aspirin, afford a higher level of analgesia than does either agent given alone (Beaver, 1988).

Absorption, Fate, and Excretion.   Following oral administration, concentrations of propoxyphene in plasma reach their highest values at 1 to 2 hours. There is great variability between subjects in the rate of clearance and the plasma concentrations that are achieved. The average half-life of propoxyphene in plasma after a single dose is from 6 to 12 hours, which is longer than that of codeine. In human beings, the major route of metabolism is *N*-demethylation to yield norpropoxyphene.

The half-life of norpropoxyphene is about 30 hours, and its accumulation with repeated doses may be responsible for some of the observed toxicity (*see* Chan and Matzke, 1987).

Toxicity.   Given orally, propoxyphene is approximately one-third as potent as orally administered codeine in depressing respiration. Moderately toxic doses usually produce CNS and respiratory depression, but with still-larger doses the clinical picture may be complicated by convulsions in addition to respiratory depression. Delusions, hallucinations, confusion, cardiotoxicity, and pulmonary edema also have been noted. Respiratory-depressant effects are significantly enhanced when ethanol or sedative-hypnotics are ingested concurrently. Naloxone antagonizes the respiratory-depressant, convulsant, and some of the cardiotoxic effects of propoxyphene.

Tolerance and Dependence.   Very large doses [800 mg of *propoxyphene hydrochloride* (DARVON, others) or 1200 mg of the napsylate (DARVON-N) per day] reduce the intensity of the morphine withdrawal syndrome somewhat less effectively than do 1500-mg doses of codeine. Maximal tolerated doses are equivalent to daily doses of 20 to 25 mg of morphine, given subcutaneously. The use of higher doses of propoxyphene is prevented by untoward side effects and the occurrence of toxic psychoses. Very large doses produce some respiratory depression in morphine-tolerant addicts, suggesting that cross-tolerance between propoxyphene and morphine is incomplete. Abrupt discontinuation of chronically administered propoxyphene hydrochloride (up to 800 mg per day, given for almost 2 months) results in mild abstinence phenomena, and large oral doses (300 to 600 mg) produce subjective effects that are considered pleasurable by postaddicts. The drug is quite irritating when administered either intravenously or subcutaneously, so that abuse by these routes results in severe damage to veins and soft tissues.

Therapeutic Uses.   Propoxyphene is recommended for the treatment of mild-to-moderate pain. Given acutely, the commonly prescribed combination of 32 mg of propoxyphene with aspirin may not produce more analgesia than aspirin alone, and doses of 65 mg of the hydrochloride or 100 mg of the napsylate are suggested. Propoxyphene is most often given in combination with aspirin or acetaminophen. The wide popularity of propoxyphene in clinical situations in which codeine was once used is largely a result of unrealistic overconcern about the addictive potential of codeine.

ACUTE OPIOID TOXICITY

Acute opioid toxicity may result from clinical overdosage, accidental overdosage in addicts, or attempts at suicide. Occasionally, a delayed type of toxicity may occur from the injection of an opioid into chilled skin areas or in patients with low blood pressure and shock. The drug is not fully absorbed, and, therefore, a subsequent dose may be given. When normal circulation is established, an excessive amount may be absorbed suddenly. It is difficult to define the exact amount of any opioid that is toxic or lethal to human beings. Recent experiences with methadone indicate that, in nontolerant individuals, serious toxicity may follow the oral ingestion of 40 to 60 mg. Older literature suggests that, in the case of morphine, a normal, pain-free adult is not likely to die after oral doses of less than 120 mg or to have serious toxicity with less than 30 mg parenterally.

Symptoms and Diagnosis.   The patient who has taken an overdose of an opioid usually is stuporous or, if a large overdose has been taken, may be in a profound coma. The respiratory rate will be very low or the patient may be apneic, and cyanosis may be present. As respiratory exchange decreases, blood pressure, at first likely to be near normal, will fall progressively. If adequate oxygenation is restored early, the blood pressure will improve; if hypoxia persists untreated, there may be capillary damage, and measures to combat shock may be required. The pupils will be symmetrical and pinpoint in size; however, if hypoxia is severe, they may be dilated. Urine formation is depressed. Body temperature falls, and the skin becomes cold and clammy. The skeletal muscles are flaccid, the jaw is relaxed, and the tongue may fall back and block the airway. Frank convulsions occasionally may be noted in infants and children. When death occurs, it is nearly always due to respiratory failure. Even if respiration is restored, death still may occur as a result of complications that develop during the period of coma, such as pneumonia or shock. Noncardiogenic pulmonary edema is seen commonly with opioid poisoning. It probably is not due to contaminants or to anaphylactoid reactions, and it has been observed following toxic doses of morphine, methadone, propoxyphene, and uncontaminated heroin.

The triad of coma, pinpoint pupils, and depressed respiration strongly suggests opioid poisoning. The finding of needle marks suggestive of addiction further supports the diagnosis. Mixed poisonings, however, are not uncommon. Examination of the urine and gastric contents for drugs may aid in diagnosis, but the results usually become available too late to influence treatment.

Treatment.   The first step is to establish a patent airway and ventilate the patient. Opioid antagonists (*see* below) can produce dramatic reversal of the severe respiratory depression, and the antagonist *naloxone* (*see* below) is the treatment of choice. However, care should be taken to avoid precipitating withdrawal in dependent patients, who may be extremely sensitive to antagonists. The safest approach is to dilute the standard naloxone dose (0.4 mg) and slowly administer it intravenously, monitoring arousal and respiratory function. With care, it usually is possible to reverse the respiratory depression without precipitating a major withdrawal syndrome. If no response is seen with the first dose, additional doses can be given. Patients should be observed for rebound increases in sympathetic nervous system activity, which may result in cardiac arrhythmias and pulmonary edema (*see* Duthie and Nimmo, 1987). For reversing opioid poisoning in children, the initial dose of naloxone is 0.01 mg/kg. If no effect is seen after a total dose of 10 mg, one can reasonably question the accuracy of the diagnosis. Pulmonary edema sometimes associated with opioid overdosage may be countered by positive-pressure respiration. Tonic-clonic seizures, occasionally seen as part of the toxic syndrome with meperidine and propoxyphene, are ameliorated by treatment with naloxone.

The presence of general CNS depressants does not prevent the salutary effect of naloxone, and in cases of mixed intoxications, the situation will be improved largely due to antagonism of the respiratory-depressant effects of the opioid. However, some evidence indicates that naloxone and naltrexone also may antagonize some of the depressant actions of sedative-hypnotics (*see* below). One need not attempt to restore the patient to full consciousness. The duration of action of the available antagonists is shorter than that of many opioids; hence, patients must be watched carefully, lest they slip back into coma. This is particularly important when the overdosage is due to methadone or *l*-acetylmethadol. The depressant effects of these drugs may persist for 24 to 72 hours, and fatalities have occurred as a result of premature discontinuation of naloxone. In cases of overdoses of these drugs, a continuous infusion of naloxone should be considered. Toxicity due to overdose of pentazocine and other opioids with mixed actions may require higher doses of naloxone. The pharmacological actions of opioid antagonists are discussed in more detail below.

OPIOID AGONIST/ANTAGONISTS AND PARTIAL AGONISTS

The drugs described in this section differ from clinically used μ-opioid receptor agonists. Drugs such as *nalbuphine* and *butorphanol* are competitive μ-receptor antagonists but exert their analgesic actions by acting as agonists at κ receptors. *Pentazocine* qualitatively resembles these drugs, but it may be a weaker μ-receptor antagonist or partial agonist while retaining its κ-agonist activity. *Buprenorphine*, on the other hand, is a partial agonist at μ receptors. The stimulus for the development of mixed agonist/antagonist drugs was a need for analgesics with less respiratory depression and addictive potential. Currently, the clinical use of these compounds is limited by undesirable side effects and by limited analgesic effects.

Pentazocine

Pentazocine was synthesized as part of a deliberate effort to develop an effective analgesic with little or no abuse potential. It has both agonistic actions and weak opioid antagonistic activity. The pharmacology of pentazocine has been reviewed by (Brogden *et al.*, 1973).

Chemistry. Pentazocine is a benzomorphan derivative with the following structural formula:

PENTAZOCINE

The compound has a large substituent on the nitrogen atom that is analogous to position 17 of morphine. This structural feature is common to a number of opioids with antagonist or agonist/antagonist activity. The analgesic and respiratory-depressant activity of the racemate is due mainly to the *l* isomer.

Pharmacological Actions. The pattern of CNS effects produced by pentazocine is generally similar to that of the morphine-like opioids, including analgesia, sedation, and respiratory depression. The analgesic effects of pentazocine are due to agonistic actions at κ-opioid receptors. Higher doses of pentazocine (60 to 90 mg) elicit dysphoric and psychotomimetic effects. The mechanisms responsible for these side effects are not known but might involve activation of supraspinal κ receptors, since it has been suggested that these untoward effects may be reversible by naloxone.

The cardiovascular responses to pentazocine differ from those seen with typical μ-receptor agonists, in that high doses cause an increase in blood pressure and heart rate. In patients with coronary artery disease, pentazocine administered intravenously elevates mean aortic pressure, left ventricular end-diastolic pressure, and mean pulmonary artery pressure and causes an increase in cardiac work (Alderman *et al.,* 1972; Lee *et al.,* 1976). A rise in the concentrations of catecholamines in plasma may account for its effects on blood pressure.

Pentazocine acts as a weak antagonist or partial agonist at μ-opioid receptors. Low doses (20 mg given parenterally) depress respiration as much as does 10 mg of morphine, but increasing the pentazocine dose does not produce a proportionate increase in respiratory depression. Pentazocine does not antagonize the respiratory depression produced by morphine. However, when given to patients dependent on morphine or other μ-receptor agonists, pentazocine may precipitate withdrawal. In patients tolerant to morphine-like opioids, pentazocine reduces the analgesia produced by their administration, even when clear-cut withdrawal symptoms are not precipitated. Ceiling effects for both analgesia and respiratory depression are observed above 50 to 100 mg of pentazocine (Bailey and Stanley, 1994).

Absorption, Fate, and Excretion. Pentazocine is well absorbed from the gastrointestinal tract and from subcutaneous and intramuscular sites. Peak analgesia occurs 15 minutes to 1 hour after intramuscular administration and 1 to 3 hours after oral administration. The half-life in plasma is 4 to 5 hours. First-pass metabolism in the liver is extensive, and somewhat less than 20% of pentazocine enters the systemic circulation. Drug action is terminated by hepatic metabolism and renal excretion.

Side Effects, Toxicity, and Precautions. The most commonly reported untoward effects are sedation, sweating, and dizziness or lightheadedness; nausea also occurs, but vomiting is less common than with morphine. Psychotomimetic effects, such as uncontrollable or weird thoughts, anxiety, nightmares, and hallucinations, occur with parenteral doses above 60 mg. Epidemiological data suggest that overdose with pentazocine alone rarely causes death. High doses produce marked respiratory depression associated with increased blood pressure and tachycardia. The respiratory depression is antagonized by naloxone. Pentazocine is irritating when administered subcutaneously or intramuscularly. Repeated injections over long periods may cause extensive fibrosis of subcutaneous and muscular tissue. Patients who have been receiving opioids on a regular basis may experience abstinence signs and symptoms when given pentazocine. After an opioid-free interval of 1 to 2 days, it is usually possible to administer pentazocine without producing such withdrawal effects.

Tolerance and Physical Dependence. With frequent and repeated use, tolerance develops to the analgesic and subjective effects of pentazocine. However, pentazocine does not prevent or ameliorate the morphine withdrawal syndrome. Instead, when high doses of pentazocine are given to subjects dependent on morphine, it precipitates withdrawal symptoms because of its antagonistic actions at the μ receptor.

After long-term administration (60 mg every 4 hours), postaddicts develop physical dependence that can be demonstrated by abrupt withdrawal or by the administration of naloxone. The withdrawal syndrome after chronic doses of more than 500 mg per day, although milder in intensity than withdrawal from morphine, includes abdominal cramps, anxiety, chills, elevated temperature, vomiting, lacrimation, and sweating. Pentazocine withdrawal symptoms can be managed by gradual reduction of pentazocine itself or by substitution of μ-receptor agonists, such as morphine or methadone. A syndrome of withdrawal from pentazocine also has been observed in neonates.

Therapeutic Uses. Pentazocine is used as an analgesic. Although the risk of drug dependence exists, it may be lower than that associated with the use of morphine-like drugs in similar circumstances. Because abuse patterns appear to be less likely to develop with oral administration, this route should be used whenever possible.

Pentazocine lactate (TALWIN) is available as a solution for injection. In an effort to reduce the use of tablets as a source of injectable pentazocine, tablets for oral use now contain *pentazocine hydrochloride* (equivalent to 50 mg of the base) and *naloxone hydrochloride* (equivalent to 0.5 mg of the base; TALWIN NX). After oral ingestion, naloxone is destroyed rapidly by the liver; however, if the material is dissolved and injected, the naloxone produces aversive effects in subjects dependent on opioids. Tablets containing mixtures of pentazocine with aspirin (TALWIN COMPOUND) or acetaminophen (TALCEN) also are available. In terms of analgesic effect, 30 to 60 mg of pentazocine given parenterally is approximately equivalent to 10 mg of morphine. An oral dose of about 50 mg of pentazocine results in analgesia equivalent to that produced by 60 mg of codeine orally.

Nalbuphine

Nalbuphine is related structurally to both naloxone and oxymorphone (*see* Table 23–5). It is an agonist/antagonist opioid with a spectrum of effects that qualitatively resembles that of pentazocine; however, nalbuphine is a more potent antagonist at μ receptors and is less likely to produce dysphoric side effects than is pentazocine.

Pharmacological Actions and Side Effects. An intramuscular dose of 10 mg of nalbuphine is equianalgesic to 10 mg of morphine, with similar onset and duration of both analgesic and subjective effects. Nalbuphine depresses respiration as much as do equianalgesic doses of morphine. However, nalbuphine exhibits a ceiling effect, such that increases in dosage beyond 30 mg produce no further respiratory depression. However, a ceiling effect for analgesia also is reached at this point. In contrast to pentazocine and butorphanol, 10 mg of nalbuphine given to patients with stable coronary artery disease does not produce an increase in cardiac index, pulmonary arterial pressure, or cardiac work, and systemic blood pressure is not significantly altered; these indices also are relatively stable when nalbuphine is given to patients with acute myocardial infarction (*see* Roth *et al.,* 1988). Its gastrointestinal effects are probably similar to those of pentazocine. Nalbuphine produces few side effects at doses of 10 mg or less; sedation, sweating, and headache are the most common. At much higher doses (70 mg), psychotomimetic side effects (dysphoria, racing thoughts, and distortions of body image) can occur. Nalbuphine is metabolized in the liver and has a half-life in plasma of 2 to 3 hours. Given orally, nalbuphine is 20% to 25% as potent as when given intramuscularly.

Tolerance and Physical Dependence. In subjects dependent on low doses of morphine (60 mg per day), nalbuphine precipitates an abstinence syndrome. Prolonged administration of nalbuphine can produce physical dependence. The withdrawal syndrome is similar in intensity to that seen with pentazocine. The potential for abuse of parenteral nalbuphine in subjects not dependent on μ-receptor agonists is probably similar to that of parenteral pentazocine.

Therapeutic Uses. *Nalbuphine hydrochloride* (NUBAIN) is used to produce analgesia. Because it is an agonist/antagonist, administration to patients who have been receiving morphine-like opioids may create difficulties unless a brief drug-free interval is interposed. The usual adult dose is 10 mg parenterally every 3 to 6 hours; this may be increased to 20 mg in nontolerant individuals.

Butorphanol

Butorphanol is a morphinan congener with a profile of actions similar to those of pentazocine. The structural formula of butorphanol is shown in Table 23–5.

Pharmacological Actions and Side Effects. In postoperative patients, a parenteral dose of 2 to 3 mg of butorphanol produces analgesia and respiratory depression approximately equal to that produced by 10 mg of morphine or 80 to 100 mg of meperidine; the onset, peak, and duration of action are similar to those that follow the administration of morphine. The plasma half-life of butorphanol is about 3 hours. Like pentazocine, analgesic

doses of butorphanol produce an increase in pulmonary arterial pressure and in the work of the heart; systemic arterial pressure is slightly decreased (Popio *et al.,* 1978).

The major side effects of butorphanol are drowsiness, weakness, sweating, feelings of floating, and nausea. While the incidence of psychotomimetic side effects is lower than that with equianalgesic doses of pentazocine, they are qualitatively similar. Physical dependence on butorphanol can occur.

Therapeutic Uses. *Butorphanol tartrate* (STADOL) is better suited for the relief of acute rather than chronic pain. Because of its side effects on the heart, it is less useful than morphine or meperidine in patients with congestive heart failure or myocardial infarction. The usual dose is between 1 and 4 mg of the tartrate given intramuscularly, or 0.5 to 2 mg given intravenously every 3 to 4 hours. A nasal formulation (STADOL NS) is available and has proven to be effective. This formulation is particularly useful for patients with severe headaches who may be unresponsive to other forms of treatment.

Buprenorphine

Buprenorphine is a semisynthetic, highly lipophilic opioid derived from thebaine (*see* Table 23–5). It is 25 to 50 times more potent than morphine.

Pharmacological Actions and Side Effects. Buprenorphine produces analgesia and other CNS effects that are qualitatively similar to those of morphine. About 0.4 mg of buprenorphine is equianalgesic with 10 mg of morphine given intramuscularly (Wallenstein *et al.,* 1986). Although variable, the duration of analgesia is usually longer than that of morphine. Some of the subjective and respiratory-depressant effects are unequivocally slower in onset and longer lasting than those of morphine. For example, peak miosis occurs about 6 hours after intramuscular injection, while maximal respiratory depression is observed at about 3 hours.

Buprenorphine appears to be a partial μ-receptor agonist. Depending on the dose, buprenorphine may cause symptoms of abstinence in patients who have been receiving μ-receptor agonists (morphine-like drugs) for several weeks. It antagonizes the respiratory depression produced by anesthetic doses of fentanyl about as well as does naloxone, without completely preventing opioid pain relief (Boysen *et al.,* 1988). Although respiratory depression has not been a major problem in clinical trials, it is not clear whether or not there is a ceiling for this effect (as seen with nalbuphine and pentazocine). The respiratory depression and other effects of buprenorphine can be prevented by prior administration of naloxone, but they are not readily reversed by high doses of naloxone once the effects have been produced. This suggests that buprenorphine dissociates very slowly from opioid receptors. The half-life for dissociation from the μ receptor is 166 minutes for buprenorphine, as opposed to 7 minutes for fentanyl (Boas and Villiger, 1985). Therefore, plasma levels of buprenorphine may not parallel clinical effects. Cardiovascular and other side effects (sedation, nausea, vomiting, dizziness, sweating, and headache) appear to be similar to those of morphine-like opioids.

Buprenorphine is relatively well absorbed by most routes. Administered sublingually, the drug (0.4 to 0.8 mg) produces satisfactory analgesia in postoperative patients. Concentrations in blood peak within 5 minutes after intramuscular injection and within 1 to 2 hours after oral or sublingual administration. While the half-life in plasma has been reported to be about 3 hours, this value bears little relationship to the rate of disappearance of effects (*see* above). Both *N*-dealkylated and conjugated metabolites are detected in the urine, but most of the drug is excreted unchanged in the feces. About 96% of the circulating drug is bound to protein.

Physical Dependence.   When buprenorphine is discontinued, a withdrawal syndrome develops that is delayed in onset for 2 days to 2 weeks; this consists of typical, but generally not very severe, morphine-like withdrawal signs and symptoms, and it persists for about 1 to 2 weeks (Bickel *et al.*, 1988; Fudala *et al.*, 1989).

Therapeutic Uses.   *Buprenorphine.* (BUPRENEX) may be used as an analgesic and also has proven to be useful as a maintenance drug for opioid-dependent subjects (Johnson *et al.*, 2000). The drug was approved provisionally for use in the treatment of heroin addiction when the Drug Addiction Treatment Act was passed by the United States Congress and signed by the President in October of 2000. Approval by the Food and Drug Administration is pending.

The usual intramuscular or intravenous dose for analgesia is 0.3 mg, given every 6 hours. Sublingual doses of 0.4 to 0.8 mg produce effective analgesia, and doses of 6 to 8 mg appear to be about equal to 60 mg of methadone as a maintenance agent.

Other Agonist/Antagonists

Meptazinol is an agonist/antagonist opioid that is about one-tenth as potent as morphine in producing analgesia. Its duration of action is somewhat shorter than that of morphine. Meptazinol also has cholinergic actions that may contribute to its analgesic effects (*see* Holmes and Ward, 1985). Nevertheless, its analgesic actions are antagonized by naloxone, and it can precipitate withdrawal in animals dependent on μ-receptor agonists. The potential for abuse of meptazinol is less than that of morphine because dysphoric side effects appear when the dose is increased. *Dezocine* (DALGAN), an aminotetralin, is another agonist/antagonist; its potency and duration of analgesic effect are similar to those of morphine. Increasing the dose above 30 mg does not produce progressively more severe respiratory depression. In postaddicts, its subjective effects are similar to those of μ-agonist opioids (Jasinski and Preston, 1985).

OPIOID ANTAGONISTS

Under ordinary circumstances, the drugs to be discussed in this section produce few effects unless opioids with agonistic actions have been administered previously. However, when the endogenous opioid systems are activated, as in shock or certain forms of stress, the administration of an opioid antagonist alone may have visible consequences. These agents have obvious therapeutic utility in the treatment of overdosage with opioids. As the understanding of the role of endogenous opioid systems in pathophysiolog-

ical states increases, additional therapeutic indications for these antagonists may develop.

Chemistry.   Relatively minor changes in the structure of an opioid can convert a drug that is primarily an agonist into one with antagonistic actions at one or more types of opioid receptors. The most common such substitution is that of a larger moiety (*e.g.*, an allyl or methylcyclopropyl group) for the *N*-methyl group that is typical of the μ-receptor agonists. Such substitutions transform morphine to *nalorphine*, levorphanol to *levallorphan*, and oxymorphone to *naloxone* or *naltrexone* (*see* Table 23–5). In some cases, congeners are produced that are competitive antagonists at μ receptors but that also have agonistic actions at κ receptors. Nalorphine and levallorphan have such properties. Other congeners, especially naloxone and naltrexone, appear to be devoid of agonistic actions and probably interact with all types of opioid receptors, albeit with widely different affinities (*see* Martin, 1983).

Nalmefene (REVIX) is a relatively pure μ-receptor antagonist that is more potent than naloxone (Dixon *et al.*, 1986). A number of other nonpeptide antagonists have been developed that are relatively selective for individual types of opioid receptors. These include *cypridime* and *β-funaltrexamine* (β-FNA) (μ), *naltrindole* (δ), and *nor-binaltorphimine* (κ) (*see* Portoghese, 1989; Pasternak, 1993).

Pharmacological Properties

If endogenous opioid systems have not been activated, the pharmacological actions of opioid antagonists depend on whether or not an opioid agonist has been administered previously, on the pharmacological profile of that opioid, and on the degree to which physical dependence on an opioid has developed.

Effects in the Absence of Opioid Drugs.   Subcutaneous doses of naloxone (NARCAN; up to 12 mg) produce no discernible subjective effects in human beings, and 24 mg causes only slight drowsiness. Naltrexone (REVIA) also appears to be a relatively pure antagonist but with higher oral efficacy and a longer duration of action. At high doses, both naloxone and naltrexone may have some special agonistic effects. However, these are of little clinical significance. At doses in excess of 0.3 mg/kg of naloxone, normal subjects show increased systolic blood pressure and decreased performance on tests of memory. High doses of naltrexone appeared to cause mild dysphoria in one study but almost no subjective effect in several others (*see* Gonzalez and Brogden, 1988).

Although high doses of antagonists might be expected to alter the actions of endogenous opioid peptides, the detectable effects are usually both subtle and limited (Cannon and Liebeskind, 1987). Most likely, this reflects the low levels of tonic activity of the opioid systems. In this regard, analgesic effects can be differentiated from endocrine effects, in which naloxone causes readily demonstrable changes in hormone levels (*see* below). It is interesting that naloxone appears to block the analgesic effects of placebo medications and acupuncture. In laboratory animals, the administration of naloxone will reverse or attenuate the hypotension associated with shock of diverse origins including that caused by anaphylaxis, endotoxin, hypovolemia, and injury to the spinal cord; opioid agonists aggravate these conditions (Amir, 1988). Naloxone apparently acts to antagonize the actions of endogenous opioids that are mobilized by pain or stress and that are involved in the regulation of blood pressure by the CNS. Although neural damage that follows trauma to the spinal cord or cerebral ischemia also appears to involve endogenous opioids, it is not certain whether opioid antagonists can prevent damage to these or other organs and/or increase rates of survival. Nevertheless, opioid antagonists can reduce the extent of injury in some animal models, perhaps by blocking κ receptors (Faden, 1988).

As noted above, endogenous opioid peptides participate in the regulation of pituitary secretion, apparently by exerting tonic inhibitory effects on the release of certain hypothalamic hormones (*see* Chapter 56). Thus, the administration of naloxone or naltrexone increases the secretion of gonadotropin-releasing hormone and corticotropin-releasing factor and elevates the plasma concentrations of LH, FSH, and ACTH, as well as the hormones produced by their target organs. Antagonists do not consistently alter basal or stress-induced concentrations of prolactin in plasma in men; paradoxically, naloxone *stimulates* the release of prolactin in women. Opioid antagonists augment the increases in plasma concentrations of cortisol and catecholamines that normally accompany stress or exercise. The neuroendocrine effects of opioid antagonists have been reviewed (Howlett and Rees, 1986). Endogenous opioid peptides probably have some role in the regulation of feeding or energy metabolism, because opioid antagonists increase energy expenditure and interrupt hibernation in appropriate species and induce weight loss in genetically obese rats. The antagonists also prevent stress-induced overeating and obesity in rats. These observations have led to the experimental use of opioid antagonists in the treatment of human obesity, especially that associated with stress-induced eating disorders. However, naltrexone does not accelerate weight loss in very obese subjects, even though short-term administration of opioid antagonists reduce food intake in both lean and obese individuals (Atkinson, 1987).

Antagonistic Actions. Small doses (0.4 to 0.8 mg) of naloxone given intramuscularly or intravenously prevent or promptly reverse the effects of μ-receptor agonists. In patients with respiratory depression, an increase in respiratory rate is seen within 1 or 2 minutes. Sedative effects are reversed, and blood pressure, if depressed, returns to normal. Higher doses of naloxone are required to antagonize the respiratory-depressant effects of buprenorphine; 1 mg of naloxone intravenously completely blocks the effects of 25 mg of heroin. Naloxone reverses the psychotomimetic and dysphoric effects of agonist/antagonist agents such as pentazocine, but much higher doses (10 to 15 mg) are required. The duration of antagonistic effects depends on

the dose but is usually 1 to 4 hours. Antagonism of opioid effects by naloxone often is accompanied by "overshoot" phenomena. For example, respiratory rate depressed by opioids transiently becomes higher than that prior to the period of depression. Rebound release of catecholamines may cause hypertension, tachycardia, and ventricular arrhythmias. Pulmonary edema also has been reported after naloxone administration.

Effects in Physical Dependence. In subjects who are dependent on morphine-like opioids, small subcutaneous doses of naloxone (0.5 mg) precipitate a moderate-to-severe withdrawal syndrome that is very similar to that seen after abrupt withdrawal of opioids, except that the syndrome appears within minutes after administration and subsides in about 2 hours. The severity and duration of the syndrome are related to the dose of the antagonist and to the degree and type of dependence. Higher doses of naloxone will precipitate a withdrawal syndrome in patients dependent on pentazocine, butorphanol, or nalbuphine. Naloxone produces "overshoot" phenomena suggestive of early acute physical dependence 6 to 24 hours after a single dose of a μ agonist (*see* Heishman *et al.*, 1989).

Tolerance and Physical Dependence. Even after prolonged administration of high doses, discontinuation of naloxone is not followed by any recognizable withdrawal syndrome, and the withdrawal of naltrexone, another relatively pure antagonist, produces very few signs and symptoms. However, long-term administration of antagonists increases the density of opioid receptors in the brain and causes a temporary exaggeration of responses to the subsequent administration of opioid agonists (Yoburn *et al.*, 1988). Naltrexone and naloxone have little or no potential for abuse.

Absorption, Fate, and Excretion. Although absorbed readily from the gastrointestinal tract, naloxone is almost completely metabolized by the liver before reaching the systemic circulation and thus must be administered parenterally. The drug is absorbed rapidly from parenteral sites of injection and is metabolized in the liver, primarily by conjugation with glucuronic acid; other metabolites are produced in small amounts. The half-life of naloxone is about 1 hour, but its clinically effective duration of action can be even less.

Compared with naloxone, naltrexone retains much more of its efficacy by the oral route, and its duration of action approaches 24 hours after moderate oral doses.

Peak concentrations in plasma are reached within 1 to 2 hours and then decline with an apparent half-life of approximately 3 hours; this value does not change with long-term use. Naltrexone is metabolized to 6-naltrexol, which is a weaker antagonist but has a longer half-life of about 13 hours. Naltrexone is much more potent than naloxone, and 100-mg oral doses given to patients addicted to opioids produce concentrations in tissues sufficient to block the euphorigenic effects of 25-mg intravenous doses of heroin for 48 hours (*see* Gonzalez and Brogden, 1988).

Therapeutic Uses

Opioid antagonists have established uses in the treatment of opioid-induced toxicity, especially respiratory depression; in the diagnosis of physical dependence on opioids; and as therapeutic agents in the treatment of compulsive users of opioids, as discussed in Chapter 24. Their potential utility in the treatment of shock, stroke, spinal cord and brain trauma, and other disorders that may involve mobilization of endogenous opioid peptides remains to be established. *Naltrexone* is approved by the United States Food and Drug Administration for treatment of alcoholism (*see* Chapters 18 and 24).

Treatment of Opioid Overdosage.   *Naloxone hydrochloride* is used to treat opioid overdose. As discussed earlier, it acts rapidly to reverse the respiratory depression associated with high doses of opioids. However, it should be used cautiously, since it also can precipitate withdrawal in dependent subjects and cause undesirable cardiovascular side effects. By carefully titrating the dose of naloxone, it usually is possible to antagonize the respiratory-depressant actions without eliciting a full withdrawal syndrome. The duration of action of naloxone is relatively short, and it often must be given repeatedly or by continuous infusion. Opioid antagonists also have been effectively employed to decrease neonatal respiratory depression secondary to the intravenous or intramuscular administration of opioids to the mother. In the neonate, the initial dose is 10 μg/kg, given intravenously, intramuscularly, or subcutaneously.

CENTRALLY ACTIVE ANTITUSSIVE AGENTS

Cough is a useful physiological mechanism that serves to clear the respiratory passages of foreign material and excess secretions. It should not be suppressed indiscriminately. There are, however, many situations in which cough

does not serve any useful purpose but may, instead, only annoy the patient or prevent rest and sleep. Chronic cough can contribute to fatigue, especially in elderly patients. In such situations the physician should use a drug that will reduce the frequency or intensity of the coughing. The cough reflex is complex, involving the central and peripheral nervous systems as well as the smooth muscle of the bronchial tree. It has been suggested that irritation of the bronchial mucosa causes bronchoconstriction, which, in turn, stimulates cough receptors (which probably represent a specialized type of stretch receptor) located in tracheobronchial passages. Afferent conduction from these receptors is *via* fibers in the vagus nerve; central components of the reflex probably involve several mechanisms or centers that are distinct from the mechanisms involved in the regulation of respiration.

The drugs that directly or indirectly can affect this complex mechanism are diverse. For example, cough may be the first or only symptom in bronchial asthma or allergy, and in such cases bronchodilators (*e.g.*, β_2-adrenergic receptor agonists; *see* Chapter 10) have been shown to reduce cough without having any significant central effects; other drugs act primarily on the central or the peripheral nervous system components of the cough reflex. The early literature on antitussives has been reviewed by Eddy *et al.* (1969).

A number of drugs are known to reduce cough as a result of their central actions, although the exact mechanisms are still not entirely clear. Included among them are the opioid analgesics discussed above (codeine and hydrocodone are the opioids most commonly used to suppress cough), as well as a number of nonopioid agents. Cough suppression often occurs with lower doses of opioids than those needed for analgesia. A 10- or 20-mg oral dose of codeine, although ineffective for analgesia, produces a demonstrable antitussive effect, and higher doses produce even more suppression of chronic cough.

In selecting a specific centrally active agent for a particular patient, the significant considerations are its antitussive efficacy against pathological cough and the incidence and type of side effects to be expected. In the majority of situations requiring a cough suppressant, liability for abuse need not be a major consideration. Most of the nonopioid agents now offered as antitussives are effective against cough induced by a variety of experimental techniques. However, the ability of these tests to predict clinical efficacy is limited.

Dextromethorphan.   *Dextromethorphan* (*d*-3-methoxy-*N*-methylmorphinan) is the *d* isomer of the codeine analog methorphan; however, unlike the *l* isomer, it has no analgesic or addictive properties and does not act through opioid receptors. The drug acts centrally to elevate the threshold for coughing. Its effectiveness in patients with pathological cough has been demonstrated in controlled studies; its potency is nearly equal to that of codeine. Compared with codeine, dextromethorphan produces fewer subjective and gastrointestinal side effects (Matthys *et al.,* 1983). In therapeutic dosages, the drug does not inhibit ciliary activity, and its antitussive effects persist for 5 to 6 hours. Its toxicity is low, but extremely high doses may produce CNS depression.

Sites that bind dextromethorphan with high affinity have been identified in membranes from various regions of the brain (Craviso and Musacchio, 1983). Although dextromethorphan is known to function as an NMDA-receptor antagonist, these binding sites are not limited to the known distribution of NMDA receptors (Elliott *et al.,* 1994). Thus, the mechanism by which dextromethorphan exerts its antitussive effects is still unclear. Two other known antitussives, carbetapentane and caramiphen, also bind avidly to this site, but codeine, levopropoxyphene, and other antitussive opioids (as well as naloxone) are not bound. Although noscapine (*see* below) enhances the affinity of dextromethorphan, it appears to interact with distinct binding sites (Karlsson *et al.,* 1988). The relationship of these binding sites to antitussive actions is not known; however, these observations, coupled with the ability of naloxone to antagonize the antitussive effects of codeine but not those of dextromethorphan, indicate that cough suppression can be achieved by a number of different mechanisms. The average adult dosage of *dextromethorphan hydrobromide* is 10 to 30 mg three to six times daily; however, as is the case with codeine, higher doses often are required. The drug is generally marketed for "over-the-counter" sale in numerous syrups and lozenges or in combinations with antihistamines and other agents.

Other Drugs. *Levopropoxyphene napsylate,* the *l*-isomer of dextropropoxyphene, in doses of 50 to 100 mg orally, appears to suppress cough to about the same degree as does 30 mg of dextromethorphan. Unlike dextropropoxyphene, levopropoxyphene has little or no analgesic activity.

Noscapine is a naturally occurring opium alkaloid of the benzylisoquinoline group; except for its antitussive effect, it has no significant actions on the CNS in doses within the therapeutic range. The drug is a potent releaser of histamine, and large doses cause bronchoconstriction and transient hypotension.

Other drugs that have been used as centrally acting antitussives include *carbetapentane, caramiphen, chlophedianol, diphenhydramine,* and *glaucine.* Each is a member of a distinct pharmacological class unrelated to the opioids. The mechanism of action of diphenhydramine, an antihistamine, is unclear. Although sedative effects are common, paradoxical excitement may be seen in infants; dryness of mucous membranes caused by anticholinergic effects and thickening of mucus may be a disadvantage. In general, the toxicity of these agents is low, but controlled clinical studies are still insufficient to determine whether or not they merit consideration as alternatives to more thoroughly studied agents.

Pholcodine [3-*O*-(2-morpholinoethyl)morphine] is used clinically in many countries outside the United States. Although structurally related to the opioids, it has no opioid-like actions because the substitution at the 3-position is not removed by metabolism. Pholcodine is at least as effective as codeine as an antitussive; it has a long half-life and can be given once or twice daily (*see* Findlay, 1988).

Benzonatate (TESSALON) is a long-chain polyglycol derivative chemically related to procaine and believed to exert its antitussive action on stretch or cough receptors in the lung, as well as by a central mechanism. It has been administered by all routes; the oral dosage is 100 mg three times daily, but higher doses have been used.

THERAPEUTIC USES OF OPIOID ANALGESICS

Sir William Osler called morphine "God's own medicine." Opioids are still the mainstay of pain treatment. However, the development of new analgesic compounds and new routes of administration have increased the therapeutic options available to clinicians, while at the same time helping to minimize undesirable side effects. In this section, we will outline guidelines for rational drug selection, discuss routes of administration other than the standard oral and parenteral methods, and outline general principles for the use of opioids in acute and chronic pain states.

Extensive efforts by many individuals and organizations have resulted in the publication of many useful guidelines for the administration of opioids. These have been developed for a number of clinical situations, including acute pain, trauma, cancer, nonmalignant chronic pain, and treatment of pain in children (Agency for Health Care Policy and Research, 1992a, 1992b, 1994; International Association for the Study of Pain, 1992; American Pain Society, 1999; Grossman *et al.,* 1999; World Health Organization, 1998; Berde *et al.,* 1990). These guidelines provide comprehensive discussions of dosing regimens and drug selection and also provide protocols for the management of complex conditions. In the case of cancer pain, adherence to standardized protocols for cancer pain management (Agency for Health Care Policy and Research, 1994) has been shown to improve pain management significantly (Du Pen *et al.,* 1999). Guidelines for the oral and parenteral dosing of commonly used opioids are presented in Table 23–6.

These guidelines are for acute pain management in opioid-naïve patients. Adjustments will need to be made for use in opioid-tolerant patients and in chronic pain states. For children under 6 months of age, especially those who are ill or premature, expert consultation should be obtained. The pharmacokinetics and potency of opioids

Table 23–6
Dosing Data for Opioid Analgesics

DRUG	APPROXIMATE EQUIANALGESIC ORAL DOSE	APPROXIMATE EQUIANALGESIC PARENTERAL DOSE	RECOMMENDED STARTING DOSE (ADULTS MORE THAN 50 kg BODY WEIGHT)		RECOMMENDED STARTING DOSE (CHILDREN AND ADULTS LESS THAN 50 kg BODY WEIGHT)[1]	
			ORAL	PARENTERAL	ORAL	PARENTERAL
Opioid Agonist						
Morphine[2]	30 mg q 3–4 hr (around-the-clock dosing) 60 mg q 3–4 hr (single dose or intermittent dosing)	10 mg q 3–4 hr	30 mg q 3–4 hr	10 mg q 3–4 hr	0.3 mg/kg q 3–4 hr	0.1 mg/kg q 3–4 hr
Codeine[3]	130 mg q 3–4 hr	75 mg q 3–4 hr	60 mg q 3–4 hr	60 mg q 2 hr (intramuscular/subcutaneous)	1 mg/kg q 3–4 hr[4]	Not recommended
Hydromorphone[2] (DILAUDID)	7.5 mg q 3–4 hr	1.5 mg q 3–4 hr	6 mg q 3–4 hr	1.5 mg q 3–4 hr	0.06 mg/kg q 3–4 hr	0.015 mg/kg q 3–4 hr
Hydrocodone (in LORCET, LORTAB, VICODIN, others)	30 mg q 3–4 hr	Not available	10 mg q 3–4 hr	Not available	0.2 mg/kg q 3–4 hr[4]	Not available
Levorphanol (LEVO-DROMORAN)	4 mg q 6–8 hr	2 mg q 6–8 hr	4 mg q 6–8 hr	2 mg q 6–8 hr	0.04 mg/kg q 6–8 hr	0.02 mg/kg q 6–8 hr
Meperidine (DEMEROL)	300 mg q 2–3 hr	100 mg q 3 hr	Not recommended	100 mg q 3 hr	Not recommended	0.75 mg/kg q 2–3 hr
Methadone (DOLOPHINE, others)	20 mg q 6–8 hr	10 mg q 6–8 hr	20 mg q 6–8 hr	10 mg q 6–8 hr	0.2 mg/kg q 6–8 hr	0.1 mg/kg q 6–8 hr
Oxycodone (ROXICODONE, also in PERCOCET, PERCODAN, TYLOX, others)[7]	30 mg q 3–4 hr	Not available	10 mg q 3–4 hr	Not available	0.2 mg/kg q 3–4 hr[4]	Not available
Oxymorphone[2] (NUMORPHAN)	Not available	1 mg q 3–4 hr	Not available	1 mg q 3–4 hr	Not recommended	Not recommended
Propoxyphene (DARVON)	130 mg[5]	Not available	65 mg q 4–6 hr[5]	Not available	Not recommended	Not recommended
Tramadol[6] (ULTRAM)	100 mg[5]	100 mg	50–100 mg q 6 hr[5]	50–100 mg q 6 hr[5]	Not recommended	Not recommended
Opioid Agonist-Antagonist or Partial Agonist						
Buprenorphine (BUPRENEX)	Not available	0.3–0.4 mg q 6–8 hr	Not available	0.4 mg q 6–8 hr	Not available	0.004 mg/kg q 6–8 hr
Butorphanol (STADOL)	Not available	2 mg q 3–4 hr	Not available	2 mg q 3–4 hr	Not available	Not recommended
Nalbuphine (NUBAIN)	Not available	10 mg q 3–4 hr	Not available	10 mg q 3–4 hr	Not available	0.1 mg/kg q 3–4 hr
Pentazocine (TALWIN, others)	150 mg q 3–4 hr	60 mg q 3–4 hr	50 mg q 4–6 hr	Not recommended	Not recommended	Not recommended

NOTE: Published tables vary in the suggested doses that are equianalgesic to morphine. Clinical response is the criterion that must be applied for each patient; titration to clinical response is necessary. Because there is not complete cross tolerance among these drugs, it is usually necessary to use a lower than equianalgesic dose when changing drugs and to retitrate to response.

Caution: Recommended doses do not apply to patients with renal or hepatic insufficiency or other conditions affecting drug metabolism and kinetics.

[1] Caution: Doses listed for patients with body weight less than 50 kg cannot be used as initial starting doses in babies less than 6 months of age. Consult the Clinical Practice Guideline for Acute Pain Management: Operative or Medical Procedures and Trauma section on management of pain in neonates for recommendations.

[2] For morphine, hydromorphone, and oxymorphone, rectal administration is an alternate route for patients unable to take oral medications, but equianalgesic doses may differ from oral and parenteral doses because of pharmacokinetic differences.

[3] Caution: Codeine doses above 65 mg often are not appropriate due to diminishing incremental analgesia with increasing doses but continually increasing constipation and other side effects.

[4] Caution: Doses of aspirin and acetaminophen in combination opioid/NSAID preparations must also be adjusted to the patient's body weight. Maximum acetaminophen dose: 4 g/day in adults, 90 mg/kg per day in children.

[5] Doses for moderate pain not necessarily equivalent to 30 mg oral or 10 mg parenteral morphine.

[6] Risk of seizures; parenteral formulation not available in the U.S.

[7] OXYCONTIN is an extended-release preparation containing up to 160 mg of oxycodone per tablet and recommended for use every 12 hours. It has been subject to substantial abuse.

ABBREVIATION: q, every.

SOURCE: Modified from Agency for Healthcare Policy and Research, 1992a, with permission.

can be substantially altered in these patients, and in some cases there is a significant risk of apnea. It also should be noted that there is substantial individual variability in responses to opioids. A standard intramuscular dose of 10 mg of morphine sulfate will relieve severe pain adequately in only 2 of 3 patients. Adjustments will have to be made based on clinical response.

In general, it is recommended that opioids always be combined with other analgesic agents, such as nonsteroidal anti-inflammatory drugs (NSAIDS) or acetaminophen. In this way, one can take advantage of additive analgesic effects and minimize the dose of opioids and thus undesirable side effects. In some situations, NSAIDS can provide analgesia equal to that produced by 60 mg of codeine. Potentiation of opioid action by NSAIDs may be due to increased conversion of arachidonic acid to 12-lipoxygenase products that facilitate effects of opioids on K^+ channels (Vaughan *et al.*, 1997). This "opioid-sparing" strategy is the backbone of the "analgesic ladder" for pain management proposed by the World Health Organization (1990). Weaker opioids can be supplanted by stronger opioids in cases of moderate and severe pain. In addition, analgesics always should be dosed in a continuous or "around the clock" fashion rather than on an as needed basis for chronic severe pain. This provides more consistent analgesic levels and avoids unnecessary suffering. Knowledge of the pharmacological profiles of analgesics allows the rational selection of dosing intervals without risk of overdosage.

Factors guiding the selection of specific opioid compounds for pain treatment include potency, pharmacokinetic characteristics, and the routes of administration available. A more potent compound could be useful when high doses of opioid are required, so the medicine can be given in a smaller volume. Duration of action also is an important consideration. For example, a long-acting opioid such as methadone may be appropriate when less-frequent dosing is desired. For short, painful procedures, a quick-acting, fast-dissipating compound such as remifentanil would be a useful choice. In special cases, where a lower addiction risk is required or in patients unable to tolerate other opioids, a partial agonist or mixed agonist/antagonist compound might be a rational choice. The properties of some commonly used orally-administered opioids are discussed in more detail below.

Morphine is available for oral use in standard and controlled-release preparations. Due to first-pass metabolism, morphine is two- to sixfold less potent orally than parenterally. This is important to remember when converting a patient from parenteral to oral medication. There is wide variability in the first-pass metabolism, and the dose should be titrated to the patient's needs. In children who weigh less than 50 kg, morphine can

be given at 0.1 mg/kg every 3 to 4 hours parenterally or at 0.3 mg/kg orally.

Codeine is widely used only due to its high oral/parenteral potency ratio. Orally, codeine at 30 mg is approximately equianalgesic to 325 to 600 mg of aspirin. Combinations of codeine with aspirin or acetaminophen usually provide additive actions, and at these doses analgesic efficacy can exceed that of 60 mg of codeine (*see* Beaver, 1988). Many drugs can be used instead of either morphine or codeine, as shown in Table 23–6. Oxycodone, with its high oral/parenteral potency ratio, is widely used in combination with aspirin (PERCODAN, others) or acetaminophen (PERCOCET 2.5/325, others), although it is available alone (ROXICODINE, others).

Heroin (diacetylmorphine) is not available for therapeutic use in the United States, although it has been used in the United Kingdom. Given intramuscularly, it is approximately twice as potent as morphine. Pharmacologically, heroin is very similar to morphine and does not appear to have any unique therapeutic advantages over the available opioids (Sawynok, 1986; Kaiko *et al.*, 1981). It also may be helpful to employ other agents (adjuvants) that enhance opioid analgesia and that may add beneficial effects of their own. For example, the combination of an opioid with a small dose of amphetamine may augment analgesia while reducing the sedative effects. Certain antidepressants, such as amitriptyline and desipramine, also may enhance opioid analgesia, and they may have analgesic actions in some types of neuropathic (deafferentation) pain (*see* McQuay, 1988). Other potentially useful adjuvants include certain antihistamines, anticonvulsants such as carbamazepine and phenytoin, and glucocorticoids.

Alternative Routes of Administration

In addition to the traditional oral and parenteral formulations for opioids, many other methods have been developed in an effort to improve therapeutic efficacy while minimizing side effects. These routes also improve the ease of use of opioids, and increase patient satisfaction.

Patient-Controlled Analgesia (PCA). With this modality, the patient has limited control of the dosing of opioid from an infusion pump within tightly mandated parameters. PCA can be used for intravenous or epidural infusion. This technique avoids any delays in administration and permits greater dosing flexibility than other regimens, better adapting to individual differences in responsiveness to pain and to opioids. It also gives the patient a greater sense of control. With shorter-acting opioids, serious toxicity or excessive use rarely occurs. An early concern that self-administration of opioids would increase the probability of addiction has not materialized. PCA is suitable for both adults and children, and it is preferred over intramuscular injections for postoperative pain control (Rodgers *et al.*, 1988).

Computer-Assisted Continuous Infusion (CACI). The idea behind this mode of administration is to enable clinicians to

Table 23–7
Intraspinal Opioids for the Treatment of Acute Pain

DRUG	SINGLE DOSE* (mg)	INFUSION RATE** (mg/hr)	ONSET (minutes)	DURATION OF EFFECT OF A SINGLE DOSE*** (hours)
Epidural				
Morphine	1–6	0.1–1.0	30	6–24
Meperidine	20–150	5–20	5	4–8
Methadone	1–10	0.3–0.5	10	6–10
Hydromorphone	1–2	0.1–0.2	15	10–16
Fentanyl	0.025–0.1	0.025–0.10	5	2–4
Sufentanil	0.01–0.06	0.01–0.05	5	2–4
Alfentanil	0.5–1	0.2	15	1–3
Subarachnoid				
Morphine	0.1–0.3		15	8–24+
Meperidine	10–30		?	10–24+
Fentanyl	0.005–0.025		5	3–6

*Low doses may be effective when administered to the elderly or when injected in the cervical or thoracic region.
**If combining with a local anesthetic, consider using 0.0625% bupivacaine.
***Duration of analgesia varies widely; higher doses produce longer duration.
SOURCE: Adapted from International Association for the Study of Pain, 1992.

titrate intravenous agents in a fashion similar to that used in delivering volatile agents (Sanford and Gutstein, 1995). CACI based on detailed pharmacokinetic models has been used successfully to administer opioids (Shafer et al., 1990; Bailey et al., 1993). However, true "closed-loop" control of opioid administration requires the capability of continuously measuring plasma opioid levels with indwelling sensors. Until such real-time measurement is available, accurate assessment of dose-effect relationships in patients is not possible.

Intraspinal Infusion. Administration of opioids into the epidural or intrathecal space provides more direct access to the first pain-processing synapse in the dorsal horn of the spinal cord. This permits the use of doses substantially lower than those required for oral or parenteral administration (see Table 23–7). Systemic side effects are thus decreased. However, epidural opioids have their own dose-dependent side effects, such as itching, nausea, vomiting, respiratory depression, and urinary retention. The use of hydrophilic opioids such as preservative-free morphine (DURAMORPH, others) permits more rostral spread of the compound, allowing it to directly affect supraspinal sites. As a consequence, after intraspinal morphine, delayed respiratory depression can be observed for as long as 24 hours after a bolus dose. While the risk of delayed respiratory depression is reduced with more lipophilic opioids, it is not eliminated. Extreme vigilance and appro-

priate monitoring are required for all patients receiving intraspinal narcotics. Nausea and vomiting also are more prominent symptoms with intraspinal morphine. However, supraspinal analgesic centers also can be stimulated, possibly leading to synergistic analgesic effects.

Analogous to the relationship between systemic opioids and NSAIDS, intraspinal narcotics often are combined with local anesthetics. This permits the use of lower concentrations of both agents, minimizing local anesthetic-induced complications of motor blockade and the opioid-induced complications listed above. Epidural administration of opioids has become popular in the management of postoperative pain and for providing analgesia during labor and delivery. Lower systemic opioid levels are achieved with epidural opioids, leading to less placental transfer and less potential for respiratory depression of the newborn (Shnider and Levinson, 1987). Intrathecal ("spinal" anesthesia) administration of opioids as a single bolus also is popular for acute pain management. Chronic intrathecal infusions generally are reserved for use in chronic pain patients.

Peripheral Analgesia. As previously mentioned, opioid receptors on peripheral nerves have been shown to respond to locally applied opioids during inflammation (Stein, 1995). Peripheral analgesia permits the use of lower doses, applied locally, than those necessary to achieve a systemic effect. The effectiveness of this technique has been demonstrated in studies of post-operative pain (Stein *et al.,* 1991). These studies also suggest that peripherally acting opioid compounds would be effective in other selected circumstances without entering the CNS to cause many undesirable side effects. Development of such compounds and expansion of clinical applications of this technique currently are active areas of research.

Rectal Administration. This route is an alternative for patients with difficulty swallowing or other oral pathology and who prefer a less-invasive route than parenteral (De Conno *et al.,* 1995). This route is not well tolerated in most children. Onset of action is seen within 10 minutes. In the United States, morphine, hydromorphone, and oxymorphone are available in rectal suppository formulation (American Pain Society, 1999).

Administration by Inhalation. Preliminary studies have shown that opioids delivered by nebulizer can be an effective means of analgesic drug delivery (Worsley *et al.,* 1990; Higgins *et al.,* 1991). However, constant supervision is required when administering the drug, and variable delivery to the lungs can cause differences in therapeutic effect. In addition, possible environmental contamination is a concern. However, development of the inhaled route could provide a more convenient and cost-effective, adjunctive method of analgesic delivery for patients experiencing chronic pain.

Oral Transmucosal Administration. Opioids can be absorbed through the oral mucosa more rapidly than through the stomach. Bioavailability is greater due to avoidance of first pass metabolism, and lipophilic opioids are better absorbed by this route than are hydrophilic compounds such as morphine (Weinberg *et al.,* 1988). A transmucosal delivery system that suspends fentanyl in a dissolvable matrix has been approved for clinical use (ACTIQ). Its primary indication is for treatment of breakthrough cancer pain (Asburn *et al.,* 1989). In this setting, transmucosal fentanyl relieves pain within 15 minutes, and patients easily can titrate the appropriate dose. Transmucosal fentanyl also has been studied as a premedicant for children. However, this technique has been largely abandoned due to a substantial incidence of undesirable side effects such as respiratory depression, sedation, nausea, vomiting, and pruritus.

Transdermal or Iontophoretic Administration. Transdermal fentanyl patches are approved for use with sustained pain. The opioid permeates the skin, and a "depot" is established in the stratum corneum layer. Unlike other transdermal systems (*i.e.,* transdermal scopolamine), anatomic position of the patch does not affect absorption. However, fever and external heat sources of heat (heating pads, hot baths) can increase absorption of fentanyl and potentially lead to an overdose (Rose *et al.,* 1993). This modality is well suited for cancer pain treatment because of its ease of use, prolonged duration of action, and stable blood levels (Portenoy *et al.,* 1993). It may take up to 12 hours to develop analgesia and up to 16 hours to observe full clinical effect. Plasma levels stabilize after two sequential patch applications, and these kinetics do not appear to change with repeated applications (Portenoy, 1993). However, there may be a great deal of variability in plasma levels after a given dose. The plasma half-life after patch removal is about 17 hours. Thus, if excessive sedation or respiratory depression is experienced, antagonist infusions may need to be maintained for an extended period (Payne, 1992). Dermatological side effects from the patches, such as rash and itching, usually are mild.

Iontophoresis is the transport of soluble ions through the skin by using a mild electric current. This technique has been employed with morphine (Ashburn *et al.,* 1992). Fentanyl and sufentanil have been chemically modified and applied by iontophoresis in rats (Thysman and Preat, 1993). Effective analgesia was achieved in less than 1 hour, suggesting that iontophoresis could be a promising modality for postoperative pain. It should be noted that increasing the applied current will increase drug delivery and could lead to overdose. However, unlike transdermal opioids, a drug reservoir does not build up in the skin, thus limiting the duration of both main and side effects.

General Principles of Opioid Use

Opioid analgesics provide symptomatic relief of pain, but the underlying disease remains. The physician must weigh the benefits of this relief against any potential risk to the patient, which may be quite different in an acute compared with a chronic disease.

In acute problems, opioids will reduce the intensity of pain. However, physical signs (such as abdominal rigidity) will generally remain. Relief of pain also can facilitate history taking, examination, and the patient's ability to tolerate diagnostic procedures. Patients should not be evaluated inadequately because of the physician's unwillingness to prescribe analgesics, nor in most cases should analgesics be withheld for fear of obscuring the progression of underlying disease.

The problems that arise in the relief of pain associated with chronic conditions are more complex. Repeated daily administration eventually will produce tolerance and some degree of physical dependence. The degree will depend on the particular drug, the frequency of administration, and the quantity administered. The decision to control any chronic symptom, especially pain, by the repeated administration of an opioid must be made carefully. When pain is due to chronic, nonmalignant disease, measures other than opioid drugs should be employed to relieve chronic pain if they are effective and available. Such measures include the use of nonsteroidal antiinflammatory agents, local nerve block, antidepressant drugs, electrical stimulation, acupuncture, hypnosis, or behavioral modification (*see* Foley, 1985). However, highly selected subpopulations of chronic nonmalignant pain patients can be adequately maintained on opioids for extended periods of time (Portenoy, 1990).

In the usual doses, morphine-like drugs relieve suffering by altering the emotional component of the painful experience as well as by producing analgesia. Control of pain, especially chronic pain, must include attention to both psychological factors and the social impact of the illness that sometimes play dominant roles in determining the suffering experienced by the patient. In addition to emotional support, the physician also must consider the substantial variability in both the patient's capacity to tolerate pain and the response to opioids. As a result, some patients may require considerably more than the average dose of a drug to experience any relief from pain; others may require dosing at shorter intervals. Some clinicians, out of an exaggerated concern for the possibility of inducing addiction, tend to prescribe initial doses of opioids that are too small or given too infrequently to alleviate pain and then respond to the patient's continued complaints with an even more exaggerated concern about drug dependence, despite the high probability that the request for more drug is only the expected consequence of the inadequate dosage initially prescribed (*see* Sriwatanakul *et al.,* 1983). It also is important to note that infants and children are probably more apt to receive inadequate treatment for pain than are adults due to communication difficulties, lack of familiarity with appropriate pain assessment methodologies, and inexperience with the use of strong opioids in children. If an illness or procedure causes pain for an adult, there is no reason to assume that it will produce less pain for a child (*see* Yaster and Deshpande, 1988).

Pain of Terminal Illness and Cancer Pain.   Opioids are not indicated in all cases of terminal illness, but the analgesia, tranquility, and even the euphoria afforded by the use of opioids can make the final days far less distressing for the patient and family. Although physical dependence and tolerance may develop, this possibility should not in any way prevent physicians from fulfilling their primary obligation to ease the patient's discomfort. The physician should not wait until the pain becomes agonizing; *no patient should ever wish for death because of a physician's reluctance to use adequate amounts of effective opioids.* This may sometimes entail the regular use of opioid analgesics in substantial doses. Such patients, while they may be physically dependent, are not "addicts" even though they may need large doses on a regular basis. Physical dependence is not equivalent to addiction (*see* Chapter 24).

Most clinicians who are experienced in the management of chronic pain associated with malignant disease or terminal illness recommend that opioids be administered at sufficiently short, fixed intervals so that pain is continually under control and patients do not dread its

return (Foley, 1993). Less drug is needed to prevent the recurrence of pain than to relieve it. Morphine remains the opioid of choice in most of these situations, and the route and dose should be adjusted to the needs of the individual patient. Many clinicians find that oral morphine is adequate in most situations. Sustained-release preparations of oral morphine are now available that can be administered at 8- to 12-hour intervals. Superior control of pain often can be achieved with fewer side effects using the same daily dose; a decrease in the fluctuation of plasma concentrations of morphine may be partially responsible.

Constipation is an exceedingly common problem when opioids are used, and the use of stool softeners and laxatives should be initiated early. Amphetamines have demonstrable mood-elevating and analgesic effects and enhance opioid-induced analgesia. However, not all terminal patients require the euphoriant effects of amphetamine, and some experience side effects, such as anorexia. Controlled studies demonstrate no superiority of oral heroin over oral morphine. Similarly, after adjustment is made for potency, parenteral heroin is not superior to morphine in terms of analgesia, effects on mood, or side effects (*see* Sawynok, 1986). Although tolerance does develop to oral opioids, many patients obtain relief from the same dosage for weeks or months. In cases where one opioid loses effectiveness, switching to another may provide better pain relief. "Cross-tolerance" among opioids exists, but, both clinically and experimentally, cross-tolerance among related μ-receptor agonists is not complete. The reasons for this are unclear, but they may relate to differences between agonists in receptor-binding characteristics and subsequent cellular signaling interactions, as discussed earlier in the chapter.

When opioids and other analgesics are no longer satisfactory, nerve block, chordotomy, or other types of neurosurgical intervention such as neurostimulation may be required if the nature of the disease permits. Epidural or intrathecal administration of opioids may be useful when administration of opioids by usual routes no longer yields adequate relief of pain (*see* above). This technique has been used with ambulatory patients over periods of weeks or months (*see* Gustafsson and Wiesenfeld-Hallin, 1988). Moreover, portable devices have been developed that permit the patient to control the parenteral administration of an opioid while remaining ambulatory (Kerr *et al.,* 1988). These devices use a pump that infuses the drug from a reservoir at a rate that can be tailored to the needs of the patient, and they include mechanisms to limit dosage and/or allow the patient to self-administer an additional "rescue" dose if there is a transient change in the intensity of pain.

Nonanalgesic Therapeutic Uses of Opioids. *Dyspnea.* Morphine is used to alleviate the dyspnea of acute left ventricular failure and pulmonary edema, and the response to intravenous morphine may be dramatic. The mechanism underlying this relief still is not clear. It may involve an alteration of the patient's reaction to impaired respiratory function and an indirect reduction of the work of the heart due to reduced fear and apprehension. However, it is more probable that the major benefit is due to cardiovascular effects, such as decreased peripheral resistance and an increased capacity of the peripheral and splanchnic vascular compartments (*see* Vismara *et al.,* 1976). Nitroglycerin, which also causes vasodilation, may be superior to morphine in this condition (*see* Hoffman and Reynolds, 1987). In patients with normal blood gases but severe breathlessness due to chronic obstruction of airflow ("pink puffers"), *drocode* (dihydrocodeine), 15 mg orally before exercise, reduces the feeling of breathlessness and increases exercise tolerance (Johnson *et al.,* 1983). Opioids are relatively contraindicated in pulmonary edema due to respiratory irritants unless severe pain also is present; relative contraindications to the use of histamine-releasing opioids in asthma already have been discussed.

Special Anesthesia. High doses of morphine or other opioids have been used as the primary anesthetic agents in certain surgical procedures. Although respiration is so depressed that physical assistance is required, patients can retain consciousness (*see* Chapter 14).

PROSPECTUS

Great strides are being made in understanding structure-function relationships between opioids and endogenous opioid peptides and their receptors. The complex signaling mechanisms and neural circuitry mediating both the salutary and undesirable effects of opioids also are beginning to be understood. The recent discovery of new μ receptor-selective endogenous opioid ligands and the opioid-related N/OFQ system also will provide opportunities to improve our understanding of opioid pharmacology and physiology. The development of new opioid analgesics and novel delivery routes are improving the care and quality of life for patients requiring opioids. Over the next several years, pursuing these lines of basic and clinical investigation should provide many valuable insights that may allow better targeting of the therapeutic effects of opioid compounds, thereby minimizing undesirable acute side effects and the potentially serious long-term consequences of tolerance and physical dependence. It also is hoped that these efforts will help overcome the less common, but devastating, problem of addiction.

BIBLIOGRAPHY

Akil, H., Mayer, D.J., and Liebeskind, J.C. Antagonism of stimulation-produced analgesia by naloxone, a narcotic antagonist. *Science,* **1976,** *191*:961–962.

Akil, H., Mayer, D.J., and Liebeskind, J.C. [Comparison in the rat between analgesia induced by stimulation of periacqueductal gray matter and morphine analgesia]. *C. R. Acad. Sci. Hebd. Seances Acad. Sci. Ser. D,* **1972,** *274*:3603–3605.

Akil, H., Shiomi, H., and Matthews, J. Induction of the intermediate pituitary by stress: synthesis and release of a nonopioid form of beta-endorphin. *Science,* **1985,** *227*:424–426.

Alderman, E.L., Barry, W.H., Graham, A.F., and Harrison, D.C. Hemodynamic effects of morphine and pentazocine differ in cardiac patients. *N. Engl. J. Med.,* **1972,** *287*:623–627.

Ashburn, M.A., Fine, P.G., and Stanley, T.H. Oral transmucosal fentanyl citrate for the treatment of breakthrough cancer pain: a case report. *Anesthesiology,* **1989,** *71*:615–617.

Ashburn, M.A., Stephen, R.L., Ackerman, E., Petelenz, T.J., Hare, B., Pace, N.L., and Hofman, A.A. Iontophoretic delivery of morphine for postoperative analgesia. *J. Pain Symptom Manage.,* **1992,** *7*:27–33.

Atkinson, R.L. Opioid regulation of food intake and body weight in humans. *Fed. Proc.,* **1987,** *46*:178–182.

Avidor-Reiss, T., Nevo, I., Levy, R., Pfeuffer, T., and Vogel, Z. Chronic opioid treatment induces adenylyl cyclase V superactivation. Involvement of G$\beta\gamma$. *J. Biol. Chem.,* **1996,** *271*:21309–21315.

Bailey, J.M., Schwieger, I.M., and Hug, C.C. Jr. Evaluation of sufentanil anesthesia obtained by a computer-controlled infusion for cardiac surgery. *Anesth. Analg.,* **1993,** *76*:247–252.

Ballantyne, J.C., Loach, A.B., and Carr, D.B. Itching after epidural and spinal opiates. *Pain,* **1988,** *331*:149–160.

Beaver, W.T. Impact of non-narcotic oral analgesics on pain management, *Am. J. Med.,* **1988,** *84*:3–15.

Beckett, A., and Casy, A. Synthetic analgesics: stereochemical considerations. *J. Pharm. Pharmacol.,* **1954,** *6*:986–1001.

Befort, K., Mattei, M.G., Roeckel, N., and Kieffer, B. Chromosomal localization of the delta opioid receptor gene to human 1p34.3-p36.1 and mouse 4D bands by in situ hybridization. *Genomics,* **1994,** *20*:143–145.

Benson, C.J., Eckert, S.P., and McCleskey, E.W. Acid-evoked current in cardiac sensory neurons: a possible mediator of myocardial ischemic sensation. *Circ. Res.,* **1999,** 84:921–928.

Bickel, W.K., Stitzer, M.L., Bigelow, G.E., Liebson, I.A., Jasinski, D.R., and Johnson, R.E. Buprenorphine: dose-related blockade of opioid challenge effects in opioid dependent humans. *J. Pharmacol. Exp. Ther.,* **1988,** 247:47–53.

Boas, R.A., and Villiger, J.W. Clinical actions of fentanyl and buprenorphine. The significance of receptor binding. *Br. J. Anaesth.,* **1985,** 57:192–196.

Bohn, L.M., Lefkowitz, R.J., Gainetdinov, R.R., Peppel, K., Caron, M.G., and Lin, F.T. Enhanced morphine analgesia in mice lacking β-arrestin 2. *Science,* **1999,** *286*:2495–2498.

Boysen, K., Hertel, S., Chraemmer-Jorgensen, B., Risbo, A., and Poulsen, N.J. Buprenorphine antagonism of ventilatory depression following fentanyl anesthesia. *Acta Anaesthesiol. Scand.,* **1988,** 32:490–492.

Bronstein, D.M., Przewlocki, R., and Akil, H. Effects of morphine treatment on pro-opiomelanocortin systems in rat brain. *Brain Res.,* **1990,** *519*:102–111.

Bunzow, J.R., Saez, C., Mortrud, M., Bouvier, C., Williams, J.T., Low, M., and Grandy, D.K. Molecular cloning and tissue distribution of a putative member of the rat opioid receptor gene family that is not a μ, δ or κ opioid receptor type. *FEBS Lett.,* **1994,** *347*:284–288.

Caraco, Y., Sheller, J., and Wood, A.J. Impact of ethnic origin and quinidine coadministration on codeine's disposition and pharmacokinetic effects. *J. Pharmacol. Exp. Ther.,* **1999,** *290*:413–422.

Chen, Y., Fan, Y., Liu, J., Mestek, A., Tian, M., Kozak, C.A., and Yu, L. Molecular cloning, tissue distribution, and chromosomal localization of a novel member of the opioid receptor gene family. *FEBS Lett.,* **1994,** *347*:279–283.

Chen, Y., Mestek, A., Liu, J., Hurley, J.A., and Yu, L. Molecular cloning and functional expression of a μ-opioid receptor from rat brain. *Mol. Pharmacol.,* **1993,** *44*:8–12.

Chesselet, M.F., Cheramy, A., Reisine, T.D., Lubetzki, C., Desban, M., and Glowinski, J. Local and distal effects induced by unilateral striatal application of opiates in the absence or in the presence of naloxone on the release of dopamine in both caudate nuclei and substantiae nigra of the cat. *Brain Res.,* **1983,** *258*:229–242.

Chu, P., Murray, S., Lissin, D., and von Zastrow, M. δ and κ opioid receptors are differentially regulated by dynamin-dependent endocytosis when activated by the same alkaloid agonist. *J. Biol. Chem.,* **1997,** *272*:27124–27130.

Chuang, L.F., Killam, K.F. Jr., and Chuang, R.Y. Induction and activation of mitogen-activated protein kinases of human lymphocytes as one of the signaling pathways of the immunomodulatory effects of morphine sulfate. *J. Biol. Chem.,* **1997,** *272*:26815–26817.

Coombs, D.W., Saunders, R.L., Lachance, D., Savage, S., Ragnarsson, T.S., and Jensen, L.E. Intrathecal morphine tolerance: use of intrathecal clonidine, DADLE, and intraventricular morphine. *Anesthesiology,* **1985,** *62*:358–363.

Coward, P., Wada, H.G., Falk, M.S., Chan, S.D., Meng, F., Akil, H., and Conklin, B.R. Controlling signaling with a specifically designed G_i-coupled receptor. *Proc. Natl. Acad. Sci. U.S.A.,* **1998,** *95*:352–357.

Craviso, G.L., and Musacchio, J.M. High-affinity dextromethorphan binding sites in guinea pig brain. II. Competition experiments. *Mol. Pharmacol.,* **1983,** *23*:629–640.

Cvejic, S., and Devi, L.A. Dimerization of the delta opioid receptor: implications for a role in receptor internalization. *J. Biol. Chem.,* **1997,** *272*:26959–26964.

De Conno, F., Ripamonti, C., Saita, L., MacEachern, T., Hanson, J., and Bruera, E. Role of rectal route in treating cancer pain: a randomized crossover clinical trial of oral versus rectal morphine administration in opioid-naive cancer patients with pain. *J. Clin. Oncol.,* **1995,** *13*:1004–1008.

Devine, D.P., Leone, P., Pocock, D., and Wise, R.A. Differential involvement of ventral tegmental *mu, delta,* and *kappa* opioid receptors in modulation of basal mesolimbic dopamine release: *in vivo* microdialysis studies. *J. Pharmacol. Exp. Ther.,* **1993,** *266*:1236–1246.

Devine, D.P., Reinscheid, R.K., Monsma, F.J. Jr., Civelli, O., and Akil, H. The novel neuropeptide orphanin FQ fails to produce conditioned place preference or aversion. *Brain Res.,* **1996a,** *727*:225-229.

Devine, D.P., Taylor, L., Reinscheid, R.K., Monsma, F.J. Jr., Civelli, O., and Akil, H. Rats rapidly develop tolerance to the locomotor-inhibiting effects of the novel neuropeptide orphanin FQ. *Neurochem. Res.,* **1996b,** *21*:1387–1396.

Devine, D.P., Watson, S., and Akil, H. Nociceptin/orphanin FQ regulates neuroendocrine function of the limbic hypothalamic pituitary adrenal axis. *Neuroscience,* **2001,** *102*:541–553.

Devine, D.P., and Wise, R.A. Self-administration of morphine, DAMGO, and DPDPE into the ventral tegmental area of rats. *J. Neurosci.,* **1994,** *14*:1978–1984.

Di Chiara, G., and Imperato, A. Opposite effects of mu and kappa opiate agonists on dopamine release in the nucleus accumbens and in the dorsal caudate of freely moving rats. *J. Pharmacol. Exp. Ther.,* **1988,** *244*:1067–1080.

Dixon, R., Howes, J., Gentile, J., Hsu, H.B., Hsiao, J., Garg, D., Weidler, D., Meyer, M., and Tuttle, R. Nalmefene: intravenous safety and kinetics of a new opioid antagonist. *Clin. Pharmacol. Ther.,* **1986,** *39*:49–53.

Dooley, C.P., Saad, C., and Valenzuela, J.E. Studies of the role of opioids in control of human pancreatic secretion. *Dig. Dis. Sci.,* **1988,** *33*:598–604.

Dray, A., and Nunan, L. Supraspinal and spinal mechanisms in morphine-induced inhibition of reflex urinary bladder contractions in the rat. *Neuroscience,* **1987,** *22*:281–287.

Edwards, D.J., Svensson, C.K., Visco, J.P., and Lalka, D. Clinical pharmacokinetics of pethidine: 1982. *Clin. Pharmacokinet.,* **1982,** *7*: 421–433.

Eichelbaum, M., and Evert, B. Influence of pharmacogenetics on drug disposition and response. *Clin. Exp. Pharmacol. Physiol.,* **1996,** *23*: 983–985.

Elliott, K., Hynansky, A., and Inturrisi, C.E. Dextromethorphan attenuates and reverses analgesic tolerance to morphine. *Pain,* **1994,** *59*:361–368.

Emmerson, P.J., Clark, M.J., Mansour, A., Akil, H., Woods, J.H., and Medzihradsky, F. Characterization of opioid agonist efficacy in a C6 glioma cell line expressing the mu opioid receptor. *J. Pharmacol. Exp. Ther.,* **1996,** *278*:1121–1127.

Evans, C.J., Keith, D.E. Jr., Morrison, H., Magendzo, K., and Edwards, R.H. Cloning of a delta opioid receptor by functional expression. *Science,* **1992,** *258*:1952–1955.

Fields, H.L., Emson, P.C., Leigh, B.K., Gilbert, R.F., and Iversen, L.L. Multiple opiate receptor sites on primary afferent fibres. *Nature,* **1980,** *284*:351–353.

Fryer, R.M., Hsu, A.K., Nagase, H., and Gross, G.J. Opioid-induced cardioprotection against myocardial infarction and arrhythmias: mitochondrial versus sacrolemmal ATP-sensitive potassium channels. *J. Pharmacol. Exp. Ther.,* **2000,** *294*:451–457.

Fudala, P.J., and Bunker, E. Abrupt withdrawal of buprenorphine following chronic administration. *Clin. Pharmacol. Ther.,* **1989,** *45*: 186.

Gaudriault, G., Nouel, D., Dal Farra, C., Beaudet, A., and Vincent, J.P. Receptor-induced internalization of selective peptidic mu and delta opioid ligands. *J. Biol. Chem.,* **1997,** *272*:2880–2888.

Gaveriaux-Ruff, C., Matthes, H.W., Peluso, J., and Kieffer, B.L. Abolition of morphine-immunosuppression in mice lacking the μ-opioid receptor gene. *Proc. Natl. Acad. Sci. U.S.A.,* **1998,** *95*:6326–6330.

Gomez-Flores, R., and Weber, R.J. Differential effects of buprenorphine and morphine on immune and neuroendocrine fuctions following acute administration in the rat mesencephalon periaqueductal gray. *Immunopharmacology,* **2000,** *48*:145–156.

Gourlay, G.K., Cherry, D.A., and Cousins, M.J. A comparative study of the efficacy and pharmacokinetics of oral methadone and morphine in the treatment of severe pain in patients with cancer. *Pain,* **1986,** *25*:297–312.

Grevel, J., and Sadee, W. An opiate binding site in the rat brain is highly selective for 4,5-epoxymorphinans. *Science,* **1983,** *221*:1198–1201.

Grisel, J.E., Mogil, J.S., Belknap, J.K., and Grandy, D.K. Orphanin FQ acts as a supraspinal, but not a spinal, anti-opioid peptide. *Neuroreport,* **1996,** *7*:2125–2129.

Gulya, K., Pelton, J.T., Hruby, V.J., and Yamamura, H.I. Cyclic somatostatin octapeptide analogues with high affinity and selectivity toward mu opioid receptors. *Life Sci.,* **1986,** *38*:2221–2229.

Gutstein, H.B., Bronstein, D.M., and Akil, H. β-endorphin processing and cellular origins in rat spinal cord. *Pain,* **1992,** *51*:241–247.

Gutstein, H.B., Mansour, A., Watson, S.J., Akil, H., and Fields, H.L. Mu and kappa receptors in periaqueductal gray and rostral ventromedial medulla. *Neuroreport,* **1998,** *9*:1777–1781.

Handa, B.K., Land, A.C., Lord, J.A., Morgan, B.A., Rance, M.J., and Smith, C.F. Analogues of beta-LPH61-64 possessing selective agonist activity at mu-opiate receptors. *Eur. J. Pharmacol.,* **1981,** *70*:531–540.

Heimer, L., Zahm, D.S., Churchill, L., Kalivas, P.W., and Wohltmann, C. Specificity in the projection patterns of accumbal core and shell in the rat. *Neuroscience,* **1991,** *41*:89–125.

Heishman, S.J., Stitzer, M.L., Bigelow, G.E., and Liebson, I.A. Acute opioid physical dependence in postaddict humans: naloxone dose effects after brief morphine exposure. *J. Pharmacol. Exp. Ther.,* **1989,** *248*:127–134.

Herman, R.J., McAllister, C.B., Branch, R.A., and Wilkinson, G.R. Effects of age on meperidine disposition. *Clin. Pharmacol. Ther.,* **1985,** *37*:19–24.

Higgins, M.J., Asbury, A.J., and Brodie, M.J. Inhaled nebulised fentanyl for postoperative analgesia. *Anaesthesia,* **1991,** *46*:973–976.

Hoffman, J.R., and Reynolds, S. Comparison of nitroglycerin, morphine and furosemide in treatment of presumed pre-hospital pulmonary edema. *Chest,* **1987,** *92*:586–593.

Hughes, J., Smith, T.W., Kosterlitz, H.W., Fothergill, L.A., Morgan, B.A., and Morris, H.R. Identification of two related pentapeptides from the brain with potent opiate agonist activity. *Nature,* **1975,** *258*:577–580.

Jasinski, D.R., and Preston, K.L. Assessment of dezocine for morphine-like subjective effects and miosis. *Clin. Pharmacol. Ther.,* **1985,** *38*:544–548.

Jessell, T.M., and Iversen, L.L. Opiate analgesics inhibit substance P release from the rat trigeminal nucleus. *Nature,* **1977,** *268*:549–551.

Jiang, Q., Takemori, A.E., Sultana, M., Portoghese, P.S., Bowen, W.D., Mosberg, H.I., and Porreca, F. Differential antagonism of opioid delta antinociception by [D-Ala^2, Leu^5, Cys^6] enkephalin and naltrindole 5'-isothiocyananate: evidence for delta receptor subtypes. *J. Pharmacol. Exp. Ther.,* **1991,** *257*:1069–1075.

Johnson, M.A., Woodcock, A.A., and Geddes, D.M. Dihydrocodeine for breathlessness in "pink puffers." *Br. Med. J. (Clin. Res. Ed.),* **1983,** *286*:675–677.

Johnson, R.E., Chutuape, M.A., Strain, E.C., Walsh, S.L., Stitzer, M.L., and Bigelow, G.E. A comparison of levomethadyl acetate, buprenorphine, and methadone for opioid dependence. *N. Engl. J. Med.,* **2000,** *343*:1290–1297.

Jones, K.A., Borowsky, B., Tamm, J.A, Craig, D.A., Durkin, M.M., Dai, M., Yao, W.J., Johnson, M., Gunwaldsen, C., Huang, L.Y., Tang, C., Shen, Q., Salon, J.A., Morse, K., Laz, T., Smith, K.E., Nagarathnam, D., Noble, S.A., Branchek, T.A., and Gerald, C. GABA$_B$ receptors function as a heteromeric assembly of the subunits GABA$_B$R1 and GABA$_B$R2. *Nature,* **1998,** *396*:674–679.

Jordan, B.A., and Devi, L.A. G-protein-coupled receptor hetereodimerization modulates receptor function. *Nature,* **1999,** *399*:697–700.

Kaiko, R.F., Foley, K.M., Grabinski, P.Y., Heidrich, G., Rogers, A.G., Inturrisi, C.E., and Reidenberg, M.M. Central nervous system excitatory effects of meperidine in cancer patients. *Ann. Neurol.,* **1983,** *13*:180–185.

Kaiko, R.F., Wallenstein, S.L., Rogers, A.G., Grabinski, P.Y., and Houde, R.W. Analgesic and mood effects of heroin and morphine in cancer patients with postoperative pain. *N. Engl. J. Med.,* **1981,** *304*:1501–1505.

Karlsson, M., Dahlstrom, B., and Neil, A. Characterization of high-affinity binding for the antitussive [3H]noscappine in guinea pig brain tisue. *Eur. J. Pharmacol.,* **1988,** *145*:195–203.

Kayser, V., Lee, S.H., and Guilbaud, G. Evidence for a peripheral component in the enhanced antinociceptive effect of a low dose of systemic morphine in rats with peripheral mononeuropathy. *Neuroscience,* **1995,** *64*:537–545.

Keith, D.E., Murray, S.R., Zaki, P.A., Chu, P.C., Lissin, D.V., Kang, L., Evans, C.J., and von Zastrow, M. Morphine activates opioid receptors without causing their rapid internalization. *J. Biol. Chem.,* **1996,** *271*:19021–19024.

Kerr, I.G., Sone, M., Deangelis, C., Iscoe, N., MacKenzie, R., and Schueller, T. Continuous narcotic infusion with patient-controlled analgesia for chronic cancer pain in outpatients. *Ann. Intern. Med.,* **1988,** *108*:554–557.

Kieffer, B.L., Befort, K., Gaveriaux-Ruff, C., and Hirth, C.G. The delta-opioid receptor: isolation of a cDNA by expression cloning and pharmacological characterization. *Proc. Natl. Acad. Sci. U.S.A.,* **1992,** *89*:12048–12052.

Kolesnikov, Y.A., Pick, C.G., Ciszewska, G., and Pasternak, G.W. Blockade of tolerance to morphine but not to kappa opioids by a nitric oxide synthase inhibitor. *Proc. Natl. Acad. Sci. U.S.A.,* **1993,** *90*:5162–5166.

Kong, H., Raynor, K., Yano, H., Takeda, J., Bell, G.I., and Reisine, T. Agonists and antagonists bind to different domains of the cloned κ opioid receptor. *Proc. Natl. Acad. Sci. U.S.A.,* **1994,** *91*:8042–8046.

Koster, A., Montkowski, A., Schulz, S., Stube, E., Knaudt, K., Jenck, F., Moreau, J.L., Nothacker, H.P., Civelli, O., and Reinscheid, R.K. Targeted disruption of the orphanin FQ/nociceptin gene increases stress susceptibility and impairs stress adaptation in mice. *Proc. Natl. Acad. Sci. U.S.A.,* **1999,** *96*:1044–10449.

Lee, G., DeMaria, A.N., Amsterdam, E.A., Realyvasquez, F., Angel, J., Morrison, S., and Mason, D.T. Comparative effects of morphine, meperidine and pentazocine on cardiocirculatory dynamics in patients with acute myocardial infarction. *Am. J. Med.,* **1976,** *60*:949–955.

Levine, J.D., Gordon, N.C., Smith, R., and McBryde, R. Desipramine enhances opiate postoperative analgesia. *Pain,* **1986,** *27*:45–49.

Liang, B.T., and Gross, G.J. Direct preconditioning of cardiac myocytes via opioid receptors and K$_{ATP}$ channels. *Circ. Res.,* **1999,** *84*:1396–1400.

Ling, W., Klett, C.J., and Gillis, R.D. A cooperative clinical study of methadyl acetate. I. Three-times-a-week regimen. *Arch. Gen. Psychiatry,* **1978,** *35*:345–353.

Mains, R.E., Eipper, B.A., and Ling, N. Common precursor to corticotrophins and endorphins. *Proc. Natl. Acad. Sci. U.S.A.,* **1977,** *74*:3014–3018.

Manabe, T., Noda, Y., Mamiya, T., Katagiri, H., Houtani, T., Nishi, M., Noda, T., Takahashi, T., Sugimoto, T., Nabeshima, T., and Takeshima, H. Facilitation of long-term potentiation and memory in mice lacking nociceptin receptors. *Nature,* **1998,** *394*:577–581.

Manning, B.H., and Mayer, D.J. The central nucleus of the amygdala contributes to the production of morphine antinociception in the rat tail-flick test. *J. Neurosci.,* **1995a,** 8199–8213.

Manning, B.H., and Mayer, D.J. The central nucleus of the amygdala contributes to the production of morphine analgesia in the formalin test. *Pain,* **1995b,** *63*:141–152.

Manning, B.H., Morgan, M.J., and Franklin, K.B. Morphine analgesia in the formalin test: evidence for forebrain and midbrain sites of action. *Neuroscience,* **1994,** *63*:289–294.

Mansour, A., Meng, F., Meador-Woodruff, J.H., Taylor, L.P., Civelli, O., and Akil, H. Site-directed mutagenesis of the human dopamine D2 receptor. *Eur. J. Pharmacol.,* **1992,** *227*:205–214.

Mansour, A., Taylor, L.P, Fine, J.L., Thompson, R.C., Hoversten, M.T., Mosberg, H.I., Watson, S.J., and Akil, H. Key residues defining the mu-opioid receptor binding pocket: a site-directed mutagenesis study. *J. Neurochem.,* **1997,** *68*:344–353.

Martin, W.R., Eades, C.G., Thompson, J.A., Huppler, R.E., and Gilbert, P.E. The effects of morphine- and nalorphine-like drugs in nondependent and morphine-dependent chronic spinal dog, *J. Pharmacol. Exp. Ther.,* **1976,** *197*:517–532.

Matthies, B.K., and Franklin, K.B. Formalin pain is expressed in decerebrate rats but not attenuated by morphine. *Pain,* **1992,** *51*:199–206.

Matthys, H., Bleicher, B., and Bleicher, U. Dextromethorphan and codeine: objective assessment of antitussive activity in patients with chronic cough. *J. Int. Med. Res.,* **1983,** *11*:92–100.

McIntosh, M., Kane, K., and Parratt, J. Effects of selective opioid receptor agonists and antagonists during myocardial ischaemia. *Eur. J. Pharmacol.,* **1992,** *210*:37–44.

Mellon, R.D., and Bayer, B.M. Evidence for central opioid receptors in the immunomodulatory effects of morphine: review of potential mechanism(s) of action. *J. Neuroimmunol.,* **1998,** *83*:19–28.

Meng, F., Hoversten, M.T., Thompson, R.C., Taylor, L., Watson, S.J., and Akil, H. A chimeric study of the molecular basis of affinity and selectivity of the kappa and the delta opioid receptors. Potential role of extracellular domains. *J. Biol. Chem.,* **1995,** *270*:12730–12736.

Meng, F., Taylor, L.P., Hoversten, M.T., Ueda, Y., Ardati, A., Reinscheid, R.K., Monsma, F.J., Watson, S.J., Civelli, O., and Akil, H. Moving from the orphanin FQ receptor to an opioid receptor using four point mutations. *J. Biol. Chem.,* **1996,** *271*:32016–32020.

Meng, F., Xie, G.X., Thompson, R.C., Mansour, A., Goldstein, A., Watson, S.J., and Akil, H. Cloning and pharmacological characterization of a rat kappa opioid receptor. *Proc. Natl. Acad. Sci. U.S.A.,* **1993,** *90*:9954–9958.

Mestek, A., Hurley, J.H., Bye, L.S., Campell, A.D., Chen, Y., Tian, M., Liu, J., Schulman, H., and Yu, L. The human μ opioid receptor: modulation of function desensitization by calcium/calmodulin-dependent protein kinase and protein kinase C. *J. Neurosci.,* **1995,** *15*:2396–2406.

Meunier, J.-C., Mollereau, C., Toll, L., Suaudeau, C., Moisand, C., Alvinerie, P., Butour, J.-L., Guillemot, J.-C., Ferrara, P., Monsarrat, B., Mazarguil, H., Vassart, G., Parmentier, M., and Costentin, J. Isolation and structure of the endogenous agonist of opioid receptor-like ORL₁ receptor. *Nature,* **1995,** *377*:532–535.

Minami, M., Toya, T., Katao, Y., Maekawa, K., Nakamura, S., Onogi, T., Kaneko, S., and Satoh, M. Cloning and expression of cDNA for the rat κ-opioid receptor. *FEBS Lett.,* **1993,** *329*:291–295.

Mollereau, C., Parmentier, M., Mailleux, P., Butour, J.L., Moisand, C., Chalon, P., Caput, D., Vassart, G., and Meunier, J.-C. ORL1, a novel member of the opioid receptor family. Cloning, functional expression and localization. *FEBS Lett.,* **1994,** *341*:33–38.

Monaco, S., Gehrmann, J., Raivich, G., and Kreutzberg, G.W. MHC-positive, ramified macrophages in the normal and injured rat peripheral nervous system. *J. Neurocytol.,* **1992,** *21*:623–634.

Mosberg, H.I., Hurst, R., Hruby, V.J., Gee, K., Yamamura, H.I., Galligan, J.J., and Burks, T.F. Bis-penicillamine enkephalins possess highly improved specificity toward delta opioid receptors. *Proc. Natl. Acad. Sci. U.S.A.,* **1983,** *80*:5871–5874.

Mulder, A.H., Burger, D.M., Wardeh, G., Hogenboom, F., and Frankhuyzen, A.L. Pharmacological profile of various kappa-agonists at kappa-, mu- and delta-opioid receptors mediating presynaptic inhibition of neurotransmitter release in the rat brain. *Br. J. Pharmacol.,* **1991,** *102*:518–522.

Narita, M., Narita, M., Mizoguchi, H., and Tseng, L.F. Inhibition of protein kinase C, but not of protein kinase A, blocks the development of acute antinociceptive tolerance to an intrathecally administered μ-opioid receptor agonist in the mouse. *Eur. J. Pharmacol.,* **1995,** *280*:R1–R3.

Neal, C.R. Jr., Mansour, A., Reinscheid, R., Nothacker, H.P., Civelli, O., and Watson, S.J. Jr. Localization of orphanin FQ (nociceptin) peptide and messenger RNA in the central nervous system of the rat. *J. Comp. Neurol.,* **1999a,** *406*:503–547.

Neal, C.R. Jr., Mansour, A., Reinscheid, R., Nothaker, H.P., Civelli, O., Akil, H., and Watson, S.J. Jr. Opioid receptor-like (ORL1) receptor distribution in the rat central nervous system: comparison of ORL1 receptor mRNA expression with ^{125}I-(^{14}Tyr)-orphanin FQ binding. *J. Comp. Neurol.,* **1999b,** *412*:563–605.

Negri, L., Potenza, R.L., Corsi, R., and Melchiorri, P. Evidence for two subtypes of delta opioid receptors in rat brain. *Eur. J. Pharmacol.,* **1991,** *196*:335–336.

Neumann, P.B., Henriksen, H., Grosman, N., and Christensen, C.B. Plasma morphine concentrations during chronic oral administration in patients with cancer pain. *Pain,* **1982,** *13*:247–252.

Nishi, M., Houtani, T., Noda, Y., Mamiya, T., Sato, K., Doi, T., Kuno, J., Takeshima, H., Nukada, T., Nabeshima, T., Yamashita, T., Noda, T., and Sugimoto, T. Unrestrained nociceptive response and disregulation of hearing ability in mice lacking the nociceptin/orphanin FQ receptor. *EMBO J.,* **1997,** *16*:1858–1864.

Nothacker, H.P., Reinscheid, R.K., Mansour, A., Henningsen, R.A., Ardati, A., Monsma, F.J. Jr., Watson, S.J., and Civelli, O. Primary structure and tissue distribution of the orphanin FQ precursor. *Proc. Natl. Acad. Sci. U.S.A.,* **1996,** *93*:8677–8682.

Oka, T. Enkephalin receptor in the rabbit ileum. *Life Sci.,* **1980,** *38*:1889–1898.

Okuda-Ashitaka, E., Minami, T., Tachibana, S., Yoshihara, Y., Nishiuchi, Y., Kimura, T., and Ito, S. Nocistatin, a peptide that blocks nociceptin action in pain transmission. *Nature,* **1998,** *392*:286–289.

Osborne, R., Joel, S., Trew, D., and Slevin, M. Morphine and metabolite behavior after different routes of morphine administration: demonstration of the importance of the active metabolite morphine-6-glucuronide. *Clin. Pharmacol. Ther.,* **1990,** *47*:12–19.

Osborne, R.J., Joel, S.P., Trew, D., and Slevin, M.L. The analgesic activity of morphine-6-glucuronide. *Lancet,* **1988,** *1*:828.

Owen, J.A., Sitar, D.S., Berger, L., Brownell, L., Duke, P.C., and Mitenko, P.A. Age-related morphine kinetics. *Clin. Pharmacol. Ther.,* **1983,** *34*:364–368.

Pan, Y.X., Xu, J., and Pasternak, G.W. Cloning and expression of a cDNA encoding a mouse brain orphanin FQ/nociceptin precursor. *Biochem. J.,* **1996,** *315*:11–13.

Pan, Z.Z., Hirakawa, N., and Fields, H.L. A cellular mechanism for the bidirectional pain-modulating actions of orphanin FQ/nociceptin. *Neuron,* **2000,** *26*:515–522.

615

Pan, Z.Z., Tershner, S.A., and Fields, H.L. Cellular mechanism for anti-analgesic action of agonists of the κ-opioid receptor. *Nature,* **1997,** *389:*382–385.

Paul, D., Standifer, K.M., Inturrisi, C.E., and Pasternak, G.W. Pharmacological characterization of morphine-6β-glucuronide, a very potent morphine metabolite. *J. Pharmacol. Exp. Ther.,* **1989,** *251:*477–483.

Pei, G., Kieffer, B.L., Lefkowitz, R.J., and Freedman, N.J. Agonist-dependent phosphorylation of the mouse delta-opioid receptor: involvement of G protein-coupled receptor kinases but not protein kinase C. *Mol. Pharmacol.,* **1995,** *48:*173–177.

Pert, C.B., and Snyder, S.H. Opiate receptor: demonstration in nervous tissue. *Science,* **1973,** *179:*1011–1014.

Pfeiffer, A., Brantl, V., Herz, A., and Emrich, H.M. Psychotomimesis mediated by kappa opiate receptors. *Science,* **1986,** *233:*774–776.

Pick, C.G., Roques, B., Gacel, G., and Pasternak, G.W. Supraspinal mu₂-opioid receptors mediate spinal/supraspinal morphine synergy. *Eur. J. Pharmacol.,* **1992a,** *220:*275–277.

Pick, C.G., Paul, D., Eison, M.S., and Pasternak, G.W. Potentiation of opioid analgesia by the antidepressant nefazodone. *Eur. J. Pharmacol.,* **1992b,** *211:*375–381.

Pilcher, W.H., Joseph, S.A., and McDonald, J.V. Immunocytochemical localization of pro-opiomelanocortin neurons in human brain areas subserving stimulation analgesia. *J. Neurosurg.,* **1988,** *68:*621–629.

Popio, K.A., Jackson, D.H., Ross, A.M., Schreiner, B.F., and Yu, P.N. Hemodynamic and respiratory effects of morphine and butorphanol. *Clin. Pharmacol. Ther.,* **1978,** *23:*281–287.

Portenoy, R.K., Khan, E., Layman, M., Lapin, J., Malkin, M.G., Foley, K.M., Thaler, H.T., Cerbone, D.J., and Inturrisi, C.E. Chronic morphine therapy for cancer pain: plasma and cerebrospinal fluid morphine and morphine-6-glucuronide concentrations. *Neurology,* **1991,** *41:*1457–1461.

Portenoy, R.K., Southam, M.A., Gupta, S.K., Lapin, J., Layman, M., Inturrisi, C.E., and Foley, K.M. Transdermal fentanyl for cancer pain. Repeated dose pharmacokinetics. *Anesthesiology,* **1993,** *78:*36–43.

Portenoy, R.K., Thaler, H.T., Inturrisi, C.E., Friedlander-Klar, H., and Foley, K.M. The metabolite morphine-6-glucuronide contributes to the analgesia produced by morphine infusion in patients with pain and normal renal function. *Clin. Pharmacol. Ther.,* **1992,** *51:*422–431.

Portoghese, P.S., Lipowski, A.W., and Takemori, A.E. Binaltorphimine and nor-binaltorphimine, potent and selective kappa-opioid receptor antagonists. *Life Sci.,* **1987,** *40:*1287–1292.

Portoghese, P.S., Sultana, M., and Takemori, A.E. Naltrindole, a highly selective and potent non-peptide delta opioid receptor antagonist. *Eur. J. Pharmacol.,* **1988,** *146:*185–186.

Reinscheid, R.K., Nothacker, H.P., Bourson, A., Ardati, A., Henningsen, R.A., Bunzow, J.R., Grandy, D.K., Langen, H., Monsma, F.J. Jr., and Civelli, O. Orphanin FQ: a neuropeptide that activates an opioidlike G protein-coupled receptor. *Science,* **1995,** *270:*792–794.

Rodgers, B.M., Webb, C.J., Stergios, D., and Newman, B.M. Patient-controlled analgesia in pediatric surgery. *J. Pediatr. Surg.,* **1988,** *23:*259–262.

Rose, P.G., Macfee, M.S., and Boswell, M.V. Fentanyl transdermal system overdose secondary to cutaneous hyperthermia. *Anesth. Analg.,* **1993,** *77:*390–391.

Rossi, G.C., Brown, G.P., Leventhal, L., Yang, K., and Pasternak, G.W. Novel receptor mechanisms for heroin and morphine-6β-glucuronide analgesia. *Neurosci. Lett.,* **1996a,** *216:*1–4.

Rossi, G.C., Leventhal, L., Pan, Y.X., Cole, J., Su, W., Bodnar, R.J., and Pasternak, G.W. Antisense mapping of MOR-1 in rats: distinguishing between morphine and morphine-6β-glucuronide antinociception. *J. Pharmacol. Exp. Ther.,* **1997,** *281:*109–114.

Rossi, G.C., Leventhal, L., and Pasternak, G.W. Naloxone sensitive orphanin FQ-induced analgesia in mice. *Eur. J. Pharmacol.,* **1996b,** *311:*R7–R8.

Rossi, G.C., Pan, Y.X., Brown, G.P., and Pasternak, G.W. Antisense mapping the MOR-1 opioid receptor: evidence for alternative splicing and a novel morphine-6β-glucuronide receptor. *FEBS Lett.,* **1995,** *369:*192–196.

Rossi, G.C., Pasternak, G.W., and Bodnar, R.J. Synergistic brainstem interactions for morphine analgesia. *Brain Res.,* **1993,** *624:*171–180.

Roth, A., Keren, G., Gluck, A., Braun, S., and Laniado, S. Comparison of nalbuphine hydrochloride versus morphine sulfate for acute myocardial infarction with elevated pulmonary artery wedge pressure. *Am. J. Cardiol.,* **1988,** *62:*551–555.

Rothman, R.B., Long, J.B., Bykov, V., Jacobson, A.E., Rice, K.C., and Holaday, J.W. β-FNA binds irreversibly to the opiate receptor complex: in vivo and in vitro evidence. *J. Pharmacol. Exp. Ther.,* **1988,** *247:*405–416.

Sadeque, A.J., Wandel, C., He, H., Shah, S., and Wood, A.J. Increased drug delivery to the brain by P-glycoprotein inhibition. *Clin. Pharmacol. Ther.,* **2000,** *68:*231–237.

Sawe, J., Dahlstrom, B., Paalzow, L., and Rane, A. Morphine kinetics in cancer patients. *Clin. Pharmacol. Ther.,* **1981,** *30:*629–635.

Schinkel, A.H., Wagenaar, E., Mol, C.A., and van Deemter, L. P-glycoprotein in the blood-brain barrier of mice influences the brain penetration and pharmacological activity of many drugs. *J. Clin. Invest.,* **1996,** *97:*2517–2524.

Schuller, A.G., King, M.A., Zhang, J., Bolan, E., Pan, Y.X., Morgan, D.J., Chang, A., Czick, M.E., Unterwald, E.M., Pasternak, G.W., and Pintar, J.E. Retention of heroin and morphine-6β-glucuronide analgesia in a new line of mice lacking exon1 of MOR-1. *Nat. Neurosci.,* **1999,** *2:*151–156.

Schultz, J.E., Hsu, A.K., and Gross, G.J. Morphine mimics the cardioprotective effect of ischemic preconditioning via a glibenclamide-sensitive mechanism in the rat heart. *Circ. Res.,* **1996,** *78:*1100–1104.

Schulz, R., Faase, E., Wuster, M., and Herz, A. Selective receptors for beta-endorphin on the rat vas deferens. *Life Sci.,* **1979,** *24:*843–849.

Schwyzer, R., Molecular mechanism of opioid receptor selection. *Biochemistry,* **1986,** *25:*6335–6342.

Segredo, V., Burford, N.T., Lameh, J., and Sadee, W. A constitutively internalizing and recycling mutant of the mu-opioid receptor. *J. Neurochem.,* **1997,** *68:*2395–2404.

Sethna, D.H., Moffitt, E.A., Gray, R.J., Bussell, J., Raymond, M., Conklin, C., Shell, W.E., and Matloff, J.M. Cardiovascular effects of morphine in patients with coronary arterial disease. *Anesth. Analg.,* **1982,** *61:*109–114.

Shafer, S.L., Varvel, J.R., Aziz, N., and Scott, J.C. Pharmacokinetics of fentanyl administered by computer-controlled infusion pump. *Anesthesiology,* **1990,** *73:*1091–1102.

Sharma, S.K., Klee, W.A., and Nirenberg, M. Opiate-dependent modulation of adenylate cyclase. *Proc. Natl. Acad. Sci. U.S.A.,* **1977,** *74:*3365–3369.

Simon, E.J., Hiller, J.M., and Edelman, I. Stereospecific binding of the potent narcotic analgesic ³H-etorphine to rat brain homogenate. *Proc. Natl. Acad. Sci. U.S.A.,* **1973,** *70:*1947–1949.

Smith, M.T. Neuroexcitatory effects of morphine and hydromorphone: evidence implicating the 3-glucuronide metabolites. *Clin. Exp. Pharmacol. Physiol.,* **2000,** *27:*524–528.

Smith, M.T., Watt, J.A., and Cramond, T. Morphine-3-glucuronide—a potent antagonist of morphine analgesia. *Life Sci.,* **1990,** *47:*579–585.

Sofuoglu, M., Portoghese, P.S., and Takemori, A.E. Differential antagonism of delta opioid agonists by naltrindole and its benzofuran analog (NTB) in mice: evidence for delta opioid receptor subtypes. *J. Pharmacol. Exp. Ther.,* **1991,** *257*:676–680.

Sriwatanakul, K., Weis, O.F., Alloza, J.L., Kelvie, W., Weintraub, M., and Lasagna, L. Analysis of narcotic analgesic usage in the treatment of postoperative pain. *JAMA,* **1983,** *250*:926–929.

Stein, C., Comisel, K., Haimerl, E., Yassouridis, A., Lehrberger, K., Herz, A., and Peter, K. Analgesic effect of intraarticular morphine after arthroscopic knee surgery. *N. Engl. J. Med.,* **1991,** *325*:1123–1126.

Strader, C.D., Sigal, I.S., Candelore, M.R., Rands, E., Hill, W.S., and Dixon, R.A. Conserved aspartic acid residues 79 and 113 of the beta-adrenergic receptor have different roles in receptor function. *J. Biol. Chem.,* **1988,** *263*:10267–10271.

Surratt, C.K., Johnson, P.S., Moriwaki, A., Seidleck, B.K., Blaschak, C.J., Wang, J.B., and Uhl, G.R. Mu opiate receptor. Charged transmembrane domain amino acids are critical for agonist recognition and intrinsic activity. *J. Biol. Chem.,* **1994,** *269*:20548–20553.

Terenius, L. Stereospecific interaction between narcotic analgesics and a synaptic plasma membrane fraction of rat brain cortex. *Acta Pharmacol. Toxicol. (Copenh.),* **1973,** *32*:317–320.

Thomas, D.A., Williams, G.M., Iwata, K., Kenshalo, D.R. Jr., and Dubner, R. Effects of central administration of opioids on facial scratching in monkeys. *Brain Res.,* **1992,** *585*:315–317.

Thomas, D.A., Williams, G.M., Iwata, K., Kenshalo, D.R. Jr., and Dubner, R. Multiple effects of morphine on facial scratching in monkeys. *Anesth. Analg.,* **1993,** *77*:933–935.

Thompson, R.C., Mansour, A., Akil, H., and Watson, S.J. Cloning and pharmacological characterization of a rat mu opioid receptor. *Neuron,* **1993,** *11*:903–913.

Thysman, S., and Preat, V. In vivo iontophoresis of fentanyl and sufentanil in rats: pharmacokinetics and acute antinociceptive effects. *Anesth. Analg.,* **1993,** *77*:61–66.

Trafton, J.A., Abbadie, C., Marchand, S., Mantyh, P.W., and Basbaum, A.I. Spinal opioid analgesia: how critical is the regulation of substance P signaling? *J. Neurosci.,* **1999,** *19*:9642–9653.

Trapaidze, N., Keith, D.E., Cvejic, S., Evans, C.J., and Devi, L.A. Sequestration of the delta opioid receptor. Role of the C terminus in agonist-mediated internalization. *J. Biol. Chem.,* **1996,** *271*:29279–29285.

Trujillo, K.A., and Akil, H. Inhibition of morphine tolerance and dependence by the NMDA receptor antagonist MK-801. *Science,* **1991,** *251*:85–87.

Ueda, H., Miyamae, T., Hayashi, C., Watanabe, S., Fukushima, N., Sasaki, Y., Iwamura, T., and Misu, Y. Protein kinase C involvement in homologous desensitization of delta-opioid receptor coupled to G_i1-phospholipase C activation in xenopus oocytes. *J. Neurosci.,* **1995,** *15*:7485–7499.

Vaughan, C.W., Ingram, S.L., Connor, M.A., and Christie, M.J. How opioids inhibit GABA-mediated neurotransmission. *Nature,* **1997,** *390*:611–614.

Vismara, L.A., Leaman, D.M., and Zelis, R. The effects of morphine on venous tone in patients with acute pulmonary edema. *Circulation,* **1976,** *54*:335–337.

VonVoigtlander, P.F., Lahti, R.A., and Ludens, J.H. U-50,488: a selective and structurally novel non-Mu (kappa) opioid agonist. *J. Pharmacol. Exp. Ther.,* **1983,** *224*:7–12.

Wallenstein, S.L., Kaiko, R.F., Rogers, A.G., and Houde, R.W. Crossover trials in clinical analgesic assays: studies of buprenorphine and morphine. *Pharmacotherapy,* **1986,** *6*:228–235.

Wang, J.B., Johnson, P.S., Persico, A.M., Hawkins, A.L., Griffin, C.A., and Uhl, G.R. Human mu opiate receptor. cDNA and genomic clones, pharmacologic characterization and chromosomal assignment. *FEBS Lett.,* **1994,** *338*:217–222.

Wang, J.B., Imai, Y., Eppler, C.M., Gregor, P., Spivak, C.E., and Uhl, G.R. Mu opiate receptor: cDNA cloning and expression. *Proc. Natl. Acad. Sci. U.S.A.,* **1993,** *90*:10230–10234.

Watson, B., Meng, F., Thompson, R., and Akil, H. Structural studies of the mu opioid receptor using chimeric constructs. *Analgesia,* **1995,** *1*: 825–828.

Way, W., Costley, E., and Way, E. Respiratory sensitivity of the newborn infant to meperidine and fentanyl. *Clin. Pharmacol. Ther.,* **1965,** *6*:454–459.

Weihe, E., Millan, M.J., Leibold, A., Nohr, D., and Herz, A. Co-localization of proenkephalin- and prodynorphin-derived opioid peptides in laminae IV/V spinal neurons revealed in arthritic rats. *Neurosci. Lett.,* **1988,** *29*:187–192.

Weinberg, D.S., Inturrisi, C.E., Reidenberg, B., Moulin, D.E., Nip, T.J., Wallenstein, S., Houde, R.W., and Foley, K.M. Sublingual absorption of selected opioid analgesics. *Clin. Pharmacol. Ther.,* **1988,** *44*:335–342.

Welters, I.D., Menzebach, A., Goumon, Y., Cadet, P., Menges, T., Hughes, T.K., Hempelmann, G., and Stefano, G.B. Morphine inhibits NF-κB nuclear binding in human neutrophils and monocytes by a nitric oxide-dependent mechanism. *Anesthesiology,* **2000,** *92*:1677–1684.

Whistler, J.L., and von Zastrow, M. Morphine-activated opioid receptors elude desensitization by β-arrestin. *Proc. Natl. Acad. Sci. U.S.A.,* **1998,** *95*:9914–9919.

Worsley, M.H., MacLeod, A.D., Brodie, M.J., Asbury, A.J., and Clark, C. Inhaled fentanyl as a method of analgesia. *Anaesthesia,* **1990,** *45*:449–451.

Xie, Y.B., Wang, H., and Segaloff, D.L. Extracellular domain of lutropin/choriogonadotropin receptor expressed in transfected cells binds choriogonadotropin with high affinity. *J. Biol. Chem.,* **1990,** *265*:21411–21414.

Xu, X.J., Hao, J.X., and Wiesenfeld-Hallin, Z. Nociceptin or antinociceptin: potent spinal antinociceptive effect of orphanin FQ/nociceptin in the rat. *Neuroreport,* **1996,** *7*:2092–2094.

Xue, J.C., Chen, C., Zhu, J., Kunapuli, S., DeRiel, J.K., Yu, L., and Liu-Chen, L.Y. Differential binding domains of peptide and non-peptide ligands in the cloned rat kappa opioid receptor. *J. Biol. Chem.,* **1994,** *269*:30195–30199.

Yaksh, T.L., Jessell, T.M., Gamse, R., Mudge, A.W., and Leeman, S.E. Intrathecal morphine inhibits substance P release from mammalian spinal cord in vivo. *Nature,* **1980,** *286*:155–157.

Yamamoto, T., Nozaki-Taguchi, N., and Kimura, S. Analgesic effect of intrathecally administered nociceptin, an opioid receptor-like 1 receptor agonist, in the rat formalin test. *Neuroscience,* **1997,** *81*:249–254.

Yasuda, K., Espinosa, R. III, Takeda, J., Le Beau, M.M., and Bell, G.I. Localization of the kappa opioid receptor gene to human chromosome band 8q11.2. *Genomics,* **1994,** *19*:596–597.

Yasuda, K., Raynor, K., Kong, H., Breder, C.D., Takeda, J., Reisine, T., and Bell, G.I. Cloning and functional comparison of κ and δ opioid receptors from mouse brain. *Proc. Natl. Acad. Sci. U.S.A.,* **1993,** *90*:6736–6740.

Yeh, S.Y., Gorodetzky, C.W., and Krebs, H.A. Isolation and identification of morphine 3- and 6-glucuronides, morphine 3,6-diglucuronide, morphine 3-ethereal sulfate, normorphine, and normorphine 6-glucuronide as morphine metabolites in humans. *J. Pharm. Sci.,* **1977,** *66*:1288–1293.

Yoburn, B.C., Luke, M.C., Pasternak, G.W., and Inturrisi, C.E. Upregulation of opioid receptor subtypes correlates with potency changes of morphine and DADLE. *Life Sci.,* **1988,** *43*:1319–1324.

Zadina, J.E., Hackler, L., Ge, L.J., and Kastin, A.J. A potent and selective endogenous agonist for the mu-opiate receptor. *Nature,* **1997,** *386*:499–502.

Zagon, I.S., Goodman, S.R., and McLaughlin, P.J. Characterization of zeta: a new opioid receptor involved in growth. *Brain Res.,* **1989,** *482*:297–305.

Zahm, D.S., and Heimer, L. Ventral striatopallidal parts of the basal ganglia in the rat: I. Neurochemical copartmentation as reflected by the distributions of neurotensin and substance P immunoreactivity. *J. Comp. Neurol.,* **1988,** *272*:516–535.

Zimmer, E.Z., Divon, M.Y., and Vadasz, A. Influence of meperidine on fetal movements and heart rate beat-to-beat variability in the active phase of labor. *Am. J. Perinatol.,* **1988,** *5*:197–200.

Zimprich, A., Simon, T., and Hollt, V. Cloning and expression of an isoform of the rat μ opioid receptor (rMOR1B) which differs in agonist induced desensitization from rMOR1. *FEBS Lett.,* **1995,** *359*:142–146.

MONOGRAPHS AND REVIEWS

Agency for Health Care Policy and Research. *Acute Pain Management in Infants, Children, and Adolescents: Operative and Medical Procedures.* No. 92-0020. U.S. Dept. of Health and Human Services, Rockville, M.D., **1992a.**

Agency for Health Care Policy and Research. *Acute Pain Management: Operative or Medical Procedures and Trauma,* no. 92-0032. U.S. Dept. of Health and Human Services, Rockville, M.D., **1992b.**

Agency for Health Care Policy and Research. *Management of Cancer Pain,* no. 94-0592. U.S. Dept. of Health and Human Services, Rockville, M.D., **1994,** 257 pp.

Akil, H., Bronstein, D., and Mansour, A. Overview of the endogenous opioid systems: anatomical, biochemical, and functional issues. In, *Endorphins, Opiates and Behavioural Processes* (Rodgers, R.J., and Cooper, S.J., eds.) Wiley, Chichester, England, **1988,** pp. 3–17.

Akil, H., Meng, F., Devine, D.P., and Watson, S.J. Molecular and neuroanatomical properties of the endogenous opioid system: implications for treatment of opiate addiction. *Semin. Neurosci.,* **1997,** *9*:70–83.

Akil, H., Owens, C., Gutstein, H, Taylor, L., Curran, E., and Watson, S. Endogenous opioids: overview and current issues. *Drug Alcohol Depend.,* **1998,** *51*:127–140.

Akil, H., and Watson, S. Cloning of kappa opioid receptors: functional significance and future directions. In, *Neuroscience: From the Molecular to the Cognitive.* (Bloom, F.E., ed.) Elsevier, Amsterdam, **1994,** pp. 81–86.

Akil, H., Watson, S.J., Young, E., Lewis, M.E., Khachaturian, H., and Walker, J.M. Endogenous opioids: biology and function. *Annu. Rev. Neurosci.,* **1984,** *7*:223–255.

Akil, H., Young, E., Walker, J.M., and Watson, S.J. The many possible roles of opioids and related peptides in stress-induced analgesia. *Ann. N. Y. Acad. Sci.,* **1986,** *467*:140–153.

American Pain Society. *Principles of Analgesic Use in the Treatment of Acute Pain and Cancer Pain.* American Pain Society, Glenview, I.L., **1999,** 64 pp.

Amir, S. Anaphylactic shock: catecholamine actions in the response to opioid antagonists. *Prog. Clin. Biol. Res.,* **1988,** *264*:265–274.

Bailey, P.L., and Stanley, T.H. Intravenous opioid anesthetics. In, *Anesthesia,* 4th ed., vol. 1. (Miller, R.D., ed.) Churchill Livingstone, New York, **1994,** pp. 291–387.

Berde, C., Ablin, A., Glazer, J., Miser, A., Shapiro, B., Weisman, S., and Zeltzer, P. American Academy of Pediatrics Report of the Subcommittee on Disease-Related Pain in Childhood Cancer. *Pediatrics,* **1990,** *86*:818–825.

Bertorelli, R., Calo, G., Ongini, E., and Regoli, D. Nociceptin/orphanin FQ and its receptor: a potential target for drug discovery. *Trends Pharmacol. Sci.,* **2000,** *21*:233–234.

Brogden, R.N., Speight, T.M., and Avery, G.S. Pentazocine: a review of its pharmacological properties, therapeutic efficacy and dependence liability. *Drugs,* **1973,** *5*:6–91.

Burkle, H., Dunbar, S., and Van Aken, H. Remifentanil: a novel, short-acting, μ-opioid. *Anesth. Analg.,* **1996,** *83*:646-651.

Cannon, J., and Liebeskind, J. Analgesic effects of electrical brain stimulation and stress. In, *Neurotransmitters and Pain Control vol. 9: Pain and Headache.* (Akil, H., and Lewis, J.W., eds.) Karger, Basel, **1987,** pp. 283–294.

Chan, G.L., and Matzke, G.R. Effects of renal insufficiency on the pharmacokinetics and pharmacodynamics of opioid analgesics. *Drug Intell. Clin. Pharm.,* **1987,** *21*:773–783.

Christup, L.L. Morphine metabolites. *Acta Anaesthesiol. Scand.,* **1997,** *41*:116–122.

Cooper, S. Interactions between endogenous opioids and dopamine: implications for reward and aversion. In, *The Mesolimbic Dopamine System: From Motivation to Action.* (Willner, P., and Scheel-Kruger, J., eds.) Wiley, Chichester, England, **1991,** pp. 331–366.

Coupar, I.M. Opioid action on the intestine: the importance of the intestinal mucosa. *Life Sci.,* **1987,** *41*:917–925.

Duggan, A.W., and North, R.A. Electrophysiology of opioids. *Pharmacol. Rev.,* **1983,** *35*:219–281.

Du Pen, S.L., Du Pen, A.R., Polissar, N., Hansberry, J., Kraybill, B.M., Stillman, M., Panke, J., Everly, R., and Syrjala, K. Implementing guidelines for cancer pain management: results of a randomized controlled clinical trial. *J. Clin. Oncol.,* **1999,** *17*:361–370.

Duthie, D.J. Remifentanil and tramadol. *Br. J. Anaesth.,* **1998,** *81*:51–57.

Duthie, D.J., and Nimmo, W.S. Adverse effects of opioid analgesic drugs. *Br. J. Anaesth.,* **1987,** *59*:61–77.

Eddy, N.B., Friebel, H., Hahn, K.J., and Halbach, H. Codeine and its alternates for pain and cough relief. *Bull. World Health Organ.,* **1969,** *40*:639–719.

Faden, A.I. Role of thyrotropin-releasing hormone and opiate receptor antagonists in limiting central nervous system injury. *Adv. Neurol.,* **1988,** *47*:531–546.

Fields, H.L., Heinricher, M.M., and Mason, P. Neurotransmitters in nociceptive modulatory circuits. *Annu. Rev. Neurosci.,* **1991,** *14*:219–245.

Findlay, J.W. Pholcodine. *J. Clin. Pharm. Ther.,* **1988,** *13*:5–17.

Fishburne, J.I. Systemic analgesia during labor. *Clin. Perinatol.,* **1982,** *9*:29–53.

Foley, K.M. The treatment of cancer pain. *N. Engl. J. Med.,* **1985,** *313*:84–95.

Foley, K.M. Opioid analgesics in clinical pain management. In, *Handbook of Experimental Pharmacology, vol. 104/II: Opioids II.* (Herz, A., ed.) Springer-Verlag, Berlin, **1993,** pp. 693–743.

Glass, P.S., Gan, T.J., and Howell, S. A review of the pharmacokinetics and pharmacodynamics of remifentanil. *Anesth. Analg.,* **1999,** *89*:S7–S14.

Gonzalez, J.P., and Brogden, R.N. Naltrexone. A review of its pharmacodynamic and pharmacokinetic properties and therapeutic efficacy in the management of opioid dependence. *Drugs,* **1988,** *35*:192–213.

Grossman, A. Opioids and stress in man. *J. Endocrinol.,* **1988,** *119*: 377–381.

Grossman, S., Benedetti, C., Payne, R., and Syrjala, K. NCCN practice guidelines for cancer pain. *NCCN Proc.,* **1999,** *13*:33–44.

Gustafsson, L.L., and Wiesenfeld-Hallin, Z. Spinal opioid analgesia. A critical update. *Drugs,* **1988,** *35*:597–603.

Harris, J.A. Descending antinociceptive mechanisms in the brainstem: their role in the animal's defensive system. *J. Physiol. Paris,* **1996,** *90*:15–25.

Heimer, L., Switzer, R., and Hoesen, G.V. Ventral striatum and ventral pallidum. Components of the motor system? *Trends Neurosci.,* **1982,** 5:83087.

Herz, A., ed. *Handbook of Experimental Pharmacology, vol. 104/I: Opioids.* Springer-Verlag, Berlin, **1993.**

Holmes, B., and Ward, A. Meptazinol. A review of its pharmacodynamic and pharmacokinetic properties and therapeutic efficacy. *Drugs,* **1985,** *30*:285–312.

Howlett, T.A., and Rees, L.H. Endogenous opioid peptides and hypothalamo-pituitary function. *Annu. Rev. Physiol.,* **1986,** *48*:527–536.

International Association for the Study of Pain. *Management of Acute Pain: A Practical Guide.* IASP Publications, Seattle, W.A., **1992.**

Kilpatrick, G.J., Dautzenberg, F.M., Martin, G.R., and Eglen, R.M. 7TM receptors: the splicing on the cake. *Trends Pharmacol. Sci.,* **1999,** 20:294–301.

Koob, G.F., and Bloom, F.E. Cellular and molecular mechanisms of drug dependence. *Science,* **1988,** *242*:715–723.

Kreek, M.J. Methadone in treatment: physiological and pharmacological issues. In, *Handbook on Drug Abuse.* (Dupont, R.L., Goldstein, A., and O'Donnell, J., eds.) U.S. Government Printing Office, Washington, D.C., **1979,** pp. 57–86.

Kromer, W. Endogenous and exogenous opioids in the control of gastrointestinal motility and secretion. *Pharmacol. Rev.,* **1988,** *40*:121–162.

Lewis, J., Mansour, A., Khachaturian, H., Watson, S., and Akil, H. Neurotransmitters and pain control. In, *Neurotransmitters and Pain Control, vol. 9: Pain and Headache.* (Akil, H., and Lewis, J.W., eds.) Karger, Basil, **1987,** pp. 129–159.

Lewis, K.S., and Han, N.H Tramadol: a new centrally acting analgesic. *Am. J. Health Syst. Pharm.,* **1997,** *54*:643–652.

Manara, L., and Bianchetti, A. The central and peripheral influences of opioids on gastrointestinal propulsion. *Annu. Rev. Pharmacol. Toxicol.,* **1985,** *25*:249–273.

Mansour, A., Fox, C.A., Akil, H., and Watson, S.J. Opioid-receptor mRNA expression in the rat CNS: anatomical and functional implications. *Trends Neurosci.,* **1995,** *18*:22–29.

Mansour, A., Khachaturian, H., Lewis, M.E., Akil, H., and Watson, S.J. Anatomy of CNS opioid receptors. *Trends Neurosci.,* **1988,** *11*:308–314.

Martin, W.R. Pharmacology of opioids. *Pharmacol. Rev.,* **1983,** *35*:283–323.

McCleskey, E.W., and Gold, M.S. Ion channels of nociception. *Annu. Rev. Physiol.,* **1999,** *61*:835–856.

McGinty, J., and Friedman, D. Opioids in the hippocampus. *Natl. Inst. Drug Abuse Res. Monogr. Ser.,* **1988,** *82*:1–145.

McQuay, H.J. Pharmacological treatment of neuralgic and neuropathic pain. *Cancer Surv.,* **1988,** *7*:141–159.

Milne, R.W., Nation, R.L., and Somogyi, A.A. The disposition of morphine and its 3- and 6-glucuronide metabolites in humans and animals, and the importance of the metabolites to the pharmacological effects of morphine. *Drug Metab. Rev.,* **1996,** 28:345–472.

Misra, A.L. Metabolism of opiates. In, *Factors Affecting the Action of Narcotics.* (Adler, M.L., Manara, L., and Samanin, R., eds.) Raven Press, New York, **1978,** pp. 297–343.

Monk, J.P., Beresford, R., and Ward, A. Sufentanil. A review of its pharmacological properties and therapeutic use. *Drugs,* **1988,** *36*: 286–313.

Mulder, A., and Schoffelmeer, A. multiple opioid receptors and presynaptic modulation of neurotransmitter release in the brain. In, *Handbook of Experimental Pharmacology, vol. 104/I: Opioids.* (Herz, A., ed.) Springer-Verlag, Berlin, **1993,** pp. 125–144.

Nestler, E.J., and Aghajanian, G.K. Molecular and cellular basis of addiction. *Science,* **1997,** *278*:58–63.

Page, G.G., and Ben-Eliyahu, S. The immune-suppressive nature of pain. *Semin. Oncol. Nurs.,* **1997,** *13*:10–15.

Pasternak, G.W. Multiple morphine and enkephalin receptors: biochemical and pharmacological aspects. *Ann. N.Y. Acad. Sci.,* **1986,** *467*: 130–139.

Pasternak, G.W. Pharmacological mechanisms of opioid analgesics. *Clin. Neuropharmacol.,* **1993,** *16*:1–18.

Pasternak, G.W., and Standifer, K.M. Mapping of opioid receptors using antisense oligodeoxynucleotides: correlating their molecular biology and pharmacology. *Trends Pharmacol. Sci.,* **1995,** *16*:344–350.

Patel, S.S., and Spencer, C.M. Remifentanil. *Drugs,* **1996,** *52*:417–427.

Payne, R. Transdermal fentanyl: suggested recommendations for clinical use. *J. Pain Sympt. Manage.,* **1992,** *7*:S40–S44.

Portenoy, R.K. Chronic opioid therapy in nonmalignant pain. *J. Pain Sympt. Manage.,* **1990,** *5*:S46–S62.

Portoghese, P.S. Bivalent ligands and the message-address concept in the design of selective opioid receptor antagonists. *Trends Pharmacol. Sci.,* **1989,** *10*:230–235.

Risdahl, J.M., Khanna, K.V., Peterson, P.K., and Molitor, T.W. Opiates and infection. *J. Neuroimmunol.,* **1998,** *83*:4–18.

Rumore, M.M., and Schlichting, D.A. Clinical efficacy of antihistaminics as analgesics. *Pain,* **1986,** *25*:7–22.

Sanford, T., and Gutstein, H.B. Fentanyl, sufentanil, and alfentanil: comparative pharmacology. *Clin. Anesth. Updates,* **1995,** *6*:1–20.

Sawynok, J. The therapeutic use of heroin: a review of the pharmacological literature. *Can. J. Physiol. Pharmacol.,* **1986,** *64*:1–6.

Sharp, B., and Yaksh, T. Pain killers of the immune system. *Nat. Med.,* **1997,** *3*:831–832.

Shippenberg, T.S., Herz, A., Spanagel, R., Bals-Kubik, R., and Stein, C. Conditioning of opioid reinforcement: neuroanatomical and neurochemical substrates. *Ann. N. Y. Acad. Sci.,* **1992,** *654*:347–356.

Shnider, S.M., and Levinson, G. *Anesthesia for Obstetrics.* Williams & Wilkins, Baltimore, **1987.**

Stack, C.G., Rogers, P., and Linter, S.P. Monoamine oxidase inhibitors and anesthesia. A review. *Br J. Anaesth.,* **1988,** *60*:222–227.

Staritz, M. Pharmacology of the sphincter of Oddi. *Endoscopy,* **1988,** *20(suppl.)1*:171–174.

Stein, C. Peripheral mechanisms of opioid analgesia. *Anesth. Analg.,* **1993,** *76*:182–191.

Stein, C. The control of pain in peripheral tissue by opioids. *N. Engl. J. Med.,* **1995,** *332*:1685–1690.

Willner, P., Ahlenius, S., Muscat, R., and Scheel-Kruger, J. The mesolimbic dopamine system. In, *The Mesolimbic Dopamine System: From Motivation to Action.* (Willner, J., and Scheel-Kruger, J., eds.) Wiley, Chichester, England, **1991.**

World Health Organization. *Cancer Pain Relief and Palliative Care: Report of a WHO Expert Committee.* World Health Organization, Geneva, Switzerland, **1990.**

World Health Organization. *Cancer Pain Relief and Palliative Care in Children.* World Health Organization, Geneva, Switzerland, **1998.**

Yaksh, T.L. CNS mechanisms of pain and analgesia. *Cancer Surv.,* **1988,** *7*:5–28.

Yaster, M., and Deshpande, J.K. Management of pediatric pain with opioid analgesics. *J. Pediatr.,* **1988,** *113*:421–429.

Acknowledgement

The authors wish to acknowledge Drs. Terry Reisine and Gavril Pasternak, authors of this chapter in the ninth edition of *Goodman and Gilman's The Pharmacological Basis of Therapeutics,* some of whose text has been retained in this edition.

Dedication

The authors would like to dedicate this chapter to the memory of Dr. Thomas F. Burks, colleague and friend, who had a major impact on the field of opioid pharmacology.

DRUG ADDICTION AND DRUG ABUSE

Charles P. O'Brien

Drugs are so commonly used and abused in modern society that virtually everyone has some familiarity with the concepts of drug addiction and abuse. The term addiction *has entered everyday language and often is used to describe behavior that does not involve drug use. For example, the media speak of "addiction" to sex, running, shopping, or TV. While there certainly can be a superficial resemblance among many varieties of compulsive behavior, there currently is no scientific basis to lump these activities with drug abuse and addiction. These are medical diagnoses with specific criteria that provide the same level of interevaluator reliability as for other medical conditions.*

Inappropriate use of any drug can be either intentional or inadvertent. Drugs that affect behavior are particularly likely to be taken in excess when the behavioral effects are considered pleasurable. Psychosocial factors tend to be similar for diverse pharmacological agents and are of equal importance in the pathogenesis of these disorders as the unique pharmacological profiles of given drugs. Nevertheless, this chapter focuses on the pharmacological aspects of drug abuse and dependence, including legal prescription drugs, illegal drugs such as heroin or cocaine, and nonprescription drugs such as ethanol and nicotine (see also Chapters 9, 17, 18, and 23).

DRUG DEPENDENCE

There are many misunderstandings about the origins and even the definitions of drug abuse and addiction. Although many physicians are concerned about "creating addicts," very few individuals begin their drug addiction problems by misuse of prescription drugs. Confusion exists because the correct use of prescribed medications for pain, anxiety, and even hypertension commonly produces tolerance and physical dependence. These are *normal* physiological adaptations to repeated use of drugs from many different categories. Tolerance and physical dependence are explained in more detail later, but it must be emphasized that they *do not* imply abuse or addiction. This distinction is important, because patients with pain are sometimes deprived of adequate opioid medication simply because they have shown evidence of tolerance and they exhibit withdrawal symptoms if the analgesic medication is abruptly stopped.

Definitions. Abuse and addiction have been defined and redefined by several organizations over the past 30 years. The reason for these revisions and disagreements is that abuse and addiction are behavioral syndromes that exist along a continuum from minimal use to abuse to addictive use. While tolerance and physical dependence are biological phenomena that can be defined precisely in the laboratory and diagnosed accurately in the clinic, there is an arbitrary aspect to the definitions of the overall behavioral syndromes of abuse and addiction. The most influential system of diagnosis for mental disorders is that published by the American Psychiatric Association (APA) (DSM-IV, 1994). The APA diagnostic system uses the term *substance dependence* instead of *addiction* for the overall behavioral syndrome. It also applies the same general criteria to all types of drugs, regardless of their pharmacological class. Although widely accepted, this terminology can lead to confusion between *physical dependence* and *psychological dependence*. The term *addiction,* when used in this chapter, refers to compulsive drug use—the entire substance dependence syndrome as defined in DSM-IV. This should not be confused with physical dependence alone, a common error among physicians. *Addiction* is not used as a pejorative term but rather for clarity of communication; in fact, the journal *Addiction* is one of the oldest scientific journals in this therapeutic area.

The APA defines substance dependence (addiction) as a cluster of symptoms indicating that the individual continues use of the substance despite significant substance-related problems. Evidence of tolerance and withdrawal symptoms is included in the list of symptoms, but neither tolerance nor withdrawal is necessary or sufficient for a diagnosis of substance dependence. Dependence (addiction) requires three or more of the symptoms, while "abuse" can be diagnosed when only one or two symptoms are present.

Origins of Substance Dependence.   Many variables operate simultaneously to influence the likelihood of any given person becoming a drug abuser or an addict. These variables can be organized into three categories: agent (drug), host (user), and environment (*see* Table 24–1).

Table 24–1

Multiple Simultaneous Variables Affecting Onset and Continuation of Drug Abuse and Addiction

Agent (drug)
  Availability
  Cost
  Purity/potency
  Mode of administration
    Chewing (absorption *via* oral mucous membranes)
    Gastrointestinal
    Intranasal
    Subcutaneous and intramuscular
    Intravenous
    Inhalation
  Speed of onset and termination of effects
    (pharmacokinetics: combination of agent and host)
Host (user)
  Heredity
    Innate tolerance
    Speed of developing acquired tolerance
    Likelihood of experiencing intoxication as pleasure
  Metabolism of the drug (nicotine and alcohol data
    already available)
  Psychiatric symptoms
  Prior experiences/expectations
  Propensity for risk-taking behavior
Environment
  Social setting
  Community attitudes
    Peer influence, role models
  Availability of other reinforcers (sources of pleasure
    or recreation)
  Employment or educational opportunities
  Conditioned stimuli: Environmental cues become
    associated with drugs after repeated use in the
    same environment

Agent (Drug) Variables.   Drugs vary in their ability to produce immediate good feelings in the user. Drugs that reliably produce intensely pleasant feelings (euphoria) are more likely to be taken repeatedly. *Reinforcement* refers to the ability of drugs to produce effects that make the user wish to take them again. The more strongly reinforcing a drug is, the greater the likelihood that the drug will be abused. Reinforcing properties of a drug can be reliably measured in animals. Generally, animals such as rats or monkeys equipped with intravenous catheters connected to lever-regulated pumps will work to obtain injections of the same drugs in roughly the same order of potency that human beings will. Thus, medications can be screened for their potential for abuse in human beings by the use of animal models.

Reinforcing properties of drugs are associated with their ability to increase levels of the neurotransmitters in critical brain areas (*see* Chapter 12). Cocaine, amphetamine, ethanol, opioids, and nicotine all reliably increase extracellular fluid dopamine levels in the nucleus accumbens region. Brain microdialysis permits sampling of extracellular fluid while animals, usually rats, are freely moving or receiving drugs. Smaller increases in dopamine in the nucleus accumbens also are observed when the rat is presented with sweet foods or a sexual partner. In contrast, drugs that block dopamine receptors generally produce bad feelings, *i.e.,* dysphoric effects. Neither animals nor human beings will take such drugs spontaneously. Despite strong correlative findings, a causal relationship between dopamine and euphoria/dysphoria has not been established, and other findings emphasize additional roles of noradrenergic, serotonergic, opioidergic, and GABAergic mechanisms in mediating the reinforcing effects of drugs.

The abuse liability of a drug is enhanced by rapidity of onset, since effects that occur soon after administration are more likely to initiate the chain of events that lead to loss of control over drug taking. The pharmacokinetic variables that influence the time it takes the drug to reach critical receptor sites in the brain are explained in more detail in Chapter 1. The history of cocaine use illustrates the changes in abuse liability of the same compound, depending on the form and the route of administration.

Coca leaves can be chewed, and the alkaloidal cocaine is slowly absorbed through the buccal mucosa. This method produces low cocaine blood levels and correspondingly low levels in the brain. The mild stimulant effects produced by the chewing of coca leaves have a gradual onset, and this practice has produced little, if any, abuse or dependence despite use over thousands of years by natives of the Andes mountains. Beginning in the late nineteenth century, scientists isolated cocaine hydrochloride from coca leaves, and the extraction of pure cocaine became possible. Cocaine could be taken in higher doses by oral ingestion (gastrointestinal absorption) or by absorption through the nasal mucosa, producing higher cocaine levels in the blood and a more rapid onset of stimulation. Subsequently, it was found that a solution of cocaine hydrochloride could be administered *via* the intravenous route, giving the ultimate in rapidity of blood levels and speed of onset of stimulatory effects. Each newly available cocaine preparation that provided greater speed of onset and an increment in blood level was paralleled by a greater likelihood to produce addiction. In the 1980s, the availability of cocaine to the American public was increased further with the invention of crack cocaine. *Crack,* sold at a very low street price ($1 to $3 per dose), is alkaloidal cocaine (free base) that can be readily vaporized by heating. Simply inhaling the vapors produces blood levels comparable to those resulting from intravenous cocaine due to the large surface area for absorption into the pulmonary circulation following inhalation. The cocaine-containing blood then enters the left side of the heart and reaches the cerebral circulation without dilution by the systemic circulation. Inhalation of crack cocaine is thus much more likely to produce addiction than is chewing, drinking, or sniffing cocaine. This method, which rapidly delivers the drug to the brain, also is the preferred route for users of nicotine and cannabis.

Although the drug variables are important, they do not fully explain the development of abuse and addiction. Most people who experiment with drugs that have a high risk of producing addiction (addiction liability) do not intensify their drug use and lose control. The risk for developing addiction among those who try nicotine is about twice that for those who try cocaine (Table 24–2), but this does not imply that the pharmacological addiction liability of nicotine is twice that of cocaine. Rather there are other variables listed in the categories of host factors and environmental conditions that influence the development of addiction.

Host (User) Variables. In general, effects of drugs vary among individuals. Even blood levels show wide variation when the same dose of a drug on a milligram-per-kilogram basis is given to different people. Polymorphism of the genes that encode enzymes involved in absorption, metabolism, and excretion and in receptor-mediated responses may contribute to the different degrees of reinforcement or euphoria observed among individuals.

Children of alcoholics show an increased likelihood of developing alcoholism, even when adopted at birth and raised by nonalcoholic parents (Schuckit, 1999). The studies of genetic influences in this disorder show only an *increased risk* for developing alcoholism, not a 100% determinism, and this is consistent with a polygenic disorder that has multiple determinants. Even identical twins, who share the same genetic endowment, do not have 100% concordance when one twin is alcoholic. However, the concordance rate for identical twins is much higher than that for fraternal twins. Also of interest is the observation that alcohol and other drug abuse tend to run in the same families, giving rise to postulates that common mechanisms may be involved.

Innate tolerance to alcohol may represent a biological trait that contributes to the development of alcoholism. Data from a longitudinal study (Schuckit and Smith, 1996) show that sons of alcoholics have reduced sensitivity to alcohol when compared to other young men of the same age (22 years old) and drinking histories. Sensitivity to alcohol was measured by measuring the effects of two different doses of alcohol in the laboratory on motor performance and subjective feelings of intoxication. When the men were reexamined 10 years later, those who had been most tolerant (insensitive) to alcohol at age 22 were the most likely to be diagnosed as alcohol-dependent at age 32. The presence of tolerance predicted the development of alcoholism even in the group without a family history of alcoholism, but

Table 24–2
Dependence Among Users 1990–1992

	EVER USED*%	ADDICTION %	RISK OF ADDICTION %
Tobacco	75.6	24.1	31.9
Alcohol	91.5	14.1	15.4
Illicit drugs	51.0	7.5	14.7
Cannabis	46.3	4.2	9.1
Cocaine	16.2	2.7	16.7
Stimulants	15.3	1.7	11.2
Anxiolytics	12.7	1.2	9.2
Analgesics	9.7	0.7	7.5
Psychedelics	10.6	0.5	4.9
Heroin	1.5	0.4	23.1
Inhalants	6.8	0.3	3.7

*The ever-used and addiction percents are those of the general population. The risk of addiction is specific to the drug indicated and refers to the percent who met criteria for addiction among those who reported having used it at least once.
SOURCE: From Anthony *et al,* 1994, with permission.

there were far fewer tolerant men in the group with a negative family history.

Differences in alcohol metabolism also may influence the propensity for alcohol abuse. Ethanol is metabolized by alcohol dehydrogenase with the production of acetaldehyde, which is then metabolized by a mitochondrial aldehyde dehydrogenase known as ALDH2. A common mutation occurs in the gene for ALDH2, resulting in a less effective aldehyde dehydrogenase. This allele has a high frequency in Asian populations and results in an excess production of acetaldehyde after the ingestion of alcohol. Those who are heterozygous for this allele experience a very unpleasant facial flushing reaction 5 to 10 minutes after ingesting alcohol; the reaction is even more severe in individuals homozygous for the allele, and this genotype has not been found in alcoholics (Higuchi *et al.*, 1996). Similarly, individuals who inherit the gene for impaired nicotine metabolism have been found to have a lower probability of becoming nicotine-dependent. (Pianezza *et al.*, 1998).

Psychiatric disorders constitute another category of host variables. Drugs may produce immediate, subjective effects that relieve preexisting symptoms. People with anxiety, depression, insomnia, or even subtle symptoms such as shyness may find, on experimentation or by accident, that certain drugs give them relief. However, the apparent beneficial effects are transient, and repeated use of the drug may lead to tolerance and eventually compulsive, uncontrolled drug use. While psychiatric symptoms commonly are seen in drug abusers presenting for treatment, most of these symptoms started *after* the person began abusing drugs. Thus, drugs of abuse appear to produce more psychiatric symptoms than they relieve.

Environmental Variables.   Initiating and continuing illicit drug use appear to be significantly influenced by societal norms and peer pressure. Taking drugs may be seen initially as a form of rebellion against authority. In some communities, drug users and drug dealers are role models who seem to be successful and respected; thus, young people emulate them. There also may be a paucity of other options for pleasure or diversion. These factors are particularly important in communities where educational levels are low and job opportunities scarce.

Pharmacological Phenomena.   *Tolerance.*   While abuse and addiction are extremely complicated conditions combining the many variables outlined above, there are a number of relevant pharmacological phenomena that occur independently of social and psychological dimensions. First are the changes in the way the body responds to a drug with repeated use. *Tolerance* is the most common response to repetitive use of the same drug and can be defined as the reduction in response to the drug after repeated administrations. Figure 24–1 shows an idealized dose–response curve for an administered drug. As the dose of the drug increases, the observed effect of the drug increases. With repeated use of the drug, however, the curve shifts to the right (tolerance). Thus a higher dose

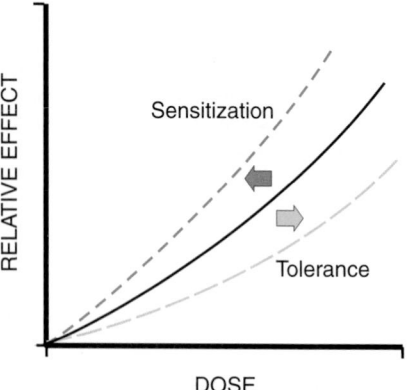

Figure 24–1. Shifts in a dose–response curve with tolerance and sensitization.

With tolerance, there is a shift of the curve to the right such that doses higher than initial doses are required to achieve the same effects. With sensitization, there is a leftward shift of the dose–response curve such that, for a given dose, there is a greater effect than seen after the initial dose.

is required to produce the same effect that was once obtained at a lower dose. Diazepam, for example, typically produces sedation at doses of 5 to 10 mg in a first-time user, but those who repeatedly use it to produce a kind of "high" may become tolerant to doses of several hundreds of milligrams; some abusers have had documented tolerance to >1000 mg/day. As outlined in Table 24–3, there are many forms of tolerance, likely arising *via* multiple mechanisms.

Tolerance develops to some drug effects much more rapidly than to other effects of the same drug. For example, tolerance develops rapidly to the euphoria produced by opioids such as heroin, and addicts tend to increase their dose in order to reexperience that elusive "high." In contrast, tolerance to the gastrointestinal effects of opiates develops more slowly. The discrepancy

Table 24–3
Types of Tolerance

Innate (preexisting sensitivity or insensitivity)
Acquired
    Pharmacokinetic (dispositional or metabolic)
    Pharmacodynamic
    Learned tolerance
        Behavioral
            Conditioned
    Acute tolerance
    Reverse tolerance (sensitization)
    Cross-tolerance

between tolerance to euphorigenic effects and tolerance to effects on vital functions, such as respiration and blood pressure, can lead to potentially fatal accidents in sedative abusers.

Innate tolerance refers to genetically determined sensitivity (or lack of sensitivity) to a drug that is observed the first time that the drug is administered. Innate tolerance is discussed above as a host variable that influences the development of abuse or addiction.

Acquired tolerance can be divided into three types: pharmacokinetic, pharmacodynamic, and learned tolerance, including a form of behavioral tolerance referred to as *conditioned tolerance*.

Pharmacokinetic or *dispositional tolerance* refers to changes in the distribution or metabolism of the drug after repeated drug administration, such that reduced concentrations are present in the blood and subsequently at the sites of drug action (*see* Chapter 1). The most common mechanism is an increase in the rate of metabolism of the drug. For example, barbiturates stimulate the production of higher levels of hepatic microsomal enzymes, causing more rapid removal and breakdown of barbiturates from the circulation. Since the same enzymes metabolize many other drugs, they too are metabolized more quickly. This results in a decrease in their plasma levels as well and thus a reduction in their effects.

Pharmacodynamic tolerance refers to adaptive changes that have taken place within systems affected by the drug, so that response to a given concentration of the drug is reduced. Examples include drug-induced changes in receptor density or efficiency of receptor coupling to signal transduction pathways (*see* Chapter 2).

Learned tolerance refers to a reduction in the effects of a drug due to compensatory mechanisms that are learned. One type of learned tolerance is called *behavioral tolerance*. This simply describes the skills that can be developed through repeated experiences with attempting to function despite a state of mild to moderate intoxication. A common example is learning to walk a straight line in spite of the motor impairment produced by alcohol intoxication. This probably involves both acquisition of motor skills and the learned awareness of one's deficit, causing the person to walk more carefully. At higher levels of intoxication, behavioral tolerance is overcome, and the deficits are obvious.

A special case of behavioral tolerance is referred to as *conditioned tolerance*. Conditioned tolerance (situation-specific tolerance) is a learning mechanism that develops when environmental cues such as sights, smells, or situations consistently are paired with the administration of a drug. When a drug affects homeostatic balance by producing sedation and changes in blood pressure, pulse rate, gut activity, *etc.*, there is usually a reflexive counteraction or adaptation that attempts to maintain the *status quo*. If a drug always is taken in the presence of specific environmental cues (smell of drug preparation, sight of syringe), these cues begin to predict the appearance of the drug. Then the adaptations begin to occur even before the drug reaches its sites of action. If the drug always is preceded by the same cues, the adaptive response to the drug will be learned, and this will prevent the full manifestation of the drug's effects (tolerance). This mechanism of conditioned tolerance production follows classical (Pavlovian) principles of learning and results in drug tolerance being evident under circumstances where the drug is "expected." When the drug is received under novel or "unexpected" circumstances, tolerance is reduced and drug effects are enhanced (Wikler, 1973; Siegel 1976).

The term *acute tolerance* refers to rapid tolerance developing with repeated use on a single occasion such as in a "binge." For example, cocaine often is used in a binge, with repeated doses over one to several hours, sometimes longer. Under binge dosing, there will be a decrease in response to subsequent doses of cocaine during the binge. This is the opposite of *sensitization,* observed with an intermittent dosing schedule, described below.

Sensitization. With stimulants such as cocaine or amphetamine, *reverse tolerance* or *sensitization* can occur. This refers to an increase in response with repetition of the same dose of the drug. Sensitization results in a shift to the left of the dose–response curve, as illustrated schematically in Figure 24–1. For example, with repeated daily administration to rats of a dose of cocaine that produces increased motor activity, the effect increases over several days, even though the dose remains constant. A conditioned response also can be a part of sensitization to cocaine. Simply putting a rat into a cage where cocaine is expected or giving a placebo injection after several days of receiving cocaine under the same circumstances produces an increase in motor activity as though cocaine actually were given—*i.e.,* a conditioned response. Sensitization, in contrast to acute tolerance during a binge, requires a longer interval between doses, usually about a day.

Sensitization has been studied in rats equipped with microdialysis cannulae for monitoring extracellular dopamine (Kalivas and Duffy, 1990; *see* Figure 24–2). The initial response to

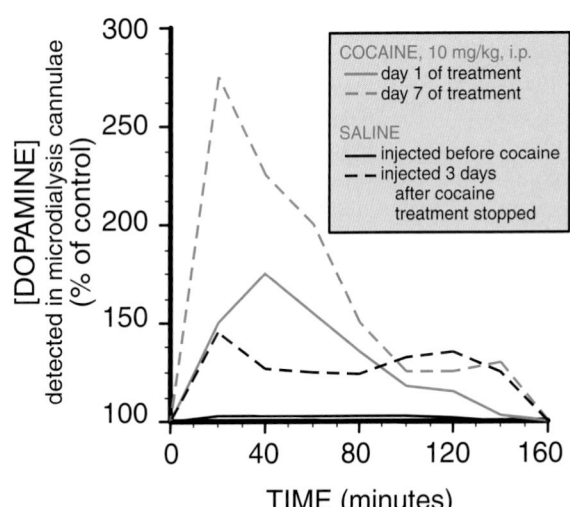

Figure 24–2. Changes in dopamine detected in the extracellular fluid of the nucleus accumbens of rats after daily intraperitoneal cocaine injections (10 mg/kg).

The first injection produces a modest increase and the last, after 7 days, produces a much greater increase in dopamine release. Note that whereas the first saline injection produces no effect on dopamine levels, the second, given 3 days after 7 days of cocaine injections, produces a significant rise in dopamine, presumably due to conditioning. (Adapted from Kalivas and Duffy, 1990, with permission.)

10 mg/kg of cocaine administered intraperitoneally is an increase in measured dopamine levels. After seven daily injections, the dopamine increase is significantly greater than on the first day, and the behavioral response also is greater. Figure 24–2 also provides an example of a conditioned response (learned drug effect), since injection of saline produced both an increase in dopamine levels and an increase in behavioral activity when it was administered 3 days after cocaine injections had stopped. Little research on sensitization has been conducted in human subjects, but the results suggest that the phenomenon can occur. It has been postulated that stimulant psychosis results from a sensitized response after long periods of use.

Cross-Tolerance.   *Cross-tolerance* refers to the fact that repeated use of drugs in a given category confers tolerance not only to the drug being used but also to other drugs in the same structural and mechanistic category. Understanding cross-tolerance is important in the medical management of persons dependent on any drug. *Detoxification* is a form of treatment for drug dependence that involves giving gradually decreasing doses of the drug to prevent withdrawal symptoms, thereby weaning the patient from the drug of dependence (*see* below). Detoxification can be accomplished with any medication that produces cross-tolerance to the initial drug of dependence. For example, users of heroin also are tolerant to other opioids. Thus the detoxification of heroin-dependent patients can be accomplished with any medication that activates opiate receptors (opioid drug; *see* Chapter 23).

Physical Dependence

Physical dependence is a *state* that develops as a result of the adaptation (tolerance) produced by a resetting of homeostatic mechanisms in response to repeated drug use. Drugs can affect numerous systems that previously were in equilibrium; these systems must find a new balance in the presence of inhibition or stimulation by a specific drug. A person in this adapted or physically dependent state requires continued administration of the drug to maintain normal function. If administration of the drug is stopped abruptly, there is another imbalance, and the affected systems must again go through a process of readjusting to a new equilibrium without the drug.

Withdrawal Syndrome.   The appearance of a withdrawal syndrome when administration of the drug is terminated is the only actual evidence of physical dependence. Withdrawal signs and symptoms occur when drug administration in a physically dependent person is abruptly terminated. Withdrawal symptoms have at least two origins: (1) removal of the drug of dependence, and (2) central nervous system hyperarousal due to readaptation to the absence of the drug of dependence. Pharmacokinetic variables are of considerable importance in the amplitude and duration of the withdrawal syndrome. Withdrawal symptoms are characteristic for a given category of drugs, and

they tend to be *opposite* to the original effects produced by the drug before tolerance developed. Thus, a drug (such as an opioid agonist) that produces meiotic (constricted) pupils and slow heart rate will result in dilated pupils and tachycardia when it is withdrawn from a dependent person.

Tolerance, physical dependence, and withdrawal are all biological phenomena. They are the natural consequences of drug use. They can be produced in experimental animals and in any human being who takes certain medications repeatedly. These symptoms in themselves do not imply that the individual is involved in abuse or addiction. *Patients who take medicine for appropriate medical indications and in the correct dose still may show tolerance, physical dependence, and withdrawal symptoms if the drug is stopped abruptly rather than gradually.* For example, a hypertensive patient receiving a β-adrenergic receptor blocker such as propranolol may have a good therapeutic response but, if the drug is stopped abruptly, may experience a withdrawal syndrome consisting of rebound increased blood pressure temporarily higher than that prior to beginning the medication.

"*Medical addict*" is a term used to describe a patient in treatment for a medical disorder who has become "addicted" to the available prescribed drugs; the patient begins taking them in excessive doses, out of control. An example would be a patient with chronic pain, anxiety, or insomnia who begins using the prescribed medication more often than directed by the physician. If the physician restricts the prescriptions, the patient may begin seeing several doctors without the knowledge of the primary physician. Such patients also may visit emergency rooms for the purpose of obtaining additional medication. This scenario rarely occurs, considering the large number of patients who receive medications capable of producing tolerance and physical dependence. *Fear of producing such medical addicts results in needless suffering among patients with pain,* as physicians needlessly limit appropriate medications. Tolerance and physical dependence are inevitable consequences of chronic treatment with opioids and certain other drugs, but tolerance and physical dependence, by themselves, do not imply "addiction."

CLINICAL ISSUES

The treatment of physically dependent individuals is discussed below with reference to the specific drug of abuse and dependence problems characteristic to each category: central nervous system (CNS) depressants, including alcohol and sedatives; nicotine and tobacco; opioids; psychostimulants, such as amphetamine and cocaine; cannabinoids; psychedelic drugs; and inhalants (volatile solvents, nitrous oxide, ethyl ether). Abuse of combinations of drugs across these categories is common. Alcohol is such a widely available drug that it is combined with practically all other categories. Some combinations reportedly are taken because of their interactive effects. An example is the combination of heroin and cocaine ("speedball"), which is described with the opioid category. When confronted with a patient exhibiting signs of overdose or withdrawal, the physician must be aware of these possible combinations, because each drug may require specific treatment.

Central Nervous System Depressants

Ethanol. The use of ethyl alcohol prepared from the fermentation of sugars, starches, or other carbohydrates dates back as early as recorded history. Experimentation with ethanol is almost universal, and a high proportion of users find the experience pleasant. Approximately 70% of American adults occasionally consume ethanol (commonly called alcohol), and the lifetime prevalence of alcohol abuse and alcohol addiction (alcoholism) in this society is 5% to 10% for men and 3% to 5% for women.

Ethanol is classed as a depressant because it indeed produces sedation and sleep. However, the initial effects of alcohol, particularly at lower doses, often are perceived as stimulation due to a suppression of inhibitory systems (*see* Chapter 18). Those who perceive only sedation from alcohol tend to choose not to drink when evaluated in a test procedure (de Wit *et al.*, 1989).

Alcohol impairs recent memory and, in high doses, produces the phenomenon of "blackouts," after which the drinker has no memory of his or her behavior while intoxicated. The effects of alcohol on memory are unclear (Mello, 1973), but evidence suggests that reports from patients about their reasons for drinking and their behavior during a binge are not reliable. Alcohol-dependent persons often say that they drink to relieve anxiety or depression. When allowed to drink under observation, however, alcoholics typically become more dysphoric as drinking continues (Mendelson and Mello, 1979), thus contradicting the tension-reduction explanation.

Tolerance, Physical Dependence, and Withdrawal. Mild intoxication by alcohol is familiar to almost everyone, but the symptoms vary among individuals. Some simply experience motor incoordination and sleepiness. Others initially become stimulated and garrulous. As the blood level increases, the sedating effects increase, with eventual coma and death at high alcohol levels. The initial sensitivity (innate tolerance) to alcohol varies greatly among individuals and is related to family history of alcoholism (Schuckit and Smith, 1997). Experience with alcohol can produce greater tolerance (acquired tolerance), such that extremely high blood levels (300 to 400 mg/dl) can be found in alcoholics who do not appear grossly sedated. In

Table 24–4
Alcohol Withdrawal Syndrome

Alcohol craving
Tremor, irritability
Nausea
Sleep disturbance
Tachycardia
Hypertension
Sweating
Perceptual distortion
Seizures (12 to 48 hours after last drink)
Delirium tremens (rare in uncomplicated withdrawal)
  Severe agitation
  Confusion
  Visual hallucinations
  Fever, profuse sweating
  Tachycardia
  Nausea, diarrhea
  Dilated pupils

these cases, the lethal dose does not increase proportionately to the sedating dose, and thus the margin of safety (therapeutic index) is decreased.

Heavy consumers of alcohol not only acquire tolerance but also inevitably develop a state of physical dependence. This often leads to drinking in the morning to restore blood alcohol levels diminished during the night. Eventually they may awaken during the night and take a drink to avoid the restlessness produced by falling alcohol levels. The alcohol withdrawal syndrome (Table 24–4) generally depends on the size of the average daily dose and usually is "treated" by resumption of alcohol ingestion. Withdrawal symptoms are experienced frequently, but they usually are not severe or life threatening until they occur in conjunction with other problems, such as infection, trauma, malnutrition, or electrolyte imbalance. In the setting of such complications, the syndrome of *delirium tremens* becomes likely (*see* Table 24–4).

Alcohol produces cross-tolerance to other sedatives such as benzodiazepines. This tolerance is operative in abstinent alcoholics, but while the alcoholic is drinking, the sedating effects of alcohol add to those of other drugs, making the combination more dangerous. This is particularly true for benzodiazepines, which are relatively safe in overdose when given alone but potentially are lethal in combination with alcohol.

The chronic use of alcohol as well as that of other sedatives is associated with the development of depression (McLellan *et al.*, 1979), and the risk of suicide among alcoholics is one of the highest of any diagnostic category. Cognitive deficits have been reported in alcoholics tested while sober. These deficits usually improve after weeks to months of abstinence (Grant, 1987). More severe recent memory impairment is associated with specific brain damage caused by nutritional deficiencies, which are common in alcoholics.

Alcohol is toxic to many organ systems. As a result, the medical complications of alcohol abuse and dependence include liver disease, cardiovascular disease, endocrine and gastrointestinal effects, and malnutrition, in addition to the CNS dysfunctions outlined above (*see* Chapter 18). Ethanol readily crosses the placental barrier, producing the *fetal alcohol syndrome,* a major cause of mental retardation (*see* Chapter 18).

Pharmacological Interventions. *Detoxification.* A patient who presents in a medical setting with an alcohol-withdrawal syndrome should be considered to have a potentially lethal condition. Although most mild cases of alcohol withdrawal never come to medical attention, severe cases require general evaluation; attention to hydration and electrolytes; vitamins, especially high-dose thiamine; and a sedating medication that has cross-tolerance with alcohol. A short-acting benzodiazepine such as *oxazepam* can be given at doses sufficient to block or diminish the symptoms described in Table 24–4; some authorities recommend a long-acting benzodiazepine unless there is demonstrated liver impairment. Anticonvulsants such as carbamazepine have been shown to be effective in alcohol withdrawal, although they appear not to relieve subjective symptoms as well as benzodiazepines. After medical evaluation, uncomplicated alcohol withdrawal can be treated effectively on an outpatient basis (Hayashida *et al.,* 1989). When there are medical problems or a history of seizures, hospitalization is required.

Other Measures. Detoxification is only the first step of treatment. Complete abstinence is the objective of long-term treatment, and this is accomplished mainly by behavioral approaches. Medications that aid in this process are being sought. *Disulfiram* (*see* Chapter 18) has been useful in some programs that focus behavioral efforts on the ingestion of the medication. Disulfiram blocks the metabolism of alcohol, resulting in the accumulation of acetaldehyde, which produces an unpleasant flushing reaction when alcohol is ingested. Knowledge of this unpleasant reaction helps the patient resist taking a drink. Although quite effective pharmacologically, disulfiram has not been found to be effective in controlled clinical trials, because so many patients failed to ingest the medication. Another FDA-approved medication used as an adjunct in

the treatment of alcoholism is *naltrexone* (*see* Chapter 18). This opiate receptor antagonist appears to block some of the reinforcing properties of alcohol and has resulted in a decreased rate of relapse to alcohol drinking in several double-blind clinical trials. It works best in combination with behavioral treatment programs that encourage adherence to medication and to remaining abstinent from alcohol.

Benzodiazepines and Other Nonalcohol Sedatives. Benzodiazepines are among the most commonly prescribed drugs worldwide; they are used mainly for the treatment of anxiety disorders and insomnia (Chapters 17 and 19). Considering their widespread use, intentional abuse of prescription benzodiazepines is relatively rare. When a benzodiazepine is taken for up to several weeks, there is little tolerance and no difficulty in stopping the medication when the condition no longer warrants its use. After several months, the proportion of patients who become tolerant increases, and reducing the dose or stopping the medication produces withdrawal symptoms (Table 24–5). It can be difficult to distinguish withdrawal symptoms from the reappearance of the anxiety symptoms that caused the benzodiazepine to be prescribed initially. Some patients may increase their dose over time, because tolerance definitely develops to the sedative effects. Many patients and their physicians, however, contend that antianxiety benefits continue to occur long after tolerance to the sedating effects. Moreover, these patients continue to take the medication for years according to medical directions without increasing their dose and are able to function very effectively as long as they take the benzodiazepine. The degree to which tolerance develops to the anxiolytic effects of benzodiazepines is a subject of controversy (Lader and File, 1987). There is, however, good evidence that significant tolerance

Table 24–5
Benzodiazepine Withdrawal Symptoms

Following moderate dose usage
   Anxiety, agitation
   Increased sensitivity to light and sound
   Paresthesias, strange sensations
   Muscle cramps
   Myoclonic jerks
   Sleep disturbance
   Dizziness
Following high-dose usage
   Seizures
   Delirium

does not develop to all benzodiazepine actions, because some effects of acute doses on memory persist in patients who have taken benzodiazepines for years (Lucki *et al.,* 1986). The American Psychiatric Association formed a task force that reviewed the issues and published guidelines on the proper medical use of benzodiazepines (American Psychiatric Association, 1990). Intermittent use when symptoms occur retards the development of tolerance and is, therefore, preferable to daily use. Patients with a history of alcohol or other drug abuse problems have an increased risk for the development of benzodiazepine abuse and should rarely, if ever, be treated with benzodiazepines on a chronic basis.

While relatively few patients who receive benzodiazepines for medical indications abuse their medication, there are individuals who specifically seek benzodiazepines for their ability to produce a "high." Among these abusers, there are differences in drug popularity, with those benzodiazepines that have a rapid onset, such as *diazepam* and *alprazolam*, tending to be the most desirable. The drugs may be obtained by simulating a medical condition and deceiving physicians or simply through illicit channels. Street drug dealers provide benzodiazepines in most major cities at a relatively low cost. Such unsupervised use can lead to the self-administration of huge quantities of such drugs and therefore tolerance to the benzodiazepine's sedating effects. For example, while 5 to 20 mg/day of diazepam is a typical dose for a patient receiving prescribed medication, abusers may take over 1000 mg/day and not appear grossly sedated.

Abusers may combine benzodiazepines with other drugs to increase the effect. For example, it is part of the "street lore" that taking diazepam 30 minutes after an oral dose of methadone will produce an augmented high that is not obtainable with either drug alone.

While there is some illicit use of benzodiazepines as a primary drug of abuse, most of the nonsupervised use seems to be by abusers of other drugs who are attempting to self-medicate the side effects or withdrawal effects of their primary drug of abuse. Thus, cocaine addicts often take diazepam to relieve the irritability and agitation produced by cocaine binges, and opioid addicts find that diazepam and other benzodiazepines relieve some of the anxiety symptoms of opioid withdrawal when they are unable to obtain their preferred drug.

Pharmacological Interventions. If patients receiving long-term benzodiazepine treatment by prescription wish to stop their medication, the process may take months of gradual dose reduction. Symptoms as listed in Table 24–5 may occur during this outpatient detoxification, but in most cases the symptoms are mild. If anxiety symptoms return, a nonbenzodiazepine such as *buspirone* may be prescribed, but this agent usually is less effective than benzodiazepines for treatment of anxiety in these patients. Some authorities recommend transferring the patient to a long-half-life benzodiazepine during detoxification; other

medications recommended include the anticonvulsants *carbamazepine* and *phenobarbital*. Controlled studies comparing different treatment regimens are lacking. Since patients who have been on low doses of benzodiazepines for years usually have no adverse effects, the physician and patient should jointly decide whether detoxification and possible transfer to a new anxiolytic is worth the effort.

The specific benzodiazepine receptor antagonist *flumazenil* has been found useful in the treatment of overdose and in reversing the effects of long-acting benzodiazepines used in anesthesia (*see* Chapter 17). It has been tried in the treatment of persistent withdrawal symptoms after cessation of long-term benzodiazepine treatment.

Deliberate abusers of high doses of benzodiazepines usually require inpatient detoxification. Frequently, benzodiazepine abuse is part of a combined dependence involving alcohol, opioids, and cocaine. Detoxification can be a complex clinical pharmacological problem, requiring knowledge of the pharmacokinetics of each drug. The patient's history may not be reliable, not simply because of lying but also because the patient frequently does not *know* the true identity of drugs purchased on the street. Medication for detoxification should not be prescribed by the "cookbook" approach but by careful titration and patient observation. The withdrawal syndrome from diazepam, for example, may not become evident until the patient develops a seizure in the second week of hospitalization. One approach to complex detoxification is to focus on the CNS-depressant drug and temporarily hold the opioid component constant with a low dose of methadone. Opioid detoxification can begin later. A long-acting benzodiazepine, such as diazepam or *clorazepate,* or a long-acting barbiturate, such as phenobarbital, can be used to block the sedative withdrawal symptoms. The phenobarbital dose should be determined by a series of test doses and subsequent observations to determine the level of tolerance. Most complex detoxifications can be accomplished using this phenobarbital loading-dose strategy (*see* Robinson *et al.,* 1981).

After detoxification, the prevention of relapse requires a long-term outpatient rehabilitation program similar to that for the treatment of alcoholism. No specific medications have been found to be useful in the rehabilitation of sedative abusers—but, of course, specific psychiatric disorders such as depression or schizophrenia, if present, require appropriate medications.

Barbiturates and Nonbenzodiazepine Sedatives. The use of barbiturates and other nonbenzodiazepine sedating medications has declined greatly in recent years due to the increased safety and efficacy of the newer medications. Abuse problems with barbiturates resemble those seen with benzodiazepines in many ways. Treatment of abuse and addiction should be handled similarly to interventions for the abuse of alcohol and benzodiazepines.

Because drugs in this category frequently are prescribed as hypnotics for patients complaining of insomnia, the physician should be aware of the problems that can develop when the hypnotic agent is withdrawn. Insomnia rarely should be treated with medication as a primary disorder except when produced by short-term stressful situations. Insomnia often is a symptom of an underlying chronic problem, such as depression, or may be due simply to a change in sleep requirements with age. Prescription of sedative medications, however, can change the physiology of sleep, with subsequent tolerance to these medication effects. When the sedative is stopped, there is a rebound effect (Kales *et al.*, 1979). This medication-induced insomnia requires detoxification by gradual dose reduction.

Nicotine

The basic pharmacology of nicotine is discussed in Chapter 9. Nicotine has complex effects that result in its self-administration. Because nicotine provides the reinforcement for the smoking of cigarettes, the most common cause of preventable death and disease in the United States, it is arguably the most dangerous dependence-producing drug. The dependence produced by nicotine can be extremely durable, as exemplified by the high failure rate among smokers who try to quit. Although more than 80% of smokers express a desire to quit, only 35% try to stop each year, and fewer than 5% are successful in unaided attempts to quit (American Psychiatric Association, 1994).

Cigarette (nicotine) addiction is influenced by multiple variables. Nicotine itself produces reinforcement; users compare nicotine to stimulants such as cocaine or amphetamine, although its effects are of lower magnitude. While there are many casual users of alcohol and cocaine, few individuals who smoke cigarettes smoke a small enough quantity (five cigarettes or fewer per day) to avoid dependence. Nicotine is absorbed readily through the skin, mucous membranes, and, of course, the lungs. The pulmonary route produces discernible CNS effects in as little as seven seconds. Thus, each puff produces some discrete reinforcement. With 10 puffs per cigarette, the one-pack-per-day smoker reinforces the habit 200 times daily. The timing, setting, situation, and preparation all become associated repetitively with the effects of nicotine.

Nicotine has both stimulant and depressant actions. The smoker feels alert, yet there is some muscle relaxation. Nicotine activates the nucleus accumbens reward system in the brain, discussed earlier; increased extracellular dopamine has been found in this region after nicotine injections in rats. Nicotine affects other systems as well, including the release of endogenous opioids and glucocorticoids.

There is evidence for tolerance to the subjective effects of nicotine. Smokers typically report that the first cigarette of the

Table 24–6
Nicotine Withdrawal Syndrome

Irritability, impatience, hostility
Anxiety
Dysphoric or depressed mood
Difficulty concentrating
Restlessness
Decreased heart rate
Increased appetite or weight gain

day after a night of abstinence gives the "best" feeling. Smokers who return to cigarettes after a period of abstinence may experience nausea if they return immediately to their previous dose. Persons naive to the effects of nicotine will experience nausea at low nicotine blood levels, and smokers will experience nausea if nicotine levels are raised above their accustomed levels.

Negative reinforcement refers to the benefits obtained from the termination of an unpleasant state. In dependent smokers, there is evidence that the urge to smoke correlates with a low nicotine blood level, as though smoking were a means to achieve a certain nicotine level and thus avoid withdrawal symptoms. Some smokers even awaken during the night to have a cigarette, which ameliorates the effect of low nicotine blood levels that could disrupt sleep. If the nicotine level is maintained artificially by a slow intravenous infusion, there is a decrease in the number of cigarettes smoked and in the number of puffs (Russell, 1987). Thus, smokers may be smoking to achieve the reward of nicotine effects, to avoid the pain of nicotine withdrawal or, most likely, a combination of the two. Nicotine withdrawal symptoms are listed in Table 24–6.

Depressed mood (dysthymic disorder, affective disorder) is associated with nicotine dependence, but it is not known whether depression predisposes one to begin smoking or depression develops during the course of nicotine dependence. Depression significantly increases during smoking withdrawal, and this is cited as one reason for relapse.

Pharmacological Interventions. The nicotine withdrawal syndrome can be alleviated by nicotine replacement therapy, available without a prescription. Figure 24–3 shows the blood nicotine concentrations achieved by different methods of nicotine delivery. Because nicotine gum and a nicotine patch do not achieve the *peak levels* seen with cigarettes, they do not produce the same magnitude of subjective effects as nicotine. These methods do, however, suppress the symptoms of nicotine withdrawal. Thus, smokers should be able to transfer their dependence to the alternative delivery system and gradually reduce the daily nicotine dose with minimal symptoms. Although this results in more smokers achieving abstinence, most resume smoking over the ensuing weeks or months. Comparisons with placebo treatment show large benefits of nicotine replacement at six weeks, but the effect diminishes with

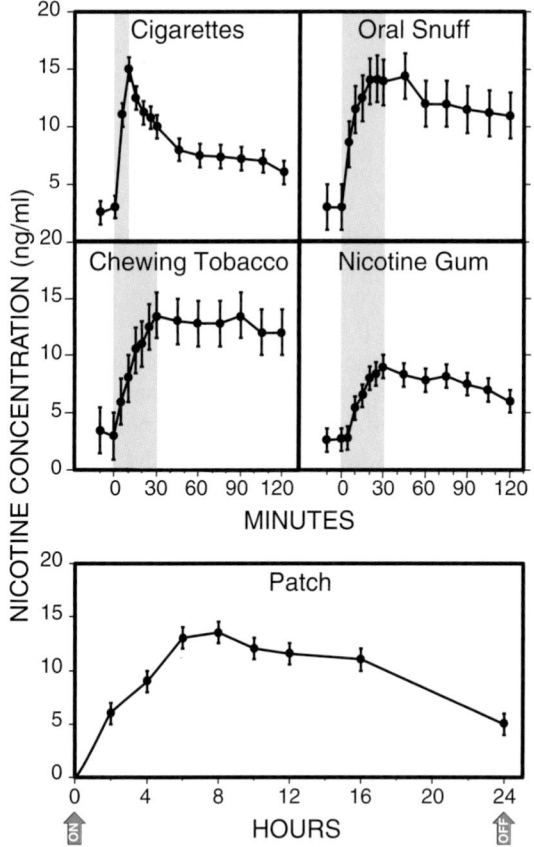

Figure 24–3. Nicotine concentrations in blood resulting from five different nicotine delivery systems.

Shaded areas indicate the periods of exposure to nicotine. The arrows in the lower panel indicate when the nicotine patch was put on and taken off. (Adapted from Benowitz *et al.,* 1988, and Srivastava *et al.,* 1991, with permission.)

time. The nicotine patch produces a steady blood level (Figure 24–3) and seems to have better patient compliance than that observed with nicotine gum. Verified abstinence rates at 12 months are reported to be in the range of 20%, which is worse than the success rate for any other addiction. The goal of complete abstinence rather than significant reduction is necessary for success; when ex-smokers "slip" and begin smoking a little, they usually relapse quickly to their prior level of dependence. *Bupropion,* an antidepressant (*see* Chapter 19), has been found to improve abstinence rates among smokers. Some smokers report that it reduces their craving for cigarettes, and controlled studies show reduced relapse in smokers randomized to this medication. The best results are in smokers receiving both nicotine patch and bupropion. Behavioral treatment in combination with medication is considered the treatment of choice.

Opioids

Opioid drugs are used primarily for the treatment of pain (*see* Chapter 23). Some of the CNS mechanisms that reduce the perception of pain also produce a state of well-being or euphoria. Thus, opioid drugs also are taken outside of medical channels for the purpose of obtaining the effects on mood. This potential for abuse has generated much research on separating the mechanism of analgesia from that of euphoria in the hope of eventually developing a potent analgesic that does not activate brain reward systems. Although this research has led to advances in understanding the physiology of pain, the standard medications for severe pain remain the derivatives of the opium poppy (opiates) and synthetic drugs that activate the same receptors (opioids). Drugs modeled after the endogenous opioid peptides may one day provide more specific treatment, but none of these currently is available for clinical use. Medications that do not act at opiate receptors, such as the nonsteroidal antiinflammatory drugs, have an important role in certain types of pain, especially chronic pain; but for acute pain and for severe chronic pain, the opioid drugs are the most effective.

A recent development in pain control stems from a greater understanding of the mechanism of tolerance to "mu" (μ)-opioid receptor–mediated analgesia, which involves *N*-methyl-D-aspartate (NMDA) receptors (Trujillo and Akil, 1991). By combining morphine with *dextromethorphan,* an NMDA receptor antagonist, tolerance is impaired and analgesia is enhanced without an increase in the dose of opioid.

The subjective effects of opioid drugs are useful in the management of acute pain. This is particularly true in high-anxiety situations, such as the crushing chest pain of a myocardial infarction, when the relaxing, anxiolytic effects complement the analgesia. Normal volunteers with no pain given opioids in the laboratory may report the effects as unpleasant because of the side effects, such as nausea, vomiting, and sedation. Patients with pain rarely develop abuse or addiction problems. Of course, patients receiving opioids develop tolerance routinely, and if the medication is stopped abruptly, they will show the signs of an opioid withdrawal syndrome, the evidence for physical dependence.

Opioids should never be withheld from patients with cancer out of fear of producing addiction. If chronic opioid medication is indicated, it is preferable to prescribe an orally active, slow-onset opioid with a long duration of action. These qualities reduce the likelihood of producing euphoria at onset of withdrawal symptoms as the medication wears off. *Methadone* is an excellent choice for the management of chronic severe pain. Controlled-release, oral *morphine* (MS CONTIN, others) or controlled-release oxycodone (OXYCONTIN) are other possibilities. Rapid-onset, short-duration opioids are excellent for acute, short-term use, such as during the postoperative period.

As tolerance and physical dependence develop, however, the patient may experience the early symptoms of withdrawal between doses, and during withdrawal, the threshold for pain decreases. Thus, for chronic administration, the long-acting opioids are recommended.

The major risk for abuse or addiction occurs in patients complaining of pain with no clear physical explanation or with evidence of a chronic disorder that is not life-threatening. Examples are chronic headaches, backaches, abdominal pain, or peripheral neuropathy. Even in these cases, an opioid might be considered as a brief emergency treatment, but long-term treatment with opioids should be used only after other alternatives have been exhausted. In those relatively rare patients who develop abuse, the transition from legitimate use to abuse often begins with patients returning to their physician earlier than scheduled to get a new prescription or visiting emergency rooms of different hospitals complaining of acute pain and asking for an opioid injection.

Heroin is the most important opioid drug that is abused. There is no legal supply of heroin for clinical use in the United States. Some claim that heroin has unique analgesic properties for the treatment of severe pain, but double-blind trials have found it to be no more effective than hydromorphone. However, heroin is widely available on the illicit market, and its price dropped sharply in the 1990s while its purity increased tenfold. For many years, heroin purchased on the streets in the United States was highly diluted. Each 100-mg bag of powder had only about 4 mg of heroin (range 0 to 8 mg), and the rest was inert or sometimes toxic adulterants such as quinine. In the mid-1990s, street heroin reached 45% to 75% purity in many large cities, with some samples testing as high as 90%. This means that the level of physical dependence among heroin addicts is relatively high and that users who interrupt regular dosing will develop more severe withdrawal symptoms. Whereas heroin previously required intravenous injection, the more potent supplies can be smoked or administered nasally (snorted), thus making the initiation of heroin use accessible to people who would not insert a needle into their veins.

There is no accurate way to count the number of heroin addicts, but based on extrapolation from overdose deaths, number of applicants for treatment, and number of heroin addicts arrested, the estimates range from 800,000 to 1 million. In national surveys, approximately three adults report having tried heroin for every one who became addicted to the drug.

Tolerance, Dependence, and Withdrawal.   Injection of a heroin solution produces a variety of sensations described as warmth, taste, or high and intense pleasure ("rush") often compared to sexual orgasm. There are some differences among the opioids in their acute effects, with

morphine producing more of a histamine-releasing effect and *meperidine* producing more excitation or confusion. Even experienced opioid addicts, however, cannot distinguish between heroin and hydromorphone in double-blind tests. Thus, the popularity of heroin may be due to its availability on the illicit market and its rapid onset. After intravenous injection, the effects begin in less than a minute. Heroin has high lipid solubility, crosses the blood-brain barrier quickly, and is deacetylated to the active metabolites, 6-monoacetyl morphine and morphine. After the intense euphoria, which lasts from 45 seconds to several minutes, there is a period of sedation and tranquility ("on the nod") lasting up to an hour. The effects of heroin wear off in 3 to 5 hours, depending on the dose. Experienced users may inject two to four times per day. Thus, the heroin addict is constantly oscillating between being "high" and feeling the sickness of early withdrawal (Figure 24–4). This produces many problems in the homeostatic systems regulated, at least in part, by endogenous opioids. For example, the hypothalamic-pituitary-gonadal axis and the hypothalamic-pituitary-adrenal axis are abnormal in heroin addicts. Women on heroin have irregular menses, and men have a variety of sexual performance problems. Mood also is affected. Heroin addicts are relatively docile and compliant after taking heroin, but during withdrawal, they become irritable and aggressive.

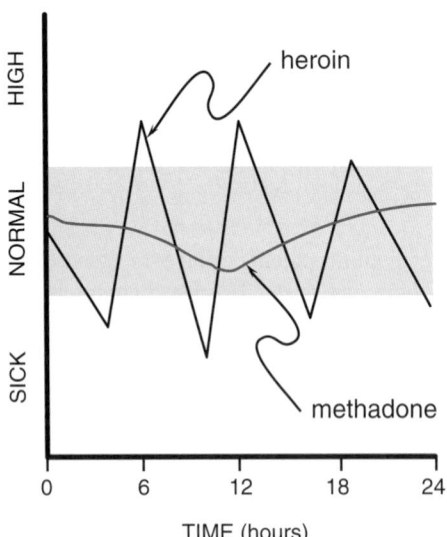

Figure 24–4. Differences in responses to heroin and methadone.

A person who injects heroin several times per day oscillates between being sick and being high. In contrast, the typical methadone patient remains in the "normal" range (*indicated in gray*) with little fluctuation after dosing once per day. The curves represent the subject's mental and physical state and not plasma levels of the drug.

Based on patient reports, tolerance develops early to the euphoria-producing effects of opioids. There also is tolerance to the respiratory depressant, analgesic, sedative, and emetic properties. Heroin users tend to increase their daily dose, depending on their financial resources and the availability of the drug. If a supply is available, the dose can be progressively increased 100-fold. Even in highly tolerant individuals, the possibility of overdose remains if tolerance is exceeded. Overdose is likely to occur when potency of the street sample is unexpectedly high or when the heroin is mixed with a far more potent opioid, such as *fentanyl,* synthesized in clandestine laboratories.

Addiction to heroin or other short-acting opioids produces behavioral disruptions and usually becomes incompatible with a productive life. There is a significant risk for opioid abuse and dependence among physicians and other health-care workers who have access to potent opioids, thus enabling unsupervised experimentation. Physicians often begin by assuming that they can manage their own dose, and they may rationalize their behavior based on the beneficial effects of the drug. Over time, however, the typical unsupervised opioid user loses control, and behavioral changes are observed by family and coworkers. Apart from the behavioral changes and the risk of overdose, especially with very potent opioids, chronic use of opioids is relatively nontoxic.

Opioids frequently are used in combinations with other drugs. A common combination is heroin and cocaine ("speedball"). Users report an improved euphoria because of the combination, and there is evidence of an interaction, because the partial opioid agonist *buprenorphine* reduces cocaine self-administration in animals (Mello *et al.,* 1989). Cocaine reduces the signs of opioid withdrawal (Kosten, 1990), and heroin may reduce the irritability seen in chronic cocaine users.

The mortality rate for street heroin users is very high. Early death comes from involvement in crime to support the habit; from uncertainty about the dose, the purity, and even the identity of what is purchased on the street; and from serious infections associated with unsterile drugs and sharing of injection paraphernalia. Heroin users commonly acquire bacterial infections producing skin abscesses, endocarditis, pulmonary infections, especially tuberculosis, and viral infections producing hepatitis and acquired immunodeficiency syndrome (AIDS).

As with other addictions, the first stage of treatment addresses physical dependence and consists of detoxification. The opioid withdrawal syndrome (Table 24–7) is very unpleasant but not life-threatening. It begins within 6 to 12 hours after the last dose of a short-acting opioid and as long as 72 to 84 hours after a very long-acting

Table 24–7
Opioid Withdrawal

SYMPTOMS	SIGNS
Regular withdrawal	
Craving for opioids	Pupillary dilation
Restlessness, irritability	Sweating
Increased sensitivity to pain	Piloerection ("gooseflesh")
	Tachycardia
Nausea, cramps	Vomiting, diarrhea
Muscle aches	Increased blood pressure
Dysphoric mood	Yawning
Insomnia, anxiety	Fever
Protracted withdrawal	
Anxiety	Cyclic changes in weight,
Insomnia	pupil size, respiratory
Drug craving	center sensitivity

opioid medication. Heroin addicts go through early stages of this syndrome frequently when heroin is scarce or expensive. Some therapeutic communities, as a matter of policy, elect not to treat withdrawal so that the addict can experience the suffering while being given group support. The duration and intensity of the syndrome are related to the clearance of the individual drug. Heroin withdrawal is brief (5 to 10 days) and intense. Methadone withdrawal is slower in onset and lasts longer. Protracted withdrawal also is likely to be longer with methadone. (*See* more detailed discussions of protracted withdrawal under "Long-Term Management," below.)

Pharmacological Interventions. Opioid withdrawal signs and symptoms can be treated by three different approaches. The first and most commonly used depends on cross-tolerance and consists of transfer to a prescription opioid medication and then gradual dose reduction. The same principles of detoxification apply as for other types of physical dependence. It is convenient to change the patient from a short-acting opioid such as heroin to a long-acting one such as *methadone.* The initial dose of methadone is typically 20 to 30 mg. This is a test dose to determine the level needed to reduce observed withdrawal symptoms. The first day's total dose then can be calculated depending on the response and then reduced by 20% per day during the course of detoxification.

A second approach to detoxification involves the use of *clonidine,* a medication approved only for the treatment of hypertension (*see* Chapter 33). Clonidine is an α_2-adrenergic agonist that decreases adrenergic neurotransmission from the locus ceruleus. Many of the autonomic symptoms of opioid withdrawal—such as nausea, vomiting, cramps, sweating, tachycardia, and hypertension—result from the loss of opioid suppression of the locus ceruleus system during the abstinence syndrome. Clonidine, acting *via* distinct receptors but by cellular mechanisms that mimic opioid effects, can alleviate many of the symptoms of opioid withdrawal. However, clonidine does not alleviate generalized aches and opioid craving characteristic of opioid withdrawal. A similar drug, *lofexidine* (not yet available in the United States), is associated with less of the hypotension that limits the usefulness of clonidine in this setting.

A third method of treating opioid withdrawal involves activation of the endogenous opioid system without medication. The techniques proposed include acupuncture and several methods of CNS activation utilizing transcutaneous electrical stimulation. While theoretically attractive, this has not yet been found to be practical.

Rapid antagonist-precipitated opioid detoxification under general anesthesia has received considerable publicity, because it promises detoxification in several hours while the patient is unconscious and thus not experiencing withdrawal discomfort. A mixture of medications has been used, and morbidity and mortality as reported in the lay press are unacceptable, with no demonstrated advantage in long-term outcome.

Long-Term Management. If patients are simply discharged from the hospital after withdrawal from opioids, there is a high probability of a quick return to compulsive opioid use. Addiction is a chronic disorder that requires long-term treatment. There are numerous factors that influence relapse. One factor is that the withdrawal syndrome does not end in 5 to 7 days. There are subtle signs and symptoms often called the *protracted withdrawal syndrome* (Table 24–7) that persist for up to 6 months. Physiological measures tend to oscillate as though a new set point were being established (Martin and Jasinski, 1969); during this phase, outpatient drug-free treatment has a low probability of success, even when the patient has received intensive prior treatment while protected from relapse in a residential program.

The most successful treatment for heroin addiction consists of stabilization on methadone. Patients who repeatedly relapse during drug-free treatment can be transferred directly to methadone without requiring detoxification. The dose of methadone must be sufficient to prevent withdrawal symptoms for at least 24 hours. *Levomethadyl acetate hydrochloride* (ORLAAM) is another maintenance option that will block withdrawal for 72 hours.

Agonist Maintenance. Patients receiving methadone or levomethadyl acetate will not experience the ups and downs they experienced while on heroin (Figure 24–4). Drug craving diminishes and may disappear. Neuroendocrine rhythms eventually are restored (Kreek, 1992). Because of cross-tolerance (from methadone to heroin), patients who inject street heroin report a reduced effect from usual heroin doses. This cross-tolerance effect is dose-related, so that higher methadone maintenance doses result in less illicit opioid use as determined by random urine testing. Patients become tolerant to the sedating effects of methadone and become able to attend school or function in a

job. Opioids also have a persistent, mild, stimulating effect noticeable after tolerance to the sedating effect, such that reaction time is quicker and vigilance is increased on a stable dose of methadone.

Antagonist Treatment. Another pharmacological option is opioid antagonist treatment. *Naltrexone* (*see* Chapter 23) is an antagonist with a high affinity for the μ-opioid receptor; it will competitively block the effects of heroin or other μ-opioid-receptor agonists. Naltrexone has almost no agonist effects of its own and will not satisfy craving or relieve protracted withdrawal symptoms. For these reasons, naltrexone treatment does not appeal to the average heroin addict, but it can be utilized after detoxification for patients with high motivation to remain opioid-free. Physicians, nurses, and pharmacists with opioid addiction problems have frequent access to opioid drugs and make excellent candidates for this treatment approach.

New Treatment Options. Two important advances in the treatment of opioid addiction are currently in clinical trials. *Buprenorphine,* a partial agonist at μ opioid receptors (*see* Chapter 23) produces minimal withdrawal symptoms, has a low potential for overdose, a long duration of action, and the ability to block heroin effects. In order to make treatment of opioid addiction more accessible, buprenorphine is proposed for use in physicians' offices rather than methadone programs. A depot formulation of naltrexone which provides 30 days of medication after a single injection is also in clinical trials. This formulation would eliminate the necessity of daily pill-taking and prevent relapse when the recently detoxified patient leaves a protected environment.

Cocaine and Other Psychostimulants

Cocaine. More than 23 million Americans are estimated to have used cocaine at some time, but the number of current users declined from an estimated 8.6 million occasional users and 5.8 million regular users to 3.6 million who still identified themselves as sometimes using cocaine in 1995. The number of frequent users (at least weekly) has remained steady since 1991 at about 640,000 persons.

Not all users become addicts, and the variables that influence this risk are discussed at the beginning of this chapter. A key factor is the widespread availability of relatively inexpensive cocaine in the alkaloidal (free base, "crack") form suitable for smoking and the hydrochloride powder form suitable for nasal or intravenous use. Drug abuse in men occurs about twice as frequently as in women. However, smoked cocaine use is particularly common in young women of childbearing age, who may use cocaine in this manner as commonly as do men.

The reinforcing effects of cocaine and cocaine analogs correlate best with their effectiveness in blocking the transporter that recovers dopamine from the synapse. This leads to increased dopaminergic stimulation at critical brain sites (Ritz *et al.,* 1987). However, cocaine also blocks both norepinephrine (NE) and serotonin (5-HT) reuptake, and chronic use of cocaine produces changes in these neurotransmitter systems as measured by reductions in the neurotransmitter metabolites MHPG (3-methoxy-4-hydroxyphenethyleneglycol) and 5-HIAA (5-hydroxyindoleacetic acid).

The general pharmacology and legitimate use of cocaine are discussed in Chapter 15. Cocaine produces a dose-dependent increase in heart rate and blood pressure accompanied by increased arousal, improved performance on tasks of vigilance and alertness, and a sense of self-confidence and well-being. Higher doses produce euphoria, which has a brief duration and often is followed by a desire for more drug. Involuntary motor activity, stereotyped behavior, and paranoia may occur after repeated doses. Irritability and increased risk of violence are found among heavy chronic users.

The half-life of cocaine in plasma is about 50 minutes, but inhalant (crack) users typically desire more cocaine after 10 to 30 minutes. Intranasal and intravenous uses also result in a "high" of shorter duration than would be predicted by plasma cocaine levels, suggesting that a declining plasma concentration is associated with termination of the high and resumption of cocaine seeking. This theory is supported by positron emission tomography imaging studies using C^{11}-labeled cocaine, which show that the time course of subjective euphoria parallels the uptake and displacement of the drug in the corpus striatum (Volkow et al., 1999).

Addiction is the most common complication of cocaine use. Some users, especially intranasal users, can continue intermittent use for years. Others become compulsive users despite elaborate methods to maintain control. Stimulants tend to be used much more irregularly than opioids, nicotine, and alcohol. Binge use is very common, and a binge may last hours to days, terminating only when supplies of the drug are exhausted.

The major route for cocaine metabolism involves hydrolysis of each of its two ester groups. Benzoylecgonine, produced upon loss of the methyl group, represents the major urinary metabolite and can be found in the urine for 2 to 5 days after a binge. As a result, benzoylecgonine tests are useful for detecting cocaine use; heavy users have been found to have detectable amounts of the metabolite in urine for up to 10 days following a binge.

Cocaine frequently is used in combination with other drugs. The cocaine-heroin combination is discussed above, with opioids. Alcohol is another drug that cocaine users take to reduce the irritability experienced during heavy cocaine use. Some develop alcohol addiction in addition to their cocaine problem. An important metabolic inter-action occurs when cocaine and alcohol are taken concurrently. Some cocaine is transesterified to cocaethylene, which is equipotent to cocaine in blocking dopamine reuptake (Hearn et al., 1991).

Toxicity.   Other risks of cocaine use, beyond the potential for addiction, involve cardiac arrhythmias, myocardial ischemia, myocarditis, aortic dissection, cerebral vasoconstriction, and seizures. Death from trauma also is associated with cocaine use (Marzuk et al., 1995). Pregnant cocaine users may experience premature labor and abruptio placentae (Chasnoff et al., 1989). Attributing the developmental abnormalities reported in infants born to cocaine-using women simply to cocaine use is confounded by the infant's prematurity, multiple drug exposure, and overall poor pre- and postnatal care.

Cocaine has been reported to produce a prolonged and intense orgasm if taken prior to intercourse, and its use is associated with compulsive and promiscuous sexual activity. Long-term cocaine use, however, usually results in reduced sexual drive; complaints of sexual problems are common among cocaine users presenting for treatment. Psychiatric disorders—including anxiety, depression, and psychosis—are common in cocaine users who request treatment. While some of these psychiatric disorders undoubtedly existed prior to the stimulant use, many develop during the course of the drug abuse (McLellan et al., 1979).

Tolerance, Dependence, and Withdrawal.   Sensitization is a consistent finding in animal studies of cocaine and other stimulants. Sensitization is produced by intermittent use and typically is measured by behavioral hyperactivity. In human cocaine users, sensitization for the euphoric effect typically is not seen. On the contrary, most experienced users report requiring more cocaine over time to obtain euphoria, i.e., tolerance. In the laboratory, tachyphylaxis (rapid tolerance) has been observed with reduced effects when the same dose is given repeatedly in one session. Sensitization may involve conditioning (Figure 24–2). Cocaine users often report a strong response on seeing cocaine before it is administered, consisting of physiological arousal and increased drug craving (O'Brien et al., 1992). Sensitization in human beings has been linked to paranoid, psychotic manifestations of cocaine use based on the observation that cocaine-induced hallucinations are typically seen after long-term exposure (mean 35 months) in vulnerable users (Satel et al., 1991). Repeated administration may be required to sensitize the patient to experience paranoia. Since cocaine typically is used intermittently, even heavy users go through frequent periods of withdrawal or "crash." The symptoms of withdrawal seen in users admitted to the hospital are listed in Table 24–8. Careful studies of cocaine users during withdrawal show gradual diminution of these symptoms over 1 to 3 weeks (Weddington

Table 24–8

Cocaine Withdrawal Symptoms and Signs

Dysphoria, depression
Sleepiness, fatigue
Cocaine craving
Bradycardia

et al., 1990). Residual depression may be seen after cocaine withdrawal and should be treated with antidepressant agents if it persists (*see* Chapter 19).

Pharmacological Interventions. Since cocaine withdrawal generally is mild, treatment of withdrawal symptoms usually is not required. The major problem in treatment is not detoxification but helping the patient to resist the urge to restart compulsive cocaine use. Rehabilitation programs involving individual and group psychotherapy based on the principles of Alcoholics Anonymous and behavioral treatments based on reinforcing, cocaine-free urine tests result in significant improvement in the majority of cocaine users (Alterman *et al.,* 1994; Higgins *et al.,* 1994). Nonetheless, there is great interest in finding a medication that can aid in the rehabilitation of cocaine addicts.

Numerous medications have been tried in clinical trials with cocaine addicts (O'Brien, 1997). While several drugs have been reported in individual studies to produce significant reductions in cocaine use, none has been found to be associated with consistent improvement in controlled clinical trials. The dopamine and serotonin systems have been the focus of many unsuccessful studies using both agonist and antagonist approaches. The concept that works well for opioid addiction, that of a long-acting agonist to satisfy drug craving and stabilize the patient so that normal function is possible, is difficult to transfer to the pharmacology of stimulants. Recent attention has been directed toward two novel approaches: a compound that competes with cocaine at the dopamine transporter and a vaccine that produces cocaine-binding antibodies. However, these should be regarded as innovative ideas that have yet to be shown to be clinically useful. For now, the treatment of choice for cocaine addiction remains behavioral, with medication indicated for specific coexisting disorders such as depression.

Other CNS Stimulants. *Amphetamine and Related Agents.* Subjective effects similar to those of cocaine are produced by *amphetamine, dextroamphetamine, methamphetamine, phenmetrazine, methylphenidate* and *diethylpropion.* Amphetamines increase synaptic dopamine primarily by stimulating presynaptic release rather than by blockade of reuptake, as is the case with cocaine. Intravenous or smoked methamphetamine produces an abuse/dependence syndrome similar to that of cocaine, although clinical deterioration may progress more rapidly. Methamphetamine can be produced in small, clandestine laboratories starting with ephedrine, a widely available nonprescription stimulant. It became a major problem in the western United States during the late 1990s. Oral stim-

ulants, such as those prescribed in weight-reduction programs, have short-term efficacy because of tolerance development. Only a small proportion of patients introduced to these appetite suppressants subsequently exhibit dose escalation or drug-seeking from various physicians. Such patients may meet diagnostic criteria for abuse or addiction. *Fenfluramine* (no longer marketed in the United States) and *phenylpropanolamine* reduce appetite with no evidence of significant abuse potential. *Mazindol* also reduces appetite, with less stimulant properties than amphetamine.

Khat is a plant material widely chewed in East Africa and Yemen for its stimulant properties; these are due to alkaloidal *cathinone,* a compound similar to amphetamine (Kalix, 1990). *Methcathinone,* a congener with similar effects, has been synthesized in clandestine laboratories throughout the midwestern United States, but widespread use in North America has not been reported.

Caffeine. Caffeine, a mild stimulant, is the most widely used psychoactive drug in the world. It is present in soft drinks, coffee, tea, cocoa, chocolate, and numerous prescription and over-the-counter drugs. It increases norepinephrine secretion and enhances neural activity in numerous brain areas. Caffeine is absorbed from the digestive tract; it is rapidly distributed throughout all tissues and easily crosses the placental barrier (*see* Chapter 28). Many of caffeine's effects are believed to occur by means of competitive antagonism at adenosine receptors. Adenosine is a neuromodulator that influences a number of functions in the CNS (*see* Chapters 12 and 28). The mild sedating effects that occur when adenosine activates particular adenosine receptor subtypes can be antagonized by caffeine.

Tolerance occurs rapidly to the stimulating effects of caffeine. Thus, a mild withdrawal syndrome has been produced in controlled studies by abrupt cessation of as little as one to two cups of coffee per day. Caffeine withdrawal consists of feelings of fatigue and sedation. With higher doses, headaches and nausea have been reported during withdrawal; vomiting is rare (Silverman *et al.,* 1992). Although a withdrawal syndrome can be demonstrated, few caffeine users report loss of control of caffeine intake or significant difficulty in reducing or stopping caffeine if desired (Dews *et al.,* 1999). Thus caffeine is not listed in the category of addicting stimulants (American Psychiatric Association, 1994).

Cannabinoids (Marijuana)

The cannabis plant has been cultivated for centuries both for the production of hemp fiber and for its presumed medicinal and psychoactive properties. The smoke from burning cannabis contains many chemicals, including 61 different cannabinoids that have been identified. One of these, Δ-9-tetrahydrocannabinol (Δ-9-THC), produces most of the characteristic pharmacological effects of smoked marijuana.

Surveys have shown that marijuana is the most commonly used nonlegal drug in the United States. Usage peaked during the late 1970s, when about 60% of high school seniors reported having used marijuana and nearly 11% reported daily use. This declined steadily among high school seniors to about 40% reporting some use during their lifetime and 2% reporting daily use in the mid-1990s, followed by a gradual increase to more than 5% reporting daily use in 1999. It must be noted that surveys among high school seniors tend to underestimate drug use because school dropouts are not surveyed.

A cannabinoid receptor has been identified in the brain (Devane *et al.*, 1988) and cloned (Matsuda *et al.*, 1990). An arachidonic acid derivative has been proposed as an endogenous ligand and named *anandamide* (Devane *et al.*, 1992). While the physiological function of these receptors or their putative endogenous ligand has not been fully elucidated, they are widely dispersed, with high densities in the cerebral cortex, hippocampus, striatum, and cerebellum (Herkenham, 1993). Specific cannabinoid receptor antagonists have been developed, and these should facilitate understanding the role of this neurotransmitter system, not only in marijuana abuse but also in normal CNS functions.

The pharmacological effects of Δ-9-THC vary with the dose, route of administration, experience of the user, vulnerability to psychoactive effects, and setting of use. Intoxication with marijuana produces changes in mood, perception, and motivation, but the effect sought after by most users is the "high" and "mellowing out." This effect is described as different from the stimulant high and the opiate high. The effects vary with dose, but the typical marijuana smoker experiences a high that lasts about two hours. During this time, there is impairment of cognitive functions, perception, reaction time, learning, and memory. Impairment of coordination and tracking behavior has been reported to persist for several hours beyond the perception of the high. These impairments have obvious implications for the operation of a motor vehicle and performance in the workplace or at school.

Marijuana also produces complex behavioral changes, such as giddiness and increased hunger. Although some users have reported increased pleasure from sex and increased insight during a marijuana high, these claims have not been substantiated. Unpleasant reactions such as panic or hallucinations and even acute psychosis may occur; several surveys indicate that 50% to 60% of marijuana users have reported at least one anxiety experience. These reactions commonly are seen with higher doses and with oral rather than smoked marijuana, because smoking permits the regulation of dose according to the effects. While there is no convincing evidence that marijuana can produce a lasting schizophrenia-like syndrome, there are numerous clinical reports that marijuana use can precipitate a recurrence in people with a history of schizophrenia.

One of the most controversial of the effects that have been claimed for marijuana is the production of an "amotivational syndrome." This syndrome is not an official diagnosis, but it has been used to describe young people who drop out of social activities and show little interest in school, work, or other goal-directed activity. When heavy marijuana use accompanies these symptoms, the drug often is cited as the cause, even though there are no data that demonstrate a causal relationship between marijuana smoking and these behavioral characteristics. There is no evidence that marijuana use damages brain cells or produces any permanent functional changes, although there are animal data indicating impairment of maze learning that persists for weeks after the last dose. These findings are consistent with clinical reports of gradual improvement in mental state after cessation of chronic high-dose marijuana use.

Several medicinal benefits of marijuana have been described. These include antinausea effects that have been applied to the relief of side effects of anticancer chemotherapy, muscle-relaxing effects, anticonvulsant effects, and reduction of intraocular pressure for the treatment of glaucoma. These medical benefits come at the cost of the psychoactive effects that often impair normal activities. Thus, there is no clear advantage of marijuana over conventional treatments for any of these indications (Institute of Medicine, 1999). With the cloning of cannabinoid receptors and the discovery of an endogenous ligand, it is hoped that medications can be developed that will produce specific therapeutic effects without the undesirable properties of marijuana.

Tolerance, Dependence, and Withdrawal.   Tolerance to most of the effects of marijuana can develop rapidly after only a few doses, but it also disappears rapidly. Tolerance to large doses has been found to persist in experimental animals for long periods after cessation of drug use. Withdrawal symptoms and signs are not typically seen in clinical populations. In fact, relatively few patients ever seek treatment for marijuana addiction. A withdrawal syndrome in human subjects has been described following close observation of marijuana users given regular oral doses of the agent on a research ward (Table 24–9). This syndrome, however, is seen clinically only in persons who use marijuana on a daily basis and then suddenly stop. Compulsive or regular marijuana users do not appear to be motivated by fear of withdrawal symptoms, although this has not been systematically studied.

Table 24–9
Marijuana Withdrawal Syndrome

Restlessness
Irritability
Mild agitation
Insomnia
Sleep EEG disturbance
Nausea, cramping

Pharmacological Interventions. Marijuana abuse and addiction have no specific treatments. Heavy users may suffer from accompanying depression and thus may respond to antidepressant medication, but this should be decided on an individual basis considering the severity of the affective symptoms after the marijuana effects have dissipated. The residual drug effects may continue for several weeks.

Psychedelic Agents

Perceptual distortions that include hallucinations, illusions, and disorders of thinking such as paranoia can be produced by toxic doses of many drugs. These phenomena also may be seen during toxic withdrawal from sedatives such as alcohol. There are, however, certain drugs that have as their primary effect the production of perception, thought, or mood disturbances at low doses with minimal effects on memory and orientation. These are commonly called *hallucinogenic drugs,* but their use does not always result in frank hallucinations. In the late 1990s, the use of "club drugs" at all-night dance parties became popular. Such drugs include *methylenedioxymethamphetamine* ("Ecstasy," MDMA), *lysergic acid diethylamide* (LSD), *phencyclidine* (PCP), and *ketamine.* They often are used in association with illegal sedatives such as *flunitrazepam* (ROHYPNOL) or *gamma hydroxybutyrate* (GHB). The latter drug has the reputation of being particularly effective in preventing memory storage, so it has been implicated in "date rapes."

The use of psychedelics received much public attention in the 1960s and 1970s, but their use waned in the 1980s. In 1989, the use of hallucinogenic drugs again began to increase in the United States. By 1993, a total of 11.8% of college students were reporting some use of these drugs during their lifetime. The increase was most striking in younger cohorts, beginning in the eighth grade.

While psychedelic effects can be produced by a variety of different drugs, major psychedelic compounds come from two main categories. The indoleamine hallucinogens include LSD, DMT (*N,N-dimethyltryptamine*),

and *psilocybin.* The phenethylamines include *mescaline, dimethoxymethylamphetamine* (DOM), *methylenedioxyamphetamine* (MDA), and MDMA. Both groups have a relatively high affinity for serotonin 5-HT$_2$ receptors (*see* Chapter 11), but they differ in their affinity for other subtypes of 5-HT receptors. There is a good correlation between the relative affinity of these compounds for 5-HT$_2$ receptors and their potency as hallucinogens in human beings (Rivier and Pilet, 1971; Titeler *et al.,* 1988). The 5-HT$_2$ receptor is further implicated in the mechanism of hallucinations by the observation that antagonists of that receptor, such as *ritanserin,* are effective in blocking the behavioral and electrophysiological effects of hallucinogenic drugs in animal models. However, LSD has been shown to interact with many receptor subtypes at nanomolar concentrations, and at present it is not possible to attribute the psychedelic effects to any single 5-HT receptor subtype (Peroutka, 1994).

LSD. LSD is the most potent hallucinogenic drug and produces significant psychedelic effects with a total dose of as little as 25 to 50 μg. This drug is more than 3000 times more potent than mescaline. LSD is sold on the illicit market in a variety of forms. A popular contemporary system involves postage stamp–sized papers impregnated with varying doses of LSD (50 to 300 μg or more). A majority of street samples sold as LSD actually contain LSD. In contrast, the samples of mushrooms and other botanicals sold as sources of psilocybin and other psychedelics have a low probability of containing the advertised hallucinogen.

The effects of hallucinogenic drugs are variable, even in the same individual on different occasions. LSD is rapidly absorbed after oral administration, with effects beginning at 40 to 60 minutes, peaking at 2 to 4 hours, and gradually returning to baseline over 6 to 8 hours. At doses of 100 μg, LSD produces perceptual distortions and sometimes hallucinations; mood changes including elation, paranoia, or depression; intense arousal; and sometimes a feeling of panic. Signs of LSD ingestion include pupillary dilation, increased blood pressure and pulse, flushing, salivation, lacrimation, and hyperreflexia. Visual effects are prominent. Colors seem more intense and shapes may appear altered. The subject may focus attention on unusual items such as the pattern of hairs on the back of the hand.

Claims about the potential of psychedelic drugs for enhancing psychotherapy and for treating addictions and other mental disorders have not been supported by controlled treatment outcome studies. Consequently, there is no current indication for these drugs as medications.

A "bad trip" usually consists of severe anxiety, although at times it is marked by intense depression and suicidal thoughts. Visual disturbances usually are prominent. The bad trip from LSD may be difficult to distinguish from reactions to anticholinergic drugs and phencyclidine. There are no documented toxic fatalities from LSD use, but fatal accidents and suicides have occurred during or shortly after intoxication.

Prolonged psychotic reactions lasting two days or more may occur after the ingestion of a hallucinogen. Schizophrenic episodes may be precipitated in susceptible individuals, and there is some evidence that chronic use of these drugs is associated with the development of persistent psychotic disorders (McLellan *et al.*, 1979).

Tolerance, Physical Dependence, and Withdrawal. Frequent, repeated use of psychedelic drugs is unusual, and thus tolerance is not commonly seen. Tolerance does develop to the behavioral effects of LSD after three to four daily doses, but no withdrawal syndrome has been observed. Cross-tolerance among LSD, mescaline, and psilocybin has been demonstrated in animal models.

Pharmacological Intervention. Because of the unpredictability of psychedelic drug effects, any use carries some risk. Dependence and addiction do not occur, but users may require medical attention because of "bad trips." Severe agitation may require medication, and *diazepam* (20 mg orally) has been found to be effective. "Talking down" by reassurance also has been shown to be effective and is the management of first choice. Neuroleptic medications (dopamine receptor antagonists; *see* Chapter 20) may intensify the experience.

A particularly troubling aftereffect of the use of LSD and similar drugs is the occurrence of episodic visual disturbances in a small proportion of former users. These originally were called "flashbacks" and resembled the experiences of prior LSD trips. There now is an official diagnostic category called the *hallucinogen persisting perception disorder* (HPPD) (American Psychiatric Association, 1994). The symptoms include false fleeting perceptions in the peripheral fields, flashes of color, geometric pseudohallucinations, and positive afterimages (Abraham and Aldridge, 1993). The visual disorder appears stable in half of the cases and represents an apparently permanent alteration of the visual system. Precipitants include stress, fatigue, entry into a dark environment, marijuana, neuroleptics, and anxiety states.

MDMA ("Ecstasy") and MDA.

MDMA and MDA are phenylethylamines that have stimulant as well as psychedelic effects. MDMA became popular during the 1980s on college campuses because of testimonials that it enhances insight and self-knowledge. It was recommended by some psychotherapists as an aid to the process of therapy, although no controlled data exist to support this contention. Acute effects are dose-dependent and include tachycardia, dry mouth, jaw clenching, and muscle aches.

At higher doses, the effects include visual hallucinations, agitation, hyperthermia, and panic attacks.

MDA and MDMA produce degeneration of serotonergic nerve cells and axons in rats. While nerve degeneration has not been demonstrated in human beings, the cerebrospinal fluid of chronic MDMA users has been found to contain low levels of serotonin metabolites (Ricaurte *et al.*, 2000). Thus there is possible neurotoxicity with no evidence that the claimed benefits of MDMA actually occur.

Phencyclidine (PCP).   PCP deserves special mention because of its widespread availability and because its pharmacological effects are different from those of the psychedelics such as LSD. PCP originally was developed as an anesthetic in the 1950s and later was abandoned because of a high frequency of postoperative delirium with hallucinations. It was classed as a dissociative anesthetic because, in the anesthetized state, the patient remains conscious with staring gaze, flat facies, and rigid muscles. PCP became a drug of abuse in the 1970s, first in an oral form and then in a smoked version enabling a better regulation of the dose. The effects of PCP have been observed in normal volunteers under controlled conditions. As little as 50 μg/kg produces emotional withdrawal, concrete thinking, and bizarre responses to projective testing. Catatonic posturing also is produced and resembles that of schizophrenia. Abusers taking higher doses may appear to be reacting to hallucinations and exhibit hostile or assaultive behavior. Anesthetic effects increase with dosage; stupor or coma may occur with muscular rigidity, rhabdomyolysis, and hyperthermia. Intoxicated patients in the emergency room may progress from aggressive behavior to coma, with elevated blood pressure and enlarged, nonreactive pupils.

PCP binds with high affinity to sites located in the cortex and limbic structures, resulting in blocking of NMDA-type glutamate receptors (*see* Chapter 12). LSD and other psychedelics do not bind NMDA receptors. There is evidence that NMDA receptors are involved in ischemic neuronal death caused by high levels of excitatory amino acids; as a result, there is interest in PCP analogs that block NMDA receptors but have fewer psychoactive effects.

Tolerance, Dependence, and Withdrawal.   PCP is reinforcing in monkeys, as evidenced by self-administration patterns that produce continuous intoxication (Balster *et al.*, 1973). Human beings tend to use PCP intermittently, but some surveys report daily use in 7% of users queried. There is evidence for tolerance to the behavioral effects of PCP in animals, but this has not been studied systematically in human beings. Signs of a PCP withdrawal syndrome were observed in monkeys after interruption of daily access to the drug. These include somnolence, tremor, seizures, diarrhea, piloerection, bruxism, and vocalizations. ***Pharmacological Intervention.*** Overdose must be treated by life support, since there is no antagonist of PCP effects and no proven way to enhance excretion, although acidification of the urine has been proposed. PCP coma may last 7 to 10 days. The agitated or psychotic state produced by PCP can be treated with *diazepam.* Prolonged psychotic behavior requires neuroleptic medication such as *haloperidol.* Because of the anticholinergic activity of PCP, neuroleptics with significant anticholinergic effects, such as *chlorpromazine,* should be avoided.

Inhalants

Abused inhalants consist of many different categories of chemicals that are volatile at room temperature and produce abrupt changes in mental state when inhaled. Examples include toluene (from airplane glue), kerosene, gasoline, carbon tetrachloride, amyl nitrite, and nitrous oxide (*see* Chapter 68 for a discussion of the toxicology of such agents). There are characteristic patterns of response for each substance. Solvents such as toluene typically are used by children. The material usually is placed in a plastic bag and the vapors inhaled. After several minutes of inhalation, dizziness and intoxication occur. Aerosol sprays containing fluorocarbon propellants are another source of solvent intoxication. Prolonged exposure or daily use may result in damage to several organ systems. Clinical problems include cardiac arrhythmias, bone marrow depression, cerebral degeneration, and damage to liver, kidney, and peripheral nerves. Death occasionally has been attributed to inhalant abuse, probably *via* the mechanism of cardiac arrhythmias, especially accompanying exercise or upper airway obstruction.

Amyl nitrite produces dilation of smooth muscle and has been used in the past for the treatment of angina. It is a yellow, volatile, flammable liquid with a fruity odor. In recent years, amyl nitrite and butyl nitrite have been used to relax smooth muscle and enhance orgasm, particularly by male homosexuals. It is obtained in the form of room deodorizers and can produce a feeling of "rush," flushing, and dizziness. Adverse effects include palpitations, postural hypotension, and headache progressing to loss of consciousness.

Anesthetic gases such as nitrous oxide or halothane are sometimes used as intoxicants by medical personnel. Nitrous oxide also is abused by food service employees, because it is supplied for use as a propellant in disposable aluminum minitanks for whipped-cream canisters. Nitrous oxide produces euphoria and analgesia and then loss of consciousness. Compulsive use and chronic toxicity rarely are reported, but there are obvious risks of overdose associated with the abuse of this anesthetic. Chronic use has been reported to cause peripheral neuropathy.

TREATMENT OF DRUG ABUSE AND ADDICTION

The management of drug abuse and addiction must be individualized according to the drugs involved and to the associated psychosocial problems of the individual patient. Pharmacological interventions have been described for each category when medications are available. An understanding of the pharmacology of the drug or combination of drugs ingested by the patient is essential to rational and effective treatment. This may be a matter of urgency for the treatment of overdose or for the detoxification of a patient who is experiencing withdrawal symptoms. It must be recognized, however, that the treatment of the underlying addictive disorder requires months or years of rehabilitation. The behavior patterns encoded during thousands of prior drug ingestions do not disappear with detoxification from the drug, even after a typical 28-day inpatient rehabilitation program. Long periods of outpatient treatment are necessary. There probably will be periods of relapse and remission. While complete abstinence is the preferred goal, in reality most patients are at risk to slip back to drug-seeking behavior and require a period of retreatment. Maintenance medication can be effective in some circumstances, such as methadone for opioid dependence. The process can best be compared to the treatment of other chronic disorders such as diabetes, asthma, or hypertension. Long-term medication may be necessary, and cures are not likely. When viewed in the context of chronic disease, the available treatments for addiction are quite successful (McLellan *et al.,* 1992; O'Brien, 1994).

Long-term treatment is accompanied by improvements in physical status as well as in mental, social, and occupational function. Unfortunately, there is general pessimism in the medical community about the benefits of treatment, so that most of the therapeutic effort is directed at the complications of addiction, such as pulmonary, cardiac, and hepatic disorders. Prevention of these complications can be accomplished by addressing the underlying addictive disorder.

For further discussion of alcoholism and drug dependency *see* Chapters 386 to 389 in *Harrison's Principles of Internal Medicine,* 14th ed., McGraw-Hill, New York, 1998.

BIBLIOGRAPHY

Alterman, A.I., O'Brien, C.P., McLellan, A.T., August, D.S., Snider, E.C., Droba, M., Cornish, J.W., Hall, C.P., Raphaelson, A.H., and Shrade, F.X. Effectiveness and costs of inpatient versus day hospital cocaine rehabilitation. *J. Nerv. Ment. Dis.,* **1994,** *182*:157–163.

Anthony, J.C., Warner, L.A., and Kessler, K.C. Comparative epidemiology of dependence on tobacco, alcohol, controlled substances and the inhalants: basic findings from the national comorbidity survey. *Exp. Clin. Psychopharmacol.,* **1994,** *2*:244–268.

Balster, R.L., Johanson, C.E., Harris, R.T., and Schuster, C.R. Phencyclidine self-administration in the rhesus monkey. *Pharmacol. Biochem. Behav.,* **1973,** *1*:167–172.

Benowitz, N.L., Porchet, H., Sheiner, L., and Jacob, P. III. Nicotine absorption and cardiovascular effects with smokeless tobacco use: comparison with cigarettes and nicotine gum. *Clin. Pharmacol. Ther.,* **1988,** *44*:23–28.

Chasnoff, I.J., Griffith, D.R., MacGregor, S., Dirkes, K., and Burns, K.A. Temporal patterns of cocaine use in pregnancy. Perinatal outcome. *JAMA,* **1989,** *261*:1741–1744.

Devane, W.A., Dysarz, F.A. III, Johnson, M.R., Melvin, L.S., and Howlett, A.C. Determination and characterization of a cannabinoid receptor in rat brain. *Mol. Pharmacol.,* **1988,** *34*:605–613.

Devane, W.A., Hanus, L., Breuer, A., Pertwee, R.G., Stevenson, L.A., Griffin, G., Gibson, D., Mandelbaum, A., Etinger, A., and Mechoulam, R. Isolation and structure of a brain constituent that binds to the cannabinoid receptor. *Science,* **1992,** *258*:1946–1949.

de Wit, H., Pierri, J., and Johanson, C.E. Assessing individual differences in alcohol preference using a cumulative dosing procedure. *Psychopharmacology,* **1989,** *98*:113–119.

Dews, P.B., Curtis, G.L., Hanford, K.J., and O'Brien, C.P. The frequency of caffeine withdrawal in a population-based survey and in a controlled, blinded pilot experiment. *J. Clin. Pharmacol.,* **1999,** *39*:1221–1232.

Hayashida, M., Alterman, A.I., McLellan, A.T., O'Brien, C.P., Purtill, J.J., Volpicelli, J.R., Raphaelson, A.H., and Hall, C.P. Comparative effectiveness and costs of inpatient and outpatient detoxification of patients with mild-to-moderate alcohol withdrawal syndrome. *N. Engl. J. Med.,* **1989,** *320*:358–365.

Hearn, W.L., Flynn, D.D., Hime, G.W., Rose, S., Cofino, J.C., Mantero-Atienza, E., Wetli, C.V., and Mash, D.C. Cocaethylene: a unique cocaine metabolite displays high affinity for the dopamine transporter. *J. Neurochem.,* **1991,** *56*:698–701.

Higgins, S.T., Budney, A.J., Bickel, W.K., Foerg, F.E., Ogden, D., and Badger, G.J. Outpatient behavioral treatment for cocaine dependence: one-year outcome. Presented at College on Problems of Drug Dependence Symposium, **1994.**

Higuchi S., Matsushita, S., Muramatsu, T., Murayama, M., and Hayashida, M. Alcohol and aldehyde dehydrogenase genetypes and drinking behavior in Japanese. *Alcohol. Clin. Exp. Res.,* **1996,** *20*:493–497.

Kales, A., Scharf, M.B., Kales, J.D., and Soldatos, C.R. Rebound insomnia: a potential hazard following withdrawal of certain benzodiazepines. *JAMA,* **1979,** *241*:1692–1695.

Kalivas, P.W., and Duffy, P. Effect of acute and daily cocaine treatment on extracellular dopamine in the nucleus accumbens. *Synapse,* **1990,** *5*:48–58.

Kosten, T.A. Cocaine attenuates the severity of naloxone-precipitated opioid withdrawal. *Life Sci.,* **1990,** *47*:1617–1623.

Lucki, I., Rickels, K., and Geller, A.M. Chronic use of benzodiazepines

and psychomotor and cognitive test performance. *Psychopharmacology (Berl.),* **1986,** *88*:426–433.

Martin, W.R., and Jasinski, D.R. Psychological parameters of morphine in man: tolerance, early abstinence, protracted abstinence. *J. Psychiatr. Res.,* **1969,** *7*:9–17.

Marzuk, P.M., Tardiff, K., Leon, A.C., Hirsch, C.S., Stajic, M., Portera, L., Hartwell, N., and Iqbal, M.I. Fatal injuries after cocaine use as a leading cause of death among young adults in New York City. *N. Engl. J. Med.,* **1995,** *332*:1753–1757.

Matsuda, L.A., Lolait, S.J., Brownstein, M.J., Young, A.C., and Bonner, T.I. Structure of a cannabinoid receptor and functional expression of the cloned cDNA. *Nature,* **1990,** *346*:561–564.

McLellan, A.T., Woody, G.E., and O'Brien, C.P. Development of psychiatric illness in drug abusers. Possible role of drug preference. *N. Engl. J. Med.,* **1979,** *301*:1310–1314.

Mello, N.K. Short-term memory function in alcohol addicts during intoxication. In, *Advances in Experimental Medicine and Biology.* Vol. 35. *Alcohol Intoxication and Withdrawal: Experimental Studies.* Proceedings of the 39th International Congress on Alcoholism and Drug Dependence. (Gross, M.M., ed.) Plenum Press, New York, **1973,** pp. 333–344.

Mello, N.K., Mendelson, J.H., Bree, M.P., and Lukas, S.E. Buprenorphine suppresses cocaine self-administration by rhesus monkeys. *Science,* **1989,** *245*:859–862.

Mendelson, J.H., and Mello, N.K. Medical progress. Biologic concomitants of alcoholism. *N. Engl. J. Med.,* **1979,** *301*:912–921.

O'Brien, C.P. A range of research-based pharmacotherapies for addiction. *Science,* **1997,** *278*:66–70.

Peroutka, S.J. 5-Hydroxytryptamine receptor interactions of *d*-lysergic acid diethylamide. In, *50 Years of LSD.* (Pletscher, A., and Ladewig, D., eds.) Parthenon Publishing, New York, **1994,** pp. 19–26.

Pianezza, M.L., Sellers, E.M., and Tyndale, R.F. Nicotine metabolism defect reduces smoking. *Nature,* **1998,** *393*:750.

Ricaurte, G.A., McCann, U.D., Szabo, Z., Scheffel, U. Toxicodynamics and long-term toxicity of the recreational drug, 3, 4-methylenedioxy methamphetamine (MDMA, "Ecstasy"). *Toxicol. Lett.,* **2000,** *112–113*:143–146.

Ritz, M.C., Lamb, R.J., Goldberg, S.R., and Kuhar, M.J. Cocaine receptors on dopamine transporters are related to self-administration of cocaine. *Science,* **1987,** *237*:1219–1223.

Rivier, P.L., and Pilet, P.-E. Composés hallucinogènes indoliques naturels. *Année Biol.,* **1971,** *10*:129–149.

Robinson G.M., Sellers, E.M., and Janecek, E. Barbiturate and hypnosedative withdrawal by a multiple oral phenobarbital loading dose technique. *Clin. Pharmacol. Ther.,* **1981,** *30*:71–76.

Russell, M.A.H. Nicotine intake and its regulation by smokers. In, *Advances in Behavioral Biology.* Vol. 31. *Tobacco Smoking and Nicotine.* (Martin, W.R., Van Loon, G.R., Iwamoto, E.T., and Davis, L., eds.) Plenum Press, New York, **1987,** pp. 25–31.

Satel, S.L., Southwick, S.M., and Gawin, F.H. Clinical features of cocaine-induced paranoia. *Am. J. Psychiatry,* **1991,** *148*:495–498.

Schuckit, M.A., and Smith, T.L. An 8-year follow-up of 450 sons of alcoholic and control subjects. *Arch. Gen. Psychol.,* **1996,** *53*:202–210.

Schuckit, M.A., and Smith, T.L. Assessing the risk for alcoholism among sons of alcoholics. *J. Study Alcohol,* **1997,** *58*:141–145.

Siegel, S. Morphine analgesic tolerance: its situation specificity supports a Pavlovian conditioning model. *Science,* **1976,** *193*:323–325.

Silverman, K., Evans, S.M., Strain, E.C., and Griffith, R.R. Withdrawal syndrome after the double-blind cessation of caffeine consumption. *N. Engl. J. Med.,* **1992,** *327*:1109–1114.

Srivastava, E.D., Russell, M.A., Feyerabend, C., Masterson, J.G., and Rhodes, J. Sensitivity and tolerance to nicotine in smokers and nonsmokers. *Psychopharmacology (Berl.),* **1991,** *105*:63–68.

Titeler, M., Lyon, R.A., and Glennon, R.A. Radioligand binding evidence implicates the brain 5-HT$_2$ receptor as a site of action for LSD and phenylisopropylamine hallucinogens. *Psychopharmacology (Berl.),* **1988,** *94*:213–216.

Trujillo, K.A., and Akil, H. Inhibition of morphine tolerance and dependence by the NMDA receptor antagonist MK-801. *Science,* **1991,** *251*:85–87.

Volkow, N.D., Wang, G.L., Fowler, J.S., Logan, J., Gatley, S.J., Wong, C., Hitzemann, R., and Pappas, N.R. Reinforcing effects of psychostimulants in humans are associated with increases in brain dopamine and occupancy of D(2) receptors. *J. Pharmacol. Exp. Ther.,* **1999,** *291*:409–415.

Weddington, W.W., Brown, B.S., Haertzen, C.A., Cone, E.J., Dax, E.M., Herning, R.I., and Michaelson, B.S. Changes in mood, craving, and sleep during short-term abstinence reported by male cocaine addicts. A controlled, residential study. *Arch. Gen. Psychiatry,* **1990,** *47*:861–868.

Wikler, A. Conditioning of successive adaptive responses to the initial effects of drugs. *Cond. Reflex,* **1973,** *8*:193–210.

MONOGRAPHS AND REVIEWS

Abraham, H.D., and Aldridge, A.M. Adverse consequences of lysergic acid diethylamide. *Addiction,* **1993,** *88*:1327–1334.

American Psychiatric Association. *Diagnostic and Statistical Manual of Mental Disorders,* 4th ed. (DSM-IV). Washington, D.C., **1994.**

American Psychiatric Association. *Benzodiazepine Dependence, Toxicity, and Abuse. A Task Force Report of the American Psychiatric Association.* Washington, D.C., **1990.**

Grant, I. Alcohol and the brain: neuropsychological correlates. *J. Consult Clin. Psychol.,* **1987,** *55*:310–324.

Herkenham, M.A. Localization of cannabinoid receptors in brain: relationship to motor and reward systems. In, *Biological Basis of Substance Abuse.* (Korenman, S.G., and Barchas, J.D., eds.) Oxford University Press, New York, **1993,** pp. 187–200.

Institute of Medicine. *Marijuana and Medicine.* National Academy Press, Washington, D.C., **1999.**

Kalix, P. Pharmacological properties of the stimulant khat. *Pharmacol. Ther.,* **1990,** *48*:397–416.

Kreek, M.J. Rationale for maintenance pharmacotherapy of opiate dependence. In, *Addictive States.* (O'Brien, C.P., and Jaffe, J.H., eds.) Raven Press, New York, **1992,** pp. 205–230.

Lader, M., and File, S. The biological basis of benzodiazepine dependence. *Psychol. Med.,* **1987,** *17*:539–547.

McLellan, A.T., O'Brien, C.P., Metzger, D., Alterman, A.I., Cornish, J., and Urschel, H. How effective is substance abuse treatment—compared to what? In, *Addictive States.* (O'Brien, C.P., and Jaffe, J., eds.) Raven Press, New York, **1992,** pp. 231–252.

O'Brien, C.P. Treatment of alcoholism as a chronic disorder. In, *Toward a Molecular Basis of Alcohol Use and Abuse. EXS.* Vol. 71. (Jansson, B., Jörnvall, H., Rydberg, U., Terenius, L., and Vallee, B.L., eds.) Birkhäuser Verlag, Basel, Switzerland, **1994,** pp. 349–359.

O'Brien, C.P., Childress, A.R., McLellan, A.T., and Ehrman, R. Classical conditioning in drug-dependent humans. *Ann. N.Y. Acad. Sci.,* **1992,** *654*:400–415.

Schuckit, M.A. New findings in the genetics of alcholism. *JAMA,* **1999,** *281*:1875–1876.

S E C T I O N   I V

AUTACOIDS; DRUG THERAPY OF INFLAMMATION

INTRODUCTION

Jason D. Morrow and L. Jackson Roberts II

The substances that are considered in this section have diverse physiological and pharmacological activities. They are grouped together in large part because they participate, at least in some settings, in physiological or pathophysiological responses to injury. At the same time, the opportunity is taken to discuss drugs that antagonize their actions or inhibit their elaboration, wherever such drugs are available. Included in Chapter 25 are discussions of histamine and bradykinin and their respective antagonists. Serotonin (5-hydroxytryptamine), another contributor to inflammatory response, is presented in Chapter 11. Chapter 26 is devoted to lipid substances that are generated by biotransformation of the products of the selective hydrolysis of membrane phospholipids—the eicosanoids (prostaglandins, thromboxanes, and leukotrienes) and platelet-activating factor. Chapter 27 deals with aspirin and aspirin-like drugs (nonsteroidal antiinflammatory agents), including selective inhibitors of the inducible cyclooxygenase, cyclooxygenase-2, which owe their therapeutic utility in large part to their capacity to inhibit the synthesis of prostaglandins and thromboxanes. Chapter 28 addresses the treatment of asthma by a variety of agents and the change in therapeutic strategy since the recognition that asthma is an inflammatory disease.

This section thus includes discussion of an array of substances that are normally present in the body or may be formed there; although these substances function in humoral regulation, they cannot be classed conveniently with other members of this broad group, such as the hormones and neurotransmitters. Because these substances usually have a brief lifetime and act near their sites of synthesis, they often have been described as local hormones. However, unlike true hormones, which reach their sites of action *via* the bloodstream, these substances often conduct their affairs closeted from the circulation, such as in the confines of an inflammatory lesion. Hence, the term *autacoid,* from the Greek *autos* ("self") and *akos* ("medicinal agent" or "remedy"), seems more appropriate and will be used in this section.

In many ways, the grouping of these substances under the rubric of "autacoids" is arbitrary. Not included here is an array of peptides that are elaborated by specialized cells within certain endocrine glands and in glands of the digestive system, whose actions are often exerted primarily on neighboring cells; these usually are described as *paracrine* hormones and include compounds such as somatostatin and gastrin. Indeed, histamine has important paracrine functions in the regulation of gastric acid secretion; these are considered in Chapter 37. Since many of these substances also are distributed by the circulation for additional actions at more distant locations, they may well deserve to be called hormones. Another omission is the burgeoning array of cytokines that mediate the complex interactions involved in humoral and cellular immune responses. In part, these substances share with autacoids their participation in inflammation and local regulatory function. Cytokines and agents that modulate their production are discussed in detail in Chapter 53. However they are defined, autacoids and related locally acting substances clearly are part and parcel of the physiological and pathological phenomena that provide the rationale for drug therapy; their existence provides numerous possibilities for therapeutic intervention by the use of drugs that mimic or antagonize their actions or interfere with their synthesis or metabolism.

HISTAMINE, BRADYKININ, AND THEIR ANTAGONISTS

Nancy J. Brown and L. Jackson Roberts II

This chapter describes the physiological role and pathophysical consequences of histamine release and provides a summary of the therapeutic use of histamine H_1-receptor antagonists. H_2-receptor antagonists are discussed in detail in Chapter 37 in the context of prevention and treatment of peptic ulcers, their principal therapeutic application. The identity and role of H_2-receptor subtypes are described briefly, as are the newly developed H_3 agonists and antagonists, although none has been approved by the U.S. Food and Drug Administration (FDA) for clinical use to date.

The second part of the chapter describes the physiology and pathophysiology of the kinins and kallidins, a subset of autacoids that contribute to the inflammatory response. The identification of at least two distinct receptors for kinins, designated B_1 and B_2, allows for the development of selective receptor antagonists, which also are discussed. Serotonin (5-hydroxytryptamine; 5-HT), another autacoid often considered in the same context as histamine and the kinin and kallidin agents, is discussed in detail in Chapter 11.

HISTAMINE

History. The history of β-aminoethylimidazole, or histamine, parallels that of acetylcholine (ACh). Both compounds were synthesized as chemical curiosities before their biological significance was recognized; both were first detected as uterine stimulants in extracts of ergot, from which they were subsequently isolated; and both proved to be contaminants of ergot that resulted from bacterial action.

When Dale and Laidlaw (1910, 1911) subjected histamine to intensive pharmacological study, they discovered that it stimulated a host of smooth muscles and had an intense vasodepressor action. Remarkably, they pointed out that the immediate signs displayed by a sensitized animal when injected with a normally inert protein closely resemble those of poisoning by histamine. These comments anticipated by many years the discovery of the presence of histamine in the body and its release during immediate hypersensitivity reactions and upon cellular injury. It was not until 1927 that Best *et al.* isolated histamine from very fresh samples of liver and lung, thereby establishing that this amine is a natural constituent of the body. Demonstrations of its presence in a variety of other tissues soon followed—hence the name *histamine* after the Greek word for tissue, *histos*.

Meanwhile, Lewis and his colleagues had amassed evidence that a substance with the properties of histamine ("H-substance") was liberated from the cells of the skin by injurious stimuli, including the reaction of antigen with antibody (Lewis, 1927). Given the chemical evidence of histamine's presence in the body, there remained little impediment to supposing that Lewis' "H-substance" was histamine itself. It is now evident that endogenous histamine plays a role in the immediate al-

lergic response and is an important regulator of gastric acid secretion. More recently, a role for histamine as a modulator of neurotransmitter release in the central and peripheral nervous systems also has emerged.

Early suspicions that histamine acts through more than one receptor have been borne out, and it is clear that there are at least three distinct classes of receptors for histamine, designated H_1 (Ash and Schild, 1966), H_2 (Black *et al.*, 1972), and H_3 (Arrang *et al.*, 1983). H_1 receptors are blocked selectively by the classical "antihistamines" (such as pyrilamine) developed around 1940. H_2-receptor antagonists were introduced in the early 1970s. The discovery of H_2 antagonists has contributed greatly to the resurgence of interest in histamine in biology and clinical medicine (*see* Chapter 37). H_3 receptors were originally discovered as a presynaptic autoreceptor on histamine-containing neurons that mediate feedback inhibition of the release and synthesis of histamine. The recent development of selective H_3-receptor agonists and antagonists has led to an increased understanding of the importance of H_3 receptors in histaminergic neurons *in vivo*. None of these H_3-receptor agonists or antagonists, however, has yet emerged as a therapeutic agent. Renewed interest in clinical use of H_1-receptor antagonists has occurred over the past 15 years due to the development of second-generation antagonists, collectively referred to as *nonsedating antihistamines*.

Chemistry. Histamine is a hydrophilic molecule comprising an imidazole ring and an amino group connected by two methylene groups. The pharmacologically active form at all histamine receptors is the monocationic $N\gamma$—H tautomer—that is, the charged form of the species depicted in Figure 25–1, although

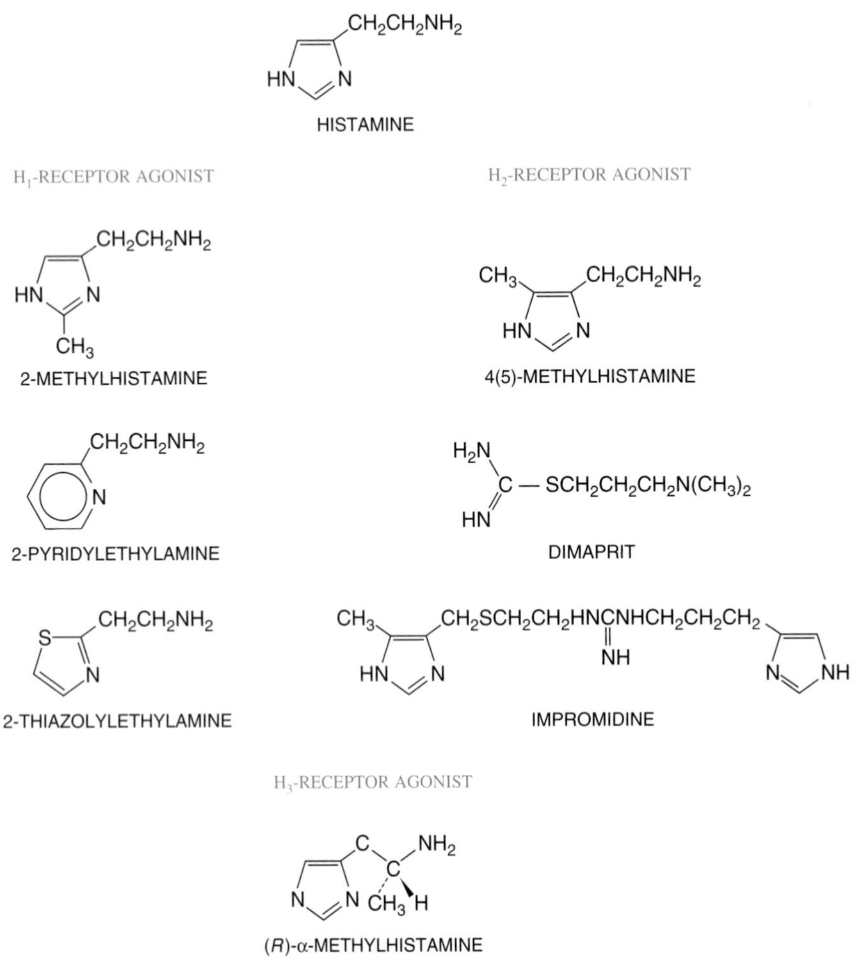

CH₂CH₂NH₂ attached to imidazole ring (HN, N)

HISTAMINE

H₁-RECEPTOR AGONIST   H₂-RECEPTOR AGONIST

CH₂CH₂NH₂ on imidazole with CH₃ (HN, N)

2-METHYLHISTAMINE

CH₃, CH₂CH₂NH₂ on imidazole (HN, N)

4(5)-METHYLHISTAMINE

CH₂CH₂NH₂ on pyridine ring (N)

2-PYRIDYLETHYLAMINE

H₂N, C—SCH₂CH₂CH₂N(CH₃)₂, HN

DIMAPRIT

CH₂CH₂NH₂ on thiazole ring (S, N)

2-THIAZOLYLETHYLAMINE

CH₃, CH₂SCH₂CH₂HNCNHCH₂CH₂CH₂, imidazole rings (HN, N ... N, NH), NH

IMPROMIDINE

H₃-RECEPTOR AGONIST

C, NH₂ on imidazole (N, N, CH₃, H)

(R)-α-METHYLHISTAMINE

Figure 25–1. Structure of histamine and some H₁, H₂, and H₃ agonists.

different chemical properties of this monocation may be involved in interactions with the H₁ and H₂ receptors (Ganellin, in Ganellin and Parsons, 1982). The three classes of histamine receptors can be activated differently by analogs of histamine (*see* Figure 25–1). Thus, 2-methylhistamine preferentially elicits responses mediated by H₁ receptors, whereas 4(5)-methylhistamine has a preferential effect on H₂ receptors (Black *et al.,* 1972). A chiral analog of histamine with restricted conformational freedom, (*R*)-α-methylhistamine, is the preferred agonist at H₃-receptor sites (Arrang *et al.,* 1987).

Distribution and Biosynthesis of Histamine

Distribution. Histamine is widely, if unevenly, distributed throughout the animal kingdom and is present in many venoms, bacteria, and plants. Almost all mammalian tissues contain histamine in amounts ranging from less than 1 μg/g to more than 100 μg/g. Concentrations in plasma and other body fluids generally are very low, but human cerebrospinal fluid contains significant amounts. The mast cell is the predominant storage site for histamine in most tissues (*see* below); the concentration of histamine is particularly high in tissues that contain large

numbers of mast cells, such as skin, the mucosa of the bronchial tree, and the intestinal mucosa. However, some tissues synthesize and turn over histamine at a remarkably fast rate, even though their steady-state content of the amine may be modest.

Synthesis, Storage, and Metabolism. Histamine, in the amounts normally ingested or formed by bacteria in the gastrointestinal tract, is rapidly metabolized and eliminated in the urine. Every mammalian tissue that contains histamine is capable of synthesizing it from histidine by virtue of its content of L-histidine decarboxylase. The chief site of histamine storage in most tissues is the mast cell; in the blood, it is the basophil. These cells synthesize histamine and store it in secretory granules. At the secretory granule pH of ~5.5, histamine is positively charged and ionically complexed with negatively charged acidic groups on other secretory granule constituents, primarily proteases and heparin or chondroitin sulfate proteoglycans (Serafin and Austen, 1987). The turnover rate of histamine in secretory granules is slow, and when tissues rich in mast cells are depleted of their stores of histamine, it may take weeks before concentrations of the autacoid return to normal levels. Non-mast-cell sites of histamine formation or storage include cells

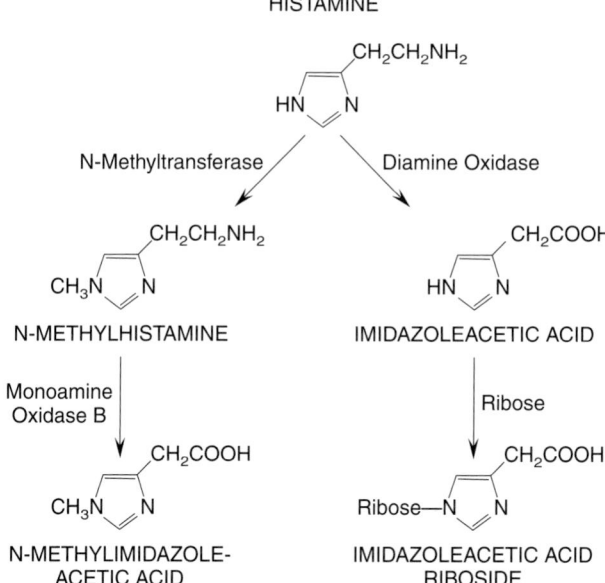

Figure 25–2. Pathways of histamine metabolism in human beings.

See text for further explanation.

of the epidermis, cells in the gastric mucosa, neurons within the central nervous system (CNS), and cells in regenerating or rapidly growing tissues. Turnover is rapid at these sites, since the histamine is continuously released rather than stored. Non-mast-cell sites of histamine production contribute significantly to the daily excretion of histamine and its metabolites in the urine. Since L-histidine decarboxylase is an inducible enzyme, the histamine-forming capacity at such non-mast-cell sites is subject to regulation by various physiological and pathophysiological factors.

There are two major paths of histamine metabolism in human beings (Figure 25–2). The more important of these involves ring methylation to form *N*-methylhistamine. This is catalyzed by histamine-*N*-methyltransferase, which is widely distributed. Most of the *N*-methylhistamine formed is then converted by monoamine oxidase (MAO) to *N*-methylimidazoleacetic acid. This reaction can be blocked by MAO inhibitors (*see* Chapter 19). Alternatively, histamine undergoes oxidative deamination catalyzed mainly by the nonspecific enzyme diamine oxidase (DAO), yielding imidazoleacetic acid, which is then converted to imidazoleacetic acid riboside. These metabolites have little or no activity and are excreted in the urine. One important aspect regarding these metabolites, however, is that it has been shown that measurement of *N*-methylhistamine in urine affords a more reliable index of endogenous histamine production than does measurement of histamine, because it circumvents the problem of artifactually elevated levels of histamine in urine that can arise from the ability of some genitourinary tract bacteria to decarboxylate histidine (Roberts and Oates, 1991). In addition, the metabolism of histamine appears to be altered in patients with mastocytosis such that measurement of histamine metabolites

has been shown to be a more sensitive diagnostic indicator of the disease than is measurement of histamine (Keyzer *et al.*, 1983).

Functions of Endogenous Histamine

Histamine has important physiological roles. Because histamine is one of the preformed mediators stored in the mast cell, its release as a result of the interaction of antigen with IgE antibodies on the mast cell surface plays a central role in immediate hypersensitivity and allergic responses. The actions of histamine on bronchial smooth muscle and blood vessels account in part for the symptoms of the allergic response. In addition, certain clinically useful drugs can act directly on mast cells to release histamine, thereby explaining some of their untoward effects. Histamine has a major role in the regulation of gastric acid secretion, and its function as a modulator of neurotransmitter release has recently become appreciated.

Role in Allergic Responses.   The principal target cells of immediate hypersensitivity reactions are mast cells and basophils (Galli, 1993; Schwartz, 1994). As part of the allergic response to an antigen, reaginic antibodies (IgE) are generated and bind to the surface of mast cells and basophils *via* high-affinity F_c receptors that are specific for IgE. This receptor, FcεRI, consists of α, β, and two γ chains, all of which have been molecularly characterized (Ravetch and Kinet, 1991). The IgE molecules function as receptors for antigens, and *via* FcεRI, interact with signal transduction systems in the membranes of sensitized cells. Atopic individuals, as opposed to those who are not, develop IgE antibodies to commonly inhaled antigens. This is a heritable trait, and a candidate gene has been identified (Cookson *et al.*, 1992; Shirakawa *et al.*, 1994). Since the candidate gene encodes the β-chain of FcεRI, an even greater interest has been generated for understanding the transmembrane signaling mechanisms of mast cells and basophils. Upon exposure, antigen bridges the IgE molecules and causes activation of tyrosine kinases and subsequent phosphorylation of multiple protein substrates within 5 to 15 seconds after contact with antigen (Scharenberg and Kinet in Symposium, 1994). Kinases implicated in this event include the *src*-related kinases lyn and syk. Prominent among the newly phosphorylated proteins are the β and γ subunits of the FcεRI itself and phospholipase Cγ1 and Cγ2. Subsequently, inositol phospholipids are metabolized, with a result being the release of Ca^{2+} from intracellular stores, thereby raising free cytosolic Ca^{2+} levels (*see* Chapter 2). These events trigger the extrusion of the contents of secretory granules by exocytosis. The secretory behavior of mast cells and basophils is similar to that of various endocrine and exocrine glands and conforms to a general pattern of stimulus-secretion coupling in which a secretagogue-induced rise in the intracellular concentration of Ca^{2+} serves to initiate exocytosis. The mechanism by which the rise in Ca^{2+} leads to fusion of the secretory granule with the plasma membrane is not fully elucidated, but is likely to involve activation of Ca^{2+}/calmodulin-dependent protein kinases and protein kinase C.

Release of Other Autacoids. The release of histamine provides only a partial explanation for all of the biological effects that ensue from immediate hypersensitivity reactions. This is because a broad spectrum of other inflammatory mediators is released upon mast cell activation.

In addition to activation of phospholipase C and the hydrolysis of inositol phospholipids, stimulation of IgE receptors also activates phospholipase A_2, leading to the production of a host of mediators, including platelet-activating factor (PAF) and metabolites of arachidonic acid. Leukotriene D_4, which is generated in this way, is a potent contractor of the smooth muscle of the bronchial tree (*see* Chapters 26 and 28). Kinins also are generated during some allergic responses (*see* below). Thus, the mast cell secretes a variety of inflammatory compounds in addition to histamine, and each contributes to varying extents to the major symptoms of the allergic response: constriction of the bronchi, decrease in blood pressure, increased capillary permeability, and edema formation (*see* below).

Regulation of Mediator Release. The wide variety of mediators released during the allergic response explains the ineffectiveness of drug therapy focused on a single mediator. Considerable emphasis has been placed on the regulation of mediator release from mast cells and basophils, and these cells do contain receptors linked to signaling systems that can enhance or block the IgE-induced release of mediators.

Agents that act at muscarinic or α-adrenergic receptors enhance the release of mediators, although this effect is of little clinical significance. Effective inhibition of the secretory response can be achieved with epinephrine and related drugs that act through β_2-adrenergic receptors. The effect is the result of accumulation of cyclic AMP. However, the beneficial effects of β-adrenergic agonists in allergic states such as asthma are due mainly to their relaxant effect on bronchial smooth muscle (*see* Chapters 10 and 28). Cromolyn sodium owes its clinical utility to its capacity to inhibit the release of mediators from mast and other cells in the lung (*see* Chapter 28).

Histamine Release by Drugs, Peptides, Venoms, and Other Agents. Many compounds, including a large number of therapeutic agents, stimulate the release of histamine from mast cells directly and without prior sensitization. Responses of this sort are most likely to occur following intravenous injections of certain categories of substances, particularly those that are organic bases. Among these bases are amides, amidines, quaternary ammonium compounds, pyridinium compounds, piperidines, alkaloids, and antibiotic bases. Tubocurarine, succinylcholine, morphine, radiocontrast media, and certain carbohydrate plasma expanders also may elicit the response. The phenomenon is one of clinical concern, for it may account for unexpected anaphylactoid reactions. Vancomycin-induced "red-man syndrome" involving upper body and facial flushing and hypotension may be mediated, at least in part if not entirely, through histamine release (Levy *et al.,* 1987).

In addition to therapeutic agents, certain experimental compounds stimulate the release of histamine as their dominant pharmacological characteristic. The archetype is the polybasic substance known as compound 48/80. This is a mixture of low-molecular-weight polymers of *p*-methoxy-*N*-methylphenethyl-amine, of which the hexamer is most active (*see* Lagunoff *et al.,* 1983).

Basic polypeptides often are effective histamine releasers, and their potency generally increases with the number of basic groups over a limited range. Polymyxin B is very active; others include bradykinin and substance P. Since basic polypeptides are released upon tissue injury or are present in venoms, they constitute pathophysiological stimuli to secretion for mast cells and basophils. Anaphylotoxins (C3a and C5a), which are low-molecular-weight peptides that are cleaved from the complement system, may act similarly.

Within seconds of the intravenous injection of a histamine liberator, human subjects experience a burning, itching sensation. This effect, most marked in the palms of the hand and in the face, scalp, and ears, is soon followed by a feeling of intense warmth. The skin reddens, and the color rapidly spreads over the trunk. Blood pressure falls, the heart rate accelerates, and the subject usually complains of headache. After a few minutes, blood pressure recovers, and crops of hives usually appear on the skin. Colic, nausea, hypersecretion of acid, and moderate bronchospasm also occur frequently. The effect becomes less intense with successive injections as the mast-cell stores of histamine are depleted. Histamine liberators do not deplete tissues of non-mast-cell histamine.

Mechanism. All of the above-mentioned histamine-releasing substances can activate the secretory response of mast cells or basophils by causing a rise in intracellular Ca^{2+}. Some are ionophores and transport Ca^{2+} into the cell; others, such as the anaphylotoxins, appear to act like specific antigens to increase membrane permeability to Ca^{2+}. Still others, such as mastoparan (a peptide from wasp venom), may bypass cell-surface receptors and directly stimulate guanine nucleotide–binding regulatory proteins (G proteins), which then activate phospholipase C (Higashijima *et al.,* 1988). Basic histamine releasers, such as compound 48/80 and polymyxin B, act principally by mobilizing Ca^{2+} from cellular stores (*see* Lagunoff *et al.,* 1983).

Histamine Release by Other Means. Clinical conditions in which release of histamine occurs in response to other stimuli include cold urticaria, cholinergic urticaria, and solar urticaria. Some of these involve specific secretory responses of the mast cells and, indeed, cell-fixed IgE. However, histamine release also occurs whenever there is nonspecific cell damage from any cause. The redness and urticaria that follow scratching of the skin is a familiar example.

Gastric Carcinoid Tumors and Increased Proliferation of Mast Cells and Basophils. In urticaria pigmentosa (cutaneous mastocytosis), mast cells aggregate in the upper corium and give rise to pigmented cutaneous lesions that urticate when stroked. In systemic mastocytosis, overproliferation of mast cells also is found in other organs. Patients with these syndromes suffer a constellation of signs and symptoms attributable to excessive histamine release, including urticaria, dermographism, pruritus, headache, weakness, hypotension, flushing of the face, and a variety of gastrointestinal effects such as peptic ulceration. Episodes of mast cell activation with attendant systemic histamine release are precipitated by a variety of stimuli, including exertion, emotional upset, and exposure to heat, and from exposure to drugs that release histamine directly or to which patients are allergic. In myelogenous leukemia, excessive numbers of basophils are present in the blood raising its histamine content to high levels, which may contribute to chronic pruritus.

Gastric carcinoid tumors secrete histamine, which is responsible for episodes of vasodilation and contributes to the patchy "geographical" flush (Roberts *et al.,* 1979).

Gastric Acid Secretion.   Histamine is a powerful gastric secretagogue and evokes a copious secretion of acid from parietal cells by acting on H_2 receptors. The output of pepsin and intrinsic factor also is increased. However, the secretion of acid also is evoked by stimulation of the vagus nerve and by the enteric hormone gastrin. In addition, there appear to be cells in the gastric mucosa that contain somatostatin, which can inhibit secretion of acid by parietal cells; the release of somatostatin is inhibited by acetylcholine. The interplay among these endogenous regulators has not been precisely defined. However, it is clear that histamine is the dominant physiological mediator of acid secretion because blockade of H_2 receptors can not only eradicate acid secretion in response to histamine, but also cause nearly complete inhibition of responses to gastrin or vagal stimulation. This is discussed in more detail in Chapter 37.

Central Nervous System.   There is substantial evidence that histamine functions as a neurotransmitter in the CNS. Histamine, histidine decarboxylase, and enzymes that catalyze the degradation of histamine are distributed nonuniformly in the CNS and are concentrated in synaptosomal fractions of brain homogenates. H_1 receptors are found throughout the CNS and are densely concentrated in the hypothalamus. Histamine increases wakefulness *via* H_1 receptors (Monti, 1993), explaining the potential for sedation by classical antihistamines. Histamine acting through H_1 receptors inhibits appetite (Ookuma *et al.,* 1993). Histamine-containing neurons may participate in the regulation of drinking, body temperature, and the secretion of antidiuretic hormone, as well as in the control of blood pressure and the perception of pain. Both H_1 and H_2 receptors seem to be involved in these responses (*see* Hough, 1988).

Pharmacological Effects: H_1 and H_2 Receptors

Once released, histamine can exert local or widespread effects on smooth muscles and glands. The autacoid contracts many smooth muscles, such as those of the bronchi and gut, but powerfully relaxes others, including those of small blood vessels. It also is a potent stimulus to gastric acid secretion. Effects attributable to these actions dominate the overall response to histamine; however, there are other effects, such as formation of edema and stimulation of sensory nerve endings. Many of these effects, such as bronchoconstriction and contraction of the gut, are mediated by H_1 receptors (Ash and Schild, 1966). Other effects, most notably gastric secretion, are the results of activation of H_2 receptors and, accordingly, can be inhibited by H_2-receptor antagonists (Black *et al.,* 1972). Some responses, such as the hypotension that results from vascular dilation, are mediated by both H_1 and H_2 receptors.

Histamine Toxicity from Ingestion.   Histamine has been identified as the toxin in food poisoning from spoiled scombroid fish, such as tuna (Morrow *et al.,* 1991). Bacteria in spoiled scombroid fish, which have a high histidine content, decarboxylate histidine to form large quantities of histamine. Ingestion of the fish causes severe nausea, vomiting, headache, flushing, and sweating. Histamine toxicity, manifested by headache and other symptoms, also can be seen following red wine consumption in persons who possibly have a diminished ability to degrade histamine (Wantke *et al.,* 1994). The symptoms of histamine poisoning can be suppressed by H_1 receptor antagonists.

Cardiovascular System.   Histamine characteristically causes dilation of small blood vessels, resulting in flushing, lowered total peripheral resistance, and a fall in systemic blood pressure. In addition, histamine tends to increase capillary permeability.

Vasodilation.   This is the characteristic action of histamine on the vasculature, and it is by far the most important vascular effect of histamine in human beings. Vasodilation involves both H_1 and H_2 receptors distributed throughout the resistance vessels in most vascular beds; however, quantitative differences are apparent in the degree of dilation that occurs in various beds. Activation of either the H_1 or H_2 type of histamine receptor can elicit maximal vasodilation, but the responses differ in their sensitivity to histamine, in the duration of the effect, and in the mechanism of their production. H_1 receptors have the higher affinity for histamine and mediate a dilator response that is relatively rapid in onset and short lived. By contrast, activation of H_2 receptors causes dilation that develops more slowly and is more sustained. As a result, H_1 antagonists effectively counter small dilator responses to low concentrations of histamine but only blunt the initial phase of larger responses to higher concentrations of the amine. H_2 receptors are located on vascular smooth muscle cells, and the vasodilator effects produced by their stimulation are mediated by cyclic AMP; H_1 receptors reside on endothelial cells, and their stimulation leads to the formation of local vasodilator substances (*see* below).

Increased "Capillary" Permeability.   This classical effect of histamine on small vessels results in outward passage of plasma protein and fluid into the extracellular spaces, an increase in the flow of lymph and its protein content, and formation of edema. H_1 receptors clearly are important for this response; whether or not H_2 receptors also participate is uncertain.

Increased permeability results mainly from actions of histamine on postcapillary venules, where histamine causes the endothelial cells to contract and separate at their boundaries and thus to expose the basement membrane, which is freely permeable to plasma protein and fluid. The gaps between endothelial cells also may permit passage of circulating cells that are recruited to the tissues during the mast-cell response. Recruitment of circulating leukocytes is promoted by H_1-receptor–mediated upregulation of leukocyte adhesion. This process involves histamine-induced expression of the adhesion molecule P-selectin on the endothelial cells (Gaboury *et al.*, 1995).

Triple Response.   If histamine is injected intradermally, it elicits a characteristic phenomenon known as the "triple response" (Lewis, 1927). This consists of (1) a localized red spot, extending for a few millimeters around the site of injection, that appears within a few seconds and reaches a maximum in about a minute; (2) a brighter red flush, or "flare," extending about 1 cm or so beyond the original red spot and developing more slowly; and (3) a wheal that is discernible in 1 to 2 minutes and occupies the same area as the original small red spot at the injection site. The red spot results from the direct vasodilatory effect of histamine, the flare is due to histamine-induced stimulation of axon reflexes that cause vasodilation indirectly, and the wheal reflects histamine's capacity to increase capillary permeability.

Constriction of Larger Vessels.   Histamine tends to constrict larger blood vessels, in some species more than in others. In rodents, the effect extends to the level of the arterioles and may overshadow dilation of the finer blood vessels. A net increase in total peripheral resistance and an elevation of blood pressure can be observed.

Heart.   Histamine has direct actions on the heart that affect both contractility and electrical events. It increases the force of contraction of both atrial and ventricular muscle by promoting the influx of Ca^{2+}, and it speeds heart rate by hastening diastolic depolarization in the SA node. It also acts directly to slow AV conduction, to increase automaticity, and, in high doses especially, to elicit arrhythmias. With the exception of slowed AV conduction, which involves mainly H_1 receptors, all these effects are largely attributable to H_2 receptors. If histamine is given intravenously, direct cardiac effects of histamine are not prominent and are overshadowed by baroreceptor reflexes elicited by the reduced blood pressure.

Histamine Shock.   Histamine given in large doses or released during systemic anaphylaxis causes a profound and progressive fall in blood pressure. As the small blood vessels dilate, they trap large amounts of blood, and as their permeability increases, plasma escapes from the circulation. Resembling surgical or traumatic shock, these effects diminish effective blood volume, reduce venous return, and greatly lower cardiac output.

Extravascular Smooth Muscle.   Histamine stimulates, or more rarely relaxes, various smooth muscles. Contraction is due to activation of H_1 receptors and relaxation (for the most part) to activation of H_2 receptors. Responses vary widely, even in individuals (*see* Parsons, in Ganellin and Parsons, 1982). Bronchial muscle of guinea pigs is exquisitely sensitive. Minute doses of histamine also will evoke intense bronchoconstriction in patients with bronchial asthma and certain other pulmonary diseases; in normal human beings the effect is much less pronounced. Although the spasmogenic influence of H_1

receptors is dominant in human bronchial muscle, H_2 receptors with dilator function also are present. Thus, histamine-induced bronchospasm *in vitro* is potentiated slightly by H_2 blockade. In asthmatic subjects in particular, histamine-induced bronchospasm may involve an additional, reflex component that arises from irritation of afferent vagal nerve endings (*see* Eyre and Chand, in Ganellin and Parsons, 1982; Nadel and Barnes, 1984).

The uterus of some species contracts to histamine; in the human uterus, gravid or not, the response is negligible. Responses of intestinal muscle also vary with species and region, but the classical effect is contraction. Bladder, ureter, gallbladder, iris, and many other smooth muscle preparations are affected little or inconsistently by histamine.

Exocrine Glands.   As mentioned above, histamine is an important physiological regulator of gastric acid secretion. This effect is mediated by H_2 receptors (*see* Chapter 37).

Nerve Endings: Pain, Itch, and Indirect Effects.   Histamine stimulates various nerve endings. Thus, when released in the epidermis, it causes itch; in the dermis, it evokes pain, sometimes accompanied by itching. Stimulant actions on one or another type of nerve ending, including autonomic afferents and efferents, have been mentioned above as factors that contribute to the "flare" component of the triple response and to indirect effects of histamine on the bronchi and other organs. In the periphery, neuronal receptors for histamine are generally of the H_1 type (*see* Rocha e Silva, 1978; Ganellin and Parsons, 1982).

Mechanism of Action.   The H_1 and H_2 receptors have been cloned and shown to belong to the superfamily of G protein–coupled receptors. H_1 receptors are coupled to phospholipase C, and their activation leads to formation of inositol-1,4,5-trisphosphate (IP_3) and diacylglycerols from phospholipids in the cell membrane; IP_3 causes a rapid release of Ca^{2+} from the endoplasmic reticulum. Diacylglycerols (and Ca^{2+}) activate protein kinase C, while Ca^{2+} activates Ca^{2+}/calmodulin-dependent protein kinases and phospholipase A_2 in the target cell to generate the characteristic response. H_2 receptors are linked to the stimulation of adenylyl cyclase and thus to the activation of cyclic AMP–dependent protein kinase in the target cell. In a species-dependent manner, adenosine receptors may interact with H_1 receptors. In the CNS of human beings, activation of adenosine A_1 receptors inhibits second messenger generation *via* H_1 receptors. A possible mechanism for this is interaction (termed *cross-talk*) between the G proteins to which the A_1 and H_1 receptors are coupled functionally (Dickenson and Hill, 1993).

In the smooth muscle of large blood vessels, bronchi, and intestine, the stimulation of H_1 receptors and the resultant IP_3-mediated release of intracellular Ca^{2+} leads to activation of the Ca^{2+}/calmodulin-dependent myosin light chain kinase.

This enzyme phosphorylates the 20,000 dalton myosin light chain, with resultant enhancement of cross-bridge cycling and contraction. The effects of histamine on sensory nerves also are mediated by H_1 receptors.

As mentioned above, the vasodilator effects of histamine are mediated by both H_1 and H_2 receptors that are located on different cell types in the vascular bed: H_1 receptors on the vascular endothelial cells and H_2 receptors on smooth muscle cells. Activation of H_1 receptors leads to increased intracellular Ca^{2+}, activation of phospholipase A_2, and the local production of endothelium-derived relaxing factor, which is nitric oxide (Palmer *et al.*, 1987). Nitric oxide diffuses to the smooth muscle cell, where it activates a soluble guanylyl cyclase and causes the accumulation of cyclic GMP. Stimulation of a cyclic GMP–dependent protein kinase and a decrease in intracellular Ca^{2+} are thought to be involved in the relaxation caused by this cyclic nucleotide. The activation of phospholipase A_2 in endothelial cells also leads to the formation of prostaglandins, predominantly prostacyclin (PGI_2); this vasodilator makes an important contribution to endothelium-mediated vasodilation in some vascular beds.

The mechanism of cyclic AMP–mediated relaxation of smooth muscle is not entirely clear, but it is presumed to involve a decrease in intracellular Ca^{2+} (*see* Taylor *et al.*, 1989). Cyclic AMP–mediated actions in the heart, mast cells, basophils, and other tissues also are understood incompletely, but the effects of histamine that are mediated by H_2 receptors obviously would be produced in the same fashion as those resulting from stimulation of β-adrenergic receptors or other receptors that are linked to the activation of adenylyl cyclase.

Clinical Uses

The practical applications of histamine are limited to uses as a diagnostic agent. Histamine (*histamine phosphate*) is used to assess nonspecific bronchial hyperreactivity in asthmatics and as a positive control injection during allergy skin testing.

H_1-RECEPTOR ANTAGONISTS

Although antagonists that act selectively at the three types of histamine receptors have been developed, this discussion is confined to the properties and clinical uses of H_1 antagonists. Specific H_2 antagonists (*e.g.*, cimetidine, ranitidine) are used extensively in the treatment of peptic ulcers; these are discussed in Chapter 37. The properties of agonists and antagonists at H_3 receptors are discussed later in this chapter. Such agents are not yet available for clinical use.

History.   Histamine-blocking activity was first detected in 1937 by Bovet and Staub in one of a series of amines with a phenolic ether function. The substance, 2-isopropyl-5-methylphenoxy-ethyldiethyl-amine, protected guinea pigs against several lethal doses of histamine, antagonized histamine-induced spasm of various smooth muscles, and lessened the symptoms of anaphylactic shock. This drug was too toxic for clinical use, but by 1944, Bovet and his colleagues had described pyrilamine maleate, which is still one of the most specific and effective his-

tamine antagonists of this category. The discovery of the highly effective histamine antagonists *diphenhydramine* and *tripelennamine* soon followed (*see* Bovet, 1950; Ganellin, in Ganellin and Parsons, 1982). In the 1980s, nonsedating H_1-histamine–receptor antagonists were developed for treatment of allergic diseases.

By the early 1950s, many compounds with histamine-blocking activity were available to physicians, but they uniformly failed to inhibit certain responses to histamine, most conspicuously gastric acid secretion. The discovery by Black and colleagues of a new class of drugs that blocked histamine-induced gastric acid secretion provided new pharmacological tools with which to explore the functions of endogenous histamine. This discovery ushered in a major new class of therapeutic agents, the H_2 receptor antagonists, including *cimetidine* (TAGAMET), *famotidine* (PEPCID), *nizatidine* (AXID), and *ranitidine* (ZANTAC) (*see* Chapter 37).

Structure–Activity Relationship.   All of the available H_1 receptor antagonists are reversible, competitive inhibitors of the interaction of histamine with H_1 receptors. Like histamine, many H_1 antagonists contain a substituted ethylamine moiety, $-\overset{|}{\underset{|}{C}}-\overset{|}{\underset{|}{C}}-N\diagup$. Unlike histamine, which has a primary amino group and a single aromatic ring, most H_1 antagonists have a tertiary amino group linked by a two- or three-atom chain to two aromatic substituents and conform to the general formula:

$$\begin{array}{c}Ar_1\\ \diagdown\\ X-\overset{|}{\underset{|}{C}}-\overset{|}{\underset{|}{C}}-N\diagup\\ \diagup\\ Ar_2\end{array}$$

where Ar is aryl and X is a nitrogen or carbon atom or a —C—O— ether linkage to the beta-aminoethyl side chain. Sometimes the two aromatic rings are bridged, as in the tricyclic derivatives, or the ethylamine may be part of a ring structure (Figure 25–3). (*see* Ganellin, in Ganellin and Parsons, 1982.)

Pharmacological Properties

Most H_1 antagonists have similar pharmacological actions and therapeutic applications and can be discussed together conveniently. Their effects are largely predictable from knowledge of the responses to histamine that involve interaction with H_1 receptors.

Smooth Muscle. H_1 antagonists inhibit most responses of smooth muscle to histamine. Antagonism of the constrictor action of histamine on respiratory smooth muscle is easily shown *in vivo* or *in vitro*. In guinea pigs, for example, death by asphyxia follows quite small doses of histamine, yet the animal may survive a hundred lethal

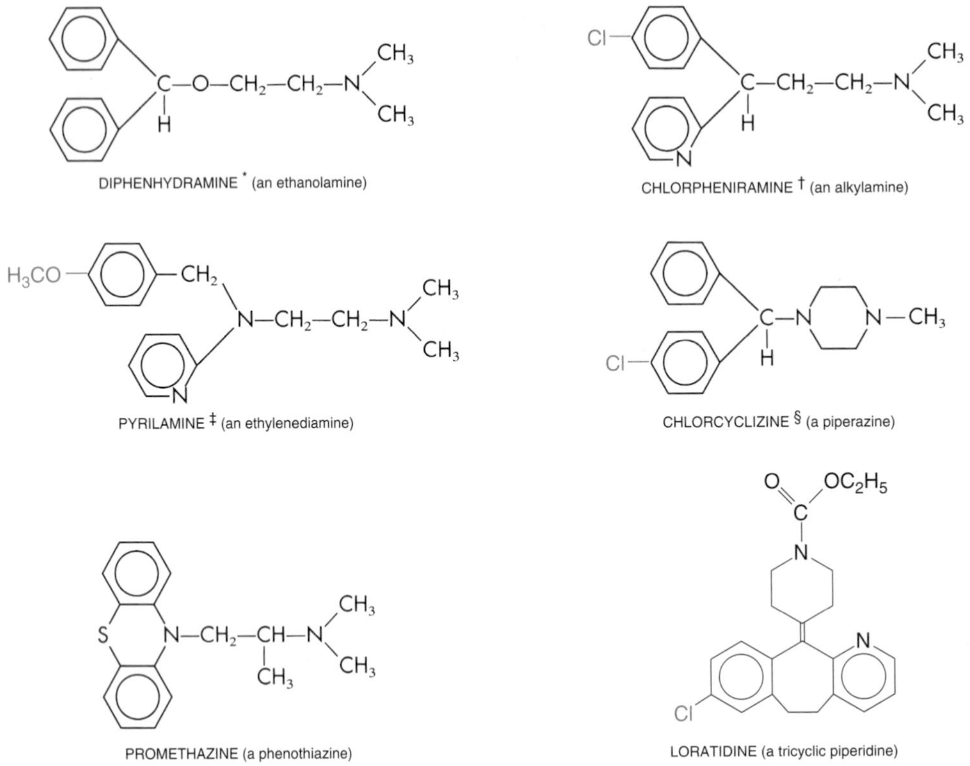

Figure 25–3. Representative H₁ antagonists.

*Dimenhydrinate is a combination of diphenhydramine and 8-chlorotheophylline in equal molecular proportions.
†Pheniramine is the same less Cl.
‡Tripelennamine is the same less H₃CO.
§Cyclizine is the same less Cl.

doses of histamine if given an H₁ antagonist. In the same species, striking protection also is afforded against anaphylactic bronchospasm. This is not so in human beings, where allergic bronchoconstriction appears to be caused by a variety of mediators such as leukotrienes and platelet activating factor (*see* Chapter 26).

Within the vascular tree, the H₁ antagonists inhibit both the vasoconstrictor effects of histamine and, to a degree, the more rapid vasodilator effects that are mediated by H₁ receptors on endothelial cells. Residual vasodilation reflects the involvement of H₂ receptors on smooth muscle and can be suppressed only by the concurrent administration of an H₂ antagonist. Effects of the histamine antagonists on histamine-induced changes in systemic blood pressure parallel these vascular effects.

Capillary Permeability.   H₁ antagonists strongly block the action of histamine that results in increased capillary permeability and formation of edema and wheal.

Flare and Itch.   The flare component of the triple response and the itching caused by intradermal injection of histamine are two different manifestations of the action of histamine on nerve endings. H₁ antagonists suppress both.

Exocrine Glands.   Gastric secretion is not inhibited at all by H₁ antagonists, and they suppress histamine-evoked salivary, lacrimal, and other exocrine secretions with variable responses. The atropine-like properties of many of these agents, however, may contribute to lessened secretion in cholinergically innervated glands and reduce ongoing secretion in, for example, the respiratory tree.

Immediate Hypersensitivity Reactions: Anaphylaxis and Allergy.   During hypersensitivity reactions, histamine is one of many potent autacoids released (*see* above), and its relative contribution to the ensuing symptoms varies widely with species and tissue. The protection afforded by histamine antagonists thus also varies accordingly. In human beings, some phenomena, such as edema formation and itch, are effectively suppressed. Others, such as hypotension, are less so. This may be explained by the existence of other mast-cell mediators, specifically prostaglandin D_2, also contributing to the vasodilation (Roberts *et al.*, 1980). Bronchoconstriction is reduced little, if at all (*see* Dahlén *et al.*, 1983).

Central Nervous System. The first-generation H_1 antagonists can both stimulate and depress the CNS. Stimulation occasionally is encountered in patients given conventional doses, who become restless, nervous, and unable to sleep. Central excitation also is a striking feature of poisoning, which commonly results in convulsions, particularly in infants. Central depression, on the other hand, is the usual accompaniment of therapeutic doses of the older H_1 antagonists. Diminished alertness, slowed reaction times, and somnolence are common manifestations. Some of the H_1 antagonists are more likely to depress the CNS than others, and patients vary in their susceptibility and responses to individual drugs. The ethanolamines (*e.g.*, diphenhydramine; *see* Figure 25–3) are particularly prone to cause sedation.

The second-generation ("nonsedating") H_1 antagonists (*e.g.*, *loratadine, cetirizine, fexofenadine*) are largely excluded from the brain when given in therapeutic doses, because they do not cross the blood–brain barrier appreciably. Their effects on objective measures of sedation such as sleep latency, EEG, and standardized performance tests are similar to those of placebo (Simons and Simons, 1994). Because of the sedation that occurs with first-generation antihistamines, these drugs cannot be tolerated or used safely by many patients. Thus, the availability of nonsedating antihistamines has been an important advance that allows the general use of these agents.

An interesting and useful property of certain H_1 antagonists is the capacity to counter motion sickness. This effect was first observed with *dimenhydrinate* and subsequently with *diphenhydramine* (the active moiety of dimenhydrinate), various piperazine derivatives, and *promethazine*. The latter drug has perhaps the strongest muscarinic blocking activity among these agents and is among the most effective of the H_1 antagonists in combating motion sickness (*see* below). Since scopolamine is the most potent drug for the prevention of motion sickness (*see* Chapter 7), it is possible that the anticholinergic properties of certain H_1 antagonists are largely responsible for this effect.

Anticholinergic Effects. Many of the first-generation H_1 antagonists tend to inhibit responses to acetylcholine that are mediated by muscarinic receptors. These atropine-like actions are sufficiently prominent in some of the drugs to be manifest during

clinical usage (*see* below). The second-generation H_1 antagonists have no effect on muscarinic receptors.

Local Anesthetic Effect. Some H_1 antagonists have local anesthetic activity, and a few are more potent than procaine. *Promethazine* (PHENERGAN) is especially active. However, the concentrations required for this effect are several orders higher than those that antagonize histamine.

Absorption, Fate, and Excretion. The H_1 antagonists are well absorbed from the gastrointestinal tract. Following oral administration, peak plasma concentrations are achieved in 2 to 3 hours and effects usually last 4 to 6 hours; however, some of the drugs are much longer acting (Table 25–1).

Extensive studies of the metabolic fate of the older H_1 antagonists are limited. Diphenhydramine, given orally, reaches a maximal concentration in the blood in about 2 hours, remains at about this level for another 2 hours, and then falls exponentially with a plasma elimination half-time of about 4 to 8 hours. The drug is widely distributed throughout the body, including the CNS. Little, if any, is excreted unchanged in the urine; most appears there as metabolites. Other first-generation H_1 antagonists appear to be eliminated in much the same way (*see* Paton and Webster, 1985).

Information on the concentrations of these drugs achieved in the skin and mucous membranes is lacking. However, significant inhibition of "wheal-and-flare" responses to the intradermal injection of histamine or allergen may persist for 36 hours or more after treatment with some longer-acting H_1 antagonists, even when concentrations of the drugs in plasma are very low. Such results emphasize the need for flexibility in the interpretation of the recommended dosage schedules (*see* Table 25–1); less frequent dosage may suffice. Doxepin, a tricyclic antidepressant (*see* Chapter 19), is one of the most potent antihistamines available; it is about 800 times more potent than diphenhydramine (Sullivan 1982; Richelson, 1979). This may account for the observation that doxepin can be effective in the treatment of chronic urticaria when other antihistamines have failed; it also is available as a topical preparation.

Like many other drugs that are metabolized extensively, H_1 antagonists are eliminated more rapidly by children than by adults and more slowly in those with severe liver disease. H_1-receptor antagonists are among the many drugs that induce hepatic microsomal enzymes, and they may facilitate their own metabolism (*see* Paton and Webster, 1985; Simons and Simons, 1988).

The second-generation H_1 antagonist loratadine is rapidly absorbed from the gastrointestinal tract and

Table 25–1

Preparations and Dosage of Representative H$_1$-Receptor Antagonists*

CLASS AND NONPROPRIETARY NAME	TRADE NAME	DURATION OF ACTION, hours	PREPARATIONS†	SINGLE DOSE (ADULT)
First-Generation Agents				
Tricyclic Dibenzoxepins				
Doxepin hydrochloride	SINEQUAN	6–24	O, L, T	10–150 mg
Ethanolamines				
Carbinoxamine maleate	RONDEC,¶ others	3–6	O, L	4–8 mg
Clemastine fumarate	TAVIST, others	12	O, L	1.34–2.68 mg
Diphenhydramine hydrochloride	BENADRYL; others	4–6	O, L, I, T	25–50 mg
Dimenhydrinate	DRAMAMINE; others	4–6	O, L, I	50–100 mg
Ethylenediamines				
Pyrilamine maleate	POLY–HISTINE-D¶	4–6	O, L, T	25–50 mg
Tripelennamine hydrochloride	PBZ	4–6	O	25–50 mg, 100 mg (sustained release)
Tripelennamine citrate	PBZ	4–6	L	37.5–75 mg
Alkylamines				
Chlorpheniramine maleate	CHLOR-TRIMETON; others	4–6	O, L, I	4 mg 8–12 mg (sustained release) 5–20 mg (injection)
Brompheniramine maleate	BROMPHEN; others	4–6	O, L, I	4 mg 8–12 mg (sustained release) 5–20 mg (injection)
Piperazines				
Hydroxyzine hydrochloride	ATARAX; others	6–24	O, L, I	25–100 mg
Hydroxyzine pamoate	VISTARIL	6–24	O, L	25–100 mg
Cyclizine hydrochloride	MAREZINE	4–6	O	50 mg
Cyclizine lactate	MAREZINE	4–6	I	50 mg
Meclizine hydrochloride	ANTIVERT; others	12–24	O	12.5–50 mg
Phenothiazines				
Promethazine hydrochloride	PHENERGAN; others	4–6	O, L, I, S	12.5–50 mg
Piperidines				
Cyproheptadine hydrochloride§	PERIACTIN	4–6	O, L	4 mg
Phenindamine tartrate	NOLAHIST	4–6	O	25 mg

Table 25–1 (continued)

CLASS AND NONPROPRIETARY NAME	TRADE NAME	DURATION OF ACTION, hours	PREPARATIONS†	SINGLE DOSE (ADULT)
Second–Generation Agents				
Alkylamines				
Acrivastine‡	SEMPREX-D¶	4–6	O	8 mg
Piperazines				
Cetirizine hydrochloride‡	ZYRTEC	12–24	O	5–10 mg
Phthalazinones				
Azelastine hydrochloride‡	ASTELIN	12–24	T	2 sprays per nostril
Piperidines				
Levocabastine hydrochloride	LIVOSTIN	6	T	One drop
Loratadine	CLARITIN	24	O, L	10 mg
Fexofenadine	ALLEGRA	12	O	60 mg

*For a discussion of phenothiazines, *see* Chapter 20.

†Preparations are designated as follows: O, oral solids; L, oral liquids; I, Injection; S, suppository; T, topical. Many H_1-receptor antagonists also are available in preparations that contain multiple drugs.

‡Has mild sedating effects.

¶Trade name drug also contains other medications.

§Also has antiserotonin properties.

metabolized in the liver to an active metabolite by the hepatic microsomal P450 system (Simons and Simons, 1994). Consequently, metabolism of this drug can be affected by competition for the P450 enzymes by other drugs. Two other second-generation H_1 antagonists that had been marketed previously, astemizole and terfenadine, also underwent P450 metabolism to active metabolites. Both of these drugs were found in rare cases to induce a potentially fatal arrhythmia, *torsades de pointes,* when their metabolism was impaired, such as by liver disease or drugs that inhibit the 3A family of P450 enzymes. This led to the withdrawal of terfenadine and astemizole from the market in 1998 and 1999. Loratadine, cetirizine (the active metabolite of hydroxyzine), fexofenadine (the active metabolite of terfenadine), and azelastine lack the propensity to prolong repolarization and induce *torsades de pointes* (DuBuske, 1999). Cetirizine, loratadine, and fexofenadine are all well absorbed and are excreted mainly in the unmetabolized form. Cetirizine and loratadine are primarily excreted into the urine, whereas fexofenadine is primarily excreted in the feces (Brogden and McTavish, 1991; Spencer *et al.,* 1993; Barnes *et al.,* 1993; Russell *et al.,* 1998).

Side Effects. *Sedation and Other Common Adverse Effects.* The side effect with the highest incidence in the first-generation H_1 antagonists, which is not a feature of the second-generation agents, is sedation. Although se-

dation may be a desirable adjunct in the treatment of some patients, it may interfere with the patient's daytime activities. Concurrent ingestion of alcohol or other CNS depressants produces an additive effect that impairs motor skills (Roehrs *et al.,* 1993). Other untoward reactions referable to central actions include dizziness, tinnitus, lassitude, incoordination, fatigue, blurred vision, diplopia, euphoria, nervousness, insomnia, and tremors.

The next most frequent side effects involve the digestive tract and include loss of appetite, nausea, vomiting, epigastric distress, and constipation or diarrhea. Their incidence may be reduced by giving the drug with meals. H_1 antagonists appear to increase appetite and cause weight gain in rare patients. Other side effects that apparently are caused by the antimuscarinic actions of some of the first-generation H_1-receptor antagonists include dryness of the mouth and respiratory passages, sometimes inducing cough, urinary retention or frequency, and dysuria. These effects are not observed with second-generation H_1 antagonists.

Mutagenicity. Results of one short-term study (Brandes *et al.,* 1994) with an unconventional mouse model indicated that melanoma and fibrosarcoma tumor lines had an increased rate of growth when injected into mice receiving certain H_1 antagonists. However, conventional studies with animals and clinical experience do not suggest carcinogenicity for H_1-receptor antagonists (Food and Drug Administration, 1994).

Other Adverse Effects.   Drug allergy may develop when H_1 antagonists are given orally, but more commonly it results from topical application. Allergic dermatitis is not uncommon; other hypersensitivity reactions include drug fever and photosensitization. Hematological complications such as leukopenia, agranulocytosis, and hemolytic anemia are very rare. Teratogenic effects have been noted in response to piperazine compounds, but extensive clinical studies have not demonstrated any association between the use of such H_1 antagonists and fetal anomalies in human beings. Since H_1 antagonists interfere with skin tests for allergy, they must be withdrawn well before such tests are performed.

In acute poisoning with H_1 antagonists, their central excitatory effects constitute the greatest danger. The syndrome includes hallucinations, excitement, ataxia, incoordination, athetosis, and convulsions. Fixed, dilated pupils with a flushed face, together with sinus tachycardia, urinary retention, dry mouth, and fever, lend the syndrome a remarkable similarity to that of atropine poisoning. Terminally, there is deepening coma with cardiorespiratory collapse and death, usually within 2 to 18 hours. Treatment is along general symptomatic and supportive lines.

Available H_1 Antagonists.   Below are summarized the therapeutic and side effects of a number of H_1 antagonists, based on their chemical structure. Representative preparations are listed in Table 25–1.

Dibenzoxepin Tricyclics (Doxepin).   Doxepin is the only drug in this class. Doxepin is marketed as a tricyclic antidepressant (*see* Chapter 19). However, it also is a remarkably potent H_1 antagonist. It can cause drowsiness and is associated with anticholinergic effects. Doxepin is much better tolerated by patients who have depression than by those who do not. In nondepressed patients, sometimes even very small doses, *e.g.,* 20 mg, may be poorly tolerated because of disorientation and confusion.

Ethanolamines (Prototype: Diphenhydramine).   The drugs in this group possess significant antimuscarinic activity and have a pronounced tendency to induce sedation. About half of those who are treated with conventional doses of these drugs experience somnolence. The incidence of gastrointestinal side effects, however, is low with this group.

Ethylenediamines (Prototype: Pyrilamine).   These include some of the most specific H_1 antagonists. Although their central effects are relatively feeble, somnolence occurs in a fair proportion of patients. Gastrointestinal side effects are quite common.

Alkylamines (Prototype: Chlorpheniramine).   These are among the most potent H_1 antagonists. The drugs are not so prone as some H_1 antagonists to produce drowsiness and are among the more suitable agents for daytime use; but again, a significant proportion of patients do experience sedation. Side effects involving CNS stimulation are more common in this than in other groups.

First-Generation Piperazines.   The oldest member of this group, *chlorcyclizine,* has a more prolonged action and produces a comparatively low incidence of drowsiness. *Hydroxyzine* is a long-acting compound that is widely used for skin allergies;

its considerable CNS-depressant activity may contribute to its prominent antipruritic action. Cyclizine and meclizine have been used primarily to counter motion sickness, although promethazine and diphenhydramine (dimenhydrinate) are more effective (as is scopolamine; *see* below).

Second-Generation Piperazines (Cetirizine).   Cetirizine is the only drug in this class. It has minimal anticholinergic effects. It also has negligible penetration into the brain but is associated with a somewhat higher incidence of drowsiness than the other second-generation H_1 antagonists.

Phenothiazines (Prototype: Promethazine).   Most drugs of this class are H_1 antagonists and also possess considerable anticholinergic activity. Promethazine, which has prominent sedative effects, and its many congeners are now used primarily for their antiemetic effects (*see* Chapter 38).

First-Generation Piperidines (Cyproheptadine, Phenindamine).   Cyproheptadine is unique in that it has both antihistamine and antiserotonin activity. Cyproheptadine and phenindamine cause drowsiness and also have significant anticholinergic effects.

Second-Generation Piperidines (Prototype: Terfenadine).   As mentioned, terfenadine and astemizole were early marketed H_1 antagonists in this class but have since been withdrawn because they induced the potentially fatal arrhythmia, *torsades de pointes*. The drugs currently marketed in this class, which are devoid of this side effect, are loratadine and fexofenadine. These agents are highly selective for H_1 receptors and are devoid of significant anticholinergic actions. These agents also penetrate poorly into the CNS. Taken together, these properties appear to account for the low incidence of side effects of piperidine agents.

Therapeutic Uses

H_1 antagonists have an established and valued place in the symptomatic treatment of various immediate hypersensitivity reactions. In addition, the central properties of some of the series are of therapeutic value for suppressing motion sickness or for sedation.

Diseases of Allergy. H_1 antagonists are most useful in acute types of allergy that present with symptoms of rhinitis, urticaria, and conjunctivitis. Their effect, however, is confined to the suppression of symptoms attributable to the histamine released by the antigen–antibody reaction. In bronchial asthma, histamine antagonists have limited beneficial effects and are not useful as sole therapy (*see* Chapter 28). In the treatment of systemic anaphylaxis, in which autacoids other than histamine play major roles, the mainstay of therapy is epinephrine, with histamine antagonists having only a subordinate and adjuvant role. The same is true for severe angioedema, in which laryngeal swelling constitutes a threat to life.

Other allergies of the respiratory tract are more amenable to therapy with H_1 antagonists. The best results are obtained in seasonal rhinitis and conjunctivitis (hay fever, pollinosis), in which these drugs relieve the sneezing, rhinorrhea, and itching of eyes, nose, and throat. A gratifying response is obtained in most patients, especially at the beginning of the season when pollen counts are low; however, the drugs are less effective when the allergens are in abundance, when exposure to them is prolonged, and when nasal congestion has become prominent. Topical preparations of antihistamines such as *levocabastine* (LIVOSTIN) have been shown to be effective in allergic conjunctivitis and rhinitis (Janssens and Vanden Bussche, 1991). A topical ophthalmic preparation of this agent is available in the United States (*see* Chapter 66) and nasal sprays are being tested.

Certain of the allergic dermatoses respond favorably to H$_1$ antagonists. Benefit is most striking in acute urticaria, although the itching in this condition is perhaps better controlled than are the edema and the erythema. Chronic urticaria is less responsive, but some benefit may occur in a fair proportion of patients. Furthermore, the combined use of H$_1$ and H$_2$ antagonists is effective for some individuals if therapy with an H$_1$ antagonist has failed. As mentioned above, doxepin is sometimes effective in the treatment of chronic urticaria that is refractory to other antihistamines. Angioedema also is responsive to treatment with H$_1$ antagonists, but the paramount importance of epinephrine in the severe attack must be reemphasized, especially in the life-threatening involvement of the larynx (*see* Chapter 10). Here, however, it may be appropriate to administer additionally an H$_1$ antagonist by the intravenous route. H$_1$ antagonists also have a place in the treatment of pruritus. Some relief may be obtained in many patients suffering atopic dermatitis and contact dermatitis (although topical corticosteroids are more effective) and in such diverse conditions as insect bites and ivy poisoning. Various other pruritides without an allergic basis sometimes respond to antihistamine therapy, usually when the drugs are applied topically but sometimes when they are given orally. However, the possibility of producing allergic dermatitis with local application of H$_1$ antagonists must be recognized. Again, doxepin may be more effective in suppressing histamine-mediated symptoms in the skin, in this case pruritus, than are other antihistamines. Since these drugs inhibit allergic dermatoses, they should be withdrawn well before skin testing for allergies.

The urticarial and edematous lesions of serum sickness respond to H$_1$ antagonists, but fever and arthralgia often do not.

Many drug reactions attributable to allergic phenomena respond to therapy with H$_1$ antagonists, particularly those characterized by itch, urticaria, and angioedema; reactions of the serum-sickness type also respond to intensive treatment. However, explosive release of histamine generally calls for treatment with epinephrine, with H$_1$ antagonists being accorded a subsidiary role. Nevertheless, prophylactic treatment with an H$_1$ antagonist may suffice to reduce symptoms to a tolerable level when a drug known to be a histamine liberator is to be given.

Common Cold.   Despite persistent popular belief, H$_1$ antagonists are without value in combating the common cold. The weak anticholinergic effects of the older agents may tend to lessen rhinorrhea, but this drying effect may do more harm than good, as may their tendency to induce somnolence.

Motion Sickness, Vertigo, and Sedation.   Although scopolamine, given orally, parenterally, or transdermally, is the most effective of all drugs for the prophylaxis and treatment of motion sickness, some H$_1$ antagonists are useful in a broad range of milder conditions and offer the advantage of fewer adverse effects. These drugs include dimenhydrinate and the piperazines (*e.g.,* cyclizine, meclizine). Promethazine, a phenothiazine, is more potent and more effective and its additional antiemetic properties may be of value in reducing vomiting, but its pronounced sedative action usually is disadvantageous. Whenever possible, the various drugs should be administered an hour or so before

the anticipated motion. Dosing after the onset of nausea and vomiting rarely is beneficial.

Some H$_1$ antagonists, notably dimenhydrinate and meclizine, are often of benefit in vestibular disturbances, such as Meniere's disease, and in other types of true vertigo. Only promethazine has usefulness in treating the nausea and vomiting subsequent to chemotherapy or radiation therapy for malignancies; however, other effective antiemetic drugs are available (*see* Chapter 38).

Diphenhydramine can be used to reverse the extrapyramidal side effects caused by phenothiazines. The anticholinergic actions of this agent also can be utilized in the early stages of treatment of patients with Parkinson's disease (*see* Chapter 22), but it is less effective than other agents such as *trihexyphenidyl* (ARTANE).

The tendency of certain of the H$_1$-receptor antagonists to produce somnolence has led to their use as hypnotics. H$_1$ antagonists, principally diphenhydramine, often are present in various proprietary remedies for insomnia that are sold over the counter. While these remedies generally are ineffective in the recommended doses, some sensitive individuals may derive benefit. The sedative and mild antianxiety activities of hydroxyzine and diphenhydramine have contributed to their use as weak anxiolytics.

H$_3$-RECEPTOR–MEDIATED ACTIONS: AGONISTS AND ANTAGONISTS

Originally the H$_3$ receptor was described as a presynaptic receptor present on histaminergic nerve terminals in the CNS that exerted feedback regulation of histamine synthesis and release (Arrang *et al.,* 1983). Since then, H$_3$ receptors have been found to function in a wide variety of tissues as feedback inhibitors not only of histamine but also of other neurotransmitters, including acetylcholine, dopamine, norepinephrine, and serotonin (Leurs *et al.,* 1998). Like H$_1$ and H$_2$ receptors, H$_3$ receptors are G protein–coupled receptors; their occupation results in a decrease of Ca^{2+} influx into the cell. (*R*)-α-*Methylhistamine* is a selective H$_3$ agonist, being approximately 1500 times more selective for the H$_3$ receptor than for the H$_2$ receptor and 3000 times more selective for the H$_3$ receptor than for the H$_1$ receptor (Timmerman, 1990). The development of this and other potent, selective agonists of the H$_3$ receptor has proven invaluable in defining the functions of the H$_3$ receptor. The H$_3$ receptor was cloned in 1999 (Lovenberg *et al.,* 1999). This important advance should now allow the development of genetically modified animals to further characterize H$_3$ receptor-mediated actions. Recently, evidence was obtained for the presence of a second isoform of the H$_3$ receptor in guinea pig brain (Tardivel-Lacome *et al.,* 2000). Whether there are two isoforms in human beings and whether the two isoforms in the guinea pig exhibit functional differences is unknown.

Many early H$_3$ antagonists such as impromidine and burimamide had mixed effects, since they also were agonists for the H$_2$ receptor. *Thioperamide* was the first specific H$_3$ antagonist available experimentally (Timmerman, 1990). This compound is still the most widely used H$_3$ antagonist and has potent pharmacological properties (*see* below). Other H$_3$ antagonists being developed include the competitive inhibitor *clobenpropit* and the irreversible inhibitor *N*-ethoxycarbonyl-2-ethoxy-1,2-dihydroquinoline (EEDQ).

H_3 receptors are known to function as feedback inhibitors in a wide variety of organ systems. In the CNS, H_3-receptor agonists cause sedation by opposing H_1-induced wakefulness (Monti, 1993). In the gastrointestinal tract, H_3 receptors antagonize H_1-induced ileal contraction as well as downregulate histamine (and thus gastrin) levels through autoregulatory actions in the gastric mucosa (Hollande *et al.,* 1993). The H_1-bronchoconstrictor response is opposed by an H_3-bronchodilatory response in the pulmonary tree.

Ishikawa and Sperelakis (1987) first documented the existence of H_3 receptors in the cardiovascular system. These authors documented that H_3-receptor agonists depressed perivascular sympathetic neurotransmission and caused vasodilation in the guinea pig mesenteric arteries. Subsequently, H_3 receptors were discovered on sympathetic nerve terminals in the human saphenous vein, where H_3-receptor agonists inhibited sympathetic outflow and norepinephrine release (Molderings *et al.,* 1992). In addition to interference with sympathetic vasoconstriction, H_3 receptors also have been shown to have negative chronotrophic effects in the atria. H_3 receptors probably have minimal effects in baseline normal states but may inhibit norepinephrine release during stresses such as ischemia (Imamura *et al.,* 1994).

Currently, much attention is focused on the therapeutic potential of ligands of the H_3 receptor in a variety of pathological situations. Agonists have potential use as gastroprotective, antiinflammatory, and anticonvulsant agents and in the treatment of septic shock, heart failure, and myocardial infarction. Antagonists have potential use in treating obesity, cognitive dysfunction, and attention-deficit–hyperactivity disorder in children (Leurs *et al.,* 2000). A number of potent, selective agonists and antagonists of H_3 receptors have been developed, but none has yet been approved for clinical use.

BRADYKININ AND KALLIDIN AND THEIR ANTAGONISTS

A variety of factors including tissue damage, allergic reactions, viral infections, and other inflammatory events activate a series of proteolytic reactions that generate bradykinin and kallidin in the tissues (*see* Wachtfogel *et al.,* 1993). These peptides are autacoids that act locally to produce pain, vasodilation, increased vascular permeability, and the synthesis of prostaglandins. Thus, they constitute a subset of the large number of mediators that contribute to the inflammatory response.

During the past several years, a number of interesting discoveries have been made concerning kinins and their receptors. Kinin metabolites that were formerly considered inactive degradation products now are considered potent mediators of inflammation and pain. These peptides interact with specific receptors whose presence is induced by tissue injury. Based on this information, novel avenues for therapeutic intervention in chronic inflammatory conditions may be possible.

History. In the 1920s and 1930s, Frey and his associates Kraut and Werle characterized a hypotensive substance in urine and showed that similar material could be obtained from saliva, plasma, and a variety of tissues. Since the pancreas was a rich source, they named this material *kallikrein* after an old Greek synonym for that organ, *kallikréas.* By 1937, Werle, Götze, and Keppler had established that kallikreins generate a pharmacologically active substance from some inactive precursor present in plasma. In 1948, Werle and Berek named the active substance *kallidin* and showed it to be a polypeptide cleaved from a plasma globulin that they termed *kallidinogen* (*see* Werle, 1970).

Interest in the field intensified when Rocha e Silva and associates (1949) reported that trypsin and certain snake venoms acted on plasma globulin to produce a substance that lowered blood pressure and caused a slowly developing contraction of the gut. Because of this slow response, they named this substance *bradykinin,* a term derived from the Greek words *bradys,* meaning "slow," and *kinein,* meaning "to move." In 1960, the nonapeptide bradykinin was isolated by Elliott and coworkers and synthesized by Boissonnas and associates. Shortly thereafter, kallidin was found to be a decapeptide—bradykinin with an additional lysine residue at the amino terminus. These substances are members of a group of polypeptides with related chemical structures and pharmacological properties that are widely distributed in nature. For the whole group, the generic term *kinins* has been adopted, and kallidin and bradykinin are referred to as plasma kinins.

In 1970, Ferreira *et al.* reported the isolation of a bradykinin-potentiating factor from the venom of the Brazilian snake, *Bothrops,* and Ondetti *et al.* (1971) subsequently reported the isolation of angiotensin converting-enzyme (ACE) inhibitors from the same venom. Later, it was shown that ACE and kininase II are the same enzyme (Erdos, 1977). ACE inhibitors (*see* Chapter 31) now are widely used in the treatment of hypertension, diabetic nephropathy, congestive heart failure, and post–myocardial infarction.

In 1980, Regoli and Barabé divided the kinin receptors into B_1 and B_2 classes based on the rank order of potency of kinin analogs. The B_1 and B_2 receptors have now been cloned. The development of first-generation kinin-receptor antagonists occurred in the mid-1980s (Vavrek and Stewart, 1985). Second-generation, receptor-specific kinin antagonists were developed in the early 1990s. These antagonists have led to increasing understanding of the actions of kinins. The development of a B_2-receptor "knockout" mouse (Borkowski *et al.,* 1995) has furthered our understanding of the role of bradykinin in the regulation of cardiovascular homeostasis.

The Endogenous Kallikrein–Kininogen–Kinin System

Synthesis and Metabolism of Kinins. Bradykinin is a nonapeptide (*see* Table 25–2). Kallidin has an additional lysine residue at the amino-terminal position and is sometimes referred to as lysyl-bradykinin. The two peptides are cleaved from α_2 globulins termed *kininogens*. There are two kininogens, high-molecular-weight (HMW) and low-molecular-weight (LMW) kininogen. A number of serine proteases will generate kinins, but the highly specific proteases that release bradykinin

Table 25–2

Structure of Kinin Agonists and Antagonists, Listed from Carboxyl Terminus

NAME	STRUCTURE	FUNCTION
Bradykinin	Arg-Pro-Pro-Gly-Phe-Ser-Pro-Phe-Arg	Agonist, $B_2 > B_1$
Kallidin	Lys-Arg-Pro-Pro-Gly-Phe-Ser-Pro-Phe-Arg	Agonist, $B_2 \simeq B_1$
des-Arg^9-bradykinin	Arg-Pro-Pro-Gly-Phe-Ser-Pro-Phe	Agonist, B_1
des-Arg^{10}-kallidin	Lys-Arg-Pro-Pro-Gly-Phe-Ser-Pro-Phe	Agonist, B_1
RMP-7	H-Arg-Pro-Hyp-Gly-Thi-Ser-Pro-4Me-Tyr(ψCH$_2$NH)-Arg-OH	Agonist, B_2
des-Arg^9-[Leu^8]-bradykinin	Arg-Pro-Pro-Gly-Phe-Ser-Pro-Leu	Antagonist, B_1
HOE 140	[D-Arg]-Arg-Pro-Hyp-Gly-Thi-Ser-Tic-Oic-Arg	Antagonist, B_2
CP 0127	B(D-Arg-Arg-Pro-Hyp-Gly-Phe-Cys-D-Phe-Leu-Arg)$_2$	Antagonist, B_2
FRI 73657	Nonpeptide	Antagonist, B_2

Hyp, *trans*-4-hydroxy-Pro; Thi, β-(2-thienyl)-Ala; Tic, [D]-1,2,3,4-tetrahydroisoquinolin-3-yl-carbonyl; Oic, (3as,7as)-octahydroindol-2-yl-carbonyl. B, bissuccimidohexane.

and kallidin from the kininogens are termed *kallikreins* (*see* Figure 25–4 and below).

Kallikreins. Bradykinin and kallidin are cleaved from high- and low-molecular-weight kininogens by plasma or tissue kallikrein, respectively. Plasma kallikrein and tissue kallikrein are distinct enzymes, and they are activated by different mechanisms (Bhoola *et al.*, 1992). Plasma prekallikrein is an inactive protein of about 88,000 daltons that is bound in a 1:1 complex with its substrate, HMW kininogen. The cascade is restrained by the protease inhibitors present in plasma. Among the most important are the inhibitor of the activated first component of complement (C1-INH) and α_2-macroglobulin. Under experimental conditions, the kallikrein-kinin system is ac-

tivated by the binding of factor XII, also known as Hageman factor, to negatively charged surfaces. Factor XII, a protease that is common to both the kinin and the intrinsic coagulation cascades (*see* Chapter 55), undergoes autoactivation and, in turn, activates kallikrein. Importantly, kallikrein further activates factor XIIa, thereby exerting a positive feedback on the system (*see* Proud and Kaplan, 1988). *In vivo*, factor XII does not undergo autoactivation upon binding to endothelial cells. Instead, the binding of a HMW kininogen/prekallikrein complex to a multiprotein receptor complex leads to activation of prekallikrein by a membrane-associated, cysteine protease. Kallikrein activates factor XII, cleaves HMW kininogen, and activates prourokinase (Schmaier *et al.*, 1999; Colman, 1999).

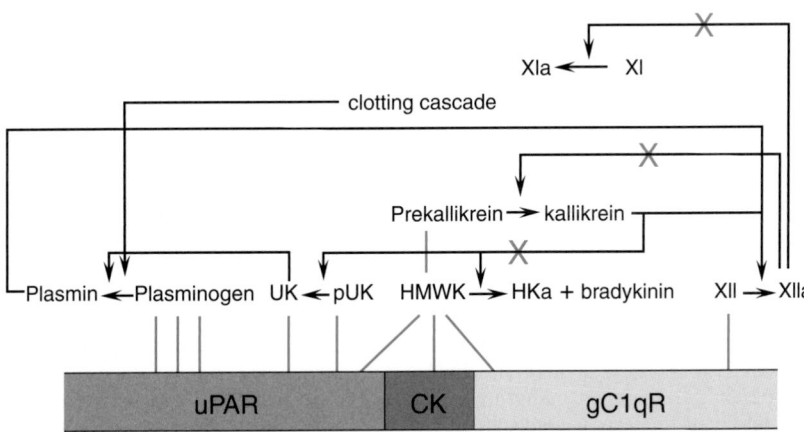

Figure 25–4. Schematic diagram of kinin production on the endothelial cell surface.

The high-molecular-weight kininogen (HMWK)–prekallikrein complex binds to a multiprotein complex, comprising the globular C1q receptor (gC1qR), cytokeratin 1 (CK), and the urokinase receptor (uPAR), on the surface of endothelial cells. This leads to activation of prekallikrein by a membrane-associated cysteine protease (not shown). Kallikrein then cleaves its substrate, HMWK, liberating kinin-free kininogen (HKa) and bradykinin from the surface. Note the relationship between kinin formation and the coagulation and fibrinolytic systems. Clotting factors are indicated by Roman numerals. Blue X's indicate the sites of inhibition by C1 esterase inhibitor (C1-INH). pUK indicates prourokinase; UK indicates urokinase. (Modified from Colman, 1999, with permission.)

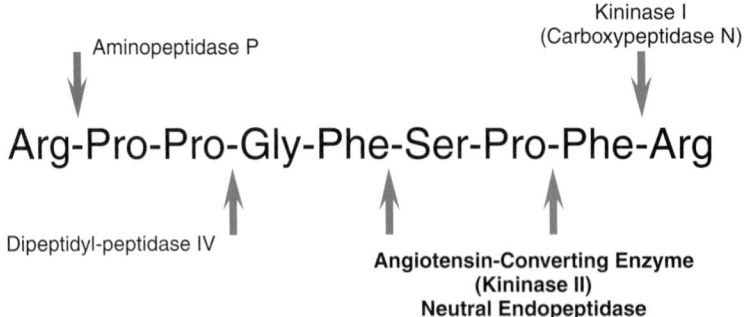

Figure 25–5. Schematic diagram of the degradation of bradykinin.

Bradykinin and kallidin are inactivated primarily by kininase II or angiotensin converting enzyme (ACE). Neutral endopeptidase also cleaves bradykinin and kallidin at the carboxyl terminus. In addition, aminopeptidase P inactivates bradykinin by hydrolyzing the N-terminal Arg[1]-Pro[2] bond, leaving bradykinin susceptible to further degradation by dipeptidyl-peptidase IV. Bradykinin and kallidin are converted to their respective des-Arg[9] metabolites by kininase I. Unlike the parent compounds, these kinin metabolites are potent ligands for B[1]-kinin receptors but not B[2]-kinin receptors.

The human tissue kallikrein family includes three members: true tissue kallikrein (hKLK1), prostate-specific antigen (PSA, hKLK3), and a PSA-like proteinase (hKLK2). Only true tissue kallikrein exhibits kininogenase activity. Compared to plasma kallikrein, tissue kallikrein is a smaller protein (molecular mass of 29,000 daltons). It is synthesized as a preproprotein in the epithelial cells or secretory cells of a number of tissues including salivary glands, pancreas, prostate, and distal nephron. Tissue kallikrein is also expressed in human neutrophils. It acts locally near its site of origin (Fukushima *et al.,* 1985; Evans *et al.,* 1988). The synthesis of tissue prokallikrein is regulated by a number of factors, including aldosterone in the kidney and salivary gland and androgens in certain other glands. The secretion of the tissue prokallikrein also may be regulated; for example, its secretion from the pancreas is enhanced by stimulation of the vagus nerve (*see* Proud and Kaplan, 1988; Margolius, 1989). The activation of tissue prokallikrein to kallikrein requires proteolytic cleavage. In human beings, the sequence of these activation events is not well delineated (Bhoola *et al.,* 1992).

Kininogens.   The two substrates for the kallikreins, HMW and LMW kininogen, are products of a single gene that arise by alternative processing of mRNA. HMW and LMW kininogen have been divided into functional domains. The HMW kininogen contains 626 amino acid residues; the internal bradykinin sequence of 9 amino acid residues, domain 4, connects an amino-terminal "heavy chain" sequence (362 amino acids) containing domains 1 through 3 and a carboxyl-terminal "light chain" sequence (255 amino acids) containing domains D5H and D6. LMW kininogen is identical to the larger form of the protein from the amino terminus through the bradykinin sequence; its short light chain differs (Takagaki *et al.,* 1985). HMW kininogen is cleaved by plasma and tissue kallikrein to yield bradykinin and kallidin, respectively. LMW kininogen is a substrate only for the tissue kallikrein and the product is kallidin (*see* Nakanishi, 1987). In addition to serving as precursors of bradykinin and kallidin, the kininogens inhibit cysteine proteinase, inhibit thrombin binding, and exhibit antiadhesive and profibrinolytic properties.

Metabolism.   The decapeptide kallidin is about as active as the nonapeptide bradykinin and need not be converted to the latter to exert its characteristic effects. Some conversion of kallidin to bradykinin occurs as the amino-terminal lysine residue is removed by a plasma aminopeptidase. However, this reaction is slow relative to the rate of inactivation by hydrolysis at the carboxyl terminus. The minimal effective structure required to elicit the classical responses is that of the nonapeptide (Figure 25–5).

The kinins have an evanescent existence—their half-life in plasma is only about 15 seconds. Moreover, in a single passage through the pulmonary vascular bed some 80% to 90% of the kinins may be destroyed (*see* Ryan, 1982). Plasma concentrations of bradykinin have been difficult to define because of its short half-life. Inadequate inhibition of kininogenases or kininases in the blood can lead to artifactual formation or degradation of bradykinin during blood collection. For this reason, physiological concentrations of bradykinin have been reported to range from picomolar to femtomolar (Pellacani *et al.,* 1992).

The principal catabolizing enzyme in the lung and in other vascular beds is the dipeptidyl carboxypeptidase kininase II, known in another context as angiotensin converting enzyme (*see* Chapter 31). Removal of the carboxyl-terminal dipeptide abolishes kinin-like activity. Neutral endopeptidase also inactivates kinins by removing the carboxyl-terminal dipeptide. A slower-acting enzyme, arginine carboxypeptidase (carboxypeptidase-N; kininase I), removes the carboxyl-terminal arginine residue producing des-Arg[9]-bradykinin and des-Arg[10]-kallidin (Table 25–2), which are themselves potent B[1]-kinin receptor agonists (Burch and Kyle, 1992; Trifilieff *et al.,* 1993). A familial carboxypeptidase-N deficiency has been described in which affected individuals with low levels of this enzyme display angioedema or urticaria (*see* below) (Mathews *et al.,* 1980). Finally, aminopeptidase-P inactivates bradykinin by cleaving the amino-terminus arginine, rendering bradykinin susceptible to further cleavage by dipeptidyl peptidase IV.

Bradykinin Receptors.   There are at least two distinct receptors for kinins, which have been designated B[1] and B[2] (Regoli and Barabé, 1980). The classical bradykinin receptor, now designated the B_2 receptor, selectively binds bradykinin and kallidin (*see* Table 25–2) and is constitutively present in most normal tissues. B_2 receptors mediate the majority of the effects of bradykinin and kallidin in the absence of inflammation. The B_1 receptor selectively binds to the carboxy-terminal des-Arg metabolites of bradykinin and kallidin (*see* Table 25–2) and is less prevalent than the B_2 receptor in most tissues. B_1 receptors are present in normal vascular smooth muscle. B_1 receptors are upregulated by inflammation and by cytokines, endotoxins, and growth factors (Regoli and Barabé, 1980; Dray and Perkins, 1993). During physiological insults such as trauma, tissue damage, or inflammation, B_1 receptor effects may predominate. The signaling mechanisms of B_1 receptors are less well characterized than are those of B_2 receptors.

The B_2 receptor is a G protein–coupled 7-transmembrane-domain receptor that activates phospholipase A_2 and phospholipase C, apparently *via* interaction with distinct G proteins. Kinin-induced phospholipase C activation through a $G_{\alpha q}$ complex leads to an increase in IP_3 (and thus cytosolic Ca^{2+}, with subsequent enhanced nitric oxide synthesis and release) and diacylglycol (and thus protein kinase C activity). Bradykinin has been shown to activate Ca^{2+}-dependent, Ca^{2+}-independent, and atypical isoforms of protein kinase C (Tippmer *et al.,* 1994). The stimulation of phospholipase A_2 *via* $G_{\alpha i}$ liberates arachidonic acid from membrane-bound phospholipids (Schrör, 1992). The liberated arachidonic acid then can be metabolized to a variety of potent inflammatory mediators and the vasodilator prostacycin (*see* Chapter 26). Binding of bradykinin to the B_2 receptor leads to internalization of the agonist-receptor complex, and to desensitization.

Based on the inability of B_1 and B_2 antagonists to compete for specific bradykinin binding in guinea pig trachea, the existence of a B_3 receptor has been suggested (Farmer *et al.,* 1989; Farmer and DeSiato, 1994). In addition, the presence of B_4 and B_5 receptors on opossum esophageal smooth muscle cells has been suggested. However, studies with more potent kinin antagonists have not supported the existence of the B_3, B_4, or B_5 receptors. These studies indicate that the guinea pig bronchoconstriction proposed as a B_3-receptor effect actually may represent previously unappreciated functions of the B_2 receptor (Regoli *et al.,* 1993).

Functions and Pharmacology of Kallikreins and Kinins

The availability of newer and more specific bradykinin antagonists and the generation of bradykinin-receptor "knockout" mice have led to significant advances in our understanding of the roles of the kinins. Of current interest is the role of these compounds in diverse areas such as pain, inflammation and chronic inflammatory diseases, the cardiovascular system, and reproduction.

Pain.   The kinins are powerful algesic agents that cause an intense, burning pain when applied to the exposed base of a blister. Bradykinin excites primary sensory neurons and provokes the release of neuropeptides such as sub-

stance P, neurokinin A, and calcitonin gene–related peptide (Geppetti, 1993). In acute pain, B_2 receptors mediate bradykinin algesia. This pain is significantly reduced by B_2 antagonists but not by B_1 antagonists. The pain of chronic inflammation appears to involve increased numbers of B_1 receptors.

Inflammation.   Injected kinins mimic inflammation. Measurement of the components of the kinin cascade and the effects of bradykinin antagonists indicates that kinins participate in a variety of inflammatory diseases. Plasma kinins increase permeability in the microcirculation. The effect, like that of histamine and serotonin in some species, is exerted on the small venules and involves separation of the junctions between endothelial cells. This, together with an increased hydrostatic pressure gradient, causes edema. Such edema, coupled with stimulation of nerve endings (*see* below), results in a "wheal-and-flare" response to intradermal injections in human beings.

Bradykinin is formed, and there is depletion of the components of the kinin cascade during episodes of swelling, laryngeal edema, and abdominal pain in hereditary angioedema (Proud and Kaplan, 1988). B_1 receptors on inflammatory cells such as macrophages can elicit production of the inflammatory mediators IL-1 and tumor necrosis factor α (TNF-α) (Dray and Perkins, 1993). Increased levels of kinins have been shown to be present in a number of chronic inflammatory diseases. These include rhinitis caused by inhalation of antigens and that associated with rhinoviral infection. Kinins also may play significant roles in conditions such as gout, disseminated intravascular coagulation, inflammatory bowel disease, rheumatoid arthritis, and asthma. The kinins also may contribute to the changes in the bones seen in chronic inflammatory states. Kinins stimulate bone resorption through B_1 and possibly B_2 receptors, perhaps by osteoblast-mediated osteoclast activation (Lerner, 1994).

Respiratory Disease.   The kinins have been implicated in the pathophysiology of allergic airway disorders such as asthma and rhinitis. Inhalation or intravenous injection of kinins causes bronchospasm in asthmatic patients but not in normal individuals. Similarly, nasal challenge with bradykinin induces sneezing and serious glandular secretions in patients with allergic rhinitis. Bradykinin-induced bronchoconstriction is blocked by anticholinergic agents but not by antihistamines or cyclooxygenase inhibitors. A bradykinin B_2-receptor antagonist also has been shown to improve pulmonary function in patients with severe asthma. Repeated inhalation of bradykinin results in an attenuated response, decreasing the bronchoconstriction in response to bradykinin as well as that in response to adenosine 5′ monophosphate (Polosa *et al.,* 1992).

Cardiovascular System.   The kallikrein-kinin system was first implicated in the regulation of blood pressure in the 1920s and 1930s when Frey and Werke identified kallikrein as a hypotensive substance in urine. Since then, numerous investigators have reported that urinary kallikrein concentrations are decreased in individuals with high blood pressure. In experimental animals and human beings, infusion of bradykinin causes vasodilation and lowers blood pressure. Bradykinin causes vasodilation through B_2-receptor-dependent effects on endothelial nitric oxide, prostacyclin, and the poorly characterized endothelium-derived hyperpolarizing factor (Vanhoutte, 1989).

The availability of specific bradykinin antagonists and genetically altered animals has greatly enhanced our understanding of the role of endogenous bradykinin in the regulation of blood pressure (Madeddu, 1993; Madeddu *et al.,* 1997). Basal blood pressure is normal in B_2-receptor antagonist–treated or B_2-receptor knockout animals. However, these animals exhibit an exaggerated blood-pressure response to salt loading or activation of the renin–angiotensin system. These data suggest that the endogenous kallikrein–kinin system plays a minor role in the regulation of blood pressure under normal circumstances, but it may play an important role in hypertensive states.

In addition to causing vasodilation, the kallikrein–kinin system appears to exert a number of cardioprotective effects. Bradykinin contributes to the protective effect of preconditioning the heart against ischemia and reperfusion injury (Linz and Schölkens, 1992). In the presence of endothelial cells, bradykinin prevents vascular smooth muscle cell growth and proliferation. Bradykinin stimulates tPA release from the vascular endothelium and may inhibit thrombin (Brown *et al.,* 1999; Hasan *et al.,* 1996). Through these mechanisms, bradykinin may contribute to the endogenous defense against cardiovascular events such as myocardial infarction and stroke.

Kinins also may increase sympathetic outflow *via* central and peripheral nervous mechanisms (Dominiak *et al.,* 1992; Schwieler and Hjemdahl, 1992; Madeddu, 1993). These findings suggest that kinins may mediate hypertension in some circumstances *via* the sympathetic nervous system, though this remains speculative.

Kidney.   Renal kinins act as paracrine hormones to regulate urine volume and composition (Saitoh *et al.,* 1995). Kallikrein is synthesized and secreted by the connecting cells of the distal nephron. Tissue kininogen and kinin

receptors are present in the cells of the collecting duct. Like other vasodilators, kinins increase renal blood flow. Bradykinin also causes natriuresis by inhibiting sodium reabsorption at the cortical collecting duct. Renal kallikreins are increased by treatment with mineralocorticoids, ACE inhibitors, and neutral endopeptidase inhibitors.

Other Effects.   The rat uterus is especially sensitive to contraction by kinins through the B_2 receptor. Kinins also function in the male reproductive system in areas such as spermatogenesis and in promoting sperm motility, possibly through a B_2 receptor on the sperm membrane (Schill and Miska, 1992). Kinins promote dilation of the fetal pulmonary artery, closure of the ductus arteriosus, and constriction of the umbilical vessels, all of which occur in the adjustment from fetal to neonatal circulation.

The kallikrein–kinin system also functions in a wide variety of other areas in the body, serving to mediate edema formation and smooth muscle contraction. The bradykinin-induced, slowly developing contraction of the isolated guinea pig ileum first prompted the name bradykinin. The kinins also have neurochemical effects in the CNS, in addition to their ability to disrupt the blood–brain barrier and allow increased CNS penetration (*see* Inamura *et al.,* 1994).

Potential Therapeutic Uses.   Bradykinin contributes to many of the effects of the widely used cardiovascular drugs, the ACE inhibitors. Aprotinin, a nonspecific kallikrein antagonist, is administered to patients undergoing coronary bypass in order to minimize bleeding and blood transfusion requirements. Kinin agonists have potential value in increasing the delivery of chemotherapeutic agents beyond the blood–brain barrier. Based on the physiology outlined above, kinin antagonists are being tested in a number of inflammatory conditions.

Kallikrein Inhibitors.   *Aprotinin* (TRASYLOL) is a natural proteinase inhibitor obtained from bovine lung. Aprotinin inhibits many of the mediators of the inflammatory response, fibrinolysis, and thrombin generation following cardiopulmonary bypass surgery, including kallikrein and plasmin. In several placebo-controlled, double-blind studies, administration of aprotinin during bypass reduced requirements for blood products in patients undergoing coronary artery bypass grafting (Levy *et al.,* 1995). Aprotinin is given as a loading dose followed by a continuous infusion during surgery. Hypersensitivity reactions, including anaphylactic or anaphylactoid reactions, may occur with aprotinin. The rate of such reactions is 2.7% in patients who have been previously exposed to aprotinin and higher in patients who have been exposed to aprotinin within the last six months. A test dose of aprotinin is recommended prior to full dosing. Aprotinin can interfere with an activated clotting time, used to determine the effectiveness of heparin anticoagulation. For this reason, alternate methods must be used to determine the degree of anticoagulation in patients treated with aprotinin during cardiopulmonary bypass. In one multicenter study of aprotinin, there was an increased closure rate of saphenous vein grafts in patients treated with aprotinin compared to those treated with placebo; there were no differences in rates of myocardial infarction or death.

Angiotensin Converting Enzyme Inhibitors. The ACE inhibitors are widely used in the treatment of hypertension and have been shown to reduce mortality in patients with diabetic nephropathy, left ventricular dysfunction, previous myocardial infarction, and coronary artery disease. ACE inhibitors block the conversion of angiotensin I to angiotensin II, a potent vasoconstrictor and growth promoter (*see* Chapter 31). Data from studies using the specific bradykinin B_2 antagonist HOE 140 demonstrate that bradykinin also contributes to many of the protective effects of ACE inhibitors. For example, in animal models, administration of HOE 140 attenuates the favorable effects of ACE inhibitors on blood pressure, on myocardial infarct size, and on ischemic preconditioning (Linz and Schölkens, 1992). Bradykinin receptor antagonism also attenuates the blood pressure–lowering effects of acute ACE inhibition in human beings (Gainer *et al.*, 1998). The contribution of bradykinin to the effects of ACE inhibitors may result not only from decreased degradation of bradykinin but also from enhanced receptor sensitivity (Marcic *et al.*, 1999).

Occasional patients receiving ACE inhibitors have experienced angioedema. This can occur at any time, but often occurs shortly after initiating therapy. This is an effect of ACE inhibitors as a group and is thought to be due to inhibition of kinin metabolism by ACE (Slater *et al.*, 1988). ACE-inhibitor-associated angioedema is more common in blacks than in Caucasians. Severe anaphylactoid reactions can occur in patients taking ACE inhibitors who are undergoing dialysis with polyacrylonitrile AN69 membranes (Schulman *et al.*, 1993; Verresen *et al.*, 1994). In these patients, kinins are produced by activation of factor XII by the negatively charged surface of the polyacrylonitrile AN69 membrane while ACE inhibition diminishes the clearance of these kinins. A more common side effect of ACE inhibitors (especially in women) is a chronic nonproductive cough that dissipates upon cessation of the ACE inhibitor. The finding that angiotensin AT_1-receptor-subtype antagonists do not cause cough has been taken as presumptive evidence for the role of bradykinin in ACE inhibitor–induced cough.

Preliminary data suggest that bradykinin also may contribute to the effects of the AT_1-receptor antagonists. During AT_1-receptor blockade, angiotensin II concentrations increase. Renal bradykinin concentrations also increase through effects of angiotensin II on the unopposed AT_2 subtype receptor (Carey *et al.*, 2000). Whether or not bradykinin contributes to the clinical effects of the AT_1-receptor antagonists remains to be determined. In addition, a new class of antihypertensive agents, the combined ACE/neutral endopeptidase inhibitors, is undergoing testing. To the extent that these drugs inhibit two kinin-degrading enzymes, bradykinin may be expected to contribute significantly to their clinical effects.

Bradykinin Antagonists. The introduction of a D-aromatic amino acid in place of the proline residue at position seven conferred antagonist activity to bradykinin and blocked the action of angiotensin converting enzyme. The addition of an N-terminal D-arginine residue also increased the half-life of these antagonists by blocking the action of aminopeptidase P. Nevertheless, the early kinin antagonists were partial agonists and had short half-lives due to enzymatic degradation by carboxypeptidase N *in vivo*. In the early 1990s, a longer-acting, more selective kinin antagonist, HOE 140, was developed by substituting synthetic amino acids at position seven [D-tetrahydroisoquinoline-3-carboxylic acid (Tic)] and position eight [octahydroindole-2-carboxylic acid (Oic)]. The substitution of the Oic residue at position eight blocked degradation by carboxypeptidase P. The availability of HOE 140 has contributed dramatically to our understanding of the role of bradykinin in human health and disease.

CP-0127, a 6-Cys substituted, cross-linked analog of bradykinin, has been tested in the treatment of sepsis in humans in a randomized prospective trial (Fein *et al.*, 1997). In a study of 504 patients with systemic inflammatory response syndrome (SIRS) and presumed sepsis, there was no effect of the bradykinin analog on 28-day survival. However, there was an improvement in risk-adjusted survival in a predefined subset of patients with gram-negative sepsis. A small pilot study in patients with edema following head trauma suggests that bradykinin-receptor antagonism may reduce intracranial pressure.

The development of orally active, nonpeptide antagonists promises to make bradykinin antagonism therapeutically feasible in the treatment of disease. The first of these, WIN64338, suffered from having muscarinic cholinergic activity. More recently, the nonpeptide antagonist FR173657 has been shown to decrease bradykinin-induced edema and hypotension in animal models.

Bradykinin Agonists. RMP-7 [H-Arg-Pro-Hyp-Gly-Thi-Ser-Pro-4Me-Tyr(ΨCH_2NH)-Arg-OH] is a bradykinin analog that has been rendered resistant to degradation by bradykinin-metabolizing enzymes by the introduction of a reduced peptide bond at the carboxyl terminus. RMP-7 increases the permeability of the blood–brain barrier, and clinical trials are evaluating its efficacy in enhancing the delivery of chemotherapeutic agents into the CNS of patients with primary brain tumors (Cloughesy *et al.*, 1993).

PROSPECTUS

The refinement of the structure–function relationships among histamine receptor subtypes has allowed the continued development of H_2-selective antagonists for the treatment of peptic ulcers (*see* Chapter 37). The further understanding of the physiological and pathophysiological roles of H_3-receptor subtypes in the CNS and elsewhere

similarly may permit the development of new and more selective therapeutic tools.

The availability of new peptide and nonpeptide bradykinin antagonists provides the tools for further elucidation of the role of the kallikrein–kinin system in health and disease. Ongoing clinical trials will determine the efficacy of bradykinin agonists in enhancing the delivery of chemotherapeutic agents across the blood–brain barrier. Clinical trials will better define the contribution of bradykinin to the cardioprotective effects of ACE inhibitors, AT_1-receptor antagonists, and combined ACE/neutral endopeptidase inhibitors.

BIBLIOGRAPHY

Arrang, J.-M., Garbarg, M., Lancelot, J.-C., Lecomte, J.-M., Pollard, H., Robba, M., Schunack, W., and Schwartz, J.-C. Highly potent and selective ligands for histamine H_3-receptors. *Nature*, **1987**, *327*:117–123.

Arrang, J.-M., Garbarg, M., and Schwartz, J.-C. Auto-inhibition of brain histamine release mediated by a novel class (H_3) of histamine receptor. *Nature*, **1983**, *302*:832–837.

Ash, A.S.F., and Schild, H.O. Receptors mediating some actions of histamine. *Br. J. Pharmacol.*, **1966**, *27*:427–439.

Barnes, C.L., McKenzie, C.A., Webster, K.D., and Poinsett-Holmes, K. Cetirizine: a new nonsedating antihistamine. *Ann. Pharmacother.*, **1993**, *27*:464–470.

Best, C.H., Dale, H.H., Dudley, J.W., and Thorpe, W.V. The nature of the vasodilator constituents of certain tissue extract. *J. Physiol. (Lond.)*, **1927**, *62*:397–417.

Black, J.W., Duncan, W.A., Durant, C.J., Ganellin, C.R., and Parsons, E.M. Definition and antagonism of histamine H_2-receptors. *Nature*, **1972**, *236*:385–390.

Borkowski, J.A., Ransom, R.W., Seabrook, G.R., Trumbauer, M., Chen, H., Hill, R.G., Strader, C.D., and Hess, J.F. Targeted disruption of a B_2 bradykinin receptor gene in mice eliminates bradykinin action in smooth muscle and neurons. *J. Biol. Chem.*, **1995**, *270*:13706–13710.

Brandes, L.J., Warrington, R.C., Arron, R.J., Bogdanovic, R.P., Fang, W., Queen, G.M., Stein, D.A., Tong, J., Zaborniak, C.L., and LaBella, F.S. Enhanced cancer growth in mice administered daily human-equivalent doses of some H_1-antihistamines: predictive *in vitro* correlates. *J. Natl. Cancer Inst.*, **1994**, *86*:770–775.

Brown, N.J., Gainer, J.V., Stein, C.M., and Vaughan, D.E. Bradykinin stimulates tissue plasminogen activator release in human vasculature. *Hypertension*, **1999**, *33*:1431–1435.

Cloughesy, T.F., Black, K.L., Gobin, Y.P., Farahani, K., Nelson, G., Villablanca, P., Kabbinavar, F., Vineula, F., and Wortel, C.H. Intra-arterial Cereport (RMP-7) and carboplatin: a dose escalation study for recurrent malignant gliomas. *Neurosurgery*, **1999**, *44*:270–278.

Cookson, W.O., Young, R.P., Sandford, A.J., Moffatt, M.F., Shirakawa, T., Sharp, P.A., Faux, J.A., Julier, C., Le Souef, P.N., Nakumura, Y., Lathrop, G.M., and Hopkin, J.M. Maternal inheritance of atopic IgE responsiveness on chromosome 11q. *Lancet*, **1992**, *340*:381–384.

Dahlén, S.-E., Hansson, G., Heqvist, P., Björck, T., Granström, E., and Dahlén, B. Allergen challenge of lung tissue from asthmatics elicits bronchial contraction that correlates with the release of leukotrienes C_4, D_4, and E_4. *Proc. Natl. Acad. Sci. U.S.A.*, **1983**, *80*:1712–1716.

Dale, H.H., and Laidlaw, P.P. The physiological action of b-imidazolylethylamine. *J. Physiol. (Lond.)*, **1910**, *41*:318–344.

Dale, H.H., and Laidlaw, P.P. Further observations on the action of β-imidazolylethylamine. *J. Physiol. (Lond.)*, **1911**, *43*:182–195.

Dominiak, P., Simon, M., Blöchl, A., and Brenner, P. Changes in peripheral sympathetic outflow of pithed spontaneously hypertensive rats after bradykinin and DesArg-bradykinin infusions: influence of converting enzyme inhibition. *J. Cardiovasc. Pharmacol.*, **1992**, *20* (suppl 9):S35–S38.

Evans, B.A., Yun, Z.X., Close, J.A., Tregear, G.W., Kitamura, N., Nakanishi, S., Callen, D.F., Baker, E., Hyland, V.J., Sutherland, G.R., and Richards, R.I. Structure and chromosomal localization of the renal kallikrein gene. *Biochemistry*, **1988**, *27*:3124–3129.

Farmer, S.G., Burch, R.M., Meeker, S.A., and Wilkins, D.E. Evidence for a pulmonary B_3 bradykinin receptor. *Mol. Pharmacol.*, **1989**, *36*:1–8.

Farmer, S.G., and DeSiato, M.A. Effects of a novel nonpeptide bradykinin B_2 receptor antagonist on intestinal and airway smooth muscle: further evidence for the tracheal B_3 receptor. *Br. J. Pharmacol.*, **1994**, *112*:461–464.

Fein, A.M., Bernard, G.R., Criner, G.J., Fletcher, E.C., Good, J.T. Jr., Knaus, W.A., Levy, H., Matuschak, G.M., Shanies, H.M., Taylor, R.W., and Rodell, T.C. Treatment of severe systemic inflammatory response syndrome and sepsis with a novel bradykinin antagonist, deltibant (CP-0127). Results of a randomized, double-blind, placebo-controlled trial. CP-0127 SIRS and Sepsis Study Group. *JAMA*, **1997**, *277*:482–487.

Ferreira, S.H., Bartelt, D.C., and Greene, L.J. Isolation of bradykinin-potentiating peptides from *Bothrops jararaca* venom. *Biochemistry*, **1970**, *9*:2583–2593.

Food and Drug Administration. FDA reviews antihistamine mouse study. *FDA TALKPaper*, May 17, **1994.**

Fukushima, D., Kitamura, N., and Nakanishi, S. Nucleotide sequence of cloned cDNA for human pancreatic kallikrein. *Biochemistry*, **1985**, *24*:8037–8043.

Gaboury, J.P., Johnston, B., Niu, X.-F., and Kubes, P. Mechanisms underlying acute mast cell–induced leukocyte rolling and adhesion *in vivo. J. Immunol.,* **1995,** *154:*804–813.

Gainer, J.V., Morrow, J.D., Loveland, A., King, D.J., and Brown, N.J. Effect of bradykinin-receptor blockade on the response to angiotensin-converting-enzyme inhibitor in normotensive and hypertensive subjects. *N. Engl. J. Med.,* **1998,** *339:*1285–1292.

Hasan, A.A., Amenta, S., and Schmaier, A.H. Bradykinin and its metabolite, Arg-Pro-Pro-Gly-Phe, are selective inhibitors of α-thrombin-induced platelet activation. *Circulation,* **1996,** *94:*517–528.

Higashijima, T., Uzu, S., Nakajima, T., and Ross, E.M. Mastoparan, a peptide toxin from wasp venom, mimics receptors by activating GTP-binding regulatory proteins (G proteins). *J. Biol. Chem.,* **1988,** *263:*6491–6494.

Hollande, F., Bali, J.-P., and Magous, R. Autoregulation of histamine synthesis through H3 receptors in isolated fundic mucosal cells. *Am. J. Physiol.,* **1993,** *265:*G1039–G1044.

Imamura, M., Poli, E., Omoniyi, A.T., and Levi, R. Unmasking of activated histamine H3 receptors in myocardial ischemia: their role as regulators of exocytotic norepinephrine release. *J. Pharmacol. Exp. Ther.,* **1994,** *271:*1259–1266.

Inamura, T., Nomura, T., Bartus, R.T., and Black K.L. Intracarotid infusion of RMP-7, a bradykinin analog: a method for selective drug delivery to brain tumors. *J. Neurosurg.,* **1994,** *81:*752–758.

Ishikawa, S., and Sperelakis, N. A novel class (H3) of histamine receptors on perivascular nerve terminals. *Nature,* **1987,** *327:*158–160.

Keyzer, J.J., deMouchy, J.G., van Doormal, J.J., and van Voorst Vader, P.C. Improved diagnosis of mastocytosis by measurement of urinary histamine metabolites. *N. Engl. J. Med.,* **1983,** *309:*1603–1605.

Levy, J.H., Kettlekamp, N., Goertz, P., Hermens, J., and Hirshman, C.A. Histamine release by vancomycin: a mechanism for hypotension in man. *Anesthesiology,* **1987,** *67:*122–125.

Levy, J.H., Pifarre, R., Schaff, H.V., Horrow, J.C., Albus, R., Spiess, B., Rosengart, T.K., Murray, J., Clark, R.E., and Smith, P. A multicenter, double-blind, placebo-controlled trial of aprotinin for reducing blood loss and the requirement for donor-blood transfusion in patients undergoing repeat coronary artery bypass grafting. *Circulation,* **1995,** *92:*2236–2244.

Lovenberg, T.W., Roland, B.L., Wilson, S.J., Jiang, X., Pyati, J., Huvar, A., Jackson, M.R., and Erlander, M.G. Cloning and functional expression of the human histamine H3 receptor. *Mol. Pharmacol.,* **1999,** *55:*1101–1105.

Madeddu, P., Varoni, M.V., Palomba, D., Emanueli, C., Demontis, M.P., Glorioso, N., Dessi-Fulgheri, P., Sarzani, R., and Anania, V. Cardiovascular phenotype of a mouse strain with disruption of bradykinin B2-receptor gene. *Circulation,* **1997,** *96:*3570–3578.

Marcic, B., Deddish, P.A., Jackman, H.L., and Erdos, E.G. Enhancement of bradykinin and resensitization of its B2 receptor. *Hypertension,* **1999,** *33:*835–843.

Mathews, K.P., Pan, P.M., Gardner, N.J., and Hugli, T.E. Familial carboxypeptidase N deficiency. *Ann. Intern Med.,* **1980,** *93:*443–445.

Molderings, G.J., Weissenborn, G., Schlicker, E., Likungu, J., and Göthert, M. Inhibition of noradrenaline release from the sympathetic nerves of the human saphenous vein by presynaptic histamine H3 receptors. *Naunyn Schmiedebergs Arch. Pharmacol.,* **1992,** *346:*46–50.

Morrow, J.D., Margolies, G.R. Rowland, J., and Roberts, L.J. II. Evidence that histamine is the causative toxin of scombroid-fish poisoning. *N. Engl. J. Med.,* **1991,** *324:*716–720.

Ondetti, M.A., Williams, N.J., Sabo, E.F., Pluscec, J., Weaver, E.R., and Kocy, O. Angiotensin-converting enzyme inhibitors from the venom of *Bothrops jararaca.* Isolation, elucidation of structure, and synthesis. *Biochemistry,* **1971,** *10:*4033–4039.

Ookuma, K., Sakata, T., Fukagawa, K., Yoshimatsu, H., Kurokawa, M., Machidori, H., and Fujimoto, K. Neuronal histamine in the hypothalamus suppresses food intake in rats. *Brain Res.,* **1993,** *628:*235–242.

Palmer, R.M., Ferrige, A.G., and Moncada, S. Nitric oxide release accounts for the biological activity of endothelium-derived relaxing factor. *Nature,* **1987,** *327:*524–526.

Pellacani, A., Brunner, H.R., and Nussberger, J. Antagonizing and measurement: approaches to understanding of hemodynamic effects of kinins. *J. Cardiovasc. Pharmacol.,* **1992,** *20(suppl 9):*S28–S34.

Polosa, R., Rajakulasingam, K., Church, M.K., and Holgate, S.T. Repeated inhalation of bradykinin attenuates adenosine 5′-monophosphate (AMP) induced bronchoconstriction in asthmatic airways. *Eur. Respir. J.,* **1992,** *5:*700–706.

Regoli, D., Jukic, D., Gobeil, F., and Rhaleb, N.E. Receptors for bradykinin and related kinins: a critical analysis. *Can. J. Physiol. Pharmacol.,* **1993,** *71:*556–567.

Richelson, E. Tricyclic antidepressants and histamine H1 receptors. *Mayo Clin. Proc.,* **1979,** *54:*669–674.

Roberts, L.J. II, Marney, S.R. Jr., and Oates, J.A. Blockade of the flush associated with metastatic gastric carcinoid syndrome by combined histamine H1 and H2 receptor antagonists: Evidence for an important role of H2 receptors in human vasculature. *N. Engl. J. Med.,* **1979,** *300:*236–238.

Roberts, L.J. II, and Oates, J.A. Biochemical diagnosis of systemic mast cell disorders. *J. Invest. Dermatol.,* **1991,** *96:*19S–25S.

Roberts, L.J. II, Sweetman, B.J., Lewis, R.A., Austen, K.F., and Oates, J.A. Marked overproduction of prostaglandin D2 in patients with mastocytosis. *N. Engl. J. Med.,* **1980,** *303:*1400–1404.

Rocha e Silva, M., Beraldo, W.T., and Rosenfeld, G. Bradykinin, a hypotensive and smooth muscle stimulating factor released from plasma globulin by snake venoms and by trypsin. *Am. J. Physiol.,* **1949,** *156:*261–273.

Roehrs, T., Zwyghuizen-Doorenbos, A., and Roth, T. Sedative effects and plasma concentrations following single dose of triazolam, diphenhydramine, ethanol, and placebo. *Sleep,* **1993,** *16:*301–305.

Russell, T., Stolz, M., and Weir, S. Pharmacokinetics, pharmacodynamics, and tolerance of single- and multiple-dose fexofenadine hydrochloride in healthy male volunteers. *Clin. Pharmacol. Ther.,* **1998,** *64:*612–621.

Saitoh, S., Scicli, A.G., Peterson, E., and Carretero, O.A. Effect of inhibiting renal kallikrein on prostaglandin E2, water, and sodium excretion. *Hypertension,* **1995,** *25:*1008–1013.

Schulman, G., Hakim, R., Arias, R., Silverberg, M., Kaplan, A.P., and Arbeit, L. Bradykinin generation by dialysis membranes: possible role in anaphylactic reaction. *J. Am. Soc. Nephrol.,* **1993,** *3:*1563–1569.

Serafin, W.E., and Austen, K.F. Mediators of immediate hypersensitivity reactions. *N. Engl. J. Med.,* **1987,** *317:*30–34.

Shirakawa, T., Li, A., Dubowitz, M., Dekker, J.W., Shaw, A.E., Faux, J.A., Ra, C., Cookson, W.O., and Hopkin, J.M. Association between atopy and variants of the β subunit of the high-affinity immunoglobulin E receptor. *Nat. Genet.,* **1994,** *7:*125–129.

Simons, F.E., and Simons, K.J. H1 receptor antagonist treatment of chronic rhinitis. *J. Allergy Clin. Immunol.,* **1988,** *81:*975–980.

Sullivan, T.J. Pharmacologic modulation of the whealing response to histamine in human skin: identification of doxepin as a potent *in vivo* inhibitor. *J. Allergy Clin. Immunol.,* **1982,** *69:*260–267.

Takagaki, Y., Kitamura, N., and Nakanishi, S. Cloning and sequence analysis of cDNAs for human high molecular weight and low molecular weight prekininogens. Primary structures of two human prekininogens. *J. Biol. Chem.,* **1985,** *260:*8601–8609.

Tardivel-Lacombe, J., Rouleau, A., Heron, A., Morisset, S., Pillot, C., Cochois, V., Schwartz, J.C., and Arrang, J.M. Cloning and cerebral expression of the guinea pig histamine H₃ receptor: evidence for two isoforms. *Neuroreport,* **2000,** *11:*755–759.

Taylor, D.A., Bowman, B.F., and Stull, J.T. Cytoplasmic Ca^{2+} is a primary determinant for myosin phosphorylation in smooth muscle cells. *J. Biol. Chem.,* **1989,** *264:*6207–6213.

Tippmer, S., Quitterer, U., Kolm, V., Faussner, A., Roscher, A., Mosthaf, L., Müller-Esterl, W., and Häring, H. Bradykinin induces translocation of the protein kinase C isoforms α, ε, and ζ. *Eur. J. Biochem.,* **1994,** *225:*297–304.

Vavrek, R.J., and Stewart, J.M. Competitive antagonists of bradykinin. *Peptides,* **1985,** *6:*161–164.

Verresen, L., Fink, E., Lemke, H.-D., and Vanrenterghem, Y. Bradykinin is a mediator of anaphylactoid reactions during hemodialysis with AN69 membranes. *Kidney Int.,* **1994,** *45:*1497–1503.

Wantke, F., Götz, M., and Jarish, R. The red wine provocation test: intolerance to histamine as a model for food intolerance. *Allergy Proc.,* **1994,** *15:*27–32.

MONOGRAPHS AND REVIEWS

Bhoola, K.D., Figueroa C.D., and Worthy, K. Bioregulation of kinins: kallikreins, kininogens, and kininases. *Pharmacol. Rev.,* **1992,** *44:*1–80.

Bovet, D. Introduction to antihistamine agents and Antergan derivatives. *Ann. N.Y. Acad. Sci.,* **1950,** *50:*1089–1126.

Brogden, R.N., and McTavish, D. Acrivastine. A review of its pharmacological properties and therapeutic efficacy in allergic rhinitis, urticaria and related disorders. *Drugs,* **1991,** *41:*927–940.

Burch, R.M., and Kyle, D.J. Recent developments in the understanding of bradykinin receptors. *Life Sci.,* **1992,** *50:*829–838.

Carey, R.M., Wang, Z.Q., and Siragy, H.M. Role of the angiotensin type 2 receptor in the regulation of blood pressure and renal function. *Hypertension,* **2000,** *35:*155–163.

Colman, R.W. Biologic activities of the contact factors *in vivo*—potentiation of hypotension, inflammation, and fibrinolysis, and inhibition of cell adhesion, angiogenesis and thrombosis. *Thromb. Haemost.,* **1999,** *82:*1568–1577.

Dickenson, J.M., and Hill, S.J. Interactions between adenosine A₁- and histamine H₁-receptors. *Int. J. Biochem.,* **1994,** *26:*959–969.

Dray, A., and Perkins, M. Bradykinin and inflammatory pain. *Trends Neurosci.,* **1993,** *16:*99–104.

DuBuske, L.M. Second-generation antihistamines: the risk of ventricular arrhythmias. *Clin. Ther.,* **1999,** *21:*281–295.

Erdos, E.G. The angiotensin I converting enzyme. *Fed. Proc.,* **1977,** *36:*1760–1765.

Galli, S.J. New concepts about the mast cell. *N. Engl. J. Med.,* **1993,** *328:*257–265.

Ganellin, C.R., and Parsons, M.E., eds. *Pharmacology of Histamine Receptors.* PSG, Bristol, MA, **1982.**

Geppetti, P. Sensory neuropeptide release by bradykinin: mechanisms and pathophysiological implications. *Regul. Pept.,* **1993,** *47:*1–23.

Hough, L.B. Cellular localization and possible functions for brain histamine: recent progress. *Prog. Neurobiol.,* **1988,** *30:*469–505.

Janssens, M.M., and Vanden Bussche, G. Levocabastine: an effective topical treatment of allergic rhinoconjunctivitis. *Clin. Exp. Allergy,* **1991,** *21(suppl 2):*29–36.

Lagunoff, D., Martin, T.W., and Read, G. Agents that release histamine from mast cells. *Annu. Rev. Pharmacol. Toxicol.,* **1983,** *23:*331–351.

Lerner, U.H. Regulation of bone metabolism by the kallikrein-kinin system, the coagulation cascade, and the acute-phase reactants. *Oral Surg. Oral Med. Oral Pathol.,* **1994,** *78:*481–493.

Leurs, R., Blandina, P., Tedford, C., and Timmerman, H. Therapeutic potential of histamine H₃ receptor agonists and antagonists. *Trends Pharmacol. Sci.,* **1998,** *19:*177–183.

Lewis, T. *The Blood Vessels of the Human Skin and Their Responses.* Shaw & Sons, Ltd., London, **1927.**

Lichtenstein, L.M., Kapey-Sobotka, A., and Gleich, G.J. The Role of Basophils and Eosinophils in Human Disease. Proceedings of a meeting. Cabo San Lucas, Mexico, March 10–13, 1994. *J. Allergy Clin. Immunol.* **1994,** *94:*1103–1326.

Linz, W., and Schölkens, B.A. Role of bradykinin in the cardiac effects of angiotensin-converting enzyme inhibitors. *J. Cardiovasc. Pharmacol.,* **1992,** *20(suppl 9):*S83–S90.

Madeddu, P. Receptor antagonists of bradykinin: a new tool to study the cardiovascular effects of endogenous kinins. *Pharmacol. Res.,* **1993,** *28:*107–128.

Margolius, H.S. Theodore Cooper Memorial Lecture. Kallikreins and kinins. Some unanswered questions about system characteristics and roles in human disease. *Hypertension,* **1995,** *26:*221–229.

Margolius, H.S. Tissue kallikreins and kinins: regulation and roles in hypertensive and diabetic diseases. *Annu. Rev. Pharmacol. Toxicol.,* **1989,** *29:*343–364.

Monti, J.M. Involvement of histamine in the control of the waking state. *Life Sci.,* **1993,** *53:*1331–1338.

Nadel, J.A., and Barnes, P.J. Autonomic regulation of the airways. *Annu. Rev. Med.,* **1984,** *35:*451–467.

Nakanishi, S. Substance P precursor and kininogen: their structures, gene organizations, and regulation. *Physiol. Rev.,* **1987,** *67:*1117–1142.

Paton, D.M., and Webster, D.R. Clinical pharmacokinetics of H₁-receptor antagonists (the antihistamines). *Clin. Pharmacokinet.,* **1985,** *10:*477–497.

Proud, D., and Kaplan, A.P. Kinin formation: mechanisms and role in inflammatory disorders. *Annu. Rev. Immunol.,* **1988,** *6:*49–83.

Ravetch, J.V., and Kinet, J.P. Fc receptors. *Annu. Rev. Immunol.,* **1991,** *9:*457–492.

Regoli, D., and Barabé, J. Pharmacology of bradykinin and related kinins. *Pharmacol. Rev.,* **1980,** *32:*1–46.

Rocha e Silva, M., ed. *Histamine II and Anti-Histaminics: Chemistry, Metabolism and Physiological and Pharmacological Actions.* [*Handbuch der Experimentellen Pharmakologie*], Vol. 18, Pt. 2. Springer-Verlag, Berlin, **1978.**

Ryan, J.W. Processing of the endogenous polypeptides by the lungs. *Annu. Rev. Physiol.,* **1982,** *44:*241–255.

Schill, W.-B., and Miska, W. Possible effects of the kallikrein-kinin system on male reproductive functions. *Andrologia,* **1992,** *24:*69–75.

Schmaier, A.H., Rojkjaer, R., and Shariat-Madar, Z. Activation of the plasma kallikrein/kinin system on cells: a revised hypothesis. *Thromb. Haemost.,* **1999,** *82:*226–233.

Schrör, K. Role of prostaglandins in the cardiovascular effects of bradykinin and angiotensin-converting enzyme inhibitors. *J. Cardiovasc. Pharmacol.,* **1992,** *20(suppl 9):*S68–S73.

Schwartz, L.B. Mast cells: function and contents. *Curr. Opin. Immunol.,* **1994,** *6:*91–97.

Schwieler, J.H., and Hjemdahl, P. Influence of angiotensin-converting enzyme inhibition on sympathetic neurotransmission: possible roles of bradykinin and prostaglandins. *J. Cardiovasc. Pharmacol.,* **1992,** *20(suppl 9):*S39–S46.

Simons, F.E., and Simons, K.J. The pharmacology and use of H₁-receptor-antagonist drugs. *N. Engl. J. Med.,* **1994,** *330*:1663–1670.

Slater, E.E., Merrill, D.D., Guess, H.A., Roylance, P.J., Cooper, W.D., Inman, W.H., and Ewan, P.W. Clinical profile of angioedema associated with angiotensin-converting enzyme inhibition. *JAMA,* **1988,** *260*:967–970.

Spencer, C.M., Faulds, D., and Peters, D.H. Cetirizine. A reappraisal of its pharmacological properties and therapeutic use in selected allergic disorders. *Drugs,* **1993,** *46*:1055–1080.

Symposium. The Role of Basophils and Eosinophils in Human Disease. Proceedings of a meeting. Cabo San Lucas, Mexico, March 10–13, 1994. *J. Allergy Clin. Immunol.,* **1994,** *94*:1103–1326.

Timmerman, H. Histamine H₃ ligands: just pharmacological tools or potential therapeutic agents? *J. Med. Chem.,* **1990,** *33*:4–11.

Trifilieff, A., Da Silva, A., and Gies, J.-P. Kinins and respiratory tract diseases. *Eur. Respir. J.,* **1993,** *6*:576–587.

Vanhoutte, P.M. Endothelium and control of vascular function. State of the art lecture. *Hypertension,* **1989,** *13*:658–667.

Wachtfogel, Y.T., DeLa Cadena, R.A., and Colman, R.W. Structural biology, cellular interactions and pathophysiology of the contact system. *Thromb. Res.,* **1993,** *72*:1–21.

Werle, E. Discovery of the most important kallikreins and kallikrein inhibitors. In, *Bradykinin, Kallidin and Kallikrein.* (Erdös, E.G., ed.) *[Handbuch der Experimentellen Pharmakologie],* Vol. 25. Springer-Verlag, Berlin, **1970,** pp. 1–6.

Acknowledgment

The authors wish to acknowledge Drs. Kenneth S. Babe, Jr., and William E. Serafin, authors of this chapter in the ninth edition of *Goodman and Gilman's The Pharmacological Basis of Therapeutics,* some of whose text we have retained in this edition.

LIPID-DERIVED AUTACOIDS

Eicosanoids and Platelet-Activating Factor

Jason D. Morrow and L. Jackson Roberts II

Few biological substances have been the focus of such intense research efforts over the past half-century as have lipid-derived autacoids. Two distinct families of autacoids derived from membrane phospholipids have been identified: the eicosanoids, *which are formed from certain polyunsaturated fatty acids (principally arachidonic acid), include the prostaglandins, prostacyclin, thromboxane A_2, and the leukotrienes; and* modified phospholipids, *represented by platelet-activating factor (PAF). The eicosanoids are extremely prevalent and have been detected in almost every tissue and body fluid. Their production increases in response to diverse stimuli, and they produce a broad spectrum of biological effects. Although its precursors are widely distributed, PAF is formed by a smaller number of cell types, principally circulating leukocytes and platelets and endothelial cells. However, because of the wide distribution of these cells, the actions of PAF can be manifest in virtually every organ and tissue of the body. These lipids contribute to a number of physiological and pathological processes including inflammation, smooth muscle tone, hemostasis, thrombosis, parturition, and gastrointestinal secretion. Several classes of drugs, most notably the nonsteroidal antiinflammatory agents, owe their therapeutic effects to blockade of the formation of eicosanoids. This chapter reviews the synthesis, metabolism, and mechanism of action of eicosanoids and PAF and also introduces the therapeutic value of selective inhibitors of eicosanoid synthesis and action. The therapeutic role of these inhibitors is expanded upon in Chapter 27, concerning antipyretic and antiinflammatory agents, and in Chapter 54, concerning antiplatelet drugs.*

EICOSANOIDS

History. In 1930 Kurzrok and Lieb, two American gynecologists, observed that strips of human uterus relax or contract when exposed to human semen. A few years later, Goldblatt in England and von Euler in Sweden independently reported smooth muscle–contracting and vasodepressor activity in seminal fluid and accessory reproductive glands. Von Euler identified the active material as a lipid-soluble acid, which he named *prostaglandin* (*see* von Euler, 1973). More than twenty years passed before the demonstration that prostaglandin was in fact a family of unique compounds; the structures of two of these, prostaglandin E_1 (PGE$_1$) and prostaglandin $F_{1\alpha}$ (PGF$_{1\alpha}$), were elucidated in 1962. More prostaglandins soon were characterized, and these, like the others, proved to be 20-carbon unsaturated carboxylic acids with a cyclopentane ring. When the general structure of the prostaglandins became apparent, their kinship with essential fatty acids was recognized. In 1964 Bergström and coworkers and van Dorp and associates independently achieved the biosynthesis of PGE$_2$ from arachidonic acid using homogenates of sheep seminal vesicle (*see* Samuelsson, 1972).

Realization that the "classically known" prostaglandins constitute only a fraction of the physiologically active products of arachidonate metabolism resulted from the discovery of thromboxane A_2 (TXA$_2$) (Hamberg *et al.*, 1975), prostacyclin (PGI$_2$) (Moncada *et al.*, 1976), and the leukotrienes (Samuelsson, 1983). The discovery by Vane, Smith, and Willis in 1971 that aspirin and related drugs inhibit prostaglandin biosynthesis provided insight into the mechanism of action of these drugs as well as an important tool for investigation of the role of these autacoids (*see* Vane, 1971).

The families of prostaglandins, leukotrienes, and related compounds are called *eicosanoids* because they are derived from 20-carbon essential fatty acids that contain three, four, or five double bonds: 8,11,14-eicosatrienoic acid (dihomo-γ-linolenic acid); 5,8,11,14-eicosatetraenoic acid (arachidonic acid) (*see* Figure 26–1); and 5,8,11,14,17-eicosapentaenoic acid. In human beings, arachidonate is the most abundant precursor, and it is either derived from dietary linoleic acid (9,12-octadecadienoic acid) or ingested as a dietary constituent. 5,8,11,14,17-Eicosapentaenoic acid is found in large amounts in fish oils. Arachidonate is esterified to the phospholipids of cell membranes or other complex lipids. Since the concentration of free

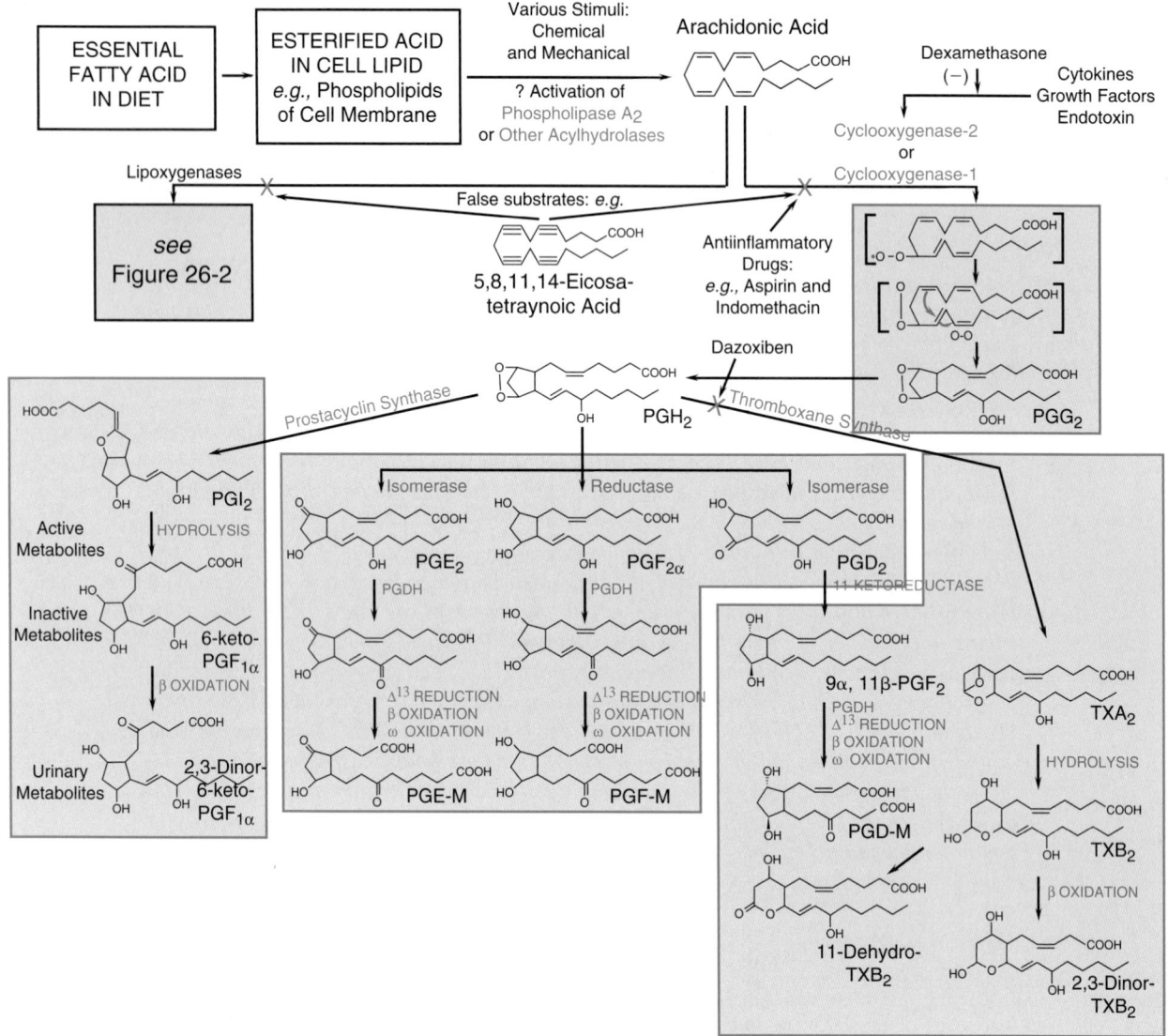

Figure 26–1. Biosynthesis of the products of arachidonic acid.

Two major routes of metabolism of arachidonic acid are shown. Lipoxygenase pathways lead to HPETEs, HETEs, and the leukotrienes (shown in Figure 26–2); the cyclooxygenase pathway leads to the cyclic endoperoxides (PGG and PGH) and subsequent metabolic products (*see* text). Cyclooxygenase-1 (COX-1) is constitutively expressed. Cyclooxygenase-2 (COX-2) is induced by cytokines, growth factors, and endotoxin, an effect that is blocked by glucocorticoids. Compounds such as aspirin and indomethacin inhibit the cyclooxygenases but not the lipoxygenases, while 5,8,11,14-eicosatetraynoic acid inhibits both pathways. Dazoxiben and other agents are selective inhibitors of thromboxane synthase. *See* text for other abbreviations.

arachidonate in the cell is very low, the biosynthesis of eicosanoids depends primarily upon the availability of arachidonate to the eicosanoid-synthesizing enzymes; this results from its release from cellular stores of lipid by acylhydrolases, most notably phospholipase A_2. The enhanced biosynthesis of the eicosanoids is closely regulated and occurs in response to widely divergent physical, chemical, and hormonal stimuli.

Biosynthesis. Hormones, autacoids, and other substances augment the biosynthesis of eicosanoids by interacting with (presumably) plasma membrane–bound receptors that are coupled to GTP-binding regulatory proteins (G proteins; *see* Chapter 2). This results either in the direct activation of phospholipases or in elevated cytosolic concentrations of Ca^{2+}, which also can activate these enzymes. Physical stimuli are believed to cause an influx of Ca^{2+} by perturbing the cell membrane, thereby activating phospholipase A_2. Phospholipase A_2 hydrolyzes the *sn*-2 ester bond of membrane phospholipids (particularly phosphatidylcholine and phosphatidylethanolamine) with the release of arachidonate. Several different phospholipase A_2s have been characterized. Cytosolic phospholipase A_2 is likely the major phospholipase involved in agonist-stimulated arachidonate release and prostaglandin production (Lin *et al.,* 1992). Other phospholipases, however, may contribute to the release of arachidonic acid in various cell types (Okazaki *et al.,* 1981; Reddy *et al.,* 1997). Once released, a portion of the arachidonate is metabolized rapidly to oxygenated products by several distinct enzyme systems, including *cyclooxygenases* or one of several *lipoxygenases* or *cytochrome P450s.*

Products of Cyclooxygenases.   The prostaglandins and thromboxanes can be considered analogs of the unnatural compounds with the trivial names *prostanoic acid* and *thrombanoic acid,* respectively, the structures of which are as follows:

PROSTANOIC ACID

THROMBANOIC ACID

They fall into several main classes, designated by letters and distinguished by substitutions on the cyclopentane ring.

Prostaglandins of the E and D series are hydroxy ketones, while the Fα prostaglandins are 1,3-diols (*see* Figure 26–1). They are products of the metabolism of prostaglandins G (PGG) and H (PGH), cyclic endoperoxides. PGA, PGB, and PGC are unsaturated ketones that arise nonenzymatically from PGE during extraction procedures; it is unlikely that they occur biologically. PGJ_2 and related compounds result from the dehydration of PGD_2. Firm evidence for their formation *in vivo* is lacking. Prostacyclin (PGI_2) has a double-ring structure; in addition to a cyclopentane ring, a second ring is formed by an oxygen bridge between carbons 6 and 9. Thromboxanes (TXs) contain a six-member oxane ring instead of the cyclopentane ring of the prostaglandins. Both PGI_2 and the thromboxanes also result from the metabolism of PGG and PGH (*see* Figure 26–1). The main classes are further subdivided in accord with the number of double bonds in the side chains. This is indicated by subscript 1, 2, or 3, and reflects the fatty acid precursor in most instances. Dihomo-γ-linolenic acid is the precursor of the one series, arachidonic acid for the two series, and 5,8,11,14,17-eicosapentaenoic acid for the three series. Prostaglandins derived from arachidonate carry the subscript 2 and are the major prostaglandins in mammals. There is little evidence that prostaglandins of the 1 or 3 series are made in adequate amounts to be important under normal circumstances.

Synthesis of prostaglandins is accomplished in a stepwise manner by a ubiquitous complex of microsomal enzymes. The first enzyme in this synthetic pathway is prostaglandin endoperoxide synthase, also called *fatty acid cyclooxygenase.* There are two isoforms of this enzyme, cyclooxygenase-1 and -2, dubbed COX-1, COX-2 (*see* Smith *et al.,* 1996; DuBois *et al.,* 1998). The former is constitutively expressed in most cells. In contrast, COX-2 is normally not present but may be induced by certain serum factors, cytokines, and growth factors, an effect that is inhibited by treatment with glucocorticoids such as dexamethasone.

The cyclooxygenases have two distinct activities: an endoperoxide synthase activity that oxygenates and cyclizes the unesterified precursor fatty acid to form the cyclic endoperoxide PGG, and a peroxidase activity that converts PGG to PGH (*see* Hamberg *et al.,* 1974). PGG and PGH are chemically unstable, but they can be transformed enzymatically into a variety of products, including PGI, TXA, PGE, PGF, or PGD (*see* Figure 26–1; Samuelsson *et al.,* 1975; Needleman *et al.,* 1986; Sigal, 1991). Isomerases for the synthesis of PGE_2 and PGD_2 have been identified. A reductase that catalyzes the conversion of PGH_2 to $PGF_{2\alpha}$ has been characterized.

The endoperoxide PGH_2 also is metabolized into two unstable and highly active compounds (Figure 26–1). Thromboxane A_2 (TXA_2) is formed by *thromboxane synthase;* TXA_2 breaks down nonenzymatically ($t_{1/2} = 30$ seconds) into the stable but inactive thromboxane B_2 (TXB_2). PGI_2 is formed from PGH_2 by *prostacyclin synthase;* it is hydrolyzed nonenzymatically ($t_{1/2} = 3$ minutes) to the inactive 6-keto-$PGF_{1\alpha}$.

Although most tissues are able to synthesize the PGG and PGH intermediates from free arachidonate, their fate varies in each tissue and depends on the complement of enzymes present and on their relative abundance. For example, lung and spleen are able to synthesize the whole range of products. In contrast, platelets contain thromboxane synthase as the principal enzyme that metabolizes PGH, while endothelial cells contain primarily prostacyclin synthase.

Products of Lipoxygenases.   Lipoxygenases are a family of cytosolic enzymes that catalyze the oxygenation of polyenic fatty acids to corresponding lipid hydroperoxides (*see* Samuelsson, 1983; Needleman *et al.,* 1986; Brash, 1999). The enzymes require a fatty acid substrate with two *cis* double bonds separated by a methylene group. Arachidonate, which contains several double bonds in this configuration, is metabolized to a number of products with the hydroperoxy group in different positions. For arachidonate, these metabolites are called hydroperoxyeicosatetraenoic acids (HPETEs). Lipoxygenases differ in their specificity for placing the hydroperoxy group, and tissues differ in the lipoxygenase(s) that they contain (*see* Brash, 1999). For example, platelets have only 12-lipoxygenase and synthesize 12-HPETE, whereas leukocytes contain both 5-lipoxygenase and 12-lipoxygenase and produce both 5-HPETE and 12-HPETE (*see* Figure 26–2). Other lipoxygenases that also catalyze the formation of 15-HPETE and 8-HPETE have been reported in human beings and laboratory animals.

The HPETEs are unstable intermediates, analogous to PGG or PGH, and are further metabolized by a variety of enzymes. All HPETEs may be converted to their corresponding hydroxy fatty acid (HETE) either by a peroxidase or nonenzymatically. 12-HPETE also can undergo a catalyzed molecular rearrangement to epoxy-hydroxyeicosatrienoic acids called *hepoxilins.* Similarly, leukocytes convert 15-HPETE to trihydroxylated metabolites called *lipoxins.*

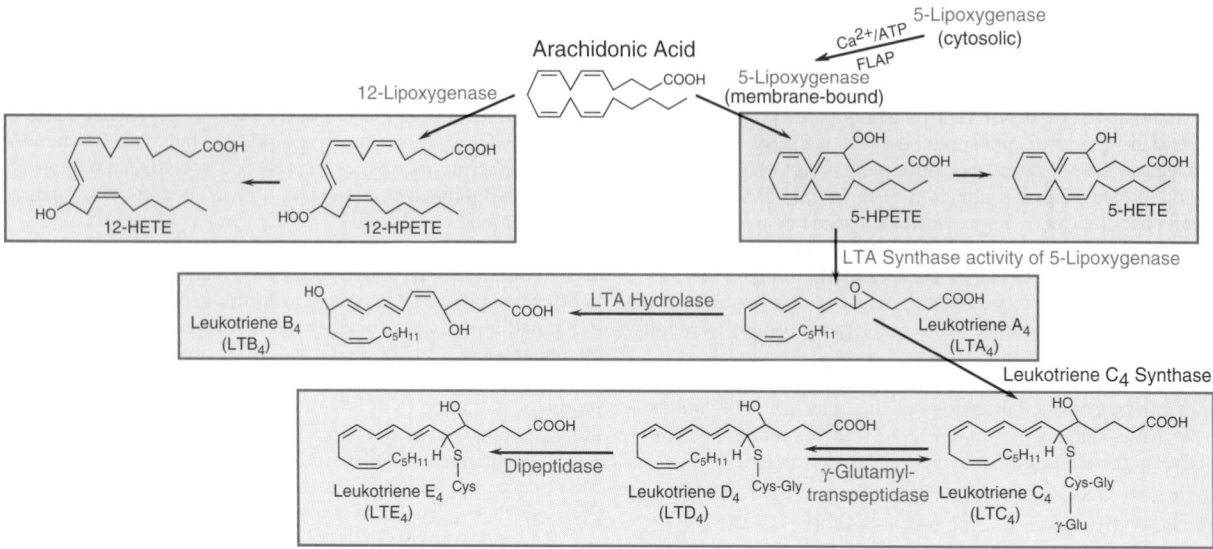

Figure 26–2. *Representative lipoxygenase pathways and structures of leukotrienes.* (See *text for abbreviations.*)

Zileuton inhibits the 5-lipoxygenase enzyme.

The 5-lipoxygenase is one of the most important of the lipoxygenases, since it leads to the synthesis of the *leukotrienes* (LTs) (Figure 26–2; *see* Samuelsson, 1983; Samuelsson *et al.,* 1987; Sigal, 1991). As with the prostaglandins, a subscript is used to indicate the number of double bonds in the fatty acid. Arachidonic acid is the precursor of the four series of leukotrienes and 5,8,11,14,17-eicosapentaenoic acid of the five series. When cells are activated, 5-lipoxygenase translocates to the nuclear membrane and associates with 5-lipoxygenase activating protein (FLAP), an integral membrane protein essential for leukotriene biosynthesis. FLAP appears to act as an arachidonic acid transfer protein that presents the substrate to the 5-lipoxygenase (*see* Brash, 1999). An experimental drug, MK-886, binds to FLAP and blocks leukotriene production. The 5-lipoxygenase catalyzes a two-step reaction: oxygenation of arachidonate at the fifth carbon to form 5-HPETE followed by dehydration of 5-HPETE to an unstable 5,6-epoxide, known as leukotriene A_4 (LTA$_4$) (Peters-Golden, 1998; Borgeat and Samuelsson, 1979). LTA$_4$ may be transformed by LTA hydrolase to a 5,12-dihydroxyeicosatetraenoic acid known as leukotriene B_4 (LTB$_4$); alternatively, it may be conjugated with reduced glutathione by LTC$_4$ synthase to form LTC$_4$ (Murphy *et al.,* 1979). Leukotriene D$_4$ (LTD$_4$) is produced by the removal of glutamic acid from LTC$_4$, and LTE$_4$ results from the subsequent cleavage of glycine (*see* Samuelsson, 1983; Piper, 1984; Samuelsson *et al.,* 1987). LTC$_4$, LTD$_4$, and LTE$_4$ often are referred to as *cysteinyl leukotrienes.* It is now generally accepted that a mixture of LTC$_4$, LTD$_4$, and LTE$_4$ makes up the material originally known as the "slow-reacting substance of anaphylaxis" (SRS-A), first described by Feldberg and Kellaway (1938).

Products of Cytochrome P450.   Arachidonate is metabolized by enzymes that contain cytochrome P450 to a variety of metabolites including 19- or 20-hydroxy arachidonate and epoxyeicosatrienoic acids (*see* Fitzpatrick and Murphy, 1988; Capdevila *et al.,* 2000). While these metabolites have potent vascular,

endocrine, renal, and ocular effects, the physiological importance of this pathway remains to be clarified.

Other Pathways.   A nonenzymatic pathway of arachidonate conversion also has been discovered, giving rise to a novel series of agents termed *isoprostanes* (Morrow *et al.,* 1990). These compounds, while having structures similar to cyclooxygenase-derived PGs, arise *in vivo* from the free radical–catalyzed peroxidation of arachidonate independent of the cyclooxygenase. Unlike the cyclooxygenase-derived eicosanoids, the isoprostanes identified to date are formed completely *in situ* on phospholipids and subsequently released preformed. Consequently, their production is not blocked *in vivo* by agents that suppress metabolism of free arachidonate, such as aspirin or nonsteroidal antiinflammatory agents, or by agents that suppress expression of the inducible COX-2 enzyme, such as steroidal antiinflammatory drugs. It is postulated that these agents might contribute to the pathophysiology of inflammatory responses insensitive to currently available steroidal or nonsteroidal antiinflammatory agents. Of importance is that this pathway of eicosanoid formation links free radical–mediated tissue injury with bioactive lipid-derived autacoid generation (Morrow *et al.,* 1999).

In the brain, arachidonate is coupled to ethanolamine to give arachidonylethanolamide, also called *anandamide* (Devane *et al.,* 1992). A similar reaction occurs with other unsaturated fatty acids. Anandamide binds to cannabinoid receptors and displays biochemical and behavioral effects very similar to those of Δ^9-tetrahydrocannabinol, including inhibition of adenylyl cyclase, inhibition of L-type calcium channels, analgesia, and hypothermia. Anandamide may be an endogenous ligand for the cannabinoid receptors (Martin *et al.,* 1999).

Inhibitors of Eicosanoid Biosynthesis.   A number of the biosynthetic steps described above can be inhibited by drugs. Inhibition of phospholipase A$_2$ decreases the release of the precursor fatty acid and thus the synthesis of all metabolites derived therefrom. Since phospholipase A_2 is activated by Ca^{2+} and calmodulin, it may be inhibited by drugs that reduce the availability of Ca^{2+}. Glucocorticoids also inhibit phospholipase A_2, but they appear to do so indirectly by inducing the synthesis of a group of proteins termed *annexins* (formerly, *lipocortins*), which modulate phospholipase A_2 activity (Flower, 1990). Glucocorticoids, however, also regulate expression of COX-2, but not of COX-1 (Masferrer *et al.*, 1994; Smith *et al.*, 1996). It is therefore conceivable that therapeutically effective doses of glucocorticoids as antiinflammatory agents correlate more closely with their potency in suppressing cytokine-induced COX-2 expression than with their potency in inhibiting phospholipase.

Aspirin and related nonsteroidal antiinflammatory drugs originally were found to prevent the synthesis of prostaglandins from arachidonate in tissue homogenates (Vane, 1971). It is now known that these drugs inhibit cyclooxygenase and, as a result, inhibit the synthesis of PGG_2, PGH_2, and all that flows therefrom. However, these drugs do not inhibit the metabolism of arachidonate by lipoxygenases. In fact, inhibition of cyclooxygenase theoretically could lead to increased formation of leukotrienes by increasing the amount of arachidonate that is available to the lipoxygenases (*see* Piper, 1984). Inhibition of cyclooxygenase provides an important basis for understanding many of the therapeutic and other effects of these agents (*see* Chapter 27).

COX-1 and -2 differ in their sensitivity to inhibition by certain antiinflammatory drugs (*see* Vane *et al.*, 1998; Marnett *et al.*, 1999). This observation has led to the recent development of clinically useful agents that selectively inhibit COX-2 (*see* Chapter 27). These drugs show distinct therapeutic advantages over nonselective nonsteroidal antiinflammatory agents, since COX-2 is the predominant cyclooxygenase at sites of inflammation but not at sites such as the gastrointestinal tract. Thus, as has been largely borne out by clinical trials, COX-2 inhibitors are antiinflammatory but do not possess many of the adverse side effects of nonselective cyclooxygenase inhibitors.

Since different metabolites of PGH_2 sometimes produce opposite biological effects (*see* below), there are theoretical advantages in compounds that preferentially inhibit one or another of the enzymes that metabolize PGH_2 (*see* Moncada and Vane, 1978). For example, there had been significant interest in the development of agents that inhibit thromboxane synthase and thus block platelet aggregation and induce vasodilation. Although these drugs block thromboxane production *in vitro* and *in vivo*, they have largely failed to produce clinical benefits in a wide variety of disorders. The lack of clinical efficacy of these agents may reflect other vasoactive mediators contributing

to the pathophysiology of disorders that were studied or that, following thromboxane synthesis inhibition, there is an accumulation of PGH_2, which shares some of the biological effects of TXA_2. Similar disappointing results have been obtained in clinical studies with combined thromboxane synthase/thromboxane receptor antagonists.

Analogs of the natural fatty acid precursors can serve as competitive inhibitors of the formation of both prostaglandins and the products of lipoxygenases. One such inhibitor is the acetylenic analog of arachidonic acid, 5,8,11,14-eicosatetraynoic acid (*see* Figure 26–1). Since leukotrienes function as inflammatory mediators, recent efforts have focused on development of leukotriene receptor antagonists and selective inhibitors of lipoxygenase synthesis. *Zileuton*, an inhibitor of 5-lipoxygenase, has proven to be useful in the treatment of asthma and possibly other inflammatory diseases. In addition, cysteinyl leukotriene receptor antagonists, including *zafirlukast, pranlukast*, and *montelukast*, are useful in the therapy of asthma (*see* Chapter 28).

Eicosanoid Catabolism. Efficient mechanisms exist for the catabolism and inactivation of most eicosanoids. About 95% of infused PGE_2 is inactivated during one passage through the pulmonary circulation. Because of the unique position of the lungs between the venous and arterial circulation, the pulmonary vascular bed constitutes an important filter for many substances (including some prostaglandins) that act locally prior to their release into the venous circulation. Broadly speaking, the enzymatic catabolic reactions are of two types: an initial (relatively rapid) step, catalyzed by widely distributed prostaglandin-specific enzymes, wherein prostaglandins lose most of their biological activity, and a second (relatively slow) step in which these metabolites are oxidized by enzymes probably identical with those responsible for the β and ω oxidation of most fatty acids. The initial step is the oxidation of the 15-OH group to the corresponding ketone by prostaglandin 15-OH dehydrogenase (PGDH). The 15-keto compound is then reduced to the 13,14-dihydro derivative, a reaction catalyzed by prostaglandin Δ^{13}-reductase. Subsequent steps consist of β and ω oxidation of the side chains of the prostaglandins, giving rise to a polar dicarboxylic acid, which is excreted in the urine as the major metabolite of both PGE_1 and PGE_2 (*see* Figure 26–1); these reactions take place particularly in the liver.

Unlike PGE_2, PGD_2 is initially reduced *in vivo* to the F-ring prostaglandin $9\alpha 11\beta$-PGF_2, which possesses significant biological activity. Subsequently, this compound undergoes metabolism similar to that of other eicosanoids (Figure 26–1).

The metabolism of TXA_2 in human beings is inferred from investigation of the fate of TXB_2. Although up to twenty metabolites have been identified in urine, by far the most abundant are 2,3-dinor-TXB_2 and 11-dehydro-TXB_2 (Uedelhoven *et al.*, 1989; *see* Figure 26–1).

The degradation of PGI_2 apparently begins with its spontaneous hydrolysis in blood to 6-keto-$PGF_{1\alpha}$. The metabolism of this compound in human beings involves the same steps as those for PGE_2 and $PGF_{2\alpha}$ (Rosenkranz *et al.*, 1980).

The degradation of LTC_4 occurs in the lungs, kidney, and liver (Denzlinger *et al.*, 1986). The initial steps involve its conversion to LTE_4, and this results in a loss in biological activity. Leukotriene C_4 also may be inactivated by oxidation of its cysteinyl sulfur to a sulfoxide. The principal route of inactivation of LTB_4 is by ω oxidation.

Pharmacological Properties of Eicosanoids

No other autacoids show more numerous and diverse effects than do prostaglandins and other metabolites of arachidonate. It would be overly confusing to present all of the pharmacological effects that have been ascribed to these substances and even more so to delve into the activities of their synthetic analogs. This discussion is limited to activities that are thought to be the most important.

Cardiovascular System. *Prostaglandins.* In the vascular beds of human beings and most animals, the PGEs are potent vasodilators. The dilation appears to involve arterioles, precapillary sphincters, and postcapillary venules; large veins are not affected by PGEs. However, PGEs are not universally vasodilatory; constrictor effects have been noted at selected sites (*see* Bergström *et al.*, 1968).

PGD$_2$ similarly causes both vasodilation and vasoconstriction; however, in most vascular beds, including the mesenteric, coronary, and renal, vasodilation occurs at lower concentrations than does vasoconstriction. An exception is the pulmonary circulation in which PGD$_2$ causes only vasoconstriction. Responses to PGF$_{2\alpha}$ vary with species and vascular bed. It is a potent constrictor of both pulmonary arteries and veins in human beings (Spannhake *et al.*, 1981; Giles and Leff, 1988).

Systemic blood pressure generally falls in response to PGEs, and blood flow to most organs, including the heart, mesentery, and kidney, is increased. These effects are particularly striking in some hypertensive patients. Blood pressure is increased by PGF$_{2\alpha}$ in some experimental animals due to venoconstriction; however, in human beings, PGF$_{2\alpha}$ does not alter blood pressure.

Cardiac output generally is increased by prostaglandins of the E and F series. Weak, direct inotropic effects have been noted in various isolated preparations. In the intact animal, however, increased force of contraction as well as increased heart rate is in large measure a reflex consequence of a fall in total peripheral resistance.

Prostaglandin endoperoxides have variable effects in vascular beds. Their major effects are a result of intrinsic vasoconstrictor activity coupled with vasodilation due to rapid conversion to PGI$_2$, which is a vasodilator. PGH$_2$ is rapidly converted to PGI$_2$ during passage through the lungs.

The intravenous administration of PGI$_2$ causes prominent hypotension; it is about five times more potent than PGE$_2$ in producing this effect. The reduction in blood pressure is accompanied by a reflex increase in heart rate. The compound relaxes vascular smooth muscle, and it is thought to be a physiological modulator of vascular tone that functions to oppose the actions of vasoconstrictors.

Thromboxane A$_2$. Thromboxane A$_2$ is a potent vasoconstrictor. It contracts vascular smooth muscle *in vitro* (Bhagwat *et al.*, 1985) and is a vasoconstrictor in the whole animal and in isolated vascular beds.

Leukotrienes. In human beings, LTC$_4$ and LTD$_4$ cause hypotension (*see* Feuerstein, 1984; Piper, 1984). This may result in part from a decrease in intravascular volume and in cardiac contractility that is secondary to a marked, leukotriene-induced reduction in coronary blood flow. Although LTC$_4$ and LTD$_4$ have little effect on most large arteries or veins, coronary arteries and distal segments of the pulmonary artery are contracted by nanomolar concentrations of these agents (Berkowitz *et al.*, 1984). The renal vasculature is resistant to this constrictor action, but the mesenteric vasculature is not.

The leukotrienes have prominent effects on the microvasculature. LTC$_4$ and LTD$_4$ appear to act on the endothelial lining of postcapillary venules to cause exudation of plasma; they are more than a thousandfold more potent than histamine in this regard (*see* Feuerstein, 1984; Piper, 1984). In higher concentrations, LTC$_4$ and LTD$_4$ constrict arterioles and reduce exudation of plasma.

Blood. Eicosanoids modify the function of the formed elements of the blood; in some instances, these actions reflect their physiological roles. The prostaglandins and related products modulate platelet function. PGI$_2$ inhibits the aggregation of human platelets *in vitro* at concentrations between 1 and 10 nM. This fact and the observation that PGI$_2$ is synthesized by the vascular endothelium have led to the suggestion that PGI$_2$ controls the aggregation of platelets *in vivo* and contributes to the antithrombogenic properties of the intact vascular wall (*see* Moncada and Vane, 1978).

TXA$_2$ is a major product of arachidonate metabolism in platelets (Hamberg *et al.*, 1975) and, as a powerful inducer of platelet aggregation and the platelet release reaction, is a physiological mediator of platelet aggregation. Pathways of platelet aggregation that are dependent on the generation of TXA$_2$ are sensitive to the inhibitory action of aspirin (*see* Chapters 27 and 55; Moncada and Vane, 1978).

LTB$_4$ is a potent chemotactic agent for polymorphonuclear leukocytes, eosinophils, and monocytes; other leukotrienes do not share this action (*see* Piper, 1984). Its potency is comparable with that of various chemotactic peptides and PAF. In higher concentrations, LTB$_4$ stimulates the aggregation of polymorphonuclear leukocytes and promotes degranulation and the generation of superoxide. LTB$_4$ promotes adhesion of neutrophils to vascular endothelial cells and their transendothelial migration; application of LTB$_4$ to the skin promotes the local accumulation of neutrophils. Prostaglandins inhibit lymphocyte function and proliferation and suppress the immunological response. PGE$_2$ inhibits the differentiation of B lymphocytes into antibody-secreting plasma cells to depress the humoral antibody response. It also inhibits mitogen-stimulated proliferation of T lymphocytes and the release of lymphokines by sensitized T lymphocytes.

Smooth Muscle. Prostaglandins contract or relax many smooth muscles beside those of the vasculature. The leukotrienes (*e.g.*, LTD$_4$) contract most smooth muscles.

Bronchial and Tracheal Muscle. In general, PGFs and PGD$_2$ contract and PGEs relax bronchial and tracheal muscle. Although both PGE$_1$ and PGE$_2$ can produce bronchodilation when given to such patients by aerosol, bronchoconstriction sometimes is observed. Prostaglandin endoperoxides and TXA$_2$ constrict human bronchial smooth muscle. PGI$_2$ causes bronchodilation in most species; human bronchial tissue is particularly sensitive, and PGI$_2$ antagonizes bronchoconstriction that is induced by other agents.

LTC$_4$ and LTD$_4$ are bronchoconstrictors in many species, including human beings (*see* Piper, 1984; Drazen and Austen, 1987). They act principally on smooth muscle in peripheral airways and are a thousand times more potent than histamine both *in vitro* and *in vivo*. They also stimulate bronchial mucus secretion and cause mucosal edema.

Uterus. Strips of nonpregnant human uterus are contracted by PGFs and TXA$_2$ but are relaxed by PGEs. The contractile response is most prominent before menstruation, whereas relaxation is greatest at midcycle (*see* Bergström *et al.*, 1968). Uterine strips from pregnant women are uniformly contracted by PGFs *and* by low concentrations of PGE$_2$; PGI$_2$ and high concentrations of PGE$_2$ produce relaxation. The intravenous infusion of PGE$_2$ or PGF$_{2\alpha}$ to pregnant women produces a dose-dependent increase in uterine tone as well as the frequency and intensity of rhythmic uterine contraction. Uterine responsiveness to prostaglandins increases as pregnancy progresses; however, the increase is far less than that to oxytocin.

Gastrointestinal Muscle. The main longitudinal muscle from stomach to colon is contracted by both PGEs and PGFs, while circular muscle generally relaxes in response to PGEs and contracts in response to PGFs. Prostaglandin endoperoxides, TXA$_2$, and PGI$_2$ produce contraction but are less active than the PGEs or PGFs on gastrointestinal smooth muscle. The leukotrienes have potent contractile effects. Prostaglandins reduce transit times in the small intestine and colon. Diarrhea, cramps, and reflux of bile have been noted in response to oral PGE; these are common side effects (along with nausea and vomiting) in patients given prostaglandins for abortion.

Gastric and Intestinal Secretions. PGEs and PGI$_2$ inhibit gastric acid secretion stimulated by feeding, histamine, or gastrin. Volume of secretion, acidity, and content of pepsin all are reduced, probably by an action exerted directly on the secretory

cells. In addition, these prostaglandins are vasodilators in the gastric mucosa, and PGI$_2$ may be involved in the local regulation of blood flow. Mucus secretion in the stomach and small intestine is increased by PGEs. These effects help to maintain the integrity of the gastric mucosa and are referred to as the cytoprotectant properties of PGEs. Furthermore, PGEs and their analogs inhibit gastric damage caused by a variety of ulcerogenic agents and promote healing of duodenal and gastric ulcers (*see* Chapter 37). PGEs and PGFs stimulate the movement of water and electrolytes into the intestinal lumen. Such effects may underlie the watery diarrhea that follows the oral or parenteral administration of prostaglandins. By contrast, PGI$_2$ does not induce diarrhea; indeed, it prevents that provoked by other prostaglandins.

Kidney and Urine Formation. Prostaglandins influence renal salt and water excretion by alterations in renal blood flow and by direct effects on renal tubules. PGE$_2$ and PGI$_2$ infused directly into the renal arteries of dogs increase renal blood flow and provoke diuresis, natriuresis, and kaliuresis; there is little change in the rate of glomerular filtration (*see* Dunn and Hood, 1977). TXA$_2$ decreases renal blood flow, decreases the rate of glomerular filtration, and participates in tubuloglomerular feedback. PGEs inhibit water reabsorption induced by antidiuretic hormone (ADH). PGE$_2$ also inhibits chloride reabsorption in the thick ascending limb of the loop of Henle in the rabbit. In addition, PGI$_2$, PGE$_2$, and PGD$_2$ cause the secretion of renin from the renal cortex, apparently through a direct effect on the granular juxtaglomerular cells.

Central Nervous System. Although a large number of observations have been made on the effects of prostaglandins in the central nervous system (CNS), evidence for a clear-cut physiological role has yet to emerge.

Both stimulant and depressant effects of prostaglandins on the CNS have been reported following their injection into the cerebral ventricles, and the firing rates of individual brain cells may be increased or decreased after iontophoretic application of these agents. The release of PGE$_2$ in the brain likely explains the genesis of pyrogen-induced fever (Coceani and Akarsu, 1998). PGD$_2$ has been proposed as a mediator responsible for sleep (Urade *et al.*, 1999).

Afferent Nerves and Pain. PGEs cause pain when injected intradermally; these effects are generally not as immediate or intense as those caused by bradykinin or histamine, but they outlast those caused by the other autacoids. PGEs and PGI$_2$ sensitize the afferent nerve endings to the effects of chemical or mechanical stimuli by lowering the threshold of the nociceptors. Hyperalgesia also is produced by LTB$_4$. The release of these prostaglandins and of LTB$_4$ during the inflammatory process thus serves as an amplification system for the pain mechanism (*see* Moncada *et al.*, 1978). The role of PGE$_2$ and PGI$_2$ in inflammation is discussed in Chapter 27.

Table 26–1
Characteristics of Prostaglandin (PG) Receptors*

PG RECEPTOR SUBTYPE	PLATELET AGGREGATION	SMOOTH MUSCLE TONE	NATURAL AGONIST	G PROTEIN	SECOND MESSENGER
DP	−	+/−	PGD_2	G_s	cAMP(↑)
EP_1		+	PGE_2	G_q (?)	Ca^{2+}; IP_3/DAG (?)
EP_2		−	PGE_2	G_s	cAMP(↑)
EP_3		+	PGE_2	G_i, G_s, G_q	cAMP(↑/↓); IP_3/DAG/Ca^{2+}
EP_4		−	PGE_2	G_s	cAMP(↑)
FP		+	$PGF_{2\alpha}$	G_q	IP_3/DAG/Ca^{2+}
IP	−	−	$PGI_2(PGE_1)$	G_s	cAMP(↑)
TP	+	+	TXA_2, PGH_2	G_q	IP_3/DAG/Ca^{2+}

*This table lists the major classes of prostanoid receptors and their biochemical and functional characteristics. Different splice variants exist for the EP_3 and TP receptors (Narumiya et al., 1999; Austin and Funk, 1999). Stimulation of aggregation is indicated by a +, while inhibition is indicated by a −. Increase in smooth muscle tone is indicated by a +, while inhibition is denoted by a −. cAMP, adenosine 3′,5′-monophosphate (cyclic AMP); IP_3, inositol-1,4,5-trisphosphate; DAG, diacylglycerol. See text for other abbreviations.

Endocrine System. A variety of endocrine tissues respond to prostaglandins. In a number of species, the systemic administration of PGE_2 increases circulating concentrations of ACTH, growth hormone, prolactin, and the gonadotropins. Other effects include stimulation of steroid production by the adrenals, stimulation of insulin release, thyrotropin-like effects on the thyroid, and LH-like effects on isolated ovarian tissue, causing increased progesterone secretion from the corpus luteum. This last effect, observed in vitro, contrasts with the luteolytic effects of prostaglandins in vivo in many species but not in pregnant women. This property is possessed especially but not uniquely by $PGF_{2\alpha}$.

Lipoxygenase metabolites of arachidonate also have endocrine effects. 12-HETE stimulates the release of aldosterone from the adrenal cortex and mediates a portion of the aldosterone release stimulated by angiotensin II but not that by ACTH.

Metabolic Effects. PGEs inhibit the basal rate of lipolysis from adipose tissue in vitro and also lipolysis stimulated by exposure to catecholamines or other lipolytic hormones. Such effects also have been noted in vivo in various species, including human beings, but are more capricious. PGEs have some insulin-like effects on carbohydrate metabolism and exert parathyroid hormone-like effects that result in mobilization of Ca^{2+} from bone in tissue culture.

Mechanism of Action of Eicosanoids. *Prostaglandin Receptor Diversity.* The diversity of the effects of prostanoids is explained by the existence of a number of distinct receptors that mediate their actions. One scheme for classifying these receptors in platelets and smooth muscle is based primarily on the pattern of effects and the relative potencies of natural and synthetic agonists. This scheme has been largely substantiated by ligand-binding studies, cloning of the receptors, the discovery of relatively selective antagonists, and the development of mice possessing disruptions of genes encoding the eicosanoid receptors (see Coleman et al., 1994; Austin and Funk, 1999; Narumiya et al., 1999). This scheme is summarized in Table 26–1. The receptors have been named for the natural prostaglandin for which they have the greatest apparent affinity and have been divided into five main types, designated DP (PGD_2), FP (PGF_2), IP (PGI_2), TP (TXA_2), and EP (PGE_2). The EP receptors have been further subdivided into EP_1, EP_2, EP_3, and EP_4, based on physiological and molecular cloning information (Coleman et al., 1994; Narumiya et al., 1999). There are several splice variants of EP_3 that appear to have different signal transduction mechanisms (Narumiya et al., 1999). Previous pharmacological studies suggested the existence of a heterogeneous population of TP receptors, and two splice variants have been characterized (Raychowdhury et al., 1994). However, only one TP gene has been found to date, and evidence from targeted disruption of this gene implies that most of the known functions of TXA_2 are mediated through products of a single TP locus. Table 26–1 also indicates the effects of the natural prostaglandins on smooth muscle tone and platelet aggregation when the various prostaglandin receptors are stimulated.

Cell Signaling Pathways. All prostanoid receptors identified to date are coupled to effector mechanisms through G proteins (*see* Coleman *et al.,* 1994; Narumiya *et al.,* 1999). Two second-messenger systems have been associated with the action of prostanoids in platelets and smooth muscle—namely, stimulation of adenylyl cyclase (enhanced accumulation of cyclic AMP), inhibition of adenylyl cyclase (reduced accumulation of cyclic AMP), and stimulation of phospholipase C (enhanced formation of diacylglycerols and inositol-1,4,5-trisphosphate leading to an increase in cytosolic Ca^{2+}) (*see* Table 26–1).

The actions of prostanoids have been extensively studied in platelets. The prostaglandin endoperoxides and TXA_2 stimulate the TP receptors and thereby activate platelet aggregation, a response associated with activation of phospholipase C. Subsequent release of intracellular Ca^{2+} promotes aggregation and production of additional TXA_2. PGI_2 binds to IP receptors and activates adenylyl cyclase in the platelet, resulting in inhibition of aggregation. PGD_2 interacts with a distinct receptor (DP) that also stimulates adenylyl cyclase. PGE_1 appears to act through IP receptors.

Leukotriene Receptors. Receptors have been identified for both LTB_4 and the cysteinyl leukotrienes LTC_4 and LTD_4 in various cells and tissues. At least two classes of receptors exist for the cysteinyl leukotrienes and are termed $cysLT_1$ and $cysLT_2$ (Nicosia *et al.,* 1999). The leukotriene receptors are coupled to G proteins, and their activation increases intracellular Ca^{2+} concentrations.

Other Agents. Other metabolites of the lipoxygenase and cytochrome P450 pathways (*e.g.,* HETEs, epoxyeicosatrienoic acids, lipoxins, hepoxilins) have potent biological activities, and there is evidence for the existence of receptors for some of these substances. It is possible that some of these metabolites also function as intracellular second messengers. Recently, it has been proposed that certain eicosanoids, including PGI_2, the J-series prostaglandin, 15-deoxy-$\Delta^{12,14}$-PGJ_2, and LTB_4 are endogenous ligands for a family of nuclear receptors, called *peroxisome proliferator–activated receptors* (PPARs), that regulate lipid metabolism and cellular proliferation and differentiation (Forman *et al.,* 1995; Devchand *et al.,* 1996). Affinities of prostanoids at these receptors, however, are significantly less than for cell surface eicosanoid receptors. Thus, the physiological relevance of these observations remains to be established.

Receptor Antagonists. There are as yet no potent, selective antagonists of prostanoid receptors that are in routine clinical use. Previously, there was significant interest in the development of TP receptor antagonists for use in human disorders associated with excessive TXA_2-mediated platelet aggregation or vasoconstriction. Agents developed included *sultroban, vapiprost,* and others. Although occasionally effective in animal models of human disease such as atherosclerosis or in small clinical trials, these drugs have been supplanted by other, more effective compounds that act to prevent or ameliorate disease *via* other biochemical pathways. TP antagonists have proven useful

in vitro, however, in elucidating the role of TXA_2 in cellular processes.

Subtype-selective antagonists for EP receptors have been developed. Compounds include SC 19220, AH 6809, and SC 51089 for EP_1 receptors and AH 23848B for EP_4 receptors. Further clinical development likely will await clarification of which EP receptor subtype prevails in which physiological or pathophysiological setting.

Orally active antagonists of leukotriene C_4 and D_4 have been approved for the treatment of asthma (*see* Chapter 28). These agents act by binding to the $cysLT_1$ receptor and include *montelukast* and *zafirlukast.* In patients with mild to moderately severe asthma, they cause bronchodilation, reduce the bronchoconstriction caused by exercise and exposure to antigen, and decrease the patient's requirement for the use of β_2-adrenergic agonists (*see* Drazen, 1997). Their effectiveness in patients with aspirin-induced asthma also has been shown.

Endogenous Prostaglandins, Thromboxanes, and Leukotrienes: Possible Functions in Physiological and Pathological Processes

Because eicosanoids can be formed by virtually every cell, it is not unreasonable to suspect that each pharmacological effect may reflect a physiological or pathophysiological function. Such suspicions have been nurtured and presented in countless hypotheses bearing on just about every bodily function. Further insights into the roles of eicosanoids in biological processes have been gleaned by the development of mice with targeted disruptions of genes regulating eicosanoid biosynthesis or action (*see* Austin and Funk, 1999), corroborating and extending earlier work that utilized pharmacological approaches.

Platelets. An area in which there has been considerable interest is the elucidation of the role played by prostaglandin endoperoxides and TXA_2 in platelet aggregation and thrombosis and by PGI_2 in the prevention of these events. It is generally accepted that stimulation of platelet aggregation leads to activation of membrane phospholipases, with the consequent release of arachidonate and its transformation into prostaglandin endoperoxides and TXA_2. These substances induce platelet aggregation. However, this pathway is not the only mechanism for the induction of platelet aggregation, since, for example, thrombin aggregates platelets without the release of arachidonate. However, the importance of the thromboxane pathway in platelets is implied by the fact that aspirin and antagonists of TP receptors inhibit the second phase of platelet aggregation and induce a mild hemostatic defect in human beings (Hamberg *et al.,* 1974; Patrono, 1994). Additionally, the platelet thromboxane pathway is activated markedly in acute coronary artery syndromes, and aspirin is beneficial in the secondary prevention, and in some cases primary prevention, of coronary and cerebrovascular diseases (*see* Antiplatelet Trialists' Collaboration, 1994; Patrono, 1994).

PGI$_2$ that is generated in the vessel wall may be the physiological antagonist of this system; it inhibits platelet aggregation and contributes to the nonthrombogenic properties of the endothelium. According to this concept, PGI$_2$ and TXA$_2$ represent biologically opposite poles of a mechanism for regulating platelet–vessel wall interaction and the formation of hemostatic plugs and intraarterial thrombi (*see* Moncada and Vane, 1978).

Reproduction and Parturition.   Much interest is attached to the possible involvement of prostaglandins in reproductive physiology. Their very high concentrations in human semen, coupled with the substantial absorption of prostaglandins by the vagina, have encouraged speculation that prostaglandins deposited during coitus may facilitate conception by actions on the cervix, uterine body, fallopian tubes, and transport of semen. Although there is some correlation between lowered concentrations of prostaglandins in semen and certain cases of male infertility, the role of the eicosanoids in semen remains obscure.

With menstruation, there is disruption of uterine membranes, the release of arachidonate, and stimulation of prostaglandin synthesis. The concentrations of prostaglandins are elevated in menstrual fluid. These prostaglandins are thought to contract uterine and gastrointestinal smooth muscle and sensitize afferent pain fibers and thereby contribute to the symptoms of primary dysmenorrhea. Inhibitors of cyclooxygenase are more effective than narcotic analgesics in relieving the symptoms of this condition.

During pregnancy in the human female, the capacity of the fetal membranes to elaborate prostaglandins rises progressively. Concentrations of prostaglandins in blood and amniotic fluid are elevated during labor, but it is not certain whether this is a major determinant of the onset of labor or only serves to sustain uterine contractions that have been initiated by oxytocin. In any event, inhibitors of cyclooxygenase increase the length of gestation, prolong the duration of spontaneous labor, and interrupt premature labor.

Additional evidence for a role of prostaglandins in reproduction and parturition is the fact that targeted disruption of the genes encoding both COX enzymes, the EP$_2$ receptor, and the FP receptor in mice results in various defects in reproduction and parturition (*see* Austin and Funk, 1999).

PGF$_{2\alpha}$, produced in the uterus, is a luteolytic hormone in some subprimate species. This knowledge has led to the development of prostaglandin analogs for veterinary use in synchronizing estrus in farm animals in order to simplify breeding procedures; they also are used to provide safe, early abortions before the animals are sent to market.

Prostaglandins and prostaglandin analogs also are useful in ripening the cervix for delivery and as abortifacients (*see* below).

Vascular and Pulmonary Smooth Muscle.   Locally generated PGE$_2$ and PGI$_2$ modulate vascular tone. Produced by the vascular endothelium, PGI$_2$ is released by shear stress and by both vasoconstrictor and vasodilator autacoids. PGI$_2$ appears to counteract the effects of circulating vasoconstrictor autacoids, to maintain blood flow to vital organs, and to mediate a portion of the dilation by other autacoids. The importance of these vascular actions is emphasized by the participation of PGI$_2$ and PGE$_2$ in the hypotension associated with septic shock. These prostaglandins also have been implicated in the

maintenance of patency of the ductus arteriosus. This hypothesis has been strengthened by the fact that nonsteroidal antiinflammatory drugs induce closure of a patent ductus in neonates (*see* Chapter 27; Coceani *et al.*, 1980). Prostaglandins also may play a role in the maintenance of placental blood flow.

A complex mixture of autacoids is released when sensitized lung tissue is challenged by the appropriate antigen. Various prostaglandins and leukotrienes are prominent components of this mixture. While both bronchodilator (PGE$_2$) and bronchoconstrictor (*e.g.*, PGF$_{2\alpha}$, TXA$_2$, PGD$_2$, LTC$_4$) substances are released, responses to the peptidoleukotrienes probably dominate during allergic constriction of the airway (*see* Piper, 1984). Included in the evidence for this conclusion is the ineffectiveness of inhibitors of cyclooxygenase and of histaminergic antagonists in the treatment of human asthma and the protection afforded by leukotriene antagonists in antigen-induced bronchoconstriction. Moreover, the relatively slow metabolism of the leukotrienes in lung tissue contributes to the long-lasting bronchoconstriction that follows challenge with antigen and may be a factor in the high bronchial tone that is observed in asthmatics in periods between acute attacks (*see* Chapter 28).

Kidney.   Prostaglandins modulate renal blood flow and may serve to regulate urine formation by both renovascular and tubular effects. Additional roles in the regulation of the secretion of renin also are likely. The elaboration of PGE$_2$ and PGI$_2$ is increased by factors that reduce renal blood flow (*e.g.*, stimulation of sympathetic nerves and angiotensin). Under these circumstances, inhibitors of cyclooxygenase augment the renovasoconstriction that is produced by such stimuli. In addition, the effects of ADH on the reabsorption of water may be restrained by the concomitant production and action of PGE$_2$.

Increased biosynthesis of prostaglandins has been associated with Bartter's syndrome. This is a rare disease characterized by low-to-normal blood pressure, decreased sensitivity to angiotensin, hyperreninemia, hyperaldosteronism, and excessive loss of K$^+$. There also is an increased excretion of prostaglandins in the urine. After long-term administration of cyclooxygenase inhibitors, sensitivity to angiotensin, plasma renin values, and the concentration of aldosterone in plasma return to normal. Although plasma K$^+$ rises, it remains low, and urinary wasting of K$^+$ persists. Whether an increase in prostaglandin biosynthesis is the cause of Bartter's syndrome or a reflection of a more basic physiological defect is not yet known (*see* Clive, 1995).

Inflammatory and Immune Responses.   Prostaglandins and leukotrienes are released by a host of mechanical, thermal, chemical, bacterial, and other insults, and they contribute importantly to the genesis of the signs and symptoms of inflammation (*see* Moncada *et al.*, 1978; Samuelsson, 1983). The peptidoleukotrienes have powerful effects on vascular permeability, while LTB$_4$ is a potent chemoattractant for polymorphonuclear leukocytes and can promote exudation of plasma by mobilizing this source of additional inflammatory mediators. Although prostaglandins do not appear to have direct effects on vascular permeability, both PGE$_2$ and PGI$_2$ markedly enhance edema formation and leukocyte infiltration by promoting blood flow in the inflamed region. Moreover, they potentiate the pain-producing activity of bradykinin and other autacoids. However, PGEs inhibit the participation of lymphocytes in delayed hypersensitivity reactions. Moreover, they inhibit the release of hydrolases and lysosomal enzymes from human neutrophils as well as from mouse peritoneal macrophages. The use of cyclooxygenase inhibitors as antiinflammatory agents is a primary focus of Chapter 27.

Some experimental tumors in animals and certain spontaneous human tumors (medullary carcinoma of the thyroid, renal-cell adenocarcinoma, carcinoma of the breast) are accompanied by increased concentrations of local or circulating prostaglandins, bone metastasis, and hypercalcemia. Since the PGEs have potent osteolytic activity, it has been suggested that they are implicated in some cases of hypercalcemia. Some studies have implicated the effects of prostaglandins and HETEs on either the hematogenous metastasis of tumors or tumor angiogenesis. Pretreatment of animals with COX inhibitors or inhibitors of thromboxane synthase reduces the formation of tumor colonies or new blood vessel formation.

There has been significant interest in the role of prostaglandins and the inducible cyclooxygenase, COX-2, in the development of malignancies, particularly colon cancer. Various prostaglandins induce proliferation of colon cancer cells, and COX inhibitors reduce colon tumor formation in experimental animals. In large epidemiological studies, regular use of aspirin is associated with a decreased incidence of colon cancer in human beings. Furthermore, in patients with familial colon polyposis syndromes, cyclooxygenase inhibitors significantly decrease polyp formation (*see* Williams *et al.,* 1999).

Therapeutic Uses

The use of eicosanoids or eicosanoid derivatives as therapeutic agents is limited, even though these compounds have been the focus of intense research efforts. Part of the reason for this is that systemic administration of prostanoids is frequently associated with significant adverse side effects. This is not surprising given that eicosanoids have an array of biological activities in diverse cell types and tissues. Another factor limiting the use of these compounds as therapeutic agents is their short half-lives in the circulation. Thus, in some cases, continuous systemic administration of eicosanoids is required to achieve therapeutic efficacy. Despite these limitations, however, several prostanoids are of clinical utility in situations discussed below.

Therapeutic Abortion. As described above, there has been intense interest in the effects of the prostaglandins on the female reproductive system. Their action as *abortifacients* when given early in pregnancy is established. However, initial hopes that they might provide a simple, convenient means of postimplantation "contraception," perhaps given as a vaginal suppository, have not been fulfilled. Moreover, the abortifacient action of prostaglandins may be inconstant and often incomplete and may be accompanied by side effects. Prostaglandins appear, however, to be of value in missed abortion and molar gestation, and they have been widely used for the induction of midtrimester abortion. While PGE_2 or $PGF_{2\alpha}$ can induce labor at term, they may

have more value when used to facilitate labor by promoting ripening and dilation of the cervix.

In the United States, PGE_2, or *dinoprostone,* is approved by the FDA for use in cervical ripening in the form of a cervical gel (PREPIDIL) containing 0.5 mg of PGE_2 per 3 g gel. PGE_2 also is approved for the induction of therapeutic midtrimester abortion as a vaginal suppository (PROSTIN E2) containing 20 mg of PGE_2.

Several studies also have shown that systemic or intravaginal administration of the PGE_1 analog *misoprostol* in combination with *mifepristone* (RU486; Peyron *et al.,* 1993) or methotrexate (Hausknecht, 1995; Christin-Maitre *et al.,* 2000) is highly effective in the termination of early pregnancy.

Gastric Cytoprotection. The capacity of several prostaglandin analogs to suppress gastric ulceration is a property of therapeutic importance. Of these, *misoprostol* (CYTOTEC), a PGE_1 analog, is available for general use; its structure is as follows:

MISOPROSTOL

When given in doses that suppress gastric acid secretion, misoprostol appears to heal gastric ulcers about as effectively as the H_2 antagonists (*see* Chapter 37); however, relief of ulcerogenic pain and healing of duodenal ulcers has not been achieved consistently with misoprostol. In what may be considered replacement therapy, the drug currently is used primarily for the prevention of ulcers that often occur during long-term treatment with nonsteroidal antiinflammatory drugs. In this setting, misoprostol appears to be as effective as the proton pump inhibitor *omeprazole*. The major adverse effect of misoprostol is diarrhea. Although frequently observed, it is mild and usually does not force discontinuation of therapy. Misoprostol is rapidly absorbed, with peak blood concentrations occurring at 30 minutes. It is converted to the active misoprostol acid with a half-time of 30 to 60 minutes (*see* Monk and Clissold, 1987; Walt, 1992). Misoprostol is available for oral administration for the prevention of gastric ulcers in patients who are at risk for development of such ulcers during long-term therapy with nonsteroidal antiinflammatory drugs. The recommended dosage is 200 μg four times daily. The drug should not be administered to pregnant women because of its uterotonic activity. In this regard, misoprostol has been found to be effective alone or in combination with either mifepristone or methotrexate as an abortifacient (*see* above).

Impotence. PGE_1 (*alprostadil*) may be used in the treatment of impotence. Intracavernous injection of PGE_1 causes complete or partial erection in impotent patients who do not have disorders of the vascular system or cavernous body damage. The erection lasts for one to three hours and is sufficient for sexual intercourse. PGE_1 is more effective than papaverine. The agent is available as a sterile powder that is reconstituted with water for injections (CARVERJECT).

Maintenance of Patent Ductus Arteriosus. The ductus arteriosus in neonates is highly sensitive to vasodilation by PGE_1. Patency of the ductus may be necessary to maintain in some neonates with congenital heart disease. For palliative, but not definitive, therapy to temporarily maintain patency until surgery can be performed, PGE_1 (alprostadil, PROSTIN VR PEDIATRIC) is highly effective. Alprostadil usually is infused intravenously at an initial rate of 0.05 to 0.1 $\mu g/kg$ per minute, with subsequent reductions to the lowest dosage that maintains the response. Apnea is observed in about 10% of neonates so treated, particularly in those who weigh less than 2 kg at birth.

Primary Pulmonary Hypertension. Primary pulmonary hypertension is a rare, idiopathic disease mainly observed in young adults that leads to right heart failure and is frequently fatal. Lung or lung-heart transplantation has been the treatment previously. Long-term therapy with PGI_2 (*epoprostenol;* FLOLAN) recently has been found to be highly effective and has either delayed or avoided the need for transplantation in a number of patients. In addition, many affected individuals have had a marked improvement in symptoms after receiving treatment with PGI_2. The agent is administered by continuous intravenous infusion through a central venous catheter using a portable infusion pump. Adverse effects can include nausea, vomiting, headache, and flushing (McLaughlin *et al.,* 1998).

PLATELET-ACTIVATING FACTOR

History. In 1971, Henson demonstrated that a soluble factor was released from leukocytes and caused platelets to aggregate. Benveniste and his coworkers confirmed these observations and named the substance *platelet-activating factor* (PAF); their research indicated that the compound was a polar lipid. During this period, Muirhead described an antihypertensive polar renal lipid (APRL) produced by interstitial cells of the renal medulla. Sufficient evidence had accumulated by 1979 to conclude that PAF and APRL were identical. Hanahan and coworkers then synthesized acetylglyceryletherphosphorylcholine (AGEPC) and determined that this phospholipid had chemical and biological properties identical with those of PAF (Demopoulos *et al.,* 1979). Subsequently, the structures of PAF and APRL were determined independently and were found to be identical with that of AGEPC (Hanahan *et al.,* 1980; Polonsky *et al.,* 1980). Of the names for the compound, platelet-activating factor has gained the greatest acceptance, despite the fact that the lipid has many biological actions in addition to those on platelets (Snyder, 1989; Koltai *et al.,* 1991).

Chemistry and Biosynthesis. PAF is 1-*O*-alkyl-2-acetyl-*sn*-glycero-3-phosphocholine. Its structure is as follows:

PLATELET-ACTIVATING FACTOR (*n* = 11 TO 17)

In contrast to the two long-chain acyl groups that are present in phosphatidylcholine, PAF contains a long-chain alkyl group

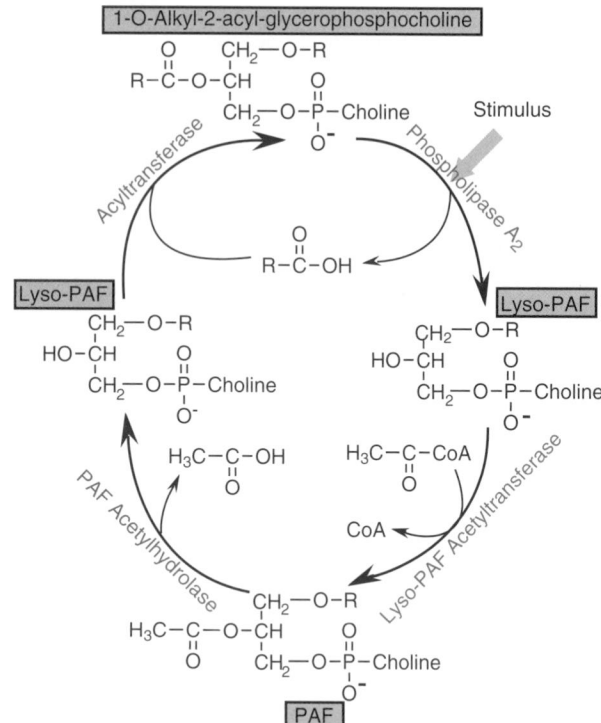

Figure 26–3. Synthesis and degradation of platelet-activating factor (PAF).

RCOOH is a mixture of fatty acids but is enriched in arachidonic acid; it may be metabolized to eicosanoids. CoA represents coenzyme A.

joined to the glycerol backbone in an ether linkage at position 1 and an acetyl group at position 2. PAF actually represents a family of phospholipids, because the alkyl group at position 1 can vary in length from 12 to 18 carbon atoms. In human neutrophils, PAF consists predominantly of a mixture of the 16- and 18-carbon ethers, but its composition may change when cells are stimulated.

Like the eicosanoids, PAF is not stored in cells but is synthesized in response to stimulation. The major pathway by which PAF is generated involves the precursor 1-*O*-alkyl-2-acyl-glycerophosphocholine, a lipid found in high concentrations in the membranes of many types of cells. The 2-acyl substituents include an abundance of arachidonate. PAF is synthesized from this substrate in two steps (*see* Figure 26–3). The first involves the action of phospholipase A_2, with the formation of 1-*O*-alkyl-2-lyso-glycerophosphocholine (lyso-PAF) and a free fatty acid (usually arachidonate) (Chilton *et al.,* 1984). In some cells, this reaction may represent a major source of the arachidonate that is metabolized to prostaglandins and leukotrienes. In the second step, lyso-PAF is acetylated by acetyl coenzyme A in a reaction catalyzed by lyso-PAF acetyltransferase. This represents the rate-limiting step. The synthesis of PAF may be stimulated during antigen-antibody reactions or by a variety of agents, including chemotactic peptides, thrombin, collagen, and other autacoids; PAF also can stimulate its own formation.

Both the phospholipase and acetyltransferase are Ca^{2+}-dependent enzymes, and PAF synthesis is regulated by the availability of Ca^{2+}.

The inactivation of PAF also occurs in two steps (see Figure 26–3; Chilton et al., 1983; Stafforini et al., 1997). Initially, the acetyl group of PAF is removed by PAF acetylhydrolase to form lyso-PAF; this enzyme is present in both cells and plasma. Lyso-PAF is then converted to a 1-O-alkyl-2-acyl-glycerophosphocholine by an acyltransferase.

PAF is synthesized by platelets, neutrophils, monocytes, mast cells, eosinophils, renal mesangial cells, renal medullary cells, and vascular endothelial cells. In most instances, stimulation of PAF synthesis results in the release of PAF and lyso-PAF from the cell. However, in some cells (e.g., endothelial cells) PAF is not released and appears to exert its effects intracellularly (Prescott et al., 1990).

In addition to the generation of PAF enzymatically, PAF-like molecules can be formed from the oxidative fragmentation of membrane phospholipids (Patel et al., 1992). They are structurally different from PAF in that they contain a fatty acid at the sn-1 position of glycerol joined through an ester bond and various short-chain acyl groups at the sn-2 position. They mimic the structure of PAF closely enough to bind to its receptor and thus elicit the same responses. They are also substrates for PAF acetylhydrolase. An important distinction between PAF and these PAF-like oxidized lipids is that the synthesis of PAF is highly controlled, whereas the oxidized PAF-like phospholipids are produced in an apparently unregulated manner. The role that these latter compounds play in settings of oxidant stress is under investigation.

Pharmacological Properties. *Cardiovascular System.* PAF is a potent vasodilator, and it lowers peripheral vascular resistance and systemic blood pressure when injected intravenously. PAF-induced vasodilation is independent of effects on the sympathetic innervation or arachidonate metabolism (Sybertz et al., 1985). However, the effects of PAF on the coronary circulation are a mixture of direct and indirect actions. The intracoronary administration of small amounts of PAF increases coronary blood flow by a mechanism that involves the release of a platelet-derived vasodilator. At higher doses, coronary blood flow is decreased by the formation of intravascular aggregates of platelets and/or the formation of TXA_2 (Sybertz et al., 1985). The pulmonary vasculature also is constricted by PAF, and a similar mechanism is thought to be involved. Intradermal injection of PAF causes an initial vasoconstriction followed by a typical wheal and flare.

PAF increases vascular permeability and promotes the movement of fluid out of the vasculature (McManus et al., 1981). As with substances such as histamine and bradykinin, the increase in permeability is due to contraction of venular endothelial cells, but PAF is thousandfold more potent than histamine or bradykinin.

Platelets. PAF is a potent stimulator of in vitro platelet aggregation that is accompanied by the release of TXA_2 and the granular contents of the platelet; however, PAF does not require the presence of TXA_2 or other aggregating agents to produce this effect. The intravenous injection of PAF causes formation of intravascular platelet aggregates and thrombocytopenia.

Leukocytes. PAF stimulates polymorphonuclear leukocytes to aggregate, to release leukotrienes and lysosomal enzymes, and

to generate superoxide. Since LTB_4 is more potent in inducing leukocyte aggregation, it may mediate the effects of PAF. Similarly, PAF promotes aggregation of monocytes and degranulation of eosinophils.

PAF is a chemotactic factor for eosinophils, neutrophils, and monocytes. It also promotes the adherence of neutrophils to endothelial cells and their diapedesis. When given systemically, PAF causes leukocytopenia, with neutrophils showing the greatest decline. Intradermal injection causes the accumulation of neutrophils and mononuclear cells at the site of injection, and inhaled PAF increases the infiltration of eosinophils into the airways.

Smooth Muscle. PAF generally contracts gastrointestinal, uterine, and pulmonary smooth muscle. PAF enhances the amplitude of spontaneous uterine contractions; quiescent muscle contracts rapidly in a phasic fashion. These contractions are inhibited by inhibitors of prostaglandin synthesis. PAF does not affect tracheal smooth muscle but contracts the smooth muscle of peripheral airways. Although controversial, most evidence suggests that another autacoid (e.g., LTC_4 or TXA_2) mediates this effect of PAF. When given by aerosol, PAF increases airway resistance as well as the responsiveness to other bronchoconstrictors (Cuss et al., 1986). This bronchial hyperresponsiveness occurs after a delay of up to three days in human beings and may persist for 1 to 4 weeks. PAF also increases mucus secretion and the permeability of pulmonary microvessels; this results in fluid accumulation in the mucosal and submucosal regions of the trachea and bronchi.

Stomach. In addition to contracting the fundus of the stomach, PAF is the most potent known ulcerogen. When given intravenously, it causes hemorrhagic erosions of the gastric mucosa that extend into the submucosa.

Kidney. When infused intrarenally in animals, PAF decreases renal blood flow, glomerular filtration rate, urine volume, and excretion of Na^+ (Schlondorff and Neuwirth, 1986). These effects are not due to the formation of platelet aggregates but are the result of a direct action on the renal circulation. PAF also stimulates the release of vasodilator prostaglandins, which tends to counteract the renal vasoconstriction.

Mechanism of Action of PAF. Extracellular PAF exerts its actions by stimulating a G protein–linked cell surface receptor that has been detected in the plasma membranes of a number of cell types (Chao and Olson, 1993). Lyso-PAF is inactive, and biological activity is markedly reduced by relatively small changes in structure. The human PAF receptor has been cloned. When stimulated, it activates multiple signaling pathways, including phospholipase A_2, phospholipase C, and phospholipase D, with resultant formation of inositol phosphates and diacylglycerol and release of arachidonate (Peplow, 1999). The arachidonate released by PAF is converted to prostaglandins, TXA_2, or leukotrienes, which may function as extracellular mediators of the effects of PAF.

PAF also may exert actions without exiting the cell. The clearest example is provided by the endothelial cell. Synthesis of PAF is stimulated by a variety of factors, but it is not released extracellularly (McIntyre et al., 1986). Accumulation of PAF intracellularly is associated with the adhesion of neutrophils to the surface of the endothelial cells, apparently because PAF promotes the expression or exposure of surface proteins that recognize and bind neutrophils.

Receptor Antagonists.   Many compounds have been described that selectively inhibit the actions of PAF *in vivo* and *in vitro* (Koltai *et al.*, 1991; Negro Alvarez *et al.*, 1997). These drugs inhibit the binding of PAF to its receptor and block its actions selectively. Driving the development of these agents was the expectation that they would be potent antiinflammatory agents that might be useful in the therapy of disorders such as asthma, sepsis, and other diseases in which PAF is postulated to play a role. Two general classes of agents have been studied: (1) those that are natural compounds and include terpenes, lignans, and gliotoxins and (2) synthetic compounds with structures either related or unrelated to PAF. In animal models of sepsis and other diseases, various PAF antagonists gave encouraging results. In human trials, however, the results have been disappointing, with at least three recent studies failing to confirm any reduction of mortality in sepsis with either TCV-309 or BN 52501, two synthetic PAF receptor antagonists (Heller *et al.*, 1998). Inconsistent results have been obtained in trials involving patients with asthma and psoriasis. Thus, after encouraging animal studies, it appears as though currently available PAF antagonists are of little benefit in human disease.

Physiological and Pathological Functions of PAF.   Unlike the eicosanoids, PAF is synthesized by a select assortment of cells; this is presumed to limit its participation in various physiological and pathological processes.

Platelets.   Since PAF is synthesized by platelets and promotes aggregation, it was proposed to be the mediator of cyclooxygenase inhibitor–resistant, thrombin-induced aggregation. However, PAF antagonists fail to block thrombin-induced aggregation, even though they prolong bleeding time and prevent thrombus formation in some experimental models. Thus, PAF does not function as an independent mediator of aggregation but contributes to thrombus formation in a manner analogous to TXA_2 and ADP.

Reproduction and Parturition.   PAF may be involved in ovulation, implantation, and parturition. Rupture of the follicle is inhibited in experimental animals by the PAF antagonist ginkgolide B (Abisogun *et al.*, 1989); the administration of PAF restores ovulation. Following ovulation and subsequent fertilization, the embryo begins to produce PAF, which promotes platelet aggregation and the release of platelet factors that appear to stimulate activation and implantation of the blastocyst.

PAF is found in the amniotic fluid only after labor commences; PAF is thought to contribute to parturition by several mechanisms. It may cause contraction of the myometrium directly, or it may promote the release of PGE_2 (and additional PAF) from amnion cells and promote uterine contractions indirectly. In any event, the importance of PAF is indicated by the delay in parturition induced by PAF antagonists in experimental animals.

Inflammatory and Allergic Responses.   PAF is elaborated by leukocytes and mast cells and exerts proinflammatory effects. For example, intradermal injection of PAF duplicates many of the signs and symptoms of inflammation, including increased vascular permeability, hyperalgesia, edema, and infiltration of neutrophils. PAF also produces effects that suggest its importance in asthma. When inhaled, it is a potent bronchoconstrictor, promotes the accumulation of eosinophils in the lung, causes tracheal and bronchial edema, and stimulates the secretion of

mucus. Moreover, PAF produces long-lasting bronchial hyperresponsiveness. The plasma concentration of PAF is increased in experimental anaphylactic shock, and the administration of PAF reproduces many of its signs and symptoms, suggesting a role for the autacoid in this condition. In addition, mice overexpressing the PAF receptor exhibit bronchial hyperreactivity and increased lethality when treated with endotoxin (Ishii *et al.*, 1997). Despite the broad implications of these observations, the effects of PAF antagonists in the treatment of inflammatory and allergic disorders have been disappointing (*see* above). Although they reverse the bronchoconstriction of anaphylactic shock and improve survival, the impact of PAF antagonists on animal models of asthma and inflammation is marginal. Similarly, in patients with asthma, PAF antagonists partially inhibit the bronchoconstriction induced by antigen challenge but not challenges to methacholine, exercise, or inhalation of cold air. These results may reflect the complexity of these pathological conditions and the fact that other mediators likely contribute to the inflammation associated with these disorders.

PROSPECTUS

The past decade has witnessed an explosion of information regarding the role of eicosanoids in human physiology and pathophysiology. Much of this has been fueled by basic scientific advances utilizing molecular approaches. Many of the genes regulating eicosanoid biosynthesis and action have been "knocked out" in mice, providing tools to define the precise role of various prostanoids in biological processes. This work is complemented by the recent development of several clinically useful inhibitors of eicosanoid action: selective COX-2 inhibitors, leukotriene biosynthesis inhibitors, and cysteinyl leukotriene receptor antagonists. COX-2 inhibitors, in particular, represent a major advance in the therapy of inflammatory processes, and their use as agents to prevent or treat other disorders associated with COX-2 overexpression, such as colon cancer, is an area of intense current interest.

The molecular delineation of the EP receptor subtypes and the recent observations that different subtypes contribute to different disease processes suggest that development of subtype-selective agonists and antagonists could be of use both as research tools and as treatments of human pathophysiology.

Development of clinically useful antagonists of other autocoid receptors, including those for PAF and TXA_2, has been disappointing. Again, however, the generation of mice with altered expression of these receptors may allow a more careful determination of the probable roles of these molecules in human disease.

The recent findings that some eicosanoids may be ligands for certain nuclear receptors, such as the peroxisome proliferator–activated receptors, extend the biological relevance of prostanoids to areas not historically considered to be eicosanoid-related. These observations also provide potentially novel therapeutic strategies for the generation of agonists or antagonists to regulate gene transcription and lipid metabolism.

In addition to the development of agents to inhibit the actions of eicosanoids, the use of several prostanoids or prostanoid analogs in the treatment of select human disorders represents a major therapeutic advance. In particular, the treatment of primary pulmonary hypertension with intravenous PGI_2 has significantly altered the course of this disorder. However, limiting the use of this agent and other eicosanoids in disease therapy are issues related to bioavailability and side effects. Future research aimed at altering these properties of clinically useful prostanoids could have important therapeutic consequences.

BIBLIOGRAPHY

Abisogun, A.O., Braquet, P., and Tsafriri, A. The involvement of platelet activating factor in ovulation. *Science*, **1989**, *243*:381–383.

Antiplatelet Trialists' Collaboration. Collaborative overview of randomised trials of antiplatelet therapy—I: Prevention of death, myocardial infarction, and stroke by prolonged antiplatelet therapy in various categories of patients. *Br. Med. J.*, **1994**, *308*:81–106.

Berkowitz, B.A., Zabko-Potapovich, B., Valocik, R., and Gleason, J.G. Effects of the leukotrienes on the vasculature and blood pressure of different species. *J. Pharmacol. Exp. Ther.*, **1984**, *229*:105–112.

Bhagwat, S.S., Hamann, P.R., Still, W.C., Bunting, S., and Fitzpatrick, F.A. Synthesis and structure of the platelet aggregation factor thromboxane A_2. *Nature*, **1985**, *315*:511–513.

Borgeat, P., and Samuelsson, B. Arachidonic acid metabolism in polymorphonuclear leukocytes: unstable intermediate in formation of dihydroxy acids. *Proc. Natl. Acad. Sci. U.S.A.*, **1979**, *76*:3213–3217.

Chilton, F.H., Ellis, J.M., Olson, S.C., and Wykle, R.L. 1-O-alkyl-2-arachidonoyl-*sn*-glycero-3-phosphocholine: a common source of platelet-activating factor and arachidonate in polymorphonuclear leukocytes. *J. Biol. Chem.*, **1984**, *259*:12014–12019.

Chilton, F.H., O'Flaherty, J.T., Ellis, J.M., Swendsen, C.L., and Wykle, R.L. Metabolic fate of platelet-activating factor in neutrophils. *J. Biol. Chem.*, **1983**, *258*:6357–6361.

Cuss, F.M., Dixon, C.M.S., and Barnes, P.J. Effects of inhaled platelet activating factor on pulmonary function and bronchial responsiveness in man. *Lancet*, **1986**, *2*:189–192.

Demopoulos, C.A., Pinckard, R.N., and Hanahan, D.J. Platelet activating factor: evidence for 1-O-alkyl-2-acetyl-*sn*-glyceryl-3-phosphorylcholine as the active component (a new class of lipid chemical mediators). *J. Biol. Chem.*, **1979**, *254*:9355–9358.

Denzlinger, C., Guhlmann, A., Scheuber, P.H., Wilker, D., Hammer, D.K., and Keppler, D. Metabolism and analysis of cysteinyl leukotrienes in the monkey. *J. Biol. Chem.*, **1986**, *261*:15601–15606.

Devane, W.A., Hanus, L., Breuer, A., Pertwee, R.G., Stevenson, L.A., Griffin, G., Gibson, D., Mandelbaum, A., Etinger, A., and Mechoulam, R. Isolation and structure of a brain constituent that binds to the cannabinoid receptor. *Science*, **1992**, *258*:1946–1949.

Devchand, P.R., Keller, H., Peters, J.H., Vazques, M., Gonzales, F.J., and Wahli, W. The $PPAR_\alpha$-leukotriene B_4 pathway to inflammation control. *Nature*, **1996**, *384*:39–43.

Feldberg, W., and Kellaway, C.H. Liberation of histamine and formation of lysocithin-like substances by cobra venom. *J. Physiol.*, **1938**, *94*:187–226.

Forman, B.M., Tontonoz, P., Chen, J., Brun, R.P., Speigelman, B.M., and Evans, R.M. 15-deoxy$\Delta^{12,14}$-prostaglandin J_2 is a ligand for the adipocyte determination factor $PPAR_\gamma$. *Cell*, **1995**, *83*:803–812.

Hamberg, M., Svensson, J., and Samuelsson, B. Thromboxanes: a new group of biologically active compounds derived from prostaglandin endoperoxides. *Proc. Natl. Acad. Sci. U.S.A.*, **1975**, *72*:2994–2998.

Hamberg, M., Svensson, J., Wakabayashi, T., and Samuelsson, B. Isolation and structure of two prostaglandin endoperoxides that cause platelet aggregation. *Proc. Natl. Acad. Sci. U.S.A.*, **1974**, *71*:345–349.

Hanahan, D.J., Demopoulos, C.A., Liehr, J., and Pinckard, R.N. Identification of platelet activating factor isolated from rabbit basophils as acetyl glyceryl ether phosphorylcholine. *J. Biol. Chem.*, **1980**, *255*:5514–5516.

Hausknecht, R.U. Methotrexate and misoprostol to terminate early pregnancy. *N. Engl. J. Med.*, **1995**, *333*:537–540.

Ishii, S., Nagase, T., Tashiro, F., Ikuta, K., Sato, S., Waga, I., Kume, K., Miyazaki, J., and Shimizu, T. Bronchial hyperactivity, increased endotoxin lethality, and melanocytic tumorigenesis in transgenic mice overexpressing platelet-activating factor receptor. *EMBO J.*, **1997**, *16*:131–142.

Lin, L.L., Lin, A.Y., and Knopf, J.L. Cytosolic phospholipase A_2 is coupled to hormonally regulated release of arachidonic acid. *Proc. Natl. Acad. Sci. U.S.A.*, **1992**, *89*:6147–6151.

McIntyre, T.M., Zimmerman, G.A., and Prescott, S.M. Leukotrienes C_4 and D_4 stimulate human endothelial cells to synthesize platelet-activating factor and bind neutrophils. *Proc. Natl. Acad. Sci. U.S.A.*, **1986**, *83*:2204–2208.

McLaughlin, V.V., Genthner, D.E., Panella, M.M., and Rich, S. Reduction in pulmonary vascular resistance with long-term epoprostenol (prostacyclin) therapy in primary pulmonary hypertension. *N. Engl. J. Med.* **1998**, *338*:273–277.

McManus, L.M., Pinckard, R.N., Fitzpatrick, F.A., O'Rourke, R.A., Crawford, M.H., and Hanahan, D.J. Acetyl glyceryl ether phosphorylcholine: intravascular alterations following intravenous infusion into the baboon. *Lab. Invest.*, **1981**, *45*:303–307.

Masferrer, J.L., Reddy, S.T., Zweifel, B.S., Seibert, K., Needleman, P., Gilbert, R.S., and Herschman, H.R. *In vivo* glucocorticoids regulate cyclooxygenase-2 but not cyclooxygenase-1 in peritoneal macrophages. *J. Pharmacol. Exp. Ther.*, **1994**, *270*:1340–1344.

Moncada, S., Gryglewski, R., Bunting, S., and Vane, J.R. An enzyme isolated from arteries transforms prostaglandin endoperoxides to an unstable substance that inhibits platelet aggregation. *Nature*, **1976**, *263*:663–665.

Morrow, J.D., Hill, K.E., Burk, R.F., Nammour, T.M., Badr, K., and Roberts, L.J. II. A series of prostaglandin F_2-like compounds are produced *in vivo* in humans by a noncyclooxygenase, free radical–catalyzed mechanism. *Proc. Natl. Acad. Sci. U.S.A.*, **1990**, *87*:9383–9387.

Murphy, R.C., Hammarstrom, S., and Samuelsson, B. Leukotriene C: a slow-reacting substance from murine mastocytoma cells. *Proc. Natl. Acad. Sci. U.S.A.,* **1979,** *76*:4275–4279.

Nicosia, S., Capra, V., Accomazzo, M.R., Ragnuni, D., Ravasi, S., Caiani, A., Jommi, L., Saponara, R., Mezzetti, M., and Rovati, G.E. Receptors for cysteinyl-leukotrienes in human cells. *Adv. Exp. Med. Biol.,* **1999,** *447*:165–170.

Okazaki, T., Sagawa, N., Okita, J.R., Bleasdale, J.E., MacDonald, P.C., and Johnston, J.M. Diacylglycerol metabolism and arachidonic acid release in human fetal membranes and decidua vera. *J. Biol. Chem.,* **1981,** *256*:7316–7321.

Patel, K.D., Zimmerman, G.A., Prescott, S.M., and McIntyre, T.M. Novel leukocyte agonists are released by endothelial cells exposed to peroxide. *J. Biol. Chem.,* **1992,** *267*:15168–15175.

Peyron, R., Aubeny, E., Targosz, V., Silvestre, L., Renault, M., Elkik, F., Leclerc, P., Ulmann, A., and Baulieu, E.E. Early termination of pregnancy with mifepristone (RU486) and the orally active prostaglandin misoprostol. *N. Engl. J. Med.,* **1993,** *328*:1509–1513.

Polonsky, J., Tence, M., Varenne, P., Das, B.C., Lunel, J., and Benveniste, J. Release of 1-O-alkylglyceryl 3-phosphorylcholine, O-deacetyl platelet-activating factor, from leukocytes: chemical ionization mass spectrometry of phospholipids. *Proc. Natl. Acad. Sci. U.S.A.,* **1980,** *77*:7019–7023.

Raychowdhury, M.K., Yukawa, M., Collins, L.J., McGrail, S.J., Kent, K.C., and Ware, J.A. Alternative splicing produces a divergent cytoplasmic tail in the human endothelial thromboxane A_2 receptor. *J. Biol. Chem.,* **1994,** *269*:19256–19261.

Reddy, S.T., Winstead, M.V., Tischfield, J.A., and Herschman, H.R. Analysis of the secretory phospholipase A_2 that mediates prostaglandin production in mast cells. *J. Biol. Chem.,* **1997,** *272*:13591–13596.

Rosenkranz, B., Fischer, C., Weimer, K.E., and Frolich, J.C. Metabolism of prostacyclin and 6-keto-prostaglandin $F_{1\alpha}$ in man. *J. Biol. Chem.,* **1980,** *255*:10194–10198.

Sybertz, E.J., Watkins, R.W., Baum, T., Pula, K., and Rivelli, M. Cardiac, coronary, and peripheral vascular effects of acetyl glyceryl ether phosphorylcholine in the anesthetized dog. *J. Pharmacol. Exp. Ther.,* **1985,** *232*:156–162.

Uedelhoven, W.M., Meese, C.O., and Weber, P.C. Analysis of the major urinary thromboxane metabolites, 2,3-dinorthromboxane B_2 and 11-dehydrothromboxane B_2, by gas chromatography–mass spectrometry and gas chromatography–tandem mass spectrometry. *J. Chromatogr.,* **1989,** *497*:1–16.

Vane, J.R. Inhibition of prostaglandin synthesis as a mechanism of action for aspirin-like drugs. *Nature New Biol.,* **1971,** *231*:232–235.

MONOGRAPHS AND REVIEWS

Austin, S.C., and Funk, C.D. Insight into prostaglandin, leukotriene, and other eicosanoid functions using mice with targeted gene disruptions. *Prostaglandins Other Lipid Mediators,* **1999,** *58*:231–252.

Bergström, S., Carlson, L.A., and Weeks, J.R. The prostaglandins: a family of biologically active lipids. *Pharmacol. Rev.,* **1968,** *20*:1–48.

Brash, A.R. Lipoxygenases: occurrence, functions, catalysis, and acquisition of substrate. *J. Biol. Chem.,* **1999,** *274*:23679–23682.

Capdevila, J.H., Falck, J.R., and Harris, R.C. Cytochrome P450 and arachidonic acid bioactivation: molecular and functional properties of the arachidonate monooxygenase. *J. Lipid Res.,* **2000,** *41*:163–181.

Chao, W., and Olson, M.S. Platelet-activating factor: receptors and signal transduction. *Biochem. J.,* **1993,** *292*:617–629.

Christin-Matire, S., Bourchard, P., and Spitz, I.M. Drug therapy: medical termination of pregnancy. *N. Engl. J. Med.,* **2000,** *342*:946–956.

Clive, D.M. Bartter's syndrome: the unsolved puzzle. *Am. J. Kidney Dis.,* **1995,** *25*:813–825.

Coceani, F., and Akarsu, E.S. Prostaglandin E_2 in the pathogenesis of fever: an update. *Ann. N.Y. Acad. Sci.* **1998,** *856*:76–82.

Coceani, F., Olley, P.M., and Lock, J.E. Prostaglandins, ductus arteriosus, pulmonary circulation: current concepts and clinical potential. *Eur. J. Clin. Pharmacol.,* **1980,** *18*:75–81.

Coleman, R.A., Smith, W.L., and Narumiya, S. International Union of Pharmacology classification of prostanoid receptors: properties, distribution, and structure of the receptors and their subtypes. *Pharmacol. Rev.,* **1994,** *46*:205–229.

Drazen, J.M. Pharmacology of leukotriene receptor antagonists and 5-lipoxygenase inhibitors in the management of asthma. *Pharmacotherapy,* **1997,** *17*:22S–30S.

Drazen, J.M., and Austen, K.F. Leukotrienes and airway responses. *Am. Rev. Respir. Dis.,* **1987,** *136*:985–998.

DuBois, R.N., Abramson, S.B., Crofford, L., Gupta, R.A., Simon, L.S., Van de Putte, L.B., and Lipsky, P.E. Cyclooxygenase in biology and disease. *FASEB J.,* **1998,** *12*:1063–1073.

Dunn, M.J., and Hood, V.L. Prostaglandins and the kidney. *Am. J. Physiol.,* **1977,** *233*:F169–F184.

Feuerstein, G. Leukotrienes and the cardiovascular system. *Prostaglandins,* **1984,** *27*:781–802.

Fitzpatrick, F.A., and Murphy, R.C. Cytochrome P-450 metabolism of arachidonic acid: formation and biological actions of "epoxygenase"-derived eicosanoids. *Pharmacol. Rev.,* **1988,** *40*:229–241.

Flower, R.J. Lipocortin. *Prog. Clin. Biol. Res.,* **1990,** *349*:11–25.

Giles, H., and Leff, P. The biology and pharmacology of PGD_2. *Prostaglandins,* **1988,** *35*:277–300.

Heller, A., Koch, T., Schmeck, J., and van Ackern, K. Lipid mediators in inflammatory disorders. *Drugs,* **1998,** *55*:487–496.

Koltai, M., Hosford, D., Guinot, P., Esanu, A., and Braquet, P. Platelet-activating factor (PAF): a review of its effects, antagonists, and future clinical implications. *Drugs,* **1991,** *42*:9–29, 174–204.

Marnett, L.J., Rowlinson, S.W., Goodwin, D.C., Kalgutkar, A.S., and Lanzo, C.A. Arachidonic acid oxygenation by COX-1 and COX-2: Mechanisms of catalysis and inhibition. *J. Biol. Chem.,* **1999,** *274*:22903–22906.

Martin, B.R., Mechoulam, R., and Razdan, R.K. Discovery and characterization of endogenous cannabinoids. *Life Sci.,* **1999,** *65*:573–595.

Moncada, S., Ferreira, S.H., and Vane, J.R. Pain and inflammatory mediators. In, *Inflammation.* (Vane, J.R., and Ferreira, S.H., eds.) *Handbook of Experimental Pharmacology,* Vol. 50-1. Springer-Verlag, Berlin, **1978,** pp. 588–616.

Moncada, S., and Vane, J.R. Pharmacology and endogenous roles of prostaglandin endoperoxides, thromboxane A_2, and prostacyclin. *Pharmacol. Rev.,* **1978,** *30*:293–331.

Monk, J.P., and Clissold, S.P. Misoprostol: a preliminary review of its pharmacodynamic and pharmacokinetic properties, and therapeutic efficacy in the treatment of peptic ulcer disease. *Drugs,* **1987,** *33*:1–30.

Morrow, J.D., Chen, Y., Brame, C.J., Yang, J., Sanchez, S.C., Xu, J., Zackart, W.E., Awad, J.A., and Roberts, L.J. The isoprostanes: unique prostaglandin-like products of free radical-initiated lipid peroxidation. *Drug Metab. Rev.,* **1999,** *31*:117–139.

Narumiya, S., Sugimoto, Y., and Ushikubi, F. Prostanoid receptors: structures, properties, and functions. *Physiol. Rev.,* **1999,** *79*:1193–1226.

Needleman, P., Turk, J., Jakschik, B.A., Morrison, A.R., and Lefkowith, J.B. Arachidonic acid metabolism. *Annu. Rev. Biochem.*, **1986**, *55*:69–102.

Negro Alvarez, J.M., Miralles Lopez, J.C., Ortiz Martinez, J.L., Abellan Aleman, A., and Rubio del Barrio, R. Platelet-activating factor antagonists. *Allergol. Immunopathol. (Madr.)*, **1997**, *25*:249–258.

Patrono, C. Aspirin as an antiplatelet drug. *N. Engl. J. Med.*, **1994**, *330*:1287–1294.

Peplow, P.V. Regulation of platelet-activating factor (PAF) activity in human diseases by phospholipase A_2 inhibitors, PAF acetylhydrolases, PAF receptor antagonists, and free-radical scavengers. *Prostaglandins, Leukotrienes, Essential Fatty Acids*, **1999**, *61*:65–82.

Peters-Golden, M. Molecular mechanisms of leukotriene synthesis: the changing paradigm. *Clin. Exp. Allergy*, **1998**, *28*:1059–1065.

Piper, P.J. Formation and actions of leukotrienes. *Physiol. Rev.*, **1984**, *64*:744–761.

Prescott, S.M., Zimmerman, G.A., and McIntyre, T.M. Platelet-activating factor. *J. Biol. Chem.*, **1990**, *265*:17381–17384.

Samuelsson, B. Biosynthesis of prostaglandins. *Fed. Proc.*, **1972**, *31*:1442–1450.

Samuelsson, B. Leukotrienes: mediators of immediate hypersensitivity reactions and inflammation. *Science*, **1983**, *220*:568–575.

Samuelsson, B., Dahlen, S.E., Lindgren, J.A., Rouzer, C.A., and Serhan, C.N. Leukotrienes and lipoxins: structures, biosynthesis, and biological effects. *Science*, **1987**, *237*:1171–1176.

Samuelsson, B., Granstrom, E., Green, K., Hamberg, M., and Hammarstrom, S. Prostaglandins. *Annu. Rev. Biochem.*, **1975**, *44*:669–695.

Schlondorff, D., and Neuwirth, R. Platelet-activating factor and the kidney. *Am. J. Physiol.*, **1986**, *251*:F1–F11.

Sigal, E. The molecular biology of mammalian arachidonic acid metabolism. *Am. J. Physiol.*, **1991**, *260*:L13–L28.

Smith, W.L., Garavito, R.M., and DeWitt, D.L. Prostaglandin endoperoxide H synthases (cyclooxygenases)-1 and -2. *J. Biol. Chem.* **1996**, *271*:33157–33160.

Snyder, D.W., and Fleisch, J.H. Leukotriene receptor antagonists as potential therapeutic agents. *Annu. Rev. Pharmacol. Toxicol.*, **1989**, *29*:123–143.

Snyder, F. Biochemistry of platelet-activating factor: a unique class of biologically active phospholipids. *Proc. Soc. Exp. Biol. Med.*, **1989**, *190*:125–135.

Spannhake, E.W., Hyman, A.L., and Kadowitz, P.J. Bronchoactive metabolites of arachidonic acid and their role in airway function. *Prostaglandins*, **1981**, *22*:1013–1026.

Stafforini, D.M., McIntyre, T.M., Zimmerman, G.A., and Prescott, S.M. Platelet-activating factor acetylhydrolases. *J. Biol. Chem.* **1997**, *272*:17895–17898.

Urade, Y., and Hayaishi, O. Prostaglandin D_2 and sleep regulation. *Biochim. Biophys. Acta*, **1999**, *1436*:606–615.

Vane, J.R., Bakhle, Y.S., and Botting, R.M. Cyclooxygenases 1 and 2. *Annu. Rev. Pharmacol. Toxicol.*, **1998**, *38*:97–120.

von Euler, U.S. Some aspects of the actions of prostaglandins. The First Heymans Memorial Lecture. *Arch. Int. Pharmacodyn. Ther.*, **1973**, *202(suppl)*:295–307.

Walt, R.P. Misoprostol for the treatment of peptic ulcer and anti-inflammatory drug-induced gastroduodenal ulceration. *N. Engl. J. Med.*, **1992**, *327*:1575–1580.

Williams, C.S., Mann, M., and DuBois, R.N. The role of cyclooxygenases in inflammation, cancer, and development. *Oncogene*, **1999**, *18*:7908–7916.

Acknowledgment

The authors wish to acknowledge Drs. William B. Campbell and Perry V. Halushka, authors of this chapter in the ninth edition of *Goodman & Gilman's The Pharmacological Basis of Therapeutics*, some of whose text we have retained in this edition.

ANALGESIC-ANTIPYRETIC AND ANTIINFLAMMATORY AGENTS AND DRUGS EMPLOYED IN THE TREATMENT OF GOUT

L. Jackson Roberts II and Jason D. Morrow

This chapter describes drugs used to treat the symptoms and signs of inflammation and drugs used for gout. Most currently available nonsteroidal antiinflammatory drugs (NSAIDs) inhibit both cyclooxygenase-1 (COX-1; constitutive) and cyclooxygenase-2 (COX-2; induced in settings of inflammation) activities, and thereby synthesis of prostaglandins and thromboxane. The inhibition of COX-2 is thought to mediate, at least in part, the antipyretic, analgesic, and antiinflammatory action of NSAIDs, but the simultaneous inhibition of COX-1 results in unwanted side effects, particularly those leading to gastric ulcers, that result from decreased prostaglandin formation. The potential therapeutic advantage of selective COX-2 inhibitors is discussed. NSAIDs include aspirin, which irreversibly acetylates cyclooxygenase, and several other classes of organic acids, including propionic acid derivatives (ibuprofen, naproxen, etc.), acetic acid derivatives (e.g., indomethacin and others), and enolic acids (e.g., piroxicam), all of which compete with arachidonic acid at the active site of cyclooxygenase. Acetaminophen is a very weak antiinflammatory drug but is effective as an antipyretic and analgesic agent and lacks certain side effects of NSAIDs, such as gastric ulceration and blockade of platelet aggregation. Gold salts, primarily used as second-line drugs to treat patients with unremitting and chronic forms of rheumatoid arthritis, also are discussed. Also covered in this chapter are agents used in prophylaxis of acute gout (e.g., colchicine) or treatment of chronic gout (allopurinol, uricosuric agents), a disorder caused by deposition of crystals of sodium urate in joints and other sites. Some agents used to treat inflammation are discussed elsewhere in this textbook, including glucocorticoids (see Chapter 60) and immunosuppressants (see Chapter 53).

NSAIDS: NONSTEROIDAL ANTIINFLAMMATORY DRUGS

The antiinflammatory, analgesic, and antipyretic drugs are a heterogeneous group of compounds, often chemically unrelated (although most of them are organic acids), which nevertheless share certain therapeutic actions and side effects. The prototype is aspirin; hence these compounds are often referred to as aspirin-like drugs; they also are frequently called *nonsteroidal antiinflammatory drugs,* or NSAIDs, an abbreviation that is used throughout this chapter to refer to these agents.

There has been substantial progress in elucidating the mechanism of action of NSAIDs. Inhibition of cyclooxy-genase (COX), the enzyme responsible for the biosynthesis of the prostaglandins and certain related autacoids, generally is thought to be a major facet of the mechanism of NSAIDs. Some of the shared properties of NSAIDs are considered first; then the more important drugs are discussed in some detail.

History. The medicinal effect of the bark of willow and certain other plants has been known to several cultures for centuries. In England in the mid-eighteenth century, Reverend Edmund Stone described in a letter to the president of the Royal Society "an account of the success of the bark of the willow in the cure of agues" (fever). Since the willow grew in damp or wet areas "where agues chiefly abound," Stone reasoned that it would probably possess curative properties appropriate to that condition.

The active ingredient in the willow bark was a bitter glycoside called salicin, first isolated in a pure form in 1829 by Leroux, who also demonstrated its antipyretic effect. On hydrolysis, salicin yields glucose and salicylic alcohol. The latter can be converted into salicylic acid, either *in vivo* or by chemical manipulation. Sodium salicylate was first used for the treatment of rheumatic fever and as an antipyretic in 1875, and the discovery of its uricosuric effects and of its usefulness in the treatment of gout soon followed. The enormous success of this drug prompted Hoffman, a chemist employed by Bayer, to prepare acetylsalicylic acid based on the earlier, but forgotten, work of Gerhardt in 1853. After demonstration of its antiinflammatory effects, this compound was introduced into medicine in 1899 by Dreser under the name of aspirin. The name is said to have been derived from *Spiraea,* the plant species from which salicylic acid was once prepared.

The synthetic salicylates soon displaced the more expensive compounds obtained from natural sources. By the early years of this century, the chief therapeutic benefits of aspirin were known. Toward the end of the nineteenth century, other drugs were discovered that shared some or all of these actions; among these, only derivatives of *para*-aminophenol (*e.g.,* acetaminophen) are used today. Beginning with the introduction of indomethacin for the treatment of rheumatoid arthritis in 1963, a host of other agents with similar actions have been introduced over the years, culminating in the recent development of selective inhibitors of COX-2 (*see* below).

Mechanism of Action of NSAIDs

Although NSAIDs had been known to inhibit a wide variety of reactions *in vitro,* no convincing relationship could be established with their known antiinflammatory, antipyretic, and analgesic effects until 1971, when Vane and associates and Smith and Willis demonstrated that low concentrations of aspirin and indomethacin inhibited the enzymatic production of prostaglandins (*see* Chapter 26). There was, at that time, some evidence that prostaglandins participated in the pathogenesis of inflammation and fever, and this reinforced the hypothesis that inhibition of the biosynthesis of these autacoids could explain a number of the clinical actions of the drugs (*see* Higgs *et al.,* in Symposium, 1983a). Numerous subsequent observations have reinforced this point of view, including the observations that prostaglandins are released whenever cells are damaged, they appear in inflammatory exudates, and NSAIDs inhibit the biosynthesis of prostaglandins in all cells tested. However, NSAIDs generally do not inhibit the formation of eicosanoids such as the leukotrienes, which also contribute to inflammation, nor do they affect the synthesis of numerous other inflammatory mediators. There are differences of opinion as to whether or not NSAIDs may have other actions that contribute to their therapeutic effects (*see* below; Abramson and Weissman, 1989; Vane, 1994).

Inflammation.   The inflammatory process involves a series of events that can be elicited by numerous stimuli (*e.g.,* infectious agents, ischemia, antigen–antibody interactions, and thermal or other physical injury). Each type of stimulus provokes a characteristic pattern of response that represents a relatively minor variation on a theme. At a macroscopic level, the response usually is accompanied by the familiar clinical signs of erythema, edema, tenderness (hyperalgesia), and pain. Inflammatory responses occur in three distinct phases, each apparently mediated by different mechanisms: (1) an acute transient phase, characterized by local vasodilation and increased capillary permeability; (2) a delayed, subacute phase, most prominently characterized by infiltration of leukocytes and phagocytic cells; and (3) a chronic proliferative phase, in which tissue degeneration and fibrosis occur. Many different mechanisms are involved in the inflammatory process (Gallin *et al.,* 1992; Kelly *et al.,* 1993). The ability to mount an inflammatory response is essential for survival in the face of environmental pathogens and injury, although in some situations and diseases the inflammatory response may be exaggerated and sustained for no apparent beneficial reason.

Several classes of leukocytes play an essential role in inflammation. Although earlier ideas emphasized the promotion of migration of cells out of the microvasculature, recent studies have examined the role of the endothelial cell and of cell adhesion molecules, including E-, P-, and L-selectins, intercellular adhesion molecule 1 (ICAM-1), vascular cell adhesion molecule 1 (VCAM-1), and leukocyte integrins in the adhesion of leukocytes, platelets, and endothelium at sites of inflammation (*see* Kishimoto and Anderson, Lasky and Rosen in Gallin *et al.,* 1992; Bevilacqua and Nelson, 1993; and Cronstein and Weissmann, 1993). Activated endothelial cells play a key role in "targeting" circulating cells to inflammatory sites. Expression of the various adhesion molecules varies among different cell types involved in the inflammatory response. For example, expression of E-selectin is restricted primarily to endothelial cells and is enhanced at sites of inflammation. P-selectin is expressed predominantly on platelets and on endothelial cells and is enhanced by cytokines. L-selectin, in contrast, is a receptor for P-selectin, and L-selectin is expressed on leukocytes and is shed when these cells are activated. Cell adhesion appears to occur by recognition of cell-surface glycoprotein and carbohydrates on circulating cells by the adhesion molecules whose expression has been enhanced on resident cells. Thus, endothelial activation results in adhesion of leukocytes by their interaction with newly expressed L-selectin and P-selectin, whereas endothelial-expressed E-selectin interacts with sialylated Lewis X and other glycoproteins on the leukocyte surface; endothelial ICAM-1 interacts with leukocyte integrins. NSAIDs may inhibit expression or activity of certain of these cell adhesion molecules. Such effects have been described for some NSAIDs and not others, suggesting that interference with action of cell adhesion molecules is not a common mechanism of action of all NSAIDs (*see* Diaz-Gonzalez and Sanchez-Madrid, 1998). Nonetheless, effects on adhesion molecules may contribute in part to the antiinflammatory actions of some NSAIDs. Novel classes of antiinflammatory drugs directed against cell adhesion molecules are under active development (*see,* for example, Kavanaugh *et al.,* 1994; Rao *et al.,* 1994; Endemann *et al.,* 1997).

The recruitment of inflammatory cells to sites of injury involves the concerted interactions of several types of soluble mediators in addition to the cell adhesion molecules outlined above. These include the complement factor C5a, platelet activating factor, and leukotriene B_4. All can act as chemotactic agonists. Several different cytokines also appear to play an essential role in orchestrating the inflammatory process, especially interleukin 1 (IL-1) and tumor necrosis factor (TNF; see Dinarello, 1992). Both IL-1 and TNF are derived from mononuclear cells and macrophages (as well as other cell types) and induce expression of numerous genes to promote the synthesis of a variety of proteins that contribute to inflammatory events. IL-1 and TNF are considered principal mediators of biological responses to bacterial lipopolysaccharides (endotoxins) and many other infectious stimuli. IL-1 and TNF appear to work in concert with each other and with growth factors (such as granulocyte/macrophage colony stimulating factor, GM-CSF) and other cytokines, such as IL-8 and related chemotactic cytokines (chemokines), which can promote neutrophil infiltration and activation.

IL-1 comprises two distinct polypeptides (IL-1α and IL-1β) that bind to the same cell surface receptor and produce similar biological responses. Plasma IL-1 levels are increased in patients with certain inflammatory processes (e.g., active rheumatoid arthritis). IL-1 can bind to two types of receptors, an 80,000 dalton IL-1 receptor type 1 and a 68,000 dalton IL-1 receptor type 2, which are present on different types of cells.

TNF, originally termed "cachectin" because of its ability to produce a wasting syndrome, is composed of two closely related proteins: mature TNF (TNFα) and lymphotoxin (TNFβ), both of which are recognized by the same cell-surface receptor. There are two types of TNF receptors, a 75-kDa type 1 and a 55-kDa type 2.

IL-1 and TNF produce many of the same proinflammatory responses, which include induction of fever, sleep, and anorexia; mobilization and activation of polymorphonuclear leukocytes; induction of cyclooxygenase and lipoxygenase enzymes; increase in adhesion molecule expression; activation of B cells, T cells, and natural killer cells; and stimulation of production of other cytokines. Other actions of these agents likely contribute to the fibrosis and tissue degeneration of the chronic proliferative phase of inflammation: stimulation of fibroblast proliferation, induction of collagenase, and activation of osteoblasts and osteoclasts. Both IL-1 and TNF increase expression of many types of genes, probably in part via the activation of transcription factors, such as NFκB and AP-1.

A naturally occurring IL-1 receptor antagonist (IL-1ra), a 17-kDa protein, competes with IL-1 for receptor binding, blocks IL-1 activity in vitro and in vivo, and can prevent death in animals induced by administration of bacteria or bacterial lipopolysaccharide (Arend, 1993). IL-1ra often appears to achieve high levels in patients with various infections or inflammatory conditions. Thus, the balance between IL-1 and IL-1ra may contribute to the extent of an inflammatory response. Studies are in progress to assess whether IL-1ra or other IL-1 antagonists are beneficial as novel types of antiinflammatory agents.

Other cytokines and growth factors (e.g., IL-2, IL-6, IL-8, and GM-CSF) contribute to manifestations of the inflammatory response. The concentrations of many of these factors are increased in the synovia of patients with arthritides, such as rheumatoid arthritis. The concentration of peptides, such as substance P, which promotes firing of pain fibers, also is increased at such sites. To counter the effects of proinflammatory mediators, other cytokines and growth factors have been implicated

as having antiinflammatory activity. These include transforming growth factor-β_1 (TGF-β_1, which increases extracellular matrix formation but also acts as an immunosuppressant), IL-10 (which has inhibitory effects on monocytes, including decreased cytokine and prostaglandin E_2 formation), and interferon gamma (which possesses myelosuppressive activity and inhibits collagen synthesis and collagenase production by macrophages).

Histamine was one of the earliest mediators of the inflammatory process identified. Although several H_1 histamine-receptor antagonists are available, they are useful only for the treatment of vascular events in the early transient phase of inflammation (see Chapter 25). Bradykinin and 5-hydroxytryptamine (serotonin, 5-HT) also may play a role in mediating inflammation, but their antagonists ameliorate only certain types of inflammatory responses (see Chapter 25). Specific inhibitors of leukotriene synthesis, (zileuton, a 5-lipoxygenase inhibitor) and cysteinyl leukotriene-receptor antagonists (montelukast and zafirlukast) exert antiinflammatory actions and have been approved for the treatment of asthma (see Chapter 28). Another lipid autacoid, platelet-activating factor (PAF), has been implicated as an important mediator of inflammation, and inhibitors of its synthesis and action are under study (see Chapter 26).

The effects produced by intradermal, intravenous, or intraarterial injections of small amounts of prostaglandins are strongly reminiscent of inflammation. Prostaglandin E_2 (PGE$_2$) and prostacyclin (PGI$_2$) cause erythema and an increase in local blood flow. With PGE$_2$, such effects may persist for up to 10 hours, and they include the capacity to counteract the vasoconstrictor effects of substances such as norepinephrine and angiotensin. These properties are not generally shared by other inflammatory mediators. In contrast to their long-lasting effects on cutaneous vessels and superficial veins, prostaglandin-induced vasodilation in other vascular beds vanishes within a few minutes.

Although PGE$_1$ and PGE$_2$ (but not PGF$_{2\alpha}$) cause edema when injected into the hind paw of rats, it is not clear if they can increase vascular permeability (leakage) in the postcapillary and collecting venules without the participation of other inflammatory mediators (e.g., bradykinin, histamine, leukotriene C_4). Furthermore, PGE$_1$ is not produced in significant quantities in human beings in vivo, except under rare circumstances, such as essential fatty acid deficiency. Prostaglandins are unlikely to be directly involved in chemotactic responses, even though they may promote the migration of leukocytes into an inflamed area by increasing blood flow. One potent chemotactic substance, leukotriene B_4, is a product of the 5-lipoxygenase pathway of arachidonate metabolism (see Chapter 26). Although high concentrations of NSAIDs can inhibit cell migration, this is not due to an ability of these drugs to inhibit 5-lipoxygenase and thus leukotriene B_4 formation.

Rheumatoid Arthritis. Although the pathogenesis of rheumatoid arthritis is largely unknown, it appears to be an autoimmune disease driven primarily by activated T cells, giving rise to T cell–derived cytokines, such as IL-1 and TNF. Although activation of B cells and the humoral response also are evident, most of the antibodies generated are IgG of unknown specificity, apparently elicited by polyclonal activation of B cells rather than from a response to a specific antigen.

Many cytokines, including IL-1 and TNF, have been found in the rheumatoid synovium. Of the available antiinflammatory drugs, only the adrenocorticosteroids are known to interfere with the synthesis and/or actions of cytokines such as IL-1 or TNF (see Chapter 60). Although some of the actions of these cytokines are accompanied by the release of prostaglandins and/or thromboxane A_2, only their pyrogenic effects are blocked by inhibitors of cyclooxygenase (see below). In addition, many of the actions of the prostaglandins are inhibitory to the immune response, including suppression of the function of helper T cells and B cells and inhibition of the production of IL-1. Thus, it is difficult to ascribe the antirheumatoid effects of aspirin-like drugs solely to inhibition of prostaglandin synthesis. It has been proposed that salicylate and certain other NSAIDs can directly inhibit the activation and function of neutrophils, perhaps by inhibition of membrane-associated processes, independent of their ability to inhibit prostaglandin synthesis (see Abramson and Weissmann, 1989). Furthermore, as mentioned previously, some NSAIDs can inhibit leukocyte adhesion by a mechanism that seems to be independent of their ability to inhibit prostaglandin biosynthesis.

Pain. NSAIDs usually are classified as mild analgesics, but this classification is not altogether correct. A consideration of the type of pain as well as its intensity is important in the assessment of analgesic efficacy. In some forms of postoperative pain, for example, the NSAIDs can be superior to the opioid analgesics. Moreover, they are particularly effective in settings in which inflammation has caused sensitization of pain receptors to normally painless mechanical or chemical stimuli. Pain that accompanies inflammation and tissue injury probably results from local stimulation of pain fibers and enhanced pain sensitivity (hyperalgesia), in part a consequence of increased excitability of central neurons in the spinal cord ("central sensitization"; see Konttinen et al., 1994).

Bradykinin, released from plasma kininogen, and cytokines, such as $TNF\alpha$, IL-1, and IL-8, appear to be particularly important in eliciting the pain of inflammation. These agents liberate prostaglandins and probably other mediators that promote hyperalgesia. Neuropeptides, such as substance P and calcitonin gene-related peptide, also may be involved in eliciting pain.

Large doses of PGE_2 or $PGF_{2\alpha}$, given in the past to women by intramuscular or subcutaneous injection to induce abortion, cause intense local pain. Prostaglandins also can cause headache and vascular pain when infused intravenously. The capacity of prostaglandins to sensitize pain receptors to mechanical and chemical stimulation appears to result from a lowering of the threshold of the polymodal nociceptors of C fibers. In general, NSAIDs do not affect the hyperalgesia or the pain caused by direct action of prostaglandins, consistent with the notion that the analgesic effects of these agents are due to inhibition of prostaglandin synthesis. However, some data have suggested that relief of pain by these compounds may occur via mechanisms other than inhibition of prostaglandin synthesis, including antinociceptive effects at peripheral or central neurons (see Gebhart and McCormack, 1994; Konttinen et al., 1994).

Fever. Regulation of body temperature requires a delicate balance between the production and loss of heat; the hypothalamus regulates the set point at which body temperature is maintained (see Saper and Breder, 1994). In fever, this set point is elevated, and NSAIDs promote its return to normal. These drugs do not influence body temperature when it is elevated by such factors as exercise or increases in the ambient temperature.

Fever may be a result of infection or one of the sequelae of tissue damage, inflammation, graft rejection, malignancy, or other disease states. A common feature of these conditions is the enhanced formation of cytokines such as IL-1β, IL-6, interferons alpha and beta, and $TNF\alpha$. The cytokines increase the synthesis of PGE_2 in circumventricular organs in and near to the preoptic hypothalamic area, and PGE_2, via increases in cyclic AMP, triggers the hypothalamus to elevate body temperature by promoting increases in heat generation and decreases in heat loss. NSAIDs suppress this response by inhibiting the synthesis of PGE_2 (Dascombe, 1985). The evidence for this scenario includes the ability of prostaglandins, especially PGE_2, to produce fever when infused into the cerebral ventricles or when injected into the hypothalamus. In addition, fever is a frequent side effect of prostaglandins when they are administered to women as abortifacients. NSAIDs do not inhibit fever caused by prostaglandins when prostaglandins are administered directly, but they do inhibit fever caused by agents that enhance the synthesis of IL-1 and other cytokines, which presumably cause fever at least in part by inducing the endogenous synthesis of prostaglandins.

Inhibition of Prostaglandin Biosynthesis by NSAIDs. Since the principal therapeutic effects of NSAIDs derive from their ability to inhibit prostaglandin production, the enzymatic activities involved in prostaglandin synthesis are described here briefly (see also Chapter 26). The mechanisms by which varying NSAIDs interfere with prostaglandin synthesis then are outlined. The first enzyme in the prostaglandin synthetic pathway is prostaglandin endoperoxide synthase, or fatty acid cyclooxygenase. This enzyme converts arachidonic acid to the unstable intermediates PGG_2 and PGH_2. It is now appreciated that there are two forms of cyclooxygenase, termed cyclooxygenase-1 (COX-1) and cyclooxygenase-2 (COX-2) (see Vane et al., 1998). COX-1 is a constitutive isoform found in most normal cells and tissues, while COX-2 is induced in settings of inflammation by cytokines and inflammatory mediators (Seibert et al., 1997). However, COX-2 also is constitutively expressed in certain areas of kidney and brain (Breder et al., 1995; Harris et al., 1994). Importantly, COX-1, but not COX-2, is constitutively expressed in the stomach. This accounts for the markedly reduced occurrence of gastric toxicity with the use of selective inhibitors of COX-2 (*see* below).

The fate of PGG_2/PGH_2 cyclooxygenase products differs from tissue to tissue, depending on the particular PGG_2/PGH_2-metabolizing enzymatic activities present (*see* Figure 26–1). Arachidonic acid also can be converted, *via* the 5-lipoxygenase pathway, to a variety of leukotrienes. Aspirin and NSAIDs inhibit the cyclooxygenase enzyme and prostaglandin production; they do not inhibit lipoxygenase pathways and, hence, do not suppress leukotriene formation. Glucocorticoids suppress the expression of COX-2 and thus COX-2-mediated prostaglandin production (Masferrer *et al.*, 1994a). This effect may contribute in part to the antiinflammatory actions of glucocorticoids.

Table 27–1 provides a classification of NSAIDs and other analgesic and antipyretic agents based on chemical categories. Structures of these agents are given in subsequent sections describing their therapeutic effects. Individual agents inhibit cyclooxygenase by differing mechanisms.

Aspirin covalently modifies both COX-1 and COX-2, thus resulting in an irreversible inhibition of cyclooxygenase activity. This is an important distinction for aspirin, as the duration of the effects of aspirin is related to the turnover rate of cyclooxygenases in different target tissues. In the structure of COX-1, aspirin acetylates serine 530, preventing the binding of arachidonic acid to the active site of the enzyme and thus the ability of the enzyme to make prostaglandins. In COX-2, aspirin acetylates a homologous serine at position 516. Although covalent modification of COX-2 by aspirin also blocks the cyclooxygenase activity of this isoform, an interesting property of COX-2, not shared by COX-1, is that acetylated COX-2 now synthesizes 15(*R*)-hydroxyeicosatetraenoic acid (15(*R*)-HETE) (Lecomte *et al.*, 1994; O'Neill *et al.*, 1994). Interestingly,

Table 27–1

Chemical Classification of Analgesic, Antipyretic, and Nonsteroidal Antiinflammatory Drugs

Nonselective COX Inhibitors

Salicylic acid derivatives
  Aspirin, sodium salicylate, choline magnesium trisalicylate, salsalate, diflunisal, sulfasalazine, olsalazine
Para-aminophenol derivatives
  Acetaminophen
Indole and indene acetic acids
  Indomethacin, sulindac
Heteroaryl acetic acids
  Tolmetin, diclofenac, ketorolac
Arylpropionic acids
  Ibuprofen, naproxen, flurbiprofen, ketoprofen, fenoprofen, oxaprozin
Anthranilic acids (fenamates)
  Mefenamic acid, meclofenamic acid
Enolic acids
  Oxicams (piroxicam, meloxicam)
Alkanones
  Nabumetone

Selective COX-2 Inhibitors

Diaryl-substituted furanones
  Rofecoxib
Diaryl-substituted pyrazoles
  Celecoxib
Indole acetic acids
  Etodolac
Sulfonanilides
  Nimesulide

this aspirin-induced product can undergo transcellular metabolism by the 5-lipoxygenase enzyme to yield 15-epi-lipoxin A_4, which exerts potent antiinflammatory actions and therefore may potentiate the antiinflammatory action of aspirin (Claria and Serhan, 1995; Serhan *et al.*, 1999).

Platelets are especially susceptible to prolonged, aspirin-mediated, irreversible inactivation of cyclooxygenase because they have little or no capacity for protein biosynthesis and thus cannot regenerate the cyclooxygenase enzyme. In practical terms, this means that a single dose of aspirin will inhibit the platelet cyclooxygenase for the life of the platelet (8 to 11 days); in human beings, a daily dose of aspirin as small as 40 mg is sufficient to produce this effect. The ability of platelets to be inhibited by such low doses of aspirin is related to the presystemic inhibition of the cyclooxygenase in the portal circulation before the aspirin is deacetylated to salicylate in the liver. In contrast to aspirin, salicylic acid has no acetylating capacity. Nevertheless, it, like aspirin, reduces the synthesis of prostaglandins *in vivo*, but whether this is due to a direct effect on cyclooxygenase and/or an indirect effect due to an ability of salicylate to inhibit the activation of NFκB remains controversial (Higgs *et al.*, 1987; Yin *et al.*, 1998).

The vast majority of NSAIDs listed in Table 27–1 are organic acids and, in contrast to aspirin, act as reversible, competitive inhibitors of cyclooxygenase activity. Even the nonacidic parent drug, nabumetone, is converted to an active acetic acid derivative *in vivo*. As organic acids, the compounds generally are well absorbed orally, highly bound to plasma proteins, and excreted either by glomerular filtration or by tubular secretion. In contrast to aspirin, whose duration of action is determined by the rate of synthesis of new cyclooxygenase enzyme, the duration of action of all other NSAIDs, which are reversible inhibitors of cyclooxygenase, is primarily related to the pharmacokinetic clearance of the drugs from the body. NSAIDs can be roughly divided into two groups, those with short (<6 hours) and those with long (>10 hours) half-lives (Brooks and Day, 1991). Because aspirin and other NSAIDs are organic acids, they accumulate at sites of inflammation, which is an attractive pharmacokinetic property of drugs intended as antiinflammatory agents.

Most NSAIDs developed before the availability of selective COX-2 inhibitors inhibit both COX-1 and COX-2 with little selectivity or have modest selectivity for the constitutive COX-1 isoform. The hope that it would be possible to retain the antiinflammatory effects of aspirin-like drugs with a lower ulcerogenic potential has propelled efforts to design NSAIDs with greater selectivity for COX-2 *versus* COX-1 (Meade *et al.*, 1993; Mitchell *et al.*, 1993; Massferrer *et al.*, 1994b; O'Neill *et al.*, 1994). These

efforts have led to the recent introduction of highly selective COX-2 inhibitors (*rofecoxib* and *celecoxib*) and the recognition that two previously marketed NSAIDs that have very low gastric toxicity (*etodolac* and *nimesulide*) also have a high degree of selectivity for inhibition of COX-2. The relative COX-isozyme selectivity of most of the NSAIDs available has been described in detail (Warner *et al.*, 1999).

There is good evidence that therapeutic doses of aspirin and other NSAIDs reduce prostaglandin biosynthesis in human beings, and there is a reasonably good rank order correlation between the potency of these drugs as inhibitors of cyclooxygenase and their antiinflammatory activity (Vane and Botting, 1987). There are some exceptions to this, but these exceptions may in part be attributed to the experimental conditions used, which do not always mimic the *in vivo* situation. For example, potencies of compounds to inhibit purified enzyme compared to enzymes contained in cells sometimes have been found to be different (Mitchell *et al.*, 1993). Moreover, *in vitro* conditions do not take into account factors such as binding of the drugs to plasma proteins. Furthermore, in addition to inhibiting cyclooxygenase, some drugs have been found to exert other effects that are antiinflammatory (Yamamoto *et al.*, 1999; Yin *et al.*, 1998). Nonetheless, many findings are consistent with inhibition of prostaglandin synthesis as the principal basis for the therapeutic actions of NSAIDs.

An example of other lines of evidence linking cyclooxygenase inhibition to antiinflammatory activity is the high degree of stereoselectivity among several pairs of enantiomers of α-methyl arylacetic acids for inhibition of cyclooxygenase and suppression of inflammation; in each instance the *d* or (+) isomer is more potent in both inhibiting cyclooxygenase and suppressing inflammation. Similarly, sulindac is a prodrug that is only weakly active as an antiinflammatory agent but is converted *in vivo* to a highly active antiinflammatory metabolite that also is a potent inhibitor of cyclooxygenase.

Acetaminophen, which is a very weak antiinflammatory agent, is a weak inhibitor of cyclooxygenase. Moreover, acetaminophen appears to inhibit the enzyme only in an environment that is low in peroxide (*e.g.*, the hypothalamus; *see* Marshall *et al.*, 1987; Hanel and Lands, 1982), which may in part explain the poor antiinflammatory activity of acetaminophen, since sites of inflammation usually contain increased concentrations of peroxides generated by leukocytes.

Shared Therapeutic Activities and Side Effects of NSAIDs

Therapeutic Effects. All NSAIDs, including selective COX-2 inhibitors (Morrison *et al.*, 1999; Malmstrom *et al.*, 1999), are antipyretic, analgesic, and antiinflammatory. One important exception is acetaminophen, which is antipyretic and analgesic but is largely devoid of antiin-flammatory activity. This can be explained by the fact that acetaminophen effectively inhibits cyclooxygenases in the brain but not at sites of inflammation in peripheral tissues (*see* above).

When employed as analgesics, these drugs usually are effective only against pain of low-to-moderate inten-sity, such as dental pain. Although their maximal effects are much lower, they lack the unwanted effects of the opi-oids on the central nervous system (CNS), including respi-ratory depression and the development of physical depen-dence. NSAIDs do not change the perception of sensory modalities other than pain. Chronic postoperative pain or pain arising from inflammation is particularly well con-trolled by NSAIDs, whereas pain arising from the hollow viscera usually is not relieved.

As antipyretics, NSAIDs reduce the body tempera-ture in febrile states. The fact that selective COX-2 in-hibitors are effective antipyretic agents indicates that the COX isoform predominantly involved in thermoregulation is COX-2.

NSAIDs find their chief clinical application as anti-inflammatory agents in the treatment of musculoskele-tal disorders, such as rheumatoid arthritis, osteoarthritis, and ankylosing spondylitis. Chronic treatment of patients with rofecoxib and celecoxib has been shown to be effec-tive in suppressing inflammation without the gastric tox-icity that is associated with treatment with nonselective NSAIDs (Simon *et al.*, 1998, 1999; Bensen *et al.*, 1999; Emery *et al.*, 1999; Hawkey *et al.*, 2000; Schnitzer *et al.*, 1999; Ehrich *et al.*, 1999; Laine *et al.*, 1999). In general, NSAIDs provide only symptomatic relief from the pain and inflammation associated with the disease and do not arrest the progression of pathological injury to tissue.

Some other uses of NSAIDs also depend upon their capacity to block prostaglandin biosynthesis. Prostaglan-dins have been implicated in the maintenance of patency of the ductus arteriosus, and indomethacin and related agents have been used in neonates to close the ductus when it has remained patent. On the other hand, admin-istration of nonselective NSAIDs to pregnant women can cause premature contraction of the ductus *in utero*. In fetal lambs, production of vasodilatory prostaglandins by both COX-1 and COX-2 appear to participate in maintaining patency of the ductus arteriosus (Clyman *et al.*, 1999). Although it remains to be established which isoform(s) is involved in maintaining patency of the fetal ductus *in utero* in human beings, it is prudent to exercise caution in the use of selective COX-2 inhibitors in pregnant women.

The release of prostaglandins by the endometrium during menstruation may be a cause of severe cramps and other symptoms of primary dysmenorrhea; treatment of this condition with NSAIDs has met with considerable success (*see* Shapiro, 1988). A recent study revealed that the selective COX-2 inhibitor rofecoxib is as effective as the nonselective NSAID sodium naproxen in the treatment of dysmenorrhea (Morrison *et al.*, 1999). Therefore, it is anticipated that there will be an increase in the use of selective COX-2 inhibitors for this condition.

Prostaglandin D_2 released from mast cells in large amounts has been found to be the major mediator of se-vere episodes of vasodilation and hypotension in patients with systemic mastocytosis. Treatment of these patients with antihistamines alone is usually ineffective, whereas addition of an NSAID usually leads to effective preven-tion of these episodes (Roberts *et al.*, 1980; Roberts and Oates, 1991; Metcalf, 1991).

Prostaglandin E_2 also has been implicated in the hu-moral hypercalcemia associated with some neoplasms, and treatment with NSAIDs can effectively suppress serum calcium levels in some cancer patients (Brenner *et al.*, 1982; Robertson, 1981).

Bartter's syndrome is characterized hypokalemia, hy-perreninemia, hyperaldosteronism, juxtaglomerular hyper-plasia, normotension, and resistance to the pressor effect of angiotensin II. Excessive production of renal prosta-glandins has been implicated in the pathogenesis of some of the metabolic abnormalities in this syndrome, and NSAIDs have been found to be useful in the treatment of this disorder (Dunn, 1981). A rare, complex syndrome occurs in infants resembling a Bartter's syndrome–like tubulopathy with systemic features including fever, diar-rhea, and osteopenia with hypercalciuria. This syndrome is associated with marked overproduction of prostaglandin E_2, and it has been termed hyperprostaglandin E syn-drome. Most of these abnormalities can be effectively controlled with long-term treatment with indomethacin (Seyberth *et al.*, 1987).

An important area where the use of NSAIDs is emerg-ing is in the prevention of colon cancer. Epidemiological studies suggested that frequent use of aspirin is associated with a striking reduction (approximately 50%) in the in-cidence of colon cancer (Thun *et al.*, 1991; Giovannucci *et al.*, 1995). Interestingly, this reduction occurred with in-gestion of as little as four to six 325-mg tablets per week. These observations have stimulated intense investigation into the mechanism(s) involved in the reduction of colon cancer incidence. NSAIDs, in particular sulindac sulfide, have been found to suppress significantly polyp formation in patients with familial polyposis coli and in mice bearing a mutation in the same *APC* gene. Whether or not these ef-fects of NSAIDs are due to a cyclooxygenase-independent

Table 27–2

Side Effects Shared by Nonselective COX Inhibitors and Selective COX-2 Inhibitors

SIDE EFFECT	SHARED BY NONSELECTIVE COX INHIBITORS	SHARED BY SELECTIVE COX-2 INHIBITORS
Gastric ulceration and intolerance	Yes*	No
Inhibition of platelet function	Yes*	No
Inhibition of induction of labor	Yes	Yes
Alterations in renal function	Yes	Yes
Hypersensitivity reactions	Yes*	Unknown

*Less pronounced with nonacetylated salicylates and *p*-aminophenol derivatives.

effect of NSAIDs has been questioned (Wu, 2000). Nevertheless, there is a compelling body of evidence suggesting that the effect of NSAIDs on colon cancer is mediated by inhibition of COX-2, which is strikingly upregulated in colon tumors (Gupta and Dubois, 1998). Controlled, randomized, prospective trials currently are under way to evaluate aspirin and selective COX-2 inhibitors as chemopreventive agents for sporadic colon cancer.

Large doses of niacin (nicotinic acid) effectively lower serum cholesterol levels, reduce LDL, and raise HDL (*see* Chapter 36). However, niacin is poorly tolerated because it induces intense flushing. This flushing has been shown to be mediated by a release of prostaglandin D_2 from the skin, which can be inhibited by treatment with low doses of aspirin (Morrow *et al.,* 1989; Morrow *et al.,* 1992).

Side Effects of NSAID Therapy. In addition to sharing many therapeutic activities, NSAIDs share several unwanted side effects, outlined in Table 27–2 (*see also* Borda and Koff, 1992). The most common is a propensity to induce gastric or intestinal ulceration that sometimes can be accompanied by anemia from the resultant blood loss. The notable exception to this is that highly selective COX-2 inhibitors lack the propensity to cause gastric ulceration. Patients who use nonselective NSAIDs on a chronic basis have about three times greater relative risk for serious adverse gastrointestinal events compared to nonusers (Gabriel *et al.,* 1991). Nonselective NSAIDs vary considerably in their tendency to cause such erosions and ulcers (*see* individual sections). Gastric damage by these agents can be brought about by at least two distinct mechanisms. Although local irritation by orally administered drugs allows back diffusion of acid into the gastric mucosa and induces tissue damage, parenteral administration also can cause damage and bleeding, correlated with inhibition of the biosynthesis of gastric prostaglandins,

especially PGI_2 and PGE_2, that serve as cytoprotective agents in the gastric mucosa (*see* articles by Ivey and by Isselbacher, in Symposium, 1988a). These eicosanoids inhibit acid secretion by the stomach, enhance mucosal blood flow, and promote the secretion of cytoprotective mucus in the intestine; inhibition of their synthesis may render the stomach more susceptible to damage. All of the NSAIDs discussed in this chapter, with the exception of *p*-aminophenol derivatives and the highly selective COX-2 inhibitors, have a strong tendency to cause gastrointestinal side effects ranging from mild dyspepsia and heartburn to ulceration of the stomach or duodenum, sometimes with fatal results. Administration of the PGE_1 analog *misoprostol* along with these NSAIDs can be beneficial in the prevention of duodenal and gastric ulceration produced by these drugs (Graham *et al.,* 1993). It also is possible that enhanced generation of lipoxygenase products contributes to ulcerogenicity in patients treated with NSAIDs and that there may be an association with *Helicobacter pylori* infection (*see* Borda in Borda and Koff, 1992).

Other side effects of these drugs that result from blockade of the synthesis of endogenous prostaglandins and thromboxane A_2 include disturbances in platelet function, the prolongation of gestation or spontaneous labor, premature closure of the patent ductus, and changes in renal function.

Platelet function is impaired because NSAIDs prevent the formation by the platelets of thromboxane A_2 (TXA_2), a potent aggregating agent. This accounts for the ability of these drugs to increase the bleeding time. Aspirin is a particularly effective inhibitor of platelet function, because, as discussed above, the irreversible effects of aspirin on cyclooxygenase activity require new platelet production for restoration of enzyme activity. This "side effect" has been exploited in the prophylactic treatment of thromboembolic disorders (*see* Chapter 55). Acute administration of 400 mg and 800 mg of the selective COX-2 inhibitor celecoxib to human beings has been found to suppress PGI_2 production by about 80%, without inhibiting TXA_2 production and platelet aggregation (McAdam *et al.*, 1999). Similar results were obtained with rofecoxib. This finding suggests that COX-2 is a major source of PGI_2 production *in vivo*. Since an important action of PGI_2 is thought to be suppression of platelet activation, alteration of the TXA_2/PGI_2 ratio that accompanies selective inhibition of COX-2 is theoretically prothrombotic. It remains to be determined whether or not this possibility is clinically relevant. Nonetheless, it may be prudent to consider these findings when choosing an NSAID for the treatment of patients who are particularly prone to thrombotic events.

Prolongation of gestation by NSAIDs has been demonstrated in both experimental animals and women. Prostaglandins of the E and F series are potent uterotropic agents, and their biosynthesis by the uterus increases dramatically in the hours before parturition. This increase in prostanoid production is thought to result from induction of COX-2 expression (Slater *et al.*, 1999). Prostaglandins are thus postulated to have a major role in the initiation and progression of labor and delivery. Accordingly, some NSAIDs have been used as tocolytic agents to inhibit preterm labor, including selective COX-2 inhibitors (Sawdy *et al.*, 1997). However, as mentioned previously, administration of nonselective COX inhibitors can cause premature closure of the ductus arteriosus *in utero,* and evidence obtained in fetal lambs suggests that selective COX-2 inhibitors also may cause this effect.

Clinically relevant, adverse effects on renal function have been well recognized with the use of nonselective NSAIDs; recent evidence suggests that selective COX-2 inhibitors also have the propensity to cause such effects (Brater, 1999). NSAIDs have little effect on renal function in normal human subjects, presumably because the production of vasodilatory prostaglandins has only a minor role in sodium-replete individuals. However, these drugs decrease renal blood flow and the rate of glomerular filtration in patients with congestive heart failure, hepatic cirrhosis with ascites, chronic renal disease, or in those who are hypovolemic (*see* Clive and Stoff, 1984; Patrono and Dunn, 1987; Oates *et al.*, 1988; Wilson and Carruthers in Borda and Koff, 1992); acute renal failure may be precipitated under these circumstances. In individuals with these clinical conditions, renal perfusion is more dependent than in normal individuals upon prostaglandins that cause vasodilation and thus oppose the increased vasoconstrictive influences of norepinephrine and angiotensin II that result from the activation of pressor reflexes.

In addition to their hemodynamic effects in the kidney, NSAIDs promote the retention of salt and water by reducing the prostaglandin-induced inhibition of both the reabsorption of chloride and the action of antidiuretic hormone. This may cause edema in some patients who are treated with NSAIDs; it also may reduce the effectiveness of antihypertensive regimens (*see* Patrono and Dunn, 1987; Oates *et al.*, 1988). These drugs promote hyperkalemia by several mechanisms, including enhanced reabsorption of K^+ as a result of decreased availability of Na^+ at distal tubular sites and suppression of the prostaglandin-induced secretion of renin. The latter effect may account in part for the usefulness of NSAIDs in the treatment of Bartter's syndrome, which is characterized by hypokalemia, hyperreninemia, hyperaldosteronism, juxtaglomerular hyperplasia, normotension, and resistance to the pressor effect of angiotensin II. Excessive production of renal prostaglandins may play an important part in the pathogenesis of this syndrome.

Although nephropathy is uncommonly associated with the long-term use of individual NSAIDs, the abuse of analgesic mixtures has been linked to the development of renal injury, including papillary necrosis and chronic interstitial nephritis (*see* Kincaid-Smith, 1986). The injury often is insidious in onset, is usually manifest initially as reduced tubular function and concentrating ability, and may progress to irreversible renal insufficiency if misuse of analgesics continues. Females are involved more frequently than are males, and often there is a history of recurring urinary tract infection. Emotional disturbances are common, and other drugs may be abused concurrently. Despite numerous clinical observations and experimental studies in laboratory animals and human beings, insights concerning the mechanisms underlying NSAID-fostered renal injury are lacking. Phenacetin was suggested to be the nephrotoxic component of older analgesic mixtures (commonly, aspirin–phenacetin–caffeine, or "APC") and, therefore, was removed from these products. Although the incidence of analgesic nephropathy in some countries has subsequently declined, this has not been a universal result, especially in Australia. It is thus possible that chronic abuse of a variety of different NSAIDs or analgesic mixtures may cause renal injury in the susceptible individual (Sandler *et al.*, 1989). An acute interstitial nephritis also can occur as a rare complication of the use of NSAIDs.

Certain individuals display intolerance to aspirin and most NSAIDs; this is manifest by symptoms that range from vasomotor rhinitis with profuse watery secretions, angioneurotic edema, generalized urticaria, and bronchial asthma to laryngeal edema and bronchoconstriction, flushing, hypotension, and shock. Although less common in children, this syndrome may occur in 10% to 25% of patients with asthma, nasal polyps, or chronic urticaria and can occur when these patients receive even small amounts (<80 mg) of aspirin. A subset of patients with mastocytosis also exhibits adverse reactions with the use of aspirin. Despite the resemblance to anaphylaxis, this reaction does not appear to be immunological in nature. These reactions are not limited to aspirin. Almost without exception, an individual who exhibits intolerance to aspirin also will react when given any of the other NSAIDs, despite their chemical diversity. Although nonacetylated salicylates and acetaminophen are less likely to produce these reactions in individuals who react to other NSAIDs, they can produce severe reactions in some, especially if high doses are administered. [Such patients also may react if they ingest tartrazine (FD&C Yellow No. 5 dye), which is found in many foods and beverages.] The underlying mechanism for this hypersensitivity reaction to NSAIDs is not known, but a common factor appears to be the ability of the drugs to inhibit cyclooxygenase activity. This has prompted the hypothesis that the reaction reflects the diversion of arachidonic acid metabolism toward the formation of increased amounts of leukotrienes and other products of lipoxygenase pathways. This view is as yet unproven, and it does not explain why only a minority of patients with asthma or other predisposing conditions display the reaction. Even so, results in a small number of patients suggest that blockade of 5-lipoxygenase with the drug zileuton may prevent symptoms and signs of aspirin intolerance (Israel *et al.*, 1993). *Hypersensitivity to aspirin is a contraindication to therapy with any of the drugs discussed in this chapter; administration of any one of these could provoke a life-threatening reaction reminiscent of anaphylactic shock (see above).*

Choice of an NSAID in Varying Clinical Situations.
The choice of an agent as an antipyretic or analgesic is seldom a problem. It is in the field of rheumatology that the decision becomes complex (*see* Brooks and Day, 1991). The choice among NSAIDs for the treatment of arthritides is largely empirical. A drug may be chosen and given for a week or more; if the therapeutic effect is adequate, treatment should be continued unless toxicity occurs. Large variations are possible in the response of individuals to different NSAIDs, even when the drugs are structurally similar members of the same chemical family. Thus, a patient may do well on one propionic acid derivative (such as ibuprofen) but not on another. Initially, fairly low doses of the agent chosen should be prescribed to determine the effect of the drug and patient tolerance. When the patient has problems sleeping because of pain or morning stiffness, a larger single dose of the drug may be given at night. A week is generally long enough to determine the effect of a given drug. If the drug is effective, treatment should be continued, reducing the dose if possible and stopping it altogether if it is no longer necessary. Side effects usually appear in the first weeks of therapy, although gastric ulceration usually takes much longer to develop. If the patient does not achieve therapeutic benefit from one NSAID, another compound should be tried, since, as noted above, there is a marked variation in the response of individuals to different but closely related drugs. Discussion of principles of the use of NSAIDs also is provided in earlier reviews (Symposium, 1983a; Lewis and Furst, 1987).

For mild arthropathies, the scheme outlined above, together with rest and physical therapy, probably will be effective. However, patients with a more debilitating disease may not respond adequately. In such cases, more aggressive therapy should be initiated with aspirin or another agent. It is best to avoid continuous combination therapy with more than one NSAID; there is little evidence of extra benefit to the patient, and the incidence of side effects generally is additive.

The choice of drugs for children is considerably restricted, and only drugs that have been extensively tested in children should be used. This commonly means that only aspirin, naproxen, or tolmetin should be prescribed. However, the association of Reye's syndrome in children with the administration of aspirin for the treatment of febrile viral illnesses precludes its use in this setting. Although some controversy remains regarding whether there is a causative link between aspirin use in children and the development of Reye's syndrome, the epidemiologic evidence for this was so compelling that labeling of aspirin and aspirin-containing medications to indicate Reye's syndrome as a risk in children was mandated in 1986 (*see*

Hurwitz, 1989). The use of aspirin in children has declined dramatically, and Reye's syndrome has almost disappeared (Belay *et al.*, 1999; Monto, 1999). Acetaminophen has not been implicated in Reye's syndrome and can be substituted for aspirin for antipyresis in children.

The use of any of the NSAIDs in pregnant women generally is not recommended. If such a drug must be given to a pregnant woman, low doses of aspirin are probably the safest. Although toxic doses of salicylates cause teratogenic effects in animals, there is no evidence to suggest that salicylates in moderate doses have teratogenic effects on the human fetus. In any case, aspirin and other NSAIDs should be discontinued prior to the anticipated time of parturition to avoid complications such as prolongation of labor, increased risk of postpartum hemorrhage, and intrauterine closure of the ductus arteriosus.

Many NSAIDs are highly bound to plasma proteins and thus may displace certain other drugs from the binding sites. Such interactions can occur in patients given salicylates or other NSAIDs together with warfarin, sulfonylurea hypoglycemic agents, or methotrexate; the dosage of such agents may require adjustment, or concurrent administration should be avoided. The problem with warfarin is accentuated, because almost all NSAIDs suppress normal platelet function. Numerous other drug interactions are observed with NSAIDs (*see* Brooks and Day, 1991).

For the seriously debilitated patient who cannot tolerate these drugs or in whom they are not adequately effective, other forms of therapy should be considered. Gold, hydroxychloroquine, and penicillamine are discussed in a separate section of this chapter. Other relevant drugs include immunosuppressive agents (Chapter 53) and glucocorticoids (Chapter 60).

A final important consideration in the selection of an NSAID for a patient is the cost of therapy, particularly since these agents frequently are used on a long-term basis. Generally speaking, aspirin is very inexpensive; the cost of the newer, nonselective NSAIDs and selective COX-2 inhibitors drugs is much higher.

THE SALICYLATES

Despite the introduction of many new drugs, aspirin (acetylsalicylic acid) is still the most widely prescribed analgesic-antipyretic and antiinflammatory agent and is the standard for the comparison and evaluation of the others. Prodigious amounts of the drug are consumed in the United States; some estimates place the quantity as high as 10,000 to 20,000 tons annually. Aspirin is the common household analgesic; yet, because the drug is so generally

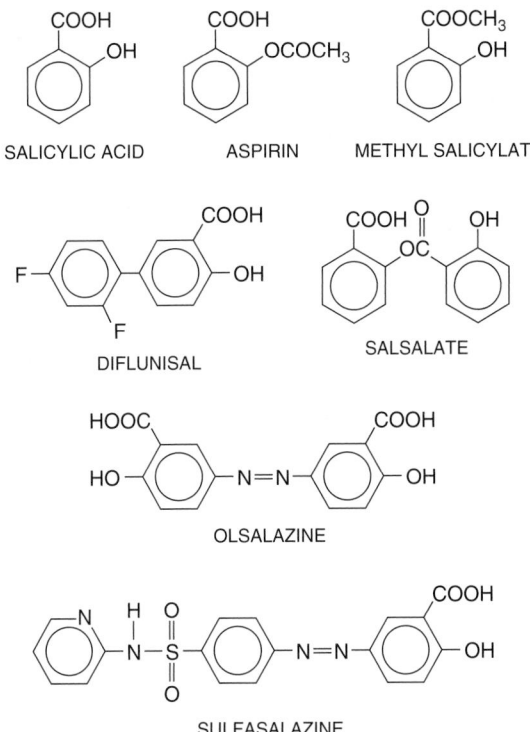

Figure 27–1. Structural formulas of the salicylates.

available, the possibility of misuse and serious toxicity is probably underappreciated, and it can be a common cause of poisoning in children, which can be fatal. Reviews of some of the clinical pharmacology of salicylate appear in several Symposia (1983a, 1983b) and in a monograph (Rainsford, 1985a).

Chemistry. Salicylic acid (orthohydroxybenzoic acid) is so irritating that it can be used only externally; therefore, various derivatives of this acid have been synthesized for systemic use. These comprise two large classes, namely, esters of salicylic acid obtained by substitution in the carboxyl group and salicylate esters of organic acids, in which the carboxyl group of salicylic acid is retained and substitution is made in the hydroxyl group. For example, aspirin is an ester of acetic acid. In addition, there are salts of salicylic acid. The chemical relationships can be seen from the structural formulas shown in Figure 27–1.

Structure-Activity Relationships. Salicylates generally act by virtue of their content of salicylic acid, although some of the unique effects of aspirin are due to its capacity to acetylate proteins, as described earlier. Substitutions on the carboxyl or hydroxyl groups change the potency or toxicity of salicylate agents. The ortho position of the hydroxyl group is an important feature for the action of salicylate. The effects of simple substitutions on the benzene ring have been extensively studied, and new salicylate derivatives still are being synthesized. A difluorophenyl derivative, *diflunisal,* also is available for clinical use.

Pharmacological Properties

Analgesia. As noted above, the types of pain usually relieved by salicylates are those of low intensity that arise from integumental structures rather than from viscera, especially headache, myalgia, and arthralgia. The salicylates are more widely used for pain relief than are any other classes of drugs. Long-term use does not lead to tolerance or addiction, and toxicity is lower than that of opioid analgesics. The salicylates alleviate pain by virtue of a peripheral action; direct effects on the CNS also may be involved.

Antipyresis. As discussed above, salicylates usually lower elevated body temperatures rapidly and effectively. However, moderate doses that produce this effect also increase oxygen consumption and metabolic rate. In toxic doses, these compounds have a pyretic effect that results in sweating; this enhances the dehydration that occurs in salicylate intoxication (*see* below).

Miscellaneous Neurological Effects. In high doses, salicylates have toxic effects on the CNS, consisting of stimulation (including convulsions) followed by depression. Confusion, dizziness, tinnitus, high-tone deafness, delirium, psychosis, stupor, and coma may occur. The tinnitus and hearing loss caused by salicylate poisoning are due to increased labyrinthine pressure or an effect on the hair cells of the cochlea, perhaps secondary to vasoconstriction in the auditory microvasculature. Tinnitus is typically observed at plasma salicylate concentrations of 200 to 450 μg/ml, and there is a close relationship between the extent of hearing loss and plasma salicylate concentration. An occasional patient may note tinnitus at lower plasma concentrations of salicylate. The symptoms are completely reversible within 2 or 3 days after withdrawal of the drug.

Salicylates induce nausea and vomiting, which result from stimulation of sites that are accessible from the cerebrospinal fluid (CSF), probably in the medullary chemoreceptor trigger zone. In human beings, centrally induced nausea and vomiting generally appear at plasma salicylate concentrations of about 270 μg/ml, but these same effects may occur at much lower plasma levels as a result of local gastric irritation.

Respiration. The effects of salicylate on respiration are important, because they contribute to the serious acid–base balance disturbances that characterize poisoning by this class of compounds. Salicylates stimulate respiration directly and indirectly. Full therapeutic doses of salicylates increase oxygen consumption and CO_2 production (especially in skeletal muscle); these effects are a result of salicylate-induced uncoupling of oxidative phosphorylation. The increased production of CO_2 stimulates respiration. The increased alveolar ventilation balances the increased CO_2 production, and thus plasma CO_2 tension (P_{CO_2}) does not change. The initial increase in alveolar ventilation is characterized mainly by an increase in depth of respiration and only a slight increase in rate. If the respiratory response to CO_2 has been depressed by the administration of a barbiturate or an opioid, salicylates will cause a marked increase in plasma P_{CO_2} and respiratory acidosis.

Salicylate directly stimulates the respiratory center in the medulla. This results in marked hyperventilation, characterized by an increase in depth and a pronounced increase in rate. Patients with salicylate poisoning may have prominent increases in respiratory minute volume, and respiratory alkalosis ensues. Plasma salicylate concentrations of 350 μg/ml are nearly always associated with hyperventilation in human beings, and marked hyperpnea occurs when the level approaches 500 μg/ml.

A depressant effect of salicylate on the medulla appears after high doses or after prolonged exposure. Toxic doses of salicylates cause central respiratory depression as well as circulatory collapse secondary to vasomotor depression. Since enhanced CO_2 production continues, respiratory acidosis ensues.

Acid–Base Balance and Electrolyte Pattern. Therapeutic doses of salicylate produce definite changes in the acid–base balance and electrolyte pattern. The initial event, as discussed above, is respiratory alkalosis. Compensation for the respiratory alkalosis is achieved by increased renal excretion of bicarbonate, which is accompanied by increased Na^+ and K^+ excretion; plasma bicarbonate is thus lowered, and blood pH returns toward normal. This is the stage of compensated respiratory alkalosis. This stage is most often seen in adults given intensive salicylate therapy and seldom proceeds further.

Subsequent changes in acid–base status generally occur only when toxic doses of salicylates are ingested by infants and children and occasionally after large doses in adults. In infants and children, the phase of respiratory alkalosis may not be observed, since the child with salicylate intoxication is rarely seen early enough. Instead, the stage of acid–base toxicity usually presented clinically is characterized by a decrease in blood pH, a low plasma bicarbonate concentration, and a normal or nearly normal plasma P_{CO_2}; except for the P_{CO_2} value, these changes resemble those of metabolic acidosis. However, in reality there is a combination of respiratory acidosis and metabolic acidosis produced as follows: the enhanced production of CO_2 outstrips its alveolar excretion because of direct salicylate-induced depression of respiration; consequently, plasma P_{CO_2} increases and blood pH decreases. Since the concentration of bicarbonate in plasma already is low because of increased renal bicarbonate excretion, the acid–base status at this stage is essentially an uncompensated respiratory acidosis. Superimposed, however, is a true metabolic acidosis caused by accumulation of acids as a result of three processes. First, toxic concentrations of salicylates displace about 2 to 3 meq per liter of plasma bicarbonate. Second, vasomotor depression caused by toxic doses of salicylate impairs renal function with consequent accumulation of strong acids of metabolic origin, namely, sulfuric and phosphoric acids. Third, organic acids accumulate secondary to salicylate-induced derangement of carbohydrate metabolism, especially pyruvic, lactic, and acetoacetic acids.

The series of events that produces acid–base disturbances in salicylate intoxication also causes alterations of water and electrolyte balance. The low plasma P_{CO_2} leads to decreased renal tubular reabsorption of bicarbonate and increased renal excretion of Na^+, K^+, and water. In addition, water is lost by salicylate-induced sweating and hyperventilation; dehydration rapidly occurs. Since more water than electrolyte is lost through the lungs and by sweating, the dehydration is associated with hypernatremia. Prolonged exposure to high doses of salicylate also causes depletion of K^+ due to both renal and extrarenal factors.

Cardiovascular Effects. Ordinary therapeutic doses of salicylates have no important direct cardiovascular actions. The peripheral vessels tend to dilate after large doses because of a direct effect on their smooth muscle. Toxic amounts depress the circulation both directly and by central vasomotor paralysis.

In patients given large doses of sodium salicylate or aspirin, such as the doses used in acute rheumatic fever, the circulating plasma volume increases (about 20%), the hematocrit falls, and cardiac output and work are increased. Consequently, in patients with clear evidence of carditis, such alterations can cause congestive failure and pulmonary edema. High doses of salicylates also can produce noncardiogenic pulmonary edema, particularly in older patients who are ingesting salicylates regularly over a prolonged duration.

Gastrointestinal Effects. The ingestion of salicylate may result in epigastric distress, nausea, and vomiting. The mechanism of the emetic effect is discussed above. Salicylate also may cause gastric ulceration; exacerbation of peptic ulcer symptoms (heartburn, dyspepsia), gastrointestinal hemorrhage, and erosive gastritis all have been reported in patients on high-dose therapy but also may occur even when low doses are administered. These adverse effects occur primarily with acetylated salicylate (aspirin). This is because nonacetylated salicylates are much weaker cyclooxygenase inhibitors than aspirin, because they lack the ability to acetylate the enzyme and thus irreversibly inhibit its activity.

Aspirin-induced gastric bleeding sometimes is painless and, if unrecognized, may lead to an iron-deficiency anemia. The daily ingestion of 4 or 5 g of aspirin, a dose that produces plasma salicylate concentrations in the usual range for antiinflammatory therapy (120 to 350 μg/ml), results in an average fecal blood loss of about 3 to 8 ml per day as compared with approximately 0.6 ml per day in untreated subjects (Leonards and Levy, 1973). Gastroscopic examination in aspirin-treated subjects reveals discrete ulcerative and hemorrhagic lesions of the gastric mucosa; in many cases, multiple hemorrhagic lesions with sharply demarcated areas of focal necrosis are observed. The incidence of bleeding is highest with salicylates that dissolve slowly and deposit as particles in the gastric mucosal folds.

Hepatic and Renal Effects. Salicylates can cause hepatic injury. This usually occurs in patients treated with high doses of salicylate that result in plasma salicylate concentrations above 150 μg/ml. The injury is not an acute effect; the onset characteristically occurs after several months of treatment. The majority of cases occur in patients with connective tissue disorders. There usually are no symptoms, but some patients note right upper quadrant abdominal discomfort and tenderness. Serum levels of hepatocellular enzymes are increased, but overt jaundice is uncommon. The injury usually is reversible upon discontinuation of salicylates. For these and other reasons, restriction of salicylates has been advised in patients with chronic liver disease. As discussed above, considerable evidence implicates the use of salicylates as an important factor in the severe hepatic injury and encephalopathy observed in Reye's syndrome.

Salicylates can cause retention of salt and water as well as acute reduction of renal function in patients with congestive heart failure, renal disease, or hypovolemia (see above). Although long-term use of salicylates alone rarely is associated with nephrotoxicity, the prolonged and excessive ingestion of analgesic mixtures containing salicylates in combination with other compounds can produce papillary necrosis and interstitial nephritis.

Uricosuric Effects.   The effects of salicylates on uric acid excretion are markedly dependent on dose (*see* "Uricosuric Agents," below). Low doses (1 or 2 g per day) may decrease urate excretion and elevate plasma urate concentrations; intermediate doses (2 or 3 g per day) usually do not alter urate excretion; large doses (over 5 g per day) induce uricosuria and lower plasma urate levels. Such large doses are poorly tolerated. Even small doses of salicylate can block the effects of probenecid and other uricosuric agents that decrease tubular reabsorption of uric acid.

Effects on the Blood.   Ingestion of aspirin by healthy individuals causes a prolongation of the bleeding time. For example, a single dose of 0.65 g of aspirin (2 tablets) approximately doubles the mean bleeding time of normal persons for a period of 4 to 7 days. This effect is due to irreversible acetylation of platelet cyclooxygenase and the consequent reduced formation of TXA_2 until production of unmodified platelets from megakaryocyte precursors occurs.

Patients with severe hepatic damage, hypoprothrombinemia, vitamin K deficiency, or hemophilia should avoid aspirin because the inhibition of platelet hemostasis can result in hemorrhage. If conditions permit, aspirin therapy should be stopped at least 1 week prior to surgery; care also should be exercised in the use of aspirin during long-term treatment with oral anticoagulant agents because of the possible danger of blood loss from the gastric mucosa as well as from hemorrhage at other sites. However, aspirin is used for the prophylaxis of thromboembolic disease, especially in the coronary and cerebral circulation (*see* Willard *et al.,* 1992; Patrono, 1994; *see* Chapter 55).

Salicylates do not ordinarily alter the leukocyte or platelet count, the hematocrit, or the hemoglobin content. However, doses of 3 to 4 g per day markedly decrease plasma iron concentration and shorten erythrocyte survival time. Aspirin is included among the drugs that can cause a mild degree of hemolysis in individuals with a deficiency of glucose-6-phosphate dehydrogenase.

Effects on Rheumatic, Inflammatory, and Immunological Processes and on Connective Tissue Metabolism.   For almost 100 years, the salicylates have retained their preeminent position in the treatment of the rheumatic diseases. Although they suppress the clinical signs and even improve the histological picture in acute rheumatic fever, subsequent tissue damage such as cardiac lesions and other visceral involvement is unaffected. In addition to their action on prostaglandin biosynthesis, the mechanism of action of the salicylates in rheumatic disease also may involve effects on other cellular and immunological processes in mesenchymal and connective tissues.

Because of the known relationship between rheumatic fever and immunological processes, attention has been directed to the capacity of salicylates to suppress a variety of antigen–antibody reactions. These include the inhibition of antibody production, of antigen–antibody aggregation, and of antigen-induced release of histamine. Salicylates also induce a nonspecific stabilization of capillary permeability during immunological insults. The concentrations of salicylates needed to produce these effects are high, and the relationship of these effects to the antirheumatic efficacy of salicylates is unclear.

Salicylates also can influence the metabolism of connective tissue, and these effects may be involved in their antiinflamma-

tory action. For example, salicylates can affect the composition, biosynthesis, or metabolism of connective tissue mucopolysaccharides in the ground substance that provides barriers to spread of infection and inflammation.

Metabolic Effects.   The salicylates have multiple effects on metabolic processes, some of which already have been discussed. Only a few pertinent aspects will be presented here. In general, these effects are minimal at usual recommended doses. *Oxidative Phosphorylation.*   The uncoupling of oxidative phosphorylation by salicylate is similar to that induced by 2,4-dinitrophenol. The effect may occur with doses of salicylate used in the treatment of rheumatoid arthritis and can result in the inhibition of a number of adenosine triphosphate (ATP)-dependent reactions. Other consequences include the salicylate-induced increase in oxygen uptake and carbon dioxide production described above, the depletion of hepatic glycogen, and the pyretic effect of toxic doses of salicylate. Salicylate in toxic doses may decrease aerobic metabolism as a result of inhibition of various dehydrogenases, by competing with the pyridine nucleotide coenzymes, and inhibition of some oxidases that require nucleotides as coenzymes, such as xanthine oxidase. *Carbohydrate Metabolism.*   Large doses of salicylates may cause hyperglycemia and glycosuria and deplete liver and muscle glycogen; these effects partly are explained by the release of epinephrine. Such doses also reduce aerobic metabolism of glucose, increase glucose-6-phosphatase activity, and promote the secretion of glucocorticoids. *Nitrogen Metabolism.*   Salicylate in toxic doses causes a significant negative nitrogen balance, characterized by an aminoaciduria. Adrenocortical activation may contribute to the negative nitrogen balance by enhancing protein catabolism. *Fat Metabolism.*   Salicylates reduce lipogenesis by partially blocking incorporation of acetate into fatty acids; they also inhibit epinephrine-stimulated lipolysis in fat cells and displace long-chain fatty acids from binding sites on human plasma proteins. The combination of these effects leads to increased entry and enhanced oxidation of fatty acids in muscle, liver, and other tissues, and to decreased plasma concentrations of free fatty acids, phospholipid, and cholesterol; the oxidation of ketone bodies also is increased.

Endocrine Effects.   Very large doses of salicylate stimulate steroid secretion by the adrenal cortex through an effect on the hypothalamus and transiently increase plasma concentrations of free adrenocorticosteroids by displacement from plasma proteins. However, it is clear that the antiinflammatory effects of salicylate are independent of these effects. Long-term administration of salicylate decreases thyroidal uptake and clearance of iodine but increases oxygen consumption and rate of disappearance of thyroxine and triiodothyronine from the circulation. These effects probably are due to the competitive displacement by salicylate of thyroxine and triiodothyronine from transthyretin and the thyroxine-binding globulin in plasma and usually are of minimal clinical significance.

Salicylates and Pregnancy.   There is no evidence that moderate therapeutic doses of salicylates are teratogenic in human beings; however, babies born to women who ingest salicylates for long periods may have significantly reduced weights at birth. There also is an increase in perinatal mortality, anemia, antepartum and postpartum hemorrhage, prolonged gestation, and complicated deliveries. These effects occur when aspirin is administered during the third trimester, and thus its use during this period should be avoided. As mentioned previously, administration of NSAIDs during the third trimester of pregnancy also can cause premature closure of the ductus arteriosus.

Local Irritant Effects. Salicylic acid is quite irritating to skin and mucosa and destroys epithelial cells. The keratolytic action of the free acid is employed for the local treatment of warts, corns, fungal infections, and certain types of eczematous dermatitis. The tissue cells swell, soften, and desquamate. Methyl salicylate (oil of wintergreen) is irritating to both skin and gastric mucosa and is used only externally.

Pharmacokinetics and Metabolism. Aspirin and other salicylates have several unique pharmacokinetic features that must be considered in patients receiving these drugs.

Absorption. Orally ingested salicylates are absorbed rapidly, partly from the stomach but mostly from the upper small intestine. Appreciable concentrations are found in plasma in less than 30 minutes; after a single dose, a peak value is reached in about 1 hour and then gradually declines. Rate of absorption is determined by many factors, particularly the disintegration and dissolution rates if tablets are given, the pH at the mucosal surfaces, and gastric emptying time.

Salicylate absorption occurs by passive diffusion primarily of nondissociated salicylic acid or acetylsalicylic acid across gastrointestinal membranes and hence is influenced by gastric pH. Even though salicylate is more ionized as the pH is increased, a rise in pH also increases the solubility of salicylate and thus dissolution of the tablets. The overall effect is to enhance absorption. As a result, there is little meaningful difference between the rates of absorption of sodium salicylate, aspirin, and the numerous buffered preparations of salicylates. The presence of food delays absorption of salicylates.

Rectal absorption of salicylate usually is slower than oral absorption and is incomplete and unreliable; rectal administration therefore is not advisable when high plasma concentrations of the drug are required.

Salicylic acid is rapidly absorbed from the intact skin, especially when applied in oily liniments or ointments, and systemic poisoning has occurred from its application to large areas of skin. Methyl salicylate is likewise speedily absorbed when applied cutaneously; its gastrointestinal absorption may be delayed many hours, and, therefore, gastric lavage should be performed even in cases of poisoning that are seen late.

Distribution. After absorption, salicylate is distributed throughout most body tissues and most transcellular fluids, primarily by pH-dependent passive processes. Salicylate is actively transported by a low-capacity, saturable system out of the CSF across the choroid plexus. The drug readily crosses the placental barrier.

The volumes of distribution of usual doses of aspirin and sodium salicylate in normal subjects average about 170 ml/kg of body weight; at high therapeutic doses, this volume increases to about 500 ml/kg because of saturation of binding sites on plasma proteins. Ingested aspirin mainly is absorbed as such, but some enters the systemic circulation as salicylic acid, because of hydrolysis by esterases in the gastrointestinal mucosa and the liver. Aspirin can be detected in the plasma only for a short

time as a result of hydrolysis in plasma, liver, and erythrocytes; for example, 30 minutes after a dose of 0.65 g, only 27% of the total plasma salicylate is in the acetylated form. As a result, plasma concentrations of aspirin are always low and rarely exceed 20 μg/ml at ordinary therapeutic doses. Methyl salicylate also is rapidly hydrolyzed to salicylic acid, mainly in the liver.

At concentrations encountered clinically, from 80% to 90% of the salicylate is bound to plasma proteins, especially albumin; the proportion of the total that is bound declines as plasma concentrations are increased. In addition, hypoalbuminemia, as may occur in rheumatoid arthritis, is associated with a proportionately higher level of free salicylate in the plasma. Salicylate competes with a variety of compounds for plasma protein binding sites; these include thyroxine, triiodothyronine, penicillin, phenytoin, sulfinpyrazone, bilirubin, uric acid, and other NSAIDs, such as naproxen. Aspirin is bound to a more limited extent; however, it acetylates human plasma albumin *in vivo* by reaction with the ε-amino group of lysine; this acetylation may change the binding of drugs to albumin. Hormones, DNA, and hemoglobin and other proteins also are acetylated.

Biotransformation and Excretion. The biotransformation of salicylate takes place in many tissues, but particularly in the hepatic endoplasmic reticulum and mitochondria. The three chief metabolic products are salicyluric acid (the glycine conjugate), the ether or phenolic glucuronide, and the ester or acyl glucuronide. In addition, a small fraction is oxidized to gentisic acid (2,5-dihydroxybenzoic acid) and to 2,3-dihydroxybenzoic and 2,3,5-trihydroxybenzoic acids; gentisuric acid, the glycine conjugate of gentisic acid, also is formed.

Salicylates are excreted in the urine as free salicylic acid (10%), salicyluric acid (75%), salicylic phenolic (10%) and acyl glucuronides (5%), and gentisic acid (<1%). However, excretion of free salicylate is extremely variable and depends upon both the dose and the urinary pH. In alkaline urine, more than 30% of the ingested drug may be eliminated as free salicylate, whereas in acidic urine this may be as low as 2%.

The plasma half-life for aspirin is approximately 15 minutes; that for salicylate is 2 to 3 hours in low doses and about 12 hours at usual antiinflammatory doses. The half-life of salicylate may be as long as 15 to 30 hours at high therapeutic doses or when there is intoxication. Thus, *small increases in dose can result in disproportionate increases in plasma levels of salicylate.* Failure to recognize this phenomenon can lead to salicylate toxicity. This dose-dependent elimination is the result of the limited ability of the liver to form salicyluric acid and the phenolic glucuronide, and a larger proportion of unchanged drug is excreted in the urine at higher doses.

Aspirin is one of the NSAIDs for which plasma level determinations can provide a means to monitor therapy and toxicity. The plasma concentration of salicylate is increased by conditions that decrease glomerular filtration rate or reduce its secretion by the proximal tubule, such as renal disease or the presence of inhibitors that compete for the transport system (*e.g.,* probenecid). Changes in urinary pH also have significant effects on salicylate excretion; for example, the clearance of salicylate is about four times as great at pH 8.0 as at pH 6.0, and it is well above the glomerular filtration rate at pH 8.0. High rates of urine flow decrease tubular reabsorption, whereas the opposite is true in oliguria. The conjugates of salicylic acid with glycine and glucuronic acid do not readily back diffuse across the renal tubular cells. Their excretion, therefore, is both by glomerular filtration and proximal tubular secretion and is not pH dependent.

Diflunisal, a difluorophenyl derivative of salicylic acid (*see* Figure 27–1) is almost completely absorbed after oral administration, and peak concentrations occur in plasma within 2 to 3 hours. It is extensively bound to plasma albumin (99%). Diflunisal appears in the milk of lactating women. About 90% of the drug is excreted as glucuronides, and its rate of elimination is dependent upon dosage. At the usual analgesic dose (500 to 750 mg per day) the plasma half-life ranges between 8 and 12 hours. (For reviews, *see* Davies, 1983; van Winzum *et al.,* in Symposium, 1983a.)

Therapeutic Uses

There are many systemic and a few local uses of the salicylates. Several are based on tradition and empirical results rather than on a clear understanding of the mechanism of therapeutic benefit. Salicylates are used commonly to treat inflammation in a wide variety of settings, including rheumatoid and other types of arthritis, musculoskeletal injury, and acute rheumatic fever. Therapy often is of a symptomatic nature in terms of alleviating fever, pain, and other signs of inflammation.

Systemic Uses. The two most commonly used preparations of salicylate for systemic effects are sodium salicylate and aspirin (acetylsalicylic acid). The dose of salicylate depends on the condition being treated.

Other salicylates are available for systemic use. These include *salsalate (salicylsalicylic acid;* DISALCID, others), which is hydrolyzed to salicylic acid during and after absorption. Sodium thiosalicylate (injection), choline salicylate (oral liquid; ARTHROPAN), and magnesium salicylate (tablets; MAGAN, others) also are available. A combination of choline and magnesium salicylates (TRILISATE, others) also is available. *Diflunisal* is discussed below.

Antipyresis. Antipyretic therapy is reserved for patients in whom fever in itself may be deleterious and for those who experience considerable relief when a fever is lowered. Little is known about the relationship between fever and the acceleration of inflammatory or immune processes; it may at times be a protective physiological mechanism. The course of the patient's illness may be obscured by the relief of symptoms and the reduction of fever from the use of antipyretic drugs. The antipyretic dose of salicylate for adults is 325 to 650 mg orally every 4 hours; for children, 50 to 75 mg/kg per day is given in four to six divided doses, not to exceed a total daily dose of 3.6 g. The route of administration nearly always is oral; parenteral administration is rarely necessary. The rectal administration of aspirin suppositories may be necessary in infants or when oral medication is not retained.

Analgesia. Salicylate is valuable for the nonspecific relief of certain types of pain, for example, headache, arthritis, dysmenorrhea, neuralgia, and myalgia. For this purpose, it is prescribed in the same doses and manner as for antipyresis.

Rheumatoid Arthritis. Although aspirin is regarded as the standard with which other drugs should be compared for the treatment of rheumatoid arthritis, many clinicians favor the use of drugs other than aspirin because of a lower incidence of side effects, in particular gastrointestinal effects. In addition to the analgesia that allows more effective therapeutic exercises, there is improvement in appetite, a feeling of well-being, and a reduction in the inflammation in joint tissues and surrounding structures. Damage to joints is the most difficult aspect of rheumatoid arthritis to manage, and any agent that reduces the inflammation is important in lessening or delaying the development of crippling diseases. Salicylates and other NSAIDs can be shown to produce objectively measurable antiinflammatory changes when given in large doses for long periods to patients with active rheumatoid disease. Large doses of salicylates, such as those used for rheumatic fever (4 to 6 g daily), are advised, but some patients respond well to less.

The majority of patients with rheumatoid arthritis can be controlled with salicylates alone or with other NSAIDs. Some patients with progressive or resistant disease require therapy with more toxic drugs, sometimes termed *second-line drugs,* such as gold salts, hydroxychloroquine, penicillamine, glucocorticoids, or immunosuppressive agents, in particular methotrexate. In the United States, methotrexate is the most frequently used second-line drug, while in Europe, sulfasalazine is generally the preferred second-line drug (Cash and Klippel, 1994).

Other Uses. Because of the potent and long-lasting effect of low doses of aspirin on platelet function, this drug is used in the treatment or prophylaxis of diseases associated with platelet hyperaggregability, such as coronary artery disease and postoperative deep-vein thrombosis (*see* Patrono, 1994 and Chapter 55). The maximal effectiveness of such therapy appears to depend upon selective blockade of TXA_2 synthesis by platelets without preventing production of PGI_2 by endothelial cells (*see* Chapters 26 and 55). Although the optimal dosage to prevent thrombotic events has not been firmly established, selective antiplatelet action appears to be best achieved when the dose of aspirin is 40 to 80 mg per day, while higher doses also inhibit PGI_2 production.

A relative excess of TXA_2 over PGI_2 has been implicated in the genesis of preeclampsia and hypertension induced by pregnancy (*see* Lubbe, 1987). The administration of 60 to 100 mg of aspirin per day to pregnant women who have a high risk of developing hypertension lowers the incidence of hypertension and also may prevent preeclampsia in patients with higher blood pressure (Imperiale and Petrulis, 1991; Sibai *et al.,* 1993).

Relationship of Plasma Salicylate Concentration to Therapeutic Effect and Toxicity. For optimal antiinflammatory effect for patients with rheumatic diseases, plasma salicylate concentrations of 150 to 300 μg/ml are required. In the lower part of this range, the clearance of the drug is nearly constant (despite the fact that saturation of metabolic capacity is approached) because the fraction of drug that is free and thus available for metabolism or excretion increases as binding sites on plasma proteins are saturated. The total concentration of salicylate in plasma is thus a relatively linear function of dose at lower concentrations, but at higher concentrations, as metabolic pathways of disposition become saturated, small increments in dose can result in disproportionate increases in plasma salicylate concentration. It is important to individualize the total dose of aspirin, especially because the range of plasma salicylate concentrations needed for optimal antiinflammatory effects may overlap that at which tinnitus is noted. Tinnitus may be a reliable index of therapeutic plasma concentration in patients with normal hearing but obviously not in those with a preexisting hearing loss. Hyperventilation generally occurs at concentrations greater than 350 μg/ml, and other signs of intoxication, such as acidosis, at concentrations greater than 460 μg/ml. Single analgesic-antipyretic doses of salicylate usually yield plasma concentrations below 60 μg/ml.

The plasma concentration of salicylate generally is little affected by other drugs, but concurrent administration of aspirin lowers the concentrations of indomethacin, naproxen, ketoprofen, and fenoprofen, at least in part by displacement from plasma proteins. Important adverse interactions of aspirin with warfarin and methotrexate are mentioned above. Other interactions of aspirin include the antagonism of spironolactone-induced natriuresis and the blockade of the active transport of penicillin from CSF to blood.

Local Uses. *Inflammatory Bowel Disease. Mesalamine* (5-aminosalicylic acid) is a salicylate that is used for its local effects in the treatment of inflammatory bowel disease. The drug is not effective orally because it is poorly absorbed and is inactivated before reaching the lower intestine. It is currently available as a suppository and rectal suspension enema (ROWASA) for treatment of mild-to-moderate proctosigmoiditis; two oral formulations that deliver drug to the lower intestine, *olsalazine* (sodium azodisalicylate, a dimer of 5-aminosalicylate linked by an azo bond; DIPENTUM) and mesalamine formulated in a pH-sensitive polymer-coated oral preparation (ASACOL), have been efficacious in treatment of inflammatory bowel disease, in particular ulcerative colitis. Sulfasalazine (salicylazosulfapyridine; AZULFIDINE) contains mesalamine linked covalently to sulfapyridine (*see* Chapter 44; Figure 27–1); it is poorly absorbed after oral administration, but it is cleaved to its active components by bacteria in the colon. The drug is of benefit in the treatment of inflammatory bowel disease, principally because of the local actions of mesalamine. Sulfasalazine and more recently olsalazine also have been used in the treatment of rheumatoid arthritis and ankylosing spondylitis (*see* Symposium, 1988b; Felson *et al.,* 1992).

Toxic Effects of Salicylates

As a result of their wide use and ready availability, salicylates frequently are the cause of intoxication. Poisoning or serious intoxication often occurs in children and is sometimes fatal. The drugs should not be viewed as harmless household remedies.

Salicylate Intoxication.   The fatal dose varies with the preparation of salicylate. From 10 to 30 g of sodium salicylate or aspirin has caused death in adults, but much larger amounts (130 g of aspirin, in one case) have been ingested without fatal outcome. The lethal dose of methyl salicylate (oil of wintergreen, sweet birch oil, gautheria oil, betula oil) is considerably less than that of sodium salicylate. As little as 4 ml (4.7 g) of methyl salicylate may be fatal in children.

Symptoms and Signs.   Mild chronic salicylate intoxication is termed *salicylism.* When fully developed, the syndrome includes headache, dizziness, ringing in the ears, difficulty in hearing, dimness of vision, mental confusion, lassitude, drowsiness, sweating, thirst, hyperventilation, nausea, vomiting, and occasionally diarrhea. A more severe degree of salicylate intoxication is characterized by more pronounced CNS disturbances (including generalized convulsions and coma), skin eruptions, and marked alterations in acid–base balance. Fever is usually prominent, especially in children. Dehydration often occurs as a result of hyperpyrexia, sweating, vomiting, and the loss of water vapor during hyperventilation. Gastrointestinal symptoms often are present; about 50% of individuals with plasma salicylate concentrations of more than 300 μg/ml experience nausea.

A prominent feature of salicylate intoxication is the disturbance in acid–base balance and electrolyte composition of the plasma described above. The most severe metabolic disturbances, in particular acidosis, occur in infants and very young children who become intoxicated.

Hemorrhagic phenomena occasionally are seen during salicylate poisoning, the mechanism and significance of which have been discussed. Petechial hemorrhages are a prominent postmortem feature. Thrombocytopenic purpura is a rare complication. While hyperglycemia may occur during salicylate intoxication, hypoglycemia may be a serious consequence of toxicity in young children. It should be seriously considered in any young child with coma, convulsions, or cardiovascular collapse.

Severe toxic encephalopathy may be a prominent feature of salicylate poisoning and may be difficult to differentiate from rheumatic encephalopathy. As poisoning progresses, central stimulation is replaced by increasing depression, stupor, and coma. Cardiovascular collapse and respiratory insufficiency ensue, and terminal asphyxial convulsions and pulmonary edema sometimes appear. Death usually results from respiratory failure after a period of unconsciousness.

Salicylate toxicity in adults may not be diagnosed readily, because such patients usually become intoxicated from their therapeutic regimen; there is no history of acute overdosage. Prominent features of toxicity in this group are noncardiogenic pulmonary edema, nonfocal neurological abnormalities, and laboratory findings that include acid–base abnormalities, unexplained ketosis, and a prolonged prothrombin time.

Symptoms of poisoning by methyl salicylate differ little from those described for aspirin. Central excitation, intense hyperpnea, and hyperpyrexia are prominent features. The odor of the drug can easily be detected on the breath and in the urine and vomitus. Poisoning by salicylic acid differs only in the increased prominence of gastrointestinal symptoms due to the marked local irritation.

Treatment.   Salicylate poisoning represents an acute medical emergency, and death may result despite all recommended procedures. The treatment is directed at cardiovascular and respiratory support and correction of acid–base abnormalities plus use of measures to accelerate excretion of salicylate. Salicylate medication is withdrawn as soon as intoxication is suspected. Blood should be obtained for plasma salicylate determinations and acid–base and electrolyte studies. The salicylate concentration is reasonably well correlated with clinical severity, when corrected for the duration of the intoxication, and is of value in assessing the type of therapy to be instituted. Since absorption of salicylate from the gastrointestinal tract may be delayed for many hours after an overdose, measures to reduce such absorption always should be employed. Use of activated charcoal is the currently preferred method to accomplish this.

Hyperthermia and dehydration are the immediate threats to life, and the initial therapy must be directed to their correction and to the maintenance of adequate renal function. Adequate amounts of intravenous fluids must be given promptly. The type and amount of solutions to be employed depend upon the interpretation of the laboratory data on acid–base balance. If the patient presents with an acidosis, correction of the low blood pH is essential, especially since acidosis results in a shift of salicylate from plasma into brain and other tissues. Bicarbonate solution should be infused intravenously in sufficient quantity to maintain alkaline diuresis. Correction of ketosis and hypoglycemia by administration of glucose also is essential for complete control of the metabolic acidosis; however, the ketosis clears only slowly. If K^+ deficiency occurs during salicylate intoxication, it should be treated by adding the cation to the intravenous fluids once it has been determined that urine formation is adequate. Plasma transfusion may be beneficial, especially if shock intervenes. Hemorrhagic phenomena may necessitate blood transfusion and vitamin K (*phytonadione*).

Measures to rid the body of salicylate rapidly should be undertaken immediately. Forced diuresis with alkalinizing solution appears not to be better than alkali alone. In severe intoxication, hemodialysis is the most effective measure available for the removal of salicylate and for the correction of the electrolyte and acid–base disturbances. Hemodialysis should be considered in patients with salicylate concentrations above 1000 μg/ml, in those with severe acid–base disturbances whose clinical condition is deteriorating despite otherwise-appropriate therapy, and in those who have associated serious disease, particularly cardiac, pulmonary, or renal disease. (*See* Meredith and Vale, 1986.)

Aspirin Hypersensitivity. Aspirin hypersensitivity or intolerance is discussed above. It is important to recognize this syndrome even though it is rather uncommon, since the administration of aspirin and many other NSAIDs may result in severe and possibly fatal reactions. The nonacetylated salicylates appear to be considerably less apt to produce these reactions than are aspirin and other NSAIDs. Treatment of such responses does not differ from that ordinarily employed in acute anaphylactic reactions; epinephrine is the drug of choice.

Diflunisal

Diflunisal (DOLOBID) is a difluorophenyl derivative of salicylic acid (*see* Figure 27–1); it is not converted to salicylic acid *in vivo*. Diflunisal is more potent than aspirin in antiinflammatory tests in animals and appears to be a competitive inhibitor of cyclooxygenase. However, it is largely devoid of antipyretic effects, perhaps because of poor penetration into the CNS. The drug has been used primarily as an analgesic in the treatment of osteoarthritis and musculoskeletal strains or sprains; in these circumstances it is about three to four times more potent than aspirin. The usual initial dose is 500 to 1000 mg, followed by 250 to 500 mg every 8 to 12 hours. For rheumatoid arthritis or osteoarthritis, 250 to 500 mg is administered twice daily; maintenance dosage should not exceed 1.5 g per day. Diflunisal does not produce auditory side effects and appears to cause

fewer and less intense gastrointestinal and antiplatelet effects than does aspirin.

PARA-AMINOPHENOL DERIVATIVES: ACETAMINOPHEN

Acetaminophen (paracetamol; *N*-acetyl-*p*-aminophenol; TYLENOL, others) is the active metabolite of phenacetin, a so-called coal tar analgesic. Acetaminophen is an effective alternative to aspirin as an analgesic-antipyretic agent; however, unlike aspirin, its antiinflammatory activity is weak and thus it is not a useful agent to treat inflammatory conditions. Because acetaminophen is well tolerated, lacks many of the side effects of aspirin, and is available without prescription, it has earned a prominent place as a common household analgesic. However, acute overdosage causes fatal hepatic damage, and the number of self-poisonings and suicides with acetaminophen has grown alarmingly in recent years. In addition, many individuals, physicians included, seem unaware of the poor antiinflammatory activity of acetaminophen.

History. Acetanilide is the parent member of this group of drugs. It was introduced into medicine in 1886 under the name of antifebrin by Cahn and Hepp, who had accidentally discovered its antipyretic action. However, acetanilide proved to be excessively toxic. In the search for less toxic compounds, para-aminophenol was tried in the belief that the body oxidized acetanilide to this compound. Toxicity was not lessened, however, and a number of chemical derivatives of para-aminophenol were then tested. One of the more satisfactory of these was phenacetin (acetophenetidin). It was introduced into therapy in 1887 and was extensively employed in analgesic mixtures until it was implicated in analgesic-abuse nephropathy (*see* above). Phenacetin no longer is available in the United States. Discussion of its pharmacology can be found in earlier editions of this textbook.

Acetaminophen was first used in medicine by von Mering in 1893. However, it has gained popularity only since 1949, after it was recognized as the major active metabolite of both acetanilide and phenacetin.

Pharmacological Properties. Acetaminophen has analgesic and antipyretic effects that do not differ significantly from those of aspirin. However, as mentioned, it has only weak antiinflammatory effects. Minor metabolites contribute significantly to the toxic effects of acetaminophen. The pharmacological properties of acetaminophen have been reviewed by Clissold (1986).

The failure of acetaminophen to exert antiinflammatory activity may be attributed to the fact that acetaminophen is only a weak inhibitor of cyclooxygenase in the presence of the high concentrations of peroxides that are found in inflammatory lesions. In contrast, its antipyretic effect may be explained by its ability to inhibit cyclooxygenase in the brain, where peroxide tone is low (Marshall *et al.,* 1987; Hanel and Lands, 1982). Further, acetaminophen does not inhibit neutrophil activation as do other NSAIDs (Abramson and Weissmann, 1989).

Single or repeated therapeutic doses of acetaminophen have no effect on the cardiovascular and respiratory systems. Acid–base changes do not occur, nor does the drug produce the gastric irritation, erosion, or bleeding that may occur after administration of salicylates. Acetaminophen has no effects on platelets, bleeding time, or the excretion of uric acid.

Pharmacokinetics and Metabolism. Acetaminophen is rapidly and almost completely absorbed from the gastrointestinal tract. The concentration in plasma reaches a peak in 30 to 60 minutes, and the half-life in plasma is about 2 hours after therapeutic doses. Acetaminophen is relatively uniformly distributed throughout most body fluids. Binding of the drug to plasma proteins is variable; only 20% to 50% may be bound at the concentrations encountered during acute intoxication. After therapeutic doses, 90% to 100% of the drug may be recovered in the urine within the first day, primarily after hepatic conjugation with glucuronic acid (about 60%), sulfuric acid (about 35%), or cysteine (about 3%); small amounts of hydroxylated and deacetylated metabolites also have been detected. Children have less capacity for glucuronidation of the drug than do adults. A small proportion of acetaminophen undergoes cytochrome P450–mediated *N*-hydroxylation to form *N*-acetyl-benzoquinoneimine, a highly reactive intermediate. This metabolite normally reacts with sulfhydryl groups in glutathione. However, after ingestion of large doses of acetaminophen, the metabolite is formed in amounts sufficient to deplete hepatic glutathione (*see* below).

Therapeutic Uses. Acetaminophen is a suitable substitute for aspirin for analgesic or antipyretic uses; it is particularly valuable for patients in whom aspirin is contraindicated (*e.g.,* those with peptic ulcer) or when the prolongation of bleeding time caused by aspirin would be a disadvantage. The conventional oral dose of acetaminophen is 325 to 1000 mg (650 mg rectally); the total daily dose should not exceed 4000 mg. For children, the single dose is 40 to 480 mg, depending upon age and weight; no more than five doses should be administered in 24 hours. A dose of 10 mg/kg also may be used.

Toxic Effects. In recommended therapeutic dosage, acetaminophen usually is well tolerated. Skin rash and other allergic reactions occur occasionally. The rash is usually erythematous or urticarial, but sometimes it is more serious and may be accompanied by drug fever and mucosal lesions. Patients who show hypersensitivity reactions to the salicylates only rarely exhibit sensitivity to acetaminophen. In a few isolated cases, the use of acetaminophen has been associated with neutropenia, thrombocytopenia, and pancytopenia.

The most serious adverse effect of acute overdosage of acetaminophen is a dose-dependent, potentially fatal hepatic necrosis (*see* Thomas, 1993). Renal tubular necrosis and hypoglycemic coma also may occur. The mechanism by which overdosage with acetaminophen leads to hepatocellular injury and death involves its conversion to a toxic reactive metabolite (*see also* Chapter 4). Minor pathways of acetaminophen elimination are *via* conjugation with glucuronide and sulfate. The major pathway of metabolism is *via* cytochrome P450s to the intermediate, *N*-acetyl-*para*-benzoquinonimine, which is very electrophilic. Under normal circumstances, this intermediate is eliminated by conjugation with glutathione (GSH) and then further metabolized to a mercapturic acid and excreted into the urine. However, in the setting of acetaminophen overdose, hepatocellular levels of GSH become depleted. Two consequences ensue as result of depletion of GSH. Since GSH is an important factor in antioxidant defense, hepatocytes are rendered highly susceptible to oxidant injury. Depletion of GSH also allows the reactive intermediate to bind covalently to cell macromolecules, leading to dysfunction of enzymatic systems.

Hepatotoxicity. In adults, hepatotoxicity may occur after ingestion of a single dose of 10 to 15 g (150 to 250 mg/kg) of acetaminophen; doses of 20 to 25 g or more are potentially fatal. Alcoholics can have hepatotoxicity with much lower doses, even with doses in the therapeutic range. The mechanism of this effect is discussed above (*see also* Chapter 4). Symptoms that occur during the first 2 days of acute poisoning by acetaminophen may not reflect the potential seriousness of the intoxication. Nausea, vomiting, anorexia, diaphoresis, and abdominal pain occur during the initial 24 hours and may persist for a week or more. Clinical indications of hepatic damage become manifest within 2 to 4 days of ingestion of toxic doses. Plasma aminotransferases are elevated (sometimes markedly so), and the concentration of bilirubin in plasma may be increased; in addition, the prothrombin time is prolonged. Perhaps 10% of poisoned patients who do not receive specific treatment develop severe liver damage; of these, 10% to 20% eventually die of hepatic failure. Acute renal failure also occurs in some patients. Biopsy of the liver reveals centrilobular necrosis with sparing of the periportal area. In nonfatal cases, the hepatic lesions are reversible over a period of weeks or months.

Severe liver damage (with levels of aspartate aminotransferase activity in excess of 1000 IU per liter of plasma) occurs in 90% of patients with plasma concentrations of acetaminophen greater than 300 μg/ml at 4 hours or 45 μg/ml at 15 hours after the ingestion of the drug. Minimal hepatic damage can be anticipated when the drug concentration is less than 120 μg/ml at 4 hours or 30 μg/ml at 12 hours after ingestion. The potential severity of hepatic necrosis also can be predicted from the half-life of acetaminophen observed in the patient; values greater than 4 hours imply that necrosis will occur, while values greater than 12 hours suggest that hepatic coma is likely. The nomogram provided in Figure 27–2 relates the plasma levels of acetaminophen and time after ingestion to the predicted severity of liver injury (*see* Rumack *et al.,* 1981).

Early diagnosis is vital in the treatment of overdosage with acetaminophen, and methods are available for the rapid determination of concentrations of the drug in plasma. However, therapy should not be delayed while awaiting laboratory results if the history suggests a significant overdosage. Vigorous supportive therapy is essential when intoxication is severe. Gastric lavage should be performed in all cases, preferably within 4 hours of the ingestion.

The principal antidotal treatment is the administration of sulfhydryl compounds, which probably act, in part, by replenishing hepatic stores of glutathione. *N-acetylcysteine* (MUCOMYST, MUCOSIL) is effective when given orally or intravenously. An intravenous form is available in Europe, where it is considered the treatment of choice. When given orally, the *N*-acetylcysteine solution (which has a foul smell and taste) is diluted with water

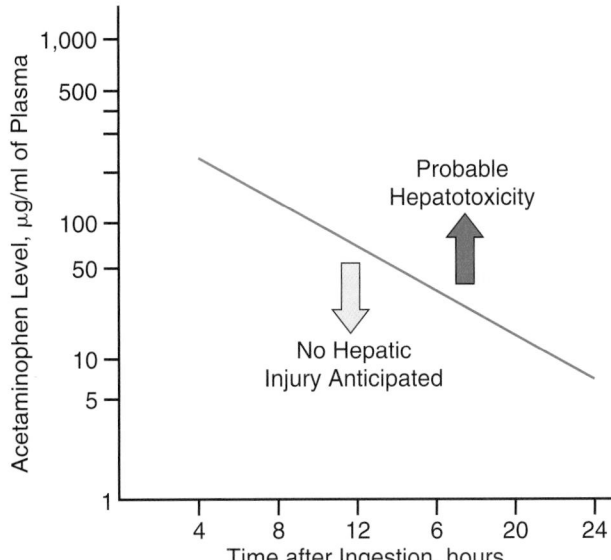

Figure 27–2. Relationship of plasma levels of acetaminophen and time after ingestion to hepatic injury.

(Adapted from Rumack *et al.*, 1981, with permission.)

or soft drinks to achieve a 5% solution and should be consumed within 1 hour of preparation. The drug is recommended if less than 36 hours has elapsed since ingestion of acetaminophen, although treatment with *N*-acetylcysteine is more effective when given less than 10 hours after ingestion (Smilkstein *et al.,* 1988). An oral loading dose of 140 mg/kg is given, followed by the administration of 70 mg/kg every 4 hours for 17 doses. Treatment is terminated if assays of acetaminophen in plasma indicate that the risk of hepatotoxicity is low. Adverse reactions to *N*-acetylcysteine include skin rash (including urticaria, which does not require one to discontinue treatment), nausea, vomiting, diarrhea, and anaphylactoid reactions. Assistance in treatment of patients with acetaminophen overdose can be obtained from the Rocky Mountain Poison Center, Denver, Colorado (telephone number: 800-525-6115; *see* Smilkstein *et al.,* 1988; Thomas, 1993).

INDOMETHACIN, SULINDAC, AND ETODOLAC

Indomethacin was the product of a laboratory search for drugs with antiinflammatory properties. It was introduced in 1963 for the treatment of rheumatoid arthritis and related disorders. Although indomethacin is used widely and is effective, toxicity often limits its use. *Sulindac* was developed in an attempt to find a less toxic but effective congener of indomethacin. The development, chemistry, and pharmacology of both drugs have been reviewed by Rhymer and Gengos (*in* Symposium, 1983a) and by Shen (*in* Rainsford, 1985a). *Etodolac* is one of the more recent

antiinflammatory drugs approved for use in the United States. Details of its pharmacology have been reviewed by Balfour and Buckley (1991). While indomethacin and sulindac exhibit little selectivity for inhibition of the cyclooxygenase isoenzymes, etodolac has been found to be a somewhat selective inhibitor of COX-2.

Indomethacin

Chemistry.   The structural formula of indomethacin, a methylated indole derivative, is shown below:

INDOMETHACIN

Pharmacological Properties.   Indomethacin has prominent antiinflammatory and analgesic-antipyretic properties similar to those of the salicylates.

The antiinflammatory effects of indomethacin are evident in patients with rheumatoid and other types of arthritis, including acute gout. Although indomethacin is more potent than aspirin, doses that are tolerated by patients with rheumatoid arthritis usually do not produce effects that are superior to those of salicylate. Indomethacin has analgesic properties distinct from its antiinflammatory effects, and there is evidence for both a central and a peripheral action; it also is an antipyretic.

Indomethacin is a potent inhibitor of the cyclooxygenases; it also inhibits the motility of polymorphonuclear leukocytes. Like many other NSAIDs, indomethacin uncouples oxidative phosphorylation at supratherapeutic concentrations and depresses the biosynthesis of mucopolysaccharides.

Pharmacokinetics and Metabolism.   Indomethacin is rapidly and almost completely absorbed from the gastrointestinal tract after oral ingestion. The peak concentration in plasma is attained within 1 to 2 hours in the fasting subject but may be somewhat delayed when the drug is taken after meals. The concentrations in plasma required for an antiinflammatory effect have not been definitely determined but are probably less than 1 μg/ml. Steady-state concentrations in plasma after long-term administration are approximately 0.5 μg/ml. Indomethacin is 90% bound to plasma proteins and also extensively bound to tissues. The concentration of the drug in the CSF is low, but its concentration in synovial fluid is equal to that in plasma within 5 hours of administration.

Indomethacin is converted primarily to inactive metabolites, including those formed by *O*-demethylation (about 50%), conjugation with glucuronic acid (about 10%), and *N*-deacylation. Some of these metabolites are detectable in plasma, and free and conjugated metabolites are eliminated in the urine, bile, and feces. There is enterohepatic cycling of the conjugates and probably of indomethacin itself. Between 10% and 20% of the drug is excreted unchanged in the urine, in part by tubular secretion. The half-life in plasma is variable, perhaps because of enterohepatic cycling, but averages about 2.5 hours.

Drug Interactions.   The total plasma concentration of indomethacin plus its inactive metabolites is increased by concurrent administration of probenecid, possibly because of reduced tubular secretion of the former. However, it has not been determined whether or not the dosage of indomethacin must be adjusted when the two drugs are employed together. Indomethacin does not interfere with the uricosuric effect of probenecid. Indomethacin is said not to modify the effect of the oral anticoagulant agents. However, concurrent administration could be hazardous because of the increased risk of gastrointestinal bleeding. Indomethacin antagonizes the natriuretic and antihypertensive effects of furosemide; the antihypertensive effects of thiazide diuretics, β-adrenergic blocking agents, or inhibitors of angiotensin converting enzyme also may be reduced.

Therapeutic Uses.   Because of the high incidence and severity of side effects associated with long-term administration, *indomethacin* (INDOCIN) is not commonly used for therapy as an analgesic or antipyretic. However, it has proven to be useful as an antipyretic in certain settings (*e.g.,* Hodgkin's disease) when the fever has been refractory to other agents.

Clinical trials of indomethacin as an antiinflammatory agent have been reviewed by Rhymer and Gengos (*in* Symposium, 1983a). The majority of these trials have demonstrated that indomethacin relieves pain, reduces swelling and tenderness of the joints, increases grip strength, and decreases the duration of morning stiffness. In these actions, the drug is superior to placebo, and estimates of its potency relative to salicylates vary between 10 and 40 times higher. Overall, about two-thirds of patients benefit from treatment with indomethacin, typically with treatment initiated at 25 mg two or three times daily. However, if 75 to 100 mg of the drug fails to provide benefit within 2 to 4 weeks, alternative therapy must be considered. The incidence and severity of side effects with indomethacin can limit its therapeutic utility; however, since the side effects of indomethacin appear to be better tolerated when taken at night, a useful way to take advantage of the effectiveness of indomethacin and to minimize untoward side effects is to give a large single dose (up to 100 mg) at bedtime, perhaps in combination with other and better-tolerated NSAIDs for daytime therapy. This enables the patient to obtain a better-quality sleep, reduces the severity and length of morning stiffness, and provides good analgesia until midmorning.

Indomethacin often is more effective than aspirin in the treatment of ankylosing spondylitis and osteoarthrosis. It also is very effective in the treatment of acute gout, although it is not uricosuric.

Patients with Bartter's syndrome have been treated successfully with indomethacin, as well as with other inhibitors of prostaglandin synthesis. The results are frequently dramatic; however, the condition of the patients may deteriorate rapidly when therapy is discontinued, and the long-term therapy necessary to control the disease requires administration of a drug that is better tolerated.

Indomethacin has at least two uses in obstetrics and neonatal medicine. It can be used as a tocolytic agent to suppress uterine contractions in women with preterm labor. In addition, cardiac failure in neonates caused by a patent ductus arteriosus may be controlled by the administration of indomethacin. A typical regimen involves the intravenous administration of 0.1 to 0.2 mg/kg every 12 hours for three doses. Successful closure can be expected in more than 70% of neonates who are treated with the drug. Such therapy is indicated primarily in premature infants who weigh between 500 and 1750 g, who have a hemodynamically significant patent ductus arteriosus, and in whom other supportive maneuvers have been attempted. Unexpectedly, treatment with indomethacin also may decrease the incidence and severity of intraventricular hemorrhage in low birth weight neonates (Ment *et al.,* 1994). The principal limitation of treating neonates is renal toxicity, and therapy is stopped if the output of urine falls below 0.6 ml/kg per hour. Renal failure, enterocolitis, thrombocytopenia, or hyperbilirubinemia contraindicates the use of indomethacin.

Toxic Effects.   A very high percentage (35% to 50%) of patients receiving usual therapeutic doses of indomethacin experience untoward symptoms, and about 20% must discontinue its use. Most adverse effects are dose related.

Gastrointestinal complaints and complications consist of anorexia, nausea, and abdominal pain. Single ulcers or multiple ulceration of the entire upper gastrointestinal tract, sometimes with perforations and hemorrhage, have been reported. Occult blood loss may lead to anemia in the absence of ulceration. Acute pancreatitis also has been reported. Diarrhea may occur and is sometimes associated with ulcerative lesions of the bowel. Hepatic involvement is rare, although some fatal cases of hepatitis and jaundice have been reported. The most frequent CNS effect (indeed, the most common side effect) is severe frontal headache, occurring in 25% to 50% of patients who take the drug for long periods. Dizziness, vertigo, light-headedness, and mental confusion also are frequent. Severe depression, psychosis, hallucinations, and suicide have occurred.

Hematopoietic reactions include neutropenia, thrombocytopenia, and, rarely, aplastic anemia. As is common with other nonselective inhibitors of the cyclooxygenases, platelet function is impaired, and reactions predictably occur in patients who exhibit hypersensitivity reactions to aspirin. Indomethacin should not be used in pregnant women, nursing mothers, persons operating machinery, or patients with psychiatric disorders, epilepsy, or Parkinsonism. Indomethacin also is contraindicated in individuals with renal disease or ulcerative lesions of the stomach or intestines.

Sulindac

Chemistry.   Sulindac is closely related to indomethacin; its structural formula is as follows:

SULINDAC

Sulindac is essentially a prodrug. Little if any of the antiinflammatory activity is due to the parent drug, sulindac sulfoxide; most of its pharmacological activity resides in its sulfide metabolite.

Pharmacological Properties. Sulindac exhibits the classical activities of NSAIDs. In all tests, sulindac is less than half as potent as indomethacin.

Because sulindac is a prodrug, it appears to be either inactive or relatively weak in *in vitro* tests because it is not metabolized to its active sulfide metabolite. The sulfide metabolite is more than 500 times more potent than sulindac as an inhibitor of cyclooxygenase. These observations may help to explain the somewhat lower incidence of gastrointestinal toxicity of sulindac as compared with indomethacin, since the gastric or intestinal mucosa is not exposed to high concentrations of an active drug during oral administration. Nevertheless, gastrointestinal toxicity is more common with sulindac than with many other NSAIDs. Sulindac also may be unusual in that some clinical studies indicate that it does not alter the urinary excretion of prostaglandins or alter renal function, perhaps because of the kidney's ability to regenerate the parent sulfoxide from active sulfide metabolites (*see* Wilson and Carruthers *in* Borda and Koff, 1992). However, "renal-sparing" is apparently only relative and dose dependent (Waslen *et al.,* 1989; Kulling *et al.,* 1995); the drug therefore must be used with caution in patients who are dependent upon the synthesis of prostaglandins in the kidney for maintenance of renal function.

Pharmacokinetics and Metabolism. The metabolism and pharmacokinetics of sulindac are complex and vary enormously among species. After oral administration in human beings, about 90% of the drug is absorbed. Peak concentrations of sulindac in plasma are attained within 1 to 2 hours, while those of the sulfide metabolite occur about 8 hours after the oral administration of sulindac.

Sulindac undergoes two major biotransformations in addition to conjugation reactions. It is oxidized to the sulfone and then reversibly reduced to the sulfide. It is this latter metabolite that is the active moiety, although all three compounds are found in comparable concentrations in human plasma. The half-life of sulindac itself is about 7 hours, but the active sulfide has a half-life of as long as 18 hours. Sulindac and its metabolites undergo extensive enterohepatic circulation. Sulindac and the sulfone and sulfide metabolites are all extensively bound to plasma protein.

Little of the sulfide or its conjugates is found in urine. The principal components that are excreted in the urine are the sulfone and its conjugate, which account for nearly 30% of an administered dose; sulindac and its conjugates account for about 20%. Up to 25% of an oral dose may appear as metabolites in the feces.

Therapeutic Uses. *Sulindac* (CLINORIL) has been used mainly for the treatment of rheumatoid arthritis, osteoarthrosis, and ankylosing spondylitis. The drug also has been used with success in the treatment of acute gout. The analgesic and antiinflammatory effects exerted by sulindac (400 mg per day) are comparable to those achieved with aspirin (4 g per day), ibuprofen (1200 mg per day), and indomethacin (125 mg per day) (*see* Rhymer, *in* Symposium, 1983a). Although dosage should be optimized for each individual, the most common dosage for adults is 150 to 200 mg twice a day. The drug usually is given with food to reduce gastric discomfort, although this may delay absorption and reduce concentration in plasma. Sulindac, like indomethacin, has been used for tocolytic therapy. A novel use

of sulindac is as treatment to reduce the number and size of adenomas in the large bowel in patients with familial adenomatous polyposis (Giardiello *et al.,* 1993). Its effectiveness in this situation may be attributed in part to the fact that reduction of sulindac to its active sulfide is mediated primarily by microflora in the gut acting on sulindac excreted in the bile (Strong *et al.,* 1985).

Toxic Effects. Although the incidence of toxicity is lower than with indomethacin, untoward reactions to sulindac are common.

Gastrointestinal side effects are seen in nearly 20% of patients, although these are generally mild. Abdominal pain and nausea are the most frequent complaints. CNS side effects are seen in up to 10% of patients, with drowsiness, dizziness, headache, and nervousness being those most frequently reported. Skin rash and pruritus occur in 5% of patients. Transient elevations of hepatic enzymes in plasma are less common.

Etodolac

Etodolac is an inhibitor of cyclooxygenase and possesses antiinflammatory activity. However, there is an unusually large difference between doses that produce antiinflammatory effects and those that cause gastric irritation in experimental animals. This can be explained by the fact that etodolac has been shown to be a selective inhibitor of COX-2 (Warner *et al.,* 1999). This selectivity also explains the findings that chronic treatment of human beings with etodolac does not reduce gastric mucosal prostaglandin production, and the incidence of gastric toxicity is not different from placebo and is much less than seen with naproxen (Laine *et al.,* 1995). The drug appears to be uricosuric. The structure of etodolac is as follows:

ETODOLAC

Pharmacokinetics and Metabolism. Etodolac is rapidly and well absorbed orally, and it is about 99% bound to plasma proteins. It is actively metabolized by the liver to various metabolites that are largely excreted in the urine. The drug may undergo enterohepatic circulation in human beings; its half-life in plasma is about 7 hours.

Therapeutic Uses. A single oral dose (200 to 400 mg) of *etodolac* (LODINE) provides postoperative analgesia that typically lasts for 6 to 8 hours. Etodolac also is effective in the treatment of osteoarthritis and rheumatoid arthritis. A sustained-release preparation (LODINE XL) is available, allowing once-a-day administration.

Toxic Effects. As mentioned above, gastric toxicity is much lower than with nonselective COX inhibitors. About 5% of patients who have taken the drug for up to 1 year discontinue treatment because of side effects, which include skin rashes and CNS effects.

THE FENAMATES

The fenamates are a family of NSAIDs that are derivatives of *N*-phenylanthranilic acid. They include *mefenamic, meclofenamic,* and *flufenamic acids.*

Although the biological activity of this group of drugs was discovered in the 1950s, the fenamates have not gained widespread clinical acceptance. Therapeutically, they have no clear advantages over several other NSAIDs and frequently cause side effects, such as diarrhea.

As an analgesic agent, *mefenamic acid* (PONSTEL) has been used to relieve pain arising from rheumatic conditions, soft tissue injuries, other painful musculoskeletal conditions, and dysmenorrhea. Toxicity limits its usefulness, and it appears to offer no advantage over other analgesic agents. As antiinflammatory agents, mefenamic acid and *meclofenamate sodium* have been tested mainly in short-term trials in the treatment of osteoarthritis and rheumatoid arthritis and appear to offer no advantage over other NSAIDs. These drugs are not recommended for use in children or pregnant women.

Mefenamic acid and meclofenamate are the only members of the series available in the United States. The use of mefenamic acid is indicated only for analgesia and for relief of the symptoms of primary dysmenorrhea. While meclofenamate is employed in the treatment of rheumatoid arthritis and osteoarthritis, it is not recommended as initial therapy. Flufenamic acid is used in many other countries, as is mefenamic acid, for its antiinflammatory effects.

Chemistry. Mefenamic acid and meclofenamate are both *N*-substituted phenylanthranilic acids. Their structures are as follows:

MEFENAMIC ACID   MECLOFENAMATE SODIUM

Pharmacological Properties. The fenamates have antiinflammatory, antipyretic, and analgesic properties. In tests of analgesia, mefenamic acid was the only fenamate to display a central as well as a peripheral action.

The fenamates appear to owe these properties primarily to their capacity to inhibit cyclooxygenase. Unlike the other NSAIDs, some of the fenamates (especially meclofenamic acid) also may antagonize certain effects of prostaglandins.

Pharmacokinetic Properties. Peak concentrations in plasma are reached in 0.5 to 2 hours after a single oral dose of meclofenamate and in 2 to 4 hours for mefenamic acid. The two agents have similar half-lives in plasma (2 to 4 hours). In human beings, approximately 50% of a dose of mefenamic acid is excreted in the urine, primarily as the conjugated 3-hydroxymethyl metabolite and the 3-carboxyl metabolite and its conjugates. Twenty percent of the drug is recovered in the feces, mainly as the unconjugated 3-carboxyl metabolite.

Toxic Effects and Precautions. The most common side effects (occurring in approximately 25% of all patients) involve the gastrointestinal system. Usually these take the form of dyspepsia or upper gastrointestinal discomfort, although diarrhea, which may be severe and associated with steatorrhea and inflammation of the bowel, also is relatively common. A potentially serious side effect seen in isolated cases is a hemolytic anemia, which may be of an autoimmune type.

The fenamates are contraindicated in patients with a history of gastrointestinal disease. If diarrhea or skin rash appears, the drug should be stopped at once. The physician and patient should watch for signs of hemolytic anemia.

TOLMETIN, KETOROLAC, AND DICLOFENAC

Tolmetin and *ketorolac* are structurally related heteroaryl acetic acid derivatives with different pharmacological features. *Diclofenac* is a phenylacetic acid derivative that was developed specifically as an antiinflammatory agent.

Tolmetin

Tolmetin is an antiinflammatory, analgesic, and antipyretic agent that was introduced into clinical practice in the United States in 1976. Tolmetin, in recommended doses, appears to be approximately equivalent in efficacy to moderate doses of aspirin; it is usually better tolerated. Its structure is given below:

TOLMETIN

Pharmacological Properties. Tolmetin is an effective antiinflammatory agent that also exerts antipyretic and analgesic effects. Like most of the other drugs considered in this chapter, tolmetin causes gastric erosions and prolongs bleeding time. The pharmacology of tolmetin has been reviewed by Ehrlich (*in* Symposium, 1983a) and by Wong (*in* Rainsford, 1985b).

Pharmacokinetics and Metabolism. Tolmetin is rapidly and completely absorbed after oral administration. Peak concentrations are achieved 20 to 60 minutes after oral administration, and the half-life in plasma is about 5 hours. Accumulation of the drug in synovial fluid begins within 2 hours and persists for up to 8 hours after a single oral dose.

After absorption, tolmetin is extensively (99%) bound to plasma proteins. Virtually all of the drug can be recovered in the urine after 24 hours; some is unchanged but most is conjugated or otherwise metabolized. The major metabolic transformation involves oxidation of the para-methyl group to a carboxylic acid.

Therapeutic Uses. Tolmetin (*tolmetin sodium;* TOLECTIN) is approved in the United States for the treatment of osteoarthritis, rheumatoid arthritis, and the juvenile form of the disease; it also has been used in the treatment of ankylosing spondylitis. In rheumatoid arthritis, many investigators have compared tolmetin (0.8 to 1.6 g per day) with aspirin (4 to 4.5 g per day) or indomethacin (100 to 150 mg per day). In general, there has been little difference in therapeutic efficacy. Tolmetin may be tolerated somewhat better than aspirin in equally effective doses. The maximum recommended dose is 2 g per day, typically given in divided doses with meals, milk, or antacids to lessen abdominal discomfort. However, peak plasma concentrations and bioavailability are reduced when the drug is taken with food.

Toxic Effects. Side effects occur in 25% to 40% of patients who take tolmetin, and 5% to 10% discontinue use of the drug. Gastrointestinal side effects are the most common, with epigastric pain (15% incidence), dyspepsia, nausea, and vomiting being the chief manifestations. Gastric and duodenal ulceration also have been observed. CNS side effects, including nervousness, anxiety, insomnia, drowsiness, and visual disturbance, are less common and are said to be neither as frequent nor as severe as those caused by indomethacin. Similarly, the incidence of tinnitus, deafness, and vertigo is less than with aspirin.

Ketorolac

Ketorolac is a potent analgesic but only a moderately effective antiinflammatory drug. It is one of the few NSAIDs approved for parenteral administration. The structure of ketorolac is given below:

KETOROLAC

Pharmacological Properties. Ketorolac inhibits prostaglandin biosynthesis. It has antipyretic, antiinflammatory, and analgesic activity, but in assays of inflammation it has greater systemic analgesic than antiinflammatory activity. Unlike opioid agonists, ketorolac is not associated with tolerance, withdrawal effects, or respiratory depression. Ketorolac also has antiinflammatory activity when topically administered in the eye. Ketorolac inhibits platelet aggregation and promotes gastric ulceration. The pharmacology of ketorolac has been reviewed (Buckley and Brogden, 1990).

Pharmacokinetics and Metabolism. Ketorolac is rapidly absorbed whether given orally or intramuscularly, achieving peak plasma concentration in 30 to 50 minutes. Oral bioavailability is about 80%. Almost totally bound to plasma proteins, it is excreted with an elimination half-life of 4 to 6 hours. Urinary excretion accounts for about 90% of eliminated drug, with about 10% excreted unchanged and the remainder as a glucuronidated conjugate. The rate of elimination is reduced in the elderly and in patients with renal failure.

Therapeutic Uses. *Ketorolac* (administered as the tromethamine salt TORADOL) is used for postoperative pain, as an alternative to opioid agents, and is administered intramuscularly, intravenously, or orally. Typical intramuscular doses are 30 to 60 mg; intravenous doses are 15 to 30 mg; and oral doses are 5 to 30 mg. Ketorolac probably should not be used for obstetric analgesia. The drug is indicated only for short-term treatment of pain (no longer than 5 days) and should not be used for minor or chronic pain. Topical ketorolac may be useful for inflamma-

tory conditions in the eye and is approved for the treatment of seasonal allergic conjunctivitis and ocular inflammation.

Toxic Effects. Side effects occur about twice as often with ketorolac as with placebo. These side effects include somnolence, dizziness, headache, gastrointestinal pain, dyspepsia and nausea, and pain at the site of injection.

Diclofenac

Diclofenac is an antiinflammatory agent approved for several uses in the United States. Details of its pharmacology are discussed in the proceedings of a symposium (Symposium, 1986) and in a review by Liauw and associates (*in* Lewis and Furst, 1987). The structure of diclofenac is given below:

DICLOFENAC

Pharmacological Properties. Diclofenac has analgesic, antipyretic, and antiinflammatory activities. It is an inhibitor of cyclooxygenase, and its potency is substantially greater than that of indomethacin, naproxen, or several other agents. In addition, diclofenac appears to reduce intracellular concentrations of free arachidonate in leukocytes, perhaps by altering the release or uptake of the fatty acid.

Pharmacokinetics and Metabolism. Diclofenac is rapidly and completely absorbed after oral administration; peak concentrations in plasma are reached within 2 to 3 hours. Administration with food slows the rate but does not alter the extent of absorption. There is a substantial first-pass effect, such that only about 50% of diclofenac is available systemically. The drug is extensively bound to plasma proteins (99%), and its half-life in plasma is 1 to 2 hours. Diclofenac accumulates in synovial fluid after oral administration, which may explain the duration of therapeutic effect that is considerably longer than the plasma half-life. Diclofenac is metabolized in the liver by a cytochrome P450 isozyme of the CYP2C subfamily to 4-hydroxydiclofenac, the principal metabolite, and other hydroxylated forms; after glucuronidation and sulfation, the metabolites are excreted in the urine (65%) and bile (35%).

Therapeutic Uses. *Diclofenac sodium* is approved in the United States for the long-term symptomatic treatment of rheumatoid arthritis, osteoarthritis, and ankylosing spondylitis. Three formulations are available: an intermediate release form (CATAFLAM), a delayed-release form (VOLTARIN), and an extended-release form (VOLTARIN-XR). The usual daily dosage for those indications is 100 to 200 mg, given in several divided doses. It also may be useful for short-term treatment of acute musculoskeletal injury, acute painful shoulder (bicipital tendinitis and subdeltoid bursitis), postoperative pain, and dysmenorrhea. Diclofenac (50 mg and 75 mg, enteric-coated tablet) and misoprostol, a prostaglandin E_1 analog (200 μg), have been formulated together in a preparation (ARTHROTEC) (*see* Symposium 1993a). This

Table 27–3

Propionic Acid Derivatives: Available Formulations and Recommendations for Antiinflammatory Therapy

NONPROPRIETARY NAME	TRADE NAME	FORMULATION	USUAL ANTIINFLAMMATORY DOSE
Ibuprofen	MOTRIN, others	Tablets	400–800 mg, three to four times a day
Naproxen	NAPROSYN, others	Tablets; suspension	250–500 mg, twice daily
Naproxen sodium	ANAPROX, others	Tablets	275–550 mg, twice daily
Fenoprofen	NALFON	Tablets; capsules	300–600 mg, three to four times a day
Ketoprofen	ORUDIS	Capsules	50–75 mg, three to four times a day
Flurbiprofen	ANSAID, others	Tablets	50–75 mg, two to four times a day
Oxaprozin	DAYPRO	Tablets	600–1200 mg, once daily

preparation is designed to retain the efficacy of diclofenac while reducing the frequency of gastrointestinal ulcers and erosions. In addition, an ophthalmic solution of diclofenac is available for treatment of postoperative inflammation after cataract extraction.

Toxic Effects. Diclofenac produces side effects in about 20% of patients, and approximately 2% of patients discontinue therapy as a result. Gastrointestinal effects are the most common; bleeding and ulceration or perforation of the intestinal wall have been observed. Elevation of hepatic aminotransferase activities in plasma occurs in about 15% of patients. Although usually moderate, these values may increase more than threefold in a small percentage of patients—often those who are being treated for osteoarthritis. The elevations in aminotransferase usually are reversible. Another member of this phenylacetic acid family of NSAIDs, bromfenac, was withdrawn from the market because of its association with severe, irreversible liver injury in some patients. Therefore, aminotransferase activities should be evaluated during the first 8 weeks of therapy with diclofenac, and the drug should be discontinued if abnormal values persist or if other signs or symptoms develop. Other untoward responses to diclofenac include CNS effects, skin rashes, allergic reactions, fluid retention and edema, and rarely, impairment of renal function. The drug is not recommended for children, nursing mothers, or pregnant women.

PROPIONIC ACID DERIVATIVES

Arylpropionic acid derivatives represent a group of effective, useful NSAIDs. They may offer significant advantages over aspirin and indomethacin for many patients, since they usually are better tolerated. Nevertheless, propionic acid derivatives share all of the detrimental features of the entire class of drugs. Furthermore, their rapid proliferation in number and the heavy promotion of these drugs make it difficult for the physician to choose ratio-

nally among members of the group and between propionic acid derivatives and the more established agents. The similarities among drugs in this class (and certain of the others discussed above) are far more striking than are the differences.

The approved indications for the use of one or another of the propionic acid derivatives include the symptomatic treatment of rheumatoid arthritis, osteoarthritis, ankylosing spondylitis, and acute gouty arthritis; they also are used as analgesics, for acute tendinitis and bursitis, and for primary dysmenorrhea. Information regarding dosage forms and usual antiinflammatory doses is shown in Table 27–3.

Clinical studies indicate that the propionic acid derivatives are comparable to aspirin for the control of the signs and symptoms of rheumatoid arthritis and osteoarthritis. In patients with rheumatoid arthritis, there is a reduction in joint swelling, pain, and duration of morning stiffness. By objective measurements, strength, mobility, and stamina are improved. In general, the intensity of untoward effects is less than that associated with the ingestion of indomethacin or high doses of aspirin. However, aspirin is less expensive than most of the propionic derivatives for those who can tolerate it.

Ibuprofen, naproxen, flurbiprofen, fenoprofen, ketoprofen, and *oxaprozin* are described individually below. These drugs currently are available in the United States. Several additional agents in this class are in use or under study in other countries. These include *fenbufen, carprofen, pirprofen, indobufen,* and *tiaprofenic acid.*

Ibuprofen was the first member of the propionic acid class of NSAIDs to come into general use, so experience

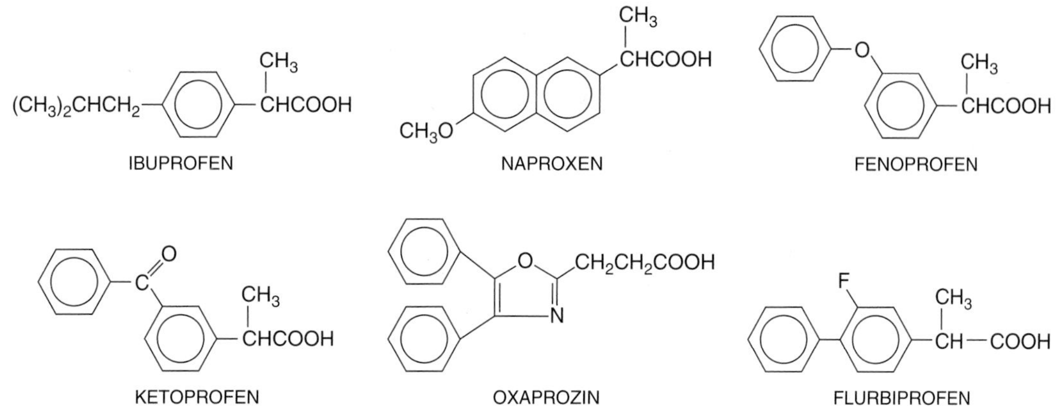

Figure 27–3. Structural formulas of antiinflammatory propionic acid derivatives.

with this drug is greater. It is available for sale without a prescription in the United States. Naproxen has a longer half-life than most of the other structurally and functionally similar agents, making twice-daily administration of it feasible. This drug also is available without a prescription in the United States. Oxaprozin also has a long half-life and can be given once daily. The structural formulas of these drugs are shown in Figure 27–3.

Pharmacological Properties.   The pharmacodynamic properties of the propionic acid derivatives do not differ significantly. All are effective cyclooxygenase inhibitors, although there is considerable variation in their potency. For example, naproxen is approximately 20 times more potent than aspirin, while ibuprofen, fenoprofen, and aspirin are roughly equipotent as cyclooxygenase inhibitors. All of these agents alter platelet function and prolong bleeding time, and it should be assumed that any patient who is intolerant of aspirin also will experience a severe reaction after administration of one of these drugs. Some of the propionic acid derivatives have prominent inhibitory effects on leukocyte function; naproxen is particularly potent in this regard. While the compounds do vary in potency, this is not of obvious clinical significance. All are effective antiinflammatory agents in various experimental animal models of inflammation; all have useful antiinflammatory, analgesic, and antipyretic activities in human beings. Although all of these compounds can cause gastric toxicity in patients, these are usually less severe than with aspirin.

It is difficult to find data on which to base a rational choice among the members of the propionic acid derivatives, if in fact one can be made. However, in relatively small clinical studies that compared the activity of several members of this group, patients preferred naproxen in terms of analgesia and relief of morning stiffness (*see*

Huskisson, *in* Symposium, 1983a; Hart and Huskisson, 1984). With regard to side effects, naproxen was the best tolerated, followed by ibuprofen and fenoprofen. There was considerable interpatient variation in the preference for a single drug and also between the designations of the best and the worst drug. Unfortunately, it is probably impossible to predict *a priori* which drug will be most suitable for any given individual. Nevertheless, more than 50% of patients with rheumatoid arthritis probably will achieve adequate symptomatic relief from the use of one or another of the propionic acid derivatives, and many clinicians favor their use instead of aspirin in such patients.

Drug Interactions.   The potential adverse drug interactions of particular concern with propionic acid derivatives result from their high degree of binding to albumin in plasma. However, the propionic acid derivatives do not alter the effects of the oral hypoglycemic drugs or warfarin. Nevertheless, the physician should be prepared to adjust the dosage of warfarin because these drugs impair platelet function and may cause gastrointestinal lesions.

Ibuprofen

Ibuprofen is supplied as tablets containing 200 to 800 mg; only the 200-mg tablets (ADVIL, NUPRIN, others) are available without a prescription.

For rheumatoid arthritis and osteoarthritis, daily doses of up to 3200 mg in divided portions may be given, although the usual total dose is 1200 to 1800 mg. It also may be possible to reduce the dosage for maintenance purposes. For mild-to-moderate pain, especially that of primary dysmenorrhea, the usual dosage is 400 mg every 4 to 6 hours as needed. The drug may be given with milk or food to minimize gastrointestinal side effects. Ibuprofen has been discussed in detail by Kantor (1979) and by Adams and Buckler (*in* Symposium, 1983a).

Pharmacokinetics and Metabolism.   Ibuprofen is rapidly absorbed after oral administration, and peak concentrations in plasma are observed after 15 to 30 minutes. The half-life in plasma is about 2 hours.

Ibuprofen is extensively (99%) bound to plasma proteins, but the drug occupies only a fraction of the total drug-binding sites at usual concentrations. Ibuprofen passes slowly into the synovial spaces and may remain there in higher concentration as the concentrations in plasma decline. In experimental animals, ibuprofen and its metabolites pass easily across the placenta.

The excretion of ibuprofen is rapid and complete. More than 90% of an ingested dose is excreted in the urine as metabolites or their conjugates. The major metabolites are a hydroxylated and a carboxylated compound.

Toxic Effects.   Ibuprofen has been used in patients with a history of gastrointestinal intolerance to other NSAIDs. Nevertheless, therapy usually must be discontinued in 10% to 15% of patients because of intolerance to the drug.

Gastrointestinal side effects are experienced by 5% to 15% of patients taking ibuprofen; epigastric pain, nausea, heartburn, and sensations of "fullness" in the gastrointestinal tract are the usual difficulties. However, the incidence of these side effects is less with ibuprofen than with aspirin or indomethacin.

Other side effects of ibuprofen have been reported less frequently. They include thrombocytopenia, skin rashes, headache, dizziness and blurred vision, and, in a few cases, toxic amblyopia, fluid retention, and edema. Patients who develop ocular disturbances should discontinue the use of ibuprofen. Ibuprofen is not recommended for use by pregnant women, or by those who are breast-feeding their infants.

Naproxen

The pharmacological properties and therapeutic uses of *naproxen* (ALEVE, NAPROSYN, others) have been reviewed by Segre (*in* Symposium, 1983a), Allison and colleagues (*in* Rainsford, 1985b), and Todd and Clissold (1990).

Pharmacokinetics and Metabolism.   Naproxen is fully absorbed when administered orally. The rapidity, but not the extent, of absorption is influenced by the presence of food in the stomach. Peak concentrations in plasma occur within 2 to 4 hours and are somewhat more rapid after the administration of naproxen sodium. Absorption may be accelerated by the concurrent administration of sodium bicarbonate or reduced by magnesium oxide or aluminum hydroxide. Naproxen also is absorbed rectally, but peak concentrations in plasma are achieved more slowly. The half-life of naproxen in plasma is about 14 hours; this value is increased about twofold in elderly subjects and may necessitate adjustment of dosage.

Metabolites of naproxen are almost entirely excreted in the urine. About 30% of the drug undergoes 6-demethylation, and most of this metabolite, as well as naproxen itself, is excreted as the glucuronide or other conjugates.

Naproxen is almost completely (99%) bound to plasma proteins following normal therapeutic doses. Naproxen crosses the placenta and appears in the milk of lactating women at approximately 1% of the maternal plasma concentration.

Toxic Effects.   Although the incidence of gastrointestinal and CNS side effects is about equal to that caused by indomethacin, naproxen is better tolerated in both regards. Gastrointestinal complications have ranged from relatively mild dyspepsia, gas-

tric discomfort, and heartburn to nausea, vomiting, and gastric bleeding. CNS side effects range from drowsiness, headache, dizziness, and sweating to fatigue, depression, and ototoxicity. Less common reactions include pruritus and a variety of dermatological problems. A few instances of jaundice, impairment of renal function, angioneurotic edema, thrombocytopenia, and agranulocytosis have been reported.

Fenoprofen

The pharmacological properties and therapeutic uses of *fenoprofen* (NALFON) have been reviewed by Burt and coworkers (Symposium, 1983a).

Pharmacokinetics and Metabolism.   Oral doses of fenoprofen are readily, but incompletely (85%) absorbed. The presence of food in the stomach retards absorption and lowers peak concentrations in plasma, which are usually achieved within 2 hours. The concomitant administration of antacids does not seem to alter the concentrations that are achieved.

After absorption, fenoprofen is almost completely (99%) bound to plasma albumin. The drug is extensively (>90%) metabolized and excreted almost entirely in the urine. Fenoprofen undergoes metabolic transformation to the 4-hydroxy analog. The glucuronic acid conjugate of fenoprofen itself and 4-hydroxy fenoprofen are formed in almost equal amounts and together account for 90% of the excreted drug. The half-life of fenoprofen in plasma is about 3 hours.

Toxic Effects.   The most frequently reported side effects have been gastrointestinal ones; abdominal discomfort and dyspepsia occur in about 15% of patients. These side effects are almost always less intense than with equieffective doses of aspirin and force discontinuation of therapy in a small percentage of patients. Other side effects include skin rash and, less frequently, CNS effects such as tinnitus, dizziness, lassitude, confusion, and anorexia.

Ketoprofen

Ketoprofen (ORUDIS, ORUVAIL) shares the pharmacological properties of other propionic acid derivatives; these have been reviewed by Harris and Vávra (*in* Rainsford, 1985b) and Vávra (*in* Lewis and Furst, 1987). Although it is a cyclooxygenase inhibitor, ketoprofen is said to stabilize lysosomal membranes and may antagonize the actions of bradykinin.

Pharmacokinetics and Metabolism.   Ketoprofen is rapidly absorbed after oral administration and maximal concentrations in plasma are achieved within 1 to 2 hours; food reduces the rate but not the extent of absorption. The drug is extensively bound to plasma proteins (99%), and it has a half-life in plasma of about 2 hours; slightly longer half-lives are observed in elderly subjects. Ketoprofen is conjugated with glucuronic acid in the liver, and the conjugate is excreted in the urine. Patients with impaired renal function eliminate the drug more slowly.

Toxic Effects.   Dyspepsia and other gastrointestinal side effects have been observed in about 30% of patients, but these side effects are generally mild and are less frequent than those in patients treated with aspirin; untoward effects are reduced when the drug is taken with food, milk, or antacids. Ketoprofen can cause fluid retention and increased plasma concentrations of creatinine. These effects are generally transient and occur in the absence of symptoms, but they are more common in patients who are receiving diuretics or in those over the age of 60. Renal function should be monitored in such patients.

Flurbiprofen

The pharmacological properties, therapeutic indications, and adverse effects of *flurbiprofen* (ANSAID) are similar to those of other antiinflammatory derivatives of propionic acid (*see* Smith *et al.*, *in* Rainsford, 1985b). Flurbiprofen also has been used in trials in Europe as antiplatelet therapy. The drug is well absorbed orally, and peak plasma concentrations occur within 1 to 2 hours. Flurbiprofen is extensively metabolized by hydroxylation and conjugation in the liver; its half-life in plasma is about 6 hours. The drug also is under study for treatment of soft tissue lesions, administered as a transcutaneous patch.

Oxaprozin

Oxaprozin (DAYPRO) is unique among propionic acid derivatives because it can be administered once daily. Its other pharmacological properties, adverse effects, and therapeutic uses are similar to those of other propionic acid derivatives (*see* Todd and Brogden, 1986).

Oxaprozin is well absorbed orally, with peak plasma concentrations achieved in 3 to 6 hours. The drug is metabolized in the liver and primarily eliminated by urinary excretion. The half-life is 40 to 60 hours, and this increases with age.

ENOLIC ACIDS (OXICAMS)

Piroxicam

Piroxicam is one of the oxicam derivatives, a class of enolic acids that have antiinflammatory, analgesic, and antipyretic activity. In recommended doses, piroxicam appears to be the equivalent of aspirin, indomethacin, or naproxen for the long-term treatment of rheumatoid arthritis or osteoarthritis. It may be tolerated better than aspirin or indomethacin. The principal advantage of piroxicam is its long half-life, which permits the administration of a single daily dose. The pharmacological properties and therapeutic uses of piroxicam have been reviewed by Wiseman (*see* Rainsford, 1985b), and by Lombardino and Wiseman (*in* Lewis and Furst, 1987). The structural formula of piroxicam is as follows:

PIROXICAM

Pharmacological Properties. Piroxicam is an effective antiinflammatory agent; it is about equal in potency to indomethacin as an inhibitor of prostaglandin biosynthesis *in vitro*. Piroxicam also can inhibit activation of neutrophils independent of its ability to inhibit the cyclooxygenase; hence, additional modes of antiinflammatory action have been proposed, including inhibition of proteoglycanase and collagenase in cartilage (Abramson and Weissman, 1989; Lombardino and Wiseman, *in* Lewis and Furst, 1987). Piroxicam exerts antipyretic and analgesic effects in experimental animals and human beings. As with other NSAIDs, piroxicam can cause gastric erosions and it prolongs bleeding time.

Pharmacokinetics and Metabolism. Piroxicam is completely absorbed after oral administration; peak concentrations in plasma occur within 2 to 4 hours. Antacids do not alter the rate or extent of absorption, but food may alter the rate. There is enterohepatic cycling of piroxicam, and estimates of the half-life in plasma have been variable; a mean value appears to be about 50 hours.

After absorption, piroxicam is extensively (99%) bound to plasma proteins. At steady state (*e.g.*, after 7 to 12 days), concentrations of piroxicam in plasma and synovial fluid are approximately equal. Less than 5% of the drug is excreted in the urine unchanged. The major metabolic transformation in human beings is cytochrome P450-mediated hydroxylation of the pyridyl ring (predominantly by an isozyme of the CYP2C subfamily), and this inactive metabolite and its glucuronide conjugate account for about 60% of the drug excreted in the urine and feces.

Therapeutic Uses. *Piroxicam* (FELDENE) is approved in the United States for the treatment of rheumatoid arthritis and osteoarthritis. The usual daily dose is 20 mg, sometimes given in two doses. Because of the long period required to achieve steady state, maximal therapeutic responses should not be expected for 2 weeks. It also has been used in the treatment of ankylosing spondylitis, acute musculoskeletal disorders, dysmenorrhea, postoperative pain, and acute gout.

Toxic Effects. The reported incidence of adverse effects in patients who take piroxicam is about 20%; approximately 5% of patients stop using the drug because of side effects. Gastrointestinal reactions are the most common; the incidence of peptic ulcer is less than 1%. Piroxicam and some other NSAIDs can reduce the renal excretion of lithium to a clinically significant extent.

Meloxicam

Another oxicam, *meloxicam* (MOBIC), recently was approved by the FDA for use in treating osteoarthritis. Its pharmacokinetics have been described in detail (Turck *et al.*, 1996). The structure of meloxicam is given below:

MELOXICAM

The recommended dose for meloxicam is 7.5 mg once daily for osteoarthritis; in severe cases, this dose can be increased to 15 mg. The recommended dose for cases of rheumatoid arthritis is 15 mg once daily.

Meloxicam has been suggested to be a selective COX-2 inhibitor based on *in vitro* studies. However, when tested *in vivo* in human beings, its selectivity to inhibit COX-2 compared to COX-1 was only about 10-fold, and there was some inhibition of platelet COX-1-mediated thromboxane production after oral treatment with both 7.5 mg/day and 15 mg/day (Panara *et al.*, 1999). In clinical trials, less gastrointestinal side effects had been found with meloxicam compared to nonselective COX inhibitors. However, in a study where endoscopy scores of gastric injury were evaluated, there was significantly less gastric injury compared to piroxicam (20 mg/day) in subjects treated with 7.5 mg/day of meloxicam but not with 15 mg/day (Patoia *et al.*, 1996). Collectively, these findings suggest that the extent of inhibition of COX-1 with meloxicam is largely a function of dose and interindividual variability of drug levels. Further clinical trials and post-marketing clinical experience will be needed to assess whether currently reported short-term benefits in suppression of inflammatory responses without gastrointestinal complications are paralleled by long-term efficacy without toxicity.

Other Oxicams

A number of other oxicam derivatives are under study or in use outside of the United States. These include several prodrugs of piroxicam (*ampiroxicam, droxicam,* and *pivoxicam*), which have been designed to reduce gastrointestinal irritation. However, as with the use of sulindac, any diminution in gastric toxicity with the use of prodrugs of nonselective COX inhibitors is only relative, because circulating concentrations of such agents can inhibit COX-1 in the stomach. Other oxicam derivatives under study or in use outside the United States include *lornoxicam, cinnoxicam, sudoxicam,* and *tenoxicam.* The efficacy and toxicity of these drugs are similar to those of piroxicam.

NABUMETONE

Nabumetone is an antiinflammatory agent approved in 1991 for use in the United States. Details of its pharmacology are discussed by Friedel *et al.* (1993). The structure of nabumetone is as follows:

NABUMETONE

Clinical trials with *nabumetone* (RELAFEN) have indicated substantial efficacy in the treatment of rheumatoid arthritis and osteoarthritis, with a relatively low incidence of side effects. The dose typically is 1000 mg given once daily. The drug also appears to be effective in the short-term treatment of soft tissue injuries.

Pharmacological Properties.   Nabumetone is a weak inhibitor of cyclooxygenase *in vitro,* but it is an active antiinflammatory drug that possesses antipyretic and analgesic activities. In experimental animals, nabumetone appears to cause less gastric damage than do other antiinflammatory agents.

Pharmacokinetics and Metabolism.   Nabumetone is absorbed rapidly and is converted in the liver to one or more active metabolites, principally 6-methoxy-2-naphthylacetic acid, a potent

inhibitor of cyclooxygenase. This metabolite is inactivated by *O*-demethylation in the liver, is then conjugated before excretion, and is eliminated with a half-life of about 24 hours.

Toxic Effects.   Side effects of treatment with nabumetone include lower bowel complaints, skin rash, headache, dizziness, heartburn, tinnitus, and pruritus. The incidence of gastrointestinal ulceration appears to be lower with nabumetone than with other NSAIDs (Scott and Palmer, 2000). This may result, in part, from the fact that nabumetone is a prodrug, and an active compound is metabolically generated only after absorption of the administered drug. Differential inhibition of cyclooxygenases is unlikely, because the active metabolite of nabumetone, 6-methoxy-2-naphthylacetic acid, is not a selective inhibitor of COX-2 (Patrignani *et al.*, 1994).

PYRAZOLON DERIVATIVES

This group of drugs includes *phenylbutazone, oxyphenbutazone, antipyrine, aminopyrine,* and *dipyrone.* These drugs have been in clinical use for many years. With the exception of antipyrine, which is used in analgesic otic drop preparations, these agents are not available in the United States because of their propensity to cause irreversible agranulocytosis. Dipyrone was banned in the United States and some European nations in the 1970s after reports of agranulocytosis among users. However, dipyrone continues to be used in several European, Asian, and Latin American countries. It was reintroduced in Sweden in 1995 because of epidemiologic data suggesting that the overall risk of serious adverse effects and death associated with dipyrone is very low; the risk is similar to that with acetaminophen and lower than that with aspirin, primarily due to a much lower incidence of gastrointestinal bleeding (Andrade *et al.*, 1998). However, it has been recommended that oral dipyrone only be used when other analgesics have failed (Arellano and Sacristan, 1990). Properties of other pyrazolon derivatives were discussed in previous editions of this book.

DIARYL SUBSTITUTED FURANONES

The only member of this class currently available is *rofecoxib* (VIOXX), a selective COX-2 inhibitor that was introduced in 1999. Details of its pharmacodynamics, pharmacokinetics, therapeutic efficacy, and toxicity have been reviewed by Scott and Lamb (1999).

Chemistry.   The structure of rofecoxib is as follows:

ROFECOXIB

Pharmacological Properties.   Rofecoxib exhibits antiinflammatory, antipyretic, and analgesic activities. These properties have been attributed to selective inhibition of COX-2. At therapeutic concentrations in human beings, rofecoxib does not inhibit COX-1 and does not alter platelet function. The incidence of gastric ulceration seen with endoscopy during treatment with rofecoxib (25 mg and 50 mg daily) is significantly less than that in subjects treated with ibuprofen (2400 mg daily). Clinical studies have not ruled out some increase in the occurrence of ulcers with rofecoxib compared to placebo. Fecal blood loss, however, has not been found to be significantly different from placebo. Rofecoxib appears to significantly inhibit endogenous production of prostaglandins in human beings, as do other selective COX-2 inhibitors (McAdam *et al.,* 1999; Cullen *et al.,* 1998).

Pharmacokinetics and Metabolism.   Rofecoxib is readily absorbed following oral administration and is highly bound to plasma proteins. Metabolism of rofecoxib occurs primarily by cytosolic reductases producing dihydro derivatives. Most of the drug is excreted in the urine as metabolites; 14% is excreted in the feces as unchanged drug. There appears to be saturable metabolism at therapeutic doses. The effective half-life is approximately 17 hours. Renal insufficiency does not alter the pharmacokinetics of the drug, but it is not recommended for use in patients with advanced renal disease, because the safety of the drug in this patient population has not been established. Limited information is available regarding the influence of significant hepatic insufficiency on the pharmacokinetics of the drug. Significant interactions have been identified with rifampin, methotrexate, and warfarin but not with ketoconazole, prednisone/prednisolone, oral contraceptives, or digoxin.

Toxic Effects.   Whether or not the greater safety of rofecoxib regarding gastric injury is sustained during long-term treatment remains to be established. Effects attributed to inhibition of prostaglandin production in the kidney, hypertension and edema, occur with nonselective COX inhibitors and also with rofecoxib. Therefore, rofecoxib should be used with caution in patients with hypertension and congestive heart failure. Whether or not patients with aspirin hypersensitivity reactions also exhibit hypersensitivity reactions following administration of selective COX-2 inhibitors has not been investigated. Until the safety of selective COX-2 inhibitors in this patient population has been established, the use of rofecoxib in these patients is contraindicated.

Therapeutic Uses.   Rofecoxib is approved by the United States Food and Drug Administration for the treatment of osteoarthritis, acute pain in adults, and dysmenorrhea. The drug has efficacy similar to that of nonselective COX inhibitors in reducing dental pain, postoperative pain, and pain associated with primary dysmenorrhea. The recommended starting dose for osteoarthritis is 12.5 mg once daily, increasing to a maximum of 25 mg once daily if necessary. For acute pain and dysmenorrhea, 50 mg per day is the recommended dose; treatment at this dose for more than 5 days has not been studied.

DIARYL SUBSTITUTED PYRAZOLES

The only member of this class currently available is *celecoxib* (CELEBREX). It is one of the selective COX-2 inhibitors and was approved for marketing in the United States in 1998. Details of its pharmacology are summarized by Davies *et al.* (2000).

Chemistry.   The structure of celecoxib is as follows:

CELECOXIB

Pharmacokinetics and Metabolism.   The rate of absorption after oral administration is moderate, with peak plasma levels occurring after 2 to 4 hours; the extent of absorption is not known. Celecoxib is extensively bound to plasma proteins. Little drug is excreted unchanged; most is excreted as carboxylic acid and glucuronide metabolites in the urine and feces. The elimination half-life is approximately 11 hours. Plasma concentrations are lower in patients with renal insufficiency, in whom there is a 47% increase in apparent clearance. Plasma concentrations are increased by approximately 40% to 180% in patients with mild and moderate hepatic impairment, respectively. Significant interactions occur with fluconazole and lithium but not with ketoconazole or methotrexate. Celecoxib is metabolized by CYP2C9, so clinical vigilance is necessary during coadministration of other substrates or inhibitors of this enzyme.

Pharmacologic Properties, Toxic Effects, and Therapeutic Uses.   The pharmacological properties and toxic effects of celecoxib are essentially the same as those of rofecoxib (*see* above). Celecoxib is approved in the United States for the treatment of osteoarthritis and rheumatoid arthritis. The recommended dose for treating osteoarthritis is 200 mg per day as a single dose or as two 100-mg doses. In the treatment of rheumatoid arthritis, the recommended dose is 100 to 200 mg twice per day.

OTHER NONSTEROIDAL ANTIINFLAMMATORY DRUGS

A large number of antiinflammatory agents are under development or clinical study. Although many are members of classes of drugs discussed above, others have novel structures and apparently different mechanisms of action. Two such agents are *apazone* and *nimesulide.*

Apazone (Azapropazone)

Apazone is an NSAID that is antiinflammatory, analgesic, and antipyretic but is only a weak inhibitor of cyclooxygenase. In addition, apazone is a potent uricosuric agent and is particularly useful for the treatment of acute gout. The antiinflammatory effects of apazone may be due in part to an ability of the drug to inhibit neutrophil migration, degranulation, and superoxide production (Mackin *et al.*, 1986). The drug is not currently available in the United States. The structural formula of apazone is as follows:

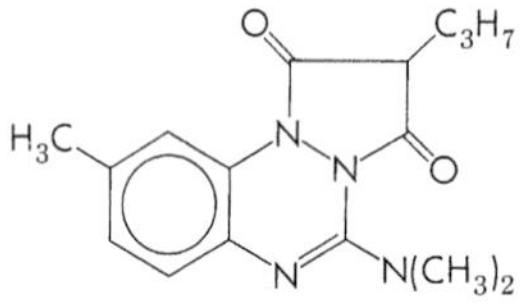

APAZONE

Apazone has been used for the treatment of rheumatoid arthritis, osteoarthritis, and gout. Clinical experience to date suggests that apazone is well tolerated. Mild gastrointestinal side effects (nausea, epigastric pain, dyspepsia) and skin rashes occur in about 3% of patients, while CNS effects (headache, vertigo) are reported less frequently. The overall incidence of untoward reactions is probably 6% to 10%.

Because apazone is an inhibitor of cyclooxygenase, albeit less active than other NSAIDs, all precautions discussed above for the group are applicable.

Nimesulide

Nimesulide is a sulfonanilide compound (*see* Symposium, 1993b) which is not available in the United States but is marketed in European countries. Its structure is as follows:

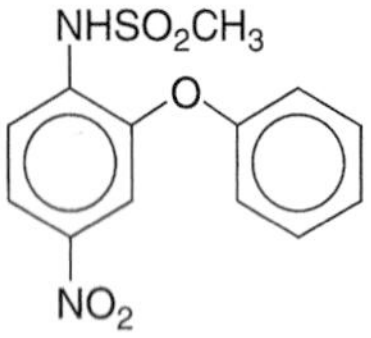

NIMESULIDE

Nimesulide is antiinflammatory, analgesic, and antipyretic. It exerts some actions in addition to inhibiting cyclooxygenase that may contribute to its antiinflammatory effects; it inhibits neutrophil activation and exhibits antioxidant properties. Nimesulide has been found to be a selective COX-2 inhibitor *in vivo* in human beings at clinically recommended doses (Cullen *et al.*, 1998). Consistent with this is the finding that nimesulide is associated with a very low incidence of adverse side effects, especially in the gastrointestinal tract (Rainsford, 1999; Bjarnason and Thjodleifsson, 1999).

GOLD

Gold, in elemental form, has been employed for centuries as an antipruritic to relieve the itching palm. In more modern times, the observation by Robert Koch in 1890 that gold inhibited *Mycobacterium tuberculosis in vitro* led to trials in arthritis and lupus erythematosus, thought by some to be tuberculous manifestations. Later observations of success in treating chronic arthritis stimulated interest in gold therapy (chrysotherapy). At present, gold is employed in the treatment of rheumatoid arthritis; usually it is reserved for patients with progressive disease who do not obtain satisfactory relief from therapy with NSAIDs. However, gold compounds are among the agents that are used in an attempt to arrest the progress of the disease and to induce remissions; these are sometimes called disease-modifying drugs, although this is probably a misnomer (Edmonds *et al.*, 1993). Since degenerative lesions do not regress once formed, there is an increasing tendency to attempt to induce remission early in the course of the disease. Such therapy is often initiated with gold, which although potentially beneficial, causes a high incidence of toxicity (Felson *et al.*, 1992; Cash and Klippel, 1994).

Chemistry.   The significant preparations of gold are all compounds in which the gold is attached to sulfur. The more water-soluble compounds employed in therapy contain hydrophilic groups in addition to the aurothio group. The structural formulas of aurothioglucose, gold sodium thiomalate, and auranofin are as follows:

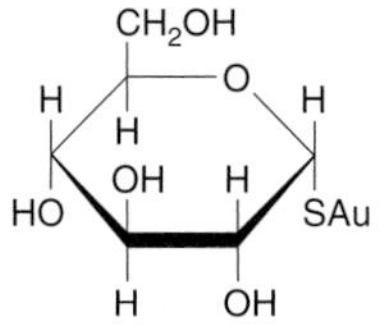

AUROTHIOGLUCOSE 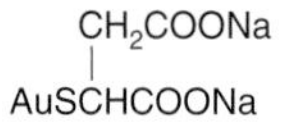   GOLD SODIUM THIOMALATE

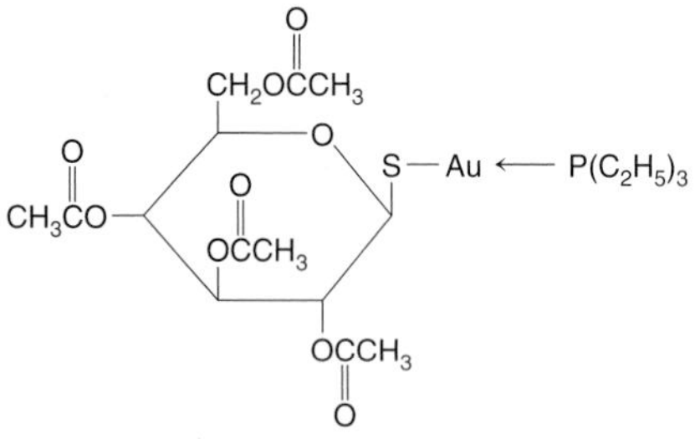

AURANOFIN

Monovalent gold has a relatively strong affinity for sulfur, weak affinities for carbon and nitrogen, and almost no affinity for oxygen, except in chelates. The high affinity for sulfur and the inhibitory effect of gold salts on various enzymes have suggested that the therapeutic effects of gold salts might derive from inhibition of sulfhydryl systems. However, other sulfhydryl inhibitors do not appear to have therapeutic actions in common with gold.

Pharmacological Properties.   Gold compounds can suppress or prevent, but not cure, experimental arthritis and synovitis due to a number of infectious and chemical agents. Gold compounds have minimal antiinflammatory effects in other circumstances and cause only a gradual reduction of the signs and symptoms of inflammation associated with rheumatoid arthritis. Although many effects of these drugs have been observed, which, if any, are related to the therapeutic effects of gold in rheumatoid arthritis is unknown. Perhaps the best hypotheses relate to the capacity of gold compounds to inhibit the maturation and function of mononuclear phagocytes and of T cells, thereby suppressing immune responsiveness. Decreased concentrations of rheumatoid factor and immunoglobulins often are observed in patients who are treated with gold.

In experimental animals, gold is sequestered in organs that are rich in mononuclear phagocytes, and it selectively accumulates in the lysosomes of type A synovial cells and other macrophages within the inflamed synovium of patients who are treated with gold compounds. Moreover, the administration of gold thiomalate to animals depresses the migration and phagocytic activity of macrophages in inflammatory exudates, and chrysotherapy reduces the augmented phagocytic capacity of blood monocytes from patients with rheumatoid arthritis. Other mechanisms of action of gold compounds have been suggested, but none is generally accepted. These include inhibition of prostaglandin synthesis, interference with complement activation, cross-linking of collagen, and inhibition of the activity of lysosomal and other enzymes, including protein kinase C, in T cells.

Absorption, Distribution, and Excretion. *Aurothioglucose and Gold Sodium Thiomalate.* These more water-soluble gold compounds are rapidly absorbed after intramuscular injection, and peak concentrations in blood are reached in 2 to 6 hours. These agents are absorbed erratically when administered orally. Tissue distribution depends not only on the type of compound administered but also on the time after administration and probably on the duration of treatment. Early in the course of therapy, several percent of the total body content of gold is in the blood, where it is first bound (about 95%) to albumin. The concentration in synovial fluid eventually reaches about half that in plasma. With continued therapy, the concentration of gold in the synovium of affected joints is about ten times that of skeletal muscle, bone, or fat. Gold deposits also are found in macrophages of many tissues, as well as in proximal tubular epithelium, seminiferous tubules, hepatocytes, and adrenocortical cells.

The pharmacokinetic properties of gold in these compounds are complex and vary with the dose and the duration of treatment. The plasma half-life is about 7 days for a 50-mg dose. With successive doses, the half-life lengthens, and values of weeks or months may be observed after prolonged therapy, reflecting the avid binding of gold in tissues. After a cumulative dose of 1 g of gold, about 60% of the amount administered is retained in the body. After termination of treatment, urinary excretion of gold can be detected for as long as a year, even though concentrations in blood fall to the normal trace amounts in about 40 to 80 days. Substantial quantities of gold have been found in the liver and skin of patients many years after the

cessation of therapy. The excretion of gold is 60% to 90% renal and 10% to 40% fecal, the latter probably mostly by biliary secretion. Sulfhydryl agents, such as dimercaprol, penicillamine, and N-acetylcysteine, increase the excretion of gold.

Auranofin. Auranofin is a more hydrophobic gold-containing compound that is absorbed more readily after oral administration (to the extent of about 25%). Steady-state concentrations of gold in plasma are proportional to the doses administered and are reached after 8 to 12 weeks of treatment. Therapeutic doses of auranofin (6 mg per day) lead to concentrations of gold in plasma that typically are lower than those achieved with conventional parenteral therapy, and the accumulation of gold during a 6-month course of treatment with auranofin is only about 20% of that found with injectable gold compounds. Studies in animals suggest that auranofin binds to tissues to a lesser extent than does gold sodium thiomalate. After cessation of treatment, the half-life of gold in the body is about 80 days. Auranofin is predominantly excreted in the feces.

Toxic Effects. The most common toxic effects associated with the therapeutic use of gold are those that involve the skin and the mucous membranes, usually of the mouth. These occur in about 15% of all patients. While clearly dose-related, these effects do not correlate well with the concentration of gold in plasma. Cutaneous reactions may vary in severity from simple erythema to severe exfoliative dermatitis. Lesions of the mucous membranes include stomatitis, pharyngitis, tracheitis, gastritis, colitis, and vaginitis; glossitis is fairly common. A gray-to-blue pigmentation (chrysiasis) may occur in the skin and mucous membranes, especially in areas exposed to light.

In 5% to 10% of patients receiving gold, kidney function also may be affected. Transient and mild proteinuria occurs in more than 50% of patients during therapy. Heavy albuminuria and microscopic hematuria occur in 1% to 3% of cases. The site of damage is usually the proximal tubules. In addition, a gold-induced nephrosis can occur; the predominant lesion is membranous glomerulonephritis that is usually reversible by cessation of treatment.

Severe blood dyscrasias also may occur. Thrombocytopenia is observed in about 1% of patients. Most often this appears to be an immunological disturbance that results in an accelerated degradation of platelets. Occasionally the thrombocytopenia is a consequence of effects upon the bone marrow. In either case, withdrawal of the drug usually leads to recovery, but fatalities have occurred. Leukopenia, agranulocytosis, and aplastic anemia also may occur; aplastic anemia is rare but often fatal.

Auranofin appears to be better tolerated than are the injectable gold compounds, and the incidence and severity of mucocutaneous and hematological side effects are less. However, auranofin produces a high incidence of gastrointestinal disturbances, which lead to discontinuation of therapy by about 5% of patients receiving the drug. About half of patients have a change in bowel habits (more frequent or loose stools often associated with abdominal cramping). Proteinuria is less common with auranofin than with parenteral preparations, and the incidence of nephrotoxicity also may be less.

Gold may cause a variety of other severe toxic reactions, including encephalitis, peripheral neuritis, hepatitis, pulmonary infiltrates, and nitritoid (vasomotor) crisis. Fortunately, these reactions are infrequent and, when encountered, usually result from failure to discontinue therapy when earlier, less serious symptoms occur.

Avoidance and Treatment. Regular examination of the skin, buccal mucosa, urine, and blood, including cell and platelet counts, should be made. It is the practice in many arthritis clinics to initiate therapy with small doses of gold and to increase the dose gradually. Although untoward effects are not eliminated by this procedure, the severity of the reactions that occur early is somewhat reduced. If an untoward response occurs, therapy should be withheld until the adverse effect subsides completely. If the reaction is a rash or stomatitis, antihistamines and glucocorticoids may be administered, the latter systemically and/or topically. Glucocorticoids also are also indicated in gold-induced nephrosis.

If the reaction to gold therapy is not serious, injections of parenteral gold preparations may be cautiously resumed 2 or 3 weeks after the toxic reaction has subsided. Maintenance dosage should be two-thirds to three-fourths that previously planned. However, many experts decline to use the drug again once toxicity has occurred. For auranofin, a decrease in dosage also can be attempted, but therapeutic responses may not be obtained.

If a severe reaction to gold occurs or if the above-mentioned steps fail to control the toxic effects, treatment with dimercaprol and glucocorticoid should be instituted. Dimercaprol chelates gold and the chelate is then excreted. Accordingly, the administration of dimercaprol may shorten a therapeutic remission induced by gold.

Therapeutic Uses. Gold compounds find their chief therapeutic application in rheumatoid arthritis. In part because these compounds can cause serious toxicity, and, in the case of oral gold, perhaps less efficacy, the use of gold compounds as second-line therapy for rheumatoid arthritis has declined in recent years (Cash and Klippel, 1994).

At present, gold is used in early, active arthritis, particularly for disease that progresses despite an adequate regimen of NSAIDs, rest, and physical therapy. Both subjective and objective manifestations of rheumatoid arthritis are improved. Gold compounds often arrest, at least temporarily, the progression of the disease in involved joints; prevent involvement of unaffected joints; improve grip strength and morning stiffness; and decrease the erythrocyte sedimentation rate and abnormal plasma glycoprotein and fibrinogen levels. Gold should not be used if the disease is mild, and it usually is of little benefit when the disease is advanced.

The optimal intramuscular dosage schedule for the treatment of rheumatoid arthritis is still debated. The usual dose is 10 mg of *aurothioglucose* (SOLGANAL) or *gold sodium thiomalate,* in the first week as a test dose, followed by 25 mg in the second and third weeks. Thereafter, either 25 to 50 mg (gold sodium thiomalate) or 50 mg (aurothioglucose) is administered at weekly intervals until the cumulative dose reaches 1 g. A favorable response may not be evident for a few months. If a remission occurs, treatment is continued, but the dose is reduced or the dosage interval is increased.

For oral therapy of active rheumatoid arthritis, the daily dosage is 3 to 6 mg of *auranofin* (RIDAURA), which is given in one or two portions; some patients may require 9 mg daily in three divided doses. This higher dosage should not be instituted until the lower dosage has been given for 6 months, and therapy should be discontinued after 3 additional months if the response is still inadequate. Although patients have been maintained

successfully on auranofin for several years, the optimal duration of therapy has not been determined.

Therapy with gold is sometimes beneficial in juvenile rheumatoid arthritis, palindromic rheumatism, psoriatic arthritis, Sjögren's syndrome, nondisseminated lupus erythematosus, and pemphigus. Except for injectable preparations in the treatment of juvenile forms of arthritis, the use of gold in these conditions has not been approved in the United States.

Contraindications. Gold therapy is contraindicated in patients with renal disease, hepatic dysfunction or a history of infectious hepatitis, or hematological disorders. Gold should not be readministered to patients who have developed severe hematological or renal toxicity during a course of chrysotherapy; auranofin should not be administered after the occurrence of several additional gold-induced disorders, including pulmonary fibrosis, necrotizing enterocolitis, and exfoliative dermatitis. Gold is contraindicated during pregnancy or breast-feeding. Patients who recently have had radiation should not receive gold because of its depressant action on hematopoietic tissue. Concomitant use of antimalarials, immunosuppressants, penicillamine, or dipyrone is contraindicated because of the potential of these drugs to cause blood dyscrasias. Urticaria, eczema, and colitis also are considered to be contraindications to the use of gold. Finally, gold is poorly tolerated by elderly individuals.

OTHER DRUGS FOR RHEUMATOID ARTHRITIS

In addition to nonsteroidal antiinflammatory agents and gold, other drugs also are used for the treatment of rheumatoid arthritis. These include immunosuppressive agents [*e.g., cyclosporine, azathioprine* (*see* Chapter 53), *leflunomide,* and the folate antagonist, *methotrexate* (*see* Chapters 52 and 53)], *glucocorticoids* (*see* Chapter 60), *penicillamine,* and *hydroxychloroquine.* With the exception of glucocorticoids, sulfasalazine, and, perhaps, methotrexate, these drugs do not possess antiinflammatory or analgesic properties. In general, their therapeutic effects become evident only after several weeks or months of treatment. They are reserved for patients who are refractory to therapeutic regimens that include rest, physiotherapy, and NSAIDs.

Although glucocorticoids often can produce dramatic symptomatic improvement, these agents do not arrest the progress of rheumatoid arthritis and are used only as adjuvants to other treatment because of their long-term toxicity (*see* Chapter 60). Immunosuppressants sometimes relieve joint inflammation, but each of these drugs has its unique and significant toxicities (*see* Chapter 53). Of the cytotoxic immunosuppressants, only azathioprine and low oral doses of methotrexate have been approved for the treatment of rheumatoid arthritis. Methotrexate appears to be a particularly useful drug for second-line therapy in rheumatoid arthritis (Felson *et al.,* 1992). Cyclosporine also has been shown to be effective in many patients, but its use is commonly associated with nephrotoxicity, especially in patients receiving concomitant treatment with NSAIDs (*see* Chapter 53 and Faulds *et al.,* 1993).

Even though their mechanisms of action are not understood, hydroxychloroquine and penicillamine are useful, orally effective alternatives to gold in the treatment of patients with early, mild, and nonerosive disease. Penicillamine is more apt to produce serious toxicity, including various cutaneous lesions, blood dyscrasias, and a number of autoimmune syndromes (*see* Chapter 67).

Hydroxychloroquine shares the toxicity of other 4-amino-quinoline antimalarials (*see* Chapter 40). Of greatest concern during the long-term treatment of rheumatoid arthritis is the danger of producing irreversible retinal damage. The risk of corneal deposits and ocular toxicity appears to be less for hydroxychloroquine than for chloroquine at the usual antirheumatic doses (200 to 400 mg daily). Even so, ophthalmological examinations should be performed before treatment is begun and every 3 to 6 months thereafter.

DRUGS EMPLOYED IN THE TREATMENT OF GOUT

An acute attack of gout occurs as a result of an inflammatory reaction to crystals of sodium urate (the end product of purine metabolism in human beings) that are deposited in the joint tissue. The inflammatory response involves local infiltration of granulocytes, which phagocytize the urate crystals. Lactate production is high in synovial tissues and in the leukocytes associated with the inflammatory process, and this favors a local decrease in pH that fosters further deposition of uric acid. Deposition of urate crystals occurs in patients with hyperuricemia, which is caused by increased production or decreased excretion of uric acid.

Several therapeutic strategies can be used to counter attacks of gout. *Uricosuric drugs* increase the excretion of uric acid, thus reducing concentrations in plasma. *Colchicine,* although associated with a high frequency of toxicity, is specifically efficacious in gout, probably secondary to an effect on the mobility of granulocytes. Allopurinol is a selective inhibitor of the terminal steps of the biosynthesis of uric acid. Although prostaglandins may be implicated in the pain and inflammation, there is no evidence that they contribute to the pathogenesis of gout; nevertheless, nonsalicylate-containing NSAIDs afford symptomatic relief, and some of them are uricosuric as well.

The pharmacology of NSAIDs is described in a previous section. Discussion in this section is limited to colchicine, allopurinol, and the uricosuric agents.

Colchicine

Colchicine is a unique antiinflammatory agent in that it is largely effective only against gouty arthritis. It provides dramatic relief of acute attacks of gout, and is an effective prophylactic agent against such attacks.

History. Colchicine is an alkaloid of *Colchicum autumnale* (autumn crocus, meadow saffron). Although the poisonous action of colchicum was known to Dioscorides, preparations of the plant were not recommended for pain of articular origin until the sixth century A.D. Colchicum was introduced for the therapy of acute gout by von Störck in 1763, and its specificity for this syndrome soon resulted in its incorporation in a number of "gout mixtures" popularized by charlatans. Benjamin Franklin, himself a sufferer from gout, is reputed to have introduced colchicum therapy in the United States. The alkaloid colchicine was isolated from colchicum in 1820 by Pelletier and Caventou.

Chemistry. The structural formula of colchicine is as follows:

COLCHICINE

The structure–activity relationship of colchicine and related agents has been discussed by Wallace (1961).

Pharmacological Properties. The antiinflammatory effect of colchicine in acute gouty arthritis is relatively selective for this disorder. Colchicine is only occasionally effective in other types of arthritis; it is not an analgesic and does not provide relief of other types of pain.

Colchicine is an antimitotic agent and is widely employed as an experimental tool in the study of cell division and function.

Effect in Gout. Colchicine does not influence the renal excretion of uric acid or its concentration in blood. By virtue of its ability to bind to tubulin, colchicine interferes with the function of the mitotic spindles and causes depolymerization and disappearance of the fibrillar microtubules in granulocytes and other motile cells. This action is apparently the basis for the beneficial effect of colchicine, namely, the inhibition of the migration of granulocytes into the inflamed area and a decreased metabolic and phagocytic activity of granulocytes. This reduces the release of lactic acid and proinflammatory enzymes that occurs during phagocytosis and breaks the cycle that leads to the inflammatory response.

Neutrophils exposed to urate crystals ingest them and produce a glycoprotein, which may be the causative agent of acute gouty arthritis. Injected into joints, this substance produces a profound arthritis that is histologically indistinguishable from that caused by direct injection of urate crystals. Colchicine appears to prevent the elaboration by leukocytes of this glycoprotein.

Effect on Cell Division. Colchicine can arrest plant and animal cell division *in vitro* and *in vivo*. Mitosis is arrested in metaphase, due to failure of spindle formation. Cells with the highest rates of division are affected earliest. High concentrations may completely prevent cells from entering mitosis, and they often die. The action also is characteristic of the vinca alkaloids (*vincristine* and *vinblastine*), *podophyllotoxin,* and *griseofulvin.*

Other Effects. Colchicine inhibits the release of histamine-containing granules from mast cells, the secretion of insulin from beta cells of pancreatic islets, and the movement of melanin granules in melanophores. Although it is questionable whether or not these effects occur at clinically achieved concentrations of colchicine, all of these processes may involve the translocation of granules by the microtubular system.

Colchicine also exhibits a variety of other pharmacological effects. It lowers body temperature, increases the sensitivity to central depressants, depresses the respiratory center, enhances the response to sympathomimetic agents, constricts blood vessels, and induces hypertension by central vasomotor stimulation. It enhances gastrointestinal activity by neurogenic stimulation but depresses it by a direct effect, and alters neuromuscular function.

Pharmacokinetics and Metabolism. Colchicine is rapidly absorbed after oral administration, and peak concentrations occur in plasma by 0.5 to 2 hours. Large amounts of the drug and metabolites enter the intestinal tract in the bile and intestinal secretions, and this fact, plus the rapid turnover of intestinal epithelium, probably explains the prominence of intestinal manifestations in colchicine poisoning. The kidney, liver, and spleen also contain high concentrations of colchicine, but it is apparently largely excluded from heart, skeletal muscle, and brain. The drug can be detected in leukocytes and in the urine for at least 9 days after a single intravenous dose.

Colchicine is metabolized to a mixture of compounds *in vitro.* Most of the drug is excreted in the feces; however, in normal individuals, 10% to 20% of the drug is excreted in the urine. In patients with liver disease, hepatic uptake and elimination are reduced and a greater fraction of the drug is excreted in the urine.

Toxic Effects. The most common side effects reflect the action of colchicine on the rapidly proliferating epithelial cells in the gastrointestinal tract, especially in the jejunum. Nausea, vomiting, diarrhea, and abdominal pain are the most common and earliest untoward effects of colchicine overdosage. To avoid more serious toxicity, administration of the drug should be discontinued as soon as these symptoms occur. There is a latent period of several hours or more between the administration of the drug and the onset of symptoms. This interval is not altered by dosage or route of administration. For this reason, and because of individual variation, adverse effects may be unavoidable during an initial course of medication with colchicine. However, since patients often remain relatively consistent in their response to a given dose of the drug, toxicity can be reduced or avoided during subsequent courses of therapy by reducing the dose. The drug is equally effective when given intravenously; the onset of the therapeutic effect may be faster, and the gastrointestinal side effects may be almost completely avoided.

In acute poisoning with colchicine, there is hemorrhagic gastroenteritis, extensive vascular damage, nephrotoxicity, muscular depression, and an ascending paralysis of the CNS.

Colchicine produces a temporary leukopenia that is soon replaced by a leukocytosis, sometimes due to a striking increase in the number of basophilic granulocytes. The site of action is apparently directly on the bone marrow. Myopathy and neuropathy also have been noted with colchicine treatment, especially in patients with decreased renal function. Long-term administration of colchicine entails some risk of agranulocytosis, aplastic anemia, myopathy, and alopecia; azoospermia also has been described.

Therapeutic Uses. Colchicine provides dramatic relief from acute attacks of gout. The effect is sufficiently selective that the drug has been used for diagnostic purposes, but the test is not infallible. Colchicine also has an established role to prevent and to abort acute attacks of gout. However, its toxicity and the availability of alternative agents that are less toxic have substantially lessened its usefulness.

Acute Attacks. When colchicine is given promptly within the first few hours of an attack, fewer than 5% of patients fail to obtain relief. Pain, swelling, and redness abate within 12 hours and are completely gone within 48 to 72 hours. Although for many years colchicine was administered orally, current practice is to administer the drug intravenously (*see* Wallace and Singer, 1988). Although a number of regimens have been used, a single dose of 2 mg, diluted in 10 to 20 ml of 0.9% sodium chloride solution, usually is adequate; a total dose of 4 mg should not be exceeded. To avoid cumulative toxicity, treatment with colchicine should not be repeated within 7 days.

Great care should be exercised in prescribing colchicine for elderly patients, and for those with cardiac, renal, hepatic, or gastrointestinal disease. In these patients and in those who do not tolerate or respond to colchicine, indomethacin or another NSAID is preferred.

Prophylactic Uses. For patients with chronic gout, colchicine has established value as a prophylactic agent, especially when there is frequent recurrence of attacks. Prophylactic medication also is indicated upon initiation of long-term medication with allopurinol or the uricosuric agents, since acute attacks often increase in frequency during the early months of such therapy.

The prophylactic dose of colchicine depends upon the frequency and severity of prior attacks. As small an oral dose as 0.5 mg two to four times a week may suffice; as much as 1.8 mg per day may be required by some patients. Colchicine should be taken in larger abortive doses immediately upon the first twinge of articular pain or the appearance of any prodrome of an acute attack. Before and after surgery in patients with gout, colchicine should be given for 3 days (0.5 or 0.6 mg, three times a day); this greatly reduces the very high incidence of acute attacks of gouty arthritis precipitated by operative procedures.

Daily administration of colchicine is useful for the prevention of attacks of familial Mediterranean fever (familial paroxysmal polyserositis) and for prevention and treatment of amyloidosis in such patients (Zemer *et al.,* 1991). Colchicine appears to benefit patients with primary biliary cirrhosis in terms of improvement of liver function tests and perhaps of survival (Warnes, 1991). Colchicine also has been employed to treat a variety of skin disorders, including psoriasis and Behçet's syndrome.

Allopurinol

Allopurinol is effective for the treatment of both the primary hyperuricemia of gout and that secondary to hematological disorders or antineoplastic therapy. In contrast to the uricosuric agents that increase the renal excretion of urate, allopurinol inhibits the terminal steps in uric acid biosynthesis. Since overproduction of uric acid is a contributing factor in most patients with gout and a characteristic of most types of secondary hyperuricemia, allopurinol represents a rational approach to therapy.

History. The introduction of allopurinol by Hitchings, Elion, and associates provides an elegant example of the development of a drug on a rational biochemical basis. Originally synthesized as a candidate for an antineoplastic agent, allopurinol was found to lack antimetabolite activity, but it proved to be a substrate for and an inhibitor of xanthine oxidase. Allopurinol delays inactivation of mercaptopurine by xanthine oxidase and reduces the plasma concentration and renal excretion of uric acid. Subsequent clinical study for treatment of gout by Rundles and coworkers was successful and quickly confirmed.

Chemistry and Pharmacological Properties. Allopurinol, an analog of hypoxanthine, has the following structural formula:

ALLOPURINOL

Both allopurinol and its primary metabolite, oxypurinol (alloxanthine), are inhibitors of xanthine oxidase. Inhibition of this enzyme accounts for the major pharmacological effects of allopurinol.

In human beings, uric acid is formed primarily by the xanthine oxidase–catalyzed oxidation of hypoxanthine and xanthine. At low concentrations, allopurinol is a substrate for and competitive inhibitor of the enzyme; at high concentrations, it is a noncompetitive inhibitor. Oxypurinol, the metabolite of allopurinol formed by the action of xanthine oxidase, is a noncompetitive inhibitor of the enzyme; the formation of this compound, together with its long persistence in tissues, is responsible for much of the pharmacological activity of allopurinol. Inhibition of uric acid biosynthesis reduces its plasma concentration and urinary excretion and increases the plasma concentrations and renal excretion of the more soluble oxypurine precursors.

In the absence of allopurinol, the urinary content of purines is almost solely uric acid. During treatment with allopurinol, the urinary purines are divided among hypoxanthine, xanthine, and uric acid. Since each has its independent solubility, the concentration of uric acid in plasma is reduced without exposing the urinary tract to an excessive load of uric acid and the likelihood of calculus formation. By lowering the uric acid concentration in plasma below its limit of solubility, allopurinol facilitates the dissolution of tophi and prevents the development or progression of chronic gouty arthritis. The formation of uric acid stones virtually disappears with therapy, and this prevents the development of nephropathy. Although it appears that gouty nephropathy can be reversed by allopurinol if administered before renal function is severely compromised, there is little evidence of improvement in advanced renal disease. The incidence of acute attacks of gouty arthritis may increase during the early months of therapy as a consequence of mobilization of tissue stores of uric acid. Coadministration of colchicine helps suppress such acute attacks. Following reduction of excess tissue stores of uric acid, the incidence of acute attacks decreases.

Tissue deposition of xanthine and hypoxanthine usually does not occur during allopurinol therapy because the renal clearance of the oxypurines is rapid; their plasma concentrations are only slightly increased and do not exceed their solubility. Although xanthine constitutes about 50% of total oxypurine excreted in the urine and is relatively insoluble, xanthine stone formation during allopurinol therapy has occurred only occasionally in patients with very high uric acid production prior to treatment. The risk can be minimized by alkalinization of the urine and by increasing the daily fluid intake during the administration of allopurinol. In some patients, the allopurinol-induced increase in excretion of oxypurines is less than the reduction in uric acid excretion; this disparity is primarily a result of reutilization of oxypurines and feedback inhibition of *de novo* purine biosynthesis.

Pharmacokinetics and Metabolism. Allopurinol is absorbed relatively rapidly after oral ingestion, and peak plasma concentrations are reached within 60 to 90 minutes. About 20% is excreted in the feces in 48 to 72 hours, presumably as unabsorbed drug. Allopurinol is rapidly cleared from plasma with a half-time of 1 to 2 hours, primarily by conversion to oxypurinol. Less than 10% of a single dose or about 30% of the drug ingested during long-term medication is excreted unchanged in the urine. Oxypurinol is slowly excreted in the urine by the net balance of glomerular filtration and probenecid-sensitive tubular reabsorption. The plasma half-life of oxypurinol is 18 to 30 hours in patients with normal renal function and increases in proportion to the reduction of glomerular filtration in patients with renal impairment.

Allopurinol and its active metabolite oxypurinol are distributed in total tissue water, with the exception of brain, in which their concentration is about one-third that in other tissues. Neither compound is bound to plasma proteins. The plasma concentrations of the two compounds do not correlate well with therapeutic or toxic effects.

Drug Interactions. Allopurinol increases the half-life of probenecid and enhances its uricosuric effect, while probenecid increases the clearance of oxypurinol, thereby increasing dose requirements of allopurinol. Allopurinol decreases metabolism and clearance of mercaptopurine (and its derivative azathioprine); thus the dosage of mercaptopurine and azathioprine should be reduced when coadministered with allopurinol. Allopurinol also may interfere with the hepatic inactivation of other drugs, including the oral anticoagulant agents. Although the effect is variable and of clinical significance only in some patients, increased monitoring of prothrombin activity is recommended in patients receiving both medications.

Whether the increased incidence of skin rash in patients receiving concurrent allopurinol–ampicillin medication, compared with that observed when these agents are administered individually, should be ascribed to allopurinol or to hyperuricemia remains to be established. Hypersensitivity reactions have been reported in patients with compromised renal function, especially those who are receiving a combination of allopurinol and a thiazide diuretic. The concomitant administration of allopurinol and theophylline leads to increased accumulation of an active metabolite of theophylline, 1-methylxanthine; the concentration of theophylline in plasma also may be increased (*see* Chapter 28).

Therapeutic Uses.   *Allopurinol* (ZYLOPRIM, ALOPRIM, others) is available for oral use and provides effective therapy for both the primary hyperuricemia of gout and that secondary to polycythemia vera, myeloid metaplasia, or other blood dyscrasias.

Allopurinol is contraindicated in patients who have exhibited serious adverse effects or hypersensitivity skin rash from the medication, nursing mothers, and children, except those with malignancy or certain inborn errors of purine metabolism.

In gout, allopurinol generally is used in the severe chronic forms characterized by one or more of the following conditions: gouty nephropathy, tophaceous deposits, renal urate stones, impaired renal function, or hyperuricemia not readily controlled by the uricosuric drugs.

The aim of therapy is to reduce the plasma uric acid concentration below 6 mg/dl (equivalent to 360 μM). Medication must not be initiated during an acute attack of gouty arthritis, and it is started at low doses to minimize the risk of precipitating such attacks. Concurrent prophylactic administration of colchicine also is recommended during and sometimes beyond the initial months of therapy. Fluid intake should be sufficient to maintain daily urinary volume above 2 liters; slightly alkaline urine is preferred. An initial daily dose of 100 mg is increased by 100-mg increments at weekly intervals to a maximum of 800 mg per day. The usual daily maintenance dose for adults is 200 to 300 mg for those with mild gout and 400 to 600 mg for patients with moderately severe tophaceous gout. Daily doses in excess of 300 mg should be given in divided portions. Dosage must be reduced in patients with renal impairment in proportion to the reduction in glomerular filtration (Hande *et al.*, 1984).

Allopurinol also is administered prophylactically to reduce the hyperuricemia and to prevent urate deposition or renal calculi in patients with leukemias, lymphomas, or other malignancies, particularly when antineoplastic or radiation therapy is initiated. A dose of 600 to 800 mg daily for 2 to 3 days is advisable, together with a high fluid intake. In children with secondary hyperuricemias associated with malignancies, the usual daily dose is 150 to 300 mg, depending upon age.

Allopurinol inhibits the enzymatic inactivation of mercaptopurine and its derivative azathioprine by xanthine oxidase. Thus, when allopurinol is used concomitantly with oral mercaptopurine or azathioprine, dosage of the antineoplastic agent must be reduced to one-fourth to one-third of the usual dose (*see* Chapter 52). The risk of bone-marrow suppression also is increased when allopurinol is administered with cytotoxic agents that are not metabolized by xanthine oxidase, particularly cyclophosphamide.

The iatrogenic hyperuricemia sometimes induced by the thiazides and other drugs can be prevented or reversed by concurrent allopurinol medication, although this is rarely necessary.

Allopurinol also is useful in lowering the high plasma concentrations of uric acid in patients with Lesch-Nyhan syndrome and thereby prevents the complications resulting from hyperuricemia; there is no evidence that it alters the progressive neurological and behavioral abnormalities characteristic of the disease.

Toxic Effects.   Allopurinol is well tolerated by most patients. The most common adverse effects are hypersensitivity reactions. They may occur even after months or years of medication. The effects usually subside within a few days after medication is discontinued. Serious reactions preclude further use of the drug.

Attacks of acute gout may occur more frequently during the initial months of allopurinol medication and may require concurrent prophylactic therapy with colchicine (*see* above).

The cutaneous reaction caused by allopurinol is predominantly a pruritic, erythematous, or maculopapular eruption, but occasionally the lesion is urticarial or purpuric. In rare patients, toxic epidermal necrolysis or Stevens-Johnson syndrome occurs, which can be fatal. This risk for Stevens-Johnson syndrome is primarily limited to the first 2 months of treatment (Roujeau *et al.*, 1995). Fever, malaise, and muscle aching also may occur. Such effects are noted in about 3% of patients with normal renal function but more frequently in those with renal impairment. Since the onset of skin rash may be followed by severe hypersensitivity reactions, allopurinol should be discontinued by patients who develop such rashes.

Transient leukopenia or leukocytosis and eosinophilia are rare reactions but may require cessation of therapy. Hepatomegaly and elevated levels of aminotransferase activities in plasma and progressive renal insufficiency also may occur.

URICOSURIC AGENTS

A uricosuric agent is a drug that increases the rate of excretion of uric acid. There is perhaps no other class of therapeutic agents for which the observations in their entirety appear so inconsistent and at times contradictory. This results from the complexity of the transport mechanisms, as well as the marked species variation of individual mechanisms and their sensitivity to drug action. Birds, reptiles, and some mammals demonstrate net secretion of urate; in some mammalian species both net secretion and net reabsorption can be observed; and in others, including human beings, net reabsorption is found almost invariably. In human beings and in other species that demonstrate net reabsorption, the reabsorptive process is mediated by a specific transporter and it is inhibitable. Finally, in all species that have been studied thoroughly, the major transport mechanism, either secretion or reabsorption, is opposed by a smaller flux operating in the opposite direction; that is, there is bidirectional transport. As a consequence of all these factors, a drug that is uricosuric in one species may produce urate retention in another; within one species a drug may cause either urate retention or uricosuria, depending on the dose; and one uricosuric drug may either add to or inhibit the action of another.

In human beings, uric acid is largely reabsorbed; the amount excreted is usually about 10% of that filtered. Studies with proximal tubule brush-border membranes indicate that the first step in reabsorption is the uptake of urate from tubular fluid by a transporter that can act as an anion exchanger. Thus, urate in the tubular fluid can be exchanged for either an organic or an inorganic anion moving in the opposite direction. It has been suggested that the anionic compositions of luminal and intracellular fluids are such that reabsorption of urate is favored. The exit step for urate at the basolateral membrane also is mediated by an anion exchanger. Uricosuric drugs, when present in the lumen or when tested in isolated brush-border members, compete with urate for the brush-border transporter, thereby inhibiting its reabsorption *via* the urate–anion exchanger system.

The *paradoxical effect of uricosuric agents* refers to the fact that, depending on dosage, a drug may either decrease or increase the excretion of uric acid. Decreased excretion usually occurs at a low dosage, while increased excretion is observed at a higher dosage. Not all agents show this phenomenon. With some drugs, such as salicylate, the biphasic effect may be seen within the normal dosage range. Two mechanisms for a drug-induced decrease in excretion of urate have been advanced; they are not mutually exclusive. The first presumes that the small secretory movement of urate is mediated by a mechanism that is thought to be extremely sensitive to low concentrations of compounds such as salicylate. Higher concentrations may inhibit urate reabsorption in the usual manner. The second proposal suggests that the urate-retaining anionic drug gains access to the intracellular fluid by an independent mechanism and promotes reabsorption of urate across the brush border by anion exchange.

There are two mechanisms by which one drug may nullify the uricosuric action of another. First, the drug may inhibit the secretion of the uricosuric agent, thereby denying it access to its site of action, the luminal aspect of the brush border. Second, the inhibition of urate secretion by one drug may counterbalance the inhibition of urate reabsorption by the other (Fanelli and Weiner, 1979). There are situations in which two uricosuric agents administered together almost completely nullify each other's actions (*see,* for example, Yü *et al.,* 1963). In such an instance, one of the drugs (A) must have a strong paradoxical action. Drug B inhibits the secretion of A, thereby preventing its uricosuric action but not its urate-retaining action. The latter effect balances the uricosuric action of drug B.

There are a great many compounds that have uricosuric activity, but only a few are prescribed for this purpose. *Probenecid* and *sulfinpyrazone* are the two uricosuric drugs available in the United States; *benzbromarone* is a uricosuric agent that is not available in the United States but is used in Europe. Some drugs have other primary pharmacological actions, and their ability to increase urate excretion is either incidental or unexpected. In all instances the active compound is probably either an anionic drug or an anionic metabolite. On the other hand, there are a number of drugs and toxins that cause retention of urate. Both classes of compounds have been reviewed by Emmerson (1978).

Probenecid

History. Probenecid was developed as a result of a planned approach to achieve a specific objective. When penicillin was first introduced, it was in critically short supply and the rapid renal excretion of the antibiotic was thus of practical significance. For this reason, Beyer and associates began a study to find an organic acid that would depress the tubular secretion of penicillin in the manner described above. The first compound to be evaluated clinically was *carinamide*. It proved to be effective, but the drug was secreted by the renal tubules fairly rapidly and it was necessary to give frequent doses. This problem was overcome with the discovery of probenecid (Beyer *et al.,* 1951).

Chemistry. Probenecid is a highly lipid-soluble benzoic acid derivative (pKa 3.4) with the following structural formula:

$$CH_3CH_2CH_2 \diagdown \qquad CH_3CH_2CH_2 \diagup NSO_2 \text{—} \bigcirc \text{—COOH}$$

PROBENECID

Pharmacological Actions. *Inhibition of Inorganic Acid Transport.* The actions of probenecid are confined largely to inhibition of the transport of organic acids across epithelial barriers. This is most important for the renal tubule, in which tubular secretion of many drugs and drug metabolites is inhibited. The renal action of probenecid reduces the concentrations of certain compounds in urine and raises them in plasma. This is a desirable therapeutic effect in the case of penicillin and related antibiotics that have a beneficial systemic action, but it may be undesirable with an agent such as nitrofurantoin when it is employed as a urinary antiseptic. When tubular secretion of a substance is inhibited, its final concentration in the urine is determined by the degree of filtration, which in turn is a function of binding to plasma protein, and by the degree of reabsorption. The significance of each of these factors varies widely with different compounds.

Uric acid is the only important endogenous compound whose excretion is known to be increased by probenecid. This results from inhibition of its reabsorption (*see* above). The uricosuric action of probenecid is blunted by the administration of salicylates.

Inhibition of Transport of Miscellaneous Substances. Probenecid inhibits the tubular secretion of a number of drugs, such as methotrexate and the active metabolite of clofibrate, but there is no clinical indication for the coadministration of probenecid in most instances. Probenecid inhibits renal secretion of the glucuronides of NSAIDs such as naproxen, ketoprofen, and indomethacin and thereby can increase plasma concentrations of such compounds. However, these metabolites are inactive. In the case of a number of endogenous or exogenous organic acids whose rate of excretion is determined for diagnostic purposes, misleading values may be obtained if the patient is receiving probenecid.

Inhibition of Monoamine Transport to CSF. Probenecid inhibits the transport of 5-hydroxyindoleacetic acid (5-HIAA) and other acidic metabolites of cerebral monoamines from the sub-arachnoid space to the plasma. The transport of drugs such as penicillin G also may be affected.

Inhibition of Biliary Excretion. Since probenecid and some of its metabolites may be secreted into the bile, it is not surprising that probenecid depresses the biliary secretion of other compounds, including the diagnostic agents indocyanine green and sulfobromophthalein (BSP). The inhibition of biliary secretion also has implications in the use of rifampin for the treatment of tuberculosis. Higher concentrations of the antibiotic are achieved in plasma if probenecid is administered concurrently.

Absorption, Fate, and Excretion. Probenecid is completely absorbed after oral administration. Peak concentrations in plasma are reached in 2 to 4 hours. The half-life of the drug in plasma is dose-dependent and varies from less than 5 hours to more than 8 hours over the therapeutic range. Between 85% and 95% of the drug is bound to plasma albumin. The small unbound portion gains access to the glomerular filtrate; a much larger portion is actively secreted by the proximal tubule. The high lipid solubility of the undissociated form results in virtually complete absorption by back diffusion unless the urine is markedly alkaline. A small amount of probenecid glucuronide appears in the urine. It is also hydroxylated to metabolites that retain their carboxyl function and have uricosuric activity.

Toxic Effects. Probenecid is well tolerated by most patients. Some degree of gastrointestinal irritation is experienced by at least 2% of patients; the incidence is considerably higher after large doses. Caution is advised in administering probenecid to patients with a history of peptic ulcer. Most reports place the incidence of hypersensitivity reactions, usually mild skin rashes, between 2% and 4%. More serious hypersensitivity reactions occur, but they are rare. The appearance of a rash during the concurrent administration of probenecid and penicillin G or a congener presents the physician with an awkward diagnostic dilemma. Huge overdosage of probenecid results in stimulation of the central nervous system, convulsions, and death from respiratory failure.

Therapeutic Use. *Probenecid* is marketed for oral administration. In the treatment of chronic gout, 250 mg is given twice daily for 1 week, following which 500 mg is administered twice daily. In some patients it may be necessary to increase the daily dosage gradually to a maximum of 2 g, given in four divided portions. Liberal fluid intake should be maintained throughout therapy because of the tendency of probenecid to produce uric acid stones. For this reason, probenecid should not be used in gouty patients with nephrolithiasis or with overproduction of uric acid. In addition, an acute gouty attack may be precipitated in up to 20% of gouty patients treated with probenecid alone. Thus, concomitant therapy should include colchicine or an NSAID. To block the renal excretion of penicillin effectively, a total daily dose of 2 g is employed in adults. This is administered in four divided doses. For children weighing less than 50 kg, an initial dose of 25 mg/kg is followed by maintenance doses of 10 mg/kg given four times daily.

Adjunct in Penicillin Therapy. The oral administration of probenecid in conjunction with penicillin G results in higher and more prolonged concentrations of the antibiotic in plasma than when penicillin is given alone. The elevation in the plasma

level is at least twofold and sometimes much greater. Although the reduction of a daily dose of penicillin G from 1 million to 500,000 units has very little significance, a reduction by 50% or more may be of importance for convenience in the treatment of resistant infections that may require the administration of penicillin G in very large doses. This combined regimen also may be useful to minimize the amount of K^+ that is administered to some patients who receive very large doses of penicillin. Probenecid also is included in certain regimens that can be completed during one visit to the physician for the treatment and prophylaxis of gonococcal infections (*see* Chapter 46).

Sulfinpyrazone

History. Despite its therapeutic efficacy as an antiinflammatory and uricosuric agent, phenylbutazone (*see* above) had undesirable side effects severe enough to preclude its continuous use. For this reason, a number of congeners were evaluated for uricosuric and antiinflammatory activity. One of these, in which a phenylthioethyl configuration replaces the butyl side chain of the parent compound, displayed promising activity. When the metabolites of the new compound were studied, it was found that side chain oxidation *in vivo* led to the formation of the sulfoxide, sulfinpyrazone, which was a potent uricosuric agent.

Chemistry. The chemical structure of sulfinpyrazone is as follows:

SULFINPYRAZONE

It is a strong organic acid (p*Ka* 2.8) that readily forms soluble salts.

Pharmacological Actions. Sulfinpyrazone in sufficient dosage is a potent inhibitor of the renal tubular reabsorption of uric acid. As with other uricosuric agents, small doses may reduce the excretion of uric acid. Like probenecid, sulfinpyrazone reduces the renal tubular secretion of many other organic anions. The drug may induce hypoglycemia by inhibiting the metabolism of the sulfonylurea oral hypoglycemic agents; hepatic metabolism of warfarin also is impaired. The uricosuric action of sulfinpyrazone is additive to that of probenecid but is mutually antagonistic to that of salicylates (Yü *et al.*, 1963).

Sulfinpyrazone lacks the antiinflammatory and analgesic properties of its congener, phenylbutazone. The inhibitory effect of sulfinpyrazone on platelet function is discussed in Chapter 55.

Absorption, Fate, and Excretion. Sulfinpyrazone is well absorbed after oral administration. It is strongly bound to plasma albumin (98% to 99%) and displaces other anionic drugs that have their highest affinity for the same binding site (site I) (Sudlow *et al.*, 1975). The half-life of the drug in plasma after its intravenous injection is about 3 hours. After oral administration, however, its uricosuric effect may persist for as long as 10 hours. Although little sulfinpyrazone is available for filtration at the glomerulus, it is secreted by the proximal tubule and undergoes little passive back diffusion. Approximately half of the orally administered dose appears in the urine within 24 hours. Most of the drug (90%) in the urine is unchanged; the remainder is eliminated as the N^1-p-hydroxyphenyl metabolite, which also is a potent uricosuric substance.

Toxic Effects.   Gastrointestinal irritation occurs in 10% to 15% of all patients receiving sulfinpyrazone, and occasionally a patient may require discontinuance of its use. Gastric distress is lessened when the drug is taken in divided doses with meals. Sulfinpyrazone should be given to patients with a history of peptic ulcer only with the greatest caution. Hypersensitivity reactions, usually a rash with fever, do occur, but less frequently than with probenecid. The severe blood dyscrasias and salt and water retention, hazards of phenylbutazone therapy, have not been observed during sulfinpyrazone therapy. However, depression of hematopoiesis has been demonstrated experimentally, and periodic blood-cell counts therefore are advised during prolonged therapy.

Therapeutic Use.   *Sulfinpyrazone* (ANTURANE) is available for oral administration. For the treatment of chronic gout, the initial dosage is 100 to 200 mg given twice daily. After the first week, the dosage may be gradually increased until a satisfactory lowering of plasma uric acid is achieved and maintained. This may require from 200 to 800 mg per day, divided in two to four doses and preferably given with meals or milk; a liberal fluid intake should be maintained. Larger doses are poorly tolerated and unlikely to produce a further uricosuric effect in the resistant patient.

Benzbromarone

This is a potent uricosuric agent that is used in Europe. It has the following structural formula:

BENZBROMARONE

The drug is readily absorbed after oral ingestion, and peak concentrations in blood are achieved in about 4 hours. It is metabolized to the monobromine and dehalogenated derivatives, both of which have uricosuric activity, and is excreted primarily in the bile. The uricosuric action is blunted by aspirin or sulfinpyrazone. No paradoxical retention of urate has been observed. At clinically effective doses, there is no effect on the synthesis of urate. Therefore, benzbromarone probably reduces the concentration of urate in plasma solely by inhibiting its tubular reabsorption.

Benzbromarone is of interest as a member of a newer chemical class of uricosuric agents. It is a potent and reversible inhibitor of the urate–anion exchanger in the proximal tubule (Dan and Koga, 1990). As the micronized powder it is effective

in a single daily dose of 40 to 80 mg, which makes it significantly more potent than other uricosuric drugs. It may be useful clinically in patients who are either allergic or refractory to other drugs used for the treatment of gout or in patients with renal insufficiency. Preparations that combine allopurinol and benzbromarone are more effective than either drug alone in lowering serum uric acid levels, in spite of the fact that benzbromarone lowers plasma levels of oxypurinol, the active metabolite of allopurinol.

TREATMENT OF GOUT AND HYPERURICEMIA

The use of probenecid and sulfinpyrazone for the mobilization of uric acid in chronic gout is well established. In about two-thirds of patients, these agents cause uric acid to be excreted at a rate sufficient to exceed that of formation and thereby promptly lower the plasma uric acid concentration. Continuous oral administration to patients with tophaceous gout approximately doubles the daily excretion of urates, prevents the formation of new tophi, and causes gradual shrinkage, or even disappearance, of old tophi. In gouty arthritis, there is a reduction in the swelling of chronically enlarged joints, and a dramatic degree of rehabilitation may be achieved in patients who suffer severe pain and limitation of joint movement. In patients who do not respond well to uricosuric agents because of impaired renal function, allopurinol is especially useful, as described above. In patients with gouty nephropathy, allopurinol offers an additional advantage over the uricosuric agents in that the daily excretion of uric acid is reduced rather than increased. Its administration is compatible with the simultaneous use of the uricosuric agents if necessary.

Neither the uricosuric agents nor allopurinol alters the course of acute attacks of gout or supplants the use of antiinflammatory agents in their management. Indeed, the acute attacks may increase in frequency or severity during the early months of therapy when urate is being mobilized from affected joints. Therefore, therapy with uricosuric agents should not be initiated during an acute attack but may be continued if already begun. Colchicine in small doses (0.5 to 1.8 mg per day) may be administered at this period to reduce the frequency of attacks. When an acute attack occurs, it is treated with an antiinflammatory drug such as indomethacin or naproxen. The use of salicylates is contraindicated both because they can elevate uric acid levels and they antagonize the action of probenecid and sulfinpyrazone.

In the treatment of gout, the uricosuric drugs are given continually in the lowest dose that will maintain satisfactory plasma uric acid concentrations. Since the pKa of uric acid is 5.6 and the solubility of the undissociated form is very low, maintaining the output of a large volume of alkaline urine minimizes its intrarenal deposition. This precaution is essential during the early weeks of therapy when uric acid excretion is large, especially in patients with a history of renal disease associated with the passage of urate stones or gravel. Eventual improvement in renal function in patients with gouty nephropathy has been reported, but it is uncommon. The use of allopurinol permits a more favorable prognosis in such patients.

Acute attacks of gout can be treated effectively with colchicine or a nonsalicylate-containing NSAID, as discussed above. Because of the greater frequency of toxicity with colchicine, use of NSAIDs is the preferred treatment of acute gout. After the acute arthritis has responded to therapy, the patient should be evaluated in order to select a rational regimen for long-term management. Elevated concentrations of uric acid in plasma and the observation of crystals of urate in the aspirated fluid from an affected joint establish the diagnosis of hyperuricemia and symptomatic gout. When evaluated on a diet that is low in purines, patients with hyperuricemia can be categorized with regard to quantities of uric acid excreted in the urine. About 80% to 90% of such individuals excrete less than 600 mg of uric acid daily; the remainder excrete more than this amount due to excessive synthesis of urate. The former group can be managed effectively with uricosuric agents; the latter, however, is logically treated with allopurinol. If deposits of urate are evident as tophi, renal stones, or renal insufficiency, allopurinol is the preferred drug. During the first several months of treatment with allopurinol, colchicine may be given simultaneously to prevent acute attacks of gout. Patients with mild-to-moderate hyperuricemia (7 to 9 mg/dl; equivalent of 420 to 530 μM) who do not have arthritis should be advised to drink large amounts of fluids, follow a diet low in purines, and limit alcohol consumption.

Drug-induced hyperuricemia most commonly is caused by diuretics (see Chapter 29); acute attacks of gout are only rarely caused by such agents. However, hyperuricemia that accompanies chemotherapy or radiotherapy for various neoplasms may be considerably more severe and usually is treated prophylactically with allopurinol and hydration.

PROSPECTUS

Nonsteroidal antiinflammatory drugs are efficacious in providing symptomatic relief, but all available agents have associated, and sometimes severe, toxicity. These agents have been highly useful for treatment of acute, self-limited inflammatory conditions. However, their ability to modify disease progression in chronic inflammatory settings is not well documented and remains an area of continuing controversy. In contrast is the efficacy of agents, such as allopurinol, in the treatment of patients with gout in whom not only is there a regression of signs and symptoms but also an arrest of disease progression.

Advances in understanding the pathobiology of the inflammatory process have suggested several novel approaches for development of drugs to block this process. These include: (1) cytokine inhibitors, (2) inhibitors of cell adhesion molecules, (3) phospholipase A_2 inhibitors, (4) inhibitors of lipoxygenase and leukotriene receptors, and (5) isoform specific–inhibitors of cyclooxygenase.

Agents that modify the production or action of "proinflammatory" cytokines, such as IL-1, TNF, IL-8, and others, are under study. Multiple approaches are in development or clinical trial, including use of antibodies or antibody fragments, molecules to block cytokine generation, and endogenous (e.g., IL-1ra) and synthetic receptor antagonists. The molecular cloning of receptors for many of the cytokines may provide structure-based therapeutic agents. For example, tenidap sodium, a drug already in clinical studies, appears to be an IL-1–synthesis inhibitor and/or IL-1–receptor antagonist, although it probably has other activities as well. Antagonists to various peptides that contribute to cytokine-mediated responses (e.g., substance P, bradykinin) also are in development.

Inhibition of cell adhesion molecules is a fertile area for development of new types of antiinflammatory agents. Multiple approaches are under investigation. These include soluble fragments of receptors to bind cell adhesion molecules and use of antibodies, peptides, and carbohydrate moieties to block cell adhesion molecules (see Bevilacqua and Nelson, 1993; Rao et al., 1994).

Most available NSAIDs have been directed against cyclooxygenase. Although some agents have been developed that inhibit lipoxygenase or leukotriene receptors, the possibility of developing agents that block both proteins by structural modification of known cyclooxygenase inhibitors is being pursued. In addition, efforts continue to identify agents that will be directed against lipases involved in generation of free arachidonic acid or their regulatory proteins. The goal is to develop compounds whose antiinflammatory activity will resemble the glucocorticoids but whose toxicity will be less frequent and severe than that of the steroids (see Bomalaski and Clark, 1993).

One of the most important advancements in antiinflammatory drugs has been the identification of selective inhibitors of COX-2, the inflammation-induced form of the enzyme. The notion that blockade of COX-1 is responsible for many of the side effects of currently available NSAIDs while blockade of COX-2 mediates the antiinflammatory activity of the drugs has spurred efforts to develop COX-2-specific agents. In addition to the COX-2-selective drugs discussed in this chapter, several other second-generation agents with more favorable pharmacokinetics and/or higher selectivity are under development. The currently available drugs appear to have a high degree of safety, especially in regards to gastric toxicity. Postmarketing surveillance and further studies should shed light on whether or not the safety of these drugs is sustained during chronic long-term therapy and whether or not the ability of these agents to significantly inhibit

prostacyclin production might have clinical relevance in some situations.

It is important to remember that inflammation represents a series of homeostatic events that have evolved to aid in our survival in the face of pathogens and tissue injury. Viewed in this context, "better" antiinflammatory therapy runs the risk of blocking such events and thereby doing more harm than good. Beyond the global issue of survival, blockade of physiologically important mechanisms (such as prostaglandin-, leukotriene-, cell adhesion molecule-, or cytokine-mediated events) likely will be associated with some degree of cellular and organ system toxicity. Thus, it may be difficult, or impossible, to avoid toxicity with antiinflammatory drugs targeted against such mechanisms.

For further discussion of rheumatoid arthritis, osteoarthritis, and gout, *see* Chapters 313, 322, and 344, respectively, in *Harrison's Principles of Internal Medicine,* 14th ed., McGraw-Hill, New York, 1998.

BIBLIOGRAPHY

Arellano, F., and Sacristan, J.A. Metamizole: reassessment of its therapeutic role. *Eur. J. Clin. Pharmacol.,* **1990,** *38:*617–619.

Belay, E.D., Bresee, J.S., Holman, R.C., Khan, A.S., Shahriari, A., and Schonberger, L.B. Reye's syndrome in the United States from 1981 through 1997. *N. Engl. J. Med.,* **1999,** *340:*1377–1382.

Bensen, W.G., Fiechtner, J.J., McMillen, J.I., Zhao, W.W., Yu, S.S., Woods, E.M., Hubbard, R.C., Isakson, P.C., Verburg, K.M., and Geis, G.S. Treatment of osteoarthritis with celecoxib, a cyclooxygenase-2 inhibitor: a randomized controlled trial. *Mayo Clin. Proc.,* **1999,** *74:*1095–1105.

Beyer, K.H., Russo, H.F., Tillson, E.K., Miller, A.K., Verwey, W.F., and Gass, S.R. BENEMID, *p*-(di-*n*-propylsulfamyl)-benzoic acid: its renal affinity and its elimination. *Am. J. Physiol.,* **1951,** *166:*625–640.

Bjarnason, I., and Thjodleifsson, B. Gastrointestinal toxicity of nonsteroidal anti-inflammatory drugs: the effect of nimesulide compared with naproxen on the human gastrointestinal tract. *Rheumatology (Oxford),* **1999,** *38*(suppl 1):24–32.

Breder, C.D., Dewitt, D., and Kraig, R.P. Characterization of inducible cyclooxygenase in rat brain. *J. Comp. Neurol.,* **1995,** *355:*296–315.

Brenner, D.E., Harvey, H.A., Lipton, A., and Demers, L. A study of prostaglandin E2, parathormone, and response to indomethacin in patients with hypercalcemia of malignancy. *Cancer,* **1982,** *49:*556–561.

Claria, J., and Serhan, C.N. Aspirin triggers previously undescribed eicosanoids by human endothelial cell-leukocyte interactions. *Proc. Natl. Acad. Sci. U.S.A.,* **1995,** *92:*9475–9479.

Clyman, R.I., Hardy, P., Waleh, N., Chen, Y.Q., Mauray, F., Fouron, J.C., and Chemtob, S. Cyclooxygenase-2 plays a significant role in regulating the tone of the fetal lamb ductus arteriosus. *Am. J. Physiol.,* **1999,** *276:*R913–R921.

Cullen, L., Kelly, L., Connor, S.O., and Fitzgerald, D.J. Selective cyclooxygenase-2 inhibition by nimesulide in man. *J. Pharmacol. Exp. Ther.,* **1998,** *287:*578–582.

Dan, T., and Koga, H. Uricosurics inhibit urate transporter in rat renal brush border membrane vesicles. *Eur. J. Pharmacol.,* **1990,** *187:*303–312.

Davies, N.M., McLachlan, A.J., Day, R.O., and Williams, K.M. Clinical pharmacokinetics and pharmacodynamics of celecoxib: a selective cyclooxygenase-2 inhibitor. *Clin. Pharmacokinet.,* **2000,** *38:*225–242.

Diaz-Gonzalez, F., and Sanchez-Madrid, F. Inhibition of leukocyte adhesion: an alternative mechanism for action for anti-inflammatory drugs. *Immunol. Today,* **1998,** *19:*169–172.

Edmonds, J.P., Scott, D.L., Furst, D.E., Brooks, P., and Paulus, H.E. Antirheumatic drugs: a proposed new classification. *Arthritis Rheum.,* **1993,** *36:*336–339.

Ehrich, E.W., Schnitzer, T.J., McIlwain, H., Levy, R., Wolfe, F., Weisman, M., Zeng, Q., Morrison, B., Bolognese, J., Seidenberg, B., and Gertz, B.J. Effect of specific COX-2 inhibition in osteoarthritis of the knee: a 6 week double-blind, placebo-controlled pilot study of rofecoxib. Rofecoxib Osteoarthritis Pilot Study Group. *J. Rheumatol.,* **1999,** *26:*2438–2447.

Emery, P., Zeidler, H., Kvien, T.K., Guslandi, M., Naudin, R., Stead, H., Verburg, K.M., Isakason, P.C., Hubbard, R.C., and Geis, G.S. Celecoxib versus diclofenac in long-term management of rheumatoid arthritis: randomised double-blind comparison. *Lancet,* **1999,** *354:*2106–2111.

Endemann, G., Abe, Y., Bryant, C.M., Feng, Y., Smith, C.W., and Liu, D.Y. Novel anti-inflammatory compounds induce shedding of L-selectin and block primary capture of neutrophils under flow conditions. *J. Immunol.,* **1997,** *158:*4879–4885.

Fanelli, G.M. Jr., and Weiner, I.M. Urate excretion: drug interactions. *J. Pharmacol. Exp. Ther.,* **1979,** *210:*186–195.

Felson, D.T., Anderson, J.J., and Meenan, R.F. Use of short-term efficacy/toxicity tradeoffs to select second-line drugs in rheumatoid arthritis. A metaanalysis of published clinical trials. *Arthritis Rheum.*, **1992**, *35*:1117–1125.

Gabriel, S.E., Jaakkimainen, L., and Bombardier, C. Risk for serious gastrointestinal complications related to use of nonsteroidal anti-inflammatory drugs. A meta-analysis. *Ann. Intern. Med.*, **1991**, *115*:787–796.

Giardiello, F.M., Hamilton, S.R., Krush, A.J., Piantadosi, S., Hylind, L.M., Celano, P., Booker, S.V., Robinson, C.R., and Offerhaus, G.J. Treatment of colonic and rectal adenomas with sulindac in familial adenomatous polyposis. *N. Engl. J. Med.*, **1993**, *328*:1313–1316.

Giovannucci, E., Egan, K.M., Hunter, D.J., Stampfer, M.J., Colditz, G.A., Willett, W.C., and Speizer, F.E. Aspirin and the risk of colorectal cancer in women. *N. Engl. J. Med.*, **1995**, *333*:609–614.

Graham, D.Y., White, R.H., Moreland, L.W., Schubert, T.T., Katz, R., Jaszewski, R., Tindall, E., Triadafilopoulos, G., Stromatt, S.C., and Teoh, L.S. Duodenal and gastric ulcer prevention with misoprostol in arthritis patients taking NSAIDs. Misoprostol Study Group. *Ann. Intern. Med.*, **1993**, *119*:257–262.

Hande, K.R., Noone, R.M., and Stone, W.J. Severe allopurinol toxicity. Description and guidelines for prevention in patients with renal insufficiency. *Am. J. Med.*, **1984**, *76*:47–56.

Hanel, A.M., and Lands, W.E. Modification of anti-inflammatory drug effectiveness by ambient lipid peroxides. *Biochem. Pharmacol.*, **1982**, *31*:3307–3311.

Harris, R.C., McKanna, J.A., Akai, Y., Jacobson, H.R., Dubois, R.N., and Breyer, M.D. Cylooxygenase-2 is associated with the macula densa of rat kidney and increases with salt restriction. *J. Clin. Invest.*, **1994**, *94*:2504–2510.

Hawkey, C., Laine, L., Simon, T., Beaulieu, A., Maldonado-Cocco, J., Acevedo, E., Shahane, A., Quan, H., Bolognese, J., and Mortensen, E. Comparison of the effect of rofecoxib (a cyclooxygenase-2 inhibitor), ibuprofen, and placebo on the gastroduodenal mucosa of patients with osteoarthritis: a randomized, double-blind, placebo-controlled trial. The Rofecoxib Osteoarthritis Endoscopy Multinational Study Group. *Arthritis Rheum.*, **2000**, *43*:370–377.

Higgs, G.A., Salmon, J.A., Henderson, B., and Vane, J.R. Pharmacokinetics of aspirin and salicylate in relation to inhibition of arachidonate cyclooxygenase and antiinflammatory activity. *Proc. Natl. Acad. Sci. U.S.A.*, **1987**, *84*:1417–1420.

Imperiale, T.F., and Petrulis, A.S. A meta-analysis of low-dose aspirin for the prevention of pregnancy-induced hypertensive disease. *JAMA*, **1991**, *266*:260–264.

Israel, E., Fischer, A.R., Rosenberg, M.A., Lilly, C.M., Callery, J.C., Shapiro, J., Cohn, J., Rubin, P., and Drazen, J.M. The pivotal role of 5-lipoxygenase products in the reaction of aspirin-sensitive asthmatics to aspirin. *Am. Rev. Respir. Dis.*, **1993**, *148*:1447–1451.

Kavanaugh, A.F., Davis, L.S., Nichols, L.A., Norris, S.H., Rothlein, R., Scharschmidt, L.A., and Lipsky, P.E. Treatment of refractory rheumatoid arthritis with a monoclonal antibody to intercellular adhesion molecule 1. *Arthritis Rheum.*, **1994**, *37*:992–999.

Kulling, P.E., Backman, E.A., and Skagius, A.S. Renal impairment after acute dicofenac, naproxen, and sulindac overdoses. *J. Toxicol. Clin. Toxicol.*, **1995**, *33*:173–177.

Laine, L., Harper, S., Simon, T., Bath, R., Johanson, J., Schwartz, H., Stern, S., Quan, H., and Bolognese, J. A randomized trial comparing the effect of rofecoxib, a cyclooxygenase 2-specific inhibitor, with that of ibuprofen on the gastrointestinal mucosa of patients with osteoarthritis. Rofecoxib Osteoarthritis Endoscopy Study Group. *Gastroenterology*, **1999**, *117*:776–783.

Laine, L., Sloane, R., Ferretti, M., and Cominelli, F. A randomized double-blind comparison of placebo, etodolac, and naproxen

on gastrointestinal injury and prostaglandin production. *Gastrointest. Endosc.*, **1995**, *42*:428–433.

Lecomte, M., Laneuville, O., Ji, C., DeWitt, D.L., and Smith, W.L. Acetylation of human prostaglandin endoperoxide synthase-2 (cyclooxygenase-2) by aspirin. *J. Biol. Chem.*, **1994**, *269*:13207–13215.

Leonards, J.R., Levy, G., and Niemczura, R. Gastrointestinal blood loss during prolonged aspirin administration. *N. Engl. J. Med.*, **1973**, *289*:1020–1022.

McAdam, B.F., Catella-Lawson, F., Mardini, I.A., Kapoor, S., Lawson, J.A., and FitzGerald, G.A. Systemic biosynthesis of prostacyclin by cyclooxygenase (COX)-2: the human pharmacology of a selective inhibitor of COX-2. *Proc. Natl. Acad. Sci. U.S.A.*, **1999**, *96*:272–277.

Mackin, W.M., Rakich, S.M., and Marshall, C.L. Inhibition of rat neutrophil functional responses by azapropazone, an anti-gout drug. *Biochem. Pharmcol.*, **1986**, *35*:917–922.

Malmstrom, K., Daniels, S., Kotey, P., Seidenberg, B.C., and Desjardins, P.J. Comparison of rofecoxib and celecoxib, two cyclooxygenase-2 inhibitors, in postoperative dental pain: a randomized, placebo- and active-comparator-controlled trial. *Clin. Ther.*, **1999**, *21*:1653–1663.

Marshall, P.J., Kulmacz, R.J., and Lands, W.E. Constraints on prostaglandin biosynthesis in tissues. *J. Biol. Chem.*, **1987**, *262*:3510–3517.

Masferrer, J.L., Reddy, S.T., Zweifel, B.S., Seibert, K., Needleman, P., Gilbert, R.S., and Herschmann, H.R. *In vivo* glucocorticoids regulate cyclooxygenase-2 but not cyclooxygenase-1 in peritoneal macrophages. *J. Pharmacol. Exp. Ther.*, **1994a**, *270*:1340–1344.

Masferrer, J.L., Zweifel, B.S., Manning, P.T., Hauser, S.D., Leahy, K.M., Smith, W.G., Isakson, P.C., and Seibert, K. Selective inhibition of inducible cyclooxygenase-2 *in vivo* is antiinflammatory and nonulcerogenic. *Proc. Natl. Acad. Sci. U.S.A.*, **1994b**, *91*:3228–3232.

Meade, E.A., Smith, W.L., and DeWitt, D.L. Differential inhibition of prostaglandin endoperoxide synthase (cyclooxygenase) isozymes by aspirin and other non-steroidal anti-inflammatory drugs. *J. Biol. Chem.*, **1993**, *268*:6610–6614.

Ment, L.R., Oh, W., Ehrenkranz, R.A., Philip, A.G., Vohr, B., Allan, W., Duncan, C.C., Scott, D.T., Taylor, K.J., Katz, K.H., Schneider, K.C., and Makuch, R.W. Low-dose indomethacin and prevention of intraventricular hemorrhage: a multicenter randomized trial. *Pediatrics*, **1994**, *93*:543–550.

Mitchell, J.A., Akarasereenont, P., Thiemermann, C., Flower, R.J., and Vane, J.R. Selectivity of nonsteroidal antiinflammatory drugs as inhibitors of constitutive and inducible cyclooxygenase. *Proc. Natl. Acad. Sci. U.S.A.*, **1993**, *90*:11693–11697.

Morrison, B.W., Daniels, S.E., Kotey, P., Cantu, N., and Seidenberg, B. Rofecoxib, a specific cylooxygenase-2 inhibitor, in primary dysmenorrhea: a randomized controlled trial. *Obstet. Gynecol.*, **1999**, *94*:504–508.

Morrow, J.D., Awad, J.A., Oates, J.A., and Roberts, L.J. II. Identification of skin as the major site of prostaglandin D_2 release following oral administration of niacin in humans. *J. Invest. Dermatol.*, **1992**, *98*:812–815.

Morrow, J.D., Parsons, W.G. III, and Roberts, L.J. II. Release of markedly increased quantities of prostaglandin D_2 *in vivo* following administration of nicotinic acid. *Prostaglandins*, **1989**, *38*:263–274.

O'Neill, G.P., Mancini, J.A., Kargman, S., Yergey, J., Kwan, M.Y., Falgueyret, J.P., Abramovitz, M., Kennedy, B.P., Ouellet, M., Cromlish, W., Culp, S., Evans, J.F., Ford-Hutchinson, A.W., and Vickers, P.J. Overexpression of human prostaglandin G/H synthase-1 and -2 by recombinant vaccine virus: inhibition by nonsteroidal anti-inflammatory drugs and biosynthesis of 15-hydroxyeicosatetraenoic acid. *Mol. Pharmacol.,* **1994,** *45:*245–254.

Panara, M.R., Renda, G., Sciulli, M.G., Santini, G., Di Giamberardino, M.D., Rotondo, M.T., Tacconelli, S., Seta, F., Patrono, C., and Patrignani, P. Dose-dependent inhibition of platelet cyclooxygenase-1 and monocyte cyclooxygenase-2 by meloxicam in healthy subjects. *J. Pharmacol. Exp. Ther.,* **1999,** *290:*276–280.

Patoia, L., Santucci, L., Furno, P., Dionisi, M.S., Dell'Orso, S., Romagnoli, M., Sattarinia, A., and Marini, M.G. A 4-week, double-blind, parallel-group study to compare the gastrointestinal effects of meloxicam 7.5 mg, meloxicam 15 mg, piroxicam 20 mg and placebo by means of faecal blood loss, endoscopy and symptom evaluation in healthy volunteers. *Br. J. Rheumatol.,* **1996,** *35*(suppl 1):61–67.

Patrignani, P., Panara, M.R., Greco, A., Fusco, O., Natoli, C., Iacobelli, S., Cipollone, F., Ganci, A., Creminon, C., and Maclouf, J. Biochemical and pharmacological characterization of the cyclooxygenase activity of human blood prostaglandin endoperoxide synthases. *J. Pharmacol. Exp. Ther.,* **1994,** *271:*1705–1712.

Rainsford, K.D. Relationship of nimesulide safety to its pharmacokinetics: assessment of adverse reactions. *Rheumatology (Oxford),* **1999,** *38*(suppl 1):4–10.

Rao, B.N., Anderson, M.B., Musser, J.H., Gilbert, J.H., Schaefer, M.E., Foxall, C., and Brandley, B.K. Sialyl Lewis X mimics derived from a pharmacophore search are selectin inhibitors with anti-inflammatory activity. *J. Biol. Chem.,* **1994,** *269:*19663–19666.

Roberts, L.J. II, Sweetman, B.J., Lewis, R.A., Austen, K.F., and Oates, J.A. Increased production of prostaglandin D_2 in patients with systemic mastocytosis. *N. Engl. J. Med.,* **1980,** *303:*1400–1404.

Roujeau, J.-C., Kelly, J.P., Naldi, L., Rzany, B., Stern, R.S., Anderson, T., Auquier, A., Bastuji-Garin, S., Correia, O., Locati, F., Mockenhaupt, M., Paoletti, C., Shapiro, S., Shear, N., Schopf, E., and Kaufman, D.W. Medication use and the risk of Stevens-Johnson syndrome or toxic epidermal necrolysis. *N. Engl. J. Med.,* **1995,** *333:*1600–1607.

Rumack, B.H., Peterson, R.C., Koch, G.G., and Amara, I.A. Acetaminophen overdose. 662 cases with evaluation of oral acetylcysteine treatment. *Arch. Intern. Med.,* **1981,** *141:*380–385.

Sandler, D.P., Smith, J.C., Weinberg, C.R., Buckalew, V.M. Jr., Dennis, V.W., Blythe, W.B., and Burgess, W.P. Analgesic use and chronic renal disease. *N. Engl. J. Med.,* **1989,** *320:*1238–1243.

Sawdy, R., Slater, D., Fisk, N., Edmonds, D.K., and Bennet, P. Use of a cyclo-oxygenase type-2-selective non-steroidal anti-inflammatory drug to prevent preterm delivery. *Lancet,* **1997,** *350:*265–266.

Schnitzer, T.J., Truitt, K., Fleischmann, R., Dalgin, P., Block, J., Zeng, Q., Bolognese, J., Seidenberg, B., and Ehrich, E.W. The safety profile, tolerability, and effective dose range of rofecoxib in the treatment of rheumatoid arthritis. Phase II Rofecoxib Rheumatoid Arthritis Study Group. *Clin. Ther.,* **1999,** *21:*1688–1702.

Scott, D.L., and Palmer, R.H. Safety and efficacy of nabumetone in osteoarthritis: emphasis on gastrointestinal safety. *Aliment. Pharmacol. Ther.,* **2000,** *14:*443–452.

Serhan, C.N., Takano, T., and Maddox, J.F. Aspirin-triggered 15-epi-lipoxin A4 and stable analogs of lipoxin A4 are potent inhibitors of acute inflammation. Receptors and pathways. *Adv. Exp. Med. Biol.,* **1999,** *447:*133–149.

Seyberth, H.W., Koniger, S.J., Rascher, W., Kuhl, P.G., and Schweer, H. Role of prostaglandins in hyperprostaglandin E syndrome and in selected renal tubular disorders. *Pediatr. Nephrol.,* **1987,** *1:*491–497.

Sibai, B.M., Caritis, S.N., Thom, E., Klebanoff, M., McNellis, D., Rocco, L., Paul, R.H., Romero, R., Witter, F., Rosen, M., Depp,

R., and The National Institute of Child Health and Human Development Network of Maternal-Fetal Medicine Units. Prevention of preeclampsia with low-dose aspirin in healthy nulliparous pregnant women. *N. Engl. J. Med.,* **1993,** *329:*1213–1218.

Simon, L.S., Lanza, F.L., Lipsky, P.E., Hubbard, R.C., Talwalker, S., Schwartz, B.D., Isakson, P.C., and Geis, G.S. Preliminary study of the safety and efficacy of SC-58635, a novel cyclooxygenase 1 inhibitor: efficacy and safety in two placebo-controlled trials in osteoarthritis and rheumatoid arthritis, and studies of gastrointestinal and platelet effects. *Arthritis Rheum.,* **1998,** *41:*1591–1602.

Simon, L.S., Weaver, A.L., Graham, D.Y., Kivitz, A.J., Lipsky, P.E., Hubbard, R.C., Isakson, P.C., Verburg, K.M, Yu, S.S., Zhao, W.W., and Geis, G.S. Anti-inflammatory and upper gastrointestinal effects of celecoxib in rheumatoid arthritis: a randomized, controlled trial. *JAMA,* **1999,** *282:*1921–1928.

Slater, D.M., Dennes, W.J., Campa, J.S., Poston, L., and Bennett, P.R. Expression of cyclo-oxygenase types-1 and -2 in human myometrium throughout pregnancy. *Mol. Hum. Reprod.,* **1999,** *5:*880–884.

Smilkstein, M.J., Knapp, G.L., Kulig, K.W., and Rumack, B.H. Efficacy of oral N-acetylcysteine in the treatment of acetaminophen overdose. Analysis of the national multicenter study (1976 to 1985). *N. Engl. J. Med.,* **1988,** *319:*1557–1562.

Strong, H.A., Warner, N.J., Renwick, A.G., and George, C.F. Sulindac metabolism: the importance of an intact colon. *Clin. Pharmacol. Ther.,* **1985,** *38:*387–393.

Sudlow, G., Birkett, D.J., and Wade, D.N. The characterization of two specific drug binding sites on human serum albumin. *Mol. Pharmacol.,* **1975,** *11:*824–832.

Thun, M.J., Namboodiri, M.M., and Heath, C.W. Jr. Aspirin use and reduced risk of fatal colon cancer. *N. Engl. J. Med.,* **1991,** *325:*1593–1596.

Vane, J., and Botting, R. Inflammation and the mechanism of action of antiinflammatory drugs. *FASEB J.,* **1987,** *1:*89–96.

Wallace, S.L. Colchicine: clinical pharmacology in acute gouty arthritis. *Am. J. Med.,* **1961,** *30:*439–448.

Warner, T.D., Giuliano, F., Vojnovic, I., Bukasa, A., Mitchell, J.A., and Vane, J.R. Nonsteroid drug selectivities for cyclo-oxygenase-1 rather than cyclo-oxygenase-2 are associated with human gastrointestinal toxicity: a full *in vitro* analysis. *Proc. Natl. Acad. Sci. U.S.A.,* **1999,** *96:*7563–7568.

Waslen, T.A., McCauley, F.A., and Wilson, T.W. Sulindac does not spare renal prostaglandins. *Clin. Invest. Med.,* **1989,** *12:*77–81.

Yamamoto, Y., Yin, M.J., Lin, K.M., and Gaynor, R.B. Sulindac inhibits activation of the NFκB pathway. *J. Biol. Chem.,* **1999,** *274:*27307–27314.

Yin, M.J., Yamamoto, Y., and Gaynor, R.B. The anti-inflammatory agents aspirin and salicylate inhibit the activity of I(kappa)B kinase-beta. *Nature,* **1998,** *396:*77–80.

Zemer, D., Livneh, A., Danon, Y.L., Pras, M., and Sohar, E. Long-term colchicine treatment in children with familial Mediterranean fever. *Arthritis Rheum.,* **1991,** *34:*973–977.

MONOGRAPHS AND REVIEWS

Abramson, S.B., and Weissmann, G. The mechanisms of action of nonsteroidal antiinflammatory drugs. *Arthritis Rheum.,* **1989,** *32:* 1–9.

Andrade, S.E., Martinez, C., and Walker, A.M. Comparative safety evaluation of non-narcotic analgesics. *J. Clin. Epidemiol.,* **1998,** *51:*1357–1365.

Arend, W.P. Interleukin-1 receptor antagonist. *Adv. Immunol.,* **1993,** *54*:167–227.

Balfour, J.A., and Buckley, M.M. Etodolac. A reappraisal of its pharmacology and therapeutic use in rheumatic diseases and pain states. *Drugs,* **1991,** *42*:274–299.

Battistini, B., Botting, R., and Bakhle, Y.S. COX-1 and COX-2: toward the development of more selective NSAIDs. *Drug News Perspect.,* **1994,** *8*:501–512.

Bevilacqua, M.P., and Nelson, R.M. Selectins. *J. Clin. Invest.,* **1993,** *91*:379–387.

Bomalaski, J.S., and Clark, M.A. Phospholipase A2 and arthritis. *Arthritis Rheum.,* **1993,** *36*:190–198.

Borda, I.T., and Koff, R.S., eds. *NSAIDs: A Profile of Adverse Effects.* Hanley & Belfus, Philadelphia, **1992.**

Brater, D.C. Effects of nonsteroidal anti-inflammatory drugs on renal function: focus on cyclooxygenase-2-selective inhibition. *Am. J. Med.,* **1999,** *107*:65S–70S.

Brooks, P.M., and Day, R.O. Nonsteroidal antiinflammatory drugs—differences and similarities. *N. Engl. J. Med.,* **1991,** *324*:1716–1725.

Buckley, M.M., and Brogden, R.N. Ketorolac. A review of its pharmocodynamic and pharmacokinetic properties, and therapeutic potential. *Drugs,* **1990,** *39*:86–109.

Cash, J.M., and Klippel, J.H. Second-line drug therapy for rheumatoid arthritis. *N. Engl. J. Med.,* **1994,** *330*:1368–1375.

Clissold, S.P. Paracetamol and phenacetin. *Drugs,* **1986,** *32*(suppl 4):46–59.

Clive, D.M., and Stoff, J.S. Renal syndromes associated with non-steroidal antiinflammatory drugs. *N. Engl. J. Med.,* **1984,** *310*:563–572.

Cronstein, B.N., and Weissmann, G. The adhesion molecules of inflammation. *Arthritis Rheum.,* **1993,** *36*:147–157.

Dascombe, M.J. The pharmacology of fever. *Prog. Neurobiol.,* **1985,** *25*:327–373.

Davies, R.O. Review of the animal and clinical pharmacology of diflunisal. *Pharmacotherapy,* **1983,** *3*:9S–22S.

Dinarello, C.A. Role of interleukin-1 and tumor necrosis factor in systemic responses to infection and inflammation. In, *Inflammation: Basic Principles and Clinical Correlates,* 2nd ed. (Gallin, J.I., Goldstein, I.M., and Snyderman, R., eds.) Raven Press, New York, **1992,** pp. 211–232.

Dunn, M.J. Prostaglandins and Bartter's syndrome. *Kidney Int.,* **1981,** *19*:86–102.

Emmerson, B.T. Abnormal urate excretion associated with renal and systemic disorders, drugs, and toxins. In, *Uric Acid.* (Kelley, W.N., and Weiner, I.M., eds.) *Handbook of Experimental Pharmacology,* Vol. 51. Springer-Verlag, Berlin, **1978,** pp. 287–324.

Faulds, D., Goa, K.L., and Benfield, P. Cyclosporin. A review of its pharmacodynamic and pharmacokinetic properties, and therapeutic use in immunoregulatory disorders. *Drugs,* **1993,** *45*:953–1040.

Friedel, H.A., Langtry, H.D., and Buckley, M.M. Nabumetone. A reappraisal of its pharmacology and therapeutic use in rheumatic diseases. *Drugs,* **1993,** *45*:131–156.

Gallin, J.I., Goldstein, I.M., and Snyderman, R., eds. *Inflammation: Basic Principles and Clinical Correlates,* 2nd ed. Raven Press, New York, **1992.**

Gebhart, G.F., and McCormack, K.J. Neuronal plasticity. Implication for pain therapy. *Drugs,* **1994,** *47*(suppl 5):1–47.

Gupta, R.A., and DuBois, R.N. Aspirin, NSAIDs, and colon cancer prevention: mechanisms? *Gastroenterology,* **1998,** *114*:1095–1098.

Hart, F.D., and Huskisson, E.C. Non-steroidal anti-inflammatory drugs. Current status and rational therapeutic use. *Drugs,* **1984,** *27*:232–255.

Hurwitz, E.S. Reye's syndrome. *Epidemiol. Rev.,* **1989,** *11*:249-253.

Kantor, T.G. Ibuprofen. *Ann. Intern. Med.,* **1979,** *91*:877–882.

Kelley, W.N., Harris, E.D. Jr., Ruddy, S., and Sledge, C.B., eds. *Textbook of Rheumatology,* 4th ed., W.B. Saunders, Philadelphia, **1993.**

Kincaid-Smith, P. Effects of non-narcotic analgesics on the kidney. *Drugs,* **1986,** *32*(suppl 4):109–128.

Konttinen, Y.T., Kemppinen, P., Segerberg, M., Hukkanen, M., Rees, R., Santavirta, S., Sorsa, T., Pertovaara, A., and Polak, J.M. Peripheral and spinal neural mechanisms in arthritis, with particular reference to treatment of inflammation and pain. *Arthritis Rheum.,* **1994,** *37*:965–982.

Lewis, A.J., and Furst, D.W., eds. *Nonsteroidal Anti-Inflammatory Drugs: Mechanisms and Clinical Use.* Marcel Dekker, New York, **1987.**

Lubbe, W.F. Low-dose aspirin in prevention of toxemia of pregnancy. Does it have a place? *Drugs,* **1987,** *34*:515–518.

Meredith, T.J., and Vale, J.A. Non-narcotic analgesics. Problems of overdosage. *Drugs,* **1986,** *32*(suppl 4):177–205.

Metcalf, D.D. The treatment of mastocytosis: an overview. *J. Invest. Dermatol.,* **1991,** *96*:55S–59S.

Monto, A.S. The disappearance of Reye's syndrome—a public health triumph. *N. Engl. J. Med.,* **1999,** *340*:1423–1424.

Oates, J.A., FitzGerald, G.A., Branch, R.A., Jackson, E.K., Knapp, H.R., and Roberts, L.J. II. Clinical implications of prostaglandin and thromboxane A2 formation. *N. Engl. J. Med.,* **1988,** *319*:689–698, 761–767.

Patrono, C. Aspirin as an antiplatelet drug. *N. Engl. J. Med.,* **1994,** *330*:1287–1294.

Patrono, C., and Dunn, M.J. The clinical significance of inhibition of renal prostaglandin synthesis. *Kidney Int.,* **1987,** *32*:1–12.

Rainsford, K.D., ed. *Inflammation Mechanisms and Actions of Traditional Drugs.* Vol. I, *Anti-Inflammatory and Anti-Rheumatic Drugs.* CRC Press, Boca Raton, FL, **1985a.**

Rainsford, K.D., ed. *Newer Anti-Inflammatory Drugs.* Vol. II, *Anti-Inflammatory and Anti-Rheumatic Drugs.* CRC Press, Boca Raton, FL, **1985b.**

Roberts, L.J. II, and Oates, J.A. Biochemical diagnosis of systemic mast cell disorders. *J. Invest. Dermatol.,* **1991,** *96*:19S–25S.

Robertson, R.P. Prostaglandins and hypercalcemia of cancer. *Med. Clin. North Am.,* **1981,** *65*:845-853.

Saper, C.B., and Breder, C.D. The neurologic basis of fever. *N. Engl. J. Med.,* **1994,** *330*:1880–1886.

Scott, L.J., and Lamb, H.M. Rofecoxib. *Drugs,* **1999,** *58*:499–505.

Seibert, K., Zhang, Y., Leahy, K., Hauser, S., Masferrer, J., and Isakson, P. Distribution of COX-1 and COX-2 in normal and inflamed tissues. *Adv. Exp. Med. Biol.,* **1997,** *400A*:167–170.

Shapiro, S.S. Treatment of dysmenorrhoea and premenstrual syndrome with non-steroidal anti-inflammatory drugs. *Drugs,* **1988,** *36*:475–490.

Symposium. (various authors). Arthrotec Investigators Meeting. *Drugs,* **1993a,** *45*(suppl 1):1–37.

Symposium. (various authors). Nimesulide: a multifactorial therapeutic approach to the inflammatory process? A 7-year clinical experience. Proceedings of an international congress, Berlin, October 1–3, 1992. *Drugs,* **1993b,** *46*(suppl 1):1–283.

Symposium. (various authors). *Anti-Rheumatic Drugs.* (Huskisson, E.C., ed.) Praeger Publishers, New York, **1983a.**

Symposium. (various authors). New perspectives on aspirin therapy. Proceedings of a symposium co-sponsored by the Aspirin Foundation of America, Inc., and Tulane University Medical Center. *Am. J. Med.,* **1983b,** *74:*1–109.

Symposium. (various authors). Inflammatory disease and the role of Voltaren (diclofenac sodium). Proceedings of a symposium, May 14-15, 1985, Tahiti. *Am. J. Med.,* **1986,** *80:*1–87.

Symposium. (various authors). Nonsteroidal anti-inflammatory drug-induced gastrointestinal damage. Current insights into patient management. Proceedings of a symposium. June 13, 1987, Washington, D.C. *Am. J. Med.,* **1988a,** *84:*1–52.

Symposium. (various authors). Sulfasalazine in rheumatic diseases. *J. Rheumatol.,* **1988b,** *15*(suppl 16):1–42.

Thomas, S.H. Paracetamol (acetaminophen) poisoning. *Pharmacol. Ther.,* **1993,** *60:*91–120.

Todd, P.A., and Brogden, R.N. Oxaprozin. A preliminary review of its pharmacodynamic and pharmacokinetic properties, and therapeutic efficacy. *Drugs,* **1986,** *32:*291–312.

Todd, P.A., and Clissold, S.P. Naproxen. A reappraisal of its pharmacology, and therapeutic use in rheumatic diseases and pain states. *Drugs,* **1990,** *40:*91–137.

Turck, D., Roth, W., and Busch, U. A review of the clinical pharmacokinetics of meloxicam. *Br. J. Rheumatol.,* **1996,** *35*(suppl 1): 13–16.

Vane, J. Towards a better aspirin. *Nature,* **1994,** *367:*215–216.

Vane, J. R., Bakhle, Y.S., and Botting, R.M. Cyclooxygenases 1 and 2. *Annu. Rev. Pharmacol. Toxicol.,* **1998,** *38:*97–120.

Vane, J.R., and Botting, R.M. New insights into the mode of action of anti-inflammatory drugs. *Inflamm. Res.,* **1995,** *44:*1–10.

Wallace, S.L., and Singer, J.Z. Review: systemic toxicity associated with intravenous administration of colchicine—guidelines for use. *J. Rheumatol.,* **1988,** *15:*495–499.

Warnes, T.W. Colchicine in primary biliary cirrhosis. *Aliment. Pharmacol. Ther.,* **1991,** *5:*321–379.

Willard, J.E., Lange, R.A., and Hillis, L.D. The use of aspirin in ischemic heart disease. *N. Engl. J. Med.,* **1992,** *327:*175–181.

Wu, G.D. A nuclear receptor to prevent colon cancer. *N. Engl. J. Med.,* **2000,** *342:*651–653.

Yü, T.-F., Dayton, P.G., and Gutman, A.B. Mutual suppression of the uricosuric effects of sulfinpyrazone and salicylate: a study in interactions between drugs. *J. Clin. Invest.,* **1963,** *42:*1330–1339.

Acknowledgment

The authors wish to acknowledge Dr. Paul A. Insel, the author of this chapter in the ninth edition of *Goodman and Gilman's The Pharmacological Basis of Therapeutics,* some of whose text we have retained in this edition.

C H A P T E R 2 8

DRUGS USED IN THE
TREATMENT OF ASTHMA

Bradley J. Undem and Lawrence M. Lichtenstein

Asthma is an extremely common disorder, accounting for 1% to 3% of all office visits, 500,000 hospital admissions per year, and more pediatric hospital admissions than any other single illness. Annually, more than 5000 children and adults die of asthma attacks in the United States. This number could be reduced with appropriate therapy. In the past decade, substantial progress has been made in understanding the pathophysiology of asthma. Asthma no longer can be viewed simply as reversible airway obstruction or "irritable airways." Asthma should be viewed primarily as an inflammatory illness with bronchial hyperreactivity and bronchospasm as a result. This view has led to changes in the recommendations regarding prevention and treatment of asthma. Recent clinical trials comparing the benefits of antiinflammatory treatment with those of simple bronchodilator therapy have shown the usefulness of addressing the inflammatory component as the underlying problem and reserving bronchodilators primarily for symptomatic use.

In this chapter, the data identifying inflammation as the primary pathophysiological process in asthmatic bronchoconstriction are examined. Therapy for bronchoconstriction per se, including β-adrenergic agonists and ipratropium (see also Chapters 7 and 10), is summarized. The chapter also reviews the drugs used to address the underlying asthmatic inflammation, primarily glucocorticoids (see also Chapter 60). Pharmacological treatments of allergic rhinitis and chronic obstructive pulmonary disease (COPD) are discussed because of their similarities to the treatment of asthma. The use of methylxanthines and leukotriene inhibitors in the treatment of asthma also is described.

ASTHMA AS AN
INFLAMMATORY ILLNESS

The recognition that asthmatic airway narrowing, both at baseline and during disease exacerbations, is due to inflammation is based on studies involving bronchial lavage and lung biopsies. Increased numbers of inflammatory cells, including eosinophils, basophils, macrophages, and lymphocytes, can be found in bronchoalveolar lavage fluid from asthmatic patients. Even asthmatics with normal baseline lung function and no recent asthma exacerbations have increased numbers of inflammatory cells in their airways. After challenge with allergen, there is a further increase in the numbers of inflammatory cells.

Lung biopsies have been performed on normal and asthmatic subjects. Asthmatic subjects have increased airway thickness and an increased number of basophils and other inflammatory cells in lung tissues. The basis for this inflammation is not entirely clear. Most children and

adults have clearly defined allergen exposures that are partially or substantially responsible for their asthmatic inflammation. Presumably, these reactions can be at a smoldering level, resulting in continuous mild to moderate inflammation but not overt bronchoconstriction. Epidemiologic studies show that there is a correlation between increasing immunoglobulin E (IgE) levels and prevalence of asthma (Burrows *et al.*, 1989). Figure 28–1 depicts basophil and mast-cell activation by exposure to allergen. Allergen-specific IgE is bound to the mast cell *via* Fc receptors. When allergen crosslinks two IgE molecules, basophils and mast cells are activated and release a large number of inflammatory mediators. The mechanisms of this release are now well established and involve dumping of granule contents and synthesis of various lipid mediators (Table 28–1). Immunological stimulation of basophils also leads to the synthesis of several proinflammatory cytokines, such as interleukin (IL)-4 and IL-13 (Schroeder and MacGlashan, 1997). Which cytokines are generated

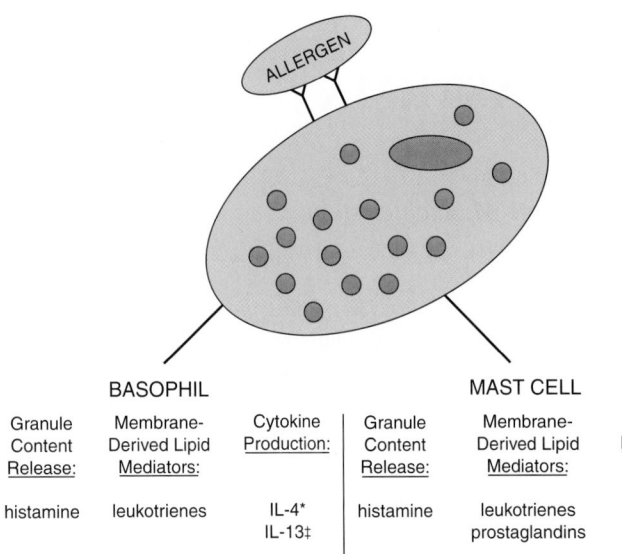

Figure 28–1. Inflammatory mediators released by activated mast cells and basophils.

IL = interleukin
∗ = over 1–4 hours
‡ = over 6–24 hours;

BASOPHIL			MAST CELL		
Granule Content Release:	Membrane-Derived Lipid Mediators:	Cytokine Production:	Granule Content Release:	Membrane-Derived Lipid Mediators:	Cytokine Production:
histamine	leukotrienes	IL-4∗ IL-13‡	histamine	leukotrienes prostaglandins	see text

by mast cells in the airways is not yet clear. The salient feature of this scheme is that an enormous variety of mediators is released, each having more than one potent effect on airway inflammation.

The result of the vasodilation, increased vasopermeability, and an increased display of endothelial leukocytic adhesion molecules is an influx of inflammatory cells from the circulation into the tissues. Lymphocytes, eosinophils, and basophils predominate. Once these newly recruited cells reach the lung, they release their own mediators, which have further inflammatory effects (Table 28–2). While histamine and leukotriene come from mast cells in an acute reaction, these mediators, together with IL-4 and IL-13, come from basophils in chronic disease. Asthmatic inflammation is characterized by bronchial hyperreactivity and therefore differs from the inflammation found in other conditions, such as pneumonia. The chronic results are airway edema, smooth muscle hypertrophy, epithelial shedding, and bronchial hyperreactivity to nonspecific stimuli such as strong odors, cold air, pollutants, and histamine. Asthmatic airway inflammation may cause increased parasympathetic tone, with resulting bronchial narrowing.

The above scheme predicts that a drug affecting only one mediator is unlikely to be of substantial benefit, simply because there are so many mediators participating.

Table 28–1

Mast Cell Mediators of Inflammatory Processes

CLASS	MEDIATOR	EFFECTS
Preformed	Histamine	Vasodilation, vasopermeability, itch, cough, bronchoconstriction, rhinorrhea
	Proteases	Vasodilation, vasopermeability, bronchoconstriction
	Heparin	?
Lipid-derived	LTC_4	Bronchoconstriction, vasodilation, vasopermeability
	LTB_4	Leukocyte chemotaxis
	PGD_2	Vasodilation, vasopermeability, bronchoconstriction, mucus secretion
	PAF	Bronchoconstriction, leukocyte chemotaxis

Abbreviations: LT, leukotriene; PG, prostaglandin; PAF, platelet activating factor.

Table 28–2
Cells Recruited During Asthmatic Inflammation

CELL	MEDIATORS	EFFECTS
Eosinophil	Major basic protein, ECP, EDNT, LTC$_4$, IL-1, IL-6, GM-CSF, superoxide	Epithelial shedding, bronchoconstriction, promotion of inflammation
T lymphocyte	Various cytokines	Promotion of inflammation
Basophil	Histamine, LTC$_4$, IL-4	Bronchoconstriction
Macrophage	TNF-α, superoxide, proteases, LTB$_4$, PGD$_2$	Tissue damage, chemotaxis, bronchoconstriction, mucus secretion

Abbreviations: ECP, eosinophil cationic protein; EDNT, eosinophil-derived neurotoxin; LT, leukotriene; IL, interleukin; GM-CSF, granulocyte/macrophage colony-stimulating factor; TNF, tumor necrosis factor; PG, prostaglandin.

For example, histamine clearly is released during allergic asthmatic reactions (Murray *et al.,* 1986), but antihistamines are of little or no benefit in allergic asthma (Holgate, 1994). In contrast, leukotriene inhibitors or an IL-4–receptor antagonist have clear effects. One also can predict that drugs that more broadly address asthmatic inflammation (*i.e.,* glucocorticoids) could be of greater therapeutic benefit than agents that address only bronchoconstriction *per se.*

TREATMENT OF ASTHMA

Aerosol Delivery of Drugs

Topical application of drugs to the lungs can be accomplished by use of aerosols. In theory, this approach should produce a high local concentration in the lungs with a low systemic delivery, thereby significantly improving the therapeutic ratio by minimizing systemic side effects. The most commonly used drugs in the treatment of asthma, β_2-adrenergic receptor agonists and glucocorticoids, have potentially serious side effects when delivered systemically. Since the pathophysiology of asthma appears to involve the respiratory tract alone, the theoretical advantages of aerosol treatments with limited systemic effects are substantial. Indeed, in clinical practice, probably more than 90% of asthmatic patients who are capable of manipulating inhaler devices can be managed by aerosol treatments alone. Because of the specialized nature of aerosol delivery and the substantial effects that these systems have on the therapeutic index, the principles of this delivery method are important to review.

A review of the chemistry and physics of aerosol delivery systems is available (Taburet and Schmit, 1994). A schematic diagram of the fate of therapeutic agents delivered by this route is shown in Figure 28–2. The critical determinant of the delivery of any particulate matter to the lungs is the size of the particles. Particles larger than 10 μm will be deposited primarily in the mouth and oropharynx, while particles smaller than 0.5 μm are inhaled to the alveolae and subsequently exhaled without being deposited in the lungs. Particles with a diameter of 1 to 5 μm allow deposition of drugs in the small airways and are therefore the most effective. Unfortunately, no aerosol system in clinical use can produce uniform particles limited to the appropriate size range. A number of

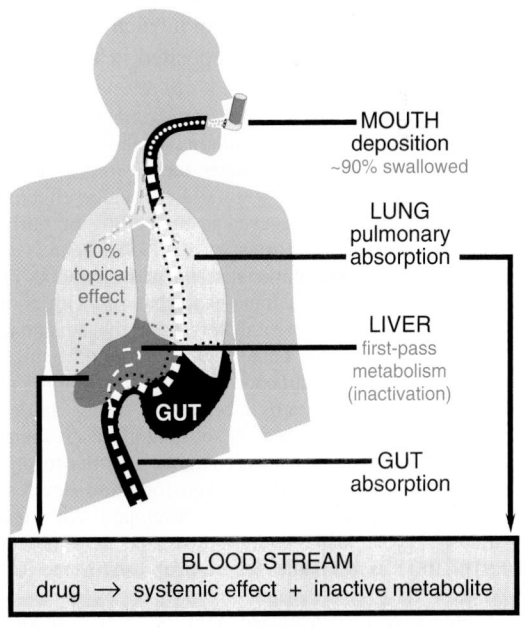

Figure 28–2. Schematic representation of the disposition of inhaled drugs.

(Modified from Taburet and Schmit, 1994 with permission.)

factors in addition to particle size determine effective deposition of drugs in the bronchial tree, including the rate of breathing and breath-holding after inhalation. It is recommended that a slow, deep breath be taken and held for 5 to 10 seconds when administering drugs to the lungs.

As depicted in Figure 28–2, even under ideal circumstances only a small fraction of the aerosolized drug is deposited in the lungs, typically 2% to 10%. Most of the remainder is swallowed. Therefore, to have minimal systemic effects, an aerosolized drug should be either poorly absorbed from the gastrointestinal system or rapidly inactivated *via* first-pass hepatic metabolism. Furthermore, any maneuvers that result in a higher percentage of deposition in the lungs and a lower percentage of drug reaching the gastrointestinal system should improve the therapeutic index. For example, with metered-dose inhalers, a large-volume "spacer" can be attached to the inhaler. A spacer is a tube or expandable bellows that fits between the inhaler and the patient's mouth; the inhaler discharges into it, and the patient inhales from it. A spacer can improve markedly the ratio of inhaled to swallowed drug by limiting the amount of larger particles (>10 μm) that reach the mouth and by reducing the need for the patient to coordinate accurately inhalation with inhaler activation (Bryant and Shimizu, 1988). The latter is not a trivial concern, since multiple studies have shown that more than 50% of patients using inhalers do not use proper technique (Epstein *et al.*, 1979; Macfarlane and Lane, 1980) and thereby markedly reduce the amount of drug inhaled into the lungs while not reducing the amount deposited in the mouth.

The two types of devices used for providing aerosol therapy are *metered-dose inhalers* and *nebulizers*. Both devices provide a range of particle sizes that includes the desired 1- to 5-μm range. When used appropriately, they are equally effective in delivery of drug to the lungs, even in the setting of fairly severe asthma exacerbations (Turner *et al.*, 1988; Benton *et al.*, 1989). Nevertheless, some clinicians and many patients prefer to use nebulizers for severe asthma exacerbations with poor inspiratory ability. Metered-dose inhalers offer the advantage of being cheaper and portable; nebulizers offer the advantages of not requiring hand/breathing coordination. In addition, nebulizer therapy can be delivered by facemask to young children or older patients who are confused. A substantial disadvantage of metered-dose inhalers is that most contain chlorofluorocarbons. Temporary exemptions have been given for these devices until alternative, safe propellants can be developed. An albuterol metered-dose inhaler using hydrofluoroalkane as a propellant (PROVENTIL HFA) is available for clinical use in the United States.

An alternative to aerosolized delivery is the use of *dry-powder inhalers*. These typically use lactose or glucose powders to carry the drugs. One disadvantage of these devices is that a relatively high airflow is needed to suspend properly the powder. Young children, the elderly, and those suffering from

a significant asthma exacerbation may not be able to generate such air flow rates. The dry powder can be irritating when inhaled. Storage of dry-powder inhalers in areas where there are wide temperature fluctuations or high humidity can affect their performance.

β-Adrenergic Receptor Agonists

The history, chemistry, pharmacological properties, and mechanisms of action of the β-adrenergic agonists are discussed in Chapter 10. The discussion of these agents in this chapter is restricted to their uses in asthma.

Mechanism of Action and Use in Asthma. The β-adrenergic receptor agonists available for the treatment of asthma are selective for the β_2-receptor subtype. With few exceptions, these are delivered directly to the airways *via* inhalation. The agonists can be classified as short- and long-acting. This subclassification is useful from a pharmacological perspective, because short-acting agonists are used only for symptomatic relief of asthma, whereas long-acting agonists are used prophylactically in the treatment of the disease.

Short-Acting β-Adrenergic Receptor Agonists. Drugs in this class include *albuterol* (PROVENTIL, VENTOLIN), *levalbuterol* [XOPENEX, the (R)-enantiomer of albuterol], *metaproterenol* (ALUPENT), *terbutaline* (BRETHAIRE), and *pirbuterol* (MAXAIR). These drugs are used for acute inhalation treatment of bronchospasm. Terbutaline (BRETHINE, BRICANYL), albuterol, and metaproterenol also are available in oral dosage form. Each of the inhaled drugs has an onset of action within 1 to 5 minutes and produces a bronchodilation that lasts for about 2 to 6 hours. When given in oral dosage forms, the duration of action is somewhat longer (oral terbutaline, for example, has a duration of action of 4 to 8 hours). Although there are slight differences in the relative β_2/β_1-receptor potency ratios among the drugs, all of them are selective for the β_2 subtype.

The mechanism of the antiasthmatic action of short-acting β-adrenergic receptor agonists is undoubtedly linked to the direct relaxation of airway smooth muscle and consequent bronchodilation. Although human bronchial smooth muscle receives little or no catecholaminergic sympathetic innervation, it nevertheless contains large numbers of β_2-adrenergic receptors. Stimulating these receptors leads to activation of adenylyl cyclase, increases in cellular cyclic AMP, and consequent reduction of muscle tone (*see* Johnson and Coleman, 1995). β_2-Adrenergic receptor agonists also have been shown to increase the conductance of potassium channels in airway muscle cells leading to membrane hyperpolarization and relaxation. This occurs, in part, by mechanisms independent of adenylyl cyclase activity and cyclic AMP production (Kume *et al.*, 1994).

The most effective drugs in relaxing airway smooth muscle and reversing bronchoconstriction are short-acting β_2-adrenergic receptor agonists. They are the preferred treatment for rapid symptomatic relief of dyspnea associated with asthmatic bronchoconstriction (Fanta *et al.,* 1986; Rossing *et al.,* 1980; Nelson, 1995). Although these drugs are prescribed on an as-needed basis, it is imperative that guidelines be given to the patient so that reliance on relief of symptoms during times of deteriorating asthma does not occur. When the asthma symptoms become persistent, the patient should be reevaluated, so that drugs aimed at controlling, in addition to reversing, the disease can be prescribed.

Long-Acting β-Adrenergic Receptor Agonists. *Salmeterol xinafoate* (SEREVENT) is a long-lasting adrenergic agonist with very high selectivity for the β_2-receptor subtype (Cheung *et al.,* 1992; D'Alonzo *et al.,* 1994; Kamada *et al.,* 1994). Inhalation of salmeterol provides persistent bronchodilation lasting over 12 hours. The mechanism underlying the therapeutic effect of salmeterol is not yet fully understood. The extended side chain on salmeterol renders it 10,000 times more lipophilic than albuterol (Brittain, 1990). The lipophilicity regulates the diffusion rate away from the receptor by determining the degree of partitioning in the lipid bilayer of the membrane. Subsequent to binding the receptor, the less lipophilic, short-acting agonists are rapidly removed from the receptor environment by diffusion in the aqueous phase. Unbound salmeterol, by contrast, persists in the membrane and only slowly dissociates from the receptor environment. *Bitolterol* (TORNALATE) is a highly selective β-adrenergic receptor agonist that also has a relatively long duration of action, although it has a rapid onset of action and is approved in the United States for acute treatment and not prophylaxis of bronchospasm. The mechanism underlying its persistent action is related to the fact that the biological action of bitolterol is dependent on metabolism within the lung to the active metabolite *colterol* (Friedel and Brogden, 1988).

Long-acting β-adrenergic receptor agonists relax airway smooth muscle and cause bronchodilation by the same mechanisms as do short-duration agonists. There are β_2-adrenergic receptors on cell types in the airways other than bronchial smooth muscle. Of particular interest are the observations that stimulation of β_2-adrenergic receptors inhibits the function of numerous inflammatory cells including mast cells, basophils, eosinophils, neutrophils, and lymphocytes. In general, stimulating β_2-adrenergic receptors in these cell types leads to elevations in cellular cyclic AMP, causing a signaling cascade leading to inhibition of inflammatory mediator and cytokine release (Lichtenstein and Margolis, 1968; Barnes, 1999). Chronic treatment with a receptor agonist often leads to receptor desensitization and a diminution of effect. The rate and degree of

β_2-adrenergic receptor desensitization is dependent on the cell type. For example, the β_2 receptors on human bronchial smooth muscle are relatively resistant to desensitization, whereas receptors on mast cells and lymphocytes are rapidly desensitized following agonist exposure (Chong and Peachell, 1999; Johnson and Coleman, 1995). This may help to explain why there is little evidence that these drugs are effective in inhibiting airway inflammation associated with asthma.

There are relatively few studies evaluating the antiinflammatory effect of adding long-acting β_2-adrenergic receptor agonist therapy to inhaled glucocorticoid treatment. In one such study, symptomatic asthmatic subjects taking inhaled glucocorticoid therapy were given either salmeterol or fluticasone. In the salmeterol group, there was a significant reduction of eosinophils in the airway wall, suggesting an antiinflammatory effect (Li *et al.,* 1999).

Chronic treatment with long-acting β_2-adrenergic receptor agonists has been shown to improve lung function, decrease asthma symptoms, decrease use of short-acting inhaled β_2-adrenergic agonists, and decrease nocturnal asthma. This was not associated with a marked decrease in airway inflammation. Therefore, in a report issued by the National Heart, Lung, and Blood Institute (Publication # 95-3659, 1996), it is suggested that treatment of chronic, persistent asthma with a long-acting β_2-adrenergic receptor agonist should be accompanied by antiinflammatory medications. For patients with chronic asthma who are not controlled adequately by inhaled glucocorticoid therapy, the physician either can increase the dose of steroid or add another class of drug to the regimen. Clinical studies have provided evidence in favor of adding a long-acting β_2-adrenergic agonist over doubling the dose of steroid in these patients (Greening *et al.,* 1994; Woolcock *et al.,* 1996). A fixed-dosage combination of salmeterol and the steroid fluticasone (ADVAIR) has been approved for treatment of asthma in Europe and is pending approval in the United States.

Salmeterol should not be used to reverse acute symptoms of asthma. Rather, physicians prescribing salmeterol also should prescribe a short-acting β_2-adrenergic receptor agonist for symptomatic relief. Use of short-acting agonists as "rescue" medication should be monitored. If the patient requires four or more inhalations a day for two or more consecutive days of a rescue medication, then the patient should be advised to see a physician for a reevaluation.

Toxicity.   Owing to their β_2-receptor selectivity and topical delivery, inhaled β-adrenergic receptor agonists, at recommended doses, have relatively few side effects. A portion of inhaled drug is inevitably absorbed into the systemic circulation. At higher doses, therefore, these drugs may lead to increased heart rate, cardiac arrhythmias, and central nervous system effects associated with β-adrenergic receptor activation as described in Chapter 10. This can become of particular concern in poorly controlled asthma, where there may be excessive and inappropriate reliance on symptomatic treatment with short-acting β-receptor agonists.

Oral Therapy with β-Adrenergic Receptor Agonists. The use of orally administered adrenergic agonists for bronchodilation has not gained wide acceptance, largely because of the greater risk of producing side effects, especially tremulousness, muscle cramps, cardiac tachyarrhythmias, and metabolic disturbances (*see* Chapter 10). There are two situations in which oral β-adrenergic agonists are used frequently. First, in young children (<5 years old) who cannot manipulate metered-dose inhalers yet have occasional wheezing with viral upper respiratory infections, brief courses of oral therapy (albuterol or metaproterenol syrups) are well tolerated and effective. Second, in some patients with severe asthma exacerbations, any aerosol, whether delivered *via* a metered-dose inhaler or a nebulizer, can be irritating and cause a worsening of cough and bronchospasm. In this circumstance, oral therapy with β_2-adrenergic agonists (albuterol, metaproterenol, or terbutaline tablets) can be effective. However, the frequency of adverse systemic side effects with orally administered agents is higher in adults than in children.

Even though stimulation of β-adrenergic receptors has been shown to inhibit the release of inflammatory mediators from mast cells, long-term administration of β_2-adrenergic agonists, either orally or by inhalation, does not reduce bronchial hyperresponsiveness. Thus, other approaches for the treatment of chronic symptoms are preferred.

Glucocorticoids

The history, chemistry, pharmacological properties, and mechanisms of action of glucocorticoids are discussed in Chapter 60. Here, the discussion is restricted to their uses in asthma. Barnes and Pedersen (1993) have provided a thorough review of this subject.

Systemic glucocorticoid administration long has been employed to treat severe chronic asthma or severe, acute exacerbations of asthma (McFadden, 1993; Greenberger, 1992). The development of aerosol formulations significantly improved the safety of glucocorticoid treatment, allowing it to be used for moderate asthma (Busse, 1993). Asthmatic subjects who require inhaled β_2-adrenergic agonists four or more times weekly are viewed as candidates for inhaled glucocorticoids (Anonymous, 1991; Israel and Drazen, 1994; Barnes, 1995).

Mechanism of Action in Asthma. Asthma is a disease associated with airway inflammation, airway hyperreactivity, and acute bronchoconstriction. Glucocorticoids do not relax airway smooth muscle and thus have little effect on acute bronchoconstriction. By contrast, these agents are singularly effective in inhibiting airway inflammation. Very few mechanisms that lead to the inflammatory reaction escape the inhibitory effects of these drugs (Schleimer, 1998). The mechanisms that contribute to the antiinflammatory effect of glucocorticoid therapy in asthma include modulation of cytokine and chemokine production, inhibition of eicosanoid synthesis, marked inhibition of accumulation of basophils, eosinophils, and other leukocytes in lung tissue, and decreased vascular permeability (Schleimer, 1998). The profound and generalized antiinflammatory action of this class of drugs explains why they are the most effective drugs used in the treatment of asthma at present.

Inhaled Glucocorticoids. Glucocorticoids have long been known to be effective in controlling asthma, but treatment with systemic glucocorticoids comes with the cost of considerable unwanted side effects. A major advance in asthma therapy was the development of glucocorticoids that could be delivered to the lungs *via* inhalation. This allowed for the targeting of the drug directly to the relevant site of inflammation. In so doing, the therapeutic index of the drugs has been greatly enhanced by substantially diminishing the number and degree of side effects, without sacrificing clinical efficacy. There are currently five glucocorticoids available in the United States for inhalation therapy: *beclomethasone dipropionate* (BECLOVENT, VANCERIL), *triamcinolone acetonide* (AZMACORT), *flunisolide* (AEROBID), *budesonide* (PULMICORT), and *fluticasone propionate* (FLOVENT). A sixth drug, *mometasone* (ASMANEX), is pending approval by the United States Food and Drug Administration for use in asthma. These drugs differ markedly in their affinity for the glucocorticoid receptor, with fluticasone and budesonide having much higher affinity than beclomethasone. Mechanistically, however, there are no differences among the available choices, and, with the appropriate dose, they all are effective in controlling asthma. Few studies have directly assessed the relative therapeutic index of the various formulations of inhaled steroids in the treatment of asthma, but available data indicate that one does not clearly stand out with a far superior therapeutic index (O'Byrne and Pedersen, 1998).

Inhaled glucocorticoids are used prophylactically to control asthma, rather than to acutely reverse asthma symptoms. As with all prophylactic therapies, compliance is a significant concern. Issues relating to drug compliance, therefore, become relevant when choosing among the various steroid formulations. Having highly potent glucocorticoid action, the newer drugs can be effective with as little as one or two puffs administered twice or even once daily.

This more convenient dosage regimen may be preferred by patients, which in turn translates to better compliance and therefore better asthma control. The appropriate dose of steroid must be determined empirically. Important variables that influence the effective dose include the severity of disease, the particular steroid used, and the device used for drug delivery, as it determines the actual quantity of drug delivered to the lungs (Smaldone, 1997). When determining the optimal dose, it should be kept in mind that maximal improvement in lung function may not occur until after several weeks of treatment.

Asthmatic patients maintained on inhaled glucocorticoids show improvement in symptoms and lowered requirements for "rescue" with β-adrenergic agonists (Laitinen *et al.*, 1992; Haahtela *et al.*, 1994). Beneficial effects may be seen within 1 week; however, improvement, in terms of reduced bronchial hyperreactivity, may continue for several months (Juniper *et al.*, 1990). When directly compared to regular use of inhaled β-adrenergic agonists, inhaled glucocorticoids provide better symptom control (Laitinen *et al.*, 1992). One study showed that, during treatment with inhaled budesonide (600 μg twice daily) for 2 years, bronchial hyperreactivity remained improved throughout the study (Haahtela *et al.*, 1994). After 2 years, most patients were able to reduce their dose of budesonide to 200 μg twice daily without loss of control of their asthma. Upon complete discontinuation of budesonide, bronchial hyperreactivity returned, and symptoms usually worsened, although one-third of patients were able to discontinue completely their budesonide inhalers without symptomatic worsening after prolonged treatment. Based on these findings, periodic attempts to discontinue inhaled glucocorticoids should be considered in patients who are extremely well controlled.

Systemic Glucocorticoids.   Systemic glucocorticoids are used for acute asthma exacerbations and chronic, severe asthma. Substantial doses of glucocorticoids (*e.g.*, 40 to 60 mg of prednisone daily for 5 days; 1 to 2 mg/kg per day for children) often are used to treat acute exacerbations of asthma (Weinberger, 1987). Although an additional week of therapy at somewhat reduced dosage may be required, the steroids can be withdrawn abruptly once control of the symptoms by other medications has been restored; any suppression of adrenal function appears to dissipate within 1 to 2 weeks. More protracted bouts of severe asthma may require longer treatment and a slow tapering of the dose to avoid exacerbating asthma symptoms and suppressing pituitary/adrenal function. In persistent asthma, alternate-day therapy with oral prednisone was common in the past. Now, most patients considered for this regimen likely can be treated better with high-dose inhaled glucocorticoids.

Toxicity.   *Inhaled Glucocorticoids.*   While there is a great deal of enthusiasm for inhaled glucocorticoids in asthma, local and systemic adverse effects remain a concern (Table 28–3). Some portion of any inhaled drug is swallowed. Therefore, inhaled drugs can reach the circulation by direct absorption from the lung or by absorption from the gastrointestinal tract. The newer glucocorticoids have extremely low oral bioavailability due to extensive first-pass metabolism by the liver. These reach the circulation almost exclusively by absorption from the lung (Brattsand and Axelsson, 1997). In contrast to the beneficial effects on asthma, which reach a plateau at about 1600 μg/day, the probability of adverse effects continues to increase at higher doses. Oropharyngeal candidiasis and, more frequently, dysphonia can be encountered. The incidence of candidiasis can be reduced substantially by rinsing the mouth and throat with water after each use and by employing spacer or reservoir devices attached to the dispenser to decrease the deposition of drug in the oral cavity (Johnson, 1987). Appreciable suppression of the

Table 28–3
Potential Adverse Effects Associated with Inhaled Glucocorticoids

ADVERSE EFFECT	RISK
Hypothalamic-pituitary-adrenal axis suppression	No significant risk until dosages of budesonide or beclomethasone increased to >1500 μg/day in adults or >400 μg/day in children
Bone resorption	Modest but significant effects at doses possibly as low as 500 μg/day
Carbohydrate and lipid metabolism	Minor, clinically insignificant changes occur with dosages of beclomethasone >1000 μg/day
Cataracts	Anecdotal reports, risk unproven
Skin thinning	Dosage-related effect with beclomethasone dipropionate over a range of 400 to 2000 μg/day
Purpura	Dosage-related increase in occurrence with beclomethasone over a range of 400 to 2000 μg/day
Dysphonia	Usually of little consequence
Candidiasis	Incidence <5%, reduced by use of spacer device
Growth retardation	Difficult to separate effect of disease from effect of treatment, but no discernible effects on growth when all studies are considered

SOURCE: Modified from Pavord and Knox (1993) and Barnes (1995).

hypothalamic-pituitary-adrenal axis is difficult to document at doses below 800 μg/day and probably is rarely of physiologic importance even at doses up to 1600 μg/day. Modest but statistically significant decreases in bone mineral density do occur in female asthmatics receiving inhaled steroids, possibly even when doses as low as 500 μg/day are employed (Ip *et al.*, 1994). Others have shown increases in markers for bone mineral turnover (serum osteocalin and urine hydroxyproline levels) during treatment with inhaled glucocorticoids (Pavord and Knox, 1993; Israel and Drazen, 1994). The clinical relevance of these bone metabolism findings remains to be determined, but they do argue that inhaled glucocorticoid treatment should be reserved for moderate and severe asthma, since such treatment is likely to last for many years (Israel and Drazen, 1994). Nonetheless, it has been suggested that the small risk of adverse effects at high doses of inhaled glucocorticoids is outweighed by the risks of not controlling severe asthma adequately (Barnes, 1995).

Systemic Glucocorticoids. The adverse effects of systemic administration of adrenocortical steroids are well known (*see* Chapter 60), but treatment for brief periods (5 to 10 days) causes relatively little dose-related toxicity. The most common adverse effects during a brief course are mood disturbances, increased appetite, loss of glucose control in diabetics, and candidiasis.

Leukotriene-Receptor Antagonists and Leukotriene-Synthesis Inhibitors

Zafirlukast (ACCOLATE) and *montelukast* (SINGULAIR) are leukotriene-receptor antagonists. *Zileuton* (ZYFLO) is an inhibitor of 5-lipoxygenase, which catalyzes the formation of leukotrienes from arachidonic acid.

History. The history of leukotrienes can be traced back to the classical pharmacological studies in the late 1930s by Kellaway and Trethewie (1940). Upon investigating antigen-induced responses in guinea pigs sensitized to egg albumin, they discovered a *slow-reacting*, smooth-muscle-stimulating *substance*. They named the substance SRS based on its pharmacological activity and concluded that it was a unique substance found only in immunologically sensitized tissues subsequently challenged with antigen. Decades later, Brocklehurst (1960) renamed SRS as *slow-reacting substance* of *anaphylaxis*, or SRS-A.

Two pivotal discoveries were required before the importance of SRS-A in allergic responses was proven. First was the discovery in 1973 by scientists at Fisons pharmaceutical company of an SRS-A antagonist called FPL 55712 (Augstein *et al.*, 1973), and second was the elucidation by Samuelsson and colleagues of the structure of SRS-A as a 5-lipoxygenase product of arachidonic acid, which they termed *cysteinyl leukotriene* (Murphy *et al.*, 1979; *see* Chapter 26). Soon thereafter, an enormous effort was undertaken by the pharmaceutical industry to discover novel inhibitors of leukotrienes as potential therapeutic agents for asthma. The strategies taken were either to reduce the synthesis of leukotrienes by inhibiting the 5-lipoxygenase enzyme, or to antagonize the effects of leukotrienes at their receptors. This effort bore fruit in the 1990s with the development

of three new drugs now available for the treatment of asthma in the United States. These drugs are the leukotriene-receptor antagonists zafirlukast (Krell *et al.*, 1990), and montelukast (Jones *et al.*, 1995), and the leukotriene-synthesis inhibitor zileuton (Carter *et al.*, 1991).

Chemistry. The chemical structures of zafirlukast, montelukast, and zileuton are shown below.

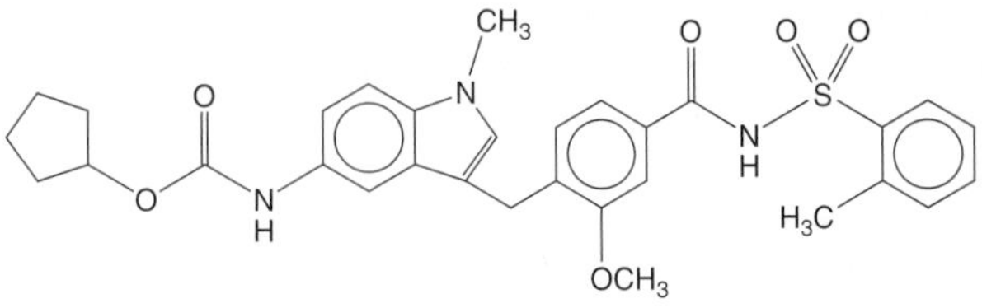

ZAFIRLUKAST

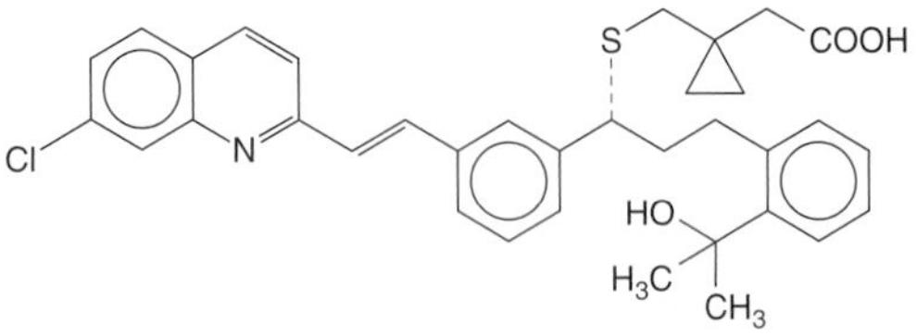

MONTELUKAST

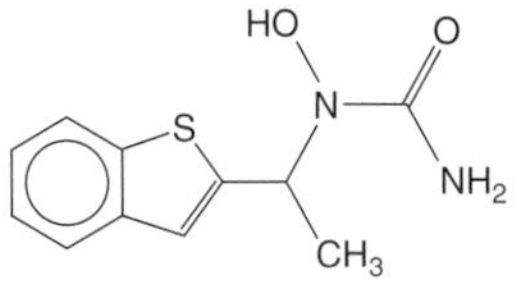

ZILEUTON

Pharmacokinetics and Metabolism. Each of the three leukotriene-modifying drugs is available for oral administration in tablet form. Zafirlukast is rapidly absorbed, with greater than 90% bioavailability. At therapeutic plasma concentrations, it is over 99% protein bound. Zafirlukast is extensively metabolized by the liver cytochrome P450 isozyme CYP2C9. The parent drug is responsible for the drug action with metabolites being less than 10% effective. The half-life of zafirlukast is approximately 10 hours.

Montelukast is rapidly absorbed, with about 60% to 70% bioavailability. At therapeutic concentrations, it is highly protein bound (99%). It is extensively metabolized by cytochrome P450 isozymes CYP3A4 and CYP2C9. The half-life of montelukast is between 3 and 6 hours.

Zileuton is rapidly absorbed upon oral administration and is extensively metabolized by cytochrome P450 isozymes and by UDP-glucuronosyltransferases. The parent molecule is responsible for the therapeutic action. Zileuton is a short-acting drug, with a half-life of

these include bronchospasm, cough or wheezing, laryngeal edema, joint swelling and pain, angioedema, headache, rash, and nausea. Such reactions have been reported at a frequency of less than 1 in 10,000 patients (*see* Murphy and Kelly, 1987). Very rare instances of anaphylaxis also have been documented. Nedocromil and cromolyn can cause a bad taste.

Use in Asthma. The main use of cromolyn (INTAL) and nedocromil (TILADE) is in the treatment of mild to moderate bronchial asthma to prevent asthmatic attacks. These agents are ineffective in treating ongoing bronchoconstriction. When inhaled several times daily, cromolyn will inhibit both the immediate and the late asthmatic responses to antigenic challenge or to exercise. With regular use for more than 2 to 3 months, there is evidence of reduced bronchial hyperreactivity, as measured by response to challenge with histamine or methacholine (*see* Murphy and Kelly, 1987; Hoag and McFadden, 1991). Nedocromil generally is more effective than cromolyn in animal models and human studies (Brogden and Sorkin, 1993). Nedocromil is approved for use in asthmatic patients 12 years old and older; cromolyn is approved for all ages.

Compared to inhaled glucocorticoids, cromolyn and nedocromil are less potent in controlling asthma. Cromolyn, 2 mg inhaled four times daily, was not as effective as beclomethasone, 200 μg twice daily (Svendsen *et al.*, 1987), and was less effective than nedocromil, 4 mg four times daily (Brogden and Sorkin, 1993). In terms of lung function measurements, 4 mg of nedocromil inhaled twice daily was approximately as effective as 200 μg of beclomethasone inhaled twice daily, but nedocromil was not as effective in controlling symptoms, reducing bronchodilator use, or improving bronchial hyperreactivity (Svendsen *et al.*, 1989). In a second study, 4 mg of nedocromil four times daily was as effective as 100 μg of beclomethasone four times daily (Bel *et al.*, 1990). In a thorough review, Brogden and Sorkin (1993) concluded that nedocromil is useful in patients with mild to moderate asthma as added therapy, as an alternative to regularly administered oral and inhaled β-adrenergic agonists and oral methylxanthines, and possibly as an alternative to low-dose, inhaled glucocorticoids.

The use of cromolyn or nedocromil in addition to inhaled glucocorticoids in moderately severe asthma has been investigated. Several studies have shown that the addition of cromolyn to inhaled glucocorticoid therapy yields no additional benefit (Toogood *et al.*, 1981). Nedocromil may allow a reduction of steroids in patients receiving high doses of inhaled steroids (Brogden and Sorkin, 1993). These studies were short term; whether or not long-term reduction in steroid doses is possible remains to be determined. In one study, the addition of nedocromil, 4 mg four times daily, to high-dose, inhaled glucocorticoid treatment resulted in modest improvements when administered for 8 weeks to patients with moderately severe asthma (Svendsen and Jorgensen, 1991). Because of its limited potency, the use of cromolyn is decreasing.

In patients with systemic mastocytosis who have gastrointestinal symptoms due to an excessive number of mast cells

in the gastrointestinal mucosa, an oral preparation of cromolyn (GASTROCROM) is effective in reducing symptoms (Horan *et al.*, 1990). The benefits are derived from the topical application rather than systemic absorption; cromolyn is poorly absorbed, and only the gastrointestinal symptoms are improved in the treated patients.

Theophylline

Theophylline, a methylxanthine, is among the least expensive drugs used to treat asthma, and consequently it remains a commonly used drug for this indication in many countries. In industrialized countries, the advent of inhaled glucocorticoids, β-adrenergic receptor agonists, and leukotriene-modifying drugs have significantly diminished the extent to which theophylline is used. In the United States, theophylline for the most part has been relegated to a third-line treatment, used in patients whose asthma is otherwise difficult to control.

Source and History. Theophylline, caffeine, and theobromine are three closely related alkaloids that occur in plants widely distributed geographically. At least half the population of the world consumes tea (containing caffeine and small amounts of theophylline and theobromine), prepared from the leaves of *Thea sinensis,* a bush native to southern China and now extensively cultivated in other countries. Cocoa and chocolate, from the seeds of *Theobroma cacao,* contain theobromine and some caffeine. Coffee, the most important source of caffeine in the American diet, is extracted from the fruit of *Coffea arabica* and related species. Cola-flavored drinks usually contain considerable amounts of caffeine, in part because of their content of extracts of the nuts of *Cola acuminata* (the guru nuts chewed by the natives of the Sudan) and in part because of the addition of caffeine as such in their production (*see* Graham, 1978).

The basis for the popularity of all the caffeine-containing beverages is the ancient belief that they have stimulant and antisoporific actions that elevate mood, decrease fatigue, and increase capacity for work. For example, legend credits the discovery of coffee to a prior of an Arabian convent. Shepherds reported that goats that had eaten the berries of the coffee plant gamboled and frisked about all through the night instead of sleeping. The prior, mindful of the long nights of prayer that he had to endure, instructed the shepherds to pick the berries so that he might make a beverage from them.

Classical pharmacological studies, principally of caffeine, during the first half of this century confirmed these experiences and revealed that methylxanthines possess other important pharmacological properties as well. These properties were exploited for a number of years in a variety of therapeutic applications, in many of which caffeine has now been replaced by more effective agents. However, in recent years there has been a resurgence of interest in the natural methylxanthines and their synthetic derivatives, principally as a result of increased knowledge of their cellular basis of action.

Chemistry. Theophylline, caffeine, and theobromine are methylated xanthines. Xanthine itself is a dioxypurine and is structurally related to uric acid. Caffeine is 1,3,7-trimethyl-xanthine; theophylline, 1,3-dimethylxanthine; and theobromine, 3,7-dimethylxanthine. The structural formulas of xanthine and the three naturally occurring xanthine derivatives are as follows:

XANTHINE   CAFFEINE

THEOPHYLLINE   THEOBROMINE

The solubility of the methylxanthines is low and is much enhanced by the formation of complexes (usually 1:1) with a wide variety of compounds. The most notable of these complexes is that between theophylline and ethylenediamine (to form *aminophylline*). The formation of complex double salts (*e.g.,* caffeine and sodium benzoate) or true salts [*e.g., choline theophyllinate (oxtriphylline)*] also enhances aqueous solubility. These salts or complexes dissociate to yield the parent methylxanthines when dissolved in aqueous solution and should not be confused with covalently modified derivatives such as *dyphylline* [1,3-dimethyl-7-(2, 3-dihydroxypropyl)xanthine].

A large number of derivatives of the methylxanthines have been prepared and examined for their ability to inhibit cyclic nucleotide phosphodiesterases (Beavo and Reifsnyder, 1990) and to antagonize receptor-mediated actions of adenosine (Daly, 1982; Linden, 1991), the two best-characterized cellular actions of the methylxanthines. In general, both activities are reduced in derivatives that lack substituents at position 1 or contain substituents at position 7, as compared with the corresponding 1,3-dialkylxanthine. For example, the order of potency for the naturally occurring methylxanthines is theophylline > caffeine > theobromine. Congeners of theophylline with larger nonpolar substituents at positions 1 and 3 usually display enhancement of both activities (Choi *et al.,* 1988). Addition of aromatic, cyclohexyl, or cyclopentyl groups at position 8 usually markedly increases affinity for adenosine receptors but reduces inhibition of cyclic nucleotide phosphodiesterases (Martinson *et al.,* 1987). Although neither caffeine nor theophylline discriminates among the subtypes of adenosine receptors (*see* below), certain 8-substituted derivatives of 1, 3-dipropylxanthine display marked selectivity for A_1 receptors, while some analogs of caffeine display appreciable selectivity for A_2 receptors. In addition, certain tricyclic nonxanthine compounds are potent antagonists at adenosine receptors (Linden, 1991).

Mechanism of Action.   Theophylline inhibits cyclic nucleotide phosphodiesterase enzymes (PDEs). PDEs catalyze the breakdown of cyclic AMP and cyclic GMP

to 5′-AMP and 5′-GMP, respectively. Inhibition of PDEs will lead to an accumulation of cyclic AMP and cyclic GMP, thereby increasing the signal transduction through these pathways. It is now recognized that cyclic nucleotide PDEs are members of a superfamily of at least eleven families of genetically distinct enzymes (Soderling and Beavo, 2000). Theophylline and related methylxanthines are relatively nonselective in the PDE subtypes they inhibit.

The potency and efficacy of PDE inhibitors in affecting cell function is dependent on the basal level of cyclic nucleotide production. Cyclic AMP and cyclic GMP production in cells is regulated by endogenous receptor-ligand interactions leading to activation of adenylyl cyclase and guanylyl cyclase, respectively (*see* Chapter 2). Diffusable mediators such as nitric oxide and related molecules also may lead to increases in cyclic GMP by direct interaction with guanylyl cyclase. Inhibitors of PDEs therefore can be thought of as drugs that enhance the activity of endogenous autacoids, hormones, and neurotransmitters that signal *via* cyclic nucleotide messengers. This may explain why the *in vivo* potency often is increased relative to that observed *in vitro*.

Theophylline also is a competitive antagonist at adenosine receptors (Fredholm and Persson, 1982). Adenosine can act as an autacoid and transmitter with myriad biological actions. Of particular relevance to asthma are the observations that adenosine can cause bronchoconstriction in asthmatics and potentiate immunologically induced mediator release from human lung mast cells (Cushley *et al.,* 1984; Peachell *et al.,* 1988). Inhibition of the actions of adenosine must therefore also be considered when attempting to explain the mechanism of action of theophylline (Feoktistov *et al.,* 1998).

Pulmonary System.   Theophylline effectively relaxes airway smooth muscle and thus can be classified as a bronchodilator. This likely contributes to the acute therapeutic efficacy in asthma. Evidence supports a role for both adenosine receptor antagonism and PDE inhibition in the bronchodilating effect of theophylline. Adenosine does not directly contract human isolated bronchial smooth muscle, but when inhaled acts as a potent bronchoconstrictor in asthmatic subjects (Cushley *et al.,* 1984). Therefore, inhibition of this function of adenosine may contribute to theophylline-induced bronchodilation in some asthmatic subjects. Inhibition of PDE isozymes type III and IV effectively relaxes human isolated bronchial smooth muscle (Torphy *et al.,* 1993). It thus seems likely that inhibition of PDEs also contributes to the bronchodilating effect of theophylline. Also seeming to support a role for PDE inhibition in the mechanism of bronchodilator action of theophylline have been studies with a related methylxanthine drug, *enprofylline* (3-propylxanthine), which has been extensively studied in Europe for use in the treatment of asthma. Enprofylline is more potent than theophylline as a bronchodilator, but is much less potent than theophylline as an antagonist at most types of adenosine receptors (Pauwels *et al.,* 1985). The latter point, however, needs to be interpreted cautiously. Activation of the A_{2B} subtype of adenosine receptor causes several proinflammatory effects, and both theophylline and enprofylline are potent competitive antagonists of A_{2B} adenosine receptors (Feoktistov *et al.,* 1998).

Theophylline also inhibits synthesis and secretion of inflammatory mediators from numerous cell types including mast cells and basophils (Page, 1999). This effect of theophylline likely is due to PDE inhibition and can be mimicked in large part with drugs that selectively inhibit the PDE IV isozymes (Torphy and Undem, 1991). It has been argued that, at therapeutic concentrations, the antiinflammatory effect of theophylline may be more relevant to the drug's therapeutic actions than is direct bronchodilation, but this remains unproven (Page, 1999).

A discussion of pharmacological properties of theophylline and other methylxanthines involving other organ systems can be found in previous editions of this book.

Absorption, Fate, and Excretion.   The methylxanthines are absorbed readily after oral, rectal, or parenteral administration. Absorption from rectal suppositories is slow and unreliable. Theophylline administered in liquids or uncoated tablets is rapidly and completely absorbed. Absorption also is complete from some, but not all, sustained-release formulations (*see* Hendeles and Weinberger, 1982). In the absence of food, solutions or uncoated tablets of theophylline produce maximal concentrations in plasma within 2 hours; caffeine is more rapidly absorbed, and maximal plasma concentrations are achieved within 1 hour. Numerous sustained-release preparations of theophylline are available, designed for dosing intervals of 8, 12, or 24 hours. These preparations cause marked interpatient variability with regard to the rate and extent of absorption and especially the effect of food and time of administration on these parameters (*see* Symposium, 1986a). Thus, it has become necessary to calibrate a given preparation in a given patient and to avoid substituting one apparently similar product for another.

Food ordinarily slows the rate of absorption of theophylline but does not limit its extent. With sustained-release preparations, food may decrease the bioavailability of theophylline within some products but may increase it with others. High-carbohydrate, low-protein diets decrease theophylline elimination, whereas low-carbohydrate, high-protein diets and consumption of "char-broiled" meat increase elimination. Recumbency or sleep also may reduce the rate or extent of absorption to an important degree. These factors make it difficult to maintain relatively constant concentrations of theophylline in plasma throughout the day. Fortunately, it also has become apparent that the concentrations required to alleviate asthmatic symptoms do not remain constant, and the emphasis has shifted toward designing dosing regimens that ensure peak concentrations in the early morning hours, when symptoms frequently worsen (*see* Symposium, 1988a).

Methylxanthines are distributed into all body compartments; they cross the placenta and pass into breast milk. The apparent volumes of distribution for caffeine and theophylline are similar and usually are between 0.4 and 0.6 liter/kg. These values are considerably higher in premature infants. Theophylline is bound to plasma proteins to a greater extent than is caffeine, and the fraction bound declines as the concentration of methylxanthine increases. At therapeutic concentrations, the protein binding of theophylline averages about 60%, but it is decreased to about 40% in newborn infants and in adults with hepatic cirrhosis (*see* Hendeles and Weinberger, 1982).

Methylxanthines are eliminated primarily by metabolism in the liver. Less than 15% and 5% of administered theophylline and caffeine, respectively, are recovered in the urine unchanged. Caffeine has a half-life in plasma of 3 to 7 hours; this increases by about twofold in women during the later stages of pregnancy or with long-term use of oral contraceptive steroids. In premature infants, the rate of elimination of both methylxanthines is quite slow. The average half-life for caffeine is more than 50 hours, while the mean values for theophylline obtained in various studies range between 20 and 36 hours. However, the latter values include the extensive conversion of theophylline to caffeine in these infants (*see* Symposium, 1981; Roberts, 1984).

There is marked interindividual variation in the rate of elimination of theophylline, due to both genetic and environmental factors; fourfold differences are not uncommon (*see* Lesko, *in* Symposium, 1986a). The half-life averages about 3.5 hours in young children, while values of 8 or 9 hours are more typical of adults. In most patients the drug obeys first-order elimination kinetics within the therapeutic range. However, at higher concentrations zero-order kinetics becomes evident because of saturation of metabolic enzymes. This prolongs the decline of theophylline concentrations to nontoxic levels.

The disposition of methylxanthines also is influenced by the presence of other agents or of disease (*see* Jonkman, *in* Symposium, 1986a). For example, the clearance of theophylline is increased nearly twofold during the administration of phenytoin or barbiturates; cigarette smoking or the administration of rifampin or oral contraceptives produces smaller but appreciable increases in theophylline clearance. By contrast, the administration of cimetidine or certain macrolide antibiotics (*e.g.,* erythromycin) reduces the clearance of theophylline. Although there have been reports to the contrary, neither glucocorticoids nor immunization with purified subvirion influenza vaccine appear to have a significant effect, although acute viral infections and interferon can reduce theophylline clearance. The half-life of theophylline can be quite prolonged in patients with hepatic cirrhosis, congestive heart failure, or acute pulmonary congestion, and values of more than 60 hours have been observed.

Although scarcely detectable in adults, the conversion of theophylline to caffeine is an important metabolic pathway in preterm infants (*see* Symposium, 1981; Roberts, 1984). Caffeine accumulates in plasma to a concentration approximately 25% that of theophylline and is one of the urinary products. About 50% of the theophylline administered to such infants appears in the urine unchanged; the excretion of 1,3-dimethyluric acid, 1-methyluric acid, and caffeine accounts for nearly all of the remainder.

Toxicology.   Fatal intoxications with theophylline have been much more frequent than with caffeine. Rapid intravenous administration of therapeutic doses of *aminophylline* (500 mg) sometimes results in sudden death that is probably due to cardiac arrhythmias, and the drug should be injected slowly over 20 to 40 minutes to avoid severe toxic symptoms. These include headache, palpitation, dizziness, nausea, hypotension, and precordial pain. Additional symptoms of toxicity are tachycardia, severe restlessness, agitation, and emesis; these effects are associated with plasma concentrations of more than 20 μg/ml. Focal and generalized seizures also can occur, sometimes without prior signs of toxicity.

Most toxicity is the result of repeated administration of theophylline by either oral or parenteral routes. Although convulsions and death have occurred at plasma concentrations as low as 25 μg/ml, seizures are relatively rare at concentrations below 40 μg/ml (*see* Goldberg *et al., in* Symposium, 1986a). Patients with long-term theophylline intoxication appear to be much more prone to seizures than those who experience short-term overdoses. Such a dependence upon the history of exposure to theophylline may contribute to the difficulty in establishing a relationship between the severity of toxic symptoms and the concentration of the drug in plasma (Aitken and Martin, 1987; Bertino and Walker, 1987), and greater caution is advised in treating intoxicated patients who have been ingesting theophylline regularly (*see* Paloucek and Rodvold, 1988). Treatment may include prophylactic administration of diazepam, perhaps together with phenytoin or phenobarbital; phenytoin also may be a useful alternative to lidocaine in the treatment of serious ventricular arrhythmias. Once seizures appear, they may be refractory to anticonvulsant therapy, and it may be necessary to resort to general anesthesia and other measures used in the treatment of status epilepticus (*see* Goldberg *et al., in* Symposium, 1986a).

The widespread use of sustained-release preparations of theophylline has renewed emphasis on measures to prevent continued absorption, particularly the use of oral activated charcoal and of sorbitol as a cathartic (Goldberg *et al.,* 1987); multiple doses of oral charcoal also will accelerate clearance of theophylline. However, when plasma concentrations exceed 100 μg/ml, invasive measures usually are required, especially hemoperfusion through charcoal cartridges (*see* Paloucek and Rodvold, 1988).

Behavioral Toxicity.   As noted above, moderate doses of caffeine can provoke intense feelings of anxiety, fear, or panic in some individuals. Even subjects with a history of light-to-moderate use of caffeine experience tension, anxiety, and dysphoria after ingesting 400 mg or more of the drug (*see* Griffiths and Woodson, *in* Symposium, 1988b). In infants who have received treatment for apnea of prematurity, theophylline may produce persistent changes in sleep-wake patterns (Thoman *et al.,* 1985), but long-term effects on behavior or cognitive development have yet to be identified (*see* Aranda *et al., in* Symposium, 1986a). There has been mounting concern that the treatment of asthmatic children with theophylline might produce depression, hyperactivity, or other behavioral toxicity. However, a study of academic performance of asthmatic children treated or not with theophylline showed equal academic performance in asthmatic and nonasthmatic children (Lindgren *et al.,* 1992). Even though it is difficult to factor out specific effects of theophylline from those caused by the illness or by other features of the treatment regimen, many investigators believe that most children will benefit from the use of alternative means of controlling their symptoms.

Use in Asthma.   Theophylline has proven efficacy as a bronchodilator in asthma and formerly was considered first-line therapy. It now has been relegated to a far less prominent role, primarily because of the modest benefits it affords, its narrow therapeutic window, and the required monitoring of drug levels (Stoloff, 1994; Nasser and Rees, 1993). Nocturnal asthma can be improved with slow-release theophylline preparations (Self *et al.,* 1992), but other interventions such as inhaled glucocorticoids or salmeterol are probably more effective (Meltzer *et al.,* 1992). Some pediatricians favor theophylline over inhaled glucocorticoids because of the theoretic potential for growth suppression. However, in most circumstances, mild or moderate asthma that can be controlled with theophylline likely can be controlled with cromolyn or nedocromil, thus avoiding potential glucocorticoid side effects. There are few data to support the routine use of theophylline in the treatment of acute, severe bronchospasm (Fanta *et al.,* 1986; Rossing *et al.,* 1980). Some chronic asthmatic patients benefit from control of nocturnal symptoms with slow-release theophylline preparations.

Therapy is usually initiated by the administration of 12 to 16 mg/kg per day of theophylline (calculated as the free base) up to a maximum of 400 mg per day for at least 3 days (Weinberger, 1987). Children <1 year old require considerably less; the dose in mg/kg per day may be calculated as 0.2 X (age in weeks) + 5.0. Starting with these low doses minimizes the early side effects of nausea, vomiting, nervousness, and insomnia, which often subside with continued therapy, and virtually eliminates the possibility of exceeding concentrations of 20 μg/ml in the plasma of patients over the age of 1 year who do not have compromised hepatic or cardiac function. Thereafter, the dosage is increased in two successive stages to between 16 to 20 and, subsequently, 18 to 22 mg/kg per day (up to a maximum of 800 mg per day), depending on the age and clinical response of the patient, allowing at least 3 days between adjustments. The plasma concentration of theophylline is determined before a further adjustment in dosage is made. Although extended-release preparations of theophylline usually allow twice-daily dosing, variations in the rate and extent of absorption of such preparations require individualized calibration of dosing regimens for each patient and preparation.

Apnea of Preterm Infants.   Episodes of prolonged apnea, lasting more than 15 seconds and accompanied by bradycardia, are not infrequent occurrences in premature infants. They pose the threat of recurrent hypoxemia and neurologic damage. Although they often are associated with serious systemic illness, no specific cause is found in many instances. Beginning with the work of Kuzemko and Paala (1973), methylxanthines have undergone numerous clinical trials for the treatment of apnea of undetermined origin. The oral or intravenous administration of methylxanthines can eliminate episodes of apnea that last more than 20 seconds, and markedly reduces the number of episodes of shorter duration (*see* Symposium, 1981; Roberts, 1984; Aranda *et al.,* in Symposium, 1986a). Satisfactory responses may occur with plasma concentrations of theophylline of 4 to 8 μg/ml, but concentrations of nearly 13 μg/ml are more frequently required (Muttitt *et al.,* 1988). Still higher concentrations may produce a more regular pattern of respiration without further reduction in the frequency of episodes of apnea and bradycardia, and these usually are associated with a definite tachycardia. Therapeutic concentrations are achieved with loading doses of about 5 mg/kg of theophylline (calculated as the free base) and can be maintained with 2 mg/kg given every 12 or 24 hours (*see* Roberts, 1984). Although caffeine initially was used less frequently than theophylline, some physicians now prefer it because the dosing regimens are simpler and more predictable. Moreover, the administration of theophylline leads to the accumulation of substantial amounts of caffeine in these infants (*see* above). Somewhat higher concentrations are required, but the available data indicate that caffeine is equally effective. The recommended loading dose is 10 mg/kg of caffeine, with maintenance doses of 2.5 mg/kg per day (*see* Roberts, 1984).

Although effects on the growth or development of infants following treatment with methylxanthines have not been detected, the evidence is far from definitive. Therapy is thus continued for as brief a period as possible, usually only a few weeks.

Anticholinergic Agents

There is a long history of the use of anticholinergic agents in the treatment of asthma. These agents are discussed in detail in Chapter 7. With the advent of inhaled β-adrenergic agonists, use of anticholinergic agents declined. However, renewed interest in anticholinergic agents has paralleled both the more recent realization that parasympathetic pathways are important in bronchospasm in some asthmatics and the availability of *ipratropium bromide* (ATROVENT), a quaternary anticholinergic agent, which has better pharmacological properties than prior drugs. A particularly good response to ipratropium may be seen in the subgroup of asthmatic patients who experience psychogenic exacerbations (Neild and Cameron, 1985; Rebuck and Marcus, 1979).

The bronchodilation produced by ipratropium in asthmatic subjects develops more slowly and is usually less intense than that produced by adrenergic agonists. Some asthmatic patients may experience a useful response lasting up to 6 hours. The variability in the response of asthmatic subjects to ipratropium presumably reflects differences in the strength of parasympathetic tone and in the degree to which reflex activation of cholinergic pathways participates in generating symptoms in individual patients. Hence, the utility of ipratropium must be assessed on an individual basis by a therapeutic trial. The pharmacolog-

ical properties and therapeutic uses of ipratropium have been reviewed by Gross (1988) (*see* also Symposium, 1986b).

Combined treatment with ipratropium and β_2-adrenergic agonists results in slightly greater and more prolonged bronchodilation than with either agent alone in baseline asthma (Bryant and Rogers, 1992). In acute bronchoconstriction, the combination of a β_2-adrenergic agonist and ipratropium is more effective than either agent alone and more effective than simply giving more β_2-adrenergic agonist (Bryant, 1985; Bryant and Rogers, 1992). A large multicenter study confirmed these findings and showed that the asthmatic subjects with the worst initial lung function benefited most from this combination of agents (Rebuck *et al.,* 1987). Thus, the combination of a selective β_2-adrenergic agonist and ipratropium should be considered in acute treatment of severe asthma exacerbations. Ipratropium is available in metered-dose inhalers and as a nebulizer solution. A metered-dose inhaler containing a mixture of ipratropium and albuterol (COMBIVENT) also is available in the United States. In Europe, metered-dose inhalers containing a mixture of ipratropium and fenoterol are available (DUOVENT, BERODUAL).

Drug Therapy of Asthma in Special Circumstances

Pediatric Asthma. The pathophysiology of asthma in children appears similar to that in adults (Hill *et al.,* 1992). International guidelines (Rachelefsky and Warner, 1993) and thorough reviews (Van Bever and Stevens, 1992; Moffitt *et al.,* 1994) dealing with the treatment of asthma in children have been published. In general, treatment strategies for children do not differ substantively from those for adults, except that more emphasis is placed on a trial of antileukotriene therapy, nedocromil (age 12 and greater), or cromolyn (Van Bever and Stevens, 1992) to avoid possible complications from glucocorticoids. Although inhaled glucocorticoids may impair growth velocity, a large meta-analysis found that final adult height appears to be unaffected by use of these agents (Allen *et al.,* 1994). Indeed, good control of asthma probably is important in allowing good growth, since poorly controlled asthma itself inhibits growth. Use of oral prednisone in asthma is associated with slightly diminished growth, in terms of attaining final predicted height (Allen *et al.,* 1994). Metered dose inhalers require substantial dexterity and cannot be used by children younger than 5 years of age. This limitation dictates use of either nebulized solutions or parenteral therapy in this patient population.

Emergency-Room Patients. β-Adrenergic agonists are the only drugs that have been proven to be effective in the immediate treatment of severe asthma exacerbations. Several studies (Fanta *et al.,* 1986; Fanta *et al.,* 1982; Rossing *et al.,* 1980) compared the use of β-adrenergic agonists and aminophylline for emergency treatment of asthma. Patients responded better to inhaled β-adrenergic agonists alone than to aminophylline alone. Addition of aminophylline infusions to inhaled β-adrenergic agonists did not improve patients' lung function or symptoms. Another study found that emergency-department patients treated for wheezing with aminophylline infusions did not differ from control subjects in terms of spirometry, symptoms, or global physician assessment, but the treated patients were less likely to be admitted to the hospital than those receiving placebo (Wrenn *et al.*, 1991). Before theophylline therapy can be considered standard emergency treatment, further studies confirming lower hospitalization rates will be required (McFadden, 1991). When glucocorticoids were administered systemically during emergency-room visits for asthma, the rate of hospitalization both during the visit and after discharge were reduced (Chapman *et al.*, 1991). Glucocorticoids take a minimum of 6 to 12 hours to be effective. Oral dosing is as rapid in onset as parenteral administration. For most adult and many pediatric asthmatic patients whose exacerbations require emergency-room visits, a short course of glucocorticoids, for example, 40 to 60 mg/day of prednisone orally (1 mg/kg per day for 5 days), is indicated.

Hospitalized Patients.   In addition to regular use of inhaled β-adrenergic agonists for bronchodilator therapy, hospitalized asthmatic patients should be treated with substantial doses of systemic glucocorticoids (McFadden, 1993). Most physicians recommend 30 to 120 mg of methylprednisolone intravenously every 6 hours. If the patient is able to take medications orally, prednisone and other glucocorticoid preparations are well absorbed and are as effective as intravenous preparations (Ratto *et al.*, 1988; McFadden, 1993). The optimal dose and frequency of administration of glucocorticoids have not been well established. A synopsis of 20 different studies has been published (McFadden, 1993). Reasonable investigations have shown that 30 mg of methylprednisolone every 6 hours is probably as effective as higher doses. While the beneficial effects of glucocorticoids may reach a plateau at 30 to 45 mg of methylprednisolone intravenously every 6 hours (equivalent to 40 to 60 mg prednisone every 6 hours), the adverse effects continue to escalate at higher dose levels. Most authors would agree with erring toward the higher doses for treatment of seriously ill asthmatic patients, but doses higher than 120 mg of methylprednisolone every 6 hours are not recommended. Prophylaxis for gastric and duodenal ulcerations using H_2-histamine receptor antagonists is recommended when using high-dose systemic glucocorticoids for asthma exacerbations.

Asthma exacerbations requiring hospitalization are handled essentially no differently in children than in adults; treatment with systemic glucocorticoids is required. The dose recommended is 1 to 2 mg/kg per day, divided into four doses. The once-common practice of instituting continuous isoproterenol infusions in children with asthma exacerbations has not been proven to be effective. Maguire *et al.* (1986) showed that such infusions in children are associated with detectable levels of cardiac-specific creatinine kinase in serum. These infusions also can be associated with tachyarrythmias. At present there is little to recommend such infusions.

Asthma During Pregnancy and Lactation.   Poorly controlled asthma can adversely affect the outcome of pregnancy and even cause maternal or fetal death. Asthma affects up to 5% of pregnant women. In the past, asthma frequently caused significant difficulty during pregnancies. With the recognition by patient and physician of the need for excellent preventive control of asthma during pregnancy, complications of pregnancy by asthma should be rare. A consensus conference published its recommendations concerning the treatment of asthma during pregnancy (NIH, 1993). In general, essentially the same guidelines should be used for treating pregnant asthmatic patients as for treating nonpregnant asthmatic patients. Although most drugs used to treat asthma are FDA category C (not proven to be safe for use during pregnancy), some are in category B (cromolyn, nedocromil, terbutaline, leukotriene modifiers), and there is a large clinical experience with inhaled $β_2$-adrenergic agonists and inhaled glucocorticoids in pregnant women. In general, the known adverse effects of poorly controlled asthma are thought to outweigh the theoretical possibility of drug-induced fetal abnormalities.

Except for a few studies in animals in which high systemic drug doses were used, there is no evidence that $β_2$-adrenergic agonists produce fetal abnormalities. Not all animal studies revealed adverse effects, even at high doses, and clinical experience does not suggest any fetal developmental abnormalities associated with use of $β_2$-adrenergic agonists. During acute bronchospasm, inhaled $β_2$-adrenergic agonists are indicated to improve maternal respiratory function and prevent fetal distress. Maternal and fetal adverse effects are rare when inhaled $β_2$-adrenergic agonists are used at the recommended doses. Systemic $β_2$-adrenergic agonists can cause fetal tachycardia and neonatal tachycardia, hypoglycemia, and tremor. There has been concern that nonselective agonists, such as epinephrine, may cause uterine vasoconstriction due to an $α$-adrenergic effect. In practice, the use of epinephrine for severe asthma exacerbation appears unlikely to cause significant fetal or maternal injury. However, inhaled $β_2$-adrenergic agonists appear to be more effective and do not carry the risk of uterine vasoconstriction. There is no contraindication to the use of inhaled β-adrenergic agonists during lactation.

Antiinflammatory treatment to prevent asthma exacerbations is indicated whenever pregnant asthmatic patients require daily inhaled $β_2$-adrenergic agonists for control of symptoms. Inhaled cromolyn is considered particularly safe in pregnancy, because it is extremely poorly absorbed from the gastrointestinal tract. There is little experience with the use of nedocromil in pregnancy. Inhaled glucocorticoids also are considered relatively safe in pregnancy. The largest and longest experience with inhaled glucocorticoids in pregnancy is with beclomethasone, and some authors favor its use for those reasons (NIH, 1993). Although high doses of systemic glucocorticoids given to pregnant rats consistently have been associated with palate defects in the pups, the doses used have far exceeded those typically prescribed for human asthma. Chronic maternal administration of systemic corticosteroids has been associated with a mild decrease in birth weight in human beings. Neither systemic nor inhaled corticosteroids are a contraindication to breast feeding (NIH, 1993).

Despite a long history of successful use of theophylline preparations in pregnancy, this drug is now infrequently used, in part because of its limited effectiveness and narrow therapeutic window. Theophylline elimination is affected by pregnancy, but to a variable degree. The increased glomerular filtration rate associated with pregnancy increases the rate of elimination of theophylline; conversely, metabolic elimination of theophylline by the liver is decreased. In the last trimester of pregnancy, the overall effect is an approximately 30% diminished rate of elimination of theophylline. Because of marked interindividual variability and the changes associated with progression of pregnancy, frequent drug level monitoring is required. When maternal levels exceed 20 μg/ml, fetal tachycardia can occur. Neonatal levels greater than 10 μg/ml are associated with jitteriness, vomiting, and tachycardia and are most often seen when maternal plasma drug levels are greater than 12 μg/ml at delivery. In practice, theophylline should be limited to third-line therapy after inhaled antiinflammatory agents and β_2-adrenergic agonists, because of the above difficulties in its administration and the potential for serious adverse effects. Theophylline is not contraindicated during lactation.

Use of Asthma Drugs in Rhinitis

Seasonal allergic rhinitis—hay fever—is caused by deposition of allergens on the nasal mucosa, resulting in an immediate hypersensitivity reaction. This reaction usually is not accompanied by asthma, because the allergens usually are contained in particles too large to be inhaled into the lower airways (*e.g.*, pollens). Treatment for allergic rhinitis is similar to that for asthma. Topical glucocorticoids (*beclomethasone, mometasone, budesonide, flunisolide, fluticasone, triamcinolone acetonide*) or *cromolyn* can be highly effective with minimal side effects, particularly if treatment is instituted immediately prior to the allergy season. Topical glucocorticoids can be administered twice daily (beclomethasone, flunisolide) or even once daily (budesonide, mometasone, fluticasone, triamcinolone). Cromolyn usually requires dosing three to six times daily for full effects. Rare instances of local candidiasis have been reported with glucocorticoids and probably can be avoided by rinsing the mouth after use. Unlike in asthma, antihistamines (Chapter 25) afford considerable, though incomplete, symptom relief in allergic rhinitis. Nasal decongestants rely on α-adrenergic agonists (pseudoephedrine, phenylephrine) as vasoconstrictors and are discussed in Chapter 10.

Perennial allergic rhinitis, caused by exposure to allergens present year-round, such as dust mites or animal dander, can be treated similarly. However, since this situation requires continuous exposure to medicines such as topical glucocorticoids, alternatives such as modifying the patient's environment and using immunotherapy (allergen desensitization) should be considered.

Use of Asthma Drugs in Chronic Obstructive Pulmonary Disease

Emphysema can be prevented or its progression slowed by the patient's ceasing to smoke (Ferguson and Cherniack,

1993). Pharmacological interventions can help patients to stop smoking. Nicotine gum and transdermal patches are moderately useful when combined with other interventions such as support groups and physician encouragement. Clonidine may be helpful in reducing the craving for cigarettes. Treatment of nicotine addiction is discussed in Chapter 24.

The pharmacological treatment of established emphysema resembles that of asthma largely because the inflammatory/bronchospastic component of a patient's disease is the aspect amenable to therapy (Ferguson and Cherniack, 1993). For patients with emphysema who have a significant degree of active inflammation with bronchospasm and excessive mucus production, symptomatic use of inhaled ipratropium or a β_2-adrenergic agonist may be helpful. Ipratropium usually produces about the same modest degree of bronchodilation in patients with chronic obstructive pulmonary disease (COPD) as do maximal doses of β_2-adrenergic agonists. As in asthmatic patients, continuous use of bronchodilators is controversial, with some studies suggesting that it is associated with an unfavorable course of COPD (van Schayck *et al.*, 1991). A subgroup of patients may respond favorably to short courses of oral glucocorticoids. It is not possible to predict whether or not a particular patient will respond to glucocorticoids without a treatment trial. Response to oral glucocorticoids may predict those patients who will respond to inhaled glucocorticoids. However, except for the treatment of acute bronchospastic episodes, glucocorticoids have given mixed results in the treatment of COPD (American Thoracic Society, 1987; Dompeling *et al.*, 1993). In some patients, theophylline may be effective (Murciano *et al.*, 1989); in others who have a profound response to β_2-adrenergic agonists, theophylline fails to produce additional bronchodilation beyond that achieved by maximal doses of the inhaled drug.

In fact, there are many patients who have nearly pure emphysema, without a significant degree of reversible inflammation or bronchoconstriction. Nevertheless, these patients often receive prolonged courses of ipratropium, β_2-adrenergic agonists, glucocorticoids, and/or theophylline, with little likelihood for benefit and all of the usual possibilities for adverse effects.

α_1-*Antiproteinase Deficiency.*   In a minority of patients, emphysema results from a genetic deficiency of the plasma proteinase inhibitor α_1-antiproteinase (also called α_1-antitrypsin) (Crystal, 1990). Lung tissue destruction is caused by the unopposed action of neutrophil elastase and other proteinases. Purified α_1-antiproteinase (PROLASTIN) from human plasma has become available for intravenous replacement. Clinical efficacy studies have not been performed except to show that intravenous administration of α_1-antiproteinase does lead to serum levels thought to be protective against development of emphysema in nonsmokers. The recommended dose is 60 mg/kg administered intravenously once weekly. This dosage regimen should maintain α_1-antitrypsin concentrations above the threshold serum concentration of 80 mg/dl to provide adequate antielastase activity in the lung epithelial lining fluid. Transgenic sheep secreting human α_1-antiproteinase in their milk have been created and may be a safer and less expensive source for α_1-antiproteinase in the future. No trials have been conducted using α_1-antiproteinase in cigarette-induced emphysema.

Recombinant DNAse (dornase alfa, PULMOZYME) is available as a nebulizer solution for treatment of cystic fibrosis. In cystic fibrosis, inspissated secretions containing large numbers of inflammatory cells lodge in the smaller airways, causing obstruction. A substantial portion of the viscosity of the purulent material is due to the DNA from the nuclei of lysed cells. Inhaled DNAse has been shown to aid in clearing these secretions and improving pulmonary function in patients with cystic fibrosis (Harris and Wilmott, 1994; Wilmott and Fiedler, 1994). Efficacy trials are currently underway to assess DNAse treatment in adult COPD exacerbations, where purulent bronchial secretions also contribute to airway obstruction.

PROSPECTUS

Over the past decade, the hypothesis that there may be a more selective and thus safer approach to controlling airway inflammation than glucocorticoid therapy has motivated much of the drug discovery effort in asthma research. In various stages of development are agents aimed at inhibiting certain cytokines, chemokines, or adhesion molecules and thereby selectively decreasing the influx of eosinophils and other leukocytes into the airways. Other approaches have targeted the atopic reaction for selective intervention. Monoclonal antibodies aimed at inhibiting the binding of immunoglobulin E (IgE) to receptors on mast cells and basophils are in clinical trials for asthma and other allergic diseases. These antibodies, in theory, would inhibit the immediate hypersensitivity reaction at its earliest stage, thus preventing allergic inflammation in the airways. Neuropeptide receptor antagonists, particularly antagonists at neurokinin receptors, are under development to inhibit neurogenic components of inflammation. These agents also may inhibit reflex activity in the airways. Another strategy to quell the inflammation associated with asthma and chronic obstructive pulmonary disease is to develop drugs that are isozyme-selective phosphodiesterase (PDE) inhibitors. The finding that the predominant PDEs in inflammatory cells are members of the PDE-IV family has led to the development of drugs that are PDE-IV–selective inhibitors. This type of drug may provide antiinflammatory actions without many of the side effects associated with nonselective PDE inhibitors such as theophylline.

For further discussion of asthma, *see* Chapter 252 in *Harrison's Principles of Internal Medicine,* 14th ed., McGraw-Hill, New York, 1998.

BIBLIOGRAPHY

Aitken, M.L., and Martin, T.R. Life-threatening theophylline toxicity is not predictable by serum levels. *Chest,* **1987,** *91*:10–14.

Augstein, J., Farmer, J.B., Lee, T.B., Sheard, P., and Tattersall, M.L. Selective inhibitor of slow reacting substance of anaphylaxis. *Nat. New Biol.,* **1973,** *245*:215–217.

Barnes, N.C., and Miller, C.J. Effect of leukotriene receptor antagonist therapy on the risk of asthma exacerbations in patients with mild to moderate asthma: an integrated analysis of zafirlukast trials. *Thorax,* **2000,** *55*:478–483.

Bel, E.H., Timmers, M.C., Hermans, J., Dijkman, J.H., and Sterk, P.J. The long-term effects of nedocromil sodium and beclomethasone dipropionate on bronchial responsiveness to methacholine in nonatopic asthmatic subjects. *Am. Rev. Respir. Dis.,* **1990,** *141*:21–28.

Benton, G., Thomas, R.C., Nickerson, B.G., McQuitty, J.C., and Okikawa, J. Experience with a metered dose inhaler with a spacer in the pediatric emergency department. *Am. J. Dis. Child.,* **1989,** *143*:678–681.

Bertino, J.S. Jr., and Walker, J.W. Reassessment of theophylline toxicity. Serum concentrations, clinical course, and treatment. *Arch. Intern. Med.,* **1987,** *147*:757–760.

Brittain, R.T. Approaches to a long-acting, selective beta 2-adrenoceptor stimulant. *Lung,* **1990,** *168* (suppl.):111–114.

Brocklehurst, W.E. The release of histamine and formation of a slow reacting substance (SRS-A) during anaphylactic shock. *J. Physiol.,* **1960,** *151*:416–435.

Bryant, D.H., and Rogers, P. Effects of ipratropium bromide nebulizer solution with and without preservatives in the treatment of acute and stable asthma. *Chest,* **1992,** *102*:742–747.

Bryant, E.E., and Shimizu, I. *Sample Design, Sampling Variance, and Estimation Procedures for the National Ambulatory Medical Care Survey.* DHHS Publication No. (PHS) 88-1382, U.S. Dept. of Health and Human Services, Hyattsville, MD., **1988.**

Buckner, C.K., Krell, R.D., Laravuso, R.B., Coursin, D.B., Bernstein, P.R., and Will, J.A. Pharmacological evidence that human intralobar airways do not contain different receptors that mediate contractions to leukotriene C4 and leukotriene D4. *J. Pharmacol. Exp. Ther.,* **1986,** *237:*558–562.

Burrows, B., Martinez, F.D., Halonen, M., Barbee, R.A., and Cline, M.G. Association of asthma with serum IgE levels and skin-test reactivity to allergens. *N. Engl. J. Med.,* **1989,** *320:*271–277.

Calhoun, W.J., Lavins, B.J., Minkwitz, M.C., Evans, R., Gleich, G.J., and Cohn, J. Effect of zafirlukast (Accolate) on cellular mediators of inflammation: bronchoalveolar lavage fluid findings after segmental antigen challenge. *Am. J. Respir. Crit. Care Med.,* **1998,** *157:*1381–1389.

Carter, G.W., Young, P.R., Albert, D.H., Bouska, J., Dyer, R., Bell, R.L., Summers, J.B., and Brooks, D.W. 5-Lipoxygenase inhibitory activity of zileuton. *J. Pharmacol. Exp. Ther.,* **1991,** *256:*929–937.

Chapman, K.R., Verbeek, P.R., White, J.G., and Rebuck, A.S. Effect of a short course of prednisone in the prevention of early relapse after the emergency room treatment of acute asthma. *N. Engl. J. Med.,* **1991,** *324:*788–794.

Cheung, D., Timmers, M.C., Zwinderman, A.H., Bel, E.H., Dijkman, J.H., and Sterk, P.J. Long-term effects of a long-acting β_2-adrenoreceptor agonist, salmeterol, on airway hyperresponsiveness in patients with mild asthma. *N. Engl. J. Med.,* **1992,** *327:*1198–1203.

Choi, O.H., Shamim, M.T., Padgett, W.L., and Daly, J.W. Caffeine and theophylline analogues: correlation of behavioral effects with activity as adenosine receptor antagonists and as phosphodiesterase inhibitors. *Life Sci.,* **1988,** *43:*387–398.

Chong, L.K., and Peachell, P.T. Beta-adrenoceptor reserve in human lung: a comparison between airway smooth muscle and mast cells. *Eur. J. Pharmacol.,* **1999,** *378:*115–122.

Cushley, M.J., Tattersfield, A.E., and Holgate, S.T. Adenosine-induced bronchoconstriction in asthma. Antagonism by inhaled theophylline. *Am. Rev. Respir. Dis.,* **1984,** *129:*380–384.

Dahlen, S.E., Hedqvist, P., Hammarstrom, S., and Samuelsson, B. Leukotrienes are potent constrictors of human bronchi. *Nature,* **1980,** *288:*484–486.

D'Alonzo, G.E., Nathan, R.A., Henochowicz, S., Morris, R.J., Ratner, P., and Rennard, S.I. Salmeterol xinafoate as maintenance therapy compared with albuterol in patients with asthma. *JAMA,* **1994,** *271:*1412–1416.

Dompeling, E., van Schayck, C.P., van Grunsven, P.M., van Herwaarden, C.L., Akkermans, R., Molema, J., Folgering, H., and van Weel, C. Slowing the deterioration of asthma and chronic obstructive pulmonary disease observed during bronchodilator therapy by adding inhaled corticosteroids. A 4-year prospective study. *Ann. Intern. Med.,* **1993,** *118:*770–778.

Epstein, S.W., Manning, C.P., Ashley, M.J., and Corey, P.N. Survey of the clinical use of pressurized aerosol inhalers. *Can. Med. Assoc. J.,* **1979,** *120:*813–816.

Fanta, C.H., Rossing, T.H., and McFadden, E.R. Jr. Emergency room treatment of asthma. Relationships among therapeutic combinations, severity of obstruction and time course of response. *Am. J. Med.,* **1982,** *72:*416–422.

Fanta, C.H., Rossing, T.H., and McFadden, E.R. Jr. Treatment of acute asthma. Is combination therapy with sympathomimetics and methylxanthines indicated? *Am. J. Med.,* **1986,** *80:*5–10.

Feoktistov, I., Polosa, R., Holgate, S.T., and Biaggioni, I. Adenosine A2B receptors: a novel therapeutic target in asthma? *Trends Pharmacol. Sci.,* **1998,** *19:*148–153.

Fredholm, B.B., and Persson, C.G. Xanthine derivatives as adenosine receptor antagonists. *Eur. J. Pharmacol.,* **1982,** *81:*673–676.

Fuller, R.W., Dixon, C.M., Cuss, F.M., and Barnes, P.J. Bradykinin-induced bronchoconstriction in humans. Mode of action. *Am. Rev. Respir. Dis.,* **1987,** *135:*176–180.

Goldberg, M.J., Spector, R., Park, G.D., Johnson, G.F., and Roberts, P. The effect of sorbitol and activated charcoal on serum theophylline concentrations after slow-release theophylline. *Clin. Pharmacol. Ther.,* **1987,** *41:*108–111.

Gorenne, I., Ortiz, J.L., Labat, C., Abram, T., Tudhop, S., Cuthbert, N., Norman, P., Gardiner, P., Morcillo, E., and Brink, C. Antagonism of leukotriene responses in human airways by BAY x7195. *Eur. J. Pharmacol.,* **1995,** *275:*207–212.

Greening, A.P., Ind, P.W., Northfield, M., and Shaw, G. Added salmeterol versus higher-dose corticosteroid in asthma patients with symptoms on existing inhaled corticosteroid. Allen & Hanburys Limited UK Study. *Lancet,* **1994,** *344:*219–224.

Haahtela, T., Jarvinen, M., Kava, T., Kiviranta, K., Koskinen, S., Lehtonen, K., Nikander, K., Persson, T., Selroos, O., Sovijärvi, A., Stenius-Aarniala, B., Svahn, T., Tammivaara, R., and Laitinen, L.A. Effects of reducing or discontinuing inhaled budesonide in patients with mild asthma. *N. Engl. J. Med.,* **1994,** *331:*700–705.

Hargreaves, M.R., and Benson, M.K. Inhaled sodium cromoglycate in angiotensin-converting enzyme inhibitor cough. *Lancet,* **1995,** *345:*13–16.

Horan, R.F., Sheffer, A.L., and Austen, K.F. Cromolyn sodium in the management of systemic mastocytosis. *J. Allergy Clin. Immunol.,* **1990,** *85:*852–855.

Hoshino, M., and Nakamura, Y. The effect of inhaled sodium cromoglycate on cellular infiltration into the bronchial mucosa and the expression of adhesion molecules in asthmatics. *Eur. Respir. J.,* **1997,** *10:*858–865.

Ip, M., Lam, K., Yam, L., Kung, A., and Ng, M. Decreased bone mineral density in premenopausal asthma patients receiving long-term inhaled steroids. *Chest,* **1994,** *105:*1722–1727.

Jones, T.R., Labelle, M., Belley, M., Champion, E., Charette, L., Evans, J., Ford-Hutchinson, A.W., Gauthier, J.Y., Lord, A., Masson, P., McAuliffe, M., McFarlane, C.S., Metters, K.M., Pickett, C., Piechuta, H., Rochette, C., Rodger, I.W., Sawyer, N., Young, R.N., Zamboni, R., and Abraham, W.M. Pharmacology of montelukast sodium (Singulair), a potent and selective leukotriene D4 receptor antagonist. *Can. J. Physiol. Pharmacol.,* **1995,** *73:*191–201.

Juniper, E.F., Kline, P.A., Vanzeileghem, M.A., Ramsdale, E.H., O'Byrne, P.M., and Hargreave, F.E. Effect of long-term treatment with an inhaled corticosteroid (budesonide) on airway hyperresponsiveness and clinical asthma in nonsteroid-dependent asthmatics. *Am. Rev. Respir. Dis.,* **1990,** *142:*832–836.

Kamada, A.K., Spahn, J.D., and Blake, K.V. Salmeterol: its place in asthma management. *Ann. Pharmacother.,* **1994,** *28:*1100–1102.

Kay, A.B., Walsh, G.M., Moqbel, R., MacDonald, A.J., Nagakura, T., Carroll, M.P., and Richerson, H.B. Disodium cromoglycate inhibits activation of human inflammatory cells *in vitro. J. Allergy Clin. Immunol.,* **1987,** *80:*1–8.

Kellaway, C.H., and Trethewie, E.R. The liberation of a slow reacting smooth-muscle stimulating substance in anaphylaxis. *Q. J. Exp. Physiol.,* **1940,** *30:*121–145.

Krell, R.D., Aharony, D., Buckner, C.K., Keith, R.A., Kusner, E.J., Snyder, D.W., Bernstein, P.R., Matassa, V.G., Yee, Y.K., Brown, F.J., Hesp, B., and Giles, R.E. The preclinical pharmacology of ICI 204,219. A peptide leukotriene antagonist. *Am. Rev. Respir. Dis.,* **1990,** *141:*978–987.

Kume, H., Hall, I.P., Washabau, R.J., Takagi, K., and Kotlikoff, M.I. Beta-adrenergic agonists regulate KCa channels in airway smooth muscle by cAMP-dependent and -independent mechanisms. *J. Clin. Invest.*, **1994**, *93*:371–379.

Kuzemko, J.A., and Paala, J. Apnoeic attacks in the newborn treated with aminophylline. *Arch. Dis. Child.*, **1973**, *48*:404–406.

Laitinen, L.A., Laitinen, A., and Haahtela, T. A comparative study of the effects of an inhaled corticosteroid, budesonide, and a β_2 agonist, terbutaline, on airway inflammation in newly diagnosed asthma: a randomized, double-blind, parallel-group controlled trial. *J. Allergy Clin. Immunol.*, **1992**, *90*:32–42.

Laitinen, L.A., Naya, I.P., Binks, S., Harris, A. Comparative efficacy of zafirlukast and low-dose steroids in asthmatics on pm β_2 agonists. *Eur. Respir. J.*, **1997**, *10*(suppl 4):4195–4205.

Li, X., Ward, C., Thien, F., Bish, R., Bamford, T., Bao, X., Bailey, M., Wilson, J.W., and Haydn-Walters, E. An antiinflammatory effect of salmeterol, a long-acting beta(2) agonist, assessed in airway biopsies and bronchoalveolar lavage in asthma. *Am. J. Respir. Crit. Care Med.*, **1999**, *160*:1493–1499.

Lichtenstein, L.M., and Margolis, S. Histamine release in vitro: inhibition by catecholamines and methylxanthines. *Science,* **1968**, *161*:902–903.

Lindgren, S., Lokshin, B., Stromquist, A., Weinberger, M., Nassif, E., McCubbin, M., and Frasher, R. Does asthma or treatment with theophylline limit children's academic performance? *N. Engl. J. Med.*, **1992**, *327*:926–930.

Lofdahl, C.G., Reiss, T.F., Leff, J.A., Israel, E., Noonan, M.J., Finn, A.F., Seidenberg, B.C., Capizzi, T., Kundu, S., and Godard, P. Randomised, placebo-controlled trial of effect of a leukotriene receptor antagonist, montelukast, on tapering inhaled corticosteroids in asthmatic patients. *Br. Med. J.,* **1999**, *319*:87–90.

Lynch, K.R., O'Neill, G.P., Liu, Q., Im, D.S., Sawyer, N., Metters, K.M., Coulombe, N., Abramovitz, M., Figueroa, D.J., Zeng, Z., Connolly, B.M., Bai, C., Austin, C.P., Chateauneuf, A., Stocco, R., Greig, G.M., Kargman, S., Hooks, S.B., Hosfield, E., Williams, D.L. Jr., Ford-Hutchinson, A.W., Caskey, C.T., and Evans, J.F. Characterization of the human cysteinyl leukotriene CysLT1 receptor. *Nature,* **1999**, *399*:789-793.

Macfarlane, J.T., and Lane, D.J. Irregularities in the use of regular aerosol inhalers. *Thorax,* **1980**, *35*:477–478.

Maguire, J.F., Geha, R.S., and Umetsu, D.T. Myocardial specific creatine phosphokinase isoenzyme elevation in children with asthma treated with intravenous isoproterenol. *J. Allergy Clin. Immunol.,* **1986**, *78*:631–636.

Malmstrom, K., Rodriguez-Gomez, G., Guerra, J., Villaran, C., Pineiro, A., Wei, L.X., Seidenberg, B.C., and Reiss, T.F. Oral montelukast, inhaled beclomethasone, and placebo for chronic asthma. A randomized, controlled trial. Montelukast/Beclomethasone Study Group. *Ann. Intern. Med.,* **1999**, *130*:487–495.

Martinson, E.A., Johnson, R.A., and Wells, J.N. Potent adenosine receptor antagonists that are selective for the A_1 receptor subtype. *Mol. Pharmacol.,* **1987**, *31*:247–252.

Meltzer, E.O., Orgel, H.A., Ellis, E.F., Eigen, H.N., and Hemstreet, M.P. Long-term comparison of three combinations of albuterol, theophylline, and beclomethasone in children with chronic asthma. *J. Allergy Clin. Immunol.,* **1992**, *90*:2–11.

Moqbel, R., Cromwell, O., Walsh, G.M., Wardlaw, A.J., Kurlak, L., and Kay, A.B. Effects of nedocromil sodium (Tilade) on the activation of human eosinophils and neutrophils and the release of histamine from mast cells. *Allergy,* **1988**, *43*:268–276.

Murciano, D., Auclair, M.H., Pariente, R., and Aubier, M. A randomized, controlled trial of theophylline in patients with severe chronic obstructive pulmonary disease. *N. Engl. J. Med.,* **1989**, *320*:1521–1525.

Murphy, R.C., Hammarstrom, S., and Samuelsson, B. Leukotriene C: a slow-reacting substance from murine mastocytoma cells. *Proc. Natl. Acad. Sci. U.S.A.,* **1979**, *76*:4275–4279.

Murray, J.J., Tonnel, A.B., Brash, A.R., Roberts, L.J. II, Gosset, P., Workman, R., Capron, A., and Oates, J.A. Release of prostaglandin D_2 into human airways during acute antigen challenge. *N. Engl. J. Med.,* **1986**, *315*:800–804.

Muttitt, S.C., Tierney, A.J., and Finer, N.N. The dose response of theophylline in the treatment of apnea of prematurity. *J. Pediatr.,* **1988**, *112*:115–121.

Neild, J.E., and Cameron, I.R. Bronchoconstriction in response to suggestion: its prevention by an inhaled anticholinergic agent. *Br. Med. J. (Clin. Res. Ed.),* **1985**, *290*:674.

O'Byrne, P.M., and Pedersen, S. Measuring efficacy and safety of different inhaled corticosteroid preparations. *J. Allergy Clin. Immunol.,* **1998**, *102*:879–886.

Paloucek, F.P., and Rodvold, K.A. Evaluation of theophylline overdoses and toxicities. *Ann. Emerg. Med.,* **1988**, *17*:135–144.

Pauwels, R., Van Renterghem, D., Van der Straeten, M., Johannesson, N., and Persson, C.G. The effect of theophylline and enprofylline on allergen-induced bronchoconstriction. *J. Allergy Clin. Immunol.,* **1985**, *76*:583–590.

Peachell, P.T., Columbo, M., Kagey-Sobotka, A., Lichtenstein, L.M., and Marone, G. Adenosine potentiates mediator release from human lung mast cells. *Am. Rev. Respir. Dis.,* **1988**, *138*:1143–1151.

Pedersen, K.E., Bochner, B.S., and Undem, B.J. Cysteinyl leukotrienes induce P-selectin expression in human endothelial cells *via* a non-CysLT1 receptor-mediated mechanism. *J. Pharmacol. Exp. Ther.,* **1997**, *281*:655–662.

Ratto, D., Alfaro, C., Sipsey, J., Glovsky, M.M., and Sharma, O.P. Are intravenous corticosteroids required in status asthmaticus? *JAMA,* **1988**, *260*:527–529.

Rebuck, A.S., Chapman, K.R., Abboud, R., Pare, P.D., Kreisman, H., Wolkove, N., and Vickerson, F. Nebulized anticholinergic and sympathomimetic treatment of asthma and chronic obstructive airways disease in the emergency room. *Am. J. Med.,* **1987**, *82*:59–64.

Rebuck, A.S., and Marcus, H.I. SCH 1000 in psychogenic asthma. *Scand. J. Respir. Dis. Suppl.,* **1979**, *103*:186–191.

Rossing, T.H., Fanta, C.H., Goldstein, D.H., Snapper, J.R., and McFadden, E.R. Jr. Emergency therapy of asthma: comparison of the acute effects of parenteral and inhaled sympathomimetics and infused aminophylline. *Am. Rev. Respir. Dis.,* **1980**, *122*:365–371.

Svendsen, U.G., Frolund, L., Madsen, F., and Nielsen, N.H. A comparison of the effects of nedocromil sodium and beclomethasone dipropionate on pulmonary function, symptoms, and bronchial responsiveness in patients with asthma. *J. Allergy Clin. Immunol.,* **1989**, *84*:224–231.

Svendsen, U.G., Frolund, L., Madsen, F., Nielsen, N.H., Holstein-Rathlou, N.H., and Weeke, B. A comparison of the effects of sodium cromoglycate and beclomethasone dipropionate on pulmonary function and bronchial hyperreactivity in subjects with asthma. *J. Allergy Clin. Immunol.,* **1987**, *80*:68–74.

Svendsen, U.G., and Jorgensen, H. Inhaled nedocromil sodium as additional treatment to high dose inhaled corticosteroids in the management of bronchial asthma. *Eur. Respir. J.,* **1991**, *4*:992–999.

Thoman, E.B., Davis, D.H., Raye, J.R., Philipps, A.F., Rowe, J.C., and Denenberg, V.H. Theophylline affects sleep-wake state development in premature infants. *Neuropediatrics,* **1985**, *16*:13–18.

Toogood, J.H., Jennings, B., and Lefcoe, N.M. A clinical trial of combined cromolyn/beclomethasone treatment for chronic asthma. *J. Allergy Clin. Immunol.,* **1981**, *67*:317–324.

Torphy, T.J., Undem, B.J., Cieslinski, L.B., Luttmann, M.A., Reeves, M.L., and Hay, D.W. Identification, characterization, and functional role of phosphodiesterase isozymes in human airway smooth muscle. *J. Pharmacol. Exp. Ther.,* **1993,** *265*:1213–1223.

Turner, J.R., Corkery, K.J., Eckman, D., Gelb, A.M., Lipavsky, A., and Sheppard, D. Equivalence of continuous flow nebulizer and metered-dose inhaler with reservoir bag for treatment of acute airflow obstruction. *Chest,* **1988,** *93*:476–481.

van Schayck, C.P., Dompeling, E., van Herwaarden, C.L., Folgering, H., Verbeek, A.L., van der Hoogen, H.J., and van Weel, C. Bronchodilator treatment in moderate asthma or chronic bronchitis: continuous or on demand? A randomised controlled study. *Br. Med. J.,* **1991,** *303*:1426–1431.

Woolcock, A., Lundback, B., Ringdal, N., and Jacques, L.A. Comparison of addition of salmeterol to inhaled steroids with doubling of the dose of inhaled steroids. *Am. J. Respir. Crit. Care Med.,* **1996,** *153*:1481–1488.

Wrenn, K., Slovis, C.M., Murphy, F., and Greenberg, R.S. Aminophylline therapy for acute bronchospastic disease in the emergency room. *Ann. Intern. Med.,* **1991,** *115*:241–247.

MONOGRAPHS AND REVIEWS

Allen, D.B., Mullen, M., and Mullen, B. A meta-analysis of the effect of oral and inhaled corticosteroids on growth. *J. Allergy Clin. Immunol.,* **1994,** *93*:967–976.

American Thoracic Society. Standards for the diagnosis and care of patients with chronic obstructive pulmonary disease (COPD) and asthma. *Am. Rev. Respir. Dis.,* **1987,** *136*:225–244.

Anonymous. Executive summary: guidelines for the diagnosis and management of asthma. NIH Publication No. 91-3042A. NIH, Bethesda, MD **1991,** pp. 1–44.

Barnes, P.J. Effect of beta-agonists on inflammatory cells. *J. Allergy Clin. Immunol.,* **1999,** *104*:S10–S17.

Barnes, P.J. Inhaled glucocorticoids for asthma. *N. Engl. J. Med.,* **1995,** *332*:868–875.

Barnes, P.J., and Pedersen, S. Efficacy and safety of inhaled corticosteroids in asthma. Report of a workshop held in Eze, France, October 1992. *Am. Rev. Respir. Dis.,* **1993,** *148*:S1–S26.

Beavo, J.A., and Reifsnyder, D.H. Primary sequence of cyclic nucleotide phosphodiesterase isozymes and the design of selective inhibitors. *Trends Pharmacol. Sci.,* **1990,** *11*:150–155.

Brattsand, R., and Axelsson, B.I. Basis of airway selectivity of inhaled glucocorticoids. In, *Inhaled Glucocorticoids in Asthma: Mechanisms and Clinical Actions.* (Schleimer, R.P., Busse, W.W., and O'Bryne, P., eds.) Marcel Dekker, New York, **1997,** pp. 351–379.

Brogden, R.N., and Sorkin, E.M. Nedocromil sodium. An updated review of its pharmacological properties and therapeutic efficacy in asthma. *Drugs,* **1993,** *45*:693–715.

Bryant, D.H. Nebulized ipratropium bromide in the treatment of acute asthma. *Chest,* **1985,** *88*:24–29.

Busse, W.W. What role for inhaled steroids in chronic asthma? *Chest,* **1993,** *104*:1565–1571.

Crystal, R.G. α1-Antitrypsin deficiency, emphysema, and liver disease. Genetic basis and strategies for therapy. *J. Clin. Invest.,* **1990,** *85*:1343–1352.

Daly, J.W. Adenosine receptors: targets for future drugs. *J. Med. Chem.,* **1982,** *25*:197–207.

Ferguson, G.T., and Cherniack, R.M. Management of chronic obstructive pulmonary disease. *N. Engl. J. Med.,* **1993,** *328*:1017–1022.

Friedel, H.A., and Brogden, R.N. Bitolterol. A preliminary review of its pharmacological properties and therapeutic efficacy in reversible obstructive airways disease. *Drugs,* **1988,** *35*:22–41.

Graham, D.M. Caffeine—its identity, dietary sources, intake, and biological effects. *Nutr. Rev.,* **1978,** *36*:97–102.

Greenberger, P.A. Corticosteroids in asthma. Rationale, use, and problems. *Chest,* **1992,** *101*:418S–421S.

Gross, N.J. Ipratropium bromide. *N. Engl. J. Med.,* **1988,** *319*:486–494.

Harris, C.E., and Wilmott, R.W. Inhalation-based therapies in the treatment of cystic fibrosis. *Curr. Opin. Pediatr.,* **1994,** *6*:234–238.

Hay, D.W., Torphy, T.J., and Undem, B.J. Cysteinyl leukotrienes in asthma: old mediators up to new tricks. *Trends Pharmacol. Sci.,* **1995,** *16*:304–309.

Hendeles, L., and Weinberger, M. Improved efficacy and safety of theophylline in the control of airways hyperreactivity. *Pharmacol. Ther.,* **1982,** *18*:91–105.

Hill, M., Szefler, S.J., and Larsen, G.L. Asthma pathogenesis and the implications for therapy in children. *Pediatr. Clin. North Am.,* **1992,** *39*:1205–1224.

Hoag, J.E., and McFadden, E.R. Jr. Long-term effect of cromolyn sodium on nonspecific bornchial hyperresponsiveness: a review. *Ann. Allergy,* **1991,** *66*:53–63.

Holgate, S.T. Antihistamines in the treatment of asthma. *Clin. Rev. Allergy.,* **1994,** *12*:65–78.

Israel, E., and Drazen, J.M. Treating mild asthma—when are inhaled steroids indicated? *N. Engl. J. Med.,* **1994,** *331*:737–739.

Jarvis, B., and Markham, A. Montelukast: a review of its therapeutic potential in persistent asthma. *Drugs,* **2000,** *59*:891–928.

Johnson, C.E. Aerosol corticosteroids for the treatment of asthma. *Drug Intell. Clin. Pharm.,* **1987,** *21*:784–790.

Johnson, M., and Coleman, R.A. Mechanisms of action of beta2-adrenoceptor agonists. In, *Asthma and Rhinitis.* (Busse, W.W., and Holgate, S.T., eds.) Blackwell Scientific Publications, Cambridge, **1995,** pp. 1278–1295.

Linden, J. Structure and function of A$_1$ adenosine receptors. *FASEB J.,* **1991,** *5*:2668–2676.

McFadden, E.R. Jr. Dosages of corticosteroids in asthma. *Am. Rev. Resp. Dis.,* **1993,** *147*:1306–1310.

McFadden, E.R. Jr. Methylxanthines in the treatment of asthma: the rise, the fall, and the possible rise again. *Ann. Intern. Med.,* **1991,** *115*:323–324.

Moffitt, J.E., Gearhart, J.G., and Yates, A.B. Management of asthma in children. *Am. Fam. Physician.,* **1994,** *50*:1039–1050, 1053–1055.

Murphy, S., and Kelly, H.W. Cromolyn sodium: a review of mechanisms and clinical use in asthma. *Drug Intell. Clin. Pharm.,* **1987,** *21*:22–35.

Nasser, S.S., and Rees, P.J. Theophylline. Current thoughts on the risks and benefits of its use in asthma. *Drug Saf.,* **1993,** *8*:12–18.

Nelson, H.S. β-Adrenergic bronchodilators. *N. Engl. J. Med.,* **1995,** *333*:499–506.

NIH. *Management of Asthma during Pregnancy.* NIH Publication No. 93-3279, NIH, Bethesda, MD, **1993.**

Page, C.P. Recent advances in our understanding of the use of theophylline in the treatment of asthma. *J. Clin. Pharmacol.,* **1999,** *39*:237–240.

Pavord, I., and Knox, A. Pharmacokinetic optimisation of inhaled steroid therapy in asthma. *Clin. Pharmacokinet.,* **1993,** *25*:126–135.

Pearce, F.L., Al-Laith, M., Bosman, L., Brostoff, J., Cunniffe, T.M., Flint, K.C., Hudspith, B.N., Jaffar, Z.H., Johnson, N.M.,

Kassessinoff, T.A., Lau, H.Y.A., Lee, P.Y., Leung, K.B.P., Liu, W.L., and Tainsh, K.R. Effects of sodium cromoglycate and nedocromil sodium on histamine secretion from mast cells from various locations. *Drugs,* **1989,** *37(suppl 1)*:37–43.

Rachelefsky, G.S., and Warner, J.O. International consensus on the management of pediatric asthma: a summary statement. *Pediatr. Pulmonol.,* **1993,** *15*:125–127.

Roberts, R.J. *Drug Therapy in Infants: Pharmacologic Principles and Clinical Experience.* W.B. Saunders, Philadelphia, **1984.**

Schleimer, R.P. Glucocorticosteroids: their mechanisms of action and use in allergic diseases. In, *Allergy: Principles and Practice,* 5th ed. (Middleton, E. Jr., Ellis, E.F., Yunginger, J.W., Reed, C.E., Adkinson, N.F., and Busse, W., eds.) Mosby, St. Louis, **1998,** pp. 638–660.

Schroeder, J.T., and MacGlashan, D.W. Jr. New concepts: the basophil. *J. Allergy Clin. Immunol.,* **1997,** *99*:429–433.

Self, T.H., Rumbak, M.J., Kelso, T.M., and Nicholas, R.A. Reassessment of the role of theophylline in the current therapy for nocturnal asthma. *J. Am. Board Fam. Pract.,* **1992,** *5*:281–288.

Shapiro, G.G., and König, P. Cromolyn sodium: a review. *Pharmacotherapy,* **1985,** *5*:156–170.

Smaldone, G.C. Determinants of dose and response to inhaled therapeutic agents in asthma. In, *Inhaled Glucocorticoids in Asthma: Mechanisms and Clinical Actions.* (Schleimer, R.P., Busse, W.W., and O'Bryne, P., eds.) Marcel Dekker, New York, **1997,** pp. 447–477.

Soderling, S.H., and Beavo, J.A. Regulation of cAMP and cGMP signaling: new phosphodiesterases and new functions. *Curr. Opin. Cell. Biol.,* **2000,** *12*:174–179.

Stoloff, S.W. The changing role of theophylline in pediatric asthma. *Am. Fam. Physician,* **1994,** *49*:839–844.

Symposium. Asthma: a nocturnal disease. January 21 to 24, 1988, Laguna Niguel, California. Proceedings. (McFadden, E.R. Jr., ed.) *Am. J. Med.,* **1988a,** *85*:1–70.

Symposium. Cholinergic pathway in obstructive airways disease. (Bergofsky, E.H., ed.) *Am. J. Med.,* **1986b,** *81*:1–192.

Symposium. Developmental pharmacology of the methylxanthines. Introduction (Soyka, L.F., ed.) *Semin. Perinatol.,* **1981,** *5*:303–304.

Symposium. Progress in understanding the relationship between the adenosine receptor system and actions of methylxanthines. (Carney, J.M., and Katz, J.L., eds.) *Pharmacol. Biochem. Behav.,* **1988b,** *29*:407–441.

Symposium. Update on theophylline. (Grant, J.A., and Ellis, E.F., eds.) *J. Allergy Clin. Immunol.,* **1986a,** *78*:669–824.

Taburet, A.-M., and Schmit, B. Pharmacokinetic optimisation of asthma treatment. *Clin. Pharmacokinet.,* **1994,** *26*:396–418.

Torphy, T.J., and Undem, B.J. Phosphodiesterase inhibitors: new opportunities for the treatment of asthma. *Thorax,* **1991,** *46*:512–523.

Van Bever, H.P., and Stevens, W.J. Pharmacotherapy of childhood asthma. An inflammatory disease. *Drugs,* **1992,** *44*:36–46.

Wasserman, S.I. A review of some recent clinical studies with nedocromil sodium. *J. Allergy Clin. Immunol.,* **1993,** *92*:210–215.

Weinberger, M. Pharmacologic management of asthma. *J. Adolesc. Health Care.,* **1987,** *8*:74–83.

Wilmott, R.W., and Fiedler, M.A. Recent advances in the treatment of cystic fibrosis. *Pediatr. Clin. North Am.,* **1994,** *41*:431–451.

Acknowledgment

The authors wish to acknowledge Theodore W. Rall and William E. Serafin, the authors of this chapter in the eighth and ninth editions of *Goodman and Gilman's The Pharmacological Basis of Therapeutics,* respectively, some of whose text has been retained in this edition.

SECTION V

DRUGS AFFECTING RENAL AND CARDIOVASCULAR FUNCTION

C H A P T E R   2 9

DIURETICS

Edwin K. Jackson

Diuretics increase the rate of urine flow and sodium excretion and are used to adjust the volume and/or composition of body fluids in a variety of clinical situations, including hypertension, heart failure, renal failure, nephrotic syndrome, and cirrhosis. The objective of this chapter is to provide the reader with unifying concepts as to how the kidney operates and how diuretics modify renal function. The chapter begins with a description of renal anatomy and physiology, as this information is prerequisite to a discussion of diuretic pharmacology. Categories of diuretics are introduced and then described with regard to chemistry, mechanism of action, site of action, effects on urinary composition, and effects on renal hemodynamics. Near the end of the chapter, diuretic pharmacology is integrated with a discussion of mechanisms of edema formation and the role of diuretics in clinical medicine. Therapeutic applications of diuretics are expanded upon in Chapters 33 (hypertension) and 34 (heart failure).

RENAL ANATOMY AND PHYSIOLOGY

Renal Anatomy. The main renal artery branches close to the renal hilum into segmental arteries, which, in turn, subdivide to form interlobar arteries that pierce the renal parenchyma. The interlobar arteries curve at the border of the renal medulla and cortex to form arc-like vessels known as arcuate arteries. Arcuate arteries give rise to perpendicular branches, called interlobular arteries, which enter the renal cortex and supply blood to the afferent arterioles. A single afferent arteriole penetrates the glomerulus of each nephron and branches extensively to form the glomerular capillary nexus. These branches coalesce to form the efferent arteriole. Efferent arterioles of superficial glomeruli ascend toward the kidney surface before splitting into peritubular capillaries that service the tubular elements of the renal cortex. Efferent arterioles of juxtamedullary glomeruli descend into the medulla and divide to form the descending vasa recta, which supply blood to the capillaries of the medulla. Blood returning from the medulla *via* the ascending vasa recta drains directly into the arcuate veins, and blood from the peritubular capillaries of the cortex enters the interlobular veins, which, in turn, connect with the arcuate veins. Arcuate veins drain into interlobar veins, which in turn drain into segmental veins, and blood leaves the kidney *via* the main renal vein.

The basic urine-forming unit of the kidney is the nephron, which consists of a filtering apparatus, the glomerulus, connected to a long tubular portion that reabsorbs and conditions the glomerular ultrafiltrate. Each human kidney is composed of approximately 1 million nephrons. The nomenclature for segments of the tubular portion of the nephron has become increasingly complex as renal physiologists have subdivided the nephron into shorter and shorter named segments. These subdivisions initially were based on the axial location of the segments but increasingly have been based on the morphology of the epithelial cells lining the various nephron segments. Figure 29–1

illustrates the currently accepted subdivision of the nephron into 14 subsegments. Commonly encountered names that refer to these subsegments and to combinations of subsegments are included.

Glomerular Filtration. In the glomerular capillaries, a portion of the plasma water is forced through a filter that has three basic components: the fenestrated capillary endothelial cells, a basement membrane lying just beneath the endothelial cells, and the filtration slit diaphragms formed by the epithelial cells that cover the basement membrane on its urinary space side. Solutes of small size flow with filtered water (solvent drag) into the urinary (Bowman's) space, whereas formed elements and macromolecules are retained by the filtration barrier. For each nephron unit, the rate of filtration (single-nephron glomerular filtration rate, SNGFR) is a function of the hydrostatic pressure in the glomerular capillaries (P_{GC}), the hydrostatic pressure in Bowman's space (which can be equated with pressure in the proximal tubule, P_T), the mean colloid osmotic pressure in the glomerular capillaries (Π_{GC}), the colloid osmotic pressure in the proximal tubule (Π_T), and the ultrafiltration coefficient (K_f), according to the equation:

$$\text{SNGFR} = K_f[(P_{GC} - P_T) - (\Pi_{GC} - \Pi_T)] \qquad (29\text{--}1)$$

If $P_{GC} - P_T$ is defined as the transcapillary hydraulic pressure difference (ΔP), and if Π_T is negligible (as it usually is since little protein is filtered), then:

$$\text{SNGFR} = K_f(\Delta P - \Pi_{GC}) \qquad (29\text{--}2)$$

This latter equation succinctly expresses the three major determinants of SNGFR. However, each of these three determinants can be influenced by a number of other variables. K_f

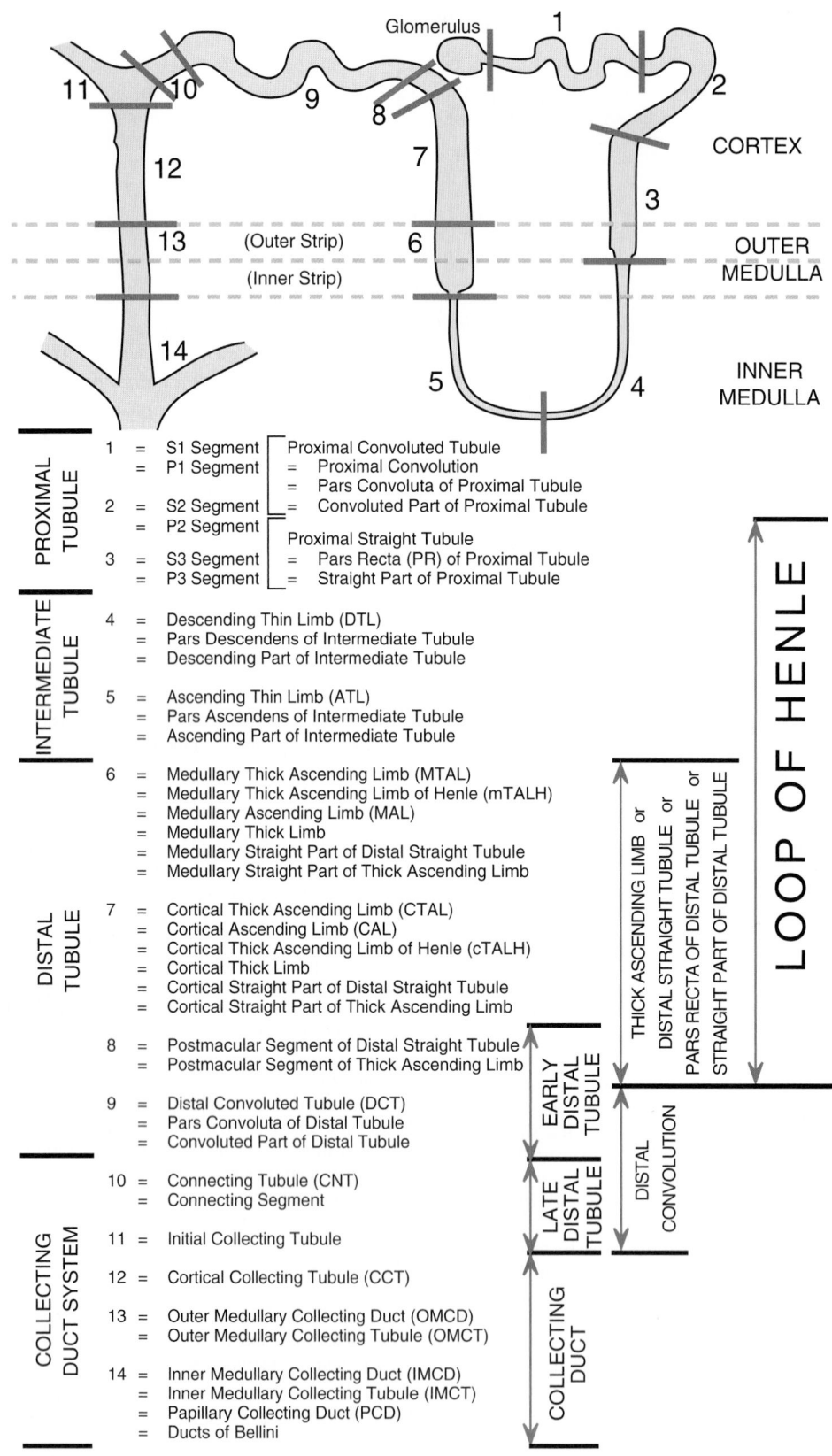

Figure 29–1. Anatomy and nomenclature of the nephron.

is determined by the physicochemical properties of the filtering membrane and by the surface area available for filtration. ΔP is determined primarily by the arterial blood pressure and by the proportion of the arterial pressure that is transmitted to the glomerular capillaries. This is governed by the relative resistances of preglomerular and postglomerular vessels. Π_{GC} is determined by two variables, *i.e.,* the concentration of protein in the arterial blood entering the glomerulus and the single-nephron blood flow (Q_A). Q_A influences Π_{GC} because, as blood transverses the glomerular capillary bed, filtration concentrates proteins in the capillaries, causing Π_{GC} to rise with distance along the glomerular bed. When Q_A is high, this effect is reduced; however, when Q_A is low, Π_{GC} may increase to the point that $\Pi_{GC} = \Delta P$ and filtration ceases (a condition known as *filtration equilibrium; see* Deen *et al.,* 1972).

Overview of Nephron Function.   Approximately 120 ml of ultrafiltrate is formed each minute, yet only 1 ml/min of urine is produced. Therefore, greater than 99% of the glomerular ultrafiltrate is reabsorbed at a staggering energy cost. The kidneys consume 7% of total-body oxygen intake despite the fact that the kidneys make up only 0.5% of body weight. The kidney is designed to filter large quantities of plasma, reabsorb those substances that the body must conserve, and leave behind and/or secrete substances that must be eliminated.

The proximal tubule is contiguous with Bowman's capsule and takes a tortuous path until finally forming a straight portion that dives into the renal medulla. The proximal tubule has been subdivided into S1, S2, and S3 segments based on the morphology of the epithelial cells lining the tubule. Normally, approximately 65% of filtered Na^+ is reabsorbed in the proximal tubule, and since this part of the tubule is highly permeable to water, reabsorption is essentially isotonic.

Between the outer and inner strips of the outer medulla, the tubule abruptly changes morphology to become the descending thin limb (DTL), which penetrates the inner medulla, makes a hairpin turn, and then forms the ascending thin limb (ATL). At the juncture between the inner and outer medulla, the tubule once again changes morphology and becomes the thick ascending limb, which is made up of three segments: a medullary portion (MTAL), a cortical portion (CTAL), and a postmacular segment. Together, the proximal straight tubule, DTL, ATL, MTAL, CTAL, and postmacular segment are known as the *loop of Henle.* The DTL is highly permeable to water, yet its permeability to NaCl and urea is low. In contrast, the ATL is permeable to NaCl and urea but is impermeable to water. The thick ascending limb actively reabsorbs NaCl but is impermeable to water and urea. Approximately 25% of filtered Na^+ is reabsorbed in the loop of Henle, mostly in the thick ascending limb, which has a large reabsorptive capacity.

The thick ascending limb passes between the afferent and efferent arterioles and makes contact with the afferent arteriole *via* a cluster of specialized columnar epithelial cells known as the *macula densa.* The macula densa is strategically located to sense concentrations of NaCl leaving the loop of Henle. If the concentration of NaCl is too high, the macula densa sends a chemical signal (perhaps adenosine) to the afferent arteriole of the same nephron, causing it to constrict. This in turn causes a reduction in P_{GC} and Q_A and decreases SNGFR. This homeostatic mechanism, known as *tubuloglomerular feedback* (TGF),

serves to protect the organism from salt and volume wasting. Besides causing a TGF response, the macula densa also regulates renin release from the adjacent juxtaglomerular cells in the wall of the afferent arteriole.

Approximately 0.2 mm past the macula densa, the tubule changes morphology once again to become the distal convoluted tubule (DCT). The postmacular segment of the thick ascending limb and the distal convoluted tubule often are referred to as the *early distal tubule.* Like the thick ascending limb, the DCT actively transports NaCl and is impermeable to water. Since these characteristics impart the ability to produce a dilute urine, the thick ascending limb and the DCT are collectively called the *diluting segment of the nephron,* and the tubular fluid in the DCT is hypotonic regardless of hydration status. However, unlike the thick ascending limb, the DCT does not contribute to the countercurrent-induced hypertonicity of the medullary interstitium (*see* below).

The collecting duct system (connecting tubule + initial collecting tubule + cortical collecting duct + outer and inner medullary collecting duct) is an area of fine control of ultrafiltrate composition and volume. It is here that final adjustments in electrolyte composition are made, a process modulated by the adrenal steroid, aldosterone. In addition, permeability of this part of the nephron to water is modulated by antidiuretic hormone (ADH; *see* Chapter 30).

The more distal portions of the collecting duct pass through the renal medulla, where the interstitial fluid is markedly hypertonic. In the absence of ADH, the collecting duct system is impermeable to water, and a dilute urine is excreted. However, in the presence of ADH, the collecting duct system is permeable to water, so that water is reabsorbed. The movement of water out of the tubule is driven by the steep concentration gradient that exists between the tubular fluid and the medullary interstitium.

The hypertonicity of the medullary interstitium plays a vital role in the ability of mammals and birds to concentrate urine and is therefore a key adaptation necessary for living in a terrestrial environment. This is accomplished *via* a combination of the unique topography of the loop of Henle and the specialized permeability features of the loop's subsegments. Although the precise mechanism giving rise to the medullary hypertonicity has remained elusive, the passive countercurrent multiplier hypothesis of Kokko and Rector (1972) is an intuitively attractive model that is qualitatively accurate (*see* Sands and Kokko, 1996). According to this hypothesis, the process begins with active transport in the thick ascending limb, which concentrates NaCl in the interstitium of the outer medulla. Since this segment of the nephron is impermeable to water, active transport in the ascending limb dilutes the tubular fluid. As the dilute fluid passes into the collecting duct system, water is extracted if and only if ADH is present. Since the cortical and outer medullary collecting ducts have a low permeability to urea, urea is concentrated in the tubular fluid. The inner medullary collecting duct, however, is permeable to urea, so that urea diffuses into the inner medulla where it is trapped by countercurrent exchange in the vasa recta. Since the DTL is impermeable to salt and urea, the high urea concentration in the inner medulla extracts water from the DTL and concentrates NaCl in the tubular fluid of the DTL. As the tubular fluid enters the ATL, NaCl diffuses out of the salt-permeable ATL, thus contributing to the hypertonicity of the medullary interstitium.

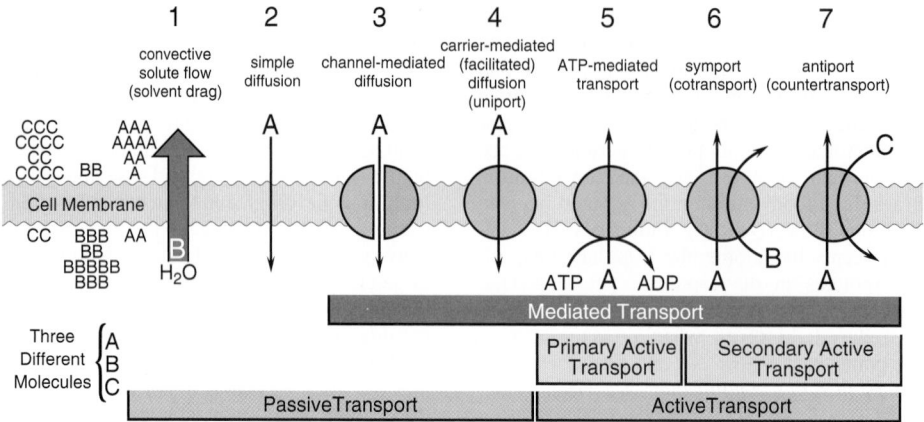

Figure 29–2. Seven basic mechanisms for transmembrane transport of solutes.

1, convective flow in which dissolved solutes are "dragged" by bulk water flow; 2, simple diffusion of lipophilic solute across membrane; 3, diffusion of solute through pore; 4, transport of solute by carrier protein down electrochemical gradient; 5, transport of solute by carrier protein against electrochemical gradient with ATP hydrolysis providing driving force; 6 and 7, cotransport and countertransport, respectively, of solutes with one solute traveling "uphill" against an electrochemical gradient and the other solute traveling down an electrochemical gradient.

General Mechanism of Renal Epithelial Transport. Figure 29–2 illustrates seven mechanisms by which solute crosses renal epithelial cell membranes. If bulk water flow occurs across a membrane, solute molecules will be transferred by convection across the membrane, a process known as *solvent drag*. Solutes with sufficient lipid solubility may also dissolve in the membrane and diffuse across the membrane down their electrochemical gradients (simple diffusion). Many solutes, however, have limited lipid solubility, and transport must rely on integral proteins embedded in the cell membrane. In some cases, the integral protein merely provides a conductive pathway (pore) through which the solute may diffuse passively (*channel-mediated diffusion*). In other cases, the solute may bind to the integral protein and, due to a conformational change in the protein, be transferred across the cell membrane down an electrochemical gradient (*carrier-mediated* or *facilitated diffusion,* also called *uniport*). However, this process will not result in net movement of solute against an electrochemical gradient. If solute must be moved "uphill" against an electrochemical gradient, then either primary active transport or secondary active transport is required. With primary active transport, ATP hydrolysis is coupled directly to conformational changes in the integral protein, thus providing the necessary free energy (*ATP-mediated transport*). Often, ATP-mediated transport is used to create an electrochemical gradient for a given solute, and the free energy of that solute gradient is then released to drive the "uphill" transport of other solutes. This process requires *symport* (cotransport of solute species in the same direction) or *antiport* (countertransport of solute species in opposite directions) and is known as *secondary active transport.*

The kinds of transport achieved in a particular nephron segment depend mainly on which transporters are present and whether they are embedded in the luminal or basolateral membrane. A general model of renal tubular transport is shown in

Figure 29–3 and can be summarized as follows:

1. Na^+,K^+–ATPase (sodium pump) in the basolateral membrane hydrolyzes ATP, which results in the transport of Na^+ into the intercellular and interstitial spaces and the movement of K^+ into the cell. Although other ATPases exist in selected renal epithelial cells and participate in the transport of specific solutes (*e.g.,* Ca^{2+}–ATPase and H^+–ATPase), the bulk of all transport in the kidney is due to the abundant supply of Na^+,K^+–ATPase in the basolateral membranes of the renal epithelial cells.

2. Na^+ may diffuse across the luminal membrane *via* Na^+ channels into the epithelial cell down the electrochemical gradient for Na^+ that is established by the basolateral Na^+,K^+–ATPases. In addition, the free energy available in the electrochemical gradient for Na^+ is tapped by integral proteins in the luminal membrane, resulting in cotransport of various solutes against their electrochemical gradients by symporters (*e.g.,* Na^+–glucose, Na^+–P_i, Na^+–amino acid). This process results in movement of Na^+ and cotransported solutes out of the tubular lumen into the cell. Also, antiporters (*e.g.,* Na^+–H^+) countertransport Na^+ out of and some solutes into the tubular lumen.

3. Na^+ exits the basolateral membrane into the intercellular and interstitial spaces *via* the Na^+ pump or *via* symporters or antiporters in the basolateral membrane.

4. The action of Na^+-linked symporters in the luminal membrane causes the concentration of substrates for these symporters to rise in the epithelial cell. These electrochemical gradients then permit simple diffusion or mediated transport (symporters, antiporters, uniporters, and channels) of solutes into the intercellular and interstitial spaces.

5. Accumulation of Na^+ and other solutes in the intercellular space creates a small osmotic pressure differential across

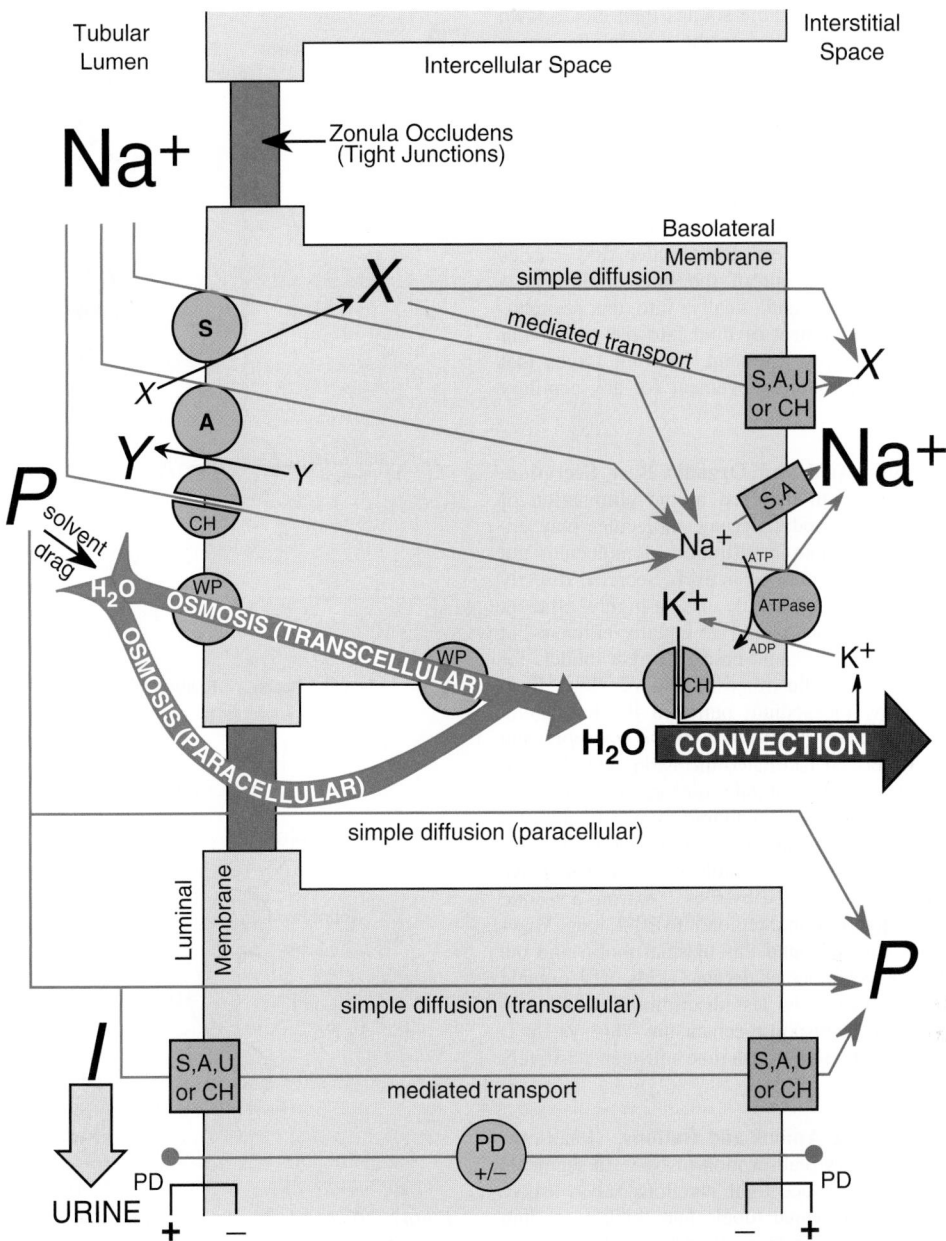

Figure 29–3. Generic mechanism of renal epithelial cell transport (see text for details).

S, symporter; A, antiporter; CH, ion channel; WP, water pore; U, uniporter; ATPase, Na^+, K^+-ATPase (sodium pump); *X* and *Y,* transported solutes; *P,* membrane-permeable (reabsorbable) solutes; *I,* membrane-impermeable (nonreabsorbable) solutes; PD, potential difference across indicated membrane or cell.

the epithelial cell. In water-permeable epithelium, water moves into the intercellular spaces driven by the osmotic pressure differential. Water moves through aqueous pores in both the luminal and the basolateral cell membranes as well as through the tight junctions (paracellular pathway).

Bulk water flow carries some solutes into the intercellular space by solvent drag.

6. Movement of water into the intercellular space concentrates other solutes in the tubular fluid, resulting in an electrochemical gradient for these substances across the

epithelium. Membrane-permeable solutes then move down their electrochemical gradients into the intercellular space *via* both the transcellular (simple diffusion, symporters, antiporters, uniporters, and channels) and paracellular pathways. Membrane-impermeable solutes remain in the tubular lumen and are excreted in the urine with an obligatory amount of water.

7. As water and solutes accumulate in the intercellular space, the hydrostatic pressure increases, thus providing a driving force for bulk water flow. Bulk water flow carries solute (solute convection) out of the intercellular space into the interstitial space and, finally, into the peritubular capillaries. The movement of fluid into the peritubular capillaries is governed by the same Starling forces that determine transcapillary fluid movement for any capillary bed.

Mechanism of Organic Acid and Organic Base Secretion. The kidney is a major organ involved in the elimination of organic chemicals from the body. Organic molecules may enter the renal tubules by glomerular filtration of molecules not bound to plasma proteins or may be actively secreted directly into the tubules. The proximal tubule has a highly efficient transport system for organic acids and an equally efficient but separate transport system for organic bases. Current models for these secretory systems are illustrated in Figure 29–4. Both systems are powered by the sodium pump in the basolateral membrane, involve secondary and tertiary active transport, and utilize a poorly characterized facilitated-diffusion step. The antiporter that exchanges α-ketoglutarate for organic acids has been cloned from several species, including human beings (Lu *et al.*, 1999). The optimal substrate for transport by the organic acid secretory mechanism is a molecule with a negative or partial negative charge, separated by 6 to 7 Å from a second negative charge, and a hydrophobic region 8 to 10 Å long. However, much flexibility exists around this optimal motif, and the system transports a large variety of organic acids. The organic base secretory mechanism is even less discriminating and may involve a family of related transport mechanisms. This system(s) transports many drugs containing an amine nitrogen positively charged at physiological pH.

Renal Handling of Specific Anions and Cations. Reabsorption of Cl^- generally follows reabsorption of Na^+. In segments of the tubule with low-resistance tight junctions (*i.e.,* "leaky" epithelium), such as the proximal tubule and thick ascending limb, Cl^- movement can occur paracellularly. With regard to transcellular Cl^- flux, Cl^- crosses the luminal membrane *via* antiport with formate and oxalate (proximal tubule), symport with Na^+/K^+ (thick ascending limb), symport with Na^+ (DCT), and antiport with HCO_3^- (collecting duct system). Cl^- crosses the basolateral membrane *via* symport with K^+ (proximal tubule and thick ascending limb), antiport with Na^+/HCO_3^- (proximal tubule), and Cl^- channels (thick ascending limb, DCT, collecting duct system).

Eighty to ninety percent of filtered K^+ is reabsorbed in the proximal tubule (diffusion and solvent drag) and thick ascending limb (diffusion), largely *via* the paracellular pathway. In contrast, the DCT and collecting duct system secrete variable amounts of K^+ *via* a conductive (channel-mediated) pathway. Modulation of the rate of K^+ secretion in the collecting duct system, particularly by aldosterone, allows urinary excretion of

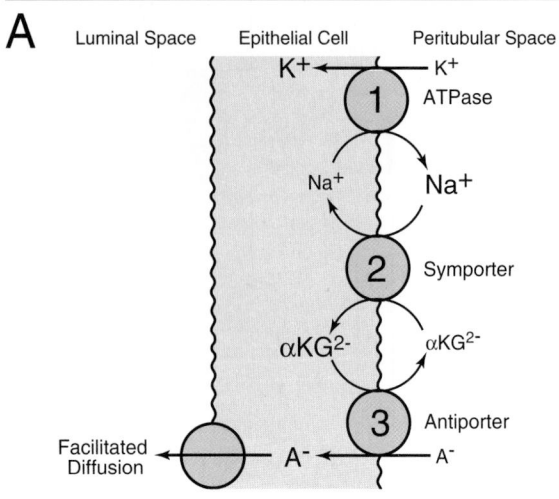

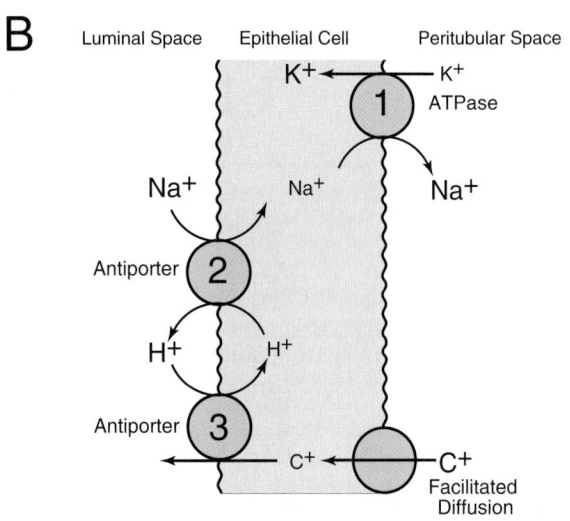

Figure 29–4. Mechanisms of organic acid (A) and organic base (B) secretion in the proximal tubule.

The numbers 1, 2, and 3 refer to primary, secondary, and tertiary active transport. A^-, organic acid (anion); C^+, organic base (cation); αKG^{2-}, α-ketoglutarate, but also other dicarboxylates.

K^+ to be matched with dietary intake. The transepithelial potential difference (V_T), lumen-positive in the thick ascending limb and lumen-negative in the collecting duct system, provides an important driving force for K^+ reabsorption and secretion, respectively.

Most of the filtered Ca^{2+} (approximately 70%) is reabsorbed by the proximal tubule by passive diffusion, probably *via* a paracellular route. Another 25% of filtered Ca^{2+} is reabsorbed by the thick ascending limb, mostly *via* a paracellular route driven by the lumen-positive V_T, although a component of active Ca^{2+} reabsorption also may exist. The remaining Ca^{2+} is reabsorbed in the distal convoluted tubule and the connecting tubule *via* a transcellular pathway that is modulated by parathyroid hormone (PTH; *see* Chapter 62). PTH appears to increase Ca^{2+} channels in the luminal membrane, thereby facilitating the passive movement of Ca^{2+} into the epithelial cell. Ca^{2+} is extruded across the basolateral membrane by a Ca^{2+}–ATPase and *via* Na^+–Ca^{2+} antiport.

Inorganic phosphate (P_i) is largely reabsorbed (80% of filtered load) by the proximal tubule. A Na^+–P_i symporter uses the free energy of the Na^+ electrochemical gradient to effect secondary active transport of P_i into the cell. The Na^+–P_i symporter is inhibited by PTH. P_i exits the basolateral membrane down its electrochemical gradient by a poorly understood transport system.

Only 20% to 25% of Mg^{2+} is reabsorbed in the proximal tubule, and only 5% is reabsorbed by the DCT and collecting duct system. The bulk of Mg^{2+} is reabsorbed in the thick ascending limb *via* a paracellular pathway driven by the lumen-positive V_T. However, transcellular movement of Mg^{2+} also may occur with basolateral exit *via* Na^+–Mg^{2+} antiport or *via* a Mg^{2+}–ATPase.

The renal tubules play an extremely important role in the reabsorption of HCO_3^- and secretion of protons (tubular acidification) and thus participate critically in the maintenance of acid–base balance. A description of these processes is presented in the section on carbonic anhydrase inhibitors.

PRINCIPLES OF DIURETIC ACTION

By definition, diuretics are drugs that increase the rate of urine flow; however, clinically useful diuretics also increase the rate of excretion of Na^+ (natriuresis) and of an accompanying anion, usually Cl^-. NaCl in the body is the major determinant of extracellular fluid volume, and most clinical applications of diuretics are directed toward reducing extracellular fluid volume by decreasing total-body NaCl content. A sustained imbalance between dietary Na^+ intake and Na^+ loss is incompatible with life. A sustained positive Na^+ balance would result in volume overload with pulmonary edema, and a sustained negative Na^+ balance would result in volume depletion and cardiovascular collapse. Although continued administration of a diuretic causes a sustained net deficit in total-body Na^+, the time course of natriuresis is finite as renal compensatory mechanisms bring Na^+ excretion in line with Na^+ intake, a phenomenon known as "diuretic braking." These compensatory, or braking, mechanisms include activation of the sympathetic nervous system, activation of the renin–angiotensin–aldosterone axis, decreased arterial blood pressure (which reduces pressure-natriuresis), hypertrophy of renal epithelial cells, increased expression of renal epithelial transporters, and perhaps

alterations in natriuretic hormones such as atrial natriuretic peptide.

Historically, the classification of diuretics was based on a mosaic of ideas such as site of action (loop diuretics), efficacy (high-ceiling diuretics), chemical structure (thiazide diuretics), similarity of action with other diuretics (thiazide-like diuretics), effects on potassium excretion (potassium-sparing diuretics), etc. However, since the mechanism of action of each of the major classes of diuretics is now reasonably well understood, a classification scheme based on mechanism of action is now possible and is used in this chapter.

Diuretics not only alter the excretion of Na^+, but also may modify renal handling of other cations (*e.g.*, K^+, H^+, Ca^{2+}, and Mg^{2+}), anions (*e.g.*, Cl^-, HCO_3^-, and $H_2PO_4^-$), and uric acid. In addition, diuretics may indirectly alter renal hemodynamics. Table 29–1 gives a comparison of the general effects of the major classes of diuretics.

INHIBITORS OF CARBONIC ANHYDRASE

Acetazolamide (DIAMOX) is the prototype of a class of agents that have limited usefulness as diuretics but have played a major role in the development of fundamental concepts of renal physiology and pharmacology.

Chemistry. When sulfanilamide was introduced as a chemotherapeutic agent, metabolic acidosis was recognized as a side effect. This observation led to *in vitro* and *in vivo* studies demonstrating that sulfanilamide is an inhibitor of carbonic anhydrase. Subsequently, an enormous number of sulfonamides were synthesized and tested for the ability to inhibit carbonic anhydrase; of these compounds, acetazolamide has been most extensively studied. Table 29–2 lists the chemical structures of the three carbonic anhydrase inhibitors currently available in the United States—acetazolamide, *dichlorphenamide* (DARANIDE), and *methazolamide* (NEPTAZANE). The common molecular motif of available carbonic anhydrase inhibitors is an unsubstituted sulfonamide moiety.

Mechanism and Site of Action. Proximal tubular epithelial cells are richly endowed with the zinc metalloenzyme carbonic anhydrase, which is found in the luminal and basolateral membranes (type IV carbonic anhydrase, an enzyme tethered to the membrane by a glycosylphosphatidylinositol linkage) as well as in the cytoplasm (type II carbonic anhydrase). Davenport and Wilhelmi (1941) were the first to discover this enzyme in the mammalian kidney, and subsequent studies revealed the key role played by carbonic anhydrase in $NaHCO_3$ reabsorption and acid secretion (*see* Maren, 1967 and 1980).

Table 29–1
Excretory and Renal Hemodynamic Effects of Diuretics*

	CATIONS					ANIONS			URIC ACID		RENAL HEMODYNAMICS			
	Na^+	K^+	$H^{+\dagger}$	Ca^{2+}	Mg^{2+}	Cl^-	HCO_3^-	$H_2PO_4^-$	Acute	Chronic	RBF	GFR	FF	TGF
Inhibitors of carbonic anhydrase (primary site of action is proximal tubule)	+	++	–	NC	V	(+)	++	++	I	–	–	–	NC	+
Osmotic diuretics (primary site of action is loop of Henle)	++	+	I	+	++	+	+	+	+	I	+	NC	–	I
Inhibitors of Na^+-K^+-$2Cl^-$ symport (primary site of action is thick ascending limb)	++	++	+	++	++	++	+‡	+‡	+	–	V(+)	NC	V(–)	–
Inhibitors of Na^+-Cl^- symport (primary site of action is distal convoluted tubule)	+	++	+	V	V(+)	+	+‡	+‡	+	–	NC	V(–)	V(–)	NC
Inhibitors of renal epithelial sodium channels (primary site of action is late distal tubule and collecting duct)	+	–	–	–	–	+	(+)	NC	I	–	NC	NC	NC	NC
Antagonists of mineralocorticoid receptors (primary site of action is late distal tubule and collecting duct)	+	–	–	I	–	+	(+)	I	I	–	NC	NC	NC	NC

*Except for uric acid, changes are for acute effects of diuretics in the absence of significant volume depletion, which would trigger complex physiological adjustments; ++, +, (+), –, NC, V, V(+), V(–), and I indicate marked increase, mild to moderate increase, slight increase, decrease, no change, variable effect, variable increase, variable decrease, and insufficient data, respectively. For cations and anions, the indicated effects refer to absolute changes in fractional excretion. RBF, renal blood flow; GFR, glomerular filtration rate; FF, filtration fraction; TGF, tubuloglomerular feedback.

†H^+, titratable acid and NH_4^+.

‡In general, these effects are restricted to those individual agents that inhibit carbonic anhydrase. However, there are notable exceptions in which symport inhibitors increase bicarbonate and phosphate (e.g., metozalone, bumetanide) (see Puschett and Winaver, 1992).

Table 29–2
Inhibitors of Carbonic Anhydrase

DRUG	STRUCTURE	RELATIVE POTENCY	ORAL AVAILABILITY	$t_{1/2}$ (HOURS)	ROUTE OF ELIMINATION
Acetazolamide	CH_3CONH — S — SO_2NH_2 ; N — N	1	~100%	6–9	R
Dichlorphenamide	SO_2NH_2 ; Cl , SO_2NH_2 ; Cl	30	ID	ID	ID
Methazolamide	CH_3CON — S — SO_2NH_2 ; N — N ; H_3C	>1 <10	~100%	~14	~25% R, ~75% M

Abbreviations: R, renal excretion of intact drug; M, metabolism; ID, insufficient data.

In the proximal tubule, the free energy in the Na^+ gradient established by the basolateral Na^+ pump is used by a Na^+–H^+ antiporter (also referred to as a Na^+–H^+ exchanger or NHE) in the luminal membrane to transport H^+ into the tubular lumen in exchange for Na^+ (Figure 29–5). In the lumen, H^+ reacts with filtered HCO_3^- to form H_2CO_3, which rapidly decomposes to CO_2 and water in the presence of carbonic anhydrase in the brush border. Normally the reaction between CO_2 and water occurs slowly, but carbonic anhydrase reversibly accelerates this reaction several thousandfold. CO_2 is lipophilic and rapidly diffuses across the luminal membrane into the epithelial cell where it reacts with water to form H_2CO_3, a reaction catalyzed by cytoplasmic carbonic anhydrase. (The actual reaction catalyzed by carbonic anhydrase is $OH^- + CO_2 \rightleftharpoons HCO_3^-$; however, $H_2O \rightleftharpoons OH^- + H^+$ and $HCO_3^- + H^+ \rightleftharpoons H_2CO_3$, so that the net reaction is $H_2O + CO_2 \rightleftharpoons H_2CO_3$.) Continued operation of the Na^+–H^+ antiporter maintains a low proton concentration in the cell, so that H_2CO_3 spontaneously ionizes to form H^+ and HCO_3^-, creating an electrochemical gradient for HCO_3^- across the basolateral membrane. The electrochemical gradient for HCO_3^- is used by a Na^+–HCO_3^- symporter (also called Na^+–HCO_3^- cotransporter or NBC) in the basolateral membrane to transport $NaHCO_3$ into the interstitial space. The net effect of this process is transport of $NaHCO_3$ from the tubular lumen to the interstitial

PROXIMAL TUBULE

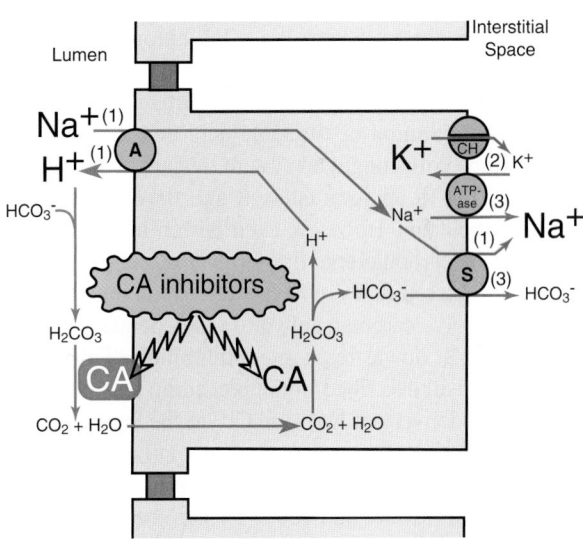

Figure 29–5. *NaHCO_3 reabsorption in proximal tubule and mechanism of diuretic action of carbonic anhydrase (CA) inhibitors.*

A, antiporter; S, symporter; CH, ion channel. (The actual reaction catalyzed by carbonic anhydrase is $OH^- + CO_2 \rightleftharpoons HCO_3^-$; however, $H_2O \rightleftharpoons OH^- + H^+$, and $HCO_3^- + H^+ \rightleftharpoons H_2CO_3$, so that the net reaction is $H_2O + CO_2 \rightleftharpoons H_2CO_3$.) Numbers in parentheses indicate stoichiometry.

space followed by movement of water (isotonic reabsorption). Removal of water concentrates Cl^- in the tubular lumen, and consequently Cl^- diffuses down its concentration gradient into the interstitium *via* the paracellular pathway.

Carbonic anhydrase inhibitors potently inhibit (IC_{50} for acetazolamide is 10 nM) both the membrane-bound and cytoplasmic forms of carbonic anhydrase, resulting in nearly complete abolition of $NaHCO_3$ reabsorption in the proximal tubule (Cogan *et al.*, 1979). Studies with a high-molecular-weight carbonic anhydrase inhibitor that only inhibits luminal enzyme because of limited cellular permeability indicate that inhibition of both the membrane-bound and cytoplasmic pools of carbonic anhydrase contributes to the diuretic activity of carbonic anhydrase inhibitors (Maren *et al.*, 1997). Because of the large excess of carbonic anhydrase in proximal tubules, a high percentage of enzyme activity must be inhibited before an effect on electrolyte excretion is observed. Although the proximal tubule is the major site of action of carbonic anhydrase inhibitors, carbonic anhydrase also is involved in secretion of titratable acid in the collecting duct system (a process that involves a proton pump); therefore the collecting duct system is a secondary site of action for this class of drugs.

Effects on Urinary Excretion. Inhibition of carbonic anhydrase is associated with a rapid rise in urinary HCO_3^- excretion to approximately 35% of filtered load. This, along with inhibition of titratable acid and ammonia secretion in the collecting duct system, results in an increase in urinary pH to approximately 8 and development of a metabolic acidosis. However, even with a high degree of inhibition of carbonic anhydrase, 65% of HCO_3^- is rescued from excretion by poorly understood mechanisms that may involve carbonic anhydrase–independent HCO_3^- reabsorption at downstream sites. Inhibition of the transport mechanism described in the preceding section results in increased delivery of Na^+ and Cl^- to the loop of Henle, which has a large reabsorptive capacity and captures most of the Cl^- and a portion of the Na^+. Thus, only a small increase in Cl^- excretion occurs, HCO_3^- being the major anion excreted along with the cations Na^+ and K^+. The fractional excretion of Na^+ may be as much as 5%, and the fractional excretion of K^+ can be as much as 70%. The increased excretion of K^+ is secondary to increased delivery of Na^+ to the distal nephron. The mechanism by which increased distal delivery of Na^+ enhances K^+ excretion is described in the section on inhibitors of sodium channels. Carbonic anhydrase inhibitors also increase phosphate excretion (mechanism unknown), but have little or no effect on the excretion of Ca^{2+} or Mg^{2+}. The effects of carbonic

anhydrase inhibitors on renal excretion are self-limiting, probably because, as metabolic acidosis develops, the filtered load of HCO_3^- decreases to the point that the uncatalyzed reaction between CO_2 and water is sufficient to achieve HCO_3^- reabsorption.

Effects on Renal Hemodynamics. By inhibiting proximal reabsorption, carbonic anhydrase inhibitors increase delivery of solutes to the macula densa. This triggers tubuloglomerular feedback (TGF), which increases afferent arteriolar resistance and reduces renal blood flow (RBF) and glomerular filtration rate (GFR) (Persson and Wright, 1982).

Other Actions. Carbonic anhydrase is present in a number of extrarenal tissues including the eye, gastric mucosa, pancreas, central nervous system (CNS), and red blood cells (RBCs). Carbonic anhydrase in the ciliary processes of the eye mediates the formation of large amounts of HCO_3^- in aqueous humor. For this reason, inhibition of carbonic anhydrase decreases the rate of formation of aqueous humor and consequently reduces intraocular pressure. Acetazolamide frequently causes paresthesias and somnolence, suggesting an action of carbonic anhydrase inhibitors in the CNS. The efficacy of acetazolamide in epilepsy is in part due to the production of metabolic acidosis; however, direct actions of acetazolamide in the CNS also contribute to its anticonvulsant action. Due to interference with carbonic anhydrase activity in RBCs, carbonic anhydrase inhibitors increase CO_2 levels in peripheral tissues and decrease CO_2 levels in expired gas. Large doses of carbonic anhydrase inhibitors reduce gastric acid secretion, but this has no therapeutic applications.

Absorption and Elimination. The oral bioavailability, plasma half-life, and route of elimination of the three currently available carbonic anhydrase inhibitors are listed in Table 29–2. Carbonic anhydrase inhibitors are avidly bound by carbonic anhydrase and, accordingly, tissues rich in this enzyme will have higher concentrations of carbonic anhydrase inhibitors following systemic administration.

Toxicity, Adverse Effects, Contraindications, Drug Interactions. Serious toxic reactions to carbonic anhydrase inhibitors are infrequent; however, these drugs are sulfonamide derivatives and, like other sulfonamides, may cause bone-marrow depression, skin toxicity, and sulfonamide-like renal lesions and may cause allergic reactions in patients hypersensitive to sulfonamides. With large doses, many patients exhibit drowsiness and paresthesias. Most adverse effects, contraindications, and drug interactions are secondary to urinary alkalinization or metabolic acidosis, including: (1) diversion of ammonia of renal origin from urine into the systemic circulation, a process that may induce hepatic encephalopathy (the drugs are contraindicated in patients with hepatic cirrhosis); (2) calculus formation and ureteral colic due to precipitation of calcium phosphate salts in an alkaline urine; (3) worsening of metabolic or respiratory acidosis (the drugs are contraindicated in patients with hyperchloremic acidosis or severe chronic obstructive pulmonary disease); (4) interference with the urinary tract antiseptic methenamine; and (5) reduction of the urinary excretion rate of weak organic bases.

Therapeutic Uses. Although acetazolamide is used for treatment of edema, the efficacy of carbonic anhydrase inhibitors as single agents is low, and carbonic anhydrase inhibitors are not widely employed in this regard. However, studies by Knauf and Mutschler (1997) indicate that the combination of acetazolamide with diuretics that block Na^+ reabsorption at more distal sites in the nephron causes a marked natriuretic response in patients with low basal fractional excretion of Na^+ ($<0.2\%$) who are resistant to diuretic monotherapy. Even so, the long-term usefulness of carbonic anhydrase inhibitors often is compromised by development of metabolic acidosis.

The major indication for carbonic anhydrase inhibitors is open-angle glaucoma. Carbonic anhydrase inhibitors also may be employed for secondary glaucoma and preoperatively in acute angle-closure glaucoma to lower ocular pressure before surgery (*see* Chapter 66). Acetazolamide also is used for the treatment of epilepsy (*see* Chapter 21). The rapid development of tolerance, however, may limit the usefulness of carbonic anhydrase inhibitors for epilepsy. Acetazolamide may provide symptomatic relief in patients with acute mountain sickness; however, it is more appropriate to give acetazolamide as a prophylactic measure (Coote, 1991). Acetazolamide also is useful in patients with familial periodic paralysis (Links *et al.*, 1988). The mechanism for the beneficial effects of acetazolamide in mountain sickness and familial periodic paralysis is not clear, but it may be related to the induction of a metabolic acidosis. Finally, carbonic anhydrase inhibitors can be useful for correcting a metabolic alkalosis, especially an alkalosis caused by diuretic-induced increases in H^+ excretion.

OSMOTIC DIURETICS

Osmotic diuretics are agents that are freely filtered at the glomerulus, undergo limited reabsorption by the renal tubule, and are relatively inert pharmacologically. Osmotic diuretics are administered in large enough doses to increase significantly the osmolality of plasma and tubular fluid. Table 29–3 gives the molecular structures of

Table 29–3
Osmotic Diuretics

DRUG	STRUCTURE	ORAL AVAILABILITY	$t_{1/2}$ (HOURS)	ROUTE OF ELIMINATION
Glycerin	HO‑‑‑OH / OH	Orally active	0.5–0.75	~80% M ~20% U
Isosorbide	HO H H O O H H OH	Orally active	5–9.5	R
Mannitol	OH OH OH OH OH OH	Negligible	0.25–1.7*	~80% R ~20% M + B
Urea	O H₂N NH₂	Negligible	ID	R

*In renal failure, 6–36.

Abbreviations: R, renal excretion of intact drug; M, metabolism; B, excretion of intact drug into bile; U, unknown pathway of elimination; ID, insufficient data.

the four currently available osmotic diuretics—*glycerin, isosorbide, mannitol,* and *urea.*

Mechanism and Site of Action. For many years it was thought that osmotic diuretics act primarily in the proximal tubule (Wesson and Anslow, 1948). By acting as nonreabsorbable solutes, it was reasoned that osmotic diuretics limit the osmosis of water into the interstitial space and thereby reduce luminal Na^+ concentration to the point that net Na^+ reabsorption ceases. Indeed, early micropuncture studies supported this concept (Windhager *et al.,* 1959). However, subsequent studies suggest that this mechanism, while operative, may be of only secondary importance. For instance, mannitol only slightly increases the delivery of Na^+ and moderately increases the delivery of water out of the proximal tubule (Seely and Dirks, 1969), and urea does not alter proximal tubular reabsorption in rats at the time of a large osmotic diuresis (Kauker *et al.,* 1970). Mannitol, on the other hand, markedly increases the delivery of Na^+ and water out of the loop of Henle (Seely and Dirks, 1969), suggesting that the major site of action is the loop of Henle.

By extracting water from intracellular compartments, osmotic diuretics expand the extracellular fluid volume, decrease blood viscosity, and inhibit renin release. These effects increase RBF, and the increase in renal medullary blood flow removes NaCl and urea from the renal medulla, thus reducing medullary tonicity. Also, under some circumstances, prostaglandins may contribute to the renal vasodilation and medullary washout induced by osmotic diuretics (Johnston *et al.,* 1981). A reduction in medullary tonicity causes a decrease in the extraction of water from the DTL, which in turn limits the concentration of NaCl in the tubular fluid entering the ATL. This latter effect diminishes the passive reabsorption of NaCl in the ATL. In addition, the marked ability of osmotic diuretics to inhibit reabsorption of Mg^{2+}, a cation that is mainly reabsorbed in the thick ascending limb, suggests that osmotic diuretics also interfere with transport processes in the thick ascending limb. The mechanism of this effect is unknown.

In summary, osmotic diuretics act both in the proximal tubule and the loop of Henle, with the latter being the primary site of action. Also, osmotic diuretics probably act by an osmotic effect in the tubules and by reducing medullary tonicity.

Effects on Urinary Excretion. Osmotic diuretics increase the urinary excretion of nearly all electrolytes, including Na^+, K^+, Ca^{2+}, Mg^{2+}, Cl^-, HCO_3^-, and phosphate.

Effects on Renal Hemodynamics. As indicated in the preceding section, osmotic diuretics increase RBF by a variety of mechanisms. Osmotic diuretics dilate the afferent arteriole, which increases P_{GC}, and dilute the plasma, which decreases Π_{GC}. These effects would increase GFR were it not for the fact that osmotic diuretics also increase P_T. In general, superficial SNGFR is increased but total GFR is little changed.

Absorption and Elimination. The oral bioavailability, plasma half-life, and route of elimination of the four currently available osmotic diuretics are listed in Table 29–3. Glycerin and isosorbide can be given orally, whereas mannitol and urea must be administered intravenously.

Toxicity, Adverse Effects, Contraindications, Drug Interactions. Osmotic diuretics are distributed in the extracellular fluid and contribute to the extracellular osmolality. Thus, water is extracted from intracellular compartments, and the extracellular fluid volume becomes expanded. In patients with heart failure or pulmonary congestion, this may cause frank pulmonary edema. Extraction of water also causes hyponatremia, which may explain common adverse effects, including headache, nausea, and vomiting. On the other hand, loss of water in excess of electrolytes can cause hypernatremia and dehydration. In general, osmotic diuretics are contraindicated in patients who are anuric due to severe renal disease or who are unresponsive to test doses of the drugs. Urea may cause thrombosis or pain if extravasation occurs, and it should not be administered to patients with impaired liver function because of the risk of elevation of blood ammonia levels. Both mannitol and urea are contraindicated in patients with active cranial bleeding. Glycerin is metabolized and can cause hyperglycemia.

Therapeutic Uses. A rapid decrease in GFR, *i.e.,* acute renal failure (ARF), is a serious medical condition that occurs in 5% of hospitalized patients and is associated with a significant mortality rate. ARF can be caused by diverse conditions both extrinsic (prerenal and postrenal failure) and intrinsic to the kidney. Acute tubular necrosis (ATN), *i.e.,* damage to tubular epithelial cells, accounts for the majority of cases of intrinsic ARF. In animal models, mannitol is effective in attenuating the reduction in GFR associated with ATN when administered before the ischemic insult or offending nephrotoxin. The renal protection afforded by mannitol may be due to removal of obstructing tubular casts, dilution of nephrotoxic substances in the tubular fluid, and/or reduction of swelling of tubular elements *via* osmotic extraction of water. Although prophylactic mannitol is effective in animal models of ATN, the clinical efficacy of mannitol is less well established. Most published clinical studies have been uncontrolled, and controlled studies have not shown a benefit over hydration *per se* (*see* Kellum, 1998). In patients with mild-to-moderate renal insufficiency, hydration with 0.45% sodium chloride is as good as or better than either mannitol or furosemide in protection against decreases in GFR induced by radiocontrast agents (Soloman *et al.,* 1994). Studies of prophylactic mannitol indicate effectiveness in jaundiced patients undergoing surgery (Dawson, 1965). However, in vascular and open heart surgery, prophylactic mannitol maintains urine flow but not GFR. In established ATN, mannitol will increase urine volume in some patients, and those patients converted from oliguric to nonoliguric ATN appear to recover more rapidly and require less dialysis compared with patients who do not respond to mannitol (Levinsky and Bernard, 1988). However, it is not clear whether these benefits are due to the diuretic or whether "responders" have lesser degrees of renal damage from the outset compared with "nonresponders." Repeated administration of mannitol to nonresponders is not recommended, and nowadays loop diuretics are more frequently used to convert oliguric to nonoliguric ATN.

Another use for mannitol and urea is in the treatment of dialysis disequilibrium syndrome. Too rapid a removal of solutes from the extracellular fluid by hemodialysis or peritoneal dialysis results in a reduction in the osmolality of the extracellular fluid. Consequently, water moves from the extracellular compartment into the intracellular compartment, causing hypotension and CNS symptoms (headache, nausea, muscle cramps, restlessness, CNS depression, and convulsions). Osmotic diuretics increase the osmolality of the extracellular fluid compartment and thereby shift water back into the extracellular compartment.

By increasing the osmotic pressure of the plasma, osmotic diuretics extract water from the eye and brain. All four osmotic diuretics are used to control intraocular pressure during acute attacks of glaucoma and for short-term reductions in intraocular pressure, both preoperatively and postoperatively, in patients who require ocular surgery. Also, mannitol and urea are used to reduce cerebral edema and brain mass before and after neurosurgery.

INHIBITORS OF Na^+–K^+–$2Cl^-$ SYMPORT (LOOP DIURETICS; HIGH-CEILING DIURETICS)

Inhibitors of Na^+–K^+–$2Cl^-$ symport are a group of diuretics that have in common an ability to block the Na^+–K^+–$2Cl^-$ symporter in the thick ascending limb of the loop of Henle; hence these diuretics also are referred to as *loop diuretics*. Although the proximal tubule reabsorbs approximately 65% of the filtered Na^+, diuretics acting only in the proximal tubule have limited efficacy because the thick ascending limb has a great reabsorptive capacity and reabsorbs most of the rejectate from the proximal tubule. Diuretics acting predominantly at sites past the thick ascending limb also have limited efficacy, because only a small percentage of the filtered Na^+ load reaches these more distal sites. In contrast, inhibitors of Na^+–K^+–$2Cl^-$ symport are highly efficacious, and for this reason they often are called *high-ceiling diuretics*. The efficacy of inhibitors of Na^+–K^+–$2Cl^-$ symport in the thick ascending limb of the loop of Henle is due to a combination of two factors: (1) Approximately 25% of the filtered Na^+ load normally is reabsorbed by the thick ascending limb; and (2) nephron segments past the thick ascending limb do not possess the reabsorptive capacity to rescue the flood of rejectate exiting the thick ascending limb.

Chemistry. Inhibitors of Na^+–K^+–$2Cl^-$ symport are a chemically diverse group of drugs (*see* Table 29–4). Furosemide, bumetanide, azosemide, piretanide, and tripamide all contain a sulfonamide moiety, whereas ethacrynic acid is a phenoxyacetic acid derivative. Muzolimine has neither of these structural features, and torsemide is a sulfonylurea. Only *furosemide* (LASIX), *bumetanide* (BUMEX), *ethacrynic acid* (EDECRIN), and *torsemide* (DEMADEX) are available currently in the United States.

Mechanism and Site of Action. Inhibitors of Na^+–K^+–$2Cl^-$ symport act primarily in the thick ascending limb. Micropuncture of the DCT demonstrates that loop diuretics increase the delivery of solutes out of the loop of Henle (Dirks and Seely, 1970). Also, *in situ* microperfusion of the loop of Henle (Morgan *et al.,* 1970) and *in vitro* microperfusion of the CTAL (Burg *et al.,* 1973) indicate inhibition of transport by low concentrations of furosemide in the perfusate. Some inhibitors of Na^+–K^+–$2Cl^-$ symport may have additional effects in the proximal tubule; however, the significance of these effects is unclear.

It was initially thought that Cl^- was transported by a primary active electrogenic transporter in the luminal membrane independent of Na^+. Discovery of furosemide-sensitive Na^+–K^+–$2Cl^-$ symport in other tissues caused Greger (1981) to investigate more carefully the Na^+ dependence of Cl^- transport in the isolated perfused rabbit CTAL. By scrupulously removing Na^+ from the luminal perfusate, Greger demonstrated the dependence of Cl^- transport on Na^+. It is now well accepted that, in the thick ascending limb, flux of Na^+, K^+, and Cl^- from the lumen into the epithelial cell is mediated by a Na^+–K^+–$2Cl^-$ symporter (*see* Figure 29–6). This symporter captures the free energy in the Na^+ electrochemical gradient

Table 29–4

Inhibitors of $Na^+–K^+–2Cl^-$ Symport (Loop Diuretics; High-Ceiling Diuretics)

DRUG	STRUCTURE	RELATIVE POTENCY	ORAL AVAILABILITY	$t_{1/2}$ (HOURS)	ROUTE OF ELIMINATION
Furosemide		1	~60%	~1.5	~65% R, ~35% M
Bumetanide		40	~80%	~0.8	~62% R, ~38% M
Ethacrynic acid		0.7	~100%	~1	~67% R, ~33% M
Torsemide		3	~80%	~3.5	~20% R, ~80% M
Azosemide*		ID	ID	ID	ID
Muzolimine*		ID	ID	ID	ID
Piretanide*		3	~80%	0.6–1.5	~50% R, ~50% M
Tripamide*		ID	ID	ID	ID

*Not available in the United States.

Abbreviations: R, renal excretion of intact drug; M, metabolism; ID, insufficient data.

THICK ASCENDING LIMB

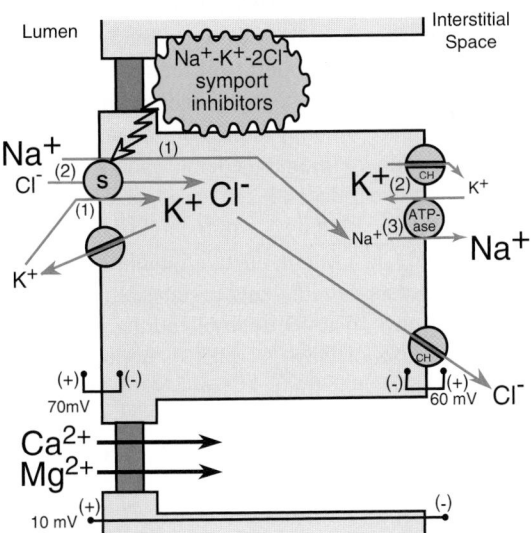

Figure 29–6. NaCl reabsorption in thick ascending limb and mechanism of diuretic action of Na^+–K^+–$2Cl^-$ symport inhibitors.

S, symporter; CH, ion channel. Numbers in parentheses indicate stoichiometry. Designated voltages are the potential differences across the indicated membrane or cell.

established by the basolateral Na^+ pump and provides for "uphill" transport of K^+ and Cl^- into the cell. K^+ channels in the luminal membrane (called ROMK) provide a conductive pathway for the apical recycling of this cation (Ho *et al.*, 1993; Kohda *et al.*, 1998), and basolateral Cl^- channels (called CLCN) provide a basolateral exit mechanism for Cl^-. The luminal membranes of epithelial cells in the thick ascending limb have conductive pathways (channels) only for K^+; therefore the apical membrane voltage is determined by the equilibrium potential for K^+ (E_K). In contrast, the basolateral membrane has channels for both K^+ and Cl^-, so that the basolateral membrane voltage is less than E_K; *i.e.*, conductance for Cl^- depolarizes the basolateral membrane. Depolarization of the basolateral membrane results in a transepithelial potential difference of approximately 10 mV, with the lumen positive with respect to the interstitial space. This lumen-positive potential difference repels cations (Na^+, Ca^{2+}, and Mg^{2+}) and thereby provides an important driving force for the paracellular flux of these cations into the interstitial space.

As the name implies, inhibitors of Na^+–K^+–$2Cl^-$ symport bind to the Na^+–K^+–$2Cl^-$ symporter in the thick ascending limb (Koenig *et al.*, 1983) and block its function, bringing salt transport in this segment of the nephron to a virtual standstill (Burg *et al.*, 1973). The molecular

mechanism by which this class of drugs blocks the Na^+–K^+–$2Cl^-$ symporter is unknown, but evidence suggests that these drugs attach to the Cl^-–binding site (Hannafin *et al.*, 1983) located in the symporter's transmembrane domain (Isenring and Forbush, 1997). Inhibitors of Na^+–K^+–$2Cl^-$ symport also inhibit Ca^{2+} and Mg^{2+} reabsorption in the thick ascending limb by abolishing the transepithelial potential difference that is the dominant driving force for reabsorption of these cations.

Na^+–K^+–$2Cl^-$ symporters are an important family of transport molecules found in many secretory and absorbing epithelia. The rectal gland of the dogfish shark is a particularly rich source of the protein, and a cDNA encoding a Na^+–K^+–$2Cl^-$ symporter was isolated from a cDNA library obtained from the dogfish shark rectal gland by screening with antibodies to the shark symporter (Xu *et al.*, 1994). Molecular cloning revealed a deduced amino acid sequence of 1191 residues containing 12 putative membrane-spanning domains flanked by long N and C termini in the cytoplasm. Expression of this protein resulted in Na^+–K^+–$2Cl^-$ symport that was sensitive to bumetanide. The shark rectal gland Na^+–K^+–$2Cl^-$ symporter cDNA subsequently was used to screen a human colonic cDNA library, and this provided Na^+–K^+–$2Cl^-$ symporter cDNA probes from this tissue. These latter probes were used to screen rabbit renal cortical and renal medullary libraries, which allowed cloning of the rabbit renal Na^+–K^+–$2Cl^-$ symporter (Payne and Forbush, 1994). This symporter is 1099 amino acids in length, is 61% identical to the dogfish shark secretory Na^+–K^+–$2Cl^-$ symporter, has 12 predicted transmembrane helices, and contains large N- and C-terminal cytoplasmic regions. Subsequent studies demonstrated that Na^+–K^+–$2Cl^-$ symporters are of two varieties (*see* Kaplan *et al.*, 1996). The "absorptive" symporter (called ENCC2, NKCC2, or BSC1) is expressed only in the kidney, is localized to the apical membrane of the thick ascending limb, and is regulated by cyclic AMP (Obermüller *et al.*, 1996; Kaplan *et al.*, 1996; Nielsen *et al.*, 1998; Plata *et al.*, 1999). At least six different isoforms of the absorptive symporter are generated by alternative mRNA splicing (Mount *et al.*, 1999). The "secretory" symporter (called ENCC3, NKCC1, or BSC2) is a "housekeeping" protein that is widely expressed and, in epithelial cells, is localized to the basolateral membrane. A model of Na^+–K^+–$2Cl^-$ symport has been proposed based on ordered binding of ions to the symporter (Lytle *et al.*, 1998). Mutations in the genes coding for the absorptive Na^+–K^+–$2Cl^-$ symporter, the apical K^+ channel, or the basolateral Cl^- channel give rise to Bartter's syndrome (inherited hypokalemic alkalosis with salt wasting and hypotension) (*see* Simon and Lifton, 1998).

Effects on Urinary Excretion. Due to blockade of the Na^+–K^+–$2Cl^-$ symporter, loop diuretics cause a profound increase in the urinary excretion of Na^+ and Cl^- (*i.e.*, up to 25% of the filtered load of Na^+). Abolition of the transepithelial potential difference also results in marked increases in the excretion of Ca^{2+} and Mg^{2+}. Some (*e.g.*, furosemide), but not all (*e.g.*, bumetanide and piretanide), sulfonamide-based loop diuretics have weak carbonic anhydrase–inhibiting activity. Those drugs with carbonic anhydrase–inhibiting activity increase the urinary excretion of HCO_3^- and phosphate. The mechanism by which inhibition of carbonic anhydrase increases phosphate excretion is not known. All inhibitors of Na^+–K^+–$2Cl^-$ symport increase the urinary excretion of K^+ and titratable acid. This effect is due in part to increased delivery of Na^+ to the distal tubule. The mechanism by which increased distal delivery of Na^+ enhances excretion of K^+ and H^+ is discussed in the section on inhibitors of Na^+ channels. Acutely, loop diuretics increase the excretion of uric acid, whereas chronic administration of these drugs results in reduced excretion of uric acid. The chronic effects of loop diuretics on uric acid excretion may be due to enhanced transport in the proximal tubule secondary to volume depletion, leading to increased uric acid reabsorption, or to competition between the diuretic and uric acid for the organic acid secretory mechanism in the proximal tubule, leading to reduced uric acid secretion.

By blocking active NaCl reabsorption in the thick ascending limb, inhibitors of Na^+–K^+–$2Cl^-$ symport interfere with a critical step in the mechanism that produces a hypertonic medullary interstitium. Therefore, loop diuretics block the kidney's ability to concentrate urine during hydropenia. Also, since the thick ascending limb is part of the diluting segment, inhibitors of Na^+–K^+–$2Cl^-$ symport markedly impair the kidney's ability to excrete a dilute urine during water diuresis.

Effects on Renal Hemodynamics. If volume depletion is prevented by replacing fluid losses, inhibitors of Na^+–K^+–$2Cl^-$ symport generally increase total RBF and redistribute RBF to the midcortex (Stein *et al.*, 1972). However, the effects on RBF are variable. The mechanism of the increase in RBF is not known, but prostaglandins have been implicated (Williamson *et al.*, 1974). In fact, nonsteroidal antiinflammatory drugs (NSAIDs) attenuate the diuretic response to loop diuretics, most likely by preventing prostaglandin-mediated increases in RBF (Brater, 1985). Loop diuretics block TGF by inhibiting salt transport into the macula densa, so that the macula densa no longer can "sense" NaCl concentrations in the tubular fluid. Therefore, unlike carbonic anhydrase inhibitors, loop diuretics do not decrease GFR by activating TGF. Loop diuretics are powerful stimulators of renin release. This effect is due to interference with NaCl transport by the macula densa and, if volume depletion occurs, to reflex activation of the sympathetic nervous system and to stimulation of the intrarenal baroreceptor mechanism. Prostaglandins, particularly prostacyclin, may play an important role in mediating the renin release response to loop diuretics (Oates *et al.*, 1979).

Other Actions. Loop diuretics may cause direct vascular effects (*see* Dormans *et al.*, 1996). Loop diuretics, particularly furosemide, acutely increase systemic venous capacitance and thereby decrease left ventricular filling pressure. This effect, which may be mediated by prostaglandins and requires intact kidneys (Johnston *et al.*, 1983), benefits patients with pulmonary edema even before diuresis ensues. Furosemide and ethacrynic acid can inhibit Na^+, K^+–ATPase, glycolysis, mitochondrial respiration, the microsomal Ca^{2+} pump, adenylyl cyclase, phosphodiesterase, and prostaglandin dehydrogenase; however, these effects do not have therapeutic implications. *In vitro*, high doses of inhibitors of Na^+–K^+–$2Cl^-$ symport can inhibit electrolyte transport in many tissues. Only in the inner ear, where alterations in the electrolyte composition of endolymph may contribute to drug-induced ototoxicity, is this effect clinically important.

Absorption and Elimination. The oral bioavailability, plasma half-life, and route of elimination of the four inhibitors of Na^+–K^+–$2Cl^-$ symport available in the United States are listed in Table 29–4. Because furosemide, bumetanide, ethacrynic acid, and torsemide are extensively bound to plasma proteins, delivery of these drugs to the tubules by filtration is limited. However, they are efficiently secreted by the organic acid transport system in the proximal tubule and thereby gain access to their binding sites on the Na^+–K^+–$2Cl^-$ symport in the luminal membrane of the thick ascending limb. Probenecid shifts the plasma concentration–response curve to furosemide to the right by competitively inhibiting furosemide secretion by the organic acid transport system (Brater, 1983). The most recent loop diuretic to receive FDA approval is torsemide, which has a longer half-life than the other loop diuretics available in the United States (Brater, 1991: *see* Knauf and Mutschler, 1997).

Toxicity, Adverse Effects, Contraindications, Drug Interactions. Adverse effects unrelated to the diuretic efficacy are rare, and most adverse effects are due to abnormalities of fluid and electrolyte balance. Overzealous use of loop diuretics can cause serious depletion of total body Na^+. This may be manifest as hyponatremia and/or extracellular fluid volume depletion associated with hypotension, reduced GFR, circulatory collapse, thromboembolic episodes, and, in patients with liver disease, hepatic encephalopathy. Increased delivery of Na^+ to the distal tubule, particularly when combined with activation of the renin–angiotensin system, leads to increased urinary excretion of K^+ and H^+, causing a hypochloremic alkalosis. If dietary K^+ intake is not sufficient, hypokalemia may develop, and this may induce cardiac arrhythmias, particularly in patients taking cardiac glycosides. Increased Mg^{2+} and Ca^{2+} excretion may result in hypomagnesemia (a risk factor for cardiac arrhythmias) and hypocalcemia (rarely leading to tetany).

Loop diuretics can cause ototoxicity that manifests itself as tinnitus, hearing impairment, deafness, vertigo, and a sense of fullness in the ears. Hearing impairment and deafness are usually, but not always, reversible. Ototoxicity occurs most frequently with rapid intravenous administration and least frequently with oral administration. Ethacrynic acid appears to induce ototoxicity more often than do other loop diuretics. Loop diuretics also can cause hyperuricemia (rarely leading to gout) and hyperglycemia (rarely precipitating diabetes mellitus) and can increase plasma levels of low-density lipoprotein (LDL) cholesterol and triglycerides, while decreasing plasma levels of high-density lipoprotein (HDL) cholesterol. Other adverse effects include skin rashes, photosensitivity, paresthesias, bone marrow depression, and gastrointestinal disturbances.

Contraindications to the use of loop diuretics include severe Na^+ and volume depletion, hypersensitivity to sulfonamides (for sulfonamide-based loop diuretics), and anuria unresponsive to a trial dose of loop diuretic.

Drug interactions may occur when loop diuretics are coadministered with: (1) aminoglycosides (synergism of ototoxicity caused by both drugs); (2) anticoagulants (increased anticoagulant activity); (3) digitalis glycosides (increased digitalis-induced arrhythmias); (4) lithium (increased plasma levels of lithium); (5) propranolol (increased plasma levels of propranolol); (6) sulfonylureas (hyperglycemia); (7) cisplatin (increased risk of diuretic-induced ototoxicity); (8) NSAIDs (blunted diuretic response; salicylate toxity when given with high doses of salicylates); (9) probenecid (blunted diuretic response); (10) thiazide diuretics (synergism of diuretic activity of both drugs leading to profound diuresis); and (11) amphotericin B (increased potential for nephrotoxicity and toxicity and intensification of electrolyte imbalance).

Therapeutic Uses. A major use of loop diuretics is in the treatment of acute pulmonary edema. A rapid increase in venous capacitance in conjunction with a brisk natriuresis reduces left ventricular filling pressures and thereby rapidly relieves pulmonary edema. Loop diuretics also are widely used for the treatment of chronic congestive heart failure when diminution of extracellular fluid volume is desirable to minimize venous and pulmonary congestion (*see* Chapter 34). Diuretics are widely used for the treatment of hypertension (*see* Chapter 33), and controlled clinical trials demonstrating reduced morbidity and mortality have been conducted with $Na^+–Cl^-$ symport (thiazides and thiazide-like diuretics), but not $Na^+–K^+–2Cl^-$

symport, inhibitors. Nonetheless, $Na^+–K^+–2Cl^-$ symport inhibitors appear to lower blood pressure as effectively as $Na^+–Cl^-$ symport inhibitors while causing smaller perturbations in the lipid profile (van der Heijden *et al.*, 1998). The edema of nephrotic syndrome often is refractory to other classes of diuretics, and loop diuretics often are the only drugs capable of reducing the massive edema associated with this renal disease. Loop diuretics also are employed in the treatment of edema and ascites of liver cirrhosis; however, care must be taken not to induce encephalopathy or hepatorenal syndrome. In patients with a drug overdose, loop diuretics can be used to induce a forced diuresis to facilitate more rapid renal elimination of the offending drug. Loop diuretics—combined with isotonic saline administration to prevent volume depletion—are used to treat hypercalcemia. Loop diuretics interfere with the kidney's ability to produce a concentrated urine. Consequently, loop diuretics combined with hypertonic saline are useful for the treatment of life-threatening hyponatremia. Loop diuretics also are used to treat edema associated with chronic renal insufficiency. However, animal studies have demonstrated that loop diuretics increase P_{GC} by activating the renin–angiotensin system, an effect that could accelerate renal injury (Lane *et al.*, 1998). Most patients with ARF receive a trial dose of a loop diuretic in an attempt to convert oliguric ARF to nonoliguric ARF. However, there is no evidence that loop diuretics prevent ATN or improve outcome in patients with ARF (*see* Kellum, 1998).

INHIBITORS OF $Na^+–Cl^-$ SYMPORT (THIAZIDE AND THIAZIDE-LIKE DIURETICS)

The benzothiadiazides were synthesized in an effort to enhance the potency of inhibitors of carbonic anhydrase. However, unlike carbonic anhydrase inhibitors, which primarily increase $NaHCO_3$ excretion, benzothiadiazides were found predominantly to increase NaCl excretion (Beyer, 1958), an effect shown to be independent of carbonic anhydrase inhibition. *Chlorothiazide* was the first serious challenge to the mercurial diuretics, a now-obsolete class of organometallic compounds that dominated diuretic therapy for more than thirty years.

Chemistry. Inhibitors of $Na^+–Cl^-$ symport are sulfonamides (*see* Table 29–5) and many are analogs of 1,2,4-benzothiadiazine-1,1-dioxide. Because the original inhibitors of $Na^+–Cl^-$ symport were benzothiadiazine derivatives, this class of diuretics became known as thiazide diuretics. Subsequently, drugs that are pharmacologically similar to thiazide diuretics but are not thiazides were developed and are called *thiazide-like diuretics*. The term *thiazide diuretics* often is used to refer to all members

Table 29–5
Inhibitors of Na$^+$–K$^+$ Symport (Thiazide and Thiazide-like Diuretics)

DRUG	STRUCTURE	RELATIVE POTENCY	ORAL AVAILABILITY	$t_{\frac{1}{2}}$ (HOURS)	ROUTE OF ELIMINATION
Bendroflumethiazide (NATURETIN)	R_2 = H, R_3 = CH_2—⟨phenyl⟩, R_6 = CF_3	10	~100%	3–3.9	~30% R, ~70% M
Chlorothiazide (DIURIL)	R_2 = H, R_3 = H, R_6 = Cl (Unsaturated between C3 and N4)	0.1	9–56% (dose-dependent)	~1.5	R
Hydrochlorothiazide (HYDRODIURIL)	R_2 = H, R_3 = H, R_6 = Cl	1	~70%	~2.5	R
Hydroflumethiazide (SALURON)	R_2 = H, R_3 = H, R_6 = CF_3	1	~50%	~17	40–80% R, 20–60% M
Methyclothiazide (ENDURON)	R_2 = CH_3, R_3 = CH_2Cl, R_6 = Cl	10	ID	ID	M
Polythiazide (RENESE)	R_2 = CH_3, R_3 = $CH_2SCH_2CF_3$, R_6 = Cl	25	~100%	~25	~25% R, ~75% U
Trichlormethiazide	R_2 = H, R_3 = $CHCl_2$, R_6 = Cl	25	ID	2.3–7.3	R
Chlorthalidone (HYGROTON)		1	~65%	~47	~65% R, ~10% B, ~25% U
Indapamide (LOZOL)		20	~93%	~14	M
Metolazone (MYKROX, ZAROXOLYN)		10	~65%	ID	~80% R, ~10% B, ~10% M
Quinethazone (HYDROMOX)		1	ID	ID	ID

Abbreviations: R, renal excretion of intact drug; M, metabolism; B, excretion of intact drug into bile; U, unknown pathway of elimination: ID, insufficient data.

of the class of inhibitors of Na$^+$–Cl$^-$ symport, and this usage is employed in the present chapter.

Mechanism and Site of Action. Some studies using split-droplet and stationary-microperfusion techniques have described reductions in proximal tubule reabsorption by thiazide diuretics; however, free-flow micropuncture studies have not consistently demonstrated increased solute delivery out of the proximal tubule following administration of thiazides. In contrast, micropuncture (Kunau *et al.,* 1975) and *in situ* microperfusion studies (Costanzo and Windhager, 1978) clearly indicate that thiazide diuretics inhibit NaCl transport in the DCT. Furthermore, the renal cortex has a high-affinity receptor for thiazide diuretics (Beaumont *et al.,* 1988), and binding of thiazides localizes to the DCT (Beaumont *et al.,* 1989). It is now well accepted that the primary site of action of thiazide diuretics is the DCT, whereas the proximal tubule may represent a secondary site of action.

Figure 29–7 illustrates the current model of electrolyte transport in the DCT. As with other nephron segments, transport is powered by a Na$^+$ pump in the basolateral membrane. The free energy in the electrochemical gradient for Na$^+$ is harnessed by a Na$^+$–Cl$^-$ symporter in the luminal membrane, which moves Cl$^-$ into the epithelial cell against its electrochemical gradient. Cl$^-$ then passively exits the basolateral membrane *via* a Cl$^-$ channel. Thiazide diuretics inhibit the Na$^+$–Cl$^-$ symporter, perhaps by competing for the Cl$^-$ binding site (Beaumont *et al.,* 1988).

DISTAL CONVOLUTED TUBULE

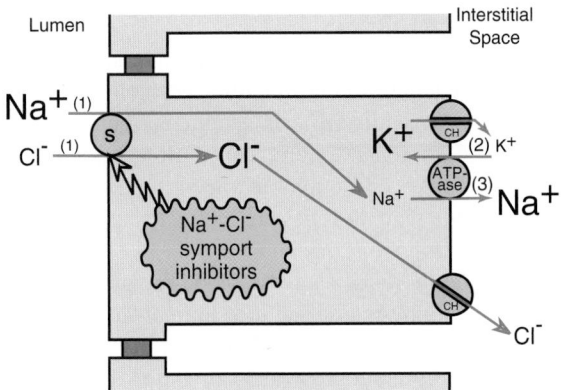

Figure 29–7. NaCl reabsorption in distal convoluted tubule and mechanism of diuretic action of Na$^+$–Cl$^-$ symport inhibitors.

S, symporter; CH, ion channel. Numbers in parentheses indicate stoichiometry.

Using a functional expression strategy (Cl$^-$-dependent Na$^+$ uptake in *Xenopus* oocytes), Gamba *et al.* (1993) isolated a cDNA clone from the urinary bladder of the winter flounder that codes for a Na$^+$–Cl$^-$ symporter. This Na$^+$–Cl$^-$ symporter is inhibited by a number of thiazide diuretics (but not by furosemide, acetazolamide, or an amiloride derivative), has 12 putative membrane-spanning domains, and its sequence is 47% identical to the cloned dogfish shark rectal gland Na$^+$–K$^+$–2Cl$^-$ symporter. Subsequently, Gamba *et al.* (1994) cloned the rat and Mastroianni *et al.* (1996) cloned the human Na$^+$–Cl$^-$ symporter. The Na$^+$–Cl$^-$ symporter (called ENCC1 or TSC) is expressed predominantly in the kidney (Chang *et al.,* 1996) and is localized to the apical membrane of DCT epithelial cells (Bachmann *et al.,* 1995; Obermüller *et al.,* 1995; Plotkin *et al.,* 1996). Expression of the Na$^+$–Cl$^-$ symporter is regulated by aldosterone (Velázquez *et al.,* 1996; Kim *et al.,* 1998; Bostonjoglo *et al.,* 1998). Mutations in the Na$^+$–Cl$^-$ symporter cause a form of inherited hypokalemic alkalosis called Gitelman's syndrome (*see* Simon and Lifton, 1998).

Effects on Urinary Excretion. As would be expected from their mechanism of action, inhibitors of Na$^+$–Cl$^-$ symport increase Na$^+$ and Cl$^-$ excretion. However, thiazides are only moderately efficacious (*i.e.,* maximum excretion of filtered load of Na$^+$ is only 5%), since approximately 90% of the filtered Na$^+$ load is reabsorbed before reaching the DCT. Some thiazide diuretics also are weak inhibitors of carbonic anhydrase, an effect that increases HCO$_3^-$ and phosphate excretion and probably accounts for the weak proximal tubular effects of some thiazide diuretics. Like inhibitors of Na$^+$–K$^+$–2Cl$^-$ symport, inhibitors of Na$^+$–Cl$^-$ symport increase the excretion of K$^+$ and titratable acid due to increased delivery of Na$^+$ to the distal tubule. Acute administration of thiazides increases the excretion of uric acid. However, uric acid excretion is reduced following chronic administration by the same mechanisms discussed for loop diuretics. The acute effects of inhibitors of Na$^+$–Cl$^-$ symport on Ca^{2+} excretion are variable; when administered chronically, thiazide diuretics decrease Ca^{2+} excretion. The mechanism is unknown but may involve increased proximal reabsorption due to volume depletion as well as direct effects of thiazides to increase Ca^{2+} reabsorption in the DCT. Thiazide diuretics may cause a mild magnesuria by a poorly understood mechanism, and there is increasing awareness that long-term use of thiazide diuretics may cause magnesium deficiency, particularly in the elderly (Martin and Milligan, 1987). Since inhibitors of Na$^+$–Cl$^-$ symport inhibit transport in the cortical diluting segment, thiazide diuretics attenuate the ability of the kidney to excrete a dilute urine during water diuresis. However, since the DCT is not involved in the mechanism that generates a hypertonic medullary interstitium, thiazide diuretics do not alter the kidney's ability to concentrate urine during hydropenia.

Effects on Renal Hemodynamics. In general, inhibitors of Na^+–Cl^- symport do not affect RBF and only variably reduce GFR due to increases in intratubular pressure. Since thiazides act at a point past the macula densa, they have little or no influence on TGF.

Other Actions. Thiazide diuretics may inhibit phosphodiesterase, mitochondrial oxygen consumption, and renal uptake of fatty acids; however, these effects are not of clinical significance.

Absorption and Elimination. The relative potency, oral bioavailability, plasma half-life, and route of elimination of inhibitors of Na^+–Cl^- symport currently used in the United States are listed in Table 29–5. Of special note is the wide range of half-lives for this class of drugs. Sulfonamides are organic acids and therefore are secreted into the proximal tubule by the organic acid secretory pathway. Since thiazides must gain access to the tubular lumen to inhibit the Na^+–Cl^- symporter, drugs such as probenecid can attenuate the diuretic response to thiazides by competing for transport into the proximal tubule. However, plasma protein binding varies considerably among thiazide diuretics, and this parameter determines the contribution that filtration makes to tubular delivery of a specific thiazide.

Toxicity, Adverse Effects, Contraindications, Drug Interactions. Thiazide diuretics rarely cause CNS (vertigo, headache, paresthesias, xanthopsia, weakness), gastrointestinal (anorexia, nausea, vomiting, cramping, diarrhea, constipation, cholecystitis, pancreatitis), hematological (blood dyscrasias), and dermatological (photosensitivity, skin rashes) disorders. The incidence of sexual dysfunction (*i.e.,* erection problems) is greater with Na^+–Cl^- symport inhibitors than with several other antihypertensive agents (β-adrenergic receptor antagonists, calcium channel blockers, angiotensin converting enzyme inhibitors, α_1-receptor antagonists) (Grimm *et al.,* 1997), but usually is tolerable. However, like loop diuretics, most serious adverse effects of thiazides are related to abnormalities of fluid and electrolyte balance. These adverse effects include extracellular volume depletion, hypotension, hypokalemia, hyponatremia, hypochloremia, metabolic alkalosis, hypomagnesemia, hypercalcemia, and hyperuricemia. Thiazide diuretics have caused fatal or near fatal hyponatremia, and some patients are at recurrent risk of hyponatremia when rechallenged with thiazides.

Thiazide diuretics also decrease glucose tolerance, and latent diabetes mellitus may be unmasked during therapy. The mechanism of the reduced glucose tolerance is not completely understood but appears to involve reduced insulin secretion and alterations in glucose metabolism. Hyperglycemia may be related in some way to K^+ depletion, in that hyperglycemia is reduced when K^+ is given along with the diuretic (Tannen, 1985). Thiazide diuretics also may increase plasma levels of LDL cholesterol, total cholesterol, and total triglycerides. Thiazide diuretics are contraindicated in individuals who are hypersensitive to sulfonamides.

With regard to drug interactions, thiazide diuretics may diminish the effects of anticoagulants, uricosuric agents used to treat gout, sulfonylureas, and insulin and may increase the effects of anesthetics, diazoxide, digitalis glycosides, lithium, loop diuretics, and vitamin D. The effectiveness of thiazide diuretics may be reduced by NSAIDs, bile acid sequestrants (reduced absorption of thiazides), and methenamines (alkalinization of urine may decrease effectiveness of thiazides). Amphotericin B and corticosteroids increase the risk of hypokalemia induced by thiazide diuretics.

A potentially lethal drug interaction warranting special emphasis is that involving thiazide diuretics with quinidine (Roden, 1993). Prolongation of the QT-interval by quinidine can lead to the development of polymorphic ventricular tachycardia (*torsades de pointes*) due to triggered activity originating from early afterdepolarizations (*see* Chapter 35). Although usually self-limiting, *torsades de pointes* may deteriorate into fatal ventricular fibrillation. Hypokalemia increases the risk of quinidine-induced *torsades de pointes,* and thiazide diuretics cause hypokalemia. It is likely, therefore, that thiazide diuretic–induced K^+ depletion accounts for many cases of quinidine-induced *torsades de pointes.*

Therapeutic Uses. Thiazide diuretics are used for treatment of the edema associated with heart (congestive heart failure), liver (hepatic cirrhosis), and renal (nephrotic syndrome, chronic renal failure, acute glomerulonephritis) disease. With the exceptions of metolazone and indapamide, most thiazide diuretics are ineffective when GFR is <30 to 40 ml/min.

Thiazide diuretics decrease blood pressure in hypertensive patients by increasing the slope of the renal pressure–natriuresis relationship (Saito and Kimura, 1996), and thiazide diuretics are widely used for the treatment of hypertension, either alone or in combination with other antihypertensive drugs (*see* Chapter 33). In this regard, thiazide diuretics are inexpensive, as efficacious as other classes of antihypertensive agents, and well tolerated. Thiazides can be administered once daily, do not require dose titration, and have few contraindications. Moreover,

Table 29–6
Inhibitors of Renal Epithelial Na$^+$ Channels (K$^+$-Sparing Diuretics)

DRUG	STRUCTURE	RELATIVE POTENCY	ORAL AVAILABILITY	$t_{1/2}$ (HOURS)	ROUTE OF ELIMINATION
Amiloride		1	15–25%	~21	R
Triamterene		0.1	~50%	~4.2	M

Abbreviations: R, renal excretion of intact drug; M, metabolism; however, triamterene is transformed into an active metabolite that is excreted in the urine.

thiazides have additive or synergistic effects when combined with other classes of antihypertensive agents. Although thiazides may marginally increase the risk of sudden death (*see* Hoes and Grobbee, 1996) and renal cell carcinoma (Grossman *et al.,* 1999), in general these agents are safe and reduce cardiovascular morbidity and mortality in hypertensive patients. Because the adverse effects of thiazides increase progressively in severity at doses higher than maximally effective antihypertensive doses, only low doses should be prescribed for hypertension (*see* Ramsey, 1999). Thiazide diuretics, which reduce urinary excretion of Ca^{2+}, sometimes are employed to treat calcium nephrolithiasis and may be useful for the treatment of osteoporosis (*see* Chapter 62). Thiazide diuretics are also the mainstay for treatment of nephrogenic diabetes insipidus, reducing urine volume by up to 50%. The mechanism of this paradoxical effect remains unknown (Grønbeck *et al.,* 1998). Since other halides are excreted by renal processes similar to those for Cl$^-$, thiazide diuretics may be useful for the management of Br$^-$ intoxication.

INHIBITORS OF RENAL EPITHELIAL Na$^+$ CHANNELS (K$^+$-SPARING DIURETICS)

Triamterene (DYRENIUM, MAXZIDE) and *amiloride* (MIDAMOR) are the only two drugs of this class in clinical use. Both drugs cause small increases in NaCl excretion and usually are employed for their antikaluretic actions to offset the effects of other diuretics that increase K$^+$ excretion. Consequently, triamterene and amiloride, along with spironolactone (*see* next section), often are classified as *potassium (K$^+$)-sparing diuretics*.

Chemistry.   Amiloride is a pyrazinoylguanidine derivative, and triamterene is a pteridine (Table 29–6). Both drugs are organic bases and are transported by the organic base secretory mechanism in the proximal tubule.

Mechanism and Site of Action.   Available data suggest that triamterene and amiloride have similar mechanisms of action. Of the two, amiloride has been studied much more extensively, so its mechanism of action is known with a higher degree of certainty. As illustrated in Figure 29–8, principal cells in the late distal tubule and collecting duct have in their luminal membranes a Na$^+$ channel that provides a conductive pathway for the entry of Na$^+$ into the cell down the electrochemical gradient created by the basolateral Na$^+$ pump. The higher permeability of the luminal membrane for Na$^+$ depolarizes the luminal membrane, but not the basolateral membrane, creating a lumen-negative transepithelial potential difference. This transepithelial voltage provides an important driving force for the secretion of K$^+$ into the lumen *via* K$^+$ channels (ROMK) in the luminal membrane. Carbonic anhydrase inhibitors, loop diuretics, and thiazide diuretics increase the delivery of Na$^+$ to the late distal tubule and collecting duct, a situation that is often associated with increased K$^+$ and H$^+$ excretion. It is likely that the elevation in luminal Na$^+$ concentration in the distal nephron induced by such diuretics augments depolarization of the luminal membrane and thereby enhances the lumen-negative V_T, which facilitates K$^+$ excretion. In addition to principal cells, the collecting duct also contains type A intercalated cells that mediate the secretion of H$^+$ into the tubular lumen. Tubular acidification is driven by a luminal H$^+$–ATPase (proton pump), and this pump is aided by the lumen-negative transepithelial voltage. However, increased distal delivery

LATE DISTAL TUBULE AND COLLECTING DUCT

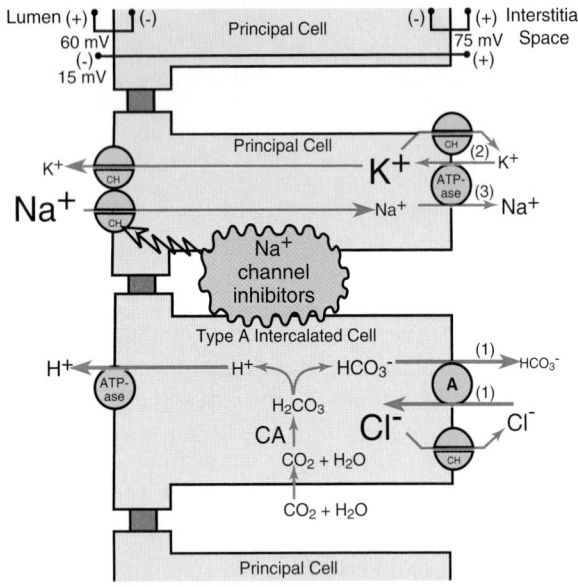

Figure 29–8. ***Na$^+$ reabsorption in late distal tubule and collecting duct and mechanism of diuretic action of epithelial Na$^+$-channel inhibitors.***

Cl$^-$ reabsorption (*not shown*) occurs both paracellularly and transcellularly, and precise mechanism of Cl$^-$ transport appears to be species specific. A, antiporter; CH, ion channel; CA, carbonic anhydrase. Numbers in parentheses indicate stoichiometry. Designated voltages are the potential differences across the indicated membrane or cell.

of Na$^+$ is not the only mechanism by which diuretics increase K$^+$ and H$^+$ excretion. Activation of the renin–angiotensin–aldosterone axis by diuretics also contributes to diuretic-induced K$^+$ and H$^+$ excretion by a mechanism explained in the section on mineralocorticoid antagonists.

Considerable evidence indicates that amiloride blocks Na$^+$ channels in the luminal membrane of principal cells in the late distal tubule and collecting duct. This evidence includes data from epithelia of nonrenal origin (amphibian skin and toad bladder) (Garty and Palmer, 1997) as well as a number of electrophysiological studies in isolated mammalian collecting ducts (O'Neil and Boulpaep, 1979). Amiloride produces half-maximal inhibition at concentrations <1 mM and, depending on the study, amiloride may interact with Na$^+$ in the channel either competitively or noncompetitively. It is important, however, to bear in mind that renal epithelial Na$^+$ channels inhibited by this class of diuretics are not the same as voltage-gated Na$^+$ channels found in many cell types (for instance, neurons and myocytes).

Molecular cloning studies have revealed that the amiloride-sensitive Na$^+$ channel (called ENaC) consists of three subunits (α, β, γ) (Canessa *et al.*, 1994). Although the α subunit is sufficient for channel activity, maximal Na$^+$ permeability is induced when all three subunits are coexpressed in the same cell, suggesting a minimal oligomeric structure in which one copy of each subunit is associated in a heterotrimeric protein. Studies in *Xenopus* oocytes expressing ENaC suggest that triamterene and amiloride bind to ENaC by similar mechanisms (Busch *et al.*, 1996). Liddle's syndrome (pseudohyperaldosteronism) is an autosomal dominant form of low-renin, volume-expanded hypertension that is due to mutations in the β or γ subunits, leading to increased basal activity of ENaC (Ismailov *et al.*, 1999).

Effects on Urinary Excretion. Since the late distal tubule and collecting duct have a limited capacity to reabsorb solutes, blockade of Na$^+$ channels in this part of the nephron results in only a mild increase in the excretion rates of Na$^+$ and Cl$^-$ (approximately 2% of filtered load). Blockade of Na$^+$ channels hyperpolarizes the luminal membrane, reducing the lumen-negative transepithelial voltage. Since the lumen-negative potential difference normally opposes cation reabsorption and facilitates cation secretion, attenuation of the lumen-negative voltage decreases the excretion rates of K$^+$, H$^+$, Ca^{2+}, and Mg^{2+}. Volume contraction may increase reabsorption of uric acid in the proximal tubule; hence, chronic administration of amiloride and triamterene may decrease uric acid excretion.

Effects on Renal Hemodynamics. Amiloride and triamterene have little or no effect on renal hemodynamics and do not alter TGF.

Other Actions. Amiloride, at concentrations higher than needed to elicit therapeutic effects, also blocks the Na$^+$–H$^+$ and Na$^+$–Ca^{2+} antiporters and inhibits the Na$^+$ pump.

Absorption and Elimination. The relative potency, oral bioavailability, plasma half-life, and route of elimination for amiloride and triamterene are listed in Table 29–6. Amiloride is eliminated predominantly by urinary excretion of intact drug. Triamterene is extensively metabolized to an active metabolite, 4-hydroxytriamterene sulfate, and this metabolite is excreted in the urine. The pharmacological activity of 4-hydroxytriamterene sulfate is comparable to that of the parent drug. Therefore, the toxicity of triamterene may be enhanced in both hepatic disease (decreased metabolism of triamterene) and renal failure (decreased urinary excretion of active metabolite).

Toxicity, Adverse Effects, Contraindications, Drug Interactions. The most dangerous adverse effect of Na$^+$-channel inhibitors is hyperkalemia, which can be life-threatening. Consequently, amiloride and triamterene are contraindicated in patients with hyperkalemia as well as in patients at increased risk of developing hyperkalemia (*e.g.,* patients with renal failure, patients receiving other K^+-sparing diuretics, patients taking angiotensin converting enzyme inhibitors, or patients taking K^+ supplements). Even NSAIDs can increase the likelihood of hyperkalemia in patients receiving Na^+-channel inhibitors. Cirrhotic patients are prone to megaloblastosis because of folic acid deficiency, and triamterene, a weak folic acid antagonist, may increase the likelihood of this adverse event. Triamterene also can reduce glucose tolerance and induce photosensitization and has been associated with interstitial nephritis and renal stones. Both drugs can cause CNS, gastrointestinal, musculoskeletal, dermatological, and hematological adverse effects. The most common adverse effects of amiloride are nausea, vomiting, diarrhea, and headache; those of triamterene are nausea, vomiting, leg cramps, and dizziness.

Therapeutic Uses.   Because of the mild natriuresis induced by Na^+-channel inhibitors, these drugs seldom are used as sole agents in the treatment of edema or hypertension. Rather, their major utility is in *combination* with other diuretics. Coadministration of a Na^+-channel inhibitor augments the diuretic and antihypertensive response to thiazide or loop diuretics. More importantly, the ability of Na^+-channel inhibitors to reduce K^+ excretion tends to offset the kaliuretic effects of thiazide and loop diuretics; consequently, the combination of a Na^+-channel inhibitor with a thiazide or loop diuretic tends to result in normal values of plasma K^+ (Hollenberg and Mickiewicz, 1989). Liddle's syndrome can be treated effectively with Na^+-channel inhibitors. Aerosolized amiloride has been shown to improve mucociliary clearance in patients with cystic fibrosis (Zahaykevich, 1991). By inhibiting Na^+ absorption from the surface of airway epithelial cells, amiloride augments hydration of respiratory secretions and thereby improves mucociliary clearance. Amiloride also is useful for lithium-induced nephrogenic diabetes insipidus because it blocks Li^+ transport into the cells of the collecting tubules.

ANTAGONISTS OF MINERALOCORTICOID RECEPTORS (ALDOSTERONE ANTAGONISTS; K^+-SPARING DIURETICS)

Mineralocorticoids cause retention of salt and water and increase the excretion of K^+ and H^+ by binding to specific mineralocorticoid receptors. Kagawa *et al.* (1957) observed that some spirolactones block the effects of mineralocorticoids; this finding led to the synthesis of specific antagonists for the mineralocorticoid receptor (MR). *Spironolactone* (ALDACTONE), a 17-spirolactone, is the only member of this class available in the United States (Table 29–7).

Mechanism of Action.   Epithelial cells in the late distal tubule and collecting duct contain cytoplasmic MRs that have a high affinity for aldosterone. This receptor is a member of the superfamily of receptors for steroid hormones, thyroid hormones, vitamin D, and retinoids (*see* Chapter 2). Aldosterone enters the epithelial cell from the basolateral membrane and binds to MRs; the MR–aldosterone complex translocates to the nucleus, where it binds to specific sequences of DNA (hormone-responsive elements) and thereby regulates the expression of multiple gene products called aldosterone-induced proteins (AIPs). Figure 29–9 illustrates some of the proposed effects of AIPs, including: activation of "silent" Na^+ channels and "silent" Na^+ pumps that preexist in the cell membrane; alterations in the cycling of Na^+ channels and Na^+ pumps between the cytosol and cell membrane so that more channels and pumps are located in the membrane; increased expression of Na^+ channels and Na^+ pumps; changes in permeability of the tight junctions; and increased activity of enzymes in the mitochondria that are involved in ATP production. The precise mechanisms by which AIPs alter transport are incompletely understood. However, the net effect of AIPs is to increase Na^+ conductance of the luminal membrane and sodium pump activity of the basolateral membrane. Consequently, transepithelial NaCl transport is enhanced and the lumen-negative transepithelial voltage is increased. The latter effect increases the driving force for secretion of K^+ and H^+ into the tubular lumen.

Drugs such as spironolactone competitively inhibit the binding of aldosterone to the MR (Marver *et al.,* 1974). Unlike the MR–aldosterone complex, the MR–spironolactone complex is not able to induce the synthesis of AIPs. Since spironolactone and other drugs in this class block the biological effects of aldosterone, these agents also are referred to as *aldosterone antagonists.*

Effects on Urinary Excretion.   The effects of spironolactone on urinary excretion are very similar to those induced by renal epithelial Na^+-channel inhibitors. However, unlike that of the Na^+-channel inhibitors, the clinical efficacy of spironolactone is a function of endogenous levels of aldosterone. The higher the levels of endogenous aldosterone, the greater the effects of spironolactone on urinary excretion.

Table 29–7

Mineralocorticoid Receptor Antagonists (Aldosterone Antagonists; Potassium-Sparing Diuretics)

DRUG	STRUCTURE	ORAL AVAILABILITY	$t_{1/2}$ (HOURS)	ROUTE OF ELIMINATION
Spironolactone		~65%	~1.6	M
Canrenone*		ID	~16.5	M
Potassium canrenoate*		ID	ID	M

*Not available in United States.
Abbreviations: M, metabolism; ID, insufficient data.

Effects on Renal Hemodynamics. Spironolactone has little or no effect on renal hemodynamics and does not alter TGF.

Other Actions. High concentrations of spironolactone have been reported to interfere with steroid biosynthesis by inhibiting 11β- and 18-, 21-, and 17α-hydroxylase. These effects have limited clinical relevance (*see* Chapter 60).

Absorption and Elimination. Spironolactone is partially absorbed (approximately 65%), is extensively metabolized (even during its first passage through the liver), undergoes enterohepatic recirculation, is highly protein-bound, and has a short half-life (approximately 1.6 hours). However, an active metabolite of spironolactone, canrenone, has a half-life of approximately 16.5 hours, which prolongs the biological effects of spironolactone. Although not available in the United States, canrenone and the K$^+$ salt of canrenoate also are in clinical use. Canrenoate is not active *per se* but is converted to canrenone in the body. MR antagonists are the only diuretics that do not require access to the tubular lumen to induce a diuresis.

Toxicity, Adverse Effects, Contraindications, Drug Interactions. As with other K$^+$-sparing diuretics, spironolactone may cause life-threatening hyperkalemia. Therefore, spironolactone is contraindicated in patients with hyperkalemia and in patients at increased risk of developing hyperkalemia, either because of disease or because of administration of other medications. Spironolactone also can induce metabolic acidosis in cirrhotic patients. Salicylates may reduce the tubular secretion of canrenone and decrease the diuretic efficacy of spironolactone, and spironolactone may alter the clearance of digitalis glycosides. Due to its steroid structure, spironolactone may cause gynecomastia, impotence, decreased libido, hirsutism, deepening of the voice, and menstrual irregularities.

LATE DISTAL TUBULE
AND COLLECTING DUCT

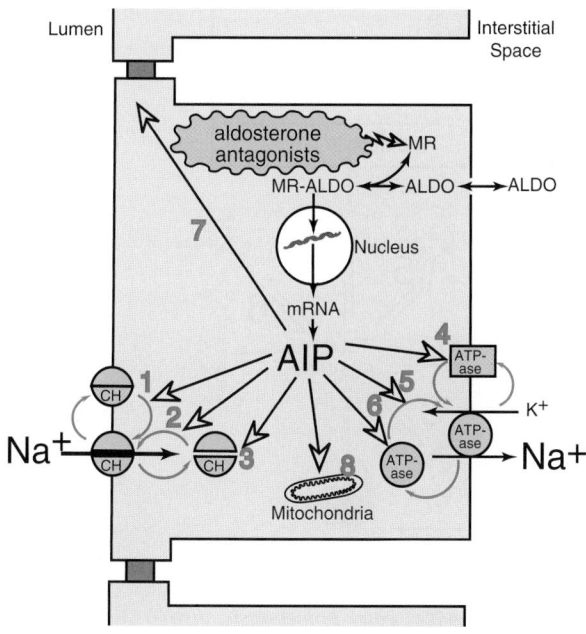

Figure 29–9. Effects of aldosterone on late distal tubule and collecting duct and diuretic mechanism of aldosterone antagonists.

AIP, aldosterone-induced proteins; ALDO, aldosterone; MR, mineralocorticoid receptor; CH, ion channel; 1, activation of membrane-bound Na^+ channels; 2, redistribution of Na^+ channels from cytosol to membrane; 3, *de novo* synthesis of Na^+ channels; 4, activation of membrane-bound Na^+,K^+–ATPase; 5, redistribution of Na^+,K^+–ATPase from cytosol to membrane; 6, *de novo* synthesis of Na^+,K^+–ATPase; 7, changes in permeability of tight junctions; 8, increased mitochondrial production of ATP.

Spironolactone also may induce diarrhea, gastritis, gastric bleeding, and peptic ulcers (the drug is contraindicated in patients with peptic ulcers). CNS adverse effects include drowsiness, lethargy, ataxia, confusion, and headache. Spironolactone may cause skin rashes and, rarely, blood dyscrasias. Breast cancer has occurred in patients taking spironolactone chronically (cause and effect not established), and high doses of spironolactone have been associated with malignant tumors in rats. Whether or not therapeutic doses of spironolactone can induce malignancies remains an open question.

Therapeutic Uses. As with other K^+-sparing diuretics, spironolactone often is coadministered with thiazide or loop diuretics in the treatment of edema and hypertension. Such combinations result in increased mobilization

of edema fluid while causing lesser perturbations of K^+ homeostasis. Spironolactone is particularly useful in the treatment of primary hyperaldosteronism (adrenal adenomas or bilateral adrenal hyperplasia) and of refractory edema associated with secondary aldosteronism (cardiac failure, hepatic cirrhosis, nephrotic syndrome, severe ascites). Spironolactone is considered the diuretic of choice in patients with hepatic cirrhosis. Pitt *et al.* (1999) have reported that spironolactone, when added to standard therapy, substantially reduces morbidity and mortality in patients with New York Heart Association (NYHA) class III and class IV heart failure (*see* Chapter 34).

MECHANISMS OF EDEMA
FORMATION AND THE ROLE OF
DIURETICS IN CLINICAL
MEDICINE

Mechanism of Edema Formation. A complex set of interrelationships (Figure 29–10) exists among the cardiovascular system, the kidneys, the CNS (Na^+ appetite, thirst regulation), and the tissue capillary beds [distribution of extracellular fluid volume (ECFV)], so that perturbations at one of these sites can affect all of the remaining sites. A primary law of the kidney is that Na^+ excretion is a steep function of mean arterial blood pressure (MABP) such that small increases in MABP cause marked increases in Na^+ excretion (Guyton, 1991). Over any given time interval, the net change in total body Na^+ (either positive or negative) is simply the dietary Na^+ intake minus the urinary excretion rate minus other losses (*e.g.,* sweating, fecal losses, vomiting). When a net positive Na^+ balance occurs, the concentration of Na^+ in the ECF will increase, stimulating water intake (thirst) and reducing urinary water output (*via* ADH release). Opposite changes occur during a net negative Na^+ balance. Changes in water intake and output adjust ECFV concentration toward normal, thereby expanding or contracting total ECFV. Total ECFV is distributed among many body compartments; however, since the volume of extracellular fluid on the arterial side of the circulation pressurizes the arterial tree, it is this fraction of ECFV that determines MABP, and it is this fraction of ECFV that is "sensed" by the cardiovascular system and kidneys. Since MABP is a major determinant of Na^+ output, a closed loop is established (Figure 29–10). This loop cycles until net Na^+ accumulation is zero; *i.e.,* in the long run, Na^+ intake must equal Na^+ loss.

The above discussion implies that three fundamental types of perturbations contribute to venous congestion

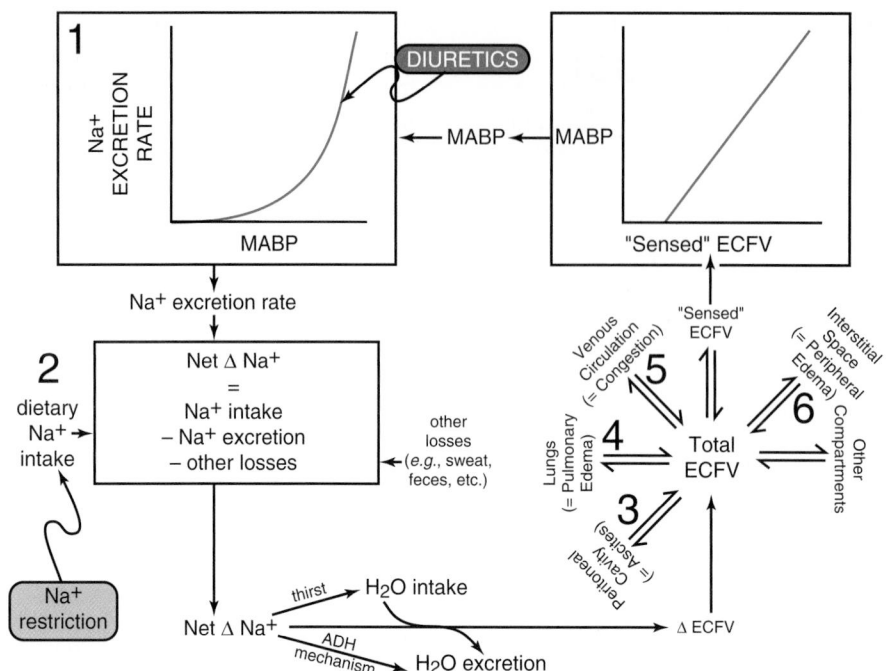

Figure 29–10. Interrelationships among renal function, Na$^+$ intake, water homeostasis, distribution of extracellular fluid volume (ECFV), and mean arterial blood pressure (MABP).

Pathophysiological mechanisms of edema formation: 1, rightward shift of renal–pressure natriuresis curve; 2, excessive dietary Na$^+$ intake; 3, increased distribution of ECFV to peritoneal cavity (*e.g.,* liver cirrhosis with increased hepatic sinusoidal hydrostatic pressure) leading to ascites formation; 4, increased distribution of ECFV to lungs (*e.g.,* left heart failure with increased pulmonary capillary hydrostatic pressure) leading to pulmonary edema; 5, increased distribution of ECFV to venous circulation (*e.g.,* right heart failure) leading to venous congestion; 6, peripheral edema caused by altered Starling forces causing increased distribution of ECFV to interstitial space (*e.g.,* diminished plasma proteins in nephrotic syndrome, severe burns, liver disease).

and/or edema formation: (1) A shift to the right in the renal pressure–natriuresis relationship (*e.g.,* chronic renal failure) causes reduced Na$^+$ excretion for any level of MABP. If all other factors remain constant, this would increase total body Na$^+$, ECFV, and MABP. The additional ECFV would be distributed throughout various body compartments, according to the state of cardiac function and prevailing Starling forces, and would predispose toward venous congestion and/or edema. Even so, in the absence of any other predisposing factors for venous congestion and/or edema, a rightward shift in the renal pressure–natriuresis curve generally causes hypertension with only a slight (usually immeasurable) increase in ECFV. As elucidated by Guyton and coworkers (Guyton, 1991), ECFV expansion triggers the following series of events: expanded ECFV → augmented cardiac output → enhanced vascular tone (*i.e.,* total body autoregulation) → increased total peripheral resistance → elevated MABP → pressure natriuresis → reduction of ECFV and cardiac output toward

normal. Most likely, a sustained rightward shift in the renal pressure–natriuresis curve is a necessary and sufficient condition for long-term hypertension but is only a predisposing factor for venous congestion and/or edema. (2) An increase in dietary Na$^+$ intake would have the same effects as a rightward shift in the renal pressure–natriuresis relationship (*i.e.,* increased MABP and predisposition to venous congestion/edema). However, changes in salt intake may have minimal or large effects depending on the shape of the patient's renal pressure–natriuresis curve. (3) Any pathophysiological alterations in the forces that govern the distribution of ECFV among the various body compartments would cause abnormal amounts of ECFV to be trapped at the site of altered forces. This would deplete the "sensed" ECFV, which would be restored back to normal by the mechanisms described in the preceding paragraph. ECFV may be trapped at several sites by different mechanisms. For instance, cirrhosis of the liver increases lymph in the space of Disse, leading to spillover *via* the glissonian wall into the peritoneal cavity (ascites). Left heart failure, both acute and chronic, increases hydrostatic pressure in the lung capillaries, leading to pulmonary edema. Chronic right heart failure redistributes ECFV from the arterial to the venous circulation, resulting in venous, hepatic, and splenic congestion and peripheral tissue edema. Decreased levels of plasma protein, particularly albumin (*e.g.,* in nephrotic syndrome, severe burns, hepatic disease), increase the distribution of ECFV into the interstitial spaces, causing generalized peripheral edema. Peripheral edema also may be "idiopathic" due to unknown alterations in the Starling forces at the capillary bed.

The Role of Diuretics in Clinical Medicine. Another implication of the mechanisms illustrated in Figure 29–10 is that three fundamental strategies exist for mobilizing edema fluid—correct the underlying disease, restrict Na^+ intake, or administer diuretics. The most desirable course of action would be to correct the primary disease; however, this is often impossible. For instance, the increased hepatic sinusoidal pressure in cirrhosis of the liver and the urinary loss of protein in nephrotic syndrome are due to structural alterations in the portal circulation and glomeruli, respectively, which may not be remediable. Restriction of Na^+ intake is the favored nonpharmacological approach for the treatment of edema and hypertension and should usually be attempted; however, compliance is a major obstacle.

Diuretics, therefore, remain the cornerstone for the treatment of edema or volume overload, particularly that due to congestive heart failure, ascites, chronic renal failure, and nephrotic syndrome. With regard to heart failure, diuretics reduce pulmonary edema and venous congestion, and it may be possible to manage mild cardiac failure with diuretics alone. However, most patients ultimately will require additional therapy with digitalis and/or angiotensin converting enzyme inhibitors (Chapter 34). Periodic administration of diuretics to cirrhotic patients with ascites may eliminate the necessity for or reduce the interval between paracenteses, adding to patient comfort and sparing protein reserves that are lost by paracenteses. Although diuretics can reduce the edema associated with chronic renal failure, increased doses of the more powerful loop diuretics may be required. In the nephrotic syndrome, the response to diuretics often is disappointing.

Whether a patient should receive diuretics and, if so, what therapeutic regimen should be used (*i.e.,* type of diuretic, route of administration, and speed of mobilization of edema fluid) depends on the clinical situation. Massive pulmonary edema in patients with acute left heart failure is a medical emergency requiring rapid, aggressive therapy including intravenous administration of a loop

diuretic. In this setting, use of oral diuretics or diuretics with lesser efficacy is inappropriate. On the other hand, mild pulmonary and venous congestion associated with chronic heart failure is best treated with an oral loop diuretic, the dosage of which should be titrated carefully to maximize the benefit-to-risk ratio. In many situations, edema will not pose an immediate health risk. Even so, uncomfortable, oppressive, and/or disfiguring edema can greatly reduce quality of life, and the decision to treat will be based in part on quality-of-life issues. In such cases, only partial removal of edema fluid should be attempted, and the fluid should be mobilized slowly using a diuretic regimen that accomplishes the task with minimal perturbation of normal physiology. Brater (1998) has provided an algorithm for diuretic therapy (specific recommendations for drug, dose, route, and drug combinations) in patients with edema caused by renal, hepatic, or cardiac disorders.

In many clinical situations, edema is not caused by an abnormal intake of Na^+ or by an altered renal handling of Na^+. Rather, edema is the result of altered Starling forces at the capillary beds, *i.e.,* a "Starling trap." Use of diuretics in these clinical settings represents a judicious compromise between the edematous state and the hypovolemic state. In such conditions, reducing total ECFV with diuretics will decrease edema but also will cause depletion of "sensed" ECFV, possibly leading to hypotension, malaise, and asthenia.

Diuretic resistance refers to edema that is or has become refractory to a given diuretic. If diuretic resistance develops against a less efficacious diuretic, a more efficacious diuretic should be substituted, *e.g.,* a loop diuretic for a thiazide. However, resistance to loop diuretics is not uncommon and can be due to several causes (Brater, 1985). NSAIDs block prostaglandin-mediated increases in RBF, resulting in resistance to loop diuretics. In chronic renal failure, a reduction in RBF decreases the delivery of diuretics to the kidney, and accumulation of endogenous organic acids competes with loop diuretics for transport at the proximal tubule. Consequently, the concentration of diuretic at the active site in the tubular lumen is diminished. In nephrotic syndrome, urinary protein binds diuretics and thereby limits the response. In hepatic cirrhosis or heart failure, the kidney may have a diminished responsiveness to diuretics because of increased proximal tubular Na^+ reabsorption, leading to diminished delivery of Na^+ to the distal nephron segments (Knauf and Mutschler, 1997).

Faced with resistance to loop diuretics, the clinician has several options:

1. Bed rest may restore drug responsiveness by improving the renal circulation.

2. An increase in the dose of loop diuretic may restore responsiveness.

3. Administration of smaller doses more frequently or a continuous intravenous infusion of a loop diuretic (Rudy *et al.,* 1991; Dormans *et al.,* 1996; Ferguson *et al.,* 1997) will increase the length of time that an effective concentration of the diuretic is at the active site.

4. Use of combination therapy to sequentially block more than one site in the nephron may result in a synergistic interaction between two diuretics. For instance, a combination of a loop diuretic with a K^+-sparing or a thiazide diuretic may improve therapeutic response; however, nothing is gained by the administration of two drugs of the same type. Thiazide diuretics with significant proximal tubular effects, *e.g.,* metolazone, are particularly well suited for sequential blockade when coadministered with a loop diuretic.

5. Scheduling of diuretic administration shortly before food intake will provide effective concentrations of diuretic in the tubular lumen when the salt load is highest.

PROSPECTUS

All currently available diuretics perturb K^+ homeostasis. However, studies in animals have established that blockade of adenosine A_1 receptors induces a brisk natriuresis without significantly increasing urinary K^+ excretion (Kuan *et al.,* 1993). Two clinical studies with FK453, a highly selective A_1-receptor antagonist, confirm that blockade of A_1 receptors induces natriuresis in human beings with minimal effects on K^+ excretion (Balakrishnan *et al.,* 1993; van Buren *et al.,* 1993). The natriuretic mechanism of this novel class of diuretics has been partially elucidated (Takeda *et al.,* 1993). Endogenous adenosine acts on A_1 receptors in the proximal tubule to inhibit adenylyl cyclase. As cyclic AMP inhibits basolateral Na^+–HCO_3^- symport activity, a reduced level of cyclic AMP increases Na^+–HCO_3^- symport activity in the basolat-

eral membrane. Blockade of A_1 receptors prevents the inhibition of adenylyl cyclase by endogenous adenosine, increases epithelial cyclic AMP levels, and consequently decreases Na^+–HCO_3^- symport activity in the basolateral membrane of the proximal tubule. Because A_1 receptors are involved in TGF, A_1-receptor antagonists uncouple increased distal delivery of Na^+ from activation of TGF (Wilcox *et al.,* 1999). Other mechanisms, including an effect in the collecting tubules, contribute to the natriuretic response to A_1-receptor antagonists; however, it is not known why this class of diuretics has little effect on K^+ excretion. An A_1-receptor antagonist is under clinical development for the treatment of edema due to heart failure.

Recently, the water channels of the proximal tubule (aquaporin 1) and of the collecting duct (aquaporins 2, 3, and 4) were cloned and their functional characteristics examined (Agre *et al.,* 1993; Fushimi *et al.,* 1993; *see* Yamamoto and Sasaki, 1998). The cloning of these proteins represents an important step in our understanding of water homeostasis. Currently, there are no specific inhibitors of aquaporins; however, these proteins are important targets for the development of novel diuretics. Inhibition of water channels in the proximal tubule would greatly diminish the flux of water across proximal tubular epithelial cells, which would reduce luminal Na^+ concentration to the point where Na^+ reabsorption would cease. Therefore, inhibitors of proximal tubular aquaporin 1 may be useful natriuretic diuretics. On the other hand, inhibitors of collecting duct aquaporins 2, 3, and 4 would prevent water reabsorption in the collecting duct and therefore would be highly efficacious "aquaretic" diuretics, *i.e.,* diuretics with a predominant effect on water, rather than on Na^+, excretion. Since aquaporin 2 is regulated by the vasopressin V_2 receptor, another potential class of aquaretic diuretics would be nonpeptide, orally active V_2-receptor antagonists. Exciting progress has been made, and this subject is developed in Chapter 30. Finally, apical K^+ channels (ROMK) are another potential molecular target for the development of K^+-sparing diuretics with high efficacy.

BIBLIOGRAPHY

Bachmann, S., Velázquez, H., Obermüller, N., Reilly, R.F., Moser, D., and Ellison, D.H. Expression of the thiazide-sensitive Na-Cl cotransporter by rabbit distal convoluted tubule cells. *J. Clin. Invest.,* **1995,** *96:*2510–2514.

Balakrishnan, V.S., Coles, G.A., and Williams, J.D. A potential role for

endogenous adenosine in control of human glomerular and tubular function. *Am. J. Physiol.,* **1993,** *265:*F504–F510.

Beaumont, K., Vaughn, D.A., and Fanestil, D.D. Thiazide diuretic drug receptors in rat kidney: identification with [³H] metolazone. *Proc. Natl. Acad. Sci. U.S.A.,* **1988,** *85:*2311–2314.

Beaumont, K., Vaughn, D.A., and Healy, D.P. Thiazide diuretic receptors: autoradiographic localization in rat kidney with [³H] metolazone. *J. Pharmacol. Exp. Ther.,* **1989,** *250*:414–419.

Beyer, K. The mechanism of action of chlorothiazide. *Ann. N. Y. Acad. Sci.,* **1958,** *71*:363–379.

Bostonjoglo, M., Reeves, W.B., Reilly, R.F., Velázquez, H., Robertson, N., Litwack, G., Morsing, P., Dørup, J., Bachmann, S., and Ellison, D.H. 11 β-Hydroxysteroid dehydrogenase, mineralcorticoid receptor, and thiazide-sensitive Na-Cl cotransporter expression by distal tubules. *J. Am. Soc. Nephrol.,* **1998,** *9*:1347–1358.

Burg, M., Stoner, L., Cardinal, J., and Green, N. Furosemide effect on isolated perfused tubules. *Am. J. Physiol.,* **1973,** *225*:119–124.

Busch, A.E., Suessbrich, H., Kunzelmann, K., Hipper, A., Greger, R., Waldegger, S., Mutschler, E., Lindemann, B., and Lang, F. Blockade of epithelial Na⁺ channels by triamterenes—underlying mechanisms and molecular basis. *Pflügers Arch.,* **1996,** *432*:760–766.

Canessa, C., Schild, L., Buell, G., Thorens, B., Gautschi, I., Horisberger, J.D., and Rossier, B.C. Amiloride-sensitive epithelial Na⁺ channel is made of three homologous subunits. *Nature,* **1994,** *367*:463–467.

Chang, H., Tashiro, K., Hirai, M., Ikeda, K., Kurokawa, K., and Fujita, T. Identification of a cDNA encoding a thiazide-sensitive sodium-chloride cotransporter from the human and its mRNA expression in various tissues. *Biochem. Biophys. Res. Commun.,* **1996,** *223*:324–328.

Cogan, M.G., Maddox, D.A., Warnock, D.G., Lin, E.T., and Rector, F.C., Jr. Effect of acetazolamide on bicarbonate reabsorption in the proximal tubule of the rat. *Am. J. Physiol.,* **1979,** *237*:F447–F454.

Costanzo, L.S., and Windhager, E.E. Calcium and sodium transport by the distal convoluted tubule of the rat. *Am. J. Physiol.,* **1978,** *235*:F492–F506.

Davenport, H.W., and Wilhelmi, A.E. Renal carbonic anhydrase. *Proc. Soc. Exp. Biol. Med.,* **1941,** *48*:53–56.

Dawson, J.L. Post-operative renal function in obstructive jaundice: effect of a mannitol diuresis. *Br. Med. J.,* **1965,** *5127*:82–86.

Deen, W.M., Robertson, C.R., and Brenner, B.M. A model of glomerular ultrafiltration in the rat. *Am. J. Physiol.,* **1972,** *223*:1178–1183.

Dirks, J.H., and Seely, J.F. Effect of saline infusions and furosemide on the dog distal nephron. *Am. J. Physiol.,* **1970,** *219*:114–121.

Dormans, T.P.J., van Meyel, J.J.M., Gerlag, P.G.G., Tan, Y., Russell, F.G.M., and Smits, P. Diuretic efficacy of high dose furosemide in severe heart failure: bolus injection versus continuous infusion. *J. Am. Coll. Cardiol.,* **1996,** *28*:376–382.

Ferguson, J.A., Sundblad, K.J., Becker, P.K., Gorski, J.C., Rudy, D.W., and Brater, D.C. Role of duration of diuretic effect in preventing sodium retention. *Clin. Pharmacol. Ther.,* **1997,** *62*:203–208.

Fushimi, K., Uchida, S., Hara, Y., Hirata, Y., Marumo, F., and Sasaki, S. Cloning and expression of apical membrane water channel of rat kidney collecting tubule. *Nature,* **1993,** *361*:549–552.

Gamba, G., Miyanoshita, A., Lombardi, M., Lytton, J., Lee, W.S., Hediger, M.A., and Hebert, S.C. Molecular cloning, primary structure and characterization of two members of the mammalian electroneutral sodium-(potassium)-chloride cotransporter family expressed in kidney. *J. Biol. Chem.,* **1994,** *269*:17713–17722.

Gamba, G., Saltzberg, S.N., Lombardi, M., Miyanoshita, A., Lytton, J., Hediger, M.A., Brenner, B.M., and Hebert, S.C. Primary structure and functional expression of a cDNA encoding the thiazide-sensitive, electroneutral sodium-chloride cotransporter. *Proc. Natl. Acad. Sci. U.S.A.,* **1993,** *90*:2749–2753.

Greger, R. Chloride reabsorption in the rabbit cortical thick ascending limb of the loop of Henle. A sodium-dependent process. *Pflügers Arch.,* **1981,** *390*:38–43.

Grimm, R.H., Jr., Grandits, G.A., Prineas, R.J., McDonald, R.H., Lewis, C.E., Flack, J.M., Yunis, C., Svendsen, K., Liebson, P.R., Elmer, P.J., and Stamler, J., for the TOMHS Research Group. Long-term effects on sexual function of five antihypertensive drugs and nutritional hygienic treatment in hypertensive men and women. Treatment of mild hypertension study (TOMHS). *Hypertension,* **1997,** *29*:8–14.

Grønbeck, L., Marples, D., Nielsen, S., and Christensen, S. Mechanism of antidiuresis caused by bendroflumethiazide in conscious rats with diabetes insipidus. *Br. J. Pharmacol.,* **1998,** *123*:737–745.

Grossman, E., Messerli, F.H., and Goldbourt, U. Does diuretic therapy increase the risk of renal cell carcinoma? *Am. J. Cardiol.,* **1999,** *83*:1090–1093.

Hannafin, J., Kinne-Saffran, E., Friedman, D., and Kinne, R. Presence of a sodium-potassium chloride cotransport system in the rectal gland of *Squalus acanthias. J. Membr. Biol.,* **1983,** *75*:73–83.

Ho, K., Nichols, C.G., Lederer, W.J., Lytton, J., Vassilev, P.M., Kanazirska, M.V., and Herbert, S.C. Cloning and expression of an inwardly rectifying ATP-regulated potassium channel. *Nature,* **1993,** *362*:31–38.

Hollenberg, N.K., and Mickiewicz, C.W. Postmarketing surveillance in 70,898 patients treated with a triamterene/hydrochlorothiazide combination (Maxide). *Am. J. Cardiol.,* **1989,** *63*:37B–41B.

Isenring, P., and Forbush, B. III. Ion and bumetanide binding by the Na-K-Cl cotransporter. *J. Biol. Chem.,* **1997,** *272*:24556–24562.

Ismailov, I.I., Shlyonsky, V.G., Serperu, E.H., Fuller, C.M., Cheung, H.C., Muccio, D., Berdiev, B.K., and Benos, D.J. Peptide inhibition of ENaC. *Biochemistry,* **1999,** *38*:354–363.

Johnston, G.D., Hiatt, W.R., Nies, A.S., Payne, N.A., Murphy, R.C., and Gerber, J.G. Factors modifying the early nondiuretic vascular effects of furosemide in man. The possible role of renal prostaglandins. *Circ. Res.,* **1983,** *53*:630–635.

Johnston, P.A., Bernard, D.B., Perrin, N.S., and Levinsky, N.G. Prostaglandins mediate the vasodilatory effect of mannitol in the hypoperfused rat kidney. *J. Clin. Invest.,* **1981,** *68*:127–133.

Kagawa, C.M., Cella, J.A., and Van Arman, C.G. Action of new steroids in blocking effects of aldosterone and deoxycorticosterone on salt. *Science,* **1957,** *126*:1015–1016.

Kaplan, M.R., Plotkin, M.D., Lee, W.S., Xu, Z.C., Lytton, J., and Herbert, S.C. Apical localization of the Na-K-Cl cotransporter, *rBSC1,* on rat thick ascending limbs. *Kidney Int.,* **1996,** *49*:40–47.

Kauker, M.L., Lassiter, W.E., and Gottschalk, C.W. Micropuncture study of effects of urea infusion on tubular reabsorption in the rat. *Am. J. Physiol.,* **1970,** *219*:45–50.

Kim, G.H., Masilamani, S., Turner, R., Mitchell, C., Wade, J.B., and Knepper, M.A. The thiazide-sensitive Na-Cl cotransporter is an aldosterone-induced protein. *Proc. Natl. Acad. Sci. U.S.A.,* **1998,** *95*:14552–14557.

Knauf, H., and Mutschler, E. Sequential nephron blockade breaks resistance to diuretics in edematous states. *J. Cardiovasc. Pharmacol.,* **1997,** *29*:367–372.

Koenig, B., Ricapito, S., and Kinne, R. Chloride transport in the thick ascending limb of Henle's loop: potassium dependence and stoichiometry of the NaCl cotransport system in plasma membrane vesicles. *Pflügers Arch.,* **1983,** *399*:173–179.

Kohda, Y., Ding, W., Phan, E., Housini, I., Wang, J., Star, R.A., and Huang, C.L. Localization of the ROMK potassium channel to the apical membrane of distal nephron in rat kidney. *Kidney Int.,* **1998,** *54*:1214–1223.

Kuan, C.J., Herzer, W.A., and Jackson, E.K. Cardiovascular and renal effects of blocking A₁ adenosine receptors. *J. Cardiovasc. Pharmacol.,* **1993,** *21*:822–828.

Kunau, R.T., Jr., Weller, D.R., and Webb, H.L. Clarification of the site of action of chlorothiazide in the rat nephron. *J. Clin. Invest.,* **1975,** *56*:401–407.

Lane, P.H., Tyler, L.D., and Schmitz, P.G. Chronic administration of furosemide augments renal weight and glomerular capillary pressure in normal rats. *Am. J. Physiol.,* **1998,** *275*:F230–F234.

Links, T.P., Zwarts, M.J., and Oosterhuis, H.J. Improvement of muscle strength in familial hypokalaemic periodic paralysis with acetazolamide. *J. Neurol. Neurosurg. Psychiatry,* **1988,** *51*:1142–1145.

Lu, R., Chan, B.S., and Schuster, V.L. Cloning of the human kidney PAH transporter: narrow substate specificity and regulation by protein kinase C. *Am. J. Physiol.,* **1999,** *276*:F295–F303.

Lytle, C., McManus, T.J., and Haas, M. A model of Na-K-2Cl cotransport based on ordered ion binding and glide symmetry. *Am. J. Physiol.,* **1998,** *274*:C299–C309.

Maren, T.H., Conroy, C.W., Wynns, G.C., and Godman, D.R. Renal and cerebrospinal fluid formation pharmacology of a high molecular weight carbonic anhydrase inhibitor. *J. Pharmacol. Exp. Ther.,* **1997,** *280*:98–104.

Martin, B.J., and Milligan, K. Diuretic-associated hypomagnesemia in the elderly. *Arch. Intern. Med.,* **1987,** *147*:1768–1771.

Marver, D., Stewart, J., Funder, J.W., Feldman, D., and Edelman, I.S. Renal aldosterone receptors: studies with [^{3}H] aldosterone and the anti-mineralocorticoid [^{3}H] spirolactone (SC-26304). *Proc. Natl. Acad. Sci. U.S.A.,* **1974,** *71*:1431–1435.

Mastroianni, N., De Fusco, M., Zollo, M., Arrigo, G., Zuffardi, O., Bettinelli, A., Ballabio, A., and Casari, G. Molecular cloning, expression pattern, and chromosomal localization of the human Na-Cl thiazide-sensitive cotransporter (SLC12A3). *Genomics,* **1996,** *35*:486–493.

Morgan, T., Tadokoro, M., Martin, D., and Berliner, R.W. Effect of furosemide on Na$^+$ and K$^+$ transport studied by microperfusion of the rat nephron. *Am. J. Physiol.,* **1970,** *218*:292–297.

Mount, D.B., Baekgaard, A., Hall, A.E., Plata, C., Xu, J., Beier, D.R., Gamba, G., and Hebert, S.C. Isoforms of the Na-K-2Cl cotransponder in murine TAL: I. Molecular characterization and intrarenal localization. *Am. J. Physiol.,* **1999,** *276*:F347–F358.

Nielsen, S., Maunsbach, A.B., Ecelbarger, C.A., and Knepper, M.A. Ultrastructural localization of the Na-K-2Cl cotransporter in thick ascending limb and macula densa of rat kidney. *Am. J. Physiol.,* **1998,** *275*:F885–F893.

Obermüller, N., Bernstein, P., Velázquez, H., Reilly, R., Moser, D., Ellison, D.H., and Bachmann, S. Expression of the thiazide-sensitive Na-Cl cotransporter in rat and human kidney. *Am. J. Physiol.,* **1995,** *269*:F900–F910.

Obermüller, N., Kunchaparty, S., Ellison, D.H., and Bachmann, S. Expression of the Na-K-2Cl cotransporter by macula densa and thick ascending limb cells of rat and rabbit nephron. *J. Clin. Invest.,* **1996,** *98*:635–640.

O'Neil, R.G., and Boulpaep, E.L. Effect of amiloride on the apical cell membrane cation channels of a sodium-absorbing, potassium-secreting renal epithelium. *J. Membr. Biol.,* **1979,** *50*:365–387.

Payne, J.A., and Forbush, B. III. Alternatively spliced isoforms of the putative renal Na-K-Cl cotransporter are differentially distributed within the rabbit kidney. *Proc. Natl. Acad. Sci. U.S.A.,* **1994,** *91*:4544–4548.

Persson, A.E.G., and Wright, F.S. Evidence for feedback mediated reduction of glomerular filtration rate during infusion of acetazolamide. *Acta Physiol. Scand.,* **1982,** *114*:1–7.

Pitt, B., Zannad, F., Remme, W.J., Cody, R., Castaigne, A., Perez, A.,

Palensky, J., and Wittes, J. for the Randomized Aldactone Evaluation Study Investigators. The effect of spironolactone on morbidity and mortality in patients with severe heart failure. *N. Engl. J. Med.,* **1999,** *341*:709–717.

Plata, C., Mount, D.B., Rubio, V., Hebert, S.C., and Gamba, G. Isoforms of the Na-K-2Cl cotransporter in murine TAL: II. Functional characterization and activation by cAMP. *Am. J. Physiol.,* **1999,** *276*:F359–F366.

Plotkin, M.D., Kaplan, M.R., Verlander, J.W., Lee, W.S., Brown, D., Poch, E., Gullans, S.R., and Hebert, S.C. Localization of the thiazide sensitive Na-Cl cotransporter, rTSC1, in the rat kidney. *Kidney Int.,* **1996,** *50*:174–183.

Rudy, D.W., Voelker, J.R., Greene, P.K., Esparza, F.A., and Brater, D.C. Loop diuretics for chronic renal insufficiency: a continuous infusion is more efficacious than bolus therapy. *Ann. Intern. Med.,* **1991,** *115*:360–366.

Saito, F., and Kimura, G. Antihypertensive mechanism of diuretics based on pressure-natriuresis relationship. *Hypertension,* **1996,** *27*:914–918.

Seely, J.F., and Dirks, J.H. Micropuncture study of hypertonic mannitol diuresis in the proximal and distal tubule of the dog kidney. *J. Clin. Invest.,* **1969,** *48*:2330–2340.

Solomon, R., Werner, C., Mann, D., D'Elia, J., and Silva, P. Effects of saline, mannitol, and furosemide on acute decreases in renal function induced by radiocontrast agents. *N. Engl. J. Med.,* **1994,** *331*:1416–1420.

Stein, J.H., Mauk, R.C., Boonjarern, S., and Ferris, T.F. Differences in the effect of furosemide and chlorothiazide on the distribution of renal cortical blood flow in the dog. *J. Lab. Clin. Med.,* **1972,** *79*:995–1003.

Takeda, M., Yoshitomi, K., and Imai, M. Regulation of Na$^+$–3HCO$_3^-$ cotransport in rabbit proximal convoluted tubule via adenosine A$_1$ receptor. *Am. J. Physiol.,* **1993,** *265*:F511–F519.

van Buren, M., Bijlsma, J.A., Boer, P., van Rijn, H.J.M., and Koomans, H.A. Natriuretic and hypotensive effect of adenosine-1 blockade in essential hypertension. *Hypertension,* **1993,** *22*:728–734.

van der Heijden, M., Donders, S.H., Cleophas, T.J., Niemeyer, M.G., van der Meulen, J., Bernick, P.J., de Planque, B.A., and van der Wall, E.E. for the BUFUL Study Group. A randomized, placebo-controlled study of loop diuretics in patients with essential hypertension: the bumetanide and furosemide on lipid profile (BUFUL) clinical study report. *J. Clin. Pharmacol.,* **1998,** *38*:630–635.

Velázquez, H., Bartiss, A., Bernstein, P., and Ellison, D. H. Adrenal steroids stimulate thiazide-sensitive NaCl transport by rat renal distal tubules. *Am. J. Physiol.,* **1996,** *270*:F211–F219.

Wesson, L.G., Jr., and Anslow, W.P., Jr. Excretion of sodium and water during osmotic diuresis in the dog. *Am. J. Physiol.,* **1948,** *153*:465–474.

Wilcox, C.S., Welch, W.J., Schreiner, G.F., and Belardinelli, L. Natriuretic and diuretic actions of a highly selective A$_1$ receptor antagonist. *J. Am. Soc. Nephrol.,* **1999,** *10*:714–720.

Williamson, H.E., Bourland, W.A., and Marchand, G.R. Inhibition of ethacrynic acid induced increase in renal blood flow by indomethacin. *Prostaglandins,* **1974,** *8*:297–301.

Windhager, E.E., Whittembury, G., Oken, D.E., Schatzmann, H.J., and Solomon, A.K. Single proximal tubules of the Necturus kidney: III. Dependence of H$_2$O movement on NaCl concentration. *Am. J. Physiol.,* **1959,** *197*:313–318.

Xu, J.C., Lytle, C., Zhu, T.T., Payne, J.A., Benz, E., Jr., and Forbush, B. III. Molecular cloning and functional expression of the bumetanide-sensitive Na-K-Cl cotransporter. *Proc. Natl. Acad. Sci. U.S.A.,* **1994,** *91*:2201–2205.

MONOGRAPHS AND REVIEWS

Agre, P., Preston, G.M., Smith, B.L., Jung, J.S., Raina, S., Moon, C., Guggino, W.B., and Nielsen, S. Aquaporin CHIP: the archetypal molecular water channel. *Am. J. Physiol.,* **1993,** *265*:F463–F476.

Brater, D.C. Pharmacodynamic considerations in the use of diuretics. *Annu. Rev. Pharmacol. Toxicol.,* **1983,** *23*:45–62.

Brater, D.C. Resistance to loop diuretics: why it happens and what to do about it. *Drugs,* **1985,** *30*:427–443.

Brater, D.C. Clinical pharmacology of loop diuretics. *Drugs,* **1991,** *41*:14–22.

Brater, D.C. Diuretic therapy. *N. Engl. J. Med.,* **1998,** *339*:387–395.

Coote, J.H. Pharmacological control of altitude sickness. *Trends Pharmacol. Sci.,* **1991,** *12*:450–455.

Dormans, T.P.J., Pickkers, P., Russel, F.G.M., and Smits, P. Vascular effects of loop diuretics. *Cardiovasc. Res.,* **1996,** *32*:988–997.

Garty, H., and Palmer, L.G. Epithelial sodium channels: function, structure, and regulation. *Physiol. Rev.,* **1997,** *77*:359–396.

Guyton, A.C. Blood pressure control—special role of the kidneys and body fluids. *Science,* **1991,** *252*:1813–1816.

Hoes, A.W., and Grobbee, D.E. Diuretics and risk of sudden death in hypertension—evidence and potential implications. *Clin. Exp. Hypertens.,* **1996,** *18*:523–535.

Kaplan, M.R., Mount, D.B., and Delpire, E. Molecular mechanisms of NaCl cotransport. *Annu. Rev. Physiol.,* **1996,** *58*:649–668.

Kellum, J.A. Use of diuretics in the acute care setting. *Kidney Int. Suppl.,* **1998,** *66*:S67–S70.

Knauf, H., and Mutschler, E. Clinical pharmacokinetics and pharmacodynamics of torasemide. *Clin. Pharmacokinet.,* **1998,** *34*:1–24.

Kokko, J.P., and Rector, F.C., Jr. Countercurrent multiplication system without active transport in inner medulla. *Kidney Int.,* **1972,** *2*:214–223.

Levinsky, N.G., and Bernard, D.B. Mannitol and loop diuretics in acute renal failure. In, *Acute Renal Failure,* 2nd ed. (Brenner, B.M., and Lazarus, J.M., eds.) Churchill Livingstone, New York, **1988** pp. 841–856.

Maren, T.H. Carbonic anhydrase: chemistry, physiology, and inhibition. *Physiol. Rev.,* **1967,** *47*:595–781.

Maren, T.H. Current status of membrane-bound carbonic anhydrase. *Ann. NY Acad. Sci.,* **1980,** *341*:246–258.

Oates, J.A., Whorton, A.R., Gerkens, J.F., Branch, R.A., Hollifield, J.W., and Frölich, J.C. The participation of prostaglandins in the control of renin release. *Fed. Proc.,* **1979,** *38*:72–74.

Puschett, J.B., and Winaver, J. Effects of diuretics on renal function. In, *Handbook of Physiology.* Sec. 8, Vol. 2. (Windhager, E.E., ed.) Oxford University Press, New York and Oxford, **1992** pp. 2335–2404.

Ramsay, L.E. Thiazide diuretics in hypertension. *Clin. Exp. Hypertens.,* **1999,** *21*:805–814.

Roden, D.M. Torsade de pointes. *Clin. Cardiol.,* **1993,** *16*:683–686.

Sands, J.M., and Kokko, J.P. Current concepts of the countercurrent multiplication system. *Kidney Int. Suppl.,* **1996,** *57*:S93–S99.

Simon, D.B., and Lifton, R.P. Mutations in Na(K)Cl transporters in Gitleman's and Bartter's syndromes. *Curr. Opin. Cell Biol.,* **1998,** *10*:450–454.

Tannen, R.L. Diuretic-induced hypokalemia. *Kidney Int.,* **1985,** *28*:988–1000.

Yamamoto, T., and Sasaki, S. Aquaporins in the kidney: emerging new aspects. *Kidney Int.,* **1998,** *54*:1041–1051..

Zahaykevich, A. Amiloride for lung disease in cystic fibrosis. *D.I.C.P.,* **1991,** *25*:1340–1341.

C H A P T E R   3 0

VASOPRESSIN AND OTHER AGENTS AFFECTING THE RENAL CONSERVATION OF WATER

Edwin K. Jackson

Precise regulation of body fluid osmolality is essential. It is controlled by a finely tuned, intricate homeostatic mechanism that operates by adjusting both the rate of water intake and the rate of solute-free water excretion by the kidneys—i.e., water balance. Abnormalities in this homeostatic system can be caused by genetic diseases, acquired diseases, or drugs and may result in serious and potentially life-threatening deviations in plasma osmolality. The goals of this chapter are to describe the physiological mechanisms that regulate plasma osmolality, to discuss the diseases that perturb those mechanisms, and to examine pharmacological approaches for treating disorders of water balance.

Arginine vasopressin (the antidiuretic hormone in human beings) is the main hormone involved in regulation of body fluid osmolality. Many diseases of water homeostasis and many pharmacological strategies for correcting such disorders pertain to vasopressin. Accordingly, vasopressin is the major focus of this chapter and is discussed with regard to: (1) chemistry (including the chemistry of vasopressin agonists and antagonists); (2) physiology (including anatomical considerations; the synthesis, transport, and storage of vasopressin and the regulation of vasopressin secretion); (3) basic pharmacology (including vasopressin receptors and their signal transduction pathways, renal actions of vasopressin, pharmacological modification of the antidiuretic response to vasopressin, and nonrenal actions of vasopressin); (4) diseases affecting the vasopressin system (diabetes insipidus, syndrome of inappropriate secretion of antidiuretic hormone, and other water-retaining states); and (5) clinical pharmacology of vasopressin peptides (therapeutic uses, pharmacokinetics, toxicities, adverse effects, contraindications, and drug interactions). A small number of other drugs can be used to treat abnormalities of water balance; a discussion of these agents is integrated into the section on diseases affecting the vasopressin system.

INTRODUCTION TO VASOPRESSIN

Immunoreactive vasopressin has been observed in neurons from organisms belonging to the first animal phylum with a nervous system (*e.g., Hydra attenuata*), and vasopressin-like peptides have been isolated and characterized from both mammalian and nonmammalian vertebrates as well as from invertebrates (Table 30–1). Genes encoding vasopressin-like peptides probably evolved more than 700 million years ago.

With the emergence of life on land, vasopressin became the mediator of a remarkable regulatory system for the conservation of water. The hormone is released by the posterior pituitary whenever water deprivation causes an increased plasma osmolality or whenever the cardiovascular system is challenged by hypovolemia and/or hypotension. In amphibians, the target organs for vasopressin are skin and the urinary bladder, whereas in other vertebrates, including human beings, the site of action is primarily the renal collecting duct. In each of these target tissues, vasopressin acts by increasing the permeability

789

of the cell membrane to water, thus permitting water to move passively down an osmotic gradient across skin, bladder, or collecting duct into the extracellular compartment.

In view of the long evolutionary history of vasopressin, it is not surprising that vasopressin acts at sites in the nephron other than the collecting duct and on tissues other than the kidney. Vasopressin is a potent vasopressor, and its name was originally chosen in recognition of its vasoconstrictor action. Vasopressin is a neurotransmitter; among its actions in the central nervous system (CNS) are apparent roles in the secretion of adrenocorticotropic hormone (ACTH) and in the regulation of the cardiovascular system, temperature, and other visceral functions. Vasopressin also promotes the release of coagulation factors

by the vascular endothelium and increases platelet aggregability; therefore, it may play a role in hemostasis.

CHEMISTRY OF VASOPRESSIN RECEPTOR AGONISTS AND ANTAGONISTS

Chemistry of Vasopressin Receptor Agonists. du Vigneaud and coworkers (1954) determined the structures of vasopressin and oxytocin and accomplished the complete synthesis of each. A number of vasopressin-like peptides occur naturally (Table 30–1). All are nonapeptides; contain cysteine residues in positions 1 and 6; have an intramolecular disulfide bridge between the two cysteine

Table 30–1
Vasopressin Receptor Agonists

I. NATURALLY OCCURRING VASOPRESSIN-LIKE PEPTIDES	A	W	X	Y	Z
A. *Vertebrates*					
1. Mammals					
Arginine vasopressin* (AVP) (human beings & other mammals)	NH_2	Tyr	Phe	Gln	Arg
Lypressin* (pigs, marsupials)	NH_2	Tyr	Phe	Gln	Lys
Phenypressin (macropodids)	NH_2	Phe	Phe	Gln	Arg
2. Nonmammalian vertebrates					
Vasotocin	NH_2	Tyr	Ile	Gln	Arg
B. *Invertebrates*					
1. Arginine conopressin (*Conus striatus*)	NH_2	Ile	Ile	Arg	Arg
2. Lysine conopressin (*Conus geographicus*)	NH_2	Phe	Ile	Arg	Lys
3. Locust subesophageal ganglia peptide	NH_2	Leu	Ile	Thr	Arg
II. SYNTHETIC VASOPRESSIN PEPTIDES					
A. *V₁-selective agonists*					
1. V_{1a}-Selective Agonist [Phe², Ile³, Orn⁸]AVP	NH_2	Phe	Ile	Gln	Orn
2. V_{1b}-Selective Agonist Deamino [D-3-(3′-pyridyl)-Ala²]AVP	H	D-3-(3′-pyridyl)-Ala²	Phe	Gln	Arg
B. *V₂-selective agonists*					
1. Desmopressin* (DDAVP)	H	Tyr	Phe	Gln	D-Arg
2. Deamino[Val⁴, D-Arg⁸]AVP	H	Tyr	Phe	Val	D-Arg

*Available for clinical use.

residues (essential for agonist activity); have additional conserved amino acids in positions 5, 7, and 9 (asparagine, proline, and glycine, respectively); contain a basic amino acid in position 8; and are amidated on the carboxyl terminus. In all mammals except swine, the neurohypophyseal peptide is 8-arginine vasopressin, and the terms *vasopressin, arginine vasopressin* (AVP), and *antidiuretic hormone* (ADH) are used interchangeably. The chemical structure of oxytocin is closely related to that of vasopressin, *i.e.*, oxytocin is [Ile^3, Leu^8]AVP. Oxytocin binds to specific oxytocin receptors on myoepithelial cells in the mammary gland and on smooth muscle cells in the uterus, causing milk ejection and uterine contraction, respectively. Inasmuch as vasopressin and oxytocin are structurally similar, it is not surprising that vasopressin and oxytocin agonists and antagonists can bind to each other's receptors. Therefore, most of the available peptide vasopressin agonists and antagonists have some affinity for oxytocin receptors; at high doses, they may block or mimic the effects of oxytocin (Manning and Sawyer, 1989).

With the advent of solid-phase peptide synthesis, many vasopressin analogs were synthesized with the goal of increasing duration of action and selectivity for vasopressin receptor subtypes (V$_1$ *versus* V$_2$ vasopressin receptors, which mediate pressor responses and antidiuretic responses, respectively). In 1967, Zaoral and coworkers announced the synthesis of desmopressin: 1-deamino-8-D-arginine vasopressin (DDAVP) (Table 30–1). Deamination at position 1 increases duration of action and increases antidiuretic activity without increasing vasopressor activity. Substitution of D-arginine for L-arginine greatly reduces vasopressor activity without reducing antidiuretic activity. Thus, the antidiuretic-to-vasopressor ratio for desmopressin is approximately 3000-fold greater than that for vasopressin, and desmopressin now is the preferred drug for the treatment of central diabetes insipidus (Robinson, 1976). Substitution of valine for glutamine in position 4 further increases the antidiuretic selectivity, and the antidiuretic-to-vasopressor ratio for deamino[Val^4, D-Arg^8]AVP (Table 30–1) is approximately 11,000-fold greater than that for vasopressin. Increasing V$_1$ selectivity has proved more difficult than increasing V$_2$ selectivity (Thibonnier, 1990). However, a limited number of agonists have been developed with modest selectivity for V$_1$ receptors (*see* Table 30–1).

Vasopressin receptors in the adenohypophysis that mediate vasopressin-induced ACTH release are neither classical V$_1$ nor V$_2$ receptors. Since the vasopressin receptors in the adenohypophysis appear to share a common signal transduction mechanism with classical V$_1$ receptors, and since many vasopressin analogs with vasoconstrictor activity release ACTH, V$_1$ receptors have been

subclassified into V$_{1a}$ (vascular/hepatic) and V$_{1b}$ (pituitary) receptors (Jard *et al.*, 1986). Vasopressin agonists selective for both V$_{1a}$ (Thibonnier, 1990) and V$_{1b}$ receptors (Schwartz *et al.*, 1991) have been described (*see* Table 30–1).

Chemistry of Vasopressin Receptor Antagonists. The impetus for the development of specific vasopressin receptor antagonists is the belief that such drugs may be useful in a number of clinical settings. Selective V$_{1a}$ antagonists may be beneficial when total peripheral resistance is increased (*e.g.*, congestive heart failure and hypertension); selective V$_2$ antagonists could be useful whenever reabsorption of solute-free water is excessive (*e.g.*, the syndrome of inappropriate secretion of antidiuretic hormone and hyponatremia associated with a reduced effective blood volume). Combined V$_{1a}$/V$_2$ receptor antagonists might be beneficial in diseases associated with a combination of increased peripheral resistance and dilutional hyponatremia (*e.g.*, congestive heart failure).

Shortly after the synthesis of vasopressin, du Vigneaud and coworkers began designing antagonists of vasopressin's pharmacological effects. Since that time, numerous vasopressin receptor antagonists have been synthesized (Manning *et al.*, 1993; László *et al.*, 1991). Highly selective V$_1$ and V$_2$ peptide antagonists that are structural analogs of vasopressin have been synthesized (*see* Table 30–2 for examples), including both cyclic and linear peptides. [1-(β-mercapto-β,β-cyclopentamethyleneproprionic acid),2-O-methyltyrosine]. Arginine vasopressin, also known as d(CH$_2$)$_5$[Tyr(Me)^2]AVP, has a greater affinity for V$_{1a}$ receptors than for either V$_{1b}$ or V$_2$ receptors; this antagonist has been widely employed in physiological and pharmacological studies (Manning and Sawyer, 1989). Although [1-deaminopenicillamine, 2-O-methyltyrosine] arginine vasopressin, also called dP[Tyr(Me)^2]AVP, is a potent V$_{1b}$ receptor antagonist with little affinity for the V$_2$ receptor, it also blocks V$_{1a}$ receptors. No truly selective V$_{1b}$ receptor antagonist currently is available. Peptide antagonists currently available have limited oral activity, and the potency of peptide V$_2$ antagonists is species-dependent. Also, with prolonged infusion, peptide V$_2$ antagonists appear to express significant agonist activity (Kinter *et al.*, 1993). However, in the early 1990s a nonpeptide, orally active V$_1$-selective antagonist (OPC-21268) (Yamamura *et al.*, 1991) and a nonpeptide, orally active V$_{1a}$-/V$_2$-selective antagonist (OPC-31260) (Yamamura *et al.*, 1992) were synthesized. Neither compound had partial agonist activity. Other highly potent nonpeptide vasopressin receptor antagonists, such as SR 49059, SR 121463A, VPA-985, and YM 087 (Mayinger and Hensen, 1999) have been synthesized (*see* Table 30–2).

Table 30–2
Vasopressin Receptor Antagonists

I. PEPTIDE ANTAGONISTS

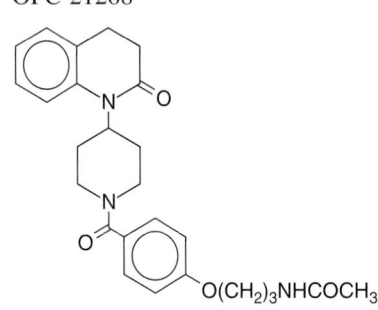

A. V_1-selective antagonists	X	Y	Z
V_{1a}-Selective Antagonist d(CH$_2$)$_5$[Tyr(Me)^2]AVP	Tyr | OMe	Gln	Gly (NH$_2$)
V_{1b}-Selective Antagonist dP [Tyr(Me)^2]AVP*○	Tyr | OMe	Gln	Gly (NH$_2$)

B. V_2-selective antagonists[†]

	X	Y	Z
1. des Gly-NH$_2$^{9}-d(CH$_2$)$_5$[D-Ile^2, Ile^4]AVP	D-Ile	Ile	—
2. d(CH$_2$)$_5$[D-Ile^2, Ile^4, Ala-NH$_2$^{9}]AVP	D-Ile	Ile	Ala (NH$_2$)

II. NONPEPTIDE ANTAGONISTS

A. V_{1a}-selective antagonists

OPC-21268

SR 49059

B. V_2-selective antagonists

SR 121463A

VPA-985

Table 30–2
Vasopressin Receptor Antagonists *(Continued)*

C. V_{1a}-/V_2-selective antagonists

OPC-31260

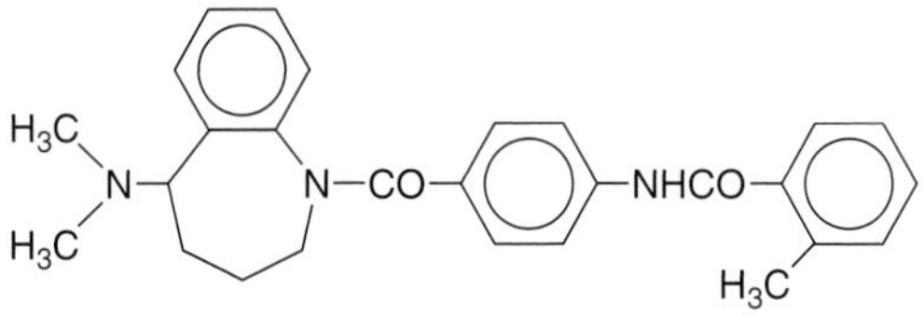

YM 087

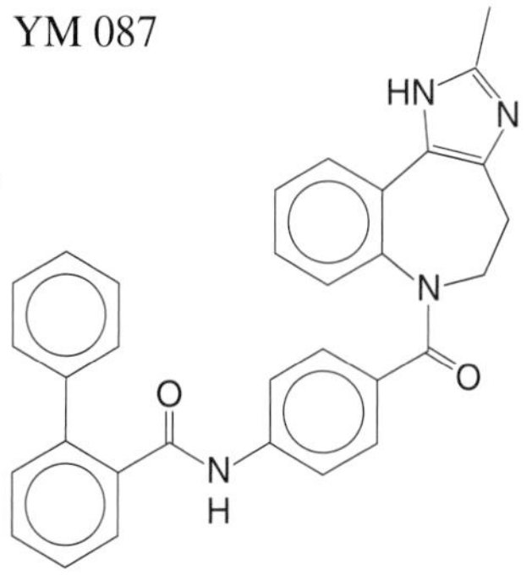

*Also blocks V_{1a} receptor, (structure) rather than (structure).

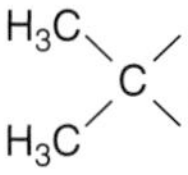

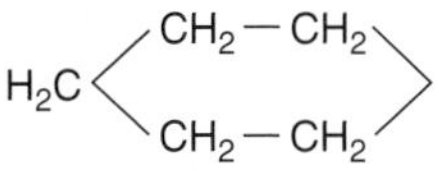

[†]V_2 antagonistic activity in rats; however, antagonistic activity may be less or nonexistent in other species. Also, with prolonged infusion may exhibit significant agonist activity.

PHYSIOLOGY OF VASOPRESSIN

Anatomy. The antidiuretic mechanism in mammals involves two anatomical components: a CNS component for the synthesis, transport, storage, and release of vasopressin, and a renal collecting duct system composed of epithelial cells that respond to vasopressin by increasing their permeability to water. The relevant anatomy of the renal collecting duct system is described in Chapter 29. The CNS component of the antidiuretic mechanism is called the *hypothalamiconeurohypophyseal* system and consists of neurosecretory neurons with perikarya located predominantly in two specific hypothalamic nuclei, the supraoptic nucleus (SON) and the paraventricular nucleus (PVN). The long axons of neurons in the SON and PVN traverse the supraopticohypophyseal tract to terminate in the median eminence and pars nervosa of the posterior pituitary.

Synthesis. Vasopressin and oxytocin are synthesized in the perikarya of magnocellular neurons in the SON and PVN; the two hormones are synthesized predominantly in separate neurons. Vasopressin synthesis appears to be regulated solely at the transcriptional level (Robinson and Fitzsimmons, 1993), and the molecular mechanism of vasopressin synthesis has been elucidated in considerable detail (Archer, 1993). In human beings, a 168-amino-acid preprohormone (Figure 30–1) is synthesized, and a signal peptide (residues -23 to -1) assures incorporation of the nascent polypeptide into ribosomes. During synthesis, the signal peptide is removed to form the vasopressin prohormone, and vesicle-mediated translocations maneuver the prohormone through the rough endoplasmic reticulum and *cis-*, *medial-*, and *trans*-Golgi compartments, so that the prohormone emerges incorporated into large (0.1- to 0.3-micron) membrane-enclosed granules. The prohormone consists of three domains: vasopressin (residues 1 to 9), vasopressin (VP)–neurophysin

(residues 13 to 105), and VP–glycopeptide (residues 107 to 145). The vasopressin domain is linked to the VP–neurophysin domain through a glycine–lysine–arginine processing signal, and the VP–neurophysin domain is linked to the VP–glycopeptide domain by an arginine-processing signal. In the secretory granules, an endopeptidase, exopeptidase, monooxygenase, and lyase act sequentially on the prohormone to produce vasopressin, VP–neurophysin (sometimes referred to as neurophysin II or MSEL–neurophysin), and VP–glycopeptide (sometimes called copeptin). The synthesis and transport of vasopressin are dependent on the conformation of the preprohormone. In particular, VP–neurophysin binds vasopressin and is critical to the correct processing, transport, and storage of vasopressin (Breslow, 1993). Genetic mutations in either the signal peptide or VP–neurophysin give rise to central diabetes insipidus (Raymond, 1994).

Transport and Storage. The process of axonal transport of vasopressin-containing granules is rapid, and newly synthesized neurohypophyseal hormones arrive at the posterior lobe within 30 minutes of a stimulus. The axons involved in transport of granules have two destinations, carrying vasopressin not only to classical storage sites in the neurohypophysis but also to the external zone of the median eminence, where vasopressin enters the adenohypophyseal portal circulation and plays a role as a corticotropin-releasing factor.

Maximal release of vasopressin occurs when impulse frequency is approximately 12 spikes per second for 20 seconds. Higher frequencies or longer periods of stimulation lead to diminished hormone release (fatigue). Appropriately, vasopressin-releasing cells demonstrate an atypical pattern of spike activity characterized by rapid phasic bursts (5 to 12 spikes per second for 15 to 60 seconds) separated by quiescent periods (15 to 60 seconds in duration). This pattern is orchestrated by

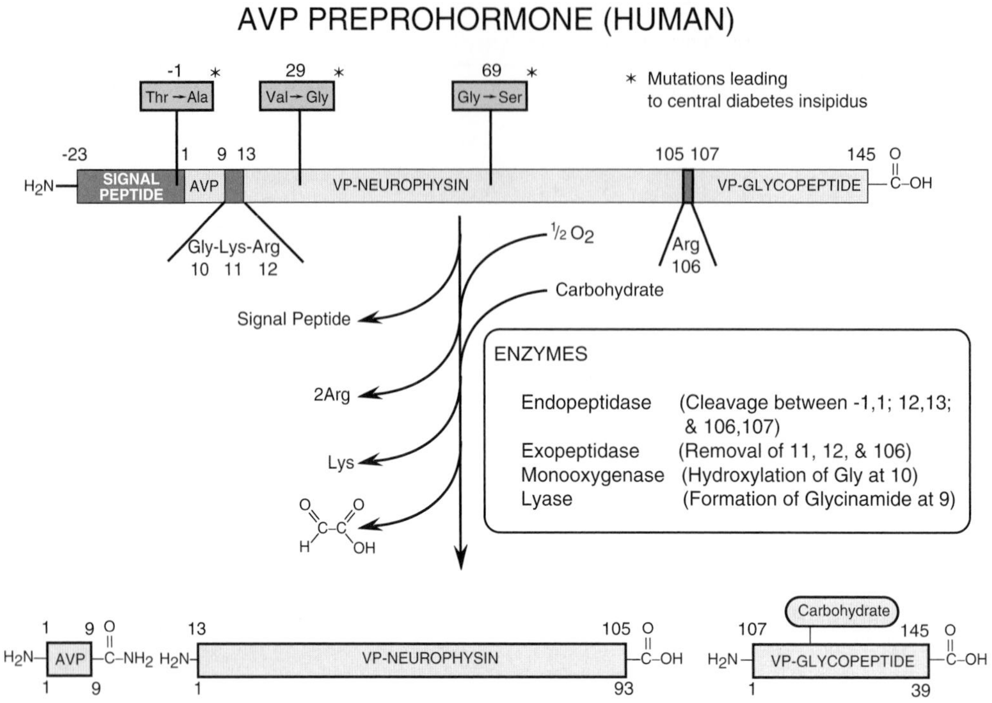

AVP PREPROHORMONE (HUMAN)

Figure 30–1. Processing of the 168–amino acid human 8-arginine vasopressin (AVP) prepro-hormone to AVP, vasopressin (VP)–neurophysin, and VP–glycopeptide.

activation and inactivation of ion channels in the magnocellular neurons and provides for optimal release of vasopressin (Leng *et al.,* 1992).

Vasopressin Synthesis Outside of the CNS.   Vasopressin also is synthesized by the heart (Hupf *et al.,* 1999) and adrenal gland (Guillon *et al.,* 1998). In the heart, elevated wall stress increases vasopressin synthesis several-fold. Cardiac synthesis of vasopressin is predominantly vascular and perivascular and may contribute to impaired ventricular relaxation and coronary vasoconstriction. Vasopressin synthesis in the adrenal medulla stimulates catecholamine secretion from chromaffin cells and may promote adrenal cortical growth and stimulate aldosterone synthesis.

Regulation of Vasopressin Secretion.   An increase in plasma osmolality is the principal physiological stimulus for vasopressin secretion. Severe hypovolemia/hypotension also is a powerful stimulus for vasopressin release. In addition, pain, nausea, and hypoxia can stimulate vasopressin secretion, and several endogenous hormones and pharmacological agents can modify vasopressin release.

Hyperosmolality.   The relationship between plasma osmolality and plasma vasopressin concentration is shown in Figure 30–2A, and the relationship between plasma vasopressin levels and urine osmolality is illustrated in Figure 30–2B. The osmolality threshold for secretion is approximately 280 mOsm/kg. Below the threshold, vasopressin is

barely detectable in plasma, and above the threshold, vasopressin levels are a steep and linear function of plasma osmolality. In fact, a 2% elevation in plasma osmolality causes a two- to threefold increase in plasma vasopressin levels. Therefore, a small increase in plasma osmolality leads to enhanced vasopressin secretion, which, in turn, causes increased solute-free water reabsorption (as evidenced by the increased urine osmolality). Increases in plasma osmolality (due to insensible water losses) above 290 mOsm/kg lead to an intense desire for water (thirst). Thus, the vasopressin system affords the organism longer thirst-free periods and, in the event that water is unavailable, allows the organism to survive longer periods of water deprivation. It is important to point out, however, that above a plasma osmolality of approximately 290 mOsm/kg, plasma levels of vasopressin exceed 5 pM. Since urinary concentration is maximal (about 1200 mOsm/kg) when vasopressin levels exceed 5 pM, further defense against hypertonicity is entirely dependent on water intake rather than on decreases in water loss.

Several CNS structures are involved in osmotic stimulation of vasopressin release; these structures are collectively referred to as the *osmoreceptive complex.* Although magnocellular neurons in the SON and PVN are osmosensitive, afferent inputs from other components of

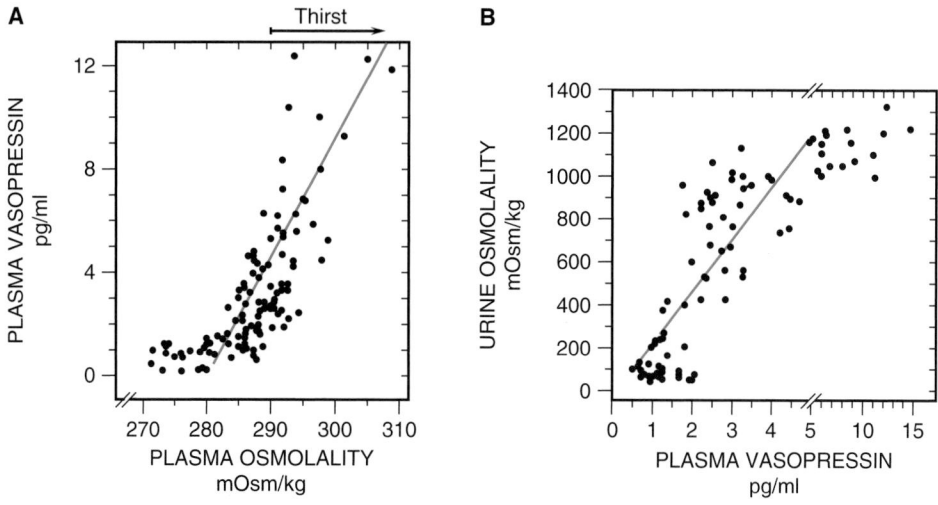

Figure 30–2.

A. The relationship between plasma osmolality and plasma vasopressin levels. Plasma osmolality associated with thirst is indicated by arrow. *B.* The relationship between plasma vasopressin levels and urine osmolality. (From Robertson *et al.,* 1977, and Kovacs and Robertson, 1992, with permission.)

the osmoreceptive complex are required for a normal vasopressin response. The SON and PVN receive projections from the subfornical organ (SFO) and the organum vasculosum of the lamina terminalis (OVLT) either directly or indirectly [*via* the median preoptic nucleus (MnPO)]. Subgroups of neurons in the SFO, OVLT, and MnPO are either osmoreceptors or osmoresponders (*i.e.,* are stimulated by osmoreceptive neurons located at other sites). Thus, a web of interconnecting neurons contributes to osmotically induced vasopressin secretion.

Aquaporin 4, a water-selective channel, is associated with CNS structures involved in osmoregulation and may confer osmosensitivity. In the CNS, aquaporin 4 resides on glial and ependymal cells rather than neurons, suggesting that osmotic status may be communicated to neuronal cell by a glial–neuron interaction (Wells, 1998).

Hypovolemia and Hypotension.   Vasopressin secretion also is regulated hemodynamically by changes in effective blood volume and/or arterial blood pressure (Robertson, 1992). Reductions in effective blood volume and/or arterial blood pressure, regardless of the cause (*e.g.,* hemorrhage, sodium depletion, diuretics, heart failure, hepatic cirrhosis with ascites, adrenal insufficiency, hypotensive drugs), may be associated with high circulating concentrations of vasopressin. However, unlike osmoregulation, hemodynamic regulation of vasopressin secretion is exponential, *i.e.,* small decreases (5% to 10%) in blood volume and/or pressure have little effect on vasopressin secretion, whereas larger decreases (20% to 30%) can increase vasopressin levels to 20 to 30 times normal levels (exceeding the concentration of vasopressin required to induce maximal antidiuresis). Vasopressin is one of the most potent vasoconstrictors known,

and the vasopressin response to hypovolemia or hypotension serves as a mechanism to stave off cardiovascular collapse during periods of severe blood loss and/or hypotension. Importantly, hemodynamic regulation of vasopressin secretion does not disrupt osmotic regulation; rather, hypovolemia/hypotension alters the setpoint and slope of the plasma osmolality–plasma vasopressin relationship (Figure 30–3).

The neuronal pathways that mediate hemodynamic regulation of vasopressin release are completely different from those involved in osmoregulation. Baroreceptors in the left atrium, left

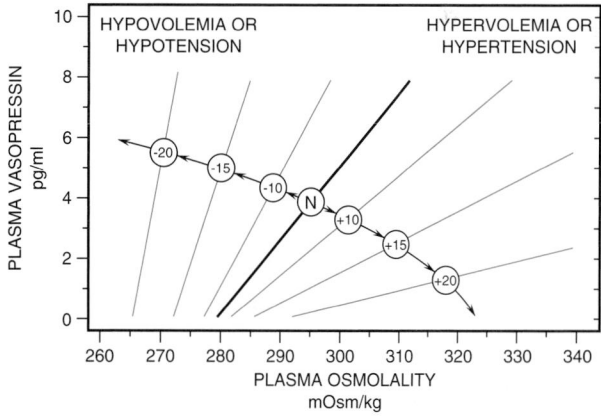

Figure 30–3. Interactions between osmolality and hypovolemia/hypotension.

Numbers in circles refer to percentage increase (+) or decrease (−) in blood volume or arterial blood pressure. N indicates normal blood volume/blood pressure. (From Robertson, 1992, with permission.)

ventricle, and pulmonary veins sense blood volume (filling pressures), and baroreceptors in the carotid sinus and aorta monitor arterial blood pressure. Nerve impulses reach brainstem nuclei predominantly through the vagus and glossopharyngeal nerves; these signals are relayed to the nucleus of the solitary tract, then to the A_1-noradrenergic cell group in the caudal ventrolateral medulla, and finally to the SON and PVN (Cunningham and Sawchenko, 1991).

Hormones and Neurotransmitters. There is a large, sometimes contradictory, body of literature on modulation of vasopressin secretion by hormones and neurotransmitters (Renaud and Bourque, 1991). Vasopressin-synthesizing magnocellular neurons have a large array of receptors on both perikarya and nerve terminals; therefore, vasopressin release can be accentuated or attenuated by chemical agents acting at both ends of the magnocellular neuron. Also, hormones and neurotransmitters can modulate vasopressin secretion by stimulating or inhibiting neurons in nuclei that project, either directly or indirectly, to the SON and PVN. Because of these complexities, the results of any given investigation may depend critically on the route of administration of the agent and on the experimental paradigm. In many cases, the precise mechanism by which a given agent modulates vasopressin secretion is either unknown or controversial, and the physiological relevance of modulation of vasopressin secretion by most hormones and neurotransmitters is unclear.

Nonetheless, several agents are known to stimulate vasopressin secretion, including acetylcholine (*via* nicotinic receptors), histamine (*via* H_1 receptors), dopamine (*via* both D_1 and D_2 receptors), glutamine, aspartate, cholecystokinin, neuropeptide Y, substance P, vasoactive intestinal polypeptide, prostaglandins, and angiotensin II. Inhibitors of vasopressin secretion include atrial natriuretic peptide, gamma-aminobutyric acid, and opioids (particularly dynorphin *via* κ receptors). Of all the aforementioned hormones/neurotransmitters, angiotensin II has received the most attention (Phillips, 1987). Angiotensin II, when applied directly to magnocellular neurons in the SON and PVN, increases neuronal excitability; when applied to the MnPO, angiotensin II indirectly stimulates magnocellular neurons in the SON and PVN. In addition, angiotensin II stimulates angiotensin-sensitive neurons in the OVLT and SFO (circumventricular nuclei lacking a blood–brain barrier) that project to the SON/PVN. Thus, both angiotensin II synthesized in the brain and that formed in the circulation may stimulate vasopressin release. Inhibition of the conversion of angiotensin II to angiotensin III blocks angiotensin II–induced vasopressin release, suggesting that angiotensin III is the main effector peptide of the brain renin–angiotensin system controlling vasopressin release (Zini *et al.*, 1996).

Pharmacological Agents. A number of drugs alter the osmolality of urine. It has been hypothesized that the action of many agents involves stimulation or inhibition of the secretion of vasopressin (Robertson, 1992). In some cases, the mechanism by which a drug alters vasopressin secretion involves direct effects on one or more CNS structures involved in the regulation of vasopressin secretion. In other cases, vasopressin secretion is indirectly altered by the effects of a drug on blood volume, arterial blood pressure, pain, or nausea. In most cases, the mechanism is not known. Stimulators of vasopressin secretion include vincristine, cyclophosphamide, tricyclic antidepressants, nicotine, epinephrine, and high doses of morphine.

Lithium, which inhibits the renal effects of vasopressin, also enhances vasopressin secretion. Inhibitors of vasopressin secretion include ethanol, phenytoin, low doses of morphine, glucocorticoids, fluphenazine, haloperidol, promethazine, oxilorphan, and butorphanol. Carbamazepine has a renal action to produce antidiuresis in patients with central diabetes insipidus but actually inhibits vasopressin secretion *via* a central action.

BASIC PHARMACOLOGY OF VASOPRESSIN

Vasopressin Receptors. The cellular effects of vasopressin are mediated by interactions of the hormone with the two principal types of receptors, V_1 and V_2. V_1 receptors have been subclassified further as V_{1a} and V_{1b}. The V_{1a} receptor is the most widespread subtype of vasopressin receptor; it is found in vascular smooth muscle, the adrenal gland, myometrium, the bladder, adipocytes, hepatocytes, platelets, renal medullary interstitial cells, vasa recta in the renal microcirculation, epithelial cells in the renal cortical collecting duct, spleen, testis, and in many CNS structures. The adenohypophysis and the adrenal medulla are known to contain V_{1b} receptors, whereas V_2 receptors are located predominantly in principal cells of the renal collecting duct system. Although originally defined by pharmacological criteria, V_{1a} (Morel *et al.*, 1992), V_{1b} (Sugimoto *et al.*, 1994), and V_2 receptors (Birnbaumer *et al.*, 1992; Lolait *et al.*, 1992) have been cloned, and vasopressin receptors now are defined by their primary amino acid sequences. The cloned vasopressin receptors are typical G protein–coupled receptors containing seven transmembrane-spanning domains. Manning and coworkers (1999) have synthesized novel, hypotensive vasopressin peptide agonists that do not interact with V_{1a}, V_{1b}, or V_2 receptors and may stimulate a putative vasopressin vasodilatory receptor.

V_1 Receptor–Effector Coupling. Considerable progress has been made in defining the mechanisms by which vasopressin receptors are coupled to biological responses (Thibonnier *et al.*, 1993; Holtzman and Ausiello, 1994). Figure 30–4 summarizes the current model of V_1 receptor–effector coupling. When vasopressin binds to V_1 receptors, a G protein–mediated activation of several membrane-bound phospholipases ensues. Activation of phospholipase C-β, probably *via* G_q, is responsible for hydrolysis of phosphatidylinositol-1,4,5-bisphosphate with the resultant generation of inositol-1,4,5-trisphosphate (IP_3) and diacylglycerol (DAG). IP_3 binds to a receptor located on Ca^{2+}-release channels in intracellular IP_3-sensitive Ca^{2+} stores, an event that triggers intracellular release of Ca^{2+}. Although the mechanism is unclear, V_1 receptors also cause Ca^{2+} influx from the extracellular compartment *via* Ca^{2+} channels located on the cell membrane. Ca^{2+} binds to and activates a number of intracellular proteins that contribute to the ultimate cellular response.

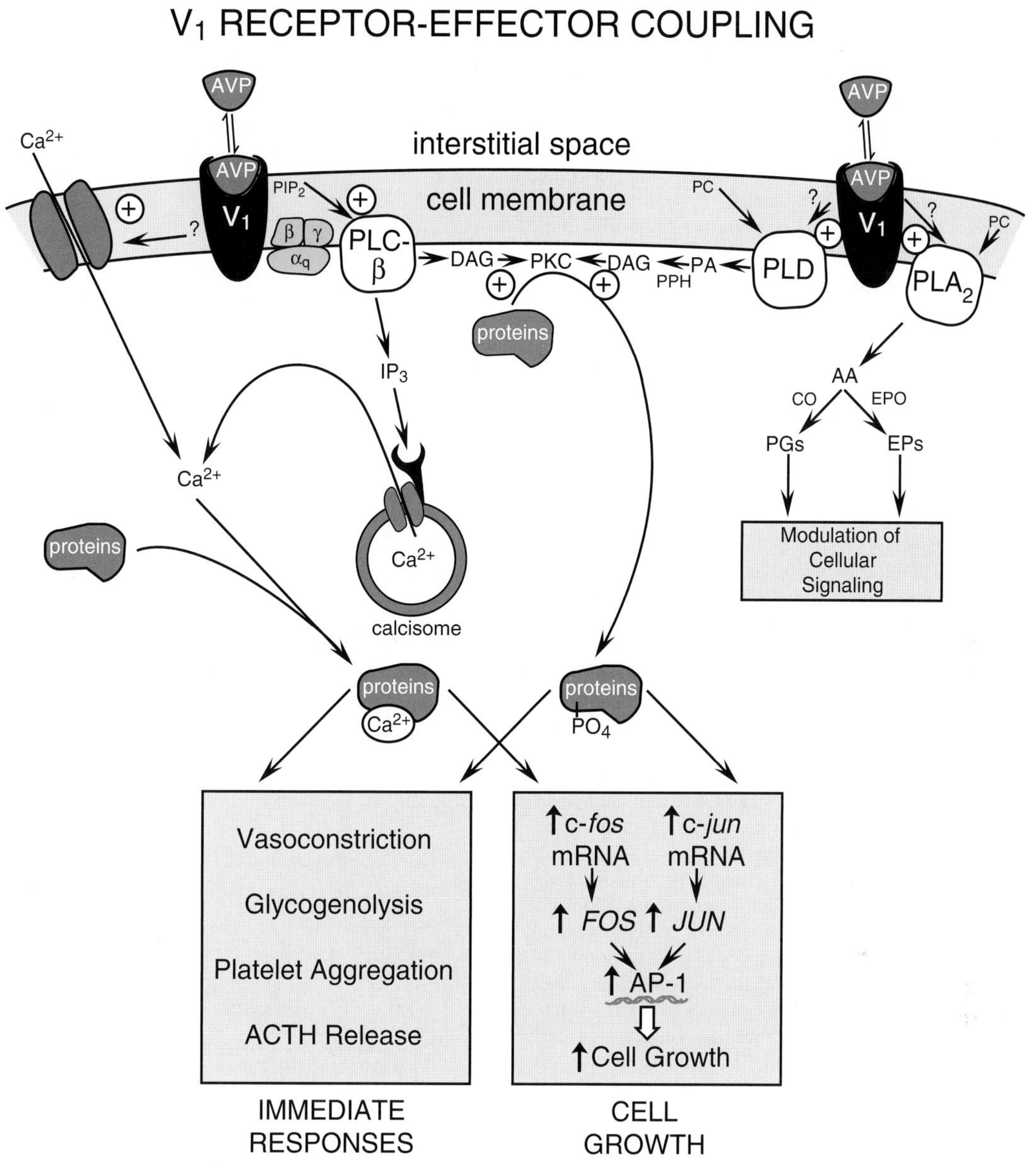

V₁ RECEPTOR-EFFECTOR COUPLING

Figure 30–4. Mechanism of V₁ receptor–effector coupling.

See text for details. "?" indicates that mechanism of coupling is unclear. V_1, V_1 vasopressin receptor; AVP, 8-arginine vasopressin; α_q, β, γ, subunits of G protein; PLD, phospholipase D; PLC-β, phospholipase C-β; PLA_2, phospholipase A_2; DAG, 1,2-diacylglycerol; PKC, protein kinase C; PIP_2, phosphatidyl-inositol-4-5-bisphosphate; IP_3, 1,4,5-inositol trisphosphate; PA, phosphatidic acid; PPH, phosphatidate phosphohydrolase; PC, phosphatidylcholine; AA, arachidonic acid; PGs, prostaglandins; EPs, epoxyeicosatrienoic acids; CO, cyclooxygenase; EPO, epoxygenase; AP-1, transcription factor consisting of heterodimer of FOS and JUN; c-*fos* and c-*jun* are proto-oncogenes; FOS and JUN are products of c-*fos* and c-*jun* gene expression, respectively.

Stimulation of phospholipase D by V_1 receptors mediates the hydrolysis of other phospholipids to produce phosphatidic acid, which is further metabolized to DAG. G protein–coupled receptors, such as the V_1 receptor, may activate phospholipase D *via* Ca^{2+}, protein kinase C, or small GTP-binding proteins such as ARF and Rho. Activation of protein kinase C by DAG leads to the phosphorylation of key proteins, and these phosphoproteins also contribute to the biological response. Finally, stimulation of phospholipase A_2, either in the membrane or in cytosol, mobilizes arachidonic acid from phospholipids, which is metabolized to various prostaglandins and epoxyeicosatrienoic acids *via* cyclooxygenase and epoxygenase, respectively (Chapter 26). Metabolites of arachidonic acid modulate biological responses to vasopressin at least in part by stimulating their own eicosanoid receptors. The biological effects mediated by the V_1 receptor include vasoconstriction, glycogenolysis, platelet aggregation, ACTH release, and growth of vascular smooth muscle cells. The effects of vasopressin on cell growth appear to involve increased expression of the proto-oncogenes c-*fos* and c-*jun*. The products of these proto-oncogenes, Fos and Jun, activate the transcription of other genes involved in the regulation of cellular growth.

V_2 Receptor–Effector Coupling.   Principal cells in the renal collecting duct have V_2 receptors on their basolateral membranes that are coupled to adenylyl cyclase *via* the timulatory G protein G_s (*see* Figure 30–5). Consequently, when vasopressin binds to V_2 receptors, adenylyl cyclase is stimulated, and intracellular levels of cyclic AMP are increased. Activation of cyclic AMP–dependent protein kinase (protein kinase A) mediates the hydroosmotic effects of vasopressin (Snyder *et al.,* 1992) *via* protein phosphorylation. In this regard, protein kinase A–mediated protein phosphorylation triggers an increased rate of exocytosis of water channel–containing vesicles (WCVs) into the apical membrane and a decreased rate of endocytosis of WCVs from the apical membrane. The distribution of WCVs between the cytosolic compartment and the apical membrane compartment is thus shifted in favor of the apical membrane compartment (Knepper and Nielsen, 1993; Nielsen *et al.,* 1999). Because WCVs contain preformed, functional water channels (aquaporin 2) their increased rate of insertion into and decreased rate of removal from the apical membrane greatly increases the water permeability of the apical membrane.

Aquaporins are a family of water channel proteins that allow water molecules to cross biological membranes (Nielsen *et al.,* 1999; Marples *et al.,* 1999). Aquaporins have six membrane domains connected by five loops (A to E). Loops B and E dip into the cell membrane, and the asparagine-proline-alanine sequences in each B and E loop interact to form a water pore. Aquaporins generally form tetrameric complexes in cell membranes. Of the nine cloned mammalian aquaporins, six are found in the kidney. Aquaporin 1 is present in the apical and basolateral membrane of the proximal tubule and in the thin descending limb. Aquaporin 2 resides in the apical membrane and WCVs of the collecting duct principal cells, whereas aquaporins 3 and 4 are present in the basolateral membrane of principal cells. Aquaporin 7 is in the apical brush border of the straight proximal tubule. Although aquaporin 6 is found in the kidney, its distribution is unknown. Aquaporin 2, the water channel in WCVs, is phosphorylated on serine 256 by protein kinase A, and this is the first step leading to vasopressin-induced insertion of WCVs into apical membranes (Nishimoto *et al.,* 1999). In addition to increasing the insertion of aquaporin 2 into apical membranes in collecting duct principal cells, vasopressin also increases the expression of aquaporin 2 mRNA and protein (Marples *et al.,* 1999). This effect is mediated by protein kinase A phosphorylation of cyclic AMP–response element binding protein (CREB). Phosphorylated CREB is a transcription factor that binds to the cyclic AMP–response element (CRE) in the 5'-untranslated region of the gene encoding aquaporin 2 and increases its transcription. Thus, chronic dehydration leads to

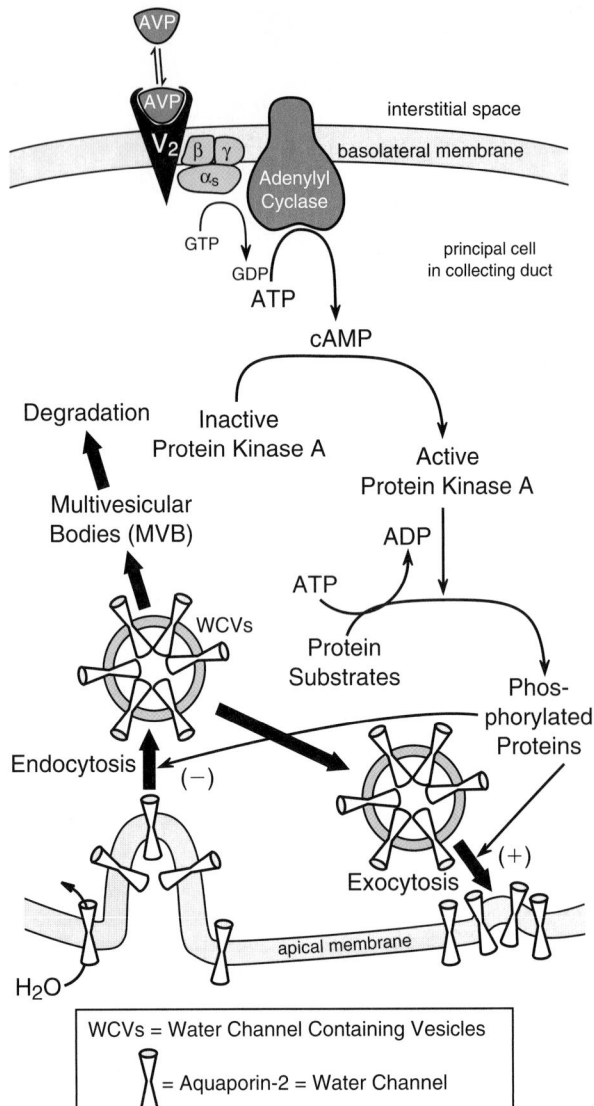

V_2 RECEPTOR-EFFECTOR COUPLING

Figure 30–5. Mechanism of V_2 receptor–effector coupling.

See text for details. V_2, V_2 vasopressin receptor; AVP, 8-arginine vasopressin; α_s, β, and γ, subunits of G protein; ATP, adenosine triphosphate; ADP, adenosine diphosphate; cAMP, adenosine 3',5'-monophosphate (cyclic AMP).

long-term upregulation of aquaporin 2 and water transport in the collecting duct.

For maximum concentration of urine, large amounts of urea must be deposited in the interstitium of the inner medullary collecting duct. It is not surprising, therefore, that V_2 receptor activation also increases urea permeability by 400% in the terminal portions of the inner medullary collecting duct. The mechanism by which V_2 receptors increase urea permeability involves activation of a vasopressin-regulated urea transporter (termed VRUT, UT1, or UT-A1), most likely by protein kinase A–induced phosphorylation (Star *et al.,*1988; Sands, 1999). The kinetics of vasopressin-induced water and urea permeability are different (Nielsen and Knepper, 1993), and vasopressin-induced regulation of VRUT does not entail vesicular trafficking to the plasma membrane (Inoue *et al.,* 1999).

In addition to increasing the permeability of the collecting duct to water and the permeability of the inner medullary collecting duct to urea, V_2 receptor activation also increases both short- and long-term NaCl transport in the thick ascending limb. Increased transport in the thick ascending limb augments the countercurrent multiplication system and thereby increases the osmolality of the medullary interstitium and the reabsorption of water (Knepper *et al.,* 1999). This effect, which is most likely mediated by cyclic AMP and protein kinase A–induced

phosphorylation, involves the immediate stimulation of Na^+–K^+–$2Cl^-$ symporter expression (Kim *et al.,* 1999). The multiple mechanisms by which vasopressin increases water reabsorption are summarized in Figure 30–6.

Renal Actions of Vasopressin. There are several sites of vasopressin action in the kidney involving both V_1 and V_2 receptors. V_1 receptors mediate contraction of mesangial cells in the glomerulus and contraction of vascular smooth muscle cells in the vasa recta and efferent arteriole (Edwards *et al.,* 1989). Indeed, V_1 receptor–mediated reduction in inner medullary blood flow contributes to the maximum concentrating capacity of the kidney (Franchini and Cowley, 1996) (*see* Figure 30–6). V_1 receptors also

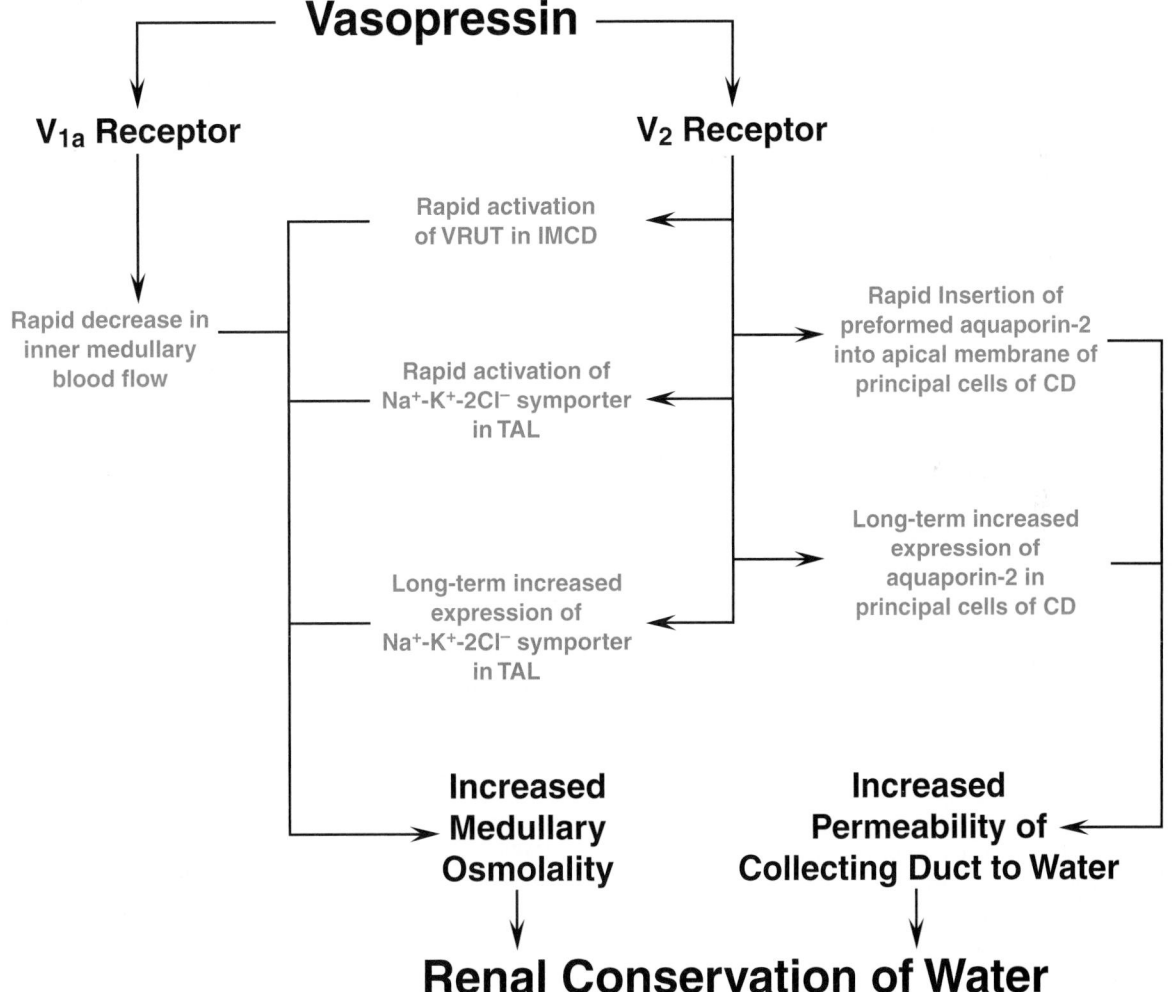

Figure 30–6. Mechanisms by which vasopressin increases the renal conservation of water.

IMCD, inner medullary collecting duct; CD, collecting duct; TAL, thick ascending limb; VRUT, vasopressin-regulated urea transporter.

stimulate prostaglandin synthesis by medullary interstitial cells. Since prostaglandin E_2 inhibits adenylyl cyclase in the collecting duct, stimulation of prostaglandin synthesis by V_1 receptors may function to restrain V_2 receptor–mediated antidiuresis (Sonnenberg and Smith, 1988). V_1 receptors on principal cells in the cortical collecting duct (Burnatowska-Hledin and Spielman, 1989) may directly inhibit V_2 receptor–mediated water flux *via* activation of protein kinase C (Schlondorff and Levine, 1985).

Without question, V_2 receptors mediate the most prominent response to vasopressin, *i.e.,* increased water permeability of the collecting duct. Indeed, vasopressin can increase water permeability in the collecting duct at concentrations as low as 50 fM. Thus, V_2 receptor-mediated effects of vasopressin occur at concentrations far lower than are required to engage the V_1 receptor-mediated actions; however, this differential sensitivity may not be due to differences in receptor affinities, since cloned rat V_{1a} and V_2 receptors have similar affinities for vasopressin ($K_d = 0.7$ and 0.4 nM, respectively). The differential sensitivity may instead be due to differential amplification of signal transduction pathways evoked by these receptors.

The collecting duct system is critical for the conservation of water. By the time tubular fluid arrives at the cortical collecting duct, it has been rendered hypotonic by the upstream diluting segments of the nephron that reabsorb NaCl without reabsorbing water. In the well-hydrated subject, plasma osmolality is in the normal range, concentrations of vasopressin are low, the entire collecting duct is relatively impermeable to water, and the urine is dilute. Under conditions of dehydration, plasma osmolality is increased, concentrations of vasopressin are elevated, and the collecting duct becomes permeable to water. The osmotic gradient between the dilute tubular urine and the hypertonic renal interstitial fluid (which becomes progressively more hypertonic in deeper regions of the renal medulla) provides for the osmotic flux of water out of the collecting duct. The final osmolality of urine may be as high as 1200 mOsm/kg in human beings, and a significant saving of solute-free water is thus possible.

Other renal actions mediated by V_2 receptors include increased urea transport in the inner medullary collecting duct and increased NaCl transport in the thick ascending limb; both effects contribute to the urine-concentrating ability of the kidney. V_2 receptors also increase Na^+ transport in the cortical collecting duct (Schafer and Troutman, 1990).

Pharmacological Modification of the Antidiuretic Response to Vasopressin.   Nonsteroidal antiinflammatory drugs (NSAIDs) (*see* Chapter 27), particularly indo-

methacin, enhance the antidiuretic response to vasopressin. Since prostaglandins attenuate antidiuretic responses to vasopressin and NSAIDs inhibit prostaglandin synthesis, reduced prostaglandin production probably accounts for the potentiation of vasopressin's antidiuretic response. Other drugs that enhance the antidiuretic effects of vasopressin include carbamazepine and chlorpropamide; however, the mechanisms by which these agents potentiate the antidiuretic response to vasopressin are not known. In rare instances, chlorpropamide can induce water intoxication.

A number of drugs inhibit the antidiuretic actions of vasopressin. Lithium is of particular importance because of its wide use in the treatment of manic-depressive disorders. Lithium-induced polyuria is usually, but not always, reversible (Ramsey and Cox, 1982). Acutely, lithium appears to reduce V_2 receptor–mediated stimulation of adenylyl cyclase. The mechanism of this effect may involve attenuation of G_s-mediated activation of adenylyl cyclase (Cogan and Abramow, 1986; Goldberg *et al.,* 1988) and/or enhancement of G_i-mediated inhibition of adenylyl cyclase (Yamaki *et al.,* 1991). Also, lithium increases plasma levels of parathyroid hormone, and parathyroid hormone is a partial antagonist to vasopressin (Carney *et al.,* 1996). In most patients, the antibiotic demeclocycline attenuates the antidiuretic effects of vasopressin, and this action of demeclocycline is probably due to decreased accumulation and action of cyclic AMP (Singer and Rotenberg, 1973).

Nonrenal Actions of Vasopressin.   Vasopressin and related peptides are ancient hormones in evolutionary terms, and they are found in species that do not concentrate urine. It is thus not surprising that vasopressin has nonrenal actions in mammals. *Cardiovascular System.*   The cardiovascular effects of vasopressin are complex, and vasopressin's role in physiological situations is ill-defined. Vasopressin is a potent vasoconstrictor (V_1 receptor–mediated), and resistance vessels throughout the circulation may be affected (László *et al.,* 1991). Vascular smooth muscle in the skin, skeletal muscle, fat, pancreas, and thyroid gland appear most sensitive, with significant vasoconstriction also occurring in the gastrointestinal tract, coronary vessels, and brain (Liard *et al.,* 1982). However, despite the potency of vasopressin as a direct vasoconstrictor, vasopressin-induced pressor responses *in vivo* are minimal and occur only with concentrations of vasopressin significantly higher than those required for maximal antidiuresis. To a large extent, this is due to circulating vasopressin that acts on V_1 receptors to inhibit sympathetic efferents and potentiate baroreflexes (Abboud *et al.,* 1990). In addition, in some blood vessels, V_2 receptors cause vasodilation, perhaps *via* release of nitric oxide (a potent vasodilator) from the vascular endothelium (Aki *et al.,* 1994), and studies by Manning and coworkers (1999) suggest the existence of a unique vasopressin vasodilator receptor.

A large body of data from experimental animals supports the conclusion that vasopressin helps maintain arterial blood pressure during episodes of severe hypovolemia/hypotension

(László *et al.,* 1991). However, antagonism of V_1 receptors does not alter the hypotensive response to lower-body negative pressure in normal subjects despite a fivefold elevation in circulating vasopressin levels (Hirsch *et al.,* 1993). Vasopressin also may increase total peripheral resistance in heart failure, and administration of a peptide V_1 receptor antagonist improves hemodynamic function in such patients (Thibonnier, 1988). At present, there is no convincing evidence for a role of vasopressin in essential hypertension in human beings (Kawano *et al.,* 1997).

The effects of vasopressin on the heart (reduced cardiac output and heart rate) are largely indirect and are the result of coronary vasoconstriction, decreased coronary blood flow, and alterations in vagal and sympathetic tone (László *et al.,* 1991). In human beings, the effects of vasopressin on coronary blood flow can be easily demonstrated, especially if large doses are employed. The cardiac actions of the hormone are of more than academic interest. Some patients with coronary insufficiency experience anginal pain even in response to the relatively small amounts of vasopressin required to control diabetes insipidus, and vasopressin-induced myocardial ischemia has led to severe reactions and even death.

Central Nervous System. It is likely that vasopressin plays a role as a neurotransmitter and/or neuromodulator (Gash *et al.,* 1987; Jolles, 1987). Vasopressin may participate in the acquisition of certain learned behaviors (Dantzer and Bluthé, 1993), in the development of some complex social processes (Insel *et al.,* 1993; Young *et al.,* 1998), and in the pathogenesis of specific psychiatric diseases (Legros *et al.,* 1993). However, the physiological/pathophysiological relevance of these findings is controversial, and some of the actions of vasopressin on memory and learned behavior may be due to visceral autonomic effects. In 1931, Cushing reported on the antipyretic effects of pituitary extracts injected into the lateral ventricle of febrile patients. Since then, many studies have supported a physiological role for vasopressin as a naturally occurring antipyretic factor (Kasting, 1989; Cridland and Kasting, 1992). Although vasopressin can modulate CNS autonomic systems controlling heart rate, arterial blood pressure, respiration rate, and sleep patterns, the physiological significance of these actions is unclear. Finally, secretion of ACTH is enhanced by vasopressin that is delivered to the anterior pituitary *via* a neuronal pathway leading to secretion of peptide into the hypophyseal portal blood. However, vasopressin is not the principal corticotropin-releasing factor. The CNS effects of vasopressin appear to be mediated predominantly by V_1 receptors.

Blood Coagulation. Activation of V_2 receptors by desmopressin or vasopressin increases circulating levels of procoagulant factor VIII and of von Willebrand factor (David, 1993). This effect is mediated by extrarenal V_2 receptors (Bernat *et al.,* 1997). Presumably, vasopressin stimulates the secretion of von Willebrand factor and of factor VIII from storage sites in vascular endothelium. However, since release of von Willebrand factor does not occur when desmopressin is applied directly to cultured endothelial cells or to isolated blood vessels, intermediate factors are likely to be involved. In this regard, it has been hypothesized that desmopressin releases interleukin 1 (IL-1) from monocytes, and IL-1 can then release von Willebrand factor (Breit and Green, 1988).

Other Nonrenal Effects of Vasopressin. At high concentrations, vasopressin stimulates uterine (*via* oxytocin receptors) and gastrointestinal (*via* V_1 receptors) smooth muscle. Vasopressin

is stored in platelets, and V_1 receptors stimulate platelet aggregation (Inaba *et al.,* 1988). Also, V_1 receptors located on hepatocytes stimulate glycogenolysis (Keppens and de Wulf, 1975). The physiological significance of these effects of vasopressin is not known.

DISEASES AFFECTING THE VASOPRESSIN SYSTEM

Diabetes Insipidus (DI). DI is a disease of impaired renal conservation of water due either to an inadequate secretion of vasopressin from the neurohypophysis (central or cranial DI) or to an insufficient renal response to vasopressin (nephrogenic DI). Very rarely, DI can be caused by an abnormally high rate of degradation of vasopressin by circulating vasopressinases (Durr *et al.,* 1987). Pregnancy may accentuate or reveal central and/or nephrogenic DI by increasing plasma levels of vasopressinase and by reducing the renal sensitivity to vasopressin. Patients with DI excrete large volumes (more than 30 ml/kg per day) of dilute (less than 200 mOsm/kg) urine and, if their thirst mechanism is functioning normally, are polydipsic. In contrast to the sweet urine excreted by patients with diabetes mellitus, urine from patients with DI is tasteless, hence the name, *insipidus.* Fortunately, the urinary taste test for DI devised by Willis in the seventeenth century has been supplanted by the more palatable approach of simply observing whether the patient is able to reduce urine volume and increase urine osmolality after a period of carefully observed fluid deprivation. Central DI can be distinguished from nephrogenic DI by administration of desmopressin, which will increase urine osmolality in patients with central DI but have little or no effect in patients with nephrogenic DI. DI can be differentiated from primary polydipsia by measuring plasma osmolality, which will be low to low-normal in patients with primary polydipsia and high to high-normal in patients with DI. For a more complete discussion of diagnostic procedures, see Vokes and Robertson (1988).

Central DI. Head injury, either surgical or traumatic, in the region of the pituitary and/or hypothalamus may cause central DI. Postoperative central DI may be transient, permanent, or triphasic (recovery followed by permanent relapse) (Seckl and Dunger, 1992). Other causes include hypothalamic or pituitary tumors, cerebral aneurysms, CNS ischemia, and brain infiltrations and infections. Finally, central DI may be idiopathic or familial. Familial central DI is usually autosomal dominant (chromosome 20) and has been associated with point mutations in the signal peptide and VP-neurophysin (*see* Figure 30–1), leading to defects in the synthesis, processing, and transport of the preprohormone complex (Raymond, 1994). Since familial central DI is autosomal dominant, the defective preprohormone coded by the mutant allele must interfere in some way with the synthesis of hormone coded by the normal allele.

Antidiuretic peptides are the primary treatment for central DI, with desmopressin being the peptide of choice. (*See* "Clinical Pharmacology of Vasopressin Peptides," below, for discussion of antidiuretic peptides in the treatment of central DI.) For patients with central DI who cannot tolerate antidiuretic peptides because of side effects or allergic reactions, other treatment options are available. *Chlorpropamide,* an oral sulfonylurea that potentiates the action of small or residual amounts of circulating vasopressin, will cause a reduction in urine volume in more than half of all patients with central DI at a dose of 125 to 500 mg daily and is particularly effective in patients with partial central DI, where it potentiates the action of low levels of circulating vasopressin. If polyuria is not satisfactorily controlled with chlorpropamide alone, addition of a thiazide diuretic (Chapter 29) to the regimen usually results in an adequate reduction in the volume of urine. *Carbamazepine* (800 to 1000 mg daily in divided doses) and *clofibrate* (1 to 2 g daily in divided doses) also reduce urine volume in patients with central DI. Long-term use of these agents may induce serious adverse effects; therefore carbamazepine and clofibrate are rarely used to treat central DI. The antidiuretic mechanism(s) of chlorpropamide, carbamazepine, and clofibrate are not clear. These agents are not effective in nephrogenic DI, which indicates that functional V_2 receptors are required for the antidiuretic mechanism to be expressed. Since carbamazepine inhibits and chlorpropamide has little effect on vasopressin secretion, it is likely that carbamazepine and chlorpropamide act directly on the kidney to enhance V_2 receptor–mediated antidiuresis.

Nephrogenic DI. Nephrogenic DI may be acquired or genetic. Hypercalcemia, hypokalemia, postobstructive renal failure, lithium, and demeclocycline can induce nephrogenic DI. As many as one in three patients treated with lithium may develop nephrogenic DI. Familial, X-linked, recessive nephrogenic DI is caused by mutations in the gene coding for the V_2 receptor (a gene located in the q28 region of the X chromosome). A number of missense, nonsense, and frame-shift mutations in the gene encoding the V_2 receptor have been identified in patients with familial, X-linked nephrogenic DI (Oksche and Rosenthal, 1998; Morello *et al.*, 2000). Of all mutant alleles reported to date, mutations encoded result predominantly in abnormal synthesis, processing, or intracellular transport of V_2 receptors. Autosomal recessive nephrogenic DI is caused

by inactivating mutations in aquaporin 2 (13 different mutations have been identified to date). These findings indicate that aquaporin 2 is essential for the antidiuretic effect of vasopressin in human beings (Deen *et al.*, 1994).

Although the mainstay of treatment of nephrogenic DI is assurance of an adequate intake of water, drugs also can be used to reduce polyuria. *Amiloride* (Chapter 29) blocks the uptake of lithium by the sodium channel in the collecting duct system and is therefore the drug of choice for lithium-induced nephrogenic DI. Paradoxically, thiazide diuretics cause a reduction in the polyuria of patients with DI and often are used to treat nephrogenic DI. The use of thiazide diuretics in infants with nephrogenic DI may be crucially important, since uncontrolled polyuria may exceed the child's capacity to imbibe and absorb fluids. The antidiuretic mechanism of thiazides in DI is incompletely understood. It is possible that the natriuretic action of thiazides and resultant depletion of extracellular fluid volume play an important role in the thiazide-induced antidiuresis in DI. In this regard, whenever extracellular fluid volume is reduced, compensatory mechanisms increase reabsorption of NaCl in the proximal tubule, with a resultant reduction of volume delivered to the distal tubule. Consequently, less free water can be formed, and this should diminish polyuria. However, recent studies in rats with vasopressin-deficient DI seriously challenge this hypothesis (Grønbeck *et al.*, 1998). Nonetheless, the antidiuretic effects appear to parallel the ability of thiazides to cause natriuresis, and the drugs are given in doses similar to those used for mobilization of edema fluid. In patients with DI, a 50% reduction of urine volume is a good response to thiazides. Moderate restriction of sodium intake can enhance the antidiuretic effectiveness of thiazides.

A number of case reports describe the effectiveness of indomethacin in the treatment of nephrogenic DI (Libber *et al.*, 1986); however, other prostaglandin synthase inhibitors (*e.g.*, ibuprofen) appear to be less effective. The mechanism of the effects of indomethacin is unclear but may involve a decrease in glomerular filtration rate, an increase in medullary solute concentration, and/or enhanced proximal reabsorption of fluid (Seckl and Dunger, 1992). Also, since prostaglandins attenuate vasopressin-induced antidiuresis in patients with at least a partially intact V_2 receptor system, a portion of the antidiuretic response to indomethacin may be due to enhancement of the effects of vasopressin on the principal cells of the collecting duct.

Syndrome of Inappropriate Secretion of Antidiuretic Hormone (SIADH).   SIADH is a disease of impaired water excretion with accompanying hyponatremia and hypoosmolality caused by the *inappropriate* secretion of vasopressin. The clinical manifestations of plasma hypotonicity resulting from SIADH may include lethargy, anorexia, nausea/vomiting, muscle cramps, coma, convulsions, and death. A multitude of disorders can induce SIADH (Zerbe *et al.*, 1980) including malignancies, pulmonary diseases, CNS injuries/diseases (head trauma, infections, tumors), general surgery, and drugs (*e.g.*, cisplatin, vinca alkaloids, cyclophosphamide, chloropropamide, thiazide diuretics, phenothiazines, carbamazepine, clofibrate, nicotine, narcotics, and tricyclic antidepressants). In a normal individual, an elevation in plasma vasopressin levels *per se* does not induce plasma hypotonicity, because the person simply stops drinking due to an osmotically induced aversion to fluids. Therefore, plasma hypotonicity only occurs when excessive fluid intake (oral or intravenous) accompanies inappropriate secretion of vasopressin. Treatment of hypotonicity in the setting of SIADH includes water restriction, intravenous administration of hypertonic saline, loop diuretics (which interfere with the concentrating ability of the kidneys), and drugs that inhibit the ability of vasopressin to increase water permeability in the collecting ducts. To inhibit vasopressin's action in the collecting ducts, *demeclocycline* is the preferred drug (however, *see* "Prospectus," below).

Although lithium can inhibit the renal actions of vasopressin, it is effective in only a minority of patients, may induce irreversible renal damage when used chronically, and has a low therapeutic index. Therefore, lithium should be used only in patients with symptomatic SIADH who cannot be controlled by other means or in whom tetracyclines are contraindicated, *e.g.*, patients with liver disease. It is important to stress that the majority of patients with SIADH do not require therapy because plasma Na^+ stabilizes in the range of 125 to 132 mM; such patients usually are asymptomatic. Only when symptomatic hypotonicity ensues, generally when plasma Na^+ levels drop below 120 mM, should therapy with demeclocycline be initiated. Since hypotonicity, which causes an influx of water into cells with resulting cerebral swelling, is the cause of symptoms, the goal of therapy is simply to increase plasma osmolality toward normal. For a more complete description of the diagnosis and treatment of SIADH, see Kovacs and Robertson (1992).

Other Water-Retaining States.   In patients with congestive heart failure, liver cirrhosis, and nephrotic syndrome, effective blood volume often is reduced, and hypovolemia is frequently exacerbated by the liberal use of diuretics in such patients. Since hypovolemia stimulates vasopressin release, patients may become hyponatremic due to vasopressin-mediated retention of water. The development

of potent, orally active V_2 receptor antagonists and specific inhibitors of water channels in the collecting duct would provide an effective therapeutic strategy, not only in patients with SIADH but also in the much more common setting of hyponatremia in patients with heart failure, liver cirrhosis, and nephrotic syndrome.

CLINICAL PHARMACOLOGY OF VASOPRESSIN PEPTIDES

Therapeutic Uses.   Only three antidiuretic peptides are available for clinical use in the United States. (1) Vasopressin (synthetic 8-L-arginine vasopressin; PITRESSIN SYNTHETIC) is available as a sterile aqueous solution; it may be administered subcutaneously, intramuscularly, or intranasally. (2) *Lypressin* (synthetic 8-lysine vasopressin; DIAPID) is supplied as an aqueous nasal spray. (3) *Desmopressin acetate* (DDAVP) is available as a sterile aqueous solution packaged for intravenous or subcutaneous injection, in a nasal solution for intranasal administration with either a nasal spray pump or rhinal tube delivery system, and in tablets for oral administration. The therapeutic uses of vasopressin and its congeners can be divided into two main categories according to the type of vasopressin receptor involved.

V_1 receptor–mediated therapeutic applications are based on the rationale that V_1 receptors cause contraction of gastrointestinal and vascular smooth muscle. V_1 receptor–mediated contraction of gastrointestinal smooth muscle is useful to treat postoperative ileus and abdominal distension and to dispel intestinal gas before abdominal roentgenography to avoid interfering gas shadows. V_1 receptor–mediated vasoconstriction of the splanchnic arterial vessels reduces blood flow to the portal system and thereby attenuates pressure and bleeding in esophageal varices (Burroughs, 1998). Although endoscopic sclerotherapy is the treatment of choice for bleeding esophageal varices, V_1 receptor agonists can be used in an emergency setting until endoscopy can be performed. Simultaneous administration of nitroglycerin with vasopressin has been reported to reverse the cardiotoxic effects of vasopressin while enhancing the beneficial splanchnic effects of the drug (Gimson *et al.*, 1986). Also, V_1 receptor agonists can be used during abdominal surgery in patients with portal hypertension to diminish the risk of hemorrhage during the procedure. Finally, V_1 receptor–mediated vasoconstriction of the gastric vascular bed reduces bleeding in acute hemorrhagic gastritis (Peterson, 1989). 8-Arginine vasopressin should be used for all V_1 receptor–mediated therapeutic applications. Although not yet available in the

United States, *terlipressin* (GLYPRESSIN) appears to be effective for bleeding esophageal varices, with reduced side effects compared with vasopressin (Soederlund, 1993).

V_2 receptor–mediated therapeutic applications are based on the rationale that V_2 receptors cause water conservation and release of blood coagulation factors. Central, but not nephrogenic, DI can be treated with V_2 receptor agonists, and polyuria and polydipsia are usually well controlled. Some patients experience transient DI (*e.g.*, in head injury or surgery in the area of the pituitary); however, for most patients with DI, therapy is lifelong. Desmopressin is the drug of choice for the vast majority of patients, and numerous clinical trials (Robinson, 1976; Cobb *et al.*, 1978) have demonstrated that desmopressin is an effective agent in both adults and children and has few side effects. The duration of effect from a single intranasal dose is from 6 to 20 hours, and twice-daily administration has proven to be effective in most patients. There is considerable variability in the intranasal dose of desmopressin required to maintain normal urine volume, and the dosage must be individually tailored. The usual intranasal dosage range in adults is 10 to 40 μg daily, either as a single dose or divided into two or three doses. In view of the high cost of the drug and the importance of avoiding water intoxication, the schedule of administration should be adjusted to determine the minimal amount required. An initial dose of 2.5 μg can be used, and therapy should first be directed toward the control of nocturia. An equivalent or higher morning dose controls daytime polyuria in most patients, although a third dose occasionally may be needed in the afternoon. In some patients, chronic allergic rhinitis or other nasal pathology may preclude reliable absorption of the peptide following nasal administration. Oral administration of desmopressin in doses 10 to 20 times the intranasal dose provides adequate blood levels of desmopressin and controls polyuria (Fjellestad-Paulsen *et al.*, 1993). Subcutaneous administration of 1 to 2 μg daily of desmopressin also is effective in central DI.

Lypressin nasal spray also can be used to treat central DI; however, lypressin's duration of action is short (4 to 6 hours), making it less convenient than desmopressin. Also, lypressin, like vasopressin, can induce V_1 receptor–mediated adverse effects. Nonetheless, for patients refractory to desmopressin or who experience side effects with desmopressin, lypressin provides an alternative. 8-Arginine vasopressin has little if any place in the long-term therapy of DI because of its short duration of action and V_1 receptor–mediated side effects. Vasopressin can be used as an alternative to desmopressin in the initial diagnostic evaluation of patients with suspected DI and to control polyuria in patients with DI who have recently undergone surgery or experienced head trauma. Under these circumstances, polyuria may be transient, and long-acting agents may produce water intoxication.

An additional V_2 receptor–mediated therapeutic application is the use of desmopressin in bleeding disorders (Mannucci, 1997; Sutor, 1998). In most patients with type I von Willebrand's disease (vWD) and in some with type IIN vWD, desmopressin will elevate von Willebrand factor and shorten bleeding time. However, desmopressin is generally ineffective in patients with types IIa, IIb, and III vWD. Desmopressin may cause a marked, transient thrombocytopenia in individuals with type IIb vWD and may be dangerous in such patients. Desmopressin also increases factor VIII levels in patients with moderately severe hemophilia A. Desmopressin is not indicated in patients with severe hemophilia A, those with hemophilia B, or those with factor VIII antibodies. The response of any given patient with type I vWD or hemophilia A to desmopressin should be determined at the time of diagnosis or 1 to 2 weeks before elective surgery to assess the extent of increase in factor VIII or von Willebrand factor. Desmopressin is employed widely to treat the hemostatic abnormalities induced by uremia (Mannucci *et al.*, 1983). In patients with renal insufficiency, desmopressin shortens bleeding time and increases circulating levels of factor VIII coagulant activity, factor VIII–related antigen, and ristocetin cofactor. It also induces the appearance of larger von Willebrand factor multimers. Desmopressin is effective in some patients with liver cirrhosis–induced or drug–induced (heparin, hirudin, antiplatelet agents) bleeding disorders. Desmopressin, given intravenously at a dose of 0.3 μg/kg, increases factor VIII and von Willebrand factor for more than 6 hours. Desmopressin can be given at intervals of 12 to 24 hours, depending on the clinical response and the severity of bleeding. Tachyphylaxis to desmopressin usually occurs after several days (due to depletion of factor VIII and von Willebrand factor storage sites) and limits its usefulness to preoperative preparation, postoperative bleeding, excessive menstrual bleeding, and emergency situations.

Another V_2 receptor–mediated therapeutic application is the use of desmopressin for primary nocturnal enuresis (Sukhai, 1993). In this regard, desmopressin should be used only intranasally and may be used alone or in combination with behavioral conditioning. Finally, desmopressin has been found to relieve post–lumbar puncture headache, probably by causing water retention and thereby facilitating rapid fluid equilibration in the CNS.

Pharmacokinetics. When vasopressin, lypressin, and desmopressin are given orally, they are quickly inactivated by trypsin, which cleaves the peptide bond between amino acids 8 and 9. Inactivation by peptidases in various tissues (particularly the liver and kidneys) results in a plasma half-life of vasopressin of 17 to 35 minutes. The plasma half-life of desmopressin has two components, a fast component of 6.5 to 9 minutes and a slow component of 30 to 117 minutes.

Toxicity, Adverse Effects, Contraindications, Drug Interactions. Most adverse effects are mediated through the V_1 receptor acting on vascular and gastrointestinal smooth muscle; consequently such adverse effects are much less common and less severe with desmopressin than with vasopressin or lypressin. After the injection of large doses of vasopressin, marked facial pallor as a result of cutaneous vasoconstriction commonly is observed. Increased intestinal activity is likely to cause nausea, belching, cramps, and an urge to defecate. Most serious, however, is the effect on the coronary circulation. Vasopressin and lypressin should be administered only at low doses and with extreme caution in individuals suffering from vascular disease, especially disease of the coronary arteries. Other cardiac complications include arrhythmia and decreased cardiac output. Peripheral vasoconstriction and gangrene have been encountered in patients receiving large doses of vasopressin.

The major V_2 receptor–mediated adverse effect is water intoxication, which can occur with desmopressin, lypressin, or vasopressin. In this regard, carbamazepine, chlorpropamide, and NSAIDs can potentiate the antidiuretic effects of these peptides. Desmopressin, lypressin, and vasopressin should be used cautiously in disease states in which a rapid increase in extracellular water may impose risks (*e.g.*, in angina, hypertension, heart failure) and should not be used in patients with acute renal failure. Also, it is imperative that these peptides not be administered to patients with primary or psychogenic polydipsia, because severe hypotonic hyponatremia will ensue.

Allergic reactions, ranging from urticaria to anaphylaxis, may occur with desmopressin, lypressin, or vasopressin. Intranasal administration may cause local adverse effects in the nasal passages, such as edema, scarring, rhinorrhea, congestion, irritation, pruritus, and ulceration.

PROSPECTUS

It is likely that nonpeptide, orally active V_2-selective receptor antagonists will become available in the near future for the treatment of dilutional hyponatremia induced by heart failure, liver cirrhosis, nephrotic syndrome, and SIADH (Schrier *et al.*, 1998; Mayinger and Hensen, 1999). In addition, orally active combined V_{1a}-/V_2-selective antagonists may become available for diseases such as congestive heart failure, in which both increased peripheral vascular resistance and dilutional hyponatremia are present (Yatsu *et al.*, 1999). Whether or not sporadic administration of membrane-permeant, nonpeptide V_2 receptor antagonists will achieve successful *in vivo* cell surface-receptor delivery of certain alleles of X-linked nephrogenic DI, as demonstrated *in vitro*, remains to be ascertained in clinical trials (Morello *et al.*, 2000).

Several important new clinical applications of the ancient hormone vasopressin are under active investigation. Vasopressin may prove superior to epinephrine as a pressor agent in cardiopulmonary resuscitation (Chugh *et al.*, 1997), and it may be particularly effective in refractory hypotension after cardiopulmonary bypass (Overland and Teply, 1998). Vasopressin levels in patients with septic shock are inappropriately low, and septic shock patients are extraordinarily sensitive to the pressor actions of vasopressin (Landry *et al.*, 1997). Vasopressin also reverses intractable hypotension in the late phase of hemorrhagic shock (Morales *et al.*, 1999). Thus, vasopressin may become the preferred pressor agent in emergency and critical care medicine.

BIBLIOGRAPHY

Aki, Y., Tamaki, T., Kiyomoto, H., He, H., Yoshida, H., Iwao, H., and Abe, Y. Nitric oxide may participate in V_2 vasopressin-receptor-mediated renal vasodilation. *J. Cardiovasc. Pharmacol.,* **1994,** *23*:331–336.

Bernat, A., Hoffmann, T., Dumas, A., Serradeil-Le Gal, C., Raufaste, D., and Herbert, J.M. V_2 receptor antagonism of DDAVP-induced release of hemostatis factors in conscious dogs. *J. Pharmacol. Exp. Ther.,* **1997,** *282*:597–602.

Birnbaumer, M., Seibold, A., Gilbert, S., Ishido, M., Barberis, C., Antaramian, A., Brabet, P., and Rosenthal, W. Molecular cloning of the receptor for human antidiuretic hormone. *Nature,* **1992,** *357*:333–335.

Breit, S.N., and Green, I. Modulation of endothelial cell synthesis of von Willebrand factor by mononuclear cell products. *Haemostasis,* **1988,** *18*:137–145.

Burnatowska-Hledin, M.A., and Spielman, W.S. Vasopressin V_1 receptors on the principal cells of the rabbit cortical collecting tubule. Stimulation of cytosolic free calcium and inositol phosphate production *via* coupling to a pertussis toxin substrate. *J. Clin. Invest.,* **1989,** *83*:84–89.

Carney, S.L., Ray, C., and Gillies, A.H.B. Mechanism of lithium-induced polyuria in the rat. *Kidney Int.,* **1996,** *50:*377–383.

Cobb, W.E., Spare, S., and Reichlin, S. Neurogenic diabetes insipidus: management with dDAVP (1-desamino-8-D arginine vasopressin). *Ann. Intern. Med.,* **1978,** *88:*183–188.

Cogan, E., and Abramow, M. Inhibition by lithium of the hydroosmotic action of vasopressin in the isolated perfused cortical collecting tubule of the rabbit. *J. Clin. Invest.,* **1986,** *77:*1507–1514.

Cridland, R.A., and Kasting, N.W. A critical role for central vasopressin in regulation of fever during bacterial infection. *Am. J. Physiol.,* **1992,** *263:*R1235–R1240.

Cushing, H. The reaction to posterior pituitary extract (pituitrin) when introduced into the cerebral ventricles. *Proc. Natl. Acad. Sci. U.S.A.,* **1931,** *17:*163–170.

Deen, P.M.T., Verdijk, M.A.J., Knoers, N.V.N.M., Wieringa, B., Monnens, L.A.H., van Os, C.H., and van Oost, B. A. Requirement of human renal water channel aquaporin-2 for vasopressin-dependent concentration of urine. *Science,* **1994,** *264:*92–95.

Durr, J.A., Hoggard, J.G., Hunt, J.M., and Schrier, R.W. Diabetes insipidus in pregnancy associated with abnormally high circulating vasopressinase activity. *N. Engl. J. Med.,* **1987,** *316:*1070–1074.

du Vigneaud, V., Gish, D.T., and Katsoyannis, P.G. A synthetic preparation possessing biological properties associated with arginine vasopressin. *J. Am. Chem. Soc.,* **1954,** *76:*4751–4752.

Edwards, R.M., Trizna, W., and Kinter, L.B. Renal microvascular effects of vasopressin and vasopressin antagonists. *Am. J. Physiol.,* **1989,** *256:*F274–F278.

Franchini, K.G., and Cowley, A.W., Jr. Renal cortical and medullary blood flow responses during water restriction: role of vasopressin. *Am. J. Physiol.,* **1996,** *270:*R1257–R1264.

Gimson, A.E.S., Westaby, D., Hegarty, J., Watson, A., and Williams, R. A randomized trial of vasopressin and vasopressin plus nitroglycerin in the control of acute variceal hemorrhage. *Hepatology,* **1986,** *6:*410–413.

Goldberg, H., Clayman, P., and Skorecki, K. Mechanism of Li inhibition of vasopressin-sensitive adenylate cyclase in cultured renal epithelial cells. *Am. J. Physiol.,* **1988,** *255:*F995–F1002.

Grønbeck, L., Marples, D., Nielsen, S., and Christensen, S. Mechanism of antidiuresis caused by bendroflumethiazide in conscious rats with diabetes insipidus. *Br. J. Pharmacol.,* **1998,** *123:*737–745.

Hirsch, A. T., Majzoub, J.A., Ren, C.J., Scales, K.M., and Creager, M.A. Contribution of vasopressin to blood pressure regulation during hypovolemic hypotension in humans. *J. Appl. Physiol.,* **1993,** *75:*1984–1988.

Hupf, H., Grimm, D., Riegger, G.A.J., and Schunkert, H. Evidence for a vasopressin system in the rat heart. *Circ. Res.,* **1999,** *84:*365–370.

Inaba, K., Umeda, Y., Yamane, Y., Urakami, M., and Inada, M. Characterization of human platelet vasopressin receptor and the relation between vasopressin-induced platelet aggregation and vasopressin binding to platelets. *Clin. Endocrinol.,* **1988,** *29:*377–386.

Inoue, T., Terris, J., Ecelbarger, C.A., Chou, C.-L., Nielsen, S., and Knepper, M.A. Vasopressin regulates apical targeting of aquaporin-2 but not of UT1 urea transporter in renal collecting duct. *Am. J. Physiol.,* **1999,** *276:*F559–F566.

Jard, S., Gaillard, R.C., Guillon, G., Marie, J., Schoenenberg, P., Muller, A.F., Manning, M., and Sawyer, W.H. Vasopressin antagonists allow demonstration of a novel type of vasopressin receptor in the rat adenohypophysis. *Mol. Pharmacol.,* **1986,** *30:*171–177.

Kawano, Y., Matsuoka, H., Nishikimi, T., Takishita, S., and Omae, T. The role of vasopressin in essential hypertension. Plasma levels and effects of the V_1 receptor antagonist OPC-21268 during different dietary sodium intakes. *Am. J. Hypertens.,* **1997,** *10:*1240–1244.

Keppens, S., and de Wulf, H. The activation of liver glycogen phosphorylase by vasopressin. *FEBS Lett.,* **1975,** *51:*29–32.

Kim, G.-H., Ecelbarger, C.A., Mitchell, C., Packer, R.K., Wade, J.B., and Knepper, M.A. Vasopressin increases Na-K-2Cl cotransporter expression in thick ascending limb of Henle's loop. *Am. J. Physiol.,* **1999,** *276:*F96–F103.

Knepper, M.A., and Nielsen, S. Kinetic model of water and urea permeability regulation by vasopressin in collecting duct. *Am. J. Physiol.,* **1993,** *265:*F214–F224.

Landry, D.W., Levin, H.R., Gallant, E.M., Ashton, R.C., Jr., Seo, S., D'Alessandro, D., Oz, M.C., and Oliver, J.A. Vasopressin deficiency contributes to the vasodilation of septic shock. *Circulation,* **1997,** *95:*1122–1125.

Liard, J.F., Deriaz, O., Schelling, P., and Thibonnier, M. Cardiac output distribution during vasopressin infusion or dehydration in conscious dogs. *Am. J. Physiol.,* **1982,** *243:*H663–H669.

Libber, S., Harrison, H., and Spector, D. Treatment of nephrogenic diabetes insipidus with prostaglandin synthesis inhibitors. *J. Pediatr.,* **1986,** *108:*305–311.

Lolait, S.J., O'Carroll, A.-M., McBride, O.W., Konig, M., Morel, A., and Brownstein, M.J. Cloning and characterization of a vasopressin V_2 receptor and possible link to nephrogenic diabetes insipidus. *Nature,* **1992,** *357:*336–339.

Mannucci, P.M., Remuzzi, G., Pusineri, F., Lombardi, R., Valsecchi, C., Mecca, G., and Zimmerman, T.S. Deamino-8-D-arginine vasopressin shortens the bleeding time in uremia. *N. Engl. J. Med.,* **1983,** *308:*8–12.

Morales, D., Madigan, J., Cullinane, S., Chen, J., Heath, M., Oz, M., Oliver, J.A., and Landry, D.W. Reversal by vasopressin of intractable hypotension in the late phase of hemorrhagic shock. *Circulation,* **1999,** *100:*226–229.

Morel, A., O'Carroll, A.-M., Brownstein, M.J., and Lolait, S.J. Molecular cloning and expression of a rat Vla arginine vasopressin receptor. *Nature,* **1992,** *356:*523–526.

Morello, J-P., Salahpour, A., Laperriere, A., Bernier, V., Arthus, M-F., Lonergan, M., Petäjä-Repo, U., Angers, S., Morin, D., Bichet, D.G., and Bouvier, M. Pharmacological chaperones rescue cell-surface expression and function of misfolded V_2 vasopressin receptor mutants. *J. Clin. Invest.,* **2000,** *105:*887–895.

Nielsen, S., and Knepper, M.A. Vasopressin activates collecting duct urea transporters and water channels by distinct physical processes. *Am. J. Physiol.,* **1993,** *265:*F204–F213.

Nishimoto, G., Zelenina, M., Li, D., Yasui, M., Aperia, A., Nielsen, S., and Nairn, A.C. Arginine vasopressin stimulates phosphorylation of aquaporin-2 in rat renal tissue. *Am. J. Physiol.,* **1999,** *276:*F254–F259.

Overand, P.T., and Teply, J.F. Vasopressin for the treatment of refractory hypotension after cardiopulmonary bypass. *Anesth. Analg.,* **1998,** *86:*1207–1209.

Robinson, A.G. DDAVP in the treatment of central diabetes insipidus. *N. Engl. J. Med.,* **1976,** *294:*507–511.

Schafer, J.A., and Troutman, S.L. cAMP mediates the increase in apical membrane Na^+ conductance produced in rat CCD by vasopressin. *Am. J. Physiol.,* **1990,** *259:*F823–F831.

Schlondorff, D., and Levine, S.D. Inhibition of vasopressin-stimulated water flow in toad bladder by phorbol myristate acetate, dioctanoylglycerol, and RHC-80267. Evidence for modulation of action of vasopressin by protein kinase C. *J. Clin. Invest.,* **1985,** *76:*1071–1078.

Schwartz, J., Derdowska, I., Sobocinska, M., and Kupryszewski, G. A potent new synthetic analog of vasopressin with relative agonist specificity for the pituitary. *Endocrinology,* **1991,** *129:*1107–1109.

Singer, I., and Rotenberg, D. Demeclocycline-induced nephrogenic diabetes insipidus. In vivo and in vitro studies. *Ann. Intern. Med.,* **1973,** *79:*679–683.

Snyder, H.M., Noland, T.D., and Breyer, M.D. cAMP-dependent protein kinase mediates hydroosmotic effect of vasopressin in collecting duct. *Am. J. Physiol.,* **1992,** *263:*C147–C153.

Sonnenburg, W.K., and Smith, W.L. Regulation of cyclic AMP metabolism in rabbit cortical collecting tubule cells by prostaglandins. *J. Biol. Chem.,* **1988,** *263:*6155–6160.

Star, R.A., Nonoguchi, H., Balaban, R., and Knepper, M.A. Calcium and cyclic adenosine monophosphate as second messengers for vasopressin in the rat inner medullary collecting duct. *J. Clin. Invest.,* **1988,** *81:*1879–1888.

Sugimoto, T., Saito, M., Mochizuki, S., Watanabe, Y., Hashimoto, S., and Kawashima, H. Molecular cloning and functional expression of a cDNA encoding the human V_{1b} vasopressin receptor. *J. Biol. Chem.,* **1994,** *269:*27088–27092.

Yamaki, M., Kusano, E., Tetsuka, T., Takeda, S., Homma, S., Murayama, N., and Asano, Y. Cellular mechanism of lithium-induced nephrogenic diabetes insipidus in rats. *Am. J. Physiol.,* **1991,** *261:*F505–F511.

Yamamura, Y., Ogawa, H., Chihara, T., Kondo, K., Onogawa, T., Nakamura, S., Mori, T., Tominaga, M., and Yabuuchi, Y. OPC-21268, an orally effective, nonpeptide vasopressin V_1 receptor antagonist. *Science,* **1991,** *252:*572–574.

Yamamura, Y., Ogawa, H., Yamashita, H., Chihara, T., Miyamoto, H., Nakamura, S., Onogawa, T., Yamashita, T., Hosokawa, T., Mori, T., Tominaga, M., and Yabuuchi, Y. Characterization of a novel aquaretic agent, OPC-31260, as an orally effective, nonpeptide vasopression V_2 receptor antagonist. *Br. J. Pharmacol.,* **1992,** *105:*787–791.

Yatsu, T., Tomura, Y., Tahara, A., Wada, K., Kusayama, T., Tsukada, J., Tokioka, T., Uchida, W., Inagaki, O., Iizumi, Y., Tanaka, A., and Honda, K. Cardiovascular and renal effects of conivaptan hydrochloride (YM087), a vasopressin V_{1A} and V_2 receptor antagonist, in dogs with pacing-induced congestive heart failure. *Eur. J. Pharmacol.,* **1999,** *376:*239–246.

Zaoral, M., Kole, J., and Sorm, F. Amino acids and peptides. LXXI. Synthesis of 1-deamino-8-D-aminobutyrine-vasopressin, 1-deamino-8-D-lysine vasopressin, and 1-deamino-8-D-arginine vasopressin. *Coll. Czech. Chem. Commun.,* **1967,** *32:*1250–1257.

Zini, S., Fournie-Zaluski, M.C., Chauvel, E., Roques, B.P., Corvol, P., and Llorens-Cortes, C. Identification of metabolic pathways of brain angiotensin II and III using specific aminopeptidase inhibitors: predominant role of angiotensin III in the control of vasopressin release. *Proc. Natl. Acad. Sci. U.S.A.,* **1996,** *93:*11968–11973.

MONOGRAPHS AND REVIEWS

Abboud, F.M., Floras, J.S., Aylward, P.E., Guo, G.B., Gupta, B.N., and Schmid, P.G. Role of vasopressin in cardiovascular and blood pressure regulation. *Blood Vessels,* **1990,** *27:*106–115.

Archer, R. Neurohypophysial peptide systems: processing machinery, hydroosmotic regulation, adaptation and evolution. *Regul. Pept.,* **1993,** *45:*1–13.

Breslow, E. Structure and folding properties of neurophysin and its peptide complexes: biological implications. *Regul. Pept.,* **1993,** *45:*15–19.

Burroughs, A.K. Pharmacological treatment of acute variceal bleeding. *Digestion,* **1998,** *59:*28–36.

Chugh, S.S., Lurie, K.G., and Lindner, K.H. Pressor with promise. Using vasopressin in cardiopulmonary arrest. *Circulation,* **1997,** *96:*2453–2454.

Cunningham, E.T. Jr., and Sawchenko, P.E. Reflex control of magnocellular vasopressin and oxytocin secretion. *Trends Neurosci.,* **1991,** *14:*406–411.

Dantzer, R., and Bluthé, R.-M. Vasopressin and behavior: from memory to olfaction. *Regul. Pept.,* **1993,** *45:*121–125.

David, J.-L. Desmopressin and hemostasis. *Regul. Pept.,* **1993,** *45:*311–317.

Fjellestad-Paulsen, A., Paulsen, O., d'Agay-Abensour, L., Lundin, S., and Czernichow, P. Central diabetes inspidus: oral treatment with DDAVP. *Regul. Pept.,* **1993,** *45:*303–307.

Gash, D.M., Herman, J.P., and Thomas, G.J. Vasopressin and animal behavior. In, *Vasopressin: Principles and Properties.* (Gash, D.M., and Boer, G.J., eds.) Plenum Press, New York, **1987,** pp. 517–547.

Guillon, G., Grazzini, E., Andrez, M., Breton, C., Trueba, M., Serradeil-LeGal, C., Boccara, G., Derick, S., Chouinard, L., and Gallo-Payet, N. Vasopressin: a potent autocrine/paracrine regulator of mammal adrenal functions. *Endocr. Res.,* **1998,** *24:*703–710.

Holtzman, E.J., and Ausiello, D.A. Nephrogenic diabetes insipidus: causes revealed. *Hosp. Pract.,* **1994,** *29:*89–104.

Insel, T.R., Winslow, J.T., Williams, J.R., Hastings, N., Shapiro, L.E., and Carter, C.S. The role of neurohypophyseal peptides in the central mediation of complex social processes—evidence from comparative studies. *Regul. Pept.,* **1993,** *45:*127–131.

Jolles, J. Vasopressin and human behavior. In, *Vasopressin: Principles and Properties.* (Gash, D.M., and Boer, G.J., eds.) Plenum Press, New York, **1987,** pp. 549–578.

Kasting, N.W. Criteria for establishing a physiological role for brain peptides. A case in point: the role of vasopressin in thermoregulation during fever and antipyresis. *Brain Res. Rev.,* **1989,** *14:*143–153.

Kinter, L.B., Caltabiano, S., and Huffman, W.F. Anomalous antidiuretic activity of antidiuretic hormone antagonists. *Biochem. Pharmacol.,* **1993,** *45:*1731–1737.

Knepper, M.A., Kim, G.-H., Fernandez-Llama, P., and Ecelbarger, C.A. Regulation of thick ascending limb transport by vasopressin. *J. Am. Soc. Nephrol.,* **1999,** *10:*628–634.

Kovacs, L., and Robertson, G.L. Syndrome of inappropriate antidiuresis. *Endocrinol. Metab. Clin. North Am.,* **1992,** *21:*859–875.

László, F.A., László, F., Jr., and De Wied, D. Pharmacology and clinical perspectives of vasopressin antagonists. *Pharmacol. Rev.,* **1991,** *43:*73–108.

Legros, J.-J., Ansseau, M., and Timsit-Berthier, M. Neurohypophyseal peptides and psychiatric diseases. *Regul. Pept.,* **1993,** *45:*133–138.

Leng, G., Dyball, R.E.J., and Luckman, S.M. Mechanisms of vasopressin secretion. *Horm. Res.,* **1992,** *37:*33–38.

Manning, M., Chan, W.Y., and Sawyer, W.H. Design of cyclic and linear peptide antagonists of vasopressin and oxytocin: current status and future directions. *Regul. Pept.,* **1993,** *45:*279–283.

Manning, M., and Sawyer, W.H. Discovery, development, and some uses of vasopressin and oxytocin antagonists. *J. Lab. Clin. Med.,* **1989,** *114:*617–632. [Published erratum in *J. Lab. Clin. Med.,* **1990,** *115:*530. (Corrections to structure of vasopressin; headings in Table VII; and heading in text, p. 624.)]

Manning, M., Stoev, S, Cheng, L.L., Wo, N.C., and Chan, W.Y. Discovery and design of novel vasopressin hypotensive peptide agonists. *J. Recept. Signal Transduct. Res.,* **1999,** *19:*631–644.

Mannucci, P.M. Desmopressin (DDAVP) in the treatment of bleeding disorders: the first 20 years. *Blood,* **1997,** *90*:2515–2521.

Marples, D., Frøkiaer, J., and Nielsen, S. Long-term regulation of aquaporin in the kidney. *Am. J. Physiol.,* **1999,** *276*:F331–F339.

Mayinger, B., and Hensen, J. Nonpeptide vasopressin antagonists: a new group of hormone blockers entering the scene. *Exp. Clin. Endocrinol. Diabetes,* **1999,** *107*:157–165.

Nielsen, S., Kwon, T.-H., Christensen, B.M., Promeneur, D., Frøkiaer, J., and Marples, D. Physiology and pathophysiology of renal aquaporins. *J. Am. Soc. Nephrol.,* **1999,** *10*:647–663.

Oksche, A., and Rosenthal, W. The molecular basis of nephrogenic diabetes insipidus. *J. Mol. Med.,* **1998,** *76*:326–337.

Peterson, W.L. Gastrointestinal bleeding. In, *Gastrointestinal Disease.* Vol. 1. (Sleisenger, M.H., and Fordtran, J.S., eds.) W.B. Saunders Co., Philadelphia, **1989,** pp. 397–427.

Phillips, M.I. Functions of angiotensin in the central nervous system. *Annu. Rev. Physiol.,* **1987,** *49*:413–435.

Ramsey, T.A., and Cox, M. Lithium and the kidney: a review. *Am. J. Psychiatry,* **1982,** *139*:443–449.

Raymond, J.R. Hereditary and acquired defects in signaling through the hormone-receptor-G protein complex. *Am. J. Physiol.,* **1994,** *266*:F163–F174.

Renaud, L.P., and Bourque, C.W. Neurophysiology and neuropharmacology of hypothalamic magnocellular neurons secreting vasopressin and oxytocin. *Prog. Neurobiol.,* **1991,** *36*:131–169.

Robertson, G.L. Regulation of vasopressin secretion. In, *The Kidney: Physiology and Pathophysiology.* 2nd ed., Vol. 2. (Seldin, D.W., and Giebisch, G., eds.) Raven Press, New York, **1992,** pp. 1595–1613.

Robertson, G.L., Athar, S., and Shelton, R.L. Osmotic control of vasopressin function. In, *Disturbances in Body Fluid Osmolality.* (Andreoli, T.E., Grantham, J.J., and Rector, F.C., eds.) American Physiological Society, Bethesda, MD, **1977,** pp. 125–148.

Robinson, A.G., and Fitzsimmons, M.D. Vasopressin homeostasis: coordination of synthesis, storage and release. *Regul. Pept.,* **1993,** *45*:225–230.

Sands, J.M. Regulation of renal urea transporters. *J. Am. Soc. Nephrol.,* **1999,** *10*:635–646.

Schrier, R.W., Ohara, M., Rogachev, B., Xu, L., and Knotek, M. Aquaporin-2 water channels and vasopressin antagonists in edematous disorders. *Mol. Genet. Metab.,* **1998,** *65*:255–263.

Seckl, J.R., and Dunger, D.B. Diabetes insipidus. Current treatment recommendations. *Drugs,* **1992,** *44*:216–224.

Soederlund, C. Terlipressin (glypressin) in the treatment of bleeding esophageal varices. State of the art. *Regul. Pept.,* **1993,** *45*:299–302.

Sukhai, R.N. Enuresis nocturna: long-term use and safety aspects of minrin (desmopressin) spray. *Regul. Pept.,* **1993,** *45*:309–310.

Sutor, A.H. Desmopressin (DDAVP) in bleeding disorders of childhood. *Semin. Thromb. Hemost.,* **1998,** *24*:555–566.

Thibonnier, M. Vasopressin and blood pressure. *Kidney Int. Suppl.,* **1988,** *25*:S52–S56.

Thibonnier, M. Vasopressin agonists and antagonists. *Horm. Res.,* **1990,** *34*:124–128.

Thibonnier, M., Bayer, A.L., and Leng, Z. Cytoplasmic and nuclear signaling pathways of V_1-vascular vasopressin receptors. *Regul. Pept.,* **1993,** *45*:79–84.

Vokes, T.J., and Robertson, G.L. Disorders of antidiuretic hormone. *Endocrinol. Metab. Clin. North Am.,* **1988,** *17*:281–299.

Wells, T. Vesicular osmometers, vasopressin secretion and aquaporin-4: a new mechanism for osmoreception? *Mol. Cell. Endocrinol.,* **1998,** *136*:103–107.

Young, L.J., Wang, Z., and Insel, T.R. Neuroendocrine bases of monogamy. *Trends Neurosci.,* **1998,** *21*:71–75.

Zerbe, R., Stopes, L., and Robertson, G. Vasopressin function in the syndrome of inappropriate antidiuresis. *Annu. Rev. Med.,* **1980,** *31*:315–327.

C H A P T E R   3 1

RENIN AND ANGIOTENSIN

Edwin K. Jackson

In the early 1970s, pharmacological interruption of the renin–angiotensin system was considered sensible only for patients with high-renin hypertension. In the ensuing years, however, an extraordinary expansion of clinical indications for pharmacological interruption of the renin–angiotensin system occurred, beginning in the late 1970s with the advent of angiotensin converting enzyme (ACE) inhibitors. Surprisingly, ACE inhibitors proved to be effective not only in patients with high-renin hypertension, but also in many patients with essential hypertension who have normal levels of plasma renin activity. More recently, ACE inhibitors have gained widespread use in patients with congestive heart failure, myocardial infarction, and diabetic nephropathy. The realization that the renin–angiotensin system participates significantly in the pathophysiology of several highly prevalent diseases has led to an enormous effort to explore all aspects of the renin–angiotensin system and to devise new approaches for inhibiting its actions. These efforts have paid off handsomely, particularly in recent years, and knowledge concerning the renin–angiotensin system and pharmacological methods for manipulating it have grown impressively. The objective of this chapter is to provide an up-to-date account of: (1) the biochemistry, molecular and cellular biology, and physiology of the renin–angiotensin system; (2) the pharmacology of drugs that interrupt the renin–angiotensin system; and (3) the clinical utility of inhibitors of the renin–angiotensin system. Therapeutic applications of drugs covered in this chapter also are discussed in Chapters 32, 33, and 34.

THE RENIN–ANGIOTENSIN SYSTEM

History. In 1898, Tiegerstedt and Bergman found that crude saline extracts of the kidney contained a pressor substance, which they named *renin*. Their discovery had an obvious bearing on the problem of arterial hypertension and its relation to kidney disease that had been posed by Richard Bright's work some 60 years earlier. However, relatively little interest was generated until 1934, when Goldblatt and his colleagues showed convincingly that it was possible to produce persistent hypertension in dogs by constricting the renal arteries. In 1940, Braun-Menéndez and his colleagues in Argentina and Page and Helmer in the United States reported that renin was an enzyme that acted on a plasma protein substrate to catalyze the formation of the actual pressor material, a peptide, which was named *hypertensin* by the former group and *angiotonin* by the latter. These two terms persisted for nearly 20 years, until it was agreed to rename the pressor substance *angiotensin* and to call the plasma substrate *angiotensinogen*. In the mid-1950s, two forms of angiotensin were recognized, the first a decapeptide (angiotensin I) and the second an octapeptide (angiotensin II) formed by enzymatic cleavage of angiotensin I by another enzyme, termed *angiotensin converting enzyme* (ACE). The octapeptide was shown to be the more active form, and its synthesis in 1957 by Schwyzer and by Bumpus made the material available for intensive study.

Further progress came in 1958, when Gross suggested that the renin–angiotensin system was involved in the regulation of aldosterone secretion. It was soon shown that the kidneys are important for such regulation and that synthetic angiotensin, in minute amounts, stimulates the production of aldosterone in human beings. Moreover, elevated rates of renin secretion were noted upon experimental depletion of Na^+ (Gross, 1968). Thus, the renin–angiotensin system came to be recognized as a mechanism to stimulate aldosterone synthesis and secretion and an important physiological mechanism in the homeostatic regulation of blood pressure and electrolyte composition of body fluids.

In the early 1970s, polypeptides (not orally active) were discovered that either inhibited the formation of angiotensin II or blocked angiotensin II receptors, and experimental studies with these inhibitors revealed important physiological and pathophysiological roles for the renin–angiotensin system. These findings inspired the development of a new and broadly efficacious class of antihypertensive drugs, the orally active ACE inhibitors. Subsequent experimental and clinical studies with ACE inhibitors uncovered additional roles for the renin–angiotensin system in the pathophysiology of hypertension, heart failure, vascular disease, and renal failure, findings that provided further impetus for the development of additional classes of drugs that inhibit the renin–angiotensin system. In patents granted in 1982 (Furakawa *et al.*, 1982), it was reported that derivatives of imidazole-5-acetic acid attenuated vasoconstriction induced by angiotensin II. Two of these compounds, S-8307 and S-8308, subsequently were shown to be selective and competitive antagonists of angiotensin II receptors. These lead compounds rapidly were improved upon and gave rise to losartan, an orally active, highly selective, and potent nonpeptide angiotensin II receptor antagonist (Carini and Duncia, 1988). Subsequently, many other angiotensin II receptor antagonists have been developed.

Overview

The renin–angiotensin system is an important participant in both the short- and long-term regulation of arterial blood pressure. Factors that decrease arterial blood pressure, such as decreases in effective blood volume (caused by, for example, a low-sodium diet, diuretics, blood loss, congestive heart failure, liver cirrhosis, or nephrotic syndrome) or reductions in total peripheral resistance (caused by, for example, vasodilators), activate renin release from the kidneys.

Renin is an enzyme that acts on angiotensinogen (renin substrate) to catalyze the formation of the decapeptide angiotensin I. This decapeptide is then cleaved by ACE to yield the octapeptide angiotensin II. A representation of the biochemical pathways of the renin–angiotensin system is shown in Figure 31–1.

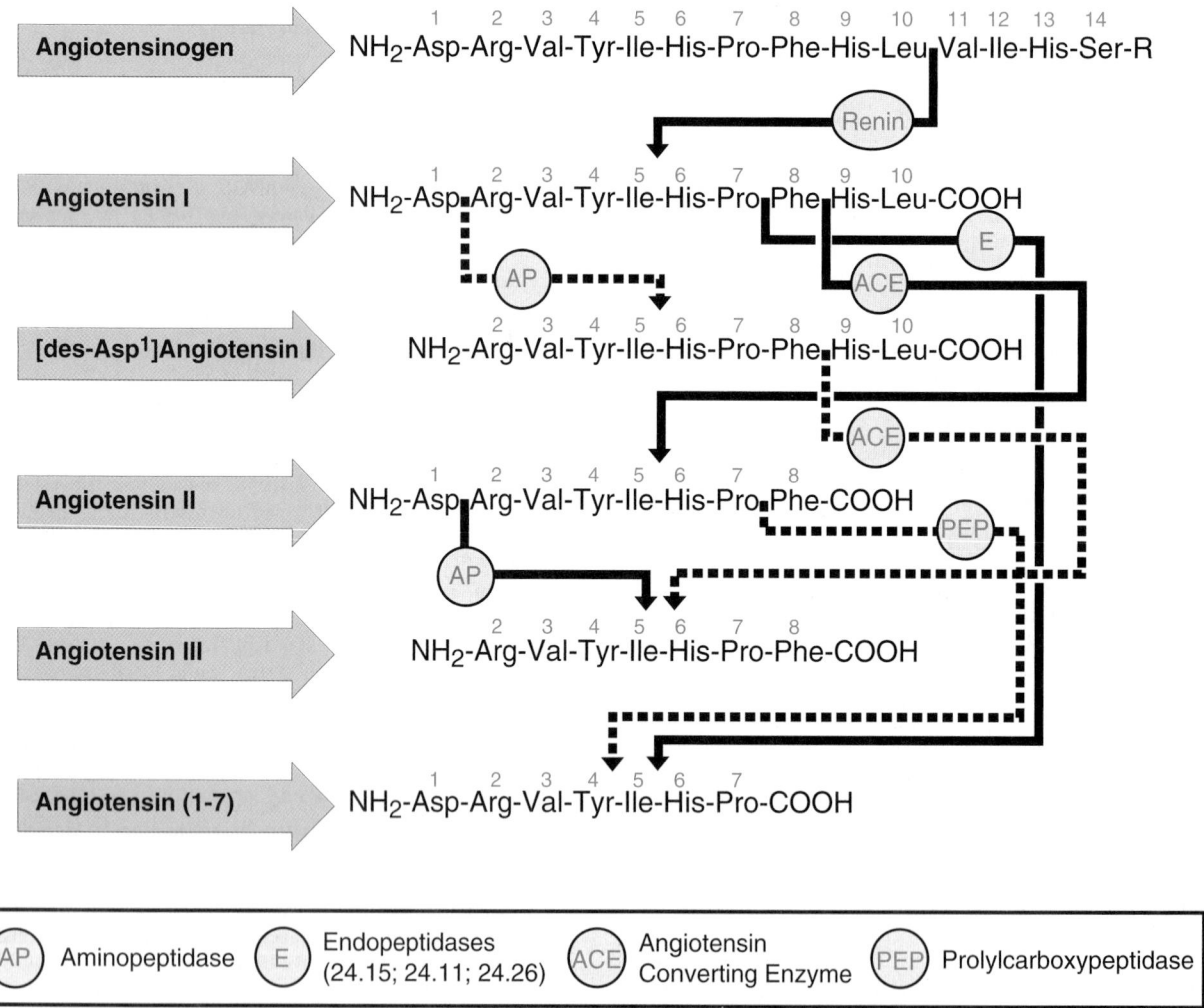

Figure 31–1. Formation of angiotensin peptides.

The solid arrows show the classical pathways, and the dashed arrows indicate minor alternative pathways. The structures of the angiotensins shown are those found in human beings, horse, rat, and pig; the bovine form has valine in the 5 position. The N-terminal sequence of human angiotensinogen is depicted.

Angiotensin II acts *via* diverse, yet coordinated, mechanisms to raise arterial blood pressure toward normal. The peptide acts in several ways to increase total peripheral resistance and thereby contributes to the short-term regulation of arterial blood pressure. Perhaps more important is the ability of angiotensin II to inhibit excretion of Na^+ and water by the kidneys. Angiotensin II–induced changes in renal function play an important role in long-term stabilization of arterial blood pressure in the face of large swings in dietary Na^+ intake (Hall *et al.,* 1980). As with its effects on peripheral resistance, the renal actions of angiotensin II also involve multiple interacting mechanisms (*see* below).

Components of the Renin–Angiotensin System

Renin. The major determinant of the rate of angiotensin II production is the amount of renin released by the kidney. Renin is synthesized, stored, and secreted into the renal arterial circulation by the granular juxtaglomerular cells that lie in the walls of the afferent arterioles as they enter the glomeruli. There is morphological and functional evidence that renin is secreted by exocytosis of storage granules, and studies by Friis *et al.* (1999) provide direct evidence of exocytosis in isolated juxtaglomerular cells.

Renin is an aspartyl protease that attacks a restricted number of substrates. Its principal natural substrate is a circulating α_2-globulin, angiotensinogen. Renin cleaves the bond between residues 10 and 11 at the amino terminus of this protein to generate angiotensin I. The active form of renin is a glycoprotein that contains 340 amino acids. It is synthesized as a preproenzyme of 406 amino acid residues that is processed to prorenin, a mature but inactive form of the protein (Imai *et al.,* 1983). Prorenin is finally activated by an as yet uncharacterized enzyme that removes 43 amino acids from the amino terminus of prorenin. Similar to other aspartyl proteases, renin has a bilobal structure with a cleft that forms the active site (Inagami, 1989; Sielecki *et al.,* 1989). A truncated, nonsecreted form of renin is expressed in the brain as a result of an alternative promoter within intron I of the renin gene (Lee-Kirsch *et al.,* 1999).

Renin and prorenin both are stored in the juxtaglomerular cells and, when released, circulate in the blood. The concentration of prorenin in the circulation is approximately tenfold greater than that of the active enzyme. The half-life of circulating renin is approximately 15 minutes. The physiological status of circulating prorenin is unclear.

***Control of Renin Secretion* (See *Figure 31–2*).** The secretion of renin from juxtaglomerular cells is controlled predominantly by three pathways: two acting locally within the kidney, and the third acting through the central nervous system (CNS) and mediated by norepinephrine release from renal noradrenergic nerves.

One intrarenal mechanism controlling renin release is called the *macula densa pathway* (top of Figure 31–2A). The macula densa lies adjacent to the juxtaglomerular cells and is composed of specialized columnar epithelial cells located in the wall of that portion of the cortical thick ascending limb that passes between the afferent and efferent arterioles of the glomerulus

(*see* Figure 29–1). A change in NaCl reabsorption by the macula densa results in the transmission to nearby juxtaglomerular cells of chemical signals that modify renin release. Increases in NaCl flux across the macula densa inhibit renin release, and decreases in NaCl flux stimulate renin release. The chemical signals mediating the macula densa pathway involve both adenosine (Itoh *et al.,* 1985; Weihprecht *et al.,* 1990) and prostaglandins (Gerber *et al.,* 1981; Greenberg *et al.,* 1993), with the former being released when NaCl transport increases and the latter being released when NaCl transport decreases. In this regard, adenosine, acting *via* an A_1 adenosine receptor, inhibits renin release (Jackson, 1991), and prostaglandins stimulate renin release (Jackson *et al.,* 1982).

Several lines of evidence suggest a critical role for inducible cyclooxygenase (COX-2) and neuronal nitric oxide synthase (nNOS) in the mechanism of macula densa–stimulated renin release. Although constitutive cyclooxygenase (COX-1) is the most abundant cyclooxygenase isoform in the mammalian kidney, inducible COX-2 is the only cyclooxygenase form expressed in the macula densa, and the amount of COX-2 in the macula densa is upregulated by chronic dietary sodium restriction (Harris *et al.,* 1994). Moreover, selective inhibition of COX-2 blocks macula densa–mediated renin release (Traynor *et al.,* 1999). Like COX-2, nNOS is expressed in the macula densa; nNOS expression in the macula densa is upregulated by dietary sodium restriction (Singh *et al.,* 1996), and selective inhibition of nNOS reduces renin release in response to chronic dietary sodium restriction (Beierwaltes, 1997). Together, these findings suggest a biochemical interplay between COX-2 and nNOS in the mechanism of macula densa–mediated renin release. Since nitric oxide reacts with superoxide anion to generate peroxynitrite, and peroxynitrite markedly activates cyclooxygenase activity (Landino *et al.,* 1996), it is conceivable that activation of macula densa–mediated renin release by sodium depletion involves the following events: upregulation of nNOS and COX-2 in the macula densa by sodium depletion; increased nitric oxide, and hence peroxynitrite, biosynthesis in the macula densa; peroxynitrite-induced activation of COX-2 in the macula densa; increased prostaglandin production in the macula densa; activation of prostaglandin receptors in the juxtaglomerular cells by prostaglandins released from the macula densa. Possible mechanisms by which the macula densa regulates renin release are summarized in Figure 31–2B.

Although a change in NaCl transport by the macula densa is the key event that modulates the macula densa pathway, regulation of this pathway is more dependent on the luminal concentration of Cl^- than Na^+. NaCl transport into the macula densa is mediated by the Na^+–K^+–2 Cl^- symporter, and the half-maximal concentrations of Na^+ and Cl^- required for transport *via* this symporter are 2 to 3 mEq/liter and 40 mEq/liter, respectively. Since the luminal concentration of Na^+ at the macula densa is usually much greater than the level required for half-maximal transport, physiological variations in luminal Na^+ concentrations at the macula densa have little effect on renin release (*i.e.,* the symporter remains saturated with respect to Na^+). On the other hand, physiological changes in Cl^- concentration at the macula densa have profound effects on macula densa–mediated renin release (Lorenz *et al.,* 1991).

The second intrarenal mechanism controlling renin release is called the *intrarenal baroreceptor pathway* (middle of Figure 31–2A). Increases and decreases in blood pressure in the

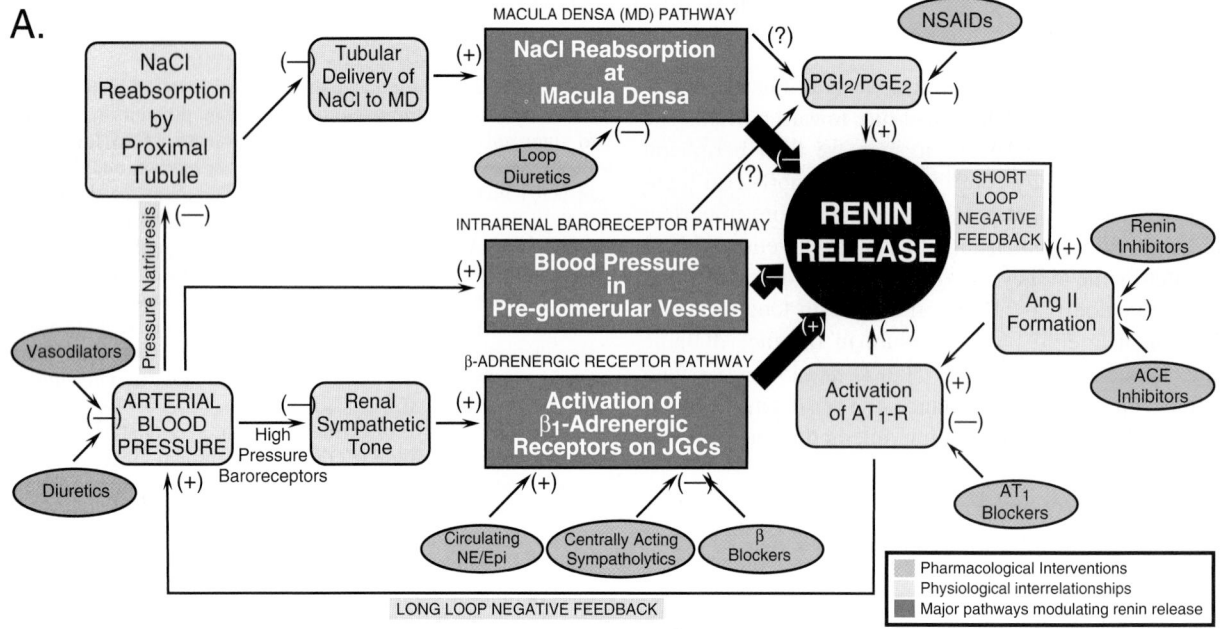

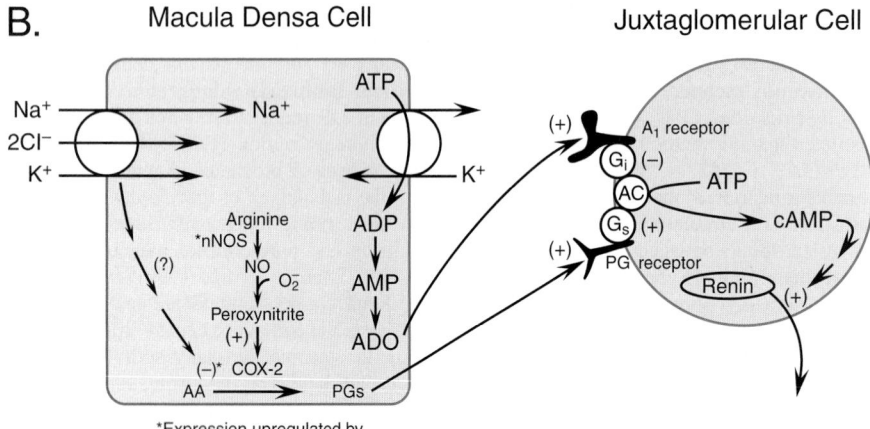

*Expression upregulated by
chronic sodium depletion

*Figure 31–2. A. A schematic portrayal of the three major physiological pathways regulating
renin release.*

See text for details. MD, macula densa; PGI_2, prostaglandin I_2; PGE_2, prostaglandin E_2; NSAIDs,
nonsteroidal antiinflammatory drugs; Ang II, angiotensin II; ACE, angiotensin converting enzyme,
AT_1-R, angiotensin subtype 1 receptor; NE/Epi, norepinephrine/epinephrine; β-blockers, β-adrenergic
receptor antagonists; AT_1 blockers, AT_1-R antagonists; JGCs, juxtaglomerular cells.

B. Possible mechanisms by which the macula densa regulates renin release.

Chronic sodium depletion upregulates neuronal nitric oxide synthase (nNOS) and inducible cyclooxygenase (COX-2) in the macula densa. nNOS increases nitric oxide (NO) production, and NO reacts
with superoxide anion (O_2^-) to form peroxynitrite, an activator of COX-2. In addition, COX-2 may
be rapidly although indirectly inhibited and stimulated by increases and decreases in NaCl transport,
respectively, across the macula densa. Arachidonic acid (AA) is converted to prostaglandins (PGs),
which diffuse to nearby juxtaglomerular cells to stimulate adenylyl cyclase (AC) *via* a stimulatory
G-protein (G_s). Cyclic AMP (cAMP) augments renin release. Increased NaCl transport depletes ATP
and increases adenosine (ADO) levels in the macula densa. ADO diffuses to the juxtaglomerular
cells and inhibits adenylyl cyclase *via* adenosine A_1 receptor–mediated activation of an inhibitory
G protein (G_i). Thus, both acute changes in tubular delivery of NaCl to the macula densa and chronic
changes in dietary sodium intake cause appropriate signals to be conveyed from macula densa to the
juxtaglomerular cells.

preglomerular vessels inhibit and stimulate renin release, respectively. The immediate stimulus to secretion is believed to be a reduction in the tension within the wall of the afferent arteriole. Increases and decreases in renal perfusion pressure may inhibit and stimulate, respectively, the release of renal prostaglandins, which perhaps mediate in part the intrarenal baroreceptor pathway (Data *et al.*, 1978; Linas, 1984). In fact, in renin-dependent renovascular hypertension, renin secretion and blood pressure are reduced by selective inhibition of COX-2 (Wang *et al.*, 1999). However, biomechanical coupling *via* stretch-activated ion channels may play an important role in the intrarenal baroreceptor pathway (Carey *et al.*, 1997).

The third mechanism, called the *β-adrenergic receptor pathway* (bottom of Figure 31–2A), is mediated by the release of norepinephrine from postganglionic sympathetic nerve terminals; activation of β_1-receptors on juxtaglomerular cells enhances renin secretion.

The three pathways regulating renin release are embedded in a physiological network. Increases in renin secretion enhance the formation of angiotensin II, and angiotensin II stimulates angiotensin subtype 1 (AT_1) receptors on juxtaglomerular cells to inhibit renin release. This feedback system has been termed the *short-loop negative feedback mechanism.* Angiotensin II also increases arterial blood pressure *via* stimulation of AT_1 receptors (*see* below). Increases in blood pressure inhibit renin release by: (1) activating high-pressure baroreceptors, thereby reducing renal sympathetic tone; (2) increasing pressure in the preglomerular vessels; and (3) reducing NaCl reabsorption in the proximal tubule (pressure natriuresis), which increases tubular delivery of NaCl to the macula densa. The inhibition of renin release due to angiotensin II–induced increases in blood pressure has been termed the *long-loop negative feedback mechanism.*

The physiological pathways regulating renin release can be influenced by a number of pharmacological agents. Loop diuretics (Chapter 29) stimulate renin release in part by blocking the reabsorption of NaCl at the macula densa. Nonsteroidal antiinflammatory drugs (NSAIDs; Chapter 27) inhibit the formation of prostaglandins and thereby decrease renin release (Frölich *et al.*, 1979). ACE inhibitors, AT_1 receptor blockers, and renin inhibitors interrupt both the short- and long-loop negative feedback mechanisms and therefore increase renin release. In general, diuretics and vasodilators increase renin release by decreasing arterial blood pressure. Centrally acting sympatholytic drugs as well as β-adrenergic receptor antagonists decrease renin secretion by inhibiting the β-adrenergic receptor pathway.

Angiotensinogen. The substrate for renin is angiotensinogen, an abundant globular glycoprotein (MW = 55,000 to 60,000 Da), containing 13% to 14% carbohydrate. High-molecular-weight (350,000 to 500,000 Da) angiotensinogen also circulates in plasma and represents a complex of angiotensinogen with other proteins. The relevant portion of angiotensinogen is the amino terminus, from which angiotensin I is cleaved. Molecular cloning studies (Kageyama *et al.*, 1984) demonstrate that human angiotensinogen contains 452 amino acids and is synthesized as preangiotensinogen, which has a 24– or 33–amino acid signal peptide. Angiotensinogen is synthesized primarily in the liver, although mRNA that encodes the protein also is abundant in fat, certain regions of the CNS, and kidney (Campbell and Habener, 1986; Cassis *et al.*, 1988). Angiotensinogen is continuously

synthesized and secreted by the liver, and its synthesis is stimulated by inflammation, insulin, estrogens, glucocorticoids, thyroid hormone, and angiotensin II (Ben-Ari and Garrison, 1988). During pregnancy, plasma levels of angiotensinogen increase severalfold under the influence of estrogen.

Circulating levels of angiotensinogen are approximately equal to the K_m of renin for its substrate (about 1 μM). Consequently, the rate of angiotensin II synthesis, and therefore blood pressure, can be influenced by changes in angiotensinogen levels. For instance, mice with no angiotensinogen gene are hypotensive (Tanimoto *et al.*, 1994), and there is a progressive relationship in genetically engineered mice among the number of copies of the angiotensinogen gene, plasma levels of angiotensinogen, and arterial blood pressure (Kim *et al.*, 1995). Moreover, oral contraceptives increase circulating levels of angiotensinogen and can induce hypertension. Increases in angiotensinogen levels are associated with essential hypertension (Jeunemaitre *et al.*, 1992), and there is genetic linkage between essential hypertension, angiotensinogen levels, and the angiotensinogen gene (Jeunemaitre *et al.*, 1992; Caulfield *et al.*, 1994, 1995). Furthermore, a specific mutation in the angiotensinogen gene (a methionine to threonine point mutation at position 235 of angiotensinogen) is associated with increased plasma levels of angiotensinogen and essential (Jeunemaitre *et al.*, 1992; Kunz *et al.*, 1997; Staessen *et al.*, 1999) and pregnancy-induced (Ward *et al.*, 1993) hypertension.

Angiotensin Converting Enzyme (ACE; Kininase II; Dipeptidyl Carboxypeptidase). ACE is an ectoenzyme and a glycoprotein with an apparent MW of 170,000 Da. Human ACE contains 1277 amino acid residues and has two homologous domains, each with a catalytic site and a region for binding Zn^{2+} (Soubrier *et al.*, 1988; Berstein *et al.*, 1989). ACE has a large amino-terminal extracellular domain, a short carboxyl-terminal intracellular domain, and a 17–amino acid hydrophobic stretch that anchors the ectoenzyme to the cell membrane. Circulating ACE represents membrane ACE that has undergone proteolysis at the cell surface by a secretase (Beldent *et al.*, 1995). ACE is rather nonspecific and cleaves dipeptide units from substrates with diverse amino acid sequences. Preferred substrates have only one free carboxyl group in the carboxyl-terminal amino acid, and proline must not be the penultimate amino acid; thus the enzyme does not degrade angiotensin II. Bradykinin is one of the many natural substrates for ACE, and ACE is identical to kininase II, which inactivates bradykinin and other potent vasodilator peptides. Although slow conversion of angiotensin I to angiotensin II occurs in plasma, the very rapid metabolism that occurs *in vivo* is due largely to the activity of membrane-bound ACE present on the luminal aspect of endothelial cells throughout the vascular system.

The ACE gene codes for both a somatic and a testis-specific isozyme. The testis ACE is found exclusively in developing spermatids and mature sperm and is encoded by the second half of the ACE gene, driven by a testis-specific promoter. Studies by Hagaman *et al.* (1998) demonstrate that testis ACE is involved in the transport of sperm in the oviduct and in binding of the sperm to the zonae pellucidae. These effects of testis-specific ACE are not mediated by angiotensin II.

The ACE gene contains, in intron 16, an insertion/deletion polymorphism that explains 47% of the phenotypic variance in serum ACE levels (Rigat *et al.*, 1990). The deletion allele is associated with higher levels of serum ACE and may confer an increased risk of ischemic heart disease (Cambien *et al.,* 1992; Gardemann *et al.,* 1995; Mattu *et al.,* 1995), coronary artery spasm (Oike *et al.,* 1995), restenosis after coronary stenting (Amant *et al.,* 1997; Ribichini *et al.,* 1998), vascular endothelial dysfunction (Butler *et al.,* 1999), left ventricular hypertrophy (Iwai *et al.,* 1994; Schunkert *et al.,* 1994), exercise-induced left ventricular growth (Montgomery *et al.,* 1997), carotid artery hypertrophy (Hosoi *et al.,* 1996), ischemic stroke (Kario *et al.,* 1996), hypertension in males (O'Donnell *et al.,* 1998; Fornage *et al.,* 1998), diabetic nephropathy (Marre *et al.,* 1997), deterioration of renal function in IgA nephropathy (Yoshida *et al.,* 1995), renal artery stenosis (Olivieri *et al.,* 1999), and thrombosis in patients undergoing hip arthroplasy (Philipp *et al.,* 1998). Surprisingly, however, the deletion allele is more frequent in centenarians (Schachter *et al.,* 1994), a finding that may be explained by the strong association of the deletion allele with protection against Alzheimer's disease (Kehoe *et al.,* 1999).

Angiotensin Peptides.   When given intravenously, angiotensin I is so rapidly converted to angiotensin II that the pharmacological responses of these two peptides are indistinguishable. However, angiotensin I *per se* is less than 1% as potent as angiotensin II on smooth muscle, heart, and the adrenal cortex. As shown in Figure 31–1, angiotensin III, also called [des-Asp^1] angiotensin II or angiotensin (2–8), can be formed either by the action of aminopeptidase on angiotensin II or by the action of ACE on [des-Asp^1] angiotensin I. Angiotensin III and angiotensin II cause qualitatively similar effects. Angiotensin III is approximately as potent as angiotensin II in stimulating the secretion of aldosterone; however, angiotensin III is only 25% and 10% as potent as angiotensin II in elevating blood pressure and stimulating the adrenal medulla, respectively (Peach, 1977; Bell *et al.,* 1984).

Angiotensin I can be metabolized to angiotensin (1–7) by the enzymes metalloendopeptidase 24.15, endopeptidase 24.11, and prolylendopeptidase 24.26, and angiotensin II can be converted to angiotensin (1–7) by prolylcarboxypeptidase (Ferrario *et al.,* 1997). ACE inhibitors increase, rather than decrease, tissue and plasma levels of angiotensin (1–7), because angiotensin I levels are increased and diverted away from angiotensin II formation (Figure 31–1) and because ACE contributes importantly to the plasma clearance of angiotensin (1–7) (Yamada *et al.,* 1998). The pharmacological profile of angiotensin (1–7) is distinct from that of angiotensin II. Unlike angiotensin II, angiotensin (1–7) does not cause vasoconstriction, aldosterone release, or facilitation of noradrenergic neurotransmission. Angiotensin (1–7) releases vasopressin, stimulates prostaglandin biosynthesis, elicits depressor responses when microinjected into certain brainstem nuclei, dilates some blood vessels, and exerts a natriuretic action on the kidneys. Angiotensin (1–7) also inhibits proliferation of vascular smooth muscle cells (Tallant *et al.,* 1999). The effects of angiotensin (1–7) may be mediated by a specific angiotensin (1–7) receptor (Tallant *et al.,* 1997). Ferrario *et al.* (1997) propose that angiotensin (1–7) serves to counterbalance the actions of angiotensin II. Putative receptors for angiotensin (3–8), also called angiotensin IV, are detectable in a number of tissues (Swanson *et al.,* 1992), and angiotensin (3–8) stimulates the expression of plasminogen activator inhibitor 1 in endothelial (Kerins *et al.,* 1995) and

proximal tubular (Gesualdo *et al.,* 1999) cells. The physiological significance of both angiotensin (1–7) and angiotensin (3–8) remains uncertain.

There is considerable information on the structure–activity relationships of angiotensin-related peptides (Samanen and Regoli, 1994). In general, phenylalanine in position 8 is critical for most agonist activity, and the aromatic residues in positions 4 and 6, the guanido group in position 2, and the C-terminal carboxyl are thought to be involved in binding to the receptor site. Position 1 is not critical, but replacement of aspartic acid in position 1 with sarcosine enhances binding to angiotensin receptors and slows hydrolysis by rendering the peptide refractory to a subgroup of aminopeptidases (angiotensinase A). Such a substitution, combined with that of alanine or isoleucine in place of phenylalanine in position 8, yields potent angiotensin II receptor antagonists.

Angiotensinases.   This term is applied to various peptidases that are involved in the degradation and inactivation of angiotensin peptides; none is specific. Among them are aminopeptidases, endopeptidases, and carboxypeptidases.

Local (Tissue) Renin–Angiotensin Systems.   The traditional view of the renin–angiotensin system is that of a classical endocrine system. Circulating renin of renal origin acts on circulating angiotensinogen of hepatic origin to produce angiotensin I in the plasma; circulating angiotensin I is converted by plasma ACE and by pulmonary endothelial ACE to angiotensin II; angiotensin II is then delivered to its target organs *via* the bloodstream, where it induces a physiological response. Recent evidence suggests that this traditional view is an oversimplification and should be expanded to include local (tissue) renin–angiotensin systems. In this regard, it is important to distinguish between *extrinsic* and *intrinsic,* local renin–angiotensin systems.

Extrinsic, Local Renin–Angiotensin Systems.   Since ACE is present on the luminal face of vascular endothelial cells throughout the circulation, and since circulating renin of renal origin can be taken up (sequestered) by the arterial wall as well as by other tissues, the conversion of hepatic angiotensinogen to angiotensin I and the conversion of angiotensin I (both circulating and locally produced) to angiotensin II may occur primarily within or at the surface of the blood vessel wall, not in the circulation *per se.* Indeed, studies by Danser *et al.* (1991; 1994) demonstrate that many vascular beds produce angiotensins I and II locally and that a substantial fraction of local production does not occur in the plasma as it transverses the vascular bed. In this regard, local sequestration of renal renin in both vascular and cardiac tissues participates in the local production of angiotensins (Kato *et al.,* 1993; Taddei *et al.,* 1993; Danser *et al.,* 1994). However, studies by Hu *et al.* (1998) do not support an important role for tissue binding of circulating renin.

Intrinsic, Local Renin–Angiotensin Systems.   Many tissues—including the brain, pituitary, blood vessels, heart, kidney, and adrenal gland—express mRNAs for renin, angiotensinogen, and/or ACE, and various cultured cell types from these tissues produce renin, angiotensinogen, ACE, and/or angiotensins I, II, and III (Phillips *et al.,* 1993; Saavedra, 1992; Dzau, 1993; Baker *et al.,* 1992). Therefore, it appears that local renin–angiotensin systems exist independently of the renal/hepatic-based system.

Although these local systems do not contribute significantly to circulating levels of active renin or angiotensins (Campbell *et al.*, 1991), there is evidence that the local production of angiotensin II by intrinsic, local renin–angiotensin systems influences vascular, cardiac, and renal function and structure. This hypothesis, although controversial (von Lutterotti *et al.*, 1994), is an active area of investigation.

Alternative Pathways for Angiotensin Biosynthesis. Some tissues contain nonrenin angiotensinogen-processing enzymes that convert angiotensinogen to angiotensin I (nonrenin proteases) or directly to angiotensin II (*e.g.,* cathepsin G, tonin) and non-ACE angiotensin I–processing enzymes that convert angiotensin I to angiotensin II (*e.g.,* cathepsin G, chymostatin-sensitive angiotensin II–generating enzyme, heart chymase) (Dzau *et al.*, 1993). There is mounting evidence that chymase, possibly mast cell–derived, importantly contributes to the local tissue conversion of angiotensin I to angiotensin II, particularly in the heart (Wolny *et al.*, 1997; Wei *et al.*, 1999) and kidneys (Hollenberg *et al.*, 1998); however, the role of chymase as a non-ACE angiotensin I–processing enzyme is species- and organ-dependent (Akasu *et al.*, 1998).

Angiotensin Receptors. The effects of angiotensins are exerted through specific cell surface receptors. Studies by Whitebread *et al.* (1989) and Chiu *et al.* (1989) have identified two subtypes of angiotensin receptors that are now designated AT_1 and AT_2 (Bumpus *et al.*, 1991). The AT_1 receptor has a high affinity for losartan (and related biphenyl tetrazole derivatives), a low affinity for PD 123177 (and related 1-benzyl spinacine derivatives), and a low affinity for CGP 42112A (a peptide analog). In contrast, the AT_2 receptor has a high affinity for PD 123177 and CGP 42112A but a low affinity for losartan.

Both the AT_1 (Sasaki *et al.*, 1991; Murphy *et al.*, 1991) and AT_2 (Mukoyama *et al.*, 1993) receptors are members of the G protein–coupled receptor family (*see* Chapter 2) with seven putative transmembrane regions. The AT_1 receptor is 359 amino acids long, and the AT_2 receptor is 363 amino acids long. The AT_1 and AT_2 receptors have little sequence homology. Most of the biological effects of angiotensin II are mediated by the AT_1 receptor; functional roles for the AT_2 receptor are poorly defined. Nonetheless, evidence suggests that AT_2 receptors may exert antiproliferative, proapoptotic, and vasodilatory effects (Inagami *et al.*, 1999; Ardaillou, 1999; Horiuchi *et al.*, 1999).

The AT_2 receptor is widely distributed in fetal tissues, but its distribution is more restricted in adults. In adults, some tissues contain primarily either AT_1 receptors or AT_2 receptors, whereas other tissues contain the receptor subtypes in similar amounts. In this regard, tissue and species differences are the rule, not the exception (Timmermans *et al.*, 1993). The AT_1 receptor gene contains a polymorphism (A to C transversion at position 1166) that may be associated with hypertension (Kainulainen *et al.*, 1999), hypertrophic cardiomyopathy (Osterop *et al.*, 1998), coronary artery vasoconstriction (Amant *et al.*, 1997), and aortic stiffness (Benetos *et al.*, 1996). Moreover, the C allele synergizes with the ACE deletion allele with regard to increased risk of coronary artery disease (Tiret *et al.*, 1994; Álvarez *et al.*, 1998). Preeclampsia is associated with development of agonistic autoantibodies against the AT_1 receptor (Wallukat *et al.*, 1999).

Angiotensin Receptor–Effector Coupling. AT_1 receptors activate a large array of signal transduction systems, including calcium release and influx pathways, phospholipases, mitogen-activated protein kinase pathways, Janus kinase pathways, serine/threonine protein kinases, nonreceptor tyrosine kinases, small GTP-binding proteins, inducible transcription factors, factors affecting translational efficiency, and pathways leading to the production of reactive oxygen species (Griendling *et al.*, 1997; Berk, 1999; Inagami, 1999; Blume *et al.*, 1999) (Figure 31–3). The most proximate coupling of AT_1 receptors to signal transduction systems is mediated by heterotrimeric GTP-binding proteins (G proteins; *see* Chapter 2) such as G_q, G_i, G_{12}, and G_{13}. A few proximate interactions engage a network of signal transduction systems as the initial signals fan out to include a wide array of signaling processes. Stimulation of AT_1 receptors leads to activation, *via* the G protein G_q, of phospholipase C-β. Phospholipase C-β is a membrane-bound enzyme that hydrolyzes phosphatidylinositol-4,5-bisphosphate to generate inositol-1,4,5-trisphosphate (IP_3) and diacylglycerol. IP_3 binds to receptors on Ca^{2+}-release channels in the IP_3-sensitive Ca^{2+} stores, an event that triggers the intracellular release of Ca^{2+}. Additional Ca^{2+} enters the cell from outside due to opening of voltage-sensitive Ca^{2+} channels located in the cell membrane. Ca^{2+} binds to calmodulin, and the Ca^{2+}/calmodulin complex activates a number of intracellular enzymes, such as Ca^{2+}-calmodulin–dependent protein kinases, that contribute to the ultimate cellular response. Although the initial surge of intracellular diacylglycerol is derived from phosphatidylinositol-4,5-bisphosphate, increases in diacylglycerol are sustained *via* activation of phospholipase D, which hydrolyzes phosphatidylcholine to generate phosphatidic acid. Phosphatidic acid, which has important cellular effects *per se*, is transformed into diacylglycerol by the enzyme phosphatidate phosphohydrolase. Ca^{2+} and/or diacylglycerol activate a family of serine/threonine kinases called protein kinase C. Activation of protein kinase C and increases in intracellular Ca^{2+} lead to the phosphorylation and activation of a network of signaling pathways, including nonreceptor tyrosine kinases. Nonreceptor tyrosine kinases, in turn, activate phospholipase C-γ, leading to additional IP_3 and diacylglycerol generation, and engage the mitogen-activated protein kinase pathways that participate importantly in the regulation of gene expression and mRNA translational efficiency. Some mitogen-activated protein kinases activate cytoplasmic phospholipase A_2, an enzyme that releases arachidonic acid from phospholipid stores and thereby increases the biosynthesis of biologically active substances such as prostaglandins, hydroxyeicosatetraenoic acids, leukotrienes, and epoxides and diols derived from arachidonic acid. Gene transcription also is regulated by the AT_1 receptor *via* activation of the Janus kinase/signal transducers and activators of transcription pathways. Although the precise mechanism by which the AT_1 receptor couples to this pathway is unknown, Janus kinases and signal transducers and activators of transcription physically associate with the cytoplasmic tail of the AT_1 receptor. Gene transcription results in the expression of a number of inducible transcription factors that, in turn, orchestrate changes in the expression of a host of gene products that regulate cell growth and extracellular matrix protein biosynthesis. In some cell types, AT_1 receptor activation decreases intracellular cyclic AMP by inhibiting adenylyl cyclase. This effect, which is mediated by the inhibitory G protein G_i, reduces the activity of protein kinase A and thereby decreases the phosphorylation state of substrates

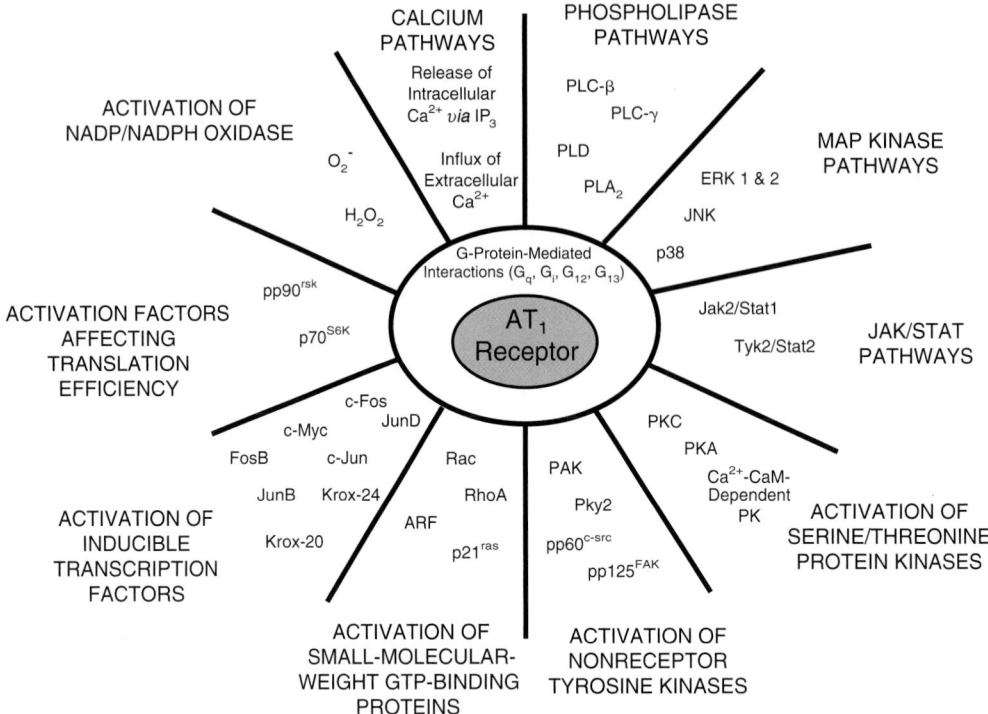

Figure 31–3. Mechanisms of AT₁ receptor–effector coupling.

The general categories of signal transduction molecules activated by the AT₁ receptor are summarized. The most proximate coupling of AT₁ receptor to signal transduction systems is mediated by heterotrimeric G proteins (such as G_q, G_i, G_{12}, and G_{13}). However, only some of the indicated systems directly couple with the AT₁ receptor *via* heterotrimeric G proteins. Rather, a few such proximate interactions engage a network of signal transduction systems as the initial signals fan out to include a wide array of signaling processes. ***Abbreviations:*** AT₁-R, angiotensin type I receptor; G_q, G_i, G_{12}, and G_{13}, different types of heterotrimeric GTP-binding proteins; RhoA, ARF, Rac, and p21ras, different types of small-molecular-weight GTP-binding proteins; PKA (protein kinase A), PKC (protein kinase C), and Ca^{2+}-CaM-dependent kinase, different types of serine/threonine protein kinases; Ca^{2+}-CaM-, calcium bound to calmodulin; PLC-β, PLC-γ, PLD, and PLA₂, different types of phospholipases; PAK, Pky2, pp60c-src, and pp125FAK, different types of nonreceptor tyrosine kinases; ERK1, ERK2, JNK, and p38, different types of mitogen-activated protein (MAP) kinases; c-Fos, FosB, c-Jun, JunB, JunD, Krox-20, Krox-24, c-Myc, family of inducible transcription factors; pp90rsk and p70s6K, S6 kinases (S6 is a protein that binds to ribosomes and regulates translation); Jak2 and Tyk2, members of the Janus kinase family of tyrosine kinases; Stat1 and Stat2, members of the family of signal transducers and activators of transcription; O₂⁻, superoxide anion.

for protein kinase A. AT₁ receptors also stimulate the activity of a membrane-bound NADH/NADPH oxidase that generates superoxide anion. Superoxide anion is transformed to hydrogen peroxide *via* catalase, and hydrogen peroxide generated by this pathway may induce important effects, such as activation of mitogen-activated protein kinase pathways and expression of monocyte chemoattractant protein-1. The relative importance of each of the aforementioned signal transduction pathways in mediating a given biological response to angiotensin II depends on the specific tissue and response under investigation. Although AT₁ receptor–effector coupling mechanisms have been studied in considerable detail, much less is known regarding AT₂ receptor–effector coupling. Signal transduction mechanisms for

the AT₂ receptor include activation of phosphatases, potassium channels, and nitric oxide production and inhibition of calcium channels (Horiuchi *et al.*, 1999). The effects of AT₂ receptors are mediated mostly by G_i.

Functions of the Renin–Angiotensin System

The renin–angiotensin system plays a major role in regulating arterial blood pressure over both the short and long term. Modest changes in plasma concentrations of angiotensin II acutely increase blood pressure; on a molar basis, angiotensin II is approximately 40 times more potent than norepinephrine in this regard. When a single moderate dose of angiotensin II is injected intravenously, systemic blood pressure begins to rise within seconds, rapidly reaches maximum, and returns to normal within minutes. This *rapid pressor response* to angiotensin II is due to a swift increase in total peripheral resistance—a response that helps maintain arterial blood pressure in the face of an acute hypotensive challenge (*e.g.,* blood loss, vasodilation). Although angiotensin II directly increases cardiac contractility (*via* opening voltage-gated Ca^{2+} channels in cardiac myocytes) and indirectly increases heart rate (*via* facilitation of sympathetic tone, enhanced noradrenergic neurotransmission, and adrenal catecholamine release), the rapid increase in arterial blood pressure activates a baroreceptor reflex that decreases sympathetic tone and increases vagal tone. Thus, angiotensin II may increase, decrease, or not change cardiac contractility, heart rate, and cardiac output, depending on the physiological state. Therefore, changes in cardiac output contribute little if at all to the rapid pressor response induced by angiotensin II.

Angiotensin II also causes a *slow pressor response* that helps stabilize arterial blood pressure over the long term. A continuous infusion of initially subpressor doses of angiotensin II gradually increases arterial blood pressure, with the maximum effect requiring days to achieve (Brown *et al.,* 1981). Most likely, the slow pressor response to angiotensin II is mediated by a decrement in renal excretory function that shifts the renal pressure–natriuresis curve to the right (*see* below). Angiotensin II–induced stimulation of endothelin-1 (Laursen *et al.,* 1997) and superoxide anion (Rajagopalan *et al.,* 1997) production mediates, in part, the slow pressor response.

In addition to buffering short- and long-term changes in arterial blood pressure, angiotensin II significantly alters the morphology of the cardiovascular system; *i.e.,* it causes hypertrophy of vascular and cardiac cells. The pathophysiological implications of this effect of the renin–angiotensin system are under intensive investigation.

The effects of angiotensin II on total peripheral resistance, renal function, and cardiovascular structure are mediated by a number of direct and indirect mechanisms. Figure 31–4 summarizes the three major effects of angiotensin II and how they are mediated.

Mechanisms by Which Angiotensin II Increases Total Peripheral Resistance.
Angiotensin II increases total peripheral resistance (TPR) *via* direct and indirect effects on blood vessels.

Direct Vasoconstriction. Angiotensin II constricts precapillary arterioles and, to a lesser extent, postcapillary venules by activating AT_1 receptors located on vascular smooth muscle cells. Angiotensin II has differential effects on the tone of vascular beds throughout the circulation. Direct vasoconstriction is strongest in the kidneys and somewhat less in the splanchnic vascular bed; blood flow in these regions falls sharply when angiotensin II is infused. Angiotensin II–induced vasoconstriction is much less in vessels of the brain and still weaker in those of the lung and skeletal muscle. In these regions, blood flow actually may increase, especially following small changes in the concentration of the peptide, because the relatively weak vasoconstrictor response is opposed by the elevated systemic blood pressure. Nevertheless, with high circulating concentrations of angiotensin II, cerebral and coronary blood flow may decrease.

Enhancement of Peripheral Noradrenergic Neurotransmission. Angiotensin II facilitates peripheral noradrenergic neurotransmission by augmenting norepinephrine release from sympathetic nerve terminals, by inhibiting the reuptake of norepinephrine into nerve terminals, and by enhancing the vascular response to norepinephrine (*see* Jackson *et al.,* 1985). High concentrations of the peptide stimulate ganglion cells directly. Facilitation of noradrenergic neurotransmission by endogenous angiotensin II occurs in animals with renin-dependent renovascular hypertension (Zimmerman *et al.,* 1987), and in human beings, intracoronary angiotensin II potentiates sympathetic nervous system–induced coronary vasoconstriction (Saino *et al.,* 1997).

Effects on the Central Nervous System. Small amounts of angiotensin II infused into the vertebral arteries cause an increase in arterial blood pressure. This effect is mediated by increased sympathetic outflow due to an effect of the hormone on circumventricular nuclei that are not protected by a blood–brain barrier (area postrema, subfornical organ, and organum vasculosum of the lamina terminalis). Blood-borne angiotensin II also attenuates baroreceptor-mediated reductions in sympathetic discharge, thereby increasing arterial pressure. The CNS is affected both by blood-borne angiotensin II and by angiotensin II formed within the brain (*see* Saavedra, 1992; Bunnemann *et al.,* 1993). The brain contains all the components of a renin–angiotensin system. Moreover, there is angiotensin-like immunoreactivity at many sites within the CNS, suggesting that angiotensin II serves as a neurotransmitter or modulator. In addition to increasing sympathetic tone, angiotensin II also causes a centrally mediated dipsogenic effect (*see* Fitzsimons, 1980) and enhances the release of vasopressin from the neurohypophysis (*see* Ganong,

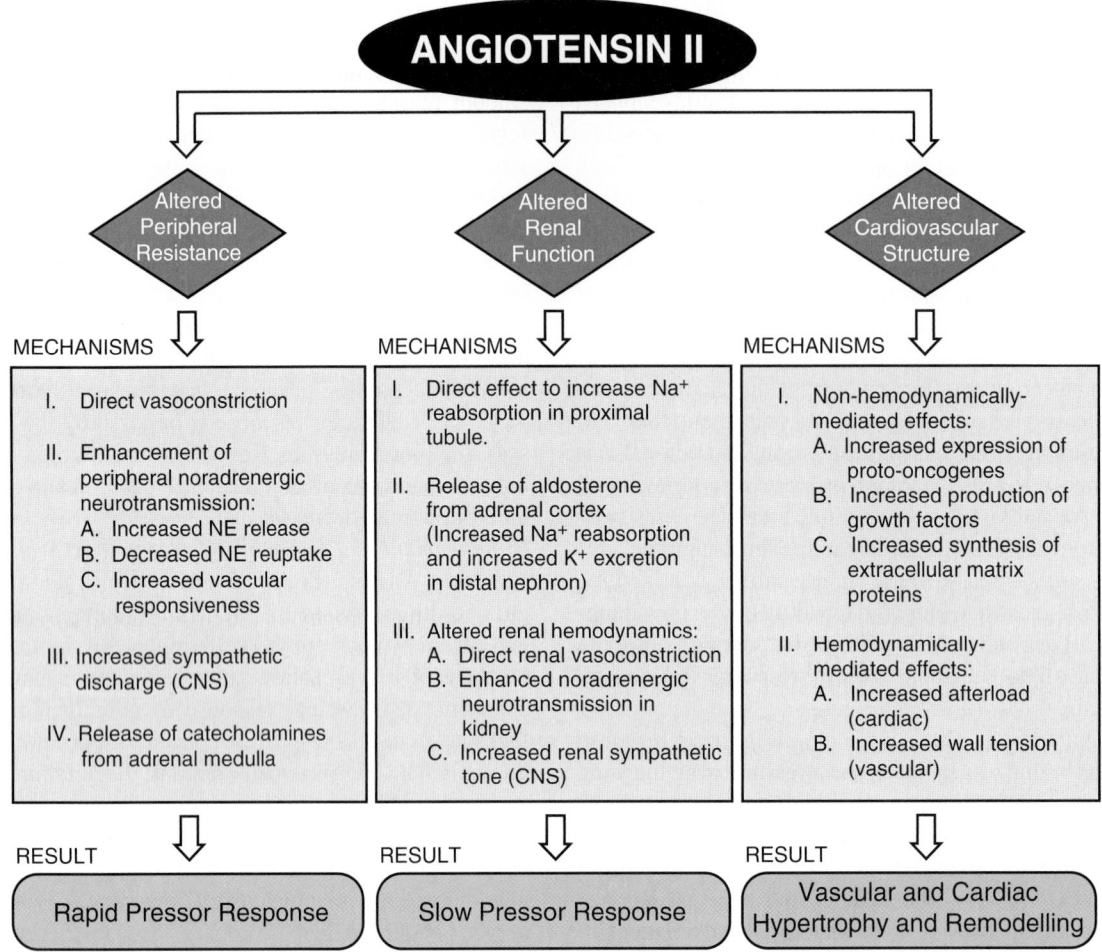

Figure 31–4. Summary of the three major effects of angiotensin II and the mechanisms that mediate them.

Abbreviation: NE, norepinephrine.

1984). Increased drinking and vasopressin secretion are produced more consistently following intraventricular than intravenous injections.

Release of Catecholamines from the Adrenal Medulla. Angiotensin II stimulates the release of catecholamines from the adrenal medulla by depolarizing chromaffin cells. Although this response is of minimal physiological importance, intense and dangerous reactions have followed the administration of angiotensin II to individuals with pheochromocytoma.

Mechanisms by Which Angiotensin II Alters Renal Function. Angiotensin II has pronounced effects on renal function to reduce the urinary excretion of Na^+ and water while increasing the excretion of K^+. The overall effect of angiotensin II on the kidneys is to shift the renal

pressure–natriuresis curve to the right (*see* below). Like the effects of angiotensin II on TPR, the effects of this peptide on renal function are multifaceted.

Direct Effects of Angiotensin II on Sodium Reabsorption in the Proximal Tubule. Very low concentrations of angiotensin II stimulate Na^+/H^+ exchange in the proximal tubule—an effect that increases Na^+, Cl^-, and bicarbonate reabsorption. Approximately 20% to 30% of the bicarbonate handled by the nephron may be affected by this mechanism (Liu and Cogan, 1987). Paradoxically, at high concentrations, angiotensin II may inhibit Na^+ transport in the proximal tubule.

Release of Aldosterone from the Adrenal Cortex. Angiotensin II stimulates the zona glomerulosa of the adrenal cortex to increase the synthesis and secretion of aldosterone, and angiotensin II exerts trophic and permissive effects that augment other stimuli (*e.g.,* ACTH and K$^+$). Increased output of aldosterone is elicited by very low concentrations of angiotensin II that have little or no acute effect on blood pressure. As described in Chapter 29, aldosterone acts on the distal and collecting tubules to cause retention of Na$^+$ and excretion of K$^+$ and H$^+$. The stimulant effect of angiotensin II on the synthesis and release of aldosterone is enhanced under conditions of hyponatremia or hyperkalemia and is reduced when concentrations of Na$^+$ and K$^+$ in plasma are altered in the opposite direction. Such changes in sensitivity are due in part to alterations in the number of receptors for angiotensin II on zona glomerulosa cells as well as to adrenocortical hyperplasia in the Na$^+$-depleted state.

Altered Renal Hemodynamics. Reductions in renal blood flow markedly attenuate renal excretory function, and angiotensin II reduces renal blood flow by directly constricting the renal vascular smooth muscle, by enhancing renal sympathetic tone (a CNS effect), and by facilitating renal noradrenergic neurotransmission (an intrarenal effect). Autoradiographic and *in situ* hybridization studies indicate a high concentration of AT$_1$ receptors in the vasa recta of the renal medulla, and angiotensin II may reduce Na$^+$ excretion in part by diminishing medullary blood flow. Angiotensin II also influences glomerular filtration rate (GFR); however, this effect of angiotensin II is variable. Angiotensin II exerts several effects that may alter GFR: (1) constriction of the afferent arterioles, which reduces intraglomerular pressure and tends to reduce GFR; (2) contraction of mesangial cells, which decreases the capillary surface area within the glomerulus available for filtration and also tends to decrease GFR; and (3) constriction of efferent arterioles, which increases intraglomerular pressure and tends to increase GFR. The outcome of these opposing effects on GFR depends on the physiological state. Normally, GFR is slightly reduced by angiotensin II; however, during renal artery hypotension, the effects of angiotensin II on the efferent arteriole predominate so that, in this setting, angiotensin II increases GFR (Hall *et al.,* 1981; Kastner *et al.,* 1984). Thus, blockade of the renin–angiotensin system may cause acute renal failure in patients with bilateral renal artery stenosis or in patients with unilateral stenosis who have only a single kidney (Hricik *et al.,* 1983).

Mechanisms by Which Angiotensin II Alters Cardiovascular Structure. Several cardiovascular diseases are accompanied by changes in the morphology of the heart and/or blood vessels, and these changes pose an increased risk of morbidity and mortality. Pathological alterations in cardiovascular structures may involve hypertrophy (an increase in tissue mass) and/or remodeling (redistribution of mass within a structure). Examples include (1) increased wall-to-lumen ratio in blood vessels (associated with hypertension); (2) cardiac concentric hypertrophy (also associated with hypertension); (3) cardiac eccentric hypertrophy and cardiac fibrosis (associated with congestive heart failure and myocardial infarction); and (4) thickening of the intimal surface of the blood vessel wall (associated with atherosclerosis and angioplasty). These morbid changes in cardiovascular structure are due to increased migration, proliferation (hyperplasia), and hypertrophy of cells as well as to increased extracellular matrix. The cells involved include vascular smooth muscle cells, cardiac myocytes, and fibroblasts. The renin–angiotensin system may contribute importantly to the aforementioned morbid changes in cardiovascular structure. In this regard, angiotensin II: (1) stimulates the migration (Bell and Madri, 1990; Dubey *et al.,* 1995), proliferation (Daemen *et al.,* 1991), and hypertrophy of vascular smooth muscle cells (Itoh *et al.,* 1993); (2) increases extracellular matrix production by vascular smooth muscle cells (Scott-Burden *et al.,* 1990); (3) causes hypertrophy of cardiac myocytes (Baker *et al.,* 1992); and (4) increases extracellular matrix production by cardiac fibroblasts (Villarreal *et al.,* 1993; Crawford *et al.,* 1994).

Nonhemodynamically Mediated Effects of Angiotensin II on Cardiovascular Structure. Angiotensin II stimulates migration, proliferation, hypertrophy, and/or synthetic capacity of vascular smooth muscle cells, cardiac myocytes, and/or fibroblasts in part by acting directly on cells to induce the expression of specific proto-oncogenes. In cell culture, angiotensin II rapidly (within minutes) increases steady-state levels of mRNA for the proto-oncogenes c-*fos,* c-*jun,* c-*myc,* and *egr*-1. FOS and JUN, the proteins coded by c-*fos* and c-*jun,* combine to form AP-1, and AP-1 alters the expression of several genes involved in stimulating cell growth (hypertrophy and hyperplasia), including basic fibroblast growth factor, platelet-derived growth factor, and transforming growth factor β. In addition, the expression of genes coding for extracellular matrix proteins, such as collagen, fibronectin, and tenascin, is increased.

Hemodynamically Mediated Effects of Angiotensin II on Cardiovascular Structure. In addition to the direct cellular effects of angiotensin II on cardiovascular structure, changes in cardiac preload (volume expansion due to Na$^+$ retention) and afterload (increased arterial blood pressure) probably contribute to cardiac hypertrophy and remodelling. Arterial hypertension also contributes to hypertrophy and remodeling of blood vessels.

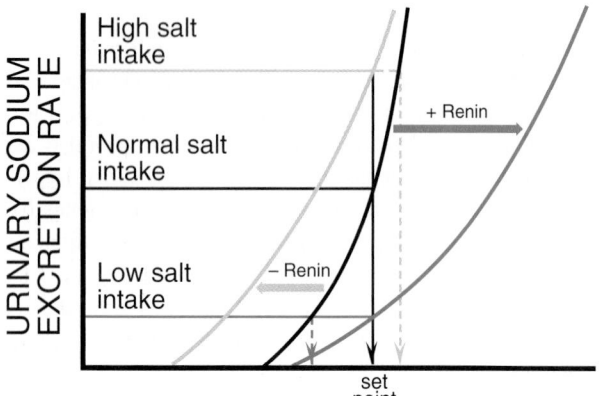

MEAN ARTERIAL BLOOD PRESSURE

Figure 31–5. Interactions among salt intake, the renal pressure–natriuresis mechanism, and the renin–angiotensin system to stabilize long-term levels of arterial blood pressure despite large variations in dietary sodium intake.

(*Modified from Jackson* et al., *1985, with permission.*)

Role of the Renin–Angiotensin System in Long-Term Maintenance of Arterial Blood Pressure Despite Extremes in Dietary Na$^+$ Intake.   Arterial blood pressure is a major determinant of Na$^+$ excretion (*see* Guyton, 1990). This can be illustrated graphically by plotting urinary Na$^+$ excretion *versus* mean arterial blood pressure (Figure 31–5), a plot known as the *renal pressure–natriuresis curve*. Over the long term, Na$^+$ excretion must equal Na$^+$ intake; therefore, the set point for long-term levels of arterial blood pressure can be obtained as the intersection of a horizontal line representing Na$^+$ intake with the renal pressure–natriuresis curve (Guyton, 1991) (Figure 31–5). If the renal pressure–natriuresis curve were fixed, then long-term levels of arterial blood pressure would be greatly affected by dietary Na$^+$ intake. However, as illustrated in Figure 31–5, the renin–angiotensin system plays a major role in maintaining a constant set point for long-term levels of arterial blood pressure despite extreme changes in dietary Na$^+$ intake. When dietary Na$^+$ intake is low, renin release is stimulated, and angiotensin II acts on the kidneys to shift the renal pressure–natriuresis curve to the right. Conversely, when dietary Na$^+$ is high, renin release is inhibited, and the withdrawal of angiotensin II causes the renal pressure–natriuresis curve to shift to the left. Consequently, the intersection of salt intake with the renal pressure–natriuresis curve remains near the same set point despite large swings in dietary Na$^+$ intake. When modulation of the renin–angiotensin system is pharmacologically prevented, changes in salt intake markedly affect long-term levels of arterial blood pressure (Hall *et al.*, 1980).

Other Roles of Renin–Angiotensin System.   Expression of the renin–angiotensin system is required for the development of normal kidney morphology, particularly the maturational growth of the renal papilla (Niimura *et al.*, 1995). Angiotensin II causes a marked anorexigenic effect and weight loss, and high circulating levels of angiotensin II may contribute to the anorexia, wasting, and cachexia of heart failure (Brink *et al.*, 1996).

INHIBITORS OF THE RENIN–ANGIOTENSIN SYSTEM

Angiotensin II itself has limited therapeutic utility and is not available for therapeutic use in the United States. Instead, clinical interest focuses on inhibitors of the renin–angiotensin system.

Angiotensin Converting Enzyme (ACE) Inhibitors

History.   In the 1960s, Ferreira and colleagues found that the venoms of pit vipers contain factors that intensify responses to bradykinin. These bradykinin-potentiating factors proved to be a family of peptides that inhibit kininase II, an enzyme that inactivates bradykinin. Erdös and coworkers established that ACE and kininase II are in fact the same enzyme, which catalyzes both the synthesis of angiotensin II, a potent pressor substance, and the destruction of bradykinin, a potent vasodilator.

Following the discovery of bradykinin-potentiating factors, the nonapeptide teprotide was synthesized and tested in human subjects. It was found to lower blood pressure in many patients with essential hypertension more consistently than did peptide angiotensin II receptor antagonists, such as saralasin, which have partial agonist activity. Teprotide also exerted beneficial effects in patients with heart failure. These key observations encouraged the search for ACE inhibitors that would be active orally.

The orally effective ACE inhibitor *captopril* (Cushman *et al.*, 1977) was developed by a rational approach that involved analysis of the inhibitory action of teprotide, inference about the action of ACE on its substrates, and analogy with carboxypeptidase A, which was known to be inhibited by D-benzylsuccinic acid. Ondetti, Cushman, and colleagues argued that inhibition of ACE might be produced by succinyl amino acids that corresponded in length to the dipeptide cleaved by ACE. This hypothesis proved to be true and led ultimately to the synthesis of a series of carboxy alkanoyl and mercapto alkanoyl derivatives that acted as potent competitive inhibitors of ACE (*see* Petrillo and Ondetti, 1982). Most active was captopril (*see* Vane, 1999, for an insider's perspective on the history of the discovery of ACE inhibitors).

Pharmacological Effects in Normal Laboratory Animals and Human Beings.   The essential effect of these agents on the renin–angiotensin system is to inhibit the conversion of the relatively inactive angiotensin I to the active angiotensin II (or the conversion of [des-Asp[1]]angiotensin I to angiotensin III). Thus, ACE inhibitors attenuate or abolish responses to angiotensin I but not to angiotensin II (*see* Figure 31–1). In this regard, ACE inhibitors are highly selective drugs. They do not interact directly with other components of the renin–angiotensin system, and the principal pharmacological and clinical effects of ACE inhibitors seem to arise from suppression of synthesis of angiotensin II. Nevertheless, ACE is an enzyme with many substrates, and inhibition of ACE therefore may induce effects unrelated to reducing the levels of angiotensin II. Since ACE inhibitors increase bradykinin levels, and since bradykinin stimulates prostaglandin biosynthesis, bradykinin and/or prostaglandins may contribute to the pharmacological effects of ACE inhibitors. Indeed, Gainer *et al.* (1998) demonstrated that blockade of bradykinin receptors in humans attenuates the acute blood pressure reduction induced by ACE inhibition. Recent studies, however, fail to demonstrate a role for bradykinin in the vascular or cardiac effects of ACE inhibitors (Davie *et al.*, 1999; Campbell *et al.*, 1999; Rhaleb *et al.*, 1999). ACE inhibitors increase by fivefold the circulating levels of the natural stem-cell regulator *N*-acetyl-seryl-aspartyl-lysyl-proline (Ac-SDKP; Azizi *et al.*, 1997); the long-term consequences of this effect are unknown. In addition, ACE inhibitors interfere with both short- and long-loop negative feedbacks on renin release (Figure 31–2A). Consequently, ACE inhibitors increase renin release and the rate of formation of angiotensin I. Since the metabolism of angiotensin I to angiotensin II is blocked by ACE inhibitors, angiotensin I is directed down alternative metabolic routes, resulting in the increased production of peptides such as angiotensin (1–7). Whether or not biologically active peptides such as angiotensin (1–7) contribute to the pharmacological effects of ACE inhibitors is unknown.

In healthy, Na^+-replete animals and human beings, a single oral dose of an ACE inhibitor has little effect on systemic blood pressure (Atlas *et al.*, 1983); but repeated doses over several days cause a small reduction in blood pressure. By contrast, even a single dose of these inhibitors lowers blood pressure substantially in normal subjects when they have been depleted of Na^+.

Clinical Pharmacology. Many ACE inhibitors have been synthesized. These drugs can be classified into three broad groups based on chemical structure: (1) sulfhydryl-containing ACE inhibitors structurally related to captopril (*e.g.*, fentiapril, pivalopril, zofenopril, alacepril); (2) dicarboxyl-containing ACE inhibitors structurally related to enalapril (*e.g.*, lisinopril, benazepril, quinapril, moexipril, ramipril, spirapril, perindopril, pentopril, cilazapril);

and (3) phosphorus-containing ACE inhibitors structurally related to fosinopril. Many ACE inhibitors are ester-containing prodrugs that are 100 to 1000 times less potent ACE inhibitors than the active metabolites but which have a much better oral bioavailability than the active molecules.

Currently 12 ACE inhibitors are approved for use (11 marketed) in the United States (*see* Figure 31–6 for chemical structures). In general, ACE inhibitors differ with regard to three properties: (1) potency; (2) whether ACE inhibition is due primarily to the drug itself or to conversion of a prodrug to an active metabolite; and (3) pharmacokinetics (*i.e.*, extent of absorption, effect of food on absorption, plasma half-life, tissue distribution, and mechanisms of elimination).

There is no compelling reason to favor one ACE inhibitor over another, since all ACE inhibitors effectively block the conversion of angiotensin I to angiotensin II and all have similar therapeutic indications, adverse-effect profiles, and contraindications. However, the Quality-of-Life Hypertension Study Group reported that, although captopril and enalapril are indistinguishable with regard to antihypertensive efficacy and safety, captopril may have a more favorable effect on quality of life (Testa *et al.*, 1993). Since hypertension usually requires lifelong treatment, quality-of-life issues are an important consideration in comparing antihypertensive drugs. ACE inhibitors differ markedly in tissue distribution, and it is possible that this difference could be exploited to inhibit some local renin–angiotensin systems while leaving others relatively intact. Whether or not site-specific inhibition actually would confer therapeutic advantages remains to be established.

With the notable exceptions of fosinopril and spirapril (which display balanced elimination by the liver and kidneys), ACE inhibitors are cleared predominantly by the kidneys. Therefore, impaired renal function significantly diminishes the plasma clearance of most ACE inhibitors, and dosages of these ACE inhibitors should be reduced in patients with renal impairment. *Elevated plasma renin activity (PRA) renders patients hyperresponsive to ACE inhibitor–induced hypotension, and initial dosages of all ACE inhibitors should be reduced in patients with high plasma levels of renin (e.g., patients with heart failure, salt-depleted patients).*

Captopril (CAPOTEN). Captopril, the first ACE inhibitor to be marketed, is a potent ACE inhibitor with a K_i of 1.7 nM. It is the only ACE inhibitor approved for use in the United States that contains a sulfhydryl moiety. Given orally, captopril is rapidly absorbed and has a bioavailability of about 75%. Peak concentrations in plasma occur within an hour, and the drug is cleared rapidly (it has a half-life of approximately 2 hours). Most of the drug

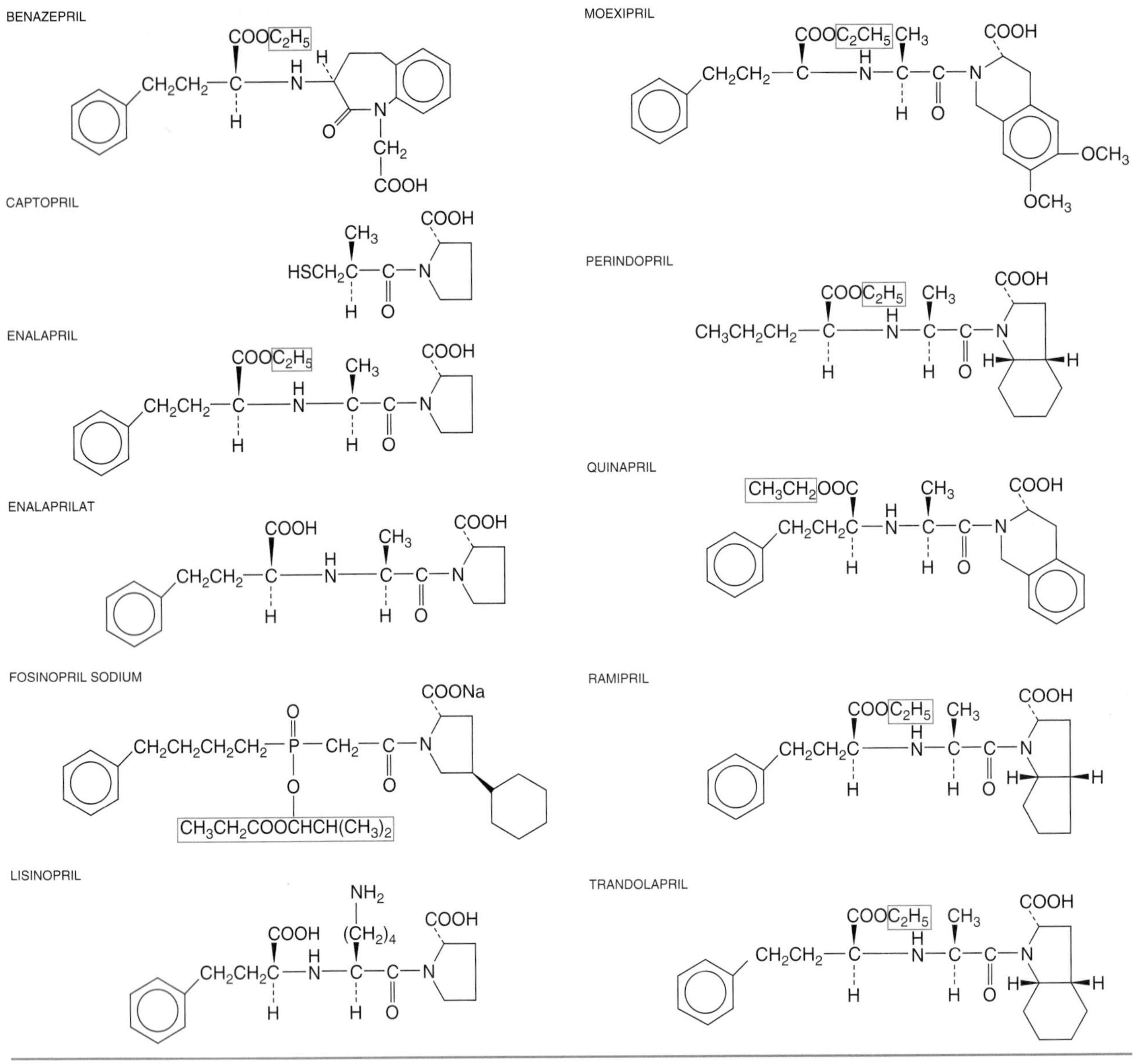

Figure 31–6. Chemical structures of selected angiotensin converting enzyme inhibitors.

Captopril, lisinopril, and enalaprilat are active molecules. Benazepril, enalapril, fosinopril, moexipril, perindopril, quinapril, ramipril, and trandolapril are relatively inactive until converted to their corresponding di-acids. The structures enclosed within blue boxes are removed by esterases and replaced with a hydrogen atom to form the active molecule *in vivo* (*e.g.,* enalapril to enalaprilat or ramipril to ramiprilat).

is eliminated in urine, 40% to 50% as captopril and the rest as captopril disulfide dimers and captopril–cysteine disulfide. The oral dose of captopril ranges from 6.25 to 150 mg two to three times daily, with 6.25 mg three times daily and 25 mg twice daily being appropriate for the initiation of therapy for heart failure and hypertension,

respectively. Most patients should not receive daily doses in excess of 150 mg. Since food reduces the oral bioavailability of captopril by 25% to 30%, the drug should be given 1 hour before meals.

Enalapril (VASOTEC). Enalapril maleate, the second ACE inhibitor approved in the United States, is a prodrug that is not highly active and must be hydrolyzed by esterases in the liver to produce the active parent dicarboxylic acid, enalaprilat. *Enalaprilat* is a highly potent inhibitor of ACE with a K_i of 0.2 nM. Although it also contains a "proline surrogate," enalaprilat differs from captopril in that it is an analog of a tripeptide rather than of a dipeptide. Enalapril is rapidly absorbed when given orally and has an oral bioavailability of about 60% (not reduced by food). Although peak concentrations in plasma occur within an hour, enalaprilat concentrations peak only after 3 to 4 hours. Enalapril has a half-life of only 1.3 hours, but enalaprilat, because of tight binding to ACE, has a plasma half-life of about 11 hours. Nearly all of the drug is eliminated by the kidneys either as intact enalapril or enalaprilat. The oral dosage of enalapril ranges from 2.5 to 40 mg daily (single or divided dosage), with 2.5 mg and 5 mg daily being appropriate for the initiation of therapy for heart failure and hypertension, respectively. The initial dose for hypertensive patients who are taking diuretics, are water- or Na^+-depleted, or have heart failure is 2.5 mg daily.

Enalaprilat (VASOTEC INJECTION). Enalaprilat is not absorbed orally but is available for intravenous administration when oral therapy is not appropriate. For hypertensive patients, the dosage is 0.625 to 1.25 mg given intravenously over 5 minutes. This dosage may be repeated every 6 hours.

Lisinopril (PRINIVIL, ZESTRIL). Lisinopril, the third ACE inhibitor approved for use in the United States, is the lysine analog of enalaprilat; unlike enalapril, lisinopril itself is active. *In vitro*, lisinopril is a slightly more potent ACE inhibitor than is enalaprilat. Lisinopril is slowly, variably, and incompletely (about 30%) absorbed after oral administration (not reduced by food); peak concentrations in plasma are achieved in about 7 hours. It is cleared as the intact compound by the kidney, and its half-life in plasma is about 12 hours. Lisinopril does not accumulate in tissues. The oral dosage of lisinopril ranges from 5 to 40 mg daily (single or divided dosage), with 5 and 10 mg daily being appropriate for the initiation of therapy for heart failure and hypertension, respectively. A daily dose of 2.5 mg is recommended for patients with heart failure who are hyponatremic or have renal impairment.

Benazepril (LOTENSIN). Cleavage of the ester moiety by hepatic esterases transforms benazepril hydrochloride, a prodrug, into benazeprilat, an ACE inhibitor that *in vitro* is more potent than captopril, enalaprilat, or lisinopril. Benazepril is rapidly, yet incompletely (37%), absorbed after oral administration (only slightly reduced by food). Benazepril is nearly completely metabolized to benazeprilat and to the glucuronide conjugates of benazepril and benazeprilat, which are excreted into both the urine and bile; peak concentrations of benazepril and benazeprilat in plasma are achieved in about 0.5 to 1 hour and 1 to 2 hours, respectively. Benazeprilat has an effective half-life in plasma of about 10 to 11 hours. With the exception of the lungs, benazeprilat does not accumulate in tissues. The oral dosage of benazepril ranges from 5 to 80 mg daily (single or divided dosage).

Fosinopril (MONOPRIL). Fosinopril sodium is the only ACE inhibitor approved for use in the United States that contains a phosphinate group that binds to the active site of ACE. Cleavage of the ester moiety by hepatic esterases transforms fosinopril, a prodrug, into fosinoprilat, an ACE inhibitor that *in vitro* is more potent than captopril yet less potent than enalaprilat. Fosinopril is slowly and incompletely (36%) absorbed after oral administration (rate but not extent reduced by food). Fosinopril is nearly completely metabolized to fosinoprilat (75%) and to the glucuronide conjugate of fosinoprilat. These are excreted in both the urine and bile; peak concentrations of fosinoprilat in plasma are achieved in about 3 hours. Fosinoprilat has an effective half-life in plasma of about 11.5 hours, and its clearance is not significantly altered by renal impairment. The oral dosage of fosinopril ranges from 10 to 80 mg daily (single or divided dosage). The dose is reduced to 5 mg daily in patients with Na^+ or water depletion or renal failure.

Trandolapril (MAVIK). Approximately 10% and 70% of an oral dose of trandolapril is bioavailable (absorption rate but not extent is reduced by food) as trandolapril and trandolaprilat, respectively. Trandolaprilat is about 8 times more potent than trandolapril as an ACE inhibitor. Trandolapril is metabolized to trandolaprilat and to inactive metabolites (mostly glucuronides of trandolapril and deesterification products), and these are recovered in the urine (33%, mostly trandolaprilat) and feces (66%). Peak concentrations of trandolaprilat in plasma are achieved in 4 to 10 hours. Trandolaprilat displays biphasic elimination kinetics with an initial half-life of about 10 hours (the major component of elimination), followed by a more prolonged half-life due to slow dissociation of trandolaprilat from tissue ACE. Plasma clearance of trandolaprilat is reduced by both renal and hepatic insufficiency. The oral dosage ranges from 1 to 8 mg daily (single or divided dosage). The initial dose is 0.5 mg in patients who are taking a diuretic or who have renal impairment.

Quinapril (ACCUPRIL). Cleavage of the ester moiety by hepatic esterases transforms quinapril hydrochloride, a prodrug, into quinaprilat, an ACE inhibitor that *in vitro* is about as potent as benazeprilat. Quinapril is rapidly absorbed (peak concentrations are achieved in 1 hour, but the peak may be delayed after food), and its rate but not extent of oral absorption (60%) may be reduced by food. Quinapril is metabolized to quinaprilat and to other minor metabolites, and quinaprilat is excreted in the urine (61%) and feces (37%). Peak concentrations of quinaprilat in plasma are achieved in about 2 hours. Conversion of quinapril to quinaprilat is reduced in patients with diminished liver function. The initial half-life of quinaprilat is about 2 hours; a prolonged terminal half-life of about 25 hours may be due to high-affinity binding of the drug to tissue ACE. The oral dosage of quinapril ranges from 5 to 80 mg daily (single or divided dosage).

Ramipril (ALTACE). Cleavage of the ester moiety by hepatic esterases transforms ramipril into ramiprilat, an ACE inhibitor that *in vitro* is about as potent as benazeprilat and quinaprilat. Ramipril is rapidly absorbed (peak concentrations of ramipril achieved in 1 hour), and the rate but not extent of its oral absorption (50% to 60%) is reduced by food. Ramipril is metabolized to ramiprilat and to inactive metabolites (glucuronides of ramipril and ramiprilat and the diketopiperazine ester and acid), and these are excreted predominantly by the kidneys. Peak concentrations of ramiprilat in plasma are achieved in about 3 hours. Ramiprilat displays triphasic elimination kinetics with half-lives of 2 to 4 hours, 9 to 18 hours, and greater than 50 hours. This triphasic elimination is due to extensive distribution to all tissues (initial half-life), clearance of free ramiprilat from plasma (intermediate half-life), and dissociation of ramiprilat from tissue ACE (terminal half-life). The oral dosage of ramipril ranges from 1.25 to 20 mg daily (single or divided dosage).

Moexipril (UNIVASC). Moexipril is another prodrug whose antihypertensive activity is almost entirely due to its deesterified metabolite, moexiprilat. Moexipril is incompletely absorbed, with bioavailability as moexiprilat of about 13%. Bioavailability is markedly decreased by food; therefore, the drug should be taken one hour before meals. The time to peak plasma concentration of moexiprilat is almost 1.5 hours, and the elimination half-life varies between 2 and 12 hours. The recommended dosage range is 7.5 to 30 mg daily in one or two divided doses. The dosage range is halved in patients who are taking diuretics or who have renal impairment.

Perindopril (ACEON). Perindopril erbumine is a prodrug, and 30% to 50% of systemically available perindopril is transformed to perindoprilat by hepatic esterases. Although the oral bioavailability of perindopril (75%) is not affected by food, the bioavailability of perindoprilat is reduced by approximately 35%. Perindopril is metabolized to perindoprilat and to inactive metabolites (glucuronides of perindopril and perindoprilat, dehydrated perindopril, and diastereomers of dehydrated perindoprilat), and these are excreted predominantly by the kidneys. Peak concentrations of perindoprilat in plasma are achieved in 3 to 7 hours. Perindoprilat displays biphasic elimination kinetics with half-lives of 3 to 10 hours (the major component of elimination) and 30 to 120 hours (due to slow dissociation of perindoprilat from tissue ACE). The oral dosage ranges from 2 to 16 mg daily (single or divided dosage).

Therapeutic Uses of ACE Inhibitors. Drugs that interfere with the renin–angiotensin system play a prominent role in the treatment of the major cause of mortality in modern societies, *i.e.,* cardiovascular disease.

ACE Inhibitors in Hypertension (**See** *Chapter 33*). Inhibition of ACE lowers systemic vascular resistance and mean, diastolic, and systolic blood pressures in various hypertensive states. The effects are readily observed in animal models of renal and genetic hypertension. In human subjects with hypertension, ACE inhibitors commonly lower blood pressure (except when high blood pressure is due to primary aldosteronism). The initial change in blood pressure tends to be positively correlated with PRA and angiotensin II plasma levels prior to treatment. However, several weeks into treatment, a greater percentage of patients show a sizable reduction in blood pressure, and the antihypertensive effect then correlates poorly or not at all with pretreatment values of PRA. It is possible that increased local (tissue) production of angiotensin II and/or increased responsiveness of tissues to normal levels of angiotensin II in some hypertensive patients make them sensitive to ACE inhibitors despite normal PRA. Regardless of the mechanisms, ACE inhibitors have a breadth of clinical utility as antihypertensive agents.

The long-term fall in systemic blood pressure observed in hypertensive individuals treated with ACE inhibitors is accompanied by a leftward shift in the renal pressure–natriuresis curve (Figure 31–5) and a reduction in total peripheral resistance in which there is variable participation by different vascular beds. The kidney is a notable exception to this variability in that there is a prominent vasodilator effect, and increased renal blood flow is a relatively constant finding. This is not surprising, since the renal vessels are exceptionally sensitive to the vasoconstrictor actions of angiotensin II. Increased renal blood flow occurs without an increase in glomerular filtration rate; in fact, the filtration fraction is reduced. Both the afferent and efferent arterioles are dilated. Blood flows in the cerebral and coronary beds, where autoregulatory mechanisms are powerful, are generally well maintained.

Besides causing systemic arteriolar dilatation, ACE inhibitors increase the compliance of large arteries, which contributes to a reduction of systolic pressure. Cardiac function in patients with uncomplicated hypertension is generally little changed, although stroke volume and cardiac output may increase slightly with sustained treatment. Baroreceptor function and cardiovascular reflexes are not compromised, and responses to postural changes and exercise are little impaired. Yet, surprisingly, even when a substantial lowering of blood pressure is achieved, heart rate and concentrations of catecholamines in plasma generally increase only slightly if at all. This perhaps reflects an alteration of baroreceptor function with increased arterial compliance and the loss of the normal tonic influence of angiotensin II on the sympathetic nervous system.

Secretion of aldosterone in the general population of hypertensive individuals is reduced but not seriously impaired by ACE inhibitors. Aldosterone secretion is maintained at adequate levels by other steroidogenic stimuli, such as adrenocorticotropic hormone and K^+. The activity of these secretagogues on the zona glomerulosa of the adrenal cortex requires, at most, only very small trophic or permissive amounts of angiotensin II, which are always present because inhibition of ACE is never complete. Excessive retention of K^+ is encountered only in patients taking supplemental K^+, in patients with renal impairment, or in patients taking other medications that reduce K^+ excretion.

ACE inhibitors alone normalize blood pressure in approximately 50% of patients with mild-to-moderate hypertension, and many consider ACE inhibitors first-line drugs for the treatment of high blood pressure except for elderly African-American patients. Ninety percent of patients with mild-to-moderate hypertension will be controlled by the combination of an ACE inhibitor with either a Ca^{2+} channel blocker, β-adrenergic receptor blocker, or diuretic (*see* Zusman, 1993). Diuretics, in particular, augment the antihypertensive response to ACE inhibitors by rendering the patient's blood pressure renin-dependent.

The goal of antihypertensive therapy is not just to lower blood pressure but, more importantly, to diminish the patient's overall risk of cardiovascular disease. Long-term clinical trials with diuretics and β-adrenergic receptor antagonists demonstrate that, while reducing blood pressure does decrease cardiovascular morbidity and mortality, the beneficial effects of lowering blood pressure are due primarily to reductions in the incidence of stroke, with only modest reductions in the incidence of myocardial infarction. This result may be due to the adverse metabolic effects of diuretics and β-adrenergic receptor antagonists and/or to the inability of these drugs to reverse the structural changes in the heart and/or blood vessels that may be mediated by the circulating (endocrine) and/or local (paracrine/autocrine/intracrine) renin–angiotensin systems.

It is possible that ACE inhibitors reduce the incidence of heart disease in hypertensive patients more than do other antihypertensive agents, and clinical trials are underway to test this hypothesis. This hypothesis is based on the lack of adverse metabolic effects of ACE inhibitors and the ability of ACE inhibitors to cause regression of left ventricular hypertrophy in hypertensive patients (DeCastro *et al.*, 1996), to prevent ventricular remodeling following myocardial infarction, and to double the life span of hypertensive rats (Linz *et al.*, 1997).

There is increasing evidence that ACE inhibitors are superior to other antihypertensive drugs in hypertensive patients with diabetes, in whom they improve endothelial function (O'Driscoll *et al.*, 1997) and reduce cardiovascular events more so than do Ca^{2+} channel blockers (Estacio *et al.*, 1998; Tatti *et al.*, 1998) or diuretics and β-adrenergic receptor antagonists (Hansson *et al.*, 1999). ***ACE Inhibitors in Left Ventricular Systolic Dysfunction (See Chapter 34).*** Left ventricular systolic dysfunction ranges from a modest, asymptomatic reduction in systolic performance to a severe impairment of left ventricular systolic function with New York Heart Association grade IV congestive heart failure. It is now clear that, unless contraindicated, ACE inhibitors should be given to all patients with impaired left ventricular systolic function whether or not they are experiencing symptoms of overt heart failure.

Several large, prospective, randomized, placebo-controlled clinical studies support the usefulness of ACE inhibitors in patients with varying degrees of left ventricular systolic dysfunction. These studies are summarized in Table 31–1 and are described in more detail in Chapter 34. The combined results of these studies strongly indicate that inhibition of ACE in patients with systolic dysfunction prevents or delays the progression of heart failure, decreases the incidence of sudden death and myocardial infarction, decreases hospitalization, and improves quality of life. The more severe the ventricular dysfunction, the greater the benefit from ACE inhibition.

Although the mechanisms by which ACE inhibitors improve outcome in patients with systolic dysfunction are not completely understood, the induction of a more favorable hemodynamic state most likely plays an important role. Inhibition of ACE commonly reduces afterload and systolic wall stress, and both cardiac output and cardiac index increase, as do indices of stroke work and stroke volume. Heart rate generally is reduced. Systemic blood pressure falls, sometimes steeply at the outset, but tends to return toward initial levels. Renovascular resistance falls sharply and renal blood flow increases. Natriuresis occurs

Table 31–1
Summary of Clinical Trials with ACE Inhibitors in Heart Disease

STUDY	REFERENCE	ACE INHIBITOR	PATIENT GROUP	OUTCOME	COMMENT
CONSENSUS	CONSENSUS Trial Study Group, 1987	Enalapril vs. placebo ($n = 257$)	NYHA IV CHF	Decreased overall mortality	Reduced pump failure
SOLVD-Treatment	SOLVD Investigators, 1991	Enalapril vs. placebo ($n = 2569$)	NYHA II & III CHF	Decreased overall mortality	Reduced pump failure
V-HeFt II	Cohn et al., 1991	Enalapril vs. hydralazine-isosorbide ($n = 804$)	NYHA II & III CHF	Decreased overall mortality	Reduced sudden death
SAVE	Pfeffer et al., 1992	Captopril vs. placebo ($n = 2231$)	MI with asymptomatic LV dysfunction	Decreased overall mortality	Reduced pump failure and recurrent MI
Kleber et al.	Kleber et al., 1992	Captopril vs. placebo ($n = 170$)	NYHA II CHF	Decreased progression of CHF	Treatment for 2.7 years
SOLVD-Prevention	SOLVD Investigators, 1992	Enalapril vs. placebo ($n = 4228$)	Asymptomatic LV dysfunction	Decreased death + hospitalization due to CHF	Treatment for 14.6 to 62 months
CONSENSUS II	Swedberg et al., 1992	Enalaprilat, then enalapril vs. placebo ($n = 6090$)	MI	No change in survival	Hypotension following iv enalaprilat
AIRE	AIRE Study Investigators, 1993	Ramipril vs. placebo ($n = 2006$)	MI with overt CHF	Decreased overall mortality	Benefit in 30 days
ISIS-4	ISIS-4 Collaborative Group, 1995	Captopril vs. placebo ($n = 58,050$)	MI	Decreased overall mortality	Treatment for 1 month
GISSI-3	GISSI-3 Investigators, 1994	Lisinopril vs. open control ($n = 19,394$)	MI	Decreased overall mortality	Treatment for 6 weeks
TRACE	Køber et al., 1995	Trandolapril vs. placebo ($n = 1749$)	MI with LV dysfunction	Decreased overall mortality	Treatment for 24 to 50 months
SMILE	Ambrosioni et al., 1995	Zofenopril vs. placebo ($n = 1556$)	MI	Decreased overall mortality	Treatment for 6 weeks
FEST	Erhart et al., 1995	Fosinopril vs. placebo ($n = 308$)	NYHA II & III CHF	Increased exercise tolerance	Treatment for 12 months
TREND	Mancini et al., 1996	Quinapril vs. placebo ($n = 105$)	CAD	Improved coronary endothelial function	Treatment for 6 months

Table 31–1
Summary of Clinical Trials with ACE Inhibitors in Heart Disease *(Continued)*

STUDY	REFERENCE	ACE INHIBITOR	PATIENT GROUP	OUTCOME	COMMENT
FAMIS	Borghi *et al.*, 1997	Fosinopril vs. placebo ($n = 285$)	MI	Decreased overall mortality and incidence of CHF	Early (<9 hours) initiation of treatment. Treatment for 3 months
QUIET	Cashin-Hemphill *et al.*, 1999	Quinapril vs. placebo ($n = 1750$)	Undergoing angioplasty	No change in progression of atherosclerosis	Treatment for 3 years
HOPE	Investigators Yusuf *et al.*, 2000	Ramipril vs. placebo ($n = 9297$)	High risk for CVD	Decreased CVD death, MI, stroke, overall mortality	Treatment for 5 years

ABBREVIATIONS: MI, myocardial infarction; CAD, coronary artery disease; CHF, congestive heart failure; CVD, cardiovascular disease; LV, left ventricular; NYHA, New York Heart Association; iv, intravenous administration

as a result of the improved renal hemodynamics, the reduced stimulus to secretion of aldosterone by angiotensin II, and the diminished direct effects of angiotensin II on the kidney. The excess volume of body fluids contracts, which reduces venous return to the right heart. A further reduction results from venodilation and an increased capacity of the venous bed. Venodilation is a somewhat unexpected effect of ACE inhibition, as angiotensin II has little acute venoconstrictor activity. Nevertheless, long-term infusion of angiotensin II increases venous tone, perhaps by central or peripheral interactions with the sympathetic nervous system (Schwartz and Chatterjee, 1983; Johns and Ayers, 1984). The response to ACE inhibitors also involves reductions of pulmonary arterial pressure, pulmonary capillary wedge pressure, and left atrial and left ventricular filling volumes and pressures. Consequently, preload and diastolic wall stress are diminished. The better hemodynamic performance results in increased exercise tolerance and suppression of the sympathetic nervous system (Grassi *et al.*, 1997). Cerebral and coronary blood flows usually are well maintained, even when systemic blood pressure is reduced (Romankiewicz *et al.*, 1983; Schwartz and Chatterjee, 1983).

The beneficial effects of ACE inhibitors in systolic dysfunction also involve improvements in ventricular geometry. In heart failure, ACE inhibitors reduce ventricular dilation and tend to restore the heart to its normal elliptical shape. ACE inhibitors may reverse ventricular remodeling *via* changes in preload/afterload, by preventing the growth effects of angiotensin II on myocytes, and/or by attenuating aldosterone-induced cardiac fibrosis.

Although the role of ACE inhibitors in left ventricular systolic dysfunction is firmly established, whether or not these drugs improve diastolic dysfunction is an important yet open question. Infusions of enalaprilat into the left coronary arteries of patients with left ventricular hypertrophy significantly improve diastolic function (Friedrich *et al.*, 1994; Kyriakidis *et al.*, 1998).

ACE Inhibitors in Acute Myocardial Infarction. Several large, prospective, randomized clinical studies involving thousands of patients (*see* Table 31–1) provide convincing evidence that ACE inhibitors reduce overall mortality when treatment is begun during the periinfarction period. The beneficial effects of ACE inhibitors in acute myocardial infarction are particularly large in hypertensive (Borghi *et al.*, 1999) and diabetic (Zuanetti *et al.*, 1997; Gustasson *et al.*, 1999) patients. Unless contraindicated (*e.g.*, cardiogenic shock or severe hypotension), ACE inhibitors should be started immediately during the acute phase of myocardial infarction and can be administered along with thrombolytics, aspirin, and β-adrenergic receptor antagonists (ACE Inhibitor Myocardial Infarction Collaborative Group, 1998). After several weeks, ACE-inhibitor therapy should be reevaluated. In high-risk patients (*e.g.*, large infarct, systolic ventricular dysfunction), ACE inhibition should be continued long-term.

ACE Inhibitors in Patients Who Are at High Risk of Cardiovascular Events. ACE inhibitors tilt the fibrinolytic balance toward a profibrinolytic state by reducing plasma levels of plasminogen activator inhibitor-1 (Vaughan *et al.*, 1997; Brown *et al.*, 1999) and improve endothelial vasomotor dysfunction in patients with coronary artery disease (Mancini *et al.*, 1996). The landmark HOPE study demonstrated that patients who were at high risk of cardiovascular events benefited considerably from treatment with ACE inhibitors (Yusuf *et al.*, 2000). In this regard, ACE inhibition significantly decreased the rate of myocardial infarction, stroke, and death in a broad range of patients who did not have left ventricular dysfunction but had evidence of vascular disease or diabetes and one other risk factor for cardiovascular disease. Thus, the HOPE study suggests that the use of ACE inhibitors should be expanded to the large population of patients at risk for ischemic cardiovascular events.

ACE Inhibitors in Chronic Renal Failure. Diabetes mellitus accounts for about one-third of all end-stage renal disease. The landmark study by Lewis *et al.* (1993) demonstrates that, in patients with type I diabetes mellitus and diabetic nephropathy, captopril prevents or delays the progression of renal disease. These findings are generalizable to other ACE inhibitors and to patients with both type I or type II diabetes regardless of baseline renal function or arterial blood pressure (Ravid *et al.*, 1993, 1996, 1998; EUCLID Study Group, 1997). The nephroprotective effects of ACE inhibitors and Ca^{2+} channel blockers in diabetes may be additive (*see* Bretzel, 1997). In addition to preventing diabetic nephropathy, ACE inhibitors also may decrease retinopathy progression in type I diabetics (Chaturvedi *et al.*, 1998). ACE inhibitors also attenuate the progression of renal insufficiency in patients with a variety of nondiabetic nephropathies (Maschio *et al.*, 1996; Gisen Group, 1997; Ruggenenti *et al.*, 1998, 1999b) and may arrest the decline in glomerular filtration rate even in patients with severe renal disease (Ruggenenti *et al.*, 1999a).

Several mechanisms participate in the renal protection afforded by ACE inhibitors. Increased glomerular capillary pressure induces glomerular injury, and ACE inhibitors reduce this parameter both by decreasing arterial blood pressure and by dilating renal efferent arterioles. ACE inhibitors increase the permeability selectivity of the filtering membrane, thereby diminishing exposure of the mesangium to proteinaceous factors that may stimulate mesangial cell proliferation and matrix production, two processes that contribute to expansion of the mesangium in diabetic nephropathy. Since angiotensin II is a growth factor, reductions in the intrarenal levels of angiotensin II may further attenuate mesangial cell growth and matrix production.

ACE Inhibitors in Scleroderma Renal Crisis. Before the use of ACE inhibitors, patients with scleroderma renal crisis generally died within several weeks. A few small, observational studies have suggested that captopril markedly improved this otherwise grim prognosis.

Adverse Effects of ACE Inhibitors. Metabolic side effects are not encountered during long-term therapy with ACE inhibitors. The drugs do not alter plasma concentrations of uric acid or Ca^{2+} (Frohlich, 1989) and may actually improve insulin sensitivity in patients with insulin resistance and decrease cholesterol levels and lipoprotein(a) levels in proteinuric renal disease. Serious untoward reactions to ACE inhibitors are rare (*see* Materson, 1992), and in general ACE inhibitors are well tolerated.

Hypotension. A steep fall in blood pressure may occur following the first dose of an ACE inhibitor in patients with elevated PRA. In this regard, care should be exercised in patients who are salt-depleted, in patients being treated with multiple antihypertensive drugs, and in patients who have congestive heart failure. In such situations, treatment should be initiated with very small doses of ACE inhibitors, or salt intake should be increased and diuretics withdrawn before beginning therapy.

Cough. In 5% to 20% of patients, ACE inhibitors induce a bothersome, dry cough; it is usually not dose-related, occurs more frequently in women than in men, usually develops between 1 week and 6 months after initiation of therapy, and sometimes requires cessation of therapy. This adverse effect may be mediated by the accumulation in the lungs of bradykinin, substance P, and/or prostaglandins. Thromboxane antagonism reduces ACE inhibitor–induced cough (Malini *et al.*, 1997). Once ACE inhibitors are stopped, the cough disappears, usually within 4 days (Israili and Hall, 1992).

Hyperkalemia. Despite some reduction in the concentration of aldosterone, significant retention of K^+ is rarely encountered in patients with normal renal function who are not taking other drugs that cause K^+ retention. However, ACE inhibitors may cause hyperkalemia in patients with renal insufficiency or in patients taking K^+-sparing diuretics, K^+ supplements, β-adrenergic receptor blockers, or NSAIDs.

Acute Renal Failure. Angiotensin II, by constricting the efferent arteriole, helps maintain adequate glomerular filtration when renal perfusion pressure is low. Consequently, inhibition of ACE can induce acute renal insufficiency in patients with bilateral renal artery stenosis, stenosis of the artery to a single remaining kidney, heart failure, or dehydration due to diarrhea or diuretics. Older patients with congestive heart failure are particularly susceptible to ACE inhibitor–induced acute renal failure. However, in nearly all patients who receive appropriate treatment, recovery of renal function occurs without sequelae (Wynckel *et al.*, 1998).

Fetopathic Potential. Although ACE inhibitors are not teratogenic during the early period of organogenesis (first trimester), continued administration of ACE inhibitors during the second and third trimesters can cause oligo-hydramnios, fetal calvarial hypoplasia, fetal pulmonary hypoplasia, fetal growth retardation, fetal death, neonatal anuria, and neonatal death. These fetopathic effects may be due in part to fetal hypotension. While ACE inhibitors are not contraindicated in women of reproductive age, *once pregnancy is diagnosed, it is imperative that ACE inhibitors be discontinued as soon as possible.* If necessary, an alternative antihypertensive regimen should be instituted. The fetus is not at risk of ACE inhibitor–induced pathology if ACE inhibitors are discontinued during the first trimester of pregnancy (Brent and Beckman, 1991).

Skin Rash. ACE inhibitors occasionally cause a maculopapular rash that may or may not itch. The rash may resolve spontaneously and may respond to a reduction in dosage or a brief course of antihistamines. This side effect was initially attributed to the presence of the sulfhydryl group in captopril; however, it also occurs with other ACE inhibitors, albeit less frequently.

Proteinuria. ACE inhibitors have been associated with proteinuria (more than 1 g/day); however, a causal relationship has been difficult to establish. In general, proteinuria is not a contraindication for ACE inhibitors, as ACE inhibitors are renoprotective in certain renal diseases associated with proteinuria, *e.g.,* diabetic nephropathy.

Angioneurotic Edema. In 0.1% to 0.2% of patients, ACE inhibitors induce a rapid swelling in the nose, throat, mouth, glottis, larynx, lips, and/or tongue. This untoward effect, called *angioneurotic edema,* apparently is not dose-related and nearly always develops within the first week of therapy, usually within the first few hours after the initial dose. Airway obstruction and respiratory distress may lead to death. Although the mechanism of angioneurotic edema is unknown, it may involve accumulation of bradykinin, induction of tissue-specific autoantibodies, or inhibition of complement 1–esterase inactivator. Once ACE inhibitors are stopped, angioneurotic edema disappears within hours; meanwhile the patient's airway should be protected, and, if necessary, epinephrine, an antihistamine, and/or a corticosteroid should be administered (Israili and Hall, 1992). African Americans have a 4.5 times greater risk of ACE inhibitor–induced angioneurotic edema than do Caucasians (Brown *et al.,* 1996).

Dysgeusia. An alteration in or loss of taste can occur in patients receiving ACE inhibitors. This adverse effect, which may occur more frequently with captopril, is reversible.

Neutropenia. Neutropenia is a rare, but serious, side effect of ACE inhibitors. Although the frequency of neutropenia is low, it occurs predominantly in hypertensive patients with collagen-vascular or renal parenchymal disease. If serum creatinine is 2 mg/dl or greater, the dose of

ACE inhibitor should be kept low, and the patient should be counseled to watch for symptoms of neutropenia (*e.g.,* sore throat, fever).

Glycosuria. An exceedingly rare and reversible side effect of ACE inhibitors is spillage of glucose into the urine in the absence of hyperglycemia (Cressman *et al.,* 1982). The mechanism is unknown.

Hepatotoxicity. Also exceedingly rare and reversible is hepatotoxicity, usually of the cholestatic variety (Hagley *et al.,* 1993). The mechanism is unknown.

Drug Interactions. Antacids may reduce the bioavailability of ACE inhibitors; capsaicin may worsen ACE inhibitor–induced cough; NSAIDs, including aspirin (Guazzi *et al.,* 1998), may reduce the antihypertensive response to ACE inhibitors; and K^+-sparing diuretics and K^+ supplements may exacerbate ACE inhibitor–induced hyperkalemia. ACE inhibitors may increase plasma levels of digoxin and lithium and may increase hypersensitivity reactions to allopurinol.

Nonpeptide Angiotensin II Receptor Antagonists

History. Attempts to develop therapeutically useful angiotensin II receptor antagonists date to the early 1970s, and these initial endeavors concentrated on angiotensin peptide analogs. Saralasin, 1-sarcosine, 8-isoleucine angiotensin II, and other 8-substituted angiotensins were potent angiotensin II receptor antagonists but were of no clinical value because of lack of oral bioavailability and because all peptide angiotensin II receptor antagonists expressed unacceptable partial agonist activity.

Although initial efforts to develop nonpeptide angiotensin receptor antagonists were unsuccessful, a breakthrough came in the early 1980s with the issuance of patents (Furakawa *et al.,* 1982) on a series of imidazole-5-acetic acid derivatives that attenuated pressor responses to angiotensin II in rats. Two of the compounds described in the patents, S-8307 and S-8308, later were found to be highly specific, albeit very weak, nonpeptide angiotensin II receptor antagonists that were devoid of partial agonist activity (Wong *et al.,* 1988; Chiu *et al.,* 1988). In an instructive example of drug design, molecular modeling of these lead compounds gave rise to the hypothesis that their structures would have to be extended to mimic more closely the pharmacophore of angiotensin II (Figure 31–7A). Through an insightful series of stepwise modifications (Figure 31–7B), the orally active, potent, and selective nonpeptide AT_1 receptor antagonist *losartan* was developed (Timmermans *et al.,* 1993). Losartan was approved for clinical use by the United States Food and Drug Administration in 1995. Since then, the Food and Drug Administration has approved five additional AT_1 receptor antagonists (Figure 31–8). Hundreds of AT_1 receptor antagonists have been synthesized, representing a diverse array of chemical structures (Weinstock and Keenan, 1994). However, AT_1 receptor antagonists approved in the United States are either biphenylmethyl derivatives or thienylmethylacrylic acid derivatives (Figure 31–8). Although approved AT_1 receptor antagonists

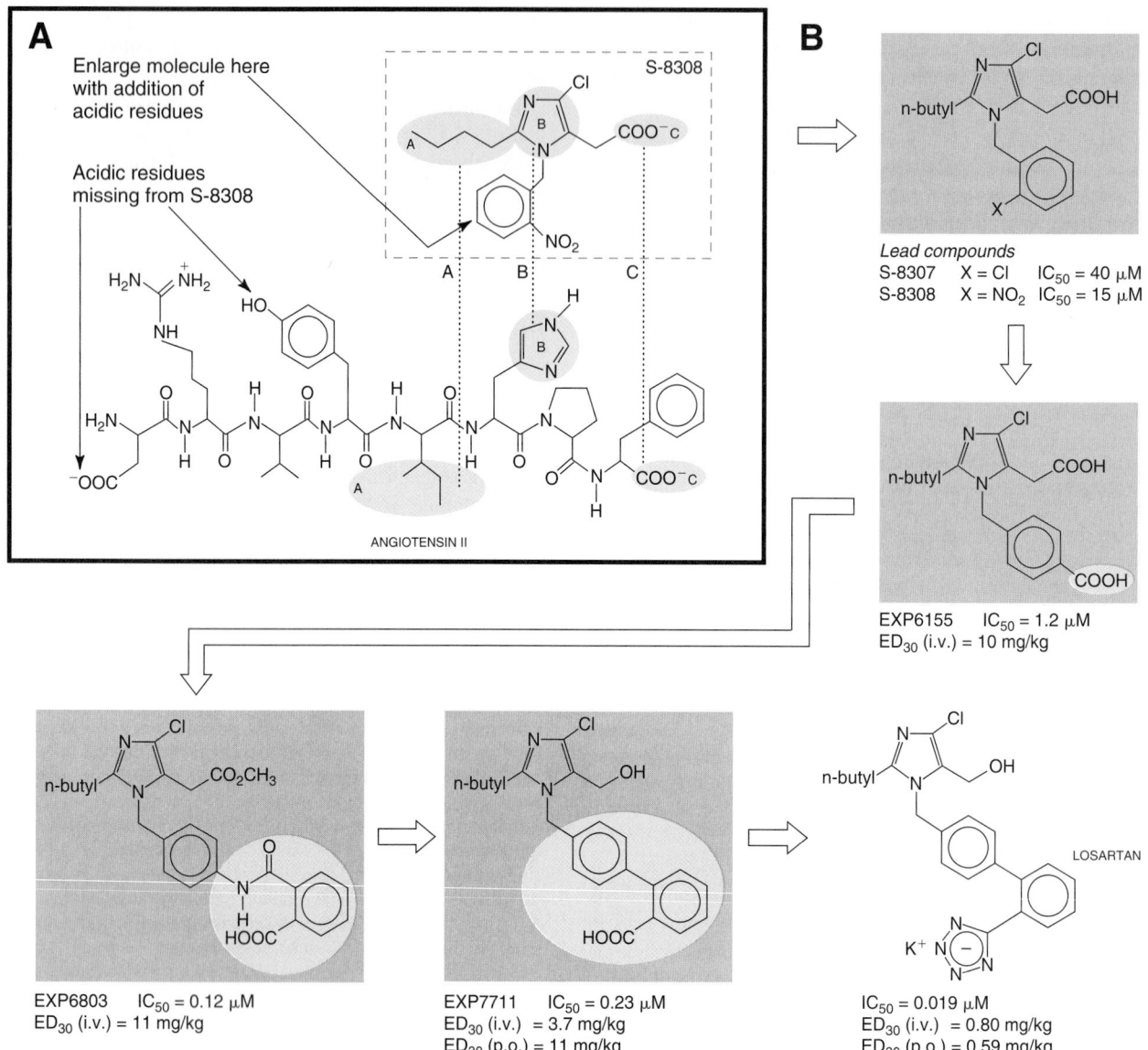

Figure 31–7. A. Hypothesized relationship between S-8308 (Takeda lead compound) and angiotensin II, and design strategies to enhance binding affinity of nonpeptide antagonists to the angiotensin II receptor. Letters indicate corresponding regions of S-8308 and angiotensin II. B. Pathway leading to the discovery of losartan.

(*Modified from Timmermans* et al., *1993, with permission.*)

are devoid of partial agonist activity, nonpeptide AT_1 receptor agonists have been synthesized, and structural modifications as minor as a methyl group can transform a potent antagonist into an agonist (Perlman *et al.,* 1997).

Pharmacological Effects. The angiotensin II receptor blockers (ARBs) available for clinical use bind to the AT_1

receptor with high affinity and are generally >10,000-fold selective for AT_1 *versus* the AT_2 receptor. The rank order affinity of the AT_1 receptor for ARBs is: candesartan > irbesartan > telmisartan = valsartan = EXP 3174 (the active metabolite of losartan) > losartan (Mimran *et al.,* 1999). Although binding of ARBs to the AT_1 receptor is competitive, the inhibition by ARBs of biological

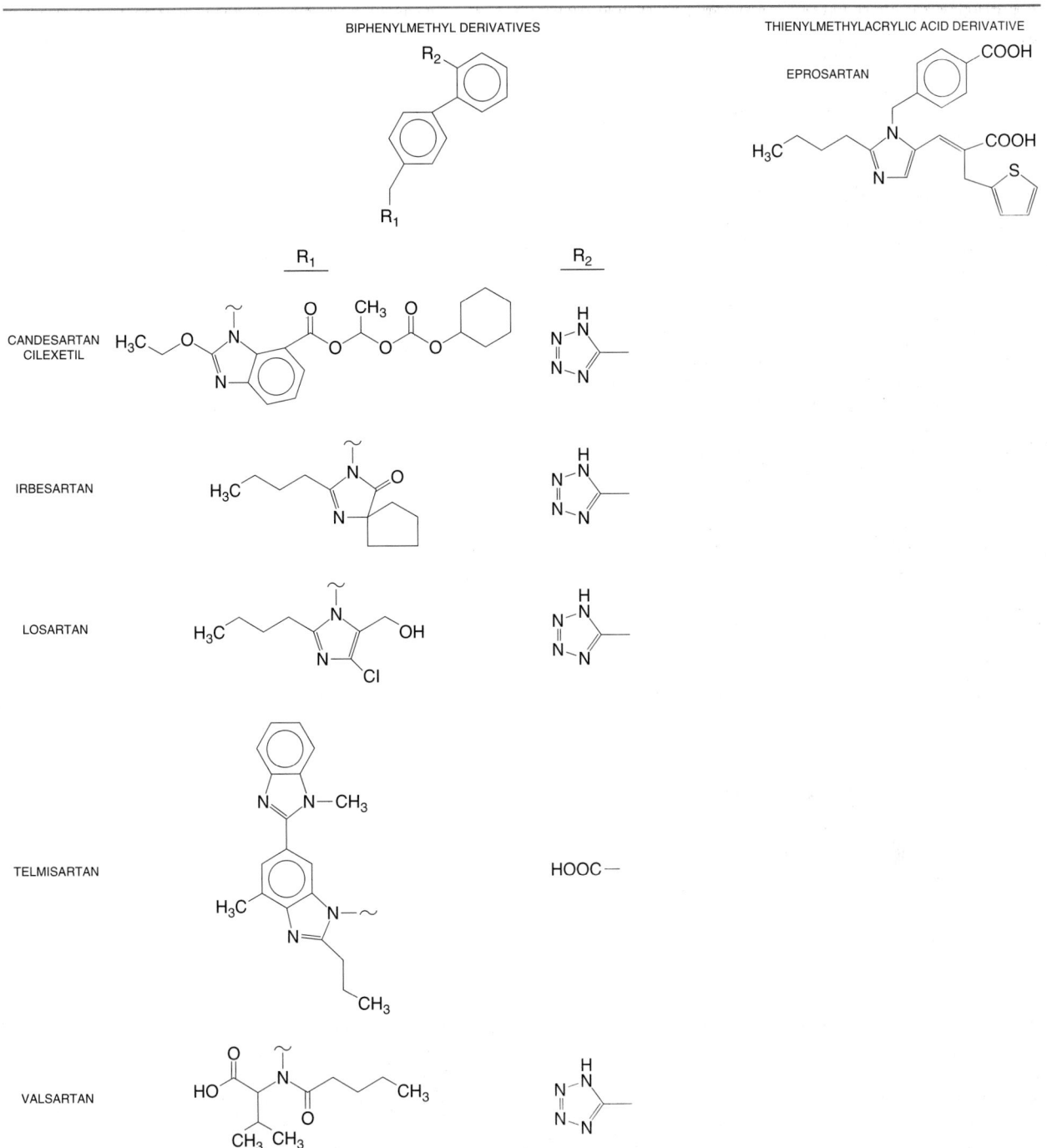

Figure 31–8. FDA-approved angiotensin II receptor antagonists.

responses to angiotensin II is often insurmountable, *i.e.,* the maximal response to angiotensin II cannot be restored in the presence of the ARB regardless of the concentration of angiotensin II added to the experimental preparation. Of the currently available ARBs, candesartan sup-

presses the maximal response to angiotensin II the most, whereas insurmountable blockade by irbesartan, eprosartan, telmisartan, and valsartan is less. Although losartan *per se* demonstrates surmountable antagonism, EXP 3174, an active metabolite of losartan, causes some degree of insurmountable blockade. The mechanism of insurmountable antagonism by ARBs may be due to slow dissociation kinetics of the compounds from the AT_1 receptor; however, a number of other factors may contribute, such as ARB-induced receptor internalization and alternative binding sites for ARBs on the AT_1 receptor (McConnaughey *et al.,* 1999). Regardless of the mechanism, insurmountable antagonism has the theoretical advantage of sustained receptor blockade even with increased levels of endogenous ligand and with missed doses of drug. Whether this theoretical advantage translates into an enhanced clinical performance remains to be determined.

The pharmacology of ARBs is well described (Timmermans *et al.,* 1993; Csajka *et al.,* 1997). ARBs potently and selectively inhibit, both *in vitro* and *in vivo,* most of the biological effects of angiotensin II, including angiotensin II-induced: (1) contraction of vascular smooth muscle; (2) rapid pressor responses; (3) slow pressor responses; (4) thirst; (5) vasopressin release; (6) aldosterone secretion; (7) release of adrenal catecholamines; (8) enhancement of noradrenergic neurotransmission; (9) increases in sympathetic tone; (10) changes in renal function; and (11) cellular hypertrophy and hyperplasia. ARBs reduce arterial blood pressure in animals with renovascular and genetic hypertension as well as in transgenic animals overexpressing the renin gene. ARBs, however, have little effect on arterial blood pressure in animals with low-renin hypertension (*e.g.,* rats with hypertension induced by NaCl and deoxycorticosterone).

A critical issue is whether or not ARBs are equivalent to ACE inhibitors with regard to therapeutic efficacy. Although both classes of drugs block the renin–angiotensin system, ARBs differ from ACE inhibitors in several important aspects: (1) *ARBs reduce activation of AT_1 receptors more effectively than do ACE inhibitors.* ACE inhibitors reduce the biosynthesis of angiotensin II produced by the action of ACE on angiotensin I, but do not inhibit alternative non-ACE angiotensin II–generating pathways. Because ARBs block the AT_1 receptor, the actions of angiotensin II *via* the AT_1 receptor are inhibited regardless of the biochemical pathway leading to angiotensin II formation. (2) In contrast to ACE inhibitors, *ARBs indirectly activate AT_2 receptors.* ACE inhibitors increase renin release; however, because ACE inhibitors block the conversion of angiotensin I to angiotensin II, ACE inhibition is not associated with increased levels of angiotensin II. ARBs also stimulate renin release; however, with ARBs, this translates into a several-fold increase in circulating levels of angiotensin II. Because AT_2 receptors are not blocked by clinically available ARBs, ARBs indirectly stimulate AT_2 receptors by increasing angiotensin II

levels. (3) *ACE inhibitors may increase angiotensin (1-7) levels more than do ARBs.* ACE is involved in the clearance of angiotensin (1-7), so inhibition of ACE may increase angiotensin (1-7) levels more so than do ARBs. (4) *ACE inhibitors increase the levels of a number of ACE substrates, including bradykinin and Ac-SDKP.* ACE is a nondiscriminating enzyme that processes a wide array of substrates; inhibiting ACE therefore increases the levels of ACE substrates and decreases the levels of their corresponding products. Whether or not the pharmacological differences between ARBs and ACE inhibitors result in significant differences in therapeutic outcomes is an open question.

Clinical Pharmacology.   Oral bioavailability of ARBs is generally low [<50%; except for irbesartan (70%)], and protein binding is high (>90%).

Candesartan Cilexetil (ATACAND).   Candesartan cilexetil is an inactive ester prodrug that is completely hydrolyzed to the active form, candesartan, during absorption from the gastrointestinal tract. Peak plasma levels are obtained 3 to 4 hours after oral administration, and the plasma half-life is about 9 hours. Plasma clearance of candesartan is due to renal elimination (33%) and biliary excretion (67%). The plasma clearance of candesartan is affected by renal insufficiency but not by mild-to-moderate hepatic insufficiency. Candesartan cilexetil should be administered orally once or twice daily for a total daily dosage of 4 to 32 mg.

Eprosartan (TEVETEN).   Peak plasma levels are obtained approximately 1 to 2 hours after oral administration, and the plasma half-life ranges from 5 to 9 hours. Eprosartan is in part metabolized to the glucuronide conjugate, and the parent compound and its glucuronide conjugate are cleared by renal elimination and biliary excretion. The plasma clearance of eprosartan is affected by both renal insufficiency and hepatic insufficiency. The recommended dosage of eprosartan is 400 to 800 mg/day in one or two doses.

Irbesartan (AVAPRO).   Peak plasma levels are obtained approximately 1.5 to 2 hours after oral administration, and the plasma half-life ranges from 11 to 15 hours. Irbesartan is in part metabolized to the glucuronide conjugate, and the parent compound and its glucuronide conjugate are cleared by renal elimination (20%) and biliary excretion (80%). The plasma clearance of irbesartan is unaffected by either renal or mild-to-moderate hepatic insufficiency. The oral dosage of irbesartan is 150 to 300 mg once daily.

Losartan (COZAAR).   Approximately 14% of an oral dose of losartan is converted to the 5-carboxylic acid metabolite, designated EXP 3174, which is more potent than losartan as an AT_1 receptor antagonist. The metabolism of losartan to EXP 3174 and to inactive metabolites is mediated by CYP2C9 and 3A4. Peak plasma levels of losartan and EXP 3174 are obtained approximately 1 to 3 hours after oral administration, respectively, and the plasma half-lives are 2.5 and 6 to 9 hours, respectively. The plasma clearances of losartan and EXP 3174 (600 and 50 ml/min, respectively) are due to renal clearance (75 and 25 ml/min, respectively) and hepatic clearance (metabolism and biliary excretion). The plasma clearance of losartan and EXP 3174 is affected by hepatic but not renal insufficiency. Losartan should be administered orally once or twice daily for a total daily dose of 25 to 100 mg.

Telmisartan (MICARDIS). Peak plasma levels are obtained approximately 0.5 to 1 hour after oral administration, and the plasma half-life is about 24 hours. Telmisartan is cleared from the circulation mainly by biliary secretion of intact drug. The plasma clearance of telmisartan is affected by hepatic, but not renal, insufficiency. The recommended oral dosage of telmisartan is 40 to 80 mg once daily.

Valsartan (DIOVAN). Peak plasma levels are obtained approximately 2 to 4 hours after oral administration, and the plasma half-life is about 9 hours. Food markedly decreases absorption. Valsartan is cleared from the circulation by the liver (about 70% of total clearance). The plasma clearance of valsartan is affected by hepatic but not renal insufficiency. The oral dosage of valsartan is 80 to 320 mg once daily.

Therapeutic Uses of Angiotensin II Receptor Antagonists. ARBs are approved only for the treatment of hypertension. The efficacy of ARBs with regard to lowering blood pressure is comparable to that of other established antihypertensive drugs, with an adverse effect profile similar to that of placebo (Mimran *et al.,* 1999). Several ARBs also are available as fixed-dose combinations with hydrochlorothiazide. Whether ARBs reduce cardiovascular morbidity and mortality as well as or better than other classes of antihypertensive drugs is unknown but under active investigation. The ongoing Losartan Intervention For Endpoint (LIFE) Reduction in Hypertension Study is a comparison of losartan with atenolol on cardiovascular morbidity and mortality in hypertensive patients with left ventricular hypertrophy (Dahlöf *et al.,* 1997).

Losartan is well tolerated in patients with heart failure and is comparable to enalapril with regard to improving exercise tolerance (Lang *et al.,* 1997). Moreover, losartan improves peak exercise capacity and attenuates symptoms in heart failure patients who have severe symptoms despite treatment with large doses of ACE inhibitors (Hamroff *et al.,* 1999). The Evaluation of Losartan in the Elderly (ELITE) study reported that, in elderly patients

with heart failure, losartan was as effective as captopril in improving symptoms and reduced mortality more than did captopril (Pitt *et al.,* 1997). However, the greater reduction in mortality by losartan was not confirmed in the larger Losartan Heart Failure Survival Study (ELITE II) trial (Pitt *et al.,* 1999); in fact, captopril tended to have a more favorable effect on several outcome measures. A similar trial comparing candesartan and an ACE inhibitor in heart failure patients (CHARM study) is in progress. Current recommendations are to use ACE inhibitors as first-line agents for the treatment of heart failure and to reserve ARBs for treatment of heart failure in patients who cannot tolerate or have an unsatisfactory response to ACE inhibitors. The ongoing Optimal Therapy in Myocardial Infarction with the Angiotensin II Antagonist Losartan (OPTIMAAL) study is comparing losartan with captopril on all-cause mortality in high-risk patients after acute myocardial infarction (Dickstein and Kjekshus, 1999).

Losartan is reported to be safe and highly effective in the treatment of portal hypertension in patients with cirrhosis and portal hypertension (Schneider *et al.,* 1999) without compromising renal function. The efficacy of ARBs in diabetic or nondiabetic patients with chronic renal insufficiency is unknown.

Adverse Effects. The incidence of discontinuation of ARBs due to adverse reactions is comparable to that of placebo. Unlike ACE inhibitors, ARBs do not cause cough, and the incidence of angioneurotic edema with ARBs is much less than with ACE inhibitors. As with ACE inhibitors, ARBs have fetopathic potential and should be discontinued before the second trimester of pregnancy. ARBs should be used cautiously in patients whose arterial blood pressure or renal function is highly dependent on the renin–angiotensin system. In such patients, ARBs can cause hypotension, oliguria, progressive azotemia, or acute renal failure. ARBs may cause hyperkalemia in patients with renal disease or in patients taking K^+ supplements or K^+-sparing drugs. ARBs enhance the blood pressure-lowering effect of other antihypertensive drugs, a desirable effect but one that may necessitate dosage adjustment.

PROSPECTUS

Vasopeptidase Inhibitors

Vasopeptidase inhibitors are drugs that inhibit enzymes that metabolize vasoactive peptides. One class of vasopeptidase inhibitors are compounds that block both ACE and neutral endopeptidase (NEP). Although ACE inhibitors are effective antihypertensive agents in high-renin and normal-renin hypertension, they are generally much less effective in hypertensive states associated with volume expansion and suppressed renin levels. NEP metabolizes various natriuretic peptides, including ANP, BNP, and CNP, as well as bradykinin. Because the secretion of natriuretic peptides is elevated by volume expansion, inhibition of NEP increases levels of natriuretic peptides during volume expansion. Thus, inhibition tends to cause natriuresis and lowers blood pressure in volume-expanded hypertension. Merging ACE and NEP inhibitory actions into a single molecular entity might afford antihypertensive drugs that, on average, lower blood pressure more and in a higher percentage of hypertensive patients than do currently available agents. These predictions recently were confirmed in hypertensive patients using the dual ACE/NEP inhibitor *omapatrilat*. Many dual ACE/NEP inhibitors are under preclinical and clinical investigation, and it is likely that such agents will become available in the near future. No doubt the efficacy of dual ACE/NEP inhibitors in patients with heart failure, myocardial infarction, and renal insufficiency, as well as in patients at high risk of cardiovascular disease, will be the focus of many outcome trials. In addition to vasopeptidase inhibitors that are dual ACE/NEP inhibitors, it is likely that other classes of vasopeptidase inhibitors will be developed and tested, such as agents that block some combination of ACE, NEP, endothelin-converting enzyme, or TNFα-converting enzyme.

Renin Inhibitors

Renin inhibitors have been the focus of drug development efforts for over two decades. Inefficient absorption and high first-pass metabolism and biliary excretion have stymied clinical development of this group of drugs. Nonetheless, development efforts continue, and some transition-state analogs of angiotensinogen hold significant promise (Lin and Frishman, 1996).

Gene Therapy for Hypertension

Many drugs now are available for the treatment of hypertension, and control of high blood pressure is no longer limited by the lack of effective drugs. However, since hypertension is usually a painless, lifelong disorder, compliance is the major obstacle to controlling hypertension in a significant percentage of patients. Consequently, the next breakthrough in hypertension research could be the development of treatments for hypertension that are semipermanent, requiring only occasional attention. Gene therapy (*see* Chapter 5) aimed at nullifying the renin–angiotensin system is a speculative, though not inconceivable, approach to the semipermanent or permanent treatment of hypertension. In this regard, two approaches have been suggested, a mutant angiotensinogen gene strategy (Jackson, 1992) and an antisense strategy; viral delivery of AT_1 receptor (Iyer *et al.*, 1996) and ACE antisense (Wang *et al.*, 1999) causes a sustained reduction of blood pressure in hypertensive animals.

For further discussion of hypertension, *see* Chapter 246 in *Harrison's Principles of Internal Medicine*, 14th ed., McGraw-Hill, New York, 1998.

BIBLIOGRAPHY

ACE Inhibitor Myocardial Infarction Collaborative Group. Indications for ACE inhibitors in the early treatment of acute myocardial infarction. Systematic overview of individual data from 100,000 patients in randomized trials. *Circulation,* **1998,** *97*:2202–2212.

AIRE Study Group. Effect of ramipril on mortality and morbidity of survivors of acute myocardial infarction with clinical evidence of heart failure. *Lancet,* **1993,** *342*:821–828.

Akasu, M., Urata, H., Kinoshita, A., Sasaguri, M., Ideishi, M., and Arakawa, K. Differences in tissue angiotensin II-forming pathways by species and organs in vitro. *Hypertension,* **1998,** *32*:514–520.

Álvarez, R., Reguero, J.R., Batalla, A., Iglesias-Cubero, G., Cortina, A., Álvarez, V., and Coto, E. Angiotensin-converting enzyme and angiotensin II receptor 1 polymorphisms: association with early coronary disease. *Cardiovasc. Res.,* **1998,** *40*:375–379.

Amant, C., Bauters, C., Bodart, J.-C., Lablanche, J.-M., Grollier, G., Danchin, N., Hamon, M., Richard, F., Helbecque, N., McFadden, E.P., Amouyel, P., and Bertrand, M.E. D allele of the angiotensin I–converting enzyme is a major risk factor for restenosis after coronary stenting. *Circulation,* **1997,** *96*:56–60.

Amant, C., Hamon, M., Bauters, C., Richard, F., Helbecque, N., McFadden, E.P., Escudero, X., Lablanche, J.-M., Amouyel, P., and Bertrand, M.E. The angiotensin II type 1 receptor gene polymorphism is associated with coronary artery vasoconstriction. *J. Am. Coll. Cardiol.,* **1997,** *29*:486–490.

Ambrosioni, E., Borghi, C., and Magnani, B. The effect of the angiotensin-converting-enzyme inhibitor zofenopril on mortality and morbidity after anterior myocardial infarction. *N. Engl. J. Med.,* **1995,** *332*:80–85.

Azizi, M., Ezan, E., Nicolet, L., Grognet, J.-M., and Ménard, J. High plasma level of *n*-acetyl-seryl-aspartyl-lysyl-proline. A new marker of chronic angiotensin-converting enzyme inhibition. *Hypertension,* **1997,** *30*:1015–1019.

Beierwaltes, W.H. Macula densa stimulation of renin is reversed by selective inhibition of neuronal nitric oxide synthase. *Am. J. Physiol.,* **1997,** *272*:R1359–R1364.

Beldent, V., Michaud, A., Bonnefoy, C., Chauvet, M.-T., and Corvol, P. Cell surface localization of proteolysis of human endothelial angiotensin I-converting enzyme. Effect of the amino-terminal domain in the solubilization process. *J. Biol. Chem.,* **1995,** *270*:28962–28969.

Bell, J.B.G., Chu, F.W., Tait, J.F., Tait, S.A.S., and Khosla, M. The use of superfusion approach with rat adrenal capsular cells to compare the steroidogenic potencies of angiotensin analogues, without the effects of peptide degradation. *Proc. R. Soc. Lond. B Biol. Sci.* **1984,** *221*:21–30.

Bell, L., and Madri, J.A. Influence of the angiotensin system on endothelial and smooth muscle cell migration. *Am. J. Physiol.,* **1990,** *137*:7–12.

Ben-Ari, E.T., and Garrison, J.C. Regulation of angiotensinogen mRNA accumulation in rat hepatocytes. *Am. J. Physiol.,* **1988,** *255*:E70–E79.

Benetos, A., Gautier, S., Ricard, S., Topouchian, J., Asmar, R., Poirier, O., Larosa, E., Guize, L., Safar, M., Soubrier, F., and Cambien, F. Influence of angiotensin-converting enzyme and angiotensin II type 1 receptor gene polymorphisms on aortic stiffness in normotensive and hypertensive patients. *Circulation,* **1996,** *94*:698–703.

Bernstein, K.E., Martin, B.M., Edwards, A.S., and Bernstein, E.A. Mouse angiotensin-converting enzyme is a protein composed of two homologous domains. *J. Biol. Chem.,* **1989,** *264*:11945–11951.

Borghi, C., Bacchelli, S., Esposti, D.D., Bignamini, A., Magnani, B., and Ambrosioni, E. Effects of the administration of an angiotensin-converting enzyme inhibitor during the acute phase of myocardial infarction in patients with arterial hypertension. SMILE Study Investigators. Survival of Myocardial Infarction Long-term Evaluation. *Am. J. Hypertens.,* **1999,** *12*:665–672.

Borghi, C., Marino, P., Zardini, P., Magnani, B., Collatina, S., and Ambrosioni, E. Post acute myocardial infarction. The Fosinopril in Acute Myocardial Infarction Study (FAMIS). *Am. J. Hypertens.,* **1997,** *10*:247S–254S.

Brink, M., Wellen, J., and Delafontaine, P. Angiotensin II causes weight loss and decreases circulating insulin-like growth factor I in rats through a pressor-independent mechanism. *J. Clin. Invest.,* **1996,** *97*:2509–2516.

Brown, A.J., Casals-Stenzel, J., Gofford, S., Lever, A.F., and Morton, J.J. Comparison of fast and slow pressor effects of angiotensin II in the conscious rat. *Am. J. Physiol.,* **1981,** *241*:H381–H388.

Brown, N.J., Agirbasli, M., and Vaughan, D.E. Comparative effect of angiotensin-converting enzyme inhibition and angiotensin II type 1 receptor antagonism on plasma fibrinolytic balance in humans. *Hypertension,* **1999,** *34*:285–290.

Brown, N.J., Ray, W.A., Snowden, M., and Griffin, M.R. Black Americans have an increased rate of angiotensin converting enzyme inhibitor-associated angioedema. *Clin. Pharmacol. Ther.,* **1996,** *60*:8–13.

Butler, R., Morris, A.D., Burchell, B., and Struthers, A.D. *DD* angiotensin-converting enzyme gene polymorphism is associated with endothelial dysfunction in normal humans. *Hypertension,* **1999,** *33*:1164–1168.

Cambien, F., Poirier, O., Lecerf, L., Evans, A., Cambou, J.P., Arveiler, D., Luc, G., Bard, J.M., Bara, L., Ricard, S., Tiret, L., Amouyel, P., Alhenc-Gelas, F., and Soubrier, F. Deletion polymorphism in the gene for angiotensin-converting enzyme is a potent risk factor for myocardial infarction. *Nature,* **1992,** *359*:641–644.

Campbell, D.J., Duncan, A.-M., and Kladis, A. Angiotensin-converting enzyme inhibition modifies angiotensin but not kinin peptide levels in human atrial tissue. *Hypertension,* **1999,** *34*:171–175.

Campbell, D.J., and Habener, J.F. Angiotensinogen gene is expressed and differentially regulated in multiple tissues of the rat. *J. Clin. Invest.,* **1986,** *78*:31–39.

Campbell, D.J., Kladis, A., Skinner, S.L., and Whitworth, J.A. Characterization of angiotensin peptides in plasma of anephric man. *J. Hypertens.,* **1991,** *9*:265–274.

Carey, R.M., McGrath, H.E., Pentz, E.S., Gomez, R.A., and Barrett, P.Q. Biomechanical coupling in renin-releasing cells. *J. Clin. Invest.,* **1997,** *100*:1566–1574.

Carini, D., and Duncia, J.V. Angiotensin II receptor blocking imidazoles. *European Patent Application 0253310,* **1988.**

Cashin-Hemphill, L., Holmvang, G., Chan, R.C., Pitt, B., Dinsmore, R.E., and Lees, R.S. Angiotensin-converting enzyme inhibition as antiatherosclerotic therapy: no answer yet. QUIET Investigators. QUinapril Ischemic Event Trial. *Am. J. Cardiol.,* **1999,** *83*:43–47.

Cassis, L.A., Saye, J., and Peach, M.J. Location and regulation of rat angiotensinogen messenger RNA. *Hypertension,* **1988,** *11*:591–596.

Caulfield, M., Lavender, P., Farrall, M., Munroe, P., Lawson, M., Turner, P., and Clark, A.J.L. Linkage of the angiotensinogen gene to essential hypertension. *N. Engl. J. Med.,* **1994,** *330*:1629–1633.

Caulfield, M., Lavender, P., Newell-Price, J., Farrall, M., Kamdar, S., Daniel, H., Lawson, M., De Freitas, P., Fogarty, P., and Clark, A.J.L. Linkage of the angiotensinogen gene locus to human essential hypertension in African Caribbeans. *J. Clin. Invest.,* **1995,** *96*: 687–692.

Chaturvedi, N., Sjolie, A.K., Stephenson, J.M., Abrahamian, H., Keipes, M., Castellarin, A., Rogulja-Pepeonik, Z., and Fuller, J.H. Effect of lisinopril on progression of retinopathy in normotensive people with type 1 diabetes. The EUCLID Study Group. EURODIAB Controlled Trial of Lisinopril in Insulin-Dependent Diabetes Mellitus. *Lancet,* **1998,** *351*:28–31.

Chiu, A.T., Carini, D.J., Johnson, A.L., McCall, D.E., Price, W.A., Thoolen, M.J.M., Wong, P.C., Taber, R.I., and Timmermans, P.B.M.W.M. Non-peptide angiotensin II receptor antagonists: II. Pharmacology of S-8308. *Eur. J. Pharmacol.,* **1988,** *157*:13–21.

Chiu, A.T., Herblin, W.F., McCall, D.E., Ardecky, R.J., Carini, D.J., Duncia, J.V., Pease, L.J., Wong, P.C., Wexler, R.R., Johnson, A.L., and Timmermans, P.B.M.W.M. Identification of angiotensin II receptor subtypes. *Biochem. Biophys. Res. Commun.,* **1989,** *165*:196–203.

Cohn, J.N., Johnson, G., Ziesche, S., Cobb, F., Francis, G., Tristani, F., Smith, R., Dunkman, W.B., Loeb, H., Wong, M., Bhat, G., Goldman, S., Fletcher, R.D., Doherty, J., Hughes, C.V., Carson, P., Cintron, G., Shabetai, R., and Haakenson, C. A comparison of enalapril with hydralazine-isosorbide dinitrate in the treatment of chronic congestive heart failure. *N. Engl. J. Med.,* **1991,** *325*:303–310.

CONSENSUS Trial Study Group. Effects of enalapril on mortality in severe congestive heart failure: results of the Cooperative North Scandinavian Enalapril Survival Study (CONSENSUS). *N. Engl. J. Med.,* **1987,** *316*:1429–1435.

Crawford, D.C., Chobanian, A.V., and Brecher, P. Angiotensin II induces fibronectin expression associated with cardiac fibrosis in the rat. *Circ. Res.,* **1994,** *74*:727–739.

Cressman, M.D., Vidt, D.G., and Acker, C. Renal glycosuria and azotemia after enalapril maleate (MK-421). *Lancet,* **1982,** *2*:440.

Cushman, D.W., Cheung, H.S., Sabo, E.F., and Ondetti, M.A. Design of potent competitive inhibitors of angiotensin-converting enzyme.

Carboxyalkanoyl and mercaptoalkanoyl amino acids. *Biochemistry,* **1977,** *16*:5484–5491.

Daemen, M.J.M.P., Lombardi, D.M., Bosman, F.T., and Schwartz, S.M. Angiotensin II induces smooth muscle cell proliferation in the normal and injured rat arterial wall. *Circ. Res.,* **1991,** *68*:450–456.

Dahlöf, B., Devereux, R., de Faire, U., Fyhrquist, F., Hedner, T., Ibsen, H., Julius, S., Kjeldsen, S., Kristianson, K., Lederballe-Pedersen, O., Lindholm, L.H., Nieminen, M.S., Omvik, P., Oparil, S., and Wedel, H. The Losartan Intervention For Endpoint reduction (LIFE) in Hypertension study. Rationale, design, and methods. The LIFE Study Group. *Am. J. Hypertens.,* **1997,** *10*:705–713.

Danser, A.H.J., Sassen, L.M.A., Admiraal, P.J.J., Derkx, F.H.M., Verdouw, P.D., and Schalekamp, M.A.D.H. Regional production of angiotensins I and II: contribution of vascular kidney-derived renin. *J. Hypertens.,* **1991,** *9*:S234–S235.

Danser, A.H.J., van Kats, J.P., Admiraal, P.J.J., Derkx, F.H.M., Lamers, J.M.J., Verdouw, P.D., Saxena, P.R., and Schalekamp, M.A.D.H. Cardiac renin and angiotensins. Uptake from plasma versus in situ synthesis. *Hypertension,* **1994,** *24*:37–48.

Danser, A.H.J.D., Koning, M.M.G., Admiraal, P.J.J., Sassen, L.M.A., Derkx, F.H.M., Verdouw, P.D., and Schalekamp, M.A.D.H. Production of angiotensins I and II at tissue sites in intact pigs. *Am. J. Physiol.,* **1992,** *263*:H429–H437.

Data, J.L., Gerber, J.G., Crump, W.J., Frölich, J.C., Hollifield, J.W., and Nies, A.S. The prostaglandin system. A role in canine baroreceptor control of renin release. *Circ. Res.,* **1978,** *42*:454–458.

Davie, A.P., Dargie, H.J., and McMurray, J.J.V. Role of bradykinin in the vasodilator effects of losartan and enalapril in patients with heart failure. *Circulation,* **1999,** *100*:268–273.

De Castro, S., Pelliccia, F., Cartoni, D., Funaro, S., Melillo, G., Beni, S., Magni, G., Migliau, G., and Fedele, F. Effects of angiotensin-converting enzyme inhibition on left ventricular geometric patterns in patients with essential hypertension. *J. Clin. Pharmacol.,* **1996,** *36*:1141–1148.

Dickstein, K., and Kjekshus, J. Comparison of the effects of losartan and captopril on mortality in patients after acute myocardial infarction: the OPTIMAAL trial design. Optimal Therapy in Myocardial Infarction with the Angiotensin II Antagonist Losartan. *Am. J. Cardiol.,* **1999,** *83*:477–481.

Dubey, R.K., Jackson, E.K., and Lüscher, T.F. Nitric oxide inhibits angiotensin II-induced migration of rat aortic smooth muscle cell: role of cyclic-nucleotides and angiotensin₁ receptors. *J. Clin. Invest.,* **1995,** *96*:141–149.

Erhardt, L., MacLean, A., Ilgenfritz, J., Gelperin, K., and Blumenthal, M. Fosinopril attenuates clinical deterioration and improves exercise tolerance in patients with heart failure. Fosinopril Efficacy/Safety Trial (FEST) Study Group. *Eur. Heart J.,* **1995,** *16*:1892–1899.

Estacio, R.O., Jeffers, B.W., Hiatt, W.R., Biggerstaff, S.L., Gifford, N., and Schrier, R.W. The effect of nisoldipine as compared with enalapril on cardiovascular outcomes in patients with non-insulin-dependent diabetes and hypertension. *N. Engl. J. Med.,* **1998,** *338*:645–652.

EUCLID Study Group. Randomised placebo-controlled trial of lisinopril in normotensive patients with insulin-dependent diabetes and normoalbuminuria or microalbuminuria. *Lancet,* **1997,** *349*:1787–1792.

Fornage, M., Amos, C.I., Kardia, S., Sing, C.F., Turner, S.T., and Boerwinkle, E. Variation in the region of the angiotensin-converting enzyme gene influences interindividual differences in blood pressure levels in young white males. *Circulation,* **1998,** *97*:1773–1779.

Friedrich, S.P., Lorell, B.H., Rousseau, M.F., Hayashida, W., Hess, O.M., Douglas, P.S., Gordon, S., Keighley, C.S., Benedict, C., Krayenbuehl, H.P., Grossman, W., and Pouleur, H. Intracardiac angiotensin-converting enzyme inhibition improves diastolic function in patients with left ventricular hypertrophy due to aortic stenosis. *Circulation,* **1994,** *90*:2761–2771.

Friis, U.G., Jensen, B.L., Aas, J.K., and Skøtt, O. Direct demonstration of exocytosis and endocytosis in single mouse juxtaglomerular cells. *Circ. Res.,* **1999,** *84*:929–936.

Frölich, J.C., Hollifield, J.W., Michelakis, A.M., Vesper, B.S., Wilson, J.P., Shand, D.G., Seyberth, H.J., Frölich, W.H., and Oates, J.A. Reduction of plasma renin activity by inhibition of the fatty acid cyclooxygenase in human subjects. Independence of sodium retention. *Circ. Res.,* **1979,** *44*:781–787.

Furakawa, Y., Kishimoto, S., and Nishikawa, K. Hypotensive imidazole derivatives and hypotensive imidazole-5-acetic acid derivatives. Patents issued to Takeda Chemical Industries Ltd. on July 20, 1982, and October 19, 1982, respectively. U.S. Patents 4,340,598 and 4,355,040, Osaka, Japan, 1982.

Gainer, J.V., Morrow, J.D., Loveland, A., King, D.J., and Brown, N.J. Effect of bradykinin-receptor blockade on the response to angiotensin-converting-enzyme inhibitor in normotensive and hypertensive subjects. *N. Engl. J. Med.,* **1998,** *339*:1285–1292.

Gardemann, A., Weiss, T., Schwartz, O., Eberbach, A., Katz, N., Hehrlein, F.W., Tillmanns, H., Waas, W., and Haberbosch, W. Gene polymorphism but not catalytic activity of angiotensin I-converting enzyme is associated with coronary artery disease and myocardial infarction in low-risk patients. *Circulation,* **1995,** *92*:2796–2799.

Gerber, J.G., Nies, A.S., and Olsen, R.D. Control of canine renin release: macula densa requires prostaglandin synthesis. *J. Physiol.,* **1981,** *319*:419–429.

Gesualdo, L., Ranieri, E., Monno, R., Rossiello, M.R., Colucci, M., Semeraro, N., Grandaliano, G., Schena, F.P., Ursi, M., and Cerullo, G. Angiotensin IV stimulates plasminogen activator inhibitor-I expression in proximal tubular epithelial cells. *Kidney Int.,* **1999,** *56*:461–470.

GISEN Group (Gruppo Italiano di Studi Epidemiologici in Nefrologia). Randomised placebo-controlled trial of effect of ramipril on decline in glomerular filtration rate and risk of terminal renal failure in proteinuric, non-diabetic nephropathy. *Lancet,* **1997,** *349*:1857–1863.

Grassi, G., Cattaneo, B.M., Seravalle, G., Lanfranchi, A., Pozzi, M., Morganti, A., Carugo, S., and Mancia, G. Effects of chronic ACE inhibition on sympathetic nerve traffic and baroreflex control of circulation in heart failure. *Circulation,* **1997,** *96*:1173–1179.

Greenberg, S.G., Lorenz, J.N., He, X.-R., Schnermann, J.B., and Briggs, J.P. Effect of prostaglandin synthesis inhibition on macula densa–stimulated renin secretion. *Am. J. Physiol.,* **1993,** *265*:F578–F583.

Gruppo Italiano per lo Studio della Sopravvivenza nell'Infarto Miocardico. GISSI-3: effects of lisinopril and transdermal glyceryl trinitrate singly and together on 6-week mortality and ventricular function after acute myocardial infarction. *Lancet,* **1994,** *343*:1115–1122.

Guazzi, M.D., Campodonico, J., Celeste, F., Guazzi, M., Santambrogio, G., Rossi, M., Trabattoni, D., and Alimento, M. Antihypertensive efficacy of angiotensin converting enzyme inhibition and aspirin counteraction. *Clin. Pharmacol. Ther.,* **1998,** *63*:79–86.

Gustafsson, I., Torp-Pedersen, C., Køber, L., Gustafsson, F., and Hildebrandt, P. Effect of the angiotensin-converting enzyme inhibitor trandolapril on mortality and morbidity in diabetic patients with left ventricular dysfunction after acute myocardial infarction. Trace Study Group. *J. Am. Coll. Cardiol.,* **1999,** *34*:83–89.

Hagaman, J.R., Moyer, J.S., Bachman, E.S., Sibony, M., Magyar, P.L., Welch, J.E., Smithies, O., Krege, J.H., and O'Brien, D.A. Angiotensin-converting enzyme and male fertility. *Proc. Natl. Acad. Sci. U.S.A.,* **1998,** *95*:2552–2557.

Hall, J.E., Coleman, T.G., Guyton, A.C., Kastner, P.R., and Granger, J.P. Control of glomerular filtration rate by circulating angiotensin II. *Am. J. Physiol.,* **1981,** *241*:R190–R197.

Hall, J.E., Guyton, A.C., Smith, M.J. Jr., and Coleman, T.G. Blood pressure and renal function during chronic changes in sodium intake: role of angiotensin. *Am. J. Physiol.,* **1980,** *239*:F271–F280.

Hamroff, G., Katz, S.D., Mancini, D., Blaufarb, I., Bijou, R., Patel, R., Jondeau, G., Olivari, M.-T., Thomas, S., and Le Jemtel, T.H. Addition of angiotensin II receptor blockade to maximal angiotensin-converting enzyme inhibition improves exercise capacity in patients with severe congestive heart failure. *Circulation,* **1999,** *99*:990–992.

Hansson, L., Lindholm, L.H., Niskanen, L., Lanke, J., Hedner, T., Niklason, A., Luomanmaki, K., Dahlof, B., de Faire, U., Morlin, C., Karlberg, B.E., Wester, P.O., and Bjorck, J.-E. Effect of angiotensin-converting-enzyme inhibition compared with conventional therapy on cardiovascular morbidity and mortality in hypertension: the Captopril Prevention Project (CAPPP) randomised trial. *Lancet,* **1999,** *353*:611–616.

Harris, R.C., McKanna, J.A., Akai, Y., Jacobson, H.R., Dubois, R.N., and Breyer, M.D. Cyclooxygenase-2 is associated with the macula densa of rat kidney and increases with salt restriction. *J. Clin. Invest.,* **1994,** *94*:2504–2510.

Hosoi, M., Nishizawa, Y., Kogawa, K., Kawagishi, T., Konishi, T., Maekawa, K., Emoto, M., Fukumoto, S., Shioi, A., Shoji, T., Inaba, M., Okuno, Y., and Morii, H. Angiotensin-converting enzyme gene polymorphism is associated with carotid arterial wall thickness in non-insulin-dependent diabetic patients. *Circulation,* **1996,** *94*:704–707.

Hricik, D.E., Browning, P.J., Kopelman, R., Goorno, W.E., Madias, N.E., and Dzau, V.J. Captopril-induced functional renal insufficiency in patients with bilateral renal-artery stenoses or renal-artery stenosis in a solitary kidney. *N. Engl. J. Med.,* **1983,** *308*:373–376.

Hu, L., Catanzaro, D.F., Pitarresi, T.-M., Laragh, J.H., and Sealey, J.E. Identical hemodynamic and hormonal responses to 14-day infusions of renin or angiotensin II in conscious rats. *J. Hypertens.,* **1998,** *16*:1285–1298.

Imai, T., Miyazaki, H., Hirose, S., Hori, H., Hayashi, T., Kageyama, R., Ohkubo, H., Nakanishi, S., and Murakami, K. Cloning and sequence analysis of cDNA for human renin precursor. *Proc. Natl. Acad. Sci. U.S.A.,* **1983,** *80*:7405–7409.

ISIS-4 (Fourth International Study of Infarct Survival) Collaborative Group. ISIS-4: a randomised factorial trial assessing early oral captopril, oral mononitrate, and intravenous magnesium sulphate in 58050 patients with suspected acute myocardial infarction. *Lancet,* **1995,** *345*:669–685.

Itoh, H., Mukoyama, M., Pratt, R.E., Gibbons, G.H., and Dzau, V.J. Multiple autocrine growth factors modulate vascular smooth muscle cell growth response to angiotensin II. *J. Clin. Invest.,* **1993,** *91*:2268–2274.

Itoh, S., Carretero, O.A., and Murray, R.D. Possible role of adenosine in the macula densa mechanism of renin release in rabbits. *J. Clin. Invest.,* **1985,** *76*:1412–1417.

Iwai, N., Ohmichi, N., Nakamura, Y., and Kinoshita, M. DD genotype of the angiotensin-converting enzyme gene is a risk factor for left ventricular hypertrophy. *Circulation,* **1994,** *90*:2622–2628.

Iyer, S.N., Lu, D., Katovich, M.J., and Raizada, M.K. Chronic control of high blood pressure in the spontaneously hypertensive rat by

delivery of angiotensin type 1 receptor antisense. *Proc. Natl. Acad. Sci. U.S.A.,* **1996,** *93*:9960–9965.

Jeunemaitre, X., Soubrier, F., Kotelevtsev, Y.V., Lifton, R.P., Williams, C.S., Charru, A., Hunt, S.C., Hopkins, P.N., Williams, R.R., Lalouel, J.M., and Corvol, P. Molecular basis of human hypertension: role of angiotensinogen. *Cell,* **1992,** *71*:169–180.

Johns, D.W., Ayers, C.R., and Williams, S.C. Dilation of forearm blood vessels after angiotensin-converting-enzyme inhibition by captopril in hypertensive patients. *Hypertension,* **1984,** *6*:545–550.

Kageyama, R., Ohkubo, H., and Nakanishi, S. Primary structure of human preangiotensinogen deduced from the cloned cDNA sequence. *Biochemistry,* **1984,** *23*:3603–3609.

Kainulainen, K., Perola, M., Terwilliger, J., Kaprio, J., Koskenvuo, M., Syvänen, A.-C., Vartiainen, E., Peltonen, L., and Kontula, K. Evidence for involvement of the type 1 angiotensin II receptor locus in essential hypertension. *Hypertension,* **1999,** *33*:844–849.

Kario, K., Kanai, N., Saito, K., Nago, N., Matsuo, T., and Shimada, K. Ischemic stroke and the gene for angiotensin-converting enzyme in Japanese hypertensives. *Circulation,* **1996,** *93*:1630–1633.

Kastner, P.R., Hall, J.E., and Guyton, A.C. Control of glomerular filtration rate: role of intrarenally formed angiotensin II. *Am. J. Physiol.,* **1984,** *246*:F897–F906.

Kato, H., Iwai, N., Inui, H., Kimoto, K., Uchiyama, Y., and Inagami, T. Regulation of vascular angiotensin release. *Hypertension,* **1993,** *21*:446–454.

Kehoe, P.G., Russ, C., McIlory, S., Williams, H., Holmans, P., Holmes, C., Liolitsa, D., Vahidassr, D., Powell, J., McGleenon, B., Liddell, M., Plomin, R., Dynan, K., Williams, N., Neal, J., Cairns, N.J., Wilcock, G., Passmore, P., Lovestone, S., Williams, J., and Owen, M.J. Variation in *DCP1,* encoding ACE, is associated with susceptibility to Alzheimer disease. *Nature Genet.,* **1999,** *21*:71–72.

Kerins, D.M., Hao, Q., and Vaughan, D.E. Angiotensin induction of PAI-1 expression in endothelial cells is mediated by the hexapeptide angiotensin IV. *J. Clin. Invest.,* **1995,** *96*:2515–2520.

Kim, H.-S., Krege, J.H., Kluckman, K.D., Hagaman, J.R., Hodgin, J.B., Best, C.F., Jennette, J.C., Coffman, T.M., Maeda, N., and Smithies, O. Genetic control of blood pressure and the angiotensinogen locus. *Proc. Natl. Acad. Sci. U.S.A.,* **1995,** *92*:2735–2739.

Kleber, F.X., Niemoller, L., and Doering, W. Impact of converting enzyme inhibition on progression of chronic heart failure: results of the Munich Mild Heart Failure Trial. *Br. Heart J.,* **1992,** *67*:289–296.

Køber, L., Torp-Pedersen, C., Carlsen, J.E., Bagger, H., Eliasen, P., Lyngborg, K., Videbaek, J., Cole, D.S., Auclert, L., Pauly, N.C., Aliopt, E., Persson, S., and Comm, A.J. A clinical trial of the angiotensin-converting-enzyme inhibitor trandolapril in patients with left ventricular dysfunction after myocardial infarction. Trandolapril Cardiac Evaluation (TRACE) Study Group. *N. Engl. J. Med.,* **1995,** *333*:1670–1676.

Kunz, R., Kreutz, R., Beige, J., Distler, A., and Sharma, A.M. Association between the angiotensinogen 235T-variant and essential hypertension in whites. A systematic review and methodological appraisal. *Hypertension,* **1997,** *30*:1331–1337.

Kyriakidis, M., Triposkiadis, F., Dernellis, J., Androulakis, A.E., Mellas, P., Kelepeshis, G.A., and Gialafos, J.E. Effects of cardiac versus circulatory angiotensin-converting enzyme inhibition on left ventricular diastolic function and coronary blood flow in hypertrophic obstructive cardiomyopathy. *Circulation,* **1998,** *97*:1342–1347.

Landino, L.M., Crews, B.C., Timmons, M.D., Morrow, J.D., and Marnett, L.J. Peroxynitrite, the coupling product of nitric oxide and superoxide, activates prostaglandin biosynthesis. *Proc. Natl. Acad. Sci. U.S.A.,* **1996,** *93*:15069–15074.

Lang, R.M., Elkayam, U., Yellen, L.G., Krauss, D., McKelvie, R.S., Vaughan, D.E., Ney, D.E., Makris, L., and Chang, P.I. Comparative effects of losartan and enalapril on exercise capacity and clinical status in patients with heart failure. The Losartan Pilot Exercise Study Investigators. *J. Am. Coll. Cardiol.,* **1997,** *30*:983–991.

Laursen, J.B., Rajagopalan, S., Galis, Z., Tarpey, M., Freeman, B.A., and Harrison, D.G. Role of superoxide in angiotensin II-induced but not catecholamine-induced hypertension. *Circulation,* **1997,** *95*: 588–593.

Lee-Kirsch, M.A., Gaudet, F., Cardoso, M.C., and Lindpaintner, K. Distinct renin isoforms generated by tissue-specific transcription initiation and alternative splicing. *Circ. Res.,* **1999,** *84*:240–246.

Lewis, E.J., Hunsicker, L.G., Bain, R.P., and Rohde, R.D. The effect of angiotensin-converting-enzyme inhibition on diabetic nephropathy. *N. Engl. J. Med.,* **1993,** *329*:1456–1462.

Linas, S.L. Role of prostaglandins in renin secretion in the isolated kidney. *Am. J. Physiol.,* **1984,** *246*:F811–F818.

Linz, W., Jessen, T., Becker, R.H.A., Schölkens, B.A., and Wiemer, G. Long-term ACE inhibition doubles lifespan of hypertensive rats. *Circulation,* **1997,** *96*:3164–3172.

Liu, F.-Y., and Cogan, M.G. Angiotensin II: a potent regulator of acidification in the rat early proximal convoluted tubule. *J. Clin. Invest.,* **1987,** *80*:272–275.

Lorenz, J.N., Weihprecht, H., Schnermann, J., Skøtt, O., and Briggs, J.P. Renin release from isolated juxtaglomerular apparatus depends on macula densa chloride transport. *Am. J. Physiol.,* **1991,** *260*: F486–F493.

Malini, P.L., Strocchi, E., Zanardi, M., Milani, M., and Ambrosioni, E. Thromboxane antagonism and cough induced by angiotensin-converting-enzyme inhibitor. *Lancet,* **1997,** *350*:15–18.

Mancini, G.B.J., Henry, G.C., Macaya, C., O'Neill, B.J., Pucillo, A.L., Carere, R.G., Wargovich, T.J., Mudra, H., Luscher, T.F., Klibaner, M.I., Haber, H.E., Uprichard, A.C., Pepine, C.J., and Pitt, B. Angiotensin-converting enzyme inhibition with quinapril improves endothelial vasomotor dysfunction in patients with coronary artery disease. The TREND (Trial on Reversing ENdothelial Dysfunction) Study. *Circulation,* **1996,** *94*:258–265.

Marre, M., Jeunemaitre, X., Gallois, Y., Rodier, M., Chatellier, G., Sert, C., Dusselier, L., Kahal, Z., Chaillous, L., Halimi, S., Muller, A., Sackmann, H., Bauduceau, B., Bled, F., Passa, P., and Alhenc-Gelas, F. Contribution of genetic polymorphism in the renin–angiotensin system to the development of renal complications in insulin-dependent diabetes. Génétique de la Néphropathie Diabétique (GENEDIAB) study group. *J. Clin. Invest.,* **1997,** *99*:1585–1595.

Maschio, G., Alberti, D., Janin, G., Locatelli, F., Mann, J.F.E., Motolese, M., Ponticelli, C., Ritz, E., and Zucchelli, P. Effect of the angiotensin-converting-enzyme inhibitor benazepril on the progression of chronic renal insufficiency. The Angiotensin-Converting-Enzyme Inhibition in Progressive Renal Insufficiency Study Group. *N. Engl. J. Med.,* **1996,** *334*:939–945.

Mattu, R.K., Needham, E.W., Galton, D.J., Frangos, E., Clark, A.J.L., and Caulfield, M. A DNA variant at the angiotensin-converting enzyme gene locus associates with coronary artery disease in the Caerphilly Heart Study. *Circulation,* **1995,** *91*:270–274.

Montgomery, H.E., Clarkson, P., Dollery, C.M., Prasad, K., Losi, M.-A., Hemingway, H., Statters, D., Jubb, M., Girvain, M., Varnava, A., World, M., Deanfield, J., Talmud, P., McEwan, J.R., McKenna, W.J., and Humphries, S. Association of angiotensin-converting enzyme gene I/D polymorphism with change in left ventricular mass in response to physical training. *Circulation,* **1997,** *96*:741–747.

Mukoyama, M., Nakajima, M., Horiuchi, M., Sasamura, H., Pratt, R.E., and Dzau, V.J. Expression cloning of type 2 angiotensin II receptor reveals a unique class of seven-transmembrane receptors. *J. Biol. Chem.,* **1993,** *268*:24539–24542.

Murphy, T.J., Alexander, R.W., Griendling, K.K., Runge, M.S., and Bernstein, K.E. Isolation of a cDNA encoding the vascular type-1 angiotensin II receptor. *Nature,* **1991,** *351*:233–236.

Niimura, F., Labosky, P.A., Kakuchi, J., Okubo, S., Yoshida, H., Oikawa, T., Ichiki, T., Naftilan, A.J., Fogo, A., Inagami, T., Hogan, B.L.M., and Ichikawa, I. Gene targeting in mice reveals a requirement for angiotensin in the development and maintenance of kidney morphology and growth factor regulation. *J. Clin. Invest.,* **1995,** *96*:2947–2954.

O'Donnell, C.J., Lindpaintner, K., Larson, M.G., Rao, V.S., Ordovas, J.M., Schaefer, E.J., Myers, R.H., and Levy, D. Evidence for association and genetic linkage of the angiotensin-converting enzyme locus with hypertension and blood pressure in men but not women in the Framingham Heart Study. *Circulation,* **1998,** *97*:1766–1772.

O'Driscoll, G., Green, D., Rankin, J., Stanton, K., and Taylor, R. Improvement in endothelial function by angiotensin converting enzyme inhibition in insulin-dependent diabetes mellitus. *J. Clin. Invest.,* **1997,** *100*:678–684.

Oike, Y., Hata, A., Ogata, Y., Numata, Y., Shido, K., and Kondo, K. Angiotensin converting enzyme as a genetic risk factor for coronary artery spasm. Implication in the pathogenesis of myocardial infarction. *J. Clin. Invest.,* **1995,** *96*:2975–2979.

Olivieri, O., Trabetti, E., Grazioli, S., Stranieri, C., Friso, S., Girelli, D., Russo, C., Pignatti, P.F., Mansueto, G., and Corrocher, R. Genetic polymorphisms of the renin–angiotensin system and atheromatous renal artery stenosis. *Hypertension,* **1999,** *34*:1097–1100.

Osterop, A.P.R.N., Kofflard, M.J.M., Sandkuijl, L.A., ten Cate, F.J., Krams, R., Schalekamp, M.A.D.H., and Danser, A.H.J. AT_1 receptor A/C^{1166} polymorphism contributes to cardiac hypertrophy in subjects with hypertrophic cardiomyopathy. *Hypertension,* **1998,** *32*:825–830.

Perlman, S., Costa-Neto, C.M., Miyakawa, A.A., Schambye, H.T., Hjorth, S.A., Paiva, A.C.M., Rivero, R.A., Greenlee, W.J., and Schwartz, T.W. Dual agonistic and antagonistic property of nonpeptide angiotensin AT_1 ligands: susceptibility to receptor mutations. *Mol. Pharmacol.,* **1997,** *51*:301–311.

Pfeffer, M.A., Braunwald, E., Moyé, L.A., Basta, L., Brown, E.J. Jr., Cuddy, T.E., Davis, B.R., Geltman, E.M., Goldman, S., Flaker, G.C., Klein, M., Lamas, G.A., Packer, M., Rouleau, J., Rouleau, J.L., Rutherford, J., Wertheimer, J.H., and Hawkins, C.M. Effect of captopril on mortality and morbidity in patients with left ventricular dysfunction after myocardial infarction. *N. Engl. J. Med.* **1992,** *327*:669–677.

Philipp, C.S., Dilley, A., Saidi, P., Evatt, B., Austin, H., Zawadsky, J., Harwood, D., Ellingsen, D., Barnhart, E., Phillips, D.J., and Hooper, W.C. Deletion polymorphism in the angiotensin-converting enzyme gene as thrombophilic risk factor after hip arthroplasty. *Thromb. Haemost.,* **1998,** *80*:869–873.

Pitt, B., and Poole-Wilson, P.A. ELITE II (Losartan Heart Failure Survival Study). Angiotensin II receptor blocker vs. ACE inhibitor in severe heart failure. Late-breaking clinical trials. Presented at the American Heart Association's 72nd Scientific Session November 7–10, **1999.**

Pitt, B., Segal, R., Martinez, F.A., Meurers, G., Cowley, A.J., Thomas, I., Deedwania, P.C., Ney, D.E., Snavely, D.B., and Chang, P.I. Randomised trial of losartan versus captopril in patients over 65 with heart failure (Evaluation of Losartan in the Elderly study, ELITE). *Lancet,* **1997,** *349*:747–752.

Rajagopalan, S., Laursen, J.B., Borthayre, A., Kurz, S., Keiser, J., Haleen, S., Giaid, A., and Harrison, D.G. Role for endothelin-1 in angiotensin II-mediated hypertension. *Hypertension*, **1997**, *30*:29–34.

Ravid, M., Brosh, D., Levi, Z., Bar-Dayan, Y., Ravid, D., and Rachmani, R. Use of enalapril to attenuate decline in renal function in normotensive, normoalbuminuric patients with type 2 diabetes mellitus. A randomized, controlled trial. *Ann. Intern. Med.*, **1998**, *128*:982–988.

Ravid, M., Lang, R., Rachmani, R., and Lishner, M. Long-term renoprotective effect of angiotensin-converting enzyme inhibition in non-insulin-dependent diabetes mellitus. A 7-year follow-up study. *Arch. Intern. Med.*, **1996**, *156*:286–289.

Ravid, M., Savin, H., Jutrin, I., Bental, T., Katz, B., and Lishner, M. Long-term stabilizing effect of angiotensin-converting enzyme inhibition on plasma creatinine and on proteinuria in normotensive type II diabetic patients. *Ann. Intern. Med.*, **1993**, *118*:577–581.

Rhaleb, N.E., Peng, H., Alfie, M.E., Shesely, E.G., and Carretero, O.A. Effect of ACE inhibitor on DOCA-salt- and aortic coarctation-induced hypertension in mice. Do kinin B2 receptors play a role? *Hypertension*, **1999**, *33*:329–334.

Ribichini, F., Steffenino, G., Dellavalle, A., Matullo, G., Colajanni, E., Camilla, T., Vado. A., Benetton, G., Uslenghi, E., and Piazza, A. Plasma activity and insertion/deletion polymorphism of angiotensin I-converting enzyme. A major risk factor and a marker of risk for coronary stent restenosis. *Circulation*, **1998**, *97*:147–154.

Rigat, B., Hubert, C., Alhenc-Gelas, F., Cambien, F., Corvol, P., and Soubrier, F. An insertion/deletion polymorphism in the angiotensin I-converting enzyme gene accounting for half the variance of serum enzyme levels. *J. Clin. Invest.*, **1990**, *86*:1343–1346.

Ruggenenti, P., Perna, A., Benini, R., Bertani, T., Zoccali, C., Maggiore, Q., Salvadori, M., and Remuzzi, G. In chronic nephropathies prolonged ACE inhibition can induce remission: dynamics of time-dependent changes in GFR. Investigators of the GISEN Group. Gruppo Italiano Studi Epidemiologici in Nefrologia. *J. Am. Soc. Nephrol.*, **1999a**, *10*:997–1006.

Ruggenenti, P., Perna, A., Gherardi, G., Garini, G., Zoccali, C., Salvadori, M., Scolari, F., Schena, F.P., and Remuzzi, G. Renoprotective properties of ACE-inhibition in non-diabetic nephropathies with non-nephrotic proteinuria. *Lancet*, **1999b**, *354*:359–364.

Ruggenenti, P., Perna, A., Gherardi, G., Gaspari, F., Benini, R., and Remuzzi, G. Renal function and requirement for dialysis in chronic nephropathy patients on long-term ramipril: REIN follow-up trial. Gruppo Italiano di Studi Epidemiologici in Nefrologia (GISEN). Ramipril Efficacy in Nephropathy. *Lancet*, **1998**, *352*:1252–1256.

Saino, A., Pomidossi, G., Perondi, R., Valentini, R., Rimini, A., Di Francesco, L., and Mancia, G. Intracoronary angiotensin II potentiates coronary sympathetic vasoconstriction in humans. *Circulation*, **1997**, *96*:148–153.

Sasaki, K., Yamano, Y., Bardhan, S., Iwai, N., Murray, J.J., Hasegawa, M., Matsuda, Y., and Inagami, T. Cloning and expression of a complementary DNA encoding a bovine adrenal angiotensin II type-1 receptor. *Nature*, **1991**, *351*:230–233.

Schachter, F., Faure-Delanef, L., Guenot, F., Rouger, H., Froguel, P., Lesueur-Ginot, L., and Cohen, D. Genetic associations with human longevity at the APOE and ACE loci. *Nature Genet.*, **1994**, *6*:29–32.

Schunkert, H., Hense, H.-W., Holmer, S.R., Stender, M., Perz, S., Keil, U., Lorell, B.H., and Riegger, G.A. Association between a deletion polymorphism of the angiotensin-converting-enzyme gene and left ventricular hypertrophy. *N. Engl. J. Med.*, **1994**, *330*:1634–1638.

Scott-Burden, T., Hahn, A.W.A., Resink, T.J., and Bühler, F.R. Modulation of extracellular matrix by angiotensin II: stimulated glyco-conjugate synthesis and growth in vascular smooth muscle cells. *J. Cardiovasc. Pharmacol.*, **1990**, *16*(suppl. 4):S36–S41.

Sielecki, A.R., Hayakawa, K., Fujinaga, M., Murphy, M.E.P., Fraser, M., Muir, A.K., Carilli, C.T., Lewicki, J.A., Baxter, J.D., and James, M.N.G. Structure of recombinant human renin, a target for cardiovascular-active drugs, at 2.5 Å resolution. *Science*, **1989**, *243*:1346–1351.

Singh, I., Grams, M., Wang, W.H., Yang, T., Killen, P., Smart, A., Schnermann, J., and Briggs, J.P. Coordinate regulation of renal expression of nitric oxide synthase, renin, and angiotensinogen mRNA by dietary salt. *Am. J. Physiol.*, **1996**, *270*:F1027–F1037.

SOLVD Investigators. Effect of enalapril on survival in patients with reduced left ventricular ejection fractions and congestive heart failure. *N. Engl. J. Med.*, **1991**, *325*:293–302.

SOLVD Investigators. Effect of enalapril on mortality and the development of heart failure in asymptomatic patients with reduced left ventricular ejection fractions. *N. Engl. J. Med.* **1992**, *327*:685–691. [Published erratum in *N. Engl. J. Med.*, **1992**, *329*:1768.]

Soubrier, F., Alhenc-Gelas, F., Hubert, C., Allegrini, J., John, M., Tregear, G., and Corvol, P. Two putative active centers in human angiotensin I-converting enzyme revealed by molecular cloning. *Proc. Natl. Acad. Sci. U.S.A.*, **1988**, *85*:9386–9390.

Staessen, J.A., Kuznetsova, T., Wang, J.G., Emelianov, D., Vlietinck, R., and Fagard, R. M235T angiotensinogen gene polymorphism and cardiovascular renal risk. *J. Hypertens.*, **1999**, *17*:9–17.

Swanson, G.N., Hanesworth, J.M., Sardinia, M.F., Coleman, J.K.M., Wright, J.W., Hall, K.L., Miller-Wing, A.V., Stobb, J.W., Cook, V.I., Harding, E.C., and Harding, J.W. Discovery of a distinct binding site for angiotensin II (3-8), a putative angiotensin IV receptor. *Regul. Pept.*, **1992**, *40*:409–419.

Swedberg, K., Held, P., Kjekshus, J., Rasmussen, K., Rydén, L., and Wedel, H. Effects of the early administration of enalapril on mortality in patients with acute myocardial infarction: results of the Cooperative New Scandinavian Enalapril Survival Study II (CONSENSUS II). *N. Engl. J. Med.*, **1992**, *327*:678–684.

Taddei, S., Virdis, A., Abdel-Haq, B., Giovannetti, R., Duranti, P., Arena, A.M., Favilla, S., and Salvetti, A. Indirect evidence for vascular uptake of circulating renin in hypertensive patients. *Hypertension*, **1993**, *21*:852–860.

Tallant, E.A., Lu, X., Weiss, R.B., Chappell, M.C., and Ferrario, C.M. Bovine aortic endothelial cells contain an angiotensin-(1-7) receptor. *Hypertension*, **1997**, *29*:388–393.

Tanimoto, K., Sugiyama, F., Goto, Y., Ishida, J., Takimoto, E., Yagami, K., Fukamizu, A., and Murakami, K. Angiotensinogen-deficient mice with hypotension. *J. Biol. Chem.*, **1994**, *269*:31334–31337.

Tatti, P., Pahor, M., Byington, R.P., Di Mauro, P., Guarisco, R., Strollo, G., and Strollo, F. Outcome results of the Fosinopril Versus Amlodipine Cardiovascular Events Randomized Trial (FACET) in patients with hypertension and NIDDM. *Diabetes Care*, **1998**, *21*:597–603.

Testa, M.A., Anderson, R.B., Nackley, J.F., Hollenberg, N.K., and the Quality-Of-Life Hypertension Study Group. Quality of life and antihypertensive therapy in men. A comparison of captopril with enalapril. *N. Engl. J. Med.*, **1993**, *328*:907–913.

Tiret, L., Bonnardeaux, A., Poirier, O., Ricard, S., Marques-Vidal, P., Evans, A., Arveiler, D., Luc, G., Kee, F., Ducimetiere, P., Soubrier, F., and Cambien, F. Synergistic effects of angiotensin-converting enzyme and angiotensin-II type 1 receptor gene polymorphisms on risk of myocardial infarction. *Lancet*, **1994**, *344*:910–913.

Traynor, T.R., Smart, A., Briggs, J.P., and Schnermann, J. Inhibition of macula densa-stimulated renin secretion by pharmacological blockade of cyclooxygenase-2. *Am. J. Physiol.*, **1999**, *277*:F706–F710.

Vaughan, D.E., Rouleau, J.-L., Ridker, P.M., Arnold, J.M.O., Menapace, F.J., and Pfeffer, M.A. Effects of ramipril on plasma fibrinolytic balance in patients with acute anterior myocardial infarction. HEART Study Investigators. *Circulation*, 1997, 96:442–447.

Villarreal, F.J., Kim, N.N., Ungab, G.D., Printz, M.P., and Dillmann, W.H. Identification of functional angiotensin II receptors on rat cardiac fibroblasts. *Circulation*, 1993, 88:2849–286l.

Wallukat, G., Homuth, V., Fischer, T., Lindschau, C., Horstkamp, B., Jüpner, A., Baur, E., Nissen, E., Vetter, K., Neichel, D., Dudenhausen, J.W., Haller, H., and Luft, F.C. Patients with preeclampsia develop agonistic autoantibodies against the angiotensin AT$_1$ receptor. *J. Clin. Invest.*, 1999, 103:945–952.

Wang, H., Katovich, M.J., Gelband, C.H., Reaves, P.Y., Phillips, M.I., and Raizada, M.K. Sustained inhibition of angiotensin I-converting enzyme (ACE) expression and long-term antihypertensive action by virally mediated delivery of ACE antisense cDNA. *Circ. Res.*, 1999, 85:614–622.

Wang, J.-L., Cheng, H.-F., and Harris, R.C. Cyclooxygenase-2 inhibition decreases renin content and lowers blood pressure in a model of renovascular hypertension. *Hypertension*, 1999, 34:96–101.

Ward, K., Hata, A., Jeunemaitre, X., Helin, C., Nelson, L., Namikawa, C., Farrington, P.F., Ogasawara, M., Suzumori, K., Tomoda, S., Berrebi, S., Sasaki, M., Corvol, P., Lifton, R.P., and Lalouel, J.-M. A molecular variant of angiotensinogen associated with preeclampsia. *Nature Genet.*, 1993, 4:59–61.

Wei, C.-C., Meng, Q.C., Palmer, R., Hageman, G.R., Durand, J., Bradley, W.E., Farrell, D.M., Hankes, G.H., Oparil, S., and Dell'Italia, L.J. Evidence for angiotensin-converting enzyme- and chymase-mediated angiotensin II formation in the interstitial fluid space of the dog heart in vivo. *Circulation*, 1999, 99:2583–2589.

Weihprecht, H., Lorenz, J., Schnermann, J.N., Skøtt, O., and Briggs, J.P. Effect of adenosine$_1$-receptor blockade on renin release from rabbit isolated perfused juxtaglomerular apparatus. *J. Clin. Invest.*, 1990, 85:1622–1628.

Whitebread, S., Mele, M., Kamber, B., and de Gasparo, M. Preliminary biochemial characterization of two angiotensin II receptor subtypes. *Biochem. Biophys. Res. Commun.*, 1989, 163:284–291.

Wolny, A., Clozel, J.-P., Rein, J., Mory, P., Vogt, P., Turino, M., Kiowski, W., and Fischli, W. Functional and biochemical analysis of angiotensin II-forming pathways in the human heart. *Circ. Res.*, 1997, 80:219–227.

Wong, P.C., Chiu, A.T., Price, W.A., Thoolen, M.J.M.C., Carini, D.J., Johnson, A.L., Taber, R.I., and Timmermans, P.B.M.W.M. Nonpeptide angiotensin II receptor antagonists: I. Pharmacological characterization of 2-n-butyl-4-chloro-1-(2-chlorobenzyl)imidazole-5-acetic acid, sodium salt (S-8307). *J. Pharmacol. Exp. Ther.*, 1988, 247:1–7.

Wynckel, A., Ebikili, B., Melin, J.-P., Randoux, C., Lavaud, S., and Chanard, J. Long-term follow-up of acute renal failure caused by angiotensin converting enzyme inhibitors. *Am. J. Hypertens.*, 1998, 11:1080–1086.

Yamada, K., Iyer, S.N., Chappell, M.C., Ganten, D., and Ferrario, C.M. Converting enzyme determines plasma clearance of angiotensin-(1-7). *Hypertension*, 1998, 32:496–502.

Yoshida, H., Mitarai, T., Kawamura, T., Kitajima, T., Miyazaki, Y., Nagasawa, R., Kawaguchi, Y., Kubo, H., Ichikawa, I., and Sakai, O. Role of the deletion of polymorphism of the angiotensin converting enzyme gene in the progression and therapeutic responsiveness of IgA nephropathy. *J. Clin. Invest.*, 1995, 96:2162–2169.

Yusuf, S., Sleight, P., Pogue, J., Bosch, J., Davies, R., and Dagenais, G. Effects of an angiotensin-converting-enzyme inhibitor ramipril, on cardiovascular events in high-risk patients. The Heart Outcomes Prevention Evaluation Study Investigators. *N. Engl. J. Med.*, 2000, 342:145–153. [Published erratum appears in *N. Engl. J. Med.*, 2000, 342:478.]

Zimmerman, J.B., Robertson, D., and Jackson, E.K. Angiotensin II-noradrenergic interactions in renovascular hypertensive rats. *J. Clin. Invest.*, 1987, 80:443–457.

Zuanetti, G., Latini, R., Maggioni, A.P., Franzosi, M., Santoro, L., and Tognoni, G. Effect of the ACE inhibitor lisinopril on mortality in diabetic patients with acute myocardial infarction. Data from the GISSI-3 study. *Circulation*, 1997, 96:4239–4245.

MONOGRAPHS AND REVIEWS

Ardaillou, R. Angiotensin II receptors. *J. Am. Soc. Nephrol.*, 1999, 10(suppl. 11):S30–S39.

Atlas, S.A., Niarchos, A.P., and Case, D.B. Inhibitors of the renin–angiotensin system. Effects on blood pressure, aldosterone secretion and renal function. *Am. J. Nephrol.*, 1983, 3:118–127.

Baker, K.M., Booz, G.W., and Dostal, D.E. Cardiac actions of angiotensin: II. Role of an intracardiac renin–angiotensin system. *Annu. Rev. Physiol.*, 1992, 54:227–241.

Berk, B.C. Angiotensin II signal transduction in vascular smooth muscle: pathways activated by specific tyrosine kinases. *J. Am. Soc. Nephrol.*, 1999, 10(suppl. 11):S62–S68.

Blume, A., Herdegen, T., and Unger, T. Angiotensin peptides and inducible transcription factors. *J. Mol. Med.*, 1999, 77:339–357.

Brent, R.L., and Beckman, D.A. Angiotensin-converting enzyme inhibitors, an embryopathic class of drugs with unique properties: information for clinical teratology counselors. *Teratology*, 1991, 43:543–546.

Bretzel, R.G. Effects of antihypertensive drugs on renal function in patients with diabetic nephropathy. *Am. J. Hypertens.*, 1997, 10:208S–217S.

Bumpus, F.M., Catt, K.J., Chiu, A.T., DeGasparo, M., Goodfriend, T., Husain, A., Peach, M.J., Taylor, D.G. Jr., and Timmermans, P.B.M.W.M. Nomenclature for angiotensin receptors. A report of the nomenclature committee of the council for high blood pressure research. *Hypertension*, 1991, 17:720–721.

Bunnemann, B., Fuxe, K., and Ganten, D. The renin–angiotensin system in the brain: an update 1993. *Regul. Pept.*, 1993, 46:487–509.

Csajka, C., Buclin, T., Brunner, H.R., and Biollaz, J. Pharmacokinetic-pharmacodynamic profile of angiotensin II receptor antagonists. *Clin. Pharmacokinet.*, 1997, 32:1–29.

Dzau, V.J. Vascular renin–angiotensin system and vascular protection. *J. Cardiovasc. Pharmacol.*, 1993, 22(suppl.)5:S1–S9.

Dzau, V.J., Sasamura, H., and Hein, L. Heterogeneity of angiotensin synthetic pathways and receptor subtypes: physiological and pharmacological implications. *J. Hypertens.*, 1993, 11:S13–S18.

Ferrario, C.M., Chappell, M.C., Tallant, E.A., Brosnihan, K.B., and Diz, D.I. Counterregulatory actions of angiotensin-(1-7). *Hypertension*, 1997, 30:535–541.

Fitzsimons, J.T. Angiotensin stimulation of the central nervous system. *Rev. Physiol. Biochem. Pharmacol.*, 1980, 87:117–167.

Frohlich, E.D. Angiotensin converting enzyme inhibitors: present and future. *Hypertension*, 1989, 13:I125–I130.

Ganong, W.F. The brain renin–angiotensin system. *Annu. Rev. Physiol.*, 1984, 46:17–31.

Griendling, K.K., Ushio-Fukai, M., Lassegue, B., and Alexander, R.W. Angiotensin II signaling in vascular smooth muscle. New concepts. *Hypertension,* **1997,** *29*:366–373.

Gross, F. The regulation of aldosterone secretion by the renin–angiotensin system under various conditions. *Acta Endocrinol. (Copenh.),* **1968,** *124*(suppl.):41–64.

Guyton, A.C. Blood pressure control—special role of the kidneys and body fluids. *Science,* **1991,** *252*:1813–1816.

Guyton, A.C. The surprising kidney-fluid mechanism for pressure control—its infinite gain! *Hypertension,* **1990,** *16*:725–730.

Hagley, M.T., Hulisz, D.T., and Burns, C.M. Hepatotoxicity associated with angiotensin-converting enzyme inhibitors. *Ann. Pharmacother.,* **1993,** *27*:228–231.

Hollenberg, N.K., Fisher, N.D.L., and Price, D.A. Pathways for angiotensin II generation in intact human tissue. Evidence from comparative pharmacological interruption of the renin system. *Hypertension,* **1998,** *32*:387–392.

Horiuchi, M., Akishita, M., and Dzau, V.J. Recent progress in angiotensin II type 2 receptor research in the cardiovascular system. *Hypertension,* **1999,** *33*:613–621.

Inagami, T. Molecular biology and signaling of angiotensin receptors: an overview. *J. Am. Soc. Nephrol.,* **1999,** *10*(suppl. 11):S2–S7.

Inagami, T. Structure and function of renin. *J. Hypertens. Suppl.,* **1989,** *7*:S3–S8.

Inamani, T., Eguchi, S., Numaguchi, K., Motley, E.D., Tang, H., Matsumoto, T., and Yamakawa, T. Cross-talk between angiotensin II receptors and the tyrosine kinases and phosphatases. *J. Am. Soc. Nephrol.,* **1999,** *10*:S57–S61.

Israili, Z.H., and Hall, W.D. Cough and angioneurotic edema associated with angiotensin-converting enzyme inhibitor therapy. A review of the literature and pathophysiology. *Ann. Intern. Med.,* **1992,** *117*:234–242.

Jackson, E.K. Adenosine: a physiological brake on renin release. *Annu. Rev. Pharmacol. Toxicol.,* **1991,** *31*:1–35.

Jackson, E.K. Gene therapy for hypertension. *Am. J. Hypertens.,* **1992,** *5*:930–932.

Jackson, E.K., Branch, R.A., Margolius, H.S., and Oates, J.A. Physiological functions of the renal prostaglandin, renin, and kallikrein systems. In, *The Kidney: Physiology and Pathophysiology.* (Seldin, D.W., and Giebisch, G.H., eds.) Raven Press, Ltd., New York, **1985,** pp. 613–644.

Jackson, E.K., Branch, R.A., and Oates, J.A. Participation of prostaglandins in the control of renin release. In, *Prostaglandins and the Cardiovascular System.* (Oates, J.A., ed.) Raven Press, Ltd., New York, **1982,** pp. 255–276.

Lin, C., and Frishman, W.H. Renin inhibition: a novel therapy for cardiovascular disease. *Am. Heart. J.,* **1996,** *131*:1024–1034.

Materson, B.J. Adverse effects of angiotensin-converting enzyme in-hibitors in antihypertensive therapy with focus on quinapril. *Am. J. Cardiol.,* **1992,** *69*:46C–53C.

McConnaughey, M.M., McConnaughey, J.S., and Ingenito, A.J. Practical considerations of the pharmacology of angiotensin receptor blockers. *J. Clin. Pharmacol.,* **1999,** *39*:547–559.

Mimran, A., Ribstein, J., and DuCailar, G. Angiotensin II receptor antagonists and hypertension. *Clin. Exp. Hypertens.,* **1999,** *21*:847–858.

Peach, M.J. Renin–angiotensin system: biochemistry and mechanisms of action. *Physiol. Rev.,* **1977,** *57*:313–370.

Petrillo, E.W. Jr., and Ondetti, M.A. Angiotensin-converting enzyme inhibitors: medicinal chemistry and biological actions. *Med. Res. Rev.,* **1982,** *2*:1–41.

Phillips, M.I., Speakman, E.A., and Kimura, B. Levels of angiotensin and molecular biology of the tissue renin angiotensin systems. *Regul. Pept.,* **1993,** *43*:1–20.

Romankiewicz, J.A., Brogden, R.N., Heel, R.C., Speight, T.M., and Avery, G.S. Captopril: an update review of its pharmacological properties and therapeutic efficacy in congestive heart failure. *Drugs,* **1983,** *25*:6–40.

Saavedra, J.M. Brain and pituitary angiotensin. *Endocr. Rev.,* **1992,** *13*:329–380.

Samanen, J., and Regoli, D. Structure-activity relationships of peptide angiotensin II receptor agonists and antagonists. In, *Angiotensin II Receptors:* Vol. 2. *Medicinal Chemistry.* (Ruffolo, R.R. Jr., ed.) CRC Press, Ann Arbor, MI, **1994,** pp. 11–97.

Schwartz, A.B., and Chatterjee, K. Vasodilator therapy in chronic congestive heart failure. *Drugs,* **1983,** *26*:148–173.

Tallant, E.A., Diz, D.I., and Ferrario, C.M. State-of-the-art lecture. Antiproliferative actions of angiotensin-(1-7) in vascular smooth muscle. *Hypertension,* **1999,** *34*:950–957.

Timmermans, P.B.M.W.M., Wong, P.C., Chiu, A.T., Herblin, W.F., Benfield, P., Carini, D.J., Lee, R.J., Wexler, R.R., Saye, J.A.M., and Smith, R.D. Angiotensin II receptors and angiotensin II receptor antagonists. *Pharmacol. Rev.,* **1993,** *45*:205–251.

Vane, J.R. The history of inhibitors of angiotensin converting enzyme. *J. Physiol. Pharmacol.,* **1999,** *50*:489–498.

von Lutterotti, N., Catanzaro, D.F., Sealey, J.E., and Laragh, J.H. Renin is not synthesized by cardiac and extrarenal vascular tissues. A review of experimental evidence. *Circulation,* **1994,** *89*:458–470.

Weinstock, J., and Keenan, R.M. Structure-activity relationships of nonpeptide angiotensin II receptor antagonists. In, *Angiotensin II Receptors:* Vol. 2. *Medicinal Chemistry.* (Ruffolo, R.R. Jr., ed.) CRC Press, Ann Arbor, MI, **1994,** pp. 161–217.

Zusman, R.M. Angiotensin-converting enzyme inhibitors: more different than alike? Focus on cardiac performance. *Am. J. Cardiol.,* **1993,** *72*:25H–36H.

DRUGS USED FOR THE TREATMENT OF MYOCARDIAL ISCHEMIA

David M. Kerins, Rose Marie Robertson,
and David Robertson

This chapter briefly reviews the pathophysiology underlying angina pectoris, the most common symptom of chronic ischemic heart disease. The causes of the myocardial ischemia that produces angina are defined in terms of the myocardial oxygen supply–demand relationship. Stable and unstable angina, silent ischemia, variant angina, and myocardial infarction are considered; the contributions of fixed atherosclerotic coronary narrowings, of active coronary vasospasm, and of intracoronary thrombosis in these syndromes are discussed to clarify the roles of antianginal agents. Also discussed is the angina of autonomic dysfunction, for which therapy must be specifically tailored to ameliorate the underlying problem of great fluctuations in coronary perfusion pressure, and in which conventional antianginal therapy is not efficacious. For each class of antianginal therapy (organic nitrates, Ca^{2+} channel antagonists, β-adrenergic receptor antagonists, and antiplatelet/antithrombotic agents), the effects of the class and its most important agents on the factors determining myocardial oxygen demand and myocardial oxygen supply are reviewed.

The use of organic nitrates (also covered in Chapter 34) in sublingual, oral, buccal, and intravenous forms is discussed, with attention to the issue of nitrate tolerance and the relationship of nitrovasodilators to endogenous endothelium-derived vasodilator(s). Interactions of organic nitrates with sildenafil also are discussed. The multiple classes of Ca^{2+} channel antagonists (also discussed in Chapter 33) have distinct effects on vascular smooth muscle and cardiac tissue, and these effects are placed in the context of the ischemic cardiac syndromes. β-Adrenergic receptor antagonists, which also are addressed in Chapters 10, 33, 34, and 35, are dealt with here in terms of their ability to improve survival in ischemic heart disease as well as their efficacy in improving exercise tolerance in stable angina. Considering unstable angina as a thrombotic disease leads to a description of the role of antiplatelet therapy in ischemic heart disease (see also Chapter 55). Agents currently under investigation and the potential role of gene-based therapy in the treatment of myocardial ischemia also are described.

The primary symptom of ischemic heart disease is angina pectoris, caused by transient episodes of myocardial ischemia. These episodes of ischemia are due to an imbalance in the myocardial oxygen supply–demand relationship and may be caused by an increase in myocardial oxygen demand (determined by heart rate, ventricular wall tension, and ventricular contractility), by a decrease in myocardial oxygen supply (primarily determined by coronary blood flow, but occasionally modified by the oxygen-carrying capacity of the blood), or sometimes by both (Friesinger and Robertson, 1985, 1986; Kaplinsky, 1992; *see* Figure 32–1). Regardless of the precipitating factors, the sensation of angina is similar in most patients. Both typical and variant (Prinzmetal's) angina are commonly experienced as a heavy, pressing, substernal discomfort (rarely called "pain"), often radiating to the left shoulder, flexor aspect of the left arm, jaw, or epigastrium, with a significant minority of patients noting discomfort in a different

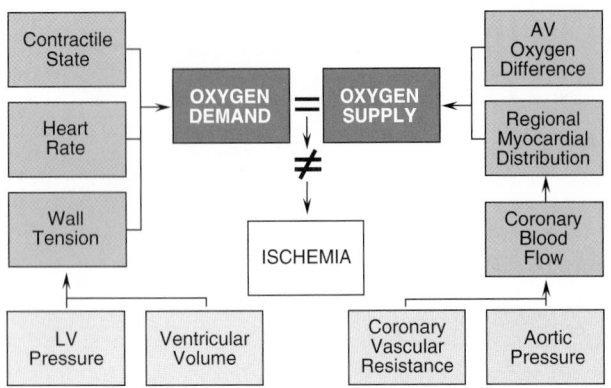

Figure 32–1. Ischemic episodes: an imbalance in the myocardial oxygen supply–demand relationship.

The figure illustrates the principal determinants of myocardial oxygen consumption and mechanisms for increasing oxygen delivery. The arteriovenous oxygen difference always is near maximum in the coronary circulation; thus, widening of the arteriovenous oxygen difference cannot significantly enhance oxygen delivery. Redistribution of regional myocardial flow probably is of major importance. (Adapted with permission from Ross, 1971.)

location or of a different character. Women, the elderly, and diabetics are more likely to have ischemia with atypical symptoms.

Angina pectoris is a common symptom, affecting 6,400,000 Americans (American Heart Association, 2001). It may occur in a stable pattern over many years or may become unstable, increasing in frequency or severity and even occurring at rest. In typical stable angina, the pathological substrate is usually fixed atherosclerotic narrowing of an epicardial coronary artery, upon which exertion, emotional stress, *etc.*, superimpose an increase in myocardial oxygen consumption. In variant angina, focal or diffuse coronary vasospasm episodically reduces coronary flow. Patients also may display a mixed pattern of angina with the addition of altered vessel tone on a background of atherosclerotic narrowing. In the majority of patients with unstable angina, rupture of an atherosclerotic plaque, with consequent platelet adhesion and aggregation, decreases coronary blood flow. Plaques with thinner fibrous caps are recognized to be more "vulnerable" to rupture (Fuster *et al.* 1996).

Myocardial ischemia also may be "silent," with electrocardiographic, echocardiographic, or radionuclide evidence of ischemia appearing in the absence of symptoms. While some patients have only silent ischemia, the majority of patients who have silent ischemia have symptomatic episodes as well. The precipitants of silent isch-

emia appear to be the same as those of symptomatic ischemia. We now know that the "ischemic burden," *i.e.,* the total time a patient is ischemic each day, is greater in many patients than was recognized previously. The agents that are efficacious in conventional angina appear, in most trials, to be efficacious in reducing silent ischemia. β-Adrenergic receptor antagonists appear to be more effective than the Ca^{2+} channel blockers in the prevention of episodes. Therapy directed at abolishing all silent ischemia has not been shown to be of additional benefit over conventional therapy.

An unusual form of angina is seen in patients with autonomic dysfunction and faulty control of the circulation in the upright posture (Hines *et al.* 1981). The marked orthostatic hypotension seen in these patients can reduce coronary perfusion pressure sufficiently to cause myocardial ischemia even in patients with normal coronary arteries. As this form of angina is precipitated by upright posture and is relieved when the blood pressure and coronary perfusion pressure rise with sitting or lying, it may appear to be typical exertional angina if the history is not taken carefully and the blood pressure determined in the upright posture. The specific therapy needed for this form of angina is discussed below.

This chapter describes the pharmacological agents used in the treatment of angina. The major drugs are nitrovasodilators (*see also* Chapter 34), β-adrenergic receptor antagonists (*see also* Chapter 10), Ca^{2+} channel antagonists (*see also* Chapter 33), and, in both stable and unstable angina, antiplatelet agents (*see* Chapters 27 and 55) as well as 3-hydroxy-3-methylglutaryl coenzyme A (HMG-CoA) reductase inhibitors, which may have a role in stabilizing the vulnerable plaque (*see* Chapter 36). All approved antianginal agents function by improving the balance of myocardial oxygen supply and demand: increasing supply by dilating the coronary vasculature or decreasing demand by reducing cardiac work (*see* Figure 32–1). Increasing the cardiac extraction of oxygen from the blood is not a practical therapeutic goal. Agents used in typical angina either increase blood flow to the heart; decrease left ventricular wall tension, heart rate, and/or contractility; or do both. In variant or vasotonic angina, prevention of coronary vasospasm is the therapeutic aim. In unstable angina, correcting the tendency to intracoronary thrombosis is the most important therapeutic maneuver.

Antianginal agents may provide prophylactic or symptomatic treatment, but β-adrenergic receptor antagonists appear, in addition, to reduce mortality by decreasing the incidence of sudden cardiac death associated with myocardial ischemia and infarction. The treatment of cardiac risk factors can reduce the progression or even lead to the regression of atherosclerosis. Aspirin is used routinely in patients with myocardial ischemia, and lipid-lowering agents also have been demonstrated to reduce the incidence of clinical events (Gibbons *et al.,* 1999). Coronary artery bypass surgery and percutaneous coronary interventions such as angioplasty, atherectomy, and stent deployment are alternatives to pharmacological treatment; in some subsets of patients, bypass surgery and other forms of revascularization have been demonstrated to have a survival advantage over medical treatment alone. Novel therapies modifying the expression of vascular or myocardial cell genes are expected to be an important part of the therapy of ischemic heart disease in the future.

ORGANIC NITRATES

History. *Nitroglycerin* was first synthesized in 1846 by Sobrero, who observed that a small quantity of the oily substance placed on the tongue elicited a severe headache. Constantin Hering, in 1847, developed the sublingual dosage form. In 1857, the eminent physician T. Lauder Brunton of Edinburgh administered amyl nitrite, a known vasodepressor, by inhalation and noted that anginal pain was relieved within 30 to 60 seconds. The action of amyl nitrite was transitory, however, and the dosage was difficult to adjust. Subsequently, William Murrell decided that the action of nitroglycerin mimicked that of amyl nitrite, and he established the use of sublingual nitroglycerin for relief of the acute anginal attack and as a prophylactic agent to be taken prior to exertion (Murrell, 1879). The empirical observation that organic nitrates could be used safely for the rapid, dramatic alleviation of the symptoms of angina pectoris led to their widespread acceptance by the medical profession. Basic investigations led to an understanding of the role of nitric oxide (Moncada *et al.,* 1988) in both the vasodilation produced by nitrates and endogenous vasodilation. The importance of nitric oxide as a signaling molecule in the cardiovascular system and elsewhere was recognized by the awarding of the Nobel Prize in Medicine or Physiology to Furchgott, Ignarro, and Murad in 1998.

Chemistry. Organic nitrates are polyol esters of nitric acid, whereas organic nitrites are esters of nitrous acid (Table 32–1). Nitrate esters (—C—O—NO_2) and nitrite esters (—C—O—NO) are characterized by a sequence of carbon–oxygen–nitrogen, whereas nitro compounds possess carbon–nitrogen bonds (C—NO_2). Thus, *glyceryl trinitrate* is not a nitro compound, and it is erroneously called *nitroglycerin;* however, this nomenclature is both widespread and official. *Amyl nitrite* is a highly volatile liquid that is administered by inhalation. Organic nitrates of low molecular mass (such as nitroglycerin) are moderately volatile, oily liquids, whereas the high-molecular-mass nitrate esters (*e.g., erythrityl tetranitrate, pentaerythritol tetranitrate, isosorbide dinitrate*) are solids. The fully nitrated polyols are lipid soluble, whereas their incompletely nitrated metabolites are more soluble in water. In the pure form (without an inert carrier such as lactose), nitroglycerin is explosive. The organic nitrates and nitrites and several other compounds that are capable of denitration to release nitric oxide (NO) have been collectively termed *nitrovasodilators.* Nitric oxide activates guanylyl cyclase, increasing intracellular levels of cyclic guanosine 3′,5′-monophosphate (cyclic GMP), and thereby produces vasodilation (Murad, 1986; Molina *et al.,* 1987; Thadani, 1992). Endogenous NO is formed when L-arginine is converted to citrulline by nitric oxide synthases. Both constitutive and inducible forms of these synthases are found in vascular endothelial and smooth muscle cells as well as in other cell types throughout the body, including the central nervous system (Lowenstein *et al.,* 1994). In the setting of human atherosclerosis, the expression of endothelial nitric oxide synthase and the production of NO are reduced (Oemar *et al.,* 1998).

Pharmacological Properties

Cardiovascular Effects. *Hemodynamic Effects.* The nitrovasodilators relax most smooth muscle, including that in arteries and veins. Low concentrations of nitroglycerin produce dilation of the veins that predominates over that of arterioles. Venodilation results in decreased left and right ventricular chamber size and end-diastolic pressures but little change in systemic vascular resistance. Systemic arterial pressure may fall slightly, and heart rate is unchanged or slightly increased reflexly. Pulmonary vascular resistance and cardiac output both are slightly reduced. Even doses of nitroglycerin that do not alter systemic arterial pressure often produce arteriolar dilation in the face and neck, resulting in a flush, or dilation of meningeal arterial vessels, causing headache. There is an enrichment of the enzyme that converts nitroglycerin to NO in venous compared to arterial smooth muscle cells, likely the basis of the partially venoselective properties of the nitrates (Bauer and Fung, 1996).

Higher doses of organic nitrates cause further venous pooling and may decrease arteriolar resistance as well, decreasing systolic and diastolic blood pressure and cardiac output and resulting in pallor, weakness, dizziness, and activation of compensatory sympathetic reflexes. The resultant tachycardia and peripheral arteriolar vasoconstriction tend to restore systemic vascular resistance; this is superimposed on sustained venous pooling. Coronary blood flow may increase transiently as a result of coronary vasodilation, but with a subsequent decrease if cardiac output and blood pressure decrease sufficiently.

In patients with autonomic dysfunction and an inability to increase sympathetic outflow (multiple-system atrophy and pure autonomic failure are the most common forms), the fall in blood pressure consequent to the venodilation produced by nitrates cannot be compensated. Nitrates

Table 32–1
Organic Nitrates Available for Clinical Use

NONPROPRIETARY NAMES AND TRADE NAMES	CHEMICAL STRUCTURE	PREPARATIONS, USUAL DOSES, AND ROUTES OF ADMINISTRATION*
Amyl nitrite (isoamyl nitrite)	H_3C $\diagdown$ $CHCH_2CH_2ONO$ H_3C $\diagup$	Inh: 0.3 ml, inhalation
Nitroglycerin (glyceryl trinitrate; NITRO-BID, NITROSTAT, NITROL, NITRO-DUR, others)	H_2C—O—NO_2 HC—O—NO_2 H_2C—O—NO_2	T: 0.3 to 0.6 mg as needed S: 0.4 mg per spray as needed C: 2.5 to 9 mg two to four times daily B: 1 mg every 3 to 5 h O: 2.5 to 5 cm (1 to 2 in.), topically to skin every 4 to 8 h D: 1 disc (2.5 to 15 mg) for 12 to 24 h per day IV: 5 μg/min; increments of 5 μg/min
Isosorbide dinitrate (ISORDIL, SORBITRATE, DILATRATE-SR, others)	(structure)	T: 2.5 to 10 mg every 2 to 3 h T(C): 5 to 10 mg every 2 to 3 h T(O): 5 to 40 mg every 6 h C: 40 to 80 mg every 8 to 12 h
Isosorbide-5-mononitrate (IMDUR, ISMO, others)	(structure)	T: 10 to 40 mg twice daily C: 60 to 120 mg daily
Erythrityl tetranitrate (CARDILATE)	H_2C—O—NO_2 HC—O—NO_2 HC—O—NO_2 H_2C—O—NO_2	T: 5 to 10 mg as needed T(O): 10 mg three times daily

*B, buccal (transmucosal) tablet; C, sustained-release capsule or tablet; D, transdermal disc or patch; Inh, inhalant; IV, intravenous injection; O, ointment; S, lingual spray; T, tablet for sublingual use; T(C), chewable tablet; T(O), oral tablet or capsule.

may reduce arterial pressure and coronary perfusion pressure significantly and actually aggravate angina in addition to producing potentially life-threatening hypotension. The correct therapy in patients with orthostatic angina and normal coronary arteries is to correct the orthostatic hypotension by increasing volume retention (fludrocortisone and a high-sodium diet) by preventing venous pooling with fit-

ted support garments and by the carefully titrated use of oral vasopressors. As patients with autonomic dysfunction occasionally may have coexistent coronary artery disease, the coronary anatomy should be defined before therapy is undertaken.

Effects on Total and Regional Coronary Blood Flow.
Ischemia is a powerful stimulus to coronary vasodilation,

and regional blood flow is adjusted by autoregulatory mechanisms. In the presence of atherosclerotic coronary narrowing, ischemia distal to the lesion is a stimulus for vasodilation, and, if the degree of narrowing is severe, much of the capacity to dilate is utilized to maintain resting blood flow. When situations arise that increase demand, further dilation may not be possible. After demonstration of direct coronary vasodilation in experimental animals, it became generally accepted that nitrates relieved anginal pain by dilating coronary arteries and thereby increasing coronary blood flow. This hypothesis was questioned by Gorlin and associates (1959), who were unable to demonstrate increases in coronary blood flow in patients with angina pectoris following the administration of nitroglycerin. However, organic nitrates do appear to cause redistribution of blood flow in the heart when the coronary circulation is partially occluded. Under these circumstances, there is a disproportionate reduction in blood flow to the subendocardial regions of the heart, which are subjected to the greatest extravascular compression during systole; organic nitrates tend to restore blood flow in these regions toward normal (Horwitz et al., 1971).

The hemodynamic mechanisms responsible for these effects are not entirely clear. Most hypotheses have focused on the ability of organic nitrates to cause dilation and prevent vasoconstriction of large epicardial vessels without impairing autoregulation in the small vessels, which are responsible for about 90% of the overall coronary vascular resistance. The vessel diameter is an important determinant of the response to nitroglycerin; vessels larger than 200 μm in diameter are highly responsive, whereas those less than 100 μm are minimally responsive (Sellke et al., 1990). Experimental evidence in patients undergoing coronary bypass surgery indicates that nitrates do have a relaxant effect on large coronary vessels. Collateral flow to ischemic regions also is increased (Goldstein et al., 1974). Moreover, analyses of coronary angiograms in human beings have shown that sublingual nitroglycerin can dilate epicardial stenoses and reduce the resistance to flow through such areas (Brown et al., 1981; Feldman et al., 1981). The resultant increase in blood flow would be distributed preferentially to ischemic myocardial regions as a consequence of vasodilation induced by autoregulation. An important indirect mechanism for a preferential increase in subendocardial blood flow is the nitroglycerin-induced reduction in intracavitary systolic and diastolic pressures that oppose blood flow to the subendocardium (see below). To the extent that organic nitrates decrease myocardial requirements for oxygen (see below), the increased blood flow in ischemic regions could be balanced by decreased flow in nonisch-

emic areas, and an overall increase in coronary blood flow need not occur. Recent studies suggest that dilation of cardiac veins may result in an improvement in the perfusion of the coronary microcirculation (Darius, 1999). Redistribution of blood flow to subendocardial tissue is *not* typical of all vasodilators. *Dipyridamole,* for example, dilates resistance vessels nonselectively by distorting autoregulation; it is ineffective in patients with typical angina.

In patients with angina due to coronary spasm, the ability of organic nitrates to dilate epicardial coronary arteries, and particularly regions affected by spasm, may be the primary mechanism by which they are of benefit.

Effects on Myocardial Oxygen Requirements. By their effects on the systemic circulation, the organic nitrates also can reduce myocardial oxygen demand. The major determinants of myocardial oxygen consumption include left ventricular wall tension, heart rate, and the contractility of the myocardium. Ventricular wall tension is affected by a number of factors that may be considered under the categories of "preload" and "afterload." *Preload* is determined by the diastolic pressure that distends the ventricle (ventricular end-diastolic pressure). Increasing end-diastolic volume augments the ventricular wall tension (by the law of Laplace, tension is proportional to pressure × radius). Increasing venous capacitance with nitrates decreases venous return to the heart, decreases ventricular end-diastolic volume, and thereby decreases oxygen consumption. An additional benefit of reducing preload is that it increases the pressure gradient for perfusion across the ventricular wall; this favors subendocardial perfusion (Parratt, 1979). *Afterload* is the impedance against which the ventricle must eject. In the absence of aortic valvular disease, afterload is related to peripheral resistance. Decreasing peripheral arteriolar resistance reduces afterload and thus myocardial work and oxygen consumption.

Organic nitrates do not directly alter the inotropic or chronotropic state of the heart. They do decrease both preload and afterload as a result of respective dilation of venous capacitance and arteriolar resistance vessels. Since the primary determinants of oxygen demand are reduced by the nitrates, their net effect usually is to decrease myocardial consumption of oxygen. In addition, an improvement in the lusitropic state of the heart may be seen, with more rapid early diastolic filling (Breisblatt et al., 1988). This may be secondary to the relief of ischemia, rather than primary, or may be due to a reflex increase in sympathetic activity. Nitrovasodilators also increase cyclic GMP in platelets with consequent inhibition of platelet function (De Caterina et al., 1988; Lacoste et al., 1994) and decreased deposition of platelets in animal models of arterial wall injury (Lam *et al.*, 1988). While this may contribute to their antianginal efficacy, the effect appears to be modest and may in some settings be confounded by the potential of nitrates to alter the pharmacokinetics of heparin, reducing its antithrombotic effect.

When nitroglycerin is injected or infused directly into the coronary circulation of patients with coronary artery disease, anginal attacks (induced by electrical pacing) are not aborted, even when coronary blood flow is increased. However, sublingual administration of nitroglycerin does relieve anginal pain in the same patients (Ganz and Marcus, 1972). Furthermore, venous phlebotomy that is sufficient to reduce left ventricular end-diastolic pressure can mimic the beneficial effect of nitroglycerin.

Patients are able to exercise for considerably longer periods after the administration of nitroglycerin. Nevertheless, angina occurs, with or without nitroglycerin, at the same value of the "triple product" (aortic pressure × heart rate × ejection time is proportional to the myocardial consumption of oxygen). The observation that angina occurs at the same level of myocardial oxygen consumption suggests that the beneficial effects of nitroglycerin are the result of a reduced cardiac oxygen demand, rather than an increase in the delivery of oxygen to ischemic regions of myocardium. However, these results do not preclude the possibility that a favorable redistribution of blood flow to ischemic subendocardial myocardium may contribute to relief of pain in a typical anginal attack, nor do they preclude the possibility that direct coronary vasodilation may be the major effect of nitroglycerin in situations where vasospasm compromises myocardial blood flow.

Mechanism of Relief of Symptoms of Angina Pectoris. Brunton ascribed the nitrate-induced relief of anginal pain to a decrease in cardiac work secondary to the fall in systemic arterial pressure. As described above, the ability of nitrates to dilate epicardial coronary arteries, even in areas of atherosclerotic stenosis, is modest, and the bulk of evidence continues to favor a reduction in myocardial work and thus in myocardial oxygen demand as their primary effect in chronic stable angina.

Paradoxically, high doses of organic nitrates may reduce blood pressure to such an extent that coronary flow is compromised; reflex tachycardia and adrenergic enhancement of contractility also occur. These effects may override the salutary action of the drugs on myocardial oxygen demand and can aggravate ischemia. Additionally, sublingual nitroglycerin administration may produce bradycardia and hypotension, probably due to activation of the Bezold-Jarisch reflex (Gibbons *et al.*, 1999).

Other Effects.   The nitrovasodilators act on almost all smooth muscle. Bronchial smooth muscle is relaxed irrespective of the cause of the preexisting tone. The muscles of the biliary tract, including those of the gallbladder, biliary ducts, and sphincter of Oddi, are effectively relaxed. Smooth muscle of the gastrointestinal tract, including that of the esophagus, can be relaxed and its spontaneous motility decreased by nitrates both *in vivo* and *in vitro*. The effect may be transient and incomplete *in vivo,* but abnormal "spasm" frequently is reduced. Indeed, many incidences of atypical chest pain and "angina" are due to biliary or esophageal spasm, and these too can be relieved by nitrates. Similarly, nitrates can relax ureteral and uterine smooth muscle, but these effects are somewhat unpredictable.

Mechanism of Action.   Nitrites, organic nitrates, nitroso compounds, and a variety of other nitrogen oxide–containing substances (including nitroprusside; *see* Chapter 33) lead to the formation of the reactive free radical nitric oxide (NO), which can activate guanylyl cyclase and increase the synthesis of cyclic GMP in smooth muscle and other tissues (*see* Murad, 1986; Molina *et al.*, 1987). The exact mechanism(s) of denitration of the organic nitrates, with the subsequent liberation of NO, is controversial (Harrison and Bates, 1993). A cyclic GMP–dependent protein kinase catalyzes the phosphorylation of various proteins in smooth muscle. Eventually, the light chain of myosin is dephosphorylated (Waldman and Murad, 1987). Phosphorylation of the myosin light chain regulates the maintenance of the contractile state in smooth muscle. The pharmacological and biochemical effects of the nitrovasodilators appear to be identical to those of an endothelium-derived relaxing factor, which has been shown to be NO (Moncada *et al.*, 1988, Ignarro *et al.*, 1987; Murad, 1996; Furchgott, 1996). The relationship of endogenous nitric oxide to its precursor, L-arginine, has been reviewed (Moncada and Higgs, 1993). Nitric oxide appears to function as a biological signal in many cell types (Lowenstein *et al.*, 1994; Vane, 1994).

Absorption, Fate, and Excretion

The biotransformation of organic nitrates is the result of reductive hydrolysis catalyzed by the hepatic enzyme glutathione–organic nitrate reductase. The enzyme converts the lipid-soluble organic nitrate esters into more water-soluble denitrated metabolites and inorganic nitrite. The partially denitrated metabolites are considerably less potent vasodilators than are the parent compounds. However, under certain conditions their activity may become important. Since the liver has an enormous capacity to catalyze the reduction of organic nitrates, their biotransformation is a major factor in determining oral bioavailability and duration of action. The pharmacokinetic properties of nitroglycerin and isosorbide dinitrate have been studied in the greatest detail.

Nitroglycerin.   One molecule of nitroglycerin reacts with two molecules of reduced glutathione to produce 1,3- or 1,2-glyceryl dinitrate and oxidized glutathione (Needleman, 1975). A comparison of the maximal velocities of metabolism of the clinically used nitrates by this reductase indicates that erythrityl tetranitrate is degraded three times faster than is nitroglycerin, while isosorbide dinitrate and pentaerythritol tetranitrate are denitrated at one-sixth and one-tenth the rate of nitroglycerin.

In human beings, peak concentrations of nitroglycerin are found in plasma within 4 minutes of sublingual administration; the drug has a half-life of 1 to 3 minutes. The onset of action of nitroglycerin may be more rapid if it is delivered as a sublingual spray, rather than as a sublingual tablet (Ducharme *et al.*, 1999). Dinitrate metabolites, which are about ten times less potent as vasodilators, appear to have a half-life of about 40 minutes.

Isosorbide Dinitrate.   The major route of metabolism of isosorbide dinitrate in human beings is by enzymatic denitration followed by formation of glucuronide conjugates. Sublingual administration produces maximal concentrations of the drug in plasma by 6 minutes, and the fall in concentration is rapid (half-life approximately 45 minutes). The primary initial metabolites, isosorbide-2-mononitrate and isosorbide-5-mononitrate, have longer half-lives (3 to 6 hours) and are presumed to be responsible, at least in part, for the therapeutic efficacy of the drug.

Isosorbide-5-Mononitrate.   This agent is available in tablet form. It has excellent bioavailability after oral administration as it does not undergo significant first-pass metabolism. It has a significantly longer half-life than does isosorbide dinitrate and has been formulated as a plain tablet and as a sustained-release preparation; both of which have longer durations of action than the corresponding dosage forms of isosorbide dinitrate.

Correlation of Plasma Concentrations of Drug and Biological Activity.

Intravenous administration of nitroglycerin or the long-acting nitrates (isosorbide dinitrate, pentaerythritol tetranitrate, and erythrityl tetranitrate) in anesthetized animals produces the same transient (1 to 4 minutes) decrease in blood pressure. Relative to nitroglycerin, the potency of erythrityl tetranitrate as a vasodepressor in dogs is about 12% and that of isosorbide dinitrate 3.5%. Since denitration markedly reduces the activity of the organic nitrates, their rapid clearance from blood indicates that the transient duration of action under these conditions correlates with the concentrations of the parent compounds. The rate of hepatic denitration is characteristic of each nitrate and is influenced by hepatic blood flow or the presence of hepatic disease. In experimental animals, injection of moderate amounts of organic nitrates into the portal vein results in little or no vasodepressor activity, indicating that a substantial fraction of drug can be metabolized during its first circulation through the liver (isosorbide mononitrate is an exception).

Tolerance

Sublingual organic nitrates should be taken at the time of an anginal attack or in anticipation of exercise or stress.

Such intermittent treatment results in reproducible cardiovascular effects. However, frequently repeated or continuous exposure to high doses of organic nitrates leads to a marked attenuation in the magnitude of most of their pharmacological effects (Anonymous, 1992; Thadani, 1992). The magnitude of tolerance is a function of dosage and the frequency of administration of the preparation.

Tolerance may result from an inability of the vascular smooth muscle to convert nitroglycerin to NO, "true vascular tolerance," or to the activation of mechanisms extraneous to the vessel wall, "pseudotolerance" (Munzel *et al.*, 1996). Multiple mechanisms have been proposed to account for nitrate tolerance, including volume expansion, neurohumoral activation, cellular depletion of sulfhydryl groups, and the generation of free radicals (Thadani, 1992; Rutherford, 1995; Parker and Parker 1998). The administration of organic nitrates to healthy volunteers is associated within 24 hours with the activation of the renin-angiotensin-aldosterone system and with increases in plasma norepinephrine (Parker *et al.*, 1991). Clinical data relating to the ability of agents that modify the renin-angiotensin-aldosterone system to prevent nitrate tolerance are contradictory (Dakak *et al.*, 1990; Muiesan *et al.*, 1993; Parker and Parker 1993; Pizzulli *et al.*, 1996; Heitzer *et al.*, 1998). Important factors that may influence the ability of angiotensin converting enzyme (ACE) inhibitors to prevent nitrate tolerance and that can influence the interpretation of clinical trials include the dose, treatment with the ACE inhibitors prior to the initiation of nitrates, and the tissue specificity of the agent. Despite the rationale for the depletion of sulfhydryl groups leading to impaired biotransformation of nitrates to NO and thereby resulting in nitrate tolerance, experimental results to date with sulfhydryl donors have been disappointing. A more recent proposal has linked nitroglycerin tolerance to endothelium-derived superoxide generation (Munzel *et al.*, 1995b). In the setting of patients with congestive heart failure, administration of *carvedilol*, but not metoprolol, doxazosin, or placebo, has resulted in the prevention of tolerance to the effects of nitroglycerin on forearm blood flow (Watanabe *et al.*, 1998). In addition to its properties as an α- and β-adrenergic receptor antagonist, carvedilol possesses antioxidant properties. A similar effect on vascular superoxide generation in the reduction of nitrate tolerance has been proposed for *hydralazine* (Elkayam *et al.*, 1998). Other changes that are observed in the setting of nitroglycerin tolerance include an enhanced response to vasocontrictors such as angiotensin II, serotonin, and phenylephrine. This increased sensitivity to vasoconstrictors may result from a priming effect of endothelin-1 derived from the vasculature (Munzel *et al.*, 1995a). Administration of nitroglycerin is associated with plasma volume expansion, which may be reflected by a decrease in hematocrit. Although diuretic therapy with hydrochlorothiazide can improve a patient's exercise duration, appropriately designed crossover trials have failed to demonstrate an effect of diuretics on nitrate tolerance (Parker *et al.,* 1996). In contrast to these adjunctive approaches, a more effective approach is to interrupt therapy for 8 to 12 hours each day, which allows the return of efficacy. It is usually most convenient to omit dosing at night in patients with exertional angina, either by adjusting dosing intervals of oral or buccal preparations or by removing cutaneous nitroglycerin. However, patients who have angina in a pattern suggesting its precipitation by increased left ventricular filling pressures (*i.e.,* occurring with or near episodes of orthopnea or paroxysmal nocturnal dyspnea) may benefit from continuing nitrates at night and omitting them during a quiet period during the day. Tolerance to isosorbide dinitrate may be minimized by giving this drug two or three times daily, at 7 A.M. and noon or at 7 A.M., noon, and 5 P.M., respectively (Parker *et al.,* 1987). Although it was thought that tolerance might be less of a problem with isosorbide-5-mononitrate, tolerance has been seen with this agent as well; an eccentric (7 or 8 A.M. and 2 or 3 P.M.) twice-daily dosing schedule appears to maintain efficacy (Parker, 1993; Thadani *et al.,* 1994).

While these approaches appear to be effective, some patients develop an increased frequency of nocturnal angina when a nitrate-free interval is employed using nitroglycerin patches; such patients may need to receive another class of antianginal agent during this period. In addition, a phenomenon referred to as the "zero-hour effect" has added to the complexity of designing an appropriate dosing regimen. In a 29-day study, the early morning exercise tolerance (before patch application) of patients using intermittent patch therapy was less than that of patients using placebo patches, though the antianginal efficacy of the patch itself was maintained (DeMots and Glasser, 1989). The clinical significance of this finding and its applicability to other dosage forms of nitroglycerin are not known. Tolerance does not appear to be a uniform phenomenon, as in some patients only partial tolerance seems to develop.

The problem of anginal rebound during nitrate-free intervals is especially troublesome in the treatment of unstable angina with intravenous nitroglycerin. If coverage of the interval with other agents is ineffective, an alternative approach that often is used is to increase gradually the dose of intravenous nitroglycerin in an attempt to overcome tolerance. This approach has not been studied carefully.

A special aspect of tolerance has been observed among individuals exposed to nitroglycerin in the manufacture of explosives. If protection is inadequate, workers may experience severe headaches, dizziness, and postural weakness during the first several days of employment. Tolerance then develops, but headache and other symptoms may reappear after a few days away from the job—the "Monday disease." The most serious effect of chronic exposure is a form of organic nitrate dependence. Workers without demonstrable organic vascular disease have been reported to have an increase in the incidence of acute coronary syndromes during the 24- to 72-hour periods away from the work environment (Morton, 1977, Parker *et al.,* 1995). Coronary and digital arteriospasm during withdrawal and its relaxation by nitroglycerin also have been demonstrated radiographically. Because of the potential problem of nitrate dependence, it seems prudent not to withdraw nitrates abruptly from a patient who has received such therapy chronically.

Toxicity and Untoward Responses

Untoward responses to the therapeutic use of organic nitrates are almost all secondary to actions on the cardiovascular system. Headache is common and can be severe. It usually decreases over a few days if treatment is continued and often can be controlled by decreasing the dose. Transient episodes of dizziness, weakness, and other manifestations associated with postural hypotension may develop, particularly if the patient is standing immobile, and may occasionally progress to loss of consciousness. This reaction appears to be accentuated by alcohol. It may be seen with very low doses of nitrates in patients with autonomic dysfunction. Even in the most severe nitrate syncope, positioning and other procedures to facilitate venous return are the only therapeutic measures required. It was widely believed that nitrates can increase intraocular pressure and precipitate glaucoma, but this fear appears to be unfounded (Robertson and Stevens, 1977). All of the organic nitrates occasionally can produce drug rash.

Interaction of Nitrates with Sildenafil. Erectile dysfunction is a frequently encountered problem, risk factors for which parallel those of coronary artery disease [diabetes mellitus, hypertension, known heart disease (Johannes *et al.,* 2000) and a low level of high-density lipoprotein (Feldman *et al.,* 1994)]. Thus, it is likely that many men requiring therapy for erectile dysfunction already may be receiving (or may require, especially if they increase physical activity) antianginal therapy. The past decade has seen remarkable advances in our understanding of the physiology of penile erection (Andersson and Wagner, 1995). Cells in the corpus cavernosum produce nitric oxide during sexual arousal in response to nonadrenergic, noncholinergic neurotransmission (Kim *et al.,*

1991; Rajfer *et al.,* 1992; and Burnett *et al.,* 1992). Nitric oxide stimulates the formation of cyclic GMP, which leads to relaxation of smooth muscle of the corpus cavernosum and penile arteries. The accumulation of cyclic GMP can be enhanced by inhibition of the cyclic GMP-specific phopshophodiesterase-5 (PDE5) family (Beavo *et al.,* 1994). *Sildenafil* (VIAGRA) was developed as an inhibitor of PDE5 (Boolell *et al.,* 1996) and has been demonstrated to improve erectile function in patients with various causes of erectile dysfunction (Goldstein *et al.,* 1998).

The side effects of sildenafil are largely predictable on the basis of its effects on PDE5. Headache, flushing, and rhinitis may be observed, as may dyspepsia due to relaxation of the lower esophageal sphincter, all thought to be consequences of the inhibition of PDE5. Sildenafil also is a weak inhibitor of PDE6, the isoenzyme involved in photoreceptor signal transduction (Beavo *et al.,* 1994), and sildenafil has been associated with visual disturbances, most notably changes in the perception of color hue or brightness (Wallis *et al.,* 1999; Goldstein *et al.,* 1998). Sildenafil's most important toxicity is hemodynamic. When given alone to men with severe coronary artery disease, sildenafil has modest effects on blood pressure, producing less than a 10% fall in systolic, diastolic, and mean systemic pressures and in pulmonary artery systolic and mean pressures (Herrman *et al.,* 2000). However, it has a significant and potentially dangerous interaction with nitrates. As discussed above, the therapeutic actions of organic nitrates are mediated *via* their conversion to NO with resultant increases in cyclic GMP. In the presence of a PDE5 inhibitor, nitrates cause profound increases in cyclic GMP and can produce dramatic reductions in blood pressure. Healthy male subjects pretreated with sildenafil exhibited a much greater decrease in systolic blood pressure when treated with sublingual glyceryl trinitrate, and in many a fall of more than 25 mm Hg was detected (Webb *et al.,* 1999). This interaction between sildenafil and nitrates is the basis for the warning that sildenafil should not be prescribed to patients receiving any form of nitrate (Cheitlen *et al.,* 1999) and dictates that patients should be questioned about the use of sildenafil within 24 hours before nitrates are administered. A period of longer than 24 hours may be needed after sildenafil for safe use of nitrates. In the event that patients develop significant hypotension following combined administration of sildenafil and a nitrate, fluids and α-adrenergic receptor agonists, if needed, should be used for support (Cheitlin *et al.,* 1999).

Sildenafil is metabolized *via* CYP3A4, and its toxicity may be enhanced in patients who receive other substrates of this enzyme, including macrolide and imidazole antibiotics, some HMG-CoA reductase inhibitors, and highly active antiretroviral therapy (HAART; *see* Chapter 51) (Hall and Ahmad, 1999). Sildenafil also has been demonstrated to prolong cardiac repolarization by blocking the I_{Kr} (Geelen *et al.,* 2000). Although these interactions and effects are clinically important, the overall incidence and profile of adverse events observed with sildenafil, when used without nitrates, are consistent with the expected background frequency of the same events in the treated population (Zusman *et al.,* 1999). In patients with coronary artery disease who are not currently taking nitrates and whose exercise capacity indicates that usual sexual activity is unlikely to precipitate angina, the use of sildenafil can be considered. Such therapy needs to be individualized and appropriate warnings given about the risk of toxicity if nitrates are taken during the next 24 hours for angina. Alternative nonnitrate antianginal therapy, such as β-adrenergic receptor antagonists, should be used during this time period (Cheitlin *et al.,* 1999).

Therapeutic Uses

Angina. Diseases that predispose to angina should be treated as part of a comprehensive therapeutic program with the primary goal being to prolong life. Such conditions as hypertension, anemia, thyrotoxicosis, obesity, heart failure, cardiac arrhythmias, and acute anxiety can precipitate anginal symptoms in many patients. The patient should be asked to stop smoking and overeating, hypertension and hyperlipidemia should be corrected (*see* Chapters 33 and 36), and daily aspirin (or a thienopyridine such as clopidogrel or ticlopidine, if aspirin is not tolerated; *see* Chapter 55) should be prescribed. Exposure to sympathomimetic agents (*e.g.,* those in nasal decongestants) should be avoided. The use of drugs that modify the perception of pain is a poor approach to the treatment of angina, since the underlying myocardial ischemia is not relieved. *See* Table 32–1 for preparations and dosages of the nitrites and organic nitrates. The rapidity of onset, the duration of action, and the likelihood of developing tolerance are related to the method of administration.

Sublingual Administration. Because of its rapid action, long-established efficacy, and low cost, nitroglycerin is the most useful drug among the organic nitrates that can be given sublingually. The onset of action is within 1 to 2 minutes, but the effects are undetectable by 1 hour after administration. An initial dose of 0.3 mg of nitroglycerin often will relieve pain within 3 minutes. Absorption may be limited in patients with dentures or with dry mouths. Tablets of nitroglycerin are stable but should be dispensed in glass containers and protected from moisture, light, and extremes of temperature. Active tablets usually produce a burning sensation under the tongue, but the absence of a burning sensation does not reliably predict loss of activity. Patients, especially elderly ones, differ in the ability to detect the burning sensation. Anginal pain may be prevented when the drug is used prophylactically immediately prior to exercise or stress. The smallest effective dose should be prescribed. Patients should be taught to seek medical attention immediately when three tablets taken over a 15-minute period do not relieve a sustained attack, since this situation may be indicative of myocardial infarction or another cause of the pain. The patient also should be advised that there is no virtue in trying to avoid taking sublingual nitroglycerin for anginal pain. Other nitrates that can be taken sublingually do not appear to be longer acting than nitroglycerin, as their half-lives depend only on the rate at which they are delivered to the liver. They are not more effective than nitroglycerin and often are more expensive.

Oral Administration.   Oral nitrates often are used to provide prophylaxis against anginal episodes in patients who have more than occasional angina. They must be given in sufficient dosage to provide effective plasma levels after first-pass hepatic degradation. At low doses (*e.g.,* 5 to 10 mg of isosorbide dinitrate) they are no more effective than placebo in decreasing the frequency of angina or increasing the patient's exercise tolerance. Clinical studies that have used higher doses of either isosorbide dinitrate (*e.g.,* 20 mg or more orally every 4 hours) or sustained-release preparations of nitroglycerin indicate that such regimens decrease the frequency of attacks of angina and improve exercise tolerance. Effects peak at 60 to 90 minutes and last for 3 to 6 hours. Under these circumstances, the activities of less potent metabolites also may contribute to the therapeutic effect. Chronic oral administration of isosorbide dinitrate (120 to 720 mg daily) results in persistence of the parent compound and higher concentrations of metabolites in plasma. However, these doses are more likely to cause troublesome side effects and tolerance. Significant, prolonged (up to 4 hours) improvement of exercise tolerance also can be demonstrated with a sustained-release oral form of nitroglycerin, but high doses (*e.g.,* 6.5 mg) of nitroglycerin are required.

Cutaneous Administration.   Application of nitroglycerin ointment can relieve angina, prolong exercise capacity, and reduce ischemic ST depression with exercise for 4 hours or more. Nitroglycerin ointment (2%) is applied to the skin [2.5 to 5 cm (1 to 2 in.) as it is squeezed from the tube; it is then spread in a uniform layer]; the dosage must be adjusted for each patient. Effects are apparent within 30 to 60 minutes (although absorption is variable) and last for 4 to 6 hours. The ointment is particularly useful for controlling nocturnal angina, which commonly develops within 3 hours after the patient goes to sleep. Transdermal nitroglycerin discs utilize a nitroglycerin-impregnated polymer (bonded to an adhesive bandage) that permits gradual absorption and a continuous plasma nitrate concentration over 24 hours. The onset of action is slow, with peak effects occurring at 1 to 2 hours. To avoid tolerance and loss of the therapeutic effect, therapy should be interrupted for at least 8 hours each day. With

this regimen, long-term prophylaxis of ischemic episodes often can be attained.

Transmucosal or Buccal Nitroglycerin.   This formulation is inserted under the upper lip above the incisors, where it adheres to the gingiva and gradually dissolves in a uniform manner. Hemodynamic effects are seen within 2 to 5 minutes, and it is therefore useful for short-term prophylaxis of angina. Nitroglycerin continues to be released into the circulation for a prolonged period, and exercise tolerance may be enhanced for up to 5 hours.

Congestive Heart Failure.   The utility of nitrovasodilators to relieve pulmonary congestion and to increase cardiac output in congestive heart failure is well established and is addressed in Chapter 34.

Unstable Angina.   Unstable angina has been considered a single entity in most therapeutic trials; it has included patients with new-onset exertional angina, with an increase in their usual pattern of angina, and with rest angina, with or without a preceding history of exertional angina. The electrocardiogram (ECG) may show either elevation or depression of the ST segment, with variable T-wave abnormalities. In patients with left main or three-vessel disease, revascularization leads to improved survival (Multicenter Study, 1978). In the remainder of patients, and in all patients prior to determination of the coronary anatomy, appropriate medical therapy provides important benefits. The pathophysiology in most patients studied involves thrombosis overlying a ruptured atherosclerotic plaque. However, there is some variability in the anatomic substrate of unstable angina, with gradually progressive atherosclerosis accounting for some cases of new-onset exertional angina, and vasospasm occurring in minimally atherosclerotic coronary vessels accounting for some cases where rest angina has never been preceded by or associated with exertional angina. It is likely that this variability accounts for the differences in therapeutic response seen in studies with differing inclusion criteria.

Multiple agents are employed in the acute phase of treatment, although few have been demonstrated conclusively to reduce mortality. Aspirin (*see* below), by inhibiting platelet aggregation, has been shown clearly to improve survival (Kerins and FitzGerald, 1991). Heparin (either unfractionated or low-molecular-weight heparin) also appears to reduce angina and prevent infarction. These and related agents are discussed in detail in Chapters 27 and 55. Nitrates are useful in reducing vasospasm and controlling angina; their administration should be initiated intravenously. Intravenous administration of nitroglycerin allows high concentrations of drug to be attained rapidly. As nitroglycerin is promptly degraded, the plasma concentration can be titrated quickly and safely using this route. If coronary vasospasm is present, intravenous nitroglycerin is likely to be effective, although the addition of a Ca^{2+} channel blocker is required to achieve complete control in some patients. Because of the potential risks of profound hypotension, nitrates should be withheld and alternate antianginal therapy administered if patients have consumed sildenafil within the prior 24 hours (*see* above).

Myocardial Infarction.   Therapeutic maneuvers in myocardial infarction are directed at reducing the ultimate size of the infarct and preserving or retrieving viable tissue by reducing the oxygen demand of the myocardium. Since the proximate cause of myocardial infarction is intracoronary thrombosis, reperfusion therapies are critically important and include thrombolytic agents and direct percutaneous coronary angioplasty (Ryan *et al.,* 1999). Thrombolytic and antiplatelet therapy are discussed in Chapter 55. A drug that favorably alters the oxygen balance could decrease the area of myocardial damage if it were given soon after infarction.

In the past, nitroglycerin was considered to be contraindicated for use in patients with acute myocardial infarction because of its ability to induce hypotension and reflex tachycardia, although it may be highly efficacious if the infarction is due to prolonged coronary spasm. Nevertheless, evidence that nitrates improve mortality in myocardial infarction is sparse. Nitrates may be most helpful in patients in whom reperfusion does not occur, despite thrombolytic agents, and may prevent adverse remodeling. The effects of nitrates in patients with acute myocardial infarction were assessed in two large trials (GISSI-3, 1994, and ISIS-4 Collaborative Group, 1995). In the GISSI-3 study, 19,394 patients with acute myocardial infarction were randomized to receive either transdermal nitroglycerin (10 mg daily with a 10-hour nitrate-free interval overnight) or placebo for 6 weeks. There were no significant effects of nitroglycerin on mortality, reinfarction, revascularization procedures, or renal dysfunction. There was a slight reduction in postinfarction angina in the nitroglycerin-treated group (20.7% vs. 19.7%). A similar lack of benefit on mortality was observed in the ISIS-4 study of 58,050 patients, some of whom were randomized to receive an oral controlled-release form of isosorbide mononitrate, 60 mg each morning for 28 days, or placebo. In the ISIS-4 study there was no effect of the nitrate on postinfarction angina. Thus transdermal or oral nitrates are safe and well tolerated in the setting of myocardial infarction and may have a beneficial effect on pain, but they do not provide a survival advantage.

Variant (Prinzmetal's) Angina.   The large coronary arteries normally contribute little to coronary resistance. However, in variant angina, coronary constriction results in reduced blood flow and ischemic pain. Multiple mechanisms have been hypothesized to be involved in the initiation of vasospasm, including endothelial cell injury (Freisinger and Robertson, 1986). It does not seem likely that abnormalities of sympathetic input are etiologic (Robertson *et al.,* 1979), and β-adrenergic receptor antagonists can be deleterious (Robertson *et al.,* 1982). Despite the presence of abnormal coronary anatomy in all cases that have come to autopsy, it does not appear that active intravascular platelet aggregation is a precipitating factor, and aspirin does not appear to provide benefit (Robertson *et al.,* 1981). Whereas long-acting nitrates alone are occasionally efficacious in abolishing episodes of variant angina, more often additional therapy with Ca^{2+} channel blockers is required. Because Ca^{2+} channel blockers, but not nitrates, have been shown to favorably influence mortality and the incidence of myocardial infarction in variant angina, they should be included in therapy.

Ca^{2+} CHANNEL ANTAGONISTS

History.   The work in the 1960s of Fleckenstein, Godfraind, and their colleagues led to the concept that drugs can alter cardiac and smooth muscle contraction by blocking the entry of Ca^{2+} into myocytes. Godfraind and associates showed that the ability of the diphenylpiperazine analogs *cinnarizine* and *lidoflazine* to prevent vascular smooth muscle contraction induced by some agonists could be overcome by raising the concentration of Ca^{2+} in the extracellular medium; they used the term "calcium antagonist" to describe these agents (*see* Godfraind and Kaba, 1972; Godfraind *et al.,* 1986).

Hass and Hartfelder reported in 1962 that *verapamil,* a putative coronary vasodilator, possessed negative inotropic and chronotropic effects that were not seen with other vasodilatory agents, such as nitroglycerin. In 1967, Fleckenstein suggested that the negative inotropic effect resulted from inhibition of excitation–contraction coupling and that the mechanism involved reduction of the movement of Ca^{2+} into cardiac myocytes (*see* Fleckenstein, 1983). A derivative of verapamil, *gallopamil,* and other compounds, such as *nifedipine* (Kohlhardt and Fleckenstein, 1977), also were shown to block the movement of Ca^{2+} through the cardiac myocyte Ca^{2+} channel, or the slow channel (*see* Chapter 35), and thereby alter the plateau phase of the cardiac action potential. Subsequently, many drugs in several chemical classes have been shown to alter cardiac and smooth muscle contraction by blocking or "antagonizing" the entry of Ca^{2+} through channels in the myocyte membrane.

Chemistry.   The ten Ca^{2+} channel antagonists that have been approved for clinical use in the United States have diverse chemical structures. Five classes of compounds have been examined: phenylalkylamines, dihydropyridines, benzothiazepines, diphenylpiperazines, and a diarylaminopropylamine. At present, *verapamil* (a phenylalkylamine); *diltiazem* (a benzothiazepine); *nicardipine, nifedipine, isradipine, amlodipine, felodipine, nisoldipine,* and *nimodipine* (dihydropyridines); and *bepridil* (a diarylaminopropylamine ether) are approved for clinical use in the United States. Their structures are shown in Table 32–2.

Pharmacological Properties

Cardiovascular Effects.   *Actions in Vascular Tissue.*
Although there is some involvement of Na^+ currents, depolarization of vascular smooth muscle cells is primarily dependent on the influx of Ca^{2+} (Bolton, 1979). At least three distinct mechanisms may be responsible for contraction of vascular smooth muscle cells. First, voltage-sensitive Ca^{2+} channels open in response to depolarization of the membrane, and extracellular Ca^{2+} moves down its electrochemical gradient into the cell. After closure of Ca^{2+} channels, a finite period of time is required before the channels can open again in response to a stimulus. Second, agonist-induced contractions that occur without depolarization of the membrane result from the hydrolysis of membrane phosphatidylinositol with the formation of inositol trisphosphate, which acts as a second messenger to release intracellular Ca^{2+} from the sarcoplasmic reticulum (*see* Berridge, 1993). This receptor-mediated release of intracellular Ca^{2+} may trigger further influx of extracellular Ca^{2+}. Third, receptor-operated Ca^{2+} channels

Table 32–2

Ca^{2+} Channel Blockers: Chemical Structures and Some Relative Cardiovascular Effects*

CHEMICAL STRUCTURE (NONPROPRIETARY AND TRADE NAMES)	VASODILATION (CORONARY FLOW)	SUPPRESSION OF CARDIAC CONTRACTILITY	SUPPRESSION OF AUTOMATICITY (SA NODE)	SUPPRESSION OF CONDUCTION (AV NODE)
Amlodipine (NORVASC)	NR	NR	NR	NR
Bepridil (VASCOR)	NR	NR	NR	NR
Diltiazem (CARDIZEM, DILACOR-XR, others)	3	2	5	4
Felodipine (PLENDIL)	NR	NR	NR	NR
Isradipine (DYNACIRC)	NR	NR	NR	NR

Table 32–2

Ca^{2+} Channel Blockers: Chemical Structures and Some Relative Cardiovascular Effects* *(Continued)*

CHEMICAL STRUCTURE (NONPROPRIETARY AND TRADE NAMES)	VASODILATION (CORONARY FLOW)	SUPPRESSION OF CARDIAC CONTRACTILITY	SUPPRESSION OF AUTOMATICITY (SA NODE)	SUPPRESSION OF CONDUCTION (AV NODE)
Nicardipine (CARDENE, others)	5	0	1	0
Nifedipine (ADALAT, PROCARDIA)	5	1	1	0
Nimodipine (NIMOTOP)	5	1	1	0
Nisoldipine (SULAR)	NR	NR	NR	NR
Verapamil (CALAN, ISOPTIN, VERELAN, COVERA-HS)	4	4	5	5

*The relative cardiovascular effects are ranked from no effect (0) to most prominent (5). NR, not ranked. (Modified from Julian, 1987; Taira, 1987.)

allow the entry of extracellular Ca^{2+} in response to receptor occupancy.

An increase in cytosolic Ca^{2+} results in enhanced binding of Ca^{2+} to the protein calmodulin. The Ca^{2+}–calmodulin complex in turn activates myosin light-chain kinase, with resultant phosphorylation of the light chain of myosin. Such phosphorylation promotes interaction between actin and myosin and contraction of smooth muscle. Ca^{2+} channel antagonists or blockers inhibit the voltage-dependent Ca^{2+} channels in vascular smooth muscle at significantly lower concentrations than are required to interfere with the release of intracellular Ca^{2+} or to block receptor-operated Ca^{2+} channels. All Ca^{2+} channel blockers relax arterial smooth muscle, but they have little effect on most venous beds and hence do not affect cardiac preload significantly.

Actions in Cardiac Cells. The mechanisms involved in excitation–contraction coupling in the heart differ from those in vascular smooth muscle in that a portion of the two inward currents is carried by Na^+ through the fast channel in addition to that carried by Ca^{2+} through the slow channel. In the sinoatrial (SA) and atrioventricular (AV) nodes, depolarization is largely dependent on the movement of Ca^{2+} through the slow channel. Within the cardiac myocyte, Ca^{2+} binds to troponin, the inhibitory effect of troponin on the contractile apparatus is relieved, and actin and myosin interact to cause contraction. Thus, Ca^{2+} channel blockers can produce a negative inotropic effect. Although this is true of all classes of Ca^{2+} channel blockers, the greater degree of peripheral vasodilation seen with the dihydropyridines is accompanied by sufficient baroreflex-mediated increase in sympathetic tone to overcome the negative inotropic effect. Diltiazem also may inhibit mitochondrial Na^+–Ca^{2+} exchange (Schwartz, 1992).

The effect of a Ca^{2+} channel blocker on atrioventricular conduction and on the rate of the sinus node pacemaker is dependent on whether or not the agent delays the recovery of the slow channel (Henry, 1983). Although nifedipine reduces the slow inward current in a dose-dependent manner, it does not affect the rate of recovery of the slow Ca^{2+} channel (Kohlhardt and Fleckenstein, 1977). The channel blockade caused by nifedipine and related dihydropyridines also shows little dependence on the frequency of stimulation. At doses used clinically, nifedipine does not affect conduction through the node. In contrast, verapamil not only reduces the magnitude of the Ca^{2+} current through the slow channel but also decreases the rate of recovery of the channel. In addition, channel blockade caused by verapamil (and to a lesser extent by diltiazem) is enhanced as the frequency of stimulation increases, a phenomenon known as "frequency dependence" or "use dependence." Verapamil and diltiazem depress the rate of the sinus node pacemaker and slow AV conduction; the latter effect is the basis for their use in the treatment of supraventricular tachyarrhythmias (*see* Chapter 35). Bepridil, like verapamil, inhibits both slow inward Ca^{2+} current and fast inward Na^+ current. It has a direct negative inotropic effect. Its electrophysiologic properties lead to slowing of the heart rate, prolongation of the AV nodal effective refractory period, and, importantly, prolongation of the QTc interval. Particularly in the setting of hypokalemia, the last effect can be associated with *torsades de pointes,* a potentially lethal ventricular arrhythmia (*see* Chapter 35).

Hemodynamic Effects. All of the Ca^{2+} channel blockers that have been approved for clinical use decrease coronary vascular resistance and increase coronary blood flow. The dihydropyridines are more potent vasodilators *in vivo* and *in vitro* than is verapamil, which is more potent than diltiazem. The hemodynamic effects of each of these agents vary, depending on the route of administration and the extent of left ventricular dysfunction.

Nifedipine given intravenously increases forearm blood flow with little effect on venous pooling; this indicates a selective dilation of arterial resistance vessels. The decrease in arterial blood pressure elicits sympathetic reflexes, with resultant tachycardia and positive inotropy. Nifedipine also has direct negative inotropic effects *in vitro*. However, nifedipine relaxes vascular smooth muscle at significantly lower concentrations than those required for prominent direct effects on the heart. Thus, arteriolar resistance and blood pressure are lowered, contractility and segmental ventricular function are improved, and heart rate and cardiac output are increased modestly (Serruys *et al.,* 1981; Theroux *et al.,* 1980). After oral administration of nifedipine, arterial dilation increases peripheral blood flow; venous tone does not change.

The other dihydropyridines—nicardipine, amlodipine, isradipine, felodipine, nisoldipine, and nimodipine—share many of the cardiovascular effects of nifedipine. There may be some selectivity of nicardipine for coronary vessels compared with peripheral vessels (Pepine and Lambert, 1988); in comparative studies, nicardipine appears to produce fewer side effects, such as dizziness, than does nifedipine but has equivalent antianginal efficacy (DeWood and Wohlbach, 1990). Intravenous or oral administration of nicardipine results in decreases in systolic and diastolic blood pressure that are accompanied by an increase in cardiac output because of the reduction in afterload and compensatory increases in heart rate and ejection fraction. It also appears to reduce left ventricular diastolic dysfunction (Hanet *et al.,* 1990). Nicardipine decreases the frequency of anginal attacks and improves exercise tolerance in patients with effort-induced angina (Pepine and Lambert, 1988). Amlodipine is a dihydropyridine that has slow absorption and a prolonged effect. With a plasma half-life of 35 to 50 hours, plasma levels and effect increase over 7 to 10 days of therapy. Amlodipine produces both peripheral arterial vasodilation and coronary dilation, with a hemodynamic profile similar to that of nifedipine. However, there is less reflex tachycardia with amlodipine, possibly because the long half-life produces minimal peaks and troughs in plasma concentrations (van Zwieten and Pfaffendorf, 1993; Taylor, 1994; Lehmann *et al.,* 1993). Felodipine appears to have even greater vascular specificity than does nifedipine or amlodipine. At concentrations producing vasodilation, there is no negative inotropic effect. Like nifedipine, felodipine produces activation of the sympathetic nervous system, leading to an increase in heart rate (Todd and Faulds, 1992). Isradipine also produces the typical peripheral vasodilation seen with other dihydropyridines, but because of its inhibitory effect on the SA node, little or no rise in heart rate is seen. This inhibitory effect does not extend to the myocardium, however, as no cardiodepressant effect is seen. Despite the negative chronotropic effect, isradipine appears to have little effect on the AV node, so it may be used in patients with AV block or combined with a β-adrenergic receptor antagonist. In general, because of their lack of myocardial depression and, to a greater or lesser extent, lack of negative chronotropic effect, dihydropyridines are less effective as monotherapy in stable angina than are verapamil, diltiazem, or a β-adrenergic receptor antagonist. Nisoldipine is more than 1000-times as potent in preventing contraction of human vascular smooth muscle than in preventing contraction of human cardiac muscle *in vitro,* suggesting a very high degree of vascular selectivity (Godfraind *et al.,* 1992). This selectivity has been confirmed by *in vitro* studies. Although nisoldipine has a short elimination half-life, a sustained-release preparation has been developed, nisoldipine coat-core, that has been demonstrated to be as effective an antianginal agent as amlodipine or diltiazem (Langtry and Spencer, 1997). Nimodipine, because of its high lipid solubility, was developed as an agent to relax the cerebral vasculature. It is effective in inhibiting cerebral vasospasm and is used primarily to treat patients with neurological defects thought to be caused by vasospasm after subarachnoid hemorrhage.

Bepridil has been demonstrated to reduce blood pressure and heart rate in patients with stable exertional angina. It also produces an increase in left ventricular performance in patients with angina, but its side-effect profile (*see* below) limits its use to truly refractory patients (Zusman *et al.,* 1993; Hollingshead *et al.,* 1992).

Verapamil is a less potent vasodilator *in vivo* than are the dihydropyridines. Like the latter agents, verapamil causes little effect on venous resistance vessels at concentrations that produce arteriolar dilation. With doses of verapamil sufficient to produce peripheral arterial vasodilation, there are more direct negative chronotropic, dromotropic, and inotropic effects than with the dihydropyridines. Intravenous verapamil causes a decrease in arterial blood pressure due to a decrease in vascular resistance, but the reflex tachycardia is blunted or abolished by the direct negative chronotropic effect of the drug. The intrinsic negative inotropic effect of verapamil is partially offset by both a decrease in afterload and the reflex increase in adrenergic tone. Thus, in patients without congestive heart failure, ventricular performance is not impaired and may actually improve, especially if ischemia is limiting performance. In contrast, in patients with congestive heart failure, intravenous verapamil can cause a marked decrease in contractility and left ventricular function. Oral administration of verapamil results in reduction of peripheral vascular resistance and blood pressure with no change in heart rate (Theroux *et al.,* 1980). The relief of pacing-induced angina seen with verapamil is due primarily to a reduction in myocardial oxygen demand (Rouleau *et al.,* 1983).

Intravenous administration of diltiazem can result initially in a marked decrease in peripheral vascular resistance and arterial blood pressure, which elicits a reflex increase in heart rate and cardiac output. Heart rate then falls below initial levels because of the direct negative chronotropic effect of the agent. Oral administration of diltiazem results in a sustained fall in both heart rate and mean arterial blood pressure (Theroux *et al.,* 1980). Despite the fact that diltiazem and verapamil produce similar effects on the SA and AV nodes, the negative inotropic effect of diltiazem is more modest.

The effect of Ca^{2+} channel blockers on diastolic ventricular relaxation (the lusitropic state of the ventricle) is complex. The direct effect of several of these agents, assessed when they are given by the intracoronary route, is to impair relaxation (Rousseau *et al.,* 1980; Amende *et al.,* 1983; Serruys *et al.,* 1983; Walsh and O'Rourke, 1985). Although several clinical studies have suggested an improvement in peak left ventricular filling rates when verapamil, nifedipine, nisoldipine, or nicardipine was given systemically (Bonow *et al.,* 1982; Paulus *et al.,* 1983; Rodrigues *et al.,* 1987; DEFIANT-II Research Group, 1997), one must be cautious in extrapolating this change in filling rates to enhancement of relaxation. Indeed, in studies by Nishimura *et al.* (1993), verapamil increased peak filling rate but also increased left ventricular end-diastolic pressure. Because ventricular relaxation is modulated at several levels (Brutsaert *et al.*, 1993), the effect of even a single agent may be complex. If reflex stimulation of sympathetic tone increases myocardial cyclic AMP levels, increased lusitropy will result and may outweigh a direct negative lusitropic effect. Likewise, a reduction in afterload will improve the lusitropic state. In addition, if ischemia is improved, the negative lusitropic effect of asymmetrical left ventricular contraction will be reduced. However, in any given patient, the sum total of these effects cannot be determined *a priori*. Thus, caution should be exercised in the use of Ca^{2+} channel blockers for this purpose; it is ideal if the end result can be determined objectively before committing the patient to therapy.

Mechanisms of Action.   Increased concentrations of cytosolic Ca^{2+} cause increased contraction of cardiac and vascular smooth muscle cells. The entry of extracellular Ca^{2+} is more important in initiating the contraction of myocardial cells, while the release of Ca^{2+} from intracellular storage sites also participates in contraction of vascular smooth muscle, particularly in some vascular beds. In addition, the entry of extracellular Ca^{2+} can trigger the release of additional Ca^{2+} from intracellular stores.

Cytosolic Ca^{2+} concentrations may be increased by various contractile stimuli. Thus, many hormones and neurohormones increase Ca^{2+} influx through so-called receptor-operated channels, while high external concentrations of K^+ and depolarizing electrical stimuli increase Ca^{2+} influx through voltage-sensitive, or "potential-operated," channels (Bevan *et al.*, 1982).

Voltage-sensitive channels contain domains of homologous sequence that are arranged in tandem within a single large subunit. In addition to the major channel-forming subunit (termed α_1), Ca^{2+} channels contain several other associated subunits (termed α_2, β, γ, and δ; *see* Schwartz, 1992).

Voltage-sensitive Ca^{2+} channels have been divided into at least three subtypes based on their conductances and sensitivities to voltage (Schwartz, 1992; Tsien *et al.*, 1988). The channels best characterized to date are the L, N, and T subtypes, although P/Q and R channels have been identified. Only the L-type channel is sensitive to the dihydropyridine Ca^{2+} channel blockers. Large divalent cations such as Cd^{2+} and Mn^{2+} block a wider range of Ca^{2+} channels. All approved Ca^{2+} channel blockers bind to the α_1 subunit of the L-type calcium channel, which is the main pore-forming unit of the channel. This 200,000- to 250,000-dalton subunit is associated with a disulfide-linked $\alpha_2\delta$ subunit of approximately 140,000 daltons and an intracellular β subunit of 55,000 to 72,000 daltons. The α_1 subunits share a common topology of four homologous domains (I, II, III and IV), each of which is composed of six putative transmembrane segments (S1–S6). The $\alpha_2\delta$ and β subunits modulate the α_1 subunit. The phenylalkylamine Ca^{2+} channel blockers bind to transmembrane segment 6 of domain IV (IVS6), the benzothiazepine Ca^{2+} channel blockers bind to the cytoplasmic bridge between domain III (IIIS) and domain IV (IVS), and the dihydropyridine Ca^{2+} channel blockers bind to transmembrane segment of both domain III (IIIS6) and domain IV (IVS6). These three separate

receptor sites are allosterically linked (Hockerman *et al.*, 1997, Abernethy and Schwartz, 1999).

The vascular and cardiac effects of some of the Ca^{2+} channel blockers are summarized below and in Table 32–2.

Absorption, Fate, and Excretion

Although the absorption of these agents is nearly complete after oral administration, their bioavailability is reduced, in some cases markedly, because of first-pass hepatic metabolism. The effects of these drugs are evident within 30 to 60 minutes of an oral dose, with the exception of the more slowly absorbed and longer-acting agents amlodipine, isradipine, and felodipine. For comparison, peak effects of verapamil occur within 15 minutes of its intravenous administration. These agents all are bound to plasma proteins to a significant extent (70% to 98%); their elimination half-lives are widely variable and may range from 1.3 to 64 hours. During repeated oral administration, bioavailability and half-life may increase because of saturation of hepatic metabolism. A major metabolite of diltiazem is desacetyldiltiazem, which has about one-half of diltiazem's potency as a vasodilator. *N*-Demethylation of verapamil results in production of norverapamil, which is biologically active but much less potent than the parent compound. The half-life of norverapamil is about 10 hours. The metabolites of the dihydropyridines are inactive or weakly active. In patients with hepatic cirrhosis, the bioavailabilities and half-lives of the Ca^{2+} channel blockers may be increased, and dosage should be decreased accordingly. The half-lives of these agents also may be longer in older patients. Except for diltiazem and nifedipine, all of the Ca^{2+} channel blockers are administered as racemic mixtures (Abernethy and Schwartz, 1999).

Toxicity and Untoward Responses

The most common side effects caused by the Ca^{2+} channel antagonists, particularly the dihydropyridines, are due to excessive vasodilation. These effects may be expressed as dizziness, hypotension, headache, flushing, digital dysesthesia, and nausea. Patients also may experience constipation, peripheral edema, coughing, wheezing, and pulmonary edema. Nimodipine may produce muscular cramps when given in the large doses required for a beneficial effect in patients with subarachnoid hemorrhage. Less common side effects include rashes, somnolence, and occasional minor elevations of liver function tests. These side effects usually are benign and may abate with time or with adjustment of the dose. Aggravation of myocardial ischemia has been observed in two studies with the dihydropyridine nifedipine (Schulz *et al.*, 1985; Egstrup and Anderson, 1993). In both of these studies, worsening of angina was observed in patients with an angiographically demonstrable coronary collateral circulation. The worsening of angina may have resulted from excessive hypotension and decreased coronary perfusion, selective coronary vasodilation in nonischemic regions of the myocardium (*i.e.,* coronary steal, since vessels perfusing ischemic regions may already be maximally dilated), or an increase in oxygen demand owing to increased sympathetic tone and excessive tachycardia. In a study of monotherapy with an immediate-release formulation of nisoldipine, the dihydropyridine was not superior to placebo therapy and was associated with a trend toward an increased incidence of serious adverse events (Thadani *et al.,* 1991), a process described by Waters (1991) as *proischemia.*

Although bradycardia, transient asystole, and exacerbation of heart failure have been reported with verapamil, these responses usually have occurred after intravenous administration of verapamil, in patients with disease of the SA node or AV nodal conduction disturbances, or in the presence of β-adrenergic receptor blockade. The use of intravenous verapamil with a β-adrenergic receptor antagonist is contraindicated because of the increased propensity for atrioventricular block and/or severe depression of ventricular function. Patients with ventricular dysfunction, SA or AV nodal conduction disturbances, and systolic blood pressures below 90 mm Hg should not be treated with verapamil or diltiazem, particularly intravenously. Some Ca^{2+} channel antagonists can cause an increase in the concentration of digoxin in plasma, although toxicity from the cardiac glycoside rarely develops. The use of verapamil to treat digitalis toxicity is thus contraindicated; AV nodal conduction disturbances may be exacerbated. Bepridil, because of its antiarrhythmic properties and its ability to prolong the QTc interval, can produce serious arrhythmic side effects. Especially in the setting of hypokalemia and/or bradycardia, polymorphic ventricular tachycardia (*torsades de pointes*), a potentially lethal arrhythmia, can be seen. Agranulocytosis also has been reported. Because of these serious side effects, this agent should be reserved for patients refractory to all other appropriate medical and surgical therapy (Hollingshead *et al.,* 1992).

A novel Ca^{2+} channel blocker, *mibefradil,* is an example of an agent that inhibits both the T- and L-type Ca^{2+} channels. The T-type Ca^{2+} channel contributes to the spontaneous contractile function of smooth muscle cells (Mishra and Hermsmyer, 1994). Mibefradil was demonstrated to be effective in reducing the frequency and duration of asymptomatic ischemic episodes in patients with stable exertional angina pectoris and asymptomatic

ischemia (Braun *et al.,* 1996) and received approval from the United States Food and Drug Administration (FDA) for use as an antianginal agent. However, it subsequently was withdrawn from the market due to adverse drug interactions, possibly due to its dual inhibition of both the P-glycoprotein and CYP3A systems (Wandel *et al.,* 2000).

Recent observational studies and a metaanalysis have raised concerns about the long-term safety of the Ca^{2+} channel blockers, and in particular, short-acting nifedipine preparations (Psaty *et al.,* 1995; Pahor *et al.,* 1995; Furberg *et al.,* 1995). Authors of a recent analysis based on a total of 100 clinical studies of Ca^{2+} channel blockers concluded that observational studies and randomized clinical trials give concordant evidence linking adverse safety effects to short-acting Ca^{2+} channel blockers, specifically to short-acting nifedipine (Opie *et al.,* 2000). The proposed hypothesis for this adverse effect lies in abrupt vasodilation with reflex sympathetic activation. A similar conclusion was reached by Stason *et al.* (1999), who performed a systematic review of the literature on nifedipine and determined that adverse effects were observed in patients on monotherapy with an immediate-release formulation of nifedipine.

Therapeutic Uses

Variant Angina. Variant angina is a direct result of a reduction in flow, not the result of an increase in oxygen demand. Controlled clinical trials have demonstrated efficacy of the Ca^{2+} channel blocking agents for the treatment of variant angina (Antman *et al.,* 1980; Severi *et al.,* 1980). These drugs can attenuate ergonovine-induced vasospasm in patients with variant angina, which suggests that protection in variant angina is due to coronary dilation rather than to alterations in peripheral hemodynamics (Waters *et al.,* 1981).

Exertional Angina. Ca^{2+} channel antagonists also are effective in the treatment of exertional, or exercise-induced, angina. The utility of these agents may result from an increase in blood flow due to coronary arterial dilation, from a decrease in myocardial oxygen demand (secondary to a decrease in arterial blood pressure, heart rate, or contractility), or from both. Numerous double-blind placebo-controlled studies have shown that these drugs decrease the number of anginal attacks and attenuate exercise-induced depression of the ST segment.

The "double product," which is calculated as heart rate × systolic blood pressure, is an indirect measure of myocardial oxygen demand. Since these agents reduce the level of the double product (or oxygen demand) at a given external work load, and the value of the double product at peak exercise is not altered, the beneficial effect of Ca^{2+} channel blockers likely is due primarily to a decrease in oxygen demand rather than to an increase in coronary flow.

As described above, Ca^{2+} channel antagonists, particularly the dihydropyridines, may aggravate anginal symptoms in some patients when used without a β-adrenergic receptor antagonist. This adverse effect is not prominent with verapamil or diltiazem because of their limited ability to induce marked peripheral vasodilation and reflex tachycardia. Concurrent therapy with nifedipine and the β-adrenergic receptor antagonist propranolol, or with amlodipine and any of several β-adrenergic receptor antagonists, has proven more effective than either agent given alone in exertional angina, presumably because the β-adrenergic receptor antagonist suppresses reflex tachycardia (Bassan *et al.,* 1982; Lehmann *et al.,* 1993). This concurrent drug therapy is particularly attractive, since the dihydropyridines, unlike verapamil and diltiazem, do not delay atrioventricular conduction and will not enhance the negative dromotropic effects associated with β-adrenergic receptor blockade. Although concurrent administration of verapamil or diltiazem with a β-adrenergic receptor antagonist also may reduce angina, the potential for atrioventricular block, severe bradycardia, and decreased left ventricular function requires that these combinations be used judiciously (Packer, 1989), especially if left ventricular function is compromised prior to therapy. Amlodipine produces less reflex tachycardia than does nifedipine, probably because of a flatter plasma concentration profile. Isradipine, approximately equivalent to nifedipine in enhancing exercise tolerance, also produces less rise in heart rate, possibly because of its slow onset of action.

Unstable Angina. Medical therapy for unstable angina involves the administration of aspirin, which reduces mortality, and nitrates, β-adrenergic receptor blocking agents, and heparin, which are effective in controlling pain and ischemic episodes. Since vasospasm occurs in some patients with unstable angina (Hugenholtz *et al.,* 1981), Ca^{2+} channel blockers offer an additional approach to the treatment of unstable angina. However, there is insufficient evidence to assess whether or not such treatment actually decreases mortality except in patients in whom the principal mechanism is vasospasm. In a randomized, double-blind, clinical trial, the short-acting dihydropyridine nifedipine was found to be less effective than was metoprolol (Muller *et al.,* 1984), and there are no studies supporting the administration of a dihydropyridine to patients with unstable angina. One small study of 121 patients reported a benefit of intravenous diltiazem, compared to nitroglycerin, on the end-points of refractory angina or event-free survival (Göbel *et al.,* 1995). In contrast, therapy directed toward reduction of platelet function and thrombotic episodes clearly decreases morbidity and mortality in patients with unstable angina (*see* Chapters 27 and 55).

Myocardial Infarction. There is no evidence that Ca^{2+} channel antagonists are of benefit in the early treatment or secondary prevention of acute myocardial infarction, and in several trials, the short-acting formulation of the dihydropyridine nifedipine appears to have had a detrimental effect on mortality at higher doses (Kloner, 1995; Opie and Messerli, 1995; Yusuf, 1995; Furberg *et al.,* 1995). Diltiazem and verapamil may reduce the incidence of reinfarction in patients with a first non-Q-wave infarction who are not candidates for a β-adrenergic receptor antagonist (Ryan *et al.,* 1999).

Other Uses. The use of Ca^{2+} channel antagonists as antiarrhythmic agents is discussed in Chapter 35, and their use for the treatment of hypertension is discussed in Chapter 33. Clinical trials are under way to evaluate the capacity of Ca^{2+} channel blockers to slow the progression of renal failure and to protect the transplanted kidney. Verapamil has been demonstrated to improve left ventricular outflow obstruction and symptoms in patients with hypertrophic cardiomyopathy. Verapamil also has been used in the prophylaxis of migraine headaches. While several studies suggest that dihydropyridines may suppress the progression of mild atherosclerosis, there is no evidence that this alters mortality or reduces the incidence of ischemic events. Nimodipine has been approved for use in patients with neurological deficits secondary to cerebral vasospasm after the rupture of a congenital intracranial aneurysm. Nifedipine, diltiazem, and felodipine have been shown to provide symptomatic relief in Raynaud's disease.

Ca^{2+} channel antagonists cause relaxation of the myometrium *in vitro* and markedly inhibit the amplitude of spontaneous and oxytocin-induced contractions. Clinical studies have shown Ca^{2+} channel blockers to be effective in stopping preterm uterine contractions (Murray *et al.,* 1992; Childress and Katz, 1994; Evidence Report/Technology Assessment, 2000). In studies comparing nifedipine with the β_2-adrenergic receptor agonist *ritodrine,* nifedipine has been found to be at least as effective as ritodrine in stopping contractions and to be associated with fewer maternal side effects and a lower incidence of neonatal morbidity (Koks *et al.,* 1998; Garcia-Velasco and Gonzalez Gonzalez, 1998; Oei *et al.,* 1999; Papatsonis *et al.,* 2000).

β-ADRENERGIC RECEPTOR ANTAGONISTS

The β-adrenergic receptor antagonists are effective in reducing the severity and frequency of attacks of exertional angina and improve survival in patients who have had a myocardial infarction. In contrast, these agents are not useful for vasospastic angina and, if used in isolation, may worsen the condition (Robertson *et al.,* 1982). Most β-adrenergic receptor antagonists appear to be equally effective in the treatment of exertional angina (Thadani *et al.,* 1980). *Timolol, metoprolol, atenolol,* and *propranolol* have been shown to exert cardioprotective effects. The effectiveness of β-adrenergic receptor antagonists in the treatment of exertional angina is attributable primarily to a fall in myocardial oxygen consumption at rest and during exertion, although there also is some tendency for increased flow toward ischemic regions. The decrease in myocardial oxygen consumption is due to a negative chronotropic effect (particularly during exercise), a negative inotropic effect, and a reduction in arterial blood pressure (particularly systolic pressure) during exercise. Not all the actions of β-adrenergic receptor antagonists are beneficial in all patients. The decrease in heart rate and contractility causes an increase in the systolic ejection period and an increase in left ventricular end-diastolic volume; this tends to increase oxygen consumption. However, the net effect of β-adrenergic blockade is usually to decrease myocardial oxygen consumption, particularly during exercise. Nevertheless, in patients with limited cardiac reserve who are critically dependent on adrenergic stimulation, β-adrenergic receptor blockade can result in profound decreases in left ventricular function. Despite this, several β-adrenergic receptor antagonists have been shown to reduce mortality in patients with congestive heart failure (see Chapter 34). Numerous β-adrenergic receptor antagonists are approved for clinical use in the United States. They are considered in detail in Chapter 10.

Therapeutic Uses

Unstable Angina. β-Adrenergic receptor antagonists are effective in reducing recurrent episodes of ischemia and reduce the risk of progression to acute myocardial infarction (Braunwald et al., 2000). Currently available results of clinical trials have not had sufficient statistical power to define effects of β-adrenergic receptor antagonists on mortality. On the other hand, if the underlying pathophysiology is coronary vasospasm, nitrates and Ca^{2+} channel blockers will be effective, and β-adrenergic receptor antagonists should not be used alone. In some patients, there is a combination of severe fixed disease and superimposed vasospasm; if adequate antiplatelet therapy and vasodilation have been provided by other agents and angina continues, the addition of a β-adrenergic receptor antagonist may be helpful.

Myocardial Infarction. β-Adrenergic receptor antagonists that do not have intrinsic sympathomimetic activity have been demonstrated clearly to improve mortality in myocardial infarction. They should be given early and continued for 2 to 3 years in all patients who can tolerate them (Ryan et al., 1999).

COMPARISON OF ANTIANGINAL THERAPEUTIC STRATEGIES

In evaluating trials in which different forms of antianginal therapy are compared, careful attention must be paid to the patient population studied, including the pathophysiology and stage of the disease. It also is important to realize that an important placebo effect may be seen in these trials. The efficacy of antianginal treatment will depend on the severity of angina, on the presence of coronary vasospasm, and on the factors underlying myocardial oxygen demand. It also is most helpful if the dose of each agent is titrated to maximum benefit.

Considering the precipitants of angina in a given patient often is helpful. In patients with normal left ventricular function who have predictable angina with exertion despite nitrate therapy, β-adrenergic receptor antagonists often will be beneficial due to their effects on heart rate and blood pressure. However, in patients with impaired ventricular performance and severe coronary disease, β-adrenergic receptor blockade may lead to further elevation of end-diastolic pressure and an increase in oxygen demand. Task forces from the European Society of Cardiology (Anonymous, 1997) and both the American College of Cardiology (ACC) and the American Heart Association (AHA) (Gibbons et al., 1999) have developed current guidelines that are useful in the selection of an appropriate initial form of therapy

for patients with chronic stable angina pectoris. Table 32–3 summarizes the issues that the ACC/AHA task force considered to be relevant in choosing between β-adrenergic receptor antagonists and Ca^{2+} channel blockers in patients with angina and other medical conditions. A recent metaanalysis of publications that compared two or more antianginal therapies has been conducted by Heidenreich et al., (1999). From the comparison of β-adrenergic receptor antagonists with Ca^{2+} channel blockers (72 studies), the authors concluded that β-adrenergic receptor antagonists were associated with fewer episodes of angina per week and a lower rate of withdrawal because of adverse events. However, there were no overall differences in effects on time to ischemia during exercise, and in the rate of adverse events when Ca^{2+} channel blockers other than nifedipine were compared with β-adrenergic receptor antagonists. There were no significant differences in outcome between the studies comparing long-acting nitrates and Ca^{2+} channel blockers and the studies comparing long-acting nitrates with β-adrenergic receptor antagonists.

Combination Therapy. Since the different categories of antianginal agents utilize different mechanisms of action, it has been suggested that combinations of these agents would allow the use of lower doses, increasing effectiveness and reducing the incidence of side effects. However, despite the potential advantages, combination therapy in practice rarely fully achieves this potential and may be accompanied by serious side effects. *Nitrates and β-Adrenergic Receptor Antagonists.* The concurrent use of organic nitrates and β-adrenergic receptor antagonists can be very effective in the treatment of typical exertional angina. The additive efficacy is primarily a result of one drug blocking the adverse effects of the other agent on net myocardial oxygen consumption. β-Adrenergic receptor antagonists can block the reflex tachycardia and positive inotropic effects that are sometimes associated with nitrates. Nitrates can attenuate the increase in left ventricular end-diastolic volume associated with β-adrenergic blockade by increasing venous capacitance. Concurrent administration of nitrates also can alleviate the increase in coronary vascular resistance associated with blockade of β-adrenergic receptors.
Ca^{2+} Channel Blockers and β-Adrenergic Receptor Antagonists. When angina is not adequately controlled by nitrates and a β-adrenergic receptor antagonist, additional improvement sometimes can be achieved by the addition of a Ca^{2+} channel blocker, especially if there is a component of coronary vasospasm. If the patient already is being treated with maximal doses of verapamil or diltiazem, it is difficult to demonstrate any additional benefit of β-adrenergic blockade, and excessive bradycardia, heart block, or heart failure may ensue. However, in patients treated with a dihydropyridine, such as nifedipine, or with nitrates, there often is substantial reflex tachycardia that limits the effectiveness of these agents. A β-adrenergic receptor antagonist may be a helpful addition in this situation, resulting in a lower heart rate and blood pressure with exercise. The efficacy of amlodipine also has been shown to be improved by combination with a β-adrenergic receptor antagonist. However, in the Total Ischaemic Burden European Trial (TIBET), which compared the effects of atenolol, a sustained-release form of nifedipine, and their combination on exercise parameters and ambulatory ischemia in 608 patients with mild angina, there were no differences between the agents, either singly or in

Table 32–3
Recommended Drug Therapy for Angina in Patients with Other Medical Conditions

CONDITION	RECOMMENDED TREATMENT (AND ALTERNATIVES) FOR ANGINA	DRUGS TO AVOID
Medical Conditions		
Systemic hypertension	β-adrenergic receptor antagonists (calcium channel antagonists)	
Migraine or vascular headaches	β-adrenergic receptor antagonists (calcium channel antagonists)	
Asthma or chronic obstructive pulmonary disease with bronchospasm	Verapamil or diltiazem	β-adrenergic receptor antagonists
Hyperthyroidism	β-adrenergic receptor antagonists	
Raynaud's syndrome	Long-acting, slow-release calcium channel antagonists	β-adrenergic receptor antagonists
Insulin-dependent diabetes mellitus	β-adrenergic receptor antagonists (particularly if prior MI) or long-acting, slow-release calcium channel antagonists	
Non-insulin-dependent diabetes mellitus	β-adrenergic receptor antagonists or long-acting, slow-release calcium channel antagonists	
Depression	Long-acting, slow-release calcium channel antagonists	β-adrenergic receptor antagonists
Mild peripheral vascular disease	β-adrenergic receptor antagonists or calcium channel antagonists	
Severe peripheral vascular disease with rest ischemia	Calcium channel antagonists	β-adrenergic receptor antagonists
Cardiac Arrhythmias and Conduction Abnormalities		
Sinus bradycardia	Long-acting, slow-release calcium channel antagonists that do not decrease heart rate	β-adrenergic receptor antagonists, diltiazem, verapamil
Sinus tachycardia (not due to heart failure)	β-adrenergic receptor antagonists	
Supraventricular tachycardia	Verapamil, diltiazem, or β-adrenergic receptor antagonists	
Atrioventricular block	Long-acting, slow-release calcium channel antagonists that do not slow A-V conduction	β-adrenergic receptor antagonists, verapamil, diltiazem
Rapid atrial fibrillation (with digitalis)	Verapamil, diltiazem, or β-adrenergic receptor antagonists	
Ventricular arrhythmias	β-adrenergic receptor antagonists	
Left Ventricular Dysfunction		
Congestive heart failure		
Mild (LVEF ≥ 40%)	β-adrenergic receptor antagonists	
Moderate to severe (LVEF < 40%)	Amlodipine or felodipine (nitrates)	Verapamil, diltiazem
Left-sided valvular heart disease		
Mild aortic stenosis	β-adrenergic receptor antagonists	
Aortic insufficiency	Long-acting, slow-release dihydropyridines	
Mitral regurgitation	Long-acting, slow-release dihydropyridines	
Mitral stenosis	β-adrenergic receptor antagonists	
Hypertrophic cardiomyopathy	β-adrenergic receptor antagonists, non-dihydropyridine calcium channel antagonists	Nitrates, dihydropyridine calcium channel antagonists

SOURCE: Modified from Gibbons *et al.*, 1999. MI = myocardial infarction; LVEF = left ventricular ejection fraction.

combination, on any of the measured ischemic parameters (Fox *et al.*, 1996). On the other hand, in two studies of patients with more severe but still stable angina, atenolol and propranolol were shown to be superior to nifedipine, and the combination of propranolol and nifedipine was more effective than nifedipine alone (Fox *et al.*, 1993). In the IMAGE trial, the combination of metoprolol and sustained–release nifedipine was compared to each agent alone (Savonitto *et al.*, 1996). Although an additional effect was observed in the group of patients receiving combination therapy, this was the result of an increase in exercise tolerance in individual patients who had not exhibited an increase during monotherapy; this recruitment effect was more marked in the patients in whom metoprolol was added to nifedipine.

Fluctuations in coronary tone long have been recognized as primary in variant angina. It also is likely that increased tone superimposed on fixed disease plays a role in the variable anginal threshold seen in many patients with otherwise chronic stable angina and possibly in ischemic episodes precipitated by cold and by emotion (Zeiher *et al.*, 1991). Increased coronary tone also may be important in the anginal episodes occurring early after myocardial infarction (Bertrand *et al.*, 1982) and after coronary angioplasty, and it probably accounts for those patients with unstable angina who respond to dihydropyridines (Hugenholtz *et al.*, 1981). Atherosclerotic arteries have abnormal vasomotor responses to a number of stimuli (Kaplinsky, 1992; Oemar *et al.*, 1998), including exercise, other forms of sympathetic activation, and cholinergic agonists; in such vessels, stenotic segments actually may become more severely stenosed during exertion. This implies that the normal exercise-induced increase in coronary flow is lost in atherosclerosis. Similar exaggerated vascular contractile responses are seen in hyperlipidemia, even before anatomic evidence of atherosclerosis develops. Because of this, coronary vasodilators (nitrates and/or Ca^{2+} channel blockers) are an important part of the therapeutic program in the majority of patients with ischemic heart disease.

Ca^{2+} Channel Blockers and Nitrates. In severe exertional or vasospastic angina, the combination of a nitrate and a Ca^{2+} channel blocker may provide additional relief over that obtained with either type of agent alone. Since nitrates primarily reduce preload, whereas Ca^{2+} channel blockers reduce afterload, the net effect on reduction of oxygen demand should be additive. However, excessive vasodilation and hypotension can occur. The concurrent administration of a nitrate and nifedipine has been advocated in particular for patients with exertional angina with heart failure, the sick-sinus syndrome, or AV nodal conduction disturbances, but excessive tachycardia may be seen.

Ca^{2+} Channel Blockers, β-Adrenergic Receptor Antagonists, and Nitrates. In patients with exertional angina that is not controlled by the administration of two types of antianginal agents, the use of all three may provide improvement, although the incidence of side effects increases significantly (Tolins *et al.*, 1984; Asirvatham *et al.*, 1998). The dihydropyridines and nitrates dilate epicardial coronary arteries; the dihydropyridines decrease afterload; the nitrates decrease preload; and the β-adrenergic receptor antagonists decrease heart rate and myocardial contractility. Therefore, there is theoretical, and sometimes real, benefit with their combination. Combining verapamil or diltiazem with a β-adrenergic receptor antagonist greatly increases the risk of conduction system and left ventricular dysfunction-related side effects, and should be undertaken only with extreme caution and only if no other alternatives exist.

ANTIPLATELET AND ANTITHROMBOTIC AGENTS

Unlike other antianginal agents, aspirin clearly has been demonstrated to reduce mortality in patients with unstable angina, reducing the incidence of myocardial infarction and death. In addition, low doses of aspirin appear to reduce the incidence of myocardial infarction in patients with chronic stable angina, and aspirin, given in doses of 160 to 325 mg at the onset of treatment of myocardial infarction, clearly reduces mortality, presumably by inhibiting the increased platelet aggregation that accompanies thrombolytic therapy (Kerins and FitzGerald, 1991). *Heparin,* in its unfractionated form and as low-molecular-weight heparin, also has been shown to reduce angina and prevent infarction in unstable angina. More direct thrombin inhibitors, such as *hirudin,* which directly inhibit even clot-bound thrombin, are not affected by circulating inhibitors, and function independently of antithrombin III, are being investigated. A metaanalysis of the GUSTO-IIB, TIMI-9B, OASIS-1, and OASIS-2 trials showed that in patients with acute myocardial ischemia without ST segment elevation there was a modest reduction in the risk of death or myocardial infarction at 35 days when hirudin was compared with unfractionated heparin, but an increase in bleeding, with the majority of the benefit occurring in patients not receiving thrombolytic agents (OASIS-2 Investigators, 1999). Further studies seem warranted. Thrombolytic agents, on the other hand, have been shown to be of no benefit in unstable angina (Anonymous, 1992). Intravenous inhibitors of the platelet glycoprotein IIb/IIIa receptor (*abciximab, tirofiban,* and *eptifibatide*) have proven to be effective in preventing the complications of percutaneous coronary interventions and in the treatment of patients presenting with acute coronary syndromes (Bhatt and Topol, 2000). In contrast, orally active platelet glycoprotein IIb/IIIa antagonists have not proven to be effective in the chronic treatment of patients with ischemic heart disease and may result in worse outcomes. It is possible that there are subsets of patients with unstable angina who have different response profiles.

PROSPECTUS

It is anticipated that new therapeutic agents in ischemic heart disease will fall into two categories. The first will include agents that modify cellular actions *via* cell surface or intracellular receptors but have no effect on gene expression. The second will include agents that either permanently or transiently alter gene expression, either by enhancing or inhibiting the production of a normal cell product, or by rendering the cell capable of producing an entirely new product. This *gene-based therapy* (*see* Chapter 5) will assume increasing importance in the treatment of ischemic heart disease.

Emerging agents in the nitrate category include *molsidomine*, a nitrate-like agent that appears to produce vascular smooth muscle relaxation utilizing mechanisms similar to those of the nitrates themselves.

A number of Ca^{2+} channel antagonists are under development in the classes of dihydropyridines (*nitrendipine*), phenylalkylamines (*gallopamil*, a verapamil derivative), and piperazines (*flunarizine,* which is marketed in some countries outside the United States, *trimetazidine,* and *ranolazine*). Whereas the first two agents share the general pharmacological characteristics of their classes, the piperazines exhibit some cytoprotective effects on myocardial energy metabolism and, in early studies, appear to exert an antianginal effect in the absence of significant hemodynamic effects. Although the first agent to block the T-type Ca^{2+} channel was withdrawn due to adverse drug interactions, the antianginal efficacy of this agent supports the future development of other members of this class.

K^+ channel activators, such as *cromakalim, pinacidil,* and *nicorandil,* have been proposed for use as direct coronary vasodilators in the treatment of both vasospastic and chronic stable angina (Hamilton and Weston, 1989; Why and Richardson, 1993; Lablanche *et al.,* 1993). Studies of *nicorandil* (Kukovetz *et al.,* 1992) demonstrate that its relaxant effect on coronary arterioles is inhibited by the K^+ channel blocker, glyburide, and thus is likely due to K^+ channel activation, with attendant cellular hyperpolarization of vascular smooth muscle. However, this agent also exerts a nitrate-like effect, stimulating guanylyl cyclase to increase cyclic GMP, primarily in epicardial coronary arteries, including stenotic segments. The relative importance of these separate effects in human beings is not known. In studies of relatively small sample size, nicorandil had antianginal efficacy similar to that of nitrates; the β-adrenergic receptor antagonists atenolol, metoprolol, and propranolol; and the Ca^{2+} channel blockers amlodipine, diltiazem, and nifedipine (Markham *et al.,* 2000). Drugs that have their primary site of vasodilation at the arteriolar level generally are not of benefit in the treatment of angina (Anonymous, 1992). The efficacy of nicorandil may be primarily due to its nitrate-like effect.

Angiotensin converting enzyme (ACE) inhibitors (*see* Chapters 31, 33, and 34) are useful not only in the treatment of hypertension but also in reducing morbidity and mortality in symptomatic and asymptomatic congestive heart failure (Cohn *et al.,* 1986; CONSENSUS Trial Study Group, 1987; Pitt, 1994). It also has been suggested that

these agents may have a beneficial effect in angina pectoris over and above their effects on blood pressure, but it has been difficult to demonstrate this effect in normotensive patients. In addition to the ability of these agents to reduce blood pressure, which would be expected to have a favorable effect on ventricular wall stress, they also may reduce the coronary vascular response to angiotensin II and may prevent deleterious ventricular remodeling. Lisinopril has been suggested to reduce mortality when used in the treatment of acute infarction in the GISSI-III trial. However, if coronary perfusion pressure is lowered, ACE inhibitors have the potential to have a deleterious effect on angina; this may account for the patients who have become worse with these drugs in some trials (Vogt *et al.,* 1993). In the HOPE trial, the ACE inhibitor *rampiril* resulted in a reduction in myocardial infarction and death from cardiovascular causes in patients with vascular disease or with diabetes plus one other cardiovascular risk factor, but without conventional indications for the use of an ACE inhibitor (Yusuf *et al.,* 2000).

Our appreciation of the role of inflammation in the development and progression of atherosclerosis and of unstable coronary syndromes is evolving (Libby, 2000; Ridker *et al.,* 2000). Clinical studies are in progress that will address the ability of *antibiotics, antiinflammatory agents,* and *HMG-CoA reductase inhibitors* to retard the atherosclerotic process and reduce cardiac events.

There has been great interest in evaluating the therapeutic utility of angiogenic factors, stem cells, and endothelial progenitor cells to facilitate growth of new vessels in areas of ischemia (Asahara *et al.,* 2000; Isner, 2000; Kalka *et al.,* 2000). Promising results have been achieved using *vascular endothelial growth factor (VEGF)* and related agents in human patients (Schumacher *et al.,* 1998; Hendel *et al.,* 2000).

Several problems in the treatment of myocardial ischemia lend themselves to the use of *gene-based therapies.* Because coronary angioplasty is so commonly followed by restenosis (30% to 40% of cases) and because conventional pharmacological therapy has not abolished this problem, the concept of altering the biology of the cellular response to angioplasty has emerged. Techniques for delivering vectors to localized segments of peripheral and coronary vessels and vein grafts have been developed, and functional genes have been transferred (Chapman *et al.,* 1992; Lemarchand *et al.,* 1993; Nabel, 1995; Duckers and Nabel, 2000; O'Blenes *et al.,* 2000). In animal models, the tendency for restenosis has been significantly inhibited (Ohno *et al.,* 1994), and clinical trials are planned. Building on the success with angiogenic factors mentioned above, studies with animals have demonstrated that transferring the gene coding for VEGF also is efficacious (Isner, 2000), and trials in human beings are under way. In an attack on one mechanism underlying the development of atherosclerosis, it recently has been shown that retroviral therapy restores apo-E levels in apo-E deficient mice and reduces the extent of atherosclerosis (Hasty *et al.*, 1999). Alternatively, disruption of the 12/15-lipoxygenase gene also was protective in this mouse model, consistent with a role for inflammation in the atherosclerotic process (Cyrus *et al.*, 1999). These areas of rapid progress suggest that therapy with genotypic strategies will play a significant role in the future.

For further discussion of acute myocardial infarction and ischemic heart disease *see* Chapters 243 and 244 in *Harrison's Principles of Internal Medicine*, 14th ed., McGraw-Hill, New York, 1998.

BIBLIOGRAPHY

Amende, I., Simon, R., Hood, W.P. Jr., Hetzer, R., and Lichtlen, P.R. Intracoronary nifedipine in human beings: magnitude and time course of changes in left ventricular contraction/relaxation and coronary sinus blood flow. *J. Am. Coll. Cardiol.*, **1983**, *2*:1141–1145.

Anonymous. Optimizing antianginal therapy: consensus guidelines. *Am. J. Cardiol.*, **1992**, *70*:72G–76G.

Anonymous. Management of stable angina pectoris. Recommendations of the Task Force of the European Society of Cardiology. *Eur. Heart. J.*, **1997**, *18*:394–413.

Antman, E., Muller, J., Goldberg, S., MacAlpin, R., Reubenfire, M., Tabatznik, B., Liang, C.S., Heupler, F., Achuff, S., Reichek, N., Geltman, E., Kerin N.Z., Neff, R.K., and Braunwald, E. Nifedipine therapy for coronary-artery spasm. Experience in 127 patients. *N. Engl. J. Med.*, **1980**, *302*:1269–1273.

Bassan, M., Weiler-Raveil, D., and Shalev, O. The additive antianginal action of oral nifedipine in patients receiving propranolol: magnitude and duration of effect. *Circulation*, **1982**, *66*:710–716.

Bauer, J.A., and Fung, H.L. Arterial versus venous metabolism of nitroglycerin to nitric oxide: a possible explanation of organic nitrate venoselectivity. *J. Cardiovasc. Pharmacol.*, **1996**, *28*:371–374.

Bertrand, M.E., LaBlanche, J.M., Tilmant, P.Y., Thieuleux, F.A., Delforge, M.R., Carre, A.G., Asseman, P., Berzin, B., Libersa, C., and Laurent, J.M. Frequency of provoked coronary arterial spasm in 1089 consecutive patients undergoing coronary arteriography. *Circulation*, **1982**, *65*:1299–1306.

Bevan, J.A., Bevan, R.D., Huo, J.J., Owen, M.P., Tayo, F.M., and Winquist, R.J. Calcium, extrinsic and intrinsic (myogenic) vascular tone. In, *International Symposium on Calcium Modulators*. (Godfraind, T., Albertini, A., and Paoletti, R., eds.) Elsevier Biomedical Press, Amsterdam, **1982**, pp. 125–132.

Bonow, R.O., Leon, M.B., Rosing, D.R., Kent, K.M., Lipson, L.C., Bacharach, S.L., Green, M.V., and Epstein, S.E. Effects of verapamil and propranolol on left ventricular systolic function and diastolic filling in patients with coronary artery disease: radionuclide angiographic studies at rest and during exercise. *Circulation*, **1982**, *65*:1337–1350.

Boolell, M., Gepi-Attee, S., Gingell, J.C., and Allen, M.J. Sildenafil, a novel effective oral therapy for male erectile dysfunction. *Br. J. Urol.*, **1996**, *78*:257–261.

Braun, S., van der Wall, E.E., Emanuelsson, H., and Kobrin, I. Effects of a new calcium antagonist, mibefradil (Ro 40-5967), on silent ischemia in patients with stable chronic angina pectoris: a multicenter placebo-controlled trial. The Mibefradil International Study Group. *J. Am. Coll. Cardiol.*, **1996**, *27*:317–322.

Breisblatt, W.M., Vita, N.A., Armuchastegui, M., Cohen, L.S., and Zaret, B.L. Usefulness of serial radionuclide monitoring during graded nitroglycerin infusion for unstable angina pectoris for determining left ventricular function and individualized therapeutic dose. *Am. J. Cardiol.*, **1988**, *61*:685–690.

Brown, B.G., Bolson, E., Petersen, R.B., Pierce, C.D., and Dodge, H.T. The mechanism of nitroglycerin action: stenosis vasodilatation as a major component of the drug response. *Circulation*, **1981**, *64*:1089–1097.

Brutsaert, D.L., Sys, S.U., and Gillebert, T.C. Diastolic failure: pathophysiology and therapeutic implications. *J. Am. Coll. Cardiol.*, **1993**, *22*:318–325.

Burnett, A.L., Lowenstein, C.J., Bredt, D.S., Chang, T.S., and Snyder, S.H. Nitric oxide: a physiologic mediator of penile erection. *Science*, **1992**, *257*:401–403.

Chapman, G.D., Lim, C.S., Gammon, R.S., Culp, S.C., Desper, J.S., Bauman, R.P., Swain, J.L., and Stack, R.S. Gene transfer into coronary arteries of intact animals with a percutaneous balloon catheter. *Circ. Res.*, **1992**, *71*:27–33.

Cohn, J.N., Archibald, D.G., Ziesche, S., Franciosa, J.A., Harston, W.E., Tristani, F.E., Dunkman, W.B., Jacobs, W., Francis, G.S., Flohr, K.H., Goldman, S., Cobb, F.R., Shah, P.M., Saunders, R., Fletcher, R.D., Loeb, H.S., Hughes, V.C., and Baker, B. Effect of vasodilator therapy on mortality in chronic congestive heart failure. Results of a Veterans Administration Cooperative Study. *N. Engl. J. Med.*, **1986**, *314*:1547–1552.

CONSENSUS Trial Study Group. Effects of enalapril on mortality in severe congestive heart failure. Results of the Cooperative North Scandinavian Enalapril Survival Study (CONSENSUS). *N. Engl. J. Med.*, **1987**, *316*:1429–1435.

Cyrus, T., Witztum, J.L, Rader, D.J., Tangirala, R., Fazio, S., Linton, M.F., and Funk, C.D. Disruption of the 12/15-lipoxygenase gene diminishes atherosclerosis in apo E-deficient mice. *J. Clin. Invest.*, **1999**, *103*:1597–1604.

Dakak, N., Makhoul, N., Flugelman, M.Y., Merdler, A., Shehadeh, H., Schneeweiss, A., Halon, D.A., and Lewis, B.S. Failure of captopril to prevent nitrate tolerance in congestive heart failure secondary to coronary artery disease. *Am. J. Cardiol.*, **1990**, *66*:608–613.

De Caterina, R., Giannessi, D., Mazzone, A., and Bernini, W. Mechanisms for the in vivo antiplatelet effects of isosorbide dinitrate. *Eur. Heart. J.,* **1988,** *9(suppl. A)*:45–49.

Deedwania, P.C., and Carbajal, E.V. Role of beta blockade in the treatment of myocardial ischemia. *Am. J. Cardiol.,* **1997,** *80*:23J–28J.

DEFIANT-II Research Group. Doppler flow and echocardiography in functional cardiac insufficiency: assessment of nisoldipine therapy. Results of the DEFIANT-II Study. *Eur. Heart J.,* **1997,** *18*:31–40.

DeMots, H., and Glasser, S.P. Intermittent transdermal nitroglycerin therapy in the treatment of chronic stable angina. *J. Am. Coll. Cardiol.,* **1989,** *13*:786–795.

DeWood, M.A., and Wolbach, R.A. Randomized double-blind comparison of side effects of nicardipine and nifedipine in angina pectoris. The Nicardipine Investigators Group. *Am. Heart J.,* **1990,** *119*:468–478.

Ducharme, A., Dupuis, J., McNicoll, S., Harel, F., and Tardif, J.C. Comparison of nitroglycerin lingual spray and sublingual tablet on time of onset and duration of brachial artery vasodilation in normal subjects. *Am. J. Cardiol.,* **1999,** *84*:952–954.

Egstrup, K., and Andersen, P.E., Jr. Transient myocardial ischemia during nifedipine therapy in stable angina pectoris, and its relation to coronary collateral flow and comparison with metoprolol. *Am. J. Cardiol.,* **1993,** *71*:177–183.

Elkayam, U., Canetti, M., Wani, O.R., Karaalp, I.S., and Tummala, P.P. Hydralazine-induced prevention of nitrate tolerance: experimental and clinical evidence and potential mechanisms. *Am. J. Cardiol.,* **1998,** *81*:44A–48A.

Evidence Report/Technology Assessment: Number 18. Management of preterm labor. Summary. AHRQ Publication No. 01-E020, October, 2000. Agency for Healthcare Research and Quality, Rockville, MD. Available at: http://www.ahrq.gov/clinic/pretermsum.htm. Accessed January 24, 2001.

Feldman, H.A., Goldstein, I., Hatzichristou, D.G., Krane, R.J., and McKinlay, J.B. Impotence and its medical and psychological correlates: results of the Massachusetts Male Aging Study. *J. Urol.,* **1994,** *151*:54–61.

Feldman, R.L., Pepine, C.J., and Conti, C.R. Magnitude of dilatation of large and small coronary arteries of nitroglycerin. *Circulation,* **1981,** *64*:324–333.

Fox, D.M., Mulcahy, D., Findlay, I., Ford, I., and Dargie, H.J. The Total Ischaemic Burden European Trial (TIBET). Effects of atenolol, nifedipine SR and their combination on the exercise test and the total ischaemic burden in 608 patients with stable angina. The TIBET Study Group. *Eur. Heart J.,* **1996,** *17*:96–103.

Furberg, C.D., Psaty, B.M., and Meyer, J.V. Nifedipine. Dose-related increase in mortality in patients with coronary heart disease. *Circulation,* **1995,** *92*:1326–1331.

Furchgott, R.F. The 1996 Albert Lasker Medical Research Awards. The discovery of endothelium-derived relaxing factor and its importance in the identification of nitric oxide. *JAMA,* **1996,** *276*:1186–1188.

Ganz, W., and Marcus, H.S. Failure of intracoronary nitroglycerin to alleviate pacing-induced angina. *Circulation,* **1972,** *46*:880–889.

Garcia-Velasco, J.A., and Gonzalez Gonzalez, A. A prospective, randomized trial of nifedipine vs. ritodrine in threatened preterm labor. *Int. J. Gynaecol. Obstet.,* **1998,** *61*:239–244.

Geelen, P., Drolet, B., Rail, J., Berube, J., Daleau, P., Rousseau, G., Cardinal, R., O'Hara, G.E., and Turgeon, J. Sildenafil (Viagra) prolongs cardiac repolarization by blocking the rapid component of the delayed rectifier potassium current. *Circulation,* **2000,** *102*:275–277.

Göbel, E.J., Hautvast, R.W., van Gilst, W.H., Spanjaard, J.N., Hillege, H.L., DeJongste, M.J.L., Molhoek, G.P., and Lie, K.I. Randomised, double-blind trial of intravenous diltiazem versus glyceryl trinitrate for unstable angina pectoris. *Lancet,* **1995,** *346*:1653–1657.

Godfraind, T., and Kaba, A. The role of calcium in the action of drugs on vascular smooth muscle. *Arch. Int. Pharmacodyn. Ther.,* **1972,** *196*(suppl.):35–49.

Godfraind, T., Salomone, S., Dessy, C., Verhelst, B., Dion, R., and Schoevaerts, J.C. Selectivity scale of calcium antagonists in the human cardiovascular system based on in vitro studies. *J. Cardiovasc. Pharmacol.,* **1992,** *20*(suppl. 5):S34–S41.

Goldstein, I., Lue, T.F., Padma-Nathan, H., Rosen, R.C., Steers, W.D., and Wicker, P.A. Oral sildenafil in the treatment of erectile dysfunction. Sildenafil Study Group. *N. Engl. J. Med.,* **1998,** *338*:1397–1404.

Goldstein, R.E., Stinson, E.B., Scherer, J.L., Seningen, R.P., Grehl, T.M., and Epstein, S.E. Intraoperative coronary collateral function in patients with coronary occlusive disease. Nitroglycerin responsiveness and angiographic correlations. *Circulation,* **1974,** *49*:298–308.

Gorlin, R., Brachfield, N., MacLeod, C., and Bopp, P. Effect of nitroglycerin on the coronary circulation in patients with coronary disease or increased left ventricular work. *Circulation,* **1959,** *19*:705–718.

Hall, M.C., and Ahmad, S. Interaction between sildenafil and HIV-1 combination therapy. *Lancet,* **1999,** *353*:2071–2072.

Hanet, C., Rousseau, M.F., van Eyll, C., and Pouleur, H. Effects of nicardipine on regional diastolic left ventricular function in patients with angina pectoris. *Circulation,* **1990,** *81*:III48–III54.

Hasty, A.H., Linton, M.F., Brandt, S.J., Babaev, V.R., Gleaves, L.A., and Fazio, S. Retroviral gene therapy in ApoE-deficient mice: ApoE expression in the artery wall reduces early foam cell lesion formation. *Circulation,* **1999,** *99*:2571–2576.

Heidenreich, P.A., McDonald, K.M., Hastie, T., Fadel, B., Hagan, V., Lee, B.K., and Hlatky, M.A. Meta-analysis of trials comparing beta-blockers, calcium antagonists, and nitrates for stable angina. *JAMA,* **1999,** *281*:1927–1936.

Heitzer, T., Just, H., Brockhoff, C., Meinertz, T., Olschewski, M., and Munzel, T. Long-term nitroglycerin treatment is associated with supersensitivity to vasoconstrictors in men with stable coronary artery disease: prevention by concomitant treatment with captopril. *J. Am. Coll. Cardiol.,* **1998,** *31*:83–88.

Hendel, R.C., Henry, T.D., Rocha-Singh, K., Isner, J.M., Kereiakes, D.J., Giordano, F.J., Simons, M., and Bonow, R.O. Effect of intracoronary recombinant human vascular endothelial growth factor on myocardial perfusion: evidence for a dose-dependent effect. *Circulation,* **2000,** *101*:118–121.

Herrmann, H.C., Chang, G., Klugherz, B.D., and Mahoney, P.D. Hemodynamic effects of sildenafil in men with severe coronary artery disease. *N. Engl. J. Med.,* **2000,** *342*:1622–1626.

Hines, S., Houston, M., and Robertson, D. The clinical spectrum of autonomic dysfunction. *Am. J. Med.,* **1981,** *70*:1091–1096.

Horwitz, L.D., Gorlin, R., Taylor, W.J., and Kemp, H.G. Effects of nitroglycerin on regional myocardial blood flow in coronary artery disease. *J. Clin. Invest.,* **1971,** *50*:1578–1584.

Hugenholtz, P.G., Michels, H.R., Serruys, P.W., and Brower, R.W. Nifedipine in the treatment of unstable angina, coronary spasm and myocardial ischemia. *Am. J. Cardiol.,* **1981,** *47*:163–173.

ISIS-4 Collaborative Group. ISIS-4: a randomised factorial trial assessing early oral captopril, oral mononitrate, and intravenous magnesium sulphate in 58,050 patients with suspected acute myocardial infarction. *Lancet,* **1995,** *345*:669–685.

Johannes, C.B., Araujo, A.B., Feldman, H.A., Derby, C.A., Kleinman, K.P., and McKinlay, J.B. Incidence of erectile dysfunction in men

40 to 69 years old: longitudinal results from the Massachusetts male aging study. *J. Urol.*, **2000**, *163*:460–463.

Kalka, C.V., Masuda, H., Takahashi, T., Gordon, R., Tepper, O., Gravereaux, E., Pieczek, A., Iwaguro, H., Hayahashi, S.I., Isner, J.M., and Ashahara, T. Vascular endothelial growth factor (165) gene transfer augments circulating endothelial progenitor cells in human subjects. *Circ. Res.*, **2000**, *86*:1198–1202.

Kim, N., Azadzoi, K.M., Goldstein, I., and Saenz de Tejada, I. A nitric oxide-like factor mediates nonadrenergic-noncholinergic neurogenic relaxation of penile corpus cavernosum smooth muscle. *J. Clin. Invest.*, **1991**, *88*:112–118.

Kloner, R.A. Nifedipine in ischemic heart disease. *Circulation*, **1995**, *92*:1074–1078.

Kohlhardt, M., and Fleckenstein, A. Inhibition of the slow inward current by nifedipine in mammalian ventricular myocardium. *Naunyn Schmiedebergs Arch. Pharmacol.*, **1977**, *298*:267–272.

Koks, C.A., Brolmann, H.A., de Kleine, M.J., and Manger, P.A. A randomized comparison of nifedipine and ritodrine for suppression of preterm labor. *Eur. J. Obstet. Gynecol. Reprod. Biol.*, **1998**, *77*:171–176.

Kukovetz, W.R., Holzmann, S., and Poch, G. Molecular mechanism of action of nicorandil. *J. Cardiovasc. Pharmacol.*, **1992**, *20*(suppl. 3):S1–S7.

Lacoste, L.L., Theroux, P., Lidon, R.M., Colucci, R., and Lam, J.Y. Antithrombotic properties of transdermal nitroglycerin in stable angina pectoris. *Am. J. Cardiol.*, **1994**, *73*:1058–1062.

Lam, Y.T., Chesebro, J.H, and Fuster, V. Platelets, vasoconstriction, and nitroglycerin during arterial wall injury. A new antithrombotic role for an old drug. *Circulation*, **1988**, *78*:712–716.

Lehmann, G., Reiniger, G., Beyerle, A., and Rudolph, W. Pharmacokinetics and additional anti-ischaemic effectiveness of amlodipine, a once-daily calcium antagonist, during acute and long-term therapy of stable angina pectoris in patients pre-treated with a beta-blocker. *Eur. Heart J.*, **1993**, *14*:1531–1535.

Lemarchand, P., Jones, M., Yamada, I., and Crystal, R.G. In vivo gene transfer and expression in normal uninjured blood vessels using replication-deficient recombinant adenovirus vectors. *Circ. Res.*, **1993**, *72*:1132–1138.

MIAMI Trial Research Group. Metoprolol in acute myocardial infarction (MIAMI). A randomised placebo-controlled international trial. *Eur. Heart J.*, **1985**, *6*:199–226.

Mishra, S.K., and Hermsmeyer, K. Selective inhibition of the T-type Ca^{2+} channels by Ro 40-5967. *Circ. Res.*, **1994**, *75*:144–148.

Molina, C., Andresen, J.W., Rapoport, R.M., Waldman, S.A., and Murad, F. Effects of in vivo nitroglycerin therapy on endothelium-dependent and independent vascular relaxation and cyclic GMP accumulation in rat aorta. *J. Cardiovasc. Pharmacol.*, **1987**, *10*:371–378.

Morton, W.E. Occupational habituation to aliphatic nitrates and the withdrawal hazards of coronary artery disease and hypertension. *J. Occup. Med.*, **1977**, *19*:197–200.

Muisan, M.L., Boni, E., Castellano, M., Beschi, M., Cefis, G., Cerri, B., Verdecchia, P., Porcellati, C., Pollavini, G., and Agabiti-Rosei, E. Effects of transdermal nitroglycerin in combination with an ACE inhibitor in patients with chronic stable angina pectoris. *Eur. Heart J.*, **1993**, *14*:1701–1708.

Muller, J.E., Morrison, J., Stone, P.H., Rude, R.E., Rosner, B., Roberts, R., Pearle, D.L., Turi, Z.G., Schneider, J.F., Serfas, D.H., Tate, C., Shceiner, E., Sobel, B.E., Hennekens, C.H., and Braunwald, E. Nifedipine therapy for patients with threatened and acute myocardial infarction: a randomized, double-blind, placebo-controlled comparison. *Circulation*, **1984**, *69*:740–747.

Multicenter Study. Unstable angina pectoris: National Cooperative Study Group to Compare Surgical and Medical Therapy. II. In-hospital experience and initial follow-up results in patients with one, two, and three vessel disease. *Am. J. Cardiol.*, **1978**, *42*:839–848.

Münzel, T., Giaid, A., Kurz, S., Stewart, D.J., and Harrison, D.G. Evidence for a role of endothelin 1 and protein kinase C in nitroglycerin tolerance. *Proc. Natl. Acad. Sci. U.S.A.*, **1995a**, *92*:5244–5248.

Münzel, T., Sayegh, H., Freeman, B.A., Tarpey, M.M., and Harrison, D.G. Evidence for enhanced vascular superoxide anion production in nitrate tolerance. A novel mechanism underlying tolerance and cross-tolerance. *J. Clin. Invest.*, **1995b**, *95*:187–194.

Murray, C., Haverkamp, A.D., Orleans, M., Berga, S., and Pecht, D. Nifedipine for treatment of preterm labor: a historic prospective study. *Am. J. Obstet. Gynecol.*, **1992**, *167*:52–56.

Murrell, W. Nitroglycerin as a remedy for angina pectoris. *Lancet*, **1879**, *1*:80–81.

Nishimura, R.A., Schwartz, R.S., Holmes, D.R., Jr., and Tajik, A.J. Failure of calcium channel blockers to improve ventricular relaxation in humans. *J. Am. Coll. Cardiol.*, **1993**, *21*:182–188.

OASIS-2 Investigators. Effects of recombinant hirudin (lepirudin) compared with heparin on death, myocardial infarction, refractory angina, and revascularisation procedures in patients with acute myocardial ischaemia without ST elevation: a randomised trial. Organisation to Assess Strategies for Ischemic Syndromes (OASIS-2) Investigators. *Lancet*, **1999**, *353*:429–438.

O'Blenes, S.B., Zaidi, S.H., Cheah, A.Y., McIntyre, B., Kaneda, Y., and Rabinovitch, M. Gene transfer of the serine elastase inhibitor elafin protects against vein graft degeneration. *Circulation*, **2000**, *102*:III289–III295.

Oei, S.G., Mol, B.W., de Kleine, M.J., and Brolmann, H.A. Nifedipine versus ritodrine for suppression of preterm labor; a meta-analysis. *Acta Obstet. Gynecol. Scand.*, **1999**, *78*:783–788.

Oemar, B.S., Tschudi, M.R., Godoy, N., Brovkovich, V., Malinski, T., and Lüscher, T.F. Reduced endothelial nitric oxide synthase expression and production in human atherosclerosis. *Circulation*, **1998**, *97*:2494–2498.

Ohno, T., Gordon, D., San, H., Pompili, V.J., Imperiale, M.J., Nabel, G.J., and Nabel, E.G. Gene therapy for vascular smooth muscle cell proliferation after arterial injury. *Science*, **1994**, *265*:781–784.

Opie, L.H., and Messerli, F.H. Nifedipine and mortality. Grave defects in the dossier. *Circulation*, **1995**, *92*:1068–1073.

Opie, L.H., Yusuf, S., and Kübler, W. Current status of safety and efficacy of calcium channel blockers in cardiovascular disease: a critical analysis based on 100 studies. *Prog. Cardiovasc. Dis.*, **2000**, *43*:171–196.

Pahor, M., Guralnik, J.M., Corti, M.C., Foley, D.J., Carbonin, P., and Havlik, R.J. Long-term survival and use of antihypertensive medications in older persons. *J. Am. Geriatr. Soc.*, **1995**, *44*:1191–1197.

Papatsonis, D.N., Kok, J.H., van Geijn, H.P., Blecker, O.P., Ader, H.J., and Dekker, G.A. Neonatal effects of nifedipine and ritodrine for preterm labor. *Obstet. Gynecol.*, **2000**, *95*:477–481.

Parker, J.D., Farrell, B., Fenton, T., Cohanim, M., and Parker, J.O. Counter-regulatory responses to continuous and intermittent therapy with nitroglycerin. *Circulation*, **1991**, *84*:2336–2345.

Parker, J.D., and Parker, J.O. Effects of therapy with an angiotensin-converting enzyme inhibitor on hemodynamic and counterregulatory responses during continuous therapy with nitroglycerin. *J. Am. Coll. Cardiol.*, **1993**, *21*:1445–1453.

Parker, J.D., Parker, A.B., Farrell, B., and Parker, J.O. Intermittent transdermal nitroglycerin therapy. Decreased anginal threshold during the nitrate-free interval. *Circulation*, **1995**, *91*:973–978.

Parker, J.D., Parker, A.B., Farrell, B., and Parker, J.O. Effects of diuretic therapy on the development of tolerance to nitroglycerin and exercise capacity in patients with chronic stable angina. *Circulation,* **1996,** *93*:691–696.

Parker, J.O. Eccentric dosing with isosorbide-5-mononitrate in angina pectoris. *Am. J. Cardiol.,* **1993,** *72*:871–876.

Parker, J.O., Farrell, B., Lahey, K.A., and Moe, G. Effect of intervals between doses on the development of tolerance to isosorbide dinitrate. *N. Engl. J. Med.,* **1987,** *316*:1440–1444.

Paulus, W.J., Lorell, B.H., Craig, W.E., Wynne, J., Murgo, J.P., and Grossman, W. Comparison of the effects of nitroprusside and nifedipine on diastolic properties in patients with hypertrophic cardiomyopathy: altered left ventricular loading or improved muscle inactivation? *J. Am. Coll. Cardiol.,* **1983,** *2*:879–886.

Pepine, C.J., and Lambert, C.R. Effects of nicardipine on coronary blood flow. *Am. Heart J.,* **1988,** *116*:248–254.

Pizzulli, L., Hagendorff, A., Zirbes, M., Fehske, W., Ewig, S., Jung, W., and Lüderitz, B. Influence of captopril on nitroglycerin-mediated vasodilation and development of nitrate tolerance in arterial and venous circulation. *Am. Heart. J.,* **1996,** *131*:342–349.

Psaty, B.M., Heckbert, S.R., Koepsell, T.D., Siscovick, D.S., Ragunathan, D.S., Weiss, T.E., Rosendaal, F.R., Lemaitre, R.N., Smith, N.L., Wahl, P.W., Wagner, E.H., and Furberg, C.D. The risk of myocardial infarction associated with antihypertensive drug therapies. *JAMA,* **1995,** *274*:620–625.

Rajfer, J., Aronson, W.J., Bush, P.A., Dorey, F.J., and Ignarro, L.J. Nitric oxide as a mediator of relaxation of the corpus cavernosum in response to nonadrenergic, noncholinergic neurotransmission. *N. Engl. J. Med.,* **1992,** *326*:90–94.

Ridker, P.M., Hennekens, C.H., Buring, J.E., and Rifai, N. C-reactive protein and other markers of inflammation in the prediction of cardiovascular disease in women. *N. Engl. J. Med.,* **2000,** *342*:836–843.

Robertson, D., Robertson, R.M., Nies, A.S., Oates, J.A., and Friesinger, G.C. Variant angina pectoris: investigation of indexes of sympathetic nervous system function. *Am. J. Cardiol.,* **1979,** *43*:1080–1085.

Robertson, D., and Stevens, R.M. Nitrates and glaucoma. *JAMA,* **1977,** *237*:117.

Robertson, R.M., Robertson, D., Roberts, L.J., Maas, R.L., FitzGerald, G.A., Friesinger, G.C., and Oates, J.A. Thromboxane A2 in vasotonic angina pectoris: evidence from direct measurements and inhibitor trials. *N. Engl. J. Med.,* **1981,** *304*:998–1003.

Robertson, R.M., Wood, A.J.J., Vaughn, W.K., and Robertson, D. Exacerbation of vasotonic angina pectoris by propranolol. *Circulation,* **1982,** *65*:281–285.

Rodrigues, E.A., Lahiri, A., and Raftery, E.B. Improvement in left ventricular diastolic function in patients with stable angina after chronic treatment with verapamil and nicardipine. *Eur. Heart J.,* **1987,** *8*:624–629.

Ross, R.S. Pathophysiology of coronary circulation. *Br. Heart J.,* **1971,** *33*:173–184.

Rouleau, J.L., Chatterjee, K., Ports, T.A., Doyle, M.B., Hiramatsu, B., and Parmley, W.W. Mechanism of relief of pacing-induced angina with oral verapamil: reduced oxygen demand. *Circulation,* **1983,** *67*:94–100.

Rousseau, M.F., Veriter, C., Detry, J.M., Brasseur, L., and Pouleur, H. Impaired early left ventricular relaxation in coronary artery disease: effects of intracoronary nifedipine. *Circulation,* **1980,** *62*:764–772.

Savonitto, S., Ardissiono, D., Egstrup, K., Rasmussen, K., Bae, E.A., Omland, T., Schjelderup-Mathiesen, P.M., Marraccini, P., Wahlqvist, N., Merlini, A., and Rehnqvist, N. Combination therapy with meto-

prolol and nifedipine versus monotherapy in patients with stable angina pectoris. Results of the International Multicenter Angina Exercise (IMAGE) Study. *J. Am. Coll. Cardiol.,* **1996,** *27*:311–316.

Schulz, W., Jost, S., Kober, G., and Kaltenbach, M. Relation of antianginal efficacy of nifedipine to degree of coronary arterial narrowing and to presence of coronary collateral vessels. *Am. J. Cardiol.,* **1985,** *55*:26–32.

Schumacher, B., Pecher, P., von Specht, B.U., and Stegman, T. Induction of neoangiogenesis in ischemic myocardium by human growth factors: first clinical results of a new treatment of coronary heart disease. *Circulation,* **1998,** *97*:645–650.

Sellke, F.W., Myers, P.R., Bates, J.N., and Harrison, D.G. Influence of vessel size on the sensitivity of porcine coronary microvessels to nitroglycerin. *Am. J. Physiol.,* **1990,** *258*:H515–H520.

Serruys, P.W., Brower, R.W., ten Katen, H.J., Bom, A.H., and Hugenholtz, P.G. Regional wall motion from radiopaque markers after intravenous and intracoronary injections of nifedipine. *Circulation,* **1981,** *63*:584–591.

Serruys, P.W., Hooghoudt, T.E., Reiger, J.H., Slager, C., Brower, R.W., and Hugenholtz, P.G. Influence of intracoronary nifedipine on left ventricular function, coronary vasomotility, and myocardial oxygen consumption. *Br. Heart. J.,* **1983,** *49*:427–441.

Severi, S., Davies, G., Maseri, A., Marzullo, P., and L'Abbate, A. Long-term prognosis of "variant" angina with medical treatment. *Am. J. Cardiol.,* **1980,** *46*:226–232.

Stason, W.B., Schmid, C.H., Niedzwiecki, D., Whiting, G.W., Caubet, J.F., Cory, D., Luo, D., Ross, S.D., and Chalmers, T.C. Safety of nifedipine in angina pectoris: a meta-analysis. *Hypertension,* **1999,** *33*:24–31.

Thadani, U., Davidson, C., Singleton, W., and Taylor, S.H. Comparison of five beta-adrenoreceptor antagonists with different ancillary properties during sustained twice daily therapy in angina pectoris. *Am. J. Med.,* **1980,** *68*:243–250.

Thadani, U., Maranda, C.R., Amsterdam, E., Spaccavento, L., Friedman, R.G., Chernoff, R., Zellner, S., Gorwit, J., and Hinderaker, P.H. Lack of pharmacologic tolerance and rebound angina pectoris during twice-daily therapy with isosorbide-5-mononitrate. *Ann. Intern. Med.,* **1994,** *120*:353–359.

Thadani, U., Zellner, S.R., Glasser, S., Bittar, N., Montoro, R., Miller, A.B., Chaitman, B., Schulman, P., Stahl, A., DiBianco, R., Bray, J., Means, W.E., Morledge, J., and coinvestigators. Double-blind, dose-response, placebo-controlled multicenter study of nisoldipine. A new second-generation calcium channel blocker in angina pectoris. *Circulation,* **1991,** *84*:2398–2408.

Theroux, P., Waters, D.D., Debaisieux, J.C., Szlachcic, J., Mizgala, H.F., and Bourassa, M.G. Hemodynamic effects of calcium ion antagonists after acute myocardial infarction. *Clin. Invest. Med.,* **1980,** *3*:81–85.

Tolins, M., Weir, E.K., Chesler, E., and Pierpont, G.L. "Maximal" drug therapy is not necessarily optimal in chronic angina pectoris. *J. Am. Coll. Cardiol.,* **1984,** *3*:1051–1057.

Tsien, R.W., Lipscombe, D., Madison, D.V., Bley, K.R., and Fox, A.P. Multiple types of neuronal calcium channels and their selective modulation. *Trends Neurosci.,* **1988,** *11*:431–438.

Wallis, R.M., Corbin, J.D., Francis, S.H., and Ellis, P. Tissue distribution of phosphodiestase families and the effects of sildenafil on tissue cyclic nucleotides, platelet function, and the contractile responses of trabeculae carneae and aortic rings in vitro. *Am. J. Cardiol.,* **1999,** *83*:3C–12C.

Walsh, R.A., and O'Rourke, R.A. Direct and indirect effects of calcium entry blocking agents on isovolumic left ventricular relaxation in conscious dogs. *J. Clin. Invest.,* **1985,** *75*:1426–1434.

Wandel, C., Kim, R.B., Guengerich, F.P., and Wood, A.J. Mibefradil is a P-glycoprotein substrate and a potent inhibitor of both P-glycoprotein and CYP3A in vitro. *Drug Metab. Dispos.,* **2000,** *28*:895–898.

Watanabe, H., Kakihana, M., Ohtsuka, S., and Sugshita, Y. Randomized, double-blind, placebo-controlled study of carvedilol on the prevention of nitrate tolerance in patients with chronic heart failure. *J. Am. Coll. Cardiol.,* **1998,** *32*:1194–1200.

Waters, D.D., Theroux, P., Szlachcic, J., and Dauwe, F. Provocative testing with ergonovine to assess the efficacy of treatment with nifedipine, diltiazem and verapamil in variant angina. *Am. J. Cardiol.,* **1981,** *48*:123–130.

Webb, D.J., Freestone, S., Allen, M.J., and Muirhead, G.J. Sildenafil citrate and blood-pressure-lowering drugs: results of drug interaction studies with an organic nitrate and a calcium antagonist. *Am. J. Cardiol.,* **1999,** *83*:21C–28C.

Yusuf, S. Calcium antagonists in coronary artery disease and hypertension. Time for reevaluation? *Circulation,* **1995,** *92*:1079–1082.

Yusuf, S., Sleight, P., Pogue, J., Bosch, J., Davies, R., and Dagenais, G. Effects of an angiotensin-converting-enzyme inhibitor, ramipril, on cardiovascular events in high-risk patients. The Heart Outcomes Prevention Evaluation Study Investigators. *N. Engl J. Med.,* **2000,** *342*:145–153.

Zeiher, A.M., Drexler, H., Wollschlager, H., and Just, H. Modulation of coronary vasomotor tone in humans. Progressive endothelial dysfunction with different early stages of coronary atherosclerosis. *Circulation,* **1991,** *83*:391–401.

Zusman, R.M., Higgins, J., Christensen, D., and Boucher, C.A. Bepridil improves left ventricular performance in patients with angina pectoris. *J. Cardiovasc. Pharmacol.,* **1993,** *22*:474–480.

MONOGRAPHS AND REVIEWS

Abernethy, D.R., and Schwartz, J.B. Calcium-antagonist drugs. *N. Engl. J. Med.,* **1999,** *341*:1447–1457.

American Heart Association. 2001 Heart and Stroke Statistical Update. Available at: http://www.americanheart.org/statistics/index.html. Accessed January 24, 2001.

Andersson, K.E., and Wagner, G. Physiology of penile erection. *Physiol. Rev.,* **1995,** *75*:191–236.

Asahara, T., Kalka, C., and Isner, J.M. Stem cell therapy and gene transfer for regeneration. *Gene Ther.,* **2000,** *7*:451–457.

Asirvatham, S., Sebastian, C., and Thadani, U. Choosing the most appropriate treatment for stable angina. Safety considerations. *Drug Saf.,* **1998,** *19*:23–44.

Beavo, J.A., Conti, M., and Heaslip, R.J. Multiple cyclic nucleotide phosphodiesterases. *Mol. Pharmacol.,* **1994,** *46*:399–405.

Berridge, M. Inositol trisphosphate and calcium signalling. *Nature,* **1993,** *361*:315–325.

Bhatt, D.L., and Topol, E.J. Current role of platelet glycoprotein IIb/IIIa inhibitors in acute coronary syndromes. *JAMA,* **2000,** *284*:1549–1558.

Bolton, T.B. Mechanisms of action of transmitters and other substances on smooth muscle. *Physiol. Rev.,* **1979,** *59*:606–718.

Braunwald, E., Antman, E.M., Beasley, J.W., Califf, R.M., Cheitlin, M.D., Hochman, J.S., Jones, R.H., Kereiakes, D., Kupersmith, J., Levin, T.N., Pepine, C.J., Schaeffer, J.W., Smith, E.E. III, Steward, D.E., Theroux, P., Alpert, J.S., Eagle, K.A., Faxon, D.P., Fuster, V., Gardner, T.J., Gregoratos, G., Russell, R.O., and Smith, S.C., Jr. ACC/AHA guidelines for the management of patients with unstable angina and non-ST-segment elevation myocardial infarction. A report of the American College of Cardiology/American Heart Association

Task Force on Practice Guidelines (Committee on the Management of Patients with Unstable Angina). *J. Am. Coll. Cardiol.,* **2000,** *36*:970–1062.

Cheitlin, M.D., Hutter, A.M., Brindis, R.G., Ganz, P., Kaul, S., Russell, R.O., Jr., and Zusman, R.M. ACC/AHA expert consensus document. Use of sildenafil (Viagra) in patients with cardiovascular disease. American College of Cardiology/American Heart Association. *J. Am. Coll. Cardiol.,* **1999,** *33*:273–282.

Childress, C.H., and Katz, V.L. Nifedipine and its indications in obstetrics and gynecology. *Obstet. Gynecol.,* **1994,** *83*:616–624.

Darius, H. Role of nitrates for the therapy of coronary artery disease patients in the years beyond 2000. *J. Cardiovasc. Pharmacol.,* **1999,** *34*(suppl. 2):S15–S20.

Duckers, H.J., and Nabel, E.G. Prospects for genetic therapy of cardiovascular disease. *Med. Clin. North Am.,* **2000,** *84*:199–213.

Fleckenstein, A. History of calcium antagonists. *Circ. Res.,* **1983,** *52*:I3–I16.

Fox, K.M., Mulcahy, D., and Purcell, H. Unstable and stable angina. *Eur. Heart. J.,* **1993,** *14*(suppl. F):15–17.

Friesinger, G.C., and Robertson, R.M. Hemodynamics in stable angina pectoris. In, *Angina Pectoris,* 2nd ed. (Julian, D.G., ed.) Churchill-Livingstone, New York, **1985,** pp. 25–37.

Friesinger, G.C., and Robertson, R.M. Vasospastic angina: a continuing search for mechanism(s). *J. Am. Coll. Cardiol.,* **1986,** *7*:30–31.

Fuster, V., Badimon, J., Chesebro, J.H., and Fallon, J.T. Plaque rupture, thrombosis, and therapeutic implications. *Haemostasis,* **1996,** *26*(*suppl. 4*):269–284.

Gibbons, R.J., Chatterjee, K., Daley, J., Douglas, J.S., Fihn, S.D., Gardin, J.M., Grunwald, M.A., Levy, D., Lytle, B.W., O'Rourke, R.A., Schafer, W.P., Williams, S.V., Ritchie, J.L., Cheitlin, M.D., Eagle, K.A., Gardner, T.J., Garson, A. Jr., Russell, R.O., Ryan, T.J., and Smith, S.C., Jr. ACC/AHA/ACP-ASIM guidelines for the management of patients with chronic stable angina: a report of the American College of Cardiology/American Heart Association Task Force on Practice Guidelines. *J. Am. Coll. Cardiol.,* **1999,** *33*:2092–2197.

Godfraind, T., Miller, R., and Wibo, M. Calcium antagonism and calcium entry blockade. *Pharmacol. Rev.,* **1986,** *38*:321–416.

Hamilton, T.C., and Weston, A.H. Cromokalim, nicorandil and pinacidil: novel drugs which open potassium channels in smooth muscle. *Gen. Pharmacol.,* **1989,** *20*:1–9.

Harrison, D.G., and Bates, J.N. The nitrovasodilators. New ideas about old drugs. *Circulation,* **1993,** *87*:1461–1467.

Henry, P.D. Mechanisms of action of calcium antagonists in cardiac and smooth muscle. In, *Calcium Channel Blocking Agents in the Treatment of Cardiovascular Disorders.* (Stone, P.H., and Antman, E.M., eds.) Futura, Mount Kisco, NY, **1983,** pp. 107–154.

Hockerman, G.H., Peterson, B.Z., Johnson, B.D., and Catterall, W.A. Molecular determinants of drug binding and action on L-type calcium channels. *Annu. Rev. Pharmacol. Toxicol.,* **1997,** *37*:361–396.

Hollingshead, L.M., Faulds, D., and Fitton, A. Bepridil. A review of its pharmacological properties and therapeutic use in stable angina pectoris. *Drugs,* **1992,** *44*:835–857.

Ignarro, L.J., Buga, G.M., Wood, K.S., Byrns, R.E., and Chaudhuri, G. Endothelium-derived relaxing factor produced and released from artery and vein is nitric oxide. *Proc. Natl. Acad. Sci. U.S.A.,* **1987,** *84*:9265–9269.

Isner, J.M. Mechanism of angiogenesis and prospects for angiogenic therapy. *FASEB J.,* **2000,** *14*:D12.

Julian, D.G. Symposium—concluding remarks. *Am. J. Cardiol.,* **1987,** *59*:37J.

Kaplinsky, E. Management of angina pectoris. Modern concepts. *Drugs,* **1992,** *43*(suppl. 1):9–14.

Kerins, D.M., and FitzGerald, G.A. The current role of platelet-active drugs in ischaemic heart disease. *Drugs,* **1991,** *41*:665–671.

Lablanche, J.M., Bauters, C., McFadden, E.P., Quandalle, P., and Bertrand, M.E. Potassium channel activators in vasospastic angina. *Eur. Heart J.,* **1993,** *14*(*suppl. B*):22–24.

Langtry, H.D., and Spencer, C.M. Nisoldipine coat-core. A review of its pharmacodynamic and pharmacokinetic properties and clinical efficacy in the management of ischaemic heart disease. *Drugs,* **1997,** *53*:867–884.

Libby, P. Coronary artery injury and the biology of atherosclerosis: inflammation, thrombosis, and stabilization. *Am. J. Cardiol.,* **2000,** *86*:3J–8J.

Lowenstein, C.J., Dinerman, J.L., and Snyder, S.H. Nitric oxide: a physiologic messenger. *Ann. Intern. Med.,* **1994,** *120*:227–237.

Markham, A., Plosker, G.L., and Goa, K.L. Nicorandil. An updated review of its use in ischaemic heart disease with emphasis on its cardioprotective effects. *Drugs,* **2000,** *60*:955–974.

Moncada, S., and Higgs, A. Mechanisms of disease: The L-arginine–nitric oxide pathway. *N. Engl. J. Med.,* **1993,** *329*:2002–2012.

Moncada, S., Radomski, M.W., and Palmer, R.M. Endothelium-derived relaxing factor. Identification as nitric oxide and role in the control of vascular tone and platelet function. *Biochem. Pharmacol.,* **1988,** *37*:2495–2501.

Münzel, T., Kurz, S., Heitzer, T., and Harrison, D.G. New insights into mechanisms underlying nitrate tolerance. *Am. J. Cardiol.,* **1996,** *77*:24C–30C.

Murad, F. Cyclic guanosine monophosphate as a mediator of vasodilation. *J. Clin. Invest.,* **1986,** *78*:1–5.

Murad, F. The 1996 Albert Lasker Medical Research Awards. Signal transduction using nitric oxide and cyclic guanosine monophosphate. *JAMA,* **1996,** *276*:1189–1192.

Nabel, E.G. Gene therapy for cardiovascular disease. *Circulation,* **1995,** *91*:541–548.

Needleman, P. Biotransformation of organic nitrates. In, *Organic Nitrates.* (Needleman, P., ed.) *Handbuch der Experimentellen Pharmakologie.* Vol 40. Springer-Verlag, Berlin, **1975,** pp. 57–96.

Packer, M. Drug therapy. Combined beta-adrenergic and calcium-entry blockade in angina pectoris. *N. Engl. J. Med.,* **1989,** *320*:709–718.

Parker, J.D., and Parker, J.O. Nitrate therapy for stable angina pectoris. *N. Engl. J. Med.,* **1998,** *338*:520–531.

Parratt, J.R. Nitroglycerin—the first one hundred years: new facts about an old drug. *J. Pharm. Pharmacol.,* **1979,** *31*:801–809.

Pitt, B. Blockade of the renin-angiotensin system. Effect on mortality in patients with left ventricular systolic dysfunction. *Cardiol. Clin.,* **1994,** *12*:101–114.

Rutherford, J.D. Nitrate tolerance in angina therapy. How to avoid it. *Drugs,* **1995,** *49*:196–199.

Ryan, T.J., Antman, E.M., Brooks, N.H., Califf, R.M., Hillis, L.D., Hiratzka, L.F., Rapaport, E., Riegel, B., Russell, R.O., Smith, E.E. III, and Weaver, W.D. 1999 update. ACC/AHA guidelines for the management of patients with acute myocardial infarction. A report of the American College of Cardiology/American Heart Association Task Force on Practice Guidelines (Committee on Management of Acute Myocardial Infarction). Available at: http://www.acc.org/clinical/guidelines/nov96/1999/index.htm and http://www.americanheart.org/scientific/statements/1999/AMI/edits. Accessed January 24, 2001.

Schwartz, A. Molecular and cellular aspects of calcium channel antagonism. *Am. J. Cardiol.,* **1992,** *70*:6F–8F.

Taira, N. Differences in cardiovascular profile among calcium antagonists. *Am. J. Cardiol.,* **1987,** *59*:24B–29B.

Taylor, S.H. Usefulness of amlodipine for angina pectoris. *Am. J. Cardiol.,* **1994,** *73*:28A–33A.

Thadani, U. Role of nitrates in angina pectoris. *Am. J. Cardiol.,* **1992,** *70*:43B–53B.

Todd, P.A., and Faulds, D. Felodipine. A review of the pharmacology and therapeutic uses of the extended release formulation in cardiovascular disorders. *Drugs,* **1992,** *44*:251–277.

Vane, J.R. The Croonian Lecture, 1993. The endothelium: maestro of the blood circulation. *Philos. Trans. R. Soc. Lond. B Biol. Sci.,* **1994,** *343*:225–246.

van Zwieten, P.A., and Pfaffendorf, M. Similarities and differences between calcium antagonists: pharmacological aspects. *J. Hypertens. Suppl.,* **1993,** *11*:S3–S11.

Vogt, M., Motz, W., and Strauer, B.E. ACE-inhibitors in coronary artery disease? *Basic Res. Cardiol.,* **1993,** *88*(*suppl. 1*):43–64.

Waldman, S.A., and Murad, F. Cyclic GMP synthesis and function. *Pharmacol. Rev.,* **1987,** *39*:163–196.

Waters, D. Proischemic complications of dihydroperidine calcium channel blockers. *Circulation,* **1991,** *84*:2598–2600.

Why, H.J., and Richardson, P.J. A potassium channel opener as monotherapy in chronic stable angina pectoris: comparison with placebo. *Eur. Heart J.,* **1993,** *14*(suppl. B):25–29.

Zusman, R.M., Morales, A., Glasser, D.B., and Osterloh, I.H. Overall cardiovascular profile of sildenafil citrate. *Am. J. Cardiol.,* **1999,** *83*:35C–44C.

ANTIHYPERTENSIVE AGENTS AND THE DRUG THERAPY OF HYPERTENSION

John A. Oates and Nancy J. Brown

Arterial pressure is the product of cardiac output and peripheral vascular resistance. Drugs lower pressure by actions on either the peripheral resistance or the cardiac output or both. The cardiac output may be reduced by drugs that either inhibit myocardial contractility or decrease ventricular filling pressure. Many of the antihypertensive drugs that affect adrenergic receptors, the renin-angiotensin system, Ca^{2+} channels, and Na^+ and water balance are also discussed in Chapters 9, 10, 29, 31, 32, and 34. The pharmacology of antihypertensive agents that are not discussed elsewhere is presented here; in addition, the properties of all of the major drugs that are particularly relevant to their use in hypertension are reviewed, and an overview of the therapy of hypertension is provided.

Hypertension is the most common cardiovascular disease. As many as 43 million adults in the United States have systolic and/or diastolic blood pressure above 140/90.

Elevated arterial pressure causes pathological changes in the vasculature and hypertrophy of the left ventricle. As a consequence, hypertension is the principal cause of stroke, leads to disease of the coronary arteries with myocardial infarction and sudden cardiac death, and is a major contributor to cardiac failure, renal insufficiency, and dissecting aneurysm of the aorta.

Hypertension is defined conventionally as blood pressure ≥140/90; this serves to characterize a group of patients who carry a risk of hypertension-related cardiovascular disease that is high enough to merit medical attention. However, from the standpoint of health promotion, it should be noted that the risk of both fatal and nonfatal cardiovascular disease in adults is lowest with systolic blood pressures of less than 120 mm Hg and diastolic of less than 80 mm Hg; these risks increase progressively with higher levels of both systolic and diastolic blood pressure. Although many of the clinical trials classify the severity of hypertension by diastolic pressure, progressive elevations of systolic pressure are similarly predictive of adverse cardiovascular events; at every level of diastolic pressure, risks are greater with higher levels of systolic blood pressure. Indeed, in elderly patients, systolic blood pressure predicts outcome better than diastolic blood pressure.

At very severe levels of hypertension (systolic ≥210 and/or diastolic ≥120), a subset of patients develops ful-

minant arteriolopathy characterized by endothelial injury and a marked proliferation of cells in the intima, leading to intimal thickening and ultimately to arteriolar occlusion. This is the pathological basis of the syndrome of malignant hypertension, which is associated with rapidly progressive microvascular occlusive disease in the kidney (with renal failure), brain (hypertensive encephalopathy), retina (hemorrhages, exudates, and discedema), and other organs. The severe endothelial disruption can lead to microangiopathic hemolytic anemia. Untreated malignant hypertension is rapidly fatal and requires in-hospital management on an emergency basis.

The presence of certain target organ changes confers on a patient a worse prognosis than that for a patient with the same level of blood pressure lacking these findings. Thus, retinal hemorrhages, exudates, and discedema indicate a far worse short-term prognosis for a given level of blood pressure. Left ventricular hypertrophy defined by electrocardiogram, or more accurately by echocardiography, is associated with a substantially worse long-term outcome that includes a higher risk of sudden cardiac death. The risk of cardiovascular disease, disability, and death in hypertensive patients also is increased markedly by concomitant cigarette smoking and by elevated low-density lipoprotein; the coexistence of hypertension with these risk factors increases cardiovascular morbidity and mortality to an extent that is supraadditive.

Robust evidence from multiple controlled trials indicates that pharmacological treatment of patients with diastolic pressures of 95 mm Hg or greater will reduce morbidity, disability, and mortality from cardiovascular disease. Effective antihypertensive therapy will almost completely prevent the hemorrhagic strokes, cardiac failure, and renal insufficiency due to hypertension. There is a marked reduction in total strokes. Moreover, several recent clinical trials suggest that reduction of diastolic blood pressure to 85 mm Hg confers a greater therapeutic benefit than reduction to 90 mm Hg, particularly in patients with diabetes (Hansson *et al.*, 1998).

The usual approach to patients with diastolic blood pressure in the range of 85 to 94 mm Hg is to use non-pharmacological therapy as an initial strategy. Because blood pressures in this range predict a clear increase in cardiovascular risk, the recommendations for nonpharmacological therapy should be accompanied by careful observation; in addition to the value of regular follow-up visits to maintain surveillance of blood pressure, they also afford an opportunity to assist and support patients in their efforts to achieve the changes in lifestyle required for effective nonpharmacological reduction in blood pressure.

Antihypertensive drugs can be classified according to their sites or mechanisms of action (*see* Table 33–1). As arterial pressure is the product of cardiac output and pe-

Table 33–1
Classification of Antihypertensive Drugs by Their Primary Site or Mechanism of Action

Diuretics (Chapter 29)
1. Thiazides and related agents (hydrochlorothiazide, chlorthalidone, *etc.*)
2. Loop diuretics (furosemide, bumetanide, torsemide, ethacrynic acid)
3. K^+-sparing diuretics (amiloride, triamterene, spironolactone)

Sympatholytic Drugs (Chapters 9, 10, 34)
1. Centrally acting agents (methyldopa, clonidine, guanabenz, guanfacine)
2. Adrenergic neuron blocking agents (guanadrel, reserpine)
3. β-Adrenergic antagonists (propranolol, metoprolol, *etc.*)
4. α-Adrenergic antagonists (prazosin, terazosin, doxazosin, phenoxybenzamine, phentolamine)
5. Mixed adrenergic antagonists (labetalol, carvedilol)

Vasodilators (Chapter 34)
1. Arterial (hydralazine, minoxidil, diazoxide, fenoldopam)
2. Arterial and venous (nitroprusside)

Ca^{2+}-*Channel Blockers* (Chapters 32, 34, 35) (verapamil, diltiazem, nifedipine, nimodipine, felodipine, nicardipine, isradipine, amlodipine)
Angiotensin Converting Enzyme Inhibitors (Chapters 31, 32) (captopril, enalapril, lisinopril, quinapril, ramipril, benazepril, fosinopril, moexipril, perindopril, trandolapril)
Angiotensin II–Receptor Antagonists (Chapters 31, 34) (losartan, candesartan, irbesartan, valsartan, telmisartan, eprosartan)

ripheral vascular resistance, it can be lowered by actions of drugs on either the peripheral resistance or the cardiac output, or both. Drugs may reduce the cardiac output by either inhibiting myocardial contractility or decreasing ventricular filling pressure. Reduction in ventricular filling pressure may be achieved by actions on the venous tone or on blood volume *via* renal effects. Drugs can reduce peripheral resistance by acting on smooth muscle to cause relaxation of resistance vessels or by interfering with the activity of systems that produce constriction of resistance vessels (*e.g.*, the sympathetic nervous system).

The hemodynamic consequences of long-term treatment with antihypertensive agents are presented in Table 33–2, which also provides a framework for potential complementary effects of concurrent therapy with two or more drugs. The simultaneous use of drugs with similar mechanisms of action and hemodynamic effects often produces little additional benefit. However, concurrent use of drugs from different classes is a strategy for achieving effective control of blood pressure while minimizing dose-related adverse effects.

DIURETICS

One of the earliest strategies for the management of hypertension was to alter Na^+ balance by restriction of salt in the diet. Pharmacological alteration of Na^+ balance became practical in the 1950s with the development of the orally active thiazide diuretics (*see* Chapter 29). These and related diuretic agents have antihypertensive effects when used alone, and they enhance the efficacy of virtually all other antihypertensive drugs.

The exact mechanism for reduction of arterial blood pressure by diuretics is not certain. Initially, the drugs decrease extracellular volume and cardiac output. However, the hypotensive effect is maintained during long-term therapy because of reduced vascular resistance; cardiac output returns to pretreatment values and extracellular volume remains somewhat reduced. Because of the persistent reduction in vascular resistance, some investigators have postulated that the diuretics have a direct effect on vascular smooth muscle that is independent of their saluretic effect. However, substantial data indicate that this is not the case. Thus, anephric patients and nephrectomized animals do not show a reduction in blood pressure when given diuretics (Bennett *et al.*, 1977); a high salt intake or an infusion of saline (but not dextran) to counteract the net negative Na^+ balance produced by diuretics reverses the antihypertensive effect; during effective therapy, plasma volume remains about 5% below pretreatment values and the plasma renin activity remains elevated, confirming a persistent reduction in body Na^+ (Shah *et al.*, 1978); diuretics do not relax vascular smooth muscle *in vitro*; and the hemodynamic effects of the diuretics to reduce vascular resistance are reproduced by restriction of salt (Freis, 1983).

Table 33–2
Hemodynamic Effects of Long-Term Administration of Antihypertensive Agents[*]

	HEART RATE	CARDIAC OUTPUT	TOTAL PERIPHERAL RESISTANCE	PLASMA VOLUME	PLASMA RENIN ACTIVITY
Diuretics	↔	↔	↓	−↓	↑
Sympatholytic agents					
Centrally acting	−↓	−↓	↓	−↑	−↓
Adrenergic neuron blockers	−↓	↓	↓	↑	−↑
α-Adrenergic antagonists	−↑	−↑	↓	−↑	↔
β-Adrenergic antagonists					
No ISA[†]	↓	↓	−↓	−↑	↓
ISA	↔	↔	↓	−↑	−↓
Arteriolar vasodilators	↑	↑	↓	↑	↑
Ca^{2+}-channel blockers	↓ or ↑	↓ or ↑	↓	−↑	−↑
ACE inhibitors	↔	↔	↓	↔	↑
ATRA	↔	↔	↓	↔	↑

[*]Changes are indicated as follows: ↑, increased; ↓, decreased; −↑, increased or no change; −↓, decreased or no change; ↔, unchanged.
[†]ISA, intrinsic sympathomimetic activity. ACE, angiotensin converting enzyme. ATRA, angiotensin II-receptor antagonists.

Potential mechanisms for reduction of vascular resistance by a persistent, albeit small, reduction in body Na^+ include a decrease in interstitial fluid volume; a fall in smooth muscle Na^+ concentration that may secondarily reduce the intracellular Ca^{2+} concentration, such that the cells are more resistant to contractile stimuli; and a change in the affinity and response of cell surface receptors to vasoconstrictor hormones (Insel and Motulsky, 1984).

Benzothiadiazines and Related Compounds

Benzothiadiazines ("thiazides") and related diuretics make up the most frequently used class of antihypertensive agents in the United States. Following the discovery of chlorothiazide, the first benzothiadiazine, a number of oral diuretics were developed that have an aryl-sulfonamide structure and block the Na^+-Cl^- symporter. Some of these are not benzothiadiazines, but because they have structural features and molecular functions that are similar to the original benzothiadiazine compounds, they have been designated as members of the "thiazide class" of diuretics. For example, chlorthalidone, one of the nonbenzothiadiazines in the thiazide class of diuretics, is widely used in the treatment of hypertension. Because the thiazide class of drugs has the same pharmacological effects, they are generally interchangeable with appropriate adjustment of dosage (*see* Chapter 29).

Regimen for Administration of the Thiazide-Class Diuretics in Hypertension. When a thiazide-class diuretic is utilized as the sole antihypertensive drug (mono-

therapy), it should be administered in a low dose. Further, there is mounting evidence that the administration of these diuretics in the long-term treatment of hypertension should be in conjunction with a K^+-sparing agent.

Antihypertensive effects can be achieved in many patients with as little as 12.5 mg of *chlorthalidone* (HYGROTON) or *hydrochlorothiazide* (HYDRODIURIL) daily. This should be the initial dose in most elderly patients who do not require urgent reduction of pressure. Furthermore, when used as monotherapy, the maximal daily dose of thiazide-class diuretics usually should not exceed 25 mg of hydrochlorothiazide or chlorthalidone (or equivalent). Even though more diuresis can be achieved with higher doses of these diuretics, abundant evidence indicates that doses higher than this are not required for monotherapy of hypertension and probably are not as safe.

A large study comparing 25 and 50 mg hydrochlorothiazide daily in an elderly population did not show a greater decrease in blood pressure with the larger dose (MRC Working Party, 1987). In the randomized, controlled trials of antihypertensive therapy in the elderly (SHEP Cooperative Research Group, 1991; Dahlöf *et al.*, 1991; MRC Working Party, 1992) that demonstrate the best outcomes in cardiovascular morbidity and mortality, 25 mg of hydrochlorothiazide or chlorthalidone was the maximum dose given; if greater reduction of blood pressure than achieved with this dose was required, treatment with a second drug was initiated. With respect to safety, a case-control study (Siscovick *et al.*, 1994) found a dose-dependent increase in the occurrence of sudden death at doses of hydrochlorothiazide greater than 25 mg daily. This finding supports the hypothesis engendered by a retrospective analysis of the Multiple Risk Factor Intervention Trial

(Multiple Risk Factor Intervention Trial Research Group, 1982), suggesting that increased cardiovascular mortality is associated with higher diuretic doses. Further, the drug-specific metabolic effects of the thiazide-class diuretics, as well as the side effects perceived by patients, are to some degree dose-dependent, providing additional reasons not to administer more than the 25-mg dose of hydrochlorothiazide/chlorthalidone required to achieve nearly maximum blood pressure reduction. Taken together, clinical studies to date indicate that, if adequate blood pressure reduction is not achieved with the 25-mg daily dose of hydrochlorothiazide or chlorthalidone, a second drug should be added rather than increasing the dose of diuretic.

When used in the treatment of hypertension, thiazide-class diuretics usually should be administered in conjunction with a K^+-sparing agent. Attenuation of the kaliuretic effect of the thiazide-class diuretics can be achieved by drugs that block the Na^+ channels in the late distal tubule and collecting duct (amiloride and triamterene), or by inhibition of aldosterone action (spironolactone). Oral K^+ supplementation in the usual doses is not as effective as these K^+-sparing agents. At this time, the data from clinical trials most strongly support the use of amiloride in combination with a thiazide-class diuretic. In the two large clinical trials that demonstrate the best results in terms of cardiovascular morbidity and mortality (Dahlöf et al., 1991; MRC Working Party, 1992), amiloride was the drug employed together with hydrochlorothiazide, used in a ratio of 1 mg amiloride/10 mg hydrochlorothiazide.

Angiotensin converting enzyme inhibitors and angiotensin receptor antagonists will attenuate diuretic-induced loss of potassium to some degree, and this is a consideration if a second drug is required to achieve further blood pressure reduction beyond that attained with the diuretic alone. Because the diuretic and hypotensive effects of these drugs are greatly enhanced when they are given in combination, care should be taken to initiate combination therapy with low doses of each of these drugs. Administration of angiotensin converting enzyme inhibitors or angiotensin receptor antagonists together with other K^+-sparing agents or with K^+ supplements requires caution; combination of K^+-sparing agents with each other or with K^+ supplementation can cause serious hyperkalemia in occasional patients.

In contrast with the limitation on dose of thiazide-class diuretics used as monotherapy, the treatment of severe hypertension that is unresponsive to three or more drugs may require larger doses of the thiazide-class diuretics. Indeed, hypertensive patients may become refractory to drugs that block the sympathetic nervous system or to vasodilator drugs, because these drugs engender a state in which the blood pressure is very volume-dependent. Therefore, it is appropriate to consider the use of thiazide-class diuretics in doses of 50 mg of daily hydrochlorothiazide equivalent when treatment with appropriate combinations and doses of three or more drugs fails to yield adequate control of the blood pressure. Dietary Na^+ restriction is a valuable adjunct to the management of such refractory patients and will minimize the dose of diuretic that is required. This can be achieved by a modest restriction of Na^+ intake to 2 g daily. A more strict Na^+ restriction is not feasible for most patients. Since the degree of K^+ loss relates to the amount of Na^+ delivered to the distal tubule, such restriction of Na^+ can minimize the development of hypokalemia and alkalosis. The effectiveness of the thiazide class of drugs as diuretic or antihypertensive agents is progressively diminished when the glomerular filtration rate falls below 30 ml/min. One exception is metolazone, which retains efficacy in patients with this degree of renal insufficiency.

Most patients will respond to the thiazide class of diuretics with a reduction in blood pressure within 2 to 4 weeks, although a minority will not achieve maximum reduction in arterial pressure for up to 12 weeks on a given dose. Therefore, doses should not be increased more often than every 2 to 4 weeks. Although the blood pressure of patients who have suppressed plasma renin activity is almost uniformly sensitive to diuretics in the thiazide class, most other patients also respond. There is no way to predict the antihypertensive response from the duration or severity of the hypertension in a given patient, although diuretics are unlikely to be effective as a sole therapy in patients with severe hypertension. Since the effect of the thiazide class of diuretics is additive with that of other antihypertensive drugs, combination regimens that include these diuretics are common and rational. Diuretics also have the advantage of minimizing the retention of salt and water that is commonly caused by vasodilators and some sympatholytic drugs.

Adverse Effects and Precautions.   The adverse effects of diuretics are discussed in Chapter 29. Some of these are effects that determine whether patients can tolerate and comply with diuretic treatment. Sexual impotence is the most common troublesome side effect of the thiazide-class diuretics, and physicians should inquire specifically regarding its occurrence in conjunction with treatment with these drugs. Gout may be a consequence of the hyperuricemia induced by these diuretics. The occurrence of either of these adverse effects is a reason for considering alternative approaches to therapy. Muscle cramps also are related to diuretic therapy in a dose-dependent manner. Other effects of the thiazide-class diuretics are laboratory observations that are of concern primarily because they are putative surrogate markers for adverse drug effects on morbidity and mortality.

Surrogate markers are factors that, in epidemiological studies, have been found to correlate with disease outcomes and therefore are used in investigations of drug therapy as a surrogate of the actual effect of a drug on disease outcome. Thus, reduction in systolic blood pressure is an example of a surrogate marker for the reduction of stroke by antihypertensive therapy that has been extensively validated (SHEP Cooperative Research Group, 1991). In contrast, the epidemiological evidence linking frequent ventricular ectopic depolarizations to sudden cardiac death had suggested that these ventricular arrhythmias might be surrogate markers for a beneficial effect of antiarrhythmic drugs on sudden cardiac death. However, reduction of ventricular ectopic depolarizations and nonsustained ventricular tachycardia by the antiarrhythmic drugs encainide and flecainide was associated with an increase in sudden cardiac death, demonstrating the fallibility of using surrogate markers to predict the outcome of a specific pharmacological intervention (CAST Investigators, 1989). Accordingly, the effect of drugs on surrogate markers cannot be considered as convincing evidence; rather, surrogate markers form the basis for hypotheses that require testing with controlled clinical trials. Until such trials are carried out, however, the effect of drugs on surrogate markers that predict adverse outcomes do cause concern and influence decisions regarding dose.

The effects of diuretic drugs on several surrogate markers for adverse outcomes merit consideration. The K^+ depletion produced by thiazide-class diuretics is dose-dependent over a wide range of doses and is variable among individuals, such that a subset of patients may become substantially K^+-depleted on diuretic drugs. Even small doses given chronically, however, lead to some K^+ depletion.

There are two types of ventricular arrhythmia that are thought to be enhanced by K^+ depletion. One of these is polymorphic ventricular tachycardia (*torsades de pointes*), which is induced by a number of drugs, including quinidine. Such drug-induced polymorphic ventricular tachycardia is an arrhythmia initiated by abnormal ventricular repolarization, and it is markedly enhanced by drugs that produce K^+ depletion, which elicits abnormal repolarization (*see* Chapter 35). Accordingly, thiazide diuretics should not be given together with drugs that can cause polymorphic ventricular tachycardia.

The most important concern regarding K^+ depletion is its influence on ischemic ventricular fibrillation, the leading cause of sudden cardiac death and a major contributor to cardiovascular mortality in treated hypertensive patients. Studies in experimental animals have demonstrated that K^+ depletion lowers the threshold for electrically induced ventricular fibrillation in the ischemic myocardium and also increases spontaneous ischemic ventricular fibrillation (Curtis and Hearse, 1989; Yano *et al.*, 1989). A case-control study of hypertensive patients has found a positive correlation between diuretic dose and sudden cardiac death and an inverse correlation between

the use of adjunctive K^+-sparing agents and sudden cardiac death (Siscovick *et al.*, 1994). One controlled clinical trial has demonstrated a significantly greater occurrence of sudden cardiac death in patients treated with 50 mg of hydrochlorothiazide daily in comparison with the β-adrenergic antagonist metoprolol (MRC Working Party, 1992). Controlled clinical trials comparing the effect of diuretics with other antihypertensive drugs on cardiovascular mortality are now under way and should further illuminate this question. In the meantime, the available data on sudden cardiac death support the limitation of diuretic dose as monotherapy to 25 mg of hydrochlorothiazide daily (or equivalent) and the use of an adjunctive K^+-sparing agent.

The thiazide class of diuretics elevates the levels of low-density lipoprotein (LDL) and increases the ratio of LDL/high-density lipoprotein (HDL). A linkage between increased LDL and increased coronary heart disease has been demonstrated in epidemiological studies and in investigations of lipid-lowering drugs, justifying the consideration that LDL is a surrogate marker for coronary heart disease morbidity and mortality. Whether the increase in the LDL/HDL ratio caused by diuretics is in fact predictive of increased coronary heart disease in patients on diuretics is not presently known, and until adequate morbidity and mortality trials comparing antihypertensive drugs are completed, the effect of the thiazide-class diuretics on plasma lipids can be a basis for concern but not for definitive recommendations regarding the choice of these drugs relative to other antihypertensive agents.

In epidemiological studies, left ventricular hypertrophy is a powerful predictor of an increase in cardiac death in hypertensive patients. The thiazide-class diuretics are less effective in reducing left ventricular hypertrophy than are other antihypertensive drugs such as the angiotensin converting enzyme inhibitors (Dahöf *et al.*, 1992).

The thiazide-class diuretics increase glycosylated hemoglobin in patients with diabetes mellitus (Gall *et al.*, 1992). This finding, taken together with evidence that angiotensin converting enzyme inhibitors delay the deterioration of renal function in diabetic patients, suggests that thiazide-class diuretics are not the first drugs of choice in the monotherapy of hypertensive patients with diabetes mellitus.

All of the thiazide-like drugs cross the placenta, but they have not been found to have direct adverse effects on the fetus. However, if administration of a thiazide is begun during pregnancy, there is a risk of transient volume depletion that may result in placental hypoperfusion. Since the thiazides appear in breast milk, they should be avoided by nursing mothers.

The Choice of a Thiazide-Type Diuretic as the Initial Drug in the Treatment of Hypertension. Few issues in hypertension are more controversial than whether or not patients should be placed on a diuretic as the initial or only drug for the treatment of hypertension (Joint National Committee, 1997; Tobian *et al.*, 1994). A definitive answer to this question awaits the completion of a large clinical trial (the ALLHAT trial) conducted by the National Institutes of Health comparing a thiazide-class diuretic with other antihypertensive drugs as the initial or only therapeutic agents. In the interim, decisions will be made based on interpretations of the available data. There are several general types of data, from which interpretations have been inferred, but none provides convincing evidence.

One set of data is the group of metabolic effects of the thiazide-class of diuretics discussed above: the increase in LDL, depletion of K^+, impairment of diabetes control, and a reduction of left ventricular hypertrophy that is less than achieved with other drugs. The case-control study demonstrating a dose-dependent linkage of these diuretics to sudden cardiac death strengthens the inference that K^+ depletion is not benign (Siscovick *et al.*, 1994).

Another type of data is that obtained from the clinical trials that have established the benefit of antihypertensive therapy. In controlled clinical trials conducted before 1991 in predominantly middle-aged patients, the beneficial effect of antihypertensive therapy on coronary heart disease and cardiac death was found to be less than the effect on stroke. Long-term prospective observational studies predict that a decrease of 5 to 6 mm Hg in diastolic pressure should lead to a 35% to 40% reduction in stroke; indeed, an overview of 14 randomized trials of pharmacological therapy (Collins *et al.*, 1990) reveals that the prevalence of fatal plus nonfatal stroke is lowered by 42% ($p<0.0002$) as a consequence of that change in diastolic pressure. Whereas the observational studies predict a 20% to 25% reduction in fatal plus nonfatal coronary heart disease with a difference of 5 to 6 mm Hg in diastolic pressure, reduction of pressure to this degree with antihypertensive treatment lowered total coronary heart disease by only 14% ($p<0.01$). Fatal stroke was lowered by 45% ($p<0.0001$), whereas fatal coronary heart disease was reduced by only 11% (not significant) during antihypertensive treatment. The failure of antihypertensive therapy to yield the expected reduction in coronary heart disease, and particularly coronary heart disease mortality, has led to considerable speculation, including the possibility that the diuretic drugs that were the primary agents used in these trials may impose adverse effects on coronary heart disease, including sudden cardiac death. These disappointing results in terms of coronary heart disease were obtained in trials on mostly middle-aged patients that predominantly employed hydrochlorothiazide or chlorthalidone in doses up to 50 mg without a K^+-sparing agent.

Subsequent to this meta-analysis of the 14 controlled trials, 2 trials in elderly patients that used a low dose of hydrochlorothiazide (25 mg daily) together with the K^+-sparing agent amiloride demonstrated more favorable trends in reducing coronary mortality, lowering it by 50% (Dahlöf *et al.*, 1991)

and 40% (MRC Working Party, 1992). In the latter study, the reduction in stroke and coronary events was significant on diuretic therapy, whereas no significant reductions in these endpoints were seen in a comparison group randomized to the β-adrenergic blocker atenolol.

The following approach to selection of a diuretic as the initial drug is derived from the data above. In elderly patients (age 65 or greater), selection of a thiazide-class diuretic as the initial drug is rational if it is given in doses in the range of 12.5 to 25 mg of hydrochlorothiazide (or equivalent) daily and together with a K^+-sparing agent. This is based on the high level of efficacy in the clinical trials with such regimens, the relatively low profile of side effects, and the fact that elderly patients are likely to have a good response to diuretic therapy.

In patients under age 65, a greater individualization of choice of the initial antihypertensive drug seems warranted. The earlier clinical trials (conducted in this age group with high doses of the thiazide-class drug given without K^+-sparing agents) provide neither reassurance regarding the thiazide-class diuretics nor rejection of them. Individualization of initial drug choice can consider several factors. In diabetic patients, angiotensin converting enzyme inhibitors attenuate the decline in renal function, making these drugs preferable to diuretics, which may impair glucose tolerance in diabetes. Other drugs, particularly the angiotensin converting enzyme inhibitors, are more effective than diuretics in reducing left ventricular mass in patients with left ventricular hypertrophy. Caucasian race, age less than 65, and a high or normal renin status at baseline predict an antihypertensive response to an angiotensin converting enzyme inhibitor or a β-adrenergic receptor antagonist that is superior to that with a diuretic.

Other Diuretic Antihypertensive Agents

The thiazide-type diuretics are more effective antihypertensive agents than are the loop diuretics, such as furosemide and bumetanide, in patients who have normal renal function (Ram *et al.*, 1981). This differential effect is most likely related to the short duration of action of loop diuretics, such that a single daily dose does not cause a significant net loss of Na^+ for an entire 24-hour period. The spectacular efficacy of the loop diuretics in producing a rapid and profound natriuresis is a potential detriment for the treatment of hypertension. When a loop diuretic is given twice daily, the acute diuresis can be excessive and lead to more side effects than occur with a slower-acting, milder thiazide diuretic. The loop diuretics produce hypercalciuria, rather than the hypocalciuria associated with the thiazides. However, other metabolic consequences of the thiazides are shared with the loop diuretics, including hypokalemia, hyperuricemia, glucose intolerance, and potentially adverse effects on plasma concentrations of lipids. Loop diuretics may be particularly useful in patients with azotemia and in patients with severe edema associated with a vasodilator such as minoxidil.

Although spironolactone in doses up to 100 mg per day is equivalent to hydrochlorothiazide in its hypotensive effect (Jeunemaitre *et al.*, 1988), higher doses produce an unacceptable incidence of side effects (Schrijver and Weinberger, 1979). Spironolactone may be particularly useful for individuals with clinically significant hyperuricemia, hypokalemia, or glucose intolerance, and it is the agent of choice for management of primary aldosteronism. In contrast to thiazide diuretics, spironolactone does not affect plasma concentrations of Ca^{2+} or glucose. The effects of spironolactone on plasma lipids have not been studied extensively, but data indicate that the changes in triglycerides, LDL cholesterol, and total cholesterol are less than those seen with the thiazides. However, spironolactone may decrease the concentration of HDL cholesterol (Falch and Schreiner, 1983). The other K^+-sparing diuretics, triamterene and amiloride, are used primarily to reduce the kaliuresis and potentiate the hypotensive effect of a thiazide (De Carvalho *et al.*, 1980; Multicenter Diuretic Cooperative Study Group, 1981). These agents should be used cautiously with frequent measurements of K^+ concentrations in plasma in patients predisposed to hyperkalemia. Patients taking spironolactone, amiloride, or triamterene should be cautioned regarding the possibility that concurrent use of K^+-containing "salt substitutes" could produce hyperkalemia. Renal insufficiency is a relative contraindication to the use of K^+-sparing diuretics.

Diuretic-Associated Drug Interactions

Since the antihypertensive effects of diuretics are frequently additive with those of other antihypertensive agents, a diuretic commonly is used in combination with other drugs. As discussed above, the concurrent administration of diuretics with quinidine and other drugs that cause polymorphic ventricular tachycardia greatly increases the risk of this drug-induced arrhythmia. The K^+- and Mg^{2+}-depleting effects of the thiazide-like and loop diuretics also can potentiate arrhythmias that arise from digitalis toxicity. Corticosteroids can amplify the hypokalemia produced by the diuretics. All diuretics can decrease the clearance of Li^+, resulting in increased plasma concentrations of Li^+ and potential toxicity (Amdisen, 1982). Nonsteroidal antiinflammatory drugs (*see* Chapter 27) that inhibit the synthesis of prostaglandins reduce the antihypertensive effects of diuretics. It is not known if this interaction is due to Na^+ retention resulting from blockade of the natriuretic effect of the diuretic by the antiinflammatory agent or is related to inhibition of vascular synthesis of prostaglandins (Webster, 1985). Based on recent studies, it would appear that the effects of selective COX-2 inhibitors on renal prostaglandin synthesis and function are similar to those of the nonselective nonsteroidal antiinflammatory drugs. Nonsteroidal antiinflammatory drugs, β-adrenergic receptor antagonists, and angiotensin converting enzyme inhibitors reduce plasma concentrations of aldosterone and can potentiate the hyperkalemic effects of a K^+-sparing diuretic.

SYMPATHOLYTIC AGENTS

Since the demonstration in 1940 that bilateral excision of the thoracic sympathetic chain could lower blood pressure, the search for effective chemical sympatholytic agents has been intensive. Many compounds were tolerated poorly because they produced symptomatic orthostatic hypotension, sexual dysfunction, diarrhea, and fluid retention, with subsequent reduction of the antihypertensive effect. However, newer agents and rational combinations of these drugs with diuretics and vasodilators have overcome many of these difficulties. The subgroups of sympatholytic agents are shown in Table 33–1.

Methyldopa

Methyldopa (ALDOMET) is a centrally acting antihypertensive agent. It is a prodrug that exerts its antihypertensive action *via* an active metabolite.

Methyldopa (α-methyl-3,4-dihydroxy-L-phenylalanine), an analog of 3,4-dihydroxyphenylalanine (DOPA), is metabolized by the L-aromatic amino acid decarboxylase in adrenergic neurons to α-methyldopamine, which then is converted to α-methylnorepinephrine (Figure 33–1). α-Methylnorepinephrine is stored in the neurosecretory vesicles of adrenergic neurons, substituting for norepinephrine itself. Thus, when the adrenergic neuron discharges its neurotransmitter, α-methylnorepinephrine is released instead of norepinephrine.

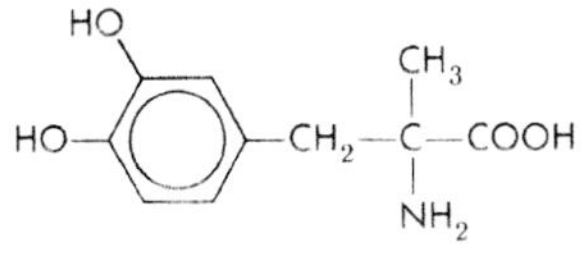

METHYLDOPA

Because α-methylnorepinephrine is as potent as norepinephrine as a vasoconstrictor, its substitution for norepinephrine in peripheral adrenergic neurosecretory vesicles does not alter the vasoconstrictor response to peripheral adrenergic neurotransmission. Rather, α-methylnorepinephrine acts in the brain to inhibit adrenergic

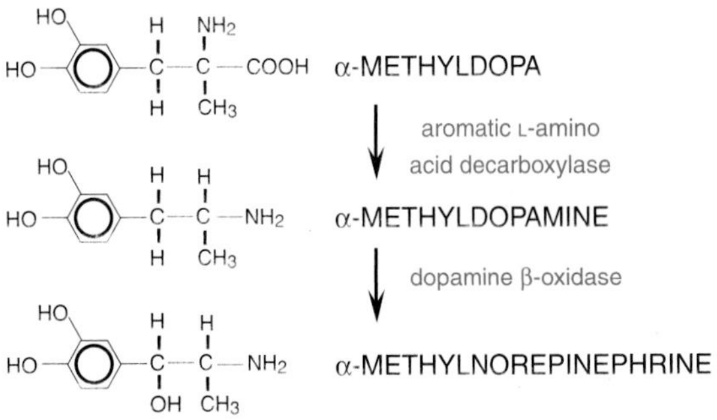

Figure 33–1. The metabolism of methyldopa in adrenergic neurons. α-Methylnorepinephrine replaces norepinephrine in neurosecretory vesicles.

neuronal outflow from the brainstem, and this central effect is principally responsible for its antihypertensive action. It is probable that methylnorepinephrine acts as an α_2-adrenergic receptor agonist in the brainstem to attenuate the output of vasoconstrictor adrenergic signals to the peripheral sympathetic nervous system.

A body of evidence supports the conclusion that methyldopa acts in the brain *via* an active metabolite to lower blood pressure (Bobik *et al.*, 1988; Granata *et al.*, 1986; Reid, 1986). In experimental animals, the hypotensive effect of methyldopa is blocked by DOPA decarboxylase inhibitors that have access to the brain, but not by inhibitors that are excluded from the central nervous system (CNS). The hypotensive effect also is abolished by inhibitors of dopamine β-hydroxylase and by centrally acting α-adrenergic receptor antagonists. Small doses of methyldopa that do not lower blood pressure when injected systemically elicit a hypotensive effect when injected into the vertebral artery. Selective microinjection of α-methylnorepinephrine into the C-1 area of the rostral ventrolateral medulla of the rat elicits a hypotensive response that is prevented by α-adrenergic receptor blockade. It is presumed that methylnorepinephrine inhibits the neurons in this area that are responsible for maintaining tonic discharge of peripheral sympathetic nerves and also for transmission of baroreflex-initiated tone. The excess α-adrenergic inhibition of sympathetic output may be a consequence of the accumulation of methylnorepinephrine in quantities larger than the norepinephrine that it displaces; this could result from the fact that the methylnorepinephrine is not a substrate for monoamine oxidase, the enzyme principally responsible for norepinephrine disposition in the brain. In addition to the α-adrenergic receptor–mediated inhibition of sympathetic output by methylnorepinephrine in the C-1 area of the rostral ventrolateral medulla, it also may exert inhibitory effects at other sites such as the nucleus tractus solitarius.

Pharmacological Effects.   Methyldopa reduces vascular resistance without causing much change in cardiac output or heart rate in younger patients with uncomplicated essential hypertension. In older patients, however, cardiac output may be decreased as a result of a reduction in heart rate and stroke volume; this is secondary to relaxation of veins and a reduction in preload. The fall in arterial pressure is maximal 6 to 8 hours after an oral or intravenous dose. Although the decrease in supine blood pressure is less than that in the upright position, symptomatic orthostatic hypotension is less common with methyldopa than with drugs that act exclusively on peripheral adrenergic neurons or autonomic ganglia; this is because methyldopa attenuates but does not completely block baroreceptor-mediated vasoconstriction. For this reason, it is well tolerated during surgical anesthesia. Any severe hypotension is reversible with volume expansion. Renal blood flow is maintained and renal function is unchanged during treatment with methyldopa.

Plasma concentrations of norepinephrine fall in association with the reduction in arterial pressure, and this reflects the decrease in sympathetic tone. Renin secretion also is reduced by methyldopa, but this is not a major effect of the drug and is not necessary for its hypotensive effects. Salt and water often are gradually retained with prolonged use of methyldopa, and this tends to blunt the antihypertensive effect. This has been termed "pseudotolerance," and it can be overcome with concurrent use of a diuretic. Of interest, treatment with methyldopa may reverse left ventricular hypertrophy within 12 weeks without any apparent relationship to the degree of change of arterial pressure (Fouad *et al.*, 1982).

Absorption, Metabolism, and Excretion.   Since methyldopa is a prodrug that is metabolized in the brain to the active form, its concentration in plasma has less relevance for its effects than is true for many other drugs. When administered orally, methyldopa is absorbed by an active amino acid transporter. Peak concentrations in plasma occur after 2 to 3 hours. The drug is distributed in a relatively small apparent volume (0.4 liter/kg) and is eliminated with a half-life of about 2 hours. The transport of methyldopa into the CNS is apparently also an active process (Bobik *et al.*, 1986). Methyldopa is excreted in the urine primarily as the sulfate conjugate (50% to 70%) and as the parent drug (25%). The remaining fraction is excreted as other metabolites, including methyldopamine, methylnorepinephrine, and O-methylated products of these catecholamines (Campbell *et al.*, 1985). The half-life of methyldopa is prolonged to 4 to 6 hours in patients with renal failure.

In spite of its rapid absorption and short half-life, the peak effect of methyldopa is delayed for 6 to 8 hours, even after intravenous administration, and the duration of action of a single dose is usually about 24 hours; this permits once- or twice-daily dosing (Wright *et al.*, 1982). The discrepancy between the effects of methyldopa and the measured concentrations of the drug in plasma is most likely related to the time required for transport into the CNS, conversion to the active metabolites, and accumulation of these metabolites in central adrenergic neurons. Patients with renal failure are more sensitive to the antihypertensive effect of methyldopa, but it is not known if this is due to alteration in excretion of the drug or to an increase in transport into the CNS.

Adverse Effects and Precautions.   In addition to lowering blood pressure, the active metabolites of methyldopa act on α_2-adrenergic receptors in the brainstem to inhibit the centers that are responsible for wakefulness and alertness. Thus, methyldopa produces sedation that is largely transient. A diminution in psychic energy may be a persistent effect in some patients, and depression occurs occasionally. Medullary centers that control salivation also are inhibited by α-adrenergic receptors, and methyldopa may produce dryness of the mouth. Other side effects that are related to the pharmacological effects in the CNS include a reduction in libido, parkinsonian signs, and hyperprolactinemia that may become sufficiently pronounced to cause gynecomastia and galactorrhea. In individuals who have sinoatrial node dysfunction, methyldopa may precipitate severe bradycardia and sinus arrest, including that which occurs with carotid sinus hypersensitivity.

Methyldopa also produces some adverse effects that are not related to its pharmacological action. Hepatotoxicity, sometimes associated with fever, is an uncommon but potentially serious toxic effect of methyldopa. Prompt diagnosis of hepatotoxicity requires a low threshold for considering the drug as a cause for hepatitis-like symptoms (e.g., nausea, anorexia) and screening for hepatotoxicity (e.g., with determination of gamma-glutamyl transpeptidase or alanine aminotransferase) at about 3 weeks and again at about 3 months following initiation of treatment with this drug. The incidence of methyldopa-induced hepatitis is unknown, but about 5% of patients will have transient increases in alanine aminotransferase activity in plasma. Hepatic dysfunction usually is reversible with prompt discontinuation of the drug, but it will recur if methyldopa is given again, and a few cases of fatal hepatic necrosis have been reported. Hepatitis may occur only after long-term therapy with methyldopa, but it usually appears within 3 months of starting the drug. It is advisable to avoid the use of methyldopa in patients with hepatic disease.

Methyldopa can cause hemolytic anemia. At least 20% of patients who receive methyldopa for a year develop a positive Coombs test (antiglobulin test) that is due to autoantibodies directed against the Rh locus on the patients' erythrocytes. The development of a positive Coombs test per se, however, is not an indication to stop treatment with methyldopa; 1% to 5% of these patients will develop a hemolytic anemia which requires prompt discontinuation of the drug. The Coombs test may remain positive for as long as a year after discontinuation of methyldopa, but the hemolytic anemia usually resolves within a matter of weeks. Severe hemolysis may be attenuated by treatment with glucocorticoids. Adverse effects that are even more rare include leukopenia, thrombocytopenia, red cell aplasia, lupus erythematosus–like syndrome, lichenoid and granulomatous skin eruptions,

myocarditis, retroperitoneal fibrosis, pancreatitis, diarrhea, and malabsorption.

Therapeutic Uses. Methyldopa is an effective antihypertensive agent when given in conjunction with a diuretic. It is generally well tolerated by patients with ischemic heart disease and by those with diastolic dysfunction, in whom it reduces left ventricular mass. However, frequent side effects and the potential for immunological abnormalities and organ toxicity are such that it is not used as the initial drug in monotherapy but is reserved for patients in whom it may have special value. Methyldopa is the preferred drug for treatment of hypertension during pregnancy based on its effectiveness and safety for both mother and fetus.

The usual initial dose of methyldopa is 250 mg twice daily, and there is little additional effect with doses above 2 g per day. Administration of a single daily dose of methyldopa at bedtime minimizes sedative effects, but administration twice daily may be required for some patients. A parenteral preparation of the ethyl ester of methyldopa, *methyldopate hydrochloride* (ALDOMET), also is available. It is usually given by intermittent intravenous infusion of 250 to 500 mg every 6 hours. The rate of deesterification of the methyldopate is variable among patients, and the doses given intravenously may deliver less methyldopa to the circulation than the same dose given orally.

Clonidine, Guanabenz, and Guanfacine

The detailed pharmacology of the α_2-adrenergic agonists *clonidine* (CATAPRES), *guanabenz* (WYTENSIN), and *guanfacine* (TENEX), is discussed in Chapter 10. These drugs stimulate the α_{2A} subtype of α_2-adrenergic receptors in the brainstem, resulting in a reduction in sympathetic outflow from the CNS (Sattler and van Zwieten, 1967; Langer et al., 1980; MacMillan et al., 1996). The decrease in plasma concentrations of norepinephrine is correlated directly with the hypotensive effect (Goldstein et al., 1985; Sorkin and Heel, 1986). Patients who have had a spinal cord transection above the level of the sympathetic outflow tracts do not display a hypotensive response to clonidine (Reid et al., 1977). At doses higher than those required to stimulate central α_{2A}-adrenergic receptors, these drugs can activate the α_{2B} subtype of α_2-adrenergic receptors on vascular smooth muscle cells (Link et al., 1996; MacMillan et al., 1996). This effect accounts for the initial vasoconstriction that is seen when overdoses of these drugs are taken, and it has been postulated to be responsible for the loss of therapeutic effect that is observed with high doses (Frisk-Holmberg et al., 1984; Frisk-Holmberg and Wibell, 1986).

Pharmacological Effects. The α_2-adrenergic agonists lower arterial pressure by an effect on both cardiac output and peripheral resistance. In the supine position, when the sympathetic tone to the vasculature is low, the major effect is to reduce both heart rate and stroke volume; however, in the upright position, when sympathetic outflow to the vasculature is normally increased, these drugs reduce vascular resistance. Some degree of orthostatic hypotension always occurs because of a reduction in venous return (secondary to systemic venodilatation), but symptomatic postural hypotension is uncommon in the absence of volume depletion. Sympathetic reflexes are damped but not entirely inhibited, and the sympathetic responses that are associated with the use of arteriolar vasodilators such as hydralazine and minoxidil are blunted. However, the α_2-adrenergic agonists do not interfere with the hemodynamic response to exercise, and exercise-induced hypotension is unusual. The decrease in cardiac sympathetic tone leads to a reduction in myocardial contractility and heart rate. Renal blood flow and glomerular filtration rate are maintained. Secretion of renin often is reduced, although it will respond to volume depletion or maintenance of an upright posture; there is no correlation between the hypotensive response and the effect on plasma renin activity. Retention of salt and water may occur with the α_2-adrenergic agonists, and it may be necessary to use a diuretic concurrently. Centrally acting α_2-adrenergic agonists have either no effect on plasma lipids or produce a slight reduction of total cholesterol, LDL cholesterol, and triglycerides (Lardinois and Neuman, 1988).

When guanabenz was first introduced, there was considerable interest in observations that the drug could be natriuretic in experimental animals. However, studies in human subjects have given variable results. With long-term therapy, there is usually a small loss of weight with no clinically significant changes in salt and water balance, suggesting that the "pseudotolerance" (Na^+ retention) seen with methyldopa and guanadrel may not occur with guanabenz. Nonetheless, the antihypertensive effects of diuretics and guanabenz are additive. If individuals are given guanabenz after a salt load, the drug has a natriuretic effect, and a new steady-state of Na^+ balance is attained by 1 week. This short-term effect is thought to be related to a reduction in renal sympathetic stimulation, with a consequent reduction in Na^+ reabsorption in the proximal nephron (Gehr et al., 1986). Guanabenz also has been shown to cause a water diuresis in some situations, which may be due to inhibition of the release and the renal actions of vasopressin (Strandhoy, 1985). Stimulation of renal α_2-adrenergic receptors by guanabenz may inhibit vasopressin-induced accumulation of cyclic AMP (Gellai and Edwards, 1988).

Adverse Effects and Precautions. Although the α_2-adrenergic agonists rarely cause life-threatening adverse reactions, many patients experience annoying and some-

times intolerable side effects. Sedation and xerostomia occur in at least 50% of patients upon initiation of therapy with clonidine and guanabenz and in 25% of patients who receive guanfacine (Wilson et al., 1986). Although these symptoms may diminish after several weeks of therapy, at least 10% of patients discontinue the drug because of persistence of these effects or because of impotence, nausea, or dizziness. The xerostomia may be accompanied by dry nasal mucosa, dry eyes, and parotid gland swelling and pain. Clonidine may produce a lower incidence of dry mouth and sedation when given transdermally, perhaps because high peak concentrations are avoided. Less common CNS side effects include sleep disturbances with vivid dreams or nightmares, restlessness, and depression. Cardiac effects related to the sympatholytic action of these drugs include symptomatic bradycardia and sinus arrest in patients with dysfunction of the sinoatrial node and atrioventricular (AV) block in patients with AV nodal disease or in patients taking other drugs that depress the AV node. Some 15% to 20% of patients who receive transdermal clonidine may develop contact dermatitis.

Sudden discontinuation of clonidine and related α_2-adrenergic agonists may cause a withdrawal syndrome consisting of headache, apprehension, tremors, abdominal pain, sweating, and tachycardia. The arterial blood pressure may rise to levels above those that were present prior to treatment, but the syndrome may occur in the absence of an overshoot in pressure. Symptoms typically occur 18 to 36 hours after the drug is stopped, and they are associated with increased sympathetic discharge, as evidenced by elevated plasma and urine concentrations of catecholamines. The exact incidence of the withdrawal syndrome is not known, but it is dose-related, occurring rarely in patients taking 0.3 mg or less daily of clonidine and more frequently and severely upon discontinuation of higher doses. It has been reported with all of the drugs of this class, but it may be milder with guanfacine, perhaps because of this drug's longer half-life. Rebound hypertension also has been seen after discontinuation of transdermal administration of clonidine (Metz et al., 1987).

Treatment of the withdrawal syndrome depends on the urgency of reducing the arterial blood pressure. In the absence of hypertensive encephalopathy, patients can be treated with their usual dose of antihypertensive drug, which should reduce the pressure within 2 hours. If a more rapid effect is required, sodium nitroprusside or a combination of an α- and β-adrenergic blocker is appropriate. β-Adrenergic blocking agents should not be used alone in this setting, since they will accentuate the hypertension by allowing unopposed α-adrenergic vasoconstriction caused by the elevated circulating concentrations of epinephrine.

Because perioperative hypertension has been described in patients when clonidine was withdrawn the night before surgery, surgical patients who are being treated with an α_2-adrenergic agonist either should be switched to another drug prior to elective surgery or should receive their morning dose and/or transdermal clonidine prior to the procedure. All patients who receive one of these drugs should be apprised of the potential danger of discontinuing the drug abruptly, and patients suspected of being noncompliant with medications should not be given α_2-adrenergic agonists for hypertension.

Adverse drug interactions with α_2-adrenergic agonists are rare. Diuretics potentiate the hypotensive effect of these drugs in a predictable manner. Tricyclic antidepressants may inhibit the antihypertensive effect of clonidine, but the mechanism of this interaction is not known.

Overdosage with an α_2-adrenergic agonist causes depression of the sensorium and transient hypertension followed by hypotension, bradycardia, and respiratory depression. The depressed respiration (with miosis) resembles the effects of an opioid. Treatment consists of ventilatory support, atropine or a sympathomimetic for bradycardia, and circulatory support with expansion of the blood volume and dopamine or dobutamine if needed.

Therapeutic Uses. The α_2-adrenergic agonists are usually used in conjunction with diuretics for the treatment of hypertension, but they may be effective when given alone; all of the drugs in this class are equally efficacious (Holmes *et al.*, 1983). The CNS effects are such that this class of drugs is not a leading option for monotherapy of hypertension, nor is it the first choice for use together with a diuretic. These drugs also are effective in blunting the reflex increase in sympathetic activity produced by vasodilators, and they may be used instead of a β-adrenergic antagonist for this purpose. Because the clonidine withdrawal syndrome occurs predominantly in patients taking higher doses of the drug, clonidine at doses of more than 0.3 mg daily is not optimal therapy for patients with severe hypertension.

Clonidine also has been used in hypertensive patients for the diagnosis of pheochromocytoma. The lack of suppression of the plasma concentration of norepinephrine to less than 500 pg/ml 3 hours after an oral dose of 0.3 mg of clonidine suggests the presence of such a tumor. A modification of this test, wherein overnight urinary excretion of norepinephrine and epinephrine is measured after administration of a 0.3-mg dose of clonidine at bedtime, may be useful when results based on plasma norepinephrine concentrations are equivocal (MacDougall *et al.*, 1988). Other uses for α_2-adrenergic agonists are discussed in Chapters 10, 14, and 24.

Guanadrel

Guanadrel (HYLOREL) specifically inhibits the function of peripheral postganglionic adrenergic neurons. The struc-

ture of guanadrel, which contains the strongly basic guanidine group, is as follows:

GUANADREL

Locus and Mechanism of Action. Guanadrel is targeted uniquely to the peripheral adrenergic neuron, where it inhibits sympathetic function. The drug reaches its site of action by active transport into the neuron by the same transporter that is responsible for the reuptake of norepinephrine (*see* Chapter 6). In the neuron, guanadrel is concentrated within the neurosecretory vesicles, where it replaces norepinephrine. During chronic administration, guanadrel acts as a "substitute neurotransmitter," in that it is present in storage vesicles, it depletes the normal transmitter, and it can be released by stimuli that normally release norepinephrine. This replacement of norepinephrine with an inactive transmitter is probably the principal mechanism of its neuron-blocking action.

When given intravenously, guanadrel initially can release norepinephrine in an amount sufficient to increase arterial blood pressure. This does not occur with oral administration, since norepinephrine is released only slowly from the vesicles under this circumstance and is degraded within the neuron by monoamine oxidase. Nonetheless, because of the potential for norepinephrine release, guanadrel is contraindicated in patients with pheochromocytoma.

During adrenergic neuron blockade with guanadrel, effector cells become supersensitive to norepinephrine. The supersensitivity is similar to that produced by postganglionic sympathetic denervation.

Pharmacological Effects. Essentially all of the therapeutic and adverse effects of guanadrel result from sympathetic blockade. The antihypertensive effect is achieved by a reduction in peripheral vascular resistance that results from inhibition of sympathetically mediated vasoconstriction. Thus, the arterial pressure is reduced modestly in the supine position when sympathetic activity is normally low, but the pressure can fall to a greater extent during situations where reflex sympathetic activation is a mechanism for maintaining arterial pressure, such as assumption of the upright posture, exercise, and depletion of plasma volume. Renal blood flow and glomerular filtration rate are modestly decreased during therapy with guanadrel, but this is without clinical consequence; renin secretion is not reduced. Plasma volume often becomes expanded, which may diminish the antihypertensive efficacy of guanadrel and require administration of diuretic to restore the antihypertensive effect.

Absorption, Distribution, Metabolism, and Excretion. Guanadrel is rapidly absorbed, leading to maximal levels in plasma at 1 to 2 hours. Because guanadrel must be transported into and accumulate in adrenergic neurons, the maximum effect on blood pressure is not seen until 4 to 5 hours. Although the β-phase of its elimination has an estimated half-life of 5 to 10 hours, this almost certainly does not reflect the longer half-life of drug stored at its site of action in the neurosecretory vesicles of adrenergic neurons. The half-life of the pharmacological effect of guanadrel is determined by the drug's persistence in this neuronal pool, and that is probably at least 10 hours. Guanadrel is administered in a regimen of twice-daily doses.

Guanadrel is cleared from the body by both renal and nonrenal disposition. Its elimination is impaired in patients with renal insufficiency; total-body clearance was reduced by 4- to 5-fold in a group of patients with a clearance of creatinine averaging 13 ml per minute.

Adverse Effects. Guanadrel produces undesirable effects that are related entirely to sympathetic blockade. Symptomatic hypotension during standing, exercise, ingestion of alcohol, or hot weather is the result of the lack of sympathetic compensation for these stresses. A general feeling of weakness and lassitude is partially, but not entirely, related to postural hypotension. Rarely, guanadrel can precipitate congestive heart failure in patients with limited cardiac reserve as a result of drug-induced fluid retention. Sexual dysfunction usually presents as delayed or retrograde ejaculation. Diarrhea also may occur.

Because guanadrel is actively transported to its site of action, drugs that block neuronal uptake of norepinephrine will inhibit the effect of guanadrel. Such drugs include the tricyclic antidepressants, cocaine, chlorpromazine, ephedrine, phenylpropanolamine, and amphetamine.

Therapeutic Uses. Because of the availability of a number of drugs that lower blood pressure without producing orthostatic hypotension, guanadrel is not employed in the monotherapy of hypertension, and is used chiefly as an additional agent in patients who have not achieved a satisfactory antihypertensive effect on two or more other agents. The usual starting dose is 10 mg daily, and side effects can be minimized by not exceeding 20 mg daily.

Reserpine

Reserpine is an alkaloid extracted from the root of *Rauwolfia serpentina* (Benth.), a climbing shrub indigenous to India. Descriptions of the medicinal use of the root of this plant are present in ancient Hindu Ayurvedic writings. "Modern" use of the whole root for the treatment of hypertension and psychoses was described in the Indian literature in 1931 (Sen and Bose, 1931). However, rauwolfia alkaloids were not used in western medicine until the mid-1950s. Reserpine was the first drug that was found to interfere with the function of the sympathetic nervous system in human beings, and its use began the modern era of effective pharmacotherapy of hypertension. The structure of reserpine is as follows:

RESERPINE

Locus and Mechanism of Action. Reserpine binds tightly to storage vesicles in central and peripheral adrenergic neurons, and the drug remains at such sites for prolonged periods of time (Giachetti and Shore, 1978). The storage vesicles are rendered dysfunctional as a result of their interaction with reserpine, and nerve endings lose their ability to concentrate and store norepinephrine and dopamine. Catecholamines leak into the cytoplasm, where they are destroyed by intraneuronal monoamine oxidase, and little or no active transmitter is discharged from nerve endings when they are depolarized. A similar process occurs at storage sites for 5-hydroxytryptamine. Reserpine-induced depletion of biogenic amines correlates with evidence of sympathetic dysfunction and antihypertensive effects. Recovery of sympathetic function requires synthesis of new storage vesicles, which takes days to weeks after discontinuation of the drug. Since reserpine depletes amines in the CNS as well as in the peripheral adrenergic neuron, it is probable that its antihypertensive effects are related to both a central and a peripheral action; it is certain that many of the side effects of reserpine are related to its effects in the CNS.

Pharmacological Effects. Both cardiac output and peripheral vascular resistance are reduced during long-term therapy with reserpine. Orthostatic hypotension may occur but does not usually cause symptoms. Heart rate and renin secretion fall. Salt and water are retained, which commonly results in "pseudotolerance."

Absorption, Metabolism, and Excretion. Few data are available on the pharmacokinetic properties of reserpine because of the lack of an assay capable of detecting low concentrations of the drug or its metabolites. Reserpine that is bound to isolated storage vesicles cannot be removed by dialysis, indicating that the binding is not in equilibrium with the surrounding medium. Because of the irreversible nature of reserpine binding, the amount of drug in plasma is unlikely to bear any consistent relationship to drug concentration at the site of action. Reserpine is entirely metabolized, and none of the parent drug is excreted unchanged.

Toxicity and Precautions. Most of the adverse effects of reserpine are due to its effect on the CNS. Sedation and inability to concentrate or perform complex tasks are the most common adverse effects. More serious is the occasional psychotic depression that can lead to suicide. Depression usually appears insidiously over many weeks or months and may not be attributed to the drug because of the delayed and gradual onset of symptoms. Reserpine must be discontinued at the first sign of depression, and the drug should never be given to patients with a history of depression. Reserpine-induced depression may last several months after the drug is discontinued. Depression appears to be uncommon, but not unknown, with doses of 0.25 mg per day or less. Other side effects include nasal stuffiness and exacerbation of peptic ulcer disease, which is uncommon with small oral doses.

Therapeutic Uses. Reserpine was the sympatholytic drug used in the landmark Veterans Administration Cooperative Study that demonstrated the beneficial effects of treatment of hypertension (Veterans Administration Cooperative Study Group on Antihypertensive Agents, 1967, 1970), but with the availability of newer drugs that are both effective and well tolerated, the use of reserpine has diminished because of its CNS side effects. However, in comparative studies, low doses of reserpine given concurrently with a diuretic were as well tolerated as combinations of a diuretic with propranolol or methyldopa. The major advantage of reserpine is that it is much less expensive than other antihypertensive drugs. Reserpine is used once daily with a diuretic, and several weeks are necessary to achieve a maximum effect. The daily dose should be limited to 0.25 mg or less, and as little as 0.05 mg per day may be efficacious when a diuretic is also used.

Metyrosine

Metyrosine (DEMSER) is (-)-α-methyl-L-tyrosine. It has the structure shown below. Metyrosine is an inhibitor of tyrosine hydroxylase, the enzyme that catalyzes the conversion of tyrosine to DOPA; this is the rate-limiting step in catecholamine biosynthesis (*see* Chapter 6). At a dose of 1 to 4 g per day, metyrosine decreases catecholamine biosynthesis by 35% to 80% in patients with pheochromocytoma. The maximal decrease in synthesis occurs only after several days, and the effect may be assessed by measurements of urinary catecholamines and their metabolites.

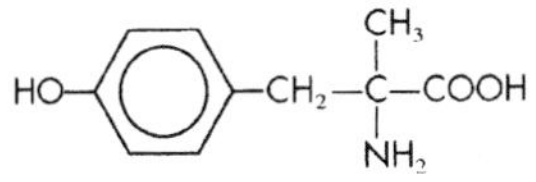

METYROSINE

Metyrosine is used as an adjuvant to phenoxybenzamine and other α-adrenergic blocking agents for the management of malignant pheochromocytoma and in the preoperative preparation of patients for resection of pheochromocytoma (Brogden *et al.*, 1981). Metyrosine carries a risk of crystalluria, which can be minimized by maintaining a daily urine volume of more than 2 liters. Other adverse effects include orthostatic hypotension, sedation, extrapyramidal signs, diarrhea, anxiety, and psychic disturbances. Doses must be titrated carefully to achieve significant inhibition of catecholamine biosynthesis and yet minimize these substantive side effects.

β-Adrenergic Receptor Antagonists

β-Adrenergic receptor blocking drugs were not expected to have antihypertensive effects when they were first investigated in patients. However, pronethalol, a drug that was never marketed, was found to reduce arterial blood pressure in hypertensive patients with angina pectoris. This antihypertensive effect was subsequently demonstrated for propranolol and all other β-adrenergic receptor antagonists. The pharmacology of these drugs is discussed in Chapter 10; characteristics relevant to their use in hypertension will be described here.

Locus and Mechanism of Action. Antagonism of β-adrenergic receptors affects the regulation of the circulation through a number of mechanisms, including a reduction in myocardial contractility and cardiac output. An important consequence of blocking β-adrenergic receptors is reduction in the secretion of renin with a resulting fall in the levels of angiotensin II. The weight of the evidence supports the concept that the reduction in angiotensin II, with its multiple effects on circulatory control and on aldosterone, contributes importantly to the antihypertensive action of this class of drugs, acting in concert with the cardiac effects. There clearly are effects of β-adrenergic blockers, particularly in higher doses, that do not seem to be dependent on renin. A number of mechanisms have been postulated to account for a non-renin-dependent reduction in blood pressure, including alteration of the control of the sympathetic nervous system at the level of the CNS, a change in baroreceptor sensitivity, an alteration in peripheral adrenergic neuron function, and an increase in prostacyclin biosynthesis. Because all β-adrenergic antagonists are effective antihypertensive agents and (+)-propranolol, which has little β-adrenergic receptor blocking activity, has no effect on blood pressure, the antihypertensive therapeutic effect of these agents is undoubtedly related to blockade of β-adrenergic receptors.

Pharmacological Effects. The β-adrenergic blockers vary in their lipid solubility, selectivity for the β_1-adrenergic receptor subtype, presence of partial agonist or intrinsic sympathomimetic activity, and membrane-stabilizing properties. Regardless of these differences, all of the β-adrenergic receptor antagonists are equally effective as antihypertensive agents. Drugs without intrinsic sympathomimetic activity produce an initial reduction in cardiac output and a reflex-induced rise in peripheral resistance with no net change in arterial pressure. In patients who respond with a reduction in blood pressure, peripheral resistance returns to pretreatment values in a few hours to a few days. It is this delayed normalization of vascular resistance in the face of a persistently reduced cardiac output that accounts for the reduction in arterial pressure (van den Meiracker *et al.*, 1988). Drugs with intrinsic sympathomimetic activity produce less of an effect on resting heart rate and cardiac output, and the fall in arterial pressure is correlated with a fall in vascular resistance below pretreatment levels, possibly because of stimulation of vascular β_2-adrenergic receptors that mediate vasodilation.

Renal blood flow is reduced in the short term by most β-adrenergic antagonists, but reports of deterioration of renal function associated with long-term administration of these drugs are rare. Nevertheless, small reductions in renal plasma flow and glomerular filtration rate may persist, particularly with the nonselective drugs that block both β_1- and β_2-adrenergic receptors.

Adverse Effects and Precautions. The adverse effects of β-adrenergic blocking agents are discussed in Chapter 10. These drugs should be avoided in patients with reactive airway disease (asthma) or with sinoatrial or atrioventricular nodal dysfunction. β-Adrenergic receptor antagonists should not be the initial drugs employed in hypertensive patients with cardiac failure because of the deleterious combination of a drop in myocardial contractility in conjuction with a rise in peripheral vascular resistance. After the cardiac failure has been addressed diagnostically and therapeutically, including the reduction of peripheral vascular resistance with another drug, β-blockers may then be considered as rational components of long-term antihypertensive therapy. Patients with insulin-dependent diabetes also are better treated with other drugs.

β-Adrenergic receptor antagonists without intrinsic sympathomimetic activity increase concentrations of triglycerides in plasma and lower those of HDL cholesterol without changing total cholesterol concentrations. β-Adrenergic blocking agents with intrinsic sympathomimetic activity have little or no effect on blood lipids or increase HDL cholesterol. The long-term consequences of these effects are unknown.

Sudden discontinuation of some β-adrenergic blockers can produce a withdrawal syndrome that is reminiscent of sympathetic hyperactivity; this can exacerbate the symptoms of coronary artery disease. Rebound hypertension to levels higher than those that existed before treatment has been noted with discontinuation of β-adrenergic receptor antagonists in hypertensive patients (Houston and Hodge, 1988). Thus, β-adrenergic blockers should not be discontinued abruptly except under close observation; dosage should be tapered over 10 to 14 days prior to discontinuation.

Nonsteroidal antiinflammatory drugs such as indomethacin can blunt the antihypertensive effect of propranolol and probably other β-adrenergic receptor antagonists. This effect may be related to inhibition of vascular synthesis of prostacyclin, as well as to retention of Na^+ (Beckmann et al., 1988).

Epinephrine can produce severe hypertension and bradycardia when a nonselective β-adrenergic receptor antagonist is present. This is due to the unopposed stimulation of α-adrenergic receptors when vascular β_2-receptors are blocked, and the bradycardia is the result of reflex vagal stimulation. Such "paradoxical" hypertensive responses to β-adrenergic receptor antagonists have been observed in patients with hypoglycemia or pheochromocytoma or during withdrawal from clonidine or administration of epinephrine as a therapeutic agent.

Therapeutic Uses. The β-adrenergic receptor antagonists provide effective therapy for all grades of hypertension. Despite marked differences in their pharmacokinetic properties, the antihypertensive effect of all the β blockers is of sufficient duration to permit twice daily administration. Populations that have a lesser antihypertensive response to β-blocking agents include the elderly and African Americans, but some individuals in these groups may have an excellent response. The β-adrenergic receptor antagonists do not usually cause retention of salt and water, and administration of a diuretic is not necessary to avoid edema or the development of tolerance. However, diuretics do have additive antihypertensive effects when combined with β blockers. The combination of a β-adrenergic receptor antagonist, a diuretic, and a vasodilator is effective for patients who require a third drug. When minoxidil is the vasodilator, this combination can control the arterial pressure of most patients, even if they are resistant to other regimens.

α_1-Adrenergic Receptor Antagonists

The development of drugs that selectively block α_1-adrenergic receptors without affecting α_2-adrenergic receptors has added another group of antihypertensive agents. The pharmacology of these drugs is discussed in detail in Chapter 10. *Prazosin* (MINIPRESS), *terazosin* (HYTRIN), and *doxazosin* (CARDURA) are the agents that are available for the treatment of hypertension. Additionally, investigational drugs such as ketanserin, indoramin, and urapidil may owe a major portion of their antihypertensive effects to blockade of α_1-adrenergic receptors (Cubeddu, 1988).

Pharmacological Effects. Initially, the α_1-adrenergic receptor antagonists reduce arteriolar resistance and venous capacitance; this causes a sympathetically mediated reflex increase in heart rate and plasma renin activity. During long-term therapy, vasodilation persists, but cardiac output, heart rate, and plasma renin activity return to normal. Renal blood flow is unchanged during therapy with an α_1-adrenergic receptor antagonist. The α_1-adrenergic blockers cause a variable amount of postural hypotension, depending on the plasma volume. Retention of salt and water occurs in many patients during continued administration, and this attenuates the postural hypotension. α_1-Adrenergic receptor antagonists reduce plasma concentrations of triglycerides and total and LDL cholesterol and increase HDL cholesterol. These potentially favorable effects on lipids persist when a thiazide-type diuretic is given concurrently. The long-term consequences of these small, drug-induced changes in lipids are unknown.

Adverse Effects. The use of doxazosin as monotherapy for hypertension increases the risk for developing congestive heart failure. There is every reason to assume that this is a "class effect" and represents an adverse effect of all of the α_1-adrenergic receptor antagonists.

A major precaution regarding the use of the α_1-adrenergic receptor antagonists for hypertension is the so-called first-dose phenomenon—symptomatic orthostatic hypotension that occurs within 90 minutes of the initial dose of the drug or when the dosage is increased rapidly. This effect may be seen in up to 50% of patients, and it is particularly likely to occur in patients who are already receiving a diuretic or a β-adrenergic receptor antagonist. After the first few doses, patients develop a tolerance to this marked hypotensive response.

Therapeutic Uses. Because α_1-adrenergic receptor antagonists increase the risk of cardiac failure, they are not recommended as monotherapy for hypertensive patients. Thus, they are used primarily in conjunction with diuretics, β-adrenergic receptor blockers, and other antihypertensive agents. β-Adrenergic receptor antagonists enhance the efficacy of the α_1 blockers. α_1-Adrenergic receptor antagonists are not the drugs of choice in patients with pheochromocytoma, because a vasoconstrictor response to epinephrine can still result from activation of unblocked vascular α_2-adrenergic receptors.

Combined α_1- and β-Adrenergic Receptor Antagonists

Labetalol (NORMODYNE, TRANDATE) (*see* Chapter 10) is an equimolar mixture of four stereoisomers. One isomer is an α_1-adrenergic receptor antagonist (like prazosin), another is a nonselective β-adrenergic receptor antagonist with partial agonist activity (like pindolol), and the other two isomers are inactive. The isomer that is the β-adrenergic receptor antagonist has been under development as a separate drug (*dilevalol*) (Lund-Johansen, 1988). Labetalol lowers arterial pressure by reducing vascular resistance as a consequence of blockade of α_1-adrenergic receptors and stimulation of β_2-adrenergic receptors. Cardiac output at rest is not reduced. Because of its capacity to block α_1-adrenergic receptors, labetalol given intravenously can reduce pressure sufficiently rapidly to be useful for the treatment of hypertensive emergencies. Given over the long term, labetalol has efficacy and side effects that would be expected with any combination of β- and α_1-adrenergic receptor antagonists; it also has the disadvantages that are inherent in fixed-dose combination products.

Carvedilol (COREG) (*see* Chapter 10) is a β-adrenergic receptor antagonist with α_1-adrenergic receptor antagonist activity that has been approved for the treatment of essential hypertension and for the treatment of symptomatic heart failure. The ratio of α_1- to β-adrenergic receptor antagonist potency for carvedilol is 1:10. Carvedilol undergoes oxidative metabolism and glucuronidation in the liver; the oxidative metabolism oc-

curs *via* cytochrome CYP2D6. Carvedilol has been shown to reduce mortality in patients with systolic dysfunction and New York Heart Association class I, II, or III symptoms when used as an adjunct to therapy with diuretics and angiotensin converting enzyme inhibitors. It should not be given to those patients with decompensated heart failure who are dependent on sympathetic stimulation. As with labetalol, the long-term efficacy and side effects of carvedilol in hypertension are predictable based on its properties as a β- and α_1-adrenergic receptor antagonist. In addition, mild reversible hepatocellular injury has been reported with carvedilol.

VASODILATORS

Hydralazine

Hydralazine (APRESOLINE) was one of the first orally active antihypertensive drugs to be marketed in the United States; however, the drug initially was used infrequently because of tachycardia and tachyphylaxis. With a better understanding of the compensatory cardiovascular responses that accompany use of arteriolar vasodilators, hydralazine was combined with sympatholytic agents and diuretics with greater therapeutic success. Numerous phthalazines have been synthesized in the hope of producing vasoactive agents, but only those with hydrazine moieties in the 1 or 4 position of the ring have vasodilatory activity (Reece, 1981). None of the analogs has any advantage over hydralazine. Hydralazine (1-hydrazinophthalazine) has the following structural formula:

HYDRALAZINE

Locus and Mechanism of Action. Hydralazine causes direct relaxation of arteriolar smooth muscle. The molecular mechanism of this effect is not known. It is not a dilator of capacitance vessels (*e.g.,* the epicardial coronary arteries) and does not relax venous smooth muscle. Hydralazine-induced vasodilation is associated with powerful stimulation of the sympathetic nervous system, which results in increased heart rate and contractility, increased plasma renin activity, and fluid retention; all of these effects counteract the antihypertensive effect of hydralazine. Although most of the sympathetic activity is due to a baroreceptor-mediated reflex, hydralazine may stimulate the release of norepinephrine from sympathetic nerve terminals and augment myocardial contractility directly (Azuma *et al.,* 1987).

Pharmacological Effects. Most of the effects of hydralazine are confined to the cardiovascular system. The decrease in blood pressure after administration of hydralazine is associated with a selective decrease in vascular resistance in the coronary, cerebral, and renal circulations, with a smaller effect in skin and muscle. Because of preferential dilation of arterioles over veins, postural hypotension is not a common problem; hydralazine lowers blood pressure equally in the supine and upright positions. Although hydralazine lowers pulmonary vascular resistance, the greater increase in cardiac output can cause mild pulmonary hypertension. It is difficult to predict which patients will respond in this manner, but the increase in cardiac output can be attenuated by the use of β-adrenergic receptor blocking agents.

Absorption, Metabolism, and Excretion. Hydralazine is *N*-acetylated in the bowel and/or the liver. The rate of acetylation is genetically determined; about half of the people in the United States acetylate rapidly and half do so slowly. Since the acetylated compound is inactive, the dose necessary to produce a systemic effect is larger in fast acetylators. Hydralazine is well absorbed through the gastrointestinal tract, but the systemic bioavailability is low (16% in fast acetylators and 35% in slow acetylators). The half-life of hydralazine is 1 hour, and the systemic clearance of the drug is about 50 ml/kg per minute. Since the systemic clearance exceeds hepatic blood flow, extrahepatic metabolism must occur. Indeed, hydralazine rapidly combines with circulating α-keto acids to form hydrazones, and the major metabolite recovered from the plasma is hydralazine pyruvic acid hydrazone. This metabolite has a longer half-life than hydralazine, but it does not appear to be very active (Reece *et al.*, 1985). Although the rate of acetylation is an important determinant of the bioavailability of hydralazine, it does not play a role in the systemic elimination of the drug, probably because the hepatic clearance is so high that systemic elimination is principally a function of hepatic blood flow.

The peak concentration of hydralazine in plasma and the peak hypotensive effect of the drug occur within 30 to 120 minutes of ingestion. Although its half-life in plasma is about an hour, the duration of the hypotensive effect of hydralazine can last as long as 12 hours. There is no clear explanation for this discrepancy.

Toxicity and Precautions. Two types of side effects occur after the use of hydralazine. The first, which are extensions of the pharmacological effects of the drug, include headache, nausea, flushing, hypotension, palpitation, tachycardia, dizziness, and angina pectoris. Myocardial ischemia occurs because of the increased oxygen demand imposed by the baroreflex-induced stimulation of the sympathetic nervous system and also because hydralazine does not dilate the epicardial coronary arteries; thus, the arteriolar dilation it produces may cause a "steal" of blood flow away from the ischemic region. Following parenteral administration to patients with coronary artery disease, the myocardial ischemia may be sufficiently severe and protracted to cause frank myocardial infarction. For this reason, parenteral administration of hydralazine is contraindicated in hypertensive patients with coronary artery disease and inadvisable for most hypertensive patients over 40 years old. In addition, if the drug is used alone, there may be salt retention with development of high-output congestive heart failure. These symptoms were common during the early clinical use of hydralazine; because tachyphylaxis developed, the daily dose of the drug was frequently increased to 400 to 1000 mg. When combined with a β-adrenergic receptor blocker and a diuretic, hydralazine is better tolerated, although side effects such as headache are still commonly described and may necessitate discontinuation of the drug.

The second type of side effect is caused by immunological reactions, of which the drug-induced lupus syndrome is the most common. Administration of hydralazine also can result in an illness that resembles serum sickness, hemolytic anemia, vasculitis, and rapidly progressive glomerulonephritis. The mechanism of these autoimmune reactions is unknown, but hydralazine has been shown to inhibit methylation of DNA and induce self-reactivity in T cells (Cornacchia *et al.*, 1988).

The drug-induced lupus syndrome usually occurs after at least 6 months of continuous treatment with hydralazine, and its incidence is related to dose, sex, acetylator phenotype, and race (Perry, 1973). In one study, after three years of treatment with hydralazine, drug-induced lupus occurred in 10.4% of patients who received 200 mg daily, 5.4% who received 100 mg daily, and none who received 50 mg daily (Cameron and Ramsay, 1984). The incidence is four times higher in women than in men, and the syndrome is seen more commonly in Caucasians than in African Americans. The rate of conversion to a positive antinuclear antibody test is faster in slow acetylators than in rapid acetylators, suggesting that the native drug or a nonacetylated metabolite is responsible. However, since the majority of patients with positive antinuclear antibody tests do not develop the drug-induced lupus syndrome, hydralazine need not be discontinued unless clinical features of the syndrome appear. These features are similar to those of other drug-induced lupus syndromes and consist mainly of arthralgia, arthritis, and fever. Pleuritis and pericarditis may be present, and pericardial effusion can occasionally cause cardiac tamponade. Discontinuation of the drug is all that is necessary for most patients with the hydralazine-induced lupus syndrome, but symptoms may persist in a few patients and administration of corticosteroids may be necessary.

Hydralazine also can produce a pyridoxine-responsive polyneuropathy. The mechanism appears to be related to the ability of hydralazine to combine with pyridoxine to form a hydrazone. This side effect is very unusual with doses up to 200 mg per day.

Therapeutic Uses.   Hydralazine generally is not used as the sole drug for the long-term treatment of hypertension because of the development of tachyphylaxis secondary to an increase in cardiac output and fluid retention. In addition, the drug should be used with the greatest of caution in elderly patients and in hypertensive patients with coronary artery disease because of the possibility of precipitation of myocardial ischemia. The usual oral dosage of hydralazine is 25 to 100 mg twice daily. Twice-daily administration is as effective as administration four times a day for control of blood pressure, regardless of acetylator phenotype. The maximum recommended dose of hydralazine is 200 mg per day to minimize drug-induced lupus syndrome. Slow acetylators show a better response to this dosage than do fast acetylators because of the greater bioavailability of the drug.

Hydralazine has been used widely to treat hypertension that occurs during pregnancy. However, the drug should be used cautiously during early pregnancy, since hydralazine can combine with DNA and cause a positive Ames test (Williams *et al.,* 1980). Parenteral administration of hydralazine has been used for the treatment of hypertensive emergencies in pregnancy, but is not recommended for the treatment of hypertensive emergencies in patients in the age range for coronary artery disease. The drug is contraindicated for the short-term production of hypotension in patients with dissecting aortic aneurysm or in those with symptomatic ischemic heart disease.

Minoxidil

The discovery in 1965 of the hypotensive action of *minoxidil* (LONITEN) was a significant advance in the treatment of hypertension, since the drug has proven to be efficacious in patients with the most severe and drug-resistant forms of hypertension. The chemical structure of minoxidil is as follows:

MINOXIDIL

Locus and Mechanism of Action.   Minoxidil is not active *in vitro* but must be metabolized by hepatic sulfotransferase to the active molecule, minoxidil *N-O* sulfate (McCall *et al.,* 1983); the formation of this active metabolite is a minor pathway in the metabolic disposition of minoxidil. Minoxidil sulfate relaxes vascular smooth muscle in isolated systems where the parent drug is inactive. Minoxidil sulfate activates the ATP-modulated potassium channel. By opening potassium channels in smooth muscle and thereby permitting potassium efflux, it causes hyperpolarization and relaxation of smooth muscle (Leblanc *et al.,* 1989).

Pharmacological Effects.   Minoxidil produces arteriolar vasodilation with essentially no effect on the capacitance vessels; the drug resembles hydralazine and diazoxide in this regard. Minoxidil increases blood flow to skin, skeletal muscle, the gastrointestinal tract, and the heart more than to the CNS. The disproportionate increase in blood flow to the heart may have a metabolic basis, in that administration of minoxidil is associated with a reflex increase in myocardial contractility and in cardiac output. The cardiac output can increase markedly, as much as three- to fourfold. The principal determinant of the elevation in cardiac output is the action of minoxidil on peripheral vascular resistance to enhance venous return to the heart; by inference from studies with other drugs, the increased venous return probably results from enhancement of flow in the regional vascular beds with a fast time constant for venous return to the heart (Ogilvie, 1985). The adrenergically mediated increase in myocardial contractility contributes to the increased cardiac output, but is not the predominant causal factor.

The effects of minoxidil on the kidney are complex. Minoxidil is a renal vasodilator, but systemic hypotension produced by the drug occasionally can decrease renal blood flow. However, in the majority of patients who take minoxidil for the treatment of hypertension, renal function improves, especially if renal dysfunction is secondary to hypertension (Mitchell *et al.,* 1980). Minoxidil is a very potent stimulator of renin secretion; this effect is mediated by a combination of renal sympathetic stimulation and activation of the intrinsic renal mechanisms for regulation of renin release.

Absorption, Metabolism, and Excretion.   Minoxidil is well absorbed from the gastrointestinal tract. Although peak concentrations of minoxidil in blood occur 1 hour after oral administration, the maximal hypotensive effect of the drug occurs later, possibly because formation of the active metabolite is delayed. Only about 20% of the absorbed drug is excreted unchanged in the urine, and the main route of elimination is by hepatic metabolism. The major metabolite of minoxidil is the glucuronide conjugate at the *N*-oxide position in the pyrimidine ring. This metabolite is less active than minoxidil, but it persists longer in the body. The extent of biotransformation of minoxidil to its active metabolite, minoxidil *N-O* sulfate, has not been evaluated in human beings. Minoxidil has a half-life in plasma of 3 to 4 hours, but its duration of action is 24 hours or occasionally even longer. It has been proposed that persistence of minoxidil in vascular smooth muscle is responsible for this discrepancy. However, without knowledge of the pharmacokinetic properties of the active metabolite, an explanation for the prolonged duration of action cannot be given.

Adverse Effects and Precautions.   The adverse effects of minoxidil are predictable and can be divided into three major categories: fluid and salt retention, cardiovascular effects, and hypertrichosis.

Retention of salt and water results from increased proximal renal tubular reabsorption, which is in turn secondary to reduced renal perfusion pressure and to reflex stimulation of renal tubular α-adrenergic receptors. Similar antinatriuretic effects can be observed with the other arteriolar dilators (*e.g.,* diazoxide and hydralazine). Although administration of minoxidil causes increased secretion of renin and aldosterone, this is not an important mechanism for retention of salt and water in this case. Fluid retention usually can be controlled by the administration of a diuretic. However, thiazides may not be sufficiently efficacious, and it may be necessary to use a loop diuretic. This is especially true if the patient has any degree of renal dysfunction.

The cardiac consequences of the baroreceptor-mediated activation of the sympathetic nervous system during minoxidil therapy are similar to those seen with hydralazine; there is an increase in heart rate, myocardial contractility, and myocardial oxygen consumption. Thus, myocardial ischemia can be induced by minoxidil in patients with coronary artery disease. The cardiac sympathetic responses are attenuated by concurrent administration of a β-adrenergic blocker. The adrenergically induced increase in renin secretion also can be ameliorated by a β-adrenergic receptor antagonist or an angiotensin converting enzyme inhibitor, with enhancement of the blood pressure control.

The increased cardiac output evoked by minoxidil has particularly adverse consequences in those hypertensive patients who have left ventricular hypertrophy and diastolic dysfunction. Such poorly compliant ventricles

respond suboptimally to increased volume loads, with a resulting increase in left ventricular filling pressure. This probably is a major contributor to the increased pulmonary artery pressure seen with minoxidil (and hydralazine) therapy in hypertensive patients, and is compounded by the retention of salt and water caused by minoxidil. Cardiac failure can result from minoxidil therapy in such patients; the potential for this complication can be reduced but not prevented by effective diuretic therapy. Pericardial effusion is an uncommon but serious complication of minoxidil. Although more commonly described in patients with cardiac failure and renal failure, pericardial effusion can occur in patients with normal cardiovascular and renal function. Mild and asymptomatic pericardial effusion is not an indication for discontinuing minoxidil, but the situation should be monitored closely to avoid progression to tamponade. Effusion usually clears when the drug is discontinued, but it will recur if treatment with minoxidil is resumed (Reichgott, 1981).

Flattened and inverted T waves frequently are observed in the electrocardiogram following the initiation of minoxidil treatment. These are not ischemic in origin and are seen with other drugs that activate potassium channels. These drugs accelerate myocardial repolarization, shorten the refractory period, and one of them, pinacidil, lowers the ventricular fibrillation threshold and increases spontaneous ventricular fibrillation in the setting of myocardial ischemia (Chi *et al.,* 1990). The effect of minoxidil on the refractory period and ischemic ventricular fibrillation has not been investigated; whether or not such findings enhance the risk of ventricular fibrillation in human myocardial ischemia is unknown.

Hypertrichosis occurs in all patients who receive minoxidil for an extended period and is probably a consequence of potassium channel activation. Growth of hair occurs on the face, back, arms, and legs and is particularly offensive to women. Frequent shaving or depilatory agents can be used to manage this problem. Topical minoxidil (ROGAINE) is now marketed for the treatment of male-pattern baldness. The topical use of minoxidil can cause measurable cardiovascular effects in some individuals (Leenen *et al.,* 1988).

Other side effects of the drug are rare and include rashes, Stevens–Johnson syndrome, glucose intolerance, serosanguinous bullae, formation of antinuclear antibodies, and thrombocytopenia.

Therapeutic Uses.   Minoxidil is best reserved for the treatment of severe hypertension that responds poorly to other antihypertensive medications (Campese, 1981). It has been used successfully in the treatment of hypertension in both adults and children. Minoxidil should never be used alone; it must be given concurrently with a diuretic to avoid fluid retention and with a sympatholytic drug (usually a β-adrenergic receptor antagonist) to control reflex cardiovascular effects. The drug usually is administered either once or twice a day, but some patients may require more frequent dosage for adequate control of blood pressure. The initial daily dose of minoxidil may be as little as 1.25 mg, which can be increased gradually to 40 mg in one or two daily doses.

Sodium Nitroprusside

Although *sodium nitroprusside* has been known since 1850 and its hypotensive effect in human beings was described in 1929, its safety and usefulness for the short-term control of severe hypertension were not demonstrated until the mid-1950s. Several investigators subsequently demonstrated that sodium nitroprusside also was effective in improving cardiac function in patients with left ventricular failure (*see* Chapter 34). The structural formula of sodium nitroprusside is as follows:

$$2Na^+ \left[\begin{array}{c} CN \\ NC-Fe-CN \\ ON \end{array} \begin{array}{c} CN \\ CN \\ CN \end{array} \right]^{--}$$

SODIUM NITROPRUSSIDE

Locus and Mechanism of Action. Nitroprusside is a nitrovasodilator. It is metabolized by blood vessels to its active metabolite, nitric oxide. Nitric oxide activates guanylyl cyclase, leading to the formation of cyclic GMP and vasodilation (Murad, 1986). The metabolic activation of nitroprusside is catalyzed by a different nitric oxide–generating system than that for nitroglycerin, probably accounting for the difference in the potency of these drugs at different vascular sites and the fact that tolerance develops to nitroglycerin but not to nitroprusside (Kowaluk *et al.*, 1992).

Pharmacological Effects. Nitroprusside dilates both arterioles and venules, and the hemodynamic response to its administration results from a combination of venous pooling and reduced arterial impedance. Because of its effect on venules, the hypotensive effect of sodium nitroprusside is greater when the patient is upright. In subjects with normal left ventricular function, venous pooling affects cardiac output more than does the reduction of afterload; cardiac output thus tends to fall. In contrast, in patients with severely impaired left ventricular function

and diastolic ventricular distention, the reduction of arterial impedance is the predominant effect, leading to a rise in cardiac output (*see* Chapter 34).

Sodium nitroprusside is a nonselective vasodilator, and regional distribution of blood flow is little affected by the drug. In general, renal blood flow and glomerular filtration are maintained, and plasma renin activity increases. Unlike minoxidil, hydralazine, diazoxide, and other arteriolar vasodilators, sodium nitroprusside usually causes only a modest increase in heart rate and an overall reduction in myocardial demand for oxygen.

Absorption, Metabolism, and Excretion. Sodium nitroprusside is an unstable molecule that decomposes under strongly alkaline conditions and when exposed to light. The drug must be given by continuous intravenous infusion to be effective. Its onset of action is within 30 seconds; the peak hypotensive effect occurs within 2 minutes, and when the infusion of the drug is stopped, the effect disappears within 3 minutes.

The metabolism of nitroprusside by smooth muscle is initiated by its reduction, which is followed by the release of cyanide and then nitric oxide (Bates *et al.*, 1991; Ivankovich *et al.*, 1978). Cyanide is further metabolized by liver rhodanase to thiocyanate, which is eliminated almost entirely in the urine. The mean elimination half-time for thiocyanate is 3 days in patients with normal renal function, and it can be much longer in patients with renal insufficiency.

Toxicity and Precautions. The short-term side effects of nitroprusside are due to excessive vasodilation, with hypotension and the consequences thereof. Close monitoring of blood pressure and the use of a continuous variable-rate infusion pump will prevent an excessive hemodynamic response to the drug in the majority of cases. Less commonly, toxicity may result from conversion of nitroprusside to cyanide and thiocyanate. Toxic accumulation of cyanide leading to severe lactic acidosis can occur usually if sodium nitroprusside is infused at a rate greater than 5 μg/kg per minute, but such toxicity can occur in some patients receiving doses about 2 μg/kg per minute. The limiting factor in the metabolism of cyanide appears to be the availability of sulfur-containing substrates in the body (mainly thiosulfate). The concomitant administration of sodium thiosulfate can prevent accumulation of cyanide in patients who are receiving higher than usual doses of sodium nitroprusside; the efficacy of the drug is unchanged (Schulz, 1984). The risk of thiocyanate toxicity increases when sodium nitroprusside is infused for more than 24 to 48 hours, especially if renal function is impaired. Signs and symptoms of thiocyanate toxicity include anorexia, nausea, fatigue, disorientation, and toxic psychosis. The plasma concentration of thiocyanate should be monitored during prolonged infusions of nitroprusside and should not be allowed to exceed 0.1 mg/ml. Rarely, excessive concentrations of thiocyanate may cause hypothyroidism by inhibiting iodine uptake by the thyroid gland. In patients with renal failure, thiocyanate can be removed readily by hemodialysis.

Nitroprusside can worsen arterial hypoxemia in patients with chronic obstructive pulmonary disease because the drug interferes with hypoxic pulmonary vasoconstriction and therefore promotes mismatching of ventilation with perfusion. Rebound hypertension may occur after abrupt cessation of short-term nitroprusside infusions (Packer *et al.,* 1979); this may be caused by persistently elevated concentrations of renin in the plasma.

Therapeutic Uses. Sodium nitroprusside is used primarily to treat hypertensive emergencies, but the drug can be used in many situations when short-term reduction of cardiac preload and/or afterload is desired. Thus, nitroprusside has been used to lower blood pressure during acute aortic dissection, to increase cardiac output in congestive heart failure (*see* Chapter 34), and to decrease myocardial oxygen demand after acute myocardial infarction. In addition, nitroprusside is the drug most often used to induce controlled hypotension during anesthesia in order to reduce bleeding in surgical procedures. In the treatment of acute aortic dissection, it is important to administer a β-adrenergic receptor antagonist with nitroprusside, since reduction of blood pressure with nitroprusside alone can increase the rate of rise in pressure in the aorta as a result of increased myocardial contractility, thereby enhancing propagation of the dissection.

Sodium nitroprusside is available in vials that contain 50 mg. The contents of the vial should be dissolved in 2 to 3 ml of 5% dextrose in water. Addition of this solution to 250 to 1000 ml of 5% dextrose in water produces a concentration of 50 to 200 μg/ml. Because the compound decomposes in light, only fresh solutions should be used, and the bottle should be covered with an opaque wrapping. The drug must be administered as a controlled, continuous infusion, and the patient must be closely observed. The majority of hypertensive patients respond to an infusion of 0.25 to 1.5 μg/kg per minute. Higher rates of infusion are necessary to produce controlled hypotension in normotensive patients under surgical anesthesia. Infusion of nitroprusside at rates exceeding 5 μg/kg per minute over a prolonged period can cause cyanide and/or thiocyanate poisoning. Patients who are receiving other antihypertensive medications usually require less nitroprusside to lower blood pressure. If infusion rates of 10 μg/kg per minute do not produce adequate reduction of blood pressure within 10 minutes, the rate of

administration of nitroprusside should be reduced to minimize potential toxicity.

Diazoxide

Diazoxide (HYPERSTAT IV) is used in the treatment of hypertensive emergencies. Sodium nitroprusside is the drug of choice for this indication, but diazoxide maintains a place in the treatment of hypertensive emergencies in situations in which accurate infusion pumps are not available and/or close monitoring of blood pressure is not feasible. The drug is a benzothiadiazine derivative, like the thiazide diuretics, but it does not cause diuresis, apparently because it lacks a sulfonamido group. Its structural formula is as follows:

DIAZOXIDE

Mechanism of Action and Pharmacological Effects. Diazoxide hyperpolarizes arterial smooth muscle cells by activating ATP-sensitive K^+ channels; this causes relaxation of the vascular smooth muscle (Standen *et al.,* 1989). The effect of the drug *in vivo* is exclusively arteriolar, with negligible effect on capacitance vessels. This produces substantial reflex activation of the sympathetic nervous system. Cardiac output may double from stimulation of heart rate and myocardial contractility. The avid retention of salt and water is probably a result of stimulation of renal sympathetic nerves and changes in intrarenal hemodynamics, as with other arteriolar vasodilators. Diazoxide increases coronary blood flow, and cerebral and renal blood flows are maintained by autoregulation. Renin secretion is enhanced, and the combination of an increased cardiac output, salt and water retention, and elevated concentrations of angiotensin II counteract the antihypertensive effects of diazoxide.

Absorption, Metabolism, and Excretion. Although well absorbed orally, diazoxide is administered only intravenously for the treatment of severe hypertension. Approximately 20% to 50% of the drug is eliminated as such by the kidney, and the rest is metabolized in the liver to the 3-hydroxymethyl and 3-carboxy derivatives (Pruitt *et al.,* 1974). Although the plasma half-life of diazoxide is 20 to 60 hours, the duration of the hypotensive response to the drug is variable and can be as short as 4 hours or as long as 20 hours; the development of a brisk rise in renin secretion may antagonize the early hypotensive effect of diazoxide.

The main indication for the use of diazoxide is for the treatment of hypertensive emergencies. Injection of an intravenous bolus lowers blood pressure within 30 seconds, and a maximum effect is achieved within 3 to 5 minutes. Although initial recommendations were to administer a 300-mg bolus of diazoxide, excessive hypotension with resultant cerebral and cardiovascular damage has resulted from this practice. Hypotension can be minimized by the administration of a "minibolus" of 50 to 150 mg at intervals of 5 to 15 minutes until the desired blood pressure is achieved (Wilson and Vidt, 1978). Diazoxide also can be given by slow intravenous infusion at a rate of 15 to 30 mg per minute (Garrett and Kaplan, 1982). Prior administration of a β-adrenergic receptor antagonist will enhance the hypotensive effect of the drug. Diazoxide should not be used to treat hypertension associated with aortic coarctation, arteriovenous shunts, or aortic dissection. Similarly, risks outweigh benefits in its use for acute pulmonary edema and ischemic heart disease.

Adverse Effects and Precautions. The most common side effects caused by diazoxide are myocardial ischemia, salt and water retention, and hyperglycemia. Myocardial ischemia may be precipitated or aggravated by diazoxide, and it results from the reflex adrenergic stimulation of the heart and from increased flow to nonischemic regions that "steal" blood flow from the regions supplied by stenotic vessels. Retention of fluid can be avoided by restriction of salt and water. The routine use of diuretic agents with diazoxide is not recommended because patients with malignant hypertension are frequently volume-depleted. Hyperglycemia results from diazoxide's capacity to inhibit the secretion of insulin from pancreatic β cells. This effect also appears to result from stimulation of ATP-sensitive K^+ channels (Zünkler et al., 1988). The drug does not alter the response to administration of insulin. Thus, hyperglycemia is mainly a problem in non-insulin-dependent diabetic patients who are being treated with oral hypoglycemic agents. Severe hyperglycemia with hyperosmolar, nonketotic coma has been described. Cerebral ischemia may be caused by excessive hypotension. Diazoxide relaxes uterine smooth muscle and may arrest labor when used to treat the hypertensive crisis of eclampsia. Rare side effects include gastrointestinal disturbances, flushing, local pain and inflammation after extravasation, altered ability to taste and smell, excessive salivation, and dyspnea.

Ca^{2+}-CHANNEL ANTAGONISTS

Ca^{2+}-channel blocking agents are an important group of drugs for the treatment of hypertension. The general pharmacology of these drugs is presented in Chapter 32; their use in heart failure is discussed in Chapter 34; and their use in cardiac arrhythmia is covered in Chapter 35. The logic behind their use in hypertension comes from the understanding that fixed hypertension is the result of increased peripheral vascular resistance. Since contraction of vascular smooth muscle is dependent on the free intracellular concentration of Ca^{2+}, inhibition of transmembrane movement of Ca^{2+} should decrease the total amount of Ca^{2+} that reaches intracellular sites. Indeed, all of the Ca^{2+}-channel blockers lower blood pressure by relaxing arteriolar smooth muscle and decreasing peripheral vascular resistance (Lehmann et al., 1983). As a consequence of a decrease in peripheral vascular resistance, the Ca^{2+}-channel blockers evoke a baroreceptor-mediated sympathetic discharge. In the case of the dihydropyridines, mild to moderate tachycardia ensues from the adrenergic stimulation of the sinoatrial node, whereas tachycardia is minimal to absent with verapamil and diltiazem because of the direct negative chronotropic effect of these two drugs.

The increased adrenergic stimulation of the heart serves to counter the negative inotropic effect of Ca^{2+}-channel blockers such as *verapamil, diltiazem,* and *nifedipine;* the importance of this compensatory support of myocardial contractility should be considered in decisions regarding possible concurrent use of β-adrenergic receptor antagonists, particularly in patients who may be prone to hypertensive cardiac failure. The adrenergic reflex response to Ca^{2+}-channel blockers also acts to attenuate the hypotensive effect of these drugs; thus, when the reflex vasoconstriction is diminished, as in the elderly or during treatment with α-adrenergic receptor antagonists, the hypotensive effect of the Ca^{2+}-channel blockers is increased, sometimes excessively.

In considering the cardiovascular effects of the Ca^{2+}-channel blockers, it is essential to evaluate both the hemodynamic effects in the normal heart and the interaction of these drugs with cardiac disease, given that both cardiac failure and coronary artery diseases are important consequences of hypertension and that left ventricular hypertrophy is a harbinger for sudden cardiac death in hypertensive patients. As a consequence of the peripheral vasodilation, Ca^{2+}-channel blockers may increase venous return, which will result in an increased cardiac output except in the case of those that exert substantial negative inotropic effects (e.g., verapamil and diltiazem). The increased venous return is not as great as with minoxidil or hydralazine, but is a consideration in the management of patients with diastolic dysfunction due to hypertensive cardiomyopathy who are at risk of left ventricular failure. The Ca^{2+}-channel blockers do not improve the diastolic function of the ventricle. Although earlier noninvasive studies had demonstrated that peak filling rates of the left ventricle of hypertensive patients were shortened by Ca^{2+}-channel blockers, direct hemodynamic evaluation of ventricular function has demonstrated that verapamil causes an increase in left ventricular end-diastolic pressure, an undesirable hemodynamic consequence that occurs in conjunction with, and probably as a contributor to, the acceleration of peak filling rate (Nishimura et al., 1993).

In addition to these findings that Ca^{2+}-channel blockers do not improve and have the potential for worsening the hemodynamics in diastolic dysfunction, the long-term effects of the Ca^{2+}-channel blockers on left ventricular hypertrophy, a major contributor to diastolic dysfunction, should be considered. An overview of all trials evaluating the effects of antihypertensive agents on left ventricular mass concludes that, although Ca^{2+}-channel blockers do reduce left ventricular mass and do so more effectively than diuretics, they are less effective than angiotensin converting enzyme inhibitors and methyldopa (Dalhöf *et al.,* 1993). Based on the sum of this evidence, Ca^{2+}-channel blockers probably are not the first choice as the initial drug in the treatment of patients whose hypertension is accompanied by left ventricular hypertrophy nor as the predominant drug in a combination for their treatment.

All Ca^{2+}-channel blockers are equally effective when used alone for the treatment of mild to moderate hypertension; and in comparative trials, Ca^{2+}-channel blockers are as effective in lowering blood pressure as β-adrenergic receptor antagonists or diuretics (Doyle, 1983; Inouye *et al.,* 1984).

The presence of ischemic heart disease in conjunction with hypertension raises a special set of concerns regarding some of the Ca^{2+}-channel blockers. Dihydropyridine Ca^{2+}-channel blockers do not improve survival in patients following myocardial infarction. Neither verapamil nor diltiazem improves mortality in the entire group of postinfarction patients. Data suggesting that diltiazem may exert a favorable effect on mortality in the subset of patients who exhibit no abnormality in systolic ventricular function does not form a strong basis for its use in such patients because of the *post hoc* selection of this group for analysis (Multicenter Diltiazem Postinfarction Trial Research Group, 1988). This is in contrast to the clear benefit to the survival of patients after myocardial infarction that is conferred by treatment with β-adrenergic receptor antagonists and angiotensin converting enzyme inhibitors. Accordingly, the Ca^{2+}-channel blockers are not the initial or even the second drugs to be used in the treatment of the hypertension in patients who have had a myocardial infarction.

In diabetic patients with hypertension, the available evidence favors an angiotensin converting enzyme inhibitor as the initial antihypertensive drug (Estacio *et al.,* 1998), following which it is appropriate to consider adding a Ca^{2+}-channel blocker if a second drug is required.

The profile of adverse reactions to the Ca^{2+}-channel blockers varies among the drugs in this class, but only a small fraction of patients discontinue these drugs because of perceived adverse reactions. The dihydropyridines cause the highest incidence of vascular side effects. Approximately 10% of patients receiving the standard formulation of nifedipine (immediate-release capsules) develop headache, flushing, dizziness, and peripheral edema. Dizziness and flushing are much less of a problem with the sustained-release formulations and with the dihydropyridines having a long half-life and relatively constant concentrations of drug in plasma. The edema usually is not the result of fluid retention; it most likely results from increased hydrostatic pressure in the lower extremities owing to precapillary dilation and reflex postcapillary con-

striction. Contraction of the lower esophageal sphincter is inhibited by the Ca^{2+}-channel blockers. Accordingly, all Ca^{2+}-channel blockers can cause gastroesophageal reflux. Constipation is a common side effect of verapamil, but it occurs less frequently with other Ca^{2+}-channel blockers. Inhibition of sinoatrial node function by diltiazem and verapamil can lead to bradycardia and even sinoatrial node arrest, particularly in patients with sinoatrial node dysfunction; this effect is exaggerated by concurrent use of β-adrenergic receptor antagonists.

Oral administration of nifedipine as an approach to urgent reduction of blood pressure has been abandoned. Sublingual administration does not achieve the maximum plasma concentration any more quickly than does oral administration. Moreover, in the absence of deleterious consequences of high arterial pressure, data do not support the rapid lowering of blood pressure. Short-acting, parenterally administered agents should be used in the setting of hypertensive emergency. Nifedipine is a suboptimal choice for treatment of hypertensive pulmonary edema; nitroprusside produces a greater reduction in left ventricular end-diastolic pressure than do equihypotensive doses of nifedipine (Aroney *et al.,* 1991), and the magnitude of nitroprusside's pharmacological effect can be regulated more effectively. There is no place in the treatment of hypertension for the use of nifedipine or other dihydropyridine Ca^{2+}-channel blockers with short half-lives when administered in a standard (immediate release) formulation, because of the oscillation in blood pressure and concurrent surges in sympathetic reflex activity within each dosage interval.

Ca^{2+}-channel blockers are versatile drugs with proven efficacy in all types of patients (Kiowski *et al.,* 1985). They seem to be especially efficacious in low-renin hypertension. Compared with other classes of antihypertensive agents, there is a greater frequency of achieving blood pressure control with Ca^{2+}-channel blockers as monotherapy in elderly subjects and in African Americans, population groups in which the low renin status is more prevalent. Long-acting dihydropyridine Ca^{2+}-channel blockers have been found to reduce cardiovascular mortality in older patients (Staessen *et al.,* 1997). The efficacy of Ca^{2+}-channel blockers is enhanced by the concomitant use of an angiotensin converting enzyme inhibitor, methyldopa, or β-adrenergic receptor antagonists. When β-adrenergic receptor antagonists are administered concurrently, the preferred Ca^{2+}-channel blocker would be one from the group that is relatively vasoselective (*e.g.,* amlodipine, isradipine, nicardipine). Diuretics also may enhance the efficacy of Ca^{2+}-channel blockers, but the data have not been consistent.

Significant drug–drug interactions may be encountered when Ca^{2+}-channel blockers are used to treat hypertension. Verapamil blocks the drug transporter, P-glycoprotein. Both the renal and hepatic disposition of digoxin occur *via* this transporter. Accordingly, verapamil inhibits the elimination of digoxin and other drugs that are cleared from the body by the P-glycoprotein (*see* Chapter 1) (Pedersen *et al.,* 1981). When used with quinidine, Ca^{2+}-channel blockers may cause excessive hypotension, particularly in patients with idiopathic hypertrophic subaortic stenosis.

Ca^{2+}-channel blockers should not be used in patients with SA or AV nodal abnormalities or in patients with overt congestive heart failure. These drugs usually are safe, however, in hypertensive patients with asthma, hyperlipidemia, diabetes mellitus, and renal dysfunction. Unlike β-adrenergic receptor antagonists, Ca^{2+}-channel blockers do not alter exercise tolerance; nor do they alter plasma concentrations of lipids, uric acid, or electrolytes.

ANGIOTENSIN CONVERTING ENZYME INHIBITORS

Angiotensin II is an important regulator of cardiovascular function (*see* Chapter 31). The ability to reduce levels of angiotensin II with orally effective inhibitors of angiotensin converting enzyme (ACE) represents an important advance in the treatment of hypertension. *Captopril* (CAPOTEN) was the first such agent to be developed for the treatment of hypertension. Since then, *enalapril* (VASOTEC), *lisinopril* (PRINIVIL), *quinapril* (ACCUPRIL), *ramipril* (ALTACE), *benazepril* (LOTENSIN), *moexipril* (UNIVASC), *fosinopril* (MONOPRIL), *trandolapril* (MAVIK), and *perindopril* (ACEON) also have become available. These drugs have proven to be very useful for the treatment of hypertension because of their efficacy and their very favorable profile of side effects, which enhances compliance.

The angiotensin converting enzyme inhibitors appear to confer a special advantage in the treatment of patients with diabetes, slowing the development of diabetic glomerulopathy. They also have been shown to be effective in slowing the progression of other forms of chronic renal disease, such as glomerulosclerosis, and many of these patients also have hypertension. An angiotensin converting enzyme inhibitor is probably the preferred initial agent in the treatment of hypertensive patients with left ventricular hypertrophy. Patients with hypertension and ischemic heart disease are candidates for treatment with angiotensin converting enzyme inhibitors; this includes

treatment in the immediate post–myocardial infarction period which has been shown to lead to improved ventricular function and reduced morbidity and mortality (*see also* Chapter 34).

The endocrine consequences of inhibiting the biosynthesis of angiotensin II are of importance in a number of facets of hypertension treatment. Because angiotensin converting enzyme inhibitors blunt the normal aldosterone response to Na$^+$ loss, the normal role of aldosterone to oppose diuretic-induced natriuresis is diminished. Thus, angiotensin converting enzyme inhibitors enhance the efficacy of diuretic drugs. This means that even very small doses of diuretics may substantially improve the antihypertensive efficacy of angiotensin converting enzyme inhibitors; and on the other end of the spectrum, the use of high doses of diuretics together with angiotensin converting enzyme inhibitors may lead to excessive reduction in blood pressure and to Na$^+$ loss in some patients.

The attenuation of aldosterone production by the angiotensin converting enzyme inhibitors also influences K$^+$ homeostasis. There is only a very small and clinically unimportant rise in serum K$^+$ when angiotensin converting inhibitors are used alone in patients with normal renal function. However, substantial retention of K$^+$ can occur in some patients with renal insufficiency. Furthermore, the potential for developing hyperkalemia should be considered when angiotensin converting enzyme inhibitors are used with other drugs that can cause K$^+$ retention; these include the K$^+$-sparing diuretics (amiloride, triamterene, spironolactone), nonsteroidal antiinflammatory drugs, K$^+$ supplements, and β-adrenergic receptor antagonists.

There are several cautions in the use of angiotensin converting enzyme inhibitors in patients with hypertension. Angioedema is an infrequent but serious and potentially fatal adverse effect of all of the angiotensin converting enzyme inhibitors. Thus, patients starting treatment with these drugs should be explicitly warned to discontinue their use with the advent of any signs of angioedema. The angiotensin converting enzyme inhibitors should not be used during pregnancy, a fact that should be communicated to patients of childbearing age.

In most patients there is no appreciable change in glomerular filtration rate following the administration of a converting enzyme inhibitor. However, in renovascular hypertension, the glomerular filtration rate is maintained as the result of increased resistance in the postglomerular arteriole caused by angiotensin II. Accordingly, in patients with bilateral renal artery stenosis or stenosis in a sole kidney, the administration of a converting enzyme inhibitor will reduce the filtration fraction and cause a substantial reduction in glomerular filtration rate.

Converting enzyme inhibitors lower the blood pressure to some extent in most patients with hypertension. Following the initial dose of a converting enzyme inhibitor, there may be a considerable fall in blood pressure in some patients; this response to the initial dose is a function of pretreatment plasma renin activity. The potential for a large initial drop in blood pressure is the reason for using a low dose for initiating therapy. On continuing treatment, there usually is a progressive fall in blood pressure that in most patients does not reach a maximum for about one week. The level of blood pressure seen during chronic treatment is not strongly correlated with the level of pretreatment plasma renin activity. Young and middle-aged Caucasian patients have a higher probability of responding to the angiotensin converting enzyme inhibitors. Elderly African-American patients as a group are more resistant to the hypotensive effect of these drugs, but concurrent use of a diuretic in low doses overcomes this relative resistance. These drugs are discussed in detail in Chapter 31.

ANGIOTENSIN II–RECEPTOR ANTAGONISTS

The importance of angiotensin II in regulating cardiovascular function has led to the development of nonpeptide antagonists of the angiotensin II receptor for clinical use. *Losartan* (COZAAR), *candesartan* (ATACAND), *irbesartan* (AVAPRO), *valsartan* (DIOVAN), *telmisartan* (MICARDIS), and *eprosartan* (TEVETEN) have been approved for the treatment of hypertension. By preventing effects of angiotensin II, these agents relax smooth muscle and thereby promote vasodilation, increase renal salt and water excretion, reduce plasma volume, and decrease cellular hypertrophy. Angiotensin II–receptor antagonists also theoretically overcome some of the disadvantages of ACE inhibitors, which not only prevent conversion of angiotensin I to angiotensin II but also prevent ACE-mediated degradation of bradykinin and substance P. Cough, an adverse effect of ACE inhibitors, has not been associated with angiotensin II–receptor antagonists. Angioedema occurs rarely.

Two distinct subtypes of angiotensin II receptors have been cloned, designated as type 1 (AT_1) and type 2 (AT_2). The AT_1 angiotensin II receptor subtype is located predominantly in vascular and myocardial tissue and also in brain, kidney, and adrenal glomerulosa cells, which secrete aldosterone (*see* Chapter 31). The AT_2 subtype of angiotensin II receptor is found in the adrenal medulla, kidney, and in the CNS, and may play a role in vascular development (Horiuchi *et al.*, 1999). Because the AT_1 receptor mediates feedback inhibition of renin release, renin and angiotensin II concentrations are increased during AT_1-receptor antagonism. The clinical consequences of increased angiotensin II effects on an uninhibited AT_2 receptor are unknown; however, emerging data suggest that the AT_2 receptor may elicit antigrowth and antiproliferative responses.

Adverse Effects and Precautions. The adverse effects of AT_1-receptor antagonists may be considered in the context of those known to be associated with the ACE inhibitors. ACE inhibitors cause problems of two major types, those related to a diminished level of angiotensin II and those due to molecular actions independent of abrogating the function of angiotensin II.

Adverse effects of ACE inhibitors that result from inhibiting angiotensin II-related functions (*see* above) occur also with AT_1-receptor antagonists. These include hypotension, hyperkalemia, and reduced renal function, including that associated with bilateral renal artery stenosis and stenosis in the artery of a solitary kidney. Hypotension is most likely to occur in patients in whom the blood pressure is highly dependent on angiotensin II, including those with volume depletion (*e.g.,* with diuretics), renovascular hypertension, cardiac failure, and cirrhosis; in such patients initiation of treatment with low doses and attention to blood volume is essential. Hyperkalemia will occur only in conjunction with other factors that alter K^+ homeostasis, such as renal insufficiency, ingestion of excess K^+, and the use of drugs that promote K^+ retention.

In contrast with ACE inhibitors, the AT_1-receptor antagonists do not cause cough. Angioedema has been reported, but it is not clear whether or not the rate of angioedema in patients taking the AT_1-receptor antagonists is any higher than that in the general population. Hepatic dysfunction has been reported with the AT_1-receptor antagonists.

AT_1-receptor antagonists should not be administered during the second or third trimester of pregnancy and should be discontinued as soon as pregnancy is detected. Although it is not yet known whether or not AT_1-receptor antagonists are secreted in human breast milk, significant amounts are detected in the milk of animals; consequently, AT_1-receptor antagonists should not be administered to patients who are breast-feeding.

Therapeutic Uses. When given in adequate doses, the AT_1-receptor antagonists appear to be as effective as ACE inhibitors in the treatment of hypertension. As with ACE inhibitors, these drugs may be less effective in African-American and low-renin patients.

The full effect of AT_1-receptor antagonists on blood pressure typically is not observed until 3 to 6 weeks after the initiation of therapy. If blood pressure is not controlled by an AT_1-receptor antagonist alone, a low dose of a hydrochlorothiazide or other diuretic may be added. In several randomized, double-blind studies of patients with mild to severe hypertension, the addition of hydrochlorothiazide to an AT_1-receptor antagonist produced significant additional reductions in blood pressure in patients who demonstrated an insufficient response to hydrochlorothiazide alone. A smaller initial dosage is preferred for patients who have already received diuretics and therefore have an intravascular volume depletion, and for other patients whose blood pressure is highly dependent on angiotensin II.

Ongoing clinical trials should shed light on the relative efficacy of ACE inhibitors and AT_1-receptor antagonists in patients with diabetic nephropathy, coronary artery disease, and left ventricular dysfunction (Pitt *et al.*, 1999a). Given the different mechanisms by which they act, there is no assurance that the effects of ACE inhibitors and antagonists of the AT_1 receptor will be equivalent.

NONPHARMACOLOGICAL THERAPY OF HYPERTENSION

Nonpharmacological approaches to the reduction of blood pressure generally are advisable as the initial approach to treatment of patients with diastolic blood pressures in the range of 90 to 95 mm Hg. Further, these approaches will augment the effectiveness of pharmacological therapy in patients with higher levels of blood pressure. Also, for patients with diastolic blood pressures in the range of 85 to 90 mm Hg, the epidemiological data on cardiovascular risks support the institution of nonpharmacological therapy. To maintain compliance with a therapeutic regimen, the intervention should not lessen the quality of life. All drugs have side effects. If minor alterations of normal activity or diet can reduce blood pressure to a satisfactory level, the complications of drug therapy can be avoided. In addition, nonpharmacological methods to lower blood pressure allow the patient to participate actively in the management of his or her disease. Reduction of weight, restriction of salt, and moderation in the use of alcohol may reduce blood pressure and improve the efficacy of drug treatment. In addition, regular isotonic exercise also lowers blood pressure in hypertensive patients.

Smoking *per se* does not cause hypertension. However, smokers do have a higher incidence of malignant hypertension (Isles *et al.*, 1979), and smoking is a major risk factor for coronary heart disease. Hypertensive patients have an exceptionally great incentive to stop smoking. Consumption of caffeine can raise blood pressure and elevate plasma concentrations of norepinephrine, but long-term consumption of caffeine causes tolerance to these effects and has not been associated with the development of hypertension. An increased intake of Ca^{2+} has been reported by some investigators to lower blood pressure. The mechanism of this effect is not understood, but suppression of the secretion of parathyroid hormone apparently is involved. However, supplemental Ca^{2+} does not lower blood pressure when populations of hypertensive subjects are studied. Although it is possible that there are some hypertensive patients who have a hypotensive response to Ca^{2+}, there is no easy way to identify such individuals. Supplemental use of Ca^{2+} for this purpose cannot be recommended at the present time (Kaplan, 1988).

Reduction of Body Weight. Obesity and hypertension are closely associated, and the degree of obesity is positively correlated with the incidence of hypertension. Obese hypertensives may lower their blood pressure by losing weight regardless of a change in salt consumption (Maxwell *et al.*, 1984). The mechanism by which obesity causes hypertension is unclear, but increased secretion of insulin in obesity could result in insulin-mediated enhancement of renal tubular reabsorption of Na^+ and an expansion of extracellular volume. Obesity also is associated with increased activity of the sympathetic nervous system; this is reversed by weight loss. Maintenance of weight loss is difficult for many. A combination of aerobic physical exercise and dietary counseling may enhance compliance.

Sodium Restriction. Severe restriction of salt will lower the blood pressure in most hospitalized hypertensive patients; this treatment method was advocated prior to the development of effective antihypertensive drugs (Kempner, 1948). However, severe salt restriction is not practical from a standpoint of compliance. Several studies have shown that moderate restriction of salt intake to approximately 5 g per day (2 g Na^+) will, on average, lower blood pressure by 12 mm Hg systolic and 6 mm Hg diastolic. The higher the initial blood pressure, the greater the response. In addition, subjects over 40 years of age are more responsive to the hypotensive effect of moderate restriction of salt (Grobbee and Hofman, 1986). Even though not all hypertensive patients respond to restriction of salt, this intervention is benign and can easily be advised as an initial approach in all patients with mild hypertension. An additional benefit of salt restriction is improved responsiveness to some antihypertensive drugs.

Alcohol Restriction. Consumption of alcohol can raise blood pressure, but it is unclear how much alcohol must be consumed to observe this effect (MacMahon *et al.*, 1984). Heavy consumption of alcohol increases the risk of cerebrovascular accidents but not coronary heart disease (Kagan *et al.*, 1985). In fact, small amounts of ethanol have been found to protect against the development of coronary artery disease. The mechanism by which alcohol raises blood pressure is unknown, but it may involve increased transport of Ca^{2+} into vascular smooth muscle cells. Excessive intake of alcohol also may result in poor compliance with antihypertensive regimens. All hypertensive patients should be advised to restrict consumption of ethanol to no more than 30 ml per day.

Physical Exercise. Increased physical activity lowers rates of cardiovascular disease in men (Paffenbarger *et al.,* 1986). It is not known if this beneficial effect is secondary to an antihypertensive response to exercise. Lack of physical activity is associated with a higher incidence of hypertension (Blair *et al.,* 1984). Although consistent changes in blood pressure are not always observed, meticulously controlled studies have demonstrated that regular isotonic exercise reduces both systolic and diastolic blood pressures by approximately 10 mm Hg (Nelson *et al.,* 1986). The mechanism by which exercise can lower blood pressure is not clear, but several hemodynamic and humoral changes have been documented. Regular isotonic exercise reduces blood volume and plasma catecholamines and elevates plasma concentrations of atrial natriuretic factor. The beneficial effect of exercise can occur in subjects who demonstrate no change in body weight or salt intake during the training period.

Relaxation and Biofeedback Therapy. The fact that long-term stressful stimuli can cause sustained hypertension in animals has given credence to the possibility that relaxation therapy will lower blood pressure in some hypertensive patients. A few studies have generated positive results but, in general, relaxation therapy has inconsistent and modest effects on blood pressure (Jacob *et al.,* 1986). In addition, the long-term efficacy of such treatment has been difficult to demonstrate, presumably in part because patients must be highly motivated to respond to relaxation and biofeedback therapy. Only those few patients with mild hypertension who wish to use this method should be encouraged to try, and these patients should be closely followed and receive pharmacological treatment if necessary.

Potassium Therapy. There is a positive correlation between total body Na^+ and blood pressure and a negative correlation between total body K^+ and blood pressure in hypertensive patients (Lever *et al.,* 1981). In addition, dietary intake, plasma concentrations, and urinary excretion of K^+ are reduced in various populations of hypertensive subjects. Increased intake of K^+ might reduce blood pressure by increasing excretion of Na^+, suppressing renin secretion, causing arteriolar dilation (possibly by stimulating Na^+, K^+-ATPase activity and decreasing intracellular concentrations of Ca^{2+}), and impairing responsiveness to endogenous vasoconstrictors. In hypertensive rats, supplementation with K^+ decreases blood pressure and reduces the incidence of stroke, irrespective of blood pressure (Tobian, 1986). In mildly hypertensive patients, oral K^+ supplements of 48 mmol per day reduce both systolic and diastolic blood pressure (Siana *et al.,* 1987). Supplementation with K^+ also may protect against ventricular ectopy and stroke (Khaw and Barrett-Connor, 1987). Based on all of these data, it seems prudent to use a high-K^+ diet in conjunction with moderate restriction of Na^+ in the nonpharmacological treatment of hypertension. However, a high-K^+ diet should not be recommended for patients on angiotensin converting enzyme inhibitors.

PROSPECTUS

The most anticipated development in antihypertensive therapy is the new knowledge expected from clinical trials comparing the effectiveness of drugs on the important endpoints of morbidity and mortality. One clinical trial addressing these endpoints has been launched by the National Heart, Lung, and Blood Institute (Davis *et al.,* 1996). It is the Antihypertensive and Lipid Lowering treatment to prevent Heart Attack Trial (ALLHAT) and is comparing the outcomes of treatment with a thiazide-class diuretic (chlorthalidone), an angiotensin converting enzyme inhibitor (lisinopril), a Ca^{2+}-channel blocker (amlodipine), and an α_1-adrenergic receptor antagonist (doxazosin). This trial is evaluating the effects of these drugs in patients over the age of 55 who are at high risk for vascular occlusive events. Concurrently, the benefit of a cholesterol-lowering drug, pravastatin, is being assessed in the same population. The Losartan Intervention for Endpoint Reduction in Hypertension (LIFE) study is comparing the AT_1-receptor antagonist losartan and β-adrenergic receptor blocker atenolol on cardiovascular mortality and morbidity in patients, aged 55 to 88 years, with hypertension and left ventricular hypertrophy (Dahlöf *et al.,* 1998). The African-American Study of Kidney Disease (AASK) will determine the efficacy of two different levels of blood pressure control and three different antihypertensive regimens on the progression of renal disease in African Americans with hypertensive nephropathy (Wright *et al.,* 1996).

A growing recognition of the contribution of the renin-angiotensin-aldosterone system (RAAS) to the development and progression of hypertensive end-organ damage promises to bring a number of studies examining new strategies for interrupting the RAAS. For example, studies comparing the efficacy of ACE inhibition, AT_1-receptor antagonism, and the combination of ACE inhibition and AT_1-receptor antagonism are ongoing. The finding that the addition of an aldosterone antagonist decreases mortality in patients with congestive heart failure treated with an ACE inhibitor (Pitt *et al.,* 1999b) has sparked a renewed interest in aldosterone antagonists in the treatment of hypertension. These studies, if they are successful, could profoundly influence the approach to treating hypertension.

For further discussion of hypertension, *see* Chapter 246 in *Harrison's Principles of Internal Medicine,* 14th ed., McGraw-Hill, New York, 1998.

BIBLIOGRAPHY

Aroney, C.N., Semigran, M.J., Dec, G.W., Boucher, C.A., and Fifer, M.A. Left ventricular diastolic function in patients with left ventricular systolic dysfunction due to coronary artery disease and effect of nicardipine. *Am. J. Cardiol.,* **1991,** *67*:823–829.

Azuma, J., Sawamura, A., Harada, H., Awata, N., Kishimoto, S., and Sperelakis, N. Mechanism of direct cardiostimulating actions of hydralazine. *Eur. J. Pharmacol.,* **1987,** *135*:137–144.

Bates, J.N., Baker, M.T., Guerra, R. Jr., and Harrison, D.G. Nitric oxide generation from nitroprusside by vascular tissue. Evidence that reduction of the nitroprusside anion and cyanide loss are required. *Biochem. Pharmacol.,* **1991,** *42*:S157–S165.

Beckmann, M.L., Gerber, J.G., Byyny, R.L., LoVerde, M., and Nies, A.S. Propranolol increases prostacyclin synthesis in patients with essential hypertension. *Hypertension,* **1988,** *12*:582–588.

Bennett, W.M., McDonald, W.J., Kuehnel, E., Hartnett, M.N., and Porter, G.A. Do diuretics have antihypertensive properties independent of natriuresis? *Clin. Pharmacol. Ther.,* **1977,** *22*:499–504.

Blair, S.N., Goodyear, N.N., Gibbons, L.W., and Cooper, K.H. Physical fitness and incidence of hypertension in healthy normotensive men and women. *JAMA,* **1984,** *252*:487–490.

Bobik, A., Jennings, G., Jackman, G., Oddie, C., and Korner, P. Evidence for a predominantly central hypotensive effect of alpha-methyldopa in humans. *Hypertension,* **1986,** *8*:16–23.

Bobik, A., Oddie C., Scott P., Mill, G., and Korner, P. Relationships between the cardiovascular effects of α-methyldopa and its metabolism in pontomedullary noradrenergic neurons of the rabbit. *J. Cardiovasc. Pharmacol.,* **1988,** *11*:529–537.

Cameron, H.A., and Ramsay, L.E. The lupus syndrome induced by hydralazine: a common complication with low dose treatment. *Br. Med. J. [Clin. Res. Ed.],* **1984,** *289*:410–412.

Campbell, N.R., Sundaram, R.S., Werness, P.G., Van Loon, J., and Weinshilboum, R.M. Sulfate and methyldopa metabolism: metabolite patterns and platelet phenol sulfotransferase activity. *Clin. Pharmacol. Ther.,* **1985,** *37*:308–315.

CAST Investigators. Preliminary report: effect of encainide and flecainide on mortality in a randomized trial of arrhythmia suppression after myocardial infarction. The Cardiac Arrhythmia Suppression Trial (CAST) Investigators. *N. Engl. J. Med.,* **1989,** *321*:406–412.

Chi, L., Uprichard, A.C., and Lucchesi B.R. Profibrillatory actions of pinacidil in a conscious canine model of sudden coronary death. *J. Cardiovasc. Pharmacol.,* **1990,** *15*:452–464.

Collins, R., Peto, R., MacMahon S., Hebert, P., Fiebach, N.H., Eberlein, K.A., Godwin, J., Qizilbash, N., Taylor, J.O., and Hennekens, C.H. Blood pressure, stroke and coronary heart disease. Part 2, Short-term reductions in blood pressure: overview of randomised drug trials in their epidemiological context. *Lancet,* **1990,** *335*:827–838.

Cornacchia, E., Golbus, J., Maybaum, J., Strahler, J., Hanash, S., and Richardson, B. Hydralazine and procainamide inhibit T cell DNA methylation and induce autoreactivity. *J. Immunol.,* **1988,** *140*:2197–2200.

Curtis, M.J., and Hearse, D.J. Ischaemia-induced and reperfusion-induced arrhythmias differ in their sensitivity to potassium: implications for mechanisms of initiation and maintenance of ventricular fibrillation. *J. Mol. Cell. Cardiol.,* **1989,** *21*:21–40.

Dahlöf, B., Devereux, R.B., Julius, S., Kjeldsen, S.E., Beevers, G., de Faire, U., Fyhrquist, F., Hedner, T., Ibsen, H., Kristianson, K., Lederballe-Pedersen, O., Lindholm, L.H., Nieminen, M.S., Omvik, P., Oparil, S., and Wedel, H. Characteristics of 9194 patients with left ventricular hypertrophy: the LIFE study. Losartan Intervention For Endpoint Reduction in Hypertension. *Hypertension,* **1998,** *32*:989–997.

Dahlöf, B., Lindholm, L.H., Hansson, L., Schersten, B., Ekbom, T., and Wester, P.O. Morbidity and mortality in the Swedish Trial in Old Patients with Hypertension (STOP-Hypertension). *Lancet,* **1991,** *338*:1281–1285.

Dahlöf, B., Pennert K., and Hansson, L. Reversal of left ventricular hypertrophy in hypertensive patients. A metaanalysis of 109 treatment studies. *Am. J. Hypertens.,* **1992,** *5*:95–110.

Davis, B.R., Cutler, J.A., Gordon, D.J., Furberg, C.D., Wright, J.T. Jr., Cushman, W.C., Grimm, R.H., LaRosa, J., Whelton, P.K., Perry, H.M., Alderman, M.H., Ford, C.E., Oparil, S., Francis, C., Proschan, M., Pressel, S., Black, H.R., and Hawkins, C.M. Rationale and design for the Antihypertensive and Lipid Lowering Treatment to Prevent Heart Attack Trial (ALLHAT). ALLHAT Research Group. *Am. J. Hypertens.,* **1996,** *9*:342–360.

DeCarvalho, J.G., Emery, A.C., Jr., and Frohlich, E.D. Spironolactone and triamterene in volume-dependent essential hypertension. *Clin. Pharmacol. Ther.,* **1980,** *27*:53–56.

Estacio, R.O., Jeffers, B.W., Hiatt, W.R., Biggerstaff, S.L., Gifford, N., and Schrier, R.W. The effect of nisoldipine as compared with enalapril on cardiovascular outcomes in patients with non-insulin-dependent diabetes and hypertension. *N. Engl. J. Med.,* **1998,** *338*:645–652.

Falch, D.K., and Schreiner, A. The effect of spironolactone on lipid, glucose and uric acid levels in blood during long-term administration to hypertensives. *Acta Med. Scand.,* **1983,** *213*:27–30.

Fouad, F.M., Nakashima, Y., Tarazi, R.C., and Salcedo, E.E. Reversal of left ventricular hypertrophy in hypertensive patients treated with methyldopa. Lack of association with blood pressure control. *Am. J. Cardiol.,* **1982,** *49*:795–801.

Frisk-Holmberg, M., Paalzow, L., and Wibell, L. Relationship between the cardiovascular effects and steady-state kinetics of clonidine in hypertension. Demonstration of a therapeutic window in man. *Eur. J. Clin. Pharmacol.,* **1984,** *26*:309–313.

Frisk-Holmberg, M., and Wibell, L. Concentration-dependent blood pressure effects of guanfacine. *Clin. Pharmacol. Ther.,* **1986,** *39*:169–172.

Gall, M.A., Rossing, P., Skøtt, P., Hommel, E., Mathiesen, E.R., Gerdes, L.U., Lauritzen, M., Vølund, A., Færgeman, O., Beck-Nielsen, H., and Parving, H.H. Placebo-controlled comparison of captopril, metoprolol, and hydrochlorothiazide therapy in non-insulin-dependent diabetic patients with primary hypertension. *Am. J. Hypertens.,* **1992,** *5*:257–265.

Garrett, B.N., and Kaplan, N.M. Efficacy of slow infusion of diazoxide in the treatment of severe hypertension without organ hypoperfusion. *Am. Heart J.,* **1982,** *103*:390–394.

Gehr, M., MacCarthy, E.P., and Goldberg, M. Guanabenz: a centrally acting, natriuretic antihypertensive drug. *Kidney Int.,* **1986,** *29*:1203–1208.

Gellai, M., and Edwards, R.M. Mechanism of α_2-adrenoceptor agonist-induced diuresis. *Am. J. Physiol.,* **1988,** *255*:F317–F323.

Giachetti, A., and Shore, P.A. The reserpine receptor. *Life Sci.,* **1978,** *23*:89–92.

Goldstein, D.S., Levinson, P.D., Zimlichman, R., Pitterman, A., Stull, R., and Keiser, H.R. Clonidine suppression testing in essential hypertension. *Ann. Intern. Med.,* **1985,** *102*:42–49.

Granata, A.R., Numao, Y., Kumada, M., and Reis, D.J. A1 noradrenergic neurons tonically inhibit sympathoexcitatory neurons of C1 area
in rat brainstem. *Brain Res.,* **1986,** *377:*127–146.

Hansson, L., Zanchetti, A., Carruthers, S.G., Dahlöf, B., Elmfeldt, D.,
Julius, S., Menard, J., Rahn, K.H., Wedel, H., and Westerling, S.
Effects of intensive blood-pressure lowering and low-dose aspirin in
patients with hypertension: principal results of the Hypertension Optimal Treatment (HOT) randomised trial. HOT Study Group. *Lancet,*
1998, *351:*1755–1762.

Horiuchi, M., Akishita, M., and Dzau, V.J. Recent progress in angiotensin II type 2 receptor research in the cardiovascular system.
Hypertension, **1999,** *33:*613–621.

Inouye, I.K., Massie, B.M., Benowitz, N., Simpson, P., and Loge,
D. Antihypertensive therapy with diltiazem and comparison with
hydrochlorothiazide. *Am. J. Cardiol.,* **1984,** *53:*1588–1592.

Isles, C., Brown, J.J., Cumming, A.M., Lever, A.F., McAreavey, D.,
Robertson, J.I., Hawthorne, V.M., Stewart, G.M., Robertson, J.W.,
and Wapshaw, J. Excess smoking in malignant-phase hypertension.
Br. Med. J., **1979,** *1:*579–581.

Jacob, R.G., Shapiro, A.P., Reeves, R.A., Johnsen, A.M., McDonald,
R.H., and Coburn, P.C. Relaxation therapy for hypertension. Com-
parison of effects with concomitant placebo, diuretic, and β-blocker.
Arch. Intern. Med., **1986,** *146:*2335–2340.

Jeunemaitre, X., Charru, A., Chatellier, G., Degoulet, P., Julien, J.,
Plouin, P.-F., Corvol, P., and Menard, J. Long-term metabolic effects
of spironolactone and thiazides combined with potassium-sparing
agents for treatment of essential hypertension. *Am. J. Cardiol.,* **1988,**
*62:*1072–1077.

Joint National Committee. The sixth report of the Joint National Committee on prevention, detection, evaluation and treatment of high
blood pressure. *Arch. Intern. Med.,* **1997,** *157:*2413–2446.

Kagan, A., Popper, J.S., Rhoads, G.G., and Yano, K. Dietary and
other risk factors for stroke in Hawaiian Japanese men. *Stroke,*
1985, *16:*390–396.

Kempner, W. Treatment of hypertensive vascular disease with rice diet.
Am. J. Med., **1948,** *4:*545–577.

Khaw, K.-T., and Barrett-Connor, E. Dietary potassium and stroke
associated mortality. A 12 year prospective population study. *N. Engl.
J. Med.,* **1987,** *316:*235–240.

Kowaluk, E.A., Seth, P., and Fung, H.L. Metabolic activation of sodium
nitroprusside to nitric oxide in vascular smooth muscle. *J. Pharmacol. Exp. Ther.,* **1992,** *262:*916–922.

Leblanc, N., Wilde, D.W., Keef, K.D., and Hume, J.R. Electrophysiological mechanisms of minoxidil sulfate-induced vasodilation of
rabbit portal vein. *Circ. Res.,* **1989,** *65:*1102–1111.

Leenen, F.H., Smith, D.L., and Unger, W.P. Topical minoxidil: cardiac
effects in bald man. *Br. J. Clin. Pharmacol.,* **1988,** *26:*481–485.

Lever, A.F., Beretta-Piccoli, C., Brown, J.J., Davies, D.L., Fraser, R.,
and Robertson, J.I. Sodium and potassium in essential hypertension.
Br. Med. J. [Clin. Res. Ed.], **1981,** *283:*463–468.

Link, R.E., Desai, K., Hein, L., Stevens, M.E., Chruscinski, A., Bernstein, D., Barsh, G.S., and Kobilka, B.K. Cardiovascular regulation
in mice lacking α_2-adrenergic receptor subtypes b and c. *Science,*
1996, *273:*803–805.

McCall, J.M., Aiken, J.W., Chidester, C.G., DuCharme, D.W., and
Wendling, M.G. Pyrimidine and triazine 3-oxide sulfates: a new
family of vasodilators. *J. Med. Chem.,* **1983,** *26:*1791–1793.

Macdougall, I.C., Isles, C.G., Stewart, H., Inglis, G.C., Finlayson, J.,
Thomson, I., Lees, K.R., McMillan, N.C., Morley, P., and Ball, S.G.
Overnight clonidine suppression test in the diagnosis and exclusion
of pheochromocytoma. *Am. J. Med.,* **1988,** *84:*993–1000.

MacMahon, S.W., Blacket, R.B., Macdonald, G.J., and Hall, W. Obesity, alcohol consumption and blood pressure in Australian men and
women. The National Heart Foundation of Australia Risk Factor
Prevalence Study. *J. Hypertens.,* **1984,** *2:*85–91.

MacMillan, L.B., Hein, L., Smith, M.S., Piascik, M.T., and Limbird,
L.E. Central hypotensive effects of the α_{2A}-adrenergic receptor subtype. *Science,* **1996,** *273:*801–803.

Maxwell, M.H., Kushiro, T., Dornfeld, L.P., Tuck, M.L., and Waks,
A.U. BP changes in obese hypertensive subjects during rapid weight
loss. Comparison of restricted v. unchanged salt intake. *Arch. Intern.
Med.,* **1984,** *144:*1581–1584.

Medical Research Council Working Party. Comparison of the antihypertensive efficacy and adverse reactions to two doses of bendrofluazide
and hydrochlorothiazide and the effect of potassium supplementation on the hypotensive action of bendrofluazide: substudies of the
Medical Research Council's trials of treatment of mild hypertension:
Medical Research Council Working Party. *J. Clin. Pharmacol.,* **1987,**
*27:*271–277.

Medical Research Council Working Party. Medical Research Council
trial of treatment of hypertension in older adults: principal results.
MRC Working Party. *Br. Med. J.,* **1992,** *304:*405–412.

Metz, S., Klein, C., and Morton, N. Rebound hypertension after discontinuation of transdermal clonidine therapy. *Am. J. Med.,* **1987,**
*82:*17–19.

Mitchell, H.C., Graham, R.M., and Pettinger, W.A. Renal function
during long-term treatment of hypertension with minoxidil: comparison of benign and malignant hypertension. *Ann. Intern. Med.,* **1980,**
*93:*676–681.

Multicenter Diltiazem Postinfarction Trial Research Group. The effect
of diltiazem on mortality and reinfarction after myocardial infarction.
N. Engl. J. Med., **1988,** *319:*385–392.

Multicenter Diuretic Cooperative Study Group. Multiclinic comparison of amiloride, hydrochlorothiazide, and hydrochlorothiazide
plus amiloride in essential hypertension. *Arch. Intern. Med.,* **1981,**
*141:*482–486.

Multiple Risk Factor Intervention Trial Research Group. Multiple risk
factor intervention trial. Risk factor changes and mortality results.
JAMA, **1982,** *248:*1465–1477.

Murad, F. Cyclic guanosine monophosphate as a mediator of vasodilation. *J. Clin. Invest.,* **1986,** *78:*1–5.

Nelson, L., Jennings, G.L., Esler, M.D., and Korner, P.I. Effect of
changing levels of physical activity on blood-pressure and haemo-
dynamics in essential hypertension. *Lancet,* **1986,** *2:*473–476.

Nishimura, R.A., Schwartz, R.S., Holmes, D.R. Jr., Tajik, A.J. Failure
of calcium channel blockers to improve ventricular relaxation in
humans. *J. Am. Coll. Cardiol.,* **1993,** *21:*182–188.

Ogilvie, R.I. Comparative effects of vasodilator drugs on flow distribution and venous return. *Can. J. Physiol. Pharmacol.,* **1985,**
*63:*1345–1355.

Packer, M., Meller, J., Medina, N., Gorlin, R., and Herman, M.V.
Rebound hemodynamic events after the abrupt withdrawal of nitro-
prusside in patients with severe chronic heart failure. *N. Engl. J.
Med.,* **1979,** *301:*1193–1197.

Paffenbarger, R.S. Jr., Hyde, R.T., Wing, A.L., and Hsieh, C.-C. Physical activity, all-cause mortality, and longevity of college alumni.
N. Engl. J. Med., **1986,** *314:*605–613.

Pedersen, K.E., Dorph-Pedersen, A., Hvidt, S., Klitgaard, N.A., and
Nielsen-Kudsk, F. Digoxin-verapamil interaction. *Clin. Pharmacol.
Ther.,* **1981,** *30:*311–316.

Pitt, B., Poole-Wilson, P., Segal, R., Martinez, F.A., Dickstein, K.,
Camm, A.J., Konstam, M.A., Riegger, G., Klinger, G.H., Neaton, J.,

Sharma, D., and Thiyagarajan, B. Effects of losartan versus captopril on mortality in patients with symptomatic heart failure: rationale, design, and baseline characteristics of patients in the Losartan Heart Failure Survival Study—ELITE II. *J. Card. Fail.,* **1999a,** 5:146–154.

Pitt, B., Zannad, F., Remme, W.J., Cody, R., Castaigne, A., Perez, A., Palensky, J., and Wittes, J. The effect of spironolactone on morbidity and mortality in patients with severe heart failure. Randomized Aldactone Evaluation Study Investigators. *N. Engl. J. Med.,* **1999b,** 341:709–717.

Pruitt, A.W., Faraj, B.A., and Dayton, P.G. Metabolism of diazoxide in man and experimental animals. *J. Pharmacol. Exp. Ther.,* **1974,** 188:248–256.

Ram, C.V., Garrett, B.N., and Kaplan, N.M. Moderate sodium restriction and various diuretics in the treatment of hypertension. *Arch. Intern. Med.,* **1981,** 141:1015–1019.

Reece, P.A., Stafford, I., Prager, R.H., Walker, G.J., and Zacest, R. Synthesis, formulation, and clinical pharmacological evaluation of hydralazine pyruvic acid hydrazone in two healthy volunteers. *J. Pharm. Sci.,* **1985,** 74:193–196.

Reichgott, M.J. Minoxidil and pericardial effusion: an idiosyncratic reaction. *Clin. Pharmacol. Ther.,* **1981,** 30:64–70.

Reid, J.L., Wing, L.M., Mathias, C.J., Frankel, H.L., and Neill, E. The central hypotensive effect of clonidine. Studies in tetraplegic subjects. *Clin. Pharmacol. Ther.,* **1977,** 21:375–381.

Sattler, R.W., and van Zwieten, P.A. Acute hypotensive action of 2-(2,6-dichlorophenylamino)-2-imidazoline hydrochloride (St 155) after infusion into the cat's vertebral artery. *Eur. J. Pharmacol.,* **1967,** 2:9–13.

Schrijver, G., and Weinberger, M.H. Hydrochlorothiazide and spironolactone in hypertension. *Clin. Pharmacol. Ther.,* **1979,** 25:33–42.

Sen, G., and Bose, K.C. *Rauwolfia serpentina,* a new Indian drug for insanity and high blood pressure. *Indian Med. World,* **1931,** 2:194–201.

Shah, S., Khatri, I., and Freis, E.D. Mechanism of antihypertensive effect of thiazide diuretics. *Am. Heart J.,* **1978,** 95:611–618.

SHEP Cooperative Research Group. Prevention of stroke by antihypertensive drug treatment in older persons with isolated systolic hypertension. Final results of the Systolic Hypertension in the Elderly Program (SHEP). *JAMA,* **1991,** 265:3255–3264.

Siani, A., Strazzullo, P., Russo, L., Guglielmi, S., Iacoviello, L., Ferrara, L.A., and Mancini, M. Controlled trial of long-term oral potassium supplements in patients with mild hypertension. *Br. Med. J. [Clin. Res. Ed.],* **1987,** 294:1453–1456.

Siscovick, D.S., Raghunathan, T.E., Psaty, B.M., Koepsell, T.D., Wicklund, K.G., Lin, X., Cobb, L., Rautaharju, P.M., Copass, M.K., and Wagner, E.H. Diuretic therapy for hypertension and the risk of primary cardiac arrest. *N. Engl. J. Med.,* **1994,** 330:1852–1857.

Staessen, J.A., Fagard, R., Thijs, L., Celis, H., Arabidze, G.G., Birkenhager, W.H., Bulpitt, C.J., de Leeuw, P.W., Dollery, C.T., Fletcher, A.E., Forette, F., Leonetti, G., Nachev, C., O'Brien, E.T., Rosenfeld, J., Rodicio, J.L., Tuomilehto, J., and Zanchetti, A. Randomised double-blind comparison of placebo and active treatment for older patients with isolated systolic hypertension. The Systolic Hypertension in Europe (Syst-Eur) Trial Investigators. *Lancet,* **1997,** 350:757–764.

Standen, N.B., Quayle, J.M., Davies, N.W., Brayden, J.E., Huang, Y., and Nelson, M.T. Hyperpolarizing vasodilators activate ATP-sensitive K⁺ channels in arterial smooth muscle. *Science,* **1989,** 245:177–180.

Tobian, L. High potassium diets markedly protect against stroke deaths and kidney disease in hypertensive rats, a possible legacy from prehistoric times. *Can. J. Physiol. Pharmacol.,* **1986,** 64:840–848.

Tobian, L., Brunner, H.R., Cohn J.N., Gavras, H., Laragh J.H., Materson, B.J., and Weber, M.A. Modern strategies to prevent coronary sequelae and stroke in hypertensive patients differ from the JNC V Consensus Guidelines. *Am. J. Hypertens.,* **1994,** 7:859–872.

van den Meiracker, A.H., Man in't Veld, A.J., van Eck, H.J., Boomsma, F., and Schalekamp, M.A. Hemodynamic and hormonal adaptations to β-adrenoceptor blockade. A 24-hour study of acebutolol, atenolol, pindolol, and propranolol in hypertensive patients. *Circulation,* **1988,** 78:957–968.

Veterans Administration Cooperative Study Group on Hypertensive Agents. Effects of treatment on morbidity in hypertension. Results in patients with diastolic blood pressure averaging 115 through 129 mm Hg. *JAMA,* **1967,** 202:1028–1034.

Veterans Administration Cooperative Study Group on Hypertensive Agents. Effects of treatment on morbidity in hypertension. II. Results in patients with diastolic blood pressure averaging 90 through 114 mm Hg. *JAMA,* **1970,** 213:1143–1152.

Williams, G.M., Mazue, G., McQueen, C.A., and Shimada, T. Genotoxicity of the antihypertensive drugs hydralazine and dihydralazine. *Science,* **1980,** 210:329–330.

Wilson, D.J., and Vidt, D.G. Control of severe hypertension with pulse doses of diazoxide. *Clin. Pharmacol. Ther.,* **1978,** 23:135–140.

Wilson, M.F., Haring, O., Lewin, A., Bedsole, G., Stepansky, W., Fillingim, J., Hall, D., Roginsky, M., McMahon, F.G., Jagger, P., and Strauss, M. Comparison of guanfacine versus clonidine for efficacy, safety and occurrence of withdrawal syndrome in step-2 treatment of mild to moderate essential hypertension. *Am. J. Cardiol.,* **1986,** 57:43E–49E.

Wright, J.M., Orozco-Gonzalez, M., Polak, G., and Dollery, C.T. Duration of effect of single daily dose methyldopa therapy. *Br. J. Clin. Pharmacol.,* **1982,** 13:847–854.

Wright, J.T. Jr., Kusek, J.W., Toto, R.D., Lee, J.Y., Agodoa, L.Y., Kirk, K.A., Randall, O.S., and Glassock, R. Design and baseline characteristics of participants in the African-American Study of Kidney Disease and Hypertension (AASK) Pilot Study. *Control. Clin. Trials,* **1996,** 17:3S–16S.

Yano, K., Hirata, M., Matsumoto, Y., Hano, O., Mori, M., Ahmed, R., Mitsuoka, T., and Hashiba, K. Effects of chronic hypokalemia on ventricular vulnerability during acute myocardial ischemia in the dog. *Jpn. Heart J.,* **1989,** 30:205–217.

Zünkler, B.J., Lenzen, S., Männer, K., Panten, U., and Trube, G. Concentration-dependent effects of tolbutamide, meglitinide, glipizide, glibenclamide and diazoxide on ATP-regulated K⁺ currents in pancreatic B-cells. *Naunyn Schmiedebergs Arch. Pharmacol.,* **1988,** 337:225–230.

MONOGRAPHS AND REVIEWS

Amdisen, A. Lithium and drug interactions. *Drugs,* **1982,** 24:133–139.

Brogden, R.N., Heel, R.C., Speight, T.M., and Avery, G.S. α-Methyl-p-tyrosine: a review of its pharmacology and clinical use. *Drugs,* **1981,** 21:81–89.

Campese, V.M. Minoxidil: a review of its pharmacological properties and therapeutic use. *Drugs,* **1981,** 22:257–278.

Cubeddu, L.X. New α₁-adrenergic receptor antagonists for the treatment of hypertension: role of vascular alpha receptors in the control of peripheral resistance. *Am. Heart J.,* **1988,** 116:133–162.

Doyle, A.E. Comparison of beta-adrenoceptor blockers and calcium antagonists in hypertension. *Hypertension,* **1983,** 5:II103–II108.

Freis, E.D. How diuretics lower blood pressure. *Am. Heart J.,* **1983,** 106:185–187.

Grobbee, D.E., and Hofman, A. Does sodium restriction lower blood pressure? *Br. Med. J. [Clin. Res.Ed.]*, **1986,** *293*:27–29.

Holmes, B., Brogden, R.N., Heel, R.C., Speight, T.M., and Avery, G.S. Guanabenz. A review of its pharmacodynamic properties and therapeutic efficacy in hypertension. *Drugs,* **1983,** *26*:212–229.

Houston, M.C., and Hodge, R. Beta-adrenergic blocker withdrawal syndromes in hypertension and other cardiovascular diseases. *Am. Heart J.,* **1988,** *116*:515–523.

Insel, P.A., and Motulsky, H.J. A hypothesis linking intracellular sodium, membrane receptors, and hypertension. *Life Sci.,* **1984,** *34*:1009–1013.

Ivankovich, A.D., Miletich, D.J., and Tinker, J.H. Sodium nitroprusside: metabolism and general considerations. *Int. Anesthesiol. Clin.,* **1978,** *16*:1–29.

Kaplan, N.M. Calcium and potassium in the treatment of essential hypertension. *Semin. Nephrol.,* **1988,** *8*:176–184.

Kiowski, W., Bühler, F.R., Fadayomi, M.O., Erne, P., Müller, F.B., Hulthén, U.L., and Bolli, P. Age, race, blood pressure and renin: predictors for antihypertensive treatment with calcium antagonists. *Am. J. Cardiol.,* **1985,** *56*:81H–85H.

Langer, S.Z., Cavero, I., and Massingham, R. Recent developments in noradrenergic neurotransmission and its relevance to the mechanism of action of certain antihypertensive agents. *Hypertension,* **1980,** *2*:372–382.

Lardinois, C.K., and Neuman, S.L. The effects of antihypertensive agents on serum lipids and lipoproteins. *Arch. Intern. Med.,* **1988,** *148*:1280–1288.

Lehmann, H.-U., Hochrein, H., Witt, E., and Mies, H.W. Hemodynamic effects of calcium antagonists. Review. *Hypertension,* **1983,** *5*:II66–II73.

Lund-Johansen, P. Hemodynamic effects of β-blocking compounds possessing vasodilating activity: a review of labetalol, prizidilol, and dilevalol. *J. Cardiovasc. Pharmacol.,* **1988,** *11(suppl. 2)*:S12–S17.

Perry, H.M. Jr. Late toxicity to hydralazine resembling systemic lupus erythematosus or rheumatoid arthritis. *Am. J. Med.,* **1973,** *54*:58–72.

Reece, P.A. Hydralazine and related compounds: chemistry, metabolism, and mode of action. *Med. Res. Rev.,* **1981,** *1*:73–96.

Reid, J.L. Alpha-adrenergic receptors and blood pressure control. *Am. J. Cardiol.,* **1986,** *57*:6E–12E.

Schulz, V. Clinical pharmacokinetics of nitroprusside, cyanide, thiosulphate and thiocyanate. *Clin. Pharmacokinet.,* **1984,** *9*:239–251.

Sorkin, E.M., and Heel, R.C. Guanfacine. A review of its pharmacodynamic and pharmacokinetic properties, and therapeutic efficacy in the treatment of hypertension. *Drugs,* **1986,** *31*:301–336.

Strandhoy, J.W. Role of alpha-2 receptors in the regulation of renal function. *J. Cardiovasc. Pharmacol.,* **1985,** *7(suppl. 8)*:S28–S33.

Webster, J. Interactions of NSAIDs with diuretics and β-blockers mechanisms and clinical implications. *Drugs,* **1985,** *30*:32–41.

C H A P T E R   3 4

PHARMACOLOGICAL TREATMENT
OF HEART FAILURE

Henry Ooi and Wilson S. Colucci

Heart failure is one of the most common causes of death and disability in industrialized nations and is among the syndromes most commonly encountered in clinical practice. Over 4.6 million patients in the United States alone carry this diagnosis, and it is the cause of death in several hundred thousand patients each year (American Heart Association, 1999). The diagnosis of heart failure carries a risk of mortality comparable to that of the major malignancies. Patients with newly diagnosed heart failure have an average five-year survival of only 35%. In the past 20 years, advances in understanding the pathophysiology of heart failure and new developments in pharmacotherapy have added substantially to the physician's ability to alleviate the symptoms of this disease and slow the natural progression of the underlying myocardial process.

This chapter deals with drug therapy of heart failure due to systolic and/or diastolic ventricular dysfunction. Systolic dysfunction due to idiopathic dilated or ischemic cardiomyopathies usually is characterized by large, dilated ventricular chambers. Diastolic dysfunction due to long-standing hypertension, stenotic valvular disease, or a primary hypertrophic cardiomyopathy generally leads to thickened, poorly compliant ventricular walls with small ventricular volumes. In reality, many patients exhibit abnormal hemodynamics comprising significant degrees of both systolic and diastolic dysfunction. Treatment must therefore be tailored to the underlying pathophysiological process in the individual patient.

The basic pharmacology of many of the classes of drugs described in this chapter is discussed in detail in other chapters and cross-referenced in the text. Therefore, the pharmacology of these agents is discussed here only in the context of the treatment of heart failure. The main elements in the pharmacotherapy of heart failure are angiotensin converting enzyme inhibitors (see Chapter 31) and β-adrenergic receptor antagonists (see Chapter 10). Accordingly, their use is discussed in detail in this chapter.

GOALS OF THERAPY

Relief of Symptoms.   A primary goal in the treatment of heart failure is the alleviation of symptoms, which, in turn, are a direct result of the underlying hemodynamic disorder. Intravascular volume expansion and elevated ventricular filling pressures result in systemic and pulmonary venous hypertension, which causes dyspnea on exertion and orthopnea. Reduced cardiac output results in fatigue and decreased exercise capacity.

In the short term, symptomatic treatment is directed at improving hemodynamic function through the use of drugs that increase cardiac output and reduce ventricular filling pressures. In the patient hospitalized because of severe symptoms of heart failure, rapid treatment may in-

clude the use of intravenous diuretics, positive inotropic agents (*e.g.,* β-adrenergic receptor agonists or phosphodiesterase inhibitors) and vasodilators (*e.g.,* nitroprusside or nitroglycerin). In the ambulatory patient in whom there is less urgency, similar goals are approached through the use of oral diuretics, digitalis, and vasodilators [*e.g.,* angiotensin converting enzyme (ACE) inhibitors].

Myocardial Remodeling.   Even in the absence of recurrent damage to the heart, the severity of the underlying myocardial dysfunction often is progressive. This is due to ventricular "remodeling," a process that results in progressive maladaptive changes in the structure and function of the ventricle (Cohn, 1995). Therefore, a second major

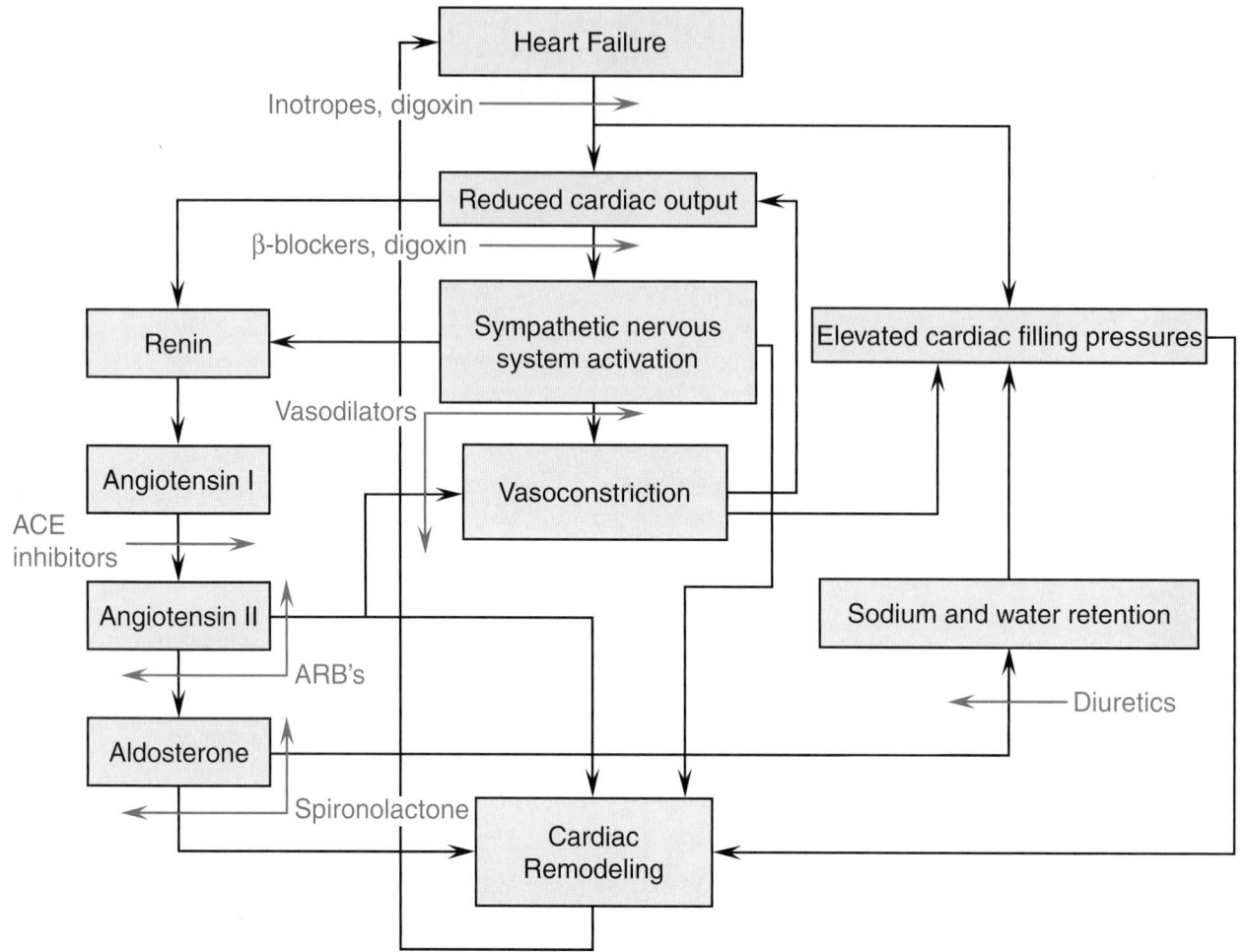

Figure 34–1. Pathophysiological mechanisms of heart failure and major sites of drug action.

Heart failure is accompanied by compensatory neurohormonal responses including activation of the sympathetic nervous and renin–angiotensin systems. Although these responses initially help to maintain cardiovascular function by increasing ventricular preload and systemic vascular tone, with time they contribute to the progression of myocardial failure. Increased ventricular afterload, due to systemic vasoconstriction and chamber dilation, causes a depression in systolic function. In addition, increased afterload and the direct effects of angiotensin and norepinephrine on the ventricular myocardium cause pathological remodeling characterized by progressive chamber dilation and loss of contractile function. The figure illustrates several mechanisms that appear to play an important role in the pathophysiology of heart failure, and the sites of action of pharmacological therapies that have been shown to be of clinical value. ACE, angiotensin converting enzyme; ARB, angiotensin-receptor blocker.

goal of therapy is to slow or prevent the progression of myocardial remodeling.

Initially, myocardial dysfunction causes intravascular volume expansion and the activation of neurohormonal systems, particularly the sympathetic nervous and renin–angiotensin systems. These primitive, compensatory responses defend the perfusion of vital organs by increasing left ventricular preload, stimulating myocardial contrac-

tility, and increasing arterial tone. However, with time each plays a role in the pathophysiology of the disease by promoting the progression of the underlying myocardial dysfunction. Expansion of the intravascular volume results in elevated ventricular filling pressures which increase ventricular wall stresses. Neurohormonal activation causes arterial and venous constriction which also leads to increased ventricular wall stresses. In addition, some neurohormones (*e.g.*, norepinephrine and angiotensin) may act directly on the myocardium to promote remodeling by causing myocyte apoptosis, abnormal gene expression, and/or alterations in the extracellular matrix (Colucci and Braunwald, 2000).

Drugs that reduce ventricular wall stresses (*e.g.*, vasodilators) and/or inhibit the renin–angiotensin system (*e.g.*, angiotensin converting enzyme inhibitors) or the sympathetic nervous system (*e.g.*, β-adrenergic receptor antagonists) have been found to decrease pathological ventricular remodeling, and are therefore a mainstay in the long-term treatment for heart failure. Some agents that slow progression also exert an immediate beneficial effect on hemodynamic function and symptoms (*e.g.*, vasodilators and angiotensin converting enzyme inhibitors). Other drugs that slow the progression of myocardial remodeling (*e.g.*, β-adrenergic receptor antagonists), may actually exert an adverse effect on hemodynamic function and can worsen symptoms in the short term. Figure 34–1 provides an overview of the pathophysiological mechanisms of heart failure and the sites of action of the major drug classes used in treatment.

The pharmacotherapeutic management of patients with heart failure is described in two sections. The first describes the use of oral drugs in ambulatory patients. The second describes intravenously administered agents primarily used for the treatment of hospitalized patients.

ORAL DRUGS FOR THE MANAGEMENT OF AMBULATORY HEART FAILURE

Diuretics

For several decades, and especially following the introduction of "loop" diuretics, this group of drugs has played a central role in the pharmacological management of the "congestive" symptoms in heart failure. Diuretics are discussed in detail in Chapter 29. Therefore, only those aspects of their pharmacology that are relevant to the treatment of heart failure will be dealt with in this chapter. The importance of these drugs is due to the central role of the kidney as the target organ for many of the hemodynamic, hormonal, and autonomic nervous system changes that occur in response to a failing myocardium. The net effect of these changes is the retention of salt and water and expansion of the extracellular fluid volume, which serves in the short run to sustain cardiac output and tissue perfusion by allowing the heart to operate higher on its ventricular function (*i.e.*, Frank–Starling) curve (Figure 34–2). However,

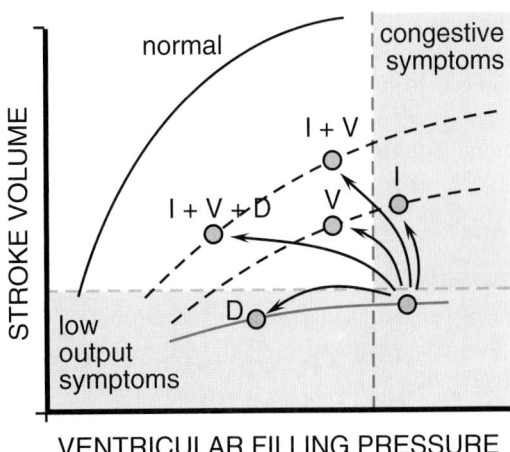

Figure 34–2. Hemodynamic responses to pharmacological interventions in heart failure.

The relationships between diastolic filling pressure (or preload) and stroke volume (or ventricular performance) are illustrated for a normal heart (*black line*) and for a patient with heart failure due to predominant systolic dysfunction (*blue line*). Note that positive inotropic agents, such as cardiac glycosides or dobutamine, move patients to a higher ventricular function curve (*dashed line*), resulting in greater cardiac work for a given level of ventricular filling pressure. Vasodilators, such as angiotensin converting enzyme inhibitors or nitroprusside, also move patients to improved ventricular function curves while reducing cardiac filling pressures. Diuretics improve symptoms of congestive heart failure by moving patients to lower cardiac filling pressures along the same ventricular function curve. Combinations of drugs often will yield additive effects on hemodynamics.

this response incurs the cost of higher end-diastolic filling pressures and increasing ventricular chamber dimensions and wall stress, which eventually limit any further increase in cardiac output and also result in pulmonary venous congestion and peripheral edema.

Diuretics act to reduce extracellular fluid volume and ventricular filling pressures (or "preload") but usually do not cause a clinically important reduction in cardiac output, particularly in patients with advanced heart failure who have an increased left ventricular filling pressure, unless there has been a profound and sustained natriuresis that results in a rapid decline in intravascular volume. Despite the clear efficacy of diuretics in controlling congestive symptoms and improving exercise capacity, it is worth noting that, with the exception of low-dose spironolactone, the use of diuretics has not been demonstrated to improve survival in heart failure. Indeed, monotherapy with a diuretic may cause increased neurohormonal activation due to volume depletion, with potentially deleterious effects on the progression of heart failure. For this reason, it may be preferable to avoid the use of diuretics in the subset of patients who have mild heart failure without evidence of fluid retention.

Dietary Sodium Restriction.   All patients with clinically significant ventricular dysfunction, regardless of whether or not they are symptomatic, should be advised to limit dietary intake of NaCl. Most patients will tolerate moderate reductions in salt intake (2 to 3 g/day total intake). More stringent salt restriction is seldom necessary and may be counterproductive in many heart-failure patients as it may lead to hyponatremia, hypokalemia, and a metabolic alkalosis due to chloride depletion when combined with loop diuretics, as well as loss of lean body mass due to reduced appetite.

Loop Diuretics.   Of the loop diuretics currently available, only *furosemide* (LASIX), *bumetanide* (BUMEX), and *torsemide* (DEMADEX) are indicated in the treatment of most patients with heart failure. Due to the increased risk of ototoxicity, ethacrynic acid should be reserved for patients who are allergic to sulfonamides or who have developed interstitial nephritis on alternative drugs.

Loop diuretics act to inhibit a specific ion transport protein, the Na^+–K^+–$2Cl^-$ symporter (*see* Chapter 29; Gamba *et al.*, 1994) on the apical membrane of renal epithelial cells in the ascending limb of Henle's loop. They rely for their efficacy on adequate renal plasma flow and proximal tubular secretion to deliver the diuretics to their site of action. These drugs also reduce the tonicity of the medullary interstitium by preventing the resorption of solute in excess of water in the thick ascending limb of the loop of Henle, and this may contribute to the development of hyponatremia in heart-failure patients. The increased delivery of Na^+ and fluid to distal nephron segments also markedly enhances K^+ secretion, particularly in the presence of elevated aldosterone levels, as is typically the case in heart failure.

The bioavailability of orally administered furosemide ranges from 40% to 70%, and adjustments in dosage may be required before it is deemed ineffective. In contrast, bumetanide and torsemide have oral bioavailabilities of more than 80% and provide more consistent absorption, albeit at a considerably greater cost. Furosemide and bumetanide are short-acting drugs. Avid renal Na^+ retention by all nephron segments following a decline in renal tubular diuretic levels can limit or prevent a negative Na^+ balance. In many patients with heart failure, this necessitates the use of two or more daily doses of these diuretics to induce and sustain a negative salt balance. This is an acceptable strategy for outpatient management of heart failure, provided that there is adequate monitoring of daily weights and blood electrolyte levels.

Thiazide Diuretics.   The principal site of action of the thiazide diuretics is now known to be the Na^+–Cl^- cotransporter (*see* Chapter 29) present in renal tubular epithelial cells in the distal convoluted tubule. The thiazide diuretics generally are useful as single drugs for the therapy of volume retention only in patients with relatively mild heart failure, largely because their site of action in the distal nephron permits rapid adjustment of water and solute absorption by other, more proximal nephron segments. Thiazide diuretics also are ineffective at glomerular filtration rates below 30 ml/minute. However, these drugs exhibit true synergism with loop diuretics (*i.e.*, a natriuresis that is greater than the sum of either class of drugs given individually). This is useful when patients become refractory to loop diuretics (*see* "Diuretic Resistance in Heart Failure," below).

K^+-Sparing Diuretics. K^+-sparing diuretics (*see* Chapter 29) are divided into those agents that inhibit apical membrane Na^+ conductance channels in epithelial cells of the collecting duct (*e.g., amiloride, triamterene*) and aldosterone antagonists that also have their principal pharmacological effect in the collecting duct (*e.g., spironolactone, canrenone*). Although these agents generally are not effective as diuretic agents when used alone, they may be useful in limiting renal K^+ and Mg^{2+} wasting and/or in augmenting the response to other classes of diuretics. As discussed below, there is evidence that a low dose of spironolactone may improve survival in patients with advanced symptoms of heart failure, apparently *via* a mechanism independent of diuresis (Pitt *et al.*, 1999).

Use of Diuretics in Clinical Practice.   The majority of patients with heart failure will require the chronic administration of a loop diuretic to maintain euvolemia. In patients with fluid retention, furosemide typically is started at a dose of 40 mg once or twice per day, and the dosage is increased until an adequate diuresis (increased urine output and weight loss of 0.5 to 1.5 kg daily) is achieved. A larger initial dose may be required if there is significant renal impairment, or in severe heart failure. Serum electrolytes and renal function should be monitored, especially if there is preexisting renal insufficiency or a brisk diuresis is desirable in a severely symptomatic patient. Once fluid retention has resolved, the dose of diuretic should be reduced to the minimum necessary to maintain euvolemia. Electrolyte abnormalities or worsening azotemia may supervene before euvolemia is achieved. Hypokalemia may occur and may be corrected by potassium supplementation or addition of a potassium-sparing diuretic. In general, diuresis should be slowed only if azotemia or renal impairment become progressive or the patient is symptomatic.

Diuretic Resistance in Heart Failure. The response to diuretics frequently is impaired in heart failure. Following prolonged administration of a loop diuretic, a process of adaptation occurs in which there is a compensatory increase in sodium reabsorption in the distal nephron and blunting of net sodium and water loss. Furthermore, while there may be a brisk response following a single dose of diuretic, a compensatory increase in sodium reabsorption for the remaining part of the 24-hour period may prevent effective diuresis. Patients who have impaired renal function typically require higher doses of diuretic to ensure adequate delivery of the diuretic to its site of action. A poor response to diuretics also may be due to edema and decreased motility of the bowel wall as well as to reduced splanchnic blood flow. This may cause slowed absorption and a delay in the peak effect of orally administered diuretics, although the total amount absorbed usually is unchanged.

The more common causes of diuretic resistance are listed in Table 34–1. It often is difficult to determine clinically whether an increasing diuretic requirement is due to intravascular volume depletion following aggressive diuretic and vasodilator therapy or to a decrease in cardiac output and blood pressure due to the underlying cardiac failure. Invasive monitoring to determine the left ventricular filling pressure may be required to make this distinction. However, a more marked decline in urea clearance than in creatinine clearance (resulting in an increase in the BUN to creatinine ratio) suggests intravascular volume depletion. Vasodilators commonly employed as "unloading" agents in heart failure may reduce renal blood flow despite an increase in cardiac output, thereby reducing diuretic effectiveness. Also, since some patients with heart failure also may have renal arterial atherosclerotic disease, vasodilator therapy may lower renal perfusion pressure below that necessary to maintain normal autoregulation and glomerular filtration.

The caveats about vasodilators also apply to ACE inhibitors and to angiotensin II type 1 receptor (*i.e.,* AT_1 receptor) antagonists (*see* Chapter 31). However, because of the unique role of angiotensin II as an intrarenal signaling autocoid, these drugs can either augment the effectiveness of diuretics by mechanisms independent of their ability to reduce systemic vascular resistance or diminish their effectiveness by reducing the transglomerular perfusion pressure to the point that the glomerular filtration rate declines abruptly. The latter response is observed most commonly in patients with decreased renal arterial perfusion pressure, due either to renal artery stenosis and/or a limited cardiac output, for whom a high angiotensin II–mediated glomerular efferent arteriolar tone is necessary to maintain glomerular filtration. This cause of diuretic resistance generally is accompanied by a decline in creatinine clearance and should be distinguished from the more modest, limited rise in serum creatinine levels and improved responsiveness to diuretics that commonly accompany ACE-inhibitor administration.

Diuretic resistance due primarily to poor cardiac function generally improves when cardiac output is increased by the use of positive inotropic agents (*e.g.,* dobutamine) or vasodilators. Decreased responsiveness to loop diuretics in patients otherwise receiving optimal medical management should be managed initially by increasing the frequency of doses and by more stringent dietary salt restriction. If this is ineffective, a thiazide diuretic (*e.g., hydrochlorothiazide* or *metolazone*) administered with the loop diuretic often is effective (Ellison, 1991). However, this diuretic combination can result in an unpredictable and at times excessive diuresis, which can cause intravascular volume depletion and renal K^+ wasting; the combination therefore should be used cautiously. *Spironolactone* also may be effective in these patients when combined with a loop diuretic. For a detailed discussion on the subject of diuretic resistance, the reader is referred to a recent comprehensive review (Ellison, 1999).

Metabolic Consequences of Diuretic Therapy. The side effects of diuretic agents are discussed in Chapter 29 and

Table 34–1
Causes of Diuretic Resistance in Heart Failure

Noncompliance with medical regimen and/or excess dietary Na^+ intake

Decreased renal perfusion and glomerular filtration rate due to:

  Excessive intravascular volume depletion and hypotension due to aggressive diuretic and/or vasodilator therapy

  Decline in cardiac output due to worsening heart failure, arrhythmias, or other primary cardiac causes

  Selective reduction in glomerular perfusion pressure following initiation (or dose increase) of angiotensin converting enzyme inhibitor therapy

Nonsteroidal anti-inflammatory drugs

Primary renal pathology (*e.g.,* cholesterol emboli, renal artery stenosis, drug-induced interstitial nephritis, obstructive uropathy)

Reduced or impaired diuretic absorption due to gut wall edema and reduced splanchnic blood flow in recent overviews of diuretic use (*e.g.,* Brater, 1998). With regard to diuretic use in heart failure, the most important adverse sequelae of diuretics are electrolyte abnormalities, including hyponatremia, hypokalemia, and hypochloremic metabolic alkalosis. The clinical importance, or even the existence, of significant Mg^{2+} deficiency with chronic diuretic use remains controversial (Bigger, 1994; Davies and Fraser, 1993). Both hypokalemia and renal Mg^{2+} wasting can be limited by administration of oral KCl supplements or a K^+-sparing diuretic.

Aldosterone Antagonists

One of the principal features of heart failure is marked activation of the renin-angiotensin-aldosterone system with elevation of the plasma aldosterone concentration to as much as 20 times the normal level. As mentioned above, when used alone spironolactone exerts only a very weak diuretic effect in patients with heart failure. However, aldosterone has a range of biological effects in addition to salt retention (*see* Table 34–2), and it has been suggested that antagonism of aldosterone, *per se,* may be beneficial in patients with heart failure. For a review of the subject of aldosterone and spironolactone in heart failure, see the recent review by Struthers (1999).

Clinical Use of Spironolactone in Heart Failure.   The Randomized Aldactone Evaluation Study (RALES) randomized patients with moderate to severe heart failure [New York Heart Association (NYHA) class III to IV] to receive 25 mg daily of spironolactone or placebo in addition to conventional therapy, which included, in the large majority of patients, an ACE inhibitor (Pitt, 1999). Patients with serum creatinine concentrations greater than

2.5 mg/dl (221 μM) were excluded from the study, and only a very small number of patients received 50 mg of spironolactone daily. Patients randomized to spironolactone had a significant 30% reduction in mortality and hospitalization for heart failure. The decrease in the risk of death was due to reductions in both progressive heart failure and sudden cardiac death and, notably, was achieved in the apparent absence of a measurable diuretic effect. Treatment was generally well tolerated, and although 10% of men in the spironolactone group developed gynecomastia, withdrawal of treatment was necessary in less than 2%. Severe hyperkalemia occurred in only 2% of patients on spironolactone, and there were no clinically important effects on renal function.

The RALES trial suggests that the beneficial effects of spironolactone are additive to those of ACE inhibitors, and its use should be considered in patients with NYHA class III to IV heart failure. However, caution should be exercised in its use when significant renal impairment is present. Treatment should be initiated at a dose of 12.5 or 25 mg daily. Higher doses should be avoided, as they may lead to hyperkalemia, particularly in patients receiving an ACE inhibitor. Serum potassium levels and electrolytes should be checked after initiation of treatment, and vigilance should be exercised for potential drug interactions and medical disorders that may cause elevations in serum potassium concentration (*e.g.,* potassium supplements, ACE inhibitors, and worsening renal function).

Vasodilators

Although several classes of drugs exhibit vasodilator activity and may improve symptoms in heart failure (Table 34–3), only *ACE inhibitors* and the *hydralazine–isosorbide dinitrate combination* have been shown to improve survival in prospective randomized trials. Some classes of

Table 34–2

Potential Roles of Aldosterone in the Pathophysiology of Heart Failure

MECHANISM	PATHOPHYSIOLOGICAL EFFECT
Increased sodium and water retention	Edema, elevated cardiac filling pressures
Potassium and magnesium loss	Arrhythmogenesis and risk of sudden cardiac death
Reduced myocardial norepinephrine uptake	Potentiation of norepinephrine effects–myocardial remodeling and arrhythmogenesis
Reduced baroreceptor sensitivity	Reduced parasympathetic activity and risk of sudden cardiac death
Myocardial fibrosis, fibroblast proliferation	Remodeling and ventricular dysfunction
Alterations in sodium channel expression	Increased excitability and contractility of cardiac myocytes

Table 34–3

Vasodilator Drugs Used to Treat Heart Failure

DRUG CLASS	EXAMPLES	MECHANISM OF VASODILATING ACTION	PRELOAD REDUCTION	AFTERLOAD REDUCTION
Organic nitrates	Nitroglycerin, isosorbide dinitrate	Nitric oxide–mediated vasodilation	+++	+
Nitric oxide donors	Nitroprusside	Nitric oxide–mediated vasodilation	+++	+++
Angiotensin converting enzyme inhibitors	Captopril, enalapril, lisinopril	Inhibition of angiotensin generation, decreased bradykinin degradation	++	++
Angiotensin receptor blockers	Iosartan, candesartan	Blockade of angiotensin receptors	++	++
Phosphodiesterase inhibitors	Milrinone, inamrinone	Inhibition of cyclic AMP degradation	++	++
Direct-acting	Hydralazine, minoxidil	Unknown	+	+++
Subtype-selective α_1-adrenergic receptor antagonists	Doxazosin, prazosin	Selective α_1-adrenergic receptor blocker	+++	++
Non-subtype-selective α-adrenergic receptor antagonists	Phentolamine	Non-selective α-adrenergic receptor blockade	+++	+++
Vasodilating β/α_1 adrenergic receptor antagonists	Carvedilol, labetalol	Selective α_1-adrenergic receptor blockade	++	++
Ca^{2+} channel blocking drugs	Amlodipine, nifedipine, felodipine	Inhibition of L-type Ca^{2+} channels	+	+++
β-adrenergic receptor agonists	Isoproterenol	Stimulation of vascular β_2-adrenergic receptors	+	++

drugs, such as α_1-adrenergic antagonists, have no demonstrated effect on mortality, while other agents, such as prostacyclin and flosequinan, appear to decrease long-term survival. The basic and clinical pharmacology of most of the vasodilators discussed in this chapter are considered in more detail in Chapters 32 and 33.

The rationale for the use of drugs with vasodilatory activity in heart failure grew out of experience with parenteral phentolamine and nitroprusside in patients with severe heart failure. Cohn and Franciosa, in an influential article in 1977, reviewed the evidence supporting this approach. Studies of ACE inhibitors in the following decade showed that these drugs generally were well tolerated and effective in improving symptoms in heart failure, while

two randomized, prospective trials verified the effectiveness of an isosorbide dinitrate–hydralazine combination (Cohn et al., 1986) and enalapril (CONSENSUS, 1987) in reducing mortality in patients with heart failure. Subsequent clinical trials have reinforced the results of these two trials and have provided evidence supporting expanded indications for the use of ACE inhibitors to patients with ventricular dysfunction but without overt symptoms of heart failure (see below).

Principles of Vasodilator Therapy.   The principles of vasodilator therapy in heart failure are reviewed in detail in texts of cardiovascular medicine and physiology (e.g., Smith et al., 1997). Briefly, the hemodynamic responses to heart failure are similar in some respects to those that accompany a fall in blood pressure due to hypovolemia; they include tachycardia and an increase in venous and arterial vasoconstriction, with shunting of blood toward the thorax and brain and away from the periphery and splanchnic and renal vascular beds. While this provides a clear evolutionary advantage to the organism to survive dehydration or hemorrhage, it is maladaptive and deleterious in chronic heart failure. The concepts of preload and afterload reduction provide a convenient framework in which to address treatment options in heart failure, which, in many respects, attempt to overcome these inappropriate compensatory hemodynamic responses. While this discussion focuses on heart failure due to left ventricular dysfunction, the general principles of preload and afterload reduction are applicable to failure of either ventricle despite differences in the specific drugs or other forms of therapy that can be employed.

Although drugs may be classified as either "arterial" or "venous" vasodilators, most vasodilators exhibit activity on both vascular beds. Also, classes of vasodilators differ in the specific arterial beds that are affected. This has important implications in preserving, for example, renal blood flow and diuretic effectiveness and may explain, in part, the superior efficacy of certain classes of vasodilator agents in heart failure.

Preload Reduction.   The principle of preload reduction can be expressed in the form of the Frank–Starling relationship illustrated in Figure 34–2. In early heart failure, increases in intraventricular volume and pressure, as well as heart rate, compensate for a decline in ventricular systolic performance due to underlying cardiac disease. In more advanced heart failure, there may be little or no further augmentation of stroke volume with increasing filling pressures (*i.e.*, a "flat Frank–Starling curve"), while the transmission of increased pressure into the pulmonary and systemic venous beds produces congestive symptoms. This usually is accompanied by worsening myocardial energetics due to an increase in ventricular wall stress and a decrease in diastolic coronary blood flow. Agents that reduce ventricular filling pressures by decreasing intravascular volume (*e.g.*, diuretics) or by increasing venous capacitance (*e.g.*, venodilators) decrease pulmonary venous congestion and may improve myocardial metabolism with minimal effects on stroke volume and cardiac output. While these measures clearly improve symptoms due to systolic ventricular dysfunction, they also benefit patients with congestive symptoms due to impaired diastolic compliance (*i.e.*, "diastolic dysfunction"), whether due to ischemia or structural changes in the myocardium. However, patients with poorly compliant hypertrophied ventricles due, for example, to aortic stenosis, often require elevated end-diastolic filling pressures to support an adequate forward stroke volume. An excessive decrease in preload may markedly reduce cardiac output in these patients.

Afterload Reduction.   The importance of systemic arterial vasodilation in improving cardiac hemodynamics in heart failure was succinctly described by Cohn and Franciosa (1977). *Afterload,* the sum of forces opposing ventricular emptying during systole, is dependent on aortic and aortic outflow tract (including valvular) impedance, systemic vascular resistance, ventricular–vascular coupling (*i.e.*, the harmonics of reflected arterial pressure waves during systole), and the volume of blood in the ventricle at the initiation of systole. Hypertrophy of ventricular muscle is a compensatory mechanism that reduces wall stress and preserves ventricular systolic function despite a primary abnormality in one or more of the determinants of afterload (*e.g.*, a stenotic aortic valve). In the failing heart, as illustrated

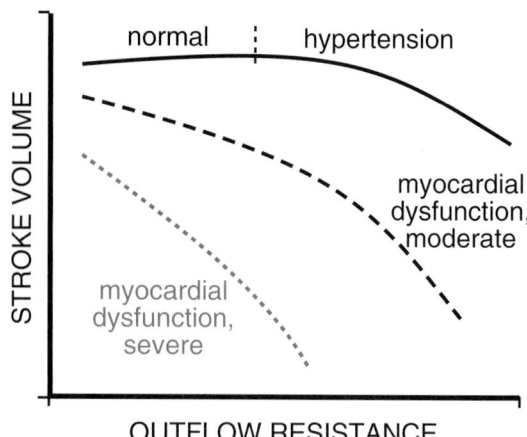

Figure 34–3. Relationship between ventricular outflow resistance and stroke volume in patients with systolic ventricular dysfunction.

An increase in ventricular outflow resistance, a principal determinant of "afterload," has little effect on stroke volume in normal hearts, as illustrated by the relatively flat curve. In contrast, in patients with systolic ventricular dysfunction, an increase in outflow resistance often is accompanied by a sharp decline in stroke volume. With more severe ventricular dysfunction, this curve becomes steeper. Because of this relationship, a reduction in systemic vascular resistance, one component of outflow resistance, following administration of an arterial vasodilator may markedly increase stroke volume in patients with severe myocardial dysfunction. The resultant increase in stroke volume may be sufficient to offset the decrease in systemic vascular resistance, thereby preventing a fall in systemic arterial pressure. (Adapted from Cohn and Franciosa, 1977, with permission.)

in Figure 34–3, any reduction in ventricular wall stress during systole, whether achieved by corrective surgery, intraaortic balloon counterpulsation, or vasodilator drugs, results in improved systolic contractile function. In addition, any reduction in aortic or arterial determinants of afterload will improve forward stroke volume and improve signs and symptoms of mitral regurgitation, which is often present in patients with severe heart failure due to systolic dysfunction, even in the absence of primary disease of the mitral valve.

Inhibition of the Renin–Angiotensin System.   The renin–angiotensin system has a central role in the pathophysiology of heart failure (for detailed description of the renin–angiotensin system, *see* Chapter 31). Angiotensinogen is cleaved by kidney-derived renin to form the decapeptide angiotensin I; ACE converts angiotensin I to the octapeptide angiotensin II (*see* Figure 34–4). Angiotensin II is a potent arterial vasoconstrictor which promotes sodium and water retention through its role in the regulation of renal hemodynamics and release from the adrenal cortex of aldosterone. Additionally, angiotensin II potentiates

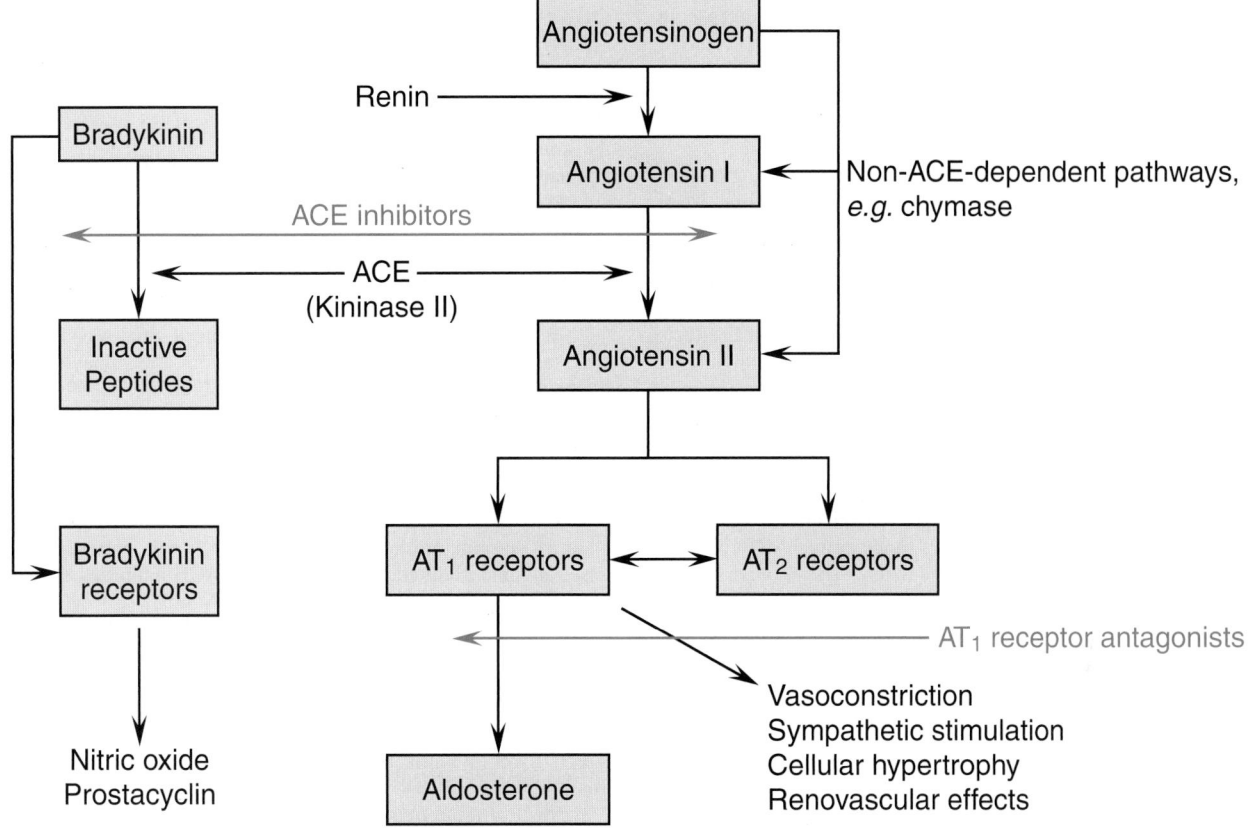

Figure 34–4. The renin-angiotensin-aldosterone system.

Angiotensin II is formed through the cleavage of angiotensin I by angiotensin converting enzyme (ACE). Most of the known biological effects of angiotensin II are mediated by the type 1 angiotensin receptor (AT$_1$). In general, the type 2 angiotensin receptor (AT$_2$) appears to counteract the actions of the AT$_1$ receptor. Angiotensin II also may be formed through non-ACE-dependent pathways. These pathways, and possibly incomplete inhibition of tissue ACE, may account for persistence of angiotensin in patients treated with ACE inhibitors. AT$_1$ receptor antagonists have been postulated to provide more complete blockade of the renin-angiotensin-aldosterone system than ACE inhibition alone. ACE also is a kininase, and therefore ACE inhibition reduces bradykinin degradation, thus enhancing its levels and biological effects including the release of nitric oxide and prostacyclin. It has been suggested that bradykinin may mediate many of the important biological effects of ACE inhibitors.

catecholamine release, is arrhythmogenic, promotes vascular hyperplasia and pathologic myocardial hypertrophy, and stimulates myocyte death. These actions of angiotensin II contribute to the pathophysiology of heart failure and, in many cases, to pathological remodeling of the myocardium leading to disease progression.

ACE inhibitors have been shown to suppress angiotensin II and aldosterone production, decrease sympathetic nervous system activity, and potentiate the effects of diuretics in heart failure. However, angiotensin II levels frequently return to baseline values following chronic treatment with ACE inhibitors (Juillerat *et al.*, 1990). This is believed to be due to production of angiotensin II through non-ACE-dependent pathways—for example, through the action of chymase, a tissue protease. The

sustained clinical effectiveness of ACE inhibitors despite failure to maintain angiotensin II suppression has raised the possibility that there may be additional or alternate mechanisms by which ACE inhibitors work in heart failure. ACE is identical to kininase II, which degrades bradykinin and other kinins; bradykinin stimulates production of nitric oxide, cyclic GMP and vasoactive prostaglandins which result in vasodilation and oppose the effects of angiotensin II on vascular- and myocardial-cell growth. Thus, it has been suggested that increased levels of bradykinin as a result of ACE inhibition may play an important role in the hemodynamic and antiremodeling effects of ACE inhibitors.

ACE inhibitors cause both arterial and venous dilation. There are reductions in systemic and pulmonary arterial resistances. Mean arterial pressure may be unchanged or decrease, but heart rate usually is unchanged, even when there is a decrease in systemic pressure, perhaps due to a decrease in sympathetic nervous system activity. The decrease in left ventricular afterload results in an increase in cardiac output due to increases in stroke volume and ejection fraction. Venodilation results in decreases in right and left heart filling pressures and end-diastolic volumes.

An alternative means of inhibiting the renin–angiotensin system is through inhibition of angiotensin receptors. Most of the known clinical actions of angiotensin II, including its deleterious effects in heart failure, are mediated through the type 1 angiotensin receptor (AT_1). Type 2 angiotensin receptors (AT_2) also are present throughout the cardiovascular system, where they are believed to counterbalance the biological effects of AT_1-receptor stimulation. Due to their more distal site of action, AT_1 angiotensin-receptor blockers (ARBs) theoretically may allow more complete interruption of angiotensin's actions than can be obtained with ACE inhibitors. Furthermore, since AT_1-receptor blockade has been associated with a compensatory increase in angiotensin II levels, AT_2-receptor stimulation is increased, potentially enhancing the beneficial effects of ARBs. On the other hand, a theoretical drawback of the ARBs is their failure to increase bradykinin production. The relative merits of these possible mechanisms of action remain to be seen, as does the value of combined therapy with an ACE inhibitor and an ARB, which has the potential to provide more complete renin–angiotensin system blockade while increasing bradykinin production.

Angiotensin Converting Enzyme Inhibitors. The first orally active ACE inhibitor, *captopril* (CAPOTEN), was introduced in 1977, and currently five other ACE inhibitors—*enalapril* (VASOTEC), *ramipril* (ALTACE), *lisinopril* (PRINIVIL, ZESTRIL), *quinapril* (ACCUPRIL), and *fosinopril* (MONOPRIL), are approved by the U.S. Food and Drug Administration (FDA) for the treatment of heart failure. ACE inhibitors are now indicated for the treatment of heart failure of any severity, including asymptomatic left ventricular dysfunction.

ACE-inhibition therapy should be initiated at a low dose (*e.g.,* 6.25 mg of captopril or 5 mg of lisinopril), as some patients may experience an abrupt drop in blood pressure, particularly if they are volume depleted. Unacceptable hypotension usually can be reversed by intravascular volume expansion, although this may be counterproductive in patients with symptomatic heart failure. ACE inhibitor doses are customarily titrated upwards over several days in hospitalized patients or a few weeks in ambulatory patients, with careful observation of blood pressure, serum electrolytes, and serum creatinine levels.

There is no precisely defined relationship between dose and long-term clinical effectiveness of these drugs. The target doses of these drugs in several large prospective trials in which a positive effect was demonstrated on mortality and other endpoints were 50 mg of captopril three times a day (Pfeffer *et al.,* 1992); 10 mg of enalapril twice daily (SOLVD Investigators, 1991; Cohn *et al.,* 1991); 10 mg of lisinopril once

daily (GISSI-3 Investigators, 1994); or 5 mg twice daily of ramipril (AIRE Study Investigators, 1993). The question of optimal dosage of ACE inhibitor was addressed in the Assessment of Treatment with Lisinopril and Survival (ATLAS) study (Packer, 1999). High-dose lisinopril (32.5 or 35 mg) reduced the combined endpoint of mortality and hospitalization when compared to a low dose (2.5 or 5 mg). Based on the available evidence, the initial dosage of an ACE inhibitor should be titrated to the dosage that was shown to be of benefit in the major heart-failure trials. In patients who have not achieved an adequate clinical response, further uptitration to higher doses, as tolerated, may be of value.

In patients with heart failure and reduced renal blood flow, ACE inhibitors, unlike other vasodilators, limit the kidney's ability to autoregulate glomerular perfusion pressure due to their selective effects on efferent arteriolar tone. If this occurs, the dose of ACE inhibitor should be reduced or another class of vasodilator added or substituted. Rarely, worsening of renal function following initiation of therapy with an ACE inhibitor will be due to the presence of bilateral renal artery stenosis. Another class of vasodilator should be substituted if this occurs. Likewise, angioneurotic edema secondary to ACE inhibitors should prompt immediate cessation of therapy. A small rise in serum potassium levels occurs frequently with ACE inhibitors; this may infrequently be substantial, especially in patients with renal impairment. Mild hyperkalemia is best managed by institution of a low potassium diet, but may require adjustment of dosage. A troublesome cough may occur, believed related to the effects of bradykinin. Substitution of an ARB often alleviates this problem.

Effect of ACE Inhibitors on Survival in Heart Failure. A number of placebo-controlled trials have demonstrated that ACE inhibitors improve survival in patients with overt heart failure due to systolic ventricular dysfunction regardless of the etiology or severity of symptoms. The Cooperative Northern Scandinavian Enalapril Survival Study (CONSENSUS, 1987) demonstrated a 40% reduction in mortality after 6 months in patients with severe heart failure randomized to enalapril rather than placebo. These results were confirmed by a 16% reduction in mortality in the treatment arm of the Studies On Left Ventricular Dysfunction (SOLVD Investigators, 1991) trial, in which patients with symptomatic mild to moderate heart failure and left ventricular ejection fractions less than 35% were randomized to receive either enalapril or placebo. The second Veterans Administration Cooperative Vasodilator–Heart Failure Trial (V-HeFT II; Cohn *et al.,* 1991) showed a small but clear survival benefit in patients with mild to moderate heart failure who were randomized to enalapril rather than the combination of hydralazine and isosorbide dinitrate. A smaller randomized trial comparing captopril to hydralazine and isosorbide dinitrate in patients with moderate to severe heart failure also demonstrated a significant survival advantage to patients receiving the ACE inhibitor (Fonarow *et al.,* 1992).

These data convinced many clinicians that ACE inhibitors clearly improved survival of patients with symptomatic heart failure. The prevention arm of the SOLVD trial subsequently examined whether or not asymptomatic patients with left ventricular systolic dysfunction also derive a survival benefit (SOLVD Investigators, 1992). Although this study failed to demonstrate a statistically significant reduction in mortality among enalapril-treated patients, there was a significant (29%) reduction in the combined end point of the development of symptomatic heart failure and death due to any cause.

ACE inhibitors also may prevent the development of clinically significant ventricular dysfunction and mortality following myocardial infarction. The Survival And Ventricular Enlargement trial (SAVE; Pfeffer *et al.,* 1992), which examined patients with recent, acute anterior myocardial infarction and ejection fractions of 40% or less, showed a 20% reduction in mortality and a 36% reduction in the rate of progression to severe heart failure in the captopril-treated group after 12 months of follow-up. Both the SOLVD trials (Konstam *et al.,* 1992) and the SAVE trial (St. John Sutton *et al.,* 1994) also demonstrated that enalapril and captopril, respectively, markedly reduced or prevented the increases in left ventricular end-diastolic and end-systolic volumes and decline in ejection fraction observed in patients randomized to receive placebo. The Acute Infarction Ramipril Efficacy trial (AIRE Investigators, 1993), which had a study design similar to that of the SAVE trial, also demonstrated a significant (27%) reduction in mortality in the ACE inhibitor–treated group. These studies attest to the safety and efficacy of ACE-inhibitor therapy initiated early in the postinfarct period regardless of whether clinically significant left ventricular dysfunction is present at the time of randomization.

Angiotensin II Receptor Antagonists. Six orally active ARBs now have been approved for the treatment of hypertension, but none has been approved for use in heart failure. ARBs are discussed in detail in Chapter 31 and a recent review (Burnier and Brunner, 2000).

In patients with heart failure, ARBs exert hemodynamic effects similar to those of the ACE inhibitors; however, there is much less information about their effects on long-term outcomes such as hospitalization and survival. The Evaluation of Losartan in the Elderly (ELITE) trial was primarily designed to examine the effects of the ARB *losartan* (COZAAR) on renal function in elderly patients with heart failure (Pitt *et al.,* 1997). Patients were randomized to receive either the ACE inhibitor captopril, 50 mg three times daily, or losartan, 50 mg once daily; there were no significant differences in renal function between the two groups, but an unexpected reduction in mortality and hospitalizations from heart failure was noted in the losartan group. This was followed by the much larger ELITE II study which, like ELITE I, compared losartan and captopril in elderly patients, but had mortality as the primary end point (Pitt *et al.,* 2000). In contrast to the findings in ELITE I, no significant difference in outcome was noted between the treatment groups. However, treatment with the ARB was better tolerated and associated with fewer adverse effects than treatment with the ACE inhibitor. Thus, ELITE II failed to confirm the superiority of an ARB over an ACE inhibitor. In addition, this study was not designed to test the equivalence of these two drug classes, and its interpretation has been confounded by concern that the dosage of losartan studied was not sufficient to achieve adequate blockade of AT_1 receptors.

Thus, until further data are available, the much larger body of data showing the benefits of ACE inhibitors in heart failure supports their routine use as first line agents. Conversely, although the present data do not allow the conclusion that ARBs

are equivalent to ACE inhibitors, it appears reasonable to use ARBs as an alternative in patients intolerant to ACE inhibitors. Large trials are in progress that should provide more definitive data regarding the relative roles of ACE inhibitors and ARBs in the treatment of heart failure.

The use of ACE inhibitors and ARBs in combination offers the interesting possibility of additive therapeutic effects due to their different modes of action on the renin–angiotensin system. Preliminary results suggest that combined therapy with the ARB *candesartan* and the ACE inhibitor enalapril had favorable effects on hemodynamics, ventricular remodeling, and neurohormonal profile compared to therapy with either agent alone (McKelvie *et al.,* 1999). Again, more definitive data are required before combination therapy is routinely applied in clinical practice.

Nitrovasodilators. Nitrovasodilators are among the oldest and most widely used vasodilators in clinical practice. The mechanism underlying the ability of these drugs to activate soluble guanylyl cyclase and relax vascular smooth muscle has become apparent only in the past 15 years. These drugs mimic the activity of nitric oxide (NO), an intracellular and paracrine signaling autocoid that is formed by the conversion of arginine to citrulline mediated by a family of enzymes termed *nitric oxide synthases.* This family of enzymes is found in endothelial and smooth muscle cells throughout the vasculature as well as in many other cell types. The basis for the differential sensitivity of selected regions of the vasculature to specific nitrovasodilators (*e.g.,* the sensitivity of the epicardial coronary arteries to *nitroglycerin,* for example) remains controversial. Unlike *nitroprusside,* which is spontaneously converted to nitric oxide by reducing agents such as glutathione, nitroglycerin and other organic nitrates undergo a more complex enzymatic biotransformation to nitric oxide or bioactive *S*-nitrosothiols. The activities of specific enzyme(s) and cofactors required for this biotransformation, while not yet clearly identified, appear to differ within the vascular beds among organs and at different levels of the vasculature within an organ (Kelly and Smith, 1996). The basic pharmacology of the organic nitrates is discussed in Chapter 32.

Organic Nitrates. Organic nitrate preparations, most commonly *isosorbide dinitrate* (ISORDIL, DILATRATE, SORBITRATE), intravenous nitroglycerin, and nitroglycerin ointment, sublingual tablets, transdermal patch, and lingual spray, are relatively safe and effective agents in reducing ventricular filling pressures in acute as well as chronic congestive heart failure. The predominant effect at conventional doses is preload reduction due to an increase in peripheral venous capacitance. Nitrates also will cause a decline in pulmonary and systemic vascular resistance, particularly at higher doses, although this response is less marked and less predictable than with nitroprusside. Due to their relatively selective vasodilating effects on the epicardial coronary vasculature, these drugs may enhance systolic and diastolic ventricular function by increasing coronary flow in patients with underlying ischemia.

Isosorbide dinitrate has been shown to be more effective than placebo in improving exercise capacity and in reducing symptoms when administered chronically to heart-failure patients. However, limited effects on systemic vascular resistance and the problem of pharmacological tolerance have restricted the use of organic nitrates as single agents in the pharmacotherapy of heart failure. In a number of smaller trials, isosorbide dinitrate has been shown to increase the clinical effectiveness of other vasodilators such as hydralazine, resulting in a sustained improvement in hemodynamics that exceeded those of either drug given alone. Importantly, the combination of isosorbide dinitrate (20 mg four times daily) and hydralazine in the V-HeFT I trial reduced overall mortality compared to either placebo or the α_1-adrenergic receptor antagonist prazosin in patients with mild to moderate heart failure concurrently treated with digoxin and diuretics (Cohn et al., 1986).

Nitrate tolerance limits the long-term effectiveness of these drugs when administered throughout the day for heart-failure symptoms. Blood levels of these drugs should be permitted to fall to negligible levels for at least 6 to 8 hours each day. The timing of nitrate withdrawal (e.g., removal of a transdermal nitroglycerin patch or skipping a dose of isosorbide dinitrate) can be adjusted to the patient's symptoms. Patients with recurrent orthopnea or paroxysmal nocturnal dyspnea, for example, would probably benefit most by using nitrates at night. Orally bioavailable compounds containing sulfhydryl groups, such as N-acetylcysteine, may diminish tolerance to the hemodynamic effects of nitrates in heart failure (Mehra et al., 1994). Likewise, hydralazine may decrease nitrate tolerance by a strong antioxidant effect reducing superoxide formation (which reacts rapidly with nitric oxide) and hence increasing bioavailability of nitric oxide (Gogia et al., 1995).

Hydralazine. The vasodilator activity of *hydralazine* (APRESOLINE) is not mediated by any known neural or hormonal agent, and its cellular mechanism of action in vascular smooth muscle remains poorly understood. Hydralazine is an effective antihypertensive drug (Chapter 33), particularly when combined with other agents that blunt compensatory increases in sympathetic tone and salt and water retention. In heart failure, hydralazine reduces right and left ventricular afterload by reducing systemic and pulmonary vascular resistance. This results in an augmentation of forward stroke volume and a reduction in ventricular systolic wall stress and regurgitant fraction in mitral

insufficiency. Hydralazine also appears to have moderate "direct" positive inotropic activity in cardiac muscle unrelated to afterload reduction. Hydralazine has minimal effects on venous capacitance and therefore is most effective when combined with agents with venodilating activity (e.g., organic nitrates). Importantly, hydralazine is effective in reducing renal vascular resistance and in increasing renal blood flow to a greater degree than are most other vasodilators, with the exception of ACE inhibitors. Therefore, hydralazine may be useful in heart-failure patients with renal dysfunction who cannot tolerate an ACE inhibitor.

The combination of hydralazine (300 mg/day) and isosorbide dinitrate was less effective than enalapril in reducing mortality in heart-failure patients in the V-HeFT II trial (Cohn et al., 1991), although this combination of agents did increase survival compared to placebo or the α_1-adrenergic antagonist prazosin in V-HeFT I (Cohn et al., 1986). This is an important point, because a number of promising vasodilator drugs, some of which also have direct effects on cardiac contractility, have been shown to increase mortality (e.g., milrinone, flosequinan, prostacyclin) in heart failure. Hydralazine, with or without nitrates, may provide additional hemodynamic improvement for patients with advanced heart failure who already are being treated with conventional doses of an ACE inhibitor, digoxin, and diuretics (Cohn, 1994).

Side effects that may necessitate dose adjustment or withdrawal of hydralazine are common. Twenty percent of patients in the V-HeFT I trial (Cohn et al., 1986) complained of symptoms that could have been related to hydralazine, although the most common complaints, headache and dizziness, also could have been due to the concomitantly administered nitrates. Usually, the symptoms diminish with time or respond to a reduction in dose. The oral bioavailability and pharmacokinetics of elimination of hydralazine do not appear to be importantly affected by heart failure unless there is severe hepatic congestion or hypoperfusion. Intravenous hydralazine is available but provides little practical advantage over oral formulations except for urgent use during pregnancy, in which relative contraindications exist for most other vasodilators. Hydralazine is typically started at a dose of 10 to 25 mg three times a day and the dosage titrated to 100 mg three times a day over several days as clinical needs dictate and side effects allow.

Ca^{2+} Channel Antagonists. The Ca^{2+} channel antagonists are effective arterial vasodilators that have been widely used to treat hypertension (see Chapter 33). Although these agents offer theoretical advantages in the management of heart failure, the clinical experience has been disappointing. The use of the first-generation Ca^{2+} channel antagonists (verapamil, diltiazem, nifedipine) has not been shown to produce sustained improvement in symptoms in patients with predominant systolic ventricular dysfunction. Indeed, these drugs may worsen symptoms and increase mortality in patients with systolic dysfunction, including patients with heart failure due to ischemic disease (Elkayam et al., 1993). The reason for this adverse effect of Ca^{2+} channel blockers in heart failure is unclear, but may be related to their known negative inotropic effects or to reflex neurohumoral activation. *Amlodipine* (NORVASC) and *felodipine* (PLENDIL) are second-generation dihydropyridines with greater vascular selectivity, and hence, fewer negative inotropic effects than the first-generation agents. In the Prospective Randomized Amlodipine Survival Evaluation Study (PRAISE), 1153 patients with severe heart failure were randomized to receive amlodipine (up to 10 mg daily) or placebo (Packer *et al.*, 1996a). A trend toward a decrease in mortality was noted in the amlodipine group, with a more pronounced survival benefit in the subgroup of patients with nonischemic cardiomyopathy. Therefore, PRAISE II further evaluated amlodipine in patients with nonischemic cardiomyopathy; preliminary results of this study, however, do not suggest a survival benefit with amlodipine, but confirmed its safety in this patient population. Similarly, felodipine was shown to have a neutral effect on survival and exercise tolerance in the third Vasodilator-Heart Failure Trial (V-HeFT III) (Cohn *et al.*, 1997). The aforementioned Ca^{2+} channel antagonists act on the voltage-sensitive L-type channel. In contrast, *mibefradil* is a Ca^{2+} channel antagonist that is selective for the non-voltage-regulated, T-type channel. Although this agent does not appear to have clinically significant negative inotropic activity, its use was associated with an increased risk of death (believed secondary to major adverse drug interactions) that prompted its withdrawal from the market.

The available clinical evidence does not support the routine use of Ca^{2+} channel antagonists as first-line therapy in patients with heart failure. However, the use of amlodipine or felodipine may be considered in certain circumstances in which additional control of blood pressure or afterload reduction is required, or if other vasodilators (*e.g.*, ACE inhibitors, angiotensin receptor antagonists or hydralazine) are contraindicated or poorly tolerated.

In contrast to results in patients with predominant systolic dysfunction, Ca^{2+} channel antagonists appear to be useful agents for the treatment of heart failure due predominantly to diastolic dysfunction, such as hypertensive or idiopathic hypertrophic cardiomyopathies. By slowing heart rate, which is an important determinant of diastolic filling time, verapamil and diltiazem may facilitate diastolic relaxation and lower diastolic filling pressures. These agents also can be useful in the acute management of patients in heart failure due to most supraventricular tachyarrhythmias in the absence of severe right or left ventricular systolic dysfunction, or a known or suspected extranodal atrioventricular accessory pathway (Wolff-Parkinson-White syndrome).

Other Vasodilators. As noted in Table 34–3, other vasodilator drugs are effective in reducing ventricular preload and afterload and improving symptoms in heart failure. None of these agents, however, has been shown to improve survival in heart-failure patients. Their use should be restricted to the treatment of patients who are intolerant to, or not adequately treated by, the agents discussed above. For the treatment of acute or chronic decompensated heart failure refractory to standard drug regimens and not complicated by significant aortic insufficiency, a mechanical aortic counterpulsation device (*i.e.*, intraaortic balloon pump) often provides the most effective short-term means to reduce left ventricular afterload and directly increase cardiac output.

β-Adrenergic Receptor Antagonists

The pharmacology of β-adrenergic receptor antagonists is discussed in detail in Chapter 10. The initial use of these agents for the treatment of heart failure was based largely on empirical evidence from small clinical trials, despite clinical and experimental animal data that these drugs can exert a negative inotropic effect and thereby worsen ventricular function. In the 1970s, Waagstein and associates in Sweden reported that β-adrenergic antagonists (most commonly, the relatively β_1-selective adrenergic receptor antagonist *metoprolol*) improved symptoms, exercise tolerance, and several measures of ventricular function over a period of several months in patients with heart failure due to idiopathic dilated cardiomyopathy (reviewed by Swedberg, 1993). With few exceptions, a number of small clinical trials over the next decade reinforced these initial observations (Bristow, 2000). Although none of these studies was sufficiently large to be definitive regarding symptoms, effort tolerance, or mortality, they did demonstrate a consistent increase in left ventricular ejection fraction (Figure 34–5). Serial measurements have shown that, immediately after starting a β-receptor antagonist in such patients, there is a decrease in systolic function as reflected by a decrease in ejection fraction. However, with continued treatment over the ensuing 2 to 4 months, systolic function gradually recovers and then improves beyond the baseline level (Hall *et al.*, 1995). Since this time-dependent effect of β-receptor antagonist therapy cannot be attributed to a direct hemodynamic action, it has been suggested that improved ventricular function with chronic β-receptor antagonist therapy is due to prevention of adverse effects of norepinephrine on the myocardium that are mediated by β-adrenergic receptors (Eichhorn and Bristow, 1996).

Early Outcome Trials. The Metoprolol in Dilated Cardiomyopathy (MDC) trial (Waagstein *et al.*, 1993) was a multicenter, prospective, randomized trial that examined metoprolol versus placebo in 383 patients with mild to moderate idiopathic dilated cardiomyopathy (*i.e.*, patients with clinically evident coronary artery disease or active myocarditis were excluded) who already were receiving optimal medical management including ACE inhibitors. Although there was no difference in mortality at 12 months of follow-up between the placebo- and metoprolol-treated groups, 19 patients receiving placebo deteriorated to the point of being listed for cardiac transplantation, a primary end point of the trial, compared to 2 patients receiving metoprolol. There was significant improvement in left ventricular ejection fraction, exercise tolerance, NYHA classification status, and the

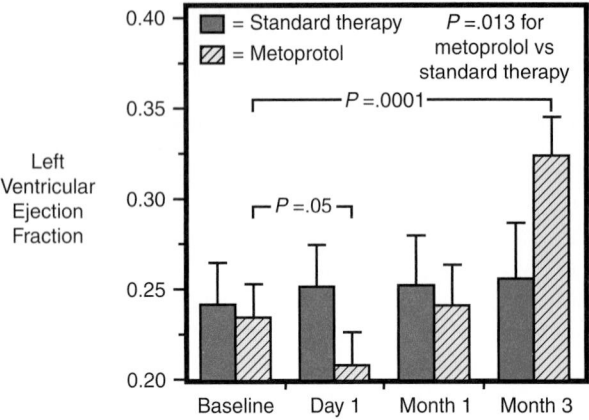

Figure 34–5. Time-dependent effects of metoprolol on left ventricular ejection fraction in patients with heart failure.

In patients with severe left ventricular dysfunction, the initial administration of a low dose of metoprolol caused an immediate depression in ejection fraction (day 1). However, over time and despite uptitration of metoprolol to full therapeutic levels, ejection fraction returned to baseline (1 month) and by 3 months was significantly higher than at baseline. In the group given standard therapy, ejection fraction did not change significantly. An increase in left ventricular systolic function between 2 and 4 months after initiation of therapy is seen consistently with a variety of β-adrenergic receptor antagonists used in patients with heart failure. This observation confirms that the direct hemodynamic effect of a β-receptor antagonist in patients with heart failure is to depress contractile function. Thus, the improvement in function with chronic therapy cannot be attributed to a direct hemodynamic effect, and likely reflects a beneficial effect of treatment on the biology of the myocardium. (Adapted from Hall *et al.,* 1995, with permission.)

patients' own assessment of their quality of life (Waagstein *et al.,* 1993; Andersson *et al.,* 1994). The mean dose of metoprolol achieved was approximately 100 mg/day following a 6-week period of gradual upward titration beginning at 10 mg/day. Subsequently, the Cardiac Insufficiency Bisoprolol (CIBIS) trial examined the effect of another β_1-selective antagonist, *bisoprolol,* in 641 patients with both ischemic and nonischemic dilated cardiomyopathy. This trial also failed to find an effect on overall mortality (Cibis Investigators, 1994). However, as in the MDC trial, there was evidence of symptomatic and functional improvement.

Carvedilol. *Carvedilol* (COREG) is a nonselective β-adrenergic receptor antagonist and an α_1-selective α-adrenergic receptor antagonist. The U.S. Carvedilol Trial randomized 1094 patients with ischemic and nonischemic dilated cardiomyopathy and an ejection fraction <35% to carvedilol (target dose of 25 mg twice per day) or placebo (Packer *et al.,* 1996b). All of the patients were ambulatory, clinically stable (essentially all were in NYHA class II or III), and receiving an angiotensin converting enzyme inhibitor. In patients randomized to carvedilol

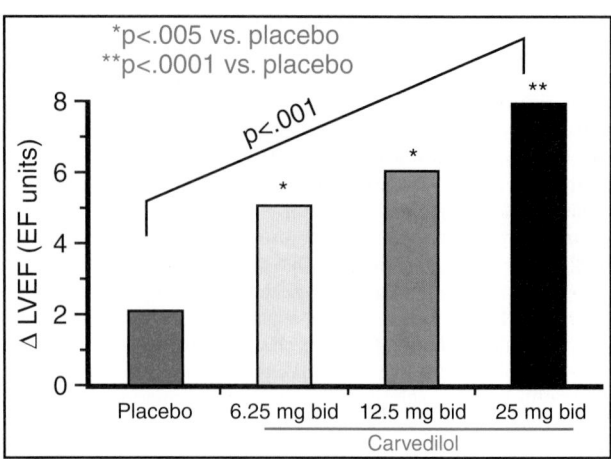

Figure 34–6. Dose-dependent effect of carvedilol on left ventricular ejection fraction.

In the U.S. Carvedilol Trials Program a subgroup of patients were randomized to placebo or carvedilol in the standard dose (25 mg twice per day [bid]) or in a reduced dose of 12.5 or 6.25 mg twice per day. After 6 months of treatment, left ventricular ejection fraction (Δ LVEF) increased with all three doses of carvedilol, but not with placebo. Of note, the increase in ejection fraction was strongly related to the dose of carvedilol. These data emphasize the importance of titrating doses of β-adrenergic receptor antagonists to the target or the highest tolerated dose. (Adapted from Bristow, 1996, with permission.)

there was a 65% reduction in all-cause mortality which was independent of age, gender, etiology of heart failure, or ejection fraction. The mortality benefit was due primarily to a decrease in deaths due to refractory pump failure, and to a lesser extent, sudden deaths. In a portion of the patients who were randomized to three dose levels of carvedilol (6.25, 12.5, or 25 mg twice per day), there was a strong relationship between the dose of carvedilol and the improvements in mortality and ejection fraction (Figure 34–6) (Bristow et al, 1996). Patient- and physician-reported symptoms were improved, and there was a 27% decrease in hospitalizations, although exercise function, as assessed by a 6-minute walk test, was not improved. In this trial, the effect of carvedilol on disease progression was assessed in a subgroup of 366 patients with good exercise function and mild symptoms at baseline (Colucci *et al.,* 1996). Approximately 85% of these patients were in NYHA class II and the rest were in class III. The primary end point of clinical progression was defined as the occurrence of death due to heart failure, hospitalization for heart failure, or the need for a sustained increase in heart-failure medications. Carvedilol caused a 48% decrease in clinical progression, so defined, due to parallel reductions in death, hospitalization, and medication increase. The Australia/New Zealand Carvedilol Trial, which enrolled 415 patients with mild heart failure due to ischemic cardiomyopathy, likewise found a 26% reduction in the combined end point of all-cause mortality and hospitalization over a follow-up period of 18 to 24 months (Australia/New Zealand Heart Failure Research Collaborative Group, 1997). Based largely on these trials, in 1997 the FDA approved carvedilol for the treatment of patients with NYHA class II or III symptoms of heart failure and an ejection fraction <35%.

Bisoprolol (ZEBETA). CIBIS-II, a follow-up trial to CIBIS I (discussed above), enrolled 2647 patients with moderate to severe heart-failure symptoms due to ischemic or nonischemic dilated cardiomyopathy (CIBIS-II Investigators, 1999). This trial found a 34% reduction in all-cause mortality in bisoprolol-treated patients that was due primarily to a decrease in sudden deaths (44% reduction) and, to a lesser extent, a decrease in pump failure (26% reduction). Because of the way deaths were classified, many patients with pump failure may have been placed in the "unknown" category, which accounted for a large fraction of all deaths. The mortality benefit of bisoprolol was independent of the etiology of heart failure and was associated with an approximately 36% decrease in hospitalizations for heart failure.

Metoprolol (LOPRESSOR, TOPROL XL). The Metoprolol Randomized Intervention Trial in Congestive Heart Failure (MERIT-HF) randomized 3991 patients with NYHA functional class II to IV symptoms and an ejection fraction <40% to metoprolol (target dose, 200 mg/day) or placebo (MERIT-HF Study Group, 1999). Metoprolol caused a 34% decrease in all-cause mortality, which was attributable to similar reductions in sudden death (41% decrease) and death from worsening heart failure (49% decrease). As in the U.S. Carvedilol and CIBIS II trials, the beneficial effects of treatment on mortality were independent of age, gender, etiology of heart failure, or ejection fraction.

Mechanism of Action. It is not completely clear how β-adrenergic receptor antagonists exert their benefits in heart failure. Although initial theories focused on resensitization of the β-adrenergic pathway, this appears not to be critical, since some β-receptor antagonists that have proven to be of clinical utility (e.g., carvedilol) do not cause this effect. A consistent finding in the large mortality trials is a reduction in the incidence of sudden death, presumably reflecting a decrease in malignant ventricular arrhythmias. Thus, an antiarrhythmic benefit seems likely. However, another consistent finding is an improvement in left ventricular structure and function with a decrease in chamber size and an increase in ejection fraction. This apparent antiremodeling action may reflect favorable effects on the molecular and cellular processes that underlie pathological remodeling. In support of this thesis, it has been shown that β-adrenergic stimulation can cause apoptosis of cardiac myocytes (Communal et al., 1998), and that mice overexpressing the $β_1$-adrenergic receptor in the myocardium develop a dilated cardiomyopathy associated with myocyte apoptosis (Bisognano et al., 2000). Likewise, β-adrenergic receptors may affect remodeling through their effects on gene expression and the turnover of extracellular matrix in the myocardium. It also has been suggested that β-receptor antagonists could improve myocardial energetics (Eichhorn et al., 1994) and/or reduce oxidative stress in the myocardium (Sawyer and Colucci, 2000).

Clinical Use of β-Adrenergic Receptor Antagonists in Heart Failure. The extensive body of data regarding the

use of β-receptor antagonists in chronic heart failure, reflecting more than 15,000 patients enrolled in controlled trials, has provided compelling evidence that β-adrenergic receptor antagonists improve symptoms, reduce hospitalization, and decrease mortality in patients with mild and moderate heart failure. Accordingly, β-receptor antagonists are now recommended for routine use in patients with an ejection fraction <35% and NYHA class II or III symptoms despite standard therapy with diuretics and an ACE inhibitor. This seemingly broad recommendation should be tempered by certain limitations in the experimental database. First, the large majority of the data that underlie this recommendation were obtained in relatively stable patients with mild to moderate symptoms. Therefore, the role of β-receptor antagonists in patients with more severe symptoms, or with recent decompensation, is not yet clear. Likewise, the utility of β-receptor blockade in patients with asymptomatic left ventricular dysfunction has not been studied. Finally, although it appears likely that the beneficial effects of these drugs is related to β-receptor blockade, it cannot be assumed that all β-receptor antagonists will exert similar effects. Thus, as discussed in Chapter 10, within this general class of drugs there is marked heterogeneity in pharmacological characteristics such as β-adrenergic receptor selectivity, direct or receptor-mediated vasodilation, and other nonreceptor-mediated actions (e.g., antioxidant effects). These properties may play a role determining the overall efficacy and utility of a given β-receptor antagonist.

Since β-receptor antagonists have the potential to worsen both ventricular function and symptoms in patients with heart failure, several caveats should be remembered. First, β-receptor antagonists should be initiated at very low doses, generally less than a tenth of the final target dose. Second, these drugs should be titrated upward slowly, over the course of weeks, and under careful supervision. The rapid institution of the usual β-receptor-blocking doses used for hypertension or coronary artery disease may cause decompensation in many patients who otherwise would be able to tolerate a slower uptitration. Even when therapy is initiated with low doses of a β-receptor antagonist, there may be an increased tendency to retain fluid that will require adjustments in the diuretic regimen. Third, although limited experience with NYHA class IIIB and IV patients suggests that they may tolerate β-receptor blockers and benefit from their use, this group of patients should be approached with a high level of caution. Fourth, there is almost no experience in patients with new-onset, recently decompensated heart failure. There are theoretical reasons for caution in such patients, and at present they should not be treated with

β-receptor blockers until after they have stabilized for several days to weeks.

Cardiac Glycosides

The cardiac glycosides possess a common molecular motif, a steroid nucleus containing an unsaturated lactone at the C 17 position and one or more glycosidic residues at C 3 (see Figure 34–7). *Digoxin* (LANOXIN, LANOXICAPS) and *digitoxin* (CRYSTODIGIN) are both orally active, but only digoxin is in widespread clinical use today. Digitoxin differs from digoxin only by the absence of a hydroxyl group at C 12, resulting in a less hydrophilic compound with altered pharmacokinetics compared to digoxin. The cardiac glycosides have been used for centuries as therapeutic agents. The beneficial effects in heart failure were believed to derive from a positive inotropic effect on failing myocardium and efficacy in controlling the ventricular rate response to atrial fibrillation. However, it is now recognized that the cardiac glycosides also modulate sympathetic nervous system activity, an additional mechanism that may contribute importantly to their efficacy in heart failure.

Mechanisms of Action.   *Inhibition of Na$^+$, K$^+$–ATPase.* All cardiac glycosides are potent and highly selective inhibitors of the active transport of Na$^+$ and K$^+$ across cell membranes, by binding to a specific site on the extracytoplasmic face of the α subunit of Na$^+$, K$^+$–ATPase, the enzymatic equivalent of the cellular "Na$^+$ pump." The binding of cardiac glycosides to Na$^+$, K$^+$–ATPase and inhibition of the cellular ion pump is reversible and en-

tropically driven. These drugs bind preferentially to the enzyme following phosphorylation at a β-aspartate on the cytoplasmic face of the α subunit and stabilize this conformation (known as E$_2$P). Extracellular K$^+$ promotes dephosphorylation of the enzyme as an initial step in this cation's active translocation into the cytosol, thereby decreasing the affinity of the enzyme for binding cardiac glycosides. This provides one explanation for why increased extracellular K$^+$ reverses some of the toxic effects of these drugs. The regulation of Na$^+$, K$^+$–ATPase by digitalis has been reviewed in detail (Eisner and Smith, 1992).

Positive Inotropic Effect.   Both Na$^+$ and Ca^{2+} ions enter cardiac muscle cells during each cycle of depolarization, contraction, and repolarization (Figure 34–8). Ca^{2+} that enters the cell *via* the L-type Ca^{2+} channel during depolarization triggers the release of additional Ca^{2+} into the cytosol from an intracellular compartment, the sarcoplasmic reticulum (SR). The greater the amount of activating Ca^{2+}, the greater the force of contraction. During myocyte repolarization and relaxation, Ca^{2+} is pumped back into the SR by a Ca^{2+}–ATPase and also is removed from the cell by the Na$^+$–Ca^{2+} exchanger and by a sarcolemmal Ca^{2+}–ATPase.

Importantly, the capacity of the exchanger to extrude Ca^{2+} from the cell depends on the intracellular Na$^+$ concentration. Binding of cardiac glycosides to the sarcolemmal Na$^+$, K$^+$–ATPase and inhibition of cellular Na$^+$ pump activity results in a reduction in the rate of active Na$^+$ extrusion and a rise in cytosolic Na$^+$. This increase in intracellular Na$^+$ reduces the transmembrane Na$^+$ gradient driving the extrusion of intracellular Ca^{2+} during myocyte repolarization. Hence, some incremental Ca^{2+} is taken up into the SR to be made available to the contractile elements during the subsequent cell depolarization cycle, and contractility of the myocardium is augmented.

Electrophysiological Actions.   (see also Chapter 35) Atrial and ventricular muscle and specialized cardiac pacemaker and conduction fibers exhibit differing responses and sensitivities to cardiac glycosides that are a summation of the direct effects of these drugs on cardiac cells and their indirect, neurally mediated effects. At therapeutic, nontoxic serum or plasma concentrations (*i.e.*, 1.0 to 2.0 ng/ml), digoxin decreases automaticity and increases maximal diastolic resting membrane potential predominantly in atrial and atrioventricular (AV) nodal tissues, due to an increase in vagal tone and a decrease in sympathetic nervous system activity. There also is a prolongation of the effective refractory period and a decrease in conduction velocity in AV nodal tissue. At higher concentrations, this may cause sinus bradycardia or arrest and/or prolongation of AV conduction or heart block. In addition, cardiac glycosides

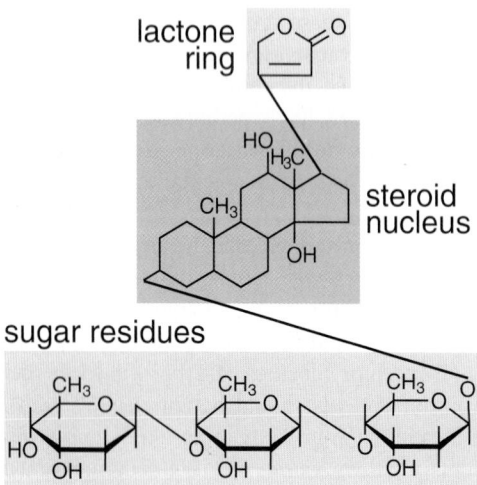

Figure 34–7. Structure of digoxin.

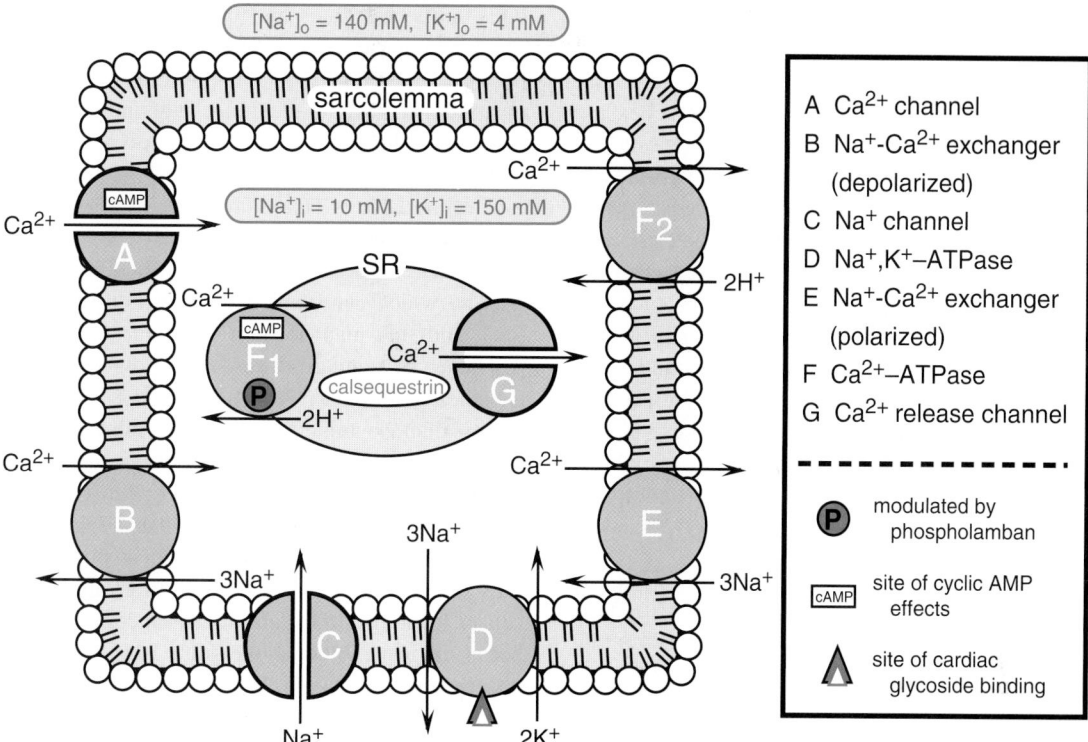

Figure 34–8. Sarcolemmal exchange of Na⁺ and Ca²⁺ during cell depolarization and repolarization.

Na⁺ and Ca²⁺ ions enter mammalian cardiac muscle cells during each cycle of membrane depolarization, triggering the release, through Ca²⁺ release channels (G), of larger amounts of Ca²⁺ from internal stores in the sarcoplasmic reticulum (SR). The resulting increase in intracellular Ca²⁺ interacts with troponin C and hence is responsible for activating the cross-bridge interactions between actin filaments and myosin cross-bridges that result in sarcomere shortening. The electrochemical gradient for Na⁺ across the sarcolemma is maintained by active (*i.e.*, ATP-consuming) transport of Na⁺ out of the cell by the sarcolemmal Na⁺, K⁺–ATPase (D). Na⁺ is actively extruded by Na⁺, K⁺–ATPase, while the bulk of cytosolic Ca²⁺ is pumped back into the SR by a Ca²⁺–ATPase (F_1), where it is bound by the protein calsequestrin, and the remainder is removed from the cell by either a plasma membrane Ca²⁺–ATPase (F_2) or a high capacity Na⁺–Ca²⁺ cation exchange protein (B, E). This sarcolemmal membrane protein exchanges 3 Na⁺ ions for every Ca²⁺ ion, using the electrochemical potential of Na⁺ to drive Ca²⁺ extrusion. Note that the direction of cation transport may reverse briefly during depolarization (B), when the electrical gradient across the sarcolemma is transiently reversed. *β*-Adrenergic receptor agonists and phosphodiesterase inhibitors, by increasing intracellular cyclic AMP levels, activate protein kinase A, which enhances the contractile state by phosphorylating target proteins, including phospholamban and the *α* subunit of the L-type Ca²⁺ channel. (Adapted from Smith *et al.,* 1992, with permission.)

at higher concentrations can increase sympathetic nervous system activity and directly affect automaticity in cardiac tissue, actions that contribute to the generation of atrial and ventricular arrhythmias. Increased intracellular Ca²⁺ loading and increased sympathetic tone result in an increase in the spontaneous (phase 4) rate of diastolic depolarization as well as delayed afterdepolarizations that may reach the threshold for generation of a propagated action potential. This simultaneous nonuniform increase in au-

tomaticity and depression of conduction in His–Purkinje and ventricular muscle fibers predisposes to arrhythmias that may lead to ventricular tachycardia or fibrillation.

Regulation of Sympathetic Nervous System Activity. An increase in sympathetic nervous system activity is one of the physiological responses to a decline in heart function below that required for maintenance of a cardiac output adequate to meet the metabolic demands of body tissues (*i.e.,* heart failure). This is due, in part, to a reduction in the sensitivity of the arterial baroreflex response to blood pressure, resulting in a decline in tonic baroreflex suppression of CNS-directed sympathetic activity (Ferguson *et al.*, 1989). This desensitization of the normal baroreflex arc also is thought to be responsible in part for the sustained elevation in plasma norepinephrine, renin, and vasopressin levels in heart failure, as well as other indices of systemic neurohumoral activation that are characteristically observed in patients with heart failure. Increased sympathetic nervous system activity initially helps to maintain blood pressure and cardiac output by *increasing* heart rate, contractility, and systemic vascular resistance, and by *decreasing* the excretion of salt and water by the kidneys. However, when sustained chronically, these effects of sympathetic overactivity contribute to the pathophysiology of heart failure and progression of the underlying myocardial disease.

A direct effect of cardiac glycosides on carotid baroreflex responsiveness to changes in carotid sinus pressure has been demonstrated in isolated baroreceptor preparations from animals with experimental heart failure (Wang *et al.*, 1990). In addition, Ferguson *et al.* (1989) demonstrated in patients with moderate to advanced heart failure that infusion of the cardiac glycoside deslanoside increased forearm blood flow and cardiac index and decreased heart rate, while markedly decreasing skeletal muscle sympathetic nerve activity, an indicator of the centrally mediated sympathetic nervous system tone. This was unlikely to have been due predominantly to a direct inotropic effect of the drug, since dobutamine, a sympathomimetic drug that increases cardiac output to a comparable extent, did not affect muscle sympathetic nerve activity in these patients. A reduction in neurohumoral activation could represent an important additional mechanism contributing to the efficacy of cardiac glycosides in the treatment of heart failure.

Pharmacokinetics.   The elimination half-life for digoxin is 36 to 48 hours in patients with normal or near-normal renal function. This permits once-a-day dosing for patients with normal or mildly impaired renal function, and near steady-state blood levels are achieved 1 week after initiation of maintenance therapy. Digoxin is excreted for the most part unchanged with a clearance rate that is proportional to the glomerular filtration rate. In patients with congestive heart failure and marginal cardiac reserve, an increase in cardiac output and renal blood flow with vasodilator therapy or sympathomimetic agents may increase renal digoxin clearance, necessitating adjustment of daily maintenance doses. Nevertheless, digoxin is not removed effectively by peritoneal or hemodialysis due to the drug's large (4 to 7 liters/kg) volume of distribution. The principal tissue reservoir is skeletal muscle and not adipose tissue and, thus, dosing should be based on estimated lean

body mass. Neonates and infants tolerate and appear to require higher doses of digoxin for an equivalent therapeutic effect than do older children or adults, although absorption and renal clearance rates are similar. Digoxin does cross the placenta, and drug levels in maternal and umbilical vein blood are similar.

Most digoxin tablets average 70% to 80% oral bioavailability; however, approximately 10% of the general population harbors the enteric bacterium *Eubacterium lentum*, which can convert digoxin into inactive metabolites, and this may account for some cases of apparent resistance to standard doses of oral digoxin. Liquid-filled capsules of digoxin (LANOXICAPS) have a higher bioavailability than do tablets and require dosage adjustment if a patient is switched from one dosage form to the other. Parenteral digoxin is available for intravenous administration, and maintenance doses can be given by intravenous injection when oral dosing is impractical. Intramuscular digoxin administration is erratically absorbed, causes local discomfort, and is not recommended. A number of drug interactions (*see* Table 34–4) and clinical conditions can alter digoxin's pharmacokinetics or alter a patient's susceptibility to toxic manifestations of these drugs. Chronic renal failure, for example, decreases digoxin's volume of distribution, necessitating a decrease in maintenance dosage of the drug. Electrolyte disturbances, especially hypokalemia, acid base imbalances, and type of underlying heart disease also may alter a patient's susceptibility to toxic manifestations of digoxin.

Clinical Use of Digoxin in Heart Failure.   Since at least the turn of the century, there has been controversy surrounding the efficacy of cardiac glycosides in the treatment of patients with heart failure who are in sinus rhythm. Despite widespread use of digoxin, objective data from randomized, controlled trials on the safety and efficacy of digoxin had been lacking until the 1990s.

The PROVED (Prospective Randomized study Of Ventricular failure and Efficacy of Digoxin; Uretsky *et al.*, 1993) and RADIANCE (Randomized Assessment of Digoxin on Inhibition of Angiotensin Converting Enzyme; Packer *et al.*, 1993) trials examined the effects of withdrawal of digoxin in patients with stable mild to moderate heart failure (*i.e.*, NYHA class II and III) and systolic ventricular dysfunction (left ventricular ejection fraction <0.35). All patients studied were in normal sinus rhythm. Withdrawal of digoxin resulted in a significant worsening of heart-failure symptoms in patients who received placebo compared with patients who continued to receive active drug. Maximal treadmill exercise tolerance also declined significantly in patients withdrawn from digoxin in both trials despite continuation of other medical therapies for heart failure.

Table 34–4
Drug Interactions with Digoxin

DRUG	MECHANISM	CHANGE IN DIGOXIN BLOOD LEVEL[*]	SUGGESTED CLINICAL MANAGEMENT
Pharmacokinetic			
Cholestyramine, kaolin–pectin, neomycin, sulfasalazine	Decrease absorption	25% decrease	Give digoxin 8 hours before agent or use solution or liquid-filled capsule form of digoxin
Antacids	Not known	25% decrease	Temporal dispersion of doses
Bran	Decreases absorption	25% decrease	Temporal dispersion of doses
Propafenone, quinidine, quinine verapamil, amiodarone	Decrease renal digoxin clearance, volume of distribution, or both	70%–100% increase	Decrease digoxin dose by 50% and monitor serum digoxin levels as necessary
Thyroxine	Increases volume of distribution and renal clearance	Variable decreases in digoxin blood levels	Monitor serum digoxin levels
Erythromycin, omeprazole, tetracycline	Increase digoxin absorption	40%–100% increase	Monitor serum digoxin levels
Albuterol	Increase volume of distribution	30% decrease	Monitor serum digoxin levels
Captopril, diltiazem, nifedipine, nitrendipine	Variable moderate decrease in digoxin clearance and/or volume of distribution	Variable increase in blood levels	Monitor serum digoxin levels
Cyclosporine	May decrease renal function and, indirectly, digoxin clearance	Variable increase in blood levels	Monitor serum digoxin levels more frequently if renal function impaired
Pharmacodynamic			
β-adrenergic receptor antagonists, verapamil, diltiazem, flecainide, disopyramide, bepridil	Decreased sinoatrial (SA) or atrioventricular (AV) junctional conduction or automaticity		Monitor ECG for evidence of SA or AV block
Kaliuretic diuretics	Decreased serum and tissue K^+, increased automaticity, promotes inhibition of Na^+, K^+–ATPase by digoxin		Monitor ECG for arrhythmias consistent with digoxin toxicity
Sympathomimetic drugs	Increased automaticity		Monitor ECG for arrhythmia
Verapamil, diltiazem, β-adrenergic receptor antagonists	Diminished cardiac contractile state		Discontinue or lower dose of Ca^{2+} channel blocker or β-adrenergic receptor antagonist

[*]Approximation only, to be monitored as clinically appropriate.
Abbreviations: ECG, electrocardiogram; SA, sinoatrial; AV, atrioventricular.

A

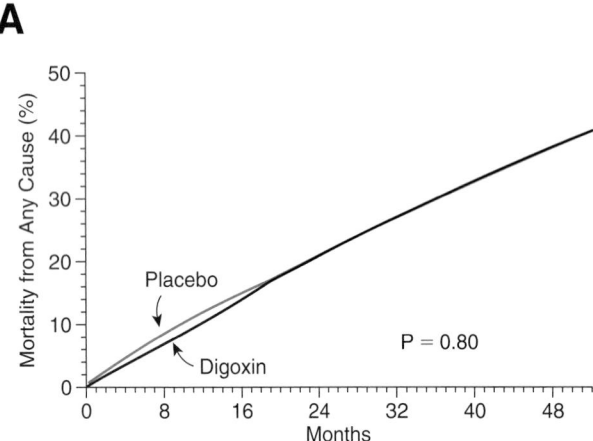

B

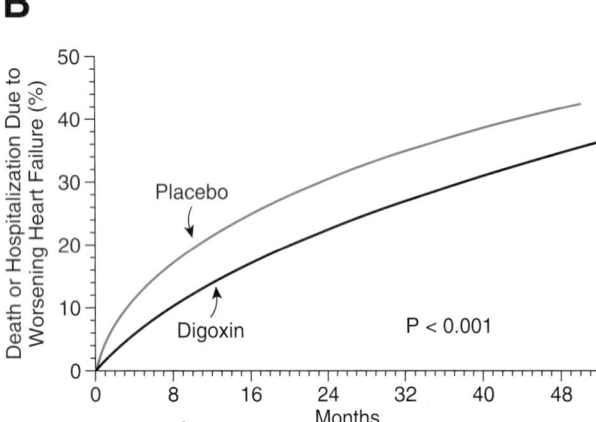

Figure 34–9. Effect of digoxin on survival and hospitalization for heart failure in the Digoxin Investigators Group (DIG) trial.

> In the DIG trial, 6800 patients with New York Heart Association class II to III symptoms of heart failure and a left ventricular ejection fraction <0.45 were randomized to digoxin or placebo in addition to standard therapy including ACE inhibitors. There was no difference in mortality between the treatment groups (*Panel A*). However, fewer patients in the digoxin group were hospitalized due to worsening heart failure (*Panel B*). (Adapted from the Digoxin Investigation Group, 1997, with permission.)

The much larger Digoxin Investigators' Group (DIG) trial was designed to detect an effect of digoxin therapy on the survival of patients with heart failure (The Digitalis Investigation Group, 1997). In this randomized, double-blind trial, 6,800 patients with predominantly mild to moderate (NYHA class II to III) heart failure and a left ventricular ejection fraction <0.45 were assigned to receive either digoxin or placebo in addition to standard therapy including ACE inhibitors. A trend was seen toward a decrease in the risk of death attributed to worsen-

ing heart failure in the digoxin-treated group. However, this was balanced by a small increase in the risk of death due to other cardiac causes (presumed to result from arrhythmia), and overall, no difference in mortality was seen between the treatment groups (*see* Figure 34–9). However, fewer patients in the digoxin group were hospitalized due to worsening heart failure. This benefit was seen at all levels of ejection fraction but was greatest in patients with more severe degrees of heart failure. Interestingly, in a predefined substudy of patients with normal ejection fraction (*i.e.,* presumed to have diastolic dysfunction), a similar pattern of benefit was seen with digoxin. Based on these data, it is recommended that digoxin be reserved for patients with heart failure who are in atrial fibrillation, or for patients in sinus rhythm who remain symptomatic despite therapy with adequate dosages of ACE inhibitors and β-adrenergic receptor antagonists.

Doses of Digoxin in Clinical Practice and Monitoring of Serum Levels. Using indices of ventricular function, most studies suggest that the greatest increase in contractility is apparent at serum levels of digoxin around 1.4 ng/ml (1.8 nM) (Kelly and Smith, 1992a). The neurohormonal effects of digoxin may occur at lower serum levels, between 0.5 and 1.0 ng/ml; higher serum concentrations than this are not associated with further decreases in neurohormonal activation or with increased clinical benefit. Furthermore, a subgroup analysis of the DIG trial (The Digitalis Investigation Group, 1997) showed an apparent increased risk of death with increasing serum concentrations, even for values within the traditional therapeutic range. Therefore, many authorities advocate maintaining digoxin levels below 1.0 ng/ml.

A common approach for initiating digoxin therapy is to begin at 0.125 to 0.25 mg/day, depending on lean body mass and creatinine clearance, and to measure serum digoxin levels a week later when a steady-state has been achieved. The blood sample should be obtained at least 6 hours following the last digoxin dose. Routine surveillance monitoring of digoxin levels need not be carried out, unless a significant deterioration in renal function occurs, or a new drug (*e.g.,* amiodarone) which substantially alters digoxin pharmacokinetics, is started. Oral or intravenous loading with digoxin, while generally safe, is rarely necessary as other safer and more effective drugs exist for short-term inotropic support.

Digoxin Toxicity. The incidence and severity of digoxin toxicity have declined substantially in the past two decades, due in part to the development of alternative drugs for the treatment of supraventricular arrhythmias and heart failure, to the increased understanding of digoxin pharmacokinetics, to the monitoring of serum digoxin levels, and to the identification of important interactions between digoxin and many commonly used drugs. Nevertheless, the recognition of digoxin toxicity remains an important consideration in the differential diagnosis of arrhythmias and/or neurological and gastrointestinal symptoms in patients receiving cardiac glycosides (Table 34–5).

Vigilance for and early recognition of disturbances of impulse formation, conduction, or both are critically

Table 34–5
Signs and Symptoms of Cardiac Glycoside Toxicity

Psychiatric
  Delirium, fatigue, malaise, confusion, dizziness,
    abnormal dreams
Visual
  Blurred or yellow vision, halos
Gastrointestinal
  Anorexia, nausea, vomiting, abdominal pain
Respiratory
  Enhanced ventilatory response to hypoxia
Cardiac arrhythmias
  Atrial and ventricular ectopic arrhythmias
Conduction disturbances
  Sinoatrial and atrioventricular node conduction
    disturbances

important. Among the more common electrophysiological manifestations are ectopic beats of AV junctional or ventricular origin, first-degree AV block, an excessively slow ventricular rate response to atrial fibrillation, or an accelerated AV junctional pacemaker. These often require only a dosage adjustment and appropriate monitoring. Sinus bradycardia, sinoatrial arrest or exit block, and second- or third-degree AV conduction delay usually respond to atropine, although temporary ventricular pacing may be necessary. Potassium administration should be considered for patients with evidence of increased AV junctional or ventricular automaticity, even when the serum K^+ is in the normal range, unless high-grade AV block also is present. Lidocaine or phenytoin, which have minimal effects on AV conduction, may be used for the treatment of worsening ventricular arrhythmias that threaten hemodynamic compromise. Electrical cardioversion carries increased risk of inducing severe rhythm disturbances in patients with overt digitalis toxicity, and it should be used with particular caution.

Antidigoxin Immunotherapy. An effective antidote for digoxin or digitoxin toxicity is now available in the form of antidigoxin immunotherapy with purified Fab fragments from ovine antidigoxin antisera (DIGIBIND). A full neutralizing dose of Fab based on either the estimated total dose of drug ingested or the total body digoxin burden (Table 34–6) can be administered intravenously in saline solution over 30 to 60 minutes. For a more comprehensive review of the treatment of digitalis toxicity, *see* Kelly and Smith (1992b).

Table 34–6
Calculation of Dose of Antidigoxin Immunotherapy

The calculation of the amount of polyclonal antidigoxin Fab antibody fragments to be administered is based on a dose of Fab that is stoichiometrically equivalent to the total body burden of digoxin.

I. Estimation of total body digoxin burden (mg):

A.
$$\begin{bmatrix} \text{Total drug in body (in mg)} \\ \text{(following acute} \\ \text{digoxin ingestion)} \end{bmatrix} = \begin{bmatrix} \text{Amount} \\ \text{ingested} \\ \text{(in mg)} \end{bmatrix} \times \begin{bmatrix} \text{Average oral bioavailability} \\ \text{of tablet formulations} \\ \text{(0.8 for digoxin)} \end{bmatrix}$$

or B.
$$\begin{bmatrix} \text{Known or suspected} \\ \text{toxicity during chronic} \\ \text{digoxin therapy} \end{bmatrix} = \frac{\begin{bmatrix} \text{Serum digoxin} \\ \text{concentration} \\ \text{(in ng/ml or } \mu\text{g/l)} \end{bmatrix} \times \begin{bmatrix} \text{Volume of} \\ \text{distribution} \\ \text{(5.6 liters/kg)} \end{bmatrix} \times \begin{bmatrix} \text{Weight} \\ \text{(in kg)} \end{bmatrix}}{1000}$$

II. Calculation of Fab fragment dose:

$$\begin{bmatrix} \text{Dose of} \\ \text{Fab fragments} \\ \text{(in mg)} \end{bmatrix} = \frac{\begin{bmatrix} \text{Molecular mass of} \\ \text{Fab fragments} \\ \text{(50,000 daltons)} \end{bmatrix} \times \begin{bmatrix} \text{Total body} \\ \text{digoxin content} \\ \text{(in mg)} \end{bmatrix}}{\begin{bmatrix} \text{Molecular mass of} \\ \text{digoxin} \\ \text{(781 daltons)} \end{bmatrix}}$$

Chronic Positive Inotropic Therapy

Several oral inotropic agents have been developed, some with vasodilating properties. Although many of these agents cause a marked improvement in hemodynamic function and may alleviate symptoms and improve exercise capacity, their effect on mortality with long-term treatment has been disappointing. The dopaminergic agonist *ibopamine,* the cyclic AMP phosphodiesterase (PDE) inhibitors *milrinone, inamrinone* (formerly *amrinone*) and *vesnarinone,* and the benzimidazoline PDE inhibitor with calcium-sensitizing properties, *pimobendan,* have been associated with increased mortality (Hampton *et al.,* 1997; Packer *et al.,* 1991; Cohn *et al.,* 1998). This increased mortality has been attributed to an increased risk of arrhythmia with these agents, and it underscores the observation that effects of a drug on hemodynamic function and survival need not be directly related. Therefore, digoxin remains the only oral inotropic agent that should be used in patients with heart failure.

Continuous or intermittent outpatient therapy with dobutamine or milrinone, administered by a portable or home-based infusion pump through a central venous catheter, has been evaluated in patients with end-stage heart failure and symptoms refractory to other classes of drugs. There is as yet no convincing evidence that chronic parenteral inotropic therapy improves the quality or length of life. Furthermore, there are concerns that this form of therapy may actually hasten death (reviewed by Gheorghiade, 2000). Outpatient inotropic therapy may be useful in patients with intractable heart failure who are awaiting heart transplantation or who are not candidates for further management in hospital. The use of parenteral inotropic agents in hospitalized patients with heart failure is discussed later in this chapter.

Anticoagulation and Antiplatelet Drugs in Heart Failure

Patients with heart failure have a significantly higher incidence of stroke and thromboembolism. Nonetheless, the rate of embolic events remains relatively low, and retrospective analyses have shown conflicting evidence of benefit from anticoagulation in patients who remain in sinus rhythm. Anticoagulation with *warfarin* (COUMADIN; *see* Chapter 55) is recommended for patients who have atrial fibrillation or a history of a previous embolic event, if there is evidence of a left ventricular thrombus, or possibly, if left ventricular dysfunction is severe and the ventricles are markedly dilated.

Similarly, while aspirin therapy is effective in reducing the incidence of ischemic events in patients with coronary artery disease, concerns have been raised that aspirin may attenuate the benefits from ACE inhibitors in patients with heart failure (Nguyen *et al.,* 1997; Al-Khadra *et al.,* 1998). A potential mechanism for this postulated adverse interaction is antagonism of bradykinin-mediated prostaglandin generation by aspirin. Synthesis of vasodilatory prostaglandins and other potentially beneficial molecules is reduced, thereby attenuating the favorable effects of ACE inhibition. In support of this thesis is the finding that the vasodilatory effects of enalapril may be blunted by concomitant administration of aspirin (Hall *et al.,* 1992). Furthermore, a recent study has shown a trend toward greater morbidity and mortality in patients with heart failure receiving aspirin compared to those receiving placebo or warfarin (Cleland, 1999). Accordingly, until more definitive data are available on the use of aspirin in heart failure, it should be reserved for patients who have a clear indication for its use (*e.g.,* the presence of known or suspected coronary artery disease).

Alternative antiplatelet agents that do not appear to interfere with prostaglandin metabolism are now available in the form of the adenosine diphosphate antagonists *ticlopidine* (TICLID) and *clopidogrel* (PLAVIX). While both agents have been demonstrated to be effective in the prevention of ischemic events, there are as yet few data on their use in patients who have heart failure.

Antiarrhythmic Drugs in Heart Failure

Sudden cardiac death accounts for a significant proportion of the mortality due to heart failure. In the majority of cases, these deaths have been attributed to a ventricular tachyarrhythmia. However, ventricular arrhythmias are common in patients in heart failure, and are usually asymptomatic. Antiarrhythmic drugs, while effective in suppressing ventricular arrhythmias, may be associated with an increased risk of mortality, believed related to the proarrhythmic and negative inotropic properties common to many of these agents (Echt *et al.,* 1991) (*see* Chapter 35). Therefore, indiscriminate use of antiarrhythmic drugs is not recommended in patients with heart failure who have ventricular arrhythmias.

A possible exception is *amiodarone* (CORDARONE; *see* Chapter 35), an antiarrhythmic agent that has additional β-adrenergic suppressing properties which may contribute to its beneficial effect in heart failure. Initial studies using amiodarone were promising, suggesting its use improved survival in patients with heart failure (Doval *et al.,* 1994); however, this has not been confirmed in later studies (Singh *et al.,* 1995; Buxton *et al.,* 1999). In the Multicenter Unsustained Tachycardia Trial

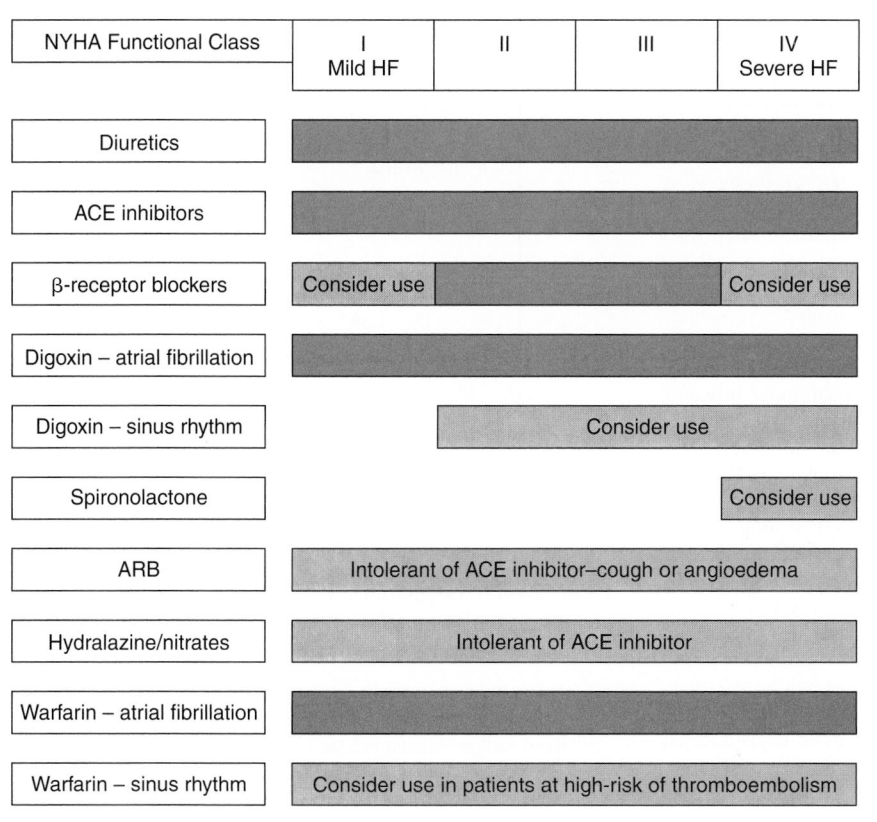

NYHA Functional Class	I Mild HF	II	III	IV Severe HF
Diuretics				
ACE inhibitors				
β-receptor blockers	Consider use			Consider use
Digoxin – atrial fibrillation				
Digoxin – sinus rhythm		Consider use		
Spironolactone				Consider use
ARB	Intolerant of ACE inhibitor–cough or angioedema			
Hydralazine/nitrates	Intolerant of ACE inhibitor			
Warfarin – atrial fibrillation				
Warfarin – sinus rhythm	Consider use in patients at high-risk of thromboembolism			

Figure 34–10. Guidelines for pharmacological management of ambulatory patients with heart failure.

As the number of options for the drug therapy of heart failure increases, it has become more important to determine, based in most cases on evidence from clinical trials, the optimal usage of these drugs. Shown are recommendations for the pharmacological management of left ventricular systolic dysfunction as formulated by the Heart Failure Society of America. Blue boxes represent groups in which drugs should be routinely administered. Gray boxes represent groups in whom drug use should be considered. (ACE inhibitor = angiotensin-converting enzyme inhibitor; ARB = angiotensin receptor blocker; HF = heart failure) (Adapted from Heart Failure Society of America, 1999, with permission.)

(MUSTT), patients with heart failure and asymptomatic ventricular tachycardia who had inducible ventricular arrhythmias documented during an electrophysiological study were randomized to receive either amiodarone, an implanted cardiac defibrillator (ICD), or routine management. Improved survival was demonstrated in patients who received an ICD compared to those receiving routine management; in contrast, no benefit was seen with amiodarone therapy (Buxton *et al.,* 1999).

Thus, the available evidence does not support the routine use of amiodarone to suppress ventricular arrhythmias in patients with heart failure. Patients who have experienced a life-threatening ventricular arrhythmia should receive an ICD as treatment of first choice, with amiodarone being reserved as alternative therapy for patients who are unable to receive an ICD. However, amiodarone is effective in preventing the recurrence of atrial fibrillation or other supraventricular arrhythmias in patients who have ventricular dysfunction.

Guidelines for the Treatment of Ambulatory Heart Failure

As the number of proven therapeutic interventions in heart failure grows, the complexity of managing these patients has correspondingly increased. A number of guidelines for the management of patients with heart failure have been published by learned societies. The main points of the most recent set of guidelines (Heart Failure Society of America, 1999) are summarized in Figure 34–10.

PARENTERAL DRUGS FOR THE TREATMENT OF HOSPITALIZED PATIENTS WITH HEART FAILURE

General Considerations. Patients with heart failure are commonly hospitalized because of increased dyspnea and peripheral edema due to pulmonary and systemic congestion. Fatigue also is a frequent complaint and is related to a reduction in cardiac output and perfusion of skeletal muscle. Accordingly, relief of congestion through the use of diuretics and possibly venodilators is often a priority in patients hospitalized for heart failure. Treatment also is directed at improving ventricular function and increasing cardiac output by lowering ventricular afterload and enhancing myocardial contractility. Wherever possible, precipitating factors (*e.g.,* fever, infection) should be identified and removed, and the underlying cause of heart failure (*e.g.,* ischemia, valvular disease) corrected.

Diuretics

As discussed in the treatment of ambulatory heart failure, diuretics are important for the alleviation of intravascular and extravascular fluid overload. In patients with decompensated heart failure of sufficient severity to warrant admission to a hospital, it is generally desirable to initiate an effective diuresis by using intravenous doses of a *loop diuretic*. Intravenous administration provides a more rapid and predictable diuresis than does the oral route, which is susceptible to delayed or impaired gut absorption, particularly in patients with marked fluid accumulation. The loop diuretic may be administered as repetitive boluses which are titrated against the desired response, or by constant infusion. An advantage of the latter approach is that the same total daily dose of diuretic, when given as a continuous infusion, can result in a more sustained and continuous natriuresis due to maintenance of high diuretic drug levels within the lumen of renal tubules. In addition, the constant infusion helps to decrease the risk of ototoxicity that occurs with transient, high blood levels of the drug following repetitive intermittent loop diuretic dosing (Lahav *et al.*, 1992). A typical continuous *furosemide* infusion is initiated with a 40-mg bolus injection followed by a constant infusion of 10 mg/hour, with upward titration of the infusion as necessary. When there is a poor response to diuretics due to reduced renal perfusion, the short-term administration of sympathomimetic drugs or phosphodiesterase inhibitors to increase cardiac output may be necessary to achieve a response. Another useful approach (*see* section on Diuretic Resistance) is the intravenous administration of dopamine at so-called "low" doses (*i.e.*, less than 2 μg/kg per minute, based on estimated lean body weight) that can cause selective dopaminergic receptor stimulation, thereby causing a selective increase in renal blood flow without causing systemic and venous constriction *via* α-adrenergic receptor stimulation, as may occur at higher infusion rates.

Parenteral Vasodilators

Sodium Nitroprusside. *Sodium nitroprusside* (NITRO-PRESS) is a potent vasodilator that is effective in reducing both ventricular filling pressures and systemic and arterial resistance. It has a rapid onset of action, within 2 to 5 minutes, is quickly metabolized to cyanide and nitric oxide, and its dose usually can be titrated expeditiously to achieve an optimal and predictable hemodynamic effect. For these reasons, nitroprusside is commonly used in intensive-care settings for rapid control of hypertension (*see* Chapter 33) and for the management of acutely decompensated heart failure.

Nitroprusside reduces ventricular filling pressures by directly increasing venous compliance, resulting in a redistribution of blood volume from central to peripheral veins. Nitroprusside is among the most effective afterload-reducing drugs by virtue of the spectrum of pharmacodynamic actions the drug has on different vascular beds (*see* Figure 34–11). It causes a fall in peripheral vascular resistance as well as an increase in aortic wall compliance and, at optimal doses, improves ventricular–vascular coupling. These effects decrease left-ventricular after-

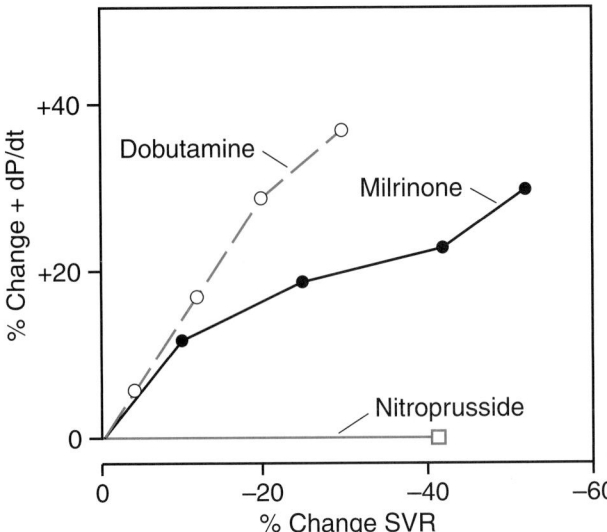

Figure 34–11. Comparative effects of dobutamine, milrinone, and nitroprusside on left ventricular contractility and systemic vascular resistance.

Dobutamine, milrinone, and nitroprusside are parenteral agents used in the management of patients with severe heart failure. Shown are the effects of these drugs on left ventricular contractility, as reflected by left ventricular peak contractility (+dP/dt), and systemic vascular resistance (SVR) in patients with heart failure. Dobutamine and milrinone both increase left ventricular contractility due to their positive inotropic actions on the myocardium. Milrinone, and to a lesser extent dobutamine, also decreased SVR indicating that they also exert a vasodilatory action. However, for a comparable increase in contractility, milrinone causes a greater decrease in SVR. Nitroprusside, a pure vasodilator, decreases SVR but had no effect on contractility. (Adapted from Colucci *et al.*, 1986, with permission.)

load, resulting in an increase in cardiac output. Nitroprusside also dilates pulmonary arterioles and reduces right ventricular afterload. This combination of preload- and afterload-reducing effects improves myocardial energetics by reducing wall stress, provided that blood pressure does not fall to the point of compromising diastolic coronary artery flow or of activating a marked reflex increase in sympathetic nervous system tone. Following the rapid withdrawal of nitroprusside infusion, there may be a transient deterioration in ventricular function associated with a "rebound" increase in systemic vascular resistance that is thought to reflect activation of neurohormonal systems. Nitroprusside is particularly effective in patients with congestive heart failure due to mitral regurgitation or left-to-right shunts through a ventricular septal defect.

The most common adverse effect of nitroprusside, as with most vasodilators, is hypotension. The increase in renal blood flow that accompanies an increase in cardiac output following initiation of nitroprusside in patients with severe heart failure may improve glomerular filtration and diuretic effectiveness. However, the redistribution of blood flow from central organs to peripheral vascular beds may limit or prevent an increase in renal blood flow in some patients. Cyanide produced during the biotransformation of nitroprusside is rapidly metabolized by the liver to thiocyanate, which is cleared by the kidney. Thiocyanate and/or cyanide toxicity is uncommon but may occur in the face of hepatic or renal failure, or following prolonged high-dose infusions of nitroprusside. Typical symptoms include unexplained abdominal pain, mental status changes, convulsions or lactic acidosis. Methemoglobinemia is another unusual complication of prolonged, high-dose nitroprusside infusion.

Nitroglycerin. *Nitroglycerin,* like nitroprusside, is a potent vasodilator (*see* previous section on the treatment of ambulatory heart failure and Chapter 32). In contrast to nitroprusside, nitroglycerin is relatively selective for veins, particularly at low infusion rates. Thus, intravenous nitroglycerin is most often used in the treatment of acute heart failure when a decrease in ventricular filling pressures is desired. At higher infusion rates, nitroglycerin also causes decreases in the systemic and pulmonary arterial resistance, thereby decreasing ventricular afterload. The use of nitroglycerin may be limited by headache and the development of nitrate tolerance, although the latter is generally overcome by uptitration of the infusion rate to the desired response. Since nitroglycerin is administered in ethanol, high infusion rates can be associated with significant blood-alcohol levels.

β-Adrenergic and Dopamine Receptor Agonists

Dopamine and dobutamine are the positive inotropic agents most often used for the short-term support of the circulation in advanced heart failure. Isoproterenol, epinephrine, and norepinephrine, although useful in specific circumstances, have little role in the treatment of most cases of severe heart failure. The basic pharmacology of these and other adrenergic agonists is discussed in Chapter 10.

Dobutamine. *Dobutamine* (DOBUTREX), in the formulation available for clinical use, is a racemic mixture that stimulates both β_1- and β_2-adrenergic receptor subtypes. In addition, the $(-)$ enantiomer is an agonist for α-adrenergic receptors, whereas the $(+)$ enantiomer is a very weak partial agonist. At clinical infusion rates that result in a positive inotropic effect in humans, the β_1-adrenergic effect in the myocardium predominates. In the vasculature, the α-adrenergic agonist effect of the $(-)$ enantiomer appears to be negated by the partial agonism of the $(+)$ enantiomer and the vasodilatory action due to β_2-receptor stimulation. Thus, the net pharmacological effect of dobutamine is to increase stroke volume due to a

positive inotropic action. At doses that increase cardiac output, there is relatively little increase in heart rate. Dobutamine also generally causes a modest decrease in systemic resistance and venous filling pressures (*see* Figure 34–12). Of note, dobutamine does not activate dopaminergic receptors at any dose. Therefore, the increase in renal blood flow with dobutamine is due to an increase in renal blood flow that is proportional to the increase in cardiac output.

Continuous infusions of dobutamine for up to several days generally are well tolerated, although pharmacological tolerance may limit the efficacy during long-term use. Infusion rates usually are initiated at 2 to 3 μg/kg per minute, without a loading dose, and titrated upward according to the patient's symptoms, the hemodynamic goals, and the responsiveness to diuretics. Blood pressure may increase, not change, or fall, depending on the relative effects on vascular tone and cardiac output achieved. Heart rate often declines due to reflex withdrawal of sympathetic tone in response to improved cardiovascular function. Measurement of pulmonary capillary wedge pressure and cardiac output using a pulmonary artery catheter often allows more effective use of dobutamine alone or in conjunction with other vasodilators and diuretics. The major side effects of dobutamine are excessive tachycardia and arrhythmias, which may require a reduction in dosage. Tolerance may occur after prolonged usage, necessitating switching to an intravenous class III cyclic AMP phosphodiesterase inhibitor (*e.g.,* milrinone; *see* below). Likewise, in patients who have been receiving a β-adrenergic receptor antagonist, the initial response to dobutamine may be attenuated until the β-receptor blocker has been metabolized.

Dopamine. *Dopamine,* an endogenous catecholamine, has limited utility in the treatment of most patients with systolic ventricular dysfunction who are not in shock due to primary cardiac failure, hemorrhage, dehydration, or toxicity from vasodilatory drugs. The pharmacological and hemodynamic effects of dopamine are strongly dose-related. At *low doses* of less than or equal to 2 μg/kg per minute (based on estimated lean body weight), dopamine causes vasodilation by direct stimulation of dopaminergic postsynaptic type 1 and presynaptic type 2 (*i.e.,* D_1 and D_2) receptors in the peripheral vasculature and relatively selective vasodilation of splanchnic and renal arterial beds. This effect may prove useful in promoting renal blood flow and maintaining glomerular filtration rate in patients who are refractory to diuretics or whose glomerular filtration rate has begun to decline due to marginal renal perfusion. Dopamine also has direct effects on renal tubular epithelial cells that promote natriuresis.

At *intermediate* infusion rates (2 to 5 μg/kg per minute), dopamine directly stimulates β-adrenergic receptors in the heart and induces norepinephrine release from vascular sympathetic neurons. At *higher* infusion rates (5 to 15 μg/kg per minute),

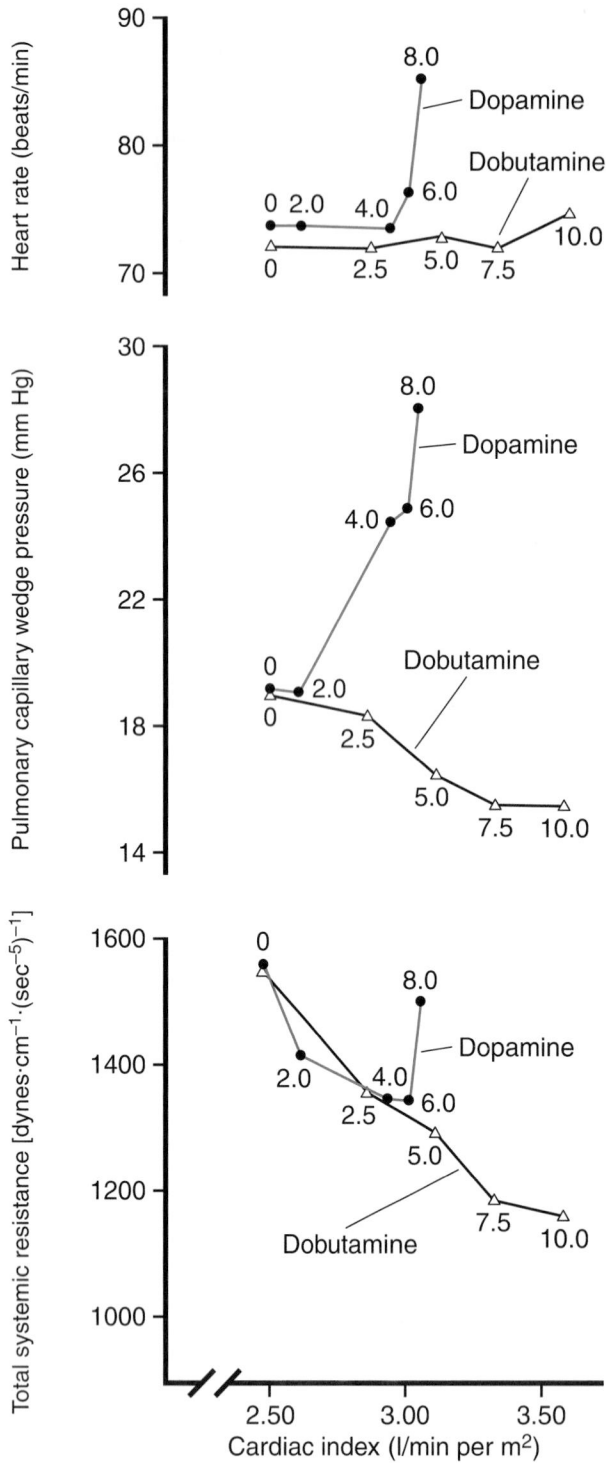

Figure 34–12. Comparative hemodynamic effects of dopamine and dobutamine in patients with heart failure.

Dopamine and dobutamine were titrated over the usual clinical doses in patients with severe heart failure. The numbers shown on the figures are infusion rates in μg/kg per minute. Dobutamine increased cardiac output due to an increase in stroke volume (not shown). This effect was associated with modest decreases in pulmonary capillary wedge pressure and systemic vascular resistance, reflecting both direct vasodilation due to stimulation of β_2-adrenergic receptors and reflex withdrawal of sympathetic tone in response to improved cardiovascular function. At infusion rates that exceeded 2 to 4 μg/kg per minute, dopamine exerted a potent vasoconstrictor effect as evidenced by the increase in systemic vascular resistance. Pulmonary capillary wedge pressure also increased with dopamine due to venoconstriction and a decrease in left ventricular function caused by the increase in afterload. (Adapted from Stevenson and Colucci, 1996, with permission.)

peripheral arterial and venous constriction caused by α-adrenergic receptor stimulation occurs, which may be desirable for support of a critically reduced arterial pressure, but which otherwise may further suppress ventricular systolic function due to

the increase in afterload. Even with intermediate infusion rates, some patients may have an increase in systemic vascular resistance. Tachycardia, which is more pronounced with dopamine than with dobutamine, may provoke ischemia in patients with coronary artery disease. It should be emphasized that the dosing ranges noted above are based on estimated lean body weight, not on the patient's actual weight. Unexplained tachycardia or newly apparent arrhythmias in a patient receiving, among other drugs, "renal range" dopamine should make the clinician suspect an inappropriately high dopamine infusion rate.

Phosphodiesterase Inhibitors

The cyclic AMP PDE inhibitors mimic the effects of adenylyl cyclase activation by inhibiting the breakdown of cyclic AMP. Increased levels of cyclic AMP result in increased myocardial contractility and vasodilation in the venous and arterial circulation. Although agents such as theophylline and caffeine had been identified as nonspecific cyclic GMP and cyclic AMP PDE inhibitors more than 30 years ago, the use of these drugs at hemodynamically effective doses is plagued by side effects. During the 1980s, amrinone (now called inamrinone), milrinone, and other PDE inhibitors with isoenzyme selectivity became available, largely alleviating these problems.

Inamrinone and Milrinone. Parenteral formulations of *inamrinone* (INOCOR) and *milrinone* (PRIMACOR) have been approved for short-term support of the circulation in advanced heart failure. Both drugs are bipyridine derivatives and relatively selective inhibitors of the cyclic GMP-inhibited, cyclic AMP PDE (type III) family. These drugs cause direct stimulation of myocardial contractility and acceleration of myocardial relaxation. In addition, they cause balanced arterial and venous dilation with a consequent fall in systemic and pulmonary vascular resistances, and left and right heart filling pressures. Cardiac output increases due to the stimulation of myocardial contractility and the decrease in left ventricular afterload. As a result of this dual mechanism of action, the increase in cardiac output with milrinone, when compared at comparable decreases in systemic pressure, is greater than with the pure vasodilator nitroprusside; and conversely, the arterial and venous dilator effects of milrinone are greater, when compared for comparable increases in cardiac output, than with dobutamine (Colucci *et al.*, 1986) (*see* Figure 34–11).

Both drugs are effective when given either as single agents or, more commonly, in combination with other oral and/or intravenous drugs for short-term treatment of patients with severe heart failure due to systolic right or left ventricular dysfunction. Intravenous infusions of either drug should be initiated by a loading dose followed by a continuous infusion. For inamrinone, typically a 0.75-mg/kg bolus injection over 2 to 3 minutes is followed by a 2- to 20-μg/kg per minute infusion. Milrinone is approximately 10-fold more potent than inamrinone. A loading dose of milrinone is usually 50 μg/kg, and the continuous infusion rate ranges from 0.25 to 1.0 μg/kg per minute. The elimination half-lives of inamrinone and milrinone in healthy subjects are 2 to 3 hours and 30 to 60 minutes, respectively, and are approximately doubled in patients with severe heart failure. Clinically significant thrombocytopenia occurs in 10% of patients receiving inamrinone but is rare with milrinone. Because of its greater selectivity for PDE III isoenzymes, shorter half-life, and fewer side effects, *milrinone* is the agent of choice among currently available PDE inhibitors for short-term, parenteral inotropic support in severe heart failure.

General Guidelines for the Use of Parenteral Drugs

In general, initial therapy in the patient with symptomatic pulmonary congestion should include diuresis to alleviate pulmonary and systemic vascular congestion (*see* Figure 34–13). The administration of an oral or intravenous nitrate preparation may provide additional rapid symptomatic relief of pulmonary congestion by causing venodilation. Cardiac output may be optimized by a variety of agents, the selection of which may be guided in part by the arterial pressure, or ideally, by knowledge of the systemic vascular resistance (SVR) as provided by a pulmonary artery catheter.

In patients with an elevated arterial pressure, afterload reduction with nitroprusside may be very effective. Nitroprusside also may be effective when there is an elevated SVR, despite the presence of a low arterial pressure. On the other hand, in patients in whom the SVR is not elevated, afterload reduction may result in an excessive fall in arterial pressure. In such patients, increasing myocardial contractility with a positive inotropic agent such as dobutamine often is preferable. Milrinone, which exerts both inotropic and vasodilatory actions, may be tolerated in some patients who do not tolerate a pure vasodilator, and conversely, may provide better relief of pulmonary congestion than dobutamine. Likewise, in patients in whom the left ventricular filling pressure is known (or suspected) not to be markedly elevated, treatment with dobutamine may avoid an excessive decrease in preload that can occur with vasodilators.

When heart failure is severe, in patients who fail to respond to standard therapy, or if there is progressive renal insufficiency in the face of persistent signs of elevated filling pressures, placement of a pulmonary artery catheter and hemodynamic monitoring may be important for guidance of drug selection and dosing. Once hemodynamic monitoring is established, therapy is directed at optimization of hemodynamics and improvement in clinical status of the patient; afterload and cardiac filling pressures

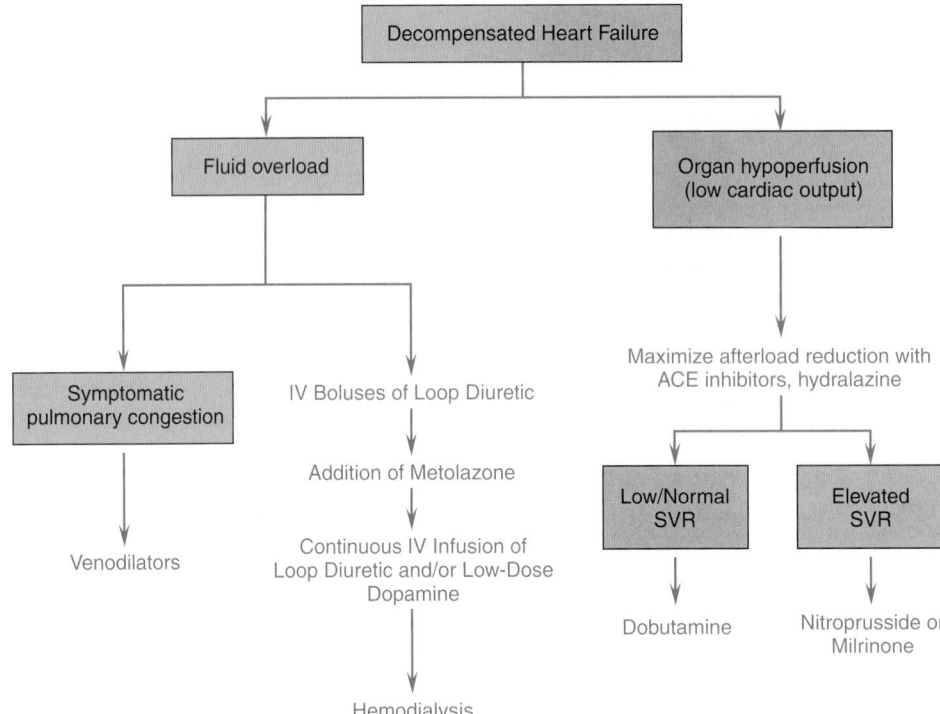

Figure 34–13. General approach to the treatment of patients hospitalized with decompensated heart failure.

Fluid overload is a common feature in patients hospitalized for decompensated heart failure. Therefore, the initial management of such patients generally involves the use of loop diuretics administered intravenously as boluses or continuous infusions. In patients who do not respond to loop diuretics alone, the addition of a thiazide diuretic (*e.g.,* metolazone) or a low-dose infusion of dopamine may facilitate diuresis. Venodilators (*e.g.,* nitroglycerin) may provide rapid alleviation of pulmonary congestion. Poor diuretic responsiveness and other sequelae of reduced organ hypoperfusion may respond to an increase in cardiac output caused by a positive inotropic agent (*e.g.,* dobutamine or milrinone) and/or a vasodilator that reduces left ventricular afterload (*e.g.,* nitroprusside or milrinone). Although it frequently is possible to use parenteral agents without invasive monitoring, in many patients therapy is best guided by knowledge of the left and right heart filling pressures and systemic vascular resistance (SVR). ACE = angiotensin converting enzyme.

should be reduced to target levels, and cardiac output augmented where necessary to ensure adequate perfusion of vital organs.

PROSPECTUS

Since the publication of the previous edition of this textbook, there has been continuing evolution in the drug treatment of heart failure. Several large randomized trials have shown consistent evidence of benefit and have firmly established the central role of β-adrenergic receptor antagonism alongside ACE inhibition in the therapy of ambulatory patients with heart failure. Although neutral with regard to mortality, the efficacy of cardiac glycosides

in improving symptoms and reducing hospitalization for heart failure has been reaffirmed. Finally, an old drug has found new life with the revival of spironolactone as a useful adjunctive therapy in patients with severe heart failure.

Despite these and other recent advances in the pharmacotherapy of heart failure, the mortality rate remains high. Thus, preventive strategies including aggressive control of risk factors for cardiovascular disease continue to be of great importance. Further insights into the cellular and molecular abnormalities that underlie the contractile, hemodynamic, and neurohormonal disturbances of heart failure have cleared the way for the development of innovative therapeutic agents that may impact positively on outcomes. New therapeutic strategies include agents that block or stimulate endogenous signaling pathways. *Endothelin receptor blockers* have been shown to exert beneficial hemodynamic effects in patients with heart failure during short-term administration and are being evaluated with regard to long-term effects on morbidity and mortality. *Antagonists of the inflammatory cytokine, tumor necrosis factor-α*, which have been shown to be both safe and effective in the treatment of inflammatory conditions such as rheumatoid arthritis and enteritis, are being evaluated for the treatment of heart failure. The *natriuretic peptides* are endogenous molecules that cause vasodila-

tion and oppose the renin–angiotensin system. *Nesiritide,* a recombinant, human-brain natriuretic peptide, exerts favorable vasodilatory effects with short-term infusion and may be of value in the treatment of patients hospitalized with heart failure. *Omapatrilat,* an orally active neutral endopeptidase inhibitor which blocks both ACE and the degradation of natriuretic peptides, has been shown to exert beneficial clinical effects in patients with chronic heart failure. Ultimately, the role of these and other new pharmacologic approaches will need to be established through controlled trials that determine their efficacy and safety.

For further discussion of normal and abnormal cardiac function and of heart failure *see* Chapters 232 and 233 in *Harrison's Principles of Internal Medicine,* 14th ed., McGraw-Hill, New York, 1998.

BIBLIOGRAPHY

Acute Infarction Ramipril Efficacy (AIRE) Study Investigators. Effect of ramipril on mortality and morbidity of survivors of acute myocardial infarction with clinical evidence of heart failure. *Lancet,* **1993,** *342*:821–828.

Al-Khadra, A.S., Salem, D.N., Rand, W.M., Udelson, J.E., Smith, J.J., and Konstam, M.A. Antiplatelet agents and survival: a cohort analysis from the Studies of Left Ventricular Dysfunction (SOLVD) trial. *J. Am. Coll. Cardiol.,* **1998,** *31*:419–425.

American Heart Association. *2000 Heart and Stroke Statistical Update,* A.H.A., Dallas, **1999.**

Andersson, B., Hamm, C., Persson, S., Wikstrom, G., Sinagra, G., Hjalmarson, A., and Waagstein, F. Improved exercise hemodynamic status in dilated cardiomyopathy after beta-adrenergic blockade treatment. *J. Am. Coll. Cardiol.,* **1994,** *23*:1397–1404.

Australia/New Zealand Heart Failure Research Collaborative Group. Randomised, placebo-controlled trial of carvedilol in patients with congestive heart failure due to ischemic heart disease. *Lancet,* **1997,** *349*:375–380.

Bisognano, J.D., Weinberger, H.D., Bohlmeyer, T.J., Pende, A., Raynolds, M.V., Sastravaha, A., Roden, R., Asano, K., Blaxall, B.C., Wu, S.C., Communal, C., Singh, K., Colucci, W., Bristow, M.R., and Port, D.J. Myocardial-directed overexpression of the human beta(1)-adrenergic receptor in transgenic mice. *J. Mol. Cell. Cardiol.,* **2000,** *32*:817–830.

Bristow, M.R., Gilbert, E.M., Abraham, W.T., Adams, K.F., Fowler, M.B., Hershberger, R.E., Kubo, S.H., Narahara, K.A., Ingersoll, H., Krueger, S., Young, S., and Shusterman, N. Carvedilol produces dose-related improvements in left ventricular function and survival in subjects with chronic heart failure. MOCHA Investigators. *Circulation,* **1996,** *94*:2807–2816.

Buxton, A.E., Lee, K.L., Fisher, J.D., Josephson, M.E., Prystowsky, E.N., and Hafley, G. A randomized study of the prevention of sudden death in patients with coronary artery disease. Multicenter Unsustained Tachycardia Trial Investigators. *N. Engl. J. Med.,* **1999,** *341*:1882–1890.

CIBIS Investigators and Committees. A randomized trial of β-blockade in heart failure. The Cardiac Insufficiency Bisoprolol Study (CIBIS). *Circulation,* **1994,** *90*:1765–1773.

The Cardiac Insufficiency Bisoprolol Study II (CIBIS II): a randomized trial. CIBIS-II Investigators and Committee. *Lancet,* **1999,** *355*:9–13.

Cleland, J.G.F. The WASH study. Presented at the XXIst Congress of the European Society of Cardiology. Barcelona, Spain: Aug. 28–Sept. 1, **1999.**

Cohn, J.N., Archibald, D.G., Ziesche, S., Franciosa, J.A., Harston, W.E., Tristani, F.E., Dunkman, W.B., Jacobs, W., Francis, G.S., Flohr, K.H., Goldman, S., Cobb, F.R., Shah, P.M., Saunders, R., Fletcher, R.D., Loeb, H.S., Hughes, V.C., and Baker, B. Effect of vasodilator therapy on mortality in chronic congestive heart failure. Results of a Veterans Administration Cooperative Study. *N. Engl. J. Med.,* **1986,** *314*:1547–1552.

Cohn, J.N., Goldstein, S.O., Greenberg, B.H., Lorell, B.H., Bourge, R.C., Jaski, B.E., Gottlieb, S.O., McGrew, F. III, DeMets, D.L., and White, B.G. A dose-dependent increase in mortality with vesnarinone among patients with severe heart failure. Vesnarinone Trial Investigators. *N. Engl. J. Med.,* **1998,** *339*:1810–1816.

Cohn, J.N., Johnson, G., Ziesche, S., Cobb, F., Francis, G., Tristani, F., Smith, R., Dunkman, W.B., Loeb, H., Wong, M., Bhat, G., Goldman, S., Fletcher, R.D., Doherty, J., Hughes, C.V., Carson, P., Cintron, G., Shabetai, R., and Haakenson, C. A comparison of enalapril with hydralazine-isosorbide dinitrate in the treatment of chronic congestive heart failure. *N. Engl. J. Med.,* **1991,** *325*:303–310.

Cohn, J.N., Ziesche, S., Smith, R., Anand, I., Dunkman, W.B., Loeb, H., Cintron, G., Boden, W., Baruch, L., Rochin, P., and Loss, L. Effect of the calcium antagonist felodipine as supplementary vasodilator therapy in patients with chronic heart failure treated with enalapril: V-HeFT III. Vasodilator-Heart Failure Trial (V-HeFT) Study Group. *Circulation,* **1997,** *96*:856–863.

Colucci, W.S., Wright, R.F., Jaski, B.E., Fifer, M.A., and Braunwald, E. Milrinone and dobutamine in severe heart failure: differing hemodynamic effects and individual patient responsiveness. *Circulation,* **1986,** *73*(suppl III):175–183.

Colucci, W.S., Packer, M., Bristow, M.R., Gilbert, E.M., Cohn, J.N., Fowler, M.B., Krueger, S.K., Hershberger, R., Uretsky, B.F., Bowers, J.A., Sackner-Bernstein, J.D., Young, S.T., Holcslaw, T.L., and Lukas, M.A. Carvedilol inhibits clinical progression in patients with mild symptoms of heart failure. U.S. Carvedilol Heart Failure Study Group. *Circulation,* **1996,** *94*:2800–2806.

Communal, C., Singh, K., Pimentel, D.R., and Colucci, W.S. Norepinephrine stimulates apoptosis in adult rat ventricular myocytes by activation of the β-adrenergic pathway. *Circulation,* **1998,** *98*:1329–1334.

CONSENSUS Trial Study Group. Effects of enalapril on mortality in severe congestive heart failure. Results of the Cooperative North Scandinavian Enalapril Survival Group (CONSENSUS). *N. Engl. J. Med.,* **1987,** *316*:1429–1435.

Davies, D.L., and Fraser, R. Do diuretics cause magnesium deficiency? *Br. J. Clin. Pharmacol.,* **1993,** *36*:1–10.

The Digitalis Investigation Group. The effect of digoxin on mortality and morbidity in patients with heart failure. *N. Engl. J. Med.,* **1997,** *336*:525–533.

Doval, H.C., Nul, D.R., Grencelli, H.O., Perrone, S.V., Bortman, G.R., and Curiel, R. Randomised trial of low-dose amiodarone in severe congestive heart failure. Grupo de Estudio de la Sobrevida en la Insuficiencia Cordiaca en Argentina. *Lancet,* **1994,** *344*:493–498.

Echt, D.S., Liebson, P.R., Mitchell, L.B., Peters, R.W., Obias-Manno, D., Barker, A.H., Arensberg, D., Baker, A., Friedman, L., Greene, H.L., Huther, M.L., and Richardson, D.W. Mortality and morbidity in patients receiving encainide, flecainide, or placebo. The Cardiac Arrhythmia Suppression Trial. *N. Engl. J. Med.,* **1991,** *324*:781–788.

Eichhorn, E.J., Heesch, C.M., Barnett, J.H., Alvarez, L.G., Fass, S.M., Grayburn, P.A., Hatfield, B.A., Marcoux, L.G., and Malloy, C.R. Effect of metoprolol on myocardial function and energetics in patients with nonischemic dilated cardiomyopathy: a randomized, double-blind, placebo-controlled study. *J. Am. Coll. Cardiol.,* **1994,** *24*:1310–1320.

Ellison, D.H. The physiologic basis of diuretic synergism: its role in treating diuretic resistance. *Ann. Intern. Med.,* **1991,** *114*:886–894.

Elkayam, U., Shotan, A., Mehra, A., and Ostrzega, E. Calcium channel blockers in heart failure. *J. Am. Coll. Cardiol.,* **1993,** *22*:139A–144A.

Ferguson, D.W., Berg, W.J., Sanders, J.S., Roach, P.J., Kempf, J.S., and Kienzle, M.G. Sympathoinhibitory responses to digitalis glycosides in heart failure patients. Direct evidence from sympathetic neural recordings. *Circulation,* **1989,** *80*:65–77.

Fonarow, G.C., Chelimsky-Fallick, C., Stevenson L.W., Luu, M., Hamilton, M.A., Moriguchi, J.D., Tillisch, J.H., Walden, J.A., and Albanese, E. Effect of direct vasodilation with hydralazine versus angiotensin-converting enzyme inhibition with captopril on mortality in advanced heart failure: the Hy-C trial. *J. Am. Coll. Cardiol.,* **1992,** *19*:842–850.

Gamba, G., Miyanoshita, A., Lombardi, M., Lytton, J., Lee, W.-S., Hediger, M.A., and Hebert, S.C. Molecular cloning, primary structure, and characterization of two members of the mammalian electroneutral sodium-(potassium)-chloride cotransporter family expressed in kidney. *J. Biol. Chem.,* **1994,** *269*:17713–17722.

Gogia, H., Mehra, A., Parikh, S., Raman, M., Ajit-Uppal, J., Johnson, J.V., and Elkayam, U. Prevention of tolerance to hemodynamic effects of nitrates with concomitant use of hydralazine in patients with chronic heart failure. *J. Am. Coll. Cardiol.,* **1995,** *26*:1575–1580.

Gruppo Italiano per lo Studio della Sopravvivenza nell'infarto Mio-

cardico. GISSI-3: effects of lisinopril and transdermal glyceryl trinitrate singly and together on 6-week mortality and ventricular function after acute myocardial infarction. *Lancet,* **1994,** *343*:1115–1122.

Hall, D., Zeitler, H., and Rudolph, W. Counteraction of the vasodilator effects of enalapril by aspirin in severe heart failure. *J. Am. Coll. Cardiol.,* **1992,** *20*:1549–1555.

Hall, S.A., Cigarroa, C.G., Marcoux, L., Risser, R.C., Grayburn, P.A., and Eichhorn, E.J. Time course of improvement in left ventricular function, mass and geometry in patients with congestive heart failure treated with beta-adrenergic blockade. *J. Am. Coll. Cardiol.,* **1995,** *25*:1154–1161.

Hampton, J.R., van Veldhuisen, D.J., Kleber, F.X., Cowley, A.J., Ardia, A., Block, P., Cortina, A., Cserhalmi, L., Follath, F., Jensen, G., Kayanakis, J., Lie, K.I., Mancia, G., and Skene, A.M. Randomised study of effect of ibopamine on survival in patients with advanced severe heart failure. Second Prospective Randomised Study of Ibopamine on Mortality and Efficacy (PRIME II) Investigators. *Lancet,* **1997,** *349*:971–977.

Heart Failure Society of America (HFSA) practice guidelines. HFSA guidelines for management of patients with heart failure caused by left ventricular systolic dysfunction—pharmacological approaches. *J. Card. Fail.,* **1999,** *5*:357–382.

Juillerat, L., Nussberger, J., Menard, J., Mooser, V., Christen, Y., Waeber, B., Graf, P., and Brunner, H.R. Determinants of angiotensin II generation during converting enzyme inhibition. *Hypertension,* **1990,** *16*:564–572.

Kelly, R.A., and Smith, T.W. Use and misuse of digitalis blood levels. *Heart Dis. Stroke,* **1992a,** *1*:117–122.

Kelly, R.A., and Smith, T.W. Recognition and management of digitalis toxicity. *Am. J. Cardiol.,* **1992b,** *69*:1086–1196.

Konstam, M.A., Rousseau, M.F., Kronenberg, M.W., Udelson, J.E., Melin, J., Stewart, D., Dolan, N., Edens, T.R., Ahn, S., Kinan, D., Howe, D.M., Kilcoyne, L., Metherall, J., Benedict, C., Yusuf, S., and Pouleur, H. Effects of the angiotensin converting enzyme inhibitor enalapril on the long-term progression of left ventricular dysfunction in patients with heart failure. SOLVD Investigators. *Circulation,* **1992,** *86*:431–438.

Lahav, M., Regev, A., Ra'anani, P., and Theodor, E. Intermittent administration of furosemide vs continuous infusion preceded by a loading dose for congestive heart failure. *Chest,* **1992,** *102*:725–731.

McKelvie, R.S., Yusuf, S., Pericak, D., Avezum, A., Burns, R.J., Probstfield, J., Tsuyuki, R.T., White, M., Rouleau, J., Latini, R., Maggioni, A., Young, J., and Pogue, J. Comparison of candesartan, enalapril, and their combination in congestive heart failure: randomized evaluation of strategies for left ventricular dysfunction (RESOLVD) pilot study. The RESOLVD Pilot Study Investigators. *Circulation,* **1999,** *100*:1056–1064.

Mehra, A., Shotan, A., Ostrzega, E., Hsueh, W., Vasquez-Johnson, J., and Elkayam, U. Potentiation of isosorbide dinitrate effects with *N*-acetylcysteine in patients with chronic heart failure. *Circulation,* **1994,** *89*:2595–2600.

MERIT-HF Study Group. Effect of metoprolol CR/XL in chronic heart failure: Metoprolol CR/XL Randomised Intervention Trial in Congestive Heart Failure (MERIT-HF). *Lancet,* **1999,** *353*:2001–2007.

Nguyen, K.N., Aursnes, I., and Kjekshus, J. Interaction between enalapril and aspirin on mortality after acute myocardial infarction: subgroup analysis of the Cooperative New Scandinavian Enalapril Survival Study II. *Am. J. Cardiol.,* **1997,** *79*:115–119.

Packer, M., Bristow, M.R., Cohn, J.N., Colucci, W.S., Fowler, M.B., Gilbert, E.M., and Shusterman, N.H. The effect of carvedilol on morbidity and mortality in patients with chronic heart failure. U.S. Carvedilol Heart Failure Study Group. *N. Engl. J. Med.,* **1996b,** *334*:1349–1355.

Packer, M., Carver, J.R., Rodeheffer, R.J., Ivanhoe, R.J., DiBianco, R., Zeldis, S.M., Hendrix, G.H., Bommer, W.J., Elkayam, U., Kukin, M.L., Mallis, G.I., Sollano, J.A., Shannon, J., Tandon, P.K., and DeMets, D.L. Effect of oral milrinone on mortality in severe chronic heart failure. PROMISE Study Research Group. *N. Engl. J. Med.,* **1991,** *325*:1468–1475.

Packer, M., Gheorghiade, M., Young, J.B., Costantini, P.J., Adams, K.F., Cody, R.J., Smith, L.K., Van Voorhees, L., Gourley, L.A., and Jolly, M.K. Withdrawal of digoxin from patients with chronic heart failure treated with angiotensin-converting-enzyme inhibitors. RADIANCE Study. *N. Engl. J. Med.,* **1993,** *329*:1–7.

Packer, M., O'Connor, C.M., Ghali, J.K., Pressler, M.L., Carson, P.E., Belkin, R.N., Miller, A.B., Neuberg, G.W., Frid, D., Wertheimer, J.H., Cropp, A.B., and DeMets, D.L. Effect of amlodipine on morbidity and mortality in severe chronic heart failure. Prospective Randomized Amlodipine Survival Evaluation Study Group. *N. Engl. J. Med.,* **1996a,** *335*:1107–1114.

Packer, M., Poole-Wilson, P.A., Armstrong, P.W., Cleland, J.G., Horowitz, J.D., Massie, B.M., Rydén, L., Thygesen, K., and Uretsky, B.F. Comparative effects of low and high doses of the angiotensin converting enzyme inhibitor, lisinopril, on morbidity and mortality in chronic heart failure. ATLAS Study Group. *Circulation,* **1999,** *100*:2312–2318.

Pfeffer, M.A., Braunwald, E., Moye, L.A., Basta, L., Brown, E.J. Jr., Cuddy, T.E., Davis, B.R., Geltman, E.M., Goldman, S., Flaker, G.C., Klein, M., Lamas, G.A., Packer, M., Rouleau, J., Rouleau, J.L., Rutherford, J., Wertheimer, J.H., and Hawkins, C.M. Effect of captopril on mortality and morbidity in patients with left ventricular dysfunction after myocardial infarction. Results of the survival and ventricular enlargement trial. The SAVE Investigators. *N. Engl. J. Med.,* **1992,** *327*:669–677.

Pitt, B., Poole-Wilson, P.A., Segal, R., Martinez, F.A., Dickstein, K., Camm, A.J., Konstam, M.A., Riegger, G., Klinger, G.H., Neaton, J., Sharma, D., and Thiyagarajan, B. Effect of losartan compared with captopril on mortality in patients with symptomatic heart failure: randomised trial—the Losartan Heart Failure Survival Study ELITE II. *Lancet,* **2000,** *355*:1582–1587.

Pitt, B., Segal, R., Martinez, F.A., Meurers, G., Cowley, A.J., Thomas, I., Deedwania, P.C., Ney, D.E., Snavely, D.B., and Chang, P.I. Randomised trial of losartan versus captopril in patients over 65 with heart failure. *Lancet,* **1997,** *349*:747–752.

Pitt, B., Zannad, F., Remme, W.J., Cody, R., Castaigne, A., Perez, A., Palensky, J., and Wittes, J. The effect of spironolactone on morbidity and mortality in patients with severe heart failure. Randomized Aldactone Evaluation Study Investigators. *N. Engl. J. Med.,* **1999,** *341*:709–717.

St. John Sutton, M., Pfeffer, M.A., Plappert, T., Rouleau, J.-L., Moye, L.A., Dagenais, G.R., Lamas, G.A., Klein M., Sussex, B., Goldman, S., Menapace, F.J. Jr., Parker, J.O., Lewis, S., Sestier, F., Gordon, D.F., McEwan, P., Bernstein, V., and Braunwald, E. Quantitative two-dimensional echocardiographic measurements are major predictors of adverse cardiovascular events after acute myocardial infarction. The protective effects of captopril. *Circulation,* **1994,** *89*:68–75.

Sawyer, D.B., and Colucci, W.S. Mitochondrial oxidative stress in heart failure: "oxygen wastage" revisited. *Circ. Res.,* **2000,** *86*:119–120.

Singh, S.N., Fletcher, R.D., Fisher, S.G., Singh, B.N., Lewis, H.D.,

Deedwania, P.C., Massie, B.M., Colling, C., and Lazzeri, D. Amiodarone in patients with congestive heart failure and asymptomatic ventricular arrhythmia. Survival Trial of Antiarrhythmic Therapy in Congestive Heart Failure. *N. Engl. J. Med.,* **1995,** *33*:77–82.

Smith, T.W., Braunwald, E., and Kelly, R.A. The management of heart failure. In, *Heart Disease,* 4th ed. (Braunwald, E., ed.) Saunders, Philadelphia, **1992,** pp. 464–519.

SOLVD Investigators. Effect of enalapril on survival in patients with reduced left ventricular ejection fractions and congestive heart failure. *N. Engl. J. Med.,* **1991,** *325*:293–302.

SOLVD Investigators. Effect of enalapril on mortality and the development of heart failure in asymptomatic patients with reduced left ventricular ejection fractions. *N. Engl. J. Med.,* **1992,** *327*:685–691. [Published erratum in *N. Engl. J. Med.,* **1992,** *329*:1768.]

Uretsky, B.F., Young, J.B., Shahidi, F.E., Yellen, L.G., Harrison, M.C., and Jolly, M.K. Randomized study assessing the effect of digoxin withdrawal in patients with mild to moderate chronic congestive heart failure: results of the PROVED trial. PROVED Investigative Group. *J. Am. Coll. Cardiol.,* **1993,** *22*:955–962.

Waagstein, F., Bristow, M.R., Swedberg, K., Camerini, F., Fowler, M.B., Silver, M.A., Gilbert, E.M., Johnson, M.R., Goss, F.G., and Hjalmarson, A. Beneficial effects of metoprolol in idiopathic dilated cardiomyopathy. Metoprolol in Dilated Cardiomyopathy (MDC) Trial Study Group. *Lancet,* **1993,** *342*:1441–1446.

Wang, W., Chen, J.-S., and Zucker, I.H. Carotid sinus baroreceptor sensitivity in experimental heart failure. *Circulation,* **1990,** *81*:1959–1966.

MONOGRAPHS AND REVIEWS

Bigger, J.T. Jr. Diuretic therapy, hypertension, and cardiac arrest. *N. Engl. J. Med.,* **1994,** *330*:1899–1900.

Brater, D.C. Diuretic therapy. *N. Engl. J. Med.,* **1998,** *339*:387–395.

Bristow, M.R. Beta-adrenergic receptor blockade in chronic heart failure. *Circulation,* **2000,** *101*:558–569.

Cohn, J.N., and Franciosa, J.A. Vasodilator therapy of cardiac failure. *N. Engl. J. Med.,* **1977,** *297*:27–31, 254–258.

Burnier, M., Brunner, H.R. Angiotensin II receptor antagonists. *Lancet,* **2000,** *355*:637–645.

Cohn, J.N. Treatment of infarct related heart failure: vasodilators other than ACE inhibitors. *Cardiovasc. Drugs Ther.,* **1994,** *8*:119–122.

Cohn, J.N. Structural basis for heart failure. Ventricular remodeling and its pharmacological inhibition. *Circulation,* **1995,** *91*:2504–2507.

Colucci, W.S., and Braunwald E. Pathophysiology of heart failure. In, *Heart Disease,* 6th ed. (Braunwald, E., ed.) Saunders, Philadelphia, **2000,** in press.

Eichhorn, E.J., and Bristow, M.R. Medical therapy can improve the biological properties of the chronically failing heart. A new era in the treatment of heart failure. *Circulation,* **1996,** *94*:2285–2296.

Eisner, D.A., and Smith, T.W. The Na-K pump and its effectors in cardiac muscle. In, *The Heart and Cardiovascular System: Scientific Foundations,* 2nd ed. (Fozzard, H.A., Haber, E., Jennings, R.B., Katz, A.M., and Morgan, H.E., eds.) Raven Press, New York, **1991,** pp. 863–902.

Ellison, D.H. Diuretic resistance: physiology and therapeutics. *Semin. Nephrol.,* **1999,** *19*:581–597.

Gheorghiade, M., Cody, R.J., Francis, G.S., McKenna, W.J., Young, J.B., and Bonow, R.O. Current medical therapy for advanced heart failure. *Heart Lung,* **2000,** *29*:16–32.

Kelly, R.A., and Smith, T.W. Nitric oxide and nitrovasodilators: similarities, differences, and interactions. *Am. J. Cardiol.,* **1996,** *77*:2C–7C.

Smith, T.W., Kelly, R.A., Stevenson, L.W., Braunwald, E. Management of heart failure. In, *Heart Disease,* 5th ed. (Braunwald, E., ed.) Saunders, Philadelphia, **1997,** pp. 492–514.

Stevenson, L.W., Colucci, W.S. Management of patients hospitalized with heart failure. In, *Cardiovascular Therapeutics: A Companion to Braunwald's Heart Disease* (Smith, T.W., ed.) Saunders, Philadelphia, **1996,** pp. 199–209.

Struthers, A.D. Why does spironolactone improve mortality over and above an ACE inhibitor in chronic heart failure? *Br. J. Clin. Pharmacol.,* **1999,** *47*:479–482.

Swedberg, K. Initial experience with beta blockers in dilated cardiomyopathy. *Am. J. Cardiol.,* **1993,** *71*:30C–38C.

Acknowledgment

The authors wish to acknowledge Drs. Ralph A. Kelley and Thomas W. Smith, the authors of this chapter in the ninth edition of *Goodman and Gilman's The Pharmacological Basis of Therapeutics,* some of whose text has been retained in this edition.

C H A P T E R 3 5

ANTIARRHYTHMIC DRUGS

Dan M. Roden

Individual cardiac cells undergo depolarization and repolarization to form cardiac action potentials about sixty times per minute. The shape and duration of each action potential are determined by the activity of ion channel protein complexes on the surface of individual cells, and the genes encoding many of these proteins have now been identified. Thus, each heartbeat is the result of the highly integrated electrophysiological behavior of multiple gene products on multiple cardiac cells. Ion channel function can be perturbed by factors such as acute ischemia, sympathetic stimulation, or myocardial scarring to create abnormalities of cardiac rhythm, or arrhythmias. Available antiarrhythmic drugs suppress arrhythmias by blocking flow through specific ion channels or by altering autonomic function.

Arrhythmias can range from incidental, asymptomatic clinical findings to life-threatening abnormalities. Mechanisms underlying cardiac arrhythmias have been identified in cellular and animal experiments. In some human cases, precise mechanisms are known, and treatment targeted against those mechanisms can be used. In other cases, mechanisms can be only inferred, and the choice of drugs is based largely on results of prior experience. Antiarrhythmic drug therapy can have two goals: termination of an ongoing arrhythmia or prevention of an arrhythmia. It is now well recognized that antiarrhythmic drugs not only help to control arrhythmias but also can cause them, especially during long-term therapy. Thus, prescribing antiarrhythmic drugs requires that precipitating factors be excluded or minimized, that a precise diagnosis of the type of arrhythmia (and its possible mechanisms) be made, that the prescriber has reason to believe that drug therapy will be beneficial, and that the risks of drug therapy be minimized.

In this chapter, the principles underlying normal and abnormal cardiac electrophysiology are outlined. Then, the mechanisms by which drugs modulate cardiac electrophysiology are presented, followed by a description of the important properties of individual agents.

PRINCIPLES OF CARDIAC ELECTROPHYSIOLOGY

The flow of charged ions across cell membranes results in the ionic currents that make up cardiac action potentials. The factors that determine the magnitude of individual currents and how these are modified by drugs now can be elucidated at the cellular and molecular levels (Fozzard and Arnsdorf, 1991; Snyders *et al.*, 1991; Priori *et al.*, 1999). However, the action potential is a highly integrated entity: changes in one current almost inevitably produce secondary changes in other currents. Most antiarrhythmic drugs affect more than one ion current, and many exert ancillary effects such as modification of cardiac contractility or autonomic nervous system function. Thus, antiarrhythmic drugs usually exert multiple actions and can be beneficial or harmful in individual patients (Roden, 1994; Priori *et al.*, 1999).

The Cardiac Cell at Rest: A K^+-Permeable Membrane

Ions move across cell membranes in response to electrical and concentration gradients, not through the lipid bilayer but through specific ion channels or transporters. The normal cardiac cell at rest maintains a transmembrane potential approximately 80 to 90 mV negative to the exterior; this gradient is established by pumps, especially Na^+,K^+–ATPase, and fixed anionic charges within cells. There is both an electrical and a concentration gradient that would move Na^+ ions into resting cells (Figure 35–1). However, Na^+ channels, which allow Na^+ to move along this gradient, are closed at negative transmembrane potentials, so Na^+ does not enter normal resting cardiac cells. In contrast, a specific type of K^+ channel protein (the inward rectifier channel) is in an open conformation at negative potentials: *i.e.,* K^+ can move across the cell membrane at negative potentials in response

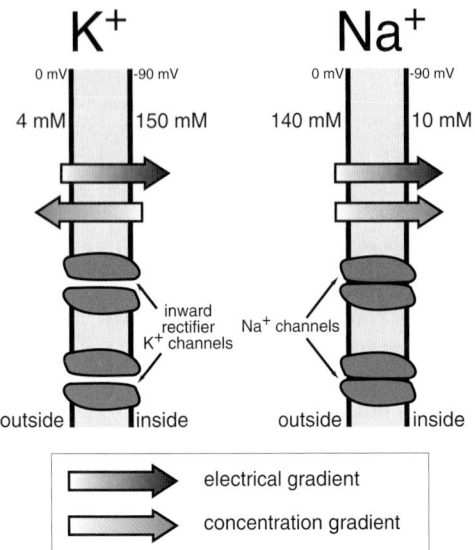

Figure 35–1. Electrical and chemical gradients for K^+ and for Na^+ in a resting cardiac cell.

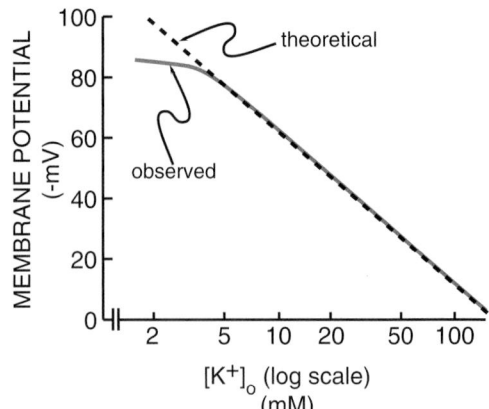

Figure 35–2. The influence of extracellular K^+ on theoretical E_K (dotted line) and on measured transmembrane potential (solid line).

At values of extracellular K^+ >4 mM, the two lines are identical, indicating that extracellular K^+ is the major factor influencing resting potential.

Inward rectifier K^+ channels are open (*left*), allowing K^+ ions to move across the membrane and the transmembrane potential to approach E_K. In contrast, Na^+ does not enter the cell despite a large net driving force because Na^+ channel proteins are in the closed conformation (*right*) in resting cells.

to either electrical or concentration gradients (Figure 35–1). For each individual ion, there is an equilibrium potential E_x at which there is no net driving force for the ion to move across the membrane. E_x can be calculated using the Nernst equation:

$$E_x = -61 \log([x]_i/[x]_o) \qquad (35\text{–}1)$$

where $[x]_o$ is the extracellular concentration of the ion and $[x]_i$ is the intracellular concentration. For usual values for K^+, $[K]_o = 4$ mM and $[K]_i = 140$ mM, the calculated K^+ equilibrium potential E_K is -94 mV. There is thus no net force driving K^+ ions into or out of a cell when the transmembrane potential is -94 mV, which is close to the resting potential. If $[K]_o$ is elevated to 10 mM, as might occur in diseases such as renal failure or myocardial ischemia, the calculated E_K rises to -70 mV. In this situation, K^+ will tend to move down its concentration gradient. In fact, there is excellent agreement between changes in theoretical E_K due to changes in $[K]_o$ and the actual measured transmembrane potential (Figure 35–2), indicating that the normal cardiac cell at rest is permeable to K^+ (because inward rectifier channels are open) and that the concentration of K^+ in the extracellular space is the major determinant of resting potential.

Na$^+$ Channel Opening Initiates the Action Potential: Ion Currents

If a cardiac cell at rest is depolarized above a threshold potential, Na^+ channel proteins change conformation from the

"closed" (or rest) to the conducting ("open") state, allowing up to 10^7 Na^+ ions per second to enter each cell and moving the transmembrane potential towards E_{Na} (+65 mV). This surge of Na^+ ion movement lasts only about a millisecond, after which the Na^+ channel protein rapidly changes conformation from the "open" state to an "inactivated," nonconducting state. Measuring Na^+ current directly is technically demanding; therefore many studies report the maximum upstroke slope of phase 0 (dV/dt_{max}, or V_{max}) of the action potential (Figure 35–3), which is proportional to Na^+ current. The traditional view is that Na^+ channels, once inactivated, cannot reopen until they reassume the rested, or closed, conformation. Electrophysiological techniques capable of measuring the behavior of individual ion channel proteins are now revealing some of the detailed mechanisms of these state transitions, and the findings obtained are changing some traditional views. For example, a small population of Na^+ channels may continue to open during the action potential plateau in some cells (Figure 35–3). In fact, a defect in the structural region of the Na^+ channel protein that has been implicated in control of channel inactivation is responsible for one form of the congenital long QT syndrome, a disease associated with abnormal repolarization and serious arrhythmias (Roden and Spooner, 1999). In general, however, as the cell membrane repolarizes, the changes in membrane potential to which Na^+ channel proteins are subject moves them from inactivated to "closed" conformations. The relationship between Na^+ channel availability and transmembrane potential is an important determinant of conduction and of refractoriness in many cells, as discussed below.

The changes in transmembrane potential generated by the inward Na^+ current produce, in turn, a series of openings (and in some cases subsequent inactivation) of other channels (Figure 35–3). For example, when a cell from the epicardium or the His–Purkinje conducting system is depolarized by the Na^+ current, "transient outward" K^+ channels change conformation to enter an open, or conducting, state; since the transmembrane

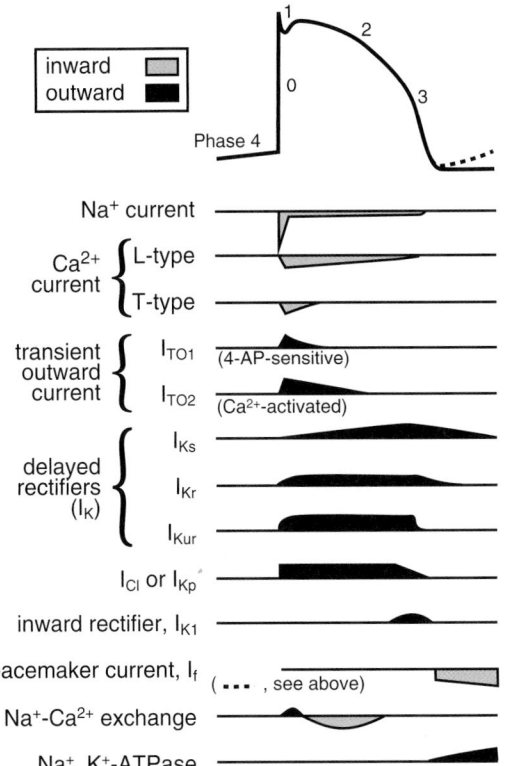

Figure 35–3. The relationship between a hypothetical action potential from the conducting system and the time course of the currents that generate it.

The current magnitudes are not to scale; the Na$^+$ current is ordinarily 50-fold larger than any other current, although the portion that persists into the plateau (phase 2) is small. Multiple types of Ca^{2+} current, transient outward current (I_{TO}), and delayed rectifier (I_K) have been identified; it is likely that each represents a different channel protein. 4-AP (4-aminopyridine) is a widely used *in vitro* blocker of K$^+$ channels. I_{TO2} may be a Cl$^-$ current in some species. Components of I_K have been separated on the basis of how rapidly they activate: slowly (I_{Ks}), rapidly (I_{Kr}), or ultrarapidly (I_{Kur}). The voltage-activated, time-independent current may be carried by Cl$^-$ (I_{Cl}) or K$^+$ (I_{Kp}, "p" for plateau). For all currents shown here (with the possible exception of I_{TO2}), the genes encoding the major pore-forming proteins have been cloned. (Adapted from Task Force of the Working Group on Arrhythmias of the European Society of Cardiology, 1991, with permission.)

potential at the end of phase 0 is positive to E_K, the opening of transient outward channels results in an outward, or repolarizing, K$^+$ current (termed I_{TO}), which contributes to the phase 1 "notch" seen in some action potentials. Transient outward K$^+$ channels, like Na$^+$ channels, rapidly inactivate. During the phase 2 plateau of a normal cardiac action potential, an inward, depolarizing current primarily through Ca^{2+} chan-

nels is balanced by an outward, repolarizing current primarily through K$^+$ ("delayed rectifier") channels. Delayed rectifier currents (termed I_K) increase with time, while Ca^{2+} currents inactivate (and so decrease with time); the result is repolarization of the cardiac cell (phase 3) several hundred milliseconds after the initial Na$^+$ channel opening. Mutations in the genes encoding repolarizing K$^+$ channels are responsible for other forms of the congenital long QT syndrome (Roden and Spooner, 1999). Identification of these specific channels has allowed more precise characterization of the pharmacological effects of antiarrhythmic drugs. A common mechanism whereby drugs prolong cardiac action potentials is inhibition of specific delayed rectifier current, I_{Kr}.

Differing Action Potential Behaviors Among Cardiac Cells

This general description of the action potential and the currents that underlie it must be modified for certain cell types (Figure 35–4), presumably because of variability in the number or products of ion channel genes expressed in individual cells. Endocardial ventricular cells lack a prominent transient outward current, while cells from the subendocardial His–Purkinje conducting system (and in some species from the midmyocardium) have very long action potentials (Antzelevitch *et al.*, 1991). Atrial cells have very short action potentials, probably because I_{TO} is larger, and an additional repolarizing K$^+$ current, activated by the neurotransmitter acetylcholine, is present. As a result, vagal stimulation further shortens atrial action potentials. Cells of the sinus and atrioventricular (AV) nodes lack substantial Na$^+$ currents. In addition, these cells, as well as cells from the conducting system, normally display the phenomenon of spontaneous diastolic, or phase 4, depolarization and thus spontaneously reach threshold for regeneration of action potentials. The rate of spontaneous firing usually is fastest in sinus node cells, which therefore serve as the natural pacemaker of the heart. Specialized K$^+$ channels underlie the pacemaker current in heart.

Modern molecular biological and electrophysiological techniques, by which the behavior of single ion channel proteins in an isolated patch of membrane can be studied, have refined the description of ion channels important for the normal functioning of cardiac cells and have identified channels that may be particularly important under pathological conditions. For example, it is now established that transient outward and delayed rectifier currents actually result from multiple ion channel subtypes (Figure 35–3; Tseng and Hoffman, 1989; Sanguinetti and Jurkiewicz, 1990), and that acetylcholine-evoked hyperpolarization results from activation of a K$^+$ channel formed by hetero-oligomerization of multiple, distinct channel proteins (Krapivinsky *et al.*, 1995).

The understanding that molecularly diverse entities subserve regulation of the cardiac action potential is important because drugs may target one channel subtype selectively. Furthermore, ancillary function-modifying proteins (the products of diverse genes) have been identified for most ion channels. In addition to the usual ("L-type") Ca^{2+} channels, a second type of Ca^{2+} channel, which is most prominent at relatively negative potentials, has been identified in some cardiac cells (Bean, 1985). This "T-type" Ca^{2+} channel may be important

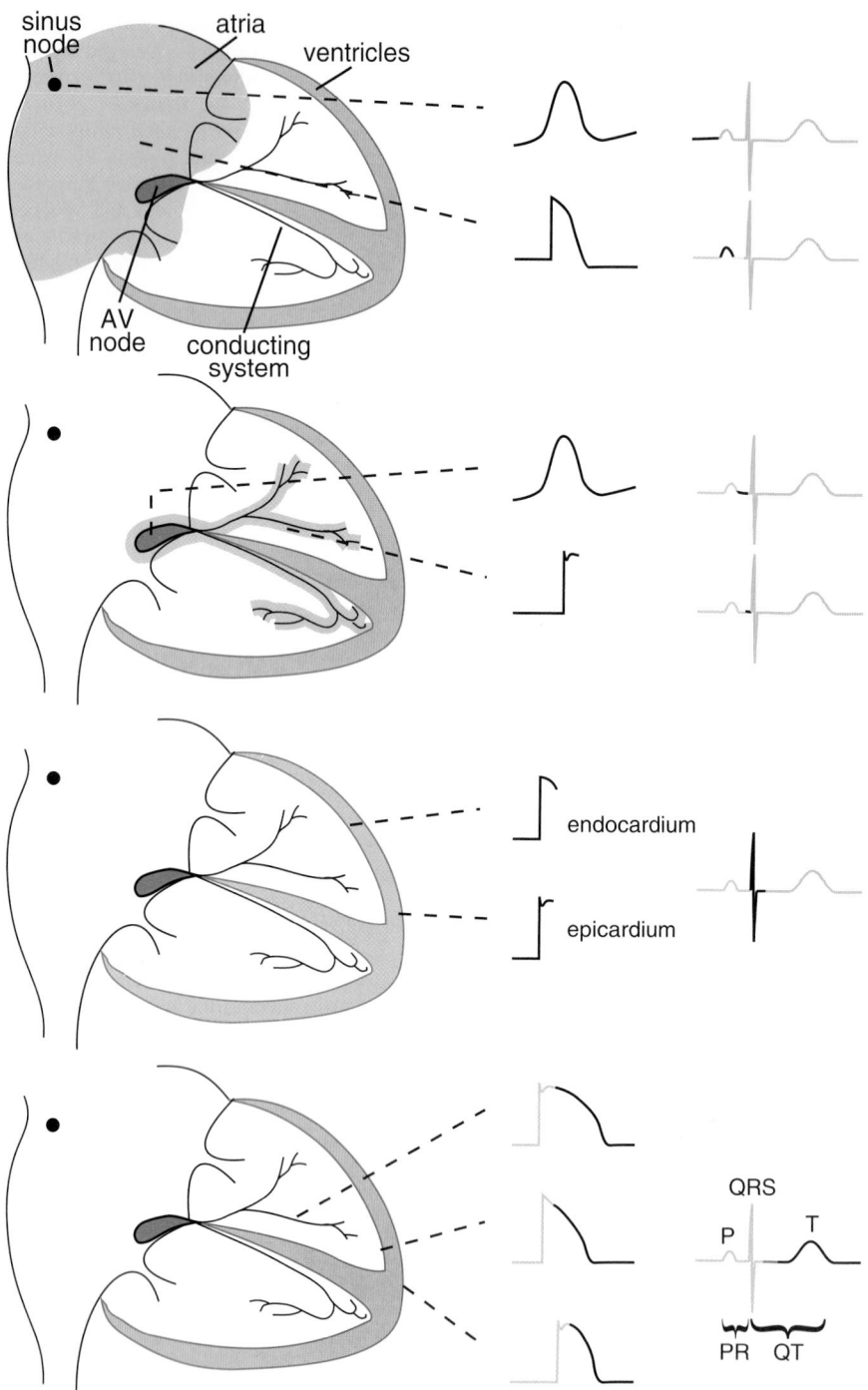

Figure 35–4. Normal impulse propagation.

Action potentials from different regions of the heart are shown. In each panel, tissue that is depolarized is shown in light blue and the portion of the electrocardiogram to which it contributes is shown in black.

in diseases such as hypertension and may play a role in pacemaker activity in some cells. A T-type–selective antihypertensive agent, mibefradil, was available briefly in the late 1990s but was withdrawn because it was involved in many serious, undesirable drug–drug interactions. Specific channels that transport Cl⁻ ions and result in repolarizing currents (I_{Cl}) have been iden-

tified in many species (Hume and Harvey, 1991); some of these are observed only under pathophysiological conditions, such as adrenergic stimulation. Some K^+ channels are quiescent when intracellular ATP stores are normal and become active when these stores are depleted. Such ATP-inhibited K^+ channels may become particularly important in repolarizing cells during states of metabolic stress such as myocardial ischemia (Weiss *et al.*, 1991; Wilde and Janse, 1994).

Maintenance of Intracellular Homeostasis

With each action potential, the cell interior gains Na^+ ions and loses K^+ ions. An ATP-requiring Na^+–K^+ exchange mechanism, or pump, is activated in most cells to maintain intracellular homeostasis. This Na^+,K^+–ATPase extrudes three Na^+ ions for every two K^+ ions shuttled from the exterior of the cell to the interior; as a result, the act of pumping itself generates a net outward (repolarizing) current.

Normally, intracellular Ca^{2+} is maintained at very low levels (<100 nM). In heart cells, the entry of Ca^{2+} during each action potential is a signal to the sarcoplasmic reticulum to release its Ca^{2+} stores. The resultant increase in intracellular Ca^{2+} then allows Ca^{2+}-dependent contractile processes to occur. Removal of intracellular Ca^{2+} occurs by both an ATP-dependent Ca^{2+} pump (which moves Ca^{2+} ions back to storage sites in the sarcoplasmic reticulum) and an electrogenic Na^+–Ca^{2+} exchange mechanism on the cell surface, which exchanges three Na^+ ions from the exterior for each Ca^{2+} ion extruded. The initial rise in Ca^{2+}, which serves as the trigger for Ca^{2+} release from intracellular stores, is a result of the opening of Ca^{2+} channels in the cell membrane or of Ca^{2+} entry through Na^+–Ca^{2+} exchange; *i.e.*, in response to phase 0 entry of Na^+, the Na^+–Ca^{2+} exchange protein may transiently extrude Na^+ ions in exchange for Ca^{2+} ions (Figure 35–3).

Impulse Propagation and the Electrocardiogram

Normal cardiac impulses originate in the sinus node. Impulse propagation in the heart depends on two factors: the magnitude of the depolarizing current (usually Na^+ current) and the geometry of cell–cell electrical connections. Cardiac cells are long and thin and well coupled through specialized gap junction proteins at their ends, whereas lateral ("transverse") gap junctions are sparser. As a result, impulses spread along cells two to three times faster than across cells. This "anisotropic" (direction-dependent) conduction may be a factor in the genesis of certain arrhythmias described below (Priori *et al.*, 1999). Once impulses leave the sinus node, they propagate rapidly throughout the atria, resulting in atrial systole and the P wave of the surface electrocardiogram (ECG; Figure 35–4). Propagation slows markedly through the AV node, where the inward current (through Ca^{2+} channels) is much smaller than the Na^+ current in atria, ventricles, or the subendocardial conducting system. This conduction delay allows the atrial contraction to propel blood into the ventricle, thereby optimizing cardiac output. Once impulses exit from the AV node, they enter the conducting system, where Na^+ currents are larger than in any other tissue. Hence, propagation is correspondingly faster, up to 0.75 meter/second longitudinally, allowing coordinated ventricular contraction, the QRS complex on the ECG, as impulses spread from the endocardium to the epicardium. Ventricular repolarization results in the T wave of the ECG. The ECG can be used as a rough guide to some cellular properties of cardiac tissue (Figure 35–4): (1) heart rate reflects sinus node automaticity, (2) PR interval duration reflects AV nodal conduction time,

(3) QRS duration reflects conduction time in the ventricle, and (4) the QT interval is a measure of ventricular action potential duration.

Refractoriness: Fast-Response Versus Slow-Response Tissue

If a single action potential, such as that shown in Figure 35–3, is restimulated very early during the plateau, no Na^+ channels are available to open, so no inward current results and no action potential is generated: the cell is refractory. If, on the other hand, an extrastimulus occurs after the cell has repolarized completely, Na^+ channels have recovered from inactivation, and a normal Na^+ channel–dependent upstroke results (Figure 35–5A). When an extrastimulus occurs during phase 3 of the action potential, the magnitude of the resultant Na^+ current is dependent on the number of Na^+ channels that have recovered from inactivation (Figure 35–5A), which, in turn, is dependent on the voltage at which the extrastimulus was applied. Thus, in atrial, ventricular, and His–Purkinje cells ("fast-response cells"), refractoriness is determined by the voltage-dependent recovery of Na^+ channels from inactivation. Refractoriness also frequently

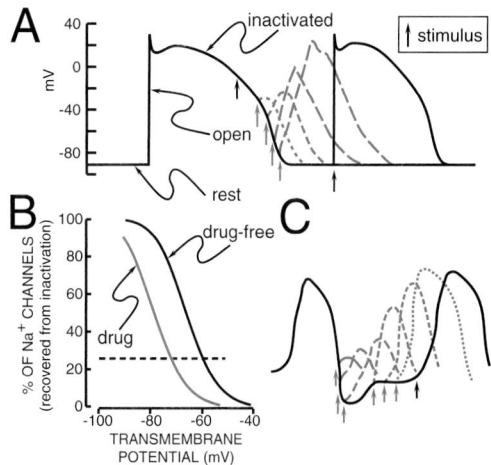

Figure 35–5. Qualitative differences in responses of fast- and slow-response tissues to premature stimuli.

A. With a very early premature stimulus (*black arrow*) in fast-response tissue, all Na^+ channels are still in the inactivated state, and no upstroke results. As the action potential repolarizes, Na^+ channels recover from the inactivated to the rest state, from which opening can occur. The phase 0 upstroke slope of the premature action potentials (*blue*) are greater with later stimuli because recovery from inactivation is voltage-dependent. **B.** The relationship between transmembrane potential and degree of recovery of Na^+ channels from inactivation. The dotted line indicates 25% recovery. Most Na^+ channel–blocking drugs shift this relationship to the left. **C.** In slow-response tissues, premature stimuli delivered even after full repolarization of the action potential are depressed; recovery from inactivation is time-dependent.

is measured by assessing whether premature stimuli applied to tissue preparations (or the whole heart) result in propagated impulses. While the magnitude of the Na^+ current is one major determinant of such propagation, cellular geometry (*see* above) also is important in multicellular preparations. Ordinarily, each cell is connected to many neighbors, so that impulses spread rapidly, and the heart acts like a single large cell, a "syncytium." However, if the geometric arrangement is such that a single cell must supply depolarizing current to many neighbors, conduction can fail. The effective refractory period (ERP) is the shortest interval at which a premature stimulus results in a propagated response and is often used to describe drug effects in intact tissue.

The situation is different in Ca^{2+} channel–dependent ("slow-response") tissue such as the AV node. The major factor controlling recovery from inactivation of Ca^{2+} channels is time (Figure 35–5C). Thus, even after a Ca^{2+} channel–dependent action potential has repolarized back to its initial resting potential, Ca^{2+} channels are not all available for reexcitation. Therefore, an extrastimulus applied shortly after repolarization is complete results in a reduced Ca^{2+} current, which may propagate slowly to adjacent cells prior to extinction. An extrastimulus applied later will result in a larger Ca^{2+} current and faster propagation. Thus, in Ca^{2+} channel–dependent tissues, which include not only the AV node but also tissues whose underlying characteristics have been altered by factors such as myocardial ischemia, refractoriness is time-dependent, and propagation occurs slowly. Conduction that exhibits such dependence on the timing of premature stimuli is termed "decremental." By contrast, conduction velocity is independent of prematurity in fast-response tissues until a stimulus shorter than the effective refractory period is applied, when it fails completely ("all-or-none" response). Slow conduction in the heart, a critical factor in the genesis of reentrant arrhythmias (below), also can occur when Na^+ currents are depressed by disease or membrane depolarization (*e.g.*, elevated $[K]_o$), resulting in decreased steady-state Na^+ channel availability (Figure 35–5B).

MECHANISMS OF CARDIAC ARRHYTHMIAS

When the normal sequence of impulse initiation and propagation is perturbed, an arrhythmia occurs. Failure of impulse initiation may result in slow heart rates (bradyarrhythmias), and failure of impulses to propagate normally from atrium to ventricle results in dropped beats or "heart block," which usually reflects an abnormality in either the AV node or the His–Purkinje system. These abnormalities may be caused by drugs (Table 35–1) or by structural heart disease; in the latter case, permanent cardiac pacing may be required.

Abnormally rapid heart rhythms (tachyarrhythmias) are common clinical problems that may be treated with antiarrhythmic drugs. Three major underlying mechanisms have been identified: enhanced automaticity, triggered automaticity, and reentry.

Enhanced Automaticity

Enhanced automaticity may occur in cells that normally display spontaneous diastolic depolarization—the sinus and AV

nodes and the His–Purkinje system. β-Adrenergic stimulation, hypokalemia, and mechanical stretch of cardiac muscle cells increase phase 4 slope and so accelerate pacemaker rate, whereas acetylcholine reduces pacemaker rate both by decreasing phase 4 slope and by hyperpolarization (making the maximum diastolic potential more negative). In addition, automatic behavior may occur in sites that ordinarily lack spontaneous pacemaker activity; for example, depolarization of ventricular cells (*e.g.*, by ischemia) may produce such "abnormal" automaticity. When impulses propagate from a region of enhanced normal or abnormal automaticity to excite the rest of the heart, arrhythmias result.

Afterdepolarizations and Triggered Automaticity

Under some pathophysiological conditions, a normal cardiac action potential may be interrupted or followed by an abnormal depolarization (Figure 35–6). If this abnormal depolarization reaches threshold, it may, in turn, give rise to secondary upstrokes which then can propagate and create abnormal rhythms. These abnormal secondary upstrokes occur only after an initial normal, or "triggering," upstroke and so are termed *triggered rhythms*. Two major forms of triggered rhythms are recognized: (1) Under conditions of intracellular Ca^{2+} overload (myocardial ischemia, adrenergic stress, digitalis intoxication), a normal action potential may be followed by a "delayed afterdepolarization" (DAD; Figure 35–6A). If this afterdepolarization reaches threshold, a secondary triggered beat or beats may occur. DAD amplitude is increased *in vitro* by rapid pacing, and clinical arrhythmias thought to correspond to DAD-mediated triggered beats are more frequent when the underlying cardiac rate is rapid (Rosen and Reder, 1981). (2) The key abnormality in the second type of triggered activity is marked prolongation of the cardiac action potential. When this occurs, phase 3 repolarization may be interrupted by an "early afterdepolarization" (EAD; Figure 35–6B). EAD-mediated triggering *in vitro* and clinical arrhythmias are most common when the underlying heart rate is slow, extracellular K^+ is low, and certain drugs (antiarrhythmics and others) that prolong action potential duration are present. EADs represent, by definition, an increase in net inward current during repolarization. However, it is not certain through which channel(s) current flows to generate EADs. When an EAD is present, sympathetic stimulation (α- or β-adrenergic) can increase the likelihood of triggered beats. EAD-related triggered upstrokes probably reflect inward current through Na^+ or Ca^{2+} channels. When cardiac repolarization is markedly prolonged, polymorphic ventricular tachycardia with a long QT interval, known as the *torsades de pointes* syndrome, may occur and is thought to be caused by early afterdepolarizations and resultant triggering (Roden and Hoffman, 1985; Jackman *et al.*, 1988). As mentioned above, the congenital long QT syndrome, a disease in which *torsades de pointes* are common, is now known to be caused by mutations in the genes encoding the Na^+ channels or the channels underlying the repolarizing currents I_{Kr} and I_{Ks} (Roden and Spooner, 1999).

Reentry

Anatomically Defined Reentry.   The principles of cardiac reentry were first described early in the 1900s. Reentry can occur

Table 35–1

Drug-Induced Cardiac Arrhythmias

ARRHYTHMIA	DRUG	LIKELY MECHANISM	TREATMENT*	CLINICAL FEATURES
Sinus bradycardia AV block	Digitalis	↑Vagal tone	Antidigitalis antibodies Temporary pacing	Atrial tachycardia may also be present
Sinus bradycardia AV block	Verapamil Diltiazem	Ca^{2+} channel block	Ca^{2+} Temporary pacing	
Sinus bradycardia AV block	β-Blockers Clonidine Methyldopa	Sympatholytic	Isoproterenol Temporary pacing	
Sinus tachycardia Any other tachycardia	β-Blocker withdrawal	Upregulation of β-receptors with chronic therapy; more receptors available for agonist after withdrawal of blocker	β-Blockade	Hypertension, angina also possible
↑ Ventricular rate in atrial flutter	Quinidine Flecainide Propafenone	Conduction slowing in atrium, with enhanced (quinidine) or unaltered AV conduction	AV nodal blockers	QRS complexes often widened at fast rates
↑ Ventricular rate in atrial fibrillation in patients with WPW syndrome	Digitalis Verapamil	↓ accessory pathway refractoriness	IV procainamide DC cardioversion	Ventricular rate can exceed 300/min
Multifocal atrial tachycardia	Theophylline	?↑ Intracellular Ca^{2+} and DADs	Withdraw theophylline ?Verapamil	Often in advanced lung disease
Polymorphic VT with ↑ QT interval (*torsades de pointes*)	Quinidine Sotalol Procainamide Disopyramide Dofetilide Ibutilide "Noncardioactive" drugs (*see* text) Amiodarone (rare)	EAD-related triggered activity	Cardiac pacing Isoproterenol Magnesium	Hypokalemia, bradycardia frequent Related to ↑ plasma concentrations, except for quinidine
Frequent or difficult to terminate VT ("incessant" VT)	Flecainide Propafenone Quinidine (rarer)	Conduction slowing in reentrant circuits	Na^+ bolus reported effective in some cases	Most often in patients with advanced myocardial scarring
Atrial tachycardia with AV block; ventricular bigeminy and others	Digitalis	DAD-related triggered activity (±↑ vagal tone)	Antidigitalis antibodies	Coexistence of abnormal impulses with abnormal sinus or AV nodal function
Ventricular fibrillation	Inappropriate use of IV verapamil	Severe hypotension and/or myocardial ischemia	Cardiac resuscitation (DC cardioversion)	Misdiagnosis of VT as PSVT → inappropriate use of verapamil

*In each of these cases, recognition and withdrawal of the offending drug(s) are mandatory.

ABBREVIATIONS: AV, atrioventricular; DAD, delayed afterdepolarization; DC, direct current; EAD, early afterdepolarization; WPW, Wolff–Parkinson–White; VT, ventricular tachycardia; PSVT, paroxysmal supraventricular tachycardia; IV, intravenous; ↑, increase; ↓, decrease; ?, *unclear;* β-blockers, β-adrenergic receptor antagonists.

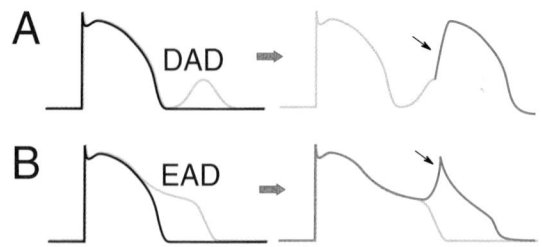

Figure 35–6. Afterdepolarizations and triggered activity.

A. Delayed afterdepolarization (DAD) arising after full repolarization. A DAD that reaches threshold results in a triggered upstroke (*black arrow, right*). **B.** Early afterdepolarization (EAD) interrupting phase 3 repolarization. Under some conditions, triggered beat(s) can arise from an EAD (*black arrow, right*).

when impulses propagate by more than one pathway between two points in the heart and those pathways have heterogeneous electrophysiological properties. An "experiment of nature" is the Wolff–Parkinson–White (WPW) syndrome, described in the 1930s. Patients with WPW have accessory connections between the atrium and ventricle (Figure 35–7). With each sinus node depolarization, impulses can excite the ventricle *via* the

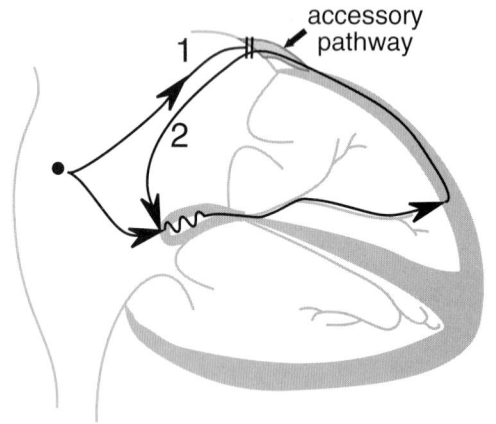

Figure 35–7. Atrioventricular reentrant tachycardia in the Wolff–Parkinson–White syndrome.

In these patients, an accessory atrioventricular connection is present (*light blue*). A premature atrial impulse blocks in the accessory pathway (1), and propagates slowly through the AV node and conducting system. Upon reaching the (by now no longer refractory) accessory pathway, it reenters the atrium (2), where it can then reenter the ventricle *via* the AV node and become self-sustaining (Figure 35–9C). AV nodal blocking drugs readily terminate this tachycardia. Recurrences can be prevented by drugs that prevent atrial premature beats, by drugs that alter the electrophysiological characteristics of tissue in the circuit (*e.g.,* they prolong AV nodal refractoriness), or by nonpharmacological techniques that section the accessory pathway.

normal structures (AV node) or the accessory pathway. However, the electrophysiological properties of the AV node and accessory pathways are different: accessory pathways consist of fast-response tissue, whereas the AV node is composed of slow-response tissue. Thus, with a premature atrial beat, conduction may fail in the accessory pathway and continue to conduct, albeit slowly, in the AV node and then through the His–Purkinje system, where the propagating impulse may encounter the ventricular end of the accessory pathway when it is no longer refractory. Note that the likelihood that the accessory pathway is no longer refractory increases as AV nodal conduction slows. When the impulse reenters the atrium, it can then reenter the ventricle *via* the AV node, reenter the atrium *via* the accessory pathway, and so on (Figure 35–7). Reentry of this type is therefore determined by (1) the presence of an anatomically defined circuit, (2) heterogeneity in refractoriness among regions in the circuit, and (3) slow conduction in one part of the circuit. Similar "anatomically defined" reentry commonly occurs in the region of the AV node (AV nodal reentrant tachycardia) and in the atrium (atrial flutter). The term *paroxysmal supraventricular tachycardia* (PSVT) includes both AV reentry and AV nodal reentry, which share many clinical features. In some of these cases, it is now possible to identify and nonpharmacologically ablate critical portions of reentrant pathways (or automatic foci), thus curing the patient and obviating the need for long-term drug therapy. The procedure is carried out through a catheter advanced to the interior of the heart and requires minimal convalescence.

Functionally Defined Reentry. Reentry also may occur in the absence of a distinct, anatomically defined pathway (Figure 35–8). For example, alterations in cell–cell coupling following acute myocardial infarction in dogs result in reentrant ventricular tachycardia (VT) whose circuit is dependent not only on postinfarction scarring but also on the rapid longitudinal and slow transverse conduction properties of cardiac tissue (Wit *et al.,* 1990). If ischemia or other electrophysiological perturbations result in an area of sufficiently slow conduction in the ventricle, impulses exiting from that area may find the rest of the myocardium reexcitable, in which case fibrillation may ensue. Atrial or ventricular fibrillation is an extreme example of "functionally defined" (or "leading circle") reentry: cells are reexcited as soon as they are repolarized sufficiently to allow enough Na^+ channels to recover from inactivation. In this setting, neither organized activation patterns nor coordinated contractile activity is present.

Common Arrhythmias and Their Mechanisms

The primary tool for diagnosis of arrhythmias is the electrocardiogram, although more sophisticated approaches, such as recording from specific regions of the heart during artificial induction of arrhythmias by specialized pacing techniques, sometimes are used. Table 35–2 lists common arrhythmias, their likely mechanisms, and approaches that should be considered for their acute termination and for long-term therapy to prevent recurrence. Examples of some arrhythmias discussed here are shown in Figure 35–9. Some arrhythmias, notably ventricular fibrillation (VF), are best treated not with drugs but with

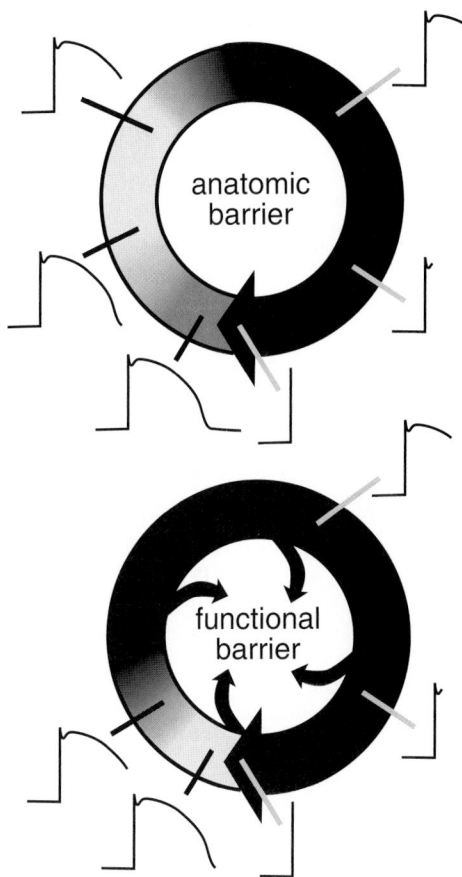

Figure 35–8. Two types of reentry.

The border of a propagating wavefront is denoted by a heavy black arrowhead. In anatomically defined reentry (*top*), a fixed pathway is present (*e.g.,* Figure 35–7). The black area denotes tissue in the reentrant circuit that is completely refractory because of the recent passage of the propagating wavefront; the gray area denotes tissue in which depressed upstrokes can be elicited (*see* Figure 35–5A), and the dark blue area represents tissue in which restimulation would result in action potentials with normal upstrokes. The dark blue area is termed an *excitable gap.* In functionally defined, or "leading circle," reentry (*bottom*), there is no anatomic pathway and no excitable gap. Rather, the circulating wavefront creates an area of inexcitable tissue at its core. In this type of reentry, the circuit does not necessarily remain in the same anatomic position during consecutive beats, and multiple such "rotors" may be present.

DC cardioversion—the application of a large electric current across the chest. This technique also can be used to immediately restore normal rhythm in less serious cases; if the patient is conscious, a brief period of general anesthesia is required. Implantable cardioverter/defibrillators (ICDs), devices that are capable of detecting VF and automatically delivering a defibrillating shock, increasingly are being used in patients who have

been resuscitated from one episode of VF. Often drugs are used with these devices to reduce the need for defibrillating shocks.

MECHANISMS OF ANTIARRHYTHMIC DRUG ACTION

Drug effects that may be antiarrhythmic can be demonstrated *in vitro* or in animal models, but the relationship between the multiple effects these drugs produce in patients and their effects on arrhythmias (whose mechanisms are only sometimes known) can be complex. A single arrhythmia may result from multiple mechanisms; for example, an automatic or triggered beat may result in a sustained reentrant arrhythmia in a patient with a potential reentrant circuit. Drugs may be antiarrhythmic by suppressing the initiating mechanism or by altering the reentrant circuit. In some cases, however, drugs also may suppress the initiator but nonetheless promote reentry (*see* below).

Drugs may slow automatic rhythms by altering one of the four determinants of spontaneous pacemaker discharge (Figure 35–10): maximum diastolic potential, phase 4 slope, threshold potential, or action potential duration. Block of Na^+ or Ca^{2+} channels usually results in altered threshold, block of cardiac K^+ channels prolongs action potential, adenosine and acetylcholine may increase maximum diastolic potential, and β-adrenergic receptor antagonists (β-blockers; *see* Chapter 10) may decrease phase 4 slope.

Antiarrhythmic drugs may block arrhythmias due to DADs or EADs through two major mechanisms: (1) inhibition of the development of afterdepolarizations or (2) interference with the inward current (usually through Na^+ or Ca^{2+} channels), which is responsible for the upstroke. Thus, for example, arrhythmias due to digitalis-induced DADs may be inhibited by *verapamil* (which blocks the development of DAD) or by *quinidine* (which blocks Na^+ channels, thus elevating the threshold required to produce the abnormal upstroke). Similarly, two approaches are used in arrhythmias thought to be related to EAD-induced triggered beats (Tables 35–1 and 35–2). EADs can be inhibited by shortening action potential duration; in practice, heart rate is accelerated by isoproterenol infusion or by pacing. Triggered beats arising from EADs can be inhibited by Mg^{2+}, without normalizing repolarization *in vitro* or QT interval in patients, through mechanisms that are not well understood. In patients with a congenitally prolonged QT interval, *torsades de pointes* often occur with adrenergic stress; preventive treatment

Table 35–2

A Mechanistic Approach to Antiarrhythmic Therapy

ARRHYTHMIA	COMMON MECHANISM	ACUTE THERAPY[a]	CHRONIC THERAPY[a]
Premature atrial, nodal, or ventricular depolarizations	Unknown	None indicated	None indicated
Atrial fibrillation	Disorganized "functional" reentry Continual AV node stimulation → irregular, often rapid, ventricular rate	1. Control ventricular response: AV nodal block[b] 2. Restore sinus rhythm: DC cardioversion	1. Control ventricular response: AV nodal block[b] 2. Maintain normal rhythm: K[+] channel block Na[+] channel block with $\tau_{recovery} > 1$ second
Atrial flutter	Stable reentrant circuit in the right atrium Ventricular rate often rapid and irregular	Same as atrial fibrillation	Same as atrial fibrillation AV nodal blocking drugs especially desirable to avoid ↑ ventricular rate Ablation in selected cases[c]
Atrial tachycardia	Enhanced automaticity, DAD-related automaticity, or reentry within the atrium	Same as atrial fibrillation	Same as atrial fibrillation Ablation of tachrycardia "focus"[c]
AV nodal reentrant tachycardia (PSVT)	Reentrant circuit within or near AV node	*Adenosine AV nodal block Less commonly: ↑ vagal tone (digitalis, edrophonium, phenylephrine)	*AV nodal block Flecainide Propafenone *Ablation[c]
Arrhythmias associated with WPW syndrome: 1. AV reentry (PSVT)	Reentry (Figure 35–7)	Same as AV nodal reentry	K[+] channel block Na[+] channel block with $\tau_{recovery} > 1$ second Ablation[c]
2. Atrial fibrillation with atrioventricular conduction *via* accessory pathway	Very rapid rate due to nondecremental properties of accessory pathway	*DC cardioversion *Procainamide	Ablation[c] K[+] channel block Na[+] channel block with $\tau_{recovery} > 1$ second (AV nodal blocking drugs occasionally harmful)
VT in patients with remote myocardial infarction	Reentry near the rim of the healed myocardial infarction	Lidocaine Amiodarone Procainamide Bretylium DC cardioversion	*ICD[d] *Amiodarone K[+] channel block Na[+] channel block
VT in patients without structural heart disease	DADs triggered by ↑ sympathetic tone	Adenosine[e] Verapamil[e] β-Blockers[e] DC cardioversion	Verapamil[e] β-Blockers[e]

(*Continued*)

Table 35–2

A Mechanistic Approach to Antiarrhythmic Therapy *(Continued)*

ARRHYTHMIA	COMMON MECHANISM	ACUTE THERAPY[a]	CHRONIC THERAPY[a]
VF	Disorganized reentry	*DC cardioversion Lidocaine Amiodarone Procainamide Bretylium	*ICD[d] *Amiodarone K^+ channel block Na^+ channel block
Torsades de Pointes, congenital or acquired (often drug-related)	EAD-related triggered activity	Pacing Magnesium Isoproterenol	β-Blockade Pacing

*Indicates treatment of choice.

[a] Acute drug therapy is administered intravenously; chronic therapy implies long-term oral use.

[b] AV nodal block can be achieved clinically by adenosine, Ca^{2+} channel block, β-adrenergic receptor blockade, or increased vagal tone (a major antiarrhythmic effect of digitalis glycosides).

[c] Ablation is a procedure in which tissue responsible for the maintenance of a tachycardia is identified by specialized recording techniques and then selectively destroyed, usually by high-frequency radio waves delivered through a catheter placed in the heart.

[d] ICD, implanted cardioverter/defibrillator. A device that can sense VT or VF and deliver pacing and/or cardioverting shocks to restore normal rhythm.

[e] These may be harmful in reentrant VT and so should be used for acute therapy only if the diagnosis is secure.

DAD, delayed afterdepolarization; EAD, early afterdepolarization; WPW, Wolff–Parkinson–White; PSVT, paroxysmal supraventricular tachycardia; VT, ventricular tachycardia; VF, ventricular fibrillation; β-blockers, β-adrenergic receptor antagonists.

includes β-adrenergic blockade (which does not shorten the QT interval) as well as pacing.

In anatomically determined reentry, drugs may terminate the arrhythmia by blocking propagation of the action potential. Conduction usually fails in a "weak leak" in the circuit. In the example of the WPW-related arrhythmia described above, the weak link is the AV node, and drugs that prolong AV nodal refractoriness and slow AV nodal conduction, such as Ca^{2+} channel blockers, β-adrenergic receptor antagonists, or digitalis glycosides, are likely to be effective. On the other hand, conduction slowing in functionally determined reentrant circuits may produce only a change in the pathway without extinguishing the circuit. In fact, slow conduction generally promotes the development of reentrant arrhythmias, and the approach that is most likely to terminate functionally determined reentry is prolongation of refractoriness (Task Force, 1991). In fast-response tissues, refractoriness is prolonged by delaying the recovery of Na^+ channels from inactivation. Drugs that act by blocking Na^+ channels generally shift the voltage dependence of recovery from block (Figure 35–5B) and so prolong refractoriness (Figure 35–11). Also, drugs that increase action potential duration (achieved without direct action on Na^+ channels, *e.g.*, by blocking delayed rectifier currents) also will prolong refractoriness (Figure 35–11; Singh, 1993). In slow-response tissues, Ca^{2+} channel block prolongs refractoriness. Drugs that interfere with

cell–cell coupling also theoretically should increase refractoriness in multicellular preparations; amiodarone may exert this effect in diseased tissue (Levine *et al.*, 1988). Acceleration of conduction in an area of slow conduction also could be antiarrhythmic in reentry; lidocaine may exert such an effect under some experimental conditions (Arnsdorf and Bigger, 1972).

State-Dependent Ion Channel Block

A key concept in understanding differences in the clinical actions among antiarrhythmic drugs is state-dependent block. Experimental evidence strongly supports the idea that ion channel–blocking drugs bind to specific receptor-like sites on the ion channel proteins to modify function (*e.g.*, decrease current) and that, as an ion channel protein shuttles among functional conformations (or ion channel "states"), the affinity of the ion channel protein for the drug on its target site will vary (Hille, 1977; Hondeghem and Katzung, 1984; Snyders *et al.*, 1991). Drugs are thought to gain access to target sites by at least two routes: through the pore (the "hydrophilic" pathway) and through the lipid bilayer (the "hydrophobic" pathway). Physicochemical characteristics, such as molecular weight or lipid solubility, are important determinants of state-dependent binding. State-dependent binding has been studied most extensively in the case of Na^+

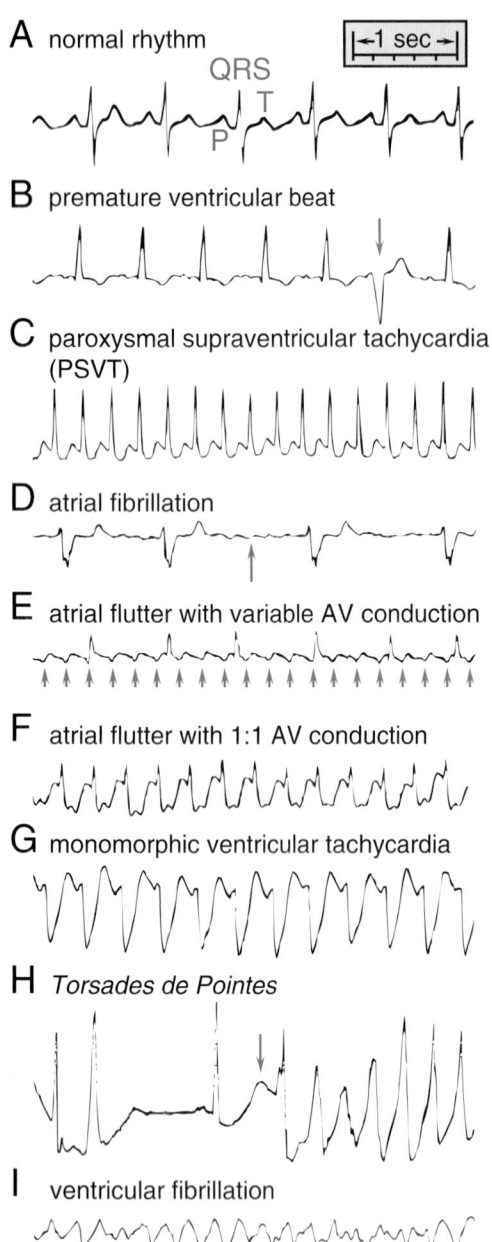

Figure 35–9. ECGs showing normal and abnormal cardiac rhythms.

The P, QRS, and T waves in normal sinus rhythm are shown in panel A. Panel B shows a premature beat arising in the ventricle (*arrow*). Paroxysmal supraventricular tachycardia (PSVT) is shown in panel C; this is most likely reentry utilizing an accessory pathway (Figure 35–7) or reentry within or near the AV node. In atrial fibrillation (panel D), there are no P waves and the QRS complexes occur irregularly (and at a slow rate in this example); electrical activity between QRS complexes shows small undulations (*arrow*), corresponding to fibrillatory activity in the atria. In atrial flutter (panel E), the atria beat rapidly, approximately 250 beats per minute (*arrows*) in this example, and the ventricular rate is irregular. If a drug that slows the rate of atrial flutter is administered, 1:1 atrioventricular conduction (panel F) can occur. In monomorphic ventricular tachycardia (VT, panel G), identical, wide QRS complexes occur at a regular rate, 180 per minute. The electrocardiographic features of the *torsades de pointes* syndrome (panel H) include a very long QT interval (>600 ms in this example, *arrow*) and ventricular tachycardia in which each successive beat has a different morphology (polymorphic VT). Panel I shows the disorganized electrical activity characteristic of ventricular fibrillation.

channel–blocking drugs. Most useful agents of this type block open and/or inactivated Na^+ channels and have very little affinity for channels in the resting state. Thus, with each action potential, drugs bind to Na^+ channels (and block them), and with each diastolic interval, drugs dissociate and "unblock." Block may be due to a drug binding within the conduction pore or to binding at a remote site that then induces changes in the ability of the channel protein to form a pore (an "allosteric" effect). As illustrated in Figure 35–12, the unblocking rate is a key determi-

nant of steady-state block of Na^+ channels. When heart rate increases, the time available for unblocking decreases, and steady-state Na^+ channel block increases. The rate of recovery from block also slows as cells are depolarized, as in ischemia (Chen *et al.,* 1975). This provides the basis for the finding that Na^+ channel blockers depress Na^+ current, and hence conduction, to a greater extent in ischemic tissues than in normal tissues. Open-versus inactivated-state block also may be important in determining the effects of some drugs. For example, increased

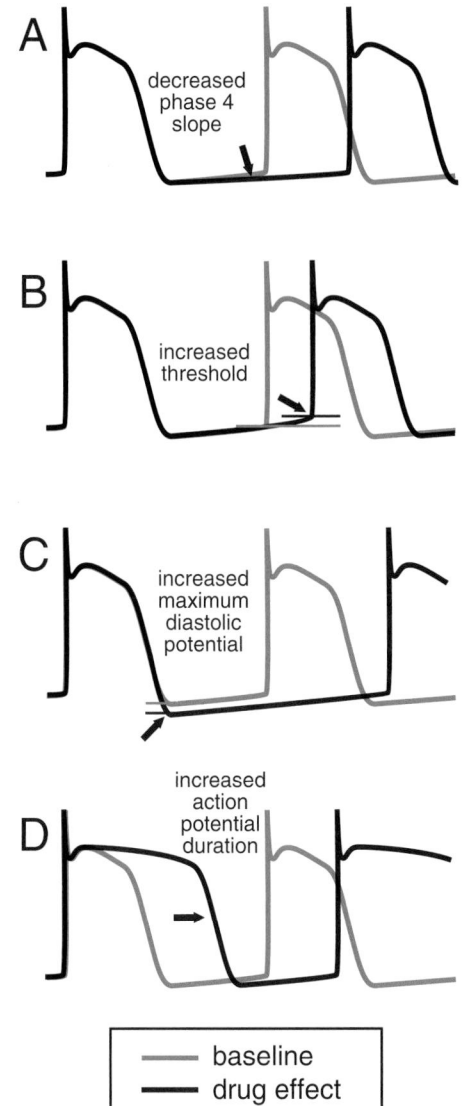

Figure 35–10. Four ways to reduce the rate of spontaneous discharge in automatic tissues.

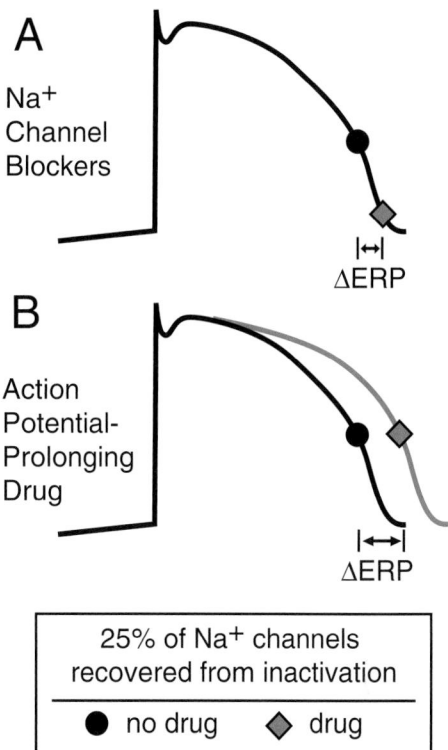

Figure 35–11. Two ways to increase refractoriness in fast-response cells.

In this figure, the black dot indicates the point at which a sufficient number of Na^+ channels (an arbitrary 25%, Figure 35–5B) have recovered from inactivation to allow a premature stimulus to produce a propagated response in the absence of a drug. Block of Na^+ channels (**A**) shifts voltage-dependence of recovery (Figure 35–5B) and so delays the point at which 25% of channels have recovered (*blue diamond*), prolonging refractoriness. Note that, if the drug also dissociates slowly from the channel (*see* Figure 35–12), refractoriness in fast-response tissues actually can extend beyond full repolarization ("postrepolarization refractoriness"). Drugs that prolong the action potential (**B**) also will extend the point at which an arbitrary percentage of Na^+ channels have recovered from inactivation, even without directly interacting with Na^+ channels.

action potential duration, which results in a relative increase in time spent in the inactivated state, may increase block by drugs such as lidocaine or amiodarone, which bind to inactivated channels (Hondeghem and Katzung, 1984).

The rate of recovery from block often is expressed as a time constant ($\tau_{recovery}$, the time required for ~63% of an exponentially determined process to be complete; Courtney, 1987). In the case of some drugs such as *lidocaine*, $\tau_{recovery}$ is so short (≪1 second) that recovery from block is very rapid, and substantial Na^+ channel block occurs only in rapidly driven tissues, particu-

larly in ischemia. At the other end of the spectrum are drugs such as *flecainide,* with such long $\tau_{recovery}$ (>10 seconds) that roughly the same number of Na^+ channels are blocked during systole and diastole. As a result, marked slowing of conduction occurs even in normal tissues, at normal rates. State-dependent block also can be demonstrated for Ca^{2+} or K^+ channel–blocking drugs, but the clinical relevance of these findings still is being evaluated.

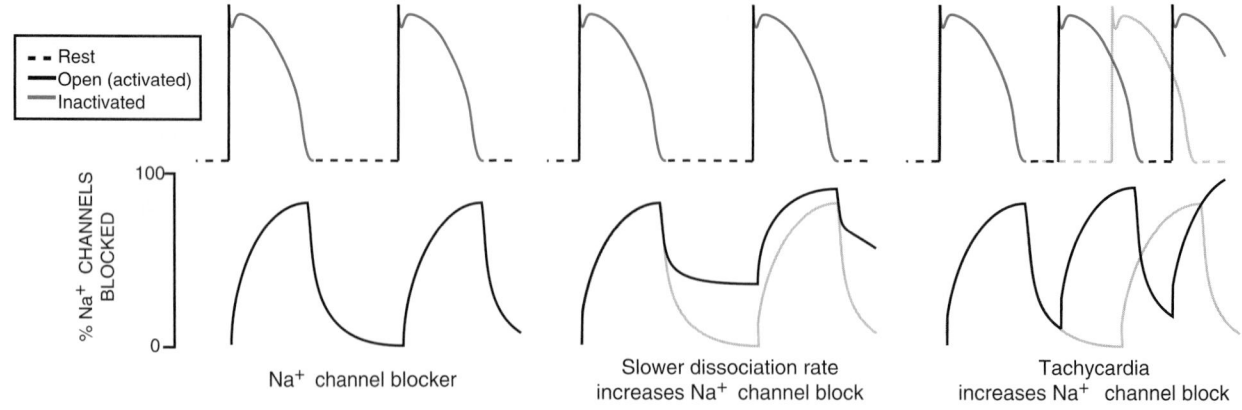

Figure 35–12. Recovery from block of Na⁺ channels during diastole.

This recovery is the critical factor determining extent of steady-state Na$^+$ channel block. Na$^+$ channel blockers bind to (and block) Na$^+$ channels in the open and/or inactivated states, resulting in phasic changes in the extent of block during the action potential. As shown in the middle panel, a decrease in the rate of recovery from block increases the extent of block. Different drugs have different rates of recovery, and depolarization reduces the rate of recovery. The right panel shows that increasing heart rate, which results in relatively less time spent in the rest state, also increases the extent of block. (Modified from Roden *et al.*, 1993, with permission.)

Classifying Antiarrhythmic Drugs

Classifying drugs by common electrophysiological properties emphasizes the connection between basic electrophysiological actions and antiarrhythmic effects (Vaughan Williams, 1992). To the extent that the clinical actions of drugs can be predicted from their basic electrophysiological properties, such classification schemes have some merit. However, as each compound is better characterized in a range of *in vitro* and *in vivo* test systems, it becomes apparent that, even among drugs that share the same classification, differences in pharmacological effects occur, some of which may be responsible for the observed clinical differences in responses to drugs of the same broad "class" (Table 35–3). An alternative way of approaching antiarrhythmic therapy is to attempt to classify arrhythmia mechanisms and then to target drug therapy to the electrophysiological mechanism most likely to terminate or prevent the arrhythmia (Table 35–2; Task Force, 1991).

Na⁺ Channel Block. The extent of Na$^+$ channel block is critically dependent on heart rate and membrane potential as well as on drug-specific physicochemical characteristics that determine $\tau_{recovery}$ (Figure 35–12). The following description applies when Na$^+$ channels are blocked, *i.e.*, at rapid rates in diseased tissue with a rapid-recovery drug such as *lidocaine* or even at normal rates in normal tissues with a slow-recovery drug such as *flecainide*. When Na$^+$ channels are blocked, threshold for excitability is decreased, *i.e.*, greater membrane depolarization is required to bring Na$^+$ channels from the rest to open states. This

change in threshold probably contributes to the clinical findings that Na$^+$ channel blockers tend to increase both pacing threshold and the energy required to defibrillate the fibrillating heart (Echt *et al.*, 1989). These deleterious effects may be important if antiarrhythmic drugs are used in patients with pacemakers or implanted defibrillators. Na$^+$ channel block decreases conduction velocity in fast-response tissue and increases QRS duration. Usual doses of flecainide prolong QRS intervals by 25% or more during normal rhythm, whereas lidocaine increases QRS intervals only if they are measured at very fast heart rates. Drugs with $\tau_{recovery}$ values >10 seconds (*e.g.*, flecainide) also tend to prolong the PR interval; it is not known whether this represents additional Ca^{2+} channel block (*see* below) or block of fast-response tissue in the region of the AV node. Drug effects on the PR interval also are highly modified by autonomic effects. For example, quinidine actually tends to shorten the PR interval, largely as a result of its vagolytic properties. Action potential duration is either unaffected or shortened by Na$^+$ channel block; some Na$^+$ channel–blocking drugs do prolong cardiac action potentials, but by other mechanisms, usually K$^+$ channel block (Table 35–3).

By increasing threshold, Na$^+$ channel block decreases automaticity (Figure 35–10B) and can inhibit triggered activity arising from delayed afterdepolarizations (DADs) or early afterdepolarizations (EADs). Many Na$^+$ channel blockers also decrease phase 4 slope (Figure 35–10A). In anatomically defined reentry, Na$^+$ channel blockers may decrease conduction sufficiently to extinguish the propagating reentrant wavefront. However, as described above, conduction slowing due to Na^+ channel block may exacerbate reentry. Block of Na^+ channels also shifts the voltage dependence of recovery from inactivation (Figure 35–5B) to more negative potentials, thereby tending to increase refractoriness. Thus, whether a given drug exacerbates or suppresses a reentrant arrhythmia depends on the balance between its effects on refractoriness and on conduction in a particular reentrant circuit. In most studies, Na^+ channel blockers prevent recurrence of reentrant ventricular tachycardia in 20% to 40% of patients. Combining drugs with fast and slow rates of recovery from Na^+ channel block (*e.g., mexiletine* plus *quinidine*) can be effective, with fewer adverse effects, when neither drug alone is effective. Lidocaine and similar agents (*mexiletine, tocainide, phenytoin*) with short $\tau_{recovery}$ values are not useful in atrial fibrillation or flutter, whereas quinidine, flecainide, *propafenone*, and similar agents are effective in some patients. Many of these agents owe part of their antiarrhythmic activity to blockade of K^+ channels.

Na^+ Channel Blocker Toxicity.   Conduction slowing in potential reentrant circuits can account for toxicity due to Na^+ channel block (Table 35–1). For example, Na^+ channel block decreases conduction velocity and hence slows atrial flutter rate. Normal AV nodal function permits a greater number of impulses to penetrate the ventricle, and heart rate actually may increase (Figure 35–9). Thus, atrial flutter rate may drop from 300 per minute, with 2:1 or 4:1 atrioventricular conduction (*i.e.,* a heart rate of 75 or 150 per minute), to 220 per minute, but with 1:1 transmission to the ventricle (*i.e.,* a heart rate of 220 per minute). This form of drug-induced arrhythmia is especially common during treatment with quinidine because the drug also increases AV nodal conduction through its vagolytic properties; flecainide and propafenone also have been implicated. Therapy with Na^+ channel blockers in patients with reentrant ventricular tachycardia after a myocardial infarction can increase the frequency and severity of arrhythmic episodes, presumably because conduction slowing allows persistence of the reentrant wavefront within the tachycardia circuit. Such drug-exacerbated arrhythmia can be very difficult to manage, and deaths due to intractable drug-induced ventricular tachycardia have been reported. Some studies suggest Na^+ infusion may be beneficial. Several Na^+ channel blockers (*procainamide,* quinidine) have been reported to exacerbate neuromuscular paralysis by *d*-tubocurarine (see Chapter 9).

Action Potential Prolongation.   Most drugs producing this effect do so by blocking K^+ channels, although enhanced inward Na^+ current also can prolong action potentials. Enhanced inward current may underlie QT prolongation (and arrhythmia suppression) by *ibutilide*. Block

of cardiac K^+ channels increases action potential duration and reduces normal automaticity (Figure 35–10D). Increased action potential duration, seen as an increase in QT interval, increases refractoriness (Figure 35–11), which should be an effective way of treating reentry (Task Force, 1991; Singh, 1993). Some studies have shown that K^+ channel block reduces heterogeneity of refractoriness, an effect that also should prevent reentrant arrhythmias. Experimentally, K^+ channel block produces a series of desirable effects: reduced defibrillation energy requirement, inhibition of ventricular fibrillation due to acute ischemia, and increased contractility (Echt *et al.,* 1989; Roden, 1993). As shown in Table 35–3, most K^+ channel blocking drugs also interact with β-adrenergic receptors (*sotalol*) or other channels (*e.g., amiodarone,* quinidine). Amiodarone and sotalol appear to be at least as effective as drugs with predominant Na^+ channel–blocking properties in both atrial and ventricular arrhythmias. "Pure" action potential–prolonging drugs *dofetilide,* ibutilide) recently have become available (Murray, 1998; Torp-Pedersen *et al.,* 1999).

Toxicity of Drugs That Prolong QT Interval.   Most of these agents prolong cardiac action potentials to a disproportionate extent when underlying heart rate is slow; this effect, in turn, results in EADs and related triggered activity *in vitro,* and can cause *torsades de pointes* (Table 35–1; Figure 35–9). In patients being treated for atrial fibrillation, *torsades de pointes* occur after conversion to sinus rhythm. For unknown reasons, this form of antiarrhythmic drug toxicity is significantly more common in women (Makkar *et al.,* 1993).

Ca^{2+} Channel Block.   The major electrophysiological effects resulting from block of cardiac Ca^{2+} channels are in slow-response tissues, the sinus and AV nodes. Dihydropyridines, such as *nifedipine,* commonly used in angina and hypertension (Chapters 32 and 33), preferentially block Ca^{2+} channels in vascular smooth muscle; their cardiac electrophysiological effects, such as heart rate acceleration, are indirect and attributable to sympathetic activation. Only *verapamil, diltiazem,* and *bepridil* block Ca^{2+} channels in cardiac cells at clinically used doses. With these drugs, heart rate generally is slowed (Figure 35–10A), although hypotension, if marked, can cause reflex sympathetic activation and tachycardia. AV nodal conduction velocity decreases, so the PR interval increases. AV nodal block occurs as a result of decremental conduction as well as increased AV nodal refractoriness. These latter effects form the basis of the antiarrhythmic actions of Ca^{2+} channel blockers in reentrant arrhythmias whose circuit involves the AV node, such as AV reentrant tachycardia (Figure 35–7).

Table 35–3
Major Electrophysiological Actions of Antiarrhythmic Drugs

DRUG	Na$^+$ CHANNEL BLOCK		↑APD	Ca^{2+} CHANNEL BLOCK	AUTONOMIC EFFECTS	OTHER EFFECTS
	$\tau_{recovery}{}^1$, seconds	State-dependence^1				
Lidocaine	0.1	I > O				
Phenytoin	0.2	I				
Mexiletine*	0.3					
Tocainide*	0.4	O > I				
Procainamide	1.8	O	✔		Ganglionic blockade (especially intravenous)	✔: Metabolite prolongs APD
Quinidine	3	O	✔	(x)	α-Blockade, vagolytic	
Disopyramide†	9	O	✔		Anticholinergic	
Moricizine	~10	O ≈ I				
Propafenone†	11	O ≈ I	✔		β-Blockade (variable clinical effect)	
Flecainide*	11	O	(x)	(x)		
β-Blockers:					β-Blockade	
Propanolol†					β-Blockade	Na$^+$ channel block *in vitro*
Sotalol†			✔		β-Blockade	
Bretylium			✔		Adrenergic stimulation followed by ganglionic blockade	↓ Dispersion of repolarization in ischemia
Amiodarone	1.6	I	✔	(x)	Noncompetitive β-blockade	Antithyroid action
Dofetilide			✔			
Ibutilide			✔			

Another important antiarrhythmic action is reduction of ventricular rate in atrial flutter or fibrillation. Rare forms of ventricular tachycardia appear to be DAD-mediated and respond to verapamil (Sung *et al.,* 1983). Unlike β-adrenergic receptor antagonists, Ca^{2+} channel blockers have not been shown to reduce mortality in patients convalescing from myocardial infarction (Singh, 1990). In contrast to other Ca^{2+} channel blockers, bepridil increases action potential duration in many tissues and can exert an antiarrhythmic effect in atria and ventricles. However, because of the incidence of *torsades de pointes* following the administration of bepridil, the drug is not widely prescribed.

Verapamil and Diltiazem. The major adverse effect of intravenous verapamil or diltiazem is hypotension, particularly with bolus doses. This is a particular problem if the drugs are mistakenly used in patients with ventricular tachycardia (in which Ca^{2+} channel blockers are not usually effective) misdiagnosed as AV nodal reentrant tachycardia (Stewart *et al.,* 1986). Hypotension also is frequent

Table 35–3
Major Electrophysiological Actions of Antiarrhythmic Drugs *(Continued)*

DRUG	Na$^+$ CHANNEL BLOCK $\tau_{recovery}$[1], *seconds*	*State-dependence*[1]	↑APD	Ca^{2+} CHANNEL BLOCK	AUTONOMIC EFFECTS	OTHER EFFECTS
Verapamil*				✔		
Diltiazem*				✔		
Digitalis					✔:Vagal stimulation	✔: Inhibition of Na$^+$,K$^+$–ATPase
Adenosine				✔	✔:Adenosine receptor activation	✔: Activation of outward K$^+$ current
Magnesium				? ✔		Mechanism not well understood

✔ indicates an effect that is important in mediating the clinical action of a drug.
(x) indicates a demonstrable effect whose relationship to drug action in patients is less well established.
*indicates drugs prescribed as racemates, and the enantiomers are thought to exert similar electrophysiological effects.
†indicates racemates for which clinically relevant differences in the electrophysiological properties of individual enantiomers have been reported
  (*see* text).

One approach to classifying drugs is:

Class	Major action
I	Na$^+$ channel block
II	β-blockade
III	action potential prolongation (usually by K$^+$ channel block)
IV	Ca^{2+} channel block

Drugs are listed here according to this scheme. It is important to bear in mind, however, that many drugs exert multiple effects which contribute to their clinical actions. It is occasionally clinically useful to subclassify Na$^+$ channel blockers by their rates of recovery from drug-induced block ($\tau_{recovery}$) under physiological conditions. Since this is a continuous variable and can be modulated by factors such as depolarization of the resting potential, these distinctions can become blurred: class Ib, $\tau_{recovery} < 1$ s; class Ia, $\tau_{recovery}$ 1–10 s; class Ic, $\tau_{recovery} > 10$ s. These class and subclass effects are associated with distinctive ECG changes, characteristic "class" toxicities, and efficacy in specific arrhythmia syndromes (*see* text).

[1]These data are dependent on experimental conditions, including species and temperature. The $\tau_{recovery}$ values cited here are from Courtney (1987), with the exception of moricizine, which was found by Lee and Rosen (1991) to have a value slightly less than that for flecainide. The state-dependence is from Snyders *et al.*, (1991).

O, Open state blocker; I, inactivated state blocker; APD, action potential duration; β-blockade, β-adrenergic receptor blockade.

in patients receiving other vasodilators, including quinidine, and in patients with underlying left ventricular dysfunction, which the drugs can exacerbate. Severe sinus bradycardia or heart block also occurs, especially in susceptible patients, such as those also receiving β-blockers. With oral therapy, these adverse effects tend to be less severe. Constipation can occur with oral verapamil.

Verapamil (CALAN, ISOPTIN, VERELAN, COVERA-HS) is prescribed as a racemate. *l*-Verapamil is a more potent calcium channel blocker than is *d*-verapamil. However, with oral therapy, the *l*-enantiomer undergoes more extensive first-pass hepatic metabolism. For this reason, a given concentration of verapamil prolongs the PR interval to a greater extent when the drug is administered intravenously (where concentrations of the *l*- and *d*-enantiomers are equivalent) than when it is administered orally (Echizen

et al., 1985). *Diltiazem* (CARDIZEM, TIAZAC, DILACOR XR, and others) also undergoes extensive first-pass hepatic metabolism, and both drugs have metabolites that exert Ca^{2+} channel–blocking actions. In clinical practice, adverse effects during therapy with verapamil or diltiazem are determined largely by underlying heart disease and concomitant therapy; plasma concentrations of these agents are not routinely measured during therapy. Both drugs can increase serum digoxin concentration, although the magnitude of this effect is variable; excess slowing of ventricular response in patients with atrial fibrillation can occur.

Block of β-Adrenergic Receptors. β-Adrenergic stimulation increases the magnitude of the Ca^{2+} current and slows its inactivation, increases the magnitude of repolarizing K^+ and Cl^- currents (Sanguinetti *et al.*, 1991; Hume and Harvey, 1991), increases pacemaker current (thereby increasing sinus rate; DiFrancesco, 1993), and— under pathophysiological conditions—can increase both DAD- and EAD-mediated arrhythmias. Also, increases in plasma epinephrine associated with severe stress, such as acute myocardial infarction or resuscitation from cardiac arrest, lower serum K^+, especially in patients receiving chronic diuretic therapy (Brown *et al.*, 1983). Thus, β-adrenergic receptor antagonists (often referred to as β-blockers), which inhibit these effects, can be antiarrhythmic by reducing heart rate, decreasing intracellular Ca^{2+} overload, and inhibiting afterdepolarization-mediated automaticity. Epinephrine-induced hypokalemia appears to be mediated by β_2-adrenergic receptors and is blocked by "noncardioselective" antagonists such as propranolol (*see* Chapter 10). In acutely ischemic tissue, β-blockers increase the energy required to fibrillate the heart, an antiarrhythmic action (Anderson *et al.*, 1983). These effects may contribute to the reduction in mortality observed in trials of chronic therapy with β-blockers— including propranolol, timolol, and metoprolol—after myocardial infarction (Singh, 1990), although the precise mechanism underlying this effect has not been established. Atenolol and metoprolol have been shown to decrease mortality in the first week following myocardial infarction.

As with Ca^{2+} channel blockers and digitalis, a major effect of β-blocker therapy is increased AV nodal conduction time (increased PR interval) and prolonged AV nodal refractoriness. Hence, β-blockers are useful in terminating reentrant arrhythmias that involve the AV node and in controlling ventricular response in atrial fibrillation or flutter. In many (but not all) patients with the congenital long QT syndrome, as well as in many other patients, arrhythmias are triggered by physical or emotional stress; β-blockers may be useful in these cases (Schwartz *et al.*, 2000; Roden and Spooner, 1999). β-Adrenergic receptor antagonists also have been reported to be effective in controlling arrhythmias due to Na^+ channel blockers; this effect may be due in part to slowing of the heart rate, which then decreases the extent of rate-dependent conduction slowing by Na^+ channel block (Myerburg *et al.*, 1989). As described further in Chapter 10, adverse effects due to β-blocker therapy include fatigue, bronchospasm, impotence, depression, aggravation of heart failure, worsening of symptoms due to peripheral vascular disease, and inhibition of the symptoms of hypoglycemia in diabetic patients. In patients with arrhythmias due to excess sympathetic stimulation (*e.g.*, pheochromocytoma, clonidine withdrawal), β-blockers may in theory result in unopposed α-adrenergic stimulation, with resultant severe hypertension and/or α-adrenergic–mediated arrhythmias. In such patients, arrhythmias should be treated with both α- and β-adrenergic antagonists. Abrupt discontinuation of chronic β-blocker therapy can lead to "rebound" symptoms including hypertension, increased angina, and arrhythmias (*see* Chapter 33).

Selected β-Adrenergic Receptor Blockers. It is likely that most β-adrenergic antagonists share antiarrhythmic properties. Some, such as *propranolol,* can be shown to exert Na^+ channel-blocking ("membrane stabilizing") effects at high concentrations *in vitro* (Davis and Temte, 1968), but whether or not this is important in patients is uncertain. Similarly, drugs with intrinsic sympathomimetic activity may be less useful as antiarrhythmics, at least in theory (Singh, 1990). *Acebutolol* is as effective as quinidine in suppressing ventricular ectopic beats, an arrhythmia that many clinicians now do not treat. *Sotalol* (*see* below) is more effective for many arrhythmias than are other β-blockers, probably because of its additional K^+ channel–blocking actions. *Esmolol* (Frishman *et al.*, 1988) is a cardioselective agent that is metabolized by red cell esterases and so has a very short elimination half-life (9 minutes). Although methanol is a metabolite, methanol intoxication has not been a clinical problem. Intravenous esmolol is useful in clinical situations in which immediate β-adrenergic blockade is desired (*e.g.*, for rate control of rapidly conducted atrial fibrillation). Because of esmolol's very rapid elimination, adverse effects due to β-adrenergic blockade—should they occur—dissipate rapidly when the drug is stopped. With most β-blockers, intravenous therapy can produce transient hypertension due to unopposed α-adrenergic stimulation; with intravenous esmolol, hypotension is more common.

PRINCIPLES IN THE CLINICAL USE OF ANTIARRHYTHMIC DRUGS

Drugs that modify cardiac electrophysiology often have a very narrow margin between the doses required to produce a desired effect and those associated with adverse effects. Moreover, adverse effects from antiarrhythmic drug therapy can include induction of new arrhythmias, with possibly fatal consequences. Nonpharmacological treatments, such as cardiac pacing, electrical defibrillation, or ablation of targeted regions (Morady, 1999), are indicated for some arrhythmias; in other cases no therapy is required even though an arrhythmia is detected. Therefore, the fundamental principles of therapeutics described here must be applied to optimize antiarrhythmic therapy.

1. Identify and Remove Precipitating Factors

Factors that commonly precipitate cardiac arrhythmias include hypoxia, electrolyte disturbances (especially hypokalemia), myocardial ischemia, and certain drugs. Antiarrhythmics, including digitalis glycosides, are not the only drugs that can precipitate arrhythmias (Table 35–1). For example, *theophylline* is a common cause of multifocal atrial tachycardia, which sometimes can be managed simply by reducing the dose of theophylline. *Torsades de pointes* can arise not only during therapy with action potential-prolonging antiarrhythmics, but also with other drugs not ordinarily classified as having effects on ion channels. These include the antihistamines *terfenadine* and *astemizole* (Chapter 25); the antibiotic, *erythromycin* (Chapter 47); the antiprotozoal, *pentamidine* (Chapter 41); some antipsychotics, notably *thioridazine* (Chapter 20); and certain tricyclic antidepressants (Chapter 19).

2. Establish the Goals of Treatment

Some Arrhythmias Should Not Be Treated: The CAST Example. Abnormalities of cardiac rhythm are readily detectable by a variety of recording methods. However, the mere detection of an abnormality should not be equated with the need for therapy. This was best illustrated in the Cardiac Arrhythmias Suppression Trial (CAST). The presence of asymptomatic ventricular ectopic beats is known to be a marker for an increased risk of sudden death due to ventricular fibrillation in patients convalescing from a myocardial infarction. In the CAST, patients in whom ventricular ectopic beats were suppressed by the potent Na^+ channel blockers encainide (no longer marketed) or flecainide were randomly assigned to receive those drugs or a matching placebo. Unexpectedly, the mortality rate was two- to threefold higher among patients treated with the drugs than those treated with placebo (CAST Investigators, 1989). While the explanation of this effect is not known, a number of lines of evidence suggest that, in the presence of these drugs, transient episodes of myocardial ischemia and/or sinus tachycardia can cause marked conduction slowing (because these drugs have a very long $\tau_{recovery}$), resulting in fatal reentrant ventricular tachyarrhythmias (Ruskin, 1989; Ranger *et al.*, 1989; Akiyama *et al.*, 1991). One consequence of this very important clinical trial was to reemphasize the concept that therapy should be initiated only when a clear benefit to the patient can be identified. When symptoms are obviously attributable to an ongoing arrhythmia, there usually is not much doubt that termination of the arrhythmia will be beneficial; when chronic therapy is used to prevent recurrence of an arrhythmia, risks may be greater (Roden, 1994). Among the antiarrhythmic drugs discussed here, only β-adrenergic blockers, and to a lesser extent amiodarone (Connolly, 1999), have been shown to reduce mortality during long-term therapy.

Symptoms Due to Arrhythmias. Some patients with an arrhythmia may be asymptomatic; in this case, establishing any benefit for treatment will be very difficult. Some patients may present with presyncope, syncope, or even cardiac arrest, which may be due to brady- or tachyarrhythmias. Other patients may present with a sensation of irregular heartbeats, which can be minimally symptomatic in some individuals and incapacitating in others. The irregular heartbeats may be due to intermittent premature contractions or to sustained arrhythmias such as atrial fibrillation (which results in an irregular ventricular rate; Figure 35–9). Finally, patients may present with symptoms due to decreased cardiac output attributable to arrhythmias. The most common symptom is breathlessness at rest or on exertion. Rarely, patients with sustained tachycardias will present with congestive heart failure, which can be controlled by treating the arrhythmia.

Choosing Among Therapeutic Approaches. Establishing the goals of therapy is especially important when different therapeutic options are available. For example, in patients with atrial fibrillation, three options are available: (1) Reduce the ventricular response, using AV nodal blocking agents such as digitalis, verapamil, diltiazem, or β-adrenergic antagonists (Table 35–1); (2) restore and maintain normal rhythm, using drugs such as quinidine, flecainide, or amiodarone; or (3) decide not to implement antiarrhythmic therapy, which may be the appropriate approach if the patient truly is asymptomatic. Most patients with atrial fibrillation also benefit from anticoagulation to reduce stroke incidence, regardless of symptoms (Singer, 1996; *see* Chapter 55).

Factors that contribute to choice of therapy include not only symptoms but also the type and extent of structural heart disease, the QT interval prior to drug therapy, the coexistence of conduction system disease, and the presence of noncardiac diseases (Table 35–4). In the rare patient with the WPW syndrome and atrial fibrillation, the ventricular response can be extremely rapid and can be paradoxically accelerated by AV nodal blocking drugs such as digitalis or Ca^{2+} channel blockers; deaths due to drug therapy have been reported under these circumstances.

Frequency and reproducibility of arrhythmia should be established prior to initiating therapy, since inherent variability in the occurrence of arrhythmias can be confused with a beneficial or adverse drug effect. Techniques for this assessment include recording cardiac rhythm for prolonged periods or evaluating the response of the heart to artificially induced premature beats. It also is important to recognize that drug therapy may be only partially effective: a marked decrease in the duration of paroxysms of atrial fibrillation may be sufficient to render a patient asymptomatic, even if an occasional episode still can be detected.

3. Minimize Risks

Antiarrhythmic Drugs Can Cause Arrhythmias. One increasingly well-recognized risk of antiarrhythmic therapy is the possibility of provoking new arrhythmias, with potentially life-threatening consequences. Mechanistically distinct syndromes of arrhythmia provocation by antiarrhythmic drugs have been described (Table 35–1). These drug-provoked arrhythmias must be recognized, since further treatment with antiarrhythmic drugs often exacerbates the problem, whereas withdrawal of the causative agent often is curative. In addition, specific therapies targeted toward underlying mechanisms of these arrhythmias may be indicated. It also is critical to establish a precise diagnosis. For example, treating a ventricular tachycardia with verapamil not only may be ineffective but also can cause catastrophic cardiovascular collapse (Stewart *et al.*, 1986).

Monitoring of Plasma Concentration. Some adverse effects of antiarrhythmic drugs are related to excessively elevated

Table 35–4
Patient-Specific Antiarrhythmic Drug Contraindications

CONDITION	EXCLUDE/USE WITH CAUTION
Cardiac:	
Heart failure	Disopyramide, flecainide
Sinus or AV node dysfunction	Digitalis, verapamil, diltiazem, β-adrenergic receptor antagonists, amiodarone
Wolff–Parkinson–White syndrome (risk of extremely rapid rate if atrial fibrillation develops)	Digitalis, verapamil, diltiazem
Infranodal conduction disease	Na^+ channel blockers, amiodarone
Aortic/subaortic stenosis	Bretylium
History of myocardial infarction	Flecainide
Prolonged QT interval	Quinidine, procainamide, disopyramide, sotalol, dofetilide, ibutilide
Cardiac transplant	Adenosine
Noncardiac:	
Diarrhea	Quinidine
Prostatism, glaucoma	Disopyramide
Arthritis	Chronic procainamide
Lung disease	Amiodarone
Tremor	Mexiletine, tocainide
Constipation	Verapamil
Asthma, peripheral vascular disease, hypoglycemia	β-Adrenergic blockers, propafenone

plasma drug concentration. Thus, measuring plasma concentration and adjusting the dose to maintain the concentration within a prescribed therapeutic range may be a useful way of minimizing some adverse effects. In many patients, the occurrence of serious adverse reactions appears to be related to interactions involving drug (often at usual plasma concentrations), transient factors such as electrolyte disturbances or myocardial ischemia, and the type and extent of the underlying heart disease (Ruskin, 1989; Morganroth et al., 1986; Roden, 1994). Factors such as generation of unmeasured active metabolites, variability in elimination of enantiomers (which may exert differing pharmacological effects), and disease- or enantiomer-specific abnormalities in drug binding to plasma proteins can complicate the interpretation of routine monitoring of plasma drug concentrations (see Chapter 1).

Patient-Specific Contraindications. Another way of minimizing the adverse effects of antiarrhythmic drugs is to avoid certain drugs in certain patient subsets altogether. For example, patients with a history of congestive heart failure are particularly prone to develop heart failure during disopyramide therapy. Often, adverse effects of drugs may be difficult to distinguish from exacerbations of underlying disease. Amiodarone may cause

interstitial lung disease; its use is therefore undesirable in a patient with advanced pulmonary disease in whom the development of this potentially fatal adverse effect would be difficult to detect. Specific diseases that constitute relative or absolute contraindications to specific drugs are listed in Table 35–4.

4. The Electrophysiology of the Heart as a "Moving Target"

Cardiac electrophysiology varies in a highly dynamic fashion in response to external influences such as changing autonomic tone, myocardial ischemia, or myocardial stretch. For example, myocardial ischemia results in changes in extracellular K^+ that, in turn, make the resting potential less negative, inactivate Na^+ channels, decrease Na^+ current, and slow conduction (Weiss et al., 1991). In addition, myocardial ischemia can result in the release of "metabolites of ischemia," such as lysophosphatidylcholine, which can alter ion channel function (DaTorre et al., 1991); ischemia also may activate channels that otherwise are quiescent, such as the ATP-inhibited K^+ channels (Wilde and Janse, 1994). Thus, a normal heart may display, in response to myocardial ischemia, changes in resting potential, conduction velocity, intracellular Ca^{2+} concentrations, and repolarization, any one of which may then create arrhythmias or alter response to antiarrhythmic therapy.

ANTIARRHYTHMIC DRUGS

Summaries of important electrophysiological and pharmacokinetic features of the drugs considered here are presented in Tables 35–3 and 35–5. Ca^{2+} channel blockers and β-adrenergic antagonists have been considered above and in Chapters 32 and 10, respectively. The drugs are presented in alphabetical order.

Adenosine. *Adenosine* (ADENOCARD) is a naturally occurring nucleoside which is administered as a rapid intravenous bolus for the acute termination of reentrant supraventricular arrhythmias (Lerman and Belardinelli, 1991). Rare cases of ventricular tachycardia in patients with otherwise normal hearts are thought to be DAD-mediated and can be terminated by adenosine. Adenosine also has been used to produce controlled hypotension during some surgical procedures and in the diagnosis of coronary artery disease. Intravenous ATP appears to produce effects similar to those of adenosine.

ADENOSINE

Pharmacological Effects. The effects of adenosine are mediated by its interaction with specific G protein–coupled adenosine receptors. Adenosine activates acetylcholine-sensitive K^+ current in the atrium and sinus and AV nodes, resulting in shortening of action potential duration, hyperpolarization, and slowing of normal automaticity (Figure 35–10C). Adenosine also inhibits the electrophysiological effects of increased intracellular cyclic AMP, which occur with sympathetic stimulation. Because adenosine thereby reduces Ca^{2+} currents, it can be antiarrhythmic by increasing AV nodal refractoriness and by inhibiting DADs elicited by sympathetic stimulation.

Administration of an intravenous bolus of adenosine to human beings transiently slows sinus rate and AV nodal conduction velocity and increases AV nodal refractoriness. It has been shown that a bolus dose of adenosine can produce transient sympathetic activation by interacting with carotid baroreceptors (Biaggioni *et al.,* 1991); when a continuous infusion of the drug is administered, hypotension results.

Adverse Effects. A major advantage of adenosine therapy is that adverse effects are short-lived, since the drug is eliminated so rapidly. Transient asystole (lack of any cardiac rhythm whatsoever) is common but usually lasts <5 seconds and is in fact the therapeutic goal. Most patients feel a sense of chest fullness and dyspnea when therapeutic doses (6 to 12 mg) of adenosine are administered. Rarely, an adenosine bolus can precipitate atrial fibrillation, presumably by heterogeneously shortening atrial action potentials, or bronchospasm.

Clinical Pharmacokinetics. Adenosine is eliminated with a half-life of seconds by carrier-mediated uptake, which occurs in most cell types including the endothelium, and subsequent metabolism by adenosine deaminase. Adenosine probably is the only drug whose efficacy requires a rapid bolus dose, preferably through a large central intravenous line; slow administration results in elimination of the drug prior to its arrival at the heart.

The effects of adenosine are potentiated in patients receiving *dipyridamole,* an adenosine-uptake inhibitor, and in patients with cardiac transplants, due to denervation hypersensitivity. Methylxanthines (*see* Chapter 28) such as theophylline and caffeine block adenosine receptors; therefore larger-than-usual doses are required to produce an antiarrhythmic effect in patients who have consumed these agents in beverages or as therapy.

Amiodarone. *Amiodarone* (CORDARONE, PACERONE) exerts a multiplicity of pharmacological effects, none of which is clearly linked to its arrhythmia-suppressing properties (Mason, 1987). Amiodarone is a structural analog of thyroid hormone, and some of its antiarrhythmic actions and its toxicity may be attributable to interaction with nuclear thyroid hormone receptors. Amiodarone is highly lipophilic, is concentrated in many tissues, and is eliminated extremely slowly; consequently, adverse effects may be very slow to resolve. In the United States, the drug currently is indicated for oral therapy in patients with recurrent ventricular tachycardia or fibrillation resistant to other drugs. Controlled clinical trials indicate that oral amiodarone also is effective in maintaining sinus rhythm in patients with atrial fibrillation (Connolly, 1999). An intravenous form has been approved in the United States for the acute termination of ventricular tachycardia or fibrillation

Table 35-5

Pharmacokinetic Characteristics and Doses of Antiarrhythmic Drugs

DRUG	BIOAVAILABILITY Reduced: ↓ absorption	BIOAVAILABILITY Reduced: 1st pass metabolism >80%	PROTEIN BINDING >80%	ELIMINATION Renal	ELIMINATION Hepatic	ELIMINATION Other	$t_{1/2}$ <2 Hours	$t_{1/2}$ Hours	$t_{1/2}$ >24 Hours	ACTIVE METABOLITE(S)	THERAPEUTIC PLASMA CONCENTRATION[†]	USUAL DOSES[‡] Loading doses	USUAL DOSES[‡] Maintenance doses
Adenosine	✓	✓				✓	<10 s					6–12 mg (IV only)	
Amiodarone	✓		✓		✓	✓			weeks	✓	0.5–2 μg/ml	800–1600 mg/day × 2–4 weeks (IV: 100–300 mg)	100–400 mg/day
Bretylium				✓				7–15				150–300 mg (IV)	1–4 mg/min (IV)
Digoxin		~80%		✓					36 h		0.5–2.0 ng/ml	1 mg over 12–24 h	0.125–0.375 mg q24h
Digitoxin			✓		✓				7–9 days	(Digoxin)	10–30 ng/ml		0.05–0.3 mg q24h
Diltiazem	✓				✓			4		(x)		0.25–0.35 mg/kg over 10 min (IV)	5–15 mg/h (IV); 30–90 mg q6h; 120–300 mg q24h¶
Disopyramide			✓	✓				4–10		(x)	2–5 μg/ml		100–200 mg q6h; 200–400 mg q12h¶
Dofetilide			✓	✓	(x)			7–10					0.25–0.5 mg q12h¶¶
Esmolol						✓	5–10 min					500 μg/kg/min; may repeat × 2 (IV)	50–200 μg/kg/min (IV)
Flecainide			✓	✓	✓			10–18			0.2–1 μg/ml		50–200 mg q12h
Ibutilide	✓				✓			6				1 mg (IV) over 10 min; may repeat once 10 min later	
Lidocaine	✓		✓		✓		120 min			(x)	1.5–5 μg/ml	3–4 mg/kg over 20–30 min (IV)	1–4 mg/min (IV)
Mexiletine	✓				✓			9–15			0.5–2 μg/ml		100–300 mg q8h
Moricizine	✓		✓		✓			2–3		(x)			200–300 mg q8h
Phenytoin	✓		✓		✓				7–42 h		10–20 μg/ml	1 g (IV), given at <50 mg/min	100 mg q8h

*ELIMINATION $t_{1/2}$

Table 35–5

Pharmacokinetic Characteristics and Doses of Antiarrhythmic Drugs (Continued)

DRUG	BIOAVAILABILITY Reduced: ↓ absorption	BIOAVAILABILITY Reduced: 1st pass metabolism	BIOAVAILABILITY >80%	PROTEIN BINDING >80%	ELIMINATION Renal	ELIMINATION Hepatic	ELIMINATION Other	ELIMINATION $t_{1/2}$* <2 Hours	ELIMINATION $t_{1/2}$* Hours	ELIMINATION $t_{1/2}$* >24 Hours	ACTIVE METABOLITE(S)	THERAPEUTIC† PLASMA CONCENTRATION	USUAL DOSES‡ Loading doses	USUAL DOSES‡ Maintenance doses
Procainamide			✓		✓	✓			3–4		✓	4–8 µg/ml	1 g (IV), given at 20 mg/min	1–4 mg/min (IV); 250–750 mg q3h; 500–1000 mg q6h¶
(N–Acetyl procainamide)			(✓)		(✓)				(6–10)			(10–20 µg/ml)		
Propafenone		✓				✓			2–32		✓	<1 µg/ml		150–300 mg q8h
Propranolol		✓		✓		✓			4				1–3 mg (IV)	10–80 mg q6–8h; 80–240 mg q24h¶
Quinidine			✓	~80%	(x)	✓			4–10		✓	2–5 µg/ml		324–648 mg (gluconate) q8h
Sotalol			✓		✓				8			<5 µg/ml (?)		80–320 mg q12h
Tocainide			✓		✓				15			3–11 µg/ml		400–600 mg q8h
Verapamil		✓		✓		✓			3–7		✓		5–10 mg (IV)	80–120 mg q8h; 120–240 mg q24h¶

(x): metabolite or route of elimination probably of minor clinical importance.

*The elimination half-life is one, but not the only, determinant of how frequently a drug must be administered to maintain a therapeutic effect and avoid toxicity (Chapter 3). For some drugs with short elimination half-lives, infrequent dosing is nevertheless possible, e.g., propranolol or verapamil. Formulations that allow slow release into the gastrointestinal tract of a rapidly eliminated compound (available for many drugs including procainamide, disopyramide, verapamil, diltiazem, and propranolol) also allow infrequent dosing.

†The therapeutic range is bounded by a plasma concentration below which no therapeutic effect is likely, and an upper concentration above which the risk of adverse effects increases. As discussed in the text, many serious adverse reactions to antiarrhythmic drugs can occur at "therapeutic" concentrations in susceptible individuals. When only an upper limit is cited, a lower limit has not been well defined. Variable generation of active metabolites may further complicate the interpretation of plasma concentration data (Chapters 1 and 3).

‡Oral doses are presented unless otherwise indicated. Doses are presented as suggested ranges in adults of average build; lower doses are less likely to produce toxicity. Lower maintenance dosages may be required in patients with renal or hepatic disease. Loading doses are only indicated when a therapeutic effect is desired before maintenance therapy would bring drug concentrations into a therapeutic range, i.e., for acute therapy (e.g., lidocaine, verapamil, adenosine) or when the elimination half-life is extremely long (amiodarone).

¶Indicates suggested dosage using slow-release formulation.

¶¶This drug is available only in a restricted distribution system (see text).

IV, intravenous; q, every.

(Kowey *et al.*, 1995). Trials of oral amiodarone in patients convalescing from acute myocardial infarction have shown a modest beneficial effect on mortality (Amiodarone Trials Meta-Analysis Investigators, 1997). The drug is nevertheless not widely prescribed in this population, perhaps because of concerns about its potential for long-term toxicity.

AMIODARONE

Pharmacological Effects. Studies of the acute effects of amiodarone in *in vitro* systems are complicated by its insolubility in water, necessitating the use of solvents such as dimethyl sulfoxide. It has been suggested that amiodarone's effects are mediated by perturbation of the lipid milieu in which ion channels are placed (Herbette *et al.*, 1988). Amiodarone blocks inactivated Na^+ channels and has a relatively rapid (time constant ~1.6 seconds) rate of recovery from block. It also decreases Ca^{2+} current and transient outward, delayed rectifier and inward rectifier K^+ currents and exerts a noncompetitive (*see* Chapter 10) adrenergic blocking effect. Amiodarone is a potent inhibitor of abnormal automaticity, and, in most tissues, it prolongs action potential duration. Amiodarone decreases conduction velocity by Na^+ channel block as well as by a poorly understood effect on cell–cell coupling that may be especially important in diseased tissue (Levine *et al.*, 1988). PR, QRS, and QT prolongations and sinus bradycardia are frequent during chronic therapy. Amiodarone prolongs refractoriness in all cardiac tissues; Na^+ channel block, delayed repolarization due to K^+ channel block, and inhibition of cell–cell coupling all may contribute to this effect of amiodarone.

Adverse Effects. Hypotension due to vasodilation and depression of myocardial performance is frequent with the intravenous form of amiodarone, and may be due in part to the solvent. While depression of contractility can occur during long-term therapy, it is unusual. During oral drug-loading regimens, which usually take place over several weeks, adverse effects are unusual, despite administration of high dosages that would cause serious toxicity if continued long-term. Occasional patients develop nausea, which responds to a decrease in daily dose during the loading phase.

Adverse effects during long-term therapy have been related to both the size of daily maintenance doses as well as to cumulative dose (*i.e.*, to duration of therapy), suggesting tissue accumulation may be responsible. The most

serious adverse effect during chronic amiodarone therapy is pulmonary fibrosis, which can be rapidly progressive and fatal. Underlying lung disease, doses ≥ 400 mg/day, and recent pulmonary insults such as pneumonia appear to be risk factors (Dusman *et al.*, 1990). Serial chest X-rays or pulmonary function studies may detect early amiodarone toxicity, but monitoring plasma concentrations has not been useful. With low doses, such as ≤ 200 mg/day used in atrial fibrillation, pulmonary toxicity is extremely unusual. Other adverse effects during long-term therapy include corneal microdeposits (which often are asymptomatic), hepatic dysfunction, hypo- or hyperthyroidism, neuromuscular symptoms (most commonly peripheral neuropathy or proximal muscle weakness), and photosensitivity. Treatment consists of withdrawal of the drug and supportive measures, including corticosteroids, for life-threatening toxicity; reduction of dosage may be sufficient if the drug is deemed necessary and the adverse effect is not life-threatening. Despite the marked QT prolongation and bradycardia typical of chronic amiodarone therapy, *torsades de pointes* and other drug-induced tachyarrhythmias are unusual.

Clinical Pharmacokinetics. Amiodarone is incompletely (~30%) bioavailable, presumably because of poor absorption. This reduced bioavailability is important in calculating equivalent dosing regimens when converting from intravenous to oral therapy. The drug is distributed in lipid; for example, heart tissue to plasma concentration ratios >20:1 and lipid to plasma ratios >300:1 have been reported. After the initiation of amiodarone therapy, increases in refractoriness, a marker of pharmacological effect, require several weeks to develop. Amiodarone undergoes hepatic metabolism by cytochrome P450 3A4 (CYP3A4) to desethyl-amiodarone, a metabolite with pharmacological effects similar to those of the parent drug. When amiodarone therapy is withdrawn from a patient who has been receiving therapy for several years, plasma concentrations decline with a half-life of weeks to months. The mechanism whereby amiodarone and desethyl-amiodarone are eliminated is not well established.

A therapeutic plasma amiodarone concentration range of 0.5 to 2.0 μg/ml has been proposed. However, efficacy appears to depend as much on duration of therapy as on plasma concentration, and elevated plasma concentrations are not useful in predicting toxicity (Dusman *et al.*, 1990). Because of amiodarone's slow accumulation in tissue, a high-dose oral loading regimen (*e.g.*, 800 to 1600 mg/day) is usually administered for several weeks and then maintenance therapy started. Maintenance dose is adjusted on the basis of adverse effects and the arrhythmias being treated. If the presenting arrhythmia is life-threatening,

dosages >300 mg/day normally are used unless clear toxicity occurs. On the other hand, maintenance doses of
≤200 mg/day are used if recurrence of an arrhythmia
would be tolerated, as in patients with atrial fibrillation.
Because of the drug's very slow elimination, amiodarone
is administered once daily, and omission of one or two
doses during chronic therapy rarely results in recurrence
of arrhythmia.

Dose adjustments are not required in conditions such
as hepatic, renal, or cardiac dysfunction. Amiodarone is a
potent inhibitor of the hepatic metabolism or renal elimination of many compounds. Mechanisms identified to
date include inhibition of CYP3A4 and CYP2C9 and of
P-glycoprotein (*see* Chapter 1). Dosages of warfarin, other
antiarrhythmics (flecainide, procainamide, quinidine), or
digoxin usually require reduction during amiodarone
therapy.

Bretylium. *Bretylium* (bretylium tosylate; BRETYLOL) is
a quaternary ammonium compound that prolongs cardiac
action potentials and interferes with reuptake of norepinephrine by sympathetic neurons; both actions may be
antiarrhythmic (Heissenbuttel and Bigger, 1979). Bretylium
loading and maintenance infusions are used to treat ventricular fibrillation and prevent its recurrence (*see* Table
35–5 for loading and maintenance doses).

BRETYLIUM

Pharmacological Effects. Bretylium prolongs action potentials in normal Purkinje cells to a greater extent than in
cells that have survived a recent ischemic insult (in which
action potentials already are prolonged abnormally). Thus,
bretylium reduces heterogeneity of repolarization times,
an effect that may suppress reentry (Cardinal and
Sasyniuk, 1978). The mechanism whereby bretylium prolongs cardiac action potentials has not been established,
although block of K^+ channels seems likely. Bretylium
has no effect on Na^+ channels, except at high concentrations, and no direct effect on automaticity. In animals and
human beings, administration of bretylium initially results
in increased norepinephrine release from sympathetic neurons and inhibition of subsequent reuptake.

Adverse Effects. As a result of norepinephrine release,
bretylium can produce transient hypertension and increased
arrhythmias; this effect rarely is observed, since bretylium
is used in critically ill patients who often are hemodynam-

ically unstable. In theory, bretylium should be avoided in
patients who are especially prone to increased arrhythmias with norepinephrine release, such as those with digitalis intoxication. In contrast, hypotension due to inhibition of norepinephrine reuptake is a common problem
during bretylium therapy. Bretylium-induced hypotension
should be managed with judicious fluid replacement if
possible. Since bretylium effectively results in sympathetic
denervation, the administration of normal doses of catecholamines such as dopamine may cause marked hypertension. Bretylium should be used only with great caution
when the drug's vasodilating effects may be particularly
hazardous, as in patients with aortic stenosis, carotid occlusive disease, or hypertrophic cardiomyopathy. The occurrence of *torsades de pointes* is unusual during bretylium
therapy.

Clinical Pharmacokinetics. Bretylium is excreted unchanged by the kidneys without undergoing significant
hepatic metabolism. Reduction of a maintenance infusion
rate has been recommended in patients with renal failure,
although adverse effects due to accumulation of bretylium
in plasma have not been seen. A lag time of ~2 hours has
been reported between peak plasma bretylium concentrations and peak prolongation of ventricular refractoriness
after an intravenous dose in dogs (Anderson *et al.*, 1980).
This lag time suggests that bretylium is distributed to sites
in peripheral tissues prior to exerting its pharmacological
effect.

An oral formulation has been investigated, but hypotension and reduced bioavailability (~35%), presumably
because of poor absorption, are problems. The hypotensive
effects of bretylium can be inhibited by coadministration
of tricyclic antidepressants such as *protriptyline,* which
blocks bretylium's effects on sympathetic norepinephrine
release and reuptake (Woosley *et al.*, 1982). Results of a
limited number of studies suggest that the antiarrhythmic
effects of bretylium may be preserved during coadministration of tricyclic antidepressants.

Digitalis Glycosides. *Pharmacological Effects.* Digitalis glycosides exert positive inotropic effects and are
widely used in heart failure (Chapter 34). Their inotropic
action is the result of increased intracellular Ca^{2+} (Smith,
1988), which also forms the basis for arrhythmias related to digitalis intoxication. Digitalis glycosides increase
phase 4 slope (*i.e.*, increase the rate of automaticity), especially if $[K]_o$ is low. Digitalis glycosides also exert prominent vagotonic actions, resulting in inhibition of Ca^{2+}
currents in the AV node and activation of acetylcholine-
mediated K^+ currents in the atrium. Thus, the major "indirect" electrophysiological effects of digitalis glycosides

are hyperpolarization, shortening of atrial action potentials, and increases in AV nodal refractoriness. The latter action accounts for the utility of digitalis in termination of reentrant arrhythmias involving the AV node, and in controlling ventricular response in patients with atrial fibrillation. Digitalis preparations may be especially useful in the latter situation, since many such patients have heart failure, which can be exacerbated by other AV nodal blocking drugs such as Ca^{2+} channel blockers or β-adrenergic receptor antagonists. However, in many patients with advanced heart failure, sympathetic drive is markedly increased, so digitalis is not very effective in decreasing the rate; on the other hand, even a modest decrease in rate can sometimes help ameliorate heart failure. Similarly, in other conditions in which high sympathetic tone drives rapid atrioventricular conduction (e.g., chronic lung disease, thyrotoxicosis), digitalis therapy may be only marginally effective in slowing the rate. Increased sympathetic activity and hypoxia can potentiate digitalis-induced changes in automaticity and DADs, thus increasing the risk of digitalis toxicity. A further complicating feature in thyrotoxicosis is increased digoxin clearance. The major ECG effects of cardiac glycosides are PR prolongation and a nonspecific alteration in ventricular repolarization (the ST segment), whose underlying mechanism is not well understood.

Adverse Effects.   Digitalis intoxication is a common clinical problem (*see also* Chapter 34). Arrhythmias, nausea, disturbances of cognitive function, and blurred or yellow vision are the usual manifestations. Often, these are not immediately recognized, since they occur frequently in patients with advanced illnesses receiving multiple drugs. Elevated serum concentrations of digitalis, hypoxia (e.g., due to chronic lung disease), and hypokalemia, hypomagnesemia, and hypercalcemia predispose patients to digitalis-induced arrhythmias. While digitalis intoxication can cause virtually any arrhythmia, certain types of arrhythmias are characteristic. Arrhythmias that should raise a strong suspicion of digitalis intoxication are those in which DAD-related tachycardias occur along with impairment of sinus node or AV nodal function. Atrial tachycardia with AV block is "classic," but ventricular bigeminy (sinus beats alternating with beats of ventricular origin), "bidirectional" ventricular tachycardia (a very rare entity), AV junctional tachycardias, and various degrees of AV block also can occur. With advanced intoxication (e.g., with suicidal ingestion), severe hyperkalemia due to poisoning of Na^+,K^+–ATPase and profound bradyarrhythmias, which may be unresponsive to pacing therapy, are seen. In patients with elevated serum digitalis blood levels, the risk of precipitating ventricular fibrillation by

DC cardioversion probably is increased; in those with therapeutic blood levels, DC cardioversion can be used safely.

Minor forms of digitalis intoxication may require no specific therapy beyond monitoring cardiac rhythm until symptoms and signs of toxicity resolve. Sinus bradycardia and AV block often respond to intravenous atropine, but the effect is transient. Mg^{2+} has been used successfully in some cases of digitalis-induced tachycardia (Seller, 1971). Any serious arrhythmia should be treated with antidigoxin Fab fragments, which are highly effective in binding digoxin and digitoxin, greatly enhancing the renal excretion of these drugs (*see* Chapter 34). Serum glycoside concentrations rise markedly with antidigitalis antibodies, but these represent bound (nonpharmacologically active) drug. Temporary cardiac pacing may be required for advanced sinus node or AV node dysfunction. Other forms of antidotal therapy that have been used in the past, but have been largely supplanted by the use of Fab fragments, include lidocaine, phenytoin, or the cautious administration of K^+ for ventricular arrhythmias; K^+ can exacerbate AV block. Digitalis exerts direct arterial vasoconstrictor effects, which can be especially deleterious in patients with advanced atherosclerosis who receive intravenous drug; ischemia in the intestinal or coronary beds has been reported.

Clinical Pharmacokinetics.   The most commonly used digitalis glycoside in the United States is *digoxin* (LANOXIN), although *digitoxin* (CRYSTODIGIN) is also used for chronic oral therapy. Digoxin tablets are incompletely (75%) bioavailable, but capsules are >90% bioavailable. In some patients, intestinal microflora may metabolize digoxin, causing a marked reduction in drug bioavailability. In these patients, higher-than-usual doses are required for clinical efficacy to be achieved; toxicity is a serious risk if antibiotics such as tetracycline or erythromycin, which destroy intestinal microflora, are administered. Inhibition of P-glycoprotein (*see* below) also may play a role. Digoxin is 20% to 30% protein-bound. The antiarrhythmic effects of digoxin can be achieved with intravenous or oral therapy. However, digoxin undergoes relatively slow distribution to effector site(s); therefore, even with intravenous therapy, there is a lag of several hours between drug administration and the development of measurable pharmacological effects such as PR interval prolongation or slowing of the ventricular rate in atrial fibrillation. To avoid digitalis intoxication, a loading regimen of ~1 to 1.5 mg given over 24 hours is administered. Measurement of postdistribution serum digoxin concentration and adjusting the daily dose (0.125 to 0.375 mg) to maintain concentrations of 0.5 to 2 ng/ml are useful during chronic digoxin therapy (*see* Table 35–5). Some patients may require and tolerate higher concentrations, but with an increased risk of adverse effects.

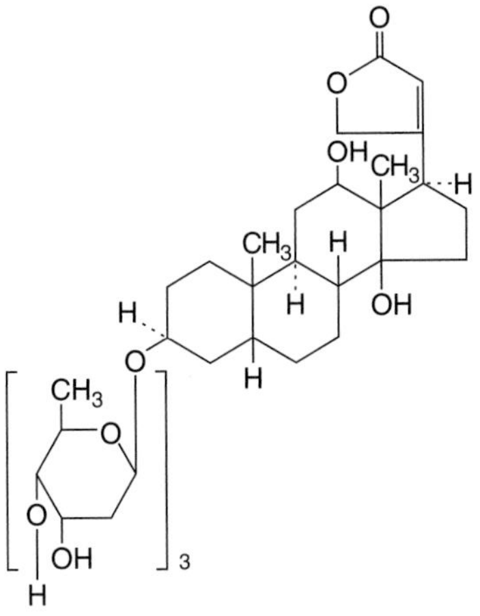

DIGOXIN

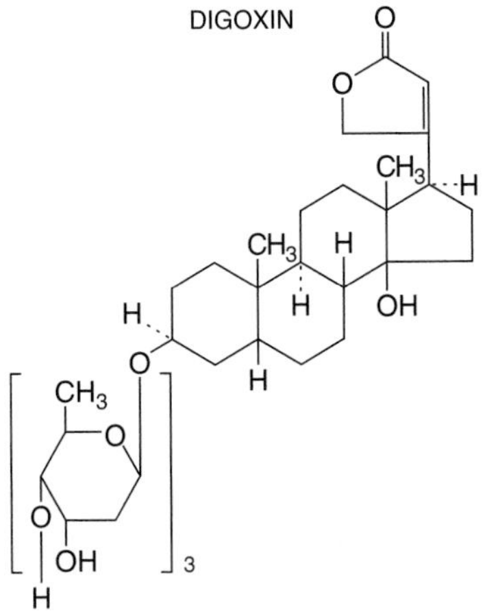

DIGITOXIN

The elimination half-life of digoxin ordinarily is ~36 hours, so maintenance doses are administered once daily. Renal elimination of unchanged drug accounts for <80% of digoxin elimination. Digoxin doses should be reduced (or dosing interval increased) and serum concentrations closely monitored in patients with impaired excretion due to renal failure or in patients who are hypothyroid. Digitoxin undergoes primarily hepatic metabolism and may be useful in patients with fluctuating or advanced renal dysfunction. Digitoxin metabolism is accelerated by drugs such as phenytoin or rifampin that induce hepatic metabolism (Chapter 1). Digitoxin's elimination half-life is even longer than that of digoxin (about 7 days); it is highly protein-bound, and its therapeutic range is 10 to 30 ng/ml.

Quinidine elevates serum digoxin concentrations by decreasing clearance and volume of distribution; new

steady-state digoxin concentrations are approached in 4 to 5 digoxin elimination half-lives, *i.e.,* in about a week (Leahey *et al.,* 1978). A similar effect has been reported with digitoxin when serum concentrations were monitored for sufficiently long periods. Digitalis toxicity results so often when quinidine is being administered that it is routine to decrease the dose of digoxin if quinidine is started. Other drugs that increase serum digoxin concentration include verapamil, diltiazem, amiodarone, cyclosporine, itraconazole, propafenone, flecainide, and spironolactone. In these cases, the effect is less predictable, and digoxin concentrations regularly are measured and the dose adjusted only if necessary. One common mechanism underlying digoxin clearance appears to involve P-glycoprotein–mediated transport. Inhibition of this transport has been implicated as the mechanism whereby quinidine and other interacting drugs decrease digoxin clearance (Fromm *et al.,* 1999). Hypokalemia, which can be caused by many drugs (*e.g., diuretics, amphotericin B, corticosteroids*), will potentiate digitalis-induced arrhythmias.

Disopyramide.   *Disopyramide* (NORPACE, others; Morady *et al.,* 1982) exerts electrophysiological effects very similar to those of quinidine, but the drugs have different adverse-effect profiles. Disopyramide is used for the maintenance of sinus rhythm in patients with atrial flutter or atrial fibrillation and for the prevention of recurrence of ventricular tachycardia or ventricular fibrillation. Disopyramide is prescribed as a racemate. Its structure is given below.

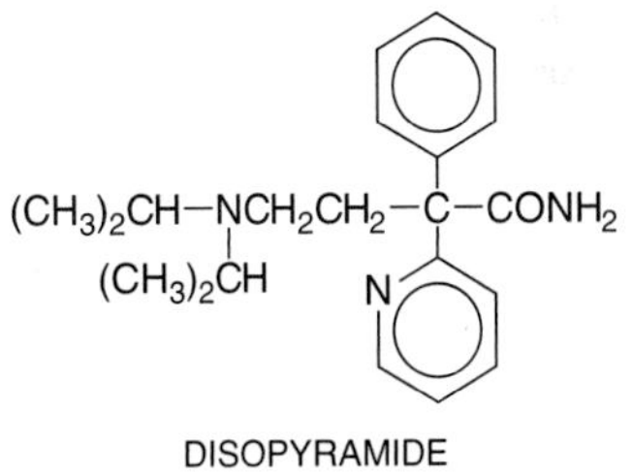

DISOPYRAMIDE

Pharmacological Actions and Adverse Effects.   The *in vitro* electrophysiological actions of S-(+)-disopyramide are similar to those of quinidine (Mirro *et al.,* 1981). The R-(−)-enantiomer produces similar Na^+ channel block but does not prolong cardiac action potentials. Unlike quinidine, racemic disopyramide is not an α-adrenergic receptor antagonist, but it does exert prominent anticholinergic actions, which account for many of its adverse effects. These include precipitation of glaucoma, constipation, dry mouth, and urinary retention; the latter is most common in males with prostatism but can occur in females.

Disopyramide commonly depresses contractility and can precipitate heart failure (Podrid *et al.*, 1980), and it can cause *torsades de pointes*.

Clinical Pharmacokinetics. Disopyramide is well absorbed. Binding to plasma proteins is concentration-dependent, so a small increase in total concentration may represent a proportionately larger increase in free drug concentration (Lima *et al.*, 1981). Disopyramide is eliminated by both hepatic metabolism (to a weakly active metabolite) and renal excretion of unchanged drug. The dose should be reduced in patients with renal dysfunction. Higher-than-usual dosages may be required in patients receiving drugs that induce hepatic metabolism, such as phenytoin.

Dofetilide. *Dofetilide* (TIKOSYN) is a potent and "pure" I_{Kr} blocker. As a result of this specificity, it has virtually no extracardiac pharmacological effects. Dofetilide is effective in maintaining sinus rhythm in patients with atrial fibrillation. In the DIAMOND studies (Torp-Pedersen *et al.*, 1999), dofetilide did not affect mortality in patients with advanced heart failure or in those convalescing from acute myocardial infarction. Dofetilide currently is available through a restricted distribution system that includes only those physicians, hospitals, and other institutions that have received special educational programs covering proper dosing and treatment initiation.

DOFETILIDE

Adverse Effects. *Torsades de pointes* occurred in 1% to 3% of patients in clinical trials, in whom strict exclusion criteria (*e.g.*, hypokalemia) were applied and continuous ECG monitoring was used to detect marked QT prolongation in the hospital. The incidence of this adverse effect during more widespread use of the drug, marketed in 2000, is unknown. Other adverse effects are no more common than with placebo.

Clinical Pharmacokinetics. Most of a dose of dofetilide is excreted unchanged by the kidneys. In patients with mild to moderate renal failure, decreases in dosage based on creatinine clearance are required to minimize the risk of *torsades de pointes*. The drug should not be used in patients with advanced renal failure and should not be used with inhibitors of renal cation transport. Dofetilide also undergoes minor hepatic metabolism.

Flecainide. The effects of *flecainide* (TAMBOCOR) therapy are thought to be attributable to the drug's very long $\tau_{recovery}$ from Na^+ channel block (Roden and Woosley, 1986a). In the CAST study, flecainide increased mortality in patients convalescing from myocardial infarction (CAST Investigators, 1989). However, it continues to be approved for the maintenance of sinus rhythm in patients with supraventricular arrhythmias, including atrial fibrillation, in whom structural heart disease is absent (Anderson *et al.*, 1989; Henthorn *et al.*, 1991). Encainide, a drug with very similar electrophysiological actions, is no longer available.

FLECAINIDE

Pharmacological Effects. Flecainide blocks Na^+ current and delayed rectifier K^+ current (I_{Kr}) at similar concentrations *in vitro*, 1 to 2 μM (Ikeda *et al.*, 1985; Follmer and Colatsky, 1990). It also blocks Ca^{2+} currents *in vitro*. Action potential duration is shortened in Purkinje cells (probably due to block of late-opening Na^+ channels) but prolonged in ventricular cells, probably due to block of delayed rectifier current (Ikeda *et al.*, 1985). Flecainide does not cause EADs *in vitro* or *torsades de pointes*. In atrial tissue, flecainide prolongs action potentials disproportionately at fast rates, an especially desirable antiarrhythmic drug effect; this effect contrasts with that of quinidine, which prolongs atrial action potentials to a greater extent at slower rates (Wang *et al.*, 1990). Flecainide prolongs the duration of PR, QRS, and QT, even at normal heart rates.

Adverse Effects. Flecainide produces few subjective complaints in most patients; dose-related blurred vision is the most common noncardiac adverse effect. It can exacerbate congestive heart failure in patients with depressed left ventricular performance. The most serious adverse effects are provocation or exacerbation of potentially lethal arrhythmias. These include acceleration of ventricular rate in patients with atrial flutter, increased frequency of episodes of reentrant ventricular tachycardia, and increased mortality in patients convalescing from myocardial infarction (Morganroth *et al.*, 1986; Crijns *et al.*, 1988; CAST Investigators, 1989; Ranger *et al.*, 1989). As discussed above, it is likely that all these effects can be attributed to Na^+ channel block. Flecainide also can cause heart block in patients with conduction system disease.

Clinical Pharmacokinetics. Flecainide is well absorbed. The elimination half-life is shorter with urinary acidification (10 hours) than with urinary alkalinization (17 hours), but it is nevertheless sufficiently long to allow dosing twice daily (*see* Table 35–5). Elimination occurs by both renal excretion of unchanged drug and hepatic metabolism to inactive metabolites. The latter is mediated by the polymorphically distributed enzyme CYP2D6 (Chapter 1) (Gross *et al.,* 1989). However, even in patients in whom this pathway is absent because of genetic polymorphism or inhibition by other drugs (*i.e.,* quinidine, fluoxetine), renal excretion ordinarily is sufficient to prevent drug accumulation. In the rare patient with renal dysfunction and lack of active CYP2D6, flecainide may accumulate to toxic plasma concentrations. Flecainide is a racemate, but there are no differences in the electrophysiological effects or disposition kinetics of its enantiomers (Kroemer *et al.,* 1989). Some reports have suggested that plasma flecainide concentrations >1000 ng/ml should be avoided to minimize the risk of flecainide toxicity; however, in susceptible patients, the adverse electrophysiological effects of flecainide therapy can occur at therapeutic plasma concentrations.

Ibutilide. *Ibutilide* (CORVERT; Murray, 1998) is an I_{Kr} blocker that in some systems also activates an inward Na^+ current. The action potential-prolonging effect of the drug may arise from either mechanism. Ibutilide is administered as a rapid infusion (1 mg over 10 minutes) for the immediate conversion of atrial fibrillation or flutter to sinus rhythm. The drug's efficacy rate is higher in patients with atrial flutter (50% to 70%) than in those with atrial fibrillation (30% to 50%). In atrial fibrillation, the conversion rate is lowest in those in whom the arrhythmia has been present for weeks or months compared with those in whom it has been present for days. The major toxicity with ibutilide is *torsades de pointes,* which occur in up to 6% of patients and requires immediate cardioversion in up to one-third of these. The drug undergoes extensive first-pass metabolism and so is not used orally. It is eliminated by hepatic metabolism and has a half-life of 2 to 12 hours (average of 6 hours).

IBUTILIDE

Lidocaine. *Lidocaine* (XYLOCAINE) is a local anesthetic that also is useful in the acute intravenous therapy of ventricular arrhythmias. When lidocaine was administered to all patients with suspected myocardial infarction, the incidence of ventricular fibrillation was reduced (Lie *et al.,* 1974). However, survival to hospital discharge tended to be decreased (Hine *et al.,* 1989), perhaps because of lidocaine-exacerbated heart block or congestive heart failure. Lidocaine is therefore no longer routinely administered to all patients in coronary care units.

LIDOCAINE

Pharmacological Effects. Lidocaine blocks both open and inactivated cardiac Na^+ channels. Findings from *in vitro* studies suggest that lidocaine-induced block reflects an increased likelihood that the Na^+ channel protein assumes a nonconducting conformation in the presence of drug (Balser *et al.,* 1996). Recovery from block is very rapid, so lidocaine exerts greater effects in depolarized (*e.g.,* ischemic) and/or rapidly driven tissues. Lidocaine is not useful in atrial arrhythmias, possibly because atrial action potentials are so short that the Na^+ channel is in the inactivated state only briefly compared with diastolic (recovery) times, which are relatively long (Hondeghem and Katzung, 1984). In some studies, lidocaine increased current through inward rectifier channels, but the clinical significance of this effect is not known. Lidocaine can hyperpolarize Purkinje fibers depolarized by low $[K]_o$ or stretch (Arnsdorf and Bigger, 1972); the resultant increased conduction velocity may be antiarrhythmic in reentry.

Lidocaine decreases automaticity by reducing the slope of phase 4 and altering the threshold for excitability. Action potential duration usually is unaffected or is shortened; such shortening may be due to block of the few Na^+ channels that inactivate late during the cardiac action potential. Lidocaine usually exerts no significant effect on PR or QRS duration; QT is unaltered or slightly shortened. The drug exerts little effect on hemodynamic function, although rare cases of lidocaine-associated exacerbations of heart failure have been reported, especially in patients with very poor left ventricular function.

Adverse Effects. When a large intravenous dose of lidocaine is administered rapidly, seizures can occur. When plasma concentrations of the drug rise slowly above the therapeutic range, as may occur during maintenance therapy, tremor, dysarthria, and altered levels of consciousness are more common. Nystagmus is an early sign of lidocaine toxicity.

Clinical Pharmacokinetics.   Lidocaine is well absorbed, but undergoes extensive, though variable, first-pass hepatic metabolism (Thompson *et al.,* 1973); thus, oral use of the drug is inappropriate. In theory, therapeutic plasma concentrations of lidocaine may be maintained by intermittent intramuscular administration, but the intravenous route is preferred (*see* Table 35–5). Lidocaine's metabolites, glycine xylidide (GX) and mono-ethyl GX (MEGX), are less potent as Na^+ channel blockers than the parent drug. GX and lidocaine appear to compete for access to the Na^+ channel, suggesting that, with infusions during which GX accumulates, lidocaine's efficacy may be diminished (Bennett *et al.,* 1988). With infusions lasting longer than 24 hours, the clearance of lidocaine falls—an effect that has been attributed to competition between parent drug and metabolites for access to hepatic drug-metabolizing enzymes (LeLorier *et al.,* 1977; Suzuki *et al.,* 1984).

Plasma concentrations of lidocaine decline biexponentially after a single intravenous dose, indicating that a multicompartment model (Chapter 1) is necessary to analyze lidocaine disposition. The initial drop in plasma lidocaine following intravenous administration occurs rapidly, with a half-life of ~8 minutes, and represents distribution from the central compartment to peripheral tissues. The terminal elimination half-life, usually ~100 to 120 minutes, represents drug elimination by hepatic metabolism. Lidocaine's efficacy depends on maintenance of therapeutic plasma concentrations in the central compartment. Therefore, the administration of a single bolus dose of lidocaine can result in transient arrhythmia suppression, but this effect dissipates rapidly as the drug is distributed and concentrations in the central compartment fall. To avoid this distribution-related loss of efficacy, a loading regimen of 3 to 4 mg/kg over 20 to 30 minutes is used—*e.g.,* an initial 100 mg followed by 50 mg every 8 minutes for three doses. Subsequently, stable concentrations can be maintained in plasma with an infusion of 1 to 4 mg/min, which replaces drug removed by hepatic metabolism. The time to steady-state lidocaine concentrations is ~8 to 10 hours. If the chosen maintenance infusion rate is too low, arrhythmias may recur hours after the institution of apparently successful therapy. On the other hand, if the rate is too high, toxicity may result. In either case, routine measurement of plasma lidocaine concentration at the time of expected steady state is useful in adjusting maintenance infusion rate.

In heart failure, the central volume of distribution is decreased, so the total loading dose should be decreased

(Thompson *et al.,* 1973). Since lidocaine clearance also is decreased, the rate of the maintenance infusion should be decreased. Lidocaine clearance is also reduced in hepatic disease (Thompson *et al.,* 1973), during treatment with cimetidine or β-blockers, and during prolonged infusions (Nies *et al.,* 1976; LeLorier *et al.,* 1977; Feely *et al.,* 1982). Frequent measurement of plasma lidocaine concentration and dose adjustment to ensure that plasma concentrations remain within the therapeutic range (1.5 to 5 μg/ml) are necessary to minimize toxicity in these settings. Lidocaine is bound to the acute phase reactant, α_1-acid glycoprotein. Diseases such as acute myocardial infarction are associated with increases in α_1-acid glycoprotein and protein binding, and hence a decreased proportion of free drug. These findings may explain why some patients require and tolerate higher-than-usual total plasma lidocaine concentrations to maintain antiarrhythmic efficacy (Alderman *et al.,* 1974; Kessler *et al.,* 1984).

Magnesium.   The intravenous administration of 1 to 2 g of $MgSO_4$ has been reported to be effective in preventing recurrent episodes of *torsades de pointes,* even if serum Mg^{2+} is normal (Tzivoni *et al.,* 1988). However, controlled studies of this effect have not been performed. The mechanism of action is unknown; since QT interval is not shortened, an effect on the inward current, possibly a Ca^{2+} current, responsible for the triggered upstroke arising from EADs (black arrow, Figure 35–6*B*) is possible (Jackman *et al.,* 1988; Roden, 1991b). Intravenous Mg^{2+} also has been used successfully in arrhythmias related to digitalis intoxication (Seller, 1971). Large, placebo-controlled trials of intravenous magnesium to improve outcome in acute myocardial infarction have yielded conflicting results (Woods and Fletcher, 1994; ISIS-4 Collaborative Group, 1995). While oral Mg^{2+} supplements may be useful in preventing hypomagnesemia, there is no evidence that chronic Mg^{2+} ingestion exerts a direct antiarrhythmic action.

Mexiletine and Tocainide.   *Mexiletine* (MEXITIL) and *tocainide* (TONOCARD) are analogs of lidocaine with structures that have been modified to reduce first-pass hepatic metabolism to make chronic oral therapy effective (Roden and Woosley, 1986b; Campbell, 1987). Their electrophysiological actions are similar to those of lidocaine. Tremor and nausea are the major dose-related adverse effects; these can be minimized by taking the drugs with food. Because tocainide can cause potentially fatal bone marrow aplasia and pulmonary fibrosis, it is rarely used.

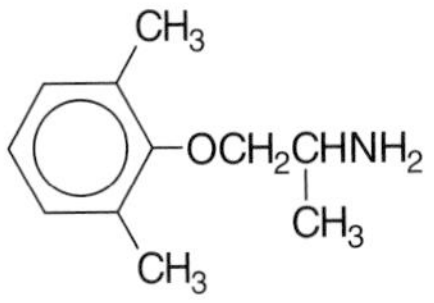

MEXILETINE

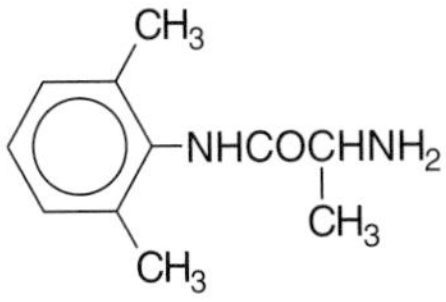

TOCAINIDE

Mexiletine undergoes hepatic metabolism, which is inducible by drugs such as phenytoin. Tocainide, on the other hand, is eliminated by renal excretion. Thus, in patients with renal disease, the dose of tocainide should be decreased. Both agents have been used for ventricular arrhythmias; combinations of mexiletine or tocainide with quinidine or sotalol may increase efficacy while reducing adverse effects. *In vitro* studies and clinical anecdotes have suggested a role for mexiletine (or flecainide) in correcting the molecular defect in the form of congenital long QT syndrome caused by abnormal Na^+ channel inactivation (Shimizu and Antzelevitch, 1997).

Moricizine.   *Moricizine* (ETHMOZINE) is a phenothiazine analog with Na^+ channel–blocking properties used in the chronic treatment of ventricular arrhythmias (Clyne *et al.*, 1992). In a randomized, double-blind trial (CAST II), moricizine increased mortality in patients shortly after a myocardial infarction and did not improve survival during long-term therapy (Cardiac Arrhythmia Suppression Trial II Investigators, 1992). Moricizine undergoes extensive first-pass hepatic metabolism; despite its short elimination half-life, its antiarrhythmic effect can persist for many hours after a single dose, suggesting that some of its metabolites may be active.

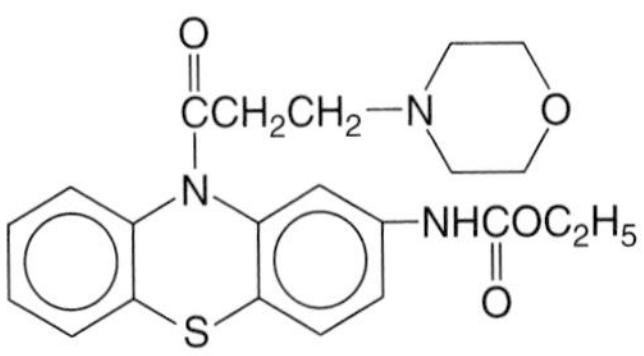

MORICIZINE

Phenytoin.   The anticonvulsant *phenytoin* (DILANTIN; Chapter 21) also is a blocker of inactivated cardiac Na^+

channels. It has been used in the acute and chronic suppression of ventricular arrhythmias and in digitalis intoxication (Atkinson and Davison, 1974). Phenytoin has a short $\tau_{recovery}$, and little QRS prolongation is observed during chronic therapy. Phenytoin undergoes extensive, saturable, first-pass hepatic metabolism; therefore, small increases in dose can produce large increases in plasma concentration and toxicity (Richens, 1979). Phenytoin is highly bound to plasma proteins, but the extent of its binding may vary. For example, in patients with renal disease, phenytoin binding falls from 90% to 80%, effectively doubling the free fraction of drug. Phenytoin toxicity may ensue if doses are adjusted on the basis of total rather than free drug concentrations. Symptoms of phenytoin toxicity include CNS complaints, such as ataxia, nystagmus, or mental confusion, and gingival hyperplasia; serious dermatological and bone marrow reactions can occur. With intravenous use, hypotension and ventricular fibrillation have been reported. Phenytoin is an inducer of the hepatic metabolism of many other drugs, including quinidine, mexiletine, digitoxin, estrogens, theophylline, and vitamin D (Richens, 1979).

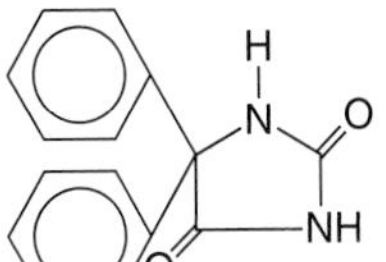

PHENYTOIN

Procainamide.   *Procainamide* (PROCAN SR; others) is an analog of the local anesthetic, procaine. It exerts electrophysiological effects similar to those of quinidine, but lacks quinidine's vagolytic and α-adrenergic blocking activity. Procainamide is better tolerated than quinidine when given intravenously. Loading and maintenance intravenous infusions are used in the acute therapy of many supraventricular and ventricular arrhythmias. However, long-term oral treatment is often stopped because of adverse effects.

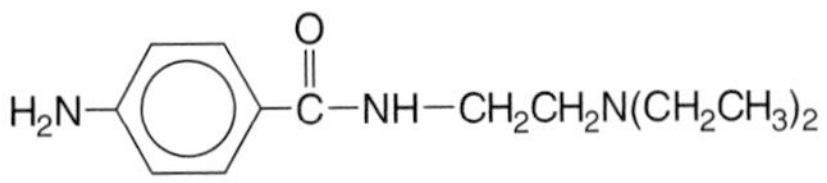

PROCAINAMIDE

Pharmacological Effects.   Procainamide is a blocker of open Na^+ channels, with an intermediate time constant of recovery from block. It also prolongs cardiac action potentials in most tissues, probably by blocking outward K^+ current(s). Procainamide decreases automaticity, increases refractory periods, and slows conduction. The major metabolite, *N*-acetyl procainamide, lacks the Na$^+$ channel–blocking activity of the parent drug but is equipotent in prolonging action potentials (Dangman and Hoffman, 1981). As the plasma concentrations of *N*-acetyl procainamide often exceed those of procainamide, increased refractoriness and QT prolongation during chronic procainamide therapy can be attributed at least in part to the metabolite. However, it is the parent drug that slows conduction and produces QRS interval prolongation. Although hypotension may occur at high plasma concentrations, this effect usually is attributable to ganglionic blockade rather than to any negative inotropic effect, which is minimal.

Adverse Effects. Hypotension and marked slowing of conduction are major adverse effects of high concentrations (>10 μg/ml) of procainamide, especially during intravenous use. Dose-related nausea is frequent during oral therapy and may be attributable in part to high plasma concentrations of *N*-acetyl procainamide. *Torsades de pointes* can occur, particularly when plasma concentrations of *N*-acetyl procainamide rise to >30 μg/ml. Procainamide produces potentially fatal bone marrow aplasia in 0.2% of patients; the mechanism is not known, but high plasma drug concentrations are not suspected.

During long-term therapy, most patients will develop biochemical evidence of the drug-induced lupus syndrome, such as circulating antinuclear antibodies (Woosley *et al.*, 1978). Therapy need not be interrupted merely because of the presence of antinuclear antibodies. However, many patients, perhaps as many as 25% to 50%, eventually will develop symptoms of the lupus syndrome; common early symptoms are rash and small-joint arthralgias. Other symptoms of lupus, including pericarditis with tamponade, can occur, although renal involvement is unusual.

Clinical Pharmacokinetics. Procainamide is rapidly eliminated ($t_{1/2} = 3$ to 4 hours) by both renal excretion of unchanged drug as well as by hepatic metabolism. The major pathway for hepatic metabolism is conjugation by *N*-acetyl transferase (*see* Chapter 1) to form *N*-acetyl procainamide. *N*-Acetyl procainamide is eliminated by renal excretion ($t_{1/2} = 6$ to 10 hours) and is not significantly converted back to procainamide. Because of the relatively rapid elimination rates of both the parent drug and its major metabolite, procainamide usually is administered as a slow-release formulation. In patients with renal failure, procainamide and/or *N*-acetyl procainamide can accumulate to potentially toxic plasma concentrations (Drayer *et al.*, 1977). Reduction of procainamide dose and dosing frequency and monitoring of plasma concentrations of both compounds are required in this situation. Because the parent drug and metabolite exert different pharma-

cological effects, the practice of using the sum of their concentrations to guide therapy is inappropriate.

In individuals who are slow acetylators the procainamide-induced lupus syndrome develops more often and earlier during treatment than among rapid acetylators (Woosley *et al.*, 1978). In addition, the symptoms of procainamide-induced lupus resolve during treatment with *N*-acetyl procainamide. Both of these findings support results of *in vitro* studies suggesting that it is chronic exposure to the parent drug (or an oxidative metabolite) that results in the lupus syndrome; these findings also provided one rationale for the further development of *N*-acetyl procainamide and its analogs as antiarrhythmic agents (Roden, 1993).

Propafenone. *Propafenone* (RYTHMOL) is a Na$^+$ channel blocker with a relatively slow time constant for recovery from block (Funck-Brentano *et al.*, 1990). Some data suggest that, like flecainide, propafenone also blocks K$^+$ channels. Its major electrophysiological effect is to slow conduction in fast-response tissues. The drug is prescribed as a racemate; while the enantiomers do not differ in their Na$^+$ channel–blocking properties, *S*-(+)-propafenone is a β-adrenergic receptor antagonist *in vitro* and in some patients. Propafenone prolongs PR and QRS durations. Chronic therapy with oral propafenone is used to maintain sinus rhythm in patients with supraventricular tachycardias, including atrial fibrillation; it also can be used in ventricular arrhythmias but, like other Na$^+$ channel blockers, it is only modestly effective.

PROPAFENONE

Adverse effects during propafenone therapy include acceleration of ventricular response in patients with atrial flutter, increased frequency or severity of episodes of reentrant ventricular tachycardia, exacerbation of heart failure, and the adverse effects of β-adrenergic blockade such as sinus bradycardia and bronchospasm (*see* above and Chapter 10).

Clinical Pharmacokinetics. Propafenone is well absorbed and is eliminated by both hepatic and renal routes. The activity of cytochrome P450 2D6 (CYP2D6), an enzyme that functionally is absent in $\sim$7% of Caucasians and African-Americans (Chapter 1), is a major determinant of plasma propafenone concentration, and thus the clinical action of the drug. In most subjects ("extensive metabolizers"), propafenone undergoes extensive first-pass hepatic metabolism to 5-hydroxy propafenone, a metabolite equipotent to propafenone as a Na^+ channel blocker but much less potent as a β-adrenergic receptor antagonist. A second metabolite, N-desalkyl propafenone, is formed by non-CYP2D6-mediated metabolism and is a less potent blocker of Na^+ channels and β-adrenergic receptors. CYP2D6-mediated metabolism of propafenone is saturable, so small increases in dose can lead to disproportionate increases in plasma propafenone concentration. In "poor metabolizer" subjects, in whom functional CYP2D6 is absent, the extent of first-pass hepatic metabolism is much less than in extensive metabolizers, and plasma propafenone concentrations are much higher. The incidence of adverse effects during propafenone therapy is significantly higher in poor than in extensive metabolizers. CYP2D6 activity can be markedly inhibited by a number of drugs, including quinidine and fluoxetine. In extensive metabolizer subjects receiving such inhibitors or in poor metabolizer subjects, plasma propafenone concentrations >1 μg/ml are associated with clinical effects of β-adrenergic receptor blockade, such as reduction of exercise heart rate (Lee et al., 1990; Mörike and Roden, 1994). It is recommended that dosage in patients with moderate to severe liver disease should be reduced to approximately 20% to 30% of the usual dose, with careful monitoring. It is not known if propafenone doses must be decreased in patients with renal disease.

Quinidine. As early as the eighteenth century, the bark of the cinchona plant was used to treat "rebellious palpitations" (Levy and Azoulay, 1994). Studies in the early twentieth century identified *quinidine,* a diastereomer of the antimalarial quinine, as the most potent of the antiarrhythmic substances extracted from the cinchona plant, and by the 1920s quinidine was used as an antiarrhythmic agent (Wenckebach, 1923). Quinidine is used for the maintenance of sinus rhythm in patients with atrial flutter or atrial fibrillation and in the prevention of recurrence of ventricular tachycardia or ventricular fibrillation (Grace and Camm, 1998).

QUINIDINE

Pharmacological Effects. Quinidine (QUINAGLUTE, QUINIDEX, others) blocks Na^+ current and multiple cardiac K^+ currents. It is an open-state blocker of Na^+ channels, with a time constant of recovery in the intermediate (~3 seconds) range; as a consequence, QRS duration increases modestly, usually from 10% to 20%, at therapeutic dosages. At therapeutic concentrations, quinidine routinely prolongs QT interval up to 25%, but the effect is highly variable. At concentrations as low as 1 μM, quinidine blocks Na^+ current and the rapid component of delayed rectifier (I_{Kr}); higher concentrations block the slow component of delayed rectifier, inward rectifier, transient outward current, and L-type Ca^{2+} current.

Quinidine's Na^+ channel-blocking properties result in an increased threshold for excitability and decreased automaticity. As a consequence of its K^+ channel–blocking actions, quinidine prolongs action potentials in most cardiac cells. This effect is most prominent at slow rates. In some cells, such as midmyocardial cells and Purkinje cells, quinidine consistently elicits EADs at slow heart rates, particularly when $[K]_o$ is low (Roden and Hoffman, 1985). Quinidine prolongs refractoriness in most tissues, probably as a result of both prolongation of action potential duration and its Na^+ channel blockade.

In the intact animal and in human beings, quinidine also produces α-adrenergic receptor blockade and vagal inhibition. Thus, the intravenous use of quinidine is associated with marked hypotension and sinus tachycardia. Quinidine's vagolytic effects tend to inhibit its direct depressant effect on AV nodal conduction, so that the effect of drug on the PR interval is variable. Moreover, quinidine's vagolytic effect can result in increased AV nodal transmission of atrial tachycardias such as atrial flutter (Table 35–1).

Adverse Effects. *Noncardiac.* Diarrhea is the most common adverse effect during quinidine therapy, occurring in 30% to 50% of patients. The mechanism is not known. Diarrhea usually occurs within the first several days of quinidine therapy, but can occur later. In mild cases of diarrhea in which quinidine therapy is deemed vital, antidiarrheal drugs can be used. Diarrhea-induced hypokalemia may potentiate *torsades de pointes* due to quinidine.

A number of immunological reactions can occur during quinidine therapy. The most common is thrombocytopenia, which can be severe but which resolves rapidly with discontinuation of the drug. Hepatitis, bone marrow depression, and a lupus syndrome occur rarely. None of these effects is related to elevated plasma quinidine concentrations.

Quinidine also can produce cinchonism, a symptom complex that includes headache and tinnitus. In contrast to other adverse events during quinidine therapy, cinchonism usually is related to elevated plasma quinidine concentrations, and can be managed by dose reduction.

Cardiac.   It is estimated that 2% to 8% of patients who receive quinidine therapy will develop marked QT-interval prolongation and *torsades de pointes*. In contrast to effects of sotalol, *N*-acetyl procainamide, and many other drugs, quinidine-associated *torsades de pointes* generally occur at therapeutic, or even subtherapeutic, plasma concentrations (Jackman *et al.,* 1988; Roden, 1991). The reasons for individual susceptibility to this adverse effect are not known.

At high plasma concentrations of quinidine, marked Na^+ channel block can occur, with resultant ventricular tachycardia. This adverse effect formerly occurred when very high doses of quinidine were used to try to convert atrial fibrillation to normal rhythm, but this aggressive approach to quinidine dosing has now been abandoned, and quinidine-induced ventricular tachycardia due to excess Na^+ channel block is unusual.

Quinidine can exacerbate heart failure or conduction system disease. However, in most patients with congestive heart failure, quinidine is well tolerated, perhaps because of its vasodilating actions.

Clinical Pharmacokinetics.   Quinidine is well absorbed and is 80% bound to plasma proteins including albumin and, like lidocaine, the acute phase reactant, α_1-acid glycoprotein. As with lidocaine, greater-than-usual doses (and total plasma quinidine concentrations) may be required to maintain therapeutic concentrations of free quinidine in high-stress states such as acute myocardial infarction (Kessler *et al.,* 1984). Quinidine undergoes extensive hepatic oxidative metabolism, and ~20% is excreted unchanged by the kidneys. One metabolite, 3-hydroxyquinidine, is nearly as potent as quinidine in blocking cardiac Na^+ channels or prolonging cardiac action potentials. Concentrations of unbound 3-hydroxyquinidine equal to or exceeding those of quinidine are tolerated by some patients. Other metabolites are less potent than quinidine, and their plasma concentrations are lower; thus, it is unlikely that they contribute significantly to the clinical effects of quinidine.

There is substantial individual variability in the range of dosages required to achieve therapeutic plasma concentrations of 2 to 5 μg/ml. Some of this variability may be assay-dependent, since not all assays have excluded quinidine metabolites. Among patients with advanced renal disease or advanced congestive heart failure, quinidine clearance is only modestly decreased. Thus, dosage requirements in these patients are similar to those in other patients.

Drug Interactions.   Quinidine is a potent inhibitor of CYP2D6. As a result, the administration of quinidine to patients receiving drugs that undergo extensive CYP2D6-mediated metabolism may result in altered drug effects due to accumulation of parent drug and failure of metabolite formation. For example, inhibition of CYP2D6-mediated metabolism of codeine to its active metabolite, morphine, results in decreased analgesia. On the other hand, inhibition of CYP2D6-mediated metabolism of propafenone results in elevated plasma propafenone concentrations and increased β-adrenergic receptor blockade. Quinidine reduces the clearance of digoxin and digitoxin; inhibition of P-glycoprotein–mediated digoxin transport has been implicated (Fromm *et al.,* 1999). This interaction is particularly important during the initiation of quinidine therapy in patients with atrial fibrillation, many of whom also are receiving digoxin (Leahey *et al.,* 1978).

Quinidine metabolism is inducible by drugs such as phenobarbital or phenytoin (Data *et al.,* 1976). In patients receiving these agents, very high doses of quinidine may be required to achieve therapeutic concentrations. It is important to note that, if therapy with the inducing agent is then stopped, quinidine concentrations may rise to very high levels, and its dosage must be adjusted downward. Cimetidine and verapamil elevate plasma quinidine concentrations, but these effects usually are modest.

Sotalol.   *Sotalol* (BETAPACE) is a nonselective β-adrenergic receptor antagonist that also prolongs cardiac action potentials by inhibiting delayed rectifier and possibly other K^+ currents (Hohnloser and Woosley, 1994). Sotalol is prescribed as a racemate; the *l*-enantiomer is a much more potent β-adrenergic receptor antagonist than the *d*-enantiomer, but the two are equipotent as K^+ channel blockers. Its structure is shown below:

$$CH_3SO_2NH-\langle\bigcirc\rangle-\overset{\overset{\displaystyle OH}{|}}{C}HCH_2NHCH(CH_3)_2$$

SOTALOL

In the United States, racemic sotalol is approved for use in patients with both ventricular tachyarrhythmias and atrial fibrillation or flutter. Clinical trials suggest that it is at least as effective as most Na^+ channel blockers in ventricular arrhythmias (Mason, 1993).

Sotalol prolongs action potential duration throughout the heart and QT interval on the ECG. It decreases automaticity, slows AV nodal conduction, and prolongs

AV refractoriness both by K^+ channel block and block of β-adrenergic receptors, but it exerts no effect on conduction velocity in fast-response tissue. Sotalol causes EADs and triggered activity *in vitro* (Strauss *et al.*, 1970) and can cause *torsades de pointes,* especially when serum K^+ is low. Unlike the situation with quinidine, the incidence of *torsades de pointes* seems to depend on the dose of sotalol, and in fact *torsades de pointes* are the major toxicity with sotalol overdose. Occasional cases occur at low dosages, often in patients with renal dysfunction, since sotalol is eliminated by renal excretion of unchanged drug. The other adverse effects of sotalol therapy are those associated with β-adrenergic receptor blockade (*see* above and Chapter 10).

PROSPECTUS

Recent and continuing elucidation of the mechanisms underlying normal and abnormal cardiac electrical behavior, along with clinical investigations clearly delineating the dangers of indiscriminate use of potent ion channel–blocking drugs in large groups of patients, have significantly altered therapeutic strategies for the treatment of arrhythmias. In some instances, nonpharmacological therapies are increasingly used to avoid the dangers of chronic drug therapy. Techniques for ablation of areas critical for the genesis of arrhythmias are now sufficiently well developed that chronic drug therapy can be avoided in many patients. When arrhythmia recurrence would be lethal and drugs may be incompletely effective, as in patients resuscitated from an episode of ventricular fibrillation, implanted defibrillators often are an appropriate choice. Among drugs discussed here, only β-blockers (and, to a lesser extent, amiodarone) reduce the incidence of sudden death. By contrast, while drugs with predominant ion channel–blocking properties can acutely terminate arrhythmias, long-term therapy has either increased or not altered the incidence of sudden death. Basic genetic, molecular, and cellular studies continue to improve our understanding of arrhythmia mechanisms; it is likely that this new knowledge will identify novel drug targets to intervene in specific ways to alleviate particular arrhythmic events and thus supplant currently available drugs.

For further discussion of cardiac arrhythmias, *see* Chapters 230 and 231 in *Harrison's Principles of Internal Medicine,* 14th ed., McGraw-Hill, New York, 1998.

BIBLIOGRAPHY

Akiyama, T., Pawitan, Y., Greenberg, H., Kuo, C.S., and Reynolds-Haertle, R.A. Increased risk of death and cardiac arrest from encainide and flecainide in patients after non-Q-wave acute myocardial infarction in the Cardiac Arrhythmia Suppression Trial. The CAST Investigators. *Am. J. Cardiol.,* **1991,** *68*:1551–1555.

Alderman, E.L., Kerber, R.E., and Harrison, D.C. Evaluation of lidocaine resistance in man using intermittent large-dose infusion techniques. *Am. J. Cardiol.,* **1974,** *34*:342–349.

Amiodarone Trials Meta-Analysis Investigators. Effect of prophylactic amiodarone on mortality after acute myocardial infarction and in congestive heart failure—meta-analysis of individual data from 6500 patients in randomised trials. *Lancet,* **1997,** *350*:1417–1424.

Anderson, J.L., Patterson, E., Conlon, M., Pasyk, S., Pitt, B., and Lucchesi, B.R. Kinetics of antifibrillatory effects of bretylium: correlation with myocardial drug concentrations. *Am. J. Cardiol.,* **1980,** *46*:583–592.

Anderson, J.L., Rodier, H.E., and Green, L.S. Comparative effects of beta-adrenergic blocking drugs on experimental ventricular fibrillation threshold. *Am. J. Cardiol.,* **1983,** *51*:1196–1202.

Anderson, J.L., Gilbert, E.M., Alpert, B.L., Henthorn, R.W., Waldo, A.L., Bhandari, A.K., Hawkinson, R.W., and Pritchett, E.L. Prevention of symptomatic recurrences of paroxysmal atrial fibrillation in patients initially tolerating antiarrhythmic therapy. A multicenter, double-blind, crossover study of flecainide and placebo with transtelephonic monitoring. Flecainide Supraventricular Tachycardia Study Group. *Circulation,* **1989,** *80*:1557–1570.

Antzelevitch, C., Sicouri, S., Litovsky, S.H., Lukas, A., Krishnan, S.C., Di Diego, J.M., Gintant, G.A., and Liu, D.W. Heterogeneity within the ventricular wall: electrophysiology and pharmacology of epicardial, endocardial, and M cells. *Circ. Res.,* **1991,** *69*:1427–1449.

Arnsdorf, M.F., and Bigger, J.T. Jr. Effect of lidocaine hydrochloride on membrane conductance in mammalian cardiac Purkinje fibers. *J. Clin. Invest.,* **1972,** *51*:2252–2263.

Balser, J.R., Nuss, H.B., Orias, D.W., Johns, D.C., Marban, E., Tomaselli, G.F., and Lawrence, J.H. Local anesthetics as effectors of allosteric gating. Lidocaine effects on inactivation-deficient rat skeletal muscle Na channels. *J. Clin. Invest.,* **1996,** *98*:2874–2886.

Bean, B.P., Two kinds of calcium channels in canine atrial cells. Differences in kinetics, selectivity, and pharmacology. *J. Gen. Physiol.,* **1985,** *86*:1–30.

Bennett, P.B., Woosley, R.L., and Hondeghem, L.M. Competition between lidocaine and one of its metabolites, glycylxylidide, for cardiac sodium channels. *Circulation,* **1988,** *78*:692–700.

Biaggioni, I., Killian, T.J., Mosqueda-Garcia, R., Robertson, R.M., and Robertson, D. Adenosine increases sympathetic nerve traffic in humans. *Circulation,* **1991,** *83*:1668–1675.

Brown, M.J., Brown, D.C., and Murphy, M.B. Hypokalemia from beta$_2$-receptor stimulation by circulating epinephrine. *N. Engl. J. Med.,* **1983,** *309:*1414–1419.

Cardiac Arrhythmia Suppression Trial II Investigators. Effect of the antiarrhythmic agent moricizine on survival after myocardial infarction. *N. Engl. J. Med.,* **1992,** *327:*227–233.

Cardinal, R., and Sasyniuk, B.I. Electrophysiological effects of bretylium tosylate on subendocardial Purkinje fibers from infarcted canine hearts. *J. Pharmacol. Exp. Ther.,* **1978,** *204:*159–174.

CAST Investigators. Preliminary report: effect of encainide and flecainide on mortality in a randomized trial of arrhythmia suppression after myocardial infarction. *N. Engl. J. Med.,* **1989,** *321:*406–412.

Chen, C.M., Gettes, L.S., and Katzung, B.G. Effect of lidocaine and quinidine on steady-state characteristics and recovery kinetics of (dV/dt)max in guinea pig ventricular myocardium. *Circ. Res.,* **1975,** *37:*20–29.

Crijns, H.J., van Gelder, I.C., and Lie, K.I. Supraventricular tachycardia mimicking ventricular tachycardia during flecainide treatment. *Am. J. Cardiol.,* **1988,** *62:*1303–1306.

Dangman, K.H., and Hoffman, B.F. In vivo and in vitro antiarrhythmic and arrhythmogenic effects of *N*-acetyl procainamide. *J. Pharmacol. Exp. Ther.,* **1981,** *217:*851–862.

Data, J.L., Wilkinson, G.R., and Nies, A.S. Interaction of quinidine with anticonvulsant drugs. *N. Engl. J. Med.,* **1976,** *294:*699–702.

DaTorre, S.D., Creer, M.H., Pogwizd, S.M., and Corr, P.B. Amphipathic lipid metabolites and their relation to arrhythmogenesis in the ischemic heart. *J. Mol. Cell Cardiol.,* **1991,** *23(Suppl 1):*11–22.

Davis, L.D., and Temte, J.V. Effects of propranolol on the transmembrane potentials of ventricular muscle in Purkinje fibers of the dog. *Circ. Res.,* **1968,** *22:*661–677.

Drayer, D.E., Lowenthal, D.T., Woosley, R.L., Nies, A.S., Schwartz, A., and Reidenberg, M.M. Cumulation of *N*-acetylprocainamide, an active metabolite of procainamide, in patients with impaired renal function. *Clin. Pharmacol. Ther.,* **1977,** *22:*63–69.

Dusman, R.E., Stanton, M.S., Miles, W.M., Klein, L.S., Zipes, D.P., Fineberg, N.S., and Heger, J.J. Clinical features of amiodarone-induced pulmonary toxicity. *Circulation,* **1990,** *82:*51–59.

Echizen, H., Vogelgesang, B., and Eichelbaum, M. Effects of *d,l*-verapamil on atrioventricular conduction in relation to its stereoselective first-pass metabolism. *Clin. Pharmacol. Ther.,* **1985,** *38:*71–76.

Echt, D.S., Black, J.N., Barbey, J.T., Coxe, D.R., and Cato, E. Evaluation of antiarrhythmic drugs on defibrillation energy requirements in dogs: sodium channel block and action potential prolongation. *Circulation,* **1989,** *79:*1106–1117.

Feely, J., Wilkinson, G.R., McAllister, C.B., and Wood, A.J. Increased toxicity and reduced clearance of lidocaine by cimetidine. *Ann. Intern. Med.,* **1982,** *96:*592–594.

Follmer, C.H., and Colatsky, T.J. Block of delayed rectifier potassium current, I_K, by flecainide and E-4031 in cat ventricular myocytes. *Circulation,* **1990,** *82:*289–293.

Fromm, M.F., Kim, R.B., Stein, C.M., Wilkinson, G.R., and Roden, D.M. Inhibition of P-glycoprotein-mediated drug transport: a unifying mechanism to explain the interaction between digoxin and quinidine. *Circulation,* **1999,** *99:*552–557.

Gross, A.S., Mikus, G., Fischer, C., Hertrampf, R., Gundert-Remy, U., and Eichelbaum, M. Stereoselective disposition of flecainide in relation to sparteine/debrisoquine metaboliser phenotype. *Br. J. Clin. Pharmacol.,* **1989,** *28:*555–566.

Heissenbuttel, R.H., and Bigger, J.T. Jr. Bretylium tosylate: a newly available antiarrhythmic drug for ventricular arrhythmias. *Ann. Intern. Med.,* **1979,** *90:*229–238.

Henthorn, R.W., Waldo, A.L., Anderson, J.L., Gilbert, E.M., Alpert, B.L., Bhandari, A.K., Hawkinson, R.W., and Pritchett, E.L. Flecainide acetate prevents recurrence of symptomatic paroxysmal supraventricular tachycardia. The Flecainide Supraventricular Tachycardia Study Group. *Circulation,* **1991,** *83:*119–125.

Herbette, L.G., Trumbore, M., Chester, D.W., and Katz, A.M. Possible molecular basis for the pharmacokinetics and pharmacodynamics of three membrane-active drugs: propranolol, nimodipine and amiodarone. *J. Mol. Cell Cardiol.,* **1988,** *20:*373–378.

Hille, B. Local anesthetics: hydrophilic and hydrophobic pathways for the drug-receptor reaction. *J. Gen. Physiol.,* **1977,** *69:*497–515.

Hine, L.K., Laird, N., Hewitt, P., and Chalmers, T.C. Meta-analytic evidence against prophylactic use of lidocaine in acute myocardial infarction. *Arch. Intern. Med.,* **1989,** *149:*2694–2698.

Hume, J.R., and Harvey, R.D. Chloride conductance pathways in heart. *Am. J. Physiol.,* **1991,** *261:*C399–C412.

Ikeda, N., Singh, B.N., Davis, L.D., and Hauswirth, O. Effects of flecainide on the electrophysiologic properties of isolated canine and rabbit myocardial fibers. *J. Am. Coll. Cardiol.,* **1985,** *5:*303–310.

ISIS-4 Collaborative Group. ISIS-4: a randomised factorial trial assessing early oral captopril, oral mononitrate, and intravenous magnesium sulphate in 58,050 patients with suspected acute myocardial infarction. ISIS-4 (Fourth International Study of Infarct Survival) Collaborative Group. *Lancet,* **1995,** *345:*669–685.

Kessler, K.M., Kissane, B., Cassidy, J., Pefkaros, K.C., Kozlovskis, P., Hamburg, C., and Myerburg, R.J. Dynamic variability of binding of antiarrhythmic drugs during the evolution of acute myocardial infarction. *Circulation,* **1984,** *70:*472–478.

Kowey, P.R., Levine, J.H., Herre, J.M., Pacifico, A., Lindsay, B.D., Plumb, V.J., Janosik, D.L., Kopelman, H.A., and Scheinman, M.M. Randomized, double-blind comparison of intravenous amiodarone and bretylium in the treatment of patients with recurrent, hemodynamically destabilizing ventricular tachycardia or fibrillation. The Intravenous Amiodarone Multicenter Investigators Group. *Circulation.,* **1995,** *92:*3255–3263.

Krapivinsky, G., Gordon, E.A., Wickman, K., Velimirovic, B., Krapivinsky, L., and Clapham, D.E. The G protein–gated atrial K$^+$ channel I_{KACh} is a heteromultimer of two inwardly rectifying K$^+$-channel proteins. *Nature,* **1995,** *374:*135–141.

Kroemer, H.K., Turgeon, J., Parker, R.A., and Roden, D.M. Flecainide enantiomers: disposition in human subjects and electrophysiologic actions in vitro. *Clin. Pharmacol. Ther.,* **1989,** *46:*584–590.

Leahey, E.B., Jr., Reiffel, J.A., Drusin, R.E., Heissenbuttel, R.H., Lovejoy, W.P., and Bigger, J.T., Jr. Interaction between quinidine and digoxin. *J.A.M.A.,* **1978,** *240:*533–534.

Lee, J.H., and Rosen, M.R. Use-dependent actions and effects on transmembrane action potentials of flecainide, encainide, and ethmozine in canine Purkinje fibers. *J. Cardiovasc. Pharmacol.,* **1991,** *18:*285–292.

Lee, J.T., Kroemer, H.K., Silberstein, D.J., Funck-Brentano, C., Lineberry, M.D., Wood, A.J., Roden, D.M., and Woosley, R.L. The role of genetically determined polymorphic drug metabolism in the beta-blockade produced by propafenone. *N. Engl. J. Med.,* **1990,** *322:*1764–1768.

LeLorier, J., Grenon, D., Latour, Y., Caillé, G., Dumont, G., Brosseau, A., and Solignac, A. Pharmacokinetics of lidocaine after prolonged intravenous infusions in uncomplicated myocardial infarction. *Ann. Intern. Med.,* **1977,** *87:*700–706.

Lerman, B.B., and Belardinelli, L. Cardiac electrophysiology of adenosine: basic and clinical concepts. *Circulation,* **1991,** *83:*1499–1509.

Levine, J.H., Moore, E.N., Kadish, A.H., Weisman, H.F., Balke, C.W., Hanich, R.F., and Spear, J.F. Mechanisms of depressed conduction from long-term amiodarone therapy in canine myocardium. *Circulation,* **1988,** *78:*684–691.

Lie, K.I., Wellens, H.J., van Capelle, F.J., and Durrer, D. Lidocaine in the prevention of primary ventricular fibrillation. A double-blind, randomized study of 212 consecutive patients. *N. Engl. J. Med.,* **1974,** *291:*1324–1326.

Lima, J.J., Boudoulas, H., and Blanford, M. Concentration-dependence of disopyramide binding to plasma protein and its influence on kinetics and dynamics. *J. Pharmacol. Exp. Ther.,* **1981,** *219:*741–747.

Makkar, R.R., Fromm, B.S., Steinman, R.T., Meissner, M.D., and Lehmann, M.H. Female gender as a risk factor for torsades de pointes associated with cardiovascular drugs. *J.A.M.A.,* **1993,** *270:*2590–2597.

Mason, J.W. A comparison of seven antiarrhythmic drugs in patients with ventricular tachyarrhythmias. Electrophysiologic Study versus Electrocardiographic Monitoring Investigators. *N. Engl. J. Med.,* **1993,** *329:*452–458.

Mirro, M.J., Watanabe, A.M., and Bailey, J.C. Electrophysiological effects of the optical isomers of disopyramide and quinidine in the dog. Dependence on stereochemistry. *Circ. Res.,* **1981,** *48:*867–874.

Morganroth, J., Anderson, J.L., and Gentzkow, G.D. Classification by type of ventricular arrhythmia predicts frequency of adverse cardiac events from flecainide. *J. Am. Coll. Cardiol.,* **1986,** *8:*607–615.

Mörike, K.E., and Roden, D.M. Quinidine-enhanced beta-blockade during treatment with propafenone in extensive metabolizer human subjects. *Clin. Pharmacol. Ther.,* **1994,** *55:*28–34.

Myerburg, R.J., Kessler, K.M., Cox, M.M., Huikuri, H., Terracall, E., Interian, A., Jr., Fernandez, P., and Castellanos, A. Reversal of proarrhythmic effects of flecainide acetate and encainide hydrochloride by propranolol. *Circulation,* **1989,** *80:*1571–1579.

Nies, A.S., Shand, D.G., and Wilkinson, G.R. Altered hepatic blood flow and drug disposition. *Clin. Pharmacokinet.,* **1976,** *1:*135–155.

Podrid, P.J., Schoeneberger, A., and Lown, B. Congestive heart failure caused by oral disopyramide. *N. Engl. J. Med.,* **1980,** *302:*614–617.

Ranger, S., Talajic, M., Lemery, R., Roy, D., and Nattel, S. Amplification of flecainide-induced ventricular conduction slowing by exercise. A potentially significant clinical consequence of use-dependent sodium channel blockade. *Circulation.,* **1989,** *79:*1000–1006.

Richens, A. Clinical pharmacokinetics of phenytoin. *Clin. Pharmacokinet.,* **1979,** *4:*153–169.

Roden, D.M., and Hoffman, B.F. Action potential prolongation and induction of abnormal automaticity by low quinidine concentrations in canine Purkinje fibers. Relationship to potassium and cycle length. *Circ. Res.,* **1985,** *56:*857–867.

Rosen, M.R., and Reder, R.F. Does triggered activity have a role in the genesis of cardiac arrhythmias? *Ann. Intern. Med.,* **1981,** *94:*794–801.

Ruskin, J.N. The cardiac arrhythmia suppression trial (CAST). *N. Engl. J. Med.,* **1989,** *321:*386–388.

Sanguinetti, M.C., and Jurkiewicz, N.K. Two components of cardiac delayed rectifier K$^+$ current: differential sensitivity to block by class III antiarrhythmic agents. *J. Gen. Physiol.,* **1990,** *96:*195–215.

Sanguinetti, M.C., Jurkiewicz, N.K., Scott, A., and Siegl, P.K. Isoproterenol antagonizes prolongation of refractory period by the class III antiarrhythmic agent E-4031 in guinea pig myocytes. Mechanism of action. *Circ. Res.,* **1991,** *68:*77–84.

Seller, R.H. The role of magnesium in digitalis toxicity. *Am. Heart J.,* **1971,** *82:*551–556.

Shimizu, W., and Antzelevitch, C. Sodium channel block with mexiletine is effective in reducing dispersion of repolarization and preventing torsade des pointes in LQT2 and LQT3 models of the long-QT syndrome. *Circulation,* **1997,** *96:*2038–2047.

Singer, D.E. Anticoagulation for atrial fibrillation: epidemiology informing a difficult clinical decision. *Proc. Assoc. Am. Physicians,* **1996,** *108:*29–36.

Stewart, R.B., Bardy, G.H., and Greene, H.L. Wide complex tachycardia: misdiagnosis and outcome after emergent therapy. *Ann. Intern. Med.,* **1986,** *104:*766–771.

Strauss, H.C., Bigger, J.T., Jr., and Hoffman, B.F. Electrophysiological and beta-receptor blocking effects of MJ 1999 on dog and rabbit cardiac tissue. *Circ. Res.,* **1970,** *26:*661–678.

Sung, R.J., Shapiro, W.A., Shen, E.N., Morady, F., and Davis, J. Effects of verapamil on ventricular tachycardias possibly caused by reentry, automaticity, and triggered activity. *J. Clin. Invest.,* **1983,** *72:*350–360.

Suzuki, T., Fujita, S., and Kawai, R. Precursor-metabolite interaction in the metabolism of lidocaine. *J. Pharm. Sci.,* **1984,** *73:*136–138.

Thompson, P.D., Melmon, K.L., Richardson, J.A., Cohn, K., Steinbrunn, W., Cudihee, R., and Rowland, M. Lidocaine pharmacokinetics in advanced heart failure, liver disease and renal failure in humans. *Ann. Intern. Med.,* **1973,** *78:*499–508.

Torp-Pedersen, C., Moller, M., Bloch-Thomsen, P.E., Kober, L., Sandoe, E., Egstrup, K., Agner, E., Carlsen, J., Videbaek, J., Marchant, B., and Camm, A.J. Dofetilide in patients with congestive heart failure and left ventricular dysfunction. Danish Investigations of Arrhythmia and Mortality on Dofetilide Study Group. *N. Engl. J. Med.,* **1999,** *341:*857–865.

Tseng, G.N., and Hoffman, B.F. Two components of transient outward current in canine ventricular myocytes. *Circ. Res.,* **1989,** *64:*633–647.

Tzivoni, D., Banai, S., Schuger, C., Benhorin, J., Keren, A., Gottlieb, S., and Stern, S. Treatment of torsade de pointes with magnesium sulfate. *Circulation,* **1988,** *77:*392–397.

Wang, Z.G., Pelletier, L.C., Talajic, M., and Nattel, S. Effects of flecainide and quinidine on human atrial action potentials. Role of rate-dependence and comparison with guinea pig, rabbit, and dog tissues. *Circulation,* **1990,** *82:*274–283.

Weiss, J.N., Nademanee, K., Stevenson, W.G., and Singh, B. Ventricular arrhythmias in ischemic heart disease. *Ann. Intern. Med.,* **1991,** *114:*784–797.

Wenckebach, K.F. Cinchona derivates in the treatment of heart disorders. *J.A.M.A.,* **1923,** *81:*472–474.

Wilde, A.A., and Janse, M.J. Electrophysiological effects of ATP sensitive potassium channel modulation: implications for arrhythmogenesis. *Cardiovasc. Res.,* **1994,** *28:*16–24.

Wit, A.L., Dillon, S.M., Coromilas, J., Saltman, A.E., and Waldecker, B. Anisotropic reentry in the epicardial border zone of myocardial infarcts. *Ann. N.Y. Acad. Sci.,* **1990,** *591:*86–108.

Woods, K.L., and Fletcher, S. Long-term outcome after intravenous magnesium sulphate in suspected acute myocardial infarction: the second Leicester Intravenous Magnesium Intervention Trial (LIMIT-2). *Lancet,* **1994,** *343:*816–819.

Woosley, R.L., Drayer, D.E., Reidenberg, M.M., Nies, A.S., Carr, K., and Oates, J.A. Effect of acetylator phenotype on the rate at which procainamide induces antinuclear antibodies and the lupus syndrome. *N. Engl. J. Med.,* **1978,** *298:*1157–1159.

Woosley, R.L., Reele, S.B., Roden, D.M., Nies, A.S., and Oates, J.A. Pharmacologic reversal of hypotensive effect complicating antiarrhythmic therapy with bretylium. *Clin. Pharmacol. Ther.,* **1982,** *32:*313–321.

MONOGRAPHS AND REVIEWS

Atkinson, A.J., Jr., and Davison, R. Diphenylhydantoin as an antiarrhythmic drug. *Annu. Rev. Med.,* **1974,** *25*:99–113.

Campbell, R.W. Mexiletine. *N. Engl. J. Med.,* **1987,** *316*:29–34.

Clyne, C.A., Estes, N.A. III, and Wang, P.J. Moricizine. *N. Engl. J. Med.,* **1992,** *327*:255–260.

Courtney, K.R. Progress and prospects for optimum antiarrhythmic drug design. *Cardiovasc. Drugs Ther.,* **1987,** *1*:117–123.

Connolly, S.J. Evidence-based analysis of amiodarone efficacy and safety. *Circulation,* **1999,** *100*:2025–2034.

DiFrancesco, D. Pacemaker mechanisms in cardiac tissue. *Annu. Rev. Physiol.,* **1993,** *55*:455–472.

Fozzard, H.A., and Arnsdorf, M.F. Cardiac electrophysiology In, *The Heart and Cardiovascular System: Scientific Foundations.* (Fozzard, H.A., Haber, E., Jennings, R.B., Katz, A.M., and Morgan, H.E., eds.) Raven Press, New York, **1991,** pp. 63–98.

Frishman, W.H., Murthy, S., and Strom, J.A. Ultra-short-acting beta-adrenergic blockers. *Med. Clin. North Am.,* **1988,** *72*:359–372.

Funck-Brentano, C., Kroemer, H.K., Lee, J.T., and Roden, D.M. Propafenone. *N. Engl. J. Med.,* **1990,** *322*:518–525.

Grace, A.A., and Camm, J. Quinidine. *N. Engl. J. Med.,* **1998,** *338*: 35–45.

Hohnloser, S.H., and Woosley, R.L. Sotalol. *N. Engl. J. Med.,* **1994,** *331*:31–38.

Hondeghem, L.M., and Katzung, B.G. Antiarrhythmic agents: the modulated receptor mechanism of action of sodium and calcium channel-blocking drugs. *Annu. Rev. Pharmacol. Toxicol.,* **1984,** *24*:387–423.

Jackman, W.M., Friday, K.J., Anderson, J.L., Aliot, E.M., Clark, M., and Lazzara, R. The long QT syndromes: a critical review, new clinical observations and a unifying hypothesis. *Prog. Cardiovasc. Dis.,* **1988,** *31*:115–172.

Levy, S., and Azoulay, S. Stories about the origin of quinquina and quinidine. *J. Cardiovasc. Electrophysiol.,* **1994,** *5*:635–636.

Mason, J.W. Amiodarone. *N. Engl. J. Med.,* **1987,** *316*:455–466.

Morady, F. Radio-frequency ablation as treatment for cardiac arrhythmias. *N. Engl. J. Med.,* **1999,** *340*:534–544.

Morady, F., Scheinman, M.M., and Desai, J. Disopyramide. *Ann. Intern. Med.,* **1982,** *96*:337–343.

Murray, K.T. Ibutilide. *Circulation,* **1998,** *97*:493–497.

Priori, S.G., Barhanin, J., Hauer, R.N., Haverkamp, W., Jongsma, H.J., Kleber, A.G., McKenna, W.J., Roden, D.M., Rudy, Y., Schwartz, K., Schwartz, P.J., Towbin, J.A., and Wilde, A. Genetic and molecular basis of cardiac arrhythmias; impact on clinical management. Study group on molecular basis of arrhythmias of the Working Group on Arrhythmias of the European Society of Cardiology. *Eur. Heart J.,* **1999,** *20*:174–195.

Roden, D.M. Long QT syndrome and torsades de pointes: basic and clinical aspects. In, *Cardiac Pacing and Electrophysiology* (El-Sherif, N., and Samet, P. eds.) W.B. Saunders, Philadelphia, **1991,** pp. 265–284.

Roden, D.M. Current status of class III antiarrhythmic drug therapy. *Am. J. Cardiol.,* **1993,** *72*:44B–49B.

Roden, D.M. Risks and benefits of antiarrhythmic therapy. *N. Engl. J. Med.,* **1994,** *331*:785–791.

Roden, D.M., Echt, D.S., Lee, J.T, and Murray, K.T. Clinical Pharmacology of antiarrhythmic agents. In, *Sudden Cardiac Death.* (Josephson, M.E., ed.) Blackwell Scientific, London, **1993,** pp. 182–185.

Roden, D.M., and Spooner, P.M. Inherited long QT syndromes: a paradigm for understanding arrhythmogenesis. *J. Cardiovasc. Electrophysiol.,* **1999,** *10*:1664–1683.

Roden, D.M., and Woosley, R.L. Drug therapy. Flecainide. *N. Engl. J. Med.,* **1986a,** *315*:36–41.

Roden, D.M., and Woosley, R.L. Drug therapy. Tocainide. *N. Engl. J. Med.,* **1986b,** *315*:41–45.

Schwartz, P.J., Priori, S.G., and Napolitano, C. Long QT syndrome. In, *Cardiac Electrophysiology: From Cell to Bedside.* 3rd ed. (Zipes, D.P., and Jalife, J., eds.) W.B. Saunders, Philadelphia, **2000,** pp. 615–640.

Singh, B.N. Advantages of beta blockers versus antiarrhythmic agents and calcium antagonists in secondary prevention after myocardial infarction. *Am. J. Cardiol.,* **1990,** *66*:9C–20C.

Singh, B.N. Arrhythmia control by prolonging repolarization: the concept and its potential therapeutic impact. *Eur. Heart J.,* **1993,** *14* (suppl H):14–23.

Smith, T.W. Digitalis. Mechanisms of action and clinical use. *N. Engl. J. Med.,* **1988,** *318*:358–365.

Snyders, D.J., Hondeghem, L.M., and Bennett, P.B. Mechanisms of drug-channel interaction. In, *The Heart and Cardiovascular System: Scientific Foundations.* (Fozzard, H.A., Haber, E., Jennings, R.B., Katz, A.M., and Morgan, H.E., eds.) Raven Press, New York, **1991,** pp. 2165–2193.

Task Force of the Working Group on Arrhythmias of the European Society of Cardiology. The Sicilian Gambit: a new approach to the classification of antiarrhythmic drugs based on their actions on arrhythmogenic mechanisms. *Circulation,* **1991,** *84*:1831–1851.

Vaughan Williams, E.M. Classifying antiarrhythmic actions: by facts or speculation. *J. Clin. Pharmacol.,* **1992,** *32*:964–977.

DRUG THERAPY FOR HYPERCHOLESTEROLEMIA AND DYSLIPIDEMIA

Robert W. Mahley and Thomas P. Bersot

Hyperlipidemia is a major cause of atherosclerosis and atherosclerosis-associated conditions, such as coronary heart disease, ischemic cerebrovascular disease, and peripheral vascular disease. This chapter covers the normal metabolism of lipoproteins, the pathophysiology of dyslipidemia and atherosclerosis, and drugs used to treat dyslipidemia. Drugs covered include HMG-CoA reductase inhibitors—the statins—which are the most effective and best-tolerated drugs currently in use for treating dyslipidemia; bile acid–binding resins; nicotinic acid (niacin); and fibric acid derivatives. The chapter concludes with a brief discussion of potential new classes of antidyslipidemic drugs that are undergoing clinical or preclinical evaluation.

Although the incidence of atherosclerosis-related vascular disease events is declining in the United States, coronary heart disease (CHD), ischemic cerebrovascular disease, and peripheral vascular disease still account for the majority of morbidity and mortality among middle-aged and older adults. Hyperlipidemia (hypercholesterolemia) is a major cause of increased atherogenic risk, and both genetic disorders and diets enriched in saturated fat and cholesterol contribute to the elevated lipid levels of our population and many other developed countries around the world.

Recognition of hypercholesterolemia as a risk factor has led to the development of drugs that reduce cholesterol levels. These drugs have been used in well-controlled studies of patients with high cholesterol levels caused primarily by elevated levels of low-density lipoproteins (LDL). The results of these trials indicate that CHD mortality is reduced by as much as 30% to 40% and that nonfatal events are similarly reduced when hypercholesterolemic patients are treated with moderate doses of hypolipidemic drugs [Scandinavian Simvastatin Survival Study Group, 1994; Shepherd *et al.,* 1995; The Long-Term Intervention with Pravastatin in Ischaemic Disease (LIPID) Study Group, 1998].

Clinical trial data support extending the benefit of lipid-lowering therapy to high-risk patients whose major lipid risk factor is a reduced plasma level of high-density-lipoprotein cholesterol (HDL-C) even if the LDL cholesterol (LDL-C) levels of these patients do not meet the existing threshold values for initiating hypolipidemic drug therapy (The Expert Panel, 1993). In patients with low HDL-C and average LDL-C levels, appropriate drug therapy reduced CHD endpoint events by 20% to 35% (Downs *et al.,* 1998; Rubins *et al.,* 1999). Since 40% of patients with CHD in the United States have low HDL-C levels, it is of obvious importance to include low-HDL patients in management guidelines for dyslipidemia, even if their LDL-C levels are in the "normal" range (Rubins *et al.,* 1995).

Hypertriglyceridemia (elevated levels of triglycerides), if severe (>1000 mg/dl), requires therapy to prevent pancreatitis. Moderately elevated triglyceride levels (150 to 400 mg/dl) also are of concern because they often occur as part of a syndrome distinguished by insulin resistance, obesity, hypertension, and substantially increased CHD risk. The atherogenic dyslipidemia in patients with this insulin resistance or metabolic syndrome is characterized by moderately elevated triglycerides, low HDL-C levels, and lipid-depleted LDL (sometimes referred to as "small, dense LDL") (Reaven, 1995; Grundy, 1998a). The metabolic syndrome is common in CHD patients; hence, identification of moderate hypertriglyceridemia in a patient, even if the total cholesterol level is normal, should trigger an evaluation to identify this disorder (National Cholesterol Education Program Expert Panel, 2001).

Hyperlipidemia (elevated levels of triglycerides or cholesterol) and reduced HDL-C levels occur as a consequence of several factors that affect the concentrations of the various plasma lipoproteins. These factors may be lifestyle or behavioral (*e.g.,* diet or exercise), genetic (*e.g.,* mutations in a gene regulating lipoprotein levels), or metabolic conditions (*e.g.,* diabetes mellitus) that influence plasma lipoprotein metabolism. An understanding of these factors requires a brief description of lipoprotein metabolism. More detailed descriptions can be found elsewhere (Breslow, 1994; Ginsberg and Goldberg, 1998; Mahley *et al.,* 1998).

PLASMA LIPOPROTEIN METABOLISM

Lipoproteins are macromolecules that contain lipids and proteins known as apolipoproteins or apoproteins. The lipid constituents include free and esterified cholesterol, triglycerides, and phospholipids. The apoproteins are very important since they provide structural stability to the lipoproteins, and a number of apoproteins function as ligands in lipoprotein–receptor interactions or are cofactors in enzymatic processes that regulate lipoprotein metabolism. In all spherical lipoproteins, the most water-insoluble lipids (cholesteryl esters and triglycerides) are core components, and the more polar, water-soluble components (apoproteins, phospholipids, and unesterified cholesterol) are located on the surface. Table 36–1 lists the major classes of lipoproteins and describes a number of their properties.

Table 36–2 provides information about apoproteins that have well-defined roles in plasma lipoprotein metabolism. These apolipoproteins include apolipoprotein (apo) A-I, apoA-II, apoA-IV, apoB-100, apoB-48, apoC-I, apoC-II, apoC-III, apoE, and apo(a). Except for apo(a), the lipid-binding regions of all apoproteins contain structural features called amphipathic helices that interact with the polar, hydrophilic lipids (such as surface phospholipids) and with the aqueous plasma environment in which the lipoproteins circulate. Differences in the non-lipid-binding regions are responsible for the functional specificities of the apolipoproteins.

Chylomicrons. Chylomicrons are synthesized from the fatty acids of dietary triglycerides and cholesterol absorbed from the small intestine by epithelial cells. Triglyceride synthesis is regulated by diacylglycerol transferase, an enzyme that regulates triglyceride synthesis in many tissues (Farese *et al.,* 2000). After they are synthesized in the endoplasmic reticulum, triglycerides are transferred by microsomal triglyceride transfer protein (MTP) to the site where newly synthesized apoB-48 is available to form chylomicrons. Dietary cholesterol is esterified by one of two forms of the enzyme acyl coenzyme A:cholesterol

acyltransferase (ACAT). This enzyme, ACAT-2, is found in the intestine and in the liver, where cellular free cholesterol is esterified before triglyceride-rich lipoproteins [chylomicrons and very-low-density lipoproteins (VLDL)] are assembled. In the intestine, ACAT-2 regulates the absorption of dietary cholesterol, and it may be a potential pharmacological target for reducing blood cholesterol levels (Cases *et al.,* 1998). [A second ACAT enzyme, ACAT-1, is expressed in macrophages, including foam cells, adrenocortical cells, and skin sebaceous glands. Although ACAT-1 esterifies cholesterol and promotes foam-cell development, ACAT-1 knockout mice do not have a reduced susceptibility for developing atherosclerosis (Accad *et al.,* 2000).]

Chylomicrons are the largest of the plasma lipoproteins and are the only lipoproteins that float to the top of a tube of plasma that has been allowed to stand undisturbed for 12 hours. The buoyancy of chylomicrons reflects their 98% to 99% fat content, of which 85% is dietary triglyceride. In chylomicrons, the ratio of triglycerides to cholesterol is ~10 or greater. In normolipidemic individuals, chylomicrons are present in plasma for 3 to 6 hours after a fat-containing meal has been ingested. After a fast of 10 to 12 hours, no chylomicrons remain.

The apolipoproteins of chylomicrons include some (apoB-48, apoA-I, and apoA-IV) that are synthesized by intestinal epithelial cells and others (apoE and apoC-I, C-II, and C-III) acquired from HDL after chylomicrons have been secreted into the lymph and enter the plasma (Table 36–2). The apoB-48 of chylomicrons is one of two forms of apoB present in lipoproteins. ApoB-48, synthesized only by intestinal epithelial cells, is unique to chylomicrons, whereas apoB-100 is synthesized by the liver and incorporated into VLDL and intermediate-density lipoproteins (IDL) and LDL, which are products of VLDL catabolism. The apparent molecular weight of apoB-48 is 48% that of apoB-100, which accounts for the name "apoB-48." This is because the amino acid sequence of apoB-48 is identical to the first 2152 of the 4536 residues of apoB-100. An RNA editing mechanism unique to the intestine accounts for the premature termination of the translation of the apoB-100 mRNA (Innerarity *et al.,* 1996). ApoB-48 does not contain the portion of the sequence of apoB-100 that allows apoB-100 to bind to the LDL receptor, so apoB-48 appears to function primarily as a structural component of chylomicrons.

After gaining entry to the circulation *via* the thoracic duct, chylomicrons are metabolized initially at the capillary luminal surface of tissues that synthesize lipoprotein lipase (LPL), a triglyceride hydrolase (Figure 36–1). These tissues include adipose tissue, skeletal and cardiac muscle, and breast tissue of lactating women. As the triglycerides are hydrolyzed by LPL, the resulting free fatty acids are taken up and utilized by the adjacent tissues. The interaction of chylomicrons and LPL requires apoC-II as an absolute cofactor that mediates the interaction of LPL and chylomicron triglycerides. The absence of functional LPL or functional apoC-II prevents the hydrolysis of triglycerides in chylomicrons and results in severe hypertriglyceridemia and pancreatitis during childhood or even infancy (chylomicronemia syndrome). Recently, a variety of new, potentially atherogenic roles for LPL have been identified that affect the metabolism and uptake of atherogenic lipoproteins by the liver, the arterial wall, and the dyslipidemia of insulin resistance (Mead *et al.,* 1999).

The concentration of chylomicrons can be controlled only by reducing dietary fat consumption. There is no current therapeutic

Table 36–1
Characteristics of Plasma Lipoproteins

LIPOPROTEIN CLASS	DENSITY OF FLOTATION, g/ml	MAJOR LIPID CONSTITUENT	TG/CHOL RATIO	SIGNIFICANT APOPROTEINS	SITE OF SYNTHESIS	MECHANISM(S) OF CATABOLISM
Chylomicrons and remnants	<<1.006	Dietary triglycerides and cholesterol	10:1	B-48, E, A-I, A-IV, C-I, C-II, C-III	Intestine	Triglyceride hydrolysis by lipoprotein lipase ApoE-mediated remnant uptake by liver
VLDL	<1.006	"Endogenous" or hepatic triglycerides	5:1	B-100, E, C-I, C-II, C-III	Liver	Triglyceride hydrolysis by lipoprotein lipase
IDL	1.006–1.019	Cholesteryl esters and "endogenous" triglycerides	1:1	B-100, E, C-II, C-III	Catabolic product of VLDL	50% converted to LDL mediated by hepatic lipase 50% apoE-mediated uptake by liver
LDL	1.019–1.063	Cholesteryl esters	NS	B-100	Catabolic product of VLDL	ApoB-100-mediated uptake by LDL receptor (~75% in liver)
HDL	1.063–1.21	Phospholipids, cholesteryl esters	NS	A-I, A-II, E, C-I, C-II, C-III	Intestine, liver, plasma	Complex: Transfer of cholesteryl ester to VLDL and LDL Uptake of HDL cholesterol by hepatocytes
Lp(a)	1.05–1.09	Cholesteryl esters	NS	B-100, apo(a)	Liver	Unknown

Abbreviations: apo, apolipoprotein; CHOL, cholesterol; HDL, high-density lipoproteins; IDL, intermediate-density lipoproteins; Lp(a), lipoprotein(a); LDL, low-density lipoproteins; NS, not significant (triglyceride is less than 5% of LDL and HDL); TG, triglyceride; VLDL, very-low-density lipoproteins.

Table 36–2
Apolipoproteins

APOLIPOPROTEIN	AVERAGE CONCENTRATION, mg/dl	CHROMOSOME	MOLECULAR MASS, kDa	SITES OF SYNTHESIS	FUNCTIONS
ApoA-I	130	11	~29	Liver, intestine	Structural in HDL; LCAT cofactor; ligand for HDL receptor; reverse cholesterol transport
ApoA-II	40	1	~17	Liver	Forms $-S-S-$ complex with apoE-2 and E-3, which inhibits E-2 and E-3 binding to lipoprotein receptors
ApoB-100	85	2	~513	Liver	Structural protein of VLDL, IDL, LDL; LDL receptor ligand
ApoB-48	Fluctuates according to dietary fat intake	2	~241	Intestine	Structural protein of chylomicrons
ApoC-I	6	19	~6.6	Liver	LCAT activator. Modulates receptor binding of remnants
ApoC-II	3	19	8.9	Liver	Lipoprotein lipase cofactor
ApoC-III	12	11	8.8	Liver	Modulates receptor binding of remnants
ApoE	5	19	34	Liver, brain, skin, gonads, spleen	Ligand for LDL receptor and receptors binding remnants; reverse cholesterol transport (HDL with apoE)
Apo(a)	Variable (under genetic control)	6	Variable	Liver	Modulator of fibrinolysis

Abbreviations: apo, apolipoprotein; HDL, high-density lipoproteins; IDL, intermediate-density lipoproteins; LCAT, lecithin:cholesterol acyltransferase; LDL, low-density lipoproteins; VLDL, very-low-density lipoproteins.

approach that will enhance chylomicron catabolism except for insulin replacement in patients with type I diabetes mellitus (insulin has a "permissive effect" on LPL-mediated triglyceride hydrolysis).

Chylomicron Remnants. After LPL-mediated removal of much of the dietary triglycerides, the chylomicron remnants, which still contain all of the dietary cholesterol, detach from the capillary surface and within minutes are removed from the circulation by the liver in a multistep process mediated by apoE (Figure 36–1) (Mahley and Ji, 1999). First, the remnants are sequestered by the interaction of apoE with heparan sulfate proteoglycans on the surface of hepatocytes and are processed by hepatic lipase (HL), which further reduces the remnant triglyceride content. Next, apoE mediates remnant uptake by interacting with the hepatic LDL receptor or the LDL receptor–related protein (LRP) (Krieger and Herz, 1994). The LRP is a receptor with multiple functions that recognizes a variety of ligands—including apoE, HL, and LPL—and several ligands unrelated to lipid metabolism. In plasma lipid metabolism, the LRP is important because it is the backup receptor responsible for the uptake of apoE-enriched remnants of chylomicrons and VLDL. Cell-surface heparan sulfate proteoglycans facilitate the interaction of apoE-containing remnant lipoproteins with the LRP, which mediates uptake by hepatocytes (Mahley and Huang, 1999). Inherited absence of either functional HL (very rare) or functional apoE impedes remnant clearance by the LDL receptor and the LRP, resulting in a hyperlipidemia characterized by an increase of triglyceride- and cholesterol-rich remnant lipoproteins in the plasma (type III hyperlipoproteinemia) (Mahley and Rall, 2001).

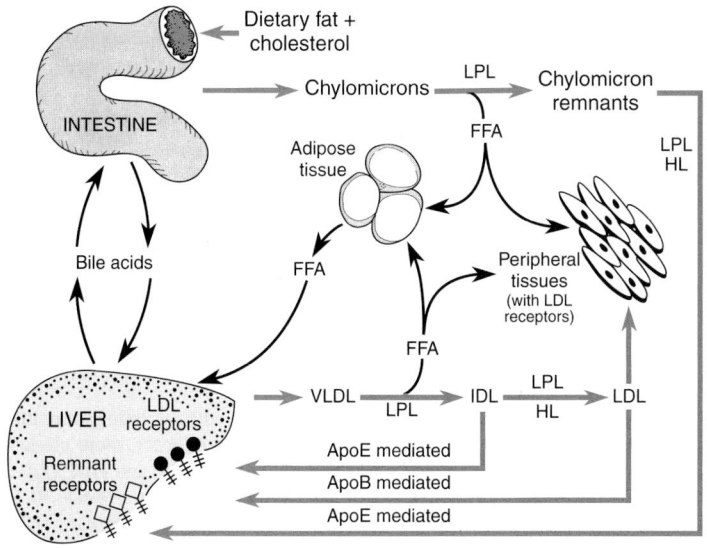

Figure 36–1. Summary of the major pathways involved in the metabolism of chylomicrons synthesized by the intestine and VLDL synthesized by the liver.

Chylomicrons are converted to chylomicron remnants by the hydrolysis of their triglycerides by LPL. Chylomicron remnants are rapidly cleared from the plasma by the liver. FFA released by LPL are used by muscle tissue as an energy source or taken up and stored by adipose tissue. FFA, free fatty acid; HL, hepatic lipase, IDL, intermediate-density lipoproteins; LDL, low-density lipoproteins; LPL, lipoprotein lipase; VLDL, very-low-density lipoproteins.

Chylomicron remnants are not precursors of LDL. However, during the initial hydrolysis of chylomicron triglycerides by LPL, apoA-I and phospholipids are shed from the surface of chylomicrons and remain in the plasma. This is one mechanism by which nascent (precursor) HDL are generated.

Very-Low-Density Lipoproteins. VLDL are produced in the liver and are synthesized when triglyceride production is stimulated by an increased flux of free fatty acids or by increased *de novo* synthesis of fatty acids by the liver. The VLDL are 400 to 1000 Å in diameter and are large enough to cause plasma turbidity, but VLDL particles, unlike chylomicrons, do not float spontaneously to the top of a tube of plasma that is allowed to stand undisturbed for 12 hours.

ApoB-100, apoE, and apoC-I, C-II, and C-III are synthesized constitutively by the liver and incorporated into VLDL (Table 36–2). If triglycerides are not available to form VLDL, the newly synthesized apoB-100 is degraded by hepatocytes. Triglycerides are synthesized in the endoplasmic reticulum and, along with other lipid constituents, are transferred by MTP to the site in the endoplasmic reticulum where newly synthesized apoB-100 is available to form nascent (precursor) VLDL. The nascent VLDL incorporate small amounts of apoE and the C apoproteins within the liver before secretion, but most of these apoproteins are acquired from plasma HDL after the VLDL are secreted by the liver.

Without MTP, hepatic triglycerides cannot be transferred to apoB-100. As a consequence, patients with dysfunctional MTP fail to make any of the apoB-containing lipoproteins (VLDL, IDL, or LDL). MTP also plays a key role in the synthesis of chylomicrons in the intestine, and mutations of MTP that result in the inability of triglycerides to be transferred to either apoB-100 in the liver or apoB-48 in the intestine prevent VLDL and chylomicron production and cause the genetic disorder abetalipoproteinemia (Gregg and Wetterau, 1994).

Plasma VLDL are then catabolized by LPL in the capillary beds in a process similar to the lipolytic processing described

for chylomicrons (Figure 36–1). When triglyceride hydrolysis is nearly complete, the VLDL remnants, usually termed IDL, are released from the capillary endothelium and reenter the circulation. ApoB-100–containing small VLDL and IDL (VLDL remnants), which have a half-life of less than 30 minutes, have two potential fates. About 40% to 60% are bound by LDL receptors or the LRP, which recognizes ligands (apoB-100 and apoE) on the remnants, and are cleared from the plasma primarily by the liver. The remainder of the IDL are further acted upon by LPL and HL—which remove additional triglycerides, C apoproteins, and apoE—and are converted to plasma LDL. Virtually all LDL particles in the plasma are derived from VLDL.

ApoE plays a major role in the metabolism of triglyceride-rich lipoproteins (chylomicrons, chylomicron remnants, VLDL, and IDL) and has a number of major functions related to the binding and uptake of plasma lipoproteins and to the redistribution of lipids locally among cells (Mahley and Rall, 2000; Mahley, 1988; Mahley and Huang, 1999). About half of the apoE in the plasma of fasting subjects is associated with triglyceride-rich lipoproteins, and the other half is a constituent of HDL. ApoE controls the catabolism of the apoE-containing lipoproteins by mediating their binding to cell-surface heparan sulfate proteoglycans (especially in the liver) and to LDL receptors and the LRP (Mahley and Ji, 1999).

About three-fourths of the apoE in plasma is synthesized by the liver and the remainder by a variety of tissues. The brain is the second most abundant site of apoE mRNA synthesis, which occurs primarily in astrocytes. ApoE also is synthesized by macrophages, where it appears to play a role in modulating cholesterol accumulation. In transgenic mice, overexpression of apoE by macrophages inhibits hypercholesterolemia-induced atherogenesis (Bellosta *et al.*, 1995; Hasty *et al.*, 1999).

There are three commonly occurring alleles of the apoE gene (designated ε2, ε3, and ε4) that occur with a frequency of ~8%, 77%, and 15%, respectively. These alleles code for the three major forms of apoE: E2, E3, and E4. Consequently, there are three homozygous apoE phenotypes (E2/2, E3/3, and E4/4) and three heterozygous phenotypes (E2/3, E2/4, and

E3/4). Approximately 60% of the population is homozygous for apoE3.

Single amino acid substitutions result from the genetic polymorphisms in the apoE gene (Mahley and Rall, 2000; Mahley, 1988). ApoE2, with a cysteine at residue 158, differs from apoE3, which has arginine at this site. ApoE3, with a cysteine at residue 112, differs from apoE4, which has arginine at this site. These single amino differences affect both receptor binding and lipid binding of the three apoE isoforms. Both apoE3 and apoE4 can bind to the LDL receptor, but apoE2 binds much less effectively and, as a consequence, causes the remnant lipoprotein dyslipidemia of type III hyperlipoproteinemia. ApoE2 and apoE3 bind preferentially to the phospholipids of HDL, whereas apoE4 binds preferentially to VLDL triglycerides.

Low-Density Lipoproteins.   The LDL particles arising from the catabolism of IDL have a half-life of 1.5 to 2 days, which accounts for the higher plasma concentration of LDL than of VLDL and IDL. In subjects without hypertriglyceridemia, two-thirds of plasma cholesterol is found in the LDL. Plasma clearance of LDL particles is mediated primarily by LDL receptors; a small component is mediated by nonreceptor clearance mechanisms (Brown and Goldstein, 1986). Defective or absent LDL receptors cause high levels of plasma LDL and familial hypercholesterolemia (Brown and Goldstein, 1986; Hobbs et al., 1992). ApoB-100, the only apoprotein of LDL, is the ligand that binds LDL to its receptor. Residues 3000 to 3700 in the carboxyl-terminal sequence are critical for binding. Mutations in this region disrupt binding and are a cause of hypercholesterolemia (familial defective apoB-100) (Innerarity et al., 1990; Pullinger et al., 1995).

The liver expresses a large complement of LDL receptors and removes ~75% of all LDL from the plasma (Dietschy et al., 1993). Consequently, manipulation of hepatic LDL receptor expression is a most effective way to modulate plasma LDL and cholesterol levels. Thyroxine and estrogen enhance LDL receptor gene expression, which explains the LDL-C-lowering effects of these hormones (Windler et al., 1980; Wiseman et al., 1993).

The most effective dietary (decreased consumption of saturated fat and cholesterol) and pharmacological (treatment with statins) treatments of hypercholesterolemia act by enhancing hepatic LDL receptor expression (Bilheimer et al., 1983; Woollett and Dietschy, 1994). Regulation of LDL receptor expression is part of a complex process by which cells regulate their free cholesterol content. This regulatory process is mediated by transcription factors called sterol regulatory binding element proteins (SREBPs) (Brown and Goldstein, 1998). SREBPs enhance LDL receptor expression when cellular cholesterol content is reduced.

LDL become atherogenic when they are modified by oxidation (Steinberg, 1997), a required step for LDL uptake by the scavenger receptors of macrophages. This process leads to foam-cell formation in arterial lesions. At least two scavenger receptors (SRs) are involved (SR-AI/II and CD36). Knocking out either receptor in transgenic mice retards the uptake of oxidized LDL by macrophages. Expression of the two receptors is differentially regulated; SR-AI/II appears to be more important in early atherogenesis, and CD36 more important as foam cells form during lesion progression (Nakata et al., 1999; Dhaliwal and Steinbrecher, 1999).

High-Density Lipoproteins.   The metabolism of HDL is complex because of the multiple mechanisms by which HDL particles are modified in the plasma compartment and by which HDL particles are synthesized (Breslow, 1994; Segrest et al., 2000; Tall et al., 2000). ApoA-I is the major HDL apoprotein, and its plasma concentration is a more powerful inverse predictor of CHD risk than is the HDL-C level (Maciejko et al., 1983).

ApoA-I synthesis is required for normal production of HDL. Mutations in the apoA-I gene that cause HDL deficiency are variable in their clinical expression and often are associated with accelerated atherogenesis (Assmann et al., 2001). Conversely, overexpression of apoA-I in transgenic mice protects against experimentally induced atherogenesis (Plump et al., 1994).

Mature HDL can be separated by ultracentrifugation into HDL_2 (d = 1.063 to 1.125 g/ml), which are larger, more cholesterol-rich lipoproteins (70 to 100 Å in diameter), and HDL_3 (d = 1.125 to 1.21 g/ml), which are smaller particles (50 to 70 Å in diameter). In addition, two major subclasses of mature HDL particles in the plasma can be differentiated by their content of the major HDL apoproteins, apoA-I and apoA-II (Duriez and Fruchart, 1999). Mature HDL particles have α electrophoretic mobility. Some α-migrating HDL particles contain only apoA-I and no apoA-II and are called LpA-I HDL particles. Others contain both apoA-I and apoA-II and are called LpA-I/A-II HDL particles. These two particles usually are separated by electroimmunoassay and quantitated by assessment of their apoA-I content (Duriez and Fruchart, 1999). LpA-I particles are larger than LpA-I/A-II and are primarily associated with HDL_2. LpA-I/A-II particles are smaller and are primarily associated with HDL_3. Patients with reduced HDL-C levels and CHD have lower levels of LpA-I, but not of LpA-I/A-II, than subjects with normal HDL-C levels (Duriez and Fruchart, 1999). This finding suggests that HDL particles containing apoA-I and apoA-II may not be atheroprotective. In fact, overexpression of apoA-II in transgenic mice enhances susceptibility to atherosclerosis (Schultz et al., 1993). ApoA-II deficiency is not associated with any apparent deleterious effects in human beings (Deeb et al., 1990).

The precursor of most of the plasma HDL is a discoidal particle containing apoA-I and phospholipid, called pre-β1 HDL because of its pre-β1 electrophoretic mobility. Pre-β1 HDL are synthesized by the liver and the intestine, and they also arise when surface phospholipids and apoA-I of chylomicrons and VLDL are lost as the triglycerides of these lipoproteins are hydrolyzed. Phospholipid transfer protein plays an important role in the transfer of phospholipids to HDL (Tall et al., 2000).

Discoidal pre-β1 HDL can then acquire free (unesterified) cholesterol from the cell membranes of tissues, such as arterial wall macrophages, by an interaction with the class B, type I scavenger receptor (SR-BI), to which the apoA-I of HDL docks, so that free cholesterol can be transferred to or from the HDL particle (Williams et al., 1999). SR-BI facilitates the movement of excess free cholesterol from cells with excess cholesterol (e.g., arterial wall foam cells) (Williams et al., 1999). In the liver, SR-BI facilitates the uptake of cholesteryl esters from the HDL without internalizing and degrading the lipoproteins. In mice, overexpression of SR-BI reduces susceptibility to atherosclerosis, and elimination of SR-BI significantly increases atherosclerosis (Krieger and Kozarsky, 1999).

A homologue of SR-BI, CLA-1, has been identified in human beings (Dhaliwal and Steinbrecher, 1999). Modulation of CLA-1 expression may offer new avenues for the management of atherogenesis (Krieger, 1999).

The membrane transporter ATP-binding cassette protein 1 (ABC-1) facilitates the transfer of free cholesterol from cells to HDL (Young and Fielding, 1999; Oram and Vaughan, 2000). When ABC-1 is defective, the acquisition of cholesterol by HDL is greatly diminished, and HDL levels are markedly reduced because poorly lipidated nascent HDL are metabolized rapidly. Dysfunctional mutants of ABC-1 cause the defect observed in Tangier disease, a genetic disorder characterized by extremely low levels of HDL and cholesterol accumulation in the liver, spleen, tonsils, and neurons of peripheral nerves.

After free cholesterol is acquired by the pre-β1 HDL, it is esterified by lecithin:cholesterol acyltransferase. The newly esterified and nonpolar cholesterol moves into the core of the discoidal HDL. As the cholesteryl ester content increases, the HDL particle becomes spherical and less dense. These newly formed spherical HDL particles (HDL$_3$) further enlarge by accepting more free cholesterol, which is in turn esterified by lecithin:cholesterol acyltransferase. In this way, HDL$_3$ are converted to HDL$_2$, which are larger and less dense than HDL$_3$.

As the cholesteryl ester content of the HDL$_2$ increases, the cholesteryl esters of these particles begin to be exchanged for triglycerides derived from any of the triglyceride-containing lipoproteins (chylomicrons, VLDL, remnant lipoproteins, and LDL). This exchange is mediated by the cholesteryl ester transfer protein and, in human beings, accounts for the removal of about two-thirds of the cholesterol associated with HDL. The transferred cholesterol subsequently is metabolized as part of the lipoprotein into which it was transferred. The triglyceride that is transferred into HDL$_2$ is hydrolyzed in the liver by HL, a process that regenerates smaller, spherical HDL$_3$ particles that recirculate and acquire additional free cholesterol from tissues containing excess free cholesterol.

HL activity is regulated and modulates HDL-C levels. Both androgens and estrogens affect HL gene expression, but with opposite effects (Haffner et al., 1983; Brinton, 1996). Androgens increase HL activity, which accounts for the lower HDL-C values observed in men than in women. Estrogens reduce HL activity, but their impact on HDL-C levels in women is substantially less than that of androgens on HDL-C levels in men. HL appears to have a pivotal role in regulating HDL-C levels, as HL activity is increased in many patients with low HDL-C levels.

HDL are protective lipoproteins that decrease the risk of CHD; thus, high levels of HDL are desirable. This protective effect may result from the participation of HDL in reverse cholesterol transport, the process by which excess cholesterol is acquired from cells and transferred to the liver for excretion. HDL also may inhibit oxidative modification of LDL through the action of paraoxonase, an HDL-associated antioxidant protein.

Lipoprotein(a).   Lipoprotein(a) [Lp(a)] is composed of an LDL particle that has a second apoprotein in addition to apoB-100 (Berg, 1994). The second apoprotein, apo(a), is attached to apoB-100 by at least one disulfide bond and does not function as a lipid-binding apoprotein. Apo(a) of Lp(a) is structurally related to plasminogen and appears to be atherogenic by interfering with fibrinolysis of thrombi on the surface of plaques.

HYPERLIPIDEMIA AND ATHEROSCLEROSIS

Despite a continuing decline in the incidence of atherosclerosis-related deaths in the past 35 years, deaths from CHD, cerebrovascular disease, and peripheral vascular disease accounted for 30% of the 2.3 million deaths in the United States during 1997. Two-thirds of atherosclerosis deaths were due to CHD. About 85% of CHD deaths occurred in individuals over 65 years of age. Among the 15% dying prematurely (below age 65), 80% died during their first CHD event. Among those dying of sudden cardiac death in 1997, 50% of the men and 63% of the women had been previously asymptomatic (American Heart Association, 1999).

These statistics illustrate the importance of identifying and managing risk factors for CHD. The major known risk factors are elevated LDL-C, reduced HDL-C, cigarette smoking, hypertension, type 2 diabetes mellitus, advancing age, and a family history of premature (men < 55 years; women < 65 years) CHD events in a first-degree relative. Control of the modifiable risk factors is especially important in preventing premature CHD (events in men below 55 years or in women below 65 years). Observational studies suggest that modifiable risk factors account for 85% of excess risk (risk over and above that of individuals with optimal risk-factor profiles) for premature CHD (Stamler et al., 1986; Wilson et al., 1998). Furthermore, these studies indicate that, when total cholesterol levels are below 160 mg/dl, CHD risk is markedly attenuated, even in the presence of additional risk factors (Grundy et al., 1998). This pivotal role of hypercholesterolemia in atherogenesis gave rise to the almost universally accepted cholesterol-diet-CHD hypothesis (Thompson and Barter, 1999).

The cholesterol-diet-CHD hypothesis states that elevated plasma cholesterol levels cause CHD, that diets rich in saturated fat (animal fat) and cholesterol raise cholesterol levels, and that the lowering of cholesterol levels reduces CHD risk. Although the relationship between cholesterol, diet, and CHD was recognized nearly 50 years ago, proof that cholesterol lowering was safe and prevented CHD death required extensive epidemiological studies and clinical trials.

Epidemiological Studies.   Epidemiological studies have demonstrated the importance of the relationship between excess saturated fat consumption and elevated cholesterol levels. Reducing the consumption of dietary saturated fat and cholesterol is the cornerstone of population-based approaches to the management of hypercholesterolemia (National Cholesterol Education Program, 1990). In addition, it is clearly established that the higher the cholesterol level, the higher the CHD risk (Stamler et al., 1986).

Clinical Trials. Studies of the efficacy of cholesterol lowering began in the 1960s. However, it was not until the advent of powerful cholesterol-reducing drugs known as *statins* that clear-cut evidence of the benefit of cholesterol lowering became available (Illingworth and Durrington, 1999). Several important trials in the 1970s and 1980s showed that average cholesterol reductions of about 10% resulted in 20% reductions in nonfatal CHD events, but these trials were not large enough to detect an effect on mortality (Lipid Research Clinics Program, 1984a; Committee of Principal Investigators, 1984; Frick *et al.,* 1987; Durrington and Illingworth, 1998). In fact, increases in noncardiac mortality in these trials raised concerns about the safety of cholesterol-lowering therapy (Wysowski and Gross, 1990).

In 1994, the Scandinavian Simvastatin Survival Study (4S), a secondary prevention trial, proved for the first time that lowering cholesterol levels with *simvastatin* reduced total mortality among CHD patients with normal HDL levels and high mean baseline LDL-C levels (188 mg/dl). Simvastatin therapy reduced LDL-C by an average of 35%, CHD mortality by 42%, nonfatal CHD events by 40%, and total mortality by 30%. Simvastatin therapy did not increase noncardiac mortality from any cause (Scandinavian Simvastatin Survival Study Group, 1994).

Subsequently, the efficacy and safety of statin therapy in patients with established CHD at baseline was evaluated in the Cholesterol and Recurrent Events (CARE) trial and the Long-Term Intervention with Pravastatin in Ischaemic Disease (LIPID) study [Sacks *et al.,* 1996; The Long-Term Intervention with Pravastatin in Ischaemic Disease (LIPID) Study Group, 1998]. In CARE and LIPID, the average baseline LDL-C and HDL-C levels (139 and 39 mg/dl in CARE and 150 and 36 mg/dl in LIPID) were lower than in 4S. Treatment with *pravastatin* reduced LDL-C levels by 25% (CARE) and 28% (LIPID) and was associated with a 24% reduction in CHD death in LIPID and 29% and 28% reductions in nonfatal myocardial infarctions in LIPID and CARE, respectively.

The results of the 4S, CARE, and LIPID trials indicated that CHD patients with baseline LDL-C values above 130 mg/dl benefit from lipid-lowering therapy. Subgroup analyses of patients in these trials with baseline LDL-C levels between 100 and 130 mg/dl did not consistently show a benefit from cholesterol-lowering drug therapy (Grundy, 1998b). More recently, however, the Veterans Affairs High Density Lipoprotein Intervention Trial (VA HIT) showed that CHD patients with LDL-C ≥ 104 mg/dl benefited from *gemfibrozil* therapy (Rubins *et al.,* 1999). **Taken together, however, the results of these four trials suggest that hypolipidemic drug therapy is beneficial in CHD patients with baseline LDL-C levels >100 mg/dl and that the goal of treatment of patients with CHD should be to reduce LDL-C to less than 100 mg/dl.**

There also have been clinical trials of lipid lowering in patients who had no evidence of vascular disease at baseline (primary prevention trials). The West of Scotland Coronary Prevention Study (WOSCOPS) (Shepherd *et al.,* 1995) demonstrated a benefit of *pravastatin* therapy in male patients with baseline LDL-C >155 mg/dl. The average LDL-C in WOSCOPS was high (192 mg/dl), and the mean HDL-C level was 44 mg/dl. The average on-treatment LDL-C was 142 mg/dl, a 26% decrease from baseline, and this resulted in a 31% reduction in CHD death and nonfatal myocardial infarction.

The second major statin trial in patients without vascular disease was the Air Force/Texas Coronary Atherosclerosis Pre-

vention Study (AFCAPS/TexCAPS) (Downs *et al.,* 1998). This trial included men and women who at baseline had only moderately elevated levels of LDL-C (average, 156 mg/dl) and who were primarily at risk because of age (men >45 years of age; women >55 years of age) and because of low HDL-C levels (average, 37 mg/dl). In this trial, *lovastatin* reduced LDL-C by 26% and primary endpoint events (fatal and nonfatal myocardial infarction and unstable angina pectoris) by 37%.

The trials described above provided evidence that supported the 2001 revision of the National Cholesterol Education Program (NCEP) guidelines for the management of dyslipidemic patients. These trials demonstrated efficacy in the prevention of vascular disease events and provided convincing evidence for the short-term (~5 years) safety of hypolipidemic therapy.

National Cholesterol Education Program Guidelines for Treatment: Managing Patients with Dyslipidemia

The current NCEP guidelines for management of patients with lipid disorders are of two types. One is a population-based approach, which is intended to lower blood cholesterol by dietary recommendations: Reduce total calories from fat to less than 30% and from saturated fat to less than 10%; consume less than 300 mg of cholesterol per day; and maintain desirable body weight (National Cholesterol Education Program, 1990). The second is the patient-based approach described in the 2001 report of the NCEP Adult Treatment Panel III, which continues to focus on lowering LDL-C levels as the primary goal of therapy (National Cholesterol Education Program Expert Panel, 2001). The 2001 Adult Treatment Panel III guidelines for the management of adults 20 years and older recommend a complete lipoprotein profile (total cholesterol, LDL-C, HDL-C, and triglycerides) rather than screening for total cholesterol and HDL-C alone. Fasting for 12 hours is required to accurately measure the triglyceride and LDL-C levels [LDL-C = total cholesterol − (triglyceride ÷ 5) − HDL-C]. The classification of lipid levels is shown in Table 36-3. If the values for total cholesterol, LDL-C, and triglycerides are in the lowest category and the HDL-C level is not low, lifestyle recommendations (diet and exercise) should be made to ensure maintenance of a normal lipid profile. Other vascular disease risk factors (Table 36-4), if present, should be assessed and treated individually. For patients with elevated levels of total cholesterol, LDL-C, or triglycerides, or reduced HDL-C values, further treatment is based on the patient's risk-factor status (Table 36-4) and LDL-C levels (Table 36-5).

All patients should receive instruction about dietary restriction of saturated fat and cholesterol. Patients with CHD or a CHD equivalent (symptomatic peripheral or

Table 36–3
Classification of Plasma Lipid Levels*

Total Cholesterol

<200 mg/dl	Desirable
200–239 mg/dl	Borderline high
≥240 mg/dl	High

HDL-C

<40 mg/dl	Low (consider <50 mg/dl as low for women)
>60 mg/dl	High

LDL-C

<100 mg/dl	Optimal
100–129 mg/dl	Near optimal
130–159 mg/dl	Borderline high
160–189 mg/dl	High
≥190 mg/dl	Very high

Triglycerides

<150 mg/dl	Normal
150–199 mg/dl	Borderline high
200–499 mg/dl	High
≥500 mg/dl	Very high

Abbreviations: HDL-C, high-density-lipoprotein cholesterol, LDL-C, low-density-lipoprotein cholesterol.
*2001 National Cholesterol Education Program guidelines.

Table 36–4
Risk Factors for Coronary Heart Disease*

Age
   Male > 45 years or female > 55 years

Family history of premature CHD
   A first-degree relative (male below 55 years or female below 65 years when the first CHD clinical event occurs)

Current cigarette smoking
Hypertension
   Blood pressure ≥ 140/90 or use of antihypertensive medication, irrespective of blood pressure

Low HDL-C
   < 40 mg/dl (consider < 50 mg/dl as "low" for women)

Obesity†
   Body mass index > 25 kg/m² and waist circumference above 40 inches (men) or 35 inches (women)

Abbreviations: CHD, coronary heart disease; HDL-C, high-density-lipoprotein cholesterol.
*Diabetes mellitus is considered to be a CHD-equivalent disorder; therefore, the lipid management of diabetes patients is the same as that for patients with established vascular disease (American Diabetes Association, 1999).
†Obesity was returned to the list of CHD risk factors in 1998, although it was not included as a risk factor in the 2001 National Cholesterol Education Program guidelines (Pi-Sunyer *et al.,* 1998).

Table 36–5
Treatment Based on LDL-C Levels (2001 National Cholesterol Education Program Guidelines)

	ADULTS	
	INITIATION LEVEL, mg/dl	GOAL, mg/dl
Lifestyle Modification		
No CHD and 0–1 other risk factor	> 160	< 160
No CHD plus 2 other risk factors	> 130	< 130
With CHD, or CHD equivalent	> 100	< 100
Drug Therapy		
No CHD and 0–1 risk factor	≥ 190	< 160
No CHD and 2+ risk factors		
<10% ten-year risk*	≥ 160	< 130
10%–20% ten-year risk*	≥ 130	< 130
CHD or CHD equivalent	> 100†	< 100

Abbreviations: CHD, coronary heart disease; CHD equivalent, peripheral vascular disease, abdominal aortic aneurysm, symptomatic carotid artery disease, >20% ten-year CHD risk, or diabetes mellitus; LDL-C, low-density-lipoprotein cholesterol.
*Ten-year risk calculated according to Framingham Risk Scoring Tables.
†Some experts require LDL-C ≥130 mg/dl to initiate drug therapy in CHD patients.

Table 36–6
Secondary Causes of Dyslipidemia

DISORDER	MAJOR LIPID EFFECT
Diabetes mellitus	Triglycerides > cholesterol; low HDL-C
Nephrotic syndrome	Triglycerides usually > cholesterol
Alcohol use	Triglycerides > cholesterol
Contraceptive use	Triglycerides > cholesterol
Estrogen use	Triglycerides > cholesterol
Glucocorticoid excess	Triglycerides > cholesterol
Hypothyroidism	Cholesterol > triglycerides
Obstructive liver disease	Cholesterol > triglycerides

Abbreviation: HDL-C, high-density-lipoprotein cholesterol.

carotid vascular disease, abdominal aortic aneurysm, >20% ten-year CHD risk or diabetes mellitus) should immediately start appropriate lipid-lowering therapy. Patients without CHD or CHD equivalent should be managed with lifestyle advice (diet, exercise, weight management) for 3 to 6 months before drug therapy is implemented.

Before drug therapy is initiated, however, secondary causes of hyperlipidemia should be excluded. Most secondary causes (Table 36–6) can be excluded by ascertaining the patient's medication history and by measuring serum creatinine, liver function tests, fasting glucose, and thyroid-stimulating hormone levels. Treatment of the disorder causing secondary dyslipidemia may preclude the necessity of treatment with hypolipidemic drugs.

Risk Assessment Using Framingham Risk Scores

The 2001 NCEP guidelines and those of the European Atherosclerosis Society (Wood *et al.,* 1998) employ risk assessment tables devised from the Framingham Heart Study in an attempt to match the intensity of treatment to the severity of CHD risk in patients without a prior history of symptomatic atherosclerotic vascular disease. High risk or "CHD equivalent" status is defined as >20% chance of sustaining a CHD event in the next ten years. The tables used to determine a patient's absolute risk do not take into account risk associated with a family history of premature CHD or obesity. As a consequence, the risk may be seriously underestimated, resulting in insufficiently aggressive management. After calculation of the risk score, more aggressive therapy should be considered for obese patients or for patients with a family history of premature CHD.

Arterial Wall Biology and Plaque Stability

More effective lipid-lowering agents and a better understanding of atherogenesis have helped to prove that aggressive lipid-lowering therapy has many beneficial effects over and above those obtained by simply decreasing lipid deposition in the arterial wall. Arteriographic trials have shown that, although aggressive lipid lowering results only in very small increases in lumen diameter, it promptly decreases acute coronary events (Brown *et al.,* 1993). Lesions causing less than 60% occlusion are responsible for more than two-thirds of the acute events. Aggressive lipid-lowering therapy may prevent acute events through its positive effects on the arterial wall; it corrects endothelial dysfunction, corrects abnormal vascular reactivity (spasms), and improves plaque stability.

Atherosclerotic lesions containing a large lipid core, large numbers of macrophages, and a poorly formed fibrous cap (Brown *et al.,* 1993; Gutstein and Fuster, 1999) are prone to plaque rupture and acute thrombosis. Aggressive lipid lowering appears to alter plaque architecture, resulting in less lipid, fewer macrophages, and a larger collagen and smooth muscle cell–rich fibrous cap. Stabilization of plaque susceptibility to thrombosis appears to be a direct result of LDL-C lowering or an indirect result of changes in cholesterol and lipoprotein metabolism or arterial wall biology (*see* below, "Potential Cardioprotective Effects Other Than LDL Lowering?").

Who and When to Treat?

Large-scale trials with statins have provided new insights into which patients with dyslipidemia should be treated and when treatment should be initiated.

Gender. Both men and women benefit from lipid-lowering therapy. In fact, CARE and AFCAPS/TexCAPS showed greater benefit in women. Statins, rather than hormone-replacement therapy, are now recommended by the American Heart Association and the American College of Cardiology as the first-line drug therapy for lowering lipids in postmenopausal women. This recommendation reflects the increased CHD morbidity in older women with established CHD who were treated with hormone-replacement therapy (Hulley *et al.,* 1998; Mosca *et al.,* 1999).

Age. Age >45 years in men and >55 years in women is considered to be a CHD risk factor. The statin trials have shown that patients >65 years of age benefit from therapy as much as do younger patients. Old age *per se* is not a reason to withhold drug therapy in an otherwise healthy person.

Cerebrovascular Disease Patients. In most studies of patients with cerebrovascular disease, plasma cholesterol levels correlate positively with risk of ischemic stroke. In clinical trials, statins reduced stroke and/or transient ischemic attacks in patients with and without CHD (Hebert *et al.*, 1997).

Peripheral Vascular Disease Patients. Statins have proved beneficial in patients with peripheral vascular disease.

Hypertensive Patients and Smokers. The risk reduction for coronary events in hypertensive patients and in smokers is similar to that in subjects without these risk factors.

Type 2 Diabetes Mellitus. Patients with type 2 diabetes benefit very significantly from aggressive lipid lowering (*see* "Treatment of Type 2 Diabetes," below).

Post–Myocardial Infarction or Revascularization Patients. As soon as CHD is diagnosed, it is essential to begin lipid-lowering therapy (NCEP guidelines: LDL-C < 100 mg/dl). Compliance with drug therapy is greatly enhanced if treatment is initiated in the hospital (Fonarow and Gawlinski, 2000). It remains to be determined if statin therapy alters restenosis after angioplasty; however, the NHLBI Post Coronary Artery Bypass Graft trial showed that statin therapy improved the long-term outcome after bypass surgery and that the lower the LDL-C, the better (The Post Coronary Artery Bypass Graft Trial Investigators, 1997).

Can Cholesterol Levels Be Lowered Too Much?

Are there total and LDL cholesterol levels below which adverse health consequences begin to increase? Observational studies initially were confusing. In the United States and western Europe, low cholesterol levels appeared to be associated with an increase in noncardiac mortality from chronic pulmonary disease, chronic liver disease, cancer (many primary sites), and hemorrhagic stroke. However, more recent data indicate that it is the noncardiac diseases that cause the low plasma cholesterol levels and not the low cholesterol levels that cause the noncardiac diseases (Law *et al.*, 1994). One exception may be hemorrhagic stroke. In the Multiple Risk Factor Intervention Trial (MRFIT), hemorrhagic stroke occurred more frequently in hypertensive patients with total cholesterol levels below 160 mg/dl; however, the increased incidence of hemorrhagic stroke was more than offset by reduced CHD risk due to the low cholesterol levels (Neaton *et al.*, 1992). In addition, in a study of the Chinese population, in which cholesterol levels rarely exceeded 160 mg/dl, lower levels of total cholesterol were not associated with increases in hemorrhagic stroke or any other cause of noncardiac mortality (Chen *et al.*, 1991).

Abetalipoproteinemia and hypobetalipoproteinemia, two rare disorders in human beings that are associated with extremely low total cholesterol levels, are instructive because affected individuals have reduced CHD risk and no increase in noncardiac mortality (Welty *et al.*, 1998). Patients who are homozygous for the mutations that cause these disorders have total cholesterol levels below 50 mg/dl and triglyceride levels below 25 mg/dl.

Individuals consuming very low levels of total fat (less than 5% of total calories) and vegetarians, who consume no animal fat, usually have total cholesterol levels below 150 mg/dl and have no increase in noncardiac mortality (Appleby *et al.*, 1999).

Based on the lack of harm associated with low total cholesterol levels in these various groups, reducing cholesterol levels to similarly low levels with drugs does not appear to be contraindicated. With the advent of more efficacious cholesterol-lowering agents, it soon may be possible to test the benefits and risks of lowering total cholesterol levels below 150 mg/dl.

Will Greater Lipid Lowering Further Reduce CHD?

Despite the remarkable results of the statin trials (a 25% to 40% reduction in events), there are still 60% to 75% as many events in the treatment groups of the statin trials as in the placebo groups. Do these results suggest that even more aggressive lipid lowering is required (Grundy, 1998b)? The investigators who conducted the AFCAPS/TexCAPS trial suggested that the 1993 NCEP guidelines are still too conservative for high-risk subjects without CHD, like those enrolled in the AFCAPS/TexCAPS study (Downs *et al.*, 1998). They state that drug therapy—along with a prudent diet, regular exercise, and risk factor modification—should be used to lower the risk of the first acute major coronary event in primary prevention candidates who are older (men ≥45 years, women ≥55 years), have HDL-C ≤50 mg/dl, and have LDL-C ≥130 mg/dl. However, subgroup analysis of baseline HDL-C levels in AFCAPS/TexCAPS indicated that only patients with HDL-C <40 mg/dl benefited, suggesting that it may not be cost-effective to treat patients with risk factor profiles like those in AFCAPS/TexCAPS if HDL-C exceeds 40 mg/dl. The 2001 NCEP guidelines would not initiate treatment of many patients like those in AFCAPS/TexCAPS unless the LDL-C was >160 mg/dl in patients without CHD, and the 2001 NCEP guidelines have a higher target LDL-C level than AFCAPS/TexCAPS (130 *versus* <110 mg/dl).

As more effective lipid-lowering drugs and better combinations of therapies are developed, we will be able to lower lipid levels more effectively. But will lower cholesterol levels translate into a further reduction of clinical events (Figure 36–2)? Many researchers believe that the answer is *yes*. In addition, as statins become generic drugs, more aggressive treatment of wider segments of the population will become more cost-effective.

Treatment of Type 2 Diabetes

Diabetes mellitus is an independent predictor of high risk for CHD. CHD morbidity is two to four times higher in patients with diabetes than in nondiabetics, and the mortality from CHD is up to 100% higher in diabetic patients than in nondiabetics over a 6-year period (Grundy *et al.*, 1999). Glucose control is essential, but this provides only minimal benefit with respect to CHD prevention. Aggressive

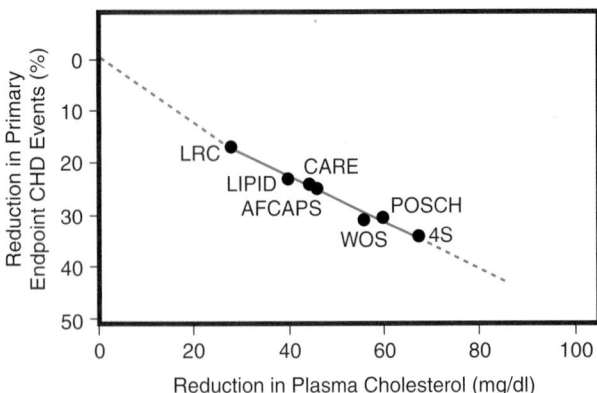

Figure 36–2. Reduction in coronary heart disease events in clinical trials is associated with the extent of cholesterol lowering. As more potent cholesterol-reducing agents become available, will it be possible to reduce events by 50% or more in a typical 5-year trial? (Adapted from Thompson and Barter, 1999, and used by permission of Lippincott Williams & Wilkins.)

AFCAPS, Air Force/Texas Coronary Atherosclerosis Prevention Study; CARE, Cholesterol and Recurrent Events trial; LIPID, Long-Term Intervention with Pravastatin in Ischaemic Disease (LIPID) study; LRC, Lipid Research Clinics Coronary Primary Prevention Trial; POSCH, Program on the Surgical Control of the Hyperlipidemias; 4S, Scandinavian Simvastatin Survival Study; WOS, West of Scotland Coronary Prevention Study.

treatment of diabetic dyslipidemia through diet, weight control, and drugs (in most cases) is critical in reducing risk.

Diabetic dyslipidemia is usually characterized by high triglycerides, low HDL-C, and moderate elevations of total cholesterol and LDL-C. Recent recommendations from the American Heart Association and the American Diabetes Association indicate that the treatment guidelines for diabetic patients should be the same as for patients with CHD (Grundy *et al.*, 1999). The revised 2001 NCEP guidelines also will reflect this recommendation. Haffner *et al.* (1998) reported that diabetics without diagnosed CHD are at the same level of risk as nondiabetics with established CHD. This is consistent with the recommendation to reduce plasma LDL-C levels of all diabetics to <100 mg/dl, irrespective of whether they have had a prior ischemic vascular disease event. The American Diabetes Association further recommends that the first line of treatment for a diabetic dyslipidemia usually should be a statin (Grundy *et al.*, 1999).

Clinical trials with simvastatin, pravastatin, and lovastatin have clearly established in *post hoc* analyses that diabetics profit from cholesterol lowering as much as other

subgroups or even more. For example, diabetics in the 4S, CARE, AFCAPS/TexCAPS, and LIPID trials had 55%, 25%, 43%, and 19% reductions in events, respectively. The Diabetes Atherosclerosis Intervention Study recently showed a significant benefit of treating type 2 diabetics with *fenofibrate*. This 3-year arteriographic study demonstrated a 40% decrease of focal coronary stenoses ($p = 0.029$) (Diabetes Atherosclerosis Intervention Study Investigators, 2001).

Metabolic Syndrome

The 2001 NCEP guidelines recognize the increased CHD risk associated with the insulin-resistant, prediabetic state described under the rubric of "metabolic syndrome." This syndrome consists of a constellation of five CHD risk factors (Table 36–7). The 2001 NCEP guidelines arbitrarily define the presence of three or more of these risk factors as indicating that a patient is affected. Treatment should focus on weight loss and increased physical activity since overweight and obesity usually preclude optimal risk factor reduction. Specific treatment of increased LDL-C and triglyceride levels and low HDL-C levels should be undertaken as well.

Table 36–7
Clinical Identification of the Metabolic Syndrome

Risk Factor	Defining Level
Abdominal obesity*	Waist circumference†
Men	>102 cm (>40 in)
Women	>88 cm (>35 in)
Triglycerides	≥150 mg/dl
HDL-C	
Men	<40 mg/dl
Women	<50 mg/dl
Blood pressure	≥130/≥85 mm Hg
Fasting glucose	>110 mg/dl†

Abbreviation: HDL-C, high-density-lipoprotein cholesterol.

*Overweight and obesity are associated with insulin resistance and the metabolic syndrome. However, the presence of abdominal obesity is more highly correlated with the metabolic risk factors than is an elevated body mass index. Therefore, the simple measurement of waist circumference is recommended to identify the body weight component of the metabolic syndrome.

†Some male patients can develop multiple metabolic risk factors when the waist circumference is only marginally increased [e.g., 94–102 cm (37–39 in)]. Such patients may have a strong genetic contribution to insulin resistance, and like men with categorical increases in waist circumference, they should benefit from changes in life habits.

Treatment of Hypertriglyceridemia

The 2001 NCEP guidelines reflect the increased CHD risk associated with the presence of triglyceride levels above 150 mg/dl. Three categories of hypertriglyceridemia are recognized (Table 36–3), and treatment is recommended based on the degree of elevation. Weight loss, increased exercise, and alcohol restriction are important for all hyper-triglyceridemic patients. The LDL-C goal should be ascertained based on each patient's risk factor or CHD status (Table 36–5). If triglycerides remain above 200 mg/dl after the LDL-C goal is reached, further reduction in triglyc-erides may be achieved by increasing the dose of a statin or of niacin. Combination therapy (statin plus niacin or statin plus fibrate) may be required, but caution is necessary with these combinations to avoid myopathy (see Statins in Combination with Other Lipid-lowering Drugs, below).

Treatment of Low HDL-C

The most frequent risk factor for premature CHD is low HDL-C. In a study of 321 men with angiographically doc-umented CHD, ~60% had HDL-C levels of <35 mg/dl and only 25% had LDL-C >160 mg/dl (Genest *et al.*, 1991). In a separate study of more than 8500 older men with CHD, 38% had HDL-C levels <35 mg/dl (Rubins *et al.*, 1995). Data from the Framingham Heart Study demonstrate that subjects with "normal" cholesterol levels of <200 mg/dl but with low HDL-C (<40 mg/dl) have as much CHD risk as subjects with higher total cholesterol levels (230 to 260 mg/dl) and more normal HDL-C (40 to 49 mg/dl) (Castelli *et al.*, 1986).

In low-HDL-C patients, the total cholesterol/HDL-C ratio is a particularly useful predictor of CHD risk. The Framingham data indicate that the ideal ratio is ≤3.5 and a ratio of >4.5 is associated with increased risk (Castelli, 1994). American men, who are a high-risk group, have a typical ratio of ~4.5. Patients with low HDL-C may have what are considered to be "normal" total and LDL cholesterol levels and would not qualify for therapy, but—because of the low HDL-C—may be at high risk based on the total cholesterol/HDL-C ratio (*e.g.,* a total cholesterol of 180 mg/dl and an HDL-C of 30 mg/dl yields a ratio of 6.0). A desirable total cholesterol level in low-HDL-C patients may be considerably lower than 200 mg/dl. This is especially true because many low-HDL-C patients also have moderately elevated triglycerides, which may re-flect increased levels of atherogenic remnant lipoproteins (Grundy, 1998a).

Results from AFCAPS/TexCAPS (a primary preven-tion trial) and VA HIT (a secondary prevention trial) are particularly relevant. Patients in these trials had average or low LDL-C, low HDL-C, and high total cholesterol/HDL-C ratios and treatment greatly reduced clinical events in both trials. The 2001 NCEP guidelines extend treatment to include some, but not all, patients typical of those who benefited in AFCAPS/TexCAPS and VA HIT. See Table 36–8 for a summary of trial results (Downs *et al.*, 1998; Rubins *et al.*, 1999).

The treatment of low HDL-C patients according to the 2001 NCEP guidelines is focused on lowering LDL-C to the target level based on the patient's risk factor or CHD status (Table 36–5) *and* a reduction of VLDL cholesterol (estimated by dividing the plasma triglyceride level by 5) below 30 mg/dl. If this strategy results in a ratio of total cholesterol/HDL-C that is ~4.0 or less, it will be optimal. Patients with higher total cholesterol/HDL-C ra-tios (>4.5) will still be at risk even if their "non-HDL-C"

Table 36–8

Benefit of Lipid-lowering Therapy in Patients with Low HDL-C and "Normal" LDL-C Levels

	AFCAPS/TexCAPS (Lovastatin, 30 mg Once Daily)		VA HIT (Gemfibrozil, 0.6 g Twice Daily)	
	BASELINE	ON TREATMENT	BASELINE	ON TREATMENT
Total cholesterol (mg/dl)	228	184	175	170
LDL-C (mg/dl)	156	115	111	115
HDL-C (mg/dl)	37	39	32	35
Triglycerides (mg/dl)	163	143	161	122
Total cholesterol/HDL-C ratio	6.3	4.8	5.5	4.9
Primary event reduction	37%		22%	

Abbreviations: AFCAPS/TexCAPS, Air Force/Texas Coronary Atherosclerosis Prevention Study; HDL-C, high-density-lipoprotein cholesterol; LDL-C, low-density-lipoprotein cholesterol; VA HIT, Veterans Affairs High Density Lipoprotein Intervention Trial.

levels (LDL-C and VLDL cholesterol) are at the goal values recommended by the 2001 NCEP guidelines.

DRUG THERAPY OF DYSLIPIDEMIA

In addition to the present discussion, the topic of drug therapy for dyslipidemia has been extensively reviewed by Durrington and Illingworth (1998).

Statins

The statins are the most effective and best-tolerated agents for treating dyslipidemia. These drugs are competitive inhibitors of 3-hydroxy-3-methylglutaryl coenzyme A (HMG-CoA) reductase, which catalyzes an early, rate-limiting step in cholesterol biosynthesis. Higher doses of the more potent statins (*e.g., atorvastatin* and *simvastatin*) also can reduce triglyceride levels caused by elevated VLDL levels. Some statins also are indicated for raising HDL-C levels, although the clinical significance of these effects on HDL-C remains to be proven.

   Five large, well-controlled clinical trials have documented the efficacy and safety of simvastatin, pravastatin, and lovastatin in reducing fatal and nonfatal CHD events, strokes, and total mortality [Scandinavian Simvastatin Survival Study Group, 1994; Shepherd *et al.,* 1995; Sacks *et al.,* 1996; Downs *et al.,* 1998; The Long-Term Intervention with Pravastatin in Ischaemic Disease (LIPID) Study Group, 1998]. Rates of adverse events in all five trials were the same in the placebo groups and in the groups receiving active drug. This was true with regard to noncardiac illness and the two laboratory tests, hepatic transaminases and creatine kinase (CK), that have been most frequently used to monitor patients taking statins.

History. Statins were isolated from a mold, *Penicillium citrinium,* and identified as inhibitors of cholesterol biosynthesis in 1976 by Endo and colleagues (Endo *et al.,* 1976). Subsequently, Brown *et al.,* (1978) established that statins act by inhibiting HMG-CoA reductase. The first statin studied in human beings was *compactin,* renamed *mevastatin,* which demonstrated the therapeutic potential of this class of drugs (Yamamoto *et al.,* 1984). However, Alberts and colleagues at Merck developed the first statin (*lovastatin;* formerly known as mevinolin) that was approved for use in human beings, which was isolated from *Aspergillus terreus* (Alberts *et al.,* 1980; Bilheimer *et al.,* 1983). Since the approval of lovastatin by the United States Food and Drug Administration (FDA) in 1987, five other statins have been approved. Two of these, *pravastatin* and simvastatin, are chemically modified derivatives of lovastatin (*see* Figure 36–3). The more recently approved statins—atorvastatin, *fluvastatin,* and

cerivastatin—are synthetic compounds. More statins are under development.

Chemistry. The structural formulas of the original statin (mevastatin) and the six statins currently available in the United States are shown in Figure 36–3 along with the reaction (conversion of HMG-CoA to mevalonate) catalyzed by HMG-CoA reductase, the enzyme they competitively inhibit. The statins possess a side group that is structurally similar to HMG-CoA. Mevastatin, lovastatin, simvastatin, and pravastatin are fungal metabolites, and each contains a hexahydronapthalene ring. Lovastatin differs from mevastatin in having a methyl group at carbon 3. There are two major side chains. One is a methylbutyrate ester (lovastatin and pravastatin) or a dimethylbutyrate ester (simvastatin). The other contains a hydroxy acid that forms a six-membered analog of the intermediate compound in the HMG-CoA reductase reaction (Figure 36–3). Fluvastatin, atorvastatin, and cerivastatin are entirely synthetic compounds containing a heptanoic acid side chain that forms a structural analog of the HMG-CoA intermediate.

   As a result of their structural similarity to HMG-CoA, statins are reversible competitive inhibitors of the enzyme's natural substrate, HMG-CoA. The inhibition constant (K_i) of cerivastatin is 0.01 nM (Bischoff *et al.,* 1997); all other statins have a K_i in the 1-nM range. The dissociation constant of HMG-CoA is three orders of magnitude higher than this value. Lovastatin and simvastatin are lactone prodrugs that are modified in the liver to active hydroxy acid forms. Since they are lactones, they are less soluble in water than are the other statins, a difference that appears to have little if any clinical significance. Pravastatin (an acid in the active form), fluvastatin and cerivastatin (sodium salts), and atorvastatin (a calcium salt), are all administered in the active, open-ring form.

Mechanism of Action. Statins exert their major effect—reduction of LDL levels—through a mevalonic acid–like moiety that competitively inhibits HMG-CoA reductase by product inhibition (Alberts *et al.,* 1980).

   Statins affect blood cholesterol levels by inhibiting cholesterogenesis in the liver, which results in increased expression of the LDL receptor gene. In response to the reduced free cholesterol content within hepatocytes, membrane-bound SREBPs are cleaved by a protease and translocated to the nucleus. The transcription factors are then bound by the sterol-responsive element of the LDL receptor gene, enhancing transcription and ultimately increasing the synthesis of LDL receptors (Brown and Goldstein, 1998). Degradation of LDL receptors also is reduced (Brown *et al.,* 1978). The greater number of LDL receptors on the surface of hepatocytes results in increased removal of LDL from the blood (Bilheimer *et al.,* 1983), thereby lowering LDL-C levels.

   Some studies suggest that statins also can reduce LDL levels by enhancing the removal of LDL precursors (VLDL and IDL) and by decreasing hepatic VLDL production (Grundy and Vega, 1985; Arad *et al.,* 1990; Aguilar-Salinas *et al.,* 1998). Since VLDL remnants and IDL are enriched in apoE, a statin-induced increase in the number of LDL receptors, which recognize both apoB-100 and apoE, enhances the clearance of these LDL precursors (Gaw *et al.,* 1993). The reduction in hepatic VLDL production induced by statins is thought to be mediated by reduced synthesis of cholesterol, a required component of

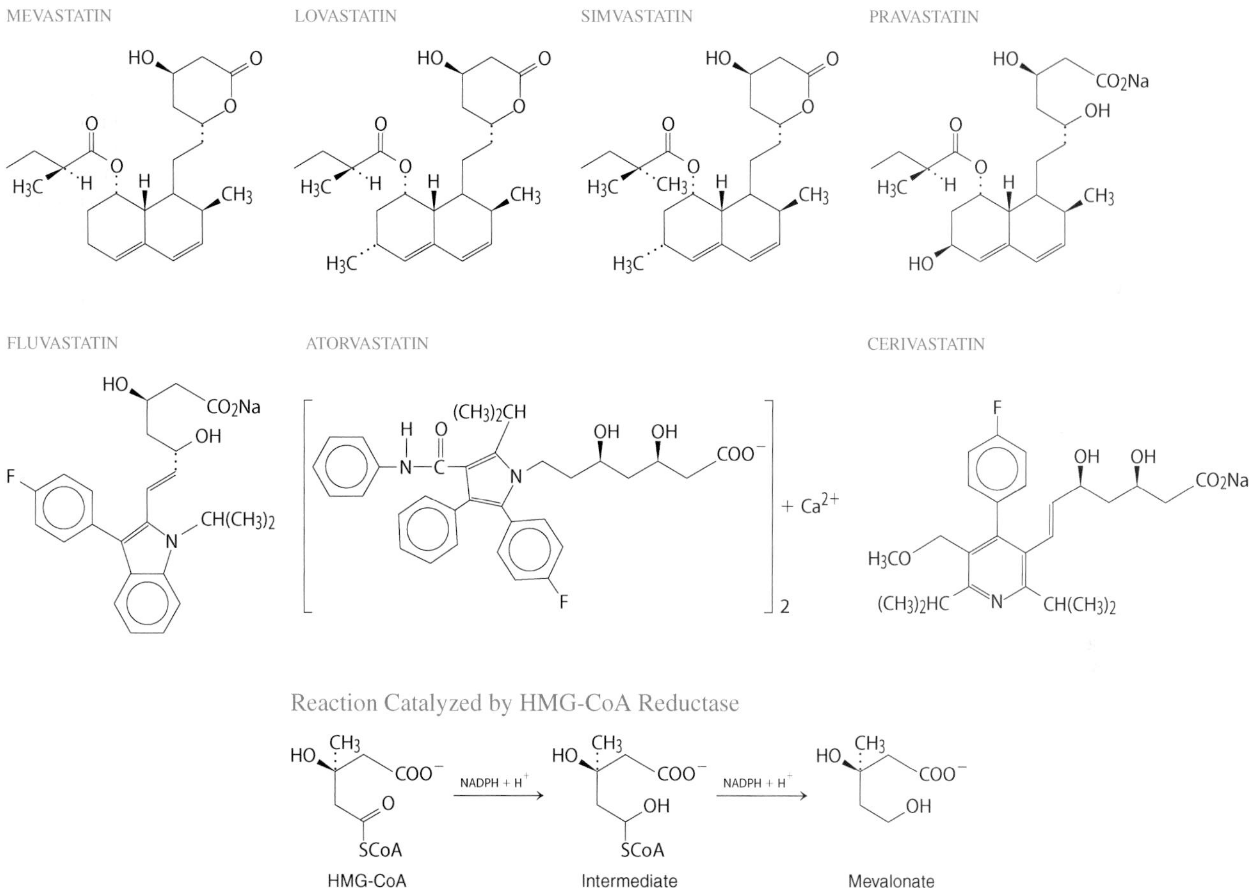

Figure 36–3. Chemical structures of the statins and the reaction catalyzed by 3-hydroxy-3-methylglutaryl coenzyme A (HMG-CoA) reductase.

VLDL (Thompson *et al.,* 1996). This mechanism also likely accounts for the triglyceride-lowering effect of statins (Ginsberg, 1998) and may account for the approximately 25% reduction of LDL-C levels in patients with homozygous familial hypercholesterolemia treated with 80 mg of either atorvastatin or simvastatin (Raal *et al.,* 1997, 2000).

Triglyceride Reduction by Statins.   Triglyceride levels greater than 250 mg/dl are reduced substantially by statins, and the percent reduction achieved is similar to the percent reduction in LDL-C (Stein *et al.,* 1998). Accordingly, hypertriglyceridemic patients taking the highest doses (80 mg/day) of two of the most potent statins (simvastatin, atorvastatin) experience a 35% to 45% reduction in LDL-C and a similar reduction in fasting triglyceride levels (Bakker-Arkema *et al.,* 1996; Ose *et al.,* 2000). If baseline triglyceride levels are below 250 mg/dl, reductions in triglycerides do not exceed 25% irrespective of the dose or statin used (Stein *et al.,* 1998). Similar reductions (35% to 45%) in triglycerides can be accomplished with usual doses of fibrates or niacin (*see* below), although these drugs do not reduce LDL-C to the same extent as 80-mg doses of atorvastatin or simvastatin.

Effect of Statins on HDL-C Levels.   Most studies of patients treated with statins have systematically excluded patients with low HDL-C levels. In studies of patients with elevated LDL-C levels and gender-appropriate HDL-C levels (40 to 50 mg/dl for men; 50 to 60 mg/dl for women), an increase in HDL-C of 5% to 10% was observed, irrespective of the dose or statin employed. However, in patients with reduced HDL-C levels (<35 mg/dl), preliminary studies suggest that statins differ in their effects on HDL-C levels. Simvastatin, at its highest dose of 80 mg, increases HDL-C and apoA-I levels more than a comparable dose of atorvastatin (Crouse *et al.,* 1999; Crouse *et al.,* 2000). However, more studies are needed to ascertain the effects of statins on HDL-C in patients with low HDL-C levels and to determine if statin effects on HDL-C are clinically meaningful.

Effects of Statins on LDL-C Levels.   Statins lower LDL-C by 20% to 55%, depending on the dose and statin used. In large trials comparing the effects of the various statins, equivalent doses appear to be 5 mg of simvastatin = ~15 mg of lovastatin = ~15 mg of pravastatin = ~40 mg of fluvastatin (Pedersen and Tobert, 1996); 20 mg of simvastatin = ~10 mg of atorvastatin (Jones *et al.,* 1998; Crouse *et al.,* 1999), and

Table 36–9

**Doses (mg) of Statins Required to Achieve Various Reductions
in Low-Density-Lipoprotein Cholesterol from Baseline**

	20%–25%	26%–30%	31%–35%	36%–40%	41%–50%	51%–55%
Atorvastatin	—	—	10	20	40	80
Cerivastatin	0.2	0.3	0.4	0.8		
Fluvastatin	20	40	80			
Lovastatin	10	20	40	80		
Pravastatin	10	20	40			
Simvastatin	—	10	20	40	80	

20 mg of simvastatin = ~0.4 mg of cerivastatin. Analysis of dose-response relationships for all statins demonstrate that the efficacy of LDL-C lowering is log linear; LDL-C is reduced by ~6% (from baseline) with each doubling of the dose (Pedersen and Tobert, 1996; Jones *et al.*, 1998). Maximal effects on plasma cholesterol levels are achieved within 7 to 10 days.

Table 36–9 provides information regarding the doses of the various statins that are required to reduce LDL-C by 20% to 55%. The percent reductions achieved with the various doses are the same regardless of the absolute value of the baseline LDL-C level. The statins are effective in virtually all patients with high LDL-C levels. The exception is patients with homozygous familial hypercholesterolemia, who have very attenuated responses to the usual doses of statins, because both alleles of the LDL receptor gene code for dysfunctional LDL receptors; the partial response in these patients is due to a reduction in hepatic VLDL synthesis associated with the inhibition of HMG-CoA reductase–mediated cholesterol synthesis (Raal *et al.*, 1997, 2000). Statin therapy does not reduce Lp(a) levels (Kostner *et al.*, 1989).

Potential Cardioprotective Effects Other Than LDL Lowering? Although the statins clearly exert their major effects on CHD by lowering LDL-C and improving the lipid profile as reflected in plasma cholesterol levels (Thompson and Barter, 1999) (Figure 36–2), a multitude of potentially cardioprotective effects are being ascribed to these drugs (Davignon and Laaksonen, 1999), largely on the basis of *in vitro* and *ex vivo* data. However, the mechanisms of action for nonlipid roles of statins have not been established, and it is not known whether these potential pleiotropic effects represent a class-action effect, differ among statins, or are biologically relevant. Until these questions are resolved, selection of a specific statin should not be based on any one of these effects. Nevertheless, the potential importance of the nonlipid roles of statins requires some discussion.
Statins and Endothelial Function. A variety of studies have established that the vascular endothelium plays a dynamic role in vasoconstriction/relaxation and that hypercholesterolemia modulates these processes directly. Acetylcholine-induced vasodilation of coronary arteries is depressed in patients with hypercholesterolemia and in patients with vascular disease (Treasure *et al.*, 1995). Statin therapy improves coronary vasodilation in response to acetylcholine. The vasomotor response is controlled by nitric oxide, which is synthesized by endothelial cell nitric

oxide synthase. Statins stabilize endothelial cell nitric oxide synthase mRNA, thereby enhancing synthesis of endothelial cell nitric oxide (Laufs *et al.*, 1998). Statin therapy reverses endothelial dysfunction as monitored by vasoactivity within as short a period as one month (O'Driscoll *et al.*, 1997), but similar results have been observed after a single acute reduction of LDL levels by apheresis (Tamai *et al.*, 1997). In nonhuman primates fed a high-cholesterol diet, statin therapy improved endothelial function independently of significant changes in plasma cholesterol levels (Williams *et al.*, 1998).
Statins and Plaque Stability. As discussed earlier, the vulnerability of plaques to rupture and thrombosis is of greater clinical relevance than the degree of stenosis they cause (Gutstein and Fuster, 1999). Statins may affect plaque stability in a variety of ways. There are reports that statins inhibit monocyte infiltration into the artery wall in a rabbit model (Bustos *et al.*, 1998) and inhibit macrophage secretion of matrix metalloproteinases *in vitro* (Bellosta *et al.*, 1998). The metalloproteinases degrade all extracellular matrix components and thus weaken the fibrous cap of atherosclerotic plaques.

Statins also appear to modulate the cellularity of the artery wall by inhibiting proliferation of smooth muscle cells and enhancing apoptotic cell death (Corsini *et al.*, 1998). It is debatable whether these effects would be beneficial or harmful if they occurred *in vivo*. Reduced proliferation of smooth muscle cells and enhanced apoptosis could retard initial hyperplasia and restenosis but also could weaken the fibrous cap and destabilize the lesion. Interestingly, statin-induced suppression of cell proliferation and the induction of apoptosis have been extended to tumor biology. The effects of statins on isoprenoid biosynthesis and protein prenylation associated with reduced availability of mevalonate may alter the development of malignancies (Davignon and Laaksonen, 1999).
Statins and Inflammation. Appreciation of the importance of inflammatory processes in atherogenesis is growing (Ross, 1999), and statins have been suggested to have an antiinflammatory role (Rossen, 1997). In a retrospective analysis of blood samples from the CARE trial, Ridker *et al.* (1998) demonstrated that the C-reactive protein concentration was a marker for high CHD risk and that statin therapy decreased baseline C-reactive protein levels and risk of CHD independently of cholesterol lowering. It remains to be determined whether the C-reactive protein is simply a marker of inflammation or it contributes to the pathogenesis of atherosclerosis.

Statins and Lipoprotein Oxidation. Oxidative modification of LDL appears to play a key role in mediating the uptake of lipoprotein cholesterol by macrophages and in other processes, including cytotoxicity within lesions (Steinberg, 1997). Statins reduce the susceptibility of lipoproteins to oxidation both *in vitro* and *ex vivo* (Kleinveld *et al.*, 1993; Hussein *et al.*, 1997b). Furthermore, atorvastatin has been reported to stabilize or increase the plasma level of paraoxonase, the antioxidation enzyme associated with plasma HDL (Aviram *et al.*, 1998).

Statins and Coagulation. Statins reduce platelet aggregation (Hussein *et al.*, 1997a), and *in vitro* model systems indicate that statins reduce the deposition of platelet thrombi on porcine aorta (Lacoste *et al.*, 1995). In addition, the different statins have variable effects on fibrinogen levels, the significance of which remains to be determined (Rosenson and Tangney, 1998). Elevated plasma fibrinogen levels are associated with an increase in the incidence of CHD (Ernst and Resch, 1993). However, it remains to be determined whether fibrinogen is involved in the pathogenesis or is a marker of disease.

Statins in Combination with Other Lipid-Lowering Drugs.

Statins plus the bile acid–binding resins *cholestyramine* and *colestipol* (*see* below) produce 20% to 30% greater reductions in LDL-C than can be achieved with statins alone (Tikkanen, 1996). Preliminary data indicate that *colesevelam hydrochloride* plus a statin lowers LDL-C by 8% to 16% more than do statins alone. *Niacin* also can enhance the effect of statins, but the occurrence of myopathy increases when statin doses greater than 25% of maximum (*e.g.*, 20 mg of simvastatin or atorvastatin) are used with niacin (Guyton and Capuzzi, 1998). A fibrate (clofibrate, gemfibrozil, or fenofibrate; *see* below) plus a statin is particularly useful in patients with hypertriglyceridemia and a high LDL-C level. This combination does increase the risk of myopathy, but it usually is safe to use a fibrate at its usual maximal dose plus no more than 25% of each statin's maximal dose (Tikkanen, 1996; Athyros *et al.*, 1997). Triple therapy with resins, niacin, and statins can reduce LDL-C by up to 70% (Malloy *et al.*, 1987).

Absorption, Fate, and Excretion.

All the statins are administered as the active β-hydroxy acid form except for lovastatin and simvastatin, which are administered in the lactone form and must be hydrolyzed *in vivo* to the corresponding β-hydroxy acid. All the statins are subject to extensive first-pass metabolism by the liver. Less than 5% to 20% of a dose reaches the general circulation. Greater than 95% of most of these drugs and their active metabolites, the β-hydroxy acids, are bound to plasma proteins. After an oral dose, plasma concentrations peak in 1 to 4 hours. The liver biotransforms all statins, resulting in low systemic availability of the parent compounds. About 70% of statin metabolites are excreted by the liver (Corsini *et al.*, 1999).

Lovastatin and simvastatin are administered as prodrugs and are converted to their active hydroxy acid forms in the liver. About 30% of lovastatin and up to 85% of simvastatin are absorbed. About 50% of the active metabolites are protein bound. The liver is the primary route of excretion.

Pravastatin is administered in its active β-hydroxy acid form as a sodium salt, and 34% of oral doses are absorbed. There is extensive first-pass metabolism, and about 50% of the circulating drug is protein bound. Its metabolites possess little HMG-CoA reductase inhibitory activity. Pravastatin is excreted without extensive metabolic modification; the liver is the major route of excretion, although up to 20% can be excreted in the urine (Quion and Jones, 1994; Corsini *et al.*, 1999).

Fluvastatin also is administered in its active form as a sodium salt and is almost completely absorbed. The drug is metabolized (50% to 80%) to inactive metabolites, and >90% of its excretion is hepatic (Corsini *et al.*, 1999). Fluvastatin is the only statin with saturable first-pass hepatic metabolism; consequently, it is the only statin to achieve peak plasma concentrations in the micromolar range. However, the clinical relevance of this is unclear, as fluvastatin and its metabolites have the shortest elimination half-life of available statins (Dain *et al.*, 1993; Corsini *et al.*, 1999).

Atorvastatin is administered as a calcium salt. It is extensively transformed in the liver to ortho- and parahydroxylated derivatives, which account for about 70% of the circulating inhibitory activity of HMG-CoA reductase. Atorvastatin and its active metabolites are metabolized principally in the liver, where they are excreted into the bile. Atorvastatin has a half-life of about 20 hours, but the half-life of plasma HMG-CoA reductase inhibitory activity is up to 30 hours. All of the other statins have half-lives of only 1 to 4 hours. The clinical significance, if any, of the prolonged half-life of atorvastatin is unclear, but it is thought to play a role in the greater efficacy of atorvastatin compared with the other statins (Christians *et al.*, 1998; Corsini *et al.*, 1999).

Cerivastatin is given in its active form as a sodium salt. Absorption is greater than 98%. In the liver, cerivastatin is transformed into two major and two minor active metabolites. About 70% of these metabolites are excreted in the feces, and the remainder is excreted in the urine (Corsini *et al.*, 1999).

Adverse Effects and Drug Interactions. *Hepatotoxicity.*

The initial postmarketing surveillance studies of the various statins revealed up to 1% incidence of elevations in hepatic transaminase to values greater than three times the upper limit of normal. The incidence appears to be dose related. However, in the placebo-controlled outcome trials, in which 20- to 40-mg doses of simvastatin, lovastatin, or pravastatin were used, the incidence of threefold elevations in hepatic transaminases was not significantly increased in the active drug treatment groups [Scandinavian Simvastatin Survival Study Group, 1994; Shepherd *et al.*, 1995; Sacks *et al.*, 1996; Downs *et al.*, 1998; The Long-Term Intervention with Pravastatin in Ischaemic Disease (LIPID) Study Group, 1998]. Serious hepatopathy must be rare, although it appears to occur (Nakad *et al.*, 1999). Primarily because of the safety data from the clinical trials, it is reasonable to measure alanine aminotransferase (ALT) at baseline and 3 to 6 months after therapy is initiated or after increasing the dose. If the ALT values are normal, it is not necessary to repeat the ALT test more than every 6 to 12 months.

Myopathy.   The only major adverse effect of clinical significance associated with statin use is myopathy. All statins have
been associated with myopathy and rhabdomyolysis (Pogson
et al., 1999; *Physicians' Desk Reference*, 2001). The incidence
of myopathy is low (<0.1%) in patients taking statins without
concomitant administration of drugs that enhance the risk of myopathy. Two classes of drugs, fibrates (gemfibrozil, clofibrate,
and fenofibrate) and niacin, also are lipid-lowering drugs and
can cause myopathy by themselves (*see* below). When statins are
administered with fibrates or niacin, the myopathy is probably
caused by an enhanced inhibition of skeletal muscle sterol synthesis (a pharmacodynamic interaction) (Christians *et al.*, 1998).
The other drugs are those that, like most statins, are metabolized by the 3A4 isoform of cytochrome P450 (CYP3A4) and
include certain macrolide antibiotics (*e.g.*, erythromycin), azole
antifungals (*e.g.*, itraconazole), cyclosporine, a phenylpiperazine
antidepressant, nefazodone, and protease inhibitors (Christians
et al., 1998; Fichtenbaum *et al.*, 2000; Dresser *et al.*, 2000).
This interaction is pharmacokinetic and is associated with increased plasma concentrations of statins and their active metabolites (Christians *et al.*, 1998). Atorvastatin, cerivastatin, lovastatin, and simvastatin are primarily metabolized by CYP3A4,
but cerivastatin also can be metabolized by CYP2C8. Recently,
cerivastatin plus gemfibrozil therapy has been contraindicated
because of a number of case reports of myopathy (*Physicians'
Desk Reference*, 2001). Fluvastatin is mostly (50% to 80%)
metabolized by CYP2C9 to inactive metabolites, but CYP3A4
and CYP2C8 also contribute to the metabolism of fluvastatin.
Pravastatin, however, is not metabolized to any appreciable extent by the CYP system (Corsini *et al.*, 1999) but is excreted
unchanged in the urine. Pravastatin and fluvastatin, which are
not extensively metabolized by the CYP3A4 system, may be
less likely to cause myopathy when used with one of the predisposing drugs. However, because cases of myopathy have
been reported with both drugs, the benefits of combined therapy
with any statin should be carefully weighed against the risk of
myopathy.

The myopathy syndrome is characterized by intense myalgia, first in the arms and thighs and then in the entire body
(similar to flu-related myalgia) along with fatigue. The symptoms progress as long as patients continue to take the drug or
drugs that induce the myopathy. Myoglobinuria and renal failure
have been reported (Pogson *et al.*, 1999). Serum creatine kinase
(CK) levels in affected patients typically are 10-fold higher than
the upper limit of normal. As soon as myopathy is suspected,
a blood sample should be drawn to document the presence of
a 10-fold elevation of CK, as many patients complain of muscle pain that is not due to true statin-induced myopathy. The
statin, and any other drug suspected of contributing to myopathy, should be discontinued if true myopathy is suspected,
even if it is not possible to measure CK activity to document
the presence of myopathy. Rhabdomyolysis should be excluded
and renal function monitored.

Since myopathy rarely occurs in the absence of combination therapy, routine CK monitoring is not recommended unless
the statins are used with one of the predisposing drugs. Such
monitoring is not sufficient to protect patients, as myopathy
can occur months to years after combined therapy is initiated.
As a rule, statins may be used in combination with one of
these predisposing drugs with reduced risk of myopathy if the
statin is administered at no more than 25% of its maximal dose
(Christians *et al.*, 1998).

Although cataracts were a concern initially, careful monitoring of patients in the early days of statin use failed to document any statin-induced eye pathology (Bradford *et al.*, 1991).
Differences in the solubility of the statins (hydrophilic *versus*
hydrophobic) prompted speculation that the more lipid-soluble
drugs might be more likely to penetrate the central nervous
system. However, cerebrospinal fluid concentrations of the two
lipid-soluble statins, lovastatin and simvastatin, are very low,
which is probably due to extensive plasma protein binding of
these drugs. Differences in lipid solubility among statins do not
appear to be clinically relevant.

Pregnancy.   *The safety of statins during pregnancy has not
been established.* Women wishing to conceive should not take
statins. During their childbearing years, women taking statins
should use highly effective contraceptive procedures. Nursing
mothers also are advised to avoid taking statins.

Therapeutic Uses.   Each statin has a low recommended
starting dose that reduces LDL-C by 20% to 30%. Since
studies have documented that a majority of dyslipidemic
patients remain on their initial dose and are not titrated
to achieve their target LDL-C level, this approach leads
to undertreatment. For this reason, it is advisable to start
patients on a dose that will achieve the patient's target
goal for LDL-C lowering. For example, a patient with a
baseline LDL-C of 150 mg/dl and a goal of 100 mg/dl
requires a 33% reduction in LDL-C and should be started
on a dose that will provide it (*see* Table 36–9).

The manufacturer's initial recommended dose of lovastatin (MEVACOR) is 20 mg and is slightly more effective
if taken with the evening meal than if it is taken at bedtime.
If it is more convenient, bedtime dosing is preferable to
missing doses. The statins that have half-lives of 4 hours
or less should be given in the evening because hepatic
cholesterol synthesis is maximal between midnight and
2:00 a.m. The dose may be increased every 3 to 6 weeks
up to a maximum of 80 mg per day. The 80-mg dose is
slightly (2% to 3%) more effective if given as 40 mg twice
daily.

The FDA-approved starting dose of simvastatin
(ZOCOR) for most patients is 20 mg at bedtime unless the
required LDL-C reduction exceeds 45%, in which case
a 40-mg starting dose is indicated. The maximal dose is
80 mg, and the drug should be taken at bedtime. In patients taking cyclosporine, fibrates, or niacin, the daily
dose should not exceed 20 mg.

Pravastatin (PRAVACHOL) therapy is initiated with a
10- or 20-mg dose that may be increased to 40 mg. This
drug should be taken at bedtime. Since pravastatin is a
hydroxy acid, it is bound by bile-acid sequestrants, which
reduces its absorption. Practically, this is rarely a problem

since the resins should be taken before meals and prava-statin should be taken at bedtime.

The starting dose of fluvastatin (LESCOL) is 20 or 40 mg, and the maximum is 80 mg per day. Like prava-statin, it is administered as a hydroxy acid and should be taken at bedtime, several hours after ingesting a bile-acid sequestrant.

Atorvastatin (LIPITOR) has a long half-life, which al-lows administration of this statin at any time of the day. The starting dose is 10 mg, and the maximum is 80 mg per day.

Cerivastatin (BAYCOL) is available in doses ranging between 0.2 and 0.4 mg. It should be taken at bedtime and several hours after a dose of a bile-acid sequestrant. The maximal FDA-approved dose is 0.8 mg.

The choice of statins should be based on efficacy and cost. Can the dose of a particular statin reduce the patient's LDL-C to the target level? Cost should be the next discriminating factor. However, three drugs (lova-statin, simvastatin, and pravastatin) have been used safely in clinical trials involving thousands of subjects for 5 or more years. The documented safety records of these statins should be considered, especially when initiating therapy in younger patients. Once drug treatment is initiated, it is almost always lifelong. Baseline determinations of ALT and repeat testing at 3 to 6 months are recommended. If ALT is normal after the initial 3 to 6 months, then it need not be repeated more than once every 6 to 12 months. CK measurements are not routinely necessary unless the patient also is taking a drug that enhances the risk of myopathy. However, even if CK levels are monitored ev-ery 3 to 4 months, patients receiving combined therapy may develop myopathy months to years after starting the therapy.

Bile-Acid Sequestrants

The two established bile-acid sequestrants or resins (*chole-styramine* and *colestipol*) are among the oldest of the hy-polipidemic drugs, and they are probably the safest, since they are not absorbed from the intestine (West *et al.*, 1980; Groot *et al.*, 1983). These resins are the only hypo-cholesterolemic drugs currently recommended for children 11 to 20 years of age, although data now are emerging that document the safety of statin therapy of children in this age range (National Cholesterol Education Program, 1991; Stein *et al.*, 1999). Because statins are so effective as monotherapy, the resins are most often used as sec-ond agents if statin therapy does not lower LDL-C lev-els sufficiently. When used with a statin, cholestyramine

and colestipol usually are prescribed at submaximal doses. Maximal doses can reduce LDL-C by up to 25% but are associated with unacceptable gastrointestinal side effects (bloating and constipation) that limit compliance. *Cole-sevelam* is a new bile-acid sequestrant that is prepared as an anhydrous gel and taken as a tablet. It lowers LDL-C by 18% at its maximum dose. The safety and efficacy of colesevelam have not been studied in pediatric patients or pregnant women.

Cholestyramine was used in the Coronary Primary Prevention Trial, one of the first studies to document that lowering LDL-C prevents heart disease events (Lipid Re-search Clinics Program, 1984a; Lipid Research Clinics Program, 1984b). Cholestyramine therapy reduced total cholesterol and LDL-C by 13% and 20%, respectively, compared with diet-induced reductions of 5% in total cho-lesterol and 8% in LDL-C. CHD events (fatal and nonfa-tal) were reduced by 19%, suggesting that a 1% reduction in total cholesterol is associated with at least a 2% reduc-tion in CHD events.

Chemistry.   Cholestyramine and colestipol are anion-exchange resins. Cholestyramine, a polymer of styrene and divinylben-zene with active sites formed from trimethylbenzylammonium groups, is a quaternary amine (Figure 36–4). Colestipol, a co-polymer of diethylenetriamine and 1-chloro-2,3-epoxypropane, is a mixture of tertiary and quaternary diamines (Figure 36–4). Cholestyramine and colestipol are hygroscopic powders admin-istered as chloride salts and are insoluble in water. Coleseve-lam is a polymer, poly(allylamine hydrochloride), cross-linked with epichlorohydrin and alkylated with 1-bromodecane and (6-bromohexyl)-trimethylammonium bromide (Figure 36–4). It is a hydrophilic gel and insoluble in water.

Mechanism of Action.   The bile-acid sequestrants are highly positively charged and bind negatively charged bile acids. Be-cause of their large size, resins are not absorbed, and the bound bile acids are excreted in the stool. Since over 95% of bile acids are normally reabsorbed, interruption of this process de-pletes the liver's pool of bile acids, and hepatic bile-acid syn-thesis increases. As a result, hepatic cholesterol content de-clines, stimulating the production of LDL receptors, an effect similar to that of statins (Bilheimer *et al.*, 1983). The increase in hepatic LDL receptors increases LDL clearance and lowers LDL-C levels, but this effect is partially offset by the enhanced cholesterol synthesis caused by upregulation of HMG-CoA re-ductase (Shepherd *et al.*, 1980; Reihnér *et al.*, 1990). Inhibition of reductase activity by a statin substantially increases the ef-fectiveness of the resins. The resin-induced increase in bile-acid production is accompanied by an increase in hepatic triglyceride synthesis, which is of consequence in patients with significant hypertriglyceridemia (baseline triglyceride level >250 mg/dl). In such patients, bile-acid sequestrant therapy may cause strik-ing increases in triglyceride levels. An initial report suggests that colesevelam may not raise triglyceride levels significantly; however, baseline triglyceride levels in the patients studied were

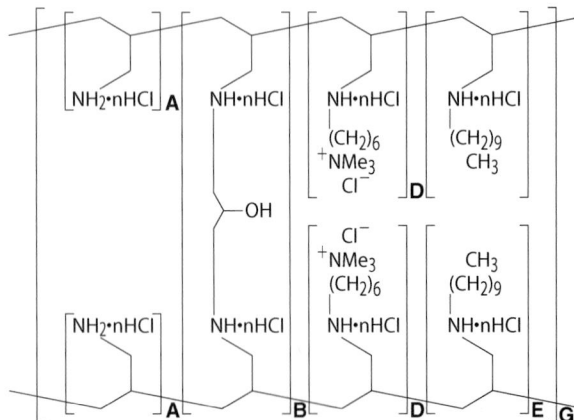

Cholestyramine

Colestipol

Colesevelam

A = Primary Amines
B = Cross-linked Amines
D = Quaternary Ammonium Alkylated Amines
E = Decyalkylated Amines
n = Fraction of Protonated Amines
G = Extended Polymeric Network

Figure 36–4. Structures of cholestyramine, colestipol, and colesevelam.

not elevated (Davidson *et al.*, 1999). Consequently, use of colesevelam to lower LDL-C levels in hypertriglyceridemic patients should be accompanied by frequent (every 1 to 2 weeks) monitoring of fasting triglyceride levels until the triglyceride level is stable, or its use should be avoided until data are published supporting the use of colesevelam in these patients.

Effects on Lipoprotein Levels. The reduction in LDL-C is dose-dependent. Doses of 8 to 12 g of cholestyramine or 10 to 15 g of colestipol are associated with 12% to 18% reductions

in LDL-C (Casdorph, 1975; Hunninghake *et al.*, 1981). Maximal doses (24 g of cholestyramine or 30 g of colestipol) may reduce LDL-C by as much as 25%, but cause gastrointestinal side effects and are poorly tolerated by most patients. One to two weeks is sufficient to attain maximal LDL-C reduction by a given resin dose. In patients with normal triglyceride levels, triglycerides may increase transiently and then return to baseline. HDL-C levels increase 4% to 5% (Witztum *et al.*, 1979). Statins plus resins or niacin plus resins can reduce LDL-C by as much as 40% to 60% (Kane *et al.*, 1981; Illingworth *et al.*, 1981; Davignon and Pearson, 1998). Colesevelam in doses of 3.0 to 3.75 g reduces LDL-C levels significantly in a dose-dependent manner by 9% to 19%.

Adverse Effects and Drug Interactions. The resins are quite safe, as they are not systemically absorbed (West *et al.*, 1980). Since they are administered as a chloride salt, rare instances of hyperchloremic acidosis have been reported. Severe hypertriglyceridemia is a contraindication to the use of cholestyramine and colestipol since these resins increase triglyceride levels (Crouse, 1987). At present, there are insufficient data on the effect of colesevelam on triglyceride levels.

Cholestyramine and colestipol both are available as a powder that must be mixed with water and drunk as a slurry. The gritty sensation is objectionable to patients initially but can be tolerated easily. Colestipol is available in a tablet form that reduces the complaint of grittiness but not the gastrointestinal symptoms. Colesevelam is available as a hard capsule that absorbs water and creates a soft, gelatinous material that allegedly minimizes the potential for gastrointestinal irritation.

The main objections of patients taking cholestyramine and colestipol are bloating and dyspepsia. However, these symptoms can be substantially reduced if the drug is completely suspended in liquid several hours before ingestion. For example, evening doses can be mixed in the morning and refrigerated; morning doses can be mixed the previous evening and refrigerated. Constipation still may occur but sometimes can be prevented by adequate daily water intake and psyllium, if necessary. Fecal impaction has been reported. Limited data from 106 patients treated with colesevelam for six weeks suggest that it may not cause the dyspepsia, bloating, and constipation observed in patients treated with cholestyramine or colestipol (Davidson *et al.*, 1999).

Cholestyramine and colestipol bind many other drugs and interfere with their absorption. Drugs affected include, but are not limited to, some thiazides, furosemide, propranolol, *l*-thyroxine, some cardiac glycosides, coumarin anticoagulants, and some of the statins (Farmer and Gotto, 1994). The effect of cholestyramine and colestipol on the absorption of most drugs has not been studied. For this reason, it is wise to administer all drugs either 1 hour before or 3 to 4 hours after a dose of cholestyramine or colestipol. Colesevelam does not appear to interfere with the absorption of fat-soluble vitamins or of drugs such as digoxin, lovastatin, warfarin, metoprolol, quinidine, and valproic acid. However, the maximum concentration and the area under the curve of sustained-release verapamil were reduced by 31% and 11%, respectively, when coadministered with colesevelam. Since the effect of colesevelam on the absorption of other drugs has not been tested, it seems prudent to recommend that patients take other medications 1 hour before or 3 or 4 hours after a dose of colesevelam.

Therapeutic Uses. *Cholestyramine resin* (QUESTRAN, QUESTRAN LIGHT, LOCHOLEST LIGHT, PREVALITE) is available in bulk (with scoops that measure a 4-g dose) or in individual packets of 4 g. Additional flavorings are added to increase palatability. The "light" preparations contain artificial sweeteners rather than sucrose. *Colestipol hydrochloride* (COLESTID, FLAVORED COLESTID) is available in bulk, in individual packets containing 5 g of colestipol, or as 1-g tablets.

The powdered forms of cholestyramine (4 g per dose) and colestipol (5 g per dose) are either mixed with a fluid (water or juice) and drunk as a slurry or mixed with crushed ice in a blender. Each patient should be instructed to determine the most palatable slurry. Resins should never be taken in the dry form. Ideally, patients should take the resins before breakfast and before supper, starting with one scoop or packet twice daily, and then increase the number of scoops or packets after several weeks or longer as needed and as tolerated. Most studies that have carefully monitored patients using resins have found that patients generally will not take more than two doses (scoops or packets) twice a day.

Colesevelam hydrochloride (WELCHOL) is available as a solid tablet containing 0.625 g of colesevelam. The starting dose is either 3 tablets taken twice daily with meals or all 6 tablets taken with a meal. The tablets should be taken with a liquid. The maximum daily dose is 7 tablets (4.375 g).

Nicotinic Acid (Niacin)

Nicotinic acid (niacin, pyridine-3-carboxylic acid) is one of the oldest drugs used to treat dyslipidemia and is the most versatile in that it favorably affects virtually all lipid parameters (Altschul *et al.*, 1955; Knopp, 1998). Niacin is a water-soluble B-complex vitamin that functions as a vitamin only after its conversion to nicotinamide adenine dinucleotide (*see* Chapter 63). Oral nicotinamide may be used as a source of niacin for its vitamin functions, but nicotinamide does not affect lipid levels. The hypolipidemic effects of niacin require larger doses than are required for its vitamin effects. Niacin is the best agent available for increasing HDL-C (increments of 30% to 40%); it also lowers triglycerides by 35% to 45% (as effectively as fibrates and the more potent statins) and reduces LDL-C levels by 20% to 30% (Knopp *et al.*, 1985; Vega and Grundy, 1994; Martin-Jadraque *et al.*, 1996). Niacin also is the only lipid-lowering drug that reduces Lp(a) levels significantly, by about 40% (Carlson *et al.*, 1989). However, adequate control of other lipid abnormalities renders an elevation of Lp(a) harmless (Maher *et al.*, 1995). The only other drugs that significantly lower Lp(a) levels are estrogen and neomycin (Gurakar *et al.*, 1985; Espeland *et al.*, 1998; Shlipak *et al.*, 2000). Despite its salutary effect on lipids, niacin has side effects that limit its use (*see* "Adverse Effects," below).

Mechanism of Action. Niacin has multiple effects on lipoprotein metabolism. In adipose tissue, niacin inhibits the lipolysis of triglycerides by hormone-sensitive lipase, which reduces transport of free fatty acids to the liver and decreases hepatic triglyceride synthesis (Grundy *et al.*, 1981). In the liver, niacin reduces triglyceride synthesis by inhibiting both the synthesis and esterification of fatty acids, effects that increase apoB degradation (Jin *et al.*, 1999). Reduction of triglyceride synthesis reduces hepatic VLDL production, which accounts for the reduced LDL levels. Niacin also enhances LPL activity, which promotes the clearance of chylomicrons and VLDL triglycerides. Niacin raises HDL-C levels by decreasing the fractional clearance of apoA-I in HDL rather than by enhancing HDL synthesis (Blum *et al.*, 1977). This effect is due to a reduction in the hepatic clearance of HDL-apoA-I, but not of cholesteryl esters, thereby increasing the apoA-I content of plasma and augmenting reverse cholesterol transport (Jin *et al.*, 1997).

Effects on Plasma Lipoprotein Levels. Niacin in doses of 2 to 6 g per day reduces triglycerides by 35% to 50%, and the maximal effect occurs within 4 to 7 days (Figge *et al.*, 1988). Reductions of 25% in LDL-C levels are possible with doses of 4.5 to 6 g per day, but 3 to 6 weeks are required for maximal LDL reductions to be observed. HDL-C increases less in patients with low HDL-C levels (<35 mg/dl) than in those with higher levels. Average increases of 15% to 30% occur in patients with low HDL-C levels; greater increases may occur in patients with normal HDL-C levels at baseline (Vega and Grundy, 1994). Combination therapy with resins can reduce LDL-C levels by as much as 40% to 60% (Malloy *et al.*, 1987).

Absorption, Fate, and Excretion. The pharmacological doses of regular (crystalline) niacin (>1 g per day) used to treat dyslipidemia are almost completely absorbed, and peak plasma concentrations (up to 0.24 mM) are achieved within 30 to 60 minutes. The half-life is about 60 minutes, which accounts for the necessity of twice or thrice daily dosing. At lower doses, most niacin is taken up by the liver; only the major metabolite, nicotinuric acid, is found in the urine. At higher doses, a greater proportion of the drug is excreted in the urine as unchanged nicotinic acid (Iwaki *et al.*, 1996).

Adverse Effects. Two of niacin's side effects, flushing and dyspepsia, limit patient compliance. The cutaneous effects include flushing and pruritus of the face and upper trunk, skin rashes, and acanthosis nigricans. Flushing and associated pruritus are prostaglandin mediated (Stern *et al.*, 1991). Flushing is worse when therapy is initiated or the dosage is increased, but after 1 to 2 weeks of a stable dose, most patients no longer flush. Taking an aspirin each day alleviates the flushing in many patients. Flushing recurs if only one or two doses are missed, and the flushing is more likely to occur when niacin is consumed with hot beverages (coffee, tea) or with ethanol-containing beverages. Flushing is minimized if therapy is initiated with low doses (100 to 250 mg twice daily) and if the drug is taken after breakfast or supper. Dry skin, a frequent complaint, can be dealt with by using skin moisturizers, and acanthosis nigricans can be dealt with by using lotions or creams containing salicylic acid. The dyspepsia and rarer episodes of nausea, vomiting, and diarrhea are less likely to occur if the drug is taken after a meal. Patients with a history (even a remote history) of peptic ulcer disease should not take niacin because it reactivates ulcer disease.

The most common, medically serious side effects are hepatotoxicity, which causes elevated serum transaminases, and hyperglycemia. Both regular (crystalline) niacin and sustained-release niacin, which was developed to reduce flushing and itching, have been reported to cause severe liver toxicity, and sustained-released niacin can cause fulminant hepatic failure (Christensen *et al.*, 1961; Mullin *et al.*, 1989; McKenney *et al.*, 1994; Tatò *et al.*, 1998). A newer preparation of sustained-release niacin (NIASPAN) appears to be less likely to cause severe hepatotoxicity (Capuzzi *et al.*, 1998), perhaps simply because it is administered once daily instead of more frequently (Guyton *et al.*, 1998). The incidence of flushing and pruritus with this preparation is not substantially different from that with regular niacin. Patients using sustained-release niacin may develop hepatic toxicity at any time, but severe toxicity appears to occur when patients take more than 2 g of sustained-release, over-the-counter preparations. Affected patients experience flu-like fatigue and weakness. Usually, aspartate transaminase and ALT are elevated, serum albumin levels decline, and all serum lipid levels decline substantially. In fact, concurrent reductions in LDL-C and HDL-C in a patient taking niacin should prompt concern about niacin toxicity.

In patients with diabetes mellitus, niacin-induced insulin resistance can cause severe hyperglycemia, and the drug usually is not recommended for use in these patients (Knopp *et al.*, 1985; Henkin *et al.*, 1991; Schwartz, 1993). In fact, niacin use in patients with diabetes mellitus often mandates a change to insulin therapy. If niacin is prescribed for patients with known or suspected diabetes, blood glucose levels should be monitored at least once a week until proven to be stable. Niacin also elevates uric acid levels and may reactivate gout. A history of gout is a relative contraindication for niacin use. More rare side effects include toxic amblyopia and toxic maculopathy,

which are reversible. Atrial tachyarrhythmias and atrial fibrillation have been reported, more commonly in elderly patients. *Niacin, at doses used in human beings, has been associated with birth defects in experimental animals and should not be taken by pregnant women.*

Therapeutic Uses.   Niacin is indicated for hypertriglyceridemia and elevated LDL-C; it is especially useful in patients with both hypertriglyceridemia and low HDL-C levels. There are two commonly available forms of niacin. Crystalline niacin (immediate-release or regular) refers to niacin tablets that dissolve quickly after ingestion. Sustained-release niacin refers to preparations that continuously release niacin for 6 to 8 hours after ingestion.

Crystalline niacin tablets do not require a prescription and are available in a variety of strengths from 50-mg to 500-mg tablets. To minimize the flushing and pruritus, it is best to start with a low dose (*e.g.*, 100 mg twice daily taken after breakfast and supper). The dose may be increased stepwise every 7 days by 100 to 200 mg to a total daily dose of 1.5 to 2.0 g. After 2 to 4 weeks at this dose, transaminases, serum albumin, fasting glucose, and uric acid levels should be measured. Lipid levels should be checked and the dose increased further until the desired effect on plasma lipids is achieved. After a stable dose is attained, blood should be drawn every 3 to 6 months to monitor for the various toxicities.

Since concurrent use of niacin and statins can cause myopathy, the dose of the statin should be maintained at no more than 25% of each particular statin's maximal dose. Patients also should be instructed to expect flu-like muscle aches throughout the body if myopathy occurs. Routine measurement of CK in patients taking niacin and statins does not assure that severe myopathy will be prevented or detected, as patients have developed myopathy after several years of concomitant use of niacin with a statin.

Over-the-counter, sustained-release niacin preparations are effective up to a total daily dose of 2.0 g per day. All doses of sustained-release niacin, but particularly doses above 2 g per day, have been reported to cause hepatotoxicity, which may occur soon after beginning therapy or after several years of use (Knopp *et al.*, 1985). Although the exact incidence of hepatotoxicity from use of sustained-release niacin is unknown because it can be purchased without a prescription, the potential for severe liver damage should preclude its use in most patients, including those who have taken an equivalent dose of crystalline niacin safely for many years and are considering switching to a sustained-release preparation (Mullin *et al.*, 1989).

Fibric Acid Derivatives

History. Thorp and Waring (1962) reported that ethyl chlorophenoxyisobutyrate lowered lipid levels in rats. In 1967, the ester form (*clofibrate*) was approved for use in the United States and was, for a number of years, the most widely prescribed hypolipidemic drug. Its use declined dramatically, however, after the results of the World Health Organization (WHO) trial were published in 1978. This trial found that, despite a 9% reduction in cholesterol levels, clofibrate treatment did not reduce fatal cardiovascular events, although nonfatal infarcts were reduced (Committee of Principal Investigators, 1978). Total mortality was significantly greater in the clofibrate group. The increased mortality was due to multiple causes, including cholelithiasis. Interpretation of these negative results was clouded by failure to analyze the data according to the intention-to-treat principle. A later analysis demonstrated that the apparent increase in noncardiac mortality did not persist in the clofibrate-treated patients after discontinuation of the drug (Heady *et al.,* 1992). Clofibrate use was virtually abandoned after the 1978 WHO trial publication, although it, as well as two other fibrates, *gemfibrozil* and *fenofibrate,* remain available in the United States.

Two subsequent trials, the Helsinki Heart Study and the Veterans Affairs HDL Intervention Trial, have reported favorable effects of gemfibrozil therapy on fatal and nonfatal cardiac events without an increase in morbidity or mortality (Frick *et al.,* 1987; Rubins *et al.,* 1999).

Chemistry. Clofibrate, the prototype of the fibric acid derivatives, is the ethyl ester of *p*-chlorophenoxyisobutyrate. Gemfibrozil is a nonhalogenated phenoxypentanoic acid and thus is distinct from the halogenated fibrates. A number of fibric acid analogs (*e.g., fenofibrate, bezafibrate,* and *ciprofibrate*) have been developed and are used in Europe and elsewhere (*see* Figure 36–5 for structural formulas).

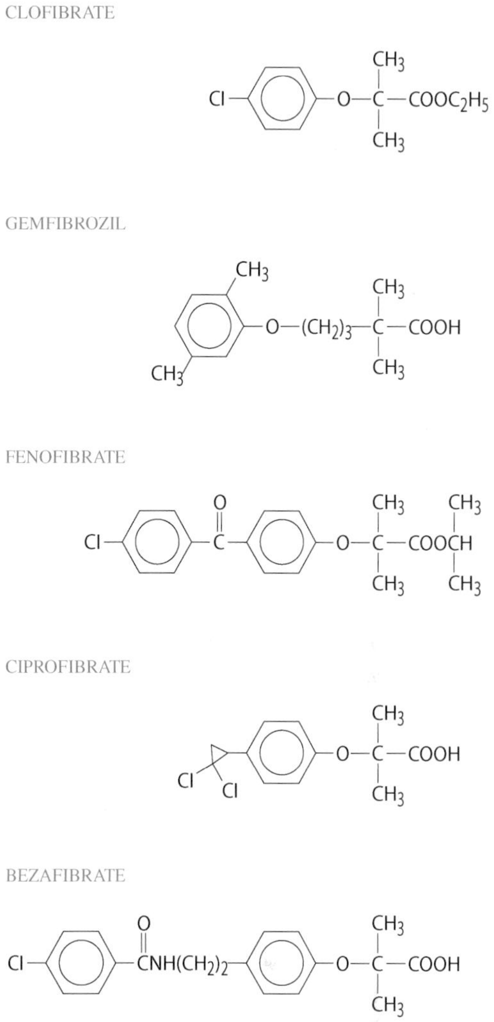

Mechanism of Action. Despite extensive studies in human beings, the mechanisms by which fibrates lower lipoprotein levels, or raise HDL levels, remain unclear (Grundy and Vega, 1987; Illingworth, 1991). Recent studies suggest that many of the effects of these compounds on blood lipids are mediated by their interaction with peroxisome proliferator–activated receptors (PPARs) (Kersten *et al.,* 2000), which regulate gene transcription. Three PPAR isotypes (α, β, and γ) have been identified. Fibrates bind to PPARα, which is expressed primarily in the liver and brown adipose tissue and to a lesser extent in the kidney, heart, and skeletal muscle. Fibrates reduce triglycerides through PPARα-mediated stimulation of fatty acid oxidation, increased LPL synthesis, and reduced expression of apoC-III. An increase in LPL would enhance the clearance of triglyceride-rich lipoproteins. A reduction in hepatic production of apoC-III, which serves as an inhibitor of lipolytic processing and receptor-mediated clearance, would enhance the clearance of VLDL. Fibrate-mediated increases in HDL-C are due to PPARα stimulation of apoA-I and apoA-II expression (Staels and Auwerx, 1998), which increases HDL levels.

LDL levels rise in many patients, especially hypertriglyceridemic patients, treated with gemfibrozil. However, LDL levels are unchanged or fall in others, especially those whose

CLOFIBRATE

GEMFIBROZIL

FENOFIBRATE

CIPROFIBRATE

BEZAFIBRATE

Figure 36–5. Structures of the fibric acids.

triglyceride levels are not elevated or who are taking a second-generation agent, such as fenofibrate, bezafibrate, or ciprofibrate. The fall of LDL levels may be due in part to changes in the cholesterol and triglyceride contents of LDL that are mediated by cholesteryl ester transfer protein activity; such changes can alter the affinity of LDL for the LDL receptor (Eisenberg *et al.,* 1984). There also is evidence that a PPARα-mediated increase in hepatic SREBP-1 production enhances hepatic expression of LDL receptors (Kersten *et al.,* 2000). Lastly, gemfibrozil reduces the plasma concentration of small, dense, more easily oxidized LDL particles (Yuan *et al.,* 1994).

Most of the fibric acid agents have potential antiatherothrombotic effects, including inhibition of coagulation and enhancement of fibrinolysis. These salutary effects also could alter cardiovascular outcomes by mechanisms unrelated to any hypolipidemic activity (Watts and Dimmitt, 1999).

Effects on Lipoprotein Levels. The effects of the fibric acid agents on lipoprotein levels differ widely depending on the starting lipoprotein profile, the presence or absence of a genetic hyperlipoproteinemia, the associated environmental influences, and the drug used.

Patients with type III hyperlipoproteinemia (dysbetalipoproteinemia) are among the most sensitive responders to fibrates (Mahley and Rall, 2001). Elevated triglyceride and cholesterol levels are dramatically lowered, and tuberoeruptive and palmar xanthomas may regress completely. Angina and intermittent claudication also improve (Kuo et al., 1988).

In patients with mild hypertriglyceridemia (e.g., triglycerides <400 mg/dl), fibrate treatment decreases triglyceride levels by up to 50% and increases HDL-C concentrations about 15%; LDL-C levels may be unchanged or increase. The second-generation agents, such as fenofibrate, bezafibrate, and ciprofibrate, lower VLDL levels to a degree similar to that produced by gemfibrozil, but they also are more likely to decrease LDL levels by 15% to 20%. In patients with more marked hypertriglyceridemia (e.g., 400 to 1000 mg/dl), a similar fall in triglycerides occurs, but LDL increases of 10% to 30% are seen frequently. Normotriglyceridemic patients with heterozygous familial hypercholesterolemia usually experience little change in LDL levels with gemfibrozil; with the other fibric acid agents, reductions as great as 20% may occur in some patients.

Fibrates usually are the drugs of choice for treating severe hypertriglyceridemia and the chylomicronemia syndrome. While the primary therapy is to remove alcohol and as much fat from the diet as possible, fibrates help both by increasing triglyceride clearance and by decreasing hepatic triglyceride synthesis. In patients with chylomicronemia syndrome, fibrate maintenance therapy and a low-fat diet keep triglyceride levels well below 1000 mg/dl and thus prevent episodes of pancreatitis.

Gemfibrozil was used in the Helsinki Heart Study, a primary prevention trial of 4081 hyperlipidemic men who received either placebo or gemfibrozil for 5 years (Frick et al., 1987). Gemfibrozil reduced total cholesterol by 10% and LDL-C by 11%, raised HDL-C levels by 11%, and decreased triglycerides by 35%. Overall, there was a 34% decrease in fatal and nonfatal cardiovascular events without any effect on total mortality. No increased incidence of gallstones or cancers was observed. Subgroup analysis suggested that the greatest benefit occurred in the subjects with the highest levels of VLDL or combined VLDL and LDL and in those with the lowest HDL-C levels (<35 mg/dl). It also is possible that gemfibrozil affected the outcome by influencing platelet function, coagulation factor synthesis, or LDL size. In a recent secondary prevention trial, gemfibrozil reduced fatal and nonfatal CHD events by 22% despite a lack of effect on LDL-C levels. HDL-C levels increased by 6%, which may have contributed to the favorable outcome (Rubins et al., 1999).

Absorption, Fate, and Excretion. All of the fibrate drugs are absorbed rapidly and efficiently (>90%) when given with a meal but less efficiently when taken on an empty stomach. The ester bond is hydrolyzed rapidly, and peak plasma concentrations are attained within 1 to 4 hours. More than 95% of these drugs in plasma are bound to protein, nearly exclusively to albumin. The half-lives of fibrates differ significantly (Miller and Spence, 1998), ranging from 1.1 hours (gemfibrozil) to 20 hours (fenofibrate). The drugs are widely distributed through-

out the body, and concentrations in liver, kidney, and intestine exceed the plasma level. Gemfibrozil is transferred across the placenta. The fibrate drugs are excreted predominantly as glucuronide conjugates; 60% to 90% of an oral dose is excreted in the urine, with smaller amounts appearing in the feces. Excretion of these drugs is impaired in renal failure, though excretion of gemfibrozil was reported to be less severely compromised in renal insufficiency than was excretion of other fibrates (Evans et al., 1987). Nevertheless, the use of fibrates is contraindicated in patients with renal failure.

Adverse Effects and Drug Interactions. Fibric acid compounds usually are well tolerated (Miller and Spence, 1998). Side effects may occur in 5% to 10% of patients but most often are not sufficient to cause discontinuation of the drug. Gastrointestinal side effects occur in up to 5% of patients. Other side effects are reported infrequently and include rash, urticaria, hair loss, myalgias, fatigue, headache, impotence, and anemia. Minor increases in liver transaminases and decreases in alkaline phosphatase have been reported. Clofibrate, bezafibrate, and fenofibrate have been reported to potentiate the action of oral anticoagulants, in part by displacing them from their binding sites on albumin. Careful monitoring of the prothrombin time and reduction in dosage of the anticoagulant may be appropriate when treatment with a fibrate is begun.

A myositis flu-like syndrome occasionally occurs in subjects taking clofibrate, gemfibrozil, and fenofibrate, and may occur in up to 5% of patients treated with a combination of an HMG-CoA reductase inhibitor and gemfibrozil, if higher doses of the reductase inhibitor are used. Patients on this combination should be instructed to be aware of the potential symptoms and should be followed at 3-month intervals with careful history and determination of CK values until a stable pattern is established. Use of fibrates with cerivastatin should be avoided because a number of cases of rhabdomyolysis have resulted from combined gemfibrozil-cerivastatin therapy (Guyton et al., 1999; Alexandridis et al., 2000).

All of the fibrates increase the lithogenicity of bile. In the Coronary Drug Project and the WHO trial, clofibrate use was associated with increased risk of gallstone formation. However, no significant increase was seen in the Helsinki Heart Study with the use of gemfibrozil or in the VA HIT. Placebo-controlled clinical trial data for fenofibrate are not available.

Renal failure is a relative contraindication to the use of fibric acid agents, as is hepatic dysfunction. Combined statin-fibrate therapy should be avoided in patients with compromised renal function. Gemfibrozil should be used with caution and at a reduced dosage to treat the hyperlipidemia of renal failure. Fibrates should not be used by children or pregnant women.

Therapeutic Uses. Clofibrate (ATROMID-S) is available for oral administration. The usual dose is 2 g per day in divided doses. This compound is little used, but it still may be useful in patients who do not tolerate gemfibrozil or fenofibrate. Gemfibrozil (LOPID) is usually administered as a 600-mg dose taken twice a day 30 minutes before the morning and evening meals. Fenofibrate (TRI-COR) is available as single-dose capsules of 67, 134, and 200 mg.

Fibrates are the drugs of choice for treating hyperlipidemic subjects with type III hyperlipoproteinemia as well as subjects with severe hypertriglyceridemia (triglycerides >1000 mg/dl), who are at risk for pancreatitis. Based on the VA HIT results, fibrates appear to have an important role in subjects with familial combined hyperlipidemia, who predominantly have elevated VLDL levels and low HDL-C levels. When fibrates are used in such patients, the LDL levels need to be monitored; if LDL levels rise, the addition of a low dose of a statin may be needed. Alternatively, many experts now treat such patients first with a statin, and only subsequently add a 600-mg dose of gemfibrozil once or twice a day to further lower VLDL levels. If this combination is used, there should be careful monitoring for myositis.

PROSPECTUS

New Lipid-Lowering Agents

Statins. More potent statins capable of lowering LDL-C by >65% are being developed. Some of these agents also may have greater efficacy in reducing triglycerides and raising HDL-C. A new statin, ZD4522, in developmental clinical trials has been reported to reduce LDL-C by 65% (Olsson et al., 2000).

MTP Inhibitor. MTP transfers triglycerides and other nonpolar lipids to the apolipoproteins of nascent lipoproteins as they form in the intestine and liver and is required for the synthesis and secretion of chylomicrons and VLDL. For example, an MTP inhibitor targeted to the liver would decrease VLDL production, thereby decreasing plasma triglyceride levels and ultimately reducing LDL production from VLDL. One such MTP inhibitor, BMS-201038, is in clinical trials (Wetterau et al., 1998).

Dietary and Biliary Cholesterol Absorption Inhibitor. *Ezetimibe* is an azetidione-based cholesterol absorption inhibitor that blocks the intestinal absorption of cholesterol, resulting in lowered plasma total cholesterol and LDL-C levels (van Heek et al., 2000). The drug under-

goes glucuronidation in the intestine, and the absorbed glucuronide, an active metabolite, is excreted into the bile by the liver. Due to its enterohepatic circulation, the half-life of the active metabolite is 22 hours in human beings, which indicates that once daily dosing is sufficient (Zhu et al., 2000). The maximum effective dose is 10 mg daily, which provides a 19% reduction in LDL-C (Lipka et al., 2000). A 19% reduction of LDL-C by ezetimibe is equivalent to three doublings of a statin from its baseline dose, since each doubling of a statin dose after the starting dose provides an additional 6% decrease in LDL-C (Pedersen and Tobert, 1996). In human beings, the combination of simvastatin (20 mg; the starting dose of simvastatin) plus ezetimibe (10 mg) provides a 52% reduction in LDL-C (Kosoglou et al., 2000). This 50% reduction achieved with low-dose simvastatin plus ezetimibe (10 mg) is equivalent to that of 80 mg of simvastatin alone. Since there is virtually no myopathy when statins are used at their starting doses, the combination of ezetimibe plus low-dose statin promises an additional margin of safety. Early studies suggest that there are no dangerous interactions between ezetimibe and statins, but further investigations are required to adequately document this initial impression.

ACAT Inhibitors. To date, ACAT inhibitors have failed to reach the marketplace. However, the recognition that there are at least two forms of this enzyme with specific tissue sites of expression suggests that it may be possible to develop an inhibitor that specifically inhibits the assimilation of dietary cholesterol.

ACAT-1 is expressed in several tissues, including macrophages (Chang et al., 1993). *Avasimibe,* an inhibitor of this enzyme, appears to reduce macrophage and cholesteryl ester contents of lesions in cholesterol-fed rabbits and could affect atherosclerotic lesion development, an effect that could stabilize lesions (Bocan et al., 2000). Avasimibe reduced plasma triglycerides and LDL-C levels by up to 50% in miniature swine; however, hepatic triglyceride content increased two- to sevenfold in a dose-dependent manner (Burnett et al., 1999). Interestingly, ACAT-1 knockout mice did not have reduced susceptibility to developing atherosclerosis (Accad et al., 2000).

ACAT-2 is expressed in the liver and intestine and appears to play a role in cholesteryl ester formation for VLDL and chylomicron production (Cases et al., 1998). An inhibitor of this form of ACAT could reduce plasma lipids.

For further discussion of hyperlipoproteinemias and other disorders of lipid metabolism, *see* Chapters 75, 242, and 341 in *Harrison's Principles of Internal Medicine,* 14th ed., McGraw-Hill, New York, 1998.

BIBLIOGRAPHY

Accad, M., Smith, S.J., Newland, D.L., Sanan, D.A., King, L.E. Jr., Linton, M.F., Fazio, S., and Farese, R.V. Jr. Massive xanthomatosis and altered composition of atherosclerotic lesions in hyperlipidemic mice lacking acyl CoA:cholesterol acyltransferase 1. *J. Clin. Invest.,* **2000,** *105*:711–719.

Aguilar-Salinas, C.A., Barrett, H., and Schonfeld, G. Metabolic modes of action of the statins in the hyperlipoproteinemias. *Atherosclerosis,* **1998,** *141*:203–207.

Alberts, A.W., Chen, J., Kuron, G., Hunt, V., Huff, J., Hoffman, C., Rothrock, J., Lopez, M., Joshua, H., Harris, E., Patchett, A., Monaghan, R., Currie, S., Stapley, E., Albers-Schonberg, G., Hensens, O., Hirshfield, J., Hoogsteen, K., Liesch, J., and Springer, J. Mevinolin: a highly potent competitive inhibitor of hydroxymethyl-glutaryl-coenzyme A reductase and a cholesterol-lowering agent. *Proc. Natl. Acad. Sci. U.S.A.,* **1980,** *77*:3957–3961.

Alexandridis, G., Pappas, G.A., and Elisaf, M.S. Rhabdomyolysis due to combination therapy with cerivastatin and gemfibrozil. *Am. J. Med.,* **2000,** *109*:261–262.

Altschul, R., Hoffer, A., and Stephen, J.D. Influence of nicotinic acid on serum cholesterol in man. *Arch. Biochem. Biophys.,* **1955,** *54*:558–559.

American Diabetes Association. Management of dyslipidemia in adults with diabetes. *Diabetes Care,* **1999,** *22(suppl. 1)*:S56–S59.

American Heart Association. *2000 Heart and Stroke Statistical Update.* American Heart Association, Dallas, **1999.**

Appleby, P.N., Thorogood, M., Mann, J.I., and Key, T.J.A. The Oxford Vegetarian Study: an overview. *Am. J. Clin. Nutr.,* **1999,** *70(3 suppl.)*: 525S–531S.

Arad, Y., Ramakrishnan, R., and Ginsberg, H.N. Lovastatin therapy reduces low density lipoprotein apoB levels in subjects with combined hyperlipidemia by reducing the production of apoB-containing lipoproteins: implications for the pathophysiology of apoB production. *J. Lipid Res.,* **1990,** *31*:567–582.

Athyros, V.G., Papageorgiou, A.A., Hatzikonstandinou, H.A., Didangelos, T.P., Carina, M.V., Kranitsas, D.F., and Kontopoulos, A.G. Safety and efficacy of long-term statin-fibrate combinations in patients with refractory familial combined hyperlipidemia. *Am. J. Cardiol.,* **1997,** *80*:608–613.

Aviram, M., Rosenblat, M., Bisgaier, C.L., and Newton, R.S. Atorvastatin and gemfibrozil metabolites, but not the parent drugs, are potent antioxidants against lipoprotein oxidation. *Atherosclerosis,* **1998,** *138*:271–280.

Bakker-Arkema, R.G., Davidson, M.H., Goldstein, R.J., Davignon, J., Isaacsohn, J.L., Weiss, S.R., Keilson, L.M., Brown, W.V., Miller, V.T., Shurzinske, L.J., and Black, D.M. Efficacy and safety of a new HMG-CoA reductase inhibitor, atorvastatin, in patients with hypertriglyceridemia. *JAMA,* **1996,** *275*:128–133.

Bellosta, S., Mahley, R.W., Sanan, D.A., Murata, J., Newland, D.L., Taylor, J.M., and Pitas, R.E. Macrophage-specific expression of human apolipoprotein E reduces atherosclerosis in hypercholesterolemic apolipoprotein E–null mice. *J. Clin. Invest.,* **1995,** *96*:2170–2179.

Bellosta, S., Via, D., Canavesi, M., Pfister, P., Fumagalli, R., Paoletti, R., and Bernini, F. HMG-CoA reductase inhibitors reduce MMP-9 secretion by macrophages. *Arterioscler. Thromb. Vasc. Biol.,* **1998,** *18*:1671–1678.

Bilheimer, D.W., Grundy, S.M., Brown, M.S., and Goldstein, J.L. Mevinolin and colestipol stimulate receptor-mediated clearance of low density lipoprotein from plasma in familial hypercholesterolemia heterozygotes. *Proc. Natl. Acad. Sci. U.S.A.,* **1983,** *80*:4124–4128.

Bischoff, H., Angerbauer, R., Bender, J., Bischoff, E., Faggiotto, A., Petzinna, D., Pfitzner, J., Porter, M.C., Schmidt, D., and Thomas, G. Cerivastatin: pharmacology of a novel synthetic and highly active HMG-CoA reductase inhibitor. *Atherosclerosis,* **1997,** *135*:119–130.

Blum, C.B., Levy, R.I., Eisenberg, S., Hall, M. III, Goebel, R.H., and Berman, M. High density lipoprotein metabolism in man. *J. Clin. Invest.,* **1977,** *60*:795–807.

Bocan, T.M.A., Krause, B.R., Rosebury, W.S., Mueller, S.B., Lu, X., Dagle, C., Major, T., Lathia, C., and Lee, H. The ACAT inhibitor avasimibe reduces macrophages and matrix metalloproteinase expression in atherosclerotic lesions of hypercholesterolemic rabbits. *Arterioscler. Thromb. Vasc. Biol.,* **2000,** *20*:70–79.

Bradford, R.H., Shear, C.L., Chremos, A.N., Dujovne, C., Downton, M., Franklin, F.A., Gould, A.L., Hesney, M., Higgins, J., Hurley, D.P., Langendorfer, A., Nash, D.T., Pool, J.L., and Schnaper, H. Expanded Clinical Evaluation of Lovastatin (EXCEL) Study results. I. Efficacy in modifying plasma lipoproteins and adverse event profile in 8245 patients with moderate hypercholesterolemia. *Arch. Intern. Med.,* **1991,** *151*:43–49.

Brinton, E.A. Oral estrogen replacement therapy in postmenopausal women selectively raises levels and production rates of lipoprotein A-I and lowers hepatic lipase activity without lowering the fractional catabolic rate. *Arterioscler. Thromb. Vasc. Biol.,* **1996,** *16*:431–440.

Brown, B.G., Zhao, X.-Q., Sacco, D.E., and Albers, J.J. Lipid lowering and plaque regression. New insights into prevention of plaque disruption and clinical events in coronary disease. *Circulation,* **1993,** *87*:1781–1791.

Brown, M.S., Faust, J.R., and Goldstein, J.L. Induction of 3-hydroxy-3-methylglutaryl coenzyme A reductase activity in human fibroblasts incubated with compactin (ML-236B), a competitive inhibitor of the reductase. *J. Biol. Chem.,* **1978,** *253*:1121–1128.

Brown, M.S., and Goldstein, J.L. A receptor-mediated pathway for cholesterol homeostasis. *Science,* **1986,** *232*:34–47.

Burnett, J.R., Wilcox, L.J., Telford, D.E., Kleinstiver, S.J., Barrett, P.H.R., Newton, R.S., and Huff, M.W. Inhibition of ACAT by avasimibe decreases both VLDL and LDL apolipoprotein B production in miniature pigs. *J. Lipid Res.,* **1999,** *40*:1317–1327.

Bustos, C., Hernández-Presa, M.A., Ortego, M., Tuñón, J., Ortega, L., Pérez, F., Díaz, C., Hernández, G., and Egido, J. HMG-CoA reductase inhibition by atorvastatin reduces neointimal inflammation in a rabbit model of atherosclerosis. *J. Am. Coll. Cardiol.,* **1998,** *32*:2057–2064.

Capuzzi, D.M., Guyton, J.R., Morgan, J.M., Goldberg, A.C., Kreisberg, R.A., Brusco, O.A., and Brody, J. Efficacy and safety of an extended-release niacin (Niaspan): a long-term study. *Am. J. Cardiol.,* **1998,** *82*:74U–81U.

Carlson, L.A., Hamsten, A., and Asplund, A. Pronounced lowering of serum levels of lipoprotein Lp(a) in hyperlipidaemic subjects treated with nicotinic acid. *J. Intern. Med.,* **1989,** *226*:271–276.

Casdorph, H.R. The single dose method of administering cholestyramine. *Angiology,* **1975,** *26*:671–682.

Cases, S., Novak, S., Zheng, Y.-W., Myers, H.M., Lear, S.R., Sande, E., Welch, C.B., Lusis, A.J., Spencer, T.A., Krause, B.R., Erickson, S.K., and Farese, R.V. Jr. ACAT-2, a second mammalian acyl-CoA:cholesterol acyltransferase. Its cloning, expression, and characterization. *J. Biol. Chem.,* **1998,** *273*:26755–26764.

Castelli, W.P., Garrison, R.J., Wilson, P.W.F., Abbott, R.D., Kalousdian, S., and Kannel, W.B. Incidence of coronary heart disease and lipoprotein cholesterol levels. The Framingham Study. *JAMA,* **1986,** *256:*2835–2838.

Chang, C.C.Y., Huh, H.Y., Cadigan, K.M., and Chang, T.Y. Molecular cloning and functional expression of human acyl-coenzyme A:cholesterol acyltransferase cDNA in mutant Chinese hamster ovary cells. *J. Biol. Chem.,* **1993,** *268:*20747–20755.

Chen, Z., Peto, R., Collins, R., MacMahon, S., Lu, J., and Li, W. Serum cholesterol concentration and coronary heart disease in population with low cholesterol concentrations. *BMJ,* **1991,** *303:*276–282.

Christensen, N.A., Achor, R.W.P., Berge, K.G., and Mason, H.L. Nicotinic acid treatment of hypercholesteremia. Comparison of plain and sustained-action preparations and report of two cases of jaundice. *JAMA,* **1961,** *177:*76–80.

Christians, U., Jacobsen, W., and Floren, L.C. Metabolism and drug interactions of 3-hydroxy-3-methylglutaryl coenzyme A reductase inhibitors in transplant patients: are the statins mechanistically similar? *Pharmacol. Ther.,* **1998,** *80:*1–34.

Committee of Principal Investigators. A co-operative trial in the primary prevention of ischaemic heart disease using clofibrate. Report from the Committee of Principal Investigators. *Br. Heart J.,* **1978,** *40:*1069–1118.

Committee of Principal Investigators. WHO cooperative trial on primary prevention of ischaemic heart disease with clofibrate to lower serum cholesterol: final mortality follow-up. Report of the Committee of Principal Investigators. *Lancet,* **1984,** *2:*600–604.

Corsini, A., Bellosta, S., Baetta, R., Fumagalli, R., Paoletti, R., and Bernini, F. New insights into the pharmacodynamic and pharmacokinetic properties of statins. *Pharmacol. Ther.,* **1999,** *84:*413–428.

Corsini, A., Pazzucconi, F., Arnaboldi, L., Pfister, P., Fumagalli, R., Paoletti, R., and Sirtori, C.R. Direct effects of statins on the vascular wall. *J. Cardiovasc. Pharmacol.,* **1998,** *31:*773–778.

Crouse, J.R. III. Hypertriglyceridemia: a contraindication to the use of bile acid binding resins. *Am. J. Med.,* **1987,** *83:*243–248.

Crouse, J.R. III, Frolich, J., Ose, L., Mercuri, M., and Tobert, J.A. Effects of high doses of simvastatin and atorvastatin on high-density lipoprotein cholesterol and apolipoprotein A-I. *Am. J. Cardiol.,* **1999,** *83:*1476–1477.

Crouse, J.R. III, Kastelein, J., Isaacsohn, J., Corsetti, L., Liu, M., Melino, M., Mercuri, L.M., O'Grady, L., and Ose, L. A large, 36-week study of the HDL-C raising effects and safety of simvastatin *versus* atorvastatin. *Atherosclerosis,* **2000,** *151:*8–9 (abstr.).

Dain, J.G., Fu, E., Gorski, J., Nicoletti, J., and Scallen, T.J. Biotransformation of fluvastatin sodium in humans. *Drug Metab. Dispos.,* **1993,** *21:*567–572.

Davidson, M.H., Dillon, M.A., Gordon, B., Jones, P., Samuels, J., Weiss, S., Isaacsohn, J., Toth, P., and Burke, S.K. Colesevelam hydrochloride (Cholestagel): a new, potent bile acid sequestrant associated with a low incidence of gastrointestinal side effects. *Arch. Intern. Med.,* **1999,** *159:*1893–1900.

Davignon, J., and Laaksonen, R. Low-density lipoprotein-independent effects of statins. *Curr. Opin. Lipidol.,* **1999,** *10:*543–559.

Davignon, J., and Pearson, T.A. Beyond LDL-cholesterol: can further reductions in CAD risk be achieved by considering triglycerides? *Can. J. Cardiol.,* **1998,** *14(suppl. B):*2B.

Deeb, S.S., Takata, K., Peng, R.L., Kajiyama, G., and Albers, J.J. A splice-junction mutation responsible for familial apolipoprotein A-II deficiency. *Am. J. Hum. Genet.,* **1990,** *46:*822–827.

Dhaliwal, B.S., and Steinbrecher, U.P. Scavenger receptors and oxidized low density lipoproteins. *Clin. Chim. Acta,* **1999,** *286:*191–205.

Diabetes Atherosclerosis Intervention Study Investigators. Effect of fenofibrate on progression of coronary-artery disease in type 2 diabetes: The Diabetes Atherosclerosis Intervention Study, a randomised study. *Lancet,* **2001,** *357:*905–910.

Dietschy, J.M., Turley, S.D., and Spady, D.K. Role of liver in the maintenance of cholesterol and low density lipoprotein homeostasis in different animal species, including humans. *J. Lipid Res.,* **1993,** *34:*1637–1659.

Downs, J.R., Clearfield, M., Weis, S., Whitney, E., Shapiro, D.R., Beere, P.A., Langendorfer, A., Stein, E.A., Kruyer, W., and Gotto, A.M. Jr. Primary prevention of acute coronary events with lovastatin in men and women with average cholesterol levels. Results of AFCAPS/TexCAPS. *JAMA,* **1998,** *279:*1615–1622.

Dresser, G.K., Spence, J.D., and Bailey, D.G. Pharmacokinetic-pharmacodynamic consequences and clinical relevance of cytochrome P450 3A4 inhibition. *Clin. Pharmacokinet.,* **2000,** *38:*41–57.

Duriez, P., and Fruchart, J.C. High-density lipoprotein subclasses and apolipoprotein A-I. *Clin. Chim. Acta,* **1999,** *286:*97–114.

Eisenberg, S., Gavish, D., Oschry, Y., Fainaru, M., and Deckelbaum, R.J. Abnormalities in very low, low and high density lipoproteins in hypertriglyceridemia. Reversal toward normal with bezafibrate treatment. *J. Clin. Invest.,* **1984,** *74:*470–482.

Endo, A., Kuroda, M., and Tsujita, Y. ML-236A, ML-236B, and ML-236C, new inhibitors of cholesterogenesis produced by *Penicillium citrinum. J. Antibiot. (Tokyo),* **1976,** *29:*1346–1348.

Espeland, M.A., Marcovina, S.M., Miller, V., Wood, P.D., Wasilauskas, C., Sherwin, R., Schrott, H., and Bush, T.L. Effect of postmenopausal hormone therapy on lipoprotein(a) concentration. PEPI Investigators. Postmenopausal Estrogen/Progestin Interventions. *Circulation,* **1998,** *97:*979–986.

Evans, J.R., Forland, S.C., and Cutler, R.E. The effect of renal function on the pharmacokinetics of gemfibrozil. *J. Clin. Pharmacol.,* **1987,** *27:*994–1000.

The Expert Panel. Summary of the second report of the National Cholesterol Education Program (NCEP) Expert Panel on Detection, Evaluation, and Treatment of High Blood Cholesterol in Adults (Adult Treatment Panel II). *JAMA,* **1993,** *269:*3015–3023.

Farese, R.V. Jr., Cases, S., and Smith, S.J. Triglyceride synthesis: insights from the cloning of diacylglycerol acyltransferase. *Curr. Opin. Lipidol.,* **2000,** *11:*229–234.

Fichtenbaum, C., Gerber, J., Rosenkranz, S., Segal, Y., Blaschke, T., Aberg, J., Royal, M., Burning, W., Lamb, K., Ferguson, E., Alston, B., and Aweeka, F., and the ACTG A5047 Team. Pharmacokinetic interactions between protease inhibitors and selected HMG-CoA reductase inhibitors. *7th Conference on Retroviruses and Opportunistic Infections.* San Francisco, **2000.** Available at: http://www.retroconference.org/2000/abstracts/lb6.htm. Accessed January 15, 2001.

Fonarow, G.C., and Gawlinski, A. Rationale and design of the Cardiac Hospitalization Atherosclerosis Management Program at the University of California Los Angeles. *Am. J. Cardiol.,* **2000,** *85:*10A–17A.

Frick, M.H., Elo, O., Haapa, K., Heinonen, O.P., Heinsalmi, P., Helo, P., Huttunen, J.K., Kaitaniemi, P., Koskinen, P., Manninen, V., Mäenpää, H., Mälkönen, M., Mänttäri, M., Norola, S., Pasternack, A., Pikkarainen, J., Romo, M., Sjöblom, T., and Nikkilä, E.A. Helsinki Heart Study: primary-prevention trial with gemfibrozil in middle-aged men with dyslipidemia. Safety of treatment, changes in risk factors, and incidence of coronary heart disease. *N. Engl. J. Med.,* **1987,** *317:*1237–1245.

Gaw, A., Packard, C.J., Murray, E.F., Lindsay, G.M., Griffin, B.A., Caslake, M.J., Vallance, B.D., Lorimer, A.R., and Shepherd, J.

Effects of simvastatin on apoB metabolism and LDL subfraction distribution. *Arterioscler. Thromb.,* **1993,** *13*:170–189.

Genest, J.J., McNamara, J.R., Salem, D.N., and Schaefer, E.J. Prevalence of risk factors in men with premature coronary artery disease. *Am. J. Cardiol.,* **1991,** *67*:1185–1189.

Ginsberg, H.N. Effects of statins on triglyceride metabolism. *Am. J. Cardiol.,* **1998,** *81*:32B–35B.

Gregg, R.E., and Wetterau, J.R. The molecular basis of abetalipoproteinemia. *Curr. Opin. Lipidol.,* **1994,** *5*:81–86.

Groot, P.H., Dijkhuis-Stoffelsma, R., Grose, W.F., Ambagtsheer, J.J., and Fernandes, J. The effects of colestipol hydrochloride on serum lipoprotein lipid and apolipoprotein B and A-I concentrations in children heterozygous for familial hypercholesterolemia. *Acta Paediatr. Scand.,* **1983,** *72*:81–85.

Grundy, S.M., Balady, G.J., Criqui, M.H., Fletcher, G., Greenland, P., Hiratzka, L.F., Houston-Miller, N., Kris-Etherton, P., Krumholz, H.M., LaRosa, J., Ockene, I.S., Pearson, T.A., Reed, J., Washington, R., and Smith, S.C. Primary prevention of coronary heart disease: guidance from Framingham: a statement for healthcare professionals from the AHA Task Force on Risk Reduction. American Heart Association. *Circulation,* **1998,** *97*:1876–1887.

Grundy, S.M., Benjamin, I.J., Burke, G.L., Chait, A., Eckel, R.H., Howard, B.V., Mitch, W., Smith, S.C., Jr., and Sowers, J.R. Diabetes and cardiovascular disease: a statement for healthcare professionals from the American Heart Association. *Circulation,* **1999,** *100*:1134–1146.

Grundy, S.M., Mok, H.Y.I., Zech, L., and Berman, M. Influence of nicotinic acid on metabolism of cholesterol and triglycerides in man. *J. Lipid Res.,* **1981,** *22*:24–36.

Grundy, S.M., and Vega, G.L. Influence of mevinolin on metabolism of low density lipoproteins in primary moderate hypercholesterolemia. *J. Lipid Res.,* **1985,** *26*:1464–1475.

Grundy, S.M., and Vega, G.L. Fibric acids: effects on lipids and lipoprotein metabolism. *Am. J. Med.,* **1987,** *83*:9–20.

Gurakar, A., Hoeg, J.M., Kostner, G., Papadopoulos, N.M., and Brewer, H.B., Jr. Levels of lipoprotein Lp(a) decline with neomycin and niacin treatment. *Atherosclerosis,* **1985,** *57*:293–301.

Gutstein, D.E., and Fuster, V. Pathophysiology and clinical significance of atherosclerotic plaque rupture. *Cardiovasc. Res.,* **1999,** *41*:323–333.

Guyton, J.R., and Capuzzi, D.M. Treatment of hyperlipidemia with combined niacin-statin regimens. *Am. J. Cardiol.,* **1998,** *82*:82U–84U.

Guyton, J.R., Dujovne, C.A., and Illingworth, D.R. Dual hepatic metabolism of cerivastatin—clarifications. *Am. J. Cardiol.,* **1999,** *84*:497.

Guyton, J.R., Goldberg, A.C., Kreisberg, R.A., Sprecher, D.L., Superko, H.R., and O'Connor, C.M. Effectiveness of once-nightly dosing of extended-release niacin alone and in combination for hypercholesterolemia. *Am. J. Cardiol.,* **1998,** *82*:737–743.

Haffner, S.M., Kushwaha, R.S., Foster, D.M., Applebaum-Bowden, D., and Hazzard, W.R. Studies on the metabolic mechanism of reduced high density lipoproteins during anabolic steroid therapy. *Metabolism,* **1983,** *32*:413–420.

Haffner, S.M., Lehto, S., Rönnemaa, T., Pyörälä, K., and Laakso, M. Mortality from coronary heart disease in subjects with type 2 diabetes and in nondiabetic subjects with and without prior myocardial infarction. *N. Engl. J. Med.,* **1998,** *339*:229–234.

Hasty, A.H., Linton, M.F., Brandt, S.J., Babaev, V.R., Gleaves, L.A., and Fazio, S. Retroviral gene therapy in apoE-deficient mice: apoE expression in the artery wall reduces early foam cell lesion formation. *Circulation,* **1999,** *99*:2571–2576.

Heady, J.A., Morris, J.N., and Oliver, M.F. WHO clofibrate/cholesterol trial: clarifications. *Lancet,* **1992,** *340*:1405–1406.

Henkin, Y., Oberman, A., Hurst, D.C., and Segrest, J.P. Niacin revisited: clinical observations on an important but underutilized drug. *Am. J. Med.,* **1991,** *91*:239–246.

Hobbs, H.H., Brown, M.S., and Goldstein, J.L. Molecular genetics of the LDL receptor gene in familial hypercholesterolemia. *Hum. Mutat.,* **1992,** *1*:445–466.

Hulley, S., Grady, D., Bush, T., Furberg, C., Herrington, D., Riggs, B., and Vittinghoff, E. Randomized trial of estrogen plus progestin for secondary prevention of coronary heart disease in postmenopausal women. Heart and Estrogen/progestin Replacement Study (HERS) Research Group. *JAMA,* **1998,** *280*:605–613.

Hunninghake, D.B., Probstfield, J.L., Crow, L.O., and Isaacson, S.O. Effect of colestipol and clofibrate on plasma lipid and lipoproteins in type IIa hyperlipoproteinemia. *Metabolism,* **1981,** *30*:605–609.

Hussein, O., Rosenblat, M., Schlezinger, S., Keidar, S., and Aviram, M. Reduced platelet aggregation after fluvastatin therapy is associated with altered platelet lipid composition and drug binding to the platelets. *Br. J. Clin. Pharmacol.,* **1997a,** *44*:77–84.

Hussein, O., Schlezinger, S., Rosenblat, M., Keidar, S., and Aviram, M. Reduced susceptibility of low density lipoprotein (LDL) to lipid peroxidation after fluvastatin therapy is associated with the hypocholesterolemic effect of the drug and its binding to the LDL. *Arteriosclerosis,* **1997b,** *128*:11–18.

Illingworth, D.R., Phillipson, B.E., Rapp, J.H., and Connor, W.E. Colestipol plus nicotinic acid in treatment of heterozygous familial hypercholesterolaemia. *Lancet,* **1981,** *1*:296–298.

Innerarity, T.L., Borén, J., Yamanaka, S., and Olofsson, S.-O. Biosynthesis of apolipoprotein B48-containing lipoproteins. Regulation by novel post-transcriptional mechanisms. *J. Biol. Chem.,* **1996,** *271*:2353–2356.

Innerarity, T.L., Mahley, R.W., Weisgraber, K.H., Bersot, T.P., Krauss, R.M., Vega, G.L., Grundy, S.M., Friedl, W., Davignon, J., and McCarthy, B.J. Familial defective apolipoprotein B-100: a mutation of apolipoprotein B that causes hypercholesterolemia. *J. Lipid Res.,* **1990,** *31*:1337–1349.

Iwaki, M., Ogiso, T., Hayashi, H., Tanino, T., and Benet, L.Z. Acute dose-dependent disposition studies of nicotinic acid in rats. *Drug Metab. Dispos.,* **1996,** *24*:773–779.

Jin, F.Y., Kamanna, V.S., and Kashyap, M.L. Niacin decreases removal of high-density lipoprotein apolipoprotein A-I but not cholesterol ester by Hep G2 cells. Implication for reverse cholesterol transport. *Arterioscler. Thromb. Vasc. Biol.,* **1997,** *17*:2020–2028.

Jin, F.Y., Kamanna, V.S., and Kashyap, M.L. Niacin accelerates intracellular apoB degradation by inhibiting triacylglycerol synthesis in human hepatoblastoma (HepG2) cells. *Arterioscler. Thromb. Vasc. Biol.,* **1999,** *19*:1051–1059.

Jones, P., Kafonek, S., Laurora, I., and Hunninghake, D. Comparative dose efficacy study of atorvastatin *versus* simvastatin, pravastatin, lovastatin, and fluvastatin in patients with hypercholesterolemia (the CURVES study). *Am. J. Cardiol.,* **1998,** *81*:582–587.

Kane, J.P., Malloy, M.J., Tun, P., Phillips, N.R., Freedman, D.D., Williams, M.L., Rowe, J.S., and Havel, R.J. Normalization of low-density lipoprotein levels in heterozygous familial hypercholesterolemia with a combined drug regimen. *N. Engl. J. Med.,* **1981,** *304*:251–258.

Kersten, S., Desvergne, B., and Wahli, W. Roles of PPARs in health and disease. *Nature,* **2000,** *405*:421–424.

Kleinveld, H.A., Demacker, P.N.M., De Haan, A.F.J., and Stalenhoef, A.F.H. Decreased *in vitro* oxidizability of low-density lipoprotein in hypercholesterolaemic patients treated with 3-hydroxy-3-methyl-glutaryl-CoA reductase inhibitors. *Eur. J. Clin. Invest.*, **1993**, *23*:289–295.

Knopp, R.H. Clinical profiles of plain *versus* sustained-release niacin (Niaspan) and the physiologic rationale for nighttime dosing. *Am. J. Cardiol.*, **1998**, *82*:24U–28U.

Knopp, R.H., Ginsberg, J., Albers, J.J., Hoff, C., Ogilvie, J.T., Warnick, G.R., Burrows, E., Retzlaff, B., and Poole, M. Contrasting effects of unmodified and time-release forms of niacin on lipoproteins in hyperlipidemic subjects: clues to mechanism of action of niacin. *Metabolism*, **1985**, *34*:642–650.

Kosoglou, T., Meyer, I., Musiol, B., Mellars, L., Statkevich, P., Miller, M.F., Soni, P.P., and Affrime, M.B. Pharmacodynamic interaction between the new selective cholesterol absorption inhibitor ezetimibe and simvastatin. *Atherosclerosis*, **2000**, *151*:135 (abstr.).

Kostner, G.M., Gavish, D., Leopold, B., Bolzano, K., Weintraub, M.S., and Breslow, J.L. HMG CoA reductase inhibitors lower LDL cholesterol without reducing Lp(a) levels. *Circulation*, **1989**, *80*:1313–1319.

Krieger, M., and Herz, J. Structures and functions of multiligand lipoprotein receptors: macrophage scavenger receptors and LDL receptor-related protein (LRP). *Annu. Rev. Biochem.*, **1994**, *63*:601–637.

Krieger, M., and Kozarsky, K. Influence of the HDL receptor SR-BI on atherosclerosis. *Curr. Opin. Lipidol.*, **1999**, *10*:491–497.

Kuo, P.T., Wilson, A.C., Kostis, J.B., Moreyra, A.B., and Dodge, H.T. Treatment of type III hyperlipoproteinemia with gemfibrozil to retard progression of coronary artery disease. *Am. Heart J.*, **1988**, *116*:85–90.

Lacoste, L., Lam, J.Y.T., Hung, J., Letchacovski, G., Solymoss, C.B., and Waters, D. Hyperlipidemia and coronary disease. Correction of the increased thrombogenic potential with cholesterol reduction. *Circulation*, **1995**, *92*:3172–3177.

Laufs, U., La Fata, V., Plutzky, J., and Liao, J.K. Upregulation of endothelial nitric oxide synthase by HMG-CoA reductase inhibitors. *Circulation*, **1998**, *97*:1129–1135.

Law, M.R., Thompson, S.G., and Wald, N.J. Assessing possible hazards of reducing serum cholesterol. *BMJ*, **1994**, *308*:373–379.

Lipid Research Clinics Program. The Lipid Research Clinics Coronary Primary Prevention Trial results: I. Reduction in incidence of coronary heart disease. *JAMA*, **1984a**, *251*:351–364.

Lipid Research Clinics Program. The Lipid Research Clinics Coronary Primary Prevention Trial results. II. The relationship of reduction in incidence of coronary heart disease to cholesterol lowering. *JAMA*, **1984b**, *251*:365–374.

Lipka, L.J., LeBeaut, A.P., Veltri, E.P., Mellars, L.E., Bays, H.L., and Moore, P.B. Reduction of LDL-cholesterol and elevation of HDL-cholesterol in subjects with primary hypercholesterolemia by SCH 58235: pooled analysis of two phase II studies. *J. Am. Coll. Cardiol.*, **2000.**, *35*(*suppl. A*):257A (abstr.).

The Long-Term Intervention with Pravastatin in Ischaemic Disease (LIPID) Study Group. Prevention of cardiovascular events and death with pravastatin in patients with coronary heart disease and a broad range of initial cholesterol levels. *N. Engl. J. Med.*, **1998**, *339*:1349–1357.

Maciejko, J.J., Holmes, D.R., Kottke, B.A., Zinsmeister, A.R., Dinh, D.M., and Mao, S.J.T. Apolipoprotein A-I as a marker of angiographically assessed coronary-artery disease. *N. Engl. J. Med.*, **1983**, *309*:385–389.

Maher, V.M., Brown, B.G., Marcovina, S.M., Hillger, L.A., Zhao, X.-Q., and Albers, J.J. Effects of lowering elevated LDL cholesterol on the cardiovascular risk of lipoprotein(a). *JAMA*, **1995**, *274*:1771–1774.

Mahley, R.W., and Ji, Z.S. Remnant lipoprotein metabolism: key pathways involving cell-surface heparan sulfate proteoglycans and apolipoprotein E. *J. Lipid Res.*, **1999**, *40*:1–16.

Malloy, M.J., Kane, J.P., Kunitake, S.T., and Tun, P. Complementarity of colestipol, niacin, and lovastatin in treatment of severe familial hypercholesterolemia. *Ann. Intern. Med.*, **1987**, *107*:616–623.

Martin-Jadraque, R., Tato, F., Mostaza, J.M., Vega, G.L., and Grundy, S.M. Effectiveness of low-dose crystalline nicotinic acid in men with low high-density lipoprotein cholesterol levels. *Arch. Intern. Med.*, **1996**, *156*:1081–1088.

McKenney, J.M., Proctor, J.D., Harris, S., and Chinchili, V.M. A comparison of the efficacy and toxic effects of sustained- vs immediate-release niacin in hypercholesterolemic patients. *JAMA*, **1994**, *271*:672–677.

Mead, J.R., Cryer, A., and Ramji, D.P. Lipoprotein lipase, a key role in atherosclerosis? *FEBS Lett.*, **1999**, *462*:1–6.

Miller, D.B., and Spence, J.D. Clinical pharmacokinetics of fibric acid derivatives (fibrates). *Clin. Pharmacokinet.*, **1998**, *34*:155–162.

Mosca, L., Grundy, S.M., Judelson, D., King, K., Limacher, M., Oparil, S., Pasternak, R., Pearson, T.A., Redberg, R.F., Smith, S.C., Jr., Winston, M., and Zinberg, S. Guide to preventive cardiology for women. AHA/ACC Scientific Statement Consensus panel statement. *Circulation*, **1999**, *99*:2480–2484.

Mullin, G.E., Greenson, J.K., and Mitchell, M.C. Fulminant hepatic failure after ingestion of sustained-release nicotinic acid. *Ann. Intern. Med.*, **1989**, *111*:253–255.

Nakad, A., Bataille, L., Hamoir, V., Sempoux, C., and Horsmans, Y. Atorvastatin-induced acute hepatitis with absence of cross-toxicity with simvastatin. *Lancet*, **1999**, *353*:1763–1764.

Nakata, A., Nakagawa, Y., Nishida, M., Nozaki, S., Miyagawa, J.I., Nakagawa, T., Tamura, R., Matsumoto, K., Kameda-Takemura, K., Yamashita, S., and Matsuzawa, Y. CD36, a novel receptor for oxidized low-density lipoproteins, is highly expressed on lipid-laden macrophages in human atherosclerotic aorta. *Arterioscler. Thromb. Vasc. Biol.*, **1999**, *19*:1333–1339.

National Cholesterol Education Program. *Report of the Expert Panel on Population Strategies for Blood Cholesterol Reduction.* U.S. Department of Health & Human Services, NIH Publi. No. 90-3046, Bethesda, MD, **1990.**

National Cholesterol Education Program. *Report of the Expert Panel on Blood Cholesterol Levels in Children and Adolescents.* U.S. Department of Health and Human Services, NIH Publi. No. 91-2732, Bethesda, MD, **1991.**

National Cholesterol Education Program Expert Panel. Executive summary of the third report of the National Cholesterol Education Program (NCEP) Expert Panel on Detection, Evaluation, and Treatment of High Blood Cholesterol in Adults (Adult Treatment Panel III). *J. Am. Med. Assoc.*, **2001**, *285*:2486–2497.

Neaton, J.D., Blackburn, H., Jacobs, D., Kuller, L., Lee, D.J., Sherwin, R., Shih, J., Stamler, J., and Wentworth, D. Serum cholesterol level and mortality findings for men screened in the Multiple Risk Factor Intervention Trial. Multiple Risk Factor Intervention Trial Research Group. *Arch. Intern. Med.*, **1992**, *152*:1490–1500.

O'Driscoll, G., Green, D., and Taylor, R.R. Simvastatin, an HMG–coenzyme A reductase inhibitor, improves endothelial function within 1 month. *Circulation*, **1997**, *95*:1126–1131.

Olsson, A.G., Pears, J.S., McKellar, J., Caplan, R.J., and Raza, A. Pharmacodynamics of new HMG-CoA reductase inhibitor ZD4522 in patients with primary hypercholesterolaemia. *Atherosclerosis*, **2000**, *151*:39 (abstr.).

Oram, J.F., and Vaughan, A.M. ABCA1-mediated transport of cellular cholesterol and phospholipids to HDL apolipoproteins. *Curr. Opin. Lipidol.*, **2000**, *11*:253–260.

Ose, L., Davidson, M.H., Stein, E.A., Kastelein, J.J.P., Scott, R.S., Hunninghake, D.B., Campodonico, S., Insull, W., Escobar, I.D., Schrott, H.G., Stepanavage, M.E., Wu, M., Tate, A.C., Melino, M.R., Mercuri, M., and Mitchel, Y.B. Lipid-altering efficacy and safety of simvastatin 80 mg/day: long-term experience in a large group of patients with hypercholesterolemia. World Wide Expanded Dose Simvastatin Study Group. *Clin. Cardiol.*, **2000**, *23*: 39–46.

Pedersen, T.R., and Tobert, J.A. Benefits and risks of HMG-CoA reductase inhibitors in the prevention of coronary heart disease: a reappraisal. *Drug Saf.*, **1996**, *14*:11–24.

Physicians' Desk Reference, 54th ed. Medical Economics Company, Montvale, NJ, **2000**, p. 2022.

Physicians' Desk Reference, 55th ed. Medical Economics Company, Montvale, NJ, **2001**, pp. 843–846.

Pi-Sunyer, F.X., Becker, D.M., Bouchard, C., Carleton, R.A., Colditz, G.A., Dietz, W.H., Foreyt, J.P., Garrison, R.J., Grundy, S.M., Hansen, B.C., Higgins, M., Hill, J.O., Howard, B.V., Klesges, R.C., Kuczmarski, R.J., Kumanyika, S., Legako, R.D., Prewitt, T.E., Rocchini, A.P., Smith, P.L., Snetselaar, L.G., Sowers, J.R., Weintraub, M., Williamson, D.F., and Wilson, G.T. *Clinical Guidelines on the Identification, Evaluation, and Treatment of Overweight and Obesity in Adults. The Evidence Report.* U.S. Department of Health and Human Services, Public Health Service, National Institutes of Health, NIH Publ. No. 98-4083, Bethesda, MD, **1998**, pp. 58–59.

Plump, A.S., Scott, C.J., and Breslow, J.L. Human apolipoprotein A-I gene expression increases high density lipoprotein and suppresses atherosclerosis in the apolipoprotein E-deficient mouse. *Proc. Natl. Acad. Sci. U.S.A.*, **1994**, *91*:9607–9611.

Pogson, G.W., Kindred, L.H., and Carper, B.G. Rhabdomyolysis and renal failure associated with cerivastatin-gemfibrozil combination therapy. *Am. J. Cardiol.*, **1999**, *83*:1146.

The Post Coronary Artery Bypass Graft Trial Investigators. The effect of aggressive lowering of low-density lipoprotein cholesterol levels and low-dose anticoagulation on obstructive changes in saphenous-vein coronary-artery bypass grafts. *N. Engl. J. Med.*, **1997**, *336*:153–162.

Pullinger, C.R., Hennessy, L.K., Chatterton, J.E., Liu, W., Love, J.A., Mendel, C.M., Frost, P.H., Malloy, M.J., Schumaker, V.N., and Kane, J.P. Familial ligand-defective apolipoprotein B. Identification of a new mutation that decreases LDL receptor binding affinity. *J. Clin. Invest.*, **1995**, *95*:1225–1234.

Quion, J.A.V., and Jones, P.H. Clinical pharmacokinetics of pravastatin. *Clin. Pharmacokinet.*, **1994**, *27*:94–103.

Raal, F.J., Pappu, A.S., Illingworth, D.R., Pilcher, G.J., Marais, A.D., Firth, J.C., Kotze, M.K., Heinonen, T.M., and Black, D.M. Inhibition of cholesterol synthesis by atorvastatin in homozygous familial hypercholesterolemia. *Atherosclerosis*, **2000**, *150*:421–428.

Raal, F.J., Pilcher, G.J., Illingworth, D.R., Pappu, A.S., Stein, E.A., Laskarzewski, P., Mitchel, Y.B., and Melino, M.R. Expanded-dose simvastatin is effective in homozygous familial hypercholesterolaemia. *Atherosclerosis*, **1997**, *135*:249–256.

Reihnér, E., Rudling, M., Ståhlberg, D., Berglund, L., Ewerth, S., Björkhem, I., Einarsson, K., and Angelin, B. Influence of pravastatin, a specific inhibitor of HMG-CoA reductase, on hepatic metabolism of cholesterol. *N. Engl. J. Med.*, **1990**, *323*:224–228.

Ridker, P.M., Rifai, N., Pfeffer, M.A., Sacks, F.M., Moye, L.A.,

Goldman, S., Flaker, G.C., and Braunwald, E. Inflammation, pravastatin, and the risk of coronary events after myocardial infarction in patients with average cholesterol levels. Cholesterol and Recurrent Events (CARE) Investigators. *Circulation,* **1998**, *98*:839–844.

Rosenson, R.S., and Tangney, C.C. Antiatherothrombotic properties of statins: implications for cardiovascular event reduction. *JAMA,* **1998**, *279*:1643–1650.

Rubins, H.B., Robins, S.J., Collins, D., Fye, C.L., Anderson, J.W., Elam, M.B., Faas, F.H., Linares, E., Schaefer, E.J., Schectman, G., Wilt, T.J., and Wittes, J. Gemfibrozil for the secondary prevention of coronary heart disease in men with low levels of high-density lipoprotein cholesterol. Veterans Affairs High-Density Lipoprotein Cholesterol Intervention Trial Study Group. *N. Engl. J. Med.,* **1999**, *341*:410–418.

Rubins, H.B., Robins, S.J., Collins, D., Iranmanesh, A., Wilt, T.J., Mann, D., Mayo-Smith, M., Faas, F.H., Elam, M.B., Rutan, G.H., Anderson, J.W., Kashyap, M.L., and Schectman, G. Distribution of lipids in 8,500 men with coronary artery disease. Department of Veterans Affairs HDL Intervention Trial Study Group. *Am. J. Cardiol.,* **1995**, *75*:1196–1201.

Sacks, F.M., Pfeffer, M.A., Moye, L.A., Rouleau, J.L., Rutherford, J.D., Cole, T.G., Brown, L., Warnica, J.W., Arnold, J.M.O., Wun, C.-C., Davis, B.R., and Braunwald, E. The effect of pravastatin on coronary events after myocardial infarction in patients with average cholesterol levels. Cholesterol and Recurrent Events Trial investigators. *N. Engl. J. Med.,* **1996**, *335*:1001–1009.

Scandinavian Simvastatin Survival Study Group. Randomised trial of cholesterol lowering in 4444 patients with coronary heart disease: the Scandinavian Simvastatin Survival Study (4S). *Lancet,* **1994**, *344*: 1383–1389.

Schultz, J.R., Verstuyft, J.G., Gong, E.L., Nichols, A.V., and Rubin, E.M. Protein composition determines the anti-atherogenic properties of HDL in transgenic mice. *Nature,* **1993**, *365*:762–764.

Schwartz, M.L. Severe reversible hyperglycemia as a consequence of niacin therapy. *Arch. Intern. Med.,* **1993**, *153*:2050–2052.

Segrest, J.P., Li, L., Anantharamaiah, G.M., Harvey, S.C., Liadaki, K.N., and Zannis, V. Structure and function of apolipoprotein A-I and high-density lipoprotein. *Curr. Opin. Lipidol.,* **2000**, *11*:105–115.

Shepherd, J., Cobbe, S.M., Ford, I., Isles, C.G., Lorimer, A.R., MacFarlane, P.W., McKillop, J.H., and Packard, C.J. Prevention of coronary heart disease with pravastatin in men with hypercholesterolemia. West of Scotland Coronary Prevention Study Group. *N. Engl. J. Med.,* **1995**, *333*:1301–1307.

Shepherd, J., Packard, C.J., Bicker, S., Lawrie, T.D., and Morgan, H.G. Cholestyramine promotes receptor-mediated low-density-lipoprotein catabolism. *N. Engl. J. Med.,* **1980**, *302*:1219–1222.

Shlipak, M.G., Simon, J.A., Vittinghoff, E., Lin, F., Barrett-Connor, E., Knopp, R.H., Levy, R.I., and Hulley, S.B. Estrogen and progestin, lipoprotein(a), and the risk of recurrent coronary heart disease events after menopause. *JAMA,* **2000**, *283*:1845–1852.

Staels, B., and Auwerx, J. Regulation of apo A-I gene expression by fibrates. *Atherosclerosis,* **1998**, *137*:S19–S23.

Stamler, J., Wentworth, D., and Neaton, J.D. Is relationship between serum cholesterol and risk of premature death from coronary heart disease continuous and graded? Findings in 356,222 primary screenees of the Multiple Risk Factor Intervention Trial (MRFIT). *JAMA,* **1986**, *256*:2823–2828.

Stein, E.A., Illingworth, D.R., Kwiterovich, P.O. Jr., Liacouras, C.A., Siimes, M.A., Jacobson, M.S., Brewster, T.G., Hopkins, P., Davidson, M., Graham, K., Arensman, F., Knopp, R.H., DuJovne, C., Williams, C.L., Isaacsohn, J.L., Jacobsen, C.A., Laskarzewski, P.M., Ames, S., and Gormley, G.J. Efficacy and safety of lovastatin in adolescent males with heterozygous familial hypercholesterolemia: a randomized controlled trial. *JAMA,* **1999,** *281:*137–144.

Stein, E.A., Lane, M., and Laskarzewski, P. Comparison of statins in hypertriglyceridemia. *Am. J. Cardiol.,* **1998,** *81:*66B–69B.

Steinberg, D. Low density lipoprotein oxidation and its pathobiological significance. *J. Biol. Chem.,* **1997,** *272:*20963–20966.

Stern, R.H., Spence, J.D., Freeman, D.J., and Parbtani, A. Tolerance to nicotinic acid flushing. *Clin. Pharmacol. Ther.,* **1991,** *50:*66–70.

Tall, A.R., Jiang, X.-C., Luo, Y., and Silver, D. 1999 George Lyman Duff memorial lecture: lipid transfer proteins, HDL metabolism, and atherogenesis. *Arterioscler. Thromb. Vasc. Biol.,* **2000,** *20:*1185–1188.

Tamai, O., Matsuoka, H., Itabe, H., Wada, Y., Kohno, K., and Imaizumi, T. Single LDL apheresis improves endothelium-dependent vasodilation in hypercholesterolemic humans. *Circulation,* **1997,** *95:*76–82.

Tatò, F., Vega, G.L., and Grundy, S.M. Effects of crystalline nicotinic acid-induced hepatic dysfunction on serum low-density lipoprotein cholesterol and lecithin cholesteryl acyl transferase. *Am. J. Cardiol.,* **1998,** *81:*805–807.

Thompson, G.R., Naoumova, R.P., and Watts, G.F. Role of cholesterol in regulating apolipoprotein B secretion by the liver. *J. Lipid Res.,* **1996,** *37:*439–447.

Thorp, J.M., and Waring, W.S. Modification of metabolism and distribution of lipids by ethyl chlorophenoxyisobutyrate. *Nature,* **1962,** *194:*948–949.

Tikkanen, M.J. Statins: within-group comparisons, statin escape and combination therapy. *Curr. Opin. Lipidol.,* **1996,** *7:*385–388.

Treasure, C.B., Klein, J.L., Weintraub, W.S., Talley, J.D., Stillabower, M.E., Kosinski, A.S., Zhang, J., Boccuzzi, S.J., Cedarholm, J.C., and Alexander, R.W. Beneficial effects of cholesterol-lowering therapy on the coronary endothelium in patients with coronary artery disease. *N. Engl. J. Med.,* **1995,** *332:*481–487.

van Heek, M., Farley, C., Compton, D.S., Hoos, L., Alton, K.B., Sybertz, E.J., and Davis, H.R. Jr. Comparison of the activity and disposition of the novel cholesterol absorption inhibitor, SCH58235, and its glucuronide, SCH60663. *Br. J. Pharmacol.,* **2000,** *129:*1748–1754.

Vega, G.L., and Grundy, S.M. Lipoprotein responses to treatment with lovastatin, gemfibrozil, and nicotinic acid in normolipidemic patients with hypoalphalipoproteinemia. *Arch. Intern. Med.,* **1994,** *154:*73–82.

Welty, F.K., Lahoz, C., Tucker, K.L., Ordovas, J.M., Wilson, P.W., and Schaefer, E.J. Frequency of apoB and apoE gene mutations as causes of hypobetalipoproteinemia in the Framingham offspring population. *Arterioscler. Thromb. Vasc. Biol.,* **1998,** *18:*1745–1751.

West, R.J., Lloyd, J.K., and Leonard, J.V. Long-term follow-up of children with familial hypercholesterolaemia treated with cholestyramine. *Lancet,* **1980,** *2:*873–875.

Wetterau, J.R., Gregg, R.E., Harrity, T.W., Arbeeny, C., Cap, M., Connolly, F., Chu, C.-H., George, R.J., Gordon, D.A., Jamil, H., Jolibois, K.G., Kunselman, L.K., Lan, S.-J., Maccagnan, T.J., Ricci, B., Yan, M., Young, D., Chen, Y., Fryszman, O.M., Logan, J.V.H., Musial, C.L., Poss, M.A., Robl, J.A., Simpkins, L.M., Slusarchyk, W.A., Sulsky, R., Taunk, P., Magnin, D.R., Tino, J.A., Lawrence, R.M., Dickson, J.K., Jr., and Biller, S.A. An MTP inhibitor that normalizes atherogenic lipoprotein levels in WHHL rabbits. *Science,* **1998,** *282:*751–754.

Williams, D.L., Connelly, M.A., Temel, R.E., Swarnakar, S., Phillips, M.C., de la Llera-Moya, M., and Rothblat, G.H. Scavenger receptor BI and cholesterol trafficking. *Curr. Opin. Lipidol.,* **1999,** *10:*329–339.

Williams, J.K., Sukhova, G.K., Herrington, D.M., and Libby, P. Pravastatin has cholesterol-lowering independent effects on the artery wall of atherosclerotic monkeys. *J. Am. Coll. Cardiol.,* **1998,** *31:*684–691.

Wilson, P.W.F., D'Agostino, R.B., Levy, D., Belanger, A.M., Silbershatz, H., and Kannel, W.B. Prediction of coronary heart disease using risk-factor categories. *Circulation,* **1998,** *97:*1837–1847.

Windler, E.E., Kovanen, P.T., Chao, Y.-S., Brown, M.S., Havel, R.J., and Goldstein, J.L. The estradiol-stimulated lipoprotein receptor of rat liver. A binding site that mediates the uptake of rat lipoproteins containing apoproteins B and E. *J. Biol. Chem.,* **1980,** *255:*10464–10471.

Wiseman, S.A., Powell, J.T., Humphries, S.E., and Press, M. The magnitude of the hypercholesterolemia of hypothyroidism is associated with variation in the low density lipoprotein receptor gene. *J. Clin. Endocrinol. Metab.,* **1993,** *77:*108–112.

Witztum, J.L., Schonfeld, G., Weidman, S.W., Giese, W.E., and Dillingham, M.A. Bile sequestrant therapy alters the compositions of low-density and high-density lipoproteins. *Metabolism,* **1979,** *28:*221–229.

Wood, D., De Backer, G., Faergeman, O., Graham, I., Mancia, G., and Pyörälä, K. Prevention of coronary heart disease in clinical practice. Recommendations of the Second Joint Task Force of European and other Societies on coronary prevention. *Eur. Heart J.,* **1998,** *19:*1434–1503.

Woollett, L.A., and Dietschy, J.M. Effect of long-chain fatty acids on low-density-lipoprotein-cholesterol metabolism. *Am. J. Clin. Nutr.,* **1994,** *60:*991S–996S.

Wysowski, D.K., and Gross, T.P. Deaths due to accidents and violence in two recent trials of cholesterol-lowering drugs. *Arch. Intern. Med.,* **1990,** *150:*2169–2172.

Yamamoto, A., Yamamura, T., Yokoyama, S., Sudo, H., and Matsuzawa, Y. Combined drug therapy—cholestyramine and compactin—for familial hypercholesterolemia. *Int. J. Clin. Pharmacol. Ther. Toxicol.,* **1984,** *22:*493–497.

Young, S.G., and Fielding, C.J. The ABCs of cholesterol efflux. *Nat. Genet.,* **1999,** *22:*316–318.

Yuan, J., Tsai, M.Y., and Hunninghake, D.B. Changes in composition and distribution of LDL subspecies in hypertriglyceridemic and hypercholesterolemic patients during gemfibrozil therapy. *Atherosclerosis,* **1994,** *110:*1–11.

Zhu, Y., Statkevich, P., Schuessler, D., Maxwell, S.E., Patrick, J., Kosoglou, T., and Batra, V. Pharmacokinetics of ezetimibe in rats, dogs and humans. *AAPS Pharm. Sci.,* **2000,** *2*(suppl.). Available at: http://www.pharmsci.org/scientificjournals/pharmsci/am_abstracts/2000/1101.html. Accessed February 14, 2001.

MONOGRAPHS AND REVIEWS

Assmann, G., von Eckardstein, A., and Brewer, H.B. Jr. Familial analphalipoproteinemia: Tangier disease. In, *The Metabolic and Molecular Bases of Inherited Disease,* 8th ed. Vol. 2. (Scriver, C.R., Beaudet, A.L., Sly, W.S., Valle, D., Childs, B., Kinzler, K.W., and Vogelstein, B., eds.) McGraw-Hill, New York, **2001,** pp. 2937–2960.

Berg, K. Lp(a) lipoprotein: an overview. *Chem. Phys. Lipids,* **1994,** *67/68:*9–16.

Breslow, J.L. Insights into lipoprotein metabolism from studies in transgenic mice. *Annu. Rev. Physiol.,* **1994,** *56:*797–810.

Brown, M.S., and Goldstein, J.L. Sterol regulatory element binding proteins (SREBPs): controllers of lipid synthesis and cellular uptake. *Nutr. Rev.,* **1998,** *56:*S1–S3.

Castelli, W.P. The folly of questioning the benefits of cholesterol reduction. *Am. Fam. Physician,* **1994,** *49*:567–574.

Durrington, P.N., and Illingworth, R. Lipid-lowering drugs: who gets what? *Curr. Opin. Lipidol.,* **1998,** *9*:289–294.

Ernst, E., and Resch, K.L. Fibrinogen as a cardiovascular risk factor: a meta-analysis and review of the literature. *Ann. Intern. Med.,* **1993,** *118*:956–963.

Farmer, J.A., and Gotto, A.M. Jr. Antihyperlipidaemic agents. Drug interactions of clinical significance. *Drug Saf.,* **1994,** *11*:301–309.

Figge, H.L., Figge, J., Souney, P.F., Mutnick, A.H., and Sacks, F. Nicotinic acid: a review of its clinical use in the treatment of lipid disorders. *Pharmacotherapy,* **1988,** *8*:287–294.

Ginsberg, H.N., and Goldberg, I.J. Disorders of lipoprotein metabolism. In, *Harrison's Principles of Internal Medicine,* 14th ed. (Fauci, A.S., Braunwald, E., Isselbacher, K.J., Wilson, J.D., Martin, J.B., Kasper, K.L., Hauser, S.L., and Longo, D.L., eds.) McGraw-Hill, New York, **1998,** pp. 2138–2149.

Grundy, S.M. Hypertriglyceridemia, atherogenic dyslipidemia, and the metabolic syndrome. *Am. J. Cardiol.,* **1998a,** *81*:18B–25B.

Grundy, S.M. Statin trials and goals of cholesterol-lowering therapy. *Circulation,* **1998b,** *97*:1436–1439.

Hebert, P.R., Gaziano, J.M., Chan, K.S., and Hennekens, C.H. Cholesterol lowering with statin drugs, risk of stroke, and total mortality. An overview of randomized trials. *JAMA,* **1997,** *278*:313–321.

Illingworth, D.R. Fibric acid derivatives. In, *Drug Treatment of Hyperlipidemia.* (Rifkind, B.M., ed.) Marcel Dekker, New York, **1991,** pp. 103–138.

Illingworth, D.R., and Durrington, P.N. Dyslipidemia and atherosclerosis: how much more evidence do we need? *Curr. Opin. Lipidol.,* **1999,** *10*:383–386.

Krieger, M. Charting the fate of the "good cholesterol": identification and characterization of the high-density lipoprotein receptor SR-BI. *Annu. Rev. Biochem.,* **1999,** *68*:523–558.

Mahley, R.W. Apolipoprotein E: cholesterol transport protein with expanding role in cell biology. *Science,* **1988,** *240*:622–630.

Mahley, R.W., and Huang, Y. Apolipoprotein E: from atherosclerosis to Alzheimer's disease and beyond. *Curr. Opin. Lipidol.,* **1999,** *10*:207–217.

Mahley, R.W., and Rall, S.C. Jr. Apolipoprotein E: far more than a lipid transport protein. *Annu. Rev. Genomics Hum. Genet.,* **2000,** *1*:507–537.

Mahley, R.W., and Rall, S.C. Jr. Type III hyperlipoproteinemia (dysbetalipoproteinemia): the role of apolipoprotein E in normal and abnormal lipoprotein metabolism. In, *The Metabolic and Molecular Bases of Inherited Disease,* 8th ed. Vol. 2. (Scriver, C.R., Beaudet, A.L., Sly, W.S., Valle, D., Childs, B., Kinzler, K.W., and Vogelstein, B., eds.) McGraw-Hill, New York, **2001,** pp. 2835–2862.

Mahley, R.W., Weisgraber, K.H., and Farese, R.V. Jr. Disorders of lipid metabolism. In, *Williams Textbook of Endocrinology,* 9th ed. (Wilson, J.D., Foster, D.W., Kronenberg, H.M., and Larsen, P.R., eds.) Saunders, Philadelphia, **1998,** pp. 1099–1153.

Reaven, G.M. Pathophysiology of insulin resistance in human disease. *Physiol. Rev.,* **1995,** *75*:473–486.

Ross, R. Atherosclerosis—an inflammatory disease. *N. Engl. J. Med.,* **1999,** *340*:115–126.

Rossen, R.D. HMG-CoA reductase inhibitors: a new class of antiinflammatory drugs? *J. Am. Coll. Cardiol.,* **1997,** *30*:1218–1219.

Thompson, G.R., and Barter, P.J. Clinical lipidology at the end of the millennium. *Curr. Opin. Lipidol.,* **1999,** *10*:521–526.

Watts, G.F., and Dimmitt, S.B. Fibrates, dyslipoproteinaemia and cardiovascular disease. *Curr. Opin. Lipidol.,* **1999,** *10*:561–574.

SECTION VI

DRUGS AFFECTING GASTROINTESTINAL FUNCTION

AGENTS USED FOR CONTROL OF GASTRIC ACIDITY AND TREATMENT OF PEPTIC ULCERS AND GASTROESOPHAGEAL REFLUX DISEASE

Willemijntje A. Hoogerwerf and Pankaj J. Pasricha

The term acid-peptic disorders *encompasses a variety of relatively specific medical conditions in which injury by gastric acid (and activated pepsin) is thought to play an important role. These disorders include gastroesophageal reflux disease (GERD), benign "peptic" ulcers of the stomach and duodenum, ulcers secondary to the use of conventional nonsteroidal antiinflammatory drugs (NSAIDs), and ulcers due to the rare Zollinger-Ellison syndrome. It appears that exposure of the involved tissue to acid is essential to the development of clinical symptoms in most instances of these diseases. Control of gastric acidity is therefore a cornerstone of therapy in these disorders, even though this approach may not address the fundamental pathophysiological process.*

Mankind has lived with peptic ulcers since ancient times. Perhaps the first description of this malady is the one inscribed on the pillars of the temple of Aesculapius at Epidaurus from around the fourth century B.C.: *"A man with an ulcer in his stomach. He incubated and saw a vision; the god seemed to order his followers to seize and hold him, that he might incise his stomach. So he fled, but they caught and tied him to the doorknocker. Then Asklepios opened his stomach, cut out the ulcer, sewed him up again, and loosed his bonds." Many prominent people have suffered from indigestion and ulcers, including the Roman emperor Marcus Aurelius, whose death has been attributed by some to a perforated ulcer and whose physician was none other than Galen himself. Acid neutralization was recognized as effective treatment more than 12 centuries ago by Paulus Aeginata, who prescribed a mixture of Samian and Lemnian earths and milk, not unlike the milk-antacid regimens of the mid-twentieth century (Smith and Rivers, 1953).*

Since then, of course, considerable advances in understanding the pathogenesis and in the treatment of acid-peptic conditions have occurred, culminating in the discovery of Helicobacter pylori *and proton pump inhibitors. We now know that eradication of* H. pylori *effectively promotes healing of peptic ulcers and prevents their recurrence in most cases. Proton pump inhibitors have become the drugs of choice in promoting healing from erosive esophagitis and peptic ulcer disease because of their ability to nearly completely suppress acid production. Although several clinical challenges still need to be met in this area, it is reasonable to conclude that the battle against the ravages of gastric acid is finally turning in our favor. This chapter covers some of the principal therapeutic agents in this area and strategies for their use.*

PHYSIOLOGY OF GASTRIC SECRETION

Gastric acid secretion is a complex, continuous process controlled by multiple central (neural) and peripheral (endocrine and paracrine) factors. Each factor attributes to a common final physiological event—the secretion of H^+ by parietal cells, which are located in the body and fundus of the stomach. Neuronal (acetylcholine, ACh), paracrine (histamine), and endocrine

(gastrin) factors all play important roles in the regulation of acid secretion (Figure 37–1). Their respective specific receptors (M_3, H_2, CCK_2 receptors) have been anatomically and/or pharmacologically localized to the basolateral membrane of the parietal cell. Two major signaling pathways are present within the parietal cell: the cyclic AMP–dependent pathway and the Ca^{2+}–dependent pathway. Histamine uses the first pathway, while gastrin and ACh exert their effect *via* the latter. The cyclic AMP–dependent pathway results in phosphorylation of parietal-cell effector proteins and the Ca^{2+}–dependent pathway leads to an

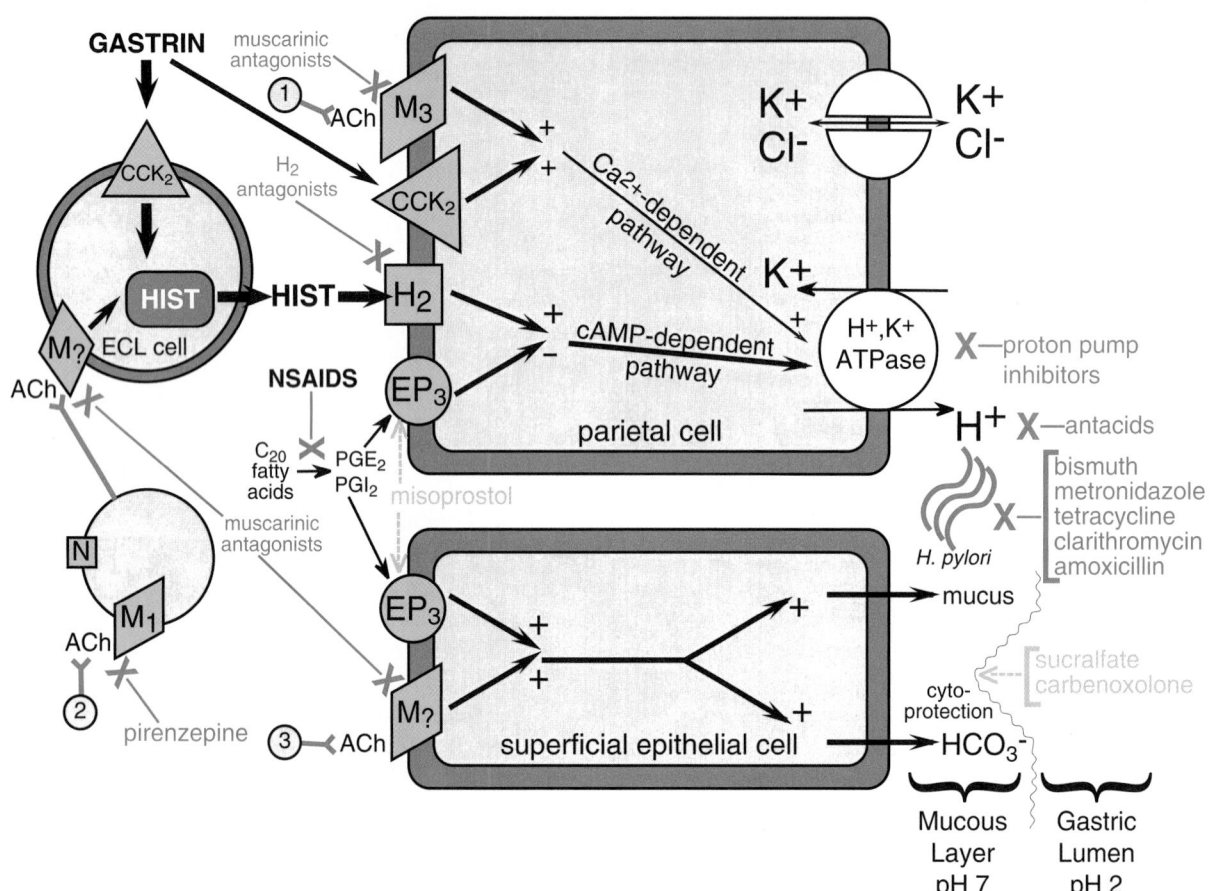

Figure 37–1. Physiological and pharmacological regulation of gastric secretions: the basis for therapy of peptic ulcer disease.

This schematic shows the interactions among an endocrine cell that secretes histamine [enterochromaffin-like (ECL) cell], an acid-secreting cell (parietal cell), and a cell that secretes the cytoprotective factors mucus and bicarbonate (superficial epithelial cell). Physiological pathways are in solid black and may be stimulated (+) or inhibited (−). Physiological agonists stimulate transmembrane receptors: muscarinic (M) and nicotinic (N) receptors for acetylcholine (ACh); CCK_2, gastrin (and cholecystokinin) receptor; H_2, histamine (HIST) receptor; EP_3, prostaglandin E_2 receptor. Actions of drugs are indicated by dashed lines. A blue X indicates a point of pharmacological antagonism. A light blue dashed line and arrow indicate a drug action that mimics or enhances a physiological pathway. Drugs currently used in treating peptic ulcer disease and discussed in this chapter are shown in dark blue. NSAIDs are nonsteroidal antiinflammatory drugs such as aspirin and are ulcerogenic. ① and ③ indicate possible input by cholinergic postganglionic fibers. ② shows neural input from the vagus nerve. *See* the text for detailed descriptions of these pathways and of therapeutic interventions.

increase in cytosolic Ca^{2+}. Both pathways activate the H^+,K^+–ATPase (the proton pump). The H^+,K^+–ATPase consists of a large α-subunit and a smaller β-subunit. This pump generates the largest ion gradient known in vertebrates, with an intracellular pH of about 7.3 and an intracanalicular pH of about 0.8.

The most important structures in the central nervous system (CNS) involved in central stimulation of gastric acid secretion are the dorsal motor nucleus of the vagal nerve (DMNV), the hypothalamus, and the nucleus tractus solitarius (NTS). Efferent fibers originating in the DMNV descend to the stomach *via* the vagus nerve and synapse with ganglion cells of the enteric nervous system (ENS). ACh release from postganglionic vagal fibers can stimulate directly gastric acid secretion through a specific muscarinic cholinergic receptor subtype, M_3, located on the basolateral membrane of the parietal cells. The CNS probably modulates the activity of the ENS with ACh as its main regulatory neurotransmitter. The CNS generally is thought of as the main contributor to the initiation of gastric acid secretion in response to the sight, smell, taste, and anticipation of food ("cephalic phase"). ACh also indirectly affects the parietal cell through the stimulation of histamine release from the enterochromaffin-like (ECL) cells in the fundus and the stimulation of gastrin release from the G cells in the gastric antrum.

Histamine is released from ECL cells through multifactorial pathways and is a critical regulator of acid production through the H_2 subtype of receptor. ECL cells usually are found in close proximity to parietal cells. Histamine activates the parietal cell in a paracrine fashion; it diffuses from its release site to the parietal cell. Its involvement in gastric acid secretion (whether or not as the final, common, effector hormone) has been convincingly demonstrated by the inhibition of acid secretion with the use of H_2-receptor antagonists. The ECL cells are the sole source of gastric histamine involved in acid secretion.

Gastrin primarily is present in the antral G cells. As with histamine, the release of gastrin is regulated through multifactorial pathways involving, among other factors, central neural activation, local distention, and chemical components of the gastric content. Gastrin stimulates acid secretion predominantly in an indirect manner by causing the release of histamine from ECL cells; a less-important, direct effect of gastrin on parietal cells also is seen.

Somatostatin, localized in the antral D cells, may inhibit gastrin secretion in a paracrine matter, but its exact role in the inhibition of gastric acid secretion remains to be defined. There appears to be a decrease in D cells in patients with *Helicobacter pylori* infection, and this may lead to excess gastrin production due to a reduced inhibition by somatostatin.

Gastric Defense. The stomach protects itself from damage by gastric acid through several mechanisms such as the presence of intercellular tight junctions between the gastric epithelial cells, the presence of a mucin layer overlying the gastric epithelial cells, the presence of prostaglandins in the gastric mucosa, and secretion of bicarbonate ions into the mucin layer. Prostaglandins E_2 and I_2 inhibit gastric acid secretion by a direct effect on the parietal cell mediated by the EP_3 receptor (*see* section entitled "Prostaglandin Analogs," below). In addition, prostaglandins enhance mucosal blood flow and stimulate secretion of mucus and bicarbonate.

AGENTS USED FOR SUPPRESSION OF GASTRIC ACID PRODUCTION

Figure 37–1 provides the rationale and pharmacological basis for the classes of drugs currently used to combat acid-peptic diseases. The most commonly used agents at present are the proton pump inhibitors and the histamine H_2-receptor antagonists.

Proton Pump Inhibitors

Chemistry, Mechanism of Action, and Pharmacological Properties.   The most effective suppressors of gastric acid secretion undoubtedly are the gastric H^+,K^+–ATPase (proton pump) inhibitors. They are the most effective drugs used in antiulcer therapy and have found worldwide popularity over the past decade. Currently, there are several different proton pump inhibitors available for clinical use: *omeprazole* (PRILOSEC), *lansoprazole* (PREVACID), *rabeprazole* (ACIPHEX), and *pantoprazole* (PROTONIX). They are α-pyridylmethylsulfinyl benzimidazoles with different substitutions on the pyridine or the benzimidazole groups; their pharmacological properties are similar. Proton pump inhibitors are "prodrugs," requiring activation in an acid environment. These agents enter the parietal cells from the blood and, because of their weak basic nature, accumulate in the acidic secretory canaliculi of the parietal cell, where they are activated by a proton-catalyzed process that results in the formation of a thiophilic sulfenamide or sulfenic acid (Figure 37–2). This activated form reacts by covalent binding with the sulfhydryl group of cysteines from the extracellular domain of the H^+,K^+–ATPase. Binding to cysteine 813, in particular, is essential for inhibition of acid production, which is irreversible for that pump molecule. Proton pump inhibitors have profound effects on acid production. When given in a sufficient dose (*e.g.,* 20 mg of omeprazole a day for seven days), the daily production of acid can be diminished by more than 95%. Secretion of acid resumes only after new molecules of the pump are inserted into the luminal membrane. Omeprazole also selectively inhibits gastric mucosal carbonic anhydrase, which may contribute to its acid suppressive properties.

Pharmacokinetics.   Proton pump inhibitors are unstable at a low pH. The oral dosage forms ("delayed release") are supplied as enteric-coated granules encapsulated in a gelatin shell (omeprazole and lansoprazole) or as enteric-coated tablets (pantoprazole and rabeprazole). The granules dissolve only at an alkaline pH, thus preventing degradation of the drugs by acid in the esophagus and stomach. Proton pump inhibitors are rapidly

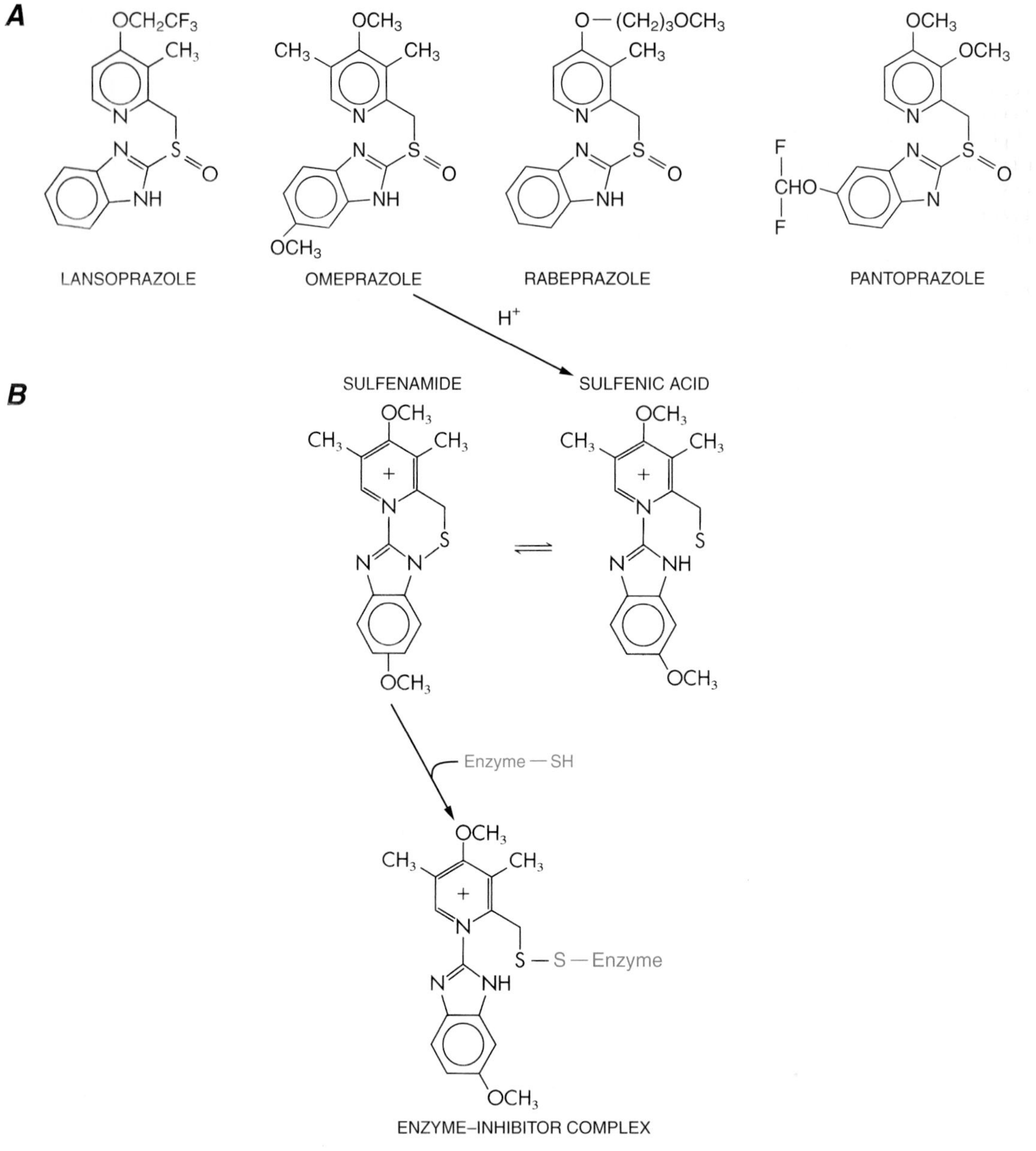

Figure 37–2. Proton pump inhibitors.

A. Structures of four inhibitors of the gastric H^+,K^+–ATPase (proton pump).

B. Conversion of omeprazole to a sulfenamide in the acidic canaliculi of the parietal cell. The other three proton pump inhibitors undergo analogous conversions. The sulfenamides interact covalently with sulfhydryl groups in the extracellular domain of the proton pump, thereby inhibiting its activity.

absorbed, highly protein bound, and extensively metabolized in the liver by the cytochrome P450 system (particularly CYP2C19 and CYP3A4). Their sulfated metabolites are excreted in the urine or feces. Their plasma half-lives are about 1 to 2 hours, but their durations of action are much longer (*see* below). Chronic renal failure and liver cirrhosis do not appear to lead to drug accumulation with once-a-day dosing of the drugs. Hepatic dis-

ease reduces the clearance of lansoprazole substantially, and dose reduction should be considered in patients with severe hepatic disease.

The requirement for enteric coating poses a challenge to the routine use of oral proton pump inhibitors in critically ill patients or in patients unable to swallow adequately. Intravenous H_2-receptor antagonists have been preferred in patients with contraindications to oral ingestion, but this picture is expected to change with the advent of intravenous preparations of proton pump inhibitors. *Pantoprazole,* a relatively more acid-stable compound, is the first such preparation to be approved in the United States. A single intravenous bolus of 80 mg can inhibit acid production by 80% to 90% within an hour, an effect that can last up to 21 hours. Therefore, once-daily dosing of intravenous proton pump inhibitors (in doses similar to those used orally) may be sufficient to achieve the desired degree of hypochlorhydria. The clinical utility of these formulations in the above situations will require further study but is expected to be equal to if not greater than that of intravenous H_2-receptor antagonists.

The requirement for acid to activate these drugs within the parietal cells has several important consequences. The drugs should be taken with or before a meal, since food will stimulate acid production by parietal cells; conversely, coadministration of other acid-suppressing agents such as H_2-receptor antagonists may diminish the efficacy of proton pump inhibitors. Since not all pumps or all parietal cells are functional at the same time, it takes several doses of the drugs to result in maximal suppression of acid secretion. With once-a-day dosing, steady-state inhibition, affecting about 70% of pumps, may take 2 to 5 days (*see* Sachs, 2000). Achieving steady-state inhibition may be accelerated somewhat by more frequent dosing initially (*e.g.,* twice daily). Since the binding of the drugs' active metabolites to the pump is irreversible, inhibition of acid production will last for 24 to 48 hours or more, until new enzyme is synthesized. The duration of action of these drugs, therefore, is not directly related to their plasma half-lives.

Adverse Effects and Drug Interactions. Proton pump inhibitors inhibit the activity of some hepatic cytochrome P450 enzymes and therefore may decrease the clearance of benzodiazepines, warfarin, phenytoin, and many other drugs. When disulfiram is coadministered with a protein pump inhibitor, toxicity has been reported. Proton pump inhibitors usually cause few adverse effects; nausea, abdominal pain, constipation, flatulence, and diarrhea are the most common side effects. Subacute myopathy, arthralgias, headaches, and skin rashes also have been reported.

Chronic treatment with omeprazole decreases the absorption of vitamin B_{12}, but insufficient data exist to demonstrate whether or not this leads to a clinically relevant deficiency. Hypergastrinemia (>500 ng/liter) occurs in approximately 5% to 10% of long-term omeprazole users. Gastrin is a trophic factor for epithelial cells, and there is a theoretical concern that elevations in gastrin can promote the growth of different kinds of tumors in the gastrointestinal tract. In rats undergoing long-term administration of proton pump inhibitors, there has been development of enterochromaffin-like cell hyperplasia and gastric carcinoid tumors secondary to sustained hypergastrinemia; this has raised concerns about the possibility of similar complications in human beings. There are conflicting data on the risk and clinical implications of enterochromaffin-like cell hyperplasia in patients on long-term proton pump inhibitor therapy. These drugs now have a track record of more than 15 years of use worldwide, and no major new issues regarding safety have emerged (Klinkenberg-Knol *et al.,* 1994; Kuipers and Meuwissen, 2000). There is as yet no reason to believe, therefore, that hypergastrinemia should be a trigger for discontinuation of therapy or that gastrin levels should be monitored routinely in patients on long-term proton pump inhibitor therapy. However, the development of a hypergastrinemic state may predispose the patient to rebound hypersecretion of gastric acid following discontinuation of therapy.

Proton pump inhibitors have not been associated with a major teratogenic risk when used during the first trimester of pregnancy; caution, however, is still warranted.

Therapeutic Uses. Proton pump inhibitors are used principally to promote healing of gastric and duodenal ulcers and to treat *g*astric *e*sophageal *r*eflux *d*isease (GERD) that is either complicated or unresponsive to treatment with H_2-receptor antagonists (*see* below). Proton pump inhibitors also are the mainstay in the treatment of Zollinger-Ellison syndrome. Therapeutic applications of proton pump inhibitors are further discussed later in this chapter, under "Specific Acid-Peptic Disorders and Therapeutic Strategies."

HISTAMINE H_2-RECEPTOR ANTAGONISTS

The description of selective histamine H_2-receptor blockade by Black in 1970 was a landmark in the history of pharmacology and set the stage for the modern approach to the treatment of acid-peptic disease, which until then had relied almost entirely on acid neutralization in the lumen of the stomach (*see* Black, 1993; Feldman and Burton, 1990a,b). Equally impressive has been the safety record of H_2-receptor antagonists, a feature that eventually led to their availability without a prescription. Increasingly, however, these agents are being replaced by the more efficacious albeit more expensive proton pump inhibitors.

Chemistry, Mechanism of Action, and Pharmacological Properties. Four different H_2-receptor antagonists are currently on the market in the United States: *cimetidine* (TAGAMET), *ranitidine* (ZANTAC), *famotidine* (PEPCID), and *nizatidine* (AXID) (Figure 37–3). Their different chemical structures do not alter the drugs' clinical efficacies as much as they determine interactions with other drugs and change the side-effect profiles. H_2-receptor antagonists inhibit acid production by reversibly competing with histamine for binding to H_2 receptors on the basolateral membrane of parietal cells.

The most prominent effects of H_2-receptor antagonists are on basal acid secretion; less profound but still significant is suppression of stimulated (feeding, gastrin, hypoglycemia, or vagal stimulation) acid production. These agents thus are particularly effective in suppressing

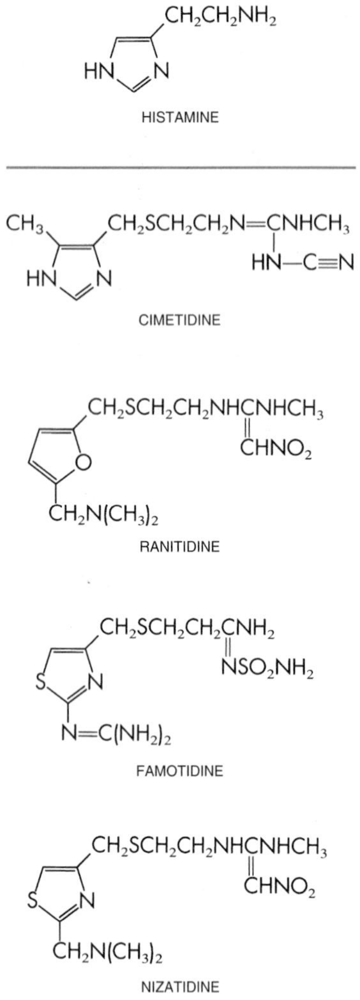

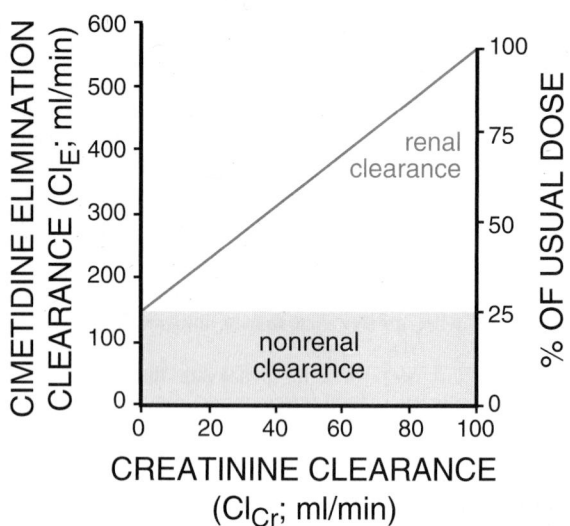

Figure 37–3. *Structures of histamine and H$_2$-receptor antagonists.*

Figure 37–4. *Relationship between creatinine clearance (CL$_{Cr}$), cimetidine elimination clearance (CL$_E$), and appropriate cimetidine dose reduction for patients with impaired renal function. (Adapted from Atkinson and Craig, 1990, with permission.)*

nocturnal acid secretion, which reflects mainly basal parietal cell activity. This fact has clinical relevance in that the most important determinant of duodenal ulcer healing is the level of nocturnal acidity. Therefore, duodenal ulcers can be healed with once-daily dosing of H$_2$-receptor antagonists given between supper and bedtime. In addition, some patients with reflux esophagitis who are being treated with proton pump inhibitors may continue to produce acid at night (so-called nocturnal acid breakthrough) and could benefit from the addition of an H$_2$-receptor antagonist at night.

Pharmacokinetics. H$_2$-receptor antagonists are absorbed rapidly after oral administration, with peak serum concentrations reached within 1 to 3 hours. Unlike proton pump inhibitors, only a small percentage of H$_2$-receptor antagonists is protein-bound. Small amounts (from <10% to ~35%) of these drugs undergo metabolism in the liver. Both metabolized and unmetabolized products are excreted by the kidney by both filtration and renal tubular secretion. It is important to reduce doses of H$_2$-receptor antagonists in patients with decreased creatinine clearance. Figure 37–4 provides a useful nomogram to guide the dosage adjustment for cimetidine when renal clearance is impaired. Hemodialysis and peritoneal dialysis clear only very small amounts of the drugs. Liver disease *per se* is not an indication for dose adjustment; however, in advanced liver disease with decreased renal clearance, reduced dosing is indicated (*see* Table 37–1 and Appendix II for pharmacokinetic properties of these drugs).

All four H$_2$-receptor antagonists are available in dosage forms for oral administration; intravenous and intramuscular preparations of cimetidine, ranitidine, and famotidine also are available. Therapeutic levels are achieved quickly after intravenous dosing and are maintained for several hours (4 to 5 hours for cimetidine, 6 to 8 hours for ranitidine, and 10 to 12 hours for famotidine). In clinical practice, these drugs can be given in intermittent boluses or by continuous infusion (Table 37–2).

Adverse Reactions and Drug Interactions. The overall incidence of adverse effects of H$_2$-receptor antagonists is low (<3%). Side effects usually are minor and include diarrhea, headache, drowsiness, fatigue, muscular pain, and constipation. Less-common side effects include those affecting the CNS (confusion, delirium, hallucinations, slurred speech, and headaches), which occur primarily with intravenous administration of the drugs. Gynecomastia in men and galactorrhea in women may occur due to the binding of cimetidine to androgen receptors and inhibition of the cytochrome P450-catalyzed hydroxylation of estradiol. Reductions in sperm count and reversible impotence have been reported in men. These effects are mainly seen with long-term use of cimetidine in high doses. Several reports have associated H$_2$-receptor antagonists with various cytopenias,

Table 37–1
Comparison of Properties of Histamine H_2–Receptor Antagonists

	CIMETIDINE	RANITIDINE	FAMOTIDINE	NIZATIDINE
Bioavailability (%)	80	50	40	>90
Relative potency	1	5–10	32	5–10
Plasma half-life (hours)	1.5–2.3	1.6–2.4	2.5–4	1.1–1.6
Approximate duration of therapeutic effect (hours)	6	8	12	8
Relative effect on cytochrome P450 activity	1	0.1	0	0

Modified from Wolfe and Sachs, 2000.

including reductions in platelet count. H_2-receptor antagonists cross the placenta and are excreted in breast milk. Although no major teratogenic risk has been associated with these agents, caution is nevertheless warranted when they are used in pregnancy. All agents that inhibit gastric acid secretion may alter the rate of absorption and subsequent bioavailability of the H_2-receptor antagonists (*see* "Antacids," below).

Drug interactions with H_2-receptor antagonists can be expected mainly with cimetidine, and these are an important factor in the preferential use of other H_2-receptor antagonists. Cimetidine inhibits cytochrome P450 more so than do the other agents in this class (Table 37–1) and can thereby alter the metabolism and increase the levels of drugs that are substrates for the cytochrome P450 system. Such drugs include warfarin, phenytoin, certain β-adrenergic receptor antagonists, quinidine, caffeine, some benzodiazepines, tricyclic antidepressants, theophylline, chlordiazepoxide, carbamazepine, metronidazole, calcium channel blockers, and sulfonylureas. Cimetidine can inhibit renal tubular secretion of procainamide, increasing the plasma concentrations of procainamide and of its cardioactive metabolite, *N*-acetylprocainamide. Special care should be taken with the concomitant use of other drugs whose metabolism can be altered by cimetidine and with the use of cimetidine in elderly patients with decreased creatinine clearance.

Therapeutic Uses.   The major therapeutic indications for H_2-receptor antagonists are for promoting healing of gastric and duodenal ulcers, for treatment of uncomplicated GERD, and for prophylaxis of stress ulcers. More information about the therapeutic applications of H_2-receptor antagonists is provided in the section of this chapter entitled "Specific Acid-Peptic Disorders and Therapeutic Strategies."

PROSTAGLANDIN ANALOGS: MISOPROSTOL

Chemistry, Mechanism of Action, and Pharmacological Properties.   Prostaglandin (PG)E_2 and PGI_2 are the major prostaglandins synthesized by the gastric mucosa; they inhibit acid production by binding to the EP_3 receptor on parietal cells (*see* Chapter 26). Prostaglandin binding to the receptor results in inhibition of adenylyl cyclase and decreased levels of intracellular cyclic AMP. PGE also can prevent gastric injury by its so-called cytoprotective effects, which include stimulation of secretion of mucin and bicarbonate and improvement in mucosal blood flow; however, acid suppression appears to be its more critical effect (Wolfe *et al.*, 1999). Although smaller doses than required for acid suppression may be protective for the gastric mucosa in laboratory animals, this has not been convincingly demonstrated in human beings. Since NSAIDs inhibit prostaglandin formation, the synthetic prostaglandins provide a rational approach to reducing NSAID-related mucosal damage. *Misoprostol* (15-deoxy-16-hydroxy-16-methyl-PGE_1; CYTOTEC) is a synthetic analog of prostaglandin E_1 with an additional methyl ester group at C1 (resulting in an increase in

Table 37–2
Intravenous Doses of Histamine H_2–Receptor Antagonists

	CIMETIDINE	RANITIDINE	FAMOTIDINE
Intermittent bolus	300 mg every 6 to 8 hours	50 mg every 6 to 8 hours	20 mg every 12 hours
Continuous infusion	37.5–100 mg/hour	6.25–12.5 mg/hour	1.7–2.1 mg/hour

potency and in the duration of the antisecretory effect) and a switch of the hydroxy group from C15 to C16 along with an additional methyl group (resulting in improved activity when given orally, increased duration of action, and improved safety profile). The degree of inhibition of gastric acid secretion by misoprostol is directly related to dose; oral doses of 100 to 200 μg produce significant inhibition of basal acid secretion (decreased by 85% to 95%) or food-stimulated acid secretion (decreased by 75% to 85%).

Pharmacokinetics. Misoprostol is rapidly absorbed and undergoes extensive and rapid first-pass metabolism (deesterification) to form misoprostol acid (the free acid), the principal and active metabolite of the drug. Some of this conversion may in fact occur in the parietal cells. After a single dose, inhibition of acid production can be seen within 30 minutes, peaks at 60 to 90 minutes, and lasts for up to 3 hours. Food and antacids decrease the rate of absorption of misoprostol, resulting in delayed and decreased peak plasma concentrations of misoprostol acid. The elimination half-life of the free acid, which is excreted mainly in the urine, is about 20 to 40 minutes.

Adverse Effects. The most frequently reported side effect of misoprostol is diarrhea, with or without abdominal pain and cramps, which can occur in up to 30% of patients. Diarrhea, which appears to be a dose-dependent response, is seen about 2 weeks after initiating therapy and often resolves spontaneously within a week. It can be severe, however, in some patients, requiring discontinuation. Misoprostol can cause clinical exacerbations in patients with inflammatory bowel disease (*see* Chapter 39) and hence should be avoided in these patients. **Misoprostol is contraindicated during pregnancy,** since it can cause abortion by increasing uterine contractility.

Therapeutic Use. Misoprostol currently is approved by the United States Food and Drug Administration (FDA) for use in preventing mucosal injury caused by nonsteroidal antiinflammatory drugs.

SUCRALFATE

Chemistry, Mechanism of Action, and Pharmacological Properties. In the presence of acid-induced damage, pepsin-mediated hydrolysis of mucosal proteins contributes to mucosal erosion and ulcerations. This process can be inhibited by sulfated polysaccharides. *Sucralfate* (CARAFATE) consists of the octasulfate of sucrose to which aluminum hydroxide has been added. In an acid environment (pH < 4), it undergoes extensive cross-linking and polymerization to produce a viscous, sticky gel that adheres strongly to epithelial cells and even more strongly to ulcer craters for as long as 6 hours after a single dose. In addition to inhibition of hydrolysis of mucosal pro-

teins by pepsin, sucralfate may have additional cytoprotective effects, including stimulation of local production of prostaglandin and epidermal growth factor (EGF). Sucralfate also binds bile salts, accounting for its use in some patients with esophagitis or gastritis in whom reflux of bile is thought by some to play a role in pathogenesis (the existence of such syndromes remains controversial). The role of sucralfate in the treatment of acid-peptic disease clearly has diminished in recent years. It still may be useful in the prophylaxis of stress ulcers (*see* below), where its use may be associated with a lower incidence of nosocomial pneumonia compared to acid-suppressing therapy with its tendency to promote gastric bacterial colonization.

Since it is activated by acid, it is recommended that sucralfate be taken on an empty stomach one hour before meals rather than after; the use of antacids within 30 minutes of a dose of sucralfate should be avoided.

Adverse Effects. The most commonly reported side effect is constipation (2%). Small amounts of aluminum can be absorbed with the use of sucralfate, and special attention needs to be given to patients with renal failure, who are at risk for aluminum overload. Aluminum-containing antacids should not be used with sucralfate in patients with renal failure. Since sucralfate forms a viscous layer in the stomach, it may inhibit absorption of other drugs and change their bioavailability. These include phenytoin, digoxin, cimetidine, ketoconazole, and fluoroquinolone antibiotics. It is therefore recommended that sucralfate be taken at least 2 hours after the intake of other drugs.

ANTACIDS

Although their use has been hallowed by tradition, antacids now are seldom part of regimens prescribed by physicians because of the availability of more effective and convenient drugs. Nevertheless, they continue to be used by patients for a variety of indications, and some knowledge of their pharmacological properties is essential for the medical professional. The usefulness of antacids is influenced by the rate of dosage-form dissolution, by their reactivity with acid, by physiological effects of the cation, by water solubility, and by the presence or absence of food in the stomach (*see* Table 37–3 for a comparison of some commonly used antacid preparations). The very water-soluble $NaHCO_3$ is rapidly cleared from the stomach and presents both an alkali and a sodium load. $CaCO_3$ can neutralize HCl rapidly (depending on particle size and crystal structure) and effectively; however, it can cause abdominal distention and belching with acid reflux. Combinations of Mg^{2+} and Al^{3+} hydroxides provide a relatively fast and sustained neutralizing capacity. Magaldrate is a hydroxymagnesium aluminate complex that is rapidly converted in

Table 37–3

Composition and Neutralizing Capacities of Some Popular Antacid Preparations

PRODUCT	CONTENTS, mg PER TABLET OR PER 5 ml				ACID-NEUTRALIZING CAPACITY, mEq PER TABLET OR PER 5 ml
	$Al(OH)_3$	$Mg(OH)_2$	$CaCO_3$	SIMETHICONE	
Tablets					
GELUSIL II	400	400	0	30	21
MAALOX QUICK DISSOLVE	0	0	600	0	11
MYLANTA	0	150	350	0	12
RIOPAN PLUS DOUBLE STRENGTH	Magaldrate, 1080			20	30
ROLAIDS	0	110	550	0	14
TUMS-EX	0	0	750	0	15
Liquids					
GELUSIL II	400	400	0	30	24
KUDROX	500	450	0	40	28
MAALOX TC	600	300	0	0	28
Milk of Magnesia	0	400	0	0	14
MYLANTA EXTRA STRENGTH	400	400	0	40	25
RIOPAN PLUS DOUBLE STRENGTH	Magaldrate, 1080			40	30

gastric acid to $Mg(OH)_2$ and $Al(OH)_3$, which are poorly absorbed and thus provide a sustained antacid effect with balanced effects on intestinal motility. Simethicone, a surfactant that may decrease foaming and hence esophageal reflux, is included in many antacid preparations.

The presence of food alone elevates gastric pH to about 5 for approximately 1 hour and prolongs the neutralizing effects of antacids for about 2 hours. Alkalinization of the gastric contents increases gastric motility, through the action of gastrin. Al^{3+} can relax gastric smooth muscle, producing delayed gastric emptying and constipation, effects that are opposed by those of Mg^{2+}. Thus, $Al(OH)_3$ and $Mg(OH)_2$ taken concurrently have relatively little effect on gastric emptying or bowel function. Because of its capacity to enhance secretion and to form insoluble compounds, $CaCO_3$ has unpredictable effects on gastrointestinal motility. The release of CO_2 from bicarbonate and carbonate-containing antacids can cause belching, occasional nausea, abdominal distention, and flatulence. Belching may cause exacerbation of gastroesophageal reflux.

Antacids are cleared from the empty stomach in about 30 minutes and vary in the extent to which they are absorbed. Antacids that contain aluminum, calcium, or magnesium are less completely absorbed than are those that contain $NaHCO_3$. In persons with normal renal function, the modest accumulations of Al^{3+} and Mg^{2+} do not pose a problem; with renal insufficiency, however, absorbed Al^{3+} can contribute to osteoporosis, encephalopathy, and proximal myopathy. About 15% of orally administered Ca^{2+} is absorbed, causing a transient hypercalcemia. Although not a problem in normal patients, the hypercalcemia from as little as 3 to 4 g per day can be problematic in patients with uremia. Absorption of unneutralized $NaHCO_3$ will cause alkalosis. Neutralized antacids also may cause alkalosis by permitting the absorption of endogenous $NaHCO_3$ spared by the addition of exogenous neutralizing equivalents into the gastrointestinal tract. These disturbances of acid-base balance by antacids usually are transient and clinically insignificant in persons with normal renal function. In the past, when large doses of $NaHCO_3$ and/or $CaCO_3$ were commonly administered with milk or cream for the management of peptic ulcer, the *milk-alkali syndrome* occurred frequently. This syndrome results from large quantities of Ca^{2+} and absorbable alkali; effects consist of hypercalcemia, reduced secretion of parathyroid hormone, retention of phosphate, precipitation of Ca^{2+} salts in the kidney, and renal insufficiency. Therapeutic regimens emphasizing the use of dairy products seldom are employed in current practice.

By altering gastric and urinary pH, antacids may alter rates of dissolution and absorption, the bioavailability, and renal elimination of a number of drugs. Al^{3+} and Mg^{2+} compounds also are notable for their propensity to adsorb drugs and to form insoluble complexes that are not absorbed. Unless bioavailability also is affected, altered rates of absorption have little clinical significance when drugs are given chronically in multiple doses. In general, it is prudent to avoid concurrent administration of antacids and drugs intended for systemic absorption. Most interactions can be avoided by taking antacids 2 hours before or after ingestion of other drugs.

OTHER AGENTS

Drugs That Suppress Acid Production. The anticholinergic compounds *pirenzepine* and *telenzepine* (*see* Chapter 7) can reduce basal acid production by 40% to 50% and have been used in countries other than the United States for many decades to treat patients with peptic ulcer. They are classically thought to be antagonists of the M_1 cholinergic receptor and may act to suppress neural stimulation of acid production (the receptor on the parietal cell itself is of the M_3 subtype). Because of their relatively poor efficacy and significant and undesirable anticholinergic side effects, their use is mainly of historical concern. Antagonists of the gastrin receptor on parietal cells (CCK_2 receptor) currently are under study.

Cytoprotective Agents. *Rebamipide* (2-(4-chlorobenzoyl-amino)-3-[2(1*H*)-quinolinon-4-yl]-propionic acid), is available as an antiulcer agent in parts of Asia. It appears to exert its cytoprotective effect by increasing prostaglandin generation in gastric mucosa as well as by scavenging reactive oxygen species. *Ecabet* (12-sulfodehydroabietic acid monosodium) is another antiulcer agent mainly used in Japan, which appears to increase the formation of PGE_2 and PGI_2. *Carbenoxolone,* a component of licorice root and a derivative of glycyrrhizic acid, has been used in Europe as an antiulcer compound for many years with modest efficacy. Its exact mechanism of action is not clear, but it may alter the composition and quantity of mucin. Unfortunately, it is a steroid congener, and its use may be limited by its significant mineralocorticoid activity. *Bismuth compounds* (*see* Chapter 39) may be as effective as cimetidine in patients with peptic ulcer. They have many potentially therapeutic effects in this regard. They bind to the base of the ulcer, promote mucin and bicarbonate production, and have significant antibacterial effects. They are an important component of many anti-*Helicobacter* regimens (*see* below). However, they are seldom used by themselves anymore, given the availability of more effective agents.

SPECIFIC ACID-PEPTIC DISORDERS AND THERAPEUTIC STRATEGIES

Drugs that suppress gastric acid production have proven their efficacy in a variety of conditions in which acid plays a major role in injury to the gastrointestinal mucosa. In addition, these drugs also are employed in combination with antibiotics to treat infection with *H. pylori* (*see* "Treatment of *Helicobacter pylori* Gastritis," below). The success of these drugs is critically dependent upon their ability to keep intragastric pH above a certain level; the target pH varies to some extent with the disease being treated (Figure 37–5). The overall therapeutic strategy and role of various drugs in individual syndromes is discussed in the following sections (*see* also DeVault, 1999; Richardson *et al.,* 1998; Sachs, 1997; Lew, 1999; Welage and Berardi, 2000; Wolfe and Sachs, 2000).

Gastroesophageal Reflux Disease

Gastroesophageal reflux disease (GERD) is common in the United States, where it is estimated that one in five adults has symptoms of heartburn and/or regurgitation at least once a week. Although most of these cases are not associated with significant damage to the esophageal lining, it is clear that, in some individuals, GERD can cause severe esophagitis with sequelae that include stricture formation and Barrett's metaplasia or Barrett's esophagus (replacement of squamous by columnar epithelium of varying degrees of specialization), which in turn is associated with a small but significant risk of adenocarcinoma. The incidence of GERD has been rising over the past several

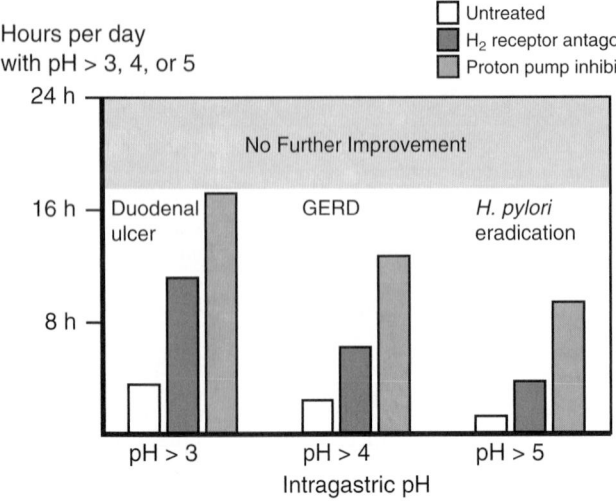

Figure 37–5.

The relative success of treatment with a proton pump inhibitor (given once daily) and an H_2-receptor antagonist (given twice daily) in obtaining an 18-hour elevation in intragastric pH to target levels of pH 3.0 for duodenal ulcer, pH 4.0 for gastroesophageal reflux disease (GERD), and pH 5.0 for *H. pylori* eradication with antibiotics. Twice-daily administration further improves the elevation in intragastric pH. (*Adapted from Wolfe and Sachs, 2000, with permission.*)

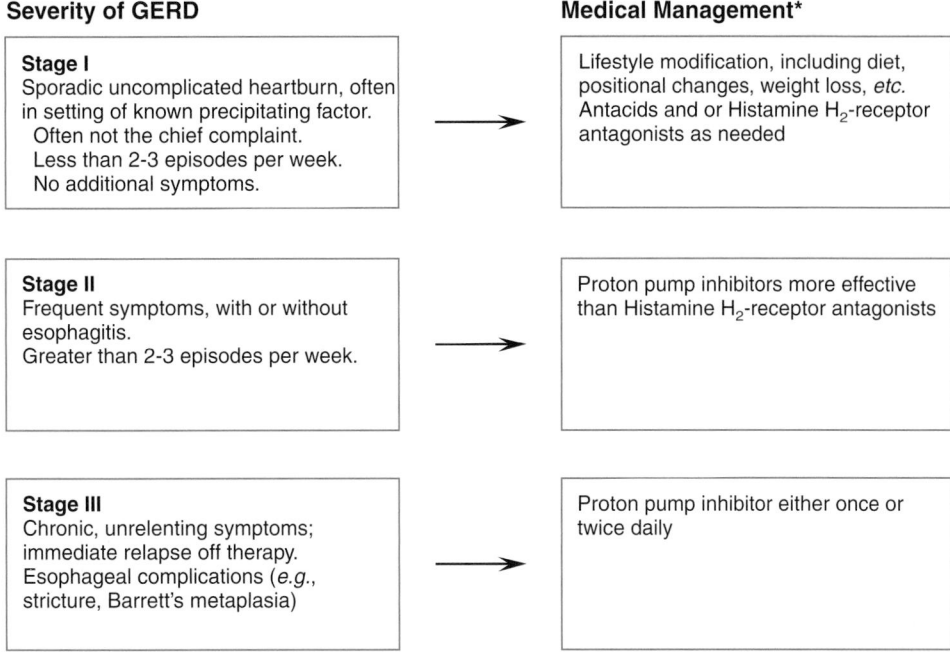

Figure 37–6. General guidelines for medical management of gastroesophageal reflux disease (GERD).

Only acid production–suppressing and acid-neutralizing medication included. (Adapted from Wolfe and Sachs, 2000, with permission.)

decades; so has the incidence of esophageal adenocarcinoma, particularly in white males. An association has been suggested between GERD symptoms and the incidence of esophageal adenocarcinoma (Lagergren *et al.,* 1999). An increasing number of reports also link GERD and tracheopulmonary symptoms such as chronic laryngitis and asthma, although a cause-and-effect relationship is still somewhat controversial. Finally, it should be borne in mind that GERD is a chronic disorder that requires long-term therapy (DeVault, 1999).

Although the pathophysiology of GERD has more to do with a disturbance of gastrointestinal motility (*see* Chapter 38), most of the symptoms are due to the injurious effects of the acid-peptic refluxate on the esophageal epithelium. This provides the rationale for the current pharmacotherapeutic approach to treating this syndrome, which is based on suppression of gastric acid. Traditional prokinetic agents have been of limited efficacy, but more specific agents currently are being developed and may hold greater promise (Chapter 38).

Treatment of Acute GERD Symptoms.   The goals of GERD therapy are complete resolution of symptoms and healing of esophagitis. Proton pump inhibitors are clearly more effective than H₂-receptor antagonists in achieving both of these goals. Healing rates after 4 weeks and 8 weeks of therapy with protein pump inhibitors are around 80% and 90%, respectively; healing rates with H₂-receptor antagonists are 50% and 75%. Indeed, protein pump inhibitors are so effective that their empirical use has been advocated as a therapeutic trial in patients in whom GERD is suspected to play a role in the pathogenesis of

symptoms. The "omeprazole test" involves giving omeprazole for a period of 12 weeks to patients with noncardiac chest pain. Expensive diagnostic tests are instituted only if such a trial fails (Fass *et al.,* 1998). Because of the wide clinical spectrum associated with GERD, the therapeutic approach is best tailored to the level of severity in the individual patient (Figure 37–6). In general, the optimal dose for each individual patient should be determined based upon symptom control. Only in patients with complicated GERD and/or Barrett's esophagus is documentation of complete acid control with 24-hour pH monitoring indicated.

Regimens for the treatment of GERD with proton pump inhibitors and histamine H₂-receptor antagonists are listed in Table 37–4. Although some patients with mild GERD symptoms may be managed by nocturnal doses of H₂-receptor antagonists, dosing two or more times a day generally is required. In patients with severe symptoms or extraintestinal manifestations of GERD, twice-daily dosing with a proton pump inhibitor may be needed. It has been shown, though, that nocturnal acid breakthrough can occur even with twice-daily proton pump inhibitor dosing in healthy subjects and that this can be controlled by the addition of an H₂-receptor antagonist at bedtime (Peghini *et al.,* 1998). The clinical importance of this finding for GERD patients with poorly responsive symptoms to standard dosing of proton pump inhibitors needs further evaluation.

A popular approach to GERD therapy, encouraged by managed-care companies, consists of a "step-up" regimen, beginning with an H₂-receptor antagonist and only progressing to one of the proton pump inhibitors if symptoms fail to respond. While theoretically appealing, this approach carries the risk of

Table 37–4
Drug Regimens for Treatment of Gastroesophageal Reflux Disease (GERD)

Histamine H$_2$–Receptor Antagonists
Nonerosive GERD
   Cimetidine 400 mg twice/day
   Ranitidine or nizatidine 150 mg twice/day
   Famotidine 20 mg twice/day
   Therapy should be individualized to fit patient's requirements; often effective when
     doses are administered between breakfast and lunch, and between the evening
     meal and bedtime.

Erosive GERD
   Cimetidine 400 mg every 6 hours
   Ranitidine or nizatidine 150 mg every 6 hours
   Famotidine 40 mg every 12 hours

Proton-Pump Inhibitors
Nonerosive or erosive GERD
   Omeprazole 20 mg daily or 20 mg twice/day
   Lansoprazole 30 mg daily or 30 mg twice/day
   Rabeprazole 20 mg daily or 20 mg twice/day
   Pantoprazole 40 mg daily or 40 mg twice/day
   All administered daily before breakfast; second dose, if necessary, should be given
     before evening meal.

SOURCE: Adapted from Wolfe and Sachs, 2000, with permission.

delaying the resolution of symptoms and or healing and eventually may be counterproductive because of the higher costs associated with ineffective therapy.

Antacids currently are recommended only for the patient with mild, infrequent episodes of heartburn. Their use, of course, is entrenched in the public mind, and it is rare for a patient with GERD not to have tried several of these medications before seeking medical help. In general, prokinetic agents (*see* Chapter 38) seldom form the mainstay of treatment for GERD, particularly since questions have been raised about the safety of cisapride. It also is doubtful that there is any value in using them in combination with acid-suppressant medications (Vigneri *et al.*, 1995).

Maintenance Therapy of GERD. Reflux esophagitis is a chronic disease with a high relapse rate after discontinuation of therapy. Acid suppressant drugs have been the mainstay of therapy. Again, "step-down" approaches are advocated by some, namely to try and maintain symptomatic remission by either decreasing the dose of the proton pump inhibitor or switching to an H$_2$-receptor antagonist. However, many patients will maintain their requirement for proton pump inhibitors. Several studies suggest that proton pump inhibitors are better than H$_2$-receptor antagonists for maintaining remission in reflux esophagitis (Hallerbäck *et al.*, 1994; Vigneri *et al.*, 1995).

Therapy for Complications of GERD. Strictures associated with GERD respond better to proton pump inhibitors than to H$_2$-receptor antagonists; indeed, the use of proton pump inhibitors has been shown to reduce the requirement for esophageal dila-

tion (Marks *et al.*, 1994). Unfortunately, one of the other complications of GERD, Barrett's esophagus, appears to be more permanent, as neither acid suppression nor antireflux surgery has been shown convincingly to produce regression of metaplasia. The role of acid suppression by proton pump inhibitors as adjuvants in ablative therapy of Barrett's esophagus currently is under investigation. It also appears that a subgroup of GERD patients with extraesophageal symptoms such as asthma and laryngitis may respond to trials of proton pump inhibitors, usually given in higher doses and more frequently than for the usual heartburn sufferer.

Peptic Ulcer Disease

The pathophysiology of peptic ulcer disease is best understood in terms of an imbalance between mucosal defense factors (bicarbonate, mucin, prostaglandin, nitric oxide, other peptides and growth factors) and aggressive factors (acid and pepsin). Patients with duodenal ulcer on average produce more acid than do control subjects, particularly at night (basal secretion). Although patients with gastric ulcers have normal or even lower acid production than control subjects, ulcers rarely if ever occur in the complete absence of acid ("no acid, no ulcer"). In these gastric ulcer patients, even the lower levels of acid can produce injury, presumably due to weakened mucosal defense and reduced bicarbonate production. Both *H. pylori* and exogenous agents such as nonsteroidal antiinflammatory drugs (NSAIDs) interact with these factors in complex ways, leading to an ulcer diathesis. Up to 80% to 90% of ulcers may be associated with *H. pylori* infection of the stomach. This infection may lead to impaired production of somatostatin by D cells and, in time, decreased inhibition of gastrin production, with a resulting higher acid production as well as impaired duodenal bicarbonate production. NSAIDs also are very frequently associated with peptic ulcers (in up to 60% of patients, particularly those with complications such as bleeding). Topical injury by the luminal presence of the drug appears to play a minor role in the pathogenesis of these ulcers, as evidenced by the fact that ulcers can occur with very low doses of aspirin (10 mg) or with parenteral administration of NSAIDs. The effects of these drugs are instead mediated systemically, with the critical element being suppression of the constitutive form of cyclooxygenase (COX)-1 in the mucosa and a consequent reduction in cytoprotective prostaglandins, PGE_2 and PGI_2.

Although antacids have been used historically and have proven to be somewhat effective, their use is inconvenient because of the need for multiple daily doses. They also may be associated with undesirable side effects (*see* "Antacids," above). It is clear that drugs causing suppression of acid production form the mainstay of peptic ulcer treatment (Table 37–5). Individual settings for their use are discussed below.

Table 37–5

Current Recommendations for Treatment of Gastroduodenal Ulcers

Active ulcer

H_2-receptor antagonists
   Cimetidine 800 mg
   Ranitidine or nizatidine 300 mg
   Famotidine 40 mg
   All administered between evening meal and bedtime

Proton-Pump Inhibitors
   Omeprazole 20 mg
   Lansoprazole 30 mg
   Rabeprazole 20 mg
   All administered daily before breakfast

Maintenance therapy[*]

H_2-receptor antagonists
   Cimetidine 400 mg
   Ranitidine or nizatidine 150 mg
   Famotidine 20 mg
   All administered between the evening meal and
      bedtime

Proton-Pump Inhibitors
   As above

Prevention of nonsteroidal antiinflammatory drug-induced ulcers

Misoprostol
   At least 200 μg 3 times/day
Proton-Pump Inhibitors
   As above

SOURCE: Adapted from Wolfe and Sachs, 2000, with permission.
[*]*See also* Table 37–6.

Uncomplicated Ulcers: Acute Symptoms and Healing.   Proton pump inhibitors promote more rapid relief of duodenal ulcer symptoms and more rapid healing than do H_2-receptor antagonists (McFarland *et al.,* 1990), although both classes of drugs are very effective in this setting.

Complicated Ulcers: Acute Gastrointestinal Bleeding.   Acid-suppressive therapy has a long history of use in patients presenting to the hospital with signs of acute upper gastrointestinal bleeding and is almost routinely prescribed. The theoretical benefits of acid-suppressive agents in this setting include acceleration of healing of the underlying ulcer. In addition, clot formation is enhanced and its dissolution retarded at a high pH (Peterson and Cook, 1998). Isolated studies suggest an improved outcome with the use of omeprazole in certain populations of patients with ulcer-related bleeding (Khuroo *et al.,* 1997). Despite such studies and the results of meta-analysis, the benefits from empiric acid-suppressive therapy in patients with acute gastrointestinal bleeding remain somewhat controversial. Although proton pump inhibitors are probably more effective than H_2-receptor antagonists in this setting, the availability of intravenous preparations of H_2-receptor antagonists has led to their widespread use. This practice probably will change with the recent introduction of intravenous proton pump inhibitors.

Uncomplicated Ulcers: Maintenance Therapy and Prophylaxis with Acid-Suppressive Agents.   With the demonstration that *H. pylori* plays a major etiopathogenic role in the majority of peptic ulcers (*see* below), prophylaxis against relapses is focused on eliminating this organism from the stomach. Chronic acid-suppressive therapy, once the mainstay of ulcer prevention, now is used mainly in patients who are *H. pylori*–negative or, in some cases, in patients with life-threatening complications.

Treatment of *Helicobacter pylori* Infection.   *H. pylori*, a gram-negative rod, has been associated with gastritis and subsequent development of gastric and duodenal ulcers, gastric adenocarcinoma and gastric B-cell lymphoma (Veldhuyzen and Lee, 1999). Because of its critical role in the pathogenesis of peptic ulcers in the majority of cases, it has become standard care to eradicate this infection in patients with gastric or duodenal ulcers (Graham, 1997; Chiba *et al.,* 2000). Such a strategy almost completely eliminates the risk of ulcer recurrence, provided patients are not taking NSAIDs. Eradication of *H. pylori* also is indicated in the treatment of MALT-lymphoma of the stomach, as this can regress significantly after such treatment.

Treatment of *H. pylori* infection is not straightforward, however, and many important factors need to be considered in the choice of a treatment regimen (Graham, 2000) (Table 37–6). Single antibiotic regimens are ineffective in treating *H. pylori* infection and lead to resistance. In addition, a proton pump inhibitor or H_2-receptor antagonist significantly enhances the effectiveness of regimens containing pH-dependent antibiotics such as amoxicillin or clarithromycin. Third, 10 to 14 days of treatment appear to be better than shorter treatment regimens; in the United States, a 14-day course generally is preferred. Finally, antibiotic resistance is increasingly being recognized as an important factor in the failure to eradicate *H. pylori*. Antibiotic resistance is a complex issue, with different underlying mechanisms and clinical implications. *Clarithromycin* resistance is related to ribosomal mutations that prevent the binding of the antibiotic and is an all-or-none phenomenon. On the other hand,

Table 37–6
Preferred Therapies for *Helicobacter pylori* infection

Twice a day PPI or ranitidine bismuth citrate (TRITEC)
  triple therapies*
  A PPI or 400 mg of rantidine bismuth citrate twice
    a day
  Plus 2 of: Amoxicillin, 1 g; clarithromycin, 500 mg;
    or metronidazole, 500 mg (each twice a day)
Quadruple therapy
  A PPI twice a day
  Tetracycline HCl 500 mg 4 times a day
  Bismuth subsalicylate or subcitrate 4 times a day
  Metronidazole 500 mg 3 times a day

*There seems to be no difference between ranitidine bismuth citrate and
  PPI triple therapies when the *H. pylori* are sensitive. There may
  be a slight advantage for ranitidine bismuth citrate triple therapies
  when resistant *H. pylori* are present.
PPI, proton pump inhibitor.
SOURCE: From Graham, 2000, with permission.

metronidazole resistance is relative rather than absolute and may
involve several different changes in the bacteria. Despite *in vitro*
resistance, however, a 14-day quadruple drug regimen generally
is effective therapy (Huang and Hunt, 1999).

Whether or not *H. pylori* infection should be treated in patients with GERD is controversial. An argument has been made
to treat all of these patients because of concerns about the development of atrophic gastritis with the use of acid-suppressive
therapy in the setting of *H. pylori* infection. However, the magnitude of this risk is unclear. On the other hand, GERD symptoms
and esophagitis have been reported to be worse after *H. pylori*
eradication in patients with ulcers. This is felt to be a consequence of the improvement in *H. pylori*–related inflammation
and increased acid secretion, which trigger the development of
GERD symptoms in this subset of patients (O'Connor, 1999).

H. pylori appears to play a minor role, if any, in the development of NSAID-induced ulcers, although its elimination
probably is done routinely (Hawkey *et al.*, 1998b). Similarly,
although often practiced, eradication of *H. pylori* does not improve the clinical symptoms in patients with nonulcer dyspepsia
(Talley *et al.*, 1999).

NSAID-Related Ulcers.   Chronic NSAID users have a 2% to
4% risk of developing a symptomatic ulcer, gastrointestinal
bleeding, or even perforation (La Corte *et al.*, 1999; Wolfe
et al., 1999). Ideally, conventional NSAIDs should be discontinued if at all possible and/or replaced with a selective COX-2
inhibitor (*see* Chapter 27). Nevertheless, healing of ulcers despite continued NSAID use is possible with the use of acid-
suppressant agents, usually at higher doses and for a considerably longer duration than with standard regimens (*e.g.*, 8
weeks or longer). Again, proton pump inhibitors are superior to
H_2-receptor antagonists and misoprostol in promoting healing
of active ulcers (80% to 90% healing rates compared to 60% to
75%) as well as in preventing recurrence (while on NSAIDs) of
both gastric ulcers (5% to 13% *versus* 10% to 16% recurrence

rates) and duodenal ulcers (0.5% to 3% *versus* 4% to 10% recurrence rate) (Hawkey *et al.*, 1998a; Lanza, 1998; Yeomans
et al., 1998).

Stress-Related Ulcers.   Stress ulcers are ulcers of the stomach or duodenum that usually occur in the context of a major
systemic or CNS illness or trauma (ASHP Therapeutic Guidelines on Stress Ulcer Prophylaxis, 1999). The etiology of stress-
related ulcers is somewhat different from that of other peptic
ulcers and involves acid as well as mucosal ischemia. Reduction of gastric acidity to a pH above 5 appears to be important
in preventing the activation of pepsin and subsequent mucosal
injury. This can be achieved by any of the acid production–
suppressing agents as well as antacids (Cook *et al.*, 1998). Because of limitations on the use of oral drugs in many patients
with stress-related ulcers, intravenous H_2-receptor antagonists
currently are the preferred agents and have been shown to reduce the incidence of gastrointestinal hemorrhage due to stress
ulcers. Now that intravenous preparations of proton pump inhibitors are becoming available, it is possible that their use will
prove to be equally if not more beneficial. There is a concern
over the risk of pneumonia secondary to gastric bacterial colonization in an alkaline milieu, and this has led to the use of
sucralfate slurries (*via* nasogastric tube), which also appears to
provide reasonable prophylaxis against bleeding, but is more
inconvenient. In a meta-analysis that compared H_2-receptor antagonists with sucralfate and placebo as prophylactic agents for
clinically important gastrointestinal bleeding, both sucralfate and
H_2-receptor antagonists were found to reduce the incidence of
overt bleeding compared to placebo or no therapy. There was a
trend toward a lower incidence of nosocomial pneumonia with
the use of sucralfate, but later studies have not confirmed this
finding (Cook *et al.*, 1996).

Zollinger-Ellison Syndrome.   Patients with this syndrome develop gastrinomas that drive the secretion of large amounts of
acid. This can lead to severe gastroduodenal ulceration and
other consequences of the uncontrolled hyperchlorhydria. Proton pump inhibitors are clearly the drugs of choice and are
usually given at twice the dosage for routine ulcers, with the
goal of therapy being to reduce acid secretion in the range of
1 to 10 mmol/hour.

Nonulcer Dyspepsia.   This term refers to ulcer-like symptoms in patients who are without overt gastroduodenal ulceration (American Gastroenterological Association position statement, 1998). This may occur with gastritis (with or without
H. pylori) or with NSAID use, but the pathogenesis of this
syndrome remains unclear. Although empirical treatment with
acid-suppressive agents is used routinely in patients with nonulcer dyspepsia, there is no convincing evidence of their benefit
in controlled trials. This disorder is best regarded as a regional
manifestation of the same general type of visceral hyperalgesia
seen in patients with irritable bowel syndrome (*see* Chapter 38).

PROSPECTUS

Impressive advances have been made in the pharmacological treatment of acid-peptic disorders. These have been
made possible largely by the availability of the proton

pump inhibitors and the discovery of *H. pylori* and its role in acid-peptic disorders. Another, somewhat indirect contribution has been made by the new selective COX-2 inhibitors, which are expected to reduce significantly the incidence of NSAID-induced ulcers. New drug discovery in this area will address specific therapeutic problems such as bleeding from gastrointestinal ulcers. Other advances should result from a greater understanding of the pathophysiology of GERD. Such understanding may eventually lead to treatments that correct the underlying defect in antireflux sphincteric mechanisms and provide alternatives to long-term treatment with acid-suppressive agents.

For further discussion of gastroesophageal reflux disease and peptic ulcer and related disorders, *see* Chapters 283 and 284 in *Harrison's Principles of Internal Medicine,* 14th ed., McGraw-Hill, New York, 1998.

BIBLIOGRAPHY

American Gastroenterological Association medical position statement: evaluation of dyspepsia. *Gastroenterology, 1998, 114*:579–581.

ASHP Therapeutic Guidelines on Stress Ulcer Prophylaxis. ASHP Commission on Therapeutics and approved by the ASHP Board of Directors on November 14, 1998. *Am. J. Health Syst. Pharm., 1999, 56*:347–379.

Black, J. Reflections on the analytical pharmacology of histamine H_2-receptor antagonists. *Gastroenterology, 1993, 105*:963–968.

Cook, D., Guyatt, G., Marshall, J., Leasa, D., Fuller, H., Hall, R., Peters, S., Rutledge, F., Griffith, L., McLellan, A., Wood, G., and Kirby, A. A. comparison of sucralfate and ranitidine for the prevention of upper gastrointestinal bleeding in patients requiring mechanical ventilation. Canadian Critical Care Trials Group. *N. Engl. J. Med., 1998, 338*:791–797.

Cook, D.J., Reeve, B.K., Guyatt, G.H., Heyland, D.K., Griffith, L.E., Buckingham, L., and Tryba, M. Stress ulcer prophylaxis in critically ill patients. Resolving discordant meta-analyses. *JAMA, 1996, 275*:308–314.

Fass, R., Fennerty, M.B., Ofman, J.J., Gralnek, I.M., Johnson, C., Camargo, E., and Sampliner, R.E. The clinical and economic value of a short course of omeprazole in patients with noncardiac chest pain. *Gastroenterology, 1998, 115*:42–49.

Hallerbäck, B., Unge, P., Carling, L., Edwin, B., Glise, H., Havu, N., Lyrenäs, E., and Lundberg, K. Omeprazole or ranitidine in long-term treatment of reflux esophagitis. The Scandinavian Clinics for United Research Group. *Gastroenterology, 1994, 107*:1305–1311.

Hawkey, C.J., Karrasch, J.A., Szczepanski, L., Walker, D.G., Barkun, A., Swannell, A.J., and Yeomans, N. Omeprazole compared with misoprostol for ulcers associated with nonsteroidal antiinflammatory drugs. Omeprazole versus Misoprostol for NSAID-induced Ulcer Management (OMNIUM) Study Group. *N. Engl. J. Med., 1998a, 338*:727–734.

Hawkey, C.J., Tulassay, Z., Szczepanski, L., van Rensburg, C.J., Filipowicz-Sosnowska, A., Lanas, A., Wason, C.M., Peacock, R.A., and Gillon, K.R. Randomised controlled trial of *Helicobacter pylori* eradication in patients on non-steroidal anti-inflammatory drugs: HELP NSAIDs study. Helicobacter Eradication for Lesion Prevention. *Lancet, 1998b, 352*:1016–1021.

Huang, J., and Hunt, R.H. The importance of clarithromycin dose in the management of *Helicobacter pylori* infection: a meta-analysis of triple therapies with proton pump inhibitor, clarithromycin and amox-

icillin or metronidazole. *Aliment. Pharmacol. Ther., 1999, 13*:719–729.

Khuroo, M.S., Yattoo, G.N., Javid, G., Khan, B.A., Shah, A.A., Gulzar, G.M., and Sodi, J.S. A comparison of omeprazole and placebo for bleeding peptic ulcer. *N. Engl. J. Med., 1997, 336*:1054–1058.

Klinkenberg-Knol, E.C., Festen, H.P., Jansen, J.B., Lamers, C.B., Nelis, F., Snel, P., Lückers, A., Dekkers C.P., Havu, N., and Meeuwissen, S.G. Long-term treatment with omeprazole for refractory esophagitis: efficacy and safety. *Ann. Intern. Med., 1994, 121*:161–167.

Kuipers, E.J., and Meuwissen, S.G. The efficacy and safety of long-term omeprazole treatment for gastroesophageal reflux disease. *Gastroenterology, 2000, 118*:795–798.

Lagergren, J., Bergström, R., Lindgren, A., and Nyrén, O. Symptomatic gastroesophageal reflux disease as a risk factor for esophageal adenocarcinoma. *N. Engl. J. Med., 1999, 340*:825–831.

Lanza, F.L. A guideline for the treatment and prevention of NSAID-induced ulcers. Members of the Ad Hoc Committee on Practice Parameters of the American College of Gastroenterology. *Am. J. Gastroenterol., 1998, 93*:2037–2046.

McFarland, R.J., Bateson, M.C., Green J.R., O'Donoghue, D.P., Dronfield, M.W., Keeling, P.W., Burke, G.J., Dickinson, R.J., Shreeve, D.R., and Peers, E.M. Omeprazole provides quicker symptom relief and duodenal ulcer healing than ranitidine. *Gastroenterology, 1990, 98*:278–283.

Marks, R.D., Richter, J.E., Rizzo, J., Koehler, R.E., Spinney, J.G., Mills, T.P., and Champion, G. Omeprazole versus H_2-receptor antagonists in treating patients with peptic stricture and esophagitis. *Gastroenterology, 1994, 106*:907–915.

Peghini, P.L., Katz, P.O., and Castell, D.O. Ranitidine controls nocturnal gastric acid breakthrough on omeprazole: a controlled study in normal subjects. *Gastroenterology, 1998, 115*:1335–1339.

Peterson, W.L., and Cook, D.J. Antisecretory therapy for bleeding peptic ulcer. *JAMA, 1998, 280*:877–878.

Talley, N.J., Vakil, N., Ballard, E.D. II, and Fennerty, M.B. Absence of benefit of eradicating *Helicobacter pylori* in patients with nonulcer dyspepsia. *N. Engl. J. Med., 1999, 341*:1106–1111.

Vigneri, S., Termini, R., Leandro, G., Badalamenti, S., Pantalena, M., Savarino, V., Di Mario, F., Battaglia, G., Mela, G.S., Pilotto, A., Plebani, M., and Davi, G. A comparison of five maintenance therapies for reflux esophagitis. *N. Engl. J. Med., 1995, 333*:1106–1110.

Yeomans N., Tulassay, Z., Juhász, L., Rácz, I., Howard, J.M., van Rensburg, C.J., Swannenell, A.J., and Hawkey, C.J. A comparison of omeprazole with ranitidine for ulcers associated with nonsteroidal antinflammatory drugs. Acid Suppression Trial: Ranitidine versus Omeprazole for NSAID-associated Ulcer Treatment (ASTRONAUT) Study Group. *N. Engl. J. Med.,* **1998,** *338*:719–726.

MONOGRAPHS AND REVIEWS

Atkinson, A.J. Jr., and Craig, R.M. Therapy of peptic ulcer disease. In, *Peptic Ulcer Disease. Mechanisms of Management.* (Molinoff, P.B., ed.) Healthpress Publishing Group, Rutherford, NJ, **1990,** pp. 83–112.

Chiba, N., Thomson, A.B., and Sinclair, P. From bench to bedside to bug: an update of clinically relevant advances in the care of persons with *Helicobacter pylori*–associated diseases. *Can. J. Gastroenterol.,* **2000,** *14*:188–198.

DeVault, K.R. Overview of medical therapy for gastroesophageal reflux disease. *Gastroenterol. Clin. North Am.,* **1999,** *28*:831–845.

Feldman, M., and Burton, M.E. Histamine$_2$-receptor antagonists. Standard therapy for acid-peptic disease. First part. *N. Engl. J. Med.,* **1990a,** *323*:1672–1680.

Feldman, M., and Burton, M.E. Histamine$_2$-receptor antagonists. Standard therapy for acid-peptic disease. Second part. *N. Engl. J. Med.,* **1990b,** *323*:1749–1755.

Graham, D.Y. Antibiotic resistance in *Helicobacter pylori*: implications for therapy. *Gastroenterology,* **1998,** *115*:1272–1277.

Graham, D.Y. *Helicobacter pylori* infection in the pathogenesis of duodenal ulcer and gastric cancer: a model. *Gastroenterology,* **1997,** *113*:1983–1991.

Graham, D.Y. Therapy of *Helicobacter pylori*: current status and issues. *Gastroenterology,* **2000,** *118*:S2–S8.

La Corte, R., Caselli, M., Castellino, G., Bajocchi, G., and Trotta, F. Prophylaxis and treatment of NSAID-induced gastroduodenal disorders. *Drug Saf.,* **1999,** *20*:527–543.

Lew, E.A. Review article: pharmacokinetic concerns in the selection of anti-ulcer therapy. *Aliment. Pharmacol. Ther.,* **1999,** *13*(*suppl. 5*):11–16.

O'Connor, H.J. Review article: *Helicobacter pylori* and gastrooesophageal reflux disease—clinical implications and management. *Aliment. Pharmacol. Ther.,* **1999,** *13*:117–127.

Richardson, P., Hawkey, C.J., and Stack, W.A. Proton pump inhibitors. Pharmacology and rationale for use in gastrointestinal disorders. *Drugs,* **1998,** *56*:307–335.

Sachs, G. Molecular targets in therapy of acid-related disorders. In, *Therapy of Digestive Disorders: A Companion to Sleisenger and Fordtran's Gastrointestinal and Liver Disease.* (Wolfe, M.M., ed.) Saunders, Philadelphia, **2000,** p. 72.

Sachs, G. Proton pump inhibitors and acid-related diseases. *Pharmacotherapy,* **1997,** *17*:22–37.

Smith, L.A., and Rivers, A.B. History. In, *Peptic Ulcer: Pain Patterns, Diagnosis and Medical Treatment.* Appleton-Century-Crofts, New York, **1953,** pp. 1–10.

Veldhuyzen van zanten, S.J., and Lee, A. The role of *Helicobacter pylori* infection in duodenal and gastric ulcer. *Curr. Top. Microbiol. Immunol.,* **1999,** *241*:47–56.

Welage, L.S., and Berardi, R.R. Evaluation of omeprazole, lansoprazole, pantoprazole, and rabeprazole in the treatment of acid-related diseases. *J. Am. Pharm. Assoc. (Wash.),* **2000,** *40*:52–62.

Wolfe, M.M., Lichtenstein, D.R., and Singh, G. Gastrointestinal toxicity of nonsteroidal antiinflammatory drugs. *N. Engl. J. Med.,* **1999,** *340*:1888–1899.

Wolfe, M.M., and Sachs, G. Acid suppression: optimizing therapy for gastroduodenal ulcer healing, gastroesophageal reflux disease, and stress-related erosive syndrome. *Gastroenterology,* **2000,** *118*:S9–S31.

Acknowledgment

The authors wish to acknowledge Laurence R. Brunton, author of this chapter in the ninth edition of *Goodman and Gilman's the Pharmacological Basis of Therapeutics,* some of whose text has been retained in this edition.

PROKINETIC AGENTS, ANTIEMETICS, AND AGENTS USED IN IRRITABLE BOWEL SYNDROME

Pankaj Jay Pasricha

"The longer I live, the more I am convinced that... half the unhappiness in the world proceeds from little stoppages, from a duct choked up, from food pressing in the wrong place, from a vexed duodenum or an agitated pylorus."

(Sydney Smith, 1771–1845)

This chapter covers a variety of conditions that, variably and often inaccurately, have been labeled as disorders of gastrointestinal motility. These include specific diseases (such as achalasia), pathophysiologic syndromes (such as gastroparesis), and symptom complexes (dyspepsia, irritable bowel syndrome). Often, no overt structural abnormalities can be detected on clinical routine investigation of the patient, giving rise to the term "functional bowel disorders," which commonly is used to describe many of these conditions. However, this definition clearly is not static, and it changes with improvements in our ability to discover subtle but real biological derangements underlying these disorders. Further, although these conditions traditionally have been viewed as abnormalities in gastrointestinal motility or motor function (either excessive or ineffective), it is becoming increasingly clear that many of them may, in fact, represent primary abnormalities in sensory or afferent neuronal function. As a group, these disorders are poorly understood, and their treatment remains one of the major challenges in gastrointestinal pharmacology.

This chapter also covers agents used for nausea and vomiting, an area where there has been considerably more therapeutic progress, matching the significant gains in knowledge about underlying neurophysiological mechanisms for these responses.

OVERVIEW OF GASTROINTESTINAL MOTILITY

The gastrointestinal tract is in a state of continuous contractile (and secretory) activity. The control of these activities is complicated, with contributions by the muscle itself, the local nerves (*i.e.,* the enteric nervous system, ENS), and the central nervous system (mediated *via* both autonomic and somatic innervation as well as humoral pathways) (*see* Kunze and Furness, 1999). However, most of the functions of the gut are autonomous and are controlled almost entirely by the ENS. Autonomous motor activity of the gut, best illustrated in the intestine, displays two broad patterns. One of these is the MMC (*migrating myoelectric complex* when referring to electrical activity and *migrating motor complex* when referring to the accompanying contractions). The MMC occurs in the fasting (interdigestive) state, during which it helps sweep debris away (hence, it also is sometimes called the intestinal "housekeeper"). It consists of a series of four phasic activities, the most characteristic of which is phase III, consisting of clusters of rhythmic contractions that occupy short segments of the intestine for a period of 6 to 10 minutes before proceeding caudally. One whole MMC cycle (all four phases) takes about 80 to 110 minutes before it repeats itself. Cycling of the MMC occurs continually in continuously feeding animals but is interrupted in intermittently feeding animals such as human beings by another pattern of contractions (the fed pattern). This consists of high-frequency (12 to 15 per minute) contractions that are either propagated for short segments (*propulsive*) or are irregular and not propagated (*mixing*). Propulsive activity in the intestine generally is considered to be synonymous with the term *peristalsis* (*see* below). Both these patterns of movement are under the dominant control of the ENS, which is an autonomous collection of nerves within the wall of the gastrointestinal tract. The ENS programs iterative activity such as the MMC as well as coordinated peristaltic or mixing movements in response to input from both the local

ORAL   ANAL

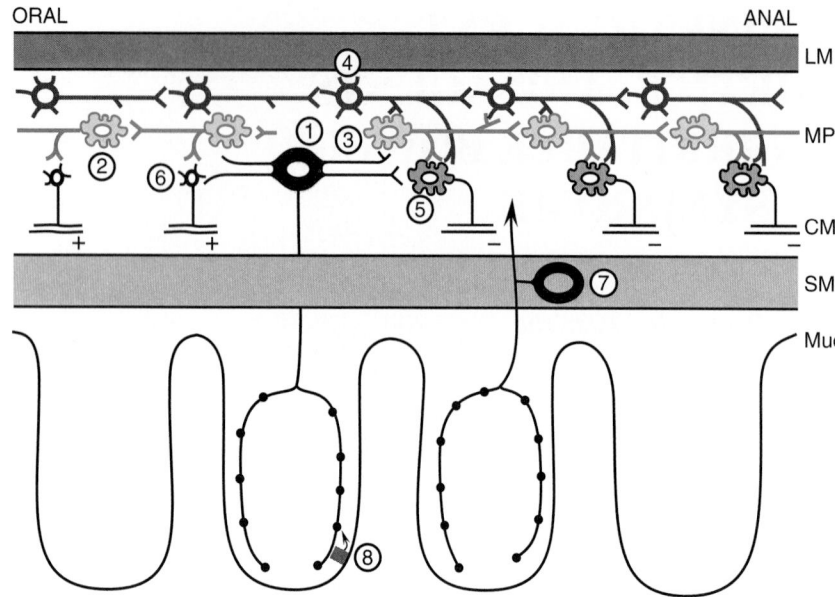

Figure 38–1. The neuronal network responsible for initiation and generation of the peristaltic reflex.

Mucosal stimulation leads to release of serotonin by enterochromaffin cells (8), which excites the intrinsic primary afferent neuron (1), which then communicates with both ascending (2) and descending (3) interneurons in the local reflex pathways. The reflex results in contraction at the oral end *via* the excitatory motor neuron (6) and aboral relaxation *via* the inhibitory motor neuron (5). The migratory myoelectric complex (*see* text) is shown here as being conducted by a different chain of interneurons (4). Another intrinsic primary afferent neuron with its cell body in the submucosa also is shown here (7). MP = myenteric plexus; CM = circular muscle; LM = longitudinal muscle; SM = submucosa; Muc = mucosa. (*Adapted from Kunze and Furness, 1999, with permission.*)

environment and the central nervous system. The ENS is organized into two plexi (connected networks of neurons): the *myenteric (Auerbach's) plexus,* found between the circular and longitudinal muscle layers, and the *submucosal (Meissner's) plexus,* found below the epithelium. The former is responsible for motor control, while the latter regulates secretion, fluid transport, and vascular flow.

A useful, if somewhat simplistic, way to view the functional elements of the myenteric plexus is from the perspective of the peristaltic reflex. Physiologically, peristalsis can be defined as a series of reflexes in response to a bolus in the lumen of a given segment of the intestine, the ascending excitatory reflex resulting in contraction of the circular muscle on the oral side of the bolus and the descending inhibitory reflex resulting in relaxation on the anal side. The net pressure gradient creates forward movement of the bolus. Three neural elements, responsible for sensory, relay, and effector functions, are required to produce these reflexes (Figure 38–1). Luminal factors stimulate sensory elements in the mucosa, leading to a coordinated pattern of muscle activity. This is under the direct control of the motor neurons of the myenteric plexus, which provide the effector component of the peristaltic reflex. These neurons receive input from both ascending and descending interneurons (which constitute the relay system) and are of two broad types: excitatory and inhibitory. The primary neurotransmitter of the excitatory motor neurons is acetylcholine (ACh), although tachykinins, coreleased by these neurons, also play a role. The principal neurotransmitter in the inhibitory motor neurons appears to be nitric oxide (NO), although important contributions may be made by ATP, vasoactive intestinal peptide, and pituitary adenylyl cyclase–activating peptide (PACAP), which are variably coexpressed with nitric oxide synthase.

It has become clear in recent years that the current view of nerve–muscle interaction within the gastrointestinal tract may be an oversimplification. Evidence is accruing rapidly that another cell type, the interstitial cell of Cajal, may play a signifi-

cant role in mediating neurogenic influence on gastrointestinal smooth muscle. These cells are found in the muscle layer and are responsive to various nerve-derived neurotransmitters including NO, ACh, and substance P. It appears that these cells may translate or modulate neuronal communication with the muscle, although the mechanisms responsible for this have yet to be worked out.

Excitation-Contraction Coupling in Gastrointestinal Smooth Muscle

Control of tension in gastrointestinal smooth muscle is in large part dependent on the intracellular Ca^{2+} concentration. In general, there are two types of excitation-contraction coupling based on the type of mechanism responsible for changes in Ca^{2+} concentration. *Electromechanical coupling* requires changes in membrane potential, due to either an action potential or a slow wave, which in turn activate voltage-dependent Ca^{2+} channels to trigger an influx of Ca^{2+}. Conversely, hyperpolarization of the membrane is associated with relaxation of the muscle due to inhibition of action potentials or closure of voltage-dependent Ca^{2+} channels. In smooth muscle, there are other stimuli, usually of a chemical nature, that act *via* specific receptors and can produce changes in tension without necessarily first affecting membrane potential. This is called *pharmacomechanical coupling* and also can be both excitatory and inhibitory in nature. Excitatory receptors involved in this mechanism often are linked to heterotrimeric G proteins such as those that can activate phospholipase C, which produces diacylglycerol (DAG) and inositol trisphosphate (IP_3). IP_3 acts on specific receptors on the sarcoplasmic reticulum causing release of Ca^{2+}, while DAG activates protein kinase C with subsequent phosphorylation (and modulation) of several important proteins, including ion channels, involved in the generation of muscle tone. Inhibitory receptors also exist on smooth muscle and generally

Table 38–1
Classification of Prokinetic Agents

GENERAL PHARMACOLOGICAL CLASS	SUBCLASS	EXAMPLES OF SPECIFIC DRUGS	MECHANISM OF ACTION
Cholinergic agents	Choline derivatives	Bethanechol and others	Muscarinic receptor activation
	Acetylcholinesterase inhibitors	Neostigmine and others	Increased availability of acetylcholine
Dopamine receptor antagonists	Benzimidazole derivatives	Domperidone	Dopamine (D_2) receptor antagonism
Serotonin (5-HT) receptor modulation	Substituted benzamides	Cisapride† (Renzapride, zacopride, ecabapide)‡	5-HT$_4$ receptor activation; 5-HT$_3$ receptor antagonism*
		Metoclopramide	5-HT$_4$ receptor activation; Dopamine (D_2) receptor antagonism*
Motilin-like agents	Macrolides	Erythromycin	Motilin receptor activation

*Minor effect.
†No longer generally available.
‡Under development.

act *via* cyclic AMP– and cyclic GMP–dependent kinases, which phosphorylate proteins and channels and eventually lead to decreased intracellular Ca^{2+} concentrations. As an example, NO is thought to induce relaxation *via* activation of guanylyl cyclase, generation of cyclic GMP, and opening of several different types of K^+ channels.

PROKINETIC AGENTS

Prokinetic agents are medications that enhance coordinated gastrointestinal motility and transit of material in the gastrointestinal tract (Reynolds and Putnam, 1992; Tonini, 1996). These agents are pharmacologically and chemically diverse (Table 38–1). Although ACh, when released from primary motor neurons in the myenteric plexus, is the principal immediate mediator of muscle contractility, most of the clinically useful prokinetic agents in fact act "upstream" of this point. These drugs may act at receptor sites on the motor neuron itself, or even more indirectly, on neurons one or two orders removed from it (Figure 38–2). Direct activation of muscarinic receptors, such as with the older cholinomimetic agents (*see*

Chapter 7), has not been a very effective strategy for treating gastrointestinal motility disorders, because contractions are enhanced globally in a relatively uncoordinated fashion, producing little or no net propulsive activity. By contrast, newer prokinetic agents enhance the release of acetylcholine at the nerve muscle junction without apparently interfering with the normal physiological pattern and rhythm of motility. Coordination of activity among the various segments of the gut, necessary for propulsion of luminal contents, therefore is maintained.

Cholinergic Agents

Choline Derivatives. The effects of ACh on smooth muscle are mediated in large part by two types of muscarinic receptors, M_2 and M_3 (*see* Chapter 7), present in a 4:1 ratio. Activation of these receptors results in an increase in intracellular Ca^{2+}, an effect mediated by inositol trisphosphate acting on internal calcium stores. ACh itself is not used pharmacologically because it affects all classes of cholinergic receptors (nicotinic and muscarinic) and is rapidly degraded by acetylcholinesterase. Modifications of the structure of acetylcholine have led to increased

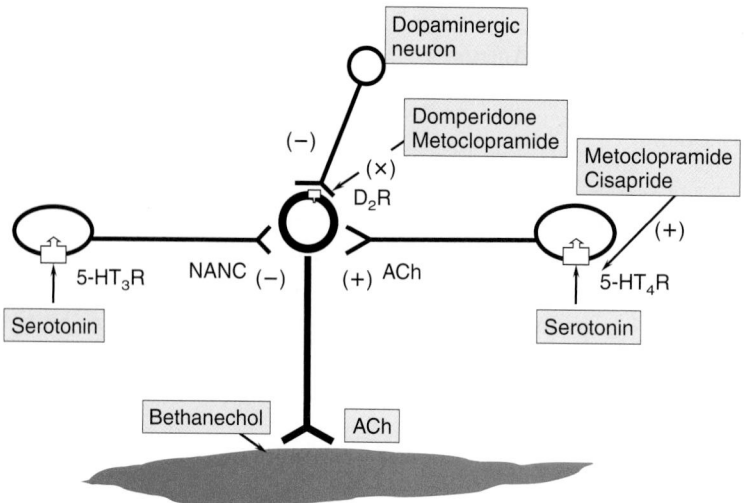

Figure 38–2. Conceptual model to explain the action of prokinetic agents.

In the center is shown the primary motor neuron in the myenteric plexus that induces smooth muscle contraction *via* the release of acetylcholine (ACh) when excited. The activity of this motor neuron can be modulated by several other neurons: as shown here, nonadrenergic, noncholinergic (NANC) and dopaminergic neurons are inhibitory, while cholinergic neurons are facilitatory. In turn the activity of the modulatory neurons can be affected by various neurotransmitters such as serotonin acting on specific receptor subtypes. Agents such as bethanechol mimic the action of ACh at the neuromuscular junction. Other prokinetic agents act more indirectly *via* the modulation of motor neuron activity and their connecting neurons. Thus, the major effect of cisapride and metoclopramide appears to be *via* the activation of 5-HT$_4$ receptors (5-HT$_4$R) on cholinergic facilitatory neurons. Domperidone and metoclopramide can act as antagonists at dopamine D$_2$ receptors (D$_2$R) and thus antagonize inhibition of the motor neuron by dopamine also resulting in net facilitation of its activity. Antagonism of the 5-HT$_3$ receptor (5-HT$_3$R), as shown here, also should have a similar facilitatory effect by dampening the activity of the inhibitory neuron. This mechanism is probably of minor importance in the effects of known prokinetic agents (*see* text for details).

receptor selectivity and resistance to enzymatic hydrolysis and have yielded drugs such as *carbachol* and *bethanechol*. Bethanechol, once widely used, is now largely of historical importance in gastroenterology. In addition to its lack of real prokinetic efficacy (*see* above), the drug is further limited by significant side effects resulting from its broad muscarinic effects on both contractility and secretion in the gastrointestinal tract and other organs. These include bradycardia, flushing, diarrhea and cramps, salivation, and blurred vision.

Acetylcholinesterase Inhibitors.   These drugs inhibit the degradation of ACh by its esterase (*see* Chapter 8), thereby allowing ACh to accumulate at sites of release. *Neostigmine* has been shown to be useful in some gastroenterological disorders, particularly those associated with colonic pseudoobstruction and paralytic ileus (Ponec *et al.,* 1999).

Dopamine-Receptor Antagonists

Dopamine is present in significant amounts in the gastrointestinal tract and has several inhibitory effects on gastroin-

testinal motility, including reduction of lower esophageal sphincter and intragastric pressure. These effects appear to result from suppression of ACh release from myenteric motor neurons and are mediated by the D$_2$ subtype of dopamine receptors (Figure 38–2). By antagonizing the effect of dopamine on myenteric motor neurons, dopamine-receptor antagonists were therefore felt to hold promise as prokinetic agents. An additional advantage of such a strategy for the treatment of gastrointestinal disorders is the relief of emesis by antagonism of dopamine receptors in the chemoreceptor trigger zone (CTZ). Examples of such agents traditionally have included *metoclopramide* and *domperidone*. However, it has become clear that the major mechanism of the prokinetic effect of metoclopramide involves activation of serotonin receptors, with antagonism of dopamine receptors playing a minor role (*see* below). Domperidone, on the other hand, appears to have a predominantly antidopaminergic effect. It is not available for use in the United States but has been used elsewhere in the world and has modest prokinetic activity (Barone, 1999). Although it does not readily cross the blood-brain barrier (hence, patients are spared the risk of extrapyramidal side effects), domperidone still can exert effects on those parts of the central nervous system (CNS) that do not possess this barrier, such as those regulating emesis, temperature, and prolactin release (dopamine inhibits prolactin release). Other D_2-receptor antagonists currently are being explored, and with some promise, as prokinetic agents, including *levosulpiride*, the levoenantiomer of sulpiride.

Serotonin-Receptor Modulators

Serotonin (5-HT) is an extremely important substance in the gastrointestinal tract and is present in both enterochromaffin cells of the mucosa and neurons of the myenteric plexus; it affects both secretion and motor activity (*see* Chapter 11 for a thorough discussion of the physiology and pharmacology of serotonin). In the mucosa, 5-HT can act as a local hormone (autocoid) and initiate the peristaltic reflex in response to local stimulation (Figure 38–1). The effects of 5-HT as a neurotransmitter within the myenteric plexus are complex and involve a variety of receptor subtypes and intracellular mechanisms. These actions appear to be mediated principally *via* 5-HT$_3$ and 5-HT$_4$ receptors, which are present on inhibitory and excitatory interneurons that synapse with cholinergic primary motor neurons (Figure 38–2). Thus, antagonism of the 5-HT$_3$ receptor on inhibitory interneurons is expected to enhance the responsiveness of the motor neurons, an effect that also can be achieved by agonists of the 5-HT$_4$ receptor on excitatory interneurons. Most of the currently useful prokinetic agents, including *cisapride* and *metoclopramide*, are considered to act predominantly as agonists at 5-HT$_4$ receptors (Briejer *et al.*, 1995).

Cisapride. Cisapride (PROPULSID) is a substituted piperidinyl benzamide that appears to stimulate 5-HT$_4$ receptors and increase adenylyl cyclase activity within neurons. Until recently, it was one of the most commonly used prokinetic agents for a variety of disorders, particularly gastroesophageal reflux disease (GERD) and gastroparesis. Its beneficial effects in GERD are thought to result from an increase in lower esophageal sphincter pressure, acceleration of gastric emptying (and hence decreased intragastric pressure), and possibly from improvements in esophageal peristalsis. In several trials, cisapride has been shown to be as effective as the histamine H$_2$-receptor antagonists ranitidine or cimetidine in patients with GERD. However, in general, prokinetic agents by themselves are seldom considered adequate for the treatment of clinically significant GERD (*see* Chapter 37). Although they may be useful additives to a regimen involving H$_2$-receptor antagonists for patients with

severe symptoms, the availability of the more efficacious proton pump inhibitors (*see* Chapter 37) has made such combination therapy largely unnecessary. Clinically, one of the greatest needs for prokinetic agents is in patients with delayed gastric emptying. Cisapride accelerates gastric emptying for both solids and liquids and improves symptoms in patients with gastroparesis due to a variety of causes. As a "true" prokinetic agent, it acts *via* enhancement of coordinated antroduodenal contractions. However, like metoclopramide (*see* below), it seldom normalizes gastric emptying, and relief of symptoms usually is only modest. The efficacy of cisapride in other functional bowel diseases such as nonulcer dyspepsia is unclear, although this drug has been used empirically for many of these patients. Similarly, although it has demonstrable effects on the small bowel and colon in experimental preparations, cisapride's usefulness in patients with paralytic ileus, intestinal pseudoobstruction, and chronic constipation have not been established with any certainty.

Cisapride is no longer generally available in the United States. The drug is available only through an investigational, limited-access program to patients who have failed all standard therapeutic modalities and who have undergone a thorough diagnostic evaluation, including an electrocardiographic evaluation. The main reason for withdrawal of cisapride from the open market has been its potential for serious cardiac adverse effects (Tonini *et al.*, 1999). The drug has been shown to block selectively the rapid component of the delayed rectifying K$^+$ current, which leads to a lengthening of the action potential and QT interval on the electrocardiogram. Serious cardiac arrhythmias and deaths from ventricular tachycardia, ventricular fibrillation, *torsades de pointes*, and QT prolongation have been reported in patients taking cisapride, particularly when used with other drugs that inhibit cytochrome P450 3A4. These include antibiotics such as erythromycin, clarithromycin, and troleandomycin; antidepressants such as nefazodone; antifungals such as fluconazole, itraconazole, and ketoconazole; and HIV protease inhibitors such as indinavir and ritonavir.

Metoclopramide. *Chemistry and Pharmacological Effects.* Metoclopramide (REGLAN) and other substituted benzamides are derivatives of *para*-aminobenzoic acid and are structurally related to *procainamide*. The chemical structure of metoclopramide is shown below.

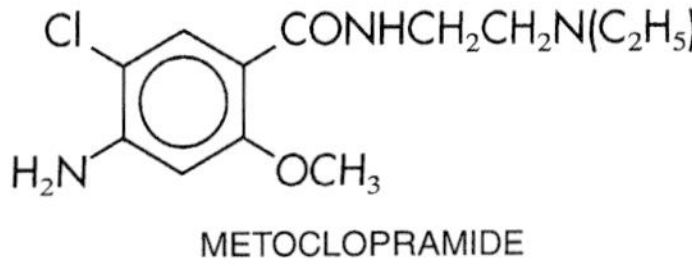

METOCLOPRAMIDE

Metoclopramide is one of the oldest true prokinetic agents; its administration results in coordinated contractions that enhance transit. Its effects are confined largely to the upper digestive tract, where it increases lower esophageal sphincter tone and stimulates antral and small intestinal contractions. Despite having *in vitro* effects on the contractility of colonic smooth muscle, the drug has no clinically significant effects on motility of the large bowel.

Mechanism of Action.   The mechanism of action of metoclopramide is complex (Figure 38–2). In general, agents of this class facilitate ACh release from enteric neurons, an action that may be mediated indirectly by several different mechanisms, including suppression of inhibitory interneurons by antagonism of 5-HT$_3$ receptors and stimulation of excitatory neurons *via* activation of 5-HT$_4$ receptors. In addition, metoclopramide is distinguished from agents such as cisapride by having both central and peripheral antidopaminergic effects. The former is responsible for its antinauseant and antiemetic effects, while the latter contributes to its prokinetic activity by counteracting the inhibitory effects of dopamine, mediated *via* dopamine D$_2$ receptors, on cholinergic enteric neurons (Figure 38–2).

Pharmacokinetics.   Metoclopramide is absorbed rapidly after oral ingestion, undergoes sulfation and glucuronide conjugation by the liver, and is excreted principally in the urine, with a half-life of 4 to 6 hours. Peak concentrations occur within about 1 hour after a single oral dose with a duration of action that lasts 1 to 2 hours.

Therapeutic Use.   Metoclopramide has been used in patients with GERD; it can produce symptomatic relief without necessarily promoting healing of associated esophagitis. It is clearly less effective than modern acid-suppressive medications such as proton pump inhibitors or even histamine H$_2$-receptor antagonists and now rarely is used for treating GERD. Metoclopramide is indicated more often in symptomatic patients with gastroparesis, in whom it may cause mild to modest improvements of gastric emptying. Metoclopramide injection also can be used as an adjunctive measure in medical or diagnostic procedures such as intestinal intubation or contrast radiography of the gastrointestinal tract. Although it has been used in patients with postoperative ileus, its effects on improving transit in disorders of small-bowel motility appear to be limited. In general, its greatest utility lies in its ability to ameliorate the nausea and vomiting that often accompany gastrointestinal dysmotility syndromes. This effect is mediated by dopamine-receptor antagonism within the chemoreceptor trigger zone (*see* below). Metoclopramide also has been used in the treatment of persistent hiccups, but its efficacy in this condition is equivocal at best.

Metoclopramide is available in oral dosage forms (tablets and solution) and as a parenteral preparation for intravenous or intramuscular use. The usual oral dose range is 10 to 20 mg three times a day, 30 minutes before a meal. The onset of action is within 30 to 60 minutes after an oral dose. In patients with severe nausea, an initial dose of 10 mg can be given intramuscularly (onset of action 10 to 15 minutes) or intravenously (onset

of action 1 to 3 minutes). Intravenous dosing for patients undergoing chemotherapy can be given as an infusion of 1 to 2 mg per kg of body weight, administered over at least 15 minutes, beginning 30 minutes before the chemotherapy is begun and repeated as needed every two or three hours. Alternatively, a continuous intravenous infusion may be given (3 mg per kg of body weight before chemotherapy, followed by 0.5 mg per kg of body weight per hour for eight hours). The usual pediatric dose for gastroparesis is 0.1 to 0.2 mg per kg of body weight per dose, given 30 minutes before meals and at bedtime.

Adverse Effects.   The major side effects of metoclopramide, although rare, can be serious and include extrapyramidal effects such as those seen with the phenothiazines (*see* Chapter 20). Dystonias, usually occurring acutely after intravenous administration, and parkinsonism-like symptoms, which may occur several weeks after initiation of therapy, generally respond to treatment (with anticholinergic or antihistaminic drugs) and are reversible after discontinuation of the drug. Tardive dyskinesia also can occur with chronic treatment (months to years) but may be irreversible. Extrapyramidal effects appear to occur more commonly in children and young adults, particularly at higher doses. Like domperidone and other dopamine antagonists, metoclopramide also can cause galactorrhea, but this is infrequent. Methemoglobinemia has been reported occasionally in premature and full-term neonates receiving metoclopramide.

Other Serotonin-Receptor Modulators.   *Ondansetron* (*see* below), a commonly used antiemetic, also has modest gastric prokinetic activity, which is attributed to its ability to act as an antagonist at 5-HT$_3$ receptors. It also may prolong colonic transit time, possibly by increasing colonic tone (Wilde and Markham, 1996). However, ondansetron does not appear to be a clinically useful prokinetic agent and is seldom if ever used in this capacity. Other 5-HT-receptor modulators with much greater promise as prokinetic agents currently are under evaluation. These drugs, which include *tegaserod* and *prucalopride,* are potent agonists at the 5-HT$_4$ receptor and appear to have relatively selective effects on the colon. Prucalopride is a benzofuran derivative and a specific 5-HT$_4$-receptor agonist that has been shown to facilitate cholinergic neurotransmission. It enhances colonic contractility in experimental animals, and preliminary studies suggest that it accelerates colonic transit in human beings (Bouras *et al.,* 1999). Tegaserod is an amino guanidine-indole with selective and partial 5-HT$_4$-receptor agonist activity (Scot and Perry, 1999). In addition to its prokinetic effects on the colon, tegaserod also appears to reduce visceral sensitivity (*see* "Irritable Bowel Syndrome," below) and thus has therapeutic potential for patients with constipation-dominant irritable bowel syndrome. Tegaserod (ZELMAC) may be approved by the United States Food and Drug Administration (FDA) in the near future.

Motilin: Macrolides and Erythromycin

Chemistry, Pharmacological Effects, and Mechanism of Action. Motilin is a 22–amino acid peptide hormone found in the gastrointestinal M cells as well as in some enterochromaffin cells of the upper small bowel. Motilin levels fluctuate in association with the MMC and appear to be responsible for the amplification, if not the actual induction, of phase III MMC activity (*see* "Overview of Gastrointestinal Motility," above). In addition, motilin receptors are found on smooth muscle cells, and motilin is a potent contractile agent of the upper gastrointestinal tract. Research on the prokinetic effects of motilin has been stimulated by the demonstration that these effects can be mimicked by *erythromycin,* a discovery that was based on the frequent occurrence of gastrointestinal side effects with the use of this antibiotic (Otterson and Sarna, 1990; Reynolds and Putnam, 1992; Faure *et al.,* 2000). Subsequent studies showed that erythromycin could induce phase III MMC activity in dogs and increase smooth muscle contractility. This property is shared to varying extents by other macrolide antibiotics (*see* Chapter 47), including *oleandomycin, azithromycin,* and *clarithromycin.* In addition to its motilin-like effects, erythromycin also may act *via* other poorly defined mechanisms, possibly involving cholinergic facilitation (Coulie *et al.,* 1998).

Erythromycin has a variety of effects on upper gastrointestinal motility, including increases in lower esophageal pressure and stimulation of gastric and small-bowel contractility. By contrast, it appears to have little or no effect on colonic motility.

Therapeutic Use. The best described use of erythromycin as a prokinetic is in patients with diabetic gastroparesis, where it can improve gastric emptying in the short term. Erythromycin-stimulated gastric contractions can be intense and result in "dumping" of relatively undigested food into the small bowel. This can be a disadvantage, but it has been exploited clinically to clear the stomach of undigestible residue such as plastic tubes or bezoars. Erythromycin also has been of anecdotal benefit in patients with small-bowel dysmotility such as that seen in scleroderma, ileus, or pseudoobstruction. Rapid development of tolerance to erythromycin, possibly by downregulation of the motilin receptor, and its undesirable (in this context) antibiotic effects have limited the practical use of this drug as a prokinetic agent. However, a variety of nonantibiotic synthetic analogs of erythromycin as well as peptide analogs of motilin currently are under evaluation; simulation of motilin's actions by these agents may represent a viable prokinetic option in the future.

A standard dose of erythromycin used for gastric stimulation is 3 mg/kg intravenously or 200 to 250 mg orally every 8 hours. However, a smaller dose (40 mg intravenously) may be more useful for small-bowel stimulation, where higher doses may actually retard motility (Medhus *et al.,* 2000; DiBaise and Quigley, 1999).

Miscellaneous Agents That Can Modulate Gastrointestinal Motility

Octreotide (SANDOSTATIN) is a long-acting somatostatin analog (*see* Chapters 39 and 56) that has complex effects on gastrointestinal motility, including inhibition of antral motor activity and colon tone (Camilleri, 1996). However, octreotide also can rapidly induce phase III MMC activity in the small bowel, and this induced phase III activity appears to last longer with faster contractions than those occurring spontaneously. Octreotide can accelerate gastric emptying of mixed meals and, paradoxically, prolong small-bowel and mouth-to-cecum transit time. These opposing effects may limit its potential as a clinically useful prokinetic agent. Nevertheless, its use has been shown to result in improvement in selected patients with scleroderma and small-bowel dysfunction. Its greatest utility, however, may be with the "dumping syndrome" seen in some patients after gastric surgery and pyloroplasty. In this condition, octreotide inhibits the release of hormones (triggered by rapid passage of food into the small intestine) that are responsible for several distressing local and systemic effects.

The gastrointestinal hormone cholecystokinin (CCK) is released from the intestine in response to meals and slows down gastric emptying. *Loxiglumide* is a CCK_1- (or CCK-A)–receptor antagonist that can improve gastric emptying and is being investigated in patients with gastroparesis.

SPECIFIC MOTILITY DISORDERS AND THERAPEUTIC STRATEGIES

Gastrointestinal motility disorders are a complex and heterogeneous group of syndromes whose pathophysiology is at best incompletely understood (McCallum, 1999; Pandolfino *et al.,* 2000). This term also traditionally has included disorders such as irritable bowel syndrome (*see* below) and noncardiac chest pain, where disturbances in pain processing or sensory function may be more important than any associated motor patterns. As a group, these disorders cause a heavy burden of suffering, but therapeutic developments in this area have been erratic, with a paucity of truly effective pharmacological agents. In most instances, the treatment approach remains empirical and symptom-based. Thus, prokinetic agents such as metoclopramide and cisapride have modest if any effects on gastric emptying in patients with gastroparesis and have only limited ability to improve symptoms (Koch, 1999; Sturm *et al.,* 1999). Chronic constipation (Chapter 39) is another syndrome of dysmotility where physicians rely predominantly on a nonspecific therapeutic approach. Clearly, with advances in understanding the physiology of gastrointestinal motility and dysmotility, better and more specific drugs will become available. Some of these, such as newer serotonin-receptor antagonists, currently are under development and offer new hope for the treatment of some of these conditions.

In some disorders of motility, effective treatment does not necessarily require a "neuroenteric" approach. An example is that of GERD. The pathophysiology of GERD is poorly defined but appears to involve a disturbance in the normal antireflux barrier composed of the lower esophageal sphincter (LES) and perhaps the diaphragmatic crura. Transient lower esophageal sphincter relaxations (tLESRs) are prolonged relaxations of the LES that occur in the absence of a swallow and appear to be the dominant factor in reflux in most patients. By contrast, a low resting LES pressure by itself does not appear to be as important unless it is less than 10 mm Hg. Anatomical factors such as hiatal hernia also can contribute to the impaired integrity of the antireflux barrier. Other factors that may play a role are delayed gastric emptying, gastric distention, and poor esophageal clearance due to impaired peristalsis. Thus, it appears that GERD is predominantly the result of problems with gastrointestinal motility and is not generally associated with hypersecretion of gastric acid. Nevertheless, the damage to the esophagus is ultimately inflicted by acid, and the most effective therapy for GERD remains the suppression of acid production by the stomach (*see* Chapter 37). Neither metoclopramide nor cisapride by itself is particularly effective in this condition. However, a new approach currently under investigation relies on the suppression of tLESRs and may hold promise. This can be achieved by CCK_1-receptor antagonists (such as loxiglumide), GABA agonists (such as baclofen), and inhibitors of nitric oxide synthesis.

By contrast with the above, some motility disorders are treated by agents that reduce contractility. These include disorders such as achalasia, in which the LES fails to relax, resulting in a functional obstruction to the passage of food and severe difficulty in swallowing. Smooth muscle relaxants such as organic nitrates and calcium channel antagonists (*see* Chapter 32) often can lead to temporary if partial relief of symptoms. A more recent approach relies on the use of *botulinum toxin,* injected directly into the LES *via* an endoscope, in doses of 80 to 200 U. This potent agent (*see* Chapter 9) causes inhibition of release of ACh from nerve endings and can produce partial paralysis of the sphincter muscle, with significant improvements in symptoms and esophageal clearance (Pasricha *et al.,* 1995). However, its effects wear off over a period of several months, requiring repetitive injections. It also is being used increasingly in other gastrointestinal conditions such as chronic anal fissures (Hoogerwerf and Pasricha, 1999).

In addition to organic nitrates and calcium channel antagonists, other agents that decrease smooth muscle contractility include the traditional anticholinergic agents ("spasmolytics" or "antispasmodics"), which often are used in patients with irritable bowel syndrome (*see* below).

Current and investigational pharmacological approaches to disorders of gastrointestinal motility are summarized in Table 38–2.

Table 38–2
Potential Target Actions and Applications of Gastrointestinal Motility-Altering Agents

DISORDER	TARGET ACTION	CURRENTLY USED MEDICATIONS	EXPERIMENTAL OR DEVELOPMENTAL AGENTS
Achalasia Esophageal spasm "Nutcracker" esophagus	Diminish LES pressure and/or peristaltic amplitude	Calcium channel antagonists Nitrites Botulinum toxin	L-Arginine
GERD (nonspecific treatment)	Augment LES pressure and/or peristaltic amplitude	Metoclopramide Cisapride	Domperidone $5\text{-}HT_3$-receptor antagonists/ $5\text{-}HT_4$-receptor agonists
GERD (specific treatment)	Attenuate tLESRs		CCK_1-receptor antagonists NO synthase inhibitors $GABA_B$ receptor agonists
Gastroparesis (nonspecific treatment)	Augment gastric emptying	Metoclopramide Cisapride Erythromycin	CCK_1-receptor antagonists Opioid receptor modifiers
Gastroparesis (specific treatment)	Stimulate phase III of MMC	Erythromycin	Motilides
IBS	Diminish colonic muscle contraction	Anticholinergics Smooth muscle relaxants	
Constipation Pseudoobstruction	Augment colonic muscle contractility	Cisapride Erythromycin Neostigmine	Misoprostol $5\text{-}HT_3$-receptor antagonists/$5\text{-}HT_4$-receptor agonists (prucalopride, tegaserod)

ABBREVIATIONS: LES = lower esophageal sphincter; GERD = gastroesophageal reflux disease; IBS = irritable bowel syndrome; tLESRs = transient lower esophageal sphincter relaxations; CCK = cholecystokinin; 5-HT = serotonin; MMC = migrating motor complex.
SOURCE: From Pandolfino *et al.,* 2000, with permission.

ANTINAUSEA AND ANTIEMETIC AGENTS

Nausea and Vomiting

The act of emesis and the sensation of nausea that accompanies it generally are thought to be protective reflexes that serve to rid the stomach and intestine of toxic substances and prevent their further ingestion. Vomiting is a complex process and consists of a preejection phase (gastric relaxation and retroperistalsis), retching (rhythmic action of respiratory muscles preceding vomiting and consisting of contraction of abdominal, intercostal, and diaphragmatic muscles against a closed glottis), and ejection (intense contraction of the abdominal muscle and relaxation of the upper esophageal sphincter). All this is accompanied by multiple autonomic phenomena including salivation, shivering, and vasomotor changes. During prolonged episodes, marked behavioral changes including lethargy, depression, and withdrawal may occur. The process appears to be coordinated by a central emesis center in the lateral reticular formation of the mid-brainstem adjacent to the CTZ in the area postrema (AP) at the bottom of the fourth ventricle and the nucleus tractus solitarius (NTS) of the vagus nerve. The lack of a blood-brain barrier allows the CTZ to monitor blood and cerebrospinal fluid constantly for toxic substances and to relay information to the emesis center to trigger nausea and/or vomiting. The emesis center also receives information from the gut, principally by the vagus nerve (*via* the NTS) but also by splanchnic afferents. Two additional inputs of importance to the emesis center come from the cerebral cortex (particularly in anticipatory nausea or vomiting) and the vestibular apparatus (in motion sickness). In turn, the center sends out efferents to the nuclei responsible for respiratory, salivary, and vasomotor activity as well as to both striated and smooth muscle involved in the act. The CTZ has high concentrations of serotonin (5-HT$_3$), dopamine (D$_2$), and opioid receptors, while the NTS is rich in enkephalin, histamine, and cholinergic receptors and also contains 5-HT$_3$ receptors. As can be imagined, a variety of neurotransmitters are involved in this complex process (Andrews *et al.,* 1998; Rizk and Hesketh, 1999); an understanding of their nature has allowed a rational approach to the pharmacological treatment of nausea and vomiting (Figure 38–3; Tables 38–3 and 38–4; *see* ASHP Therapeutic Guidelines, 1999; Mazzotta *et al.,* 1998).

5-HT$_3$-Receptor Antagonists

Chemistry, Pharmacological Effects, and Mechanism of Action. *Ondansetron* (ZOFRAN) is the prototypical drug in this

class; since its introduction in the early 1990s, it and other 5-HT$_3$-receptor antagonists have become some of the most widely used drugs for chemotherapy-induced emesis (Gregory and Ettinger, 1998; Hesketh, 2000). Other agents in this class now are available, including *granisetron* (KYTRIL), *dolasetron* (ANZEMET), and *tropisetron* (available in some countries but not in the United States). The differences among these agents are mainly related to their chemical structures, 5-HT$_3$–receptor affinities, and pharmacokinetic profile (Table 38–5). The chemical structures of the three agents currently available in the United States are shown below.

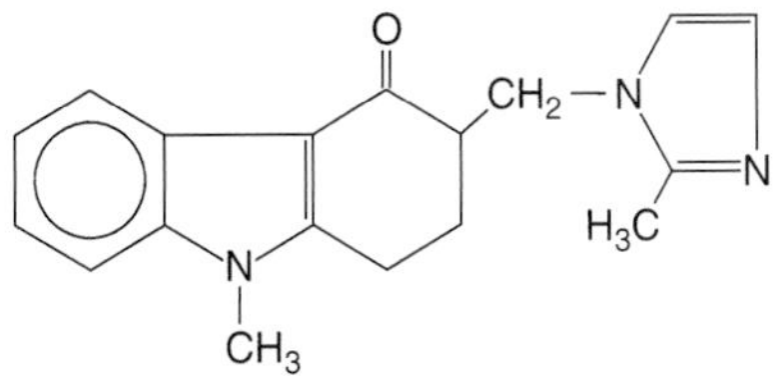

ONDANSETRON

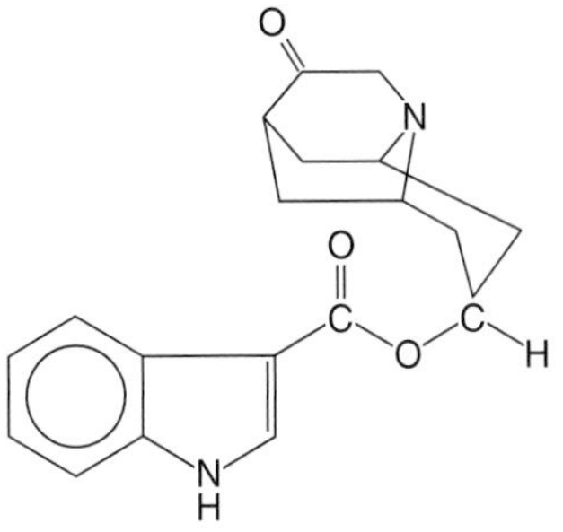

DOLASETRON

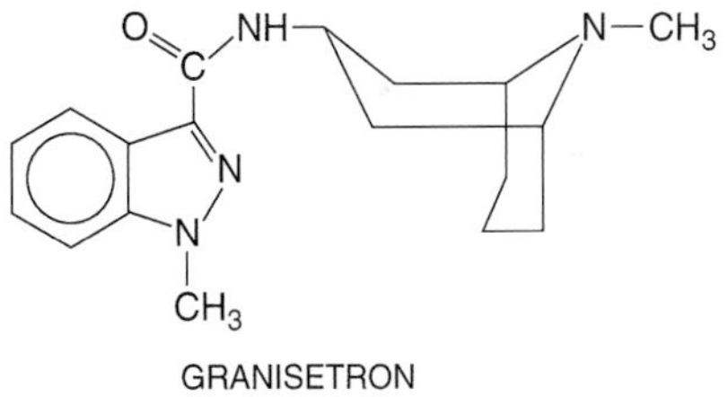

GRANISETRON

Whether the main site of action of these drugs is central or peripheral is not clear; there is evidence that effects at both locations contribute to their efficacy. 5-HT$_3$ receptors are present in several critical sites involved in emesis, including vagal afferents, the NTS (which receives signals from vagal afferents), and the area postrema itself. Serotonin is released by the enterochromaffin cells of the small intestine in response to chemotherapeutic agents and may stimulate vagal afferents (*via* 5-HT$_3$ receptors) to initiate the vomiting reflex. Experimentally, vagotomy has been shown to prevent cisplatin-induced emesis. However, the highest concentrations of 5-HT$_3$ receptors in the CNS are found in the NTS and CTZ, and antagonists of 5-HT$_3$ receptors also may suppress nausea and vomiting by acting at these sites.

Pharmacokinetics. The differences in plasma half-lives of these agents (Table 38–5) are not very meaningful in practice, as the antiemetic effects persist long after the drugs disappear

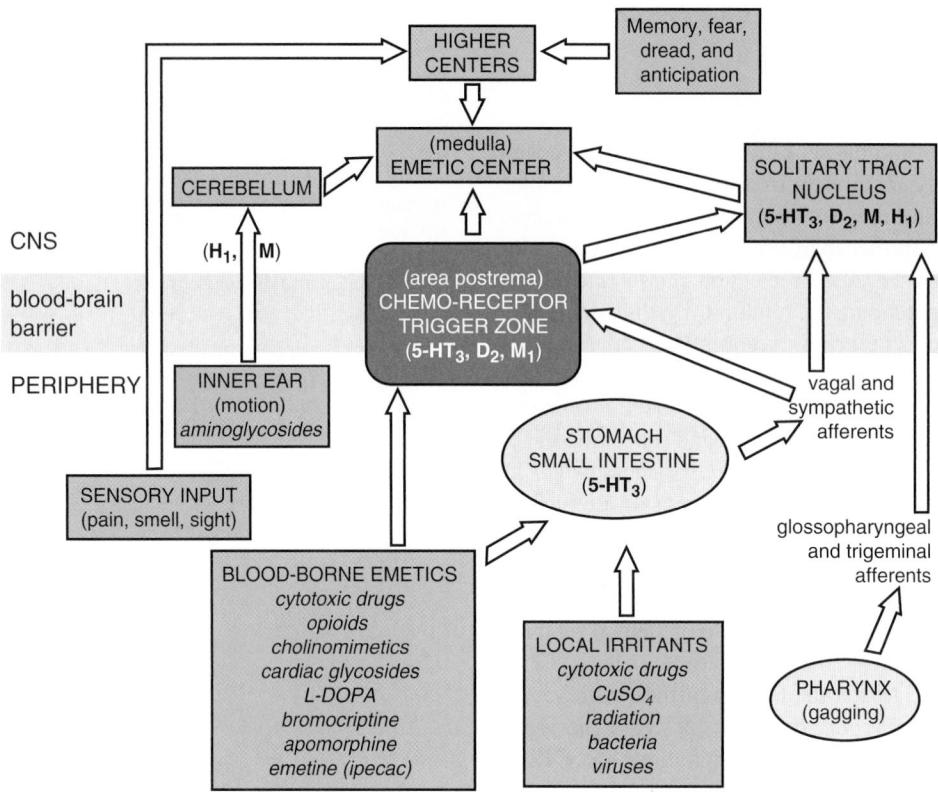

Figure 38–3. Pharmacologist's view of emetic stimuli.

Myriad signaling pathways lead from the periphery to the emetic center. Stimulants of these pathways are noted in *italics*. These pathways involve specific neurotransmitters and their receptors (**bold** text). Receptors are shown for: dopamine, D; acetylcholine (muscarinic), M; histamine, H; and 5-hydroxytryptamine, 5-HT. Some of these receptor types also may mediate signaling in the emetic center. This knowledge offers a rationale for current antiemetic therapy. Vomiting in response to stimulation of the emetic center is a complex response and is described in the text.

from the circulation, suggesting their continuing interaction at the receptor level. In fact, all of these drugs can be effectively administered just once a day.

These agents are well absorbed from the gastrointestinal tract. Ondansetron is extensively metabolized by the liver by a cytochrome P450 pathway, followed by glucuronide or sulfate conjugation. Patients with liver dysfunction have a reduction in plasma clearance, and some adjustment in the dosage is advisable. Although some reduction in ondansetron clearance also is seen in elderly patients, no adjustment in dosage for age is recommended. Granisetron also is predominantly metabolized by the liver, a process that appears to involve the CYP3A family of enzymes, as it is inhibited by ketoconazole. Dolasetron is converted rapidly by the plasma enzyme carbonyl reductase to its active metabolite, *hydroxydolasetron* (hydrodolasetron). A portion of this compound then undergoes subsequent biotransformation by CYP2D6 and CYP3A4 in the liver, while about one-third of it is excreted unchanged in the urine.

Therapeutic Use. These agents are most effective in treating chemotherapy-induced nausea and in treating

nausea secondary to upper abdominal irradiation, where all three agents appear to be equally efficacious. They also are effective against hyperemesis of pregnancy and, although to a lesser extent, postoperative nausea, but not against motion sickness.

These agents are available as tablets, oral solution (ondansetron), and intravenous preparations for injection. For patients on cancer chemotherapy, these drugs can be given in a single intravenous dose (Table 38–5) infused over 15 minutes, beginning 30 minutes before chemotherapy, or in 2 to 3 divided doses, with the first usually given 30 minutes before and subsequent doses at various intervals after chemotherapy. The drugs also can be used intramuscularly or orally.

Adverse Effects. In general, these drugs are very well tolerated, with the most common adverse effects being constipation or diarrhea, headache, and light-headedness. As a class, these agents have been shown experimentally to induce minor

Table 38–3
General Classification of Antiemetic Agents

ANTIEMETIC CLASS	EXAMPLES	TYPE OF VOMITING MOST EFFECTIVE AGAINST
5-HT$_3$–receptor antagonists*	Ondansetron	Cytotoxic drug-induced emesis
Centrally acting dopamine–receptor antagonists	Metoclopramide*† Promethazine‡	Cytotoxic drug-induced emesis
Histamine H$_1$–receptor antagonists	Cyclizine	Vestibular (motion sickness)
Muscarinic-receptor antagonists	Hyoscine (scopolamine)	Motion sickness
Neurokinin-receptor antagonists	Investigational	Cytotoxic drug–induced emesis (delayed vomiting)
Cannabinoid-receptor agonists	Dronabinol	Cytotoxic drug–induced emesis

*The most effective agents for chemotherapy-induced nausea and vomiting are the 5-HT$_3$ antagonists and metoclopramide. In addition to their individual use, they are often combined with other agents to improve efficacy as well as reduce the incidence of side effects.
†Also has some peripheral activity at 5-HT$_3$ receptors.
‡Also has some antihistaminic and anticholinergic activity.

electrocardiographic changes, but these are not felt to be clinically significant in most cases.

Dopamine-Receptor Antagonists

Phenothiazines such as *prochlorperazine, thiethylperazine,* and *chlorpromazine* (Chapter 20) are among the most commonly used "general purpose" antinauseants and antiemetics in clinical practice. Their effects in this regard are complex, but their principal mechanism of action is dopamine D$_2$-receptor antagonism at the CTZ. Compared to metoclopramide or ondansetron, these drugs do not appear to be as uniformly effective in cancer chemotherapy–induced emesis. On the other hand, they also possess antihistaminic and anticholinergic activities, which are of value in other forms of nausea such as motion sickness.

For many years, the standard for drugs used to treat chemotherapy-induced nausea was metoclopramide, a D$_2$-receptor antagonist acting on the CTZ. In recent years, an additional mechanism involving 5-HT$_3$-receptor antagonism has been found (*see* above). The prokinetic effects of metoclopramide may contribute to its effectiveness in chemotherapy-induced nausea. *Domperidone* is another D$_2$-receptor antagonist with antinauseant and prokinetic effects. Its principal advantage over metoclopramide is the lack of CNS side effects because of its poor penetration

into the brain. This drug, however, is not approved for general use in the United States.

Antihistamines

Histamine H$_1$-receptor antagonists are primarily useful for motion sickness and postoperative emesis (Kovac, 2000). They act on vestibular afferents and within the brain stem. *Cyclizine, hydroxyzine, promethazine,* and *diphenhydramine* are examples of this class of agents. Cyclizine has additional anticholinergic effects that may be useful for patients with abdominal cancer. For a detailed discussion of these drugs, *see* Chapter 25.

Anticholinergic Agents

The most commonly used muscarinic receptor antagonist is *scopolamine* (hyoscine), which can be injected as the hydrobromide but is administered usually as the free base in the form of a transdermal patch (TRANSDERM-SCOP). Its principal utility is in the prevention and treatment of motion sickness, although it has been shown to have some activity in postoperative nausea and vomiting as well. In general, anticholinergic agents have no role in chemotherapy-induced nausea. For a detailed discussion of these drugs, *see* Chapter 7.

DRONABINOL

Dronabinol (delta-9-tetrahydrocannabinol; MARINOL) is a naturally occurring cannabinoid that can be synthesized chemically or extracted from the marijuana plant, *Cannabis sativa.* Its structure is shown below. The exact mechanism of action of dronabinol is not known but probably is related to stimulation

Table 38–4

A. Some Antiemetic Regimens Used in Cancer Chemotherapy

ANTIEMETIC AGENT	INITIAL DOSE
For Severe Chemotherapy-Induced Emesis (Several Antiemetic Agents Used in Combination)	
Dexamethasone	20 mg IV
Metoclopramide	3 mg/kg body weight IV every 2 hr × 2
Diphenhydramine	25–50 mg IV every 2 hr × 2
Lorazepam	1–2 mg IV
Dexamethasone	20 mg IV
Ondansetron	32 mg IV daily, in divided doses
For Moderate Chemotherapy-Induced Emesis (Antiemetic Agents Used Singly)	
Prochlorperazine	5–10 mg orally or IV, or 25 mg by rectal suppository
Thiethylperazine	10 mg orally, IM, or by rectal suppository
Dexamethasone	10–20 mg IV
Ondansetron	8 mg orally or 10 mg IV
Dronabinol	10 mg orally

B. Useful Combinations of Antiemetic Agents for Improved Antiemetic Effect

PRIMARY AGENT	SUPPLEMENTAL AGENT
5-HT$_3$-receptor antagonist	Corticosteroid, phenothiazine, butyrophenone
Substituted benzamide	Corticosteroid ± muscarinic-receptor antagonist
Phenothiazine/butyrophenone	Corticosteroid
Corticosteroid	Benzodiazepine
Cannabinoid	Corticosteroid

C. Useful Combinations of Antiemetic Agents Providing Decreased Toxicity of the Primary Agent

PRIMARY AGENT	SUPPLEMENTAL AGENT
Substituted benzamide	H$_1$-receptor antagonist, corticosteroid, benzodiazepine
Phenothiazine/butyrophenone	H$_1$-receptor antagonist
Cannabinoid	Phenothiazine

ABBREVIATIONS: H, histamine, 5-HT, serotonin; IV, intravenous; IM, intramuscular.
SOURCE: All combination regimens are from Grunberg and Hasbeth, 1993, with permission.

Table 38–5

Properties of Antiemetic Serotonin-Receptor Antagonists

DRUG	CHEMICAL CLASS	PHARMACOLOGICAL CLASS	T$_{1/2}$ (hours)	INTRAVENOUS DOSE (mg/kg)
Ondansetron	Carbazole derivative	5-HT$_3$-receptor antagonist Weak 5-HT$_4$-receptor antagonist	3–4	0.15
Granisetron	Indazole derivative	5-HT$_3$-receptor antagonist	5–9	0.01
Dolasetron (Hydroxydolasetron)	Indole derivative	5-HT$_3$-receptor antagonist	7–9	0.6–3.0

5-HT, serotonin

of the CB_1 subtype of cannabinoid receptors on neurons in and around the vomiting center.

DRONABINOL

Pharmacokinetics.   Dronabinol is a highly lipid-soluble compound that is readily absorbed after oral administration; its onset of action occurs within an hour, and peak levels are achieved within 2 to 4 hours. It undergoes extensive first-pass metabolism with limited systemic bioavailability after single doses (only 10% to 20%). Both active and inactive metabolites are formed in the liver, the principal example of the former being 11-OH-delta-9-tetrahydrocannabinol. These metabolites are excreted primarily *via* the biliary-fecal route, with only 10% to 15% being excreted in the urine. Both dronabinol and its metabolites are highly bound (>95%) to plasma proteins. Because of its large volume of distribution, a single dose of dronabinol can result in detectable levels of metabolites for several weeks.

Therapeutic Use.   Dronabinol is a useful prophylactic agent in patients receiving cancer chemotherapy when other antiemetic medications are not effective. It also can stimulate the appetite and has been used in patients with acquired immunodeficiency syndrome (AIDS) and anorexia. As an antiemetic agent, it is administered at an initial dose of 5 mg/m^2 given 1 to 3 hours before chemotherapy and then every 2 to 4 hours afterward for a total of 4 to 6 doses. If this is not adequate, incremental increases in dose can be made up to a maximum of 15 mg/m^2. Most patients with anorexia will respond to 2.5 mg taken before lunch and dinner; doses up to 10 mg twice a day may be tolerated.

Adverse Effects.   Dronabinol has complex effects on the central nervous system, including a prominent central sympathomimetic activity. This can lead to tachycardia and conjunctival injection. Marijuana-like "highs" (changes in mood, easy laughing, *etc.*) can occur, as can more disturbing effects such as paranoid reactions and thinking abnormalities. Following abrupt withdrawal of dronabinol, an abstinence syndrome—manifest by irritability, insomnia, and restlessness—can occur. Because of the high affinity of dronabinol for plasma proteins, it can displace other plasma protein-bound drugs, whose doses may have to be adjusted. Dronabinol should be prescribed with great caution to persons with a history of substance abuse (alcohol, drugs) as it also may be abused by these patients.

Glucocorticoids and Antiinflammatory Agents

Glucocorticoids such as *dexamethasone* can be useful adjuncts (*see* Table 38–4) in the treatment of nausea in patients with widespread cancer, possibly by suppressing peritumoral inflammation and prostaglandin production. A similar mechanism has been invoked to explain beneficial effects of nonsteroidal antiinflammatory drugs in the nausea and vomiting induced by systemic irradiation. For a detailed discussion of these drugs, *see* Chapters 27 and 60.

Benzodiazepines

Benzodiazepines, such as *lorazepam* and *alprazolam,* by themselves are not very effective antiemetics, but their sedative, amnesic, and antianxiety effects can be helpful in reducing the anticipatory component of nausea and vomiting in patients. For a detailed discussion of these drugs, *see* Chapter 17.

Substance P Receptor Antagonists

The nausea and vomiting associated with cisplatin (*see* Chapter 52) has two components: an acute phase that is universally experienced (within 24 hours after chemotherapy) and a delayed phase that affects only some patients (on days 2 to 5). Serotonin-receptor antagonists are not very effective against delayed emesis, which currently is treated with a combination of a serotonin-receptor antagonist or metoclopramide with dexamethasone (Kris *et al.,* 1998). Antagonists of the NK1 subtype of substance P receptors have been shown to have antiemetic effects (Rupniak and Kramer, 1999). Recently, a synthetic, nonpeptide antagonist of the NK1 receptor was found to be effective as a single agent in the prevention of delayed nausea after cisplatin therapy (Navari *et al.,* 1999). Substance P belongs to the tachykinin family of neurotransmitters and is found in vagal afferent fibers innervating the NTS and area postrema. The tachykinins therefore represent a novel, promising target for new antinauseant drugs.

IRRITABLE BOWEL SYNDROME

Irritable bowel syndrome (IBS), a condition that affects up to 15% of the United States population, is perhaps one of the most challenging nonfatal illnesses seen by gastroenterologists. Patients may complain of a variety of symptoms, the most characteristic of which is recurrent abdominal pain associated with altered bowel movements (Drossman *et al.,* 1997).

Although the pathophysiology of this condition is far from clear, it appears to result from a varying combination of disturbances in visceral motor and sensory function, often associated with significant affective disorders. The disturbances in bowel function (which can be either constipation or diarrhea or both at different times) have led to the classical interpretation of IBS as being a "motility disorder." However, it is clear that motor disturbances may be subtle and, even when present, cannot explain the entire clinical picture. In recent years, more emphasis has been devoted to the pathogenesis of pain in these patients, and there is now considerable evidence to suggest a specific enhancement of visceral (as opposed to somatic) sensitivity to noxious as well as physiological stimuli in this syndrome. The etiopathogenesis of this visceral hypersensitivity is probably multifactorial; a popular hypothesis is that transient visceral injury in genetically predisposed individuals leads to long-lasting sensitization of the neural pain circuit despite complete resolution of the initiating event. Increasingly, this concept is being extended to other so-called functional disorders of the gut characterized by unexplained pain, including noncardiac chest pain and nonulcer dyspepsia. These disorders, also considered for many years to arise from motor disturbances, may in fact represent part of a spectrum of a new syndrome of "visceral hyperalgesia" (Mayer and Gebhart, 1994).

Many patients can be managed satisfactorily with a strong patient-physician relationship, simple counseling, and adjunctive measures including dietary restrictions and fiber supplementation. Overt psychological abnormalities are treated appropriately. Despite these measures, a significant proportion of patients remain plagued by severe symptoms, and drug therapy is almost invariably attempted. However, there are very few effective pharmacological options for these patients, a situation that in part reflects our limited understanding of the pathogenesis of this syndrome.

The pharmacological approach to IBS reflects the multifaceted nature of this syndrome. Treatment of bowel symptoms (either diarrhea or constipation) is predominantly symptomatic and nonspecific. Patients with mild symptoms often are started on fiber supplements; this approach may work for both constipation and diarrhea (by binding water; see Chapter 39). Patients with episodic, discrete pain episodes often are treated with agents that may reduce smooth muscle contractility in the gut. These so-called antispasmodics include anticholinergic agents, calcium channel antagonists, and peripheral opioid-receptor antagonists. The use of most such drugs is hallowed by years of tradition, but it seldom has been subjected to critical assessment; indeed, many reports suggest that they are no better than placebo. However, a meta-analysis of 26 studies showed that at least some such drugs may have some clinical efficacy in IBS (Poynard et al., 1994).

In recent years, an increasing emphasis is being placed on the pharmacological treatment of visceral sensitivity (Mayer et al., 1999). Although the biological basis of visceral hyperalgesia in IBS patients is not known, a possible role for serotonin has been suggested, based on its known involvement in sensitization of nociceptor neurons in inflammatory conditions. Insight into the role of serotonin receptors in mediating visceral motor responses (see above) has prompted a great deal of interest in the development of specific antagonists of serotonin receptors for the treatment of IBS (Maxton et al., 1996; Scarpignato and Pelosini, 1999). Another class of agents that has been useful in this regard includes antidepressants (see Chapter 19), which can have neuromodulatory and analgesic properties independent of their antidepressant effect. The most widely studied drugs in this class have been the tricyclic agents. Although selective serotonin-reuptake inhibitors increasingly are being used, there have been no randomized trials of these agents in patients with irritable bowel syndrome. In general, it appears that selective serotonin-reuptake inhibitors are not as effective as the tricyclic antidepressants in patients with neuropathic pain or with chronic unexplained pain (Jackson et al., 2000).

Alosetron (LOTRONEX) is a potent and highly selective 5-HT$_3$–receptor antagonist that can antagonize 5-HT$_3$ receptors on vagal afferents in laboratory animals as well as inhibit the vasomotor response to colorectal distention. In patients with IBS but not in healthy volunteers, the drug was shown to increase rectal compliance and the threshold at which pain is felt and to reduce colonic transit. Although serotonin plays several roles in the gut, including stimulation of gastrointestinal motility and secretion and possibly the transmission of painful impulses, the mechanism and site of action of alosetron are far from established. Adding to the confusion is the fact that other highly selective 5-HT$_3$–receptor antagonists have produced variable effects on visceral sensitivity. Thus, granisetron but not ondansetron can reduce sensation thresholds for visceral distention in laboratory animals and human beings. Nevertheless, alosetron was shown to be modestly effective in reducing overall symptoms as well as diarrhea in female but not male patients with diarrhea-predominant IBS and was approved by the FDA in February 2000 for use in female patients. In November 2000, however, the manufacturer withdrew the drug from the market because of cases of severe constipation and ischemic colitis, including several deaths, with use of alosetron.

Buspirone and *sumatriptan* are serotonin 5-HT$_1$–receptor agonists (see Chapter 11) that can reduce gastric and colonic sensitivity to distention and are being evaluated in clinical trials. α_2-Adrenergic receptor agonists such as *clonidine* (see Chapter 10) and other agents also can increase visceral compliance and reduce distention-induced pain. *Mianserin* (see Chapter 19) is an antidepressant with 5-HT$_3$–receptor and α_2-adrenergic receptor antagonistic activity that also may have some potential value for these patients. The somatostatin analog *octreotide* (see above) has selective inhibitory effects on peripheral afferent nerves projecting from the gut to the spinal cord in healthy human beings and has been shown to blunt the perception of rectal distention in patients with IBS (Hasler et al., 1994). *Fedotozine* is a recently developed opioid that appears to be a peripherally active, selective κ-receptor antagonist and produces marginal improvement in symptoms in patients with IBS and functional dyspepsia (Read et al., 1997). The lack of a CNS effect is an advantage in such patients in whom chronic medication use is anticipated. Other agents being developed include the CCK receptor antagonist *loxiglumide* and the 5-HT$_4$–receptor agonists *prucalopride* and *tegaserod* (*see* above). Other agents of unproven value include *leuprolide,* a gonadotrophin-releasing hormone analog (*see* Chapter 56).

PROSPECTUS

The discovery of the 5-HT$_3$–receptor antagonists has led to a major advance in the treatment of nausea and vomiting, especially in the postchemotherapy setting. By contrast, treatment of the "functional bowel disorders" remains problematic. These conditions are surprisingly common and their symptoms often intractable. As a group, these disorders represent the most difficult therapeutic challenge in the field of gastroenterology. Although recognition of the key roles of molecules such as serotonin has led to some advances in both prokinetic and analgesic therapy, these advances have solved only a small part of the puzzle. The enteric nervous system and the visceral sensory system are very complicated and poorly understood; much more research needs to be done before a truly rational approach to drug development can occur. Fortunately, this challenge is being increasingly taken up by academic researchers and pharmaceutical companies. Knowledge of the pain pathways in both somatic and visceral systems is increasing rapidly, and future therapeutic advances will almost certainly include specific and effective analgesics for use in conditions such as IBS and dyspepsia. The future development of a truly effective prokinetic agent is more uncertain because of our current ignorance of the pathophysiology of most of the target symptomology for such drugs.

For further information about gastrointestinal disorders covered in this chapter, *see* Chapters 41, 283, and 287 in *Harrison's Principles of Internal Medicine,* 14th ed., McGraw-Hill, New York, 1998.

BIBLIOGRAPHY

Bouras, E.P., Camilleri, M., Burton, D.D., and McKinzie, S. Selective stimulation of colonic transit by the benzofuran 5HT$_4$ agonist, prucalopride, in healthy humans. *Gut,* **1999,** *44*:682–686.

Coulie, B., Tack, J., Peeters, T., and Janssens, J. Involvement of two different pathways in the motor effects of erythromycin on the gastric antrum in humans. *Gut,* **1998,** *43*:395–400.

DiBaise, J.K., and Quigley, E.M. Efficacy of prolonged administration of intravenous erythromycin in an ambulatory setting as treatment of severe gastroparesis: one center's experience. *J. Clin. Gastroenterol.,* **1999,** *28*:13–134.

Faure, C., Wolff, V.P., and Navarro, J. Effect of meal and intravenous erythromycin on manometric and electrogastrographic measurements of gastric motor and electrical activity. *Dig. Dis. Sci.,* **2000,** *45*:525–528.

Grunberg, S.J., and Hesketh, P.M. Control of chemotherapy-induced emesis. *N. Engl. J. Med.,* **1993,** *329*:1790–1796.

Hasler, W.L., Soudah, H.C., and Owyang, C. Somatostatin analog inhibits afferent response to rectal distention in diarrhea-predominant irritable bowel patients. *J. Pharmacol. Exp. Ther.,* **1994,** *268*:1206–1211.

Hoogerwerf, W.A., and Pasricha, P.J. Botulinum toxin for spastic gastrointestinal disorders. *Baillières Best Pract. Res. Clin. Gastroenterol.,* **1999,** *13*:131–143.

Jackson, J.L., O'Malley, P.G., Tomkins, G., Balden, E., Santoro, J., and Kroenke, K. Treatment of functional gastrointestinal disorders with antidepressant medications: a meta-analysis. *Am. J. Med.,* **2000,** *108*:65–72.

Medhus, A.W., Bondi, J., Gaustad, P., and Husebye, E. Low-dose intravenous erythromycin: effects on postprandial and fasting motility of the small bowel. *Aliment. Pharmacol. Ther.,* **2000,** *14*:233–240.

Navari, R.M., Reinhardt, R.R., Gralla, R.J., Kris, M.G., Hesketh, P.J., Khojasteh, A., Kindler, H., Grote, T.H., Penergrass, K., Grunberg, S.M., Carides, A.D., and Gertz, B.J. Reduction of cisplatin-induced emesis by a selective neurokinin-1-receptor antagonist. L-754,030 Antiemetic Trials Group. *N. Engl. J. Med.,* **1999,** *340*:190–195.

Pasricha, P.J., Ravich, W.J., Hendrix, T.R., Sostre, S., Jones, B., and Kalloo, A.N. Intrasphincteric botulinum toxin for the treatment of achalasia. *N. Engl. J. Med.,* **1995,** *332*:774–778.

Ponec, R.J., Saunders, M.D., and Kimmey, M.B. Neostigmine for the treatment of acute colonic pseudo-obstruction. *N. Engl. J. Med.,* **1999,** *341*:137–141.

Poynard, T., Naveau, S., Mory, B., and Chaput, J.C. Meta-analysis of smooth muscle relaxants in the treatment of irritable bowel syndrome. *Aliment. Pharmacol. Ther.,* **1994,** *8*:499–510.

Read, N.W., Abitbol, J.L., Bardhan, K.D., Whorwell, P.J., and Fraitag, B. Efficacy and safety of the peripheral kappa agonist fedotozine versus placebo in the treatment of functional dyspepsia. *Gut,* **1997,** *41*:664–668.

MONOGRAPHS AND REVIEWS

Andrews, P.L., Naylor, R.J., and Joss, R.A. Neuropharmacology of emesis and its relevance to anti-emetic therapy. Consensus and controversies. *Support Care Cancer,* **1998,** *6*:197–203.

ASHP Therapeutic Guidelines on the Pharmacologic Management of Nausea and Vomiting in Adult and Pediatric Patients Receiving

Chemotherapy or Radiation Therapy or Undergoing Surgery. *Am. J. Health Syst. Pharm.,* **1999,** *56:*729–764.

Barone, J.A. Domperidone: a peripherally acting dopamine2-receptor antagonist. *Ann. Pharmacother.,* **1999,** *33:*429–440.

Briejer, M.R., Akkermans, L.M., and Schuurkes, J.A. Gastrointestinal prokinetic benzamides: the pharmacology underlying stimulation of motility. *Pharmacol. Rev.,* **1995,** *47:*631–651.

Camilleri, M. Effects of somatostatin analogues on human gastrointestinal motility. *Digestion,* **1996,** *57*(suppl 1):90–92.

Drossman, D.A., Whitehead, W.E., and Camilleri, M. Irritable bowel syndrome: a technical review for practice guideline development. *Gastroenterology,* **1997,** *112:*2120–2137.

Gregory, R.E., and Ettinger, D.S. 5-HT$_3$ receptor antagonists for the prevention of chemotherapy-induced nausea and vomiting. A comparison of their pharmacology and clinical efficacy. *Drugs,* **1998,** *55:*173–189.

Hesketh, P.J. Comparative review of 5-HT$_3$ receptor antagonists in the treatment of acute chemotherapy-induced nausea and vomiting. *Cancer Invest.,* **2000,** *18:*163–173.

Koch, K.L. Diabetic gastropathy: gastric neuromuscular dysfunction in diabetes mellitus: a review of symptoms, pathophysiology, and treatment. *Dig. Dis. Sci.,* **1999,** *44:*1061–1075.

Kovac, A.L. Prevention and treatment of postoperative nausea and vomiting. *Drugs,* **2000,** *59:*213–243.

Kris, M.G., Roila, F., De Mulder, P.H., and Marty, M. Delayed emesis following anticancer chemotherapy. *Support Care Cancer,* **1998,** *6:*228–232.

Kunze, W.A., and Furness, J.B. The enteric nervous system and regulation of intestinal motility. *Annu. Rev. Physiol.,* **1999,** *61:*117–142.

Maxton, D.G., Morris, J., and Whorwell, P.J. Selective 5-hydroxytryptamine antagonism: a role in irritable bowel syndrome and funtional dyspepsia? *Aliment. Pharmacol. Ther.,* **1996,** *10:*595–599.

Mayer, E.A., and Gebhart, G.F. Basic and clinical aspects of visceral hyperalgesia. *Gastroenterology,* **1994,** *107:*271–293.

Mayer, E.A., Lembo, T., and Chang, L. Approaches to the modulation of abdominal pain. *Can. J. Gastroenterol.,* **1999,** *13*(suppl A):65A–70A.

Mazzotta, P., Gupta, A., Maltepe, C., Koren, G., Magee, L. Pharmacologic treatment of nausea and vomiting during pregnancy. *Can. Fam. Physician,* **1998,** *44:*1455–1457.

McCallum, R.W. Pharmacologic modulation of motility. *Yale J. Biol. Med.,* **1999,** *72:*173–180.

Otterson, M.F., and Sarna, S.K. Gastrointestinal motor effects of erythromycin. *Am. J. Physiol.,* **1990,** *259:*G355–G363.

Pandolfino, J.E., Howden, C.W., and Kahrilas, P.J. Motility-modifying agents and management of disorders of gastrointestinal motility. *Gastroenterology,* **2000,** *118:*S32–S47.

Reynolds, J.C., and Putnam, P.E. Prokinetic agents. *Gastroenterol. Clin. North Am.,* **1992,** *21:*567–596.

Rizk, A.N., and Hesketh, P.J. Antiemetics for cancer chemotherapy-induced nausea and vomiting. A review of agents in development. *Drugs R.D.,* **1999,** *2:*229–235.

Rupniak, N.M., and Kramer, M.S. Discovery of the antidepressant and anti-emetic efficacy of substance receptor (NK1) antagonists. *Trends Pharmacol. Sci.,* **1999,** *20:*485–490.

Scarpignato, C., and Pelosini, I. Management of irritable bowel syndrome: novel approaches to the pharmacology of gut motility. *Can. J. Gastroenterol.,* **1999,** *13*(suppl A):50A–65A.

Scott, L.J., and Perry, C.M. Tegaserod. *Drugs,* **1999,** *58:*491–496.

Sturm, A., Holtmann, G., Goebell, H., and Gerken, G. Prokinetics in patients with gastroparesis: a systematic analysis. *Digestion,* **1999,** *60:*422–427.

Tonini, M. Recent advances in the pharmacology of gastrointestinal prokinetics. *Pharmacol. Res.,* **1996,** *33:*217–226.

Tonini, M., De Ponti, F., Di Nucci, A., and Crema, F. Review article: cardiac adverse effects of gastrointestinal prokinetics. *Aliment. Pharmacol. Ther.,* **1999,** *13:*1585–1591.

Wilde, M.I., and Markham, A. Ondansetron. A review of its pharmacology and preliminary clinical findings in novel applications. *Drugs,* **1996,** *52:*773–794.

Acknowledgment

The author wishes to acknowledge Laurence L. Brunton, author of this chapter in the ninth edition of *Goodman and Gilman's The Pharmacological Basis of Therapeutics,* some of whose text has been retained in this edition.

C H A P T E R 3 9

AGENTS USED FOR DIARRHEA, CONSTIPATION, AND INFLAMMATORY BOWEL DISEASE; AGENTS USED FOR BILIARY AND PANCREATIC DISEASE

Syed Jafri and Pankaj J. Pasricha

Diarrhea and constipation are among the most ancient of human maladies; not surprisingly, their remedies occupy a special place in the annals of medicine. Antidiarrheal preparations of opium were used as early as 3000 B.C. by Sumerian physicians; just as old is the use of the plant alkaloid berberine (benzyl tetrahydroxy quinolone), derived from Berberis aristata, *in India and China. The seed of* Ricinus communis, *from which castor oil is derived, was well known to ancient Egyptians for treatment of constipation. However, despite this long history, the pharmacological approach to disturbances in bowel movements remains largely empirical. This is especially true with constipation, as a true colonic prokinetic agent has yet to be found. More progress has been made in specific diarrheal diseases, such as inflammatory bowel disease, where advances in understanding the pathophysiology have led to an increasingly rational approach to therapy. Drugs used in treating diarrhea, constipation, and inflammatory bowel disease are the main topics dealt with in this chapter. This chapter also covers miscellaneous drugs such as choleretic agents (bile acids) used in biliary diseases as well as enzymes and other agents used for pancreatic disorders.*

OVERVIEW OF GASTROINTESTINAL WATER AND ELECTROLYTE FLUX

Fluid content is the principal determinant of stool volume and consistency; water normally accounts for 70% to 85% of total stool weight. Net stool fluid content reflects a balance between luminal input (ingestion and secretion of water and electrolytes) and output (absorption) along the length of the gastrointestinal tract. The daily challenge for the gut is to extract water, minerals, and nutrients from the luminal contents, leaving behind a manageable pool of fluid for proper expulsion of waste material *via* the process of defecation. Normally about 8 to 9 liters of fluid enters the small intestine daily from both exogenous and endogenous sources (Figure 39–1). Net absorption of the water occurs in the small intestine in response to osmotic gradients that result from the uptake and secretion of ions and the absorption of nutrients (mainly sugars and amino acids), with only

about 1 to 1.5 liters crossing the ileocecal valve. The colon then extracts most of the remaining fluid, leaving about 100 ml of fecal water daily.

Under normal circumstances, these quantities are well within the range of the total absorptive capacity of the small bowel (about 16 liters) and colon (4 to 5 liters). Neurohumoral mechanisms, pathogens, and drugs can alter these processes, resulting in changes in either secretion or absorption of fluid by the intestinal epithelium. Altered motility also contributes in a general way to this process, as the extent of absorption parallels transit time. When the capacity of the colon to absorb fluid is exceeded, diarrhea will occur. On the other hand, excessive reabsorption will lead to decreased stool volume and constipation. Defecatory disorders resulting from neuromuscular or structural disturbances of the evacuation function of the rectum are additional causes of constipation, even though stool volume may not be diminished.

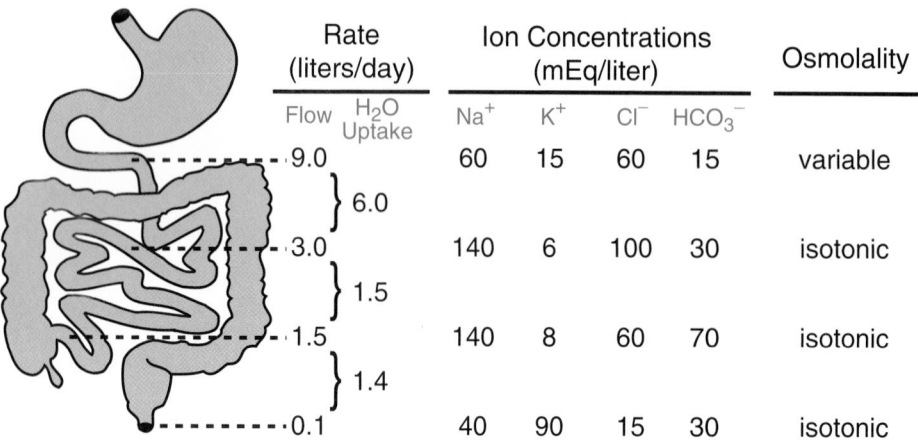

	Rate (liters/day)		Ion Concentrations (mEq/liter)				Osmolality
	Flow	H$_2$O Uptake	Na$^+$	K$^+$	Cl$^-$	HCO$_3^-$	
	9.0		60	15	60	15	variable
		6.0					
	3.0		140	6	100	30	isotonic
		1.5					
	1.5		140	8	60	70	isotonic
		1.4					
	0.1		40	90	15	30	isotonic

Figure 39–1. The approximate volume and composition of fluid that traverses the small and large intestines daily.

Of the 9 liters of fluid presented to the small intestine each day, 2 liters are from the diet and 7 liters are from secretions (salivary, gastric, pancreatic, and biliary). The absorptive capacity of the colon is 4 to 5 liters per day. For details of absorptive and secretory processes in the gastrointestinal tract, *see* Sellin, 1993.

DIARRHEA: GENERAL CONSIDERATIONS AND NONSPECIFIC TREATMENTS

Diarrhea (Greek and Latin: *dia,* through, and *rheein,* to flow or run) does not require any definition to people who suffer from "the too-rapid evacuation of too-fluid stools." However, with their love for quantification, scientists usually define diarrhea as excessive fluid weight, with 200 g per day representing the upper limit of normal stool water weight for healthy adults in the western world. Since stool weight is largely determined by stool water, most cases of diarrhea result from disorders of intestinal water and electrolyte transport. From a mechanistic perspective, diarrhea can be caused by an increased osmotic load within the intestine (resulting in retention of water within the lumen); excessive secretion of electrolytes and water into the intestinal lumen; exudation of protein and fluid from the mucosa; and altered intestinal motility, resulting in rapid transit. In most instances, multiple processes are simultaneously affected, leading to a net increase in stool volume and weight accompanied by changes in percent water content.

An appreciation and knowledge of the underlying causative process(es) in diarrhea enables the clinician to develop the most effective treatment. Many patients with sudden onset of diarrhea have a benign, self-limited illness requiring no treatment or evaluation. In severe cases, dehydration and electrolyte imbalances are the principal risk, particularly in infants, children, and frail elderly patients. Oral rehydration therapy is therefore a cornerstone for patients with acute illnesses resulting in significant diarrhea. This is of particular importance in developing countries, where the use of such therapy saves many thousands of lives every year. This therapy exploits the fact that nutrient-linked cotransport of water and electrolytes remains intact in the small bowel in most cases of acute diarrhea. Sodium and chloride absorption is linked to glucose uptake by the enterocyte; this is followed by move-

ment of water in the same direction. A balanced mixture of glucose and electrolytes in volumes matched to losses therefore can prevent dehydration. World Health Organization–recommended formulas for oral rehydration solutions are ideal; other mixtures or home remedies may not be as balanced (Table 39–1).

Pharmacotherapy of diarrhea (Schiller, 1995) should be reserved for patients with significant or persistent symptoms. Nonspecific antidiarrheal agents typically do not address the underlying pathophysiology responsible for the diarrhea; their principal utility is in the provision of symptomatic relief in mild cases of acute diarrhea. Many of these agents act by decreasing intestinal motility and should be avoided as far as possible in acute diarrheal illnesses caused by invasive organisms. In such cases, these agents may mask the clinical picture, delay clearance of organisms, and increase the risk of systemic invasion by the infectious organisms as well as local complications such as toxic megacolon.

Intraluminal Agents

Bulk-Forming and Hydroscopic Agents. Hydrophilic colloids such as *psyllium* (METAMUCIL, others), *polycarbophil* (FIBERCON, FIBERALL, others), and *carboxymethylcellulose* absorb water and increase stool bulk. They usually are used for constipation (*see* below) but are sometimes useful in mild chronic diarrheas in patients suffering with irritable bowel syndrome. The mechanism of this effect is unclear, but it may involve texture modification, *i.e.,* alterations in stool viscosity and a perception of decreased stool fluidity. Some of these agents also may bind bacterial toxins and bile salts. Clays such as *kaolin* (a hydrated aluminum silicate) and other silicates such as *attapulgite* (magnesium aluminum disilicate; DIASORB) bind

Table 39–1
Oral Rehydration Solutions for Treatment of Diarrhea[*]

SOLUTION	Na$^+$	K$^+$	Cl$^-$(chloride)	CITRATE	BICARBONATE	GLUCOSE
WHO[†] solution	90	20	80	30		111
PEDIALYTE	45	20	35	10		140
RESOL	50	20	50			111
INFALYTE	50	25	45		30	111
GATORADE	23.5	<1	17			(40)
COCA-COLA	1.6	<1			13	(100)
Apple juice	<1	25	30			(120)
Tea	0	0	0	0	0	0
Chicken soup	250	8	250	0	0	0

[*]All values are given as millimoles per liter except those in parentheses, which are given in grams per liter.
[†]World Health Organization.
SOURCE: From Korman, 1994, with permission.

water avidly and also may bind enterotoxins. A mixture of kaolin and pectin (a plant polysaccharide) is a popular over-the-counter remedy (KAOPECTOLIN) and may provide useful symptomatic relief of mild diarrhea.

Cholestyramine. *Cholestyramine* (QUESTRAN) is an anion-exchange resin that effectively binds bile acids and some bacterial toxins. It is useful in the treatment of bile salt–induced diarrhea, as in patients with resection of the distal ileum. In these patients, there is partial interruption of the normal enterohepatic circulation of bile salts, resulting in excessive concentrations reaching the colon and stimulating water and electrolyte secretion. Patients with extensive ileal resection (usually more than 100 cm) eventually develop net bile salt depletion, which can produce steatorrhea because of inadequate micellar formation required for fat absorption. In such patients, the use of cholestyramine will aggravate the diarrhea. The drug also has had a historic role in treating mild antibiotic-associated diarrhea and mild colitis due to *Clostridium difficile*. However, its use in infectious diarrheas generally is to be discouraged, as it may decrease clearance of the pathogen from the bowel. Cholestyramine also binds medications and vitamins (*see* Chapter 36) and should not be given within a few hours of the administration of other drugs. In patients suspected of having bile salt-induced diarrhea, a trial of cholestyramine can be given at a dose of 9 g four times a day and the dose titrated down to achieve a desired stool frequency.

Bismuth. Bismuth compounds have been used to treat a variety of gastrointestinal diseases and symptoms for centuries, although their mechanism of action remains poorly understood. PEPTO-BISMOL (bismuth subsalicylate) is an over-the-counter preparation estimated to be used by 60% of American households. It is a crystal complex consisting of trivalent bismuth and salicylate suspended in a mixture of magnesium aluminum silicate clay. In the low pH of the stomach, the bismuth subsalicylate reacts with hydrochloric acid to form bismuth oxychloride and salicylic acid. The latter is absorbed in the stomach and small intestine, leaving 99% of the bismuth to pass unaltered and unabsorbed into the feces.

Bismuth is thought to have antisecretory, antiinflammatory, and antimicrobial effects; nausea and abdominal cramps also may be relieved. The clay in PEPTO-BISMOL also may have some additional benefits, but this is not clear. Bismuth subsalicylate has best been used effectively for the prevention and treatment of traveler's diarrhea, but it also may be effective in other forms of nonsyndromic, episodic diarrhea. A recommended dose of the liquid bismuth subsalicylate preparation contains approximately equal amounts of bismuth and salicylate (250 to 300 mg each). It is taken up to eight times a day and appears to be extremely safe at recommended doses, although impaction may occur in infants and debilitated patients. Bismuth sulfide is the black, solid agent responsible for the darkening of the stool (mistaken by some for melena!) that is associated with bismuth subsalicylate use. Likewise, a darkening of the tongue occurs because of a reaction between the drug and sulfides produced by bacteria in the mouth. The most common antibacterial use of this agent is in the treatment of *Helicobacter pylori* (*see* Chapter 37).

Antimotility and Antisecretory Agents

Opioids. Opioids continue to be widely used in the treatment of diarrhea and may act by several different mechanisms, mediated principally by either μ- or δ-opioid receptors on enteric nerves, epithelial cells, and muscle (*see* Chapter 23). These include effects on intestinal motility (μ receptors), intestinal secretion (δ receptors), or absorption (both μ and δ receptors). Commonly used antidiarrheals such as *diphenoxylate, difenoxin,* and *loperamide* act principally *via* peripheral μ-opioid receptors and are preferred to other agents because of their limited ability to penetrate the central nervous system (CNS).

Loperamide. Loperamide (IMODIUM, IMODIUM A-D, others), a piperidine butyramide derivative, is an orally active antidiarrheal agent (Daugherty, 1990). The drug is 40 to 50 times more potent than morphine as an antidiarrheal agent and penetrates the CNS poorly. It increases small intestinal transit time as well as mouth-to-cecum transit time. Loperamide also increases anal sphincter tone, an effect that may be of therapeutic use in some patients who suffer from anal incontinence. In addition to above actions, it has antisecretory activity against cholera toxin and some forms of *E. coli* toxin.

Because of its effectiveness and safety profile, loperamide now is marketed for over-the-counter distribution and is available in capsule, solution, and chewable forms. It acts quickly following an oral dose, with peak plasma levels being achieved within 3 to 5 hours. It has a half-life of about 11 hours and undergoes extensive hepatic metabolism. The usual adult dose is 4 mg initially followed by 2 mg after each subsequent loose stool, up to 16 mg per day. Recommended maximum daily doses for children are 3 mg for ages 2 to 5 years, 4 mg for ages 6 to 8 years, and 6 mg for ages 8 to 12 years. Loperamide should not be used in children younger than 2 years of age.

Loperamide has been shown to be effective against *traveler's diarrhea,* used either alone or in combination with antimicrobial agents (*trimethoprim, trimethoprim–sulfamethoxazole,* or a *fluoroquinolone*). If clinical improvement in *acute* diarrhea does not occur within 48 hours, loperamide should be discontinued. However, loperamide also has been used as adjunct treatment in almost all forms of chronic diarrheal disease. Very few adverse effects have been reported worldwide with loperamide. Loperamide lacks significant abuse potential and is more effective in treating diarrhea than diphenoxylate (*see* below). Overdosage, however, can result in CNS depression and paralytic ileus. Children may be more sensitive than adults to the CNS-depressant effects of loperamide. In patients with active inflammatory disease of the colon, loperamide should be used with great caution, if at all, to prevent development of toxic megacolon.

Loperamide N-*oxide,* an investigational agent, is a site-specific prodrug; it is chemically designed for controlled release of loperamide in the intestinal lumen, reducing systemic absorption.

Diphenoxylate and Difenoxin. *Diphenoxylate* and *difenoxin* (diphenoxylic acid) are piperidine derivatives that are structurally related to meperidine. Difenoxin is the active metabolite of diphenoxylate and also is used as such to treat diarrhea. As antidiarrheal agents, diphenoxylate and difenoxin are somewhat more potent than morphine. Both compounds are extensively absorbed after oral administration, with peak levels achieved within 1 to 2 hours. Diphenoxylate is rapidly deesterified to difenoxin, which is eliminated with a half-life of about 12 hours. Both these drugs can produce CNS effects when used in higher doses (40 to 60 mg per day) and therefore have a potential for abuse and/or addiction. They are available in preparations containing small doses of atropine (considered subtherapeutic) to discourage abuse and deliberate overdosage. These preparations contain 25 μg of atropine sulfate per tablet with either 2.5 mg diphenoxylate hydrochloride (LOMOTIL) or 1 mg of difenoxin hydrochloride (MOTOFEN). The usual dosage is two tablets initially, then one tablet every 3 to 4 hours. With excessive use or overdose, constipation and (in inflammatory conditions of the colon) toxic megacolon may develop. In high doses, these drugs also cause CNS effects as well as anticholinergic effects from the atropine (dry mouth, blurred vision, *etc.; see* Chapter 7).

Other opioids, including codeine, and opium-containing compounds such as paregoric (camphorated tincture of opium, containing 0.4 mg/ml of morphine) and deodorized tincture of opium (containing 10 mg/ml of morphine), are mainly of historical importance in the treatment of diarrhea because of their potential for addiction and CNS side effects. The two tinctures sometimes were confused in prescribing and dispensing, leading to dangerous overdoses.

Acetorphan (*racecadotril*) represents a new class of drugs under investigation (Matheson and Noble, 2000). It is an enkephalinase inhibitor that increases local levels of enkephalins, with consequent stimulation of both μ- and δ-opioid receptors to produce an antidiarrheal effect. Moreover, unlike loperamide, racecadotril does not prolong transit time in the small intestine or colon and may have a relatively specific antisecretory effect.

α_2-Adrenergic Receptor Agonists. α_2-Adrenergic receptor agonists can stimulate absorption and inhibit secretion of fluid and electrolytes as well as increase intestinal transit time by interacting with specific receptors on multiple sites including enteric neurons and enterocytes

(DiJoseph *et al.,* 1984). These agents may have a special role in diabetics with chronic diarrhea, in whom autonomic neuropathy can lead to loss of noradrenergic innervation. Oral clonidine (beginning at 0.1 mg twice a day) has been used in these patients; the use of a topical preparation (*e.g.,* CATAPRES TTS, two patches a week) may result in more steady plasma levels of the drug. Clonidine also may be useful in patients with diarrhea caused by opiate withdrawal. Side effects such as hypotension, depression, and perceived fatigue may be major limiting factors.

Octreotide.   *Octreotide* (SANDOSTATIN; *see* Chapters 38 and 56) is an octapeptide analog of somatostatin and is effective in inhibiting the severe secretory diarrhea brought about by hormone-secreting tumors of the pancreas and the gastrointestinal tract (Beglinger and Drewe, 1999). Its mechanism of action appears to involve inhibition of hormone secretion rather than a proabsorptive effect. It also is effective in patients with the dumping syndrome (due to rapid emptying of gastric contents, usually seen in the postoperative setting). Octreotide has been used, with varying degrees of success, in other forms of secretory diarrhea such as chemotherapy-induced diarrhea, diarrhea associated with human immunodeficiency virus (HIV), and diabetic diarrhea (Fried, 1999).

Octreotide has a longer half-life (1 to 2 hours) than does somatostatin (1 to 2 minutes) and therefore can be administered either subcutaneously or intravenously as a bolus dose. Standard initial therapy with octreotide is 50 to 100 μg, given subcutaneously 2 or 3 times a day, with titration to a maximum dose of 500 μg three times a day, based on clinical and biochemical responses. A long-acting preparation of octreotide acetate enclosed in biodegradable microspheres (SANDOSTATIN, LAR DEPOT) is available for use in the treatment of diarrheas associated with carcinoid tumors and vasoactive intestinal peptide–secreting tumors as well as in the treatment of acromegaly. This preparation is injected intramuscularly once per month in a dose of 20 mg. Side effects of octreotide are dependent on the duration of therapy. Short-term therapy leads to transient nausea, bloating, or pain at sites of injection. Long-term therapy can lead to gallstone formation and hypo- or hyperglycemia. Another long-acting somatostatin analog, *lanreotide,* is available in Europe but not in the United States; another one, *vapreotide,* is under development.

Use in Variceal Bleeding.   Vasoactive agents have been used to control variceal bleeding for 40 years. Traditionally, vasopressin has been used, but its significant side effects—such as myocardial ischemia, peripheral vascular disease, and the release of plasminogen activator and factor VIII—have led to its decline in popularity. Somatostatin and octreotide are effective in reducing hepatic blood flow, wedged hepatic venous pressure, and azygos blood flow. These agents cause splanchnic arteriolar constriction by a direct action on vascular smooth muscle as well as by inhibiting the release of peptides contributing to the hyperdynamic circulatory syndrome of portal hypertension. It also is possible that octreotide may act through the autonomic nervous system. These agents can control bleeding acutely and decrease bleeding-related mortality, with an efficacy that is comparable to endoscopic therapy or balloon tamponade. The major advantage of somatostatin and octreotide over vasopressin is their safety. Because of the short half-life of somatostatin, it can be given only by intravenous infusion (250 μg bolus dose followed by 250 μg hourly). For patients with variceal bleeding, therapy with octreotide usually is initiated while the patient is awaiting endoscopy. It is given intravenously as an infusion of 25 to 50 μg/hour for 48 hours after a bolus of 100 μg. Some clinicians give 100 μg subcutaneously every 6 to 8 hours for an additional 72 hours until the patient has had the second endoscopic treatment.

Other Agents.   Calcium channel blockers such as *verapamil* and *nifedipine* (*see* Chapter 32) reduce motility and may promote intestinal electrolyte and water absorption. Constipation, in fact, is a significant side effect of these drugs. However, because of their systemic effects and the availability of other agents, they are seldom if ever used for diarrheal illnesses.

Berberine is a plant alkaloid and may exert an antidiarrheal effect through antimicrobial as well as antisecretory and antimotility activity. There are few controlled studies to attest to its efficacy as a routine antidiarrheal therapy. *Alosetron,* a selective 5-HT$_3$–receptor antagonist, is indicated for the treatment of irritable bowel syndrome in female patients whose predominant symptom is diarrhea (*see* Chapter 38). Chloride channel blockers are effective antisecretory agents *in vitro* but are too toxic for human use and have not proven to be effective antidiarrheal agents *in vivo*. Calmodulin inhibitors, which include chlorpromazine, also are antisecretory. *Zaldaride maleate,* a new drug in this class, may be effective in traveler's diarrhea.

CONSTIPATION AND ITS TREATMENT

The principal functions of the colon relate to solidification, storage, and proper and timely evacuation of stools. The efficiency of these processes is determined both by the nature of luminal contents as well as the integrity of normal colonic absorptive and neuromuscular function. Constipation (Latin: *con,* together; *stipare,* to cram or pack) is a symptom complex the definition of which has baffled patients and clini... tific definitions rely mostly on stool num... found the normal stool frequency on a ... 3 times a week. However, it is clear th... proach and does not take into accou... of difficulty in evacuation or change... spite a normal frequency. Patients us... decreased frequency, difficulty in in... of firm or small-volume feces, or a... uation. By questionnaire, 25% of ... States may complain of constipat... and elderly people. Although ge... vere constipation can lead to sig... few patients, including urinary ... lapse. Fecal impaction in the elde... lead to soiling and stercoral ulcers.

There are many reversible or secondary causes of con... stipation, including lack of dietary fiber, drugs, hormonal disturbances, neurogenic disorders, and systemic illnesses. However, in most cases of chronic constipation, no specific cause is found. In these patients, attempts usually are made to categorize the underlying pathophysiology either as a disorder of delayed colonic transit ("slow transit idiopathic constipation," "colonic inertia") because of an underlying defect in colonic motility, or, less commonly, as an isolated disorder of defecation or evacuation (outlet disorder) because of dysfunction of the neuromuscular apparatus of the rectoanal region. However, given the paucity of data on the underlying mechanisms of chronic constipation, this classification is far from satisfactory and does not, in most cases, lead to specific therapeutic approaches. Colonic motility is responsible for mixing luminal contents to promote absorption of water and moving them from the proximal to distal segments by means of propulsive contractions. Mixing is accomplished in the colon in a way similar to that in the small bowel, by short- or long-duration, stationary (nonpropulsive) contractions, the electrical counterparts of which are short- or long-spike bursts (SSBs or LSBs). Propulsive contractions in the colon are of two kinds: (1) long-duration propulsive contractions (accompanied electrically by LSBs) that assist in local propulsion of feces from one segment to the next and (2) giant migrating contractions, also known as colonic mass actions or mass movements, which propagate caudally over extended lengths in the colon and evoke mass transfer of feces from the right to the left colon once or twice a day. There is evidence that some patients with constipation have increased SSBs correlated with prolongation of the intestinal transit time. Disturbances in motility therefore may have complex effects on bowel movements. Both "decreased motility" of the mass action type as well as "increased motility" of the nonpropulsive type may lead to constipation. In any given patient, which one of these factors is predominant often is not obvious. Consequently, the pharmacological approach to constipation remains empirical and is based, in most cases, on nonspecific principles.

Many individuals have preconceived ideas of what a normal bowel habit should be. They have unusual notions regarding the frequency, consistency, or quantity of stool; if they are not "satisfied," they resort to self-prescribed laxatives to achieve this goal. Abuse of laxatives includes

...ives frequently are used by ...rs. A survey of bowel habits ...ates showed that 18% of re... ...least once a month, but nearly ...t have constipation. Approxi... ...ian visits per year are attributed ...ual expenditures on laxatives in ...imated at $1 billion.

...stipation can be corrected by ad... ...(20 to 30 g daily) diet, plenty of ...riate bowel habits and training. Im... ...activity and attention to psychoso... ...ctors and similar measures often help ...of constipation. Constipation related to ... be corrected by use of alternatives, where possible, or adjustment of drug dosage. If nonpharmacological measures alone are inadequate or unrealistic (e.g., because of elderly age or infirmity), they may be supplemented with bulk-forming agents. When stimulant laxatives are used, they should be administered at the least-effective dosage and for the shortest period of time to avoid abuse. In addition to perpetuating dependence on drugs, the laxative habit may lead to excessive loss of water and electrolytes; secondary aldosteronism may occur if volume depletion is prominent. Steatorrhea and protein-losing enteropathy with hypoalbuminemia have been reported, as have excessive excretion of calcium in the stool and osteomalacia of the vertebral column.

In addition to treating constipation, laxatives frequently are employed prior to surgical, radiological, and endoscopic procedures where an empty colon is desirable. Laxatives also can help maintain soft stools in patients with anorectal disorders such as hemorrhoids and in patients with irritable bowel syndrome and diverticulosis.

AGENTS USED TO TREAT CONSTIPATION: GENERAL CONSIDERATIONS

The terms *laxatives, cathartics, purgatives, aperients,* and *evacuants* often are used interchangeably. Strictly speaking, however, there is a distinction between laxation (the evacuation of formed fecal material from the rectum) and catharsis (the evacuation of unformed, usually watery fecal material from the entire colon). Most of the commonly used agents promote laxation, but some actually are cathartics, which, at low doses, are used as laxatives.

General Mechanisms of Action. Laxatives generally have been thought to act in one of the following ways:

Table 39–2

Classification of Agents Used for Constipation

1. Luminally active agents

    a. Hydrophilic colloids; bulk-forming agents (bran, psyllium, *etc.*)

    b. Osmotic agents (nonabsorbable inorganic salts or sugars)

    c. Stool-wetting agents (surfactants) and emollients (docusate, mineral oil)

2. Nonspecific stimulants or irritants (with effects on both fluid secretion and motility)

    Diphenylmethanes (bisacodyl)

    Anthraquinones (senna and cascara)

    Castor oil

3. Prokinetic agents (acting primarily on motility)

    $5\text{-}HT_4$-receptor agonists

    Opioid-receptor antagonists

(1) retention of intraluminal fluid, by hydrophilic or osmotic mechanisms; (2) decreased net absorption of fluid, by effects on small and large bowel fluid and electrolyte transport; or (3) effects on motility by either inhibiting segmenting (nonpropulsive) contractions or stimulating propulsive contractions. Based on the above, laxatives usually have been classified as shown in Table 39–2; their known effects on motility and secretion are listed in Table 39–3. Another, perhaps more practical way to classify laxatives is by the pattern of effects produced by the usual clinical dosage (Table 39–4).

Classification of laxatives as represented in Table 39–2 may have to be revised, as recent studies indicate considerable overlap among these traditional categories. Thus, information on the roles of biological factors such as platelet activating factor (PAF) and nitric oxide (NO) paints a far more complex picture of the effects of laxatives than previously thought (Izzo *et al.*, 1998). PAF is a phospholid proinflammatory mediator, and it produces significant stimulation of colonic secretion and gastrointestinal motility. NO also may be involved in stimulation of intestinal secretion *via* prostaglandin- and cyclic GMP–dependent mechanisms. In addition, NO may inhibit segmenting contractions in the colon, promoting laxation. Agents that reduce the expression of NO synthase or its activity can prevent the laxative effects of castor oil, cascara, bisacodyl (but not senna), as well as magnesium sulfate. A variety of laxatives, both osmotic agents and stimulants, have been found to increase the activity of NO synthase and to increase the biosynthesis of PAF in the gut (*see* Izzo *et al.*, 1998).

Dietary Fiber and Supplements

Under normal circumstances, the bulk, softness, and hydration of feces are highly dependent on the fiber content of the diet. Dietary fiber may be defined as that part of food that is resistant to enzymatic digestion and hence is presented to the colon largely unchanged. Colonic bacteria produce fermentation of fiber to varying degrees, depending on the chemical nature and water solubility of different fiber subtypes. Fermentation of fiber has two important effects: (1) it produces short chain fatty acids (SCFAs) that are trophic for colonic epithelium, and (2) it increases bacterial mass. Although fermentation of fiber generally decreases stool water, SCFAs also may have a prokinetic

Table 39–3

Summary of Effects of Some Laxatives on Bowel Function

	Small Bowel		*Colon*		
AGENT	TRANSIT TIME	MIXING CONTRACTIONS	PROPULSIVE CONTRACTIONS	MASS ACTIONS	STOOL WATER
Dietary fiber	↓	?	↑	?	↑
Magnesium	↓	–	↑	↑	↑↑
Lactulose	↓	?	?	?	↑↑
Metoclopramide	↓	?	↑	?	–
Cisapride	↓	?	↑	?	↑
Erythromycin	↓	?	?	?	?
Naloxone	↓	↓	–	–	↑
Anthraquinones	↓	↓	↑	↑	↑↑
Diphenylmethanes	↓	↓	↑	↑	↑↑
Docusates	–	?	?	?	–

KEY: ↑ = increased, ↓ = decreased, ? = no data available, – = no effect on this parameter.
SOURCE: Modified from Kreek, 1994, with permission.

Table 39–4
Classification and Comparison of Representative Laxatives

Laxative Effect and Latency in Usual Clinical Dosage

SOFTENING OF FECES, 1 TO 3 DAYS	SOFT OR SEMIFLUID STOOL, 6 TO 8 HOURS	WATERY EVACUATION, 1 TO 3 HOURS

Bulk-forming laxatives
  Bran
  Psyllium preparations
  Methylcellulose
  Calcium polycarbophil
	Stimulant laxatives
	  Diphenylmethane
	    derivatives
	  Bisacodyl
		Osmotic laxatives*
		  Sodium phosphates
		  Magnesium sulfate
		  Milk of magnesia
		  Magnesium citrate

Surfactant laxatives
  Docusates
  Poloxamers
Lactulose
	Anthraquinone
	  derivatives
	  Senna
	  Cascara sagrada
		Castor oil

*Employed in high dosage for rapid cathartic effect and in lower dosage for laxative effect.

effect, and increased bacterial mass may contribute to increased stool volume. On the other hand, fiber that is not fermented can attract water and increase stool bulk. The net effect on bowel movement therefore varies with different compositions of dietary fiber (Table 39–5). In general, insoluble, poorly fermentable fibers such as lignin are the most effective in increasing stool bulk and transit.

Bran is the residue left when flour is made from cereals and contains more than 40% dietary fiber. Wheat bran, with its high lignin content, is most effective in increasing stool weight. Fruits and vegetables contain more *pectins* and *hemicelluloses,* which are more readily fermentable and produce less effect on stool transit. *Psyllium husk,* derived from the plantago seed, is a component of many commercial products for constipation (METAMUCIL, others), some available as wafers. Psyllium husk contains a hydrophilic mucilloid that undergoes significant fermentation in the colon, leading to an increase in colonic bac-

terial mass. The usual dosage is 2.5 to 4 g (1 to 3 teaspoonfuls in 250 ml of fruit juice). A variety of semisynthetic celluloses—*e.g., methylcellulose* (CITRUCEL, others) and *polycarbophils* (FIBERCON, others)—also are available. These poorly fermentable compounds are able to absorb water and increase fecal bulk.

Fiber is contraindicated in patients with obstructive symptoms and in those with megacolon or megarectum. Fecal impaction should be treated before initiating fiber supplementation. Bloating and abdominal pain are the most common side effects of fiber but usually decrease with time. Calcium polycarbophil preparations release Ca^{2+} in the gastrointestinal tract and should thus be avoided by patients who must restrict their intake of calcium or who are taking tetracycline. Sugar-free bulk laxatives may contain aspartame and are contraindicated in patients with phenylketonuria. Allergic reactions have been reported with psyllium.

Table 39–5
Properties of Different Dietary Fibers

TYPE OF FIBER	WATER SOLUBILITY	% FERMENTED
Nonpolysaccharides		
Lignin	Poor	0
Cellulose	Poor	15
Noncellulose polysaccharides		
Hemicellulose	Good	56–87
Mucilages and gums	Good	85–95
Pectins	Good	90–95

Osmotically Active Agents

Saline Laxatives (Magnesium Sulfate, Magnesium Hydroxide, Magnesium Citrate, Sodium Phosphate). Laxatives containing magnesium cations or phosphate anions are commonly called *saline laxatives.* Their cathartic action is believed to result from osmotically mediated water retention, which then stimulates peristalsis. However, other mechanisms may contribute to their effects, including the production of inflammatory mediators (*see* above). It also has been suggested that magnesium-containing laxatives stimulate the release of cholecystokinin, which leads to intraluminal fluid and electrolyte accumulation as well as to increased intestinal motility. It is estimated that, for every additional mEq of Mg^{2+} in the intestinal lumen, fecal weight increases by about 7 g. The usual dose of magnesium salts contains 40 to 120 mEq of Mg^{2+} and produces 300 to 600 ml of stool within 6 hours. The intensely bitter taste of some preparations may induce nausea and can be masked with citrus juices.

Phosphate salts are better absorbed than magnesium-based agents and therefore need to be given in larger doses to effect catharsis. The most frequently employed preparation of sodium phosphate is an oral solution (FLEET PHOSPHO-SODA), which contains 1.8 g of dibasic sodium phosphate and 4.8 g of monobasic sodium phosphate in 10 ml. The usual adult dose is 20 to 30 ml taken with ample water. Magnesium- and phosphate-containing preparations are tolerated reasonably well by most patients. However, they need to be used with caution or avoided in patients with renal insufficiency, cardiac disease, or preexisting electrolyte abnormalities and in patients on diuretic therapy. Under these circumstances, there should be monitoring for hypermagnesemia, hyperphosphatemia, hyperkalemia, hypernatremia, and hypocalcemia. Sodium phosphate also can be given as an enema. Phosphate-containing enemas are known to alter the appearance of rectal mucosa.

Nondigestible Sugars and Alcohols (Glycerin, Lactulose, Sorbitol, and Mannitol).

Glycerin is a trihydroxy alcohol (*see* structure below) that is absorbed orally, but acts as a hygroscopic agent and lubricant when given rectally. The water retention stimulates peristalsis and usually produces a bowel movement in less than an hour. Glycerin is for rectal use only and is given in a single daily dose as a 2- or 3-g suppository or as 5 to 15 ml of an 80% solution in enema form. It may cause rectal discomfort, burning, or local hyperemia with minimal bleeding. Some glycerin suppositories contain sodium stearate, which can cause local irritation.

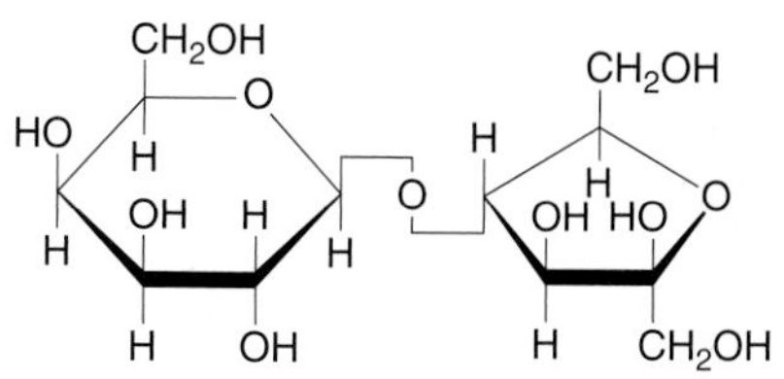

$$HOCH_2 - \underset{\underset{OH}{|}}{\overset{\overset{H}{|}}{C}} - \underset{\underset{OH}{|}}{\overset{\overset{H}{|}}{C}} - \underset{\underset{H}{|}}{\overset{\overset{OH}{|}}{C}} - \underset{\underset{H}{|}}{\overset{\overset{OH}{|}}{C}} - CH_2OH$$

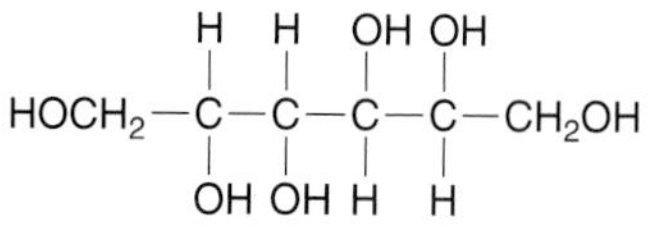

MANNITOL

$$\begin{array}{c} H_2C-OH \\ | \\ HC-OH \\ | \\ H_2C-OH \end{array}$$

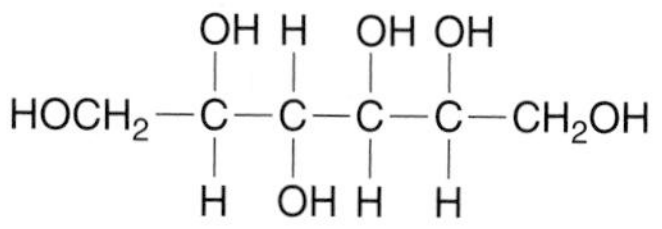

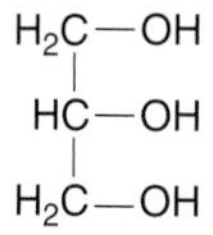

GLYCERIN
(GLYCEROL)

Lactulose (CHRONULAC, others), *sorbitol,* and *mannitol,* whose structures are shown above, are nonabsorbable sugars that are hydrolyzed in the intestine to organic acids, which acidify the luminal contents and osmotically draw water into the lumen, stimulating colonic propulsive motility. Sorbitol and lactulose appear to be equally efficacious in the treatment of constipation caused by opioids and vincristine, of constipation in the elderly, and of idiopathic chronic constipation. These agents are available as 70% solutions, which are given in doses of 15 to 30 ml at night with increases as needed up to 60 ml per day in divided doses. Effects may not be seen for 24 to 48 hours after dosing is begun. Abdominal discomfort or distention and flatulence are relatively common in the first few days of treatment; these symptoms usually subside with continued administration. A few patients dislike the sweet taste of the preparations; dilution with water or administering the preparation with fruit juice can mask the taste.

Lactulose also is used for the treatment of hepatic encephalopathy (marketed for this purpose as CEPHULAC, others). Patients with severe liver disease have an impaired capacity to detoxify ammonia coming from the colon, where it is produced by bacterial metabolism of fecal urea. The drop in luminal pH induced by lactulose results in "trapping" of the ammonia by its conversion to the polar ammonium ion. Combined with the increases in colonic transit, this results in significantly lower circulating ammonia levels. The goal of therapy in this condition is to give sufficient amounts of lactulose (usually 20 to 30 gm 3 to 4 times per day) to produce 2 to 3 soft stools a day with a pH of 5 to 5.5.

Polyethylene Glycol (PEG)-Electrolyte Solutions (COLYTE, GOLYTELY, others).

Long-chain PEGs are poorly absorbed and retain added water by virtue of their high osmotic nature. To avoid net transfer of ions across the intestinal wall, they are prepared with an isotonic mixture of sodium sulfate, sodium bicarbonate, sodium chloride, and potassium chloride. Although widely used as cathartics

LACTULOSE

$$HOCH_2 - \underset{\underset{H}{|}}{\overset{\overset{OH}{|}}{C}} - \underset{\underset{OH}{|}}{\overset{\overset{H}{|}}{C}} - \underset{\underset{H}{|}}{\overset{\overset{OH}{|}}{C}} - \underset{\underset{H}{|}}{\overset{\overset{OH}{|}}{C}} - CH_2OH$$

SORBITOL

prior to bowel procedures (4 liters of this solution over 3 to 4 hours), they are increasingly being used in smaller doses (250 to 500 ml daily) for the treatment of constipation in difficult cases. A powder form of polyethylene glycol 3350 (MIRALAX) is now available for the short-term treatment of occasional constipation. The usual dose is 17 g of powder per day in 8 ounces of water.

Stool-Wetting Agents and Emollients

Docusate salts are anionic surfactants that lower the surface tension of stool to allow mixing of aqueous and fatty substances. This softens the stool and permits easier defecation. However, these agents also stimulate intestinal fluid and electrolyte secretion (possibly by increasing mucosal cyclic AMP) and alter intestinal mucosal permeability. *Docusate sodium* (diocytl sodium sulfosuccinate; COLACE, DOXINATE, others), *docusate calcium* (dioctyl calcium sulfosuccinate; SURFAK, others), and *docusate potassium* (dioctyl potassium sulfosuccinate; KASOF, others) are available in several dosage forms. Despite their widespread use, these agents have marginal, if any, efficacy in most cases of constipation.

Mineral oil is a mixture of aliphatic hydrocarbons obtained from petrolatum. The oil is indigestible and absorbed only to a limited extent. When taken for 2 to 3 days, it penetrates and softens the stool and may interfere with absorption of water. The side-effect profile of mineral oil precludes its regular usage. Side effects include interference with absorption of fat-soluble substances, elicitation of foreign-body reactions in the intestinal mucosa and in other tissues, and leakage of oil past the anal sphincter. Rare complications such as lipid pneumonitis due to aspiration also can occur, so mineral oil should not be taken at bedtime.

Stimulant (Irritant) Laxatives

Stimulant laxatives have direct effects on enterocytes, enteric neurons, and muscle that are only now beginning to be understood (*see* "Diarrhea: General Considerations," above). They probably induce a limited low-grade inflammation in the small and large bowel to promote accumulation of water and electrolytes and stimulate intestinal motility. Important mediators of these effects include activation of prostaglandin/cyclic AMP and nitric oxide/cyclic GMP pathways and perhaps inhibition of Na^+,K^+–ATPase. Included in this group are *diphenylmethane derivatives, anthraquinones,* and *ricinoleic acid.*

Diphenylmethane Derivatives (Bisacodyl, Phenolphthalein). *Bisacodyl* and *phenolphthalein* have similar pharmacological characteristics. Phenolphthalein, once among the most popular components of laxatives, has been withdrawn from the market in the United States because of potential carcinogenicity. Oxyphenisatin, another older drug, was withdrawn due to hepatotoxicity. Effective doses of the diphenylmethane derivatives vary as much as four-to eightfold in individual patients. Consequently, recommended doses may be ineffective in some patients but may produce cramps and excessive fluid excretion in others. Bisacodyl is available in an enteric-coated preparation given once daily, the usual oral dose for which is 10 to 15 mg for adults and 5 to 10 mg for children 6 to 12 years old. Since the drug requires hydrolysis in the bowel for activation, the laxative effects after an oral dose usually are not produced in less than 6 hours. It is therefore frequently taken at bedtime to produce its effect the next morning. Suppositories, however, can work much more rapidly, within 30 to 60 minutes. Due to the drug's side-effect profile, its use should not exceed 10 consecutive days.

Bisacodyl is mainly excreted in the stool; about 5% is absorbed and excreted in the urine as a glucuronide. Overdosage can lead to catharsis and fluid and electrolyte deficits. The diphenylmethanes can damage the mucosa and initiate an inflammatory response in the small bowel and colon. To avoid activation of the drug in the stomach and consequent gastric irritation and cramping, patients should swallow tablets without chewing or crushing and avoid milk or antacid medications within one hour of their ingestion.

Anthraquinone Laxatives. These are derivatives of plants such as *aloe, cascara,* and *senna,* whose use has been enshrined by time. The active agents share a tricyclic anthracene nucleus with hydroxyl, methyl, or carboxyl groups to form monoanthrones, such as rhein and frangula. Monoanthrones are irritant to the oral mucosa; however, the process of aging or drying converts them to more innocuous dimeric (dianthrones) or glycoside forms. This process is reversed by bacterial action in the colon with the formation of the active forms. Senna is obtained from the dried leaflets on pods of *Cassia acutifolia* or *Cassia angustifolia* and contains the rhein dianthrone glycosides, *sennoside A* and *B. Cascara sagrada* (sacred bark) is obtained from the bark of the buckthorn tree and contains the glycosides *barbaloin* and *chrysaloin.* Barbaloin also is found in aloe. Rhubarb is another plant that produces anthraquinone compounds that have been used as laxatives. Anthraquinones also can be synthesized; however, the synthetic monoanthrone danthron has been withdrawn because of concerns over carcinogenicity.

These agents can produce giant migrating colonic contractions as well as induce water and electrolyte secretion. They are poorly absorbed in the small bowel, but because they require activation in the colon, the laxative effect is not noted until 6 to 12 hours after ingestion. Active compounds are absorbed to a variable degree from the colon and excreted in the bile, saliva, milk, and urine.

The consequences of long-term use of these agents have been controversial (Muller-Lissner, 1993). A melanotic pigmentation of the colonic mucosa (melanosis coli) has been observed in the colon in patients using anthraquinone laxatives for long periods (at least 4 to 9 months). Histologically this is caused by the presence of pigment-laden macrophages within the lamina propria. The source of the pigment is not clear. It may be a degenerative product of cells or possibly derived from the extracts themselves. In any case, it is now well established that the condition is benign and reversible on discontinuation of the laxative. What is not so clear is whether or not these agents can cause the more serious condition called "cathartic colon," which can be seen in patients (typically women) who have a long-standing history (typically years) of laxative abuse. The colon in typical cases is dilated and ahaustral; histology reveals loss of myenteric plexus neurons and atrophy of the muscularis propria. Discontinuation of laxatives may reverse some of these abnormalities. Regardless of whether or not a definitive causal relationship can be demonstrated between the use of these agents and colonic pathology, it is clear that these agents should not be recommended for chronic or long-term use.

Ricinoleic Acid (Castor Oil). An age-old home remedy, castor oil is derived from the bean of the castor plant, *Ricinus communis,* and contains two well known noxious ingredients: an extremely toxic protein, *ricin,* and an oil composed chiefly of the triglyceride of *ricinoleic acid.* The triglyceride is hydrolyzed in the small bowel by the action of lipases into glycerol and the active agent, ricinoleic acid, which acts primarily in the small intestine, where it stimulates secretion of fluid and electrolytes and speeds intestinal transit. As little as 4 ml of castor oil, when taken on an empty stomach, may produce a laxative effect within 1 to 3 hours. However, the usual dose for a cathartic effect is 15 to 60 ml for adults. Because of its unpleasant taste as well as its potential toxic effects on intestinal epithelium and enteric neurons, castor oil is now seldom recommended.

Prokinetic and Other Agents for Constipation

Although several of the agents described above stimulate motility, they do so in nonspecific or indirect ways. By contrast, the term *prokinetic* is generally reserved for agents that produce enhancement of gastrointestinal transit *via* interaction with specific receptors involved in the regulation of motility (*see* Chapter 38). Currently available prokinetic agents are not very useful in the treatment of constipation. However, it is expected that newer agents, particularly the more potent 5-HT$_4$-receptor agonists (*see* Chapter 38), may be of considerable promise. Another potentially useful agent is *misoprostol,* a synthetic prostaglandin analog primarily used for protection against gastrointestinal ulcers resulting from the use of nonsteroidal antiinflammatory agents (*see* Chapter 37). Prostaglandins can stimulate colonic

contractions, particularly on the left side, and this may account for the diarrhea that occurs when misoprostol is used at high doses. This property may be utilized for therapeutic gain in patients with intractable constipation.

Enemas

Enemas still are used widely for nonmedicinal purposes. They also are commonly employed by themselves or as adjuncts to bowel preparation regimens, with the primary purpose of emptying the distal colon or rectum of retained solid material. Bowel distention by any means will produce an evacuation reflex in most people, and almost any form of enema, including normal saline solution, can achieve this. Specialized enemas contain additional substances that either are osmotically active or irritant; however, their safety and efficacy have not been studied in a rigorous manner. Repeated enemas with tap water or other hypotonic solutions can cause hyponatremia, and repeated enemas with sodium phosphate–containing solution can cause hypocalcemia.

AGENTS USED IN INFLAMMATORY BOWEL DISEASE

The term *inflammatory bowel disease* (IBD) refers to a group of diseases that principally affect the small and large intestines and are characterized by chronic inflammation of unknown etiology. The two major and relatively well-defined clinical entities are ulcerative colitis and Crohn's disease. Additional forms that are less common and less understood include the microscopic colitides (lymphocytic and collagenous colitis). Although ulcerative colitis and Crohn's disease have several overlapping features, they generally are distinguished on the basis of several clinical and pathological features. Ulcerative colitis is confined to the colon and is characterized by a chronic but superficial inflammatory process that always involves the distal portion and extends in a continuous fashion for a variable length proximally. Crohn's disease can affect both the small and large bowel in a given patient as well as, less commonly, any other segment of the gastrointestinal tract. Inflammation is focal but can affect all layers of the bowel wall and can be associated with several transluminal complications including abscesses and fistulae.

An appreciation of the pathogenesis of IBD as it relates to therapy is essential to understanding the treatment options available. Although the pathogenesis remains to be defined, it is postulated that bowel inflammation and injury are the result of a cascade of events and processes initiated by a putative antigen or antigens in genetically susceptible individuals. This antigen-driven response may be an appropriate one, directed against an unrecognized pathogen, or an inappropriate response to an otherwise innocuous antigen. The host response to these intestinal responses is secretory diarrhea, ulceration, and exudation with protein-losing enteropathy, bleeding, and malabsorption. Immune activation is followed by an inflammatory response that is mediated and amplified by several factors, prominent among which are various cytokines, oxygen radicals, and metabolites of arachidonic acid such as the lipooxygenase product leukotriene B$_4$ (LTB$_4$).

The pharmacological approach to the treatment of IBD is complex because of the unknown nature of the inciting agent(s), the chronic and variable nature of the inflammation, and the need to incorporate variations in pharmacokinetics of drugs related to patient characteristics such as genetic composition, age, and severity of disease (Sands, 2000). It also is important to note that the treatment of IBD in any given patient may have several different goals, such as relief of symptoms, induction of remission (in patients with active disease), prevention of relapse (*i.e.,* maintenance therapy), healing of fistulae, and avoidance of emergent surgery (Table 39–6). No single drug is effective for all these goals.

5-Aminosalicylates

The parent compound of this class of agents, *sulfasalazine* (AZULFIDINE), is among the oldest drugs used for IBD (Allgayer, 1992). This compound is a conjugate of *mesalamine* (5-aminosalicylic acid, 5-ASA) linked to sulfapyridine by a diazo bond, which is split into its components by bacterial azoreductases in the colon (Figure 39–2). The 5-ASA component is now accepted as being the main active therapeutic moiety, with a minor, if any, contribution by sulfapyridine. Sulfapyridine, however, is responsible for most of the significant adverse effects of the preparation.

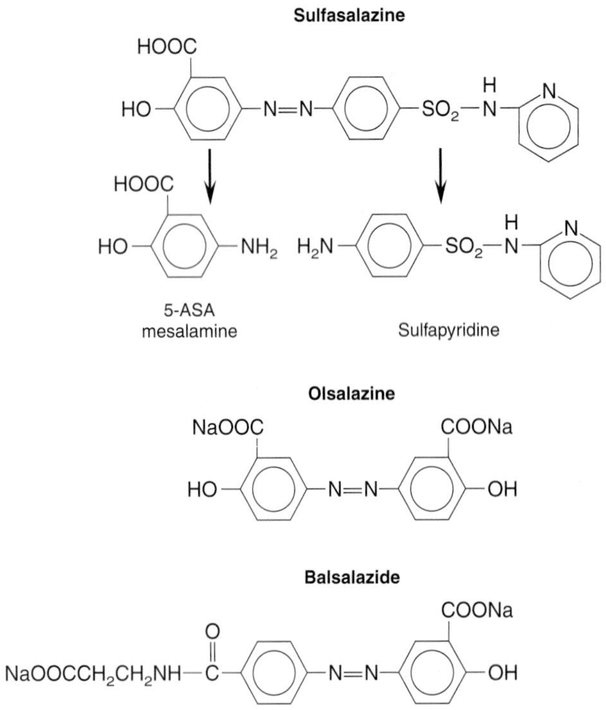

Figure 39–2. *Structure of sulfasalazine and related agents.*

Mesalamine inhibits the cyclooxygenase and 5-lipoxygenase pathways of arachidonic acid metabolism; the latter pathway is felt to be more important in IBD and results in the reduction of LTB_4 and hydroxyeicosatetraenoic acid (5-HETE) levels. Mesalamine also may act as a scavenger of reactive oxygen metabolites, reduce neutrophil and macrophage chemotaxis and phagocytosis, and inhibit cytokine production and immunoglobulin secretion by peripheral blood and intestinal mononuclear cells (Table 39–7).

Oral use of sulfasalazine is of proven value in patients with mild or moderate active ulcerative colitis, with response rates in the range of 60% to 80%. The usual dose is about 4 g per day in 4 divided doses with food; this is achieved gradually, beginning at 500 mg twice a day to avoid adverse effects. Higher doses (up to 6 g per day) can be used but are associated with an increased incidence of side effects. For patients with severe colitis, sulfasalazine is of less-certain value, even though it is often added as an adjunct to systemic glucocorticoids. Regardless of the severity, once remission has been achieved, the drug plays a useful role in the prevention of relapses.

In contrast to ulcerative colitis, Crohn's disease is much less responsive to sulfasalazine. The drug is now seldom used for this condition, having been replaced by newer 5-ASA preparations (*see* below).

Approximately 20% to 30% of orally administered sulfasalazine is absorbed in the small intestine. Much of this is taken up by the liver and excreted unmetabolized in the bile; the rest (about 10%) is excreted unchanged in the urine. About 70% enters the colon, where, if cleavage by bacterial enzymes is complete, 400 mg of mesalamine is produced from every gram of the parent compound. Thereafter, the daughter compounds follow different metabolic pathways. Sulfapyridine, which is highly lipid soluble, is rapidly absorbed from the colon, and undergoes extensive hepatic metabolism, including acetylation and hydroxylation, followed by conjugation with glucuronic acid and excretion in the urine. The acetylation phenotype of the patient determines plasma levels of sulfapyridine and the probability of side effects, with rapid acetylators having lower levels of the drug and less adverse effects. By contrast, only 25% of mesalamine is absorbed from the colon, and most of the drug is expelled with the stool. The small amount that is absorbed is acetylated in the intestinal mucosal wall and the liver and excreted in the urine. Intraluminal concentrations of mesalamine are therefore very high (around 1500 μg/ml in patients taking 3 g of the drug per day).

Side effects of sulfasalazine are common, being reported in 10% to 45% of patients with ulcerative colitis. Several of these are dependent on plasma levels of sulfapyridine and therefore related to both dose and acetylation status of the patient. They include fever and malaise,

Table 39–6

Medications Commonly Used to Treat Inflammatory Bowel Disease

CLASS/DRUG	Crohn's Disease					Ulcerative Colitis			
	Active Disease			Maintenance		Active disease			MAINTENANCE
	MILD-MODERATE	MODERATE-SEVERE	FISTULA	MEDICAL REMISSION	SURGICAL REMISSION	DISTAL COLITIS	MILD-MODERATE	MODERATE-SEVERE	
Mesalamine									
Enema	+[a]	−	−	−	−	+	+[b]	−	+
Oral	+	−	−	+/−	+[c]	+	+	−	+
Antibiotics (metronidazole, ciprofloxacin, others)	+	+	+	?	+[c]	−	−	−	+[c]
Corticosteroids, classic and novel									
Enema, foam, suppository	+[a]	−	−	−	−	+	+[b]	−	−
Oral	+	+	−	−	−	+	+	+	−
Intravenous	−	+	−	−	−	+[d]	−	+	−
Immunomodulators									
6-MP/AZA	−	+	+	+	+[c]	+[d]	−	+[d]	+[d]
Methotrexate	−	+	?	?	?	−	−	−	−
Cyclosporine	−	+[d]	+[d]	−	−	+[d]	−	+[d]	−
Biological response modifiers									
Infliximab	+[d]	+	+	+[c]	?	?	?	?	?

[a]Distal colonic disease only.
[b]For adjunctive therapy.
[c]Some data to support use; remains controversial.
[d]Selected patients.
ABBREVIATIONS: 6-MP, 6-mercaptopurine; AZA, azathioprine.
SOURCE: From Sands, 1999, with permission.

Table 39–7

In Vitro Effects of Mesalazine in Human Colonic Epithelial Cells and in Isolated Human Peripheral Blood Cells*

Eicosanoids
$\downarrow$ LTB$_4$ production
$\downarrow/\leftrightarrow$ PGE$_2$ production

Cytokines
$\downarrow$ IFN-γ–induced HLA-DR expression and $\uparrow$ cellular permeability
$\downarrow$ IFN-γ binding to colonic epithelial cells
$\downarrow$ IL-1/1β production and release
$\downarrow$ IL-2 production, IL-2 receptor α-chain expression and IL-2 mRNA steady-state levels
$\leftrightarrow$ IL-6 production
$\downarrow/\leftrightarrow$ TNF-α production

Oxygen-Derived Free Radicals
$\downarrow$ O$_2$$^-$ production
$\downarrow$ Membrane lipid peroxidation
$\downarrow$ HOCl production
$\downarrow$ PN-induced apoptosis

ABBREVIATIONS: HLA-DR, major histocompatibility gene complex D–related; HOCl, hypochlorous acid; ICAM, intercellular adhesion molecule; IFN, interferon; IL, interleukin; LT, leukotriene, O$_2$$^-$, superoxide anion; PG, prostaglandin; PN, peroxynitrite; TNF, tumor necrosis factor; $\downarrow$, significant decrease; $\uparrow$, significant increase; $\leftrightarrow$, absence of effect versus controls.

*Data obtained from colonic biopsy specimens from patients with active inflammatory bowel disease or patients with normal colons or from cultures of human colonic epithelial cell lines (such as HT29, HT29:19A, and T84).

SOURCE: From Prakash and Markham, 1999, with permission.

nausea, vomiting, headaches, epigastric discomfort, and diarrhea and may be partially overcome by gradual increments of the dose. Megaloblastic anemia and low sperm counts, supposedly due to impaired folic acid absorption, also can occur, and some physicians advocate the routine coadministration of folate supplements. Allergic reactions (not related to plasma levels) can include arthralgias, hemolysis, agranulocytosis, thrombocytopenia, red cell aplasia, and a variety of skin manifestations such as rash, urticaria, and a bluish discoloration. Most serious but rare are toxic epidermal necrolysis and Stevens–Johnson syndrome, pancreatitis, eosinophilic pneumonia, bronchospasm, fibrosing alveolitis, drug-induced lupus, and neurotoxicity.

The fact that most of the side effects of sulfalsalazine are related to the relatively inactive sulfapyridine component spurred the development of the newer 5-ASA preparations. However, the azo bond joining sulfapyridine to mesalamine does serve an important function—namely, the prevention of early absorption of the aminosalicylate from the upper small bowel, allowing high concentrations to be achieved intraluminally in the colon (this is the so-called "carrier hypothesis"). To achieve this goal without the use of the sulfonamide moiety, several innovative approaches have been developed (Table 39–8). In general, the efficacy of these newer oral forms of mesalamine is comparable to that of sulfasalazine for treatment and maintenance in patients with ulcerative colitis. The usual doses for treatment of active disease are 800 mg three times a day for ASACOL and 1 g four times a day for PENTASA. Lower doses are used for maintenance (*e.g.*, ASACOL, 800 mg twice a day). The newer forms of mesalamine represent a modest gain over sulfasalazine in patients with active Crohn's disease and appear to be effective in inducing remission in about 45% of patients, although higher doses than are used in ulcerative colitis are required (Camma *et al.*, 1997). These agents also may be useful in preventing recurrences of Crohn's disease, particularly in the postoperative setting.

Mesalamine formulations generally are well tolerated, with side effects that are relatively infrequent and minor. Headache, dyspepsia, and skin rash are the most common. Diarrhea appears to be particularly common with *olsalazine* (10% to 20% of patients); this may be related to its ability to stimulate chloride and fluid secretion in the small bowel. Nephrotoxicity is a more serious concern, although it is rare, and the precise role of the drug in its pathogenesis is controversial. Patients with preexisting renal disease should be monitored carefully. Both sulfasalazine and its metabolites cross the placental barrier but do not appear to exert a harmful effect on the fetus. The newer derivatives also appear to be safe in pregnancy, although they have not been studied as thoroughly. In general, the risks to the fetus from the consequences of uncontrolled IBD in pregnant women may be more serious than risks associated with the therapeutic use of these agents.

Topical aminosalicylate preparations—mesalamine suspended in wax matrix (ROWASA suppository) or in a suspension enema (ROWASA enema) are effective in active proctitis and distal ulcerative colitis, respectively. They appear to be superior to topical hydrocortisone in this setting with a response rate of 75% to 90%. Mesalamine enema (4 g per 60 ml) should be used at bedtime and retained for at least 8 hours; the suppository (500 mg) should be used 2 to 3 times a day with the objective of retaining it for at least 3 hours. Response to local therapy with mesalamine may occur within 3 to 21 days; however, the usual course of therapy is from 3 to 6 weeks. Once remission has occurred, lower doses may be used for maintenance.

Table 39-8
Non-Sulfonamide-Containing Formulations of Mesalamine and Sites of Drug Release

GENERIC NAME	FORMULATION	TRADE NAME	SOLUBILITY	SITE OF RELEASE	URINARY RECOVERY
Mesalamine	Eudragit S* enteric coating	ASACOL	pH ≥ 7	Delayed release: Terminal ileum, colon	20%–35%
	Eudragit L* enteric coating	CLAVERSA[†] SALOFALK[†]	pH ≥ 6	Delayed release: Jejunum, ileum, colon	25%–45%
	Microgranules individually coated with a semipermeable membrane of ethylcellulose and contained in a capsule	PENTASA	Prolonged release of drug through semipermeable membrane	Sustained release: Duodenum, jejunum, ileum, colon	30%–55%
Olsalazine	Two molecules of mesalamine bound together with an azo bond. Gelatin capsules	DIPENTUM	pH-independent bacterial azoreduction in the colon	Colon	13%–27%
Balsalazide	Mesalamine linked to an inert carrier (4-amino-benzoyl-β-alanine)	COLAZIDE	pH-independent bacterial azoreduction in the colon	Colon	Not available
Mesalamine	Mesalamine in wax matrix in suppository or enema form	ROWASA		Local release: Rectum	10%–30%

*Acrylic resin preparations: Eudragit S, methacrylic acid and methyl methacrylic acid in 1:2 ratio; Eudragit L, methacrylic acid and methyl methacrylic acid in 1:1 ratio.
[†]Not available in the United States.
SOURCE: Adapted from Prakash and Markham, 1999, with permission.

Topical 4-aminosalicylate preparations (derivatives of *para*-aminosalicylic acid) also have been used to a limited extent in distal ulcerative colitis, but they are not generally available. Their mechanism of action may be different from that of 5-ASA and principally related to their ability to act as scavengers of free radicals.

Glucocorticoids

Glucocorticoids have been the mainstay of treatment for acute severe exacerbations of IBD since 1955, when Truelove and Witt first convincingly showed their efficacy in ulcerative colitis. The effects of glucocorticoids on the inflammatory responses are numerous and well documented (*see* Chapter 60). These agents can be given orally or intravenously, and result in remission in up to 90% of patients with ulcerative colitis. Oral *prednisone* is the preferred agent, and a dose of 40 mg once a day is considered standard. Higher doses have not been shown to improve efficacy. Most patients improve substantially within 5 days of initiating treatment; others go into remission during the next 6 weeks. For more severe cases, glucocorticoids can be given intravenously. These steroids also are effective in inducing remission in 60% to 90% of patients with active Crohn's disease. However, their use in this condition is exercised with considerably more caution, since symptoms in these patients may be caused by fibrosis or strictures (which will not respond to antiinflammatory measures alone) or by local complications such as abscesses (in which case the use of steroids may lead to uncontrolled sepsis).

Glucocorticoid enemas also have been shown to be of value in treating patients with inflammation limited to the rectum (proctitis) and left colon. Hydrocortisone is available as a retention enema (100 mg/60 ml), and the usual dose is one 60-ml enema per night for 2 or 3 weeks. When optimally administered, the drug can reach all the way to the descending colon or higher. Patients with distal disease usually respond within 3 to 7 days. Absorption is less than with oral preparations but is still considerable, up to 50% to 75%. Hydrocortisone also is available in a foam suspension [each application of a 10% preparation (CORTIFOAM) delivering 80 mg of hydrocortisone] that can be useful in patients with very short areas of distal proctitis and difficulty retaining fluid. The usual dose is one application once or twice a day.

Newer synthetic steroids are being developed with the aim of limiting their activity to the lumen (Lofberg, 1995). These agents include poorly absorbed steroids and/or steroids with a high first-pass metabolism such as topical *prednisolone methasulfobenzoate, tixocortol pivalate, fluticasone propionate* and *beclomethasone dipropionate. Budesonide* is another such steroid and is available outside the United States in enema form and in a controlled ileal release formulation for treatment of distal colitis and Crohn's disease, respectively (Greenberg *et al.,* 1994). Its topical potency is 200 times higher than that of hydrocortisone, but its oral bioavailability is only 10% to 20%. When absorbed, budesonide undergoes extensive first-pass metabolism, yielding metabolites that are far less active. It is hoped that the use of these newer agents will minimize the occurrence of classic glucocorticoid side effects (*see* Chapter 60), but their use will not improve either the short- or long-term efficacy of steroid therapy.

Immunosuppressive Agents

Thioguanine Derivatives. The cytotoxic thioguanine derivatives *6-mercaptopurine* (6-MP) and *azathioprine* (IMURAN; AZA) (*see* Chapters 52 and 53) are second-line agents in the treatment of patients with severe IBD or those who are steroid-resistant or -dependent (Pearson *et al.,* 1995). AZA is a prodrug, yielding 6-MP. The two drugs can be used interchangeably. These agents and their active metabolite, 6-thioguanine (6-TG), suppress lymphocyte proliferation and may have several additional antiinflammatory properties including depression of natural killer (NK) cytotoxicity.

The use of these drugs for patients with IBD is limited by their slow onset of action, sometimes taking 3 to 6 months. In some earlier trials, with short observation periods, it was concluded that these drugs were ineffective in IBD. However, more recent trials and meta-analyses have shown that these agents are indeed effective in the long term, reducing the requirement for steroids in patients as well as maintaining patients with both ulcerative colitis and Crohn's disease in remission. AZA generally is given in a dose of 2.0 to 2.5 mg/kg body weight per day, whereas 6-MP is most often given in a dose of 1.5 mg/kg body weight per day. Attempts to shorten the time to onset of action with intravenous loading have been unsuccessful.

The most common side effect of these drugs is bone marrow suppression, which requires close monitoring of blood counts, particularly when initiating therapy. Both clinical efficacy and side effects are related to 6-TG levels, which are determined by dose as well as by activity of the enzyme thiopurine methyltransferase (TPMT), which varies with the genetic makeup of the patient. Consequently, TPMT genotyping and monitoring of 6-TG levels have been advocated, but the value of this approach is yet to be demonstrated convincingly. The risk of long-term complications such as the development of opportunistic infection or lymphomas is controversial. These drugs are teratogenic in laboratory animals, and their use in patients who are contemplating motherhood generally is not recommended. The risk for patients wishing to be fathers is not clear, but the use of these drugs probably should be avoided in such individuals.

Methotrexate. *Methotrexate* (*see* Chapter 52), an inhibitor of dihydrofolate reductase, is a cytotoxic agent with pronounced immune-suppressive and antiinflammatory properties. Its onset of action is more rapid than that of 6-MP or AZA. Intramuscular methotrexate appears to be effective in steroid-dependent Crohn's disease but not in ulcerative colitis (Feagan *et al.,* 1995). The usual dose administered intramuscularly in clinical trials has been 15 to 25 mg weekly.

Cyclosporine. *Cyclosporine* (SANDIMMUNE, NEORAL), an inhibitor of calcineurin, causes pronounced suppression of proinflammatory transcription factors (*see* Chapter 53). Its greatest value is in the treatment of acute, severe ulcerative colitis that does not appear to be responding adequately to glucocorticoids (Kornbluth *et al.,* 1997). The drug is administered as a continuous infusion (4 mg/kg per day) and has been shown to be effective in up to 80% of such patients, thus avoiding an emergent colectomy. However, it does not reduce the rate of relapse and is not effective as maintenance therapy. Its use therefore is considered to be temporizing while more definitive treatment that may include elective colectomy or long-term immunosuppressive therapy with AZA/6-MP is planned. Careful monitoring of cyclosporine levels by monoclonal radioimmunoassay is necessary, maintaining the therapeutic range between 300 and 400 ng/ml of whole blood.

Other immunomodulators currently being evaluated in patients with IBD include *tacrolimus* and *mycophenolate mofetil* (*see* Chapter 53).

Antibiotics

Despite the postulated important role of bacteria in the pathogenesis of IBD, particularly Crohn's disease, there is a paucity of data regarding the role of antibiotics in IBD therapy. Antibiotics appear to have little effect on ulcerative colitis, and their use should be confined largely to adjunctive therapy with severe, refractory colitis. By contrast, clinical benefit has been shown with *metronidazole* (*see* Chapter 41) and/or *ciprofloxacin* (*see* Chapter 44) in treating mild to moderately active Crohn's disease, particularly in patients with colonic disease. These antibiotics also may possess immunomodulatory activity. Other indications for the use of antibiotics in Crohn's disease include perineal and perianal disease and bacterial overgrowth, and as adjuncts to drainage therapy for abscesses and fistulae.

Biological Response Modifiers: Infliximab

Tumor necrosis factor alpha (TNF-α), a product of monocytes, macrophages, and T cells, is thought to be a critical cytokine in the pathogenesis of inflammation. Consequently, there has been a great deal of interest in the development of therapeutic approaches to antagonize the effects of this protein. *Infliximab* (REMICADE, cA2) is a chimeric (25% mouse, 75% human) immunoglobulin that binds to TNF and neutralizes its activity. The United States Food and Drug Administration has approved it for use in moderate to severe Crohn's disease. About two-thirds of patients respond to a single infusion of this agent. Repeated dosing may be useful as maintenance therapy (Rutgeerts *et al.*, 1999), although the safety and efficacy of this approach has yet to be demonstrated unequivocally. The greatest value of this agent may be in promoting the healing of fistulae in Crohn's disease, for which few therapeutic options are available (Present *et al.*, 1999).

Infliximab is given as an intravenous infusion; for nonfistulous disease, a single infusion of 5 mg/kg is recommended. For fistulous disease, the initial infusion should be followed with additional doses at 2 and 6 weeks. The short-term safety profile seems to be favorable. Upper respiratory infections are seen more commonly with treatment and delayed hypersensitivity reactions have been noted. Antinuclear antibody formation has been noted in patients treated with infliximab, but the long-term risk of developing clinical syndromes such as lupus is unknown. Similarly, concern has been raised over the possible development of lymphomas in these patients, but, as with the use of 6-MP/AZA, the long-term risk of this complication is controversial.

Many issues relating to the use of infliximab remain to be clarified before its final role in the treatment of IBD is defined. Nevertheless, this drug is a promising first example of a new generation of agents being developed for the treatment of IBD.

CDP571 is an experimental humanized antibody against TNF that has been shown to be effective in short-term studies in patients with active Crohn's disease. The theoretical advantage of using human antibodies is the reduced risk of antigenicity.

Novel and Experimental Treatments Under Development for IBD

There has been much interest in recent years in the development of novel treatments for IBD with greater efficacy and fewer side effects (Sands, 1999b). Some of these therapeutic strategies are based on insights into the pathogenesis of inflammation, whereas others are more empirical, although still promising. Many of these are biological response modifiers (Table 39–9) and have shown considerable promise in early clinical trials (Ehrenpreis *et al.*, 1999; Pullan *et al.*, 1994; Sands *et al.*, 1999; Sands, 1999; Targan *et al.*, 1997; Van Deventer *et al.*, 1997, van Dullemen *et al.*, 1995).

Supportive Therapy in IBD

Analgesic, anticholinergic, and *antidiarrheal* agents play a supportive role in reducing patients' symptoms and improving their quality of life. These drugs should be individualized based on a patient's symptoms and are supplementary to antiinflammatory medications. Oral *iron, folate,* and *vitamin B$_{12}$* should be administered as indicated. *Loperamide* or *diphenoxylate* (*see* "Opioids," above) are useful in patients with mild disease to reduce the frequency of bowel movements and relieve rectal urgency. They are contraindicated in patients with severe disease, as they may predispose to the development of toxic megacolon. *Cholestyramine* can be used to prevent bile salt-induced colonic secretion in patients who have undergone limited ileocolic resections (*see* "Cholestyramine," above). Anticholinergic agents (*clidinium bromide, dicyclomine hydrochloride, tincture of belladonna, etc.; see* Chapter 7) are useful to reduce abdominal cramps, pain, and rectal urgency. As with the antidiarrheal agents, anticholinergic agents are contraindicated in severe disease and when obstruction is suspected. Care should be taken to differentiate exacerbation of inflammatory bowel disease from symptoms that may be related to coexistent functional bowel disease.

MISCELLANEOUS GASTROINTESTINAL AGENTS

Bile Acids

Bile acids and their conjugates are essential components of bile. They are natural steroids synthesized from cholesterol in the liver. The physiological effects of bile acids include induction of bile flow, feedback inhibition of cholesterol synthesis, elimination of cholesterol (bile acids are water-soluble products

Table 39–9

New and Experimental Forms of Therapy for Inflammatory Bowel Disease (IBD)

AGENT	DESCRIPTION	RATIONALE	TYPE OF IBD
ISIS-2302	Antisense oligonucleotide to ICAM-1	Downregulation of ICAM-1 prevents local recruitment of white blood cells	Crohn's disease
IL-10	Th2 cytokine	IL-10 suppresses production of IL-2 and IFN-γ and interferes with macrophage function	Crohn's disease
IL-11	Cytokine derived from mesenchymal cells	Improves intestinal mucosal integrity	Crohn's disease
Anti-α4 antibody	Humanized antibody to α4 integrin	Antagonism of α4 integrin may prevent homing of lymphocytes to site of inflammation	Crohn's disease and ulcerative colitis
Nicotine		Possible inhibition of IL-2 and TNF production; persons who quit smoking more at risk for development of ulcerative colitis	Moderately severe ulcerative colitis
Heparin	Anticoagulant	Improvement in patients with ulcerative colitis on heparin therapy; mechanism unknown	Ulcerative colitis
Thalidomide	Immune modulator	Anti-TNF effects; inhibition of neutrophil activity	Crohn's disease
Fish oil and ω-3 fatty acids		Inhibition of leukotriene B synthesis	Crohn's disease and ulcerative colitis

ABBREVIATIONS: ICAM-1, intercellular adhesion molecule-1; IL, interleukin; IFN, interferon; TNF, tumor necrosis factor.

of cholesterol in bile and promote intestinal cholesterol excretion), and facilitation of dispersion and absorption of lipids and fat-soluble vitamins. After secretion in bile, bile acids are largely (95%) reabsorbed in the intestine (mainly in the terminal ileum), returned to the liver, and then resecreted in bile as part of an enterohepatic circulation. *Cholic acid, chenodeoxycholic acid,* and *deoxycholic acid* (Figure 39–3) constitute 95% of bile acids. Lithocholic acid and ursodeoxycholic acid are minor constituents. The bile acids exist largely as glycine and taurine conjugates, the salts of which are called *bile salts.* Primary bile acids (cholic and chenodeoxycholic acid) are deconjugated and then dehydroxylated to secondary acids (mainly deoxycholic and lithocholic acid) by colonic bacteria. The secondary acids are absorbed in the colon and cycle with the primary acids.

Dried bile from the Himalayan bear (Yutan) has been used in liver disease for centuries by the Chinese. Ursodeoxycholic acid (UDCA; ursodiol; ACTIGALL) is a hydrophilic, dehydroxylated bile acid that also is present in very small quantities as a secondary bile acid in human beings (1% to 3% of the total bile acid pool); it is formed by epimerization of the primary bile acid chenodeoxycholic acid (CDCA; chenodiol) in the gut by intestinal bacteria. Litholytic bile acids such as CDCA and UDCA, when given therapeutically, can alter relative concentrations of bile acids, decrease biliary lipid secretion, and reduce the cholesterol content of the bile so that it is no longer as lithogenic (Broughton, 1994). UDCA may have additional cytoprotective effects on hepatocytes as well as on the immune system, accounting for some of its benefits in cholestatic liver diseases.

Bile acids were first used therapeutically for gallstone dissolution, which requires a functional gallbladder, as the modified bile must be able to enter the gallbladder to

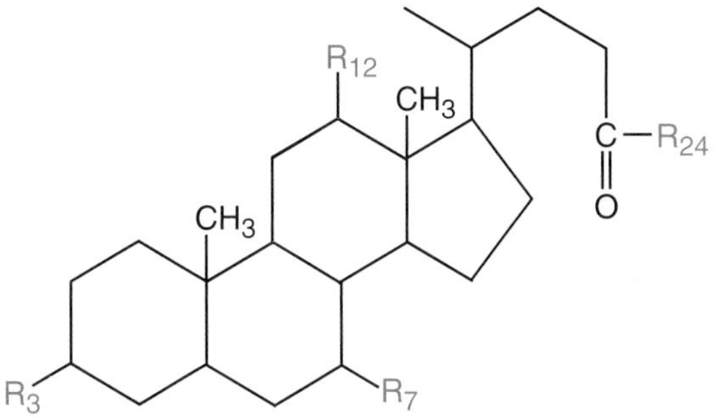

Bile Acid	R_3	R_7	R_{12}	R_{24}
Cholic acid	–OH	–OH	–OH	
Chenodeoxycholic acid	–OH	–OH	–H	glycine (75%)
Deoxycholic acid	–OH	–H	–OH	taurine (24%)
Lithocholic acid	$-SO_3^-$ / –OH	–H	–H	–OH (<1%)
Ursodeoxycholic acid	–OH	◄OH	–H	

Figure 39–3. Major bile acids in adults.

interact with gallstones. The gallstones must be composed of cholesterol monohydrate crystals to be dissolvable. Gallstones of more than 15 mm in diameter in general are not suitable for bile-acid therapy alone (because of their unfavorable ratio of surface to size). For these reasons, the overall efficacy of litholytic bile acids in the treatment of gallstones has been disappointing (dissolution occurs in about 40% to 60% of patients completing therapy and is complete in only about a third or half of these). The combination of CDCA and UDCA is probably better than either agent alone. As a single agent, UDCA is the preferred agent because of its greater efficacy and less frequent side effects.

UDCA also has been shown to improve biochemical and some immunological features of primary biliary cirrhosis (PBC)—a chronic, progressive, cholestatic liver disease of unknown etiology, most often diagnosed in middle-aged to elderly women. Continuous administration of 13 to 15 mg/kg per day (in two divided doses) has induced marked changes in plasma bile-acid composition and distribution in PBC. This dosage gives an optimal enrichment (about 60%) of circulatory bile acids in UDCA, as well as a reduction in the bile concentration of primary bile acids. UDCA also has been used in a variety of other cholestatic liver diseases including primary sclerosing cholangitis as well as in cystic fibrosis, but in general it appears to be less effective in these conditions than in PBC.

Pancreatic Enzymes

Chronic pancreatitis is a debilitating syndrome that results in symptoms from loss of glandular function (both exocrine and endocrine) and inflammation (pain). Since there is no cure for chronic pancreatitis, the goals of pharmacological therapy are prevention of malabsorption and palliation of pain. The cornerstone of therapy of either of these symptoms remains the appropriate use of a pancreatic enzyme formulation (Forsmark and Toskes, 2000). Another major use for pancreatic enzymes is in the prevention of malnutrition in patients with cystic fibrosis, which causes pancreatic insufficiency.

Enzyme Formulations.   The two major enzymatic components of these preparations are a lipase and a protease. The preparations come in both uncoated and enteric-coated forms; the latter designed to withstand gastric acid (lipase is inactivated by acid). Familiarity with these two different classes of preparations is important clinically (Table 39–10).

Table 39–10
Comparison of Uncoated and Enteric-Coated Pancreatic Enzyme Preparations*

	UNCOATED PREPARATIONS	ENTERIC-COATED PREPARATIONS
Number of tablets or capsules required per dose	2–8	2–3
Acid suppression required	Yes	No
Site of delivery	Duodenum	More distal small bowel and beyond
Symptoms relieved	Pain; malabsorption	Malabsorption

*The major components of these preparations are a lipase and a protease (*see* Table 39–11).

Table 39–11
Pancreatic Enzyme Formulations

BRAND NAME	LIPASE*	PROTEASE*
Conventional (uncoated)		
VIOKASE	8,000	30,000
COTAZYM	8,000	30,000
KUZYME HP	8,000	30,000
Enteric coated		
COTAZYM-S	5,000	20,000
PANCREASE MT 4	4,000	12,000
MT 10	10,000	30,000
MT 16	16,000	48,000
CREON 5	5,000	18,750
10	10,000	37,500
20	20,000	75,000
ULTRASE MT 12	12,000	39,000
MT 18	18,000	58,500
MT 20	20,000	65,000

*U.S. Pharmacopeia units per tablet or capsule.
SOURCE: From Forsmark and Toskes, 2000, with permission.

Replacement Therapy for Malabsorption. Fat malabsorption (steatorrhea) and protein maldigestion occur when the pancreas loses more than 90% of its ability to produce digestive enzymes. The resultant diarrhea and malabsorption can be managed reasonably well if 30,000 USP units of pancreatic lipase are delivered to the duodenum during a 4-hour period with and after a meal; this represents about 10% of the normal pancreatic output. Currently available preparations of pancreatic enzymes (Table 39–11) contain up to 20,000 U of lipase and 75,000 U of protease. The loss of pancreatic amylase does not present a problem because of other sources of this enzyme (e.g., salivary glands). Patients using uncoated preparations require concomitant pharmacological control of gastric acid production with a proton pump inhibitor.

Enzymes for Pain. Pain is the other cardinal symptom of chronic pancreatitis. The rationale for its treatment with pancreatic enzymes is based on the principle of negative feedback inhibition of the pancreas by the presence of duodenal proteases. The release of cholecystokinin (CCK), the principal secretagogue for pancreatic enzymes, is triggered by CCK-releasing monitor peptide in the duodenum, which is normally denatured by pancreatic trypsin. In chronic pancreatitis, trypsin insufficiency leads to persistent activation of this peptide and an increased release of CCK. This is thought to cause pancreatic pain, presumably because of continuous stimulation of pancreatic

enzyme output and increased intraductal pressure. Delivery of active proteases to the duodenum (which can be done reliably only with uncoated preparations) therefore is important for the interruption of this loop. In accordance with this hypothesis, clinical trials have shown modest improvements in pain with the use of uncoated preparations but not with enteric-coated formulations of proteases.

In general, pancreatic enzyme preparations are extremely well tolerated by patients. For patients with hypersensitivity to pork protein, bovine enzymes are available. Hyperuricosuria in patients with cystic fibrosis can occur, and malabsorption of folate and iron has been reported. In the past, products with higher lipase content were available, but these were withdrawn following reports associating their use with the development of colonic strictures in patients with cystic fibrosis.

Octreotide (see "Octreotide," above, and Chapter 38) also may decrease refractory abdominal pain in patients with chronic pancreatitis, possibly by suppressing pancreatic secretion as well as by an independent, visceral analgesic effect (Jenkins and Berein, 1995; Uhl et al., 1999). In the future, CCK antagonists also may have a therapeutic role.

PROSPECTUS

Our knowledge of the pathophysiology of diarrheal diseases is increasing rapidly, especially in conditions such as inflammatory bowel disease. As discussed in this chapter, this growth of knowledge already has led to the development of significant new treatments using a rational pharmacological approach. Future pharmacological developments eventually should lead to the control of most symptoms of IBD. However, specific problems in these patients still will pose major therapeutic challenges, such as the long-term safety of biological agents and the prevention of fibrosis and cancer in patients with long-standing inflammation. While more effective agents for treating constipation also are being developed, progress has been slower because of our limited understanding of normal and colonic motility. Until we have a better understanding of the pathophysiology of colonic function, specific treatment of difficult constipation will remain elusive in most cases. Other disease areas covered in this chapter also are clearly in need of more effective therapy. The advent of minimally invasive surgery has reduced the interest in bile stone dissolution therapy, but pharmacologically induced improvements in bile flow can be beneficial in a variety of cholestatic diseases. Finally, the treatment of painful, chronic pancreatitis remains unsatisfactory with available enzyme formulations that offer modest relief at best. Improvement in treatment will require much research on the pathogenesis of pain in this condition.

For further information on diarrhea, constipation, inflammatory bowel disease, gallbladder and bile duct disorders, and pancreatic disorders, *see* Chapters 42, 286, 302, and 304 in *Harrison's Principles of Internal Medicine,* 14th ed., McGraw-Hill, New York, 1998.

BIBLIOGRAPHY

Ehrenpreis, E.D., Kane, S.V., Cohen, L.B., Cohen, R.D., and Hanauer, S.B. Thalidomide therapy for patients with refractory Crohn's disease: an open-label trial. *Gastroenterology,* **1999,** *117*:1271–1277.

Feagan, B.G., Rochon, J., Fedorak, R.N., Irvine, E.J., Wild, G., Sutherland, L., Steinhart, A.H., Greenberg, G.R., Gillies, R., Hopkins, M., Hanauer, S.B., and McDonald, J.W.D. Methotrexate for the treatment of Crohn's disease. The North American Crohn's Study Group Investigators. *N. Engl. J. Med.,* **1995,** *332*:292–297.

Greenberg, G.R., Feagan, B.G., Martin, F., Sutherland, L.R., Thomson, A.B., Williams, C.N., Nilsson, L.G., and Persson, T. Oral budesonide for active Crohn's disease. Canadian Inflammatory Bowel Disease Study Group. *N. Engl. J. Med.,* **1994,** *331*:836–841.

Pearson, D.C., May, G.R., Fick, G.H., and Sutherland, L.R. Azathioprine and 6-mercaptopurine in Crohn's disease. A meta-analysis. *Ann. Intern. Med.,* **1995,** *123*:132–142.

Present, D.H., Rutgeerts, P., Targan, S., Hanauer, S.B., Mayer, L., van Hogezand, R.A., Podolsky, D.K., Sands, B.E., Braakman, T., DeWoody, K.L., Schaible, T.F., and van Deventer, S.J. Infliximab for the treatment of fistulas in patients with Crohn's disease. *N. Engl. J. Med.,* **1999,** *340*:1398–1405.

Pullan, R.D., Rhodes, J., Ganesh, S., Mani, V., Morris, J.S., Williams, G.T., Newcombe, R.G., Russell, M.A.H., Feyerabend, C., Thomas, G.A.O., and Sawe, U. Transdermal nicotine for active ulcerative colitis. *N. Engl. J. Med.,* **1994,** *330*:811–815.

Rutgeerts, P., D'Haens, G., Targan, S., Vasiliauskas, E., Hanauer, S.B., Present, D.H., Mayer, L., Van Hogezand, R.A., Braakman, T., DeWoody, K.L., Schaible, T.F., and van Deventer, S.J. Efficacy and safety of retreatment with anti-tumor necrosis factor antibody (infliximab) to maintain remission in Crohn's disease. *Gastroenterology,* **1999,** *117*:761–769.

Sands, B.E., Bank, S., Sninsky, C.A., Robinson, M., Katz, S., Singleton, J.W., Miner, P.B., Safdi, M.A., Galandiuk, S., Hanauer, S.B., Varilek, G.W., Buchman, A.L., Rodgers, V.D., Salzberg, B., Cai, B., Loewy, J., DeBruin, M.F., Rogge, H., Shapiro, M., and Schwertschlag, U.S. Preliminary evaluation of safety and activity of recombinant human interleukin 11 in patients with active Crohn's disease. *Gastroenterology,* **1999a,** *117*:58–64.

Targan, S.R., Hanauer, S.B., van Deventer, S.J., Mayer, L., Present, D.H., Braakman, T., DeWoody, K.L., Schaible, T.F., and Rutgeerts, P.J. A short-term study of chimeric monoclonal antibody cA2 to tumor necrosis factor α for Crohn's disease. Crohn's Disease cA2 Study Group. *N. Engl. J. Med.,* **1997,** *337*:1029–1035.

van Deventer, S.J., Elson, C.O., and Fedorak, R.N. Multiple doses of intravenous interleukin 10 in steroid-refractory Crohn's disease. Crohn's Disease Study Group. *Gastroenterology,* **1997,** *113*:383–389.

van Dullemen, H.M., van Deventer, S.J., Hommes, D.W., Bijl, H.A., Jansen, J., Tytgat, G.N., and Woody, J. Treatment of Crohn's disease with anti-tumor necrosis factor chimeric monoclonal antibody (cA2). *Gastroenterology,* **1995,** *109*:129–135.

MONOGRAPHS AND REVIEWS

Allgayer, H. Sulfasalazine and 5-ASA compounds. *Gastroenterol. Clin. North Am.,* **1992,** *21*:643–658.

Beglinger, C., and Drewe, J. Somatostatin and octreotide: physiological background and pharmacological application. *Digestion,* **1999,** *60* (suppl. 2):2–8.

Broughton, G. II. Chenodeoxycholate: the bile acid. The drug. A review. *Am. J. Med. Sci.,* **1994,** *307*:54–63.

Camma, C., Giuta, M., Rosselli, M., and Cottone, M. Mesalamine in the maintenance treatment of Crohn's disease: a meta-analysis adjusted for confounding variables. *Gastroenterology,* **1997,** *113*:1465–1473.

Daugherty, L.M. Loperamide hydrochloride. *Am. Pharm.,* **1990,** *NS30*:45–48.

DiJoseph, J.F., Taylor, J.A., and Mir, G.N. Alpha-2 receptors in the gastrointestinal system: a new therapeutic approach. *Life Sci.,* **1984,** *35*:1031–1042.

Forsmark, C.E., and Toskes, P.P. Treatment of chronic pancreatitis. In, *Therapy of Digestive Disorders: A Companion to Sleisenger and Fordtran's Gastrointestinal and Liver Disease.* (Wolfe, M.M., and Cohen, S., eds.) Saunders, Philadelphia, **2000,** pp. 235–245.

Fried, M. Octreotide in the treatment of refractory diarrhea. *Digestion,* **1999,** *60(suppl. 2)*:42–46.

Izzo, A.A., Gaginella, T.S., Mascolo, N., and Capasso, F. Recent findings on the mode of action of laxatives: the role of platelet activating factor and nitric oxide. *Trends Pharmacol. Sci.,* **1998,** *19*:403–405.

Jenkins, S.A., and Berein, A. Review article: the relative effectiveness of somatostatin and octreotide therapy in pancreatic disease. *Aliment. Pharmacol. Ther.,* **1995,** *9*:349–361.

Korman, L.Y. Secretory and miscellaneous noninfectious diarrhea. In, *A Pharmacologic Approach to Gastrointestinal Disorders.* (Lewis, J.H., ed.) Williams & Wilkins, Baltimore, **1994,** pp. 281–291.

Kornbluth, A., Present, D.H., Lichtiger, S., and Hanauer, S. Cyclosporin for severe ulcerative colitis: a user's guide. *Am. J. Gastroenterol.,* **1997,** *92*:1424–1428.

Kreek, M.J. Constipation syndromes. In, *A Pharmacologic Approach to Gastrointestinal Disorders.* (Lewis, J.H., ed.) Williams & Wilkins, Baltimore, **1994,** pp. 179–208.

Lofberg, R. New steroids for inflammatory bowel disease. *Inflamm. Bowel. Dis.,* **1995,** *1*:135–141.

Matheson, A.J., and Noble, S. Racecadotril. *Drugs,* **2000,** *59*:829–835.

Muller-Lissner, S.A. Adverse effects of laxatives: fact and fiction. *Pharmacology,* **1993,** *47*(*suppl. 1*):138–145.

Prakash, A., and Markham, A. Oral delayed release mesalazine: a review of its use in ulcerative colitis and Crohn's disease. *Drugs,* **1999,** *57*:383–408.

Sands, B.E. Novel therapies for inflammatory bowel disease. *Gastroenterol. Clin. North Am.,* **1999b,** *28*:323–351.

Sands, B.E. Therapy of inflammatory bowel disease. *Gastroenterology,* **2000,** *118*:S68–S82.

Schiller, L.R. Review article: anti-diarrhoeal pharmacology and therapeutics. *Aliment. Pharmacol. Ther.,* **1995,** *9*:87–106.

Sellin, J.H. Intestinal elecrocyte absorption and secretion. In, *Gastrointestinal Disease: Pathophysiology, Diagnosis, Management,* 5th ed. (Sleisenger, M.H., and Fordtran, J.S., eds.) Saunders, Philadelphia, **1993,** pp. 954–976.

Uhl, W., Anghelacopoulos, S.E., Friess, H., and Buchler, M.W. The role of octreotide and somatostatin in acute and chronic pancreatitis. *Digestion,* **1999,** *60*(*suppl. 2*):23–31.

Acknowledgment

The authors wish to acknowledge Laurence R. Brunton, author of this chapter in the ninth edition of *Goodman and Gilman's The Pharmacological Basis of Therapeutics,* some of whose text has been retained in this edition.

SECTION VII

CHEMOTHERAPY OF PARASITIC INFECTIONS

INTRODUCTION

James W. Tracy and Leslie T. Webster, Jr.

Parasitic infections caused by pathogenic protozoa or helminths (worms) affect more than 3 billion people worldwide and impose a substantial health and economic burden, particularly on less-developed countries where they are most prevalent. Conditions promoting these infections include poor sanitation, personal hygiene, and health education; debilitation and compromised resistance of the host; high population density; inadequate control of parasite vectors and reservoirs of infection; increased population migration, military operations, and world travel; and resistance to agents used for chemotherapy and vector control. Just a few parasitic infections, *e.g.,* malaria due to *Plasmodium falciparum,* invite attention, because without treatment, they cause high morbidity and mortality. Most are neglected, however, for financial reasons and because their effects on human health are more subtle.

Despite major efforts at vaccine development, chemotherapy remains the single most effective, efficient, and inexpensive means to control most parasitic infections. In the six decades since the first edition of this textbook was published, there have been remarkable improvements in treating human infections caused by flukes and intestinal parasites. Older, more toxic anthelmintics such as aspidium (male fern) and carbon tetrachloride have been replaced by safe and effective broad-spectrum agents including the benzimidazoles, ivermectin, and praziquantel. In contrast, many of the drugs available to treat serious protozoal infections, including African trypanosomiasis and malaria, have been in use for decades or even centuries. New or superior pharmaceuticals are urgently required to combat such systemic infections as falciparum malaria, Chagas' disease, the filariases, echinococcosis, cysticercosis, trichinosis, and toxocariasis. These compounds also are needed to counteract development of drug resistance, manifested especially by *Plasmodium* and other protozoan parasites. Protozoa develop resistance to drugs far more readily than do helminths, consistent with their more rapid proliferation in the host.

Many antiparasitic agents were developed originally for veterinary use and only later adapted to human beings. Indeed, most were discovered by random screening of natural products or synthetic compounds for efficacy against pathogenic parasites in infected animals. Improved methods for maintaining protozoan parasites *in vitro,* more successful to date with protozoa than with helminths, allow examination of organisms collected from experimental animals or human patients. This advance permits direct studies of the basic genetics, development, biochemistry, and cell biology of pathogenic parasites. Such studies can help investigators identify appropriate molecular targets for selective therapeutic attack and elucidate mechanisms of drug action and resistance. Purified candidate targets for drug action then can be used to develop rapid, automated, and inexpensive *in vitro* screening procedures to select potential drug molecules in complex mixtures of synthetic or natural compounds. This combined approach, in turn, reduces the number of candidate compounds that must be tested, first in animal models of parasitic infection and eventually in human beings.

Ultimately, antiparasitic drugs must be safe and effective in patients. The therapeutic uses of antiparasitic drugs are complex and are subject to variations in host, parasite, and environmental factors. Thus, the best drugs and optimal dose regimens often have been determined by trial and error rather than from careful pharmacokinetic and pharmacodynamic studies of patients in areas of endemic infection. For proper evaluation, population-based chemotherapy should be instituted only after appropriate epidemiological studies divulge patterns of transmission and the relationship of age-specific prevalence and intensity of infection to disease. For optimal results, chemotherapy should be combined with other public health measures appropriate for the particular infection, environment, and host population. The ideal agent for mass chemotherapy would have a broad spectrum of activity against all developmental stages of infecting parasites. It also would be safe at high therapeutic doses taken orally for one day only, be chemically stable under conditions of use, be ineffective as an inducer of drug resistance, and be inexpensive. Few available antiparasitic drugs meet these criteria. Even with excellent drugs, population compliance with therapeutic regimens will remain a major issue. Poor compliance now contributes more to the failure of control programs than do inadequate antiparasitic agents.

Despite the paucity of newly developed antiparasitic drugs, there have been substantial recent achievements. One important approach is to evaluate drugs developed as antiparasitic agents in animals for human use or, alternatively, drugs developed for other clinical indications in human beings. For example, a single oral dose of triclabendazole, a veterinary drug used against fascioliasis in sheep, has had marked efficacy against this infection in limited trials in human patients. Miltefosine, an oral phosphocholine analog originally tested against human tumors, has shown promising activity against human visceral leishmaniasis in phase 2 studies. Perhaps the greatest recent, but hardly novel, advance has been the use of two or more drugs with complementary properties to thwart other major parasitic infections of human beings. Of several different regimens, one employing an artemisinin derivative and mefloquine has been especially effective against multidrug-resistant falciparum malaria. Moreover, the use of albendazole together with either diethylcarbamazine or ivermectin has dramatically reduced the prevalence of lymphatic filariasis. Large pharmaceutical companies and multinational agencies now are cooperating with local groups to expand effective mass chemotherapy programs using several antiparasitic drugs. While evaluation of drugs developed against animal parasites or for other human indications together with multidrug antiparasitic therapy can be exploited further, these strategies do not adequately substitute for the continuous development of new and improved drugs for the treatment of parasitic infections in human populations.

The major parasitic infections of human beings and the agents that are, in the authors' opinion, currently favored for their prophylaxis or treatment are listed in Table VII–1; the pharmacology of antiprotozoal and anthelmintic drugs is presented in Chapters 40 to 42. Treatment of infections with ectoparasites is not considered here, nor is a comprehensive or exhaustive coverage of the chemotherapy of human parasitic infections intended. In addition to the current medical and scientific literature, authoritative information about this subject can be obtained from the Centers for Disease Control and Prevention (CDC), Atlanta, Georgia 30333, U.S.A., and the World Health Organization (WHO), 1211 Geneva 27, Switzerland.

Table VII–1

Drugs for Chemotherapy of Parasitic Infections

The recommendations presented here represent the best judgment not only of the authors but also of several authorities in the United States and abroad. However, this field is a dynamic one; certain of these recommendations will require modification in time.

INFECTION AND PARASITE	DRUG OF CHOICE		COMMENTS
	1st	*2nd*	
I. PROTOZOAN INFECTIONS			
Amebiasis			
Entamoeba histolytica			
Asymptomatic and mild intestinal infection	Diloxanide furoate	Iodoquinol or paromomycin	Excessive doses of iodoquinol can cause neurotoxicity.
Moderate to severe intestinal infection (amebic dysentery)	Metronidazole plus diloxanide furoate	Paromomycin plus diloxanide furoate	Iodoquinol can be substituted for diloxanide furoate.
Systemic amebiasis, including amebic abscesses	Metronidazole plus diloxanide furoate	Chloroquine plus diloxanide furoate	Although effective, emetine and dehydroemetine are *not* recommended because of potential toxicity.
Balantidiasis			
Balantidium coli	Tetracycline‡	Iodoquinol or metronidazole	—
Babesiosis			
Babesia microti (USA), *B. divergens*, *B. bovis* (Europe)	Clindamycin with quinine sulfate	—	Specific therapy is required only in severe cases and in immunocompromised hosts.
Cryptosporidiosis			
Cryptosporidium spp.	—	—	Specific drug therapy is currently unavailable. Paromomycin plus azithromycin may be of some benefit.§
Giardiasis			
Giardia lamblia	Metronidazole	Furazolidone or Paromomycin‡ or Tinidazole†	Paromomycin may be useful to treat giardiasis during pregnancy.

*Available from the Center for Infectious Disease, Centers for Disease Control and Prevention, Atlanta, GA 30333, U.S.A. *Telephone:* 404-639-3670 (8:00 A.M. to 4:30 P.M., Eastern time).

†Not available in the United States.

‡Investigational use only or not approved for this indication in the United States.

§Based on limited data.

¶Available by special request from the World Health Organization.

Table VII–1

Drugs for Chemotherapy of Parasitic Infections (*Continued*)

INFECTION AND PARASITE	DRUG OF CHOICE		COMMENTS
	1st	*2nd*	
Leishmaniasis			
Leishmania braziliensis and *L. mexicana* American cutaneous and mucocutaneous leishmaniasis	Stibogluconate sodium	Amphotericin B	Lipid-encapsulated amphotericin B is used when antimonials are ineffective or contraindicated.
L. donovani Visceral leishmaniasis (kala azar)	Stibogluconate sodium or amphotericin B	Pentamidine isethionate‡ or miltefosine§	Lipid-encapsulated amphotericin B is used when antimonials are ineffective or contraindicated.
L. tropica Cutaneous leishmaniasis (Oriental sore)	Stibogluconate sodium	—	Topical heat may be effective.
Malaria			
Plasmodium falciparum Chloroquine-sensitive strains			
a. Prophylaxis	Chloroquine phosphate	—	No chemoprophylactic regimen is always effective in preventing infection with *P. falciparum*.
b. Treatment	Chloroquine phosphate	—	
Chloroquine- or multi-drug-resistant strains a. Prophylaxis	Mefloquine	Doxycycline with or without chloroquine phosphate or Chloroquine phosphate and carry self-treatment dose of pyrimethamine-sulfadoxine or Proguanil† plus chloroquine phosphate	2nd-choice regimens should be used for mefloquine-resistant strains or when mefloquine is contraindicated. The particular regimen depends on the geographic area and other factors (*see* text). No chemotherapeutic regimen is always effective in preventing infection with *P. falciparum*.

*Available from the Center for Infectious Disease, Centers for Disease Control and Prevention, Atlanta, GA 30333, U.S.A. *Telephone:* 404-639-3670 (8:00 A.M. to 4:30 P.M., Eastern time).

†Not available in the United States.

‡Investigational use only or not approved for this indication in the United States.

§Based on limited data.

¶Available by special request from the World Health Organization.

Table VII–1
Drugs for Chemotherapy of Parasitic Infections (*Continued*)

INFECTION AND PARASITE	DRUG OF CHOICE		COMMENTS
	1st	*2nd*	
Malaria **(cont.)**			
b. Treatment	Quinidine gluconate, parenterally, in combination with either pyrimethamine-sulfadoxine or pyrimethamine-sulfadiazine or a tetracycline or clindamycin	—	Quinidine gluconate in combination with antifolates or antibiotics is the 1st choice for treatment of drug-resistant falciparum malaria for *nonimmune individuals*. If available, quinine dihydrochloride may be substituted for quinidine gluconate. Choice of regimen depends on the profile of drug resistance in the geographic area of infection (*see* Table 40–2).
	or mefloquine	—	Mefloquine can only be taken orally (*see* text).
	or artesunate followed by mefloquine	—	
	or atovaquone‡ plus proguanil†	— —	— —
P. malariae Prophylaxis and treatment	Chloroquine phosphate	—	—
P. vivax, P. ovale Prophylaxis and treatment	Chloroquine phosphate plus primaquine phosphate	—	Primaquine is used with chloroquine to prevent relapses after departure from an endemic area and to effect a "radical" cure.
Toxoplasmosis *Toxoplasma gondii*	Pyrimethamine plus sulfadiazine	Spiramycin	—

*Available from the Center for Infectious Disease, Centers for Disease Control and Prevention, Atlanta, GA 30333, U.S.A.
Telephone: 404-639-3670 (8:00 A.M. to 4:30 P.M., Eastern time).
†Not available in the United States.
‡Investigational use only or not approved for this indication in the United States.
§Based on limited data.
¶Available by special request from the World Health Organization.

Table VII–1

Drugs for Chemotherapy of Parasitic Infections (*Continued*)

INFECTION AND PARASITE	DRUG OF CHOICE		COMMENTS
	1st	*2nd*	
Trichomoniasis *Trichomonas vaginalis*	Metronidazole	Tinidazole†	—
Trypanosomiasis *Trypanosoma cruzi* South American trypanosomiasis (Chagas' disease)	Nifurtimox*	Benznidazole†	These drugs are effective only in acute infection.
T. brucei gambiense, T. brucei rhodesiense African trypanosomiasis (sleeping sickness)			
a. Early stage (no CNS involvement)	Suramin,* intravenously plus pentamidine isethionate, intramuscularly or	Pentaminide isethionate‡	This regimen is effective only against *T.b. gambiense*. Suramin alone is used for *T.b. rhodesiense* because pentamidine is ineffective.
	Eflornithine†¶	—	Eflornithine is effective only against *T.b. gambiense*. Treatment of early-stage infection is probably effective, but costly.
b. Late stage (CNS involvement)	Melarsoprol*	Eflornithine†¶	Eflornithine is effective only against *T.b. gambiense*.
	Suramin* followed by melarsoprol*	—	—

*Available from the Center for Infectious Disease, Centers for Disease Control and Prevention, Atlanta, GA 30333, U.S.A.
Telephone: 404-639-3670 (8:00 A.M. to 4:30 P.M., Eastern time).
†Not available in the United States.
‡Investigational use only or not approved for this indication in the United States.
§Based on limited data.
¶Available by special request from the World Health Organization.

Table VII–1
Drugs for Chemotherapy of Parasitic Infections (*Continued*)

INFECTION AND PARASITE	DRUG OF CHOICE		COMMENTS
	1st	*2nd*	
II. METAZOAN (HELMINTH) INFECTIONS			
A. NEMATODE (ROUNDWORM) INFECTIONS			
Ascariasis *Ascaris lumbricoides*	Mebendazole or Albendazole‡	Pyrantel pamoate or Piperazine citrate	The choice of drug is dictated by spectrum of polyparasitic infections.
Capillariasis *Capillaria philippinensis*	Albendazole‡	Mebendazole	—
Dracunculiasis *Dracunculus medinensis* (guinea worm infection)	Metronidazole‡	—	Drug therapy aids only in extraction of worms.
Enterobiasis *Enterobius (Oxyuris) vermicularis* (pinworm infection)	Pyrantel pamoate	Mebendazole‡ or albendazole‡	—
Filariasis *Wuchereria bancrofti, Brugia malayi, Dipetalonema perstans*	Diethylcarbamazine* plus albendazole or Ivermectin plus albendazole		—
Loa loa	Diethylcarbamazine*	—	Choice of drug combination depends on geographic location (*see* text). Diethylcarbamazine can cause severe reactions to dying microfilariae (*see* text).
Onchocerca volvulus	Ivermectin	Diethylcarbamazine*	Diethylcarbamazine can cause severe reactions to dying microfilariae (*see* text).

*Available from the Center for Infectious Disease, Centers for Disease Control and Prevention, Atlanta, GA 30333, U.S.A. *Telephone:* 404-639-3670 (8:00 A.M. to 4:30 P.M., Eastern time).
†Not available in the United States.
‡Investigational use only or not approved for this indication in the United States.
§Based on limited data.
¶Available by special request from the World Health Organization.

Table VII–1

Drugs for Chemotherapy of Parasitic Infections (*Continued*)

INFECTION AND PARASITE	DRUG OF CHOICE		COMMENTS
	1st	*2nd*	
Hookworm Infections			
Necator americanus, Ancylstoma duodenale	Albendazole or mebendazole	Pyrantel pamoate	—
Cutaneous larva migrans	Thiabendazole	—	—
Strongyloidiasis			
Stronglyoides stercoralis	Ivermectin	Thiabendazole or albendazole	Immunosuppressed patients are especially at risk. Efficacy of ivermectin against disseminated strongyloidiasis is not established.
Toxocariasis			
Toxocara spp. Visceral larva migrans	Diethylcarbamazine‡	Albendazole or mebendazole	Efficacy of drug therapy is questionable.
Trichinosis			
Trichinella spiralis	Albendazole‡	Mebendazole‡	Efficacy against larvae in tissues is questionable. Glucocorticoids may be of benefit in controlling symptoms of chronic infection.
Trichuriasis			
Trichuris trichiura (whipworm infection)	Mebendazole	Albendazole‡ or oxantel pamoate†	—

*Available from the Center for Infectious Disease, Centers for Disease Control and Prevention, Atlanta, GA 30333, U.S.A.
Telephone: 404-639-3670 (8:00 A.M. to 4:30 P.M., Eastern time).
†Not available in the United States.
‡Investigational use only or not approved for this indication in the United States.
§Based on limited data.
¶Available by special request from the World Health Organization.

Table VII–1
Drugs for Chemotherapy of Parasitic Infections (*Continued*)

INFECTION AND PARASITE	DRUG OF CHOICE		COMMENTS
	1st	*2nd*	
B. CESTODE (TAPEWORM) INFECTIONS **Taeniasis**			
Taenia saginata (beef tapeworm)	Praziquantel‡	Niclosamide	—
T. solium (pork tapeworm)	Praziquantel‡	—	Niclosamide should not be used for *T. solium* because of the danger of cysticercosis.
Neurocysticercosis (caused by *T. solium*)	Albendazole‡	—	Praziquantel is not effective (*see* text).
Diphyllobothriasis			
Diphyllobothrium latum (fish tapeworm)	Praziquantel‡	Niclosamide	—
Hymenolepiasis			
Hymenolepis nana (dwarf tapeworm)	Praziquantel‡	—	—
Echinococcosis			
Echinococcus granulosus Cystic hydatid disease or hydatidosis	Albendazole‡	Mebendazole‡	Treatment by surgical resection is recommended.
E. multilocularis Alveolar hydatid disease	Albendazole‡	—	Surgical resection is recommended before drug therapy. Albendazole may be only marginally effective.

*Available from the Center for Infectious Disease, Centers for Disease Control and Prevention, Atlanta, GA 30333, U.S.A.
Telephone: 404-639-3670 (8:00 A.M. to 4:30 P.M., Eastern time).
†Not available in the United States.
‡Investigational use only or not approved for this indication in the United States.
§Based on limited data.
¶Available by special request from the World Health Organization.

Table VII–1

Drugs for Chemotherapy of Parasitic Infections (*Continued*)

INFECTION AND PARASITE	DRUG OF CHOICE		COMMENTS
	1st	*2nd*	
C. TREMATODE (FLUKE) INFECTIONS **Blood Fluke Infections (Schistoso- miasis)**			
Schistosoma hematobium	Praziquantel	Metrifonate	—
S. japonicum	Praziquantel	—	—
S. mansoni	Praziquantel	Oxamniquine	—
S. mekongi	Praziquantel	—	—
Intestinal Fluke Infections			
Fasciolopsis buski	Praziquantel‡	—	—
Heterophyes heterophyes	Praziquantel‡	—	—
Metagonimus yokogawai	Praziquantel‡	—	—
Liver Fluke Infections			
Clonorchis sinensis	Praziquantel‡	—	—
Opisthorchis felineus	Praziquantel‡	—	—
O. viverrini	Praziquantel‡	—	—
Fasciola hepatica	Bithionol*	Triclabendazole†§	Praziquantel is not effective.
Lung Fluke Infections (Paragonimiasis)			
Paragonimus spp.	Praziquantel‡	—	—
P. westermani	Praziquantel‡	—	—
P. kellicotti	Praziquantel‡	—	—

*Available from the Center for Infectious Disease, Centers for Disease Control and Prevention, Atlanta, GA 30333, U.S.A. *Telephone:* 404-639-3670 (8:00 A.M. to 4:30 P.M., Eastern time).

†Not available in the United States.

‡Investigational use only or not approved for this indication in the United States.

§Based on limited data.

¶Available by special request from the World Health Organization.

DRUGS USED IN THE CHEMOTHERAPY OF PROTOZOAL INFECTIONS

Malaria

James W. Tracy and Leslie T. Webster, Jr.

Malaria, caused by four species of Plasmodium, *of which* Plasmodium falciparum *is the most dangerous, remains the world's most devastating human parasitic infection. This chapter deals with the properties and uses of important drugs used to treat and prevent this infection. Highly effective agents that act against asexual erythrocytic stages of malarial parasites responsible for clinical attacks include chloroquine, quinine, quinidine, mefloquine, atovaquone, and the artemisinin compounds. Less effective, slower-acting drugs in this category are proguanil, pyrimethamine, sulfonamides, sulfones, and the antimalarial antibiotics. Primaquine is the only drug used against latent tissue forms of* Plasmodium vivax *and* Plasmodium ovale *that cause relapsing infections. No single antimalarial agent has successfully controlled the spread of increasingly drug-resistant strains of* P. falciparum. *Instead, multidrug regimens are discussed as the optimal strategy to address this problem.*

Malaria remains the world's most devastating human parasitic infection, afflicting more than 500 million people and causing from 1.7 million to 2.5 million deaths each year (World Health Organization, 1997). Infection with *Plasmodium falciparum* causes much of this mortality, which preferentially affects children less than 5 years of age, pregnant women, and nonimmune individuals. Although mosquito-transmitted malaria virtually has been eliminated from North America, Europe, and Russia, its increasing prevalence in many parts of the tropics, especially sub-Saharan Africa, poses a major local health and economic burden and a serious risk to travelers from nonendemic areas.

Practical, inexpensive, effective, and safe drugs, insecticides, and vaccines still are needed to combat malaria. In the 1950s, attempts to eradicate this scourge from most parts of the world failed, primarily because of the development of resistance to insecticides and antimalarial drugs. Since 1960, transmission of malaria has risen in most regions where the infection is endemic; chloroquine-resistant and multidrug-resistant strains of *P. falciparum* have spread, and the degree of drug resistance has increased. More recently, chloroquine-resistant strains of *P. vivax* also have been documented in Oceania.

Nearly all antimalarial drugs were developed because of their action against asexual erythrocytic forms of malarial parasites that cause clinical illness. Efficacious, rapidly acting drugs in this category include *chloroquine, quinine, quinidine, mefloquine, atovaquone,* and the *artemisinin* compounds. *Proguanil, pyrimethamine, sulfonamides, sulfones,* and antimalarial antibiotics, such as the *tetracyclines,* are slower acting and less effective. *Primaquine* is the only drug used clinically to eradicate latent tissue forms that cause relapses of *P. vivax* and *P. ovale* infections. Due to the continuing spread of increasingly drug-resistant and multidrug-resistant strains of *P. falciparum,* no single agent successfully controls infections with these parasites. Instead, use of two or more antimalarial agents with complementary properties is recommended (*see* White, 1997, 1999).

The discovery of techniques for continuous maintenance of *P. falciparum in vitro* (Trager and Jensen, 1976) led to practical assays of susceptibility of these organisms to antimalarial drugs. This important advance, together with the imminent availability of the sequence of the entire 24.6-megabase *P. falciparum* genome (Su *et al.,* 1999), should reveal molecular targets for antimalarial drug action and resistance as well as for vaccine development.

The biology of malarial infection must be appreciated in order to understand the actions and therapeutic uses of antimalarial drugs.

BIOLOGY OF MALARIAL INFECTION

Nearly all human malaria is caused by four species of obligate intracellular protozoa of the genus *Plasmodium*. Although malaria can be transmitted by transfusion of infected blood and by sharing needles, human beings usually are infected by sporozoites injected by the bite of infected female mosquitoes (genus *Anopheles*). These parasite forms rapidly leave the circulation and localize in hepatocytes, where they transform, multiply, and develop into tissue schizonts (Figure 40–1). This primary asymp-

tomatic tissue (preerythrocytic or exoerythrocytic) stage of infection lasts for 5 to 15 days, depending on the *Plasmodium* species. Tissue schizonts then rupture, each releasing thousands of merozoites that enter the circulation, invade erythrocytes, and initiate the erythrocytic stage of cyclic infection. Once the tissue schizonts burst in *P. falciparum* and *Plasmodium malariae* infections, no forms of the parasite remain in the liver. But in *P. vivax* and *P. ovale* infections, there persist tissue parasites that can produce relapses of erythrocytic infection months to years after the primary attack. The origin of such latent tissue forms is unclear. Once plasmodia enter the erythrocytic cycle, they cannot invade other tissues; thus, there is no tissue stage of infection for human malaria contracted by transfusion. In erythrocytes, most parasites undergo asexual development from young ring forms to trophozoites and finally to mature schizonts. Schizont-containing erythrocytes rupture, each releasing 6 to 24 merozoites, depending on the *Plasmodium* species. It is this process that produces febrile clinical attacks. The released merozoites invade more erythrocytes to continue the cycle, which proceeds until death of the host or modulation by drugs or acquired partial immunity. The periodicity of parasitemia and febrile clinical manifestations thus depend on the timing of schizogony of a generation of erythrocytic parasites. For *P. falciparum, P. vivax,* and *P. ovale,* it takes about 48 hours to complete this process. Synchronous rupture of infected erythrocytes and release of merozoites into the circulation lead to typical febrile attacks on days 1 and 3, hence the designation "tertian malaria." Actually the periodic febrile pattern is less regular in falciparum malaria due to a combination of asynchronous release of parasites and segregation of infected erythrocytes in the periphery. In *P. malariae* infection, schizogony requires about 72 hours, resulting in malarial attacks on days 1 and 4, or "quartan malaria."

Some erythrocytic parasites differentiate into sexual forms known as gametocytes. After infected human blood is ingested by a female mosquito, exflagellation of the male gametocyte is followed by male gametogenesis and fertilization of the female gametocyte in the insect's gut. The resulting zygote, which develops as an oocyst in the gut wall, eventually gives rise to the infective sporozoite, which invades the salivary gland of the mosquito. The insect then can infect another human host by taking a blood meal.

Each *Plasmodium* species causes a characteristic illness and shows distinguishing morphological features in blood smears: (1) *P. falciparum* causes malignant tertian malaria, the most dangerous form of human malaria. By invading erythrocytes of any age, this species can produce

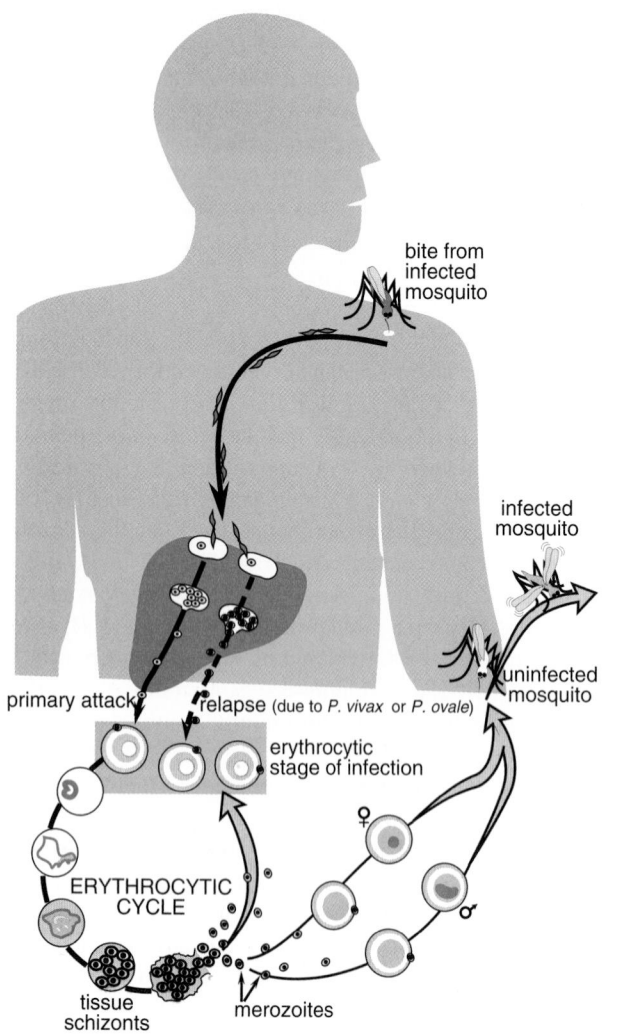

bite from
infected
mosquito

infected
mosquito

uninfected
mosquito

primary attack   relapse (due to *P. vivax* or *P. ovale*)

erythrocytic
stage of infection

ERYTHROCYTIC
CYCLE

tissue
schizonts

merozoites

Figure 40–1. Life cycle of malaria.

an overwhelming parasitemia, sequestration of infected erythrocytes in the peripheral microvasculature, hypoglycemia, hemolysis, and shock with multiorgan failure. Delay in treatment until after demonstration of parasitemia may lead to a fatal outcome even after the peripheral blood is free of parasites. If treated early, the infection usually responds with 48 hours to appropriate chemotherapy. If treatment is inadequate, *recrudescence* of infection may result from multiplication of parasites that persist in the blood. (2) *P. vivax* causes benign tertian malaria. Like the other benign malarias, it produces milder clinical attacks than does *P. falciparum,* because erythrocytes it infects are not sequestered in the peripheral microvasculature. *P. vivax* infection has a low mortality rate in untreated adults and is characterized by relapses caused by latent tissue forms. (3) *P. ovale* causes a rare malarial infection with a periodicity and relapses similar to those of *P. vivax,* but it is even milder and more readily cured. (4) *P. malariae* causes quartan malaria, an infection that is common in localized areas of the tropics. Clinical attacks may occur years after infection but are much rarer than after infection with *P. vivax.*

CLASSIFICATION OF ANTIMALARIAL AGENTS

Antimalarials can be categorized by the stage of the parasite that they affect and the clinical indication for their use. Some drugs have more than one type of antimalarial activity.

Drugs Used for Causal Prophylaxis.   These agents act on *primary tissue forms* of plasmodia within the liver, which are destined within less than a month to initiate the erythrocytic stage of infection. Invasion of erythrocytes and further transmission of infection are thereby prevented. *Proguanil* (formerly called *chloroguanide*) is the prototypic drug of this class, which has been extensively used for causal prophylaxis of falciparum malaria. Because of widespread drug resistance, however, it no longer provides reliable protection when used alone. Although primaquine also has such activity against *P. falciparum,* this potentially toxic drug is reserved for other clinical applications (*see* below).

Drugs Used to Prevent Relapse.   These compounds act on *latent tissue forms* of *P. vivax* and *P. ovale* remaining after the primary hepatic forms have been released into the circulation. Such latent tissue forms eventually mature, invade the circulation, and produce malarial attacks, *i.e.,* re-

lapsing malaria, months or years after the initial infection. Drugs active against latent tissue forms are used for *terminal prophylaxis* and for *radical cure* of relapsing malarial infections. For terminal prophylaxis, regimens with such a drug are initiated shortly before or after a person leaves an endemic area. To achieve radical cure, this type of drug is taken either during the long-term latent period of infection or during an acute attack. In the latter case, the agent is given together with an appropriate drug, usually chloroquine, to eradicate erythrocytic stages of *P. vivax* and *P. ovale.* Primaquine is the prototypical drug used to prevent *relapse,* the term reserved to specify recurring erythrocytic infection stemming from latent tissue plasmodia.

Drugs (Blood Schizontocides) Used for Clinical and Suppressive Cure.   These agents act on asexual erythrocytic stages of malarial parasites to interrupt erythrocytic schizogony and thereby terminate clinical attacks (*clinical cure*). Such drugs also may produce *suppressive cure,* which refers to complete elimination of parasites from the body by continued therapy. Inadequate therapy with blood schizontocides may result in recrudescence of infection due to erythrocytic schizogony. With the notable exception of primaquine, virtually all antimalarial drugs used clinically were developed primarily for their activity against asexual parasite stages. These agents can be divided into two groups. The rapidly acting blood schizontocides include classical antimalarial alkaloids such as chloroquine, quinine, and their related derivatives quinidine and mefloquine. Atovaquone and the artemisinin antimalarial endoperoxides also are rapidly acting agents. Slower-acting, less effective blood schizontocides are exemplified by the antimalarial antifolate and antibiotic compounds. These drugs most commonly are used in conjunction with their more rapidly acting counterparts.

Gametocytocides.   These agents act against sexual erythrocytic forms of plasmodia, thereby preventing transmission of malaria to mosquitoes. Chloroquine and quinine have gametocytocidal activity against *P. vivax, P. ovale,* and *P. malariae,* whereas primaquine displays especially potent activity against gametocytes of *P. falciparum.* However, antimalarials are not used clinically just for their gametocytocidal action.

Sporontocides.   Such drugs ablate transmission of malaria by preventing or inhibiting formation of malarial oocysts and sporozoites in infected mosquitoes. Although chloroquine prevents normal plasmodial development within the mosquito, neither this nor other antimalarial agents are used clinically for this purpose.

Regimens currently recommended for *chemoprophy-laxis* in nonimmune individuals are given in Table 40–1, whereas regimens for *treatment* of malaria in nonimmune individuals are given in Table 40–2. Properties of individual agents are discussed in more detail in a separate section.

ANTIMALARIAL DRUGS

Artemisinin and Derivatives

History. *Artemisinin* is a sesquiterpene lactone endoperoxide derived from the weed *qing hao* (*Artemisia annua*), also called sweet wormwood or annual wormwood. The Chinese have ascribed medicinal value to this plant for more than 2000 years (reviewed by Klayman, 1985). As early as 340 A.D., Ge Hong prescribed tea made from *qing hao* as a remedy for fevers, and in 1596 Li Shizhen recommended it to relieve the symptoms of malaria. By 1972, Chinese scientists had extracted and crystallized the major antimalarial ingredient, *qinghaosu,* now known as artemisinin. They synthesized three derivatives with greater antimalarial potency than artemisinin itself, namely *dihydroartemisinin,* a reduced product, *artemether,* an oil-soluble methyl ester, and *artesunate,* the water-soluble hemisuccinate salt of dihydroartemisinin. In 1979, the Chinese reported that artemisinin drugs were rapidly acting, effective, and safe for the treatment of patients with *P. vivax* or *P. falciparum* infections. More than two million people with malaria in China, Southeast Asia, and parts of Africa have since been treated with artemisinin or one of its semisynthetic derivatives without serious side effects or clinical evidence of drug resistance. These drugs are not yet available in the United States but are available in other countries. The antimalarial endoperoxides, especially when used in conjunction with a longer-acting blood schizontocide such as *mefloquine,* represent a major advance for the treatment of severe, multidrug-resistant falciparum malaria (Meshnick *et al.,* 1996; Newton and White, 1999). The chemical structures of artemisinin and some of its derivatives are shown below.

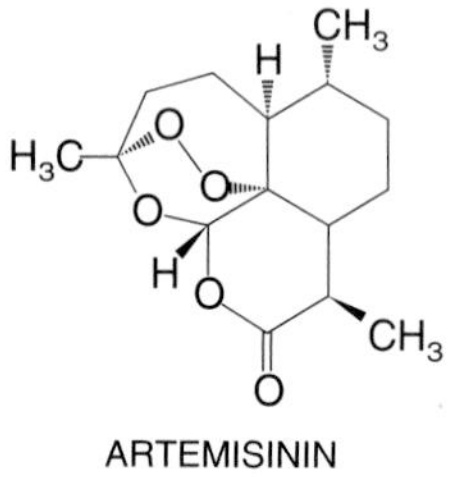

ARTEMISININ

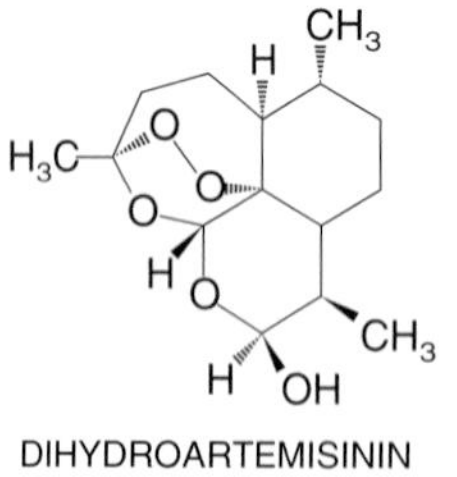

DIHYDROARTEMISININ

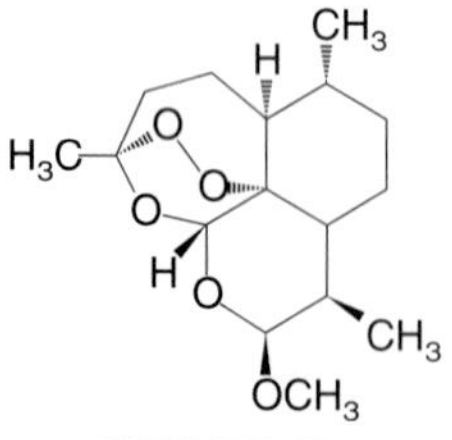

ARTEMETHER

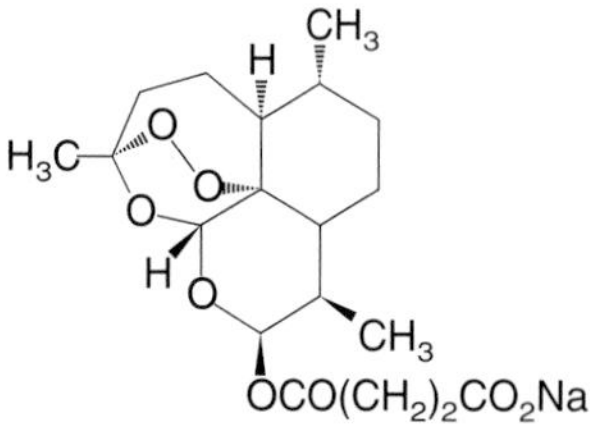

OCH$_3$

ARTESUNATE

OCO(CH$_2$)$_2$CO$_2$Na

Antiparasitic Activity. The endoperoxide moiety is required for antimalarial activity of artemisinin compounds, whereas substitutions on the lactone carbonyl group markedly increase potency. These compounds act rapidly upon asexual erythrocytic stages of *P. vivax* and chloroquine-sensitive, chloroquine-resistant, and multidrug-resistant strains of *P. falciparum.* Their potency *in vivo* is 10- to 100-fold greater than that of other antimalarial drugs (White, 1997). They have gametocytocidal activity but do not affect either primary or latent tissue stage parasites. Thus, artemisinin compounds are not useful either for chemoprophylaxis or for preventing relapses of vivax malaria. The current model of artemisinin action involves two steps. First, intraparasitic heme iron of infected erythrocytes catalyzes cleavage of the endoperoxide bridge. This is followed by intramolecular rearrangement to produce carbon-centered radicals that covalently modify and damage specific malarial proteins (*see* Meshnick *et al.,* 1996). Artemisinin and its derivatives also exhibit antiparasitic activity *in vitro* against several other protozoa including *Leishmania major* and *Toxoplasma gondii* and *in vivo* against schistosomes, but they are not used clinically to treat infections with these parasites.

Absorption, Fate, and Excretion. The disposition of the artemisinin compounds is incompletely understood due to difficulties with proper preservation of biological samples and reliable analytical assays. Indeed, few pharmacokinetic studies carried out in humans have been published (*see* Barradell and Fitton, 1995; de Vries and Dien, 1996). Time to peak plasma levels for the artemisinin compounds varies from minutes to several hours, depending on the drug formulation and its route of administration. Likewise, the profile and extent of drug binding to plasma proteins is variable. Artemether and artesunate are both converted to dihydroartemisinin. Much of the hydrolysis of artesunate to dihydroartemisinin may occur presystemically. Artemisinin itself is metabolized to at least four inactive metabolites, although it is unclear whether dihydroartemisinin is formed as an intermediate (*see* de Vries and Dien, 1996). The antimalarial effect of artemisinin compounds results primarily from dihydroartemisinin, which rapidly disappears from plasma with a half-life of about 45 minutes. Little or none of the administered drugs or dihydroartemisinin is recovered in urine. Although artemisinin can induce CYP2C19 in humans (Svensson *et al.,* 1998), there is no evidence yet of clinically important drug interactions as a consequence.

Therapeutic Uses. Artemisinin compounds are the most rapidly acting, effective, and safe drugs for the treatment of severe malaria, including infections due to chloroquine- and multidrug-resistant strains of *P. falciparum* (*see* White, 1999). They should not be used for prophylaxis of malaria or treatment of mild attacks (Meshnick *et al.,* 1996). Artemisinin drugs act more rapidly and produce less toxicity than the antimalarial alkaloids; moreover, they are just

Table 40–1

Regimens for Malaria Chemoprophylaxis and Self-Treatment in Nonimmune Individuals*

Prophylaxis for infections with chloroquine-sensitive P. falciparum†, P. vivax, P. malariae, *and* P. ovale

  Chloroquine phosphate (ARALEN) is available for oral administration. Adults take 500 mg of chloroquine phosphate (300 mg of base) weekly starting 1 week before entering an endemic area and continuing until 4 weeks after leaving. The pediatric dosage is 8.3 mg/kg of chloroquine phosphate (5 mg base per kg) taken orally by the same schedule. *Note:* Primaquine *phosphate* is used to eradicate latent tissue forms of *P. vivax* and *P. ovale* and effect a radical cure after individuals leave areas endemic for these infections (*see* Table 40–2 and text).

Prophylaxis for infections with chloroquine-resistant or multidrug-resistant strains of P. falciparum‡. *Note:* The choice of regimen depends on the local geographic profile of drug resistance and other factors (*see* text).

Preferred regimens:

  Mefloquine hydrochloride (LARIAM) is available for oral administration only. Adults and children over 45 kg body weight take one 250-mg tablet weekly starting 1 week before entering an endemic area and ending 4 weeks after leaving. Pediatric doses taken by the same schedule are: for children weighing 5 to 9 kg, 31.25 mg (0.125 tablet); 10 to 19 kg, 62.5 mg; 20 to 30 kg, 125 mg; and for those weighing 31 to 45 kg, 187.5 mg. *Note:* Mefloquine is *not* recommended for children weighing less than 5 kg or individuals with a history of seizures, severe neuropsychiatric disturbances, or sensitivity to quinoline antimalarials.

  Doxycycline hyclate (VIBRAMYCIN, others). Formulations of doxycycline are available in capsules, coated tablets, and liquid preparations for oral administration. The adult dose of doxycycline is 100 mg daily. For children over 8 years of age, the dosage is 2 mg/kg given once daily, increasing up to the daily adult dose. Prophylaxis with doxycycline should begin 1 day before travel to an endemic area and end 4 weeks after leaving. This regimen is used in geographic areas where highly multidrug-resistant strains of *P. falciparum* are prevalent. *Note:* Doxycycline use for malaria prophylaxis should not exceed 4 months; it should not be given to children less than 8 years of age or to pregnant women. Doxycycline is contraindicated in individuals who are hypersensitive to any tetracycline. Prophylaxis with doxycycline can be combined with the chloroquine phosphate regimen shown above for chloroquine-sensitive malaria. This strategy often is used in geographic areas where infection with more than one *Plasmodium* species is likely.

Other regimens:

  Use one of the mefloquine, doxycycline, or chloroquine prophylactic regimens listed above, together with a self-treatment dose of *pyrimethamine–sulfadoxine* (FANSIDAR). The latter combination is available in tablets containing pyrimethamine (25 mg) and sulfadoxine (500 mg) for oral use only. Pyrimethamine–sulfadoxine is taken just once as a single dose only if a malaria attack is suspected (febrile episode) and a physician is not available. *Medical attention must then be sought immediately.* Doses of pyrimethamine–sulfadoxine are as follows: Adults take 3 tablets. Children less than 1 year old, 0.25 tablet; 1 to 3 years (or weighing 5 to 10 kg), 0.5 tablet; 4 to 8 years (or 11 to 20 kg), 1 tablet; 9 to 14 years (or 31 to 45 kg), 2 tablets; 15 years and older (or over 45 kg), 3 tablets. (*Note:* Pyrimethamine–sulfadoxine is not recommended for infants less than 2 months old, women in the last trimester of pregnancy, or individuals who are sensitive to sulfonamides.) This regimen is ineffective in geographic areas where resistance to chloroquine and pyrimethamine–sulfadoxine is high, *e.g.*, parts of Southeast Asia, Africa, and South America.

  Proguanil hydrochloride (PALUDRINE) with *chloroquine phosphate*. The oral dose of proguanil for adults and children older than 10 years is 200 mg daily upon entry into an endemic area and continuing for 4 weeks after leaving. Pediatric doses taken by the same schedule are as follows: for children less than 2 years old, 50 mg; 2 to 6 years, 100 mg; 7 to 10 years, 150 mg. Chloroquine phosphate is taken according to the regimen outlined above for prophylaxis of chloroquine-sensitive *P. falciparum*. This regimen has been found useful in parts of sub-Saharan Africa, but resistance to proguanil is common. Failure of chemoprophylaxis also may occur because some individuals fail to convert this prodrug to its active form (*see* text). Proguanil is not available in the United States as a single-drug product, but is available in Canada and elsewhere.

  Proguanil hydrochloride and *atovaquone* in a fixed-dose combination (MALARONE) has been found effective for prophylaxis of *P. falciparum* infections (Shanks *et al.*, 1999). However, this drug combination would best be reserved for treatment of clinical attacks of falciparum malaria.

---

*No chemoprophylactic regimen is always effective in preventing infection with *P. falciparum*. Recommended drug regimens should always be used in conjunction with other protective measures to avoid mosquito bites (*see* text).

†These strains now exist only in Mexico, Central America west of the Panama Canal Zone, the Caribbean, and in parts of South America and the Middle East.

‡These strains exist in other geographic areas endemic for falciparum malaria.

Table 40–2

Regimens for Treatment of Malaria in Nonimmune Individuals

Treatment of severe malarial infections

Note: Infections with *P. falciparum* in nonimmune patients constitute medical emergencies because they can progress rapidly to a fatal outcome.† Chemotherapy should be initiated promptly and not await parasitological confirmation. Parenteral therapy with *quinidine gluconate* is advised for severely ill patients who cannot take oral medication; the regimen is identical for all species of *Plasmodium*. Exchange transfusion may benefit some patients with parasitemias of 10% or more (*see* text).

Preferred regimen:

Quinidine gluconate is given intravenously to both adults and children, starting with a loading dose of 10 mg of the salt per kg dissolved in 300 ml of normal saline and infused over 1 to 2 hours (maximum dose 600 mg of the salt). This is followed by continuous infusion at the rate of 0.02 mg of the salt per kg per minute until oral therapy with quinine sulfate is feasible. During administration of quinidine gluconate, blood pressure (for hypotension) and ECG (for widening of the QRS complex and lengthening of the QT interval) should be monitored continuously and total blood glucose (for hypoglycemia) periodically. These complications, if severe, warrant discontinuation of the drug.

    Quinine sulfate can be substituted for quinidine gluconate once patients can take oral medication. The dose for adults is 650 mg of the salt given every 8 hours. The pediatric dose is 10 mg of the salt per kg given every 8 hours. Therapy with quinidine/quinine is usually given for 3 to 7 days, depending on the species of *Plasmodium* and geographic profile of drug resistance. The dose should be reduced by 30% to 50% after 48 hours if there is no clinical improvement. Previous use of mefloquine also may mandate dosage reduction (*see* text).

Adjunctive therapy:

For optimal clinical response, any one of the following regimens should be used together with oral quinine sulfate therapy. The particular choice depends on the geographic profile of antimalarial drug resistance.

Doxycycline hyclate (VIBRAMYCIN, others). The adult dose is 100 mg taken orally every 8 hours for 7 days. For children over 8 years of age, the dosage is 2 mg/kg, increasing up to the adult dose and given by the same schedule. *Tetracycline* may be substituted if doxycycline hyclate is unavailable. Adults receive 250 mg every 6 hours for 7 days whereas the pediatric dosage is 5 mg/kg every 6 hours for 7 days. *Note:* Because of adverse effects on bones and teeth, tetracyclines should not be given to children less than 8 years old or to pregnant women. These drugs are contraindicated in individuals who are hypersensitive to any tetracycline.

Pyrimethamine-sulfadoxine (FANSIDAR). One dose (3 tablets for adults and lower doses for children, as described in Table 40–1) is given by mouth on the last day of quinine sulfate therapy.

Other oral treatment regimens for infections with chloroquine-resistant P. vivax, *and chloroquine-resistant or multidrug-resistant strains of* P. falciparum

Mefloquine hydrochloride (LARIAM, MEPHAQUINE). The adult dose is 750 mg of the salt taken by mouth followed 12 hours later by 500 mg. The corresponding pediatric dose for children weighing less than 45 kg is 15 mg of the salt per kg followed 12 hours later by 10 mg of the salt per kg. (*Note:* The pediatric dosage is not approved by the FDA.) The initial dose should be repeated *only* if vomiting occurs within the first hour. Therapeutic doses of mefloquine may induce gastrointestinal and neuropsychiatric symptoms. Because of its long half-life and potential for serious drug interactions, extreme caution is advised in using any alkaloid antimalarial (*e.g.*, quinine or chloroquine) with or shortly after mefloquine. (*See* Table 40–1 and text for further details.)

Artesunate plus *mefloquine hydrochloride*. Therapy should be initiated with artesunate given by mouth at a dose of 4 mg/kg once on the first day and 2 mg/kg daily for the next 4 days (total dose of 12 mg/kg is the same for adults and children). Mefloquine is given once on the second day at a dose of 25 mg base per kg. *Note:* Artesunate is not available in the United States.

Atovaquone (MEPRON) and *proguanil hydrochloride* (PALUDRINE). A fixed-dose combination of these drugs is available outside the United States in tablets each containing 250 mg of atovaquone and 100 mg of proguanil hydrochloride (MALARONE). The dose for adults is 1000 mg atovaquone plus 400 mg proguanil hydrochloride taken by mouth once each day for 3 days. The pediatric dose for children weighing 11 to 20 kg is 250 mg atovaquone plus 100 mg proguanil hydrochloride; 21 to 30 kg, 500 mg atovaquone plus 200 mg proguanil hydrochloride; 31 to 40 kg, 750 mg atovaquone plus 300 mg proguanil hydrochloride. These doses are given once daily for 3 days. Tablets should be crushed or chewed and taken after a fatty meal to increase drug bioavailability.

Table 40–2

Regimens for Treatment of Malaria in Nonimmune Individuals (*Continued*)

Oral treatment of infections with P. vivax, P. malariae, P. ovale, *and chloroquine-sensitive* P. falciparum

Chloroquine phosphate (ARALEN) is available in 250-mg and 500-mg tablets (equivalent to 150 mg and 300 mg base, respectively) for oral administration. The dosage for adults and children is similar on a body-weight basis. Give 16.7 mg/kg (10 mg base per kg) immediately followed by 8.3 mg/kg (5 mg base per kg) at 6, 12, 24, and 36 hours to reach a total dose of 50 mg/kg (30 mg base per kg) by 2 days. Doses of 8.3 mg/kg (5 mg base per kg) should be repeated on days 7 and 14 for infections with *P. vivax* and *P. ovale*.

Prevention of relapse:

To eradicate latent tissue forms of *P. vivax* and *P. ovale* that persist to cause relapses of infection, primaquine phosphate is supplied in tablets containing either 13.2 or 26.3 mg of the salt (7.5 mg or 15 mg base, respectively) for oral administration only. Therapy with primaquine is started after the acute attack (about day 4) at doses of 26.3 mg (15 mg base) daily for 14 days. Pediatric doses are 0.53 mg/kg (0.3 mg base per kg) daily, also for 14 days. The same primaquine regimen also can be used during the last 2 weeks of chloroquine phosphate prophylaxis for individuals who have left areas endemic for *P. vivax* or *P. ovale* infection. Alternatively, adults using chloroquine for prophylaxis against *P. vivax* or *P. ovale* may take 500 mg of chloroquine phosphate (300 mg base) together with 78.9 mg of primaquine phosphate (45 mg base), weekly for 8 weeks starting after leaving an endemic area, to achieve a "radical" cure.

†Emergency advice is available from the Division of Parasitic Diseases, Centers for Disease Control and Prevention (CDC) (telephone: 770-488-7760).

as effective against cerebral malaria. Although artemisinin and its derivatives can be used as single agents, infections often relapse unless therapy is continued for 5 to 7 days. A brief course of these agents given in tandem with a longer-acting quinoline or antibiotic antimalarial, *e.g.,* mefloquine or doxycycline, usually prevents relapses and may delay the development of drug resistance (White, 1997, 1999). Although optimal dosage regimens have yet to be standardized, one strategy is to give a course of artesunate to reduce parasite burden rapidly, followed by one or two doses of mefloquine to eradicate the infection (White, 1999; Price *et al.,* 1999; *see* Table 40–2). This approach has the advantage of reducing the frequency of side effects while retaining antimalarial efficacy. Individual endoperoxide antimalarials differ in formulation and clinical utility. Dihydroartemisinin can be given only orally. The oil-soluble artemether can be given only orally or intramuscularly. Artemisinin is effective when given orally or as a rectal suppository. Of the various artemisinin compounds, artesunate is perhaps the most versatile, because it is effective when given orally, intramuscularly, intravenously, or rectally. The intravenous formulation is particularly suitable for treating cerebral malaria, whereas suppositories are especially advantageous for treating patients with severe malaria in isolated areas.

Toxicity and Contraindications. Given for up to 7 days at therapeutic doses, the artemisinin endoperoxides appear to be surprisingly safe in human beings (*see* de Vries and Dien, 1996). Transient first-degree heart block, dose-related reversible de-

creases in reticulocyte and neutrophil counts, and temporary elevations of serum aspartate aminotransferase activity have been reported, but their clinical significance is not established. Brief episodes of drug-induced fever in human volunteers were noted in some studies but not in others. Because high doses of artemisinin drugs can produce neurotoxicity, prolongation of the QT interval, bone marrow depression, and fetal reabsorption in experimental animals, the possibility of long-term toxicity in human beings exists (*see* de Vries and Dien, 1996). But evidence thus far indicates that these effective drugs are remarkably safe for emergency treatment of severe, multidrug-resistant malaria, even in pregnant women (McGready *et al.,* 1998) and in children (Price *et al.,* 1999).

Atovaquone

History. Based on the antiprotozoal activity of certain hydroxynaphthoquinones, *atovaquone* (MEPRON) was developed as a promising synthetic derivative with potent activity against *Plasmodium* species and opportunistic pathogens (Hudson *et al.,* 1991). Subsequent clinical studies revealed that atovaquone produced good responses but high rates of relapse in patients with uncomplicated falciparum malaria (Looareesuwan *et al.,* 1996). In contrast, use of proguanil with atovaquone evoked high cure rates with few relapses and minimal toxicity (Looareesuwan *et al.,* 1996, 1999a). A fixed combination of atovaquone with *proguanil* (MALARONE) is now available in the United States (Looareesuwan *et al.,* 1999a). Atovaquone also was developed for its activity against *Pneumocystis carinii* and *T. gondii,* pathogens that cause serious opportunistic infections in AIDS patients (Hughes *et al.,* 1990). After limited clinical trials, the United States Food and Drug Administration (FDA) approved this compound in 1992 for treatment of mild to moderate *P. carinii* pneumonia in patients intolerant to trimethoprim-sulfamethoxazole (*see* Chapter 44). Atovaquone has some efficacy against human brain and eye infections with *T. gondii* and its use in combination with other antiparasitic agents is still being explored. Atovaquone has the chemical structure shown below:

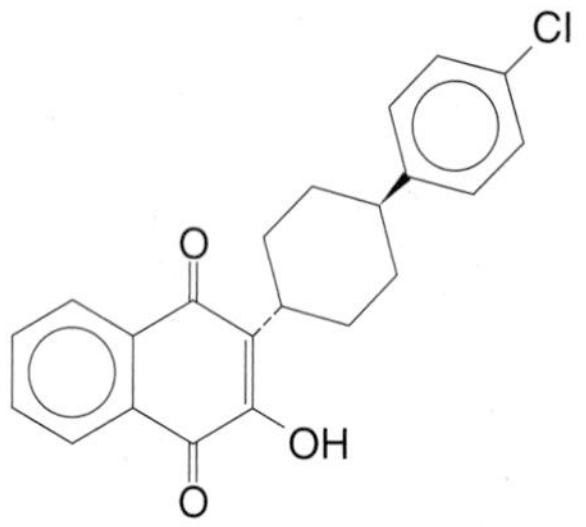

ATOVAQUONE

Antiparasitic Effects.   Atovaquone is a highly lipophilic analog of ubiquinone. In animal models and *in vitro* systems, it has potent activity against blood stages of plasmodia, tachyzoite and cyst forms of *T. gondii,* the fungus *P. carinii,* and *Babesia* species (Hughes *et al.,* 1990; Hudson *et al.,* 1991; Hughes and Oz, 1995). Atovaquone is highly potent against rodent malaria and *P. falciparum,* both in culture (IC_{50} 0.7 to 4.3 nM) and in *Aotus* monkeys (Hudson *et al.,* 1991). This compound selectively interferes with mitochondrial electron transport and related processes, such as ATP and pyrimidine biosynthesis in susceptible malaria parasites. Thus, atovaquone acts selectively at the cytochrome bc_1 complex of malaria mitochondria to inhibit electron transport and collapse the mitochondrial membrane potential (*see* Vaidya, 1998). Synergism between proguanil and atovaquone appears due to the capacity of proguanil as a biguanide to enhance the membrane-collapsing activity of atovaquone (Srivastava and Vaidya, 1999). Atovaquone likewise affects mitochondrial function in permeabilized *T. gondii* tachyzoites (Vercesi *et al.,* 1998).

Absorption, Fate, and Excretion.   Because of its low water solubility, the bioavailability of atovaquone depends on formulation. A microfine suspension shows twofold greater oral bioavailability than do tablets. Drug absorption after a single oral dose is slow, erratic, and variable; increased by 2- to 3-fold by fatty food; and dose-limited above 750 mg. More than 99% of the drug is bound to plasma protein, so its concentration in cerebrospinal spinal fluid is less than 1% of that in plasma. Plasma level–time profiles often show a double peak, albeit with considerable variability; the first peak appears in 1 to 8 hours while the second occurs 1 to 4 days after a single dose. This pattern suggests an enterohepatic circulation, as does the long half-life, averaging 1.5 to 3 days. Atovaquone is not significantly metabolized by human beings. It is excreted in bile, and more than 94% of the drug is recovered unchanged in feces; only traces appear in the urine (Rolan *et al.,* 1997). Clearance of atovaquone may vary among different ethnic populations treated for falciparum malaria (Hussein *et al.,* 1997).

Therapeutic Uses.   Atovaquone is used with a biguanide for treatment of malaria to obtain optimal clinical results and avoid emergence of drug-resistant plasmodial strains. A tablet containing a fixed dose of 250 mg of atovaquone and 100 mg of proguanil hydrochloride, taken orally, has been highly effective and safe in a 3-day regimen for treating mild to moderate attacks of chloroquine- and multidrug-resistant falciparum malaria (*see* Looareesuwan *et al.,* 1999a and Table 40–2). The same regimen followed by primaquine produced excellent results in chloroquine-resistant vivax malaria (Looareesuwan *et al.,* 1999b). To delay emergence of drug resistance, atovaquone plus proguanil is not recommended generally for prophylaxis of malaria, even though the combination is highly effective in adults and children. Such resistance develops readily when either drug is used alone. Opportunistic infections due to the fungus *P. carinii* or the protozoan *T. gondii* are especially serious threats to immunocompromised patients such as those with HIV infection and AIDS. Atovaquone remains an attractive alternative for prophylaxis and treatment of pulmonary *P. carinii* infection in patients who can take oral medication but cannot tolerate trimethoprim-sulfamethoxazole or parenteral pentamidine isethionate (*see* Chapters 44 and 49 and the 9th edition of this textbook). *T. gondii* infections in these patients, especially cerebral lesions, have shown only limited dose-related positive responses to prolonged regimens of atovaquone (Torres *et al.,* 1997). *Toxoplasma* chorioretinitis in immunocompetent patients probably responds better to this drug (Pearson *et al.,* 1999). Atovaquone may have potential use in human infections due to *Babesia* species (Hughes and Oz, 1995).

Toxicity and Contraindications.   Both in patients with acute falciparum malaria and in severely debilitated and immunocompromised patients such as those with AIDS, adverse effects directly attributable to atovaquone have been difficult to distinguish from manifestations of underlying disease. Atovaquone causes few side effects that require withdrawal of therapy. The most common reactions are rash, fever, vomiting, diarrhea, and headache. Vomiting and diarrhea may result in therapeutic failure due to decreased drug absorption. However, readministration of this drug within an hour of vomiting still may evoke a positive therapeutic response in patients with falciparum malaria (Looareesuwan *et al.,* 1999a). Dose-related maculopapular rashes occur in about 20% of treated patients, but most are mild and do not progress even when therapy is continued. Caution would dictate, however, that atovaquone not be given to patients with histories of allergic skin reactions or possible allergy to the drug. Patients treated with atovaquone only occasionally exhibit abnormalities of serum transaminase and amylase levels. Atovaquone lacks proven efficacy against bacterial, viral, and most opportunistic infections that commonly afflict immunocompromised individuals; these infections must be treated separately. On balance, the drug appears to cause few acute adverse effects, but more clinical evaluation is needed, especially to detect possible rare, unusual, or long-term toxicity. An example of the last is the association of reversible vortex keratopathy with highly lipid-soluble antiparasitic drugs like atovaquone (Shah *et al.*, 1995).

Precautions and Contraindications.   While atovaquone seems remarkably safe, the drug needs further evaluation in pediatric patients, older persons, pregnant women, and lactating mothers. Accordingly, the drug should be used with caution in these individuals. Routine tests for carcinogenicity, mutagenicity, and teratogenicity have been negative thus far, although therapeutic doses can cause maternal toxicity and interfere with normal fetal development in rabbits. Atovaquone may possibly compete with certain drugs for binding to plasma proteins, and therapy with rifampin, a potent inducer of cytochrome P450–mediated drug metabolism, can substantially reduce plasma levels of atovaquone, whereas plasma levels of rifampin are raised. Until it is known whether atovaquone induces or inhibits the hepatic metabolism or biliary uptake and elimination of other drugs, caution is advised in using the drug in patients with severe liver disease.

Chloroquine and Congeners

History.   *Chloroquine* (ARALEN) is one of a large series of 4-aminoquinolines investigated as part of the extensive cooperative program of antimalarial research in the United States during World War II. Beginning in 1943, thousands of these compounds were synthesized and tested for activity. Chloroquine eventually proved most promising and was released for field trial. When hostilities ceased, it was discovered that the compound had been synthesized and studied under the name of RESOCHIN by the Germans as early as 1934.

Chemistry.   Chloroquine has the following chemical structure:

CHLOROQUINE

Chloroquine closely resembles the obsolete 8-aminoquinoline antimalarials, pamaquine and pentaquine. It contains the same side chain as quinacrine but differs from this antimalarial in having a quinoline instead of an acridine nucleus and in lacking the methoxy moiety. The *d, l,* and *dl* forms of chloroquine have equal potency in duck malaria, but the *d* isomer is somewhat less toxic than the *l* isomer in mammals. A chlorine atom attached to position 7 of the quinoline ring confers the greatest antimalarial activity in both avian and human malarias. Research on the structure-activity relationships of chloroquine and related alkaloid compounds continues in an effort to find new, effective antimalarials with improved safety profiles that can be used successfully against chloroquine- and multidrug-resistant strains of *P. falciparum* (*see* below and, for example, Goldberg *et al.,* 1997; O'Neill *et al.,* 1998; Raynes, 1999).

Amodiaquine is a congener of chloroquine that is no longer recommended for chemoprophylaxis of falciparum malaria because its use is associated with hepatic toxicity and agranulocytosis. *Pyronaridine* is a Mannich-base antimalarial that is structurally related to amodiaquine. This compound, developed by the Chinese in the 1970s, was shown to be well tolerated and effective against falciparum and vivax malarias. However, it cannot be recommended for routine use because of a lack of standardized dosage regimens and because its possible long-term toxicity has yet to be adequately evaluated (Naisbitt *et al.,* 1998). *Hydroxychloroquine* (PLAQUENIL), in which one of the *N*-ethyl substituents of chloroquine is β-hydroxylated, is essentially equivalent to chloroquine against falciparum malaria. This analog is preferred over chloroquine for treatment of mild rheumatoid arthritis and lupus erythematosus because, given in the high doses required, it may cause less ocular toxicity than chloroquine would (Easterbrook, 1999).

Pharmacological   Effects.   *Antimalarial   Actions.* Chloroquine is highly effective against erythrocytic forms of *P. vivax, P. ovale, P. malariae,* and chloroquine-sensitive strains of *P. falciparum.* It exerts activity against gametocytes of the first three plasmodial species but not against those of *P. falciparum.* The drug has no activity against latent tissue forms of *P. vivax* or *P. ovale* and thus cannot cure infections with these species.

Other Effects.   Chloroquine or its analogs are used for therapy of conditions other than malaria. Their use to treat hepatic amebiasis is described in Chapter 41. Chloroquine and hydroxychloroquine have been used as secondary drugs to treat a variety of chronic diseases, because both alkaloids concentrate in lysosomes and have antiinflammatory properties. Thus, high doses of these compounds, often together with other agents, have clinical efficacy in rheumatoid arthritis, systemic lupus erythematosus, discoid lupus, sarcoidosis, and photosensitivity diseases such as porphyria cutanea tarda and severe polymorphous light eruption (Danning and Boumpas, 1998; Fritsch *et al.,* 1998; Baltzan *et al.,* 1999).

Mechanisms of Antimalarial Action of and Resistance to Chloroquine and Other Antimalarial Quinolines.   Asexual malaria parasites flourish in host erythrocytes by digesting hemoglobin in their acidic food vacuoles, a process that generates free radicals and heme (ferriprotoporphyrin IX) as highly reactive by-products. After nucleation aided by histidine-rich proteins and perhaps by lipids, heme polymerizes into an insoluble unreactive malarial pigment termed *hemozoin.* Quinoline blood schizontocides that behave as weak bases concentrate in food vacuoles of susceptible plasmodia, where they increase pH, inhibit the peroxidative activity of heme, and disrupt its nonenzymatic polymerization to hemozoin. Failure to inactivate heme then kills the parasites *via* oxidative damage to membranes, digestive proteases, and possibly other critical biomolecules (reviewed by Foley and Tilley, 1998). Of possible mechanisms for the action of the malarial quinolines, inhibition of heme

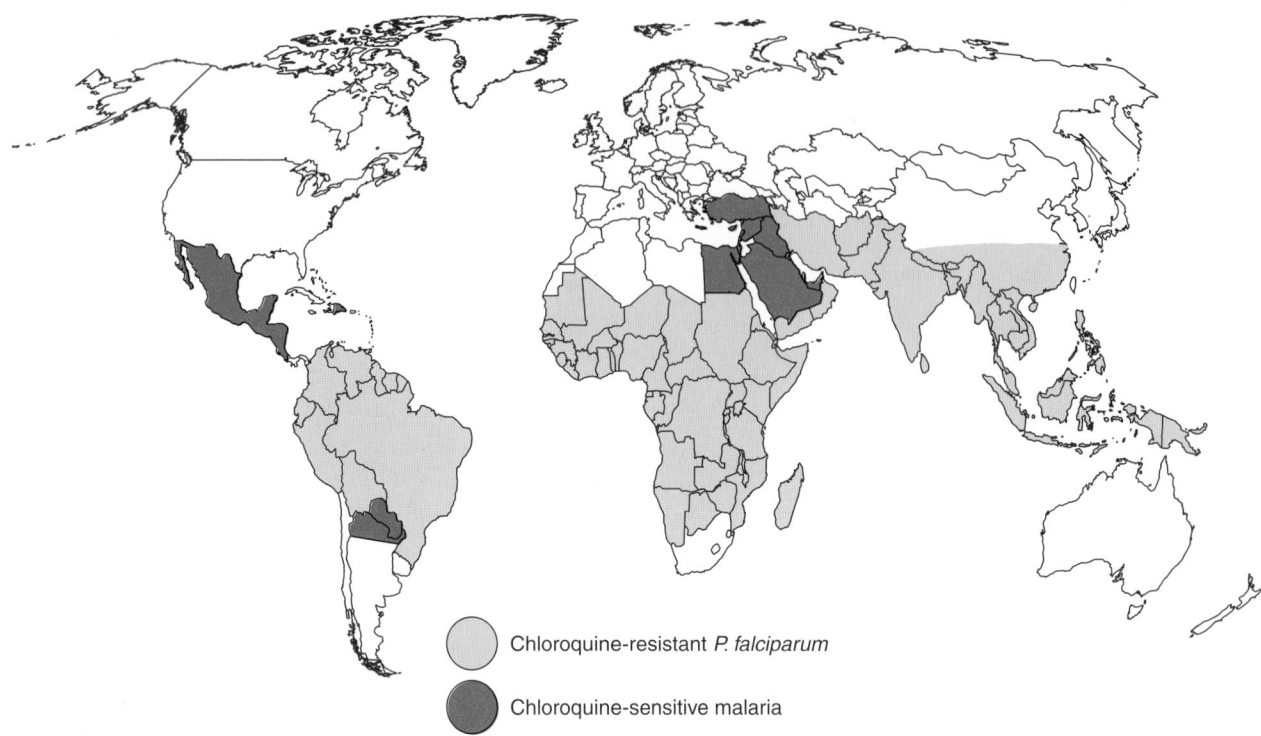

Chloroquine-resistant *P. falciparum*

Chloroquine-sensitive malaria

Figure 40–2. Distribution of malaria and chloroquine-resistant **Plasmodium falciparum,** *1993.*

Source: Centers for Disease Control and Prevention.

polymerization appears crucial. Recent kinetic studies indicate that radiolabeled chloroquine, quinidine, and mefloquine bind first to heme and then prevent further heme polymerization by incorporating as heme-quinoline complexes into growing heme polymer chains. This unifying model also may apply to amodiaquine, quinacrine, and quinine but not to primaquine (Sullivan *et al.,* 1996; Mungthin *et al.,* 1998). Whether resulting accumulation of heme, heme-quinoline complexes, or both suffices to kill the parasites or other actions of the antimalarial quinolines are required is unknown (Ginsburg *et al.,* 1998; Bray *et al.,* 1998; Loria *et al.,* 1999).

Intrinsic resistance of erythrocytic asexual forms of *P. falciparum* to antimalarial quinolines, especially chloroquine, has been slow to develop but is now common worldwide, particularly in areas of extensive antimalarial drug use (Figure 40–2). Chloroquine resistance is emphasized here even though resistance mechanisms probably differ between antimalarial quinoline classes (*see* below). More than 20 years ago, Fitch and coworkers noted that chloroquine-sensitive falciparum parasites concentrated the drug to higher levels than did chloroquine-resistant organisms (Fitch *et al.,* 1979). Reasons for the relatively reduced levels of chloroquine in food vacuoles of chloroquine-resistant parasites have yet to be completely clarified. These could include differences in plasmodial uptake and transport of chloroquine to food vacuoles as well as differences in vacuolar influx, efflux, and trapping of drug (Goldberg *et al.,* 1997; Bray *et al.,* 1998; Foley and Tilley, 1998).

Chloroquine export initially attracted attention because verapamil, an inhibitor of P-glycoprotein–mediated drug efflux by

multidrug-resistant (MDR) tumor cells, enhanced chloroquine efflux and partially restored susceptibility of resistant *P. falciparum* to this drug (*see* Foley and Tilley, 1998). Indeed, two homologues of *mdr* genes, *pfmdr1* and *pfmdr2,* were later identified in *P. falciparum* (Wilson *et al.,* 1989; Foote *et al.,* 1989). But neither gene was linked to chloroquine resistance in genetic studies (Wellems *et al.,* 1990). One, *pfmdr1,* encodes a P-glycoprotein–like protein, Pgh1, which, when overexpressed, may even confer relative sensitivity to chloroquine but resistance to antimalarial aminoalcohols such as mefloquine, halofantrine, and quinine (Cowman *et al.,* 1994). Moreover, field studies failed to link chloroquine resistance to alterations in *pfmdr1* (von Seidlein *et al.,* 1997; Póvoa *et al.,* 1998; Zalis *et al.,* 1998), and inhibitors of P-glycoprotein–mediated transport when given with chloroquine have not proven clinically effective in treating chloroquine-resistant falciparum malaria. Thus, based on evidence accumulated from both laboratory strains and clinical isolates, resistance to chloroquine, mefloquine/halofantrine, and quinine probably involves at least three nonidentical mechanisms (*see* Zalis *et al.,* 1998; Reed *et al.,* 2000).

More recently, the proposed existence of a chloroquine transporter (Sanchez *et al.,* 1997) was supported by an elegant study indicating that chloroquine resistance in a *P. falciparum* gene cross-mapped to a 36-kb segment of chromosome 7 (Su *et al.,* 1997). This segment contains *cg2,* a gene that encodes a 330,000-dalton protein with complex polymorphisms, a set of which was associated with the chloroquine-resistant phenotype in 20 of 21 progeny examined; the finding of one chloroquine-sensitive strain with the same set of polymorphisms indicated that this set was necessary but not sufficient to confer chloroquine resistance. The same genetic study supported clinical evidence that South American and Asian/African *P. falciparum* have separate origins of chloroquine resistance. The CG2 protein (the product of *cg2*) was located both at the parasite periphery and in association with hemozoin in the food vacuoles, consistent with a role in chloroquine transport (Su *et al.*, 1997). Further studies confirmed an incomplete but positive association of *cg2* polymorphisms with chloroquine resistance in clinical isolates from travelers returning from endemic regions (Durand *et al.*, 1999). Indeed, chemical probes to identify CG2 already may have been identified (Goldberg *et al.*, 1997). In summary, resistance to the antimalarial quinolines probably involves multiple mechanisms under complex multigenic control.

Absorption, Fate, and Excretion. Chloroquine is well absorbed from the gastrointestinal tract and rapidly from intramuscular and subcutaneous sites. The drug distributes relatively slowly into a very large apparent volume (over 100 liters/kg; *see* Krishna and White, 1996). This is due to extensive sequestration of chloroquine in tissues, particularly liver, spleen, kidney, lung, melanin-containing tissues, and, to a lesser extent, brain and spinal cord. Chloroquine binds moderately (60%) to plasma proteins and undergoes appreciable biotransformation *via* the hepatic cytochrome P450 system to two active metabolites, desethylchloroquine and bisdesethylchloroquine (*see* Ducharme and Farinotti, 1996). These metabolites may reach concentrations in plasma 40% and 10% of that of chloroquine, respectively. The $S(+)$ enantiomer of chloroquine exhibits both greater binding to plasma proteins and a greater metabolic clearance than the $R(-)$ enantiomer (*see* Krishna and White, 1996). The renal clearance of chloroquine is about half of its total systemic clearance. Unchanged chloroquine and its major metabolite account for more than 50% and 25% of the urinary drug products, respectively, and the renal excretion of both compounds is increased by acidification of the urine.

Both in adults and children, chloroquine exhibits complex pharmacokinetics such that plasma levels of the drug shortly after dosing are determined primarily by the rate of distribution rather than elimination (*see* Krishna and White, 1996). Because of extensive tissue binding, a loading dose is required to achieve effective concentrations in plasma. After parenteral administration, rapid entry together with slow exit of chloroquine from a small central compartment can result in transiently high and potentially lethal concentrations of the drug in plasma. Hence, chloroquine is given either slowly by constant intravenous infusion or in small divided doses by the subcutaneous or intramuscular routes (Foley and Tilley, 1998). Chloroquine is safer when given orally because the rates of absorption and distribution are more closely matched; peak plasma levels are achieved in about 3 to 5 hours after dosing by this route. The half-life of chloroquine increases from a few days to weeks as plasma levels decline, reflecting the transition from slow distribution to even slower elimination from extensive tissue stores. The terminal half-life ranges from 30 to 60 days, and traces of the drug can be found in the urine for years after a therapeutic regimen.

Therapeutic Uses. Chloroquine is the most versatile antimalarial drug available, but its usefulness has declined

in those parts of the world where strains of *P. falciparum* have emerged that are relatively or absolutely resistant to its action. The compound is superior to quinine in that it is more potent and less toxic, and it need be given only once weekly as a suppressive agent. Chloroquine has neither prophylactic nor radical curative value in human *P. vivax* or *P. ovale* malarias. However, except in Oceania and other areas where relatively resistant strains of *P. vivax* are reported (Newton and White, 1999), chloroquine is very effective in terminating or suppressing acute attacks of malaria caused by these plasmodial species. Relapses of vivax malaria may occur after chloroquine is discontinued, but intervals between their appearance are prolonged. Primaquine can either be given with chloroquine to eradicate this infection or reserved for use until after a patient leaves an endemic area. Chloroquine is highly effective for the prophylaxis and cure of malarias due to *P. malariae* and sensitive strains of *P. falciparum* that still exist in limited geographic areas (Figure 40–2). The drug rapidly controls the clinical symptoms and parasitemia of acute malarial attacks. Most patients become completely afebrile within 24 to 48 hours after receiving therapeutic doses, and thick smears of peripheral blood generally are negative by 48 to 72 hours. If patients fail to respond during the second day of chloroquine therapy, resistant strains of *P. falciparum* should be suspected and therapy instituted with quinine or another rapidly acting blood schizontocide. Although chloroquine can be given safely by parenteral routes to comatose or vomiting patients until the drug can be taken orally, quinidine gluconate usually is given. In comatose children, chloroquine is well absorbed and effective when given through a nasogastric tube. Tables 40–1 and 40–2 provide information about recommended prophylactic and therapeutic dosage regimens involving the use of chloroquine. These regimens are subject to modification according to clinical judgment and geographic patterns of chloroquine resistance. For example, persons living in areas of high endemicity often develop partial resistance to malaria and may require little or no chemotherapy.

Toxicity and Side Effects. Taken in proper doses, chloroquine is an extraordinarily safe drug. Acute chloroquine toxicity is most frequently encountered when therapeutic or high doses are administered too rapidly by parenteral routes (*see* above). Toxic manifestations relate primarily to the cardiovascular and central nervous systems. Cardiovascular effects include hypotension, vasodilation, suppressed myocardial function, cardiac arrhythmias, and eventual cardiac arrest. Confusion, convulsions, and coma indicate central nervous system dysfunction. Chloroquine doses of more than 5 g given parenterally usually are fatal. Prompt treatment with mechanical ventilation, epinephrine, and diazepam may be lifesaving.

Doses of chloroquine used for oral therapy of the acute malarial attack may cause gastrointestinal upset, headache, visual disturbances, and urticaria. Pruritus also occurs, most commonly among dark-skinned persons. Prolonged medication with suppressive doses occasionally causes side effects such as headache, blurring of vision, diplopia, confusion, convulsions, lichenoid skin eruptions, bleaching of hair, widening of the QRS interval, and T-wave abnormalities. These complications usually disappear soon after the drug is withheld. Rare instances of hemolysis and blood dyscrasias have been reported. Chloroquine may cause discoloration of nail beds and mucous membranes. Chloroquine can interfere with the immunogenicity of certain vaccines (Brachman *et al.*, 1992; Horowitz and Carbonaro, 1992; Pappaioanou *et al.*, 1986).

High daily doses (>250 mg) of chloroquine or hydroxychloroquine used for treatment of diseases other than malaria can result in irreversible retinopathy and ototoxicity. Retinopathy presumably is related to drug accumulation in melanin-rich tissues and can be avoided if the daily dose is 250 mg or less (*see* Rennie, 1993). Prolonged therapy with high doses of either 4-aminoquinoline also can cause toxic myopathy, cardiopathy, and peripheral neuropathy; these reactions improve if the drug is promptly withdrawn (Estes *et al.*, 1987). Rarely, neuropsychiatric disturbances, including suicide, may be related to overdose.

Precautions and Contraindications. This topic has been briefly reviewed by Griffin (1999). Chloroquine is not recommended for treating individuals with epilepsy or myasthenia gravis. The drug should be used cautiously if at all in the presence of hepatic disease or severe gastrointestinal, neurological, or blood disorders. If such disorders occur during the course of therapy, the drug should be discontinued. Chloroquine can cause hemolysis in patients with glucose-6-phosphate dehydrogenase deficiency (*see* "Primaquine," below). Concomitant use of gold or phenylbutazone with chloroquine should be avoided because of the tendency of all three agents to produce dermatitis. Chloroquine should not be prescribed for patients with psoriasis or other exfoliative skin conditions because it causes severe reactions. Chloroquine interacts with a variety of different agents. It should not be given with mefloquine because of increased risk of seizures. Most importantly, this antimalarial opposes the action of anticonvulsants and increases the risk of ventricular arrhythmias from coadministration with amiodarone or halofantrine. By increasing plasma levels of digoxin and cyclosporine, chloroquine also can increase the risk of toxicity from these agents. For patients receiving long-term, high-dose therapy, ophthalmological and neurological evaluation is recommended every 3 to 6 months.

Diaminopyrimidines

History. Based on their ability to antagonize folic and folinic acids in supporting the growth of *Lactobacillus casei*, a number of diaminopyrimidines were tested for inhibitory activity against other pathogenic organisms. Several 2,4-diaminopyrimidines, including *pyrimethamine* (DARAPRIM) and the antibacterial agent *trimethoprim*, exhibited significant antimalarial activity in animal models. Pyrimethamine was later found to be especially effective against plasmodia infecting human beings (*see* Symposium, 1952). The antifolate combination (FANSIDAR) of pyrimethamine and sulfadoxine, a long-acting sulfonamide, has been used extensively for prophylaxis and suppression of human malarias,

especially those caused by chloroquine-resistant strains of *P. falciparum*. Resistance to this formulation rapidly developed in Indochina and is now widespread except in parts of Africa, where the drug combination is used primarily by indigenous populations to suppress attacks of chloroquine-resistant falciparum malaria. It is no longer recommended for long-term prophylaxis because of the risk of toxicity (*see* below). Pyrimethamine has the following chemical structure:

PYRIMETHAMINE

Antiprotozoal Effects. *Antimalarial Actions.* Pyrimethamine is a slow-acting blood schizontocide with antimalarial effects *in vivo* similar to those of proguanil (*see* below). However, pyrimethamine has greater antimalarial potency because it acts directly on malarial parasites, and its half-life is much longer than that of cycloguanil, the active metabolite of proguanil. Unlike proguanil, pyrimethamine does not show marked efficacy against hepatic forms of *P. falciparum*. At therapeutic doses, pyrimethamine fails to eradicate latent tissue forms of *P. vivax* or gametocytes of any plasmodial species. The antimalarial effects of both pyrimethamine and proguanil have been reviewed by Davey (1963) and by Hill (1963).

Action against Other Protozoa. High doses of pyrimethamine given concurrently with sulfadiazine is the preferred therapy for toxoplasmosis, an infection with *Toxoplasma gondii* that can be particularly severe in infants and immunosuppressed individuals (*see* Chapter 41).

Mechanisms of Antimalarial Action and Resistance. In an elegant series of investigations, the 2,4-diaminopyrimidines were shown to act by inhibiting dihydrofolate reductase of plasmodia at concentrations far lower than those required to produce comparable inhibition of the mammalian enzymes (Ferone *et al.*, 1969). Plasmodial dihydrofolate reductase, unlike its mammalian counterparts, possesses both dihydrofolate reductase and thymidylate synthetase activities. Synergism between pyrimethamine and the sulfonamides or sulfones is explained by inhibition of two steps in an essential metabolic pathway (*see* Chapter 44). The two steps involved are the utilization of *p*-aminobenzoic acid for the synthesis of dihydropteroic acid, which is catalyzed by dihydropteroate synthase and inhibited by sulfonamides, and the reduction of dihydrofolate to tetrahydrofolate, which is catalyzed by dihydrofolate reductase and inhibited by pyrimethamine. Inhibition by antifolates is manifested late in the life cycle of malarial parasites by failure of nuclear division at the time of schizont formation in erythrocytes and liver. This mechanism is consistent with the slow onset of action of the antifolate as compared with the quinoline antimalarials. However, resistance to pyrimethamine does develop in regions of prolonged or extensive drug use. Dihydrofolate reductase–thymidylate synthetase genes have been cloned and sequenced in strains of *P. falciparum* that are either sensitive or resistant to pyrimethamine. Several different mutations have been identified that produce single amino acid changes linked to pyrimethamine resistance; these changes are thought to decrease the binding affinity of pyrimethamine for its active site on the dihydrofolate reductase moiety of the parasite enzyme. The primary change associated with pyrimethamine resistance is a substitution of asparagine for serine at position 108 (S108N). Secondary mutations associated with increasing levels of resistance result from amino acid substitutions at Arg^{50}, Ile^{51}, Arg^{59}, and Leu^{164}; of these, the Leu^{164} change most markedly enhances pyrimethamine resistance when associated with the primary S108N mutation. These and other amino acid changes in various combinations also may contribute to pyrimethamine resistance. However, the pattern of amino acid substitutions differs from that observed for resistance to cycloguanil, even though cross resistance can occur between these structurally related compounds that target plasmodial dihydrofolate reductase (*see* "Proguanil"; Cowman, 1998; Cortese and Plowe, 1998).

Absorption, Fate, and Distribution.   After oral administration pyrimethamine is slowly but completely absorbed; it reaches peak plasma levels in about 4 to 6 hours. The compound binds to plasma proteins and accumulates mainly in kidneys, lungs, liver, and spleen. It is eliminated slowly with a half-life in plasma of about 80 to 95 hours. Concentrations that are suppressive for responsive plasmodial strains remain in the blood for about 2 weeks, but these are lower in patients with malaria (Winstanley *et al.*, 1992). Several metabolites of pyrimethamine appear in the urine, but their identities and antimalarial properties have not been fully characterized. Pyrimethamine also is excreted in the milk of nursing mothers.

Therapeutic Uses.   Pyrimethamine is not a first-line antimalarial. The drug is virtually always given with either a sulfonamide or sulfone to enhance its antifolate activity, but it still acts slowly relative to the quinoline blood schizontocides, and its prolonged elimination encourages the selection of resistant parasites. The use of pyrimethamine should be restricted to the suppressive treatment of chloroquine-resistant falciparum malaria in areas, *e.g.*, parts of Africa, where resistance to antifolates has not yet fully developed. Travelers to these areas are instructed to carry a treatment dose of pyrimethamine–sulfadoxine to take in case of a presumed malarial illness. *Medical attention should be sought as soon as possible thereafter.*

Pyrimethamine together with a short-acting sulfonamide such as sulfadiazine also may be used as an adjunct to quinine to treat an acute malarial attack. Dosage regimens for both of these indications are given in Tables 40–1 and 40–2. Pyrimethamine–sulfadoxine is no longer recommended for prophylaxis because of toxicity due to the accompanying sulfonamide (*see* below). The combination has been used with mefloquine for prophylaxis and treatment of multidrug-resistant falciparum malaria, but the regimens employed risked greater toxicity and offered little advantage over the use of mefloquine alone (*see* Palmer *et al.*, 1993).

High doses of pyrimethamine plus sulfadiazine is the treatment of choice for infections with *Toxoplasma gondii* in immunocompromised adults; if such patients are left untreated, these infections rapidly progress to a fatal outcome (*see* Kasper, 1998; Chapter 41). Initial therapy consists of an oral loading dose of 200 mg followed by 50 to 75 mg of pyrimethamine daily for 4 to 6 weeks along with 4 to 6 g of sulfadiazine daily in four divided doses. *Leucovorin* (folinic acid), 10 to 15 mg daily, should be taken for the same period to prevent bone marrow toxicity (*see* below). For subsequent long-term suppressive therapy, lower doses of pyrimethamine (25 to 50 mg daily) and sulfadiazine (2 to 4 g daily) may suffice. To deal with toxicity, pyrimethamine often has been used with agents such as *clindamycin, spiramycin,* or other *macrolides* (*see* Kasper, 1998). Infants with congenital, placentally transmitted toxoplasmosis usually respond positively to oral pyrimethamine (0.5 to 1.0 mg/kg daily) and oral sulfadiazine (100 mg/kg daily) given over a one-year period.

Toxicity, Precautions, and Contraindications.   Antimalarial doses of pyrimethamine alone cause little toxicity except occasional skin rashes and depression of hematopoiesis. Excessive doses produce a megaloblastic anemia, resembling that of folate deficiency, that responds readily to drug withdrawal or treatment with folinic acid. At very high doses pyrimethamine is teratogenic in animals, but there is no evidence for such toxicity in human beings.

Sulfonamides or sulfones, rather than pyrimethamine, usually account for the toxicity associated with coadministration of these antifolate drugs (*see* Chapter 44). The combination of pyrimethamine (25 mg) and sulfadoxine (500 mg) (FANSIDAR) is no longer recommended for antimalarial prophylaxis, because in about 1:5000 to 1:8000 individuals, it causes severe and even fatal cutaneous reactions, such as erythema multiforme, Stevens-Johnson syndrome, and toxic epidermal necrolysis. This combination also has been associated with serum-sickness-type reactions, urticaria, exfoliative dermatitis, and hepatitis. Pyrimethamine–sulfadoxine is contraindicated for individuals with previous reactions to sulfonamides, for lactating mothers, and for infants less than 2 months old. Administration of pyrimethamine with dapsone (MALOPRIM, a drug combination unavailable in the United States) occasionally has been associated with agranulocytosis. Higher doses of pyrimethamine

(75 mg daily), used along with sulfadiazine (4 to 6 g daily) to treat toxoplasmosis, produce skin rashes, bone marrow suppression, and renal toxicity in about 40% of immunocompromised patients. However, much of this toxicity is probably due to sulfadiazine (*see* Kasper, 1998, and Chapter 44).

Halofantrine

Halofantrine (HALFAN) is a phenanthrene methanol antimalarial drug with blood schizontocidal properties similar to those of the quinoline antimalarials. This compound was originally developed and has been used as an alternative to quinine and mefloquine to treat acute malarial attacks caused by chloroquine-resistant and multidrug-resistant strains of *P. falciparum*. Because halofantrine displays erratic bioavailability, potentially lethal cardiotoxicity, and extensive cross resistance with mefloquine, its use generally is not recommended. Details of the history, pharmacology, and toxicology of halofantrine are presented in the 9th edition of this textbook.

Mefloquine

History. *Mefloquine* (LARIAM) is a product of the Malaria Research Program established in 1963 by the Walter Reed Institute for Medical Research to develop promising new compounds to combat emerging strains of drug-resistant *P. falciparum*. Of many 4-quinoline-methanols tested based on their structural similarity to quinine, mefloquine displayed high antimalarial activity in animal models and emerged from clinical trials as safe and highly effective against drug-resistant strains of *P. falciparum* (Schmidt *et al.*, 1978). Mefloquine was first used to treat chloroquine-resistant falciparum malaria in Thailand, where it was formulated with pyrimethamine–sulfadoxine (FANSIMEF) to delay development of drug-resistant parasites. This strategy failed, largely because slow elimination of mefloquine fostered the selection of resistant parasites at subtherapeutic drug concentrations (*see* White, 1999). Mefloquine now is recommended for oral use exclusively for the prophylaxis and chemotherapy of chloroquine-resistant or multidrug-resistant falciparum malaria. This quinoline is most effective for treating uncomplicated drug-resistant falciparum malaria when given 48 hours after the parasite burden has been substantially reduced by prior administration of an artemisinin antimalarial (*see* "Artemisinin," above) (White, 1997, 1999). The antimalarial activity, pharmacokinetic properties, therapeutic efficacy, and side effects of this drug have been extensively reviewed (Palmer *et al.*, 1993; Schlagenhauf, 1999). The chemical structure of mefloquine is shown below:

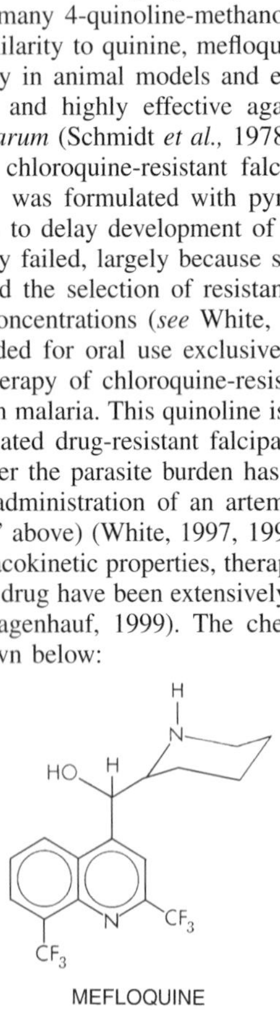

MEFLOQUINE

Antimalarial Actions. Mefloquine exists as a racemic mixture of four optical isomers with about the same anti-

malarial potency. It is a highly effective blood schizontocide, especially against mature trophozoite and schizont forms of malarial parasites. Mefloquine has no activity against early hepatic stages and mature gametocytes of *P. falciparum* or latent tissue forms of *P. vivax*. The drug may have some sporontocidal activity but is not used clinically for this purpose.

Mechanisms of Antimalarial Action and Resistance. The exact mechanism of action of mefloquine is unknown (*see* description of proposed mechanisms for quinoline action and resistance under "Chloroquine," above). As a blood schizontocide, mefloquine behaves like quinine in many respects but does not intercalate with DNA. The two compounds produce similar morphological changes in early erythrocytic ring stages of *P. falciparum* and *P. vivax* (Schmidt *et al.*, 1978). Like quinine, mefloquine competes for accumulation of chloroquine and inhibits chloroquine-induced clumping of pigment in erythrocytic plasmodia (Fitch *et al.*, 1979). Mefloquine causes swelling of the parasitic food vacuoles in *P. falciparum*. Like chloroquine, low extracellular concentrations of mefloquine raise the intravacuolar pH of plasmodia in excess of that predicted from passive distribution of a weak base. This suggests that mefloquine is concentrated in plasmodia by an unknown mechanism. Mefloquine may act by both inhibiting heme polymerization and forming toxic complexes with free heme that damage membranes and interact with other plasmodial components (*see* Palmer *et al.*, 1993; Sullivan *et al.*, 1998). The orientation of the hydroxyl and amine groups with respect to each other in mefloquine may be essential for its hydrogen bonding and antimalarial activity (Karle and Karle, 1991).

Certain isolates of *P. falciparum* exhibit resistance to mefloquine, especially those obtained from people exposed to the drug. Individuals harboring resistant parasites generally require larger than the usual doses of mefloquine to control their infections. Depending on their geographic origin and history of exposure to antimalarial drugs, many isolates of *P. falciparum* also display multidrug-resistant phenotypes. This raises the question of common or overlapping mechanisms responsible for intrinsic or acquired resistance to mefloquine and its structurally related antimalarials (*see* Palmer *et al.*, 1993). Genes in the multidrug-resistant (MDR) family can play a role in the resistance of *P. falciparum* to mefloquine. Products of this gene family lower intracellular concentrations of drugs in mammalian cells by increasing their efflux in an ATP-dependent manner; this effect is inhibited by some Ca^{2+} channel blockers but not by others. In *P. falciparum*, a gene of this family, *pfmdr1*, is usually but not always amplified, that is, the gene copy number is increased in parasites unresponsive *in vitro* to mefloquine and halofantrine (*see* Wilson *et al.*, 1993; Lim *et al.*, 1996). In contrast, there is no clear-cut association between chloroquine resistance and amplification of *pfmdr1* (Mungthin *et al.*, 1999). Patterns of resistance to mefloquine and quinine usually but not always overlap, suggesting that genetic differences aside from *pfmdr1* can play a differential role in resistance to these structurally related compounds (Zalis *et al.*, 1998). The stereoselectivity of mefloquine resistance (and action) has yet to be characterized.

Absorption, Fate, and Excretion. Mefloquine is taken orally because parenteral preparations cause severe local reactions.

The drug is well absorbed, a process enhanced by the presence of food. Probably due to extensive enterogastric and enterohepatic circulation, plasma levels of mefloquine rise in a biphasic manner to their peak in about 17 hours. The drug is widely distributed, highly bound (~98%) to plasma proteins, and slowly eliminated with a terminal half-life of about 20 days. The biotransformation of mefloquine has not been well characterized in human beings, although several metabolites are formed. Plasma levels of the inactive mefloquine 4-carboxylic acid exceed those of mefloquine itself and decline at about the same rate. In human beings, excretion is mainly by the fecal route; only about 10% of mefloquine appears unchanged in the urine. This is consistent with evidence that mefloquine undergoes biliary excretion and extensive enterohepatic circulation in animals. The (+) and (−) enantiomers of mefloquine exhibit quite different pharmacokinetic characteristics that relate to their biodisposition (Hellgren *et al.,* 1997). However, changes in the pharmacokinetics of racemic mefloquine that can occur as a result of age, ethnicity, pregnancy, and malarial illness do not substantially affect dosing regimens (*see* Palmer *et al.,* 1993; Schlagenhauf, 1999).

Therapeutic Uses. Mefloquine should be reserved for the prevention and treatment of malaria caused by chloroquine-resistant and multidrug-resistant *P. falciparum.* The drug is especially useful as a prophylactic agent for nonimmune travelers who stay for only brief periods in areas where these infections are endemic (*see* Table 40–1); prophylactic use of mefloquine for long-term residents of these regions should be avoided to prevent the selection of mefloquine-resistant parasites. Mefloquine and halofantrine are currently the only agents capable of ensuring suppression and cure of infections with multidrug-resistant *P. falciparum.* However, both medications can be given only orally, which is a major disadvantage for acutely ill patients, who are best treated with parenteral preparations of quinidine or quinine. Because of possible cross resistance, misuse of either mefloquine or halofantrine is likely to encourage the selection of falciparum parasites resistant to both drugs and possibly to quinine as well (*see* Wilson *et al.,* 1993). Clinical resistance to mefloquine can be overcome by increasing the dose, but only at the cost of increased drug toxicity. Vomiting frequently occurs when high single or divided doses of mefloquine are used to treat a malarial attack. Patients should be observed and the full dose repeated if vomiting occurs within the first hour. Typical dosage schedules for monotherapy of falciparum malaria with mefloquine are given in Table 40–2. These may be modified; for example, lower doses than shown are effective for suppression of malarial attacks in partially immune individuals. More information about this topic is provided in the review by Palmer and colleagues (1993).

To treat uncomplicated attacks of malaria due to chloroquine- and multidrug-resistant strains of *P. falciparum,* recent evidence indicates that mefloquine is most effective when used in tandem with an artemisinin compound such as artesunate (*see* "Artemisinin," above) (White, 1997, 1999). The artemisinin derivative is given first to reduce the parasite burden followed by mefloquine therapy to enhance parasite clearance and prevent recrudescence of infection. Studies have shown no clinically significant pharmacokinetic or toxic interactions between the artemisinin compounds and mefloquine when therapy with the latter is begun about 36 to 48 hours after the former. The 1250-mg adult dose of mefloquine is usually split; namely, 750 mg is given after food, followed by 500 mg 12 hours later. A similar strategy with 25 mg/kg of mefloquine, given either as a single or split dose on the second day of antimalarial therapy with artesunate, has produced excellent results in children (Price *et al.,* 1999).

Toxicity and Side Effects. The adverse effects of mefloquine were reviewed in detail by Palmer and colleagues (1993) and more recently by Schlagenhauf (1999). Mefloquine, given orally in single doses up to 1500 mg or in 250- to 500-mg doses each week, is generally well tolerated. Side effects such as nausea, late vomiting, abdominal pain, diarrhea, dysphoria, and dizziness are noted frequently. These tend to be dose-related, self-limiting, and at times difficult to distinguish from the clinical features of malarial illness. Signs of central nervous system toxicity occur in about half of the individuals taking mefloquine. Dizziness, ataxia, headache, alterations in motor function or the level of consciousness, and visual or auditory disturbances are self-limiting and usually mild. Severe neuropsychiatric reactions such as disorientation, seizures, encephalopathy, and a range of neurotic and psychotic manifestations are rare and usually reversible upon drug withdrawal and symptomatic therapy. While such complications occur more frequently in patients receiving therapeutic than prophylactic doses of mefloquine, they appear to be unrelated to plasma levels of the drug.

Contraindications and Interactions. At very high doses, mefloquine causes teratogenesis and developmental abnormalities in rodents. Prophylactic doses of mefloquine appear to cause little if any toxicity during the second and third trimesters of pregnancy, and they may even provide benefit to the fetus (Schlagenhauf, 1999). However, until more information becomes available or unless the risk of malarial infection outweighs the benefits of prophylaxis, caution dictates that mefloquine should be avoided during pregnancy, especially during the first trimester. Mefloquine should not be used in children weighing less than 5 kg. The drug is contraindicated for patients with a history of seizures, severe neuropsychiatric disturbances, or adverse reactions to quinoline antimalarials such as quinine, quinidine, and chloroquine. Use of mefloquine with these compounds must be avoided because of the increased risk of convulsions and cardiotoxicity. Although mefloquine can be taken safely 12 hours after a last dose of quinine, taking quinine shortly after mefloquine can be very hazardous because the latter is eliminated so slowly. Mefloquine is reported to increase the risk of seizures in epileptic patients controlled by valproate, and it may compromise adequate immunization by live typhoid vaccine. Until more data become available, caution is advised for use of mefloquine along with drugs that can perturb cardiac conduction. Recent studies do not indicate that mefloquine compromises the performance of tasks that require good motor coordination, for example, driving or operating machinery (Schlagenhauf, 1999).

Primaquine

History. The weak plasmodicidal activity of methylene blue, first discovered by Ehrlich in 1891, was later exploited to develop the 8-aminoquinoline antimalarials. From a large series of quinoline derivatives synthesized with methoxy and substituted 8-amino groups, pamaquine was the first introduced into medicine. During World War II the search for more potent and less toxic 8-aminoquinoline antimalarials led to the selection of pentaquine, isopentaquine, and primaquine for further evaluation (*see* earlier editions of this textbook). These compounds, in contrast with other antimalarials, act on tissue stages (exoerythrocytic) of *P. vivax* and *P. ovale* to prevent and cure relapsing malaria. Only *primaquine,* tested extensively during the Korean War, is widely used now. Unfortunately, hemolysis due to human glucose-6-phosphate dehydrogenase (G6PD) deficiency is notoriously identified with primaquine therapy, so there is a pressing need for alternatives to this important drug. The 8-aminoquinoline *tafenoquine,* formerly called WR 238605, shows promise but needs more evaluation in this regard (Walsh *et al.,* 1999). The chemical structure of primaquine is shown below:

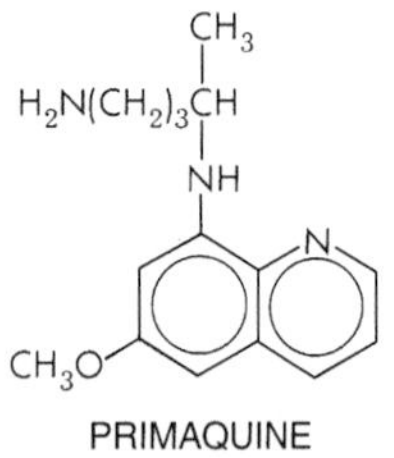

PRIMAQUINE

Antimalarial Actions. Primaquine destroys late hepatic stages and latent tissue forms of *P. vivax* and *P. ovale* and thus has great clinical value for the radical cure of relapsing malarias. The drug by itself will not suppress attacks of vivax malaria, even though it displays activity against erythrocytic stages of *P. vivax.* Though primaquine has activity against hepatic stages of *P. falciparum,* the compound is ineffective against erythrocytic stages of this parasite and hence is not used clinically to treat falciparum malaria. The 8-aminoquinolines exert a marked gametocidal effect against all four species of plasmodia that infect human beings, especially *P. falciparum.* Some strains of *P. vivax* exhibit partial resistance to the action of primaquine (Smoak *et al.,* 1997), which makes it imperative that the drug not be misused and that other antimalarials with similar properties be developed.

Mechanism of Antimalarial Action. There are as yet no methods for maintaining *P. vivax in vitro,* so little is known

about the antimalarial action of the 8-aminoquinolines, especially why they are far more active against tissue forms and gametes than asexual blood forms of plasmodia. Primaquine may be converted to electrophiles that act as oxidation-reduction mediators (*see* below and Tarlov *et al.,* 1962). Such activity could contribute to antimalarial effects by generating reactive oxygen species or interfering with electron transport in the parasite (Bates *et al.,* 1990).

Absorption, Fate, and Excretion. Primaquine causes marked hypotension after parenteral administration and therefore is given only by the oral route. Absorption from the gastrointestinal tract is nearly complete. After a single dose the plasma concentration reaches a maximum within 3 hours and then falls with an apparent elimination half-time of 6 hours (Fletcher *et al.,* 1981). The apparent volume of distribution is several times that of total body water.

Primaquine is rapidly metabolized; only a small fraction of an administered dose is excreted as the parent drug. Three identified oxidative metabolites of primaquine are 8-(3-carboxyl-1-methylpropylamino)-6-methoxyquinoline, 5-hydroxy primaquine, and 5-hydroxy-6-desmethylprimaquine. The carboxyl derivative is the major metabolite found in human plasma. After a single dose it reaches concentrations in plasma more than 10 times those of primaquine; this nontoxic metabolite also is eliminated more slowly and accumulates with multiple doses (*see* Symposium, 1987). The three metabolites of primaquine appear to have appreciably less antimalarial activity than does primaquine. However, except for the carboxyl derivative, their hemolytic activity, as assessed by formation of methemoglobin *in vitro,* is greater than that of the parent compound (Fletcher *et al.,* 1988).

Therapeutic Uses. Primaquine is reserved primarily for the terminal prophylaxis and radical cure of vivax and ovale (relapsing) malarias because of its high activity against latent tissue forms of these plasmodial species. The compound is given together with a blood schizontocide, usually chloroquine, to eradicate erythrocytic stages of these plasmodia and reduce the possibility of emerging drug resistance. For terminal prophylaxis, primaquine regimens are initiated shortly before or immediately after the patient leaves an endemic area (*see* Table 40–1). Radical cure of vivax or ovale malarias can be achieved if the drug is given either during the long-term latent period of infection or during an acute attack. Regimens for this purpose are shown in Table 40–2. Long-term use of primaquine should be avoided because of the risk of toxicity and sensitization.

Toxicity and Side Effects. Primaquine is fairly innocuous when given to Caucasians in the usual therapeutic doses. Larger doses cause occasional epigastric distress and mild-to-moderate abdominal distress in some individuals; these symptoms often are alleviated by taking the drug at mealtime. Mild anemia, cyanosis (methemoglobinemia), and leukocytosis are less common. High doses (60 to 240 mg of primaquine daily) accentuate the abdominal symptoms and cause methemoglobinemia in most subjects and leukopenia in some. Methemoglobinemia can occur even with usual doses of primaquine, chloroquine, or dapsone and can be severe in individuals with congenital deficiency of nicotinamide adenine dinucleotide (NADH) methemoglobin reductase (Coleman and Coleman, 1996). Hepatic function is unaffected. Granulocytopenia and agranulocytosis are rare complications of therapy and usually are associated with overdosage. Also rare are hypertension, arrhythmias, and symptoms referable to the central nervous system.

Therapeutic or higher doses of primaquine, *via* its oxidative metabolites, may cause acute hemolysis and hemolytic anemia in humans with G6PD deficiency. This X-linked inherited condition, primarily due to amino acid substitutions in the G6PD enzyme, affects more than 200 million people worldwide. More than 400 genetic variants have been identified that are associated with variable responses to oxidative stress. About 11% of African Americans have the A– variant of G6PD, which makes them vulnerable to hemolysis caused by prooxidant drugs such as primaquine. Sensitivity of erythrocytes to primaquine can be even more severe in some darker-hued Caucasian ethnic groups, including Sardinians, Sephardic Jews, Greeks, and Iranians. Because primaquine sensitivity is inherited by a gene on the X chromosome, hemolysis often is of intermediate severity in heterozygous females who have two populations of red cells, one normal and the other deficient in G6PD. Due to "variable penetrance," such females may be less frequently affected than predicted. Primaquine is the prototype of more than 50 drugs, including antimalarial sulfonamides, and other substances known to cause hemolysis in susceptible individuals with G6PD deficiency.

Precautions and Contraindications.   Patients should be tested for G6PD deficiency before they receive primaquine. If a daily dose of more than 30 mg of primaquine base (more than 15 mg in possibly sensitive patients) is given, repeated blood counts and at least gross examination of the urine for hemoglobin should be undertaken.

Primaquine is contraindicated for acutely ill patients suffering from systemic disease characterized by a tendency to granulocytopenia; very active forms of rheumatoid arthritis and lupus erythematosus are examples of such conditions. Primaquine should not be given to patients receiving other potentially hemolytic drugs or agents capable of depressing the myeloid elements of the bone marrow.

Proguanil

History.   *Proguanil* (PALUDRINE) is the common name for *chloroguanide,* a biguanide derivative that emerged in 1945 as a product of British antimalarial drug research. The antimalarial activity of proguanil was ascribed to cycloguanil, an active cyclic triazine metabolite shown to be a selective inhibitor of the bifunctional plasmodial dihydrofolate reductase-thymidylate synthetase. Indeed, investigation of compounds bearing a structural resemblance to cycloguanil resulted in the development of antimalarial dihydrofolate reductase inhibitors such as pyrimethamine. Accrued evidence also indicates that proguanil itself has

intrinsic antimalarial activity independent of its effect on parasite dihydrofolate reductase–thymidylate synthetase (*see* Fidock and Wellems, 1997).

Chemistry.   Proguanil and its triazine metabolite cycloguanil have the following chemical structures:

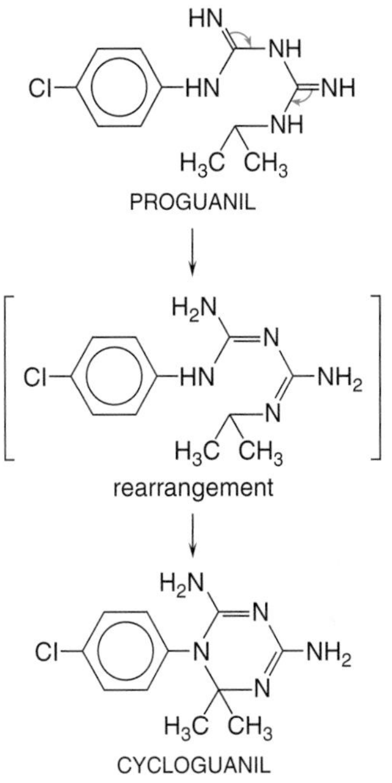

Proguanil has the widest margin of safety of a large series of antimalarial biguanide analogs examined. Dihalogen substitution in positions 3 and 4 of the benzene ring yields *chlorproguanil* (LAPUDRINE), a more potent prodrug than proguanil that also is used clinically. Cycloguanil is structurally related to pyrimethamine.

Antimalarial Actions.   Through its active metabolite, proguanil exerts causal prophylactic and suppressive activity in sporozoite-induced falciparum malaria, adequately controls the acute attack, and usually eradicates the infection. Proguanil suppresses acute attacks of vivax malaria, but because latent tissue stages of *P. vivax* are unaffected, erythrocytic forms often appear shortly after the drug is withdrawn. Proguanil treatment does not destroy gametocytes, but fertilized gametes encysted in the gut of the mosquito fail to develop normally.

Mechanisms of Antimalarial Action and Resistance.   The active triazine metabolite of proguanil selectively inhibits the bifunctional dihydrofolate reductase-thymidylate synthetase of sensitive plasmodia, causing inhibition of DNA synthesis and depletion of folate cofactors. This mechanism accounts for the slow antimalarial action of the antifolate biguanides compared to the quinoline antimalarials. By cloning and sequencing dihydrofolate reductase-thymidylate synthetase genes from sensitive and resistant *P. falciparum,* investigators found that certain amino acid changes near the dihydrofolate reductase binding site are linked to resistance to either the triazine metabolite, to pyrimethamine, or to both antimalarials. Specifically, resistance to cycloguanil (and chlorcycloguanil) can be linked to mutations leading to paired V^{16}/Thr^{108} substitutions in plasmodial dihydrofolate reductase, such resistance being especially enhanced by an additional substitution at Leu^{164}. This pattern differs from that typically observed for pyrimethamine resistance, where mutations result in a primary Asn^{108} substitution and secondary Arg^{50}, Ile^{51}, Arg^{59}, and Leu^{164} substitutions that progressively increase resistance; again resistance is increased most by a Leu^{164} substitution. However, overlapping resistance to cycloguanil and pyrimethamine indicates that mutation patterns leading to the final resistance phenotype may be quite complex. Thus, genetic analyses of resistant *P. falciparum* strains together with novel expression and assay systems represent a powerful approach for identifying and monitoring new generations of antimalarials directed at vulnerable plasmodia biochemical targets (*see,* for example, Fidock and Wellems, 1997; Cowman, 1998; Cortese and Plowe, 1998).

The presence of plasmodial dihydrofolate reductase is not required for the intrinsic antimalarial activity of proguanil or chlorproguanil (Fidock and Wellems, 1998), but the molecular basis for this activity is still unknown. Proguanil as the biguanide accentuates the mitochondrial membrane-potential-collapsing action of atovaquone against *P. falciparum* but displays no such activity by itself (*see* "Atovaquone," above) (Srivastava and Vaidya, 1999). In contrast to cycloguanil, resistance to the intrinsic antimalarial activity of proguanil itself, either alone or in combination with atovaquone, has yet to be well documented.

Absorption, Fate, and Excretion.   Proguanil is slowly but adequately absorbed from the gastrointestinal tract. After a single oral dose, peak concentrations of the drug in plasma usually are attained within 5 hours. The mean plasma elimination half-life is about 20 hours or longer depending on the rate of metabolism. Metabolism of proguanil in mammals cosegregates with mephenytoin oxidation polymorphism (Ward *et al.,* 1991) controlled by isoforms in the 2C subfamily of cytochrome P450. Only about 3% of Caucasians are deficient in this oxidation phenotype, as contrasted to about 20% of Asians and Kenyans. Proguanil is oxidized to two major metabolites, cycloguanil and an inactive 4-chlorophenyl-biguanide. On a 200-mg daily dosage regimen, extensive metabolizers develop plasma levels of cycloguanil that are above the therapeutic range, whereas poor metabolizers may not (Helsby *et al.,* 1993). Proguanil itself does not accumulate appreciably in tissues during long-term administration, except in erythrocytes, where its concentration is about three times that in plasma. Accumulation in infected erythrocytes could be critical for the intrinsic antimalarial effects of proguanil, either by itself or together with atovaquone. The inactive 4-chlorophenyl-biguanide metabolite is not readily detected in plasma but appears in increased quantities in the urine of poor proguanil metabolizers. In human beings, from 40% to 60% of the absorbed proguanil is excreted in urine either as the parent drug or the active metabolite.

Therapeutic Uses.   Proguanil together with chloroquine is used as a safe alternative to mefloquine or other regimens for the prophylaxis of falciparum malaria or mixed vivax and falciparum infections in parts of eastern, southern, and central Africa (*see* Table 40–1). This drug is not available in the United States but is prescribed in England and Europe for Caucasians traveling to those regions. Strains of *P. falciparum* resistant to proguanil emerge rapidly in areas where the drug is used exclusively, but breakthrough infections also may result from deficient conversion of this compound to its active antimalarial metabolite. Proguanil is ineffective against multidrug-resistant strains of *P. falciparum* in Thailand and New Guinea. The drug can protect against certain strains of *P. falciparum* in sub-Saharan Africa that are resistant to chloroquine and pyrimethamine-sulfadoxine.

Proguanil is effective and well tolerated when given orally once daily for three days in combination with atovaquone for treatment of malarial attacks due to chloroquine- and multidrug-resistant strains of *P. falciparum* and *P. vivax* (*see* "Atovaquone," above) (Looareesuwan *et al.,* 1999a,b). Indeed, this drug combination (MALARONE) has been successful in Southeast Asia where highly drug-resistant strains of *P. falciparum* prevail (*see* Kremsner *et al.,* 1999). While studies have shown proguanil plus atovaquone to be effective for prophylaxis, this application generally is discouraged to delay the development of drug resistance. *P. falciparum* readily develops clinical resistance to monotherapy with either proguanil or atovaquone. But resistance to the combination is uncommon unless the strain is initially resistant to atovaquone. In contrast, some strains resistant to proguanil do respond to proguanil plus atovaquone.

Toxicity and Side Effects.   In prophylactic doses of 200 to 300 mg daily, proguanil causes few untoward effects except occasional nausea and diarrhea. Large doses (1 g daily or more) may cause vomiting, abdominal pain, diarrhea, hematuria, and the transient appearance of epithelial cells and casts in the urine. Gross accidental or deliberate overdose (as much as 15 g) has been followed by complete recovery. Doses as high as 700 mg twice daily have been taken for more than 2 weeks without serious toxicity. Proguanil is considered safe for use during pregnancy. It is remarkably safe when used in conjunction with other antimalarial drugs such as chloroquine, atovaquone, tetracyclines, and other antifolates. This may bear on the use of proguanil plus atovaquone in conjunction with artemisinin derivatives to reduce parasite burden, impede transmission of infection, and further delay the development of drug resistance (van Vugt *et al.,* 1999).

Quinine

History.   The medicinal use of *quinine* dates back more than 350 years. Quinine is the chief alkaloid of cinchona, the bark of the South American cinchona tree, otherwise known as Peruvian,

Jesuit's, or Cardinal's bark. In 1633, an Augustinian monk named Calancha, of Lima, Peru, first wrote that a powder of cinchona "given as a beverage, cures the fevers and tertians." By 1640, cinchona was used to treat fevers in Europe, a fact first mentioned in the European medical literature in 1643. The Jesuit fathers were the main importers and distributors of cinchona in Europe, hence the name Jesuit's bark. Cinchona also was called Cardinal's bark because it was sponsored in Rome by the eminent philosopher Cardinal de Lugo. However, the medical establishment was slow to accept cinchona, delaying its official recognition until 1677 when it was included in the *London Pharmacopoeia* as "Cortex Peruanus" (Jarcho, 1993).

For almost two centuries the bark was employed for medicine as a powder, extract, or infusion. In 1820, Pelletier and Caventou isolated quinine and cinchonine from cinchona, and the use of the alkaloids as such gained favor rapidly. Quinine, together with secondary antimalarial antifolate or antibiotic drugs, is still the mainstay for treating attacks of chloroquine- and multidrug-resistant falciparum malaria today (*see* Table 40–2). However, multitherapy with other antimalarials may supplant the 7-day quinine regimens because of increasing resistance of *P. falciparum* to quinine together with its toxicity (*see* "Prospectus," below).

Chemistry.   Although quinine has been synthesized, the procedure is complex; quinine and the other alkaloids are, therefore, still obtained entirely from natural sources. Cinchona contains a mixture of more than 20 alkaloids. The most important of these are two pairs of optical isomers, quinine and quinidine, and cinchonidine and cinchonine. Quinine and cinchonidine are levorotatory. Quinine has the following chemical structure:

QUININE

Quinine contains a quinoline group attached through a secondary alcohol linkage to a quinuclidine ring. A methoxy side chain is attached to the quinoline ring and a vinyl to the quinuclidine. *Quinidine* has the same structure as quinine except for the steric configuration of the secondary alcohol group. Stereoisomerism at this position is relatively unimportant in the structure–activity relationship. Quinidine is both more potent as an antimalarial and more toxic than quinine (*see* Krishna and White, 1996). The many natural alkaloids related to quinine and the semisynthetic chemicals derived from quinine differ mainly in the nature of the substitutions on the side chain. These alterations cause quantitative but not qualitative changes in the pharmacological actions of the resulting compounds. The structure–activity relationships of the cinchona alkaloids are detailed in earlier editions of this textbook. Such studies provided the basis for the discovery of more effective and less toxic antimalarials, for example, *mefloquine*.

Pharmacological Effects.   *Antimalarial Actions.*   Quinine acts primarily as a blood schizontocide; it has little effect on sporozoites or preerythrocytic forms of malarial parasites. The alkaloid also is gametocidal for *P. vivax* and *P. malariae* but not for *P. falciparum*. Because of this spectrum of antimalarial activity, quinine is not used for prophylaxis. As both a suppressive and therapeutic agent, quinine is more toxic and less effective than chloroquine against malarial parasites susceptible to both drugs. However, quinine, along with its stereoisomer quinidine, is especially valuable for the treatment of severe illness due to chloroquine- and multidrug-resistant strains of *P. falciparum*, even though these strains have become more resistant to both agents in certain parts of Southeast Asia and South America.

The mechanism of the antimalarial action of quinine and related quinoline antimalarials is reviewed under "Chloroquine," above. In part because it is a weak base, quinine concentrates in the acidic food vacuoles of *P. falciparum*. The drug inhibits the nonenzymatic polymerization of the highly reactive, toxic heme molecule into a nontoxic polymer pigment called hemozoin. This is proposed to occur by a two-step process whereby the quinoline binds first to heme, and the resulting heme-drug complex binds to and saturates the heme-polymer chains (Sullivan *et al.*, 1996, 1998). Whether consequent buildup of heme itself, heme-quinoline complexes, or both kill the parasites is not established.

The basis of *P. falciparum* resistance to quinine is unknown and probably is quite complex. As discussed under "Chloroquine" in this chapter, patterns of *P. falciparum* resistance to quinine more closely resemble those of resistance to mefloquine and halofantrine rather than to chloroquine. Amplification of *pfmdr1* in *P. falciparum*, implicated in resistance to mefloquine and halofantrine, also can confer resistance to quinine *in vitro*. However, various field isolates that show resistance to mefloquine are quite sensitive to quinine and *vice versa* (*see* Meshnick, 1998; Zalis *et al.*, 1998).

Action on Skeletal Muscle.   Quinine and related cinchona alkaloids exert effects on skeletal muscle that have clinical implications. Quinine increases the tension response to a single maximal stimulus delivered to muscle directly or through nerves, but it also increases the refractory period of muscle so that the response to tetanic stimulation is diminished. The excitability of the motor end-plate region decreases so that responses to repetitive nerve stimulation and to acetylcholine are reduced. Thus, quinine can antagonize the actions of physostigmine on skeletal muscle as effectively as curare. Quinine also may produce alarming respiratory distress and dysphagia in patients with myasthenia gravis. Quinine may cause symptomatic relief of myotonia congenita. This disease is the pharmacological antithesis of myasthenia gravis, such that drugs effective in one syndrome aggravate the other.

Absorption, Fate, and Excretion. Quinine and its congeners are readily absorbed when given orally or intramuscularly. In the former case, absorption occurs mainly from the upper small intestine and is more than 80% complete, even in patients with marked diarrhea. After an oral dose, plasma levels of quinine reach a maximum in 3 to 8 hours and, after distributing into an apparent volume of about 1.5 liters per kg in healthy individuals, decline with a half-life of about 11 hours after termination of therapy. As reviewed by Krishna and White (1996), the pharmacokinetics of quinine change according to the severity of malarial infection. Values for both the apparent volume of distribution and the systemic clearance of quinine decrease, the latter more than the former, so that the average elimination half-life increases from 11 to 18 hours. After standard therapeutic doses, peak plasma levels of quinine may reach 15 to 20 mg per liter in severely ill Thai patients without causing major toxicity (see below); in contrast, levels greater than 10 mg per liter produce severe drug reactions in self-poisoning. Apparently, the high levels of plasma α_1-acid glycoproteins produced in severe malaria prevent quinine toxicity by binding the drug, thereby reducing the free fraction of quinine from about 15% down to 5% to 10% of its total concentration in plasma (see Krishna and White, 1996). As patients improve, levels of α_1-acid glycoprotein decrease, the apparent volume of distribution expands, the systemic clearance increases, and the plasma levels of quinine fall. Concentrations of quinine are lower in erythrocytes (33% to 40%) and cerebrospinal fluid (2% to 5%) than in plasma, and the drug readily reaches fetal tissues.

The cinchona alkaloids are extensively metabolized, especially by CYP3A4 in the liver (Zhao et al., 1996), so that only about 20% of an administered dose is excreted unaltered in the urine. There is no accumulation of the drugs in the body upon continued administration, because their metabolites are excreted in the urine. However, the major metabolite of quinine, 3-hydroxyquinine, retains some antimalarial activity and can accumulate and possibly cause toxicity in patients with renal failure (Newton et al., 1999). Renal excretion of quinine itself is more rapid when the urine is acidic than when it is alkaline.

Therapeutic Uses. *Treatment of Malaria.* Despite its potential toxicity, quinine remains the prototype blood schizontocide for the suppressive treatment and cure of chloroquine-resistant and multidrug-resistant falciparum malaria. In the severe illness, prompt use of loading doses of intravenous quinine (or quinidine) is imperative and can be lifesaving for nonimmune patients. Oral medication to maintain therapeutic concentrations is then given as soon as it can be tolerated and is continued for 5 to 7 days. Especially for treatment of infections with multidrug-resistant strains of *P. falciparum,* slower acting blood schizontocides such as a sulfonamide or tetracycline are given concurrently to enhance the action of quinine. Formula-

tions of quinine and quinidine and specific regimens for their use in the treatment of falciparum malaria are shown in Table 40–2.

Recommendations shown in Table 40–2 are derived from practice and should be modified as appropriate. In a series of studies over the past two decades, White and associates derived rational regimens, including the institution of loading doses, for the use of quinine and quinidine in the treatment of falciparum malaria in Southeast Asia (see Krishna and White, 1996). After full therapeutic doses, adult patients achieved very high plasma levels of quinine (15 to 20 mg per liter) with few signs of toxicity. Apparently elevated plasma α_1-acid glycoproteins during the acute phase of infection prevented quinine toxicity through binding most of the drug in plasma. Between 0.2 and 2.0 mg per liter has been estimated as the therapeutic range for "free" quinine. Regimens needed to achieve this target may vary according to age, severity of illness, and the responsiveness of *P. falciparum* to the drug. For example, lower doses are more effective in treating children in Africa than adults in Southeast Asia because the pharmacokinetics of quinine differ in the two populations, as does the susceptibility of *P. falciparum* to the drug (Krishna and White, 1996). If patients fail to respond clinically after 48 hours of treatment, therapeutic doses of quinine should be decreased by 30% to 50% to prevent untoward accumulation of the drug and toxicity (Krishna and White, 1996). Dosage regimens for quinidine are similar to those for quinine, although quinidine binds less to plasma proteins and has a larger apparent volume of distribution, greater systemic clearance, and shorter terminal elimination half-life than quinine (see Miller et al., 1989; Krishna and White, 1996).

Treatment of Nocturnal Leg Cramps. Recumbency leg muscle cramps (night cramps) have been reportedly relieved by quinine in a dose of 200 to 300 mg (available until 1995 in products that did not require a prescription) before retiring. In some individuals, only a brief period of quinine therapy has been said to be required to provide relief, but in others even large doses of the drug were ineffective. In 1995, the FDA issued a ruling that required drug manufacturers to stop marketing over-the-counter quinine products for nocturnal leg cramps. The FDA stated, as the basis for the ruling, that there were inadequate data to support the safety and effectiveness of quinine for use in treating nocturnal leg cramps.

Toxicity and Side Effects. The fatal oral dose of quinine for adults is about 2 to 8 g. Quinine is associated with a triad of dose-related toxicities when it is given at full therapeutic or excessive doses. These are cinchonism, hypoglycemia, and hypotension. Mild forms of cinchonism—consisting of tinnitus, high-tone deafness, visual disturbances, headache, dysphoria, nausea, vomiting, and postural hypotension—occur frequently and disappear soon after the drug is withdrawn. Hypoglycemia, too, is common but can be life-threatening if not promptly treated with intravenous glucose. Hypotension is rarer but also serious and most often associated with excessively rapid intravenous infusions of quinine or quinidine. Prolonged medication or high single doses also may produce gastrointestinal, cardiovascular, and dermal manifestations. These and other drug-associated toxicities are discussed in more detail below.

Hearing and vision are particularly affected. Functional impairment of the eighth nerve results in tinnitus, decreased auditory acuity, and vertigo. Visual signs consist of blurred vision, disturbed color perception, photophobia, diplopia, night blindness, constricted visual fields, scotomata, mydriasis, and even blindness (Bateman and Dyson, 1986). The visual and auditory effects are probably the result of direct neurotoxicity, although secondary vascular changes may have a role. Marked spastic constriction of the retinal vessels occurs; the retina is ischemic, the discs are pale, and retinal edema may ensue. In severe cases, optic atrophy results.

Gastrointestinal symptoms also are prominent in cinchonism. Nausea, vomiting, abdominal pain, and diarrhea result from the local irritant action of quinine, but the nausea and emesis also have a central basis. The skin often is hot and flushed, and sweating is prominent. Rashes frequently appear. Angioedema, especially of the face, occasionally is observed.

Quinine and quinidine, even at therapeutic doses, may cause hyperinsulinemia and severe hypoglycemia through their powerful stimulatory effect on pancreatic beta cells. Despite treatment with glucose infusions, this complication can be serious and possibly life-threatening, especially in pregnancy and prolonged severe infection.

Quinine rarely causes cardiovascular complications unless therapeutic plasma concentrations are exceeded (Krishna and White, 1996). However, severe hypotension is predictable when the drug is administered too rapidly by the intravenous route. Acute overdosage also may cause serious and even fatal cardiac dysrhythmias such as sinus arrest, junctional rhythms, A-V block, and ventricular tachycardia and fibrillation (Bateman and Dyson, 1986). Quinidine is even more cardiotoxic than quinine; its effects on the heart are discussed in detail in Chapter 35.

When small doses of cinchona alkaloids cause toxic manifestations, the individual usually is hypersensitive to the drug. Cinchonism may appear after a single dose of quinine, but it is usually mild. Cutaneous flushing, pruritus, skin rashes, fever, gastric distress, dyspnea, ringing in the ears, and visual impairment are the usual expressions of hypersensitivity; extreme flushing of the skin accompanied by intense, generalized pruritus is the most common form. Hemoglobinuria and asthma from quinine may occur more rarely. "Blackwater fever"—the triad of massive hemolysis, hemoglobinemia, and hemoglobinuria leading to anuria, renal failure, and even death—is a rare type of

hypersensitivity reaction to quinine therapy that occurs in pregnancy and in treatment of malaria. Quinine may cause milder hemolysis upon occasion, especially in people with glucose-6-phosphate dehydrogenase deficiency. Symptomatic thrombocytopenic purpura by an antibody- and complement-dependent mechanism also is rare, but this reaction can occur even in response to ingestion of tonic water ("cocktail purpura"). Asthma may occur in hypersensitive individuals, and other rare reactions to the drug include hypoprothrombinemia, leukopenia, and agranulocytosis. High doses of quinine used to terminate pregnancy may possibly cause fetal abnormalities.

Precautions, Contraindications, and Interactions. Quinine must be used with considerable caution, if at all, in patients who manifest hypersensitivity to the drug, especially when this takes the form of cutaneous, angioedematous, visual, or auditory symptoms. Quinine should be discontinued immediately if evidence of hemolysis appears. The drug should not be used in patients with tinnitus or optic neuritis. In patients with cardiac dysrhythmias, the administration of quinine requires the same precautions as for quinidine (see Chapter 35).

Because parenteral solutions of quinine are highly irritating, the drug should not be given subcutaneously; concentrated solutions may cause abscesses when injected intramuscularly or thrombophlebitis when infused intravenously. Absorption of quinine from the gastrointestinal tract can be delayed by antacids containing aluminum. Quinine and quinidine can delay the absorption and elevate plasma levels of digoxin and related cardiac glycosides (see Chapters 34 and 35). Likewise, the alkaloid may raise plasma levels of warfarin and related anticoagulants. The action of quinine at neuromuscular junctions will enhance the effect of neuromuscular blocking agents and oppose the action of acetylcholinesterase inhibitors (see above). The renal clearance of quinine can be decreased by cimetidine and increased by acidification of the urine.

ANTIBACTERIAL AGENTS IN ANTIMALARIAL CHEMOTHERAPY

Shortly after their introduction into therapeutics, the sulfonamides were found to have antimalarial activity, a property investigated extensively during World War II. The sulfones also were shown to be effective; the first trial of dapsone was against *P. falciparum* in 1943. The sulfonamides are used together with pyrimethamine and often in addition to quinine to treat chloroquine-resistant falciparum malaria, especially in parts of Africa. The tetracyclines are slow-acting blood schizontocides that are used alone for short-term prophylaxis and along with quinine for the treatment of malaria due to multidrug-resistant strains of *P. falciparum*.

Sulfonamides and Sulfones. The sulfonamides and sulfones are slow-acting blood schizontocides that are more active against *P. falciparum* than *P. vivax*. As *p*-aminobenzoate analogs that competitively inhibit the dihydropteroate synthase of *P. falciparum,* the sulfonamides are used together with an inhibitor of parasite dihydrofolate reductase to enhance their antiplasmodial action. For example, *sulfadiazine* and the dihydrofolate reductase inhibitor, pyrimethamine, are effective when used together with quinine to treat acute attacks of chloroquine-resistant falciparum malaria in Africa. The synergistic "antifolate" combination of *sulfadoxine,* a long-acting sulfonamide, with pyrimethamine (FANSIDAR) is used to treat malarial attacks in parts of Africa before medical advice can be obtained. The sulfone *dapsone* given with the biguanide chlorproguanil also has been effective for therapy of chloroquine-resistant falciparum malaria in Africa.

The future of the slow-acting antimalarial antifolates appears bleak unless they are used together with more effective, rapidly acting drugs, *e.g.,* an artemisinin derivative. Long-term use of pyrimethamine-sulfadoxine, for example, is no longer recommended for prophylaxis of falciparum malaria because of potentially serious toxicity from the sulfonamide (*see* "Diaminopyrimidines," above, and Chapter 44) (Bjorkman and Phillips-Howard, 1991). Moreover, resistance of *P. falciparum* to the antifolates is prevalent and develops rapidly upon exposure to these agents, rendering them ineffective in many parts of the world. Mutations that cause amino acid substitutions at several different loci in the dihydropteroate synthase of *P. falciparum* confer resistance to sulfadoxine and raise the K_i values for other sulfonamides and dapsone as well. These and other mutations that accumulate during exposure to sulfonamides, together with dihydrofolate reductase mutations associated with pyrimethamine and cycloguanil resistance, can severely compromise therapy of falciparum malaria with antifolate combinations (reviewed by Cowman, 1998).

Tetracyclines. Tetracyclines are particularly useful for the treatment of the acute malarial attack due to multidrug-resistant strains of *P. falciparum* that also show partial resistance to quinine (Chongsuphajaisiddhi *et al.,* 1986). Their relative slowness of action makes concurrent treatment with quinine mandatory for rapid control of parasitemia. Several tetracyclines appear equivalent, but tetracycline or doxycycline usually is recommended. Although tetracycline has shown marked activity against primary tissue schizonts of chloroquine-resistant *P. falciparum,* its long-term use for prophylaxis is not advised. Instead, doxycycline is used alone by travelers for short-term prophylaxis of multidrug-resistant strains. Dosage regimens for tetracyclines and doxycycline are listed in Tables 40–1 and 40–2. Because of their adverse effects on bones and teeth, tetracyclines should not be given to pregnant women or children less than 8 years old. Photosensitivity reactions or drug-induced superinfections may mandate discontinuation of therapy or prophylaxis with these agents (*see* Chapter 47).

GUIDELINES FOR PROPHYLAXIS AND CHEMOTHERAPY OF MALARIA

Pharmacological control of malaria poses a difficult challenge, because *P. falciparum,* which causes more than 85% of the cases and nearly all the deaths from human malaria, has become progressively more resistant to available antimalarial drugs. Fortunately, chloroquine is still effective against malarias caused by *P. ovale, P. malariae,* most strains of *P. vivax* (Newton and White, 1999), and chloroquine-sensitive strains of *P. falciparum* found in some geographic areas. However, chloroquine-resistant strains of *P. falciparum* now prevail in all endemic areas except Mexico, Central America west of the Panama Canal Zone, the Caribbean, and parts of South America and the Middle East (*see* Figure 40–2). Except for parts of Africa, extensive geographic overlap also exists between chloroquine resistance and resistance to pyrimethamine-sulfadoxine, an inexpensive combination of antifolate drugs used widely for the treatment of falciparum malaria. Multidrug-resistant falciparum malaria, especially prevalent and severe in Southeast Asia and Oceania, is now well established in South America and threatens Africa. These infections may not respond adequately even to toxic doses of individual antimalarial agents such as mefloquine or quinine.

Genetic studies indicate that single isolates of *P. falciparum* from patients in highly endemic areas contain many parasite clones with different drug-resistance phenotypes (Druilhe *et al.,* 1998). Any given clone may exhibit several drug-resistant traits and considerable variation in its infectious behavior. Differing and often complex genetic profiles also may be associated with a particular drug-resistant phenotype. Such findings strongly suggest that using any single agent to treat falciparum malaria encourages the selection and spread of drug-resistant strains that ultimately render such therapy both ineffective and hazardous. Indeed, parasites that had already developed drug-resistant traits might be even more prone to acquiring resistance to new unrelated antimalarial agents (Rathod *et al.,* 1997). These observations, along with evidence from dose-finding pharmacokinetic/pharmacodynamic clinical studies, strongly suggest using regimens consisting of two or more agents with complementary antimalarial actions to treat drug-resistant falciparum malaria (*see* reviews by White, 1997, 1999). Promising examples of such regimens under evaluation are an artemisinin compound followed by mefloquine; an artemisinin compound, chlorproguanil, and dapsone; and proguanil together with atovaquone. Current recommendations for drugs and dosing regimens for the prophylaxis and therapy of malaria in nonimmune individuals are shown in Tables 40–1 and 40–2. These will change and should serve only as general guidelines to be appropriately modified according to the status and habitat of the patient; the geographic origin, species, and drug resistance profile of infecting parasites; and the agents used locally for malaria control.

The following section presents an overview of the chemoprophylaxis and chemotherapy of malaria. For more details about individual drugs and their clinical applications, the reader should consult the text and references, especially reviews by Zucker and Campbell (1993) and Newton and White (1999). The latest information about malaria risk areas and prophylaxis is available from the Centers for Disease Control and Prevention (CDC) either *via* the Internet (www.cdc.gov/travel/travel.html) or by toll-free fax (888-232-3299). Consultation and emergency advice about treatment are available 24 hours a day from the duty officer, Division of Parasitic Diseases, CDC (telephone: 770-488-7760).

Importantly, drugs should not replace simple, inexpensive measures for malaria prevention. Individuals visiting malarious areas should take appropriate steps to prevent mosquito bites. Avoiding exposure to mosquitoes at dusk and dawn, usually times of maximal feeding, is one such measure. Others include wearing long-sleeved dark clothes, using insect repellents containing at least 30% *N,N'*-diethylmetatoluamide (DEET), and sleeping in well-screened rooms or under bed nets impregnated with a pyrethrin insecticide such as permethrin (Zucker and Campbell, 1993).

In areas where malaria is endemic, mefloquine is the drug of choice for prophylaxis. For those individuals who cannot take mefloquine, doxycycline represents an alternative chemoprophylactic agent. If both mefloquine and doxycycline are contraindicated, travelers must resort to less-effective regimens. In certain parts of Africa south of the Sahara, a combination of proguanil plus chloroquine is a common alternative for prophylaxis of chloroquine-resistant falciparum malaria. In areas where chloroquine-resistant *P. falciparum* is endemic, pyrimethamine-sulfadoxine is no longer recommended for prophylaxis because of potential drug toxicity. Instead, chloroquine prophylaxis along with a single therapeutic dose of pyrimethamine-sulfadoxine for emergency self-treatment of a presumed malarial attack should be used until help from a physician becomes available. But antifolate regimens may fail utterly to abort attacks with highly chloroquine-resistant or multidrug-resistant strains of *P. falciparum* such as those found in Southeast Asia. In some cases, prophylaxis with mefloquine or doxycycline may prove inadequate, and there may be no alternative but to control acute attacks with more than one course of chemotherapy if required (*see* below). In those few areas where chloroquine-sensitive strains of *P. falciparum* are found, chloroquine is still suitable for prophylaxis. It also remains the drug of choice for prophylaxis and control of infections due to *P. vivax, P. ovale,* and *P. malariae.* Attempts at radical cure of vivax malaria with primaquine should be delayed until the patient leaves an endemic area.

With the notable exception of infection due to drug-resistant strains of *P. falciparum,* the chemotherapy of an acute attack of human malaria is the same for all species of *Plasmodium;* only subsequent treatment depends on the species. A malarial attack should be viewed as a medical emergency, especially for vulnerable populations such as nonimmune travelers, pregnant women, or young children. Treatment with a rapidly acting blood schizontocide must be instituted promptly if falciparum malaria is suspected from a travel history and clinical findings. One should not wait for a definitive parasitological diagnosis in such patients because their clinical status may deteriorate rapidly. Moreover, the clinical presentation may be atypical, and thick blood smears may fail to reveal plasmodia in early stages of this infection. Chloroquine is the drug of choice for *P. vivax, P. ovale, P. malariae,* or chloroquine-sensitive strains of *P. falciparum.* The oral route of administration is used whenever possible, but chloroquine can be given intramuscularly or even intravenously if suitable precautions are taken (*see* text). Within 48 to 72 hours of initiating therapy, patients should show marked clinical improvement and a substantial decrease in parasitemia as monitored by daily thick blood smears. Lack of such a response or failure to clear parasites from the blood by 7 days is indicative of drug resistance. If chloroquine-resistant falciparum malaria is suspected, either from the travel history or lack of response to chloroquine, the preferred schizontocide is quinine despite its toxicity. For multidrug-resistant falciparum malaria, quinine is given together with other effective but slower-acting blood schizontocides such as antifolates or tetracyclines; choice of the latter drugs depends on multiple factors (*see* Table 40–2) and text). Again, the oral route of drug administration is preferred (quinine sulfate), but intravenous preparations (quinine dihydrochloride) should be given until oral medication can be taken. Quinidine gluconate, available in most hospitals in the United States, must be substituted for quinine dihydrochloride in the United States because the latter is no longer available. Exchange transfusion may be of additional value in severe falciparum malaria with high parasitemia (Miller *et al.,* 1989).

Attacks of malaria may recur during or after a course of antimalarial chemotherapy, even in the absence of reinfection. Recurrent attacks caused by *P. vivax, P. ovale,* or *P. malariae* usually are well controlled by another course of chloroquine, combined with or followed by a course of primaquine in the case of *P. vivax* or *P. ovale.* Some patients with vivax infection may require more than one course to effect a radical cure. Recrudescence of falciparum malarial attacks or parasitemia after appropriate treatment with chloroquine usually denotes infection with chloroquine-resistant plasmodia (for clinical classification of drug resistance, *see* World Health Organization, 1981). Quinine together with a slower-acting drug such as doxycycline in Southeast Asia or with antifolate antimalarials (*e.g.,* pyrimethamine-sulfadoxine) in Africa has successfully combated this problem (*see* Table 40–2). However, the 7-day course of required treatment, the toxic doses of quinine needed to overcome increasingly drug-resistant parasites, and poor patient compliance compromise the utility of these regimens. Mefloquine is a good alternative to quinine for geographic areas where resistance to both drugs is lacking. But mefloquine cannot be given parenterally, and it should not be taken with quinine. Moreover, toxic doses of mefloquine may be needed to eradicate parasites that exhibit *in vitro* cross-resistance to quinine. Especially promising compounds still undergoing evaluation for treatment of multidrug-resistant falciparum malaria are the artemisinin compounds. As the most rapidly acting and potent blood schizontocides known, these endoperoxides markedly reduce parasite burden in a single life cycle and, when used to initiate therapy, make ideal partners for other drugs such as mefloquine or chlorproguanide plus a sulfone. Parasite resistance to these relatively safe drugs has been minimal to date, probably because of their rapid action and very short half-lives (*see* text). Success against multidrug-resistant *P. falciparum* malaria also has been achieved with atovaquone together with an antimalarial biguanide such as proguanil or chlorproguanil. However, these combinations are relatively expensive and may not avoid the eventual selection of resistant parasites; strains of *P. falciparum* already exhibit resistance to either component alone.

Malarial infection, especially with *P. falciparum,* is a severe threat to children and pregnant women. With appropriate adjustments and safety precautions, the treatment of children is generally the same as for adults. However, tetracyclines should not be given except in an emergency to children less than 8 years old. Pregnant women should be urged not to travel to endemic areas if at all possible. While chloroquine, proguanil, and the artemisinin compounds may be used during pregnancy, antifolates, tetracyclines, and primaquine should be avoided (*see* text and Tables 40–1 and 40–2).

PROSPECTUS

The future of antimalarial chemotherapy, long the mainstay for malaria control, appears bleak unless prompt action is taken. As with antibiotics, extensive use of antimalarials has expedited the selection and spread of increasingly drug-resistant strains of *P. falciparum,* which cause lethal infections in human beings. Previously effective drugs such as chloroquine rapidly are becoming obsolete. The search for novel antimalarials has suffered from lack of financial resources and commitment. Even development and distribution of lifesaving alternatives such as artemisinin and its derivatives have been seriously delayed.

Ironically, the pace of relevant scientific discovery has dramatically increased. Cultivation and isolation of drug-sensitive and drug-resistant clones of *P. falciparum* from human beings and experimental animals now provide parasite materials essential for biological characterization, drug screening, and identification of molecular targets for drug action and resistance. The sequencing of the entire *P. falciparum* genome soon will be completed. Together with a rich variety of multidisciplinary experimental approaches, this achievement provides a major advance for antimalarial drug development.

Clinical evaluation of antimalarial chemotherapy must keep pace with the identification of promising new agents. To place the chemotherapy of malaria on a rational basis, combined pharmacokinetic and pharmacodynamic studies must continue to determine the optimal indications and appropriate dosing regimens for different parasite and human populations.

For further discussion of malaria, *see* chapter 216 in *Harrison's Principles of Internal Medicine,* 14th ed., McGraw-Hill, New York, 1998.

BIBLIOGRAPHY

Baltzan, M., Mehta, S., Kirkham, T.H., and Cosio, M.G. Randomized trial of prolonged chloroquine therapy in advanced pulmonary sarcoidosis. *Am. J. Respir. Crit. Care Med.,* **1999,** *160*:192–197.

Bates, M.D., Meshnick, S.R., Sigler, C.I., Leland, P., and Hollingdale, M.R. In vitro effects of primaquine and primaquine metabolites on exoerythrocytic stages of *Plasmodium berghei. Am. J. Trop. Med. Hyg.,* **1990,** *42*:532–537.

Bjorkman, A., and Phillips-Howard, P.A. Adverse reactions to sulfa drugs: implications for malaria chemotherapy. *Bull. World Health Organ.,* **1991,** *69*:297–304.

Brachman, P.S. Jr., Metchock, B., and Kozarsky, P.E. Effects of antimalarial chemoprophylactic agents on the viability of the Ty21a vaccine strain. *Clin. Infect. Dis.,* **1992,** *15*:1057–1058.

Bray, P.G., Mungthin, M., Ridley, R.G. and Ward, S.A. Access to hematin: the basis of chloroquine resistance. *Mol. Pharmacol.,* **1998,** *54*:170–179.

Cortese, J.F., and Plowe, C.V. Antifolate resistance due to new and known *Plasmodium falciparum* dihydrofolate reductase mutations expressed in yeast. *Mol. Biochem. Parasitol.,* **1998,** *94*:205–214.

Cowman, A.F., Galatis, D., and Thompson, J.K. Selection for mefloquine resistance in *Plasmodium falciparum* is linked to amplification of the *pfmdr1* gene and cross-resistance to halofantrine and quinine. *Proc. Natl. Acad. Sci. U.S.A.,* **1994,** *91*:1143–1147.

Danning, C.L., and Boumpas, D.T. Commonly used disease-modifying antirheumatic drugs in the treatment of inflammatory arthritis: an update on mechanisms of action. *Clin. Exp. Rheumatol.,* **1998,** *16*:595–604.

Druilhe, P., Daubersies, P., Patarapotikul, J., Gentil, C., Chene, L., Chongsuphajaisiddhi, T., Mellouk, S., and Langsley, G. A primary malarial infection is composed of a very wide range of genetically diverse but related parasites. *J. Clin. Invest.,* **1998,** *101*:2008–2016.

Ducharme, J., and Farinotti, R. Clinical pharmacokinetics and metabolism of chloroquine. Focus on recent advancements. *Clin. Pharmacokinet.,* **1996,** *31*:257–274.

Durand, R., Gabbett, E., di Piazza, J.P., Delabre, J.F., and Le Bras, J. Analysis of kappa and omega repeats of the *cg2* gene and chloroquine susceptibility in isolates of *Plasmodium falciparum* from sub-Saharan Africa. *Mol. Biochem. Parasitol.,* **1999,** *101*:185–197.

Easterbrook, M. Detection and prevention of maculopathy associated with antimalarial agents. *Int. Ophthalmol. Clin.*, **1999**, *39*:49–57.

Estes, M.L., Ewing-Wilson, D., Chou, S.M., Mitsumoto, H., Hanson, M., Shirey, E., and Ratliff, N.B. Chloroquine neuromyotoxicity. Clinical and pathologic perspective. *Am. J. Med.*, **1987**, *82*:447–455.

Ferone, R., Burchall, J.J., and Hitchings, G.H. *Plasmodium berghei* dihydrofolate reductase. Isolation, properties, and inhibition by antifolates. *Mol. Pharmacol.*, **1969**, *5*:49–59.

Fidock, D.A., and Wellems, T.E. Transformation with human dihydrofolate reductase renders malaria parasites insensitive to WR99210 but does not affect the intrinsic activity of proguanil. *Proc. Natl. Acad. Sci. U.S.A.*, **1997**, *94*:10931–10936.

Fitch, C.D., Chan, R.L., and Chevli, R. Chloroquine resistance in malaria: accessibility of drug receptors to mefloquine. *Antimicrob. Agents Chemother.*, **1979**, *15*:258–262.

Fletcher, K.A., Evans, D.A., Gilles, H.M., Greaves, J., Bunnag, D., and Harinasuta, T. Studies on the pharmacokinetics of primaquine. *Bull. World Health Organ.*, **1981**, *59*:407–412.

Foote, S.J., Thompson, J.K., Cowman, A.F., and Kemp, D.J. Amplification of the multidrug resistance gene in some chloroquine-resistant isolates of *P. falciparum*. *Cell*, **1989**, *57*:921–930.

Fritsch, C., Lang, K., von Schmiedeberg, S., Bolsen, K., Merk, H., Lehmann, P., and Ruzicka, T. Porphyria cutanea tarda. *Skin Pharmacol. Appl. Skin Physiol.*, **1998**, *11*:321–335.

Ginsburg, H., Famin, O., Zhang, J., and Krugliak, M. Inhibition of glutathione-dependent degradation of heme by chloroquine and amodiaquine as a possible basis for their antimalarial mode of action. *Biochem. Pharmacol.*, **1998**, *56*:1305–1313.

Goldberg, D.E., Sharma, V., Oksman, A., Gluzman, I.Y., Wellems, T.E., and Piwnica-Worms, D. Probing the chloroquine resistance locus of *Plasmodium falciparum* with a novel class of multidentate metal(III) coordination complexes. *J. Biol. Chem.*, **1997**, *272*:6567–6572.

Hellgren, U., Berggren-Palme, I., Bergqvist, Y., and Jerling, M. Enantioselective pharmacokinetics of mefloquine during long-term intake of the prophylactic dose. *Br. J. Clin. Pharmacol.*, **1997**, *44*:119–124.

Helsby, N.A., Edwards, G., Breckenridge, A.M., and Ward, S.A. The multiple dose pharmacokinetics of proguanil. *Br. J. Clin. Pharmacol.*, **1993**, *35*:653–656.

Horowitz, H., and Carbonaro, C.A. Inhibition of the *Salmonella typhi* oral vaccine strain, Ty21a, by mefloquine and chloroquine. *J. Infect. Dis.*, **1992**, *166*:1462–1464.

Hudson, A.T., Dickins, M., Ginger, C.D., Gutteridge, W.E., Holdich, T., Hutchinson, D.B., Pudney, M., Randall, A.W., and Latter, V.S. 566C80: a potent broad spectrum anti-infective agent with activity against malaria and opportunistic infections in AIDS patients. *Drugs Exp. Clin. Res.*, **1991**, *17*:427–435.

Hughes, W.T., Gray, V.L., Gutteridge, W.E., Latter, V.S., and Pudney, M. Efficacy of a hydroxynaphthoquinone, 566C80, in experimental *Pneumocystis carinii* pneumonitis. *Antimicrob. Agents Chemother.*, **1990**, *34*:225–228.

Hughes, W.T., and Oz, H.S. Successful prevention and treatment of babesiosis with atovaquone. *J. Infect. Dis.*, **1995**, *172*:1042–1046.

Hussein, Z., Eaves, J., Hutchinson, D.B., and Canfield, C.J. Population pharmacokinetics of atovaquone in patients with acute malaria caused by *Plasmodium falciparum*. *Clin. Pharmacol. Ther.*, **1997**, *61*:518–530.

Karle, J.M., and Karle, I.L. Crystal structure and molecular structure of mefloquine methylsulfonate monohydrate: implications for a malaria receptor. *Antimicrob. Agents Chemother.*, **1991**, *35*:2238–2245.

Kremsner, P.G., Looareesuwan, S., and Chulay, J.D. Atovaquone and proguanil hydrochloride for treatment of malaria. *J. Travel Med.*, **1999**, *6(suppl. 1)*:S18–S20.

Lim, A.S., Galatis, D., and Cowman, A.F. *Plasmodium falciparum*: amplification and overexpression of *pfmdr1* is not necessary for increased mefloquine resistance. *Exp. Parasitol.*, **1996**, *83*:295–303.

Looareesuwan, S., Chulay, J.D., Canfield, C.J., and Hutchinson, D.B. Malarone (atovaquone and proguanil hydrochloride): a review of its clinical development for treatment of malaria. Malarone Clinical Trials Study Group. *Am. J. Trop. Med. Hyg.*, **1999a**, *60*:533–541.

Looareesuwan, S., Viravan, C., Webster, H.K., Kyle, D.E., Hutchinson, D.B., and Canfield, C.J. Clinical studies of atovaquone, alone or in combination with other antimalarial drugs, for treatment of acute uncomplicated malaria in Thailand. *Am. J. Trop. Med. Hyg.*, **1996**, *54*:62–66.

Looareesuwan, S., Wilairatana, P., Glanarongran, R., Indravijit, K.A., Supeeranontha, L., Chinnapha, S., Scott, T.R., and Chulay, J.D. Atovaquone and proguanil hydrochloride followed by primaquine for treatment of *Plasmodium vivax* malaria in Thailand. *Trans. R. Soc. Trop. Med. Hyg.*, **1999b**, *93*:637–640.

Loria, P., Miller, S., Foley, M., and Tilley, L. Inhibition of the peroxidative degradation of haem as the basis of action of chloroquine and other quinoline antimalarials. *Biochem. J.*, **1999**, *339*:363–370.

McGready, R., Cho, T., Cho, J.J., Simpson, J.A., Luxemburger, C., Dubowitz, L., Looareesuwan, S., White, N.J., and Nosten, F. Artemisinin derivatives in the treatment of falciparum malaria in pregnancy. *Trans. R. Soc. Trop. Med. Hyg.*, **1998**, *92*:430–433.

Miller, K.D., Greenberg, A.E., and Campbell, C.C. Treatment of severe malaria in the United States with a continuous infusion of quinidine gluconate and exchange transfusion. *N. Engl. J. Med.*, **1989**, *321*:65–70.

Mungthin, M., Bray, P.G., Ridley, R.G., and Ward, S.A. Central role of hemoglobin degradation in mechanisms of action of 4-aminoquinolines, quinoline methanols, and phenanthrene methanols. *Antimicrob. Agents Chemother.*, **1998**, *42*:2973–2977.

Mungthin, M., Bray, P.G., and Ward, S.A. Phenotypic and genotypic characteristics of recently adapted isolates of *Plasmodium falciparum* from Thailand. *Am. J. Trop. Med. Hyg.*, **1999**, *60*:469–474.

Naisbitt, D.J., Williams, D.P., O'Neill, P.M., Maggs, J.L., Willock, D.J., Pirmohamed, M., and Park, B.K. Metabolism-dependent neutrophile cytotoxicity of amodiaquine: a comparison with pyronaridine and related antimalarial drugs. *Chem. Res. Toxicol.*, **1998**, *11*:1586–1595.

Newton, P., Keeratithakul, D., Teja-Isavadharm, P., Pukrittayakamee, S., Kyle, D., and White, N. Pharmacokinetics of quinine and 3-hydroxyquinine in severe falciparum malaria with acute renal failure. *Trans. R. Soc. Trop. Med. Hyg.*, **1999**, *93*:69–72.

Pappaioanou, M., Fishbein, D.B., Dreesen, D.W., Schwartz, I.K., Campbell, G.H., Sumner, J.W., Patchen, L.C., and Brown, W.J. Antibody response to preexposure human diploid-cell rabies vaccine given concurrently with chloroquine. *N. Engl. J. Med.*, **1986**, *314*:280–284.

Pearson, P.A., Piracha, A.R., Sen, H.A., and Jaffe, G.J. Atovaquone for the treatment of toxoplasma retinochoroiditis in immunocompetent patients. *Ophthalmology*, **1999**, *106*:148–153.

Povoa, M.M., Adagu, I.S., Oliveira, S.G., Machado, R.L., Miles, M.A., and Warhurst, D.C. Pfmdr1 Asn1042Asp and Asp1246Tyr polymorphisms, thought to be associated with chloroquine resistance, are present in chloroquine-resistant and -sensitive Brazilian field isolates of *Plasmodium falciparum*. *Exp. Parasitol.*, **1998**, *88*:64–68.

Price, R.N., Simpson, J.A., Teja-Isavatharm, P., Than, M.M., Luxemburger, C., Heppner, D.G., Chongsuphajaisiddhi, T., Nosten,

F., and White, N.J. Pharmacokinetics of mefloquine combined with artesunate in children with acute falciparum malaria. *Antimicrob. Agents Chemother.,* **1999,** *43*:341–346.

Rathod, P.K., McErlean, T., and Lee, P.C. Variations in frequencies of drug resistance in *Plasmodium falciparum. Proc. Natl. Acad. Sci. U.S.A.,* **1997,** *94*:9389–9393.

Raynes, K. Bisquinoline antimalarials: their role in malaria chemotherapy. *Int. J. Parasitol.,* **1999,** *29*:367–379.

Reed, M.B., Saliba, K.J., Caruana, S.R., Kirk, K., and Cowman, A.F. Pgh1 modulates sensitivity and resistance to multiple antimalarials in *Plasmodium falciparum. Nature,* **2000,** *403*:906–909.

Rolan, P.E., Mercer, A.J., Tate, E., Benjamin, I., and Posner, J. Disposition of atovaquone in humans. *Antimicrob. Agents Chemother.,* **1997,** *41*:1319–1321.

Sanchez, C.P., Wunsch, S., and Lanzer, M. Identification of a chloroquine importer in *Plasmodium falciparum.* Differences in import kinetics are genetically linked with the chloroquine-resistant phenotype. *J. Biol. Chem.,* **1997,** *272*:2652–2658.

Schmidt, L.H., Crosby, R., Rasco, J., and Vaughan, D. Antimalarial activities of various 4-quinolonemethanols with special attention to WR-142,490 (mefloquine). *Antimicrob. Agents Chemother.,* **1978,** *13*:1011–1030.

Shah, G.K., Cantrill, H.L., and Holland, E.J. Vortex keratopathy associated with atovaquone. *Am. J. Ophthalmol.,* **1995,** *120*:669–671.

Shanks, G.D., Kremsner, P.G., Sukwa, T.Y., van der Berg, J.D., Shapiro, T.A., Scott, T.R., and Chulay, J.D. Atovaquone and proguanil hydrochloride for prophylaxis of malaria. *J. Travel Med.,* **1999,** *6(suppl. 1)*:S21–S27.

Smoak, B.L., DeFraites, R.F., Magill, A.J., Kain, K.C., and Wellde, B.T. *Plasmodium vivax* infections in U.S. Army troops: failure of primaquine to prevent relapse in studies from Somalia. *Am. J. Trop. Med. Hyg.,* **1997,** *56*:231–234.

Srivastava, I.K., and Vaidya, A.B. A mechanism for the synergistic antimalarial action of atovaquone and proguanil. *Antimicrob. Agents Chemother.,* **1999,** *43*:1334–1339.

Su, X., Ferdig, M.T., Huang, Y., Huynh, C.Q., Liu, A., You, J., Wootton, J.C., and Wellems, T.E. A genetic map and recombination parameters of the human malaria parasite *Plasmodium falciparum. Science,* **1999,** *286*:1351–1353.

Su, X., Kirkman, L.A., Fujioka, H., and Wellems, T.E. Complex polymorphisms in an approximately 300-kDa protein are linked to chloroquine-resistant *P. falciparum* in Southeast Asia and Africa. *Cell,* **1997,** *91*:593–603.

Sullivan, D.J. Jr., Gluzman, I.Y., Russell, D.G., and Goldberg, D.E. On the molecular mechanism of chloroquine's antimalarial action. *Proc. Natl. Acad. Sci. U.S.A.,* **1996,** *93*:11865–11870.

Sullivan, D.J. Jr., Matile, H., Ridley, R.G., and Goldberg, D.E. A common mechanism for blockade of heme polymerization by antimalarial quinolines. *J. Biol. Chem.,* **1998,** *273*:31103–31107.

Svensson, U.S., Ashton, M., Trinh, N.H., Bertilsson, L., Dinh, X.H., Nguyen, V.H., Nguyen, T.N., Nguyen, D.S., Lykkesfeldt, J., and Le, D.C. Artemisinin induces omeprazole metabolism in human beings. *Clin. Pharmacol. Ther.,* **1998,** *64*:160–167.

Torres, R.A., Weinberg, W., Stansell, J., Leoung, G., Kovacs, J., Rogers, M., and Scott, J. Atovaquone for salvage treatment and suppression of toxoplasmic encephalitis in patients with AIDS. *Clin. Infect. Dis.,* **1997,** *24*:422–429.

Trager, W., and Jensen, J.B. Human malaria parasites in continuous culture. *Science,* **1976,** *193*:673–675.

van Vugt, M., Edstein, M.D., Proux, S., Lay, K., Ooh, M., Looareesuwan, S., White, N.J., and Nosten, F. Absence of an interaction between artesunate and atovaquone—proguanil. *Eur. J. Clin. Pharmacol.,* **1999,** *55*:469–474.

Vercesi, A.E., Rodrigues, C.O., Uyemura, S.A., Zhong, L., and Moreno, S.N. Respiration and oxidative phosphorylation in the apicomplexan parasite *Toxoplasma gondii. J. Biol. Chem.,* **1998,** *273*:31040–31047.

von Seidlein, L., Duraisingh, M.T., Drakeley, C.J., Bailey, R., Greenwood, B.M., and Pinder, M. Polymorphism of the *pfmdr1* gene and chloroquine resistance in *Plasmodium falciparum* in The Gambia. *Trans. R. Soc. Trop. Med. Hyg.,* **1997,** *91*:450–453.

Walsh, D.S., Looareesuwan, S., Wilairatana, P., Heppner, D.G. Jr., Tang, D.B., Brewer, T.G., Chokejindachai, W., Viriyavejakul, P., Kyle, D.E., Milhous, W.K., Schuster, B.G., Horton, J., Braitman, D.J., and Brueckner, R.P. Randomized dose-ranging study of the safety and efficacy of WR 238605 (Tafenoquine) in the prevention of relapse of *Plasmodium vivax* malaria in Thailand. *J. Infect. Dis.,* **1999,** *180*:1282–1287.

Ward, S.A., Helsby, N.A., Skjelbo, E., Brøsen, K., Gram, L.F., and Breckenridge, A.M. The activation of the biguanide antimalarial proguanil co-segregates with the mephenytoin oxidation polymorphism—a panel study. *Br. J. Clin. Pharmacol.,* **1991,** *31*:689–692.

Wellems, T.E., Panton, L.J., Gluzman, I.Y., do Rosario, V.E., Gwadz, R.W., Walker-Jonah, A., and Krogstad, D.J. Chloroquine resistance not linked to *mdr*-like genes in a *Plasmodium falciparum* cross. *Nature,* **1990,** *345*:253–255.

White, N.J. Antimalarial drug resistance and combination chemotherapy. *Philos. Trans. R. Soc. Lond. Biol. Sci.,* **1999,** *354*:739–749.

White, N.J. Assessment of the pharmacodynamic properties of antimalarial drugs in vivo. *Antimicrob. Agents Chemother.,* **1997,** *41*:1413–1422.

Wilson, C.M., Serrano, A.E., Wasley, A., Bogenschutz, M.P., Shankar, A.H., and Wirth, D.F. Amplification of a gene related to mammalian *mdr* genes in drug-resistant *Plasmodium falciparum. Science,* **1989,** *244*:1184–1196.

Wilson, C.M., Volkman, S.K., Thaithong, S., Martin, R.K., Kyle, D.E., Milhous, W.K., and Wirth, D.F. Amplification of *pfmdr1* associated with mefloquine and halofantrine resistance in *Plasmodium falciparum* from Thailand. *Mol. Biochem. Parasitol.,* **1993,** *57*:151–160.

Winstanley, P.A., Watkins, W.M., Newton, C.R., Nevill, C., Mberu, E., Warn, P.A., Waruiru, C.M., Mwangi, I.N., Warrell, D.A., and Marsh, K. The disposition of oral and intramuscular pyrimethamine/sulphadoxine in Kenyan children with high parasitemia but clinically non-severe falciparum malaria. *Br. J. Clin. Pharmacol.,* **1992,** *33*:143–148.

Zalis, M.G., Pang, L., Silveira, M.S., Milhous, W.K., and Wirth, D.F. Characterization of *Plasmodium falciparum* isolated from the Amazon region of Brazil: evidence for quinine resistance. *Am. J. Trop. Med. Hyg.,* **1998,** *58*:630–637.

Zhao, X.J., Yokoyama, H., Chiba, K., Wanwimolruk, S., and Ishizaki, T. Identification of human cytochrome P450 isoforms involved in the 3-hydroxylation of quinine by human liver microsomes and nine recombinant cytochromes P450. *J. Pharmacol. Exp. Ther.,* **1996,** *279*:1327–1334.

MONOGRAPHS AND REVIEWS

Barradell, L.B., and Fitton, A. Artesunate. A review of its pharmacology and therapeutic efficacy in the treatment of malaria. *Drugs,* **1995,** *50*:714–741.

Bateman, D.N., and Dyson, E.H. Quinine toxicity. *Adverse Drug React. Acute Poisoning Rev.,* **1986,** *5*:215–233.

Chongsuphajaisiddhi, T., Gilles, C.H.M., Krogstand, D.J., Salako, L.A., Warrell, D.A., White, N.J., Beales, P.F., Najera, J.A., Sheth, U.K., Spencer, H.C., and Wernsdorfer, W.H. Severe and complicated malaria. World Health Organization Malaria Action Programme. *Trans. R. Soc. Trop. Med. Hyg.,* **1986,** *80*(suppl.):3–50.

Coleman, M.D., and Coleman, N.A. Drug-induced methaemoglobin-aemia. Treatment issues. *Drug Saf.,* **1996,** *14*:394–405.

Cowman, A.F. The molecular basis of resistance to the sulfones, sulfon-amides, and dihydrofolate reductase inhibitors. In, *Malaria: Parasite Biology, Pathogenesis, and Protection.* (Sherman, I.W., ed.) ASM Press, Washington D.C., **1998,** pp. 317–330.

Davey, D.G. Chemotherapy of malaria. Part 1. Biological basis of testing methods. In, *Experimental Chemotherapy,* Vol. 1. (Schnitzer, R. J., and Hawking, F., eds.) Academic Press, New York, **1963,** pp. 487–511.

de Vries, P.J., and Dien, T.K. Clinical pharmacology and therapeutic potential of artemisinin and its derivatives in the treatment of malaria. *Drugs,* **1996,** *52*:818–836.

Foley, M., and Tilley, L. Quinoline antimalarials: mechanisms of action and resistance and prospects for new agents. *Pharmacol. Ther.,* **1998,** *79*:55–87.

Griffin, J.P. Drug interactions with antimalarial agents. *Adverse Drug React. Toxicol. Rev.,* **1999,** *18*:25–43.

Hill, J. Chemotherapy of malaria. Part 2. The antimalarial drugs. In, *Experimental Chemotherapy.* Vol. 1. (Schnitzer, R.J., and Hawking, F., eds.) Academic Press, New York, **1963,** pp. 513–601.

Jarcho, S. *Quinine's Predecessor: Francesco Torti and the Early History of Cinchona.* Johns Hopkins University Press, Baltimore, **1993.**

Kasper, L.H. *Toxoplasma* infection. In, *Harrison's Principles of Internal Medicine,* 14th ed. (Fauci, A.S., Braunwald, E., Isselbacker, K.J., Wilson, J.D., Martin, J.B., Kasper, D.L., Hauger S.L., and Longo, D.L., eds.) McGraw-Hill, New York, **1998,** pp. 1197–1202.

Klayman, D.L. Qinghaosu (artemisinin): an antimalarial drug from China. *Science,* **1985,** *228*:1049–1055.

Krishna, S., and White, N.J. Pharmacokinetics of quinine, chloroquine and amodiaquine. Clinical implications. *Clin. Pharmacokinet.,* **1996,** *30*:263–299.

Meshnick, S.R. From Quinine to Qinghaosu. In, *Malaria: Parasite Biology, Pathogenesis, and Protection* (Sherman, I.W., ed.) ASM Press, Washington D.C., **1998,** pp. 341–353.

Meshnick, S.R., Taylor, T.E., and Kamchonwongpaisan, S. Artemisinin and the antimalarial endoperoxides: from herbal remedy to targeted chemotherapy *Microbiol. Rev.,* **1996,** *60*:301–315.

Newton, P., and White, N.J. Malaria: new developments in treatment and prevention. *Annu. Rev. Med.,* **1999,** *50*:179–192.

O'Neill, P.M., Bray, P.G., Hawley, S.R., Ward, S.A., and Park, B.K. 4-Aminoquinolines—past, present, and future: a chemical perspective. *Pharmacol. Ther.,* **1998,** *77*:29–58.

Palmer, K.J., Holliday, S.M., and Brogden, R.N. Mefloquine. A review of its antimalarial activity, pharmacokinetic properties and therapeutic efficacy. *Drugs,* **1993,** *45*:430–475.

Rennie, I.G. Clinically important ocular reactions to systemic drug therapy. *Drug Saf.,* **1993,** *9*:196–211.

Schlagenhauf, P. Mefloquine for malaria chemoprophylaxis 1992–1998: a review *J. Travel Med.,* **1999,** *6*:122–133.

Symposium on DARAPRIM. (Various authors.) *Trans. R. Soc. Trop. Med. Hyg.,* **1952,** *46*:467–508.

Symposium. (Various authors.) *Primaquine: Pharmacokinetics, Metabolism, Toxicity, and Activity.* Proceedings of a meeting of the Scientific Working Group on the Chemotherapy of Malaria. (Wernsdorfer, W.H., and Trigg, P.I., eds.) Wiley, New York, **1987.**

Tarlov, A.R., Brewer, G.J., Carson, P.E., and Alving, A.S. Primaquine sensitivity. *Arch. Intern. Med.,* **1962,** *109*:209–234.

Vaidya, A.B. Mitochondrial physiology as a target for atovaquone and other antimalarials. In, *Malaria: Parasite Biology, Pathogenesis, and Protection.* (Sherman, I.W., ed.) ASM Press, Washington D.C., **1998,** pp. 355–368.

World Health Organization. *Chemotherapy of Malaria,* 2nd ed. WHO Monograph Series No. 27. (Bruce-Chwatt, L.J., and Black, R.H., eds.) WHO, Geneva, **1981.**

World Health Organization. World malaria situation in 1994. Part I. Population at risk. *Wkly. Epidemiol. Rec.,* **1997,** *72*:269–276.

Zucker, J.R., and Campbell, C.C. Malaria. Principles of prevention and treatment. *Infect. Dis. Clin. North Am.,* **1993,** *7*:547–567.

CHAPTER 41

DRUGS USED IN THE CHEMOTHERAPY OF PROTOZOAL INFECTIONS
(*Continued*)

Amebiasis, Giardiasis, Trichomoniasis, Trypanosomiasis, Leishmaniasis, and Other Protozoal Infections

James W. Tracy and Leslie T. Webster, Jr.

Human beings host a wide variety of protozoal parasites that can be transmitted by insect vectors, directly from other mammalian reservoirs, or from one person to another. Because protozoa multiply rapidly in their hosts and effective vaccines are as yet unavailable, chemotherapy has been the only practical way to both treat infected individuals and reduce transmission. The immune system plays a crucial role in protecting against the pathological consequences of protozoal infection. Thus, opportunistic infections with protozoa are prominent in infants, individuals with cancer, transplant recipients, those receiving immunosuppressive drugs or extensive antibiotic therapy, and persons with advanced human immunodeficiency virus (HIV) infection. Treatment of protozoal infections in immunocompromised individuals is especially difficult, and the outcome is often unsatisfactory.

Most antiprotozoal drugs have been in use for years despite major advances in bioscience relevant to parasite biology, host defenses, and mechanisms of disease. Satisfactory agents for treating important protozoal infections such as African trypanosomiasis *(sleeping sickness) and chronic* Chagas' disease *still are lacking. Many effective antiprotozoal drugs are toxic at therapeutic doses, a problem exacerbated by increasing drug resistance. Development of drug resistance also poses a serious threat to better-tolerated antiprotozoal agents in current use.*

This chapter briefly describes important human protozoal infections other than malaria and features the drugs used to treat them. Presented first are amebiasis, giardiasis, *and* trichomoniasis, *three cosmopolitan infections caused by anaerobic protozoa. Descriptions of* toxoplasmosis *and* cryptosporidiosis *follow: these infections especially threaten immunocompromised individuals such as those with acquired immunodeficiency syndrome (AIDS). Next are* trypanosomiasis *and* leishmaniasis, *two devastating infections caused by different* Kinetoplastidae *that affect millions of people in tropical regions. Mention is then made of far less-common protozoal infections of human beings such as* balantidiasis *and* babesiosis. *The main text deals with the properties and uses of primary drugs for these infections—i.e.,* diloxanide furoate, eflornithine, melarsoprol, metronidazole, nifurtimox, pentamidine, sodium stibogluconate, *and* suramin. *Less attention is devoted to secondary and historical drugs used for these infections—i.e.,* chloroquine, emetine/dehydroemetine, iodoquinol, quinacrine, *and the antiprotozoal antibiotics. The chapter concludes with a brief prospectus about the future of antiprotozoal chemotherapy.*

INTRODUCTION TO PROTOZOAL INFECTIONS OF HUMAN BEINGS

Amebiasis. Amebiasis affects about 10% of the world's population, causing invasive disease in about 50 million people and death in about 100,000 of these annually. Although endemic amebiasis is relatively rare in the general population of the United States, it still has a prevalence of 2% to 4%. Infection is especially common in lower socioeconomic groups and institutionalized individuals living under crowded, poorly hygienic conditions. Two morphologically identical but genetically and biochemically distinct species of *Entamoeba* (*i.e., E. histolytica* and *E. dispar*) have been isolated from infected persons. *E. dispar* accounts for about 90% of the infections and *E. histolytica* for about 10%, but only *E. histolytica* is pathogenic. Human beings are the only known hosts for these protozoa, which are transmitted exclusively by the fecal-oral route. Ingested amebic *cysts* from contaminated food or water survive acid gastric contents and transform into *trophozoites* that usually act as commensals in the large intestine—that is, they produce cysts but otherwise cause little harm. However, in about 1% of people infected with *E. histolytica,* trophozoites invade the intestinal mucosa and cause mild to severe colitis that can be acute or chronic (*amebic dysentery*). In some instances, these trophozoites also invade extraintestinal tissues, chiefly the liver and less commonly the brain, where they produce amebic abscesses and systemic disease (*see* Ravdin, 1995).

Drugs used to treat amebiasis can be categorized as *luminal, systemic,* or *mixed* amebicides. Luminal amebicides, exemplified by *diloxanide furoate, iodoquinol,* and the nonabsorbed aminoglycoside *paromomycin,* are active against only intestinal forms of amoebae. These compounds can be used successfully by themselves to treat asymptomatic or mild intestinal forms of amebiasis or after a systemic or mixed amebicide to eradicate the infection. Systemic amebicides are effective only against invasive forms of amebiasis. These agents have been employed primarily to treat severe amebic dysentery (*dehydroemetine*) or hepatic abscesses (dehydroemetine or *chloroquine*), but they are not recommended unless other drugs fail or cause unacceptable side effects. Mixed amebicides are active against both intestinal and systemic forms of amebiasis. *Metronidazole,* a nitroimidazole derivative, is the prototypical mixed amebicide available in the United States. Use of this compound and its analogs, *tinidazole* and *ornidazole,* has revolutionized the treatment of this infection. Because metronidazole is well absorbed and therefore may fail to reach the large intestine in therapeutic concentrations, it is likely to be more effective against systemic amebiasis than intestinal amebiasis. Antibiotics such as paromomycin or a *tetracycline* can be used in conjunction with metronidazole to treat severe forms of intestinal amebiasis. Treatment with metronidazole is generally followed by a luminal amebicide to effect a cure. Asymptomatic infected individuals, *i.e.,* cyst passers, should be tested for stool antigens that distinguish *E. histolytica* from *E. dispar* (Haque *et al.,* 1998), and those testing positive for *E. histolytica* should be treated with a luminal amebicide. If such tests are unavailable, treatment with a luminal amebicide still is recommended on a presumptive basis if infection with *E. histolytica* is suspected (*see* World Health Organization, 1997).

Giardiasis. Giardiasis, caused by the flagellated protozoan *Giardia lamblia,* is prevalent worldwide and is also the most commonly reported intestinal protozoal infection in the United States (*see* Farthing, 1996). Most infected individuals are asymptomatic. However, these organisms may produce either isolated cases or epidemics of diarrhea that can be transient or persistent. Indeed, nonbloody diarrhea lasting for 2 weeks or longer should suggest a diagnosis of giardiasis. Malabsorption, manifest by steatorrhea and weight loss, may occur, and the illness can be life-threatening in individuals with hypogammaglobulinemia. Infection results from ingestion of *cysts,* most commonly from fecal contamination of water or food. No intermediate host is required, although several species of mammals may serve as reservoirs for *G. lamblia.* Human-to-human transmission is especially common among children in day-care centers and nurseries, as well as among other institutionalized individuals and among male homosexuals. Because the infectious cysts persist for long periods in cold water, hikers can become infected by drinking water from contaminated lakes or streams. Community outbreaks, in contrast, usually result from contaminated central water supplies. Ingested cysts change into motile *trophozoites* in the upper small intestine, where they may or may not produce disease. The diagnosis of giardiasis is made by identification of cysts or trophozoites in fecal specimens or of trophozoites in duodenal contents. Chemotherapy with a 5-day course of *metronidazole* usually is successful, although therapy may have to be repeated or prolonged in some instances. A single dose of *tinidazole,* a nitroimidazole drug available outside the United States, probably is superior to metronidazole for treatment of giardiasis. *Furazolidone* (FUROXONE), although less effective, often is prescribed for children because the drug is available in a pleasant liquid formulation. The nonabsorbed aminoglycoside *paromomycin* has been used to treat pregnant women to avoid any possible mutagenic effects of the other drugs. Ironically, furazolidone is the only drug currently approved by the United States Food and Drug Administration (FDA) for treatment of giardiasis (*see* Ortega and Adam, 1997).

Trichomoniasis. Trichomoniasis is caused by the flagellated protozoan *Trichomonas vaginalis.* This organism inhabits the genitourinary tract of the human host, where it causes vaginitis in women and, uncommonly, urethritis in men. Transmission of the infection occurs by sexual contact, and over 200 million people worldwide become infected each year. In the United States, at least 3 million women are infected annually, and prevalence is greater among those with multiple sexual partners (*see* Heine and McGregor, 1993). Only *trophozoite* forms of *T. vaginalis* have been identified in infected secretions. Confirmed cases usually are treated successfully with a single course of *metronidazole.* Treatment failures usually result from failure to adhere to the therapeutic regimen or from reinfection by an untreated asymptomatic partner. However, the prevalence of metronidazole-resistant isolates of *T. vaginalis* is increasing, so the prospect of widespread drug resistance cannot be ignored (Sobel *et al.,* 1999). In countries other than the United States, nitroheterocyclic drugs such as *tinidazole* are preferred for therapy of trichomoniasis. However, due to emerging resistance of *T. vaginalis* to such drugs, alternatives such as vaginal application of *paromomycin* are undergoing evaluation.

Toxoplasmosis. Toxoplasmosis is a cosmopolitan zoonotic infection caused by the obligate intracellular protozoan *Toxoplasma gondii* (*see* Wong and Remington, 1993). Although cats and other feline species are the natural hosts, tissue cysts (*bradyzoites*) have been recovered from all mammalian species examined. The four most common routes of infection in human beings are (1) ingestion of undercooked meat containing tissue cysts, (2) ingestion of vegetable matter contaminated with soil containing infective *oocysts,* (3) direct oral contact with feces of cats shedding oocysts, and (4) transplacental fetal infection with *tachyzoites* from acutely infected mothers.

Toxoplasmosis produces clinical symptoms in only about 10% to 20% of immunocompetent individuals, although close to 70% of adults in the United States become seropositive. The acute illness is usually self-limiting in this population so that no treatment is required. Congenital toxoplasmosis usually presents as ocular disease (chorioretinitis), which can appear as late as 15 to 20 years after prenatal exposure. Individuals who are immunocompromised, however, are at risk of developing toxoplasmic encephalitis from reactivation of tissue cysts deposited in the brain. Toxoplasmic encephalitis is a major cause of death in AIDS patients, and it is in this group that chemotherapy is both essential and inadequate. The primary treatment for toxoplasmic encephalitis consists of the antifolates *pyrimethamine* and *sulfadiazine* given over long periods to prevent relapses (*see* Georgiev, 1994). However, therapy must be discontinued in about 50% of cases because of toxicity due primarily to the sulfa compound. In this instance, *clindamycin* is usually substituted for sulfadiazine, but other antibiotics such as *spiramycin* and *trimetrexate* have yielded comparable results in preliminary studies. *Atovaquone,* shown to be active against both the tachyzoite and cyst forms of *T. gondii,* is a less toxic alternative but also may be less effective than pyrimethamine and sulfadiazine (Torres *et al.,* 1997; *see* "Atovaquone" in Chapter 40). Because spiramycin concentrates in placental tissue, regimens using this drug have been advocated for the first 20 weeks of pregnancy to prevent congenital toxoplasmosis; spiramycin therapy then can be continued or switched to pyrimethamine and sulfadiazine for the remainder of pregnancy (*see* Georgiev, 1994).

Cryptosporidiosis. Coccidian protozoan parasites of the genus *Cryptosporidium* have been detected in mammals, birds, fish, and reptiles. Recognized as human pathogens in 1976, these enteric organisms can cause severe bouts of watery diarrhea in both domestic animals and human beings (*see* Griffiths, 1998). Infectious *oocysts* in feces may be spread either by direct human-to-human contact or by contaminated water supplies, the latter an established route of epidemic infection. Groups at risk include travelers, children in day-care facilities, male homosexuals, animal handlers, veterinarians, and other health care personnel. Immunocompromised individuals are especially vulnerable. After ingestion, the mature oocyte is digested, releasing *sporozoites* that invade host epithelial cells, penetrating the cell membrane but not actually entering the cytoplasm. In most individuals, infection is self-limited. However, in AIDS patients and other immunocompromised individuals, the severity of voluminous, secretory diarrhea usually requires hospitalization and supportive therapy to prevent severe electrolyte imbalance and dehydration. Combined therapy with *paromomycin* and *azithromycin* may be beneficial in some AIDS patients suffer-

ing from chronic cryptosporidiosis (Smith *et al.,* 1998). However, there is currently no known effective drug for treatment of cryptosporidiosis.

Trypanosomiasis. African trypanosomiasis or "sleeping sickness" is caused by subspecies of the hemoflagellate *Trypanosoma brucei* that are transmitted by bloodsucking tsetse flies of the genus *Glossinia.* Largely restricted to central Africa, where it threatens livestock (*nagana*), this infection is often fatal to human beings unless they are treated. Due to strict surveillance, vector control, and early therapy, the prevalence of African sleeping sickness declined to its nadir in the early 1960s. However, relaxation of such measures together with massive population displacement and breakdowns in societal infrastructure due to armed conflict led to a resurgence of this serious illness in the 1990s. An estimated 300,000 to 500,000 Africans carry the infection, even though it is rare in travelers returning to the United States. Early human infection without central nervous system (CNS) involvement (stage 1) is typified by a febrile illness, lymphadenopathy, splenomegaly, and occasional myocarditis that result from systemic dissemination of the parasites. Stage 2 disease is characterized by later CNS involvement. There are two types of African trypanosomiasis, the East African (Rhodesian) and West African (Gambian), caused by *T. brucei rhodesiense* and *T. brucei gambiense,* respectively. *T.b. rhodesiense* produces a progressive and usually fatal form of disease marked by early involvement of the CNS and terminal cardiac failure; *T.b. gambiense* causes illness characterized by later involvement of the CNS and a more long-term course. Standard treatment with toxic agents such as *suramin, pentamidine,* and *melarsoprol* has not changed for decades. All three compounds must be given parenterally over long periods, can cause serious toxic reactions, and may fail to produce a cure (*see* Pépin and Milord, 1994). Melarsoprol, the only one effective against late-stage CNS disease, causes a fatal reactive encephalopathy in about 10% of treated patients. Moreover, resistance to this agent is on the rise. Although *T. brucei* offers a variety of attractive molecular targets for selective pharmacological intervention, few have been turned to practical advantage despite their promise in experimental systems and animal models (reviewed by Wang, 1995 and 1997). Developed as an anticancer agent, *eflornithine* is an irreversible inhibitor of ornithine decarboxylase, a key enzyme in polyamine metabolism. This compound has shown marked efficacy against both early and late stages of human *T.b. gambiense* infection, even in some patients who failed to respond to melarsoprol therapy. However, when given in high doses intravenously and then orally for several weeks, eflornithine causes significant toxicity in nearly 40% of patients. This agent also is expensive and ineffective as monotherapy for infections of *T.b. rhodesiense* (*see* "Eflornithine," further on in this chapter). Thus, economic, pharmacokinetic, and logistical problems may limit widespread use of eflornithine (*see* Pépin and Milord, 1994).

American trypanosomiasis or *Chagas' disease,* a zoonotic infection caused by *Trypanosoma cruzi,* affects about 24 million people from southern California to Argentina and Chile (*see* Tanowitz *et al.,* 1992; Kirchhoff, 1996), where the chronic form of the disease in adults is a major cause of cardiomyopathy, megaesophagus, megacolon, and death. Bloodsucking triatomid bugs infesting poor rural dwellings most commonly transmit this infection to young children; transplacental transmission also may occur in endemic areas. Acute infection is evidenced by a raised tender skin nodule (*chagoma*) at the site of inoculation; other signs may be absent or range from fever, adenitis, skin rash, and hepatosplenomegaly to, albeit rarely, acute myocarditis and death. Invading metacyclic *trypomastigotes* penetrate host cells, especially macrophages, where they proliferate as *amastigotes*. The latter then differentiate into trypomastigotes that enter the bloodstream. Circulating trypomastigotes do not multiply until they invade other cells or are ingested by an insect vector during a blood meal. After recovery from the acute infection within a few weeks to months, individuals usually remain asymptomatic for years despite sporadic parasitemia. During this period their blood can transmit the parasites to transfusion recipients and accidentally to laboratory workers. An increasing fraction of adults develop overt chronic disease of the heart and gastrointestinal tract as they age. Progressive destruction of myocardial cells and neurons of the myenteric plexus results from the special tropism of *T. cruzi* for muscle cells. Whether or not an undefined autoimmune response also contributes to the pathogenesis of Chagas' disease is controversial, especially since recent studies with improved techniques indicate the presence of *T. cruzi* at sites of cardiac lesions (Urbina, 1999). However, immunological defenses, especially cell-mediated immunity, do play a role in modulating the course of disease. Two nitroheterocyclic drugs, *nifurtimox,* which is available from the Centers for Disease Control and Prevention (CDC), and *benznidazole,* which is not, are used to treat this infection. Both agents suppress parasitemia and may even cure the acute phase of Chagas' disease, but they are far less effective against the chronic infection (Kirchhoff, 1996). Both drugs are toxic and must be taken for long periods. Field isolates vary with respect to their susceptibility to nifurtimox and benznidazole. Moreover, resistance to both compounds can be induced in the laboratory. While both drugs can generate intracellular free radicals, their mechanisms of action and resistance are not well understood. Drug development for Chagas' disease has lagged due to lack of economic incentives, even though *T. cruzi* offers a variety of potential therapeutic targets (*see* Urbina, 1999). Indeed, alternative measures such as improved vector control and housing accommodations have substantially reduced transmission of Chagas' disease in Brazil, Chile, and Venezuela (World Health Organization, 1999).

Leishmaniasis. Leishmaniasis is a complex, vector-borne zoonosis caused by about 20 different species of obligate intramacrophage protozoa of the genus *Leishmania*. Small mammals and canines generally serve as reservoirs for these pathogens, which can be transmitted to human beings by the bites of some 30 different species of female phlebotomine sandflies. Various forms of leishmaniasis affect people in southern Europe and many tropical and subtropical regions throughout the world. Flagellated extracellular, free *promastigotes,* regurgitated by feeding flies, enter the host, where they attach to and become phagocytized by tissue macrophages. There they transform into *amastigotes,* which reside and multiply within phagolysosomes until the cell bursts. Released amastigotes then propagate the infection by invading more macrophages. Amastigotes taken up by feeding sandflies transform back into promastigotes, thereby completing the transformation cycle. The particular localized or systemic disease syndrome caused by *Leishmania* depends

on the species or subspecies of infecting parasite, the distribution of infected macrophages, and especially the host's immune response. In increasing order of systemic involvement and potential clinical severity, major syndromes of human leishmaniasis have been classified into *cutaneous, mucocutaneous, diffuse cutaneous,* and *visceral (kala azar)* forms. Leishmaniasis is becoming increasingly recognized as an AIDS-associated opportunistic infection (*see* Berman, 1997).

The classification, clinical features, course, and chemotherapy of the various human leishmaniasis syndromes have been reviewed recently, in addition to the biochemistry and immunology of the parasite and host germane to chemotherapy (*see* Herwaldt, 1999b). Cutaneous forms of leishmaniasis generally are self-limiting, whereas the mucocutaneous, diffuse cutaneous, and visceral forms are not. Initial parenteral treatment with *pentavalent antimonials,* according to regimens based on collective empirical experience, appears safe and effective in most cases, but prolonged therapy is required, and resistance to these agents is increasing. *Amphotericin B* and *pentamidine,* formerly judged as secondary drugs because of unacceptable toxicity at therapeutic doses, are now undergoing reevaluation because of improved formulations and dosage schedules. For example, in 1997 the FDA approved a lipid formulation of amphotericin B (AMBISOME; *see* Chapter 49) for therapy of visceral leishmaniasis. Now considered a first-line drug for this indication, lipid formulations of amphotericin B can be especially useful for patients who fail antimonial therapy or who cannot tolerate long courses of parenteral therapy (*see* Meyerhoff, 1999; Herwaldt, 1999b). The aminoglycoside *paromomycin* has been used parenterally as monotherapy for visceral leishmaniasis in India or together with pentavalent antimonials for treatment of this illness in other settings. Adjunctive parenteral immunotherapy with agents such as *interferon gamma* derives from observations that *Leishmania* amastigotes that replicate in quiescent macrophages are killed by macrophage activation. Intact cellular immunity, especially T1 helper-cell development and activity, plays a critical role in host protection as is illustrated by the poor responses and relapses of AIDS patients and other immunocompromised individuals to antileishmaniasis chemotherapy. As yet, no oral therapy for leishmaniasis has proven to be highly effective (Herwaldt, 1999a), although a number of different compounds, especially those interfering with parasite lipid biosynthesis, have shown promise in experimental systems and disease models (*see* Urbina, 1999).

Other Protozoal Infections. Just a few of the many less-common protozoal infections of human beings are highlighted here. The reader is referred to the *14th edition* of *Harrison's Principles of Internal Medicine* for more details and to Rosenblatt (1999) for specific therapeutic regimens.

Babesiosis, caused by either *Babesia microcoti* or *B. divergens,* is a tick-borne zoonosis that superficially resembles malaria in that the parasites invade erythrocytes, producing a febrile illness, hemolysis, and hemoglobinuria. This infection usually is mild and self-limiting but can be severe or even fatal in asplenic or severely immunocompromised individuals. The macrolide antibiotic *azithromycin* has been used successfully along with either *quinine* or *atovaquone* (*see* Chapter 40) to treat babesiosis in experimental animals and in some patients; *chloroquine* is not effective.

Gastrointestinal infections caused by a variety of pathogenic protozoa can be especially severe in immunocompromised patients such as those with AIDS. Whereas chemotherapy of cryptosporidiosis has proven to be difficult in this population, it has produced better responses in two other coccidian infections of human beings, *i.e., isosporiasis* and *cyclosporiasis.* Thus, *trimethoprim-sulfamethoxazole* has been found successful for controlling diarrhea due to *Isospora belli* in AIDS patients, even though relapses may occur and long-term maintenance therapy may be required. *Pyrimethamine* has been used to treat those patients who cannot tolerate sulfonamides. Trimethoprim-sulfamethoxazole also is effective against *Cyclospora cayatensis,* an organism that can produce prolonged or relapsing diarrhea in travelers or AIDS patients. *Microsporidiosis,* a transient infection in travelers to the tropics but a major cause of diarrhea in immunocompromised individuals, can be caused by several different genera of microsporidian parasites that respond in varying degrees to the benzimidazole anthelmintic *albendazole (see* Chapter 42), given alone or with other agents such as *furazolidone. Balantidiasis,* caused by the ciliated protozoan *Balantidium coli,* is an infection of the large intestine that may be confused with amebiasis. Unlike amebiasis, however, this infection usually responds to *tetracycline* therapy.

CHLOROQUINE

The pharmacology and toxicology of chloroquine are presented in Chapter 40. Only those features of the drug pertinent to its use in amebiasis are described here.

The unique therapeutic value of chloroquine for *extraintestinal amebiasis* in human beings relates to its direct toxic action against trophozoites of *E. histolytica* together with the fact that it is highly concentrated in liver. Chloroquine is used as a systemic amebicide to treat *hepatic amebiasis* only when treatment with metronidazole is unsuccessful or contraindicated. The clinical response to chloroquine in patients with hepatic amebiasis is usually prompt, and there is no evidence that amoebae develop resistance to this agent. The drug is far less effective in intestinal amebiasis, because it is almost completely absorbed from the small bowel and attains only low concentrations in the intestinal wall. Colonic infection with *E. histolytica* is always the source of extraintestinal amebiasis, so a drug effective in intestinal amebiasis is given routinely to all patients receiving chloroquine for hepatic amebiasis; such therapy reduces the relapse rate.

The conventional course of treatment with chloroquine phosphate for extraintestinal amebiasis in adults is 1 g daily for 2 days, followed by 500 mg daily for at least 2 to 3 weeks. Because of the low toxicity of this drug, this dose can be increased or the schedule can be repeated if necessary.

DILOXANIDE FUROATE

History. *Diloxanide* is a dichloroacetamide derivative that was identified as a result of the examination of a series of substituted acetanilides for amebicidal activity. Of the many derivatives of diloxanide prepared, the furoate ester proved to be appreciably more active than the parent compound in experimentally infected rats (Main *et al.,* 1960). The results of clinical trials showed it to be effective in cases of acute intestinal amebiasis. *Diloxanide*

furoate (FURAMIDE), which is not available in the United States, has the following chemical structure:

DILOXANIDE FUROATE

Pharmacological Effects. Diloxanide is directly amebicidal when tested *in vitro.* The furoate ester is active at 0.01 to 0.1 μg/ml and is thus considerably more potent than emetine. Little is known of its mechanism of action.

Absorption, Fate, and Excretion. After oral ingestion, the ester is largely hydrolyzed in the lumen or mucosa of the intestine to diloxanide and furoic acid; only diloxanide appears in the systemic circulation. In experimental animals, 60% to 90% of an oral dose is excreted in the urine within 48 hours, chiefly as the glucuronide. More than half of this appears within 6 hours. Excretion in the feces accounts for 4% to 9% of the dose. The blood concentration of diloxanide peaks within 1 hour but falls to a fraction of this level within 6 hours.

Therapeutic Uses. Given alone, diloxanide furoate is effective for treatment of asymptomatic passers of amebic cysts (Krogstad *et al.,* 1978). Other drugs effective in asymptomatic amebiasis are *iodoquinol* and *paromomycin* (Anonymous, 1998). Diloxanide is ineffective when administered alone in the treatment of extraintestinal amebiasis, and its efficacy when used alone in the treatment of acute amebiasis with frank dysentery is controversial. Although good results have been reported in some areas, other trials have been less successful (Suchak *et al.,* 1962). In trials carried out primarily in asymptomatic subjects passing trophozoites or cysts, or in patients with nondysenteric, symptomatic intestinal amebiasis, treatment with diloxanide furoate resulted in a high percentage of cures (Wolfe, 1973). Diloxanide furoate is used along with or after an appropriate systemic or mixed amebicide to effect a cure of invasive and extraintestinal amebiasis.

Diloxanide furoate is given orally. The recommended dose for adults is 500 mg three times daily for 10 days. If necessary, treatment can be extended to 20 days. Children should be given 20 mg/kg per day in three divided doses for 10 days.

Toxicity and Side Effects. Diloxanide furoate generally is well tolerated and side effects are mild. Flatulence is most commonly reported; nausea, vomiting, diarrhea, pruritus, and urticaria occur occasionally (*see* Wolfe, 1973).

EFLORNITHINE

History. *Eflornithine* (α-*difluoromethylornithine, DFMO;* ORNIDYL) is an irreversible catalytic (suicide) inhibitor of ornithine decarboxylase, the enzyme that catalyzes the first and rate-limiting step in the biosynthesis of polyamines (Metcalf *et al.,* 1978; reviewed by McCann and Pegg, 1992). The polyamines—putrescine, spermidine, and, in mammals, spermine—are required for cell division and for normal cell differentiation. Both in animal models and *in vitro,* eflornithine arrests the growth of several types of tumor cells, providing the basis for its initial clinical evaluation as an antitumor agent (*see* Pegg, 1988). The discovery that eflornithine cured rodent infections with *Trypanosoma brucei* first focused attention on protozoal polyamine biosynthesis as a potential target for chemotherapeutic attack (Bacchi *et al.,* 1980). Eflornithine has been used since with considerable success to treat West African (Gambian) trypanosomiasis caused by *T.b. gambiense.* The drug usually is curative, even for late CNS stages of infection resistant to arsenical trypanocides (*see* Pépin and Milord, 1994). In contrast, this compound is largely ineffective for East African trypanosomiasis (*see* below), and its high cost and marginal success as therapy for both neoplasia and *Pneumocystis carinii* pneumonia make its future uncertain (*see* McCann and Pegg, 1992). However, recent studies have sparked renewed interest in the potential of eflornithine as a chemopreventive agent for people at high risk for various types of epithelial cancer (*see* Meyskens and Gerner, 1999). Eflornithine is no longer available for systemic use in the United States but may be available for treatment of Gambian trypanosomiasis by special request from the World Health Organization (*see* Table VII–1). The chemical structure of eflornithine is shown below:

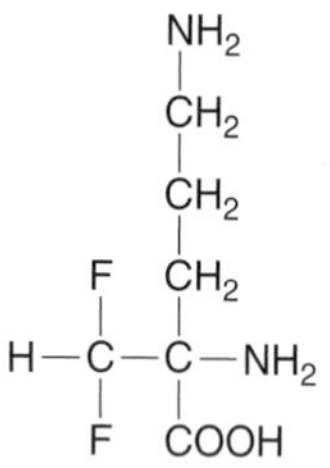

EFLORNITHINE

Antitrypanosomal Effects. The effects of eflornithine have been evaluated both on drug-susceptible and drug-resistant *T. brucei in vitro* and on infections with these parasites in rodent models. This cytostatic agent has multiple biochemical effects on trypanosomes. Not only is polyamine and trypanothione biosynthesis reduced and methionine metabolism altered, but macromolecular biosynthesis is generally depressed and cell division ceases. Trypanosomes exposed to eflornithine change from long, slender, quickly dividing bloodstream forms that avoid host defenses by rapidly synthesizing variable cell-surface glycoproteins to short, nonreplicating forms that fail to synthesize these molecules and are rapidly cleared from the circulation (Wang, 1997).

Molecular mechanisms of eflornithine action and resistance in African trypanosomes, though complex, are becoming better understood, as indeed are the reasons for the drug's greater effectiveness against *T.b. gambiense* than against *T.b. rhodesiense* (reviewed by Wang, 1997). Eflornithine irreversibly inhibits both mammalian and trypanosomal ornithine decarboxylases, thereby preventing the synthesis of putrescine, a precursor of polyamines needed for cell division. However, both the mammalian host and

T.b. rhodesiense replace the inhibited enzyme far more rapidly than *T.b. gambiense,* and *T.b. rhodesiense* has higher levels of ornithine decarboxylase activity than does *T.b. gambiense.* Both findings are consistent with the selective trypanostatic action of eflornithine in *T.b. gambiense* (*see* Wang, 1997; Iten *et al.,* 1998). The slender bloodstream forms of human trypanosomes must synthesize polyamines *de novo,* because human blood contains only very low levels of these essential compounds. Mutant bloodstream trypanosomes lacking ornithine decarboxylase or wild-type trypanosomes treated with eflornithine convert into nonreplicating, noninfectious, stationary parasites that are rapidly cleared from the blood (Li *et al.,* 1998).

Absorption, Fate, and Excretion. Eflornithine is given by either the intravenous or the oral route; its bioavailability after oral administration is about 54%. Peak plasma levels are achieved about 4 hours after an oral dose, and the elimination half-life averages about 200 minutes. The drug does not bind to plasma proteins, but it is well distributed and penetrates into the cerebrospinal fluid. The last property is especially important in late-stage African trypanosomiasis, where cerebrospinal fluid/plasma ratios exceeding 0.9 have been reported. Over 80% of eflornithine is cleared by the kidney, largely in unchanged form. There is some evidence that eflornithine displays dose-dependent pharmacokinetics at the highest doses used clinically (*see* Abeloff *et al.,* 1984; Pépin and Milord, 1994).

Therapeutic Uses. Experience with the use of eflornithine for the treatment of West African trypanosomiasis due to *T.b. gambiense* has been well summarized by van Nieuwenhove (1992) and by Pépin and Milord (1994). Most patients reported had advanced disease with CNS complications, and many had received arsenicals prior to treatment with eflornithine. The preferred regimen for adult patients was found to be 100 mg/kg given intravenously every 6 hours for 14 days. Virtually all patients improved on this regimen unless they were extremely ill; the probable cure rate exceeded 60%. Whether or not a shorter course of therapy would be equally effective is not known. Children younger than 12 years old required higher doses of eflornithine, probably because they clear the drug more rapidly than do adults and because the drug does not reach the CNS as well. To avoid early convulsions, which could be more frequent in children receiving higher doses, a regimen using the current intravenous dosage (400 mg/kg per day) in the first few days, followed by an increase for the second part of therapy, has been proposed (Milord *et al.,* 1993).

Equal doses of eflornithine were less effective when given by the oral route, probably because of limited bioavailability. The problem cannot be overcome simply by increasing the oral dose, because of ensuing osmotic diarrhea. However, the oral route can be used when intravenous therapy cannot be instituted. A relapse rate of about 15% was estimated for patients taking 100 mg orally every 6 hours for 21 to 45 days. Relapses occurred in only about 5% of patients receiving the optimal 14-day intravenous regimen.

Eflornithine has proven to be less successful for treating AIDS patients with West African trypanosomiasis, presumably because host defenses play a critical role in clearing drug-treated *T.b. gambiense* from the bloodstream. Even high doses of eflornithine failed to improve East African trypanosomiasis due to *T.b. rhodesiense*, consistent with the relatively short half-life and high activity of ornithine decarboxylase in these parasites. Eflornithine alone appears to be rather ineffective for therapy of human leishmaniasis and *P. carinii* pneumonia, even though experimental evidence indicates that this compound can deplete polyamines in *Leishmania* spp. and *P. carinii*.

Toxicity and Side Effects. Eflornithine causes a wide array of adverse effects in treated patients (*see* van Nieuwenhove, 1992; Pépin and Milord, 1994). Anemia (48%), diarrhea (39%), and leukopenia (27%) are the most common complications in patients receiving intravenous medication. Diarrhea is both dose-related and dose-limiting, especially after oral administration of the drug. Convulsions occur early in about 7% of treated patients, but they do not appear to recur despite continuation of therapy. Other complications—such as thrombocytopenia, alopecia, vomiting, abdominal pain, dizziness, fever, anorexia, and headache—occur in less than 10% of treated patients. Most of the above side effects are reversed by withdrawal of the drug. Patients are not routinely tested for hearing loss, but this reversible complication can occur after prolonged therapy with low oral doses (Pasic *et al.,* 1997). Eflornithine interferes with normal embryonic development in experimental animals.

Therapeutic doses of eflornithine are large and require coadministration of substantial volumes of intravenous fluid. This can pose practical limitations in remote settings and cause fluid overload in susceptible patients. In any event, the risks may outweigh the benefits if eflornithine therapy is continued beyond 21 days.

EMETINE AND DEHYDROEMETINE

The use of emetine, an alkaloid derived from ipecac ("Brazil root"), as a direct-acting, systemic amebicide dates from the early part of this century. Dehydroemetine (MEBADIN) has similar pharmacological properties but is considered to be less toxic. Although both drugs have been widely used to treat severe invasive intestinal amebiasis and extraintestinal amebiasis, they largely have been replaced by the mixed amebicide metronidazole, which is as effective and far safer. Thus, emetine and dehydroemetine should not be used unless metronidazole is

ineffective or contraindicated. Details of the pharmacology and toxicology of emetine and dehydroemetine are presented in the *fifth and earlier editions* of this textbook.

8-HYDROXYQUINOLINES

A number of halogenated 8-hydroxyquinolines have been synthesized and used clinically as luminal amebicides, especially to treat asymptomatic cyst passers. Such direct-acting amebicidal agents also have been used together with metronidazole to treat intestinal forms of amebiasis. *Iodoquinol (diiodohydroxyquin)* and *clioquinol (iodochlorhydroxyquin;* available in the United States for topical use only) are the best known of this class of compounds. They have been widely, and all too often indiscriminately, employed for the treatment of diarrhea. The use of these drugs, especially at doses exceeding 2 g per day for long periods, is unfortunately associated with significant risk. The most important toxic reaction, which has been ascribed primarily to clioquinol, is subacute myelooptic neuropathy. This disease is a myelitis-like illness that was first described in epidemic form (thousands of afflicted patients) in Japan; only sporadic cases have been reported elsewhere, but the actual prevalence is undoubtedly higher. Peripheral neuropathy is a less severe manifestation of neurotoxicity due to these drugs. Administration of iodoquinol in high doses to children with chronic diarrhea has been associated with optic atrophy and permanent loss of vision. Iodoquinol is thought to be safer than clioquinol (probably because the former is less well absorbed after oral administration), and it remains available as YODOXIN in the United States. Because diloxanide furoate also is available as a luminal amebicide and considered safer, routine use of iodoquinol is not uniformly recommended. Moreover, iodoquinol must be taken for 20 days, in contrast to the 10-day therapeutic regimen for diloxanide furoate. The pharmacology and toxicology of the 8-hydroxyquinolines are described in greater detail in the *fifth and earlier editions* of this textbook.

MELARSOPROL

History. In 1949, Friedheim demonstrated that melarsoprol, the dimercaptopropanol derivative of melarsen oxide, was effective in the treatment of advanced cases of trypanosomiasis. It was considerably safer than other trypanocides available at the time and has remained a first-line drug in the treatment of late (CNS) stages of both West and East African trypanosomiasis.

Chemistry and Preparation. Melarsoprol has the following chemical structure:

MELARSOPROL

Melarsoprol (*Mel B;* ARSOBAL), consisting of two stereoisomers in a 3:1 ratio (Ericsson *et al.,* 1997), is insoluble in water and is supplied as a 3.6% (w/v) solution in propylene glycol for intravenous administration. It is available in the United States only from the CDC.

Antiprotozoal Effects. It is the trivalent arsenoxide form of an organic arsenical that accounts for both its rapid lethal effect on African trypanosomes and its toxicity to the host (*see* Albert, 1979). Arsenoxides react avidly and reversibly with vicinal sulfhydryl groups, including those of proteins, and thereby inactivate a great number and variety of enzymes. The same nonspecific mechanism by which melarsoprol is lethal to parasites is probably responsible for its toxicity to host tissues. However, susceptible African trypanosomes actively concentrate melarsoprol *via* an unusual purine transporter (Carter and Fairlamb, 1993; Barrett and Fairlamb, 1999).

The basis for the trypanocidal action of melarsoprol is not understood, probably due to its high reactivity with many biomolecules. For example, melarsoprol is a potent inhibitor of pyruvate kinase (Flynn and Bowman, 1969), and disruption of energy metabolism by inhibition of glycolysis was long thought to explain its trypanocidal activity. Other evidence suggests, however, that this is not a primary effect (Van Schaftigen *et al.,* 1987; Eisenthal and Cornish-Bowden, 1998). In a series of studies, Fairlamb and coworkers found that melarsoprol reacts with an unusual trypanosomal dithiol, trypanothione, a spermidine-glutathione adduct. Trypanothione substitutes for glutathione in trypanosomes and other Kinetoplastida to maintain an intracellular reducing environment. Binding of melarsoprol to trypanothione results in formation of melarsen oxide-trypanothione adduct (*Mel T*), a compound that is a potent competitive inhibitor of trypanothione reductase, the enzyme responsible for maintaining trypanothione in its reduced form. However, critical evidence directly linking melarsoprol's action on the trypanothione system to parasite death is still lacking (*see* Barrett and Fairlamb, 1999).

At concentrations of 0.5 to 10 μM, melarsoprol causes lysis of sensitive strains of *T. brucei in vitro,* whereas arsenical-resistant strains are not lysed at concentrations exceeding 100 μM (Yarlett *et al.,* 1991). Arsenical-resistant trypanosomes do not contain increased levels of trypanothione (Yarlett *et al.,* 1991), and the trypanothione reductases from both arsenical-sensitive and resistant strains are equally inhibited by Mel T (*see* Barrett and Fairlamb, 1999).

MELARSEN OXIDE-TRYPANOTHIONE ADDUCT (*Mel T*)

Resistance to melarsoprol can result from altered drug uptake *via* an unusual purine transporter (Carter and Fairlamb, 1993). Moreover, cross-resistance between arsenicals and diamidines (pentamidine) in cloned lines of *T. brucei* suggests that these drugs are concentrated by the same transport system (*see* Barrett and Fairlamb, 1999).

Absorption, Fate, and Excretion. Melarsoprol is always administered intravenously. A small but therapeutically significant amount of the drug enters the cerebrospinal fluid and has a lethal effect on trypanosomes infecting the CNS. The compound is excreted rapidly, with 70% to 80% of the arsenic appearing in the feces (*see* Pépin and Milord, 1994).

Therapeutic Uses. Melarsoprol is the only effective drug available for treatment of the late meningoencephalitic stage of both West African (Gambian) and East African (Rhodesian) trypanosomiasis. Also effective in the early hemolymphatic stage of these infections, melarsoprol is reserved for therapy of late-stage infections because of its toxicity. Treatment of East African trypanosomiasis with melarsoprol is initiated soon after the diagnosis is made, because CNS involvement occurs early in this aggressive infection. Melarsoprol is not used for prophylaxis of trypanosomiasis because of its toxicity and rapid elimination.

The pattern of resistance to melarsoprol therapy differs between the two subspecies of *T. brucei.* Patients infected with *T.b. rhodesiense* who relapse after a course of melarsoprol usually respond to a second course of the drug. In contrast, patients infected with *T.b. gambiense* who are not cured with melarsoprol rarely benefit from repeated treatment with this drug. Such patients often respond well to *eflornithine,* which is ineffective against *T.b. rhodesiense* (Pépin and Milord, 1994).

Treatment schedules with melarsoprol were derived empirically more than 40 years ago, and they have not changed appreciably since (*see* Pépin and Milord, 1994). Melarsoprol is administered by slow intravenous injection; care must be taken to avoid leakage into the surrounding tissues, because the drug is intensely irritating. Therapeutic regimens are complex and difficult to individualize because melarsoprol has such a narrow therapeutic window (*i.e.,* low doses risk therapeutic failure, whereas higher doses can cause reactive encephalopathy in 4% to 10% of treated patients). For example, a regimen recommended for patients with advanced meningoencephalitis and those who are febrile consists of pretreatment with suramin (5 mg/kg, 10 mg/kg, and 20 mg/kg intravenously on days 1, 3, and 5) followed by four series of escalating intravenous doses of melarsoprol (0.36 mg/kg, 0.72 mg/kg, and 1.1 mg/kg on days 7, 8, and 9; 1.8 mg/kg on days 16, 17, and 18; 2.2 mg/kg on day 25; 2.9 mg/kg on day 26; 3.6 mg/kg on day 27; and 3.6 mg/kg on days 34, 35, and 36, to a total maximum daily dose of 180 mg). A shorter course of therapy with higher doses has been used for patients in generally good condition. This consists of suramin pretreatment (5 mg/kg and 10 mg/kg intravenously on days 1 and 3) followed by three series of melarsoprol doses given intravenously (1.4 mg/kg, 1.8 mg/kg, and 2.2 mg/kg on days 5, 6, and 7; 2.5 mg/kg, 2.9 mg/kg, and 3.3 mg/kg on days 14, 15, and 16; and 3.6 mg/kg on days 23, 24, and 25, to a maximum daily dose of 180 mg). Lesser doses should be given to children and debilitated patients. Unless contraindicated, pretreatment with glucocorticoids should be initiated 48 hours before suramin to decrease the incidence of reactive encephalopathy. Although 80% to 90% of patients have been cured by them, such regimens are complex, cumbersome, and difficult to administer. Moreover, based on better pharmacokinetic data, lower doses given over shorter periods may prove to be just as effective. As stated above, those with West African trypanosomiasis who relapse should be treated with eflornithine, whereas those with East African trypanosomiasis often respond favorably to a second course of melarsoprol (*see* Pépin and Milord, 1994).

Toxicity and Side Effects. Toxicity is common during treatment with melarsoprol (*see* Pépin and Milord, 1994). A febrile reaction often occurs soon after drug injection, especially if parasitemia is high. The most serious complications involve the nervous system. A reactive encephalopathy occurs in about 6% of patients, usually between the first two courses of therapy. This is more common in East African than in West African sleeping sickness and is more likely to develop in patients whose cerebrospinal fluid contains many cells and trypanosomes (Pépin *et al.*, 1995). Manifestations include convulsions associated with acute cerebral edema, rapidly progressive coma, and acute, nonlethal mental disturbances without neurological signs. The reaction often is fatal and may occur in the early hemolymphatic stages as well as in the later CNS stages of the illness. Its cause is unknown, but it may represent an immune reaction elicited by the rapid release of trypanosomal antigens from dying parasites rather than by a direct, toxic effect of the drug. Concurrent administration of prednisolone reduces the frequency of reactive encephalopathy and also can be used to control hypersensitivity reactions that occur most often during the second or subsequent courses of melarsoprol therapy. Peripheral neuropathy, noted in about 10% of patients receiving melarsoprol, probably is due to a direct, toxic effect of the drug. Hypertension and myocardial damage are not uncommon, although shock is rare. Albumin-

uria occurs frequently, and occasionally the appearance of numerous casts in the urine or evidence of hepatic disturbances may necessitate modification of treatment. Vomiting and abdominal colic also are common, but their incidence can be reduced by injecting melarsoprol slowly into the supine, fasting patient. The patient should remain in bed and not eat for several hours after the injection is given.

Precautions and Contraindications. Melarsoprol should be given only to patients under hospital supervision so that the dosage regimen may be modified if necessary. It is most important that the initial dosage be based on clinical assessment of the general condition of the patient rather than on body weight. Initiation of therapy during a febrile episode has been associated with an increased incidence of reactive encephalopathy. Administration of melarsoprol to leprous patients may precipitate erythema nodosum. The use of the drug is contraindicated during epidemics of influenza. Severe hemolytic reactions have been reported in patients with deficiency of glucose-6-phosphate dehydrogenase. Pregnancy is not a contraindication for treatment with melarsoprol.

METRONIDAZOLE

History. The isolation of the antibiotic *azomycin* (2-nitroimidazole) from a streptomycete by Maeda and collaborators in 1953 and the demonstration of its trichomonacidal properties by Horie (1956) led to the chemical synthesis and biological testing of many nitroimidazoles. One compound, 1-(β-hydroxyethyl)-2-methyl-5-nitroimidazole, now called *metronidazole* (FLAGYL, others), had especially high activity *in vitro* and *in vivo* against the anaerobic protozoa *T. vaginalis* and *E. histolytica* (Cosar *et al.*, 1961). Durel and associates (1960) reported that oral doses of the drug imparted trichomonacidal activity to semen and urine and that high cure rates could be obtained in both male and female patients with trichomoniasis. Later studies revealed that metronidazole had extremely useful clinical activity against a variety of anaerobic pathogens that included both gram-negative and gram-positive bacteria, in addition to the protozoan *G. lamblia* (*see* below and Freeman *et al.*, 1997). Other clinically effective 5-nitroimidazoles closely related in structure and activity to metronidazole are available outside the United States. These include *tinidazole* (FASIGYN, others), *secnidazole* (SECZOL-DS, others), and *ornidazole* (TIBERAL, others). *Benznidazole* (ROCHAGAN) is another 5-nitroimidazole derivative that is unusual in that it is effective in acute Chagas' disease. Metronidazole has the following chemical structure:

$$\begin{array}{c} H-C-N \\ \| \quad \quad \verb|\|C-CH_3 \\ O_2N-C-N \\ \quad \quad | \\ CH_2CH_2OH \end{array}$$

METRONIDAZOLE

Antiparasitic and Antimicrobial Effects. Metronidazole and related nitroimidazoles are active *in vitro* against a wide variety of anaerobic protozoal parasites and anaerobic bacteria (*see* Freeman *et al.,* 1997). The compound is directly trichomonacidal. Sensitive isolates of *T. vaginalis* are killed by <0.05 μg/ml of the drug under anaerobic conditions; higher concentrations are required when 1% oxygen is present or to affect isolates from patients who display poor therapeutic responses to metronidazole. The drug also has potent amebicidal activity against *E. histolytica* grown in culture by itself or in mixed culture conditions. Trophozoites of *G. lamblia* probably are directly affected by metronidazole at concentrations of 1 to 50 μg/ml *in vitro*. Recently reported structural requirements for antiprotozoal activity of 5-nitroimidazoles against sensitive and resistant strains of anaerobic parasites in culture pertain to future drug development (*see* Upcroft *et al.,* 1999). Aside from the essential nitro group at the 5 position of metronidazole, substitutions at the 2 position of the imidazole ring that enhanced the resonance conjugation of the chemical structure, especially one with a lactam ring, generally increased antiprotozoal activity. In contrast, substitution of an acyl group at the 2 position that ablated such conjugation reduced antiprotozoal activity.

Metronidazole manifests antibacterial activity against all anaerobic cocci and both anaerobic gram-negative bacilli, including *Bacteroides* species, and anaerobic spore-forming gram-positive bacilli. Nonsporulating gram-positive bacilli often are resistant, as are aerobic and facultatively anaerobic bacteria.

Metronidazole is clinically effective in trichomoniasis, amebiasis, and giardiasis, as well as in a variety of infections caused by obligate anaerobic bacteria, including *Bacteroides, Clostridium,* and *Helicobacter* species. Metronidazole may facilitate extraction of adult guinea worms in dracunculiasis, even though it has no direct effect on the parasite (*see* Chapter 42).

Mechanism of Action and Resistance. Metronidazole is a prodrug; it requires reductive activation of the nitro group by susceptible organisms. Its selective toxicity towards anaerobic and microaerophilic pathogens such as the amitochondriate protozoa, *T. vaginalis, E. histolytica,* and *G. lamblia,* and various anaerobic bacteria derives from their energy metabolism, which differs from that of aerobic cells (*see* Land and Johnson, 1997; Samuelson, 1999; Upcroft and Upcroft, 1999). These organisms, unlike their aerobic counterparts, contain electron transport components such as ferredoxins, small Fe-S proteins that have a sufficiently negative redox potential to donate electrons to metronidazole. The single electron transfer forms a highly reactive nitro radical anion that kills susceptible organisms by radical-mediated mechanisms that target DNA and possibly other vital

biomolecules. Metronidazole is catalytically recycled; loss of the active metabolite's electron regenerates the parent compound. Increasing levels of O_2 inhibit metronidazole-induced cytotoxicity, because O_2 competes with metronidazole for electrons generated by energy metabolism. Thus, O_2 can both decrease reductive activation of metronidazole and increase recycling of the activated drug. Anaerobic or microaerophilic organisms susceptible to metronidazole derive energy from the oxidative fermentation of ketoacids such as pyruvate. Pyruvate decarboxylation, catalyzed by pyruvate:ferredoxin oxidoreductase, produces electrons that reduce ferredoxin, which catalytically donates its electrons to biological electron acceptors or to metronidazole.

Clinical resistance to metronidazole is well documented for *T. vaginalis, G. lamblia,* and a variety of anaerobic bacteria but has yet to be shown for *E. histolytica*. Resistance to 5-nitroimidazole drugs *in vitro* has been studied most extensively with trichomonads, whereas data are limited for both *Giardia* and amoebae (*see* Land and Johnson, 1997; Samuelson, 1999; Kulda, 1999; Upcroft and Upcroft, 1999; Wassmann *et al.,* 1999). Resistant strains of *T. vaginalis* derived from nonresponsive patients have shown two major types of abnormalities when tested under aerobic conditions. The first correlates with impaired oxygen-scavenging capabilities, leading to higher local O_2 concentrations, decreased activation of metronidazole, and futile recycling of the activated drug (*see* above and Yarlett *et al.,* 1986). The second type is associated with lowered levels for pyruvate:ferredoxin oxidoreductase and ferredoxin, the latter due to reduced transcription of the ferredoxin gene (Quon *et al.,* 1992). That pyruvate:ferredoxin oxidoreductase and ferredoxin are not completely absent may explain why infections with such strains usually respond to higher doses of metronidazole or more prolonged therapy (Johnson, 1993). Whether or not other mechanisms of metronidazole resistance induced by drug exposure in culture actually operate *in vivo* for trichomonads and amoebae is not known (*see* Brown *et al.,* 1999; Wassmann *et al.,* 1999).

Absorption, Fate, and Excretion. The pharmacokinetic properties of metronidazole and its two major metabolites have been investigated intensively (*see* Lamp *et al.,* 1999). Preparations of metronidazole are available for oral, intravenous, intravaginal, and topical administration. The drug usually is completely and promptly absorbed after oral intake, reaching concentrations in plasma of 8 to 13 μg/ml within 0.25 to 4 hours after a single 500-mg dose. (Mean effective concentrations of the compound are 8 μg/ml or less for most susceptible protozoa and bacteria.) A linear relationship between dose and plasma concentration pertains for doses of 200 to 2000 mg. Repeated doses every 6 to 8 hours result in some accumulation of the drug; systemic clearance exhibits dose-dependence. The half-life of metronidazole in plasma is about 8 hours, and its volume of distribution is approximately that of total body water. Less than 20% of the drug is bound to plasma proteins. With the exception of placenta, metronidazole penetrates well into body tissues and fluids, including vaginal secretions, seminal fluids, saliva, and breast milk. Therapeutic concentrations also are achieved in cerebrospinal fluid.

After an oral dose, over 75% of labeled metronidazole is eliminated in the urine, largely as metabolites; only about 10% is recovered as unchanged drug. The liver is the main site of metabolism, and this accounts for over 50% of the systemic clearance of metronidazole. The two principal metabolites result from oxidation of side chains, a hydroxy derivative and an acid. The hydroxy metabolite has a longer half-life (about 12 hours) and nearly 50% of the antitrichomonal activity of metronidazole. Formation of glucuronides also is observed. Small quantities of reduced metabolites, including ring-cleavage products, are formed by the gut flora. The urine of some patients may be reddish-brown owing to the presence of unidentified pigments derived from the drug. Oxidative metabolism of metronidazole is induced by phenobarbital, prednisone, rifampin, and possibly ethanol. Cimetidine appears to inhibit hepatic metabolism of the drug.

Therapeutic Uses. The uses of metronidazole for antiprotozoal therapy have been extensively reviewed (*see* Freeman *et al.,* 1997; Johnson, 1993; Ravdin, 1995; Zaat *et al.,* 1997). Metronidazole cures genital infections with *T. vaginalis* in both females and males in more than 90% of cases. The preferred treatment regimen is 2 g of metronidazole as a single oral dose for both males and females. For patients who cannot tolerate a single 2-g dose, an alternative regimen is a 250-mg dose given three times daily or a 375-mg dose given twice daily for 7 days. When repeated courses or higher doses of the drug are required for uncured or recurrent infections, it is recommended that intervals of 4 to 6 weeks elapse between courses. In such cases, leukocyte counts should be carried out before, during, and after each course of treatment.

Lack of satisfactory response may be due to bacterial vaginosis, chronic infection of the cervical glands or of Skene's and Bartholin's glands. Reinfection by an infected partner also may cause an unsatisfactory response. Although once rare, treatment failures due to the presence of metronidazole-resistant strains of *T. vaginalis* are becoming increasingly common. Most of these cases can be treated successfully by giving a second 2-g dose to both patient and sexual partner. In addition to oral therapy, the use of topical gel containing 0.75% metronidazole or a 500 to 1000 mg vaginal suppository will increase the local concentration of drug and may be beneficial in refractory cases (Heine and McGregor, 1993).

Metronidazole is an effective amebicide and has become the agent of choice for the treatment of all symptomatic forms of amebiasis, including acute gastrointestinal infection and liver abscess. The recommended dose is 500 to 750 mg of metronidazole taken orally three times daily for 10 days. The daily dose for children is 35 to 50 mg/kg given in three divided doses for 10 days. *E. histolytica* persist in most patients who recover from acute amebiasis after metronidazole therapy, so it is recommended that all such individuals be treated with a luminal amebicide such as diloxanide furoate. Clinical re-

sistance of *E. histolytica* to metronidazole has not been confirmed, despite extensive clinical use of this drug. *Mass treatment* with a large dose of metronidazole once monthly for a few months and then in alternate months has resulted in a marked decrease in the incidence of amebic dysentery in relatively isolated communities with a high degree of endemicity.

Although effective for the therapy of giardiasis, metronidazole has yet to be approved for treatment of this infection in the United States. Favorable responses have been noted with doses the same as or lower than those used for trichomoniasis; the usual regimen is 250 mg given three times daily for 5 days for adults and 15 mg/kg given three times a day for 5 days for children. A daily dose of 2 g for 3 days also has been used successfully.

Metronidazole is a relatively inexpensive, highly versatile drug with clinical efficacy against a broad spectrum of anaerobic bacteria (*see* Freeman *et al.,* 1997). The compound is used for treatment of serious infections due to susceptible anaerobic bacteria, including *Bacteroides, Clostridium, Fusobacterium, Peptococcus, Peptostreptococcus, Eubacterium,* and *Helicobacter.* The drug also can be given along with other antimicrobial agents to treated mixed infections with aerobic and anaerobic bacteria. Due to excellent tissue penetration, metronidazole can achieve clinically effective levels at sites such as bones, joints, and the brain. Intraabdominal, gynecologic, dermal, and CNS infections with susceptible anaerobes all have responded to this drug, as have bacterial septicemia and endocarditis. Metronidazole can be given intravenously when oral administration is not indicated. A typical intravenous regimen for severe anaerobic infections is a loading dose of 15 mg/kg followed 6 hours later by a maintenance dose of 7.5 mg/kg every 6 hours, usually for 7 to 10 days. Together with other antibiotics, metronidazole has shown efficacy for prophylaxis of postsurgical mixed bacterial infections (Song and Glenny, 1998) and for treatment of gastric infections with *H. pylori* when taken in various regimens that include the proton pump inhibitors (Hopkins and Morris, 1994; Harris, 1998; Megraud and Doermann, 1998; *see* Chapter 37). Because of its low cost, the drug has also been used instead of vancomycin to treat pseudomembranous colitis.

Metronidazole and other nitroimidazoles can sensitize hypoxic tumor cells to the effects of ionizing radiation, but these drugs are not used clinically for this purpose.

Toxicity, Contraindications, and Drug Interactions. The toxicity of metronidazole has been reviewed (*see* Roe,

1977; Lau *et al.*, 1992). Side effects only rarely are severe enough to discontinue therapy. The most common are headache, nausea, dry mouth, and a metallic taste. Vomiting, diarrhea, and abdominal distress occasionally are experienced. Furry tongue, glossitis, and stomatitis occurring during therapy usually are associated with an exacerbation of moniliasis. Dizziness, vertigo, and, very rarely, encephalopathy, convulsions, incoordination, and ataxia are neurotoxic effects that warrant discontinuation of metronidazole. The drug also should be withdrawn if numbness or paresthesias of the extremities occur. Reversal of serious sensory neuropathies may be slow or incomplete. Urticaria, flushing, and pruritus are indicative of drug sensitivity that can require withdrawal of metronidazole. Dysuria, cystitis, and a sense of pelvic pressure also have been reported. Metronidazole has a well-documented disulfiram-like effect, such that some patients experience abdominal distress, vomiting, flushing, or headache if they drink alcoholic beverages during or within 3 days after therapy with this drug. Patients should be cautioned to avoid consuming alcohol during metronidazole treatment, even though the risk of a severe reaction is low. By the same token, metronidazole and disulfiram should not be taken together, because confusional and psychotic states may occur. Although related chemicals have caused blood dyscrasias, only a temporary neutropenia, reversible after discontinuation of therapy, occurs with metronidazole.

Metronidazole should be used with caution in patients with active disease of the CNS because of its potential neurotoxicity. The drug also may precipitate CNS signs of lithium toxicity in patients receiving high doses of lithium. Plasma levels of metronidazole can be elevated by drugs such as cimetidine that inhibit hepatic microsomal metabolism. Moreover, metronidazole can prolong the prothrombin time of patients receiving therapy with coumadin anticoagulants. The dosage of metronidazole should be reduced in patients with severe hepatic disease.

Given in high doses for prolonged periods, metronidazole is carcinogenic in rodents; it also is mutagenic in bacteria (*see* Lau *et al.*, 1992). Mutagenic activity is associated with metronidazole and several of its metabolites found in the urine of patients treated with therapeutic doses of the drug. However, there is no evidence that therapeutic doses of metronidazole pose any significant increased risk of cancer to human patients. There is conflicting evidence about the teratogenicity of metronidazole in animals. While metronidazole has been taken during all stages of pregnancy with no apparent adverse effects, its use during the first trimester is not advised.

NIFURTIMOX

History. Nitrofurans were known to be effective in experimental infections with American trypanosomiasis caused by *T. cruzi*, so numerous congeners were tested for their chemotherapeutic potential. Of these, one drug, *nifurtimox* (3-methyl-4(5'-nitrofurfurylideneamino)-tetrahydro-4H-1,4-thiazine-1,1-dioxide) is quite effective in treatment of acute Chagas' disease (Brener, 1979). Nifurtimox (*Bayer 2502;* LAMPIT) is no longer commercially available but can be obtained in the United States from the CDC. It has the following chemical structure:

NIFURTIMOX

Antiprotozoal Effects. Nifurtimox is trypanocidal against both the trypomastigote and amastigote forms of *T. cruzi*. Concentrations of 1 μM damage intracellular amastigotes *in vitro* and inhibit their development. Continuous exposure to this concentration of the drug considerably lengthens the intracellular cycle. Trypomastigotes are less sensitive; 10-μM concentrations of nifurtimox inhibit but do not eliminate penetration of vertebrate cells. The trypanocidal action of nifurtimox derives from its ability to undergo activation by partial reduction to nitro radical anions. Transfer of electrons from the activated drug then regenerates the native nitrofuran and forms superoxide radical anions and other reactive oxygen species, such as hydrogen peroxide and hydroxyl radical (*see* Docampo, 1990). The enzyme responsible for the reductive activation of nifurtimox remains to be identified, although *T. cruzi* trypanothione reductase has been implicated (Wang, 1997; Henderson *et al.*, 1988). *T. cruzi* appears to be deficient in enzymatic defenses against reactive oxygen species (*see* Docampo, 1990). Reaction of free radicals with cellular macromolecules results in cellular damage that includes lipid peroxidation and membrane injury, enzyme inactivation, and damage to DNA. Nifurtimox also may produce damage to mammalian tissues by formation of radicals and redox cycling (Moreno *et al.*, 1980).

Absorption, Fate, and Excretion. Nifurtimox is well absorbed after oral administration, with peak plasma levels observed after about 3.5 hours (Paulos *et al.*, 1989). Despite this, only low concentrations of the drug (10 to 20 μM) are present in plasma, and less than 0.5% of the dose is excreted in urine. The elimination half-life is only about 3 hours. High concentrations of several unidentified metabolites are found, however, and it is obvious that nifurtimox undergoes rapid biotransformation, probably *via* a presystemic, first-pass effect. Whether or not the metabolites have any trypanocidal activity is unknown.

Therapeutic Uses. Nifurtimox is employed in the treatment of American trypanosomiasis (Chagas' disease) caused by *T. cruzi*. Although the drug markedly reduces the parasitemia, morbidity, and mortality from acute Chagas' disease, it is ineffective in chronic stages of this infection. Moreover, only about half of the patients who complete a course of therapy appear cured of the parasitic infestation. Treatment with nifurtimox has no effect on irreversible organ lesions. Whether or not the cardiomyopathy associated with chronic disease actually reflects an autoimmune disease that is independent of the presence of trypanosomes is debatable (*see* Urbina, 1999). The clinical response of the acute illness to drug therapy varies with geographic region; parasite strains present in Argentina, southern Brazil, Chile, and Venezuela appear to be more susceptible than those in central Brazil. Differences in the susceptibility of various strains of *T. cruzi* to nifurtimox have been described in animal models (*see* Brener, 1979), but whether or not these account for the variable clinical outcomes is unknown. Despite these uncertainties, treatment of acutely infected individuals should be initiated as soon as possible. Therapy with nifurtimox should start promptly after exposure for persons at risk of *T. cruzi* infection from laboratory accidents or from blood transfusions.

Nifurtimox is given orally. Adults with acute infection should receive 8 to 10 mg/kg daily in four divided doses for 90 to 120 days. Children 1 to 10 years of age with acute Chagas' disease should receive 15 to 20 mg/kg per day in four divided doses for 90 days; for individuals 11 to 16 years old, the daily dose is 12.5 to 15 mg/kg given according to the same schedule. Gastric upset and weight loss can occur during treatment. If the latter occurs, dosage should be reduced. The ingestion of alcohol should be avoided during treatment, because the incidence of side effects may increase.

Toxicity and Side Effects. Children tolerate nifurtimox better than do adults. Nonetheless, drug-related side effects are common. They range from hypersensitivity reactions—such as dermatitis, fever, icterus, pulmonary infiltrates, and anaphylaxis—to dose- and age-dependent complications primarily referable to the gastrointestinal tract and both the peripheral and central nervous systems (*see* Brener, 1979). Nausea and vomiting are common, as are myalgia and weakness. Peripheral neuropathy and gastrointestinal symptoms are especially common after prolonged treatment; the latter complication may lead to weight loss and preclude further therapy. Headache, psychic disturbances, paresthesias, polyneuritis, and CNS excitability are less frequent. Leukopenia and decreased sperm counts also have been reported. The compound may suppress cell-mediated immune reactions, both *in vitro* and *in vivo* (Lelchuk *et al.,* 1977a,b). Because of the seriousness of Chagas' disease and the lack of superior drugs, there are few absolute contraindications to the use of nifurtimox.

PENTAMIDINE

History. The discovery of antiprotozoal activity in the diamidine family of drugs was a fortuitous consequence of the search for hypoglycemic compounds that might compromise parasite energy metabolism. Of the compounds tested, three were found to possess outstanding activity: *stilbamidine, pentamidine,* and *promamidine. Pentamidine* was the most useful clinically because of its relative stability, lower toxicity, and ease of administration. Although it is effective clinically against a number of pathogenic protozoa, including *Leishmania* species, pentamidine is now used primarily for the prophylaxis and treatment of pulmonary and systemic infections with *P. carinii* in patients who cannot tolerate trimethoprim-sulfamethoxazole. It continues to be used alone or combined with suramin for the treatment of early-stage West African trypanosomiasis (*see* Pépin and Milord, 1994; Pépin and Khonde, 1996). *Diminazene* (BERENIL) is a related diamidine that is used as a cheap alternative to pentamidine for the treatment of early African trypanosomiasis in some endemic areas, despite the fact that it is *approved for veterinary use only*. A number of promising analogs of pentamidine have been tested in a rat model of *P. carinii* infection (*see* Vöhringer and Arastéh, 1993), but none has been developed for human use.

Chemistry. Pentamidine has the following chemical structure:

PENTAMIDINE

Pentamidine isethionate is the preparation used clinically. It is marketed for injection (PENTAM 300) or for use as an aerosol (NEBUPENT). One milligram of pentamidine base is equivalent to 1.74 mg of the pentamidine isethionate. Solutions should be used promptly after preparation.

Antiprotozoal and Antifungal Effects. The positively charged aromatic diamidines are toxic to a number of different protozoa yet show rather marked selectivity of action. For example, the drugs are curative against *T.b. rhodesiense* and *T.b. congolense* infections in experimental animals but are ineffective in curing mice infected with *T. cruzi*. They also are capable of curing *Babesia canis* infections in puppies and *Leishmania donovani* infections in hamsters. These findings provide the basis for diamidine treatment of African trypanosomiasis and leishmaniasis in human beings.

The diamidines also are fungicidal. Activity *in vitro* against *Blastomyces dermatitidis* led to the successful therapeutic trial of these drugs in systemic blastomycoses. The use of amphotericin B, however, has reduced the value of the diamidines in the treatment of this disease. At near therapeutic levels, pentamidine kills nonreplicating forms of *P. carinii* in culture (Pifer *et al.,* 1983), but other evidence suggests that pentamidine exerts a biostatic rather than biocidal effect (*see* Vöhringer and Arastéh, 1993).

Mechanism of Action and Resistance. The mechanism of action of the diamidines is unknown. These dicationic compounds may display multiple effects on a given parasite and act by disparate mechanisms in different parasites (*see* Sands *et al.,* 1985; Wang, 1995; Barrett and Fairlamb, 1999). In *T. brucei,* for example, the diamidines are concentrated *via* an energy-dependent, high-affinity uptake system that operates more effectively in drug-sensitive than in drug-resistant strains (Damper and Patten, 1976). The diamidines utilize a transporter selective for adenine and adenosine, purines that must be imported to assure parasite survival (Barrett and Fairlamb, 1999). Melamine-based arsenicals use the same purine (P-2) transporter, which explains the cross-resistance to diamidines exhibited by certain arsenical-resistant strains of *T. brucei* (*see* Carter *et al.,* 1995; Barrett and Fairlamb, 1999; Maser *et al.,* 1999; de Koning and Jarvis, 1999). Although failure to concentrate diamidines is the usual cause of pentamidine resistance, other mechanisms could be involved (Berger *et al.,* 1995). After achieving millimolar concentrations within trypanosomes, the positively charged hydrophobic diamidines may exert their trypanocidal effects by reacting with a variety of negatively charged intracellular targets such as membrane phospholipids, enzymes, RNA, and DNA. Indeed, ribosomal aggregation, inhibition of DNA and protein synthesis, and inhibition of several enzymes—along with seeming loss of trypanosomal kinetoplast—have all been reported (*see* Barrett and Fairlamb, 1999). Inhibition of *S*-adenosyl-L-methionine decarboxylase *in vitro* suggested that pentamidine might interfere with polyamine biosynthesis, but this seems unlikely to explain the drug's action *in vitro* (Bitoni *et al.,* 1986; Berger *et al.,* 1993). Inhibition *in vitro* of trypanosomal mitochondrial topoisomerase II and plasma Ca^{2+},Mg^{2+}-ATPase also has been reported (*see* Barrett and Fairlamb, 1999). The diamidines bind to DNA at sequences composed of at least four consecutive A-T base pairs (Bailly *et al.,* 1994). Pentamidine promotes linearization of trypanosome kinetoplast DNA, consistent with its being a type II topoisomerase inhibitor (Shapiro and Englund, 1990). The drug also inhibits ATP-dependent topoisomerases in extracts of *P. carinii* (Dykstra and Tidwell, 1991).

Absorption, Fate, and Excretion. The pharmacokinetics and biodisposition of pentamidine isethionate have been studied most extensively in AIDS patients with *P. carinii* infections (*see* Vöhringer and Arastéh, 1993); information from patients with Gambian trypanosomiasis is more limited (*see* Pépin and Milord, 1994; Bronner *et al.,* 1995). Pentamidine isethionate is fairly well absorbed from parenteral sites of administration despite the formation of sterile abscesses that may occur after its use. Following a single intravenous dose, the drug disappears from plasma with an apparent half-life of several minutes to a few hours; this is followed by a slower distribution phase and a prolonged elimination phase lasting from weeks to months. Patients with African trypanosomiasis exhibit marked interindividual variations in pharmacokinetic parameters. Their mean system plasma clearance after a single dose is about 1120 ml/minute, but the volume of distribution is about 25,000 liters, a finding that accounts for the prolonged average elimination half-life of about 12 days (Bronner *et al.,* 1995). The renal clearance of pentamidine averages only about 2% to 11% of its systemic clearance (Conte, 1991; Bronner *et al.,* 1995), but whether the drug is metabolized or excreted in bile, for example, is unknown. In patients receiving multiple injections of the drug over a 13-day period for treatment of pneumocystosis, drug accumulation occurs such that no steady-state plasma concentration is attained (Conte, 1991). Extensive accumulation of pentamidine in tissues and its slow excretion during repeated administration may relate to both its therapeutic properties and its prophylactic efficacy in both pneumocystosis and African trypanosomiasis (*see* Pépin and Milord, 1994). After multiple parenteral doses, the liver, kidney, adrenal, and spleen of patients with AIDS contain the highest concentrations of drug, whereas only traces are found in the brain (Donnelly *et al.,* 1988). Lungs of such patients contain intermediate but therapeutic concentrations after five daily doses of 4 mg of base per kilogram. Higher pulmonary concentrations should be achieved by inhalation of pentamidine aerosols for prophylaxis or as adjunctive treatment for mild to moderate *P. carinii* pneumonia; delivery of drug by this route results in little systemic absorption and decreased toxicity compared with intravenous administration in both adults and children (Leoung *et al.,* 1990; Hand *et al.,* 1994). The actual dose delivered to the lungs depends on both the size of particles generated by the nebulizer and the patient's ventilatory patterns.

Therapeutic Uses. Pentamidine isethionate usually is given by intramuscular injection or by slow intravenous infusion over 60 minutes in single daily doses of 4 mg of base per kilogram. However, dosage regimens vary by disease and, in some instances, are not firmly established (*see* above).

For treatment of early lymphatic African trypanosomiasis due to *T.b. gambiense,* pentamidine can be given intramuscularly on days 1, 3, 5, 7, 13, and 17, while suramin is administered intravenously (20 mg/kg up to a maximum of 1 g) on days 1 and 13. An alternative is to give seven intramuscular doses of pentamidine alone on alternate days (*see* Pépin and Milord, 1994). Because of failure to penetrate the CNS, pentamidine is not used to treat *T.b. rhodesiense,* which affects the brain early in the course of infection. The drug also is largely ineffective in *T.b. gambiense* infections once the CNS is involved.

Pentamidine has been used successfully in courses of 12 to 15 intramuscular doses of 2 to 4 mg/kg, either daily or every other day, to treat visceral leishmaniasis (*kala azar* caused by *L. donovani*). This compound provides an alternative to antimonials or lipid formulations of amphotericin B for patients who cannot tolerate the latter agents. Pentamidine isethionate given as 4 intramuscular doses of 3 mg/kg every other day has enjoyed some success in the treatment of cutaneous leishmaniasis (*Oriental sore* caused by *L. tropica*) but is not used routinely to treat this infection (*see* Berman, 1997).

Pentamidine is one of a number of drugs and drug combinations used extensively for the prophylaxis and treatment of infections with *P. carinii*, *P. carinii* pneumonia (PCP) being the most common opportunistic infection in individuals infected with HIV. In western countries, these drugs have markedly reduced mortality from PCP, changed the spectrum of AIDS-related illnesses, and increased life expectancy in this population.

Fauci and Lane (1998) have reviewed the use of pentamidine and other drugs for the prophylaxis and treatment of *P. carinii* infections in HIV-infected adults. Prophylaxis against PCP is recommended for such persons with either a previous *P. carinii* infection, a CD4 lymphocyte count of 200 cells per microliter or less, an unexplained fever for 2 or more weeks, or a history of oropharyngeal candidiasis. Pentamidine, taken by aerosol inhalation, is no longer recommended for routine prophylaxis against PCP; instead, it is reserved for those few individuals unable to tolerate systemic therapy with more effective agents, *e.g.*, trimethoprim-sulfamethoxazole (*see* Chapter 44). The usual monthly dose is 300 mg of a 5% to 10% nebulized aqueous solution of pentamidine isethionate delivered over 30 to 45 minutes *via* a RESPIRGARD II device. Disadvantages of aerosolized pentamidine are that it lacks efficacy against extrapulmonary infections with *P. carinii* and it induces an increased incidence of pneumothorax.

For treatment of moderate to severe PCP or systemic pneumocystosis in nondebilitated, HIV-infected adults, pentamidine isethionate is the preferred alternative to trimethoprim-sulfamethoxazole when the latter cannot be tolerated. The optimal dosage regimen is 4 mg/kg of pentamidine given intravenously each day for 21 days, depending on the severity of infection and tolerance to the drug. In some instances, a lower 2- to 3-mg/kg daily dosage may be equally effective and produce substantially less toxicity (*see* Vöhringer and Arastéh, 1993). HIV-infected patients with PCP may worsen during the first 5 days of therapy, possibly from an inflammatory response to killed organisms. Treatment with corticosteroids may ameliorate this life-threatening response if instituted as soon as the diagnosis is made but no later than 72 hours thereafter. Clinical improvement usually occurs by the end of the first week of pentamidine therapy if the patient responds. A high proportion of cures can be expected even though side effects may force cessation of therapy. The prognosis is less favorable in debil-

itated patients with altered immunity or neoplastic disease, who may require more than one course of therapy. Consistent with a biostatic action of pentamidine against *P. carinii*, treatment failures, relapses, and drug toxicity and intolerance are especially prevalent in patients with AIDS. These individuals are more likely to respond favorably to trimethoprim-sulfamethoxazole if that medication is tolerated.

The use of pentamidine has reduced mortality markedly in the epidemic form of *P. carinii* infection found in debilitated and premature infants. While the feasibility of administering this drug by aerosol to infants with HIV infection has been demonstrated, the efficacy of such therapy has yet to be proven (Hand *et al.*, 1994).

Toxicity and Side Effects. At therapeutic doses (4 mg/kg per day), pentamidine causes toxicity in about 50% of patients treated, whether or not they have AIDS. The major complications of pentamidine therapy have been well reviewed (*see* Sands *et al.*, 1985; Vöhringer and Arastéh, 1993). Intravenous injection of pentamidine (and other diamidines) can be followed by alarming and sometimes dangerous reactions. These include breathlessness, tachycardia, dizziness or fainting, headache, and vomiting. These reactions probably relate to the sharp fall in blood pressure that follows too rapid intravenous administration of the drug, and they may be due in part to the release of histamine. If solutions of pentamidine cannot be given slowly by the intravenous route, the drug is well tolerated after intramuscular injection. However, the latter route is associated with formation of sterile abscesses at the injection site. Pentamidine does not appear to cause late neuropathies. Pancreatitis and hypoglycemia and, paradoxically, hyperglycemia and insulin-dependent diabetes have been documented following its administration; the hypoglycemia may be life-threatening or even fatal if not recognized (*see* Sands *et al.*, 1985). Other adverse effects include skin rashes, thrombophlebitis, thrombocytopenia, anemia, neutropenia, elevation of liver enzymes, and nephrotoxicity (*see* Vöhringer and Arastéh, 1993). Impaired renal function has been seen in 24% of patients receiving the drug, but this is usually reversible.

QUINACRINE

Quinacrine is an acridine derivative widely used during World War II as an antimalarial agent. Although it has been replaced by newer and safer antimalarial drugs (*see* Chapter 40), *quinacrine hydrochloride* is very effective against *G. lamblia,* producing cure rates of at least 90%. However, quinacrine is no longer available in the United States. For a description of the pharmacology and toxicology of quinacrine, the *fifth and earlier editions* of this textbook should be consulted.

SODIUM STIBOGLUCONATE

History.   Antimonial compounds long have been used for therapy of leishmaniasis and other protozoal infections. The first trivalent antimonial compound used to treat cutaneous leishmaniasis and kala azar was *antimony potassium tartrate (tartar emetic),* which was both toxic and difficult to administer. Tartar emetic and other trivalent arsenicals eventually were replaced by pentavalent antimonial derivatives of phenylstibonic acid. These drugs were as effective as but far less toxic than tartar emetic, thus permitting the use of larger doses and shorter periods of treatment. Later syntheses reverted to the "tartar emetic" type of compound in which trivalent antimony was replaced by pentavalent antimony. An early member of this type of compound was *sodium stibogluconate (sodium antimony gluconate;* PENTOSTAM). This drug is widely used today and, together with *meglumine antimonate* (GLUCANTIME), a pentavalent antimonial compound preferred in French-speaking countries, is the mainstay of the treatment of leishmaniasis by antimony. The history of leishmanicides has been reviewed by Steck (1974) and Berman (1988).

Chemistry.   Sodium stibogluconate has the following chemical structure:

SODIUM STIBOGLUCONATE

Clinical formulations of sodium stibogluconate actually consist of multiple uncharacterized molecular forms, some of which have higher molecular masses than the compound shown (*see* Berman, 1988). Typical preparations contain 30% to 34% pentavalent antimony by weight as well as *m*-chlorocresol added as a preservative. In the United States, sodium stibogluconate is available only from the CDC as an aqueous solution containing an equivalent of 100 mg of Sb^{5+}/ml.

Antiprotozoal Effects and Drug Resistance.   The mechanism of the antileishmanial action of sodium stibogluconate remains to be clarified. Exposure to this compound compromises the bioenergetics of *Leishmania* amastigotes (*see* Berman, 1988). Both glycolysis and fatty acid metabolism, processes primarily localized in unusual organelles termed *glycosomes,* are suppressed. Sodium stibogluconate also diminishes net generation of ATP and GTP. Whether this is a primary or a secondary drug effect is not known. Other mechanisms such as carbohydrate-directed targeting of the drug to macrophages and nonspecific binding of antimony to the sulfhydryl groups of amastigote

proteins may be involved (Roberts *et al.,* 1995). Recent studies support the old hypothesis that relatively nontoxic pentavalent antimonials act as prodrugs. These compounds are reduced to the more toxic Sb^{3+} species that kill amastigotes within the phagolysosomes of macrophages (Roberts *et al.,* 1995; Sereno and Lemesre, 1997; Sereno *et al.,* 1998). Incidentally, but perhaps importantly, the *m*-chlorocresol preservative used in formulations of sodium stibogluconate has intrinsic activity that may contribute to antileishmanial effects of the drug preparation *in vivo* (Roberts and Rainey, 1993; Sereno *et al.,* 1998).

Naturally resistant *Leishmania* or parasites made resistant to antimonial drugs in culture show several biochemical differences from drug-sensitive strains. Resistant strains have displayed elevated levels of intracellular thiols, especially trypanothione, and amplification of the ATP-binding cassette (ABC) transporter gene, *pgp A.* However, while these changes may contribute to antimonial drug resistance, they are variable and insufficient to confer the high degree of resistance noted for some strains (*see* Legare *et al.,* 1997; Haimeur *et al.,* 2000). Indeed, susceptibility of *L. donovani* to pentavalent antimonials appears to be parasite-intrinsic, stage-specific (amastigotes are more susceptible than promastigotes), and macrophage-independent (Ephros *et al.,* 1999).

Absorption, Fate, and Excretion.   The pentavalent antimonials attain much higher concentrations in plasma than do the trivalent compounds. Consequently, most of a single dose of sodium stibogluconate is excreted in the urine within 24 hours. Its pharmacokinetic behavior is similar whether the drug is given intravenously or intramuscularly (Pamplin *et al.,* 1981; Chulay *et al.,* 1988). The agent is rapidly absorbed, distributed in an apparent volume of about 0.22 liter/kg, and eliminated in two phases. The first has a short half-life of about 2 hours, and the second is much slower ($t_{1/2}$ = 33 to 76 hours). The prolonged terminal elimination phase may reflect conversion of the pentavalent antimonial (Sb^{5+}) to the more toxic trivalent (Sb^{3+}) form that is concentrated and slowly released from tissues. Indeed, about 20% of the plasma antimony is present in the trivalent form after pentavalent antimonial administration. Sequestration of antimony in macrophages also may contribute to the prolonged antileishmanial effect after plasma antimony levels have dropped below the minimal inhibitory concentration (MIC) observed *in vitro.*

Therapeutic Uses.   The changing use of sodium stibogluconate, meglumine antimonate, and other agents for the chemotherapy of leishmaniasis has been extensively reviewed (*see* Berman, 1988 and 1997). Sodium stibogluconate is given either intravenously or intramuscularly, the dosage regimen depending on the local responsiveness of a particular form of leishmaniasis to this compound.

Prolonged dosage schedules with maximally tolerated doses are now needed for successful therapy of visceral, mucosal, and some forms of cutaneous leishmaniasis, in part to overcome increasing clinical resistance to antimonial drugs. Even high-dose regimens may no longer produce satisfactory results. For example, pentavalent antimonials are no longer superior to amphotericin B for treatment of either visceral leishmaniasis (*kala azar*) in India or mucosal leishmaniasis in general.

The current recommended daily dose of sodium stibogluconate has been increased from 10 to 20 mg of pentavalent antimony per kilogram body weight, a dose that ordinarily causes minimal added risk to patients. Given intramuscularly for 10 days, this regimen has cured over 90% of individuals with cutaneous leishmaniasis. For visceral leishmaniasis, except in India, and for mucosal leishmaniasis everywhere, the same daily dose should be continued for 28 days if tolerated. This regimen produces a cure rate of about 85% to 90% for visceral disease but only about 60% for mucosal leishmaniasis (*see* Berman, 1997). Children usually tolerate the drug well, and the dose per kilogram is the same as that given to adults. Patients who respond favorably show clinical improvement within 1 to 2 weeks after initiation of therapy. The drug may be given on alternate days or for longer intervals if unfavorable reactions occur in especially debilitated individuals. Patients infected with HIV present a challenge, because they usually relapse after successful initial therapy with either pentavalent antimonials or amphotericin B. Such persons should be treated periodically with secondary agents, such as pentamidine or paromomycin, when this happens. Alternative drugs also are recommended for patients who do not respond to a full course of antimonial therapy (*see* Berman, 1997).

The incidence of treatment failures with sodium stibogluconate in visceral, mucocutaneous, and some forms of cutaneous leishmaniasis is increasing dramatically in endemic areas (Ouellette and Papadopoulou, 1993). Although many treatment failures may be attributable to reinfection or to pharmacokinetic or immunological variability in patients, resistance to sodium stibogluconate is well documented in both laboratory-derived strains and clinical isolates (Berman *et al.*, 1989; Grogl *et al.*, 1992). Indeed, assays of intracellular amastigote resistance to sodium stibogluconate *in vitro* may prove helpful in predicting the clinical response of visceral *L. donovani* infections to this drug (Lira *et al.*, 1999). However, sodium stibogluconate still remains the drug of choice for leishmaniasis. Its main disadvantages are the long courses of therapy required, the necessity for parenteral administration, and its relatively

high cost. For cases of East African and Indian *kala azar* and mucosal leishmaniasis that are unresponsive to pentavalent antimonials, lipid formulations of amphotericin B are preferred.

Toxicity and Side Effects. The toxicity of the pentavalent antimonials is best evaluated in patients without systemic disease, *i.e.,* visceral leishmaniasis. In general, high-dose regimens of sodium stibogluconate are fairly well tolerated; toxic reactions are usually reversible, and most subside despite continued therapy. Effects most commonly noted include pain at the injection site after intramuscular administration; chemical pancreatitis in nearly all patients; elevation of serum hepatic transaminase levels; bone-marrow suppression manifested by decreased red-cell, white-cell, and platelet counts in the blood; muscle and joint pain; weakness and malaise; headache; nausea and abdominal pain; and skin rashes. Changes in the electrocardiogram that include T-wave flattening and inversion and prolongation of the QT interval found in patients with systemic disease are uncommon in other forms of leishmaniasis (Navin *et al.*, 1992; Berman, 1997; Sundar *et al.*, 1998). Reversible polyneuropathy has been reported. Hemolytic anemia and renal damage are rare manifestations of antimonial toxicity, as are shock and sudden death.

SURAMIN

History. Based on the trypanocidal activity of the dyestuffs *trypan red, trypan blue,* and *afridol violet,* several years of research in Germany resulted in the introduction of *suramin* into therapy in 1920. Today the drug is used primarily for treatment of African trypanosomiasis; it has no clinical utility against American trypanosomiasis. Although suramin is effective in clearing adult filariae in *onchocerciasis,* it has been replaced by ivermectin for treatment of this condition (*see* Chapter 42). Suramin is a potent inhibitor of retroviral reverse transcriptase, but it is ineffective in HIV infection (Cheson *et al.*, 1987). Drug-associated adrenal insufficiency along with the antiproliferative activity of suramin stimulated the experimental use of high doses, alone or with other compounds, for the therapy of adrenocortical hyperfunction, adrenocortical carcinoma, and a variety of other metastatic tumors (*see,* for example, Voogd *et al.*, 1993; Bowden *et al.*, 1996; Frommel, 1997). The antiparasitic and antineoplastic properties of suramin along with its clinical uses and limitations have been the topic of numerous reviews (*see* Cheson *et al.*, 1987; Voogd *et al.*, 1993; Pépin and Milord, 1994; Barrett and Barrett, 2000).

Chemistry and Preparation. *Suramin sodium* (BAYER 205, formerly GERMANIN, others) has the chemical structure shown on the next page.

SURAMIN SODIUM

The drug is soluble in water, but solutions deteriorate quickly in air; only freshly prepared solutions should be used. In the United States, suramin is available only from the CDC.

Antiparasitic Effects. Suramin is a relatively slowly acting trypanoside (>6 hours *in vitro*) with high clinical activity against both *T.b. gambiense* and *T.b. rhodesiense* and an unknown mechanism of action (*see* Voogd *et al.,* 1993). Its delayed onset of action probably stems from slow endocytic uptake of the drug-protein complex by trypanosomes (Fairlamb and Bowman, 1977). Structural modifications of this polyanion usually result in substantial loss of trypanocidal activity. Suramin reacts reversibly with a variety of biomolecules *in vitro,* inhibiting many trypanosomal and mammalian enzymes unrelated to its antiparasitic effects (*see* Pépin and Milord, 1994; Wang, 1995 and 1997). Compartmentation protects many vital molecules, such as the glycolytic enzymes inside trypanosomal glycosomes, from suramin's action, because this compound does not cross membrane barriers by passive diffusion (Wang, 1995). However, the chemical structure of suramin may confer transport specificity, because removal of its two methyl groups results in the loss of trypanocidal activity *in vivo* but not *in vitro* (Morty *et al.,* 1998). Suramin-treated trypanosomes exhibit damage to intracellular membrane structures other than lysosomes, but whether or not this relates to the drug's primary action is unknown. Inhibition of a trypanosomal cytosolic serine oligopeptidase may account for at least part of suramin's activity (Morty *et al.,* 1998).

Suramin is the only microfilaricide used clinically, albeit rarely now, for treatment of human onchocerciasis (*see* Chapter 42). This compound displays delayed but prolonged filaricidal activity against both adult male and female worms and lesser but significant activity against microfilariae. Its mechanism of action against *Onchocerca volvulus* is unknown (*see* Voogd *et al.,* 1993).

Absorption, Fate, and Excretion. Because it is not absorbed after oral intake, suramin is given intravenously to avoid local inflammation and necrosis associated with subcutaneous or in-

tramuscular injections. After its administration, the drug displays complex pharmacokinetics with marked interindividual variability. The concentration in plasma falls fairly rapidly for a few hours, more slowly for a few days, and finally very slowly, with a terminal elimination half-life of about 90 days. The persistence of suramin in the circulation is due to extremely tight binding to plasma proteins; over 99.7% of the drug is bound after a typical 1-g dose (*see* Pépin and Milord, 1994). The drug is not appreciably metabolized, and its renal clearance of about 5 ml/hour accounts for elimination of about 80% of the compound from the body. Although the apparent volume of distribution of suramin in an adult is about 20 liters, this large polar anion does not enter cells readily, and tissue concentrations are uniformly lower than those in plasma. In experimental animals, however, the kidneys contain considerably more suramin than do other organs. Such retention may account for the fairly frequent occurrence of albuminuria following injection of the drug in human beings. Very little suramin penetrates the cerebrospinal fluid, consistent with its lack of efficacy once the CNS has been invaded by trypanosomes. The dose-dependent, prolonged persistence of suramin in the circulation explains why the drug has been used for prophylaxis of African trypanosomiasis.

Therapeutic Uses. Suramin is used to treat African trypanosomiasis but is of no value in South American trypanosomiasis caused by *T. cruzi*. Because only small amounts of the drug enter the brain, suramin is used primarily to treat early stages (before CNS involvement) of both East and West African trypanosomiasis (*see* Pépin and Milord, 1994). For therapy of early West African infections, this drug is more effective when given by intravenous regimens that also include intramuscular injections of pentamidine. In contrast, suramin alone appears superior for therapy of early East African disease. Suramin will clear the hemolymphatic system of trypanosomes even in late-stage disease, so it is often administered before initiating melarsoprol to reduce the risk of reactive encephalopathy associated with the administration of that arsenical (*see* above). In animal models, suramin has been found to display synergism with other trypanocides, including eflornithine. However, suramin-eflornithine therapy has been disappointing against late stage human *T.b. rhodesiense* infection (Clerinx *et al.,* 1998).

Suramin is given by slow intravenous injection as a 10% aqueous solution. Treatment of active African trypanosomiasis should not be started until 24 hours after diagnostic lumbar puncture, and caution is required if the patient has onchocerciasis because of the potential for eliciting a Mazzotti reaction. The normal single dose for adults with *T.b. rhodesiense* infection is 1 g. It is advisable to employ a test dose of 200 mg initially to detect sensitivity, after which the normal dose is given on days 1, 3, 7, 14, and 21. The pediatric dose is 20 mg/kg, given according to the same schedule. Patients in poor condition should be treated with lower doses during the first week. When suramin and pentamidine are used to treat early stage *T.b. gambiense* infection, Pépin and Milord (1994) recommend suramin (20 mg/kg, up to a maximum of 1 g) given intravenously on days 1 and 13, and pentamidine isethionate (4 mg/kg) given intramuscularly on days 1, 3, 5, 13, 15, and 17. However, suramin and pentamidine may lose their advantage over pentamidine alone for treatment of Gambian trypanosomiasis if there is even minimal evidence of CNS involvement (Pépin and Khonde, 1996). Patients who relapse after suramin therapy should be treated with melarsoprol (*see* Pépin and Milord, 1994).

Suramin is effective for the prophylaxis of African trypanosomiasis. Chemoprophylaxis is not recommended for travelers on occasional brief visits to endemic areas, because the risk of serious drug toxicity outweighs the risk of acquiring the disease (*see* below). For chemoprophylaxis, the single dose of 1 g is repeated weekly for 5 or 6 weeks.

Toxicity and Side Effects. Suramin can cause a variety of untoward reactions that vary in intensity and frequency and tend to be more severe in debilitated patients. Fortunately, the most serious immediate reaction consisting of nausea, vomiting, shock, and loss of consciousness is very rare (about 1 in 2000 patients). Malaise, nausea, and fatigue are common immediate reactions. Parasite destruction may cause febrile episodes and skin hypersensitivity rashes that are reduced by pretreatment with glucocorticoids; concomitant onchocerciasis optimally should be treated first with ivermectin to minimize these reactions (*see* Chapter 42). The most common problem encountered after several doses of suramin is renal toxicity, manifested by albuminuria; delayed neurological complications, including headache, metallic taste, paresthesias, and peripheral neuropathy also occur. These complications usually disappear spontaneously despite continued therapy. At higher doses over long periods of treatment used for cancer chemotherapy, suramin-induced coagu-

lopathy is the most common toxicity observed, whereas development of a severe polyradiculoneuropathy is the most serious complication (*see* Voogd *et al.*, 1993; Bowden *et al.*, 1996). Other less-prevalent reactions include vomiting, diarrhea, stomatitis, chills, abdominal pain, and edema. Laboratory abnormalities noted in 12% to 26% of patients with AIDS include leukopenia and occasional agranulocytosis, thrombocytopenia, proteinuria, and elevations of plasma creatinine, transaminases, and bilirubin, which are reversible. Unexpected findings in patients with AIDS include adrenal insufficiency and vortex keratopathy.

Precautions and Contraindications. Patients receiving suramin should be followed closely. Therapy should not be continued in patients who show intolerance to initial doses, and the drug should be employed with great caution in individuals with renal insufficiency. Moderate albuminuria is common during control of the acute phase, but persisting, heavy albuminuria calls for caution as well as modification of the treatment schedule. If casts appear, treatment with suramin should be discontinued. The occurrence of palmar-plantar hyperesthesia may presage peripheral neuritis.

ANTIPROTOZOAL ANTIBIOTICS

Numerous antibiotics have been tested for efficacy against many protozoal infections. A few of these have been shown to be of benefit, but not usually as primary drugs. Whereas *tetracycline* is recommended as first-line therapy for balantidiasis and intestinal infections with *Dientamoeba fragilis, clindamycin* is prescribed along with quinine for therapy of babesiosis. *Paromomycin* is discussed below because it has clinical efficacy against a wide spectrum of protozoal infections. Unlike some tetracyclines and erythromycin, which also have been used to treat intestinal amebiasis, paromomycin is the only antibiotic that is directly amebicidal. Other antibiotics act by interfering with the enteric flora essential for proliferation of pathogenic amoebae.

Paromomycin. This aminoglycoside antibiotic, isolated from cultures of *Streptomyces rimosus,* is structurally related to neomycin and shares most of the antibacterial properties of other antibiotics in this class (*see* Chapter 46). Indeed, paromomycin is licensed in Europe for parenteral therapy of bacterial infections that are thought to respond to aminoglycosides. Paromomycin acts directly on amebae and also has antibacterial activity against normal and pathogenic microorganisms in the gastrointestinal tract. Besides its role in the treatment of amebiasis, paromomycin may have some value in treating other protozoal infections. For example, it has been found to be effective in some cases of visceral and cutaneous leishmaniasis (*see* Berman, 1997), and it has undergone limited controlled clinical trials for the treatment of cryptosporidiosis in AIDS patients (Smith *et al.*, 1998). Other clinical uses of paromomycin include the experimental therapy of amebiasis and giardiasis in pregnancy and the treatment of infections with *D. fragilis.*

Paromomycin also is effective in the treatment of infections with various tapeworms. Its chemical structure is shown below.

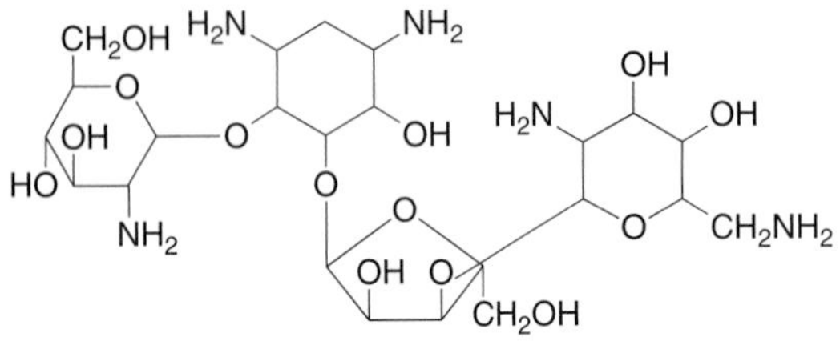

PAROMOMYCIN

The recommended dosage of *paromomycin sulfate* (HUMATIN) for intestinal amebiasis is 25 to 35 mg/kg given orally in three divided doses at mealtimes for 7 days. Higher dosages, up to 66 mg/kg, have been used by some practitioners. After oral administration, little of the drug is absorbed into the systemic circulation. Side effects are limited mainly to gastrointestinal upset and diarrhea. Marked renal damage occurs in animals treated parenterally with this drug. Human beings who are given injectable formulations of paromomycin may experience damage to both the kidney and the eighth cranial nerve if the recommended dosage is exceeded or if they also are exposed to other potentially toxic agents (*see* Berman, 1997). Experience has shown paromomycin to be effective but by no means infallible in the treatment of intestinal amebiasis; it is ineffective against extraintestinal forms of the disease (*see* Woolfe, 1965).

PROSPECTUS

Two major challenges must be faced to improve the chemoprophylaxis and therapy of human protozoal infections. The first is to find effective remedies for infections, such as Chagas' disease and East African trypanosomiasis, that respond poorly if at all to known drugs. The second is to deal successfully with increased inherent and acquired resistance of pathogenic protozoa to effective antiprotozoal agents. Examples here include increasing resistance of *T. brucei* to melarsoprol, *Leishmania* to pentavalent antimonials, and *T. vaginalis* to metronidazole. Progress in finding new antiprotozoal drugs and combating drug resistance has been hampered by lack of economic incentives and commitment to emphasize research and drug development in this field.

Several strategies may help address these problems despite economic limitations. To avoid some of the high costs associated with drug development and regulatory approval, drugs already approved for other indications could be tested for efficacy against human protozoal diseases in limited clinical trials. Ideally, this decision would be based on supportive evidence from *in vitro* experiments and animal models. Several examples illustrate the utility of this approach. *Atovaquone,* approved for treatment of infections with *P. carinii,* is now used clinically against

multidrug-resistant *falciparum* malaria and infections with *T. gondii. Eflornithine,* originally evaluated as an antineoplastic agent, is clinically effective against West African trypanosomiasis. *Miltefosine,* an alkylphospholipid originally tested for safety as an anticancer drug, shows promise as the first oral medication for treatment of visceral leishmaniasis (*see* Herwaldt, 1999a). Drugs developed to combat protozoal infections in animals provide a rich source of possible candidates for human use; such compounds often are cheap and readily available. *Diminazine* (BERENIL) is a case in point. This aromatic diamidine used to treat bovine trypanosomiasis has shown some promise for the therapy of East African trypanosomiasis. However, there is little economic incentive to develop it for human use.

Combination chemotherapy with known effective antiprotozoal agents is another approach that can prove fruitful. Ideally, a combination would be selected on the basis of known complementary antiprotozoal activities, just as was done with the antifolates. Alternatively, drugs acting on different but vital protozoal processes also may enhance each other's effect. This approach, along with the use of drugs with compatible pharmacokinetic properties, has proven to be successful, not only to improve the clinical response but also to circumvent and delay the emergence of drug resistance. Several multidrug regimens for the treatment of multidrug-resistant *falciparum* malaria amply illustrate this point (*see* Chapter 40).

The effectiveness of antiprotozoal chemotherapy is critically dependent on the status of host defense mechanisms. The worldwide AIDS epidemic is notoriously associated with exacerbations of many coexisting infections, including those with pathogenic protozoa. For example, visceral leishmaniasis as a component of AIDS has increased dramatically in southern Europe, and the latter has rendered standard antileishmanial therapy ineffective (*see* Berman, 1997). The effect of AIDS is most pronounced when a drug does not kill pathogens directly but requires host mechanisms for their removal. In addition to the intrinsic illness, toxic drugs used for antiprotozoal therapy often suppress host defenses. Investigators have tried immunotherapy in addition to chemotherapy to boost host defenses against pathogenic protozoa. In systemic forms of leishmaniasis, for example, immune responses are impaired; patients with this infection have been treated experimentally with recombinant interferon-gamma or bacillus Calmette-Guérin (BCG) to facilitate increased destruction of intracellular protozoa.

Targeted drug delivery represents yet another strategy to combat protozoal infections. This alternative is largely experimental and, as yet, too costly to be of much practical use. For instance, associating pentavalent antimony with mannan instead of sodium gluconate increases its potency against *Leishmania* amastigotes in culture, possibly by directing the antimony complexes to macrophages (Roberts *et al.,* 1995). Moreover, newer lipid formulations of amphotericin B have increased the therapeutic index of this antifungal agent, and it is now considered first-line therapy for Indian visceral leishmaniasis.

The best long-term defense against protozoan infections, however, is continued basic and clinical research directed at understanding parasite biology as it applies to the rational design and development of improved drugs and vaccines. Although the cost of this effort is high, the cost of failure is much higher.

For further discussion of protozoal infections *see* Chapters 215–220 in *Harrison's Principles of Internal Medicine,* 14th ed., McGraw-Hill, New York, 1998.

BIBLIOGRAPHY

Abeloff, M.D., Slavik, M., Luk, G.D., Griffin, C.A., Hermann, J., Blanc, O., Sjoerdsma, A., and Baylin, S.B. Phase I trial and pharmacokinetic studies of α-difluoromethylornithine—an inhibitor of polyamine biosynthesis. *J. Clin. Oncol.,* **1984,** 2:124–130.

Bacchi, C.J., Nathan, H.C., Hunter, S.H., McCann, P.P., and Sjoerdsma, A. Polyamine metabolism: a potential therapeutic target in trypanosomes. *Science,* **1980,** 210:332–334.

Bailly, C., Donkor, I.O., Gentle, D., Thornalley, M., and Waring, M.J. Sequence-selective binding to DNA of *cis-* and *trans*-butamidine analogues of the anti–*Pneumocystis carinii* pneumonia drug pentamidine. *Mol. Pharmacol.,* **1994,** 46:313–322.

Berger, B.J., Carter, N.S., and Fairlamb, A.H. Polyamine and pentamidine metabolism in African trypanosomes. *Acta Trop.,* **1993,** 54: 215–224.

Berger, B.J., Carter, N.S., and Fairlamb, A.H. Characterization of pentamidine-resistant *Trypanosoma brucei brucei. Mol. Biochem. Parasitol.,* **1995,** 69:289–298.

Berman, J.D., Edwards, N., King, M., and Grogl, M. Biochemistry of Pentostam-resistant *Leishmania. Am. J. Trop. Med. Hyg.,* **1989,** 40: 159–164.

Bitonti, A.J., Dumont, J.A., and McCann, P.P. Characterization of *Trypanosoma brucei brucei* S-adenosyl-L-methionine decarboxylase and its inhibition by Berenil, pentamidine, and methylglyoxal bis(guanylhydrazone). *Biochem. J.,* **1986,** 237:685–689.

Bowden, C.J., Figg, W.D., Dawson, N.A., Sartor, O., Bitton, R.J., Weinberger, M.S., Headlee, D., Reed, E., Myers, C.E., and Cooper, M.R. A phase I/II study of continuous infusion suramin in patients with hormone-refractory prostate cancer: toxicity and response. *Cancer Chemother. Pharmacol.,* **1996,** 39:1–8.

Bronner, U., Gustafsson, L.L., Doua, F., Ericsson, O., Miezan, T., Rais, M., and Rombo, L. Pharmacokinetics and adverse reactions after a single dose of pentamidine in patients with *Trypanosoma gambiense* sleeping sickness. *Br. J. Clin. Pharmacol.,* **1995,** 39:289–295.

Brown, D.M., Upcroft, J.A., Dodd, H.N., Chen, N., and Upcroft, P. Alternative 2-keto acid oxidoreductase activities in *Trichomonas vaginalis. Mol. Biochem. Parasitol.,* **1999,** 98:203–214.

Carter, N.S., Berger, B.J., and Fairlamb, A.H. Uptake of diamidine drugs by the P2 nucleoside transporter in melarsen-sensitive and -resistant *Trypanosoma brucei brucei. J. Biol. Chem.,* **1995,** 270:28153–28157.

Carter, N.S., and Fairlamb, A.H. Arsenical-resistant trypanosomes lack an unusual adenosine transporter. *Nature,* 1993, 361:173–176.

Cheson, B.D., Levine, A.M., Mildvan, D., Kaplan, L.D., Wolfe, P., Rios, A., Groopman, J.E., Gill, P., Volberding, P.A., Poiesz,

B.J., Gottlieb, M.S., Holden, H., Volsky, D.J., Silver, S.S., and Hawkins, M. Suramin therapy in AIDS and related disorders. Report of the U.S. Suramin Working Group. *JAMA,* **1987,** 258:1347–1351.

Chulay, J.D., Fleckenstein, L., and Smith, D.H. Pharmacokinetics of antimony during treatment of visceral leishmaniasis with sodium stibogluconate or meglumine antimoniate. *Trans. R. Soc. Trop. Med. Hyg.,* **1988,** 82:69–72.

Clerinx, J., Taelman, H., Bogaerts, J., and Vervoort, T. Treatment of late-stage rhodesiense trypanosomiasis using suramin and eflornithine: report of six cases. *Trans. R. Soc. Trop. Med. Hyg.,* **1998,** 92:449–450.

Conte, J.E., Jr. Pharmacokinetics of intravenous pentamidine in patients with normal renal function or receiving hemodialysis. *J. Infect. Dis.,* **1991,** 163:169–175.

Cosar, C., Ganter, P., and Julou, L. Etude expérimentale du métronidazole, 8823 R.P., activités trichomonacide et amoebicide. Toxicité et propriétés pharmacologiques générales. *Presse Med.,* **1961,** 69: 1069–1972.

de Koning, H.P., and Jarvis, S.M. Adenosine transporters in bloodstream forms of *Trypanosoma brucei brucei*: substrate recognition motifs and affinity for trypanocidal drugs. *Mol. Pharmacol.,* **1999,** 56:1162–1170.

Donnelly, H., Bernard, E.M., Rothkotter, H., Gold, J.W., and Armstrong, D. Distribution of pentamidine in patients with AIDS. *J. Infect. Dis.,* **1988,** 157:985–989.

Durel, P., Roiron, V., Siboulet, A., and Borel, L.J. Systemic treatment of human trichomoniasis with a derivative of nitroimidazole, 8823 R.P. *Br. J. Vener. Dis.,* **1960,** 36:21–26.

Dykstra, C.C., and Tidwell, R.R. Inhibition of topoisomerases from *Pneumocystis carinii* by aromatic dicationic molecules. *J. Protozool.,* **1991,** 38:78S–81S.

Eisenthal, R., and Cornish-Bowden, A. Prospects for antiparasitic drugs. The case for *Trypanosoma brucei,* the causative agent of African sleeping sickness. *J. Biol. Chem.,* **1998,** 273:5500–5505.

Ephros, M., Bitnun, A., Shaked, P., Waldman, E., and Zilberstein, D. Stage-specific activity of pentavalent antimony against *Leishmania donovani* axenic amastigotes. *Antimicrob. Agents Chemother.,* **1999,** 43:278–282.

Ericsson, O., Schweda, E.K., Bronner, U., Rombo, L., Friden, M., and Gustafsson, L.L. Determination of melarsoprol in biological fluids by high-performance liquid chromatography and characterisation of two stereoisomers by nuclear magnetic resonance spectroscopy. *J. Chromatogr. B Biomed. Sci. Appl.,* **1997,** 690:242–251.

Flynn, I.W., and Bowman, I.B. Further studies on the mode of action of arsenicals on trypanosome pyruvate kinase. *Trans. R. Soc. Trop. Med. Hyg.,* **1969,** *63*:121.

Friedheim, E.A.H. Mel B in the treatment of human trypanosomiasis. *Am J. Trop. Med. Hyg.,* **1949,** *29*:173–180.

Frommel, T.O. Suramin is synergistic with vinblastine in human colonic tumor cell lines: effect of cell density and timing of drug delivery. *Anticancer Res.,* **1997,** *17*:2065–2071.

Grogl, M., Thomason, T.N., and Franke, E.D. Drug resistance in leishmaniasis: its implications in systemic chemotherapy of cutaneous and mucocutaneous disease. *Am. J. Trop. Med. Hyg.,* **1992,** *47*:117–126.

Haimeur, A., Brochu, C., Genest, P., Papadopoulou, B., and Ouellette, M. Amplification of the ABC transporter gene *PGPA* and increased trypanothione levels in potassium antimonyl tartrate (SbIII) resistant *Leishmania tarentolae. Mol. Biochem. Parasitol.,* **2000,** *108*:131–135.

Hand, I.L., Wiznia, A.A., Porricolo, M., Lambert, G., and Caspe, W.B. Aerosolized pentamidine for prophylaxis of *Pneumocystis carinii* pneumonia in infants with human immunodeficiency virus infection. *Pediatr. Infect. Dis. J.,* **1994,** *13*:100–104.

Haque, R., Ali, I.K., Akther, S., and Petri, W.A., Jr. Comparision of PCR, isoenzyme analysis, and antigen detection for diagnosis of *Entamoeba histolytica* infection. *J. Clin. Microbiol.,* **1998,** *36*:449–452.

Henderson, G.B., Ulrich, P., Fairlamb, A.H., Rosenberg, I., Pereira, M., Sela, M., and Cerami, A. "Subversive" substrates for the enzyme trypanothione disulfide reductase: alternative approach to chemotherapy of Chagas' disease. *Proc. Natl. Acad. Sci. U.S.A.,* **1988,** *85*:5374–5378.

Herwaldt, B.L. Miltefosine—the long-awaited therapy for visceral leishmaniasis? *N. Engl. J. Med.,* **1999a,** *341*:1840–1842.

Hopkins, R.J., and Morris, J.G., Jr. *Helicobacter pylori:* the missing link in perspective. *Am. J. Med.,* **1994,** *97*:265–277.

Horie, H. Anti-*Trichomonas* effect of azomycin. *J. Antibiot. (Tokyo),* **1956,** *9*:168.

Iten, M., Mett, H., Evans, A., Enyaru, J.C., Brun, R., and Kaminsky, R. Alterations in ornithine decarboxylase characteristics account for tolerance of *Trypanosoma brucei rhodesiense* to D,L-α-difluoromethylornithine. *Antimicrob. Agents Chemother.,* **1998,** *41*:1922–1925.

Legare, D., Papadopoulou, B., Roy, G., Mukhopadhyay, R., Haimeur, A., Dey, S., Grondin, K., Brochu, C., Rosen, B.P., and Ouellette, M. Efflux systems and increased trypanothione levels in arsenite-resistant *Leishmania. Exp. Parasitol.,* **1997,** *87*:275–282.

Lelchuk, R., Cardoni, R.L., and Fuks, A.S. Cell-mediated immunity in Chagas' disease: alterations induced by treatment with a trypanocidal drug (nifurtimox). *Clin. Exp. Immunol.,* **1977a,** *30*:434–438.

Lelchuk, R., Cardoni, R.L., and Levis, S. Nifurtimox-induced alterations in the cell-mediated immune response to PPD in guinea pigs. *Clin. Exp. Immunol.,* **1977b,** *30*:469–473.

Leoung, S.G., Feigal, D.W., Jr., Montgomery, A.B., Corkery, K., Wardlaw, L., Adams, M., Busch, D., Gordon, S., Jacobson, M.A., Volberding, P.A., Abrams, D., and the San Francisco County Community Consortium. Aerosolized pentamidine for prophylaxis against *Pneumocystis carinii* pneumonia. The San Francisco community prophylaxis trial. *N. Engl. J. Med.,* **1990,** *323*:769–775.

Li, F., Hua, S.B., Wang, C.C., and Gottesdiener, K.M. *Trypanosoma brucei brucei:* characterization of an ODC null bloodstream form mutant and the action of α-difluoromethylornithine. *Exp. Parasitol.,* **1998,** *88*:255–257.

Lira, R., Sundar, S., Makharia, A., Kenney, R., Gam, A., Saraiva, E., and Sacks, D. Evidence that the high incidence of treatment failures in Indian kala-azar is due to the emergence of antimony-resistant strains of *Leishmania donovani. J. Infect. Dis.,* **1999,** *180*:564–567.

Main, P.T., Bristow, N.W., Oxley, P., Watkins, T.I., Williams, G.A.H., Wilmshurst, E.C., and Woolfe, G. Entamide. *Ann. Biochem. Exp. Med.,* **1960,** *20*:441–448.

Maser, P., Sutterlin, C., Kralli, A., and Kaminsky, R. A nucleoside transporter from *Trypanosoma brucei* involved in drug resistance. *Science,* **1999,** *285*:242–244.

Metcalf, B.W., Bey, P., Danzin, C., Jung, M.J., Casara, P., and Vevert, J.P. Catalytic irreversible inhibition of mammalian ornithine decarboxylase (E.C. 4.1.1.17) by substrate and product analogues. *J. Am. Chem. Soc.,* **1978,** *100*:2551–2553.

Meyerhoff, A. U.S. Food and Drug Administration approval of AmBisome (lipsomal amphotericin B) for treatment of leishmaniasis. *Clin. Infect. Dis.,* **1999,** *28*:42–48.

Milord, F., Loko, L., Éthier, L., Mpia, B., and Pépin, J. Eflornithine concentrations in serum and cerebrospinal fluid of 63 patients treated for *Trypanosoma brucei gambiense* sleeping sickness. *Trans. R. Soc. Trop. Med. Hyg.,* **1993,** *87*:473–477.

Moreno, S.N., Palmero, D.J., Eiguchi de Palmero, K., Docampo, R., and Stoppani, A.O. [Stimulation of lipid peroxidation and ultrastructural changes induced by nifurtimox in mammalian tissues.] *Medicina (B. Aires),* **1980,** *40*:553–559.

Morty, R.E., Troeberg, L., Pike, R.N., Jones, R., Nickel, P., Lonsdale-Eccles, J.D., and Coetzer, T.H. A trypanosome oligopeptidase as a target for the trypanocidal agents pentamidine, diminazene, and suramin. *FEBS Lett.,* **1998,** *433*:251–256.

Navin, T.R., Arana, B.A., Arana, F.E., Berman, J.D., and Chajón, J.F. Placebo-controlled clinical trial of sodium stibogluconate (Pentostam) versus ketoconazole for treating cutaneous leishmaniasis in Guatemala. *J. Infect. Dis.,* **1992,** *165*:528–534.

Pamplin, C.L., Desjardins, R., Chulay, J., Tramont, E., Hendricks, L., and Canfield, C. Pharmacokinetics of antimony during sodium stibogluconate therapy for cutaneous leishmaniasis. *Clin. Pharmacol. Ther.,* **1981,** *29*:270–271.

Pasic, T.R., Heisey, D., and Love, R.R. α-Difluoromethylornithine ototoxicity. Chemoprevention clinical trial results. *Arch. Otolaryngol. Head Neck Surg.,* **1997,** *123*:1281–1286.

Paulos, C., Paredes, J., Vasquez, I., Thambo, S., Arancibia, A., and Gonzalez-Martin, A. Pharmacokinetics of a nitrofuran compound, nifurtimox, in healthy volunteers. *Int. J. Clin. Pharmacol. Ther. Toxicol.,* **1989,** *27*:454–457.

Pépin, J., and Khonde, N. Relapses following treatment of early-stage *Trypanosoma brucei gambiense* sleeping sickness with a combination of pentamidine and suramin. *Trans. R. Soc. Trop. Med. Hyg.,* **1996,** *90*:183–186.

Pépin, J., Milord, F., Khonde, A.N., Niyonsenga, T., Loko, L., Mpia, B., and De Wals, P. Risk factors for encephalopathy and mortality during melarsoprol treatment of *Trypanosoma brucei gambiense* sleeping sickness. *Trans. R. Soc. Trop. Med. Hyg.,* **1995,** *89*:92–97.

Pifer, L.L., Pifer, D.D., and Woods, D.R. Biological profile and response to antipneumocystis agents of *Pneumocystis carinii* in cell culture. *Antimicrob. Agents Chemother.,* **1983,** *24*:674–678.

Quon, D.V., d'Oliveira, C.E., and Johnson, P.J. Reduced transcription of the ferredoxin gene in metronidazole-resistant *Trichomonas vaginalis. Proc. Natl. Acad. Sci. U.S.A.,* **1992,** *89*:4402–4406.

Roberts, W.L., Berman, J.D., and Rainey, P.M. In vitro antileishmanial properties of tri- and pentavalent antimonial preparations. *Antimicrob. Agents Chemother.,* **1995,** *39*:1234–1239.

Roberts, W.L., and Rainey, P.M. Antileishmanial activity of sodium stibogluconate fractions. *Antimicrob. Agents Chemother.,* **1993,** *37*:1842–1846.

Sereno, D., Cavaleyra, M., Zemzoumi, K., Maquaire, S., Ouaissi, A., and Lemesre, J.L. Axenically grown amastigotes of *Leishmania infantum* used as an in vitro model to investigate the pentavalent antimony mode of action. *Antimicrob. Agents Chemother.*, **1998**, *42*:3097–3102.

Sereno, D., and Lemesre, J.L. Axenically cultured amastigote forms as an in vitro model for investigation of antileishmanial agents. *Antimicrob. Agents Chemother.*, **1997**, *41*:972–976.

Shapiro, T.A., and Englund, P.T. Selective cleavage of kinetoplast DNA minicircles promoted by antitrypanosomal drugs. *Proc. Natl. Acad. Sci. U.S.A.*, **1990**, *87*:950–954.

Smith, N.H., Cron, S., Valdez, L.M., Chappell, C.L., and White, A.C., Jr. Combination drug therapy for cryptosporidiosis in AIDS. *J. Infect. Dis.*, **1998**, *178*:900–903.

Sobel, J.D., Nagappan, V., and Nyirjesy, P. Metronidazole-resistant vaginal trichomoniasis—an emerging problem. *N. Engl. J. Med.*, **1999**, *341*:292–293.

Suchak, N.G., Satoskar, R.S., and Sheth, U.K. Entamide furoate in the treatment of intestinal amoebiasis. *Am. J. Trop. Med. Hyg.*, **1962**, *11*:330–332.

Sundar, S., Sinha, P.R., Agrawal, N.K., Srivastava, R., Rainey, P.M., Berman, J.D., Murray, H.W., and Singh, V.P. A cluster of cases of severe cardiotoxicity among kala-azar patients treated with a high-osmolarity lot of sodium antimony gluconate. *Am. J. Trop. Med. Hyg.*, **1998**, *59*:139–143.

Torres, R.A., Weinberg, W., Stansell, J., Leoung, G., Kovacs, J., Rogers, M., and Scott, J. Atovaquone for salvage treatment and suppression of toxoplasmic encephalitis in patients with AIDS. Atovaquone/toxoplasmic Encephalitis Study Group. *Clin. Infect. Dis.*, **1997**, *24*:422–429.

Upcroft, J.A., Campbell, R.W., Benakli, K., Upcroft, P., and Vanelle, P. Efficacy of new 5-nitroimidazoles against metronidazole-susceptible and -resistant *Giardia*, *Trichomonas*, and *Entamoeba* spp. *Antimicrob. Agents Chemother.*, **1999**, *43*:73–76.

Van Schaftingen, E., Opperdoes, F.R., and Hers, H.G. Effects of various metabolic conditions and of the trivalent arsenical melarsen oxide on the intracellular levels of fructose 2,6-bisphosphate and of glycolytic intermediates in *Trypanosoma brucei*. *Eur. J. Biochem.*, **1987**, *166*:653–661.

Wassmann, C., Hellberg, A., Tannich, E., and Bruchhaus, I. Metronidazole resistance in the protozoan parasite *Entamoeba histolytica* is associated with increased expression of iron-containing superoxide dismutase and peroxidredoxin and decreased expression of ferredoxin 1 and flavin reductase. *J. Biol. Chem.*, **1999**, *274*:26051–26056.

Wolfe, M.S. Nondysenteric intestinal amebiasis. Treatment with diloxanide furoate. *JAMA*, **1973**, *224*:1601–1604.

World Health Organization. Amoebiasis. *Wkly. Epidemiol. Rec.*, **1997**, *14*:97–99.

World Health Organization. Chile and Brazil to be certified free of transmission of Chagas disease. *TDR News*, **1999**, No. *59*:10.

Yarlett, N., Goldberg, B., Nathan, H.C., Garofalo, J., and Bacchi, C.J. Differential susceptibility of *Trypanosoma brucei rhodesiense* isolates to *in vitro* lysis by arsenicals. *Exp. Parasitol.*, **1991**, *72*:205–215.

Yarlett, N., Yarlett, N.C., and Lloyd, D. Metronidazole-resistant clinical isolates of *Trichomonas vaginalis* have lowered oxygen affinities. *Mol. Biochem. Parasitol.*, **1986**, *19*:111–116.

MONOGRAPHS AND REVIEWS

Albert, A. *Selective Toxicity: The Physico-Chemical Basis of Therapy*, 6th ed. Chapman & Hall, London, **1979**.

Anonymous. Drugs for parasitic infections. *Med. Lett. Drugs Ther.*, **1998**, *40*:1–12.

Barrett, M.P., and Fairlamb, A.H. The biochemical basis of arsenical-diamidine crossresistance in African trypanosomes. *Parasitol. Today*, **1999**, *15*:136–140.

Barrett, S.V., and Barrett, M.P. Anti–sleeping sickness drugs and cancer chemotherapy. *Parasitol. Today*, **2000**, *16*:7–9.

Berger, B.J., and Fairlamb, A.H. Interactions between immunity and chemotherapy in the treatment of the trypanosomiases and leishmaniases. *Parasitology*, **1992**, *105*:S71–S78.

Berman, J.D. Chemotherapy for leishmaniasis: biochemical mechanisms, clinical efficacy, and future strategies. *Rev. Infect. Dis.*, **1988**, *10*:560–586.

Berman, J.D. Human leishmaniasis: clinical, diagnostic, and chemotherapeutic developments in the last 10 years. *Clin. Infect. Dis.*, **1997**, *24*:684–703.

Brener, Z. Present status of chemotherapy and chemoprophylaxis of human trypanosomiasis in the Western Hemisphere. *Pharmacol. Ther.*, **1979**, *7*:71–90.

Damper, D., and Patten, C.L. Pentamidine transport and sensitivity in *brucei*-group trypanosomes. *J. Protozool.*, **1976**, *23*:349–356.

Docampo, R. Sensitivity of parasites to free radical damage by antiparasitic drugs. *Chem. Biol. Interact.*, **1990**, *73*:1–27.

Fairlamb, A.H., and Bowman, I.B. *Trypanosoma brucei*: suramin and other trypanocidal compounds' effects on *sn*-glycerol-3-phosphate oxidase. *Exp. Parasitol.*, **1977**, *43*:353–361.

Farthing, M.J. Giardiasis. *Gastroenterol. Clin. North Am.*, **1996**, *25*:493–515.

Fauci, A.S., and Lane, H.C. Human immunodeficiency virus (HIV) disease: AIDS and related disorders. In, *Harrison's Principles of Internal Medicine*, 14th ed. (Fauci, A.S., Braunwald, E., Isselbacher, K.J., Wilson, J.D., Martin, J.B., Kasper, D.L., Hauser, S.L., and Longo, D.L., eds.) McGraw-Hill, New York, **1998**, pp. 1791–1856.

Freeman, C.D., Klutman, N.E., and Lamp, K.C. Metronidazole. A therapeutic review and update. *Drugs*, **1997**, *54*:679–708.

Georgiev, V.S. Management of toxoplasmosis. *Drugs*, **1994**, *48*:179–188.

Griffiths, J.K. Human cryptosporidiosis: epidemiology, transmission, clinical disease, treatment, and diagnosis. *Adv. Parasitol.*, **1998**, *40*:37–85.

Harris, A. Current regimens for treatment of *Helicobacter pylori* infection. *Br. Med. Bull.*, **1998**, *54*:195–205.

Heine, P., and McGregor, J.A. *Trichomonas vaginalis*: a reemerging pathogen. *Clin. Obstet. Gynecol.*, **1993**, *36*:137–144.

Herwaldt, B.L. Leishmaniasis. *Lancet*, **1999b**, *354*:1191–1199.

Johnson, P.J. Metronidazole and drug resistance. *Parasitol. Today*, **1993**, *9*:183–186.

Kirchhoff, L.V. American trypanosomiasis (Chagas' disease). *Gastroenterol. Clin. North Am.*, **1996**, *25*:517–533.

Krogstad, D.J., Spencer, H.C., Jr., and Healy, G.R. Current concepts in parasitology. Amebiasis. *N. Engl. J. Med.*, **1978**, *298*:262–265.

Kulda, J. Trichomonads, hydrogenosomes, and drug resistance. *Int. J. Parasitol.*, **1999**, *29*:199–212.

Lamp, K.C., Freeman, C.D., Klutman, N.E., and Lacy, M.K. Pharmacokinetics and pharmacodynamics of the nitroimidazole antimicrobials. *Clin. Pharmacokinet.*, **1999**, *36*:353–373.

Land, K.M., and Johnson, P.J. Molecular mechanisms underlying metronidazole resistance in trichomonads. *Exp. Parasitol.*, **1997**, *87*:305–308.

Lau, A.H., Lam, N.P., Piscitelli, S.C., Wilkes, L., and Danziger, L.H. Clinical pharmacokinetics of metronidazole and other nitroimidazole anti-infectives. *Clin. Pharmacokinet.*, **1992**, *23*:328–364.

McCann, P.P., and Pegg, A.E. Ornithine decarboxylase as an enzyme target for therapy. *Pharmacol. Ther.,* **1992,** *54*:195–215.

Megraud, F., and Doermann, H.P. Clinical relevance of resistant strains of *Helicobacter pylori*: a review of current data. *Gut,* **1998,** *43*:S61–S65.

Meyskens, F.L., Jr., and Gerner, E.W. Development of difluoromethylornithine (DFMO) as a chemopreventative agent. *Clin. Cancer Res.,* **1999,** *5*:945–951.

Ortega, Y.R., and Adam, R.D. Giardia: overview and update. *Clin. Infect. Dis.,* **1997,** *25*:545–550.

Ouellette, M., and Papadopoulou, B. Mechanisms of drug resistance in *Leishmania. Parasitol. Today,* **1993,** *9*:150–153.

Pegg, A.E. Polyamine metabolism and its importance in neoplastic growth as a target for chemotherapy. *Cancer Res.,* **1988,** *48*:759–774.

Pépin, J., and Milord, F. The treatment of human African trypanosomiasis. *Adv. Parasitol.,* **1994,** *33*:1–47.

Ravdin, J.I. Amebiasis. *Clin. Infect. Dis.,* **1995,** *20*:1453–1466.

Roe, F.J. Metronidazole: review of uses and toxicity. *J. Antimicrob. Chemother.,* **1977,** *3*:205–212.

Rosenblatt, J.E. Antiparasitic agents. *Mayo Clin. Proc.,* **1999,** *74*:1161–1175.

Samuelson, J. Why metronidazole is active against both bacteria and parasites. *Antimicrob. Agents Chemother.,* **1999,** *43*:1533–1541.

Sands, M., Kron, M.A., and Brown, R.B. Pentamidine: a review. *Rev. Infect. Dis.,* **1985,** *7*:625–634.

Song, F., and Glenny, A.M. Antimicrobial prophylaxis in colorectal surgery: a systematic review of randomised controlled trials. *Health Technol. Assess.,* **1998,** *2*:1–110.

Steck, E.A. The leishmaniases. *Prog. Drug Res.,* **1974,** *18*:289–351.

Tanowitz, H.B., Kirchhoff, L.V., Simon, D., Morris, S.A., Weiss, L.M., and Wittner, M. Chagas' disease. *Clin. Microbiol. Rev.,* **1992,** *5*:400–419.

Upcroft, J.A., and Upcroft, P. Keto-acid oxidoreductases in the anaerobic protozoa. *J. Eukaryot. Microbiol.,* **1999,** *46*:447–449.

Urbina, J.A. Chemotherapy of Chagas' disease: the how and the why. *J. Mol. Med.,* **1999,** *77*:332–338.

Urbina, J.A. Parasitological cure of Chagas' disease: Is it possible? Is it relevant? *Mem. Inst. Oswaldo Cruz,* **1997,** *94*(suppl. 1):349–355.

van Nieuwenhove, S. Advances in sleeping sickness therapy. *Ann. Soc. Belg. Med. Trop.,* **1992,** *72*(suppl. 1):39–51.

Vöhringer, H.F., and Arastéh, K. Pharmacokinetic optimisation in the treatment of *Pneumocystis carinii* pneumonia. *Clin. Pharmacokinet.,* **1993,** *24*:388–412.

Voogd, T.E., Vansterkenburg, E.L., Wilting, J., and Janssen, L.H. Recent research on the biological activity of suramin. *Pharmacol. Rev.,* **1993,** *45*:177–203.

Wang, C.C. Molecular mechanisms and therapeutic approaches to the treatment of African trypanosomiasis. *Annu. Rev. Pharmacol. Toxicol.,* **1995,** *35*:93–127.

Wang, C.C. Validating targets for antiparasitic chemotherapy. *Parasitology,* **1997,** *114*:S31–S44.

Wong, S.Y., and Remington, J.S. Biology of *Toxoplasma gondii. AIDS,* **1993,** *7*:299–316.

Woolfe, G. The chemotherapy of amoebiasis. In, *Progress in Drug Research.* Vol. 8. (Jucker, E., ed.) Birkhaüser Verlag, Basel, **1965,** pp. 11–52.

Zaat, J.O., Mank, T.G., and Assendelft, W.J. A systematic review on the treatment of giardiasis. *Trop. Med. Int. Health,* **1997,** *2*:63–82.

C H A P T E R 4 2

DRUGS USED IN THE CHEMOTHERAPY OF HELMINTHIASIS

James W. Tracy and Leslie T. Webster, Jr.

Helminthiasis, or infection with parasitic worms, affects over two billion people worldwide. In tropical regions, where prevalence is greatest, simultaneous infection with more than one type of helminth is common. Moreover, human beings can spread these pathogens to previously uninvolved populations through travel, migration, and military operations.

Worms pathogenic for human beings are Metazoa, classified into roundworms (nematodes) and two types of flatworms, flukes (trematodes) and tapeworms (cestodes). These biologically diverse eukaryotes vary with respect to life cycle, bodily structure, development, physiology, localization within the host, and susceptibility to chemotherapy. Immature forms invade human beings via *the skin or gastrointestinal tract and evolve into well-differentiated adult worms that have characteristic tissue distributions. With few exceptions, such as* Strongyloides *and* Echinococcus, *these organisms cannot complete their life cycles, i.e., replicate themselves, within the human host. Therefore, the extent of exposure to these parasites dictates the severity of infection, and reduction in the number of adult organisms by chemotherapy is sustained unless reinfection occurs. The prevalence of parasitic helminths typically displays a negative binomial distribution within an infected population such that relatively few persons carry heavy parasite burdens. Without treatment, those individuals are most likely to become ill and to perpetuate infection within their community.*

Anthelmintics are drugs that act either locally to expel worms from the gastrointestinal tract or systemically to eradicate adult helminths or developmental forms that invade organs and tissues. Due to discovery and development of anthelmintics, particularly for veterinary applications, physicians now have effective and, in some cases, broad-spectrum agents that will cure or control most human infections caused by either flukes or intestinal helminths. But cysticercosis, echinococcosis, filariasis, and trichinosis are examples of systemic infections caused by tissue-dwelling helminths that at best respond only partially to currently available drugs. Because metazoan parasites are generally long-lived and have relatively complex life cycles, acquired resistance to anthelmintics in human beings has yet to become a major factor limiting clinical efficacy. However, based on extensive use of anthelmintics, such as the benzimidazoles in veterinary medicine, the potential for drug resistance among human helminths cannot be discounted.

This chapter begins with brief descriptions of recommended chemotherapy for common human infections caused by parasitic helminths. The following section features properties of selected antihelmintic drugs in alphabetical order, and the chapter concludes with a prospectus about the chemotherapy of helminthiasis.

TREATMENT OF HELMINTH INFECTIONS

Nematodes (Roundworms)

Ascaris lumbricoides. *Ascaris lumbricoides,* known as the "roundworm," parasitizes more than 1.4 billion people worldwide. Although ascariasis is not uncommon in temperate climates, it may affect from 70% to 90% of persons in some tropical regions. In the United States, the prevalence of ascariasis is highest among children of poor families in the rural South. People become infected by ingesting food or soil contaminated with embryonated *A. lumbricoides* eggs.

More effective, less toxic compounds largely have replaced the older ascaricides. *Mebendazole, pyrantel pamoate,* and *albendazole* are preferred agents. *Piperazine* also is effective but is used less often because of occasional neurotoxicity and hypersensitivity reactions. Cure with any of these drugs can be achieved in nearly 100% of cases, and all infected persons should be treated. Mebendazole and albendazole are preferred for therapy of asymptomatic to moderate ascariasis. Both of these benzimidazoles are cidal and have a broad spectrum of activity against mixed infections with other gastrointestinal nematodes. Albendazole is useful against infections with some systemic nematodes and some cestodes as well (*see* Table VII–1). Both compounds should be used with caution to treat heavy *Ascaris* infections, alone or with hookworms. In rare instances, hyperactive ascarids may migrate to unusual loci and cause serious complications such as appendicitis, occlusion of the common bile duct, intestinal obstruction, and intestinal perforation with peritonitis. Therapy with noncidal agents such as pyrantel or piperazine is preferred for heavy *Ascaris* infections; pyrantel also is useful for mixed infections with hookworms. Surgery still may be required despite the use of these agents. Pyrantel and piperazine are considered safe for use during pregnancy, whereas the bendimidazoles should be avoided during the first trimester because of their teratogenic potential. Pyrantel and albendazole are considered "investigational" drugs for treatment of ascariasis in the United States, even though they are approved for other indications.

Hookworm. *Necator americanus, Ancylostoma duodenale.* These closely related hookworm species infest about 1.3 billion people, chiefly between the latitudes 30°S and 40°N. *N. americanus* predominates in the Americas and sub-Saharan Africa, whereas *A. duodenale* prevails in southern Europe, North Africa, and northern Asia. Infection also occurs farther north in unusual but relatively warm settings such as mines and large mountain tunnels, hence the term *miner's disease* and *tunnel disease.* Hookworm larvae live in the soils and penetrate exposed skin. After reaching the lungs, the larvae migrate to the oral cavity and are swallowed. After attaching to the jejunal mucosa, the derived adult worms feed on host blood and fluids. In heavily infected persons, this process causes iron deficiency anemia and malnutrition if food and iron intake are inadequate.

Treatment of hookworm disease involves two related objectives. The first is to restore the blood values to normal, and the second is to expel the intestinal parasites. Proper diet and treatment with iron usually are sufficient for the first objective, but blood transfusion is required occasionally. Albendazole and mebendazole are now agents of first choice against both *A. duodenale* and *N. americanus,* and both benzimidazoles have the advantage of effectiveness against other roundworms when there is multiple infection. However, use of these cidal drugs in heavy mixed infections with *Ascaris* may risk unwanted ascarid activation and migration (*see* "*Ascaris lumbricoides,*" above). Therapy with pyrantel, which just paralyzes ascarids, may be safe under these circumstances. Topical or oral thiabendazole is the drug of choice for treating *cutaneous larva migrans* or "creeping eruption," which is due most commonly to penetration of the skin of human beings by larvae of the dog hookworm, *A. braziliense.*

Trichuris trichiura. *Trichuris* (whipworm) infection affects nearly one billion people throughout the world, especially children in warm, humid climates, where it frequently is found along with *Ascaris* and hookworms. The infection is acquired by eating food contaminated with parasite eggs. The adult worms usually do not cause problems except in heavily infected young children, who may exhibit abdominal cramping, diarrhea, and some degree of anemia. Rarely, worms lodge in the appendix or penetrate the bowel wall to cause peritonitis. *Mebendazole* and *albendazole* are considered the safest agents and the most effective for treatment of whipworm, alone or together with *Ascaris* and hookworm infections. Pyrantel pamoate is ineffective against *Trichuris.*

Strongyloides stercoralis. *S. stercoralis,* sometimes called the threadworm or dwarf threadworm, is exceptional among helminths because it can replicate and cause cycles of larval reinfection within the human host. The organism infects more than 200 million people worldwide, most frequently in the tropics and other hot, humid locales. In the United States, strongyloidiasis is most common among children in the rural South. It also is found in institutionalized individuals living in unsanitary conditions and in immigrants, travelers, and military personnel who lived in endemic areas. Infective larvae in fecally contaminated soil penetrate the skin or mucous membranes, travel to the lungs, and ultimately mature into adult worms in the small intestine, where they reside. Most infected individuals are asymptomatic, whereas others most commonly experience skin rashes and gastrointestinal symptoms. Life-threatening, disseminated systemic disease due to massive larval autoinfection can occur in immunosuppressed persons even decades after the initial infection. Most of the deaths caused by parasites in the United States probably are due to *Strongyloides* hyperinfection. *Ivermectin* is the best drug for treating intestinal strongyloidiasis. Effective benzimidazole compounds, listed in order of decreasing efficacy, are *thiabendazole, albendazole,* and *mebendazole.* Thiabendazole shows efficacy comparable to that of ivermectin but is far more toxic.

Enterobius vermicularis. *Enterobius,* the pinworm, causes the most common helminthic infection in the United States, where more than 40 million school children are affected. The infection has a worldwide distribution but is more prevalent in temperate than in tropical climates. This parasite rarely causes serious complications; pruritus in the perianal and perineal regions, however, can be severe, and scratching may cause secondary infection. In female patients, worms may wander into the genital tract and penetrate into the peritoneal cavity. Salpingitis or even peritonitis may ensue. Because the infection is easily distributed throughout members of a family, a school, or an institution, the physician must decide whether or not to treat all individuals in close contact with an infected person, and more than one course of therapy may be required.

Pyrantel pamoate, mebendazole, and *albendazole* are highly effective. Single oral doses of each should be repeated after 2 weeks. When their use is combined with rigid standards of personal hygiene, a very high proportion of cures can be obtained. Treatment is simple and almost devoid of side effects. The benzimidazoles should not be used during pregnancy because of their teratogenic potential. Daily doses of *piperazine* for 1 week also are effective but less convenient.

Trichinella spiralis. The trichina worm is ubiquitous, regardless of climate, and can live outside its hosts. It is found in Canada, eastern Europe, and now less frequently the United States. The infection results from eating raw or insufficiently cooked flesh of trichinous animals, especially pigs. Encysted larvae, released by acid stomach contents, mature into adult worms in the intestine. Adults then produce infectious larvae that invade tissues, especially skeletal muscle and heart. Severe infection can be fatal but more typically causes marked muscle pain and cardiac complications. Fortunately, infection is readily preventable. All pork, including pork sausages, should be thoroughly cooked before being eaten. The encysted larvae are killed by exposure to heat of 60°C for 5 minutes.

Albendazole and *mebendazole* appear to be effective against the intestinal forms of *T. spiralis* that are present early in infection. The efficacy of these agents or any anthelmintic agent on larvae that have migrated to muscle is questionable. *Glucocorticoids* may be of considerable value in controlling the acute and dangerous manifestations of established infection.

Filariae. Adult worms that cause human filariasis dwell either in the lymphatic system (*Wurchereria bancrofti, Brugia malayi, Brugia timori*) or other tissues (*Loa loa, Onchocerca volvulus, Mansonella* species). Spread by the bites of infected mosquitoes, lymphatic filariasis affects nearly 90 million people, about 90% of them infected with *W. bancrofti* and most of the rest with *B. malayi. W. bancrofti* is especially a risk in central Africa, South America, India, and southern China, although it also is distributed widely throughout the tropics. *B. malayi* is restricted to Indonesia, southeast Asia, and central India, whereas *B. timori* is found in Indonesia. In bancroftian and brugian filariasis, host reactions to the adult worms initially cause lymphatic inflammation manifested by fevers, lymphangytis, and lymphadenitis; this progresses to lymphatic obstruction typified by lymphedema, hydrocele, and elephantiasis. A reaction to microfilariae, *tropical pulmonary eosinophilia,* also occurs in some persons. Transmitted by deerflies, *L. loa,* the African eyeworm, is a migrating filarial parasite found in large river regions of central and west Africa. Adult worms in subcutaneous tissues typically cause episodic "Calabar" swellings and allergic reactions but also can penetrate the conjunctivae and skin. Rarely, encephalopathy, cardiopathy, or nephropathy occur in association with heavy infection. *O. volvulus,* transmitted by blackflies near fast-flowing streams and rivers, infects some 13 million people in central Africa and less than 100,000 in parts of Mexico and South America. Inflammatory reactions, primarily to microfilariae rather than adult worms, affect the subcutaneous tissues, lymph nodes, and eyes. Onchocerciasis is the second leading cause of infectious blindness worldwide. Filariasis caused by *Mansonella* species, transmitted largely by midges, is rare and variably responsive to chemotherapy.

Diethylcarbamazine and *ivermectin* are the primary compounds used to treat lymphatic filariasis. Population-based, yearly chemotherapy with a single oral dose of either diethylcarbamazine or ivermectin together with an oral dose of *albendazole* may be more effective in markedly reducing the microfilaremia and prevalence of this infection (Ottesen *et al.,* 1999). Ivermectin is the safer primary agent for areas where bancroftian filariasis may coexist with either loiasis or onchocerciasis; diethylcarbamazine can be used with albendazole elsewhere.

The best results are achieved in *W. bancrofti* and *B. malayi* infections if chemotherapy is started early, before obstructive lesions of the lymphatics have occurred. Even in late cases, some improvement may result. In long-standing elephantiasis, surgical measures are required to improve lymph drainage and remove redundant tissue. *Diethylcarbamazine* currently is the best single drug for the treatment of loiasis, but it is advisable to start with a small initial dose to diminish host reactions that result from destruction of microfilariae. *Glucocorticoids* often are required to control acute reactions. In rare instances, serious cerebral reactions occur in the treatment of loiasis, probably due to destruction of microfilariae in the brain. If headache is severe and there is other evidence of an adult *L. loa* near the orbit, extra caution for initial dosing is advised.

Ivermectin is the best single drug for control and treatment of onchocerciasis. Diethylcarbamazine no longer is recommended. Both agents kill only microfilariae of *O. volvulus,* but ivermectin produces far milder systemic reactions and few if any ocular complications. With diethylcarbamazine, such reactions are likely to be severe, particularly in cases where there are lesions of the eye. Although suramin (*see* Chapter 41) is lethal to adult *O. volvulus,* treatment with this relatively toxic agent probably is unwarranted. Less toxic macrofilaricides are needed.

Dracunculus medinensis. Known as the guinea, dragon, or Medina worm, this parasite causes dracunculiasis, an infection in decline that is most commonly found in rural Sudan and west Africa. People become infected by drinking water containing copepods that carry infective larvae. After about one year, the adult female worms migrate and emerge through the skin, usually of the lower legs or feet.

There is no suitable anthelmintic that acts directly against *D. medinensis.* Traditional treatment for this disabling condition is to draw the live adult female worm out day by day by rolling it onto a small piece of wood. This procedure risks severe infection if rupture occurs. *Metronidazole,* 250 mg given 3 times a day for 10 days, can provide symptomatic and functional relief by facilitating removal of the worm through indirect suppression of host inflammatory responses. Strategies such as filtering drinking water and reducing contact of infected individuals with water have caused marked reductions in the transmission and prevalence of dracunculiasis in most endemic regions.

Cestodes (Flatworms)

Taenia saginata. Human beings are the definitive hosts for *Taenia saginata,* known as the beef tapeworm. This most common form of tapeworm usually is detected after passage of proglottids from the intestine. It is cosmopolitan, occurring most commonly in sub-Saharan Africa and the Middle East, where undercooked or raw beef is consumed. Preventable by cooking beef to 60°C for over 5 minutes, this infection rarely produces serious clinical disease, but it must be distinguished from that produced by *Taenia solium.*

Praziquantel is the drug of choice for treatment of infection by *T. saginata,* although *niclosamide* also is used because it is cheap and available. Both are very effective, simple to administer, and comparatively free from side effects. Assessment of cure can be difficult because the worm (segments as well as scolex) is usually passed in a partially digested state. If parasitological diagnosis is uncertain, praziquantel is the preferred drug because of the danger of cysticercosis (*see* below).

Taenia solium.   *Taenia solium,* or pork tapeworm, also has a cosmopolitan distribution; immigrant populations are a common source of infection in the United States. This cestode causes two types of infection. The intestinal form with adult tapeworms is caused by eating undercooked meat containing cysticerci; this can be prevented by proper cooking of infected meat. *Cysticercosis,* the far more dangerous systemic form that usually coexists with the intestinal form, is caused by invasive larval forms of the parasite (Garcia and Del Brutto, 2000). This autoinfection by parasite eggs usually results either from ingestion of fecally contaminated infectious material or from eggs, liberated from a gravid segment, passing upward into the duodenum, where the outer layers are digested. In either case, larvae gain access to the circulation and the tissues exactly as in their cycle in the intermediate host, usually the pig. The seriousness of the disease that results depends on the particular tissue involved. Invasion of the brain (neurocysticercosis) is common and dangerous. Epilepsy, meningitis, and increased intracranial pressure can occur, depending on the inflammatory reactions to the cysticerci and/or their size and location. *Praziquantel* is preferred for treatment of intestinal infections with *T. solium.* *Albendazole* and *praziquantel* are the drugs of choice for treating cysticercosis, although most studies suggest that albendazole is more effective. Chemotherapy is appropriate only when it is directed at live cysticerci causing pathology; pretreatment with glucocorticoids is advised strongly in this situation to minimize inflammatory reactions to dying parasites (Evans *et al.,* 1997).

Diphyllobothrium latum.   *Diphyllobothrium latum,* the fish tapeworm, is found most commonly in rivers and lakes of the northern hemisphere. In North America, the pike is the most common second intermediate host. The eating of inadequately cooked, infested fish introduces the larvae into the human intestine; the larvae can develop into adult worms up to 25 meters long. Most infected individuals are asymptomatic, but some, aside from abdominal symptoms and weight loss, may develop a megaloblastic anemia. The latter condition results from a deficiency of vitamin B_{12}, which is taken up by the parasite. Therapy with *praziquantel* readily eliminates the worm and ensures hematological remission.

Hymenolepis nana.   *Hymenolepis nana,* the dwarf tapeworm, is the smallest and most common tapeworm parasitizing human beings. Infection with this cestode is cosmopolitan, more prevalent in tropical than temperate climates, and most common among institutionalized children, including those in the southern United States. *H. nana* is the only cestode that can develop from ovum to mature adult in human beings without an intermediate host. Cysticerci develop in the villi of the intestine and then regain access to the intestinal lumen where larvae mature into adults. Treatment therefore must be adapted to this cycle of autoinfection. *Praziquantel* is effective against *H. nana* infections, but therapy may have to be repeated. Failure of treatment or reinfection is indicated by the appearance of eggs in the stool about 4 weeks after the last dose.

Echinococcus Species.   Human beings serve as one of several intermediate hosts for larval forms of *Echinococcus* species that cause "cystic" (*E. granulosus*) and "alveolar" (*E. multilocoularis* and *E. vogeli*) hydatid disease. Dogs are definitive hosts for these tapeworms. Parasite eggs from canine stools are a major worldwide cause of disease in associated livestock, *e.g.,* sheep and goats. *E. granulosus* produces unilocular, slowly growing cysts, most often in liver and lung, whereas *E. multilocularis* creates multilocular invasive cysts predominantly in the same organs. Removal of the cysts by surgery is the preferred treatment, but leakage from ruptured cysts may spread disease to other organs. Prolonged regimens of *albendazole,* either alone or as an adjunct to surgery, are reportedly of some benefit. However, some patients are not cured despite multiple courses of therapy. Treatment of infected dogs with praziquantel eradicates adult worms and interrupts transmission of these infections.

Trematodes (Flukes)

Schistosoma haematobium, Schistosoma mansoni, Schistosoma japonicum.   These are the main species of blood flukes that cause human schistosomiasis; less common species are *Schistosoma intercalatum* and *Schistosoma mekongi.* The infection affects about 200 million people, and more than 600 million are considered at risk. Schistosomiasis is widely distributed over the South American continent and certain Caribbean islands (*S. mansoni*), much of Africa and the Arabian Peninsula (*S. mansoni* and *S. haematobium*), and China, the Philippines, and Indonesia (*S. japonicum*). Infected snails act as intermediate hosts for freshwater transmission of the infection, which continues to spread as the development of agricultural and water resources increases. Schistosomal disease, which generally correlates with the intensity of infection, primarily involves the liver, spleen, and gastrointestinal tract (*S. mansoni* and *S. japonicum*) or the lower genitourinary tract (*S. haematobium*). Heavy infections with *S. haematobium* appear to be associated with squamous cell carcinoma of the bladder in some endemic regions.

Praziquantel is the drug of choice for treating all species of schistosomes that infect human beings. The drug is safe and effective when it is given in single or divided oral doses on the same day. These properties make praziquantel especially suitable for population-based chemotherapy. Although not effective clinically against *S. haematobium* and *S. japonicum,* oxamniquine is effective for treatment of *S. mansoni* infections, particularly in South America, where the sensitivity of most strains may permit single-dose therapy. However, resistance has been reported, in both the field and the laboratory, and higher doses of the drug are required to treat African than to treat Brazilian strains of *S. mansoni.* Metrifonate has been used with considerable success in the treatment of *S. haematobium* infections, but the drug is not effective against *S. mansoni* and *S. japonicum.* Metrifonate is relatively inexpensive and can be used in conjunction with oxamniquine for treatment of mixed infections with *S. haematobium* and *S. mansoni.*

Paragonimus westermani and Other Paragonimus Species. Called lung flukes, a number of *Paragonimus* species, of which *P. westermani* is the most common, are pathogenic for human beings and carnivores. Found in the Far East and on the African and South American continents, these parasites have two intermediate hosts—snails and crustaceans. Human beings become infected by eating raw or undercooked crabs or crayfish. Disease is caused by reactions to adult worms in the lungs and ectopic sites. Although these flukes are rather refractory to praziquantel *in vitro,* the drug is effective when used clinically.

Clonorchis sinensis, Opisthorchis viverrini, Opisthorchis felineus. These closely related trematodes exist in the Far East (*C. sinensis,* "the Chinese liver fluke," and *O. viverrini*) and parts of eastern Europe (*O. felineus*). Metacercariae released from poorly cooked infected fish mature into adult flukes that inhabit the human biliary system. Heavy infections can cause obstructive liver disease, inflammatory gallbladder pathology associated with cholangiocarcinoma, and obstructive pancreatitis. One-day therapy with *praziquantel* is highly effective against these parasites.

Fasciola hepatica. Human beings are only accidentally infected with *F. hepatica,* the large liver fluke that exists worldwide and primarily affects herbivorous ruminants such as cattle and sheep. Eating contaminated freshwater plants such as watercress initiates the infection. Migratory larvae penetrate the intestine, invade the liver from the peritoneum, and eventually reside in the biliary tract. The acute illness is characterized by fever, urticaria, and abdominal symptoms, whereas chronic infection resembles that caused by other hepatic flukes. However, *F. hepatica* infection is not associated with cholangiocarcinoma. Unlike infections with other flukes, fascioliasis does not usually respond to praziquantel. The current recommended drug is *bithionol,* 30 to 50 mg/kg given on alternate days for 10 to 15 doses. Bithionol may be obtained from the United States Centers for Disease Control and Prevention Drug Service. Based on limited trials, *triclabendazole,* a narrow-spectrum benzimidazole used in veterinary medicine, shows more promise for treating fascioliasis (*see* Arjone *et al.,* 1995).

Fasciolopsis buski, Heterophyes heterophyes, Metagonimus yokogawai, Nanophyetus salmincola. Obtained by eating contaminated water chestnuts and other caltrops in Southeast Asia, *F. buski* is one of the largest parasites causing human infection. Undercooked fish transmit infection with the other, much smaller gastrointestinal trematodes that are widely distributed geographically. Abdominal symptoms produced by reactions to these flukes are usually mild, but heavy infections with *F. buski* can cause intestinal obstruction and peritonitis. Infections with all the intestinal trematodes respond well to single-day therapy with praziquantel.

ANTHELMINTIC DRUGS

Benzimidazoles

History. The discovery by Brown and coworkers (1961) that thiabendazole possessed potent activity against gastrointestinal nematodes sparked development of the benzimidazoles as broad-spectrum anthelmintic agents against parasites of both veterinary and human medical importance. Of the hundreds of derivatives tested, those most therapeutically useful have modifications at the 2 and/or 5 positions of the benzimidazole ring system (*see* Townsend and Wise, 1990). Three compounds, *thiabendazole, mebendazole,* and *albendazole,* have been used extensively for the treatment of human helminthiasis. The chemical structures of these drugs are shown in Table 42–1. Thiabendazole, which contains a thiazole ring at position 2, is active against a wide range of nematodes that infect the gastrointestinal tract. However, its

Table 42–1
Structure of the Benzimidazoles

R_1	R_2	DERIVATIVE
(thiazole ring)	H—	Thiabendazole
—$NHCO_2CH_3$	(benzoyl group)	Mebendazole
—$NHCO_2CH_3$	$CH_3CH_2CH_2S$—	Albendazole

clinical use against these organisms has declined markedly because of thiabendazole's toxicity relative to that of other equally effective drugs. Mebendazole, the prototype benzimidazole carbamate, was introduced for the treatment of intestinal roundworm infections as a result of research carried out by Brugmans and collaborators (1971). Albendazole is a newer benzimidazole carbamate that is used worldwide, primarily against a variety of intestinal and tissue nematodes but also against larval forms of certain cestodes (de Silva *et al.,* 1997; Venkatesan, 1998). As to the latter, albendazole has become the drug of choice for treating cysticercosis (*see* Sotelo and Jung, 1998; Garcia and Del Brutto, 2000) and the drug of choice for cystic hydatid disease (*see* Horton, 1997). However, albendazole is not effective against *F. hepatica.* When used yearly in conjunction with either ivermectin or diethylcarbamazine, single doses of albendazole have shown considerable promise for global control of lymphatic filariasis and related tissue filarial infections (*see* Ottesen *et al.,* 1999).

Anthelmintic Action. The benzimidazoles, exemplified by mebendazole and albendazole, are versatile anthelmintic agents, particularly against gastrointestinal nematodes, where their action is not dictated by the systemic drug concentration. Appropriate doses of mebendazole and albendazole are highly effective in ascariasis, intestinal capillariasis, enterobiasis, trichuriasis, and hookworm (*Ancylostoma duodenale* and *Necator americanus*) infection as single or mixed infections. These drugs are active against both larval and adult stages of nematodes that cause these infections, and they are ovicidal for *Ascaris* and *Trichuris.* Immobilization and death of susceptible gastrointestinal parasites occur slowly, and their clearance from the gastrointestinal tract may not be complete until a few days after treatment. Albendazole is superior to mebendazole in curing hookworm infections in children (de Silva *et al.,* 1997; Bennett and Guyatt, 2000). Moreover, albendazole is more effective than mebendazole against strongyloidiasis (Liu and Weller, 1993), cystic hydatid disease caused by *Echinococcus granulosus* (Horton, 1997; Davis *et al.,* 1989), and neurocysticercosis caused by larval forms of *Taenia solium* (Evans *et al.,* 1997; Garcia and Del Brutto, 2000). The benzimidazoles probably are active against the intestinal stages of *Trichinella spiralis* in human beings but probably do not affect the larval stages in tissues. Albendazole is highly effective against the migrating forms of dog and cat hookworms that cause cutaneous larval migrans, although thiabendazole can be used topically for this purpose. Regimens in which albendazole with either ivermectin or diethylcarbamazine are given as single annual doses show great promise for controlling lymphatic filariasis occurring either alone or together with other filarial infections (*see* Ottesen *et al.*, 1999). Such combined therapy has the additional benefit of reducing intestinal roundworm infestations in school-aged children (Albonico *et al.*, 1999). Certain microsporidial species that cause intestinal infections in people with AIDS respond partially (*Enterocytozoon bieneusi*) or completely (*Encephalitozoon intestintalis* and related *Encephalitozoon* species) to albendazole; albendazole's sulfoxide metabolite appears to be especially effective against these parasites *in vitro* (*see* Katiyar and Edlind, 1997). Albendazole also has some efficacy against anaerobic protozoa such as *Trichomonas vaginalis* and *Giardia lamblia* (Ottesen *et al.*, 1999). While benzimidazoles have antifungal activity, their clinical use against human mycoses is limited.

Benzimidazoles produce many biochemical changes in susceptible nematodes, *e.g.*, inhibition of mitochondrial fumarate reductase, reduced glucose transport, and uncoupling of oxidative phosphorylation (*see* Lacey, 1988). There is strong evidence, however, that the primary action of these drugs is to inhibit microtubule polymerization by binding to β-tubulin (*see* Lacey, 1988; Lacey, 1990; Prichard, 1994). The selective toxicity of these agents derives from the fact that specific, high-affinity binding to parasite β-tubulin occurs at much lower concentrations than does binding to the mammalian protein. Studies on benzimidazole-resistant worms, such as the free-living nematode *Caenorhabditis elegans* (Driscoll *et al.*, 1989), and the sheep nematode *Haemonchus contortus* have provided insights into the mechanism of benzimidazole action (*see* Lacey, 1990; Prichard, 1994). In particular, both laboratory-derived and field-isolated strains of benzimidazole-resistant *H. contortus* display reduced high-affinity drug binding to β-tubulin (Lubega and Prichard, 1991) and alterations in β-tubulin isotype gene expression (Kwa *et al.*, 1993; Kwa *et al.*, 1995; Roos, 1997) that correlate with drug resistance. Thus, the two identified mechanisms of drug resistance in nematodes involve both a progressive loss of "susceptible" β-tubulin gene isotypes together with emergence of a "resistant" isotype with a conserved point mutation that encodes a tyrosine instead of a phenylalanine at position 200 of β-tubulin (Roos, 1997; Sangster and Gill, 1999). While this mutation may not be required for benzimidazole resistance in all parasites, *e.g.*, *G. lamblia* (*see* Upcroft *et al.*, 1996), benzimidazole resistance in parasitic nematodes is unlikely to be overcome by novel benzimidazole analogs, because tyrosine also is present at position 200 of human β-tubulin.

Absorption, Fate, and Excretion.   Benzimidazoles have only limited solubility in water; consequently, minor differences in solubility tend to have a major effect on absorption. Thiabendazole is absorbed rapidly after oral ingestion and reaches peak concentrations in plasma after about 1 hour. Most of the drug is excreted in the urine within 24 hours as 5-hydroxythiabendazole, conjugated either as the glucuronide or as the sulfate. In contrast,

tablet formulations of mebendazole are poorly and erratically absorbed, and concentrations of the drug in plasma are low and do not reflect the dosage taken (Witassek *et al.*, 1981). The low systemic bioavailability (22%) of mebendazole results from a combination of poor absorption and rapid first-pass hepatic metabolism. Mebendazole is about 95% bound to plasma proteins and is extensively metabolized. Two major metabolites, methyl-5-(α-hydroxybenzyl)-2-benzimidazole carbamate and 2-amino-5-benzoylbenzimidazole, have lower rates of clearance than does mebendazole itself (Braithwaite *et al.*, 1982). Mebendazole, rather than its metabolites, appears to be the active drug form (*see* Gottschall *et al.*, 1990). Conjugates of mebendazole and its metabolites have been found in bile, but little unchanged mebendazole appears in the urine.

Albendazole is variably and erratically absorbed after oral administration; absorption is enhanced by the presence of fatty foods and possibly by bile salts as well. After a 400-mg oral dose, albendazole cannot be detected in plasma, because the drug is rapidly metabolized in the liver and possibly in the intestine as well, to albendazole sulfoxide, which has potent anthelmintic activity (Marriner *et al.*, 1986; Moroni *et al.*, 1995; Redondo *et al.*, 1999). Both the (+) and (−) enantiomers of albendazole sulfoxide are formed, but in human beings the (+) enantiomer reaches much higher peak concentrations in plasma and is cleared much more slowly than the (−) form (Delatour *et al.*, 1991; Marques *et al.*, 1999). Total sulfoxide attains peak plasma concentrations of about 300 ng/ml, but with wide interindividual variation. Albendazole sulfoxide is about 70% bound to plasma proteins and has a highly variable plasma half-life ranging from about 4 to 15 hours (Delatour *et al.*, 1991; Jung *et al.*, 1992; Marques *et al.*, 1999). It is well distributed into various tissues, including hydatid cysts, where it reaches a concentration of about one-fifth that in plasma (Marriner *et al.*, 1986; Morris *et al.*, 1987). This probably explains why albendazole is more effective than mebendazole for treating hydatid cyst disease. Formation of albendazole sulfoxide is catalyzed by both microsomal flavin monooxygenase and isoforms of cytochrome P450 in the liver and possibly also in the intestine (Redondo *et al.*, 1999). Hepatic flavin monooxygenase activity appears associated with (+) albendazole sulfoxide formation, whereas cytochromes P450 preferentially produce the (−) sulfoxide metabolite (Delatour *et al.*, 1991). Both sulfoxide derivatives are oxidized further to the nonchiral sulfone metabolite of albendazole, which is pharmacologically inactive; this reaction favors the (−) sulfoxide and probably becomes rate limiting in determining the clearance and plasma half-life of the bioactive (+) sulfoxide metabolite (Delatour *et al.*, 1991). Induction of enzymes involved in sulfone formation from the (+) sulfoxide could account for some of the wide variation noted in plasma half-lives of albendazole sulfoxide. Indeed, in animal models, benzimidizoles can induce their own metabolism (for example, *see* Gleizes *et al.*, 1991). Albendazole metabolites are excreted mainly in the urine.

Therapeutic Uses. The introduction of *thiabendazole* (MINTEZOL) was a major advance in the therapy of cutaneous larva migrans (creeping eruption) and *S. stercoralis* infection. The majority of patients experience marked relief of symptoms of creeping eruption, and a high percentage of cures are achieved after topical treatment with 15% thiabendazole in a water-soluble cream base applied to the affected area two or three times per day for 5 days (Davies *et al.*, 1993). A common regimen for therapy of strongyloidiasis is 25 mg/kg of thiabendazole given twice daily after meals for 2 days; the total daily dose should not exceed 3 grams. This schedule should be extended for 5 to 7 days for treatment of disseminated strongyloidiasis or until the parasites have been eliminated. The thiabendazole regimen has been replaced largely by a single dose of ivermectin for treatment of intestinal strongyloidiasis (*see* "Ivermectin," below), but as yet thiabendazole is the only drug with established efficacy against disseminated strongyloidiasis (Gann *et al.*, 1994; Liu and Well, 1998). Thiabendazole given at a dosage of 25 mg/kg twice per day for 7 days may produce some benefit for early trichinosis. The drug, however, has no effect on migrating or muscle-stage larvae. Thiabendazole also is effective in gastrointestinal nematode infections, but because of its toxicity, it should no longer be used for those infections.

Mebendazole (VERMOX) is highly effective against gastrointestinal nematode infections and is particularly valuable for the treatment of mixed infections. Mebendazole is always taken orally, and the same dosage schedule applies to adults and children more than 2 years of age. For control of enterobiasis, a single 100-mg tablet is taken; a second should be given after 2 weeks. For control of ascariasis, trichuriasis, and hookworm infection, the recommended regimen is 100 mg of mebendazole taken in the morning and evening for 3 consecutive days. If the patient is not cured 3 weeks after treatment, a second course should be given. The 3-day mebendazole regimen is more effective than single doses of either mebendazole (500 mg) or albendazole (400 mg), which also have been used successfully to control these mixed infections. A 500-mg dose of mebendazole may be slightly more effective against trichuriasis than a 400-mg dose of albendazole, but the single dose of albendazole appears superior to mebendazole against hookworms (de Silva *et al.*, 1997; Bennett and Gyatt, 2000).

Infections with *Capillaria philippinensis* are more resistant to treatment with mebendazole; 400 mg of the drug has been given per day in two divided doses for at least 20 days (Cross, 1992). Mebendazole has been used to treat cystic hydatid disease, although surgery should be performed first, and chemotherapy with albendazole is now considered to be superior (*see* Horton, 1997).

Like mebendazole, *albendazole* (ALBENZA) provides safe and highly effective therapy against infections with gastrointestinal nematodes, including mixed infections of *Ascaris, Trichuria,* and hookworms. For treatment of enterobiasis, ascariasis, trichuriasis, and hookworm infections, albendazole is taken as a single oral 400-mg dose by adults and children more than 2 years of age. Cure rates for light to moderate *Ascaris* infections are typically over 97%, although heavy infections may require therapy for 2 to 3 days. A 400-mg dose of albendazole appears to be superior to a 500-mg dose of mebendazole for curing hookworm infections and reducing egg counts (Sacko *et al.*, 1999; Bennett and Guyatt, 2000). Given at a dose of 400 mg daily for 3 days, albendazole exhibits highly variable efficacy against strongyloidiasis; both thiabendazole and ivermectin are more effective in treating this infection.

Albendazole is the drug of choice for treating people with cystic hydatid disease due to *E. granulosus*. While the drug provides only a modest cure rate when used alone, it produces superior results when used before and after either surgery to remove cysts or aspiration/injection of cysts with protoscolicidal agents (*see* Horton, 1997; Schantz, 1999). A typical dosage regimen for adults is 400 mg given twice a day for 28 days, the course to be repeated as necessary. However, albendazole at 10 to 12 mg/kg per day has been given continuously for 3 to 6 months without producing serious or irreversible toxicity (Franchi *et al.*, 1999). While still the best drug available, albendazole appears to be just marginally effective against alveolar echinococcosis caused by *E. multilocularis* (*see* Venkatesen, 1998). Albendazole also is the preferred treatment of neurocysticercosis caused by larval forms of *T. solium* (*see* Evans *et al.*, 1997; Sotelo and Jung, 1998; Garcia and Del Brutto, 2000). The recommended dosage is 400 mg given twice a day for adults with therapy continued for 3 to 28 days, depending on the number, type, and location of the cysts. Glucocorticoids usually are given for several days prior to the start of albendazole therapy to reduce the incidence of side effects resulting from inflammatory reactions to dead and dying cysticerci. Such pretreatment also increases plasma levels of albendazole sulfoxide. Albendazole, 400 mg per day, has shown efficacy for therapy of microsporidial intestinal infections in patients with AIDS; *Encephalitozoon intestinalis* responds well to this drug, whereas the related *Enterocytozoon bieneusi* seems to be more refractory (*see* Vankatesan, 1999).

A notable recent advance is the use of albendazole together with either diethylcarbamazine or ivermectin in programs directed toward controlling lymphatic filariasis (reviewed by Ottesen *et al.,* 1999). Albendazole itself has delayed microfilaricidal activity but only slight macrofilarcidal activity against *W. bancrofti.* But a single dose of albendazole (400 to 600 mg) given alone with a single dose of either diethylcarbamazine (6 mg/kg) or ivermectin (0.2 to 0.4 mg/kg) markedly decreases the microfilaremia in *W. bancrofti* infection for well over a year. By annual dosing for 4 to 6 years, the strategy is to maintain the microfilaremia at such low levels that transmission cannot occur. The period of therapy is estimated to correspond to the duration of fecundity of adult worms. Albendazole is given with diethylcarbamazine to treat lymphatic filariasis in most parts of the world. However, to avoid serious reactions to dying microfilariae, the albendazole/ivermectin combination should be used in locations where filariasis coexists with either onchocerciasis or loiasis.

Toxicity, Side Effects, Precautions, and Contraindications. The clinical utility of thiabendazole is compromised by its toxicity. Side effects frequently encountered with therapeutic doses are anorexia, nausea, vomiting, and dizziness. Less frequently, diarrhea, weariness, drowsiness, giddiness, and headache occur. Occasional fever, rashes, erythema multiforme, hallucinations, sensory disturbances, and Stevens–Johnson syndrome have been reported. Angioneurotic edema, shock, tinnitus, convulsions, and intrahepatic cholestasis are rare complications of therapy. Some patients excrete a metabolite that imparts an odor to the urine much like that occurring after ingestion of asparagus. Crystalluria without hematuria has been reported on occasion; it promptly subsides with discontinuation of therapy. Transient leukopenia has been noted in a few patients on thiabendazole therapy. There are no absolute contraindications to the use of thiabendazole. Because central nervous system (CNS) side effects occur frequently, activities requiring mental alertness should be avoided during therapy. Thiabendazole has hepatotoxic potential, so it should be used with caution in patients with hepatic disease or decreased hepatic function. The effects of thiabendazole in pregnant women have not been studied adequately, so it should be used in pregnancy

only when the potential benefit justifies the potential risk.

Unlike thiabendazole, mebendazole does not cause significant systemic toxicity in routine clinical use, even in the presence of anemia and malnutrition. This probably results from its low systemic bioavailability. Transient symptoms of abdominal pain, distention, and diarrhea have occurred in cases of massive infestation and expulsion of gastrointestinal worms. Rare side effects in patients treated with high doses of mebendazole include allergic reactions, alopecia, reversible neutropenia, agranulocytosis, and hypospermia. Reversible elevation of serum transaminases is not uncommon in this population. Mebendazole is a potent embryotoxin and teratogen in laboratory animals; effects may occur in pregnant rats at single oral doses as low as 10 mg/kg. Thus, despite a lack of evidence for teratogenicity in human beings, it is advised that mebendazole not be given to pregnant women or to children less than 2 years of age. It should not be used in patients who have experienced allergic reactions to the agent.

Like mebendazole, albendazole produces few side effects when used for short-term therapy of gastrointestinal helminthiasis, even in patients with heavy worm burdens. Transient abdominal pain, diarrhea, nausea, dizziness, and headache occur on occasion. Even when used for long-term therapy of cystic hydatid disease and neurocysticercosis, albendazole is well tolerated by most patients. The most common side effect is an increase in serum aminotransferase activity; in rare instances, jaundice or chemical cholestasis may be noted, but enzyme activities return to normal after therapy is completed. Routine liver function should be monitored during protracted albendazole therapy, and the drug is not recommended for patients with hepatic cirrhosis (Davis *et al.,* 1989). Especially if not pretreated with glucocorticoids, some patients with neurocysticercosis may experience serious neurological sequelae that depend on the location of inflamed cysts with dying cysticerci. Other side effects reported during extended therapy include gastrointestinal pain, severe headaches, fever, fatigue, loss of hair, leukopenia, and thrombocytopenia. Albendazole is teratogenic and embryotoxic in animals. Thus, it should not be given to pregnant women. The safety of albendazole in children less than 2 years of age has not been established.

The benzimidazoles as a group display remarkably few clinically significant interactions with other drugs. The most versatile of this family, albendazole, probably induces its own metabolism, and plasma levels of its sulfoxide metabolites can be increased by coadministration of glucocorticoids and possibly praziquantel. Caution is advised when using high doses of albendazole together with general inhibitors of hepatic cytochromes P450.

Diethylcarbamazine

History. Over 1500 cases of filariasis in American military personnel during World War II stimulated the search for effective filaricides. The most promising group of antifilarial compounds to emerge were piperazine derivatives, of which diethylcarbamazine is the most important (Hawking, 1979; Mackenzie and Kron, 1985). Diethylcarbamazine is a first-line agent for control and treatment of lymphatic filariasis and for therapy of tropical pulmonary eosinophilia caused by *W. bancrofti* and *B. malayi* (*see* Ottesen and Ramachandran, 1995). Although this agent is effective against onchocerciasis and loiasis, it can cause serious reactions to affected microfilariae in both infections. For this reason, ivermectin has replaced diethylcarbamazine for therapy of onchocerciasis. Despite its toxicity, diethylcarbamazine remains the best drug available to treat loiasis. Programs that feature annual single doses of both dietnylcarbamazine and albendazole show considerable promise for the control of lymphatic filariasis in geographic regions where onchocerciasis and loiasis are not endemic (*see* Ottesen *et al.*, 1999).

Chemistry. Diethylcarbamazine (HETRAZAN) is formulated as the water-soluble citrate salt containing 51% by weight of the active base. Because the compound is tasteless, odorless, and stable to heat, it also can be taken in the form of fortified table salt containing 0.2% to 0.4% by weight of the base. The drug is available outside the United States. In the United States it can be obtained from the Centers for Disease Control and Prevention Drug Service (telephone: 404-639-3670). Diethylcarbamazine has the following chemical structure:

DIETHYLCARBAMAZINE

Anthelmintic Action. Microfilarial forms of susceptible filarial species are most affected by diethylcarbamazine, which elicits rapid disappearance of these developmental forms of *W. bancrofti*, *B. malayi*, and *L. loa* from human blood. The drug causes microfilariae of *O. volvulus* to disappear from skin but does not kill microfilariae in nodules that contain the adult (female) worms. It does not affect the microfilariae of *W. bancrofti* in a hydrocele, despite penetration into the fluid. The mechanism of action of diethylcarbamazine on susceptible microfilariae is not well understood (*see* Martin *et al.*, 1997; de Silva *et al.*, 1997). The drug exerts little effect *in vitro*, whereas it acts rapidly *in vivo*. One possibility is that diethylcarbamazine may perturb arachidonic acid metabolism in both microfilariae and host endothelial cells with resulting vasoconstriction and aggregation of host platelets and granulocytes around membrane-damaged parasites. The compound does not appear to activate adaptic immune responses in the host, but innate immune response(s) could be involved (Maizels and Denham, 1992; Maizels *et al.*, 1993). There is evidence that diethylcarbamazine kills worms of adult *L. loa* and probably adult *W. bancrofti* and *B. malayi* as well. However, it has little action against adult *O. volvulus*. The mechanism of filaricidal action of diethylcarbamazine against adult worms is unknown (*see* Hawking, 1979). Some studies suggest that diethylcarbamazine compromises intracellular processing and transport of certain macromolecules to the plasma membrane (Spiro *et al.*, 1986). The drug also may affect specific immune and inflammatory responses of the host by as yet undefined mechanisms (*see* Mackenzie and Kron, 1985; Martin *et al.*, 1997).

Absorption, Fate, and Excretion. Diethylcarbamazine is absorbed rapidly from the gastrointestinal tract. Peak plasma levels occur within 1 to 2 hours after a single oral dose, and the plasma half-life of this base varies from 2 to 10 hours, depending on the urinary pH. Metabolism is both rapid and extensive (Faulkner and Smith, 1972). A major metabolite, diethylcarbamazine-*N*-oxide, is bioactive. Diethylcarbamazine is excreted by both urinary and extraurinary routes; over 50% of an oral dose appears in acidic urine as the unchanged drug, but this value is decreased when the urine is alkaline (Edwards *et al.*, 1981). Indeed, alkalinizing the urine can elevate plasma levels, prolong the plasma half-life, and increase both the therapeutic effect and toxicity of diethylcarbamazine (Awadzi *et al.*, 1986). Therefore, dosage reduction may be required for people with renal dysfunction or sustained alkaline urine.

Therapeutic Uses. Dosages of *diethylcarbamazine citrate* used to prevent or treat filarial infections have evolved empirically and vary according to local experience. Recommended regimens differ according to whether the drug is used for population-based chemotherapy, control of filarial disease, or prophylaxis against infection.

W. bancrofti, B. malayi, and B. timori. For mass treatment with the objective of reducing microfilaremia to subinfective levels for mosquitoes, the recent introduction of diethylcarbamazine into table salt (0.2% to 0.4% by weight of the base) has markedly reduced the prevalence, severity, and transmission of lymphatic filariasis in many endemic areas (Gelband, 1994). Moreover, single 6-mg/kg doses given orally every 6 to 12 months have proven just as effective as former prolonged daily dosage regimens. A major discovery was that diethylcarbamazine given annually as a single oral dose of 6 mg/kg was most effective in reducing microfilaremia when given along with a single dose of another antifilarial agent (*see* Ottesen *et al.*, 1999). Initial studies were done with ivermectin as the partner drug, but more recent evidence indicates that 400 mg of albendazole taken orally in addition to diethylcarbamazine is an even more appropriate choice for mass chemotherapy (*see* "Benzimidazoles," above). Adverse reactions to microfilarial destruction, greater after the oral diethylcarbamazine tablet than the table salt preparation, usually are well tolerated. However, mass chemotherapy with diethylcarbamazine should *not* be used in regions where onchocerciasis or loiasis coexist because, even in the table salt formulation, this drug may induce especially severe reactions related to parasite burden in these infections.

Diethylcarbamazine, given in doses of 2 mg/kg three times daily for 14 days, causes rapid disappearance of symptoms of tropical eosinophilia, the pulmonary inflammatory response typical of infection with *W. bancrofti* or *B. malayi*. After taking a small test dose of 50 mg, asymptomatic individuals with microfilaremia should be treated with "standard" courses of diethylcarbamazine, *e.g.,* 6 mg/kg in 3 divided doses per day for 14 to 21 days; the 21-day period is customary for *B. malayi*. Such therapy should minimize further lymphatic and renal damage. It is largely ineffective against more advanced complications of lymphatic filariasis, such as lymphangitis and chronic obstructive lymphedema (*elephantiasis*), that respond better to antibiotics and maintenance of good local hygiene, respectively. A monthly dose of 50 mg of diethylcarbamazine is effective for prophylaxis against lymphatic filariasis.

O. volvulus and L. loa.   Diethylcarbamazine no longer is recommended for initial treatment of onchocerciasis, because it causes severe reactions related to microfilarial destruction (*see* below). Such reactions are far less severe in response to ivermectin, the drug now preferred for this infection. Diethylcarbamazine, despite its drawbacks, remains the best available drug for therapy of loiasis. Treatment is initiated with test doses of 1 mg/kg daily for 2 to 3 days, escalating to maximally tolerated daily doses of 8 to 10 mg/kg for a total of 2 to 3 weeks. Low test doses are used, often accompanied by pretreatment with glucocorticoids or antihistamines, to minimize reactions to dying microfilariae and adult worms; these reactions consist of severe allergic reactions and, occasionally, meningoencephalitis and coma from invasion of the CNS by microfilariae. Repeated courses of treatment with diethylcarbamazine, separated by 3 to 4 weeks, may be required to cure loiasis, and doses of 300 mg weekly have proven to be effective for prophylaxis against this infection. Ivermectin does not provide a good alternative to diethylcarbamazine for treatment of loiasis, but albendazole may prove to be useful in patients who either fail therapy with diethylcarbamazine or who cannot take the drug (Klion *et al.,* 1999).

Diethylcarbamazine is clinically effective against microfilariae and adult worms of *Dipetalonema streptocerca*, but filariasis due to *Mansonella perstans, M. ozzardi,* or *Dirofilaria immitis* responds minimally to this agent.

Although therapy with diethylcarbamazine, 6 mg/kg daily in divided doses for 7 to 10 days, has been recommended for treatment of toxocariasis, the drug is considered experimental for this indication.

Toxicity and Side Effects.   Unless a daily dose of 8 to 10 mg/kg is exceeded, direct toxic reactions to diethylcarbamazine are rarely severe and usually disappear within a few days despite continuation of therapy. These reactions include anorexia, nausea, headache, and, at high doses, vomiting. Major adverse effects result directly or indirectly from the host response to destruction of parasites, primarily microfilariae. Reactions are especially severe in patients heavily infected with *O. volvulus*. They usually are less serious in *B. malayi* or *L. loa* infections and usually are mild in bancroftian filariasis, but the drug occasionally induces retinal hemorrhages and severe encephalitis in patients heavily infected with *L. loa*. In patients with onchocerciasis, there usually is a typical reaction (termed a *Mazzotti reaction*) that occurs within a few hours after the first oral dose. This consists of intense itching and skin rashes, enlargement and tenderness of the lymph nodes, sometimes a fine papular rash, fever, tachycardia, arthralgia, and headache. These symptoms persist for 3 to 7 days and then subside, after which quite high doses can be tolerated. Ocular complications include limbitis, punctate keratitis, uveitis, and atrophy of the retinal pigment epithelium (Rivas-Alcala *et al.,* 1981; Dominguez-Vazquez *et al.,* 1983). In patients with bancroftian or brugian filariasis, nodular swellings may occur along the course of the lymphatics, and there is often an accompanying lymphadenitis. This reaction also subsides within a few days. Almost all patients receiving therapy exhibit a leukocytosis, first evident on the second day, reaching its peak on the fourth or fifth day, and gradually subsiding over a period of a few weeks. Reversible proteinuria may occur, and the eosinophilia so frequently observed in patients with filariasis can be intensified by therapy with diethylcarbamazine. Delayed reactions to more mature dying filarial forms include lymphangitis, swelling and lymphoid abscesses in bancroftian and brugian filariasis, and small skin weals in loiasis. Diethylcarbamazine appears to be safe for use during pregnancy.

Precautions and Contraindications.   Population-based chemotherapy with diethylcarbamazine should be avoided in areas where onchocerciasis or loiasis is endemic, even though the drug can be used to protect foreign travelers from these infections. Pretreatment with glucocorticoids and antihistamines often is undertaken to minimize indirect reactions to diethylcarbamazine that result from dying microfilariae. Dosage reduction must be considered for patients with impaired renal function or persistent alkaline urine.

Ivermectin

History. In the mid-1970s, a survey of natural products revealed that a fermentation broth of the soil actinomycete *Streptomyces avermitilis* ameliorated infection with *Nematospiroides dubius* in mice (Burg *et al.*, 1979; Egerton *et al.*, 1979; Miller *et al.*, 1979). Isolation of the anthelmintic components from cultures of this organism led to discovery of the *avermectins*, a novel class of 16-membered lactones (*see* Campbell, 1989). *Ivermectin* (MECTIZAN; STROMECTOL; 22,23-dihydroavermectin B_{1a}) is a semisynthetic analog of avermectin B_{1a} (*abamectin*), an insecticide developed for crop management. Ivermectin now is used extensively to control and treat a broad spectrum of infections caused by parasitic nematodes (roundworms) and arthropods (insects, ticks, and mites) that plague livestock and domestic animals (*see* Campbell and Benz, 1984; Campbell, 1993). In 1996, the United States Food and Drug Administration approved the use of ivermectin in human beings for treatment of onchocerciasis, the filarial infection responsible for river blindness, and for therapy of intestinal strongyloidiasis. Ivermectin taken as a single oral dose every 6 to 12 months continues to serve as the mainstay of major programs to control onchocerciasis. In addition, annual oral doses of ivermectin, either taken alone or specifically when taken together with annual oral doses of albendazole, markedly reduce microfilaremia in lymphatic filariasis due to *W. bancrofti* or *B. malayi* (Ottesen *et al.*, 1999; Plaisier *et al.*, 2000; *see* "Benzimidazoles," above). The two-drug regimen now is featured in programs to control lymphatic filariasis and it is preferred in regions where lymphatic filariasis coexists with either onchocerciasis or loiasis. Ivermectin is the drug of choice against intestinal strongyloidiasis and it is effective against several other human infections caused by intestinal nematodes (Naquira *et al.*, 1989; Gann *et al.*, 1994; de Silva *et al.*, 1997). The agent also has been used successfully against human scabies and head lice.

The *milbemycins* are macrocyclic lactone analogs of the avermectins. Some of these compounds have antiparasitic activity similar to that of the avermectins and probably act by similar mechanisms (Fisher and Mrozik, 1992; Arena *et al.*, 1995).

The chemical structure of ivermectin is shown below.

Antiparasitic Activity and Resistance. Several reviews have focused on the antiparasitic action of and resistance to the avermectins and related milbemycins (*see* Cully *et al.*, 1996; Sangster, 1996; Martin *et al.*, 1997; Sangster and Gill, 1999). Ivermectin is effective and highly potent against at least some developmental stages of many parasitic nematodes and insects that affect animals and human beings. The drug immobilizes affected organisms by inducing a tonic paralysis of the musculature. Work with the free-living nematode *Caenorhabditis elegans* indicates that avermectins act on a group of glutamate-gated Cl^- channels to produce this effect. Found only in invertebrates, these channels and two of their cloned subunits have been expressed and characterized in *Xenopus laevis* oocytes. There is close correlation among activation and potentiation by avermectins and milbemycin D of glutamate-sensitive Cl^- current, nematicidal activity, and membrane binding affinity in this system (*see* Arena *et al.*, 1995; Cully *et al.*, 1996). Moreover, glutamate-gated Cl^- channels are expressed in the pharyngeal muscle cells of these worms, consistent with the marked and potent inhibitory effect of avermectins on the feeding behavior of the organisms (*see* Sangster and Gill, 1997). The basis for resistance or relative unresponsiveness to avermectin action shown by different nematodes, especially those species parasitizing livestock, is complex. Several different avermectin-"resistant" developmental and physiological phenotypes have been described, but definitive relationships among these phenotypes and native avermectin receptor subtypes, locations, numbers, and binding affinities require clarification (*see* Sangster and Gill, 1999; Hejmadi *et al.*, 2000). Alterations in genes encoding ATP-dependent P-glycoprotein transporters that bind avermectins and in those encoding putative components of the glutamate-gated Cl^- channel have been associated with the development of resistance in *Haemonchus contortus* (Xu *et al.*, 1998; Blackhall *et al.*, 1998). A large increase in low-affinity glutamate binding has been detected in ivermectin-resistant nematodes, but how this relates to drug resistance is unclear (Hejmadi *et al.*, 2000). Glutamate-gated Cl^- channels probably serve as one site of ivermectin action in insects and crustaceans too (Duce and Scott, 1985; Scott and Duce, 1985; Zufall *et al.*, 1989). Avermectins also bind with high affinity to GABA-gated and other ligand-gated Cl^- channels in nematodes such as ascaris and in insects, but the physiological consequences are less well defined. Lack of high-affinity avermectin receptors in cestodes and trematodes may explain why these helminths are not sensitive to ivermectin (Shoop *et al.*, 1995). Avermectins do

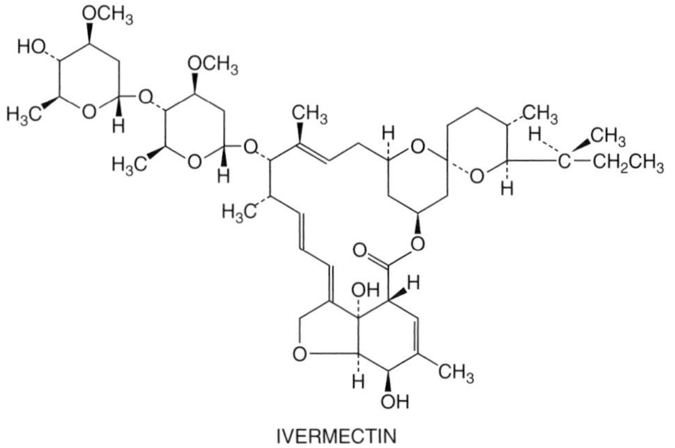

IVERMECTIN

interact with gamma-aminobutyric acid (GABA) receptors in vertebrate (mammalian) brain, but their affinity for invertebrate receptors is about 100-fold greater (*see* Schaeffer and Haines, 1989).

In human beings infected with *Onchocerca volvulus,* ivermectin causes a rapid, marked decrease in microfilarial counts in the skin and ocular tissues that lasts for 6 to 12 months (Greene *et al.,* 1987; Newland *et al.,* 1988). The drug has little discernible effect on adult parasites, but affects developing larvae and blocks egress of microfilariae from the uterus of adult female worms (Awadzi *et al.,* 1985; Court *et al.,* 1985). By reducing microfilariae in the skin, ivermectin decreases transmission to the *Simulium* black fly vector (Cupp *et al.,* 1986, 1989). Ivermectin also is effective against microfilaria but not against adult worms of *W. bancrofti, B. malayi, L. loa,* and *M. ozzardi* (*see* de Silva *et al.,* 1997). The drug exhibits excellent efficacy in human beings against *A. lumbricoides, S. stercoralis,* and cutaneous larva migrans. Other gastrointestinal nematodes are either partially affected (*T. trichuria* and *E. vermicularis*) or unresponsive (*N. americanus* and *A. duodenale*) (Naquira *et al.,* 1989; de Silva *et al.,* 1997).

Absorption, Fate, and Excretion.   In human beings, peak levels of ivermectin in plasma are achieved within 4 to 5 hours after oral administration. The long terminal half-life of about 57 hours in adults primarily reflects a low systemic clearance (about 1 to 2 liters/hour) and a large apparent volume of distribution (*see* Appendix II). Ivermectin is about 93% bound to plasma proteins (Klotz *et al.,* 1990). The drug is extensively converted by hepatic CYP3A4 to at least 10 metabolites, mostly hydroxylated and demethylated derivatives (Zeng *et al.,* 1998). Virtually no ivermectin appears in human urine in either unchanged or conjugated form (Krishna and Klotz, 1993). In animals, ivermectin is recovered in feces, nearly all as unchanged drug, and the highest tissue concentrations occur in liver and fat. Extremely low levels are found in brain, even though ivermectin would be expected to penetrate the blood-brain barrier on the basis of its lipid solubility. Studies in transgenic mice suggest, however, that a P-glycoprotein efflux pump in the blood–brain barrier prevents ivermectin from entering the CNS (Schinkel *et al.,* 1994). This and the limited affinity of ivermectin for CNS receptors may explain the paucity of CNS side effects and the relative safety of this drug in human beings.

Therapeutic Uses. Onchocerciasis.   As reviewed by Goa and colleagues (1991), single oral doses of ivermectin (150 μg/kg) given every 6 to 12 months are considered effective, safe, and practical for the control of onchocerciasis in adults and children 5 years or older. Most important, such therapy results in reversal of lymphadenopathy and acute inflammatory changes in ocular tissues and arrests the development of further ocular pathology due to

microfilariae. Marked reduction of microfilariae in the skin and ocular tissues is noted within a few days and lasts for 6 to 12 months; the dose then should be repeated. Cure is not attained, because ivermectin has little effect on adult *O. volvulus.* Ivermectin, donated by Merck and Company, has been used since 1987 as the mainstay for onchocerciasis control programs in all 34 countries in Africa and in the Middle East and Latin America where the disease is endemic. Nearly 20 million people have received at least one dose of the drug, and many have received 6 to 9 doses (Dull and Meridith, 1998). Annual doses of the drug are quite safe and can cause a substantial reduction in transmission of this infection (Brown, 1998; Boatin *et al.,* 1998). How long such therapy should continue still is unknown.

Lymphatic Filariasis.   Initial studies indicate that single annual doses of ivermectin (400 μg/kg) are both effective and safe for mass chemotherapy of infections with *W. bancrofti* and *B. malayi* (*see* Ottesen and Ramachandran, 1995). Ivermectin is as effective as diethylcarbamazine for controlling lymphatic filariasis and, unlike the latter agent, can be used in regions where onchocerciasis, loiasis, or both infections are endemic. More recent evidence indicates that a single annual dose of ivermectin (200 to 400 μg/kg) and a single annual dose of albendazole (400 mg) are even more effective in controlling lymphatic filariasis than either drug alone. The period of treatment is about 4 to 6 years based on the estimated fecundity of the adult worms. This dual drug regimen also reduces infections with intestinal nematodes. Facilitated by the donation of the drugs by Merck and Company (ivermectin) and SmithKline Beecham (albendazole), the drug combination now serves as the treatment standard for mass chemotherapy and control of lymphatic filariasis (*see* Ottesen *et al.,* 1999, and "Benzimidazoles," above).

Infections with Intestinal Nematodes.   The finding that a single dose of 150 to 200 μg/kg of ivermectin can cure human strongyloidiasis is encouraging, especially because this drug also is effective against coexisting ascariasis, trichuriasis, and enterobiasis (Naquira *et al.,* 1989). A single dose of 100 μg/kg of ivermectin is as effective as traditional treatment of intestinal strongyloidiasis with thiabendazole, and less toxic (Gann *et al.,* 1994). However, the efficacy of ivermectin against disseminated strongyloidiasis has yet to be established.

Other Indications.   Although ivermectin has activity against microfilaria but not against adult worms of *L. loa* and *M. ozzardi,* it is not used clinically for treating infections with these parasitic worms. Taken as a single 150 to 200 μg/kg oral dose, ivermectin is a first-line drug for treatment of cutaneous larva migrans caused by dog or cat hookworms. Similar doses of this compound also are safe and highly effective against human head lice and scabies, the latter even in HIV-infected individuals (*see* de Silva *et al.,* 1997).

Toxicity, Side Effects, and Precautions.   Ivermectin is well tolerated by uninfected human beings and other mammals. In animals, signs of CNS toxicity, including lethargy, ataxia, mydriasis, tremors, and eventually death, occur only at very high doses; dogs, particularly collie breeds, are especially vulnerable (Campbell and Benz, 1984). In human beings, ivermectin toxicity nearly always results from Mazzotti-like reactions to dying microfilariae; the intensity and nature of these reactions relate to the microfilarial burden and the duration and type of filarial infection. After treatment of *O. volvulus* infections with ivermectin, these side effects usually are limited to mild itching and swollen, tender lymph nodes, which arise in 5% to 35% of people, last just a few days, and are relieved by aspirin and antihistamine drugs (*see* Goa *et al.,* 1991). Rarely, more severe reactions occur that include high fever, tachycardia, hypotension, prostration, dizziness, headache, myalgia, arthralgia, diarrhea, and facial and peripheral edema; these may respond to glucocorticoid therapy. Ivermectin induces milder side effects than does diethylcarbamazine and, unlike the latter, seldom exacerbates lesions of ocular tissues in onchocerciasis. The drug can cause rare but serious side effects including marked disability and encephalopathies in patients coinfected with heavy burdens of *L. loa* microfilaria (Gardon *et al.,* 1997). There is little evidence that ivermectin is teratogenic or carcinogenic.

Because of its effects on gamma-aminobutyric acid receptors in the CNS, ivermectin is contraindicated in conditions associated with an impaired blood-brain barrier, *e.g.,* African trypanosomiasis and meningitis. Caution also is advised about coadministration of ivermectin with other agents that depress CNS activity. Possible adverse interactions of ivermectin with other drugs that are extensively metabolized by hepatic CYP3A4 have yet to be evaluated. Ivermectin has not yet been approved for use in children less than 5 years old and in pregnant women, but both populations undoubtedly have been exposed to the drug in mass treatment programs. Lactating women taking the drug secrete low levels in their milk; the consequences for nursing infants are unknown.

Metrifonate

Metrifonate (trichlorfon; BILARCIL) is an organophosphorous compound used first as an insecticide and later as an anthelmintic, especially for treatment of schistosomiasis hematobium. Metri-

fonate has the following chemical structure:

METRIFONATE

Metrifonate is a prodrug; it is converted nonenzymatically at physiological pH to *dichlorvos* (2,2-dichlorovinyl dimethyl phosphate, DDVP), a potent cholinesterase inhibitor (Hinz *et al.,* 1996). However, inhibition of cholinesterase alone is unlikely to explain the antischistosomal properties of metrifonate (Bloom, 1981). *In vitro,* dichlorvos is about equally potent as a inhibitor of both *S. mansoni* and *S. haematobium* acetylcholinesterases, yet metrifonate is effective clinically only against infections with *S. hematobium.* The molecular basis for this species-selective effect is not understood.

Peak concentrations in plasma of metrifonate (30 μM) and of dichlorvos (0.3 μM) are reached within an hour after a single oral dose of metrifonate (10 mg/kg). The half-life of both compounds in plasma is 1.5 to 2.0 hours; this value is similar to that found for the spontaneous rearrangement of metrifonate at physiological pH (Abdi and Villen, 1991).

Because of its low cost, effectiveness, and ready acceptance, metrifonate is used as an alternative to praziquantel for treatment of urinary schistosomiasis caused by *S. haematobium.* The usual dose is 7.5 to 10 mg/kg, given orally three times at intervals of 2 weeks. Recently, metrifonate has been investigated for the treatment of central cholinergic deficits associated with Alzheimer's disease (*see* Williams, 1999). Metrifonate is not an approved drug in the United States.

At therapeutic doses, metrifonate inhibits the activities of plasma cholinesterase and erythrocyte acetylcholinesterase; both recover to almost normal levels within weeks of stopping treatment. Despite these changes, metrifonate is well tolerated. Side effects such as mild vertigo, lassitude, nausea, and colic are dose-related and occur infrequently. Treated individuals should be free from recent exposure to insecticides that might add to the anticholinesterase effect. They also should not receive depolarizing neuromuscular blocking agents for at least 48 hours after treatment.

Niclosamide

Niclosamide (NICLOCIDE), a halogenated salicylanilide derivative, was introduced in the 1960s for human use as a taeniacide. This compound is considered as a second-choice drug to praziquantel for treating human intestinal infections with *T. saginata, D. latum, H. nana,* and most other cestodes because it was cheap, effective, and readily available in many parts of the world. However, therapy with niclosamide poses a risk to people infected with *T. solium,* because ova released from drug-damaged gravid worms develop into larvae that can cause cysticercosis, a dangerous infection that responds poorly to chemotherapy. Niclosamide is no longer approved for use in the United States. More complete information on the pharmacology and therapeutic uses of niclosamide can be found in the *ninth* and *earlier editions* of this textbook.

Oxamniquine

Oxamniquine (VANSIL) is a 2-aminomethyltetrahydroquinoline derivative that is used as a second-choice drug to praziquantel for the treatment of schistosomiasis. Most strains of *S. mansoni* are highly susceptible to oxamniquine, but *S. haematobium* and *S. japonicum* are virtually unaffected by therapeutic doses. Because of a low incidence of mild side effects together with normally high efficacy after a single oral dose, oxamniquine continues to be used in *S. mansoni* control programs, especially in South America. More details on the pharmacology and therapeutic uses of oxamniquine can be found in the *ninth* and *earlier editions* of this textbook.

Piperazine

The discovery of the anthelmintic properties of piperazine usually is credited to Fayard (1949), but these were first observed by Boismare, a Rouen pharmacist, whose recipe is quoted in Fayard's thesis. A large number of substituted piperazine derivatives exhibit anthelmintic activity, but apart from diethylcarbamazine, none has found a place in human therapeutics (*see* Standen, 1963). Piperazine, a cyclic secondary amine, has the following chemical structure:

PIPERAZINE

Piperazine is highly effective against both *A. lumbricoides* and *E. vermicularis*. The predominant effect of piperazine on *Ascaris* is to cause a flaccid paralysis that results in expulsion of the worm by peristalsis. Affected worms recover if incubated in drug-free medium. Piperazine acts as a GABA agonist. By increasing chloride ion conductance of *Ascaris* muscle membrane, the drug produces hyperpolarization and reduced excitability that leads to muscle relaxation and flaccid paralysis (Martin, 1985). The basis for its selectivity of action is not clear, but studies like those done on ivermectin (Arena *et al.*, 1995) could help resolve this issue. Piperazine is rapidly absorbed after an oral dose. About 20% is excreted unchanged in the urine (Fletcher *et al.*, 1982).

Piperazine citrate (MULTIFUGE), the form available in the United States, is a useful and inexpensive second-choice alternative to mebendazole or pyrantel pamoate in treating combined ascariasis and enterobius infections. Piperazine preparations (tablets or syrup) always are given orally. Prior fasting or supplementary treatment with cathartics or enemas is unnecessary. Many different dosage schedules have been investigated, and all have resulted in considerable success. In ascariasis, accepted therapy is to give 75 mg/kg, to a maximum of 3.5 grams, as a single daily dose for 2 consecutive days. Children should be treated in the same way. This dosage schedule will cure nearly all patients. In the treatment of ascariasis, piperazine has the advantage of greatly reducing the motility of the worms, thereby reducing the hazard of migration. Since the worms are usually alive when passed, there is little chance of absorption of disintegration products. Where partial intestinal obstruction is a complication of infection, conservative management together with the administration of piperazine syrup through a drainage tube may obviate the need for surgical intervention.

In enterobiasis, single daily doses of 65 mg/kg, with a maximum of 2.5 grams, given for 7 days, will result in 95% to 100% cure. Treatment of enterobiasis is complicated by the readiness with which reinfection may occur. Thus, a second course of therapy should be given to ambulatory patients 1 to 2 weeks after the first. Many authorities advocate the simultaneous treatment of the entire household with piperazine in lieu of diagnosing each member by anal swabs.

There is a large difference between effective therapeutic and overtly toxic doses of piperazine. Occasional gastrointestinal upset, transient neurological effects, and urticarial reactions have attended its use. Piperazine has been used without ill effect during pregnancy. Lethal doses cause convulsions and respiratory depression. Piperazine is contraindicated in patients with a history of epilepsy. Neurotoxic effects occur in individuals with renal dysfunction, because urinary excretion is the main route of elimination of the drug.

Praziquantel

History. *Praziquantel* (BILTRICIDE, DISTOCIDE) is a pyrazinoisoquinoline derivative developed after this class of compounds was discovered to have anthelmintic activity in 1972. In animals and human beings, infections with many different cestodes and trematodes respond favorably to this agent, whereas nematodes are unaffected (*see* Symposium, 1981; Andrews, 1985). Praziquantel has the following chemical structure:

PRAZIQUANTEL

The (−) isomer is responsible for most of the drug's anthelmintic activity.

Anthelmintic Action. After rapid and reversible uptake, praziquantel has two major effects on adult schistosomes. At the lowest effective concentrations, it causes increased muscular activity, followed by contraction and spastic paralysis. Affected worms detach from blood vessel walls, resulting in a rapid shift from the mesenteric veins to the liver. At slightly higher therapeutic concentrations, praziquantel causes tegumental damage, which exposes a number of tegumental antigens (*see* Redman *et al.*, 1996). Comparisons of stage-specific susceptibility of *S. mansoni* to praziquantel *in vitro* and *in vivo* indicate that the clinical efficacy of this drug correlates better with tegumental action (Xiao *et al.*, 1985). Studies in laboratory animals have shown that praziquantel is less effective against *S. mansoni* and *S. japonicum* in immunosuppressed mice (*see* Fallon *et al.*, 1996). Whether or not host immune status is important for clinical efficacy of praziquantel in human beings is not known.

The tegument of schistosomes seems to be the primary site of action of praziquantel. The drug causes an influx of Ca^{2+} across the tegument, and the effect is blocked in Ca^{2+}-free medium. A number of praziquantel-sensitive sites have been suggested as possible targets, but the precise molecular mechanism of action remains elusive (*see* Redman *et al.*, 1996).

Praziquantel also produces a variety of biochemical changes, but most appear to be secondary to its primary tegumental action (*see* Andrews, 1985). Nearly all available information about the action of praziquantel has come from studies on schistosomes. Although it generally is assumed that the anthelmintic action of praziquantel against other trematodes and cestodes is the same as for schistosomes, direct evidence is lacking.

Absorption, Fate, and Excretion. Praziquantel is readily absorbed after oral administration, so that maximal levels in human plasma occur in 1 to 2 hours. The pharmacokinetics of praziquantel are dose-related. Extensive first-pass metabolism to many inactive hydroxylated and conjugated products limits the bioavailability of this drug and results in plasma concentrations of metabolites at least 100-fold higher than that of praziquantel. The drug is about 80% bound to plasma proteins. Its plasma half-life is 0.8 to 3.0 hours, depending on the dose, compared with 4 to 6 hours for its metabolites, but this may be prolonged in patients with severe liver disease, including those with hepatosplenic schistosomiasis. About 70% of an oral dose of praziquantel is recovered as metabolites in the urine within 24 hours; most of the remainder is metabolized in the liver and eliminated in the bile.

Therapeutic Uses. Praziquantel is approved in the United States only for therapy of schistosomiasis and liver fluke infections, but elsewhere, this remarkably versatile and safe drug also is used to treat infections with many other trematodes and cestodes (*see* Table VII–1). Praziquantel should be stored at temperatures less than 30°C and swallowed in water without chewing because of its bitter taste.

Praziquantel is the drug of choice for treating schistosomiasis caused by all *Schistosoma* species that infect human beings. Although dosage regimens vary, a single oral dose of 40 mg/kg or three doses of 20 mg/kg each, given 4 to 6 hours apart, generally produce cure rates of 70% to 95% and consistently high reductions (over 85%) in egg counts. Strains of *S. mansoni* and *S. japonicum* resistant to praziquantel have been selected in laboratory studies (*see* Fallon *et al.,* 1996). Moreover, decreased clinical efficacy of praziquantel against infections with *S. mansoni* has been reported in two human populations, one in a focal area of high transmission in northern Senegal (Van Lieshout *et al.,* 1999) and the other in Egypt, where 1% to 2% of patients were not cured after two or three treatments with praziquantel (Ismail *et al.,* 1999). However, praziquantel-tolerant or -resistant schistosome strains currently do not limit the clinical usefulness of this drug (*see* Fallon *et al.,* 1996).

Three doses of 25 mg/kg taken 4 to 8 hours apart on the same day result in high rates of cure for infections with either the liver flukes, *C. sinensis* and *O. viverrini,* or the intestinal flukes, *Fasciolopis buski, Heterophyes heterophyes,* and *Metagonimus yokogawi.* The same three-dose regimen used for two days is highly effective against infections with the lung fluke, *Paragonimus westermani.* Infections with *Fasciola hepatica* are unresponsive to high doses, even though praziquantel penetrates this trematode. The reason for the insensitivity of *F. hepatica* to praziquantel is unknown.

Low doses of praziquantel can be used successfully to treat intestinal infections with adult cestodes, for example, a single oral dose of 25 mg/kg for *Hymenolepis nana* and 10 to 20 mg/kg for *D. latum, T. saginata,* or *T. solium.* Retreatment after 7 to 10 days is advisable for individuals heavily infected with *H. nana.* While albendazole is preferred for therapy of human cysticercosis, the tissue infection with intermediate cyst larvae of *T. solium,* prolonged high-dose therapy with praziquantel remains an alternative treatment (*see* Evans *et al.,* 1997). Neither the "cystic" nor "alveolar" hydatid diseases caused by larval stages of *Echinococcus* tapeworms respond to praziquantel; here too, albendazole is effective (*see* Horton, 1997; Schantz, 1999).

Toxicity, Precautions, and Interactions. Abdominal discomfort, particularly pain and nausea, headache, dizziness, and drowsiness may occur shortly after taking praziquantel; these direct effects are transient and dose-related. Indirect effects such as fever, pruritus, urticaria, rashes, arthralgia, and myalgia are noted occasionally. Such side effects and increases in eosinophilia often relate to parasite burden. In neurocysticercosis, inflammatory reactions to praziquantel may produce meningismus, seizures, mental changes, and cerebrospinal fluid pleocytosis. These effects usually are delayed in onset, last 2 to 3 days, and respond to appropriate symptomatic therapy such as analgesics and anticonvulsants.

Praziquantel is considered safe in children over 4 years of age, who probably tolerate the drug better than do adults. Low levels of the drug appear in the maternal milk, but there is no evidence that this compound is mutagenic or carcinogenic. High doses of praziquantel do increase abortion rates in rats, so the drug probably is best avoided during human pregnancy.

The bioavailability of praziquantel is reduced by inducers of hepatic cytochromes P450 such as carbamazepine and phenobarbital; predictably, coadministration of the cytochrome P450 inhibitor cimetidine has the opposite effect (Bittencourt *et al.,* 1992; Dachman *et al.,* 1994). Dexamethasone reduces the bioavailability of praziquantel, but the mechanism is not understood. Under certain conditions, praziquantel may increase the bioavailability of albendazole (Homeida *et al.*, 1994).

Praziquantel is contraindicated in ocular cysticercosis, because the host response can produce irreversible damage to the eye. Shortly after taking the drug, driving, operating machinery, and other tasks requiring mental alertness should be avoided. The half-life of praziquantel can be prolonged in patients with severe hepatic disease; dosage adjustment in such patients may be required (Mandour *et al.*, 1990).

Pyrantel Pamoate

Pyrantel pamoate (ANTIMINTH, others) was introduced first into veterinary practice as a broad-spectrum anthelmintic directed against pinworm, roundworm, and hookworm infections (Austin *et al.*, 1966). Its effectiveness and lack of toxicity led to its trial against related intestinal helminths in human beings (Bumbalo *et al.*, 1969). *Oxantel pamoate*, an *m*-oxyphenol analog of pyrantel, is effective for single-dose treatment of trichuriasis. Pyrantel is employed as the pamoate salt. It has the following chemical structure:

PYRANTEL

Pyrantel and its analogs are depolarizing neuromuscular blocking agents. They open nonselective cation channels and induce marked, persistent activation of nicotinic acetylcholine receptors, which results in spastic paralysis of the worm (Robertson *et al.*, 1994). Pyrantel also inhibits cholinesterases. It causes a slowly developing contracture of preparations of *Ascaris* at 1% of the concentration of acetylcholine required to produce the same effect. In single muscle cells of this helminth, pyrantel causes depolarization and increased spike-discharge frequency, accompanied by increase in tension. Pyrantel is effective against hookworm, pinworm, and roundworm; unlike its analog oxantel, it is ineffective against *T. trichiura*.

Pyrantel pamoate is poorly absorbed from the gastrointestinal tract, a property that contributes to its selective action on gastrointestinal nematodes. Less than 15% is excreted in the urine as parent drug and metabolites. The major proportion of an administered dose is recovered in the feces.

Pyrantel pamoate is an alternative to mebendazole in the treatment of ascariasis and enterobiasis. High cure rates have been achieved after a single oral dose of 11 mg/kg, to a maximum of 1 gram. Pyrantel also is effective against hookworm infections caused by *A. duodenale* and *N. americanus*, although repeated doses are needed to cure heavy infections with *N. americanus*. The drug should be used in combination with oxantel for mixed infections with *T. trichiura*. In the case of pinworm, it is wise to repeat the treatment after an interval of 2 weeks.

When given parenterally, pyrantel can produce complete neuromuscular blockade in animals; if given orally, toxic effects are produced only by very large doses. Transient and mild gastrointestinal symptoms are occasionally observed in human beings, as are headache, dizziness, rash, and fever. Pyrantel pamoate has not been studied in pregnant women. Thus, its use in pregnant patients and children less than 2 years of age is not recommended. Because pyrantel pamoate and piperazine are mutually antagonistic with respect to their neuromuscular effects on parasites, the two should not be used together.

PROSPECTUS

Eradication of helminthiasis is highly unlikely because of its close association with human poverty. Although these infections are both common and cosmopolitan, their subtle clinical course encourages neglect until disease becomes obvious. Helminthiasis flourishes especially in warm environments marked by inadequate sanitation, parasitized reservoirs and vectors, and contaminated food and water sources. Affluence, however, does not protect against these infections; young or debilitated individuals are particularly vulnerable regardless of socioeconomic status.

Chemotherapy now provides the single most efficient, practical, and inexpensive strategy to control helminth infections. Moreover, it still will be needed even if effective vaccines become available. To achieve optimal results, chemotherapy must be combined with other measures such as improved sanitation and vector and reservoir control. Even for chemotherapy itself to succeed, there must be a felt need for the drug regimen, a suitable delivery infrastructure for it, and appropriate follow-up to ensure compliance. Periodic treatment with effective agents can reduce the parasite burden to the point where transmission is affected, because few helminth species multiply within the human host.

A major challenge is to develop better drugs against systemic infections with helminths that respond inadequately to current compounds, *i.e.*, the filariases, echinococcosis, fascioliasis, trichinosis, toxocariasis, and cysticercosis. Discovery of agents effective against all developmental stages of parasitic helminths, *e.g.*, adult filarial worms instead of just microfilariae, would constitute a major advance in this context. That most effective anthelmintics have been in use for years invites eventual development of resistance to these drugs. Although the emergence of drug-resistant helminths has not yet become a problem for treatment of infections in human beings, resistance to benzimidazoles and avermectins is well established in animal infections. The specter of drug resistance mandates the search for improved anthelmintics, even for therapy of infections that now respond adequately to available drugs.

Because of lack of economic incentives, scientific knowledge relevant to drug discovery is likely to outpace drug development in this field. Broad applications to helminths of modern techniques such as genome sequencing projects and proteomics together with other approaches should accelerate identification and characterization of drug receptors and increase understanding of mechanisms of drug resistance. Understanding the relationship between avermectin resistance of helminths *in vivo* to their cloned avermectin-modulated, glutamate-gated Cl⁻ channel "receptors" is a case in point. Rapid automatic screening of compounds for reactivity with essential parasite macromolecules *in vitro* also is feasible, so components with anthelmintic activity can be identified readily in large libraries of structurally diverse synthetic compounds.

Barring development of novel drugs, what other pharmacological measures might be taken to control helminth infections of human beings? One strategy would be to improve the use of available anthelmintics. Indeed, introduction of diethylcarbamazine into table salt already has modulated lymphatic filariasis, and periodic use of anthelmintics such as praziquantel for schistosomiasis and either diethylcarbamazine or ivermectin for lymphatic filariasis has reduced the parasite burden, rate of transmission, and severity of disease in these infections. Empirical dosage regimens must undergo continuing clinical evaluation; this process already has resulted in the reduction of doses of diethylcarbamazine and ivermectin used to control the filariases. Concomitant use of current drugs with different mechanisms of action against the same organism represents a major advance in anthelmintic chemotherapy. This concept is aptly illustrated by the periodic use of albendazole together with either diethylcarbamazine or ivermectin for successful control of lymphatic filariasis. Human populations coinfected with different classes of helminths should benefit from periodic therapy with two or more broad-spectrum drugs, each with a different anthelmintic profile. This approach already has had success, *i.e.,* albendazole and ivermectin, used together to control lymphatic filariasis, are highly effective against intestinal nematodes. Praziquantel, ivermectin, and albendazole together have been advocated for periodic treatment of populations infected with several species of helminths.

At far less cost than required for development of novel drugs, profitable drugs used for veterinary purposes or even approved for other clinical indications in human beings could improve the control of human helminthiasis. Indeed, the avermectins and benzimidazoles were developed initially for veterinary use, and both ivermectin and albendazole have been donated by their respective manufacturers for control of human helminth infections. Limited studies have shown that the veterinary benzimidazole, *triclabendazole,* is probably the most effective known drug against fascioliasis in human beings. *Moxidectin,* a veterinary drug related to the avermectins, shows macrofilaricidal activity against onchocerciasis and lymphatic filariasis and is now ready for evaluation in human beings. A veterinary formulation of ivermectin administered subcutaneously to bypass hepatic metabolism might achieve higher plasma levels and greater efficacy against certain human systemic infections with marginally drug-responsive helminths. Moreover, animal models of helminthic infections provide a powerful approach to explore mechanisms of anthelmintic drug resistance.

Ultimately, society will be forced to pay the high cost of developing novel anthelmintic drugs for human use. The technology is either available now or soon will be. Both drugs and vaccines may be needed to combat helminth infections that now exact a heavy toll on human health and productivity.

For further discussion of helminth infections, *see* Chapters 214 and 221–225 in *Harrison's Principles of Internal Medicine,* 14th ed., McGraw-Hill, New York, 1998.

BIBLIOGRAPHY

Abdi, Y.A., and Villen, T. Pharmacokinetics of metrifonate and its rearrangement product dichlorvos in whole blood. *Pharmacol. Toxicol.,* **1991,** *68*:137–139.

Arena, J.P., Liu, K.K., Paress, P.S., Frazier, E.G., Cully, D.F., Mrozik, H., and Schaeffer, J.M. The mechanism of action of avermectins in *Caenorhabditis elegans:* correlation between activation of glutamate-sensitive chloride current, membrane binding, and biological activity. *J. Parasitol.,* **1995,** *81*:286–294.

Arjona, R., Riancho, J.A., Aguado, J.M., Salesa, R., and González-Macías, J. Fascioliasis in developed countries: a review of classic and aberrant forms of the disease. *Medicine (Baltimore),* **1995,** *74*:13–23.

Austin, W.C., Courtney, W., Danilewicz, J.C., Morgan, D.H., Conover, L.H., Howes, H.L. Jr., Lynch, J.E., McFarland, J.W., Cornwall, R.L., and Theodorides, V.J. Pyrantel tartrate, a new anthelmintic effective against infections of domestic animals. *Nature,* **1966,** *212*:1273–1274.

Awadzi, K., Adjepon-Yamoah, K.K., Edwards, G., Orme, M.L., Breckenridge, A.M., and Gilles, H.M. The effect of moderate urine alkalinisation on low dose diethycarbamazine therapy in patients with onchocerciasis. *Br. J. Clin. Pharmacol.,* **1986,** *21*:669–676.

Awadzi, K., Dadzie, K.Y., Shulz-Key, H., Haddock, D.R., Gilles, H.M., and Aziz, M.A. The chemotherapy of onchocerciasis X. An assessment of four single dose treatment regimes of MK-933 (ivermectin) in human onchocerciasis. *Ann. Trop. Med. Parasitol.,* **1985,** *79*:63–78.

Bittencourt, P.R., Gracia, C.M., Martins, R., Fernandes, A.G., Diekmann, H.W., and Jung, W. Phenytoin and carbamazepine decreased oral bioavailability of praziquantel. *Neurology,* **1992,** *42*:492–496.

Blackhall, W.J., Liu, H.Y., Xu, M., Prichard, R.K., and Beech, R.N. Selection at a P-glycoprotein gene in ivermectin- and moxidectin-selected strains of *Haemonchus contortus. Mol. Biochem. Parasitol.,* **1998,** *95*:193–201.

Bloom, A. Studies of the mode of action of metrifonate and DDVP in schistosomes—cholinesterase activity and the hepatic shift. *Acta Pharmacol. Toxicol. (Copenh.),* **1981,** *49*(*suppl 5*):109–113.

Boatin, B.A., Hougard, J.M., Alley, E.S., Akpoboua, L.K., Yameogo, L., Dembele, N., Seketeli, A., and Dadzie, K.Y. The impact of Mectizan on the transmission of onchocerciasis. *Ann. Trop. Med. Parasitol.,* **1998,** *92*(*suppl 1*):S46–S60.

Braithwaite, P.A., Roberts, M.S., Allan, R.J., and Watson, T.R. Clinical pharmacokinetics of high dose mebendazole in patients treated for cystic hydatid disease. *Eur. J. Clin. Pharmacol.,* **1982,** *22*:161–169.

Brown, H.D., Matzuk, A.R., Ilves, I.R., Peterson, L.H., Harris, S.A., Sarett, L.H., Egerton, J.R., Yakstis, J.J., Campbell, W.C., and Cuckler, A.C. Antiparasitic drugs. IV. 2-(4′-thiazolyl)-benzimidazole, a new anthelmintic. *J. Am. Chem. Soc.,* **1961,** *83*:1764–1765.

Brugmans, J.P., Thienpont, D.C., van Wijngaarden, I., Vanparijs, O.F., Schuermans, V.L., and Lauwers, H.L. Mebendazole in enterobiasis. Radiochemical and pilot clinical study in 1,278 subjects. *JAMA,* **1971,** *217*:313–316.

Bumbalo, T.S., Fugazzotto, D.J., and Wyczalek, J.V. Treatment of enterobiasis with pyrantel pamoate. *Am. J. Trop. Med. Hyg.,* **1969,** *18*:50–52.

Burg, R.W., Miller, B.M., Baker, E.E., Birnbaum, J., Currie, S.A., Hartman, R., Kong, Y.L., Monaghan, R.L., Olson, G., Putter, I., Tunac, J.B., Wallick, H., Stapley, E.O., Oiwa, R., and Omura, S. Avermectins, new family of potent anthelmintic agents: producing organism and fermentation. *Antimicrob. Agents Chemother.,* **1979,** *15*:361–367.

Court, J.P., Bianco, A.E., Townson, S., Ham, P.J., and Friedheim, E. Study on the activity of antiparasitic agents against *Onchocerca lienalis* third stage larvae *in vitro. Trop. Med. Parasitol.,* **1985,** *36*:117–119.

Cupp, E.W., Bernardo, M.J., Kiszewski, A.E., Collins, R.C., Taylor, H.R., Aziz, M.A., and Greene, B.M. The effects of ivermectin on transmission of *Onchocerca volvulus. Science,* **1986,** *231*:740–742.

Cupp, E.W., Onchoa, A.O., Collins, R.C., Ramberg, F.R., and Zea, G. The effect of multiple ivermectin treatments on infection of *Simulium ochraceum* with *Onchocerca volvulus. Am. J. Trop. Med. Hyg.,* **1989,** *40*:501–506.

Dachman, W.D., Adubofour, K.O., Bikin, D.S., Johnson, C.H., Mullin, P.D., and Winograd, M. Cimetidine-induced rise in praziquantel levels in a patient with neurocysticercosis being treated with anticonvulsants. *J. Infect. Dis.,* **1994,** *169*:689–691.

Davies, H.D., Sakuls, P., and Keystone, J.S. Creeping eruption. A review of clinical presentation and management of 60 cases presenting to a tropical disease unit. *Arch. Dermatol.,* **1993,** *129*:588–591.

Davis, A., Dixon, H., and Pawlowski, Z.S. Multicentre clinical trials of benzimidazole-carbamates in human cystic echinococcosis (phase 2). *Bull. World Health Organ.,* **1989,** *67*:503–508.

Delatour, P., Benoit, E., Besse, S., and Boukraa, A. Comparative enantioselectivity in the sulfoxidation of albendazole in man, dogs and rats. *Xenobiotica,* **1991,** *21*:217–221.

Dominguez-Vazquez, A., Taylor, H.R., Greene, B.M., Ruvalcaba-Macias, A.M., Rivas-Alcala, A.R., Murphy, R.P., and Beltran-Hernandez, F. Comparison of flubendazole and diethylcarbamazine in treatment of onchocerciasis. *Lancet,* **1983,** *1*:139–143.

Driscoll, M., Dean, E., Reilly, E., Bergholz, E., and Chalfie, M. Genetic and molecular analysis of *Caenorhabditis elegans* β-tubulin that conveys benzimidazole sensitivity. *J. Cell Biol.,* **1989,** *109*:2993–3003.

Duce, I.R., and Scott, R.H. Actions of dihydroavermectin B_{1a} on insect muscle. *Br. J. Pharmacol.,* **1985,** *85*:395–401.

Edwards, G., Breckenridge, A.M., Adjepon-Yamoah, K.K., Orme, M.L., and Ward, S.A. The effect of variations in urinary pH on the pharmacokinetics of diethylcarbamazine. *Br. J. Clin. Pharmacol.,* **1981,** *12*:807–812.

Egerton, J.R., Ostlind, D.A., Blair, L.S., Eary, C.H., Suhayda, D., Cifelli, S., Riek, R.F., and Campbell, W.C. Avermectins, new family of potent anthelmintic agents: efficacy of the B_{1a} component. *Antimicrob. Agents Chemother.,* **1979,** *15*:372–378.

Faulkner, J.K., and Smith, K.J. Dealkylation and N-oxidation in the metabolism of 1-diethylcarbamyl-4-methylpiperazine in the rat. *Xenobiotica,* **1972,** *2*:59–68.

Fayard, C. Ascaridiose et piperazine. Thesis, Paris, **1949.** (Quoted from *Semin. Hop. Paris,* **1949,** *35*:1778.)

Fletcher, K.A., Evans, D.A., and Kelly, J.A. Urinary piperazine excretion in healthy Caucasians. *Ann. Trop. Med. Parasitol.,* **1982,** *76*:77–82.

Franchi, C., Di Vico, B., and Teggi, A. Long-term evaluation of patients with hydatidosis treated with benzimidazole carbamates. *Clin. Infect. Dis.,* **1999,** *29*:304–309.

Gann, P.H., Neva, F.A., and Gam, A.A. A randomized trial of single- and two-dose ivermectin *versus* thiabendazole for treatment of strongyloidiasis. *J. Infect. Dis.,* **1994,** *169*:1076–1079.

Gardon, J., Gardon-Wendel, N., Demanga-Ngangue, Kamgno, J., Chippaux, J.P., and Boussinesq, M. Serious reactions after mass treatment of onchocerciasis with ivermectin in an area endemic for *Loa loa* infection. *Lancet,* **1997,** *350*:18–22.

Gelband, H. Diethylcarbamazine salt in the control of lymphatic filariasis. *Am. J. Trop. Med. Hyg.,* **1994,** *50*:655–662.

Gleizes, C., Eeckhoutte, C., Pineau, T., Alvinerie, M., and Galtier, P. Inducing effect of oxfendazole on cytochrome P450IA2 in rabbit liver. Consequences on cytochrome P450 dependent monooxygenases. *Biochem. Pharmacol.,* **1991,** *41*:1813–1820.

Goa, K.L., McTavish, D., and Clissold, S.P. Ivermectin. A review of its antifilarial activity, pharmacokinetic properties and clinical efficacy in onchocerciasis. *Drugs,* **1991,** *42*:640–658.

Greene, B.M., White, A.T., Newland, H.S., Keyvan-Larijani, E., Dukuly, Z.D., Gallin, M.Y., Aziz, M.A., Williams, P.N., and Taylor, H.R. Single dose therapy with ivermectin for onchocerciasis. *Trans. Assoc. Am. Physicians,* **1987,** *100*:131–138.

Hejmadi, M.V., Jagannathan, S., Delany, N.S., Coles, G.C., and Wolstenholme, A.J. L-glutamate binding sites of parasitic nematodes: and association with ivermectin resistance? *Parasitology,* **2000,** *120*:535–545.

Hinz, V.C., Grewig, S., and Schmidt, B.H. Metrifonate induces cholinesterase inhibition exclusively via slow release of dichlorvos. *Neurochem. Res.,* **1996,** *21*:331–337.

Homeida, M., Leahy, W., Copeland, S., Ali, M.M., and Harron, D.W. Pharmacokinetic interaction between praziquantel and albendazole in Sudanese men. *Ann. Trop. Med. Parasitol.*, **1994,** 88:551–559.

Ismail, M., Botros, S., Metwally, A., William, S., Farghally, A., Tao, L.F., Day, T.A., and Bennett, J.L. Resistance to praziquantel: direct evidence from *Schistosoma mansoni* isolated from Egyptian villagers. *Am. J. Trop. Med. Hyg.*, **1999,** 60:932–935.

Jung, H., Hurtado, M., Sanchez, M., Medina, M.T., and Sotelo, J. Clinical pharmacokinetics of albendazole in patients with brain cysticercosis. *J. Clin. Pharmacol.*, **1992,** 32:28–31.

Katiyar, S.K., and Edlind, T.D. *In vitro* susceptibilities of the AIDS-associated microsporidian *Encephalitozoon intestinalis* to albendazole, its sulfoxide metabolite, and 12 additional benzimidazole derivatives. *Antimicrob. Agents Chemother.*, **1997,** 41:2729–2732.

Klion, A.D., Horton, J., and Nutman, T.B. Albendazole therapy for loiasis refractory to diethylcarbamazine treatment. *Clin. Infect. Dis.*, **1999,** 29:680–682.

Klotz, U., Ogbuokiri, J.E., and Okonkwo, P.O. Ivermectin binds avidly to plasma proteins. *Eur. J. Clin. Pharmacol.*, **1990,** 39:607–608.

Krishna, D.R., and Klotz, U. Determination of ivermectin in human plasma by high-performance liquid chromatography. *Arzneimittelforschung*, **1993,** 43:609–611.

Kwa, M.S., Kooyman, F.N., Boersema, J.H., and Roos, M.H. Effect of selection for benzimidazole resistance in *Haemonchus contortus* on β-tubulin isotype 1 and isotype 2 genes. *Biochem. Biophys. Res. Commun.*, **1993,** 191:413–419.

Kwa, M.S., Veenstra, J.G., Van Dijk, M., and Roos, M.H. Beta-tubulin genes from the parasitic nematode *Haemonchus contortus* modulate drug resistance in *Caenorhabditis elegans*. *J. Mol. Biol.*, **1995,** 246:500–510.

Lacey, E. The role of the cytoskeletal protein, tubulin, in the mode of action and mechanism of drug resistance to benzimidazoles. *Int. J. Parasitol.*, **1988,** 18:885–936.

Lubega, G.W., and Prichard, R.K. Beta-tubulin and benzimidazole resistance in the sheep nematode *Haemonchus contortus*. *Mol. Biochem. Parasitol.*, **1991,** 47:129–137.

Maizels, R.M., Bundy, D.A., Selkirk, M.E., Smith, D.F., and Anderson, R.M. Immunological modulation and evasion by helminth parasites in human populations. *Nature*, **1993,** 365:797–805.

Mandour, M.E., el Turabi, H., Homeida, M.M., el Sadig, T., Ali, H.M., Bennett, J.L., Leahey, W.J., and Harron, D.W. Pharmacokinetics of praziquantel in healthy volunteers and patients with schistosomiasis. *Trans. R. Soc. Trop. Med. Hyg.*, **1990,** 84:389–393.

Marques, M.P., Takayanagui, O.M., Bonato, P.S., Santos, S.R., and Lanchote, V.L. Enantioselective kinetic disposition of albendazole sulfoxide in patients with neurocysticercosis. *Chirality*, **1999,** 11:218–223.

Marriner, S.E., Morris, D.L., Dickson, B., and Bogan, J.A. Pharmacokinetics of albendazole in man. *Eur. J. Clin. Pharmacol.*, **1986,** 30:705–708.

Martin, R.J. γ-Aminobutyric acid- and piperazine-activated single-channel currents from *Ascaris suum* body muscle. *Br. J. Pharmacol.*, **1985,** 84:445–461.

Miller, T.W., Chaiet, L., Cole, D.J., Cole, L.J., Flor, J.E., Goegelman, R.T., Gullo, V.P., Joshua, H., Kempf, A.J., Krellwitz, W.R., Monaghan, R.L., Ormond, R.E., Wilson, K.E., Albers-Schonberg, G., and Putter, I. Avermectins, new family of potent anthelmintic agents: isolation and chromatographic properties. *Antimicrob. Agents Chemother.*, **1979,** 15:368–371.

Moroni, P., Buronfosse, T., Longin-Sauvageon, C., Delatour, P., and Benoit, E. Chiral sulfoxidation of albendazole by the flavin adenine

dinucleotide-containing and cytochrome P450–dependent monooxygenases from rat liver microsomes. *Drug Metab. Dispos.*, **1995,** 23:160–165.

Morris, D.L., Chinnery, J.B., Georgiou, G., Stamatakis, G., and Golematis, B. Penetration of albendazole sulfoxide into hydatid cysts. *Gut*, **1987,** 28:75–80.

Naquira, C., Jimenez, G., Guerra, J.G., Bernal, R., Nalin, D.R., Neu, D., and Aziz, M. Ivermectin for human strongyloidiasis and other intestinal helminths. *Am. J. Trop. Med. Hyg.*, **1989,** 40:304–309.

Newland, H.S., White, A.T., Greene, B.M., D'Anna, S.A., Keyvan-Larijani, E., Aziz, M.A., Williams, P.N., and Taylor, H.R. Effect of single-dose ivermectin therapy on human *Onchocerca volvulus* infection with onchocercal ocular involvement. *Br. J. Ophthalmol.*, **1988,** 72:561–569.

Plaisier, A.P., Stolk, W.A., van Oortmarssen, G.J., and Habbema, J.D. Effectiveness of annual ivermectin treatment for *Wuchereria bancrofti* infection. *Parasitol. Today*, **2000,** 16:298–302.

Redondo, P.A., Alvarez, A.I., Garcia, J.L., Larrode, O.M., Merino, G., and Prieto, J.G. Presystemic metabolism of albendazole: experimental evidence of an efflux process of albendazole sulfoxide to intestinal lumen. *Drug Metab. Dispos.*, **1999,** 27:736–740.

Rivas-Alcala, A.R., Greene, B.M., Taylor, H.R., Dominguez-Vazquez, A., Ruvalcaba-Macias, A.M., Lugo-Pfeiffer, C., Mackenzie, C.D., and Beltran, F. Chemotherapy of onchocerciasis: a controlled comparison of mebendazole, levamisole, and diethylcarbamazine. *Lancet*, **1981,** 2:485–490.

Robertson, S.J., Pennington, A.J., Evans, A.M., and Martin, R.J. The action of pyrantel as an agonist and an open-channel blocker at acetylcholine receptors in isolated *Ascaris suum* muscle vesicles. *Eur. J. Pharmacol.*, **1994,** 271:273–282.

Sacko, M., De Clercq, D., Behnke, J.M., Gilbert, F.S., Dorny, P., and Vercruysse, J. Comparison of the efficacy of mebendazole, albendazole and pyrantel in treatment of hookworm infections in the southern region of Mali, West Africa. *Trans. R. Soc. Trop. Med. Hyg.*, **1999,** 93:195–203.

Schaeffer, J.M., and Haines, H.W. Avermectin binding in *Caenorhabditis elegans*. A two-state model for the avermectin binding site. *Biochem. Pharmacol.*, **1989,** 38:2329–2338.

Schantz, P.M. Editorial response: Treatment of cystic echinococcosis—improving but still limited. *Clin. Infect. Dis.*, **1999,** 29:310–311.

Schinkel, A.H., Smit, J.J., van Tellingen, O., Beijnen, J.H., Wagenaar, E., van Deemter, L., Mol, C.A., van der Valk, M.A., Robanus-Maandag, E.C., te Riele, H.P., Berus, A.J.M., and Borst, P. Disruption of the mouse *mdr1a* P-glycoprotein gene leads to a deficiency in the blood-brain barrier and to increased sensitivity to drugs. *Cell*, **1994,** 77:491–502.

Scott, R.H., and Duce, I.R. Effects of 22,23-dihydroavermectin on locust (*Schistocerca gregaria*) muscles may involve several sites of action. *Pest. Science*, **1985,** 16:599–604.

Shoop, W.L., Ostlind, D.A., Roher, S.P., Mickle, G., Haines, H.W., Michael, B.F., Mrozik, H., and Fisher, M.H. Avermectins and milbemycins against *Fasciola hepatica: in vivo* drug efficacy and *in vitro* receptor binding. *Int. J. Parasitol.*, **1995,** 25:923–927.

Sotelo, J., and Jung, H. Pharmacokinetic optimisation of the treatment of neurocysticercosis. *Clin. Pharmacokinet.*, **1998,** 34:503–515.

Spiro, R.C., Parsons, W.G., Perry, S.K., Caulfield, J.P., Hein, A., Reisfeld, R.A., Harper, J.R., Austen, K.F., and Stevens, R.L. Inhibition of post-translational modification and surface expression of a melanoma-associated chondroitin sulfate proteoglycan by diethylcarbamazine or ammonium chloride. *J. Biol. Chem.*, **1986,** 261:5121–5129.

Upcroft, J., Mitchell, R., Chen, N., and Upcroft, P. Albendazole resistance in *Giardia* is correlated with cytoskeletal changes but not with a mutation at amino acid 200 in β-tubulin. *Microb. Drug Resist.*, **1996**, *2*:303–308.

van Lieshout, L., Stelma, F.F., Guisse, F., Falcao Ferreira, S.T., Polman, K., van Dam, G.J., Diakhate, M., Sow, S., Deelder, A., and Gryseels, B. The contribution of host-related factors to low cure rates of praziquantel for the treatment of *Schistosoma mansoni* in Senegal. *Am. J. Trop. Med. Hyg.*, **1999**, *61*:760–765.

Witassek, F., Burkhardt, B., Eckert, J., and Bircher, J. Chemotherapy of alveolar echinococcosis: comparison of plasma mebendazole concentrations in animals and man. *Eur. J. Clin. Pharmacol.*, **1981**, *20*:427–433.

Xiao, S.H., Catto, B.A., and Webster, L.T., Jr. Effects of praziquantel on different developmental stages of *Schistosoma mansoni in vitro* and *in vivo*. *J. Infect. Dis.*, **1985**, *151*:1130–1137.

Xu, M., Molento, M., Blackhall, W., Ribeiro, P., Beech, R., and Prichard, R. Ivermectin resistance in nematodes may be caused by alteration of P-glycoprotein homolog. *Mol. Biochem. Parasitol.*, **1998**, *91*:327–335.

Zeng, Z., Andrew, N.W., Arison, B.H., Luffer-Atlas, D., and Wang, R.W. Identification of cytochrome P4503A4 as the major enzyme responsible for the metabolism of ivermectin by human liver microsomes. *Xenobiotica*, **1998**, *28*:313–321.

Zufall, F., Franke, C., and Hatt, H. The insecticide avermectin B$_{1a}$ activates a chloride channel in crayfish muscle membrane. *J. Exp. Biol.*, **1989**, *142*:191–205.

MONOGRAPHS AND REVIEWS

Albonico, M., Crompton, D.W., and Savioli, L. Control strategies for human intestinal nematode infections. *Adv. Parasitol.*, **1999**, *42*:277–341.

Andrews, P. Praziquantel: mechanisms of anti-schistosomal activity. *Pharmacol. Ther.*, **1985**, *29*:129–156.

Bennett, A., and Guyatt, H. Reducing intestinal nematode infection: efficacy of albendazole and mebendazole. *Parasitol. Today*, **2000**, *16*:71–74.

Brown, K.R. Changes in the use profile of Mectizan: 1987–1997. *Ann. Trop. Med. Parasitol.*, **1998**, *92*(*suppl 1*):S61–S64.

Campbell, W.C., ed., *Ivermectin and Abamectin*. Springer-Verlag, New York, **1989**.

Campbell, W.C. Ivermectin, an antiparasitic agent. *Med. Res. Rev.*, **1993**, *13*:61–79.

Campbell, W.C., and Benz, G.W. Ivermectin: a review of efficacy and safety. *J. Vet. Pharmacol. Ther.*, **1984**, *7*:1–16.

Cross, J.H. Intestinal capillariasis. *Clin. Microbiol. Rev.*, **1992**, *5*:120–129.

Cully, D.F., Wilkinson, H., Vassilatis, D.K., Etter, A., and Arena, J.P. Molecular biology and electrophysiology of glutamate-gated chloride channels of invertebrates. *Parasitology*, **1996**, *113*(*suppl*):S191–S200.

de Silva, N., Guyatt, H., and Bundy, D. Anthelminitics. A comparative review of their clinical pharmacology. *Drugs*, **1997**, *53*:769–788.

Dull, H.B., and Meredith, S.E. The Mectizan Donation Programme—a 10-year report. *Ann. Trop. Med. Parasitol.*, **1998**, *92*(*suppl 1*):S69–S71.

Evans, C., Garcia, H.H., Gilman, R.H., and Friedland, J.S. Controversies in the management of cysticercosis. *Emerg. Infect. Dis.*, **1997**, *3*:403–405.

Fallon, P.G., Tao, L.-F., Ismail, M.M., and Bennett, J.L. Schistosome resistance to praziquantel: fact or artifact? *Parasitol. Today*, **1996**, *12*:316–320.

Fisher, M.H., and Mrozik, H. The chemistry and pharmacology of avermectins. *Annu. Rev. Pharmacol. Toxicol.*, **1992**, *32*:537–553.

Garcia, H.H., and Del Brutto, O.H. *Taenia solium* cysticercosis. *Infect. Dis. Clin. North Am.*, **2000**, *14*:97–119.

Gottschall, D.W., Theodorides, V.J., and Wang, R. The metabolism of benzimidazole anthelmintics. *Parasitol. Today*, **1990**, *6*:115–124.

Hawking, F. Diethylcarbamazine and new compounds for the treatment of filariasis. *Adv. Pharmacol. Chemother.*, **1979**, *16*:129–194.

Horton, R.J. Albendazole in treatment of human cystic echinococcosis: 12 years of experience. *Acta Trop.*, **1997**, *64*:79–93.

Lacey, E. The mode of action of benzimidazoles. *Parasitol. Today*, **1990**, *6*:112–115.

Liu, L.X., and Weller, P.F. Strongyloidiasis and other intestinal nematode infections. *Infect. Dis. Clin. North. Am.*, **1993**, *7*:655–682.

Liu, L.X., and Weller, P.F. Intestinal Nematodes. In, *Harrison's Principles of Internal Medicine*, 14th ed. (Braunwald, E., Fauci, A., Kasper, D., Jameson, J.L., and Longo, D.L., eds.) McGraw-Hill, New York, **1998**, pp.1208–1212.

Mackenzie, C.D., and Kron, M.A. Diethylcarbamazine: a review of its action in onchocerciasis, lymphatic filariasis and inflammation. *Trop. Dis. Bull.*, **1985**, *82*:R1–R37.

Maizels, R.M., and Denham, D.A. Diethylcarbamazine (DEC): immunopharmacological interactions of an anti-filarial drug. *Parasitology*, **1992**, *105*(*suppl*):S49–S60.

Martin, R.J., Robertson, A.P., and Bjorn, H. Target sites of anthelmintics. *Parasitology*, **1997**, *114*(*suppl*):S111–S124.

Ottesen, E.A., and Ramachandran, C.P. Lymphatic filariasis infection and disease: control strategies. *Parasitol. Today*, **1995**, *11*:129–131.

Ottesen, E.A., Ismail, M.M., and Horton, J. The role of albendazole in programmes to eliminate lymphatic filariasis. *Parasitol. Today*, **1999**, *15*:382–386.

Prichard, R. Anthelmintic resistance. *Vet. Parasitol.*, **1994**, *54*:259–268.

Redman, C.A., Robertson, A., Fallon, P.G., Modha, J., Kusel, J.R., Doenhoff, M.J., and Martin, R.J. Praziquantel: an urgent and exciting challenge. *Parasitol. Today*, **1996**, *12*:14–20.

Roos, M.H. The role of drugs in the control of parasitic nematode infections: must we do without? *Parasitology*, **1997**, *114*(*suppl*):S137–S144.

Sangster, N.C. Pharmacology of anthelmintic resistance. *Parasitology*, **1996**, *113*(*suppl*):S201–S216.

Sangster, N.C., and Gill, J. Pharmacology of anthelmintic resistance. *Parasitol. Today*, **1999**, *15*:141–146.

Standen, O.D. Chemotherapy of helminthic infections. In, *Experimental Chemotherapy*. Vol. I. (Schnitzer, R.J., and Hawking, F., eds.) Academic Press, New York, **1963**, pp. 701–892.

Symposium. (Various authors.) Biltricide symposium on African schistosomiasis. Nairobi, 24–26 February, 1980. (Classen, H.G., and Schramm, V., eds.) *Arzneimittelforschung*, **1981a**, *31*:535–618.

Townsend, L.B., and Wise, D.S. The synthesis and chemistry of certain anthelmintic benzimidazoles. *Parasitol. Today*, **1990**, *6*:107–112.

Venkatesan, P. Albendazole. *J. Antimicrob. Chemother.*, **1998**, *41*:145–147.

Williams, B.R. Metrifonate: a new agent for the treatment of Alzheimer's disease. *Am. J. Health Syst. Pharm.*, **1999**, *56*:427–432.

CHEMOTHERAPY OF MICROBIAL DISEASES

CHAPTER 43

ANTIMICROBIAL AGENTS

General Considerations

Henry F. Chambers

Antimicrobial agents, the general classes of these drugs, and their mechanisms of action and mechanisms of bacterial resistance are reviewed in this chapter. The principles that are important for the selection of the appropriate antibiotic, the use of antibiotic combinations, and the role of chemoprophylaxis are discussed. This chapter presents both a philosophical and a practical approach to the appropriate use of antimicrobial agents as well as a discussion of the factors that influence the outcome of such treatment. Also emphasized is the frequent misuse of antimicrobial agents due to lack of identification of the responsible microorganism, leading in some cases to superinfection.

History. Pasteur and Joubert were among the first to recognize the potential of microbial products as therapeutic agents. In 1877, they published their observations that common microorganisms could inhibit growth of anthrax bacilli in urine. The modern era of antimicrobial chemotherapy dates to 1936, with the introduction of sulfanilamide into clinical practice. Penicillin became available in quantities sufficient for clinical use in 1941. Streptomycin, chloramphenicol, and chlortetracycline were identified toward the end of or soon after World War II. Since then, numerous classes of antimicrobial agents have been discovered, and literally hundreds of drugs are available for use today. Antimicrobials are among the most commonly used of all drugs. For example, 30% or more of all hospitalized patients are treated with one or more courses of antimicrobial therapy. Death from an incurable bacterial infection came to be considered a thing of the past. However, antimicrobial agents also are among the drugs most commonly *misused* by physicians. Although antibacterial agents are universally recognized as having no antiviral activity, 50% or more of patients diagnosed with a viral respiratory tract infection are prescribed a course of antibacterial therapy. The inevitable consequence of the widespread use of antimicrobial agents has been the emergence of antibiotic-resistant pathogens, fueling an ever-increasing need for new drugs and contributing to the rising costs of medical care. Moreover, the pace of antimicrobial drug development has dramatically slowed during the last decade, with only a handful of new agents, few of which are really novel, being introduced into clinical practice each year. If the gains in the treatment of infectious diseases are to be preserved, physicians must be wiser and more selective in the use of antimicrobial agents.

Definition and Characteristics. In the strictest sense, antibiotics are substances produced by various species of microorganisms (bacteria, fungi, actinomycetes) that suppress the growth of other microorganisms. Common usage often extends the term *antibiotics* to include synthetic antimicrobial agents, such as sulfonamides and quinolones. Hundreds of antibiotics have been identified and developed to the stage where they are of value in the therapy of infectious diseases. Antibiotics differ markedly in physical, chemical, and pharmacological properties, in antibacterial spectra, and in mechanisms of action. Knowledge of molecular mechanisms of bacterial, fungal, and viral replication has greatly facilitated rational development of compounds that can interfere with the life cycles of microorganisms.

Classification and Mechanism of Action. Several schemes have been proposed to classify and group antimicrobial agents, and all are hampered by exceptions and overlaps. Historically, the most common classification has been based on chemical structure and proposed mechanism of action, as follows: (1) agents that inhibit synthesis of bacterial cell walls; these include the penicillins and cephalosporins, which are structurally similar, and dissimilar agents such as *cycloserine, vancomycin, bacitracin,* and the *azole* antifungal agents (*e.g., clotrimazole, fluconazole,* and *itraconazole*); (2) agents that act directly on the cell membrane of the microorganism, affecting permeability and leading to leakage of intracellular compounds; these include the detergents such as *polymyxin* and the polyene antifungal agents *nystatin* and *amphotericin B,* which bind to cell-wall sterols; (3) agents that affect the function of 30S or 50S ribosomal subunits to cause a reversible inhibition of protein synthesis; these bacteriostatic drugs include *chloramphenicol;* the *tetracyclines; erythromycin; clindamycin;* and *pristinamycins;*

(4) agents that bind to the 30S ribosomal subunit and alter protein synthesis, which eventually leads to cell death; these include the *aminoglycosides;* (5) agents that affect bacterial nucleic acid metabolism, such as the rifamycins (*e.g., rifampin*), which inhibit RNA polymerase, and the *quinolones,* which inhibit topoisomerases; (6) the antimetabolites, including *trimethoprim* and the *sulfonamides,* which block essential enzymes of folate metabolism; and (7) antiviral agents, which are of several classes including: (a) nucleic acid analogs, such as *acyclovir* or *ganciclovir,* that selectively inhibit viral DNA polymerase, and *zidovudine* or *lamivudine,* which inhibit reverse transcriptase; (b) nonnucleoside reverse transcriptase inhibitors, such as *nevirapine* or *efavirenz;* and (c) inhibitors of other essential viral enzymes, *e.g.,* inhibitors of HIV protease or influenza neuraminidase. Additional categories likely will emerge as more complex mechanisms are elucidated. The precise mechanism of action of some antimicrobial agents is unknown.

Factors That Determine the Susceptibility and Resistance of Microorganisms to Antimicrobial Agents.

Successful antimicrobial therapy of an infection depends on several factors. In simplest terms, the concentration of antibiotic at the site of infection must be sufficient to inhibit growth of the offending microorganism. If host defenses are intact and active, a minimum inhibitory effect, such as that provided by *bacteriostatic* agents (*i.e.,* agents that interfere with growth or replication of the microorganism, but do not kill it), may be sufficient. On the other hand, if host defenses are impaired, antibiotic-mediated killing (*i.e.,* a *bactericidal* effect) may be required to eradicate the infection. Concentration of drug at the site of infection must not only inhibit the organism, but also must remain below the level that is toxic to human cells. If this can be achieved, the microorganism is considered to be susceptible to the antibiotic. If an inhibitory or bactericidal concentration cannot be achieved safely, then the microorganism is considered resistant to that drug.

The achievable concentration for an antibiotic in serum typically guides selection of the breakpoint for designating a microorganism as either susceptible or resistant by *in vitro* susceptibility testing. However, the concentration at the site of infection may be considerably lower than achievable serum concentrations (*e.g.,* vitreous fluid of the eye or cerebrospinal fluid). Local factors (*e.g.,* low pH, high protein concentration) also may impair drug activity. Thus, the drug may be only marginally effective or ineffective in such cases even though standardized *in vitro* tests would likely report the microorganism as "sensitive."

Conversely, concentrations of drug in urine may be much higher than those in plasma. Microorganisms reported as "resistant" may thus respond to therapy when infection is limited to the urinary tract.

Bacterial Resistance to Antimicrobial Agents. For an antibiotic to be effective, it must reach its target, bind to it, and interfere with its function. Bacterial resistance to an antimicrobial agent falls into three general categories: (1) the drug does not reach its target; (2) the drug is not active; or (3) the target is altered (Davies, 1994; Nikaido, 1994; Spratt, 1994).

The outer membrane of gram-negative bacteria is a permeability barrier that excludes large polar molecules from entering the cell. Small polar molecules, including many antibiotics, enter the cell through channels made up of proteins called *porins.* Absence of, mutation in, or loss of the appropriate porin channel can slow the rate of drug entry into the cell or prevent entry altogether, reducing the effective drug concentration at the target site. If the target is intracellular and the drug requires active transport across the cell membrane, a mutation or environmental condition that shuts down this transport mechanism can confer resistance. For example, gentamicin is actively transported across the cell membrane. Energy for this process is provided by the electrochemical gradient across the cell membrane. This gradient is generated by the respiratory enzymes that couple electron transport and oxidative phosphorylation. A mutation in an enzyme in this pathway or anaerobic conditions (oxygen is the terminal electron acceptor of this pathway, and its absence reduces the potential energy across the membrane) reduces the amount of gentamicin that enters the cell, resulting in resistance. Bacteria also have efflux pumps that may transport drugs out of the cell. Resistance to tetracycline and to β-lactam antibiotics is an example of an efflux pump mechanism (Li, 1995; Okusu, 1996). Figure 43–1 depicts multiple components that can mediate bacterial resistance to β-lactam antibiotics by regulating their intracellular concentrations.

Inactivation of drug is the second general mechanism of drug resistance. Bacterial resistance to aminoglycosides and to β-lactam antibiotics often is due to production of aminoglycoside-modifying enzymes and β-lactamase, respectively. A variation of this mechanism is failure of the bacterial cell to convert an inactive drug to its active metabolite. This is the basis of the most common type of resistance to isoniazid in *Mycobacterium tuberculosis.*

Alteration of the target may be due to mutation of the natural target (fluoroquinolone resistance), target modification (ribosomal protection type of resistance to

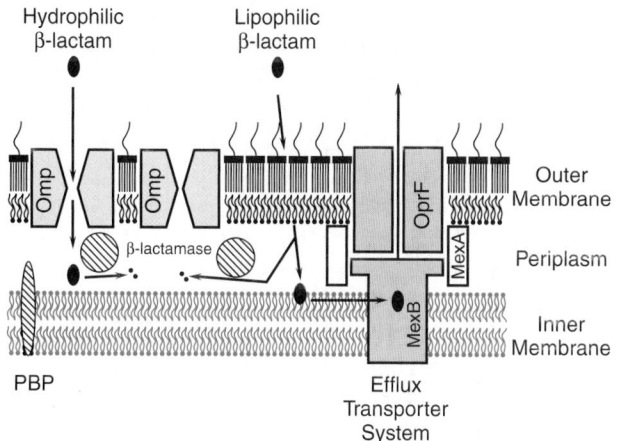

Hydrophilic
β-lactam

Lipophilic
β-lactam

Outer
Membrane

Periplasm

Inner
Membrane

PBP

Efflux
Transporter
System

Figure 43–1. Model depicting the interaction among components mediating resistance to β-lactam antibiotics in **Pseudomonas aeruginosa** *(courtesy of Hiroshi Nikaido).*

Most β-lactam antibiotics are hydrophilic and must cross the outer membrane barrier of the cell *via* outer membrane protein (Omp) channels, or porins. There is size and charge selectivity of the channel such that some Omps slow or block transit of the drug. If an Omp permitting drug entry is altered by mutation, is missing, or is deleted, then drug entry is slowed or prevented. β-Lactamase concentrated between the inner and outer membranes in the periplasmic space constitutes an enzymatic barrier that works in concert with the porin permeability barrier. If the antibiotic is a good substrate for the β-lactamase, it will be destroyed rapidly even if the outer membrane is relatively permeable to the drug. If the rate of drug entry is slow, then a relatively inefficient β-lactamase with a slow turnover rate can hydrolyze just enough drug that an effective concentration cannot be achieved. If the target (PBP, penicillin-binding protein) has low binding affinity for the drug or is altered, then the minimum concentration for inhibition is elevated, further contributing to resistance. Finally, β-lactam antibiotics (and other polar antibiotics) that enter the cell and avoid β-lactamase destruction can be taken up by an efflux transporter system (for example, MexA, MexB, and OprF) and pumped across the outer membrane, further reducing the intracellular concentration of active drug.

macrolides and tetracyclines), or substitution with a resistant alternative to the native, susceptible target (methicillin resistance in staphylococci). This mechanism of resistance is due to reduced binding of drug by the critical target or substitution of a new target that does not bind the drug for the native target.

Resistance may be acquired by mutation and selection, with passage of the trait vertically to daughter cells. For mutation and selection to be successful in generating resistance, the mutation cannot be lethal and should not appreciably alter virulence. Also, for the trait to spread, the original mutant or its progeny have to be transmitted directly; otherwise, the mutation must be "rediscovered" by an unrelated mutant within a susceptible strain.

More commonly, resistance is acquired by horizontal transfer of resistance determinants from a donor cell, often of another bacterial species, by transduction, transformation, or conjugation. Resistance that is acquired by horizontal transfer can become rapidly and widely disseminated either by clonal spread of the resistant strain itself or by further genetic transfers from the resistant strain to other susceptible strains. The staphylococcal β-lactamase gene, which is plasmid-encoded, presumably has been transferred on numerous occasions, because it is widely distributed among a large number of unrelated strains and also has been identified in enterococci (Murray, 1992). Plasmid-encoded class-A β-lactamases of gram-negative bacteria also have spread widely to *Escherichia coli, Neisseria gonorrhoeae,* and *Haemophilus* sp.

Mutations. Mutation and antibiotic selection of the resistant mutant are the molecular basis for resistance to streptomycin (ribosomal mutation), quinolones (gyrase gene mutation), and rifampin (RNA polymerase gene mutation). This mechanism underlies the drug resistance of *M. tuberculosis* to antituberculous agents. Mutations may occur in the gene encoding (1) the target protein, altering its structure so that it no longer binds the drug; (2) a protein involved in drug transport; (3) a protein important for drug activation; or (4) in a regulatory gene or promoter affecting expression of the target, a transport protein, or an inactivating enzyme. Any large population of antibiotic-susceptible bacteria is likely to contain some mutants that are relatively resistant to the drug. Mutations are not the result of exposure to the particular drug; rather, they are random events that confer a survival advantage upon reexposure to the drug. In some instances a single-step mutation results in a high degree of resistance. For example, a point mutation within the drug-binding domain in the beta subunit of bacterial RNA polymerase confers high-level resistance to rifampin. In other cases the emergence of resistant mutants may require several steps, each step conferring only slight alterations in susceptibility. High-level resistance of *E. coli.* to fluoroquinolones is due to accumulation of multiple stepwise mutations.

Transduction. Transduction is acquisition of bacterial DNA from a bacteriophage (a virus that propagates on bacteria) that has incorporated DNA from a previous host bacterium within its outer protein coat. If the DNA includes a gene for drug resistance, a newly infected bacterial cell may become resistant to the agent and capable of passing the trait on to its progeny. Transduction is particularly important in the transfer of antibiotic resistance among strains of *Staphylococcus aureus,* where some phages can carry plasmids (autonomously replicating pieces of extrachromosomal DNA) that code for penicillinase, while others transfer genes encoding resistance to erythromycin, tetracycline, or chloramphenicol.

Transformation. This method of transferring genetic information involves uptake and incorporation of DNA that is free in the environment into the host genome by homologous recombination.

Transformation is the molecular basis of penicillin resistance in pneumococci and *Neisseria* (Spratt, 1994). Penicillin-resistant pneumococci produce altered penicillin-binding proteins (PBPs) that have low-affinity binding of penicillin. Nucleotide sequence analysis of the genes encoding these altered PBPs indicates that they are mosaics in which blocks of foreign DNA from a closely related species of streptococcus have been imported and incorporated into the resident PBP gene.

Conjugation.   The passage of genes from cell to cell by direct contact through a sex pilus or bridge is termed *conjugation.* This is an extremely important mechanism for spread of antibiotic resistance, since DNA that codes for resistance to multiple drugs may be so transferred. The clinical importance of conjugation was first recognized in Japan in 1959, after an outbreak of bacillary dysentery caused by *Shigella flexneri* that was resistant to four different classes of antibiotics (Watanabe, 1966). Resistance could be easily transferred to sensitive strains of both *Shigella* and other Enterobacteriaceae. The transferable genetic material consists of two different sets of plasmid-encoded genes. One codes for the actual resistance; the second encodes genes necessary for bacterial conjugation. The two sets of genes can be present on either the same or two different plasmids. Some genes that encode resistance determinants are located on transposons, which are mobile, transposable elements that can jump from place to place in the bacterial genomic or plasmid DNA (*i.e.,* from plasmid to plasmid, from plasmid to chromosome, or from chromosome to plasmid).

Genetic transfer by conjugation is common among gram-negative bacilli, and resistance is conferred on a susceptible cell as a single event. Enterococci also contain broad host-range conjugative plasmids which are involved in the transfer and spread of resistance genes among gram-positive organisms. Vancomycin resistance in enterococci is mediated by a conjugative plasmid (Arthur and Courvalin, 1993; Murray, 2000). Conjugation with genetic exchange between nonpathogenic and pathogenic microorganisms probably occurs in the intestinal tract of human beings and in animals. The efficiency of transfer is low; however, antibiotics can exert a powerful selective pressure to allow emergence of the resistant strain. The proportion of enteric bacteria that carry plasmids for multiple-drug resistance has thus risen inexorably in the past 30 years. In some studies, more than 50% of persons have been found to carry multiply resistant coliform bacilli. Such bacteria have been isolated in large numbers from rivers containing untreated sewage and from animals. Multiply resistant Enterobacteriaceae have become a problem worldwide, creating an insatiable need for new antibiotics. In several situations where antibiotic usage has been controlled, the rate of emergence of these resistant strains was slowed; in some instances their incidence was actually reduced.

The recent emergence of antibiotic resistance in bacterial pathogens, both nosocomially and in the community setting, is a very serious development that threatens the end of the antibiotic era. Penicillin-resistant strains of pneumococci account for 50% or more of isolates in some European countries, and the proportion of such strains is rising in the United States. The worldwide emergence of *Haemophilus* and gonococci that produce β-lactamase is a major therapeutic problem. Methicillin-resistant strains of *S. aureus* are widely distributed among hospitals and are increasingly isolated from community-acquired infections. Multiple-drug-resistant strains of *S. aureus* with intermediate susceptibility to vancomycin have been reported (Hiramatsu *et al.,* 1997; Sieradski *et al.,* 1999; Smith *et al.,* 1999). There now are strains of enterococci, pseudomonas, and enterobacters that are resistant to all known drugs. Epidemics of multiple-drug-resistant strains of *M. tuberculosis* have been reported in the United States. A more responsible approach to the use of antibiotics, both those that are now available and new agents that might be developed in the future, is essential if the end of the antibiotic era is to be averted.

Selection of an Antimicrobial Agent

Optimal and judicious selection of antimicrobial agents for the therapy of infectious diseases requires clinical judgment and detailed knowledge of pharmacological and microbiological factors. Unfortunately, the decision to use antibiotics frequently is made lightly, without regard to the potential infecting microorganism or to the pharmacological features of the drug. Antibiotics are used in three general ways—as empirical therapy, as definitive therapy, and as prophylactic or preventive therapy. When used as empirical, or initial, therapy, the antibiotic must "cover" all of the likely pathogens, since the infecting organism(s) has not yet been defined. Combination therapy or treatment with a single broad-spectrum agent often is employed. However, once the infecting microorganism is identified, definitive antimicrobial therapy should be instituted—a narrow-spectrum, low-toxicity regimen to complete the course of treatment. When an antimicrobial agent is indicated, the goal is to choose a drug that is selectively active for the most likely infecting microorganism(s) and that has the least potential to cause toxicity or allergic reactions in the individual being treated (*see* Table 43–1).

The first decision to be made is whether or not administration of an antimicrobial agent is even indicated. The reflex action of many physicians is to associate fever with treatable infections and prescribe antimicrobial therapy without further evaluation. This practice is irrational and potentially dangerous. The diagnosis may be masked if appropriate cultures are not obtained prior to therapy. Antibiotics can cause serious toxicity, and injudicious use of antimicrobial agents promotes selection of resistant microorganisms. Of course, definitive identification of a bacterial infection before treatment is initiated often is not possible. In the absence of a clear indication, antibiotics often may be used if disease is severe and if it seems likely that withholding therapy will result in failure to manage a potentially life-threatening infection.

Initiation of optimal empirical antibiotic therapy requires a knowledge of the most likely infecting microorganisms and their susceptibilities to antimicrobial drugs. A number of techniques are helpful in the selection of

Table 43–1

Current Use of Antimicrobial Agents in the Therapy of Infections

Presentation of choices of specific agents for the treatment of various infections inevitably provokes discussion and disagreement because of differences in viewpoints or personal clinical experiences. Also, there may be several equally effective agents from which to choose, at times making the choice of one agent over another seem arbitrary. Patterns of sensitivity of microorganisms can vary widely depending upon the hospital or clinic in which they are isolated. The material presented in this table represents not only the practice of the author, based on experience with the management of these infections, but also that of other experts in the United States (see The choice of antibacterial drugs, 1999). These drug selections represent initial, empirical therapy only. Each choice must be verified by appropriate susceptibility testing. As more information accumulates, as recently introduced drugs are used for longer periods, and as entirely new agents are developed, some of the recommendations will require modifications not only in the order of choices but even in the specific drugs that are suggested.

			DRUG ORDER OF CHOICE		
	DISEASES		FIRST	SECOND[1]	THIRD[1]
I. GRAM-POSITIVE COCCI					
Staphylococcus aureus*	Abscesses Bacteremia Endocarditis Pneumonia Osteomyelitis Cellulitis	Methicillin-sensitive	Nafcillin or oxacillin	A cephalosporin (G1)[2] Vancomycin	Clindamycin[3] A macrolide[3] Trimethoprim-sulfamethoxazol + rifampin[4] FQ(GP)[5] + rifampin[4]
	Other	Methicillin-resistant	Vancomycin[6]	Quinupristin-dalfopristin	Linezolid
		Vancomycin-intermediate[7]	Quinupristin-dalfopristin Linezolid Vancomycin + nafcillin or oxacillin		

*All strains must be examined *in vitro* for sensitivity to various antimicrobial agents.

[1] Drugs included for second and third choices are (a) indicated in patients hypersensitive to equally or more effective agents, (b) potentially more dangerous than equally active drugs, (c) less likely to produce the desired therapeutic response, or (d) in need, in some cases, of further study to allow a valid evaluation of their efficacy.

[2] G1, G2, and G3 designate first-, second-, and third-generation cephalosporins, respectively. If no generation is specified, certain agents may be preferable to others depending upon the organism, susceptibility patterns, and the site of infection (*see* Chapter 46). Therapeutic concentrations of most cephalosporins may not be achieved in the cerebrospinal fluid (CSF) (exceptions include cefotaxime, ceftriaxone, and ceftizoxime), and alternative agents should be used to treat infections of the central nervous system (CNS).

[3] Not indicated in endocarditis, meningitis, or other CNS infections.

[4] Rifampin is highly active against most strains of *S. aureus*, including some that are resistant to methicillin. Since resistance develops rapidly (one-step mutation) during therapy, a second active drug, such as trimethoprim-sulfamethoxazole or ciprofloxacin, should be used concurrently.

[5] FQ(GP) indicates afluoroquinolone with relatively good anti–gram positive activity such as levofloxacin, moxifloxacin, or gatifloxacin.

[6] Vancomycin is the only antimicrobial agent proven to be effective for treatment of serious infections due to methicillin-resistant *S. aureus*.

[7] Agents shown have *in vitro* or *in vivo* activity against these strains; however, there are no clinical data indicating clinical efficacy.

Table 43–1
Current Use of Antimicrobial Agents in the Therapy of Infections (*Continued*)

I. GRAM-POSITIVE COCCI	DISEASES	DRUG ORDER OF CHOICE		
		FIRST	SECOND[1]	THIRD[1]
Streptococcus pyogenes (group A)	Pharyngitis Scarlet fever Otitis media, sinusitis Cellulitis Erysipelas Pneumonia Bacteremia Toxic shock–like syndrome Other systemic infections	Penicillin Amoxicillin	A cephalosporin (G1) [2,8] Vancomycin	A macrolide [3,9] Clindamycin [3]
*Streptococcus** (viridans group)	Endocarditis Bacteremia	Penicillin G [10] ± gentamicin	Ceftriaxone	Vancomycin
Streptococcus agalactiae (group B)	Bacteremia Endocarditis	Ampicillin or penicillin G [11] ± gentamicin	A cephalosporin (G1) [2]	Vancomycin
	Meningitis	Ampicillin or penicillin G [11] ± gentamicin	Ceftriaxone or cefotaxime	—
Streptococcus bovis	Endocarditis Bacteremia	See *viridans* streptococci	—	—
*Streptococcus** (anaerobic species)	Bacteremia Endocarditis Brain and other abscesses Sinusitis	Penicillin G [11]	A cephalosporin (G1) [2] Clindamycin [3]	Vancomycin
*Streptococcus pneumoniae** (pneumococcus)	Pneumonia Arthritis Sinusitis Otitis	Penicillin-sensitive (MIC < 0.1 μg/ml) or intermediately resistant (MIC ≥ 0.1 and < 1.0)	Penicillin Amoxicillin	A cephalosporin (G1) [2]	A macrolide Clindamycin Trimethoprim-sulfamethoxazole [12]
	Penicillin-resistant (MIC ≥ 1.0) [13]	Ceftriaxone or cefotaxime Vancomycin [14] Penicillin [11]	Clindamycin FQ(GP) [5]	Trimethoprim-sulfamethoxazole [12]

		Penicillin	Ceftriaxone or cefotaxime	Vancomycin[15]
Meningitis Endocarditis Other serious infection	Penicillin-sensitive (MIC < 0.1)	Penicillin	Ceftriaxone or cefotaxime	Vancomycin[15]
	Penicillin–intermediately resistant (MIC ≥ 0.1 and < 1.0)	Cefotaxime or ceftriaxone	Vancomycin[15]	—
	Penicillin G-resistant (MIC ≥ 1.0)[16]	Vancomycin + rifampin or ceftriaxone or cefotaxime	Ceftriaxone or cefotaxime + rifampin	—
Enterococcus[17] Endocarditis or other serious infection (bacteremia)	Vancomycin-susceptible	Penicillin G or ampicillin + gentamicin[18]	Vancomycin + gentamicin[18]	Chloramphenicol Doxycycline
	Vancomycin-resistant	Quinupristin-dalfopristin[19] Linezolid	—	Ciprofloxacin or FG(GP)[5]
Urinary tract infections	Vancomycin-susceptible	Amoxicillin or ampicillin or penicillin	Vancomycin	Chloramphenicol Doxycycline
	Vancomycin-resistant	Quinupristin-dalfopristin[19] Linezolid	Ampicillin or amoxicillin FQ(GP)	
II. GRAM-NEGATIVE COCCI				
Moraxella catarrhalis[20] Otitis Sinusitis Pneumonia		Amoxicillin + clavulanate Ampicillin + sulbactam Trimethoprim-sulfamethoxazole	A cephalosporin (G2 or G3)[2]	Ciprofloxacin Tetracycline Erythromycin

[8] Especially for endocarditis or bacteremia.

[9] Strains may be resistant to erythromycin and susceptibility should be documented before using erythromycin to treat serious infections.

[10] Therapy depends on host and bacteria: (a) age >65 years: penicillin G (4 weeks); (b) age <65 years, with normal auditory and renal function: penicillin G(2 weeks) + gentamicin (2 weeks); (c) nutritionally deficient strains of *viridans* streptococci or penicillin MIC ≥ 1 μg/ml: penicillin G (4 weeks) + streptomycin or gentamicin (2 weeks).

[11] Large doses of penicillin (20 million units per day) may be required.

[12] Resistance is increasing among strains of *S. pneumoniae*.

[13] Penicillin-resistant strains frequently are resistant to multiple antibiotics and documentation of susceptibility is essential whenever second- or third-line agents are used.

[14] Some authorities recommend that vancomycin be used for seriously ill or immunocompromised patients.

[15] Rifampin should be added if treating meningitis.

[16] Vancomycin, ceftriaxone, and cefotaxime are likely to be effective as single agents unless the patient has meningitis, in which case a combination regimen is recommended.

[17] Susceptibility testing is recommended because strains of enterococci may be resistant to any or all of the agents used to treat serious infections.

[18] Some gentamicin-resistant strains may be susceptible to streptomycin.

[19] Strains of *E. faecalis* are resistant to quinupristin-dalfopristin.

[20] Almost all strains produce β-lactamase.

Table 43–1
Current Use of Antimicrobial Agents in the Therapy of Infections (Continued)

		DRUG ORDER OF CHOICE		
	DISEASES	FIRST	SECOND[1]	THIRD[1]
II. GRAM-NEGATIVE COCCI				
Neisseria gonorrhoeae[21] (gonococcus)	Uncomplicated urethritis or cervicitis	Ceftriaxone Cefixime Ciprofloxacin or levofloxacin	Cefoxitin Doxycycline	Spectinomycin
Neisseria meningitidis (meningococcus)	Meningitis	Penicillin G	Ceftriaxone or cefotaxime	Chloramphenicol[22]
	Carrier state (posttreatment)	Rifampin	Ciprofloxacin	Ceftriaxone
III. GRAM-POSITIVE BACILLI				
*Bacillus anthracis**	"Malignant pustule" Pneumonia	Penicillin G	Erythromycin Doxycycline	A cephalosporin (G1)[2] Chloramphenicol
Corynebacterium diphtheriae[23]	Pharyngitis Laryngotracheitis Pneumonia Other local lesions	A macrolide	Clindamycin	A cephalosporin (G1)[2] Rifampin
	Carrier state	A macrolide	—	—
Corynebacterium species, aerobic and anaerobic (diphtheroids)	Endocarditis Infected foreign bodies Bacteremia	Penicillin G ± an aminoglycoside Vancomycin	Rifampin + penicillin G Ampicillin-sulbactam	—
Listeria monocytogenes	Meningitis	Ampicillin or penicillin G[9] ± gentamicin	Trimethoprim-sulfamethoxazole	—
	Bacteremia	Ampicillin or penicillin G[9] ± gentamicin	Trimethoprim-sulfamethoxazole	Erythromycin Chloramphenicol
Erysipelothrix rhusiopathiae	Erysipeloid	Penicillin G	Erythromycin Doxycycline	Chloramphenicol

Organism	Infection			
_Clostridium perfringens_* and other species	Gas gangrene[24]	Penicillin G	Cefoxitin, cefotetan, ceftizoxime; Clindamycin[25]	Imipenem; Chloramphenicol; Doxycycline
Clostridium tetani	Tetanus	Penicillin G[26]; Vancomycin	Clindamycin	Doxycycline
Clostridium difficile	Antibiotic-associated colitis	Metronidazole (oral)	Vancomycin (oral)	—
IV. GRAM-NEGATIVE BACILLI				
_Escherichia coli_*	Urinary tract infection[27]	Ciprofloxacin or levofloxacin (G1)[2]; A cephalosporin[2]	A penicillin + a penicillinase inhibitor[28]; An aminoglycoside	Aztreonam; Nitrofurantoin; Trimethoprim-sulfamethoxazole[29]
	Other infections; Bacteremia	Ciprofloxacin or levofloxacin (G1)[2]; A cephalosporin[2]	An aminoglycoside; A penicillin + a penicillinase inhibitor[28]	Trimethoprim-sulfamethoxazole[29]
Enterobacter species	Urinary tract[30] and other infections	Trimethoprim-sulfamethoxazole; Ciprofloxacin; Imipenem	Cefepime; An aminoglycoside	A broad-spectrum penicillin[31]
_Proteus mirabilis_*	Urinary tract[30] and other infections	Ampicillin or amoxicillin	A cephalosporin[2]; Ciprofloxacin	An aminoglycoside

[21] All strains of gonococci should be considered penicillinase-producers until proven otherwise.

[22] Chloramphenicol is indicated only for patients with life-threatening allergy to β-lactams.

[23] Antibiotics alone do not alter the clinical course of diphtheria, but drugs can eradicate the carrier state.

[24] Adequate debridement is absolutely essential.

[25] Clindamycin inhibits toxin production, which may be of additional benefit.

[26] Ten to 20 million units of penicillin G daily, with debridement and tetanus immune globulin.

[27] Trimethoprim-sulfamethoxazole, quinolones, and urinary tract antiseptics are useful for acute urinary tract infections, especially cystitis, in the patient without obstructive uropathy or in whom the disease has not become chronic. These agents also prove useful for chronic suppressive therapy in patients with recurrent urinary tract infection. In some areas, 20 to 40% of _E. coli_ infections acquired in the community are resistant to ampicillin.

[28] Amoxicillin-clavulanate, ampicillin-sulbactam, ticarcillin-clavulanate, or piperacillin-tazobactam.

[29] Resistance is increasing.

[30] Urinary tract infections caused by microorganisms other than _E. coli_ are less usual and frequently occur in the setting of obstructive uropathy or an indwelling catheter, or following recurrent infections and the use of antibiotics. Therapy must be individualized but is frequently unsuccessful unless the underlying condition is corrected.

[31] Ticarcillin, piperacillin, mezlocillin, or azlocillin.

Table 43–1
Current Use of Antimicrobial Agents in the Therapy of Infections (*Continued*)

IV. GRAM-NEGATIVE BACILLI		DRUG ORDER OF CHOICE		
DISEASES	FIRST	SECOND[1]	THIRD[1]	
Proteus, other species*	Urinary tract[30] and other infections	A cephalosporin (G3)[2] Ciprofloxacin	A penicillin + β-lactamase inhibitor[28]	Aztreonam Imipenem
Pseudomonas aeruginosa*	Urinary tract[30] infection	A broad-spectrum penicillin[31] Ceftazidime or cefepime Ciprofloxacin	Tobramycin Aztreonam	Imipenem or meropenem
	Pneumonia[32] Bacteremia[32]	A broad-spectrum penicillin[31] + tobramycin Ceftazidime[33] or cefepime + tobramycin	Ciprofloxacin + a broad-spectrum penicillin[31]	Aztreonam + tobramycin Imipenem + tobramycin
Klebsiella pneumoniae*	Urinary tract[32] infection	A cephalosporin[2]	An aminoglycoside Mezlocillin or piperacillin	Trimethoprim-sulfamethoxazole Ciprofloxacin or ofloxacin
	Pneumonia	A cephalosporin[2]	Ciprofloxacin Aztreonam	A penicillin + a penicillinase inhibitor[28] Imipenem
Salmonella*	Typhoid fever Paratyphoid fever Bacteremia	Ciprofloxacin or levofloxacin Ceftriaxone	Trimethoprim-sulfamethoxazole Ampicillin[34]	Chloramphenicol
	Acute gastroenteritis	No therapy Ciprofloxacin	No therapy or trimethoprim-sulfamethoxazole	No therapy or ampicillin[34]
Shigella*	Acute gastroenteritis	Ciprofloxacin	Trimethoprim-sulfamethoxazole	Ampicillin[34]
Serratia*	Variety of nosocomial and opportunistic infections	Imipenem Cefoxitin	A cephalosporin (G3)[2]	A broad-spectrum penicillin[31] Aztreonam
Acinetobacter*	Various nosocomial infections	Imipenem An aminoglycoside	A cephalosporin (G3)[2]	Trimethoprim-sulfamethoxazole
Haemophilus influenzae*	Otitis media Sinusitis Pneumonia	Trimethoprim-sulfamethoxazole Amoxicillin-clavulanate Cefuroxime axetil	Cefuroxime axetil Amoxicillin or ampicillin[29]	Ciprofloxacin Azithromycin

Organism	Infection			
	Epiglottitis Meningitis	Ceftriaxone or cefotaxime	Trimethoprim-sulfamethoxazole; Ampicillin-sulbactam[35]	Ciprofloxacin
Haemophilus ducreyi	Chancroid	Ceftriaxone; Trimethoprim-sulfamethoxazole; Erythromycin	Ciprofloxacin	A sulfonamide; Doxycycline
Brucella	Brucellosis	Doxycycline + gentamicin[36]; Doxycycline + rifampin; Trimethoprim + rifampin	Trimethoprim-sulfamethoxazole ± gentamicin	Chloramphenicol
Yersinia pestis	Plague	Streptomycin[37] ± a tetracycline	Doxycycline; Ciprofloxacin[38]	Chloramphenicol
Yersinia enterocolitica	Yersiniosis	Trimethoprim-sulfamethoxazole	A cephalosporin (G3)[2]	Ciprofloxacin or ofloxacin
	Sepsis	An aminoglycoside; Chloramphenicol		
Francisella tularensis	Tularemia	Streptomycin	Doxycycline	Chloramphenicol; Ciprofloxacin
Pasteurella multocida	Wound infection (animal bites) Abscesses Bacteremia Meningitis	Amoxicillin-clavulanate; Penicillin G	Doxycycline[3]	Ceftriaxone
Vibrio cholerae	Cholera	Doxycyline; Ciprofloxacin	Trimethoprim-sulfamethoxazole	Chloramphenicol
Flavobacterium meningosepticum	Meningitis	Vancomycin	Trimethoprim-sulfamethoxazole	Rifampin
Pseudomonas mallei	Glanders	Streptomycin + a tetracycline	Streptomycin + chloramphenicol	—
Pseudomonas pseudomallei	Melioidosis	Ceftazidime or ceftriaxone; Trimethoprim-sulfamethoxazole	Imipenem; Chloramphenicol	—

[32] Although single-drug therapy with an antipseudomonal β-lactam antibiotic or an aminoglycoside is adequate for some infections caused by *P. aeruginosa*, the combination of the two classes of drugs is recommended for therapy of serious infections, especially in the neutropenic patient or in the individual with pneumonia.

[33] Cephalosporins that are most active against *P. aeruginosa* include ceftazidime and cefepime, but resistance may develop during therapy.

[34] Many strains are now resistant to ampicillin.

[35] Experience with ampicillin-subactam in the treatment of meningitis is limited.

[36] Gentamicin added to therapy for approximately the first 5 days.

[37] Gentamicin is active *in vitro* and probably *in vivo*.

[38] Activity *in vitro* is good.

Table 43–1
Current Use of Antimicrobial Agents in the Therapy of Infections (*Continued*)

		DRUG ORDER OF CHOICE		
	DISEASES	FIRST	SECOND[1]	THIRD[1]
IV. GRAM-NEGATIVE BACILLI				
*Campylobacter jejuni**	Enteritis	Ciprofloxacin	A macrolide	Clindamycin
*Campylobacter fetus**	Bacteremia Endocarditis	Gentamicin Ampicillin	Ceftriaxone Imipenem	Ciprofloxacin or ofloxacin
	Meningitis	Ampicillin	Ceftriaxone	Chloramphenicol
Fusobacterium nucleatum	Ulcerative pharyngitis Lung abscess, empyema Genital infections Gingivitis	Penicillin G Clindamycin	Metronidazole A cephalosporin (G1)[2]	Erythromycin Doxycycline Chloramphenicol Cefoxitin
Calymmatobacterium granulomatis	Granuloma inguinale	Doxycycline	Trimethoprim-sulfamethoxazole	—
Streptobacillus moniliformis	Bacteremia Arthritis Endocarditis Abscesses	Penicillin G	Streptomycin Doxycycline	Erythromycin Chloramphenicol
Legionella pneumophila	Legionnaires' disease	Azithromycin A fluoroquinolone	Erythromycin or clarithromycin	Trimethoprim-sulfamethoxazole Doxycycline
V. ACID-FAST BACILLI				
Mycobacterium avium–intracellulare	Disseminated disease in AIDS	Clarithromycin + ethambutol	Rifabutin + ethambutol ± ciprofloxacin	Amikacin[39]
Mycobacterium tuberculosis[40]	Pulmonary, miliary, renal, meningeal, and other tuberculous infections	Isonazid + rifampin + pyrazinamide + ethambutol	Isonazid + rifampin	Rifampin + ethambutol + pyrazinamide
Mycobacterium leprae	Leprosy[41]	Dapsone + rifampin	Clofazimine Levofloxacin	Amoxicillin-clavulanate Clarithromycin

1154

VI. SPIROCHETES				
Treponema pallidum	Syphilis	Penicillin G	Doxycycline	—
Treponema pertenue	Yaws	Penicillin G Streptomycin	Doxycycline	—
Borrelia burgdorferi (Lyme disease)	Erythema chronica migrans—skin	Doxycycline	Amoxicillin	Ceftriaxone Azithromycin or clarithromycin
	Stage 2—neurological, cardiac, arthritis	Ceftriaxone	Penicillin G	Tetracycline
Borrelia recurrentis	Relapsing fever	Doxycycline	Erythromycin	Penicillin G
Leptospira	Weil's desease Meningitis	Penicillin G[9]	Doxycycline[42]	—
VII. ACTINOMYCETES				
Actinomyces israelii	Cervicofacial, abdominal, thoracic, and other lesions	Penicillin G[9] Ampicillin	Doxycycline	Erythromycin
Nocardia asteroides*	Pulmonary lesions Brain abscess Lesions of other organs	Trimethoprim-sulfamethoxazole	Minocycline ± a sulfonamide	Imipenem Amikacin Amoxicillin-clavulanate Ceftriaxone
VIII. MISCELLANEOUS AGENTS				
Ureaplasma urealyticum	Nonspecific urethritis	Doxycycline[43]	A macrolide	—
Mycoplasma pneumoniae	"Atypical pneumonia"	Doxycycline	A macrolide	—

[39] Amikacin should not be used as a single agent.

[40] Second- and third-choice drugs are available for the treatment of disease caused by *M. tuberculosis*; their use, which is complex, is discussed in Chapter 48. If multiple drug resistance is suspected, initial therapy should include pyrazinamide + ciprofloxacin (or ofloxacin) + amikacin.

[41] A combination of two drugs should be used for lepromatous leprosy.

[42] Some physicians favor a tetracycline over penicillin G as the drug of first choice.

[43] Some 6 to 10% of *Ureaplasma* organisms are resistant to tetracycline.

Table 43–1
Current Use of Antimicrobial Agents in the Therapy of Infections (*Continued*)

VIII. MISCELLANEOUS AGENTS	DISEASES		DRUG ORDER OF CHOICE		
			FIRST	SECOND[1]	THIRD[1]
Rickettsia	Typhus fever Murine typhus Brill's disease Rocky Mountain spotted fever Q fever Rickettsialpox		Doxycycline	Chloramphenicol	—
Chlamydia psittaci	Psittacosis (ornithosis)		Doxycycline	Chloramphenicol	—
Chlamydia trachomatis	Lymphogranuloma venereum		Doxycycline	Azithromycin Trimethoprim-sulfamethoxazole	—
	Trachoma		Azithromycin	Doxycycline[44]	—
	Inclusion conjunctivitis (blennorrhea)		Azithromycin	Doxycycline	A sulfonamide
	Nonspecific urethritis Cervicitis		Azithromycin	Doxycycline	Amoxicillin Levofloxacin
Chlamydia pneumoniae	Pneumonia		Doxycycline Azithromycin or clarithromycin	A fluoroquinolone	—
Pneumocystis carinii	Pneumonia in impaired host	Mild or moderate disease[45]	Trimethoprim-sulfamethoxazole	Trimethoprim-dapsone Clindamycin-primaquine	Atovaquone
		Moderately severe or severe disease[46]	Trimethoprim-sulfamethoxazole	Pentamidine Clindamycin-primaquine	Trimetrexate
IX. FUNGI					
Candida species	Cutaneous or vaginal thrush		Fluconazole Nystatin[47]	Itraconazole	—
	Oral thrush		Fluconazole Clotrimazole[40] Nystatin[40]	Itraconazole	—
	Deep infection		Amphotericin B	Fluconazole	—

Organism	Condition	Drug of choice		
Coccidioides immitis	Disseminated (nonmeningeal)	Amphotericin B / Fluconazole	Itraconazole	—
	Meningitis	Amphotericin B[48] / Fluconazole	Itraconazole	—
Histoplasma capsulatum	Chronic pulmonary disease	Itraconazole	Amphotericin B	Fluconazole
	Disseminated	Amphotericin B	Itraconazole	—
Blastomyces dermatitidis	All	Itraconazole	Amphotericin B	—
Paracoccidioides brasiliensis	All	Itraconazole	Amphotericin B followed by a sulfonamide	—
Sporothrix schenckii	Cutaneous	Iodide	Itraconazole	—
	Extracutaneous	Amphotericin B	Itraconazole	—
Aspergillus species	Invasive	Liposomal amphotericin B	Itraconazole	Amphotericin B
Agents of mucormycosis	All	Amphotericin B	—	—
Cryptococcus neoformans	Nonmeningeal	None or amphotericin B	—	—
	Meningitis	Amphotericin B ± flucytosine	Fluconazole	—
X. VIRUSES				
Cytomegalovirus	Retinitis in patients with AIDS	Ganciclovir	Foscarnet	Cidofovir
Hepatitis B virus	Chronic hepatitis	Interferon alfa / Lamivudine	—	—
Hepatitis C virus	Chronic hepatitis	Interferon alfa + ribavirin	Interferon alfa	—
Herpes simplex virus	Genital disease	Acyclovir	—	—
	Keratoconjunctivitis	Trifluridine	Acyclovir	Idoxuridine
	Encephalitis	Acyclovir	—	—
	Neonatal HSV	Acyclovir	—	—
	Mucocutaneous HSV in immunocompromised host	Acyclovir	Foscarnet[49]	—

[44] A tetracycline may be given orally alone, or it may be applied locally in the conjunctival sac while a sulfonamide is being administered orally.

[45] Patients with mild or moderate disease (e.g., arterial $P_{O_2} > 60$ mm Hg on room air) can be treated orally.

[46] Patients with moderately severe disease (arterial $P_{O_2} < 60$ mm Hg on room air) should be treated parenterally. Adjunctive glucocorticoids also are recommended for patients with severe disease.

[47] Topical application.

[48] Systemic and intrathecal.

[49] For acyclovir-resistant strains.

Table 43–1
Current Use of Antimicrobial Agents in the Therapy of Infections (*Continued*)

X. VIRUSES	DISEASES	DRUG ORDER OF CHOICE		
		FIRST	SECOND[1]	THIRD[1]
Human immunodeficiency virus	AIDS HIV antibody positive and CD4 count less than 500/mm^3	2 NRTIs[50] + PI[51]	2 NRTIs[50] + NNRTI[52]	NRTI[50] + NNRTI[52] + PI[51]
Human papilloma virus	Genital papilloma	Interferon alfa	—	—
Influenza A	Influenza	Rimantidine	Amantidine	Zanamivir Oseltamivir
Respiratory syncytial virus	Pneumonia and bronchiolitis of infancy	Ribavirin (aerosol)[53]	—	—
Varicella zoster virus	Herpes zoster or varicella in immunocompromised host, pregnancy	Acyclovir	Foscarnet[49,54]	—
	Varicella or herpes zoster in normal host	No therapy Acyclovir Famciclovir Valacyclovir	—	—

[50] NRTI indicates a nucleotide or nucleoside reverse transcriptase inhibitor. Zidovudine and stavudine should not be used together. Didanosine, zalcitibine, and lamivudine should not be used together.

[51] PI indicates human immunodeficiency virus protease inhibitor—*e.g.*, ritonavir, indinavir, nelfinavir.

[52] NNRTI indicates a nonnucleoside reverse transcriptase inhibitor such as delavirdine, nevirapine, and efavirenz.

[53] Use of this agent remains controversial.

[54] Safety in pregnancy not proven.

an antibiotic regimen. The clinical picture may suggest the specific microorganism. Knowledge of the microorganisms most likely to cause specific infections in a given host is essential. In addition, simple and rapid laboratory techniques are available for the examination of infected tissues. The most valuable and time-tested method for immediate identification of bacteria is the examination of the infected secretion or body fluid with Gram's stain. Tests such as this one help to narrow the list of potential pathogens and permit more rational selection of initial antibiotic therapy. However, in most situations, identification of the morphology of the infecting organism is not adequate to arrive at a specific bacteriological diagnosis, and the selection of a single narrow-spectrum antibiotic may be inappropriate, particularly if the infection is life-threatening. Broad antimicrobial coverage is then indicated, pending isolation and identification of the microorganism. *Whenever the clinician is faced with initiating therapy on a presumptive bacteriological diagnosis, cultures of the presumed site of infection and blood, if bacteremia is a possibility, should be taken prior to the institution of drug therapy.* For definitive therapy, the regimen should be changed to a more specific (narrow-spectrum) antimicrobial agent once an organism has been isolated and results of susceptibility tests are known.

Testing for Microbial Sensitivity to Antimicrobial Agents. There may be wide variations in the susceptibility of different strains of the same bacterial species to antibiotics. Information about the pattern of sensitivity of the infecting microorganism is important for appropriate drug selection. Several tests are now available for determination of bacterial sensitivity to antimicrobial agents. The most commonly used are disk-diffusion, agar- or broth-dilution tests, and automated test systems.

The disk-diffusion technique provides only qualitative or semiquantitative information on the susceptibility of a given microorganism to a given antibiotic. The test is performed by applying commercially available filter-paper disks impregnated with a specific amount of the drug onto an agar surface, over which a culture of the microorganism has been streaked. After 18 to 24 hours of incubation, the size of a clear zone of inhibition around the disk is measured. The diameter of the zone depends upon the activity of the drug against the test strain. Standardized values for zone sizes for each bacterial species and each antibiotic permit classification of the clinical isolate as resistant, intermediate, or susceptible.

Dilution tests employ antibiotics in serially diluted concentrations in solid agar or broth media containing a culture of the test microorganism. The lowest concentration of the agent that prevents visible growth after 18 to 24 hours of incubation is known as the minimal inhibitory concentration (MIC), and the lowest concentration that results in a 99.9% decline in bacterial numbers is known as the minimal bactericidal concentration (MBC). The value of the MBC as a clinical test has not been established.

Automated systems also use a broth-dilution method. The optical density of a broth culture of the clinical isolate incubated in the presence of drug is measured by absorbance densitometry. If the density of the culture exceeds a threshold optical density, then growth has occurred at that concentration of drug. The MIC is the concentration at which the optical density remains below the threshold.

Pharmacokinetic Factors. *In vitro* activity, although critical, is only a guide as to whether or not an antibiotic is likely to be effective in an infection. Successful therapy also depends upon achieving a drug concentration that is sufficient to inhibit or kill bacteria at the site of the infection without harming the host. To accomplish this therapeutic goal, several pharmacokinetic and host factors must be evaluated.

The location of the infection may, to a large extent, dictate the choice of drug and the route of administration. The minimal drug concentration achieved at the infected site should be approximately equal to the MIC for the infecting organism, although in most instances it is advisable to achieve multiples of this concentration if possible. However, there is evidence to suggest that even subinhibitory concentrations of antibiotics may enhance phagocytosis (Nosanchuk *et al.*, 1999) and may be effective. Although these and related observations may explain why some infections are cured even when inhibitory concentrations are not achieved, it should be the aim of antimicrobial therapy to produce antibacterial concentrations of drug at the site of infection during the dosing interval. This can be achieved only if the pharmacokinetic and pharmacodynamic principles presented in Chapters 1 and 2 are understood and employed.

Access of antibiotics to sites of infection depends on multiple factors. If the infection is in the cerebrospinal fluid (CSF), the drug must pass the blood-brain barrier, and many antimicrobial agents that are polar at physiological pH do so poorly; some, such as penicillin G, are actively transported out of the CSF by an anion transport mechanism in the choroid plexus. The concentrations of penicillins and cephalosporins in the CSF are usually only 0.5% to 5% of steady-state concentrations determined simultaneously in plasma. However, the integrity of the blood-brain barrier is diminished during active bacterial infection; tight junctions in cerebral capillaries open, leading to a marked increase in the penetration of even polar drugs (Quagliarello and Scheld, 1997). As the infection is eradicated and the inflammatory reaction subsides, penetration reverts toward normal. Since this may occur while viable microorganisms persist in the CSF, drug dosage should not be reduced as the patient improves until the CSF is presumed or proven to be sterile.

Penetration of drugs into infected loci almost always depends on passive diffusion. The rate of penetration is thus proportional to the concentration of free drug in the plasma or extracellular fluid. Drugs that are extensively bound to protein thus may not penetrate to the same extent as those that are bound to a lesser extent. Drugs that are highly protein bound also may have reduced activity, because only the unbound fraction of drug is free to interact with its target.

Traditionally, the dose and dosing frequency of antibiotics have been selected to achieve antibacterial activity at the site of infection for most of the dosing interval. However, controversy exists as to whether the therapeutic effect achieved from relatively constant antibacterial activity is superior to that from high peak concentrations followed by periods of subinhibitory activity. To a certain extent, this depends upon whether a drug exhibits concentration-dependent or time-dependent growth inhibition (Craig, 1998). The activity of β-lactam antibiotics, for example, is primarily time-dependent, whereas that of aminoglycosides is concentration-dependent. Activity also may depend upon the specific organism and the site of infection. Studies in animals with meningitis suggest that pulse dosing (intermittent administration) of β-lactam antibiotics may be more efficient (equivalent efficacy from less drug) (Täuber *et al.*, 1989); it appears that constant activity is superior in other experimental infections. Experimental data suggest that aminoglycosides are at least as efficacious, and are less toxic, when given in a single, large daily dose as when given more frequently (Gilbert, 1991; Barclay *et al.*, 1999). Studies in patients also suggest that continuous administration of aminoglycosides may cause unnecessary toxicity.

Knowledge of the status of the individual patient's mechanisms for elimination of drugs also is essential, especially when excessive plasma or tissue concentrations of the drugs may cause serious toxicity. Most antimicrobial agents and their metabolites are eliminated primarily by the kidneys. Specific nomograms are available to facilitate adjustment of dosage of many such agents in patients with renal insufficiency. These are discussed in the chapters dealing with the individual drugs and in Appendix II. One must be particularly careful when using aminoglycosides, vancomycin, or flucytosine in patients with impaired renal function, since these drugs are eliminated exclusively by renal mechanisms, and their toxicity appears to correlate with their concentration in plasma and tissue. If renal toxicity of a drug that is cleared by the kidney occurs and care

is not exercised, a vicious cycle may ensue. For drugs that are metabolized or excreted by the liver (erythromycin, chloramphenicol, metronidazole, clindamycin), dosages may have to be reduced in patients with hepatic failure.

Route of Administration. The discussion of choice of routes of administration that appears in Chapter 1 of course applies to antimicrobial agents. While oral administration is preferred whenever possible, parenteral administration of antibiotics usually is recommended in seriously ill patients in whom predictable concentrations of drug must be achieved. Specific factors that govern the choice of route of administration for individual agents are discussed in the chapters that follow.

Host Factors. Innate host factors can be the prime determinants not only of the type of drug selected but also of its dosage, route of administration, risk and nature of untoward effects, and therapeutic effectiveness.

Host Defense Mechanisms. A critical determinant of the therapeutic effectiveness of antimicrobial agents is the functional state of host defense mechanisms. Both humoral and cellular immunity are important. Inadequacy of type, quality, and quantity of the immunoglobulins; alteration of the cellular immune system; or a qualitative or quantitative defect in phagocytic cells may result in therapeutic failure despite the use of otherwise appropriate and effective drugs. Frequently, infection in the immunocompetent host can be cured merely by halting multiplication of the microorganisms (a bacteriostatic effect). If host defenses are impaired, bacteriostatic activity may be inadequate and a bactericidal agent may be required for cure. Examples include bacterial endocarditis, where phagocytic cells are absent from the infected site; bacterial meningitis, where phagocytic cells are ineffective because of lack of opsonins; and disseminated bacterial infections in neutropenic patients, where the total mass of phagocytic cells is reduced. Patients with acquired immunodeficiency syndrome (AIDS) have impaired cellular immune responses, and therapy for various opportunistic infections in these patients is often suppressive but not curative. For example, most AIDS patients with bacteremia due to *Salmonella* will respond to conventional therapy, but this infection will relapse even after prolonged treatment (Jacobson *et al.*, 1989), and treatment of disseminated atypical mycobacterial infection is lifelong.

Local Factors. Cure of an infection with antibiotics depends on an understanding of how local factors at the site of infection affect the antimicrobial activity of the drug. Antimicrobial activity may be significantly reduced in pus, which contains phagocytes, cellular debris, and proteins that can bind drugs or create conditions unfavorable to drug action (Bamberger *et al.,* 1993; Konig *et al.,* 1998). Large accumulations of hemoglobin in infected hematomas can bind penicillins and tetracyclines and may thus reduce the effectiveness of the drugs (Craig and Kunin, 1976). The pH in abscess cavities and in other confined infected sites (pleural space, CSF, and urine) is usually low, result-ing·in a marked loss of antimicrobial activity of aminogly-cosides, erythromycin, and clindamycin (Strausbaugh and Sande, 1978). However, some drugs, such as chlortetra-cycline, nitrofurantoin, and methenamine, are more active in such an acidic environment. The anaerobic conditions found in abscess cavities impair activity of the amino-glycosides (Verklin and Mandell, 1977). Penetration of antimicrobial agents into infected areas such as abscess cavities is impaired, because the vascular supply is re-duced. Successful therapy of abscesses usually requires drainage.

The presence of a foreign body in an infected site markedly reduces the likelihood of successful antimicro-bial therapy. Prosthetic material [*e.g.,* prosthetic cardiac valves, prosthetic joints, pacemakers, vascular grafts, and various vascular and central nervous system (CNS) shunts] is perceived by phagocytic cells as foreign. In an attempt to phagocytose and destroy it, degranulation occurs, re-sulting in the depletion of intracellular bactericidal sub-stances. Thus, these phagocytes are relatively inefficient in killing bacterial pathogens. Bacteria also may reside within phagocytes, sequestered from most antimicrobial agents (Zimmerli *et al.,* 1984). There also is evidence that bacteria adhering to prosthetic material resist killing by bactericidal agents (Chuard *et al.,* 1991). Infections asso-ciated with foreign bodies are thus characterized by fre-quent relapses and failure, even with long-term, high-dose antibiotic therapy. Successful therapy usually requires re-moval of the foreign material.

Infectious agents that reside within phagocytic cells (intracellular parasites) are protected from the action of many antimicrobial agents that penetrate into cells poorly. This may be a problem in infections with *Salmonella, Brucella, Toxoplasma, Listeria,* and *M. tuberculosis* and, in some instances, even in infections caused by *S. aureus.* Certain antibiotics—for example, fluoroquinolones, isoni-azid, trimethoprim-sulfamethoxazole, and rifampin—penetrate cells well and can achieve intracellular concen-trations that inhibit or kill pathogens residing within cells.

Age. The age of the patient is an important determinant of pharmacokinetic properties of antimicrobial agents (*see* Chapter 1). Mechanisms of elimination, especially renal excretion and he-patic biotransformation, are poorly developed in the newborn, especially the premature infant. Failure to make adjustments for such differences can have disastrous consequences (*e.g.,* see

discussion of the "gray-baby syndrome," caused by chloram-phenicol, in Chapter 47). Elderly patients may clear renally eliminated drugs less well because of reduced creatinine clear-ance. They also may metabolize drugs less rapidly, predisposing them to elevated and potentially toxic concentrations of drugs when compared to younger patients. Elderly patients often are more likely to suffer toxicity at otherwise safe concentrations of drugs, as is the case for aminoglycoside ototoxicity.

Developmental factors also may determine the type of un-toward response to a drug. Tetracyclines bind avidly to develop-ing teeth and bones, and their use in young children can result in retardation of bone growth and discoloration or hypoplasia of tooth enamel. Fluoroquinolones accumulate in cartilage of developing bone, affecting its growth. Kernicterus may follow the use of sulfonamides in newborn infants, because this class of drugs competes effectively with bilirubin for binding sites on plasma albumin. Achlorhydria in young children and in the elderly or antacid therapy may alter absorption of orally ad-ministered antimicrobial agents (*e.g.,* increased absorption of penicillin G and decreased absorption of ketoconazole).

Genetic Factors. Certain genetic or metabolic abnormalities must be considered when prescribing antibiotics. A number of drugs (*e.g.,* sulfonamides, nitrofurantoin, chloramphenicol, and nalidixic acid) may produce acute hemolysis in patients with glucose-6-phosphate dehydrogenase deficiency. Patients who acetylate isoniazid rapidly may have subtherapeutic concentra-tions of the drug in plasma.

Pregnancy. Pregnancy may impose an increased risk of reac-tion to antimicrobial agents for both mother and fetus. Hearing loss in the child has been associated with administration of streptomycin to the mother during pregnancy. Tetracyclines can affect the bones and teeth of the fetus. Pregnant women receiv-ing tetracycline may develop fatal acute fatty necrosis of the liver, pancreatitis, and associated renal damage. Pregnancy also may affect the pharmacokinetics of various antibiotics.

The lactating female can pass antimicrobial agents to her nursing child. Both nalidixic acid and sulfonamides in breast milk have been associated with hemolysis in children with glucose-6-phosphate dehydrogenase deficiency. In addition, sul-fonamides, even in the small amounts received from breast milk, may predispose the nursing child to kernicterus (Vorherr, 1974).

Drug Allergy. Antibiotics, especially β-lactams, are notorious for provoking allergic reactions. Patients with a history of atopic allergy seem particularly susceptible to the development of these reactions. The sulfonamides, trimethoprim, nitrofurantoin, and erythromycin also have been associated with hypersensitivity reactions, especially rash. A history of anaphylaxis (immediate reaction) or hives and laryngeal edema (accelerated reaction) precludes the use of the drug in all but extreme, life-threatening situations. Skin testing, particularly of the penicillins, may be of value in predicting life-threatening reactions. However, the utility of such tests is controversial. Antimicrobial agents, like other drugs, can cause "drug fever," which can be mistaken for a sign of continued infection.

Disorders of the Nervous System. Patients predisposed to seizures are at risk for localized or major motor seizures while taking high doses of penicillin G. This neurotoxicity of peni-cillin and other β-lactam antibiotics correlates with high con-centrations of drug in the CSF. It usually occurs in patients with renal insufficiency who are receiving large doses of these drugs. Decreased renal function increases concentrations of penicillin in CSF by two mechanisms: reduction of renal elimination of penicillin from plasma, which results in a higher concentration gradient for passive diffusion into CSF; and accumulation of organic acids (in the uremic state), which competitively inhibit the transport mechanism in the choroid plexus that removes penicillin and other organic acids from the CSF. Patients with myasthenia gravis or other neuromuscular problems are susceptible to the neuromuscular blocking effect of the aminoglycosides, polymyxins, and colistin. Patients undergoing general anesthesia who receive a neuromuscular blocking agent also are particularly susceptible to such antibiotic toxicity.

Therapy with Combined Antimicrobial Agents

The simultaneous use of two or more antimicrobial agents has a certain rationale and is recommended in specifically defined situations (Table 43–1). However, selection of an appropriate combination requires an understanding of the potential for interaction between the antimicrobial agents. Interactions may affect either the microorganism or the patient. Antimicrobial agents acting at different targets may enhance or impair overall antimicrobial activity. A combination of drugs may have additive or superadditive toxicities in the patient. For example, vancomycin given alone usually has minimal nephrotoxicity. However, when vancomycin is given with an aminoglycoside, the toxicity of the aminoglycoside is increased (Farber and Moellering, 1983).

Methods of Testing Antimicrobial Activity of Drug Combinations. Two methods are used to measure antimicrobial activity of drug combinations. The first employs serial twofold dilutions of antibiotics in broth inoculated with a standard number of the test microorganism in a checkerboard array, so that a large number of antibiotic concentrations in different proportions can be tested simultaneously (Figure 43–2). The concentrations of each drug, singly and in combination, that prevent visible growth are determined after an 18- to 24-hour incubation. Synergism is defined as inhibition of growth by a combination of drugs at concentrations less than or equal to 25% of the MIC of each drug acting alone. This implies that one drug is affecting the microorganism in such a way that it becomes more sensitive to the inhibitory effect of the other. If one-half of the inhibitory concentration of each drug is required to produce inhibition, the result is called additive [fractional inhibitory concentration (FIC) index = 1; see Figure 43–2], suggesting that the two drugs are working independently of each other. If more than one-half of the MIC of each drug is necessary to produce the inhibitory effect, the drugs are said to be

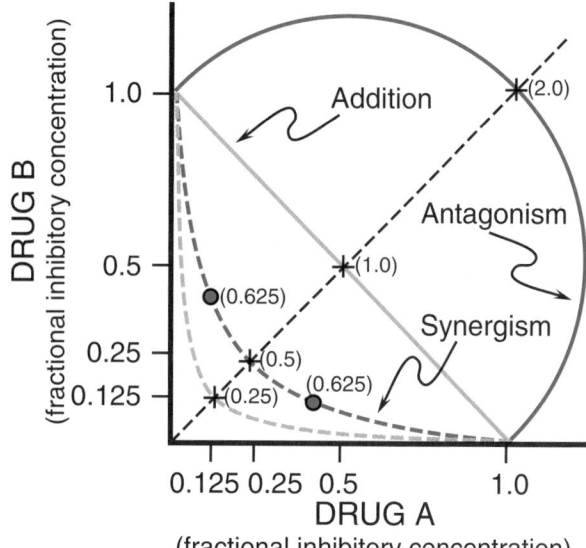

Figure 43–2. Effect of combinations of two antimicrobial agents to inhibit bacterial growth.

The effects are expressed as isobols and fractional inhibitory concentration (FIC) indices. The FIC index is equal to the sum of the values of FIC for the individual drugs:

$$\text{FIC index} = \frac{(\text{MIC of A with B})}{(\text{MIC of A alone})} + \frac{(\text{MIC of B with A})}{(\text{MIC of B alone})}$$

Points on concave isobols (FIC index <1) are indicative of synergistic interaction between the two agents, and points on convex isobols (FIC index >1) represent antagonism. The nature of the interaction is adequately revealed by testing combinations lying along the black dashed line (marked +). *See* text for further explanation.

antagonistic (FIC index >1). When the drugs are tested for a variety of proportionate drug concentrations, as with the checkerboard technique, an isobologram may be constructed (Figure 43–2). Synergism is shown by a concave curve, the additive effect by a straight line, and antagonism by a convex curve. A potential limitation of this method is that its endpoint is growth inhibition, not killing. Consequently, synergism may not indicate enhanced bactericidal effect.

The second method for evaluating drug combinations is the time-kill curve, which assays bactericidal activity. Identical cultures are incubated simultaneously with antibiotics added singly or in combination. Quantitative subcultures are taken over time to determine the number of bacteria remaining. If a combination of antibiotics is more bactericidal than either drug alone, typically defined as at least a 100-fold reduction in the inoculum for the combination compared to the most active single agent, the result is termed *synergism*. If the combination kills fewer bacteria than the most active drug alone, *antagonism* is said to occur. If the combination kills the same number of bacteria or results in less than a 100-fold reduction in the inoculum compared to the most active single drug, the result is called *indifference.*

Jawetz and Gunnison (1952) devised a simple scheme to predict synergism and antagonism from a knowledge of the action of the two drugs involved. They observed that bacteriostatic antibiotics (*e.g.,* tetracyclines, erythromycin, chloramphenicol) frequently antagonized the action of a bactericidal drug (*e.g.,* β-lactam antibiotics, vancomycin, aminoglycosides), because bacteriostatic antibiotics inhibit cell division and protein synthesis, which are required for the bactericidal effect of most bactericidal agents. They further noted that two bactericidal drugs tended to be synergistic. For example, an inhibitor of cell wall synthesis plus an aminoglycoside are synergistic against many bacterial species. Rifampin combinations appear to be an exception to this general rule. Although it is bactericidal, rifampin inhibits protein synthesis, which may account for its indifferent or antagonistic effect *in vitro* when combined with other bactericidal antibiotics. The clinical relevance of this phenomenon is not clear, because rifampin combinations are effective clinically.

Indications for the Clinical Use of Combinations of Antimicrobial Agents.

Use of a combination of antimicrobial agents may be justified (1) for empirical therapy of an infection in which the cause is unknown; (2) for treatment of polymicrobial infections; (3) to enhance antimicrobial activity (*i.e.,* synergism) for a specific infection; or (4) to prevent emergence of resistance.

Empirical Therapy of Severe Infections in Which a Cause Is Unknown. Empirical therapy of infections is probably the most common reason for using a combination of antibiotics. Knowledge of the type(s) of infection, its microbiology, and the spectrum of activity of the several potentially useful antimicrobial agents is essential for selection of a rational and effective regimen. Severe illness and less certainty as to the particular infection or the causative agent may mandate broad coverage initially. More than one agent may be required to ensure that the regimen includes an agent that is active against the potential pathogens (for example, in the treatment of community-acquired pneumonia, a macrolide for atypical organisms such as mycoplasma and cefuroxime for gram-negative pathogens). Prolonged administration of empirical, broad-spectrum coverage or multiple antibiotics, however, should be avoided. It is often unnecessary (*e.g.,* the

infection is caused by a single pathogen or no infection is documented) and unnecessarily expensive. Moreover, toxicity, superinfection, and selection of multiple-drug-resistant microorganisms may result. Inappropriately broad coverage often arises because the physician fails to obtain adequate cultures prior to the initiation of therapy or fails to discontinue the combination chemotherapy after the microorganism has been identified and its antimicrobial susceptibilities are known. Although reluctance to change antimicrobial agents is understandable when a favorable clinical response has occurred, the goal should be to use the most selectively active drug that produces the fewest adverse effects.

Treatment of Polymicrobial Infections. Treatment of intraabdominal, hepatic, and brain abscesses and some genital tract infections may require the use of a drug combination to eradicate these typically mixed aerobic-anaerobic infections. These and other mixed infections may be caused by two or more microorganisms that are sufficiently different in antimicrobial susceptibility such that no single agent can provide the required coverage.

Enhancement of Antibacterial Activity in the Treatment of Specific Infections. Antimicrobial agents administered together may produce a synergistic effect. Synergistic combinations of antimicrobial agents have been shown to be better than single-agent therapy in relatively few infections.

Perhaps the best-documented example of the utility of a synergistic combination of antimicrobial agents is in the treatment of enterococcal endocarditis (Wilson *et al.,* 1995). *In vitro,* penicillin alone is bacteriostatic against strains of *E. faecalis* or *E. faecium,* whereas a combination of penicillin and streptomycin or gentamicin is bactericidal. Treatment of enterococcal endocarditis with penicillin alone frequently results in relapses, whereas combination therapy is curative.

Penicillin and streptomycin or gentamicin also are synergistic *in vitro* against strains of *viridans* streptococci. This combination eradicates bacteria from infected valvular vegetations more rapidly than does penicillin alone in animal models. A two-week course of treatment with the combination is just as effective as a four-week penicillin-only regimen for patients with streptococcal endocarditis. Synergism *in vitro* and in experimental models *in vivo* by a combination of a penicillin and an aminoglycoside also has been demonstrated with *S. aureus.* Selected patients with tricuspid valve endocarditis caused by *S. aureus* can be treated successfully with nafcillin and a low dose of tobramycin or gentamicin administered for a total of 2 weeks, instead of the 4 to 6 weeks of nafcillin alone traditionally used to treat this disease (Chambers *et al.,* 1988).

β-Lactam antibiotic-aminoglycoside combinations have been recommended in the therapy of infections with *Pseudomonas aeruginosa. In vitro,* an antipseudomonal β-lactam plus an aminoglycoside is synergistic against most strains of *P. aeruginosa.* This combination is more active than either drug alone in animal models. Some clinical studies, although by no means all (Hilf *et al.,* 1989; Vidal *et al.,* 1996; Leibovici *et al.,* 1997), suggest survival is improved when a β-lactam plus aminoglycoside combination is used for serious pseudomonal infections. Combination chemotherapy has been advocated for treatment of infections caused by other gram-negative rods. However, the benefits of using a drug combination over a single, effective agent remains largely unproven (Barriere, 1992; Rybak and McGrath, 1996).

The combination of a sulfonamide and an inhibitor of dihydrofolate reductase, such as trimethoprim, is synergistic due to the blocking of sequential steps in microbial folate synthesis. A fixed combination of sulfamethoxazole and trimethoprim, which is active against organisms that may be resistant to sulfonamides alone, is effective for treatment of urinary tract infections, *Pneumocystis carinii* pneumonia, typhoid fever, shigellosis, and certain infections due to ampicillin-resistant *Haemophilus influenzae.*

The combination of flucytosine and amphotericin B is synergistic against *Cryptococcus neoformans in vitro* and in animal models of infection. The combination permits lowering the dose of amphotericin B and a 6-week rather than a 10-week duration of therapy with similar cure rates and less toxicity in non-HIV-infected patients with cryptococcal meningitis (Bennett *et al.,* 1979). This combination also has been shown to sterilize the CSF more rapidly than amphotericin B alone in AIDS patients with cryptococcal meningitis (van der Horst *et al.,* 1997).

Prevention of the Emergence of Resistant Microorganisms.   A combination of antibiotics may prevent selection of mutants that are resistant to a single drug. For example, if the frequency of mutation for the acquisition of resistance to one drug is 10^{-7} and that for a second drug is 10^{-6}, the probability of two simultaneous, independent mutations in a single cell is the product of the two frequencies, 10^{-13}. The number of organisms that would have to be present for such a mutant to occur is several orders of magnitude greater than that likely to be encountered clinically. This is the theoretical basis for combination chemotherapy of tuberculosis, for which a single agent is likely to fail because of emergence of resistant mutants during therapy. The concomitant use of two or more active agents vastly improves cure rates by preventing development of resistance. Other examples include infections that are treated with rifampin, such as staphylococcal osteomyelitis or prosthetic valve endocarditis (Zimmerli *et al.,* 1998), in which a second agent is added to prevent emergence of rifampin-resistant mutants, and combination therapy of *Helicobacter pylori* infection (Taylor *et al.,* 1997). Other than for these specific examples, few data document that drug combinations improve outcome by preventing emergence of resistance.

Disadvantages of Combinations of Antimicrobial Agents.   Antimicrobial combinations also can be disadvantageous due to the risk of toxicity from two or more

agents, the selection of multiple-drug-resistant microorganisms, and the increased cost to the patient. In addition, as noted above, antagonism of antibacterial effect may result when bacteriostatic and bactericidal agents are given concurrently. The clinical significance of antibiotic antagonism is not well defined. Although antagonism of one antibiotic by another has been a frequent observation *in vitro,* well-documented clinical examples of this phenomenon are relatively rare. The most notable of these involves the therapy of pneumococcal meningitis.

In 1951, Lepper and Dowling reported that the fatality rate among patients with pneumococcal meningitis who were treated with penicillin alone was 21%, while patients who received the combination of penicillin and chlortetracycline had a fatality rate of 79%. This conclusion was supported by Mathies and colleagues (1967), who reported that children with bacterial meningitis of multiple causes treated with ampicillin alone had a 4.3% mortality rate compared to a 10.5% mortality rate in children treated with the combination of ampicillin, chloramphenicol, and streptomycin.

Antagonism between antibiotics is probably relatively unimportant in most infections. For antagonism between two antibiotics to occur, both agents must be active against the infecting microorganism. Because the addition of a bacteriostatic drug to a bactericidal drug frequently results in a bacteriostatic effect, in many infections where host defenses are adequate, this is of no consequence. On the other hand, if achieving a bactericidal effect is critical for cure of the infection (*e.g.,* meningitis, endocarditis, and gram-negative infections in neutropenic patients), antagonism of this activity could adversely affect outcome.

The Prophylaxis of Infection with Antimicrobial Agents

A large percentage (from 30% to 50%) of antimicrobial agents administered in the United States is given to prevent infection rather than to treat established disease. This practice accounts for some of the most flagrant misuses of these drugs.

Chemoprophylaxis is highly effective in some clinical settings, and in others is totally without value and may be deleterious. Use of antimicrobial compounds to prevent infections remains controversial in numerous situations. *In general, if a single, effective, nontoxic drug is used to prevent infection by a specific microorganism or to eradicate an early infection, then chemoprophylaxis frequently is successful. On the other hand, if the aim of prophylaxis is to prevent colonization or infection by any or all microorganisms present in the environment of a patient, then prophylaxis often fails.*

Prophylaxis may be used to protect healthy persons from acquisition of or invasion by specific microorganisms to which they are exposed. Successful examples of this practice include the following: use of rifampin to prevent meningococcal meningitis in people who are in close contact with a case; prevention of gonorrhea or syphilis after contact with an infected person; the intermittent use of trimethoprim-sulfamethoxazole to prevent recurrent urinary tract infections usually caused by *E. coli.*

Antimicrobial prophylaxis is used to prevent a variety of infections in patients undergoing organ transplantation or receiving cancer chemotherapy. Although specific infections often can be prevented, superinfections with opportunistic fungal pathogens or multiple-drug-resistant bacteria can be a problem. Moreover, the infection rate may be apparently lowered without changing overall outcomes.

Chemoprophylaxis is recommended for patients with valvular or other structural lesions of the heart predisposing to endocarditis who are undergoing dental, surgical, or other procedures that produce a high incidence of bacteremia (Dajani *et al.,* 1997). Recent data suggesting that dental procedures have a minimal, if indeed any, role in causing endocarditis (Strom *et al.,* 1998) have called some of the recommendations for chemoprophylaxis into question, but the recommendations nevertheless remain the standard of care. A procedure that injures a mucous membrane where there are large numbers of bacteria (such as in the oropharyngeal or gastrointestinal tract) will produce transient bacteremia. Streptococci from the mouth, enterococci from the gastrointestinal or genitourinary tract, and staphylococci from the skin commonly enter the bloodstream and may adhere to an abnormal or damaged valve surface, producing endocarditis. Chemoprophylaxis is directed against these microorganisms. Therapy, generally as a single dose, should not begin until immediately before the procedure, because prolonged administration of antibiotics can lead to colonization by resistant strains. Criteria have been established for the selection of specific drugs and patients who should receive chemoprophylaxis for various procedures.

The most extensive and probably best studied use of chemoprophylaxis is to prevent wound infections after various surgical procedures (*see* Table 43–2; *see* Antimicrobial prophylaxis in surgery, 1997). Wound infection results when a critical number of bacteria are present in the wound at the time of closure. Several factors determine the size of this critical inoculum, including virulence of the bacteria, the presence of devitalized or poorly vascularized tissue, the presence of a foreign body, and the status of the host. Antimicrobial agents directed against the invading microorganisms may reduce the number of viable bacteria below the critical level and thus prevent infection.

Several factors are important for the effective and judicious use of antibiotics for surgical prophylaxis. First, antimicrobial activity must be present at the wound site at the time of its closure. Thus, the drug should be given immediately preoperatively and perhaps intraoperatively for prolonged procedures. Second, the antibiotic must be active against the most likely contaminating microorganisms. Thus, cephalosporins are commonly used in this form of chemoprophylaxis. Third, there is mounting evidence that the continued use of drugs after the surgical procedure is unwarranted and potentially harmful. No data suggest that the incidence of wound infections is lower if antimicrobial treatment is continued after the day of surgery (Rowlands *et al.,* 1982). Use beyond 24 hours not only is unnecessary, but also leads to the development of more resistant flora and superinfections caused by antibiotic-resistant strains. The risk of toxicity and the unnecessary expense are, of course, additional disadvantages.

Chemoprophylaxis should be limited to operative procedures for which there are data supporting its use. A number of studies indicate that it can be justified in dirty and contaminated surgical procedures (*e.g.,* resection of the colon), where the incidence of wound infections is high. These include less than 10% of all surgical procedures. In clean surgical procedures, which account for approximately 75% of the total, the expected incidence of wound infection is less than 5%, and antibiotics should not be used routinely. Exceptions are rational when the surgery involves insertion of a prosthetic implant (*e.g.,* prosthetic valve, vascular graft, prosthetic joint), cardiac surgery, or neurosurgical procedures; the complications of infection are so drastic that most authorities currently agree to chemoprophylaxis with these indications. Of course, the use of systemic antibiotics for chemoprophylaxis during surgical procedures does not reduce the need for sterile and skilled surgical technique.

Superinfections

All individuals who receive therapeutic doses of antibiotics undergo alterations in the normal microbial population of the intestinal, upper respiratory, and genitourinary tracts; some develop superinfection as a result of such changes. *Superinfection* may be defined as the appearance of bacteriological and clinical evidence of a new infection during the chemotherapy of a primary one. This phenomenon is relatively common and potentially very dangerous because the microorganisms responsible for the new infection are, in many cases, Enterobacteriaceae, *Pseudomonas,* and *Candida* or other fungi. These may be

Table 43–2

Guidelines for Prophylactic Antibiotics in Surgical Procedures

Antibiotics should be administered 30 to 60 minutes prior to incision and may need to be readministered to maintain effective serum drug concentrations during prolonged procedures. A single preoperative antibiotic dose is usually sufficient prophylaxis for most surgical procedures. However, continuation of antibiotics for up to 24 hours may be considered in some cases (for example, contaminated cases, surgery of long duration, implantation of prosthetic material).

NATURE OF OPERATION	PROBABLE PATHOGEN(S)	RECOMMENDED DRUG(S) (ADULT DOSAGE)	TIME OF ADMINISTRATION
I. CLEAN			
A. Thoracic, cardiac, vascular, and orthopedic surgery; neurosurgery	S. aureus*, congulase-negative staphylococci, gram-negative bacilli, Pseudomonas	Cefazolin (1.0 g IV) Vancomycin* (1.0 g IV)	At induction of anesthesia
B. Ophthalmic		Gentamicin or neomycin-gramacidin-polymixin B ophthalmic drops; multiple drugs at intervals for first 24 hours	
II. CLEAN–CONTAMINATED			
A. Head and neck surgery (potentially entering esophageal lumen)	S. aureus and oral anaerobes	Cefazolin (1 to 2 g, IV) or clindamycin (600 mg IV) ± gentamicin (1.5 mg/kg IV)	At induction of anesthesia
B. Abdominal surgery— cholecystectomy and high-risk gastroduodenal or biliary		Cefazolin (1.0 g IV)	At induction of anesthesia
C. Abdominal surgery— appendectomy		Cefoxitin or cefotetan (1.0 g IV)	At induction of anesthesia
D. Colorectal surgery Preoperative lavage also recommended in addition to antimicrobial treatment		Go-LYTELY—a polyethylene glycol electrolyte solution (4 liters)	Preoperative day
1. Oral antimicrobial prophylaxis		Erythromycin stearate (1.0 g PO) *or* metronidazole (500 mg PO) **plus** neomycin (1.0 g PO)	At 1 P.M., 2 P.M., and 11 P.M. on the preoperative day
2. Parenteral antimicrobial prophylaxis	Patients who have not received lavage and oral prophylaxis should receive parenteral antibiotics for ≤24 hours which cover aerobic enteric organisms including E. coli, Klebsiella spp., and anaerobic enteric organisms including B. fragilis, Clostridium spp., anaerobic cocci, and Fusobacterium spp.	Cefotetan (1 g every 12 hours for 2 doses) Ceftizoxime (1 g every 12 hours for 2 doses) Cefoxitin (1 g every 4 to 8 hours for 3 doses)	

Table 43–2

Guidelines for Prophylactic Antibiotics in Surgical Procedures *(Continued)*

NATURE OF OPERATION	PROBABLE PATHOGEN(S)	RECOMMENDED DRUG(S) (ADULT DOSAGE)	TIME OF ADMINISTRATION
II. CLEAN–CONTAMINATED *(Continued)*			
E. Gynecological procedures			
1. Vaginal or abdominal hysterectomy and high-risk cesarean section (following labor or ruptured membrane only)		Cefazolin (1.0 g IV)	At induction of anesthesia or postcord clamp
2. High-risk abortion, first trimester		Penicillin G (2 million units IV) *or* doxycycline (300 mg PO)	
3. High-risk abortion, second trimester		Cefazolin (1 g IV)	
F. Urology		Prophylactic antibiotics have not been shown to reduce the incidence of wound infection after urological procedures. Bacteriuria is the most common postoperative complication; only patients with evidence of infected urine should be treated with antibiotics directed against the specific pathogens isolated.	
III. TRAUMA-CONTAMINATED WOUNDS			
A. Extremity	Antimicrobial coverage for Group A streptococci, staphylococci, and *Clostridium* spp.	Cefazolin (1 g every 8 hours IV) Vancomycin (1 g every 12 hours IV)†	
B. Ruptured viscus— abdomen/bowel injury		Cefotetan (1 g every 12 hours) *or* ceftizoxime (1 g every 12 hours) *or* cefoxitin (1 g every 6 hours) *or* clindamycin (600 mg IV every 8 hours) + gentamicin (1.5 mg/kg IV every 8 hours)† for ≤5 days	
C. Bites (cat and human)	Aerobic and anaerobic streptococci from skin and oral flora. Infection of animal bites additionally may be caused by *Pasteurella multocida*, which is penicillin-sensitive.	Amoxicillin-clavulanate 750/125 mg twice a day for 5 days *or* doxycycline 100 mg PO twice a day for 5 days	

*Recommended for hospitals with a high prevalence of infections caused by methicillin-resistant staphylococci or for serious allergy to β-lactams.
†For serious β-lactam allergy.
Abbreviations: IV, intravenous administration; PO, oral administration.

very difficult to eradicate with the currently available antiinfective drugs. Superinfection by these microorganisms is due to removal of the inhibitory influence of the normal flora. Normal flora may themselves produce antibacterial substances, and they also presumably compete for essential nutrients. The more "broad" the effect of an antibiotic on microorganisms, the greater the alteration in the normal microflora and the greater the possibility that a single microorganism will become predominant, invade the host, and produce infection. Thus, the incidence of superinfection is lowest with penicillin G, higher with tetracyclines and chloramphenicol, and highest with combinations of broad-spectrum antimicrobials and the expanded-spectrum third-generation cephalosporins. It can be expected that further development and use of broad-spectrum agents will lead to more extensive alterations in the normal flora and, thus, to more superinfections. The development of agents that kill pathogens selectively while carefully preserving the normal flora would be beneficial. The most specific antimicrobial agent to treat a given infection should be chosen whenever possible. The incidence of superinfection also increases when administration of antibiotics is prolonged.

The fact that harmful effects may follow the therapeutic or prophylactic use of antiinfective agents should not discourage the physician from their administration in any situation in which they are definitely indicated. However, the physician should be hesitant to use antimicrobial drugs in instances where evidence of infection is entirely lacking or, at most, only suggestive. To do otherwise is to run the risk, at times, of converting a simple, benign, and self-limited disease into one that may be serious or even fatal.

Misuses of Antibiotics

The purpose of this introductory chapter has been to lay the groundwork for the maximally effective utilization of antimicrobial drugs. A brief discussion of the misuse and overuse of antimicrobial agents is in order.

Treatment of Untreatable Infections. A common misuse of these agents is in infections that have been proved by experimental and clinical observation to be untreatable: *i.e.,* they do not respond to treatment with antimicrobial agents (Nyquist *et al.,* 1998). The majority of the diseases caused by viruses are self-limited and do not respond to any of the currently available antiinfective compounds. Thus, antimicrobial therapy of measles, mumps, and at least 90% of infections of the upper respiratory tract and many gastrointestinal infections is ineffective and, therefore, useless.

Therapy of Fever of Unknown Origin. Fever of undetermined cause may be of two types: one that is present for only a few days to a week and another that persists for an extended period. Both of these are frequently (and inappropriately) treated with empirical antimicrobial agents. Fever of short duration, in the absence of localizing signs, is probably associated with undefined viral infections. Antimicrobial therapy is unnecessary and defervescence takes place spontaneously within a week or less. Fever persisting for two or more weeks, commonly referred to as "fever of unknown origin," has a variety of causes, of which only about one-quarter are infections (de Kleijn *et al.,* 1997). Some of these infections—for example, tuberculosis or disseminated fungal infections—may require treatment with antimicrobial agents that are not used for common bacterial infections. Others, such as occult abscesses, may require surgical drainage or prolonged courses of pathogen-specific therapy, as in the case of bacterial endocarditis. Inappropriately administered antimicrobial therapy may serve to mask an underlying infection and contribute to delay in diagnosis, and prevent establishing a microbial etiology by rendering cultures negative. The noninfectious causes—including regional enteritis, lymphoma, renal cell carcinoma, hepatitis, collagen-vascular disorders, and drug fever, to name a few—do not respond to antimicrobial agents at all. Rather than embarking on a course of empirical antimicrobial therapy for fever of unknown origin, the physician should search for its cause.

Improper Dosage. Dosing errors, which can be the wrong frequency of administration or the use of either an excessive or a subtherapeutic dose, are common. Although antimicrobial drugs are among the safest and least toxic of drugs used in medical practice, excessive amounts can result in significant toxicities, including seizures (*e.g.,* penicillin), vestibular damage (aminoglycosides), and renal failure (aminoglycosides), especially in patients with impaired drug excretion or metabolism. The use of too low a dose may result in treatment failure and is most likely to select for microbial resistance.

Inappropriate Reliance on Chemotherapy Alone. Infections complicated by abscess formation, the presence of necrotic tissue, or the presence of a foreign body often cannot be cured by antimicrobial therapy alone. Drainage, debridement, and removal of the foreign body are just as important as the choice of antimicrobial agent and in some cases more important. Two of many possible examples follow. The patient with pneumonia and empyema often fails to be cured even with administration of large doses of an effective drug unless the infected pleural fluid is drained. The patient with *S. aureus* bacteremia due to an intravascular device will continue to have fevers and positive blood cultures and be at an increased risk of dying unless the device is removed. As a general rule, when an appreciable quantity of pus, necrotic tissue, or a foreign body is present, the most effective treatment is an antimicrobial agent given in adequate dose plus a properly performed surgical procedure.

Lack of Adequate Bacteriological Information.   One-half of the courses of antimicrobial therapy administered to hospitalized patients appear to be given in the absence of supporting microbiological data. Bacterial cultures and Gram stains of infected material are obtained too infrequently, and the results, when available, are often disregarded in the selection and application of drug therapy. Frequent use of drug combinations or drugs with the broadest spectra is a cover for diagnostic imprecision. The agents are selected more likely by habit than for specific indications, and the dosages employed are routine, rather than individualized on the basis of the clinical situation, microbiological information, and the pharmacological considerations presented in this and subsequent chapters of this section.

For general information regarding infectious diseases, the reader is referred to the following chapters of *Harrison's Principles of Internal Medicine,* 14th ed., McGraw-Hill, New York, 1998: basic considerations in infectious disease (Chapters 120 and 121), issues regarding bacterial infections (Chapters 139 and 140), viral diseases (Chapter 182), fungal diseases (Chapter 202), and parasitic infections (Chapters 212 and 213).

BIBLIOGRAPHY

Arthur, M., and Courvalin, P. Genetics and mechanisms of glycopeptide resistance in enterococci. *Antimicrob. Agents Chemother.,* **1993,** *37*:1563–1571.

Bamberger, D.M., Herndon, B.L., and Suvarna, P.R. The effect of zinc on microbial growth and bacterial killing by cefazolin in a *Staphylococcus aureus* abscess milieu. *J. Infect. Dis.,* **1993,** *168*:893–896.

Barclay, M.L., Kirkpatrick, C.M., and Begg, E.J. Once daily aminoglycoside therapy. Is it less toxic than multiple daily doses and how should it be monitored? *Clin. Pharmacokinet.,* **1999,** *36*:89–98.

Bennett, J.E., Dismukes, W.E., Duma, R.J., Medoff, G., Sande, M.A., Gallis, H., Leonard, J., Fields, B.T., Bradshaw, M., Haywood, H., McGee, Z.A., Cate, T.R., Cobbs, C.G., Warner, J.F., and Alling, D.W. A comparison of amphotericin B alone and combined with flucytosine in the treatment of cryptococcal meningitis. *N. Engl. J. Med.,* **1979,** *301*:126–131.

Chambers, H.F., Miller, R.T., and Newman, M.D. Right-sided *Staphylococcus aureus* endocarditis in intravenous drug abusers: two-week combination therapy. *Ann. Intern. Med.,* **1988,** *109*:619–624.

Chuard, C., Herrmann, M., Vaudaux, P., Waldvogel, F.A., and Lew, D.P. Successful therapy of experimental chronic foreign-body infection due to methicillin-resistant *Staphylococcus aureus* by antimicrobial combinations. *Antimicrob. Agents Chemother.,* **1991,** *35*:2611–2616.

Craig, W.A. Pharmacokinetic/pharmacodynamic parameters: rationale for antibacterial dosing of mice and men. *Clin. Infect. Dis.,* **1998,** *26*:1–10.

Dajani, A.S., Taubert, K.A., Wilson, W., Bolger, A.F., Bayer, A., Ferrieri, P., Gewitz, M.H., Shulman, S.T., Nouri, S., Newburger, J.W., Hutto, C., Pallasch, T.J., Gage, T.W., Levison, M.E., Peter, G., and Zuccaro, G. Jr. Prevention of bacterial endocarditis. Recommendations by the American Heart Association. *JAMA,* **1997,** *277*:1794–1801.

Davies, J. Inactivation of antibiotics and the dissemination of resistance genes. *Science,* **1994,** *264*:375–382.

de Kleijn, E.M., Vandenbroucke, J.P., and van der Meer, J.W. Fever of unknown origin (FUO): I. A prospective multicenter study of 167 patients with epidemiologic entry criteria. The Netherlands FUO Study Group. *Medicine (Baltimore),* **1997,** *76*:392–400.

Farber, B.F., and Moellering, R.C. Jr. Retrospective study of the toxicity of preparations of vancomycin from 1974 to 1981. *Antimicrob. Agents Chemother.,* **1983,** *23*:138–141.

Gilbert, D.N. Once-daily aminoglycoside therapy. *Antimicrob. Agents Chemother.,* **1991,** *35*:399–405.

Hilf, M., Yu, V.L., Sharp, J., Zuravleff, J.J., Korvick, J.A., and Muder, R.R. Antibiotic therapy for *Pseudomonas aeruginosa* bacteremia: outcome correlations in a prospective study of 200 patients. *Am. J. Med.,* **1989,** *87*:540–546.

Hiramatsu, K., Hanaki, H., Ino, T., Yabuta, K., Oguri, T., and Tenover, F.C. Methicillin-resistant *Staphylococcus aureus* clinical strain with reduced vancomycin susceptibility. *J. Antimicrob. Chemother.,* **1997,** *40*:135–136.

Jacobson, M.A., Hahn, S.M., Gerberding, J.L., Lee, B., and Sande, M.A. Ciprofloxacin for *Salmonella* bacteremia in the acquired immunodeficiency syndrome (AIDS). *Ann. Intern. Med.,* **1989,** *110*:1027–1029.

Jawetz, E., and Gunnison, J.B. Studies on antibiotic synergism and antagonism: the scheme of combined antimicrobial activity. *Antibiot. Chemother.,* **1952,** *2*:243–248.

Konig, C., Simmen, H.P., and Blaser, J. Bacterial concentrations in pus and infected peritoneal fluid—implications for bactericidal activity of antibiotics. *J. Antimicrob. Chemother.,* **1998,** *42*:227–232.

Leibovici, L., Paul, M., Poznanski, O., Drucker, M., Samra, Z., Konigsberger, H., and Pitlik, S.D. Monotherapy versus beta-lactam-aminoglycoside combination treatment for gram-negative bacteremia:

a prospective, observational study. *Antimicrob. Agents Chemother.,* **1997,** *41*:1127–1133.

Lepper, M.H., and Dowling, H.F. Treatment of pneumococcic meningitis with penicillin plus Aureomycin: studies including observations on apparent antagonism between penicillin and Aureomycin. *Arch. Intern. Med.,* **1951,** *88*:489–494.

Li, X.Z., Nikaido, H., and Poole, K. Role of mexA-mexB-oprM in antibiotic efflux in *Pseudomonas aeruginosa. Antimicrob. Agents Chemother.,* **1995,** *39*:1948–1953.

Mathies, A.W. Jr., Leedom, J.M., Ivler, D., Wehrle, P.F., and Portnoy, B. Antibiotic antagonism in bacterial meningitis. *Antimicrob. Agents Chemother.,* **1967,** *7*:218–224.

Murray, B.E. Beta-lactamase-producing enterococci. *Antimicrob. Agents Chemother.,* **1992,** *36*:2355–2359.

Nikaido, H. Prevention of drug access to bacterial targets: permeability barriers and active efflux. *Science,* **1994,** *264*:382–388.

Nosanchuk, J.D., Cleare, W., Franzot, S.P., and Casadevall, A. Amphotericin B and fluconazole affect cellular charge, macrophage phagocytosis, and cellular morphology of *Cryptococcus neoformans* at subinhibitory concentrations. *Antimicrob. Agents Chemother.,* **1999,** *43*: 233–239.

Okusu, H., Ma, D., and Nikaido, H. AcrAB efflux pump plays a major role in the antibiotic resistance phenotype of *Escherichia coli* multiple-antibiotic-resistance (Mar) mutants. *J. Bacteriol.,* **1996,** *178*:306–308.

Pasteur, L., and Joubert, J. Charbonne et septicémie. *C. R. Acad. Sci. [D],* **1877,** *85*:101–115.

Quagliarello, V.J., and Scheld, W.M. Treatment of bacterial meningitis. *N. Engl. J. Med.,* **1997,** *336*:708–716.

Rowlands, B.J., Clark, R.G., and Richards, D.G. Single-dose intraoperative antibiotic prophylaxis in emergency abdominal surgery. *Arch. Surg.,* **1982,** *117*:195–199.

Sieradzki, K., Roberts, R.B., Haber, S.W., and Tomasz, A. The development of vancomycin resistance in a patient with methicillin-resistant *Staphylococcus aureus* infection. *N. Engl. J. Med.,* **1999,** *340*:517–523.

Smith, T.L., Pearson, M.L., Wilcox, K.R., Cruz, C., Lancaster, M.V., Robinson-Dunn, B., Tenover, F.C., Zervos, M.J., Band, J.D., White, E., and Jarvis, W.R. Emergence of vancomycin resistance in *Staphylococcus aureus.* Glycopeptide-Intermediate *Staphylococcus aureus* Working Group. *N. Engl. J. Med.,* **1999,** *340*:493–501.

Spratt, B.G. Resistance to antibiotics mediated by target alterations. *Science,* **1994,** *264*:388–393.

Strausbaugh, L.J., and Sande, M.A. Factors influencing the therapy of experimental *Proteus mirabilis* meningitis in rabbits. *J. Infect. Dis.,* **1978,** *137*:251–260.

Strom, B.L., Abrutyn, E., Berlin, J.A., Kinman, J.L., Feldman, R.S., Stolley, P.D., Levison, M.E., Korzeniowski, O.M., and Kaye, D. Dental and cardiac risk factors for infective endocarditis. A population-based, case-control study. *Ann. Intern. Med.,* **1998,** *129*:761–769.

Täuber, M.G., Kunz, S., Zak, O., and Sande, M.A. Influence of antibiotic dose, dosing interval and duration of therapy on outcome in experimental pneumococcal meningitis in rabbits. *Antimicrob. Agents Chemother.,* **1989,** *33*:418–423.

Taylor, J.L., Zagari, M., Murphy, K., and Freston, J.W. Pharmacoeconomic comparison of treatments for the eradication of *Helicobacter pylori. Arch. Intern. Med.,* **1997,** *157*:87–97.

van der Horst, C.M., Saag, M.S., Cloud, G.A., Hamill, R.J., Graybill, J.R., Sobel, J.D., Johnson, P.C., Tuazon, C.U., Kerkering, T., Moskovitz, B.L., Powderly, W.G., and Dismukes, W.E. Treatment of cryptococcal meningitis associated with the acquired immunodeficiency syndrome. National Institute of Allergy and Infectious Diseases Mycoses Study Group and AIDS Clinical Trials Group. *N. Engl. J. Med.,* **1997,** *337*:15–21.

Verklin, R.M. Jr., and Mandell, G.L. Alteration of effectiveness of antibiotics by anaerobiosis. *J. Lab. Clin. Med.,* **1977,** *89*:65–71.

Vidal, F., Mensa, J., Almela, M., Martinez, J.A., Marco, F., Casals, C., Gatell, J.M., Soriano, E., and Jimenez de Anta, M.T. Epidemiology and outcome of *Pseudomonas aeruginosa* bacteremia, with special emphasis on the influence of antibiotic treatment. Analysis of 189 episodes. *Arch. Intern. Med.,* **1996,** *156*:2121–2126.

Vorherr, H. Drug excretion in breast milk. *Postgrad. Med.,* **1974,** *56*: 97–104.

Watanabe, T. Infectious drug resistance in enteric bacteria. *N. Engl. J. Med.,* **1966,** *275*:888–894.

Wilson, W.R., Karchmer, A.W., Dajani, A.S., Taubert, K.A., Bayer, A., Kaye, D., Bisno, A.L., Ferrieri, P., Shulman, S.T., and Durack, D.T. Antimicrobial treatment of adults with infective endocarditis due to streptococci, enterococci, staphylococci, and HACEK microorganisms. American Heart Association. *JAMA,* **1995,** *274*:1706–1713.

Zimmerli, W., Lew, P.D., and Waldvogel, F.A. Pathogenesis of foreign body infection. Evidence for a local granulocyte defect. *J. Clin. Invest.,* **1984,** *73*:1191–1200.

Zimmerli, W., Widmer, A.F., Blatter, M., Frei, R., and Ochsner, P.E. Role of rifampin for treatment of orthopedic implant-related staphylococcal infections: a randomized controlled trial. Foreign-Body Infection (FBI) Study Group. *JAMA,* **1998,** *279*:1537–1541.

MONOGRAPHS AND REVIEWS

Antimicrobial prophylaxis in surgery. *Med. Lett. Drugs Ther.,* **1997,** *39*: 97–101.

Barriere, S.L. Bacterial resistance to beta-lactams, and its prevention with combination antimicrobial therapy. *Pharmacotherapy,* **1992,** *12*:397–402.

The choice of antibacterial drugs. *Med. Lett. Drugs. Ther.,* **1999,** *41*: 95–104.

Craig, W.A., and Kunin, C.M. Significance of serum protein and tissue binding of antimicrobial agents. *Annu. Rev. Med.,* **1976,** *27*:287–300.

Murray, B.E. Vancomycin-resistant enterococcal infections. *N. Engl. J. Med.,* **2000,** *342*:710–721.

Nyquist, A.C., Gonzales, R., Steiner, J.F., and Sande, M.A. Antibiotic prescribing for children with colds, upper respiratory tract infections, and bronchitis. *JAMA,* **1998,** *279*:875–877.

Rybak, M.J., and McGrath, B.J. Combination antimicrobial therapy for bacterial infections. Guidelines for the clinician. *Drugs,* **1996,** *52*:390–405.

ANTIMICROBIAL AGENTS
(*Continued*)

Sulfonamides, Trimethoprim-
Sulfamethoxazole, Quinolones, and Agents
for Urinary Tract Infections

William A. Petri, Jr.

Sulfonamides are used primarily in the treatment of urinary tract infections; in combination with trimethoprim, they also are frequently used for the treatment of otitis, bronchitis, sinusitis, and Pneumocystis carinii *pneumonia. Emergence of resistance has limited their usefulness in other settings.*

The quinolone antibiotics, by virtue of their broad spectrum of antimicrobial activity against aerobic gram-negative bacilli, staphylococci, and gram-negative cocci and their oral bioavailability, are a very important class of antibiotics. Therapeutic uses include treatment of urinary tract infections, prostatitis, several sexually transmitted diseases, osteomyelitis, and bacterial diarrhea. New agents with excellent activity against the organisms of atypical pneumonia, anaerobes, and pneumococci are available for single-agent treatment of pneumonia. Quinolone antibiotics generally are not recommended for use in children or during pregnancy because of their potential to produce arthropathy.

The urinary tract antiseptic methenamine is of value for chronic suppressive treatment of urinary tract infections.

SULFONAMIDES

The sulfonamide drugs were the first effective chemotherapeutic agents to be employed systemically for the prevention and cure of bacterial infections in human beings. The considerable medical and public health importance of their discovery and their subsequent widespread use were quickly reflected in the sharp decline in morbidity and mortality figures for treatable infectious diseases. The advent of penicillin and subsequently of other antibiotics has diminished the usefulness of the sulfonamides, and they presently occupy a relatively small place in the therapeutic armamentarium of the physician. However, the introduction in the mid-1970s of the combination of trimethoprim and sulfamethoxazole has resulted in increased use of sulfonamides for the prophylaxis and/or treatment of specific microbial infections.

History. Investigations at the I. G. Farbenindustrie resulted, in 1932, in a German patent to Klarer and Mietzsch, covering PRONTOSIL and several other azo dyes containing a sulfonamide group. Domagk, a research director of the I. G. working with Klarer and Mietzsch, was aware of the fact that synthetic azo dyes had been studied for their action against streptococci, which prompted him to test the new compounds. He quickly observed that mice with streptococcal and other infections could be protected by PRONTOSIL (Domagk, 1935). The credit for the discovery of the chemotherapeutic value of PRONTOSIL belongs to Domagk, who was awarded the Nobel Prize in Medicine for 1938. In 1933, the first clinical case study was reported by Foerster, who gave PRONTOSIL to a 10-month-old infant with staphylococcal septicemia and obtained a dramatic cure. However, no great attention was paid elsewhere to these epoch-making advances in chemotherapy until the interest of English investigators was aroused. Colebrook and Kenny (1936) as well as Buttle and coworkers (1936) reported their favorable clinical results with PRONTOSIL and its active metabolite, sulfanilamide, in puerperal sepsis and meningococcal infections. These two reports awakened the medical profession to the new field of antibacterial chemotherapy, and experimental and clinical articles soon appeared in great profusion. The development of the carbonic anhydrase inhibitor–type diuretics and the sulfonylurea hypoglycemic agents followed from observations made with the sulfonamide antibiotics.

Chemistry. The term *sulfonamide* is employed herein as a generic name for derivatives of para-aminobenzenesulfonamide

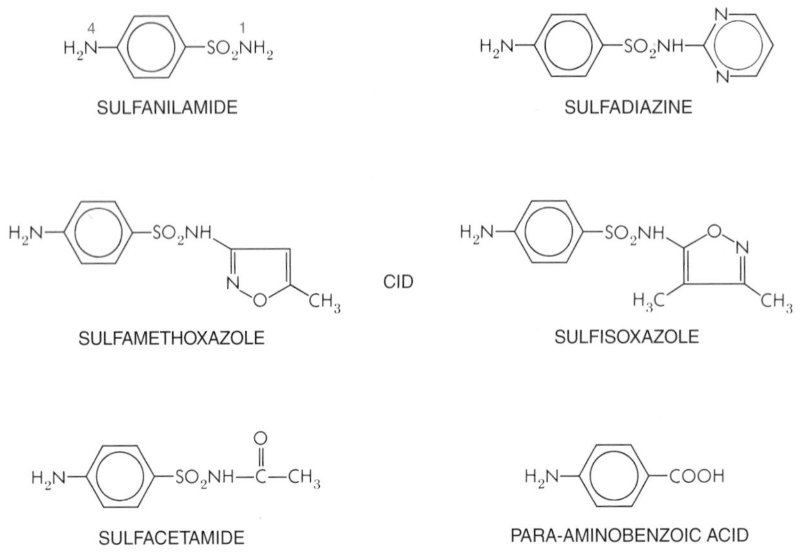

SULFANILAMIDE

SULFADIAZINE

SULFAMETHOXAZOLE   CID

SULFISOXAZOLE

SULFACETAMIDE

PARA-AMINOBENZOIC ACID

Figure 44–1. Structural formulas of selected sulfonamides and para-aminobenzoic acid.

The N of the para-NH$_2$ group is designated as N^4; that of the amide NH$_2$, as N^1.

(sulfanilamide); the structural formulas of selected members of this class are shown in Figure 44–1. Most of them are relatively insoluble in water, but their sodium salts are readily soluble. The minimal structural prerequisites for antibacterial action are all embodied in sulfanilamide itself. The –SO$_2$NH$_2$ group is not essential as such, but the important feature is that the sulfur is directly linked to the benzene ring. The para-NH$_2$ group (the N of which has been designated as N^4) is essential and can be replaced only by such radicals as can be converted *in vivo* to a free amino group. Substitutions made in the amide NH$_2$ group (the N of which has been designated as N^1) have variable effects on antibacterial activity of the molecule. However, substitution of heterocyclic aromatic nuclei at N^1 yields highly potent compounds.

Effects on Microbial Agents

Sulfonamides have a wide range of antimicrobial activity against both gram-positive and gram-negative bacteria. However, resistant strains have become common in recent years, and the usefulness of these agents has diminished correspondingly. In general, the sulfonamides exert only a bacteriostatic effect, and cellular and humoral defense mechanisms of the host are essential for the final eradication of the infection.

Antibacterial Spectrum.   Resistance to sulfonamides is increasingly a problem. Microorganisms that may be susceptible *in vitro* to sulfonamides include *Streptococcus pyogenes, Streptococcus pneumoniae, Haemophilus influenzae, Haemophilus ducreyi, Nocardia, Actinomyces, Calymmatobacterium granulomatis,* and *Chlamydia trachomatis.* Minimal inhibitory concentrations (MIC) range

from 0.1 μg/ml for *C. trachomatis* to 4 to 64 μg/ml for *Escherichia coli*. Peak plasma drug concentrations achievable *in vivo* are approximately 100 to 200 μg/ml.

Although sulfonamides were used successfully for the management of meningococcal infections for many years, the majority of isolates of *Neisseria meningitidis* of serogroups B and C in the United States and group A isolates from other countries are now resistant. A similar situation prevails with respect to *Shigella*. Strains of *E. coli* isolated from patients with urinary tract infections (community-acquired) often are resistant to sulfonamides, so that they are no longer the therapy of choice for such infections.

Mechanism of Action.   Sulfonamides are structural analogs and competitive antagonists of para-aminobenzoic acid (PABA) and thus prevent normal bacterial utilization of PABA for the synthesis of folic acid (pteroylglutamic acid; *see* Fildes, 1940; Woods, 1940). More specifically, sulfonamides are competitive inhibitors of dihydropteroate synthase, the bacterial enzyme responsible for the incorporation of PABA into dihydropteroic acid, the immediate precursor of folic acid (Figure 44–2). Sensitive microorganisms are those that must synthesize their own folic acid; bacteria that can utilize preformed folate are not affected. Bacteriostasis induced by sulfonamides is counteracted by PABA competitively. Sulfonamides do not affect mammalian cells by this mechanism, since they require preformed folic acid and cannot synthesize it. They are, therefore, comparable to sulfonamide-insensitive bacteria that utilize preformed folate.

Synergists of Sulfonamides.   One of the most active agents that exerts a synergistic effect when used with a sulfonamide is trimethoprim (*see* Bushby and Hitchings, 1968). This compound is a potent and selective competitive inhibitor of microbial

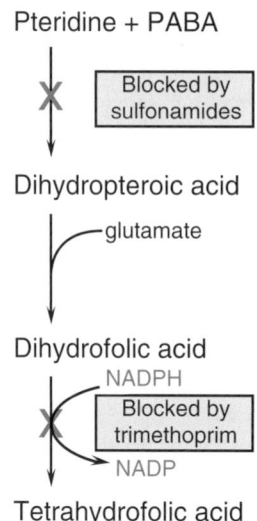

Pteridine + PABA

Dihydropteroic acid

Dihydrofolic acid

Tetrahydrofolic acid

Figure 44–2. Steps in folate metabolism blocked by sulfon-amides and trimethoprim.

dihydrofolate reductase, the enzyme that reduces dihydrofolate to tetrahydrofolate. It is this reduced form of folic acid that is required for one-carbon transfer reactions. The simultaneous administration of a sulfonamide and trimethoprim thus introduces sequential blocks in the pathway by which microorganisms synthesize tetrahydrofolate from precursor molecules. The expectation that such a combination would yield synergistic antimicrobial effects has been realized both *in vitro* and *in vivo* (*see* below).

Acquired Bacterial Resistance to Sulfonamides. Bacteria resistant to sulfonamides are presumed to originate by random mutation and selection or by transfer of resistance by plasmids (Chapter 43). Such resistance, once it is maximally developed, usually is persistent and irreversible, particularly when produced *in vivo*. Acquired resistance to sulfonamide usually does not involve cross-resistance to chemotherapeutic agents of other classes. The *in vivo* acquisition of resistance has little or no effect on either virulence or antigenic characteristics of microorganisms.

Resistance to sulfonamide is probably the consequence of an altered enzymatic constitution of the bacterial cell; the alteration may be characterized by (1) a lower affinity for sulfonamides by the enzyme that utilizes PABA, dihydropteroate synthase; (2) decreased bacterial permeability or active efflux of the drug; (3) an alternative metabolic pathway for synthesis of an essential metabolite; or (4) an increased production of an essential metabolite or drug antagonist. For example, some resistant staphylococci may synthesize 70 times as much PABA as do the susceptible parent strains. Nevertheless, an increased production of PABA is not a constant finding in sulfonamide-resistant bacteria, and resistant mutants may possess enzymes for folate biosynthesis that are less readily inhibited by sulfonamides. Plasmid-mediated resistance is due to plasmid-encoded, drug-resistant dihydropteroate synthetase.

Absorption, Fate, and Excretion

Except for sulfonamides especially designed for their local effects in the bowel, this class of drugs is rapidly absorbed from the gastrointestinal tract. Approximately 70% to 100% of an oral dose is absorbed, and sulfonamide can be found in the urine within 30 minutes of ingestion. Peak plasma levels are achieved in 2 to 6 hours, depending on the drug. The small intestine is the major site of absorption, but some of the drug is absorbed from the stomach. Absorption from other sites, such as the vagina, respiratory tract, or abraded skin, is variable and unreliable, but a sufficient amount may enter the body to cause toxic reactions in susceptible persons or to produce sensitization.

All sulfonamides are bound in varying degree to plasma proteins, particularly to albumin. The extent to which this occurs is determined by the hydrophobicity of a particular drug and its pK_a; at physiological pH, drugs with a high pK_a exhibit a low degree of protein binding, and *vice versa*.

Sulfonamides are distributed throughout all tissues of the body. The diffusible fraction of sulfadiazine is uniformly distributed throughout the total body water, while sulfisoxazole is largely confined to the extracellular space. The sulfonamides readily enter pleural, peritoneal, synovial, ocular, and similar body fluids and may reach concentrations therein that are 50% to 80% of the simultaneously determined concentration in blood. Since the protein content of such fluids usually is low, the drug is present in the unbound active form.

After systemic administration of adequate doses, sulfadiazine and sulfisoxazole attain concentrations in cerebrospinal fluid that may be effective in meningeal infections. At steady state, the concentration ranges between 10% and 80% of that in the blood. However, because of the emergence of sulfonamide-resistant microorganisms, these drugs are now used only rarely for the treatment of meningitis.

Sulfonamides readily pass through the placenta and reach the fetal circulation. The concentrations attained in the fetal tissues are sufficient to cause both antibacterial and toxic effects.

The sulfonamides undergo metabolic alterations *in vivo*, especially in the liver. The major metabolic derivative is the N^4-acetylated sulfonamide. Acetylation, which occurs to a different extent with each agent, is disadvantageous, because the resulting products have no antibacterial activity and yet retain the toxic potentialities of the parent substance.

Sulfonamides are eliminated from the body partly as the unchanged drug and partly as metabolic products. The largest fraction is excreted in the urine, and the half-life of sulfonamides in the body is thus dependent on renal function. In acid urine, the older sulfonamides are insoluble and may precipitate, causing crystalline deposits that can cause urinary obstruction (*see* below). Small amounts are eliminated in the feces and in bile, milk, and other secretions.

Pharmacological Properties of Individual Sulfonamides

The sulfonamides may be classified into three groups on the basis of the rapidity with which they are absorbed and excreted: (1) agents absorbed rapidly and excreted rapidly, such as sulfisoxazole and sulfadiazine; (2) agents absorbed very poorly when administered orally and hence active in the bowel lumen, such as sulfasalazine; (3) sulfonamides employed mainly for topical use, such as sulfacetamide, mafenide, and silver sulfadiazine; and (4) long-acting sulfonamides, such as sulfadoxine, which are absorbed rapidly but excreted slowly (Table 44–1).

Rapidly Absorbed and Rapidly Eliminated Sulfonamides. *Sulfisoxazole.* Early studies of *sulfisoxazole* (GANTRISIN, others) established that it was a rapidly absorbed and rapidly excreted sulfonamide with excellent antibacterial activity. Since its high solubility eliminates much of the renal toxicity inherent in the use of older sulfonamides, it has essentially replaced the less-soluble agents.

Sulfisoxazole is bound extensively to plasma proteins. Following an oral dose of 2 to 4 g, peak concentrations in plasma of 110 to 250 μg/ml are found in 2 to 4 hours. From 28% to 35% of sulfisoxazole in the blood and about 30% in the urine is in the acetylated form. Approximately 95% of a single dose is excreted by the kidney in 24 hours. Concentrations of the drug in urine thus greatly exceed those in blood and may be bactericidal. The cerebrospinal fluid concentration averages about a third of that in the blood.

Sulfisoxazole diolamine is available for topical use in the eye. *Sulfisoxazole acetyl* is tasteless and hence preferred for oral use in children. Sulfisoxazole also is marketed in a fixed-dose combination with phenazopyridine (sulfisoxazole, 500 mg; phenazopyridine, 50 mg) as a urinary tract antiseptic and analgesic. The urine becomes orange-red soon after ingestion of this mixture because of the presence of phenazopyridine, an orange-red dye. Sulfisoxazole acetyl also is marketed in combination with erythromycin ethylsuccinate (PEDIAZOLE, others) for use in children with otitis media.

Fewer than 0.1% of patients receiving sulfisoxazole suffer serious toxic reactions. The untoward effects produced by this agent are similar to those that follow the administration of other sulfonamides, as discussed below. Because of its relatively high solubility in the urine as compared with sulfadiazine, sulfisoxazole only infrequently produces hematuria or crystalluria (0.2% to 0.3%). Despite this, patients taking this drug should ingest an adequate quantity of water. Sulfisoxazole and all sulfonamides that are absorbed must be used with caution in patients with impaired renal function. Like all other sulfonamides, sulfisoxazole may produce hypersensitivity reactions, some of which are potentially lethal. Sulfisoxazole currently is preferred over other sulfonamides by most clinicians when a rapidly absorbed and rapidly excreted sulfonamide is indicated.

Sulfamethoxazole. *Sulfamethoxazole* is a close congener of sulfisoxazole, but its rates of enteric absorption and urinary excretion are slower. It is administered orally and employed for both systemic and urinary tract infections. Precautions must be observed to avoid sulfamethoxazole crystalluria because of the high percentage of the acetylated, relatively insoluble form of the drug in the urine. The clinical uses of sulfamethoxazole are the same as those for sulfisoxazole. It also is marketed in fixed-dose combinations with phenazopyridine as a urinary antiseptic and analgesic, and with trimethoprim (*see* below).

Sulfadiazine. *Sulfadiazine* given orally is rapidly absorbed from the gastrointestinal tract, and peak blood concentrations are reached within 3 to 6 hours after a single dose. Following an oral dose of 3 g, peak concentrations in plasma are 50 μg/ml. About 55% of the drug is bound to plasma protein at a concentration of 100 μg/ml when plasma protein levels are normal. Therapeutic concentrations are attained in cerebrospinal fluid within 4 hours after a single oral dose of 60 mg/kg.

Sulfadiazine is excreted quite readily by the kidney in both the free and the acetylated form, rapidly at first and then more slowly over a period of 2 to 3 days. It can be detected in the urine within 30 minutes after oral ingestion. About 15% to 40% of the excreted sulfadiazine is in the acetylated form. This form of the drug is excreted more readily than the free fraction, and the administration of alkali accelerates the renal clearance of both forms by further diminishing their tubular reabsorption.

In adults and children who are being treated with sulfadiazine, every precaution must be taken to ensure fluid intake adequate to produce a urine output of at least 1200 ml in adults and a corresponding quantity in children. If this cannot be accomplished, sodium bicarbonate may be given to reduce the risk of crystalluria.

Poorly Absorbed Sulfonamides. *Sulfasalazine* (AZALINE, AZULFIDINE) is very poorly absorbed from the gastrointestinal

Table 44–1
Classes of Sulfonamides

CLASS	SULFONAMIDE	SERUM HALF-LIFE, hours
Absorbed and excreted rapidly	Sulfisoxazole	5–6
	Sulfamethoxazole	11
	Sulfadiazine	10
Poorly absorbed–active in bowel lumen	Sulfasalazine	—
Topically used	Sulfacetamide	—
	Silver sulfadiazine	—
Long-acting	Sulfadoxine	100–230

tract. It is used in the therapy of ulcerative colitis and regional enteritis, but relapses tend to occur in about one-third of patients who experience a satisfactory initial response. Corticosteroids are more effective in treating acute attacks, but sulfasalazine is preferred to corticosteroids for treatment of patients mildly or moderately ill with ulcerative colitis. The drug also is being employed as the first approach to treatment of relatively mild cases of regional enteritis and granulomatous colitis. Sulfasalazine is broken down by intestinal bacteria to sulfapyridine, an active sulfonamide that is absorbed and eventually excreted in the urine, and 5-aminosalicylate, which reaches high levels in the feces. There is evidence that this latter compound is the effective agent in inflammatory bowel disease, whereas the sulfapyridine is responsible for most of the toxicity. Toxic reactions include Heinz-body anemia, acute hemolysis in patients with glucose-6-phosphate dehydrogenase deficiency, and agranulocytosis. Nausea, fever, arthralgias, and rashes occur in up to 20% of patients treated with the drug; desensitization has been effective. Sulfasalazine can cause a reversible infertility in males due to changes in sperm number and morphology. There is no evidence that the compound alters the intestinal microflora of persons with ulcerative colitis.

Sulfonamides for Topical Use. *Sulfacetamide.* *Sulfacetamide* is the N^1-acetyl-substituted derivative of sulfanilamide. Its aqueous solubility (1:140) is approximately 90 times that of sulfadiazine. Solutions of the sodium salt of the drug (ISOPTO-CETAMIDE, SODIUM SULAMYD, others) are employed extensively in the management of ophthalmic infections. Although topical sulfonamide for most purposes is discouraged because of lack of efficacy and a high risk of sensitization, sulfacetamide has certain advantages. Very high aqueous concentrations are nonirritating to the eye and are effective against susceptible microorganisms. A 30% solution of the sodium salt has a pH of 7.4, whereas the solutions of sodium salts of other sulfonamides are highly alkaline. The drug penetrates into ocular fluids and tissues in high concentration. Sensitivity reactions to sulfacetamide are rare, but the drug should not be used in patients with known hypersensitivity to sulfonamides.
Silver Sulfadiazine. (SILVADENE, others). This drug inhibits the growth *in vitro* of nearly all pathogenic bacteria and fungi, including some species resistant to sulfonamides. The compound is used topically to reduce microbial colonization and the incidence of infections of wounds from burns. It should not be used to treat an established deep infection. Silver is released slowly from the preparation in concentrations that are selectively toxic to the microorganisms. However, bacteria may develop resistance to silver sulfadiazine. While little silver is absorbed, the plasma concentration of sulfadiazine may approach therapeutic levels if a large surface area is involved. Adverse reactions are infrequent and include burning, rash, and itching. Silver sulfadiazine is considered by most authorities to be one of the agents of choice for the prevention of infection of burns.
Mafenide. This sulfonamide (α-amino-*p*-toluene-sulfonamide) is marketed as *mafenide acetate* (SULFAMYLON). When applied topically, it is effective for the prevention of colonization of burns by a large variety of gram-negative and gram-positive bacteria. It should not be used in treatment of an established deep infection. Superinfection with *Candida* occasionally may be a problem. The cream is applied once or twice daily to a thickness of 1 to 2 mm over the burned skin. Cleansing of

the wound and removal of debris should be carried out before each application of the drug. Therapy is continued until skin grafting is possible. Mafenide is rapidly absorbed systemically and converted to para-carboxybenzenesulfonamide. Studies of absorption from the burn surface indicate that peak plasma concentrations are reached in 2 to 4 hours. Adverse effects include intense pain at sites of application, allergic reactions, and loss of fluid by evaporation from the burn surface, since occlusive dressings are not used. The drug and its primary metabolite inhibit carbonic anhydrase, and the urine becomes alkaline. A metabolic acidosis with compensatory tachypnea and hyperventilation may ensue and has limited the usefulness of mafenide.

Long-Acting Sulfonamides. *Sulfadoxine* (N^1-[5,6-dimethoxy-4-pyrimidinyl] sulfanilamide) is a sulfonamide with a particularly long half-life (7 to 9 days). It is utilized in combination with *pyrimethamine* (500 mg of sulfadoxine plus 25 mg of pyrimethamine as FANSIDAR) for the prophylaxis and treatment of malaria caused by mefloquine-resistant strains of *Plasmodium falciparum* (*see* Chapter 40). Because of severe and sometimes fatal reactions, including the Stevens–Johnson syndrome, the drug should be used for prophylaxis only where the risk of resistant malaria is high.

Untoward Reactions to Sulfonamides

The untoward effects that follow the administration of sulfonamides are numerous and varied; the overall incidence of reactions is about 5%. Certain forms of toxicity may be related to individual differences in sulfonamide metabolism (Shear *et al.*, 1986).

Disturbances of the Urinary Tract. Although the risk of crystalluria was relatively high with the older, less soluble sulfonamides, the incidence of this problem is very low with more soluble agents such as sulfisoxazole. Crystalluria has occurred in dehydrated patients with AIDS who were receiving sulfadiazine for *Toxoplasma* encephalitis. Fluid intake should be such as to ensure a daily urine volume of at least 1200 ml (in adults). Alkalinization of the urine may be desirable if urine volume or pH is unusually low, since the solubility of sulfisoxazole increases greatly with slight elevations of pH.

Disorders of the Hematopoietic System. *Acute Hemolytic Anemia.* The mechanism of the acute hemolytic anemia produced by sulfonamides is not always readily apparent. In some cases, it has been thought to be a sensitization phenomenon. In other instances, the hemolysis is related to an erythrocytic deficiency of glucose-6-phosphate dehydrogenase activity. Hemolytic anemia is rare after sulfadiazine (0.05%); its exact incidence following therapy with sulfisoxazole is unknown.
Agranulocytosis. Agranulocytosis occurs in about 0.1% of patients who receive sulfadiazine; it also can follow the use of other sulfonamides. Although return of granulocytes to normal levels may be delayed for weeks or months after sulfonamide is withdrawn, most patients recover spontaneously with supportive care.
Aplastic Anemia. Complete suppression of bone-marrow activity with profound anemia, granulocytopenia, and thrombocytopenia is an extremely rare occurrence with sulfonamide

therapy. It probably results from a direct myelotoxic effect and may be fatal. However, reversible suppression of the bone marrow is quite common in patients with limited bone-marrow reserve (*e.g.,* patients with AIDS or those receiving myelosuppressive chemotherapy).

Hypersensitivity Reactions. The incidence of other hypersensitivity reactions to sulfonamides is quite variable. Among the skin and mucous membrane manifestations attributed to sensitization to sulfonamide are morbilliform, scarlatinal, urticarial, erysipeloid, pemphigoid, purpuric, and petechial rashes; and erythema nodosum, erythema multiforme of the Stevens-Johnson type, Behçet's syndrome, exfoliative dermatitis, and photosensitivity. Drug eruptions occur most often after the first week of therapy but may appear earlier in previously sensitized individuals. Fever, malaise, and pruritus are frequently present simultaneously. The incidence of untoward dermal effects is about 2% with sulfisoxazole, although patients with AIDS manifest a higher frequency of rashes with sulfonamide treatment than do other individuals. A syndrome similar to serum sickness may appear after several days of sulfonamide therapy. Drug fever is a common untoward manifestation of sulfonamide treatment; the incidence approximates 3% with sulfisoxazole.

Focal or diffuse necrosis of the liver due to direct drug toxicity or sensitization occurs in fewer than 0.1% of patients. Headache, nausea, vomiting, fever, hepatomegaly, jaundice, and laboratory evidence of hepatocellular dysfunction usually appear 3 to 5 days after sulfonamide administration is started, and the syndrome may progress to acute yellow atrophy and death.

Miscellaneous Reactions. Anorexia, nausea, and vomiting occur in 1% to 2% of persons receiving sulfonamides, and these manifestations are probably central in origin. The administration of sulfonamides to newborn infants, especially if premature, may lead to the displacement of bilirubin from plasma albumin. In newborn infants, free bilirubin can become deposited in the basal ganglia and subthalamic nuclei of the brain, causing an encephalopathy called *kernicterus*. Sulfonamides should not be given to pregnant women near term because these drugs pass through the placenta and are secreted in milk.

Drug Interactions. The most important interactions of the sulfonamides involve those with the oral anticoagulants, the sulfonylurea hypoglycemic agents, and the hydantoin anticonvulsants. In each case, sulfonamides can potentiate the effects of the other drug by mechanisms that appear to involve primarily inhibition of metabolism and, possibly, displacement from albumin. Dosage adjustment may be necessary when a sulfonamide is given concurrently.

Sulfonamide Therapy

The number of conditions for which the sulfonamides are therapeutically useful and constitute drugs of first choice has been reduced sharply by the development of more effective antimicrobial agents and by the gradual increase in the resistance of a number of bacterial species to this class of drugs. However, the use of sulfonamides has undergone a revival as a result of the introduction of the combination of trimethoprim and sulfamethoxazole.

Urinary Tract Infections. Since a significant percentage of urinary tract infections in many parts of the world are caused by sulfonamide-resistant microorganisms, these drugs are no longer a therapy of first choice. Trimethoprim–sulfamethoxazole, a quinolone, or ampicillin are the preferred agents. However, sulfisoxazole may be used effectively in areas where the prevalence of resistance is not high or when the organism is known to be sensitive. The usual dosage is 2 to 4 g initially followed by 1 to 2 g, orally, four times a day for 5 to 10 days. Patients with acute pyelonephritis with high fever and other severe constitutional manifestations are at risk of bacteremia and shock and should not be treated with a sulfonamide.

Nocardiosis. Sulfonamides are of value in the treatment of infections due to *Nocardia* species. A number of instances of complete recovery from the disease after adequate treatment with a sulfonamide have been recorded. Sulfisoxazole or sulfadiazine may be given in dosages of 6 to 8 g daily. Concentrations of sulfonamide in plasma should be 80 to 160 μg/ml. This schedule is continued for several months after all manifestations have been controlled. The administration of sulfonamide together with a second antibiotic has been recommended, especially for advanced cases, and ampicillin, erythromycin, or streptomycin has been suggested for this purpose. The clinical response and the results of sensitivity testing may be helpful in choosing a companion drug. It should be emphasized, however, that there are no clinical data to show that combination therapy is better than therapy with a sulfonamide alone. Trimethoprim–sulfamethoxazole also has been effective, and some authorities consider it to be the drug of choice.

Toxoplasmosis. The combination of pyrimethamine and sulfadiazine is the treatment of choice for toxoplasmosis (Montoya and Remington, 2000). Pyrimethamine is given as a loading dose of 75 mg followed by 25 mg orally per day, with sulfadiazine, 1 g orally every 6 hours, plus folinic acid, 10 mg orally each day, for at least 3 to 6 weeks. Patients should receive at least 2 liters of fluid intake daily to prevent crystalluria during therapy.

Use of Sulfonamides for Prophylaxis. The sulfonamides exhibit a degree of effectiveness equal to that of oral penicillin in preventing streptococcal infections and recurrences of rheumatic fever among susceptible subjects. Despite the efficacy of sulfonamides for long-term prophylaxis of rheumatic fever, their toxicity and the possibility of infection by drug-resistant streptococci make them less desirable than penicillin for this purpose. They should be used, however, without hesitation in patients who are hypersensitive to penicillin. If untoward responses occur, they usually do so during the first 8 weeks of therapy; serious reactions after this time are rare. White cell counts should be carried out once weekly during the first 8 weeks.

TRIMETHOPRIM–SULFAMETHOXAZOLE

The introduction of trimethoprim in combination with sulfamethoxazole constitutes an important advance in the development of clinically effective antimicrobial agents and represents the practical application of a theoretical consideration; that is, if two drugs act on sequential steps in the pathway of an obligate enzymatic reaction in bacteria (*see* Figure 44–2), the result of their combination will be synergistic (*see* Hitchings, 1961). In much of the world the combination is known as *co-trimoxazole.* In addition to its combination with sulfamethoxazole (BACTRIM, SEPTRA, others), trimethoprim also is available as a single entity preparation (TRIMPEX, PROLOPRIM, others).

Chemistry. Sulfamethoxazole has been discussed earlier in this chapter, and its structural formula is shown in Figure 44–1. The history of trimethoprim, a diaminopyrimidine, is discussed in Chapter 40. Its structural formula is as follows:

TRIMETHOPRIM

Antibacterial Spectrum. The antibacterial spectrum of trimethoprim is similar to that of sulfamethoxazole, although the former drug is usually 20 to 100 times more potent than the latter. Most gram-negative and gram-positive microorganisms are sensitive to trimethoprim, but resistance can develop when the drug is used alone. *Pseudomonas aeruginosa, Bacteroides fragilis,* and enterococci usually are resistant. There is significant variation in the susceptibility of Enterobacteriaceae to trimethoprim in different geographical locations because of the spread of resistance mediated by plasmids and transposons. The data presented below refer to the antimicrobial activity of the combination of trimethoprim and sulfamethoxazole.

Chlamydia diphtheriae and *N. meningitidis* are susceptible to trimethoprim–sulfamethoxazole. Although most *S. pneumoniae* are susceptible, there has been a disturbing increase in resistance (*see* below). From 50% to 95% of strains of *Staphylococcus aureus, Staphylococcus epidermidis, S. pyogenes,* the *viridans* group of streptococci, *E. coli, Proteus mirabilis, Proteus morganii, Proteus rettgeri, Enterobacter* species, *Salmonella, Shigella, Pseudomonas pseudomallei, Serratia,* and *Alcaligenes* species are inhibited. Also sensitive are *Klebsiella* species, *Brucella abortus, Pasteurella haemolytica, Yersinia pseudotuberculosis, Yersinia enterocolitica,* and *Nocardia asteroides.* Methicillin-resistant strains of *S. aureus,* although also resistant to trimethoprim or sulfamethoxazole alone, may be susceptible to the combination. A synergistic interaction between the components of the preparation is apparent even when microorganisms are resistant to sulfonamide or are resistant to sulfonamide and moderately resistant to trimethoprim. However, a maximal degree of synergism occurs when microorganisms are sensitive to both components. The activity of trimethoprim–sulfamethoxazole *in vitro* depends on the medium in which it is determined; for example, low concentrations of thymidine almost completely abolish the antibacterial activity (*see* Symposium, 1973).

Mechanism of Action. The antimicrobial activity of the combination of trimethoprim and sulfamethoxazole results from its actions on two steps of the enzymatic pathway for the synthesis of tetrahydrofolic acid. As shown earlier in Figure 44–2, sulfonamide inhibits the incorporation of para-aminobenzoic acid (PABA) into folic acid, and trimethoprim prevents the reduction of dihydrofolate to tetrahydrofolate. The latter is the form of folate essential for one-carbon transfer reactions, for example, the synthesis of thymidylate from deoxyuridylate. Selective toxicity for microorganisms is achieved in two ways. Mammalian cells utilize preformed folates from the diet and do not synthesize the compound. Furthermore, trimethoprim is a highly selective inhibitor of dihydrofolate reductase of lower organisms, with 100,000-fold more drug required to inhibit human reductase than the bacterial enzyme. This is vitally important, since this enzymatic function is a crucial one in all species.

The synergistic interaction between sulfonamide and trimethoprim is predictable from their respective mechanisms. There is an optimal ratio of the concentrations of the two agents for synergism, and this is equal to the ratio of the minimal inhibitory concentrations of the drugs acting independently. While this ratio varies for different bacteria, the most effective ratio for the greatest number of microorganisms is 20 parts of sulfamethoxazole to 1 part of trimethoprim. The combination is thus formulated to achieve a sulfamethoxazole concentration *in vivo* 20 times greater than that of trimethoprim. (*See* articles by Hitchings, Burchall, and Bushby in Symposium, 1973.) The pharmacokinetic properties of the sulfonamide chosen to be in combination with trimethoprim are thus important, since relative constancy of the concentrations of the two compounds in the body is desired.

Bacterial Resistance. Bacterial resistance to trimethoprim–sulfamethoxazole is a rapidly increasing problem, although resistance is lower than it is to either of the agents alone. Resistance often is due to the acquisition of a plasmid that codes for an altered dihydrofolate reductase. The development of resistance is a problem for treatment of many different bacterial infections. In a survey of children with otitis media in Memphis, Tennessee, 29% of isolates were penicillin-resistant, and 25% of these also were resistant to trimethoprim–sulfamethoxazole (Centers for Disease Control, 1994a). In another survey, approximately 50% of *Shigella sonnei* isolates from The Netherlands were resistant (Voogd *et al.,* 1992). Emergence of trimethoprim–sulfamethoxazole-resistant *S. aureus* and Enterobacteriaceae is a special problem in AIDS patients receiving the drug for prophylaxis of *Pneumocystis carinii* pneumonia (Martin *et al.,* 1999).

Absorption, Distribution, and Excretion. The pharmacokinetic profiles of sulfamethoxazole and trimethoprim are closely but not perfectly matched to achieve a constant ratio of 20:1 in their concentrations in blood and tissues. The ratio in blood is often greater than 20:1 and that in tissues is frequently less. After a single oral dose of the combined preparation, trimethoprim is absorbed more rapidly than sulfamethoxazole. The concurrent administration of the drugs appears to slow the absorption of sulfamethoxazole. Peak blood concentrations of trimethoprim usually occur by 2 hours in most patients, while peak concentrations of sulfamethoxazole occur by 4 hours after a single oral dose. The half-lives of trimethoprim and sulfamethoxazole are approximately 11 and 10 hours, respectively.

When 800 mg of sulfamethoxazole is given with 160 mg of trimethoprim (the conventional 5:1 ratio) twice daily, the peak concentrations of the drugs in plasma are approximately 40 and 2 μg/ml, the optimal ratio. Peak concentrations are similar (46 and 3.4 μg/ml) after intravenous infusion of 800 mg of sulfamethoxazole and 160 mg of trimethoprim over a period of 1 hour.

Trimethoprim is rapidly distributed and concentrated in tissues, and about 40% is bound to plasma protein in the presence of sulfamethoxazole. The volume of distribution of trimethoprim is almost nine times that of sulfamethoxazole. The drug readily enters cerebrospinal fluid and sputum. High concentrations of each component of the mixture also are found in bile. About 65% of sulfamethoxazole is bound to plasma protein.

About 60% of administered trimethoprim and from 25% to 50% of administered sulfamethoxazole are excreted in the urine in 24 hours. Two-thirds of the sulfonamide is unconjugated. Metabolites of trimethoprim also are excreted. The rates of excretion and the concentrations of both compounds in the urine are significantly reduced in patients with uremia.

Untoward Effects. There is no evidence that trimethoprim–sulfamethoxazole, when given in the recommended doses, induces folate deficiency in normal persons. However, the margin between toxicity for bacteria and that for human beings may be relatively narrow when the cells of the patient are deficient in folate. In such cases, trimethoprim–sulfamethoxazole may cause or precipitate megaloblastosis, leukopenia, or thrombocytopenia. In routine use, the combination appears to exert little toxicity. About 75% of the untoward effects involve the skin. These are typical of those known to be produced by sulfonamides, as already described. However, trimethoprim–sulfamethoxazole has been reported to cause up to three times as many dermatological reactions as does sulfisoxazole when given alone (5.9% *versus* 1.7%; Arndt and Jick, 1976). Exfoliative dermatitis, Stevens–Johnson syndrome, and toxic epidermal necrolysis (Lyell's syndrome) are rare, occurring primarily in older individuals. Nausea and vomiting constitute the bulk of gastrointestinal reactions; diarrhea is rare. Glossitis and stomatitis are relatively common. Mild and transient jaundice has been noted and appears to have the histological features of allergic cholestatic hepatitis. Central nervous system reactions consist of headache, depression, and hallucinations, manifestations

known to be produced by sulfonamides. Hematological reactions, in addition to those mentioned above, are various types of anemia (including aplastic, hemolytic, and macrocytic), coagulation disorders, granulocytopenia, agranulocytosis, purpura, Henoch–Schönlein purpura, and sulfhemoglobinemia. Permanent impairment of renal function may follow the use of trimethoprim–sulfamethoxazole in patients with renal disease, and a reversible decrease in creatinine clearance has been noted in patients with normal renal function (Symposium, 1973).

Patients with AIDS frequently react adversely when trimethoprim–sulfamethoxazole is administered to treat infection due to *P. carinii* (Gordin *et al.,* 1984). These adverse reactions include rash, neutropenia, Stevens-Johnson syndrome, Sweet's syndrome, and pulmonary infiltrates. It may be possible to continue therapy *via* rapid oral desensitization (Gluckstein and Ruskin, 1995).

Therapeutic Uses. *Urinary Tract Infections.* Treatment of uncomplicated lower urinary tract infections with trimethoprim–sulfamethoxazole often is highly effective for sensitive bacteria. The preparation has been shown to produce a better therapeutic effect than does either of its components given separately when the infecting microorganisms are of the family Enterobacteriaceae. Single-dose therapy (320 mg of trimethoprim plus 1600 mg of sulfamethoxazole in adults) has been effective in some cases for the treatment of acute uncomplicated urinary tract infections, but a minimum of 3 days of therapy is more likely to be effective (Zinner and Mayer, 2000; Stamm and Hooton, 1993).

The combination appears to have special efficacy in chronic and recurrent infections of the urinary tract. Small doses (200 mg of sulfamethoxazole plus 40 mg of trimethoprim per day, or two to four times these amounts once or twice per week) appear to be effective in reducing the number of recurrent urinary tract infections in adult females. This effect may be related to the presence of therapeutic concentrations of trimethoprim in vaginal secretions. Enterobacteriaceae surrounding the urethral orifice may be eliminated or markedly reduced in number, thus diminishing the chance of an ascending reinfection. Trimethoprim also is found in therapeutic concentrations in prostatic secretions, and trimethoprim–sulfamethoxazole is often effective for the treatment of bacterial prostatitis.

Bacterial Respiratory Tract Infections. Trimethoprim–sulfamethoxazole is effective for acute exacerbations of chronic bronchitis. Administration of 800 to 1200 mg of sulfamethoxazole plus 160 to 240 mg of trimethoprim twice a day appears to be effective in decreasing fever, purulence and volume of sputum, and sputum bacterial count. Trimethoprim–sulfamethoxazole should *not* be used to treat streptococcal pharyngitis, since it does not eradicate the microorganism. It is effective for acute otitis media in children and acute maxillary sinusitis in adults caused by susceptible strains of *H. influenzae* and *S. pneumoniae.*

Gastrointestinal Infections. The combination is an alternative for fluoroquinolone for treatment of shigellosis, since many strains of the causative agent are now resistant to ampicillin; however, resistance to trimethoprim–sulfamethoxazole is increasingly common. It is also a second-line drug (ceftriaxone or a fluoroquinolone is the preferred treatment) for typhoid fever, but resistance is an increasing problem. In adults, trimethoprim-sulfamethoxazole appears to be effective when the dose is 800 mg of sulfamethoxazole plus 160 mg of trimethoprim every 12 hours for 15 days.

Trimethoprim–sulfamethoxazole appears to be effective in the management of carriers of sensitive strains of *Salmonella typhi* and other species of *Salmonella.* One proposed schedule is the administration of 800 mg of sulfamethoxazole plus 160 mg of trimethoprim twice a day for 3 months; however, failures have occurred. The presence of chronic disease of the gallbladder may be associated with a high incidence of failure to clear the carrier state. Acute diarrhea due to sensitive strains of enteropathogenic *E. coli* can be treated or prevented with either trimethoprim or trimethoprim plus sulfamethoxazole (Hill and Pearson, 1988). However, antibiotic treatment (either trimethoprim–sulfamethoxazole or cephalosporin) of diarrheal illness due to enterohemorrhagic *E. coli* O157:H7 may increase the risk of hemolytic-uremic syndrome, perhaps by increasing the release of shiga toxin by the bacteria (Wong *et al.,* 2000).

Infection by **Pneumocystis carinii.** High-dose therapy (trimethoprim, 20 mg/kg per day, plus sulfamethoxazole, 100 mg/kg per day, in three or four divided doses) is effective for this severe infection in patients with AIDS. This combination compares favorably with pentamidine for treatment of this disease. Adjunctive corticosteroids should be given at the onset of antipneumocystis therapy in patients with a P_{O_2} of <70 mm Hg or an alveolar-arterial gradient of >35 mm Hg (Lane *et al.,* 1994). However, the incidence of side effects is high for both regimens (Sattler and Remington, 1981; Lane *et al.,* 1994). Lower-dose oral therapy with 800 mg of sulfamethoxazole plus 160 mg of trimethoprim (given twice daily) has been used successfully in AIDS patients with less severe pneumonia (P_{O_2} >60 mm Hg: Medina *et al.,* 1990). Prophylaxis with 800 mg of sulfamethoxazole and 160 mg of trimethoprim once daily or three times a week is effective in preventing pneumonia caused by this organism in patients with AIDS (Schneider *et al.,* 1992; Gallant *et al.,* 1994). Adverse reactions are less frequent with the lower prophylactic doses of trimethoprim–sulfamethoxazole. The most common problems are rash, fever, leukopenia, and hepatitis.

Prophylaxis in Neutropenic Patients. Several studies have demonstrated the effectiveness of low-dose therapy (150 mg/m^2 of body-surface area of trimethoprim and 750 mg/m^2 of body-surface area of sulfamethoxazole) for the prophylaxis of infection by *P. carinii* (*see* Hughes *et al.,* 1977). In addition, significant protection against sepsis caused by gram-negative bacteria was noted when 800 mg of sulfamethoxazole plus 160 mg of trimethoprim were given twice daily to severely neutropenic patients. The emergence of resistant bacteria may limit the usefulness of trimethoprim–sulfamethoxazole for prophylaxis (Gualtieri *et al.,* 1983).

Miscellaneous Infections. Nocardia infections have been treated successfully with the combination, but failures also have been reported. Although a combination of doxycycline and streptomycin or gentamicin now is considered to be the treatment of choice for brucellosis, trimethoprim–sulfamethoxazole may be an effective substitute for the doxycycline combination. Trimethoprim–sulfamethoxazole also has been used successfully in the treatment of Whipple's disease, infection by *Stenotrophomonas maltophilia,* and the intestinal parasites *Cyclospora* and *Isospora.* Wegener's granulomatosis may respond, depending on the stage of the disease.

THE QUINOLONES

Older members of this class of synthetic antimicrobial agents, particularly *nalidixic acid,* have been available for the treatment of urinary tract infections for many years. These drugs are of relatively minor significance because of their limited therapeutic utility and the rapid development of bacterial resistance. Against this backdrop, the more recent introduction of fluorinated 4-quinolones, such as *ciprofloxacin* (CIPRO) and *ofloxacin* (FLOXIN), represents a particularly important therapeutic advance, since these agents have broad antimicrobial activity and are effective after oral administration for the treatment of a wide variety of infectious diseases. Relatively few side effects appear to accompany the use of these fluoroquinolones, and microbial resistance to their action does not develop rapidly (*see* Andriole, 1993; Hooper, 2000a).

Chemistry. The compounds that are currently available for clinical use in the United States are 4-quinolones that all contain a carboxylic acid moiety in the 3 position of the basic ring structure. The newer fluoroquinolones also contain a fluorine substituent at position 6, and many of these compounds contain a piperazine moiety at position 7 (Table 44–2).

Mechanism of Action. The quinolone antibiotics target bacterial DNA gyrase and topoisomerase IV (Drlica and Zhao, 1997). For many gram-positive bacteria (such as *S. aureus*), topoisomerase IV is the primary activity inhibited by the quinolones (Ng *et al.,* 1996). In contrast, for many gram-negative bacteria (such as *E. coli*) DNA gyrase is the primary quinolone target (Hooper, 2000a; Alovero *et al.,* 2000). The two strands of double-helical DNA must be separated to permit DNA replication or transcription. However, anything that separates the strands results in "overwinding" or excessive positive supercoiling of the DNA in front of the point of separation. To combat this mechanical obstacle, the bacterial enzyme DNA gyrase is responsible for the continuous introduction of negative supercoils into DNA. This is an ATP-dependent reaction requiring that both strands of the DNA be cut to permit passage of a segment of DNA through the break; the break is then resealed.

The DNA gyrase of *E. coli* is composed of two 105,000-dalton A subunits and two 95,000-dalton B subunits encoded by the *gyrA* and *gyrB* genes, respectively. The A subunits, which carry out the strand-cutting function of the gyrase, are the site of action of the quinolones (Figure 44–3). The drugs inhibit gyrase-mediated DNA supercoiling at concentrations that correlate well with those required to inhibit bacterial growth (0.1 to 10 μg/ml). Mutations of the gene that encode the A subunit polypeptide can confer resistance to these drugs (Hooper, 2000a).

Topoisomerase IV also is composed of four subunits encoded by the *parC* and *parE* genes in *E. coli* (Drlica and Zhao, 1997; Hooper, 2000a). Topoisomerase IV separates interlinked (catenated) daughter DNA molecules that are the product of

Table 44-2
Structural Formulas of Selected Quinolones and Fluoroquinolones

CONGENER	R_1	R_6	R_7	X
Nalidixic acid	$-C_2H_5$	$-H$	$-CH_3$	$-N-$
Cinoxacin*	$-C_2H_5$	(Fused dioxolo ring)[†]		$-CH-$
Norfloxacin	$-C_2H_5$	$-F$		$-CH-$
Ciprofloxacin		$-F$		$-CH-$
Ofloxacin		$-F$		$-CH-$
Sparfloxacin‡		$-F$		
Lomefloxacin	$-C_2H_5$	$-F$		
Fleroxacin	$-CH_2-CH_2-F$	$-F$		
Pefloxacin	$-C_2H_5$	$-F$		$-CH-$
Levofloxacin		$-F$		
Trovafloxacin		$-F$		$-N-$

Table 44-2 *(Continued)*

Structural Formulas of Selected Quinolones and Fluoroquinolones

CONGENER	R_1	R_6	R_7	X
Gatifloxacin	▷	—F	—N (piperazine with CH_3, NH)	—C— with OCH_3
Moxifloxacin	▷	—F	—N (octahydropyrrolopyridine, H, H, NH)	—C— with OCH_3

*An N replaces C-2 in the basic ring structure of cinoxacin.

† [structure: C bonded to two O— groups in a ring]

‡An —NH$_2$ group is attached to the C-5 in the basic ring structure of sparfloxacin.

DNA replication. Eukaryotic cells do not contain DNA gyrase. However, they do contain a conceptually and mechanistically similar type II DNA topoisomerase that removes positive supercoils from eukaryotic DNA to prevent its tangling during replication. Quinolones inhibit eukaryotic type II topoisomerase only at much higher concentrations (100 to 1000 μg/ml).

Antibacterial Spectrum. The fluoroquinolones are potent bactericidal agents against *E. coli* and various species of *Salmonella, Shigella, Enterobacter, Campylobacter,* and *Neisseria* (*see* Eliopoulos and Eliopoulos, 1993). Minimal inhibitory concentrations of the fluoroquinolones for 90% of these strains (MIC_{90}) are usually less than 0.2 μg/ml. Ciprofloxacin is more active than *norfloxacin* (NOROXIN) against *P. aeruginosa;* values

of MIC_{90} range from 0.5 to 6 μg/ml. Fluoroquinolones also have good activity against staphylococci, including methicillin-resistant strains (MIC_{90} = 0.1 to 2 μg/ml).

Activity against streptococci is limited to a subset of the quinolones, including *grepafloxacin* (RAXAR, now withdrawn from the market), *levofloxacin* (LEVAQUIN), *gatifloxacin* (TEQUIN), *clinafloxacin,* and *moxifloxacin* (ALELOX) (Hooper, 2000a; Eliopoulos and Eliopoulos, 1993). Several intracellular bacteria are inhibited by fluoroquinolones at concentrations that can be achieved in plasma; these include species of *Chlamydia, Mycoplasma, Legionella, Brucella,* and *Mycobacterium* (including *Mycobacterium tuberculosis;* Leysen *et al.,* 1989; Alangaden and Lerner, 1997). Ciprofloxacin, ofloxacin (FLOXIN), *pefloxacin,* and *sparfloxacin* (ZAGAM) have MIC_{90} values from 0.5 to 3 μg/ml

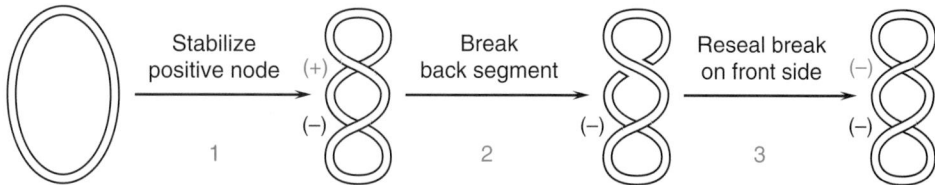

Figure 44–3. Model of the formation of negative DNA supercoils by DNA gyrase.

The enzyme binds to two segments of DNA (1), creating a node of positive (+) superhelix. The enzyme then introduces a double-strand break in the DNA and passes the front segment through the break (2). The break is then resealed (3), creating a negative (−) supercoil. Quinolones inhibit the nicking and closing activity of the gyrase and also block the decatenating activity of topoisomerase IV. (Reprinted from Cozzarelli, 1980, with permission.)

for *Mycobacterium fortuitum, Mycobacterium kansasii,* and *M. tuberculosis;* ofloxacin and pefloxacin are active in animal models of leprosy (Hooper, 2000a). However, clinical experience with these pathogens remains limited.

Several of the new fluoroquinolones have activity against anaerobic bacteria, including *trovafloxacin* (TROVAN), gatifloxacin, moxifloxacin, clinafloxacin, and *sitafloxacin* (Medical Letter, 2000).

Although *nalidixic acid* (NEGGRAM) and *cinoxacin* (CINOBAC) are bactericidal to most of the common gram-negative bacteria that cause urinary tract infections, their intrinsic activity is limited. Concentrations of nalidixic acid that approach 20 μg/ml are required to kill most enteric gram-negative bacilli; *P. aeruginosa* is resistant.

Resistance to quinolones may develop during therapy *via* mutations in the bacterial chromosomal genes encoding DNA gyrase or topoisomerase IV, or by active transport of the drug out of the bacteria (Oethinger *et al.,* 2000). No quinolone-modifying or inactivating activities have been identified in bacteria (Gold and Moellering, 1996; Ng *et al.,* 1996; Okusu *et al.,* 1996). Resistance has increased after the introduction of fluoroquinolones, especially in *Pseudomonas* and staphylococci (Pegues *et al.,* 1998; Peterson *et al.,* 1998). Increasing fluoroquinolone resistance also is being observed in *Clostridium jejuni, Salmonella, Neisseria gonorrhoeae,* and *S. pneumoniae* (Smith *et al.,* 1999; Centers for Disease Control, 1994b; Thornsberry *et al.,* 1997; Mølbak *et al.,* 1999).

Absorption, Fate, and Excretion.   The quinolones are well absorbed after oral administration and are widely distributed in body tissues. Peak serum levels of the fluoroquinolones are obtained within 1 to 3 hours of an oral dose of 400 mg, with peak levels ranging from 1.1 μg/ml for sparfloxacin to 6.4 μg/ml for levofloxacin. Relatively low serum levels are reached with norfloxacin and limit its usefulness to the treatment of urinary tract infections. Food does not impair oral absorption, but may delay the time to peak serum concentrations. Oral doses in adults are 200 to 400 mg every 12 hours for ofloxacin and *enoxacin* (PENETREX), 400 mg every 12 hours for norfloxacin and pefloxacin, 400 mg every 24 hours for *lomefloxacin* (MAXAQUIN), and 250 to 750 mg every 12 hours for ciprofloxacin. Bioavailability of the fluoroquinolones is greater than 50% for all agents and greater than 95% for several. The serum half-life ranges from 3 to 5 hours for norfloxacin and ciprofloxacin to 20 hours for sparfloxacin. The volume of distribution of quinolones is high, with concentrations of quinolones in urine, kidney, lung and prostate tissue, stool, bile, and macrophages and neutrophils higher than serum levels. Quinolone concentrations in cerebrospinal fluid, bone, and prostatic fluid are lower than in serum. Pefloxacin and ofloxacin levels in ascites fluid are close to serum levels, and ciprofloxacin, ofloxacin, and pefloxacin have been detected in human breast milk.

Routes of elimination differ among the quinolones. Renal clearance predominates for ofloxacin, lomefloxacin, and cinoxacin; pefloxacin, nalidixic acid, sparfloxacin, grepafloxacin, and trovafloxacin are predominantly eliminated nonrenally. Dose adjustments in patients with renal insufficiency are required for cinoxacin, norfloxacin, ciprofloxacin, ofloxacin, enoxacin, and lomefloxacin but not for nalidixic acid, grepafloxacin, trovafloxacin, and pefloxacin. None of the agents is efficiently removed by peritoneal or hemodialysis. A fluoroquinolone other than trovafloxacin, grepafloxacin, or pefloxacin should be used in patients with hepatic failure.

Adverse Effects.   Quinolones and fluoroquinolones are generally well tolerated (Lipsley and Baker, 1999). The most common adverse reactions involve the gastrointestinal tract, with 3% to 17% of patients reporting mostly mild nausea, vomiting, and/or abdominal discomfort. Diarrhea and antibiotic-associated colitis have been unusual. Central nervous system side effects, predominately mild headache and dizziness, have been seen in 0.9% to 11% of patients. Rarely, hallucinations, delirium, and seizures have occurred, predominantly in patients who also were receiving theophylline or a nonsteroidal antiinflammatory drug (*see* below). Nonsteroidal antiinflammatory drugs may augment displacement of gamma-aminobutyric acid (GABA) from its receptors by the quinolones (Halliwell *et al.,* 1993). Rashes, including photosensitivity reactions, also can occur. All of these agents can produce arthropathy in several species of immature animals. Traditionally, the use of quinolones in children has been contraindicated for that reason. However, children with cystic fibrosis given ciprofloxacin, norfloxacin, and nalidixic acid have had few, and reversible, joint symptoms (Burkhardt *et al.,* 1997). Therefore, in some cases the benefits may outweigh the risks of quinolone therapy in children. Arthralgias and joint swelling have developed in children receiving fluoroquinolones; therefore, these drugs are not generally recommended for use in prepubertal children or pregnant women. Ciprofloxacin, grepafloxacin, pefloxacin, and enoxacin inhibit the metabolism of theophylline, and toxicity from elevated concentrations of the methylxanthine may occur (Schwartz *et al.,* 1988). Concurrent administration of a nonsteroidal antiinflammatory drug may potentiate the central nervous system stimulant effects of the quinolones, with seizures reported in patients receiving enoxacin and fenbufen.

Leukopenia, eosinophilia, and mild elevations in serum transaminases rarely occur. Rare but serious hepatic damage, including liver failure resulting in death, was observed with patients receiving trovafloxacin. For this reason, the use of trovafloxacin has been restricted to serious or life-threatening infections where the benefits of therapy outweigh the risk (Public Health Advisory, 1999). Temafloxacin was removed from the market by the manufacturer after approximately 1 out of 5000 prescriptions resulted in hemolysis, renal failure, thrombocytopenia, and/or disseminated intravascular coagulation. These problems have rarely been seen with other quinolones. QT_c interval (QT interval, corrected for heart rate) prolongation has been observed for sparfloxacin and for grepafloxacin, which is no longer marketed.

Therapeutic Uses. *Urinary Tract Infections.* Nalidixic acid and cinoxacin are useful only for urinary tract infections caused by susceptible microorganisms. The fluoroquinolones are significantly more potent and have a much broader spectrum of antimicrobial activity. Norfloxacin is approved for use in the United States only for urinary tract infections. Comparative clinical trials indicate that norfloxacin, ciprofloxacin, ofloxacin, and trimethoprim–sulfamethoxazole are equally efficacious for the treatment of urinary tract infections (Stein *et al.,* 1987; Hooper and Wolfson, 1991).

Prostatitis. Norfloxacin, ciprofloxacin, and ofloxacin all have been effective in uncontrolled trials for the treatment of prostatitis caused by sensitive bacteria. Fluoroquinolones administered for 4 to 6 weeks appear to be effective in patients not responding to trimethoprim–sulfamethoxazole (Hooper and Wolfson, 1991).

Sexually Transmitted Diseases. Fluoroquinolones lack activity for *Treponema pallidum* but have activity *in vitro* against *N. gonorrhoeae, C. trachomatis,* and *Haemophilus ducreyi.* It is important to remember that the quinolones are contraindicated in pregnancy. For chlamydial urethritis/cervicitis, a 7-day course of ofloxacin or sparfloxacin is an alternative to a 7-day treatment with doxycycline or a single dose of azithromycin; other available quinolones have not been reliably effective. A single oral dose of a fluoroquinolone such as ofloxacin or ciprofloxacin is effective treatment for gonorrhea and is an alternative to intramuscular ceftriaxone or oral cefixime for this infection, although fluoroquinolone resistance is emerging (Centers for Disease Control, 1994b). Pelvic inflammatory disease has been treated effectively with a 14-day course of ofloxacin combined with an antibiotic with activity against anaerobes (clindamycin or metronidazole) (Centers for Disease Control and Prevention, 1998). Chancroid (infection by *H. ducreyi*) can be treated with 3 days of ciprofloxacin or enoxacin.

Gastrointestinal and Abdominal Infections. For traveler's diarrhea (frequently caused by enterotoxigenic *E. coli*), the quinolones are equal to trimethoprim-sulfamethoxazole in effectiveness, reducing the duration of loose stools by 1 to 3 days (DuPont and Ericsson, 1993). Norfloxacin, ciprofloxacin, and ofloxacin given for 5 days all have been effective in the treatment of patients with shigellosis, with even shorter courses effective in many cases (Bennish *et al.,* 1992). Norfloxacin is superior to trimethoprim-sulfamethoxazole in decreasing the duration of diarrhea in cholera (Bhattacharya *et al.,* 1990). Ciprofloxacin and ofloxacin treatment cures most patients with enteric fever caused by *S. typhi* as well as bacteremic nontyphoidal infections in AIDS patients, and it clears chronic fecal carriage. Shigellosis is effectively treated with either ciprofloxacin or azithromycin (Khan *et al.,* 1997). The *in vitro* ability of the quinolones to induce the Shiga toxin *stx2* gene in *E. coli* suggests that the quinolones should not be used for Shiga toxin-producing *E. coli* (Miedouge *et al.,* 2000). Ciprofloxacin and ofloxacin have been less effective in treating episodes of peritonitis occurring in patients on chronic ambulatory peritoneal dialysis, likely due to the higher MICs for these drugs for the coagulase-negative staphylococci that are a common cause of peritonitis in this setting.

Respiratory Tract Infections. The major limitation of the use of quinolones for the treatment of community-acquired pneumonia and bronchitis had been the poor *in vitro* activity of ciprofloxacin, ofloxacin, and norfloxacin against *S. pneumo-*

niae and anaerobic bacteria. However many of the new fluoroquinolones—including levofloxacin, trovafloxacin, gatifloxacin, clinafloxacin, and moxifloxacin—have excellent activity against *S. pneumoniae.* Initial clinical experience with some of these newer quinolones shows comparable efficacy to β-lactam antibiotics (Aubier *et al.,* 1998; File *et al.,* 1997). The fluoroquinolones have *in vitro* activity against the rest of the commonly recognized respiratory pathogens, including *H. influenzae, Moraxella catarrhalis, S. aureus, M. pneumoniae, Chlamydia pneumoniae,* and *Legionella pneumophila.* Either a fluoroquinolone (ciprofloxacin or levofloxacin) or azithromycin is the antibiotic of choice for *Legionella pneumoniae* (Yu, 2000). Fluoroquinolones have been very effective at eradicating both *H. influenzae* and *M. catarrhalis* from sputum. Mild to moderate respiratory exacerbations due to *P. aeruginosa* in patients with cystic fibrosis have responded to oral fluoroquinolone therapy. Emerging clinical data are demonstrating a clear role for the newer fluoroquinolones as single agents for treatment of community-acquired pneumonia (Hooper, 2000a). However, on the horizon is a decreasing susceptibility of *S. pneumoniae* to fluoroquinolones (Chen *et al.,* 1999; Wortmann and Bennett, 1999).

Bone, Joint, and Soft Tissue Infections. The treatment of chronic osteomyelitis requires prolonged (weeks to months) antimicrobial therapy with agents active against *S. aureus* and gram-negative rods. The fluoroquinolones, by virtue of their oral administration and appropriate antibacterial spectrum for these infections, may be appropriately used in some cases (Gentry and Rodriguez-Gomez, 1991). Higher doses of ciprofloxacin are used than for treatment of urinary tract infections; recommended doses are 500 mg every 12 hours or, if severe, 750 mg twice daily. Therapy usually is continued for 7 to 14 days; bone and joint infections may require treatment for 4 to 6 weeks or more. Dosage should be reduced for patients with severely impaired renal function. Ciprofloxacin should not be given to children or pregnant women. Clinical cures have been as high as 75% in chronic osteomyelitis in which gram-negative rods predominated (Hooper, 2000a). Failures have been associated with the development of resistance in *S. aureus, P. aeruginosa,* and *Serratia marcescens.* In diabetic foot infections, which are commonly caused by a mixture of bacteria including gram-negative rods, anaerobes, streptococci, and staphylococci, the fluoroquinolones in combination with an agent with antianaerobic activity are a reasonable choice. Ciprofloxacin as sole therapy was effective in 50% of diabetic foot infections (Peterson *et al.,* 1989).

Other Infections. The quinolones may be used as part of multiple-drug regimens for the treatment of multidrug-resistant tuberculosis and for the treatment of atypical mycobacterial infections as well as *Mycobacterium avium* complex infections in AIDS (*see* Chapter 48). In neutropenic cancer patients with fever, the combination of a quinolone with an aminoglycoside is comparable to β-lactam–aminoglycoside combinations but is less effective when used as a single drug (Meunier *et al.,* 1991). Quinolones when used as prophylaxis in neutropenic patients have decreased the incidence of gram-negative rod bacteremias (GIMEMA Infection Program, 1991). Ciprofloxacin plus amoxicillin-clavulanate recently has been shown to be effective as an oral empiric therapy for fever in low-risk patients with granulocytopenia secondary to cancer chemotherapy (Kern *et al.,* 1999; Freifeld *et al.,* 1999).

ANTISEPTIC AND ANALGESIC AGENTS FOR URINARY TRACT INFECTIONS

The urinary tract antiseptics inhibit the growth of many species of bacteria. They cannot be used to treat systemic infections because effective concentrations are not achieved in plasma with safe doses. However, because they are concentrated in the renal tubules, they can be used by oral administration to treat infections of the urinary tract. Furthermore, effective antibacterial concentrations reach the renal pelves and the bladder. Treatment with such drugs can be thought of as local therapy in that only in the kidney and bladder, with the rare exceptions mentioned below, are adequate therapeutic levels achieved (*see* Hooper, 2000b).

Methenamine.   *Methenamine* is a urinary tract antiseptic that owes its activity to formaldehyde.

Chemistry.   Methenamine is hexamethylenetetramine (hexamethyleneamine). It has the following structure:

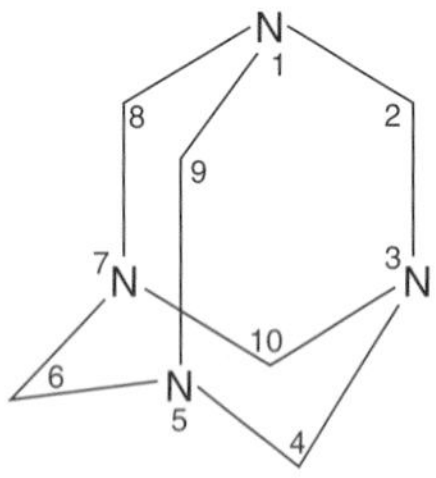

METHENAMINE

The compound decomposes in water to generate formaldehyde, according to the following reaction:

$$NH_4(CH_2)_6 + 6H_2O + 4H^+ \rightarrow 4NH_4^+ + 6HCHO$$

At pH 7.4, almost no decomposition occurs; however, 6% of the theoretical amount of formaldehyde is yielded at pH 6 and 20% at pH 5. Thus, acidification of the urine promotes the formaldehyde-dependent antibacterial action. The reaction is fairly slow, and 3 hours are required to reach 90% of completion (Strom and Jun, 1993).

Antimicrobial Activity.   Nearly all bacteria are sensitive to free formaldehyde at concentrations of about 20 μg/ml. Urea-splitting microorganisms (*e.g.,* Proteus species) tend to raise the pH of the urine and thus inhibit the release of formaldehyde. Microorganisms do not develop resistance to formaldehyde.

Pharmacology and Toxicology.   Methenamine is absorbed orally, but 10% to 30% decomposes in the gastric juice unless the drug is protected by an enteric coating. Because of the ammonia produced, methenamine is contraindicated in hepatic insufficiency. Excretion in the urine is nearly quantitative. When the urine pH is 6 and the daily urine volume is 1000 to 1500 ml, a daily dose of 2 g will yield a concentration of 18 to 60 μg/ml of formaldehyde; this is more than the MIC for most urinary tract pathogens. Various poorly metabolized acids can be used to acidify the urine. Low pH alone is bacteriostatic, so that acidification serves a double function. The acids commonly used are mandelic acid and hippuric acid (UREX, HIPREX).

Gastrointestinal distress frequently is caused by doses greater than 500 mg four times a day, even with enteric-coated tablets. Painful and frequent micturition, albuminuria, hematuria,

and rashes may result from doses of 4 to 8 g a day given for longer than 3 to 4 weeks. Once the urine is sterile, a high dose should be reduced. Because systemic methenamine has low toxicity at the typically used doses, renal insufficiency does not constitute a contraindication to the use of methenamine alone, but the acids given concurrently may be detrimental. Methenamine mandelate is contraindicated in renal insufficiency. Crystalluria from the mandelate moiety can occur. Methenamine combines with sulfamethizole and perhaps other sulfonamides in the urine, which results in mutual antagonism.

Therapeutic Uses and Status.   Methenamine is not a primary drug for the treatment of acute urinary tract infections, but it is of value for chronic suppressive treatment (Stamm and Hooton, 1993). The agent is most useful when the causative organism is *E. coli,* but it can usually suppress the common gram-negative offenders and often *S. aureus* and *S. epidermidis* as well. *Enterobacter aerogenes* and *Proteus vulgaris* are usually resistant. Urea-splitting bacteria (mostly *Proteus*) make it difficult to control the urine pH. The physician should strive to keep the pH below 5.5.

Nitrofurantoin.   *Nitrofurantoin* (FURADANTIN, MACROBID, others) is a synthetic nitrofuran that is used for the prevention and treatment of infections of the urinary tract. Its structural formula is as follows:

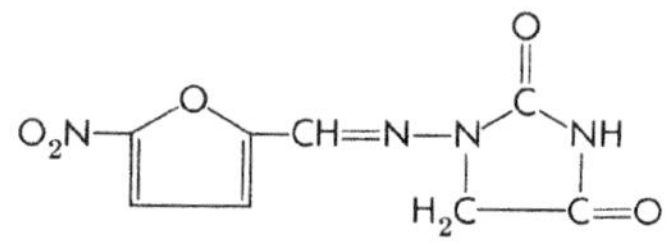

NITROFURANTOIN

Antimicrobial Activity.   Enzymes capable of reducing nitrofurantoin appear to be crucial for its activation. Highly reactive intermediates are formed, and these seem to be responsible for the observed capacity of the drug to damage DNA. Bacteria reduce nitrofurantoin more rapidly than do mammalian cells, and this is thought to account for the selective antimicrobial activity of the compound. Bacteria that are susceptible to the drug rarely become resistant during therapy. Nitrofurantoin is active against many strains of *E. coli* and enterococci. However, most species of *Proteus* and *Pseudomonas* and many of *Enterobacter* and *Klebsiella* are resistant. Nitrofurantoin is bacteriostatic for most susceptible microorganisms at concentrations of 32 μg/ml or less and is bactericidal at concentrations $\geq$100 μg/ml. The antibacterial activity is higher in an acidic urine.

Pharmacology and Toxicity.   Nitrofurantoin is rapidly and completely absorbed from the gastrointestinal tract. The macrocrystalline form of the drug is absorbed and excreted more slowly. Antibacterial concentrations are not achieved in plasma following ingestion of recommended doses, because the drug is rapidly eliminated. The plasma half-life is 0.3 to 1 hour; about 40% is excreted unchanged into the urine. The average dose of nitrofurantoin yields a concentration in urine of approximately 200 μg/ml. This amount is soluble at pH values above 5, but the urine should not be alkalinized because this reduces antimicrobial activity. The rate of excretion is linearly related to the creatinine clearance, so that, in patients with impaired glomerular function, the efficacy of the drug may be decreased and the systemic toxicity increased. Nitrofurantoin colors the urine brown.

The most common untoward effects are nausea, vomiting, and diarrhea; the macrocrystalline preparation is better tolerated. Various hypersensitivity reactions occasionally occur. These include chills, fever, leukopenia, granulocytopenia, hemolytic anemia [associated with glucose-6-phosphate dehydrogenase deficiency (Gait, 1990)], cholestatic jaundice, and hepatocellular damage. Chronic active hepatitis is an uncommon but serious side effect (Black *et al.,* 1980; Tolman, 1980). Acute pneumonitis with fever, chills, cough, dyspnea, chest pain, pulmonary infiltration, and eosinophilia may occur within hours to days of the initiation of therapy; it usually resolves within hours after discontinuation of the drug. More insidious subacute reactions also may be noted, and interstitial pulmonary fibrosis can occur in patients on chronic medication. This appears to be due to generation of oxygen radicals as a result of redox cycling of the drug in the lung. Elderly patients are especially susceptible to the pulmonary toxicity of nitrofurantoin (*see* Holmberg *et al.,* 1980). Megaloblastic anemia is rare. Various neurological disorders occasionally are observed. Headache, vertigo, drowsiness, muscular aches, and nystagmus are readily reversible, but severe polyneuropathies with demyelination and degeneration of both sensory and motor nerves have been reported; signs of denervation and muscle atrophy result. Neuropathies are most likely to occur in patients with impaired renal function and in persons on long-continued treatment. Nitrofurantoin-induced polyneuropathy has been reviewed by Toole and Parrish (1973). Certain adverse reactions may be caused by toxic reactive metabolites (Spielberg and Gordon, 1981).

The oral dosage of nitrofurantoin for adults is 50 to 100 mg four times a day, with meals and at bedtime. Alternatively, the daily dosage is better expressed as 5 to 7 mg/kg in four divided doses (not to exceed 400 mg). A single 50- to 100-mg dose at bedtime may be sufficient to prevent recurrences. The daily dose for children is 5 to 7 mg/kg, but it may be as low as 1 mg/kg for long-term therapy (Lohr *et al.,* 1977). A course of therapy should not exceed 14 days, and repeated courses should be separated by rest periods. Pregnant women, individuals with impaired renal function (creatinine clearance less than 40 ml per minute), and children less than 1 month of age should not receive nitrofurantoin.

Nitrofurantoin is approved only for the treatment of urinary tract infections caused by microorganisms known to be susceptible to the drug. Currently, bacterial resistance to nitrofurantoin is more frequent than resistance to fluoroquinolones or trimethoprim–sulfamethoxazole, making nitrofurantoin a second-line agent for treatment of urinary tract infections (Stamm and Hooton, 1993). Nitrofurantoin also is not recommended for treatment of pyelonephritis or prostatitis. However, nitrofurantoin is effective for prophylaxis of recurrent urinary tract infections (Brumfitt and Hamilton-Miller, 1995).

Phenazopyridine. *Phenazopyridine hydrochloride* (PYRIDIUM, others) is *not* a urinary antiseptic. However, it does have an analgesic action on the urinary tract and alleviates symptoms of dysuria, frequency, burning, and urgency. The usual dose is 200 mg three times daily. The compound is an azo dye, and the urine is colored orange or red; the patient should be so informed. Gastrointestinal upset is seen in up to 10% of patients and can be reduced by administering the drug with food; overdosage may result in methemoglobinemia. Phenazopyridine also is marketed in combination with sulfisoxazole and sulfamethoxazole.

PROSPECTUS

The most dramatic advance in the past decade for the group of antimicrobial agents reviewed in this chapter has been the introduction of the fluoroquinolones, such as ciprofloxacin. The attractiveness of these agents includes their bioavailability after oral administration, excellent gram-negative spectrum of activity, and relatively few side effects. Promising new fluoroquinolone agents are now being introduced and demonstrate a broader spectrum of antimicrobial activity, including, in some cases, effectiveness against gram-positive and anaerobic infections. The improved activity of newer quinolones against penicillin- and cephalosporin-resistant strains of pneumococcus and the atypical pneumonia organisms is resulting in an increasing role for these agents in the empirical treatment of pneumonia. The development and use of quinolones for the treatment of mycobacterial infections is ongoing (*see* Chapter 48).

For further information regarding particular infections for which the antimicrobial agents discussed in this chapter are useful, the reader is referred to the following chapters of *Harrison's Principles of Internal Medicine,* 14th ed., McGraw-Hill, New York, 1998: urinary tract infections, Chapter 131; sexually transmitted diseases, Chapter 129; osteomyelitis, Chapter 132; enteric infections, Chapter 128; and pneumocystis pneumonia, Chapter 211.

BIBLIOGRAPHY

Alovero, F.L., Pan, X.-S., Morris, J.E., Manzo, R.H., and Fisher, L.M. Engineering the specificity of antibacterial fluoroquinolones: benzenesulfonamide modifications at C-7 of ciprofloxacin change its primary target in *Streptococcus pneumoniae* from topoisomerase IV to gyrase. *Antimicrob. Agents Chemother.,* **2000,** *44:*320–325.

Arndt, K.A., and Jick, H. Rates of cutaneous reactions to drugs. A report from the Boston Collaborative Drug Surveillance Program. *JAMA,* **1976,** *235:*918–923.

Aubier, M., Verster, R., Reganney, C., Geslin, P., and Vercken, J.B. Once-daily sparfloxacin versus high-dosage amoxicillin in the treatment of community-acquired, suspected pneumococcal pneumonia in adults. Sparfloxacin European Study Group. *Clin. Infect. Dis.,* **1998,** *26*:1312–1320.

Bennish, M.L., Salam, M.A., Khan, W.A., and Khan, A.M. Treatment of shigellosis: III. Comparison of one- or two-dose ciprofloxacin with standard 5-day therapy. A randomized, blinded trial. *Ann. Intern. Med.,* **1992,** *117*:727–734.

Bhattacharya, S.K., Bhattacharya, M.K., Dutta, P., Dutta, D., De, S.P., Sikdar, S.N., Maitra, A., Dutta, A., and Pal, S.C. Double-blind, randomized, controlled clinical trial of norfloxacin for cholera. *Antimicrob. Agents Chemother.,* **1990,** *34*:939–940.

Black, M., Rabin, L., and Schatz, N. Nitrofurantoin-induced chronic active hepatitis. *Ann. Intern. Med.,* **1980,** *92*:62–64.

Brumfitt, W., and Hamilton-Miller, J.M. A comparative trial of low dose cefaclor and macrocrystallline nitrofurantoin in the prevention of recurrent urinary tract infection. *Infection,* **1995,** *23*:98–102.

Burkhardt, J.E., Walterspeil, J.N., and Schaad, U.B. Quinolone arthropathy in animals versus children. *Clin. Infect. Dis.,* **1997,** *25*:1196–1204.

Bushby, S.R., and Hitchings, G.H. Trimethoprim, a sulphonamide potentiator. *Br. J. Pharmacol.,* **1968,** *33*:72–90.

Buttle, G.A.H., Gray, W.H., and Stephenson, D. Protection of mice against streptococcal and other infections by *p*-aminobenzene-sulphonamide and related substances. *Lancet,* **1936,** *1*:1286–1290.

Centers for Disease Control. Drug-resistant *Streptococcus pneumoniae*—Kentucky and Tennessee, 1993. *M.M.W.R. Morb. Mortal. Wkly. Rep.,* **1994a,** *43*:23–26 and 31.

Centers for Disease Control. Decreased susceptibility of *Neisseria gonorrhoeae* to fluoroquinolones—Ohio and Hawaii, 1992–1994. *M.M.W.R. Morb. Mortal. Wkly. Rep.,* **1994b,** *43*:325–327.

Centers for Disease Control and Prevention. 1998 guidelines for treatment of sexually transmitted diseases. *M.M.W.R. Morb. Mortal. Wkly. Rep.,* **1998,** *47*:1–111.

Chen, D.K., McGeer, A., de Azavedo, J.C., and Low, D.E. Decreased susceptibility of *Streptococcus pneumoniae* to fluoroquinolones in Canada. Canadian Bacterial Surveillance Network. *N. Engl. J. Med.,* **1999,** *341*:233–239.

Colebrook, L., and Kenny, M. Treatment of human puerperal infections, and of experimental infections in mice, with PRONTOSIL. *Lancet,* **1936,** *1*:1279–1286.

Domagk, G. Ein Beitrag zur Chemotherapie der Bakteriellen Infektionen. *Dtsch. Med. Wochenschr.,* **1935,** *61*:250–253.

Eliopoulos, G.M., and Eliopoulos, C.T. Activity *in vitro* of the quinolones. In, *Quinolone Antimicrobial Agents,* 2nd ed. (Hooper, D.C., and Wolfson, J.S., eds.) American Society for Microbiology, Washington, D.C., **1993,** pp. 161–193.

Fildes, P. A rational approach to research in chemotherapy. *Lancet,* **1940,** *1*:955–957.

File, T.M., Jr., Segreti, J., Dunbar, L., Player, R., Kohler, R., Williams, R.R., Kojak, C., and Rubin, A. A multicenter, randomized study comparing the efficacy and safety of intravenous and/or oral levofloxacin versus ceftriaxone and/or cefuroxime axetil in treatment of adults with community-acquired pneumonia. *Antimicrob. Agents Chemother.,* **1997,** *41*:1965–1972.

Freifeld, A., Marchigiani, D., Walsh, T., Chanock, S., Lewis, L., Hiemenz, J., Hiemenz, S., Hicks, J.E., Gill, V., Steinberg, S.M., and Pizzo, P.A. A double-blind comparison of empirical oral and intravenous antibiotic therapy for low-risk febrile patients with neutropenia during cancer chemotherapy. *N. Engl. J. Med.,* **1999,** *341*:305–311.

Gait, J.E. Hemolytic reactions to nitrofurantoin in patients with glucose-6-phosphate dehydrogenase deficiency: theory and practice. *D.I.C.P.,* **1990,** *24*:1210–1213.

Gentry, L.O., and Rodriguez-Gomez, G. Ofloxacin versus parenteral therapy for chronic osteomyelitis. *Antimicrob. Agents Chemother.,* **1991,** *35*:538–541.

The GIMEMA Infection Program. Prevention of bacterial infection in neutropenic patients with hematologic malignancies. A randomized, multicenter trial comparing norfloxacin with ciprofloxacin. Gruppo Italiano Malattie Ematologiche Maligne dell'Adulto. *Ann. Intern. Med.,* **1991,** *115*:7–12.

Gluckstein, D., and Ruskin, J. Rapid oral desensitization to trimethoprim-sulfamethoxazole (TMP-SMZ): use in prophylaxis for *Pneumocystis carinii* pneumonia in patients with AIDS who were previously tolerant to TMP-SMZ. *Clin. Infect. Dis.,* **1995,** *20*:849–853.

Gordin, F.M., Simon, G.L., Wofsy, C.B., and Mills, J. Adverse reactions to trimethoprim-sulfamethoxazole in patients with acquired immunodeficiency syndrome. *Ann. Intern. Med.,* **1984,** *100*:495–499.

Gualtieri, R.J., Donowitz, G.R., Kaiser, D.L., Hess, C.E., and Sande, M.A. Double-blind randomized study of prophylactic trimethoprim/sulfamethoxazole in granulocytopenic patients with hematologic malignancies. *Am. J. Med.,* **1983,** *74*:934–940.

Halliwell, R.F., Davey, P.G., and Lambert, J.J. Antagonism of GABA$_A$ receptors by 4-quinolones. *J. Antimicrob. Chemother.,* **1993,** *31*:457–462.

Hitchings, G.H. A biochemical approach to chemotherapy. *Ann. N.Y. Acad. Sci.,* **1961,** *23*:700–708.

Holmberg, L., Boman, G., Bottiger, L.E., Eriksson, B.A., Spross, R., and Wessling, A. Adverse reactions to nitrofurantoin. Analysis of 921 reports. *Am. J. Med.,* **1980,** *69*:733–738.

Hughes, W.T., Kuhn, S., Chaudhary, S., Feldman, S., Verzosa, M., Aur, R.J., Pratt, C., and George, S.L. Successful chemoprophylaxis for *Pneumocystis carinii* pneumonitis. *N. Engl. J. Med.,* **1977,** *297*:1419–1426.

Kern, W.V., Cometta, A., De Bock, R., Langenaeken, J., Paesmans, M., and Gaya, H. Oral versus intravenous empirical antimicrobial therapy for fever in patients with granulocytopenia who are receiving cancer chemotherapy. International Antimicrobial Therapy Cooperative Group of the European Organization for Research and Treatment of Cancer. *N. Engl. J. Med.,* **1999,** *341*:312–318.

Khan, W.A., Seas, C., Dhar, U., Salam, M.A., and Bennish, M.L. Treatment of shigellosis: V. Comparison of azithromycin and ciprofloxacin. A double-blind, randomized, controlled trial. *Ann. Intern. Med.,* **1997,** *126*:697–703.

Leysen, D.C., Haemers, A., and Pattyn, S.R. Mycobacteria and the new quinolones. *Antimicrob. Agents Chemother.,* **1989,** *33*:1–5.

Lipsky, B.A., and Baker, C.A. Fluoroquinolone toxicity profiles: a review focusing on newer agents. *Clin. Infect. Dis.,* **1999,** *28*:352–364.

Lohr, J.A., Nunley, D.H., Howards, S.S., and Ford, R.F. Prevention of recurrent urinary tract infections in girls. *Pediatrics,* **1977,** *59*:562–565.

Martin, J.N., Rose, D.A., Hadley, W.K., Perdreau-Remington, F., Lam, P.K., and Gerberding, J.L. Emergence of trimethoprim-sulfamethoxazole resistance in the AIDS era. *J. Infect. Dis.,* **1999,** *180*:1809–1818.

Medina, I., Mills, J., Leoung, G., Hopewell, P.C., Lee, B., Modin, G., Benowitz, N., and Wofsy, C.B. Oral therapy for *Pneumocystis carinii* pneumonia (PCP) in the acquired immune deficiency syndrome. A controlled trial of trimethoprim-sulfamethoxazole versus trimethoprim-dapsone. *N. Engl. J. Med.,* **1990,** *323*:776–782.

Meunier, F., Zinner, S.H., Gaya, H., Calandra, T., Viscoli, C., Klastersky, J., and Glauser, M. Prospective randomized evaluation of ciprofloxacin versus piperacillin plus amikacin for empiric antibiotic therapy of febrile granulocytopenic cancer patients with lymphomas and solid tumors. The European Organization for Research on Treatment of Cancer International Antimicrobial Therapy Cooperative Group. *Antimicrob. Agents Chemother.,* **1991,** *35*:873–878.

Miedouge, M., Hacini, J., Grimont, F., and Watine, J. Shiga toxin-producing *Escherichia coli* urinary tract infection associated with hemolytic-uremic syndrome in an adult and possible adverse effect of ofloxacin therapy. *Clin. Infect. Dis.,* **2000,** *30*:395–396.

Mølbak, K., Baggesen, D.L., Aarestrup, F.M., Ebbesen, J.M., Engberg, J., Frydendahl, K., Gerner-Smidt, P., Petersen, A.M., and Wegener, H.C. An outbreak of multidrug-resistant, quinolone-resistant *Salmonella enterica* serotype typhimurium DT104. *N. Engl. J. Med.,* **1999,** *341*:1420–1425.

Ng, E.Y., Trucksis, M., and Hooper, D.C. Quinolone resistance mutations in topoisomerase IV: Relationship to the *flgA* locus and genetic evidence that topoisomerase IV is the primary target and DNA gyrase is the secondary target of fluoroquinolones in *Staphylococcus aureus. Antimicrob. Agents Chemother.,* **1996,** *40*:1881–1888.

Oethinger, M., Kern, W.V., Jellen-Ritter, A.S., McMurry, L.M., and Levy, S.B. Ineffectiveness of topoisomerase mutations in mediating clinically significant fluoroquinolone resistance in *Escherichia coli* in the absence of the AcrAB efflux pump. *Antimicrob. Agents Chemother.,* **2000,** *44*:10–13.

Okusu, H., Ma, D., and Nikaido, H. AcrAB efflux pump plays a major role in the antibiotic resistance phenotype of *Escherichia coli* multiple-antibiotic-resistance (Mar) mutants. *J. Bacteriol.,* **1996,** *178*:306–308.

Peterson, L.R., Lissack, L.M., Canter, K., Fasching, C.E., Clabots, C., and Gerding, D.N. Therapy of lower extremity infections with ciprofloxacin in patients with diabetes mellitus, peripheral vascular disease, or both. *Am. J. Med.,* **1989,** *86*:801–808.

Peterson, L.R., Postelnick, M., Pozdol, T.L., Reisberg, B., and Noskin, G.A. Management of fluoroquinolone resistance in *Pseudomonas aeruginosa*—outcome of monitored use in a referral hospital. *Int. J. Antimicrob. Agents,* **1998,** *10*:207–214.

Pegues, D.A., Colby, C., Hibberd, P.L., Cohen, L.G., Ausubel, F.M., Calderwood, S.B., and Hooper, D.C. The epidemiology of resistance to ofloxacin and oxacillin among clinical coagulase-negative staphylococcal isolates: analysis of risk factors and strain types. *Clin. Infect. Dis.,* **1998,** *26*:72–79.

Public Health Advisory. Trovan (trovafloxacin/alatrofloxacin mesylate) June 9, 1999. Food and Drug Administration Web site. Available at: http://www.fda.gov/cder/news/trovan. Accessed June 5, 2000.

Sattler, F.R., and Remington, J.S. Intravenous trimethoprim-sulfamethoxazole therapy for *Pneumocystis carinii* pneumonia. *Am. J. Med.,* **1981,** *70*:1215–1221.

Schneider, M.M., Hoepelman, A.I., Eeftinck Schattenkerk, J.K., Nielsen, T.L., van der Graaf, Y., Frissen, J.P., van der Ende, I.M., Kolsters, A.F., and Borleffs, J.C. A controlled trial of aerosolized pentamidine or trimethoprim-sulfamethoxazole as primary prophylaxis against *Pneumocystis carinii* pneumonia in patients with human immunodeficiency virus infection. The Dutch AIDS Treatment Group. *N. Engl. J. Med.,* **1992,** *327*:1836–1841.

Schwartz, J., Jauregui, L., Lettieri, J., and Bachmann, K. Impact of ciprofloxacin on theophylline clearance and steady-state concentrations in serum. *Antimicrob. Agents Chemother.,* **1988,** *32*:75–77.

Shear, N.H., Spielberg, S.P., Grant, D.M., Tang, B.K., and Kalow, W. Differences in metabolism of sulfonamides predisposing to idiosyncratic toxicity. *Ann. Intern. Med.,* **1986,** *105*:179–184.

Smith, K.E., Besser, J.M., Hedberg, C.W., Leano, F.T., Bender, J.B., Wicklund, J.H., Johnson, B.P., Moore, K.A., and Osterholm, M.T. Quinolone-resistant *Campylobacter jejuni* infections in Minnesota, 1992–1998. Investigation Team. *N. Engl. J. Med.,* **1999,** *340*:1525–1532.

Spielberg, S.P., and Gordon, G.B. Nitrofurantoin cytotoxicity. *In vitro* assessment of risk based on glutathione metabolism. *J. Clin. Invest.,* **1981,** *67*:37–41.

Stein, G.E., Mummaw, N., Goldstein, E.J., Boyko, E.J., Reller, L.B., Kurtz, T.O., Miller, K., and Cox, C.E. A multicenter comparative trial of three-day norfloxacin *vs.* ten-day sulfamethoxazole and trimethoprim for the treatment of uncomplicated urinary tract infections. *Arch. Intern. Med.,* **1987,** *147*:1760–1762.

Strom, J.G. Jr., and Jun, H.W. Effect of urine pH and ascorbic acid on the rate of conversion of methenamine to formaldehyde. *Biopharm. Drug Dispos.,* **1993,** *14*:61–69.

Thornsberry, C., Ogilvie, P., Kahn, J., and Mauriz, Y. Surveillance of antimicrobial resistance in *Streptococcus pneumoniae, Haemophilus influenzae,* and *Moraxella catarrhalis* in the United States in 1996–1997 respiratory season. The Laboratory Investigator Group. *Diagn. Microbiol. Infect. Dis.,* **1997,** *29*:249–257.

Tolman, K.G. Nitrofurantoin and chronic active hepatitis. *Ann. Intern. Med.,* **1980,** *92*:119–120.

Voogd, C.E., Schot, C.S., van Leeuwen, W.J., and van Klingeren, B. Monitoring of antibiotic resistance in shigellae isolated in The Netherlands 1984–1989. *Eur. J. Clin. Microbiol. Infect. Dis.,* **1992,** *11*:164–167.

Weidner, W., Schiefer, H.G., and Dalhoff, A. Treatment of chronic bacterial prostatitis with ciprofloxacin. Results of a one-year follow-up study. *Am. J. Med.,* **1987,** *82*:280–283.

Wong, C.S., Jelacic, S., Habeeb., R.L., Watkins, S.L., Tarr, P.L. The risk of the hemolytic-uremic syndrome after antibiotic treatment of *Escherichia coli* O157:H7. *N. Engl. J. Med.,* **2000,** *342*:1930–1936.

Woods, D.D. Relation of *p*-aminobenzoic acid to mechanism of action of sulphanilamide. *Br. J. Exp. Pathol.,* **1940,** *21*:74–90.

Wortmann, G.W., and Bennett, S.P. Fatal meningitis due to levofloxacin-resistant *Streptococcus pneumoniae. Clin. Infect. Dis.,* **1999,** *29*:1599–1600.

Yu, V.L. *Legionella pneumophila* (Legionnaires' disease). In, *Mandell, Douglas, and Bennett's Principles and Practice of Infectious Diseases,* 5th ed. (Mandell, G.L., Bennett, J.E., and Dolin, R., eds.) Churchill Livingstone, Inc., Philadelphia, **2000,** pp. 2424–2435.

MONOGRAPHS AND REVIEWS

Alangaden, G.J., and Lerner, S.A. The clinical use of fluoroquinolones for the treatment of mycobacterial diseases. *Clin. Infect. Dis.,* **1997,** *25*:1213–1221.

Andriole, V.T. The future of the quinolones. *Drugs,* **1993,** *45(suppl 3)*:1–7.

Cozzarelli, N.R. DNA gyrase and the supercoiling of DNA. *Science,* **1980,** *207*:953–960.

Drlica, K., and Zhao, X. DNA gyrase, topoisomerase IV, and the 4-quinolones. *Microbiol. Mol. Biol. Rev.,* **1997,** *61*:377–392.

DuPont, H.L., and Ericsson, C.D. Prevention and treatment of traveler's diarrhea. *N. Engl. J. Med.,* **1993,** *328*:1821–1827.

Gallant, J.E., Moore, R.D., and Chaisson, R.E. Prophylaxis for opportunistic infections in patients with HIV infection. *Ann. Intern. Med.,* **1994,** *120*:932–944.

Gold, H.S., and Moellering, R.C., Jr. Antimicrobial-drug resistance. *N. Engl. J. Med.,* **1996,** *335*:1445–1453.

Hill, D.R., and Pearson, R.D. Health advice for international travel. *Ann. Intern. Med.,* **1988,** *108*:839–852.

Hooper, D.C. Quinolones. In, *Mandell, Douglas, and Bennett's Principles and Practice of Infectious Diseases,* 5th ed. (Mandell, G.L., Bennett, J.E., and Dolin, R., eds.) Churchill Livingstone, Inc., Philadelphia, **2000a,** pp. 404–423.

Hooper, D.C. Urinary tract agents: nitrofurantoin and methenamine. In, *Mandell, Douglas, and Bennett's Principles and Practice of Infectious Diseases,* 5th ed. (Mandell, G.L., Bennett, J.E., and Dolin, R., eds.) Churchill Livingstone, Inc., New York, **2000b,** pp. 423–428.

Hooper, D.C., and Wolfson, J.S. Fluoroquinolone antimicrobial agents. *N. Engl. J. Med.,* **1991,** *324*:384–394.

Lane, H.C., Laughon, B.E., Falloon, J., Kovacs, J.A., Davey, R.T., Jr., Polis, M.A., and Masur, H. N.I.H. conference. Recent advances in the management of AIDS-related opportunistic infections. *Ann. Intern. Med.,* **1994,** *120*:945–955.

Medical Letter. Gatifloxacin and noxifloxacin: two new fluoroquinolones. *Med. Lett. Drugs Ther.,* **2000,** *42*:15–17.

Montoya, J.G., and Remington, J.S. *Toxoplasma gondii.* In, *Mandell, Douglas, and Bennett's Principles and Practice of Infectious Diseases,* 5th ed. (Mandell, G.L., Bennett, J.E., and Dolin, R., eds.) Churchill Livingstone, Inc., Philadelphia, **2000,** pp. 2858–2888.

Stamm, W.E., and Hooton, T.M. Management of urinary tract infection in adults. *N. Engl. J. Med.,* **1993,** *329*:1328–1334.

Symposium. (Various authors.) Trimethoprim-sulfamethoxazole. *J. Infect. Dis.,* **1973,** *128*(*suppl*):425–816.

Toole, J.F., and Parrish, M.L. Nitrofurantoin polyneuropathy. *Neurology,* **1973,** *23*:554–559.

Zinner, S.H., and Mayer, K.H. Sulfonamides and trimethoprim. In, *Mandell, Douglas, and Bennett's Principles and Practice of Infectious Diseases,* 5th ed. (Mandell, G.L., Bennett, J.E., and Dolin, R., eds.) Churchill Livingstone, Inc., Philadelphia, **2000,** pp. 394–404.

ANTIMICROBIAL AGENTS
(Continued)

Penicillins, Cephalosporins, and Other
β-Lactam Antibiotics

William A. Petri, Jr.

β-Lactam antibiotics are useful and frequently prescribed antibiotics that share a common structure and mechanism of action—inhibition of synthesis of the bacterial peptidoglycan cell wall. Important classes of penicillins include penicillins G and V, which are highly active against susceptible gram-positive cocci; penicillinase-resistant penicillins such as nafcillin, which are active against penicillinase-producing Staphylococcus aureus; *ampicillin and other agents with an improved gram-negative spectrum; and extended-spectrum penicillins with activity against* Pseudomonas aeruginosa, *such as ticarcillin and piperacillin.*

The cephalosporin antibiotics are classified by generation, with the first-generation agents having gram-positive and modest gram-negative activity; the second generation having somewhat better activity against gram negatives and including some agents with antianaerobe activity; the third generation with activity against gram-positive organisms and much more activity against the Enterobacteriaceae, with a subset active against P. aeruginosa; *and the fourth generation with a spectrum similar to the third, but having increased stability to hydrolysis by β-lactamases.*

β-Lactamase inhibitors such as clavulanate are used to extend the spectrum of penicillins against β-lactamase–producing organisms. Carbapenems have the broadest antimicrobial spectrum of any antibiotic, while the monobactams have a gram-negative spectrum resembling that of the aminoglycosides.

Bacterial resistance against the β-lactam antibiotics continues to increase at a dramatic rate. Mechanisms of resistance include not only production of β-lactamases that destroy the antibiotics but also alterations in penicillin-binding proteins and decreased entry and active efflux of the antibiotic.

THE PENICILLINS

The penicillins constitute one of the most important groups of antibiotics. Although numerous other antimicrobial agents have been produced since the first penicillin became available, these still are widely used, major antibiotics, and new derivatives of the basic penicillin nucleus still are being produced. Many of these have unique advantages, such that members of this group of antibiotics are presently the drugs of choice for a large number of infectious diseases.

History. The history of the brilliant research that led to the discovery and development of penicillin has been recorded by the chief participants. (*See* Fleming, 1946; Florey, 1946, 1949; Abraham, 1949; Chain, 1954.) In 1928, while studying *Staphylococcus* variants in the laboratory at St. Mary's Hospital in London, Alexander Fleming observed that a mold contaminating one of his cultures caused the bacteria in its vicinity to undergo lysis. Broth in which the fungus was grown was markedly inhibitory for many microorganisms. Because the mold belonged to the genus *Penicillium*, Fleming named the antibacterial substance *penicillin*.

A decade later, penicillin was developed as a systemic therapeutic agent by the concerted research of a group of investigators at Oxford University headed by Florey, Chain, and Abraham. By May 1940, the crude material then available was found to produce dramatic therapeutic effects when administered parenterally to mice with experimentally produced streptococcal infections. Despite great obstacles to its laboratory production, enough penicillin was accumulated by 1941 to conduct therapeutic trials in several patients desperately ill with staphylococcal and streptococcal infections refractory to all other therapy. At this stage, the crude, amorphous penicillin was only about 10% pure, and it required nearly 100 liters of the broth in which the mold had been grown to obtain enough of the antibiotic to treat one patient for 24 hours. Herrell (1945) records that bedpans actually were used by the Oxford group for growing cultures of *Penicillium notatum*. Case 1 in the 1941 report from Oxford was that of a policeman who was suffering from a severe mixed staphylococcal and streptococcal infection. He was treated with penicillin, some of which had been recovered from the urine of other patients who had been given the drug. It is said that an Oxford professor referred to penicillin as a remarkable substance, grown in bedpans and purified by passage through the Oxford Police Force.

A vast research program soon was initiated in the United States. During 1942, 122 million units of penicillin were made available, and the first clinical trials were conducted at Yale University and the Mayo Clinic, with dramatic results. By the spring of 1943, 200 patients had been treated with the drug. The results were so impressive that the surgeon general of the U.S. Army authorized trial of the antibiotic in a military hospital. Soon thereafter, penicillin was adopted throughout the medical services of the U.S. Armed Forces.

The deep-fermentation procedure for the biosynthesis of penicillin marked a crucial advance in the large-scale production of the antibiotic. From a total production of a few hundred million units a month in the early days, the quantity manufactured rose to over 200 trillion units (nearly 150 tons) by 1950. The first marketable penicillin cost several dollars per 100,000 units; today, the same dose costs only a few cents.

Chemistry. The basic structure of the penicillins, as shown in Figure 45–1, consists of a thiazolidine ring (A) connected to a β-lactam ring (B), to which is attached a side chain (R). The penicillin nucleus itself is the chief structural requirement for biological activity; metabolic transformation or chemical alteration of this portion of the molecule causes loss of all significant

antibacterial activity. The side chain (*see* Table 45–1) determines many of the antibacterial and pharmacological characteristics of a particular type of penicillin. Several natural penicillins can be produced, depending on the chemical composition of the fermentation medium used to culture *Penicillium*. Penicillin G (benzylpenicillin) has the greatest antimicrobial activity of these and is the only natural penicillin used clinically.

Semisynthetic Penicillins. The discovery that 6-aminopenicillanic acid could be obtained from cultures of *Penicillium chrysogenum* that were depleted of side-chain precursors led to the development of the semisynthetic penicillins. Side chains can be added that alter the susceptibility of the resultant compounds to inactivating enzymes (β-lactamases) and that change the antibacterial activity and the pharmacological properties of the drug. 6-Aminopenicillanic acid is now produced in large quantities with the aid of an amidase from *P. chrysogenum* (Figure 45–1). This enzyme splits the peptide linkage by which the side chain of penicillin is joined to 6-aminopenicillanic acid.

Unitage of Penicillin. The international unit of penicillin is the specific penicillin activity contained in 0.6 μg of the crystalline sodium salt of penicillin G. One milligram of pure penicillin G sodium thus equals 1667 U; 1.0 mg of pure penicillin G potassium represents 1595 U. The dosage and the antibacterial potency of the semisynthetic penicillins are expressed in terms of weight.

Mechanism of Action of the Penicillins and Cephalosporins. The β-lactam antibiotics can kill susceptible bacteria. Although knowledge of the mechanism of this action is incomplete, numerous researchers have supplied information that allows understanding of the basic phenomenon (*see* Tomasz, 1986; Ghuysen, 1991; Bayles, 2000).

The cell walls of bacteria are essential for their normal growth and development. Peptidoglycan is a heteropolymeric component of the cell wall that provides rigid mechanical stability by virtue of its highly cross-linked latticework structure (Figure 45–2). In gram-positive microorganisms, the cell wall is 50 to 100 molecules thick, but it is only 1 or 2 molecules thick

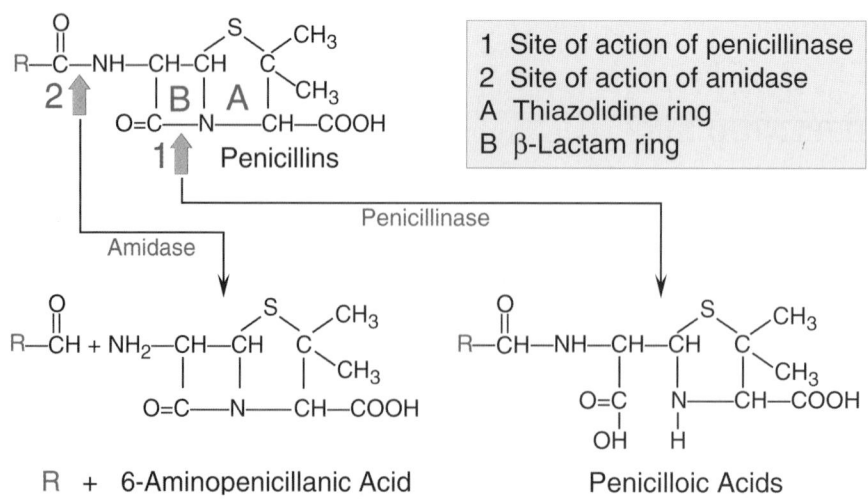

1 Site of action of penicillinase
2 Site of action of amidase
A Thiazolidine ring
B β-Lactam ring

Figure 45–1. Structure of penicillins and products of their enzymatic hydrolysis.

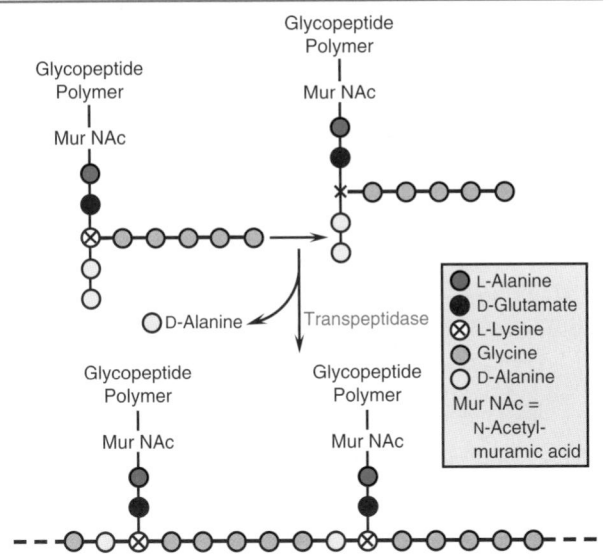

*Figure 45–2. The transpeptidase reaction in **Staphylococcus aureus** that is inhibited by penicillins and cephalosporins.*

in gram-negative bacteria (Figure 45–3). The peptidoglycan is composed of glycan chains, which are linear strands of two alternating amino sugars (N-acetylglucosamine and N-acetylmuramic acid) that are cross-linked by peptide chains.

The biosynthesis of the peptidoglycan involves about 30 bacterial enzymes and may be considered in three stages. The first stage, precursor formation, takes place in the cytoplasm. The product, uridine diphosphate (UDP)-acetylmuramyl-penta-

peptide, called a "Park nucleotide" after its discoverer (Park and Strominger, 1957), accumulates in cells when subsequent synthetic stages are inhibited. The last reaction in the synthesis of this compound is the addition of a dipeptide, D-alanyl-D-alanine. Synthesis of the dipeptide involves prior racemization of L-alanine and condensation catalyzed by D-alanyl-D-alanine synthetase. D-Cycloserine is a structural analog of D-alanine and acts as a competitive inhibitor of both the racemase and the synthetase (*see* Chapter 48).

During reactions of the second stage, UDP-acetylmuramyl-pentapeptide and UDP-acetylglucosamine are linked (with the release of the uridine nucleotides) to form a long polymer.

The third and final stage involves the completion of the cross-link. This is accomplished by a transpeptidation reaction that occurs outside the cell membrane. The transpeptidase itself is membrane-bound. The terminal glycine residue of the pentaglycine bridge is linked to the fourth residue of the pentapeptide (D-alanine), releasing the fifth residue (also D-alanine) (Figure 45–2). It is this last step in peptidoglycan synthesis that is inhibited by the β-lactam antibiotics and glycopeptide antibiotics such as vancomycin (by a different mechanism than the β-lactams; *see* Chapter 46). Stereomodels reveal that the conformation of penicillin is very similar to that of D-alanyl-D-alanine (Waxman *et al.,* 1980; Kelly *et al.,* 1982). The transpeptidase probably is acylated by penicillin; that is, penicilloyl enzyme apparently is formed, with cleavage of the —CO—N— bond of the β-lactam ring.

Although inhibition of the transpeptidase described above is demonstrably important, there are additional, related targets for the actions of penicillins and cephalosporins; these are collectively termed *penicillin-binding proteins* (PBPs; Spratt, 1980; Ghuysen, 1991). All bacteria have several such entities; for example, *S. aureus* has four PBPs, while *Escherichia coli* has at least seven. The PBPs vary in their affinities for different

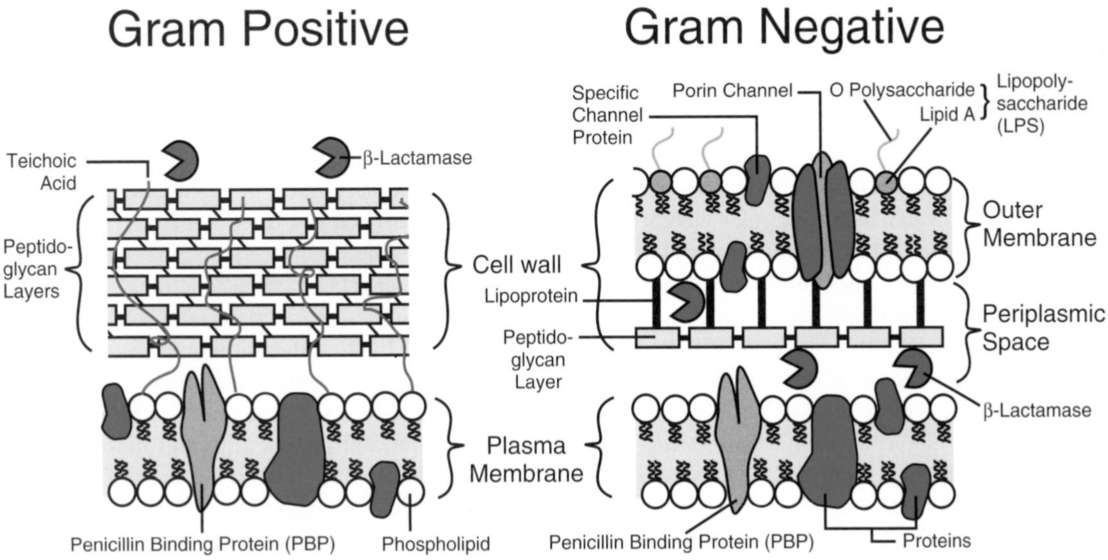

Gram Positive   Gram Negative

Figure 45–3. Comparison of the structure and composition of gram-positive and gram-negative cell walls.

(Adapted from Tortora *et al.,* 1989, with permission.)

β-lactam antibiotics, although the interactions eventually become covalent. The higher-molecular-weight PBPs of *E. coli* (PBP 1a and 1b) include the transpeptidases responsible for synthesis of the peptidoglycan. Other PBPs in *E. coli* include those that are necessary for maintenance of the rodlike shape of the bacterium and for septum formation at division. Inhibition of the transpeptidases causes spheroplast formation and rapid lysis. However, inhibition of the activities of other PBPs may cause delayed lysis (PBP 2) or the production of long, filamentous forms of the bacterium (PBP 3). The lethality of penicillin for bacteria appears to involve both lytic and nonlytic mechanisms. Penicillin's disruption of the balance between PBP-mediated peptidoglycan assembly and murein hydrolase activity results in autolysis. Nonlytic killing by penicillin may involve holin-like proteins in the bacterial membrane that collapse the membrane potential (Bayles, 2000).

Mechanisms of Bacterial Resistance to Penicillins and Cephalosporins.

Although most or all bacteria contain PBPs, β-lactam antibiotics cannot kill or even inhibit all bacteria, and various mechanisms of bacterial resistance to these agents are operative. The microorganism may be intrinsically resistant because of structural differences in the PBPs that are the targets of these drugs. Furthermore, it is possible for a sensitive strain to acquire resistance of this type by the development of high-molecular-weight PBPs that have decreased affinity for the antibiotic. Because the β-lactam antibiotics inhibit many different PBPs in a single bacterium, the affinity for β-lactam antibiotics of several PBPs must decrease for the organism to be resistant. Altered PBPs with decreased affinity for β-lactam antibiotics are acquired by homologous recombination between PBP genes of different bacterial species. Four of the five high-molecular-weight PBPs of the most highly penicillin-resistant *Streptococcus pneumoniae* isolates have decreased affinity for β-lactam antibiotics as a result of interspecies homologous recombination events (Figure 45–4). In contrast, isolates with high-level resistance to third-generation cephalosporins contain alterations of only two of the five high-molecular-weight PBPs, as the other PBPs have inherently low affinity for the third-generation cephalosporins. Penicillin resistance in *Streptococcus sanguis* and other *viridans* streptococci apparently emerged as a result of replacement of its PBPs with resistant PBPs from *S. pneumoniae* (Carratalá *et al.*, 1995). Methicillin-resistant *S. aureus* are resistant *via* acquisition of an additional high-molecular-weight PBP (*via* a transposon from an unknown organism) with a very low affinity for all β-lactam antibiotics. The gene encoding this new PBP also is present in and responsible for methicillin resistance in the coagulase-negative staphylococci (Spratt, 1994).

Other instances of bacterial resistance to the β-lactam antibiotics are caused by the inability of the agent to pene-

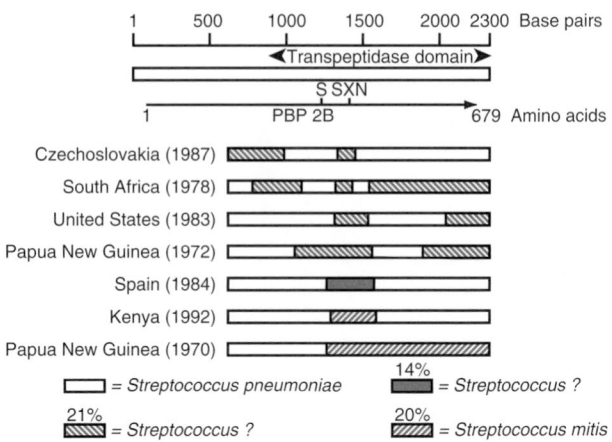

Figure 45–4. Mosaic PBP 2B genes in penicillin-resistant pneumococci.

The divergent regions in the PBP 2B genes of seven resistant pneumococci from different countries are shown. These regions have been introduced from at least three sources, one of which appears to be *Streptococcus mitis*. The approximate percent sequence divergence of the divergent regions from the PBP 2B genes of susceptible pneumococci is shown. (Reprinted from Spratt, 1994, with permission.)

trate to its site of action or by energy-dependent efflux systems for pumping the antibiotic out of the bacteria (Jacoby, 1994; Nikaido, 1998) (Figure 45–5). In gram-positive bacteria, the peptidoglycan polymer is very near the cell surface (Figure 45–3). Only surface macromolecules (capsule) are external to the peptidoglycan. The small β-lactam antibiotic molecules can penetrate easily to the outer layer of the cytoplasmic membrane and the PBPs, where the final stages of the synthesis of the peptidoglycan take place. The situation is different with gram-negative bacteria. Their surface structure is more complex, and the inner membrane (which is analogous to the cytoplasmic membrane of gram-positive bacteria) is covered by the outer membrane, lipopolysaccharide, and capsule (Figure 45–3). The outer membrane functions as an impenetrable barrier for some antibiotics (*see* Nakae, 1986). However, some small, hydrophilic antibiotics diffuse through aqueous channels in the outer membrane that are formed by proteins called *porins*. Broader-spectrum penicillins, such as ampicillin and amoxicillin, and most of the cephalosporins diffuse through the pores in the *E. coli* outer membrane significantly more rapidly than can penicillin G. The number and size of pores in the outer membrane are variable among different gram-negative bacteria. An extreme example is *P. aeruginosa,* which is intrinsically resistant to a wide variety of antibiotics by virtue of lacking the classical high-permeability porins (Nikaido, 1994). Active

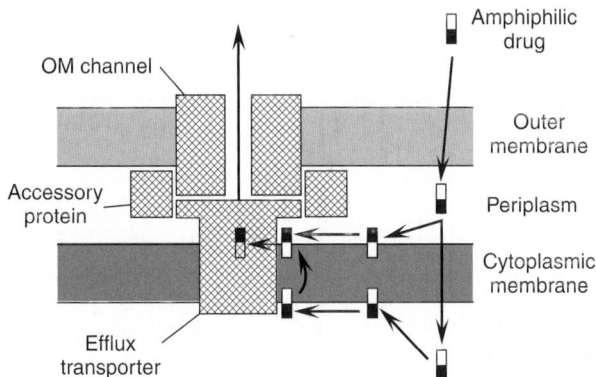

Figure 45–5. Antibiotic efflux pumps of gram negative bacteria.

Multidrug efflux pumps traverse both the inner and outer membranes of gram negative bacteria. The pumps are composed of a minimum of three proteins, and are energized by the proton motive force. Increased expression of these pumps is an important cause of antibiotic resistance (reprinted with permission from Nikaido, 1998).

efflux pumps serve as another mechanism of resistance, removing the antibiotic from its site of action before it can act (Nikaido, 1998). This is an important mechanism of β-lactam resistance in *P. aeruginosa, E. coli,* and *Neisseria gonorrhoeae.*

Bacteria can destroy β-lactam antibiotics enzymatically. While amidohydrolases may be present, these enzymes are relatively inactive and do not protect the bacteria. β-Lactamases, however, are capable of inactivating certain of these antibiotics and may be present in large quantities (*see* Figures 45–1 and 45–3). Different microorganisms elaborate a number of distinct β-lactamases, although most bacteria produce only one form of the enzyme. The substrate specificities of some of these enzymes are relatively narrow, and these often are described as either penicillinases or cephalosporinases. Other "broad-spectrum" enzymes are less discriminant and can hydrolyze a variety of β-lactam antibiotics. Individual penicillins and cephalosporins vary in their susceptibility to these enzymes.

In general, gram-positive bacteria produce a large amount of β-lactamase, which is secreted extracellularly (Figure 45–3). Most of these enzymes are penicillinases. The information for staphylococcal penicillinase is encoded in a plasmid, and this may be transferred by bacteriophage to other bacteria. The enzyme is inducible by substrates, and 1% of the dry weight of the bacterium can be penicillinase. In gram-negative bacteria, β-lactamases are found in relatively small amounts, but are located in the periplasmic space between the inner and outer cell

membranes (Figure 45–3). Since the enzymes of cell-wall synthesis are on the outer surface of the inner membrane, these β-lactamases are strategically located for maximal protection of the microbe. β-Lactamases of gram-negative bacteria are encoded either in chromosomes or in plasmids, and they may be constitutive or inducible. The plasmids can be transferred between bacteria by conjugation. These enzymes may hydrolyze penicillins, cephalosporins, or both (*see* Davies, 1994). However, there is an inconsistent correlation between the susceptibility of an antibiotic to inactivation by β-lactamase and the ability of that antibiotic to kill the microorganism. For example, penicillins that are hydrolyzed by β-lactamase (*e.g.,* carbenicillin) are able to kill certain strains of β-lactamase–producing gram-negative microbes.

Other Factors That Influence the Activity of β-Lactam Antibiotics. The density of the bacterial population and the age of an infection influence the activity of β-lactam antibiotics. The drugs may be several thousand times more potent when tested against small bacterial inocula than when tested against a dense culture. Many factors are involved. Among these are the greater number of relatively resistant microorganisms in a large population, the amount of β-lactamase produced, and the phase of growth of the culture. The clinical significance of this effect of inoculum size is uncertain. The intensity and the duration of penicillin therapy needed to abort or cure experimental infections in animals increase with the duration of the infection. The primary reason is that the bacteria are no longer multiplying as rapidly as they do in a fresh infection. These antibiotics are most active against bacteria in the logarithmic phase of growth and have little effect on microorganisms in the stationary phase, when there is no need to synthesize components of the cell wall.

The presence of proteins and other constituents of pus, low pH, or low oxygen tension does not appreciably decrease the ability of β-lactam antibiotics to kill bacteria. However, bacteria that survive inside viable cells of the host are protected from the action of the β-lactam antibiotics.

Classification of the Penicillins and Summary of Their Pharmacological Properties

It is useful to classify the penicillins according to their spectra of antimicrobial activity (*see* Table 45–1; Chambers, 2000).

1. *Penicillin G* and its close congener *penicillin V* are highly active against sensitive strains of gram-positive cocci, but they are readily hydrolyzed by penicillinase. Thus, they are ineffective against most strains of *S. aureus.*

2. The penicillinase-resistant penicillins (*methicillin, nafcillin, oxacillin, cloxacillin,* and *dicloxacillin*) have less

Table 45–1
Chemical Structures and Major Properties of Various Penicillins

SIDE CHAIN*	NONPROPRIETARY NAME	MAJOR PROPERTIES		
		Absorption After Oral Administration	*Resistance To Penicillinase*	*Useful Antimicrobial Spectrum*
⬡–CH₂–	Penicillin G	Variable (poor)	No	*Streptococcus* species,** Enterococci,** *Listeria*, *Neisseria meningitidis*, many anaerobes (not *Bacteroides fragilis*),*** spirochetes, *Actinomyces*, *Erysipelothrix* spp., *Pasteurella multocida****
⬡–OCH₂–	Penicillin V	Good	No	
(structure with OCH₃ groups)	Methicillin	Poor (not given orally)	Yes	
(isoxazolyl structure with R₁, R₂, CH₃)	Oxacillin (R₁ = R₂ = H) Cloxacillin (R₁ = Cl; R₂ = H) Dicloxacillin (R₁ = R₂ = Cl)	Good	Yes	Indicated only for non-methicillin-resistant strains of *Staphylococcus aureus* and *Staphylococcus epidermidis*. Compared to other penicillins, these penicillinase-resistant penicillins lack activity against *Listeria monocytogenes* and *Enterococcus* spp.
(naphthalene structure with OC₂H₅)	Nafcillin	Variable	Yes	
R–⬡–CH– with NH₂	Ampicillin† (R = H) Amoxicillin (R = OH)	Good Excellent	No	Extends spectrum of penicillin to include sensitive strains of Enterobacteriaceae*** *Escherichia coli*, *Proteus mirabilis*, *Salmonella*, *Shigella*, *Haemophilus influenzae*,*** and *Helicobacter pylori*.

Table 45–1 Chemical Structures and Major Properties of Various Penicillins *(Continued)*

SIDE CHAIN*	NONPROPRIETARY NAME	MAJOR PROPERTIES		
		Absorption After Oral Administration	*Resistance To Penicillinase*	*Useful Antimicrobial Spectrum*
				Superior to penicillin for treatment of *Listeria monocytogenes* and sensitive enterococci. Amoxicillin most active of all oral β-lactams against penicillin-resistant *Streptococcus pneumoniae*.
	Carbenicillin (R = H) Carbenicillin indanyl (R = 5-indanol)	Poor (not given orally) Good	No	Less active than ampicillin against *Streptococcus* species, *Enterococcus faecalis*, *Klebsiella*, and *Listeria monocytogenes*. Activity against *Pseudomonas aeruginosa* is inferior to that of mezlocillin and piperacillin
	Ticarcillin	Poor (not given orally)	No	
	Mezlocillin	Poor (not given orally)	No	
	Piperacillin	Poor (not given orally)	No	Extends spectrum of ampicillin to include *Pseudomonas aeruginosa*,‡ Enterobacteriaceae,*** Bacteroides species***

*Equivalent to R in Figure 45-1.

**Many strains are resistant due to altered penicillin-binding proteins.

***Many strains are resistant due to production of β-lactamases.

†There are other congeners of ampicillin; *see* the text.

‡ Some strains are resistant due to decreased entry or active efflux.

potent antimicrobial activity against microorganisms that are sensitive to penicillin G, but they are effective against penicillinase-producing *S. aureus* and *S. epidermidis* that are not methicillin-resistant.

3. *Ampicillin, amoxicillin, bacampicillin,* and others make up a group of penicillins whose antimicrobial activity is extended to include such gram-negative microorganisms as *Haemophilus influenzae, E. coli,* and *Proteus mirabilis.* Unfortunately, these drugs and the others listed below are hydrolyzed readily by broad-spectrum β-lactamases that are found with increasing frequency in clinical isolates of these gram-negative bacteria.

4. The antimicrobial activity of *carbenicillin,* its indanyl ester (carbenicillin indanyl), and *ticarcillin* is extended to include *Pseudomonas, Enterobacter,* and *Proteus* species. These agents are inferior to ampicillin against gram-positive cocci and *Listeria monocytogenes.*

5. *Mezlocillin, azlocillin,* and *piperacillin* have useful antimicrobial activity against *Pseudomonas, Klebsiella,* and certain other gram-negative microorganisms. Piperacillin retains the excellent activity of ampicillin against gram-positive cocci and *L. monocytogenes.*

Although the pharmacological properties of the individual drugs are discussed in detail below, certain generalizations are useful. Following absorption of orally administered penicillins, these agents are widely distributed throughout the body. Therapeutic concentrations of penicillins are achieved readily in tissues and in secretions such as joint fluid, pleural fluid, pericardial fluid, and bile. However, only low concentrations of these drugs are found in prostatic secretions, brain tissue, and intraocular fluid, and penicillins do not penetrate living phagocytic cells to a significant extent. Concentrations of penicillins in cerebrospinal fluid (CSF) are variable, but are less than 1% of those in plasma when the meninges are normal. When there is inflammation, concentrations in CSF may increase to as much as 5% of the plasma value. Penicillins are eliminated rapidly, particularly by glomerular filtration and renal tubular secretion, such that their half-lives in the body are short; values of 30 to 90 minutes are typical. Concentrations of these drugs in urine thus are high.

Penicillin G and Penicillin V

Antimicrobial Activity. The antimicrobial spectra of penicillin G *(benzylpenicillin)* and penicillin V (the phenoxymethyl derivative) are very similar for aerobic gram-positive microorganisms. However, penicillin G is five to ten times more active against *Neisseria* species sensitive to penicillins and against certain anaerobes.

Penicillin G has activity against a variety of species of gram-positive and gram-negative cocci, although many bacteria previously sensitive to the agent are now resistant. Most streptococci (but not enterococci) are very susceptible to the drug; concentrations of less than 0.01 μg/ml usually are effective. However, penicillin-resistant *viridans* streptococci (Carratalá *et al.,* 1995) and *S. pneumoniae* are becoming more common. During 1997, 13.6% of *S. pneumoniae* sterile-site isolates had high-level [minimal inhibitory concentration (MIC) ≥2.0 μg/ml)] and 11.4% of isolates had low-level (MIC ≥0.12 μg/ml) penicillin resistance, for a total of 25% of isolates (Centers for Disease Control and Prevention, 1999). Penicillin-resistant pneumococci are especially common in pediatric populations, such as children attending day care centers. Many penicillin-resistant pneumococci also are resistant to third-generation cephalosporins.

Whereas most strains of *S. aureus* were highly sensitive to similar concentrations of penicillin G when this agent was first employed therapeutically, more than 90% of strains of staphylococci isolated from individuals inside or outside of hospitals are now resistant to penicillin G. Most strains of *Staphylococcus epidermidis* also are resistant to penicillin. Unfortunately, penicillinase-producing strains of gonococci that are highly resistant to penicillin G have become widespread. With rare exceptions, meningococci are quite sensitive to penicillin G.

Although the vast majority of strains of *Corynebacterium diphtheriae* are sensitive to penicillin G, some are highly resistant. This also is true for *Bacillus anthracis.* Most anaerobic microorganisms, including *Clostridium* species, are highly sensitive. *Bacteroides fragilis* is an exception; many strains are now resistant because of elaboration of β-lactamase. Some strains of *Bacteroides melaninogenicus* also have acquired this trait. *Actinomyces israelii, Streptobacillus moniliformis, Pasteurella multocida,* and *L. monocytogenes* are inhibited by penicillin G. Most species of *Leptospira* are moderately susceptible to the drug. One of the most exquisitely sensitive microorganisms is *Treponema pallidum. Borrelia burgdorferi,* the organism responsible for Lyme disease, also is susceptible. None of the penicillins is effective against amoebae, plasmodia, rickettsiae, fungi, or viruses.

Absorption. *Oral Administration of Penicillin G.* About one-third of an orally administered dose of penicillin G is absorbed from the intestinal tract under favorable conditions. Gastric juice at pH 2 rapidly destroys the antibiotic. The decrease in gastric acid production with aging accounts for better absorption of penicillin G from the gastrointestinal tract of older individuals. Absorption is rapid, and maximal concentrations in blood are attained in 30 to 60 minutes. The peak value is approximately 0.5 U/ml (0.3 μg/ml) after an oral dose of 400,000 U (about 250 mg) in an adult. Ingestion of food may interfere with enteric absorption of all penicillins, perhaps by adsorption of the antibiotic onto food particles. Thus, oral penicillin G should be administered at least 30 minutes before a meal or 2 hours after. Despite the convenience of oral administration of penicillin G, this route should be used only in infections in which clinical experience has proven its efficacy.

Oral Administration of Penicillin V.   The virtue of penicillin V in comparison with penicillin G is that it is more stable in an acidic medium, and therefore is better absorbed from the gastrointestinal tract. On an equivalent oral-dose basis, penicillin V (K$^+$ salt PEN-VEE K, V-CILLIN K, others) yields plasma concentrations two to five times greater than those provided by penicillin G. The peak concentration in the blood of an adult after an oral dose of 500 mg is nearly 3 μg/ml. Once absorbed, penicillin V is distributed in the body and excreted by the kidney in a manner similar to that of penicillin G.

Parenteral Administration of Penicillin G.   After intramuscular injection, peak concentrations in plasma are reached within 15 to 30 minutes. This value declines rapidly, since the half-life of penicillin G is 30 minutes.

Many means for prolonging the sojourn of the antibiotic in the body and thereby reducing the frequency of injections have been explored. Probenecid blocks renal tubular secretion of penicillin, but it is rarely used for this purpose (*see* below). More commonly, repository preparations of penicillin G are employed. The two such compounds currently favored are *penicillin G procaine* (DURACILLIN, A.S., WYCILLIN, others) and *penicillin G benzathine* (BICILLIN L-A, PERMAPEN). Such agents release penicillin G slowly from the area in which they are injected and produce relatively low but persistent concentrations of antibiotic in the blood.

Penicillin G procaine suspension is an aqueous preparation of the crystalline salt that is only 0.4% soluble in water. Procaine combines with penicillin mol for mol; a dose of 300,000 U thus contains approximately 120 mg of procaine. When large doses of penicillin G procaine are given (*e.g.*, 4.8 million units), procaine may reach toxic concentrations in the plasma. If the patient is believed to be hypersensitive to procaine, 0.1 ml of 1% solution of procaine should be injected intradermally as a test. The anesthetic effect of the procaine accounts in part for the fact that injections of penicillin G procaine are virtually painless.

The injection of 300,000 U of penicillin G procaine produces a peak concentration in plasma of about 0.9 μg/ml within 1 to 3 hours; after 24 hours the concentration is reduced to 0.1 μg/ml, and by 48 hours it has fallen to 0.03 μg/ml. A larger dose (600,000 U) yields somewhat higher values that are maintained for as long as 4 to 5 days.

Penicillin G benzathine suspension is the aqueous suspension of the salt obtained by the combination of 1 mol of an ammonium base and 2 mol of penicillin G to yield *N,N'*-dibenzylethylenediamine dipenicillin G. The salt itself is only 0.02% soluble in water. The long persistence of penicillin in the blood after a suitable intramuscular dose reduces cost, need for repeated injections, and local trauma. The local anesthetic effect of penicillin G benzathine is comparable to that of penicillin G procaine.

Penicillin G benzathine is absorbed very slowly from intramuscular depots and produces the longest duration of detectable antibiotic of all the available repository penicillins. For example, in adults, a dose of 1.2 million units given intramuscularly produces a concentration in plasma of 0.09 μg/ml on the first, 0.02 μg/ml on the fourteenth, and 0.002 μg/ml on the thirty-second day after injection. The average duration of demonstrable antimicrobial activity in the plasma is about 26 days.

Distribution.   Penicillin G is distributed widely throughout the body, but the concentrations in various fluids and tissues differ widely. Its apparent volume of distribution is about 0.35 liter/kg. Approximately 60% of the penicillin G in plasma is reversibly bound to albumin. Significant amounts appear in liver, bile, kidney, semen, joint fluid, lymph, and intestine.

While probenecid markedly decreases the tubular secretion of the penicillins, this is not the only factor responsible for the elevated plasma concentrations of the antibiotic that follow its administration. Probenecid also produces a significant decrease in the apparent volume of distribution of the penicillins.

Cerebrospinal Fluid.   Penicillin does not readily enter the CSF when the meninges are normal. However, when the meninges are acutely inflamed, penicillin penetrates into the CSF more easily. Although the concentrations attained vary and are unpredictable, they are usually in the range of 5% of the value in plasma and are therapeutically effective against susceptible microorganisms.

Penicillin and other organic acids are secreted rapidly from the CSF into the bloodstream by an active transport process. Probenecid competitively inhibits this transport and thus elevates the concentration of penicillin in CSF. In uremia, other organic acids accumulate in the CSF and compete with penicillin for secretion; the drug occasionally reaches toxic concentrations in the brain and can produce convulsions.

Excretion.   Under normal conditions, penicillin G is rapidly eliminated from the body, mainly by the kidney but in small part in the bile and by other routes. Approximately 60% to 90% of an intramuscular dose of penicillin G in aqueous solution is eliminated in the urine, largely within the first hour after injection. The remainder is metabolized to penicilloic acid. The half-time for elimination of penicillin G is about 30 minutes in normal adults. Approximately 10% of the drug is eliminated by glomerular filtration and 90% by tubular secretion. Renal clearance approximates the total renal plasma flow. The maximal tubular secretory capacity for penicillin in the normal male adult is about 3 million units (1.8 g) per hour.

Clearance values are considerably lower in neonates and infants because of incomplete development of renal function; as a result, after doses proportionate to surface area, the persistence of penicillin in the blood is several times as long in premature infants as in children and adults. The half-life of the antibiotic in children less than 1 week old is 3 hours; by 14 days of age it is 1.4 hours. After renal function is fully established in young children, the rate of renal excretion of penicillin G is considerably more rapid than in adults.

Anuria increases the half-life of penicillin G from a normal value of 0.5 hour to about 10 hours. When renal function is impaired, 7% to 10% of the antibiotic may be inactivated each hour by the liver. Patients with renal shutdown who require high-dose therapy with penicillin can be treated adequately with 3 million units of aqueous penicillin G followed by 1.5 million units every 8 to 12 hours. The dose of the drug must be readjusted during dialysis and the period of progressive recovery of renal function. If, in addition to renal failure, hepatic insufficiency also is present, the half-life will be prolonged even further.

Therapeutic Uses.   *Pneumococcal Infections.* Penicillin G remains the agent of choice for the management of infections caused by sensitive strains of *S. pneumoniae.* However, strains of pneumococci resistant to usual doses of penicillin G are being more frequently isolated in several countries, including the United States (*see* Centers for Disease Control and Prevention, 1999; Fiore *et al.,* 2000).

Pneumococcal Pneumonia.   Until it is highly likely or established that the infecting isolate of pneumococcus is penicillin-sensitive, pneumococcal pneumonia should be treated with a third-generation cephalosporin or with vancomycin. For parenteral therapy of sensitive isolates of pneumococci, penicillin G or penicillin G procaine is favored. Although oral treatment with 500 mg of penicillin V given every 6 hours for treatment of pneumonia due to penicillin-sensitive isolates has been used with success in this disease, it cannot be recommended for routine initial use because of the existence of resistance. Therapy should be continued for 7 to 10 days, including 3 to 5 days after the patient's temperature has returned to normal.

Pneumococcal Meningitis.   Until it is established that the infecting pneumococcus is penicillin-sensitive, pneumococcal meningitis should be treated with a combination of vancomycin and a third-generation cephalosporin (John, 1994; Catalan *et al.,* 1994). Some authorities advocate a third-generation cephalosporin plus rifampin. Prior to the appearance of penicillin resistance, penicillin treatment reduced the death rate in this disease from nearly 100% to about 25%. The recommended therapy is 20 million to 24 million units of penicillin G daily by constant intravenous infusion or divided into boluses given every 2 to 3 hours. The usual duration of therapy is 14 days.

Streptococcal Infections.   *Streptococcal Pharyngitis (Including Scarlet Fever).*   This is the most common disease produced by *Streptococcus pyogenes* (group A β-hemolytic streptococcus). Penicillin-resistant isolates have yet to be observed for *S. pyogenes* (Tomasz, 1994). The preferred oral therapy is with penicillin V, 500 mg every 6 hours for 10 days. Equally good results

are produced by the administration of 600,000 U of penicillin G procaine intramuscularly, once daily for 10 days, or by a single injection of 1.2 million units of penicillin G benzathine. Parenteral therapy is preferred if there are questions of patient compliance. Penicillin therapy of streptococcal pharyngitis reduces the risk of subsequent acute rheumatic fever; however, current evidence suggests that the incidence of glomerulonephritis that follows streptococcal infections is not reduced to a significant degree by treatment with penicillin.

Streptococcal Pneumonia, Arthritis, Meningitis, and Endocarditis.   While uncommon, these conditions should be treated with penicillin G when they are caused by *S. pyogenes;* daily doses of 12 million to 20 million units are administered intravenously for 2 to 4 weeks. Such treatment of endocarditis should be continued for a full 4 weeks.

Infections Caused by Other Streptococci.   The *viridans* streptococci are the most common cause of infectious endocarditis. These are nongroupable α-hemolytic microorganisms that are increasingly resistant to penicillin G (MIC < 0.1 μg/ml). Since enterococci may also be α-hemolytic and certain other α-hemolytic strains may be relatively resistant to penicillin, it is important to determine quantitative microbial sensitivities to penicillin G in patients with endocarditis. Patients with penicillin-sensitive *viridans* group streptococcal endocarditis can be treated successfully with 1.2 million units of procaine penicillin G, given four times daily for 2 weeks, or with daily doses of 12 million to 20 million units of intravenous penicillin G for 2 weeks, both regimens in combination with streptomycin, 500 mg intramuscularly every 12 hours or gentamicin (1 mg/kg every 8 hours). Some physicians prefer a 4-week course of treatment with penicillin G alone.

Enterococcal endocarditis is one of the few diseases that is optimally treated with two antibiotics. The recommended therapy for penicillin- and aminoglycoside-sensitive enterococcal endocarditis is 20 million units of penicillin G or 12 grams of ampicillin daily, administered intravenously in combination with an aminoglycoside. Therapy usually should be continued for 6 weeks, but selected patients with a short duration of illness (less than 3 months) have been treated successfully in 4 weeks (Wilson *et al.,* 1984).

Infections with Anaerobes.   Many anaerobic infections are caused by mixtures of microorganisms. The majority are sensitive to penicillin G. An exception is the *B. fragilis* group, in which up to 75% of strains may be resistant to high concentrations of this antibiotic. Pulmonary and periodontal infections (with the exception of β-lactamase-producing *Prevotella melaninogenica*) usually respond well to penicillin G, although a multicenter study indicated that clindamycin is more effective than penicillin for therapy of lung abscess (Levison *et al.,* 1983). Mild-to-moderate infections at these sites may be treated with oral medication (either penicillin G or penicillin V, 400,000 U four times daily). More severe infections should be treated with 12 million to 20 million units of penicillin G intravenously. Brain abscesses also frequently contain several species of anaerobes, and most authorities prefer to treat such disease with high doses of penicillin G (20 million units per day) plus metronidazole or chloramphenicol. Some physicians add a third-generation cephalosporin for activity against aerobic gram-negative bacilli.

Staphylococcal Infections.   The vast majority of staphylococcal infections are caused by microorganisms that produce penicillinase. A patient with a staphylococcal infection who requires treatment with an antibiotic should receive one of the penicillinase-resistant penicillins—for example, nafcillin, oxacillin, or methicillin.

So-called methicillin-resistant staphylococci are resistant to penicillin G, all of the penicillinase-resistant penicillins, and the cephalosporins. Isolates occasionally may appear to be sensitive to various cephalosporins *in vitro,* but resistant populations arise during therapy and lead to failure (Chambers *et al.,* 1984). Vancomycin is the drug of choice for infections caused by these bacteria, although reduced susceptibility to vancomycin has now been observed (Centers for Disease Control and Prevention, 1997). Ciprofloxacin also may be effective, although prolonged therapy often leads to the emergence of ciprofloxacin-resistant *S. aureus.*

Meningococcal Infections. Penicillin G remains the drug of choice for meningococcal disease. Patients should be treated with high doses of penicillin given intravenously, as described for pneumococcal meningitis. Penicillin-resistant strains of *N. meningitides* have been reported in Britain and Spain but are infrequent at present. In 1997, 97% of *N. meningitides* isolates analyzed from the United States were penicillin-sensitive (Rosenstein *et al.,* 2000). The occurrence of penicillin-resistant strains should be considered in patients who are slow to respond to treatment (Sprott *et al.,* 1988, Mendelman *et al.,* 1988). It should be remembered that penicillin G does not eliminate the meningococcal carrier state, and its administration thus is ineffective as a prophylactic measure.

Gonococcal Infections. Gonococci gradually have become more resistant to penicillin G, and penicillins are no longer the therapy of choice, unless it is known that gonococcal strains in a particular geographical area are susceptible. Uncomplicated gonococcal urethritis is the most common infection, and a single intramuscular injection of 250 mg of ceftriaxone is the recommended treatment (Sparling and Handsfield, 2000).

Gonococcal arthritis, disseminated gonococcal infections with skin lesions, and gonococcemia should be treated with ceftriaxone, 1 g daily given either intramuscularly or intravenously for 7 to 10 days. Ophthalmia neonatorum also should be treated with ceftriaxone for 7 to 10 days (25 to 50 mg/kg per day intramuscularly or intravenously).

Syphilis. Therapy of syphilis with penicillin G is highly effective. Primary, secondary, and latent syphilis of less than 1 year's duration may be treated with penicillin G procaine (2.4 million units per day intramuscularly) plus probenecid (1.0 g per day orally) for 10 days or with 1 to 3 weekly intramuscular doses of 2.4 million units of penicillin G benzathine (3 doses in patients with HIV). Patients with late latent syphilis, neurosyphilis, or cardiovascular syphilis may be treated with a variety of regimens. Since these diseases are potentially lethal and their progression can be halted (but not reversed), intensive therapy with 20 million units of penicillin G daily for 10 days is recommended.

Infants with congenital syphilis discovered at birth or during the postnatal period should be treated for at least 10 days with 50,000 U/kg daily of aqueous penicillin G in two divided doses or 50,000 U/kg of procaine penicillin G in a single daily dose (*see* Tramont, 2000).

The majority (70% to 90%) of patients with secondary syphilis develop the Jarisch-Herxheimer reaction. This also may be seen in patients with other forms of syphilis. Several hours after the first injection of penicillin, chills, fever, headache,

myalgias, and arthralgias may develop. The syphilitic cutaneous lesions may become more prominent, edematous, and brilliant in color. Manifestations usually persist for a few hours, and the rash begins to fade within 48 hours. It does not recur with the second or subsequent injections of penicillin. This reaction is thought to be due to release of spirochetal antigens, with subsequent host reactions to the products. Aspirin gives symptomatic relief, and therapy with penicillin should not be discontinued.

Actinomycosis. Penicillin G is the agent of choice for the treatment of all forms of actinomycosis. The dose should be 12 million to 20 million units of penicillin G intravenously per day for 6 weeks. Some physicians continue therapy for 2 to 3 months with oral penicillin V (500 mg four times daily). Surgical drainage or excision of the lesion may be necessary before cure is accomplished.

Diphtheria. There is no evidence that penicillin or any other antibiotic alters the incidence of complications or the outcome of diphtheria; specific antitoxin is the only effective treatment. However, penicillin G eliminates the carrier state. The parenteral administration of 2 to 3 million units per day in divided doses for 10 to 12 days eliminates the diphtheria bacilli from the pharynx and other sites in practically 100% of cases. A single daily injection of penicillin G procaine for the same period produces about the same results.

Anthrax. Penicillin G is the agent of choice in the treatment of all clinical forms of anthrax. However, strains of *Bacillus anthracis* resistant to this antibiotic have been recovered from human infections. When penicillin G is used, the dose should be 12 million to 20 million units per day.

Clostridial Infections. Penicillin G is the agent of choice for gas gangrene; the dose is in the range of 12 million to 20 million units per day, given parenterally. Adequate debridement of the infected areas is essential. Antimicrobial drugs probably have no effect on the ultimate outcome of tetanus. Debridement and administration of human tetanus immune globulin may be indicated. Penicillin is administered, however, to eradicate the vegetative forms of the bacteria that may persist.

Fusospirochetal Infections. Gingivostomatitis, produced by the synergistic action of *Leptotrichia buccalis* and spirochetes that are present in the mouth, is readily treatable with penicillin. For simple "trench mouth," 500 mg of penicillin V given every 6 hours for several days is usually sufficient to clear the disease.

Rat-Bite Fever. The two microorganisms responsible for this infection, *Spirillum minor* in the Orient and *Streptobacillus moniliformis* in America and Europe, are sensitive to penicillin G, the therapeutic agent of choice. Since most cases due to *Streptobacillus* are complicated by bacteremia and, in many instances, by metastatic infections especially of the synovia and endocardium, the dose should be large; a daily dose of 12 million to 15 million units given parenterally for 3 to 4 weeks has been recommended.

Listeria *Infections.* Penicillin G or ampicillin with or without gentamicin are regarded as the drugs of choice in the management of infections due to *L. monocytogenes.* The recommended dose of penicillin G is 15 million to 20 million units parenterally per day for at least 2 weeks. When endocarditis is the problem, the dose is the same, but the duration of treatment should be no less than 4 weeks.

Lyme Disease. Although a tetracycline is the usual drug of choice for early disease, amoxicillin is effective; the dose is 500 mg three times daily for 21 days. Severe disease is treated with a third-generation cephalosporin or 20 million units of intravenous penicillin G daily for 14 days.

Erysipeloid.   The causative agent of this disease, *Erysipelothrix rhusiopathiae,* is sensitive to penicillin. The uncomplicated infection responds well to a single injection of 1.2 million units of penicillin G benzathine. When endocarditis is present, penicillin G, 12 million to 20 million units per day, has been found to be effective; therapy should be continued for 4 to 6 weeks.

Prophylactic Uses of the Penicillins.   Demonstration of the effectiveness of penicillin in eradicating microorganisms was quickly, and quite naturally, followed by attempts to prove that it also was effective in preventing infection in susceptible hosts. As a result, the antibiotic has been administered in almost every situation in which a risk of bacterial invasion has been present. As prophylaxis has been investigated under controlled conditions, it has become clear that penicillin is highly effective in some situations, useless and potentially dangerous in others, and of questionable value in still others (*see* Chapter 43).

Streptococcal Infections.   The administration of penicillin to individuals exposed to *Streptococcus pyogenes* affords protection from infection. The oral ingestion of 200,000 units of penicillin G or penicillin V twice a day or a single injection of 1.2 million units of penicillin G benzathine is effective. Indications for this type of prophylaxis include outbreaks of streptococcal disease in closed populations, such as boarding schools or military bases. Patients with extensive deep burns are at high risk of severe wound infections with *S. pyogenes;* several days of "low-dose" prophylaxis appears to be effective in reducing the incidence of this complication.

Recurrences of Rheumatic Fever.   The oral administration of 200,000 units of penicillin G or penicillin V every 12 hours produces a striking decrease in the incidence of recurrences of rheumatic fever in susceptible individuals. Because of the difficulties of compliance, parenteral administration is preferable, especially in children. The intramuscular injection of 1.2 million units of penicillin G benzathine once a month yields excellent results. In cases of hypersensitivity to penicillin, sulfisoxazole or sulfadiazine, 1 g twice a day for adults, also is effective; for children weighing under 27 kg, the dose is halved. Prophylaxis must be continued throughout the year. The duration of such treatment is an unsettled question. It has been suggested that prophylaxis should be continued for life, because instances of acute rheumatic fever have been observed in the fifth and sixth decades. However, the necessity for such prolonged prophylaxis has not been established and may be unnecessary for certain young adults judged to be low risk for recurrence (Berrios *et al.,* 1993).

Syphilis.   Prophylaxis for a contact with syphilis consists of a course of therapy as described for primary syphilis. A serological test for syphilis should be performed at monthly intervals for at least 4 months thereafter.

Surgical Procedures in Patients with Valvular Heart Disease. About 25% of cases of subacute bacterial endocarditis follow dental extractions. This observation, together with the fact that up to 80% of persons who have teeth removed experience a transient bacteremia, emphasizes the potential importance of chemoprophylaxis for those who have congenital or acquired valvular heart disease of any type and need to undergo dental procedures. Since transient bacterial invasion of the bloodstream occurs occasionally after surgical procedures (*e.g.,* tonsillectomy and genitourinary and gastrointestinal procedures) and during childbirth, these too are indications for prophylaxis in patients with valvular heart disease. Whether the incidence of bacterial endocarditis actually is altered by this type of chemoprophylaxis remains to be determined.

Detailed recommendations for both adults and children with valvular heart disease have been formulated (*see* Dajani *et al.,* 1990; Durack, 2000).

The Penicillinase-Resistant Penicillins

The penicillins described in this section are resistant to hydrolysis by staphylococcal penicillinase. Their appropriate use should be restricted to the treatment of infections that are known or suspected to be caused by staphylococci that elaborate the enzyme—the vast majority of strains of this bacterium that are encountered in the hospital or in the general community. These drugs are much less active than is penicillin G against other penicillin-sensitive microorganisms, including non-penicillinase-producing staphylococci.

The role of the penicillinase-resistant penicillins as the agents of choice for most staphylococcal disease may be changing with the increasing incidence of isolates of so-called methicillin-resistant microorganisms. As commonly used, this latter term denotes resistance of these bacteria to all of the penicillinase-resistant penicillins and cephalosporins. Such strains are usually resistant as well to the aminoglycosides, tetracyclines, erythromycin, and clindamycin. Vancomycin is considered to be the drug of choice for such infections. Some physicians use a combination of vancomycin and rifampin, especially for life-threatening infections and those involving foreign bodies. Methicillin-resistant *S. aureus* contains an additional high molecular weight PBP with a very low affinity for β-lactam antibiotics (Spratt, 1994). From 40% to 60% of strains of *S. epidermidis* also are resistant to the penicillinase-resistant penicillins by the same mechanism. As with methicillin-resistant *S. aureus,* these strains may appear to be susceptible to cephalosporins on disc sensitivity testing, but there is usually a significant population of microbes that is resistant to cephalosporins and that emerges during such therapy. Vancomycin also is the drug of choice for serious infection caused by methicillin-resistant *S. epidermidis;* rifampin is given concurrently when a foreign body is involved.

The Isoxazolyl Penicillins: Oxacillin, Cloxacillin, and Dicloxacillin.   These three congeneric semisynthetic penicillins are similar pharmacologically and are thus conveniently considered together. Their structural formulas are shown in Table 45–1. All are relatively stable in an acidic medium and are adequately absorbed after oral administration. All are markedly resistant to cleavage by penicillinase. These drugs are not substitutes for penicillin G in the treatment of diseases amenable to it. Furthermore, because of variability in intestinal absorption, oral administration is not a substitute for the parenteral route in the treatment of serious staphylococcal infections that require a penicillin unaffected by penicillinase.

Pharmacological Properties.   The isoxazolyl penicillins are potent inhibitors of the growth of most penicillinase-producing staphylococci. This is their valid clinical use. Dicloxacillin (PATHOCIL, others) is the most active, and many strains of *S. aureus* are inhibited by concentrations of 0.05 to 0.8 μg/ml. Comparable values for cloxacillin and oxacillin are 0.1 to 3 μg/ml and 0.4 to 6 μg/ml, respectively. These differences may have little practical significance, however, since dosages (*see* below) are adjusted accordingly. These agents are, in general, less effective against microorganisms susceptible to penicillin G, and they are not useful against gram-negative bacteria.

These agents are rapidly but incompletely (30% to 80%) absorbed from the gastrointestinal tract. Absorption of the drugs is more efficient when they are taken on an empty stomach; preferably they are administered one hour before or two hours after meals to ensure better absorption. Peak concentrations in plasma are attained by 1 hour and approximate 5 to 10 μg/ml after the ingestion of 1 g of oxacillin. Slightly higher concentrations are achieved after the administration of 1 g of cloxacillin, while the same oral dose of dicloxacillin yields peak plasma concentrations of 15 μg/ml. There is little evidence that these differences are of clinical significance. All these congeners are bound to plasma albumin to a great extent (approximately 90% to 95%); none is removed from the circulation to a significant degree by hemodialysis.

The isoxazolyl penicillins are rapidly excreted by the kidney. Normally, about one-half of any of these drugs is excreted in the urine in the first 6 hours after a conventional oral dose. There also is significant hepatic elimination of these agents in the bile. The half-lives for all are between 30 and 60 minutes. Intervals between doses of oxacillin, cloxacillin, and dicloxacillin do not have to be altered for patients with renal failure. The above-noted differences in plasma concentrations produced by the isoxazolyl penicillins are related mainly to differences in rate of urinary excretion and degree of resistance to degradation in the liver.

Nafcillin.   This semisynthetic penicillin is highly resistant to penicillinase and has proven effective against infections caused by penicillinase-producing strains of *S. aureus*. Its structural formula is shown in Table 45–1.
Pharmacological Properties.   Nafcillin (UNIPEN, NALLPEN, others) is slightly more active than oxacillin against penicillin G–resistant *S. aureus* (most strains are inhibited by 0.06 to 2 μg/ml). While it is the most active of the penicillinase-resistant penicillins against other microorganisms, it is not as potent as penicillin G.

Nafcillin is inactivated to a variable degree in the acidic medium of the gastric contents. Its absorption after oral administration is irregular, regardless of whether the drug is taken with meals or on an empty stomach. Consequently, although oral preparations are available, injectable preparations should be used because of the variable absorption of nafcillin from the gastrointestinal tract. The peak plasma concentration is about 8 μg/ml 60 minutes after a 1-g intramuscular dose. Nafcillin is about 90% bound to plasma protein. Peak concentrations of nafcillin in bile are well above those found in plasma. Concentrations of the drug in CSF appear to be adequate for therapy of staphylococcal meningitis.

The Aminopenicillins: Ampicillin, Amoxicillin, and Their Congeners

These agents have similar antibacterial activity and a spectrum that is broader than the antibiotics heretofore discussed. They are all destroyed by β-lactamase (from both gram-positive and gram-negative bacteria).

Antimicrobial Activity.   Ampicillin and the related aminopenicillins are bactericidal for both gram-positive and gram-negative bacteria. The meningococci and *L. monocytogenes* are sensitive to the drug. Many pneumococcal isolates have varying levels of resistance to ampicillin. Penicillin-resistant strains should be considered ampicillin/amoxicillin-resistant. *H. influenzae* and the *viridans* group of streptococci exhibit varying degrees of resistance. Enterococci are about twice as sensitive to ampicillin, on a weight basis, as they are to penicillin G (MIC for ampicillin averages 1.5 mg/ml). Although most strains of *N. gonorrhoeae*, *E. coli*, *P. mirabilis*, *Salmonella*, and *Shigella* were highly susceptible when ampicillin was first used in the early 1960s, an increasing percentage of these species is now resistant. From 30% to 50% of *E. coli*, a significant number of *P. mirabilis*, and practically all species of *Enterobacter* are presently insensitive. Resistant strains of *Salmonella* (plasmid mediated) have been recovered with increasing frequency in various parts of the world. Most strains of *Shigella* are now resistant. Most strains of *Pseudomonas, Klebsiella, Serratia, Acinetobacter,* and indole-positive *Proteus* also are resistant to this group of penicillins; these antibiotics are less active against *B. fragilis* than is penicillin G. However, concurrent administration of a β-lactamase inhibitor such as clavulanate or sulbactam markedly expands the spectrum of activity of these drugs (*see* below).

Ampicillin.   This drug is the prototypical agent of the group. Its structural formula is shown in Table 45–1.
Pharmacological Properties.   Ampicillin (OMNIPEN, POLYCILLIN, others) is stable in acid and is well absorbed after oral administration. An oral dose of 0.5 g produces peak concentrations in plasma of about 3 μg/ml at 2 hours. Intake of food prior to ingestion of ampicillin results in less complete absorption. Intramuscular injection of 0.5 or 1 g of sodium ampicillin yields peak plasma concentrations of about 7 or 10 μg/ml, respectively, at 1 hour; these decline exponentially, with a half-time of approximately

80 minutes. Severe renal impairment markedly prolongs the persistence of ampicillin in the plasma. Peritoneal dialysis is ineffective in removing the drug from the blood, but hemodialysis removes about 40% of the body store in about 7 hours. Adjustment of the dose of ampicillin is required in the presence of renal dysfunction. Ampicillin appears in the bile, undergoes enterohepatic circulation, and is excreted in appreciable quantities in the feces.

Amoxicillin.   This drug, a penicillinase-susceptible semisynthetic penicillin, is a close chemical and pharmacological relative of ampicillin (*see* Table 45–1). The drug is stable in acid and is designed for oral use. It is more rapidly and completely absorbed from the gastrointestinal tract than is ampicillin, which is the major difference between the two. The antimicrobial spectrum of amoxicillin is essentially identical to that of ampicillin, with the important exception that amoxicillin appears to be less effective than ampicillin for shigellosis.

Peak concentrations of amoxicillin (AMOXIL, others) in plasma are two to two and one-half times greater for amoxicillin than for ampicillin after oral administration of the same dose; they are reached at 2 hours and average about 4 μg/ml when 250 mg is administered. Food does not interfere with absorption. Perhaps because of more complete absorption of this congener, the incidence of diarrhea with amoxicillin is less than that following administration of ampicillin. The incidence of other adverse effects appears to be similar. While the half-life of amoxicillin is similar to that for ampicillin, effective concentrations of orally administered amoxicillin are detectable in the plasma for twice as long as with ampicillin, again because of the more complete absorption. About 20% of amoxicillin is protein-bound in plasma, a value similar to that for ampicillin. Most of a dose of the antibiotic is excreted in an active form in the urine. Probenecid delays excretion of the drug.

Therapeutic Indications for the Aminopenicillins. *Upper Respiratory Infections.* Ampicillin and amoxicillin are active against *S. pyogenes* and many strains of *S. pneumoniae* and *H. influenzae,* which are major upper respiratory bacterial pathogens. The drugs constitute effective therapy for sinusitis, otitis media, acute exacerbations of chronic bronchitis, and epiglottitis caused by sensitive strains of these organisms. Amoxicillin is the most active of all the oral β-lactam antibiotics against both penicillin-sensitive and penicillin-resistant *S. pneumoniae* (Friedland and McCracken, 1994). Based on the increasing prevalence of pneumococcal resistance to penicillin, an increase in dose of oral amoxicillin (from 40 to 45 up to 80 to 90 mg/kg per day) for empiric treatment of acute otitis media in children is recommended (Dowell *et al.,* 1999). Ampicillin-resistant *H. influenzae* may be a problem in many areas. The addition of a β-lactamase inhibitor (amoxicillin-clavulanate or ampicillin-sulbactam) extends the spectrum to β-lactamase-producing *H. influenzae* and Enterobacteriaceae. Bacterial pharyngitis should be treated with penicillin G or penicillin V, since *S. pyogenes* is the major pathogen.

Urinary Tract Infections.   Most uncomplicated urinary tract infections are caused by Enterobacteriaceae, and *E. coli* is the most common species; ampicillin often is an effective agent, although resistance is increasingly common. Enterococcal urinary tract infections are treated effectively with ampicillin alone.
Meningitis.   Acute bacterial meningitis in children is most frequently due to *S. pneumoniae* or *N. meningitidis*. Since 20% to 30% of strains of *S. pneumoniae* now may be resistant to this antibiotic, ampicillin is not indicated for single-agent treatment of meningitis. Ampicillin has excellent activity against *L. monocytogenes,* a cause of meningitis in immunocompromised persons. Thus, the combination of ampicillin and vancomycin plus a third-generation cephalosporin is a rational regimen for empiric treatment of suspected bacterial meningitis.
Salmonella Infections.   Disease associated with bacteremia, disease with metastatic foci, and the enteric fever syndrome (including typhoid fever) respond favorably to antibiotics. A fluoroquinolone or ceftriaxone is considered by some to be the drug of choice, but the administration of trimethoprim–sulfamethoxazole or high doses of ampicillin (12 g per day for adults) also is effective. In some geographical areas, resistance to ampicillin is common. The typhoid carrier state has been eliminated successfully in patients without gallbladder disease with ampicillin, trimethoprim–sulfamethoxazole, or ciprofloxacin.

Antipseudomonal Penicillins: The Carboxypenicillins and the Ureidopenicillins

The carboxypenicillins, *carbenicillin* and *ticarcillin* and their close relatives, are active against some isolates of *P. aeruginosa* and certain indole-positive *Proteus* species that are resistant to ampicillin and its congeners. They are ineffective against most strains of *S. aureus, Enterococcus faecalis, Klebsiella,* and *L. monocytogenes. B. fragilis* is susceptible to high concentrations of these drugs, but penicillin G is actually more active on the basis of weight. The ureidopenicillins, *mezlocillin* and *piperacillin,* have superior activity against *P. aeruginosa* compared to carbenicillin and ticarcillin. In addition, mezlocillin and piperacillin are useful for treatment of infections with *Klebsiella*. The carboxypenicillins and the ureidopenicillins are sensitive to destruction by β-lactamases.

Carbenicillin and Carbenicillin Indanyl. *Carbenicillin.* This drug is a penicillinase-susceptible derivative of 6-aminopenicillanic acid. Its structural formula is shown in Table 45–1. Carbenicillin was the first penicillin with activity against *P. aeruginosa* and some *Proteus* strains that are resistant to ampicillin. It has been superseded by ticarcillin or piperacillin for most uses (*see* below).

Preparations of carbenicillin may cause adverse effects in addition to those that follow use of the other penicillins (*see* below). Congestive heart failure may result from the administration of excessive Na$^+$. Hypokalemia may occur because of obligatory excretion of cation with the large amount of nonreabsorbable anion (carbenicillin) presented to the distal renal tubule. The drug interferes with platelet function, and bleeding may occur because of abnormal aggregation of platelets.

Carbenicillin Indanyl Sodium (GEOCILLIN).   This congener is the indanyl ester of carbenicillin; it is acid-stable and is suitable for oral administration. After absorption, the ester is rapidly converted to carbenicillin by hydrolysis of the ester linkage. The antimicrobial spectrum of the drug is therefore that of carbenicillin. Although relatively low concentrations of carbenicillin are achieved in plasma, the active moiety is excreted rapidly in the urine. Thus, the only use of this drug is for the management of urinary tract infections caused by *Proteus* species other than *P. mirabilis* and by *P. aeruginosa.*

Ticarcillin (TICAR).   This semisynthetic penicillin (Table 45–1) is very similar to carbenicillin, but it is two to four times more active against *P. aeruginosa.* Ticarcillin is inferior to piperacillin and mezlocillin for the treatment of serious infections caused by *Pseudomonas.*

Mezlocillin.   This ureidopenicillin is more active against *Klebsiella* than is carbenicillin; its activity against *Pseudomonas in vitro* is similar to that of ticarcillin. It is more active than ticarcillin against *Enterococcus faecalis. Mezlocillin sodium* (MEZLIN) is available as a powder to be dissolved for injection and contains about 2 mEq of Na^+ per gram. The usual dose for adults is 6 to 18 g per day, divided into four to six portions. Mezlocillin and piperacillin (below) are excreted in bile to a significant degree. In the absence of biliary tract obstruction, high concentrations of mezlocillin in bile are achieved by intravenous administration.

Piperacillin.   Piperacillin (PIPRACIL) extends the spectrum of ampicillin to include most strains of *P. aeruginosa,* Enterobacteriaceae (non-β-lactamse-producing), and many *Bacteroides* species. In combination with a β-lactamase inhibitor (piperacillin-tazobactam, ZOSYN) it has the broadest antibacterial spectrum of the penicillins. Pharmacokinetic properties are reminiscent of the other ureidopenicillins. High biliary concentrations are achieved, as with mezlocillin.

Therapeutic Indications.   These penicillins are important agents for the treatment of patients with serious infections caused by gram-negative bacteria. Such patients frequently have impaired immunological defenses, and their infections often are acquired in the hospital. Many authorities feel that a β-lactam agent, often in combination with an aminoglycoside, should be employed for all such infections. Therefore, these penicillins find their greatest use in treating bacteremias, pneumonias, infections following burns, and urinary tract infections due to microorganisms resistant to penicillin G and ampicillin; the bacteria especially responsible include *P. aeruginosa,* indole-positive strains of *Proteus,* and *Enterobacter* species. Since *Pseudomonas* infections are common in neutropenic patients,

therapy for severe bacterial infections in such individuals should include a β-lactam antibiotic with good activity against these microorganisms.

Untoward Reactions to Penicillins

Hypersensitivity Reactions.   Hypersensitivity reactions are by far the most common adverse effects noted with the penicillins, and these agents probably are the most common cause of drug allergy. Allergic reactions complicate between 0.7% and 4% of all treatment courses. There is no convincing evidence that any single penicillin differs from the group in its potential for causing true allergic reactions. In approximate order of decreasing frequency, manifestations of allergy to penicillins include maculopapular rash, urticarial rash, fever, bronchospasm, vasculitis, serum sickness, exfoliative dermatitis, Stevens–Johnson syndrome, and anaphylaxis (Anonymous, 1988; Weiss and Adkinson, 2000). The overall incidence of such reactions to the penicillins varies from 0.7% to 10% in different studies.

Hypersensitivity reactions may occur with any dosage form of penicillin; allergy to one penicillin exposes the patient to a greater risk of reaction if another is given. On the other hand, the occurrence of an untoward effect does not necessarily imply repetition on subsequent exposures. Hypersensitivity reactions may appear in the absence of a previous known exposure to the drug. This may be caused by unrecognized prior exposure to penicillin in the environment (*e.g.,* in foods of animal origin or from the fungus producing penicillin). Although elimination of the antibiotic usually results in rapid clearing of the allergic manifestations, they may persist for 1 or 2 weeks or longer after therapy has been stopped. In some cases, the reaction is mild and disappears even while the use of penicillin is continued; in others, it necessitates immediate cessation of penicillin treatment. In a few instances, it is necessary to interdict the future use of penicillin because of the risk of death, and the patient should be so warned. It must be stressed that fatal episodes of anaphylaxis have followed the ingestion of very small doses of this antibiotic or skin testing with minute quantities of the drug.

Penicillins and breakdown products of penicillins act as haptens after their covalent reaction with proteins. The most important antigenic intermediate of penicillin appears to be the penicilloyl moiety, which is formed when the β-lactam ring is opened. This is considered to be the major (predominant) determinant of penicillin allergy. In addition, minor determinants of allergy to penicillins are present. These include the intact molecule itself and penicilloate. These products are formed *in vivo* and also can be found in solutions of penicillin prepared for administration. The terms *major determinant* and *minor determinant* refer to the frequency with which antibodies to these haptens appear to be formed. They do *not* describe the severity of the reaction that may result. In fact, anaphylactic reactions to penicillin are usually mediated by IgE antibodies against the minor determinants.

Antipenicillin antibodies are detectable in virtually all patients who have received the drug and in many who have never knowingly been exposed to it (Klaus and Fellner, 1973). Recent treatment with the antibiotic induces an increase in major-determinant-specific antibodies that are skin sensitizing. The incidence of positive skin reactors is three to four times higher in atopic than in nonatopic individuals. Clinical and immunological studies suggest that immediate allergic reactions are mediated by skin-sensitizing or IgE antibodies, usually of minor-determinant specificities. Accelerated and late urticarial reactions usually are mediated by major-determinant–specific skin-sensitizing antibodies. The recurrent-arthralgia syndrome appears to be related to the presence of skin-sensitizing antibodies of minor-determinant specificities. Some maculopapular and erythematous reactions may be due to toxic antigen-antibody complexes of major determinant–specific IgM antibodies. Accelerated and late urticarial reactions to penicillin may terminate spontaneously because of the development of blocking antibodies.

Skin rashes of all types may be caused by allergy to penicillin. Scarlatiniform, morbilliform, urticarial, vesicular, and bullous eruptions may develop. Purpuric lesions are uncommon and are usually the result of a vasculitis; thrombocytopenic purpura may occur very rarely. Henoch–Schönlein purpura with renal involvement has been a rare complication. Contact dermatitis is observed occasionally in pharmacists, nurses, and physicians who prepare penicillin solutions. Fixed-drug reactions also have occurred. More severe reactions involving the skin are exfoliative dermatitis and exudative erythema multiforme of either the erythematopapular or vesiculobullous type; these lesions may be very severe and atypical in distribution and constitute the characteristic Stevens–Johnson syndrome. The incidence of skin rashes appears to be highest following the use of ampicillin, being about 9%; rashes follow the administration of ampicillin in nearly all patients with infectious mononucleosis. When allopurinol and ampicillin are administered concurrently, the incidence of rash also increases. Ampicillin-induced skin eruptions in such patients may represent a "toxic" rather than a truly allergic reaction. Positive skin reactions to the major and minor determinants of penicillin sensitization may be absent. The

rash may clear even while administration of the drug is continued.

The most serious hypersensitivity reactions produced by the penicillins are angioedema and anaphylaxis. Angioedema with marked swelling of the lips, tongue, face, and periorbital tissues, frequently accompanied by asthmatic breathing and "giant hives," has been observed after topical, oral, or systemic administration of penicillins of various types.

Acute anaphylactic or anaphylactoid reactions induced by various preparations of penicillin constitute the most important immediate danger connected with their use. Among all drugs, the penicillins are most often responsible for this type of untoward effect. Anaphylactoid reactions may occur at any age. Their incidence is thought to be 0.004% to 0.04% in persons treated with penicillins (Kucers and Bennett, 1987). About 0.001% of patients treated with these agents die from anaphylaxis. It has been estimated that there are at least 300 deaths per year due to this complication of therapy. About 70% have had penicillin previously, and one-third of these reacted to it on a prior occasion. Anaphylaxis has most often followed the injection of penicillin, although it also has been observed after oral ingestion of the drug and even has resulted from the intradermal instillation of a very small quantity for the purpose of testing for the presence of hypersensitivity. The clinical pictures that develop vary in severity. The most dramatic is sudden, severe hypotension and rapid death. In other instances, bronchoconstriction with severe asthma; abdominal pain, nausea, and vomiting; extreme weakness and a fall in blood pressure; or diarrhea and purpuric skin eruptions have characterized the anaphylactic episodes.

Serum sickness varies from mild fever, rash, and leukopenia to severe arthralgia or arthritis, purpura, lymphadenopathy, splenomegaly, mental changes, electrocardiographic abnormalities suggestive of myocarditis, generalized edema, albuminuria, and hematuria. It is mediated by IgG antibodies. This reaction usually appears after penicillin treatment has been continued for 1 week or more; it may be delayed, however, until 1 or 2 weeks after the drug has been stopped. Serum sickness caused by penicillin may persist for a week or longer.

Vasculitis of the skin or other organs may be related to hypersensitivity to penicillin. The Coombs reaction frequently becomes positive during prolonged therapy with a penicillin or cephalosporin, but hemolytic anemia is rare. Reversible neutropenia may occur. It is not known if this is truly a hypersensitivity reaction; it has been noted with all of the penicillins and has been seen in up to 30% of patients treated with 8 to 12 g of nafcillin for longer than 21 days. The bone marrow shows an arrest of maturation.

Fever may be the only evidence of a hypersensitivity reaction to the penicillins. It may reach high levels and be maintained, remittent, or intermittent; chills occasionally occur. The febrile reaction usually disappears within 24 to 36 hours after administration of the drug is stopped but may persist for days.

Eosinophilia is an occasional accompaniment of other allergic reactions to penicillin. At times, it may be the sole abnormality, and eosinophils may reach levels of 10% to 20% or more of the total number of circulating white blood cells.

Interstitial nephritis rarely may be produced by the penicillins; methicillin has been implicated most frequently. Hematuria, albuminuria, pyuria, renal-cell and other casts in the urine, elevation of serum creatinine, and even oliguria have been noted. Biopsy shows a mononuclear infiltrate with eosinophilia and tubular damage. IgG is present in the interstitium. This reaction usually is reversible.

Management of the Patient Potentially Allergic to Penicillin.

Evaluation of the patient's history is the most practical way to avoid the use of penicillin in patients who are at the greatest risk of adverse reaction. The majority of patients who give a history of allergy to penicillin should be treated with a different type of antibiotic. Unfortunately there is no available means to confirm a history of penicillin allergy. Skin testing for IgE-mediated immediate-type responses is compromised by the lack of a commercially available minor determinant mixture and the inability of skin tests using major and minor penicillin determinants to predict confidently allergic reactions to synthetic penicillins. Radioallergosorbent tests (RAST) for IgE antipenicilloyl determinants suffer from the same limitations as skin tests (Weiss and Adkinson, 2000).

Desensitization occasionally is recommended for patients who are allergic to penicillin and who must receive the drug. This procedure consists of administering gradually increasing doses of penicillin in the hope of avoiding a severe reaction and should be performed only in an intensive-care setting. This may result in a subclinical anaphylactic discharge and the binding of all IgE before full doses are administered. Penicillin may be given in doses of 1, 5, 10, 100, and 1000 U intradermally in the lower arm, with 60-minute intervals between doses. If this is well tolerated, then 10,000 U and 50,000 U may be given subcutaneously. Desensitization also may be accomplished by the oral administration of penicillin (Sullivan *et al.,* 1982). When full doses are reached, penicillin should not be discontinued and then restarted, since immediate reactions may recur (*see* Weiss and Adkinson, 2000, for details). The patient should be observed constantly during the desensitizing procedure, an intravenous line must be in place, and epinephrine and equipment and expertise for artificial ventilation must be on hand. It must be emphasized that this procedure may be dangerous, and its efficacy is unproven.

Patients with life-threatening infections (*e.g.,* endocarditis or meningitis) may be continued on penicillin despite the development of a maculopapular rash, although alternative antimicrobial agents should be used whenever possible. The rash often clears as therapy is continued. This is thought to be due to the development of blocking antibodies of the IgG class. The rash may be treated with antihistamines or adrenocorticosteroids, although there is no evidence that this therapy is efficacious. Rarely, exfoliative dermatitis with or without vasculitis develops in these patients if therapy with penicillin is continued.

Other Adverse Reactions. The penicillins have minimal direct toxicity. Apparent toxic effects that have been reported include bone marrow depression, granulocytopenia, and hepatitis. The last-named effect is rare but is most commonly seen following the administration of oxacillin and nafcillin (Kirkwood *et al.,* 1983). The administration of penicillin G, carbenicillin, piperacillin, or ticarcillin has been associated with a potentially significant defect of hemostasis that appears to be due to an impairment of platelet aggregation; this may be caused by interference with the binding of aggregating agents to platelet receptors (Fass *et al.,* 1987).

Most common among the irritative responses to penicillin are pain and sterile inflammatory reactions at the sites of intramuscular injections—reactions that are related to concentration. Serum transaminases and lactic dehydrogenase may be elevated as a result of local damage to muscle. In some individuals who receive penicillin intravenously, phlebitis or thrombophlebitis develops. Many persons who take various penicillin preparations by mouth experience nausea, with or without vomiting, and some have mild-to-severe diarrhea. These manifestations often are related to the dose of the drug.

When penicillin is injected accidentally into the sciatic nerve, severe pain occurs and dysfunction in the area of distribution of this nerve develops and persists for weeks. Intrathecal injection of penicillin G may produce arachnoiditis or severe and fatal encephalopathy. Because of this, intrathecal or intraventricular administration of penicillins should be avoided. The parenteral administration of large doses of penicillin G (greater than 20 million units per day, or less with renal insufficiency) may produce lethargy, confusion, twitching, multifocal myoclonus, or localized or generalized epileptiform seizures. These are most apt to occur in the presence of renal insufficiency, localized lesions of the central nervous system (CNS), or hyponatremia. When the concentration of penicillin G in CSF exceeds 10 μg/ml, significant dysfunction of the CNS is frequent. The injection of 20 million units of penicillin G potassium, which contains 34 mEq of K^+, may lead to severe or even fatal hyperkalemia in persons with renal dysfunction.

Injection of penicillin G procaine may result in an immediate reaction, characterized by dizziness, tinnitus, headache, hallucinations, and sometimes seizures. This is due to the rapid liberation of toxic concentrations of procaine. It has been reported to occur in 1 of 200 patients receiving 4.8 million units of penicillin G procaine to treat their venereal disease.

Reactions Unrelated to Hypersensitivity or Toxicity. Regardless of the route by which the drug is administered, but most strikingly when it is given by mouth, penicillin changes the composition of the microflora by eliminating sensitive microorganisms. This phenomenon is usually of no clinical significance, and the normal microflora is reestablished shortly after therapy is stopped. In some persons, however, superinfection results from the changes in flora. Pseudomembranous colitis, related to overgrowth and production of a toxin by *Clostridium difficile*, has followed oral and, less commonly, parenteral administration of penicillins.

THE CEPHALOSPORINS

History and Source. *Cephalosporium acremonium,* the first source of the cephalosporins, was isolated in 1948 by Brotzu from the sea near a sewer outlet off the Sardinian coast. Crude filtrates from cultures of this fungus were found to inhibit the *in vitro* growth of *S. aureus* and to cure staphylococcal infections and typhoid fever in human beings. Culture fluids in which the Sardinian fungus was cultivated were found to contain three distinct antibiotics, which were named cephalosporin P, N, and C. With the isolation of the active nucleus of cephalosporin C, 7-aminocephalosporanic acid, and with the addition of side chains, it became possible to produce semisynthetic compounds with antibacterial activity very much greater than that of the parent substance. (For a historical review and discussion of the biochemistry of the cephalosporins, *see* Abraham, 1962; Flynn, 1972.)

Chemistry. Cephalosporin C contains a side chain derived from D-α-aminoadipic acid, which is condensed with a dihydrothiazine β-lactam ring system (7-aminocephalosporanic acid). Compounds containing 7-aminocephalosporanic acid are relatively stable in dilute acid and highly resistant to penicillinase, regardless of the nature of their side chains and their affinity for the enzyme.

Cephalosporin C can be hydrolyzed by acid to 7-aminocephalosporanic acid. This compound subsequently has been modified by the addition of different side chains to create a whole family of cephalosporin antibiotics. It appears that modifications at position 7 of the β-lactam ring are associated with alteration in antibacterial activity and that substitutions at position 3 of the dihydrothiazine ring are associated with changes in the metabolism and the pharmacokinetic properties of the drugs.

The cephamycins are similar to the cephalosporins, but have a methoxy group at position 7 of the β-lactam ring of the 7-aminocephalosporanic acid nucleus. The structural formulas of representative cephalosporins and cephamycins are shown in Table 45–2.

Mechanism of Action. Cephalosporins and cephamycins inhibit bacterial cell-wall synthesis in a manner similar to that of penicillin. This is discussed in detail above.

Classification. The explosive growth of the cephalosporins during the past decade has taxed the best of memories and makes a system of classification most desirable. Although cephalosporins may be classified by their chemical structure, clinical pharmacology, resistance to β-lactamase, or antimicrobial spectrum, the well-accepted system of classification by "generations" is very useful, although admittedly somewhat arbitrary (Table 45–3).

Classification by generations is based on general features of antimicrobial activity (*see* Karchmer, 2000). The *first-generation* cephalosporins, epitomized by *cephalothin* and *cefazolin,* have good activity against gram-positive bacteria and relatively modest activity against gram-negative microorganisms. Most gram-positive cocci (with the exception of enterococci, methicillin-resistant *S. aureus,* and *S. epidermidis*) are susceptible. Most oral cavity anaerobes are sensitive, but the *Bacteroides fragilis* group is resistant. Activity against *Moraxella catarrhalis, E. coli, K. pneumoniae,* and *P. mirabilis* is good. The *second-generation* cephalosporins have somewhat increased activity against gram-negative microorganisms, but are much less active than the third-generation agents. A subset of second-generation agents (*cefoxitin, cefotetan,* and *cefmetazole*) also is active against the *B. fragilis* group. *Third-generation* cephalosporins generally are less active than first-generation agents against gram-positive cocci, but they are much more active against the Enterobacteriaceae, including β-lactamase-producing strains. A subset of third-generation agents (*ceftazidime* and *cefoperazone*) also is active against *P. aeruginosa* but less active than other third-generation agents against gram-positive cocci (Donowitz and Mandell, 1988). *Fourth-generation* cephalosporins, such as *cefepime,* have an extended spectrum of activity compared to the third generation and have increased stability from hydrolysis by plasmid and chromosomally mediated β-lactamases. Fourth-generation agents may prove to have particular therapeutic usefulness in the treatment of infections due to aerobic gram-negative bacilli resistant to third-generation cephalosporins.

Mechanisms of Bacterial Resistance to the Cephalosporins. Resistance to the cephalosporins may be related to inability of the antibiotic to reach its sites of action; to alterations in the penicillin-binding proteins (PBPs) that are targets of the cephalosporins, such that the antibiotics bind with lower affinity; or to bacterial enzymes (β-lactamases) that can hydrolyze the β-lactam ring and inactivate the cephalosporin. Alterations in two PBPs (1A and 2X), such that they bind cephalosporins with lower affinity, are sufficient to render pneumococci resistant to third-generation cephalosporins, as the other three high-molecular-weight PBPs have inherently low affinity (Spratt, 1994).

The most prevalent mechanism of resistance to cephalosporins is destruction of the cephalosporins by hydrolysis of the β-lactam ring. Many gram-positive microorganisms release

Table 45–2

Names, Structural Formulas, Dosage, and Dosage Forms of Selected Cephalosporins and Related Compounds

$$R_1-\overset{\overset{\displaystyle O}{\|}}{C}-NH-\underset{\underset{COO^-}{\big|}}{\overset{7}{\text{...}}}\overset{\overset{1}{S}}{\text{(cephem ring)}}\,^{4}N\,R_2$$

Cephem nucleus

COMPOUND (TRADE NAMES)	R_1	R_2	DOSAGE FORMS,* ADULT DOSAGE FOR SEVERE INFECTION, AND $t_{1/2}$
First-generation			
Cephalothin (KEFLIN)	thiophene-2-yl-CH_2-	$-CH_2OC(=O)CH_3$	I: 1 to 2 g every 4 hours; $t_{1/2}=0.6$ hour
Cefazolin (ANCEF, KEFZOL, others)	tetrazol-1-yl-CH_2-	$-CH_2S$–(1,3,4-thiadiazol-2-yl)–CH_3	I: 1 to 1.5 g every 6 hours; $t_{1/2}=$ about 2 hours
Cephalexin (KEFLEX)	$C_6H_5-CH(NH_2)-$	$-CH_3$	O: 1 g every 6 hours; $t_{1/2}=0.9$ hour
Cefadroxil (DURICEF, ULTRACEF)	$HO-C_6H_4-CH(NH_2)-$	$-CH_3$	O: 1 g every 12 hours; $t_{1/2}=1.1$ hours
Second-generation			
Cefamandole (MANDOL)	$C_6H_5-CH(OH)-$	$-CH_2S$–(1-methyltetrazol-5-yl)	I: 2 g every 4 to 6 hours; $t_{1/2}=0.8$ hour
Cefoxitin† (MEFOXIN)	thiophene-2-yl-CH_2-	$-CH_2OC(=O)NH_2$	I: 2 g every 4 hours or 3 g every 6 hours; $t_{1/2}=0.7$ hour
Cefaclor (CECLOR)	$C_6H_5-CH(NH_2)-$	$-Cl$	O: 1 g every 8 hours; $t_{1/2}=0.7$ hour
Cefuroxime (KEFUROX, ZINACEF) Cefuroxime axetil‡ (CEFTIN)	furan-2-yl-$C(=N-OCH_3)-$	$-CH_2OC(=O)NH_2$	I: up to 3 g every 8 hours; $t_{1/2}=1.7$ hours; T: 500 mg every 12 hours
Loracarbef¶ (LORABID)	$C_6H_5-CH(NH_2)-$	$-Cl$	O: 200 to 400 mg every 12 hours; $t_{1/2}=1.1$ hours
Cefonicid (MONOCID)	$C_6H_5-CH(OH)-$	$-CH_2S$–(1-($CH_2SO_3^-$)tetrazol-5-yl)	I: 2 g every 24 hours; $t_{1/2}=4.4$ hours
Cefotetan (CEFOTAN)	$H_2NC(=O)$, $HOOC$, $C=C$, S-ring-$C-$	$-CH_2S$–(1-methyltetrazol-5-yl)	I: 2 to 3 g every 12 hours; $t_{1/2}=3.3$ hours

Table 45–2 (*Continued*)

Cephem nucleus

COMPOUND (TRADE NAMES)	R_1	R_2	DOSAGE FORMS,* ADULT DOSAGE FOR SEVERE INFECTION, AND $t_{1/2}$
Second-generation (cont.)			
Ceforanide (PRECEF)			I: 1 g every 12 hours $t_{1/2}$ = 2.6 hours
Third-generation			
Cefotaxime (CLAFORAN)			I: 2 g every 4 to 8 hours $t_{1/2}$ = 1.1 hours
Cefpodoxime proxetil§ (VANTIN)		$-CH_2OCH_3$	O: 200 to 400 mg every 12 hours $t_{1/2}$ = 2.2 hours
Ceftizoxime (CEFIZOX)		$-H$	I: 3 to 4 g every 8 hours $t_{1/2}$ = 1.8 hours
Ceftriaxone (ROCEPHIN)			I: 2 g every 12 to 24 hours $t_{1/2}$ = 8 hours
Cefoperazone (CEFOBID)			I: 1.5 to 4 g every 6 to 8 hours $t_{1/2}$ = 2.1 hours
Ceftazidime (FORTAZ, others)			I: 2 g every 8 hours $t_{1/2}$ = 1.8 hours
Fourth-generation			
Cefepime (MAXIPIME)			I: 2 g every 12 hours $t_{1/2}$ = 2.0 hours

*T, tablet; C, capsule; O, oral suspension; I, injection.

†Cefoxitin, a cephamycin, has a —OCH_3 group at position 7 of cephem nucleus.

‡Cefuroxime axetil is the acetyloxyethyl ester of cefuroxime.

¶Loracarbef, a carbacephem, has a carbon instead of sulfur at position 1 of cephem nucleus.

§Cefpodoxime proxetil has a —$COOCH(CH_3)OCOOCH(CH_3)_2$ group at position 4 of cephem nucleus.

Table 45–3

Cephalosporin Generations

GENERATION	EXAMPLES	USEFUL SPECTRUM[a]
First	Cefazolin (ANCEF, KEFZOL, ZOLICEF) Cephalothin (KEFLIN) Cephalexin (KEFLEX, others)	Streptococci[b]; *Staphylococcus aureus.*[c]
Second	Cefuroxime (CEFTIN, KEFUROX, ZINACEF) Cefaclor (CECLOR)	*Escherichia coli, Klebsiella, Proteus, Haemophilus influenzae, Moraxella catarrhalis.* Not as active against gram-positive organisms as first-generation agents.
	Cefoxitin (MEFOXIN) Cefotetan (CEFOTAN)	Inferior activity against *S. aureus* compared to cefuroxime but with added activity against *Bacteroides fragilis* and other *Bacteroides* spp.
Third	Cefotaxime (CLAFORAN) Ceftriaxone (ROCEPHIN) Ceftazidime (CEPTAZ, FORTAZ, TAZIDIME, others)	Enterobacteriaceae[d]; *Pseudomonas aeruginosa*[e]; *Serratia; Neisseria gonorrhoeae;* activity for *S. aureus Streptococcus pneumoniae* and *Streptococcus pyogenes*[f] comparable to first-generation agents. Activity against *Bacteroides* spp. inferior to that of cefoxitin and cefotetan.
Fourth	Cefepime (MAXIPIME)	Comparable to third-generation but more resistant to some β-lactamases.

[a]All cephalosporins lack activity against enterococci, *Listeria monocytogenes, Legionella* spp., methicillin-resistant *S. aureus, Xanthomonas maltophilia,* and *Acinetobacter* species.

[b]Except for penicillin-resistant strains.

[c]Except for methicillin-resistant strains.

[d]Resistance to cephalosporins may be induced rapidly during therapy by de-repression of bacterial chromosomal β-lactamases which destroy the cephalosporins.

[e]Ceftazidime only.

[f]Ceftazidime lacks significant gram-positive activity. Cefotaxime is most active in class against *S. aureus* and *S. pyogenes.*

relatively large amounts of β-lactamase into the surrounding medium. Although gram-negative bacteria seem to produce less β-lactamase, the location of their enzyme in the periplasmic space may make it more effective in destroying cephalosporins as they diffuse to their targets on the inner membrane, as is the case for the penicillins. The cephalosporins, however, have variable susceptibility to β-lactamase. For example, of the first-generation agents, cefazolin is more susceptible to hydrolysis by β-lactamase from *S. aureus* than is cephalothin. Cefoxitin, cefuroxime, and the third-generation cephalosporins are more resistant to hydrolysis by the β-lactamases produced by gram-negative bacteria than first-generation cephalosporins. Third-generation cephalosporins are susceptible to hydrolysis by inducible, chromosomally encoded (type I) β-lactamases. Induction of type I β-lactamases by treatment of infections due to aerobic gram-negative bacilli (especially *Enterobacter* spp., *Citrobacter freundii, Morganella, Serratia, Providencia,*

and *P. aeruginosa*) with second- or third-generation cephalosporins and/or imipenem may result in resistance to all third-generation cephalosporins. The fourth-generation cephalosporins, such as cefepime, are poor inducers of type I β-lactamases and are less susceptible to hydrolysis by type I β-lactamases than are the third-generation agents.

It is important to remember that none of the cephalosporins has reliable activity against the following bacteria: penicillin-resistant *S. pneumoniae,* methicillin-resistant *S. aureus,* methicillin-resistant *S. epidermidis* and other coagulase-negative staphylococci, *Enterococcus, L. monocytogenes, Legionella pneumophila, Legionella micdadei, C. difficile, Xanthomonas maltophilia, Campylobacter jejuni,* and *Acinetobacter* species.

General Features of the Cephalosporins. Cephalexin, cephradine, cefaclor, cefadroxil, loracarbef, cefprozil, cefixime, cefpodoxime proxetil, ceftibuten, and cefuroxime axetil are absorbed after oral administration and can be given by this route. Cephalothin and cephapirin cause pain when given by intramuscular injection and thus are usually used only intravenously. The other agents can be administered intramuscularly or intravenously.

Cephalosporins are excreted primarily by the kidney; dosage thus should be altered in patients with renal insufficiency. Probenecid slows the tubular secretion of most cephalosporins. Cefpiramide (not yet available in the United States) and cefoperazone are exceptions, because they are excreted predominantly in the bile. Cephalothin, cephapirin, and cefotaxime are deacetylated *in vivo,* and these metabolites have less antimicrobial activity than the parent compounds. The deacetylated metabolites also are excreted by the kidneys. None of the other cephalosporins appears to undergo appreciable metabolism.

Several cephalosporins penetrate into CSF in sufficient concentration to be useful for the treatment of meningitis. These include cefuroxime, cefotaxime, ceftriaxone, cefepime, and ceftizoxime (*see* "Therapeutic Uses," below). Cephalosporins also cross the placenta, and they are found in high concentrations in synovial and pericardial fluid. Penetration into the aqueous humor of the eye is relatively good after systemic administration of third-generation agents, but penetration into the vitreous humor is poor. There is some evidence that concentrations sufficient for therapy of ocular infections due to gram-positive and certain gram-negative microorganisms can be achieved after systemic administration. Concentrations in bile are usually high, with those achieved after administration of cefoperazone and cefpiramide being the highest.

Specific Agents

First-Generation Cephalosporins. *Cephalothin* is not well absorbed orally and is available only for parenteral administration. Because of pain on intramuscular injection, it usually is given intravenously. Since, among the cephalosporins, cephalothin is the most impervious to attack by staphylococcal β-lactamase, it is very effective in severe staphylococcal infections, such as endocarditis.

The antibacterial spectrum of *cefazolin* is similar to that of cephalothin. Although cefazolin is more active against *E. coli* and *Klebsiella* species, it is somewhat more sensitive to staphylococcal β-lactamase than is cephalothin. Cefazolin is relatively well tolerated after either intramuscular or intravenous administration, and concentrations of the drug in plasma are higher after intramuscular (64 μg/ml after 1 g) or intravenous injection than are concentrations of cephalothin. The half-life also is appreciably longer—1.8 hours. The renal clearance of cefazolin is lower than that of cephalothin; this is presumably related to the fact that cefazolin is excreted by glomerular filtra-

tion, whereas cephalothin also is secreted by the kidney tubule. Cefazolin is bound to plasma proteins to a great extent (about 85%). Cefazolin usually is preferred among the first-generation cephalosporins, since it can be administered less frequently because of its longer half-life.

Cephalexin is available for oral administration, and it has the same antibacterial spectrum as the other first-generation cephalosporins. However, it is somewhat less active against penicillinase-producing staphylococci. Oral therapy with cephalexin results in peak concentrations in plasma of 16 μg/ml after a dose of 0.5 g; this is adequate for the inhibition of many gram-positive and gram-negative pathogens that are sensitive to cephalothin. The drug is not metabolized, and between 70% and 100% is excreted in the urine.

Cephradine is similar in structure to cephalexin, and its activity *in vitro* is almost identical. Cephradine is not metabolized and, after rapid absorption from the gastrointestinal tract, is excreted unchanged in the urine. Cephradine can be administered orally, intramuscularly, or intravenously. When administered orally, it is difficult to distinguish cephradine from cephalexin; some authorities feel that these two drugs can be used interchangeably. Because cephradine is so well absorbed, the concentrations in plasma are nearly equivalent after oral or intramuscular administration.

Cefadroxil is the *para*-hydroxy analog of cephalexin. Concentrations of cefadroxil in plasma and urine are at somewhat higher levels than those with cephalexin. The drug may be orally administered once or twice a day for the treatment of urinary tract infections. Its activity *in vitro* is similar to that of cephalexin.

Second-Generation Cephalosporins. *Cefamandole* is more active than the first-generation cephalosporins against certain gram-negative microorganisms. It contains the methyl-tetrazole-thiomethyl (MTT) group at position 3, which is associated with disulfiram-like reactions, hypoprothrombinemia, and inhibition of vitamin K activation. Cefamandole and other second-generation cephalosporins have a broader spectrum than do the first-generation agents and are active against *Enterobacter* species, indole-positive *Proteus* species, and *Klebsiella* species. Strains of *H. influenzae* containing the plasmid β-lactamase TEM-1 are resistant to cefamandole. Most gram-positive cocci are sensitive to cefamandole. The half-life of the drug is 45 minutes, and it is excreted unchanged in the urine. Concentrations in plasma are 20 to 36 μg/ml after a dose of 1 g is given intramuscularly.

Cefoxitin is a cephamycin produced by *Streptomyces lactamdurans.* It is resistant to some β-lactamases produced by gram-negative rods (Barradell and Bryson, 1994). This antibiotic is more active than cephalothin against certain gram-negative microorganisms, although it is less active than cefamandole against *Enterobacter* species and *H. influenzae.* It also is less active than both cefamandole and the first-generation cephalosporins against gram-positive bacteria. Cefoxitin is more active than other first- or second-generation agents (except cefotetan) against anaerobes, especially *B. fragilis* (Appleman *et al.,* 1991). After an intramuscular dose of 1 g, concentrations in plasma are about 22 μg/ml. The half-life is approximately 40 minutes. Cefoxitin's special role seems to be for treatment of certain anaerobic and mixed aerobic-anaerobic infections, such as pelvic inflammatory disease and lung abscess (Sutter and Finegold, 1975; Bach *et al.,* 1977; Chow and Bednorz, 1978).

Cefaclor is used orally. The concentrations in plasma after oral administration are about 50% of those achieved after an equivalent oral dose of cephalexin. However, cefaclor is more active against *H. influenzae* and *Moraxella catarrhalis*, although some β-lactamase-producing strains of these organisms may be resistant (Jorgensen *et al.*, 1990).

Loracarbef is an orally administered carbacephin, similar in activity to cefaclor, that is more stable against some β-lactamases (Jorgensen *et al.*, 1990). The serum half-life is 1.1 hours.

Cefuroxime is very similar to cefamandole in structure and antibacterial activity *in vitro* (Smith and LeFrock, 1983), although it lacks the MTT group and its attendant toxicities and is somewhat more resistant to β-lactamases. The half-life is longer than that of cefamandole (1.7 hours versus 0.8 hour), and the drug can be given every 8 hours. Concentrations in CSF are about 10% of those in plasma, and the drug is effective (but inferior to ceftriaxone) for treatment of meningitis due to *H. influenzae* (including strains resistant to ampicillin), *N. meningitidis*, and *S. pneumoniae* (Schaad *et al.*, 1990).

Cefuroxime axetil is the 1-acetyloxyethyl ester of cefuroxime. Thirty to fifty percent of an oral dose is absorbed, and the drug is then hydrolyzed to cefuroxime; resultant concentrations in plasma are variable.

Cefonicid has antimicrobial activity *in vitro* similar to that of cefamandole. The half-life of the drug is about 4 hours, and administration once daily has been effective for certain infections caused by susceptible microorganisms (Gremillion *et al.*, 1983).

Cefotetan is a cephamycin, and, like cefoxitin, it has good activity against *B. fragilis*. It also is effective against several other species of *Bacteroides*, and it is slightly more active than cefoxitin against gram-negative aerobes. After an intramuscular dose of 1 g, peak plasma concentrations of cefotetan average 70 μg/ml. It has a half-life of 3.3 hours (Phillips *et al.*, 1983; Wexler and Finegold, 1988). Hypoprothrombinemia with bleeding has occurred in malnourished patients receiving cefotetan due to the MTT group at position 3; this is preventable if vitamin K also is administered.

Ceforanide is similar in structure and antimicrobial activity to cefamandole; however, it is less active against strains of *H. influenzae* (Barriere and Mills, 1982). Its half-life is about 2.6 hours and it is administered parenterally every 12 hours.

Cefprozil is an orally administered agent more active than first-generation cephalosporins against penicillin-sensitive streptococci, *E. coli, P. mirabilis, Klebsiella* spp., and *Citrobacter* spp. It has a serum half-life of 1.2 to 1.4 hours (Barriere, 1992).

Third-Generation Cephalosporins. *Cefotaxime* is highly resistant to many (but not the extended spectrum) of the bacterial β-lactamases and has good activity against many gram-positive and gram-negative aerobic bacteria. However, activity against *B. fragilis* is poor as compared to agents such as clindamycin and metronidazole (Neu *et al.*, 1979). Cefotaxime has a half-life in plasma of about 1 hour, and the drug should be administered every 4 to 8 hours for serious infections. The drug is metabolized *in vivo* to desacetylcefotaxime, which is less active against most microorganisms than is the parent compound. However, the metabolite acts synergistically with the parent compound against certain microbes (Neu, 1982).

Cefotaxime has been utilized effectively for meningitis caused by *H. influenzae*, penicillin-sensitive *S. pneumoniae*, and *N. meningitidis* (Landesman *et al.*, 1981; Cherubin *et al.*, 1982; Mullaney and John, 1983).

Ceftizoxime has a spectrum of activity *in vitro* very similar to that of cefotaxime, except that it is less active against *S. pneumoniae* and more active against *B. fragilis* (Haas *et al.*, 1995). The half-life is somewhat longer, 1.8 hours, and the drug can thus be administered every 8 to 12 hours for serious infections. Ceftizoxime is not metabolized, and 90% is recovered in urine (Neu *et al.*, 1982).

Ceftriaxone has activity *in vitro* very similar to that of ceftizoxime and cefotaxime. A half-life of about 8 hours is the outstanding feature. Administration of the drug once or twice daily has been effective for patients with meningitis (Del Rio *et al.*, 1983; Brogden and Ward, 1988), while dosage once a day has been effective for other infections (Baumgartner and Glauser, 1983). About half the drug can be recovered from the urine; the remainder appears to be eliminated by biliary secretion. A single dose of ceftriaxone (125 to 250 mg) is effective in the treatment of urethral, cervical, rectal, or pharyngeal gonorrhea, including disease caused by penicillinase-producing microorganisms (Rajan *et al.*, 1982; Handsfield and Murphy, 1983).

Cefixime is orally administered and, compared to orally administered second-generation agents, is less active against gram-positive cocci and more active against Enterobacteriaceae and β-lactamase–producing *H. influenzae, M. catarrhalis*, and *N. gonorrhoeae*. It has poor activity against *S. aureus*. It has a serum half-life of approximately 3 hours.

Cefpodoxime proxetil is an orally administered third-generation agent very similar in activity to cefixime, except that is it slightly more active against *S. aureus*. It has a serum half-life of 2.2 hours.

Third-Generation Cephalosporins with Good Activity Against Pseudomonas. *Cefoperazone* is less active than cefotaxime against gram-positive microorganisms and less active than cefotaxime or moxalactam against many species of gram-negative bacteria. It is more active than both of these agents against *P. aeruginosa*, but less active than ceftazidime. Unfortunately, resistant strains may emerge on treatment. Activity against *B. fragilis* is similar to that of cefotaxime. Cefoperazone is slightly less stable with β-lactamases than are the cefotaxime-like or 7-methoxycephem drugs (Klein and Neu, 1983). Only 25% of a dose of cefoperazone can be recovered from the urine, and most of the drug is eliminated by biliary excretion. The half-life is about 2 hours. Concentrations of cefoperazone in bile are higher than those achieved with other cephalosporins; concentrations in blood are two to three times higher than those found with cefotaxime. The dose of cefoperazone does not have to be altered in patients with renal insufficiency, but hepatic dysfunction or biliary obstruction affects clearance. Cefoperazone can cause bleeding due to hypoprothrombinemia secondary to the MTT group; this can be reversed by administration of vitamin K. A disulfiram-like reaction has been reported in patients who drink alcohol while taking cefoperazone.

Ceftazidime is one-quarter to one-half as active by weight against gram-positive microorganisms as is cefotaxime. Its activity against the Enterobacteriaceae is very similar, but its major distinguishing feature is excellent activity against *Pseudomonas* and other gram-negative bacteria. Ceftazidime has poor activity against *B. fragilis* (Hamilton-Miller and Brumfitt, 1981). Its half-life in plasma is about 1.5 hours, and the drug is not metabolized. Ceftazidime is more active *in vitro* against *Pseudomonas* than is cefoperazone or piperacillin (Edmond *et al.,* 1999; Sahm *et al.,* 1999).

Fourth-Generation Cephalosporins.   *Cefepime* and *cefpirome* are fourth-generation cephalosporins. Cefepime is available for use in the United States, but cefpirome is not. Cefepime is stable to hydrolysis by many of the previously identified plasmid-encoded β-lactamases (called TEM-1, TEM-2, and SHV-1). It is a poor inducer of, and relatively resistant to, the type I chromosomally encoded, and some extended-spectrum, β-lactamases. It is thus active against many Enterobacteriaceae that are resistant to other cephalosporins *via* induction of type I β-lactamases, but remains susceptible to many bacteria expressing extended-spectrum plasmid-mediated β-lactamases (such as TEM-3 and TEM-10). Against the fastidious gram-negative bacteria (*H. influenzae, Neisseria gonorrhoeae,* and *Neisseria meningitidis*), cefepime has comparable or greater *in vitro* activity than cefotaxime. For *P. aeruginosa,* cefepime has comparable activity to ceftazidime, although it is less active than ceftazidime for other *Pseudomonas* species and *X. maltophilia.* Cefepime has higher activity than ceftazidime, and comparable activity to cefotaxime, for streptococci and methicillin-sensitive *S. aureus* (Sanders, 1993). It is not active against methicillin-resistant *S. aureus,* penicillin-resistant pneumococci, enterococci, *B. fragilis, L. monocytogenes, Mycobacterium avium* complex, or *Mycobacterium tuberculosis.* Cefepime is almost 100% renally excreted, and doses should be adjusted for renal failure. Cefepime has excellent penetration into the CSF in animal models of meningitis. When given at the recommended dosage for adults of 2 g intravenously every 12 hours, peak serum concentrations in human beings range from 126 to 193 μg/ml. The serum half-life is 2 hours.

Adverse Reactions.   Hypersensitivity reactions to the cephalosporins are the most common side effects (*see* Petz, 1978), and there is no evidence that any single cephalosporin is more or less likely to cause such sensitization. The reactions appear to be identical to those caused by the penicillins, and this may be related to the shared β-lactam structure of both groups of antibiotics (Bennett *et al.,* 1983). Immediate reactions such as anaphylaxis, bronchospasm, and urticaria are observed. More commonly, maculopapular rash develops, usually after several days of therapy; this may or may not be accompanied by fever and eosinophilia.

Because of the similarity in structure of the penicillins and cephalosporins, patients who are allergic to one class of agents may manifest cross-reactivity when a member of the other class is administered. Immunological studies have demonstrated cross-reactivity in as many as 20% of patients who are allergic to penicillin (*see* Levine, 1973), but clinical studies indicate a much lower frequency

(about 1%) of such reactions (Saxon *et al.,* 1984). There are no skin tests that can reliably predict whether a patient will manifest an allergic reaction to the cephalosporins.

Patients with a history of a mild or a temporally distant reaction to penicillin appear to be at low risk of rash or other allergic reaction following the administration of a cephalosporin. However, patients who have had a recent severe, immediate reaction to a penicillin should be given a cephalosporin with great caution, if at all. A positive Coombs reaction appears frequently in patients who receive large doses of a cephalosporin. Hemolysis is not usually associated with this phenomenon, although it has been reported. Cephalosporins have produced rare instances of bone-marrow depression, characterized by granulocytopenia (Kammer, 1984).

The cephalosporins have been implicated as potentially nephrotoxic agents, although they are not nearly as toxic to the kidney as are the aminoglycosides or the polymyxins (Barza, 1978). Renal tubular necrosis has followed the administration of cephaloridine in doses greater than 4 g per day; this agent is no longer available in the United States. Other cephalosporins are much less toxic and, in recommended doses, rarely produce significant renal toxicity when used by themselves. High doses of cephalothin have produced acute tubular necrosis in certain instances, and usual doses (8 to 12 g per day) have caused nephrotoxicity in patients with preexisting renal disease (Pasternack and Stephens, 1975). There is good evidence that the concurrent administration of cephalothin and gentamicin or tobramycin act synergistically to cause nephrotoxicity (Wade *et al.,* 1978). This is especially marked in patients over 60 years of age. Diarrhea can result from the administration of cephalosporins and may be more frequent with cefoperazone, perhaps because of its greater biliary excretion. Intolerance to alcohol (a disulfiram-like reaction) has been noted with cephalosporins that contain the MTT group, including cefamandole, cefotetan, moxalactam, and cefoperazone. Serious bleeding related either to hypoprothrombinemia due to the MTT group, thrombocytopenia, and/or platelet dysfunction has been reported with several β-lactam antibiotics (Bank and Kammer, 1983; Sattler *et al.,* 1986). This appears to be a particular problem with certain patients (elderly, poorly nourished, or those with renal insufficiency) who are receiving moxalactam.

Therapeutic Uses.   The cephalosporins are widely used and therapeutically important antibiotics. Unfortunately, a wide array of bacteria are resistant to their activity. Clinical studies have shown cephalosporins to be effective as both therapeutic and prophylactic agents (Donowitz and Mandell, 1988).

The first-generation cephalosporins are excellent agents for skin and soft tissue infections due to *S. aureus* and *S. pyogenes*. A single dose of cefazolin just before surgery is the preferred prophylaxis for procedures in which skin flora are the likely pathogens. For colorectal surgery where prophylaxis for intestinal anaerobes is desired, the second-generation agents cefoxitin or cefotetan are preferred.

The second-generation cephalosporins have been displaced by third-generation agents for many infections. The second-generation agents have inferior activity against penicillin-resistant *S. pneumoniae* compared to either the third-generation agents or ampicillin, and therefore should not be used for empirical treatment of meningitis or pneumonia. The oral second-generation cephalosporins can be used to treat respiratory tract infections, although they are suboptimal for treatment of penicillin-resistant *S. pneumoniae*. In situations where facultative gram-negative bacteria and anaerobes are involved, such as intraabdominal infections, pelvic inflammatory disease, and diabetic foot infection, cefoxitin and cefotetan have been shown to be effective.

The third-generation cephalosporins, either with or without aminoglycosides, have been considered to be the drugs of choice for serious infections caused by *Klebsiella, Enterobacter, Proteus, Providencia, Serratia,* and *Haemophilus* species. Ceftriaxone is now the therapy of choice for all forms of gonorrhea and for severe forms of Lyme disease. The third-generation cephalosporins cefotaxime or ceftriaxone (as part of a 3-drug combination with vancomycin and ampicillin) are used for the initial treatment of meningitis in nonimmunocompromised adults and children older than 3 months (pending identification of the causative agent) because of their antimicrobial activity, good penetration into CSF, and record of clinical successes. They are the drugs of choice for the treatment of meningitis caused by *H. influenzae,* sensitive *S. pneumoniae, N. meningitidis,* and gram-negative enteric bacteria. Cefotaxime has failed in the treatment of meningitis due to resistant *S. pneumoniae* (Friedland and McCracken, 1994). Ceftazidime plus an aminoglycoside is the treatment of choice for *Pseudomonas* meningitis. Third-generation cephalosporins, however, lack activity against *L. monocytogenes* and penicillin-resistant pneumococci, which may cause meningitis. The antimicrobial spectrum of cefotaxime and ceftriaxone is excellent for the treatment of community-acquired pneumonia, *i.e.,* that caused by pneumococci (achievable serum concentrations exceed minimal inhibitory concentrations for many or most penicillin-resistant isolates), *H. influenzae,* or *S. aureus.*

The fourth-generation cephalosporins are indicated for the empirical treatment of nosocomial infections where antibiotic resistance due to extended-spectrum β-lactamases or chromosomally induced β-lactamases are anticipated. For example, cefepime has superior activity against nosocomial isolates of *Enterobacter, Citrobacter,* and *Serratia* spp. compared to ceftazidime and piperacillin (Jones *et al.,* 1998).

OTHER β-LACTAM ANTIBIOTICS

Important therapeutic agents with a β-lactam structure that are neither penicillins nor cephalosporins have been developed.

Carbapenems

Carbapenems are β-lactams that contain a fused β-lactam ring and a 5-membered ring system that differs from the penicillins in being unsaturated and containing a carbon atom instead of the sulfur atom. This class of antibiotics has a broader spectrum of activity than do most other β-lactam antibiotics.

Imipenem. *Imipenem* is marketed in combination with cilastatin, a drug that inhibits the degradation of imipenem by a renal tubular dipeptidase.

Source and Chemistry. Imipenem is derived from a compound produced by *Streptomyces cattleya.* The compound thienamycin is unstable, but imipenem, the *N*-formimidoyl derivative, is stable. The structural formula of imipenem is as follows:

IMIPENEM

Antimicrobial Activity. Imipenem, like other β-lactam antibiotics, binds to penicillin-binding proteins, disrupts bacterial cell-wall synthesis, and causes death of susceptible microorganisms. It is very resistant to hydrolysis by most β-lactamases.

The activity of imipenem is excellent *in vitro* for a wide variety of aerobic and anaerobic microorganisms. Streptococci (including penicillin-resistant *S. pneumoniae*), enterococci (excluding *Enterococcus faecium* and non–β-lactamase-producing penicillin-resistant strains), staphylococci (including penicillinase-producing strains), and *Listeria* are all susceptible. Although some strains of methicillin-resistant staphylococci are susceptible, many strains are not. Activity is excellent against the Enterobacteriaceae, including those organisms that are cephalosporin-resistant by virtue of expression of chromosomal or plasmid extended-spectrum β-lactamases. Most strains of *Pseudomonas* and *Acinetobacter* are inhibited. *X. maltophilia* is resistant. Anaerobes, including *B. fragilis,* are highly susceptible.

Pharmacokinetics and Adverse Reactions.   Imipenem is not absorbed orally. The drug is hydrolyzed rapidly by a dipeptidase found in the brush border of the proximal renal tubule (Kropp *et al.,* 1982). Because concentrations of active drug in urine were low, an inhibitor of the dehydropeptidase was synthesized. This compound is called *cilastatin*. A preparation has been developed that contains equal amounts of imipenem and cilastatin (PRIMAXIN).

   After the intravenous administration of 500 mg of imipenem (as PRIMAXIN), peak concentrations in plasma average 33 μg/ml. Both imipenem and cilastatin have a half-life of about 1 hour. When administered concurrently with cilastatin, approximately 70% of administered imipenem is recovered in the urine as the active drug. Dosage should be modified for patients with renal insufficiency.

   Nausea and vomiting are the most common adverse reactions (1% to 20%). Seizures also have been noted in up to 1.5% of patients, especially when high doses are given to patients with CNS lesions and to those with renal insufficiency. Patients who are allergic to other β-lactam antibiotics may have hypersensitivity reactions when given imipenem.

Therapeutic Uses.   Imipenem–cilastatin is effective for a wide variety of infections (Eron *et al.,* 1983), including urinary tract and lower respiratory infections; intraabdominal and gynecological infections; and skin, soft-tissue, bone, and joint infections. The drug combination appears to be especially useful for the treatment of infections caused by cephalosporin-resistant nosocomial bacteria, such as *Citrobacter freundii* and *Enterobacter* spp. It would be prudent to use imipenem for empiric treatment of serious infections in hospitalized patients who have recently received other β-lactam antibiotics, because of the increased risk of infection with cephalosporin- and/or penicillin-resistant bacteria. Imipenem should not be used as monotherapy for infections due to *P. aeruginosa* because of the risk of resistance developing during therapy.

Meropenem.   *Meropenem* (MERREM IV) is a dimethylcarbamoyl pyrolidinyl derivative of thienamycin. It does not require coadministration with cilastatin as it is not sensitive to renal dipeptidase. Its toxicity is similar to that of imipenem except that it may be less likely to cause seizures (0.5% of meropenem- and 1.5% of imipenem-treated patients seized). Its *in vitro* activity is similar to that of imipenem, with activity against some imipenem-resistant *P. aeruginosa* but less activity against gram-positive cocci. Clinical experience with meropenem demonstrates therapeutic equivalence with imipenem.

Aztreonam.   *Aztreonam* (AZACTAM) is a monocyclic β-lactam compound (a monobactam) isolated from *Chro-*

mobacterium violaceum (Sykes *et al.,* 1981). Its structural formula is as follows:

AZTREONAM

   Aztreonam interacts with penicillin-binding proteins of susceptible microorganisms and induces the formation of long filamentous bacterial structures. The compound is resistant to many of the β-lactamases that are elaborated by most gram-negative bacteria.

   The antimicrobial activity of aztreonam differs from those of other β-lactam antibiotics and more closely resembles that of an aminoglycoside. Gram-positive bacteria and anaerobic organisms are resistant. However, activity against Enterobacteriaceae is excellent, as is that against *P. aeruginosa.* It is also highly active *in vitro* against *H. influenzae* and gonococci.

   Aztreonam is administered either intramuscularly or intravenously. Peak concentrations of aztreonam in plasma average nearly 50 μg/ml after a 1-g intramuscular dose. The half-time for elimination is 1.7 hours, and most of the drug is recovered unaltered in the urine. The half-life is prolonged to about 6 hours in anephric patients.

   Aztreonam generally is well tolerated. Interestingly, patients who are allergic to penicillins or cephalosporins appear not to react to aztreonam (Saxon *et al.,* 1984).

   The usual dose of aztreonam for severe infections is 2 g every 6 to 8 hours. This should be reduced for patients with renal insufficiency. Aztreonam has been used successfully for the therapy of a variety of infections. One of its notable features is little allergic cross-reactivity with β-lactam antibiotics. It is therefore quite useful for treating gram-negative infections that normally would be treated with a β-lactam antibiotic, were it not for the history of a prior allergic reaction.

β-LACTAMASE INHIBITORS

Certain molecules can bind to β-lactamases and inactivate them, thus preventing the destruction of β-lactam antibiotics that are substrates for these enzymes. β-Lactamase inhibitors are most active against plasmid-encoded β-lactamases (including the extended-spectrum ceftazidime- and cefotaxime-hydrolyzing enzymes), but they are inactive at clinically achievable concentrations against the type I chromosomal β-lactamases induced in gram-negative bacilli (such as *Enterobacter, Acinetobacter,* and

Citrobacter) by treatment with second- and third-generation cephalosporins.

Clavulanic acid is produced by *Streptomyces clavuligerus;* its structural formula is as follows:

CLAVULANIC ACID

It has poor intrinsic antimicrobial activity, but it is a "suicide" inhibitor (irreversible binder) of β-lactamases produced by a wide range of gram-positive and gram-negative microorganisms (Neu and Fu, 1978). Clavulanic acid is well absorbed by mouth and also can be given parenterally. It has been combined with amoxicillin as an oral preparation (AUGMENTIN) and with ticarcillin as a parenteral preparation (TIMENTIN).

Amoxicillin plus clavulanate is effective *in vitro* and *in vivo* for β-lactamase-producing strains of staphylococci, *H. influenzae,* gonococci, and *E. coli* (Ball *et al.,* 1980; Yogev *et al.,* 1981). Amoxicillin-clavulanate plus ciprofloxacin recently has been shown to be an effective oral treatment for low-risk, febrile patients with neutropenia from cancer chemotherapy (Freifeld *et al.,* 1999; Kern *et al.,* 1999). It also is effective in the treatment of acute otitis media in children, sinusitis, animal or human bite wounds, cellulitis, and diabetic foot infections. The addition of clavulanate to ticarcillin (TIMENTIN) extends its spectrum such that it resembles imipenem to include aerobic gram-negative bacilli, *S. aureus,* and *Bacteroides* species. There is no increased activity against *Pseudomonas* species (Bansal *et al.,* 1985). The dosage should be adjusted for patients with renal insufficiency. The combination is especially useful for mixed nosocomial infections and is often used with an aminoglycoside.

Sulbactam is another β-lactamase inhibitor similar in structure to clavulanic acid. It may be given orally or parenterally along with a β-lactam antibiotic. It is available for intravenous or intramuscular use combined with ampicillin (UNASYN). Dosage must be adjusted for patients with impaired renal function. The combination has good activity against gram-positive cocci, including β-lactamase-producing strains of *S. aureus,* gram-negative aerobes (but not *Pseudomonas*), and anaerobes; it also has been used effectively for the treatment of mixed intraabdominal and pelvic infections (Reinhardt *et al.,* 1986).

Tazobactam is a penicillanic acid sulfone β-lactamase inhibitor. In common with the other available inhibitors, it has poor activity against the inducible, chromosomal β-lactamases of Enterobacteriaceae but has good activity against many of the plasmid β-lactamases, including some of the extended spectrum class. It has been combined with piperacillin as a parenteral preparation (ZOSYN, *see* Bryson and Brogden, 1994).

The combination of piperacillin plus tazobactam does not increase the activity of piperacillin against *P. aeruginosa,* as resistance is due to either chromosomal β-lactamases or decreased permeability of piperacillin into the periplasmic space. Because the currently recommended dose (3 g piperacillin/375 mg tazobactam every 4 to 8 hours) is less than the recommended dose of piperacillin when used alone for serious infections (3 to 4 g every 4 to 6 hours), concern has been raised that piperacillin/tazobactam may prove ineffective in the treatment of some *P. aeruginosa* infections that would have responded to piperacillin. The combination of piperacillin plus tazobactam should be equivalent in antimicrobial spectrum to ticarcillin plus clavulanate.

PROSPECTUS

Therapy with β-lactam antibiotics is dynamic. The prevalence of bacterial resistance to these agents continues to rise, while new and more effective agents are released for clinical use.

For further information regarding particular infections for which the antimicrobial agents discussed in this chapter are useful, the reader is referred to the following chapters of *Harrison's Principles of Internal Medicine,* 14th ed., McGraw-Hill, New York, 1998: diseases caused by gram-positive organisms (Chapters 141 to 148), diseases caused by gram-negative infections (Chapters 149 to 166), actinomycosis (Chapter 168), infections due to mixed anaerobic organisms (Chapter 169), syphilis (Chapter 174), and Lyme disease (Chapter 178).

BIBLIOGRAPHY

Anonymous. Penicillin allergy. *Med. Lett. Drug Ther.,* **1988,** *30:*79–80.

Appleman, M.D., Heseltine, P.N., and Cherubin, C.E. Epidemiology, antimicrobial susceptibility, pathogenicity, and significance of *Bacteroides fragilis* group organisms isolated at Los Angeles County–University of Southern California Medical Center. *Rev. Infect. Dis.,* **1991,** *13:*12–18.

Bach, V.T., Roy, I., and Thadepalli, H. Susceptibility of anaerobic bacteria to cefoxitin and related compounds. *Antimicrob. Agents Chemother.,* **1977,** *11:*912–913.

Ball, A.P., Geddes, A.M., Davey, P.G., Farrell, I.D., and Brookes, G.R. Clavulanic acid and amoxycillin: a clinical, bacteriological, and pharmacological study. *Lancet,* **1980,** *1:*620–623.

Bansal, M.B., Chuah, S.K., and Thadepalli, H. *In vitro* activity and *in vivo* evaluation of ticarcillin plus clavulanic acid against aerobic and anaerobic bacteria. *Am. J. Med.*, **1985,** *79:*33–38.

Barriere, S.L., and Mills, J. Ceforanide: antibacterial activity, pharmacology, and clinical efficacy. *Pharmacotherapy*, **1982,** *2:*322–327.

Barriere, S.L. Pharmacology and pharmacokinetics of cefprozil. *Clin. Infect. Dis.*, **1992,** *14 (suppl. 2):*S184–S188.

Barza, M. The nephrotoxicity of cephalosporins: an overview. *J. Infect. Dis.*, **1978,** *137:*S60–S73.

Baumgartner, J.D., and Glauser, M.P. Single daily dose treatment of severe refractory infections with ceftriaxone. Cost savings and possible parenteral outpatient treatment. *Arch. Intern. Med.*, **1983,** *143:*1868–1873.

Bennett, S., Wise, R., Weston, D., and Dent, J. Pharmacokinetics and tissue penetration of ticarcillin combined with clavulanic acid. *Antimicrob. Agents Chemother.*, **1983,** *23:*831–834.

Berrios, X., del Campo, E., Guzman, B., and Bisno, A.L. Discontinuing rheumatic fever prophylaxis in selected adolescents and young adults. A prospective study. *Ann. Intern. Med.*, **1993,** *118:*401–406.

Brogden, R.N., and Ward, A. Ceftriaxone: a reappraisal of its antibacterial activity and pharmacokinetic properties, and an update on its therapeutic use with particular reference to once-daily administration. *Drugs*, **1988,** *35:*604–645.

Carratalá, J., Alcaide, F., Fernandez-Sevilla, A., Corbella, X., Linares, J., and Gudiol, F. Bacteremia due to *viridans* streptococci that are highly resistant to penicillin: increase among neutropenic patients with cancer. *Clin. Infect. Dis.*, **1995,** *20:*1169–1173.

Catalan, M.J., Fernandez, J.M., Vazquez, A., Varela de Seijas, E., Suarez, A., and Bernaldo de Quiros, J.C. Failure of cefotaxime in the treatment of meningitis due to relatively resistant *Streptococcus pneumoniae. Clin. Infect. Dis.*, **1994,** *18:*766–769.

Centers for Disease Control and Prevention. Update: *Staphylococcus aureus* with reduced susceptibility to vancomycin—United States, 1997. *M.M.W.R., Morb. Mortal. Wkly. Rep.*, **1997,** *46:*813–815.

Centers for Disease Control and Prevention. Geographic variation in penicillin resistance in *Streptococcus pneumoniae*—selected sites, United States, 1997. *M.M.W.R., Morb. Mortal. Wkly. Rep.*, **1999,** *48:*656–661.

Chain, E.B. The development of bacterial chemotherapy. *Antibiot. Chemother.*, **1954,** *4:*215–241.

Chambers, H.F., Hackbarth, C.J., Drake, T.A., Rusnak, M.G., and Sande, M.A. Endocarditis due to methicillin-resistant *Staphylococcus aureus* in rabbits: expression of resistance to beta-lactam antibiotics *in vivo* and *in vitro. J. Infect. Dis.*, **1984,** *149:*894–903.

Chow, A.W., and Bednorz, D. Comparative *in vitro* activity of newer cephalosporins against anaerobic bacteria. *Antimicrob. Agents Chemother.*, **1978,** *14:*668–671.

Dajani, A.S., Bisno, A.L., Chung, K.J., Durack, D.T., Freed, M., Gerber, M.A., Karchmer, A.W., Millard, H.D., Rahimtoola, S., and Shulman, S.T. Prevention of bacterial endocarditis. Recommendations by the American Heart Association. *JAMA*, **1990,** *264:*2919–2922.

del Rio, M.A., Chrane, D., Shelton, S., McCracken, G.H., Jr., and Nelson, J.D. Ceftriaxone versus ampicillin and chloramphenicol for treatment of bacterial meningitis in children. *Lancet,* **1983,** *1:*1241–1244.

Dowell, S.F., Butler, J.C., Giebink, G.S., Jacobs, M.R., Jernigan, D., Musher, D.M., Rakowsky, A., and Schwartz, B. Acute otitis media: management and surveillance in an era of pneumococcal resistance—a report from the Drug-resistant *Streptococcus pneumoniae* Therapeutic Working Group. *Pediatr. Infect. Dis. J.*, **1999,** *18:*1–9.

Edmond, M.B., Wallace, S.E., McClish, D.K., Pfaller, M.A., Jones, R.N., and Wenzel, R.P. Nosocomial bloodstream infections in United States hospitals: a three-year analysis. *Clin. Infect. Dis.*, **1999,** *29:*239–244.

Eron, L.J., Hixon, D.L., Park, C.H., Goldenberg, R.I., and Poretz, D.M. Imipenem versus moxalactam in the treatment of serious infections. *Antimicrob. Agents Chemother.*, **1983,** *24:*841–846.

Fass, R.J., Copelan, E.A., Brandt, J.T., Moeschberger, M.L., and Ashton, J.J. Platelet-mediated bleeding caused by broad-spectrum penicillins. *J. Infect. Dis.*, **1987,** *155:*1242–1248.

Fiore, A.E., Moroney, J.F., Farley, M.M., Harrison, L.H., Patterson, J.E., Jorgensen, J.H., Cetron, M., Kolczak, M.S., Breiman, R.F., and Schuchat, A. Clinical outcomes of meningitis caused by *Streptococcus pneumoniae* in the era of antibiotic resistance. *Clin. Infect. Dis.*, **2000,** *30:*71–77.

Freifeld, A., Marchigiani, D., Walsh, T., Chanock, S., Lewis, L., Hiemenz, J., Hiemenz, S., Hicks, J.E., Gill, V., Steinberg, S.M., and Pizzo, P.A. A double-blind comparison of empirical oral and intravenous antibiotic therapy for low-risk febrile patients with neutropenia during cancer chemotherapy. *N. Engl. J. Med.,* **1999,** *341:*305–311.

Friedland, I.R., and McCracken, G.H., Jr. Management of infections caused by antibiotic-resistant *Streptococcus pneumoniae. N. Engl. J. Med.,* **1994,** *331:*377–382.

Gremillion, D.H., Winn, R.E., and Vandenbout, E. Clinical trial of cefonicid for treatment of skin infections. *Antimicrob. Agents Chemother.*, **1983,** *23:*944–946.

Haas, D.W., Stratton, C.W., Griffin, J.P., Weeks, L., and Alls, S.C. Diminished activity of ceftizoxime in comparison to cefotaxime and ceftriaxone against *Streptococcus pneumoniae. Clin. Infect. Dis.*, **1995,** *20:*671–676.

Hamilton-Miller, J.M., and Brumfitt, W. Activity of ceftazidime (GR 20263) against nosocomially important pathogens. *Antimicrob. Agents Chemother.*, **1981,** *19:*1067–1069.

Handsfield, H.H., and Murphy, V.L. Comparative study of ceftriaxone and spectinomycin for treatment of uncomplicated gonorrhoea in men. *Lancet*, **1983,** *2:*67–70.

John, C.C. Treatment failure with use of a third-generation cephalosporin for penicillin-resistant pneumococcal meningitis: case report and review. *Clin. Infect. Dis.*, **1994,** *18:*188–193.

Jones, R.N., Pfaller, M.A., Doern, G.V., Erwin, M.E., and Hollis, R.J. Antimicrobial activity and spectrum investigation of eight broad-spectrum β-lactam drugs: a 1997 surveillance trial in 102 medical centers in the United States. Cefepime Study Group. *Diagn. Microbiol. Infect. Dis.*, **1998,** *30:*215–228.

Jorgensen, J.H., Doern, G.V., Maher, L.A., Howell, A.W., and Redding, J.S. Antimicrobial resistance among respiratory isolates of *Haemophilus influenzae, Moraxella catarrhalis,* and *Streptococcus pneumoniae* in the United States. *Antimicrob. Agents Chemother.,* **1990,** *34:*2075–2080.

Kelly, J.A., Moews, P.C., Knox, J.R., Frere, J.M., and Ghuysen, J.M. Penicillin target enzyme and the antibiotic binding site. *Science,* **1982,** *218:*479–481.

Kern, W.V., Cometta, A., De Bock, R., Langenaeken, J., Paesmans, M., and Gaya, H. Oral versus intravenous empirical antimicrobial therapy for fever in patients with granulocytopenia who are receiving cancer chemotherapy. International Antimicrobial Therapy Cooperative Group of the European Organization for Research and Treatment of Cancer. *N. Engl. J. Med.,* **1999,** *341:*312–318.

Kirkwood, C.F., Smith, L.L., Rustagi, P.K., and Schentag, J.J. Neutropenia associated with β-lactam antibiotics. *Clin. Pharmacol.,* **1983,** *2:*569–578.

Klaus, M.V., and Fellner, M.J. Penicilloyl-specific serum antibodies in man. Analysis in 592 individuals from the newborn to old age. *J. Gerontol.*, **1973**, *28:*312–316.

Klein, J.O., and Neu, H.C. Empiric therapy for bacterial infections. Evaluation of cefoperazone. A symposium, Geneva, Switzerland, October 4–5, 1981. *Rev. Infect. Dis.*, **1983**, *5:*S1–S209.

Kropp, H., Sundelof, J.G., Hajdu, R., and Kahan, F.M. Metabolism of thienamycin and related carbapenem antibiotics by the renal dipeptidase, dehydropeptidase. *Antimicrob. Agents Chemother.*, **1982**, *22:*62–70.

Landesman, S.H., Corrado, M.L., Shah, P.M., Armengaud, M., Barza, M., and Cherubin, C.E. Past and current roles for cephalosporin antibiotics in treatment of meningitis. Emphasis on use in gram-negative bacillary meningitis. *Am. J. Med.*, **1981**, *71:*693–703.

Levine, B.B. Antigenicity and cross reactivity of penicillins and cephalosporins. *J. Infect. Dis.*, **1973**, *128* (*suppl.*):S364–S366.

Levison, M.E., Mangura, C.T., Lorber, B., Abrutyn, E., Pesanti, E.L., Levy, R.S., MacGregor, R.R., and Schwartz, A.R. Clindamycin compared with penicillin for the treatment of anaerobic lung abscess. *Ann. Intern. Med.*, **1983**, *98:*466–471.

Mendelman, P.M., Campos, J., Chaffin, D.O., Serfass, D.A., Smith, A.L., and Saez-Nieto, J.A. Relative penicillin G resistance in *Neisseria meningitidis* and reduced affinity of penicillin-binding protein 3. *Antimicrob. Agents Chemother.*, **1988**, *32:*706–709.

Mullaney, D.T., and John, J.F. Cefotaxime therapy. Evaluation of its effect on bacterial meningitis, CSF drug levels, and bactericidal activity. *Arch. Intern. Med.*, **1983**, *143:*1705–1708.

Neu, H.C. Antibacterial activity of desacetylcefotaxime alone and in combination with cefotaxime. *Rev. Infect. Dis.*, **1982**, *4* (*suppl.*): S374–S378.

Neu, H.C., Aswapokee, N., Aswapokee, P., and Fu, K.P. HR 756, a new cephalosporin active against gram-positive and gram-negative aerobic and anaerobic bacteria. *Antimicrob. Agents Chemother.*, **1979**, *15:*273–281.

Neu, H.C., and Fu, K.P. Clavulanic acid, a novel inhibitor of β-lactamases. *Antimicrob. Agents Chemother.*, **1978**, *14:*650–655.

Neu, H.C., Turck, M., and Phillips, I. Ceftizoxime, a broad-spectrum beta-lactamase stable cephalosporin. *J. Antimicrob. Chemother.*, **1982**, *10* (*suppl. C*): 1–355.

Nikaido, H. Antibiotic resistance caused by gram-negative multidrug efflux pumps. *Clin. Infect. Dis.*, **1998**, *27* (*suppl. I*):S32–S41.

Park, J.T., and Strominger, J.L. Mode of action of penicillin. *Science*, **1957**, *125:*99–101.

Pasternack, D.P., and Stephens, B.G. Reversible nephrotoxicity associated with cephalothin therapy. *Arch. Intern. Med.*, **1975**, *135:*599–602.

Petz, L.D. Immunologic cross-reactivity between penicillins and cephalosporins: a review. *J. Infect. Dis.*, **1978**, *137* (*suppl.*):S74–S79.

Phillips, I., Wise, R., and Leigh, D.A. Cefotetan: a new cephamycin. *J. Antimicrob. Chemother.*, **1983**, *11* (*suppl.*):1–239.

Rajan, V.S., Sng, E.H., Thirumoorthy, T., and Goh, C.L. Ceftriaxone in the treatment of ordinary and penicillinase-producing strains of *Neisseria gonorrhoeae*. *Br. J. Vener. Dis.*, **1982**, *58:*314–316.

Reinhardt, J.F., Johnston, L., Ruane, P., Johnson, C.C., Ingram-Drake, L., MacDonald, K., Ward, K.W., Mathisen, G., George, W.L., and Finegold, S.M. et al. A randomized, double-blind comparison of sulbactam/ampicillin and clindamycin for the treatment of aerobic and aerobic-anaerobic infections. *Rev. Infect. Dis.*, **1986**, *8* (*suppl. 5*):S569–S575.

Rosenstein, N.E., Stocker, S.A., Popovic, T., Tenover, F.C., and Perkins, B.A. Antimicrobial reisistance of *Neisseria meningitidis* in the United States, 1997. The Active Bacterial Core Surveillance (ABCs) Team. *Clin. Infect. Dis.*, **2000**, *30:*212–213.

Sahm, D.F., Marsilio, M.K., and Piazza, G. Antimicrobial resistance in key bloodstream bacterial isolates: electronic surveillance with the Surveillance Network Database—USA. *Clin. Infect. Dis.*, **1999**, *29:*259–263.

Sanders, C.S. Cefepime: the next generation? *Clin. Infect. Dis.*, **1993**, *17:*369–379.

Sattler, F.R., Weitekamp, M.R., and Ballard, J.O. Potential for bleeding with the new beta-lactam antibiotics. *Ann. Intern. Med.*, **1986**, *105:*924–931.

Saxon, A., Hassner, A., Swabb, E.A., Wheller, B., and Adkinson, N.F., Jr. Lack of cross-reactivity between aztreonam, a monobactam antibiotic, and penicillin in penicillin-allergic subjects. *J. Infect. Dis.*, **1984**, *149:*16–22.

Schaad, U.B., Suter, S., Gianella-Borradori, A., Pfenninger, J., Auckenthaler, R., Bernath, O., Chesaux, J.J., and Wedgwood, J. A comparison of ceftriaxone and cefuroxime for the treatment of bacterial meningitis in children. *N. Engl. J. Med.*, **1990**, *322:*141–147.

Smith, B.R., and LeFrock, J.L. Cefuroxime: antimicrobial activity, pharmacology, and clinical efficacy. *Ther. Drug Monit.*, **1983**, *5:*149–160.

Spratt, B.G. Biochemical and genetical approaches to the mechanism of action of penicillin. *Philos. Trans. R. Soc. Lond. B. Biol. Sci.*, **1980**, *289:*273–283.

Sprott, M.S., Kearns, A.M., and Field, J.M. Penicillin-insensitive *Neisseria meningitidis*. *Lancet*, **1988**, *1:*1167.

Sullivan, T.J., Yecies, L.D., Shatz, G.S., Parker, C.W., and Wedner, H.J. Desensitization of patients allergic to penicillin using orally administered β-lactam antibiotics. *J. Allergy Clin. Immunol.*, **1982**, *69:*275–282.

Sutter, V.L., and Finegold, S.M. Susceptibility of anaerobic bacteria to carbenicillin, cefoxitin, and related drugs. *J. Infect. Dis.*, **1975**, *131:*417–422.

Sykes, R.B., Cimarusti, C.M., Bonner, D.P., Bush, K., Floyd, D.M., Georgopapadakou, N.H., Koster, W.M., Liu, W.C., Parker, W.L., Principe, P.A., Rathnum, M.L., Slusarchyk, W.A., Trejo, W.H., and Wells, J.S. Monocyclic β-lactam antibiotics produced by bacteria. *Nature*, **1981**, *291:*489–491.

Tomasz, A. Penicillin-binding proteins and the antibacterial effectiveness of β-lactam antibiotics. *Rev. Infect. Dis.*, **1986**, *8* (*suppl. 3*): S260–S278.

Wade, J.C., Smith, C.R., Petty, B.G., Lipsky, J.J., Conrad, G., Ellner, J., and Leitman, P.S. Cephalothin plus an aminoglycoside is more nephrotoxic than methicillin plus an aminoglycoside. *Lancet*, **1978**, *2:*604–606.

Waxman, D.J., Yocum, R.R., and Strominger, J.L. Penicillins and cephalosporins are active site-directed acylating agents: evidence in support of the substrate analogue hypothesis. *Philos. Trans. R. Soc. Lond. B. Biol. Sci.*, **1980**, *289:*257–271.

Wexler, H.M., and Finegold, S.M. *In vitro* activity of cefotetan compared with that of other antimicrobial agents against anaerobic bacteria. *Antimicrob. Agents Chemother.*, **1988**, *32:*601–604.

Wilson, W.R., Wilkowske, C.J., Wright, A.J., Sande, M.A., and Geraci, J.E. Treatment of streptomycin-susceptible and streptomycin-resistant enterococcal endocarditis. *Ann. Intern. Med.*, **1984**, *100:*816–823.

Yogev, R., Melick, C., and Kabat, W.J. *In vitro* and *in vivo* synergism between amoxicillin and clavulanic acid against ampicillin-resistant *Haemophilus influenzae* type b. *Antimicrob. Agents Chemother.*, **1981**, *19:*993–996.

MONOGRAPHS AND REVIEWS

Abraham, E.P. The action of antibiotics on bacteria. In, *Antibiotics,* Vol. II. (Florey, H.W. *et al.,* authors.) Oxford University Press, New York, **1949,** pp. 1438–1496.

Abraham, E.P. The cephalosporins. *Pharmacol. Rev.,* **1962,** *14:*473–500.

Bank, N.U., and Kammer, R.B. Hematologic complications associated with beta-lactam antibiotics. *Rev. Infect. Dis.,* **1983,** *5:*S380–S398.

Barradell, L.B., and Bryson, H.M. Cefepime: a review of its antibacterial activity, pharmacokinetic properties and therapeutic use. *Drugs,* **1994,** *47:*471–505.

Bayles, K.W. The bactericidal action of penicillin: new clues to an unsolved mystery. *Trends Microbiol.,* **2000,** 81274–81278.

Bryson, H.M., and Brogden, R.N. Piperacillin/tazobactam. A review of its antibacterial activity, pharmacokinetic properties and therapeutic potential. *Drugs,* **1994,** *47:*506–535.

Chambers, H.F. Penicillins. In, *Mandell, Douglas, and Bennett's Principles and Practice of Infectious Diseases,* 5th ed. (Mandell, G.L., Bennett, J.E., and Dolin, R., eds.) Churchill Livingstone, Inc., Philadephia **2000,** pp. 261–274.

Cherubin, C.E., Neu, H.C., and Turck, M. Current status of cefotaxime sodium: a new cephalosporin. A symposium. Phoenix, Arizona, January 12–13, 1981. *Rev. Infect. Dis.,* **1982,** *4 (suppl.):* S281–S488.

Davies, J. Inactivation of antibiotics and the dissemination of resistance genes. *Science,* **1994,** *264:*375–382.

Donowitz, G.R., and Mandell, G.L. Beta-lactam antibiotics. *N. Engl. J. Med.,* **1988,** *318:*419–426, 490–500.

Durack, D.T. Prophylaxis of infective endocarditis. In, *Mandell, Douglas, and Bennett's Principles and Practice of Infectious Diseases,* 5th ed. (Mandell, G.L., Bennett, J.E., and Dolin, R., eds.) Churchill Livingstone, Inc., Philadephia, **2000,** pp. 917–925.

Fleming, A. History and development of penicillin. In, *Penicillin: Its Practical Application.* (Fleming, A., ed.) The Blakiston Co., Philadelphia, **1946,** pp. 1–33.

Florey, H.W. The use of micro-organisms for therapeutic purposes. *Yale J. Biol. Med.,* **1946,** *19:*101–118.

Florey, H.W. Historical introduction. In, *Antibiotics.* Vol. I. (Florey, H.W., *et al.,* authors.) Oxford University Press, New York, **1949,** pp. 1–73.

Flynn, E.H. (ed.). *Cephalosporins and Penicillins: Chemistry and Biology.* Academic Press, Inc., New York, **1972.**

Ghuysen, J.M. Serine beta-lactamases and penicillin-binding proteins. *Annu. Rev. Microbiol.,* **1991,** *45:*37–67.

Herrell, W.E. *Penicillin and Other Antibiotic Agents.* W.B. Saunders Co., Philadelphia, **1945.**

Jacoby, G.A. Prevalence and resistance mechanisms of common bacterial respiratory pathogens. *Clin. Infect. Dis.,* **1994,** *18:*951–957.

Kammer, R.B. Host effects of beta-lactam antibiotics. In, *Contemporary Issues in Infectious Diseases.* Vol. 1. *New Dimensions in Antimicrobial Therapy.* (Root, R.K., and Sande, M.A., eds.) Churchill Livingstone, Inc., New York, **1984,** pp. 101–119.

Karchmer, A.W. Cephalosporins. In, *Mandell, Douglas, and Bennett's Principles and Practice of Infectious Diseases,* 5th ed. (Mandell, G.L., Bennett, J.E., and Dolin, R., eds.) Churchill Livingstone, Inc., Philadelphia, **2000,** pp. 274–291.

Kucers, A., and Bennett, N.M. *The Use of Antibiotics: A Comprehensive Review with Clinical Emphasis.* J.B. Lippincott, Philadelphia, **1987.**

Nakae, T. Outer-membrane permeability of bacteria. *Crit. Rev. Microbiol.,* **1986,** *13:*1–62.

Nikaido, H. Prevention of drug access to bacterial targets: permeability barriers and active efflux. *Science,* **1994,** *264:*382–388.

Sparling, P.F. and Handsfield, H.H. *Neisseria gonorrhoeae.* In, *Mandell, Douglas, and Bennett's Principles and Practice of Infectious Diseases,* 5th ed. (Mandell, G.L., Bennett, J.E., and Dolin, R., eds.) Churchill Livingstone, Inc., Philadelphia, **2000,** pp. 2242–2258.

Spratt, B.G. Resistance to antibiotics mediated by target alterations. *Science,* **1994,** *264:*388–393.

Tomasz, A. Multiple-antibiotic-resistant pathogenic bacteria. A report on the Rockefeller University Workshop. *N. Engl. J. Med.,* **1994,** *330:*1247–1251.

Tortora, G.J., Funke, B.R., and Case, C.L. *Microbiology. An Introduction,* 3rd ed. Benjamin/Cummings, New York, **1989,** p. 83.

Tramont, E.C. *Treponema pallidum* (syphilis). In, *Mandell, Douglas, and Bennett's Principles and Practice of Infectious Diseases,* 5th ed. (Mandell, G.L., Bennett, J.E., and Dolin, R., eds.) Churchill Livingstone, Inc., Philadelphia, **2000,** pp. 2474–2490.

Weiss, M.E., and Adkinson, N.F., Jr. Beta-lactam allergy. In, *Mandell, Douglas, and Bennett's Principles and Practice of Infectious Diseases,* 5th ed. (Mandell, G.L., Bennett, J.E., and Dolin, R., eds.) Churchill Livingstone, Inc., Philadelphia, **2000,** pp. 299–305.

C H A P T E R 4 6

ANTIMICROBIAL AGENTS
(Continued)
The Aminoglycosides

Henry F. Chambers

Aminoglycosides, which are aminoglycosidic aminocyclitols, are bactericidal inhibitors of protein synthesis. Although relatively toxic compared with other classes of antibiotics, they remain useful primarily in the treatment of infections caused by aerobic gram-negative bacteria. Streptomycin is an important agent for treatment of tuberculosis. This chapter covers the antibacterial spectrum, pharmacokinetics, and toxicity of this general class of drugs and the therapeutic uses of the individual agents—gentamicin, tobramycin, amikacin, netilmicin, kanamycin, streptomycin, and neomycin.

Aminoglycosides contain amino sugars linked to an aminocyclitol ring by glycosidic bonds. They are polycations, and their polarity is in part responsible for pharmacokinetic properties shared by all members of the group. For example, none is absorbed adequately after oral administration, inadequate concentrations are found in cerebrospinal fluid, and all are excreted relatively rapidly by the normal kidney.

The aminoglycosides are used primarily to treat infections caused by aerobic gram-negative bacteria; they interfere with protein synthesis in susceptible microorganisms. In contrast to most inhibitors of microbial protein synthesis, which are bacteriostatic, the aminoglycosides are bactericidal. Mutations affecting proteins in the bacterial ribosome, the target for these drugs, can confer marked resistance to their action. Resistance most commonly results from the acquisition of plasmids or transposon-encoding genes for aminoglycoside-metabolizing enzymes or from impaired transport of drug into the cell. There can be cross-resistance between some members of the class.

Although they are widely used and important agents, serious toxicity is a major limitation to the usefulness of the aminoglycosides. The same spectrum of toxicity is shared by all members of the group. Most notable are nephrotoxicity and ototoxicity, which can involve both the auditory and vestibular functions of the eighth cranial nerve.

History and Source. The development of streptomycin was the result of a well-planned, scientific search for antibacterial

substances. Stimulated by the discovery of penicillin, Waksman and coworkers examined a number of soil actinomycetes between 1939 and 1943. In 1943, a strain of *Streptomyces griseus* was isolated that elaborated a potent antimicrobial substance, *streptomycin,* which was shown to inhibit the growth of the tubercle bacillus and a number of aerobic gram-positive and gram-negative microorganisms. In less than two years, extensive bacteriological, chemical, and pharmacological investigations of streptomycin had been carried out, and its clinical usefulness was established (Waksman, 1949). However, streptomycin-resistant gram-negative bacilli and gram-positive cocci (enterococci) have emerged, limiting its clinical usefulness. It is now rarely used except for the treatment of certain types of streptococcal or enterococcal endocarditis, tularemia, and plague, and for treatment of tuberculosis.

In 1949, Waksman and Lechevalier isolated a soil organism, *Streptomyces fradiae,* which produced a group of antibacterial substances that were named *neomycin.* One component, *neomycin B,* is still used topically or given orally for its local effect on bowel flora, because it causes severe renal toxicity and ototoxicity when administered parenterally.

Kanamycin, an antibiotic elaborated by *Streptomyces kanamyceticus,* was first produced and isolated by Umezawa and coworkers at the Japanese National Institutes of Health in 1957. Because of toxicity and the emergence of resistant microorganisms, kanamycin has been replaced almost entirely by the newer aminoglycosides.

Gentamicin and *netilmicin* are both broad-spectrum antibiotics derived from species of the actinomycete *Micromonospora.* The difference in spelling (-*micin*) as compared with that of the other aminoglycoside antibiotics (-*mycin*) reflects this difference in origin. Gentamicin was first studied and described by Weinstein and coworkers in 1963. It has a broader spectrum of activity than kanamycin and currently is used widely. *Tobramycin* and *amikacin* were introduced into clinical practice in the 1970s. Tobramycin is one of several components of

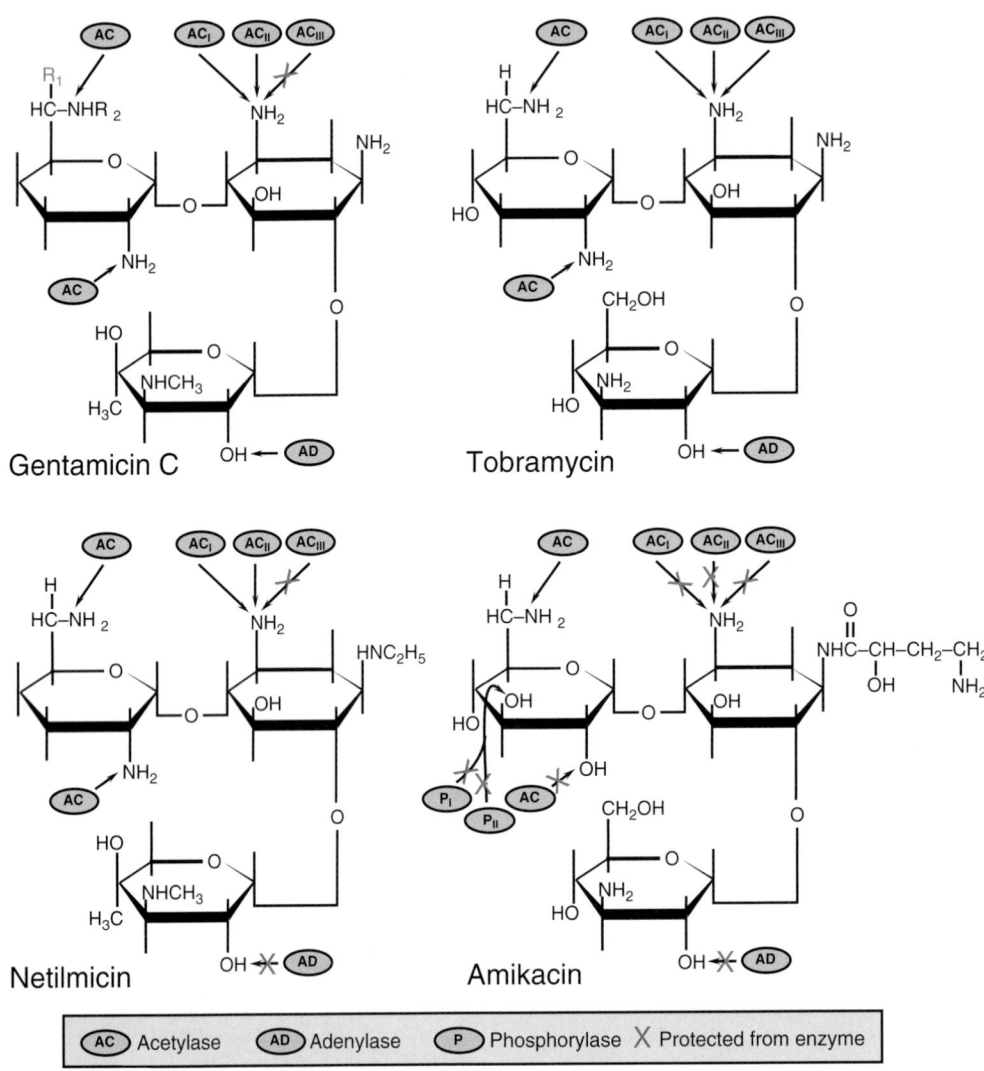

Figure 46–1. *Sites of activity of various plasmid-mediated enzymes capable of inactivating amino-glycosides.*

The symbol "X" indicates regions of the molecules that are protected from the designated enzyme. In gentamicin C_1, $R_1 = R_2 = CH_3$; in gentamicin C_2, $R_1 = CH_3$, $R_2 = H$; in gentamicin C_{1a}, $R_1 = R_2 = H$. (Modified from Moellering, 1977. Courtesy of the *Medical Journal of Australia*.)

an aminoglycoside complex (nebramycin) that is produced by *Streptomyces tenebrarius* (Higgins and Kastner, 1967). It is most similar in antimicrobial activity and toxicity to gentamicin. In contrast to the other aminoglycosides, amikacin and netilmicin are semisynthetic products. Amikacin, which is a derivative of kanamycin, was described by Kawaguchi and coworkers (1972); netilmicin is a derivative of sisomicin. Other aminoglycoside antibiotics have been developed (*e.g., arbekacin, isepamicin, sisomicin*). These have not been introduced into clinical practice in the United States, because numerous potent, less toxic alternatives (*e.g.,* broad-spectrum β-lactam antibiotics and quinolones) are available.

Chemistry. The aminoglycosides consist of two or more amino sugars joined in glycosidic linkage to a hexose nucleus, which is usually in a central position (*see* Figure 46–1). This hexose, or aminocyclitol, is either streptidine (found in streptomycin) or 2-deoxystreptamine (all other available aminoglycosides). These compounds are thus aminoglycosidic aminocyclitols, although the simpler term *aminoglycoside* is commonly used to describe them. An additional drug, *spectinomycin,* is an aminocyclitol that does not contain amino sugars; it is discussed in Chapter 47.

The aminoglycoside families are distinguished by the amino sugars attached to the aminocyclitol. In the neomycin family, which includes neomycin B and *paromomycin,* an aminoglycoside used orally for the treatment of intestinal parasitic infections, there are three amino sugars attached to the central 2-deoxystreptamine. The kanamycin and gentamicin families have only two such amino sugars. Neomycin B has the following structural formula:

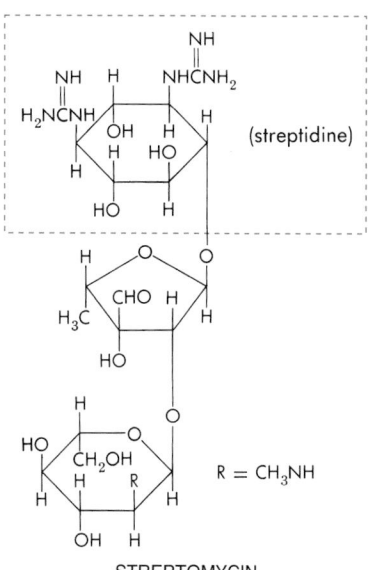

NEOMYCIN B

In the kanamycin family, which includes kanamycins A and B, amikacin, and tobramycin, two amino sugars are linked to a centrally located 2-deoxystreptamine moiety; one of these is a 3-aminohexose (*see* Figure 46–1). The structural formula of kanamycin A, which is the major component of the commercial product, is as follows:

KANAMYCIN A

Amikacin is a semisynthetic derivative prepared from kanamycin A by acylation of the 1-amino group of the 2-deoxystreptamine moiety with 2-hydroxy-4-aminobutyric acid.

The gentamicin family, which includes gentamicin C_1, C_{1a}, and C_2, sisomicin, and netilmicin (the 1-*N*-ethyl derivative of sisomicin), contains a different 3-amino sugar (garosamine). Variations in methylation of the other amino sugar result in the different components of gentamicin (Figure 46–1). These modifications appear to have little effect on biological activity.

Streptomycin and dihydrostreptomycin (the latter is no longer available because of excessive ototoxicity) differ from the other aminoglycoside antibiotics in that they contain strepti-

dine rather than 2-deoxystreptamine, and their aminocyclitol is not in a central position. The structural formula of streptomycin is as follows:

STREPTOMYCIN

Mechanism of Action. The aminoglycoside antibiotics are rapidly bactericidal. Bacterial killing is concentration-dependent: the higher the concentration, the greater the rate at which bacteria are killed. A postantibiotic effect, that is, residual bactericidal activity persisting after the serum concentration has fallen below the minimum inhibitory concentration, also is characteristic of aminoglycoside antibiotics, and the duration of this effect is concentration-dependent. These properties probably account for the efficacy of once-daily dosing regimens of aminoglycosides. Although much is known about their capacity to inhibit protein synthesis and decrease the fidelity of translation of mRNA at the ribosome (Shannon and Phillips, 1982), the precise mechanism responsible for the rapidly lethal effect of aminoglycosides on bacteria is unknown.

Aminoglycosides diffuse through aqueous channels formed by porin proteins in the outer membrane of gram-negative bacteria to enter the periplasmic space (Nakae and Nakae, 1982). Transport of aminoglycosides across the cytoplasmic (inner) membrane depends on electron transport, in part because of a requirement for a membrane electrical potential (interior negative) to drive permeation of these antibiotics (Bryan and Kwan, 1983). This phase of transport has been termed *energy-dependent phase I*. It is rate-limiting and can be blocked or inhibited by divalent cations (*e.g.*, Ca^{2+} and Mg^{2+}), hyperosmolarity, a reduction in pH, and anaerobiasis. The last two of these

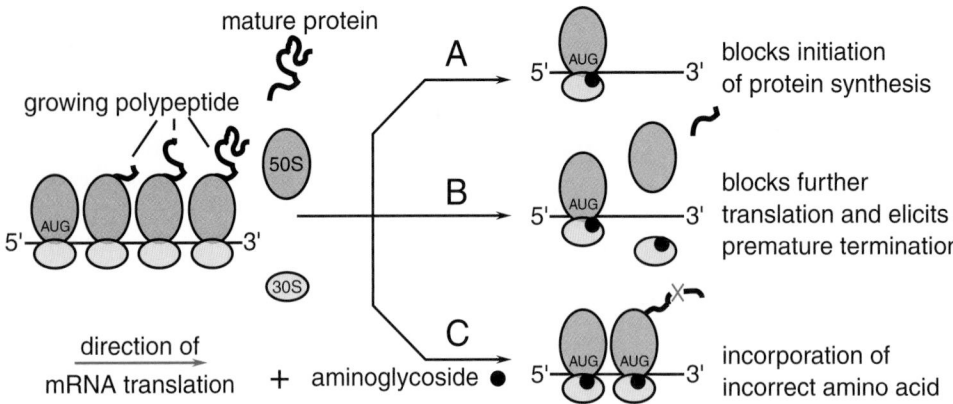

Figure 46–2. Effects of aminoglycosides on protein synthesis.

A. Aminoglycoside (represented by closed circles) binds to the 30 S ribosomal subunit and interferes with initiation of protein synthesis by fixing the 30 S–50 S ribosomal complex at the start codon (AUG) of mRNA. As 30 S–50 S complexes downstream complete translation of mRNA and detach, the abnormal initiation complexes, so-called streptomycin monosomes, accumulate, blocking further translation of message. Aminoglycoside binding to the 30 S subunit also causes misreading of mRNA, leading to *B.* premature termination of translation with detachment of the ribosomal complex and incompletely synthesized protein, or *C.* incorporation of incorrect amino acids (indicated by the "X"), resulting in the production of abnormal or nonfunctional proteins.

conditions impair the ability of the bacteria to maintain the membrane potential, which is the driving force necessary for transport. Thus, the antimicrobial activity of aminoglycosides is reduced markedly in the anaerobic environment of an abscess, in hyperosmolar acidic urine, and so forth. Once inside the cell, aminoglycosides bind to polysomes and interfere with protein synthesis by causing misreading and premature termination of translation of mRNA (*see* Figure 46–2). The aberrant proteins produced may be inserted into the cell membrane, leading to altered permeability and further stimulation of aminoglycoside transport (Busse *et al.,* 1992). This phase of aminoglycoside transport, termed *energy-dependent phase II* (EDP₂), is poorly understood; however, it has been suggested that EDP₂ is in some way linked with disruption of the structure of the cytoplasmic membrane, perhaps by the aberrant proteins. This concept is consistent with the observed progression of the leakage of small ions, followed by larger molecules and, eventually, by proteins from the bacterial cell prior to aminoglycoside-induced death. This progressive disruption of the cell envelope, as well as other vital cell processes, may help to explain the lethal action of aminoglycosides (Bryan, 1989).

The primary intracellular site of action of the aminoglycosides is the 30 S ribosomal subunit, which consists of 21 proteins and a single 16 S molecule of RNA. At least three of these proteins and perhaps the 16 S ribosomal RNA as well contribute to the streptomycin binding site, and alterations of these

molecules markedly affect the binding and subsequent action of streptomycin. For example, a single amino acid substitution of asparagine for lysine at position 42 of one ribosomal protein (S₁₂) prevents binding of the drug; the resultant mutant is totally resistant to streptomycin. Another mutant, in which glutamine is the amino acid at this position, is dependent on streptomycin, which is actually required for survival. The other aminoglycosides also bind to the 30 S ribosomal subunit; however, they also appear to bind to several sites on the 50 S ribosomal subunit (Davis, 1988).

Aminoglycosides disrupt the normal cycle of ribosomal function by interfering, at least in part, with the initiation of protein synthesis, leading to the accumulation of abnormal initiation complexes or "streptomycin monosomes," shown schematically in Figure 46–2*B* (Luzzatto *et al.,* 1969). Another effect of the aminoglycosides is their capacity to induce misreading of the mRNA template, causing incorrect amino acids to be incorporated into the growing polypeptide chains (*see* Tai *et al.,* 1978). The aminoglycosides vary in their capacity to cause misreading, and this property presumably depends on differences in their affinities for specific ribosomal proteins. Although there appears to be a strong correlation between bactericidal activity and the ability to induce misreading (Hummel and Böck, 1989), it remains to be established that this is the primary mechanism of aminoglycoside-induced cell death.

Microbial Resistance to the Aminoglycosides. Bacteria may be resistant to the antimicrobial activity of the aminoglycosides because of failure of permeation of the antibiotic, low affinity of the drug for the bacterial ribosome, or inactivation of the drug by microbial enzymes. Drug inactivation is by far the most important explanation for the acquired microbial resistance to aminoglycosides that is encountered in clinical practice.

Penetration of drug through the pores in the outer membrane of gram-negative microorganisms into the periplasmic space may be retarded; resistance of this type is unimportant clinically. Once the aminoglycoside does reach the periplasmic space, it may be altered by microbial enzymes that phosphorylate, adenylate, or acetylate specific hydroxyl or amino groups (Figure 46–1). The genes for these enzymes are acquired primarily by conjugation and the transfer of DNA as plasmids and resistance transfer factors (Davies, 1994; see Chapter 43). These plasmids have become widespread in nature (especially in hospital environments), and they code for a large number of enzymes (more than 20) that have markedly reduced the clinical usefulness of aminoglysides. Amikacin is less vulnerable to these inactivating enzymes because of protective molecular side chains (Figure 46–1); thus, this drug has a particularly important role in certain hospital settings. The metabolites of the aminoglycosides may compete with the unaltered drug for intracellular transport, but they are incapable of binding effectively to ribosomes and interfering with protein synthesis.

Acquisition of aminoglycoside-inactivating enzymes by enterococci has become a source of concern. In several centers, a significant percentage of clinical isolates of these organisms (both *Enterococcus faecalis* and *Enterococcus faecium*) are highly resistant to all aminoglycosides because of this mechanism (Spera and Farber, 1992; Vemuri and Zervos, 1993). Because different enzymes are responsible for inactivation of gentamicin and streptomycin, a smal proportion of gentamicin-resistant strains of enterococci will be susceptible to streptomycin. Resistance to gentamicin indicates resistance to tobramycin, amikacin, kanamycin, and netilmicin, because the inactivating enzyme is bifunctional and modifies all of these aminoglycosides (Murray, 1991). The synergistic bactericidal effect of penicillin or vancomycin and an aminoglycoside on enterococci is lost. Enterococci also have acquired plasmids that code for β-lactamases (Murray and Mederski-Samaroj, 1983) and vancomycin resistance (Leclercq et al., 1988). These factors could make serious enterococcal infections extremely difficult to treat. Strains of *E. faecium* that are resistant to virtually all clinically important antibiotics have emerged as pathogens in intensive care units in hospitals across the United States.

Another common form of natural resistance to aminoglycosides is caused by failure of the drug to penetrate the cytoplasmic (inner) membrane. As mentioned above, the transport of aminoglycosides across the cytoplasmic membrane is an oxygen-dependent, active process. Strictly anaerobic bacteria are thus resistant to these drugs, since they lack the necessary transport system. Similarly, facultative bacteria become resistant when they are grown under anaerobic conditions (Mates et al., 1983). The significance of this transport defect for resistance to aminoglycosides among aerobic gram-negative bacilli is not known. Natural resistance to amikacin by *Pseudomonas maltophilia* and certain other microorganisms appears to have a similar basis, as does the low-level resistance of some gram-positive cocci to aminoglycosides.

Resistance that results from alterations in ribosomal structure is relatively uncommon for aminoglycosides other than streptomycin. Single-step mutations in *Escherichia coli* that result in the substitution of an amino acid in a crucial ribosomal protein may prevent binding of the drug. Although such strains of *E. coli* are highly resistant to streptomycin, they are not widespread in nature. Similarly, only 5% of strains of *Pseudomonas aeruginosa* exhibit such ribosomal resistance to streptomycin. It has been estimated that approximately half of the streptomycin-resistant strains are ribosomally resistant (Eliopoulos et al., 1984). There is no synergistic effect of penicillin and streptomycin against these strains demonstrable *in vitro*. Because ribosomal resistance often is specific for streptomycin, these strains of enterococci generally are sensitive to a combination of penicillin and gentamicin *in vitro*.

Antibacterial Activity of the Aminoglycosides. The antibacterial activity of gentamicin, tobramycin, kanamycin, netilmicin, and amikacin is primarily directed against aerobic, gram-negative bacilli. Kanamycin, like streptomycin, has a more limited spectrum compared with other aminoglycosides, and in particular it should not be used to treat infections caused by *Serratia* or *P. aeruginosa*. As noted above, these antibiotics have little activity against anaerobic microorganisms or facultative bacteria under anaerobic conditions. Their action against most gram-positive bacteria is limited. *Streptococcus pneumoniae* and *Streptococcus pyogenes* are resistant, and, in fact, gentamicin has been added to blood-agar plates to aid in the isolation of these microorganisms from sputum and pharyngeal secretions. Although not active when used alone, either streptomycin or gentamicin in combination with a cell wall–active agent, such as a penicillin or vancomycin, is active against "sensitive" strains of enterococci and streptococci at concentrations that can be achieved clinically. Such combinations result in a more rapid bactericidal effect than is produced by either drug alone (*i.e.*, they are synergistic). Both gentamicin and tobramycin are active *in vitro* against more than 90% of strains of *Staphylococcus*

Table 46–1

Typical Minimal Inhibitory Concentrations of Aminoglycosides That Will Inhibit 90% (MIC_{90}) of Clinical Isolates for Several Species

SPECIES	MIC_{90}, $\mu g/ml$				
	KANAMYCIN	GENTAMICIN	NETILMICIN	TOBRAMYCIN	AMIKACIN
Citrobacter freundii	8	0.5	0.25	0.5	1
Enterobacter spp.	4	0.5	0.25	0.5	1
Escherichia coli	16	0.5	0.25	0.5	1
Klebsiella pneumoniae	32	0.5	0.25	1	1
Proteus mirabilis	8	4	4	0.5	2
Providencia stuartii	128	8	16	4	2
Pseudomonas aeruginosa	>128	8	32	4	2
Serratia spp.	>64	4	16	16	8
Enterococcus faecalis	—	32	2	32	≥64
Staphylococcus aureus	2	0.5	0.25	0.25	16

SOURCE: Adapted with permission from Wiedemann and Atkinson, 1991.

aureus and 75% of strains of *Staphylococcus epidermidis*. The clinical efficacy of aminoglycosides alone in the treatment of serious staphylococcal infections has not been documented, and they should not be used. Gentamicin-resistant mutant strains of staphylococci emerge rapidly during exposure to the drug. Moreover, staphylococcal resistance that is mediated by conjugative plasmids that code for aminoglycoside-modifying enzymes is common among methicillin-resistant strains of staphylococci.

The aerobic gram-negative bacilli vary in their susceptibility to the aminoglycosides as shown in Table 46–1. "Sensitive" microorganisms are defined as those inhibited by concentrations that can be achieved clinically in plasma without a high incidence of toxicity; when given at 8- or 12-hour intervals, these therapeutic peak values range from 4 to 12 $\mu g/ml$ for gentamicin, tobramycin, and netilmicin and 20 to 35 $\mu g/ml$ for amikacin and kanamycin. Tobramycin and gentamicin exhibit similar activity against most gram-negative bacilli, although tobramycin usually is more active against *P. aeruginosa* and against some strains of *Proteus* species. Many gram-negative bacilli that are resistant to gentamicin because of plasmid-mediated inactivating enzymes also will inactivate tobramycin. Nosocomial flora have shown a gradual increase in resistance to gentamicin and tobramycin over the last 20 to 30 years. The relative frequency of these changes varies dramatically—even in different units within a single hospital (Cross *et al.,* 1983). Fortunately, amikacin and, in some instances, netilmicin have retained their activity in this setting, probably due to resistance of the drugs to many of the aminoglycoside-inactivating enzymes. These agents thus have a broad spectrum of activity and are particularly valuable in treating nosocomial infections.

ABSORPTION, DISTRIBUTION, DOSING, AND ELIMINATION OF THE AMINOGLYCOSIDES

Absorption.   The aminoglycosides are highly polar cations and therefore are very poorly absorbed from the gastrointestinal tract. Less than 1% of a dose is absorbed following either oral or rectal administration. The drugs are not inactivated in the intestine, and they are eliminated quantitatively in the feces. However, long-term oral or rectal administration may result in accumulation of aminoglycosides to toxic concentrations in patients with renal impairment. Absorption of gentamicin from the gastrointestinal tract may be increased by gastrointestinal disease (ulcers, inflammatory bowel disease; Breen *et al.,* 1972). Instillation of these drugs into body cavities with serosal surfaces may result in rapid absorption and unexpected toxicity, *i.e.,* neuromuscular blockade. Similarly, intoxication may occur when aminoglycosides are applied topically for long periods to large wounds, burns, or cutaneous ulcers, particularly if there is renal insufficiency.

All of the aminoglycosides are absorbed rapidly from intramuscular sites of injection. Peak concentrations in plasma occur after 30 to 90 minutes and are similar to those observed 30 minutes after completion of an intravenous infusion of an equal dose over a 30-minute period. In critically ill patients, especially those in shock, absorption of drug may be reduced from intramuscular sites because of poor perfusion.

Distribution.   Because of their polar nature, the aminoglycosides largely are excluded from most cells, from the central nervous system, and from the eye. Except for streptomycin, there is negligible binding of aminoglycosides to plasma albumin. The apparent volume of distribution of these drugs is 25% of lean body weight and approximates the volume of extracellular fluid (Barza *et al.*, 1975).

Concentrations of aminoglycosides in secretions and tissues are low. High concentrations are found only in the renal cortex and in the endolymph and perilymph of the inner ear; this may contribute to the nephrotoxicity and ototoxicity caused by these drugs. Concentrations in bile approach 30% of those found in plasma as a result of active hepatic secretion, but this represents a very minor excretory route for the aminoglycosides. Penetration into respiratory secretions is poor (Levy, 1986). Diffusion into pleural and synovial fluid is relatively slow, but concentrations that approximate those in the plasma may be achieved after repeated administration. Inflammation increases the penetration of aminoglycosides into peritoneal and pericardial cavities.

Concentrations of aminoglycosides in cerebrospinal fluid (CSF) that are achievable with parenteral administration of drug usually are subtherapeutic. In experimental animals and human beings, concentrations in CSF are less than 10% of those in plasma in the absence of inflammation; this value may approach 25% when there is meningitis (Strausbaugh *et al.*, 1977). The concentrations achieved are therefore inadequate for the treatment of gram-negative bacillary meningitis in adults. Intrathecal or intraventricular administration of aminoglycosides has been used to achieve therapeutic levels, but the availability of third-generation cephalosporins has now made this unnecessary in most cases. There is no proven benefit of either intrathecal or intraventricular injection of aminoglycosides to neonates with meningitis, perhaps because of the immaturity of the blood-brain barrier (McCracken *et al.*, 1980). Penetration of aminoglycosides into ocular fluids is so poor that effective therapy of bacterial endophthalmitis requires periocular and intraocular injections of the drugs (Barza, 1978).

Administration of aminoglycosides to women late in pregnancy may result in accumulation of drug in fetal plasma and amniotic fluid. Streptomycin can cause hearing loss in children born to women who receive the drug during pregnancy (Warkany, 1979), as can tobramycin. Insufficient data are available regarding the other aminoglycosides; it is thus recommended that they be used with caution in pregnancy and only for strong clinical indications in the absence of suitable alternatives.

Dosing. Recommended doses of individual aminoglycosides in the treatment of specific infections are given in later sections of this chapter. Traditionally, the total daily dose of aminoglycosides is administered as two or three equally divided doses. Administration of the total dose once daily, however, appears to be less toxic and just as effective (Verpooten *et al.*, 1989; Gilbert, 1991; Prins *et al.*, 1993; The International Antimicrobial Therapy Cooperative Group of the European Organization for Research and Treatment of Cancer, 1993; Charnas *et al.*, 1997; Urban and Craig, 1997; Gilbert *et al.*, 1998; Rybak *et al.*, 1999). Toxicity results from accumulation of drug in the inner ear and kidney. The amount of drug that accumulates increases with higher plasma concentrations and longer periods of exposure. Elimination (or washout) of aminoglycoside from these organs occurs more slowly than from plasma and is retarded by high plasma concentrations (Tran Ba Huy *et al.*, 1983), accounting for the association between toxicity and high plasma trough concentrations (Swan, 1997). Toxicity, then, can be considered as a threshold phenomenon, more likely to occur the longer the

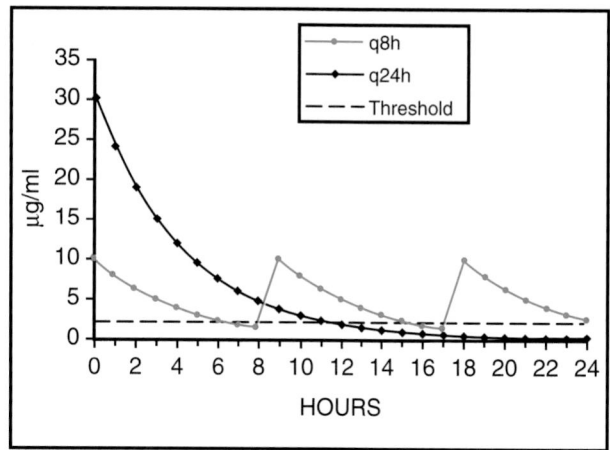

Figure 46–3. Plasma concentrations (μg/ml) after administration of 5.1 mg/kg of gentamicin intravenously to a hypothetical patient either as a single dose (q24h) or as three divided doses (q8h).

The threshold for toxicity has been chosen to correspond to a plasma concentration of 2 μg/ml, the maximum recommended. The q24h regimen produces a threefold higher plasma concentration, which enhances efficacy that might otherwise be compromised due to prolonged sub-MIC concentrations later in the dosing interval, compared to the q8h regimen. The 12-hour period of the q24h regimen during which plasma concentrations are below the threshold for toxicity minimizes the toxicity that might otherwise result from the high plasma concentrations early on. The q8h regimen, in contrast, provides only a brief period during which plasma concentrations are below the threshold for toxicity.

plasma concentration exceeds a relatively safe upper limit (*e.g.*, above a recommended trough concentration) (Figure 46–3). A once-daily dosing regimen, despite the higher peak concentration, provides a longer period when concentrations are below the threshold for toxicity than does a multiple-dosing regimen (12 hours *versus* less than 3 hours total in the example shown in the figure), accounting for its lower toxicity. Aminoglycoside bactericidal activity, on the other hand, is directly related to the concentration achieved, because aminoglycosides have concentration-dependent killing and a concentration-dependent postantibiotic effect. This enhanced activity at higher concentrations probably accounts for the equivalent efficacy of a once-daily regimen compared to a multiple-dosing regimen despite the relatively prolonged periods of time that plasma concentrations are "subtherapeutic," *i.e.*, below the minimum inhibitory concentration (MIC).

Numerous studies in a variety of clinical settings employing virtually every commonly used aminoglycoside have demonstrated that once-daily regimens are just as safe as or safer than multiple-dosing regimens and as efficacious (Barza *et al.*, 1996; Deaney and Tate, 1996; Ferriols-Lisart and Alos-Alminana, 1996; Freeman and Strayer, 1996; Ali and Goetz, 1997; Bailey *et al.*, 1997; Charnas *et al.*, 1997; Freeman *et al.*, 1997; Deamer, 1998). Once-daily dosing also costs less and

Table 46–2

Algorithm for Dose Reduction of Aminoglycosides Based on Calculated Creatinine Clearance

CREATININE CLEARANCE, ml/min	% OF MAXIMUM DAILY DOSE*	FREQUENCY OF DOSING
100	100	Every 24 hours
75	75	Every 24 hours
50	50	Every 24 hours
25	25	Every 24 hours
20	80	Every 48 hours
10	60	Every 48 hours
<10	40	Every 48 hours

*The maximum adult daily dose for amikacin, kanamycin, and streptomycin is 15 mg/kg; for gentamicin and tobramycin, 5.5 mg/kg; and for netilmicin, 6.5 mg/kg.

is more easily administered. Administration of aminoglycosides as a single daily dose is for these reasons generally preferred with few exceptions. Exceptions are use in pregnancy, neonatal infections, and low-dose combination therapy of bacterial endocarditis, because data documenting equivalent safety and efficacy are inadequate. Once-daily dosing should also be avoided in patients with creatinine clearances less than 20 to 25 ml/min, because accumulation is likely to occur. Less frequent dosing (*e.g.*, every 48 hours) is more appropriate for these patients.

Whether once-daily or multiple-daily dosing is chosen, the dose must be adjusted for patients with creatinine clearances below 80 to 100 ml/min (Table 46–2). If it is anticipated that the patient will be treated with an aminoglycoside for more than three to four days, then plasma concentrations should be monitored to avoid accumulation of the drug. In addition, an aminoglycoside in general should not be used as a single agent except for urinary tract infections because of relatively poor tissue penetration and poorer outcome compared to combination regimens or other classes of antibiotics (Bodey *et al.*, 1985; Leibovici *et al.*, 1997).

For twice-daily or three-times-daily dosing regimens, both trough and peak plasma concentrations are determined. The trough sample is obtained just prior to a dose, and the peak sample is obtained thirty minutes following intramuscular injection or thirty minutes after an intravenous infusion given over thirty minutes. The peak concentration is used to document that the dose produces therapeutic concentrations, generally accepted to be 4 to 10 μg/ml for gentamicin, netilmicin, and tobramycin and 15 to 30 μg/ml for amikacin and streptomycin (Gilbert *et al.*, 1999). The trough concentration is used to avoid toxicity by monitoring for accumulation of drug. Trough concentrations should be less than 1 to 2 μg/ml for gentamicin, netilmicin, and tobramycin and 5 to 10 μg/ml for amikacin and streptomycin.

Monitoring of aminoglycoside plasma concentrations also is important when using a once-daily dosing regimen, although peak concentrations are not routinely determined (these will be three to four times higher than the peak achieved with a multiple-daily-dosing regimen). Several approaches may be used to determine that drug is being cleared and not accumulating. The simplest method is to obtain a trough sample 24 hours after dosing and adjust the dose to achieve the recommended plasma concentration, *e.g.*, below 1 to 2 μg/ml in the case of

gentamicin or tobramycin. This approach is probably the least desirable. An undetectable trough concentration could reflect grossly inadequate dosing with prolonged periods (perhaps well over half of the dosing interval), during which concentrations are subtherapeutic in patients who rapidly clear the drug. In contrast, a 24-hour trough concentration target of 1 to 2 μg/ml would actually increase aminoglycoside exposure compared to a multiple-daily-dosing regimen (Barclay *et al.*, 1999). This defeats the goal of providing a washout with concentrations of 0 to 1 μg/ml between 18 to 24 hours after a dose. A second approach relies on nomograms to target a range of concentration in a sample obtained earlier in the dosing interval. For example, if the plasma concentration from a sample obtained 8 hours after a dose of gentamicin is between 1.5 and 6 μg/ml, then the concentration at 18 hours will be <1 μg/ml (Chambers *et al.*, 1998). A target range of 1 to 1.5 μg/ml for gentamicin at 18 hours for patients with creatinine clearances above 50 ml/min and 1 to 2.5 μg/ml for clearances below 50 ml/min also has been used (Gilbert *et al.*, 1998). The most accurate method for monitoring plasma levels for dose adjustment is to measure the concentration in two plasma samples drawn several hours apart (*e.g.*, at 2 and 12 hours after a dose). The clearance then can be calculated and the dose adjusted to achieve the desired target range.

Elimination. The aminoglycosides are excreted almost entirely by glomerular filtration, and concentrations in the urine of 50 to 200 μg/ml are achieved. A large fraction of a parenterally administered dose is excreted unchanged during the first 24 hours, with most of this appearing in the first 12 hours. The half-lives of the aminoglycosides in plasma are similar and vary between 2 and 3 hours in patients with normal renal function. Renal clearance of aminoglycosides is approximately two-thirds of the simultaneous creatinine clearance; this observation suggests some tubular reabsorption of these drugs.

Following a single dose of an aminoglycoside, disappearance from the plasma exceeds renal excretion by 10% to 20%; however, after 1 to 2 days of therapy, nearly 100% of subsequent doses is eventually recovered in the urine. This lag period probably represents saturation of binding sites in tissues. The rate of elimination of drug from these sites is considerably longer than from plasma; the half-life for tissue-bound aminoglycoside has been estimated to range from 30 to 700 hours (Schentag and Jusko, 1977). For this reason, small amounts of aminoglycosides can be detected in the urine for 10 to 20 days after drug administration is discontinued. Aminoglycoside bound to renal tissue exhibits antibacterial activity and protects experimental animals against bacterial infections of the kidney, even when the drug no longer can be detected in serum (Bergeron *et al.,* 1982).

The concentration of aminoglycoside in plasma produced by the initial dose is dependent only on the volume of distribution of the drug. Since the elimination of aminoglycosides is almost entirely dependent on the kidney, a linear relationship exists between the concentration of creatinine in plasma and the half-life of all aminoglycosides in patients with moderately compromised renal function. In anephric patients, the half-life varies from 20 to 40 times that determined in normal individuals. *Because the incidence of nephrotoxicity and ototoxicity is related to the concentration to which an aminoglycoside accumulates, it is critical to reduce the maintenance dosage of these drugs in patients with impaired renal function.* The size of the individual dose, the interval between doses, or both, can be altered. There is no conclusive information on the best approach, and even the currently accepted therapeutic range has been questioned (McCormack and Jewesson, 1992). The most consistent plasma concentrations are achieved when the loading dose is given in milligrams per kilogram of body weight; and since aminoglycosides are minimally distributed in fatty tissue, the lean or expected body weight should be used. Methods for calculation of dosage are described in Appendix II.

There are obvious difficulties in utilizing any of these approaches for ill patients with rapidly changing renal function (Lesar *et al.,* 1982). In addition, even when known factors are taken into consideration, concentrations of aminoglycosides achieved in plasma after a given dose vary widely among patients (Barza *et al.,* 1975). If the extracellular volume is expanded, the volume of distribution is increased and concentrations will be reduced. For unknown reasons, the clearances are increased, and the half-lives of the aminoglycosides are reduced in patients with cystic fibrosis; the volume of distribution is increased in patients with leukemia (Rosenthal *et al.,* 1977; Spyker *et al.,* 1978). Patients with anemia (hematocrit <25%) have a concentration in plasma that is higher than expected, probably because of a reduction in the number of binding sites on red blood cells (Siber *et al.,* 1975).

Determination of the concentration of drug in plasma is an essential guide to the proper administration of aminoglycosides. In patients with life-threatening systemic infections, aminoglycoside concentrations should be determined several times per week (more frequently if renal function is changing) and always should be determined within 24 hours after a change in dosage.

Aminoglycosides are removed from the body by either hemodialysis or peritoneal dialysis. Approximately 50% of the administered dose is removed in 12 hours by hemodialysis, which has been used for the treatment of overdosage. As a general rule, a dose equal to half the loading dose administered after each hemodialysis should maintain the plasma concentration in the desired range; however, a number of variables make this a rough approximation at best. Continuous arteriovenous hemofiltration (CAVH) and continuous venovenous hemofiltration (CVVH) will result in aminoglycoside clearances approximately equivalent to 15 ml/min and 15 to 30 ml/min of creatinine clearance, respectively, depending on the flow rate. The amount of aminoglycoside removed can be replaced by administering approximately 15% to 30% of the maximum daily dose (Table 46–2) each day. Frequent monitoring of drug concentrations in plasma is again crucial.

Peritoneal dialysis is less effective than hemodialysis in removing aminoglycosides. Clearance rates are approximately 5 to 10 ml per minute for the various drugs, but are highly variable. If a patient who requires dialysis has bacterial peritonitis, a therapeutic concentration of the aminoglycoside probably will not be achieved in the peritoneal fluid, since the ratio of the concentration in plasma to that in peritoneal fluid may be 10 to 1 (Smithivas *et al.,* 1971). It is thus recommended that antibiotic be added to the dialysate to achieve concentrations equal to those desired in plasma. For intermittent dosing *via* peritoneal dialysate, 2 mg/kg of amikacin is added to the bag once a day. The corresponding dose for gentamicin, netilmicin, or tobramycin is 0.6 mg/kg. For continuous dosing, the dose of amikacin is 12 mg per liter (25 mg/l loading dose in the first bag) and the dose of gentamicin, netilmicin, or tobramycin is 4 mg per liter in each bag (8 mg/l loading dose). This should be preceded by administration of a loading dose, either parenterally or in dialysis fluid.

Although excretion of aminoglycosides is similar in adults and children over 6 months of age, half-lives of the drugs may be significantly prolonged in the newborn. Newborn infants who weigh less than 2 kg have half-lives for aminoglycosides of 8 to 11 hours during the first week of life, while those who weigh over 2 kg eliminate these drugs with half-lives of about 5 hours (Yow, 1977). It is thus critically important to monitor concentrations of aminoglycosides during treatment of neonates (Philips *et al.,* 1982).

Aminoglycosides can be inactivated by various penicillins *in vitro* (Konishi *et al.,* 1983) and in patients with end-stage renal failure (Blair *et al.,* 1982), thus making dosage recommendations even more difficult. Amikacin appears to be the least affected by this interaction.

UNTOWARD EFFECTS OF THE AMINOGLYCOSIDES

All aminoglycosides have the potential to produce reversible and irreversible vestibular, cochlear, and renal toxicity. These side effects complicate the use of these compounds and make their proper administration difficult.

Ototoxicity. Both vestibular and auditory dysfunction can follow the administration of any of the aminoglycosides. Studies of both animals and human beings have documented progressive accumulation of these drugs in the perilymph and endolymph of the inner ear (Tran Ba Huy *et al.,* 1983). Accumulation occurs predominantly when concentrations in plasma are high. Diffusion back into the bloodstream is slow; the half-lives of the aminoglycosides are five to six times longer in the otic fluids than in plasma. Back-diffusion is concentration-dependent and is facilitated at the trough concentration of drug in plasma. Ototoxicity is more likely to occur in patients with persistently elevated concentrations of drug in plasma. However, even a single dose of tobramycin has been reported to produce slight temporary cochlear dysfunction during periods when the concentration in plasma is at its peak (Wilson and Ramsden, 1977). The relationship of this observation to permanent loss of hearing is not known.

Ototoxicity is largely irreversible and results from progressive destruction of vestibular or cochlear sensory cells, which are highly sensitive to damage by aminoglycosides (Brummett, 1983). Studies in guinea pigs exposed to large doses of gentamicin reveal degeneration of the type I sensory hair cells in the central part of the crista ampullaris (vestibular organ) and fusion of individual sensory hairs into giant hairs (Wersäll et al., 1973). Similar studies with gentamicin and tobramycin also demonstrate loss of hair cells in the cochlea of the organ of Corti (Theopold, 1977). With increasing dosage and prolonged exposure, damage progresses from the base of the cochlea, where high-frequency sounds are processed, to the apex, which is necessary for the perception of low frequencies. While these histological changes correlate with the ability of the cochlea to generate an action potential in response to sound, the biochemical mechanism for ototoxicity is poorly understood. Early changes induced by aminoglycosides have been shown in experimental ototoxicity to be reversible by Ca^{2+}. Once sensory cells are lost, however, regeneration does not occur; retrograde degeneration of the auditory nerve follows, resulting in irreversible hearing loss. It has been suggested that aminoglycosides interfere with the active transport system essential for the maintenance of the ionic balance of the endolymph (Neu and Bendush, 1976). This would lead to alteration in the normal concentrations of ions in the labyrinthine fluids, with impairment of electrical activity and nerve conduction. Eventually, the electrolyte changes, or perhaps the drugs themselves, damage the hair cells irreversibly. Interest also has centered on the interaction of aminoglycosides with membrane phospholipids, particularly phosphatidylinositol and its phosphorylated derivatives, which are the precursors of the intracellular second messengers inositol 1,4,5-trisphosphate and diacylglycerol.

The degree of permanent dysfunction correlates with the number of destroyed or altered sensory hair cells and is thought to be related to sustained exposure to the drug. Repeated courses of aminoglycosides, each resulting in the loss of more cells, can lead to deafness. Since there is a decrease in the number of cells with age, older patients may be more susceptible to ototoxicity. Drugs such as *ethacrynic acid* and *furosemide* potentiate the ototoxic effects of the aminoglycosides in animals (Brummett, 1983); data implicating furosemide are less convincing in human beings (Moore et al., 1984a). Hearing loss also is more

likely to develop in patients with preexisting auditory impairment following exposure to these agents.

Although all aminoglycosides are capable of affecting both cochlear and vestibular function, some preferential toxicity is evident. Streptomycin and gentamicin produce predominantly vestibular effects, whereas amikacin, kanamycin, and neomycin primarily affect auditory function; tobramycin affects both equally. The incidence of ototoxicity is extremely difficult to determine. Data from audiometry suggest that the incidence may be as high as 25% (Moore et al., 1984a). The relative incidence appears to be equal for tobramycin, gentamicin, and amikacin. Initial studies in laboratory animals and human beings suggested that netilmicin is less ototoxic than other aminoglycosides (Lerner et al., 1983); however, the incidence of ototoxicity from netilmicin is not negligible—such complications developed in 10% of patients in one clinical trial of netilmicin (Trestman et al., 1978).

The incidence of vestibular toxicity is particularly high in patients receiving streptomycin; nearly 20% of individuals who received 500 mg twice daily for 4 weeks for enterococcal endocarditis developed clinically detectable, irreversible vestibular damage (Wilson et al., 1984). In addition, up to 75% of patients who received 2 g of streptomycin for more than 60 days showed evidence of nystagmus or postural imbalance.

It is recommended that patients receiving high doses and/or prolonged courses of aminoglycosides be monitored carefully for ototoxicity, since the initial symptoms may be reversible; however, deafness may occur several weeks after therapy is discontinued.

Clinical Symptoms of Cochlear Toxicity. A high-pitched tinnitus often is the first symptom of toxicity. If the drug is not discontinued, auditory impairment may develop after a few days. The tinnitus may persist for several days to 2 weeks after therapy is stopped. Since perception of sound in the high-frequency range (outside the conversational range) is lost first, the affected individual is not always aware of the difficulty, and it will not be detected unless careful audiometric examination is carried out. If the loss of hearing progresses, the lower sound ranges are affected, and conversation becomes difficult.

Clinical Symptoms of Vestibular Toxicity. Moderately intense headache lasting 1 or 2 days may precede the onset of labyrinthine dysfunction. This is immediately followed by an acute stage, in which nausea, vomiting, and difficulty with equilibrium develop and persist for 1 to 2 weeks. Vertigo in the upright position, inability to perceive termination of movement ("mental past pointing"), and difficulty in sitting or standing without visual cues are prominent symptoms. Drifting of the eyes at the end of a movement so that focusing and reading are difficult, positive Romberg test, and rarely pendular trunk movement and spontaneous nystagmus are outstanding signs. The acute stage ends suddenly and is followed by the appearance of manifestations consistent with chronic labyrinthitis, in which, although symptomless while in bed, the patient has difficulty when attempting to walk or make sudden movements; ataxia is the most prominent feature. The chronic phase persists for approximately 2 months; it is gradually superseded by a compensatory stage, in which symptoms are latent and appear only when the eyes are closed. Adaptation to the impairment of labyrinthine function is accomplished by the use of visual cues and deep proprioceptive sensation for determining movement and position. It is more adequate in the young than in the old, but may not be sufficient to permit the high degree of coordination required in many special trades. Recovery from this phase may require 12 to 18 months, and most patients have some permanent residual damage. Although there is no specific treatment for the vestibular deficiency, early discontinuation of the drug may permit recovery prior to irreversible damage of the hair cells.

Nephrotoxicity.   Approximately 8% to 26% of patients who receive an aminoglycoside for more than several days will develop mild renal impairment that is almost always reversible (Smith *et al.,* 1977, 1980). The toxicity results from accumulation and retention of aminoglycoside in the proximal tubular cells (Aronoff *et al.,* 1983; Lietman and Smith, 1983). The initial manifestation of damage at this site is excretion of enzymes of the renal tubular brush border (Patel *et al.,* 1975). After several days, there is a defect in renal concentrating ability, mild proteinuria, and the appearance of hyaline and granular casts. The glomerular filtration rate is reduced after several additional days (Schentag *et al.,* 1979). The nonoliguric phase of renal insufficiency has been postulated to be due to the effects of aminoglycosides on the distal portion of the nephron. They are thought by some investigators to decrease the sensitivity of the collecting-duct epithelium to endogenous antidiuretic hormone (Appel, 1982). While severe acute tubular necrosis may occur rarely, the most common significant finding is a mild rise in plasma creatinine (0.5 to 2.0 mg/dl; 40 to 175 μM). Hypokalemia, hypocalcemia, and hypophosphatemia are seen very infrequently. The impairment in renal function is almost always reversible, since the proximal tubular cells have the capacity to regenerate.

Several variables appear to influence nephrotoxicity from aminoglycosides. Toxicity correlates with the total amount of drug administered. Consequently toxicity is more likely to be encountered with longer courses of therapy. Continuous infusion is more nephrotoxic in dogs and rats than is intermittent dosing (Reiner *et al.,* 1978; Powell *et al.,* 1983), and constant concentrations of drug in plasma above a critical level, which is manifest by elevated trough serum concentrations, correlate with toxicity in human beings (Keating *et al.,* 1979).

The nephrotoxic potential varies among individual aminoglycosides. The relative toxicity correlates with the concentration of drug found in the renal cortex in experimental animals. Neomycin, which concentrates to the greatest degree, is highly nephrotoxic in human beings and should not be administered systemically. Streptomycin does not concentrate in the renal cortex and is the least nephrotoxic. Most of the

controversy has concerned the relative toxicities of gentamicin and tobramycin. Gentamicin is concentrated in the kidney to a greater degree than is tobramycin, but several controlled clinical trials have given different estimates of their relative nephrotoxicities (Smith *et al.,* 1977, 1980; Fong *et al.,* 1981; Keys *et al.,* 1981). If differences between the renal toxicity of these two aminoglycosides do exist in human beings, they appear to be slight. Comparative studies with amikacin, sisomicin, and netilmicin are not conclusive. Other drugs, such as *amphotericin B, vancomycin, cisplatin,* and *cyclosporine,* may potentiate aminoglycoside-induced nephrotoxicity (Wood *et al.,* 1986). Several studies suggest that *cephalothin* aggravates the nephrotoxicity produced by aminoglycosides (Klastersky *et al.,* 1975; Wade *et al.,* 1978). *Furosemide* enhances the nephrotoxicity of aminoglycosides in rats if there is concurrent fluid depletion (Mitchell *et al.,* 1977). It has been suggested that the diuretic-induced loss of K^+ might be responsible for this toxicity. Clinical studies have not proven conclusively that furosemide aggravates nephrotoxicity (Smith and Lietman, 1983); however, both volume depletion and wasting of K^+ have been incriminated.

Advanced age, liver disease, and septic shock have been suggested as risk factors for the development of nephrotoxicity from aminoglycosides, but data are not convincing (Moore *et al.,* 1984b). It should be emphasized, however, that renal function is overestimated in the elderly patient from measurement of creatinine concentration in plasma, and overdosing will occur if this value is used as the only guide in this patient population.

Whereas aminoglycosides consistently alter the structure and function of renal proximal tubular cells, these effects usually are reversible. The most important result of this toxicity may be reduced excretion of the drug, which, in turn, predisposes ototoxicity. Monitoring drug concentrations in plasma is useful, particularly during prolonged and/or high-dose therapy. However, it never has been proven that toxicity can be prevented by avoiding excessive peak or trough concentrations of aminoglycosides. In fact, experience with once-daily dosing regimens strongly suggests that high peaks (*e.g.,* 25 μg/ml or higher) do not increase toxicity.

The biochemical events leading to tubular cell damage and glomerular dysfunction are poorly understood, but they may involve perturbations of the structure of cellular membranes. Aminoglycosides inhibit various phospholipases, sphingomyelinases, and ATPases, and they alter the function of mitochondria and ribosomes (Silverblatt, 1982; Queener *et al.,* 1983; Humes *et al.,* 1984). Because of the ability of cationic aminoglycosides to interact with anionic phospholipids, these drugs may impair the generation of membrane-derived autacoids and intracellular second messengers such as prostaglandins, inositol phosphates, and diacylglycerol. Derangements of prostaglandin metabolism might explain the relationship between tubular damage and reduction in glomerular filtration rate. Others have observed morphological changes in glomerular endothelial cells (decreased number of endothelial fenestrations) in animals receiving aminoglycosides (Luft and Evan, 1980) and drug-induced reduction in the glomerular capillary ultrafiltration coefficient (Baylis *et al.,* 1977).

Ca^{2+} has been shown to inhibit the uptake and binding of aminoglycosides to the renal brush-border luminal membrane *in vitro,* and supplementary dietary Ca^{2+} attenuates experimental nephrotoxicity (Bennett *et al.,* 1982). Aminoglycosides eventually are internalized by pinocytosis. Morphologically, there is clear evidence of accumulation of drug in liposomes, a means by which aminoglycosides are trapped, concentrated (up to 50 times the plasma concentration; Aronoff *et al.,* 1983), and prepared for extrusion into the urine as multilamellar, phospholipid structures called *myeloid bodies* (Silverblatt, 1982).

Neuromuscular Blockade. An unusual toxic reaction of acute neuromuscular blockade and apnea has been attributed to the aminoglycosides. A review of 83 reports of prolonged muscular paralysis implicated neomycin as the most frequent cause (Pittinger *et al.,* 1970). The order of decreasing potency for blockade is neomycin, kanamycin, amikacin, gentamicin, and tobramycin.

In human beings, neuromuscular blockade generally has occurred after intrapleural or intraperitoneal instillation of large doses of an aminoglycoside; however, the reaction can follow intravenous, intramuscular, and even the oral administration of these agents (Holtzman, 1976). Most episodes have occurred in association with anesthesia or the administration of other neuromuscular blocking agents. Patients with myasthenia gravis are particularly susceptible to neuromuscular blockade by aminoglycosides.

Animal studies indicate that the aminoglycosides inhibit prejunctional release of acetylcholine while also reducing postsynaptic sensitivity to the transmitter (Pittinger and Adamson, 1972; Sokoll and Gergis, 1981). Ca^{2+} overcomes the effect of the aminoglycoside at the neuromuscular junction, and the intravenous administration of a calcium salt is the preferred treatment for this toxicity (Singh *et al.,* 1978). Inhibitors of cholinesterase (edrophonium, neostigmine) also have been used with varying degrees of success. Since physicians have become aware of this complication, it is now relatively uncommon.

Other Effects on the Nervous System. The administration of streptomycin in particular may produce dysfunction of the optic nerve. Scotomas, presenting as enlargement of the blind spot, have been associated with the drug.

Among the less common toxic reactions to streptomycin is peripheral neuritis. This may be due either to accidental injection of a nerve during the course of parenteral therapy or to toxicity involving nerves remote from the site of antibiotic administration. Paresthesia, most commonly perioral but also present in other areas of the face or in the hands, occasionally follows the use of the antibiotic and usually appears within 30 to 60 minutes after injection of the drug. It may persist for several hours.

Other Untoward Effects. In general, the aminoglycosides have little allergenic potential; both anaphylaxis and rash are unusual. Rare hypersensitivity reactions—including skin rashes, eosinophilia, fever, blood dyscrasias, angioedema, exfoliative dermatitis, stomatitis, and anaphylactic shock—have been reported. Parenterally administered aminoglycosides are not associated with pseudomembranous colitis, probably because they do not disrupt the normal anaerobic flora. Other reactions that have been attributed to individual drugs are discussed below.

STREPTOMYCIN

Streptomycin is used today for the treatment of certain unusual infections, generally in combination with other antimicrobial agents. It is in general less active than other members of the class against aerobic gram-negative rods. It therefore has fallen into disuse, and for a time the drug was unavailable in the United States. Streptomycin is administered by deep intramuscular injection, although it can be administered safely intravenously as well. Intramuscular injections often are painful with hot, tender masses developing at the site of injection. The dose of streptomycin is 15 mg/kg per day for patients with creatinine clearances above 80 ml/min. It is typically administered as a 1000 mg single daily dose or 500 mg twice daily, resulting in peak serum concentrations of approximately 50 to 60 μg/ml and 15 to 30 μg/ml and trough concentrations of less than 1 and 5 to 10 μg/ml, respectively. The total daily dose should be reduced in direct proportion to the reduction in creatinine clearance for creatinine clearances above 30 ml/min (Table 46–2).

Therapeutic Uses. *Bacterial Endocarditis.* Streptomycin and penicillin produce a synergistic bactericidal effect *in vitro* and in animal models of infection against strains of enterococci, group D streptococci, and the various oral streptococci of the viridans group. Many authorities recommend a combination of such antibiotics (although gentamicin has almost entirely replaced streptomycin) for treatment of endocarditis caused by these microorganisms. Penicillin G alone is ineffective in the therapy of enterococcal endocarditis, and either streptomycin

(500 mg twice daily) or gentamicin (1 mg/kg three times daily) also must be given to ensure cure. Gentamicin is preferred when the strain is resistant to streptomycin (MIC > 2000 μg/ml). Both penicillin G and the aminoglycoside are administered for 4 to 6 weeks. Treatment for 4 weeks has been successful in patients who had symptoms for less than 3 months prior to therapy (Wilson *et al.,* 1984). Some authorities prefer gentamicin for all cases of enterococcal endocarditis, since its toxicity is primarily renal and reversible while that of streptomycin is vestibular and irreversible. Unfortunately, gentamicin-resistant strains of enterococci have now appeared (Eliopoulos *et al.,* 1988). Because the enzymes that inactivate gentamicin and streptomycin are distinct, a small proportion of gentamicin-resistant strains will be susceptible to streptomycin.

Endocarditis caused by penicillin-sensitive streptococci (MIC < 0.1 μg/ml) has been treated successfully with penicillin G alone for 4 weeks (relapse rate 1% to 2%; Karchmer *et al.,* 1979), penicillin G plus streptomycin (0.5 g twice a day) for 2 weeks (relapse rate 1% to 2%, Wilson *et al.,* 1978), or penicillin G for 4 weeks combined with streptomycin for the first 2 weeks of therapy (relapse rate 0%; Wolfe and Johnson, 1974). The clinician thus has several options, one of which can be chosen based on the needs of the individual patient. For example, the elderly patient with streptococcal endocarditis due to a penicillin-sensitive strain probably should receive penicillin alone for 4 weeks because of the increased toxicity from streptomycin in this age group. The short, 2-week course of therapy is indicated for uncomplicated cases (Bisno *et al.,* 1989). However, if the infection is on a prosthetic valve, is caused by a relatively resistant strain (MIC of penicillin >0.2 μg/ml), or is caused by nutritionally deficient streptococci, a longer duration of therapy is recommended.

Tularemia. Patients with tularemia benefit dramatically from the administration of streptomycin (Evans *et al.,* 1985). The best results are obtained when therapy is instituted early; however, chronicity does not exclude the possibility of complete cure. Most cases respond to the administration of 1 to 2 g (15 to 25 mg/kg) of streptomycin per day (in divided doses) for 7 to 10 days. The tetracyclines also are highly effective in tularemia and are preferred by some physicians for milder forms of the disease.

Plague. Streptomycin is one of the most effective agents for the treatment of all forms of plague. The tetracyclines and chloramphenicol also are beneficial in this disease. When streptomycin is used, a dose of 1 to 4 g per day may be given in two to four divided doses for 7 to 10 days.

Tuberculosis. In treatment of tuberculosis, streptomycin always should be used in combination with at least one or two other drugs to which the causative strain is susceptible. The dose for patients with normal renal function is 15 mg/kg per day as a single intramuscular injection for two to three months, then two or three times a week thereafter.

GENTAMICIN

Gentamicin is an important agent for the treatment of many serious gram-negative bacillary infections. It is the aminoglycoside of first choice because of its low cost and its reliable activity against all but the most resistant gram-negative aerobes. However, emergence of resistant microorganisms in some hospitals has become a serious problem and may limit the future use of this agent.

Therapeutic Uses of Gentamicin and Other Aminoglycosides. Gentamicin, tobramycin, amikacin, and netilmicin can be used interchangeably for the treatment of most of the following infections and are therefore discussed together. For most indications, gentamicin is the preferred agent because of long experience with its use and its relatively low cost.

The recommended intramuscular or intravenous dose of *gentamicin sulfate* (GARAMYCIN) for adults is a loading dose of 2 mg/kg, then 3 to 5 mg/kg per day, one-third being given every 8 hours when administered as a multiple-daily-dosing regimen. The once-daily dose is 5.1 mg/kg given over 30 to 60 minutes for patients with normal renal function. Several dosage schedules have been suggested for infants: 2 to 2.5 mg/kg every 8 hours has been found to be safe for children up to 2 years of age; 5 mg/kg daily, divided into two equally spaced injections, has been recommended for neonates with severe infections. Peak plasma concentrations range from 4 to 10 μg/ml and 16 to 24 μg/ml with 1.7 mg/kg every 8 hours and 5.1 mg/kg once-daily dosing, respectively. It should be emphasized that the recommended doses of gentamicin do not always yield desired concentrations. Periodic determinations of the plasma concentration of aminoglycosides are recommended strongly, especially in seriously ill patients, to confirm that drug concentrations are in the desired range (*see* sections on dosing, above, for more details). Although it has not been established exactly what plasma concentration is toxic, trough concentrations that exceed 2 μg/ml for longer than 10 days have been associated with toxicity.

A large variety of infections have been treated successfully with these aminoglycosides; however, due to their toxicities, prolonged use should be restricted to the therapy of life-threatening infections and those for which a less toxic agent is contraindicated or less effective.

These antibiotics frequently are used (often in combination with a penicillin or a cephalosporin) for the therapy of proven or suspected serious gram-negative microbial infections—especially those due to *P. aeruginosa, Enterobacter, Klebsiella, Serratia,* and other species resistant to less toxic antibiotics—urinary tract infections, bacteremia, infected burns, osteomyelitis, pneumonia, peritonitis, and otitis.

Penicillins and aminoglycosides must never be mixed in the same bottle because the penicillin inactivates the aminoglycoside to a significant degree. Similar incompatibilities exist *in vitro* to different degrees between gentamicin and heparin, amphotericin B, and the various cephalosporins.

Urinary Tract Infections. Aminoglycosides usually are not indicated for the treatment of uncomplicated urinary tract infections, although a single intramuscular dose of gentamicin (5 mg/kg) has been effective in curing over 90% of uncomplicated infections of the lower urinary tract (Varese *et al.,* 1980). In the seriously ill patient with pyelonephritis, an aminoglycoside alone or in combination with a β-lactam antibiotic offers broad and effective initial coverage. Once the microorganism is isolated and its sensitivities to antibiotics are determined, the aminoglycoside should be discontinued if the infecting microorganism is sensitive to less toxic antibiotics. The antibacterial activity of aminoglycosides is markedly reduced by low pH (Strausbaugh and Sande, 1978) and hyperosmolarity (Papapetropoulou *et al.,* 1983); however, the very high concentrations achieved in urine in patients with normal renal function usually are sufficient to eradicate sensitive microorganisms. The prolonged release of gentamicin from the renal cortex following discontinuation of therapy has been shown to produce a therapeutic effect for several months in experimental pyelonephritis in rats (Bergeron *et al.,* 1982).

Pneumonia. The frequency of pneumonia caused by various gram-negative bacilli is increasing, especially in hospitalized patients, patients on respirators, and those with impaired defenses (especially granulocytopenia). Selection of an antibiotic depends on the sensitivity of the microorganism. The majority of organisms that cause community-acquired pneumonia will be susceptible to broad-spectrum β-lactam antibiotics, and it usually is not necessary to add an aminoglycoside. Therapy with an aminoglycoside alone is not very effective because therapeutic concentrations are difficult to achieve owing to relatively poor penetration of drug into inflamed tissues and the associated conditions of low oxygen tension and low pH, both of which interfere with aminoglycoside antibacterial activity. An aminoglycoside in combination with a β-lactam antibiotic is indicated for empirical therapy of hospital-acquired pneumonia in which multiple-drug-resistant, gram-negative aerobes are a likely causative agent. Combination therapy also is recommended for treatment of pneumonia caused by *P. aeruginosa.*

Gentamicin- and tobramycin-resistant strains of *Klebsiella, Enterobacter, Serratia, Proteus,* and *Pseudomonas* have emerged in many hospitals, particularly in burn units and intensive care units, where these drugs are used extensively. Critically ill patients with tracheostomies and impaired host defenses and those with indwelling intravenous and urinary catheters frequently are colonized or infected by resistant bacteria.

Aminoglycosides are ineffective for treatment of pneumonia due to anaerobes or *S. pneumoniae,* which are common causes of community-acquired pneumonia. They should not be considered as effective single-drug therapy for any aerobic gram-positive cocci (including *S. aureus* or streptococci), the microorganisms commonly responsible for suppurative pneumonia or lung abscess. Thus, gentamicin (or other aminoglycosides) should never be used as the sole agent to treat pneumonia acquired in the community or as the initial treatment for pneumonia acquired in the hospital (Kunin, 1977).

Meningitis. Availability of third-generation cephalosporins, especially *cefotaxime* and *ceftriaxone,* has reduced the need for treatment with aminoglycosides in most cases of meningitis, except for infections caused by gram-negative organisms that are resistant to β-lactam antibiotics (*e.g.,* species of *Pseudomonas* and *Acinetobacter*). If therapy with an aminoglycoside is necessary, direct administration of gentamicin (or other aminoglycoside) into the cerebral ventricles has been suggested, using 0.03 mg of gentamicin or tobramycin per ml of CSF or 0.1 mg of amikacin per ml of CSF every 24 hours (McGee and Baringer, 1990). In one study, however, children with gram-negative bacillary meningitis failed to show a beneficial effect from direct administration of gentamicin into the cerebral ventricles.

Peritonitis. Patients who develop peritonitis as a result of peritoneal dialysis may benefit from therapy with an aminoglycoside. Since suboptimal intraperitoneal concentrations of the antibiotic may follow intramuscular or intravenous administration in patients undergoing dialysis, the procedure should be continued with fluids containing an appropriate concentration of the aminoglycoside.

Gram-Positive Infections. Although there are very few indications for the use of aminoglycosides for gram-positive bacterial infections, at times it may be necessary and lifesaving. In cases of enterococcal endocarditis, up to 50% of isolates of enterococci are not killed by penicillin plus streptomycin; these strains, however, are nearly always sensitive to penicillin plus gentamicin. This is not revealed by testing for sensitivity to a standard dose of gentamicin, and the breakpoint for resistance is defined as 500 μg/ml. Gentamicin (or tobramycin) also may be used in a two-week regimen in combination with nafcillin for the treatment of selected cases of staphylococcal tricuspid valve endocarditis in injection drug users (Chambers *et al.,* 1988).

Sepsis. When a patient has granulocytopenia and infection (sepsis) with *P. aeruginosa* is suspected, the administration of an antipseudomonal penicillin in combination with gentamicin, tobramycin, amikacin, or netilmicin is recommended. Treatment of gram-negative bacillary sepsis, especially in neutropenic patients, has been improved by the use of such synergistic combinations (Klastersky, 1987).

Topical Applications. Gentamicin is very slowly absorbed when applied in an ointment, but absorption may be more rapid when a cream is used topically. When the antibiotic is applied to large areas of denuded body surface, as may be the case in burned patients, plasma concentrations can reach 4 μg/ml, and 2% to 5% of the drug used may appear in the urine.

Untoward Effects. The untoward effects of gentamicin are similar to those of other aminoglycosides. The most important and serious side effects of the use of gentamicin are nephrotoxicity and irreversible ototoxicity. Intrathecal or intraventricular administration may cause local inflammation and can result in radiculitis and other complications and therefore is rarely used (*see* above).

TOBRAMYCIN

The antimicrobial activity and pharmacokinetic properties of *tobramycin* (NEBCIN) are very similar to those of gentamicin. Tobramycin may be given either intramuscularly or intravenously. Dosages and serum concentrations are identical with those for gentamicin. Toxicity is most common at minimal (trough) concentrations that exceed 2 μg/ml for a prolonged period. The latter observation usually suggests impairment of renal function and requires reduction of dosage.

Tobramycin (TOBREX) also is available in ophthalmic ointments and solutions.

Therapeutic Uses.   Indications for the use of tobramycin are essentially identical with those for gentamicin. The superior activity of tobramycin against *P. aeruginosa* may make it desirable in the treatment of bacteremia, osteomyelitis, and pneumonia caused by *Pseudomonas* species. It usually should be used concurrently with an antipseudomonal β-lactam antibiotic.

In contrast to gentamicin, tobramycin shows poor activity in combination with penicillin against many strains of enterococci. Most strains of *E. faecium* are highly resistant (Moellering *et al.*, 1979). Tobramycin is ineffective against mycobacteria (Gangadharam and Candler, 1977).

Untoward Effects.   Tobramycin, like other aminoglycosides, causes both nephrotoxicity and ototoxicity, as discussed above. Studies in experimental animals suggest that tobramycin may be less toxic to hair cells in the cochlear and vestibular end organs and cause less renal tubular damage than does gentamicin. However, clinical data are less convincing.

AMIKACIN

The spectrum of antimicrobial activity of *amikacin* (AMIKIN) is the broadest of the group, and because of its unique resistance to the aminoglycoside-inactivating enzymes, it has a special role in hospitals where gentamicin- and tobramycin-resistant microorganisms are prevalent. Amikacin is similar to kanamycin in dosage and pharmacokinetic properties.

The recommended dose of amikacin is 15 mg/kg per day, as a single daily dose or divided into two or three equal portions. The individual dose or the interval between doses must be altered in patients with renal failure. The drug is rapidly absorbed after intramuscular injection, and peak concentrations in plasma approximate 20 μg/ml after injection of 7.5 mg/kg. An intravenous infusion of the same dose over a 30-minute period produces a peak concentration in plasma of nearly 40 μg/ml at the end of the infusion, which falls to about 20 μg/ml 30 minutes later. The concentration 12 hours after a 7.5-mg/kg dose typically is between 5 and 10 μg/ml. A 15-mg/kg once-daily dose produces peak concentrations that are between 50 and 60 μg/ml and a trough of <1 μg/ml.

Therapeutic Uses.   Amikacin has become the preferred agent for initial treatment of serious nosocomial gram-negative bacillary infections in hospitals where resistance to gentamicin and tobramycin has become a significant problem. Some hospitals have restricted its use to avoid emergence of resistant strains, although some suggest that this is not likely (Betts *et al.*, 1984).

Because of its unique resistance to aminoglycoside-inactivating enzymes, amikacin is active against the vast majority of aerobic gram-negative bacilli in both the community and the hospital. This includes most strains of *Serratia, Proteus,* and *P. aeruginosa*. It is active against nearly all strains of *Klebsiella, Enterobacter,* and *E. coli* that are resistant to gentamicin and tobramycin. Most resistance to amikacin is found among strains of *Acinetobacter, Providencia,* and *Flavobacter* and strains of *Pseudomonas* other than *P. aeruginosa*. These are all unusual pathogens. Like tobramycin, amikacin is less active than gentamicin against enterococci and should not be used. Amikacin is not active against the majority of gram-positive anaerobic bacteria. It is effective against *M. tuberculosis* (99% of strains inhibited by 4 μg/ml) and certain atypical mycobacteria (Gangadharam and Candler, 1977) and has been used in the treatment of disseminated atypical mycobacterial infection in AIDS patients.

Untoward Effects.   Like the other aminoglycosides, amikacin causes both ototoxicity and nephrotoxicity. Auditory deficits are most commonly produced, as discussed above.

NETILMICIN

Netilmicin (NETROMYCIN) is the latest of the aminoglycosides to be marketed. It is similar to gentamicin and tobramycin in its pharmacokinetic properties and dosage. Its antibacterial activity is broad against aerobic gram-negative bacilli. Like amikacin, it is not metabolized by the majority of the aminoglycoside-inactivating enzymes, and it may be active against certain bacteria that are resistant to gentamicin.

The recommended dose of netilmicin for complicated urinary tract infections in adults is 1.5 to 2 mg/kg every 12 hours. For other serious systemic infections, a total daily dose of 4 to 6.5 mg/kg is administered as a single dose or divided into two or three portions. Children should receive 3.0 to 7.5 mg/kg per day in two to three divided doses; neonates receive 4 to 6.5 mg/kg per day in two divided doses. The distribution and elimination of netilmicin, gentamicin, and tobramycin are very similar. An intravenous infusion of 2 mg/kg netilmicin, given over a 60-minute period, results in a peak plasma concentration of approximately 11 μg/ml (Luft *et al.*, 1978). The half-time for elimination is usually 2.0 to 2.5 hours in adults and increases with renal insufficiency.

Therapeutic Uses.   Netilmicin is a useful antibiotic for the treatment of serious infections due to susceptible Enterobacteriaceae and other aerobic gram-negative bacilli. It has been shown to be effective against certain gentamicin-resistant pathogens, except enterococci (Panwalker *et al.*, 1978).

Untoward Effects. Like other aminoglycosides, netilmicin also may produce ototoxicity and nephrotoxicity. Although studies in animals have suggested that netilmicin may be less toxic (Luft *et al.,* 1976), this remains to be proven in human beings (Trestman *et al.,* 1978; Bock *et al.,* 1980).

KANAMYCIN

The use of kanamycin has declined markedly because its spectrum of activity is limited compared with other aminoglycosides, and it is among the most toxic.

Kanamycin sulfate (KANTREX) is available for injection and oral use. The parenteral dose for adults is 15 mg/kg per day (two to four equally divided and spaced doses), with a maximum of 1.5 g per day. Children may be given up to 15 mg/kg per day.

Therapeutic Uses. Kanamycin is all but obsolete, and there are few indications for its use. Kanamycin has been employed to treat tuberculosis in combination with other effective drugs. Because the therapy of this disease is protracted and involves the administration of large total doses of the drug, with the risk of ototoxicity and nephrotoxicity, kanamycin should be used only to treat patients who harbor microorganisms that are resistant to the more commonly used agents (*see* Chapter 48).

Prophylactic Uses. Kanamycin can be administered orally as adjunctive therapy in cases of hepatic coma. The rationale for such therapy is described under neomycin (*see* below). The dose usually employed for these purposes is 4 to 6 g per day for 36 to 72 hours; quantities as large as 12 g per day (in divided doses) have been given. The effect on intestinal bacteria may not be sustained even when such large doses of kanamycin are administered.

Untoward Effects. The untoward effects of the oral administration of aminoglycosides are considered under neomycin, below.

NEOMYCIN

Neomycin is a broad-spectrum antibiotic. Susceptible microorganisms usually are inhibited by concentrations of 5 to 10 μg/ml or less. Gram-negative species that are highly sensitive are *E. coli, Enterobacter aerogenes, Klebsiella pneumoniae,* and *Proteus vulgaris.* Gram-positive microorganisms that are inhibited include *S. aureus* and *E. faecalis. M. tuberculosis* also is sensitive to neomycin. Strains of *P. aeruginosa* are resistant to neomycin.

Neomycin sulfate (MYCIFRADIN) is available for topical and oral administration. Neomycin and *polymyxin B* have been used for bladder irrigation in solutions containing 40 mg of neomycin and 200,000 units of polymyxin B per milliliter (NEOSPORIN G.U. IRRIGANT). One milliliter of this preparation is added to 1000 ml of 0.9% sodium chloride solution and is used for continuous irrigation of the urinary bladder through appropriate catheter systems. The goal is to prevent bacteriuria and bacteremia associated with the use of indwelling catheters. The bladder usually is irrigated at the rate of 1000 ml every 24 hours.

Neomycin currently is available in many brands of creams, ointments, and other products both alone and in combination with polymyxin, bacitracin, other antibiotics, and a variety of corticosteroids. There is no evidence that these topical preparations shorten the time required for healing of wounds or that those containing a steroid are more effective.

Therapeutic Uses. Neomycin has been widely used for topical application in a variety of infections of the skin and mucous membranes caused by microorganisms susceptible to the drug. These include infections associated with burns, wounds, ulcers, and infected dermatoses. However, such treatment does not eradicate bacteria from the lesions.

The oral administration of neomycin (usually in combination with erythromycin base) has been employed primarily for "preparation" of the bowel for surgery. As an adjunct to the therapy of hepatic coma, a daily dose of 4 to 12 g (in divided doses) by mouth can be given without difficulty to patients, provided renal function is normal. Because severe renal insufficiency may develop in the late stages of hepatic failure, treatment with neomycin must be followed with the greatest care and stopped if evidence of ototoxicity or further injury to the kidney appears. Lactulose is a much less toxic agent for treatment of hepatic coma, and neomycin is used rarely for this condition.

Absorption and Excretion. Neomycin is poorly absorbed from the gastrointestinal tract and is excreted by the kidney, as are the other aminoglycosides. An oral dose of 3 g produces a peak plasma concentration of only 1 to 4 μg/ml; a total daily intake of 10 g for 3 days yields a blood concentration below that associated with systemic toxicity if renal function is normal. Patients with renal insufficiency may accumulate the drug. About 97% of an oral dose of neomycin escapes absorption and is eliminated unchanged in the feces. Although neomycin can be given orally to very young children, in doses as high as 100 mg/kg per day, its use in such patients for longer than 3 weeks should be avoided because of partial absorption from the intestinal tract, especially if it is the site of disease.

Untoward Effects. Hypersensitivity reactions, primarily skin rashes, occur in 6% to 8% of patients when neomycin is applied topically. Individuals sensitive to this agent may develop cross-reactions when exposed to other aminoglycosides. The most important toxic effects of neomycin are renal damage and nerve deafness. These were most frequent when relatively large quantities of the antibiotic were used parenterally and are the reason the drug is no longer used in this way. Toxicity has even occurred in patients with normal renal function following topical application or irrigation of wounds with 0.5%

neomycin solution. Neuromuscular blockade with respiratory paralysis also has occurred after irrigation of wounds or serosal cavities.

The most important adverse effects resulting from the oral administration of neomycin are intestinal malabsorption and superinfection. Individuals treated with 4 to 6 g of the drug by mouth per day sometimes develop a spruelike syndrome with diarrhea, steatorrhea, and azotorrhea. Overgrowth of yeasts in the intestine also may occur; this is not associated with diarrhea or other symptoms in most cases. The oral administration of even large doses of neomycin usually has no effect on blood levels of prothrombin.

For further information regarding particular infections for which the antimicrobial agents discussed in this chapter are useful, the reader is referred to the following chapters of *Harrison's Principles of Internal Medicine,* 14th ed. (McGraw-Hill, New York, 1998): diseases caused by gram-negative enteric bacilli and *P. aeruginosa* (Chapters 155 and 157); tularemia (Chapter 163); plague (Chapter 164); tuberculosis (Chapter 171).

BIBLIOGRAPHY

Ali, M.Z., and Goetz, M.B. A meta-analysis of the relative efficacy and toxicity of single daily dosing *versus* multiple daily dosing of aminoglycosides. *Clin. Infect. Dis.,* **1997,** *24*:796–809.

Appel, G.B. Aminoglycoside nephrotoxicity: physiologic studies of the sites of nephron damage. In, *The Aminoglycosides: Microbiology, Clinical Use, and Toxicity.* (Whelton, A., and Neu, H.C., eds.) Marcel Dekker, Inc., New York 1982, pp. 269–282.

Aronoff, G.R., Pottratz, S.T., Brier, M.E., Walker, N.E., Fineberg, N.S., Glant, M.D., and Luft, F.C. Aminoglycoside accumulation kinetics in rat renal parenchyma. *Antimicrob. Agents Chemother.,* **1983,** *23*:74–78.

Bailey, T.C., Little, J.R., Littenberg, B., Reichley, R.M., and Dunagan, W.C. A meta-analysis of extended-interval dosing versus multiple daily dosing of aminoglycosides. *Clin. Infect. Dis.,* **1997,** *24*:786–795.

Barclay, M.L., Kirkpatrick, C.M., and Begg, E.J. Once daily aminoglycoside therapy. Is it less toxic than multiple daily doses and how should it be monitored? *Clin. Pharmacokinet.,* **1999,** *36*:89–98.

Barza, M. Factors affecting the intraocular penetration of antibiotics. The influence of route, inflammation, animal species, and tissue pigmentation. *Scand. J. Infect. Dis. Suppl.,* **1978,** *14*:151–159.

Barza, M., Brown, R.B., Shen, D., Gibaldi, M., and Weinstein, L. Predictability of blood levels of gentamicin in man. *J. Infect. Dis.,* **1975,** *132*:165–174.

Barza, M., Ioannidis, J.P., Cappelleri, J.C., and Lau, J. Single or multiple daily doses of aminoglycosides: a meta-analysis. *BMJ.,* **1996,** *312*:338–345.

Baylis, C., Rennke, H.R., and Brenner, B.M. Mechanisms of the defect in glomerular ultrafiltration associated with gentamicin administration. *Kidney Int.,* **1977,** *12*:344–353.

Bennett, W.M., Elliott, W.C., Houghton, D.C., Gilbert, D.N., DeFehr, J., and McCarron, D.A. Reduction of experimental gentamicin nephrotoxicity in rats by dietary calcium loading. *Antimicrob. Agents Chemother.,* **1982,** *22*:508–512.

Bergeron, M.G., Bastille, A., Lessard, C., and Gagnon, P.M. Significance of intrarenal concentrations of gentamicin for the outcome of experimental pyelonephritis in rats. *J. Infect. Dis.,* **1982,** *146*:91–96.

Betts, R.F., Valenti, W.M., Chapman, S.W., Chonmaitree, T., Mowrer, G., Pincus, P., Messner, M., and Robertson, R. Five-year surveillance of aminoglycoside usage in a university hospital. *Ann. Intern. Med.,* **1984,** *100*:219–222.

Bisno, A.L., Dismukes, W.E., Durack, D.T., Kaplan, E.L., Karchmer, A.W., Kaye, D., Rahimtoola, S.H., Sande, M.A., Sanford, J.P., Watanakunakorn, C., and Wilson, W.R. Antimicrobial treatment of infective endocarditis due to viridans streptococci, enterococci, and staphylococci. *JAMA,* **1989,** *261*:1471–1477.

Blair, D.C., Duggan, D.O., and Schroeder, E.T. Inactivation of amikacin and gentamicin by carbenicillin in patients with end-stage renal failure. *Antimicrob. Agents Chemother.,* **1982,** *22*:376–379.

Bock, B.V., Edelstein, P.H., and Meyer, R.D. Prospective comparative study of efficacy and toxicity of netilmicin and amikacin. *Antimicrob. Agents Chemother.,* **1980,** *17*:217–225.

Bodey, G.P., Jadeja, L., and Elting, L. *Pseudomonas* bacteremia. Retrospective analysis of 410 episodes. *Arch. Intern. Med.,* **1985,** *145*:1621–1629.

Breen, K.J., Bryant, R.E., Levinson, J.D., and Schenker, S. Neomycin absorption in man. Studies of oral and enema administration and effect of intestinal ulceration. *Ann. Intern. Med.,* **1972,** *76*:211–218.

Brummett, R.E. Animal models of aminoglycoside antibiotic ototoxicity. *Rev. Infect. Dis.,* **1983,** 5(suppl. 2):S294–S303.

Bryan, L.E., and Kwan, S. Roles of ribosomal binding, membrane potential, and electron transport in bacterial uptake of streptomycin and gentamicin. *Antimicrob. Agents Chemother.,* **1983,** *23*:835–845.

Busse, H.J., Wöstmann, C., and Bakker, E.P. The bactericidal action of streptomycin: membrane permeabilization caused by the insertion of mistranslated proteins into the cytoplasmic membrane of *Escherichia coli* and subsequent caging of the antibiotic inside the cells due to degradation of these proteins. *J. Gen. Microbiol.,* **1992,** *138*:551–561.

Chambers, H.F., Miller, R.T., and Newman, M.D. Right-sided *Staphylococcus aureus* endocarditis in intravenous drug abusers: two-week combination study. *Ann. Intern. Med.,* **1988,** *109*:619–624.

Charnas, R., Luthi, A.R., and Ruch, W. Once daily ceftriaxone plus amikacin vs. three times daily ceftazidime plus amikacin for treatment of febrile neutropenic children with cancer. Writing Committee for the International Collaboration on Antimicrobial Treatment of Febrile Neutropenia in Children. *Pediatr. Infect. Dis. J.,* **1997,** *16*:346–353.

Cross, A.S., Opal, S., and Kopecko, D.J. Progressive increase in antibiotic resistance of gram-negative bacterial isolates. Walter Reed Hospital, 1976 to 1980: specific analysis of gentamicin, tobramycin, and amikacin resistance. *Arch. Intern. Med.,* **1983,** *143*:2075–2080.

Deamer, R.L. Single daily dosing of aminoglycosides. *Am. Fam. Physician,* **1998,** *58*:1747–1750.

Deaney, N.B., and Tate, H. A meta-analysis of clinical studies of imipenem-cilastatin for empirically treating of febrile neutropenic patients. *J. Antimicrob. Chemother.,* **1996,** 37:975–986.

Eliopoulos, G.M., Farber, B.F., Murray, B.E., Wennersten, C., and Moellering, R.C., Jr. Ribosomal resistance of clinical enterococcal to streptomycin isolates. *Antimicrob. Agents Chemother.,* **1984,** 25:398–399.

Eliopoulos, G.M., Wennersten, C., Zighelboim-Daum, S., Reiszner, E., Goldmann, D., and Moellering, R.C. Jr. High-level resistance to gentamicin in clinical isolates of *Streptococcus (enterococcus) faecium.* *Antimicrob. Agents Chemother.,* **1988,** 32:1528–1532.

Evans, M.E., Gregory, D.W., Schaffner, W., and McGee, Z.A. Tularemia: a 30-year experience with 88 cases. *Medicine (Baltimore),* **1985,** 64:251–269.

Ferriols-Lisart, R., and Alos-Alminana, M. Effectiveness and safety of once-daily aminoglycosides: a meta-analysis. *Am. J. Health Syst. Pharm.,* **1996,** 53:1141–1150.

Fong, I.W., Fenton, R.S., and Bird, R. Comparative toxicity of gentamicin versus tobramycin: a randomized prospective study. *J. Antimicrob. Chemother.,* **1981,** 7:81–88.

Freeman, C.D., Nicolau, D.P., Belliveau, P.P., and Nightingale, C.H. Once-daily dosing of aminoglycosides: review and recommendations for clinical practice. *J. Antimicrob. Chemother.,* **1997,** 39:677–686.

Freeman, C.D., and Strayer, A.H. Mega-analysis of meta-analysis: an examination of meta-analysis with an emphasis on once-daily aminoglycoside comparative trials. *Pharmacotherapy,* **1996,** 16:1093–1102.

Gangadharam, P.R., and Candler, E.R. *In vitro* antimycobacterial activity of some new amino-glycoside antibiotics. *Tubercle,* **1977,** 58:35–38.

Gilbert, D.N., Lee, B.L., Dworkin, R.J., Leggett, J.L., Chambers, H.F., Modin, G., Tauber, M.G., and Sande, M.A. A randomized comparison of the safety and efficacy of once-daily gentamicin or thrice-daily gentamicin in combination with ticarcillin-clavulanate. *Am. J. Med.,* **1998,** 105:182–191.

Higgins, C.E., and Kastner, R.E. Nebramycin, a new broad-spectrum antibiotic complex. II. Description of *Streptomyces tenebrarius. Antimicrob. Agents Chemother.,* **1967,** 7:324–331.

Holtzman, J.L. Gentamicin and neuromuscular blockade (letter). *Ann. Intern. Med.,* **1976,** 84:55.

Humes, H.D., Sastrasinh, M., and Weinberg, J.M. Calcium is a competitive inhibitor of gentamicin-renal membrane binding interactions, and dietary calcium supplementation protects against gentamicin nephrotoxicity. *J. Clin. Invest.,* **1984,** 73:134–147.

Hummel, H., and Böck, A. Ribosomal changes resulting in antimicrobial resistance. In, *Microbial Resistance to Drugs,* (Bryan, L.E., ed.) *Handbook of Experimental Pharmacology.* Vol. 91. Springer-Verlag, Berlin, **1989,** pp. 193–226.

The International Antimicrobial Therapy Cooperative Group of the European Organization for Research and Treatment of Cancer. Efficacy and toxicity of single daily doses of amikacin and ceftriaxone versus multiple daily doses of amikacin and ceftazidime for infection in patients with cancer and granulocytopenia. *Ann. Intern. Med.,* **1993,** *119*:584–593.

Karchmer, A.W., Moellering, R.C., Jr., Maki, D.G., and Swartz, M.N. Single-antibiotic therapy for streptococcal endocarditis. *JAMA,* **1979,** *241*:1801–1806.

Kawaguchi, H., Naito, T., Nakagawa, S., and Fugisawa, K.I. BB-K8, a new semisynthetic aminoglycoside antibiotic. *J. Antibiot. (Tokyo),* **1972,** 25:695–708.

Keating, M.J., Bodey, G.P., Valdivieso, M., and Rodriguez, V. A randomized comparative trial of three aminoglycosides—comparison of continuous infusions of gentamicin, amikacin, and sisomicin combined with carbenicillin in the treatment of infections in neutropenic patients with malignancies. *Medicine (Baltimore),* **1979,** 58:159–170.

Keys, T.F., Kurtz, S.B., Jones, J.D., and Muller, S.M. Renal toxicity during therapy with gentamicin or tobramycin. *Mayo Clin. Proc.,* **1981,** 56:556–559.

Klastersky, J., Hensgens, C., and Debusscher, L. Empiric therapy for cancer patients: comparative study of ticarcillin-tobramycin, ticarcillin-cephalothin, and cephalothin-tobramycin. *Antimicrob. Agents Chemother.,* **1975,** 7:640–645.

Konishi, H., Goto, M., Nakamoto, Y., Yamamoto, I., and Yamashina, H. Tobramycin inactivation by carbenicillin, ticarcillin, and piperacillin. *Antimicrob. Agents Chemother.,* **1983,** 23:653–657.

Kunin, C.M. Blunder drug for pneumonia (letter). *N. Engl. J. Med.,* **1977,** 297:113–114.

Leclercq, R., Derlot, E., Duval, J., and Courvalin, P. Plasmid-mediated resistance to vancomycin and teicoplanin in *Enterococcus faecium. N. Engl. J. Med.,* **1988,** 319:157–161.

Leibovici, L., Paul, M., Poznanski, O., Drucker, M., Samra, Z., Konigsberger, H., and Pitlik, S.D. Monotherapy *versus* beta-lactam-aminoglycoside combination treatment for gram-negative bacteremia: a prospective, observational study. *Antimicrob. Agents Chemother.,* **1997,** *41*:1127–1133.

Lerner, A.M., Reyes, M.P., Cone, L.A., Blair, D.C., Jansen, W., Wright, G.E., and Lorber, R.R. Randomised, controlled trial of the comparative efficacy, auditory toxicity, and nephrotoxicity of tobramycin and netilmicin. *Lancet,* **1983,** *1*:1123–1126.

Lesar, T.S., Rotschafer, J.C., Strand, L.M., Solem, L.D., and Zaske, D.E. Gentamicin dosing errors with four commonly used nomograms. *JAMA,* **1982,** *248*:1190–1193.

Levy, J. Antibiotic activity in sputum. *J. Pediatr.,* **1986,** *108*:841–846.

Lietman, P.S., and Smith, C.R. Aminoglycoside nephrotoxicity in humans. *J. Infect. Dis.,* **1983,** *5*(suppl. 2):S284–S292.

Luft, F.C., Brannon, D.R., Stropes, L.L., Costello, R.J., Sloan, R.S., and Maxwell, D.R. Pharmacokinetics of netilmicin in patients with renal impairment and in patients on dialysis. *Antimicrob. Agents Chemother.,* **1978,** 14:403–407.

Luft, F.C., and Evan, A.P. Comparative effects of tobramycin and gentamicin on glomerular ultrastructure. *J. Infect. Dis.,* **1980,** *142*:910–914.

Luft, F.C., Yum, M.N., and Kleit, S.A. Comparative nephrotoxicities of netilmicin and gentamicin in rats. *Antimicrob. Agents Chemother.,* **1976,** 10:845–849.

Luzzatto, L., Apirion, D., and Schlessinger, D. Polyribosome depletion and blockage of the ribosome cycle by streptomycin in *Escherichia coli. J. Mol. Biol.,* **1969,** 42:315–335.

Mates, S.M., Patel, L., Kaback, H.R., and Miller, M.H. Membrane potential in anaerobically growing *Staphylococcus aureus* and its relationship to gentamicin uptake. *Antimicrob. Agents Chemother.,* **1983,** 23:526–530.

McCormack, J.P., and Jewesson, P.J. A critical reevaluation of the "therapeutic range" of aminoglycosides. *Clin. Infect. Dis.,* **1992,** 14:320–339.

McCracken, G.H., Jr., Mize, S.G., and Threlkeld, N. Intraventricular gentamicin therapy in gram-negative bacillary meningitis of infancy. Report of the Second Neonatal Meningitis Cooperative Study Group. *Lancet,* **1980,** *1*:787–791.

Mitchell, C.J., Bullock, S., and Ross, B.D. Renal handling of gentamicin and other antibiotics by the isolated perfused rat kidney: mechanism of nephrotoxicity. *J. Antimicrob. Chemother.,* **1977,** 3:593–600.

Moellering, R.C. Jr., Korzeniowski, O.M., Sande, M.A., and Wennersten, C.B. Species-specific resistance to antimicrobial synergism in *Streptococcus faecium* and *Streptococcus faecalis. J. Infect. Dis.,* **1979,** 140:203–208.

Moore, R.D., Smith, C.R., and Lietman, P.S. Risk factors for the development of auditory toxicity in patients receiving aminoglycosides. *J. Infect. Dis.,* **1984a,** 149:23–30.

Moore, R.D., Smith, C.R., Lipsky, J.J., Mellits, E.D., and Lietman, P.S. Risk factors for nephrotoxicity in patients with aminoglycosides. *Ann. Intern. Med.,* **1984b,** 100:352–357.

Murray, B.E., and Mederski-Samaroj, B. Transferable β-lactamase: a new mechanism for *in vitro* penicillin resistance in *Streptococcus faecalis. J. Clin. Invest.,* **1983,** 72:1168–1171.

Nakae, R., and Nakae, T. Diffusion of aminoglycoside antibiotics across the outer membrane of *Escherichia coli. Antimicrob. Agents Chemother.,* **1982,** 22:554–559.

Panwalker, A.P., Malow, J.B., Zimelis, V.M., and Jackson, G.G. Netilmicin: clinical efficacy, tolerance, and toxicity. *Antimicrob. Agents Chemother.,* **1978,** 13:170–176.

Papapetropoulou, M., Papavassiliou, J., and Legakis, N.J. Effect of the pH and osmolality of urine on the antibacterial activity of gentamicin. *J. Antimicrob. Chemother.,* **1983,** 12:571–575.

Patel, V., Luft, F.C., Yum, M.N., Patel, B., Zeman, W., and Kleit, S.A. Enzymuria in gentamicin-induced kidney damage. *Antimicrob. Agents Chemother.,* **1975,** 7:364–369.

Philips, J.B. III, Satterwhite, C., Dworsky, M.E., and Cassady, G. Recommended amikacin doses in newborns often produce excessive serum levels. *Pediatr. Pharmacol. (New York),* **1982,** 2:121–125.

Powell, S.H., Thompson, W.L., Luthe, M.A., Stern, R.C., Grossniklaus, D.A., Bloxham, D.D., Groden, D.L., Jacobs, M.R., DiScenna, A.O., Cash, H.A., and Klinger, J.D. Once-daily vs. continuous aminoglycoside dosing: efficacy and toxicity in animal and clinical studies of gentamicin, netilmicin, and tobramycin. *J. Infect. Dis.,* **1983,** 147:918–932.

Prins, J.M., Buller, H.R., Kuijper, E.J., Tange, R.A., and Speelman, P. Once versus thrice daily gentamicin in patients with serious infections. *Lancet,* **1993,** 341:335–339.

Queener, S.F., Luft, F.C., and Hamel, F.G. Effect of gentamicin treatment on adenylate cyclase and Na$^+$, K$^+$-ATPase activities in renal tissues of rats. *Antimicrob. Agents Chemother.,* **1983,** 24:815–818.

Reiner, N.E., Bloxham, D.D., and Thompson, W.L. Nephrotoxicity of gentamicin and tobramycin given once daily or continuously in dogs. *J. Antimicrob. Chemother.,* **1978,** 4(suppl. A):85–101.

Rosenthal, A., Button, L.N., and Khaw, K.T. Blood volume changes in patients with cystic fibrosis. *Pediatrics,* **1977,** 59:588–594.

Rybak, M.J., Abate, B.J., Kang, S.L., Ruffing, M.J., Lerner, S.A., and Drusano, G.L. Prospective evaluation of the effect of an aminoglycoside dosing regimen on rates of observed nephrotoxicity and ototoxicity. *Antimicrob. Agents Chemother.,* **1999,** 43:1549–1555.

Schentag, J.J., Gengo, F.M., Plaut, M.E., Danner, D., Mangione, A., and Jusko, W.J. Urinary casts as an indicator of renal tubular damage in patients receiving aminoglycosides. *Antimicrob. Agents Chemother.,* **1979,** 16:468–474.

Schentag, J.J., and Jusko, W.J. Renal clearance and tissue accumulation of gentamicin. *Clin. Pharmacol. Ther.,* **1977,** 22:364–370.

Siber, G.R., Echeverria, P., Smith, A.L., Paisley, J.W., and Smith, D.H. Pharmacokinetics of gentamicin in children and adults. *J. Infect. Dis.,* **1975,** 132:637–651.

Singh, Y.N., Harvey, A.L., and Marshall, I.G. Antibiotic-induced paralysis of the mouse phrenic nerve—hemidiaphragm preparation and

reversibility by calcium and by neostigmine. *Anesthesiology,* **1978,** 48:418–424.

Smith, C.R., Baughman, K.L., Edwards, C.Q., Rogers, J.F., and Lietman, P.S. Controlled comparison of amikacin and gentamicin. *N. Engl. J. Med.,* **1977,** 296:349–353.

Smith, C.R., and Lietman, P.S. Effect of furosemide on aminoglycoside-induced nephrotoxicity and auditory toxicity in humans. *Antimicrob. Agents Chemother.,* **1983,** 23:133–137.

Smith, C.R., Lipsky, J.J., Laskin, O.L., Hellman, D.B., Mellits, E.D., Longstreth, J., and Lietman, P.S. Double-blind comparison of the nephrotoxicity and auditory toxicity of gentamicin and tobramycin. *N. Engl. J. Med.,* **1980,** 302:1106–1109.

Smithivas, T., Hyams, P.J., Matalon, R., Simberkoff, M.S., and Rahal, J.J., Jr. The use of gentamicin in peritoneal dialysis. I. Pharmacologic results. *J. Infect. Dis.,* **1971,** 124(suppl):77–83.

Spera, R.V. Jr., and Farber, B.F. Multiply-resistant *Enterococcus faecium.* The nosocomial pathogen of the 1990s. *JAMA,* **1992,** 268:2563–2564.

Spyker, D.A., Sande, M.A., and Mandell, G.L. Tobramycin pharmacokinetics in patients with cystic fibrosis and leukemia. In, *Eighteenth Interscience Conference on Antimicrobial Agents and Chemotherapy.* American Society for Microbiology, Washington, D.C., **1978,** p. 345.

Strausbaugh, L.J., Mandaleris, C.D., and Sande, M.A. Comparison of four aminoglycoside antibiotics in the therapy of experimental *E. coli* meningitis. *J. Lab. Clin. Med.,* **1977,** 89:692–701.

Strausbaugh, L.J., and Sande, M.A. Factors influencing the therapy of experimental *Proteus mirabilis* meningitis in rabbits. *J. Infect. Dis.,* **1978,** 137:251–260.

Tai, P.C., Wallace, B.J., and Davis, B.D. Streptomycin causes misreading of natural messenger by interacting with ribosomes after initiation. *Proc. Natl Acad. Sci. U.S.A.,* **1978,** 75:275–279.

Theopold, H.M. Comparative surface studies of ototoxic effects of various aminoglycoside antibiotics on the organ of Corti in the guinea pig. A scanning electron microscopic study. *Acta Otolaryngol. (Stockh.),* **1977,** 84:57–64.

Tran Ba Huy, P., Meulemans, A., Wassef, M., Manuel, C., Sterkers, O., and Amiel, C. Gentamicin persistence in rat endolymph and perilymph after a two-day constant infusion. *Antimicrob. Agents Chemother.,* **1983,** 23:344–346.

Trestman, I., Parsons, J., Santoro, J., Goodhart, G., and Kaye, D. Pharmacology and efficacy of netilmicin. *Antimicrob. Agents Chemother.,* **1978,** 13:832–836.

Varese, L.A., Graziolo, F., Viretto, A., and Antoniola, P. Single-dose (bolus) therapy with gentamicin in management of urinary tract infection. *Int. J. Pediatr. Nephrol.,* **1980,** 1:104–105.

Vemuri, R.K., and Zervos, M.J. Enterococcal infections. The increasing threat of nosocomial spread and drug resistance. *Postgrad. Med J.,* **1993,** 93:121–124, 127–128.

Verpooten, G.A., Giuliano, R.A., Verbist, L., Eestermans, G., and De Broe, M.E. Once-daily dosing decreases renal accumulation of gentamicin and netilmicin. *Clin. Pharmacol. Ther.,* **1989,** 45: 22–27.

Wade, J.C., Smith, C.R., Petty, B.G., Lipsky, J.J., Conrad, G., Ellner, J., and Lietman, P.S. Cephalothin plus an aminoglycoside is more nephrotoxic than methicillin plus an aminoglycoside. *Lancet,* **1978,** 2:604–606.

Warkany, J. Antituberculous drugs. *Teratology,* **1979,** 20:133–138.

Wersäll, J., Bjorkroth, B., Flock, A., and Lundquist, P.G. Experiments on the ototoxic effects of antibiotics. *Adv. Otorhinolaryngol.,* **1973,** 20:14–41.

Wiedemann, B., and Atkinson, B.A. Susceptibility to antibiotics: species incidence and trends. In, *Antibiotics in Laboratory Medicine,* 3rd ed. (Lorian, V., ed.) Williams & Wilkins, Baltimore, **1991,** pp. 962–1208.

Wilson, P., and Ramsden, R.T. Immediate effects of tobramycin on human cochlea and correlation with serum tobramycin levels. *Br. Med. J.,* **1977,** *1:*259–261.

Wilson, W.R., Geraci, J.E., Wilkowske, C.J., and Washington, J.A. II. Short-term intramuscular therapy with procaine penicillin plus streptomycin for infective endocarditis due to viridans streptococci. *Circulation,* **1978,** *57:*1158–1161.

Wilson, W.R., Wilkowske, C.J., Wright, A.J., Sande, M.A., and Geraci, J.E. Treatment of streptomycin-susceptible and streptomycin-resistant enterococcal endocarditis. *Ann. Intern. Med.,* **1984,** *100:*816–823.

Wolfe, J.C., and Johnson, W.D. Penicillin-sensitive streptococcal endocarditis. *In vitro* and clinical observations on penicillin-streptomycin therapy. *Ann. Intern. Med.,* **1974,** *81:*178–181.

Wood, C.A., Kohlhepp, S.J., Kohnen, P.W., Houghton, D.C., and Gilbert, D.N. Vancomycin enhancement of experimental tobramycin nephrotoxicity. *Antimicrob. Agents Chemother.,* **1986,** *30:*20–24.

Yow, M.D. An overview of pediatric experience with amikacin. *Am. J. Med.,* **1977,** *62:*954–958.

MONOGRAPHS AND REVIEWS

Bryan, L.E. Cytoplasmic membrane transport and antimicrobial resistance. In, *Microbial Resistance to Drugs.* (Bryan, L.E., ed.) *Handbook of Experimental Pharmacology.* Vol. 91. Springer-Verlag, Berlin, **1989,** pp. 35–57.

Chambers, H.F., Hadley, W.K., and Jawetz, E. Aminoglycosides and spectinomycin. In, *Basic and Clinical Pharmacology,* 7th ed. (Katzung, B.G., ed.) Appleton & Lange, Stamford, CT, **1998,** pp. 752–760.

Davies, J. Inactivation of antibiotics and the dissemination of resistance genes. *Science,* **1994,** *264:*375–382.

Davis, B.B. The lethal action of aminoglycosides. *J. Antimicrob. Chemother.,* **1988,** *22:*1–3.

Gilbert, D.N. Once-daily aminoglycoside therapy. *Antimicrob. Agents Chemother.,* **1991,** *35:*399–405.

Gilbert, D.N., Moellering, R.C., Jr., and Sande, M.A. *The Sanford Guide to Antimicrobial Therapy 1999,* 29th ed. Antimicrobial Therapy Inc., Hyde Park, VT, **1999.**

Klastersky, J.A. Fever in the compromised host. In, *Internal Medicine,* 2nd ed. (Stein, J.H., ed.) Little, Brown & Co., Boston, **1987,** pp. 1467–1472.

McGee, Z.A., and Baringer, J.R. Acute meninigitis. In, *Principles and Practice of Infectious Diseases,* 3rd ed. (Mandell, G.L., Douglass, R.G., and Bennett, J.E., eds.) Churchill Livingstone, New York, **1990,** pp. 741–755.

Moellering, R.C. Jr. Microbiological considerations in the use of tobramycin and related aminoglycosidic aminocyclitol antibiotics. *Med. J. Aust.,* **1977,** *2*(suppl):4–8.

Murray, B.E. New aspects of antimicrobial resistance and the resulting therapeutic dilemmas. *J. Infect. Dis.,* **1991,** *163:*1184–1194.

Neu, H.C., and Bendush, C.L. Ototoxicity of tobramycin: a clinical overview. *J. Infect. Dis.,* **1976,** *134:*S206–S218.

Pittinger, C., and Adamson, R. Antibiotic blockade of neuromuscular function. *Annu. Rev. Pharmacol.,* **1972,** *12:*169–184.

Pittinger, C.B., Eryasa, Y., and Adamson, R. Antibiotic-induced paralysis. *Anesth. Analg.,* **1970,** *49:*487–501.

Shannon, K., and Phillips, I. Mechanisms of resistance to aminoglycosides in clinical isolates. *J. Antimicrob. Chemother.,* **1982,** *9:*91–102.

Silverblatt, F. Pathogenesis of nephrotoxicity of cephalosporins and aminoglycosides: a review of current concepts. *Rev. Infect. Dis.,* **1982,** *4:*S360–S365.

Sokoll, M.D., and Gergis, S.D. Antibiotics and neuromuscular function. *Anesthesiology,* **1981,** *55:*148–159.

Swan, S.K. Aminoglycoside nephrotoxicity. *Semin. Nephrol.,* **1997,** *17:*27–33.

Urban, A.W., and Craig, W.A. Daily dosage of aminoglycosides. *Curr. Clin. Top. Infect. Dis.,* **1997,** *17:*236–255.

Waksman, S.A. (ed.). *Streptomycin: Nature, and Practical Applications.* The Williams & Wilkins Co., Baltimore, **1949.**

ANTIMICROBIAL AGENTS
(*Continued*)

Protein Synthesis Inhibitors and
Miscellaneous Antibacterial Agents

Henry F. Chambers

The antimicrobial agents discussed in this chapter are: (1) bacteriostatic, protein-synthesis inhibitors that act principally by binding to ribosomes; (2) non-β-lactam inhibitors of cell-wall synthesis; or (3) a miscellaneous group of compounds acting by diverse mechanisms that have limited indications. Included within the first group are tetracyclines, chloramphenicol, macrolides, clindamycin, streptogramins, and linezolid. The tetracyclines are broad-spectrum antibiotics with activity against aerobic and anaerobic gram-positive and gram-negative organisms, rickettsiae, mycoplasmas, and chlamydiae. However, resistance to tetracyclines has reduced their clinical usefulness over the last decade. Chloramphenicol is recommended only for treatment of life-threatening infections (for example, bacterial meningitis when alternative drugs cannot be used, or rickettsial infections) because of its potential for causing aplastic anemia. The macrolides, erythromycin, clarithromycin, and azithromycin, are used primarily for treatment of respiratory tract infections because of their activity against Streptococcus pneumoniae *and agents of atypical pneumonia. Clarithromycin and azithromycin are effective for prophylaxis and treatment of nontuberculous mycobacterial infections. Clindamycin, a lincosamide antibiotic, exerts a potent bacteriostatic effect against streptococci, staphylococci, and anaerobic organisms, including* Bacteroides fragilis. *Clindamycin also has been found to be useful in the treatment of* Pneumocystis carinii *and* Toxoplasma gondii *infections. Quinupristin-dalfopristin is a streptogramin combination. It is a parenteral agent indicated for treatment of infections caused by multiple-drug-resistant gram-positive bacteria, particularly vancomycin-resistant strains of* Enterococcus faecium. *Linezolid is a member of the oxazolidinone class of compounds. It acts at an earlier step in protein synthesis than other inhibitors, and there is no cross resistance between it and other agents. It is active against vancomycin-resistant strains of enterococci and methicillin-resistant strains of* Staphylococcus aureus. *Vancomycin, the only glycopeptide antibiotic currently approved for use in the United States, is active against staphylococci (including all strains of* Staphylococcus aureus—*except those rare strains that exhibit intermediate susceptibility—and virtually all strains of coagulase-negative staphylococci), streptococci, and enterococci. Teicoplanin is available in Europe, but offers little advantage over vancomycin, except that it can be administered intramuscularly. Bacitracin is active against aerobic gram-positive bacteria and is used only in topical preparations because of nephrotoxicity with parenteral use. Spectinomycin, an aminocyclitol, is used exclusively for treatment of* Neisseria gonorrhoeae *in patients who have contraindications to first-line therapies. Polymyxin B, which is active against aerobic gram-negative bacilli, including* Pseudomonas aeruginosa, *is limited to use in ointments and irrigation solutions because of its extreme nephrotoxicity when administered systemically. These agents and issues related to their appropriate selection for therapy represent the focus of this chapter.*

TETRACYCLINES

History. Tetracycline antibiotics were discovered by systematic screening of soil specimens collected from many parts of the world for antibiotic-producing microorganisms. The first of these compounds, chlortetracycline, was introduced in 1948. Tetracyclines were found to be highly effective against rickettsiae, a number of gram-positive and gram-negative bacteria, and *Chlamydia,* and hence became known as "broad-spectrum" antibiotics. With establishment of their *in vitro* antimicrobial activity, effectiveness in experimental infections, and pharmacological properties, the tetracyclines rapidly became widely used in therapy.

Although there are specific and useful differences among the tetracyclines currently available in the United States, they are sufficiently similar to permit discussion as a group.

Source and Chemistry. *Chlortetracycline* and *oxytetracycline* are elaborated by *Streptomyces aureofaciens* and *Streptomyces rimosus,* respectively. *Tetracycline* is produced semisynthetically from chlortetracycline. *Demeclocycline* is the product of a mutant strain of *Strep. aureofaciens,* and *methacycline, doxycycline,* and *minocycline* are all semisynthetic derivatives.

The tetracyclines are close congeners of polycyclic naphthacenecarboxamide. Their structural formulas are shown in Table 47–1.

Effects on Microorganisms. The tetracyclines are active against a wide range of aerobic and anaerobic gram-positive and gram-negative bacteria. They also are effective against some microorganisms that are resistant to cell-wall-active antimicrobial agents, such as *Rickettsia, Coxiella burnetii, Mycoplasma pneumoniae, Chlamydia* spp., *Legionella* spp., *Ureaplasma,* some atypical mycobacteria, and *Plasmodium* spp. They are not active against fungi. Demeclocycline, tetracycline, oxytetracycline, minocycline, and doxycycline are available in the United States for systemic use. Chlortetracycline and oxytetracycline are used in ophthalmic preparations. Methacycline is not available. Other derivatives are available in other countries.

The more lipophilic drugs, minocycline and doxycycline, usually are the most active by weight, followed by tetracycline. Resistance of a bacterial strain to any one member of the class usually results in cross-resistance to other tetracyclines. Most bacterial strains that are inhibited by ≤ 4 μg/ml of tetracycline are considered sensitive. Exceptions to this minimal inhibitory concentration (MIC) are *Haemophilus influenzae* and *Streptococcus pneumoniae,* both of which are considered sensitive at ≤ 2 μg/ml, and *Neisseria gonorrhoeae,* considered sensitive at ≤ 0.25 μg/ml. Tetracyclines are bacteriostatic agents.

Bacteria. In general, tetracyclines are more active against gram-positive than gram-negative microorganisms. Problems of resistance and the availability of superior antimicrobial agents limit the use of tetracyclines for treatment of infections caused by many gram-positive bacteria. Most strains of enterococci are resistant to tetracycline; group B streptococci are 50% susceptible, and only 65% or less of *Staphylococcus aureus* remain susceptible (Standiford, 2000). Both tetracycline and doxycycline are quite active against most strains of *S. pneumoniae,* although penicillin-resistant strains also are often resistant to tetracyclines (Doern *et al.,* 1998).

Although the tetracyclines initially were useful for treatment of infections with aerobic gram-negative organisms, many Enterobacteriaceae are now relatively resistant. However, more than 90% of strains of *H. influenzae* still may be sensitive to doxycycline (Doern *et al.,*

Table 47–1

Structural Formulas of the Tetracyclines

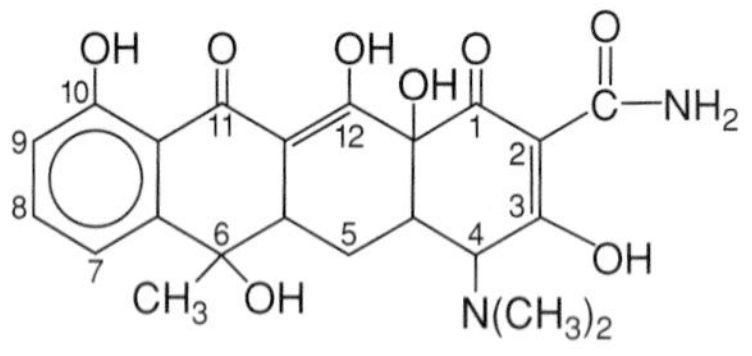

TETRACYCLINE

CONGENER	SUBSTITUENT(S)	POSITION(S)
Chlortetracycline	—Cl	(7)
Oxytetracycline	—OH,—H	(5)
Demeclocycline	—OH,—H; —Cl	(6; 7)
Methacycline	—OH,—H; ═CH$_2$	(5; 6)
Doxycycline	—OH,—H; —CH$_3$, —H	(5; 6)
Minocycline	—H,—H; —N(CH$_3$)$_2$	(6; 7)

1997). Although all strains of *Pseudomonas aeruginosa* are resistant, 90% of strains of *Pseudomonas pseudomallei* (the cause of melioidosis) are sensitive. Most strains of *Brucella* also are susceptible. Tetracyclines are particularly useful for infections caused by *Haemophilus ducreyi* (chancroid), *Brucella,* and *Vibrio cholerae.* These drugs also inhibit the growth of *Legionella pneumophila, Campylobacter jejuni, Helicobacter pylori, Yersinia pestis, Yersinia enterocolitica, Francisella tularensis,* and *Pasteurella multocida.* Strains of *N. gonorrhoeae* and *Neisseria meningitidis,* once uniformly susceptible to tetracycline, generally are resistant (Harnett *et al.,* 1997).

The tetracyclines are active against many anaerobic and facultative microorganisms, and their activity against *Actinomyces* is particularly relevant. The MIC breakpoint for susceptible anaerobic bacteria is 8 μg/ml. A variable number of anaerobes (*i.e., Bacteroides* spp.) are sensitive to doxycycline, the most active congener of tetracycline. However, doxycycline is much less active against *Bacteroides fragilis* than are chloramphenicol, clindamycin, metronidazole, and certain β-lactam antibiotics. Grampositive anaerobes also vary in sensitivity, with *Propionibacterium* the most susceptible and *Peptococcus* the least susceptible.

Rickettsiae. Like chloramphenicol, all of the tetracyclines are highly effective against the rickettsiae responsible for Rocky Mountain spotted fever, murine typhus, epidemic typhus, scrub typhus, rickettsialpox, and Q fever (*C. burnetii*).

Miscellaneous Microorganisms. The tetracyclines are active against many spirochetes, including *Borrelia recurrentis, Borrelia burgdorferi* (Lyme disease), *Treponema pallidum* (syphilis), and *Treponema pertenue.* The activity of tetracyclines against *Chlamydia* and *Mycoplasma* has become particularly important. Strains of *Mycobacterium marinum* also are susceptible.

Effects on Intestinal Flora. Many of the tetracyclines are incompletely absorbed from the gastrointestinal tract, such that high concentrations are reached in the bowel, and therefore the enteric flora is markedly altered. Many aerobic and anaerobic coliform microorganisms and grampositive spore-forming bacteria are sensitive and may be suppressed markedly during long-term tetracycline regimens before resistant strains reappear. The stools become softer and odorless and acquire a yellow-green color. However, as the fecal coliform count declines, overgrowth of tetracycline-resistant microorganisms occurs, particularly of yeasts (*Candida* spp.), enterococci, *Proteus,* and *Pseudomonas.* Tetracycline occasionally produces pseudomembranous colitis caused by toxin from *Clostridium difficile.*

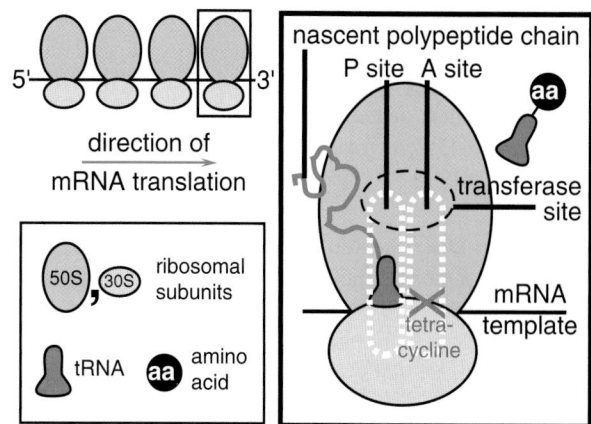

Figure 47–1. Inhibition of bacterial protein synthesis by tetracyclines.

Messenger RNA (mRNA) becomes attached to the 30 S subunit of bacterial ribosomal RNA. The P (peptidyl) site of the 50 S ribosomal RNA subunit contains the nascent polypeptide chain; normally, the aminoacyl tRNA charged with the next amino acid (aa) to be added to the chain moves into the A (acceptor) site, with complementary base pairing between the anticodon sequence of tRNA and the codon sequence of mRNA. Additional details of bacterial protein synthesis are given in Chapter 46. *Tetracyclines* inhibit bacterial protein synthesis by binding to the 30 S subunit, which blocks tRNA binding to the A site.

Mechanism of Action. Tetracyclines inhibit bacterial protein synthesis by binding to the 30 S bacterial ribosome and preventing access of aminoacyl tRNA to the acceptor (A) site on the mRNA-ribosome complex (*see* Figure 47–1). They enter gram-negative bacteria by passive diffusion through the hydrophilic channels formed by the porin proteins of the outer cell membrane, and active transport by an energy-dependent system that pumps all tetracyclines across cytoplasmic membrane. Although permeation of these drugs into gram-positive bacteria is less well understood, it also is energy requiring.

At high concentrations, these compounds impair protein synthesis in mammalian cells. However, because mammalian cells lack the active transport system found in bacteria, and the ribosomal target is less sensitive, tetracyclines are selectively active against bacteria.

Resistance to the Tetracyclines. Microorganisms that have become resistant to one tetracycline frequently are resistant to the others. Resistance to the tetracyclines in *Escherichia coli* and probably in other bacterial species is primarily plasmid-mediated and is an inducible trait. The three main resistance mechanisms are: (1) decreased accumulation of tetracycline as a result of either decreased antibiotic influx or acquisition of an energy-dependent efflux pathway; (2) decreased access of tetracycline to the ribosome because of the presence of ribosome protection proteins; and (3) enzymatic inactivation of tetracyclines (Speer *et al.,* 1992).

Absorption, Distribution, and Excretion. *Absorption.* Absorption of most tetracyclines from the gastrointestinal tract is incomplete. The percentage of an oral dose that is absorbed (when the stomach is empty) is lowest for chlortetracycline (30%); intermediate for oxytetracycline, demeclocycline, and tetracycline (60% to 80%); and high for doxycycline (95%) and minocycline (100%) (Barza and Scheife, 1977). The percentage of unabsorbed drug rises as the dose increases. Most absorption takes place from the stomach and upper small intestine and is greater in the fasting state. Absorption of tetracyclines is impaired by the concurrent ingestion of dairy products; aluminum hydroxide gels; calcium, magnesium, and iron or zinc salts; and bismuth subsalicylate. The mechanism responsible for the decreased absorption appears to be chelation of divalent and trivalent cations.

The wide range of plasma concentrations present in different individuals following the oral administration of the various tetracyclines is related to the variability of their absorption. These drugs can be divided into three groups based on the dosage and frequency of oral administration required to produce effective plasma concentrations.

Oxytetracycline and tetracycline are incompletely absorbed. After a single oral dose, the peak plasma concentration is attained in 2 to 4 hours. These drugs have half-lives in the range of 6 to 12 hours and are frequently administered two to four times daily. The administration of 250 mg every 6 hours produces peak plasma concentrations of 2 to 2.5 μg/ml. Increasing the dosage above 1 g every 6 hours does not produce significantly higher plasma concentrations.

Demeclocycline, which also is incompletely absorbed, usually is administered in lower daily dosages than are the above-mentioned congeners, because its half-life of about 16 hours permits effective plasma concentrations lasting for 24 to 48 hours.

Doxycycline and minocycline should be administered in even lower daily dosages by the oral route, since their half-lives are long (16 to 18 hours) and they are better absorbed (90% to 100%) than tetracycline, oxytetracycline, or demeclocycline. After an oral dose of 200 mg of doxycycline, a maximum plasma concentration of 3 μg/ml is achieved at 2 hours, and the plasma concentration is maintained above 1 μg/ml for 8 to 12 hours. Plasma concentrations are equivalent when doxycycline is given by the oral or parenteral route. Food does not interfere with the absorption of doxycycline or minocycline.

Distribution. Tetracyclines distribute widely throughout the body and into tissues and secretions, including the urine and prostate. They accumulate in the reticuloen-

dothelial cells of the liver, spleen, and bone marrow, and in bone, dentine, and the enamel of unerupted teeth (*see* below).

Inflammation of the meninges is not a prerequisite for the passage of tetracyclines into the cerebrospinal fluid (CSF). Penetration of these drugs into most other fluids and tissues is excellent. Concentrations in synovial fluid and the mucosa of the maxillary sinus approach that in plasma. Tetracyclines cross the placenta and enter the fetal circulation and amniotic fluid. Concentrations of tetracycline in umbilical-cord plasma reach 60%, and in amniotic fluid 20%, of those in the circulation of the mother. Relatively high concentrations of these drugs also are found in breast milk.

Excretion. The primary route of elimination for most tetracyclines is the kidney (doxycycline being an important exception), although they are also concentrated in the liver and excreted by way of the bile into the intestines, where they are partially reabsorbed *via* enterohepatic recirculation. Elimination *via* the intestinal tract occurs even when the drugs are given parenterally, as a result of excretion into the bile. Minocycline is an exception and is significantly metabolized by the liver.

Since renal clearance of these drugs is by glomerular filtration, their excretion is significantly affected by the renal function status of the patient (*see* below). From 20% to 60% of an intravenous 0.5-g dose of tetracycline is excreted in the urine during the first 24 hours; from 20% to 55% of an oral dose is excreted by this route. Approximately 10% to 35% of a dose of oxytetracycline is excreted in active form in the urine, in which it is detectable within 30 minutes and reaches a peak concentration about 5 hours after it is administered. The rate of renal clearance of demeclocycline is less than half that of tetracycline. About 50% of methacycline is excreted unchanged in the urine. Decreased hepatic function or obstruction of the common bile duct reduces the biliary excretion of these agents, resulting in longer half-lives and higher plasma concentrations. Because of their enterohepatic circulation, the tetracyclines may be present in the body for a long time after cessation of therapy.

Minocycline is recoverable from both urine and feces in significantly lower amounts than are the other tetracyclines, and it appears to be metabolized to a considerable extent. Renal clearance of minocycline is low. The drug persists in the body after its administration is stopped; this may be due to retention in fatty tissues. The half-life of minocycline is not prolonged in patients with hepatic failure.

With conventional doses, doxycycline is not eliminated *via* the same pathways as are other tetracyclines, and it does not accumulate significantly in patients with renal failure. It is thus one of the safest of the tetracyclines for the treatment of extrarenal infections in such individuals. The drug is excreted in the feces, largely as an inactive conjugate or perhaps as a chelate; for this reason it has less impact on the intestinal microflora (Nord and Heimdahl, 1988). The half-life of doxycycline may be shortened from approximately 16 to 7 hours in patients who are receiving long-term treatment with barbiturates or phenytoin.

Routes of Administration and Dosage. The tetracyclines are available in a wide variety of forms for oral, parenteral, and topical administration. As indicated earlier, only tetracycline (ACHROMYCIN, others), oxytetracycline (TERRAMYCIN, others), demeclocycline (DECLOMYCIN), minocycline (MINOCIN, others), doxycycline (VIBRAMYCIN, others), and chlortetracycline (AUREOMYCIN) are available in the United States.

Oral Administration. The appropriate oral dose of the tetracyclines varies with the nature and the severity of the infection being treated. For tetracycline, it ranges from 1 to 2 g per day in adults. Children over 8 years of age should receive 25 to 50 mg/kg daily in two to four divided doses. The recommended dose of demeclocycline is somewhat lower, being 150 mg every 6 hours or 300 mg every 12 hours for adults. The daily dose for children over 8 years of age is 6 to 12 mg/kg in two to four divided portions. Demeclocycline, however, is rarely used as an antimicrobial agent because of its higher risks of photosensitivity reactions and diabetes insipidus syndrome (*see* below). The dose of doxycycline for adults is 100 mg every 12 hours during the first 24 hours, followed by 100 mg once a day, or twice daily when severe infection is present. Children over 8 years of age should receive doxycycline, 4 to 5 mg/kg per day, divided into two equal doses given every 12 hours the first day, after which half this amount (2 to 2.5 mg/kg) should be given as a single daily dose. In serious disease, the 2 to 2.5 mg/kg dose is given every 12 hours. The dose of minocycline for adults is 200 mg initially, followed by 100 mg every 12 hours; for children it is 4 mg/kg initially, followed by 2 mg/kg every 12 hours.

Gastrointestinal distress, nausea, and vomiting can be minimized by administration of the tetracyclines with food (but not dairy products). Dairy products; antacids containing calcium, aluminum, zinc, magnesium, or silicate; vitamins with iron; sulcralfate (which contains aluminum); and bismuth subsalicylate will chelate and therefore interfere with the absorption of tetracyclines and should not be ingested at the same time. Cholestyramine and colestipol also bind orally administered tetracyclines and interfere with their absorption.

Parenteral Administration. Doxycycline is the preferred parenteral tetracycline in the United States. It is used in severe illness, in patients unable to ingest medication, or when the drug causes significant nausea and vomiting if given orally. Because of local irritation and poor absorption, intramuscular administration of these tetracyclines is generally unsatisfactory and is not recommended.

The usual intravenous dose of doxycycline is 200 mg in one or two infusions on the first day and 100 to 200 mg on subsequent days. The dose for children who weigh less than 45 kg is 4.4 mg/kg on the first day, after which it is reduced correspondingly. The total daily dose of intravenous tetracycline (where available) for most acute infections is 500 mg to 1 g, usually administered in equally divided doses at 6-hour or 12-hour intervals. Up to 2 g per day may be given in severe infections. This dose should not be exceeded and may cause difficulty in some patients (*see* "Toxic Effects," below). Parenteral preparations of tetracycline no longer are available in the United States. The intravenous dose of minocycline for adults is 200 mg, followed by 100 mg every 12 hours. Children over 8 years of age should receive an initial dose of 4 mg/kg, followed by 2 mg/kg every 12 hours. Each 100 mg of minocycline must be diluted with 500 ml to 1 liter of compatible fluid and is slowly administered over 6 hours to minimize toxicity.

Local Application. Except for local use in the eye, topical use of the tetracyclines is not recommended. Ophthalmic preparations include *chlortetracycline hydrochloride, tetracycline hydrochloride,* and *oxytetracycline hydrochloride;* they are available as ophthalmic ointments or suspensions. Their use in ophthalmic therapy is discussed in Chapter 66.

Therapeutic Uses. The tetracyclines have been used extensively both for the treatment of infectious diseases and as an additive to animal feeds to facilitate growth. Both uses have resulted in dramatically increased bacterial resistance to these drugs, and their use has declined. Tetracyclines are especially useful in diseases caused by rickettsiae, mycoplasmas, and chlamydiae. The status of the tetracyclines for the therapy of various infections is given in Table 43–1.

Rickettsial Infections. The tetracyclines and chloramphenicol are effective and may be life-saving in rickettsial infections, including Rocky Mountain spotted fever, recrudescent epidemic typhus (Brill's disease), murine typhus, scrub typhus, rickettsialpox, and Q fever. Clinical improvement often is evident within 24 hours after initiation of therapy.

Mycoplasma Infections. *Mycoplasma pneumoniae* is sensitive to the tetracyclines. Treatment of pneumonia with either tetracycline or erythromycin results in a shorter duration of fever, cough, malaise, fatigue, pulmonary rales, and radiological changes in the lungs. Mycoplasma may persist in the sputum following cessation of therapy, despite rapid resolution of the active infection.

Chlamydia. *Lymphogranuloma Venereum.* Doxycycline (100 mg twice daily for 21 days) is first-line therapy for treatment of this infection (Prevention, 1998). Decided reduction in the size of buboes occurs within 4 days, and inclusion and elementary bodies entirely disappear from the lymph nodes within 1 week. Lymphogranulomatous proctitis is improved promptly. Rectal pain, discharge, and bleeding are decreased markedly. When relapses occur, treatment is resumed with full doses and is continued for longer periods.

Pneumonia, bronchitis, or sinusitis caused by *Chlamydia pneumoniae* responds to tetracycline therapy. The tetracyclines also are of value in cases of psittacosis. Drug therapy for 10 to 14 days usually is adequate.

Trachoma. Doxycycline (100 mg twice daily for 14 days) or tetracycline (250 mg four times daily for 14 days) is effective for this infection. However, this disease is important in early childhood, and tetracyclines therefore often are contraindicated (*see* "Untoward Effects," below). Azithromycin (*see* section on macrolides), which is effective as a single dose, is preferred.

Nonspecific Urethritis. Nonspecific urethritis is often due to *Chlamydia trachomatis.* One hundred mg of doxycycline every 12 hours for 7 days is effective, although azithromycin, which can be given as a single 1-g dose, is preferred because of improved compliance.

Sexually Transmitted Diseases. Tetracyclines have been effective for uncomplicated gonococcal infections. Doxycycline (100 mg twice daily for 7 days) is still recommended for treatment of gonorrhea, although cefixime, ceftriaxone (*see* Chapter 45), or a fluoroquinolone (*see* Chapter 44), each of which is effective as a single dose, is preferred (Centers for Disease Control and Prevention, 1998). Because coinfection with *N. gonorrhoeae* and *C. trachomatis* is common, doxycycline or azithromycin should be administered empirically in addition to one of these other agents when treating gonorrhea.

C. trachomatis often is a coexistent pathogen in acute pelvic inflammatory disease, including endometritis, salpingitis, parametritis, and/or peritonitis (Walker *et al.,* 1993). Doxycycline, 100 mg intravenously twice daily, is recommended for at least 48 hours after substantial clinical improvement, followed by oral therapy at the same dosage to complete a 14-day course. Doxycycline usually is combined with cefoxitin or cefotetan (*see* Chapter 45) to cover anaerobes and facultative aerobes.

Acute epididymitis is caused by infection with *C. trachomatis* or *N. gonorrhoeae* in men less than 35 years of age. Effective regimens include a single injection of cef-

triaxone (250 mg) plus doxycycline, 100 mg orally twice daily for 10 days. Sexual partners of patients with any of the above conditions should also be treated.

Nonpregnant, penicillin-allergic patients who have primary, secondary, or latent syphilis can be treated with a tetracycline regimen such as doxycycline 100 mg orally twice daily for 2 weeks (Centers for Disease Control and Prevention, 1998). Tetracyclines should not be used for treatment of neurosyphilis.

Bacillary Infections. *Brucellosis.* Tetracyclines are effective for acute and chronic infections caused by *Brucella melitensis, Brucella suis,* and *Brucella abortus.* Combination therapy with doxycycline, 200 mg per day, plus rifampin (*see* Chapter 48), 600 to 900 mg daily for 6 weeks, is recommended by the World Health Organization for the treatment of acute brucellosis (World Health Organization, 1986). Relapses usually respond to a second course of therapy. The combination of doxycycline given with streptomycin (1 g daily, intramuscularly) also is effective and may be more efficacious than doxycycline-rifampin in patients with spondylitis (Ariza *et al.,* 1992).

Tularemia. Although streptomycin (*see* Chapter 48) is preferable, treatment with the tetracyclines also produces prompt results in tularemia. Both the ulceroglandular and typhoidal types of the disease respond well. Fever, toxemia, and clinical signs and symptoms all are improved.

Cholera. Doxycycline (300 mg as a single dose) is effective in reducing stool volume and eradicating *Vibrio cholerae* from the stool within 48 hours. Antimicrobial agents, however, are not substitutes for fluid and electrolyte replacement in this disease. In addition, some strains of *V. cholerae* are resistant to tetracyclines (Khan *et al.,* 1996).

Other Bacillary Infections. Therapy with the tetracyclines is often ineffective in infections caused by *Shigella, Salmonella,* or other Enterobacteriaceae because of a high prevalence of drug-resistant strains in many areas. Doxycycline has been used successfully to reduce the incidence of travelers' diarrhea, but a high prevalence of resistance in enteric bacteria limits the usefulness of the drug for this indication.

Coccal Infections. Because of the emergence of resistance, the tetracyclines are no longer indicated for infections caused by staphylococci, streptococci, or meningococci. Approximately 85% of strains of *S. pneumoniae* are susceptible to tetracyclines. Doxycycline remains an effective agent for empirical therapy of community-acquired pneumonia (Ailani *et al.,* 1999; Bartlett *et al.,* 1998).

Urinary Tract Infections. Tetracyclines are no longer recommended for routine treatment of urinary tract infections, because many enteric organisms, including *E. coli,* that cause these infections are resistant.

Other Infections. Actinomycosis, although most responsive to penicillin G, may be successfully treated with a tetracycline. Minocycline has been suggested as an alternative for the treatment of nocardiosis, but a sulfonamide should be used concurrently. Yaws and relapsing fever respond favorably to the tetracyclines. Tetracyclines have been shown to be useful in the acute treatment and for prophylaxis of leptospirosis (*Leptospira* spp.). *Borrelia* spp., including *B. recurrentis* (relapsing fever) and *B. burgdorferi* (Lyme disease), respond to therapy with a tetracycline. The tetracyclines have been used to treat atypical mycobacterial pathogens when susceptible, including *M. marinum.*

Acne. Tetracyclines have been used for the treatment of acne. These drugs may act by inhibiting propionibacteria, which reside in sebaceous follicles and metabolize lipids into irritating free fatty acids. Tetracycline seems to be associated with few side effects when given in relatively low doses of 250 mg orally twice a day.

Untoward Effects. *Toxic Effects.* *Gastrointestinal.* The tetracyclines all produce gastrointestinal irritation to varying degrees in some but not all individuals; such effects are more common after oral administration of the drugs. Epigastric burning and distress, abdominal discomfort, nausea, and vomiting may occur. Gastric distress can be reduced by administering the drug with food, but tetracyclines should not be taken with dairy products. Esophagitis and esophageal ulcers have been reported (Winckler, 1981; Amendola and Spera, 1985), as has an association with pancreatitis (Elmore and Rogge, 1981). Diarrhea also may result from the irritative effects of the tetracyclines given orally. *Pseudomembranous colitis caused by overgrowth of* Clostridium difficile *is a potentially life-threatening complication (see* below).

Photosensitivity. Demeclocycline, doxycycline, and, to a lesser extent, other derivatives may produce mild to severe photosensitivity reactions in the skin of treated individuals exposed to sunlight. Onycholysis and pigmentation of the nails may develop with or without accompanying photosensitivity.

Hepatic Toxicity. Oxytetracycline and tetracycline appear to be the least hepatotoxic of these agents. Most hepatic toxicity develops in patients receiving 2 g or more of drug per day parenterally; however, this effect also may occur when large quantities are administered orally. Pregnant women appear to be particularly susceptible to severe tetracycline-induced hepatic damage. Jaundice appears first, and azotemia, acidosis, and irreversible shock may follow.

Renal Toxicity. Tetracyclines may aggravate uremia in patients with renal disease by inhibiting protein synthesis and provoking a catabolic effect. Doxycycline has fewer renal side effects than do other tetracyclines. Nephrogenic diabetes insipidus has been observed in some patients receiving demeclocycline, and this phenomenon has been exploited for the treatment of chronic inappropriate secretion of antidiuretic hormone (*see* Chapter 30).

A clinical syndrome characterized by nausea, vomiting, polyuria, polydipsia, proteinuria, acidosis, glycosuria, and gross aminoaciduria—a form of the Fanconi syndrome—has been observed in patients ingesting outdated and degraded tetracycline. It results from a toxic effect on proximal renal tubules.

Effects on Teeth. Children receiving long- or short-term therapy with a tetracycline may develop brown discoloration of the teeth. The larger the dose of drug relative to body weight, the more intense the discoloration of enamel. This discoloration is permanent. The duration of therapy appears to be less important than the total quantity of antibiotic administered. The risk of this untoward effect is highest when the tetracycline is given to neonates and babies prior to the first dentition. However, pigmentation of the permanent dentition may develop if the drug is given between the ages of 2 months and 5 years, when these teeth are being calcified. The deposition of the drug in the teeth and bones probably is due to its chelating property and the formation of a tetracycline–calcium orthophosphate complex.

Treatment of pregnant patients with tetracyclines may produce discoloration of the teeth in their children. The period of greatest danger to the teeth is from midpregnancy to about 4 to 6 months of the postnatal period for the deciduous anterior teeth, and from a few months to 5 years of age for the permanent anterior teeth, the periods when the crowns of the teeth are being formed. However, children up to 8 years old may be susceptible to this complication of tetracycline therapy.

Miscellaneous Effects. Tetracyclines are deposited in the skeleton during gestation and throughout childhood. A 40% depression of bone growth, as determined by measurement of fibulas, has been demonstrated in premature infants treated with these agents (Cohlan *et al.,* 1963). This depression is readily reversible if the period of exposure to the drug is short.

Thrombophlebitis frequently follows intravenous administration, especially when a single vein is used for repeated infusion. This irritative effect of tetracyclines has been used therapeutically in patients with malignant pleural effusions, where drug is instilled into the pleural space.

Long-term therapy with tetracyclines may produce changes in the peripheral blood. Leukocytosis, atypical lymphocytes, toxic granulation of granulocytes, and thrombocytopenic purpura have been observed.

The tetracyclines may cause increased intracranial pressure and tense bulging of the fontanels (pseudotumor cerebri) in young infants, even when given in the usual therapeutic doses. Except for the elevated pressure, the spinal fluid is normal. Discontinuation of therapy results in prompt return of the pressure to normal. This complication may occur rarely in older individuals (Walters and Gubbay, 1981).

Patients receiving minocycline may experience vestibular toxicity, manifested by dizziness, ataxia, nausea, and vomiting. The symptoms occur soon after the initial dose and generally disappear within 24 to 48 hours after drug administration is stopped. The frequency of this side effect is directly related to the dose, and the effect has been noted more often in women than in men (Fanning *et al.*, 1977).

Hypersensitivity Reactions.   Various skin reactions, including morbilliform rashes, urticaria, fixed drug eruptions, and generalized exfoliative dermatitis, may follow the use of any of the tetracyclines, but they are rare. Among the more severe allergic responses are angioedema and anaphylaxis; anaphylactoid reactions can occur even after the oral use of these agents. Other effects that have been attributed to hypersensitivity are burning of the eyes, cheilosis, atrophic or hypertrophic glossitis, pruritus ani or vulvae, and vaginitis; these effects often persist for weeks or months after cessation of tetracycline therapy. The exact cause of these reactions is unknown. Fever of varying degrees and eosinophilia may occur when these agents are administered. Asthma also has been observed. Cross-sensitization among the various tetracyclines is common.

Biological Effects Other Than Allergic or Toxic.   Like all antimicrobial agents, the tetracyclines administered orally or parenterally may lead to the development of superinfections caused by strains of bacteria or yeasts resistant to these agents. Vaginal, oral, and even systemic infections with yeasts and fungi are observed. The incidence of these infections appears to be much higher with the tetracyclines than with the penicillins.

Pseudomembranous colitis, due to an overgrowth of toxin-producing *C. difficile,* is characterized by severe diarrhea, fever, and stools containing shreds of mucous membrane and a large number of neutrophils. The toxin is cytotoxic to mucosal cells and causes shallow ulcerations that can be seen by sigmoidoscopy. Discontinuation of the drug, combined with the oral administration of metronidazole, usually is curative.

To decrease the incidence of toxic effects, the following precautions should be observed in the use of the tetracyclines. They should not be given to pregnant patients; they should not be employed for treatment of common infections in children under the age of 8 years; and unused supplies of these antibiotics should be discarded.

CHLORAMPHENICOL

History and Source.   *Chloramphenicol* is an antibiotic produced by *Streptomyces venezuelae,* an organism first isolated in 1947 from a soil sample collected in Venezuela (Bartz, 1948). When the relatively simple structure of the crystalline material was determined, the antibiotic was prepared synthetically. Late in 1947, the small amount of available chloramphenicol was employed to treat an outbreak of epidemic typhus in Bolivia, with dramatic results. It was then tried with excellent success in

cases of scrub typhus on the Malay peninsula. By 1948, chloramphenicol was available for general clinical use. By 1950, however, it became evident that the drug could cause serious and fatal blood dyscrasias. For this reason, use of the drug is reserved for patients with serious infections, such as meningitis, typhus, and typhoid fever, who cannot take safer alternatives because of resistance or allergies. It also is an effective therapy for Rocky Mountain spotted fever.

Chemistry.   Chloramphenicol has the following structural formula:

$$O_2N-\bigcirc-\underset{\underset{\text{CHORAMPHENICOL}}{}}{\overset{\overset{\displaystyle OH}{|}}{CHCH}}-\overset{\overset{\displaystyle CH_2OH}{|}}{}NH-\overset{\overset{\displaystyle O}{\parallel}}{C}-CHCl_2$$

CHLORAMPHENICOL

The antibiotic is unique among natural compounds in that it contains a nitrobenzene moiety and is a derivative of dichloroacetic acid. The biologically active form is levorotatory.

Mechanism of Action.   Chloramphenicol inhibits protein synthesis in bacteria and, to a lesser extent, in eukaryotic cells. The drug readily penetrates bacterial cells, probably by facilitated diffusion. Chloramphenicol acts primarily by binding reversibly to the 50 S ribosomal subunit (near the site of action of the macrolide antibiotics and clindamycin, which it inhibits competitively). Although binding of tRNA at the codon recognition site on the 30 S ribosomal subunit is thus undisturbed, the drug appears to prevent the binding of the amino acid–containing end of the aminoacyl tRNA to the acceptor site on the 50 S ribosomal subunit. The interaction between peptidyltransferase and its amino acid substrate cannot occur, and peptide bond formation is inhibited (*see* Figure 47–2).

Chloramphenicol also can inhibit mitochondrial protein synthesis in mammalian cells, perhaps because mitochondrial ribosomes resemble bacterial ribosomes (both are 70 S) more than they do the 80 S cytoplasmic ribosomes of mammalian cells. The peptidyltransferase of mitochondrial ribosomes, but not cytoplasmic ribosomes, is susceptible to the inhibitory action of chloramphenicol. Mammalian erythropoietic cells seem to be particularly sensitive to the drug.

Antimicrobial Actions.   Chloramphenicol possesses a wide spectrum of antimicrobial activity. Strains are considered sensitive if they are inhibited by concentrations of 8 μg/ml or less, except *N. gonorrhoeae, S. pneumoniae,* and *H. influenzae,* which have lower MIC breakpoints. Chloramphenicol is primarily bacteriostatic, although it may be bactericidal to certain species, such as *H. influenzae, N. meningitidis,* and *S. pneumoniae.* More than 95% of strains of the following

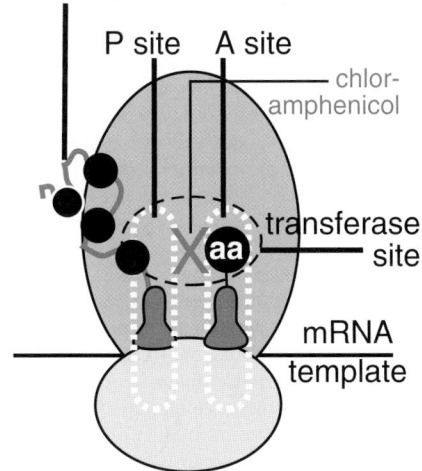

nascent polypeptide chain

Figure 47–2. Mechanism of inhibition of bacterial protein synthesis by chloramphenicol.

Chloramphenicol binds to the 50 S ribosomal subunit at the peptidyltransferase site and inhibits the transpeptidation reaction. Chloramphenicol binds to the 50 S ribosomal subunit near the site of action of clindamycin and the macrolide antibiotics. These agents interfere with the binding of chloramphenicol and thus may interfere with each other's actions if given concurrently. *See* Figure 47–1 and its legend for additional information.

gram-negative bacteria are inhibited *in vitro* by 8.0 μg/ml or less of chloramphenicol: *H. influenzae, N. meningitidis, N. gonorrhoeae, Brucella* spp., and *Bordetella pertussis.* Likewise, most anaerobic bacteria, including gram-positive cocci and *Clostridium* spp., and gram-negative rods including *B. fragilis,* are inhibited by this concentration of the drug. Some aerobic gram-positive cocci, including *Streptococcus pyogenes, Streptococcus agalactiae* (group B streptococci) and *S. pneumoniae,* are sensitive to 8 μg/ml. Strains of *S. aureus* tend to be less susceptible, with MICs greater than 8 μg/ml (Standiford, 2000). Chloramphenicol is active against *Mycoplasma, Chlamydia,* and *Rickettsia.*

The Enterobacteriaceae have a variable sensitivity to chloramphenicol. Most strains of *E. coli* (75% or more) and *Klebsiella pneumoniae* are susceptible. Approximately 50% of strains of *Proteus mirabilis* and indole-positive *Proteus* spp. are susceptible (Standiford, 2000). *P. aeruginosa* is resistant to even very high concentrations of chloramphenicol. Strains of *V. cholerae* have remained largely susceptible to chloramphenicol. Strains of *Shigella* and *Salmonella* resistant to multiple drugs, including chloramphenicol, are on the rise (Prats *et al.,* 2000; Replogle *et al.,* 2000). Of special concern is the increasing prevalence of multiple-drug-resistant strains of *Salmonella* serotype typhi, particularly for strains acquired outside the United States (Prats *et al.,* 2000; Ackers *et al.,* 2000).

Resistance to Chloramphenicol.   Resistance to chloramphenicol usually is caused by a plasmid-encoded acetyltransferase that inactivates the drug. At least three types of enzyme have been characterized (Gaffney and Foster, 1978). Acetylated derivatives of chloramphenicol fail to bind to bacterial ribosomes. Plasmid-mediated resistance to chloramphenicol in *Salmonella* serotype typhi first emerged as a significant problem during the epidemic of 1972 through 1973 in Mexico and the United States (Baine *et al.,* 1977). The prevalence of chloramphenicol acetyltransferase-mediated resistance of staphylococci has increased. It varies from one hospital to another and is as high as 50% or more in some, with the high frequency found in methicillin-resistant stains of staphylocci. Although resistance to chloramphenicol usually is due to acetylation of the drug, both decreased permeability of the microorganisms (which has been found in *E. coli* and *Pseudomonas*) and mutation to ribosomal insensitivity also have been described.

Absorption, Distribution, Fate, and Excretion.   Chloramphenicol (CHLOROMYCETIN) has been available for oral administration in two forms: the active drug itself and the inactive prodrug, chloramphenicol palmitate (which was used to prepare an oral suspension). The palmitate form no longer is available in the United States. Chloramphenicol is absorbed rapidly from the gastrointestinal tract, and peak concentrations of 10 to 13 μg/ml occur within 2 to 3 hours after the administration of a 1-g dose.

The preparation of chloramphenicol for parenteral use is the water-soluble, inactive prodrug sodium succinate preparation (*chloramphenicol succinate*). Similar concentrations of chloramphenicol succinate in plasma are achieved after intravenous and intramuscular administration (Shann *et al.,* 1985). It is unclear where the hydrolysis of chloramphenicol succinate occurs *in vivo,* but esterases of the liver, kidneys, and lungs all may be involved. Chloramphenicol succinate itself is rapidly cleared from plasma by the kidneys. This renal clearance of the prodrug may affect the overall bioavailability of chloramphenicol, because up to 20% to 30% of the dose may be excreted prior to hydrolysis. Poor renal function in the neonate and other states of renal insufficiency result in increased plasma concentrations of chloramphenicol succinate and of chloramphenicol (Slaughter *et al.,* 1980; Mulhall *et al.,* 1983). Decreased esterase activity has been observed in the plasma of neonates and infants. This results in a prolonged period to reach peak concentrations of active chloramphenicol (up to 4 hours) and a longer period over which renal clearance of chloramphenicol succinate can occur.

Chloramphenicol is well distributed in body fluids and readily reaches therapeutic concentrations in CSF, where values are approximately 60% of those in plasma (range, 45% to 99%) in the presence or absence of meningitis (Friedman *et al.,* 1979). The drug actually may accumulate in brain tissue (Kramer *et al.,* 1969). Chloramphenicol is present in bile, is secreted into milk, and readily traverses the placental barrier. It also penetrates into the aqueous humor after subconjunctival injection.

The major route of elimination of chloramphenicol is hepatic metabolism to the inactive glucuronide. This metabolite, as well as chloramphenicol itself, is excreted in the urine by filtration and secretion. Over a 24-hour period, 75% to 90% of an orally administered dose is so excreted; about 5% to 10% is in the biologically active form. Patients with hepatic cirrhosis or otherwise impaired hepatic function have decreased metabolic clearance, and dosage should be adjusted in these individuals.

The half-life of chloramphenicol has been correlated with plasma bilirubin concentrations (Koup *et al.*, 1979). About 50% of chloramphenicol is bound to plasma proteins; such binding is reduced in cirrhotic patients and in neonates. The half-life of the active drug (4 hours) is not altered significantly by renal insufficiency, and dosage adjustment is not required. The extent to which hemodialysis removes chloramphenicol from plasma does not appear to warrant adjustment of dosage. However, if the dose of chloramphenicol has been reduced because of cirrhosis, clearance in the patient receiving hemodialysis may be significant. This effect can be avoided by administering the maintenance dosing at the end of hemodialysis. The variability in the metabolism and pharmacokinetic parameters of chloramphenicol in neonates, infants, and children necessitates monitoring of drug concentrations in plasma, especially when an agent that enhances its metabolism (*e.g.*, phenobarbital, phenytoin, or rifampin) is administered concomitantly (McCracken *et al.*, 1987).

Therapeutic Uses. *Therapy with chloramphenicol must be limited to infections for which the benefits of the drug outweigh the risks of the potential toxicities. When other antimicrobial drugs are available that are equally effective and potentially less toxic than chloramphenicol, they should be used* (Standiford, 2000).

Typhoid Fever. Although chloramphenicol is an important drug for the treatment of typhoid fever and other types of systemic salmonella infections, other, safer drugs are available. Also, infections and epidemics in developing countries have been due to strains of *Salmonella* serotype typhi highly resistant to chloramphenicol (Miller *et al.*, 1995; Ackers, 2000). Third-generation cephalosporins and quinolones are drugs of choice for the treatment of this disease.

The adult dose of chloramphenicol for typhoid fever is 1 g every 6 hours for 4 weeks. Although both intravenous and oral routes have been used, the response is more rapid with oral administration. Relapses usually respond satisfactorily to retreatment; microorganisms isolated during recurrences are usually still sensitive to the antibiotic *in vitro*.

Bacterial Meningitis. Treatment with chloramphenicol produces excellent results in *H. influenzae* meningitis, equal to or better than those achieved with ampicillin (Jones and Hanson, 1977; Koskiniemi *et al.*, 1978). Although chloramphenicol is bacteriostatic against most microorganisms, it is bactericidal for many meningeal pathogens, such as *H. influenzae* (Rahal and Simberkoff, 1979). The total daily dose for children should be 50 to 75 mg per kilogram of body weight, divided into four equal doses given intravenously every 6 hours for 2 weeks. However, third-generation cephalosporins are less toxic and have replaced chloramphenicol as initial therapy for meningitis when *H. influenzae* is suspected. Chloramphenicol remains an alternative drug for the treatment of meningitis caused by *N. meningitidis* and *S. pneumoniae* in patients who have severe allergy to β-lactams. Third-generation cephalosporins also are efficacious, and they are preferred to chloramphenicol for this indication as well (*see* Chapter 45). Results with chloramphenicol used for meningitis caused by *S. pneumoniae* frequently are unsatisfactory, because some strains are inhibited but not killed. Moreover, penicillin-resistant strains frequently also are resistant to chloramphenicol. In the rare situation in which chloramphenicol must be used, lumbar puncture should be repeated 2 to 3 days after treatment has been initiated to ensure that an adequate response has occurred (Scheld *et al.*, 1979). Higher doses of chloramphenicol (100 mg/kg per day) may be required in some instances.

Anaerobic Infections. Chloramphenicol is quite effective against most anaerobic bacteria, including *Bacteroides* spp. It is effective for treatment of serious intraabdominal infections or brain abscesses, both of which are commonly caused by anaerobes. However, numerous equally effective and less toxic alternatives are available, and chloramphenicol is rarely indicated.

Rickettsial Diseases. The tetracyclines usually are the preferred agents for the treatment of rickettsial diseases. However, in patients sensitized to these drugs, in those with reduced renal function, in pregnant women, in children less than 8 years of age, and in certain patients who require parenteral therapy because of severe illness, chloramphenicol is the drug of choice. Either tetracycline or chloramphenicol produces a favorable clinical response early in the course of Rocky Mountain spotted fever (Saah, 1995). Epidemic, murine, scrub, and recrudescent typhus as well as Q fever respond well to chloramphenicol. The same dose schedule is applicable in all the rickettsial diseases. For adults, 50 mg/kg per day is recommended. Oral therapy is preferable whenever possible. The daily dose of chloramphenicol for children with these diseases is 75 mg per kilogram of body weight, divided into equal portions and given every 6 to 8 hours; if chloramphenicol palmitate is used, the daily maintenance dose may be as high as 100 mg/kg, given at the same intervals. Therapy should be continued until the general condition has improved and fever has been absent for 24 to 48 hours. The duration of illness and the incidence of relapses and complications are greatly reduced.

Brucellosis. Chloramphenicol is not as effective as the tetracyclines in the treatment of brucellosis. When a tetracycline is contraindicated, 750 mg to 1 g of chloramphenicol orally every 6 hours may produce a beneficial effect in both the acute and chronic forms of the disease. Relapses usually respond to retreatment.

Untoward Effects. Chloramphenicol inhibits the synthesis of proteins of the inner mitochondrial membrane that are synthesized in mitochondria, probably by inhibiting the ribosomal peptidyltransferase. These include subunits of cytochrome c oxidase, ubiquinone-cytochrome c reductase, and the proton-translocating ATPase. Much of the toxicity observed with this drug can be attributed to these effects.

Hypersensitivity Reactions. Although relatively uncommon, macular or vesicular skin rashes occur as a result of hypersensitivity to chloramphenicol. Fever may appear simultaneously or be the sole manifestation. Angioedema is a rare complication. Jarisch-Herxheimer reactions have been observed shortly after institution of chloramphenicol therapy for syphilis, brucellosis, and typhoid fever.

Hematological Toxicity. The most important adverse effect of chloramphenicol is on the bone marrow. Chloramphenicol affects the hematopoietic system in two ways: by a dose-related toxic effect that presents as anemia, leukopenia, or thrombocytopenia, and by an idiosyncratic response manifested by aplastic anemia, leading in many cases to fatal pancytopenia. The latter response is not dose-related. It seems to occur more commonly in individuals who undergo prolonged therapy and especially in those who are exposed to the drug on more than one occasion. A genetic predisposition is suggested by the occurrence of pancytopenia in identical twins. Although the incidence of the reaction is low—1 in approximately 30,000 or more courses of therapy—the fatality rate is high when bone-marrow aplasia is complete, and there is a higher risk of acute leukemia in those who recover (Shu *et al.,* 1987). Aplastic anemia accounts for approximately 70% of cases of blood dyscrasias due to chloramphenicol. Hypoplastic anemia, agranulocytosis, thrombocytopenia, and bone-marrow inhibition made up the remainder.

Absence of reported instances of aplastic anemia following parenteral administration of chloramphenicol suggested that absorption of a toxic breakdown product from the gastrointestinal tract might be responsible (Holt, 1967). Subsequently, a few cases of aplastic anemia have been described in patients who received parenteral chloramphenicol. However, some of these patients also had received other drugs known to affect the bone marrow (phenylbutazone and glutethimide). The issue thus remains unsettled. The structural feature of chloramphenicol that is responsible for aplastic anemia is hypothesized to be the nitro group, which might be metabolized by intestinal bacteria to a toxic intermediate (Jimenez *et al.,* 1987). However, the exact biochemical mechanism has not yet been elucidated.

The risk of aplastic anemia does not contraindicate the use of chloramphenicol in situations in which it is necessary. The drug should never be used, however, in undefined situations or in diseases readily, safely, and effectively treatable with other antimicrobial agents.

A second, and dose-related, toxic hematologic effect of chloramphenicol is a common and predictable (but reversible) erythroid suppression of the bone marrow, which is probably due to an inhibitory action of the drug on mitochondrial protein synthesis, which in turn impairs iron incorporation into heme (Ward, 1966). Leukopenia and thrombocytopenia also may occur. The incidence and severity of this syndrome are related to dose. It occurs regularly when plasma concentrations are 25 μg/ml or higher and is observed with the use of large doses of chloramphenicol, prolonged treatment, or both. Dose-related suppression of the bone marrow may progress to fatal aplasia. Some patients who developed chronic bone marrow hypoplasia after chloramphenicol treatment subsequently developed acute myeloblastic leukemia.

The administration of chloramphenicol in the presence of hepatic disease frequently results in depression of erythropoiesis. About one-third of patients with severe renal insufficiency exhibit the same reaction.

Toxic and Irritative Effects. Nausea, vomiting, unpleasant taste, diarrhea, and perineal irritation may follow the oral administration of chloramphenicol. Among the rare toxic effects produced by this antibiotic are blurring of vision and digital paresthesias. Optic neuritis occurs in 3% to 5% of children with mucoviscidosis who are given chloramphenicol; there is symmetrical loss of ganglion cells from the retina and atrophy of the fibers in the optic nerve (Godel *et al.,* 1980).

Fatal chloramphenicol toxicity may develop in neonates, especially premature babies, when they are exposed to excessive doses of the drug. The illness, the *gray baby syndrome,* usually begins 2 to 9 days (average, 4 days) after treatment is started. The manifestations in the first 24 hours are vomiting, refusal to suck, irregular and rapid respiration, abdominal distention, periods of cyanosis, and passage of loose, green stools. All the children are severely ill by the end of the first day and, in the next 24 hours, become flaccid, turn an ashen-gray color, and become hypothermic. A similar "gray syndrome" condition also has been reported in adults who were accidentally given excessive quantities of the drug. Death occurs in about 40% of patients within 2 days of initial symptoms. Those who recover usually exhibit no sequelae.

Two mechanisms are apparently responsible for chloramphenicol toxicity in neonates (Craft *et al.,* 1974): (1) failure of the drug to be conjugated with glucuronic acid, owing to inadequate activity of glucuronyl transferase in the liver, which is characteristic of the first 3 to 4 weeks of life; and (2) inadequate renal excretion of unconjugated drug in the newborn. At the time of onset of the clinical syndrome, the chloramphenicol concentrations in plasma usually exceed 100 μg/ml, although they may be as low as 75 μg/ml. Excessive plasma concentrations of the glucuronide conjugate also are present, despite its low rate of formation, because tubular secretion, the pathway of excretion of this compound, is underdeveloped in the neonate. Children 2 weeks of age or younger should receive chloramphenicol in a daily dose no larger than 25 mg per kilogram of body weight; after this age, full-term infants may be given daily quantities up to 50 mg/kg. Toxic effects have not been observed in the newborn when as much as 1 g of the antibiotic has been given every 2 hours to women in labor.

Chloramphenicol is removed from the blood only to a very small extent by either peritoneal dialysis or traditional hemodialysis. However, both exchange transfusion and charcoal hemoperfusion have been used to treat overdose with chloramphenicol in infants (Freundlich *et al.*, 1983).

Other organ systems that have a high rate of oxygen consumption also may be affected by the action of chloramphenicol on mitochondrial enzyme systems; encephalopathic changes have been observed (Levine *et al.*, 1970), and cardiomyopathy also has been reported (Biancaniello *et al.*, 1981).

Drug Interactions. Chloramphenicol inhibits hepatic microsomal cytochrome P450 enzymes (Halpert, 1982), and thus may prolong the half-lives of drugs that are metabolized by this system. Such drugs include warfarin, dicumarol, phenytoin, chlorpropamide, antiretroviral protease inhibitors, rifabutin, and tolbutamide. Severe toxicity and death have occurred because of failure to recognize such effects.

Conversely, other drugs may alter the elimination of chloramphenicol. Chronic administration of phenobarbital or acute administration of rifampin shortens the half-life of the antibiotic, presumably because of enzyme induction, and may result in subtherapeutic concentrations of the drug.

MACROLIDES (ERYTHROMYCIN, CLARITHROMYCIN, AND AZITHROMYCIN)

History and Source. Erythromycin was discovered in 1952 by McGuire and coworkers in the metabolic products of a strain of *Streptomyces erythreus*, originally obtained from a soil sample collected in the Philippine archipelago. Clarithromycin

and azithromycin are semisynthetic derivatives of erythromycin (Alvarez-Elcoro and Enzler, 1999).

Chemistry. Macrolide antibiotics, are so named because they contain a many-membered lactone ring (14-membered ring for erythromycin and clarithromycin and 15-membered ring for azithromycin) to which are attached one or more deoxy sugars. Clarithromycin differs from erythromycin only by methylation of the hydroxyl group at the 6 position, and azithromycin differs by the addition of a methyl-substituted nitrogen atom into the lactone ring. These structural modifications improve acid stability and tissue penetration and broaden the spectrum of activity. The structural formulas of the macrolides are as follows:

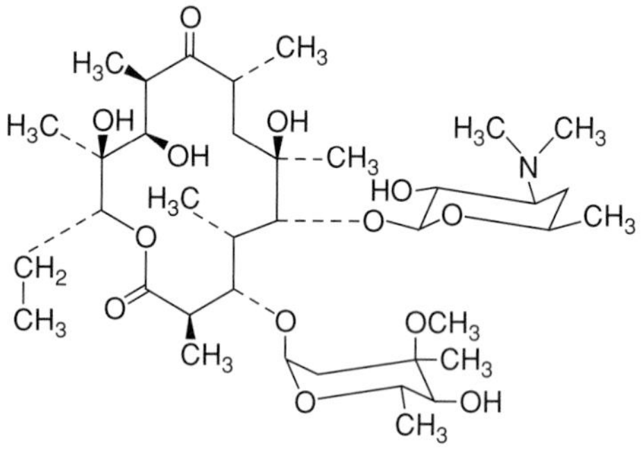

ERYTHROMYCIN

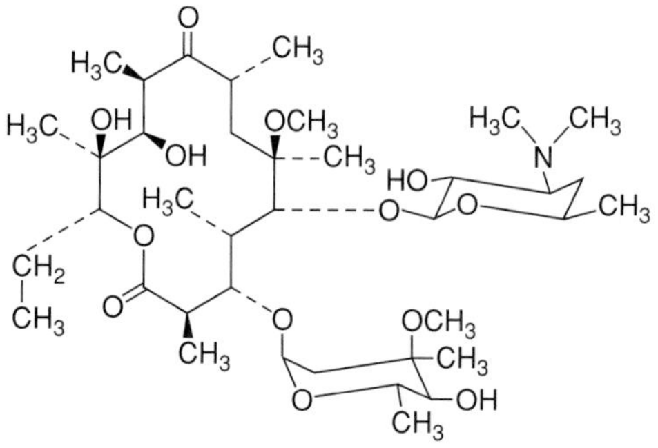

CLARITHROMYCIN

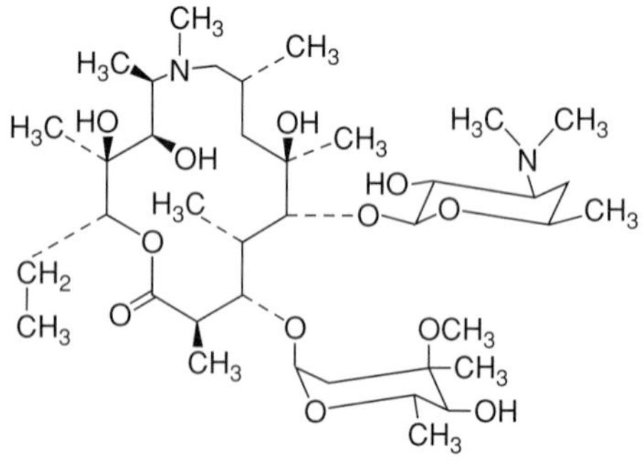

AZITHROMYCIN

Antibacterial Activity. Erythromycin is usually bacteriostatic, but can be bactericidal in high concentrations against very susceptible organisms. The antibiotic is most effective *in vitro* against aerobic gram-positive cocci and bacilli (Steigbigel, 2000). Susceptible strains of *S. pyogenes* and *S. pneumoniae* have MIC ranges from 0.015 to 1.0 μg/ml. Strains of streptococci that are resistant to erythromycin may be on the rise. Because the mechanisms producing resistance to erythromycin affect all macrolides, cross-resistance among them is complete. The prevalence of macrolide resistance among Group A streptococcal isolates, which can be as high as 40%, is related to consumption of macrolide antibiotics within the population (Seppala *et al.*, 1997; Esposito *et al.*, 1998). Macrolide resistance among *S. pneumoniae* is associated with resistance to penicillin. Only 5% of penicillin-susceptible strains are macrolide-resistant, whereas 60% of penicillin-resistant strains are macrolide-resistant (Thornsberry *et al.*, 1997; Thornsberry *et al.*, 1999). Viridans streptococci often are inhibited by 0.06 to 3.1 μg/ml. Although some staphylococci are sensitive to erythromycin, the range of inhibitory concentrations is very high (MIC for *S. epidermidis*, 8 to >32 μg/ml, and for *S. aureus*, 0.12 to >128 μg/ml). Macrolide-resistant strains of *S. aureus* are frequently encountered in hospitals, and resistance may emerge during treatment of an individual patient. Macrolide-resistant strains of *S. aureus* may be cross-resistant to clindamycin as well (Fass, 1993). Many other gram-positive bacilli also are sensitive to erythromycin; values of MIC are 1 μg/ml for *Clostridium perfringens*, from 0.2 to 3 μg/ml for *Corynebacterium diphtheriae*, and from 0.25 to 4 μg/ml for *Listeria monocytogenes*.

Erythromycin is not active against most aerobic enteric gram-negative bacilli. However, it has modest activity *in vitro* against other gram-negative organisms, including *H. influenzae* (MIC, 1 to 32 μg/ml) and *N. meningitidis* (MIC, 0.4 to 1.6 μg/ml), and good activity against most strains of *N. gonorrhoeae* (MIC, 0.12 to 2.0 μg/ml) (Steigbigel, 2000). Useful antibacterial activity also is observed against *Pasteurella multocida*, *Borrelia* spp., and *Bordetella pertussis*. Resistance is common for *B. fragilis* (the MIC ranging from 2.0 to 32 μg/ml). It is usually active against *Campylobacter jejuni* (MIC, 0.5 to 4 μg/ml). Erythromycin is effective against *M. pneumoniae* (MIC, 0.004 to 0.02 μg/ml) and *Legionella pneumophila* (MIC, 0.01 to 2.0 μg/ml). Most strains of *C. trachomatis* are inhibited by 0.06 to 2.0 μg/ml of erythromycin. Some of the atypical mycobacteria, including *M. scrofulaceum*, are sensitive to erythromycin *in vitro*; *M. kansasii* and *M. avium-intracellulare* vary in sensitivity (Molavi and Weinstein, 1971). *M. fortuitum* is resistant. Macrolides have no effect on viruses, yeasts, and fungi.

Clarithromycin is more slightly potent against erythromycin-sensitive strains of streptococci and staphylococci, and has modest activity against *H. influenzae* and

N. gonorrhoeae. Clarithromycin has good activity against *M. catarrhalis*, *Chlamydia* spp., *L. pneumophila*, *B. burgdorferi*, and *Mycoplasma pneumoniae*.

Azithromycin generally is less active than erythromycin against gram-positive organisms (*Streptococcus* spp. and enterococci) and is slightly more active than either erythromycin or clarithromycin against *H. influenzae* and *Campylobacter* spp. (Peters *et al.*, 1992). Azithromycin is very active against *M. catarrhalis*, *P. multocida*, *Chlamydia* spp., *M. pneumoniae*, *L. pneumophila*, *B. burgdorferi*, *Fusobacterium* spp., and *N. gonorrhoeae*.

In general, organisms are considered susceptible to these newer agents at a minimal inhibitory concentration (MIC breakpoint) of ≤ 2 μg/ml. An exception is *H. influenzae*, with MIC breakpoints of ≤ 8 μg/ml and ≤ 4 μg/ml for clarithromycin and azithromycin, respectively.

Both azithromycin and clarithromycin have enhanced activity against *M. avium-intracellulare*, as well as against some protozoa (e.g., *Toxoplasma gondii*, *Cryptosporidium*, and *Plasmodium* spp.). Clarithromycin has good activity against *Mycobacterium leprae* (Chan *et al.*, 1994).

Mechanism of Action. Macrolide antibiotics are bacteriostatic agents that inhibit protein synthesis by binding reversibly to 50 S ribosomal subunits of sensitive microorganisms (Figure 47–3) (*see* Brisson-Noël *et al.*, 1988). Erythromycin has been shown to interfere with the binding of chloramphenicol, which also acts at this site (*see* Figure 47–2). Certain resistant microorganisms with mutational changes in components of this ribosomal subunit fail to bind the drug. It is believed that erythromycin does not inhibit peptide bond formation directly but rather inhibits the translocation step wherein a newly synthesized peptidyl tRNA molecule moves from the acceptor site on the ribosome to the peptidyl (or donor) site.

Gram-positive bacteria accumulate about 100 times more erythromycin than do gram-negative microorganisms. Cells are considerably more permeable to the nonionized form of the drug, and this fact probably explains the increased antimicrobial activity that is observed at alkaline pH (Sabath *et al.*, 1968; Vogel *et al.*, 1971).

Acquired resistance to macrolides usually results from one of three mechanisms: (1) efflux of drug by an active pump mechanism (encoded by *mrsA, mefA,* or *mefE* in staphylococci, Group A streptococci, or *S. pneumoniae*, respectively); (2) inducible or constitutive production of a methylase enzyme that modifies the ribosomal target, leading to decreased drug binding, so-called ribosomal protection mediated by expression of *ermA, ermB,* and *ermC;* and (3) hydrolysis of macrolides by esterases produced by Enterobacteriaceae (Barthélémy *et al.*, 1984). The MLS$_B$

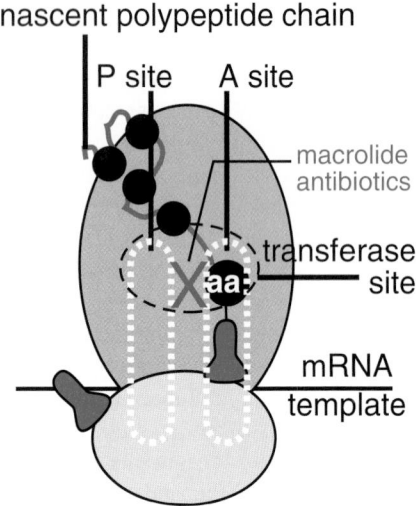

Figure 47–3. Inhibition of bacterial protein synthesis by the macrolide antibiotics erythromycin, clarithromycin, and azithromycin.

> Macrolide antibiotics are bacteriostatic agents that inhibit protein synthesis by binding reversibly to the 50 S ribosomal subunits of sensitive organisms. Erythromycin appears to inhibit the translocation step wherein the nascent peptide chain temporarily residing at the A site of the transferase reaction fails to move to the P, or donor, site. Alternatively, macrolides may bind and cause a conformational change that terminates protein synthesis by indirectly interfering with transpeptidation and translocation. *See* Figure 47–1 and its legend for additional information.

phenotype is conferred by *erm* genes, indicating resistance to macrolides, lincosamides, and type B streptogramins, all of which have the same ribosomal binding site, methylase modification of which results in resistance. Chromosomal mutations that alter a 50 S ribosomal protein is a fourth mechanism of resistance found in *Bacillus subtilis, Campylobacter* spp., and gram-positive cocci.

Absorption, Distribution, and Excretion.   *Absorption.* Erythromycin base is incompletely but adequately absorbed from the upper part of the small intestine. It is inactivated by gastric acids, and the drug is thus administered as enteric-coated tablets or as capsules containing enteric-coated pellets that dissolve in the duodenum. Food increases GI acidity and may delay absorption. Peak concentrations in plasma are only 0.3 to 0.5 μg/ml, 4 hours after oral administration of 250 mg of the base, and are 0.3 to 1.9 μg/ml after a single dose of 500 mg. Esters of erythromycin base (*i.e.,* stearate, estolate, and ethylsuccinate) have been formulated to attempt to improve acid

stability and facilitate absorption. *Erythromycin estolate* is less susceptible to acid than is the base and is better absorbed than other formulations. Its bioavailability is not appreciably altered by food. A single oral 250-mg dose of the erythromycin estolate produces peak concentrations in plasma of approximately 1.5 μg/ml after 2 hours, and a 500-mg dose produces peak concentrations of 4 μg/ml. These peak values include both the inactive ester and the free base, the latter comprising 20% to 35% of the total. Thus, the actual concentration of microbiologically active erythromycin base in plasma may be similar for the three preparations. *Erythromycin ethylsuccinate* is another ester that is adequately absorbed after oral administration. Peak concentrations in plasma are 1.5 μg/ml (0.5 μg/ml of base) 1 to 2 hours after administration of a 500-mg dose.

High concentrations of erythromycin can be achieved by intravenous administration. Values are approximately 10 μg/ml 1 hour after intravenous administration of 500 to 1000 mg of erythromycin lactobionate or glucepate.

Clarithromycin is absorbed rapidly from the gastrointestinal tract after oral administration, but its bioavailability is reduced to 50% to 55% because of rapid first-pass metabolism. Peak concentrations occur approximately 2 hours after drug administration. The standard formulation of clarithromycin may be given with or without food. The extended-release form of clarithromycin, which is given as a once-daily 1-g dose, should be administered with food, which improves bioavailability. Steady-state peak concentrations in plasma are 2 to 3 μg/ml after 2 hours from a regimen of 500 mg every 12 hours (Fraschini *et al.,* 1993) or 2 to 4 hours after two 500-mg extended-release tablets given once daily.

Azithromycin administered orally is absorbed rapidly and distributes widely throughout the body, except to cerebrospinal fluid. Concomitant administration of aluminum and magnesium hydroxide antacids will decrease the peak serum drug concentrations although not the overall bioavailability; however, it should not be administered with food. The peak plasma drug concentration after a 500 mg loading dose is approximately 0.4 μg/ml. When this loading dose is followed by 250 mg once daily for 4 days, the steady-state peak drug concentration is 0.24 μg/ml. Azithromycin also is available in a formulation for intravenous administration. Plasma concentrations of 3 to 4 μg/ml are achieved at the end of a one-hour infusion of 500 mg of azithromycin.

Distribution.   Erythromycin diffuses readily into intracellular fluids, and antibacterial activity can be achieved at essentially all sites except the brain and CSF. Erythromycin penetrates into prostatic fluid, achieving concentrations approximately 40% of those in plasma. Concentrations in middle ear exudate reach only 50% of serum concentrations, and thus may be too low for the treatment of otitis media caused by *H. influenzae*. Protein binding is approximately 70% to 80% for erythromycin base and even higher, 96%, for the estolate. Erythromycin traverses the placental barrier, and concentrations of the drug in fetal plasma are about 5% to 20% of those in the maternal circulation. Concentrations in breast milk also are significant (50% of those in serum).

After absorption, clarithromycin undergoes rapid first-pass metabolism to its active metabolite, 14-hydroxyclarithromycin. Both of these agents distribute widely throughout the body and achieve high intracellular concentrations. Tissue concentrations generally exceed serum concentrations. Concentrations in middle ear fluid are 50% higher than simultaneous serum concentrations for both clarithromycin and the active metabolite. Protein binding of clarithromycin has been shown to range from 40% to 70% and is concentration-dependent.

Azithromycin's unique pharmacokinetic properties include extensive tissue distribution and high drug concentrations within cells (including phagocytes), resulting in much greater tissue or secretion drug concentrations compared to simultaneous serum concentrations. Tissue fibroblasts act as the natural reservoir for drug *in vivo,* and transfer of drug to phagoctyes is easily accomplished (McDonald and Pruul, 1991). Protein binding is low (51% at very low plasma concentrations) and appears to be concentration-dependent, decreasing with increasing concentrations.

Elimination. Only 2% to 5% of orally administered erythromycin is excreted in active form in the urine; this value is from 12% to 15% after intravenous infusion. The antibiotic is concentrated in the liver and is excreted as the active form in the bile, which may contain as much as 250 μg/ml when plasma concentrations are very high. The plasma elimination half-life of erythromycin is approximately 1.6 hours. Although some reports suggest a prolonged half-life in patients with anuria, dosage reduction is not routinely recommended in renal-failure patients. The drug is not removed significantly by either peritoneal dialysis or hemodialysis.

Clarithromycin is eliminated by renal and nonrenal mechanisms. It is metabolized in the liver to several metabolites, the active 14-hydroxy metabolite being the most significant. The rate of metabolism appears to be saturable and probably accounts for the nonlinear pharmacokinetics with higher dosages (Chu *et al.,* 1992). Primary metabolic pathways are oxidative *N*-demethylation and stereospecific hydroxylation at the 14 position. Formation

of the *R*- and *S*-epimers occurs *in vivo,* with the *R*-epimer present to a greater degree and with greater biological activity. The elimination half-lives of clarithromycin and 14-hydroxyclarithromycin are approximately 3 to 7 hours and 5 to 9 hours, respectively. Longer half-lives are observed after larger doses. The amount of clarithromycin excreted unchanged in the urine ranges from 20% to 40%, depending on the dose administered and the formulation (tablet versus oral suspension). An additional 10% to 15% of a dose is excreted in the urine as 14-hydroxyclarithromycin. Although the pharmacokinetics of clarithromycin are altered in patients with either hepatic or renal dysfunction, dosage adjustment is not necessary unless a patient has severe renal dysfunction (creatine clearance of less than 30 ml per minute).

The exact biodisposition of azithromycin still is being elucidated. The drug undergoes some hepatic metabolism to inactive metabolites, but biliary excretion is the major route of elimination. Only 12% of drug is excreted unchanged in the urine. The elimination half-life, 40 to 68 hours, is prolonged because of extensive tissue sequestration and binding.

Therapeutic Uses. The usual oral dose of erythromycin (*erythromycin base;* E-MYCIN, others) for adults ranges from 1 to 2 g per day, in equally divided and spaced amounts, usually given every 6 hours, depending on the nature and severity of the infection. Daily doses of erythromycin as large as 8 g orally, given for 3 months, have been well tolerated. Food should be avoided, if possible, immediately before or after oral administration of erythromycin base or the stearate; this precaution need not be taken when *erythromycin estolate* (ILOSONE) or *erythromycin ethylsuccinate* (E.E.S., others) is administered. The oral dose of erythromycin for children is 30 to 50 mg/kg per day, divided into four portions; this dose may be doubled for severe infections. Intramuscular administration of erythromycin is not recommended because of pain upon injection. Intravenous administration is reserved for the therapy of severe infections, such as legionellosis. The usual dose is 0.5 to 1 g every 6 hours; 1 g of erythromycin gluceptate has been given intravenously every 6 hours for as long as 4 weeks with no difficulty except for thrombophlebitis at the site of injection. *Erythromycin gluceptate* (ILOTYCIN GLUCEPTATE) and *erythromycin lactobionate* (ERYTHROCIN LACTOBIONATE-I.V.) are available for intravenous injection.

Clarithromycin (BIAXIN FILMTABS, BIAXIN XL FILMTABS, and BIAXIN granules for suspension) usually is given as a twice-daily regimen: 250 mg twice daily for children older than 12 years and adults with mild to moderate infection. Larger doses are indicated (500 mg twice daily) for more severe infection (*e.g.,* pneumonia) or when infection is caused by more resistant organisms (*e.g., H. influenzae*). Children less than 12 years old have received 7.5 mg/kg twice daily in clinical studies. The 500-mg extended-release formulation is given as two tablets once daily.

Azithromycin (ZITHROMAX tablet, oral suspension, and powder for intravenous injection) should be given 1 hour before or 2 hours after meals when administered orally. For outpatient therapy of community-acquired pneumonia, pharyngitis, or skin and skin-structure infections, a loading dose of 500 mg is given on the first day, then 250 mg per day is given for days 2 through 5. Treatment or prophylaxis of *M. avium-intracellulare* infection in AIDS patients requires higher doses: 500 mg daily in combination with one or more other agents for treatment, or 1200 mg once weekly for primary prevention. The treatment of uncomplicated nongonococcal urethritis presumed to be due to *C. trachomatis* consists of a single 1-g dose of azithromycin. A single 2-g dose is effective for gonorrhea, but is not routinely recommended (Centers for Disease Control and Prevention, 1998).

In children, the recommended dose of oral suspension for acute otitis media and pneumonia is 10 mg/kg the first day (maximum 500 mg) and 5 mg/kg (maximum 250 mg per day) on days 2 through 5. The dose for tonsillitis or pharyngitis is 12 mg/kg per day, up to 500 mg total, for 5 days.

Mycoplasma pneumoniae Infections. Erythromycin (given orally in doses of 500 mg four times daily, or, if oral administration is not tolerated, given intravenously) reduces the duration of fever caused by *M. pneumoniae*. In addition, the rate of clearing, as indicated by chest radiographs, is accelerated (Rasch and Mogabgab, 1965). Tetracycline or another macrolide is just as effective.

Legionnaires' Disease. Erythromycin has been considered as the drug of choice for treatment of pneumonia caused by *L. pneumophila, L. micdadei,* or other *Legionella* spp. Azithromycin has supplanted erythromycin as the first-line agent (along with fluoroquinlones) for treatment of legionellosis because of excellent *in vitro* activity, superior tissue concentration, the ease of administration as a single daily dose, and better tolerability compared to erythromycin (Stout et al., 1998; Garey and Amsden 1999; Yu, 2000). The recommended dose is 500 mg intravenously or orally for a total of 10 to 14 days.

Chlamydia Infections. Chlamydial infections can be treated effectively with any of the macrolides. Azithromycin is specifically recommended as an alternative to doxycycline in patients with uncomplicated urethral, endocervical, rectal, or epididymal infections (Centers for Disease Control and Prevention, 1998). Clearly the major impact of azithromycin is due to the better compliance that results from a single-dose treatment

regimen. During pregnancy, erythromycin base, 500 mg four times daily for 7 days, is recommended as first-line therapy for chlamydial urogenital infections. Azithromycin, 1 g orally as a single dose, is a suitable alternative (Centers for Disease Control and Prevention, 1998). Erythromycin base is preferred for chlamydial pneumonia of infancy and ophthalmia neonatorum (50 mg/kg per day in four divided doses for 10 to 14 days), as tetracyclines are contraindicated in this patient group.

Pneumonia caused by *Chlamydia pneumoniae* responds to macrolides, fluoroquinolones, and tetracyclines in standard doses for community-acquired pneumonia. No comparative trials have been conducted to determine which, if any, agent is most efficacious. Duration of therapy also is ill defined. A two-week duration of therapy has been recommended (Bartlett *et al.,* 1993), although in practice a specific etiological diagnosis rarely is made and length of treatment often is determined empirically based on clinical response.

Diphtheria. Erythromycin is very effective for acute infections or for eradicating the carrier state. Erythromycin estolate (250 mg four times daily for 7 days) was found to be effective in 90% of adults. The other macrolides also are likely to be effective, but clinical experience with them is lacking, and they are not FDA-approved for this indication. Neither erythromycin nor any other antibiotic alters the course of an acute infection with the diphtheria bacillus or the risk of complications. Antitoxin is indicated in the treatment of acute infection.

Pertussis. Erythromycin is the drug of choice for treating persons with *B. pertussis* disease and for post-exposure prophylaxis of all household members and other close contacts. A 7-day regimen of erythromycin estolate (40 mg/kg per day, maximum 1 g/day) is as effective as 14-day erythromycin regimens traditionally recommended (Halperin *et al.,* 1997). Clarithromycin and azithromycin appear to be just as effective, although clinical experience is limited (Aoyama *et al.,* 1996; Bace *et al.,* 1999). If administered early in the course of whooping cough, erythromycin may shorten the duration of illness. The drug has little influence on the disease once the paroxysmal stage is reached, although it may eliminate the microorganisms from the nasopharynx. Nasopharyngeal cultures should be obtained from persons with pertussis who do not improve with erythromycin therapy, as resistance has been reported (Centers for Disease Control, 1994).

Streptococcal Infections. Pharyngitis, scarlet fever, erysipelas, and cellulitis caused by *S. pyogenes* and pneumonia caused by *S. pneumoniae* respond to macrolides. They are valuable alternatives for treatment of patients who have serious allergy to penicillin. Unfortunately, macrolide-resistant strains are increasingly encountered and may cause infections that do not respond to these agents. As noted above, penicillin-resistant strains of *S. pneumoniae* are very likely also to be resistant to macrolides.

Staphylococcal Infections. Erythromycin has been an alternative agent for the treatment of relatively minor infections caused by either penicillin-sensitive or penicillin-resistant *S. aureus*. However, many strains of *S. aureus,* including community-acquired isolates, are resistant to macrolides, such that these agents no longer can be relied upon unless *in vitro* susceptibility has been documented.

Campylobacter Infections. The treatment of gastroenteritis caused by *Campylobacter jejuni* with erythromycin (250 to

500 mg orally four times a day for 7 days) hastens eradication of the microorganism from the stools and reduces the duration of symptoms (Salazar-Lindo *et al.*, 1986). Availability of fluoroquinolones, which are highly active against *Campylobacter* species and other enteric pathogens, has largely replaced the need for erythromycin for this disease in adults. Erythromycin remains useful for treatment of *Campylobacter* gastroenteritis in children.

Helicobacter pylori Infection. Clarithromycin 500 mg, in combination with omeprazole, 20 mg, and amoxicillin, 1g, each administered twice daily for 10 to 14 days is effective for treatment of peptic ulcer disease caused by *H. pylori* (Peterson *et al.*, 2000). Numerous other regimens, some effective as a seven-day treatment, have been studied and also are effective (Misiewicz *et al.*, 1997; Hunt *et al.*, 1999). The more effective regimens generally include three agents, one of which usually is clarithromycin.

Tetanus. Erythromycin (500 mg orally every 6 hours for 10 days) may be given to eradicate *Clostridium tetani* in patients with tetanus who are allergic to penicillin. However, the mainstays of therapy are debridement, physiological support, tetanus antitoxin, and drug control of convulsions.

Syphilis. Erythromycin has been used in the treatment of early syphilis in patients who are allergic to penicillin, but is no longer recommended (Centers for Disease Control and Prevention, 1998). Tetracyclines are the recommended alternative in penicillin-allergic patients. During pregnancy it is recommended that patients be desensitized to penicillin.

Mycobacterial Infections. Clarithromycin or azithromycin is recommended as first-line therapy for prophylaxis and treatment of disseminated infection caused by *M. avium-intracellulare* in AIDS patients and for treatment of pulmonary disease in non-HIV-infected patients (American Thoracic Society 1997; Kovacs and Masur 2000). Azithromycin (1200 mg once weekly) or clarithromycin (500 mg twice daily) is recommended for primary prevention for AIDS patients with less than 50 CD4 cells per mm³. Single-agent therapy should not be used for treatment of active disease or for secondary prevention in AIDS patients. First-line therapy is clarithromycin (500 mg twice daily) plus ethambutol (15 mg/kg once daily) with or without rifabutin. Azithromycin (500 mg once daily) may be used instead of clarithromycin, but clarithromycin appears to be slightly more efficacious (Ward *et al.*, 1998). Clarithromycin also has been used with minocycline for the treatment of *Mycobacterium leprae* in lepromatous leprosy (Ji *et al.*, 1993).

Other Infections. Clarithromycin and azithromycin have been used in the treatment of toxoplasmosis encephalitis (Saba *et al.*, 1993) and diarrhea due to *Cryptosporidium* (Rehg, 1991) in AIDS patients. Rigorous clinical trials demonstrating efficacy of macrolides for these infections are lacking.

Prophylactic Uses. Penicillin is the drug of choice for the prophylaxis of recurrences of rheumatic fever, but it cannot be used in individuals who are allergic to this antibiotic. Erythromycin is an effective alternative.

Erythromycin has been recommended as an alternative to penicillin in allergic patients for prevention of bacterial endocarditis following dental or respiratory-tract procedures (Dajani *et al.*, 1990). Clindamycin has replaced erythromycin for use in penicillin-allergic patients. Clarithromycin or azithromycin as a single 500-mg dose also may be used (Dajani *et al.*, 1997).

Untoward Effects. Serious untoward effects are only rarely caused by erythromycin. Among the allergic reactions observed are fever, eosinophilia, and skin eruptions, which may occur alone or in combination; each disappears shortly after therapy is stopped. Cholestatic hepatitis is the most striking side effect. It is caused primarily by erythromycin estolate and only rarely by the ethylsuccinate or the stearate (*see* Ginsburg and Eichenwald, 1976). The illness starts after about 10 to 20 days of treatment and is characterized initially by nausea, vomiting, and abdominal cramps. The pain often mimics that of acute cholecystitis, and unnecessary surgery has been performed. These symptoms are followed shortly thereafter by jaundice, which may be accompanied by fever, leukocytosis, eosinophilia, and elevated activities of transaminases in plasma. Biopsy of the liver reveals cholestasis, periportal infiltration by neutrophils, lymphocytes, and eosinophils, and, occasionally, necrosis of neighboring parenchymal cells. All manifestations usually disappear within a few days after cessation of drug therapy and rarely are prolonged. The syndrome may represent a hypersensitivity reaction to the estolate ester (*see* Tolman *et al.*, 1974). Mild elevations of serum aspartate aminotransferase enzymes also may occur (McCormack *et al.*, 1977).

Oral administration of erythromycin, especially of large doses, frequently is accompanied by epigastric distress, which may be quite severe. Intravenous administration of erythromycin may cause similar symptoms, with abdominal cramps, nausea, vomiting, and diarrhea. Erythromycin may stimulate gastrointestinal motility by acting on motilin receptors (Smith *et al.*, 2000). The gastrointestinal symptoms are dose-related and occur more commonly in children and young adults (Seifert *et al.*, 1989); they may be reduced by prolonging the infusion time to 1 hour or by pretreatment with glycopyrrolate (Bowler *et al.*, 1992). Intravenous infusion of 1-g doses, even when dissolved in a large volume, often is followed by thrombophlebitis. This can be minimized by slow rates of infusion.

Erythromycin has been reported to cause cardiac arrhythmias, including QT prolongation with ventricular tachycardia. Most patients have had underlying cardiac disease, or the arrhythmias were associated with combination drug therapies that included erythromycin (*e.g.*, cisapride or terfenadine plus erythromycin) (Brandriss *et al.*, 1994).

Transient auditory impairment is a potential complication of treatment with erythromycin; it has been observed to follow intravenous administration of large doses of the gluceptate or lactobionate (4 g per day) or oral ingestion of large doses of the estolate (Karmody and Weinstein, 1977).

Drug Interactions. Erythromycin and clarithromycin have been reported to cause clinically significant drug interactions (Periti *et al.*, 1992). Erythromycin has been reported to potentiate the effects of astemizole, carbamazapine, corticosteroids, cyclosporine, digoxin, ergot alkaloids, terfenadine, theophylline, triazolam, valproate, and warfarin, probably by interfering with cytochrome P450-mediated metabolism of these drugs (Ludden, 1985; Martell *et al.*, 1986; Honig *et al.*, 1992). Clarithromycin, which is structurally closely related to erythromycin, has a similar drug interaction profile. Azithromycin, which differs from erythromycin and clarithromycin because of its 15-membered lactone ring structure, appears to be free of these drug interactions. Caution is advised, nevertheless, when using azithromycin in conjuction with drugs known to interact with erythromycin.

CLINDAMYCIN

Chemistry. Clindamycin is a derivative of the amino acid *trans*-L-4-*n*-propylhygrinic acid, attached to a sulfur-containing derivative of an octose. It is a congener of lincomycin, and its structural formula is as follows:

CLINDAMYCIN

Mechanism of Action. Clindamycin binds exclusively to the 50 S subunit of bacterial ribosomes and suppresses protein synthesis. Although clindamycin, erythromycin, and chloramphenicol are not structurally related, they all act at sites within close proximity (*see* Figures 47–2 and 47–3), and binding by one of these antibiotics to the ribosome may inhibit the interaction of the others. There are no clinical indications for the concurrent use of these antibiotics. Macrolide resistance due to ribosomal methylation by *erm*-encoded enzymes also may produce resistance to clindamycin. However, because clindamycin is not an inducer of the methylase, there is cross-resistance only if the enzyme is produced constitutively. Clindamycin is not a substrate for macrolide efflux pumps, and strains that are resistant to macrolides by this mechanism are susceptible to clindamycin. Plasmid-mediated resistance to clindamycin (and erythromycin) has been found in *B. fragilis* (Tally *et al.*, 1979); it may be due to methylation of bacte-

rial RNA found in the 50 S ribosomal subunit (Steigbigel, 2000).

Antibacterial Activity. Bacterial strains are susceptible to clindamycin at minimal inhibitory concentrations of ≤0.5 µg/ml. In general, clindamycin is similar to erythromycin in its activity *in vitro* against susceptible strains of pneumococci, *S. pyogenes,* and viridans streptococci. Ninety percent or more of strains of streptococci, including some that are macrolide-resistant, remain susceptible to clindamycin with MICs less than 0.5 µg/ml (Carroll *et al.*, 1997; Doern *et al.*, 1998; Wisplinghoff *et al.*, 1999). Methicillin-susceptible strains of *S. aureus* usually are susceptible to clindamycin, but methicillin-resistant strains of *S. aureus* and coagulase-negative staphylococci frequently are resistant.

Clindamycin is more active than erythromycin or clarithromycin against anaerobic bacteria, especially *B. fragilis;* some strains are inhibited by <0.1 µg/ml, and more than 90% of strains are inhibited by 2 µg/ml. Minimal inhibitory concentrations for other anaerobes are as follows: *Bacteroides melaninogenicus,* 0.1 to 1 µg/ml; *Fusobacterium,* <0.5 µg/ml (although most strains of *Fusobacterium varium* are resistant); *Peptostreptococcus,* <0.1 to 0.5 µg/ml; *Peptococcus,* 1 to 100 µg/ml (with 10% of strains resistant); and *C. perfringens,* <0.1 to 8 µg/ml. From 10% to 20% of clostridial species other than *C. perfringens* are resistant. Strains of *Actinomyces israelii* and *Nocardia asteroides* are sensitive. Essentially all aerobic gram-negative bacilli are resistant.

With regard to atypical organisms and parasites, *M. pneumoniae* is resistant. *Chlamydia* spp. are variably sensitive, although the clinical relevance is not established. Clindamycin shows good activity in experimental models of *Pneumocystis carinii* pneumonia and *T. gondii* encephalitis. Clindamycin has some activity against both chloroquine-sensitive and chloroquine-resistant strains of *Plasmodium falciparum* and *Plasmodium vivax,* but a cure rate of only 50% of patients with malaria was observed in one study (Hall *et al.*, 1975; see also Seaberg *et al.*, 1984). Clindamycin has been used for treatment of babesiosis.

Absorption, Distribution, and Excretion. *Absorption.* Clindamycin is nearly completely absorbed following oral administration. Peak plasma concentrations of 2 to 3 µg/ml are attained within 1 hour after the ingestion of 150 mg. The presence of food in the stomach does not reduce absorption significantly. The half-life of the antibiotic is about 2.9 hours, and modest accumulation of drug is thus expected if it is given at 6-hour intervals.

Clindamycin palmitate, an oral preparation for pediatric use, is an inactive prodrug, but the ester is hydrolyzed rapidly *in vivo*. Its rate and extent of absorption are similar to those of clindamycin. After several oral doses at 6-hour intervals, children attain plasma concentrations of 2 to 4 μg/ml with the administration of 8 to 16 mg/kg.

The phosphate ester of clindamycin, which is given parenterally, also is rapidly hydrolyzed *in vivo* to the active parent compound. After intramuscular injection, peak concentrations in plasma are not attained until 3 hours in adults and 1 hour in children; these values approximate 6 μg/ml after a 300-mg dose and 9 μg/ml after a 600-mg dose in adults.

Distribution. Clindamycin is widely distributed in many fluids and tissues, including bone. Significant concentrations are not attained in CSF, even when the meninges are inflamed. Concentrations sufficient to treat cerebral toxoplasmosis are achievable (Gatti *et al.,* 1998). The drug readily crosses the placental barrier. Ninety percent or more of clindamycin is bound to plasma proteins (*see* Panzer *et al.,* 1972). Clindamycin accumulates in polymorphonuclear leukocytes, alveolar macrophages, and in abscesses.

Excretion. Only about 10% of the clindamycin administered is excreted unaltered in the urine, and small quantities are found in the feces. However, antimicrobial activity persists in feces for 5 or more days after parenteral therapy with clindamycin is stopped; growth of clindamycin-sensitive microorganisms in colonic contents may remain suppressed for up to 2 weeks (Kager *et al.,* 1981).

Clindamycin is inactivated by metabolism to *N*-demethylclindamycin and clindamycin sulfoxide, which are excreted in the urine and bile. Accumulation of clindamycin can occur in patients with severe hepatic failure, and dosage adjustments thus may be required.

Therapeutic Uses. The oral dose of clindamycin (*clindamycin hydrochloride;* CLEOCIN) for adults is 150 to 300 mg every 6 hours; for severe infections, it is 300 to 600 mg every 6 hours. Children should receive 8 to 12 mg/kg per day of *clindamycin palmitate hydrochloride* (CLEOCIN PEDIATRIC) in three or four divided doses (some physicians recommend 10 to 30 mg/kg per day in six divided doses) or for severe infections, 13 to 25 mg/kg per day. However, children weighing 10 kg or less should receive 1/2 teaspoonful of clindamycin palmitate hydrochloride (37.5 mg) every 8 hours as a minimal dose.

For serious infections due to aerobic gram-positive cocci and the more sensitive anaerobes (not generally including *B. fragilis, Peptococcus,* and *Clostridium* spp. other than *C. perfringens*), intravenous or intramuscular administration is recommended in dosages of 600 to 1200 mg per day, divided into two to four equal portions for adults. *Clindamycin phosphate* (CLEOCIN PHOSPHATE) is available for intramuscular or intravenous use. For more severe infections, particularly those proven or suspected to be caused by *B. fragilis, Peptococcus,* or *Clostridium* species other than *C. perfringens,* parenteral administration of 1200 to 2400 mg per day of clindamycin is suggested. Daily doses as high as 4800 mg have been given intravenously to adults. Children should receive 10 to 40 mg/kg per day in three or four divided doses. In severe infections, a minimal daily dose of 300 mg is recommended, regardless of body weight.

Although a number of infections with gram-positive cocci will respond favorably to clindamycin, the high incidence of diarrhea and the occurrence of colitis require limitation of its use to infections in which it is clearly superior to other agents. Clindamycin is particularly valuable for the treatment of infections with anaerobes, especially those due to *B. fragilis.* It has been used successfully in combination with an aminoglycoside for infections resulting from fecal spillage (intraabdominal or pelvic abscesses and peritonitis). Other drugs that are effective against anaerobes, such as metronidazole, chloramphenicol, cefoxitin, cefmetazole, cefotetan, ceftizoxime, cefotaxime, imipenem, or penicillins plus β-lactamase inhibitors (*i.e.,* ticarcillin and clavulanate, ampicillin and clavulanate, piperacillin and tazobactam, ampicillin and sulbactam), appear to be as efficacious as clindamycin in this setting (Bartlett *et al.,* 1981; DiPiro, 1995). Clindamycin is not predictably useful for the treatment of bacterial brain abscesses, since penetration into the CSF is poor; metronidazole in combination with penicillin or a third-generation cephalosporin is preferred.

One randomized, prospective trial has shown that clindamycin (600 mg intravenously every 8 hours) was superior to penicillin (1 million units intravenously every 4 hours) for the treatment of lung abscesses (Levison *et al.,* 1983). On the basis of this study, the results of which continue to be debated (Bartlett, 1993), clindamycin has become the drug of choice instead of penicillin for treatment of lung abscess and anaerobic lung and pleural space infections.

Clindamycin (600 to 1200 mg given intravenously every 6 hours) in combination with pyrimethamine (a 200-mg loading dose followed by 75 mg orally each day) and folinic acid (10 mg/day) has been shown to be effective for acute treatment of encephalitis caused by *T. gondii* in patients with AIDS (Dannemann *et al.,* 1992; Katlama *et al.,* 1996). Clindamycin (600 mg intravenously every 8 hours, or 300 to 450 orally every 6 hours for less severe disease) in combination with primaquine (15 mg of base once daily) has been shown to be useful for the treatment of mild to moderate cases of *P. carinii* pneumonia (PCP) in AIDS patients (Black *et al.*, 1994; Toma *et al.*, 1993).

Clindamycin also is available as a topical solution, gel, or lotion (CLEOCIN T, others) and as a vaginal cream (CLEOCIN). It is effective topically (or orally) for acne vulgaris and bacterial vaginosis.

Untoward Effects. The reported incidence of diarrhea associated with the administration of clindamycin ranges from 2% to 20%. A number of patients (variously reported as 0.01% to 10%) have developed pseudomembranous colitis caused by the toxin from the organism *C. difficile* (Rifkin *et al.*, 1977). This colitis is characterized by abdominal pain, diarrhea, fever, and mucus and blood in the stools. Proctoscopic examination reveals white to yellow plaques on the mucosa of the colon. *This syndrome may be lethal.* Discontinuation of the drug, combined with administration of metronidazole orally or intravenously usually is curative, but relapses occur. Agents that inhibit peristalsis, such as opioids, may prolong and worsen the condition. Although the incidence of this problem is unknown, it is clear that the therapeutic indications for clindamycin, or any antibiotic, should be considered very seriously before it is given.

Skin rashes occur in approximately 10% of patients treated with clindamycin and may be more common in patients with human immunodeficiency virus (HIV) infection. Other reactions, which are uncommon, include exudative erythema multiforme (Stevens-Johnson syndrome), reversible elevation of aspartate aminotransferase and alanine aminotransferase, granulocytopenia, thrombocytopenia, and anaphylactic reactions. Local thrombophlebitis may follow intravenous administration of the drug. Clindamycin can inhibit neuromuscular transmission and may potentiate the effect of a neuromuscular blocking agent administered concurrently (Fogdall and Miller, 1974).

QUINUPRISTIN/DALFOPRISTIN

Quinupristin/dalfopristin (SYNECID) is a combination of a streptogramin B, quinupristin, with a streptogramin A, dalfopristin, in a 30:70 ratio (Chant and Rybak 1995). These compounds are semisynthetic derivatives of naturally occurring pristinamycins, produced by *Streptomyces pristinaespiralis*. Pristinamycin has been available as an oral agent in France for more than 30 years for treatment of staphylococcal infections. Quinupristin and dalfopristin are more soluble derivatives of pristinamycin IA and pristinamycin IIA, respectively, and therefore are suitable for intravenous administration. Their chemical structures are as follows:

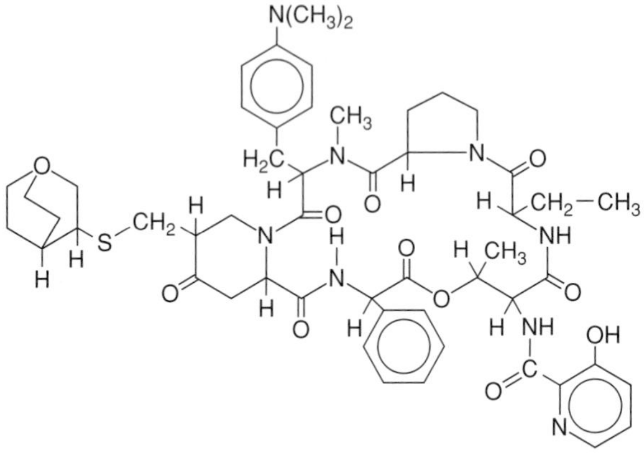

QUINUPRISTIN

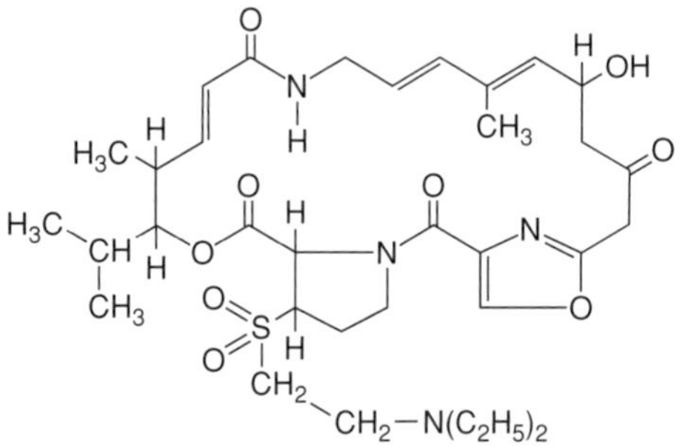

DALFOPRISTIN

Antibacterial Activity. Quinupristin/dalfopristin is active against gram-positive cocci, including *S. pneumoniae*, beta-hemolytic and alpha-hemolytic strains of streptococci, *E. faecium* (but not *E. faecalis*), and staphylococci, both coagulase-positive and coagulase-negative strains (Chang *et al.*, 1999). The combination is largely inactive against gram-negative organisms, although *Moraxella catarrhalis* and *Neiserria* spp. are susceptible. It is also active against organisms responsible for atypical pneumonia, *M. pneumoniae*, *Legionella* spp., and *Chlamydia pneumoniae* (Lamb *et al.*, 1999). The combination is bactericidal against streptococci and many strains of staphylococci, but bacteriostatic against *E. faecium*. MICs for strains of streptococci, including penicillin-susceptible and penicillin-resistant strains of *S. pneumoniae*, are 0.25 to 1 μg/ml. MICs typically are <1 μg/ml for both methicillin-susceptible and methicillin-resistant strains of staphylococci and for vancomycin-intermediate *S. aureus* strains. MICs for

E. faecium are 1 μg/ml or less for both vancomycin-susceptible and vancomycin-resistant strains, but for *E. faecalis* are 8 μg/ml or higher.

Mechanism of Action. Quinupristin and dalfopristin are protein synthesis inhibitors that bind the 50 S ribosomal subunit. Quinupristin, a type B streptogramin, binds at the same site as macrolides and has a similar effect, with inhibition of polypeptide elongation and early termination of protein synthesis. Dalfopristin binds at a site nearby, resulting in a conformational change in the 50 S ribosome, synergistically enhancing the binding of quinupristin at its target site. Dalfopristin directly interferes with polypeptide-chain formation. The net effect, in many bacterial species, of the cooperative and synergistic binding of these two molecules to the ribosome is bactericidal activity.

Resistance to quinupristin is mediated by MLS type B resistance determinants (*e.g., ermA* and *ermC* in staphylococci and *ermB* in enterococci), encoding a ribosomal methylase that prevents binding of drug to its target; or *vgb* or *vgbB*, which encode lactonases that inactivate type B streptogramins (Allignet *et al.,* 1998; Bozdogan and Leclercq, 1999). Resistance to dalfopristin is mediated by *vat, vatB, vatC, vatD,* and *satA,* which encode acetyltransferases that inactivate type A streptogramins (Allignet *et al.,* 1998; Allignet and El Solh, 1999; Soltani *et al.,* 2000); or staphylococcal genes *vga, vgb,* and *vgaB,* which encode ATP-binding efflux proteins that pump type A compounds out of the cell (Allignet *et al.,* 1998; Bozdogan and Leclercq, 1999). These resistance determinants are located on plasmids that may be transferable by conjugative mobilization (Allignet *et al.,* 1998). Resistance to quinupristin/dalfopristin always is associated with a resistance gene for type A streptogramins. Genes encoding resistance to type B streptogramins also may be present, but are not sufficient to produce resistance alone. Methylase-encoding *erm* genes, however, can render the combination bacteriostatic instead of bactericidal, rendering it ineffective in certain infections in which bactericidal activity is necessary for cure, such as endocarditis (Chambers, 1992; Fantin *et al.,* 1995).

Absorption, Distribution, and Excretion. Quinupristin/dalfopristin is administered only by intravenous infusion over at least one hour. It is incompatible with saline and heparin and should be dissolved in 5% dextrose in water. Steady-state peak serum concentrations in healthy male volunteers are approximately 3 μg/ml of quinupristin and 7 μg/ml of dalfopristin with a 7.5-mg/kg dose administered every 8 hours. The half-life is 0.85 hour for quinu-

pristin and 0.7 hours for dalfopristin. The volume of distribution is 0.87 l/kg for quinupristin and 0.71 l/kg for dalfopristin. Hepatic metabolism by conjugation is the principal means of clearance for both compounds, with 80% of an administered dose eliminated by biliary excretion. Renal elimination of active compound accounts for most of the remainder. No dosage adjustment is necessary for renal insufficiency. Pharmacokinetics are not significantly altered by peritoneal dialysis or hemodialysis (Johnson *et al.,* 1999; Moellering *et al.,* 1999). The area under the concentration curve of active component and its metabolites is increased by 180% for quinupristin and 50% for dalfopristin by hepatic insufficiency. No adjustment is recommended unless the patient is unable to tolerate the drug, in which case the dosing frequency should be reduced from 8 hours to 12 hours.

Therapeutic Uses. Quinupristin/dalfopristin is approved in the United States for treatment of infections caused by vancomycin-resistant strains of *E. faecium* and complicated skin and skin structure infections caused by methicillin-susceptible strains of *S. aureus* or *S. pyogenes* (Nichols *et al.,* 1999). In Europe it also is approved for treatment of nosocomial pneumonia and infections caused by methicillin-resistant strains of *S. aureus* (Fagon *et al.,* 2000). In open label, nonrandomized studies, clinical and microbiological cure rates for a variety of infections caused by vancomycin-resistant *E. faecium* were approximately 70% with quinupristin/dalfopristin at a dose of 7.5 mg/kg every 8 to 12 hours (Moellering *et al.,* 1999). Quinupristin/dalfopristin should be reserved for treatment of serious infections caused by multiple-drug-resistant gram-positive organisms such as vancomycin-resistant *E. faecium.*

Untoward Effects. The most common side effects are infusion-related events, such as pain and phlebitis at the infusion site and arthralgias and myalgias. Phlebitis and pain can be minimized by infusion of drug through a central venous catheter. Arthalgias and myalgias, which are more likely to be a problem in patients with hepatic insufficiency and may be due to accumulation of metabolites, is managed by reducing the infusion frequency to every 12 hours. Quinupristin/dalfopristin is an inhibitor of cytochrome P450 enzyme 3A4 (CYP3A4). Drugs that are metabolized by CYP3A4 include terfenadine, astemizole, indinavir, nevirapine, midazolam, nifedipine and other calcium channel blockers, and cyclosporine. Concomitant administration of quinupristin/dalfopristin with these or other drugs metabolized by CYP3A4 may enhance drug effects and result in significant toxicity. Appropriate caution and monitoring are recommended for drugs in which the toxic therapeutic window is narrow or for drugs that cause QTc prolongation (*e.g.,* some antihistamines).

LINEZOLID

Linezolid (ZYVOX) is a synthetic antimicrobial agent of the oxazolidinone class (Zurenko *et al.,* 1996; Diekema and Jones, 2000). Its chemical structure is:

LINEZOLID

Antibacterial Activity. Linezolid is active against gram-positive organisms including staphylococci, streptococci, enterococci, gram-positive anaerobic cocci, and gram-positive rods such as *Corynebacterium* spp. and *Listeria monocytogenes* (Jones *et al.,* 1996; Zurenko *et al.,* 1996). It has poor activity against most gram-negative aerobic or anaerobic bacteria. It is bacteriostatic against enterococci and staphylococci and bactericidal against streptococci. MICs are ≤2 μg/ml against strains of *E. faecium, E. fae-calis, S. pyogenes, S. pneumoniae,* and viridans strains of streptococci. MICs are ≤4 μg/ml for strains of *S. aureus* and coagulase-negative staphylococci. *Mycobacterium tu-berculosis* is moderately susceptible with MICs of 2 μg/ml (Cynamon *et al.,* 1999). Because of its unique mechanism of action, linezolid is active against strains that are resistant to multiple other agents, including penicillin-resistant strains of *S. pneumoniae,* methicillin-resistant and van-comycin-intermediate strains of staphylococci, and vanco-mycin-resistant strains of enterococci.

Mechanism of Action. Linezolid inhibits protein synthesis. Linezolid prevents formation of the 70 S ribosome complex that initiates protein synthesis by binding to the 23 S subunit of the 50 S subunit. Because of its unique binding site and its action at the early, ribosome-assembly step of protein synthesis, there is no cross-resistance with other drug classes. Resistance is due to mutation of the ribosomal binding site (Kloss *et al.,* 1999; Hamel *et al.,* 2000). Resistance has been reported clinically only for enterococci, although resistant mutants have been selected from strains of *S. aureus* by passage in linezolid *in vitro.*

Absorption, Distribution and Excretion. Linezolid is well absorbed after oral administration. It may be administered without regard to food. With oral bioavailability approaching 100%, dosing for oral and intravenous preparations is the same. Peak serum concentrations average 12 to 14 μg/ml 1 to 2 hours after a single 600-mg dose in adults and approximately 20 μg/ml at steady state with dosing every 12 hours. The half-life is approximately 4 to 6 hours. Linezolid is 31% protein-bound and distributes widely to well-perfused tissues, with a 0.6 to 0.7 l/kg volume of distribution.

Linezolid is metabolized by nonenzymatic oxidation to aminoethoxyacetic acid and hydroxyethyl glycine metabolites. Approximately 80% of the dose of linezolid appears in the urine, 30% as active compound, and 50% as the two primary metabolites. Ten percent of the administered dose appears as metabolites in feces. Serum concentrations and half-life of the parent compound are not appreciably altered by renal insufficiency. The metabolites accumulate in renal insufficiency, with half-lives increasing by approximately 50% to 100%. The clinical significance of this is unknown, and no dose adjustment is recommended at this time. Linezolid and its metabolites are eliminated by dialysis; therefore, the drug should be administered following hemodialysis. No data concerning the effect of peritoneal dialysis are available.

Therapeutic Uses. Linezolid is approved by the United States Food and Drug Administration for treatment of infections caused by vancomycin-resistant *E. faecium;* nosocomial pneumonia caused by methicillin-susceptible and -resistant strains of *S. aureus;* community-acquired pneumonia caused by penicillin-susceptible strains of *S. pneumoniae;* complicated skin and skin-structure infections caused by streptococci and methicillin-susceptible and -resistant strains of *S. aureus;* and uncomplicated skin and skin-structure infections (Clemett and Markham, 2000). In noncomparative studies, linezolid (600 mg twice daily) has had clinical and microbiological cure rates in the range of 85% to 90% in treatment of a variety of infections (soft tissue, urinary tract and bacteremia) caused by vancomycin-resistant *E. faecium.* A 200-mg twice-daily dose was less effective, with a clinical cure rate of approximately 75% and a microbiological cure rate of only 59%. The 600-mg twice-daily dose and not the 200-mg dose, therefore, should be used for treatment of infections caused by enterococci. A 400-mg twice-daily dosage regimen is recommended only for treatment of uncomplicated skin and skin-structure infections.

In randomized, comparative studies, cures rates with linezolid (which were about 60%) were similar to those with vancomycin for nosocomial pneumonia caused by methicillin-resistant or -susceptible *S. aureus.* Efficacy of linezolid also was similar to that of either oxacillin or vancomycin for skin and skin-structure infections, the majority of microbiologically documented cases being caused by *S. aureus*. Although relatively few patients with *S. aureus* bacteremia have been treated, linezolid appears to be comparable in efficacy to vancomycin for methicillin-resistant strains. However, linezolid is bacteriostatic for staphylococci and enterococci, and it should not be used for treatment of suspected endocarditis.

Linezolid should be reserved as an agent of last resort for treatment of infections caused by multiple-drug-resistant strains. It should not be used when alternative agents are likely to be effective (*e.g.,* community-acquired pneumonia, even though it has the indication). Indiscriminant use and overuse will hasten selection of resistant strains and the eventual loss of this valuable new agent.

Untoward Effects. Data on toxicity and side effects are extremely limited at present. The drug seems to be well tolerated, with generally minor side effects (*e.g.,* gastrointestinal complaints, headache, rash) reported at rates no different from comparator agents in clinical trials. Thrombocytopenia or a significant reduction in platelet count has been associated with linezolid. The reported incidence is 2.4%, and its occurrence is related to duration of therapy. Platelet counts should be monitored in patients with risk of bleeding, preexisting thrombocytopenia, or intrinsic or acquired disorders of platelet function (including those potentially caused by concomitant medication) and in patients receiving courses of therapy lasting beyond two weeks. Linezolid is a weak, nonspecific monoamine-oxidase inhibitor. Patients receiving concomitant therapy with an adrenergic or serotonergic agent or consuming more than 100 mg of tyramine a day may experience an enhancement of drug effect. No other significant drug interactions have been identified. Specifically, linezolid is neither a substrate nor an inhibitor of cytochrome P450 enzymes.

SPECTINOMYCIN

Source and Chemistry. *Spectinomycin* is an antibiotic produced by *Streptomyces spectabilis*. The drug is an aminocyclitol; its structural formula is as follows:

SPECTINOMYCIN

Antibacterial Activity and Mechanism. Spectinomycin is active against a number of gram-negative bacterial species, but it is inferior to other drugs to which such microorganisms are susceptible (Schoutens *et al.,* 1972). Its only therapeutic use is in the treatment of gonorrhea caused by strains resistant to first-line drugs or if there are contraindications to the use of these drugs. Resistance, although rare, does occur (Clendennen *et al.,* 1992).

Spectinomycin selectively inhibits protein synthesis in gram-negative bacteria. The antibiotic binds to and acts on the 30 S ribosomal subunit. Its action is similar to that of the aminoglycosides; however, spectinomycin is not bactericidal and does not cause misreading of messenger RNA. Bacterial resistance may develop as a result of mutation or a modifying enzyme (Clark *et al.,* 1999).

Absorption, Distribution, and Excretion. Spectinomycin is rapidly absorbed after intramuscular injection. A single dose of 2 g produces peak serum concentrations of 100 μg/ml at 1 hour. Eight hours after injection, the concentration is approximately 15 μg/ml. The drug is not significantly bound to plasma protein, and all of an administered dose is recovered in the urine within 48 hours.

Therapeutic Uses. The Centers for Disease Control and Prevention recommends ceftriaxone, cefixime, ciprofloxacin, or ofloxacin for the treatment of uncomplicated gonococcal infection. However, spectinomycin is recommended as an alternative regimen in patients who are intolerant or allergic to β-lactam antibiotics and quinolones. Spectinomycin also is useful in pregnancy when patients are intolerant to β-lactams and when quinolones are contraindicated. The recommended dose for both men and women is a single, deep intramuscular injection of 2 g. One of the disadvantages of this regimen is that spectinomycin has no effect on incubating or established syphilis, and it is not active against *Chlamydia* spp. It also is less effective for pharyngeal infections, and follow-up cultures to document cure should be obtained.

Untoward Effects. Spectinomycin, when given as a single intramuscular injection, produces few significant untoward effects (Duncan *et al.,* 1972). Urticaria, chills, and fever have been noted after single doses, as have dizziness, nausea, and insomnia. The injection may be painful.

POLYMYXIN B AND COLISTIN

Because of the extreme nephrotoxicity associated with parenteral administration of these drugs, they are now rarely if ever used except topically.

Source and Chemistry. The *polymyxins,* discovered in 1947, are a group of closely related antibiotic substances elaborated by various strains of *Bacillus polymyxa,* an aerobic spore-forming rod found in soil. Colistin (polymyxin E) is produced by *Bacillus (Aerobacillus) colistinus,* a microorganism isolated from a soil sample obtained from Fukushima Prefecture, Japan. These drugs, which are cationic detergents, are relatively simple, basic peptides with molecular masses of about 1000 daltons. The structural formula for polymyxin B, which is itself a mixture of polymyxins B_1 and B_2, is as follows:

R—L-DAB—L-Thr—L-DAB—L-DAB
L-DAB—D-Phe—L-Leu
L-Thr—L-DAB—L-DAB

Polymyxin B_1: R = (+)-6-methyloctanoyl
Polymyxin B_2: R = 6-methylheptanoyl
DAB = α,γ-diaminobutyric acid

Colistin is polymyxin E, and it has a similar structure; it is available for clinical use as colistin sulfate, for oral use, and as colistimethate sodium, a parenteral preparation.

Antibacterial Activity and Mechanism of Action. The antimicrobial activities of polymyxin B and colistin are similar and are restricted to gram-negative bacteria, including *Enterobacter, E. coli, Klebsiella, Salmonella, Pasteurella, Bordetella,* and *Shigella,* which usually are sensitive to concentrations of 0.05 to 2.0 μg/ml. Most strains of *P. aeruginosa* are inhibited by less than 8 μg/ml *in vitro*.

Polymyxins are surface-active, amphipathic agents (containing both lipophilic and lipophobic groups within the molecule). They interact strongly with phospholipids and penetrate into and disrupt the structure of cell membranes. The permeability of the bacterial membrane changes immediately on contact with the drug. Sensitivity to polymyxin B apparently is related to the phospholipid content of the cell wall–membrane complex (Brown and Wood, 1972). The cell wall of certain resistant bacteria may prevent access of the drug to the cell membrane.

Polymyxin B binds to the lipid A portion of endotoxin (the lipopolysaccharide of the outer membrane of gram-negative bacteria) and inactivates this molecule. Polymyxin B attenuates pathophysiologic consequences of the release of endotoxin in several experimental systems (Shenep *et al.,* 1984; Tauber *et al.,* 1987). The clinical utility of polymixin B for this indication has not yet been established.

Absorption, Distribution, and Excretion. Neither polymyxin B nor colistin is absorbed when given orally. They are also poorly absorbed from mucous membranes and the surface of large burns.

Therapeutic Uses. *Polymyxin B sulfate* is available for ophthalmic, otic, and topical use in combination with a variety of other compounds. Although parenteral preparations are still marketed, they are not recommended.

Infections of the skin, mucous membranes, eye, and ear due to polymyxin B-sensitive microorganisms respond to local application of the antibiotic in solution or ointment. External otitis, frequently due to *Pseudomonas,* may be cured by the topical use of the drug. *P. aeruginosa* is a common cause of infection of corneal ulcers; local application or subconjunctival injection of polymyxin B often is curative.

Untoward Effects. Polymyxin B applied to intact or denuded skin or mucous membranes produces no systemic reactions because of its almost complete lack of absorption from these sites. Hypersensitization is uncommon with topical application. Adverse effects that follow the parenteral administration of these drugs are discussed in the *fifth edition* of this textbook.

VANCOMYCIN

History and Source. Vancomycin is an antibiotic produced by *Streptococcus orientalis,* an actinomycete isolated from soil samples obtained in Indonesia and India. Structurally related antimicrobial agents and daptomycin and LY333328 are investigational agents, and teicoplanin is available in Europe (Bernareggi *et al.,* 1992; Biavasco *et al.,* 1997).

Chemistry. Vancomycin is a complex and unusual tricyclic glycopeptide with a molecular mass of about 1500 daltons. Its structural formula was determined by x-ray analysis (Sheldrick *et al.,* 1978), and is as follows:

VANCOMYCIN

Antibacterial Activity. Vancomycin is primarily active against gram-positive bacteria. Strains are considered susceptible at MICs of ≤4 μg/ml. *S. aureus* and *S. epidermidis,* including strains resistant to methicillin, usually are inhibited by concentrations of 1.0 to 4.0 μg/ml (Fekety 1995). Strains of *S. aureus* (Hiramatsu *et al.,* 1997; Sieradzki *et al.,* 1999a; Smith *et al.,* 1999) and coagulase-negative staphylococci (Schwalbe *et al.,* 1987; Del' Alamo *et al.,* 1999; Garrett *et al.,* 1999) with reduced or "intermediate" susceptibility to vancomycin (MIC = 8 μg/ml) have been isolated. Infections caused by such strains have failed to respond to vancomycin clinically and in animal models (Climo *et al.,* 1999). These strains also are resistant to methicillin and multiple other antibiotics, and their emergence is a major concern, because vancomycin had been the only antibiotic to which staphylococci were reliably susceptible. Strains of enterococci also once were uniformly susceptible to vancomycin. Vancomycin-resistant strains of enterococci, primarily *Enterococcus faecium,* have emerged as major nosocomial pathogens in hospitals in the United States (Murray, 2000). Vancomycin resistance determinants in *E. faecium* and *E. faecalis* are located on a transposon which is itself part of a conjugative plasmid, rendering it readily transferable among enterococci and potentially other gram-positive bacteria (Walsh, 1993; Arthur and Courvalin, 1993). These strains typically are resistant to multiple antibiotics, including streptomycin, gentamicin, and ampicillin, effectively eliminating these as alternative therapeutic agents. Resistance to streptomycin and gentamicin is of special concern, because the combination of an aminoglycoside with a cell-wall-synthesis inhibitor is the only reliably bactericidal regimen for treatment of enterococcal infections.

S. pyogenes, S. pneumoniae, and viridans streptococci are highly susceptible to vancomycin. *Corynebacterium* spp. (diphtheroids) are inhibited by less than 0.04 to 3.1 μg/ml of vancomycin; most species of Actinomyces by 5 to 10 μg/ml; and *Clostridium* spp. by 0.39 to 6 μg/ml. Essentially all species of gram-negative bacilli and mycobacteria are resistant to vancomycin (*see* Cunha and Ristuccia, 1983).

Mechanisms of Action and Resistance. Vancomycin inhibits the synthesis of the cell wall in sensitive bacteria by binding with high affinity to the D-alanyl-D-alanine terminus of cell wall precursor units (*see* Figure 47–4). The drug is bactericidal for dividing microorganisms.

Enterococcal resistance to vancomycin is the result of alteration of the D-alanyl-D-alanine target to D-alanyl-D-lactate or D-alanyl-D-serine (Walsh, 1993; Arias *et al.,* 2000), which bind vancomycin poorly, because a critical site for hydrogen bonding is missing. Several enzymes within the *van* gene cluster are required for this target alteration to occur.

Several phenotypes of resistance to vancomycin have been described. The Van A phenotype confers resistance to both teicoplanin and vancomycin. The trait is inducible and has been identified in *E. faecium* and *E. faecalis.* The Van B phenotype, which tends to be a lower level of resistance, also has been identified in *E. faecium* and *E. faecalis.* The trait is inducible by vancomycin but not teicoplanin, and, consequently, many strains remain susceptible to teicoplanin. The Van C phenotype, the least important clinically and least well characterized, confers resistance only to vancomycin, is constitutive, and is present in no species of enterococci other than *E. faecalis* and *E. faecium.* Van D and Van E gene clusters also have been identified and others presumably will follow. The genetic and biochemical basis of reduced susceptibility to vancomycin in *Staphylococcus* is not well understood. Several genetic elements and multiple mutations are required. Many of the genes that have been implicated encode enzymes of the cell-wall biosynthetic pathway (Hanaki *et al.,* 1998; Sieradzki and Tomasz 1999; Sieradzki *et al.,* 1999b).

Absorption, Distribution, and Excretion. Vancomycin is poorly absorbed after oral administration, and large quantities are excreted in the stool. For parenteral therapy, the drug should be administered intravenously, never intramuscularly. A single intravenous dose of 1 g in adults produces plasma concentrations of 15 to 30 μg/ml 1 hour after a 1- to 2-hour infusion. The drug has a serum elimination half-life of about 6 hours (Matzke *et al.,* 1986). Approximately 30% of vancomycin is bound to plasma protein. Vancomycin appears in various body fluids, including the CSF when the meninges are inflamed (7% to 30%); bile; and pleural, pericardial, synovial, and ascitic fluids (Levine, 1987). About 90% of an injected dose is excreted by glomerular filtration. The drug accumulates if renal function is impaired, and dosage adjustments must be made under these circumstances (Moellering *et al.,* 1981). The drug can be cleared rapidly from plasma with the newer, high-flux methods of hemodialysis (Lanese *et al.,* 1989; Quale *et al.,* 1992).

Therapeutic Uses. *Vancomycin hydrochloride* (VANCOCIN, others) is marketed for *intravenous* use as a sterile powder for solution. It should be diluted and infused over at least a 60-minute period to avoid infusion-related adverse reactions (*see* below). The dose of vancomycin for adults is 30 mg/kg per day in 2 to 4 divided doses. A

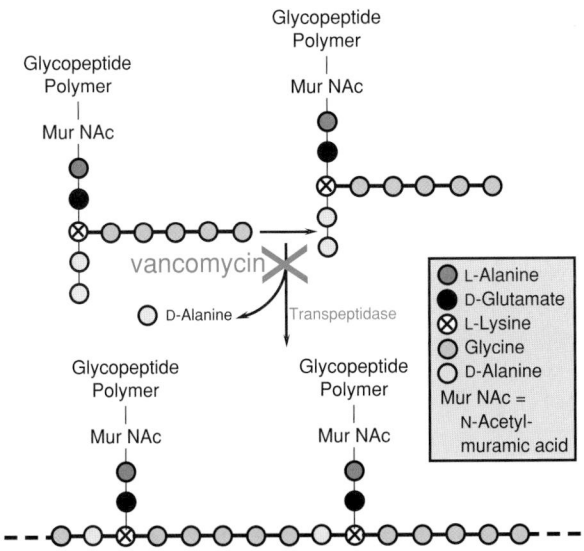

Figure 47–4. Inhibition of cell-wall synthesis in sensitive bacteria by vancomycin.

Vancomycin binds with high affinity to the D-alanyl-D-alanine terminus of cell wall precursor units, inhibits the release of the building block unit from the carrier, and thus prevents peptidoglycan synthesis. Resistance to vancomycin is due to expression of a unique enzyme that modifies the cell wall precursor so that it no longer binds vancomycin.

higher dose, 60 mg/kg per day in 4 divided doses, is recommended for meningitis (Quagliarello and Scheld, 1997). This regimen will yield an average steady-state concentration of 15 μg/ml in patients with normal renal function (*see* Moellering *et al.*, 1981). The "therapeutic range" for this agent is somewhat controversial, but a target trough concentration of 5 to 15 μg/ml is routinely recommended. It is not recommended that "peak" concentrations be monitored, as the distribution phase of the drug is long. The peak concentration should generally remain below 60 μg/ml to avoid ototoxicity.

Pediatric doses are as follows: for newborns during the first week of life, 15 mg/kg initially, followed by 10 mg/kg every 12 hours; for infants 8 to 30 days old, 15 mg/kg followed by 10 mg/kg every 8 hours; for older infants and children, 10 mg/kg every 6 hours (Schaad *et al.*, 1980). Alteration of dosage is required for patients with impaired renal function (*see* Appendix II). The drug has been used effectively in functionally anephric patients (who are being dialyzed) by the administration of 1 g (approximately 15 mg/kg) each week.

Vancomycin can be administered orally to patients with pseudomembranous colitis, although metronidazole is preferred. The dose for adults is 125 to 250 mg every 6 hours; the total daily dose for children is 40 mg/kg, given in three to four divided doses. *Vancomycin hydrochloride for oral solution* is available for this purpose, as are capsules.

Vancomycin should be employed only to treat serious infections and is particularly useful in the management of infections due to methicillin-resistant staphylococci, including pneumonia, empyema, endocarditis, osteomyelitis, and soft-tissue abscesses and in severe staphylococcal infections in patients who are allergic to penicillins and cephalosporins (Geraci, 1977). However, vancomycin is less rapidly bactericidal than any of the antistaphylococcal β-lactams (*e.g.*, nafcillin or cefazolin) and therefore may be less efficacious clinically (Levine *et al.*, 1991; Small and Chambers, 1990). Treatment with vancomycin is effective and convenient when there is disseminated staphylococcal infection or localized infection of a shunt in a patient with irreversible renal disease who is being maintained by hemodialysis or peritoneal dialysis, because the drug can be administered once weekly or in the dialysis fluid. Intraventricular administration of vancomycin (*via* a shunt or reservoir) has been necessary in a few cases of CNS infections due to susceptible microorganisms that did not respond to intravenous therapy alone (Visconti and Peter, 1979; Sutherland *et al.*, 1981).

Administration of vancomycin is an effective alternative for the treatment of endocarditis caused by viridans streptococci in patients who are allergic to penicillin. In combination with an aminoglycoside, it may be used for enterococcal endocarditis in patients with serious penicillin allergy. Vancomycin also is effective for the treatment of infections caused by *Flavobacterium* and *Corynebacterium* spp. Vancomycin has become an important antibiotic in the management of known or suspected penicillin-resistant pneumococcal infections (Friedland and McCracken, 1994).

Untoward Effects.   Among the hypersensitivity reactions produced by vancomycin are macular skin rashes and anaphylaxis. Phlebitis and pain at the site of intravenous injection are relatively uncommon. Chills, rash, and fever may occur. Rapid intravenous infusion may cause a variety of symptoms, including erythematous or urticarial reactions, flushing, tachycardia, and hypotension. The extreme flushing that can occur is sometimes called "red-neck" or "red-man" syndrome (Newfield and Roizen, 1979; Davis *et al.*, 1986).

Auditory impairment, which is frequently although not always permanent, may follow the use of this drug. Ototoxicity is associated with excessively high concentrations of the drug in plasma (60 to 100 μg/ml). Nephrotoxicity, formerly quite common probably because of less pure concentrations of the drug, has become an unusual side effect when appropriate doses are used, as judged by renal function and determinations of the concentration of the antibiotic in blood. Caution must be exercised, however, when other ototoxic or nephrotoxic drugs such as aminoglycosides are administered concurrently (Farber and Moellering, 1983), or in patients with impaired renal function.

TEICOPLANIN

Source and Chemistry.   Teicoplanin is a glycopeptide antibiotic produced by *Actinoplanes teichomyetius*. The drug actually is a mixture of six closely related compounds: one compound has a terminal hydrogen at the oxygen indicated by an asterisk; five compounds have an R substituent of either a decanoic acid [*n*-, 8-methyl-, 9-methyl-, (Z)-4-] or of a nonanoic acid [8-methyl]. Although not FDA-approved for use in the United States, it is available in Europe. It is similar to vancomycin in chemical structure, mechanism of action, spectrum of activity, and route of elimination (*i.e.*, primarily renal). Its structure is as follows:

TEICOPLANIN

Mechanisms of Action and Resistance. Teicoplanin, like vancomycin, is an inhibitor of cell-wall synthesis, and it is active only against gram-positive bacteria. It is reliably bactericidal against susceptible strains, except for enterococci. It is active against methicillin-susceptible and methicillin-resistant staphylococci, which typically have minimal inhibitory concentrations of <4 μg/ml (Wiedemann and Atkinson, 1991). Minimal inhibitory concentrations for *Listeria monocytogenes, Corynebacterium* spp., *Clostridium* spp., and anaerobic gram-positive cocci range from 0.25 to 2.0 μg/ml. Non-viridans and viridans streptococci, *S. pneumoniae,* and enterococci are inhibited by concentrations ranging from 0.01 to 1.0 μg/ml. Some strains of staphylococci, both coagulase-positive and coagulase-negative, as well as enterococci and other organisms that are intrinsically resistant to vancomycin (*i.e., Lactobacillus* spp. and *Leuconostoc* spp.) are resistant to teicoplanin.

The mechanisms of resistance to teicoplanin in strains of staphylococci have not been elucidated, but resistance can emerge in a previously susceptible strain during a course of therapy (Kaatz *et al.,* 1990). The Van A phenotype of vancomycin-resistant enterococci also determines resistance to teicoplanin. The mechanism is the same as for vancomycin: alteration of the cell wall target such that the glycopeptide does not bind. Strains of enterococci with Van B resistance often are susceptible to teicoplanin, because it is a poor inducer of the enzymes responsible for the cell wall alteration. Van C strains of enterococci, which in general are not human pathogens, are susceptible to teicoplanin (Arthur and Courvalin, 1993).

Absorption, Distribution, and Excretion. The primary differences between vancomycin and teicoplanin are that teicoplanin can be administered safely by intramuscular injection; it is highly bound by plasma proteins (90% to 95%); and it has an extremely long serum elimination half-life (up to 100 hours in patients with normal renal function). The dose of teicoplanin in adults is 6 to 30 mg/kg per day, with the higher dosages reserved for treatment of serious staphylococcal infections. Once-daily dosing is possible for the treatment of most infections because of the prolonged serum elimination half-life. As with vancomycin, teicoplanin doses must be adjusted in patients with renal insufficiency. For functionally anephric patients, administration once weekly has been appropriate, but serum drug concentrations should be monitored to determine that the therapeutic range has been maintained (*e.g.,* trough concentration of 15 to 20 μg/ml).

Therapeutic Uses. Teicoplanin has been used to treat a wide variety of infections, including osteomyelitis and endocarditis, caused by methicillin-resistant and methicillin-susceptible staphylococci, streptococci, and enterococci (Bibler *et al.,* 1987; Glupsczynski *et al.,* 1986). Teicoplanin has been found to be comparable to vancomycin in efficacy, except for treatment failures from low doses used to treat serious infections, such as endocarditis (Calain *et al.,* 1987). Teicoplanin is not as efficacious as antistaphylococcal penicillins for treating bacteremia and endocarditis caused by methicillin-susceptible *S. aureus,* with teicoplanin cure rates of 60% to 70% versus 85% to 90% for the penicillins. The efficacy of teicoplanin against *S. aureus* may be improved by the addition of an aminoglycoside (*e.g.,* gentamicin 1 mg/kg every 8 hours in patients with normal renal function) to provide a synergistic effect. Strains of streptococci are uniformly susceptible to teicoplanin. This drug has been very

effective in a once-daily regimen for patients with streptococcal osteomyelitis or endocarditis (Leport *et al.,* 1989). Teicoplanin is among the most active drugs against enterococci. Limited experience indicates that it is effective, although only bacteriostatic, for serious enterococcal infections. It should be combined with gentamicin to achieve a bactericidal effect in the treatment of enterococcal endocarditis.

Untoward Effects. The main side effect reported for teicoplanin is skin rash, which is more common in higher dosages. Hypersensitivity reactions, drug fever, and neutropenia also have been reported. Ototoxicity has occurred rarely.

BACITRACIN

History and Source. Bacitracin is an antibiotic produced by the Tracy-I strain of *Bacillus subtilis,* isolated in 1943 from the damaged tissue and street dirt debrided from a compound fracture in a young girl named Tracy; hence the name bacitracin. The history, properties, and uses of bacitracin have been reviewed by Meleney and Johnson (1949).

Chemistry. The bacitracins are a group of polypeptide antibiotics; multiple components have been demonstrated in the commercial products. The major constituent is bacitracin A. Its probable structural formula is as follows:

A unit of the antibiotic is equivalent to 26 μg of the USP standard.

Antibacterial Activity. A variety of gram-positive cocci and bacilli, *Neisseria, H. influenzae,* and *Treponema pallidum* are sensitive to 0.1 U or less of bacitracin per milliliter. *Actinomyces* and *Fusobacterium* are inhibited by concentrations of 0.5 to 5 U/ml. Enterobacteriaceae, *Pseudomonas, Candida* spp., and *Nocardia* are resistant to the drug. Bacitracin inhibits bacterial cell-wall synthesis.

Absorption, Fate, and Excretion. While bacitracin has been employed parenterally in the past and injectable products are still available, current use is restricted primarily to topical application.

Therapeutic Uses. *Bacitracin* is available in ophthalmic and dermatologic ointments; the antibiotic also is available in the form of a powder for the preparation of topical solutions. The ointments are applied directly to the involved surface one or more times daily. A number of topical preparations of bacitracin to which neomycin or polymyxin or both have been added are available, and some contain the three antibiotics plus hydrocortisone.

Topical bacitracin alone or in combination with other antimicrobial agents has no established value in the treatment of furunculosis, pyoderma, carbuncle, impetigo, and superficial and deep abscesses. For open infections such as infected eczema and infected dermal ulcers, the local application of the antibiotic may be of some help in eradicating sensitive bacteria. Bacitracin has an advantage over other antibiotics in that topical administration, even in an ointment, rarely produces hypersensitivity. Suppurative conjunctivitis and infected corneal ulcer respond well to the topical use of bacitracin when they are caused by susceptible bacteria. Bacitracin has been used with limited success for eradication of nasal carriage of staphylococci. Oral bacitracin has been used with some success for the treatment of antibiotic-associated diarrhea caused by *C. difficile* (Dudley *et al.,* 1986).

Untoward Effects.   Serious nephrotoxicity results from the parenteral use of this antibiotic. Hypersensitivity reactions result from topical application, but this is uncommon.

For further discussion of particular infections for which the antimicrobial agents discussed in this chapter are useful, see Chapters 141, 144, 149–169, and 174–181 in *Harrison's Principles of Internal Medicine,* 14th ed., McGraw-Hill, New York, 1998.

BIBLIOGRAPHY

Ackers, M.L., Puhr, N.D., Tauxe, R.V., and Mintz, E.D. Laboratory-based surveillance of *Salmonella* serotype *typhi* infections in the United States: antimicrobial resistance on the rise. *JAMA,* **2000,** *283*:2668–2673.

Ailani, R.K., Agastya, G., Ailani, R.K., Mukunda, B.N., and Shekar, R. Doxycycline is a cost-effective therapy for hospitalized patients with community-acquired pneumonia. *Arch. Intern. Med.,* **1999,** *159*:266–270.

Allignet, J., and El Solh, N. Comparative analysis of staphylococcal plasmids carrying three streptogramin-resistance genes: vat-vgb-vga. *Plasmid,* **1999,** *42*:134–138.

Allignet, J., Liassine, N., and el Solh, N. Characterization of a staphylococcal plasmid related to pUB110 and carrying two novel genes, vatC and vgbB, encoding resistance to streptogramins A and B and similar antibiotics. *Antimicrob. Agents Chemother.,* **1998,** *42*:1794–1798.

Amendola, M.A., and Spera, T.D. Doxycycline-induced esophagitis. *JAMA,* **1985,** *253*:1009–1011.

American Thoracic Society. Diagnosis and treatment of disease caused by nontuberculous mycobacteria. This official statement of the American Thoracic Society was approved by the Board of Directors, March 1997. Medical Section of the American Lung Association. *Am. J. Respir. Crit. Care Med.,* **1997,** *156*:S1–S25.

Aoyama, T., Sunakawa, K., Iwata, S., Takeuchi, Y., and Fujii, R. Efficacy of short-term treatment of pertussis with clarithromycin and azithromycin. *J. Pediatr.,* **1996,** *129*:761–764.

Arias, C.A., Courvalin, P., and Reynolds, P.E. vanC cluster of vancomycin-resistant *Enterococcus gallinarum* BM4174. *Antimicrob. Agents Chemother.,* **2000,** *44*:1660–1666.

Ariza, J., Gudiol, F., Pallares, R., Viladrich, P.F., Rufi, G., Corredoira, J., and Miravitlles, M.R. Treatment of human brucellosis with doxycycline plus rifampin or doxycycline plus streptomycin. A randomized, double-blind study. *Ann. Intern. Med.,* **1992,** *117*:25–30.

Arthur, M., and Courvalin, P. Genetics and mechanisms of glycopeptide resistance in enterococci. *Antimicrob. Agents Chemother.,* **1993,** *37*:1563–1571.

Bace, A., Zrnic, T., Begovac, J., Kuzmanovic, N., and Culig, J. Short-term treatment of pertussis with azithromycin in infants and young children. *Eur. J. Clin. Microbiol. Infect. Dis.,* **1999,** *18*:296–298.

Baine, W.B., Farmer, J.J. III, Gangarosa, E.J., Hermann, G.T., Thornsberry, C., and Rice, P.A. Typhoid fever in the United States associated with the 1972–1973 epidemic in Mexico. *J. Infect. Dis.,* **1977,** *135*:649–653.

Barthélémy, P., Autissier, D., Gerbaud, G., and Courvalin, P. Enzymatic hydrolysis of erythromycin by a strain of *Escherichia coli.* A new mechanism of resistance. *J. Antibiot. (Tokyo),* **1984,** *37*:1692–1696.

Bartlett, J.G., Breiman, R.F., Mandell, L.A., and File, T.M. Jr. Community-acquired pneumonia in adults: guidelines for management. The Infectious Diseases Society of America. *Clin. Infect. Dis.,* **1998,** *26*:811–838.

Bartz, Q.R. Isolation and characterization of chloromycetin. *J. Biol. Chem.,* **1948,** *172*:445–450.

Bernareggi, A., Borghi, A., Borgonovi, M., Cavenaghi, L., Ferrari, P., Vekey, K., Zanol, M., and Zerilli, L.F. Teicoplanin metabolism in humans. *Antimicrob. Agents Chemother.,* **1992,** *36*:1744–1749.

Biancaniello, T., Meyer, R.A., and Kaplan, S. Chloramphenicol and cardiotoxicity. *J. Pediatr.,* **1981,** *98*:828–830.

Biavasco, F., Vignaroli, C., Lupidi, R., Manso, E., Facinelli, B., and Varaldo, P.E. In vitro antibacterial activity of LY333328, a new semisynthetic glycopeptide. *Antimicrob. Agents Chemother.,* **1997,** *41*:2165–2172.

Bibler, M.R., Frame, P.T., Hagler, D.N., Bode, R.B., Staneck J.L., Thamlikitkul, V., Harris, J.E., Haregewoin, A., and Bullock, W.E. Jr. Clinical evaluation of efficacy, pharmacokinetics, and safety of teicoplanin for serious gram-positive infections. *Antimicrob. Agents Chemother.,* **1987,** *31*:207–212.

Black, J.R., Feinberg, J., Murphy, R.L., Fass, R.J., Finkelstein, D., Akil, B., Safrin, S., Carey, J.T., Stansell, J., Plouffe, J.F., He, W., Shelton, B., and Sattler, F.R. Clindamycin and primaquine therapy for mild-to-moderate episodes of *Pneumocystis carinii* pneumonia in patients with AIDS: AIDS clinical trials group 044. *Clin. Infect. Dis.,* **1994,** *18*:905–913.

Bowler, W.A., Hostettler, C., Samuelson, D., Lavin, B.S., and Oldfield, E.C. III. Gastrointestinal side effects of intravenous erythromycin: incidence and reduction with prolonged infusion time and glycopyrrolate pretreatment. *Am J Med.,* **1992,** *92*:249–253.

Bozdogan, B., and Leclercq, R. Effects of genes encoding resistance to streptogramins A and B on the activity of quinupristin-dalfopristin against *Enterococcus faecium. Antimicrob Agents Chemother.,* **1999,** *43*:2720–2725.

Brandriss, M.W., Richardson, W.S., and Barold, S.S. Erythromycin-induced QT prolongation and polymorphic ventricular tachycardia (torsades de pointes): case report and review. *Clin. Infect. Dis.,* **1994,** *18*:995–998.

Brisson-Noël, A., Trieu-Cuot, P., and Courvalin, P. Mechanism of action of spiramycin and other macrolides. *J. Antimicrob. Chemother.,* **1988,** *22 (suppl. B)*:13–23.

Brown, M.R., and Wood, S.M. Relation between cation and lipid content of cell walls of *Pseudomonas aeruginosa, Proteus vulgaris* and *Klebsiella aerogenes* and their sensitivity to polymyxin B and other antibacterial agents. *J. Pharm. Pharmacol.,* **1972,** *24*:215–218.

Calain, P., Krause, K.H., Vaudaux, P., Auckenthaler, R., Lew, D., Waldvogel, F., and Hirschel, B. Early termination of a prospective, randomized trial comparing teicoplanin and flucloxacillin for treating severe staphylococcal infection. *J. Infect. Dis.,* **1987,** *155*:187–191.

Carroll, K.C., Monroe, P., Cohen, S., Hoffman, M., Hamilton, L., Korgenski, K., Reimer, L., Classen, D., and Daly, J. Susceptibility of beta-hemolytic streptococci to nine antimicrobial agents among four medical centers in Salt Lake City, Utah, USA. *Diagn. Microbiol. Infect. Dis.,* **1997,** *27*:123–128.

Centers for Disease Control. Erythromycin-resistant *Bordetella pertussis*—Yuma County, Arizona, May–October 1994. *MMWR Morb. Mortal. Wkly. Rep.,* **1994,** *43*:807–810.

Centers for Disease Control and Prevention. 1998 guidelines for treatment of sexually transmitted diseases. *MMWR Morb. Mortal. Wkly. Rep.,* **1998,** *47*:1–111.

Chambers, H.F. Studies of RP-59500 *in vitro* and in a rabbit model of aortic valve endocarditis caused by methicillin-resistant *Staphylococcus aureus. J. Antimicrob. Chemother.,* **1992,** *30 (suppl. A)*:117–122.

Chan, G.P., Garcia-Ignacio, B.Y., Chavez, V.E., Livelo, J.B., Jimenez, C.L., Parrilla, M.L., and Franzblau, S.G. Clinical trial of clarithromycin for lepromatous leprosy. *Antimicrob. Agents Chemother.,* **1994,** *38*:515–517.

Chang, S.C., Fang, C.T., Hsueh, P.R., Luh, K.T., and Hsieh, W.C. In vitro activity of quinupristin/dalfopristin against clinical isolates of common gram-positive bacteria in Taiwan. *Diagn. Microbiol. Infect. Dis.,* **1999,** *33*:299–303.

Chu, S.-Y., Sennello, L.T., Bunnell, S.T., Varga, L.L., Wilson, D.S., and Sonders, R.C. Pharmacokinetics of clarithromycin, a new macrolide, after single ascending oral doses. *Antimicrob. Agents Chemother.,* **1992,** *36*:2447–2453.

Clark, N.C., Olsvik, O., Swenson, J.M., Spiegel, C.A., and Tenover, F.C. Detection of a streptomycin/spectinomycin adenylyltransferase gene (aadA) in *Enterococcus faecalis. Antimicrob. Agents Chemother.,* **1999,** *43*:157–160.

Clendennen, T.E., Echeverria, P., Saengeur, S., Kees, E.S., Boslego, J.W., and Wignall, F.S. Antibiotic susceptibility survey of *Neisseria gonorrhoeae* in Thailand. *Antimicrob. Agents Chemother.,* **1992,** *36*:1682–1687.

Climo, M.W., Patron, R.L., and Archer, G.L. Combinations of vancomycin and beta-lactams are synergistic against staphylococci with reduced susceptibilities to vancomycin. *Antimicrob. Agents Chemother.,* **1999,** *43*:1747–1753.

Cohlan, S.Q., Bevelander, G., and Tiamsic, T. Growth inhibition of prematures receiving tetracycline: clinical and laboratory investigation. *Am. J. Dis. Child.,* **1963,** *105*:453–461.

Craft, A.W., Brocklebank, J.T., Hey, E.N., and Jackson, R.H. The "grey toddler." Chloramphenicol toxicity. *Arch. Dis. Child.,* **1974,** *49*:235–237.

Cynamon, M.H., Klemens, S.P., Sharpe, C.A., and Chase, S. Activities of several novel oxazolidinones against *Mycobacterium tuberculosis* in a murine model. *Antimicrob. Agents Chemother.,* **1999,** *43*:1189–1191.

Dajani, A.S., Bisno, A.L., Chung, K.J., Durack, D.T., Freed, M., Gerber, M.A., Karchmer, A.W., Millard, H.D., Rahimtoola, S., Shulman, S.T., *et al.* Prevention of bacterial endocarditis. Recommendations by the American Heart Association. *JAMA,* **1990,** *264*:2919–2922.

Dajani, A.S., Taubert, K.A., Wilson, W., Bolger, A.F., Bayer, A., Ferrieri, P., Gewitz, M.H., Shulman, S.T., Nouri, S., Newburger, J.W., Hutto, C., Pallasch, T.J., Gage, T.W., Levison, M.E., Peter, G., Zuccaro, G. Jr. Prevention of bacterial endocarditis: recommendations by the American Heart Association. *Clin. Infect. Dis.,* **1997,** *25*:1448–1458.

Dannemann, B., McCutchan, J.A., Israelski, D., Antoniskis, D., Leport, C., Luft, B., Nussbaum, J., Clumeck, N., Morlat, P., Chiu, J., Vilde, J.-L., Orellana, M., Feigal, D., Bartok, A., Heseltine, P., Leedom, J., and Remington, J. Treatment of toxoplasmic encephalitis in patients with AIDS. A randomized trial comparing pyrimethamine plus clindamycin to pyrimethamine plus sulfadiazine. The California Collaborative Treatment Group. *Ann. Intern. Med.,* **1992,** *116*:33–43.

Davis, R.L., Smith, A.L., and Koup, J.R. The "red man's syndrome" and slow infusion of vancomycin. *Ann. Intern. Med.,* **1986,** *104*:285–286.

Del' Alamo, L., Cereda, R.F., Tosin, I., Miranda, E.A., and Sader, H.S. Antimicrobial susceptibility of coagulase-negative staphylococci and characterization of isolates with reduced susceptibility to glycopeptides. *Diagn. Microbiol. Infect. Dis.,* **1999,** *34*:185–191.

DiPiro, J.T. Considerations for therapy of mixed infections: focus on intraabdominal infection. *Pharmacotherapy,* **1995,** *15*:15S–21S.

Doern, G.V., Brueggemann, A.B., Pierce, G., Holley, H.P. Jr., and Rauch, A. Antibiotic resistance among clinical isolates of *Haemophilus influenzae* in the United States in 1994 and 1995 and detection of beta-lactamase-positive strains resistant to amoxicillin-clavulanate: results of a national multicenter surveillance study. *Antimicrob. Agents Chemother.,* **1997,** *41*:292–297.

Doern, G.V., Pfaller, M.A., Kugler, K., Freeman, J., and Jones, R.N. Prevalence of antimicrobial resistance among respiratory tract isolates of *Streptococcus pneumoniae* in North America: 1997 results from the SENTRY antimicrobial surveillance program. *Clin. Infect. Dis.,* **1998,** *27*:764–770.

Dudley, M.N., McLaughlin, J.C., Carrington, G., Frick, J., Nightingale, C.H., and Quintiliani, R. Oral bacitracin vs. vancomycin therapy for *Clostridium difficile*–induced diarrhea. A randomized double-blind trial. *Arch. Intern. Med.,* **1986,** *146*:1101–1104.

Duncan, W.C., Holder, W.R., Roberts, D.P., and Knox, J.M. Treatment of gonorrhea with spectinomycin hydrochloride: comparison with standard penicillin schedules. *Antimicrob. Agents Chemother.,* **1972,** *1*:210–214.

Elmore, M.F., and Rogge, J.D. Tetracycline-induced pancreatitis. *Gastroenterology,* **1981,** *81*:1134–1136.

Esposito, S., Noviello, S., Ianniello, F., and D'Errico, G. Erythromycin resistance in group A beta hemolytic streptococcus. *Chemotherapy,* **1998,** *44*:385–390.

Fagon, J., Patrick, H., Haas, D.W., Torres, A., Gibert, C., Cheadle, W.G., Falcone, R.E., Anholm, J.D., Paganin, F., Fabian, T.C., and Lilienthal, F. Treatment of gram-positive nosocomial pneumonia. Prospective randomized comparison of quinupristin/dalfopristin versus vancomycin. Nosocomial Pneumonia Group. *Am. J. Respir. Crit. Care Med.,* **2000,** *161*:753–762.

Fanning, W.L., Gump, D.W., and Sofferman, R.A. Side effects of minocycline: a double-blind study. *Antimicrob. Agents Chemother.,* **1977,** *11*:712–717.

Fantin, B., Leclercq, R., Merle, Y., Saint-Julien, L., Veyrat, C., Duval, J., and Carbon, C. Critical influence of resistance to streptogramin B-type antibiotics on activity of RP 59500 (quinupristin-dalfopristin) in experimental endocarditis due to *Staphylococcus aureus. Antimicrob. Agents Chemother.,* **1995,** *39*:400–405.

Farber, B.F., and Moellering, R.C. Jr. Retrospective study of the toxicity of preparations of vancomycin from 1974 to 1981. *Antimicrob. Agents Chemother.,* **1983,** *23*:138–141.

Fass, R.J. Erythromycin, clarithromycin, and azithromycin: use of frequency distribution curves, scattergrams, and regression analyses to compare *in vitro* activities and describe cross-resistance. *Antimicrob. Agents Chemother.,* **1993,** *37*:2080–2086.

Fogdall, R.P., and Miller, R.D. Prolongation of a pancuronium-induced neuromuscular blockade by clindamycin. *Anesthesiology,* **1974,** *41*:407–408.

Fraschini, F., Scaglione, F., and Demartini, G. Clarithromycin clinical pharmacokinetics. *Clin. Pharmacokinet.,* **1993,** *25*:189–204.

Freundlich, M., Cynamon, H., Tamer, A., Steele, B., Zilleruelo, G., and Strauss, J. Management of chloramphenicol intoxication in infancy by charcoal hemoperfusion. *J. Pediatr.,* **1983,** *103*:485–487.

Friedland, I.R., and McCracken G.H. Jr. Management of infections caused by antibiotic-resistant *Streptococcus pneumoniae. N. Engl. J. Med.,* **1994,** *331*:377–382.

Friedman, C.A., Lovejoy, F.C., and Smith, A.L. Chloramphenicol disposition in infants and children. *J. Pediatr.,* **1979,** *95*:1071–1077.

Gaffney, D.F., and Foster, T.J. Chloramphenicol acetyltransferase determined by R plasmids from gram-negative bacteria. *J. Gen. Microbiol.,* **1978,** *109*:351–358.

Garey, K.W., and Amsden, G.W. Intravenous azithromycin. *Ann. Pharmacother.,* **1999,** *33*:218–228.

Garrett, D.O., Jochimsen, E., Murfitt, K., Hill, B., McAllister, S., Nelson, P., Spera, R.V., Sall, R.K., Tenover, F.C., Johnston, J., Zimmer, B., and Jarvis, W.R. The emergence of decreased susceptibility to vancomycin in *Staphylococcus epidermidis. Infect. Control Hosp. Epidemiol.,* **1999,** *20*:167–170.

Gatti, G., Malena, M., Casazza, R., Borin, M., Bassetti, M., and Cruciani, M. Penetration of clindamycin and its metabolite N-demethylclindamycin into cerebrospinal fluid following intravenous infusion of clindamycin phosphate in patients with AIDS. *Antimicrob. Agents Chemother.,* **1998,** *42*:3014–3017.

Glupczynski, Y., Lagast, H., Van der Auwera, P., Thys, J.P., Crokaert, E., Yourassowsky, E., Meunier-Carpentier, F., Klastersky, J., Kains, J.P., Serruys-Schoutens, E., and Legrand, J.C. Clinical evaluation of teicoplanin for therapy of severe infections caused by gram-positive bacteria. *Antimicrob. Agents Chemother.,* **1986,** *29*:52–57.

Godel, V., Nemet, P., and Lazar, M. Chloramphenicol optic neuropathy. *Arch. Ophthalmol.,* **1980,** *98*:1417–1421.

Hall, A.P., Doberstyn, E.B., Nanokorn, A., and Sonkom, P. *Falciparum* malaria semiresistant to clindamycin. *Br. Med. J.,* **1975,** *2*:12–14.

Halperin, S.A., Bortolussi, R., Langley, J.M., Miller, B., and Eastwood, B.J. Seven days of erythromycin estolate is as effective as fourteen days for the treatment of *Bordetella pertussis* infections. *Pediatrics,* **1997,** *100*:65–71.

Halpert, J. Further studies of the suicide inactivation of purified rat liver cytochrome P-450 by chloramphenicol. *Mol. Pharmacol.,* **1982,** *21*:166–172.

Hanaki, H., Labischinski, H., Inaba, Y., Kondo, N., Murakami, H., and Hiramatsu, K. Increase in glutamine-non amidated muropeptides in

the peptidoglycan of vancomycin-resistant *Staphylococcus aureus* strain Mu50. *J. Antimicrob. Chemother.,* **1998,** *42*:315–320.

Harnett, N., Brown, S., Terro, R., Krishnan, C., Pauze, M., and Yeung, K.H. High-level tetracycline-resistant *Neisseria gonorrhoeae* in Ontario, Canada—investigation of a cluster of isolates, showing chromosomally mediated resistance to penicillin combined with plasmid-mediated resistance to tetracycline. *J. Infect. Dis.,* **1997,** *176*:1269–1276.

Hiramatsu, K., Aritaka, N., Hanaki, H., Kawasaki, S., Hosoda, Y., Hori, S., Fukuchi, Y., and Kobayashi, I. Dissemination in Japanese hospitals of strains of *Staphylococcus aureus* heterogeneously resistant to vancomycin. *Lancet,* **1997,** *350*:1670–1673.

Holt, R. The bacterial degradation of chloramphenicol. *Lancet,* **1967,** *1*:1259–1260.

Honig, P.K., Woosley, R.L., Zamani, K., Conner, D.P., and Cantilena, L.R. Jr. Changes in the pharmacokinetics and electrocardiographic pharmacodynamics of terfenadine with concomitant administration of erythromycin. *Clin. Pharmacol. Ther.,* **1992,** *52*:231–238.

Hunt, R.H., Fallone, C.A., and Thomson, A.B. Canadian *Helicobacter pylori* Consensus Conference update: infections in adults. Canadian *Helicobacter* Study Group. *Can. J. Gastroenterol.,* **1999,** *13*:213–217.

Ji, B., Jamet, P., Perani, E.G., Bobin, P., and Grosset, J.H. Powerful bactericidal activities of clarithromycin and minocycline against *Mycobacterium leprae* in lepromatous leprosy. *J. Infect. Dis.,* **1993,** *168*:188–190.

Jimenez, J.J., Arimura, G.K., Abou-Khalil, W.H., Isildar, M., and Yunis, A.A. Chloramphenicol-induced bone marrow injury: possible role of bacterial metabolites of chloramphenicol. *Blood,* **1987,** *70*:1180–1185.

Johnson, C.A., Taylor, C.A. III, Zimmerman, S.W., Bridson, W.E., Chevalier, P., Pasquier, O., and Baybutt, R.I. Pharmacokinetics of quinupristin-dalfopristin in continuous ambulatory peritoneal dialysis patients. *Antimicrob. Agents Chemother.,* **1999,** *43*:152–156.

Jones, F.E., and Hanson, D.R. *H. influenzae* meningitis treated with ampicillin or chloramphenicol, and subsequent hearing loss. *Dev. Med. Child Neurol.,* **1977,** *19*:593–597.

Jones, R.N., Johnson, D.M., and Erwin, M.E. In vitro antimicrobial activities and spectra of U-100592 and U-100766, two novel fluorinated oxazolidinones. *Antimicrob. Agents Chemother.,* **1996,** *40*:720–726.

Kaatz, G.W., Seo, S.M., Dorman, N.J., and Lerner, S.A. Emergence of teicoplanin resistance during therapy of *Staphylococcus aureus* endocarditis. *J. Infect. Dis.,* **1990,** *162*:103–108.

Kager, L., Liljeqvist, L., Malmborg, A.S., and Nord, C.E. Effect of clindamycin prophylaxis on the colonic microflora in patients undergoing colorectal surgery. *Antimicrob. Agents Chemother.,* **1981,** *20*:736–740.

Karmody, C.S., and Weinstein, L. Reversible sensorineural hearing loss with intravenous erythromycin lactobionate. *Ann. Otol. Rhinol. Laryngol.,* **1977,** *86*:9–11.

Katlama, C., De Wit, S., O'Doherty, E., Van Glabeke, M., and Clumeck, N. Pyrimethamine-clindamycin vs. pyrimethamine-sulfadiazine as acute and long-term therapy for toxoplasmic encephalitis in patients with AIDS. *Clin. Infect. Dis.,* **1996,** *22*:268–275.

Khan, W.A., Bennish, M.L., Seas, C., Khan, E.H., Ronan, A., Dhar, U., Busch, W., and Salam, M.A. Randomised controlled comparison of single-dose ciprofloxacin and doxycycline for cholera caused by *Vibrio cholerae* 01 or 0139. *Lancet,* **1996,** *348*:296–300.

Kloss, P., Xiong, L., Shinabarger, D.L., and Mankin, A.S. Resistance mutations in 23 S rRNA identify the site of action of the protein synthesis inhibitor linezolid in the ribosomal peptidyl transferase center. *J. Mol. Biol.,* **1999,** *294*:93–101.

Koskiniemi, M., Pettay, O., Raivio, M., and Sarna, S. *Haemophilus influenzae* meningitis. A comparison between chloramphenicol and ampicillin therapy with special reference to impaired hearing. *Acta Paediatr. Scand.,* **1978,** *67*:17–24.

Koup, J.R., Lau, A.H., Brodsky, B., and Slaughter, R.L. Chloramphenicol pharmacokinetics in hospitalized patients. *Antimicrob. Agents Chemother.,* **1979,** *15*:651–657.

Kovacs, J.A., and Masur, H. Prophylaxis against opportunistic infections in patients with human immunodeficiency virus infection. *N. Engl. J. Med.,* **2000,** *342*:1416–1429.

Kramer, P.W., Griffith, R.S., and Campbell, R.L. Antibiotic penetration of the brain. A comparative study. *J. Neurosurg.,* **1969,** *31*:295–302.

Lanese, D.M., Alfrey, P.S., and Molitoris, B.A. Rapid vancomycin removal during high flux hemodialysis necessitates supplementation to maintain therapeutic levels. *Kidney Int.,* **1989,** *35*:253.

Leport, C., Perronne, C., Massip, P., Canton, P., Leclerq, P., Bernard, E., Lutun, P., Garaud, J.J., and Vilde, J.-L. Evaluation of teicoplanin for treatment of endocarditis caused by gram-positive cocci in 20 patients. *Antimicrob. Agents Chemother.,* **1989,** *33*:871–876.

Levine, D.P., Fromm, B.S., and Reddy, B.R. Slow response to vancomycin or vancomycin plus rifampin in methicillin-resistant *Staphylococcus aureus* endocarditis. *Ann. Intern. Med.,* **1991,** *115*:674–680.

Levine, P.H., Regelson, W., and Holland, J.F. Chloramphenicol-associated encephalopathy. *Clin. Pharmacol. Ther.,* **1970,** *11*:194–199.

Levison, M.E., Mangura, C.T., Lorber, B., Abrutyn, E., Pesanti, E.L., Levy, R.S., MacGregor, R.R., and Schwartz, A.R. Clindamycin compared with penicillin for the treatment of anaerobic lung abscess. *Ann. Intern. Med.,* **1983,** *98*:466–471.

McCormack, W.M., George, H., Donner, A., Kodgis, L.F., Alpert, S., Lowe, E.W., and Kass, E.H. Hepatotoxicity of erythromycin estolate during pregnancy. *Antimicrob. Agents Chemother.,* **1977,** *12*:630–635.

McDonald, P.J., and Pruul, H. Phagocyte uptake and transport of azithromycin. *Eur. J. Clin Microbiol. Infect Dis.,* **1991,** *10*:828–833.

Martell, R., Heinrichs, D., Stiller, C.R., Jenner, M., Keown, P.A., and Dupre, J. The effects of erythromycin in patients treated with cyclosporine. *Ann. Intern. Med.,* **1986,** *104*:660–661.

Matzke, G.R., Zhanel, G.G., and Guay, D.R.P. Clinical pharmacokinetics of vancomycin. *Clin. Pharmacokinet.,* **1986,** *11*:257–282.

Misiewicz, J.J., Harris, A.W., Bardhan, K.D., Levi, S., O'Morain, C., Cooper, B.T., Kerr, G.D., Dixon, M.F., Langworthy, H., and Piper, D. One week triple therapy for *Helicobacter pylori*: a multicentre comparative study. Lansoprazole Helicobacter Study Group. *Gut,* **1997,** *41*:735–739.

Moellering, R.C. Jr., Krogstad, D.J., and Greenblatt, D.J. Vancomycin therapy in patients with impaired renal function: a nomogram for dosage. *Ann. Intern. Med.,* **1981,** *94*:343–346.

Moellering, R.C., Linden, P.K., Reinhardt, J., Blumberg, E.A., Bompart, F., and Talbot, G.H. The efficacy and safety of quinupristin/dalfopristin for the treatment of infections caused by vancomycin-resistant *Enterococcus faecium*. Synercid Emergency-Use Study Group. *J. Antimicrob. Chemother.,* **1999,** *44*:251–261.

Molavi, A., and Weinstein, L. *In-vitro* activity of erythromycin against atypical mycobacteria. *J. Infect. Dis.,* **1971,** *123*:216–219.

Mulhall, A., de Louvois, J., and Hurley, R. The pharmacokinetics of chloramphenicol in the neonate and young infant. *J. Antimicrob. Chemother.,* **1983,** *12*:629–639.

Newfield, P., and Roizen, M.F. Hazards of rapid administration of vancomycin. *Ann. Intern. Med.,* **1979,** *91*:581.

Nichols, R.L., Graham, D.R., Barriere, S.L., Rodgers, A., Wilson, S.E., Zervos, M., Dunn, D.L., and Kreter, B. Treatment of hospitalized

patients with complicated gram-positive skin and skin structure infections: two randomized, multicentre studies of quinupristin/dalfopristin versus cefazolin, oxacillin or vancomycin. Synercid Skin and Skin Structure Infection Group. *J. Antimicrob. Chemother.,* **1999,** *44*:263–273.

Nord, C.E., and Heimdahl, A. Impact of different antimicrobial agents on the colonisation resistance in the intestinal tract with special reference to doxycycline. *Scand. J. Infect. Dis. Suppl.,* **1988,** *53*:50–58.

Panzer, J.D., Brown, D.C., Epstein, W.L., Lipson, R.L., Mahaffrey, H.W., and Atkinson, W.H. Clindamycin levels in various body tissues and fluids. *J. Clin. Pharmacol. New Drugs,* **1972,** *12*:259–262.

Periti, P., Mazzei, T., Mini, E., and Novelli, A. Pharmacokinetic drug interactions of macrolides. *Clin. Pharmacokinet.,* **1992,** *23*:106–131.

Peterson, W.L., Fendrick, A.M., Cave, D.R., Peura, D.A., Garabedian-Ruffalo, S.M., and Laine, L. *Helicobacter pylori*–related disease: guidelines for testing and treatment. *Arch. Intern. Med.,* **2000,** *160*:1285–1291.

Prats, G., Mirelis, B., Llovet, T., Munoz, C., Miro, E., and Navarro, F. Antibiotic resistance trends in enteropathogenic bacteria isolated in 1985–1987 and 1995–1998 in Barcelona. *Antimicrob. Agents Chemother.,* **2000,** *44*:1140–1145.

Quale, J.M., O'Halloran, J.J., DeVincenzo, N., and Barth, R.H. Removal of vancomycin by high-flux hemodialysis membranes. *Antimicrob. Agents. Chemother.,* **1992,** *36*:1424–1426.

Rahal, J.J. Jr., and Simberkoff, M.S. Bactericidal and bacteriostatic action of chloramphenicol against meningeal pathogens. *Antimicrob. Agents Chemother.,* **1979,** *16*:13–18.

Rasch, J.R., and Mogabgab, W.J. Therapeutic effect of erythromycin on *Mycoplasma pneumoniae* pneumonia. *Antimicrob. Agents Chemother.,* **1965,** *5*:693–699.

Rehg, J.E. Activity of azithromycin against cryptosporidia in immunosuppressed rats. *J. Infect. Dis.,* **1991,** *163*:1293–1296.

Replogle, M.L., Fleming, D.W., and Cieslak, P.R. Emergence of antimicrobial-resistant shigellosis in Oregon. *Clin. Infect. Dis.,* **2000,** *30*:515–519.

Rifkin, G.D., Fekety, F.R., and Silva, J. Jr. Antibiotic-induced colitis: implication of a toxin neutralized by *Clostridium sordellii* antitoxin. *Lancet,* **1977,** *2*:1103–1106.

Saba, J., Morlat, P., Raffi, F., Hazebroucq, V., Joly, V., Leport, C., and Vilde J.L. Pyrimethamine plus azithromycin for treatment of acute toxoplasmic encephalitis in patients with AIDS. *Eur. J. Clin. Microbiol. Infect. Dis.,* **1993,** *12*:853–856.

Sabath, L.D., Gerstein, D.A., Loder, P.B., and Finland, M. Excretion of erythromycin and its enhanced activity in urine against gram-negative bacilli with alkalinization. *J. Lab. Clin. Med.,* **1968,** *72*:916–923.

Salazar-Lindo, E., Sack, R.B., Chea-Woo, E., Kay, B.A., Piscoya, Z.A., Leon-Barua, R., and Yi, A. Early treatment with erythromycin of *Campylobacter jejuni*–associated dysentery in children. *J. Pediatr.,* **1986,** *109*:355–360.

Schaad, U.B., McCracken, G.H. Jr., and Nelson, J.D. Clinical pharmacology and efficacy of vancomycin in pediatric patients. *J. Pediatr.,* **1980,** *96*:119–126.

Scheld, W.M., Brown, R.S. Jr., Fletcher, D.D., and Sande, M.A. Bactericidal versus bacteriostatic antibiotic therapy of experimental pneumococcal meningitis. *Ann. Clin. Res.,* **1979,** *27*:355a.

Schoutens, E., Peromet, M., and Yourassowsky, E. Microbiological and clinical study of spectinomycin in urinary tract infections: reevaluation with hospital strains. *Curr. Ther. Res. Clin. Exp.,* **1972,** *14*:349–357.

Schwalbe, R.S., Stapleton, J.T., and Gilligan, P.H. Emergence of vancomycin resistance in coagulase-negative staphylococci. *N. Engl. J. Med.*, **1987**, *316*:927–931.

Seaberg, L.S., Parquette, A.R., Gluzman, I.Y., Phillips, G.W. Jr., Brodasky, T.F., and Krogstad, D.J. Clindamycin activity against chloroquine-resistant *Plasmodium falciparum*. *Antimicrob. J. Infect. Dis.*, **1984**, *150*:904–911.

Seifert, C.F., Swaney, R.J., and Bellanger-McCleery, R.A. Intravenous erythromycin lactobionate-induced severe nausea and vomiting. *DICP*, **1989**, *23*:40–44.

Seppala, H., Klaukka, T., Vuopio-Varkila, J., Muotiala, A., Helenius, H., Lager, K., and Huovinen, P. The effect of changes in the consumption of macrolide antibiotics on erythromycin resistance in group A streptococci in Finland. Finnish Study Group for Antimicrobial Resistance. *N. Engl. J. Med.*, **1997**, *337*:441–446.

Shann, F., Linnemann, V., Mackenzie, A., Barker, J., Gratten, M., and Crinis, N. Absorption of chloramphenicol sodium succinate after intramuscular administration in children. *N. Engl. J. Med.*, **1985**, *313*:410–414.

Sheldrick, G.M., Jones, P.G., Kennard, O., Williams, D.H., and Smith, G.A. Structure of vancomycin and its complex with acyl-D-alanyl-D-alanine. *Nature*, **1978**, *271*:223–225.

Shenep, J.L., Barton, R.P., and Mogan, K.A. Role of antibiotic class in the rate of liberation of endotoxin during therapy for experimental gram-negative bacterial sepsis. *J. Infect. Dis.*, **1984**, *151*:1012–1018.

Shu, X.O., Gao, Y.T., Linet, M.S., Brinton, L.A., Gao, R.N., Jin, F., and Fraumeni, J.F. Jr. Chloramphenicol use and childhood leukemia in Shanghai. *Lancet*, **1987**, *2*:934–937.

Sieradzki, K., and Tomasz, A. Gradual alterations in cell wall structure and metabolism in vancomycin-resistant mutants of *Staphylococcus aureus*. *J. Bacteriol.*, **1999**, *181*:7566–7570.

Sieradzki, K., Roberts, R.B., Haber, S.W., and Tomasz, A. The development of vancomycin resistance in a patient with methicillin-resistant *Staphylococcus aureus* infection. *N. Engl. J. Med.*, **1999a**, *340*:517–523.

Sieradzki, K., Wu, S.W., and Tomasz, A. Inactivation of the methicillin resistance gene mecA in vancomycin-resistant *Staphylococcus aureus*. *Microb. Drug Resist.*, **1999b**, *5*:253–237.

Slaughter, R.L., Pieper, J.A., Cerra, F.B., Brodsky, B., and Koup, J.R. Chloramphenicol sodium succinate kinetics in critically ill patients. *Clin. Pharmacol. Ther.*, **1980**, *28*:69–77.

Small, P.M., and Chambers, H.F. Vancomycin for *Staphylococcus aureus* endocarditis in intravenous drug users. *Antimicrob. Agents Chemother.*, **1990**, *34*:1227–1231.

Smith, A.J., Nissan, A., Lanouette, N.M., Shi, W., Guillem, J.G., Wong, W.D., Thaler, H., and Cohen, A.M. Prokinetic effect of erythromycin after colorectal surgery: randomized, placebo-controlled, double-blind study. *Dis. Colon Rectum*, **2000**, *43*:333–337.

Smith, T.L., Pearson, M.L., Wilcox, K.R., Cruz, C., Lancaster, M.V., Robinson-Dunn, B., Tenover, F.C., Zervos, M.J., Band, J.D., White, E., and Jarvis, W.R. Emergence of vancomycin resistance in *Staphylococcus aureus*. Glycopeptide-Intermediate *Staphylococcus aureus* Working Group. *N. Engl. J. Med.*, **1999**, *340*:493–501.

Soltani, M., Beighton, D., Philpott-Howard, J., and Woodford, N. Mechanisms of resistance to quinupristin-dalfopristin among isolates of *Enterococcus faecium* from animals, raw meat, and hospital patients in Western Europe. *Antimicrob. Agents Chemother.*, **2000**, *44*:433–436.

Speer, B.S., Shoemaker, N.B. and Salyers, A.A. Bacterial resistance to tetracycline: mechanisms, transfer, and clinical significance. *Clin. Microbiol. Rev.*, **1992**, *5*:387–399.

Stout, J.E., Arnold, B., and Yu, V.L. Activity of azithromycin, clarithromycin, roxithromycin, dirithromycin, quinupristin/dalfopristin and erythromycin against *Legionella* species by intracellular susceptibility testing in HL-60 cells. *J. Antimicrob. Chemother.*, **1998**, *41*:289–291.

Sutherland, G.E., Palitang, E.G., Marr, J.J., and Luedke, S.L. Sterilization of Ommaya reservoir by instillation of vancomycin. *Am. J. Med.*, **1981**, *71*:1068–1070.

Tally, F.P., Snydman, D.R., Gorbach, S.L., and Malamy, M.H. Plasmid-mediated transferable resistance to clindamycin and erythromycin in *Bacteroides fragilis*. *J. Infect. Dis.*, **1979**, *139*:83–88.

Tauber, M.G., Shibl, A.M., Hackbarth, C.J., Larrick, J.W., and Sande, M.A. Antibiotic therapy, endotoxin concentration in cerebrospinal fluid, and brain edema in experimental *Escherichia coli* meningitis in rabbits. *J. Infect. Dis.*, **1987**, *156*:456–462.

Thornsberry, C., Jones, M.E., Hickey, M.L., Mauriz, Y., Kahn, J., and Sahm, D.F. Resistance surveillance of *Streptococcus pneumoniae*, *Haemophilus influenzae* and *Moraxella catarrhalis* isolated in the United States, 1997–1998. *J. Antimicrob. Chemother.*, **1999**, *44*:749–759.

Thornsberry, C., Ogilvie, P., Kahn, J., and Mauriz, Y. Surveillance of antimicrobial resistance in *Streptococcus pneumoniae*, *Haemophilus influenzae*, and *Moraxella catarrhalis* in the United States in 1996–1997 respiratory season. The Laboratory Investigator Group. *Diagn. Microbiol. Infect. Dis.*, **1997**, *29*:249–257.

Tolman, K.G., Sannella, J.J., and Freston, J.W. Chemical structure of erythromycin and hepatotoxicity. *Ann. Intern. Med.*, **1974**, *81*:58–60.

Toma, E., Fournier, S., Dumont, M., Bolduc, P., and Deschamps, H. Clindamycin/primaquine versus trimethoprim-sulfamethoxazole as primary therapy for *Pneumocystis carinii* pneumonia in AIDS: a randomized, double-blind pilot trial. *Clin. Infect. Dis.*, **1993**, *17*:178–184.

Visconti, E.B., and Peter, G. Vancomycin treatment of cerebrospinal fluid shunt infections. Report of two cases. *J. Neurosurg.*, **1979**, *51*:245–246.

Vogel, Z., Vogel, T., and Elson, D. The effect of erythromycin on peptide bond formation and the termination reaction. *FEBS Lett.*, **1971**, *15*:249–253.

Walker, C.K., Kahn, J.G., Washington A.E., Peterson, H.B., and Sweet, R.L. Pelvic inflammatory disease: metaanalysis of antimicrobial regimen efficacy. *J. Infect. Dis.*, **1993**, *168*:969–978.

Walsh, C.T. Vancomycin resistance: decoding the molecular logic. *Science*, **1993**, *261*:308–309.

Walters, B.N., and Gubbay, S.S. Tetracycline and benign intracranial hypertension: report of five cases. *Br. Med. J. (Clin. Res. Ed.)*, **1981**, *282*:19–20.

Ward, H.P. The effect of chloramphenicol on RNA and heme synthesis in bone marrow cultures. *J. Lab. Clin. Med.*, **1966**, *68*:400–410.

Ward, T.T., Rimland, D., Kauffman, C., Huycke, M., Evans, T.G., and Heifets, L. Randomized, open-label trial of azithromycin plus ethambutol vs. clarithromycin plus ethambutol as therapy for *Mycobacterium avium* complex bacteremia in patients with human immunodeficiency virus infection. Veterans Affairs HIV Research Consortium. *Clin. Infect. Dis.*, **1998**, *27*:1278–1285.

Winckler, K. Tetracycline ulcers of the oesophagus; endoscopy, histology and roentgenology in two cases, and review of the literature. *Endoscopy*, **1981**, *13*:225–228.

Wisplinghoff, H., Reinert, R.R., Cornely, O., and Seifert, H. Molecular relationships and antimicrobial susceptibilities of *viridans* group streptococci isolated from blood of neutropenic cancer patients. *J. Clin. Microbiol.*, **1999**, *37*:1876–1880.

World Health Organization. Joint FAO/WHO expert committee on brucellosis. *World Health Organ. Tech. Rep. Ser.* **1986,** *740*:1–132.

Zurenko, G.E., Yagi, B.H., Schaadt, R.D., Allison, J.W., Kilburn, J.O., Glickman, S.E., Hutchinson, D.K., Barbachyn, M.R., and Brickner, S.J. In vitro activities of U-100592 and U-100766, novel oxazolidinone antibacterial agents. *Antimicrob. Agents Chemother.,* **1996,** *40*:839–845.

MONOGRAPHS AND REVIEWS

Alvarez-Elcoro, S., and Enzler, M.J. The macrolides: erythromycin, clarithromycin, and azithromycin. *Mayo Clin. Proc.,* **1999,** *74*:613–634.

Bartlett, J.G. Anaerobic bacterial infections of the lung and pleural space. *Clin. Infect. Dis.,* **1993,** *16 (suppl. 4)*:S248–S255.

Bartlett, J.G., Breiman, R.F., Mandell, L.A., and File, T.M. Jr. Community-acquired pneumonia in adults: guidelines for management. The Infectious Diseases Society of America. *Clin. Infect. Dis.,* **1998,** *26*:811–838.

Bartlett, J.G., Louie, T.J., Gorbach, S.L., and Onderdonk, A.B. Therapeutic efficacy of 29 antimicrobial regimens in experimental intraabdominal sepsis. *Rev. Infect. Dis.,* **1981,** *3*:535–542.

Barza, M., and Scheife, R.T. Antimicrobial spectrum, pharmacology, and therapeutic use of antibiotics. IV. Aminoglycosides. *J. Maine Med. Assoc.,* **1977,** *68*:194–210.

Chant, C., and Rybak, M.J. Quinupristin/dalfopristin (RP 59500): a new streptogramin antibiotic. *Ann. Pharmacother.,* **1995,** *29*:1022–1027.

Clemett, D., and Markham, A. Linezolid. *Drugs,* **2000,** *59*:815–827; discussion 828.

Diekema, D.I., and Jones, R.N. Oxazolidinones: a review. *Drugs,* **2000,** *59*:7–16.

Ginsburg, C.M., and Eichenwald, H.F. Erythromycin: a review of its uses in pediatric practice. *J. Pediatr.,* **1976,** *86*:872–884.

Hamel, J.C., Stapert, D., Moerman, J.K., and Ford, C.W. Linezolid, critical characteristics. *Infection,* **2000,** *28*:60–64.

Lamb, H.M., Figgitt, D.P., and Faulds, D. Quinupristin/dalfopristin: a review of its use in the management of serious gram-positive infections. *Drugs,* **1999,** *58*:1061–1097.

Levine, J.F. Vancomycin: a review. *Med. Clin. North Am.,* **1987,** *71*:1135–1145.

Ludden, T.M. Pharmacokinetic interactions of the macrolide antibiotics. *Clin. Pharmacokinet.,* **1985,** *10*:63–79.

McCracken, G.H. Jr., Nelson, J.D., Kaplan, S.L., Overturf, G.D., Rodriguez, W.J., and Steele, R.W. Consensus report: antimicrobial therapy for bacterial meningitis in infants and children. *Pediatr. Infect. Dis. J.,* **1987,** *6*:501–505.

Meleney, F.L., and Johnson, B.A. Bacitracin. *Am. J. Med.,* **1949,** *7*:794–806.

Miller, S.J., Hohmann, E.L., and Pegues, D.A. Salmonella (including *Salmonella typhi*). In, *Mandell, Douglas, and Bennett's Principles and Practice of Infectious Diseases,* 4th ed. (Mandell, G.L., Bennett, J.E., and Dolin, R., eds.) Churchill Livingstone, New York, **1995,** pp. 2013–2032.

Murray, B.E. Vancomycin-resistant enterococcal infections. *N. Engl. J. Med.,* **2000,** *342*:710–721.

Peters, D.H., Friedel, H.A., McTavish, D. Azithromycin—a review of its antimicrobial activity, pharmacokientic properties, and clinical efficacy. *Drugs,* **1992,** *44*:750–799.

Quagliarello, V.J., and Scheld, W.M. Treatment of bacterial meningitis. *N. Engl. J. Med.,* **1997,** *336*:708–716.

Saah, A.J. Rickettsiosis. In, *Mandell, Douglas, and Bennett's Principles and Practice of Infectious Diseases,* 4th ed. (Mandell, G.L., Bennett, J.E., and Dolin, R., eds.) Churchill Livingstone, New York, **1995,** pp. 1719–1727.

Standiford, H.C. Tetracyclines and chloramphenicol. In, *Mandell, Douglas, and Bennett's Principles and Practice of Infectious Diseases,* 5th ed. (Mandell, G.L., Bennett, J.E., and Dolin, R., eds.) Churchill Livingstone, Philadelphia, **2000,** pp. 336–348.

Steigbigel, N.H. Macrolides and clindamycin. In, *Mandell, Douglas, and Bennett's Principles and Practice of Infectious Diseases,* 5th ed. (Mandell, G.L., Bennett, J.E., and Dolin, R., eds.) Churchill Livingstone, Philadelphia, **2000,** pp. 366–382.

Wiedemann, B., and Atkinson B.A. Susceptibility to antibiotics: species, incidence and trends. In, *Antibiotics in Laboratory Medicine,* 3rd ed. (Lorian, V., ed.) Williams & Wilkins, Philadelphia, **1991,** pp. 926–1208.

Yu, V.L. *Legionella pneumophilia* (Legionnaires' disease). In, *Mandell, Douglas, and Bennett's Principles and Practice of Infectious Diseases,* 5th ed. (Mandell, G.L., Bennett, J.E., and Dolin, R., eds.) Churchill Livingstone, Philadelphia, **2000,** pp. 2424–2435.

ANTIMICROBIAL AGENTS
(*Continued*)

Drugs Used in the Chemotherapy of Tuberculosis, *Mycobacterium avium* Complex Disease, and Leprosy

William A. Petri, Jr.

The pharmacological characteristics and the therapeutic use of each class of compounds employed in the chemotherapy of tuberculosis, diseases caused by the Mycobacterium avium *complex, and leprosy are discussed in this chapter. The increase in tuberculosis case rates in the United States associated with HIV infection has been halted, but tuberculosis remains the number one worldwide cause of death due to infectious diseases. Because the microorganisms grow slowly and the diseases often are chronic, patient compliance, drug toxicity, and the development of microbial resistance present special therapeutic problems. This chapter provides an overview of drugs used for first- and second-line treatment of tuberculosis and discusses therapeutic strategies evolving as resistance to available agents increases. Prophylaxis and treatment of* M. avium *infection in the setting of HIV coinfection are discussed. In addition, this chapter covers the five clinically recognized forms of leprosy and the drug combinations used for their treatment.*

Drugs used in the treatment of tuberculosis can be divided into two major categories (*see* Table 48–1). "First-line" agents combine the greatest level of efficacy with an acceptable degree of toxicity; these include isoniazid, rifampin, ethambutol, streptomycin, and pyrazinamide. The large majority of patients with tuberculosis can be treated successfully with these drugs. Excellent results for patients with non–drug-resistant tuberculosis can be obtained with a 6-month course of treatment; for the first 2 months, isoniazid, rifampin, and pyrazinamide are given, followed by isoniazid and rifampin for the remaining 4 months. Administration of rifampin in combination with isoniazid for 9 months also is effective therapy for all forms of disease caused by strains of *Mycobacterium tuberculosis* susceptible to both agents (Bass *et al.*, 1994). In areas where primary resistance to isoniazid occurs, therapy usually is initiated with four drugs—rifampin, isoniazid, pyrazinamide, and ethambutol (or streptomycin)—until sensitivity tests are completed. Occasionally, however, because of microbial resistance, it may be necessary to resort to "second-line" drugs in addition, so that treatment may be initiated with 5 to 6 drugs. This category of agents includes ofloxacin, ciprofloxacin, ethionamide, aminosali-cylic acid, cycloserine, amikacin, kanamycin, and capreomycin (*see* Iseman, 1993). In HIV-infected patients receiving protease inhibitors and/or nonnucleoside reverse transcriptase inhibitors, drug interactions with the rifamycins (rifampin, rifapentine, rifabutin) are an important concern. Directly observed therapy improves the outcome of tuberculosis treatment regimens (Havlir and Barnes, 1999).

Isoniazid is ineffective in the treatment of leprosy or *M. avium* complex infection. Lepromatous (multibacillary) leprosy is treated with dapsone, clofazimine, and rifampin for a minimum of 2 years, while tuberculoid (paucibacillary) leprosy is treated with dapsone and rifampin for 6 months.

Antimicrobial agents with activity against *M. avium* complex include rifabutin, clarithromycin, azithromycin, and fluoroquinolones. Clarithromycin and azithromycin are more effective than rifabutin for prophylaxis of *M. avium* complex infection in patients with AIDS. Clarithromycin or azithromycin, in combination with ethambutol (to prevent development of resistance), is effective treatment for *M. avium* complex infection in HIV-infected individuals.

Table 48–1

Drugs Used in the Treatment of Tuberculosis, *Mycobacterium avium* Complex, and Leprosy

MYCOBACTERIAL SPECIES	FIRST-LINE THERAPY	ALTERNATIVE AGENTS
M. tuberculosis	Isoniazid + rifampin* + pyrazinamide + ethambutol or streptomycin	Ciprofloxacin or ofloxacin; cycloserine; capreomycin; kanamycin; amikacin; ethionamide; clofazimine; aminosalicylic acid
M. avium complex	Clarithromycin or azithromycin + ethambutol with or without rifabutin	Rifabutin; rifampin; ethionamide; cycloserine; sparfloxacin; ofloxacin; levofloxacin
M. kansasii	Isoniazid + rifampin* + ethambutol	Ethionamide; cycloserine; clarithromycin; amikacin; streptomycin; levofloxacin
M. fortuitum complex	Amikacin + doxycycline	Cefoxitin; rifampin; a sulfonamide; ciprofloxacin; ofloxacin; clarithromycin; trimethoprim–sulfamethoxazole; imipenem
M. marinum	Rifampin + ethambutol	Trimethoprim–sulfamethoxazole; clarithromycin; minocycline; doxycycline
M. leprae	Dapsone + rifampin ± clofazimine	Minocycline; ofloxacin; clarithromycin; ethionamide

*In HIV-infected patients, the substitution of rifabutin for rifampin minimizes drug interactions with the HIV protease inhibitors and nonnucleoside reverse transcriptase inhibitors.

I. DRUGS FOR TUBERCULOSIS

ISONIAZID

Isoniazid (isonicotinic acid hydrazide; NYDRAZID, others) is still considered to be the primary drug for the chemotherapy of tuberculosis, and all patients with disease caused by isoniazid-sensitive strains of the tubercle bacillus should receive the drug if they can tolerate it.

History. The discovery of isoniazid was somewhat fortuitous. In 1945, Chorine reported that nicotinamide possesses tuberculostatic action. Examination of the compounds related to nicotinamide revealed that many pyridine derivatives possess tuberculostatic activity; among these are congeners of isonicotinic acid. Because the thiosemicarbazones were known to inhibit *M. tuberculosis,* the thiosemicarbazone of isonicotinaldehyde was synthesized and studied. The starting material for this synthesis was the methyl ester of isonicotinic acid, and the first intermediate was isonicotinylhydrazide (isoniazid). The interesting history of these chemical studies has been reviewed by Fox (1953).

Chemistry. Isoniazid is the hydrazide of isonicotinic acid; the structural formula is as follows:

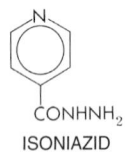

ISONIAZID

The isopropyl derivative of isoniazid, iproniazid (1-isonicotinyl-2-isopropylhydrazide), also inhibits the multiplication of the tubercle bacillus. This compound, which is a potent inhibitor of monoamine oxidase, is too toxic for use in human beings. However, its study led to the use of monoamine oxidase inhibitors for the treatment of depression (*see* Chapter 19).

Antibacterial Activity. Isoniazid is bacteriostatic for "resting" bacilli but is bactericidal for rapidly dividing microorganisms. The minimal tuberculostatic concentration is 0.025 to 0.05 μg/ml. The bacteria undergo one or two divisions before multiplication is arrested. The drug is remarkably selective for mycobacteria, and concentrations in excess of 500 μg/ml are required to inhibit the growth of other microorganisms.

Isoniazid is highly effective for the treatment of experimentally induced tuberculosis in animals and is strikingly superior to streptomycin. Unlike streptomycin, isoniazid penetrates cells with ease and is just as effective against bacilli growing within cells as it is against those growing in culture media.

Among the various nontuberculous (atypical) mycobacteria, only *M. kansasii* is usually susceptible to isoniazid. However, sensitivity always must be tested *in vitro,* since the inhibitory concentration required may be rather high.

Bacterial Resistance. When tubercle bacilli are grown *in vitro* in increasing concentrations of isoniazid, mutants are readily selected that are resistant to the drug, even when the drug is present in enormous concentrations. However, cross-resistance between isoniazid and other agents used to treat tuberculosis (except ethionamide, which is structurally related to isoniazid) does not occur. The most common mechanism of isoniazid resistance is mutations in catalase-peroxidase that decrease its activity, preventing conversion of the prodrug isoniazid to its active metabolite (Blanchard, 1996). Another mechanism of resistance is related to a missense mutation within the mycobacterial *inhA* gene involved in mycolic acid biosynthesis (Banerjee *et al.,* 1994).

As with the other agents described, treatment with isoniazid alone leads to the emergence *in vivo* of resistant strains. The shift from primarily sensitive to mainly insensitive microorganisms occasionally occurs within a few weeks after therapy is started; however, the time of appearance of this phenomenon varies considerably from one case to another. Approximately one in 10^6 tubercle bacilli will be genetically resistant to isoniazid; since tuberculous cavities may contain as many as 10^7 to 10^9 microorganisms, it is not surprising that treatment with isoniazid alone results in the selection of these resistant bacteria. The incidence of primary resistance to isoniazid in the United States until recently had been fairly stable at 2% to 5% of isolates of *M. tuberculosis*. Resistance currently is estimated at 8% of isolates, but it may be much higher in certain populations, including Asian and Hispanic immigrants and in large urban areas and coastal or border communities (Centers for Disease Control and Prevention, 1999; Iseman, 1993).

Mechanism of Action. Takayama and associates (1975) were among the first to suggest that a primary action of isoniazid is to inhibit the biosynthesis of mycolic acids, important constituents of the mycobacterial cell wall. The mechanism of action of isoniazid is complex, with resistance mapping to mutations in at least five different genes (*katG, inhA, ahpC, kasA,* and *ndh*). The preponderance of evidence points to *inhA* as the primary drug target. The *inhA* gene encodes the enoyl-ACP reductase of fatty acid synthase II, which converts Δ^2-unsaturated to saturated fatty acids on the pathway to mycolic acid biosynthesis (Vilcheze *et al.,* 2000). Because mycolic acids are unique to mycobacteria, this action explains the high degree of selectivity of the antimicrobial activity of isoniazid. Exposure to isoniazid leads to a loss of acid-fastness and a decrease in the quantity of methanol-extractable lipid of the microorganisms.

Absorption, Distribution, and Excretion. Isoniazid is readily absorbed when administered either orally or parenterally. Aluminum-containing antacids may interfere with absorption. Peak plasma concentrations of 3 to 5 μg/ml develop 1 to 2 hours after oral ingestion of usual doses.

Isoniazid diffuses readily into all body fluids and cells. The drug is detectable in significant quantities in pleural and ascitic fluids; concentrations in the cerebrospinal fluid (CSF) with inflamed meninges are similar to those in the plasma (Holdiness, 1985). Isoniazid penetrates well into caseous material. The concentration of the agent is initially higher in the plasma and muscle than in the infected tissue, but the latter retains the drug for a long time in quantities well above those required for bacteriostasis.

From 75% to 95% of a dose of isoniazid is excreted in the urine within 24 hours, mostly as metabolites. The main excretory products in human beings are the result of enzymatic acetylation (acetylisoniazid) and enzymatic hydrolysis (isonicotinic acid). Small quantities of an isonicotinic acid conjugate (probably isonicotinyl glycine),

one or more isonicotinyl hydrazones, and traces of *N*-methylisoniazid also are detectable in the urine.

Human populations show genetic heterogeneity with regard to the rate of acetylation of isoniazid (Evans *et al.,* 1960). The distribution of slow and rapid inactivators of the drug is bimodal owing to differences in the activity of an acetyltransferase (Figure 48–1). The rate of acetylation significantly alters the concentrations of the drug that are achieved in plasma and its half-life in the circulation. The half-life of the drug may be prolonged in the presence of hepatic insufficiency.

The frequency of each acetylation phenotype is dependent upon race but is not influenced by gender or age. Fast acetylation is found in Inuit and Japanese. Slow acetylation is the predominant phenotype in most Scandinavians, Jews, and North African Caucasians. The incidence of "slow acetylators" among the various racial types in the United States is about 50%. Since high acetyltransferase activity (fast acetylation) is inherited as an autosomal dominant trait, "fast acetylators" of isoniazid are either heterozygous or homozygous. The average concentration of active isoniazid in the circulation of fast acetylators is about 30% to 50% of that present in persons who acetylate the drug slowly. In the whole population, the half-life of isoniazid varies from less than 1 to more than 4 hours (Figure 48–1). The mean half-life in fast acetylators is approximately 70 minutes, whereas 2 to 5 hours is characteristic of slow acetylators. However, because isoniazid is relatively nontoxic, a sufficient amount of drug can be administered to fast acetylators to achieve a therapeutic effect equal to that seen in slow acetylators. A dosage reduction is recommended for slow acetylators with hepatic failure.

The clearance of isoniazid is dependent to only a small degree on the status of renal function, but patients who are slow inactivators of the drug may accumulate toxic concentrations if their renal function is impaired. Bowersox and colleagues (1973) have suggested that 300 mg per day of the drug can be administered safely to individuals in whom the plasma creatinine concentration is less than 12 mg/dl (1.1 mM).

Therapeutic Uses. Isoniazid is still the most important drug worldwide for the treatment of all types of tuberculosis. Toxic effects can be minimized by prophylactic therapy with *pyridoxine* and careful surveillance of the patient. The drug must be used concurrently with another agent for treatment, although it is used alone for prophylaxis.

Isoniazid is available for oral and parenteral administration. The commonly used total daily dose of isoniazid is 5 mg/kg, with a maximum of 300 mg; oral and intramuscular doses are identical. Isoniazid usually is given orally in a single daily dose but may be given in two divided doses. Although doses of 10 to 20 mg/kg, with a maximum of 600 mg, occasionally are used in severely ill patients, there is no evidence that this regimen is more effective. Children should receive 10 to 20 mg/kg per day (300 mg maximum). Isoniazid may be used as intermittent

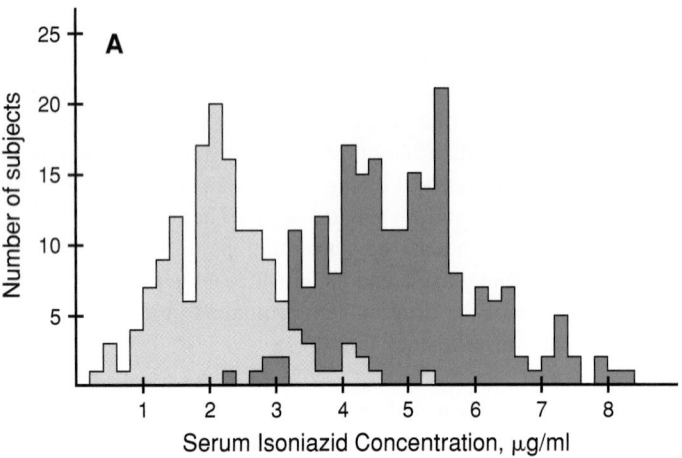

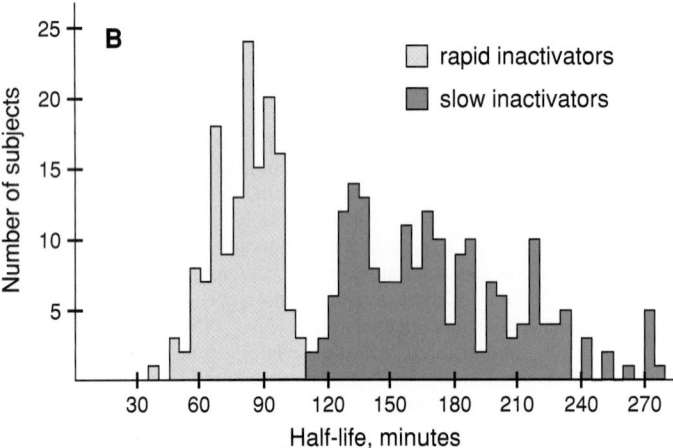

Figure 48–1. Bimodal distribution of serum isoniazid concentrations and half-lives in a large group of Finnish patients.

More than 300 patients were given intravenous injections of 5 mg/kg of isoniazid. Serum drug concentrations were assayed at multiple times after injection. *A*. The distribution of the serum concentrations of isoniazid 180 minutes after injection; the light blue histograms represent rapid inactivators, and the dark blue histograms, slow inactivators. *B*. The distribution of serum half-lives of isoniazid for patients of each group. (Reproduced with permission from Tiitinen, 1969.)

therapy for tuberculosis; after a minimum of 2 months of daily therapy of tuberculosis due to sensitive strains of *M. tuberculosis* with isoniazid, rifampin, and pyrazinamide, patients may be treated with twice-weekly doses of isoniazid (15 mg/kg orally) plus rifampin (10 mg/kg, up to 600 mg per dose) for 4 months.

Pyridoxine (15 to 50 mg per day) should be administered with isoniazid to minimize adverse reactions (*see* below) in malnourished patients and those predisposed to neuropathy (*e.g.,* the elderly, pregnant women, HIV-infected individuals, diabetics, alcoholics, and uremics; Snider, 1980).

Untoward Effects. The incidence of adverse reactions to isoniazid was estimated to be 5.4% among more than 2000 patients treated with the drug; the most prominent of these reactions were rash (2%), fever (1.2%), jaundice (0.6%), and peripheral neuritis (0.2%). Hypersensitivity to isoniazid may result in fever, various skin eruptions, hepatitis, and morbilliform, maculopapular, purpuric, and urticarial rashes. Hematological reactions also may occur (agranulocytosis, eosinophilia, thrombocytopenia, anemia). Vasculitis associated with antinuclear antibodies may appear during treatment but disappears when the drug is stopped. Arthritic symptoms (back pain; bilateral proximal interphalangeal joint involvement; arthralgia of the knees, elbows, and wrists; and the "shoulder-hand" syndrome) have been attributed to this agent.

If pyridoxine is not given concurrently, peripheral neuritis (most commonly paresthesia of feet and hands) is the most common reaction to isoniazid and occurs in about 2% of patients receiving 5 mg/kg of the drug daily. Higher doses may result in peripheral neuritis in 10% to 20% of patients. Neuropathy is more frequent in slow acetylators and in individuals with diabetes mellitus, poor nutrition, or anemia. The prophylactic administration of pyridoxine prevents the development not only of peripheral neuritis but also of most other nervous system disorders in practically all instances even when therapy lasts as long as 2 years.

Isoniazid may precipitate convulsions in patients with seizure disorders and, rarely, in patients with no history of seizures. Optic neuritis and atrophy also have occurred during therapy with the drug. Muscle twitching, dizziness, ataxia, paresthesias, stupor, and toxic encephalopathy that may be fatal are other manifestations of the neurotoxicity of isoniazid. A number of mental abnormalities may appear during the use of this drug; among these are euphoria, transient impairment of memory, separation of ideas and reality, loss of self-control, and florid psychoses.

Isoniazid is known to inhibit the parahydroxylation of phenytoin, and signs and symptoms of toxicity occur in approximately 27% of patients given both drugs, particularly in those who are slow acetylators (Miller *et al.,* 1979). Concentrations of phenytoin in plasma should be monitored and adjusted if necessary. The dosage of isoniazid should not be changed.

Although jaundice has been known for some time to be an untoward effect of exposure to isoniazid, not until the early 1970s did it become apparent that severe hepatic injury leading to death may occur in some individuals receiving this drug (Garibaldi *et al.,* 1972). Additional studies in adults and children have confirmed this observation; the characteristic pathological process is bridging and multilobular necrosis. Continuation of the drug after symptoms of hepatic dysfunction have appeared tends to increase the severity of damage. The mechanisms responsible for this toxicity are unknown, although acetylhydrazine, which is a metabolite of isoniazid, causes hepatic damage in adults. Hence, patients who are rapid acetylators of isoniazid might be expected to be more likely to develop hepatotoxicity than slow acetylators. Whether or not this is true, however, is unresolved. A contributory role of alcoholic hepatitis has been noted, but chronic carriers of the hepatitis B virus tolerate isoniazid (McGlynn *et al.,* 1986). Age appears to be the most important factor in determining the risk of isoniazid-induced hepatotoxicity. Hepatic damage is rare in patients less than 20 years old; the complication is observed in 0.3% of those 20 to 34 years old, and the incidence increases to 1.2% and 2.3% in individuals 35 to 49 and older than 50 years of age, respectively (Bass *et al.,* 1994; Comstock, 1983). Up to 12% of patients receiving isoniazid may have elevated plasma aspartate and alanine transaminase activities (Bailey *et al.,* 1974). Patients receiving isoniazid should be carefully evaluated at monthly intervals for symptoms of hepatitis (anorexia, malaise, fatigue, nausea, and jaundice) and warned to discontinue the drug if such symptoms occur. Some clinicians also prefer to determine serum aspartate aminotransferase activities at monthly intervals (Byrd *et al.,* 1979) and recommend that an elevation greater than

five times normal is cause for discontinuation of the drug. Most hepatitis occurs 4 to 8 weeks after the start of therapy. Isoniazid should be administered with great care to those with preexisting hepatic disease.

Among miscellaneous reactions associated with isoniazid therapy are dryness of the mouth, epigastric distress, methemoglobinemia, tinnitus, and urinary retention. In persons predisposed to pyridoxine-deficiency anemia, the administration of isoniazid may result in its appearance in full-blown form. Treatment with large doses of the vitamin gradually returns the blood to normal in such cases (*see* Goldman and Braman, 1972). A drug-induced syndrome resembling systemic lupus erythematosus has been reported. Overdose of isoniazid, as in attempted suicide, may result in nausea, vomiting, dizziness, slurred speech, and visual hallucinations followed by coma, seizures, metabolic acidosis, and hyperglycemia. Pyridoxine is an antidote in this setting; it should be given in a dose that approximates the amount of isoniazid ingested.

RIFAMPIN

The rifamycins (rifampin, rifabutin, rifapentine) are a group of structurally similar, complex macrocyclic antibiotics produced by *Streptomyces mediterranei* (Farr, 2000); *rifampin* (RIFADIN; RIMACTANE) is a semisynthetic derivative of one of these—rifamycin B.

Chemistry. Rifampin is soluble in organic solvents and in water at acidic pH. It has the following structure:

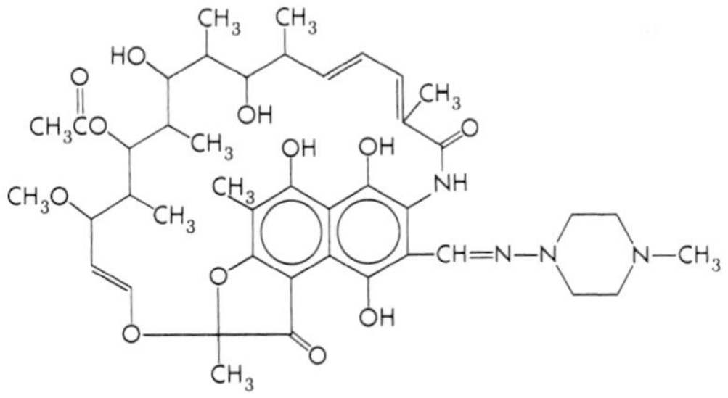

RIFAMPIN

Antibacterial Activity. Rifampin inhibits the growth of most gram-positive bacteria as well as many gram-negative microorganisms such as *Escherichia coli, Pseudomonas,* indole-positive and indole-negative *Proteus,* and *Klebsiella.* Rifampin is very active against *Staphylococcus aureus* and coagulase-negative staphylococci; bactericidal concentrations range from 3 to 12 ng/ml. The drug also is highly active against *Neisseria meningitidis* and *Haemophilus influenzae*; minimal inhibitory concentrations range from 0.1 to 0.8 μg/ml. Rifampin is very inhibitory to *Legionella* species in cell culture and in animal models.

Rifampin in concentrations of 0.005 to 0.2 μg/ml inhibits the growth of *M. tuberculosis in vitro.* Among nontuberculous mycobacteria, *Mycobacterium kansasii* is inhibited by 0.25 to 1 μg/ml. The majority of strains of *Mycobacterium scrofulaceum, Mycobacterium intracellulare,* and *M. avium* are suppressed by concentrations of 4 μg/ml, but certain strains may be resistant to 16 μg/ml. *Mycobacterium fortuitum* is highly resistant to the drug. Rifampin increases the *in vitro* activity of streptomycin and isoniazid, but not that of ethambutol, against *M. tuberculosis* (Hobby and Lenert, 1972).

Bacterial Resistance. Microorganisms, including mycobacteria, may develop resistance to rifampin rapidly *in vitro* as a one-step process, and one of every 10^7 to 10^8 tubercle bacilli is resistant to the drug. Resistance in most cases is due to mutations between codons 507 and 533 of the polymerase *rpoB* gene (Blanchard, 1996). This also appears to be the case *in vivo,* and therefore the antibiotic must not be used alone in the chemotherapy of tuberculosis. When rifampin has been used for eradication of the meningococcal carrier state, failures have been due to the appearance of drug-resistant bacteria after treatment for as little as 2 days. Microbial resistance to rifampin is due to an alteration of the target of this drug, DNA-dependent RNA polymerase. Certain rifampin-resistant bacterial mutants have decreased virulence. Tuberculosis caused by rifampin-resistant mycobacteria has been described in patients who had not received prior chemotherapy, but this is very rare (usually less than 1%; Cauthen *et al.,* 1988).

Mechanism of Action. Rifampin inhibits DNA-dependent RNA polymerase of mycobacteria and other microorganisms by forming a stable drug–enzyme complex, leading to suppression of initiation of chain formation (but not chain elongation) in RNA synthesis. More specifically, the β subunit of this complex enzyme is the site of action of the drug, although rifampin binds only to the holoenzyme. Nuclear RNA polymerase from a variety of eukaryotic cells does not bind rifampin, and RNA synthesis is correspondingly unaffected. While rifampin can inhibit RNA synthesis in mammalian mitochondria, considerably higher concentrations of the drug are required than for the inhibition of the bacterial enzyme. High concentrations of rifamycin antibiotics also inhibit viral DNA-dependent RNA polymerases and reverse transcriptases. Rifampin is bactericidal for both intracellular and extracellular microorganisms.

Absorption, Distribution, and Excretion. The oral administration of rifampin produces peak concentrations in plasma in 2 to 4 hours; after ingestion of 600 mg, this value is about 7 μg/ml, but there is considerable variability. Aminosalicylic acid may delay the absorption of rifampin, and adequate plasma concentrations may not be reached. If these agents are used concurrently, they should be given separately at an interval of 8 to 12 hours (*see* Radner, 1973).

Following absorption from the gastrointestinal tract, rifampin is eliminated rapidly in the bile, and an enterohepatic circulation ensues. During this time, the drug is progressively deacetylated, to a degree that, after 6 hours, nearly all of the antibiotic in the bile is in the deacetylated

form. This metabolite retains essentially full antibacterial activity. Intestinal reabsorption is reduced by deacetylation (as well as by food), and thus metabolism facilitates elimination of the drug. The half-life of rifampin varies from 1.5 to 5 hours and is increased in the presence of hepatic dysfunction; it may be decreased in patients receiving isoniazid concurrently who are slow inactivators of this drug. The half-life of rifampin is progressively shortened by about 40% during the first 14 days of treatment, owing to induction of hepatic microsomal enzymes with acceleration of deacetylation of the drug. Up to 30% of a dose of the drug is excreted in the urine and 60% to 65% in the feces; less than half of this may be unaltered antibiotic. Adjustment of dosage is not necessary in patients with impaired renal function.

Rifampin is distributed throughout the body and is present in effective concentrations in many organs and body fluids, including the CSF (Sippel *et al.,* 1974). This is perhaps best exemplified by the fact that the drug may impart an orange-red color to the urine, feces, saliva, sputum, tears, and sweat; patients should be so warned. (For various aspects of rifampin metabolism, *see* Furesz, 1970; Farr, 2000.)

Therapeutic Uses. Rifampin is available alone and as a fixed-dose combination with isoniazid (150 mg of isoniazid, 300 mg of rifampin; RIFAMATE) or with isoniazid and pyrazinamide (50 mg of isoniazid, 120 mg of rifampin, and 300 mg pyrazinamide; RIFATER). Rifampin and isoniazid are the most effective drugs available for the treatment of tuberculosis. The dose of rifampin for treatment of tuberculosis in adults is 600 mg, given once daily, either 1 hour before or 2 hours after a meal. Children should receive 10 mg/kg, with a daily maximum, given in the same way. Doses of 15 mg/kg or higher are associated with increased hepatotoxicity in children (Centers for Disease Control, 1980). Rifampin, like isoniazid, should never be used alone for this disease because of the rapidity with which resistance may develop. Despite the long list of untoward effects from rifampin, their incidence is low, and treatment seldom has to be interrupted.

The use of rifampin in the chemotherapy of tuberculosis is detailed below. Rifampin also is indicated for the prophylaxis of meningococcal disease and *H. influenzae* meningitis. To prevent meningococcal disease, adults may be treated with 600 mg twice daily for 2 days or 600 mg once daily for 4 days; children should receive 10 to 20 mg/kg, to a maximum of 600 mg.

Untoward Effects. Rifampin generally is well tolerated. When given in usual doses, fewer than 4% of patients with tuberculosis have significant adverse reactions; the most common are rash (0.8%), fever (0.5%), and nausea and vomiting (1.5%) (*see* Grosset and Leventis, 1983). Rarely, hepatitis and deaths due to liver failure have been observed in patients who received other hepatotoxic agents in addition to rifampin or who had preexisting liver disease. Hepatitis from rifampin rarely occurs in patients with normal hepatic function; likewise, the combination of isoniazid and rifampin appears generally safe in such patients (Gangadharam, 1986). However, chronic liver disease, alcoholism, and old age appear to increase the incidence of severe hepatic problems when rifampin is given alone or concurrently with isoniazid.

Administration of rifampin on an intermittent schedule (less than twice weekly) and/or daily doses of 1200 mg or greater is associated with frequent side effects, and the drug should not be used in this manner. A flulike syndrome with fever, chills, and myalgias develops in 20% of patients so treated. The syndrome also may include eosinophilia, interstitial nephritis, acute tubular necrosis, thrombocytopenia, hemolytic anemia, and shock (Girling and Hitze, 1979).

Because rifampin is a potent inducer of hepatic microsomal enzymes, its administration results in a decreased half-life for a number of compounds, including HIV protease and nonnucleoside reverse transcriptase inhibitors, digitoxin, digoxin, quinidine, disopyramide, mexiletine, tocainide, ketoconazole, propranolol, metoprolol, clofibrate, verapamil, methadone, cyclosporine, corticosteroids, oral anticoagulants, theophylline, barbiturates, oral contraceptives, halothane, fluconazole, and the sulfonylureas (Farr, 2000). Rifabutin has less of an effect on the metabolism of the HIV protease inhibitors indinavir and nelfinavir. The significant interaction between rifampin and oral anticoagulants of the coumarin type leads to a decrease in efficacy of these agents. This effect appears about 5 to 8 days after rifampin administration is started and persists for 5 to 7 days after it is stopped (O'Reilly, 1975). The ability of rifampin to enhance the catabolism of a variety of steroids leads to the decreased effectiveness of oral contraceptives (Skolnick *et al.*, 1976). The increased metabolism of methadone has led to reports of precipitation of withdrawal syndromes. Rifampin may reduce biliary excretion of contrast media used for visualization of the gallbladder (*see* Baciewicz *et al.*, 1987).

Gastrointestinal disturbances produced by rifampin (epigastric distress, nausea, vomiting, abdominal cramps, diarrhea) have occasionally required discontinuation of the drug. Various symptoms related to the nervous system also have been noted, including fatigue, drowsiness, headache, dizziness, ataxia, confusion, inability to concentrate, generalized numbness, pain in the extremities, and muscular weakness. Among hypersensitivity reactions are fever, pruritus, urticaria, various types of skin eruptions, eosinophilia, and soreness of the mouth and tongue. Hemolysis, hemoglobinuria, hematuria, renal insufficiency, and acute renal failure have been observed rarely; these also are thought to be hypersensitivity reactions. Thrombocytopenia, transient leukopenia, and anemia have occurred during therapy. Since the potential teratogenicity of rifampin is unknown and the drug is known to cross the placenta, it is best to avoid the use of this agent during pregnancy.

Graber and associates (1973) have noted immunoglobulin light-chain proteinuria (either kappa, lambda, or both) in about 85% of patients with tuberculosis treated with rifampin. None of the patients had symptoms or electrophoretic patterns compatible with myeloma. However, renal failure has been associated with light-chain proteinuria (Warrington *et al.*, 1977).

Rifampin is a drug of choice for chemoprophylaxis of meningococcal disease and meningitis due to *H. influenzae* in household contacts of patients with such infections. Combined with a β-lactam antibiotic or vancomycin, rifampin may be useful for therapy in selected cases of staphylococcal endocarditis (on both natural and prosthetic valves) or osteomyelitis, especially those caused by staphylococci "tolerant" to penicillin. Rifampin may be indicated for therapy of infections in patients with inadequate leukocytic bactericidal activity and for eradication of the staphylococcal nasal carrier state in patients with chronic furunculosis (Wheat *et al.*, 1983).

ETHAMBUTOL

Chemistry. Ethambutol is a water-soluble and heat-stable compound. The structural formula is as follows:

ETHAMBUTOL

Antibacterial Activity. Nearly all strains of *M. tuberculosis* and *M. kansasii* as well as a number of strains of *M. avium* complex are sensitive to ethambutol (Pablos-Méndez *et al.*, 1998). The sensitivities of other nontuberculous organisms are variable. Ethambutol has no effect on other bacteria. It suppresses the growth of most isoniazid- and streptomycin-resistant tubercle bacilli. Resistance to ethambutol develops very slowly *in vitro*.

Mycobacteria take up ethambutol rapidly when the drug is added to cultures that are in the exponential growth phase. However, growth is not significantly inhibited before about 24 hours; the drug is tuberculostatic. Ethambutol blocks arabinosyl transferases involved in cell wall biosynthesis (Takayama *et al.*, 1979). Bacterial resistance to the drug develops *in vivo via* single amino acid changes in the *embA* gene when ethambutol is given in the absence of another effective agent (Belanger *et al.*, 1996).

Absorption, Distribution, and Excretion. About 75% to 80% of an orally administered dose of ethambutol is absorbed from the gastrointestinal tract. Concentrations in plasma are maximal in human beings 2 to 4 hours after the drug is taken and are proportional to the dose. A single dose of 25 mg/kg produces a plasma concentration of 2 to 5 μg/ml at 2 to 4 hours. The drug has a half-life of 3 to 4 hours.

Within 24 hours, three-fourths of an ingested dose of ethambutol is excreted unchanged in the urine; up to 15% is excreted in the form of two metabolites, an aldehyde and a dicarboxylic acid derivative. Renal clearance of ethambutol is approximately 7 ml·min^{-1}·kg^{-1}; thus it is evident that the drug is excreted by tubular secretion in addition to glomerular filtration.

Therapeutic Uses.   Ethambutol (*ethambutol hydrochloride*; MYAMBUTOL) has been used with notable success in the therapy of tuberculosis of various forms when given concurrently with isoniazid. Because of a lower incidence of toxic effects and better acceptance by patients, ethambutol has essentially replaced aminosalicylic acid (*see* Bobrowitz, 1974).

Ethambutol is available for oral administration in tablets containing the *d* isomer. The usual adult dose of ethambutol is 15 mg/kg given once a day. Some physicians prefer to institute therapy with a dose of 25 mg/kg per day for the first 60 days and then to reduce the dose to 15 mg/kg per day, particularly for those who have received previous therapy. Ethambutol accumulates in patients with impaired renal function, and adjustment of dosage is necessary.

Ethambutol is not recommended for children under 5 years of age, in part because of concern about the ability to test their visual acuity (*see* below). Children from ages 6 to 12 years should receive 10 to 15 mg/kg per day.

The use of ethambutol in the chemotherapy of tuberculosis is described below.

Untoward Effects.   The most important side effect is optic neuritis, resulting in decrease of visual acuity and loss of ability to differentiate red from green. The incidence of this reaction is proportional to the dose of ethambutol and is observed in 15% of patients receiving 50 mg/kg per day, in 5% of patients receiving 25 mg/kg per day, and in fewer than 1% of patients receiving daily doses of 15 mg/kg (the recommended dose for treatment of tuberculosis). The intensity of the visual difficulty is related to the duration of therapy after the decrease in visual acuity first becomes apparent, and it may be unilateral or bilateral. Tests of visual acuity and red-green discrimination prior to the start of therapy and periodically thereafter are thus recommended. Recovery usually occurs when etham-

butol is withdrawn; the time required is a function of the degree of visual impairment.

Ethambutol produces very few reactions. Daily doses of 15 mg/kg are minimally toxic. Fewer than 2% of nearly 2000 patients who received 15 mg/kg of ethambutol had adverse reactions; 0.8% experienced diminished visual acuity, 0.5% had a rash, and 0.3% developed drug fever. Other side effects that have been observed are pruritus, joint pain, gastrointestinal upset, abdominal pain, malaise, headache, dizziness, mental confusion, disorientation, and possible hallucination. Numbness and tingling of the fingers owing to peripheral neuritis are infrequent. Anaphylaxis and leukopenia are rare.

Therapy with ethambutol results in an increased concentration of urate in the blood in about 50% of patients, owing to decreased renal excretion of uric acid. The effect may be detectable as early as 24 hours after a single dose or as late as 90 days after treatment is started. This untoward effect is possibly enhanced by isoniazid and pyridoxine (Postlethwaite *et al.*, 1972).

STREPTOMYCIN

A discussion of the pharmacology of *streptomycin*, including its adverse effects and its uses in infections other than tuberculosis, is presented in Chapter 46. Only features of the drug related to its antibacterial activity and therapeutic effects in the management of diseases caused by mycobacteria are considered here.

History.   Streptomycin was the first clinically effective drug to become available for the treatment of tuberculosis. At first, it was given in large doses, but problems related to toxicity and the development of resistant microorganisms seriously limited its usefulness. The antibiotic was then administered in smaller quantities, but streptomycin administered alone still proved to be far from the ideal agent for the management of all forms of the disease. However, the discovery of other compounds that, given concurrently with the antibiotic, reduced the rate at which microorganisms became drug-resistant enabled physicians to treat tuberculosis effectively with streptomycin. It is now the least used of the "first-line" agents in the therapy of tuberculosis.

Antibacterial Activity.   Streptomycin is bactericidal for the tubercle bacillus *in vitro*. Concentrations as low as 0.4 μg/ml may inhibit growth. The vast majority of strains of *M. tuberculosis* are sensitive to 10 μg/ml. *M. kansasii* is frequently sensitive, but other nontuberculous mycobacteria are only occasionally susceptible.

The activity of streptomycin *in vivo* is essentially suppressive. When the antibiotic is administered to experimental animals prior to inoculation with the tubercle bacillus, the development of disease is not prevented. Infection progresses until the animals' immunological mechanisms respond. The presence of viable microorganisms in abscesses and in the regional lymph nodes adds support to the concept that the activity of streptomycin *in vivo* is to suppress, not to eradicate, the tubercle bacillus. This property of streptomycin may be related to the observation that the drug does not readily enter living cells and thus cannot kill intracellular microbes.

Bacterial Resistance.   Large populations of all strains of tubercle bacilli include a number of cells that are markedly resistant to streptomycin because of mutation. However, primary resistance to the antibiotic is found in only 2% to 3% of isolates of *M. tuberculosis.*

Selection for resistant tubercle bacilli occurs *in vivo* as it does *in vitro.* In general, the longer therapy is continued, the greater is the incidence of resistance to streptomycin. When streptomycin was used alone, as many as 80% of patients harbored insensitive tubercle bacilli after 4 months of treatment; many of these microorganisms were not inhibited by concentrations of drug as high as 1000 μg/ml.

Therapeutic Uses.   Since other effective agents have become available, the use of streptomycin for the treatment of pulmonary tuberculosis has been sharply reduced. Many clinicians prefer to give four drugs, of which streptomycin may be one, for the most serious forms of tuberculosis, such as disseminated disease or meningitis.

For tuberculosis, adults should be given 15 mg/kg per day in divided doses given every 12 hours, not to exceed 1 g per day. Children should receive 20 to 40 mg/kg per day in divided doses every 12 to 24 hours, not to exceed 1 g per day. Therapy usually is discontinued after 2 to 3 months, or sooner if cultures become negative. Dosage schedules for various forms of tuberculosis are discussed further below.

Untoward Effects.   Untoward effects of streptomycin are considered in detail in Chapter 46. Of 515 patients with tuberculosis who were treated with this aminoglycoside, 8.2% had adverse reactions; half of these involved the auditory and vestibular functions of the eighth cranial nerve. Other relatively frequent problems included rash (in 2%) and fever (in 1.4%).

PYRAZINAMIDE

Chemistry.   *Pyrazinamide* is the synthetic pyrazine analog of nicotinamide. It has the following structural formula:

PYRAZINAMIDE

Antibacterial Activity.   Pyrazinamide exhibits bactericidal activity *in vitro* only at a slightly acidic pH. Activity at acid pH is ideal, since *M. tuberculosis* resides in an acidic phagosome within the macrophage (Jacobs, 2000). Tubercle bacilli within monocytes *in vitro* are inhibited or killed by the drug at a concentration of 12.5 μg/ml. Resistance develops rapidly if pyrazinamide is used alone. The target of pyrazinamide appears to be the mycobacterial fatty acid synthase I gene involved in mycolic acid biosynthesis (Zimhony *et al.,* 2000).

Absorption, Distribution, and Excretion.   Pyrazinamide is well absorbed from the gastrointestinal tract, and it is widely distributed throughout the body. The oral administration of 500 mg produces plasma concentrations of about 9 to 12 μg/ml at 2 hours and 7 μg/ml at 8 hours. The plasma half-life is 9 to 10 hours in patients with normal renal function. The drug is excreted primarily by renal glomerular filtration. Pyrazinamide is distributed widely— including the CNS, lungs, and liver—after oral administration. Penetration of the drug into the CSF is excellent. Pyrazinamide is hydrolyzed to pyrazinoic acid and subsequently hydroxylated to 5-hydroxypyrazinoic acid, the major excretory product.

Therapeutic Uses.   Pyrazinamide has become an important component of short-term (6-month) multiple-drug therapy of tuberculosis (British Thoracic Association, 1983; Bass *et al.,* 1994).

Pyrazinamide is available in tablets for oral administration. The daily dose for adults is 15 to 30 mg/kg orally, given as a single dose. The maximum quantity to be given is 2 g per day, regardless of weight. Children should receive 15 to 30 mg/kg per day; daily doses should not exceed 2 g. Pyrazinamide also has been safe and effective when administered twice or thrice weekly (at increased dosages).

Untoward Effects.   Injury to the liver is the most serious side effect of pyrazinamide. When a dose of 40 to 50 mg/kg is administered orally, signs and symptoms of hepatic disease appear in about 15% of patients, with jaundice in 2% to 3% and death due to hepatic necrosis in rare instances. Elevations of the plasma alanine and aspartate aminotransferases are the earliest abnormalities produced by the drug. Regimens employed currently (15 to 30 mg/kg per day) are much safer (Girling, 1978). All patients who are being treated with pyrazinamide should undergo studies of hepatic function before the drug is administered; these studies should be repeated at frequent intervals during the entire period of treatment. If evidence of significant hepatic damage becomes apparent, therapy must be stopped. Pyrazinamide should not be given to individuals with any degree of hepatic dysfunction unless this is absolutely unavoidable.

The drug inhibits excretion of urate, resulting in hyperuricemia in nearly all patients; acute episodes of gout have occurred. Other untoward effects that have been observed with pyrazinamide are arthralgias, anorexia, nausea and vomiting, dysuria, malaise, and fever. While some international organizations recommend the use of pyrazinamide in pregnancy, this is not the case in the United States because of inadequate data on teratogenicity (Bass *et al.,* 1994).

ETHIONAMIDE

Chemistry. Synthesis and study of a variety of congeners of thioisonicotinamide revealed that an alpha-ethyl derivative—*ethionamide* (TRECATOR-SC)—is considerably more effective than the parent compound. It has the following structural formula:

ETHIONAMIDE

Antibacterial Activity. The multiplication of *M. tuberculosis* is suppressed by concentrations of ethionamide ranging from 0.6 to 2.5 μg/ml. Resistance can develop rapidly *in vitro*. A concentration of 10 μg/ml or less will inhibit approximately 75% of photochromogenic mycobacteria; the scotochromogens are more resistant. Ethionamide is very effective in the treatment of experimental tuberculosis in animals, although its activity varies greatly with the animal model studied.

Absorption, Distribution, and Excretion. The oral administration of 1 g of ethionamide yields peak concentrations in plasma of about 20 μg/ml in 3 hours; the concentration at 9 hours is 3 μg/ml. The half-life of the drug is about 2 hours. Approximately 50% of patients are unable to tolerate a single dose larger than 500 mg because of gastrointestinal disturbance. Ethionamide is rapidly and widely distributed; the concentrations in the blood and various organs are approximately equal. Significant concentrations are present in CSF. Ethionamide, like aminosalicylic acid, inhibits the acetylation of isoniazid *in vitro*. Less than 1% of ethionamide is excreted in active form in the urine; there are several metabolites.

Therapeutic Uses. Ethionamide is a secondary agent, to be used concurrently with other drugs only when therapy with primary agents is ineffective or contraindicated.

Ethionamide is administered only orally. The initial dosage of ethionamide for adults is 250 mg twice daily; it is increased by 125 mg per day every 5 days until a dose of 15 to 20 mg/kg per day is achieved. The maximal dose is 1 g daily. The drug is best taken with meals in divided doses in order to minimize gastric irritation. Children should receive 15 to 20 mg/kg per day in two divided doses, not to exceed 1 g per day.

Untoward Effects. The most common reactions to ethionamide are anorexia, nausea, and vomiting. A metallic taste also may be noted. Severe postural hypotension, mental de-

pression, drowsiness, and asthenia are common. Convulsions and peripheral neuropathy are rare. Other reactions referable to the nervous system include olfactory disturbances, blurred vision, diplopia, dizziness, paresthesias, headache, restlessness, and tremors. Severe allergic skin rashes, purpura, stomatitis, gynecomastia, impotence, menorrhagia, acne, and alopecia also have been observed. Hepatitis has been associated with the use of the drug in about 5% of cases (Simon *et al.,* 1969). The signs and symptoms of hepatotoxicity clear when treatment is stopped. Hepatic function should be assessed at regular intervals in patients receiving ethionamide. The concomitant use of pyridoxine is recommended for patients being treated with ethionamide.

AMINOSALICYLIC ACID

Chemistry. The structural formula of *aminosalicylic acid* (*p*-aminosali-cylic acid, PAS) is as follows:

AMINOSALICYLIC ACID

Antibacterial Activity. Aminosalicylic acid is bacteriostatic. *In vitro,* most strains of *M. tuberculosis* are sensitive to a concentration of 1 μg/ml. The antimicrobial activity of aminosalicylic acid is highly specific, and microorganisms other than *M. tuberculosis* are unaffected. Most nontuberculous mycobacteria are not inhibited by the drug.

Studies of the treatment of experimental *M. tuberculosis* infections indicate that aminosalicylic acid exerts a beneficial effect on the disease. However, the doses required are relatively large, and the compound must be present continuously. Aminosalicylic acid alone is of little value in the treatment of tuberculosis in human beings.

Bacterial Resistance. Strains of tubercle bacilli insensitive to several hundred times the usual bacteriostatic concentration of aminosalicylic acid can be produced *in vitro*. Resistant strains of tubercle bacilli also emerge in patients treated with aminosalicylic acid, but much more slowly than with streptomycin.

Mechanism of Action. Aminosalicylic acid is a structural analog of paraaminobenzoic acid, and its mechanism of action appears to be very similar to that of the sulfonamides (*see* Chapter 44). Since the sulfonamides are ineffective against *M. tuberculosis,* and aminosalicylic acid is inactive against sulfonamide-susceptible bacteria, it is probable that the enzymes responsible for folate biosynthesis in various microorganisms may be quite exacting in their capacity to distinguish various analogs from the true metabolite.

Absorption, Distribution, and Excretion. Aminosalicylic acid is readily absorbed from the gastrointestinal tract. A single oral dose of 4 g of the free acid produces maximal concentrations in plasma of about 75 μg/ml within 1.5 to 2 hours. The sodium salt is absorbed even more rapidly. The drug appears to be distributed throughout the total body water and reaches high concentrations in pleural fluid and caseous tissue. However, values in CSF are low, perhaps because of active outward transport.

The drug has a half-life of about 1 hour, and concentrations in plasma are negligible within 4 to 5 hours after a single conventional dose. Over 80% of the drug is excreted in the urine; more than 50% is in the form of the acetylated compound. The largest portion of the remainder is made up of the free acid. Excretion of aminosalicylic acid is greatly retarded in the presence of renal dysfunction, and the use of the drug is not recommended in such patients. Probenecid decreases the renal excretion of this agent.

Therapeutic Uses. Aminosalicylic acid is a "second-line" agent. Its importance in the management of pulmonary and other forms of tuberculosis has markedly decreased since more active and better-tolerated drugs, such as rifampin and ethambutol, have been developed (*see* discussion of chemotherapy of tuberculosis, below).

Aminosalicylic acid is administered orally in a daily dose of 10 to 12 g. Because it is a gastric irritant, the drug is best administered after meals, the daily dose being divided into two to four equal portions. Children should receive 150 to 300 mg/kg per day in three to four divided doses.

Untoward Effects. The incidence of untoward effects associated with the use of aminosalicylic acid is approximately 10% to 30%. Gastrointestinal problems—including anorexia, nausea, epigastric pain, abdominal distress, and diarrhea—are predominant, and patients with peptic ulcer tolerate the drug poorly. Compliance is often poor because of gastrointestinal distress. Hypersensitivity reactions to aminosalicylic acid are seen in 5% to 10% of patients. High fever may develop abruptly, with intermittent spiking, or it may appear gradually and be low-grade. Generalized malaise, joint pains, or sore throat may be present at the same time. Skin eruptions of various types appear as isolated reactions or accompany the fever. Among the hematological abnormalities that have been observed are leukopenia, agranulocytosis, eosinophilia, lymphocytosis, an atypical mononucleosis syndrome, and thrombocytopenia. Acute hemolytic anemia may appear in some instances.

CYCLOSERINE

Cycloserine (SEROMYCIN) is a broad-spectrum antibiotic produced by *Streptococcus orchidaceus*. It was first isolated from a fermentation brew in 1955 and was later synthesized. Currently, cycloserine is used in conjunction with other tuberculostatic drugs in the treatment of pulmonary or extrapulmonary tuberculosis when primary agents (isoniazid, rifampin, ethambutol, pyrazinamide, streptomycin) have failed.

Chemistry. Cycloserine is D-4-amino-3-isoxazolidone; the structural formula is as follows:

CYCLOSERINE

The drug is stable in alkaline solution but is rapidly destroyed when exposed to neutral or acidic pH.

Antibacterial Activity and Mechanism of Action. Cycloserine is inhibitory for *M. tuberculosis* in concentrations of 5 to 20 μg/ml *in vitro*. There is no cross-resistance between cycloserine and other tuberculostatic agents. While the antibiotic is effective in experimental infections caused by other microorganisms, studies *in vitro* reveal no suppression of growth in cultures made in conventional media, which contain D-alanine; this amino acid blocks the antibacterial activity of cycloserine. The two compounds are structural analogs, and cycloserine inhibits reactions in which D-alanine is involved in bacterial cell-wall synthesis (*see* Chapter 45). The use of media free of D-alanine reveals that the antibiotic inhibits the growth *in vitro* of enterococci, *Escherichia coli, Staphylococcus aureus, Nocardia* species, and *Chlamydia*.

Absorption, Distribution, and Excretion. When given orally, 70% to 90% of cycloserine is rapidly absorbed. Peak concentrations in plasma are reached 3 to 4 hours after a single dose and are in the range of 20 to 35 μg/ml in children who receive 20 mg/kg; only small quantities are present after 12 hours. Cycloserine is distributed throughout body fluids and tissues. There is no appreciable blood–brain barrier to the drug, and CSF concentrations in all patients are approximately the same as those in plasma. About 50% of a parenteral dose of cycloserine is excreted unchanged in the urine in the first 12 hours; a total of 65% is recoverable in the active form over a period of 72 hours. Very little of the antibiotic is metabolized. The drug may accumulate to toxic concentrations in patients with renal insufficiency; it may be removed from the circulation by dialysis.

Therapeutic Uses. Cycloserine should be used only when retreatment is necessary or when microorganisms are resistant to other drugs. When cycloserine is employed to treat tuberculosis, it must be given together with other effective agents. Cycloserine is available for oral administration. The usual dose for adults is 250 to 500 mg twice daily.

Untoward Effects. Reactions to cycloserine most commonly involve the central nervous system. They tend to appear within the first 2 weeks of therapy and usually disappear when the drug is withdrawn. Among the central manifestations are somnolence, headache, tremor, dysarthria, vertigo, confusion, nervousness, irritability, psychotic states with suicidal tendencies, paranoid reactions, catatonic and depressed reactions, twitching, ankle clonus, hyperreflexia, visual disturbances, paresis, and tonic-clonic or absence seizures. Large doses of cycloserine or the ingestion of ethyl alcohol increases the risk of seizures. Cycloserine is contraindicated in individuals with a history of epilepsy.

OTHER DRUGS

The agents grouped in this section are similar in several aspects. They are all "second-line" drugs that are used only for treatment of disease caused by resistant microorganisms or by nontuberculous mycobacteria. They all must be given parenterally, and they have similar pharmacokinetics and toxicity. Since these agents are potentially ototoxic and nephrotoxic, no two drugs from this group should be employed simultaneously, and these drugs should not be used in combination with streptomycin.

Kanamycin, an aminoglycoside that is discussed in Chapter 46, inhibits the growth of *M. tuberculosis in vitro* in a concentration of 10 μg/ml or less. Small groups of patients with tuberculosis have been treated with 1 g of kanamycin daily; toxic effects have been common, including the risk of serious reactions, such as neuromuscular paralysis, respiratory depression, agranulocytosis, anaphylaxis, and nephrotoxicity.

Amikacin also is an aminoglycoside (*see* Chapter 46). It is extremely active against several mycobacterial species and has a role in the treatment of disease caused by nontuberculous mycobacteria (*see* Brown and Wallace, 2000).

Capreomycin (CAPASTAT SULFATE) is an antimycobacterial cyclic peptide elaborated by *Streptococcus capreolus.* It consists of four active components—capreomycins IA, IB, IIA, and IIB. The agent used clinically contains primarily IA and IB. Bacterial resistance to capreomycin develops when it is given alone; such microorganisms show cross-resistance with kanamycin and neomycin. Capreomycin is used only in conjunction with other appropriate antitubercular drugs in treatment of pulmonary tuberculosis when bactericidal agents cannot be tolerated or when causative organisms have become resistant.

Capreomycin must be given intramuscularly. The recommended daily dose is 15 to 30 mg/kg per day or up to 1 g for 60 to 120 days, followed by 1 g two to three times a week.

The reactions associated with the use of capreomycin are hearing loss, tinnitus, transient proteinuria, cylindruria, and nitrogen retention. Severe renal failure is rare. Eosinophilia is common. Leukocytosis, leukopenia, rashes, and fever have also been observed. Injections of the drug may be painful.

CHEMOTHERAPY OF TUBERCULOSIS

The availability of effective agents has so altered the treatment of tuberculosis that most patients are now treated in the ambulatory setting, often after diagnosis and initial therapy in a general hospital. Prolonged bed rest is not necessary or even helpful in speeding recovery. Patients must be seen at frequent intervals to follow the course of their disease and treatment. The local health department must be notified of all cases. Contacts should be investigated for the possibility of disease and for the appropriateness of prophylactic therapy with isoniazid.

The majority of cases of previously untreated tuberculosis in the United States is caused by microorganisms that are sensitive to isoniazid, rifampin, ethambutol, and streptomycin. To prevent the development of resistance to these agents that frequently occurs during the course of therapy of the individual patient, *treatment must include at least two drugs to which the bacteria are sensitive.* The standard 6-month treatment program for drug-sensitive tuberculosis usually is preferred for adults and children and consists of isoniazid, rifampin, and pyrazinamide for 2 months, followed by isoniazid and rifampin for 4 additional months. The combination of isoniazid and rifampin for 9 months is equally effective for drug-sensitive tuberculosis. Because of the increasing frequency of drug resistance, the Centers for Disease Control and Prevention (CDC) has recommended that initial therapy should be with a four-drug regimen (isoniazid, rifampin, pyrazinamide, and ethambutol or streptomycin) pending sensitivity results. Directly observed therapy is the most effective approach to ensure treatment completion rates of about 90% (Chaulk and Kazandjian, 1998).

Drug interactions are a special concern in patients receiving highly active antiretroviral therapy. The rifamycins accelerate the metabolism of protease inhibitors and nonnucleoside reverse transcriptase inhibitors. Of the rifamycins, rifabutin has the least effect on indinavir and nelfinavir serum levels.

Patients infected with the human immunodeficiency virus (HIV) may benefit from longer (9- to 12-month) treatment regimens (Havlir and Barnes, 1999). Treatment should be initiated with at least a four-drug regimen consisting of isoniazid, rifabutin, pyrazinamide, and ethambutol or streptomycin. In patients with a high likelihood of infection with multidrug-resistant strains, an initial five- or six-drug regimen may be appropriate (Lane *et al.,* 1994; Gallant *et al.,* 1994). Treatment should be continued for at least 6 months after three negative cultures have been obtained. If isoniazid or rifampin cannot be used, therapy should be continued for at least 18 months (12 months after cultures become negative). Chemoprophylaxis (*see* below) should be undertaken if a patient with HIV infection has a positive tuberculin test (induration $\geq$5 mm), a history of a positive tuberculin skin test that was not treated with chemoprophylaxis, or recent close contact with a potentially infectious patient with tuberculosis. Isoniazid does not reduce the incidence of tuberculosis in anergic patients with HIV, so the earlier recommendation to treat such patients with chemoprophylaxis has been abandoned (Gordin *et al.,* 1997).

Therapy of Specific Types of Tuberculosis. Therapy for uncomplicated drug-sensitive pulmonary tuberculosis consists of isoniazid (5 mg/kg, up to 300 mg per day), rifampin (10 mg/kg per day, up to 600 mg daily), and pyrazinamide (15 to 30 mg/kg per day or a maximum of 2 g per day). Pyridoxine, 15 to 50 mg per day, also should be included for most adults to minimize adverse reactions to isoniazid (Snider, 1980). Isoniazid, rifampin, and pyrazinamide are given for 2 months; isoniazid and rifampin are then continued for 4 additional months. Children are treated similarly; doses are isoniazid, 10 mg/kg per day (300 mg maximum); rifampin, 10 to 20 mg/kg per day (600 mg maximum); pyrazinamide, 15 to 30 mg/kg per day (2 g maximum; Bass *et al.*, 1994). Surgery is rarely indicated (Haas, 2000). The multidrug regimen of isoniazid, rifampin, and ethambutol is considered safe during pregnancy.

Certain patients should receive at least four drugs initially to ensure that the microorganisms will be susceptible to at least two of the agents. These patients include (1) those known to have been exposed to drug-resistant microorganisms; (2) Asians and Hispanics, especially if they are recent immigrants; (3) those with miliary tuberculosis or other extrapulmonary disease; (4) those with meningitis; (5) those with extensive pulmonary disease; and (6) those with HIV infection. The microorganisms should be cultured for determination of their sensitivity to antimicrobial agents, but results will not be available for several weeks. The fourth agent may be either ethambutol (usual adult dose of 15 mg/kg once per day) or streptomycin (1 g daily). The dosage of streptomycin is reduced to 1 g twice weekly after 2 months. Some physicians prefer to institute ethambutol therapy with a dose of 25 mg/kg per day for the first 60 days and then to reduce the dose to 15 mg/kg per day, particularly for those who have received previous therapy.

Clinical improvement is readily discernible in the vast majority of patients with pulmonary tuberculosis if the treatment is appropriate. Efficacy usually becomes obvious within the first 2 weeks of therapy and is evidenced by a reduction of fever, decrease in cough, gain in weight, and increase in the sense of well-being. Progressive radiological improvement also is evident. Over 90% of patients who receive optimal treatment will have negative cultures within 3 to 6 months, depending on the severity of the disease. Cultures that remain positive after 6 months frequently yield resistant microorganisms; the value of using an alternative therapeutic program should then be considered.

Failure of chemotherapy may be due to (1) irregular or inadequate therapy (resulting in persistent or resistant mycobacteria) caused by poor patient compliance during the protracted therapeutic regimen; (2) the use of a single drug, with interruption necessitated by toxicity or hypersensitivity; (3) an inadequate initial regimen; or (4) the primary resistance of the microorganism.

Problems in Chemotherapy. *Bacterial Resistance to Drugs.* One of the more important problems in the chemotherapy of tuberculosis is bacterial resistance. The primary reason for development of drug resistance is poor patient compliance. To prevent noncompliance and the attendant development of drug-resistant tuberculosis, directly observed therapy is advisable for most patients. For directly observed therapy, a health care provider observes the patient ingest the medications 2 to 5 times weekly (Barnes and Barrows, 1993; Chaulk and Kazandjian, 1998).

Where drug resistance is suspected but sensitivities are not yet known (as in patients who have undergone several courses of treatment), therapy should be instituted with five or six drugs, including two or three that the patient has not received in the past.

Such a program might include isoniazid, rifampin, ethambutol, streptomycin, pyrazinamide, and ethionamide. Some physicians include isoniazid in the therapeutic regimen, even if microorganisms are resistant, because of some evidence that disease with isoniazid-resistant mycobacteria does not "progress" during such therapy. Others prefer to discontinue isoniazid to lessen the possibility of toxicity. Therapy should be continued for at least 24 months.

Nontuberculous (Atypical) Mycobacteria. These microorganisms (not including *M. avium* complex, which is discussed later) have been recovered from a variety of lesions in human beings (Brown and Wallace, 2000). Because they frequently are resistant to many of the commonly used agents, they must be examined for sensitivity *in vitro* and drug therapy selected on this basis. In some instances, surgical removal of the infected tissue followed by long-term treatment with effective agents is necessary.

M. kansasii causes disease similar to that caused by *M. tuberculosis,* but it may be milder. The microorganisms may be resistant to isoniazid. Therapy with isoniazid, rifampin, and ethambutol has been successful (Pezzia *et al.*, 1981; Lane *et al.*, 1994). *M. marinum* causes skin lesions. A combination of rifampin and ethambutol is probably effective; minocycline (Loria, 1976) or tetracycline is active *in vitro* and is used by some physicians (Izumi *et al.*, 1977). *M. scrofulaceum* is an uncommon cause of cervical lymphadenitis. Surgical excision still seems to be the therapy of choice (Lincoln and Gilberg, 1972). Microbes of the *M. fortuitum* complex (including *Mycobacterium chelonei*) are usually saprophytes, but they may cause chronic lung disease and infections of skin and soft tissues. The microorganisms are highly resistant to most drugs, but amikacin, cefoxitin, and tetracyclines are active *in vitro* (Sanders *et al.*, 1977; Sanders, 1982).

Chemoprophylaxis of Tuberculosis. There are several approaches to the chemoprophylaxis of tuberculosis. The classical prophylaxis with 12 months of isoniazid resulted in a 75% reduction in the risk of active tuberculosis (from an incidence of 14.3% to 3.6% over 5 years). A 6-month course of isoniazid therapy was nearly as effective, with a 65% risk reduction and a lower incidence of isoniazid-induced hepatitis (IUAT, 1982). Recently, a 2-month regimen of daily rifampin and pyrazinamide was shown to be as effective as 12 months of isoniazid in one study of HIV-infected individuals (Halsey *et al.*, 1998).

Prophylactic therapy can effectively prevent the development of active tuberculosis in certain instances (Haas, 2000). There are three categories of patients for whom prophylactic therapy should be considered: those exposed to tuberculosis but who have no evidence of infection; those with infection [positive tuberculin test: more than 5 mm (HIV infected) or 10 mm (not immunocompromised) of induration to 5 units of purified protein derivative (PPD)] and no apparent disease; and those with a history of tuberculosis but in whom the disease is presently "inactive" (*see* Bass *et al.*, 1994; Stead and To, 1987; Wilkinson *et al.*, 1998; Gordin *et al.*, 1997; Gallant *et al.*,

1994). The main risk of chemoprophylaxis is isoniazid-induced hepatitis, which is much more common about the age of 35. Some authorities argue that monitored isoniazid prophylaxis minimizes the risk of toxicity even in patients over the age of 35 (Salpeter *et al.*, 1997).

Household contacts and other close associates of patients with tuberculosis who have negative tuberculin tests should receive isoniazid for at least 6 months after the contact has been broken, regardless of age. This is especially important for children. If the tuberculin skin test becomes positive, therapy should be continued for 12 months.

Persons without apparent disease whose skin test has converted from negative to positive within the preceding 2 years should probably receive isoniazid for 12 months regardless of age. These patients are considered to be "infected" but not to have clinical disease. Some authorities believe that persons with positive skin tests, no matter when they became so, who are under 35 years of age, or who are at risk of infection because of such factors as infection with HIV, immunosuppressive therapy, leukemia, lymphoma, or silicosis should receive isoniazid for 1 year (Bass *et al.*, 1994; Gallant *et al.*, 1994). For individuals over 35 years of age, the risk of isoniazid toxicity may outweigh the potential benefit of therapy.

Patients with old "inactive" tuberculosis who have not received adequate chemotherapy in the past should be considered for 1 year of treatment with isoniazid (*see* Comstock, 1983). HIV-infected intravenous drug abusers with a positive skin test have an approximately 8% chance per year of developing active tuberculosis (Selwyn *et al.*, 1989). Isoniazid prophylaxis in HIV-infected persons appears to be as effective as in nonimmunocompromised persons (Wilkinson *et al.*, 1998). The CDC recommends that isoniazid prophylaxis be continued for 12 months. Prophylaxis should be given to HIV-infected persons with more than 5 mm of induration to 5 units of PPD. A 1991 CDC recommendation that anergic HIV-infected persons from populations at risk for tuberculosis receive prophylaxis was reversed in 1997, when it was shown to be without foundation (Gordin *et al.*, 1997; Whalen *et al.*, 1997). Persons infected with HIV who are exposed to multidrug-resistant tuberculosis should receive prophylaxis with high-dose ethambutol and pyrazinamide, with or without a fluoroquinolone (Gallant *et al.*, 1994).

Prophylaxis with isoniazid is contraindicated for patients who have active hepatic disease or who have had reactions to the drug. The recent demonstration of the comparable efficacy of a 2-month course of rifampin and pyrazinamide (in HIV-infected adults) offers a potential alternative to isoniazid prophylaxis (Halsey *et al.*, 1998). In pregnant women, prophylaxis usually should be delayed until after delivery. For prophylaxis, isoniazid generally is given to adults in a daily dose of 300 mg. Children should receive 10 mg/kg to a maximal daily dose of 300 mg.

II. Drugs for *Mycobacterium avium* Complex

Before the advent of highly active antiretroviral therapy (HAART, *see* Chapter 51) and the use of prophylactic regimens, disseminated infection with *M. avium* complex (MAC) bacteria occurred in 15% to 40% of patients with HIV infection. Infections with MAC now are greatly reduced (Benson, 1997–98). Patients with *M. avium* complex infection usually are in advanced stages of HIV disease, with CD4 T-lymphocyte counts below 100/mm^3 and symptoms of fever, night sweats, weight loss, and anemia at the time of diagnosis (Masur *et al.*, 1993). In non-HIV-infected persons, MAC infection usually is limited to the lungs and presents with a chronic productive cough and chest roentgenograms showing evidence of limited, diffuse, and/or cavitary disease (Havlir and Ellner, 2000). Although standard antimycobacterial agents have little activity against MAC, new antimicrobial agents with activity against MAC recently have become available. These agents currently are in use for both the prevention and treatment of MAC in patients with AIDS.

RIFABUTIN

Rifabutin (MYCOBUTIN) is a derivative of rifamycin S. Rifabutin shares its mechanism of action with rifampin (inhibition of mycobacterial RNA polymerase), but is more active *in vitro* and in experimental murine tuberculosis than is rifampin.

Chemistry. Rifabutin is soluble in organic solvents and at low concentrations (0.19 mg/ml) in water. It has the following structure:

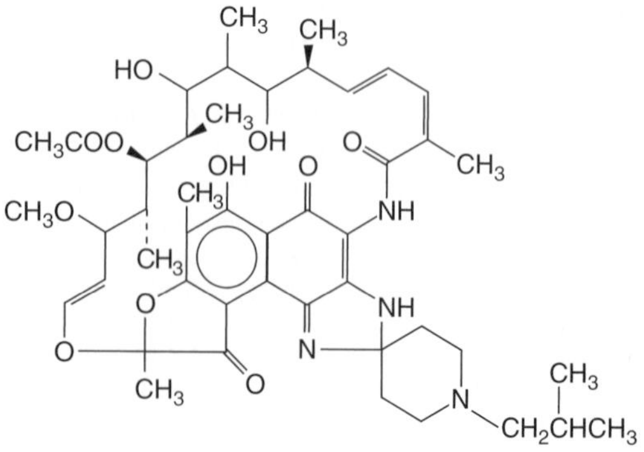

RIFABUTIN

Antibacterial Activity. Rifabutin has better activity against the MAC organisms than does rifampin. Rifabutin is active *in vitro* against MAC bacteria isolated from both HIV-infected (where the majority of MAC infections are *M. avium*) and non-HIV-infected individuals (where approximately 40% of MAC infections are *M. intracellulare*). Rifabutin inhibits the growth of most MAC isolates at concentrations ranging from 0.25 to 1.0 μg/ml. Rifabutin also inhibits the growth of many strains of *M. tuberculosis* at concentrations of $\leq$0.125 μg/ml.

Bacterial Resistance. Cross-resistance between rifampin and rifabutin occurs to some extent with both *M. avium* and *M. tuberculosis*; of 225 *M. avium* strains that were resistant to 10 μg/ml of rifampin, 80% were sensitive to 1 μg/ml rifabutin (Heifets *et al.*, 1985).

Absorption, Distribution, and Excretion. The oral administration of 300 mg of rifabutin produces a peak plasma concentration of approximately 0.4 μg/ml at 2 to 3 hours. The drug is eliminated in a biphasic manner with a mean terminal half-life of 45 hours (range of 16 to 96 hours). Because rifabutin is a lipophilic drug, concentrations are substantially higher (5- to 10-fold) in tissue than in plasma. Following absorption from the GI tract, rifabutin is eliminated in the urine and bile. Adjustment of dosage is not necessary in patients with impaired renal function.

Therapeutic Uses. Rifabutin is effective for the prevention of MAC infection in HIV-infected individuals. At a dose of 300 mg per day, rifabutin decreased the frequency of MAC bacteremia by half (Nightingale *et al.*, 1993). However, azithromycin or clarithromycin are more effective and less likely to interact with HAART drugs. Rifabutin also is commonly substituted for rifampin in the treatment of tuberculosis in HIV-infected patients, as it has a less profound interaction with indinavir and nelfinavir (Haas, 2000). Rifabutin also is used in combination with clarithromycin and ethambutol for the therapy of MAC disease (Shafran *et al.*, 1996).

Untoward Effects. Rifabutin generally is well tolerated in persons with HIV infection; primary reasons for discontinuation of therapy include rash (4%), gastrointestinal intolerance (3%), and neutropenia (2%; Nightingale *et al.*, 1993). Overall neutropenia occurred in 25% of patients with severe HIV infection who received rifabutin. Uveitis and arthralgias have occurred in patients receiving rifabutin doses greater than 450 mg daily in combination with clarithromycin or fluconazole. Patients should be cautioned to discontinue the drug if visual symptoms (pain or blurred vision) occur. Like rifampin, the drug causes an orange-tan discoloration of skin, urine, feces, saliva, tears, and contact lenses. Rarely, thrombocytopenia, a flu-like syndrome, hemolysis, myositis, chest pain, and hepatitis have occurred in patients treated with rifabutin.

Rifabutin shares with rifampin the property of inducing hepatic microsomal enzymes, with its administration decreasing the half-life of a number of different compounds, including zidovudine, prednisone, digitoxin, quinidine, ketoconazole, propranolol, phenytoin, sulfonylureas, and warfarin. It has less effect than does rifampin on serum levels of indinavir and nelfinavir.

MACROLIDES

A discussion of the pharmacology of the macrolides, including their adverse effects and uses in infections other than MAC, is presented in Chapter 47. Only features of the macrolides related to their use in the treatment of MAC infections are considered here.

Antibacterial Activity. Clarithromycin is approximately fourfold more active than azithromycin against MAC bacteria *in vitro* and is active against most nontuberculous mycobacteria with the exception of *Mycobacterium simiae* at $\leq$4 μg/ml. Azithromycin's lower potency may be compensated for *in vivo* by its greater intracellular penetration: tissue levels generally exceed plasma levels by two orders of magnitude.

Bacterial Resistance. Use of clarithromycin or azithromycin alone in the therapy of MAC infection is associated with the development of resistance after prolonged treatment. For this reason, these drugs should not be used as monotherapy of MAC infection.

Therapeutic Uses. Clarithromycin (500 mg twice daily) or azithromycin (500 mg daily) is used in combination with ethambutol, with or without rifabutin, for treatment of MAC infection (Shafran *et al.*, 1996; Masur *et al.*, 1993). Treatment should be continued throughout the lifetime of an HIV-infected individual (USPHS, 1999).

Untoward Effects. With high doses used to treat MAC infections, tinnitus, dizziness, and reversible hearing loss occasionally have occurred.

QUINOLONES

A discussion of the pharmacology of the quinolones, including their adverse effects and uses in infections other than MAC, is presented in Chapter 44. Only features of the quinolones related to their use in the treatment of MAC infections are considered here.

Antibacterial Activity. Fluoroquinolones, such as levofloxacin, ciprofloxacin, ofloxacin, fleroxacin, and sparfloxacin, have inhibitory activity against *M. tuberculosis* and MAC bacteria *in vitro* (at concentrations of $\leq$1.3 μg/ml for *M. tuberculosis* and $\leq$10 to 100 μg/ml for MAC bacteria). Minimal inhibitory concentrations for *M. fortuitum* and *M. kansasii* are ≤ 3 μg/ml for these quinolones.

Bacterial Resistance. Single-agent therapy of *M. fortuitum* infection with ciprofloxacin has been associated with the development of resistance.

Therapeutic Uses. Ciprofloxacin, 750 mg twice daily or 500 mg three times daily, has been used as part of a four-drug regimen (with clarithromycin, rifabutin, and amikacin) as salvage therapy for MAC infections in HIV-infected patients, with improvement in symptoms (Havlir and Ellner, 2000). Multidrug-resistant tuberculosis has been treated with ofloxacin, 300 or 800 mg each day, in combination with second-line agents.

CLOFAZIMINE

Discussed more fully under drugs for the treatment of leprosy, clofazimine inhibits most MAC isolates *in vitro* at levels of 1.6 to 2.0 μg/ml, although clinical experience with the drug in combination with other agents has been disappointing.

AMIKACIN

The antibacterial activity and pharmacology of amikacin are discussed fully in Chapter 46. Amikacin may have a role as a third or fourth agent in a multiple-drug regimen for MAC treatment. Most isolates of MAC are inhibited *in vitro* by 8 to 32 μg/ml of amikacin.

CHEMOTHERAPY OF *Mycobacterium avium* COMPLEX

Initial pessimism about the treatment of MAC infection has lifted with the availability of clarithromycin and azithromycin. Both of these agents have excellent activity against many strains of MAC, with clinical responses (decrease or elimination of bacteremia, resolution of fever and night sweats) demonstrated even with single-drug therapy. Single-agent therapy, however, has been associated with the emergence of resistant strains. Most clinicians are currently treating MAC infections with clarithromycin or azithromycin plus ethambutol (Haas, 2000; Shafran *et al.,* 1996). In some situations, and with unclear benefits, rifabutin, clofazimine, and/or a quinolone are added to the above regimen. Drug interactions and adverse drug reactions are common with multiple-drug regimens and necessitated drug discontinuation in 46% of patients in one study (Kemper *et al.,* 1992). Clinical improvement should be expected in the first 1 to 2 months of treatment, with sterilization of blood cultures seen as late as 3 months into therapy (Masur *et al.,* 1993). Therapy of MAC infection in HIV-infected individuals should continue for life if the therapy is associated with clinical and microbiological improvement (USPHS, 1999). Isoniazid and pyrazinamide have no role in the treatment of MAC infection.

Prophylaxis of MAC infection with clarithromycin or azithromycin should be strongly considered for HIV-infected persons whose CD4 cell count is less than 50/mm^3. Clarithromycin and azithromycin are well-tolerated medications that have proven effective at reducing the incidence of MAC infection in this population. With the advent of HAART, it would be a reasonable decision to stop prophylaxis in a patient who responds to anti-HIV therapy with a sustained CD4$^+$ T-lymphocyte count greater than 100/mm^3 and a sustained suppression of HIV plasma RNA (USPHS, 1999).

III. DRUGS FOR LEPROSY

Although leprosy (Hansen's disease) is seen rarely in the United States, it is estimated that 6 million patients worldwide have this disease. The development of effective chemotherapy for leprosy has allowed most patients to be managed outside of hospitals.

SULFONES

The sulfones, as a class, are derivatives of 4,4'-diaminodiphenylsulfone (dapsone), all of which have certain pharmacological properties in common. They are discussed here as a class; only dapsone and sulfoxone are considered individually.

History. The sulfones first attracted interest because of their chemical relationship to the sulfonamides. In the 1940s, sulfones were found to be effective in suppressing experimental infections with the tubercle bacillus and for rat leprosy; this finding was soon followed by successful clinical trials in human leprosy. The sulfones are currently the most important drugs for the treatment of this disorder.

Chemistry. All the sulfones of clinical value are derivatives of dapsone. Despite the study and development of a large variety of sulfones, this drug remains the agent most useful clinically. The structures of dapsone and sulfoxone sodium are as follows:

DAPSONE

SULFOXONE SODIUM

Antibacterial Activity. Because *Mycobacterium leprae* does not grow on artificial media, conventional methods cannot be applied to determine its susceptibility to potential therapeutic agents *in vitro*. Crude sensitivities *in vivo* can be determined by injecting microorganisms into the foot pads of mice and treating them with the agents to be tested. After 6 to 8 months, the mice are killed, the foot pads are homogenized, and microscopic counts are made of acid-fast microorganisms (Shepard *et al.,* 1976). Dapsone is bacteriostatic, but not bactericidal, for *M. leprae,* and the estimated sensitivity to the drug is between 1 and 10 ng/ml for microorganisms recovered from untreated patients (Levy and Peters, 1976). *M. leprae* may become resistant to the drug during therapy.

The mechanism of action of the sulfones is the same as that of the sulfonamides. Both possess approximately the same range of antibacterial activity and both are antagonized by paraaminobenzoic acid.

Dapsone-resistant strains of *M. leprae* are termed *secondary* if they emerge during therapy. Secondary resistance usually is seen in lepromatous (multibacillary) patients treated with a single drug. The incidence is as high as 19% (WHO Expert Committee on Leprosy, 1998). Partial-to-complete primary resistance (seen in previously untreated patients) has been described in from 2.5% to 40% of patients, depending on geographical location (Centers for Disease Control, 1982), although some authorities question the clinical significance of primary resistance (Gelber *et al.,* 1990; Gelber and Rea, 2000).

Therapeutic Uses. *Dapsone* is available for oral administration. Several dosage schedules have been recommended (*see* Trautman, 1965; Gelber and Rea, 2000). Daily therapy with 100 mg has been successful in adults. Therapy usually is begun with smaller amounts, and doses are increased to those recommended over 1 to 2 months. Therapy should be continued for at least 3 years and may be necessary for the lifetime of the patient.

Sulfoxone sodium may be substituted for dapsone in patients in whom the latter drug produces sufficient gastric distress to impede effective therapy. The recommended daily dose of sulfoxone sodium is 330 mg.

The use of sulfones in malaria resistant to the usual antimalarial drugs is discussed in Chapter 40.

Untoward Effects. The reactions induced by various sulfones are very similar. The most common untoward effect is hemolysis of varying degree. This develops in almost every individual treated with 200 to 300 mg of dapsone per day. Doses of 100 mg or less in normal healthy persons and 50 mg or less in healthy individuals with a glucose-6-phosphate dehydrogenase deficiency do not cause hemolysis. Methemoglobinemia also is common, and Heinz-body formation may occur. A genetic deficiency in the NADH-dependent methemoglobin reductase can result in severe methemoglobinemia after administration of dapsone. While diminished red-cell survival usually occurs during the use of sulfones and is presumed to be a dose-related effect of their oxidizing activity, hemolytic anemia is unusual unless the patient also has a disorder of either the erythrocytes or the bone marrow (Pengelly, 1963). The hemolysis may be so severe that manifestations of hypoxia become striking.

Anorexia, nausea, and vomiting may follow the oral administration of sulfones. Isolated instances of headache, nervousness, insomnia, blurred vision, paresthesia, reversible peripheral neuropathy (thought to be due to axonal degeneration), drug fever, hematuria, pruritus, psychosis, and a variety of skin rashes have been reported (Rapoport and Guss, 1972). An infectious mononucleosis-like syndrome, which may be fatal, occurs occasionally. The sulfones may induce an exacerbation of lepromatous leprosy by a process thought to be analogous to the Jarisch–Herxheimer reaction. This "sulfone syndrome" may develop 5 to 6 weeks after initiation of treatment in malnourished people. Its manifestations include fever, malaise, exfoliative dermatitis, jaundice with hepatic necrosis, lymphadenopathy, methemoglobinemia, and anemia.

The sulfones may be given safely for many years in doses adequate for the successful therapy of leprosy if proper precautions are observed. Treatment should be initiated with a small dose and the quantity then increased gradually. Patients must be under consistent and prolonged laboratory and clinical supervision. The reactions induced by the sulfones, especially those related to exacerbation of the leprosy, may be very severe and may require the cessation of treatment as well as the institution of specific measures to reduce the threat to life.

Absorption, Distribution, and Excretion. Dapsone is absorbed rapidly and nearly completely from the gastrointestinal tract. The disubstituted sulfones, such as sulfoxone, are absorbed incompletely when administered orally, and large amounts are excreted in the feces. Peak concentrations of dapsone in plasma are reached within 2 to 8 hours after administration; the mean half-life of elimination is about 20 to 30 hours. Twenty-four hours after oral ingestion of 100 mg, plasma concentrations range from 0.4 to 1.2 μg/ml (Shepard *et al.,* 1976), and a dose of 100 mg of dapsone per day produces an average of 2 μg of "free" dapsone per gram of blood or nonhepatic tissue. About 70% of the drug is bound to plasma protein. Concentrations in plasma following conventional doses of sulfoxone sodium are 10 to 15 μg/ml. These values fall relatively rapidly; however, appreciable quantities are still present at 8 hours.

The sulfones are distributed throughout total body water and are present in all tissues. They tend to be retained in skin and muscle and especially in liver and kidney; traces of the drug are present in these organs up to 3 weeks after therapy is stopped. The sulfones are retained in the circulation for a long time because of intestinal reabsorption from the bile; periodic interruption of treatment is advisable for this reason. Dapsone is acetylated in the liver, and the rate of acetylation is genetically determined; the same enzyme carries out the acetylation of isoniazid. Daily administration of 50 to 100 mg results in serum levels exceeding the usual minimal inhibitory concentrations, even in rapid acetylators, in whom the serum half-life of dapsone and certain other drugs is shorter than usual.

The urinary excretion of sulfones varies with the type of drug; about 70% to 80% of a dose of dapsone is so excreted. The drug is present in urine as an acid-labile mono-*N*-glucuronide and mono-*N*-sulfamate in addition to an unknown number of unidentified metabolites. Probenecid decreases the urinary excretion of the acid-labile dapsone metabolites significantly and that of free dapsone to a lesser extent (Goodwin and Sparell, 1969).

RIFAMPIN

Rifampin has been discussed above with regard to its use in tuberculosis. This antibiotic is rapidly bactericidal for *M. leprae,* and the minimal inhibitory concentration is less than 1 μg/ml. Infectivity of patients is reversed rapidly by therapy that includes rifampin (Bullock, 1983). Because of the prevalence of resistance to dapsone, the WHO Expert Committee on Leprosy

(1998) now recommends a regimen of multiple drugs, including rifampin.

CLOFAZIMINE

Clofazimine (LAMPRENE) is a phenazine dye with the following structural formula:

CLOFAZIMINE

Clofazimine appears to preferentially bind to GC-rich mycobacterial DNA (Morrison and Marley, 1976). It is weakly bactericidal against *M. intracellulare*. The drug also exerts an antiinflammatory effect and prevents the development of erythema nodosum leprosum. Clofazimine is now recommended as a component of multiple-drug therapy for leprosy (*see* below). The compound also is useful for treatment of chronic skin ulcers (Buruli ulcer) produced by *Mycobacterium ulcerans*.

Clofazimine is absorbed by the oral route and appears to accumulate in tissues. Human leprosy from which dapsone-resistant bacilli have been recovered has been treated with clofazimine with good results. However, unlike dapsone-sensitive microorganisms, in which killing occurs immediately after dapsone is administered, dapsone-resistant strains do not exhibit an appreciable effect until 50 days after initiation of therapy with clofazimine. The daily dose of clofazimine is usually 100 mg (*see* Levy *et al.*, 1972). Patients treated with clofazimine may develop red discoloration of the skin, which may be very distressing to light-skinned individuals. Eosinophilic enteritis has also been described as an adverse reaction to the drug (Mason *et al.*, 1977).

MISCELLANEOUS AGENTS

Thalidomide seems to be effective for the treatment of erythema nodosum leprosum (Iyer *et al.*, 1971). Doses of 100 to 300 mg per day have been effective. **Because of the marked teratogenicity of thalidomide, it should never be administered during pregnancy or to any woman of childbearing age.**

Ethionamide has been discussed above as an agent for treatment of tuberculosis. It can be used as a substitute for clofazimine in oral doses of 250 to 375 mg per day. New agents that appear promising based on animal trials and limited experience in patients include minocycline, clarithromycin, pefloxacin, and ofloxacin (Gelber and Rea, 2000).

CHEMOTHERAPY OF LEPROSY

Few physicians other than specialists in the field are called upon to treat leprosy. Consultation is available with physicians at the National Hansen's Disease Center (Carville, LA 70721). There-

fore, the following discussion is intended mainly to familiarize the reader with the progress that has been made in the treatment of this chronic bacterial disease, which has proven very resistant to chemotherapy.

Five clinical types of leprosy are recognized. At one end of the spectrum is *tuberculoid leprosy*. This form of the disease is characterized by skin macules with clear centers and well-defined margins; these are almost always anesthetic. *M. leprae* is rarely found in smears made from quiescent lesions but may appear during activity. Virchow cells are not demonstrable. Noncaseating foci with giant cells of the Langhans variety are present. The patient's cell-mediated immune responses are normal, and the lepromin test (intradermal injection of a suspension of heat-killed, bacillus-laden tissue) is invariably positive. The disease is characterized by prolonged remissions with periodic reactivation.

At the other end of the spectrum is the widely disseminated *lepromatous* form of the disease. Patients with this disease have markedly impaired cell-mediated immunity and are frequently anergic; the lepromin test causes no reaction. Lepromatous disease is characterized by diffuse or ill-defined, localized infiltration of the skin, which becomes thickened, glossy, and corrugated; areas of decreased sensation may appear. *M. leprae* is demonstrable in smears, and granulomas containing bacteria-laden histiocytes (Virchow cells) are present. As the disease progresses, large nerve trunks are involved and anesthesia, atrophy of skin and muscle, absorption of small bones, ulceration, and spontaneous amputations may occur. Three intermediate forms of the disease are recognized: borderline tuberculoid disease, borderline lepromatous disease, and borderline disease (Gelber and Rea, 2000).

Patients with tuberculoid leprosy may develop "reversal reactions," which are manifestations of delayed hypersensitivity to antigens of *M. leprae*. Cutaneous ulcerations and deficits of peripheral nerve function may occur. Early therapy with corticosteroids or clofazimine is effective.

Reactions in the lepromatous form of the disease (erythema nodosum leprosum) are characterized by the appearance of raised, tender, intracutaneous nodules, severe constitutional symptoms, and high fever. This reaction may be triggered by several conditions but is often associated with therapy. It is thought to be an Arthus-type reaction related to release of microbial antigens in patients harboring large numbers of bacilli. Treatment with clofazimine or thalidomide is effective.

The outlook for persons with leprosy has been remarkably altered by successful chemotherapy, surgical procedures that help to restore function and repair disfigurement, and a striking change in the attitude of the public toward patients who have this infection. The social stigma of individuals with this affliction gradually is being replaced by the attitude that considers leprosy a disease caused by a bacterium. Patients with leprosy can be classified as "infectious" or "noninfectious" on the basis of the type and duration of disease and effects of therapy. Thus, even "infectious" patients need not be hospitalized provided that adequate medical supervision and therapy are maintained, the home environment meets specific conditions, and the local health officer concurs in the disposition of the case.

Therapy, when effective, heals ulcers and mucosal lesions in months. Cutaneous nodules respond more slowly, and it may take years to eradicate bacteria from mucous membranes, skin, and nerves. The degree of residual pigmentation or depigmentation, atrophy, and scarring depends upon the extent of the initial involvement. Severe ocular lesions show little response to the sulfones. If treatment is initiated before ocular disease is evident, the latter may be prevented. Keratoconjunctivitis and corneal ulceration may be secondary to nerve involvement.

The World Health Organization now recommends therapy with multiple drugs for all patients with leprosy (WHO Expert Committee on Leprosy, 1998). The reasons for using combinations of agents include reduction in the development of resistance, the need for adequate therapy when primary resistance already exists, and reduction in the duration of therapy. Dosage recommendations for control programs take a number of practical constraints into account. For patients with large populations of bacteria (multibacillary forms)—including lepromatous disease, borderline lepromatous disease, and borderline disease—the following regimen is suggested: dapsone, 100 mg daily; plus clofazimine, 50 mg daily; plus rifampin, 600 mg and clofazimine (300 mg) once a month under supervision for 1 to 5 years. Some prefer to treat lepromatous leprosy with daily dapsone (100 mg) and daily rifampin (450 to 600 mg) (Jacobson, 1982; Gelber and Rea, 2000). All drugs are given orally. The minimal duration of therapy is 2 years, and treatment should continue until acid-fast bacilli are not detected in lesions.

Patients with a small population of bacteria (paucibacillary disease), including those with tuberculoid, borderline tuberculoid, and indeterminate disease, should be treated with dapsone, 100 mg daily, plus rifampin, 600 mg once monthly (under supervision), for a minimum of 6 months. Relapses are treated by repeating the regimen. A recent clinical trial suggests that single-dose multidrug therapy with rifampin (600 mg), ofloxacin (400 mg), and minocycline (100 mg) may be as effective (Single Lesion Multicentre Trial Group, 1997). More prolonged treatment programs are recommended for patients in the United States (*see* Hastings and Franzblau, 1988; Gilber and Rea, 2000).

PROSPECTUS

Applications of fluoroquinones in the treatment of mycobacterial disease hold promise. Wider application of directly observed therapy and the advent of HAART for HIV infection portend a continued decline in tuberculosis in the United States. Understanding of mechanisms of resistance to antimycobacterial agents may result in the development of more effective agents for infections due to resistant organisms. The use of immunomodulators, such as interferon gamma, to increase macrophage killing of the intracellular bacterium also is a potentially important new avenue for treatment.

For further information regarding particular infections for which the antimicrobial agents discussed in this chapter are useful, the reader is referred to the following chapters of *Harrison's Principles of Internal Medicine,* 14th ed., McGraw-Hill, New York, 1998: "Tuberculosis" (Chapter 171), "Leprosy" (Chapter 172), "*Mycobacterium avium* Complex and Other Nontuberculous Mycobacterial Infections" (Chapter 173).

BIBLIOGRAPHY

Baciewicz, A.M., Self, T.H., and Bekemeyer, W.B. Update on rifampin drug interactions. *Arch. Intern. Med., 1987, 147:*565–568.

Bailey, W.C., Weill, H., DeRouen, T.A., Ziskind, M.M., and Jackson, H.A. The effect of isoniazid on transaminase levels. *Ann. Intern. Med., 1974, 81:*200–202.

Banerjee A., Dubnau, E., Quemard, A., Balasubramanian, V., Um, K.S., Wilson, T., Collins, D., de Lisle, G., Jacobs, W.R., Jr. inhA, a gene encoding a target for isoniazid and ethionamide in *Mycobacterium tuberculosis. Science, 1994, 263:*227–230.

Belanger, A.E., Besra, G.S., Ford, M.E., Mikusova, K., Belisle, J.T., Brennan, P.J., and Inamine, J.M. The *embAB* genes of *Mycobacterium avium* encode an arabinosyl transferase involved in cell wall arabinan biosynthesis that is a target for the antimycobacterial drug ethambutol. *Proc. Natl. Acad. Sci. U.S.A., 1996, 93:*11919–11924.

Benson, C.A. Disseminated *Mycobacterium avium* complex infection: implications of recent chemical trials on prophylaxis and treatment. *AIDS Clin. Rev., 1997–98,* 271–287.

Bobrowitz, I.D. Ethambutol-isoniazid versus streptomycin-ethambutol-isoniazid in original treatment of cavitary tuberculosis. *Am. Rev. Respir. Dis., 1974, 109:*548–553.

Bowersox, D.W., Winterbauer, R.H., Stewart, G.L., Orme, B., and

Barron, E. Isoniazid dosage in patients with renal failure. *N. Engl. J. Med., 1973, 289:*84–87.

British Thoracic Association. A controlled trial of six months chemotherapy in pulmonary tuberculosis. Second report: results during the twenty-four months after the end of chemotherapy. *Am. Rev. Respir. Dis., 1982, 126:*460–462.

Byrd, R.B., Horn, B.R., Solomon, D.A., and Griggs, G.W. Toxic effects of isoniazid in tuberculosis chemoprophylaxis. Role of biochemical monitoring in 1,000 patients. *JAMA, 1979, 241:*1239–1241.

Cauthen, G.M., Kilburn, J.O., Kelly, G.D., and Good, R.C. Resistance to anti-tuberculosis drugs in patients with and without prior treatment: survey of 31 state and large city laboratories, 1982–1986. *Am. Rev. Respir. Dis., 1988, 137(suppl.):*260.

Centers for Disease Control. Adverse drug reactions among children treated for tuberculosis. *M.M.W.R. Morb. Mortal. Wkly. Rep., 1980, 29:*589–591.

Centers for Disease Control. Increase in prevalence of leprosy caused by dapsone-resistant *Mycobacterium leprae. M.M.W.R. Morb. Mortal. Wkly. Rep., 1982, 30:*637–638.

Centers for Disease Control and Prevention. Tuberculosis elimination revisited: obstacles, opportunities, and a renewed commitment.

Advisory Council for the Elimination of Tuberculosis (ACET). *M.M.W.R. Morb. Mortal. Wkly. Rep.,* **1999,** *48:*1–13.

Chaulk, C.P., and Kazandjian, V.A. Directly observed therapy for treatment completion of pulmonary tuberculosis: Consensus Statement of the Public Health Tuberculosis Guidelines Panel. *JAMA,* **1998,** *279:*943–948.

Comstock, G.W. New data on preventive treatment with isoniazid. *Ann. Intern. Med.,* **1983,** *98:*663–665.

Evans, D.A.P., Manley, K.A., and McKusick, V.A. Genetic control of isoniazid metabolism in man. *Br. Med. J.,* **1960,** *2:*485–491.

Furesz, S. Chemical and biological properties of rifampicin. *Antibiot. Chemother.,* **1970,** *16:*316–351.

Gangadharam, P.R. Isoniazid, rifampin, and hepatotoxicity. *Am. Rev. Respir. Dis.,* **1986,** *133:*963–965.

Garibaldi, R.A., Drusin, R.E., Ferebee, S.H., and Gregg, M.B. Isoniazid-associated hepatitis. Report of an outbreak. *Am. Rev. Respir. Dis.,* **1972,** *106:*357–365.

Gelber, R.H., Rea, T.H., Murray, L.P., Siu, P., Tsang, M., and Byrd, S.R. Primary dapsone-resistant Hansen's disease in California. Experience with over 100 *Mycobacterium leprae* isolates. *Arch. Dermatol.,* **1990,** *126:*1584–1586.

Girling, D.J. The hepatic toxicity of antituberculous regimens containing isoniazid, rifampicin and pyrazinamide. *Tubercle,* **1978,** *59:*13–32.

Girling, D.J., and Hitze, H.L. Adverse reactions to rifampicin. *Bull. World Health Organ.,* **1979,** *57:*45–49.

Goodwin, C.S., and Sparell, G. Inhibition of dapsone excretion by probenecid. *Lancet,* **1969,** *2:*884–885.

Gordin, F.M., Matts, J.P., Miller, C., Brown, L.S., Hafner, R., John, S.L., Klein, M., Vaughn, A., Besch, C.L., Perez, G., Szabo, S., and El-Sadr, W. A controlled trial of isoniazid in persons with anergy and human immunodeficiency virus infection who are at risk for tuberculosis. Terry Beirn Community Programs for Clinical Research on AIDS. *N. Engl. J. Med.,* **1997,** *337:*315–320.

Graber, C.D., Jebaily, J., Galphin, R.L., and Doering, E. Light chain proteinuria and humoral immunocompetence in tuberculous patients treated with rifampin. *Am. Rev. Respir. Dis.,* **1973,** *107:*713–717.

Grosset, J., and Leventis, S. Adverse effects of rifampin. *Rev. Infect. Dis.,* **1983,** *5:*S440–S446.

Halsey, N.A., Coberly, J.S., Desormeaux, J., Losikoff, P., Atkinson, J., Moulton, L.H., Contave, M., Johnson, M., Davis, H., Geiter, L., Johnson, E., Huebner, R., Boulos, R., and Chaisson, R.E. Randomised controlled trial of isoniazid *versus* rifampin and pyrazinamide for prevention of tuberculosis in HIV-1 infection. *Lancet,* **1998,** *351:*786–792.

Heifets, L.B., Iseman, M.D., Lindholm-Levy, P.J., and Kanes, W. Determination of ansamycin MICs for *Mycobacterium avium* complex in liquid medium by radiometric and conventional methods. *Antimicrob. Agents Chemother.,* **1985,** *28:*570–575.

Hobby, G.L., and Lenert, T.F. Observations on the action of rifampin and ethambutol alone and in combination with other antituberculous drugs. *Am. Rev. Respir. Dis.,* **1972,** *105:*292–295.

Holdiness, M.R. Cerebrospinal fluid pharmacokinetics of antituberculosis antibiotics. *Clin. Pharmacokinet.,* **1985,** *10:*532–534.

IUAT. Efficacy of various durations of isoniazid preventive therapy for tuberculosis: five years follow-up in the IUAT trial. International Union Against Tuberculosis. *Bull. World Health Organ.,* **1982,** *60:*555–564.

Iyer, C.G., Languillon, J., Ramanujam, K., Tarabini-Castellani, G., De las Aguas, J.T., Bechelli, L.M., Uemura, K., Martinez Dominguez, V., and Sundaresan, T. WHO co-ordinated short-term double-blind trial with thalidomide in the treatment of acute lepra reactions in male lepromatous patients. *Bull. World Health Organ.,* **1971,** *45:*719–732.

Izumi, A.K., Hanke, C.W., and Higaki, M. *Mycobacterium marinum* infections treated with tetracycline. *Arch. Dermatol.,* **1977,** *113:*1067–1068.

Kemper, C.A., Meng, T.C., Nussbaum, J., Chiu, J., Feigal, D.F., Bartok, A.E., Leedom, J.M., Tilles, J.G., Deresinski, S.C., and McCutchan, J.A. Treatment of *Mycobacterium avium* complex bacteremia in AIDS with a four-drug oral regimen: rifampin, ethambutol, clofazimine and ciprofloxacin. The California Collaborative Treatment Group. *Ann. Intern. Med.,* **1992,** *116:*466–472.

Levy, L., and Peters, J.H. Susceptibility of *Mycobacterium leprae* to dapsone as a determinant of patient response to acedapsone. *Antimicrob. Agents Chemother.,* **1976,** *9:*102–112.

Levy, L., Shepard, C.C., and Fasal, P. Clofazimine therapy of lepromatous leprosy caused by dapsone-resistant *Mycobacterium leprae. Am. J. Trop. Med. Hyg.,* **1972,** *21:*315–321.

Lincoln, E.M., and Gilberg, L.A. Disease in children due to mycobacteria other than *Mycobacterium tuberculosis. Am. Rev. Respir. Dis.,* **1972,** *105:*683–714.

Loria, P.R. Minocycline hydrochloride treatment for atypical acid-fast infection. *Arch. Dermatol.,* **1976,** *112:*517–519.

Mason, G.H., Ellis-Pegler, R.B., and Arthur, J.F. Clofazimine and eosinophilic enteritis. *Lepr. Rev.,* **1977,** *48:*175–180.

McGlynn, K.A., Lustabader, E.D., Sharrar, R.G., Murphy, E.C., and London, W.T. Isoniazid prophylaxis in hepatitis B carriers. *Am. Rev. Respir. Dis.,* **1986,** *134:*666–668.

Miller, R.R., Porter, J., and Greenblatt, D.J. Clinical importance of the interaction of phenytoin and isoniazid: a report from the Boston Collaborative Drug Surveillance Program. *Chest,* **1979,** *75:*356–358.

Morrison, N.E., and Marley, G.M. Clofazimine binding studies with deoxyribonucleic acid. *Int. J. Lepr. Other Mycobact. Dis.,* **1976,** *44:*475–481.

Nightingale, S.D., Cameron, D.W., Gordin, F.M., Sullam, P.M., Cohn, D.L., Chaisson, R.E., Eron, L.J., Sparti, P.D., Bihari, B., Kaufman, D.L., Stern, J.J., Pearce, D.D., Weinberg, W.G., LaMarca, A., and Siegal, F.P. Two controlled trials of rifabutin prophylaxis against *Mycobacterium avium* complex infection in AIDS. *N. Engl. J. Med.,* **1993,** *329:*828–833.

O'Reilly, R.A. Interaction of chronic daily warfarin therapy and rifampin. *Ann. Intern. Med.,* **1975,** *83:*506–508.

Pablos-Méndez, A., Raviglione, M.C., Laszlo, A., Binkin, N., Reider, H.L., Bustreo, F., Cohn, D.L., Lambregts-van Weezenbeek, C.S., Kim, S.J., Chavlet, P., and Nunn, P. Global surveillance for antituberculosis-drug resistance, 1994–1997. World Health Organization-International Union against Tuberculosis and Lung Disease Working Group on Anti-Tuberculosis Drug Resistance Surveillance. *N. Engl. J. Med.,* **1998,** *338:*1641–1649.

Pengelly, C.D.R. Dapsone-induced hemolysis. *Br. Med. J.,* **1963,** *2:*662–664.

Pezzia, W., Raleigh, J.W., Bailey, M.C., Toth, E.A., and Silverblatt, J. Treatment of pulmonary disease due to *Mycobacterium kansasii:* recent experience with rifampin. *Rev. Infect. Dis.,* **1981,** *3:*1035–1039.

Postlethwaite, A.E., Bartel, A.G., and Kelley, W.N. Hyperuricemia due to ethambutol. *N. Engl. J. Med.,* **1972,** *286:*761–762.

Radner, D.B. Toxicologic and pharmacologic aspects of rifampin. *Chest,* **1973,** *64:*213–216.

Rapoport, A.M., and Guss, S.B. Dapsone-induced peripheral neuropathy. *Arch. Neurol.,* **1972,** *27:*184–186.

Salpeter, S.R., Sanders, G.D., Salpeter, E.E., and Owens, D.K. Monitored isoniazid prophylaxis for low risk tuberculin reactors older than 35 years of age: a risk-benefit and cost-effectiveness analysis. *Ann. Intern. Med.,* **1997,** *127*:1051–1061.

Sanders, W.E., Jr. Lung infection caused by rapidly growing mycobacteria. *J. Respir. Dis.,* **1982,** *3*:30–38.

Sanders, W.E., Jr., Hartwig, E.C., Schneider, N.J., Cacciatore, R., and Valdez, H. Susceptibility of organisms in the *Mycobacterium fortuitum* complex to antituberculous and other antimicrobial agents. *Antimicrob. Agents Chemother.,* **1977,** *12*:295–297.

Selwyn, P.A., Hortel, D., Lewis, V.A., Schoenbaum, E.E., Vermund, S.H., Klein, R.S., Walker, A.T., and Friedland, G.H. A prospective study of the risk of tuberculosis among intravenous drug users with human immunodeficiency virus infection. *N. Engl. J. Med.,* **1989,** *320*:545–555.

Shafran, S.D., Singer, J., Zarowny, D.P., Phillips, P., Salit, I., Walmsey, S.L., Fong, I.W., Gill, M.J., Rachlis, A.R., Lalonde, R.G., Fanning, W.M., and Tsoukas, C.M. A comparison of two regimens for the treatment of *Mycobacterium avium* complex bacteremia in AIDS: rifabutin, ethambutol, and clarithromycin *versus* rifampin, ethambutol, clofazimine, and ciprofloxacin. Canadian HIV Trials Network Protocol 010 Study Group. *N. Engl. J. Med.,* **1996,** *335*:377–383.

Shepard, C.C., Ellard, G.A., Levy, L., Opromolla, V., Pattyn, S.R., Peters, J.H., Rees, R.J.W., and Waters, M.F.R. Experimental chemotherapy of leprosy. *Bull. World Health Organ.,* **1976,** *53*:425–433.

Simon, E., Veres, E., and Banki, G. Changes in SGOT activity during treatment with ethionamide. *Scand. J. Respir. Dis.,* **1969,** *50*:314–322.

Single Lesion Multicentre Trial Group. Efficacy of single-dose multidrug therapy for the treatment of single-lesion paucibacillary leprosy. *Lepr. Rev.,* **1997,** *68*:341–349.

Sippel, J.E., Mikhail, I.A., Girgis, N.I., and Youssef, H.H. Rifampin concentrations in cerebrospinal fluid of patients with tuberculous meningitis. *Am. Rev. Respir. Dis.,* **1974,** *109*:579–580.

Skolnick, J.L., Stoler, B.S., Katz, D.B., and Anderson, W.H. Rifampin, oral contraceptives, and pregnancy. *JAMA,* **1976,** *236*:1382.

Snider, D.E., Jr. Pyridoxine supplementation during isoniazid therapy. *Tubercle,* **1980,** *61*:191–196.

Stead, W.W., and To, T. The significance of the tuberculin skin test in elderly persons. *Ann. Intern. Med.,* **1987,** *107*:837–842.

Takayama, K., Armstrong, E.L., Kunugi, K.A., and Kilburn, J.O. Inhibition by ethambutol of mycolic acid transfer into the cell wall of *Mycobacterium smegmatis. Antimicrob. Agents Chemother.,* **1979,** *16*:240.

Takayama, K., Schnoes, H.K., Armstrong, E.L., and Boyle, R.W. Site of inhibitory action of isoniazid in the synthesis of mycolic acids in *Mycobacterium tuberculosis. J. Lipid Res.,* **1975,** *16*:308–317.

Tiitinen, H. Isoniazid and ethionamide serum levels and inactivation in Finnish subjects. *Scand. J. Resp. Dis.,* **1969,** *50*:110–124.

USPHS. 1999 USPHS/IDSA guidelines for the prevention of opportunistic infections in persons infected with human immunodeficiency virus. U.S. Public Health Service (USPHS) and Infectious Diseases Society of America (IDSA). *M.M.W.R. Morb. Mortal. Wkly. Rep.,* **1999,** *48*:1–59, 61–66.

Vilcheze, C., Morbidoni, H.R., Weisbrod, T.R., Iwamoto, H., Kuo, M., Sacchettini, J.C., and Jacobs, W.R. Jr. Inactivation of the *inhA*-encoded fatty acid synthase II (FASII) enoyl-acyl carrier protein reductase induces accumulation of the FASI end products and cell lysis of *Mycobacterium smegmatis. J. Bacteriol.,* **2000,** *182*:4059–4067.

Warrington, R.J., Hogg, G.R., Paraskevas, F., and Tse, K.S. Insidious rifampin-associated renal failure with light-chain proteinuria. *Arch. Intern. Med.,* **1977,** *137*:927–930.

Whalen, C.C., Johnson, J.L., Okwera, A., Hom, D.L., Huebner, R., Mugyenyi, P., Mugerwa, R.D., and Ellner, J.J. A trial of three regimens to prevent tuberculosis in Ugandan adults infected with the human immunodeficiency virus. Uganda-Case Western Reserve University Research Collaboration. *N. Engl. J. Med.,* **1997,** *337*:801–808.

Wheat, L.J., Kohler, R.B., Luft, F.C., and White, A. Long-term studies of the effect of rifampin on nasal carriage of coagulase-positive staphylococci. *Rev. Infect. Dis.,* **1983,** *5*:S459–S462.

Wilkinson, D., Squire, S.B., and Garner, P. Effect of preventive treatment for tuberculosis in adults infected with HIV: systematic review of randomised placebo controlled trials. *Br. Med. J.,* **1998,** *317*:625–629.

WHO Expert Committee on Leprosy. *World Health Organ. Tech. Rep. Ser.,* **1998,** *874*:1–43.

Zimhony, O., Cox, J.S., Welch, J.T., Vilcheze, C., and Jacobs, W.R. Jr. Pyrazinamide inhibits the eukaryotic-like fatty acid synthetase I (FASI) of *Mycobacterium tuberculosis. Nat. Med.,* **2000,** *6*:1043–1047.

MONOGRAPHS AND REVIEWS

Barnes, P.F., and Barrows, S.A. Tuberculosis in the 1990s. *Ann. Intern. Med.,* **1993,** *119*:400–410.

Bass, J.B., Jr., Farer, L.S., Hopewell, P.C., O'Brien, R., Jacobs, R.F., Ruben, F., Snider, D.E., Jr., and Thornton, G. Treatment of tuberculosis and tuberculosis infections in adults and children. American Thoracic Society and The Centers for Disease Control and Prevention. *Am. J. Respir. Crit. Care Med.,* **1994,** *149*:1359–1374.

Blanchard, J.S. Molecular mechanisms of drug resistance in *Mycobacterium tuberculosis. Annu. Rev. Biochem.,* **1996,** *65*:215–239.

Brown, B.A., and Wallace, R.J. Jr. Infections due to nontuberculous mycobacteria. In, *Mandell, Douglas and Bennett's Principles and Practice of Infectious Diseases,* 5th ed. (Mandell, G.L., Bennett, J.E., and Dolin, R., eds.) Churchill Livingstone, Inc., Philadephia, **2000,** pp. 2630–2636.

Farr, B.F. Rifamycins. In, *Mandell, Douglas and Bennett's Principles and Practice of Infectious Diseases,* 5th ed. (Mandell, G.L., Bennett, J.E., and Dolin, R., eds.) Churchill Livingstone, Inc., Philadephia, **2000,** pp. 348–361.

Fox, H.H. The chemical attack on tuberculosis. *Trans. N.Y. Acad. Sci.,* **1953,** *15*:234–242.

Gallant, J.E., Moore, R.D., and Chaisson, R.E. Prophylaxis for opportunistic infections in patients with HIV infection. *Ann. Intern. Med.,* **1994,** *120*:932–944.

Gelber, R.H., and Rea, T.E. *Mycobacterium leprae* (leprosy, Hansen's disease). In, *Mandell, Douglas and Bennett's Principles and Practice of Infectious Diseases,* 5th ed. (Mandell, G.L., Dolin, R., and Bennett, J.E., eds.) Churchill Livingstone, Inc., Philadelphia, **2000,** pp. 2608–2616.

Goldman, A.L., and Braman, S.S. Isoniazid: a review with emphasis on adverse effects. *Chest,* **1972,** *62*:71–77.

Haas, D.W. *Mycobacterium tuberculosis.* In, *Mandell, Douglas and Bennett's Principles and Practice of Infectious Diseases,* 5th ed. (Mandell, G.L., Dolin, R., and Bennett, J.E., eds.) Churchill Livingstone, Inc., Philadephia, **2000,** pp. 2576–2607.

Hastings, R.C., and Franzblau, S.G. Chemotherapy of leprosy. *Annu. Rev. Pharmacol. Toxicol.,* **1988,** *28*:231–245.

Havlir, D.V., and Barnes, P.F. Tuberculosis in patients with human immunodeficiency virus infection. *N. Engl. J. Med.,* **1999,** *340*:367–373.

Havlir, D.V., and Ellner, J.J. *Mycobacterium avium* complex. In, *Mandell, Douglas and Bennett's Principles and Practice of Infectious Diseases,* 5th ed. (Mandell, C.L., Dolin, R., and Bennett, J.E., eds.) Churchill Livingstone, Inc., Philadephia, **2000,** pp. 2616–2630.

Iseman, M.D. Treatment of multidrug-resistant tuberculosis. *N. Engl. J. Med.,* **1993,** *329*:784–791. [Published erratum in *N. Engl. J. Med.,* **1993,** *329*:1435 (error in Table 4).]

Jacobs, W.R., Jr. *Mycobacterium tuberculosis*: a once genetically intractable organism. In, *Molecular Genetics of Mycobacteria.* (Hatfall, G.F., and Jacobs, W.R., Jr., eds.) ASM Press, Washington D.C., **2000.**

Jacobson, R.R. The treatment of leprosy (Hansen's disease). *Hosp. Formul.* **1982,** *17*:1076–1091.

Lane, H.C., Laughon, B.E., Falloon, J., Kovacs, J.A., Davey, R.T., Jr., Polis, M.A., and Masur, H. Recent advances in the management of AIDS-related opportunistic infections. *Ann. Intern. Med.,* **1994,** *120*:945–955.

Masur, H. Recommendations on prophylaxis and therapy for disseminated *Mycobacterium avium* complex disease in patients infected with the human immunodeficiency virus. Public Health Service Task Force on Prophylaxis and Therapy for *Mycobacterium avium* Complex. *N. Engl. J. Med.,* **1993,** *329*:898–904.

Trautman, J.R. The management of leprosy and its complications. *N. Engl. J. Med.,* **1965,** *273*:756–758.

ANTIMICROBIAL AGENTS
(*Continued*)
Antifungal Agents

John E. Bennett

Fungal infections traditionally have been divided into two distinct classes: systemic and superficial. Consequently, the major antifungal agents described in this chapter are discussed under two major headings, systemic and topical, although this distinction is becoming arbitrary. For example, the imidazole, triazole, and polyene antifungal agents may be used either systemically or topically, and, similarly, many superficial mycoses can be treated either systemically or topically. Amphotericin B, fluconazole, and itraconazole are discussed in considerable detail. Although Pneumocystis carinii, *responsible for life-threatening pneumonia in immunocompromised patients, has been demonstrated to be a fungus and not a protozoan, its treatment is discussed in other chapters in this section, because currently employed agents in this setting are primarily antibacterial or antiprotozoal rather than antifungal.*

Azole antifungal agents have dominated drug development and clinical use for nearly three decades. While the antifungal spectrum, physical properties, and pharmacology differ among compounds, azoles are remarkable as a drug class for their broad spectrum, oral bioavailability, and low toxicity. New compounds are still being developed, though the innovations are becoming more marginal, and resistance to azoles is slowly emerging in species that formerly were susceptible, particularly *Candida albicans*.

Another area of antifungal drug development has been new, lipid formulations of amphotericin B. Compared with the original deoxycholate formulation (DOC), the lipid formulations have provided a major reduction in renal toxicity, with more variable reduction in infusion-related chills and fever. Oddly, none of the preparations has been evaluated prospectively in the treatment of established mycoses. Rather, they have been used to treat and are approved for use in patients who have failed or been unable to tolerate DOC, so-called salvage therapy. Although some formulations also have been studied as empiric therapy of neutropenic patients, efficacy has been extraordinarily difficult to assess in these trials. It remains unclear whether any lipid preparation is more effective in any mycosis than the DOC preparation given at full dosages, but the probable answer is no.

Determination of blood concentrations of antifungal drugs remains a research procedure except in the case of flucytosine. The toxicity of flucytosine clearly depends on

drug concentration; azotemia readily increases flucytosine to toxic levels. For the azoles and amphotericin B formulations, blood levels have not predicted either toxicity or efficacy.

The advance of systemic antifungal agents into common medical practice has made it important to define their efficacy, toxicity, and interactions with other drugs. The wider choice of topical agents has complicated the selection process for the physician and, because of new over-the-counter azole drugs, for the patient as well. Table 49–1 lists the most common mycoses and the treatments of choice.

SYSTEMIC ANTIFUNGAL AGENTS

Amphotericin B

History and Source. *Amphotericin B* was discovered in 1956 by Gold and coworkers, who were studying a strain of *Streptomyces nodosus*, an aerobic actinomycete, obtained from the Orinoco River Valley of Venezuela.

Chemistry. Amphotericin B is one of a family of some 200 polyene macrolide antibiotics. Those studied to date share the characteristics of four to seven conjugated double bonds, an internal cyclic ester, poor aqueous solubility, substantial toxicity on parenteral administration, and a common mechanism of antifungal action. Amphotericin B (*see* below for structure)

Table 49–1

Treatment of Mycoses

DEEP MYCOSES	DRUGS	SUPERFICIAL MYCOSES	DRUGS
Aspergillosis, invasive		*Candidiasis*	
Immunosuppressed	Amphotericin B	Vulvovaginal	Topical
Nonimmunosuppressed	Amphotericin B, itraconazole		Butoconazole
			Clotrimazole
			Miconazole
Blastomycosis			Nystatin
Rapidly progressive or CNS	Amphotericin B		Terconazole
Indolent, non-CNS	Itraconazole, ketoconazole		Tioconazole
			Oral
Coccidioidomycosis			Fluconazole
Rapidly progressing	Amphotericin B	Oropharyngeal	Topical
Indolent	Itraconazole, ketoconazole, fluconazole		Amphotericin B
			Clotrimazole
Meningeal	Fluconazole, intrathecal amphotericin B		Nystatin
			Oral (systemic)
			Fluconazole
			Itraconazole
			Ketoconazole
Cryptococcosis		Cutaneous	Topical
Non-AIDS and initial AIDS	Amphotericin B ±flucytosine		Amphotericin B
			Clotrimazole
Maintenance, AIDS	Fluconazole		Ciclopirox
			Econazole
Histoplasmosis			Ketoconazole
Chronic pulmonary	Itraconazole		Miconazole
Disseminated			Nystatin
Rapidly progressing or CNS	Amphotericin B	*Ringworm*	Topical
Indolent, non-CNS	Itraconazole		Clotrimazole
Maintenance, AIDS	Itraconazole		Ciclopirox
			Econazole
			Haloprogin
Mucormycosis	Amphotericin B		Ketoconazole
Pseudallescheriasis	Itraconazole		Miconazole
			Naftifine
			Oxiconazole
			Sulconazole
Sporotrichosis			Terbinafine
Cutaneous	Iodide, itraconazole		Undecylenate
Extracutaneous	Amphotericin B, itraconazole		Systemic
			Griseofulvin
			Itraconazole
			Terbinafine

AMPHOTERICIN B

is a heptaene macrolide containing seven conjugated double bonds in the trans position and 3-amino-3,6-dideoxymannose (mycosamine) connected to the main ring by a glycosidic bond. The amphoteric behavior for which the drug is named derives from the presence of a carboxyl group on the main ring and a primary amino group on mycosamine; these groups confer aqueous solubility at extremes of pH. X-ray crystallography has shown the molecule to be rigid and rod-shaped, with the hydrophilic hydroxyl groups of the macrolide ring forming an opposing face to the lipophilic polyenic portion.

Drug Formulations. Amphotericin B is insoluble in water but was formulated for intravenous infusion by complexing it with the bile salt deoxycholate. The complex is marketed as a lyophilized powder (FUNGIZONE) containing 50 mg of amphotericin B, 41 mg of deoxycholate, and a small amount of sodium phosphate buffer. The amphotericin B–deoxycholate complex (DOC) forms a colloid in water, with particles largely below 0.4 μm in diameter. Filters in intravenous infusion lines that filter out particles above 0.22 μm in diameter will remove significant amounts of drug. Addition of electrolyte to infusion solutions causes the colloid to aggregate. The resulting cloudy solution should not be infused, because the blood levels achieved are likely to be very low.

N-acyl and O-acyl derivatives of amphotericin B form water-soluble salts, but none is available commercially. The amphipathic nature of amphotericin B has made it possible to create lipid formulations for intravenous infusion. Three such formulations of amphotericin B are marketed in the United States (Wong-Beringer et al., 1998). Amphotericin B colloidal dispersion (ABCD, AMPHOTEC, AMPHOCIL) is a colloidal dispersion containing roughly equimolar amounts of amphotericin B and cholesteryl sulfate. Like DOC, ABCD forms a colloidal solution when dispersed in aqueous solution. ABCD particles are disk-shaped; they are 115 nm wide by 4 nm thick. ABCD provides much lower blood levels than DOC in mice and human beings. In mice, 41% to 80% of 14 daily doses can be recovered in the liver. In a randomized, double-blind study in patients with neutropenic fever comparing ABCD (4 mg/kg daily) with DOC (0.8 mg/kg), chills and hypoxia were significantly more common with ABCD (79.8% and 12%, respectively) than with DOC (65.4% and 2.9%), requiring withdrawal of 4.6% of the study patients receiving ABCD, compared with 0.9% of those receiving DOC (White et al., 1998). Hypoxia was associated with severe febrile reactions. Administration of the recommended ABCD dose of 3 to 4 mg/kg over 3 to 4 hours and use of premedication to reduce febrile reactions is advised, particularly with initial infusions. Unlike the situation with DOC, nephro-

toxicity rarely leads to dose reductions of ABCD, even in bone marrow transplant recipients (Noskin et al., 1999). Efficacy has been difficult to evaluate in all the published studies to date. ABCD is approved only for patients with invasive aspergillosis who are not responding to or are unable to tolerate DOC. This approval is based on open, noncomparative trials.

A small unilamellar vesicle formulation of amphotericin B (AMBISOME) also is available. Amphotericin B (50 mg) is combined with 350 mg of lipid in an approximately 10% molar ratio. The lipid contains hydrogenated soy lecithin (phosphatidylcholine), cholesterol, and distearoylphosphatidylglycerol in a 10:5:4 molar ratio. The drug is supplied as a lyophilized powder, which is reconstituted with sterile water for injection and then the dose diluted with 5% dextrose solution. With complete dispersion, particle size is about 80 nm. Blood levels following intravenous infusion are almost equivalent to those obtained with DOC, and, because AMBISOME can be given at higher doses, blood levels have been achieved that exceed those obtained with DOC. Amphotericin B accumulation in the liver and spleen is higher with AMBISOME than with DOC (de Marie et al., 1994). In a series of 23 patients receiving 3 mg/kg daily for an average of 27 days, the average serum creatinine rise was only 34%, with nephrotoxicity leading to dose reduction in only one patient (Coker et al., 1993). Nephrotoxicity, hypokalemia, and infusion-related reactions—such as fever, chills, hypoxia, hypotension, and hypertension—are less with AMBISOME than with either DOC or ABLC (see below), but they still occur (Walsh et al., 1999). Infusion-related pain in the back, abdomen, or chest occurs in occasional patients, usually with the first few doses (Johnson et al., 1998). Anaphylaxis has been reported. Most of the information about the efficacy of AMBISOME comes from open, noncomparative studies. Blinded, randomized comparisons of DOC and AMBISOME as empirical therapy or prophylaxis in febrile neutropenic patients are very helpful in comparing toxicity of the two drugs (Walsh et al., 1999; Prentice et al., 1997; Kelsey et al., 1999). By the primary endpoints of these studies, both preparations have been comparable. However, because the efficacy of DOC in these patients cannot be quantitated from historical data, the relative efficacy of AMBISOME is impossible to ascertain. Secondary analysis of mycoses emerging despite the use of AMBISOME or DOC in these trials has been limited by the rarity of this event and the tendency of investigators to reduce the DOC doses to subtherapeutic levels. AMBISOME is approved for empiric therapy of fever in the neutropenic host not responding to appropriate antibacterial agents as well as for salvage therapy of aspergillosis, cryptococcosis, and candidiasis. The recommended dose for empiric therapy is 3 mg/kg daily, and that for treatment of mycoses is 3 to 5 mg/kg intravenously. AMBISOME also is effective in visceral leishmaniasis at doses of 3 to 4 mg/kg daily. The drug is administered in 5% dextrose in water, with initial doses being infused over 2 hours. If well tolerated, infusion duration can be shortened to one hour. Although doses up to 10 mg/kg have been used in a few patients without causing death, 8 mg/kg is highly toxic in dogs (Bekersky *et al.*, 1999).

The third lipid formulation is amphotericin B lipid complex (ABLC, ABELCET). This preparation of dimyristoylphosphatidyl-choline and dimyristoylphosphatidylglycerol in a 7:3 mixture with approximately 35 mol% amphotericin B forms ribbon-like sheets which range in size from 1.6 to 11 μm. Blood levels of amphotericin B are much lower with ABLC than with the same dose of DOC. In unpublished studies, blood levels have been comparable when ABLC is given at five times the dose of DOC. In open, noncomparative trials, ABLC has seemed to be effective in a variety of mycoses with the possible exception of cryptococcal meningitis (Walsh *et al.*, 1998; Wingard, 1997; Sharkey *et al.*, 1996). Nephrotoxicity and infusion-related reactions of fever, chills, hypoxia, hypertension, and hypotension appear to be intermediate between DOC and AMBISOME. ABLC is given as 5 mg/kg in 5% dextrose in water, infused once daily over two hours. The drug is approved for salvage therapy of deep mycoses.

DOC has been mixed with a 20% lipid emulsion (INTRALIPID) and infused intravenously. Whether amphotericin B aggregates or is bound to lipid in the infusate is unknown. Nephrotoxicity appears to be less than with DOC at 1 mg/kg, but there is a suggestion that both blood levels and efficacy are also lower (Chavanet *et al.*, 1992). Intravenous infusion of DOC with lipid emulsion is not recommended.

Rational use of the lipid formulations has been problematic for hospital pharmacies and physicians. Cost of the formulations is 20 to 50 times that of DOC, raising formidable cost-benefit issues. The person making the choice must weigh the uncertainties about relative efficacy of the lipid formulations against the gravity of potential nephrotoxicity of the formulation in individual patients. In some patients, the additive burden of amphotericin B nephrotoxicity can help precipitate advanced renal failure, with attendant morbidity and financial burden (Wingard *et al.*, 1999).

Antifungal Activity. Amphotericin B has useful clinical activity against *Candida* spp., *Cryptococcus neoformans, Blastomyces dermatitidis, Histoplasma capsulatum, Sporothrix schenckii, Coccidioides immitis, Paracoccidioides braziliensis, Aspergillus* spp., *Penicillium marneffei*, and the agents of mucormycosis. Some isolates of *Candida lusitaniae* have appeared to be relatively resistant to amphotericin B.

Amphotericin B has limited activity against the protozoa *Leishmania braziliensis* and *Naegleria fowleri*. The drug has no antibacterial activity.

Mechanism of Action. The antifungal activity of amphotericin B depends at least in part on its binding to a sterol moiety, primarily ergosterol, that is present in the membrane of sensitive fungi. By virtue of their interaction with the sterols of cell membranes, polyenes appear to form pores or channels. The result is an increase in the permeability of the membrane, allowing leakage of a variety of small molecules. Additional mechanisms

of action may include oxidative damage to fungal cells, at least *in vitro*.

Fungal Resistance. Mutants selected *in vitro* for nystatin or amphotericin B resistance replace ergosterol with certain precursor sterols. The rarity of significant amphotericin B resistance arising during therapy has left it unclear whether or not ergosterol-deficient mutants retain sufficient pathogenicity to survive in deep tissue. Failure of amphotericin B to penetrate the fungal cell wall of some resistant species has been suggested by the greater susceptibility of protoplasts.

Absorption, Distribution, and Excretion. Absorption of all amphotericin B formulations from the gastrointestinal tract is negligible. Repeated daily intravenous infusions to adults of 0.5 mg/kg of DOC result in concentrations in plasma of about 1.0 to 1.5 μg/ml at the end of the infusion, which fall to about 0.5 to 1.0 μg/ml by 24 hours later. The drug is released from its complex with deoxycholate in the bloodstream, and the amphotericin B that remains in plasma is more than 90% bound to proteins, largely β-lipoprotein. Approximately 2% to 5% of each dose appears in the urine when patients are on daily therapy. Elimination of the drug appears to be unchanged in anephric patients and in patients receiving hemodialysis. Hepatic or biliary disease has no known effect on metabolism of the drug in human beings. At least one-third of an injected dose can be recovered unchanged by methanolic extraction of tissue at autopsy; the highest concentrations are found in liver and spleen, with lesser amounts in kidney and lung. Concentrations of amphotericin B (DOC) in fluids from inflamed pleura, peritoneum, synovium, and aqueous humor are approximately two-thirds of trough concentrations in plasma. Little amphotericin B penetrates into cerebrospinal fluid (CSF), vitreous humor, or normal amniotic fluid. Because of extensive binding to tissues, there is a terminal phase of elimination with a half-time of about 15 days.

Therapeutic Uses. The usual therapeutic dose of amphotericin B DOC is 0.5 to 0.6 mg/kg, administered in 5% glucose over 4 hours. *Candida* esophagitis in adults responds to 0.15 to 0.2 mg/kg daily. Rapidly progressive mucormycosis or invasive aspergillosis is treated with doses of 1.0 to 1.2 mg/kg daily until progression is arrested. Double-dose alternate day therapy may be more convenient but is not less toxic and is therefore rarely indicated. The infusion bottle need not be protected from light, as once recommended. Infusion intervals as short as one hour have been used, but, during the first 5 to 7 days of therapy, they lead to more febrile reactions.

Intrathecal infusion of amphotericin B DOC is useful in patients with meningitis caused by *Coccidioides*. The drug can be injected into the CSF of the lumbar spine, cisterna magna, or lateral cerebral ventricle. Regardless of the site of injection, the treatment is begun with 0.05 to 0.1 mg and increased on a three-times-a-week schedule to 0.5 mg, as tolerance permits. Therapy is then continued on a twice-a-week schedule. Fever and headache are common reactions and may be decreased by intrathecal administration of 10 to 15 mg of hydrocortisone. Less common but more serious problems attend the use of intrathecal injections; the nature of the problem depends on the injection site chosen. Local injections of amphotericin B into a joint or peritoneal dialysate fluid commonly produce irritation and pain. Intraocular injection following pars plana vitrectomy has been used successfully for fungal endophthalmitis.

Intravenous administration of amphotericin B is the treatment of choice for mucormycosis, invasive aspergillosis, extracutaneous sporotrichosis, cryptococcosis, fusariosis, alternariosis, trichosporonosis, and penicilliosis marneffei. Although imidazoles or triazoles are useful in many patients with blastomycosis, histoplasmosis, coccidioidomycosis, and paracoccidioidomycosis, amphotericin B is preferred when these mycoses are rapidly progressive, occur in an immunosuppressed host, or involve the central nervous system. Amphotericin B (DOC or AMBISOME) also can be useful in selected patients with profound neutropenia and fever that is unresponsive to broad-spectrum antibacterial agents. Amphotericin B given once weekly has been used to prevent relapse in patients with AIDS who have been treated successfully for cryptococcosis or histoplasmosis.

Bladder irrigation with 50 μg/ml of amphotericin B in sterile water is effective for *Candida* cystitis. Relapse is common if the catheter remains in the bladder or there is significant postvoiding residual urine. Inhalational administration of amphotericin B has not been successful in treatment of pulmonary mycoses, nor has intranasal instillation proved useful in preventing aspergillosis in neutropenic patients. Topical amphotericin B is useful only in cutaneous candidiasis (*see* below).

Untoward Effects. The major acute reaction to intravenous amphotericin B DOC is fever and chills. Sometimes hyperpnea and respiratory stridor or modest hypotension may occur, but true bronchospasm or anaphylaxis is rare. Patients with preexisting cardiac or pulmonary disease may tolerate the metabolic demands of the reaction poorly and develop hypoxia or hypotension. A test dose of 1 mg may be considered for unstable patients; the patient should be observed for two hours prior to infusing the usual therapeutic dose. Although the reaction ends spontaneously in 30 to 45 minutes, meperidine may shorten it. Pretreatment with oral acetaminophen or use of intravenous hydrocortisone hemisuccinate, 0.7 mg/kg, at the start of the infusion decreases reactions. Febrile reactions abate with subsequent infusions. Infants, children, and patients receiving therapeutic doses of corticosteroids are less prone to reactions.

Azotemia occurs in 80% of patients who receive amphotericin B for deep mycoses (Carlson and Condon, 1994). Toxicity is dose-dependent and transient and is increased by concurrent therapy with other nephrotoxic agents, such as aminoglycosides or cyclosporine. Although permanent histological damage to renal tubules occurs even during short courses, permanent functional deficits are uncommon in patients whose renal function was normal prior to treatment unless a total dose in excess of 3 to 4 g is given (to an adult). Renal tubular acidosis and renal wasting of K^+ and Mg^{2+} also may be seen during and for several weeks after therapy. Supplemental K^+ is required in

one-third of patients on prolonged therapy. An increase in intrarenal vascular resistance is the major cause of nephrotoxicity in amphotericin B–treated rats (Tolins and Raij, 1988). In patients and experimental animals, loading with sodium chloride has decreased nephrotoxicity, even in the absence of water or salt deprivation. Administration of 1 liter of saline intravenously on the day that amphotericin B is to be given has been recommended for adults who are able to tolerate the Na^+ load and who are not already receiving that amount in intravenous fluids (Branch, 1988).

Hypochromic, normocytic anemia is usual; the average hematocrit declined to 27% in one study. Decreased production of erythropoietin is the probable mechanism. Patients with low plasma erythropoietin may respond to administration of recombinant erythropoietin. Anemia reverses slowly following therapy. Headache, nausea, vomiting, malaise, weight loss, and phlebitis at peripheral infusion sites are common side effects. Encephalopathy also has been attributed to amphotericin B (Balmaceda and Walker, 1994). Thrombocytopenia or mild leukopenia is observed rarely. Hepatotoxicity is not firmly established.

Flucytosine

Chemistry. *Flucytosine* is a fluorinated pyrimidine related to fluorouracil and floxuridine. It is 5-fluorocytosine, the formula of which is as follows:

FLUCYTOSINE

Antifungal Activity. Flucytosine has clinically useful activity against *Cryptococcus neoformans, Candida* spp., and the agents of chromomycosis. Within these species, determination of susceptibility *in vitro* has been extremely dependent on the method employed, and susceptibility testing performed on isolates obtained prior to treatment has not correlated with clinical outcome.

Mechanism of Action. All susceptible fungi are capable of deaminating flucytosine to 5-fluorouracil, a potent antimetabolite (*see* Figure 49–1). Fluorouracil is metabolized first to 5-fluorouridylic acid by the enzyme uridine monophosphate (UMP) pyrophosphorylase. It can then either be incorporated into RNA (*via* synthesis of 5-fluorouridine triphosphate) or be metabolized to 5-fluorodeoxyuridylic acid, a potent inhibitor of thymidylate synthetase. DNA synthesis is impaired as the ultimate result of this latter reaction. Mammalian cells do not convert flucytosine to fluorouracil. This fact is crucial for the selective action of this compound.

Fungal Resistance. Drug resistance that arises during therapy (secondary resistance) is an important cause of therapeutic failure when flucytosine is used alone for cryptococcosis and

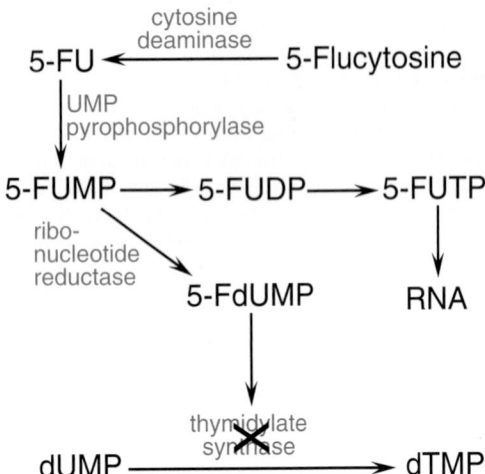

Figure 49–1. Action of flucytosine in fungi.

5-Flucytosine is transported into the fungal cell, where it is deaminated to 5-fluorouracil (5-FU). The 5-FU is then converted to 5-fluorouracil-ribose monophosphate (5-FUMP) and then is either converted to 5-FUTP and incorporated into RNA or converted by ribonucleotide reductase to 5-FdUMP, which is a potent inhibitor of thymidylate synthase.

candidiasis. In chromomycosis, resurgence of lesions after an initial response has led to the presumption of secondary drug resistance. In isolates of *Cryptococcus* and *Candida* species, secondary drug resistance has been accompanied by a change in the minimal inhibitory concentration from less than 2.5 μg/ml to more than 360 μg/ml. The mechanism for this resistance can be loss of the permease necessary for cytosine transport or decreased activity of either UMP pyrophosphorylase or cytosine deaminase (*see* Figure 49–1). In *Candida albicans,* a diploid fungus, partial resistance can occur because of heterozygous deficiency of UMP pyrophosphorylase. The clinical significance of partial resistance is unknown.

Absorption, Distribution, and Excretion.

Flucytosine is absorbed rapidly and well from the gastrointestinal tract. It is widely distributed in the body, with a volume of distribution that approximates total body water. The drug is minimally bound to plasma proteins. The peak plasma concentration in patients with normal renal function is approximately 70 to 80 μg/ml, achieved 1 to 2 hours after a dose of 37.5 mg/kg. Approximately 80% of a given dose is excreted unchanged in the urine; concentrations in the urine range from 200 to 500 μg/ml. The half-life of the drug is 3 to 6 hours in normal individuals. In renal failure, the half-life may be as long as 200 hours. The clearance of flucytosine is approximately equivalent to that of creatinine. Because of the obligate renal excretion of the drug, modification of dosage is necessary in patients with decreased renal function. It is recommended that concentrations of drug in plasma be measured periodically in patients with renal insufficiency. Peak concentrations should range between 50 and 100 μg/ml. Flucytosine is cleared by hemodialysis, and patients undergoing such treatment should receive a single dose of 37.5 mg/kg after dialysis; the drug also is removed by peritoneal dialysis.

Flucytosine is present in CSF at a concentration about 65% to 90% of that simultaneously present in the plasma. The drug also appears to penetrate into the aqueous humor.

Therapeutic Uses. Flucytosine (ANCOBON) is given orally in amounts of 100 to 150 mg/kg per day, divided into 4 doses at 6-hour intervals. Dosage must be adjusted for decreased renal function. Flucytosine is used predominantly in combination with amphotericin B. Flucytosine had a possible, though not statistically significant, benefit and no added toxicity when added to 0.7 mg/kg of amphoterin B for the initial two weeks of therapy of cryptococcal meningitis in AIDS patients (van der Horst *et al.,* 1997). An all-oral regimen of flucytosine plus fluconazole also has been advocated for therapy of AIDS patients with cyrptococcosis, but there is substantial gastrointestinal toxicity with the combination and no evidence that flucytosine adds benefit to the regimen. In cryptococcal meningitis of non-AIDS patients, in whom the goal is cure and not suppression, the role of flucytosine is more conjectural. Addition of flucytosine to six weeks or more of therapy with amphotericin B runs the risk of substantial bone marrow suppression or colitis if the flucytosine dose is not promptly adjusted downward as amphotericin B–induced azotemia occurs. More rapid culture conversion has been shown in cryptococcal meningitis of non-AIDS patients when flucytosine is added to an amphotericin B dose of 0.3 mg/kg daily but not when added to the more commonly used dosage of 0.7 mg/kg. Use of flucytosine in deep candidiasis has all but disappeared because of toxicity, absence of an intravenous formulation, and availability of other agents.

Untoward Effects. Flucytosine may depress the function of bone marrow and lead to the development of leukopenia and thrombocytopenia; patients are more prone to this complication if they have an underlying hematological disorder, are being treated with radiation or drugs that injure the bone marrow, or have a history of treatment with such agents. Other untoward effects—including rash, nausea, vomiting, diarrhea, and severe enterocolitis—have been noted. In approximately 5% of patients, plasma levels of hepatic enzymes are elevated, but this effect reverses when therapy is stopped. Toxicity is more frequent in patients with AIDS or azotemia (including those who are receiving amphotericin B concurrently) and when concentrations of the drug in plasma exceed 100 μg/ml (Stamm *et al.,* 1987). Toxicity may be the result of conversion of flucytosine to 5-fluorouracil by the microbial flora in the intestinal tract of the host.

Imidazoles and Triazoles

The azole antifungals include two broad classes, imidazoles and triazoles. Both classes share the same antifungal spectrum and mechanism of action. The systemic triazoles are more slowly metabolized and have less effect on human sterol synthesis than do the imidazoles. Because of these advantages, new congeners under development are mostly triazoles, not imidazoles. Of the drugs now on the market in the United States, clotrimazole, miconazole, ketoconazole, econazole, butoconazole, oxiconazole, and sulconazole are imidazoles; terconazole, itraconazole, fluconazole, and new azoles in clinical trials are triazoles. The topical use of azole antifungals is described in the second section of this chapter. The structure of triazole is as follows:

TRIAZOLE

Antifungal Activity. Susceptibility testing with azole antifungals has not been useful in predicting which fungal species will respond to therapy. Although individual drugs have their own useful spectrum, azoles as a group have clinically useful activity against *C. albicans, Candida tropicalis, Candida glabrata, C. neoformans, B. dermatitidis, H. capsulatum, C. immitis, Paracoccidioides brasiliensis,* and ringworm fungi (dermatophytes). *Aspergillus* spp. and *S. schenckii* are intermediate in susceptibility. *Candida krusei* and the agents of mucormycosis appear to be resistant. These drugs do not appear to have any useful antibacterial or antiparasitic activity, with the possible exception of antiprotozoal effects against *Leishmania major.*

Mechanism of Action.   At concentrations achieved during systemic use, the major effect of imidazoles and triazoles on fungi is inhibition of sterol 14-α-demethylase, a microsomal cytochrome P450–dependent enzyme system. Imidazoles and triazoles thus impair the biosynthesis of ergosterol for the cytoplasmic membrane and lead to the accumulation of 14-α-methylsterols. These methylsterols may disrupt the close packing of acyl chains of phospholipids, impairing the functions of certain membrane-bound enzyme systems such as ATPase and enzymes of the electron transport system and thus inhibiting growth of the fungi.

Some azoles, such as clotrimazole, directly increase permeability of the fungal cytoplasmic membrane, but the concentrations required are likely only obtained with topical use.

Azole resistance has emerged gradually during prolonged azole therapy and has caused clinical failure in patients with far-advanced HIV infection and oropharyngeal or esophageal candidiasis. The primary mechanism of resistance in *C. albicans* is accumulation of mutations in ERG11, the gene coding for the C14-α-sterol demethylase (Marichal *et al.,* 1999). These mutations appear to protect heme in the enzyme pocket from binding to azole but allow access of the natural substrate for the enzyme, lanosterol. Cross resistance is conferred to all azoles. Increased azole efflux by both ATP-binding cassette (ABC) and major facilitator superfamily (MFS) transporters can add to fluconazole resistance in *C. albicans* and *C. glabrata.* Increased production of C14-α-sterol demethylase is another potential cause of resistance.

Ketoconazole

Ketoconazole, administered orally, has been replaced by itraconazole for the treatment of all mycoses except when the lower cost of ketoconazole outweighs the advantage of itraconazole. Itraconazole lacks ketoconazole's hepatotoxicity and corticosteroid suppression, while retaining most of ketoconazole's pharmacological properties and expanding the antifungal spectrum. Introduction of even newer triazoles likely will reduce further the usefulness of ketoconazole. The structural formula of ketoconazole is as follows:

KETOCONAZOLE

Absorption, Distribution, and Excretion.   Oral absorption of ketoconazole varies among individuals. Since an acidic environment is required for the dissolution of ketoconazole, bioavailability is markedly depressed in patients taking H_2-histamine receptor blocking agents such as cimetidine or proton pump inhibitors. Simultaneous administration of antacids also may impair absorption, as will didanosine (an anti-HIV agent) products, which contain a buffer to neutralize gastric acid and increase the absorption of didanosine. Ingestion of food has no significant effect on the maximal concentration of the drug achieved in plasma. After oral doses of 200, 400, and 800 mg, peak plasma concentrations of ketoconazole are approximately 4, 8, and 20 μg/ml. The half-life of the drug increases with dose, and it may be as long as 7 to 8 hours when the dose is 800 mg. Ketoconazole is metabolized extensively, and the inactive products appear in the feces. Concentrations of active drug in urine are very low. In blood, 84% of ketoconazole is bound to plasma proteins, largely albumin; 15% is bound to erythrocytes; and 1% is free. Metabolism of the drug is unchanged by azotemia, hemodialysis, or peritoneal dialysis. Moderate hepatic dysfunction has no effect on the concentration of ketoconazole in blood.

Ketoconazole reaches keratinocytes efficiently, and its concentration in vaginal fluid approaches that in plasma. The concentration of ketoconazole in the CSF of patients with fungal meningitis is less than 1% of the total drug concentration in plasma.

Induction of hepatic microsomal enzymes by rifampin, isoniazid, and possibly by phenytoin accelerates the metabolic clearance of ketoconazole, and concentrations of the antifungal agent may be reduced by more than 50%. Ketoconazole raises plasma concentrations of cyclosporine, midazolam, triazolam, indinavir, and phenytoin because the drugs are metabolized by the cytochrome P450 enzyme CYP3A4. The anticoagulant effect of warfarin also may be enhanced.

Therapeutic Uses. Ketoconazole (NIZORAL) is effective in blastomycosis, histoplasmosis, coccidioidomycosis, pseudallescheriasis, paracoccidioidomycosis, ringworm, tinea versicolor, chronic mucocutaneous candidiasis, *Candida* vulvovaginitis, and oral and esophageal candidiasis. Efficacy is poor in immunosuppressed patients and in meningitis. The usual adult dose is 400 mg taken once daily. Children are given 3.3 to 6.6 mg/kg daily. Duration of therapy is 5 days for *Candida* vulvovaginitis, 2 weeks for *Candida* esophagitis, and 6 to 12 months for deep mycoses. The slow response to therapy has made ketoconazole inappropriate for patients with severe or rapidly progressive mycoses. For all of the above indications, itraconazole has replaced ketoconazole for patients who can afford the more expensive, newer product.

Untoward Effects. The most common side effects of ketoconazole are dose-dependent nausea, anorexia, and vomiting, which occur in about 20% of patients receiving 400 mg daily. Administration of the drug with food, at bedtime, or in divided doses may improve tolerance. An allergic rash occurs in about 4% of ketoconazole-treated patients and pruritus without rash in about 2%. Hair loss has also been reported.

Ketoconazole inhibits steroid biosynthesis in patients, as it does in fungi, by inhibition of cytochrome P450–dependent enzyme systems. Several endocrinologic abnormalities thus may be evident. Approximately 10% of females report menstrual irregularities. A variable number of males experience gynecomastia and decreased libido and potency. At high doses, azoospermia has been reported, but sterility has not been permanent. Doses of ketoconazole as low as 400 mg can cause a transient drop in the plasma concentrations of free testosterone and estradiol C-17β. Similar doses also can cause a transient decrease in the ACTH-stimulated plasma cortisol response and can suppress androgen production in women with polycystic ovary syndrome. Daily doses of 800 to 1200 mg of ketoconazole have been used to suppress plasma cortisol in patients with Cushing's disease. Similar doses were evaluated in patients with prostatic carcinoma. Hypertension and fluid retention have been reported and are associated with elevated concentrations of deoxycorticosterone, corticosterone, and 11-deoxycortisol. Although reports of Addison's disease due to ketoconazole are not convincing, it

would seem prudent to discontinue the drug before major surgical procedures and to avoid using high doses in patients with trauma, severe burns, or other stressful conditions.

Mild, asymptomatic elevation of aminotransferase activity in plasma is common, occurring in 5% to 10% of patients; these values revert to normal spontaneously. Symptomatic drug-induced hepatitis is rare but is potentially fatal. Hepatitis may occur after a few days of treatment, or it may be delayed for many months. The earliest symptoms are anorexia, malaise, nausea, and vomiting, with or without dull abdominal pain. Liver function tests usually mimic the pattern seen with hepatitis A, but a cholestatic or mixed picture can occur. Patients should be alerted to the symptoms and asked to return for liver function tests should this toxicity be suspected. Ketoconazole is teratogenic in animals, causing syndactyly in rats. Its use during pregnancy is not recommended, and because of secretion of the drug into breast milk, its use in nursing mothers also is unwise.

Itraconazole

This synthetic triazole is a 1:1:1:1 racemic mixture of four diastereoisomers (two enantiomeric pairs), each possessing three chiral centers. The structural formula is closely related to the imidazole, ketoconazole, as shown below:

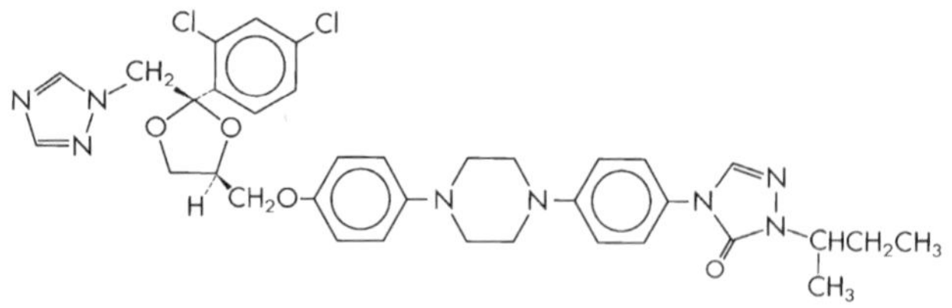

ITRACONAZOLE

Absorption, Distribution, and Excretion. *Itraconazole* (SPORONOX) is available as a capsule and two solution formulations, one for oral and one for intravenous administration. The capsule form of the drug is best absorbed in the fed state, but the oral solution is better absorbed in the fasting state and provides, under that condition, peak plasma concentrations that are more than 150% of those obtained with the capsule. Both the oral solution and intravenous formulation are solubilized in a 40:1 weight ratio of hydroxypropyl-β-cyclodextrin, so that administration of 200 mg of itraconazole provides 8 g of this excipient. Itraconazole is metabolized in the liver, primarily by the cytochrome CYP3A4 isoenzyme system, and it inhibits the metabolism of other drugs by CYP3A4. Itraconazole is present in plasma with an approximately equal concentration of a biologically active metabolite, hydroxyitraconazole. Bioassays may report up to approximately 3.3 times as much itraconazole in plasma as do physical methods such as HPLC, depending on the susceptibility of the bioassay organism to hydroxyitraconazole. Some laboratories using HPLC will also report the levels of hydroxyitraconazole as well as native drug, so the two may be added together for total antifungal drug concentration. The native drug and metabolite are 99.8% and 99.5% bound to plasma proteins, respectively. Neither appears in urine or CSF. The half-life of itraconazole in the steady state is approximately 30 to 40 hours. Steady-state levels of itraconazole are not reached for 4 days and those of hydroxyitraconazole for 7 days, for which reason loading doses are recommended when treating deep mycoses. Far advanced liver disease will increase itraconazole plasma concentrations, but azotemia and hemodialysis have no effect. Some 80% to 90% of intravenously administered hydroxypropyl-β-cyclodextrin is excreted in the urine. Intravenously administered hydroxypropyl-β-cyclodextrin accumulates is the presence of azotemia. Intravenous administration of itraconazole is contraindicated in patients with a creatinine clearance below 30 ml/min because of concern about hydroxypropyl-β-cyclodextrin concentrations. Itraconazole is not carcinogenic but is teratogenic in rats, classified as pregnancy category C, and is contraindicated during pregnancy. Hydroxypropyl-β-cyclodextrin causes pancreatic adenocarcinoma in rats but not mice. Relevance of this finding to clinical use of the oral solution is unclear.

Drug Interactions. Table 49–2 lists the known interactions of itraconazole with other drugs, but this list is still expanding. Many of the interactions can cause serious toxicity of the companion drug, as potentially fatal cardiac arrhythmias with cisapride, quinidine, or astemizole. Other interactions may decrease the itraconazole concentrations below therapeutic levels.

Therapeutic Uses. Itraconazole given as a capsule is the drug of choice for patients with indolent, nonmeningeal infections due to *B. dermatitidis*, *H. capsulatum*, *P. brasiliensis*, and *C. immitis*. This dosage form also is useful in therapy of indolent invasive aspergillosis outside the central nervous system, particularly after the infection has been stabilized with amphotericin B. The intravenous formulation is approved for the initial two weeks of therapy with blastomycosis, histoplasmosis, and indolent aspergillosis. The intravenous route would be most appropriate for patients unable to tolerate the oral formulation or unable to absorb it because of decreased gastric acid. Approximately half the patients with distal subungual onychomycosis respond well to itraconazole (Evans and Sigurgeirsson, 1999). Although not an approved use, itraconazole is often the best choice for treatment of pseudallescheriasis, an infection not responding to amphotericin B therapy, as well as cutaneous and extracutaneous sporotrichosis, tinea corporis, and extensive tinea versicolor. HIV-infected patients with disseminated histoplasmosis or *P. marneffei* infections have a decreased incidence of relapse if given prolonged itraconazole "maintenance" therapy (Wheat *et al.*, 1993; Supparatpinyo *et al.*, 1998). It is as yet unclear whether patients responding to highly active antiretroviral therapy (HAART) will require less than lifelong

Table 49–2
Interactions of Itraconazole with Other Drugs

OTHER DRUG CONCENTRATION INCREASED	ITRACONAZOLE CONCENTRATION DECREASED
Alfentanil	Drugs that decrease gastric acidity
Alprazolam	
Astemizole	H$_2$ receptor blockers
Atorvastatin	Proton pump blockers
Bromperidol	Simultaneous antacids
Buspirone	Simultaneous didanosine
Cerivastatin	(buffer)
Cisapride	Carbamazepine
Cyclosporine	Isoniazid
Delavirdine	Nevirapine
Diazepam	Phenobarbital
Digoxin	Phenytoin
Dihydropyridine calcium channel blockers	Rifampin, rifabutin
Docetaxel	
Felodipine	ITRACONAZOLE CONCENTRATION INCREASED
Indinavir	
Loratidine	Clarithromycin
Lovastatin	Indinavir
Midazolam	Ritonavir
Nisoldipine	
Phenytoin	
Pimozide	
Quinidine	
Ritonavir	
Saquinavir	
Sildenafil	
Simvastatin	
Sirolimus	
Sulfonylureas (glyburide, others)	
Tacrolimus	
Triazolam	
Verapamil	
Vinca alkaloids	
Warfarin	

therapy (*see* Chapter 51). Itraconazole is not recommended for maintenance therapy of cryptococcal meningitis in HIV-infected patients because of a high incidence of relapse. However, itraconazole prophylaxis in patients with advanced HIV infection yielded a decreased incidence of cryptococcosis as well as histoplasmosis. The incidence of mucosal candidiasis was not reduced (McKinsey *et al.*, 1999). This study was done in the pre-HAART era, and itraconazole prophylaxis is not recommended.

Long-term therapy has been used in non-HIV-infected patients with allergic bronchopulmonary aspergillosis to decrease the dose of corticosteroids and reduce attacks of acute bronchospasm (Salez *et al.*, 1999).

Itraconazole solution is effective and approved for use in oropharyngeal and esophageal candidiasis. Because the preparation has more gastrointestinal side effects than do fluconazole tablets, itraconazole solution usually is reserved for patients not responding to fluconazole (Saag *et al.*, 1999). Unfortunately, these patients are often receiving protease inhibitors and other drugs that make itraconazole contraindicated. Itraconazole capsules and oral solution are not bioequivalent and should not be used interchangeably.

Dosage. In treating deep mycoses, two 100-mg capsules are given twice daily with food. Divided doses are said to increase the area under the curve (AUC) (*see* Chapter 1) compared to once-daily dosing, even though the half-life is about 30 hours. For the first three days, 200 mg three times daily is used as a loading dose. For maintenance therapy of HIV-infected patients with disseminated histoplasmosis, 200 mg once daily is used. Onychomycosis can be treated with either 200 mg once daily for 12 weeks or as 200 mg twice daily for one week out of each month, so-called pulse therapy (Evans and Sigurgeirsson, 1999). Retention of active drug in the nail keratin permits intermittent treatment. Daily therapy is preferred by some authorities for infections likely to be more refractory but is twice the cost of pulse therapy. Once-daily terbinafine (250 mg) is slightly superior to pulse therapy with itraconazole (*see* below). Treatment is usually continued for three months. Intravenous itraconazole is reserved for seriously ill patients; it is given as an infusion over one hour of 200 mg twice daily for two days followed by 200 mg once daily for 12 days. Safety and efficacy of the intravenous regimen beyond 14 days is currently unknown. Itraconazole oral solution should be taken fasting in a dose of 100 mg in 10 ml once daily and swished vigorously in the mouth before swallowing to optimize any topical effect. Patients with fluconazole-resistant oropharyngeal or esophageal thrush are given 100 mg twice a day for 2 to 4 weeks.

Untoward Effects. Adverse effects of itraconazole therapy can occur as a result of interactions with many other drugs (*see* below). Itraconazole capsules, in the absence of interacting drugs, are well tolerated at 200 mg daily. Gastrointestinal distress occasionally prevents use of 400 mg per day. In a series of 189 patients receiving 50 to 400 mg per day, nausea and vomiting were recorded in 10%, hypertriglyceridemia in 9%, hypokalemia in 6%, increased serum aminotransferase in 5%, rash in 2%, and at least one side effect in 39%. Occasionally, hepatotoxicity or rash leads to drug discontinuation, but most adverse effects can be handled with dose reduction. Profound hypokalemia has been seen in patients receiving 600 mg or more daily (Sharkey *et al.*, 1991) and in those who recently have received prolonged amphotericin B therapy. Doses of 300 mg twice daily have led to other side effects, including adrenal insufficiency, lower limb edema, hypertension, and, in one patient, rhabdomyolysis (Sharkey *et al.*, 1991). Doses above 400 mg per day are not recommended for long-term use.

Intravenous itraconazole has been well tolerated except for chemical phlebitis. A dedicated catheter port is required. If other medications are administered through the same port at a later time, the catheter should be thoroughly flushed with normal saline. Although the volume of infusion is small, 25 ml of itraconazole in excipient plus 50 ml of saline, infusion durations less than one hour are not recommended. Toxicity of high plasma levels of hydroxypropyl-β-cyclodextrin in azotemic patients is unknown, but until this issue is clarified, the intravenous formulation is contraindicated in patients with a creatinine clearance below 30 ml/min.

The oral solution of itraconazole is well tolerated but has all the adverse effects of itraconazole capsules. Anaphylaxis has been observed rarely, as well as severe rash, including Stevens–Johnson syndrome. Some patients complain of the taste, and gastrointestinal side effects are common, though compliance is generally unimpaired. Diarrhea, abdominal cramps, anorexia, and nausea are more common than with the capsules.

Fluconazole

Fluconazole is a fluorinated bistriazole. Its structure is as follows:

FLUCONAZOLE

Absorption, Distribution, and Excretion. Fluconazole is almost completely absorbed from the gastrointestinal tract. Concentrations in plasma are essentially the same whether the drug is given orally or intravenously, and bioavailability is not altered by food or gastric acidity. Peak plasma concentrations are 4 to 8 μg/ml after repetitive doses of 100 mg. Renal excretion accounts for over 90% of elimination, and the elimination half-time is 25 to 30 hours. Fluconazole diffuses readily into body fluids, including sputum and saliva; concentrations in CSF are 50% to 90% of the simultaneous values in plasma. The dosage interval should be increased from 24 to 48 hours with a creatinine clearance of 21 to 40 ml/min and to 72 hours at 10 to 20 ml/min. A dose of 100 to 200 mg should be given after each hemodialysis. About 11% to 12% of plasma drug is protein bound.

Interactions. Fluconazole significantly increases plasma concentrations of astemizole, cisapride, cyclosporine, rifampin, rifabutin, sulfonylureas (glipizide, tolbutamide, others), theophylline, tacrolimus, and warfarin. Patients who receive more than 400 mg daily or azotemic patients who have elevated fluconazole blood levels may experience drug interactions not otherwise seen. Rifampin decreases the fluconazole AUC by about 25%, an amount that ordinarily would not be significant. Drugs that decrease gastric acidity do not significantly lower fluconazole blood levels.

Therapeutic Uses. *Candidiasis.* Fluconazole, 200 mg on the first day and then 100 mg daily for at least 2 weeks, is effective in oropharyngeal candidiasis. Esophageal candidiasis responds to 100 to 200 mg daily. This dose also has been used to decrease candiduria in high-risk patients (Sobel *et al.,* 2000). A single dose of 150 mg is effective in vaginal candidiasis. A dose of 400 mg daily decreases the incidence of deep candidiasis in allogeneic bone marrow transplant recipients and is useful in treating candidemia of nonimmunosuppressed patients. Fluconazole is not known to be effective treatment for deep candidiasis in profoundly neutropenic patients. Based on resistance *in vitro, Candida krusei* would not be expected to respond to fluconazole or other azoles.

Cryptococcosis. Fluconazole, 400 mg daily, is used for the initial 8 weeks in cryptococcal meningitis of AIDS after the patient's clinical condition has been stabilized with intravenous amphotericin B. After the 8 weeks, the dose is decreased to 200 mg daily for life. It is still unclear whether or not patients with a sustained response to HAART can stop lifelong maintenance therapy. For AIDS patients with cryptococcal meningitis who are alert and oriented and have other favorable prognostic signs, initial therapy with 400 mg daily may be considered. The role of fluconazole for non-AIDS patients with cryptococcosis is not defined.

Other Mycoses. Fluconazole has become the drug of choice for treatment of coccidioidal meningitis because of much less morbidity than with intrathecal amphotericin B. In other forms of coccidioidomycosis, fluconazole appears roughly comparable to itraconazole. Fluconazole has activity against histoplasmosis, blastomycosis, sporotrichosis, and ringworm, but response is less than with equivalent doses of itraconazole. Fluconazole is not effective in the prevention or treatment of aspergillosis. As with other azoles, there is no activity in mucormycosis.

Fluconazole (DIFLUCAN) is marketed in the United States as tablets of 50, 100, and 200 mg for oral administration, powder for oral suspension providing 10 and 40 mg/ml, and intravenous solutions containing 2 mg/ml in saline and in dextrose solution. Dosage is 50 to 400 mg once daily and is identical for oral and intravenous administration. Children are treated with 3 to 6 mg/kg once daily.

Untoward Effects. Nausea and vomiting may be seen at doses above 200 mg daily. Patients receiving 800 mg daily may require antiemetics and may need to be treated intravenously to prevent emesis, which reduces drug availability. Data provided in the package insert states that side effects in patients receiving more than 7 days of drug, irrespective of dose, include the following: nausea 3.7%, headache 1.9%, skin rash 1.8%, vomiting 1.7%, abdominal pain 1.7%, and diarrhea 1.5%. Reversible alopecia may occur with prolonged therapy at 400 mg daily. Rare cases of deaths due to hepatic failure (Jacobson *et al.,* 1994) or Stevens–Johnson syndrome have been reported. Although the relationship between these deaths and fluconazole treatment is not completely clear in these cases, it is prudent to be alert to early symptoms of these disorders and to stop fluconazole if they occur. Fluconazole is teratogenic in rodents and has been associated with skeletal and cardiac deformities in three infants born to two women taking high doses during pregnancy (Pursley *et al.,* 1996). The drug should be avoided during pregnancy.

Pneumocandins

Caspofungin acetate (CANCIDASE, MK-0991) is a water-soluble, semisynthetic lipopeptide derivative of pneumocandin B_0. Drugs of this class, also referred to as echinocandins, inhibit the formation of $\beta(1,3)$-D-glucans in the fungal cell wall. Resistance is conferred by mutations in the *FKS1* gene, which codes for a large subunit of $(1,3)\beta$-glucan synthase. Azole-resistant isolates of *C. albicans* remain susceptible to caspofungin. The drug is active in experimental animal infection with *C. albicans, Aspergillus fumigatus, P. carinii,* and *H. capsulatum.* Clinical trials are in progress with intravenous formulations of caspofungin and a similar lipopeptide, FK463, in patients with deep candidiasis, and with neutropenia and fever not responding to antibacterial therapy.

Griseofulvin

Chemistry. The structural formula of *griseofulvin* is as follows:

GRISEOFULVIN

The drug is practically insoluble in water.

Antifungal Activity. Griseofulvin is fungistatic *in vitro* for various species of the dermatophytes *Microsporum, Epidermophyton,* and *Trichophyton.* The drug has no effect on bacteria or on other fungi.

Resistance. Although failure of ringworm lesions to improve is not rare, isolates from these patients usually are still susceptible to griseofulvin *in vitro.*

Mechanism of Action. A prominent morphological manifestation of the action of griseofulvin is the production of multinucleate cells as the drug inhibits fungal mitosis. An explanation for this phenomenon appears to come from studies of the effects on mammalian cells of higher concentrations of the antibiotic. Griseofulvin causes disruption of the mitotic spindle by interacting with polymerized microtubles. Although the effects of the drug are thus similar to those of colchicine and the vinca alkaloids, its binding sites on the microtubular protein are distinct. There is evidence that griseofulvin binds to a microtubule-associated protein in addition to its binding to tubulin.

Absorption, Distribution, and Excretion. The oral administration of a 0.5-g dose of griseofulvin produces peak plasma concentrations of approximately 1 μg/ml in about 4 hours. Blood levels are quite variable. Some studies have shown improved absorption when the drug is taken with a fatty meal. Since the rates of dissolution and disaggregation limit the bioavailability of griseofulvin, microsized and ultramicrosized powders are now

..ations (FULVICIN P/G; GRISACTIN; GRIFULVIN V). ..gn the bioavailability of the ultramicrocrystalline preparation is said to be 50% greater than that of the conventional microsized powder, this may not always be true. Griseofulvin has a half-life in plasma of about 1 day, and approximately 50% of the oral dose can be detected in the urine within 5 days, mostly in the form of metabolites. The primary metabolite is 6-methylgriseofulvin. Barbiturates decrease the absorption of griseofulvin from the gastrointestinal tract.

The drug is deposited in keratin precursor cells. The antibiotic present in such cells when they differentiate is tightly bound to, and persists in, keratin and makes this substance resistant to fungal invasion. For this reason, the new growth of hair or nails is the first to become free of disease. As the fungus-containing keratin is shed, it is replaced by normal tissue. Griseofulvin is detectable in the stratum corneum of the skin within 4 to 8 hours of oral administration. Sweat and transepidermal fluid loss play an important role in the transfer of the drug in the stratum corneum. Only a very small fraction of a dose of the drug is present in body fluids and tissues.

Therapeutic Uses. Mycotic disease of the skin, hair, and nails due to *Microsporum, Trichophyton,* or *Epidermophyton* responds to griseofulvin therapy. Infections that are readily treatable with this agent include infections of the hair (tinea capitis) caused by *Microsporum canis, Microsporum audouini, Trichophyton schoenleinii,* and *Trichophyton verrucosum;* "ringworm" of the glabrous skin; tinea cruris and tinea corporis caused by *M. canis, Trichophyton rubrum, T. verrucosum,* and *Epidermophyton floccosum;* and tinea of the hands (*T. rubrum, Trichophyton mentagrophytes*) and beard (*Trichophyton* species). Griseofulvin also is highly effective in "athlete's foot" or epidermophytosis involving the skin and nails, the vesicular form of which is most commonly due to *T. mentagrophytes* and the hyperkeratotic type to *T. rubrum.* However, topical therapy is preferred (*see* below). *T. rubrum* and *T. mentagrophytes* infections may require higher-than-conventional doses. Since very high doses of griseofulvin are carcinogenic and teratogenic in laboratory animals, the drug should not be used to treat trivial infections that respond to topical therapy.

The recommended daily dose of griseofulvin is 5 to 15 mg/kg for children and 500 mg to 1 g for adults. Doses of 1.5 to 2.0 g daily may be used for short periods in severe or extensive infections. Best results are obtained when the daily dose is divided and given at 6-hour intervals, although the drug often is given twice per day. Treatment must be continued until infected tissue is replaced by normal hair, skin, or nails, which requires 1 month for scalp and hair ringworm, 6 to 9 months for fingernails, and at least a year for toenails. Itraconazole or terbinafine is preferred for onychomycosis. Griseofulvin is not effective in treatment of subcutaneous or deep mycoses.

Untoward Effects. The incidence of serious reactions associated with the use of griseofulvin is very low. One of the minor effects is headache; it is sometimes severe and usually disappears as therapy is continued. The incidence of headache may be as high as 15%. Other nervous system manifestations include peripheral neuritis, lethargy, mental confusion, impairment of performance of routine tasks, fatigue, syncope, vertigo, blurred vision, transient macular edema, and augmentation of the effects of alcohol. Among the side effects involving the

alimentary tract are nausea, vomiting, diarrhea, heartburn, flatulence, dry mouth, and angular stomatitis. Hepatotoxicity also has been observed. Hematologic effects include leukopenia, neutropenia, punctate basophilia, and monocytosis; these often disappear despite continuation of therapy. Blood studies should be carried out at least once a week during the first month of treatment or longer. Common renal effects include albuminuria and cylindruria without evidence of renal insufficiency. Reactions involving the skin are cold and warm urticaria, photosensitivity, lichen planus, erythema, erythema multiforme-like rashes, and vesicular and morbilliform eruptions. Serum sickness syndromes and severe angioedema develop rarely during treatment with griseofulvin. Estrogen-like effects have been observed in children. A moderate but inconsistent increase of fecal protoporphyrins has been noted when the drug is used for a long time.

Griseofulvin induces hepatic microsomal enzymes, thus increasing the rate of metabolism of warfarin; adjustment of the dosage of the latter agent may be necessary in some patients. The drug may reduce the efficacy of some oral contraceptive agents, probably by a similar mechanism.

Terbinafine   *LAMISIL*

Terbinafine is a synthetic allylamine, structurally similar to the topical agent naftifine. Its structural formula is shown below:

TERBINAFINE

Terbinafine is well absorbed, but bioavailability is decreased to about 40% because of first-pass metabolism in the liver. Proteins bind more than 99% of the drug in plasma. Drug accumulates in skin, nails, and fat. The initial half-life is about 12 hours but extends to 200 to 400 hours at steady state. Drug can be found in plasma for 4 to 8 weeks after prolonged therapy (Balfour and Faulds, 1992). Terbinafine is not recommended in patients with marked azotemia or hepatic failure because terbinafine plasma levels are increased by unpredictable amounts. Rifampin decreases and cimetidine increases plasma terbinafine concentrations. The drug is well tolerated, with a low incidence of gastrointestinal distress, headache, or rash. Rarely, hepatotoxicity, severe neutropenia, Stevens–Johnson syndrome, or toxic epidermal necrolysis may occur. The drug is in pregnancy category B. Its mechanism of action is probably inhibition of fungal squalene epoxidase, blocking ergosterol biosynthesis.

Terbinafine (LAMISIL), given as one 250-mg tablet daily, is at least as effective for onychomycosis of nails as 200 mg daily of itraconazole, and slightly more effective than pulse itraconazole therapy (*see* above) (Evans, 1999). Duration of treatment varies with the nail being treated but typically is 3 months. Although not approved for this use, terbinafine (250 mg daily) also is effective in ringworm elsewhere on the body. No pediatric formulation is available, so there is little experience with the drug in tinea capitis, usually a disease of children. The topical use of terbinafine is discussed in the following section.

TOPICAL ANTIFUNGAL AGENTS

Topical treatment is useful in many superficial fungal infections—that is, those confined to the stratum corneum, squamous mucosa, or cornea. Such diseases include dermatophytosis (ringworm), candidiasis, tinea versicolor, piedra, tinea nigra, and fungal keratitis. Topical administration of antifungal agents is usually not successful for mycoses of the nails (onychomycosis) and hair (tinea capitis) and has no place in the treatment of subcutaneous mycoses, such as sporotrichosis and chromomycosis. The efficacy of topical agents in the superficial mycoses depends not only on the type of lesion and the mechanism of action of the drug but also on the viscosity, hydrophobicity, and acidity of the formulation. Regardless of formulation, penetration of topical drugs into hyperkeratotic lesions often is poor. Removal of thick, infected keratin is sometimes a useful adjunct to therapy; this is, for example, the principal mode of action of Whitfield's ointment (*see* below).

A plethora of topical agents are available for the treatment of superficial mycoses. Many of the older drugs—including gentian violet, carbol-fuchsin, acrisorcin, triacetin, sulfur, iodine, and aminacrine—are now rarely indicated and are not discussed here (*see* previous editions of this textbook). Among the topical agents to be discussed, the preferred formulation for cutaneous application usually is a cream or solution. Ointments are messy and are too occlusive for macerated or fissured intertriginous lesions. The use of powders, whether applied by shake containers or aerosols, is largely confined to the feet and moist lesions of the groin and other intertriginous areas.

The systemic agents that are used for the treatment of superficial mycoses are discussed in the first section of this chapter. Some of these agents are also administered topically; their uses are described here and also in Chapter 65.

Imidazoles and Triazoles for Topical Use

As discussed above, these closely related classes of drugs are synthetic antifungal agents that are used both topically and systemically. Indications for their topical use include ringworm, tinea versicolor, and mucocutaneous candidiasis. Resistance to imidazoles or triazoles is very rare among the fungi that cause ringworm. Selection of one of these agents for topical use should be based on cost and availability, since testing *in vitro* for fungal susceptibility to these drugs is not predictive of clinical responses.

Cutaneous Application. The preparations for cutaneous use described below are effective for tinea corporis, tinea pedis, tinea cruris, tinea versicolor, and cutaneous candidiasis. They

should be applied twice a day for 3 to 6 weeks. Despite some activity *in vitro* against bacteria, this effect is not clinically useful. The cutaneous formulations are not suitable for oral, vaginal, or ocular use.

Vaginal Application. The vaginal creams, suppositories, and tablets are the preparations of choice for vaginal candidiasis. None is useful in trichomoniasis, despite some activity *in vitro*. They are all used once a day, preferably at bedtime to facilitate retention. Most vaginal creams are administered in 5-g amounts. Three vaginal formulations—clotrimazole tablets, miconazole suppositories, and terconazole cream—come in both low- and high-dose preparations. A shorter duration of therapy is recommended for the higher dose of each. Except for the 500-mg clotrimazole tablet and tioconazole ointment, which are given only once, these preparations are administered for 3 to 7 days. Approximately 3% to 10% of the vaginal dose is absorbed. Although some imidazoles are embryotoxic in rodents, no adverse effects on the human fetus have been attributed to the vaginal use of imidazoles or triazoles. The most common side effect is vaginal burning or itching. A male sexual partner may experience mild penile irritation. Cross-allergenicity among these compounds is assumed to exist, based on their structural similarities.

Oral Use. Use of the oral troche of clotrimazole is properly considered as topical therapy. The only indication for this 10-mg troche is oropharyngeal candidiasis. Antifungal activity is due entirely to the local concentration of the drug; there is no systemic effect. The patient should be told to suck on the troche until it dissolves.

Clotrimazole. *Clotrimazole* has the following structure:

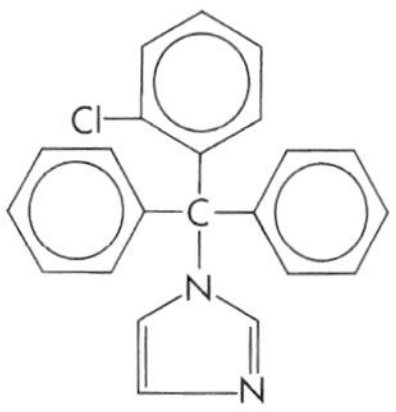

CLOTRIMAZOLE

Absorption of clotrimazole is less than 0.5% after application to the intact skin; from the vagina, it is 3% to 10%. Fungicidal concentrations remain in the vagina for as long as 3 days after application of the drug. The small amount absorbed is metabolized in the liver and excreted in bile. In adults, an oral dose of 200 mg per day will give rise initially to plasma concentrations of 0.2 to 0.35 μg/ml, followed by a progressive decline.

In a small fraction of recipients, clotrimazole on the skin may cause stinging, erythema, edema, vesication, desquamation, pruritus, and urticaria. When it is applied to the vagina, about 1.6% of recipients complain of a mild burning sensation and, rarely, of lower abdominal cramps, slight increase in urinary frequency, or skin rash. Occasionally, the sexual partner may experience penile or urethral irritation. By the oral route, clotrimazole can cause gastrointestinal irritation. In patients using troches, the incidence of this side effect is about 5%.

Therapeutic Uses. *Clotrimazole* is available as a 1% cream, lotion, and solution (LOTRIMIN, MYCELEX), 1% or 2% vaginal cream or vaginal tablets of 100, 200, or 500 mg (GYNE-LOTRIMIN, MYCELEX-G), and 10-mg troches (MYCELEX). On the skin, applications are made twice a day. For the vagina, the standard regimens are one 100-mg tablet once a day at bedtime for 7 days, one 200-mg tablet daily for 3 days, one 500-mg tablet inserted only once, or 5 g of cream once a day for 3 days (2% cream) or 7 days (1% cream). For nonpregnant females, two 100-mg tablets may be used once a day for 3 days. Troches are to be dissolved slowly in the mouth five times a day for 14 days.

Clotrimazole has been reported to cure dermatophyte infections in 60% to 100% of cases. The cure rates in cutaneous candidiasis are 80% to 100%. In vulvovaginal candidiasis, the cure rate is usually above 80% when the 7-day regimen is used. A 3-day regimen of 200 mg once a day appears to be similarly effective, as does single-dose treatment (500 mg). Recurrences are common after all regimens. The cure rate with oral troches for oral and pharyngeal candidiasis may be as high as 100% in the immunocompetent host.

Econazole. *Econazole,* the deschloro derivative of miconazole, has the following structure:

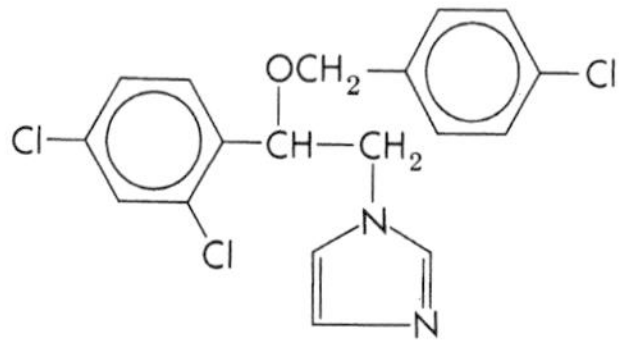

ECONAZOLE

Econazole readily penetrates the stratum corneum and is found in effective concentrations down to the mid-dermis. However, less than 1% of an applied dose appears to be absorbed into the blood. Approximately 3% of recipients have local erythema, burning, stinging, or itching.

Econazole nitrate (SPECTAZOLE) is available as a water-miscible cream (1%) to be applied twice a day.

Miconazole. *Miconazole* is a very close chemical congener of econazole, with the following structure:

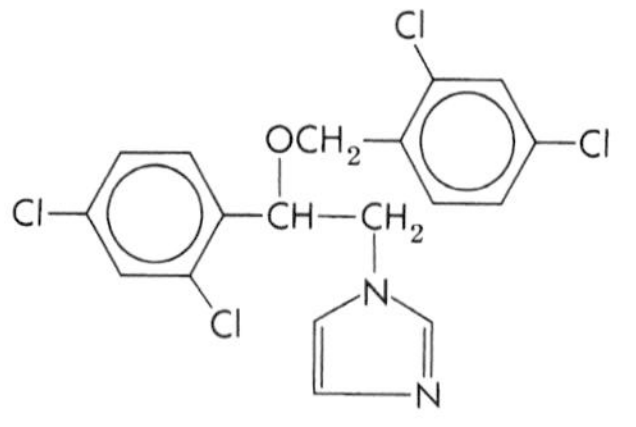

MICONAZOLE

Miconazole readily penetrates the stratum corneum of the skin and persists there for more than 4 days after application. Less than 1% is absorbed into the blood. Absorption is no more than 1.3% from the vagina.

Adverse effects from topical application to the vagina include burning, itching, or irritation in about 7% of recipients

and, infrequently, pelvic cramps (0.2%), headache, hives, or skin rash. Irritation, burning, and maceration are rare after cutaneous application. Miconazole is considered safe for use during pregnancy, although some authors believe that its vaginal use should be avoided during the first trimester.

Therapeutic Uses. *Miconazole nitrate* is available as a dermatologic ointment, cream, solution, spray, powder, or lotion (MICATIN, MONISTAT-DERM, others). To avoid maceration, only the lotion should be applied to intertriginous areas. It is available as a 2% and 4% vaginal cream, as 100-mg suppositories (MONISTAT 7), to be applied high in the vagina at bedtime for 7 days, and as 200-mg vaginal suppositories (MONISTAT 3) for 3-day therapy.

In the treatment of tinea pedis, tinea cruris, and tinea versicolor, the cure rate may be over 90%. In the treatment of vulvovaginal candidiasis, the mycologic cure rate at the end of 1 month is about 80% to 95%. Pruritus sometimes is relieved after a single application. Some vaginal infections caused by *Candida glabrata* also respond.

Terconazole and Butoconazole. *Terconazole* (TERAZOL) is a ketal triazole with structural similarities to ketoconazole. Its structure is as follows:

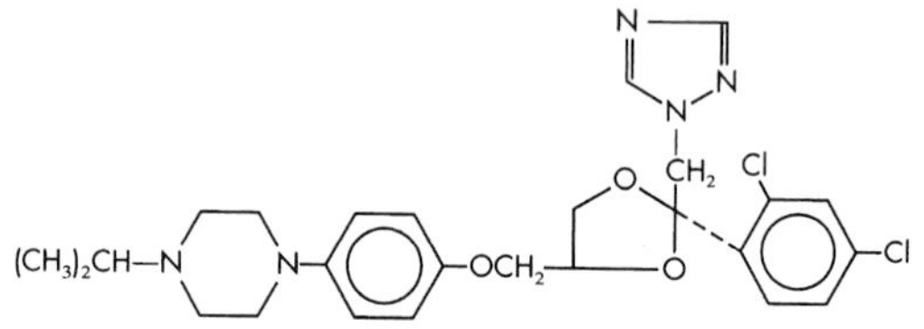

TERCONAZOLE

The mechanism of action of terconazole is similar to that of the imidazoles. The 80-mg vaginal suppository is inserted at bedtime for 3 days, while the 0.4% vaginal cream is used for 7 days and the 0.8% cream for 3 days. Clinical efficacy and patient acceptance of both preparations are at least as good as for clotrimazole in patients with vaginal candidiasis.

Butoconazole is an imidazole quite comparable to clotrimazole. Its structural formula is as follows:

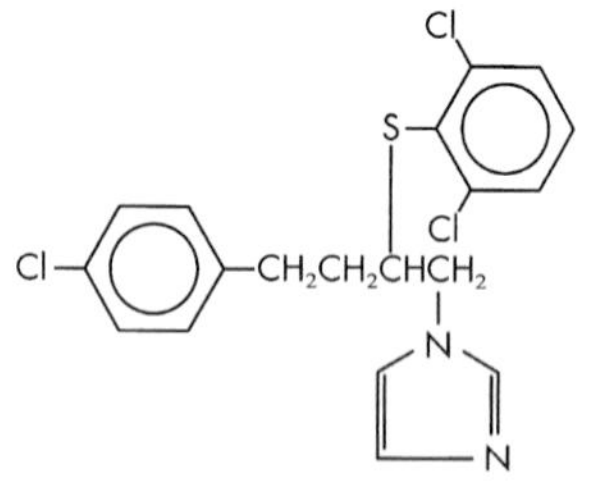

BUTOCONAZOLE

Butoconazole nitrate (FEMSTAT 3) is available as a 2% vaginal cream; it is used at bedtime for 3 days in nonpregnant females. Because of the slower response during pregnancy, a 6-day course is recommended (during the second and third trimester).

Tioconazole. *Tioconazole* (VAGISTAT 1) is an imidazole that is marketed for treatment of *Candida* vulvovaginitis. A single 4.6-g dose of ointment containing 6.5% drug is given at bedtime.

Oxiconazole and Sulconazole. Oxiconazole and sulconazole are two imidazole derivatives that are used for the topical treatment of infections caused by the common pathogenic dermatophytes. *Oxiconazole nitrate* (OXISTAT) is available as a cream and lotion; *sulconazole nitrate* (EXELDERM) is supplied as a solution and cream.

Ciclopirox Olamine

Ciclopirox olamine (LOPROX) has broad-spectrum antifungal activity. The chemical structure is as follows:

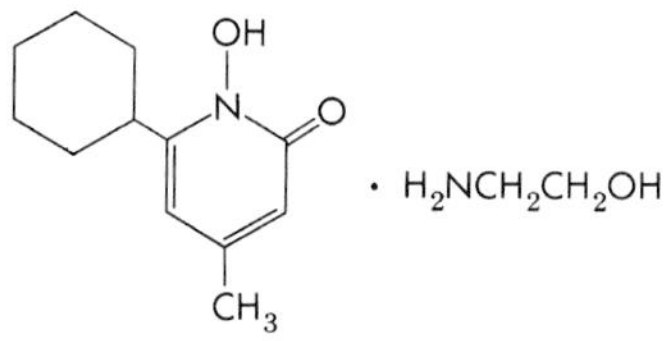

CICLOPIROX OLAMINE

It is fungicidal to *C. albicans, E. floccosum, M. canis, T. mentagrophytes,* and *T. rubrum.* It also inhibits the growth of *Malassezia furfur.* After application to the skin, it penetrates through the epidermis into the dermis, but even under occlusion, less than 1.5% is absorbed into the systemic circulation. Since the half-life is 1.7 hours, no systemic accumulation occurs. The drug penetrates into hair follicles and sebaceous glands. It can sometimes cause hypersensitivity. It is available as a 1% cream and lotion for the treatment of cutaneous candidiasis and for tinea corporis, cruris, pedis, and versicolor. Cure rates in the dermatomycoses and candidal infections have been variously reported to be 81% to 94%. No topical toxicity has been noted.

Haloprogin

Haloprogin is a halogenated phenolic ether with the following structure:

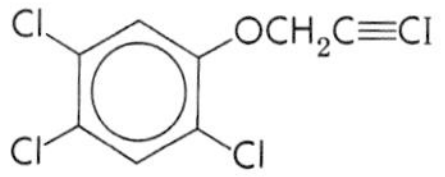

HALOPROGIN

It is fungicidal to various species of *Epidermophyton, Pityrosporum, Microsporum, Trichophyton,* and *Candida.* During treatment with this drug, irritation, pruritus, burning sensations, vesiculation, increased maceration, and "sensitization" (or exacerbation of the lesion) occasionally occur, especially on the foot if occlusive footgear is worn. Haloprogin is poorly absorbed through the skin; it is converted to trichlorophenol in the body. The systemic toxicity from topical application appears to be low.

Haloprogin (HALOTEX) cream or solution is applied twice a day for 2 to 4 weeks. Its principal use is against tinea pedis, for which the cure rate is about 80%; it is thus approximately equal in efficacy to tolnaftate (*see* below). It also is used against tinea cruris, tinea corporis, tinea manuum, and tinea versicolor.

Tolnaftate

Tolnaftate is a thiocarbamate with the following structure:

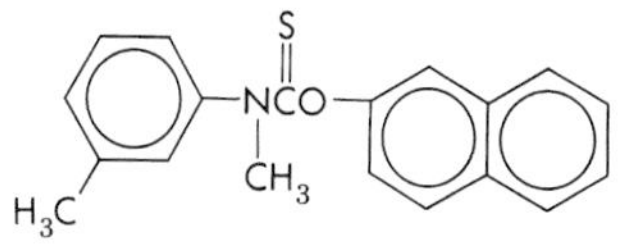

TOLNAFTATE

Tolnaftate is effective in the treatment of most cutaneous mycoses caused by *T. rubrum, T. mentagrophytes, T. tonsurans, E. floccosum, M. canis, M. audouinii, Microsporum gypseum,* and *M. furfur,* but it is ineffective against *Candida.* In tinea pedis, the cure rate is around 80%, compared with about 95% for miconazole. Toxic or allergic reactions to tolnaftate have not been reported.

Tolnaftate (AFTATE, TINACTIN, others) is available in a 1% concentration as a cream, gel, powder, aerosol powder, and topical solution, or as a topical aerosol liquid. The preparations are applied locally twice a day. Pruritus is usually relieved in 24 to 72 hours. Involution of interdigital lesions caused by susceptible fungi is very often complete in 7 to 21 days.

Naftifine

Naftifine is an allylamine with the following structure:

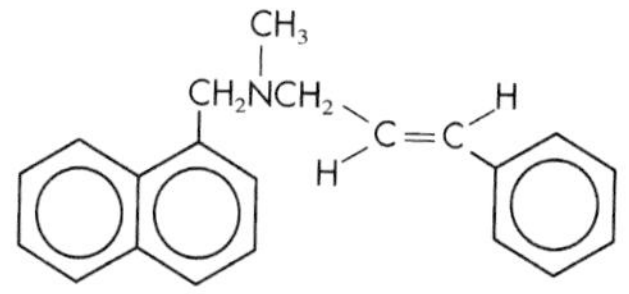

NAFTIFINE

Naftifine is representative of the allylamine class of synthetic agents that inhibit squalene-2,3-epoxidase and thus inhibit fungal biosynthesis of ergosterol. The drug has broad-spectrum fungicidal activity *in vitro. Naftifine hydrochloride* (NAFTIN) is available as a 1% cream or gel. It is effective for the topical treatment of tinea cruris and tinea corporis; twice-daily application is recommended. The drug is well tolerated, although local irritation has been observed in 3% of treated patients. Allergic contact dermatitis also has been reported. Naftifine also may be efficacious for cutaneous candidiasis and tinea versicolor, although the drug has not been approved for these uses.

Terbinafine

Terbinafine cream is applied twice daily and is effective in tinea corporis, tinea cruris, and tinea pedis. Terbinafine is less active against *Candida* species and *Malassezia furfur,* but the cream also can be used in cutaneous candidiasis and tinea versicolor. In European studies, oral terbinafine has appeared to be effective in treatment of ringworm and in some cases of onychomycosis. The systemic use of terbinafine is discussed above.

Butenafine

Butenafine hydrochloride (MENTAX) is a benzylamine derivative with a mechanism of action similar to that of terbinafine and naftifine. Its spectrum of antifungal activity and use also are similar to those of the allylamines.

Polyene Antifungal Antibiotics

Nystatin. *Nystatin* was discovered in the New York State Health Laboratory and was named accordingly; it is a tetraene macrolide produced by *Streptomyces noursei*. Nystatin is structurally similar to amphotericin B and has the same mechanism of action. Nystatin is not absorbed from the gastrointestinal tract, skin, or vagina. A liposomal formulation (NYOTRAN) is in clinical trials for candidemia.

Nystatin (MYCOSTATIN, NILSTAT, others) is useful only for candidiasis and is supplied in preparations intended for cutaneous, vaginal, or oral administration for this purpose. Infections of the nails and hyperkeratinized or crusted skin lesions do not respond. Topical preparations include ointments, creams, and powders, all of which contain 100,000 U/g. Powders are preferred for moist lesions and are applied two or three times a day. Creams or ointments are used twice daily. Combinations of nystatin with antibacterial agents or corticosteroids also are available. Allergic reactions to nystatin are very uncommon.

Vaginal tablets containing 100,000 U of the drug are inserted once daily for 2 weeks. Although the tablets are well tolerated, imidazoles or triazoles are more effective agents for vaginal candidiasis.

An oral suspension that contains 100,000 U of nystain per milliliter is given four times a day. Premature and low-birth-weight neonates should receive 1 ml of this preparation, infants 2 ml, and children or adults 4 to 6 ml per dose. Older children and adults should be instructed to swish the drug around the mouth and then swallow. If not otherwise instructed, the patient may expectorate the bitter liquid and fail to treat the infected mucosa in the posterior pharynx or esophagus. Nystatin suspension is usually effective for oral candidiasis of the immunocompetent host. Other than the bitter taste and occasional complaints of nausea, adverse effects are uncommon. Oral tablets containing 500,000 U have been used to decrease gastrointestinal colonization with *Candida* in the hope of preventing relapse of vaginal candidiasis or of protecting the neutropenic patient from gastrointestinal candidiasis. Careful studies have failed to document efficacy for these indications.

Amphotericin B. Topical amphotericin B (FUNGIZONE) also is used for cutaneous and mucocutaneous candidiasis. A lotion, cream, and ointment are marketed; these preparations all contain 3% amphotericin B and are applied to the lesion two to four times daily. The systemic use of amphotericin B is discussed above.

Miscellaneous Antifungal Agents

Undecylenic Acid. *Undecylenic acid* is 10-undecenoic acid, an 11-carbon unsaturated compound. It is a yellow liquid with a characteristic rancid odor. It is primarily fungistatic, although fungicidal activity may be observed with long exposure to high concentrations of the agent. The drug is active against a variety of fungi, including those that cause ringworm. *Undecylenic acid* (DESENEX) is available in a foam, ointment, cream, powder, spray powder, soap, and liquid. *Zinc undecylenate* is marketed in combination with other ingredients. The zinc provides an astringent action that aids in the suppression of inflammation. *Compound undecylenic acid ointment* contains both undecylenic acid (about 5%) and zinc undecylenate (about 20%). *Calcium undecylenate* (CALDESENE, CRUEX) is available as a powder.

Undecylenic acid preparations are used in the treatment of various dermatomycoses, especially tinea pedis. Concentrations of the acid as high as 10%, as well as those of the acid and salt in the compound ointment, may be applied to the skin. The preparations as formulated are usually not irritating to tissue, and sensitization to them is uncommon. It is of undoubted benefit in retarding fungal growth in tinea pedis, but the infection frequently persists despite intensive treatment with preparations of the acid and the zinc salt. At best, the clinical "cure" rate is about 50% and is thus much lower than that obtained with the imidazoles, haloprogin, or tolnaftate. The efficacy in the treatment of tinea capitis is marginal, and the drug is no longer used for that purpose. Undecylenic acid preparations also are approved for use in the treatment of diaper rash, tinea cruris, and other minor dermatologic conditions.

Benzoic Acid and Salicylic Acid. An ointment containing benzoic and salicylic acids is known as *Whitfield's ointment*. It combines the fungistatic action of benzoate with the keratolytic action of salicylate. It contains benzoic acid and salicylic acid in a ratio of 2 to 1 (usually 6% to 3%). It is used mainly in the treatment of tinea pedis. Since benzoic acid is only fungistatic, eradication of the infection occurs only after the infected stratum corneum is shed, and continuous medication is required for several weeks to months. The salicylic acid accelerates the desquamation. The ointment also is sometimes used to treat tinea capitis. Mild irritation may occur at the site of application.

Propionic Acid and Caprylic Acid. Propionic acid and sodium propionate are promoted for the treatment of the dermatomycoses. Both their low efficacy and exaggerated price make them irrational choices for treatment. They may be compounded together or with sodium caprylate or other agents. Sodium propionate is used in proprietary preparations in concentrations of 1% to 5%.

Potassium Iodide. A saturated solution of potassium iodide, containing 1 g/ml, is useful in treating cutaneous sporotrichosis. The drug has a bitter taste and causes nausea, bitter eructation, and excessive salivation. Patient acceptance is improved if the initial dosage is low, such as 10 drops in a small amount of water, taken three times daily. Drinking water or juice immediately following the dose lessens the bitter aftertaste. Dosage is increased gradually to 25 to 40 drops three times daily in children and to 40 to 50 drops three times a day in adults. Therapy is continued for at least 6 weeks and until the cutaneous lesions have flattened and any ulcerations have healed. Gradual enlargement of the salivary and lacrimal glands is usual, and adults may develop an acneiform rash over the cape area of the chest. These side effects go away after therapy is discontinued and are not a cause for drug discontinuation. Patients with true allergic rashes should be changed to itraconazole therapy.

For further discussion of fungal diseases in human beings *see* Chapters 202 to 211 in *Harrison's Principles of Internal Medicine,* 14th ed., McGraw-Hill, New York, 1998.

BIBLIOGRAPHY

Balmaceda, C.M., Walker, R.W., Castro-Malaspina, H., and Dalmau, J. Reversal of amphotericin-B-related encephalopathy. *Neurology.* **1994,** *44*:1183–1184.

Bekersky, I., Boswell, G.W., Hiles, R., Fielding, R.M., Buell, D., and Walsh, T.J. Safety and toxicokinetics of intravenous liposomal amphotericin B (AmBisome) in beagle dogs. *Pharm. Res.,* **1999,** *16*:1694–1701.

Carlson, M.A., and Condon, R.E. Nephrotoxicity of amphotericin B. *J. Am. Coll. Surg.,* **1994,** *179*:361–381.

Chavanet, P.Y., Garry, I., Charlier, N., Caillot, D., Kisterman, J.-P., D'Athis, M., and Portier, H. Trial of glucose versus fat emulsion in preparation of amphotericin for use in HIV infected patients with candidiasis. *B.M.J.,* **1992,** *305*:921–925.

Coker, R.J., Viviani, M., Gazzard, B.G., Du Pont, B., Pohle, H.D., Murphy, S.M., Atouguia, J., Champalimaud, J.L., and Harris, J.R. Treatment of cryptococcosis with liposomal amphotericin B (AmBisome) in 23 patients with AIDS. *AIDS,* **1993,** *7*:829–835.

deMarie, S., Janknegt, R., and Bakker-Woudenberg, I.A.J.M. Clinical use of liposomal and lipid-complexed amphotericin B. *J. Antimicrob. Chemother.,* **1994,** *33*:907–916.

Evans, E.G., and Sigurgeirsson, B. Double blind, randomised study of continuous terbinafine compared with intermittent itraconazole in treatment of toenail onychomycosis. The LION Study Group. *B.M.J.,* **1999,** *318*:1031–1035.

Jacobson, M.A., Hanks, D.K., and Ferrell, L.D. Fatal acute hepatic necrosis due to fluconazole. *Am. J. Med.,* **1994,** *96*:188–190.

Johnson, M.D., Drew, R.H., and Perfect, J.R. Chest discomfort associated with liposomal amphotericin B: report of three cases and review of the literature. *Pharmacotherapy,* **1998,** *18*:1053–1061.

Kelsey, S.M., Goldman, J.M., McCann, S., Newland, A.C., Scarffe, J.H., Oppenheim, B.A., and Mufti, G.J. Liposomal amphotericin (AmBisome) in the prophylaxis of fungal infections in neutropenic patients: a randomised, double-blind, placebo-controlled study. *Bone Marrow Transplant.,* **1999,** *23*:163–168.

McKinsey, D.S., Wheat, L.J., Cloud, G.A., Pierce, M., Black, J.R., Bamberger, D.M., Goldman, M., Thomas, C.J., Gutsch, H.M., Moskovitz, B., Dismukes, W.E., and Kauffman, C.A. Itraconazole prophylaxis for fungal infections in patients with advanced human immunodeficiency virus infection: randomized, placebo-controlled, double-blind study. National Institute of Allergy and Infectious Diseases Mycoses Study Group. *Clin. Infect. Dis.,* **1999,** *28*:1049–1056.

Marichal, P., Koymans, L., Willemsens, S., Bellens, D., Verhasselt, P., Luyten, W., Borgers, M., Ramaekers, F.C., Odds, F.C., and Bossche, H.V. Contribution of mutations in the cytochrome P450 14alpha-demethylase (Erg11p, Cyp51p) to azole resistance to *Candida albicans. Microbiology,* **1999,** *145*:2701–2713.

Noskin, G., Pietrelli, L., Gurwith, M., and Bowden, R. Treatment of invasive fungal infections with amphotericin B colloidal dispersion in bone marrow transplant recipients. *Bone Marrow Transplant.,* **1999,** *23*:697–703.

Prentice, H.G., Hann, I.M., Herbrecht, R., Aoun, M., Kvaloy, S., Catovsky, D., Pinkerton, C.R., Schey, S.A., Jacobs, F., Oakhill, A., Stevens, R.F., Darbyshire, P.J., and Gibson, B.E. A randomized comparison of liposomal versus conventional amphotericin B for the treatment of pyrexia of unknown origin in neutropenic patients. *Br. J. Haematol.,* **1997,** *98*: 711–718.

Pursley, T.J., Blomquist, I.K., Abraham, J., Andersen, H.F., and Bartley, J.A. Fluconazole-induced congenital abnormalities in three infants. *Clin. Infect. Dis.,* **1996,** *22*:336–340.

Saag, M.S., Fessel, W.J., Kaufman, C.A., Merrill, K.W., Ward, D.J., Moskovitz, B.L., Thomas, C., Oleka, N., Guarnieri, J.A., Lee, J., Brenner-Gati, L., and Klausner, M. Treatment of fluconazole-refractory oropharyngeal candidiasis with itraconazole oral solution in HIV-positive patients. *AIDS Res. Hum. Retroviruses,* **1999,** *15*:1413–1417.

Salez, F., Brichet, A., Desurmont, S., Grobois, J-M., Wallaert, B., and Tonnel, A-B. Effects of itraconazole therapy in allergic bronchopulmonary aspergillosis. *Chest,* **1999,** *116*:1665–1668.

Sharkey, P.K., Graybill, J.R., Johnson, E.S., Hausrath, S.G., Pollard, R.B., Kolokathis, A., Mildvan, D., Fan-Havard, P., Eng, R.H., Patterson, T.F., Pottage, J.C., Jr., Simberkoff, M.S., Wolf, J., Meyer, R.D., Gupta, R., Lee, L.W., and Gordon, D.S. Amphotericin B lipid complex compared with amphotericin B in the treatment of cryptococcal meningitis in patients with AIDS. *Clin. Infect. Dis.,* **1996,** *22*:315–321.

Sharkey, P.K., Rinaldi, M.G., Dunn, J.F., Hardin, T.C., Fetchick, R.J., and Graybill, J.R. High-dose itraconazole in the treatment of severe mycoses. *Antimicrob. Agents Chemother.,* **1991,** *35*:707–713.

Sobel, J.D., Kauffman, C.A., McKinsey, D., Zervos, M., Vazquez, J.A., Karchmer, A.W., Lee, J., Thomas, C., Panzer, H., and Dismukes, W.E. Candiduria: a randomized, double-blind study of treatment with fluconazole and placebo. National Institute of Allergy and Infectious Disease (NIAID) Mycoses Study Group. *Clin. Infect. Dis.,* **2000,** *30*:19–24.

Stamm, A.M., Diasio, R.B., Dismukes, W.E., Shadomy, S., Cloud, G.A., Bowles, C.A., Karam, G.H., and Espinel-Ingroff, A. Toxicity of amphotericin B plus flucytosine in 194 patients with cryptococcal meningitis. *Am. J. Med.,* **1987,** *83*:236–242.

Supparatpinyo, K., Perriens, J., Nelson, K.E., and Sirisanthana, T. A controlled trial of itraconazole to prevent relapse of *Penicillium marneffei* infection in patients infected with the human immunodeficiency virus. *N. Engl. J. Med.,* **1998,** *339*:1739–1743.

Tolins, J.P., and Raij, L. Adverse effect of amphotericin B administration on renal hemodynamics in the rat. Neurohumoral mechanisms and influence of calcium channel blockade. *J. Pharmacol. Exp. Ther.,* **1988,** *245*:594–599.

van der Horst, C.M., Saag, M.S., Cloud, G.A., Hamill, R.J., Graybill, J.R., Sobel, J.D., Johnson, P.C., Tuazon, C.U., Kerkering, T., Moskovitz, B.L., Powderly, W.G., and Dismukes, W.E. Treatment of cryptococcal meningitis associated with the acquired immunodeficiency syndrome.

National Institute of Allergy and Infectious Diseases Mycoses Study Group and AIDS Clinical Trials Group. *N. Engl. J. Med.,* **1997,** *337*: 15–21.

Walsh, T.J., Finberg, R.W., Arndt, C., Hiemenz, J., Schwartz, C., Bodensteiner, D., Pappas, P., Seibel, N., Greenberg, R.N., Dummer, S., Schuster, M., and Holcenberg, J.S. Liposomal amphotericin B for empirical therapy in patients with persistent fever and neutropenia. National Institute of Allergy and Infectious Diseases Mycoses Study Group. *N. Engl. J. Med.,* **1999,** *340*:764–771.

Walsh, T.J., Hiemenz, J.W., Seibel, N.L., Perfect, J.R., Horwith, G., Lee, L., Silber, J.L., DiNubile, M.J., Reboli, A., Bow, E., Lister, J., and Anaissie, E.J. Amphotericin B lipid complex for invasive fungal infections: analysis of safety and efficacy in 556 cases. *Clin. Infect. Dis.,* **1998,** *26*:1383–1396.

Wheat, J., Hafner, R., Wulfsohn, M., Spencer, P., Squires, K., Powderly, W., Wong, B., Rinaldi, M., Saag, M., Hamill, R., Murphy, R., Connolly-Stringfield, P., Briggs, N., and Owens, S. Prevention of relapse of histoplamosis with itraconazole in patients with the acquired immunodeficiency syndrome. The National Institute of Allergy and Infectious Diseases Clinical Trials and Mycoses Study Group Collaborators. *Ann. Intern. Med.,* **1993,** *118*:610–616.

White, M.H., Bowden, R.A., Sandler, E.S., Graham, M.L., Noskin, G.A., Wingard, J.R., Goldman, M., van Burik, J.A., McCabe, A., Lin, J.S., Gurwith, M., and Miller, C.B. Randomized, double-blind clinical trial of amphotericin B colloidal dispersion vs. amphotericin B in the empirical treatment of fever and neutropenia. *Clin. Infect. Dis.,* **1998,** 27:296–302.

Wingard, J.R. Efficacy of amphotericin B lipid complex injection (ABLC) in bone marrow transplant recipients with life-threatening systemic mycoses. *Bone Marrow Transplant.,* **1997,** *19*:343–347.

Wingard, J.R., Kubilis, P., Lee, L., Yee, G., White, M., Walshe, L., Bowden, R., Ainaissie, E., Hiemenz, J., and Lister, J. Clinical significance of nephrotoxicity in patients treated with amphotericin B for suspected or proven aspergillosis. *Clin. Infect. Dis.,* **1999,** *29*:1402–1407.

Wong-Beringer, A., Jacobs, R.A., and Guglielmo, B.J. Lipid formulations of amphotericin B: clinical efficacy and toxicities. *Clin. Infect. Dis.,* **1998,** *27*:603–618.

MONOGRAPHS AND REVIEWS

Balfour, J.A., and Faulds, D. Terbinafine. A review of its pharmacodynamic and pharmacokinetic properties, and therapeutic potential in superficial mycoses. *Drugs,* **1992,** *43*:259–284.

Branch, R.A. Prevention of amphotericin B-induced renal impairment. A review on the use of sodium supplementation. *Arch. Intern. Med.,* **1988,** *148*:2389–2394.

ANTIMICROBIAL AGENTS
(*Continued*)

Antiviral Agents (Nonretroviral)

Frederick G. Hayden

The number of antiviral drugs has increased dramatically over the past decade, largely in response to human immunodeficiency virus (HIV) infection and its sequelae (see reviews by Hayden, 2000; Balfour, 1999). This chapter summarizes the agents available for treatment of infections due to DNA and RNA viruses, excluding retroviruses, such as HIV. Many of the available therapeutic agents are directed toward disrupting one of the many steps in viral infection and replication. However, interferons, cytokines that evoke immunomodulating and antiproliferative actions in host cells, also are described (see also Chapter 53). Special sections on antiherpesvirus and antiinfluenza agents are included. The issues related to effective therapy against viruses, including emergence of resistance to particular agents and immunopathological responses to viral antigens, also are discussed. The use of purine and pyrimidine nucleoside analogs for treatment of neoplastic disease, rather than as antiviral agents, is discussed in Chapter 52. Antiretroviral agents are discussed in Chapter 51.

Viruses consist of either double-stranded or single-stranded DNA or RNA enclosed in a protein coat, called a *capsid*. Some viruses also possess a lipoprotein envelope that, like the capsid, may contain antigenic proteins. Most viruses contain or encode enzymes essential for viral replication inside a host cell. Since viruses have no metabolic machinery of their own, they usurp the machinery of their host cell which, depending on the virus, may be a plant, bacterium, or animal cell. Table 50–1 outlines the multiple stages of viral replication, which suggest the possibility for development of multiple classes of antiviral agents that could act at each stage of replication. Effective antiviral agents must inhibit virus-specific replicative events or preferentially inhibit virus-directed rather than host cell–directed nucleic acid or protein synthesis. The discovery of novel antiviral inhibitors often is linked to a better understanding of the molecular events in viral replication. This chapter provides information about the antiviral activity, pharmacology, and clinical uses of specific antiviral agents for non-HIV infections. Table 50–2 shows the nomenclature and dosage forms of available antiviral agents.

Figure 50–1 provides a schematic diagram of the replicative cycle of a DNA virus (*A*) and of an RNA virus (*B*). DNA viruses (and the diseases they cause) include poxviruses (smallpox), herpesviruses (chickenpox, shingles, herpes), adenoviruses (conjunctivitis, sore throat), hepadnaviruses (hepatitis B), and papillomaviruses (warts). Typically, DNA viruses enter into the host cell nucleus, where the viral DNA is transcribed into mRNA by host cell mRNA polymerase; mRNA is translated in the usual host cell fashion into virus-specific proteins. One exception to this strategy is poxvirus, which has its own RNA polymerase and consequently replicates in the host cell cytoplasm.

For RNA viruses, the replication strategy in the host cell relies either on enzymes in the virion (the whole infective viral particle) to synthesize its mRNA or on the viral RNA serving as its own mRNA. The mRNA is translated into various viral proteins, including RNA polymerase, which directs the synthesis of more viral mRNA (*see* Figure 50–1*B*). Certain RNA viruses, such as influenza, have a requirement for active transcription in the host cell nucleus. Examples of RNA viruses (and the

Table 50–1
Stages of Virus Replication and Possible Targets of Action of Antiviral Agents

STAGE OF REPLICATION	CLASSES OF SELECTIVE INHIBITORS
Cell entry	
Attachment	Soluble receptor decoys, antireceptor
Penetration	antibodies, fusion protein inhibitors
Uncoating	Ion channel blockers, capsid stabilizers
Release of viral genome	
Transcription of viral genome*	Inhibitors of viral DNA polymerase, RNA
Transcription of viral	polymerase, reverse transcriptase, helicase,
messenger RNA	primase, or integrase
Replication of viral genome	
Translation of viral proteins	Interferons, antisense oligonucleotides,
	ribozymes
Regulatory proteins (early)	Inhibitors of regulatory proteins
Structural proteins (late)	
Posttranslational modifications	
Proteolytic cleavage	Protease inhibitors
Myristoylation, glycosylation	
Assembly of virion components	Interferons, assembly protein inhibitors
Release	Neuraminidase inhibitors, antiviral
Budding, cell lysis	antibodies, cytotoxic lymphocytes

*Depends on specific replication strategy of virus, but virus-specified enzyme required for part of process.

diseases they cause) include rubella virus (German measles), rhabdoviruses (rabies), picornaviruses (poliomyelitis, meningitis, colds), arenaviruses (meningitis, Lassa fever), arboviruses (yellow fever, arthropod-borne encephalitis), orthomyxoviruses (influenza), and paramyxoviruses (measles, mumps).

One group of RNA viruses that deserve special mention are retroviruses, responsible for diseases such as acquired immunodeficiency syndrome (AIDS; see Chapter 51) and T-cell leukemias (the human T lymphotropic virus I, HTLV-I). In retroviruses, the virus contains a reverse transcriptase enzyme activity that makes a DNA copy of the viral RNA template. The DNA copy is then integrated into the host genome, at which point it is referred to as a *provirus* and is transcribed into both genomic RNA and mRNA for translation into viral proteins, giving rise to the generation of new virus particles.

Experiences from development of antiviral agents have provided useful general insights that have practical implications. (1) Although many compounds show antiviral activity *in vitro,* most affect some host cell function and are associated with unacceptable toxicity in human beings.

(2) Effective agents typically have a restricted spectrum of antiviral activity and target a specific viral protein, most often an enzyme (polymerase or transcriptase) involved in viral nucleic acid synthesis. (3) Single nucleotide changes leading to critical amino acid substitutions in a target protein often are sufficient to cause antiviral drug resistance. Indeed, the selection of a drug-resistant variant indicates that a drug has a specific antiviral mechanism of action. (4) Current agents inhibit active replication, so that viral growth may resume following drug removal. Effective host immune responses remain essential for recovery from infection. Clinical failures of antiviral therapy may occur with drug-sensitive virus in highly immunocompromised patients or following emergence of drug-resistant variants. Most drug-resistant viruses (*e.g.,* herpesviruses, HIV-1 responsible for AIDS) are recovered from immunocompromised patients with high viral replicative loads and repeated or prolonged courses of antiviral treatment, although influenza A virus is an exception. (5) Current agents do not eliminate nonreplicating or latent virus, although some drugs have been used effectively for chronic suppression of disease reactivation. (6) Clinical efficacy

Table 50–2

Nomenclature of Currently Approved Antiviral Agents (Excluding Antiretroviral Agents)

GENERIC NAME	OTHER NAMES	TRADE NAMES (USA)	DOSAGE FORMS AVAILABLE
Antiherpesvirus agents			
Acyclovir	ACV, acycloguanosine	ZOVIRAX	IV, O, T, Ophth*
Cidofovir	HPMPC	VISTIDE	IV, T*
Docosanol		ABREVA	T
Famciclovir	FCV	FAMVIR	O
Foscarnet	PFA, phosphonoformate	FOSCAVIR	IV, O*
Fomivirsen	ISIS 2922	VITRAVENE	Intravitreal
Ganciclovir	GCV, DHPG	CYTOVENE, VITRASERT	IV, O, intravitreal
Idoxuridine	IDUR	HERPLEX, DENDRID	Ophth
Penciclovir	PCV	DENAVIR	T, IV*
Trifluridine	TFT, trifluorothymidine	VIROPTIC	Ophth
Valacyclovir		VALTREX	O
Vidarabine	ara-A, adenine arabinoside	VIRA-A	Ophth, IV*
Antiinfluenza agents			
Amantadine		SYMMETREL, SYMADINE	O
Oseltamivir	GS4104	TAMIFLU	O
Rimantadine		FLUMADINE	O
Zanamivir	GC167	RELENZA	Inhaled
Other antiviral agents			
Fomivirsen		VITRAVENE	Intravitreal
Imiquimod		ALDARA	T
Interferon-alfa (alfa-2a, alfa-2b, alfa-n3, alfacon-1, alfa-n1)		ROFERON A, INTRON A, ALFERON N, INFERGEN, WELLFERON*	C/IM, Intralesional
Peginterferon alfa-2b		PEG-INTRON	SC
Peginterferon alfa-2a*		PEGASYS	SC
Lamivudine		EPIVIR	O
Ribavirin		REBETOL, VIRAZOLE	O, Inhaled, IV*

*Not currently approved for use in the United States.
KEY: IV, intravenous; O, oral; T, topical; Ophth, ophthalmic; SC, subcutaneous; IM, intramuscular

depends on achieving inhibitory concentrations at the site of infection, usually within infected cells. For example, nucleoside analogs must be taken up and phosphorylated intracellularly for activity; consequently, concentrations of critical enzymes or competing substrates influence antiviral effects in cells of different types and metabolic states. (7) *In vitro* sensitivity tests for antiviral agents are not standardized, and results depend on the assay system, cell type, viral inoculum, and laboratory. Therefore, clear relationships among drug concentrations active *in vitro,* those achieved in blood or other body fluids, and clini-

cal response have not been established for most antiviral agents.

ANTIHERPESVIRUS AGENTS

Infection with herpes simplex virus type 1 typically causes diseases of the mouth, face, skin, esophagus, or brain. Herpes simplex virus type 2 usually causes infections of the genitals, rectum, skin, hands, or meninges. In either case, the infection may be a primary one or disease can result from activation of a latent infection.

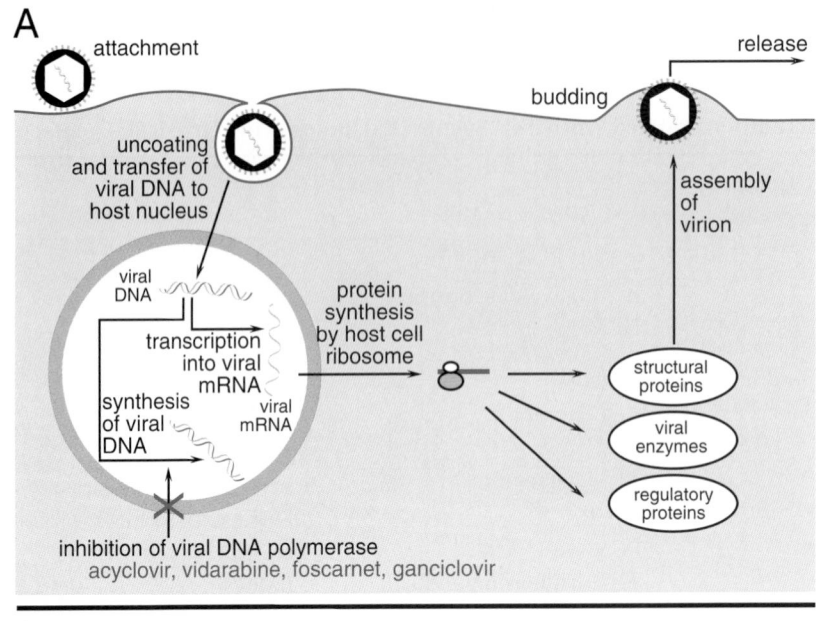

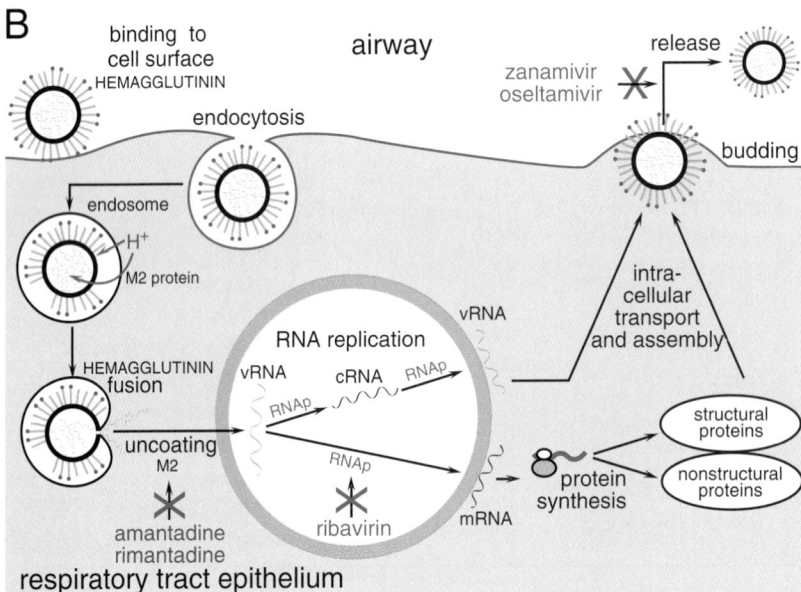

Figure 50–1. Replicative cycles of DNA (A) and RNA (B) viruses.

The replicative cycles of herpesvirus (A) and influenza (B) are given as examples of DNA-encoded and RNA-encoded viruses, respectively. Sites of action of antiviral agents also are shown. Key: mRNA, messenger RNA; cDNA, complementary DNA; vRNA, viral RNA; DNAp, DNA polymerase; RNAp, RNA polymerase; cRNA, complementary RNA. An X on top of an arrow indicates a block to virus growth.

A. Replicative cycles of herpes simplex virus, an example of a DNA virus, and the probable sites of action of antiviral agents. Herpesvirus replication is a regulated, multistep process. After infection, a small number of so-called immediate-early genes are transcribed; these genes encode proteins that regulate their own synthesis and are responsible for synthesis of so-called early genes that are involved in genome replication, such as thymidine kinases, DNA polymerases, *etc*. After DNA replication, the bulk of the herpesvirus genes (called "late" genes) are expressed and encode proteins that either are incorporated into or aid in the assembly of progeny virions.

B. Replicative cycles of influenza, an example of an RNA virus, and the loci for effects of antiviral agents. The M2 protein of influenza virus allows an influx of hydrogen ions into the virion interior, which in turn promotes dissociation of the RNP segments and release into the cytoplasm (uncoating). Influenza virus mRNA synthesis requires a primer cleared from cellular mRNA and used by the viral RNAp complex. The neuraminidase inhibitors, zanamivir and oseltamivir, specifically inhibit release of progeny virus. Small capitals indicate virus proteins.

The first systemically administered antiherpesvirus agent of proven value, *vidarabine,* was approved in 1977. However, its toxicities restricted its use to life-threatening herpes simplex virus (HSV) and varicella zoster virus (VZV) infections. The discovery and development of *acyclovir,* initially approved in 1982, provided the first effective treatment for less severe HSV and VZV infections in ambulatory patients. Subsequent trials also found that intravenous acyclovir is superior to vidarabine in regard to efficacy and/or toxicity in HSV encephalitis and in VZV infections of immunocompromised patients. Acyclovir is the prototype of a group of antiviral agents that are phosphorylated intracellularly by a viral kinase to become inhibitors of viral DNA synthesis. Other agents employing this strategy include *penciclovir* and *ganciclovir.*

Acyclovir and Valacyclovir

Chemistry and Antiviral Activity.   Acyclovir (9-[(2-hydroxyethoxy)methyl]-9H-guanine) is an acyclic guanine nucleoside analog that lacks a 3'-hydroxyl on the side chain. Acyclovir is available as capsules, as an ointment, and as a powder to be reconstituted for intravenous use. *Valacyclovir* is the L-valyl ester prodrug of acyclovir. Acyclovir's clinically useful antiviral spectrum is limited to herpesviruses. *In vitro* it is most active against HSV-1 (0.02 to 0.9 μg/ml), approximately twofold less active against HSV-2 (0.03 to 2.2 μg/ml), 10-fold less potent against VZV (0.8 to 4.0 μg/ml) or Epstein-Barr virus (EBV), and least active against cytomegalovirus (CMV) (gen-

erally >20 μg/ml) or human herpesvirus (HHV-6) (Wagstaff *et al.,* 1994). Uninfected mammalian cell growth is generally unaffected by high acyclovir concentrations (>50 μg/ml).

ACYCLOVIR

Mechanisms of Action and Resistance.   Acyclovir inhibits viral DNA synthesis *via* a mechanism outlined in Figure 50–2 (Elion, 1986). Its selectivity of action depends on interaction with two distinct viral proteins. Cellular uptake and initial phosphorylation are facilitated by HSV thymidine kinase. The affinity of acyclovir for HSV thymidine kinase is about 200-fold greater than for the mammalian enzyme. Cellular enzymes convert the monophosphate to acyclovir triphosphate, which is present in 40- to 100-fold higher concentrations in HSV-infected than in uninfected cells, and competes for endogenous deoxyguanosine triphosphate (dGTP). The immunosuppressive agent mycophenolate mofetil (*see* Chapter 53) potentiates the antiherpes activity of acyclovir and related agents by depleting intracellular dGTP pools (Neyts *et al.,* 1998). Acyclovir triphosphate competitively inhibits viral DNA polymerases and, to a much smaller extent, cellular DNA polymerases. Acyclovir triphosphate also is incorporated into viral DNA, where it acts as a chain terminator because of the lack of 3'-hydroxyl group. By a mechanism termed *suicide inactivation,* the terminated DNA template containing acyclovir binds the enzyme and leads to irreversible inactivation of the DNA polymerase.

Table 50–3
Comparative Pharmacokinetics of Selected Antiherpesvirus Agents

PARAMETER	ACYCLOVIR	FAMCICLOVIR (PENCICLOVIR)	GANCICLOVIR	CIDOFOVIR	FOSCARNET
Oral bioavailability	10%–30%	65%–77%	< 10%	< 5%	9%–17%
Effect of meals on AUC	↓ (18% heavy meal)	Negligible	↑ (20%)	Not applicable	Uncertain
Plasma $T_{1/2elim}$ (hours)	2.5–3	2	2–4	2–3	4–8 (initial)
Intracellular $T_{1/2elim}$ of triphosphate (hours)	~1	7–20	> 24	17–65	Not applicable
CSF/plasma ratio (mean)	0.5	Uncertain	0.2–0.7	Uncertain	0.7
Protein binding	9%–33%	< 20%	1%–2%	< 6%	15%
Metabolism	~15%	~5%	Negligible	Negligible	Negligible
Renal excretion (parent drug)	60%–90%	70%	> 90%	> 90%	> 80%
Dose adjustments	$CL_{cr} < 50$ (IV) $CL_{cr} < 25$ (PO)	$CL_{cr} < 60$	$CL_{cr} < 80$	$S_{cr} > 1.5$ mg/dl* $CL_{cr} < 55*$	$CL_{cr} < 58$–67

KEY: AUC, area under plasma concentration-time curve; $T_{1/2elim}$, half-life of elimination; CL_{cr}, creatinine clearance in ml/min; S_{cr}, serum creatinine;
↓, decrease; ↑ increase; CSF, cerebrospinal fluid.

*Contraindicated in renal failure

Acyclovir resistance in HSV has been linked to one of three mechanisms: absence or partial production of viral thymidine kinase, altered thymidine kinase substrate specificity (*e.g.*, phosphorylation of thymidine but not acyclovir), or altered viral DNA polymerase. Alterations in viral enzymes are caused by point mutations or base insertions or deletions in the corresponding genes. Resistant variants are present in native virus populations, and heterogeneous mixtures of viruses occur in isolates from treated patients. The most common resistance mechanism in clinical HSV isolates is deficient thymidine kinase activity (Hill *et al.*, 1991). Less common is altered thymidine kinase activity; DNA polymerase mutants are rare. Phenotypic resistance typically is defined by *in vitro* inhibitory concentrations >2 to 3 μg/ml, which predict failure of therapy in immunocompromised patients.

Acyclovir resistance in VZV isolates is caused by mutations in VZV thymidine kinase or less often by mutations in viral DNA polymerase.

Absorption, Distribution, and Elimination. Table 50–3 compares the pharmacokinetic properties of acyclovir with those of other antiherpesvirus agents. The oral bioavailability of acyclovir ranges from 10% to 30% and decreases with increasing dose (Wagstaff *et al.*, 1994). Peak plasma concentrations average 0.4 to 0.8 μg/ml after 200-mg and 1.6 μg/ml after 800-mg doses. Following intravenous dosing, peak and trough plasma concentrations average 9.8 μg/ml and 0.7 μg/ml after 5 mg/kg per 8 hours and 20.7 μg/ml and 2.3 μg/ml after 10 mg/kg per 8 hours, respectively.

Valacyclovir is converted rapidly and virtually completely to acyclovir after oral administration in healthy adults. This conversion is thought to result from first-pass intestinal and hepatic metabolism through enzymatic hydrolysis. Unlike acyclovir, valacyclovir is a substrate for intestinal and renal peptide transporters (Ganapathy *et al.*, 1998). The relative oral bioavailability of acyclovir increases three- to fivefold to approximately 70% following valacyclovir administration (Steingrimsdottir *et al.*, 2000). Peak acyclovir concentrations average 5 to 6 μg/ml following single 1000-mg doses of oral valacyclovir and occur approximately 2 hours after this dose is administered. Valacyclovir, 2000 mg four times daily, provides steady-state peak and trough acyclovir concentrations of 8.4 and 2.5 μg/ml, respectively, which approximate those observed with intravenous doses of acyclovir (Jacobson *et al.*, 1994). Peak plasma concentrations of valacyclovir are only 4% of acyclovir levels. Less than 1% of an administered dose of valacyclovir is recovered in the urine, and most is eliminated as acyclovir.

Acyclovir distributes widely in body fluids including vesicular fluid, aqueous humor, and cerebrospinal fluid. Compared to plasma, salivary concentrations are low, and vaginal secretion concentrations vary widely. Acyclovir is concentrated in breast milk, amniotic fluid, and placenta. Newborn plasma levels are similar to maternal ones (Frenkel *et al.*, 1991). Percutaneous absorption of acyclovir after topical administration is low.

The mean plasma half-life ($t_{1/2}$) of elimination of acyclovir is about 2.5 hours, with a range of 1.5 to 6 hours in adults with normal renal function. The plasma $t_{1/2}$ of elimination of acyclovir is about 4 hours in neonates and increases to 20 hours in anuric patients (Blum *et al.*, 1982). Renal excretion of unmetabolized acyclovir by glomerular filtration and tubular secretion is the principal route of elimination. Less than 15% is excreted as 9-carboxymethoxymethylguanine or minor metabolites. The pharmacokinetics of oral acyclovir and valacyclovir appear to be similar in pregnant and nonpregnant women (Kimberlin *et al.*, 1998).

Untoward Effects. Acyclovir generally is well tolerated. Topical acyclovir in a polyethylene glycol base may cause mucosal irritation and transient burning when applied to genital lesions.

Oral acyclovir has been associated infrequently with nausea, diarrhea, rash, or headache and very rarely with renal insufficiency or neurotoxicity. Valacyclovir also may be associated with headache, nausea, and diarrhea. Chronic acyclovir suppression of genital herpes has been used safely for over 5 years (Goldberg *et al.*, 1993). No excess frequency of abnormalities has been recognized in infants born to women exposed to acyclovir during pregnancy (Reiff-Eldridge *et al.*, 2000). The tolerance profile of valacyclovir appears to be similar to that of oral acyclovir. High doses of valacyclovir have been associated with confusion, hallucinosis, nephrotoxicity and, uncommonly, with severe thrombocytopenic syndromes, sometimes fatal, in immunocompromised patients (Feinberg *et al.*, 1998).

The principal dose-limiting toxicities of intravenous acyclovir are renal insufficiency and central nervous system side effects. Preexisting renal insufficiency, high doses, and high acyclovir plasma levels (>25 μg/ml) are risk factors for both. Reversible renal dysfunction occurs in approximately 5% of patients, probably related to high urine levels causing crystalline nephropathy (Sawyer *et al.*, 1988). Manifestations include nausea, emesis, flank pain, and increasing azotemia. Rapid infusion, dehydration, and inadequate urine flow increase the risk. Infusions should be given at a constant rate over at least an hour. Nephrotoxicity usually resolves with drug cessation and volume expansion. Neurotoxicity occurs in 1% to 4% of patients and may be manifested by altered sensorium, tremor, myoclonus, delirium, seizures, and/or extrapyramidal signs (Haefeli *et al.*, 1993). Hemodialysis may be useful in severe cases. Phlebitis following extravasation, rash, diaphoresis, nausea, hypotension, or interstitial nephritis has been described.

Severe somnolence and lethargy may occur with combinations of zidovudine and acyclovir. Concomitant cyclosporine and probably other nephrotoxic agents enhance the risk of nephrotoxicity. Probenecid decreases the renal clearance and prolongs the plasma $t_{1/2}$ of elimination. Acyclovir may decrease the renal clearance of other drugs eliminated by active renal secretion, such as methotrexate.

Therapeutic Uses. In immunocompetent persons, the clinical benefits of acyclovir are greater in initial HSV infections than in recurrent ones, which typically are milder in severity (Whitley and Gnann, 1992). Acyclovir is particularly useful in immunocompromised patients, because these individuals experience both more frequent and more severe HSV and VZV infections. Since VZV is less susceptible than HSV to acyclovir, higher doses must be used for treating varicella or zoster cases than for HSV infections. Oral valacyclovir is as effective as oral acyclovir in HSV infections and more effective for treating herpes zoster.

Herpes Simplex Virus Infections. In initial genital HSV infections, oral acyclovir (200 mg five times daily for 10 days) and valacyclovir (1000 mg twice daily for 10 days) are associated with significant reductions in virus shedding, symptoms, and time to healing (Fife *et al.*, 1997). Intravenous acyclovir (5 mg/kg per 8 hours) has similar effects in patients hospitalized with severe primary genital HSV infections. Topical acyclovir is much less effective than systemic administration. None of these regimens reproducibly reduces the risk of recurrent genital lesions. Patient-initiated acyclovir (200 mg 5 times daily for 5 days) or valacyclovir (500 mg or 1000 mg twice daily for 5 days) shortens the manifestations of recurrent genital HSV episodes by 1 to 2 days (Tyring *et al.*, 1998b). Topical acyclovir offers no significant clinical benefit in recurrent genital herpes. Frequently recurring genital herpes can be suppressed effectively with chronic oral acyclovir (400 mg two times daily or 200 mg three times daily) (Goldberg *et al.*, 1993) or with valacyclovir (500 or 1000 mg once daily) (Patel *et al.*, 1997). During use,

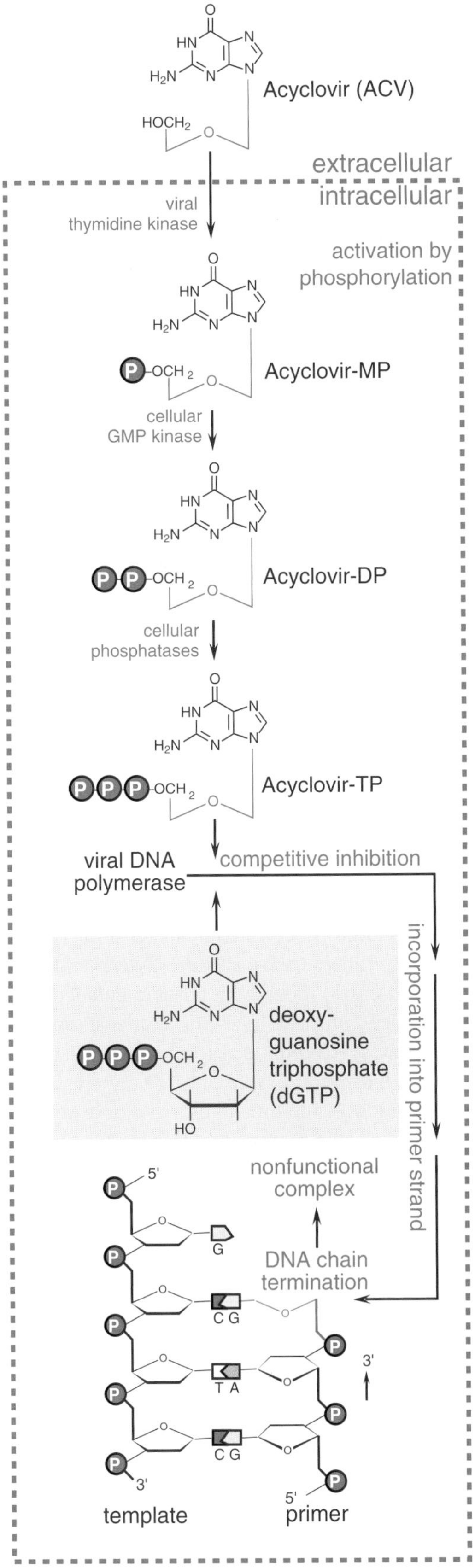

Figure 50–2. Conversion of acyclovir to acyclovir triphosphate leading to DNA chain termination.

Acyclovir is converted to the monophosphate derivative by a herpesvirus thymidine kinase. Acyclovir-MP is then phosphorylated to acyclovir-DP and acyclovir-TP by cellular enzymes. Uninfected cells convert very little or no drug to the phosphorylated derivatives. Thus, acyclovir is selectively activated in cells infected with herpesviruses that code for appropriate thymidine kinases. Incorporation of acyclovir-MP from acyclovir-TP into the primer strand during viral DNA replication leads to chain termination and formation of an inactive complex with the viral DNA polymerase. (Adapted from Elion, 1986, with permission.)

recurrences decrease by about 90%, and the majority of patients are free from symptomatic recurrences for periods up to 5 years. Asymptomatic shedding may occur during suppression, as may HSV transmission to sexual partners. Chronic suppression may be useful in those with disabling recurrences of herpetic whitlow or HSV-related erythema multiforme.

Oral acyclovir is effective in primary herpetic gingivostomatitis (600 mg/m^2 four times daily for 10 days in children) but provides modest clinical benefit in recurrent orolabial herpes. Topical acyclovir ointment is not clinically beneficial in recurrent herpes labialis. Topical acyclovir cream, not available in the United States, may be more effective in recurrent labial and genital herpes simplex virus infections. Preexposure acyclovir prophylaxis (400 mg twice daily for 1 week) reduces the overall risk of recurrence by 73% in those with sun-induced recurrences of HSV infections (Spruance et al., 1988).

In immunocompromised patients with mucocutaneous HSV infection, intravenous acyclovir (250 mg/m^2 per 8 hours for 7 days) shortens healing time, duration of pain, and the period of virus shedding (Wade et al., 1982). Oral acyclovir (800 mg five times per day) also is effective. Recurrences are common after cessation of therapy and may require long-term suppression. In those with very localized labial or facial HSV infections, topical acyclovir may provide some benefit. Intravenous acyclovir may be beneficial in viscerally disseminating HSV in immunocompromised patients and in HSV-infected burn wounds.

Systemic acyclovir prophylaxis is highly effective in preventing mucocutaneous HSV infections in seropositive patients undergoing immunosuppression. Intravenous acyclovir (250 mg/m^2 every 8 to 12 hours), begun prior to transplantation and continuing for several weeks, prevents HSV disease in bone-marrow transplant recipients. For patients who can tolerate oral medications, oral acyclovir (400 mg five times/day) is effective, and long-term oral acyclovir (200 to 400 mg three times a day for 6 months) also reduces the risk of VZV infection (Steer et al., 2000). Oral acyclovir prophylaxis also is effective in transplant patients and in those on chemotherapy.

In HSV encephalitis, acyclovir (10 mg/kg per 8 hours for a minimum of 10 days) reduces mortality by over 50% and improves overall neurologic outcome compared to vidarabine (Whitley et al., 1986). Higher doses (15 to 20 mg/kg per 8 hours and treatment to 21 days) are recommended by some experts. Intravenous acyclovir (20 mg/kg per 8 hours for 21 days) is more effective than lower doses in neonatal HSV infections (Kimberlin et al., 1999). In

neonates and immunosuppressed patients, and, rarely, in previously healthy persons, relapses of encephalitis following acyclovir indicate that longer courses of treatment are needed.

An ophthalmic formulation of acyclovir, not available in the United States, is at least as effective as topical vidarabine or trifluridine in herpetic keratoconjunctivitis.

In immunocompromised hosts, acyclovir-resistant HSV isolates can cause extensive mucocutaneous disease and rarely meningoencephalitis, pneumonitis, or visceral disease. Infection due to resistant HSV is rare in immunocompetent persons. Resistant HSV can be recovered from 6% to 17% of immunocompromised patients receiving acyclovir treatment (Christophers et al., 1998; Englund et al., 1990). Recurrences after cessation of acyclovir usually are due to sensitive virus but may be due to acyclovir-resistant virus in AIDS patients. Limited acyclovir-resistant HSV infections sometimes undergo spontaneous healing after acyclovir treatment is terminated. In patients with progressive disease, intravenous foscarnet therapy is effective, but vidarabine is not (Safrin et al., 1991).

Varicella Zoster Virus Infections. If begun within 24 hours of rash onset, oral acyclovir has therapeutic effects in varicella infections of children and adults. In children up to 40 kg body weight, acyclovir (20 mg/kg, up to 800 mg per dose, four times daily for 5 days) reduces fever and new lesion formation by about 1 day. Routine use in uncomplicated pediatric varicella is not recommended, but should be considered in those at risk of moderate to severe illness (persons over 12 years old, secondary household cases, those with chronic cutaneous or pulmonary disorders, or those receiving corticosteroids or long-term salicylates) (Committee on Infectious Diseases, 2000). In adults, early oral acyclovir (800 mg five times daily for 7 days) reduces the time to crusting of lesions by approximately 2 days, the maximum number of lesions by one-half, and the duration of fever (Wallace et al., 1992). Later treatment is not beneficial. Intravenous acyclovir appears to be effective in varicella pneumonia or encephalitis of previously healthy adults. Oral acyclovir (10 mg/kg 4 times daily) given between 7 through 14 days after exposure appears to be effective prophylaxis for varicella (Kumagai et al., 1999).

In older adults with localized herpes zoster, oral acyclovir (800 mg five times daily for 7 days) reduces pain and healing times if treatment can be initiated within 72 hours of rash onset (Wood et al., 1998). A reduction in ocular complications, particularly keratitis and anterior uveitis, occurs with treatment of zoster ophthalmicus

(Cobo *et al.*, 1986). Prolonged acyclovir and concurrent prednisone for 21 days speed zoster healing and improve quality of life measures compared to each therapy alone (Whitley *et al.*, 1996). Valacyclovir (1000 mg three times daily for 7 days) provides more prompt relief of zoster-associated pain than acyclovir in acute herpes zoster of older adults ($\geq$50 years) (Beutner *et al.*, 1995).

In immunocompromised patients with herpes zoster, intravenous acyclovir (500 mg/m^2 per 8 hours for 7 days) reduces viral shedding, healing times, the risks of cutaneous dissemination and visceral complications, as well as the length of hospitalization in disseminating zoster. In immunosuppressed children with varicella, intravenous acyclovir decreases healing times and the risk of visceral complications.

Acyclovir-resistant VZV isolates uncommonly have been recovered from HIV-infected children and adults who may manifest chronic hyperkeratotic or verrucous lesions. Meningoradiculitis due to resistant virus also has been described. Intravenous foscarnet also appears to be effective for acyclovir-resistant VZV infections.

Other Viruses. Acyclovir is ineffective therapeutically in established cytomegalovirus (CMV) infections but has been used for CMV prophylaxis in immunocompromised patients. High-dose intravenous acyclovir (500 mg/m^2 per 8 hours for 1 month) in CMV-seropositive bone-marrow transplant recipients is associated with about 50% lower risk of CMV disease and, when combined with prolonged oral acyclovir (800 mg four times daily through 6 months), improves survival (Prentice *et al.*, 1994). High-dose oral acyclovir suppression for 3 months may reduce the risk of CMV disease in certain solid-organ transplant recipients. In seronegative renal transplant patients receiving seropositive donations, valacyclovir (2000 mg 4 times daily for 90 days) prophylaxis reduces CMV disease, other infections, and acute graft rejection risk (Lowance *et al.*, 1999). Compared to acyclovir, high-dose valacyclovir reduces CMV disease in advanced HIV infection but is associated with greater toxicity and possibly shorter survival (Feinberg *et al.*, 1998).

In infectious mononucleosis, acyclovir is associated with transient antiviral effects but no clinical benefits. Epstein-Barr virus (EBV)–related oral hairy leukoplakia may improve with acyclovir.

Cidofovir

Chemistry and Antiviral Activity. *Cidofovir* (1-[(*S*)-3-hydroxy-2-(phosphonomethoxy)-propyl]cytosine dihydrate) is a cytidine nucleotide analog with inhibitory activity against human herpes, papilloma, polyoma, pox, and adenoviruses (Hitchcock *et al.*, 1996). *In vitro* inhibitory concentrations range from <0.2 to 0.7 μg/ml for CMV, 0.4 to 33 μg/ml for HSV, and 0.02 to 17 μg/ml for adenoviruses. Because cidofovir is a phosphonate that is phosphorylated by cellular but not virus enzymes, it inhibits acyclovir-resistant, thymidine kinase (TK)-deficient or -altered HSV or VZV strains; ganciclovir-resistant CMV strains with UL97 mutations but not those with DNA polymerase mutations; and some foscarnet-resistant CMV strains. Cidofovir synergistically inhibits CMV replication in combination with ganciclovir or foscarnet.

CIDOFOVIR

Mechanisms of Action and Resistance. Cidofovir inhibits viral DNA synthesis by slowing and eventually terminating chain elongation. Cidofovir is metabolized to its active diphosphate form by cellular enzymes; the levels of phosphorylated metabolites are similar in infected and uninfected cells. The diphosphate acts as both a competitive inhibitor with respect to dCTP and as an alternative substrate for viral DNA polymerase. The diphosphate has a prolonged intracellular half-life and competitively inhibits CMV and HSV DNA polymerases at concentrations 8- to 600-fold lower than those required to inhibit human DNA polymerases (Hitchcock *et al.*, 1996). A phosphocholine metabolite has a prolonged intracellular half-life ($\sim$87 hours) and may serve as an intracellular reservoir of drug. The prolonged intracellular half-life of cidofovir diphosphate allows infrequent dosing regimens, and single doses are effective in experimental HSV, varicella, and poxvirus infections.

Cidofovir resistance in CMV is due to mutations in viral DNA polymerase. Low-level resistance to cidofovir develops in a minority of patients by 3 months of therapy (Jabs *et al.*, 1998). Highly ganciclovir-resistant CMV isolates that possess DNA polymerase and UL97 kinase mutations are resistant to cidofovir, and prior ganciclovir therapy may select for cidofovir resistance. Some foscarnet-resistant CMV isolates show cross-resistance to cidofovir, and triple-drug resistant variants with DNA polymerase mutations occur (Tatarowicz *et al.*, 1992).

Absorption, Distribution, and Elimination. Cidofovir is dianionic at physiological pH and has very low oral bioavailability (Cundy, 1999). The plasma levels after intravenous dosing decline in a biphasic pattern with a terminal half-life that averages about 2.6 hours (Cundy *et al.*, 1995b). The volume of distribution approximates total body water. Penetration into the central nervous system (CNS) or eye have not been well characterized; low cerebrospinal fluid (CSF) levels were found in one patient with progressive multifocal leukoencephalopathy. Topical cidofovir gel may result in low plasma concentrations (<0.5 μg/ml) in patients with large mucocutaneous lesions (Lalezari *et al.,* 1997).

Cidofovir is cleared by the kidney *via* glomerular filtration and tubular secretion. Over 90% of the dose is recovered unchanged in the urine without significant metabolism in human beings. The probenecid-sensitive organic anion transporter 1 mediates uptake of cidofovir into proximal renal tubular epithelial cells (Ho *et al.,* 2000). High-dose probenecid (2 g 3 hours before and 1 g 2 and 8 hours after each infusion) blocks tubular transport of cidofovir and reduces renal clearance and associated nephrotoxicity. At cidofovir doses of 5 mg/kg, peak plasma concentrations increase from 11.5 to 19.6 μg/ml with probenecid, and renal clearance is reduced to the level of glomerular filtration. Elimination relates linearly to creatinine clearance, and the half-life increases to 32.5 hours in patients on chronic ambulatory peritoneal dialysis (CAPD). Both CAPD and hemodialysis remove over 50% of the administered dose (Cundy, 1999).

Untoward Effects. Nephrotoxicity is the principal dose-limiting side effect of intravenous cidofovir. Proximal tubular dysfunction includes proteinuria, azotemia, glycosuria, metabolic acidosis, and uncommonly Fanconi's syndrome. Concomitant oral probenecid (*see* above) and saline prehydration reduce the risk of renal toxicity. On maintenance doses of 5 mg/kg every two weeks, up to 50% of patients develop proteinuria, 10% to 15% elevated serum creatinine, and 15% to 20% neutropenia. Anterior uveitis, responsive to topical corticosteroids and cycloplegia, occurs commonly and ocular hypotony infrequently with intravenous cidofovir (Ambati *et al.,* 1999). Concurrent probenecid is associated with gastrointestinal upset, constitutional symptoms, and hypersensitivity reactions including fever, rash, and, uncommonly, anaphylactoid manifestations. Administration with food and pretreatment with antiemetics, antihistamines, and/or acetaminophen may improve tolerance.

Probenecid but not cidofovir alters zidovudine pharmacokinetics, such that zidovudine doses should be reduced on probenecid-administration days. The excretion of other agents affected by probenecid [*e.g.,* β-lactam antibiotics, nonsteroidal antiinflammatory drugs (NSAIDs), acyclovir, lorazepam, furosemide, methotrexate, theophylline, rifampin] may require dose adjustment. Concurrent nephrotoxic agents are contraindicated, and an interval of at least 7 days before beginning cidofovir treatment is recommended after prior aminoglycoside, intravenous pentamidine, amphotericin B, foscarnet, NSAID, or contrast dye exposure. Cidofovir and oral ganciclovir are poorly tolerated in combination at full doses.

Topical application of cidofovir is associated with dose-related application-site reactions (burning, pain, pruritus) in up to one-third of patients and occasionally ulceration (Lalezari *et al.,* 1997). Intravitreal cidofovir may cause vitreitis, hypotony, and visual loss and is contraindicated.

Preclinical studies indicate that cidofovir has mutagenic, gonadotoxic, embryotoxic, and teratogenic effects. Because cidofovir is carcinogenic in rats, although not in monkeys, this agent is considered a potential human carcinogen. It may cause infertility and is contraindicated during pregnancy.

Therapeutic Uses. Intravenous cidofovir is approved for the treatment of CMV retinitis in HIV-infected patients. Intravenous cidofovir (5 mg/kg once a week for 2 weeks followed by dosing every 2 weeks) increases the time to progression of CMV retinitis in previously untreated patients and in those failing or intolerant of ganciclovir and foscarnet therapy (Lalezari *et al.,* 1998; Safrin *et al.,* 1997). CMV viremia may persist during cidofovir administration. Maintenance doses of 5 mg/kg are more effective but less well tolerated than 3 mg/kg doses (Anonymous, 1997). Intravenous cidofovir has been used for treating acyclovir-resistant mucocutaneous HSV infection (Lalezari *et al.,* 1994), adenovirus disease in transplant recipients, and progressive multifocal leukoencephalopathy and extensive molluscum contagiosum in HIV patients.

Topical cidofovir gel eliminates virus shedding and lesions in some HIV-infected patients with acyclovir-resistant mucocutaneous HSV infections (Lalezari *et al.,* 1997) and has been used in treating anogenital warts and molluscum contagiosum in immunocompromised patients and cervical intraepithelial neoplasia in women. Intralesional cidofovir induces remissions in adults or children with respiratory papillomatosis (Snoeck *et al.,* 1998). An ophthalmic formulation is under study in adenoviral keratoconjunctivitis.

Docosanol

Docosanol is a long-chain saturated alcohol that has been approved by the United States Food and Drug Administration (FDA) as a 10% over-the-counter cream for treatment of recurrent orolabial herpes. Doconsanol inhibits the *in vitro* replication of many lipid enveloped viruses, including HSV, at millimolar concentrations. It does not directly inactivate HSV but appears to block fusion between the cellular and viral envelope membranes and inhibit viral entry into the cell (Pope *et al.,* 1998). Topical treatment beginning within 12 hours of prodromal symptoms or lesion onset reduces healing time by about one day and appears to be well tolerated (Anonymous, Medical Letter, 2000). Treatment initiation at papular or later stages provides no benefit.

Famciclovir and Penciclovir

Chemistry and Antiviral Activity. *Famciclovir* is the diacetyl ester prodrug of 6-deoxy penciclovir and lacks intrinsic antiviral activity. *Penciclovir* (9-[4-hydroxy-3-hydroxymethylbut-1-yl] guanine) is an acyclic guanine nucleoside analog. Its structure is given below:

PENCICLOVIR

Penciclovir is similar to acyclovir in its spectrum of activity and potency against HSV and VZV (Boyd *et al.*, 1993). The side chain differs structurally in that the oxygen has been replaced by a carbon and an additional hydroxymethyl group is present. The inhibitory concentrations of penciclovir depend on cell type but are usually within twofold of those of acyclovir for HSV and VZV (Boyd *et al.*, 1993). It also is inhibitory for hepatitis B virus (HBV).

Mechanisms of Action and Resistance.   Penciclovir is an inhibitor of viral DNA synthesis. In HSV- or VZV-infected cells, penciclovir is initially phosphorylated by viral thymidine kinase. Penciclovir triphosphate serves as a competitive inhibitor of viral DNA polymerase (Vere Hodge, 1993; *see also* Figure 50–2). Although penciclovir triphosphate is approximately 100-fold less potent in inhibiting viral DNA polymerase than is acyclovir triphosphate, it is present in much higher concentrations and for more prolonged periods in infected cells than acyclovir triphosphate. The prolonged intracellular $t_{1/2}$ of penciclovir triphosphate, which ranges from 7 to 20 hours, is associated with prolonged antiviral effects. Because it has a 3′-hydroxyl group, penciclovir is not an obligate chain terminator, but it does inhibit DNA elongation.

Resistant variants due to thymidine kinase or DNA polymerase mutations can be selected by passage *in vitro,* but the occurrence of resistance during clinical use is currently low. Thymidine kinase–deficient, acyclovir-resistant herpes viruses are cross-resistant to penciclovir.

Absorption, Distribution, and Elimination.   Oral penciclovir has low (5%) bioavailability. In contrast, famciclovir is well absorbed orally and rapidly converted to penciclovir by deacetylation of the side chain and oxidation of the purine ring during and following absorption from the intestine (Gill and Wood, 1996). Although poorly absorbed itself, the bioavailability of penciclovir is 65% to 77% following oral administration of famciclovir. Food slows absorption but does not reduce overall bioavailability. After single 250- or 500-mg doses of famciclovir, the peak plasma concentration of penciclovir averages 1.6 and 3.3 μg/ml, respectively. A small quantity of the 6-deoxy precursor but no famciclovir is detectable. After intravenous infusion of penciclovir at 10 mg/kg, peak plasma levels average 12 μg/ml. The volume of distribution is about twice the volume of total body water. The plasma $t_{1/2}$ of elimination of penciclovir averages about 2 hours, and over 90% is excreted unchanged in the urine, probably by both filtration and active tubular secretion. Following oral famciclovir, nonrenal clearance accounts for about 10% of each dose, primarily through fecal

excretion, but penciclovir (60% of dose) and its 6-deoxy precursor (<10% of dose) are eliminated primarily in the urine. The plasma half-life averages 9.9 hours in renal insufficiency (CL_{cr} <30 ml/minute); hemodialysis efficiently removes penciclovir. Lower peak plasma concentrations of penciclovir but no reduction in overall bioavailability occur in compensated chronic hepatic insufficiency (Boike *et al.*, 1994).

Untoward Effects.   Oral famciclovir is well tolerated but may be associated with headache, diarrhea, and nausea (Saltzman *et al.*, 1994). Its short-term tolerance is comparable to that of acyclovir. Urticaria, rash, and, predominantly in the elderly, hallucinations or confusional states have been reported. Topical penciclovir, which is formulated in 40% propylene glycol and a cetomacrogol base, is associated with application-site reactions at low rates ($\sim$1%).

Penciclovir is mutagenic at high concentrations *in vitro*. Studies in laboratory animals indicate that chronic famciclovir administration is tumorigenic and decreases spermatogenesis and fertility in rodents and dogs, but long-term administration (1 year) does not affect spermatogenesis in men (Sacks *et al.*, 1998). No teratogenic effects have been observed in animals, but safety during pregnancy has not been established.

No clinically important drug interactions have been identified to date with famciclovir or penciclovir (Gill and Wood, 1996).

Therapeutic Uses.   Oral famciclovir, topical penciclovir, and intravenous penciclovir are approved for managing HSV and VZV infections in various countries (Sacks and Wilson, 1999). Oral famciclovir (250 mg three times a day for 5 to 10 days) is as effective as acyclovir in treating first-episode genital herpes (Loveless *et al.*, 1997). In patients with recurrent genital HSV, patient-initiated famciclovir treatment (125 or 250 mg twice a day for 5 days) reduces healing time and symptoms by about 1 day. Famciclovir (250 mg twice a day for up to one year) is effective for suppression of recurrent genital HSV, but single daily doses are less effective (Diaz-Mitoma *et al.*, 1998). Higher doses (500 mg twice a day) reduce HSV recurrences in HIV-infected persons. Intravenous penciclovir (5 mg/kg per 8 or 12 hours for 7 days) is comparable to intravenous acyclovir for treating mucocutaneous HSV infections in immunocompromised hosts (Lazarus *et al.*, 1999). In immunocompetent persons with recurrent orolabial HSV, topical 1% penciclovir cream (applied every 2 hours while awake for 4 days) shortens healing time and symptoms by about 1 day (Spruance *et al.*, 1997).

In immunocompetent adults with herpes zoster of 3 days duration or less, famciclovir (500 mg three times a day for 10 days) is at least as effective as acyclovir (800 mg 5 times daily) in reducing healing time and zoster-associated pain, particularly in those aged ≥50 years

(Degreef *et al.,* 1994). Famciclovir is comparable to vala-cyclovir in treating zoster and reducing associated pain in older adults (Tyring *et al.,* 2000). Famciclovir (500 mg three times a day for 10 days) also is comparable to high-dose oral acyclovir in treating zoster in immunocompromised patients and in ophthalmic zoster (Tyring *et al.,* 1998a).

Famciclovir is associated with dose-related reductions in hepatitis B virus (HBV) DNA and transaminase levels in patients with chronic HBV hepatitis (Trepo *et al.,* 2000) and has been used for recurrent HBV infection following liver transplantation. However, it appears to be less potent than lamivudine and is ineffective in treating lamivudine-resistant HBV infections due to emergence of multiply resistant variants (Mutimer *et al.,* 2000).

Fomivirsen

Fomivirsen, a 21-mer phosphorothioate oligionucleotide, is the first FDA-approved antisense therapy for viral infections. It is complementary to the messenger RNA sequence for the major immediate-early transcriptional region of CMV and inhibits CMV replication through sequence-specific and nonspecific mechanisms, including inhibition of virus binding to cells (Anderson *et al.,* 1996). Fomivirsen is active against CMV strains resistant to ganciclovir, foscarnet, and cidofovir. CMV variants with 10-fold reduced susceptibility to fomivirsen have been selected by *in vitro* passage (Mulamba *et al.,* 1998).

Fomivirsen is given by intravitreal injection in the treatment of CMV retinitis for patients intolerant of or unresponsive to other therapies (Perry and Balfour, 1999). In monkeys, the half-life from the vitreous is about 24 hours and from the retina is up to 78 hours (Leeds *et al.,* 1998). Local metabolism by exonucleases accounts for elimination. In HIV-infected patients with refractory, sight-threatening CMV retinitis, fomivirsen injections (330 μg weekly for 3 weeks and then every 2 weeks or on days 1 and 15 followed by monthly) significantly delay time to retinitis progression. Ocular side effects include iritis in up to one-quarter of patients, which can be managed with topical corticosteroids; vitritis; cataracts; and increases in intraocular pressure in 15% to 20%. Recent cidofovir use may increase the risk of inflammatory reactions.

Foscarnet

Chemistry and Antiviral Activity. *Foscarnet* (trisodium phosphonoformate) is an inorganic pyrophosphate analog that is inhibitory for all herpesviruses and HIV (Oberg, 1989; Wagstaff

and Bryson, 1994). Its structure is given below:

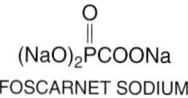

FOSCARNET SODIUM

In vitro inhibitory concentrations are generally 100 to 300 μM for CMV and 80 to 200 μM for other herpesviruses, including most ganciclovir-resistant CMV and acyclovir-resistant HSV and VZV strains. Combinations of foscarnet and ganciclovir synergistically inhibit CMV replication *in vitro.* Concentrations of 500 to 1000 μM reversibly inhibit the proliferation and DNA synthesis of uninfected cells.

Mechanisms of Action and Resistance. Foscarnet inhibits viral nucleic acid synthesis by interacting directly with herpesvirus DNA polymerase or HIV reverse transcriptase (Oberg, 1989; Chrisp and Clissold, 1991; *see* Figure 50–1*B*). It is taken up slowly by cells and does not undergo significant intracellular metabolism. Foscarnet reversibly blocks the pyrophosphate binding site of the viral polymerase in a noncompetitive manner and inhibits cleavage of pyrophosphate from deoxynucleotide triphosphates. Foscarnet has approximately 100-fold greater inhibitory effects against herpesvirus DNA polymerases than against cellular DNA polymerase α.

Herpesviruses resistant to foscarnet have point mutations in the viral DNA polymerase and are associated with three- to sevenfold reductions *in vitro* (Safrin *et al.,* 1994; Schmit and Boivin, 1999).

Absorption, Distribution, and Elimination. Oral bioavailability of foscarnet is low (*see* Table 50–3). Following an intravenous infusion of 60 mg/kg per 8 hours, peak and trough plasma concentrations are approximately 450 to 575 μM and 80 to 150 μM, respectively. Vitreous levels approximate those in plasma (Arevalo *et al.,* 1995), and CSF levels average 66% of those in plasma at steady state (Hengge *et al.,* 1993).

Over 80% of foscarnet is excreted unchanged in the urine by glomerular filtration and probably tubular secretion. Plasma clearance decreases proportionately with creatinine clearance, and dose adjustments are indicated for small decreases in renal function. Plasma elimination is complex, with initial bimodal half-lives totaling 4 to 8 hours and a prolonged terminal $t_{1/2}$ for elimination averaging 3 to 4 days. Sequestration in bone with gradual release accounts for the fate of an estimated 10% to 20% of a given dose. Foscarnet is cleared efficiently by hemodialysis (~50% of a dose).

Untoward Effects. Foscarnet's major dose-limiting toxicities are nephrotoxicity and symptomatic hypocalcemia. Increases in serum creatinine occur in up to one-half of patients but are reversible after cessation in most patients. High doses, rapid infusion, dehydration, prior renal insufficiency, and concurrent nephrotoxic drugs are risk factors. Acute tubular necrosis, crystalline glomerulopathy, nephrogenic diabetes insipidus, and interstitial nephritis have been described. Saline loading may reduce the risk of nephrotoxicity.

Foscarnet is highly ionized at physiologic pH, and metabolic abnormalities are very common. These include increases or decreases in Ca^{2+} and phosphate, hypomagnesemia, and hypokalemia. Decreased serum ionized Ca^{2+} may cause paresthesia, arrhythmias, tetany, seizures, and other central nervous system disturbances. Concomitant intravenous *pentamidine* administration increases the risk of symptomatic hypocalcemia. Parenteral magnesium sulfate does not alter foscarnet-induced hypocalcemia or symptoms (Huycke *et al.,* 2000).

CNS side effects include headache in about one-fourth of patients, tremor, irritability, seizures, and hallucinosis. Other reported side effects are generalized rash, fever, nausea or emesis, anemia, leukopenia, abnormal liver function tests, electrocardiographic (EKG) changes, infusion-related thrombophlebitis, and painful genital ulcerations. Topical foscarnet may cause local irritation and ulceration, and oral foscarnet may cause gastrointestinal disturbance. Preclinical studies indicate that high foscarnet concentrations are mutagenic and that it may cause tooth and skeletal abnormalities in developing laboratory animals. Safety in pregnancy or childhood is uncertain.

Therapeutic Uses.   Intravenous foscarnet is effective for treatment of CMV retinitis, including ganciclovir-resistant infections, and of acyclovir-resistant HSV and VZV infections. It also is effective for treating other types of CMV infections (Wagstaff and Bryson, 1994). Foscarnet is poorly soluble in aqueous solutions and requires large volumes for administration.

In CMV retinitis in AIDS patients, foscarnet (60 mg/kg per 8 hours or 90 mg/kg per 12 hours for 14 to 21 days followed by chronic maintenance at 90 to 120 mg/kg per day in one dose) is associated with clinical stabilization in about 90% of patients (Wagstaff and Bryson, 1994).

A comparative trial of foscarnet with ganciclovir found comparable control of CMV retinitis in AIDS patients but improved overall survival in the foscarnet-treated group (Studies of Ocular Complications of AIDS Research Group, 1992). This improved survival with foscarnet may be related to foscarnet's intrinsic anti-HIV activity (Bergdahl *et al.,* 1998), but patients stop taking foscarnet over three times as often as ganciclovir because of side effects. A combination of foscarnet and ganciclovir is more effective than either drug alone in refractory retinitis (Anonymous, 1996). Foscarnet benefits other CMV syndromes in AIDS or transplant patients but is ineffective as a single drug in treating CMV pneumonia in bone-marrow transplant patients (Oberg, 1989). When used for preemptive therapy of CMV antigenemia in bone-marrow transplant recipients, foscarnet (90 mg/kg per 12 hours for 15 days) is at least as effective as intravenous ganciclovir (Moretti *et al.,* 1998). When used for CMV infections, foscarnet may reduce the risk of Kaposi's sarcoma

in HIV-infected patients (Glesby *et al.,* 1996). Intravitreal injections of foscarnet have been used.

In acyclovir-resistant mucocutaneous HSV infections, lower doses of foscarnet (40 mg/kg per 8 hours for 7 days or longer) are associated with cessation of viral shedding and with complete healing of lesions in about three-quarters of patients (Safrin *et al.,* 1991). Foscarnet also appears to be effective in acyclovir-resistant VZV infections. Topical foscarnet cream is ineffective in treating recurrent genital HSV in immunocompetent persons but appears to be useful in chronic, acyclovir-resistant infections in immunocompromised patients (Javaly *et al.,* 1999).

Resistant clinical isolates of herpesviruses have emerged during therapeutic use (Birch *et al.,* 1992; Safrin *et al.,* 1994) and may be associated with poor clinical response to foscarnet treatment.

Ganciclovir and Valganciclovir

Chemistry and Antiviral Activity.   *Ganciclovir* (9-[1,3-dihydroxy-2-propoxymethyl] guanine) is an acyclic guanine nucleoside analog, similar in structure to acyclovir except in having an additional hydroxymethyl group on the acyclic side chain. *Valganciclovir* (CYMEVAL) is the L-valyl ester prodrug of ganciclovir. The structure of ganciclovir is given below:

GANCICLOVIR

This agent has inhibitory activity against all herpesviruses but is especially active against CMV (Noble and Faulds, 1998). Inhibitory concentrations are similar to those of acyclovir for HSV and VZV but 10- to 100-fold lower for human CMV strains (0.2 to 2.8 μg/ml).

Inhibitory concentrations for human bone marrow progenitor cells are similar to those inhibitory for CMV replication, a finding predictive of ganciclovir's myelotoxicity during clinical use. Inhibition of human lymphocyte blastogenic responses also occurs at clinically achievable concentrations of 1 to 10 μg/ml.

Mechanisms of Action and Resistance.   Ganciclovir inhibits viral DNA synthesis. It is monophosphorylated intracellularly by a virus-induced enzyme. Phosphorylation is catalyzed by a viral thymidine kinase during HSV infection and by a viral phosphotransferase encoded by the UL97 gene during CMV infection. Ganciclovir di- and triphosphate are formed by cellular enzymes. At least 10-fold higher concentrations of ganciclovir triphosphate are present in CMV-infected than in uninfected cells. The triphosphate is a competitive inhibitor of deoxyguanosine triphosphate incorporation into DNA and preferentially inhibits viral rather than host cellular DNA polymerases. Ganciclovir is incorporated into both viral and cellular DNA. Incorporation into viral DNA causes eventual cessation of DNA chain elongation (*see* Figure 50–1*B* and Figure 50–2).

A novel strategy of suicide gene therapy involves transduction of the HSV thymidine kinase gene into tumor cells by viral vectors. Subsequent exposure to ganciclovir induces apoptosis and cell-death receptor expression (Beltinger *et al.,* 1999).

Intracellular ganciclovir triphosphate concentrations are 10-fold higher than those of acyclovir triphosphate and decline much more slowly with an intracellular $t_{1/2}$ of elimination exceeding 24 hours (Biron *et al.,* 1985). These differences may account in part for ganciclovir's greater anti-CMV activity and provide the rationale for single daily doses in suppressing human CMV infections.

CMV can become resistant to ganciclovir by one of two mechanisms: reduced intracellular ganciclovir phosphorylation due to mutations in the viral phosphotransferase encoded by the UL97 gene and to mutations in viral DNA polymerase (Erice, 1999). Resistant CMV clinical isolates have 4- to >20-fold increases in inhibitory concentrations. Resistance has been associated primarily with impaired phosphorylation (Stanat *et al.,* 1991), but sometimes only with DNA polymerase mutations. Highly resistant variants have dual UL97 and polymerase mutations and are variably cross-resistant to cidofovir or foscarnet. Ganciclovir also is much less active against acyclovir-resistant, thymidine kinase–deficient HSV strains.

Absorption, Distribution, and Elimination. The oral bioavailability of ganciclovir averages 6% to 9% following ingestion with food and less in the fasting state. Peak and trough plasma levels are about 0.5 to 1.2 μg/ml and 0.2 to 0.5 μg/ml, respectively, after 1000-mg doses every 8 hours. Oral valganciclovir is well absorbed and rapidly hydrolyzed to ganciclovir; the bioavailability of ganciclovir averages 61% following valganciclovir. After 360-mg doses of valganciclovir, peak serum levels of ganciclovir average 3 μg/ml and only low prodrug levels are detectable (Jung and Dorr, 1999). Food increases the bioavailability of valganciclovir by about 25%. High oral valganciclovir doses in the fed state provide ganciclovir exposures comparable to intravenous dosing (Brown *et al.,* 1999). Following intravenous administration of 5-mg/kg doses of ganciclovir, peak and trough plasma concentrations average 8 to 11 μg/ml and 0.6 to 1.2 μg/ml, respectively. Following intravenous dosing, vitreous fluid levels are similar to or higher than those in plasma (Arevalo *et al.,* 1995) and average about 1 μg/ml. Vitreous levels decline with a half-life of 23 to 26 hours. Intraocular sustained release ganciclovir implants provide vitreous levels of about 4.1 μg/ml.

The plasma half-life is about 2 to 4 hours in patients with normal renal function. Over 90% of ganciclovir is eliminated unchanged by renal excretion, which occurs by glomerular filtration and tubular secretion. Consequently, the plasma half-life increases almost linearly as creatinine clearance declines and may reach 28 to 40 hours in those with severe renal insufficiency.

Untoward Effects. Myelosuppression is the principal dose-limiting toxicity of ganciclovir. Neutropenia occurs in about 15% to 40% of patients and thrombocytopenia in 5% to 20% (Faulds and Heel, 1990). Neutropenia most commonly is observed during the second week of treatment and usually is reversible within 1 week of drug cessation. Persistent fatal neutropenia has occurred. Oral ganciclovir also causes neutropenia. Oral valganciclovir is associated with headache and gastrointestinal disturbance (nausea, pain, diarrhea) in addition to the toxicities associated with ganciclovir. Recombinant granulocyte colony-stimulating factor (G-CSF, filgrastim, lenograstim) may be useful in treating ganciclovir-induced neutropenia (*see* Chapter 54).

CNS side effects occur in 5% to 15% of patients and range in severity from headache to behavioral changes to convulsions and coma. About one-third of patients have had to interrupt or prematurely stop therapy because of bone marrow or CNS toxicity. Infusion-related phlebitis, azotemia, anemia, rash, fever, liver function test abnormalities, nausea or vomiting, and eosinophilia also have been described.

Teratogenicity, embryotoxicity, irreversible reproductive toxicity, and myelotoxicity have been observed in animals at ganciclovir dosages comparable to those used in human beings.

Zidovudine (Hochster *et al.,* 1990) and probably other cytotoxic agents increase the risk of myelosuppression, as do nephrotoxic agents that impair ganciclovir excretion. Probenecid and possibly acyclovir reduce renal clearance of ganciclovir. Zalcitabine increases oral ganciclovir exposure by an average of 22%. Oral ganciclovir increases the absorption and peak plasma concentrations of didanosine by approximately twofold and that of zidovudine by about 20% (*see* Chapter 51 for discussion of zidovudine, zalcitabine, and didanosine).

Therapeutic Uses. Ganciclovir is effective for treatment and chronic suppression of CMV retinitis in immunocompromised patients and prevention of CMV disease in transplant patients. In CMV retinitis, initial induction treatment (5 mg/kg with food every 12 hours for 10 to 21 days) is associated with improvement or stabilization in about 85% of patients (Faulds and Heel, 1990; Drew, 1992). Reduced viral excretion is usually evident by 1 week, and funduscopic improvement by 2 weeks. Because of the high risk of relapse, AIDS patients with retinitis require suppressive therapy with high doses of ganciclovir (30 to 35 mg/kg per week). Oral ganciclovir (1000 mg three times daily) is effective for suppression of retinitis after initial intravenous treatment. Oral valganciclovir is comparable to intravenous dosing for initial control and sustained suppression of CMV retinitis.

Intravitreal ganciclovir injections have been used in some patients, and an intraocular sustained-release ganciclovir implant (VITRASERT) is more effective than systemic dosing in suppressing retinitis progression (Musch *et al.,* 1997).

Ganciclovir therapy (5 mg/kg per 12 hours for 14 to 21 days) may benefit other CMV syndromes in AIDS patients or solid-organ transplant recipients (Nichols and Boeckh, 2000). Response rates of 67% or higher have been found in combination with a decrease in immuno-suppressive therapy. Recurrent CMV disease occurs commonly after initial treatment. In bone-marrow transplant recipients with CMV pneumonia or gastrointestinal infection, ganciclovir alone is ineffective. However, ganciclovir combined with intravenous immunoglobulin or CMV immunoglobulin reduces the mortality of CMV pneumonia by about one-half. Ganciclovir treatment (12 mg/kg per day in 2 divided doses for 6 weeks) is associated with suppression of viuria and possibly clinical benefit in infants with congenital CMV disease (Whitley *et al.*, 1997).

Ganciclovir has been used both for prophylaxis and for suppression of CMV infections in transplant recipients. In bone-marrow transplant recipients, preemptive ganciclovir treatment (5 mg/kg per 12 hours for 7 to 14 days followed by 5 mg/kg per day to day 100 to 120 posttransplant), starting when CMV is isolated from bronchoalveolar lavage (Schmidt *et al.*, 1991) or from other sites (Goodrich *et al.*, 1991), is highly effective in preventing CMV pneumonia and appears to reduce mortality in these patients. Guidelines for patient monitoring (CMV blood levels, antigenemia) and use of ganciclovir prophylaxis have been published recently (Centers for Disease Control and Prevention, 2000). Initiation of ganciclovir at the time of engraftment also reduces CMV disease rates but does not improve survival, in part because of infections due to ganciclovir-related neutropenia (Goodrich *et al.*, 1993). Preemptive therapy (5 mg/kg two times daily for 7 days) when CMV shedding occurs also appears to be effective in solid-organ transplants or during rejection episodes (Singh *et al.*, 1994).

Intravenous ganciclovir administration reduces the risk of CMV disease in solid-organ transplant recipients (Pillay, 2000). Oral ganciclovir (1000 mg three times daily for 3 months) reduces CMV disease risk in liver transplant recipients, including high-risk patients with primary infection or those receiving antilymphocyte antibodies (Gane *et al.*, 1997). Oral ganciclovir prophylaxis is more effective than high-dose oral acyclovir in solid-organ transplant recipients (Flechner *et al.*, 1998). In advanced HIV disease, oral ganciclovir (1000 mg three times daily) may reduce the risk of CMV disease and possibly mortality in those not receiving didanosine (Spector *et al.*, 1996; Brosgart *et al.*, 1998). The addition of oral high-dose ganciclovir (1500 mg three times daily) to the intraocular ganciclovir implant further delays the time to retinitis progression and reduces the risk of new CMV disease (Martin *et al.*, 1999) and the risk of Kaposi's sarcoma.

The susceptibility of strains recovered before and after therapy in transplant patients generally is unchanged, although resistance emergence occurs in a minority of patients and is associated with poorer prognosis (Kruger *et al.*, 1999). The use of antithymocyte globulin and prolonged ganciclovir exposure are risk factors. Recovery of ganciclovir-resistant CMV isolates has been associated with progressive CMV disease in AIDS and other immunocompromised patients (Erice, 1999). Over one-quarter of retinitis patients have resistant isolates by 9 months of therapy, and resistant CMV has been recovered from cerebrospinal fluid (CSF), vitreous fluid, and visceral sites.

A ganciclovir ophthalmic gel formulation appears to be effective in treating HSV keratitis (Colin *et al.*, 1997). Oral ganciclovir reduces hepatitis B virus (HBV) DNA levels and aminotransferase levels in chronic hepatitis B (Hadziyannis *et al.*, 1999).

Systemic ganciclovir is being used in conjunction with suicide gene therapy expressing HSV thymidine kinase for treatment of brain tumors and a variety of other malignancies (Packer *et al.*, 2000).

Idoxuridine

Chemistry and Antiviral Activity. *Idoxuridine* (5-iodo-2'-deoxyuridine) is an iodinated thymidine analog that inhibits the *in vitro* replication of various DNA viruses, including herpesviruses and poxviruses (Prusoff, 1988). Its structure is given below:

IDOXURIDINE

Inhibitory concentrations for HSV-1 are 2 to 10 μg/ml, at least 10-fold higher than those of acyclovir. Idoxuridine lacks selectivity, in that low concentrations inhibit the growth of uninfected cells.

Mechanism of Action and Resistance. The antiviral mechanism of idoxuridine is not completely defined, but the phosphorylated derivatives interfere with various enzyme systems. The triphosphate inhibits viral DNA synthesis and is incorporated into both viral and cellular DNA. Such altered DNA is more susceptible to breakage and also leads to faulty transcription. Resistance to idoxuridine readily develops *in vitro* and occurs in viral isolates recovered from idoxuridine-treated patients with HSV keratitis.

Therapeutic Uses. In the United States, idoxuridine is approved only for topical treatment of HSV keratitis, although idoxuridine in dimethyl sulfoxide is available outside of the United States for treatment of herpes labialis, genitalis, and zoster. In ocular HSV infections, topical idoxuridine is more effective in epithelial infections, especially initial episodes, than in stromal infections (Kaufman, 1988). Adverse reactions include pain, pruritus, inflammation, or edema involving the eye or lids; rarely do allergic reactions occur.

Trifluridine

Trifluridine (5-trifluoromethyl-2'-deoxyuridine) is a fluorinated pyrimidine nucleoside that has *in vitro* inhibitory activity against HSV types 1 and 2, CMV, vaccinia, and, to a lesser extent, certain adenoviruses (Carmine *et al.,* 1982). Its structure is given below:

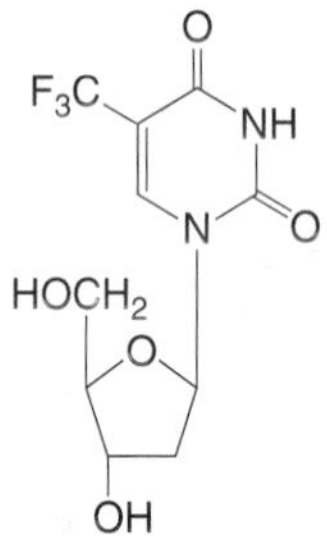

TRIFLURIDINE

Concentrations of trifluridine of 0.2 to 10 μg/ml inhibit replication of herpesviruses, including acyclovir-resistant strains (Birch *et al.,* 1992). Trifluridine also inhibits cellular DNA synthesis at relatively low concentrations.

Mechanism of Action and Resistance. The antiviral mechanism of trifluridine involves inhibition of viral DNA synthesis. Trifluridine monophosphate irreversibly inhibits thymidylate synthetase, and trifluridine triphosphate is a competitive inhibitor of thymidine triphosphate incorporation into DNA by DNA polymerases (Carmine *et al.,* 1982). Trifluridine is incorporated into viral and cellular DNA. Trifluridine-resistant HSV with altered thymidine kinase substrate specificity can be selected *in vitro,* and resistance in clinical isolates has been described.

Therapeutic Uses. Trifluridine currently is approved in the United States for treatment of primary keratoconjunctivitis and recurrent epithelial keratitis due to HSV types 1 and 2 (Kaufman, 1988; Carmine *et al.,* 1982). Topical trifluridine is more active than idoxuridine and comparable to vidarabine in HSV ocular infections. Adverse reactions include discomfort upon instillation and palpebral edema. Hypersensitivity reactions, irritation, and superficial punctate or epithelial keratopathy are uncommon. Topical tri-

fluridine also appears to be effective in some patients with acyclovir-resistant HSV cutaneous infections (Birch *et al.,* 1992).

Vidarabine

Vidarabine (9-β-D-ribofuranosyladenine) is an adenosine analog with an altered sugar (arabinose is the 2'-epimer of ribose). Its structure is given below:

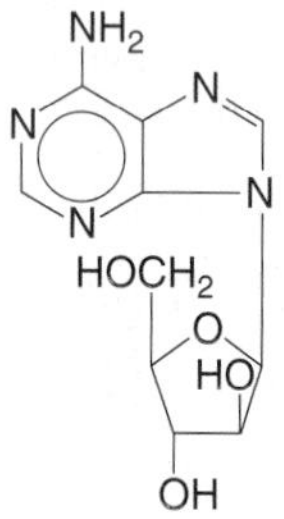

VIDARABINE

It is active against herpesviruses, poxviruses, rhabdoviruses, hepadnaviruses, and some RNA tumor viruses (Whitley *et al.,* 1980). Inhibitory concentrations are 3.0 μg/ml or less for HSV and VZV strains, including acyclovir-resistant strains.

The antiviral mechanism of vidarabine is incompletely understood, but vidarabine is an inhibitor of viral DNA synthesis. Cellular enzymes phosphorylate vidarabine to the triphosphate, which inhibits viral DNA polymerase activity in a manner that is competitive with deoxyadenosine triphosphate. Vidarabine triphosphate is incorporated into both cellular and viral DNA, where it may act as a chain terminator. Vidarabine triphosphate also inhibits ribonucleoside reductase, RNA polyadenylation, and S-adenosylhomocysteine hydrolase (SAHH), an enzyme involved in transmethylation reactions. Resistant variants due to mutations in viral DNA polymerase can be selected *in vitro.*

Intravenous vidarabine causes dose-related gastrointestinal toxicity, acute neurotoxicities, painful peripheral neuropathy, weakness, hypokalemia, rash, elevated transaminases, anemia, and leukopenia or thrombocytopenia. Vidarabine is teratogenic and oncogenic in animals.

Intravenous vidarabine once was used for treating HSV encephalitis, neonatal herpes, and zoster or varicella in immunocompromised patients, but acyclovir has replaced it for these indications. Combined administration of vidarabine and acyclovir has been used occasionally in life-threatening herpesvirus infections. In HSV keratoconjunctivitis, topical vidarabine is superior to idoxuridine (Kaufman, 1988).

ANTIINFLUENZA AGENTS

Amantadine and Rimantadine

Chemistry and Antiviral Activity. *Amantadine* (1-adamantanamine hydrochloride) and its α-methyl derivative *rimantadine* (α-methyl-1-adamantane methylamine hydrochloride) are uniquely configured tricyclic amines. The structures of the two agents are as follows:

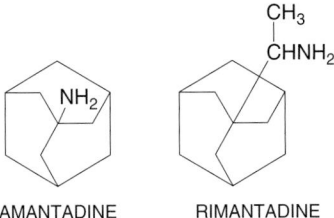

AMANTADINE   RIMANTADINE

Both agents specifically inhibit the replication of influenza A viruses at low concentrations (Hayden and Aoki, 1999). Depending on the assay method and strain, inhibitory concentrations of the drugs range from about 0.03 to 1.0 μg/ml for influenza A viruses. Rimantadine generally is 4- to 10-fold more active than amantadine. Concentrations of $\geq$10 μg/ml inhibit other enveloped viruses but are not achievable in human beings and may be cytotoxic. Rimantadine is inhibitory *in vitro* for *Trypanosoma brucei*, a cause of African sleeping sickness, at concentrations of 1 to 2.5 μg/ml (Kelly *et al.*, 1999). Neither agent inhibits hepatitis C virus (HCV) enzymes or internal ribosomal entry site-mediated translation *in vitro* (Jubin *et al.*, 2000).

Mechanisms of Action and Resistance. Amantadine and rimantadine share two mechanisms of antiviral action (Hayden and Aoki, 1999). They inhibit an early step in viral replication, probably viral uncoating; for some strains, they have an effect on a late step in viral assembly probably mediated through altering hemagglutinin processing. The primary locus of action is the influenza A virus M2 protein, an integral membrane protein that functions as an ion channel. By interfering with this function of the M2 protein, the drugs inhibit the acid-mediated dissociation of the ribonucleoprotein complex early in replication and potentiate acidic pH-induced conformational changes in the hemagglutinin during its intracellular transport later in replication.

Resistant variants are rare (<1%) in field isolates (Zieger *et al.*, 1999), but selected readily by virus passage in the presence of drug and have been recovered from treated persons. Resistance with over 100-fold increases in inhibitory concentrations has been associated with single nucleotide changes leading to amino acid substitutions in the transmembrane region of M2 (Hayden, 1996). Amantadine and rimantadine share cross-susceptibility and resistance.

Absorption, Distribution, and Elimination. Amantadine and rimantadine are well absorbed after oral administration (*see* Table 50–4) (Aoki and Sitar, 1988; Wills *et al.*, 1987). Peak plasma concentrations of amantadine average 0.5 to 0.8 μg/ml on a 100-mg twice-daily regimen in healthy young adults. Comparable doses of rimantadine give peak and trough plasma concentrations of approximately 0.4 to 0.5 μg/ml and 0.2 to 0.4 μg/ml, respectively. The elderly require only one-half of the weight-adjusted dose of amantadine needed for young adults to achieve equivalent trough plasma levels of 0.3 μg/ml (Aoki and Sitar, 1988). Similarly, rimantadine plasma concentrations in elderly residents of nursing homes average over twofold higher than those observed in healthy adults.

Both drugs have very large volumes of distribution. Nasal secretion and salivary levels of amantadine approximate those found in the serum. Amantadine is excreted in breast milk. Rimantadine concentrations in nasal mucus average 50% higher than those in plasma.

Amantadine is excreted largely unmetabolized in the urine through glomerular filtration and probably tubular secretion. The

Table 50–4
Pharmacological Characteristics of Antiinfluenza Agents

	AMANTADINE	RIMANTADINE	ZANAMIVIR	OSELTAMIVIR
Spectrum (types of influenza)	A	A	A, B	A, B
Route/formulations	Oral (tablet/capsule/syrup)	Oral (tablet/syrup)	Inhaled (powder) Intravenous*	Oral (capsule/syrup*)
Oral bioavailability	50%–90%	> 90%	< 5%‡	~ 80%†
Effect of meals on AUC§	Negligible	Negligible	Not applicable	Negligible
Plasma $t_{1/2}$, hours	12–18	24–36	2.5–5	6–10†
Protein binding, %	67%	40%	< 10%	3%†
Metabolism, %	< 10%	~ 75%	Negligible	Negligible†
Renal excretion, % (parent drug)	50%–90%	~ 25%	100%	95%†
Dose adjustments	$CL_{cr} < 80\%$¶ Age > 65 yrs	$CL_{cr} < 10$ Age > 65 years	None	$CL_{cr} < 30$

*Investigational at present.

†For antivirally active oseltamivir carboxylate.

‡Systemic absorption 4% to 17% after inhalation.

§AUC = area under the plasma concentration-time curve.

¶CL_{cr} = creatinine clearance.

plasma $t_{1/2}$ of elimination is about 12 to 18 hours in young adults. Because amantadine's elimination is highly dependent on renal function, the $t_{1/2}$ of elimination increases up to twofold in the elderly and even more in those with renal impairment (Horadam *et al.*, 1981). Dose adjustments are advisable in those with mild decrements in renal function. In contrast, rimantadine is metabolized extensively by hydroxylation, conjugation, and glucuronidation prior to renal excretion. Following oral administration, the plasma $t_{1/2}$ of elimination of rimantadine averages 24 to 36 hours, and 60% to 90% is excreted in the urine as metabolites (Wills *et al.*, 1987). Renal clearance of unchanged rimantadine is similar to creatinine clearance.

Untoward Effects. The most common side effects related to amantadine and rimantadine are minor dose-related gastrointestinal and CNS complaints (Hayden and Aoki, 1999). These include nervousness, lightheadedness, difficulty concentrating, insomnia, and loss of appetite or nausea. CNS side effects occur in approximately 5% to 33% of patients treated with amantadine at doses of 200 mg/day, but are significantly less frequent with rimantadine. Amantadine dose reductions are required in older adults (100 mg/day) because of decreased renal function, but 20% to 40% of infirm elderly will experience side effects even at this lower dose. At comparable doses of 100 mg per day, rimantadine is significantly better tolerated in nursing home residents than is amantadine (Keyser *et al.*, 2000).

High amantadine plasma concentrations (1.0 to 5.0 μg/ml) have been associated with serious neurotoxic reactions, including delirium, hallucinosis, seizures or coma, and cardiac arrhythmias. Exacerbations of preexisting seizure disorders and psychiatric symptoms may occur with amantadine and possibly with rimantadine. Amantadine is teratogenic in animals, and the safety of either drug has not been established in pregnancy.

The neurotoxic effects of amantadine appear to be increased by concomitant ingestion of antihistamines and psychotropic or anticholinergic drugs, especially in the elderly.

Therapeutic Uses. Amantadine and rimantadine are effective for prevention and treatment of influenza A virus infections. Seasonal prophylaxis with either drug (a total of 200 mg/day in 1 or 2 divided doses in young adults) is about 70% to 90% protective against influenza A illness (Hayden and Aoki, 1999). Efficacy has been shown during pandemic influenza, in preventing nosocomial influenza, and in curtailing nosocomial outbreaks. Doses of 100 mg/day are better tolerated and appear to be protective against influenzal illness. Postexposure prophylaxis with either drug provides protection of exposed family contacts, if ill young children are not concurrently treated.

Seasonal prophylaxis is an alternative in high-risk patients, if the influenza vaccine cannot be administered or may be ineffective. Prophylaxis should be started as soon as influenza is identified in a community or region and should be continued throughout the period of risk (usually 4 to 8 weeks), since any protective effects are lost several days after cessation. Alternatively, the drugs can be started in conjunction with immunization and continued for 2 weeks until protective immune responses develop.

In uncomplicated influenza A illness of adults, early amantadine or rimantadine treatment (200 mg/day for 5 days) reduces the duration of fever and systemic complaints by 1 to 2 days, speeds functional recovery, and sometimes decreases the duration of virus shedding (Hayden and Aoki, 1999). In children, rimantadine treatment may be associated with less illness and lower viral titers during the first 2 days of treatment, but rimantadine-treated children have more prolonged shedding of virus. The optimal dose and duration of therapy have not been established in children for either agent. It also is uncertain whether treatment reduces risk of complications in high-risk patients or is useful in patients with established pulmonary complications.

Resistant variants have been recovered from approximately 30% of treated children or adults by the fifth day of therapy (Hayden, 1996). Resistant variants also arise commonly when amantadine or rimantadine is used to treat influenza in immunocompromised patients (Englund *et al.*, 1998). Illnesses due to apparent transmission of resistant virus, associated with failure of drug prophylaxis, have been documented in contacts of drug-treated ill persons in households and in nursing homes. Resistant variants appear to be pathogenic and can cause typical disabling influenzal illness.

The discovery that amantadine also is useful in treating parkinsonism was due to serendipity. This application is discussed in Chapter 22. Amantadine and rimantadine have been used alone or in combination with interferon and other agents in treating chronic hepatitis C with inconsistent results to date (Younossi and Perrillo, 1999).

Oseltamivir

Chemistry and Antiviral Activity. *Oseltamivir carboxylate* [(3*R*, 4*R*, 5*S*)-4-acetylamino-5-amino-3(1-ethylpropoxyl)-1-cyclohexene-1-carboxylic acid] is a transition-state analog of sialic acid that is a potent, selective inhibitor of influenza A and B virus neuraminidases (Kim *et al.*, 1997). Its structure is shown below. Oseltamivir phosphate is an ethyl ester prodrug that lacks antiviral activity. Oseltamivir carboxylate has an antiviral spectrum and potency similar to that of zanamivir (*see* below) (Mendel *et al.*, 1998). It inhibits amantadine- and rimantadine-resistant influenza A viruses and some zanamivir-resistant variants.

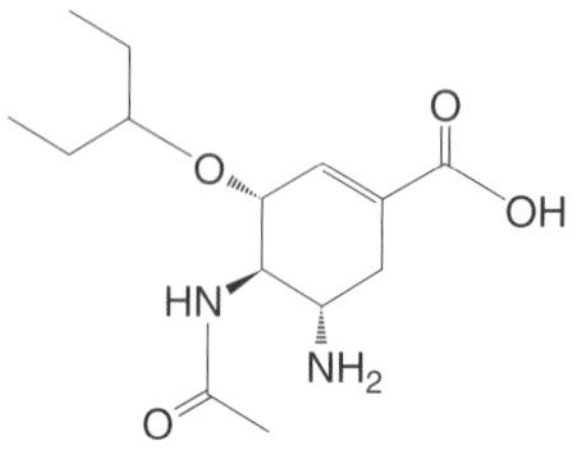

OSELTAMIVIR CARBOXYLATE

Mechanisms of Action and Resistance. Influenza neuraminidase cleaves terminal sialic acid residues and destroys the receptors recognized by viral hemagglutinin, which are present on the cell surface, progeny virions, and in respiratory secretions (Gubareva *et al.,* 2000). This enzymatic action is essential for release of virus from infected cells. Interaction of oseltamivir carboxylate with the neuraminidase causes a conformational change within the enzyme's active site and inhibition of activity. Inhibition of neuraminidase activity leads to viral aggregation at the cell surface and reduced virus spread within the respiratory tract.

Influenza variants selected *in vitro* for resistance to oseltamivir carboxylate contain hemagglutinin and/or neuraminidase mutations (McKimm-Breschkin, 2000). Resistance has not been recognized in influenza B viruses to date. The most commonly recognized variants (mutations at positions 292 or 274 of neuraminidase) have reduced infectivity and virulence *in vivo*. Oral oseltamivir therapy has been associated with recovery of resistant variants in about 1% to 2% of treated adults.

Absorption, Distribution, and Elimination. Oral oseltamivir phosphate is rapidly absorbed (about 80%; *see* Table 50–4) and cleaved by esterases in the gastrointestinal tract or liver to the antivirally active carboxylate. Low blood levels of oseltamivir phosphate are detectable, but are only 3% to 5% of those of the metabolite. The bioavailability of the carboxylate is estimated to be ~80% (He *et al.,* 1999). The time to maximum plasma concentrations of the carboxylate is about 2.5 to 5 hours. Food does not decrease bioavailability but reduces the risk of gastrointestinal intolerance. After 75-mg doses, peak plasma concentrations average 0.07 μg/ml for oseltamivir phosphate and 0.35 μg/ml for the carboxylate. The carboxylate has a volume of distribution similar to extracellular water. In animals, bronchoalveolar lavage levels are similar to plasma levels. Following oral administration, the plasma half-life of oseltamivir phosphate is 1 to 3 hours and that of the carboxylate ranges from 6 to 10 hours. Both the prodrug and active metabolite are eliminated primarily unchanged through the kidney. Probenecid doubles the plasma half-life of the carboxylate, which indicates tubular secretion by the anionic pathway.

Untoward Effects. Oral oseltamivir is associated with nausea, abdominal discomfort, and, less often, emesis, probably due to local irritation. Gastrointestinal complaints usually are mild to moderate in intensity, typically resolve despite continued dosing in 1 to 2 days, and are preventable by administration with food. The frequency of such complaints is about 10% to 15% when oseltamivir is used for treatment of influenza illness and less than 5% when used for prophylaxis. An increased frequency of headache was reported in one prophylaxis study in elderly adults.

Oseltamivir phosphate and the carboxylate do interact with the cytochrome P450 system *in vitro*. Their protein binding is low. No clinically significant drug interactions have been recognized to date. High doses of oseltamivir cause renal tubular mineralization and delayed parturition in mice; these effects are of uncertain clinical significance.

Therapeutic Uses. Oral oseltamivir is effective in the treatment and prevention of influenza. Treatment of previously healthy adults (75 mg twice daily for 5 days) or children aged 1 to 12 years (2 mg/kg twice daily for 5 days) with acute influenza reduces illness duration by about 1 to 2 days, speeds functional recovery, and reduces the risk of complications leading to antibiotic use by 40% to 50% (Treanor *et al.,* 2000; Whitley *et al.,* 2001). Efficacy in the elderly and in high-risk patients with underlying cardiopulmonary conditions is under study. When used for prophylaxis during the influenza season, oseltamivir (75 mg once daily) is effective in reducing the likelihood of influenza illness in both unimmunized working adults and in immunized nursing-home residents (Hayden *et al.,* 1999; Peters *et al.,* 1999), and short-term use (7 days) protects against influenza in household contacts.

Zanamivir

Chemistry and Antiviral Activity. *Zanamivir* (4-guanidino-2,4-dideoxy-2,3-dehydro-*N*-acetyl neuraminic acid) is a sialic acid analog that potently and specifically inhibits the neuraminidases of influenza A and B viruses (von Itzstein *et al.,* 1993). Its structure is shown below. Depending on the strain, zanamivir competitively inhibits influenza neuraminidase activity at concentrations of approximately 0.2 to 3 ng/ml (Woods *et al.,* 1993) but affects neuraminidases from other pathogens and mammalian sources only at 10^6-fold higher concentrations. Zanamivir inhibits *in vitro* replication of influenza A and B viruses, including amantadine- and rimantadine-resistant strains, and is active after topical administration in animal models of influenza.

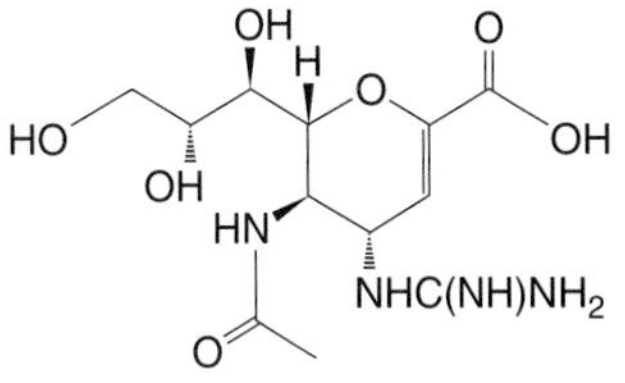

ZANAMIVIR

Mechanisms of Action and Resistance. Like oseltamivir, zanamivir inhibits viral neuraminidase and thus causes viral aggregation at the cell surface and reduced spread of virus within the respiratory tract (Gubareva *et al.,* 2000).

In vitro selection of viruses resistant to zanamivir is associated with mutations in the viral hemagglutinin and/or neuraminidase (McKimm-Breschkin, 2000). Hemagglutinin variants generally have mutations in or near the receptor binding site that make them less dependent on neuraminidase action for release from cells *in vitro*, although they may retain susceptibility *in vivo* (Woods *et al.,* 1993). Hemagglutinin variants are cross-resistant to other neuraminidase inhibitors. Neuraminidase variants contain mutations in the enzyme active site that diminish binding of zanamivir, but the altered enzymes show reduced activity or stability. Resistant variants may have decreased infectivity in animals. Resistance emergence has not been documented with zanamivir in immunocompetent hosts to date. One resistant influenza B variant containing dual hemagglutinin and neuraminidase mutations was recovered from an immunocompromised child treated with nebulized zanamivir (Gubareva *et al.,* 1998).

Absorption, Distribution, and Elimination. The oral bioavailability of zanamivir is low (<5%; *see* Table 50–4), and most clinical trials have used intranasal or dry powder inhalation delivery. The proprietary inhaler device for delivering zanamivir in a lactose carrier is breath-actuated and requires a cooperative patient. Following inhalation of the dry powder, approximately 15% is deposited in the lower respiratory tract and about 80% in the oropharynx (Cass *et al.,* 1999). Overall bioavailability is less than 20%, and plasma levels after 10-mg inhaled doses average about 35 to 100 ng/ml in adults and children (Peng *et al.,* 2000a). Median zanamivir concentrations in induced sputum samples are 1336 ng/ml at 6 hours and 47 ng/ml at 24 hours after a single 10-mg dose in healthy volunteers (Peng *et al.,* 2000b). The plasma half-life of zanamivir averages 2.5 to 5 hours after oral inhalation but only 1.7 hours following intravenous dosing. Over 90% is eliminated in the urine without recognized metabolism.

Untoward Effects. Topically applied zanamivir generally is well tolerated in ambulatory adults and children with influenza. Wheezing and bronchospasm have been reported in some influenza-infected patients without known airway disease, and acute deteriorations in lung function, including fatal outcomes, have occurred in those with underlying asthma or chronic obstructive airway disease. No significant changes in lung function or airway reactivity were found in uninfected mild to moderate asthmatics given 2 weeks of inhaled zanamivir (Cass *et al.,* 2000). Tolerability in more serious bronchopulmonary disorders or in intubated patients is uncertain. Zanamivir administration to patients with underlying airway disease requires close monitoring and availability of rapidly acting bronchodilators and should be stopped if problems develop.

Preclinical studies of zanamivir revealed no evidence of mutagenic, teratogenic, or oncogenic effects. No clinically significant drug interactions have been recognized to date. Zanamivir does not diminish the immune response to injected influenza vaccine.

Therapeutic Uses. Inhaled zanamivir is effective for prevention and treatment of acute influenza. Early zanamivir treatment (10 mg twice daily for 5 days) of febrile influenza in ambulatory adults and children aged 5 years and older shortens the time to illness resolution by 1 to 3 days (Hayden *et al.,* 1997; Hedrick *et al.,* 2000). In previously healthy adults, zanamivir treatment also reduces by 40% the risk of lower respiratory tract complications leading to antibiotic use. Once-daily inhaled, but not intranasal, zanamivir is highly protective against community-acquired influenza illness (Monto *et al.,* 1999), and when given for 10 days, it protects against household transmission (Hayden *et al.,* 2000). Intravenous zanamivir is protective against experimental human influenza but has not been studied in treating natural influenza.

OTHER ANTIVIRAL AGENTS

Interferons

Classification and Antiviral Activity. Interferons (IFNs) are potent cytokines that possess antiviral, immunomodulating, and antiproliferative actions (Baron *et al.,* 1992; *see also* Chapter 53). These proteins are synthesized by cells in response to various inducers and in turn cause biochemical changes leading to an antiviral state in cells of the same species. Three major classes of human interferons with significant antiviral activity currently are recognized: alpha (>18 individual species), beta, and gamma. Clinically used recombinant alpha interferons (Table 50–2) are nonglycosylated proteins of approximately 19,500 daltons. Preparations of natural and recombinant interferons alpha available for clinical use are referred to as interferons *alfa.*

Interferon alpha and interferon beta may be produced by nearly all cells in response to viral infection and a variety of other stimuli, including double-stranded RNA and certain cytokines (*e.g.,* interleukin 1, interleukin 2, and tumor necrosis factor). Interferon gamma production is restricted to T lymphocytes and natural killer cells responding to antigenic stimuli, mitogens, and specific cytokines. Interferons alpha and beta exhibit antiviral and antiproliferative actions; stimulate the cytotoxic activity of lymphocytes, natural killer cells, and macrophages; and upregulate class I major histocompatibility antigens (MHC) and other surface markers. Interferon gamma has less antiviral activity but more potent immunoregulatory effects, particularly macrophage activation, expression of class II MHC, and mediation of local inflammatory responses.

Most animal viruses are inhibited by the antiviral actions of interferons, although many DNA viruses are relatively insensitive. Considerable differences in potency exist among different viruses and assay systems. Interferon biological activity usually is measured in terms of antiviral effects in cell culture and generally is expressed as international units (IU) relative to reference standards.

Mechanisms of Action. Following binding to specific cellular receptors, interferons activate the JAK-STAT signal transduction pathway and lead to the nuclear translocation of a cellular protein complex that binds to genes containing an interferon-specific response element. This, in turn, leads to synthesis of over two dozen proteins that contribute to viral resistance (Stark *et al.,* 1998; Figure 50–3). The antiviral effects of interferon are mediated through inhibition of viral penetration or uncoating, synthesis of messenger RNA, translation of viral proteins, and/or viral assembly and release. Inhibition of protein

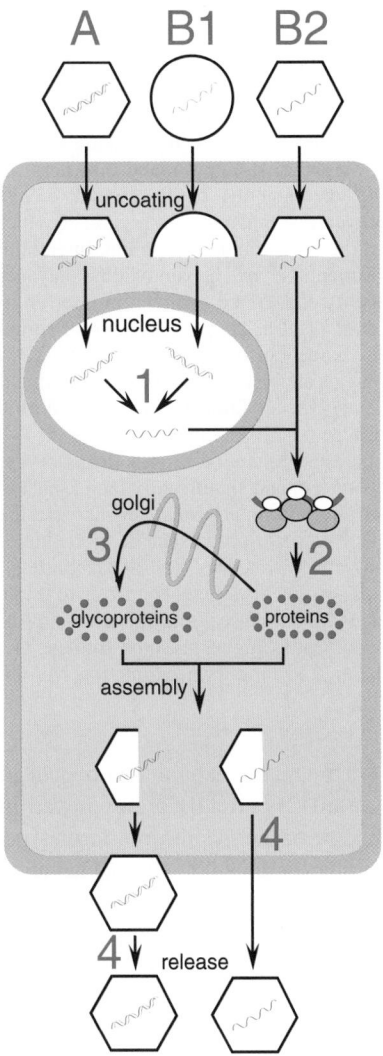

Viruses

A. DNA

B. RNA

1. orthomyxoviruses and retroviruses
2. picornaviruses and most RNA viruses

IFN Effects

1. transcription inhibition

activates Mx protein
blocks mRNA synthesis

2. translation inhibition

activates methylase —>
blocks mRNA cap methylation

activates 2'5' oligoadenylate synthetase
—> 2'5'A —> inhibits mRNA splicing
and activates RNase L —> cleaves
viral RNA

activates protein kinase P1 —> blocks
eIF-2α function —> inhibits initiation
of mRNA translation

activates phosphodiesterase —> blocks
tRNA function

3. protein processing inhibition

glycosyltransferase —> blocks protein
glycosylation

4. virus maturation inhibition

glycosyltransferase —>blocks
glycoprotein maturation

causes membrane changes —> blocks
budding

Figure 50–2. Interferon-mediated antiviral activity occurs via multiple mechanisms.

The binding of IFN to specific cell-surface receptor molecules signals the cell to produce a series of antiviral proteins. The stages of viral replication that are inhibited by various IFN-induced antiviral proteins are shown. Most of these act to inhibit the translation of viral proteins (mechanism 2), but other steps in viral replication also are affected (mechanisms 1, 3, and 4). The roles of these mechanisms in the other actions of IFNs are under study. *Key:* IFN, interferon; mRNA, messenger RNA; Mx, specific cellular protein; tRNA, transfer RNA; RNase L, latent cellular endoribonuclease; 2'5'A, 2'–5' oligoadenylates; eIF-2α, protein synthesis initiation factor. (Modified from Baron *et al.,* 1992, with permission.)

synthesis is the major inhibitory effect for many viruses. Interferon-induced proteins include 2'-5'-oligoadenylate [2-5(A)] synthetases and a protein kinase, either of which can inhibit protein synthesis in the presence of double-stranded RNA. The 2-5(A) synthetase produces adenylate oligomers that activate a latent cellular endoribonuclease (RNase L) to cleave both cellular and viral single-stranded RNAs. The protein kinase selectively phosphorylates and inactivates a protein involved in protein synthesis, eukaryotic initiation factor 2 (eIF-2). Interferon-induced protein kinase also may be an important effector of apoptosis. Interferon also induces a phosphodiesterase, which cleaves a portion of transfer RNA and thus prevents peptide elongation. A particular virus may be inhibited at several steps, and the principal inhibitory effect for a specific virus differs among virus families. In addition, certain viruses are able to counter interferon effects by blocking production or activity of selected interferon-inducible proteins. For example, interferon resistance in hepatitis C virus is attributable to inhibition of protein kinase and to other mechanisms (Francois *et al.,* 2000).

Complex interactions exist between interferons and other parts of the immune system. Interferons may ameliorate viral infections by exerting direct antiviral effects and/or by modifying the immune response to infection. For example, interferon-induced expression of major histocompatibility antigens may contribute to the antiviral actions of interferon by enhancing the lytic effects of cytotoxic T lymphocytes. In addition to contributing to controlling infection, interferons may mediate some of the systemic symptoms associated with viral infections and contribute to immunologically mediated tissue damage in certain viral diseases.

Absorption, Distribution, and Elimination. Oral administration does not result in detectable interferon levels in serum or increases in 2-5(A) synthetase activity in peripheral blood mononuclear cells (Wills, 1990). After intramuscular or subcutaneous injection of interferon alfa, absorption exceeds 80%. Plasma levels are dose-related, peaking at 4 to 8 hours and returning to baseline by 18 to 36 hours. Levels of 2-5(A) synthetase in peripheral-blood mononuclear cells, which have been used as a marker of interferon's biologic activity, show increases beginning at 6 hours and lasting through 4 days after a single injection. An antiviral state in peripheral-blood mononuclear cells peaks at 24 hours and slowly decreases to baseline by 6 days after injection. Absorption of interferon gamma is more variable, and intramuscular or subcutaneous injections of interferon beta result in negligible plasma levels, although increases in 2-5(A) synthetase levels may occur. The volume of distribution of interferon alfa averages about 31 liters. After systemic administration, low levels of interferon are detected in respiratory secretions, CSF, eye, and brain.

Because interferons induce long-lasting biological effects, their activities are not easily predictable from usual pharmacokinetic measures. After intravenous dosing, clearance of interferon from plasma occurs in a complex, multiexponential manner (Bocci, 1992). The plasma elimination half-life of interferon alfa is about 40 minutes; those of recombinant interferon beta or interferon gamma are approximately 4 hours and 0.5 hour, respectively. Elimination from the blood relates to distribution to the tissues, cellular uptake, and catabolism primarily in the kidney and liver. Negligible amounts are excreted in the urine.

Attachment of interferon proteins to large inert polyethylene glycol (PEG) molecules (pegylation) decreases the clearance substantially. Plasma concentrations of interferon are prolonged, and the extended duration of therapeutic activity allows for once-weekly dosing. Pegylation also may increase the antigenicity of the protein to which it is bonded. Two pegylated interferons have received extensive clinical testing. Peginterferon alfa-2b has a straight chain, 12,000-dalton type of PEG which increases the half-life from approximately 2 to 3 hours to about 54 hours (Glue *et al.*, 2000). Peginterferon alfa-2a consists of an ester derivative of a branched-chain 40,000-dalton PEG bonded to interferon alfa-2a and has a plasma half-life averaging 77 hours. Increasing PEG size is associated with longer half-life and less renal clearance and relative antiviral activity. About 70% of PEG interferon alfa-2b is cleared by hepatic metabolism; peginterferon alfa-2a also is cleared primarily by the liver.

Untoward Effects. Injection of interferon doses of 1 to 2 million units (MU) or greater usually is associated with an acute influenzalike syndrome beginning several hours after injection. Symptoms include fever, chills, headache, myalgia, arthralgia, nausea, vomiting, and diarrhea (Dusheiko, 1997). Fever usually resolves within 12 hours. Tolerance gradually develops in most patients. Febrile responses can be moderated by pretreatment with various antipyretics. Up to one-half of patients receiving intralesional therapy for genital warts experience the

influenzal illness initially, as well as discomfort at the injection site, and leukopenia.

The principal dose-limiting toxicities of systemic interferon are myelosuppression with granulocytopenia and thrombocytopenia; neurotoxicity manifested by somnolence, confusion, behavioral disturbance, and rarely seizures; debilitating neurasthenia with fatigue and weight loss; autoimmune disorders including thyroiditis; and, uncommonly, cardiovascular effects with hypotension and tachycardia. Elevations in hepatic enzymes and triglycerides, alopecia, proteinuria and azotemia, interstitial nephritis, autoantibody formation, and hepatotoxicity may occur. Alopecia and personality change are common in interferon-treated children (Sokal *et al.*, 1998). The development of serum neutralizing antibodies to exogenous interferons may be associated infrequently with loss of clinical responsiveness (Antonelli *et al.*, 1991). Interferon may impair fertility, and safety during pregnancy is not established.

Interferon reduces the metabolism of various drugs by the hepatic cytochrome P450 system and significantly increases levels of drugs such as theophylline. Interferons can increase the bone-marrow toxicity of myelotoxic drugs such as zidovudine.

Pegylated interferons are tolerated as well as standard interferons with discontinuation rates ranging from 6% to 11%, although the frequencies of fever, nausea, and injection-site inflammation appear to be somewhat higher in some studies. The safety of PEG accumulation and long-term circulation has not been established.

Therapeutic Uses. Recombinant, natural, and pegylated alpha interferons (Table 50–2) currently are approved in the United States, depending on the specific interferon type, for treatment of condyloma acuminatum, chronic hepatitis C, chronic hepatitis B, Kaposi's sarcoma in HIV-infected patients, other malignancies, and multiple sclerosis.

Hepatitis B Virus. In patients with chronic hepatitis B, parenteral administration of various interferons is associated with loss of hepatitis B virus (HBV) DNA, loss of HBV *e* antigen (HBeAg), and development of anti-HBe antibody, and biochemical and histological improvement in about 25% to 50% of the patients (Haria and Benfield, 1995; Main and Thomas, 1997). Lasting responses require moderately high interferon doses and prolonged administration (typically 5 MU/day or 10 MU in adults and 6 MU/m^2 in children three times per week for 4 to 6 months) (Sokal *et al.*, 1998). Plasma HBV DNA and polymerase activity decline promptly in most patients, but complete disappearance is sustained in only about one-third. Low pretherapy serum HBV DNA levels and high aminotransferase levels are predictors of response. Sustained responses are infrequent in those with vertically acquired infection, anti-HBe positivity, or concurrent immunosuppression due to HIV. Responses with seroconversion to anti-HBe usually are associated with transaminase elevations and often a hepatitis-like illness during the second or third month of therapy, likely related to immune clearance of infected hepatocytes. High-dose interferon can cause myelosuppression and clinical deterioration in those with decompensated liver disease.

Remissions in chronic hepatitis B induced by interferon are sustained in over 80% of patients treated and frequently are followed by loss of HBV surface antigen (HbsAg), histological improvement or stabilization, and reduced risk of liver-related complications and mortality (Lau *et al.*, 1997). Interferon may benefit HBV-associated nephrotic syndrome and glomerulonephritis in some patients. Antiviral effects and improvements occur in about one-half of chronic hepatitis D virus (HDV) infections, but relapse is common unless HbsAg disappears (Farci *et al.*, 1994). Interferon does not appear to be beneficial in acute HBV or hepatitis D virus (HDV) infections.

Hepatitis C Virus. In chronic HCV infection, subcutaneous interferon alfa-2b monotherapy (3 MU three times a week) is associated with an approximate 50% to 70% rate of aminotransferase normalization and loss of plasma viral RNA. However, relapse rates are high, and sustained virologic remission is observed in only about 10% to 25% of patients treated for 6 months (Main and Thomas, 1997). Prolonged treatment (12 to 18 months) and possibly higher doses increase the likelihood of sustained responses. Sustained responses are associated with long-term histologic improvement and possibly reduced risk of hepatocellular carcinoma (Yoshida *et al.*, 1999). Viral genotype and pretreatment RNA level influence response to treatment, but early viral clearance is the best predictor of sustained response (Civeira and Prieto, 1999). Those who are HCV RNA–negative at 3 months of initiating therapy generally should continue treatment for 12 months or longer (Gish, 1999).

Pegylated interferons are superior to conventional thrice-weekly interferon monotherapy in inducing sustained remissions in treatment-naïve patients. A once-weekly dosing regimen of peginterferon alfa-2a (180 μg subcutaneously for 48 weeks) doubled sustained response rates in patients with chronic hepatitis C (Zeuzem *et al.*, 2000), including those with cirrhosis (Heathcote *et al.*, 2000). Responses to peginterferon alfa-2b are dose-related, and weight-adjusted doses of 1.5 μg/kg per week are recommended. The efficacy of pegylated interferons appears to be enhanced by the addition of ribavirin to the treatment regimens, with sustained viral responses exceeding 50% (Manns *et al.*, 2000); large studies of combination therapy are ongoing. In addition, studies of prolonged (4 years) maintenance monotherapy with pegylated interferons are in progress.

Nonresponders generally do not benefit from interferon monotherapy retreatment but may respond to combined interferon and ribavirin therapy (*see* "Ribavirin," below). Patients relapsing after monotherapy may respond to interferon retreatment or more often to combined interferon-ribavirin therapy. Interferon treatment may benefit HCV–associated cryoglobulinemia and glomerulonephritis. Interferon administration during acute hepatitis C infection appears to reduce the risk of chronicity.

Papillomavirus. In refractory condylomata acuminata (genital warts), intralesional injection of various natural and recombinant interferons is associated with complete clearance of injected warts in 36% to 62% of patients (Frazer and McMillan, 1997). Relapse occurs in 20% to 30% of patients with interferon-induced remission. Verruca vulgaris may respond to intralesional interferon alfa. Intramuscular or subcutaneous administration is associated with some regression in wart size but greater toxicity, and no higher complete response rate when used as an adjunctive modality. Systemic interferon may provide adjunctive benefit in recurrent juvenile laryngeal papillomatosis and in treating laryngeal disease in older patients.

Other Viruses. Interferons have been shown to have virologic and/or clinical effects in various herpesvirus infections including genital HSV infections, localized herpes zoster of cancer patients or of older adults, and CMV infections of renal transplant patients. However, interferon generally is associated with more side effects and inferior clinical benefits compared to conventional antiviral therapies. Topically applied interferon and trifluridine combinations appear active in drug-resistant mucocutaneous HSV infections (Birch *et al.*, 1992).

In HIV-infected persons, interferons have been associated with antiretroviral effects. In advanced infection, however, the combination of zidovudine and interferon is associated with only transient benefit and excessive hematological toxicity. Interferon alfa (3 MU three times weekly) is effective for treatment of HIV-related thrombocytopenia resistant to zidovudine therapy (Marroni *et al.*, 1994).

Except for adenovirus, interferon has broad-spectrum antiviral activity against respiratory viruses *in vitro*. However, prophylactic intranasal interferon alfa is protective only against rhinovirus colds, and chronic use is limited by the occurrence of nasal side effects. Intranasal interferon is therapeutically ineffective in established rhinovirus colds.

Lamivudine

Lamivudine, the (−) enantiomer of 2′,3′-dideoxy-3′thiacytidine, is a nucleoside analog that inhibits HIV reverse transcriptase and HBV DNA polymerase. Its use as an antiretroviral agent is discussed in depth in Chapter 51. It inhibits HBV replication *in vitro* by 50% at concentrations of 4 to 7 ng/ml with negligible cellular cytotoxicity. Cellular enzymes convert lamivudine to the triphosphate, which competitively inhibits HBV DNA polymerase and causes chain termination. The intracellular $t_{1/2}$ of the triphosphate averages 17 to 19 hours in HBV-infected cells, so that infrequent dosing is possible.

HBV resistance to lamivudine is associated with from 40- to 10^4-fold reduced *in vitro* susceptibility. Resistant HBV variants recovered from treated patients have mutations in the viral DNA polymerase, particularly involving position 550/2 in the YMDD motif and often position 526/8. Some variants appear to replicate less efficiently than wild-type virus *in vitro,* and some are lamivudine-dependent (Yeh *et al.,* 2000).

Following oral administration, lamivudine is rapidly absorbed with a bioavailability of about 80% in adults (Johnson *et al.,* 1999). Peak plasma levels are observed at 0.5 to 1.5 hours after dosing and average approximately 1000 ng/ml after 100-mg doses. Lamivudine is distributed widely in a volume comparable to total body water. The plasma $t_{1/2}$ averages about 9 hours, and approximately 70% of the dose is excreted unchanged in the urine. About 5% is metabolized to an inactive *trans*-sulfoxide metabolite. In HBV-infected children, doses of 3 mg/kg per day provide plasma exposure and trough plasma levels comparable to those in adults receiving 100 mg daily (Sokal *et al.,* 2000). Dose reductions are indicated for moderate renal insufficiency (creatinine clearance <50 ml/minute). Trimethoprim decreases the renal clearance of lamivudine.

Long-term lamivudine treatment (100 mg daily for ≥1 year) of chronic hepatitis B suppresses HBV DNA levels (generally ≥2 $\log_{10}$) and is associated with biochemical normalization and histological improvements in inflammation and progression of fibrosis (Lai *et al.,* 1998; Dienstag *et al.,* 1999). However, a minority of patients develop HbeAg seroconversion (loss of HbeAg and development of anti-Hbe antibody), and in most patients, HBV viremia returns to pretreatment levels after discontinuation of lamivudine, sometimes in association with hepatitis flare. HbeAg seroconversion appears to be durable. Lamivudine therapy can benefit patients with decompensated cirrhosis and extend the transplantation-free time. Combined use of interferon alfa and lamivudine generally shows no greater efficacy than monotherapy, although the combination may be associated with a higher frequency of HbeAg seroconversion and perhaps less resistance emergence (Schalm *et al.,* 2000).

Resistance emergence with return of detectable HBV DNA occurs in 14% to 32% of immunocompetent patients treated with lamivudine (100 mg daily) by 1 year and increases over time to over 50% by three years of therapy. The clinical significance of genotypic resistance is under study. Virologic breakthroughs are often subclinical but may be associated with clinical and biochemical deterioration. Despite higher doses of lamivudine (300 mg daily), dually infected HIV patients also have high frequencies of resistance emergence. Resistance development in HBV-infected liver-transplant recipients occurs frequently and may be associated with histological worsening.

Ribavirin

Chemistry and Antiviral Activity.   *Ribavirin* (1-β-D-ribofuranosyl-1H-1,2,4-triazole-3-carboxamide) is a purine nucleoside analog with a modified base and D-ribose sugar. Its structure is given below:

RIBAVIRIN

Ribavirin inhibits the replication of a wide range of RNA and DNA viruses, including orthomyxo-, paramyxo-, arena-, bunya-, flavi-, herpes-, adeno-, pox-, and retroviruses (Gilbert and Knight, 1986; Huggins, 1989). *In vitro* inhibitory concentrations range from 3 to 10 μg/ml for influenza, parainfluenza, and respiratory syncytial (RSV) viruses. Similar concentrations may reversibly inhibit macromolecular synthesis and proliferation of uninfected cells, suppress lymphocyte responses (Heagy *et al.,* 1991), and alter cytokine profiles *in vitro.*

Mechanisms of Action and Resistance.   The antiviral mechanism of ribavirin is not fully defined but relates to alteration of cellular nucleotide pools and inhibition of viral messenger RNA synthesis (Gilbert and Knight, 1986). Intracellular phosphorylation to the mono-, di-, and triphosphate derivatives is mediated by host cell enzymes. In both uninfected and RSV-infected cells, the predominant derivative (>80%) is the triphosphate, which has an intracellular $t_{1/2}$ of elimination of less than 2 hours.

Ribavirin monophosphate competitively inhibits cellular inosine-5'-phosphate dehydrogenase and interferes with the synthesis of guanosine triphosphate (GTP) and thus nucleic acid synthesis in general. Ribavirin triphosphate also competitively inhibits the GTP-dependent 5'-capping of viral messenger RNA, and specifically influenza virus transcriptase activity. Ribavirin appears to have multiple sites of action, and some of these (*e.g.,* inhibition of GTP synthesis) may potentiate others (*e.g.,* inhibition of GTP-dependent enzymes).

Emergence of viral resistance to ribavirin has not been documented in clinical isolates, although it has been possible to select cells that do not phosphorylate it to active forms.

Absorption, Distribution, and Elimination.   Ribavirin is actively taken up by gastrointestinal nucleoside transporters located in the proximal small bowel, and oral bioavailability averages approximately 50% (Glue, 1999). Extensive accumulation occurs in plasma, and steady state is reached by about 4 weeks. Food increases plasma levels substantially, so ingestion with food may be prudent (Glue, 1999). Following single or multiple oral doses of 600 mg and 1200 mg, peak plasma concentrations average 0.8 μg/ml and 3.7 μg/ml, respectively. After intravenous doses of 1000 mg and 500 mg, plasma concentrations average approximately 24 μg/ml and 17 μg/ml, respectively. With aerosol administration, plasma levels increase with the duration of exposure and range from 0.2 to 1.0 μg/ml after 5 days (Englund *et al.,* 1994). Levels in respiratory secretions are much higher but vary up to 1000-fold.

The apparent volume of distribution is large ($\sim$10 liters/kg) due to ribavirin's uptake into cells. Plasma protein binding is negligible. The elimination of ribavirin is complex. The plasma half-life averages 30 to 40 hours after a single dose but increases to approximately 200 to 300 hours at steady state. Ribavirin triphosphate concentrates in erythrocytes, and red blood cell levels gradually decrease with a $t_{1/2}$ of about 40 days. Hepatic metabolism and renal excretion of ribavirin and its metabolites are the principal routes of elimination. Hepatic metabolism involves deribosylation and hydrolysis to yield a triazole carboxamide. Ribavirin clearance decreases 3-fold in those with advanced renal insufficiency (CL_{cr} 10 to 30 ml/minute); the drug should be used cautiously in patients with creatinine clearances of less than 50 ml/minute.

Untoward Effects. Aerosolized ribavirin may cause mild conjunctival irritation, rash, transient wheezing, and occasional reversible deterioration in pulmonary function. When used in conjunction with mechanical ventilation, equipment modifications and frequent monitoring are required to prevent plugging of ventilator valves and tubing with ribavirin. Techniques to reduce environmental exposure of health care workers are important (Shults *et al.*, 1996).

Systemic ribavirin causes dose-related reversible anemia due to extravascular hemolysis and suppression of bone marrow (Huggins, 1989). Associated increases occur in reticulocyte counts and in serum bilirubin, iron, and uric acid concentrations. High ribavirin triphosphate levels may cause oxidative damage to membranes, leading to erythrophagocytosis by the reticuloendothelial system (De Franceschi *et al.*, 2000). Bolus intravenous infusion may cause rigors. About 20% of chronic hepatitis C patients receiving combination interferon-ribavirin therapy discontinue treatment early because of side effects. In addition to interferon toxicity, oral ribavirin increases the risk of fatigue, cough, rash, pruritus, nausea, insomnia, dyspnea, depression, and, particularly, anemia. About 8% of patients require ribavirin dose reduction because of anemia.

Preclinical studies indicate that ribavirin is teratogenic, embryotoxic, oncogenic, and possibly gonadotoxic. To prevent possible teratogenic effects, up to 6 months is required for washout following cessation of long-term treatment (Glue, 1999). **Pregnant women should not directly care for patients receiving ribavirin aerosol. Ribavirin is in FDA pregnancy category X.**

Ribavirin inhibits the phosphorylation and antiviral activity of pyrimidine nucleoside HIV reverse-transcriptase inhibitors such as zidovudine and stavudine but increases the activity of purine nucleoside reverse-transcriptase inhibitors (*e.g.*, didanosine) *in vitro*.

Therapeutic Uses. Ribavirin aerosol is approved in the United States for treatment of RSV bronchiolitis and pneumonia in hospitalized children. Aerosolized ribavirin (usual dose of 20 mg/ml for 18 hours exposure per day) may reduce some illness measures, but its use is controversial (Committee on Infectious Diseases, American Academy of Pediatrics, 2000). No consistent beneficial effects on duration of hospitalization, ventilatory support equipment, mortality, or long-term pulmonary function have been found (Randolph and Wang, 1996; Long *et al.*,

1997). High-dose, reduced-duration therapy (60 mg/ml for 2 hours, three times daily) has been used (Englund *et al.*, 1994). Infants and young children at high risk for serious RSV disease (*e.g.*, those with congenital heart disease, chronic lung disease, immunodeficiency states, prematurity, age <6 weeks), and those hospitalized with severe illness may be considered for treatment (Committee on Infectious Diseases, 1996). Aerosol ribavirin combined with intravenous immunoglobulin appears to reduce mortality of RSV infection in bone-marrow transplant and other highly immunocompromised patients (Ghosh *et al.*, 2000).

Oral ribavirin in combination with injected interferon-alfa (REBETRON) is effective for treatment of chronic hepatitis C. Ribavirin monotherapy for 6 to 12 months reversibly decreases aminotransferase elevations to normal in about 30% of patients but does not affect HCV RNA levels. Combination therapy with interferon-alfa (3 million units subcutaneously three times weekly) and oral ribavirin (500 mg, or 600 mg twice daily if weight is greater than 75 kg for 24 to 48 weeks) increases the likelihood of sustained biochemical and virologic responses to about 40% depending on genotype (Battaglia and Hagmeyer, 2000). The combination is superior to interferon alone in both treatment-naïve patients (McHutchison and Poynard, 1999) and in those not responding to or relapsing after interferon monotherapy (Barbaro *et al.*, 1999). A longer duration of therapy (48 weeks) appears to benefit those with genotype 1 infections, high plasma HCV-RNA levels, or advanced fibrosis. Combined therapy has been used in the management of recurrent HCV infection after liver transplantation (Lavezzo and Rizzetto, 1999).

Intravenous and/or aerosol ribavirin has been used occasionally in treating severe influenza virus infection and in the treatment of immunosuppressed patients with adenovirus, vaccinia, parainfluenza, or measles virus infections. Aerosolized ribavirin is associated with reduced duration of fever but no other clinical or antiviral effects in influenza infections in hospitalized children (Rodriguez *et al.*, 1994). Intravenous ribavirin decreases mortality in Lassa fever and has been used in treating other arenavirus-related hemorrhagic fevers. In hemorrhagic fever with renal syndrome due to Hantaan virus infection (Huggins *et al.*, 1991), intravenous ribavirin is beneficial, and it is under study in hantavirus-associated pulmonary syndrome. Oral ribavirin has been used for treatment of Crimean-Congo hemorrhagic fever. Intravenous ribavirin is investigational in the United States.

Imiquimod

Imiquimod (1-(2-methylpropyl)-1*H*-imidazo[4,5-c]quinolin-4 amine) is a novel immunomodulatory agent that is effective for topical treatment of condylomata acuminata (Miller *et al.,* 1999). *In vitro,* it lacks direct antiviral or antiproliferative effects but rather induces interferon-alpha, tumor necrosis factor-alpha (TNF-α), and other cytokines and chemokines. Imiquimod shows antiviral activity in animal models after systemic or topical administration. When applied topically as a 5% cream to genital warts in human beings, it induces local interferon-alpha, -beta, and -gamma and TNF-α responses and causes reductions in viral load and wart size (Tyring *et al.,* 1998). When applied topically (3 times weekly for up to 16 weeks), imiquimod cream is associated with complete clearance of treated genital and perianal warts in about 50% of patients, with response rates being higher in women than men (Slade *et al.,* 1998). The median time to clearance is 8 to 10 weeks; relapses are not uncommon. Application is associated with local erythema in about 20% of patients, excoriation/flaking in 18% to 26%, itching in 10% to 20%, burning in 5% to 12%, and less often erosions or ulcerations.

NEWER AGENTS UNDER CLINICAL DEVELOPMENT

Table 50–5 summarizes a number of antiviral agents that are in clinical development, excluding agents for HIV in-

fection. Several of the more promising agents that are in advanced stages of clinical testing are discussed below.

Adefovir

Adefovir (9-[2-phosphonylmethoxyethyl]-adenine) is a phosphonate nucelotide analog of adenosine with inhibitory activity against hepadna-, retro-, and herpesviruses. *Adefovir dipivoxil* (bis-POM PMEA) is an oral prodrug active in hepatitis B and HIV infections. Adefovir inhibits hepatitis B virus at concentrations of 0.2 to 1.2 μM in cell culture and is active against lamivudine- or famciclovir-resistant variants. Host-cell enzymes phosphorylate adefovir to the active intracellular metabolite, adefovir diphosphate, which selectively inhibits viral polymerases. The diphosphate has a prolonged intracellular half-life of 12 to 30 hours, thus enabling once-daily dosing. Upon incorporation into DNA, it acts as a chain terminator of DNA synthesis. No HBV resistance has been recognized to date.

Adefovir is poorly absorbed, but the dipivoxil prodrug is absorbed rapidly and metabolized by esterases in the intestinal mucosa or blood to adefovir with bioavailability averaging over 50%. Plasma-protein binding is negligible, and the volume of distribution approximates total body water. After intravenous administration, plasma levels decline biexponentially with a mean terminal half-life of 1.6 hours (Cundy *et al.,* 1995a). The plasma adefovir half-life after oral administration of the prodrug is 5 to 7 hours. Adefovir is eliminated unchanged by the kidney; active tubular secretion accounts for approximately 60% of the clearance.

Adefovir dipivoxil causes dose-related nephrotoxicity and tubular dysfunction, manifested by hypophosphatemia and azotemia. Higher doses (30 mg and above) cause abnormalities after

Table 50–5

Examples of Antiviral Agents Undergoing Clinical Testing

VIRUS	AGENTS	CLASSIFICATION/SITE OF ACTION	ROUTE OF ADMINISTRATION
Hepatitis B virus	Adefovir	Nucleoside DNAp inhibitor	O
	Clevudine (L-FMAN)	Nucleoside DNAp inhibitor	O
	Entecavir (BMS-200475)	Nucleoside DNAp inhibitor	O
	Emtricitabine (FTC)	Nucleoside DNAp inhibitor	O
	β-L-deoxythymidine (L-dT)	Nucleoside DNAp inhibitor	O
Cytomegalovirus	Maribavir	Nucleoside UL97 inhibitor	O
	BDCRB	Nucleoside UL98 inhibitor	O
	Lobucavir	Nucleoside DNAp inhibitor	O
Papillomavirus	Afovirsen	Antisense oligonucleotide	Injected
Rhinovirus	sICAM-1	Soluble receptor decoy	Intranasal
	Pleconaril	Capsid binder	O
	AG7088	3C protease inhibitor	Intranasal
Respiratory syncytial virus	VP 14637	Fusion inhibitor	Topical (intranasal, inhaled)
	R 170591	Fusion inhibitor	Topical (intranasal, inhaled)
Enterovirus	Pleconaril	Capsid binder	O
Influenza virus	RWJ270701	Neuraminidase inhibitor	O

KEY: DNAp, DNA polymerase; UL97, viral protein kinase; UL98, viral alkaline nuclease; O, oral.

6 to 9 months of treatment, but the doses being studied for chronic HBV (10 mg daily) have been generally well tolerated. Asthenia, headache, nausea, and diarrhea occur in some patients. Pivalic acid, a product of the metabolism of the prodrug, can esterify with free carnitine and cause depletion at high doses of adefovir dipivoxil. Preclinical studies indicate that adefovir in high doses is mutagenic and causes renal tubular nephropathy, gastrointestinal and lymphoid toxicity, embryotoxicity, and elevated transaminases and creatine phosphokinase levels in certain species.

Although associated with anti-HIV effects at doses of 60 to 120 mg daily, HIV-related clinical studies have been stopped because of toxicity concerns. Reduction of HBV DNA levels occurs at low doses, and long-term trials (10 mg and 30 mg daily) in patients with chronic hepatitis B are in progress. Combinations of adefovir and lamivudine show enhanced anti-HBV activity *in vitro* (Colledge *et al.,* 2000), and trials of dual therapy are anticipated.

Entecavir

Entecavir is a novel cyclopentyl guanosine analog that potently inhibits hepatitis B virus replication and, to a much lesser extent, herpesviruses. In hepatic cell cultures, the inhibitory concentrations are approximately 3 to 5 nM, about 30-fold lower than those of lamivudine (Innaimo *et al.,* 1997). Following phosphorylation by cellular enzymes, entecavir triphosphate, which has a prolonged intracellular half-life averaging about 15 hours, competitively inhibits HBV polymerase and affects both the priming and elongation steps of hepadnaviral DNA replication. Entecavir has high oral bioavailability and inhibits hepadnaviral replication at low oral doses in experimentally infected animals. Prolonged administration in infected woodchucks is well tolerated and appears to protect against development of hepatocellular carcinoma. Short-term entecavir treatment (0.1 to 1.0 once daily for 28 days) of patients with chronic hepatitis B is generally well tolerated and associated with significant reductions in plasma HBV DNA levels (de Man *et al.,* 2000). Other clinical studies are in progress.

Pleconaril

Pleconaril (3-[3,5 dimethyl-4[[3-(3-methyl-5-isoxazoyl)propyl] oxy]phenyl]-5-(trifluoromethyl)-1,2,4-oxadiazole) is an orally active antipicornavirus agent in advanced clinical development (Rogers *et al.,* 1999). Pleconaril binds to a hydrophobic pocket within the viral capsid and inhibits viral attachment and/or uncoating of the genome. In cell culture, pleconaril inhibits replication of over 90% of the most commonly isolated enterovirus serotypes at concentrations <0.07 μg/ml (Pevear *et al.,* 1999) and approximately 90% of rhinovirus serotypes at concentrations of 1.0 μg/ml or lower. It is active in animal models of enteroviral CNS infection and experimental human coxsackie A21 virus respiratory tract infection.

Following oral administration in adults, the time to reach maximal plasma concentrations is 1.5 to 5 hours, and the terminal half-life averages 25 hours. Peak plasma concentrations average 1.1 to 1.6 and 2.0 to 2.4 μg/ml after doses of 200 or 400 mg, respectively (Abdel-Rahman and Kearns, 1999). Ingestion with food, particularly fat, markedly increases plasma concentrations. Single oral doses of 5 mg/kg in children pro-

vide maximum plasma concentrations of 1.3 μg/ml and approximately 40% lower overall drug exposure due to a larger volume of distribution and more rapid clearance with a half-life averaging 5.7 hours (Kearns *et al.,* 1999). Pleconaril generally is well tolerated but may be associated with headache, nausea, diarrhea, and stomach discomfort.

Oral pleconaril treatment results in reduced illness duration and reduced analgesic use in adults with enteroviral meningitis (Rogers *et al.,* 1999) and appears to be beneficial in rhinovirus colds. Clinical studies of picornaviral respiratory tract disease and severe and/or life threatening enteroviral syndromes such as chronic enteroviral meningoencephalitis in agammaglobulinemic patients and neonatal sepsis are in progress.

Maribavir

Maribavir is a benzimidazole ribonucleoside that selectively inhibits CMV *in vitro* at concentrations (0.1 to 0.6 μM) about 4- to 10-fold lower than those of ganciclovir (Chulay *et al.,* 1999). It also inhibits Epstein-Barr virus replication at 0.2 to 1.1 μM concentrations but is inactive against HSV and VZV. Maribavir's unique mechanism of antiviral action involves inhibition of viral DNA synthesis but without intracellular phosphorylation or effects on viral DNA polymerase. Consequently, maribavir retains activity against CMV variants resistant to ganciclovir, foscarnet, or cidofovir. Maribavir appears to inhibit phosphorylation of certain proteins and the formation of new DNA replication complexes. Variants selected for resistance to maribavir *in vitro* have a mutation in the UL97 protein kinase, which appears to mediate its antiviral effects.

Preclinical toxicology studies indicate lack of mutagenicity and good oral bioavailability. Maribavir is extensively (98.5%) but reversibly bound to human plasma proteins. Penetration into the aqueous humor of laboratory animals is limited. Oral maribavir appears to be rapidly and well absorbed; plasma levels average about 18 μg/ml after single 400-mg doses. The plasma half-life averages 3 to 5 hours. Maribavir has been generally well tolerated but causes dose-related taste perversion with bitter or metallic taste, and, less often, headache, fatigue, and gastrointestinal disturbance. Dose-related (300 to 1200 mg/day) reductions in CMV titers in semen and urine have been found in clinical trials to date.

PROSPECTUS

More satisfactory antiviral therapies likely will come in part from the identification of agents with improved pharmacokinetic properties, greater potency, and/or improved toxicity profiles compared to existing ones. New drug-delivery techniques that improve pharmacokinetic properties or target particular tissues also will be of benefit. Prodrugs that can be used to enhance oral absorption and/or avoid degradation of the parent compound are receiving particular attention in drug development.

As in other areas of antimicrobial chemotherapy, the combined use of antiviral agents has been studied as a means of increasing antiviral activity, reducing drug dosage and the associated risk of toxicity, and preventing or modifying the development of drug resistance. Because viral isolates may be mixtures of sensitive and resistant viruses or viruses with different resistance mutations, treatment with combinations of drugs may provide broader activity than treatment with single agents. Drug combinations may constrain the mutability of the virus, enhance susceptibility to a second agent, or diminish viral replicative capacity.

Future therapeutic breakthroughs probably will depend on the identification of novel molecular targets in viruses. A particularly interesting area of investigation is gene inhibition therapy (*e.g.,* antisense oligonucleotides, ribozymes). This approach not only may inhibit active

replication but potentially may eradicate latent viral infection. The first antisense oligonucleotide has been approved for a human viral infection (fomivirsen for CMV retinitis), but important problems regarding potency, selectivity, and pharmacology remain to be solved. Interesting approaches to gene therapy include expression of mutated proteins that act as transdominant inhibitors and intracellular expression of antibody fragments against critical viral proteins. Other approaches that may prove to be useful involve agents to moderate host immunopathological responses, agents to boost host immune responses, or virus-specific immunotherapies (*e.g.,* monoclonal antibodies, therapeutic vaccines) to supplement host responses.

For further discussion of viruses causing human disease, *see* Chapters 182 through 201 in *Harrison's Principles of Internal Medicine,* 14th ed., McGraw-Hill, New York, 1998.

BIBLIOGRAPHY

Abdel-Rahman, S.M., and Kearns, G.L. Single oral dose escalation pharmacokinetics of pleconaril (VP 63,843) capsules in adults. *J. Clin. Pharmacol.,* **1999,** *39*:613–618.

Ambati, J., Wynne, K.B., Angerame, M.C., and Robinson, M.R. Anterior uveitis associated with intravenous cidofovir use in patients with cytomegalovirus retinitis. *Br. J. Ophthalmol.,* **1999,** *83*:1153–1158.

Anderson, K.P., Fox, M.C., Brown-Driver, V., Martin, M.J., and Azad, R.F. Inhibition of human cytomegalovirus immediate-early gene expression by an antisense oligonucleotide complementary to immediate-early RNA. *Antimicrob. Agents Chemother.,* **1996,** *40*:2004–2011.

Anonymous. Combination foscarnet and ganciclovir therapy vs monotherapy for the treatment of relapsed cytomegalovirus retinitis in patients with AIDS. The Cytomegalovirus Retreatment Trial. The Studies of Ocular Complications of AIDS Research Group in Collaboration with the AIDS Clinical Trials Group. *Arch. Ophthalmol.,* **1996,** *114*:23–33.

Anonymous. Parenteral cidofovir for cytomegalovirus retinitis in patients with AIDS: the HPMPC peripheral cytomegalovirus retinitis trial. A randomized, controlled trial. Studies of Ocular Complications of AIDS Research Group in Collaboration with the AIDS Clinical Trials Group. *Ann. Intern. Med.,* **1997,** *126*:264–274.

Antonelli, G., Currenti, M., Turriziani, O., and Dianzani, F. Neutralizing antibodies to interferon-alpha: relative frequency in patients treated with different interferon preparations. *J. Infect. Dis.,* **1991,** *163*:882–885.

Arevalo, J.F., Gonzalez, C., Capparelli, E.V., Kirsch, L.S., Garcia, R.F., Quiceno, J.I., Connor, J.D., Gambertoglio, J., Bergeron-Lynn, G., and Freeman, W.R. Intravitreous and plasma concentrations of ganciclovir and foscarnet after intravenous therapy in patients with AIDS and cytomegalovirus retinitis. *J. Infect. Dis.,* **1995,** *172*:951–956.

Barbaro, G., Di Lorenzo, G., Belloni, G., Ferrari, L., Paiano, A., Del Poggio, P., Bacca, D., Fruttaldo, L., Mongio, F., Francavilla, R., Scotto, G., Grisorio, B., Calleri, G., Annese, M., Barelli, A., Rocchetto, P., Rizzo, G., Gualandi, G., Poltronieri, I., and Barbarini, G. Interferon alpha-2B and ribavirin in combination for patients with chronic hepatitis C who failed to respond to, or relapsed after, interferon alpha therapy: a randomized trial. *Am. J. Med.,* **1999,** *107*:112–118.

Beltinger, C., Fulda, S., Kammertoens, T., Meyer, E., Uckert, W., and Debatin, K.M. Herpes simplex virus thymidine kinase/ganciclovir-induced apoptosis involves ligand-independent death receptor aggregation and activation of caspases. *Proc. Natl Acad. Sci. U.S.A.,* **1999,** *96*:8699–8704.

Bergdahl, S., Jacobsson, B., Moberg, L., and Sonnerborg, A. Pronounced anti-HIV-1 activity of foscarnet in patients without cytomegalovirus infection. *J. Acquir. Immune Defic. Syndr. Hum. Retrovirol.,* **1998,** *18*:51–53.

Beutner, K.R., Friedman, D.J., Forszpaniak, C., Andersen, P.L., and Wood, M.J. Valaciclovir compared with acyclovir for improved therapy for herpes zoster in immunocompetent adults. *Antimicrob. Agents Chemother,* **1995,** *39*:1546–1553.

Birch, C.J., Tyssen, D.P., Tachedjian, G., Doherty, R., Hayes, K., Mijch, A., and Lucas, C.R. Clinical effects and *in vitro* studies of trifluorothymidine combined with interferon-α for treatment of drug-resistant and -sensitive herpes simplex viral infections. *J. Infect. Dis.,* **1992,** *166*:108–112.

Biron, K.K., Stanat, S.C., Sorrell, J.B., Fyfe, J.A., Keller, P.M., Lambe, C.U., and Nelson, D.J. Metabolic activation of the nucleoside analog 9-[2-hydroxy-1-(hydroxymethyl)ethoxy]methyl guanine in human diploid fibroblasts infected with human cytomegalovirus. *Proc. Natl. Acad. Sci. U.S.A.,* **1985,** *82*:2473–2477.

Boike, S.C., Pue, M., Audet, P.R., Freed, M.I., Fairless, A., Ilson, B.E., Zariffa, N., and Jorkasky, D.K. Pharmacokinetics of famciclovir in subjects with chronic hepatic disease. *J. Clin. Pharmacol.,* **1994,** *34*:1199–1207.

Brosgart, C.L., Louis, T.A., Hillman, D.W., Craig, C.P., Alston, B., Fisher, E., Abrams, D.I., Luskin-Hawk, R.L., Sampson, J.H., Ward, D.J., Thompson, M.A., and Torres, R.A. A randomized, placebo-controlled trial of the safety and efficacy of oral ganciclovir for prophylaxis of cytomegalovirus disease in HIV-infected individuals. Terry Beirn Community Programs for Clinical Research on AIDS. *AIDS,* **1998,** *12*:269–277.

Brown, F., Banken, L., Saywell, K., and Arum, I. Pharmacokinetics of valganciclovir and ganciclovir following multiple oral dosages of valganciclovir in HIV- and CMV-seropositive volunteers. *Clin. Pharmacokinet.,* **1999,** *37*:167–176.

Cass, L., Efthymiopoulos, C., and Bye, A. Pharmacokinetics of zanamivir after intravenous, oral, inhaled or intranasal administration to healthy volunteers. *Clin. Pharmacokinet.,* **1999,** *36(suppl. 1)*:1–11.

Cass, L., Gunawardena, K.A., Macmahon, M.M., and Bye, A. Pulmonary function and airway responsiveness in mild to moderate asthmatics given repeated inhaled doses of zanamivir. *Respir. Med.,* **2000,** *94*:166–173.

Centers for Disease Control and Prevention. Guidelines for preventing opportunistic infections among hematopoietic stem cell transplant recipients. *MMWR Morb. Mortal. Wkly. Rep.,* **2000,** *49*:1–125.

Christophers, J., Clayton, J., Craske, J., Ward, R., Collins, P., Trowbridge, M., and Darby, G. Survey of resistance of herpes simplex virus to acyclovir in northwest England. *Antimicrob. Agents Chemother.,* **1998,** *42*:868–872.

Civeira, M.P., and Prieto, J. Early predictors of response to treatment in patients with chronic hepatitis C. *J. Hepatol.,* **1999,** *31(suppl. 1)*: 237–243.

Cobo, L.M., Foulks, G.N., Liesegang, T., Lass, J., Sutphin, J.E., Wilhelmus, K., Jones, D.B., Chapman, S., Segreti, A.C., and King, D.H. Oral acyclovir in the treatment of acute herpes zoster ophthalmicus. *Ophthalmology,* **1986,** *93*:763–770.

Colin, J., Hoh, H.B., Easty, D.L., Herbort, C.P., Resnikoff, S., Rigal, D., and Romdana, K. Ganciclovir ophthalmic gel (Virgan; 0.15%) in the treatment of herpes simplex keratitis. *Cornea,* **1997,** *16*:393–399.

Colledge, D., Civitico, G., Locarnini, S., and Shaw, T. In vitro antihepadnaviral activities of combinations of penciclovir, lamivudine, and adefovir. *Antimicrob. Agents Chemother.,* **2000,** *44*:551–560.

Committee on Infectious Diseases. Reassessment of the indications for ribavirin therapy in respiratory syncytial virus infections. American Academy of Pediatrics Committee on Infectious Diseases. *Pediatrics,* **1996,** *97*:137–140.

Committee on Infectious Diseases, American Academy of Pediatrics. *2000 Red Book: Report of the Committee on Infectious Diseases,* 25th ed., American Academy of Pediatrics, Elk Grove Village, IL, **2000.**

Cundy, K.C., Barditch-Crovo, P., Walker, R.E., Collier, A.C., Ebeling, D., Toole, J., and Jaffe, H.S. Clinical pharmacokinetics of adefovir in human immunodeficiency virus type 1-infected patients. *Antimicrob. Agents Chemother.,* **1995a,** *39*:2401–2405.

Cundy, K.C., Petty, B.G., Flaherty, J., Fisher, P.E., Polis, M.A., Wachsman, M., Lietman, P.S., Lalezari, J.P., Hitchcock, M.J., and Jaffe, H.S. Clinical pharmacokinetics of cidofovir in human immunodeficiency virus-infected patients. *Antimicrob. Agents Chemother.,* **1995b,** *39*:1247–1252.

De Franceschi, L., Fattovich, G., Turrini, F., Ayi, K., Brugnara, C., Manzato, F., Noventa, F., Stanzial, A.M., Solero, P., and Corrocher, R. Hemolytic anemia induced by ribavirin therapy in patients with

chronic hepatitis C virus infection: role of membrane oxidative damage. *Hepatology,* **2000,** *31*:997–1004.

de Man, R.A., Wolters, L., Nevens, F., Chua, D., Sherman, M., Lai, C.L., Thomas, N., and DeHertogh, D. Safety and efficacy of oral entecavir given for 28 days in subjects with chronic hepatitis B. Abstracts of the 40th Conference on Antimicrobial Agents and Chemotherapy. Toronto, Canada, September 17–20. **2000,** pp. 273.

Degreef, H., and the Famciclovir Herpes Zoster Clinical Study Group. Famciclovir, a new oral antiherpes drug: results of the first controlled clinical study demonstrating its efficacy and safety in the treatment of uncomplicated herpes zoster in immunocompetent patients. *Int. J. Antimicrob. Agents,* **1994,** *4*:241–246.

Diaz-Mitoma, F., Sibbald, R.G., Shafran, S.D., Boon, R., and Saltzman, R.L. Oral famciclovir for the suppression of recurrent genital herpes: a randomized controlled trial. Collaborative Famciclovir Genital Herpes Research Group. *JAMA,* **1998,** *280*:887–892.

Dienstag, J.L., Schiff, E.R., Wright, T.L., Perrillo, R.P., Hann, H.W., Goodman, Z., Crowther, L., Condreay, L.D., Woessner, M., Rubin, M., and Brown, N.A. Lamivudine as initial treatment for chronic hepatitis B in the United States. *N. Engl. J. Med.,* **1999,** *341*:1256–1263.

Englund, J.A., Champlin, R.E., Wyde, P.R., Kantarjian, H., Atmar, R.L., Tarrand, J.J., Yousuf, H., Regnery, H., Klimov, A.I., Cox, N.J., and Whimbey, E. Common emergence of amantadine- and rimantadine-resistant influenza A viruses in symptomatic immunocompromised adults. *Clin. Infect. Dis.,* **1998,** *26*:1418–1424.

Englund, J.A., Piedra, P., Ahn, Y.M., Gilbert, B.E., and Hiatt, P. High-dose, short-duration ribavirin aerosol therapy compared with standard ribavirin therapy in children with suspected respiratory syncytial virus infection. *J. Pediatr.,* **1994,** *125*:635–641.

Englund, J.A., Zimmerman, M.E., Swierkosz, E.M., Goodman, J.L., Scholl, D.R., and Balfour, H.H., Jr. Herpes simplex virus resistant to acyclovir. A study in a tertiary care center. *Ann. Intern. Med.,* **1990,** *112*:416–422.

Farci, P., Mandas, A., Coiana, A., Lai, M.E., Desmet, V., Var Eyken, P., Gibo, Y., Caruso, L., Scaccabarozzi, S., Criscuolo, D., Ryff, J.-C., and Balestrieri, A. Treatment of chronic hepatitis D with interferon alfa-2a. *N. Engl. J. Med.,* **1994,** *330*:88–94.

Feinberg, J.E., Hurwitz, S., Cooper, D., Sattler, F.R., MacGregor, R.R., Powderly, W., Holland, G.N., Griffiths, P.D., Pollard, R.B., Youle, M., Gill, M.J., Holland, F.J., Power, M.E., Owens, S., Coakley, D., Fry, J., and Jacobson, M.A. A randomized, double-blind trial of valaciclovir prophylaxis for cytomegalovirus disease in patients with advanced human immunodeficiency virus infection. AIDS Clinical Trials Group Protocol 204/Glaxo Wellcome 123-014 International CMV Prophylaxis Study Group. *J. Infect. Dis.,* **1998,** *177*:48–56.

Fife, K.H., Barbarash, R.A., Rudolph, T., Degregorio, B., and Roth, R. Valaciclovir versus acyclovir in the treatment of first-episode genital herpes infection. Results of an international, multicenter, double-blind, randomized clinical trial. The Valaciclovir International Herpes Simplex Virus Study Group. *Sex. Transm. Dis.,* **1997,** *24*:481–486.

Flechner, S.M., Avery, R.K., Fisher, R., Mastroianni, B.A., Papajcik, D.A., O'Malley, K.J., Goormastic, M., Goldfarb, D.A., Modlin, C.S., and Novick, A.C. A randomized prospective controlled trial of oral acyclovir versus oral ganciclovir for cytomegalovirus prophylaxis in high-risk kidney transplant recipients. *Transplantation,* **1998,** *66*:1682–1688.

Francois, C., Duverlie, G., Rebouillat, D., Khorsi, H., Castelain, S., Blum, H.E., Gatignol, A., Wychowski, C., Moradpour, D., and Meurs, E.F. Expression of hepatitis C virus proteins interferes with the antiviral action of interferon independently of PKR-mediated control of protein synthesis. *J. Virol.,* **2000,** *74*:5587–5596.

Frenkel, L.M., Brown, Z.A., Bryson, Y.J., Corey, L., Unadkat, J.D., Hensleigh, P.A., Arvin, A.M., Prober, C.G., and Connor, J.D. Pharmacokinetics of acyclovir in the term human pregnancy and neonate. *Am. J. Obstet. Gynecol.,* **1991,** *164*:569–576.

Ganapathy, M.E., Huang, W., Wang, H., Ganapathy, V., and Leibach, F.H. Valacyclovir: a substrate for the intestinal and renal peptide transporters PEPT1 and PEPT2. *Biochem. Biophys. Res. Commun.,* **1998,** *246*:470–475.

Gane, E., Saliba, F., Valdecasas, G.J., O'Grady, J., Pescovitz, M.D., Lyman, S., and Robinson, C.A. Randomised trial of efficacy and safety of oral ganciclovir in the prevention of cytomegalovirus disease in liver-transplant recipients. The Oral Ganciclovir International Transplantation Study Group. *Lancet,* **1997,** *350*:1729–1733.

Ghosh, S., Champlin, R.E., Englund, J., Giralt, S.A., Rolston, K., Raad, I., Jacobson, K., Neumann, J., Ippoliti, C., Mallik, S., and Whimbey, E. Respiratory syncytial virus upper respiratory tract illnesses in adult blood and marrow transplant recipients: combination therapy with aerosolized ribavirin and intravenous immunoglobulin. *Bone Marrow Transplant.,* **2000,** *25*:751–755.

Glesby, M.J., Hoover, D.R., Weng, S., Graham, N.M., Phair, J.P., Detels, R., Ho, M., and Saah, A.J. Use of antiherpes drugs and the risk of Kaposi's sarcoma: data from the Multicenter AIDS Cohort Study. *J. Infect. Dis.,* **1996,** *173*:1477–1480.

Glue, P., Rouzier-Panis, R., Raffanel, C., Sabo, R., Gupta, S.K., Salfi, M., Jacobs, S., and Clement, R.P. A dose-ranging study of pegylated interferon alfa-2b and ribavirin in chronic hepatitis C. The Hepatitis C Intervention Therapy Group. *Hepatology,* **2000,** *32*:647–653.

Goldberg, L.H., Kaufman, R., Kurtz, T.O., Conant, M.A., Eron, L.J., Batenhorst, R.L., and Boone, G.S. Long-term suppression of recurrent genital herpes with acyclovir. A 5-year benchmark. Acyclovir Study Group. *Arch. Dermatol.,* **1993,** *129*:582–587.

Goodrich, J.M., Bowden, R.A., Fisher, L., Keller, C., Schoch, G., and Meyers, J.D. Ganciclovir prophylaxis to prevent cytomegalovirus disease after allogeneic marrow transplant. *Ann. Intern. Med.,* **1993,** *118*:173–178.

Goodrich, J.M., Mori, M., Gleaves, C.A., Du Mond, C., Cays, M., Ebeling, D.F., Buhles, W.C., DeArmond, B., and Meyers, J.D. Early treatment with ganciclovir to prevent cytomegalovirus disease after allogeneic bone marrow transplantation. *N. Engl. J. Med.,* **1991,** *325*:1601–1607.

Gubareva, L.V., Matrosovich, M.N., Brenner, M.K., Bethell, R., and Webster, R.G. Evidence for zanamivir resistance in an immunocompromised child infected with influenza B virus. *J. Infect. Dis.,* **1998,** *178*:1257–1262.

Hadziyannis, S.J., Manesis, E.K., and Papakonstantinou, A. Oral ganciclovir treatment in chronic hepatitis B virus infection: a pilot study. *J. Hepatol.,* **1999,** *31*:210–214.

Hayden, F.G., Atmar, R.L., Schilling, M., Johnson, C., Poretz, D., Parr, D., Huson, L., Ward, P., and Mills, R.G. Use of the selective oral neuraminidase inhibitor oseltamivir to prevent influenza. *N. Engl. J. Med.,* **1999,** *341*:1336–1343.

Hayden, F.G., Gubareva, L.V., Monto, A.S., Klein, T.C., Elliott, M.J., Hammond, J.M., Sharp, S.J., and Ossi, M.J. Inhaled zanamivir for the prevention of influenza in families. *N. Engl. J. Med.,* **2000,** *343*:1282–1289.

Hayden, F.G., Osterhaus, A.D., Treanor, J.J., Fleming, D.M., Aoki, F.Y., Nicholson, K.G., Bohnen, A.M., Hirst, H.M., Keene, O., and Wightman, K. Efficacy and safety of the neuraminidase inhibitor

zanamivir in the treatment of influenzavirus infections. GG167 Influenza Study Group. *N. Engl. J. Med.,* **1997,** *337*:874–879.

He, G., Massarella, J., and Ward, P. Clinical pharmacokinetics of the prodrug oseltamivir and its active metabolite Ro 64-0802. *Clin. Pharmacokinet.,* **1999,** *37*:471–484.

Heagy, W., Crumpacker, C., Lopez, P.A., and Finberg, R.W. Inhibition of immune functions by antiviral drugs. *J. Clin. Invest.,* **1991,** *87*:1916–1924.

Heathcote, E.J., Shiffman, M.L., Cooksley, W.G., Dusheiko, G.M., Lee, S.S., Balart, L. Reindollar, R., Reddy, R. K., Wright, T. L., Lin, A., Hoffman, J., and De Pamphilis, J. Peginterferon alfa-2a in patients with chronic hepatitis C and cirrhosis. *N. Engl. J. Med.,* **2000,** *343*:1673–1680.

Hedrick, J.A., Barzilai, A., Behre, U., Henderson, F.W., Hammond, J., Reilly, L., and Keene, O. Zanamivir for treatment of symptomatic influenza A and B infection in children five to twelve years of age: a randomized controlled trial. *Pediatr. Infect. Dis. J.,* **2000,** *19*:410–417.

Hengge, U.R., Brockmeyer, N.H., Malessa, R., Ravens, U., and Goos, M. Foscarnet penetrates the blood-brain barrier: rationale for therapy of cytomegalovirus encephalitis. *Antimicrob. Agents Chemother.,* **1993,** *37*:1010–1014.

Hill, E.L., Hunter, G.A., and Ellis, M.N. *In vitro* and *in vivo* characterization of herpes simplex virus clinical isolates recovered from patients infected with human immunodeficiency virus. *Antimicrob. Agents Chemother.,* **1991,** *35*:2322–2328.

Hitchcock, M.J., Jaffe, H.S., Martin, J.C., and Stagg, R.J. Cidofovir, a new agent with potent anti-herpesvirus activity. *Antivir. Chem. Chemother.,* **1996,** *7*:115–127.

Ho, E.S., Lin, D.C., Mendel, D.B., and Cihlar, T. Cytotoxicity of antiviral nucleotides adefovir and cidofovir is induced by the expression of human renal organic anion transporter 1. *J. Am. Soc. Nephrol.,* **2000,** *11*:383–393.

Hochster, H., Dieterich, D., Bozzette, S., Reichman, R.C., Connor, J.D., Liebes, L., Sonke, R.L., Spector, S.A., Valentine, F., Pettineli, C., and Richman, D.D. Toxicity of combined ganciclovir and zidovudine for cytomegalovirus disease associated with AIDS. An AIDS Clinical Trials Group Study. *Ann. Intern. Med.,* **1990,** *113*:111–117.

Horadam, V.W., Sharp, J.G., Smilack, J.D., McAnalley, B.H., Garriott, J.C., Stephens, M.K., Prati, R.C., and Brater, D.C. Pharmacokinetics of amantadine hydrochloride in subjects with normal and impaired renal function. *Ann. Intern. Med.,* **1981,** *94*:454–458.

Huggins, J.W., Hsiang, C.M., Cosgriff, T.M., Guang, M.Y., Smith, J.I., Wu, Z.O., LeDue, J.W., Zheng, Z.M., Meegan, J.M., Wang, Q.N., Oland, D.D., Gui, X.E., Gibbs, P.H., Yuan, G.H., and Zhang, T.M. Prospective, double-blind, concurrent, placebo-controlled clinical trial of intravenous ribavirin therapy of hemorrhagic fever with renal syndrome. *J. Infect. Dis.,* **1991,** *164*:1119–1127.

Huycke, M.M., Naguib, M.T., Stroemmel, M.M., Blick, K., Monti, K., Martin-Munley, S., and Kaufman, C. A double-blind placebo-controlled crossover trial of intravenous magnesium sulfate for foscarnet-induced ionized hypocalcemia and hypomagnesemia in patients with AIDS and cytomegalovirus infection. *Antimicrob. Agents Chemother.,* **2000,** *44*:2143–2148.

Innaimo, S.F., Seifer, M., Bisacchi, G.S., Standring, D.N., Zahler, R., and Colonno, R.J. Identification of BMS-200475 as a potent and selective inhibitor of hepatitis B virus. *Antimicrob. Agents Chemother.,* **1997,** *41*:1444–1448.

Jabs, D.A., Enger, C., Forman, M., and Dunn, J.P. Incidence of foscarnet resistance and cidofovir resistance in patients treated for cytomegalovirus retinitis. The Cytomegalovirus Retinitis and Viral

Resistance Study Group. *Antimicrob. Agents Chemother.,* **1998,** *42:*2240–2244.

Jacobson, M.A., Gallant, J., Wang, L.H., Coakley, D., Weller, S., Gary, D., Squires, L., Smiley, M.L., Blum, M.R., and Feinberg, J. Phase I trial of valaciclovir, the L-valyl ester of acyclovir, in patients with advanced human immunodeficiency virus disease. *Antimicrob. Agents Chemother.,* **1994,** *38:*1534–1540.

Javaly, K., Wohlfeiler, M., Kalayjian, R., Klein, T., Bryson, Y., Grafford, K., Martin-Munley, S., and Hardy, W.D. Treatment of mucocutaneous herpes simplex virus infections unresponsive to acyclovir with topical foscarnet cream in AIDS patients: a phase I/II study. *J. Acquir. Immune Defic. Syndr.,* **1999,** *21:*301–306.

Jubin, R., Murray, M.G., Howe, A.Y-M., Butkiewicz, N., Hong, Z., and Lau, J.Y-N. Amantadine and rimantadine have no direct inhibitory effects against hepatitis C viral protease, helicase, ATPase, polymerase, and internal ribosomal entry site-mediated translation. *J. Infect. Dis.,* **2000,** *181:*331–334.

Jung, D., and Dorr, A. Single-dose pharmacokinetics of valganciclovir in HIV- and CMV-seropositive subjects. *J. Clin. Pharmacol.,* **1999,** *39:*800–804.

Kearns, G.L., Abdel-Rahman, S.M., James, L.P., Blowey, D.L., Marshall, J.D., Wells, T.G., and Jacobs, R.F. Single-dose pharmacokinetics of a pleconaril (VP63843) oral solution in children and adolescents. Pediatric Pharmacology Research Unit Network. *Antimicrob. Agents Chemother.,* **1999,** *43:*634–638.

Kelly, J.M., Miles, M.A., and Skinner, A.C. The anti-influenza virus drug rimantadine has trypanocidal activity. *Antimicrob. Agents Chemother.,* **1999,** *43:*985–987.

Keyser, L.A., Karl, M., Nafziger, A.N., and Bertino, J.S., Jr. Comparison of central nervous system adverse effects of amantadine and rimantadine used as sequential prophylaxis of influenza A in elderly nursing home patients. *Arch. Intern. Med.,* **2000,** *160:*1485–1488.

Kim, C.U., Lew, W., Williams, M.A., Liu, H., Zhang, L., Swaminathan, S., Bischofberger, H., Chen, M.S., Mendel, D.B., Tai, C.Y., Laver, W.G., and Stevens, R.C. Influenza neuraminidase inhibitors possessing a novel hydrophobic interaction in the enzyme active site: design, synthesis, and structural analysis of carbocyclic sialic acid analogues with potent anti-influenza activity. *J. Am. Chem. Soc.,* **1997,** *119:*681–690.

Kimberlin, D.F., Weller, S., Whitley, R.J., Andrews, W.W., Hauth, J.C., Lakeman, F., and Miller, G. Pharmacokinetics of oral valacyclovir and acyclovir in late pregnancy. *Am. J. Obstet. Gynecol.,* **1998,** *179:*846–851.

Kimberlin, D.W., Jacobs, R.F., Powell, D.A., Corey, L., Gruber, W., Rathore, M., Bradley, J., Diaz, P., Kumar, M., Arvin, A.M., Shelton, M., Weiner, L.B., Sleasman, J.W., Sierra, T., Lin, C.Y., Soong, S.J., Lakeman, F.D., Whitley, R.J., and the NIAD Collaborative Antiviral Study Group (CASG). The safety and efficacy of high-dose (HD) acyclovir (ACV) in neonatal herpes simplex virus (HSV) infections. *Pediatr. Res.,* **1999,** *37:*165A.

Kruger, R.M., Shannon, W.D., Arens, M.Q., Lynch, J.P., Storch, G.A., and Trulock, E.P. The impact of ganciclovir-resistant cytomegalovirus infection after lung transplantation. *Transplantation,* **1999,** *68:*1272–1279.

Kumagai, T., Kamada, M., Igarashi, C., Yuri, K., Furukawa, H., Chiba, S., Kojima, H., Saito, A., Okui, T., and Yano, S. Varicella-zoster virus—specific cellular immunity in subjects given acyclovir after household chickenpox exposure. *J. Infect. Dis.,* **1999,** *180:*834–837.

Lai, C.L., Chien, R.N., Leung, N., Chang, T.T., Guan, R., Tai, D.I., Ng, K.Y., Wu, P.C., Dent, J.C., Barber, J., Stephenson, S.L., and

Gray, D.F. A one-year trial of lamivudine for chronic hepatitis B. Asia Hepatitis Lamivudine Study Group. *N. Engl. J. Med.,* **1998,** *339:*61–68.

Lalezari, J., Holland, G.N., Kramer, F., McKinley, G.F., Kemper, C.A., Ives, D.V., Nelson, R., Hardy, W.D., Kuppermann, B.D., Northfelt, D.W., Youle, M., Johnson, M., Lewis, R.A., Weinberg, D.V., Simon, G.L., Wolitz, R.A., Ruby, A.E., Stagg, R.J., and Jaffe, H.S. Randomized, controlled study of the safety and efficacy of intravenous cidofovir for the treatment of relapsing cytomegalovirus retinitis in patients with AIDS. *J. Acquir. Immune Defic. Syndr. Hum. Retrovirol.,* **1998,** *17:*339–344.

Lalezari, J., Schacker, T., Feinberg, J., Gathe, J., Lee, S., Cheung, T., Kramer, F., Kessler, H., Corey, L., Drew, W.L., Boggs, J., McGuire, B., Jaffe, H.S., and Safrin, S. A randomized, double-blind, placebo-controlled trial of cidofovir gel for the treatment of acyclovir-unresponsive mucocutaneous herpes simplex virus infection in patients with AIDS. *J. Infect. Dis.,* **1997,** *176:*892–898.

Lalezari, J.P., Drew, W.L., Glutzer, E., Miner, D., Safrin, S., Owen, W.J., Jr., Dawdson, J.M., Fisher, P.E., and Jaffe, H.S. Treatment with intravenous (S)-1-[3-hydroxy-2-(phosphonylmethoxy)propyl]-cytosine of acyclovir-resistant mucocutaneous infection with herpes simplex virus in a patient with AIDS. *J. Infect. Dis.,* **1994,** *170:*570–572.

Lau, D.T., Everhart, J., Kleiner, D.E., Park, Y., Vergalla, J., Schmid, P., and Hoofnagle, J.H. Long-term follow-up of patients with chronic hepatitis B treated with interferon alfa. *Gastroenterology,* **1997,** *113:*1660–1667.

Lazarus, H.M., Belanger, R., Candoni, A., Aoun, M., Jurewicz, R., and Marks, L. Intravenous penciclovir for treatment of herpes simplex infections in immunocompromised patients: results of a multicenter, acyclovir-controlled trial. The Penciclovir Immunocompromised Study Group. *Antimicrob. Agents Chemother.,* **1999,** *43:*1192–1197.

Leeds, J.M., Henry, S.P., Bistner, S., Scherrill, S., Williams, K., and Levin, A.A. Pharmacokinetics of an antisense oligonucleotide injected intravitreally in monkeys. *Drug Metab. Dispos.,* **1998,** *26:*670–675.

Long, C.E., Voter, K.Z., Barker, W.H., and Hall, C.B. Long term follow-up of children hospitalized with respiratory syncytial virus lower respiratory tract infection and randomly treated with ribavirin or placebo. *Pediatr. Infect. Dis. J.,* **1997,** *16:*1023–1028.

Loveless, M., Sacks, S.L., and Harris, R.J. Famciclovir in the management of first-episode genital herpes. *Infect. Dis. Clin. Pract.,* **1997,** *6(suppl. 1):*S12–S16.

Lowance, D., Neumayer, H., Legendre, C.M., Squifflet, J.P., Kovarik, J., Brennan, J., Norman, D., Mendez, R., Keating, M.R., Coggon, G.L., Crisp, A., and Lee, I.C. Valacyclovir for the prevention of cytomegalovirus disease after renal transplantation. International Valacyclovir Cytomegalovirus Prophylaxis Transplantation Study Group. *N. Engl. J. Med.,* **1999,** *340:*1462–1470.

McHutchison, J.G., and Poynard, T. Combination therapy with interferon plus ribavirin for the initial treatment of chronic hepatitis C. *Semin. Liver Dis.,* **1999,** *19(suppl. 1):*57–65.

Manns, M.P., McHutchison, J.G., Gordon, S., Rustgi, V, Schiffman, M.L., Lee, W.M., Ling, M.L., Cort, S., and Albrecht, J.K. Peginterferon alfa-2b plus ribavirin compared to interferon alfa-2b plus ribavirin for treatment of chronic hepatitis C: 24-week treatment analysis of a multicenter, multinational phase III randomized controlled trial. Presidential Plenary Session II. Abstract 552. Presented at the 51st Annual Meeting of American Association for the Study of Liver Diseases (AASLD), Dallas, TX, October 27–31, **2000.**

Marroni, M., Gresele, P., Londonio, G., Lazzarin, A., Coen, M., Vezza, R., Sinnone, M.S., Boschetti, E., Nosari, A.M., Stagni, G., Nenci, G.G., and Paluzzi, S. Interferon-α is effective in the treatment of HIV-1–related, severe, zidovudine-resistant thrombocytopenia. A prospective, placebo-controlled, double-blind trial. *Ann. Intern. Med.,* **1994,** *121*:423–429.

Martin, D.F., Kuppermann, B.D., Wolitz, R.A., Palestine, A.G., Li, H., and Robinson, C.A. Oral ganciclovir for patients with cytomegalovirus retinitis treated with a ganciclovir implant. Roche Ganciclovir Study Group. *N. Engl. J. Med.,* **1999,** *340*:1063–1070.

Mendel, D.B., Tai, C.Y., Escarpe, P.A., Li, W., Sidwell, R.W., Huffman, J.H., Sweat, C., Jakeman, K.J., Merson, J., Lacy, S.A., Lew, W., Williams, M.A., Zhang, L., Chen, M.S., Bischofberger, N., and Kim, C.U. Oral administration of a prodrug of the influenza virus neuraminidase inhibitor GS 4071 protects mice and ferrets against influenza infection. *Antimicrob. Agents Chemother.,* **1998,** *42*:640–646.

Miller, R.L., Gerster, J.F., Owens, M.L., Slade, H.B., and Tomai, M.A. Imiquimod applied topically: a novel immune response modifier and new class of drug. *Int. J. Immunopharmacol.,* **1999,** *21*:1–14.

Monto, A.S., Robinson, D.P., Herlocher, M.L., Hinson, J.M., Jr., Elliott, M.J., and Crisp, A. Zanamivir in the prevention of influenza among healthy adults. *JAMA,* **1999,** *282*:31–36.

Moretti, S., Zikos, P., Van Lint, M.T., Tedone, E., Occhini, D., Gualandi, F., Lamparelli, T., Mordini, N., Berisso, G., Bregante, S., Bruno, B., and Bachgalupo, A. Forscarnet vs ganciclovir for cytomegalovirus (CMV) antigenemia after allogeneic hemopoietic stem cell transplantation (HSCT): a randomised study. *Bone Marrow Transplant.,* **1998,** *22*:175–180.

Mulamba, G.B., Hu, A., Azad, R.F., Anderson, K.P., and Coen, D.M. Human cytomegalovirus mutant with sequence-dependent resistance to the phosphorothioate oligonucleotide fomivirsen (ISIS 2922). *Antimicrob. Agents Chemother.,* **1998,** *42*:971–973.

Musch, D.C., Martin, D.F., Gordon, J.F., Davis, M.D., and Kuppermann, B.D. Treatment of cytomegalovirus retinitis with a sustained-release ganciclovir implant. The Ganciclovir Implant Study Group. *N. Engl. J. Med.,* **1997,** *337*:83–90.

Mutimer, D., Pillay, D., Cook, P., Ratcliffe, D., O'Donnell, K., Dowling, D., Shaw, J., Elias, E., and Cane, P.A. Selection of multiresistant hepatitis B virus during sequential nucleoside-analogue therapy. *J. Infect. Dis.,* **2000,** *181*:713–716.

Neyts, J., Andrei, G., and De Clercq, E. The novel immunosuppressive agent mycophenolate mofetil markedly potentiates the antiherpesvirus activities of acyclovir, ganciclovir, and penciclovir in vitro and in vivo. *Antimicrob. Agents Chemother.,* **1998,** *42*:216–222.

Nichols, W.G., and Boeckh, M. Recent advances in the therapy and prevention of CMV infections. *J. Clin. Virol.,* **2000,** *16*:25–40.

Packer, R.J., Raffel, C., Villablanca, J.G., Tonn, J.C., Burdach, S.E., Burger, K., LaFond, D., McComb, J.G., Cogen, P.H., Vezina, G., and Kapcala, L.P. Treatment of progressive or recurrent pediatric malignant supratentorial brain tumors with herpes simplex virus thymidine kinase gene vector-producer cells followed by intravenous ganciclovir administration. *J. Neurosurg.,* **2000,** *92*:249–254.

Patel, R., Bodsworth, N.J., Woolley, P., Peters, B., Vejlsgaard, G., Saari, S., Gibb, A., and Robinson, J. Valaciclovir for the suppression of recurrent genital HSV infection: a placebo controlled study of once daily therapy. International Valaciclovir HSV Study Group. *Genitourin. Med.,* **1997,** *73*:105–109.

Peng, A.W., Hussey, E.K., Rosolowski, B., and Blumer, J.L. Pharmacokinetics and tolerability of a single inhaled dose of zanamivir in children. *Curr. Ther. Res. Clin. Exp.,* **2000a,** *61*:36–46.

Peng, A.W., Milleri, S., and Stein, D.S. Direct measurement of the anti-influenza agent zanamivir in the respiratory tract following inhalation. *Antimicrob. Agents Chemother.,* **2000b,** *44*:1974–1976.

Peters, P.H., Norwood, P., DeBock, V., VanCouter, T., Gibbens, M., VonPlanta, T., and Ward, P. Oseltamivir is effective in the long-term prophylaxis of influenza in vaccinated frail elderly. Abstracts of the II International Symposium on Influenza and other Respiratory Viruses, December 10–12. Grand Cayman, Cayman Islands, British West Indies, **1999.**

Pevear, D.C., Tull, T.M., Seipel, M.E., and Groarke, J.M. Activity of pleconaril against enteroviruses. *Antimicrob. Agents Chemother.,* **1999,** *43*:2109–2115.

Pillay, D. Working Party Report: Management of herpes virus infections following transplantation. *J. Antimicrob. Chemother.,* **2000,** *45*:729–748.

Pope, L.E., Marcelletti, J.F., Katz, L.R., Lin, J.Y., Katz, D.H., Parish, M.L., and Spear, P.G. The anti-herpes simplex virus activity of *n*-docosanol includes inhibition of the viral entry process. *Antiviral Res.,* **1998,** *40*:85–94.

Prentice, H.G., Gluckman, E., Powles, R.L., Ljungman, P., Milpied, N., Fernandez Ranada, J.M., Mandelli, F., Kho, P., Kennedy, L., and Bell, A.R. Impact of long-term acyclovir on cytomegalovirus infection and survival after allogeneic bone marrow transplantation. European Acyclovir for CMV Prophylaxis Study Group. *Lancet,* **1994,** *343*:749–753.

Reiff-Eldridge, R., Heffner, C.R., Ephross, S.A., Tennis, P.S., White, A.D., and Andrews, E.B. Monitoring pregnancy outcomes after prenatal drug exposure through prospective pregnancy registries: a pharmaceutical company commitment. *Am. J. Obstet. Gynecol.,* **2000,** *182*:159–163.

Rodriguez, W.J., Hall, C.B., Welliver, R., Simoes, E.A., Ryan, M.E., Stutman, H., Johnson, G., VanDyke, R., Groothuis, J.R., Arrobio, J., and Schnabel, K. Efficacy and safety of aerosolized ribavirin in young children hospitalized with influenza: a double-blind, multicenter, placebo-controlled trial. *J. Pediatr.,* **1994,** *125*:129–135.

Sacks, S.L., Sasadeusz, J.J., and Shafran, S.D. Effect of long-term famciclovir treatment on sperm parameters in patients with recurrent genital herpes. 8th International Congress on Infectious Diseases, Boston, MA, Abst. #22.022. **1998.**

Safrin, S., Crumpacker, C.S., Chatis, P., Davis, R., Hafner, R., Rush, J., Kessler, H.A., Landry, B., and Mills, J. A controlled trial comparing foscarnet with vidarabine for acyclovir-resistant mucocutaneous herpes simplex in the acquired immunodeficiency syndrome. The AIDS Clinical Trials Group. *N. Engl. J. Med.,* **1991,** *325*:551–555.

Safrin, S., Kemmerly, S., Plotkin, B., Smith, T., Weissbach, N., De Veranez, D., Phan, L.D., and Cohn, D. Foscarnet-resistant herpes simplex virus infection in patients with AIDS. *J. Infect. Dis.,* **1994,** *169*:193–196.

Saltzman, R., Jurewicz, R., and Boon, R. Safety of famciclovir in patients with herpes zoster and genital herpes. *Antimicrob. Agents Chemother.,* **1994,** *38*:2454–2457.

Sawyer, M.H., Webb, D.E., Balow, J.E., and Straus, S.E. Acyclovir-induced renal failure. Clinical course and histology. *Am. J. Med.,* **1988,** *84*:1067–1071.

Schalm, S.W., Heathcote, J., Cianciara, J., Farrell, G., Sherman, M., Willems, B., Dhillon, A., Moorat, A., Barber, J., and Gray, D.F. Lamivudine and alpha interferon combination treatment of patients with chronic hepatitis B infection: a randomised trial. *Gut,* **2000,** *46*:562–568.

Schmidt, G.M., Horak, D.A., Niland, J.C., Duncan, S.R., Forman, S.J., and Zaia, J.A. A randomized, controlled trial of prophylactic ganciclovir for cytomegalovirus pulmonary infection in recipients of allogeneic bone marrow transplants; The City of Hope-Stanford-Syntex CMV Study Group. *N. Engl. J. Med.,* **1991,** *324*:1005–1011.

Schmit, I., and Boivin, G. Characterization of the DNA polymerase and thymidine kinase genes of herpes simplex virus isolates from AIDS patients in whom acyclovir and foscarnet therapy sequentially failed. *J. Infect. Dis.,* **1999,** *180*:487–490.

Shults, R.A., Baron, S., Decker, J., Deitchman, S.D., and Connor, J.D. Health care worker exposure to aerosolized ribavirin: biological and air monitoring. *J. Occup. Environ. Med.,* **1996,** *38*:257–263.

Singh, N., Yu, V.L., Mieles, L., Wagener, M.M., Miner, R.C., and Gayowski, T. High-dose acyclovir compared with short-course pre-emptive ganciclovir therapy to prevent cytomegalovirus disease in liver transplant recipients. A randomized trial. *Ann. Intern. Med.,* **1994,** *120*:375–381.

Slade, H.B., Owens, M.L., Tomai, M.A., and Miller, R.L. Imiquimod 5% cream (Aldara). *Expert Opin. Investig. Drugs,* **1998,** *7*:437–449.

Snoeck, R., Wellens, W., Desloovere, C., Van Ranst, M., Naesens, L., De Clercq, E., and Feenstra, L. Treatment of severe laryngeal papillomatosis with intralesional injections of cidofovir [(S)-1-(3-hydroxy-2-phosphonylmethoxypropyl)cytosine]. *J. Med. Virol.,* **1998,** *54*:219–225.

Sokal, E.M., Conjeevaram, H.S., Roberts, E.A., Alvarez, F., Bern, E.M., Goyens, P., Rosenthal, P., Lachaux, A., Shelton, M., Sarles, J., and Hoofnagle, J. Interferon alfa therapy for chronic hepatitis B in children: a multinational randomized controlled trial. *Gastroenterology,* **1998,** *114*:988–995.

Sokal, E.M., Roberts, E.A., Mieli-Vergani, G., McPhillips, P., Johnson, M., Barber, J., Dallow, N., Boxall, E., and Kelly, D. A dose-ranging study of the pharmacokinetics, safety, and preliminary efficacy of lamivudine in children and adolescents with chronic hepatitis B. *Antimicrob. Agents Chemother.,* **2000,** *44*:590–597.

Spector, S.A., McKinley, G.F., Lalezari, J.P., Samo, T., Andruczk, R., Follansbee, S., Sparti, P.D., Havlir, D.V., Simpson, G., Buhles, W., Wong, R., and Stempien, M. Oral ganciclovir for the prevention of cytomegalovirus disease in persons with AIDS. Roche Cooperative Oral Ganciclovir Study Group. *N. Engl. J. Med.,* **1996,** *334*:1491–1497.

Spruance, S.L., Hamill, M.L., Hoge, W.S., Davis, L.G., and Mills, J. Acyclovir prevents reactivation of herpes simplex labialis in skiers. *JAMA,* **1988,** *260*:1597–1599.

Spruance, S.L., Rea, T.L., Thoming, C., Tucker, R., Saltzman, R., and Boon, R. Penciclovir cream for the treatment of herpes simplex labialis. A randomized, multicenter, double-blind, placebo-controlled trial. Topical Penciclovir Collaborative Study Group. *JAMA,* **1997,** *277*:1374–1379.

Stanat, S.C., Reardon, J.E., Erice, A., Jordan, M.C., Drew, W.L., and Biron, K.K. Ganciclovir-resistant cytomegalovirus clinical isolates: mode of resistance to ganciclovir. *Antimicrob. Agents Chemother.,* **1991,** *35*:2191–2197.

Steer, C.B., Szer, J., Sasadeusz, J., Matthews, J.P., Beresford, J.A., and Grigg, A. Varicella-zoster infection after allogeneic bone marrow transplantation: incidence, risk factors and prevention with low-dose aciclovir and ganciclovir. *Bone Marrow Transplant.,* **2000,** *25*:657–664.

Steingrimsdottir, H., Gruber, A., Palm, C., Grimfors, G., Kalin, M., and Eksborg, S. Bioavailability of aciclovir after oral administration of aciclovir and its prodrug valaciclovir to patients with leukopenia after chemotherapy. *Antimicrob. Agents Chemother.,* **2000,** *44*:207–209.

Studies of Ocular Complications of AIDS Research Group. Mortality in patients with the acquired immunodeficiency syndrome treated with either foscarnet or ganciclovir for cytomegalovirus retinitis. *N. Engl. J. Med.,* **1992,** *326*:213–220.

Tatarowicz, W.A., Lurain, N.S., and Thompson, K.D. A ganciclovir-resistant clinical isolate of human cytomegalovirus exhibiting cross-resistance to other DNA polymerase inhibitors. *J. Infect. Dis.,* **1992,** *166*:904–907.

Treanor, J.J., Hayden, F.G., Vrooman, P.S., Barbarash, R.A., Bettis, R., Riff, D., Singh, S., Kinnersley, N., Ward, P., and Mills, R.G. Efficacy and safety of the oral neuraminidase inhibitor oseltamivir in treating acute influenza: a randomized controlled trial. US Oral Neuraminidase Study Group. *JAMA,* **2000,** *283*:1016–1024.

Trepo, C., Jezek, P., Atkinson, G.F., Boon, R.J., and Young, C. Famciclovir in chronic hepatitis B: results of a dose-finding study. *J. Hepatol.,* **2000,** *32*:1011–1018.

Tyring, S., Engst, R., Lassonde, M.T.S., Van Slycken, S., Crann, R., Locke, L., and Palestine, A. Famciclovir for the treatment of ophthalmic herpes zoster (HZO). Abstracts of the 38th Interscience Conference on Antimicrobial Agents and Chemotherapy, San Diego, (Abst. #LB-3), **1998a.**

Tyring, S.K., Arany, I., Stanley, M.A., Tomai, M.A., Miller, R.L., Smith, M.H., McDermott, D.J., and Slade, H.B. A randomized, controlled, molecular study of condylomata acuminata clearance during treatment with imiquimod. *J. Infect. Dis.,* **1998,** *178*:551–555.

Tyring, S.K., Beutner, K., Tucker, B.A., Anderson, W.C., and Crooks, J. Antiviral therapy for herpes zoster: randomized, controlled clinical trial of valacyclovir and famciclovir therapy in immunocompetent patients 50 years and older. *Arch. Fam. Med.,* **2000,** *9*:863–869.

Tyring, S.K., Douglas, J.M. Jr., Corey, L., Spruance, S.L., and Esmann, J. A randomized, placebo-controlled comparison of oval valacyclovir and acyclovir in immunocompetent patients with recurrent genital herpes infections. The Valaciclovir International Study Group. *Arch. Dermatol.,* **1998b,** *134*:185–191.

von Itzstein, M., Wu, W.Y., Kok, G.B., Pegg, M.S., Dyason, J.C., Jin, B., Van Phan, T., Smythe, M.L., White, H.F., Oliver, S.W., Colman, P.M., Varghese, J.N., Ryan, D.M., Woods, J.M., Bethell, R.C., Hotham, V.J., Cameron, J.M., and Penn, C.R. Rational design of potent sialidase-based inhibitors of influenza virus replication. *Nature,* **1993,** *363*:418–423.

Wade, J.C., Newton, B., McLaren, C., Fluornoy, N., Keeney, R.E., and Meyers, J.D. Intravenous acyclovir to treat mucocutaneous herpes simplex infection after marrow transplantation: a double-blind trial. *Ann. Intern. Med.,* **1982,** *96*:265–269.

Wallace, M.R., Bowler, W.A., Murray, N.B., Brodine, S.K., and Oldfield, E.C. III. Treatment of adult varicella with oral acyclovir. A randomized, placebo-controlled trial. *Ann. Intern. Med.,* **1992,** *117*:358–363.

Whitley, R.J., Alford, C.A., Hirsch, M.S., Schooley, R.T., Luby, J.P., Aoki, F.Y., Hanley, D., Nahmias, A.J., and Soong, S.J., Vidarabine versus acyclovir therapy in herpes simplex encephalitis. *N. Engl. J. Med.,* **1986,** *314*:144–149.

Whitley, R.J., Cloud, G., Gruber, W., Storch, G.A., Demmler, G.J., Jacobs, R.F., Dankner, W., Spector, S.A., Starr, S., Pass, R.F., Stagno, S., Britt, W.H., Alford, C., Jr., Soong, S., Zhou, X.J., Sherrill, L., FitzGerald, J.M., and Sommadossi, J.P. Ganciclovir treatment of symptomatic congenital cytomegalovirus infection: results of a phase II study. National Institute of Allergy and Infectious Diseases Collaborative Antiviral Study Group. *J. Infect. Dis.,* **1997,** *175*:1080–1086.

Whitley, R.J., Hayden, F.G., Reisinger, K.S., Young, N., Dutkowski, R., Ipe, D., Mills, R.G., and Ward, P. Oral oseltamivir treatment of influenza in children. *Pediatr. Infect. Dis. J.,* **2001,** *20*:127–133.

Whitley, R.J., Weiss, H., Gnann, J.W., Jr., Tyring, S., Mertz, G.J., Pappas, P.G., Schleupner, C.J., Hayden, F., Wolf, J., and Soong, S.J. Acyclovir with and without prednisone for the treatment of herpes zoster. A randomized, placebo-controlled trial. The National Institute of Allergy and Infectious Diseases Collaborative Antiviral Study Group. *Ann. Intern. Med.,* **1996,** *125*:376–383.

Wills, R.J., Farolino, D.A., Choma, N., and Keigher, N. Rimantadine pharmacokinetics after single and multiple doses. *Antimicrob. Agents Chemother.,* **1987,** *31*:826–828.

Wood, M.J., Shukla, S., Fiddian, A.P., and Crooks, R.J. Treatment of acute herpes zoster: effect of early (<48 h) versus late (48–72 h) therapy with acyclovir and valaciclovir on prolonged pain. *J. Infect. Dis.,* **1998,** *178(suppl. 1)*:S81–S84.

Woods, J.M., Bethell, R.C., Coates, J.A., Healy, N., Hiscox, S.A., Pearson, B.A., Ryan, D.M., Ticehurst, J., Tilling, J., and Walcott, S.M. 4-Guanidino-2,4-dideoxy-2,3-dehydro-N-acetylneuraminic acid is a highly effective inhibitor both of the sialidase (neuraminidase) and of growth of a wide range of influenza A and B viruses in vitro. *Antimicrob. Agents Chemother.,* **1993,** *37*:1473–1479.

Yeh, C.T., Chien, R.N., Chu, C.M., and Liaw, Y.F. Clearance of the original hepatitis B virus YMDD-motif mutants with emergence of distinct lamivudine-resistant mutants during prolonged lamivudine therapy. *Hepatology,* **2000,** *31*:1318–1326.

Yoshida, H., Shiratori, Y., Moriyama, M., Arakawa, K., Ide, T., Sata, M., Inoue, O., Yano, M., Tanaka, M., Fujiyama, S., Nishiguchi, S., Kuroki, T., Imazeki, F., Yokosuka, O., Kinoyama, S., Yamada, G., and Omata, M. Interferon therapy reduces the risk for hepatocellular carcinoma: national surveillance program of cirrhotic and noncirrhotic patients with chronic hepatitis C in Japan. IHIT Study Group. Inhibition of Hepatocarcinogenesis by Interferon Therapy. *Ann. Intern. Med.,* **1999,** *131*:174–181.

Younossi, Z.M., and Perrillo, R.P. The roles of amantadine, rimantadine, ursodeoxycholic acid, and NSAIDs, alone or in combination with alpha interferons, in the treatment of chronic hepatitis C. *Semin. Liver Dis.,* **1999,** *19(suppl. 1)*:95–102.

Zabawski, E.J., Jr., and Cockerell, C.J. Topical and intralesional cidofovir: a review of pharmacology and therapeutic effects. *J. Am. Acad. Dermatol.,* **1998,** *39*:741–745.

Zeuzem, S., Feinman, V., Rasenack, J., Heathcote, J., Lai, M.Y., Gane, E., O'Grady, J., Reichen, J., Diago, M., Lin, A., Hoffman, J., and Brunda, M.J. Peginterferon alfa-2a in patients with chronic hepatitis C. *N. Engl. J. Med.,* **2000,** *343*:1666–1672.

Ziegler, T., Hemphill, M.L., Ziegler, M.L., Perez-Oronoz, G., Klimov, A.I., Hampson, A.W., Regnery, H.L., and Cox, N.J. Low incidence of rimantadine resistance in field isolates of influenza A viruses. *J. Infect. Dis.,* **1999,** *180*:935–939.

MONOGRAPHS AND REVIEWS

Anonymous. Docosanol cream (abreva) for recurrent herpes labialis. *Med. Lett. Drugs Ther.,* **2000,** *42*:108.

Aoki, F.Y., and Sitar, D.S. Clinical pharmacokinetics of amantadine hydrochloride. *Clin. Pharmacokinet.,* **1988,** *14*:35–51.

Balfour, H.H., Jr. Antiviral drugs. *N. Engl. J. Med.,* **1999,** *340*:1255–1268.

Baron, S., Coppenhaver, D.H., and Dianzani, F., et al. Introduction to the interferon system. In, *Interferon: Principles and Medical Applications.* (Baron, S., Dianzani, F., Stanton, G.J., Fleischmann, W.R., Jr., Coppenhaver, D.H., Hughes, T.K., Klimpel, G.R., Niesel, D.W., and Tyring, S.K., eds.) University of Texas Medical Branch Dept. of Microbiology, Galveston, TX, **1992,** pp. 1–15.

Battaglia, A.M., and Hagmeyer, K.O. Combination therapy with interferon and ribavirin in the treatment of chronic hepatitis C infection. *Ann. Pharmacother.,* **2000,** *34*:487–494.

Blum, R.M., Liao, S.H., and de Miranda, P. Overview of acyclovir pharmacokinetic disposition in adults and children. *Am. J. Med.,* **1982,** *73*:186–192.

Bocci, V. Pharmacokinetics and interferons and routes of administration. In, *Interferon: Principles and Medical Applications.* (Baron, S., Dianzani, F., Stanton, G.J., Fleischmann, W.R., Jr., Coppenhaver, D.H., Hughes, T.K., Klimpel, G.R., Niesel, D.W., and Tyring, S.K., eds.) University of Texas Medical Branch Dept. of Microbiology, Galveston, TX, **1992,** pp. 417–425.

Boyd, M.R., Kern, E.R., and Safrin, S. Penciclovir: a review of its spectrum of activity, selectivity, and cross-resistance pattern. *Antivir. Chem. Chemother.,* **1993,** *4(suppl. 1)*:3–11.

Carmine, A.A., Brogden, R.N., Heel, R.C., Speight, T.M., and Avery, G.S. Trifluridine: a review of its antiviral activity and therapeutic use in the topical treatment of viral eye infections. *Drugs,* **1982,** *23*:329–353.

Chrisp, P., and Clissold, S.P. Foscarnet. A review of its antiviral activity, pharmacokinetic properties and therapeutic use in immunocompromised patients with cytomegalovirus retinitis. *Drugs,* **1991,** *41*:104–129.

Chulay, J., Biron, K., Wang, L., Underwood, M., Chamberlain, S., Frick, L., Good, S., Davis, M., Harvey, R., Townsend, L., Drach, J., and Koszalka, G. Development of novel benzimidazole riboside compounds for treatment of cytomegalovirus disease. In, *Antiviral Chemotherapy,* 5th ed. (Mills, J., Volberding, P., and Corey, L., eds.) Plenum Publishers, New York, **1999,** pp. 129–134.

Cundy, K.C. Clinical pharmacokinetics of the antiviral nucleotide analogues cidofovir and adefovir. *Clin. Pharmacokinet.,* **1999,** *36*:127–143.

Drew, W.L. Cytomegalovirus infection in patients with AIDS. *Clin. Infect. Dis.,* **1992,** *14*:608–615.

Dusheiko, G. Side effects of alpha interferon in chronic hepatitis C. *Hepatology,* **1997,** *26*:112S–121S.

Elion, G.B. History, mechanism of action, spectrum and selectivity of nucleoside analogs. In, *Antiviral Chemotherapy: New Directions for Clinical Application and Research,* (Mills, J., and Corey, L., eds.) Elsevier, New York, **1986,** pp. 118–137.

Erice, A. Resistance of human cytomegalovirus to antiviral drugs. *Clin. Microbiol. Rev.,* **1999,** *12*:286–297.

Faulds, D., and Heel, R.C. Ganciclovir. A review of its antiviral activity, pharmacokinetic properties and therapeutic efficacy in cytomegalovirus infections. *Drugs,* **1990,** *39*:597–638.

Frazer, I.H., and McMillan, A.J. Papillomatosis and condylomata acuminata. In, *Clinical Applications of the Interferons.* (Stuart-Harris, R., and Penny, R.D., eds.) Chapman & Hall, London, **1997,** pp. 79–90.

Gilbert, B.E., and Knight, V. Biochemistry and clinical applications of ribavirin. *Antimicrob. Agents Chemother.,* **1986,** *30*:201–205.

Gill, K.S., and Wood, M.J. The clinical pharmacokinetics of famciclovir. *Clin. Pharmacokinet.,* **1996,** *31*:1–8.

Gish, R.G. Standards of treatment in chronic hepatitis C. *Semin. Liver Dis.,* **1999,** *19(suppl. 1)*:35–47.

Glue, P. The clinical pharmacology of ribavirin. *Semin. Liver Dis.,* **1999,** *19(suppl. 1)*:17–24.

Gubareva, L.V., Kaiser, L., and Hayden, F.G. Influenza virus neuraminidase inhibitors. *Lancet,* **2000,** *355*:827–835.

Haefeli, W.E., Schoenenberger, R.A., Weiss, P., and Ritz, R.F. Acyclovir-induced neurotoxicity: concentration-side effect relationship in acyclovir overdose. *Am. J. Med.,* **1993,** *94*:212–215.

Haria, M., and Benfield, P. Interferon-alpha-2a. A review of its pharmacological properties and therapeutic use in the management of viral hepatitis. *Drugs,* **1995,** *50*:873–896.

Hayden, F.G. Amantadine and rimantadine—clinical aspects. In, *Antiviral Drug Resistance.* (Richman, D.D., ed.) Wiley, New York, **1996,** pp. 59–77.

Hayden, F.G. Antiviral drugs (other than antiretrovirals). In, *Mandell, Douglas, and Bennett's Principles and Practice of Infectious Diseases.* (Mandell, G.L., Bennett, J.E., and Dolin, R., eds.) Churchill Livingstone, Philadelphia, **2000,** pp. 460–491.

Hayden, F.G., Aoki, F.Y. Amantadine, rimantadine, and related agents. In, *Antimicrobial Therapy and Vaccines.* (Yu, V.L., Merigan, T.C., and Barriere, S., eds.) Williams & Wilkins, Baltimore, **1999,** pp. 1344–1365.

Huggins, J.W. Prospects for treatment of viral hemorrhagic fevers with ribavirin, a broad-spectrum antiviral drug. *Rev. Infect. Dis.,* **1989,** *11*(suppl. 4):S750–S761.

Johnson, M.A., Moore, K.H., Yuen, G.J., Bye, A., and Pakes, G.E. Clinical pharmacokinetics of lamivudine. *Clin. Pharmacokinet.,* **1999,** *36*:41–66.

Kaufman, H.E. The treatment of herpetic eye infections with trifluridine and other antivirals. In, *Clinical Use of Antiviral Drugs.* (De Clercq, E., ed.) Nijhoff, Boston, **1988,** pp. 25–38.

Lavezzo, B., and Rizzetto, M. Treatment of recurrent hepatitis C virus infection after liver transplantation. *J. Hepatol.,* **1999,** *31*(suppl. 1): 222–226.

McKimm-Breschkin, J.L. Resistance of influenza viruses to neuraminidase inhibitors—a review. *Antiviral Res.,* **2000,** *47*:1–17.

Main, J., and Thomas, H. Interferon in chronic viral hepatitis. In, *Clinical Applications of the Interferons.* (Stuart-Harris, R., and Penny, R.D., eds.) Chapman & Hall, London, **1997,** pp. 53–66.

Noble, S., and Faulds, D. Ganciclovir. An update of its use in the prevention of cytomegalovirus infection and disease in transplant recipients. *Drugs,* **1998,** *56*:115–146.

Oberg, B. Antiviral effects of phosphonoformate (PFA, foscarnet sodium). *Pharmacol. Ther.,* **1989,** *40*:213–285.

Perry, C.M., and Balfour, J.A. Formivirsen. *Drugs,* **1999,** *57*:375–380.

Prusoff, W.H. Idoxuridine or how it all began. In, *Clinical Use of Antiviral Drugs.* (De Clercq, E., ed.) Nijhoff, Boston, **1988,** pp. 15–24.

Randolph, A.G., and Wang, E.E. Ribavirin for respiratory syncytial virus lower respiratory tract infection. A systematic overview. *Arch. Pediatr. Adolesc. Med.,* **1996,** *150*:942–947.

Rogers, J.M., Diana, G.D., and McKinlay, M. Pleconaril. In, *Antiviral Chemotherapy,* 5th ed. (Mills, J., Volberding, P.A., and Corey, L., eds.) Plenum Publishers, New York, **1999,** pp. 69–76.

Sacks, S.L., and Wilson, B. Famciclovir/penciclovir. *Adv. Exp. Med. Biol.,* **1999,** *458*:135–147.

Safrin, S., Cherrington, J., and Jaffe, H.S. Clinical uses of cidofovir. *Rev. Med. Virol.,* **1997,** *7*:145–156.

Sommadossi, J.P. Nucleoside analogs: similarities and differences. *Clin. Infect. Dis.,* **1993,** *16*:S7–S15.

Stark, G.R., Kerr, I.M., Williams, B.R., Silverman, R.H., and Schreiber, R.D. How cells respond to interferons. *Annu. Rev. Biochem.,* **1998,** *67*:227–264.

Vere Hodge, R.A. Review: Antiviral portraits series, Number 3. Famciclovir and penciclovir. The mode of action of famciclovir including its conversion to penciclovir. *Antivir. Chem. Chemother.,* **1993,** *4*:67–84.

Wagstaff, A.J., and Bryson, H.M. Foscarnet. A reappraisal of its antiviral activity, pharmacokinetic properties and therapeutic use in immunocompromised patients with viral infections. *Drugs,* **1994,** *48*:199–226.

Wagstaff, A.J., Faulds, D., and Goa, K.L. Aciclovir. A reappraisal of its antiviral activity, pharmacokinetic properties and therapeutic efficacy. *Drugs,* **1994,** *47*:153–205.

Whitley, R., Alford, C., Hess, F., and Buchanan, R. Vidarabine: a preliminary review of its pharmacological properties and therapeutic use. *Drugs,* **1980,** *20*:267–282.

Whitley, R.J., and Gnann, J.W., Jr. Acyclovir: a decade later. *N. Engl. J. Med.,* **1992,** *327*:782–789. Published errata appear in *N. Engl. J. Med.,* **1993,** *328*:671 and **1997,** *337*:1703.

Whitley, R.J., Hayden, F.G., Reisinger, K.S., Young, N., Dutkowski, R., Ipe, D., Mills, R.G., Ward, P. Oral oseltamivir treatment of influenza in children. *Pediatr. Infect. Dis. J.,* **2001,** *20*:127–133.

Wills, R.J. Clinical pharmacokinetics of interferons. *Clin. Pharmacokinet.,* **1990,** *19*:390–399.

ANTIMICROBIAL AGENTS
(*Continued*)
Antiretroviral Agents

Stephen Raffanti and David W. Haas

The acquired immunodeficiency syndrome (AIDS) epidemic is one of the greatest chal-lenges facing the medical community today. Infection with human immunodeficiency virus (HIV) is a dynamic process characterized by vigorous viral replication, CD4 lymphocyte depletion, and profound immunodeficiency. The error-prone nature of HIV reverse tran-scriptase promotes rapid evolution of genetic diversity and a remarkable propensity to develop resistance to antiretroviral agents. Improved understanding of viral pathogenesis as well as the genetic basis of resistance has fueled the rapid and rational development of numerous effective drugs that target either HIV reverse transcriptase or HIV protease. Various multidrug regimens have been shown to inhibit viral replication effectively, re-verse CD4 cell depletion, and reduce morbidity and mortality dramatically. Despite much progress, many patients do not benefit from antiretroviral therapy due to emergence of viral resistance, adverse effects of chronic therapy, or inability to adhere to complex reg-imens. In addition, current agents generally are not available in developing countries, where HIV has its greatest impact. This chapter addresses the pathophysiological ra-tionale for HIV therapy, considers general treatment principles, and reviews individual agents.

I. OVERVIEW OF HIV INFECTION

The hallmark of human immunodeficiency virus (HIV) in-fection is depletion of CD4 lymphocytes, leading to cel-lular immunodeficiency. Since the first reports of acquired immunodeficiency syndrome (AIDS) appeared in 1981 (Gottlieb *et al.,* 1981; Masur *et al.,* 1981), the vast major-ity of cases worldwide has been caused by HIV-1. Another retrovirus, HIV-2, is a prevalent cause of AIDS in west Africa. Mature virions contain two single-stranded RNA molecules surrounded by a nucleocapsid and an outer lipid envelope. Like all retroviruses, HIV contains three major genes (*gag, pol,* and *env*). Although HIV-1 and HIV-2 share approximately 50% amino-acid homology, individ-ual antiretroviral agents may be more active against one than the other. An entire drug class (nonnucleoside reverse transcriptase inhibitors) is not active against HIV-2.

Improved understanding of HIV pathogenesis has led to rational drug development, sound treatment principles, and decreased morbidity and mortality due to AIDS (Palella *et al.,* 1998). Therapeutic strategies evolve rapidly, and treatment errors may have dire and irreversible conse-

quences. It is therefore recommended that HIV infection be managed only by practitioners with specific training and expertise in treating the disease (HIV/AIDS Treat-ment Information Service, 2000).

HIV Pathogenesis

Development of AIDS is characterized by susceptibility to various infections and malignancies. Early in the AIDS epidemic, it was erroneously assumed that HIV had a pro-longed latent phase without viral replication and that even-tual reactivation of viral replication triggered disease pro-gression. However, sensitive viral culture and nucleic acid detection methods showed that almost all untreated pa-tients experience continuous plasma viremia (Ho *et al.,* 1989). Landmark studies demonstrated that the plasma HIV-1 RNA concentration predicts time for progression to AIDS and death (Mellors *et al.,* 1996) and that CD4 cell counts are independently prognostic (Mellors *et al.,* 1997). Such discoveries have focused research on ways to achieve durable control of HIV replication.

The development of highly effective antiretroviral agents made it possible to probe viral pathogenesis. Administering such agents disrupts the steady-state equilibrium between virion production and clearance. Studies of treatment-naïve patients demonstrated that plasma HIV-1 RNA concentrations decline by 10- to 100-fold within one week of initiating treatment with potent inhibitors of either HIV protease or reverse transcriptase. Mathematical modeling of such data established that HIV infection is extremely dynamic, with daily production of an estimated 10^9 virions (Ho *et al.*, 1995; Perelson *et al.*, 1996; Wei *et al.*, 1995).

Approximately 99% of plasma HIV arises from recently infected CD4+ lymphocytes, which have an average life span of 2.2 days (Perelson *et al.*, 1997). A second source of virus (presumably macrophages) decays with a life span of 2 weeks (Perelson *et al.*, 1996, 1997). It was predicted that complete inhibition of HIV replication for 2 to 3 years might allow all infected cells to be eradicated if these were the only reservoirs for HIV, and that infection would be cured in some patients.

Unfortunately, there is an additional long-lived pool of resting CD4+ lymphocytes cells that harbor replication-competent HIV (Chun *et al.*, 1997; Chun *et al.*, 1998; Finzi *et al.*, 1997). Although there are relatively few such cells in the body, their average life span may be months

or even years. Based on the previous strategy, greater than 100 years of complete control of viral replication would be needed to eradicate these cells! In fact, discontinuing efficacious antiretroviral therapy after years of apparently complete response invariably leads to relapse of viremia (Davey *et al.*, 1999).

The Life Cycle of HIV

HIV is an RNA retrovirus that infects CD4+ lymphocytes, macrophages, and dendritic cells. Its cellular life cycle suggests many potential drug targets (Figure 51–1). Currently approved agents target either reverse transcriptase or protease, but drugs with different targets are being developed.

The initial step in infection involves attachment and membrane fusion. Virus enters cells through interactions between HIV envelope glycoproteins (gp41 and gp120) and cell receptors (CD4 and chemokine receptors such as CCR5 and CXCR4) (He *et al.*, 1997; Sodroski, 1999). In general, only cells expressing both CD4 and chemokine receptors are susceptible. The envelope glycoprotein spike is a trimeric structure consisting of three outer gp120 molecules and three transmembrane gp41 molecules. Attachment of gp120 to CD4 and chemokine receptors brings HIV very close to the cell. Before gp120 binds to the receptor (the prefusogenic state), a region of the gp41 molecule (N36) is an α-helical coiled coil configuration. Following receptor

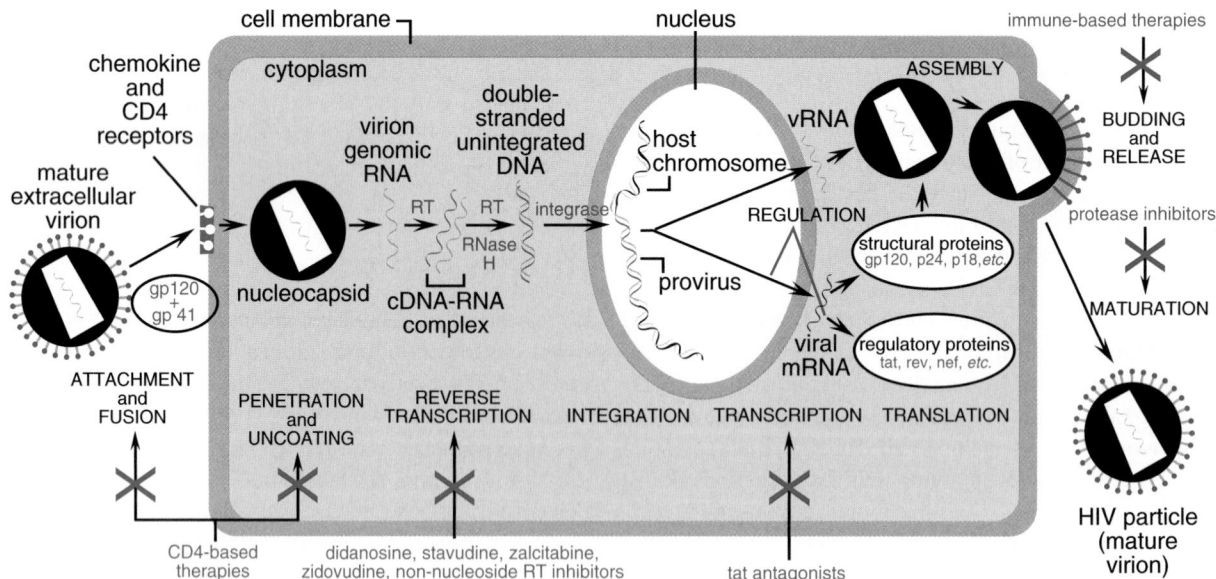

Figure 51–1. Replicative cycle of HIV-1, an example of a retrovirus, showing the sites of action of antiviral agents.

Various antiviral agents are shown in blue. Key: RT, reverse transcriptase; cDNA, complementary DNA; mRNA, messenger RNA; tat, a protein that regulates viral transcription and affects the rate of replication; RNaseH, ribonuclease H; gp120, envelope glycoprotein. (Adapted from Hirsh and D'Aquila, 1993.)

binding, another region of gp41 (C34) packs into a hydrophobic groove on the outer surface of N36, forming an extended six-helix bundle (the fusogenic state) (Sodroski, 1999). Binding of this fusion peptide to the cell membrane leads to fusion and entry of the viral core into the cytoplasm. At least one fusion inhibitor (T20) is in advanced stages of clinical development.

After entering the cytoplasm and uncoating, viral RNA serves as a template from which complementary DNA strands are transcribed. This reverse transcription is the distinguishing feature of retroviruses and is catalyzed by the HIV RNA-dependent DNA polymerase (*reverse transcriptase*). Two classes of antiretroviral agents (nucleoside reverse transcriptase inhibitors and nonnucleoside reverse transcriptase inhibitors) target this enzyme. Following reverse transcription, the double-stranded DNA circularizes and enters the nucleus. Integration of this proviral DNA into the host chromosome is mediated by a second essential viral enzyme, *integrase*. Although integrase seems an attractive target for drug treatment, the discovery of inhibitors for clinical use has been difficult because of the complex interactions between host and viral molecules during integration.

After being incorporated into the host chromosome, proviral DNA can be transcribed into HIV RNA by the cellular transcription machinery. This RNA then may be translated into viral polyproteins (including gag-pol and env) or be incorporated into immature virions during virion assembly. Immature virions then undergo a process of maturation and budding from the cell membrane. Maturation requires that the gag-pol polyprotein be cleaved by *protease,* the third essential enzyme of HIV. Mature virions may then infect other susceptible cells. Exposure of infected cells to inhibitors of HIV protease results in production of immature virions that lack a typical nucleocapsid and that are noninfectious.

GENERAL PRINCIPLES OF ANTIRETROVIRAL THERAPY

The clinical benefit of antiretroviral therapy is determined by the magnitude and duration of plasma HIV RNA suppression (Marschner *et al.*, 1998; O'Brien *et al.*, 1996). A central principle of therapy is to inhibit viral replication as completely and durably as possible while avoiding toxicity as much as possible. This requires administering multiple drugs simultaneously (HIV/AIDS Treatment Information Service, 2000). Adherence to complex regimens is difficult for many patients, and nonadherence is a major cause of therapeutic failure and death. In a study of patients for whom HIV protease inhibitors had been prescribed (mostly *indinavir, nelfinavir,* or *saquinavir/ritonavir*) plus nucleoside reverse transcriptase inhibitors, at least 95% adherence was necessary for optimal response (Paterson *et al.*, 2000).

Drug Resistance

The HIV reverse transcriptase is highly error prone. Like all polymerases that use RNA as a template, it lacks the 3' exonuclease activity needed to correct transcription errors.

With an error rate of 3.4×10^{-5} per base pair during each replication cycle and a genome of 10^4 base pairs, every mutation at every nucleotide probably occurs many times each day in untreated patients, and every double mutation may arise within 100 days (Coffin, 1995; Wain-Hobson, 1993). (The latter prediction assumes that single point mutations do not impair replication efficiency, which is likely not the case.)

Incomplete therapeutic control of replication inevitably selects for drug-resistant mutants (Havlir and Richman, 1996; Molla *et al.*, 1996). Although nonnucleoside reverse transcriptase inhibitors are very effective antiretroviral agents, a single mutation at reverse transcriptase codon 103 confers high-level resistance. Since all patients infected with HIV likely harbor such mutants prior to therapy, monotherapy with a nonnucleoside reverse transcriptase inhibitor will cause an initial plasma HIV RNA decline (inhibition of susceptible virus), followed within weeks by virologic failure (emergence of resistant virus). In contrast, nonnucleoside reverse transcriptase inhibitors can provide durable control of HIV in multidrug regimens (Staszewski *et al.*, 1999). Since only replicating HIV can accumulate mutations, complete suppression of replication will both reverse CD4 lymphocyte depletion and prevent resistance (Havlir and Richman, 1996).

Many patients who initiate antiretroviral therapy experience emergence of multidrug-resistant virus. Future treatment options always must be kept in mind when antiretroviral therapy is begun or when a regimen is changed (HIV/AIDS Treatment Information Service, 2000).

Virologic response to therapy may be improved by using HIV-resistance assay results to guide prescribing (Durant *et al.*, 1999). However, resistance testing is only one factor to consider when making treatment decisions. At least as important are prior treatment regimens, previous plasma HIV RNA responses to each regimen, comorbidities, anticipated adherence to complex regimens, and patient preference. Although virus in plasma is replaced by sensitive strains if selective drug pressure is not maintained, resistant strains may remain in tissues indefinitely (Hirsch *et al.*, 2000; Romanelli and Pomeroy, 2000). Therefore, resistance testing may falsely indicate susceptibility if the patient is no longer on the drug that selected for resistant virus. In addition, available resistance assays do not reliably detect minor resistant subpupulations. The role of HIV resistance testing is being evaluated in clinical trials.

Deciding When to Initiate Therapy

The decision to initiate treatment must be individualized and should involve consideration of both the plasma HIV-1

RNA concentration and CD4 cell count. Treatment probably should be offered to all patients with greater than 20,000 plasma HIV-1 RNA copies per milliliter (by polymerase-chain-reaction assay) or less than 350 CD4 cells per cubic millimeter. It is reasonable to defer treatment for other patients, since the short-term prognosis is excellent (Harrington and Carpenter, 2000; Mellors *et al.,* 1996; HIV/AIDS Treatment Information Service, 2000).

Monitoring Treatment Response

Periodic plasma HIV-1 RNA determinations are used to monitor therapeutic response (Marschner *et al.,* 1998). Due to biological and inherent assay variability, results of two assays using samples obtained on different days generally should be used to define the pretreatment baseline. It is essential that the patient fully understand the importance of adherence to long-term therapy and that non-adherence will promote drug resistance, limiting future options. After starting therapy, plasma HIV RNA levels should be quantified within 2 to 4 weeks to assure at least a 1.0 $\log_{10}$ HIV RNA decline, and every 3 to 4 months thereafter to assure that undetectable plasma HIV RNA levels are achieved and maintained (HIV/AIDS Treatment Information Service, 2000).

Extraordinary patients with HIV infection have no evidence of viral replication or immunodeficiency in the absence of therapy. These "long-term nonprogressors" have robust cellular immune responses to HIV, and it has been suggested that their immune systems can control HIV. If this is true, then boosting HIV-specific immunity in other patients who are receiving antiretroviral therapy might allow immunological control of virus without the need for continued medications. Current clinical trials are testing this hypothesis.

ANTIRETROVIRAL DRUG DEVELOPMENT

The very rapid discovery of effective antiretroviral agents was made possible by drug-development programs already established for other diseases including cancer, hypertension, and other viral infections. Pharmaceutical companies previously had produced many nucleoside analogs as potential antiviral and anticancer agents. The ability to grow HIV in cell culture allowed these agents to be screened for activity. Through a labor-intensive process, thousands of compounds were tested, and promising lead compounds were modified to enhance anti-HIV activity, minimize toxicity, and improve bioavailability. *Zidovudine* arose from

this process, and in 1987 it was the first drug approved by the United States Food and Drug Administration (FDA) for treating HIV infection. By 2000, five additional nucleoside reverse transcriptase inhibitors had been approved.

Although nucleoside reverse transcriptase inhibitors remain cornerstones of antiretroviral therapy, early agents had limited efficacy. They could delay only temporarily progression to AIDS and death (Fischl *et al.,* 1987). The search for more effective agents with different mechanisms of action produced the nonnucleoside reverse transcriptase-inhibitor class of drugs. *Nevirapine,* one of the first such agents, inhibited HIV-1 replication far more completely than either zidovudine or *didanosine,* another nucleoside analog. However, enthusiasm for reverse transcriptase inhibitors temporarily waned when resistance emerged rapidly when the drugs were administered in suboptimal regimens.

Concurrently with the development of nonnucleoside reverse transcriptase inhibitors, pharmaceutical companies sought inhibitors of HIV protease. The sequence of HIV-1 protease was first published in 1985, its enzymatic activity reported the following year, and its crystalline structure determined in 1989 (Navia *et al.,* 1989; Wlodawer *et al.,* 1989). Although there were no known inhibitors of HIV protease when the enzyme was first identified, the protease was known to be an aspartyl protease like renin. Hypertension researchers previously had developed nonhydrolyzable substrate analogs as renin inhibitors (transition state analogs); this approach was taken to develop HIV protease inhibitors (Dreyer *et al.,* 1989). By 1990, several groups had reported peptidic inhibitors of HIV protease. *Saquinavir,* the first HIV-1 protease inhibitor, entered clinical trials in 1992 and received FDA approval three years later.

Elucidating the three-dimensional structure of HIV protease has facilitated structure-based "rational drug design" (Frecer *et al.,* 1998; Thaisrivongs and Strohbach, 1999). Although lead protease inhibitors designed *via* these strategies were poorly absorbed due to high lipophilicity and poor water solubility, these limitations were overcome. Clinical trials demonstrated that protease inhibitors are effective inhibitors of HIV replication and that they select for resistance more slowly than do nonnucleoside reverse transcriptase inhibitors.

Measuring Antiretroviral Efficacy in Clinical Trials

The effectiveness of early antiretroviral agents was assessed by determining whether or not treatment, often as monotherapy, delayed or prevented AIDS and death in HIV-infected patients. Once it was demonstrated that plasma levels of HIV RNA and CD4 cell responses could predict clinical benefit, these laboratory tests became preferred surrogate markers of efficacy. Drugs that lowered HIV RNA the most were considered to be most efficacious.

Once the basis of drug resistance became appreciated, it was no longer acceptable to administer prolonged monotherapy. Efficacy of newer drugs thus was tested in multidrug regimens, making it difficult to assess the relative contributions of individual agents in multidrug regimens, since many regimens appear to inhibit viral replication completely based on available assays. In addition, because multidrug therapies so effectively prevent opportunistic infections, it became impractical to perform "clinical end point" studies. At present, the usual way to assess antiretroviral efficacy in phase III clinical trials is by determining the proportion of patients with plasma HIV RNA below limits of detection at 24 weeks and/or 48 weeks. The complexity of individual treatment regimens in terms of the number of pills, frequency of dosage, and dietary requirement varies. Patient adherence rather than inherent drug efficacy may explain apparent differences among regimens in comparative studies.

A review of available results of clinical trials of antiretroviral agents is beyond the scope of this chapter, and this area is evolving rapidly. Although selected important studies are cited in the text, the reader is referred elsewhere for an overview of major clinical trials (Tavel et al., 1999).

II. Drugs Used to Treat HIV Infection

NUCLEOSIDE REVERSE TRANSCRIPTASE INHIBITORS

Reverse transcriptase converts viral RNA into proviral DNA before its incorporation into the host cell chromosome. Because agents in this class act at an early and essential step in HIV replication, they prevent acute infection of susceptible cells but have little effect on cells already infected with HIV. All drugs of the nucleoside reverse transcriptase-inhibitor class are substrates for reverse transcriptase. To become active, these drugs first must be phosphorylated by host cell enzymes in the cytoplasm. Since nucleoside reverse transcriptase inhibitors lack a 3'-hydroxyl group, incorporation into DNA terminates chain elongation.

There currently are six FDA-approved nucleoside reverse transcriptase inhibitors (Table 51–1). Their chemical structures are shown in Figure 51–2. These agents differ in phosphorylation pathways utilized and in untoward effects. This class of drugs includes both early

(e.g., zidovudine and didanosine) and recently approved (e.g., abacavir) drugs for treating HIV infection. Although initially evaluated as monotherapy or in dual combinations, these agents now are most important as components of efficacious three- and four-drug regimens. Recently recognized complications include lactic acidosis and severe hepatomegaly with steatosis. A summary of the pharmacokinetic properties of these agents is presented in Table 51–2.

Zidovudine

Chemistry and Antiviral Activity. *Zidovudine* (3'-azido-3'-deoxythymidine; AZT) is a synthetic thymidine analog active against HIV-1, HIV-2, and human T-cell lymphotrophic virus (HTLV) I and II (McLeod and Hammer, 1992). Its *in vitro* 90% inhibitory concentration (IC_{90}) against laboratory and clinical isolates of HIV-1 ranges from 0.03 to 0.3 μg/ml. Zidovudine is active in lymphoblastic and monocytic cell lines but is substantially less active in chronically infected cells (Geleziunas et al., 1993).

Mechanisms of Action and Resistance. After entering the host cell, zidovudine is phosphorylated by thymidine kinase to a monophosphate, then by thymidylate kinase to the diphosphate, and finally by nucleoside diphosphate kinase to active zidovudine 5-triphosphate (Furman et al., 1986). High concentrations of the monophosphate may accumulate in the cell, and the intracellular half-life of zidovudine 5-triphosphate is approximately 3 hours. Zidovudine 5-triphosphate terminates viral DNA chain elongation by competing with thymidine triphosphate for incorporation into DNA. Zidovudine 5-triphosphate also weakly inhibits cellular DNA polymerase-α and mitochondrial polymerase-γ, and the monophosphate competitively inhibits cellular thymidylate kinase, an effect that reduces levels of thymidine triphosphate (Furman et al., 1986). These latter effects may contribute to the drug's cytotoxicity and adverse effects.

Resistance to zidovudine is associated with the mutations at reverse transcriptase codons 41, 67, 70, 215, and 219. Those at codons 41, 215, and 219 are most important. Mutations accumulate gradually, and resistance develops in one-third of patients after one year of zidovudine monotherapy. Cross-resistance to multiple nucleoside analogs has been reported following prolonged therapy and has been associated with mutations at codons 62, 75, 77, 116, and especially 151 (Richman, 1993).

Absorption, Distribution, and Elimination. Zidovudine is absorbed rapidly from the gastrointestinal tract, with peak serum levels achieved within about one hour (Dudley, 1995). The plasma half-life of the prodrug is considerably shorter than the intracellular half-life of active zidovudine 5-triphosphate. Importantly, plasma zidovudine concentrations do not correlate with intracellular triphosphate concentrations or clinical efficacy. The rate-limiting step in intracellular activation is conversion to the monophosphate. Therefore, higher plasma concentrations of zidovudine do not proportionately increase intracellular triphosphate concentrations. Zidovudine crosses the blood–brain barrier relatively well and achieves a cerebrospinal fluid (CSF)-to-plasma ratio of approximately 0.6. Zidovudine also is detectable

Table 51–1

Antiretroviral Agents Approved for Use in the United States

GENERIC NAME [TRADE NAME]	DEVELOPMENTAL OR OTHER NAMES	ESTIMATED RELATIVE ANTIVIRAL EFFECT‡
Nucleoside reverse transcriptase inhibitors		
Zidovudine [RETROVIR]* [VIDEX EC]	AZT; azidothymidine	++
Didanosine [VIDEX]	ddI; dideoxyinosine	++
Stavudine [ZERIT]	D4T	++
Zalcitabine [HIVID]	ddC; dideoxycytidine	+
Lamivudine [EPIVIR]*	3TC	++
Abacavir [ZIAGEN]*	1592U89	+++
Nonnucleoside reverse transcriptase inhibitors		
Nevirapine [VIRAMUNE]	BI-RG-587	+++
Efavirenz [SUSTIVA]	DMP266	+++
Delavirdine [RESCRIPTOR]		+++
Protease inhibitors		
Saquinavir [INVIRASE]		++
[FORTOVASE]		+++
Indinavir [CRIXIVAN]	L-735,524	+++
Ritonavir [NORVIR]	ABT-538	+++
Nelfinavir [VIRACEPT]		+++
Amprenavir [AGENERASE]	VX-478; 141W94	+++
Lopinavir$_R$ [KALETRA]†	ABT-378	+++

*A fixed-dose coformulation of zidovudine + lamivudine = [COMBIVIR]; a fixed-dose coformulation of zidovidine + lamivudine + abacavir = [TRIZIVIR].

†Lopinavir$_R$ refers to a fixed dose coformulation of lopinavir and ritonavir (KALETRA).

‡+ = least active, +++ = most active.

in breast milk, semen and fetal tissue (Gillet *et al.,* 1989; Watts *et al.,* 1991).

Zidovudine undergoes rapid first-pass hepatic metabolism by conversion to 5-glucuronyl zidovudine. This metabolite has an elimination half-life of 1 hour. Total urinary recovery of zidovudine and its major metabolite is approximately 90%. The pharmacokinetics of zidovudine generally is unaffected by pregnancy, and drug concentrations in the newborn approach those of the mother (Watts *et al.,* 1991).

Untoward Effects. Common adverse effects include anorexia, fatigue, headache, malaise, myalgia, nausea, and insomnia. Anemia may develop as early as four weeks, occurs in 7% of patients with advanced HIV disease, and probably is due to toxic effects on erythroid stem cells (Walker *et al.,* 1988). Evaluation may reveal depletion of bone marrow red-cell precursors, elevated serum erythropoietin levels, and normal serum folate and vitamin B$_{12}$ levels. Management involves replacing zidovudine with another antiretroviral agent or administering recombinant

human erythropoietin. Erythrocytic macrocytosis occurs in approximately 90% of patients but is not necessarily associated with anemia.

Neutropenia also can occur within four weeks of initiating zidovudine and is more frequent (37%) during advanced HIV disease. Management may involve replacing zidovudine with another agent or administering recombinant granulocyte or granulocyte/macrophage colony-stimulating factors (*see* Chapter 54). Chronic zidovudine administration may cause nail hyperpigmentation, myopathy (Dalakas *et al.,* 1990), hepatic toxicity with or without steatosis, and lactic acidosis (Chattha *et al.,* 1993). Zidovudine can cause muscle damage associated with reduced amounts of mitochondrial DNA, possibly by inhibiting mitochondrial DNA polymerase-γ (Arnaudo *et al.,* 1991).

Drug Interactions and Precautions. Since zidovudine may cause bone marrow suppression, it should be used

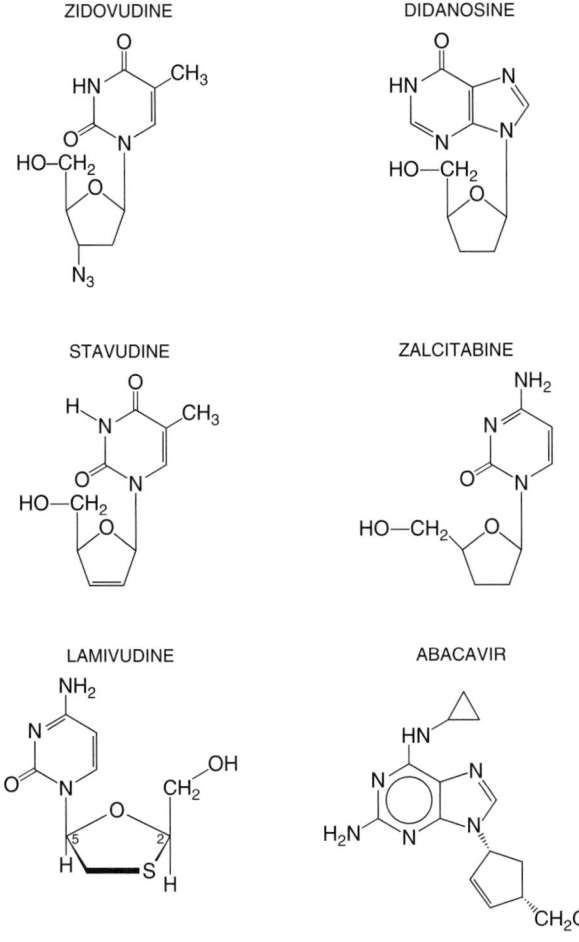

ZIDOVUDINE

DIDANOSINE

STAVUDINE

ZALCITABINE

LAMIVUDINE

ABACAVIR

Figure 51–2. Structures of nucleoside reverse transcriptase inhibitors.

cautiously in patients with preexisting granulocytopenia or anemia. Concurrent administration with other potentially marrow-suppressive agents such as ganciclovir, interferon-alfa, dapsone, flucytosine, vincristine, or vinblastine increases the risk of toxicity. Probenecid, fluconazole, atovaquone, and valproic acid administration may increase plasma zidovudine levels, but the clinical significance of these interactions is unknown, because intracellular triphosphate levels may be unchanged. Both stavudine and ribavirin compete with zidovudine for intracellular activation by common pathways. Zidovudine has been shown to decrease the efficacy of stavudine in clinical trials. Concomitant use of these drugs should be avoided.

Therapeutic Uses. Zidovudine is FDA-approved for treating adults and children with HIV infection, as monotherapy or in combination with other antiretroviral agents. It also is approved for preventing prenatal transmission of virus in pregnant women with HIV infection and is recommended for postexposure chemoprophylaxis in HIV-exposed health-care workers.

Zidovudine was the first antiretroviral agent to show clinical efficacy in treating HIV infection. Since its release in 1987, the effectiveness of zidovudine has been established in numerous clinical trails. An early monotherapy trial in patients with advanced disease showed that zidovudine improved survival over 24 weeks (Fischl *et al.,* 1987). A later study confirmed decreased risk of disease progression among patients with symptomatic and asymptomatic disease over a 12-month period but did not show a survival benefit (Fischl *et al.,* 1990).

Zidovudine plus other nucleoside reverse transcriptase inhibitors provides greater clinical benefits than zidovudine alone. Zidovudine combined with lamivudine produced a 66% reduction in disease progression. More effective

Table 51–2

Pharmacokinetic Properties of Nucleoside Reverse Transcriptase Inhibitors

PARAMETER	ZIDOVUDINE	LAMIVUDINE	STAVUDINE	DIDANOSINE	ABACAVIR	ZALCITABINE
Oral bioavailability, %	60	80	80–90	40	>70	90
Effect of meals on AUC	↓ 24 (high fat)	↔	↔	↓ 50% (acidity)	↔	↓ 15%
Plasma $t_{1/2elim}$, hours	0.8–1.9	5–7	1.4	1.0	0.8–1.5	1–2
Intracellular $t_{1/2elim}$ of triphosphate, hours	3–4	12	3.5	8–24	3	2–3
Plasma protein binding, %	20–38	<35	<5	<5	50	<5
Metabolism, %	60–80 (glucuronidation)	20–30	80	50 (Purine metabolism)	>80	20
Renal excretion of parent drug, %	15	70	40	20–50	<5	70

Abbreviations: AUC, area under plasma concentration–time curve; $t_{1/2elim}$, half-life of elimination; ↑, increase; ↓, decrease; ↔, no effect.

regimens have combined zidovudine with two nucleoside analogs (Saag *et al.,* 1998), with a protease inhibitor and a nucleoside analog (Hammer *et al.,* 1997), or with a non-nucleoside reverse transcriptase inhibitor and a nucleoside analog (Staszewski *et al.,* 1999). These regimens control viremia, substantially increase CD4 counts, and decrease morbidity and mortality. When given to pregnant HIV-infected mothers and to their newborns, zidovudine reduces the relative risk of perinatal transmission by two-thirds (Connor *et al.,* 1994). Administration to health-care workers soon after exposure to contaminated body fluids can prevent HIV transmission (Cardo *et al.,* 1997).

Didanosine

Chemistry and Antiviral Activity.   *Didanosine* (2′,3′-dideoxy-inosine; ddI) is a purine nucleoside analog active against HIV-1, HIV-2, and HTLV-1 (Hitchcock, 1993; McGowan *et al.,* 1990). Its 50% inhibitory concentration (IC_{50}) for HIV-1 is 0.24 to 0.6 mg/l in T-cell cultures and 0.002 to 0.02 mg/l in mono-cycte/macrophage cultures (Perry and Balfour, 1996).

Mechanisms of Action and Resistance.   The active intracellular metabolite of didanosine, 2′,3′-dideoxyadenosine 5′-triphosphate (ddATP), competes with cellular dATP for incorporation into viral DNA. Didanosine enters the cell *via* a nucleobase carrier and undergoes monophosphorylation by a 5′-nucleotidase. This metabolite then is converted to dideoxyadenosine monophosphate by adenylosuccinate synthetase and adenylosuccinate lyase. Phosphorylation produces the diphosphate and ultimately the active triphosphate, which accumulates with an intracellular half-life of many hours (Shelton *et al.,* 1992).

Decreased susceptibility to didanosine is associated with mutations at reverse transcriptase codon 74. This causes a 5- to 26-fold decrease in didanosine susceptibility. Additional mutations at codons 184, 65, 135, and 200 also have been associated with resistance (St. Clair *et al.,* 1991).

Absorption, Distribution, and Elimination.   Didanosine is acid labile and is degraded at low gastric pH (Burger *et al.,* 1995b). Some oral preparations include buffers to minimize degradation; delayed-release capsules do not. The chewable tablets contain calcium carbonate and magnesium hydroxide, while the powder form contains citrate-phosphate buffer. A pediatric powder formulation is available without buffer and can be reconstituted with purified water and mixed with liquid antacid preparations.

Oral bioavailability of didanosine is variable and dose-dependent (Shelton *et al.,* 1992). It is approximately 40% for the chewable tablet and somewhat less for the powder form (Cooney *et al.,* 1987). Percentage bioavailability decreases with increasing dose and in children. Food may decrease the drug's absorption (Perry and Balfour, 1996), so oral dosing should be at least one hour before or two hours after meals.

Peak plasma concentrations occur approximately one hour after oral administration of chewable tablets or powder formula-

tions and two hours after delayed-release capsules. The plasma elimination half-life ranges from 0.76 to 2.74 hours (Perry and Balfour, 1996). Didanosine is excreted both by glomerular filtration and tubular secretion (Knupp *et al.,* 1993). Purine nucleoside phosphorylase converts the active drug to hypoxanthine, which is ultimately converted to uric acid.

The mean CSF-to-plasma ratio is 0.20, but variable ratios have been reported in children (Burger *et al.,* 1995a). Didanosine has been detected in placental and fetal circulation at a small fraction of concentrations in maternal circulation (Dancis *et al.,* 1993).

Untoward Effects.   Although diarrhea is a frequent side effect, peripheral neuropathy and pancreatitis are the most serious dose-limiting toxicities of didanosine. Diarrhea has been attributed in part to the buffer in oral preparations and was reported in 16% of AIDS patients receiving didanosine through the expanded access program. However, in some controlled trials, rates of diarrhea in patients receiving chewable didanosine tablets did not differ from rates in patients receiving zidovudine (Dolin *et al.,* 1995; Kahn *et al.,* 1992).

Didanosine-associated peripheral neuropathy is dose-related and is more frequent in patients with underlying neuropathy or receiving neurotoxic drugs. It is a symmetrical, distal, sensory polyneuropathy that most frequently involves the feet and lower extremities. Patients report numbness, tingling, and painful dysthesias. The incidence of peripheral neuropathy increases with addition of stavudine and hydroxyurea to didanosine-containing regimens (Moore *et al.,* 2000).

Acute pancreatitis is a rare but potentially fatal complication of didanosine. Lactic acidosis and severe hepatomegaly with steatosis are other potentially fatal complications. In early monotherapy trials, pancreatitis occurred in 3% to 4% more patients receiving didanosine than receiving zidovudine (Rozencweig *et al.,* 1990). This is more common with advanced HIV disease. Risk factors include a previous history of pancreatitis, alcohol or illicit drug use, and hypertriglyceridemia (Hammer *et al.,* 1996). Other untoward effects include elevated liver function tests, headache, and retinal pigmentation in children (Pike and Nicaise, 1993).

Drug Interactions and Precautions.   Didanosine should be used cautiously in patients with a history of pancreatitis or neuropathy. Concurrent administration of drugs that cause pancreatitis (*e.g.,* ethambutol, pentamidine) or neuropathy (*e.g.,* ethambutol, isoniazid, vincristine, cisplatin) should be avoided. Oral ganciclovir can increase plasma didanosine concentrations by twofold. Regimens containing stavudine and/or hydroxyurea increase the risk of neuropathy (Moore *et al.*, 2000). Concurrent administration with zalcitabine is contraindicated.

Therapeutic Use.   Didanosine is FDA-approved for treating adults and children with HIV infection in combination with other antiretroviral agents. Initial studies that compared didanosine to zidovudine monotherapy demonstrated that didanosine reduced clinical progression and death (Dolin *et al.*, 1995; Kahn *et al.*, 1992; Spruance *et al.*, 1994). Several trials showed decreased clinical progression and greater viral suppression with dual nucleoside regimens containing didanosine than with zidovudine monotherapy (Anonymous, 1996; Hammer *et al.*, 1996; Katzenstein *et al.*, 1996; Saravolatz *et al.*, 1996). Multidrug regimens that include didanosine and nonnucleoside reverse transcriptase inhibitors and protease inhibitors have produced effective control of viremia and increased CD4 cell counts. Studies of the use of didanosine in children also have revealed beneficial effects (Englund *et al.*, 1997; Luzuriaga *et al.*, 1997).

Stavudine

Chemistry and Antiviral Activity.   *Stavudine* (2′,3′-didehydro-2′,3′-dideoxythymidine; d4T) is a thymidine analog reverse transcriptase inhibitor that is active *in vitro* against HIV-1 and HIV-2. Its IC_{50} in various *in vitro* cell systems ranges from 0.002 to 0.9 μg/ml (Sommadossi, 1995).

Mechanisms of Action and Resistance.   After passive diffusion into the cell, stavudine must be phosphorylated to the active form, stavudine triphosphate. It is first phosphorylated by thymidine kinase. Unlike zidovudine monophosphate, stavudine monophosphate does not accumulate in the cell. Subsequent phosphorylation events are catalyzed by thymidylate kinase and pyrimidine diphosphate kinase. Stavudine triphosphate inhibits reverse transcriptase by competing with cellular 2′-deoxythymidine-5′-triphosphate, resulting in chain DNA termination (Ho and Hitchcock, 1989). Because thymidine kinase has a higher affinity for zidovudine than for stavudine, zidovudine antagonizes the effect of stavudine (Merrill *et al.*, 1996).

Unlike the situations with other nucleoside analogs, the genetic basis of stavudine resistance is poorly understood. Exposure of HIV-1 to stavudine *in vitro* selects for mutations at codon 75, which confers modest (sevenfold) resistance, and at codon 50. However, *in vivo* resistance is not clearly associated with these mutations. Strains that are highly resistant to multiple nucleoside reverse transcriptase inhibitors are consistently resistant to stavudine (Lin *et al.*, 1994).

Absorption, Distribution, and Elimination.   Stavudine has very high oral bioavailability (Dudley *et al.*, 1992) and reaches peak plasma concentrations within 1 hour (Zhu *et al.*, 1990). The ratio of the CSF area under the concentration–time curve

(AUC) to the plasma AUC is approximately 0.40 in adults (Haas *et al.*, 2000b). Stavudine has been detected in human placental tissue and in the fetal circulation of pregnant macaques (Odinecs *et al.*, 1996).

Untoward Effects.   The major adverse effect of stavudine is dose-related peripheral neuropathy. In early high-dose studies, the cumulative incidence of peripheral neuropathy exceeded 60% among patients receiving greater than 4 mg/kg daily. At the current daily dosage of approximately 1 mg/kg, the incidence of neuropathy of any grade is 12% (Skowron, 1995). Neuropathy causes numbness, tingling, and pain of the feet and usually resolves after stopping therapy, although temporary worsening may occur. Neuropathy is more common with advanced HIV disease, preexisting neuropathy, or administration of other neurotoxic compounds (Moore *et al.*, 2000; Spruance *et al.*, 1997a).

Lactic acidosis has been associated with stavudine administration (Mokrzycki *et al.*, 2000). Moderate transaminase elevations are common during stavudine administration but rarely require discontinuation of therapy. Other, less frequent adverse events include headache, nausea, and rash. An increased risk of pancreatitis has not been demonstrated clearly (Spruance *et al.*, 1997).

Drug Interactions and Precautions.   Medications that cause neuropathy (*e.g.*, ethambutol, isoniazid, phenytoin, vincristine) should be used cautiously in patients receiving stavudine. Regimens containing stavudine, didanosine, and/or hydroxyurea are associated with an increased risk for neuropathy. Zidovudine and stavudine should not be used concomitantly because zidovudine antagonizes the effect of stavudine (*see* above).

Therapeutic Use.   Stavudine is FDA-approved for treating patients with HIV infection, in combination with other antiretroviral agents. In initial clinical trials, zidovudine-experienced patients were randomized to either continue zidovudine monotherapy or switch to stavudine. Stavudine administration delayed clinical progression compared to continued zidovudine therapy (Spruance *et al.*, 1997a). Stavudine plus lamivudine has yielded plasma HIV RNA decreases of up to 1.6 $\log_{10}$ copies per milliliter. Stavudine, in combination with didanosine and hydroxyurea, has produced median plasma HIV RNA decreases ranging from 1.2 to 1.9 $\log_{10}$ copies per milliliter. Durable suppression of viremia has been reported in three- and four-drug regimens that include stavudine plus other nucleoside reverse transcriptase inhibitors in combination with nonnucleoside reverse transcriptase inhibitors or protease inhibitors (Gisolf *et al.*, 2000; Roca *et al.*, 2000).

Zalcitabine

Chemistry and Antiviral Activity. *Zalcitabine* (2',3'-dideoxycytidine; ddC) is a cytosine analog reverse transcriptase inhibitor. It was the first antiretroviral agent licensed through the FDA's accelerated approval process and is active against HIV-1, HIV-2, and hepatitis B virus (Mitsuya and Broder, 1986; Yokota *et al.*, 1991). It is especially active against macrophage-tropic strains of HIV-1 in monocyte/macrophage cell lines. Zalcitabine inhibits HIV in peripheral blood lymphocytes at 0.5 μM and in monocyte/macrophage cell lines at 0.002 μM (Balzarini *et al.*, 1988).

Mechanisms of Action and Resistance. Zalcitabine enters the cell through carrier-mediated and non–carrier-mediated mechanisms (Cooney *et al.*, 1986; Plagemann and Woffendin, 1989; Ullman *et al.*, 1988). It is first phosphorylated by deoxycytidine kinase and further by cellular kinases to its active metabolite, dideoxycytidine 5'-triphosphate (Broder, 1990). Unlike other nucleoside analogs, zalcitabine is most efficiently triphosphorylated in resting peripheral blood mononuclear cells (Gao *et al.*, 1993). The triphosphate terminates viral DNA elongation. Zalcitabine decrease the intracellular pool of deoxycytidine triphosphate and binds somewhat to host β and γ DNA polymerases (Chen *et al.*, 1991).

High-level resistance to zalcitabine has not been reported. Low-level to moderate resistance has been associated with mutations at reverse transcriptase codons 65, 69, 74, and 184. Strains resistant to multiple nucleoside analogs including zalcitabine have demonstrated mutations at codon 151. Resistance mutations related to zalcitabine exposure develop slowly, although phenotypic cross-resistance with didanosine and lamivudine has been reported (Craig and Moyle, 1997).

Absorption, Distribution, and Elimination. Zalcitabine has high oral bioavailability and is recovered mostly unchanged in urine (Gustavson *et al.*, 1990; Klecker *et al.*, 1988). The CSF-to-plasma ratio is approximately 0.2. Pharmacokinetic properties in adults and children are similar.

Untoward Effects. The major adverse events of zalcitabine administration are peripheral neuropathy, stomatitis, rash, and pancreatitis. Zalcitabine-associated peripheral neuropathy is dose-related and more common with preexisting neuropathy and advanced disease. Alcohol consumption, diabetes, and low vitamin B_{12} levels also are associated with an increased risk of zalcitabine-induced neuropathy (Fichtenbaum *et al.*, 1995; Fischl *et al.*, 1995). Severe neuropathy occurs in up to 15% of patients. Symptoms include numbness, burning, and tingling of the feet. Symptoms may worsen after stopping the drug, then slowly improve. Stomatitis with ulcerations of buccal mucosa, soft palate, tongue, or pharynx occurs in 3% of patients (Fischl *et al.*, 1995) and may resolve with continued ther-

apy. Mild and self-limited rash is common but rarely necessitates discontinuing therapy (Yarchoan *et al.*, 1988). Pancreatitis is a rare complication of zalcitabine therapy (Saravolatz *et al.*, 1996). Other toxicities include arthragias, myalgias, and elevated serum transaminase levels (Fischl *et al.*, 1995; Saravolatz *et al.*, 1996; Yarchoan *et al.*, 1988).

Drug Interactions and Precautions. Concurrent administration of agents that cause neuropathy or pancreatitis should be avoided in patients receiving zalcitabine. Coadministration with didanosine is contraindicated. Cimetidine and probenecid decrease zalcitabine elimination, and dosage adjustment may be needed with their coadministration.

Therapeutic Use. Zalcitabine has been approved by the FDA for use in combination with other antiretroviral agents to treat HIV infection in adults. Early trials that evaluated zalcitabine monotherapy in advanced disease showed moderate increases in CD4 cell counts and decreases in HIV antigenemia (Yarchoan *et al.*, 1988). Zidovudine monotherapy was clearly superior to zalcitabine monotherapy (Fischl *et al.*, 1993). Several studies showed clinical benefit of zalcitabine in combination with zidovudine compared with zidovudine monotherapy (Anonymous, 1996; Saravolatz *et al.*, 1996).

A few trials have evaluated zalcitabine in efficacious three-drug combinations. A regimen of zalcitabine, zidovudine, and saquinavir was superior to two-drug regimens (Collier *et al.*, 1996). Since the antiretroviral efficacy of zalcitabine is less than that of other agents, this drug is prescribed relatively infrequently.

Lamivudine

Chemistry and Antiviral Activity. *Lamivudine* (2'-deody-3-thiacytidine; 3TC) is a pyrimidine analog reverse transcriptase inhibitor active against HIV-1, HIV-2, and hepatitis B virus. It was first prepared as a racemic mixture (BCH-189). Lamivudine, the ($-$) enantiomer, has less cytotoxicity and greater antiviral activity than the ($+$) enantiomer (Skalski *et al.*, 1993). The IC_{50} of lamivudine against laboratory strains of HIV-1 ranges from 4.0 to 670 nM (Coates *et al.*, 1992). It is synergistic with other antiretroviral agents including zidovudine, stavudine, didanosine, nevirapine, and delavirdine. Lamivudine antagonizes zalcitabine by interfering with its phosphorylation (Bridges *et al.*, 1996; Merrill *et al.*, 1996; Veal *et al.*, 1996).

Mechanism of Action and Resistance. Lamivudine enters cells by passive diffusion and is phosphorylated to its active metabolite, lamivudine triphosphate. Lamivudine triphosphate competes with deoxycytidine triphosphate for binding to reverse transcriptase, and incorporation into DNA results in chain termination. Lamivudine has very low affinity for human α and δ DNA polymerases, moderate affinity for β DNA polymerase, and higher affinity for γ DNA polymerase (Gao *et al.*, 1994).

High-level resistance to lamivudine, unlike other nucleoside analogs, develops rapidly (Schinazi *et al.*, 1993; Schuurman *et al.*, 1995). A single mutation at codon 184 causes high-level resistance and also may inhibit viral growth somewhat (Larder *et al.*, 1995). This codon lies in an essential amino acid motif in the active site of the enzyme. Importantly, the codon mutation restores zidovudine susceptibility to zidovudine-resistant HIV. Cross-resistance to didanosine and zalcitabine occurs, but the decreased susceptibility to these drugs is less than for lamivudine (Schinazi *et al.*, 1993).

Absorption, Distribution, and Elimination. Lamivudine has high oral bioavailability with or without food and reaches peak plasma levels within approximately 1 hour. The long intracellular half-life of the triphosphate suggests than once-daily dosing may be effective (Gao *et al.*, 1994; Heald *et al.*, 1996; Yuen *et al.*, 1995). Lamivudine is excreted primarily unchanged in the urine. The CSF-to-plasma AUC ratio is 0.15 (Haas *et al.*, 2000b; Lewis *et al.*, 1996). Lamivudine crosses the placenta and has been detected in the fetal circulation.

Untoward Effects. Significant adverse effects of lamivudine are rare. Headache and nausea have been reported at higher-than-recommended doses (Bartlett *et al.*, 1996). Pancreatitis has been reported in pediatric patients, but this has not been confirmed in controlled trials of adults or children.

Drug Interactions and Precautions. Lamivudine and zalcitabine may be antagonistic and should not be used concomitantly. Trimethoprim–sulfamethoxazole increases plasma lamivudine concentrations, but this does not require dose adjustment.

Therapeutic Use. Lamivudine is FDA-approved for treating HIV infection in adults and children, in combination with other antiretroviral agents. Before the rapid emergence of resistance was appreciated with lamivudine monotherapy, a limited number of monotherapy trials were performed (Pluda *et al.*, 1995; Schuurman *et al.*, 1995). Lamivudine in combination with zidovudine produced substantial but incomplete decreases in plasma HIV-1 RNA (Eron *et al.*, 1995; Katlama *et al.*, 1996). Many trials have confirmed the antiretroviral activity of lamivudine in three-drug regimens with other nucleoside analogs, protease inhibitors, and/or nonnucleoside reverse transcriptase inhibitors. Lamivudine has been effective in combination with other antiretroviral compounds for treating experienced or naïve patients (Gulick *et al.*, 1997; Hammer *et al.*, 1997).

Abacavir

Chemistry and Antiviral Activity. *Abacavir sulfate*—(1*S,cis*)-4-[2-amino-6-(cyclopropylamino)-9H-purin-9-yl)]-2-cyclopentene-1-methanol sulfate (salt) (2:1)—is a carbocyclic nucleoside analog that contains a novel 6-cyclopropylamino-substituted purine. The active metabolite of abacavir, carbovir triphosphate, is a potent HIV-1 reverse transcriptase inhibitor. The IC_{50} of abacavir against clinical isolates is 0.26 μM, and its IC_{50} *in vitro* against laboratory strains ranges from 0.07 to 5.8 μM (Daluge *et al.*, 1997).

Mechanisms of Action and Resistance. Abacavir undergoes intracellular phosphorylation by enzymes that do not phosphorylate other FDA-approved nucleoside reverse transcriptase inhibitors. It is monophosphorylated by a pathway involving adenosine phosphotransferase and is then di- and triphosphorylated. Carbovir triphosphate accumulates and has an intracellular half-life of 3 hours (Daluge *et al.*, 1997; Faletto *et al.*, 1997).

In vitro passage of HIV-1 in the presence of abacavir selects for modest resistance (up to 10-fold) with mutations at reverse transcriptase codons 184, 65, 74, and 115. Resistance in clinical isolates from patients who had received prior therapy with nucleoside reverse transcriptase inhibitors is associated with multiple mutations. Strains that are resistant to all other nucleoside reverse transcriptase inhibitors also are resistant to abacavir (Tisdale *et al.*, 1997), and may contain mutations at codons 41, 210, 215, or 151 or an insertion mutation at codon 69. Increasing numbers of mutations increase the likelihood of abacavir resistance (Tisdale *et al.*, 1997).

Absorption, Distribution, and Elimination. The oral bioavailability of abacavir is high with or without food (Daluge *et al.*, 1997; Chittick *et al.*, 1999); the CSF-to-plasma AUC ratio is approximately 0.3. Abacavir is partially metabolized by alcohol dehydrogenase (to form the 5'-carboxylic acid) and glucuronidation (to form the 5'-glucuronide) (Chittick *et al.*, 1999).

Untoward Effects. The most common adverse events are gastrointestinal symptoms, neurologic complaints, and a unique hypersensitivity syndrome. Nausea, vomiting, diarrhea, and abdominal pain were common in one large clinical trial, but only 10% of patients withdrew because of adverse events. Neurological complaints, including headache, dizziness, and insomnia, were less frequent. Asthenia has been reported in 40% of patients (Harrigan *et al.*, 2000).

Abacavir Hypersensitivity Reaction. A unique and potentially fatal hypersensitivity reaction occurs in 2% to 5% of patients receiving abacavir. Symptoms typically occur within the first six weeks of therapy and include fever, rash, nausea, malaise, and respiratory complaints, in various combinations. Symptoms initially may be mild but increase in severity with continued administration. Discontinuation of the medication usually resolves all signs and symptoms, but rechallenge may cause rapid onset of severe reactions, hypotension, and death. Once an abacavir hypersensitivity reaction is suspected or confirmed, it is recommended that the patient never be rechallenged with abacavir.

Drug Interactions and Precautions.   Ethanol increases plasma levels of abacavir by 41% (McDowell *et al.,* 2000). Patients who begin abacavir must be educated regarding the hypersensitivity reaction (*see* above) and instructed about what to do if this occurs. This generally involves seeking medical help immediately if they develop symptoms of hypersensitivity.

Therapeutic Use.   Abacavir is FDA-approved for treating HIV infection in adults and children in combination with other antiretroviral agents. Several studies have evaluated abacavir in combination with other nucleoside analogs, nonnucleoside reverse transcriptase inhibitors, and protease inhibitors. The combination of abacavir, zidovudine, and lamivudine has efficacious antiretroviral activity in both adults and pediatric patients. Substantially greater decreases in plasma HIV-1 RNA occurred in patients re-

ceiving this three-drug regimen *versus* zidovudine plus lamivudine. Adding abacavir to stable antiretroviral therapy may exert significant antiviral effect, but not if there are multiple, preexisting zidovudine resistance mutations. Abacavir also has been used in three- and four-drug regimens for heavily experienced patients failing previous therapies (Deeks *et al.,* 1999; Falloon *et al.,* 2000).

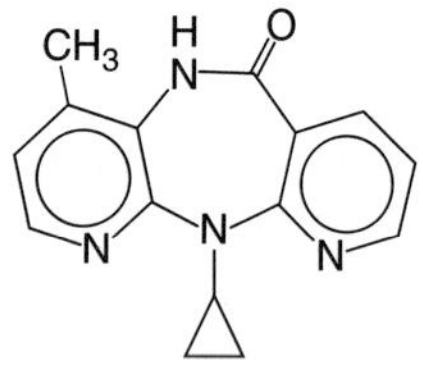

NONNUCLEOSIDE REVERSE TRANSCRIPTASE INHIBITORS

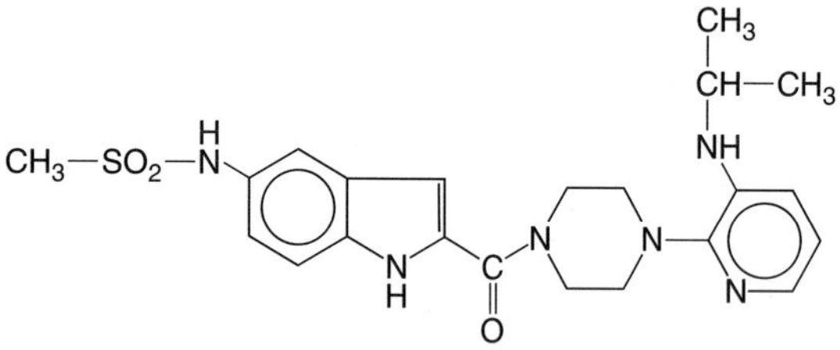

The nonnucleoside reverse transcriptase inhibitors are a class of chemically distinct synthetic compounds that block reverse transcriptase activity by binding adjacent to the enzyme's active site, inducing conformational changes in this site. These agents share not only a common mechanism of action but also some toxicities and resistance profiles. Unlike nucleoside analogs, nonnucleoside reverse transcriptase inhibitors do not undergo phosphorylation. In addition, they are active against only HIV-1, not HIV-2. All compounds in this class are metabolized by the CYP450 system and thus are prone to drug interactions.

Three nucleoside reverse transcriptase inhibitors are FDA-approved (Table 51–1). Their chemical structures are shown in Figure 51–3 and selected pharmacokinetic parameters in Table 51–3.

Nevirapine

Chemistry and Antiviral Activity.   *Nevirapine* is a nonnucleoside reverse transcriptase inhibitor with potent activity against HIV-1. It is active in several cell lines including T lymphocytes and macrophages. Infectivity of extracellular virions also can be decreased by exposure to nevirapine. The IC_{50} of nevirapine ranges from 10 to 100 nM (Zhang *et al.,* 1996). Like other compounds in this class, nevirapine does not have significant activity against HIV-2 and other retroviruses.

Mechanism of Action and Resistance.   Nevirapine diffuses into the cell and binds to reverse transcriptase adjacent to the catalytic site. This induces conformational changes that inactivate the enzyme. Resistance develops rapidly in cells exposed to nevirapine. High-level resistance is associated with mutations at reverse transcriptase codons 101, 103, 106, 108, 135, 181, 188, and 190. A single mutation at either codon 103 or 181 decreases susceptibility more than 100-fold. Cross-resistance may extend to all FDA-approved nonnucleoside reverse transcriptase inhibitors, especially with the codon 103 mutation (Casado *et al.,* 2000).

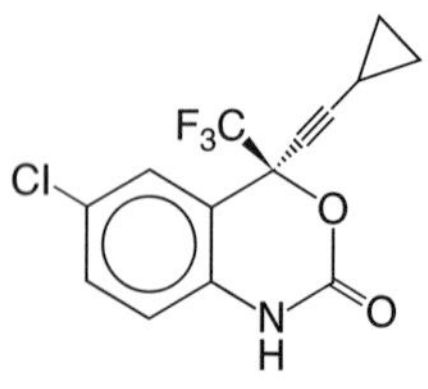

Figure 51–3. Structures of nonnucleoside reverse transcriptase inhibitors.

Absorption, Distribution, and Elimination.   Nevirapine is well absorbed orally. Neither food nor antacids affect bioavailability

Table 51–3
Pharmacokinetic Properties of Nonnucleoside Reverse Transcriptase Inhibitors

PARAMETER	NEVIRAPINE*	EFAVIRENZ*	DELAVIRDINE
Oral bioavailability, %	90	50	85
Plasma $t_{1/2elim}$, hours	25–30	40–50	2–11
Plasma protein binding, %	60	99	98
Metabolism	Hepatic	Hepatic	Hepatic
Renal excretion of parent drug, %	< 3	< 3	< 3
Autoinduction of metabolism	Yes	Yes	No

Abbreviation: $t_{1/2elim}$, half-life of elimination.
*Values after multiple doses.

(Cheeseman *et al.*, 1993, 1995). Nevirapine readily crosses the placenta and has been found in breast milk. The CSF-to-plasma ratio for nevirapine is approximately 0.45 (Mirochnick *et al.*, 1998; Zhou *et al.*, 1999).

Oxidative metabolism of nevirapine in the liver by cytochrome P450 isoforms CYP3A4 and CYP2B6 produces several metabolites including 2-, 3-, 8-, and 12-hydroxynevirapine. Glucuronidation of metabolites and urinary excretion constitute the primary elimination pathway (Erickson *et al.*, 1999; Riska *et al.*, 1999).

Nevirapine also induces the synthesis of CYP3A4, which decreases the plasma half-life of nevirapine from 45 hours following the first dose to 25 hours after 2 weeks. To compensate for this induction, initiation of nevirapine includes a 14-day initial dosing period, at the end of which the dose is increased if no adverse reactions have occurred.

Untoward Effects. The most frequent adverse events associated with nevirapine include rash, fever, fatigue, headache, somnolence, nausea, and elevated liver enzymes.

Rash occurs in approximately 16% of patients. This usually is a mild macular or papular eruption involving the trunk, face, and extremities and generally occurs within the first six weeks of therapy. Pruritus is common. Approximately 7% of patients discontinue therapy due to rash, and preemptive administration of glucocorticoids paradoxically may cause a more severe rash. Stevens–Johnson syndrome occurs with an incidence of approximately 0.3%. The incidence of nevirapine-induced hepatitis approaches 1%.

Drug Interactions and Precautions. Since nevirapine induces CYP3A4, coadministration with agents metabolized by this system may lower their plasma levels. Methadone withdrawal has been reported in patients receiving nevirapine (Altice *et al.*, 1999).

Rifampin and ketoconazole are contraindicated in patients receiving nevirapine. Plasma ethinyl estradiol levels decrease significantly with nevirapine coadministration, and alternative methods of birth control are advised. Although nevirapine can lower plasma concentrations of protease inhibitors, most such combinations do not require dose adjustment. Nevirapine levels generally are unaffected by concomitant protease inhibitors (Table 51–4).

Therapeutic Use. Nevirapine is FDA-approved for treating HIV-1 infection in adults and children, in combination with other antiretroviral agents. It can be very effective during long-term administration in multidrug regimens. Nevirapine was evaluated originally in small clinical trials as monotherapy or alternating monotherapy with zidovudine administration. Only modest, short-term improvements in laboratory markers of HIV infection were reported because of rapid emergence of resistance (Havlir *et al.*, 1995). More recent trials have evaluated nevirapine in three-drug regimens. In one large trial that examined a three-drug regimen of nevirapine, zidovudine, and didanosine in antiretroviral-naïve adults, 52% of patients had plasma HIV-1 RNA below 400 copies per milliliter (Montaner *et al.*, 1998). Many trials currently are evaluating nevirapine-containing regimens in treatment of naïve and experienced patients. Clinical trials also are addressing whether or not lipodystrophy (*see* section on untoward effects of protease inhibitors, below) resolves when a protease inhibitor is replaced by nevirapine (Raboud *et al.*, 1999; Raffi *et al.*, 1998).

Nevirapine has been evaluated in pregnant HIV-infected women. In a landmark study performed in Uganda, a single, oral intrapartum dose of nevirapine followed by a single dose to the newborn was superior to more complicated zidovudine therapy in preventing vertical transmission of HIV. Only 13% of nevirapine-treated women

Table 51–4

Drug Interactions between Nonnucleoside Reverse Transcriptase Inhibitors and HIV Protease Inhibitors

	EFFECT OF NNRTI ON PLASMA AUC OF PI (% CHANGE)			EFFECT OF PI ON PLASMA AUC OF NNRTI (% CHANGE)		
	DELAVIRDINE	NEVIRAPINE	EFAVIRENZ	DELAVIRDINE	NEVIRAPINE	EFAVIRENZ
RITONAVIR	↑ 1.7-fold	↓ 41%	↑ 1.2-fold	↔	↔	↑ 1.2-fold
INDINAVIR	↑ 1.4-fold	↓ 30%	↓ 30%	↔	↔	?
NELFINAVIR	↑ 2-fold	↑ 1.1-fold	↑ 1.2-fold	↓ 50%	↔	?
SAQUINAVIR	↑ 6-fold	↓ 25%	↓ 60%	↔	↔	↓ 10%
AMPRENAVIR	?	?	↓ 35%	?	?	↔
LOPINAVIR	?	↔	↓ 19%	?	?	↓ (slight)

Abbreviations: NNRTI, nonnucleoside reverse transcriptase inhibitor; PI, HIV protease inhibitor; AUC, area under the plasma concentration–time curve; ↑, increase, ↓, decrease; ↔, no change.

transmitted HIV compared to 21.5% of zidovudine-treated women (Guay *et al.,* 1999).

Delavirdine

Chemistry and Antiviral Activity. *Delavirdine* is a bishetero-arylpiperazine nonnucleoside reverse transcriptase inhibitor that selectively inhibits HIV-1 in several *in vitro* cell systems. Its median inhibitory concentration is 0.006 μM (Dueweke *et al.,* 1993a). Like other compounds in this class, delavirdine does not have significant activity against HIV-2 or other retroviruses (Romero *et al.,* 1991).

Mechanism of Action and Resistance. After entering the cell, delavirdine binds to a hydrophobic pocket in the p66 subunit of reverse transcriptase. This causes a conformational change to a stable, inactive form of the enzyme. The delavirdine-reverse transcriptase complex is stabilized by hydrogen bonds at residue Lys-103 and strong hydrophobic interactions with residue Pro-236 (Spence *et al.,* 1995). Much higher concentrations of delavirdine are required to inhibit cellular polymerase than reverse transcriptase (Dueweke *et al.,* 1993a).

As with other nonnucleoside reverse transcriptase inhibitors, high-level resistance to delavirdine can emerge rapidly. *In vitro* passage of HIV-1 in the presence of delavirdine selects for a mutation at reverse transcriptase codon 236, which does not confer cross-resistance to other compounds in this class. However, *in vivo* resistance rarely is associated with the 236 mutation. Most clinically derived resistant strains have mutations at reverse transcriptase codons 181 and/or 103. Resistance also has been associated with mutations at codons 100, 101, 106, and 188 (Dueweke *et al.,* 1993b). There is evidence that resistance to delavirdine may restore zidovudine susceptibility to zidovudine-resistant HIV.

Absorption, Distribution, and Elimination. Delavirdine is well absorbed, especially at pH less than 2.0. Antacids, his-

tamine H_2-receptor antagonists, achlorhydria, and high-fat meals may decrease its absorption (Barry *et al.,* 1999). Its plasma half-life increases with increasing doses (Cheng *et al.,* 1997; Freimuth, 1996).

Delavirdine binds extensively to plasma proteins and primarily is metabolized by CYP3A4. The major metabolic pathway results in *N*-dealkylation. There is considerable intersubject variability in plasma delavirdine concentrations related to differences in CYP3A activity. The CSF-to-plasma ratio is 0.02.

Untoward Effects. The most common side effect of delavirdine is rash, which develops in 18% to 36% of subjects. This typically occurs in the first few weeks of administration and often resolves despite continued therapy. The rash may be macular, papular, erythematous, or pruritic and usually involves the trunk and extremities. Rash causes discontinuation of delavirdine in less than 5% of patients and generally is less severe than the rash associated with nevirapine. Severe dermatitis, including Stevens–Johnson syndrome, is rare. Elevated liver function tests and rare cases of neutropenia have been reported (Para *et al.,* 1999).

Drug Interactions and Precautions. Delavirdine is both a substrate and inhibitor of CYP3A4, and it can alter the metabolism of other CYP3A4 substrates. Such drugs include rifampin, rifabutin, ergot derivatives, triazolam, midazolam, and cisapride. Delavirdine also inhibits CYP2C9. Carbamazepine, phenobarbital, phenytoin, rifabutin, and rifampin may decrease delavirdine levels by inducing CYP3A4. Compounds metabolized by CYP3A4 should be administered cautiously to patients receiving delavirdine. Delavirdine increases plasma levels of saquinavir, indinavir, nelfinavir, and ritonavir (Table 51–4).

Therapeutic Use.   Delavirdine is approved for the treatment of HIV-1 infection in adults in combination with other antiretroviral agents. Although delavirdine may be highly effective in multidrug regimens, initial monotherapy studies showed only transient decreases in plasma HIV-1 RNA levels due to rapid emergence of resistance. Later studies of delavirdine in combination with nucleoside analogs showed sustained decreases in HIV-1 RNA levels. Delavirdine increases plasma concentrations of indinavir, which may increase the efficacy of this combination. Current studies are evaluating the efficacy of delavirdine in three-drug regimens (Friedland *et al.*, 1999; Para *et al.*, 1999).

Efavirenz

Chemistry and Antiviral Activity.   *Efavirenz* is a 1,4-dihydro-2H-3,1-benzoxazin-2-one nonnucleoside reverse transcriptase inhibitor. Efavirenz inhibits HIV-1 reverse transcriptase both *in vitro* and *in vivo*, with an IC_{90} ranging from 3 to 9 nM (Young *et al.*, 1995). Like other compounds in this class, efavirenz does not have significant activity against HIV-2 or other retroviruses.

Mechanisms of Action and Resistance.   Efavirenz diffuses into the cell where it binds adjacent to the active site of reverse transcriptase. This produces a conformational change in the enzyme that inhibits function.

High-level resistance to efavirenz can develop *in vitro* and *in vivo*. Passage of HIV-1 in the presence of efavirenz yielded a strain with a greater than 300-fold decreased susceptibility. This strain had mutations at reverse transcriptase codons 100, 179, and 181. High-level *in vitro* resistance also was associated with mutations at codon 188 (Winslow *et al.*, 1996). The most frequent resistance-associated mutation in patients receiving efavirenz is at codon 103. Additional mutations have been reported at codons 100, 106, 188, and 190.

Absorption, Distribution, and Elimination.   Efavirenz is well absorbed from the gastrointestinal tract and reaches peak plasma concentrations within 3 to 4 hours. The proportion absorbed decreases with increasing doses; bioavailability is increased by a high-fat meal. Its long half-life allows once-daily dosing of efavirenz. Its low CSF-to-plasma ratio of 0.01 may reflect the drug being highly bound to plasma proteins (Tashima *et al.*, 1999; Villani *et al.*, 1999).

Efavirenz is a substrate for cytochrome P450 isoforms, particularly CYP3A4 and CYP2B6. The 8-hydroxy metabolite is excreted in the urine, and the glucuronide conjugate of 8-hydroxy-efavirenz is present in plasma and urine. Sixty percent of the dose is excreted in urine as the glucuronide conjugate (Villani *et al.*, 1999).

Untoward Effects.   Common side effects of efavirenz include headache, dizziness, abnormal dreams, impaired concentration, and rash. Central nervous symptoms usually occur with the first dose and may last for hours. More severe symptoms usually resolve over several weeks. As many as 52% of patients report some central nervous system or psychiatric side effects, but less than 5% discontinue drug for this reason.

Rash develops in up to 27% of patients, usually within the first 1 or 2 weeks; it is mild and rarely requires drug discontinuation. Serious rashes are uncommon. Increased liver enzymes, elevated lipid levels, and false positive screening tests for marijuana metabolites have been reported (Adkins and Noble, 1998).

Although teratotoxicity studies in rats and rabbits demonstrated no significant effects, when efavirenz was administered to pregnant cynomolgus monkeys, 25% of fetuses developed malformations. *Women of childbearing potential should use two methods of birth control to avoid pregnancy when taking efavirenz.*

Drug Interactions and Precautions.   Efavirenz may decrease levels of phenobarbital, phenytoin, carbamazepine, and methadone by inducing cytochrome P450 isoforms. Rifampin levels are unchanged by concurrent administration, but it may reduce levels of efavirenz. Rifabutin levels are reduced by efavirenz. The effect of efavirenz on protease inhibitor concentrations is variable (Table 51–4). Indinavir, saquinavir, and amprenavir levels are reduced by efavirenz, but ritonavir and nelfinavir levels are increased (Adkins and Noble, 1998). Drugs that induce CYP3A4 (*e.g.*, phenobarbital, phenytoin, carbamazepine) would be expected to increase the clearance of efavirenz and lower its plasma levels.

Therapeutic Use.   Efavirenz is approved for treating HIV-1 infection in combination with other antiretroviral agents. It was the first antiretroviral agent approved by the FDA for once-daily administration. Initial short-term monotherapy studies showed significant antiviral effects of efavirenz. Later studies evaluated efavirenz in multidrug combinations in HIV-infected adults and children. In antiretroviral-naïve patients, suppression of HIV-1 RNA to undetectable levels occurred in 70% of patients receiving efavirenz, zidovudine, and lamivudine and in 48% of those receiving indinavir plus zidovudine and lamivudine (Staszewski *et al.*, 1999). Much of this difference reflected greater patient compliance with the former regimen. Efavirenz prescribed in multiple-drug combinations also has demonstrated activity in patients failing prior regimens (Falloon *et al.*, 2000; Piketty *et al.*, 1999). When children failing prior therapy with a nucleoside analog reverse transcriptase inhibitor were treated with a combination of efavirenz, nelfinavir, and a nucleoside analog, 60% had a sustained antiviral benefit at 48 weeks (Starr *et al.,* 1999).

PROTEASE INHIBITORS

A review of available clinical trials of HIV-1 protease inhibitors is beyond the scope of this chapter (Flexner, 2000). Although selected important studies are cited in the text, the reader is referred elsewhere for a summary of many important clinical trials (Tavel *et al.,* 1999).

Shared Features

Mechanism of Action and Resistance. The HIV-1 protease is a dimer consisting of two 99-amino acid monomers; each monomer contributes an aspartic acid to form the catalytic site (Pearl and Taylor, 1987). In contrast, human aspartyl proteases (renin, gastricsin, and cathepsin D/E) contain only one polypeptide chain. Such structural differences allow the HIV protease inhibitors to have greater than 1000-fold higher affinity for HIV protease than for human aspartyl proteases. The HIV protease is essential for viral infectivity (Kohl *et al.,* 1988) and cleaves the viral polyprotein (gag-pol) into active viral enzymes (reverse transcriptase, protease, and integrase) and structural proteins (p17, p24, p9, and p7). Its preferred cleavage site is the *N*-terminal side of proline residues, especially between phenylalanine and proline. All six available protease inhibitors (amprenavir, indinavir, ritonavir, nelfinavir, nelfinavir, and lopinavir) act by binding reversibly to the active site of HIV protease. This prevents the protease from cleaving the viral precursor polypeptide and blocks subsequent viral maturation. Cells incubated in the presence of HIV protease inhibitors produce viral particles that are immature and noninfectious.

As with all antiretroviral agents, viral replication in the presence HIV protease inhibitors ultimately will select for drug-resistant virus. Suboptimal plasma protease inhibitor concentrations predispose to viral breakthrough and resistance (Schapiro *et al.,* 1996). Although each drug selects for different mutations of the protease gene, resistance to one HIV protease inhibitor often predicts less-favorable clinical responses to other subsequently prescribed protease inhibitors regardless of resistance test results.

Resistance to protease inhibitors generally occurs by stepwise accumulation of mutations of the protease gene. It is thought that initial mutations confer low-level resistance that allows the virus to replicate inefficiently in the presence of drug. Additional mutations may be compensatory, restoring more efficient replication and conferring high-level resistance. Resistance mutations also may alter the cleavage sites of gag-pol.

Almost all approved agents of this class are potent inhibitors of HIV-1 replication, and monotherapy lowers plasma HIV-1 RNA levels approximately 100- to 1000-fold within 4 to 12 weeks. The exception is a hard-gelatin capsule dosage form of saquinavir, which has poor bioavailability unless adminis-

tered with ritonavir. Otherwise, relative efficacies of individual agents are uncertain, because comparative studies generally are lacking. When any potent protease inhibitor has been administered with two nucleoside analogs during clinical trials, 60% to 95% of antiretroviral-naïve patients have achieved plasma HIV RNA levels below limits of detection. In this situation, many (if not most) therapeutic failures likely are due to poor patient adherence.

Absorption, Distribution, and Elimination. Most HIV protease inhibitors have poor systemic bioavailability. Amprenavir, indinavir, ritonavir, nelfinavir, saquinavir, and lopinavir all undergo oxidative metabolism by CYP3A4, and additional CYP isoforms metabolize individual protease inhibitors. Metabolism occurs predominantly in the liver, but metabolism by intestinal epithelial cells also may decrease bioavailability. The greater than 10- to 20-fold range in activity of various isoforms among individuals may contribute to variable drug pharmacokinetics (Rendic and Di Carlo, 1997). Only nelfinavir has an active metabolite, which is generated by CYP2C19.

All HIV protease inhibitors also are substrates for P-glycoprotein, the multidrug efflux pump encoded by *MDR 1*. This may limit cellular penetration and tissue delivery. P-glycoprotein in capillary endothelial cells of the blood–brain barrier may limit drug penetration into the brain (Kim *et al.,* 1998). P-glycoprotein also is present in bile canaliculi, small intestine epithelia, renal tubules, testes, and the placenta. Most protease inhibitors penetrate less well into semen than do nucleoside reverse transcriptase inhibitors and nonnucleoside reverse transcriptase inhibitors, although virologic response in plasma and semen usually are concordant (Taylor *et al.,* 1999).

Since little drug is excreted unchanged by the kidneys, dose adjustments for renal dysfunction are generally unnecessary (Jayasekara *et al.,* 1999). The six FDA-approved HIV protease inhibitors are listed in Table 51–1, and their chemical structures are shown in Figure 51–4. Selected pharmacokinetic parameters for individual protease inhibitors are summarized in Table 51–5.

Protein Binding. The HIV protease inhibitors bind extensively to normal plasma proteins, especially α_1-acid glycoprotein. The percentage of protein binding varies approximately as follows: (ritonavir, nelfinavir, saquinavir, lopinavir) > amprenavir > indinavir. The extent and reversibility of binding, or "on-off rate," must be considered when assessing *in vitro* binding data. The concentration of free drug may be most relevant, since only this fraction can directly exert antiviral activity. Conversely, protein binding provides a reservoir from which drug in plasma can equilibrate with drug in tissues. An early HIV-1 protease inhibitor, SC-52151, was potent *in vitro* but was inactive in clinical trials due to high-affinity binding to α_1-acid glycoprotein. In response to this lesson, all subsequent HIV protease inhibitors have been tested to assess the effect of plasma protein binding on activity. Very high concentrations of α_1-acid glycoprotein may substantially decrease the activity of some protease inhibitors.

Untoward Effects. Toxicities of protease inhibitors include nausea, vomiting, diarrhea, and paresthesias. These

SAQUINAVIR

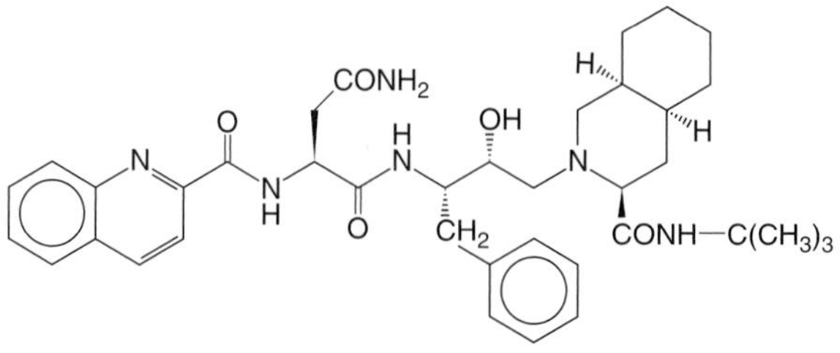

INDINAVIR

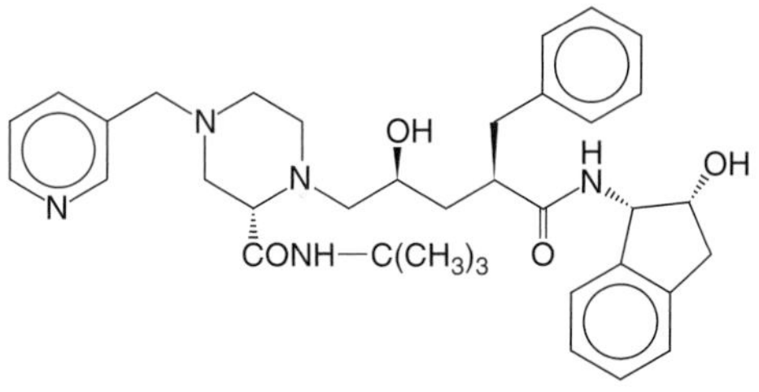

RITONAVIR

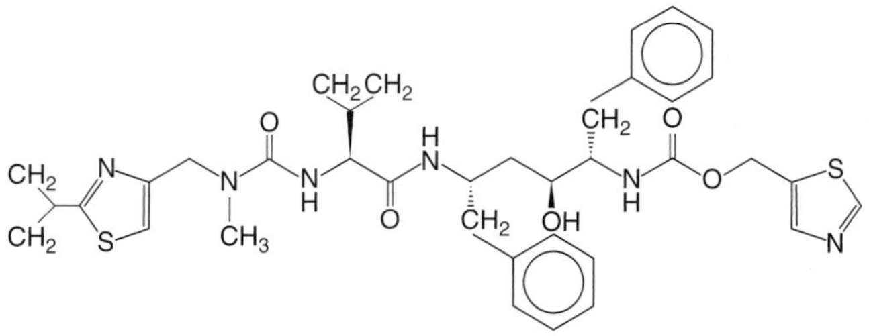

NELFINAVIR

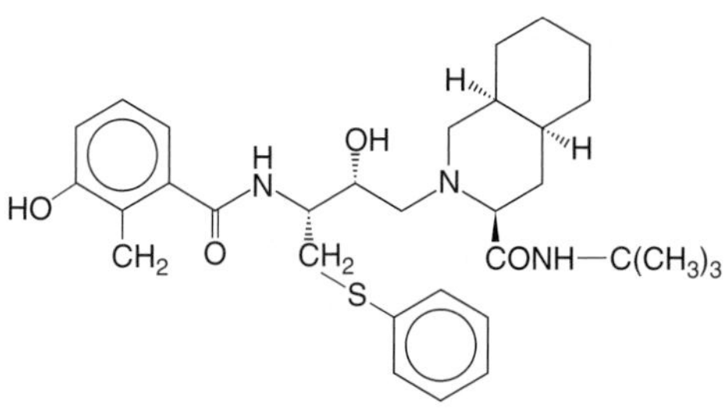

AMPRENAVIR

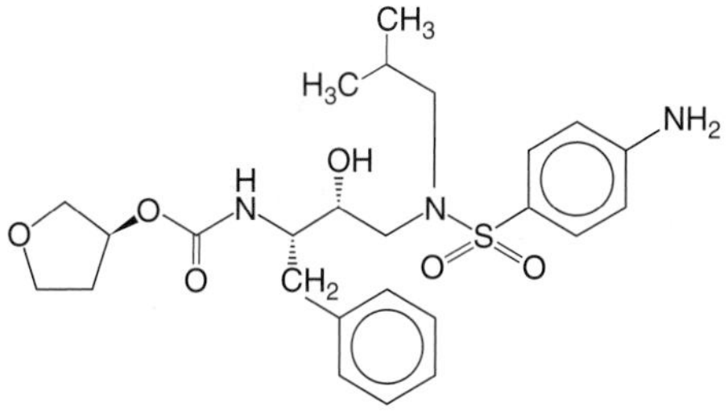

LOPINAVIR

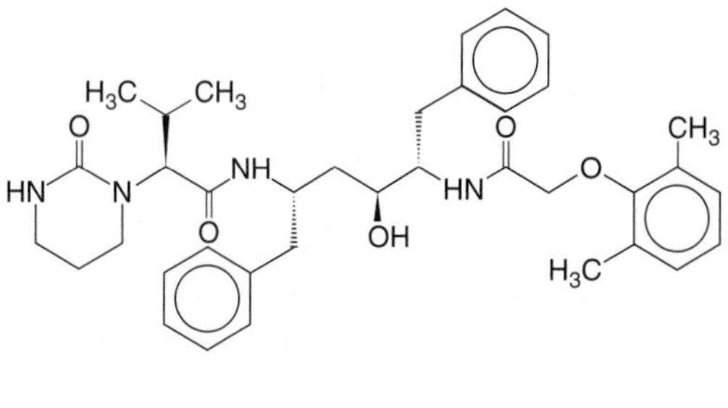

Figure 51–4. Structures of HIV protease inhibitors.

Table 51-5
Pharmacokinetic Properties of HIV-1 Protease Inhibitors

PARAMETER	AMPRENAVIR	INDINAVIR	NELFINAVIR	RITONAVIR	SAQUINAVIR*	LOPINAVIR$_R$†
Oral bioavailability, %	35–90	60–65	20–80	65–75	12	?
Effect of meals on AUC	↓21% (high fat)	↓77% (high fat)	↑200–300%	↑15% (capsule formulation)	↑600%	↑50%
Plasma $t_{1/2elim}$, hours	7–11	1.5–2	3.5–5	3–5	7–12	6–8
Plasma protein binding, %	90	60	98	98–99	98	98–99
Metabolism	CYP3A4	CYP3A4	CYP3A4>2C 19	CYP3A4>2D6 6	CYP3A4	CYP3A4
Autoinduction of metabolism	no	no	yes	yes	no	yes
Renal excretion, % (parent drug)	<3	11	1–2	3.5	<3	<3
Inhibition of CYP3A4	++	++	++	++++	+	+++

Abbreviations: AUC, area under plasma concentration-time curve; $t_{1/2elim}$, half-life of elimination; CL_{cr}, creatinine clearance in ml/min; ↑, increase; ↓, decrease. CYP, cytochrome P450.
*Saquinavir data refer to soft-gel capsule formulation.
†Lopinavir$_R$ refers to coformulation with ritonavir.

agents also may cause glucose intolerance, diabetes, hypercholesterolemia, and hypertriglyceridemia. Prolonged administration of HIV protease inhibitors has been associated with fat redistribution, especially central fat accumulation, in some patients. This includes increased visceral fat and abdominal girth, an enlarged fat pad at the base of the neck ("buffalo hump"), breast enlargement, and/or subcutaneous lipomas. Current studies are defining the epidemiology, mechanisms, and optimal management of this complication.

Precautions and Interactions. Since all HIV protease inhibitors are both substrates and inhibitors of CYP isoforms, drug interactions are common. The rank order of CYP3A4 inhibitory potency is ritonavir ≫ (indinavir, amprenavir, nelfinavir) > saquinavir. Some metabolic interactions between protease inhibitors may be beneficial, such as the use of ritonavir to increase the AUC, half-life, and trough concentrations of saquinavir, indinavir, amprenavir, or lopinavir. Concomitant administration of CYP3A4 inducers such as rifampin may yield subtherapeutic plasma concentrations of protease inhibitors. Assiduous attention must be paid to avoid detrimental drug interactions.

A summary of interactions between individual protease inhibitors is presented in Table 51–6; interactions between protease inhibitors and nonnucleoside reverse transcriptase inhibitors are summarized in Table 51–4.

Saquinavir

Chemistry and Antiviral Activity. *Saquinavir* is a peptidomimetic HIV protease inhibitor of the hydroxyethylamine class developed by rational drug design (Roberts *et al.*, 1990). Once it was recognized that some sites cleaved by HIV-1 protease were unique compared to sites cleaved by eukaryotic protease, peptides were synthesized to mimic the transition state of the phenylalanine-proline cleavage site in the viral polyprotein. Saquinavir is a potent inhibitor of both HIV-1 and HIV-2 proteases. In peripheral blood lymphocytes, its IC_{50} ranges from 3.5 to 10 nM (Craig *et al.*, 1991).

Mechanisms of Action and Resistance. HIV protease cleaves the viral polyprotein (gag-pol) into active enzymes and structural proteins. Saquinavir reversibly binds to the active site of HIV protease, preventing polypeptide processing and subsequent viral maturation. Viral particles produced in the presence of saquinavir are immature and noninfectious.

Viral replication in the presence of saquinavir selects for drug-resistant virus. Among patients treated with saquinavir, resistance has been associated with progressive accumulation of resistance mutations over time. The most common mutation associated with saquinavir resistance is at protease codon 90, followed in frequency by codon 48 (Ives *et al.*, 1997). With prolonged administration, additional mutations at positions 36, 46, 82, and 84 occur and are associated with cross-resistance to other protease inhibitors.

Absorption, Distribution, and Elimination. Oral bioavailability of the hard-gelatin capsule formulation of saquinavir (saquinavir mesylate, INVIRASE) is only 4% due to limited absorption and extensive first-pass metabolism, with considerable interpatient variability (Noble and Faulds, 1996). Limited antiviral efficacy is achieved at the approved dosage, yielding only a fivefold reduction in plasma HIV-1 RNA. A greater effect is achieved by administering 7200 mg daily in six divided doses, four times the approved dose, with a strong correlation between plasma drug concentration and therapeutic effect (Schapiro *et al.*, 1996). A soft-gelatin capsule formulation (FORTOVASE) with approximately threefold increased oral bioavailability became available in 1997 (Perry and Noble, 1998). Absorption of saquinavir may be enhanced when the drug is taken with a high-calorie, high-fat meal. Saquinavir's short half-life requires administration every 8 hours. In addition, saquinavir demonstrates a greater than dose-proportional increase in exposure. For example, tripling the oral dose of saquinavir is associated with an eightfold increase in exposure. Substances that inhibit intestinal but not hepatic CYP3A4, such as grapefruit

Table 51–6
Drug Interactions between HIV Protease Inhibitors

DRUG EXERTING EFFECT	DRUG AFFECTED (CHANGE IN PLASMA AUC)					
	RITONAVIR	INDINAVIR	NELFINAVIR	SAQUINAVIR	AMPRENAVIR	LOPINAVIR$_R$*
RITONAVIR	—	↑ 3–6-fold	↑ 2.5-fold	↑ 20-fold	↑ 3.5-fold	profound
INDINAVIR	↔	—	↑ 1.8-fold	↑ 5–8-fold	↑ 1.6-fold	?
NELFINAVIR	↔	↑ 1.5-fold	—	↑ 4–6-fold	↑ 2.5-fold	?
SAQUINAVIR	↔	↔	↑ 1.2-fold	—	↓ 30%	?
AMPRENAVIR	↔	↓ 38%	↑ 1.2-fold	↓ 18%	—	?
LOPINAVIR$_R$*	↔	?	?	?	?	?

Abbreviations: AUC, area under the plasma concentration–time curve; ↑, increase, ↓, decrease; ↔, no change.
*Coformulation of lopinavir with ritonavir.

juice, increase the saquinavir AUC by threefold at most (Flexner, 2000).

Saquinavir is metabolized primarily by hepatic CYP3A4 (Fitzsimmons and Collins, 1997). The metabolites of saquinavir are not active against HIV-1. Saquinavir and its metabolites are eliminated from the body primarily through the biliary system and feces (more than 95% of drug), with minimal urinary excretion (less than 3% of administered drug).

Untoward Effects.　The most frequent side effects of both saquinavir formulations are gastrointestinal, and include nausea, vomiting, diarrhea, and abdominal discomfort. Most side effects of saquinavir are mild. A causal relationship between other adverse effects and saquinavir is less clear.

Precautions and Interactions.　Although saquinavir is a weak inhibitor of CYP3A4, it should not be prescribed with ergot derivatives, cisapride, triazolam, or midazolam. Decreased clearance of these agents because of CYP3A4 inhibition may cause life-threatening cardiac arrhythmias or prolonged sedation, depending on the drug. Among the HIV protease inhibitors, saquinavir is particularly susceptible to increased clearance due to CYP3A4 induction. Coadministration of nevirapine or efavirenz lowers saquinavir levels considerably, so coadministration of these drugs should be avoided. The ability of nevirapine or efavirenz to lower saquinavir levels may be overcome when ritonavir is coadministered.

Coadministering ritonavir with saquinavir markedly increases plasma saquinavir concentrations, presumably by inhibiting CYP3A4 (Flexner, 2000). In a single-dose study, ritonavir increased the saquinavir AUC by 50- to 132-fold (Hsu et al., 1998). This is a commonly prescribed dual protease inhibitor combination.

Therapeutic Use.　In 1995, saquinavir became the first protease inhibitor approved by the FDA for treating HIV infection. Among patients with susceptible strains, soft-gelatin capsules of saquinavir substantially lower plasma HIV-1 RNA concentrations. In early clinical trials, hard-gelatin capsules of saquinavir mesylate (600 mg 3 times daily) demonstrated only modest virologic effect because of poor oral bioavailability. Greater activity was achieved with high-dose therapy of 1200 mg given 6 times daily (Schapiro et al., 1996). The soft-gelatin-capsule formulation (1200 mg every 8 hours) appears to have antiviral activity comparable to other HIV protease inhibitors. Saquinavir is commonly prescribed in combination with ritonavir because of a favorable pharmacokinetic interaction (see "Precautions and Interactions," above).

Indinavir

Chemistry and Antiviral Activity.　Indinavir is a peptidomimetic hydroxyethylamine HIV protease inhibitor (Plosker and Noble, 1999). It is formulated as the sulfate salt to yield more consistent plasma concentrations than with the free base following oral administration. Indinavir is tenfold more active against the protease of HIV-1 than that of HIV-2, and its 95% inhibitory concentration (IC_{95}) for wild-type HIV-1 ranges from 25 to 100 nM. The lead developmental compound for indinavir was a renin inhibitor that mimicked the phenylalanine-proline cleavage site in the viral polyprotein. Chemical modifications enhanced its antiretroviral activity and oral absorption, ultimately leading to the discovery of indinavir (Vacca et al., 1994).

Mechanisms of Action and Resistance.　Indinavir reversibly binds to the active site of HIV protease, preventing viral polypeptide processing and viral maturation. Viral particles produced in the presence of indinavir are immature and noninfectious.

Viral replication in the presence of indinavir selects for drug-resistant virus. Clinical indinavir resistance has been associated with progressive accumulation of mutations at protease codons 10, 20, 24, 46, 54, 63, 71, 82, 84, and 90. The mutations of primary importance are at positions 46 and 82. High-level resistance requires multiple mutations.

Absorption, Distribution, and Elimination.　Indinavir is rapidly absorbed after oral administration, with peak levels achieved in approximately 0.8 hour. Its aqueous solubility is much greater at pH 3.5 than at 7.4 (Lin et al., 1995). Absorption is unaffected by light, low-fat meals, but high-calorie, high-fat, high-protein meals reduce absorption by 75%. Therefore, indinavir must be taken while fasting or with a low-fat meal (e.g., corn flakes with skim milk and sugar). Its short half-life makes three-times-daily (every 8 hours) dosing necessary. Dietary restrictions and frequent dosing make patient compliance a challenge. Coadministration with ritonavir overcomes the effect of food and may allow twice-daily dosing.

Indinavir undergoes extensive hepatic metabolism by CYP3A4. Glucuronidation, oxidation, and N-acetylation produce at least six major metabolites. These achieve appreciable plasma concentrations, but none has documented antiretroviral activity. Indinavir and its metabolites are eliminated primarily in feces (81% of unchanged drug and metabolites) and urine (19% of unchanged drug and metabolites). Plasma indinavir levels increase with moderate liver disease, and dose reduction may be required.

Indinavir is only about 60% bound to plasma proteins, considerably less than other available protease inhibitors. The fact that only free drug is directly available for transfer to other compartments may explain the relatively high CSF-to-plasma AUC ratio of 0.07 for total indinavir, and 0.15 for free drug (Haas et al., 2000c). Only 5% of drug is protein bound in CSF.

Untoward Effects.　A unique adverse effect of indinavir is crystalluria. Precipitation of indinavir and its metabolites in urine may cause renal colic. Nephrolithiasis occurs in approximately 3% of patients. To reduce this risk, patients must drink sufficient fluids to maintain dilute urine. Prolonged administration of indinavir may be associated with fat redistribution in some patients. Hair and skin problems also have been observed with indinavir, including hair loss, dry skin, dry and cracked lips, and ingrown toenails (Bouscarat *et al.,* 1999, 1998). Gastrointestinal disturbances and central nervous system symptoms (headache, insomnia) also can occur.

Precautions and Interactions. Persons receiving indinavir should drink at least 72 fluid ounces of fluid daily. Indinavir-induced renal colic usually resolves with vigorous hydration and without discontinuing therapy. Some cases require drug discontinuation.

Since indinavir solubility markedly decreases at higher pH, antacids or other buffering agents should not be taken at the same time. Didanosine is coformulated with a buffer and should not be taken within one hour of indinavir. Since indinavir is metabolized by CYP3A4 and also is a modest inhibitor of the enzyme, drugs most prone to interactions with indinavir either induce, inhibit, or are metabolized by CYP3A4. Drugs that induce CYP3A4 activity may lower indinavir levels. Rifampin lowers the indinavir AUC by 90%, and is contraindicated. Efavirenz, nevirapine, and rifabutin lower indinavir levels less substantially (25% to 35%) and necessitate an increased indinavir dose. Indinavir can inhibit the metabolism of other CYP3A4 substrates. Indinavir raises rifabutin concentrations, increasing toxicity. The rifabutin daily dose in regimens containing indinavir therefore should be reduced by 50%. Indinavir may inhibit metabolism of cisapride, triazolam, and midazolam, causing cardiac arrhythmias or prolonged sedation, depending on the drug (Plosker and Noble, 1999).

Ritonavir increases the indinavir plasma AUC and trough concentrations by inhibiting CYP3A4. This may allow indinavir to be administered twice daily rather than three times daily, and may allow lower total daily doses. Delavirdine increases indinavir plasma concentrations, unlike other nonnucleoside reverse transcriptase inhibitors.

Therapeutic Use. Indinavir is indicated for treating HIV infection in adults and children. Among patients with susceptible strains of HIV-1, indinavir therapy substantially lowers plasma HIV-1 RNA levels. Large clinical trials have demonstrated both virologic and survival benefit when patients with AIDS received indinavir three times daily in combination with zidovudine and lamivudine (Gulick *et al.,* 1997; Hammer *et al.,* 1997). However, twice-daily administration of the same total daily dose was less efficacious (Haas *et al.,* 2000a). Various clinical trials currently are evaluating the use of indinavir in combination with ritonavir, since this combination is predicted to yield at

least equal efficacy with less frequent administration of indinavir.

Ritonavir

Chemistry and Antiviral Activity. Ritonavir is a peptidomimetic hydroxyethylamine HIV protease inhibitor. Ritonavir is more active against HIV-1 than against HIV-2, and its IC_{50} for wild-type HIV variants in MT4 cells in the presence of 50% human serum is approximately 45 nM.

Mechanisms of Action and Resistance. Ritonavir reversibly binds to the active site of HIV protease, preventing polypeptide processing and subsequent viral maturation. Viral particles produced in the presence of ritonavir are immature and noninfectious.

In patients treated with ritonavir, viral replication in the presence of drug selects for progressive accumulation of drug-resistance mutations (Molla *et al.,* 1996). The first ritonavir resistance mutation is usually at protease codon 82. Additional mutations associated with increasing resistance occur at codons 20, 32, 46, 54, 63, 71, 84, and 90. High-level resistance requires multiple mutations.

Absorption, Distribution, and Elimination. Absorption of ritonavir is only slightly affected by diet, and this is somewhat dependent on the formulation. The overall absorption of ritonavir from the capsule formulation may increase by 15% when taken with meals. Its half-life allows twice-daily administration. There is greater than sixfold variability in drug trough concentrations among patients given 600 mg of ritonavir every 12 hours (Danner *et al.,* 1995).

Ritonavir is metabolized primarily in the liver by cytochrome P450 isoforms, especially CYP3A and less so by CYP2D6. Ritonavir and its metabolites are eliminated from the body predominantly in the feces (86% of unchanged drug and metabolites), with minor urinary elimination (11%, mostly metabolites).

Ritonavir in Dual-Protease-Inhibitor Regimens. Ritonavir initially was developed as a potent protease inhibitor and produced clinical benefit in patients with advanced AIDS. Its pronounced inhibitory effect on CYP3A4 was viewed as a detriment, because this would reduce elimination of many drugs. For example, delayed clearance of midazolam by ritonavir causes prolonged sedation and respiratory depression. However, coadministration with ritonavir also increases the plasma AUCs, half-lives, and trough concentrations of saquinavir, indinavir, amprenavir, and lopinavir (Table 51–6) (Flexner, 2000). This effect can allow lower doses of a second protease inhibitor to be used. Using ritonavir as a "pharmacokinetic enhancer" to increase plasma concentrations of other HIV protease inhibitors has become common practice, and many clinical trials are in progress. For drugs with limited oral bioavailability, such as saquinavir and lopinavir, ritonavir markedly increases plasma drug levels and enhances anti-retroviral effect, and lopinavir is available only as a co-formulation with ritonavir. Ritonavir also overcomes the deleterious effect of food on indinavir bioavailability.

Untoward Effects. Side effects of ritonavir are dose-dependent, and include gastrointestinal complaints, such as nausea, diarrhea, anorexia, abdominal pain, and taste perversion. Peripheral and perioral paresthesias also are common. Ritonavir induces its own metabolism, and gradual dose escalation over the first two weeks minimizes early intolerance when the drug is prescribed at full dose. Ritonavir causes dose-dependent elevations in serum cholesterol and triglycerides, raising the concern that ritonavir therapy will increase the long-term risk of atherosclerosis.

Precautions and Interactions. To minimize intolerance during the initial weeks of therapy when prescribed at maximal approved doses for adults and adolescents, ritonavir should be initiated at 300 mg every 12 hours, and gradually escalated to 600 mg every 12 hours by day 14 of therapy. It is better tolerated if taken with meals.

Ritonavir potently inhibits CYP3A4, markedly increasing plasma levels of many drugs including amiodarone, propafenone, ergot derivatives, pimozide, cisapride, triazolam, and midazolam. Coadministration of ritonavir with these agents is contraindicated because it may cause life-threatening cardiac arrhythmias or prolonged sedation, depending on the drug (Plosker and Noble, 1999). Ritonavir may increase rifabutin concentrations markedly and cause toxicity. This combination therefore should be avoided. Concomitant administration of agents that induce CYP3A4 activity such as rifampin may lower ritonavir levels and also should be avoided. St. John's wort also can lower ritonavir levels. The capsule and solution formulations of ritonavir contain alcohol and may produce unpleasant reactions if administered with disulfiram or metronidazole (*see* Chapter 18).

Therapeutic Use. Ritonavir is indicated for treating HIV infection in adults and children. Among patients with susceptible strains of HIV-1, ritonavir substantially lowers plasma HIV-1 RNA levels. Clinical trials have demonstrated both virologic benefit and improved survival when patients with advanced disease were treated with ritonavir. Ritonavir was the first HIV protease inhibitor to have survival benefit (Tavel *et al.,* 1999). Numerous clinical trials have demonstrated the efficacy of ritonavir in various dual-protease-inhibitor regimens (Gisolf *et al.,* 2000).

Nelfinavir

Chemistry and Antiviral Activity. Traditional development of antiviral agents was based on screening thousands of compounds for viral activity in the laboratory. In contrast, nelfinavir was developed by rational drug design (Roberts *et al.,* 1990). Nelfinavir is a nonpeptide protease inhibitor that is active against both HIV-1 and HIV-2 and is formulated as the mesylate salt of a basic amine (Bardsley-Elliot and Plosker, 2000). The mean IC_{95} for HIV-1 in various *in vitro* assays is 59 nM.

Mechanisms of Action and Resistance. Nelfinavir inhibits protease by reversibly binding to the active site, preventing polypeptide processing and subsequent viral maturation. Viral particles produced in the presence of nelfinavir are immature and noninfectious.

Viral replication in the presence of nelfinavir can select for drug-resistant virus. The central resistance mutation associated with resistance to nelfinavir is at protease codon 30. Isolates with only this mutation still may be inhibited by other protease inhibitors. However, additional mutations are associated with decreased susceptibility to nelfinavir and to other protease inhibitors, including those at positions 35, 36, 46, 71, 77, 88, and 90.

Absorption, Distribution, and Elimination. Nelfinavir is absorbed more slowly than are other HIV-1 protease inhibitors, with peak levels achieved in 2 to 4 hours. In addition, intraindividual and interindividual variability in plasma nelfinavir levels is considerable. Administration with food increases the plasma AUC of nelfinavir two- to threefold. The drug is FDA-approved for clinical use as a three-times-daily agent, although pharmacokinetic and some clinical data suggest that it may be effective at a dose of 1250 mg given twice daily.

Nelfinavir undergoes oxidative metabolism in the liver primarily by CYP3A4, but also by CYP2C19 and CYP2D6. Its major hydroxy-*t*-butylamide metabolite (M8) has *in vitro* antiretroviral activity comparable to that of the parent drug but achieves plasma levels that are only 40% of nelfinavir levels. The M8 metabolite is generated primarily by CYP2C19. Nelfinavir and its metabolites are eliminated primarily in feces, with less than 2% of drug being excreted in the urine. Moderate or severe liver disease may prolong the half-life and increase plasma concentrations of the parent drug while lowering plasma concentrations of M8.

Nelfinavir induces CYPs involved in its metabolism, and average trough plasma concentrations after one week of therapy are approximately one-half of those at day 2 of therapy. Steady-state plasma levels may be achieved at about one week. Nelfinavir inhibits CYP3A4 less than does ritonavir and does not appear to inhibit other CYP isoforms.

Nelfinavir is greater than 98% bound to plasma proteins, mostly to albumin and α_1-acid glycoprotein. It is present in CSF at less than 1% of plasma concentrations (Aweeka *et al.,* 1999), at least in part due to its extensive binding to plasma protein but perhaps also due to the P-glycoprotein at the blood–brain barrier (Kim *et al.,* 1998). The implications of this for treating HIV in the brain are not known. There is little evidence of sequestration within red blood cells.

Untoward Effects. A common side effect of nelfinavir is diarrhea or loose stools. This is generally mild, and less than 2% of patients discontinue drug due to diarrhea. Other side effects associated with nelfinavir as well as other HIV protease inhibitors include diabetes, glucose intolerance, elevated triglycerides, and elevated cholesterol levels.

Precautions and Interactions. Since nelfinavir is metabolized by CYP3A4, concomitant administration of agents that induce CYP3A4 may be contraindicated (*e.g.,* rifampin) or may necessitate an increased nelfinavir dosage (*e.g.,* rifabutin). In addition, nelfinavir may alter plasma concentrations of drugs that are metabolized through CYP3A4. Nelfinavir lowers the delavirdine plasma AUC by 42%. In addition, levels of midazolam, triazolam, ergot derivatives, amiodarone, and quinidine may be increased by nelfinavir, and coadministration of these drugs with nelfinavir should be avoided.

Therapeutic Use. Nelfinavir is indicated for the treatment of HIV infection in adults and children. Among patients with susceptible strains of HIV-1, initial studies of nelfinavir monotherapy produced substantial decreases in plasma HIV-1 RNA concentrations. Large clinical trials have demonstrated both virologic and clinical benefit when patients naïve to HIV protease inhibitors and lamivudine received nelfinavir in combination with zidovudine and lamivudine.

Amprenavir

Chemistry and Antiviral Activity. Amprenavir is an *N, N*-disubstituted (hydroxyethyl) amino sulfonamide nonpeptide HIV protease inhibitor (Adkins and Faulds, 1998). It was developed from a structure-based drug design program that utilized the known crystal structure of HIV-1 to create progressively smaller and more potent inhibitors, and it is the only available HIV protease inhibitor that is a sulfonamide. Amprenavir is active against both HIV-1 and HIV-2, with an IC_{90} for wild-type HIV-1 of approximately 80 nM.

Mechanisms of Action and Resistance. Amprenavir acts by reversibly binding to the active site of HIV protease. This prevents polypeptide processing and subsequent viral maturation. Viral particles produced in the presence of lopinavir are immature and noninfectious.

Viral replication in the presence of amprenavir selects for drug-resistant virus. A mutation at protease codon 50 is central to amprenavir resistance and confers twofold decreased susceptibility. Accumulation of additional mutations at codons 46 and 47 greatly increase resistance (Partaledis *et al.,* 1995; Tisdale *et al.,* 1995).

Absorption, Distribution, and Elimination. Amprenavir is absorbed rapidly after oral administration. Taking amprenavir with a standard meal reduces the plasma AUC by only about 13%, but high-fat meals may have greater effects and should be avoided. Ritonavir increases amprenavir concentrations considerably by inhibiting CYP3A4 and allows lower amprenavir doses to be administered. Coadministration with low doses of ritonavir may allow the total daily dose of amprenavir to be reduced by one-half.

Amprenavir undergoes limited hepatic metabolism by CYP3A4 and is excreted primarily *via* the biliary route. Amprenavir also is a modest inhibitor of CYP3A4 and CYP2C19. In plasma, amprenavir is 90% bound to proteins, mostly α_1-acid glycoprotein. This binding is relatively weak, and physiological concentrations of α_1-acid glycoprotein increase the *in vitro* IC_{50} three- to fivefold.

Untoward Effects. The most common adverse effects associated with amprenavir are nausea, vomiting, diarrhea or loose stools, hyperglycemia, fatigue, paresthesias, and headache. In one study of amprenavir monotherapy, rash occurred in 5 of 35 patients over 24 weeks, and began within 7 to 12 days of starting therapy.

Precautions and Interactions. Drugs that induce CYP3A4 activity (*e.g.,* rifampin and efavirenz) will lower plasma amprenavir levels, whereas plasma concentrations of some agents metabolized by CYP3A4 will increase if the drugs are coadministered with amprenavir (*e.g.,* ketoconazole, carbamazepine, sildenafil, midazolam, triazolam).

Therapeutic Use. Amprenavir is indicated for the treatment of HIV infection in adults and children, in combination with other agents. Among patients with susceptible strains of HIV-1, amprenavir monotherapy substantially lowers plasma HIV-1 RNA levels. Clinical trials have demonstrated virologic benefit when patients naïve to HIV protease inhibitors and lamivudine were treated with amprenavir (1200 mg every 12 hours) in combination with zidovudine and lamivudine. A number of clinical trials are evaluating amprenavir in combination with ritonavir.

Lopinavir

Chemistry and Antiviral Activity. Lopinavir (ABT-378) is a peptidomimetic HIV protease inhibitor that is structurally similar to ritonavir, but is tenfold more potent against HIV-1 *in vitro* in the presence of human serum. Lopinavir is active against both HIV-1 and HIV-2, with an IC_{50} for wild-type HIV variants of approximately 100 nM.

Mechanisms of Action and Resistance. Lopinavir acts by binding reversibly to the active site of HIV protease, thus preventing polypeptide processing and subsequent viral maturation.

Viral particles produced in the presence of amprenavir are immature and noninfectious.

As with all antiretroviral agents, viral replication in the presence of lopinavir will select for drug-resistant virus. Lopinavir resistance mutations have not been well defined.

Absorption, Distribution, and Elimination. When administered orally without ritonavir, lopinavir plasma concentrations are very low. However, metabolism of lopinavir by CYP3A4 is exquisitely sensitive to inhibition by ritonavir. To overcome its inherent poor bioavailability, lopinavir is coformulated with ritonavir in a fixed dosage combination. (Lopinavir is available only in this coformulation, which will be referrred to hereafter as *lopinavir$_R$*.) Lopinavir is rapidly absorbed after oral administration. Although the capsules contain lopinavir/ritonavir in a fixed 4:1 ratio, the observed plasma concentration ratio following oral administration is nearly 20:1, reflecting the sensitivity of lopinavir to the inhibitory effect of ritonavir on CYP3A4.

Lopinavir undergoes extensive hepatic oxidative metabolism by CYP3A4. Most metabolites are eliminated in feces, and 89% of total drug in plasma is the parent compound. Although lopinavir is a weak inhibitor of CYP3A4, the ritonavir in the coformulated capsule strongly inhibits CYP3A4 activity.

Untoward Effects. Lopinavir$_R$ generally is very well tolerated. The most common adverse events have been gastrointestinal and include abnormal stools, diarrhea, and nausea. The most common laboratory abnormalities include elevated cholesterol and triglycerides.

Precautions and Interactions. Since lopinavir is metabolized predominantly by CYP3A4, concomitant administration of agents that strongly induce CYP3A4, such as rifampin, may lower plasma lopinavir concentrations considerably, and such drugs should be avoided. Coadministration of nevirapine or efavirenz may require increasing the dose of lopinavir$_R$. St. John's wort can lead to lower levels of lopinavir and loss of antiviral effectiveness. The ritonavir component of the formulation will increase levels of a number of drugs (*e.g.,* midazolam, triazolam, propafenone, ergot derivatives, pimozide). Coadministration of these agents should be avoided. The oral solution of lopinavir$_R$ contains alcohol and can cause unpleasant reactions if administered with disulfiram or metronidazole (*see* Chapter 18).

Therapeutic Use. Lopinavir$_R$ has been approved by the FDA for the treatment of HIV infection in adults and children. In clinical trials, lopinavir$_R$ has had antiretroviral activity at least comparable to that of other potent HIV protease inhibitors. It also has had considerable and sustained antiretroviral activity in patients who were not responding to other HIV protease inhibitors. In one study, 70 subjects who had failed therapy with one previous HIV protease inhibitor were treated for 2 weeks with lopinavir$_R$, after which nevirapine was added. These patients had relatively low baseline plasma HIV RNA levels. At 48 weeks, 60% of subjects had plasma HIV-1 RNA levels of less than 50 copies/ml, despite substantial phenotypic resistance to other HIV protease inhibitors. It has been postulated that the very high plasma levels of lopinavir overcome such resistance.

PROSPECTUS

Emergence of multidrug-resistant virus among patients treated with current anti-AIDS agents has created an urgent need for new antiretroviral agents, including ones that target molecules other than reverse transcriptase and protease. A number of agents in development are shown in Table 51–7. Potential steps to target include binding,

Table 51–7
Selected Antiretroviral Agents in Development

CLASS	AGENT
Nucleoside RT* inhibitors	FTC (2′,3′-dideoxy-5-fluoro-3′-thiacytidine)
	Emivirine (MKC-442)
	dOTC (BCH-10652)
Nucleotide RT inhibitors	Tenofovir disoproxil fumarate (PMPA)
Nonnucleoside RT inhibitors	DPC-083
	Capravirine (AG-1549)
	GW-420867X
Protease inhibitors	Tipranavir
	BMS-232632
Fusion inhibitors	T20 peptide (DP 178)

*RT, reverse transcriptase.

fusion, integration, and assembly (*see* Figure 51–1). In addition, antagonists of regulatory molecules such as *tat* possibly could be developed. It is hoped that at least some agents directed at these novel targets will control replication of drug-resistant HIV, have fewer side effects, and/or require less frequent dosing and fewer capsules or tablets than currently available agents.

Drugs that target HIV fusion with the cell membrane are furthest in clinical development. Investigators serendipitously discovered that peptides corresponding to short sequences of gp41 inhibited HIV entry into cells (Jiang *et al.,* 1993; Wild *et al.,* 1994). These peptides disrupt the interaction of the N36 and C34 sequences of the gp41 glycoprotein. One such 36-amino acid peptide known as T20 (also called DP178) binds to the hydrophobic groove on the N36 coiled coil, and effectively blocks HIV-1 entry into target cells with an IC_{50} of 50 to 60 nM (Sodroski, 1999). In the first treatment trial, administration of T20 monotherapy to 16 HIV-infected individuals reduced plasma HIV-1 RNA by a median of 2 $\log_{10}$ copies per milliliter after two weeks (Kilby *et al.,* 1998), which compares favorably with standard combination therapy (Richman, 1998; Rimsky *et al.,* 1998; Sodroski, 1999). Resistance to T20 emerged due to mutations in gp41 (Rimsky *et al.,* 1998). Studies of T20 in combination with other agents are in progress. Since T20 is a large peptide, it is not orally bioavailable and must be administered by subcutaneous or intravenous injection twice daily. Efforts to develop small, orally bioavailable HIV fusion inhibitors are under way.

BIBLIOGRAPHY

Altice, F.L., Friedland, G.H., and Cooney, E.L. Nevirapine induced opiate withdrawal among injection drug users with HIV infection receiving methadone. *AIDS,* **1999,** *13*:957–962.

Anonymous. Delta; a randomised double-blind controlled trial comparing combinations of zidovudine plus didanosine or zalcitabine with zidovudine alone in HIV-infected individuals. Delta Coordinating Committee. *Lancet,* **1996,** *348*:283–291.

Arnaudo, E., Dalakas, M., Shanske, S., Moraes, C.T., DiMauro, S., and Schon, E.A. Depletion of muscle mitochondrial DNA in AIDS patients with zidovudine-induced myopathy. *Lancet,* **1991,** *337*:508–510.

Aweeka, F., Jayewardene, A., Staprans, S., Bellibas, S.E., Kearney, B., Lizak, P., Novakovic-Agopian, T., and Price, R.W. Failure to detect nelfinavir in the cerebrospinal fluid of HIV-1–infected patients with and without AIDS dementia complex. *J. Acquir. Immune Defic. Syndr. Hum. Retrovirol.,* **1999,** *20*:39–43.

Balzarini, J., Pauwels, R., Baba, M., Herdewijn, P., de Clercq, E., Broder, S., and Johns, D.G. The in vitro and in vivo anti-retrovirus activity, and intracellular metabolism of 3′-azido-2′,3′-dideoxythymidine and 2′,3′-dideoxycytidine are highly dependent on the cell species. *Biochem. Pharmacol.,* **1988,** *37*:897–903.

Bartlett, J.A., Benoit, S.L., Johnson, V.A., Quinn, J.B., Sepulveda, G.E., Ehmann, W.C., Tsoukas, C., Fallon, M.A., Self, P.L., and Rubin, M. Lamivudine plus zidovudine compared with zalcitabine plus zidovudine in patients with HIV infection. A randomized, double-blind, placebo-controlled trial. North American HIV Working Party. *Ann. Intern. Med.,* **1996,** *125*:161–172.

Bouscarat, F., Bouchard, C., and Bouhour, D. Paronychia and pyogenic granuloma of the great toes in patients treated with indinavir. *N. Engl. J. Med.,* **1998,** *338*:1776–1777.

Bouscarat, F., Prevot, M.H., and Matheron, S. Alopecia associated with indinavir therapy. *N. Engl. J. Med.,* **1999,** *341*:618.

Bridges, E.G., Dutschman, G.E., Gullen, E.A., and Cheng, Y.C. Favorable interaction of beta-L(−) nucleoside analogues with clinically approved anti-HIV nucleoside analogues for the treatment of human immunodeficiency virus. *Biochem. Pharmacol.,* **1996,** *51*:731–736.

Burger, D.M., Kraayeveld, C.L., Meenhorst, P.L., Mulder, J.W., Hoetelmans, R.M., Koks, C.H., and Beijnen, J.H. Study on didanosine concentrations in cerebrospinal fluid. Implications for the treatment and prevention of AIDS dementia complex. *Pharm. World Sci.,* **1995a,** *17*:218–221.

Burger, D.M., Meenhorst, P.L., and Beijnen, J.H. Concise overview of the clinical pharmacokinetics of dideoxynucleoside antiretroviral agents. *Pharm. World Sci.,* **1995b,** *17*:25–30.

Cardo, D.M., Culver, D.H., Ciesielski, C.A., Srivastava, P.U., Marcus, R., Abiteboul, D., Heptonstall, J., Ippolito, G., Lot, F., McKibben, P.S., and Bell, D.M. A case-control study of HIV seroconversion in health care workers after percutaneous exposure. Centers for Disease Control and Prevention Needlestick Surveillance Group. *N. Engl. J. Med.,* **1997,** *337*:1485–1490.

Casado, J.L., Hertogs, K., Ruiz, L., Dronda, F., Van Cauwenberge, A., Arno, A., Garcia-Arata, I., Bloor, S., Bonjoch, A., Blazquez, J., Clotet, B., and Larder, B. Non-nucleoside reverse transcriptase inhibitor resistance among patients failing a nevirapine plus protease inhibitor-containing regimen. *AIDS,* **2000,** *14*:F1–F7.

Chattha, G., Arieff, A.I., Cummings, C., and Tierney, L.M., Jr. Lactic acidosis complicating the acquired immunodeficiency syndrome. *Ann. Intern. Med.,* **1993,** *118*:37–39.

Cheeseman, S.H., Hattox, S.E., McLaughlin, M.M., Koup, R.A., Andrews, C., Bova, C.A., Pav, J.W., Roy, T., Sullivan, J.L., and Keirns, J.J. Pharmacokinetics of nevirapine: initial single-rising-dose study in humans. *Antimicrob. Agents Chemother.,* **1993,** *37*:178–182.

Cheeseman, S.H., Havlir, D., McLaughlin, M.M., Greenough, T.C., Sullivan, J.L., Hall, D., Hattox, S.E., Spector, S.A., Stein, D.S., Myers, M., *et al.* Phase I/II evaluation of nevirapine alone and in combination with zidovudine for infection with human immunodeficiency virus. *J. Acquir. Immune Defic. Syndr. Hum. Retrovirol.,* **1995,** *8*:141–151.

Chen, C.H., Vazquez-Padua, M., and Cheng, Y.C. Effect of anti–human immunodeficiency virus nucleoside analogs on mitochondrial DNA and its implication for delayed toxicity. *Mol. Pharmacol.,* **1991,** *39*:625–628.

Cheng, C.L., Smith, D.E., Carver, P.L., Cox, S.R., Watkins, P.B., Blake, D.S., Kauffman, C.A., Meyer, K.M., Amidon, G.L., and Stetson, P.L. Steady-state pharmacokinetics of delavirdine in HIV-positive patients: effect on erythromycin breath test. *Clin. Pharmacol. Ther.,* **1997,** *61*:531–543.

Chittick, G.E., Gillotin, C., McDowell, J.A., Lou, Y., Edwards, K.D., Prince, W.T., and Stein, D.S. Abacavir: absolute bioavailability, bioequivalence of three oral formulations, and effect of food. *Pharmacotherapy,* **1999,** *19*:932–942.

Chun, T.W., Carruth, L., Finzi, D., Shen, X., DiGiuseppe, J.A., Taylor, H., Hermankova, M., Chadwick, K., Margolick, J., Quinn, T.C., Kuo, Y.H., Brookmeyer, R., Zeiger, M.A., Barditch-Crovo, P., and Siliciano, R.F. Quantification of latent tissue reservoirs and total body viral load in HIV-1 infection. *Nature,* **1997,** *387*:183–188.

Chun, T.W., Engel, D., Berrey, M.M., Shea, T., Corey, L., and Fauci, A.S. Early establishment of a pool of latently infected, resting CD4(+) T cells during primary HIV-1 infection. *Proc. Natl. Acad. Sci. U.S.A.,* **1998,** *95*:8869–8873.

Coates, J.A., Cammack, N., Jenkinson, H.J., Jowett, A.J., Jowett, M.I., Pearson, B.A., Penn, C.R., Rouse, P.L., Viner, K.C., and Cameron, J.M. (−)-2′-deoxy-3′-thiacytidine is a potent, highly selective inhibitor of human immunodeficiency virus type 1 and type 2 replication in vitro. *Antimicrob. Agents Chemother.,* **1992,** *36*:733–739.

Coffin, J.M. HIV population dynamics in vivo: implications for genetic variation, pathogenesis, and therapy. *Science,* **1995,** *267*:483–489.

Collier, A.C., Coombs, R.W., Schoenfeld, D.A., Bassett, R.L., Timpone, J., Baruch, A., Jones, M., Facey, K., Whitacre, C., McAuliffe, V.J., Friedman, H.M., Merigan, T.C., Reichman, R.C., Hooper, C., and Corey, L. Treatment of human immunodeficiency virus infection with saquinavir, zidovudine, and zalcitabine. AIDS Clinical Trials Group. *N. Engl. J. Med.,* **1996,** *334*:1011–1017.

Connor, E.M., Sperling, R.S., Gelber, R., Kiselev, P., Scott, G., O'Sullivan, M.J., VanDyke, R., Bey, M., Shearer, W., Jacobson, R.L., Jimenez, E., O'Neill, E., Bazin, B., Delfraissy, J.-F., Culnane, M., Coombs, R., Elkins, M., Moye, J., Stratton, P., and Balsley, J. Reduction of maternal-infant transmission of human immunodeficiency virus type 1 with zidovudine treatment. Pediatric AIDS Clinical Trials Group Protocol 076 Study Group. *N. Engl. J. Med.,* **1994,** *331*:1173–1180.

Cooney, D. A., Ahluwalia, G., Mitsuya, H., Fridland, A., Johnson, M., Hao, Z., Dalal, M., Balzarini, J., Broder, S., and Johns, D.G. Initial studies on the cellular pharmacology of 2′,3′-dideoxyadenosine, an inhibitor of HTLV-III infectivity. *Biochem. Pharmacol.,* **1987,** *36*:1765–1768.

Cooney, D.A., Dalal, M., Mitsuya, H., McMahon, J.B., Nadkarni, M., Balzarini, J., Broder, S., and Johns, D.G. Initial studies on the cellular pharmacology of 2′,3-dideoxycytidine, an inhibitor of HTLV-III infectivity. *Biochem. Pharmacol.,* **1986,** *35*:2065–2068.

Craig, J.C., Duncan, I.B., Hockley, D., Grief, C., Roberts, N.A., and Mills, J.S. Antiviral properties of Ro 31-8959, an inhibitor of human immunodeficiency virus (HIV) proteinase. *Antiviral Res.,* **1991,** *16*:295–305.

Dalakas, M.C., Illa, I., Pezeshkpour, G.H., Laukaitis, J.P., Cohen, B., and Griffin, J.L. Mitochondrial myopathy caused by long-term zidovudine therapy. *N. Engl. J. Med.,* **1990,** *322*:1098–1105.

Daluge, S.M., Good, S.S., Faletto, M.B., Miller, W.H., St. Clair, M.H., Boone, L.R., Tisdale, M., Parry, N.R., Reardon, J.E., Dornsife, R.E., Averett, D.R., and Krenitsky, T.A. 1592U89, a novel carbocyclic nucleoside analog with potent, selective anti-human immunodefi-

ciency virus activity. *Antimicrob. Agents Chemother.,* **1997,** *41*:1082–1093.

Dancis, J., Lee, J.D., Mendoza, S., and Liebes, L. Transfer and metabolism of dideoxyinosine by the perfused human placenta. *J. Acquir. Immune Defic. Syndr.,* **1993,** *6*:2–6.

Danner, S.A., Carr, A., Leonard, J.M., Lehman, L.M., Gudiol, F., Gonzales, J., Raventos, A., Rubio, R., Bouza, E., Pintado, V., Aguado, A.G., Garcia de Lomas, J., Delgado, R., Borleffs, J.C.C., Hsu, A., Valdes, J.M., Boucher, C.A.B., and Cooper, D.A. A short-term study of the safety, pharmacokinetics, and efficacy of ritonavir, an inhibitor of HIV-1 protease. European-Australian Collaborative Ritonavir Study Group. *N. Engl. J. Med.,* **1995,** *333*:1528–1533.

Davey, R.T.J., Bhat, N., Yoder, C., Chun, T.W., Metcalf, J.A., Dewar, R., Natarajan, V., Lempicki, R.A., Adelsberger, J.W., Miller, K.D., Kovacs, J.A., Polis, M.A., Walker, R.E., Falloon, J., Masur, H., Gee, D., Baseler, M., Dimitrov, D.S., Fauci, A.S., and Lane, H.C. HIV-1 and T cell dynamics after interruption of highly active antiretroviral therapy (HAART) in patients with a history of sustained viral suppression. *Proc. Natl. Acad. Sci. U.S.A.,* **1999,** *96*:15109–15114.

Deeks, S.G., Hellmann, N.S., Grant, R.M., Parkin, N.T., Petropoulos, C.J., Becker, M., Symonds, W., Chesney, M., and Volberding, P.A. Novel four-drug salvage treatment regimens after failure of a human immunodeficiency virus type 1 protease inhibitor-containing regimen: antiviral activity and correlation of baseline phenotypic drug susceptibility with virologic outcome. *J. Infect. Dis.,* **1999,** *179*:1375–1381.

Dolin, R., Amato, D.A., Fischl, M.A., Pettinelli, C., Beltangady, M., Liou, S.H., Brown, M.J., Cross, A.P., Hirsch, M.S., Hardy, W.D., Mildvan, D., Blair, D.C., Powderly, W.G., Para, M.F., Fife, K.H., Steigbigel, R.T., and Smaldone, L. Zidovudine compared with didanosine in patients with advanced HIV type 1 infection and little or no previous experience with zidovudine. AIDS Clinical Trials Group. *Arch. Intern. Med.,* **1995,** *155*:961–974.

Dreyer, G.B., Metcalf, B.W., Tomaszek, T.A, Jr., Carr, T.J., Chandler, A.C. III, Hyland, L., Fakhoury, S.A., Magaard, V.W., Moore, M.L., Strickler, J.E., *et al.* Inhibition of human immunodeficiency virus 1 protease in vitro: rational design of substrate analogue inhibitors. *Proc. Natl. Acad. Sci. U.S.A.,* **1989,** *86*:9752–9756.

Dudley, M.N., Graham, K.K., Kaul, S., Geletko, S., Dunkle, L., Browne, M., and Mayer, K. Pharmacokinetics of stavudine in patients with AIDS or AIDS-related complex. *J. Infect. Dis.,* **1992,** *166*:480–485.

Dueweke, T.J., Poppe, S.M., Romero, D.L., Swaney, S.M., So, A.G., Downey, K.M., Althaus, I.W., Reusser, F., Busso, M., Resnick, L., *et al.* U-90152, a potent inhibitor of human immunodeficiency virus type 1 replication. *Antimicrob. Agents Chemother.,* **1993a,** *37*:1127–1131.

Dueweke, T.J., Pushkarskaya, T., Poppe, S.M., Swaney, S.M., Zhao, J.Q., Chen, I.S., Stevenson, M., and Tarpley, W.G. A mutation in reverse transcriptase of bis(heteroaryl)piperazine-resistant human immunodeficiency virus type 1 that confers increased sensitivity to other nonnucleoside inhibitors. *Proc. Natl. Acad. Sci. U.S.A.,* **1993b,** *90*:4713–4717.

Durant, J., Clevenbergh, P., Halfon, P., Delgiudice, P., Porsin, S., Simonet, P., Montagne, N., Boucher, C.A., Schapiro, J.M., and Dellamonica, P. Drug-resistance genotyping in HIV-1 therapy: the VIRADAPT randomised controlled trial. *Lancet,* **1999,** *353*:2195–2199.

Englund, J.A., Baker, C.J., Raskino, C., McKinney, R.E., Petrie, B., Fowler, M.G., Pearson, D., Gershon, A., McSherry, G.D., Abrams, E.J., Schliozberg, J., and Sullivan, J.L. Zidovudine, didanosine, or both as the initial treatment for symptomatic HIV-infected children.

AIDS Clinical Trials Group (ACTG) Study 152 Team. *N. Engl. J. Med.,* **1997,** *336*:1704–1712.

Erickson, D.A., Mather, G., Trager, W.F., Levy, R.H., and Keirns, J.J. Characterization of the *in vitro* biotransformation of the HIV-1 reverse transcriptase inhibitor nevirapine by human hepatic cytochromes P-450. *Drug Metab. Dispos.,* **1999,** *27*:1488–1495.

Eron, J.J., Benoit, S.L., Jemsek, J., MacArthur, R.D., Santana, J., Quinn, J.B., Kuritzkes, D.R., Fallon, M.A., and Rubin, M. Treatment with lamivudine, zidovudine, or both in HIV-positive patients with 200 to 500 CD4+ cells per cubic millimeter. North American HIV Working Party. *N. Engl. J. Med.,* **1995,** *333*:1662–1669.

Faletto, M.B., Miller, W.H., Garvey, E.P., St. Clair, M.H., Daluge, S.M., and Good, S.S. Unique intracellular activation of the potent anti-human immunodeficiency virus agent 1592U89. *Antimicrob. Agents Chemother.,* **1997,** *41*:1099–1107.

Falloon, J., Piscitelli, S., Vogel, S., Sadler, B., Mitsuya, H., Kavlick, M.F., Yoshimura, K., Rogers, M., LaFon, S., Manion, D.J., Lane, H.C., and Masur, H. Combination therapy with amprenavir, abacavir, and efavirenz in human immunodeficiency virus (HIV)-infected patients failing a protease-inhibitor regimen: pharmacokinetic drug interactions and antiviral activity. *Clin. Infect. Dis.,* **2000,** *30*:313–318.

Fichtenbaum, C.J., Clifford, D.B., and Powderly, W.G. Risk factors for dideoxynucleoside-induced toxic neuropathy in patients with the human immunodeficiency virus infection. *J. Acquir. Immune Defic. Syndr. Hum. Retrovirol.,* **1995,** *10*:169–174.

Finzi, D., Hermankova, M., Pierson, T., Carruth, L.M., Buck, C., Chaisson, R.E., Quinn, T.C., Chadwick, K., Margolick, J., Brookmeyer, R., Gallant, J., Markowitz, M., Ho, D.D., Richman, D.D., and Siliciano, R.F. Identification of a reservoir for HIV-1 in patients on highly active antiretroviral therapy. *Science,* **1997,** *278:* 1295–1300.

Fischl, M.A., Olson, R.M., Follansbee, S.E., Lalezari, J.P., Henry, D.H., Frame, P.T., Remick, S.C., Salgo, M.P., Lin, A.H., Nauss-Karol, C., Lieberman, J., and Soo, W. Zalcitabine compared with zidovudine in patients with advanced HIV-1 infection who received previous zidovudine therapy. *Ann. Intern. Med.,* **1993,** *118*:762–769.

Fischl, M.A., Richman, D.D., Grieco, M.H., Gottlieb, M.S., Volberding, P.A., Laskin, O.L., Leedom, J.M., Groopman, J.E., Mildvan, D., Schooley, R.T., *et al.* The efficacy of azidothymidine (AZT) in the treatment of patients with AIDS and AIDS-related complex. A double-blind, placebo-controlled trial. *N. Engl. J. Med.,* **1987,** *317*:185–191.

Fischl, M.A., Richman, D.D., Hansen, N., Collier, A.C., Carey, J.T., Para, M.F., Hardy, W.D., Dolin, R., Powderly, W.G., Allan, J.D., *et al.* The safety and efficacy of zidovudine (AZT) in the treatment of subjects with mildly symptomatic human immunodeficiency virus type 1 (HIV) infection. A double-blind, placebo-controlled trial. The AIDS Clinical Trials Group. *Ann. Intern. Med.,* **1990,** *112*:727–737.

Fischl, M.A., Stanley, K., Collier, A.C., Arduino, J.M., Stein, D.S., Feinberg, J.E., Allan, J.D., Goldsmith, J.C., and Powderly, W.G. Combination and monotherapy with zidovudine and zalcitabine in patients with advanced HIV disease. The NIAD AIDS Clinical Trials Group. *Ann. Intern. Med.,* **1995,** *122*:24–32.

Fitzsimmons, M.E., and Collins, J.M. Selective biotransformation of the human immunodeficiency virus protease inhibitor saquinavir by human small-intestinal cytochrome P4503A4: potential contribution to high first-pass metabolism. *Drug Metab. Dispos.,* **1997,** *25*:256–266.

Frecer, V., Miertus, S., Tossi, A., and Romeo, D. Rational design of inhibitors for drug-resistant HIV-1 aspartic protease mutants. *Drug Des. Discov.,* **1998,** *15*:211–231.

Friedland, G.H., Pollard, R., Griffith, B., Hughes, M., Morse, G., Bassett, R., Freimuth, W., Demeter, L., Connick, E., Nevin, T., Hirsch, M., and Fischl, M. Efficacy and safety of delavirdine mesylate with zidovudine and didanosine compared with two-drug combinations of these agents in persons with HIV disease with CD4 counts of 100 to 500 cells/mm³ (ACTG 261). ACTG 261 Team. *J. Acquir. Immune Defic. Syndr.,* **1999,** *21*:281–292.

Furman, P.A., Fyfe, J.A., St. Clair, M.H., Weinhold, K., Rideout, J.L., Freeman, G.A., Lehrman, S.N., Bolognesi, D.P., Broder, S., Mitsuya, H., *et al.* Phosphorylation of 3′-azido-3′-deoxythymidine and selective interaction of the 5′-triphosphate with human immunodeficiency virus reverse transcriptase. *Proc. Natl. Acad. Sci. U.S.A.,* **1986,** *83*:8333–8337.

Gao, W.Y., Agbaria, R., Driscoll, J.S., and Mitsuya, H. Divergent anti-human immunodeficiency virus activity and anabolic phosphorylation of 2′,3′-dideoxynucleoside analogs in resting and activated human cells. *J. Biol. Chem.,* **1994,** *269*:12633–12638.

Gao, W.Y., Shirasaka, T., Johns, D.G., Broder, S., and Mitsuya, H. Differential phosphorylation of azidothymidine, dideoxycytidine, and dideoxyinosine in resting and activated peripheral blood mononuclear cells. *J. Clin. Invest.,* **1993,** *91*:2326–2333.

Geleziunas, R., Arts, E.J., Boulerice, F., Goldman, H., and Wainberg, M.A. Effect of 3′-azido-3′-deoxythymidine on human immunodeficiency virus type 1 replication in human fetal brain macrophages. *Antimicrob. Agents Chemother.,* **1993,** *37*:1305–1312.

Gillet, J.Y., Garraffo, R., Abrar, D., Bongain, A., Lapalus, P., and Dellamonica, P. Fetoplacental passage of zidovudine. *Lancet,* **1989,** *2*:269–270.

Gisolf, E.H., Jurriaans, S., Pelgrom, J., van Wanzeele, F., van der Ende, M.E., Brinkman, K., Borst, M.J., de Wolf, F., Japour, A.J., and Danner, S.A. The effect of treatment intensification in HIV-infection: a study comparing treatment with ritonavir/saquinavir and ritonavir/saquinavir/stavudine. Prometheus Study Group. *AIDS,* **2000,** *14*:405–413.

Gottlieb, M.S., Schroff, R., Schanker, H.M., Weisman, J.D., Fan, P.T., Wolf, R.A., and Saxon, A. *Pneumocystis carinii* pneumonia and mucosal candidiasis in previously healthy homosexual men: evidence of a new acquired cellular immunodeficiency. *N. Engl. J. Med.,* **1981,** *305*:1425–1431.

Guay, L.A., Musoke, P., Fleming, T., Bagenda, D., Allen, M., Nakabiito, C., Sherman, J., Bakaki, P., Ducar, C., Deseyve, M., Emel, L., Mirochnick, M., Fowler, M.G., Mofenson, L., Miotti, P., Dransfield, K., Bray, D., Mmiro, F., and Jackson, J.B. Intrapartum and neonatal single-dose nevirapine compared with zidovudine for prevention of mother-to-child transmission of HIV-1 in Kampala, Uganda: HIVNET 012 randomised trial. *Lancet,* **1999,** *354*:795–802.

Gulick, R.M., Mellors, J.W., Havlir, D., Eron, J.J., Gonzalez, C., McMahon, D., Richman, D.D., Valentine, F.T., Jonas, L., Meibohm, A., Emini, E.A., and Chodakewitz, J.A. Treatment with indinavir, zidovudine, and lamivudine in adults with human immunodeficiency virus infection and prior antiretroviral therapy. *N. Engl. J. Med.,* **1997,** *337*:734–739.

Gustavson, L.E., Fukuda, E.K., Rubio, F.A., and Dunton, A.W. A pilot study of the bioavailability and pharmacokinetics of 2′,3′-dideoxycytidine in patients with AIDS or AIDS-related complex. *J. Acquir. Immune Defic. Syndr.,* **1990,** *3*:28–31.

Haas, D.W., Arathoon, E., Thompson, M.A., de Jesus Pedro, R., Gallant, J.E., Uip, D.E., Currier, J., Noriega, L.M., Lewi, D.S., Uribe, P., Benetucci, J., Cahn, P., Paar, D., White, A.C., Jr., Ramirez-Ronda, H.C., Harvey, C., Chung, M.O., Mehrotra, D., Chodakewitz, J., and Nguyen, B.Y. Comparative studies of two-times-daily versus three-times-daily indinavir in combination with zidovudine and lamivudine. Protocol 054/069 Study Teams. *AIDS,* **2000a,** *14*:1973–1978.

Haas, D.W., Clough, L.A., Johnson, B.W., Harris, V.L., Spearman, P., Wilkinson, G.R., Fletcher, C.V., Fiscus, S., Raffanti, S., Donlon, R., McKinsey, J., Nicotera, J., Schmidt, D., Shoup, R.E., Kates, R.E., Lloyd, R.M., Jr., and Larder, B. Evidence for a source of HIV-1 within the central nervous system by ultraintensive sampling of cerebrospinal fluid and plasma. *AIDS Res. Hum. Retroviruses,* **2000b,** *16*:1491–1502.

Haas, D.W., Stone, J., Clough, L.A., Johnson, B., Spearman, P., Harris, V.L., Nicotera, J., Johnson, R.H., Raffanti, S., Zhong, L., Bergqwist, P., Chamberlin, S., Hoagland, V., and Ju, W.D. Steady-state pharmacokinetics of indinavir in cerebrospinal fluid and plasma among adults with human immunodeficiency virus type 1 infection. *Clin. Pharmacol. Ther.,* **2000c,** 68:367–374.

Hammer, S.M., Katzenstein, D.A., Hughes, M.D., Gundacker, H., Schooley, R.T., Haubrich, R.H., Henry, W.K., Lederman, M.M., Phair, J.P., Niu, M., Hirsch, M.S., and Merigan, T.C. A trial comparing nucleoside monotherapy with combination therapy in HIV-infected adults with CD4 cell counts from 200 to 500 per cubic millimeter. AIDS Clinical Trials Group Study 175 Study Team. *N. Engl. J. Med.,* *1996, 335*:1081–1090.

Hammer, S.M., Squires, K.E., Hughes, M.D., Grimes, J.M., Demeter, L.M., Currier, J.S., Eron, J.J., Jr., Feinberg, J.E., Balfour, H.H., Jr., Deyton, L.R., Chodakewitz, J.A., and Fischl, M.A. A controlled trial of two nucleoside analogues plus indinavir in persons with human immunodeficiency virus infection and CD4 cell counts of 200 per cubic millimeter or less. AIDS Clinical Trials Group 320 Study Team. *N. Engl. J. Med.,* **1997,** *337*:725–733.

Harrigan, P.R., Stone, C., Griffin, P., Najera, I., Bloor, S., Kemp, S., Tisdale, M., and Larder, B. Resistance profile of the human immunodeficiency virus type 1 reverse transcriptase inhibitor abacavir (1592U89) after monotherapy and combination therapy. CNA2001 Investigative Group. *J. Infect. Dis.,* **2000,** *181*:912–920.

Havlir, D., McLaughlin, M.M., and Richman, D.D. A pilot study to evaluate the development of resistance to nevirapine in asymptomatic human immunodeficiency virus-infected patients with CD4 cell counts of >500/mm³: AIDS Clinical Trials Group Protocol 208. *J. Infect. Dis.,* **1995,** *172*:1379–1383.

He, J., Chen, Y., Farzan, M., Choe, H., Ohagen, A., Gartner, S., Busciglio, J., Yang, X., Hofmann, W., Newman, W., Mackay, C.R., Sodroski, J., and Gabuzda, D. CCR3 and CCR5 are co-receptors for HIV-1 infection of microglia. *Nature,* **1997,** *385*:645–649.

Heald, A.E., Hsyu, P.H., Yuen, G.J., Robinson, P., Mydlow, P., and Bartlett, J.A. Pharmacokinetics of lamivudine in human immunodeficiency virus-infected patients with renal dysfunction. *Antimicrob. Agents Chemother.,* **1996,** 40:1514–1519.

Hirsch, M.S., Brun-Vezinet, F., D'Aquila, R.T., Hammer, S.M., Johnson, V.A., Kuritzkes, D.R., Loveday, C., Mellors, J.W., Clotet, B., Conway, B., Demeter, L.M., Vella, S., Jacobsen, D.M., and Richman, D.D. Antiretroviral drug resistance testing in adult HIV-1 infection: recommendations of an International AIDS Society-USA Panel. *JAMA,* **2000,** *283*:2417–2426.

HIV/AIDS Treatment Information Service. Guidelines for the use of antiretroviral agents in HIV-infected adults and adolescents (January 28, 2000). Panel on Clinical Practices for Treatment of HIV Infection. Available at: http://www.hivatis.org/guidelines/adult/text. Accessed January 15, 2001.

Ho, D.D., Moudgil, T., and Alam, M. Quantitation of human immunodeficiency virus type 1 in the blood of infected persons. *N. Engl. J. Med.,* 1989, *321*:1621–1625.

Ho, D.D., Neumann, A.U., Perelson, A.S., Chen, W., Leonard, J.M., and Markowitz, M. Rapid turnover of plasma virions and CD4 lymphocytes in HIV-1 infection. *Nature,* **1995,** *373*:123–126.

Ho, H.T., and Hitchcock, M.J. Cellular pharmacology of 2′,3′-dideoxy-2′,3′-didehydrothymidine, a nucleoside analog active against human immunodeficiency virus. *Antimicrob. Agents Chemother.,* **1989,** *33*:844–849.

Ives, K.J., Jacobsen, H., Galpin, S.A., Garaev, M.M., Dorrell, L., Mous, J., Bragman, K., and Weber, J.N. Emergence of resistant variants of HIV in vivo during monotherapy with the proteinase inhibitor saquinavir. *J. Antimicrob. Chemother.,* **1997,** *39*:771–779.

Jayasekara, D., Aweeka, F.T., Rodriguez, R., Kalayjian, R.C., Humphreys, M.H., and Gambertoglio, J.G. Antiviral therapy for HIV patients with renal insufficiency. *J. Acquir. Immune Defic. Syndr.,* **1999,** *21*:384–395.

Jiang, S., Lin, K., Strick, N., and Neurath, A.R. HIV-1 inhibition by a peptide. *Nature,* **1993,** *365*:113.

Kahn, J.O., Lagakos, S.W., Richman, D.D., Cross, A., Pettinelli, C., Liou, S.H., Brown, M., Volberding, P.A., Crumpacker, C.S., Beall, G., *et al.* A controlled trial comparing continued zidovudine with didanosine in human immunodeficiency virus infection. The NIAD AIDS Clinical Trials Group. *N. Engl. J. Med.,* **1992,** *327*:581–587.

Katlama, C., Ingrand, D., Loveday, C., Clumeck, N., Mallolas, J., Staszewski, S., Johnson, M., Hill, A.M., Pearce, G., and McDade, H. Safety and efficacy of lamivudine-zidovudine combination therapy in antiretroviral-naive patients. A randomized controlled comparison with zidovudine monotherapy. Lamivudine European HIV Working Group. *JAMA,* **1996,** *276*:118–125.

Katzenstein, D.A., Hammer, S.M., Hughes, M.D., Gundacker, H., Jackson, J.B., Fiscus, S., Rasheed, S., Elbeik, T., Reichman, R., Japour, A., Merigan, T.C., and Hirsch, M.S. The relation of virologic and immunologic markers to clinical outcomes after nucleoside therapy in HIV-infected adults with 200 to 500 CD4 cells per cubic millimeter. AIDS Clinical Trials Group Study 175 Virology Study Team. *N. Engl. J. Med.,* **1996,** *335*:1091–1098.

Kilby, J.M., Hopkins, S., Venetta, T.M., DiMassimo, B., Cloud, G.A., Lee, J.Y., Alldredge, L., Hunter, E., Lambert, D., Bolognesi, D., Matthews, T., Johnson, M.R., Nowak, M.A., Shaw, G.M., and Saag, M.S. Potent suppression of HIV-1 replication in humans by T-20, a peptide inhibitor of gp41-mediated virus entry. *Nat. Med.,* **1998,** *4*:1302–1307.

Kim, R.B., Fromm, M.F., Wandel, C., Leake, B., Wood, A.J., Roden, D.M., and Wilkinson, G.R. The drug transporter P-glycoprotein limits oral absorption and brain entry of HIV-1 protease inhibitors. *J. Clin. Invest.,* **1998,** *101*:289–294.

Klecker, R.W., Jr., Collins, J.M., Yarchoan, R.C., Thomas, R., McAtee, N., Broder, S., and Myers, C.E. Pharmacokinetics of 2′,3′-dideoxycytidine in patients with AIDS and related disorders. *J. Clin. Pharmacol.,* **1988,** *28*:837–842.

Knupp, C.A., Milbrath, R., and Barbhaiya, R.H. Effect of time of food administration on the bioavailability of didanosine from a chewable tablet formulation. *J. Clin. Pharmacol.,* **1993,** *33*:568–573.

Kohl, N.E., Emini, E.A., Schleif, W.A., Davis, L.J., Heimbach, J.C., Dixon, R.A., Scolnick, E.M., and Sigal, I.S. Active human immunodeficiency virus protease is required for viral infectivity. *Proc. Natl. Acad. Sci. U.S.A.,* **1988,** *85*:4686–4690.

Larder, B.A., Kemp, S.D., and Harrigan, P.R. Potential mechanism for sustained antiretroviral efficacy of AZT-3TC combination therapy. *Science,* **1995,** *269*:696–699.

Lewis, L.L., Venzon, D., Church, J., Farley, M., Wheeler, S., Keller, A., Rubin, M., Yuen, G., Mueller, B., Sloas, M., Wood, L., Balis, F.,

Shearer, G.M., Brouwers, P., Goldsmith, J., and Pizzo, P.A. Lamivudine in children with human immunodeficiency virus infection: a phase I/II study. The National Cancer Institute Pediatric Branch-Human Immunodeficiency Virus Working Group. *J. Infect. Dis.,* **1996,** *174*:16–25.

Lin, J.H., Chen, I.W., Vastag, K.J., and Ostovic, D. pH-dependent oral absorption of L-735,524, a potent HIV protease inhibitor, in rats and dogs. *Drug Metab. Dispos.,* **1995,** *23*:730–735.

Lin, P.F., Samanta, H., Rose, R.E., Patick, A.K., Trimble, J., Bechtold, C.M., Revie, D.R., Khan, N.C., Federici, M.E., Li, H., *et al.* Genotypic and phenotypic analysis of human immunodeficiency virus type 1 isolates from patients on prolonged stavudine therapy. *J. Infect. Dis.,* **1994,** *170*:1157–1164.

Luzuriaga, K., Bryson, Y., Krogstad, P., Robinson, J., Stechenberg, B., Lamson, M., Cort, S., and Sullivan, J.L. Combination treatment with zidovudine, didanosine, and nevirapine in infants with human immunodeficiency virus type 1 infection. *N. Engl. J. Med.,* **1997,** *336*:1343–1349.

Marschner, I.C., Collier, A.C., Coombs, R.W., D'Aquila, R.T., DeGruttola, V., Fischl, M.A., Hammer, S.M., Hughes, M.D., Johnson, V.A., Katzenstein, D.A., Richman, D.D., Smeaton, L.M., Spector, S.A., and Saag, M.S. Use of changes in plasma levels of human immunodeficiency virus type 1 RNA to assess the clinical benefit of antiretroviral therapy. *J. Infect. Dis.,* **1998,** *177*:40–47.

Masur, H., Michelis, M.A., Greene, J.B., Onorato, I., Stouwe, R.A., Holzman, R.S., Wormser, G., Brettman, L., Lange, M., Murray, H.W., and Cunningham-Rundles, S. An outbreak of community-acquired *Pneumocystis carinii* pneumonia: initial manifestation of cellular immune dysfunction. *N. Engl. J. Med.,* **1981,** *305*:1431–1438.

McDowell, J.A., Chittick, G.E., Stevens, C.P., Edwards, K.D., and Stein, D.S. Pharmacokinetic interaction of abacavir (1592U89) and ethanol in human immunodeficiency virus-infected adults. *Antimicrob. Agents Chemother.,* **2000,** *44*:1686–1690.

Mellors, J.W., Munoz, A., Giorgi, J.V., Margolick, J.B., Tassoni, C.J., Gupta, P., Kingsley, L.A., Todd, J.A., Saah, A.J., Detels, R., Phair, J.P., and Rinaldo, C.R., Jr. Plasma viral load and CD4+ lymphocytes as prognostic markers of HIV-1 infection. *Ann. Intern. Med.,* **1997,** *126*:946–954.

Mellors, J.W., Rinaldo, C.R., Jr., Gupta, P., White, R.M., Todd, J.A., and Kingsley, L.A. Prognosis in HIV-1 infection predicted by the quantity of virus in plasma. *Science,* **1996,** *272*:1167–1170.

Merrill, D.P., Moonis, M., Chou, T.C., and Hirsch, M.S. Lamivudine or stavudine in two- and three-drug combinations against human immunodeficiency virus type 1 replication in vitro. *J. Infect. Dis.,* **1996,** *173*:355–364.

Mirochnick, M., Fenton, T., Gagnier, P., Pav, J., Gwynne, M., Siminski, S., Sperling, R.S., Beckerman, K., Jimenez, E., Yogev, R., Spector, S.A., and Sullivan, J.L. Pharmacokinetics of nevirapine in human immunodeficiency virus type 1–infected pregnant women and their neonates. Pediatric AIDS Clinical Trials Group Protocol 250 Team. *J. Infect. Dis.,* **1998,** *178*:368–374.

Mitsuya, H., and Broder, S. Inhibition of the in vitro infectivity and cytopathic effect of human T-lymphotrophic virus type III/lymphadenopathy-associated virus (HTLV-III/LAV) by 2′,3′-dideoxynucleosides. *Proc. Natl. Acad. Sci. U.S.A.,* **1986,** *83*:1911–1915.

Mokrzycki, M.H., Harris, C., May, H., Laut, J., and Palmisano, J. Lactic acidosis associated with stavudine administration: a report of five cases. *Clin. Infect. Dis.,* **2000,** *30*:198–200.

Molla, A., Korneyeva, M., Gao, Q., Vasavanonda, S., Schipper, P.J., Mo, H.M., Markowitz, M., Chernyavskiy, T., Niu, P., Lyons, N., Hsu, A.,

Granneman, G.R., Ho, D.D., Boucher, C.A., Leonard, J.M., Norbeck, D.W., and Kempf, D.J. Ordered accumulation of mutations in HIV protease confers resistance to ritonavir. *Nat. Med.,* **1996,** *2*:760–766.

Montaner, J.S., Reiss, P., Cooper, D., Vella, S., Harris, M., Conway, B., Wainberg, M.A., Smith, D., Robinson, P., Hall, D., Myers, M., and Lange, J.M. A randomized, double-blind trial comparing combinations of nevirapine, didanosine, and zidovudine for HIV-infected patients: the INCAS Trial. Italy, Netherlands, Canada and Australia Study. *JAMA,* **1998,** *279*:930–937.

Moore, R.D., Wong, W.M., Keruly, J.C., and McArthur, J.C. Incidence of neuropathy in HIV-infected patients on monotherapy versus those on combination therapy with didanosine, stavudine and hydroxyurea. *AIDS,* **2000,** *14*:273–278.

Navia, M.A., Fitzgerald, P.M., McKeever, B.M., Leu, C.T., Heimbach, J.C., Herber, W.K., Sigal, I.S., Darke, P.L., and Springer, J.P. Three-dimensional structure of aspartyl protease from human immunodeficiency virus HIV-1. *Nature,* **1989,** *337*:615–620.

O'Brien, W.A., Hartigan, P.M., Martin, D., Esinhart, J., Hill, A., Benoit, S., Rubin, M., Simberkoff, M.S., and Hamilton, J.D. Changes in plasma HIV-1 RNA and CD4+ lymphocyte counts and the risk of progression to AIDS. Veterans Affairs Cooperative Study Group on AIDS. *N. Engl. J. Med.,* **1996,** *334*:426–431.

Odinecs, A., Nosbisch, C., Keller, R.D., Baughman, W.L., and Unadkat, J.D. In vivo maternal-fetal pharmacokinetics of stavudine (2′,3′-didehydro-3′-deoxythymidine) in pigtailed macaques (*Macaca nemestrina*). *Antimicrob. Agents Chemother.,* **1996,** *40*:196–202.

Palella, F.J., Jr., Delaney, K.M., Moorman, A.C., Loveless, M.O., Fuhrer, J., Satten, G.A., Aschman, D.J., and Holmberg, S.D. Declining morbidity and mortality among patients with advanced human immunodeficiency virus infection. HIV Outpatient Study Investigators. *N. Engl. J. Med.,* **1998,** *338*:853–860.

Para, M.F., Meehan, P., Holden-Wiltse, J., Fischl, M., Morse, G., Shafer, R., Demeter, L.M., Wood, K., Nevin, T., Virani-Ketter, N., and Freimuth, W.W. ACTG 260: a randomized, phase I–II, dose-ranging trial of the anti-human immunodeficiency virus activity of delavirdine monotherapy. The AIDS Clinical Trials Group Protocol 260 Team. *Antimicrob. Agents Chemother.,* **1999,** *43*:1373–1378.

Partaledis, J.A., Yamaguchi, K., Tisdale, M., Blair, E.E., Falcione, C., Maschera, B., Myers, R.E., Pazhanisamy, S., Futer, O., Cullinan, A.B., *et al.* In vitro selection and characterization of human immunodeficiency virus type 1 (HIV-1) isolates with reduced sensitivity to hydroxyethylamino sulfonamide inhibitors of HIV-1 aspartyl protease. *J. Virol.,* **1995,** *69*:5228–5235.

Paterson, D.L., Swindells, S., Mohr, J., Brester, M., Vergis, E.N., Squier, C., Wagener, M.M., and Singh, N. Adherence to protease inhibitor therapy and outcomes in patients with HIV infection. *Ann. Intern. Med.,* **2000,** *133*:21–30.

Pearl, L.H., and Taylor, W.R. A structural model for the retroviral proteases. *Nature,* **1987,** *329*:351–354.

Perelson, A.S., Essunger, P., Cao, Y., Vesanen, M., Hurley, A., Saksela, K., Markowitz, M., and Ho, D.D. Decay characteristics of HIV-1-infected compartments during combination therapy. *Nature,* **1997,** *387*:188–191.

Perelson, A.S., Neumann, A.U., Markowitz, M., Leonard, J.M., and Ho, D.D. HIV-1 dynamics in vivo: virion clearance rate, infected cell life-span, and viral generation time. *Science,* **1996,** *271*:1582–1586.

Pike, I.M., and Nicaise, C. The Didanosine Expanded Access Program: safety analysis. *Clin. Infect. Dis.,* **1993,** *16*(*suppl. 1*):S63–S68.

Piketty, C., Race, E., Castiel, P., Belec, L., Peytavin, G., Si-Mohamed, A., Gonzalez-Canali, G., Weiss, L., Clavel, F., and Kazatchkine, M.D.

Efficacy of a five-drug combination including ritonavir, saquinavir and efavirenz in patients who failed on a conventional triple-drug regimen: phenotypic resistance to protease inhibitors predicts outcome of therapy. *AIDS,* **1999,** *13*:F71–F77.

Plagemann, P.G., and Woffendin, C. Dideoxycytidine permeation and salvage by mouse leukemia cells and human erythrocytes. *Biochem. Pharmacol.,* **1989,** *38*:3469–3475.

Pluda, J.M., Cooley, T.P., Montaner, J.S., Shay, L.E., Reinhalter, N.E., Warthan, S.N., Ruedy, J., Hirst, H.M., Vicary, C.A., Quinn, J.B., *et al.* A phase I/II study of 2'-deoxy-3'-thiacytidine (lamivudine) in patients with advanced human immunodeficiency virus infection. *J. Infect. Dis.,* **1995,** *171*:1438–1447.

Raboud, J.M., Rae, S., Vella, S., Harrigan, P.R., Bucciardini, R., Fragola, V., Ricciardulli, D., and Montaner, J.S. Meta-analysis of two randomized controlled trials comparing combined zidovudine and didanosine therapy with combined zidovudine, didanosine, and nevirapine therapy in patients with HIV. INCAS study team. *J. Acquir. Immune Defic. Syndr.,* **1999,** *22*:260–266.

Raffi, F., Reliquet, V., Francois, C., Garre, M., Hascoet, C., Allavena, C., Arvieux, C., Breux, J.P., Perre, P., Rozenbaum, W., and Auger, S. Stavudine plus didanosine and nevirapine in antiretroviral-naive HIV-infected adults: preliminary safety and efficacy results. VIRGO Study Team. *Antivir. Ther.,* **1998,** *3*(suppl 4):57–60.

Richman, D.D. Nailing down another HIV target. *Nat. Med.,* **1998,** *4*:1232–1233.

Rimsky, L.T., Shugars, D.C., and Matthews, T.J. Determinants of human immunodeficiency virus type 1 resistance to gp41-derived inhibitory peptides. *J. Virol.,* **1998,** *72*:986–993.

Riska, P., Lamson, M., MacGregor, T., Sabo, J., Hattox, S., Pav, J., and Keirns, J. Disposition and biotransformation of the antiretroviral drug nevirapine in humans. *Drug Metab. Dispos.,* **1999,** *27*:895–901.

Roberts, N.A., Martin, J.A., Kinchington, D., Broadhurst, A.V., Craig, J.C., Duncan, I.B., Galpin, S.A., Handa, B.K., Kay, J., Krohn, A., *et al.* Rational design of peptide-based HIV proteinase inhibitors. *Science,* **1990,** *248*:358–361.

Roca, B., Gomez, C.J., and Arnedo, A. A randomized, comparative study of lamivudine plus stavudine, with indinavir or nelfinavir, in treatment-experienced HIV-infected patients. *AIDS,* **2000,** *14*:157–161.

Romero, D.L., Busso, M., Tan, C.K., Reusser, F., Palmer, J.R., Poppe, S.M., Aristoff, P.A., Downey, K.M., So, A.G., Resnick, L., *et al.* Nonnucleoside reverse transcriptase inhibitors that potently and specifically block human immunodeficiency virus type 1 replication. *Proc. Natl. Acad. Sci. U.S.A.,* **1991,** *88*:8806–8810.

Saag, M.S., Sonnerborg, A., Torres, R.A., Lancaster, D., Gazzard, B.G., Schooley, R.T., Romero, C., Kelleher, D., Spreen, W., and LaFon, S. Antiretroviral effect and safety of abacavir alone and in combination with zidovudine in HIV-infected adults. Abacavir Phase 2 Clinical Team. *AIDS,* **1998,** *12*:F203–F209.

St. Clair, M.H., Martin, J.L., Tudor-Williams, G., Bach, M.C., Vavro, C.L., King, D.M., Kellam, P., Kemp, S.D., and Larder, B.A. Resistance to ddI and sensitivity to AZT induced by a mutation in HIV-1 reverse transcriptase. *Science,* **1991,** *253*:1557–1559.

Saravolatz, L.D., Winslow, D.L., Collins, G., Hodges, J.S., Pettinelli, C., Stein, D.S., Markowitz, N., Reves, R., Loveless, M.O., Crane, L., Thompson, M., and Abrams, D. Zidovudine alone or in combination with didanosine or zalcitabine in HIV-infected patients with the acquired immunodeficiency syndrome or fewer than 200 CD4 cells per cubic millimeter. Investigators for the Terry Beirn Community Programs for Clinical Research on AIDS. *N. Engl. J. Med.,* **1996,** *335*:1099–1106.

Schapiro, J.M., Winters, M.A., Stewart, F., Efron, B., Norris, J., Kozal, M.J., and Merigan, T.C. The effect of high-dose saquinavir on viral load and CD4+ T-cell counts in HIV-infected patients. *Ann. Intern. Med.,* **1996,** *124*:1039–1050.

Schinazi, R.F., Lloyd, R.M., Jr., Nguyen, M.H., Cannon, D.L., McMillan, A., Ilksoy, N., Chu, C.K., Liotta, D.C., Bazmi, H.Z., and Mellors, J.W. Characterization of human immunodeficiency viruses resistant to oxathiolane-cytosine nucleosides. *Antimicrob. Agents Chemother.,* **1993,** *37*:875–881.

Schuurman, R., Nijhuis, M., van Leeuwen, R., Schipper, P., de Jong, D., Collis, P., Danner, S.A., Mulder, J., Loveday, C., Christopherson, C., *et al.* Rapid changes in human immunodeficiency virus type 1 RNA load and appearance of drug-resistant virus populations in persons treated with lamivudine (3TC). *J. Infect. Dis.,* **1995,** *171*:1411–1419.

Skalski, V., Chang, C.N., Dutschman, G., and Cheng, Y.C. The biochemical basis for the differential anti-human immunodeficiency virus activity of two cis enantiomers of 2',3'-dideoxy-3'-thiacytidine. *J. Biol. Chem.,* **1993,** *268*:23234–23238.

Spence, R.A., Kati, W.M., Anderson, K.S., and Johnson, K.A. Mechanism of inhibition of HIV-1 reverse transcriptase by nonnucleoside inhibitors. *Science,* **1995,** *267*:988–993.

Spruance, S.L., Pavia, A.T., Mellors, J.W., Murphy, R., Gathe, J., Jr., Stool, E., Jemsek, J.G., Dellamonica, P., Cross, A., and Dunkle, L. Clinical efficacy of monotherapy with stavudine compared with zidovudine in HIV-infected, zidovudine-experienced patients. A randomized, double-blind, controlled trial. Bristol-Myers Squibb Stavudine/019 Study Group. *Ann. Intern. Med.,* **1997,** *126*:355–363.

Spruance, S.L., Pavia, A.T., Peterson, D., Berry, A., Pollard, R., Patterson, T.F., Frank, I., Remick, S.C., Thompson, M., MacArthur, R.D., *et al.* Didanosine compared with continuation of zidovudine in HIV-infected patients with signs of clinical deterioration while receiving zidovudine. A randomized, double-blind clinical trial. The Bristol-Myers Squibb A1454-010 Study Group. *Ann. Intern. Med.,* **1994,** *120*:360–368.

Starr, S.E., Fletcher, C.V., Spector, S.A., Yong, F.H., Fenton, T., Brundage, R.C., Manion, D., Ruiz, N., Gersten, M., Becker, M., McNamara, J., Mofenson, L.M., Purdue, L., Siminski, S., Graham, B., Kornhauser, D.M., Fiske, W., Vincent, C., Lischner, H.W., Dankner, W.M., and Flynn, P.M. Combination therapy with efavirenz, nelfinavir, and nucleoside reverse-transcriptase inhibitors in children infected with human immunodeficiency virus type 1. Pediatric AIDS Clinical Trials Group 382 Team. *N. Engl. J. Med.,* **1999,** *341*:1874–1881.

Staszewski, S., Morales-Ramirez, J., Tashima, K.T., Rachlis, A., Skiest, D., Stanford, J., Stryker, R., Johnson, P., Labriola, D.F., Farina, D., Manion, D.J., and Ruiz, N.M. Efavirenz plus zidovudine and lamivudine, efavirenz plus indinavir, and indinavir plus zidovudine and lamivudine in the treatment of HIV-1 infection in adults. Study 006 Team. *N. Engl. J. Med.,* **1999,** *341*:1865–1873.

Tashima, K.T., Caliendo, A.M., Ahmad, M., Gormley, J.M., Fiske, W.D., Brennan, J.M., and Flanigan, T.P. Cerebrospinal fluid human immunodeficiency virus type 1 (HIV-1) suppression and efavirenz drug concentrations in HIV-1-infected patients receiving combination therapy. *J. Infect. Dis.,* **1999,** *180*:862–864.

Taylor, S., Back, D.J., Workman, J., Drake, S.M., White, D.J., Choudhury, B., Cane, P.A., Beards, G.M., Halifax, K., and Pillay, D. Poor penetration of the male genital tract by HIV-1 protease inhibitors. *AIDS,* **1999,** *13*:859–860.

Tisdale, M., Alnadaf, T., and Cousens, D. Combination of mutations in human immunodeficiency virus type 1 reverse transcriptase required for resistance to the carbocyclic nucleoside 1592U89. *Antimicrob. Agents Chemother.,* **1997,** *41*:1094–1098.

Tisdale, M., Myers, R.E., Maschera, B., Parry, N.R., Oliver, N.M., and Blair, E.D. Cross-resistance analysis of human immunodeficiency virus type 1 variants individually selected for resistance to five different protease inhibitors. *Antimicrob. Agents Chemother.,* **1995,** *39*:1704–1710.

Ullman, B., Coons, T., Rockwell, S., and McCartan, K. Genetic analysis of 2′,3′-dideoxycytidine incorporation into cultured human T lymphoblasts. *J. Biol. Chem.,* **1988,** *263*:12391–12396.

Vacca, J.P., Dorsey, B.D., Schleif, W.A., Levin, R.B., McDaniel, S.L., Darke, P.L., Zugay, J., Quintero, J.C., Blahy, O.M., Roth, E., *et al.* L-735,524: an orally bioavailable human immunodeficiency virus type 1 protease inhibitor. *Proc. Nat. Acad. Sci. U.S.A.,* **1994,** *91*:4096–4100.

Veal, G.J., Hoggard, P.G., Barry, M.G., Khoo, S., and Back, D.J. Interaction between lamivudine (3TC) and other nucleoside analogues for intracellular phosphorylation. *AIDS,* **1996,** *10*:546–548.

Villani, P., Regazzi, M.B., Castelli, F., Viale, P., Torti, C., Seminari, E., and Maserati, R. Pharmacokinetics of efavirenz (EFV) alone and in combination therapy with nelfinavir (NFV) in HIV-1 infected patients. *Br. J. Clin. Pharmacol.,* **1999,** *48*:712–715.

Walker, R.E., Parker, R.I., Kovacs, J.A., Masur, H., Lane, H.C., Carleton, S., Kirk, L.E., Gralnick, H.R., and Fauci, A.S. Anemia and erythropoiesis in patients with the acquired immunodeficiency syndrome (AIDS) and Kaposi sarcoma treated with zidovudine. *Ann. Intern. Med.,* **1988,** *108*:372–376.

Watts, D.H., Brown, Z.A., Tartaglione, T., Burchett, S.K., Opheim, K., Coombs, R., and Corey, L. Pharmacokinetic disposition of zidovudine during pregnancy. *J. Infect. Dis.,* **1991,** *163*:226–232.

Wei, X., Ghosh, S.K., Taylor, M.E., Johnson, V.A., Emini, E.A., Deutsch, P., Lifson, J.D., Bonhoeffer, S., Nowak, M.A., Hahn, B.H., *et al.* Viral dynamics in human immunodeficiency virus type 1 infection. *Nature,* **1995,** *373*:117–122.

Wild, C.T., Shugars, D.C., Greenwell, T.K., McDanal, C.B., and Matthews, T.J. Peptides corresponding to a predictive alpha-helical domain of human immunodeficiency virus type 1 gp41 are potent inhibitors of virus infection. *Proc. Natl. Acad. Sci. U.S.A.,* **1994,** *91*:9770–9774.

Winslow, D.L., Garber, S., Reid, C., Scarnati, H., Baker, D., Rayner, M.M., and Anton, E.D., Selection conditions affect the evolution of specific mutations in the reverse transcriptase gene associated with resistance to DMP 266. *AIDS,* **1996,** *10*:1205–1209.

Wlodawer, A., Miller, M., Jaskolski, M., Sathyanarayana, B.K., Baldwin, E., Weber, I.T., Selk, L.M., Clawson, L., Schneider, J., and Kent, S.B. Conserved folding in retroviral proteases: crystal structure of a synthetic HIV-1 protease. *Science,* **1989,** *245*:616–621.

Yarchoan, R., Perno, C.F., Thomas, R.V., Klecker, R.W., Allain, J.P., Wills, R.J., McAtee, N., Fischl, M.A., Dubinsky, R., McNeely, M.C., *et al.* Phase I studies of 2′,3′-dideoxycytidine in severe human immunodeficiency virus infection as a single agent and alternating with zidovudine (AZT). *Lancet,* **1988,** *1*:76–81.

Yokota, T., Mochizuki, S., Konno, K., Mori, S., Shigeta, S., and De Clercq, E. Inhibitory effects of selected antiviral compounds on human hepatitis B virus DNA synthesis. *Antimicrob. Agents Chemother.,* **1991,** *35*:394–397.

Young, S.D., Britcher, S.F., Tran, L.O., Payne, L.S., Lumma, W.C., Lyle, T.A., Huff, J.R., Anderson, P.S., Olsen, D.B., Carroll, S.S., *et al.* L-743,726 (DMP-266): a novel, highly potent nonnucleoside inhibitor of the human immunodeficiency virus type 1 reverse transcriptase. *Antimicrob. Agents Chemother.,* **1995,** *39*:2602–2605.

Yuen, G.J., Morris, D.M., Mydlow, P.K., Haidar, S., Hall, S.T., and Hussey, E.K. Pharmacokinetics, absolute bioavailability, and absorption characteristics of lamivudine. *J. Clin. Pharmacol.,* **1995,** *35*:1174–1180.

Zhang, H., Dornadula, G., Wu, Y., Havlir, D., Richman, D.D., and Pomerantz, R.J. Kinetic analysis of intravirion reverse transcription in the blood plasma of human immunodeficiency virus type 1-infected individuals: direct assessment of resistance to reverse transcriptase inhibitors in vivo. *J. Virol.,* **1996,** *70*:628–634.

Zhou, X.J., Sheiner, L.B., D'Aquila, R.T., Hughes, M.D., Hirsch, M.S., Fischl, M.A., Johnson, V.A., Myers, M., and Sommadossi, J.P. Population pharmacokinetics of nevirapine, zidovudine, and didanosine in human immunodeficiency virus-infected patients. The National Institute of Allergy and Infectious Diseases AIDS Clinical Trials Group Protocol 241 Investigators. *Antimicrob. Agents Chemother.,* **1999,** *43*:121–128.

Zhu, Z., Ho, H.T., Hitchcock, M.J., and Sommadossi, J.P., Cellular pharmacology of 2′,3′-didehydro-2′,3′-dideoxythymidine (D4T) in human peripheral blood mononuclear cells. *Biochem. Pharmacol.,* **1990,** *39*:R15–R19.

MONOGRAPHS AND REVIEWS

Adkins, J.C., and Faulds, D. Amprenavir. *Drugs,* **1998,** *55*:837–842.

Adkins, J.C., and Noble, S. Efavirenz. *Drugs,* **1998,** *56*:1055–1064.

Bardsley-Elliot, A., and Plosker, G.L. Nelfinavir: an update on its use in HIV infection. *Drugs,* **2000,** *59*:581–620.

Barry, M., Mulcahy, F., Merry, C., Gibbons, S., and Back, D. Pharmacokinetics and potential interactions amongst antiretroviral agents used to treat patients with HIV infection. *Clin. Pharmacokinet.,* **1999,** *36*:289–304.

Broder, S. Pharmacodynamics of 2′,3′-dideoxycytidine: an inhibitor of human immunodeficiency virus. *Am. J. Med.,* **1990,** *88*:2S–7S.

Craig, C., and Moyle, G. The development of HIV-1 resistance to zalcitabine. *AIDS,* **1997,** *11*:271–279.

Dudley, M.N. Clinical pharmacokinetics of nucleoside antiretroviral agents. *J. Infect. Dis.,* **1995,** *171*(suppl 2):S99–S112.

Flexner, C. Dual protease inhibitor therapy in HIV-infected patients: pharmacologic rationale and clinical benefits. *Annu. Rev. Pharmacol. Toxicol.,* **2000,** *40*:649–674.

Freimuth, W.W. Delavirdine mesylate, a potent non-nucleoside HIV-1 reverse transcriptase inhibitor. *Adv. Exp. Med. Biol.,* **1996,** *394*:279–289.

Harrington, M., and Carpenter, C.C. Hit HIV-1 hard, but only when necessary. *Lancet,* **2000,** *355*:2147–2152.

Havlir, D.V., and Richman, D.D. Viral dynamics of HIV: implications for drug development and therapeutic strategies. *Ann. Intern. Med.,* **1996,** *124*:984–994.

Hitchcock, M.J. In vitro antiviral activity of didanosine compared with that of other dideoxynucleoside analogs against laboratory strains and clinical isolates of human immunodeficiency virus. *Clin. Infect. Dis.,* **1993,** *16*(suppl 1):S16–S21.

Hsu, A., Granneman, G.R., and Bertz, R.J. Ritonavir, Clinical pharmacokinetics and interactions with other anti-HIV agents. *Clin. Pharmacokinet.,* **1998,** *35*:275–291.

Jayasekara, D., Aweeka, F.T., Rodriguez, R., Kalayjian, R.C., Humphreys, M.H., and Gambertoglio, J.G. Antiviral therapy for HIV patients with renal insufficiency. *J. Acquir. Immune Defic. Syndr.,* **1999,** *21*:384–395.

McGowan, J.J., Tomaszewski, J.E., Cradock, J., Hoth, D., Grieshaber, C.K., Broder, S., and Mitsuya, H. Overview of the preclinical development of an antiretroviral drug, 2',3'-dideoxyinosine. *Rev. Infect. Dis.,* **1990,** *12*(*suppl 5*):S513–S520.

McLeod, G.X., and Hammer, S.M. Zidovudine: five years later. *Ann. Intern. Med.,* **1992,** *117*:487–501.

Noble, S., and Faulds, D. Saquinavir. A review of its pharmacology and clinical potential in the management of HIV infection. *Drugs,* **1996,** *5*:93–112.

Perry, C.M., and Balfour, J.A. Didanosine. An update on its antiviral activity, pharmacokinetic properties and therapeutic efficacy in the management of HIV disease. *Drugs,* **1996,** *52*:928–962.

Perry, C.M., and Noble, S. Saquinavir soft-gel capsule formulation. A review of its use in patients with HIV infection. *Drugs,* **1998,** *55*:461–486.

Plosker, G.L., and Noble, S. Indinavir: a review of its use in the management of HIV infection. *Drugs, 1999, 58*:1165–1203.

Rendic, S., and Di Carlo, F.J. Human cytochrome P450 enzymes: a status report summarizing their reactions, substrates, inducers, and inhibitors. *Drug Metab. Rev.,* **1997,** *29*:413–580.

Richman, D.D. Resistance of clinical isolates of human immunodeficiency virus to antiretroviral agents. *Antimicrob. Agents Chemother.,* **1993,** *37*:1207–1213.

Romanelli, F., and Pomeroy, C. Human immunodeficiency virus drug resistance testing: state of the art in genotypic and phenotypic testing of antiretrovirals. *Pharmacotherapy, 2000, 20*:151–157.

Rozencweig, M., McLaren, C., Beltangady, M., Ritter, J., Canetta, R., Schacter, L., Kelley, S., Nicaise, C., Smaldone, L., Dunkle, L., *et al.* Overview of phase I trials of 2',3'-dideoxyinosine (ddI) conducted on adult patients. *Rev. Infect. Dis.,* **1990,** *12*(suppl 5):S570–S575.

Shelton, M.J., O'Donnell, A.M., and Morse, G.D. Didanosine. *Ann. Pharmacother.,* **1992,** *26*:660–670.

Skowron, G. Biologic effects and safety of stavudine: overview of phase I and II clinical trials. *J. Infect. Dis.,* **1995,** *171*(suppl 2):S113–S117.

Sodroski, J.G. HIV-1 entry inhibitors in the side pocket. *Cell,* **1999,** *99*:243–246.

Sommadossi, J.P. Comparison of metabolism and *in vitro* antiviral activity of stavudine versus other 2',3'-dideoxynucleoside analogues. *J. Infect. Dis.,* **1995,** *171*(*suppl 2*):S88–S92.

Tavel, J.A., Miller, K.D., and Masur, H. Guide to major clinical trials of antiretroviral therapy in human immunodeficiency virus-infected patients: protease inhibitors, non-nucleoside reverse transcriptase inhibitors, and nucleotide reverse transcriptase inhibitors. *Clin. Infect. Dis.,* **1999,** *28*:643–676.

Thaisrivongs, S., and Strohbach, J.W. Structure-based discovery of Tipranavir disodium (PNU-140690E): a potent, orally bioavailable, nonpeptidic HIV protease inhibitor. *Biopolymers,* **1999,** *51*:51–58.

Wain-Hobson, S. The fastest genome evolution ever described: HIV variation *in situ. Curr. Opin. Genet. Dev.,* **1993,** *3*:878–883.

S E C T I O N   I X

CHEMOTHERAPY OF NEOPLASTIC DISEASES

INTRODUCTION

Paul Calabresi and Bruce A. Chabner

Among the subspecialties of internal medicine, medical oncology may have had the greatest impact in changing the practice of medicine in the past four decades, as curative treatments have been identified for a number of previously fatal malignancies such as testicular cancer, lymphomas, and leukemia. New drugs have entered clinical use for disease presentations previously either untreatable or amenable to only local means of therapy, such as surgery and irradiation. At present, adjuvant chemotherapy routinely follows local treatment of breast cancer, colon cancer, and rectal cancer, and chemotherapy is employed as part of a multimodality approach to the initial treatment of many other tumors, including locally advanced stages of head and neck, lung, cervical, and esophageal cancer, soft tissue sarcomas, and pediatric solid tumors. The basic approaches to cancer treatment are constantly changing. Clinical protocols are now exploring genetic therapies, manipulations of the immune system, stimulation of normal hematopoietic elements, induction of differentiation in tumor tissues, and inhibition of angiogenesis. Research in each of these new areas has led to experimental or, in some cases, routine applications for both malignant and nonmalignant disease. The same drugs used for cytotoxic antitumor therapy have become important components of immunosuppressive regimens for rheumatoid arthritis (*methotrexate* and *cyclophosphamide*), organ transplantation (methotrexate and *azathioprine*), sickle cell anemia (*hydroxyurea*), antiinfective chemotherapy (*trimetrexate* and *leucovorin*), and psoriasis (methotrexate). Thus, a broad spectrum of medical, surgical, and pediatric specialists employ these drugs for both neoplastic and nonneoplastic disease.

At the same time, few categories of medication in common use have a narrower therapeutic index and a greater potential for causing harmful side effects than do the antineoplastic drugs. A thorough understanding of their pharmacology, drug interactions, and clinical pharmacokinetics is essential for safe and effective use in human beings.

Traditionally, cancer drugs were discovered through large-scale screening of synthetic chemicals and natural products against animal tumor systems, primarily murine leukemias. The agents discovered in the first two decades of cancer chemotherapy (1950 to 1970) largely interacted with DNA or its precursors, inhibiting the synthesis of new genetic material or causing irreparable damage to DNA itself. An overview of such agents is given in Figure IX–1. In recent years, the discovery of new agents has extended from the more conventional natural products such as *paclitaxel* and semisynthetic agents such as *etoposide,* both of which target the proliferative process, to entirely new fields of investigation that represent the harvest of new knowledge about cancer biology. The first successful applications of this knowledge include diverse drugs. One agent, *interleukin-2,* regulates the proliferation of tumor-killing T lymphocytes and so-called natural killer cells; this agent has proven able to induce remissions in a fraction of patients with malignant melanoma and renal cell carcinoma, diseases unresponsive to

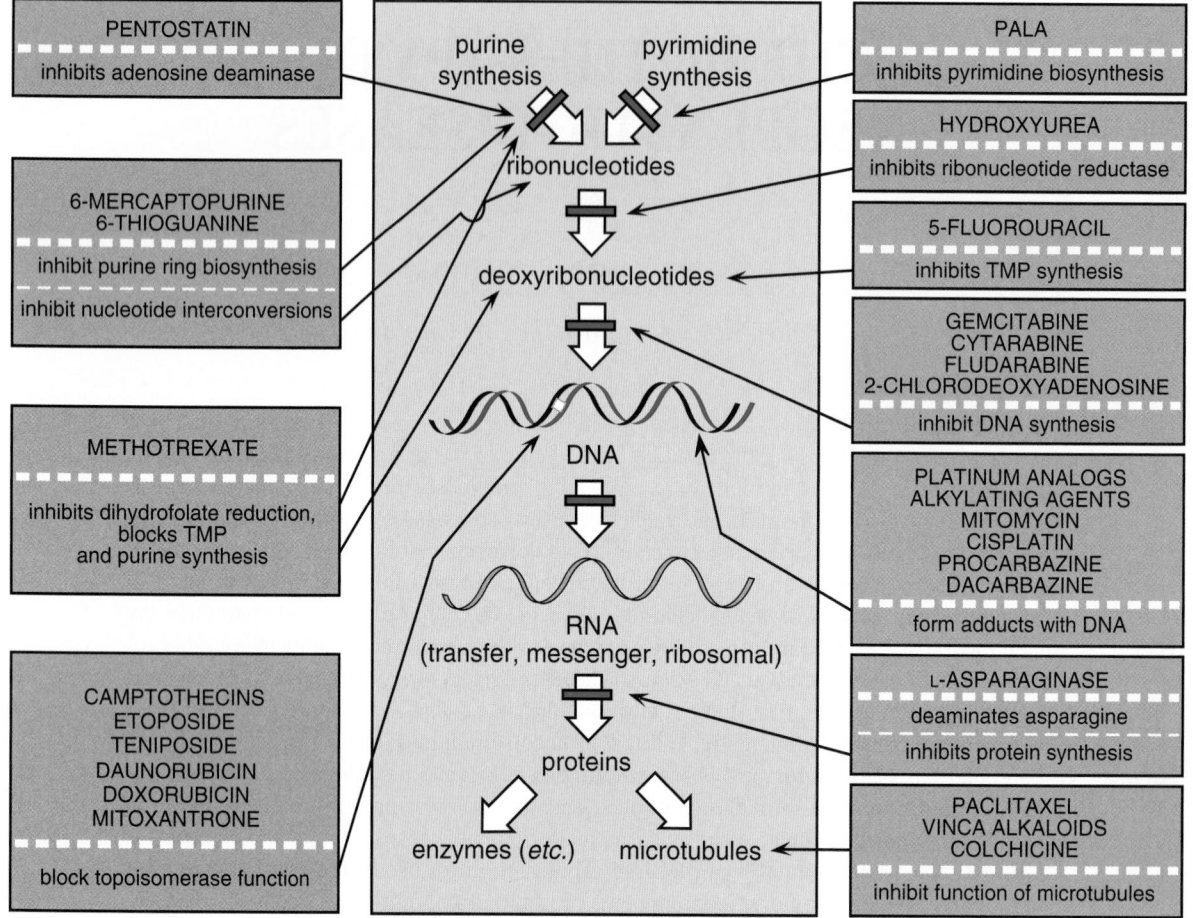

Figure IX–1. Summary of the mechanisms and sites of action of chemotherapeutic agents useful in neoplastic disease.

PALA = *N*-phosphonoacetyl-L-aspartate; TMP = thymidine monophosphate.

conventional drugs. Another agent, all-*trans*-retinoic acid, elicits differentiation and can be used to promote remission in acute promyelocytic leukemia, even after failure of standard chemotherapy. The related compound 13-*cis*-retinoic acid prevents occurrence of second primary tumors in patients with head and neck cancer. Initial success in characterizing unique tumor antigens and oncogenes has introduced new possible therapeutic opportunities based on an understanding of tumor biology. Thus the *bcr-abl* translocation in chronic myelocytic leukemia codes for a tyrosine kinase essential to cell proliferation and survival. Inhibition of the kinase by *imatinib* (STI-571), a new molecularly targeted drug, has produced a high response rate in chronic-phase patients resistant to standard therapy. In a similar, though immunological, approach tumor-associated antigens, such as the her-2/neu receptor in breast cancer cells, have become the target for monoclonal antibody therapy that has shown activity in patients. These examples emphasize that the care of cancer patients is likely to undergo revolutionary changes as entirely new treatment approaches are identified, based on new knowledge of cancer biology (Kaelin, 1999). The diversity of agents useful in treatment of neoplastic disease is summarized in Table IX–1. The classification used in Chapter 52, which follows, is a convenient framework for describing various types of agents.

Table IX–1
Chemotherapeutic Agents Useful in Neoplastic Disease

CLASS	TYPE OF AGENT	NONPROPRIETARY NAMES (OTHER NAMES)	DISEASE*
Alkylating Agents	Nitrogen Mustards	Mechlorethamine	Hodgkin's disease, non-Hodgkin's lymphomas
		Cyclophosphamide Ifosfamide	Acute and chronic lymphocytic leukemias; Hodgkin's disease; non-Hodgkin's lymphomas; multiple myeloma; neuroblastoma; breast, ovary, lung cancer; Wilms' tumor; cervix, testis cancer; soft-tissue sarcomas
		Melphalan (L-sarcolysin)	Multiple myeloma; breast, ovarian cancer
		Chlorambucil	Chronic lymphocytic leukemia, primary macroglobulinemia, Hodgkin's disease, non-Hodgkin's lymphomas
	Ethylenimines and Methylmelamines	Hexamethylmelamine	Ovarian cancer
		Thiotepa	Bladder, breast, ovarian cancer
	Alkyl Sulfonates	Busulfan	Chronic granulocytic leukemia
	Nitrosoureas	Carmustine (BCNU)	Hodgkin's disease, non-Hodgkin's lymphomas, primary brain tumors, multiple myeloma, malignant melanoma
		Streptozocin (streptozotocin)	Malignant pancreatic insulinoma, malignant carcinoid
	Triazenes	Dacarbazine (DTIC; dimethyltriazenoimidazolecarboxamide)	Malignant melanoma, Hodgkin's disease, soft-tissue sarcomas
		Temozolomide	Glioma, malignant melanoma
Antimetabolites	Folic Acid Analogs	Methotrexate (amethopterin)	Acute lymphocytic leukemia; choriocarcinoma; mycosis fungoides; breast, head and neck, lung cancer; osteogenic sarcoma
	Pyrimidine Analogs	Fluorouracil (5-fluorouracil; 5-FU) Floxuridine (fluorodeoxyuridine; FUdR)	Breast, colon, stomach, pancreas, ovarian, head and neck, urinary bladder cancer; premalignant skin lesions (topical)
		Cytarabine (cytosine arabinoside)	Acute granulocytic and acute lymphocytic leukemias
		Gemcitabine	Pancreatic cancer, ovarian cancer
	Purine analogs and related inhibitors	Mercaptopurine (6-mercaptopurine; 6-MP)	Acute lymphocytic, acute granulocytic, and chronic granulocytic leukemias

*Neoplasms are carcinomas unless otherwise indicated.

Table IX–1

Chemotherapeutic Agents Useful in Neoplastic Disease *(Continued)*

CLASS	TYPE OF AGENT	NONPROPRIETARY NAMES (OTHER NAMES)	DISEASE*
Antimetabolites *(cont.)*	Purine Analogs and Related Inhibitors	Thioguanine (6-thioguanine; TG)	Acute granulocytic, acute lymphocytic, and chronic granulocytic leukemias
		Pentostatin (2'-deoxycoformycin) Cladribine Fludarabine	Hairy cell leukemia, mycosis fungoides, chronic lymphocytic leukemia, small cell lymphoma
Natural Products	Vinca Alkaloids	Vinblastine (VLB)	Hodgkin's disease, non-Hodgkin's lymphomas, breast and testis cancer
		Vincristine	Acute lymphocytic leukemia, neuroblastoma, Wilms' tumor, rhabdomyosarcoma, Hodgkin's disease, non-Hodgkin's lymphomas, small-cell lung cancer
	Taxanes	Paclitaxel, Docetaxel	Ovarian, breast, lung, head and neck cancer
	Epipodophyllotoxins	Etoposide Teniposide	Testis, small-cell lung and other lung, breast cancer; Hodgkin's disease, non-Hodgkin's lymphomas, acute granulocytic leukemia, Kaposi's sarcoma
	Camptothecins	Topotecan Irinotecan	Ovarian cancer, small cell lung cancer Colon cancer
	Antibiotics	Dactinomycin (actinomycin D)	Choriocarcinoma, Wilms' tumor, rhabdomyosarcoma, testis, Kaposi's sarcoma
		Daunorubicin (daunomycin; rubidomycin)	Acute granulocytic and acute lymphocytic leukemias
		Doxorubicin	Soft-tissue, osteogenic, and other sarcomas; Hodgkin's disease, non-Hodgkin's lymphomas; acute leukemias; breast, genitourinary, thyroid, lung, stomach cancer; neuroblastoma
		Bleomycin	Testis, head and neck, skin, esophagus, lung, and genitourinary tract cancer; Hodgkin's disease, non-Hodgkin's lymphomas
		Mitomycin (mitomycin C)	Stomach, cervix, colon, breast, pancreas, bladder, head and neck cancer
	Enzymes	L-Asparaginase	Acute lymphocytic leukemia

*Neoplasms are carcinomas unless otherwise indicated.

Table IX–1
Chemotherapeutic Agents Useful in Neoplastic Disease (*Continued*)

CLASS	TYPE OF AGENT	NONPROPRIETARY NAMES (OTHER NAMES)	DISEASE*
Natural Products (*cont.*)	Biological Response Modifiers	Interferon-alfa Interleukin 2	Hairy cell leukemia, Kaposi's sarcoma, melanoma, carcinoid, renal cell, ovary, bladder, non-Hodgkin's lymphomas, mycosis fungoides, multiple myeloma, chronic granulocytic leukemia, Malignant melanoma, renal cell cancer
Miscellaneous Agents	Platinum Coordination Complexes	Cisplatin (*cis*-DDP) Carboplatin	Testis, ovary, bladder, head and neck, lung, thyroid, cervix and endometrium cancer; neuroblastoma, osteogenic sarcoma
	Anthracenedione	Mitoxantrone	Acute granulocytic leukemia, breast and prostate cancer
	Substituted Urea	Hydroxyurea	Chronic granulocytic leukemia, polycythemia vera, essential thrombocytosis, malignant melanoma
	Methylhydrazine Derivative	Procarbazine (*N*-methylhydrazine, MIH)	Hodgkin's disease
	Adrenocortical Suppressant	Mitotane (*o,p'*-DDD)	Adrenal cortex cancer
		Aminoglutethimide	Breast cancer
	Tyrosine kinase inhibitor	Imatinib	Chronic myelocytic leukemia
Hormones and Antagonists	Adrenocorticosteroids	Prednisone (several other equivalent preparations available; *see* Chapter 60)	Acute and chronic lymphocytic leukemias, non-Hodgkin's lymphomas, Hodgkin's disease, breast cancer
	Progestins	Hydroxyprogesterone caproate Medroxyprogesterone acetate Megestrol acetate	Endometrium, breast cancer
	Estrogens	Diethylstilbestrol Ethinyl estradiol (other preparations available; *see* Chapter 58)	Breast, prostate cancer
	Antiestrogen	Tamoxifen, Anastrozole	Breast cancer
	Androgens	Testosterone propionate Fluoxymesterone (other preparations available; *see* Chapter 59)	Breast cancer
	Antiandrogen	Flutamide	Prostate cancer
	Gonadotropin-Releasing Hormone Analog	Leuprolide	Prostate cancer

*Neoplasms are carcinomas unless otherwise indicated.

It is unlikely that new therapies will totally replace existing drugs, as these drugs have become increasingly effective and their toxicities have become more manageable and predictable in recent years. Improvements in their use are the result of a number of factors, including the following:

1. Drugs now are routinely used earlier in the course of the patient's management, often in conjunction with radiation or surgery, to treat malignancy when it is most curable and when the patient is best able to tolerate treatment. Thus, adjuvant therapy and neoadjuvant chemotherapy are used in conjunction with irradiation and surgery in the treatment of head and neck, esophageal, lung, and breast cancer patients.

2. The availability of granulocyte colony-stimulating factor (G-CSF; *see* Chapter 54) has shortened the period of leukopenia after high-dose chemotherapy, increasing the safety of bone marrow–ablative regimens and decreasing the incidence of life-threatening infection. A similar megakaryocyte growth and development factor has been cloned but has not yet achieved a useful place as an adjunct to chemotherapy.

3. A greater insight into the mechanisms of tumor cell resistance to chemotherapy has led to the more rational construction of drug regimens and the earlier use of intensive therapies.

Drug-resistant cells may be selected from the larger tumor population by exposure to low-dose, single-agent chemotherapy. The resistance that arises may be specific for the selecting agent, such as the deletion of a necessary activating enzyme (deoxycytidine kinase for cytosine arabinoside), or more general, such as the overexpression of a general drug-efflux pump such as the P-glycoprotein, a product of the *MDR* gene. This membrane protein is one of several ATP-dependent transporters that confer resistance to a broad range of natural products used in cancer treatment. More recently, it has become appreciated that mutations underlying malignant transformation, such as the loss of the p53 suppressor oncogene, may lead to drug resistance. (A suppressor gene is essential for normal control of cell proliferation; its loss or mutation allows cells to undergo malignant transformation.) Mutation of p53, or its loss, or the overexpression of the *bcl*-2 gene that is translocated in nodular non-Hodgkin's lymphomas, inactivates a key pathway of programmed cell death (apoptosis) and leads to survival of highly mutated tumor cells that have the capacity to survive DNA damage. Drug discovery efforts are now directed toward restoring apoptosis in tumor cells, as this process, or its absence, seems to have profound influence on tumor cell sensitivity to drugs. Each of these topics concerning drug resistance is covered in greater detail in Chapter 52.

In designing specific regimens for clinical use, a number of factors must be taken into account. Drugs are generally more effective in combination and may be synergistic through biochemical interactions. These interactions are useful in designing new regimens. It is more effective to use drugs that do not share common mechanisms of resistance and that do not overlap in their major toxicities. Drugs should be used as close as possible to their maximum individual doses and should be given as frequently as possible to discourage tumor regrowth and to maximize dose intensity (the dose given per unit time, a key parameter in the success of chemotherapy). Since the tumor cell population in patients with visible disease exceeds 1 g, or 10^9 cells, and since each cycle of therapy kills less than 99% of the cells, it is necessary to repeat treatments in multiple cycles to kill all the tumor cells.

The Cell Cycle. An understanding of cell-cycle kinetics is essential for the proper use of the current generation of antineoplastic agents. Many of the most potent cytotoxic agents act by damaging DNA. Their toxicity is greater during the S, or DNA synthetic, phase of the cell cycle, while others, such as the vinca alkaloids and taxanes, block the formation of the mitotic spindle in M phase. These agents have activity only against cells that are in the process of division. Accordingly, human neoplasms that are currently most susceptible to chemotherapeutic measures are those with a high percentage of cells undergoing division. Similarly, normal tissues that proliferate rapidly (bone marrow, hair follicles, and intestinal epithelium) are subject to damage by most antineoplastic drugs, and such toxicity often limits the usefulness of drugs. On the other hand, slowly growing tumors with a small growth fraction (for example, carcinomas of the colon or lung) often are unresponsive to cytotoxic drugs. Although differences in the duration of the cell cycle occur between cells of various types, all cells display a similar pattern during the division process. This cell cycle may be characterized as follows (*see* Figure IX–2): (1) There is a presynthetic phase (G_1); (2) the synthesis of DNA occurs (S); (3) an interval follows the

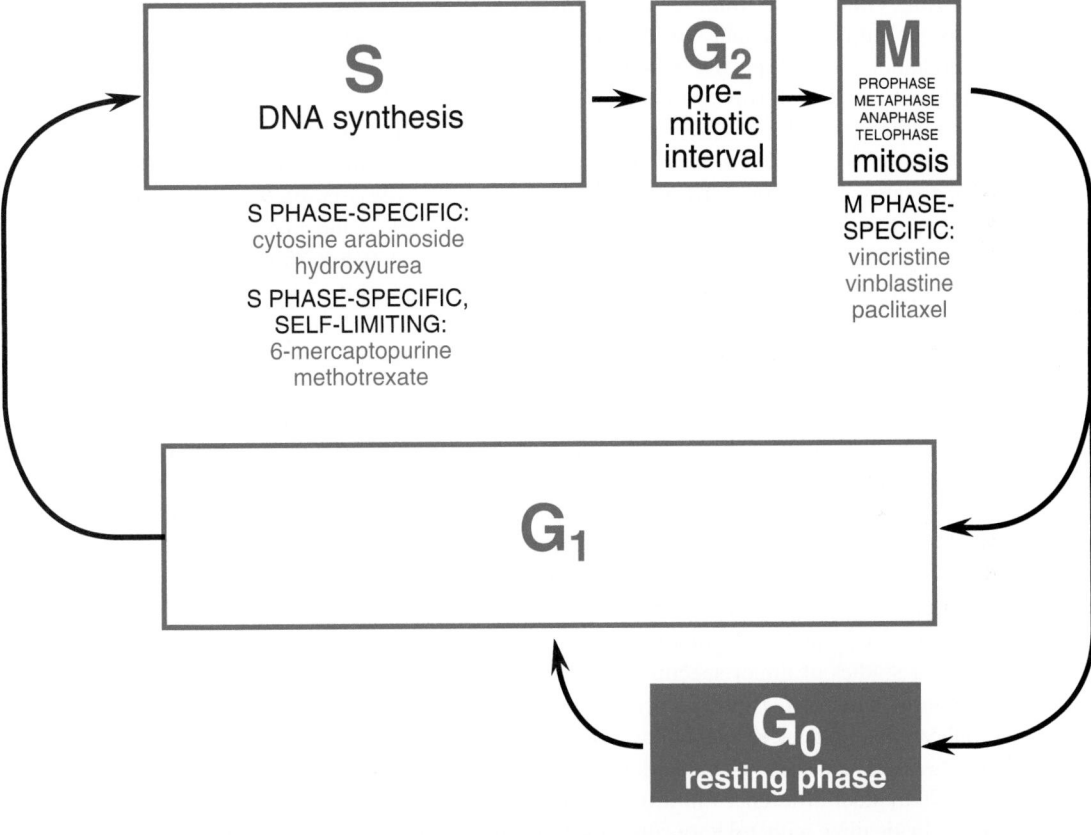

Figure IX–2. The cell cycle and the relationship of antitumor drug action to the cycle.

G_1 is the period between mitosis and the beginning of DNA synthesis. Resting cells (cells that are not preparing for cell division) are said to be in a subphase of G_1, G_0. S is the period of DNA synthesis; G_2 the premitotic interval; and M the period of mitosis. Examples of cell-cycle–dependent anticancer drugs are listed in blue below the phase in which they act. Drugs that are cytotoxic for cells at any point in the cycle are called cycle-phase-nonspecific drugs. (*Modified from* Pratt *et al., 1994 with permission.*)

termination of DNA synthesis, the postsynthetic phase (G_2); and (4) mitosis (M) ensues— the G_2 cell, containing a double complement of DNA, divides into two daughter G_1 cells. Each of these cells may immediately reenter the cell cycle or pass into a nonproliferative stage, referred to as G_0. The G_0 cells of certain specialized tissues may differentiate into functional cells that no longer are capable of division. On the other hand, many cells, especially those in slow-growing tumors, may remain in the G_0 state for prolonged periods, only to reenter the division cycle at a later time. Damaged cells that reach the G_1/S boundary undergo apoptosis, or programmed cell death, if the p53 gene is intact and if it exerts its normal checkpoint function. If the p53 gene is mutated and the checkpoint function fails, damaged cells will not be diverted to the apoptotic pathway. These cells will proceed through S phase and some will emerge as a drug-resistant population. Thus, an understanding of cell-cycle kinetics and the controls of normal and malignant cell growth is crucial to the design of current therapy regimens and the search for new drugs.

Achieving Therapeutic Balance and Efficacy.   While not the subject of this chapter, it must be emphasized that the treatment of most cancer patients requires a skillful interdigitation of multiple modalities of treatment, including surgery, irradiation, and drugs. Each of these forms of treatment carries its own risks and benefits. It is obvious that not all drugs and not all regimens are safe or appropriate for all patients. Numerous factors must be considered, such as renal and hepatic function, bone marrow reserve, and the status of general performance and accessory medical problems. Beyond those considerations, however, are less quantifiable factors such as the likely natural history of the tumor being treated, the patient's willingness to undergo harsh treatments, the patient's physical and emotional tolerance for side effects, and the likely long-term gains and risks involved.

The emphasis in Chapter 52 is placed upon the drugs, but it is essential to point out the importance of the role played by the patient. It is generally agreed that patients in good nutritional state and without severe metabolic disturbances, infections, or other complications have better tolerance for chemotherapy and have a better chance for significant improvement than do severely debilitated individuals. Ideally, the patient should have adequate renal, hepatic, and bone marrow function, the latter uncompromised by tumor invasion, previous chemotherapy, or irradiation (particularly of the spine or pelvis). Nevertheless, even patients with advanced disease have improved dramatically with chemotherapy. Although methods that would enable accurate prediction of the responsiveness of a particular tumor to a given agent are still investigational, in the future, molecular studies of tumor specimens may allow prediction of response and the rational selection of patients for specific drugs. Despite efforts to anticipate the development of complications, anticancer agents have variable pharmacokinetics and toxicity in individual patients. The causes of this variability are not always clear and often may be related to interindividual differences in drug metabolism, drug interactions, or bone marrow reserves. In dealing with toxicity, the physician must provide vigorous supportive care, including, where indicated, platelet transfusions, antibiotics, and hematopoietic growth factors (*see* Chapter 54). Other delayed toxicities affecting the heart, lungs, or kidneys may not be reversible and may lead to permanent organ damage or death. Fortunately, such toxicities will be uncommon if the physician adheres to standard protocols and respects the guidelines for drug usage detailed in the following discussion.

ANTINEOPLASTIC AGENTS

Bruce A. Chabner, David P. Ryan, Luiz Paz-Ares,
Rocio Garcia-Carbonero, and Paul Calabresi

I. ALKYLATING AGENTS

History. Although synthesized in 1854, the vesicant properties of sulfur mustard were not described until 1887. During World War I, medical attention was first focused on the vesicant action of sulfur mustard on the skin, eyes, and respiratory tract. It was appreciated later, however, that serious systemic toxicity also follows exposure. In 1919, Krumbhaar and Krumbhaar made the pertinent observation that the poisoning caused by sulfur mustard is characterized by leukopenia and, in cases that came to autopsy, by aplasia of the bone marrow, dissolution of lymphoid tissue, and ulceration of the gastrointestinal tract.

In the interval between World Wars I and II, extensive studies of the biological and chemical actions of the *nitrogen mustards* were conducted. The marked cytotoxic action on lymphoid tissue prompted Gilman, Goodman, and T.F. Dougherty to study the effect of nitrogen mustards on transplanted lymphosarcoma in mice, and in 1942 clinical studies were initiated. This launched the era of modern cancer chemotherapy (Gilman, 1963).

In their early phases, all these investigations were conducted under secrecy restrictions imposed by the use of classified chemical-warfare agents. At the termination of World War II, however, the nitrogen mustards were declassified; a general review was presented by Gilman and Philips (1946). A more recent review is provided by Ludlum and Tong (1985).

Thousands of variants of the basic chemical structure of the nitrogen mustards have been prepared, but only a few of these agents have proven more useful than the original compound in specific clinical circumstances (*see* below). At present five major types of alkylating agents are used in the chemotherapy of neoplastic diseases: (1) the nitrogen mustards, (2) the ethylenimines, (3) the alkyl sulfonates, (4) the nitrosoureas, and (5) the triazenes.

Chemistry. The chemotherapeutic alkylating agents have in common the property of becoming strong electrophiles through the formation of carbonium ion intermediates or of transition complexes with the target molecules. These reactions result in the formation of covalent linkages by alkylation of various nucleophilic moieties such as phosphate, amino, sulfhydryl, hydroxyl, carboxyl, and imidazole groups. The chemotherapeutic and cytotoxic effects are directly related to the alkylation of DNA. The 7 nitrogen atom of guanine is particularly susceptible to the formation of a covalent bond with bifunctional alkylating agents and may well represent the key target that determines their biological effects. It must be appreciated, how-

ever, that other atoms in the purine and pyrimidine bases of DNA—particularly, the 1 and 3 nitrogens of adenine, the 3 nitrogen of cytosine, and the 6 oxygen of guanine—also may be alkylated, as will be the phosphate atoms of the DNA chains and amino and sulfhydryl groups of proteins.

To illustrate the actions of alkylating agents, possible consequences of the reaction of *mechlorethamine* (nitrogen mustard) with guanine residues in DNA chains are shown in Figure 52–1. First, one 2-chloroethyl side chain undergoes a first-order (S_N1) intramolecular cyclization, with release of Cl^- and formation of a highly reactive ethyleniminium intermediate (Figure 52–1A). By this reaction, the tertiary amine is converted to an unstable quaternary ammonium compound, which can react avidly, through formation of a carbonium ion or transition complex intermediate, with a variety of sites that possess high electron density. This reaction proceeds as a second-order (S_N2) nucleophilic substitution. Alkylation of the 7 nitrogen of guanine residues in DNA (Figure 52–1B), a highly favored

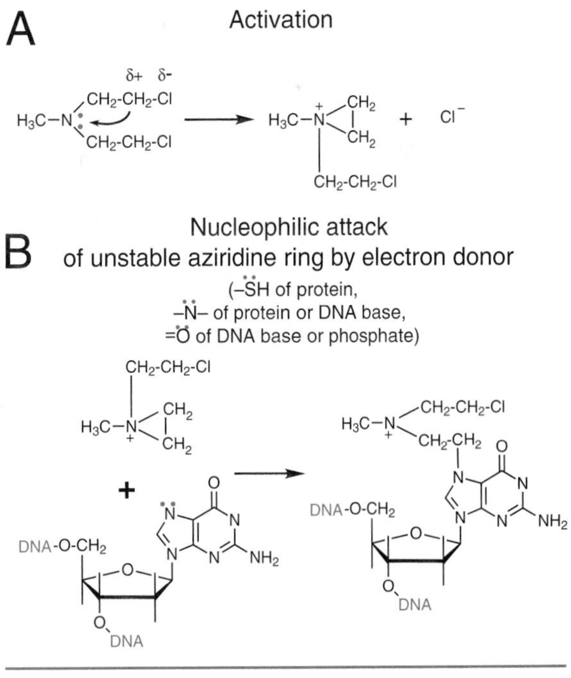

Figure 52–1. Mechanism of action of alkylating agents.

reaction, may exert several effects of considerable biological importance. Normally, guanine residues in DNA exist predominantly as the keto tautomer and readily make Watson–Crick base pairs by hydrogen bonding with cytosine residues. However, when the 7 nitrogen of guanine is alkylated (to become a quaternary ammonium nitrogen), the guanine residue is more acidic and the enol tautomer is favored. The modified guanine can mispair with thymine residues during DNA synthesis, leading to the substitution of an adenine–thymine base pair for a guanine–cytosine base pair. Second, alkylation of the 7 nitrogen labilizes the imidazole ring, making possible the opening of the imidazole ring or depurination by excision of guanine residues. Either of these seriously damages the DNA molecule and must be repaired. Third, with bifunctional alkylating agents, such as nitrogen mustard, the second 2-chloroethyl side chain can undergo a similar cyclization reaction and alkylate a second guanine residue or another nucleophilic moiety, resulting in the cross-linking of two nucleic acid chains or the linking of a nucleic acid to a protein, alterations that would cause a major disruption in nucleic acid function. Any of these effects could adequately explain both the mutagenic and the cytotoxic effects of alkylating agents. However, cytotoxicity of bifunctional alkylators correlates very closely with interstrand cross-linkage of DNA (Garcia *et al.*, 1988).

The ultimate cause of cell death related to DNA damage is not known. Specific cellular responses include cell-cycle arrest, DNA repair, and *apoptosis,* a specific form of nuclear fragmentation termed *programmed cell death* (Fisher, 1994). The p53 gene product senses DNA damage and initiates apoptosis in response to DNA alkylation. Mutations of p53 lead to alkylating-agent resistance (Kastan, 1999).

All nitrogen mustards are chemically unstable but vary greatly in their degree of instability. Therefore, the specific chemical properties of each member of this class of drugs must be considered individually in therapeutic applications. For example, mechlorethamine is very unstable, and it reacts almost completely in the body within a few minutes of its administration. By contrast, agents such as chlorambucil are sufficiently stable to permit oral administration. *Cyclophosphamide* requires biochemical activation by the cytochrome P450 system of the liver before its cytotoxicity becomes evident.

The ethylenimine derivatives such as *chlorambucil* and *melphalan* react by an S_N2 reaction; since the opening of the ethylenimine intermediate is acid-catalyzed, they are more reactive at acidic pH.

Structure–Activity Relationship.   The alkylating agents used in chemotherapy encompass a diverse group of chemicals that have in common the capacity to contribute, under physiological conditions, alkyl groups to biologically vital macromolecules such as DNA. In most instances, physical and chemical parameters, such as lipophilicity, capacity to cross biological membranes, acid dissociation constants, stability in aqueous solution, and sites of macromolecular attack, determine drug activity *in vivo*. With several of the most valuable agents (*e.g.,* cyclophosphamide and the nitrosoureas), the active alkylating moieties are generated *in vivo* after complex metabolic reactions.

The nitrogen mustards may be regarded as nitrogen analogs of sulfur mustard. The biological activity of both types of compounds is based upon the presence of the *bis*-(2-chloroethyl) grouping. While mechlorethamine has been widely used in the past, various structural modifications have resulted in compounds with greater selectivity and stability and therefore less toxicity. *Bis*-(2-chloroethyl) groups have been linked to amino acids (phenylalanine), substituted phenyl groups (aminophenyl butyric acid, as in chlorambucil), pyrimidine bases (uracil), and other chemical entities in an effort to make a more stable and orally available form. Although none of these modifications has produced an agent highly selective for malignant cells, some have unique pharmacological properties and are more useful clinically than is mechlorethamine. Their structures are shown in Figure 52–2.

The addition of substituted phenyl groups has produced a series of relatively stable derivatives that retain the ability to form reactive charged intermediates; the electron-withdrawing capacity of the aromatic ring greatly reduces the rate of cyclization and carbonium ion formation, and these compounds therefore can reach distant sites in the body before reacting with components of blood and other tissues. Chlorambucil and melphalan are the most successful examples of such aromatic mustards. These compounds can be administered orally if desired.

A classical example of the role of host metabolism in the activation of an alkylating agent is seen with cyclophosphamide—now the most widely used agent of this class. The design of this molecule was based on two considerations. First, if a cyclic phosphamide group replaced the *N*-methyl of mechlorethamine, the compound might be relatively inert, presumably because the *bis*-(2-chloroethyl) group of the molecule could not ionize until the cyclic phosphamide was cleaved at the phosphorus–nitrogen linkage. Second, it was hoped that neoplastic tissues might possess high phosphatase or phosphamidase

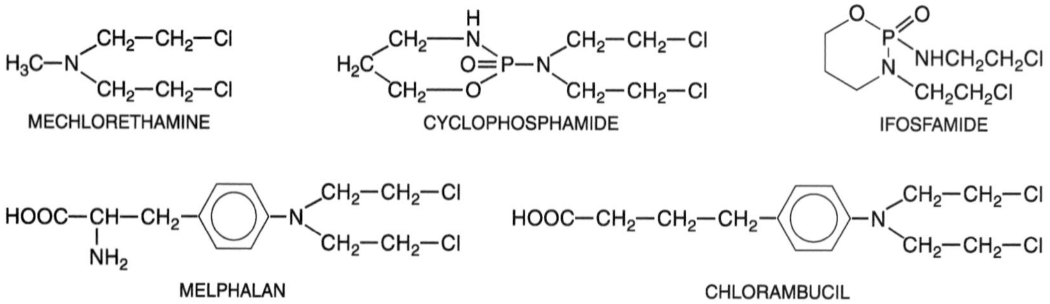

Figure 52–2. Nitrogen mustards employed in therapy.

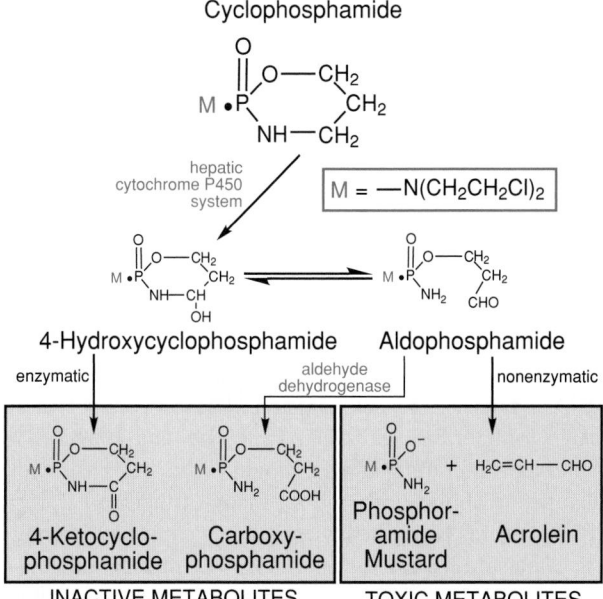

Figure 52–3. Metabolism of cyclophosphamide.

activity capable of accomplishing this cleavage, thus resulting in the selective production of an activated nitrogen mustard in the malignant cells. In accord with these predictions, the parent cyclophosphamide displays only weak cytotoxic, mutagenic, or alkylating activity *in vitro* and is relatively stable in aqueous solution. However, when administered to experimental animals or patients bearing susceptible tumors, it causes marked chemotherapeutic effects, as well as mutagenicity and carcinogenicity. The postulated role for phosphatases or phosphamidases in the mechanism of action of cyclophosphamide has proven incorrect. Rather, the drug undergoes metabolic activation (hydroxylation) by the cytochrome P450 mixed-function oxidase system of the liver (Figure 52–3), with subsequent transport of the activated intermediate to sites of action, as discussed below. The selectivity of cyclophosphamide against certain malignant tissues may result in part from the capacity of normal tissues, such as liver, to protect themselves against cytotoxicity by further degrading the activated intermediates *via* aldehyde dehydrogenase and other pathways.

Ifosfamide is an oxazaphosphorine, similar to cyclophosphamide. Cyclophosphamide has two chloroethyl groups on the exocyclic nitrogen atom, whereas one of the two chloroethyl groups of ifosfamide is on the cyclic phosphamide nitrogen of the oxazaphosphorine ring. Like cyclophosphamide, ifosfamide is activated in the liver by hydroxylation. However, the activation of ifosfamide proceeds more slowly, with greater production of dechlorinated metabolites and chloroacetaldehyde. These differences in metabolism likely account for the higher doses of ifosfamide required for equitoxic effects and the possible differences in antitumor spectrum of the two agents.

Although initially considered an antimetabolite, the triazene derivative 5-(3,3-dimethyl-1-triazeno)-imidazole-4-carboxamide, usually referred to as *dacarbazine* or DTIC, functions through

alkylation. Its structural formula is shown below:

DACARBAZINE

Dacarbazine requires initial activation by the cytochrome P450 system of the liver through an *N*-demethylation reaction. In the target cell, spontaneous cleavage of the metabolite yields an alkylating moiety, diazomethane. A related triazene, *temozolomide* undergoes spontaneous activation, and has significant activity against gliomas and melanoma in human beings (Agarwala and Kirkwood, 2000). It has the same profile of toxicity as DTIC, and is active against malignant gliomas and melanoma. Its structure is shown below:

TEMOZOLOMIDE

The nitrosoureas, which include compounds such as 1,3-bis-(2-chloroethyl)-1-nitrosourea (*carmustine,* BCNU), 1-(2-chloroethyl)-3-cyclohexyl-1-nitrosourea (*lomustine,* CCNU), and its methyl derivative (*semustine,* methyl-CCNU), as well as the antibiotic *streptozocin* (streptozotocin), exert their cytotoxicity through the spontaneous breakdown to alkylating and carbamoylating moieties. The structural formula of carmustine is as follows:

CARMUSTINE (BCNU)

The antineoplastic nitrosoureas have in common the capacity to undergo spontaneous, nonenzymatic degradation with the formation of the 2-chloroethyl carbonium ion (from CNU compounds). This strong electrophile can alkylate a variety of substances; guanine, cytidine, and adenine adducts have been identified (Ludlum, 1990). Displacement of the halogen atom can then lead to interstrand or intrastrand cross-linking of the DNA. The formation of the cross-links after the initial alkylation reaction is relatively slow and can be interrupted by the DNA repair enzyme guanine O^6-alkyl transferase (Dolan *et al.,* 1990). The same enzyme, when overexpressed in gliomas, produces resistance to nitrosoureas and various methylating agents, including DTIC, temozolomide, and procarbazine. As with the nitrogen mustards, it is generally agreed that interstrand cross-linking is associated with the cytotoxicity of nitrosoureas (Hemminki and Ludlum,

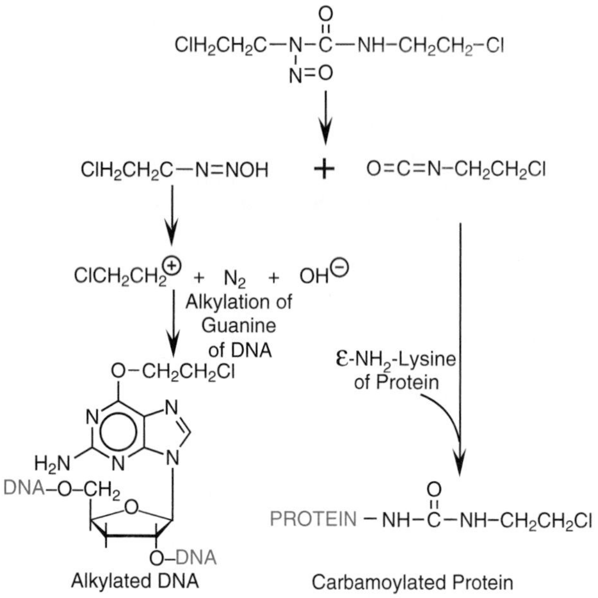

Figure 52–4. Degradation of carmustine (BCNU) with generation of alkylating and carbamoylating intermediates.

1984). In addition to the generation of carbonium ions, the spontaneous degradation of BCNU, CCNU, and methyl-CCNU liberates organic isocyanates that attach carbamoyl groups to lysine residues of proteins, a reaction that apparently can inactivate certain DNA repair enzymes. The reactions of the nitrosoureas with macromolecules are shown in Figure 52–4.

Since the formation of the ethyleniminium ion constitutes the initial reaction of the nitrogen mustards, it is not surprising that stable ethylenimine derivatives have antitumor activity. Several compounds of this type, including *triethylenemelamine* (TEM) and *triethylene thiophosphoramide* (thiotepa), have been used clinically. In standard doses, thiotepa produces little toxicity other than myelosuppression and is thus increasingly used for high-dose chemotherapy regimens. *Altretamine* (hexamethylmelamine; HMM) is mentioned here because of its chemical similarity to TEM. The methylmelamines are *N*-demethylated by hepatic microsomes, with the release of formaldehyde, and there is a relationship between the degree of the demethylation and their activity against murine tumors. Altretamine requires microsomal activation to display cytotoxicity (Friedman, 2001).

Several interesting compounds have emerged from a large group of esters of alkanesulfonic acids. One of these, *busulfan*, is of value in the treatment of chronic granulocytic leukemia and in high-dose chemotherapy; its structural formula is as follows:

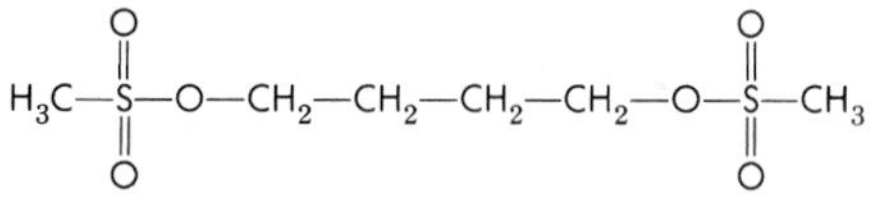

BUSULFAN

Busulfan is a member of a series of symmetrical *bis*-substituted methanesulfonic acid esters in which the length of a bridge of methylene varies from 2 to 10. The compounds of intermediate length ($n = 4$ or 5) possess the highest activi-

ties and therapeutic indices. Cross-linked guanine residues have been identified in DNA incubated *in vitro* with busulfan (Tong and Ludlum, 1980).

Pharmacological Actions

The pharmacological actions of the various groups of alkylating agents are considered together in the following discussion. Although there are many similarities, some notable differences also are evident.

Cytotoxic Actions. The most important pharmacological actions of the alkylating agents are those that disturb DNA synthesis and cell division. The capacity of these drugs to interfere with DNA integrity and function in rapidly proliferating tissues provides the basis for their therapeutic applications and for many of their toxic properties. Whereas certain alkylating agents may have damaging effects on tissues with normally low mitotic indices—for example, liver, kidney, and mature lymphocytes—they are most cytotoxic to rapidly proliferating tissues in which a large proportion of the cells are in division. These compounds may readily alkylate nondividing cells, but cytotoxicity is markedly enhanced if DNA is damaged in cells programmed to divide. Thus, DNA alkylation itself may not be a lethal event if DNA repair enzymes can correct the lesions in DNA prior to the next cellular division.

In contrast to many other antineoplastic agents, the effects of the alkylating drugs, although dependent on proliferation, are not cell-cycle–specific, and the drugs may act on cells at any stage of the cycle. However, the toxicity is usually expressed when the cell enters the S phase and progression through the cycle is blocked. While not strictly cell-cycle–specific, quantitative differences may be detected when nitrogen mustards are applied to synchronized cells at different phases of the cycle. Cells appear more sensitive in late G_1 or S than in G_2, mitosis, or early G_1. Polynucleotides are more susceptible to alkylation in the unpaired state than in the helical form; during replication of DNA, portions of the molecule are unpaired.

The actual mechanism(s) of cell death related to DNA alkylation are not well understood. There is evidence that, in normal cells of the bone marrow and intestinal epithelium, DNA damage activates a checkpoint dependent on the presence of a normal p53 gene. Cells thus blocked in the G_1/S interface either repair DNA alkylation or undergo apoptosis. Malignant cells with mutant or absent p53 fail to suspend cell-cycle progression and do not undergo apoptosis (Fisher, 1994).

The great preponderance of evidence indicates that the primary target of pharmacological doses of alkylating agents is DNA, as illustrated in Figure 52–1. A crucial distinction that must be emphasized is between the bifunctional agents, in which cytotoxic effects predominate, and the monofunctional methylating agents (procarbazine, temozolomide), which, although cytotoxic, have greater capacity for mutagenesis and carcinogenesis. This suggests that the cross-linking of DNA strands represents a much greater threat to cellular survival than do other effects, such as single-base alkylation and the resulting depurination and chain scission. On the other hand, the latter reactions may cause permanent modifications in DNA structure and sequence that are compatible with continued life of the cell and are transmissible to subsequent generations; such modifications may result in mutagenesis or carcinogenesis.

The remarkable DNA repair systems found in most cells likely play an important but as yet poorly defined role in the relative resistance of nonproliferating tissues, the selectivity of action against particular cell types, and acquired resistance to alkylating agents. Although alkylation of a single strand of DNA often may be repaired with relative ease, interstrand cross-linkages, such as those produced by the bifunctional alkylating agents, require more complex mechanisms for repair. Many of the cross-links formed in DNA by these agents at low doses also may be corrected; higher doses cause extensive cross-linkage, and DNA breakdown occurs. Specific repair enzymes for removing alkyl groups from the O-6 of guanine (guanine O^6-alkyl transferase) and the N-3 of adenine and N-7 of guanine (3-methyladenine-DNA glycosylase) have been identified (Matijasevic *et al.*, 1993). The presence of sufficient levels of guanine O^6-alkyl transferase protects cells from cytotoxic effects of nitrosoureas and methylating agents (Pegg, 1990) and confers drug resistance.

Detailed information is lacking on mechanisms of cellular uptake of alkylating agents. Mechlorethamine appears to enter murine tumor cells by means of an active transport system, the natural substrate of which is choline. Melphalan, an analog of phenylalanine, is taken up by at least two active transport systems that normally react with leucine and other neutral amino acids. The highly lipophilic drugs, including nitrosoureas, carmustine, and lomustine, diffuse into cells passively.

Mechanisms of Resistance to Alkylating Agents. Acquired resistance to alkylating agents is a common event, and the acquisition of resistance to one alkylating agent often but not always imparts cross-resistance to others; thus, there are at least theoretical reasons to combine alkylating agents in high-dose therapy. While definitive information on the biochemical mechanisms of clinical resistance is lacking, specific biochemical changes have been implicated in the development of such resistance by tumor cells. Among these changes are (1) decreased permeation of actively transported drugs (mechlorethamine and melphalan); (2) increased production of nucleophilic substances, principally thiols such as glutathione, that can conjugate with and detoxify electrophilic intermediates; (3) increased activity of the DNA repair enzymes, such as the guanine O^6-alkyl transferase, that repair nitrosourea-produced alkylation; and (4) increased rates of metabolism of the activated forms of cyclophosphamide to its inactive keto and carboxy metabolites by aldehyde dehydrogenase (*see* Figure 52–3; Tew *et al.*, 2001).

To reverse cellular changes that lead to resistance, strategies have been devised and appear to be effective in selected experimental tumors. These include the use of compounds that deplete glutathione, such as L-*buthionine-sulfoximine;* sulfhydryl compounds, such as *WR-2721,* that selectively detoxify alkylating species in normal cells and thereby prevent toxicity; compounds such as O^6-*benzylguanine* that inactivate the guanine O^6-alkyl transferase DNA repair enzyme; and compounds such as ethacrynic acid that inhibit the enzymes (glutathione transferases) that conjugate thiols with alkylating agents. While each

of these modalities has experimental evidence to support its use, the clinical efficacy has not yet been proven for these strategies. Of these, O^6-benzylguanine has advanced to phase II trials used in conjunction with carmustine (BCNU) or procarbazine against malignant gliomas (Schilsky *et al.*, 2000).

Toxicities of Alkylating Agents. The alkylating agents differ in their patterns of antitumor activity and in the sites and severity of their side effects. Most cause dose-limiting toxicity to bone marrow elements and, to a lesser extent, intestinal mucosa. Most alkylating agents, including nitrogen mustard, melphalan, chlorambucil, cyclophosphamide, and ifosfamide, produce an acute myelosuppression, with a nadir of the peripheral blood granulocyte count at 6 to 10 days and recovery in 14 to 21 days. Cyclophosphamide has lesser effects on peripheral blood platelet counts than do the other agents. Busulfan suppresses all blood elements, particularly stem cells, and may produce a prolonged and cumulative myelosuppression lasting months. For this reason, it is used as a preparative regimen in allogenic bone marrow transplantation. BCNU and other chloroethylnitrosoureas cause delayed and prolonged suppression of both platelets and granulocytes, reaching a nadir 4 to 6 weeks after drug administration and reversing slowly thereafter.

Both cellular and humoral immunity are suppressed by alkylating agents, which have been used to treat various autoimmune diseases. Immunosuppression is reversible at doses used in most anticancer protocols.

In addition to effects on the hematopoietic system, alkylating agents are highly toxic to dividing mucosal cells, leading to oral mucosal ulceration and intestinal denudation. The mucosal effects are particularly significant in high-dose chemotherapy protocols associated with bone marrow reconstitution, as they predispose to bacterial sepsis arising from the gastrointestinal tract. In these protocols, melphalan and thiotepa have the advantage of causing less mucosal damage than the other agents. In high-dose protocols, a number of toxicities not seen at conventional doses become dose-limiting. They are listed in Table 52–1.

While mucosal and bone marrow toxicities occur predictably with conventional doses of these drugs, other organ toxicities, although less common, can be irreversible and at times lethal. All alkylating agents have caused pulmonary fibrosis, and in high-dose regimens, endothelial damage that may precipitate venoocclusive disease of the liver; the nitrosoureas, after multiple cycles of therapy, may lead to renal failure; ifosfamide in high-dose regimens frequently causes a central neurotoxicity, with seizures, coma, and at times death; and all such agents are leukemogenic, particularly procarbazine (a methylating agent) and the nitrosoureas. Cyclophosphamide and ifosfamide release a nephrotoxic and urotoxic metabolite, acrolein, which causes a severe hemorrhagic cystitis, a side effect that in high-dose regimens can be prevented by coadministration of the sulfhydryl-releasing agent *mesna* (2-mercaptoethanesulfonate). Mesna, when administered with the offending agent at 60% of the drug dosage, conjugates toxic metabolites in urine.

The more unstable alkylating agents (particularly nitrogen mustard and the nitrosoureas) have strong vesicant properties, damage veins with repeated use, and, if extravasated, produce ulceration. Topical application of nitrogen mustard is an effective treatment for cutaneous neoplasms such as mycosis fungoides. Most alkylating agents cause alopecia.

Table 52–1
Dose-Limiting Extramedullary Toxicities of Single Alkylating Agents

DRUG	MTD,* mg/m^2	-FOLD INCREASE OVER STANDARD DOSE	MAJOR ORGAN TOXICITIES
Cyclophosphamide	7000	7.0	Cardiac, hepatic VOD
Ifosfamide	16,000	2.7	Renal, CNS, hepatic VOD
Thiotepa	1000	18.0	GI, CNS, hepatic VOD
Melphalan	180	5.6	GI, hepatic VOD
Busulfan	640	9.0	GI, hepatic VOD
Carmustine (BCNU)	1050	5.3	Lung, hepatic VOD
Cisplatin	200	2.0	PN, renal
Carboplatin	2000	5.0	Renal, PN, hepatic VOD

*Maximum tolerated dose (MTD; cumulative) in treatment protocols.
ABBREVIATIONS: GI, gastrointestinal; CNS, central nervous system; PN, peripheral neuropathy; VOD, venooc-clusive disease.

Central nervous system (CNS) toxicity is manifest in the form of nausea and vomiting, particularly after intravenous administration of nitrogen mustard or BCNU. Ifosfamide is the most neurotoxic of this class of agents, producing altered mental status, coma, generalized seizures, and paralysis. These side effects have been linked to the release of chloroacetaldehyde from the phosphate-linked chloroethyl side chain of ifosfamide. High-dose busulfan may cause seizures; in addition, it accelerates the clearance of phenytoin, an antiseizure medication (*see* Chapter 21).

As a class of drugs, the alkylating agents are highly leukemogenic. Acute nonlymphocytic leukemia, often associated with partial or total deletions of chromosome 5 or 7, peaks in incidence about four years after therapy and may affect up to 5% of patients treated on regimens containing alkylating drugs (Levine and Bloomfield, 1992). Melphalan, the nitrosoureas, and the methylating agent procarbazine have the greatest propensity to cause leukemia, while cyclophosphamide is less potent in this regard.

Finally, all alkylating agents have toxic effects on the male and female reproductive systems, causing an often permanent amenorrhea, particularly in perimenopausal women, and an irreversible azoospermia in men.

NITROGEN MUSTARDS

The chemistry and the pharmacological actions of the alkylating agents as a group, and of the nitrogen mustards, have been presented above. Only the unique pharmacological characteristics of the individual agents are considered below.

Mechlorethamine

Mechlorethamine, the first nitrogen mustard to be introduced into clinical medicine, is the most reactive of the drugs in this class.

Absorption and Fate. Severe local reactions of exposed tissues necessitate intravenous injection of mechlorethamine for most clinical uses. In either water or body fluids, at rates affected markedly by pH, mechlorethamine rapidly undergoes chemical transformation and combines with either water or nucleophilic molecules of cells, so that the parent drug has an extremely short mean residence time in the body.

Therapeutic Uses. *Mechlorethamine HCl* (MUSTARGEN) is used primarily in the combination chemotherapy regimen MOPP [mechlorethamine, ONCOVIN (vincristine), procarbazine, and prednisone] in patients with Hodgkin's disease (DeVita *et al.,* 1972). It is given by intravenous bolus administration in doses of 6 mg/m^2 on days 1 and 8 of the 28-day cycles of each course of treatment. It has been largely replaced in other regimens by cyclophosphamide, melphalan, and other, more stable, alkylating agents.

Clinical Toxicity. The major acute toxic manifestations of mechlorethamine are nausea, vomiting, and lacrimation as well as myelosuppression. Leukopenia and thrombocytopenia limit the amount of drug that can be given in a single course.

Like other alkylating agents, nitrogen mustard blocks reproductive function and may produce menstrual irregularities or premature menopause in women and oligospermia in men. Since fetal abnormalities can be induced, this drug as well as other alkylating agents should not be used in the first trimester of pregnancy and should be used with caution in later stages of pregnancy. Breast-feeding should be terminated before therapy with mechlorethamine is initiated.

Local reactions to extravasation of mechlorethamine into the subcutaneous tissue result in a severe, brawny, tender induration that may persist for a long time. If the local reaction is unusually severe, a slough may result. If it is obvious that extravasation has occurred, the involved area should be promptly infiltrated with a sterile isotonic solution of sodium thiosulfate (1/6 M); an ice compress then should be applied intermittently for 6 to 12 hours. Thiosulfate provides an ion that reacts avidly with the nitrogen mustard and thereby protects tissue constituents.

Cyclophosphamide

Pharmacological and Cytotoxic Actions. Although the general cytotoxic action of this drug is similar to that of other alkylating agents, there are notable differences. Thrombocytopenia is less severe, while alopecia is marked. There are no severe acute or delayed central nervous system (CNS) manifestations either in conventional doses or in high-dose regimens. Nausea and vomiting, however, may occur. The drug is not a vesicant, and there is no local irritation.

Absorption, Fate, and Excretion. Cyclophosphamide is well absorbed orally. As mentioned above, the drug is activated by the hepatic cytochrome P450 system (*see* Figure 52–3). Cyclophosphamide is first converted to 4-hydroxycyclophosphamide, which is in a steady state with the acyclic tautomer aldophosphamide. *In vitro* studies with human liver microsomes and cloned P450 isoenzymes have shown that cyclophosphamide is activated by the CYP2B group of P450 isoenzymes, while a closely related oxazaphosphorine, ifosfamide, is hydroxylated by the CYP3A system (Chang *et al.*, 1993). This difference may account for the somewhat different patterns of antitumor activity, the slower activation of ifosfamide *in vivo*, and the interpatient variability in toxicity of these two closely related molecules. 4-Hydroxycyclophosphamide may be oxidized further by aldehyde oxidase either in liver or in tumor tissue and perhaps by other enzymes, yielding the metabolites carboxyphosphamide and 4-ketocyclophosphamide, neither of which possesses significant biological activity. It appears that hepatic damage is minimized by these secondary reactions, whereas significant amounts of the active metabolites, such as 4-hydroxycyclophosphamide and its tautomer, aldophosphamide, are transported to the target sites by the circulatory system. In tumor cells, the aldophosphamide cleaves spontaneously, generating stoichiometric amounts of phosphoramide mustard and acrolein. The former is believed to be responsible for antitumor effects. The latter compound may be responsible for the hemorrhagic cystitis seen during therapy with cyclophosphamide. Cystitis can be reduced in intensity or prevented by the parenteral administration of *mesna* (MESNEX), a sulfhydryl compound that reacts readily with acrolein in the acid environment of the urinary tract (Tew *et al.*, 2001).

Pretreatment with P450 inducers such as phenobarbital enhances the rate of drug activation but does not alter toxicity or therapeutic activity in human beings.

Urinary and fecal recovery of unchanged cyclophosphamide is minimal after intravenous administration. Maximal concentrations in plasma are achieved 1 hour after oral administration, and the half-life in plasma is about 7 hours.

Therapeutic Uses. *Cyclophosphamide* (CYTOXAN, NEO-SAR) is administered orally or intravenously. Recommended doses vary widely, and published protocols for the dosage of cyclophosphamide and other chemotherapeutic agents and for the method and sequence of administration should be consulted. As a single agent, a daily dose of 100 mg/m^2 orally for 14 days has been recommended for patients with more susceptible neoplasms, such as lymphomas and chronic leukemias. A higher dosage of 500 mg/m^2 intravenously every 3 to 4 weeks in combination with other drugs often is employed in the treatment of breast cancer and lymphomas. The leukocyte count generally serves as a guide to dosage adjustments in prolonged therapy. An absolute neutrophil count between 500 and 1000 cells per cubic millimeter is recommended as the desired target. In regimens associated with bone marrow or peripheral stem cell rescue, cyclophosphamide may be given in doses of 5 to 7 g/m^2 over a 3-day period. Gastrointestinal ulceration, cystitis (counteracted by mesna and diuresis), and, less commonly, pulmonary, renal, hepatic, and cardiac toxicities may occur after high-dose therapy.

The clinical spectrum of activity for cyclophosphamide is very broad. It is an essential component of many effective drug combinations for non-Hodgkin's lymphomas. Complete remissions and presumed cures have been reported when cyclophosphamide was given as a single agent for Burkitt's lymphoma. It is frequently used in combination with methotrexate (or doxorubicin) and fluorouracil as adjuvant therapy after surgery for carcinoma of the breast.

Notable advantages of this drug are the availability of the oral route of administration and the possibility of giving fractionated doses over prolonged periods. For these reasons it possesses a versatility of action that allows an intermediate range of use, between that of the highly reactive intravenous mechlorethamine and that of oral chlorambucil. Beneficial results have been obtained in multiple myeloma; chronic lymphocytic leukemia; carcinomas of the lung, breast, cervix, and ovary; and neuroblastoma, retinoblastoma, and other neoplasms of childhood.

Because of its potent immunosuppressive properties, cyclophosphamide has received considerable attention for the control of organ rejection after transplantation and in nonneoplastic disorders associated with altered immune reactivity, including Wegener's granulomatosis, rheumatoid arthritis, and the nephrotic syndrome in children. Caution is advised when the drug is considered for use in these conditions, not only because of its acute toxic effects but also because of its potential for inducing sterility, teratogenic effects, and leukemia.

Clinical Toxicity. Nausea and vomiting, myelosuppression with platelet sparing, and alopecia are common to virtually all regimens using cyclophosphamide. Mucosal ulcerations and, less frequently, interstitial pulmonary fibrosis also may result from cyclophosphamide treatment. Extravasation of the drug into sub-cutaneous tissues does not produce local reactions, and thrombophlebitis does not complicate intravenous administration. The occurrence of sterile hemorrhagic cystitis has been reported in 5% to 10% of patients. As noted above, this has been attributed to chemical irritation produced by acrolein. Its incidence is significantly reduced by coadministration of mesna (Brock and Pohl, 1986). For routine clinical use, ample fluid intake is recommended. Administration of the drug should be interrupted at the first indication of dysuria or hematuria. The syndrome of inappropriate secretion of antidiuretic hormone (ADH) has been observed in patients receiving cyclophosphamide, usually at doses higher than 50 mg/kg (DeFronzo *et al.,* 1973). It is important to be aware of the possibility of water intoxication, since these patients usually are vigorously hydrated.

Ifosfamide

Ifosfamide, an analog of cyclophosphamide, also is activated by ring hydroxylation in the liver. Severe urinary tract toxicity limited the use of ifosfamide when it was first introduced in the early 1970s. However, adequate hydration and coadministration of mesna now permit effective use of ifosfamide.

Therapeutic Uses. Ifosfamide currently is approved for use in combination with other drugs for germ cell testicular cancer and is widely used to treat pediatric and adult sarcomas. Clinical trials also have shown ifosfamide to be active against carcinomas of the cervix and lung and against lymphomas. It is a common component of high-dose chemotherapy regimens with bone marrow or stem cell rescue; in these regimens, in total doses of 12 to 14 g/m², it may cause severe neurological toxicity, including coma and death. This toxicity is thought to result from a metabolite, chloracetaldehyde (Colvin, 1982). In addition to hemorrhagic cystitis, ifosfamide causes nausea, vomiting, anorexia, leukopenia, nephrotoxicity, and CNS disturbances (especially somnolence or confusion) (*see* Brade *et al.,* 1987).

Ifosfamide (IFEX) is infused intravenously over at least 30 minutes at a dose of 1.2 g/m² per day for 5 days. Intravenous mesna is given as bolus injections in a dosage equal to 20% of the ifosfamide dosage concomitantly and again 4 and 8 hours later, for a total mesna dose of 60% of the ifosfamide dose. Alternatively, mesna may be given in a single dose equal to the ifosfamide dose concomitantly. Patients also should receive at least 2 liters of oral or intravenous fluid daily. Treatment cycles are usually repeated every 3 to 4 weeks.

Pharmacokinetics. Ifosfamide has a half-life in plasma of approximately 15 hours after doses of 3.8 to 5.0 g/m² and a somewhat shorter half-life at lower doses.

Toxicity. Ifosfamide has virtually the same toxicity profile as does cyclophosphamide, with perhaps greater platelet suppression, neurotoxicity, and, in the absence of mesna, urothelial damage.

Melphalan

Pharmacological and Cytotoxic Actions. The general pharmacological and cytotoxic actions of melphalan, the phenylala-

nine derivative of nitrogen mustard, are similar to those of other nitrogen mustards. The drug is not a vesicant.

Absorption, Fate, and Excretion. When given orally, melphalan is absorbed in an incomplete and variable manner, and 20% to 50% of the drug is recovered in the stool. The drug has a half-life in plasma of approximately 45 to 90 minutes, and 10% to 15% of an administered dose is excreted unchanged in the urine (Alberts *et al.,* 1979b).

Therapeutic Uses. The usual oral *melphalan* (ALKERAN) dose for multiple myeloma is 6 mg daily for a period of 2 to 3 weeks, during which time the blood count should be carefully observed. A rest period of up to 4 weeks should then intervene. When the leukocyte and platelet counts are rising, maintenance therapy, ordinarily 2 to 4 mg daily, is begun. It usually is necessary to maintain a significant degree of bone marrow depression (total leukocyte count in the range of 2500 to 3500 cells per cubic millimeter) in order to achieve optimal results. The usual intravenous dose is 16 mg/m² infused over 15 to 20 minutes. Doses are repeated at 2-week intervals for four doses and then at 4-week intervals based on response and tolerance. Dosage adjustments should be considered based on blood cell counts and in patients with renal impairment.

Although the general spectrum of action of melphalan seems to resemble that of other nitrogen mustards, the advantages of administration by the oral route have made the drug useful in the treatment of multiple myeloma.

Clinical Toxicity. The clinical toxicity of melphalan is mostly hematological and is similar to that of other alkylating agents. Nausea and vomiting are infrequent. Alopecia does not occur at standard doses, and changes in renal or hepatic function have not been observed.

Chlorambucil

Pharmacological and Cytotoxic Actions. The cytotoxic effects of chlorambucil on the bone marrow, lymphoid organs, and epithelial tissues are similar to those observed with the nitrogen mustards. Although CNS side effects can occur, these have been observed only with large doses. Nausea and vomiting may result from single oral doses of 20 mg or more.

Absorption, Fate, and Excretion. Oral absorption of chlorambucil is adequate and reliable. The drug has a half-life in plasma of approximately 1.5 hours, and it is almost completely metabolized (Alberts *et al.,* 1979a).

Therapeutic Uses. The standard initial daily dosage of *chlorambucil* (LEUKERAN) is 0.1 to 0.2 mg/kg, continued for at least 3 to 6 weeks. The total daily dose, usually 4 to 10 mg, is given at one time. With a fall in the peripheral total leukocyte count or clinical improvement, the dosage is reduced; maintenance therapy (usually 2 mg daily) is feasible and may be required, depending on the nature of the disease. Other dosage schedules also are used.

At the recommended dosages, chlorambucil is the slowest-acting nitrogen mustard in clinical use. It is a standard agent for patients with chronic lymphocytic leukemia and primary (Waldenström's) macroglobulinemia.

Clinical Toxicity. In chronic lymphocytic leukemia, chlorambucil may be given orally for months or years, achieving its effects gradually and often without toxicity to a precariously compromised bone marrow. Clinical improvement comparable to that with melphalan or cyclophosphamide has been observed in some patients with plasma cell myeloma. Beneficial results also have been reported in disorders with altered immune reactivity, such as vasculitis associated with rheumatoid arthritis and autoimmune hemolytic anemia with cold agglutinins.

Although it is possible to induce marked hypoplasia of the bone marrow with excessive doses of chlorambucil administered over long periods, its myelosuppressive action is usually moderate, gradual, and rapidly reversible. Gastrointestinal discomfort, azoospermia, amenorrhea, pulmonary fibrosis, seizures, dermatitis, and hepatotoxicity may be rarely encountered. A marked increase in the incidence of leukemia and other tumors has been noted in a large controlled study of its use for the treatment of polycythemia vera by the National Polycythemia Vera Study Group, as well as in patients with breast cancer receiving long-term adjuvant chemotherapy (Lerner, 1978).

ETHYLENIMINES AND METHYLMELAMINES

Triethylenemelamine (TEM), Thiotepa (Triethylene Thiophosphoramide), and Altretamine (Hexamethylmelamine; HMM)

Pharmacological and Cytotoxic Effects. Although nitrogen mustards have largely replaced ethylenimines in general clinical practice, this class of agents continues to have specific use. *Thiotepa* (THIOPLEX) is active as an intravesicular agent in bladder cancer and is used as a component of experimental high-dose chemotherapy regimens (Kletzel *et al.,* 1992), and *altretamine* (HEXALEN), formerly known as *hexamethylmelamine,* is used in patients with advanced ovarian cancer after failure of first-line therapies.

Both thiotepa and its primary metabolite, triethylenephosphoramide (TEPA), to which it is rapidly converted by hepatic mixed-function oxygenases (Ng and Waxman, 1991), are capable of forming DNA cross-links. The aziridine rings open after protonation of the ring-nitrogen, leading to a reactive molecule.

Absorption, Fate, and Excretion. TEPA becomes the predominant form of the drug present in plasma within 5 minutes of thiotepa administration. The parent compound has a plasma half-life of 1.2 to 2 hours, as compared to a half-life of 3 to 24 hours for TEPA. Thiotepa pharmacokinetics are essentially the same in children as in adults at conventional doses (up to 80 mg/m^2), and drug and metabolite half-lives are unchanged in children receiving high-dose therapy of 300 mg/m^2 per day for 3 days (Kletzel *et al.,* 1992). Less than 10% of the administered drug appears in urine as the parent drug or the primary metabolite. The remainder is metabolized, interacts with biological molecules, or undergoes spontaneous chemical degradation.

Clinical Toxicities. The toxicities of thiotepa are essentially the same as those of the other alkylating agents, namely myelosuppression and, to a lesser extent, mucositis. Myelosuppression tends to develop somewhat later than with cyclophosphamide, with leukopenic nadirs at 2 weeks and platelet nadirs at 3 weeks.

ALKYL SULFONATES

Busulfan

Pharmacological and Cytotoxic Actions. Busulfan is unique in that, in conventional doses, it exerts few pharmacological actions other than myelosuppression. At low doses, selective depression of granulocytopoiesis is evident, leading to its primary use in the chronic phase of chronic myelogenous leukemia (CML). However, platelets and erythroid elements also may be suppressed as the dosage is raised, and in some patients a severe and prolonged pancytopenia results. In low doses, cytotoxic action does not appear to extend to either the lymphoid tissues or the gastrointestinal epithelium. In high-dose regimens, new toxicities, including pulmonary fibrosis and venoocclusive disease of the liver, become apparent.

Absorption, Fate, and Excretion. Busulfan is well absorbed after oral administration in doses of 2 to 6 mg/day, and it disappears from the blood with a half-life of 2 to 3 hours. Almost all of the drug is excreted in the urine as methanesulfonic acid. In high doses, children under 18 years of age clear the drug faster than do adults, and tolerate higher doses (Vassal *et al.,* 1993).

Therapeutic Uses. In treating chronic granulocytic leukemia, the initial oral dose of *busulfan* (MYLERAN, BUSULFEX) varies with the total leukocyte count and the severity of the disease; daily doses from 2 to 8 mg are recommended to initiate therapy and are adjusted appropriately to subsequent hematological and clinical responses, with the aim of reduction of the total leukocyte count to ≤10,000 cells per cubic millimeter. Maintenance doses of 1 to 3 mg may be given daily.

The beneficial effects of busulfan in chronic granulocytic leukemia are well established, and clinical remissions may be expected in 85% to 90% of patients after the initial course of therapy, but the drug has largely been replaced by interferon-alfa and hydroxyurea.

In CML, reduction of the leukocyte count is noted during the second or third week, and regression of splenomegaly follows. Beneficial results have been reported in other myeloproliferative disorders, including polycythemia vera and myelofibrosis with myeloid metaplasia. High doses of busulfan (640 mg/m^2) have been used effectively in combination with high doses of cyclophosphamide to prepare patients with acute myelogenous leukemia for bone marrow transplantation (Santos *et al.,* 1983). High-dose regimens are given in multiple doses over 3 to 4 days to reduce the incidence of acute CNS toxicities, including tonic-clonic seizures, which may occur several hours after each dose. As mentioned earlier, busulfan induces the metabolism of phenytoin.

Clinical Toxicity.   The major toxic effects of busulfan are related to its myelosuppressive properties, and prolonged thrombocytopenia may be a hazard. Occasional instances of nausea, vomiting, diarrhea, impotence, sterility, amenorrhea, and fetal malformation have been reported. The drug is leukemogenic. In the initial phase of chronic granulocytic leukemia treatment, hyperuricemia, resulting from extensive purine catabolism accompanying the rapid cellular destruction, and renal damage from precipitation of urates have been noted. The concurrent use of *allopurinol* is recommended to avoid this complication. A number of unusual complications have been observed in patients receiving busulfan, but their relation to the drug is poorly understood; these include a syndrome resembling Addison's disease (but without steroid deficiency), cataracts, gynecomastia, cheilosis, glossitis, anhidrosis, and pulmonary fibrosis (Tew *et al.,* 2001).

NITROSOUREAS

The nitrosoureas have an important role in the treatment of brain tumors and gastrointestinal neoplasms. They appear to function as bifunctional alkylating agents but differ in both pharmacological and toxicological properties from conventional nitrogen mustards. Carmustine (BCNU) and lomustine (CCNU) have attracted special interest because of their high lipophilicity and, thus, their capacity to cross the blood–brain barrier, an important property in the treatment of brain tumors. Unfortunately, with the exception of streptozocin, the nitrosoureas used in the clinic to date cause profound, cumulative myelosuppression that restricts their therapeutic value. In addition, long-term treatment with the nitrosoureas, especially semustine (methyl-CCNU), has resulted in renal failure. As

with other alkylating agents, the nitrosoureas are highly carcinogenic and mutagenic.

Streptozocin, originally discovered as an antibiotic, is of special interest. This compound has a methylnitrosourea (MNU) moiety attached to the 2 carbon of glucose. It has a high affinity for β cells of the islets of Langerhans and causes diabetes in experimental animals. Streptozocin is useful in the treatment of human pancreatic islet cell carcinoma and malignant carcinoid tumors. Unmodified MNU, the active moiety of streptozocin, is cytotoxic to selected human tumors and produces delayed myelosuppression. Furthermore, MNU is particularly prone to cause carbamoylation of lysine residues of proteins (*see* Figure 52–4). Unlike MNU, streptozocin is not myelosuppressive and displays little carbamoylating activity. Thus, the nitrosourea-type moiety has been attached to various carrier molecules, with alterations in crucial properties such as tissue specificity, distribution, and toxicity. *Chlorozotocin,* an agent in which the 2 carbon of glucose is substituted by the chloronitrosourea group (CNU), is not diabetogenic and, unlike many other nitrosoureas, causes little myelosuppression or carbamoylation. However, it has no clear therapeutic advantage over the other members of its class.

Carmustine (BCNU)

Pharmacological and Cytotoxic Actions.   Carmustine's major action is its alkylation of DNA at the O^6-guanine position. It kills cells in all phases of the cell cycle. This drug characteristically causes an unusually delayed myelosuppression, with a nadir of the leukocyte and platelet counts at 4 to 6 weeks. In high doses with bone marrow rescue, it produces hepatic venoocclusive disease, pulmonary fibrosis, renal failure, and secondary leukemia (Tew *et al.,* 2001).

Absorption, Fate, and Excretion.   Carmustine is unstable in aqueous solution and in body fluids. After intravenous infusion, it disappears from the plasma with a highly variable half-life of from 15 to 90 minutes or longer (*see* Levin *et al.,* 1978). Approximately 30% to 80% of the drug appears in the urine within 24 hours as degradation products. The entry of alkylating metabolites into the cerebrospinal fluid (CSF) is rapid, and their concentrations in the CSF are 15% to 30% of the concurrent plasma values (Oliverio, 1976).

Therapeutic Uses.   *Carmustine* (BICNU) usually is administered intravenously at doses of 150 to 200 mg/m^2, given by infusion over 1 to 2 hours, and it is not repeated for 6 weeks. When used in combination with other chemotherapeutic agents, the dose is usually reduced by 25% to 50%.

The spectrum of activity of carmustine is similar to that of other alkylating agents, with significant responses observed in Hodgkin's disease and a lower response rate in other lymphomas and myeloma. Because of its ability to cross the blood–brain barrier, carmustine is used as a component of multimodality treatment of malignant astrocytomas and metastatic tumors of the brain. Beneficial responses have been reported in patients with melanoma and gastrointestinal tumors.

Streptozocin

This naturally occurring nitrosourea is an antibiotic derived from *Streptomyces acromogenes*. It has been particularly useful in treating functional, malignant pancreatic islet cell tumors. It affects cells in all stages of the mammalian cell cycle.

Absorption, Fate, and Excretion. Streptozocin is administered parenterally. After intravenous infusions of 200 to 1600 mg/m^2, peak concentrations in the plasma are 30 to 40 μg/ml; the half-life of the drug is approximately 15 minutes. Only 10% to 20% of a dose is recovered in the urine (Schein *et al.*, 1973).

Therapeutic Uses. *Streptozocin* (ZANOSAR) is administered intravenously, 500 mg/m^2 once daily for 5 days; this course is repeated every 6 weeks. Alternatively, 1000 mg/m^2 can be given weekly for 2 weeks, and the weekly dose can then be increased to a maximum of 1500 mg/m^2.

Streptozocin has been used primarily in patients with metastatic pancreatic islet cell carcinoma, and beneficial responses are translated into a significant increase in 1-year survival rate and a doubling of median survival time for the responders.

Clinical Toxicity. Nausea is a frequent side effect. Renal or hepatic toxicity occurs in approximately two-thirds of cases; although usually reversible, renal toxicity is dose-related and cumulative and may be fatal, and proximal tubular damage is the most important toxic effect. Serial determinations of urinary protein are most valuable in detecting early renal effects. Streptozocin should not be given with other nephrotoxic drugs. Hematological toxicity—anemia, leukopenia, or thrombocytopenia—occurs in 20% of patients.

TRIAZENES

Dacarbazine (DTIC)

Dacarbazine functions as a methylating agent after metabolic activation in the liver. Its active metabolite is a monomethyl triazino derivative, the same metabolite formed spontaneously by its analog, temozolomide. It kills cells in all phases of the cell cycle. Dacarbazine resistance has been ascribed to the repair of methylated guanine bases in DNA by guanine O^6-alkyl transferase.

Absorption, Fate, and Excretion. Dacarbazine is administered intravenously; after an initial rapid phase of disappearance ($t_{1/2}$ of about 20 minutes), the drug is removed from plasma with a terminal half-life of about 5 hours (Loo *et al.*, 1976). The half-life is prolonged in the presence of hepatic or renal disease. Almost one-half of the compound is excreted intact in the urine by tubular secretion. Elevated urinary concentrations of 5-aminoimidazole-4-carboxamide (AIC) are derived from the catabolism of dacarbazine, rather than by inhibition of *de novo* purine biosynthesis. Concentrations of dacarbazine in CSF are approximately 14% of those in plasma (Friedman, 2001).

Therapeutic Uses. *Dacarbazine* (DTIC-DOME) is administered intravenously. The recommended regimen for malignant melanoma is to give 3.5 mg/kg per day, intravenously, for a 10-day period; this is repeated every 28 days. Alternatively, 250 mg/m^2 can be given daily for 5 days and repeated every 3 weeks. Extravasation of the drug may cause tissue damage and severe pain.

At present, dacarbazine is employed in combination regimens for the treatment of malignant melanoma, Hodgkin's disease, and adult sarcomas. *Temozolomide* (TEMODAL), the spontaneously activated analog, has shown activity in patients with malignant gliomas (Newlands *et al.*, 1992; Agarwala and Kirkwood, 2000).

Clinical Toxicity. The toxicity of both DTIC and temozolomide includes nausea and vomiting in more than 90% of patients; this usually develops 1 to 3 hours after treatment and may last up to 12 hours. Myelosuppression, with both leukopenia and thrombocytopenia, is usually mild to moderate. A flulike syndrome, consisting of chills, fever, malaise, and myalgias, may occur during treatment with DTIC. Hepatotoxicity, alopecia, facial flushing, neurotoxicity, and dermatological reactions also have been reported.

II. ANTIMETABOLITES

FOLIC ACID ANALOGS

Methotrexate

Antifolates occupy a special place in antineoplastic chemotherapy, in that they produced the first striking, although temporary, remissions in leukemia (Farber *et al.*, 1948) and the first cure of a solid tumor, choriocarcinoma (Hertz, 1963). The consistent cure of choriocarcinoma by methotrexate provided great impetus to investigations into the chemotherapy of cancer. Interest in folate antagonists further increased with the introduction of high-dose regimens with "rescue" of host toxicity by the reduced folate, *leucovorin* (folinic acid, citrovorum factor). These methods extend the usefulness of methotrexate to tumors such as osteogenic sarcoma that do not respond to lower doses.

Recognition that methotrexate, an inhibitor of dihydrofolate reductase, also directly inhibits the folate-dependent enzymes of *de novo* purine and thymidylate

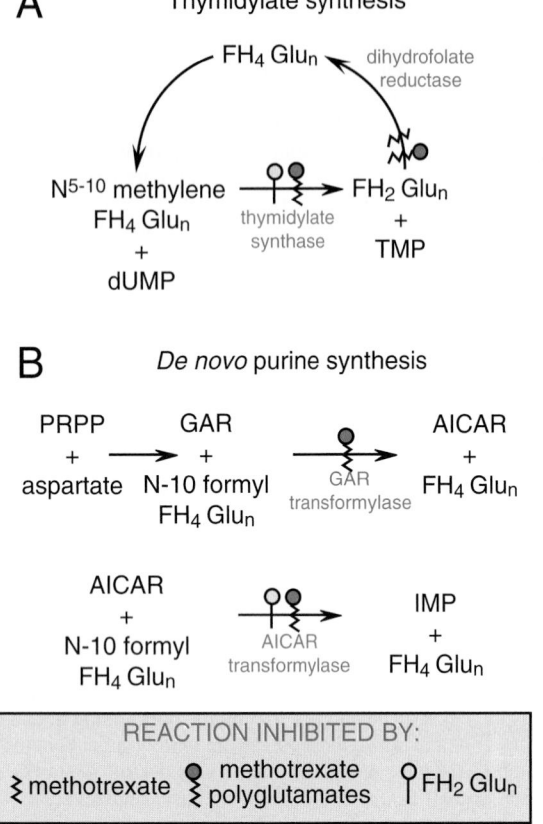

A   Thymidylate synthesis

B   *De novo* purine synthesis

Figure 52–5. Sites of action of methotrexate and its polyglutamates.

AICAR, aminoimidazole carboxamide; TMP, thymidine monophosphate; dUMP, deoxyuridine monophosphate; FH_2Glu_n, dihydrofolate polyglutamate; FH_4Glu_n, tetrahydrofolate polyglutamate; GAR, glycinamide ribonucleotide; IMP, inosine monophosphate; PRPP, 5-phosphoribosyl-1-pyrophosphate.

synthesis focused attention on the development of antifolate analogs that specifically target these other folate-dependent enzyme targets of methotrexate (*see* Figure 52–5). Replacement of the 5, 8, and/or 10 nitrogens of the pteridine ring of folate, as well as various side-chain substitutions, has generated a series of new inhibitors that preserve the common folate potential to form long-lived, intracellular polyglutamates. These new agents, however, have greater capacity for transport into tumor cells (Messmann and Allegra, 2001), and exert their primary inhibitory effect on thymidylate synthesis (*raltitrexed,* TOMUDEX), purine biosynthesis (*lometrexol*) or both [the multitargeted antifolate *permefrexed* (MTA)] (Calvete *et al.,* 1994; Beardsley *et al.,* 1986; Chen *et al.,* 1999).

Aside from its antineoplastic activity, methotrexate also has been used with benefit in the therapy of the common skin disease psoriasis (McDonald, 1981; *see* Chapter 65). Additionally, methotrexate inhibits cell-mediated immune reactions and is employed as an immunosuppressive agent, for example, in allogeneic bone marrow and organ transplantation and for the treatment of dermatomyositis, rheumatoid arthritis, Wegener's granulomatosis, and Crohn's disease (Messmann and Allegra, 2001; Feagan *et al.,* 1995; *see* Chapter 53).

Structure–Activity Relationship. Folic acid is an essential dietary factor from which is derived a series of tetrahydrofolate cofactors that provide single carbon groups for the synthesis of precursors of DNA (thymidylate and purines) and RNA (purines). A detailed description of the biological functions and therapeutic applications of folic acid appears in Chapter 54.

The enzyme dihydrofolate reductase (DHFR) is the primary site of action of most folate analogs studied to date (*see* Figures 52–5 and 52–6). Inhibition of DHFR leads to toxic effects through partial depletion of the tetrahydrofolate cofactors that are required for the synthesis of purines and thymidylate (Messmann and Allegra, 2001) and through direct inhibition of the folate-dependent enzymes of purine and thymidylate metabolism by the polyglutamates of methotrexate and the dihydrofolate polyglutamates that accumulate with DHFR inhibition (Figure 52–5) (Allegra *et al.,* 1986, 1987b). Inhibitors of DHFR differ in their relative potency for blocking enzyme from different species. Agents have been identified that have little effect on the human enzyme but have strong activity against bacterial and parasitic infections (*see* discussions of trimethoprim, Chapter 44; pyrimethamine, Chapter 40). By contrast, methotrexate is an effective inhibitor of DHFR in all species investigated. Crystallographic studies have revealed the atomic basis for the high affinity of methotrexate for DHFR (Kraut and Matthews, 1987; Schweitzer *et al.,* 1989; Bystroff and Kraut, 1991; Blakley and Sorrentino, 1998) and the species specificity of the various DHFR inhibitors (Matthews *et al.,* 1985; Stone and Morrison, 1986).

Because folic acid and many of its analogs are very polar, they cross the blood–brain barrier poorly and require specific transport mechanisms to enter mammalian cells (Elwood, 1989; Dixon *et al.,* 1994). Two inward folate transport systems are found on mammalian cells: (1) a folate receptor, which has high affinity for folic acid but lesser ability to transport methotrexate and other analogs (Elwood, 1989); and (2) the reduced folate transporter, the major transit protein for methotrexate, raltitrexed, and most analogs (Westerhof *et al.,* 1995). Once in the cell, additional glutamyl residues are added to the molecule by the enzyme folylpolyglutamate synthetase (Cichowicz and Shane, 1987). Intracellular methotrexate polyglutamates have been identified with up to six glutamyl residues. Since these higher polyglutamates cross cellular membranes poorly, if at all, this serves as a mechanism of entrapment and may account for the prolonged retention of methotrexate in tumors and normal tissues such as liver. Polyglutamylated folates and analogs have substantially greater affinity than the monoglutamate form for folate-dependent enzymes that are required for purine and thymidylate synthesis, but not for DHFR.

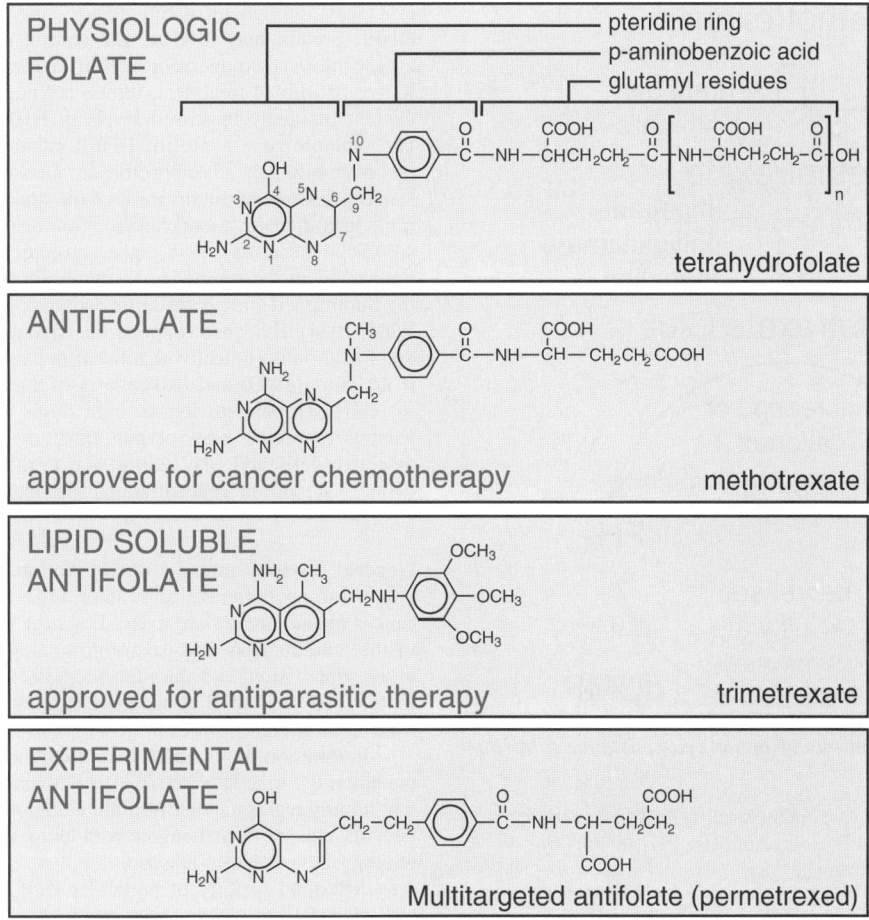

Figure 52–6. The structure–activity bases for antifolate action.

Novel folate antagonists have been identified that exploit differences between the folate influx system in certain tumors and that in normal tissues (*e.g.,* bone marrow). The analog 10-ethyl,10-deaza aminopterin (*edatrexate*) is transported into some tumor cells much more efficiently than into normal tissues and is an excellent inhibitor of DHFR. This promising compound is undergoing clinical evaluation (Grant *et al.,* 1993). In efforts to bypass the obligatory membrane transport system and facilitate penetration of the blood–brain barrier, lipid-soluble folate antagonists also have been synthesized. *Trimetrexate* (Figure 52–6) was one of the first to be tested for clinical activity. The analog was found to have modest antitumor activity, primarily in combination with leucovorin (5-formyl tetrahydrofolate) rescue. However, it has proven to be beneficial in the treatment of *Pneumocystis carinii* pneumonia (Allegra *et al.,* 1987a).

The other important new folate analog, MTA or *pemetrexed* (ALTIMA) (Figure 52–6), is a tetrahydrofolate analog. It readily converts to polyglutamates that inhibit thymidylate and purine biosynthesis, as well as dihydrofolate reductase. In early trials, it has shown activity against colon cancer, mesothelioma, and non-small cell lung cancer (Rusthoven *et al.,* 1999).

Mechanism of Action.   To function as a cofactor in one-carbon transfer reactions, folate must first be reduced by DHFR to tetrahydrofolate (FH_4). Single-carbon fragments are added enzymatically to FH_4 in various configurations and may then be transferred in specific synthetic reactions. In a key metabolic event catalyzed by thymidylate synthase (Figure 52–5), 2'-deoxyuridylate (dUMP) is converted to thymidylate, an essential component of DNA. In this reaction, a one-carbon group is transferred to dUMP from 5,10-methylene FH_4, and the reduced folate cofactor is oxidized to dihydrofolate (FH_2). To function again as a cofactor, FH_2 must be reduced to FH_4 by DHFR. Inhibitors, such as methotrexate, with a high affinity for DHFR ($K_i \sim 0.01$ to 0.2 nM) prevent the formation of FH_4, producing an acute intracellular deficiency of certain folate coenzymes and a vast accumulation of the toxic inhibitory substrate, FH_2 polyglutamate. The one-carbon transfer reactions crucial for the *de novo* synthesis of purine nucleotides and thymidylate cease, with the subsequent interruption of the synthesis of DNA and RNA (as well as other vital metabolic reactions). The toxic effects of methotrexate may be terminated by administering leucovorin (N^5-formyl FH_4; folinic acid). Leucovorin, a fully reduced folate coenzyme, enters cells *via* a specific carrier-mediated

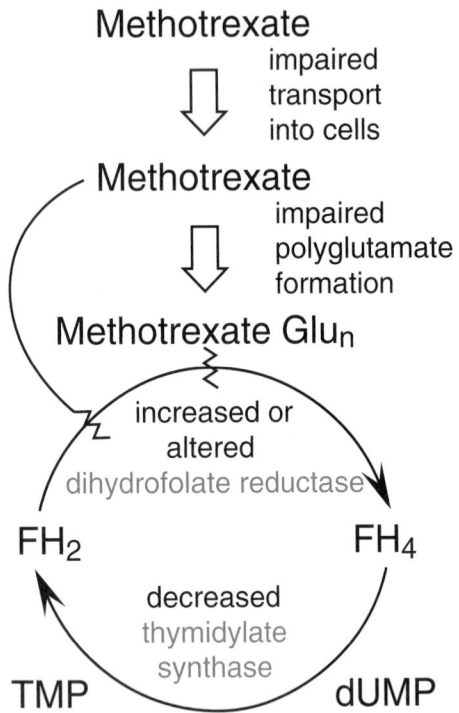

Methotrexate
⇩ impaired transport into cells

Methotrexate
⇩ impaired polyglutamate formation

Methotrexate Glu$_n$

increased or altered
dihydrofolate reductase

FH$_2$ FH$_4$

decreased
thymidylate synthase

TMP   dUMP

Figure 52–7. Mechanisms of tumor cell resistance to methotrexate.

TMP, thymidine monophosphate; dUMP, deoxyuridine monophosphate; FH$_2$, dihydrofolate; FH$_4$, tetrahydrofolate; Glu$_n$, polyglutamate.

transport system and is converted to other active folate cofactors (Boarman *et al.*, 1990).

As with most antimetabolites, methotrexate is only partially selective for tumor cells and is toxic to all rapidly dividing normal cells, such as those of the intestinal epithelium and bone marrow. Folate antagonists kill cells during the S phase of the cell cycle and are most effective when cells are in the logarithmic phase of growth.

Mechanisms of Resistance to Antifolates. In experimental systems, a vast array of biochemical mechanisms of acquired resistance to methotrexate have been demonstrated (Figure 52–7) affecting each known step in methotrexate action, including: (1) impaired transport of methotrexate into cells (Assaraf and Schimke, 1987; Trippett *et al.*, 1992); (2) production of altered forms of DHFR that have decreased affinity for the inhibitor (Srimatkandada *et al.*, 1989); (3) increased concentrations of intracellular DHFR through gene amplification or altered gene regulation (Pauletti *et al.*, 1990; Matherley *et al.*, 1997); (4) decreased ability to synthesize methotrexate polyglutamates (Li *et al.*, 1992); and (5) decreased thymidylate synthase activity (Curt *et al.*, 1985). DHFR levels in leukemic cells increase within 24 hours after treatment of patients with methotrexate; this likely reflects induction of new enzyme synthesis. Recent investigations have demonstrated that the intracellular level of DHFR protein is controlled at the level of mRNA translational

efficiency through an autoregulatory mechanism whereby the DHFR protein may bind to and control the translational efficiency of its own messenger RNA (Chu *et al.*, 1993). Over longer periods of treatment, tumor cell populations emerge that contain markedly increased levels of DHFR. These cells contain multiple gene copies of DHFR either in mitotically unstable double-minute chromosomes or in stable, homogeneously staining regions or amplisomes of the tumor cell chromosomes. First identified as an explanation for resistance to methotrexate (Schimke *et al.*, 1978), gene amplification has since been implicated in the resistance to many antitumor agents, including fluorouracil and pentostatin (2′-deoxycoformycin) (Stark and Wahl, 1984). Evidence supports the conclusion that DHFR gene amplification is clinically significant in patients with lung cancer (Curt *et al.*, 1983) and leukemia (Goker *et al.*, 1995).

To overcome resistance, high doses of methotrexate with leucovorin rescue may permit entry of drug into transport-defective cells and may permit the intracellular accumulation of methotrexate in concentrations that inactivate high levels of DHFR.

General Toxicity and Cytotoxic Action. The primary toxic effects of methotrexate and other folate antagonists used in cancer chemotherapy are exerted against rapidly dividing cells of the bone marrow and gastrointestinal epithelium. Mucositis, myelosuppression, and thrombocytopenia reach their maximum in 5 to 10 days after drug administration and—except in instances of altered drug excretion—reverse rapidly thereafter.

In addition to its acute toxicities, methotrexate can cause pneumonitis, characterized by patchy inflammatory infiltrates that rapidly regress upon discontinuation of drug. In some cases, patients can be rechallenged with drug without toxicity. The etiology is not clearly allergic.

A second toxicity of particular significance in its chronic administration in patients with psoriasis or rheumatoid arthritis is hepatic fibrosis and cirrhosis. Increased hepatic portal fibrosis is detected with higher frequency than in control patients after 6 months or longer of continuous oral methotrexate treatment of psoriasis. Its presence should lead to discontinuation of methotrexate. Acute, reversible elevation of hepatic enzymes is detected in serum after high-dose administration but is rarely associated with permanent changes.

Folic acid antagonists are toxic to developing embryos. In preliminary trials, methotrexate has been highly effective when used with the prostaglandin analog, misoprostol, in inducing abortion in first trimester pregnancy (Hausknecht, 1995).

Absorption, Fate, and Excretion. Methotrexate is readily absorbed from the gastrointestinal tract at doses of less than 25 mg/m^2, but larger doses are absorbed incompletely and are routinely administered intravenously. Peak concentrations in the plasma of 1 to 10 μM are obtained after doses of 25 to 100 mg/m^2, and concentrations of 0.1 to 1 mM are achieved after high-dose infusions of 1.5 g/m^2 or more. After intravenous administration, the drug disappears from plasma in a triphasic fashion (Sonneveld *et al.*, 1986). The rapid distributive phase is followed by a second phase, which reflects renal clearance ($t_{1/2}$ of about 2 to 3 hours). A third phase has a half-life of approximately 8 to 10 hours. This third-phase half-life, if unduly prolonged by renal failure, may be responsible for major toxic effects of the drug on the marrow and gastrointestinal tract. Distribution of methotrexate into body spaces, such as the pleural or peritoneal cavity, occurs slowly. However, if such spaces are expanded (*e.g.,* by ascites or pleural effusion), they may act as a site of storage and release of drug, with resultant prolonged elevation of plasma concentrations and more severe toxicity.

Approximately 50% of methotrexate is bound to plasma proteins and may be displaced from plasma albumin by a number of drugs, including sulfonamides, salicylates, tetracycline, chloramphenicol, and phenytoin; caution should be used if these are given concomitantly. Of the drug absorbed, about 90% is excreted unchanged in the urine within 48 hours, mostly within the first 8 to 12 hours. A small amount of methotrexate also is excreted in the stool, probably through the biliary tract. Metabolism of methotrexate in human beings is usually minimal. After high doses, however, metabolites do accumulate; these include 7-hydroxy-methotrexate, which is potentially nephrotoxic (Messmann and Allegra, 2001). Renal excretion of methotrexate occurs through a combination of glomerular filtration and active tubular secretion. Therefore, the concurrent use of drugs that reduce renal blood flow (*e.g.,* nonsteroidal anti-inflammatory agents), that are nephrotoxic (*e.g.,* cisplatin), or that are weak organic acids (*e.g.,* aspirin or piperacillin) can delay drug excretion and lead to severe myelosuppression (Stoller *et al.,* 1977; Iven and Brasch, 1988; Thyss *et al.,* 1986). Particular caution must be exercised in treating patients with renal insufficiency, and the dose should be adjusted in these patients in proportion to decreases in renal function.

Methotrexate is retained in the form of polyglutamates for long periods—for example, for weeks in the kidneys and for several months in the liver. There also is evidence for enterohepatic recirculation.

It is important to emphasize that concentrations of methotrexate in cerebrospinal fluid are only 3% of those in the systemic circulation at steady state; hence, neoplastic cells in the CNS are probably not killed by standard dosage regimens. When high doses of methotrexate are given (>1.5 g/m^2), followed by leucovorin rescue (*see* below), cytotoxic concentrations of methotrexate may be attained in the CNS.

Therapeutic Uses. Methotrexate (*methotrexate sodium; amethopterin;* FOLEX, MEXATE, RHEUMATREX, others) has been used in the treatment of severe, disabling psoriasis in doses of 2.5 mg orally for 5 days, followed by a rest period of at least 2 days, or 10 to 25 mg intravenously weekly. An initial parenteral test dose of 5 to 10 mg is recommended to detect any possible idiosyncrasy. It also is used intermittently at low dosage to induce remission in refractory rheumatoid arthritis (Hoffmeister, 1983). Complete awareness of the pharmacology and toxic potential of methotrexate is a prerequisite for its use in these nonneoplastic disorders (Weinstein, 1977).

Methotrexate is a useful drug in the management of acute lymphoblastic leukemia in children. It is of great value in remission induction and consolidation, used in high doses, and in the maintenance of remissions in leukemia. For maintenance therapy, it is administered intermittently at doses of 30 mg/m^2 intramuscularly weekly in two divided doses or in 2-day "pulses" of 175 to 525 mg/m^2 at monthly intervals. Outcome of treatment in children correlates inversely with the rate of drug clearance. During methotrexate infusion, high steady-state levels are associated with a lower leukemia relapse rate (Borsi and Moe, 1987). Methotrexate is of very limited value in the types of leukemia seen in adults, except for treatment and prevention of leukemic meningitis. The intrathecal administration of methotrexate has been employed for treatment or prophylaxis of meningeal leukemia or lymphoma and for treatment of meningeal carcinomatosis. This route of administration achieves high concentrations of methotrexate in the CSF and is effective also in patients whose systemic disease has become resistant to methotrexate, since the leukemic cells in the CNS beyond the blood–brain barrier have survived in a pharmacological sanctuary and may retain their original degree of sensitivity to the drug. The recommended intrathecal dose in all patients over 3 years of age is 12 mg (Bleyer, 1978). The dose is repeated every 4 days until malignant cells are no longer evident in the CSF. Leucovorin may be administered to counteract the toxicity of methotrexate that escapes into the systemic circulation, although this is generally not necessary. Since methotrexate administered into the lumbar space distributes poorly over the cerebral convexities, the drug may be more effectively distributed through the use of an intraventricular Ommaya reservoir. The use of 1-mg doses of methotrexate at intervals of 12 to 24 hours yields an effective regimen with reduced neurotoxicity.

Methotrexate is of established value in choriocarcinoma and related trophoblastic tumors of women; cure is achieved in approximately 75% of advanced cases treated sequentially with methotrexate and dactinomycin, and in over 90% when early diagnosis is made. In the treatment of choriocarcinoma with methotrexate, 1 mg/kg is administered intramuscularly every other day for four doses, alternating with leucovorin (0.1 mg/kg every other day). Courses are repeated at 3-week intervals, toxicity permitting, and urinary gonadotropin titers are used as a guide for persistence of disease.

Beneficial effects also are observed in patients with osteosarcoma and mycosis fungoides and when methotrexate is used as part of the combination therapy of Burkitt's and other non-Hodgkin's lymphomas and carcinomas of the breast, head and neck, ovary, and bladder. High-dose methotrexate, with leucovorin rescue, can cause substantial tumor regression in osteosarcoma and in combination therapy of leukemias and non-Hodgkin's lymphomas. A 6- to 72-hour infusion of relatively large amounts of methotrexate may be employed intermittently (from 250 mg to 7.5 g/m^2 or more), but only when leucovorin rescue is used. Such regimens produce cytotoxic concentrations of drug in the cerebrospinal fluid (CSF) and protect against leukemic meningitis. A typical regimen includes the infusion of methotrexate for 6 hours followed by leucovorin at a dose of 15 mg/m^2 every 6 hours for seven doses, with the goal of rescuing normal cells and thereby preventing toxicity. Other dosage regimens also are used. The administration of methotrexate in high dosage has the potential for serious toxicity and should be performed only by experienced chemotherapists who are able to monitor concentrations of methotrexate in plasma. If methotrexate values measured 48 hours after drug administration are 1 μM or higher, higher doses (100 mg/m^2) of leucovorin must be given until the plasma concentration of methotrexate falls below the toxic threshold of 2×10^{-8} M (Stoller et al., 1977). With appropriate precautions, these schedules are relatively free of toxicity. It is imperative to maintain the output of a large volume of alkaline urine, since methotrexate precipitates in the renal tubules in acidic urine. In the presence of malignant effusions, delayed clearance may cause severe toxicity. In patients who become oliguric, isolated reports suggest that continuous-flow hemodialysis can eliminate methotrexate at a rate approximating 50% of the clearance rate in patients with intact renal function (Wall et al., 1996). Methotrexate in high doses with leucovorin rescue has been studied clinically for many years with promising results in osteosarcoma, childhood leukemia, and non-Hodgkin's lymphoma, although the optimal timing and dose of leucovorin required and the optimal schedule of methotrexate administration remain to be established (Ackland and Schilsky, 1987).

Clinical Toxicities. As previously stated, the primary toxicities of methotrexate affect the bone marrow and the intestinal epithelium. Such patients may be at risk for spontaneous hemorrhage or life-threatening infection, and they may require prophylactic transfusion of platelets and broad-spectrum antibiotics if febrile. Side effects usually disappear within 2 weeks, but prolonged suppression of the bone marrow may occur in patients with compromised renal function who have delayed excretion of the drug. The dosage of methotrexate must be reduced in proportion to any reduction in creatinine clearance.

Additional toxicities of methotrexate include alopecia, dermatitis, interstitial pneumonitis, nephrotoxicity, defective oogenesis or spermatogenesis, abortion, and teratogenesis. Hepatic dysfunction is usually reversible but sometimes leads to cirrhosis after long-term continuous treatment, as in patients with psoriasis. Intrathecal administration of methotrexate often causes meningismus and an inflammatory response in the CSF. Seizures, coma, and death may occur rarely. Leucovorin does not reverse neurotoxicity.

PYRIMIDINE ANALOGS

This class of agents encompasses a diverse and interesting group of drugs that have in common the capacity to inhibit the biosynthesis of pyrimidine nucleotides or to mimic these natural metabolites to such an extent that the analogs interfere with the synthesis or function of nucleic acids. Analogs of deoxycytidine and thymidine have been synthesized as inhibitors of DNA synthesis, and an analog of uracil, 5-fluorouracil, effectively inhibits both RNA function and/or processing and synthesis of thymidylate (see Figure 52–8). Drugs in this group have been employed in the treatment of diverse afflictions, including neoplastic diseases, psoriasis, and infections caused by fungi and DNA-containing viruses. The pathways for metabolic activation and degradation of these compounds during systemic administration present opportunities for the development of synergistic combination therapies with other clinically effective drugs.

General Mechanism of Action. The best-characterized agents in this class are the halogenated pyrimidines, a group that includes *fluorouracil* (5-fluorouracil, or 5-FU), *floxuridine* (5-fluoro-2'-deoxyuridine, or 5-FUdR), and *idoxuridine* (5-iododeoxyuridine; see Chapter 50). If one compares the van der Waals radii of the various 5-position substituents, the dimension of the fluorine atom resembles that of hydrogen, whereas the bromine and iodine atoms are larger and close in size to the methyl group. Thus, idoxuridine behaves as an analog of thymidine, and its primary biological action results from its phosphorylation and ultimate incorporation into DNA in place of thymidylate. In 5-FU, the smaller fluorine at position 5 allows the molecule to mimic uracil biochemically. However, the fluorine–carbon bond is much tighter than that of C—H and prevents the methylation of the 5 position of 5-FU by thymidylate synthase. Instead, in the presence of the physiological cofactor 5,10-methylene tetrahydrofolate, the fluoropyrimidine locks the enzyme in an inhibited state. Thus, substitution of a halogen atom of the correct dimensions can produce a molecule that sufficiently resembles a natural pyrimidine to interact with enzymes of pyrimidine metabolism but at the same time interferes drastically with certain other aspects of pyrimidine action.

A number of 5-FU analogs have reached the clinic. The most important of these is *capecitabine* (N4-pentoxycarbonyl-5'-deoxy-5-fluorocytidine), a drug with proven activity against colon and breast cancers. This orally administered agent is converted to 5'-deoxy-5-fluorocytidine by carboxylesterase activity in liver and other normal and malignant tissues. From that point, it is converted to 5'-deoxy-fluorodeoxyuridine by cytidine deaminase. The final step in its activation occurs when thymidine

FLUOROPYRIMIDINE ANALOGS

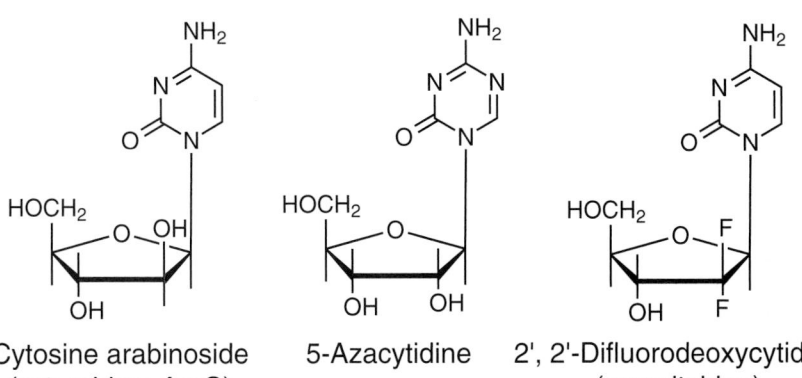

Capecitabine

5-Fluorouracil
(5-FU)

5-Fluorodeoxyuridine
(floxuridine)

5-Fluorodeoxyuridine
monophosphate
(active metabolite)

CYTIDINE ANALOGS

Cytosine arabinoside
(cytarabine; AraC)

5-Azacytidine

2', 2'-Difluorodeoxycytidine
(gemcitabine)

Figure 52–8. Structures of available pyrimidine analogs.

phosphorylase cleaves off the 5'-deoxy sugar, leaving intracellular 5-FU. Tumors with elevated thymidine phosphorylase activity seem particularly susceptible to this drug (Ishikawa *et al.,* 1998).

Nucleotides in RNA and DNA contain ribose and 2'-deoxyribose, respectively. Among the various modifications of the sugar moiety that have been attempted, the replacement of the ribose of cytidine with arabinose has yielded a useful chemotherapeutic agent, *cytarabine* (AraC). As may be seen in Figure 52–8, the hydroxyl group in this molecule is attached to the 2'-carbon in the β, or upward, configuration, as compared with the α, or downward, position of the 2'-hydroxyl in ribose. The arabinose analog is recognized enzymatically as a 2'-deoxyriboside; it is phosphorylated to a nucleoside triphosphate that competes with dCTP for incorporation into DNA (Chabner *et al.,* 2001), where it blocks elongation of the DNA strand and its template function.

Two other cytidine analogs have received extensive clinical evaluation. 5-*Azacytidine,* an inhibitor of DNA methylation as well as a cytidine antimetabolite, becomes incorporated predominantly into RNA and has antileukemic as well as differentiating actions *in vitro*. A newer analog, 2',2'-difluorodeoxycytidine (*gemcitabine*), becomes incorporated into DNA and inhibits the elongation of nascent DNA strands (*see* Figure 52–8). It has

promising activity in various human solid tumors, including pancreatic, lung, and ovarian cancer.

Fluorouracil and Floxuridine (Fluorodeoxyuridine)

Mechanism of Action. 5-FU requires enzymatic conversion to the nucleotide (ribosylation and phosphorylation) in order to exert its cytotoxic activity (Figure 52–9). Several routes are available for the formation of the 5'-monophosphate nucleotide (F-UMP) in animal cells. 5-FU may be converted to fluorouridine by uridine phosphorylase and then to F-UMP by uridine kinase, or it may react directly with 5-phosphoribosyl-1-pyrophosphate (PRPP), in a reaction catalyzed by the enzyme orotate phosphoribosyl transferase, to form F-UMP. Many metabolic pathways are available to F-UMP, including incorporation into RNA. A reaction sequence crucial for antineoplastic activity involves reduction of the diphosphate nucleotide by the enzyme ribonucleotide diphosphate reductase to the deoxynucleotide level and the eventual formation of 5-fluoro-2'-deoxyuridine-5'-phosphate (F-dUMP). 5-FU also may be converted directly to the deoxyriboside 5-FUdR by the enzyme thymidine phosphorylase and further to F-dUMP, a potent

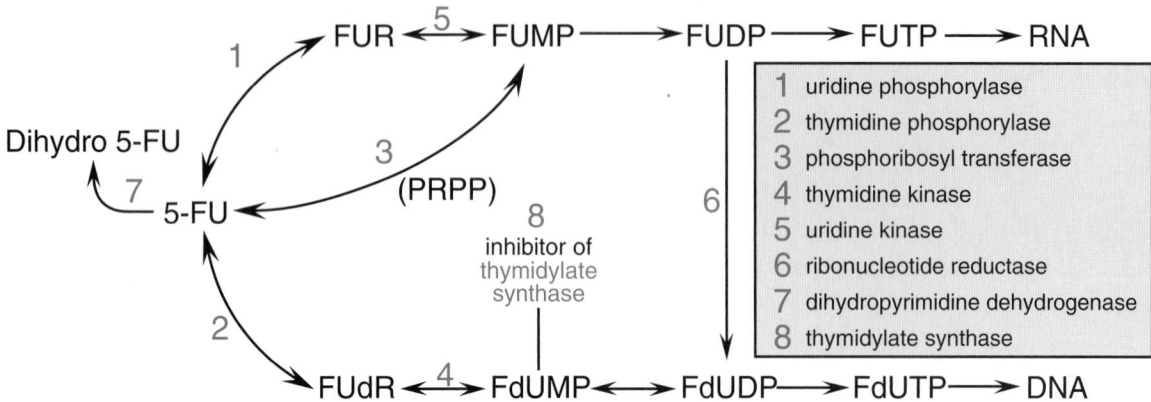

Figure 52–9. Activation pathways for 5-fluorouracil (5-FU) and 5-floxuridine (FUR).

FUDP, floxuridine diphosphate; FUMP, floxuridine monophosphate; FUTP, floxuridine triphosphate; FUdR, fluorodeoxyuridine; FdUDP, fluorodeoxyuridine diphosphate; FdUMP, fluorodeoxyuridine monophosphate; FdUTP, fluorodeoxyuridine triphosphate; PRPP, 5-phosphoribosyl-1-pyrophosphate.

inhibitor of thymidylate synthesis, by thymidine kinase. This complex metabolic pathway for the generation of F-dUMP may be bypassed through use of the deoxyribonucleoside of fluoro–uracil—floxuridine (fluorodeoxyuridine, FUdR)—which is converted directly to F-dUMP by thymidine kinase.

The interaction between F-dUMP and the enzyme thymidylate synthase leads to deletion of TTP, a necessary constituent of DNA (Figure 52–10). The folate cofactor, 5,10-methylenetetrahydrofolate, and F-dUMP form a covalently bound ternary complex with the enzyme. This inhibitory complex resembles the transition state formed during the normal enzymatic reaction when dUMP is converted to thymidylate. Although the physio-

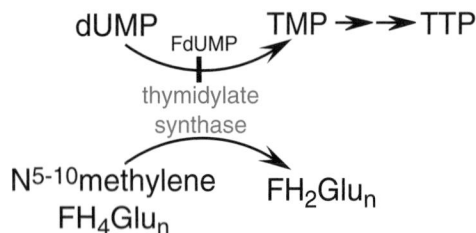

Figure 52–10. Site of action of 5-fluoro-2′-deoxyuridine-5′-phosphate (5-FdUMP).

5-FU, 5-fluorouracil; dUMP, deoxyuridine monophosphate; TMP, thymidine monophosphate; TTP, thymidine triphosphate; FdUMP, fluorodeoxyuridine monophosphate; FH_2Glu_n, dihydrofolate polyglutamate; FH_4Glu_n, tetrahydrofolate polyglutamate

logical complex progresses to the synthesis of thymidylate by transfer of the methylene group and two hydrogen atoms from folate to dUMP, this reaction is blocked in the inhibitory complex by the stability of the fluorine carbon bond on F-dUMP; sustained inhibition of the enzyme results (Santi *et al.*, 1974).

5-FU also is incorporated into both RNA and DNA. In 5-FU–treated cells, both F-dUTP and dUTP (the substrate that accumulates behind the blocked thymidylate synthase reaction) incorporate into DNA in place of the depleted physiological TTP. The significance of the incorporation of F-dUTP and dUTP into DNA is unclear (Canman *et al.*, 1993). Presumably, the incorporation of deoxyuridylate and/or fluorodeoxyuridylate into DNA would call into action the excision–repair process. This process may result in DNA strand breakage because DNA repair requires TTP, but this substrate is lacking as a result of thymidylate synthase inhibition (Mauro *et al.*, 1993). 5-FU incorporation into RNA also causes toxicity as the result of major effects on both the processing and functions of RNA (Armstrong, 1989; Danenberg *et al.*, 1990).

A number of biochemical mechanisms have been identified that are associated with resistance to the cytotoxic effects of 5-FU or floxuridine. These mechanisms include loss or decreased activity of the enzymes necessary for activation of 5-FU, decreased pyrimidine monophosphate kinase (which decreases incorporation into RNA), amplification of thymidylate synthase (Washtein, 1982), and altered thymidylate synthase that is not inhibited by F-dUMP (Barbour *et al.*, 1990). Both experimental studies and clinical trials support the position that the response to 5-FU correlates significantly with low levels of the degradative enzymes, dihydrouracil dehydrogenase and thymidine phosphorylase, and a low level of expression of the target enzyme, thymidylate synthase (van Triest *et al.*, 2000). Recent investigations have demonstrated that the level of thymidylate synthase is finely controlled by an autoregulatory feedback mechanism wherein the thymidylate synthase protein interacts with and controls the translational efficiency of its own messenger RNA. This mechanism provides for the rapid modulation of the level of thymidylate synthase necessary for cellular division and also

Table 52–2

Modulators of Cytotoxic Activity of 5-Fluorouracil (5-FU)

MODULATOR	PURPORTED MECHANISM(S) OF INTERACTION
Cisplatin	Enhanced DNA strand breaks secondary to decreased repair Enhanced thymidylate synthase inhibition
Interferon	Enhanced 5-FU anabolism Decreased "rebound" synthesis of thymidylate synthase
Leucovorin	Enhanced thymidylate synthase inhibition
Methotrexate	Enhanced 5-FU anabolism Enhanced RNA incorporation
PALA*	Enhanced 5-FU anabolism Enhanced RNA incorporation
Uridine	Diminished RNA incorporation (? selective rescue for normal cells)

*PALA, N-phosphonoacetyl-L-aspartate.

may be an important mechanism by which malignant cells become rapidly insensitive to the effects of 5-fluorouracil (Chu et al., 1991; Swain et al., 1989). Some malignant cells appear to have insufficient concentrations of 5,10-methylene tetrahydrofolate and, thus, cannot form maximal levels of the inhibited ternary complex with thymidylate synthase. Addition of exogenous folate in the form of 5-formyl-tetrahydrofolate (leucovorin) increases formation of the complex in both laboratory and clinical experiments and has enhanced responses to 5-FU in clinical trials (Ullman et al., 1978; Grogan et al., 1993). Except for inadequate intracellular folate pools, it is not established which (if any) of the other mechanisms is associated with clinical resistance to 5-FU and its derivatives (Grem et al., 1987).

In addition to leucovorin, a number of other agents have been combined with 5-FU in attempts to enhance the cytotoxic activity through biochemical modulation. These agents, along with their proposed mechanisms of interaction, are shown in Table 52–2. The most clinically interesting combinations with 5-FU include methotrexate, interferon, leucovorin, or cisplatin, all of which are currently under investigation to define their ultimate clinical roles. Agents that inhibit early steps in pyrimidine biosynthesis, such as PALA (N-phosphonoacetyl-L-aspartate), an inhibitor of aspartate transcarbamylase, provide synergistic interaction with 5-FU in experimental systems, but these combinations have no proven clinical value (Grem et al., 1988). Methotrexate, by inhibiting purine synthesis and increasing cellular pools of PRPP, enhances the activation of 5-FU and increases antitumor activity of 5-FU when given prior to but not following 5-FU. In clinical trials, the combination of cisplatin and 5-FU has yielded impressive responses in tumors of the upper aerodigestive tract, but the molecular basis of their interaction is not well understood (Grem, 2001).

Absorption, Fate, and Excretion. 5-FU and floxuridine are administered parenterally, since absorption after ingestion of

the drugs is unpredictable and incomplete. Metabolic degradation occurs in many tissues, particularly the liver. Floxuridine is converted by thymidine or deoxyuridine phosphorylases into 5-FU. 5-FU is inactivated by reduction of the pyrimidine ring; this reaction is carried out by dihydropyrimidine dehydrogenase (DPD), which is found in liver, intestinal mucosa, tumor cells, and other tissues. Inherited deficiency of this enzyme leads to greatly increased sensitivity to the drug (Lu et al., 1993; Milano et al., 1999). The rare individual who totally lacks this enzyme may experience profound drug toxicity following conventional doses of the drug. DPD deficiency can be detected either by enzymatic or molecular assays using peripheral white blood cells, or by determining the plasma ratio of 5-FU to its metabolite, 5-fluoro-5,6-dihydrouracil, which is ultimately degraded to α-fluoro-β-alanine (Heidelberger, 1975; Zhang et al., 1992).

Rapid intravenous administration of 5-FU produces plasma concentrations of 0.1 to 1.0 mM; plasma clearance is rapid ($t_{1/2}$ 10 to 20 minutes). Urinary excretion of a single dose of 5-FU given intravenously amounts to only 5% to 10% in 24 hours. Although the liver contains high concentrations of DPD, dosage does not have to be modified in patients with hepatic dysfunction, presumably because of degradation of the drug at extrahepatic sites or by vast excess of this enzyme in the liver. Given by continuous intravenous infusion for 24 to 120 hours, 5-FU achieves plasma concentrations in the range of 0.5 to 8.0 μM. 5-FU readily enters the CSF, and concentrations greater than 0.01 μM are sustained for up to 12 hours following conventional doses (Grem, 2001).

Capecitabine is well absorbed orally, yielding high plasma concentrations of 5′-deoxy-fluorodeoxyuridine (5′-dFdU), which disappears with a half-life of about 1 hour. 5-FU levels are less than 10% of those of 5′-dFdU. Liver dysfunction delays the conversion of the parent compound to 5′-dFdU and 5-FU, but there is no consistent effect on toxicity (Twelves et al., 1999).

Therapeutic Uses. *5-Fluorouracil.* Accumulated experience with 5-FU (ADRUCIL) indicates that the drug produces partial responses in 10% to 20% of patients with metastatic carcinomas of the breast and the gastrointestinal tract; beneficial effects also have been reported in carcinoma of the ovary, cervix, urinary bladder, prostate, pancreas, and oropharyngeal areas. For average-risk patients in good nutritional status with adequate hematopoietic function, the weekly dosage regimen employs 750 mg/m² alone or 500 to 600 mg/m² with leucovorin once each week for 6 of 8 weeks. Other regimens use daily doses of 500 mg/m² for 5 days, repeated in monthly cycles. When used with leucovorin, daily doses of 5-FU must be reduced to 375 to 425 mg/m² for 5 days because of mucositis and diarrhea. It also has been given as a continuous infusion for up to 21 days (300 mg/m² per day), or as a biweekly 48-hour continuous infusion (de Gramont et al., 1998).

Floxuridine (FUdR). FUdR (fluorodeoxyuridine; FUDR) is used primarily by continuous infusion into the hepatic artery for treatment of metastatic carcinoma of the colon or following resection of hepatic metastases (Kemeny *et al.*, 1999); the response rate to such infusion is 40% to 50%, or double that observed with intravenous administration. Intrahepatic arterial infusion for 14 to 21 days may be used with minimal systemic toxicity. However, there is a significant risk of biliary sclerosis if this route is used for multiple cycles of therapy (Kemeny *et al.*, 1987; Hohn *et al.*, 1986). Continuous infusion of floxuridine into the arterial blood supply of tumors at other sites, such as in the head and neck region, may provide beneficial clinical effects. With any of these regimens, treatment should be discontinued at the earliest manifestation of toxicity (usually stomatitis or diarrhea) because the maximal effects of bone marrow suppression and gut toxicity will not be evident until days 7 to 14.

Capecitabine (XELODA). Capecitabine is approved by the United States Food and Drug Administration (FDA) for the treatment of metastatic breast cancer in patients who have not responded to a regimen of paclitaxel and an anthracycline antibiotic (*see* below). The recommended dose is 2500 mg/m^2 daily, given orally in two divided doses with food, for 2 weeks followed by a rest period of 1 week. This cycle is then repeated two more times.

Combination Therapy. Higher response rates are seen when 5-FU is used in combination with other agents, such as cyclophosphamide and methotrexate (breast cancer), cisplatin (head and neck cancer), and with leucovorin in colon cancer (*see* Table 52–2). The use of 5-FU in combination regimens has improved survival in the adjuvant treatment for breast cancer (Early Breast Cancer Trialists Collaborative Group, 1988) and, with leucovorin, for colorectal cancer (Wolmark *et al.*, 1993). 5-FU is a potent radiation sensitizer and is being used with concurrent radiotherapy for primary therapy of locally advanced tumors of the head and neck, esophagus, lung, and rectum. 5-FU is used widely with very favorable results for the topical treatment of premalignant keratoses of the skin and multiple superficial basal cell carcinomas. It also is effective in severe recalcitrant psoriasis (Alper *et al.*, 1985).

Clinical Toxicities. The clinical manifestations of toxicity caused by 5-FU and floxuridine are similar and may be difficult to anticipate because of their delayed appearance. The earliest untoward symptoms during a course of therapy are anorexia and nausea; these are followed by stomatitis and diarrhea, which constitute reliable warning signs that a sufficient dose has been administered. Mucosal ulcerations occur throughout the gastrointestinal tract and may lead to fulminant diarrhea, shock, and death, particularly in patients who are receiving continuous infusions of 5-FU or in those receiving 5-FU with leucovorin. The major toxic effects of bolus-dose regimens result from the myelosuppressive action of these drugs. The nadir of leukopenia

is usually between days 9 and 14 after the first injection of drug. Thrombocytopenia and anemia also may occur. Loss of hair, occasionally progressing to total alopecia, nail changes, dermatitis, and increased pigmentation and atrophy of the skin may be encountered. Neurological manifestations, including an acute cerebellar syndrome, have been reported, and myelopathy has been observed after the intrathecal administration of 5-FU. Cardiac toxicity, particularly acute chest pain with evidence of ischemia in the electrocardiogram, also may occur. The low therapeutic indices of these agents emphasize the need for very skillful supervision by physicians familiar with the action of the fluorinated pyrimidines and the possible hazards of chemotherapy.

Capecitabine causes much the same spectrum of toxicities as 5-FU (diarrhea, myelosuppression), but also a progressive hand-foot syndrome consisting of erythema, desquamation, pain, and sensitivity to touch of the palms and soles.

Cytarabine (Cytosine Arabinoside; AraC)

Cytarabine (1-β-D-arabinofuranosylcytosine; AraC) is the most important antimetabolite used in the therapy of acute myelocytic leukemia. It is the single most effective agent for induction of remission in this disease (for review, *see* Garcia-Carbonero *et al.*, 2001).

Mechanism of Action. This compound is an analog of 2′-deoxycytidine with the 2′-hydroxyl in a position *trans* to the 3′-hydroxyl of the sugar, as shown in Figure 52–8. The 2′-hydroxyl causes steric hindrance to the rotation of the pyrimidine base around the nucleosidic bond. The bases of polyarabinonucleotides cannot stack normally, as do the bases of polydeoxynucleotides.

AraC penetrates cells by a carrier-mediated process shared by physiological nucleosides. As with most purine and pyrimidine antimetabolites, cytarabine must be "activated" by conversion to the 5′-monophosphate nucleotide (AraCMP), a reaction catalyzed by deoxycytidine kinase. AraCMP can then react with appropriate nucleotide kinases to form the diphosphate and triphosphate nucleotides (AraCDP and AraCTP). AraC competes with the physiological substrate deoxycytidine 5′-triphosphate (dCTP) for incorporation into DNA by DNA polymerases. The incorporated AraCMP residue is a potent inhibitor of DNA polymerase. The effects of AraC on DNA polymerase activity extend not only to DNA chain elongation during semiconservative DNA replication, but also to DNA repair. There is a significant relationship between inhibition of DNA synthesis and the total amount of AraC incorporated into DNA. Thus, incorporation of about five molecules of AraC per 10^4 bases of DNA decreases cellular clonogenicity by about 50%.

AraC also causes an unusual reiteration of DNA segments, thus increasing the possibility of recombination, crossover, and gene amplification. In addition, AraC is converted intracellularly to AraCDP-choline, an analog of the physiological CDP-choline, which inhibits the synthesis of membrane glycoproteins and glycolipids. Furthermore, AraCMP inhibits the transfer of galactose, *N*-acetylglucosamine, and sialic acid to cell-surface glycoproteins, and AraCTP inhibits the synthesis of CMPacetylneuraminic acid. Thus, AraC may alter membrane structure, antigenicity, and function.

AraC induces terminal differentiation of leukemic cells in tissue culture, an effect that is accompanied by decreased c-*myc* oncogene expression (Bianchi Scarra *et al.,* 1986). These changes in morphology and oncogene expression occur at concentrations above the threshold for cytotoxicity and may simply represent terminal injury of cells. However, molecular analysis of bone marrow specimens from some leukemic patients in remission after AraC therapy has revealed persistence of leukemic markers, suggesting that differentiation may have occurred.

The precise mechanism of cellular death caused by AraC is not fully understood. Fragmentation of DNA is observed in AraC-treated cells, and there is cytological and biochemical evidence for apoptosis in both tumor and normal tissues (Smets, 1994). A complex system of interacting transduction signals ultimately determines whether or not a cell exposed to a cytotoxic agent is destined to die. Exposure of leukemic cells to AraC stimulates the formation of ceramide, a potent inducer of apoptosis. On the other hand, an increase in protein kinase C (PKC) activity is observed in leukemic cells in response to AraC *in vitro*. Because PKC activation is known to oppose apoptosis in hematopoietic cells, the lethal actions of AraC may depend, at least partially, on its relative effects on the PKC and sphingomyelin pathways (Strum *et al.,* 1994). Transcriptional regulation of gene expression may be another key mechanism through which malignant cell growth and differentiation are regulated. The induction of some transcription factors, such as AP-1 (a dimer of jun-fos or jun-jun proteins) and NF-κB, has been temporarily associated with AraC-induced apoptosis (Kharbanda *et al.,* 1990). It also has been reported that induction of pRb phosphatase activity by AraC leads to a hypophosphorylated pRb that binds to and inactivates the E2F transcription factor, inhibiting the transcription of numerous genes involved in cell-cycle progression (Ikeda *et al.,* 1996).

In addition to biochemical factors that determine response, cell kinetic properties exert an important influence on the results of AraC treatment. It is likely that continued inhibition of DNA synthesis for a duration equivalent to at least one cell cycle is necessary to expose cells during the S, or DNA-synthetic, phase of the cycle. This mechanism may thus be important when AraC is administered by continuous prolonged infusion. A number of investigations have indicated that the optimal interval between bolus doses of AraC is about 8 to 12 hours. This interval may be determined by the need to maintain intracellular concentrations of AraCTP at inhibitory levels for at least one cell cycle. The mean cycle time of acute myelocytic leukemia cells is 1 to 2 days. Typical schedules for administration of AraC employ bolus doses every 12 hours for 5 to 7 days or continuous infusion for 7 days.

Mechanisms of Resistance to Cytarabine. Response to AraC is strongly influenced by the relative activities of anabolic and catabolic enzymes that determine the proportion of drug converted to AraCTP. The rate-limiting enzyme is deoxycytidine kinase, which produces AraCMP. An important degradative enzyme is cytidine deaminase, which deaminates AraC to a nontoxic metabolite, arauridine. Cytidine deaminase is found in high activity in many tissues, including some human tumors. A second degradative enzyme, dCMP deaminase, converts

AraCMP to the inactive metabolite, AraUMP. Relationships have been shown between the synthesis and retention of AraCTP in leukemic cells and the duration of complete remission in patients with acute myeloblastic leukemia (Preisler *et al.,* 1985). The ability of cells to transport AraC also appears to be an important determinant of the clinical response (Wiley *et al.,* 1985).

Because drug concentration in plasma rapidly falls below the level needed to saturate transport and activation processes, clinicians have employed high-dose regimens (2 to 3 g/m^2 every 12 hours for 6 doses) to achieve 20- to 50-fold higher serum levels with improved results in remission induction (Bishop *et al.,* 1996) and consolidation (Mayer *et al.,* 1994) for acute nonlymphocytic leukemia (ANLL).

Several biochemical mechanisms have been identified in AraC-resistant subpopulations in various murine and human tumor cell lines. Most commonly encountered is deficiency of deoxycytidine kinase (Flasshove *et al.,* 1994). Another mechanism of resistance is marked expansion of the dCTP pool due to increased CTP synthase activity (Garcia-Carbonero *et al.,* 2001). The increased concentrations of intracellular dCTP presumably can block the actions of AraCTP on DNA synthesis. Other mechanisms include increased cytidine deaminase activity and reduced affinity of DNA polymerase for AraCTP. Finally, while specific steps in AraC activation and degradation exert a strong influence on its ultimate action, the cellular response to AraC-mediated DNA damage also governs whether or not the genotoxic insult results in cell death. For example, overexpression of Bcl-2 and Bcl-x$_L$ in leukemic blasts have been associated with *in vitro* resistance to AraC-mediated apoptosis (Ibrado *et al.,* 1996). Phosphorylation of DNA-damage response factors or transcription factors also may influence the cellular response to AraC toxic insult. Recent studies have shown that phosphorylation of Bcl-2 or the AP-1 transcription factor is associated with AraC resistance in human myeloid leukemia cell lines *in vitro* (Kolla and Studzinski, 1994). At the clinical level, AraC resistance is poorly understood.

Absorption, Fate, and Excretion. Due to the presence of high concentrations of cytidine deaminase in the gastrointestinal mucosa and liver, only about 20% of the drug reaches the circulation after oral AraC administration; thus, the drug is not given orally. Peak concentrations of 2 to 50 μM are measurable in plasma after injection of 30 to 300 mg/m^2 intravenously. After intravenous administration, there is a rapid phase of disappearance of AraC ($t_{1/2} = 10$ minutes), followed by a slower phase of elimination with a half-time of about 2.5 hours. Less than 10% of the injected dose is excreted unchanged in the urine within 12 to 24 hours, while most appears as the inactive, deaminated product, arabinosyl uracil. Higher concentrations of AraC are found in CSF after continuous infusion than after rapid intravenous injection. After intrathecal administration of the drug at a dose of 50 mg/m^2, relatively little deamination occurs, even after 7 hours, and peak concentrations of 1 to 2 mM are achieved, which decline slowly with a terminal half-life of approximately 3.4 hours. Concentrations above the threshold for cytotoxicity (0.4 μM) are maintained in the CSF for 24 hours. More recently, a formulation of AraC for sustained release into the cerebrospinal fluid has been developed. Cytarabine concentration is maintained at cytotoxic levels for an average of 12 days, which avoids the need for repeated lumbar punctures. A possible benefit in terms of time to neurologic progression was suggested in a preliminary study comparing the administration of the sustained-release formulation, 50 mg every 2 weeks, with the standard intrathecal formulation in patients with lymphomatous meningitis (Glantz *et al.*, 1999).

Therapeutic Uses. Two standard dosage schedules are recommended for administration of *cytarabine* (CYTOSAR-U, TARABINE PFS): (1) rapid intravenous injection of 100 mg/m^2 every 12 hours for 5 to 7 days; or (2) continuous intravenous infusion of 100 to 200 mg/m^2 daily for 5 to 7 days. In general, children seem to tolerate higher doses than do adults. Intrathecal doses of 30 mg/m^2 every 4 days have been used to treat meningeal leukemia. The intrathecal administration of 50 mg of the liposomal formulation of cytarabine (DEPOCYT) every 2 weeks probably is at least as effective. In both pediatric and adult patients with acute nonlymphocytic leukemia, high-dose cytarabine (2 to 3 g/m^2 administered over 2 hours every 12 hours for 6 doses) has greater efficacy but greater neurotoxicity, especially in elderly patients (Mayer *et al.*, 1994).

Cytarabine is indicated for induction of remission in acute leukemia in children and adults. When used alone, remission rates of 20% to 40% have been reported. The drug is particularly useful in acute nonlymphocytic leukemia in adults. Cytarabine is most effective when used with other agents, particularly anthracyclines or mitoxantrone. The drug also is used in combination therapy for aggressive presentations of non-Hodgkin's lymphomas in adults and in children and for treatment of relapses of acute lymphocytic leukemia in both age groups.

Clinical Toxicities. Cytarabine is primarily a potent myelosuppressive agent capable of producing severe leukopenia, thrombocytopenia, and anemia with striking megaloblastic changes. Other toxic manifestations include gastrointestinal disturbances, stomatitis, conjunctivitis, mild and reversible hepatic dysfunction, pneumonitis, fever, and dermatitis. Seizures and other manifestations of neurotoxicity may occur after intrathecal administration or when high doses (particularly greater than 3 g/m^2) are administered intravenously to patients older than 40 and/or patients with poor renal function or abnormal alkaline phosphatase activity (Rubin *et al.*, 1992).

Gemcitabine

Gemcitabine (2,2 difluorodeoxycytidine; dFdC) is the most important antimetabolite to enter the clinic in recent years and is part of the first-line regimen for patients with metastatic pancreatic cancer and non-small cell lung cancer. The drug was selected for development on the basis of its impressive activity against murine solid tumors and human xenografts in nude mice (Hertel *et al.*, 1990).

Mechanism of Action. Gemcitabine retains many of the principal features of cytarabine. Influx of gemcitabine through the cell membrane occurs *via* active nucleoside transporters (Mackey *et al.*, 1998). Intracellularly, deoxycytidine kinase phosphorylates gemcitabine to produce difluorodeoxycytidine monophosphate (Heinemann *et al.*, 1988), from which point it is converted to difluorodeoxycytidine di- and triphosphate (dFdCDP, dFdCTP). While its metabolism to triphosphate status and its effects on DNA in general mimic those of cytarabine, there are differences in kinetics of inhibition, additional sites of action, incorporation in DNA, and spectrum of activity (Iwasaki *et al.*, 1997). Unlike that of cytarabine, the cytotoxicity of gemcitabine is not confined to the S phase of the cell cycle, and the drug is equally effective against confluent cells and cells in log-phase growth. The cytotoxic activity may be a result of several actions on DNA synthesis: dFdCTP competes with dCTP as a weak inhibitor of DNA polymerase; dFdCDP is a potent inhibitor of ribonucleotide reductase, resulting in depletion of deoxyribonucleotide pools necessary for DNA synthesis; and dFdCTP is incorporated into DNA and after the incorporation of one more nucleotide leads to DNA strand termination (Heinemann *et al.*, 1990; Huang *et al.*, 1991). This "extra" nucleotide may be important in hiding the dFdCTP from DNA repair enzymes, as incorporation of dFdCTP into DNA appears to be resistant to the normal mechanisms of DNA repair. The ability of cells to incorporate dFdCTP into DNA is critical for gemcitabine-induced apoptosis (Huang *et al.*, 1995).

Absorption, Fate, and Elimination. Gemcitabine is administered as an intravenous infusion. The pharmacokinetics of the parent compound are largely determined by deamination, and the predominant elimination product is difluorodeoxyuridine (dFdU). Gemcitabine has a $t_{1/2}$ of 40 to 90 minutes, depending on the age and gender of subjects. There is a biphasic elimination of dFdU, which has a $t_{1/2}\alpha$ of about 27 minutes and $t_{1/2}\beta$ of about 14 hours (Abbruzzese *et al.*, 1991). Clearance is dose-independent but can vary widely among individuals.

Similar to that of cytarabine, conversion of gemcitabine to dFdCTP by deoxycytidine kinase is saturated at infusion rates of approximately 10 mg/m^2 per minute, which produce plasma drug concentrations in the range of 15 to 20 μM (or at similar concentrations in cell culture) (Grunewald *et al.*, 1991; 1992). In an attempt to increase dFdCTP formation, the duration of infusion at this maximum concentration has been extended to 90 minutes. In contrast to a fixed infusion duration of 30 minutes, the 90-minute infusion produces a higher level of dFdCTP within peripheral blood mononuclear cells, increases the degree of myelosuppression, and may enhance activity (Tempero *et al.*, 1999).

The activity of dFdCTP on DNA repair mechanisms may allow for increased cytotoxicity of other chemotherapeutic agents, particularly platinum compounds. Preclinical studies of tumor cell lines show that cisplatin-DNA adducts are enhanced in the presence of gemcitabine, presumably through suppression of nuclear excision repair (van Moorsel *et al.*, 1999).

Therapeutic Uses. The standard dosing schedule for *gemcitabine* (GEMZAR) is a 30-minute intravenous infusion of 1000 to 1200 mg/m^2 on days 1, 8, and 15 every 28 days. Besides pancreatic cancer and non–small cell lung cancer, activity has been noted in patients with transitional cell carcinoma, cervical cancer, ovarian cancer, and breast cancer.

Clinical Toxicities. The principal toxicity of gemcitabine is myelosuppression. In general, the longer duration infusions lead to greater myelosuppression. Nonhematologic toxicities including a flu-like syndrome, asthenia, and mild elevation in liver transaminases may occur in 40% or more of patients. Although severe nonhematologic toxicities are rare, interstitial pneumonitis may occur and is responsive to steroids. Rarely, hemolytic-uremic syndrome has been reported (Aapro *et al.,* 1998).

PURINE ANALOGS

Since the pioneering studies of Hitchings and associates, begun in 1942, many analogs of natural purine bases, nucleosides, and nucleotides have been examined in a wide variety of biological and biochemical systems. These extensive investigations have led to the development of several drugs, of use not only in the treatment of malignant diseases *(mercaptopurine, thioguanine)* but also for immunosuppressive *(azathioprine)* (Schwartz, 2000) and antiviral *(acyclovir, ganciclovir, vidarabine, zidovudine)* therapy (*see* Figure 52–11). The hypoxanthine analog *allopurinol,* a potent inhibitor of xanthine oxidase, is an important by-product of this effort (*see* Chapter 27). A promising development has been the discovery of powerful inhibitors of adenosine deaminase, for example, erythro-9-(2-hydroxy-3-nonyl)-adenine (EHNA) and *pentostatin* (2'-deoxycoformycin). Recent studies have confirmed that pentostatin has clinical activity against hairy cell and chronic lymphocytic leukemias and lymphomas. In experimental systems, these inhibitors of adenosine deaminase have produced marked synergistic effects in combination with various analogs of adenosine, such as *vidarabine* (arabinosyladenine; AraA); they also show promise as immunosuppressive agents. Two drugs that are resistant to deamination by adenosine deaminase, *fludarabine phosphate* and *cladribine,* have outstanding activity in several types of leukemias and lymphomas (Beutler, 1992; Cheson, 1992; Piro, 1992; Calabresi and Schein 1993; Chabner *et al.,* 2001).

Structure–Activity Relationship. Mercaptopurine and thioguanine, both established clinical agents for the therapy of human leukemias, are analogs of the natural purines hypoxanthine and guanine, in which the keto group on carbon 6 of the purine ring is replaced by a sulfur atom. Substitution in this position by chlorine or selenium also yields antineoplastic compounds. Cytotoxicity also is observed with the β-D-ribonucleoside and β-D-2'-deoxyribonucleoside derivatives. Because these nucleoside analogs are excellent substrates for purine nucleoside phosphorylase, a highly active enzyme in many tissues, the analog

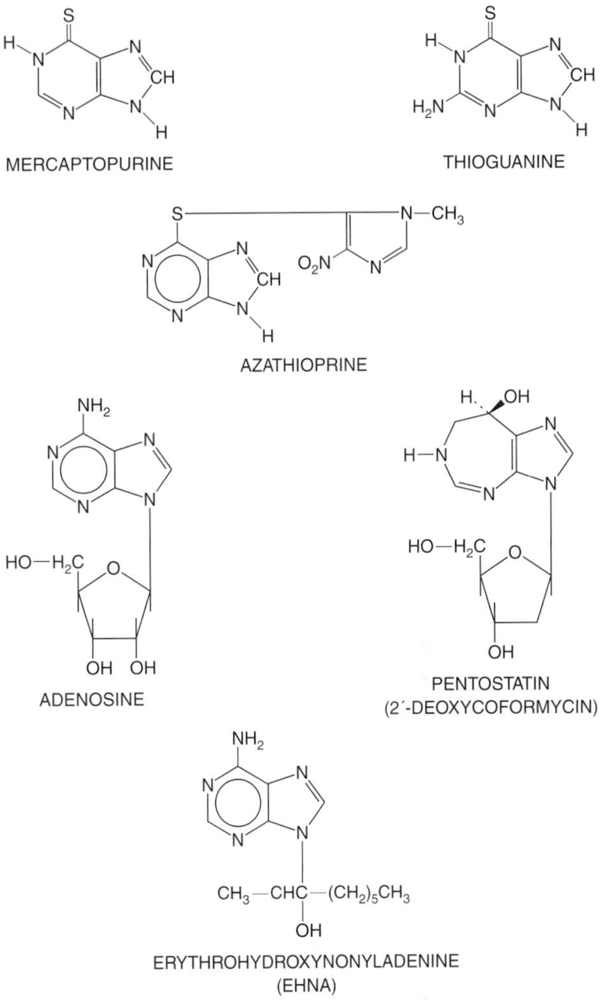

Figure 52–11. Structural formulas of adenosine and various purine analogs.

nucleosides act as prodrugs and generate respective hypoxanthine or guanine analogs in tissues. With several important exceptions, analogs of purine bases or nucleosides must undergo enzymatic conversion to the nucleotide to display cytotoxic activity.

Many attempts have been made to modify the structures of such analogs to improve their therapeutic indices or selectivity. Azathioprine (*see* Figure 52–11) was developed to decrease the rate of inactivation of 6-mercaptopurine by enzymatic *S*-methylation, nonenzymatic oxidation, or conversion to thiourate by xanthine oxidase. Azathioprine can react with sulfhydryl compounds such as glutathione (apparently nonenzymatically) and thus serves as a prodrug, permitting the slow liberation of mercaptopurine in tissues. Superior immunosuppressive activity is achieved in comparison with mercaptopurine (Elion, 1967).

An important development has been the discovery of potent inhibitors of adenosine deaminase such as pentostatin

(2'-deoxycoformycin; $K_i = 2.5$ pM) and erythro-9-(2-hydroxy-3-nonyl)-adenine (EHNA; $K_i = 2$ nM). Pentostatin (*see* Figure 52–11) is a natural product derived from *Streptomyces*. Structurally, the drug resembles the transition state of adenosine as it is hydrolyzed by adenosine deaminase. As a result, the drug has an affinity for the enzyme that is 10^7-fold greater than that of the natural substrate. The enzyme–inhibitor complex is very stable and dissociates with a $t_{1/2}$ of about 25 to 30 hours (Agarwal *et al.*, 1977; Agarwal, 1982). Thus, pentostatin blocks not only the deamination of natural nucleosides but also that of many analogs used in chemotherapy.

Mechanism of Action.   Although animal tissues have nucleoside kinases that are capable of converting adenosine or the 2'-deoxyribonucleosides of guanine, hypoxanthine, adenine, and many of their analogs to the corresponding 5'-monophosphates, similar reactions do not occur with inosine, guanosine, or their analogs. The latter compounds must first undergo phosphorolysis by purine nucleoside phosphorylase, which is present in high activity in many human tissues. The liberated bases then may be converted to the corresponding nucleotides by hypoxanthine-guanine phosphoribosyltransferase (HGPRT). Similarly, 2'-deoxyguanosine, 2'-deoxyinosine, and many related analogs may react with purine nucleoside phosphorylase, and the product of this reaction—a purine base or analog—then may be converted to the corresponding ribonucleoside 5'-monophosphate.

Both thioguanine and mercaptopurine are excellent substrates for HGPRT and are converted to the ribonucleotides 6-thioguanosine-5'-phosphate (6-thioGMP) and 6-thioinosine-5'-phosphate (T-IMP), respectively. Because T-IMP is a poor substrate for guanylyl kinase, the enzyme that converts GMP to GDP, T-IMP accumulates intracellularly. Careful studies have demonstrated, however, that mercaptopurine can be incorporated into cellular DNA in the form of thioguanine deoxyribonucleotide, indicating that slow reactions catalyzed by enzymes of guanine metabolism can operate. The accumulation of T-IMP may inhibit several vital metabolic reactions, such as the conversion of inosinate (IMP) to adenylosuccinate (AMPS) and then to adenosine-5'-phosphate (AMP) and the oxidation of IMP to xanthylate (XMP) by inosinate dehydrogenase. These reactions are crucial steps in the conversion of IMP to adenine and guanine nucleotides. On the other hand, in cells incubated with thioguanine, 6-thioGMP first accumulates; it is a poor but definite substrate for guanylyl kinase. Thus, there is slow conversion to 6-thioGDP and 6-thioGTP and entry of thioguanine nucleotides into the nucleic acids of the cell. In addition, the concentrations of 6-thioGMP achieved are sufficient to cause progressive and irreversible inhibition of inosinate dehydrogenase, presumably through the formation of disulfide bonds. Furthermore, both 6-thioGMP and T-IMP, as well as a number of other 5'-monophosphate derivatives of purine nucleoside analogs, can cause "pseudo–feedback inhibition" of the first committed step in the *de novo* pathway of purine biosynthesis, the reaction of glutamine and PRPP to form ribosylamine-5-phosphate. This enzyme is a major control point in the biosynthesis of purine nucleotides, and its activity is regulated by the intracellular concentrations of 5'-mononucleotides (natural, as well as analogs). The synthesis of PRPP also is powerfully inhibited by ADP and ATP or related analogs. Mercaptopurine also inhibits 6-phosphofructo-2-

kinase, an essential enzyme in the glycolytic pathway (Mojena *et al.*, 1992). 6-Methymercaptopurine ribonucleoside (MMPR) is produced from mercaptopurine in an *S*-methylation reaction catalyzed by 6-thiopurine methytransferase. The nucleotides of MMPR are potent inhibitors of *de novo* purine biosynthesis. MMPR has been shown to have antiangiogenic activity *in vivo* (Presta *et al.*, 1999).

Despite extensive investigations, it is still not possible to assess precisely the role of incorporation of thioguanine or mercaptopurine into cellular DNA in the production of either the therapeutic or toxic effects of these drugs (Bo *et al.*, 1999; Marathias *et al.*, 1999). The incidence of pregnancy-related complications, however, was significantly increased when fathers used mercaptopurine within 3 months of conception (Rajapakse *et al.*, 2000). These compounds can cause marked inhibition of the coordinated induction of various enzymes required for DNA synthesis, as well as potentially critical alterations in the synthesis of polyadenylate-containing RNA (Carrico and Sartorelli, 1977; Giverhaug *et al.*, 1999).

Other studies indicate that disruption of the synthesis of membrane glycoproteins may be caused by brief exposure to 6-thioguanine. These effects, which are potentially lethal to cellular survival, are likely mediated by depletion of guanosine diphosphate sugars. In view of these diverse biochemical actions, which involve vital systems such as purine biosynthesis, nucleotide interconversions, DNA and RNA synthesis, chromosomal replication, and glycoprotein synthesis, it is not possible to pinpoint a single biochemical event as the cause of thiopurine cytotoxicity. It seems likely that this class of drugs acts by multiple mechanisms (Hortelano and Bosca, 1997). Recently, a thiopurine analog, 6-methylmercaptopurine riboside also has been shown to inhibit angiogenesis (Presta *et al.*, 1999).

Of many adenosine analogs studied experimentally, *vidarabine* (arabinosyladenine, AraA) is used for the treatment of herpetic infections (*see* Chapter 50), but it has failed to produce useful antitumor activity due to its rapid deamination. A deamination-resistant analog, 2-fluoro-9-β-D-arabinosyladenine-5'-phosphate (2-F-AraAMP, *fludarabine phosphate*), has substantial activity in patients with refractory chronic lymphocytic leukemia and low-grade lymphomas. (For additional discussion and references, *see* Bloch, 1975; Chun *et al.*, 1986; Calabresi and Shein, 1993; Keating *et al.*, 1998; Chabner *et al.*, 2001; Zinzani *et al.*, 2000.)

As mentioned above, pentostatin is a potent inhibitor of adenosine deaminase. The relationship between this effect and drug-induced cytotoxicity, however, is not clear. Alterations of the usual intracellular concentrations of adenosine-containing compounds appear to cause feedback inhibition of *S*-adenosylhomocysteine hydrolase; as a result, cellular methylation reactions are impaired. The drug interferes with the synthesis of nicotinamide adenine dinucleotide. The nucleoside triphosphate analog of pentostatin can be incorporated into DNA, resulting in strand breakage (Siaw and Coleman, 1984; Johnston *et al.*, 1986; Begleiter *et al.*, 1987; Calabresi *et al.*, 1993; Chabner *et al.*, 2001).

Genetic deficiency of adenosine deaminase is associated with malfunction of both T and B lymphocytes, with little effect on other normal tissues (Giblett *et al.*, 1972). Thus, animals treated with pentostatin display marked immunosuppression. Severe and sometimes fatal opportunistic infections also have been associated with the clinical use of pentostatin. Treatment with pentostatin alone has induced remissions in T lymphocyte–related diseases, such as T-cell leukemia and mycosis fungoides. These initial trials were predicated on the observation that malignant T cells have high levels of adenosine deaminase. However, encouraging results also have been obtained in B-cell disease; 25% of patients with refractory chronic lymphocytic leukemia have responded to the drug, as have 90% of patients with hairy cell leukemia. Another purine analog that has shown potent activity in hairy cell leukemia is 2-chlorodeoxyadenosine (2-CdA, *cladribine*). Cladribine is resistant to adenosine deaminase, and after intracellular phosphorylation by deoxycytidine kinase, it is incorporated into DNA. Because of its extremely high effectiveness and lower toxicity, cladribine often is preferred to pentostatin in hairy cell leukemia. It also is active in other leukemias and lymphoma (*see* Symposium, 1984; Tritsch, 1985; Beutler, 1992; Kay *et al.*, 1992; Estey *et al.*, 1992; Saven and Piro, 1992; Hoffman *et al.*, 1994; Tallman *et al.*, 1995; Dearden *et al.*, 1999; Chabner *et al.*, 2001).

Mechanisms of Resistance to the Purine Antimetabolites. As with other tumor-inhibiting antimetabolites, acquired resistance is a major obstacle to the successful use of the purine analogs. The most commonly encountered mechanism observed *in vitro* is deficiency or complete lack of the enzyme HGPRT. In addition, resistance can result from decreases in the affinity of this enzyme for its substrates. Cells that are resistant because of these mechanisms usually show cross-resistance to analogs such as mercaptopurine, thioguanine, and 8-azaguanine.

Another mechanism of resistance identified in cells from leukemic patients is an increase in particulate alkaline phosphatase activity. Other mechanisms include (1) decreased drug transport, (2) increased rates of degradation of the drugs or their intracellular "activated" analogs, (3) alteration in allosteric inhibition of ribosylamine 5-phosphate synthase, (4) altered DNA-repair efficiency, (5) loss or alterations of the enzymes adenine phosphoribosyltransferase or adenosine kinase (for adenine or adenosine analogs and deoxycytidine kinase for fludarabine phosphate), and (6) increased activity of multidrug resistance protein 5 (Wijnholds *et al.*, 2000). However, the most important determinants of resistance to these drugs in the clinical setting remain uncertain (for review, *see* Brockman, 1974).

Mercaptopurine

The introduction of mercaptopurine by Elion and coworkers represents a landmark in the history of antineoplastic and immunosuppressive therapy. Mercaptopurine and its derivative, azathioprine, remain among the most important and most clinically useful drugs of the class (Relling *et al.*, 1999a,b; Mahoney *et al.*, 1998). Mercaptopurine is used principally in the maintenance therapy of acute lymphocytic leukemia. The structure–activity relationship and the mechanism of action and of drug resistance are discussed above. The structural formula of mercaptopurine is presented in Figure 52–11.

Absorption, Fate, and Excretion.   Absorption of mercaptopurine is incomplete after oral ingestion and bioavailability is reduced by first-pass metabolism by the liver. Oral bioavailability is only 5% to 37%, with great interpatient variability. Measurements of drug concentrations in plasma may be necessary to optimize therapy with oral mercaptopurine. Bioavailability is increased when mercaptopurine is combined with high-dose methotrexate (Innocenti *et al.*, 1996). After an intravenous dose, the half-life of the drug in plasma is relatively short (about 50 minutes in adults), due to uptake by cells, renal excretion, and rapid metabolic degradation. Restricted brain distribution of mercaptopurine is related to the efficient efflux transport system in the blood–brain barrier (Deguchi *et al.*, 2000). In addition to the HGPRT-catalyzed anabolism of mercaptopurine, there are two other pathways for its metabolism. The first involves methylation of the sulfhydryl group and subsequent oxidation of the methylated derivatives. Expression of the enzyme thiopurine methyltransferase reflects the inheritance of polymorphic alleles (Yates *et al.*, 1997; Iyer, 1999; Relling *et al.*, 1999b); up to 15% of the population of the United Kingdom have little or no enzyme activity (Weinshilboum, 1989). Low levels of erythrocyte thiopurine methyltransferase activity are associated with increased drug toxicity in individual patients. The formation of nucleotides of 6-methylmercaptopurine has been shown to occur after administration of mercaptopurine or mercaptopurine ribonucleoside. Substantial amounts of the mono-, di-, and triphosphate nucleotides of 6-methylmercaptopurine ribonucleoside (6-MMPR) have been identified in the blood and bone marrow of patients treated with mercaptopurine or azathioprine. Desulfuration of thiopurines can occur, and relatively large percentages of the administered sulfur are excreted as inorganic sulfate. The second major pathway for mercaptopurine metabolism involves the enzyme xanthine oxidase, which is present in relatively large amounts in the liver. Mercaptopurine is a good substrate for this enzyme, which oxidizes it to 6-thiouric acid, a noncarcinostatic metabolite.

An attempt to modify the metabolic inactivation of mercaptopurine by xanthine oxidase led to the development of allopurinol. This analog of hypoxanthine is a powerful inhibitor of xanthine oxidase and not only blocks the conversion of mercaptopurine to 6-thiouric acid but also interferes with the production of uric acid from hypoxanthine and xanthine (*see* Chapter 27). Because of its ability to interfere with the enzymatic oxidation of mercaptopurine and related derivatives, allopurinol increases the exposure of cells to the action of these compounds. Although it greatly potentiates the antineoplastic action of mercaptopurine in tumor-bearing mice, allopurinol increases the toxicity as well, and there is no apparent improvement in the therapeutic index (Zinner and Klastersky, 1985).

Therapeutic Uses.   The initial average daily oral dose of mercaptopurine (*6-mercaptopurine;* PURINETHOL) is 2.5 mg/kg. Starting doses usually range from 100 to 200 mg per day; with hematological and clinical improvement, the dose is diminished to an appropriate multiple of 25 mg and, in general, maintenance therapy of 1.5 to 2.5 mg/kg per day is continued. If beneficial effects have not been noted after 4 weeks, the daily dose may be increased gradually up to 5 mg/kg until evidence of toxicity is encountered. The total dose required to produce depression of the bone marrow in patients with nonhematological malignancies is about 45 mg/kg and may range from 18 to 106 mg/kg.

Hyperuricemia with hyperuricosuria may occur during treatment; the accumulation of uric acid presumably reflects the destruction of cells with release of purines that are oxidized by xanthine oxidase, as well as an inhibition of the conversion of inosinic acid to precursors of nucleic acids. This circumstance may be an indication for the use of allopurinol. Special caution must be employed if mercaptopurine or its imidazolyl derivative, azathioprine, is used with allopurinol, for reasons presented above. Patients treated simultaneously with both drugs should receive approximately 25% of the usual dose of mercaptopurine.

In the early studies with mercaptopurine, bone marrow remissions were described in more than 40% of children with acute leukemia. In adults with acute leukemia, the results have been much less impressive, but occasional remissions have been obtained. The drug has contributed to the treatment of lymphoblastic leukemia more by maintaining than by inducing remissions. Cross-resistance does not occur between mercaptopurine and other classes of antileukemic agents.

In the treatment of chronic granulocytic leukemia, maintenance therapy with mercaptopurine can be useful, but more effective agents are available. Mercaptopurine has not been of value in chronic lymphocytic leukemia, Hodgkin's disease and related lymphomas, and a wide variety of carcinomas, even at unusually high doses. Although active as an immunosuppressive agent, it has been superseded by its imidazolyl derivative, azathioprine.

Clinical Toxicities. The principal toxic effect of mercaptopurine is bone marrow depression, although, in general, this develops more gradually than with folic acid antagonists; accordingly, thrombocytopenia, granulocytopenia, or anemia may not be encountered for several weeks. When depression of normal bone marrow elements occurs, cessation of therapy with the drug usually results in prompt recovery. Anorexia, nausea, or vomiting is seen in approximately 25% of adults, but stomatitis and diarrhea are rare; manifestations of gastrointestinal effects are less frequent in children than in adults. The occurrence of jaundice in about one-third of adult patients treated with mercaptopurine has been reported; although the pathogenesis of this manifestation is obscure, it usually clears upon discontinuation of therapy. Its appearance has been associated with bile stasis and hepatic necrosis. Dermatological manifestations have been reported. The long-term complications associated with the use of mercaptopurine and its derivative, azathioprine, for immunosuppressive therapy are discussed by Schein and Winokur (1975), Kirschner (1998), and Korelitz et al. (1999). Teratogenic effects during the first trimester are associated with chronic mercap-

topurine treatment, and acute myelogenous leukemia has been reported after prolonged use of mercaptopurine for Crohn's disease (Heizer and Peterson, 1998).

Azathioprine

Azathioprine, a derivative of 6-mercaptopurine, is used as an immunosuppressive agent; its structural formula is shown in Figure 52–11. The rationale that led to its synthesis and its mechanism of action and metabolic degradation have been discussed above. Additional information is presented in Chapter 53.

Thioguanine

The synthesis of thioguanine was first described by Elion and Hitchings in 1955. It is of particular value in the treatment of acute granulocytic leukemia when given with cytarabine. The structural formula of thioguanine is shown in Figure 52–11, and its mechanism of action is discussed above.

Absorption, Fate, and Excretion. Absorption of thioguanine is incomplete and erratic, and concentrations of the drug in plasma may vary more than tenfold after oral administration. Peak concentrations in the blood are reached 2 to 4 hours after ingestion. When thioguanine is administered to human beings, the S-methylation product, 2-amino-6-methylthiopurine, rather than free thioguanine appears in the urine; inorganic sulfate and, after continuous intravenous infusion, 8-hydroxythioguanine also are major urinary metabolites (Kitchen et al., 1999). Lesser amounts of 6-thiouric acid are formed, suggesting that deamination catalyzed by the enzyme guanase does not have a major role in the metabolic inactivation of thioguanine. Since 6-thioxanthine, the deamination product of thioguanine, is inactive, thioguanine may be administered concurrently with allopurinol without reduction in dosage, unlike mercaptopurine and azathioprine.

Therapeutic Uses. *Thioguanine* (6-thioguanine, TG) is available for oral administration. The average daily dose is 2 mg/kg. If there is no clinical improvement or toxicity after 4 weeks, the dosage may be increased cautiously to 3 mg/kg daily.

Clinically, thioguanine has been used in the treatment of acute leukemia and, in conjunction with cytarabine, is one of the most effective agents for induction of remissions in acute granulocytic leukemia; it has not been useful in the treatment of patients with solid tumors. This compound has been used as an immunosuppressive agent, particularly in patients with nephrosis or with collagen-vascular disorders.

Clinical Toxicities. Toxic manifestations include bone marrow depression and gastrointestinal effects, although the latter may be less pronounced than with mercaptopurine. Hepatotoxicity also is lower for thioguanine than for mercaptopurine.

Fludarabine Phosphate

A fluorinated deamination-resistant nucleotide analog of the antiviral agent vidarabine (9-β-D-arabinofuranosyladenine), this compound is active in chronic lymphocytic leukemia and low-grade lymphomas (Calabresi et al., 1993; Chabner et al., 2001; Zinzani et al., 2000; Nagler et al., 2000; Petrus et al., 2000). After rapid dephosphorylation to the nucleoside fludarabine by membrane 5'-ectonucleotidase, it is rephosphorylated intracellularly by deoxycytidine kinase to the active triphosphate derivative. This antimetabolite inhibits DNA polymerase, DNA primase, DNA ligase, and ribonucleotide reductase and is incorporated into DNA and RNA (Brockman et al., 1980). The triphosphate nucleotide is an effective chain terminator when incorporated into DNA (Kamiya et al., 1996), and the incorporation of fludarabine into RNA results in inhibition of RNA function, RNA processing, and mRNA translation (Plunkett and Gandhi, 1992). A major effect of this drug may be its activation of apoptosis (Huang et al., 1995), and this may explain its activity against indolent lymphoproliferative disease where only a small fraction of cells are in S phase (Dighiero, 1996). Although the precise mechanism of cytotoxicity of fludarabine phosphate is not completely understood, it is capable of causing DNA chain termination and induction of apoptosis (Sandoval et al., 1996).

The structural formulas of fludarabine phosphate and a related adenosine analog, cladribine, are shown below:

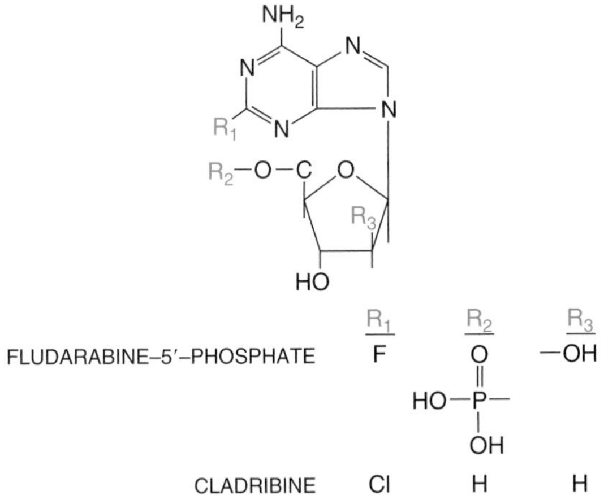

	R_1	R_2	R_3
FLUDARABINE–5′–PHOSPHATE	F	O‖HO–P–‖OH	–OH
CLADRIBINE	Cl	H	H

Absorption, Fate, and Excretion. Fludarabine phosphate is administered intravenously and is rapidly converted to fludarabine in the plasma. The terminal half-life of fludarabine is approximately 10 hours. The compound is primarily eliminated by renal excretion, and approximately 23% appears in the urine as fludarabine because of its relative resistance to deamination by adenosine deaminase.

Therapeutic Uses. *Fludarabine phosphate* (FLUDARA) is available for intravenous use. The recommended dose of fludarabine phosphate is 20 to 30 mg/m² daily for 5 days. The drug is administered intravenously by infusion during a period of 30 minutes to 2 hours. Dosage may need to be reduced in renal impairment. Treatment may be repeated every 4 weeks, and gradual improvement, at these doses, usually occurs during a period of two to three cycles.

Fludarabine phosphate is used primarily for the treatment of patients with chronic lymphocytic leukemia (CLL), although experience is accumulating that suggests effectiveness in B-cell lymphomas refractory to standard therapy. Activity also has been seen with indolent non-Hodgkin's lymphoma, promyelocytic leukemia, cutaneous T-cell lymphoma, and Waldentröm's macroglobulinemia (Chun et al., 1991). In CLL patients previously refractory to a regimen containing a standard alkylating agent, response rates of 32% to 48% have been reported. In patients with previously untreated low-grade lymphomas, fludarabine phosphate in combination with cyclophosphamide has resulted in almost 90% complete responses (Hochster et al., 1994). In combination with the anthracycline, mitoxantrone, and dexamethasone, fludarabine phosphate gives response rates greater than 90% against indolent non-Hodgkin's lymphoma (McLaughlin et al., 1996; Emmanouilides et al., 1998).

Clinical Toxicities. Toxic manifestations include myelosuppression, nausea and vomiting, and chills and fever, as well as malaise, anorexia, and weakness. Lymphopenia and thrombocytopenia are dose-limiting and possibly cumulative (Malspeis et al., 1990). CD4-positive T cells are depleted with therapy (O'Brien et al., 1993). Opportunistic infections (Cheson, 1995) and tumor lysis syndrome have been reported. Peripheral neuropathy may occur at standard doses (Cheson et al., 1999), as well as altered mental status, seizures, optic neuritis, and coma, usually at higher doses. Neurotoxicity is seen more frequently and with increased severity in older patients. In combination with pentostatin, severe or even fatal pulmonary toxicity has been encountered. Because a significant fraction of drug (about one-quarter) is eliminated in the urine, patients with compromised renal function should be treated with caution. Initial doses should be reduced in proportion to serum creatinine levels.

Pentostatin (2′-Deoxycoformycin)

Pentostatin is a transition-state analog of the intermediate stage in the adenosine deaminase (ADA) reaction and is a potent inhibitor of this enzyme. This compound, also known as 2′-deoxycoformycin (DCF), was isolated from fermentation cultures of *Streptomyces antibioticus*. Inhibition of ADA by pentostatin leads to accumulation of intracellular adenosine and deoxyadenosine nucleotides, which can block DNA synthesis by inhibiting ribonucleotide reductase. Deoxyadenosine also inactivates *S*-adenosyl homocysteine hydrolase, with resulting accumulation of *S*-adenosyl homocysteine, which is toxic to lymphocytes. Pentostatin also can inhibit RNA synthesis, and its triphosphate derivative is incorporated into DNA. In combination with 2'-deoxyadenosine, it is capable of inducing apoptosis in human monocytoid leukemia cells (Niitsu *et al.*, 1998). Although the precise mechanism of cytotoxicity is not known, it is probable that the imbalance in purine nucleotide pools accounts for its antineoplastic effect in hairy cell leukemia and T-cell lymphomas (*see* Calabresi *et al.*, 1993; Chabner *et al.*, 2001; Rafel *et al.*, 2000).

The structural formula of pentostatin (2'-deoxycoformycin) is shown in Figure 52–11.

Absorption, Fate, and Excretion. Pentostatin is administered intravenously, and a single dose of 4 mg/m² has been reported to have a distribution half-life of 11 minutes and a mean terminal half-life of 5.7 hours. The drug is eliminated almost entirely by renal excretion. Appropriate reduction of dosage is recommended in patients with renal impairment as measured by reduced creatinine clearance.

Therapeutic Uses. *Pentostatin* (NIPENT) is available for intravenous use. The recommended dosage is 4 mg/m² administered every other week. After hydration with 500 to 1000 ml of 5% dextrose in half-normal saline, the drug is administered by rapid intravenous injection or by infusion during a period of up to 30 minutes, followed by an additional 500 ml of fluids. Extravasation does not produce cellulitis, vesication, or tissue necrosis.

Pentostatin is extremely effective in producing complete remissions in hairy cell leukemia. Complete responses of 58% and partial responses of 28% have been reported even in patients who were refractory to interferon-alfa. Activity also is seen against CLL, CML, promyelocytic leukemia, cutaneous T-cell lymphoma, non-Hodgkin's lymphoma, and Langerhans-cell histiocytosis (Dillman, 1994; Cortes *et al.*, 1997). Pentostatin has no significant activity against solid tumors or multiple myeloma.

Clinical Toxicities. Toxic manifestations include myelosuppression, gastrointestinal symptoms, skin rashes, and abnormal liver function studies at standard (4 mg/m²) doses. Depletion of normal T cells occurs at these doses, and neutropenic fever and opportunistic infections have been reported (Steis *et al.*, 1991). Immunosuppression may persist for several years after discontinuation of pentostatin therapy (Kraut *et al.*, 1990). At higher doses (10 mg/m²), major renal and neurological complications are encountered. The use of pentostatin in combination with fludarabine phosphate may result in severe or even fatal pulmonary toxicity.

Cladribine

An adenosine deaminase-resistant purine analog, cladribine (2-chlorodeoxyadenosine; 2-CdA) has demonstrated potent activity in hairy cell leukemia, chronic lymphocytic leukemia, and low-grade lymphomas (Estey *et al.*, 1992; Kay *et al.*, 1992; Beutler, 1992; Dearden *et al.*, 1999; Tondini *et al.*, 2000). It appears to be safe and moderately effective in patients with progressive multiple sclerosis (Rice *et al.*, 2000). After intracellular phosphorylation by deoxycytidine kinase and conversion to cladribine triphosphate, it is incorporated into DNA. It produces DNA strand breaks and NAD and ATP depletion, as well as apoptosis in some cell lines (Piro, 1992; Beutler, 1992). Although the precise mechanism of action of cladribine is not fully understood, the drug does not require cell division to be cytotoxic.

The structural formula of cladribine is shown above with that of fludarabine-5-phosphate.

Absorption, Fate, and Excretion. Cladribine is not well absorbed orally (55% ± 17%) and is administered intravenously (Liliemark *et al.*, 1992). The drug is excreted primarily by the kidneys, with plasma half-lives of 35 minutes and 6.7 hours (Liliemark and Juliusson, 1991). Cladribine crosses the blood–brain barrier and reaches CSF concentrations of about 25% of those seen in plasma. In patients with meningeal involvement, however, CSF concentrations can exceed those in plasma.

Therapeutic Uses. *Cladribine* (LEUSTATIN) is available in an injectable dosage form. The recommended dose is a single course of 0.09 mg/kg per day for 7 days by continuous intravenous infusion.

Cladribine is considered the drug of choice in hairy cell leukemia because of its high level of effectiveness and low profile of toxicity. Complete responses have been reported in 80% of patients, and partial responses in the rest after a single course of therapy (Saven and Piro, 1992; Dearden *et al.*, 1999). The drug also is active in chronic lymphocytic leukemia, acute myelogenous leukemia, especially in pediatric patients, low-grade lymphomas, Langerhans-cell histiocytosis, cutaneous T-cell lymphomas, including mycosis fungoides and the Sézary syndrome, and Waldenström's macroglobulinemia (Piro *et al.*, 1988; Piro, 1992; Santana *et al.*, 1992; Kuzel *et al.*, 1992; Kay *et al.*, 1992; Saven *et al.*, 1992; Dimopoulos *et al.*, 1993; Robak *et al.*, 1999; Tondini *et al.*, 2000; Saen and Burian, 1999).

Clinical Toxicities. The major dose-limiting toxicity of cladribine is myelosuppression, although cumulative thrombocytopenia may occur with repeated courses. Opportunistic infections are common and are correlated with decreased CD4+

cell counts. Other toxic effects include nausea, infections, high fever, headache, fatigue, skin rashes, and tumor lysis syndrome. Neurological and immunosuppressive adverse effects are less evident than with pentostatin at clinically active doses, perhaps because cladribine is not an inhibitor of adenosine deaminase.

III. NATURAL PRODUCTS

ANTIMITOTIC DRUGS

Vinca Alkaloids

History. The beneficial properties of the Madagascar periwinkle plant, *Catharanthus roseus* (formerly called *Vinca rosea*), a species of myrtle, have been described in medicinal folklore in various parts of the world. While exploring claims that extracts of the periwinkle might have beneficial effects in diabetes mellitus, Noble and coworkers (1958) observed granulocytopenia and bone marrow suppression in rats, effects that led to purification of an active alkaloid. Other investigations, by Johnson and associates, demonstrated activity of certain alkaloidal fractions against an acute lymphocytic neoplasm in mice. Fractionation of these extracts yielded four active dimeric alkaloids: vinblastine, vincristine, vinleurosine, and vinrosidine. Two of these, *vinblastine* and *vincristine,* are important clinical agents for treatment of leukemias, lymphomas, and testicular cancer. Another agent, *vinorelbine,* has important activity against lung cancer and breast cancer (*see* Budman, 1997).

Chemistry. The vinca alkaloid antimitotic agents are asymmetrical dimeric compounds; the structures of vinblastine, vincristine, vindesine, and vinorelbine are shown opposite.

Structure–Activity Relationship. Minor differences in structure result in notable differences in toxicity and antitumor spectra among the vinca alkaloids. A number of related dimeric alkaloids are without biological activity. Removal of the acetyl group at C4 of one portion of vinblastine destroys its antileukemic activity, as does acetylation of the hydroxyl groups. Either hydrogenation of the double bond or reductive formation of carbinols reduces or destroys activity of these compounds.

Mechanism of Action. The vinca alkaloids are cell-cycle–specific agents and, in common with other drugs such as colchicine, podophyllotoxin, and taxanes, block cells in mitosis. The biological activities of these drugs can be explained by their ability to bind specifically to tubulin and to block the ability of the protein to polymerize into microtubules. When cells are incubated with vinblastine, dissolution of the microtubules occurs, and highly regular crystals are formed that contain 1 mol of bound vinblastine per mol of tubulin. Through disruption of the microtubules of the mitotic apparatus, cell division is arrested in metaphase. In the absence of an intact mitotic spindle, the chromosomes may disperse throughout the cytoplasm (exploded mitosis) or may clump in unusual groupings, such as balls or stars. The inability to segregate chromosomes correctly during mitosis presumably leads to cell death. Both normal and malignant cells exposed to vinca alkaloids undergo changes characteristic of apoptosis (Smets, 1994).

(A)

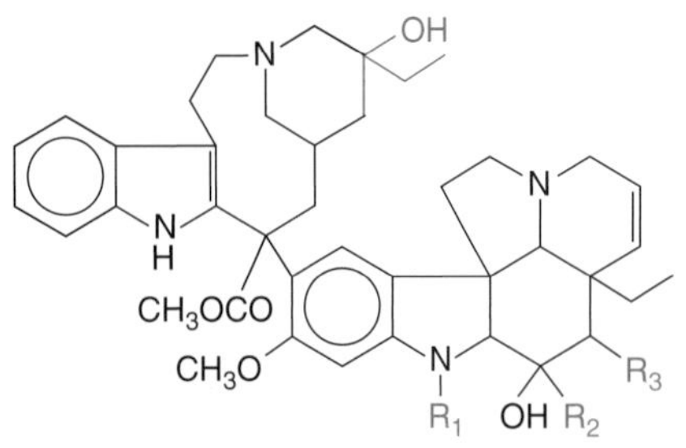

(B)

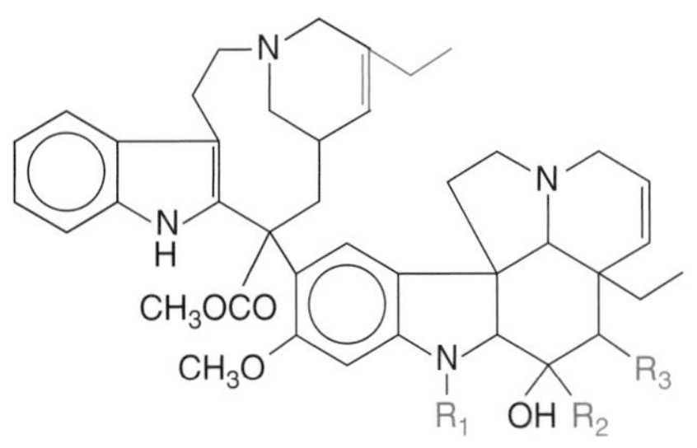

	R_1	R_2	R_3
Structure A			
VINBLASTINE	—CH₃	—C(=O)—OCH₃	—O—C(=O)—CH₃
VINCRISTINE	—CH(=O)	—C(=O)—OCH₃	—O—C(=O)—CH₃
VINDESINE	—CH₃	—C(=O)—NH₂	—OH
Structure B			
VINORELBINE	—CH₃	—C(=O)—OCH₃	—O—C(=O)—CH₃

In addition to their key role in the formation of mitotic spindles, microtubules are involved in other cellular functions such as movement, phagocytosis, and axonal transport. Side effects of the vinca alkaloids, such as their neurotoxicity, may be due to disruption of these functions.

Drug Resistance. Despite their structural similarity, cross-resistance among the individual vinca alkaloids is not absolute. For over a decade, however, attention has been drawn to the phenomenon of multidrug resistance, in which tumor cells become cross-resistant to a wide range of chemically dissimilar agents after exposure to a single (natural product) drug. Such multidrug-resistant tumor cells display cross-resistance to vinca alkaloids, the epipodophyllotoxins, anthracyclines, and taxanes. Chromosomal abnormalities consistent with gene amplification have been observed in resistant cells in culture, and the cells contain markedly increased levels of the P-glycoprotein, a membrane efflux pump that transports drugs from the cells (*see* Endicott and Ling, 1989). Ca²⁺ channel blockers, such as verapamil, can reverse resistance of this type. Other membrane transporters such as the multidrug resistance-associated protein (Kuss *et al.*, 1994) may mediate multidrug resistance; still other forms of resistance to vinca alkaloids involve mutations in tubulin that prevent the effective binding of the inhibitors to their target.

Cytotoxic Actions. Both vincristine and vinblastine, as well as the analog vinorelbine, have potent and selective antitumor effects, although their actions on normal tissue differ significantly. Vincristine is a standard component of regimens for treating pediatric leukemias and solid tumors and is frequently used in adult lymphoma treatment. Vinblastine is employed primarily in treating testicular carcinomas and lymphomas and as second-line therapy of various solid tumors. Vinorelbine has activity against non–small cell lung cancer and breast cancer, and its range of usefulness is expanding as new trials mature. The limited myelosuppressive action of vincristine makes it a valuable component of a number of combination therapy regimens for leukemia and lymphoma, while the lack of neurotoxicity of vinblastine is a decided advantage in relapsed lymphomas or in combination with cisplatin against testicular cancer. Vinorelbine, which causes a mild neurotoxicity as well as myelosuppression, has an intermediate toxicity profile.

Myelosuppression. The nadir of leukopenia following vinblastine or vinorelbine occurs 7 to 10 days following drug administration. Vincristine in standard doses, 1.4 to 2 mg/m^2, causes little reduction of formed elements in the blood. All three agents cause hair loss and local cellulitis if extravasated. A syndrome of inappropriate secretion of antidiuretic hormone occurs rarely after vincristine administration.

Neurological Toxicity. While all three derivatives may cause neurotoxic symptoms, vincristine has predictable cumulative effects. Numbness and tingling of the extremities and loss of deep tendon reflexes constitute the most common and earliest signs and are followed by motor weakness. The sensory changes do not usually warrant an immediate reduction in drug dose, but loss of motor function should lead to a reevaluation of the therapeutic plan and, under most circumstances, discontinuation of the drug. Rarely, patients may experience vocal cord paralysis or loss of extraocular muscle function. High-dose vincristine causes severe constipation or obstipation. Inadvertent intrathecal vincristine administration produces devastating and invariably fatal central neurotoxicity, with seizures and irreversible coma (Williams *et al.*, 1983).

Absorption, Fate, and Excretion. All three agents are extensively metabolized by the liver, and the conjugates and metabolites are excreted in the bile (Zhou and Rahmani, 1992; Robieux *et al.*, 1996). Only a small fraction of a dose (less than 15%) is found in the urine unchanged. In patients with hepatic dysfunction (bilirubin greater than 3 mg/dl), a 75% reduction in dose of any of the vinca alkaloids is advisable, although firm guidelines for dose adjustment have not been established. The pharmacokinetics of each of the three drugs are similar, with elimination half-lives of 1 and 20 hours for vincristine, 3 and 23 hours for vinblastine, and 1 and 45 hours for vinorelbine (Marquet *et al.*, 1992).

Vinblastine. *Therapeutic Uses.* Vinblastine sulfate (VELBAN) is given intravenously; special precautions must be taken against subcutaneous extravasation, since this may cause painful irritation and ulceration. The drug should not be injected into an extremity with impaired circulation. After a single dose of 0.3 mg/kg of body weight, myelosuppression reaches its maximum in 7 to 10 days. If a moderate level of leukopenia (approximately 3000 cells per cubic millimeter) is not attained, the weekly dose may be increased gradually by increments of 0.05 mg/kg of body weight. In regimens designed to cure testicular cancer, vinblastine is used in doses of 0.3 mg/kg every 3 weeks irrespective of blood cell counts or toxicity.

The most important clinical use of vinblastine is with bleomycin and cisplatin (*see* below) in the curative therapy of metastatic testicular tumors (Williams and Einhorn, 1985), although it has been significantly supplanted by etoposide in this disease. Beneficial responses have been reported in various lymphomas, particularly Hodgkin's disease, where significant improvement may be noted in 50% to 90% of cases. The effectiveness of vinblastine in a high proportion of lymphomas is not diminished when the disease is refractory to alkylating agents. It also is active in Kaposi's sarcoma, neuroblastoma, and Letterer–Siwe disease (histiocytosis X), as well as in carcinoma of the breast and choriocarcinoma.

Clinical Toxicities. The nadir of the leukopenia that follows the administration of vinblastine usually occurs within 7 to 10 days, after which recovery ensues within 7 days. Other toxic effects of vinblastine include neurological manifestations as described above. Gastrointestinal disturbances, including nausea, vomiting, anorexia, and diarrhea, may be encountered. The syndrome of inappropriate secretion of antidiuretic hormone has been reported. Loss of hair, mucositis of the mouth, and dermatitis occur infrequently. Extravasation during injection may lead to cellulitis and phlebitis. Local injection of hyaluronidase and application of moderate heat to the area may be of help by dispersing the drug.

Vincristine. *Therapeutic Uses.* Vincristine sulfate (ONCOVIN, VINCASAR PFS, others) used together with corticosteroids is presently the treatment of choice to induce remissions in childhood leukemia; common dosages for these drugs are vincristine, intravenously, 2 mg/m^2 of body surface area, weekly, and prednisone, orally, 40 mg/m^2, daily. Adult patients with Hodgkin's disease or non-Hodgkin's lymphomas usually receive vincristine as part of a complex protocol. When used in the MOPP regimen (*see* below), the recommended dose of vincristine is 1.4 mg/m^2. Vincristine seems to be tolerated better by children than by adults, who may experience severe, progressive neurological toxicity. Administration of the drug more frequently than every 7 days or at higher doses seems to increase the toxic manifestations without proportional improvement in the response rate. Maintenance therapy with vincristine is not recommended in children with leukemia. Precautions also should be used to avoid extravasation during intravenous administration of vincristine.

Despite their structural similarity, vincristine has a spectrum of clinical activity that differs significantly from that of vinblastine, although vincristine is effective in Hodgkin's disease and other lymphomas. It appears to be somewhat less beneficial than vinblastine when used alone in Hodgkin's disease, but when used with mechlorethamine, prednisone, and procarbazine (the so-called MOPP regimen), it was a part of the first curative treatment for the advanced stages (III and IV) of this disease (DeVita, 1981). In large-cell non-Hodgkin's lymphomas, vincristine remains an important agent, particularly when used in the CHOP regimen with cyclophosphamide, doxorubicin, and prednisone. As mentioned previously, vincristine is more useful for remission induction in lymphocytic leukemia. Vincristine also is a standard component of a number of regimens used to treat pediatric solid tumors such as Wilms' tumor, neuroblastoma, and rhabdomyosarcoma.

Clinical Toxicities. The clinical toxicity of vincristine is mostly neurological, as described above. The more severe neurological manifestations may be avoided or reversed by either suspending therapy or reducing the dosage upon occurrence of motor dysfunction. Severe constipation, sometimes resulting in colicky abdominal pain and obstruction, may be prevented by a prophylactic program of laxatives and hydrophilic agents and is usually a problem only with doses above 2 mg/m^2.

Alopecia occurs in about 20% of patients given vincristine; however, it is always reversible, frequently without cessation of therapy. Although less common than with vinblastine, leukopenia may occur with vincristine, and thrombocytopenia, anemia, polyuria, dysuria, fever, and gastrointestinal symptoms have been reported occasionally. The syndrome of hyponatremia associated with high urinary concentration of Na$^+$ and inappropriate secretion of antidiuretic hormone occasionally has been observed during vincristine therapy. In view of the rapid action of the vinca alkaloids, it is advisable to prevent hyperuricemia by the administration of allopurinol.

Vinorelbine. *Vinorelbine* (NAVELBINE) is administered in normal saline as an intravenous infusion of 30 mg/m^2 given over 6 to 10 minutes. A lower dose (20 to 25 mg/m^2) may be required for patients who have received prior chemotherapy. It is initially given every week until progression of disease or dose-limiting toxicity when used alone. When used with cisplatin for the treatment of non-small cell lung carcinoma, it is given every 3 weeks. Its primary toxicity is granulocytopenia, with only modest thrombocytopenia and less neurotoxicity than other vinca alkaloids. It may cause allergic reactions and mild, reversible changes in liver enzymes. In experimental studies, it

has been given in an oral capsule, but bioavailability is only 30% to 40% (Fumoleau *et al.*, 1993).

Paclitaxel

This compound, first isolated from the bark of the Western yew tree in 1971 (Wani *et al.*, 1971), exhibits unique pharmacological actions as an inhibitor of mitosis, differing from the vinca alkaloids and colchicine derivatives in that it promotes rather than inhibits microtubule formation. The drug has a central role in the combination therapy of cisplatin-refractory ovarian, breast, lung, esophagus, bladder, and head and neck cancers (Rowinsky *et al.*, 1993; Rowinsky and Donehower, 1995). The optimal dose, schedule, and use in drug combinations are incompletely understood.

Chemistry. Paclitaxel is a diterpenoid compound that contains a complex taxane ring as its nucleus (Figure 52–12). The side chain linked to the taxane ring at carbon 13 is essential for its antitumor activity. Modification of the side chain has led to identification of a more potent analog, *docetaxel* (TAXOTERE) (Figure 52–12), which has clinical activity against breast and ovarian cancers. Originally purified as the parent molecule from yew bark, paclitaxel can now be obtained for commercial purposes by semisynthesis from 10-desacetylbaccatin, a precursor found in yew leaves. It also has been successfully synthesized (Nicolau *et al.*, 1994) in a complex series of reactions. The molecule has very limited solubility and must be administered

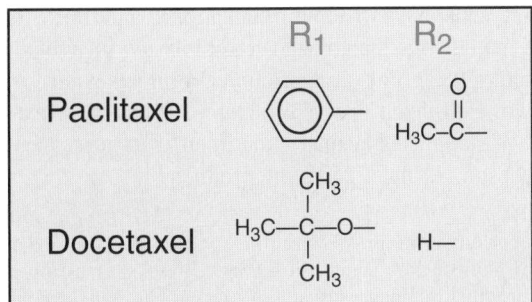

Figure 52–12. Chemical structures of paclitaxel (TAXOL) and its more potent analog, docetaxel (TAXOTERE).

Table 52–3
Paclitaxel Clearance as a Function of Drug Infusion Rate

SCHEDULE	INFUSION RATE, mg/m^2 PER HOUR	PLASMA CLEARANCE, ml/min per m^2
1. 175 mg/m^2 over 3 hours	58	212
2. 175 mg/m^2 over 24 hours	7	393
3. 140 mg/m^2 over 96 hours	1.5	471

in a vehicle of 50% ethanol and 50% polyethoxylated castor oil (Cremophor EL), a formation likely responsible for a high rate of hypersensitivity reactions in patients not protected with both a histamine H$_1$-receptor antagonist such as diphenhydramine, an H$_2$-receptor antagonist such as cimetidine (*see* Chapter 25), and a corticosteroid such as dexamethasone (*see* Chapter 60).

Mechanism of Action.   Interest in paclitaxel was stimulated by the finding that the drug possessed the unique ability to promote microtubule formation at cold temperatures and in the absence of GTP. It binds specifically to the β-tubulin subunit of microtubules and appears to antagonize the disassembly of this key cytoskeletal protein, with the result that bundles of microtubules and aberrant structures derived from microtubules appear in paclitaxel-treated cells. Arrest in mitosis follows. Cell killing is dependent on both drug concentrations and duration of cell exposure. Drugs that block the progression of cells through DNA synthesis and into mitosis antagonize the toxic effects of paclitaxel. Schedules for its optimal use alone or in combination with other drugs, including doxorubicin and cisplatin, are still in evolution. Drug interactions have been noted; the sequence of cisplatin preceding paclitaxel prolongs paclitaxel clearance and produces greater toxicity than the opposite schedule (Rowinsky *et al.,* 1991).

In cultured tumor cells, resistance to paclitaxel is associated in some lines with increased expression of the *mdr*-1 gene and its product, the P-glycoprotein; other resistant cells have β-tubulin mutations, and these latter cells may display heightened sensitivity to vinca alkaloids (Cabral, 1983). The basis of clinical drug resistance is not known. Cell death occurs by apoptosis, but the effectiveness of paclitaxel against experimental tumors does not depend on an intact p53 gene product.

Absorption, Fate, and Excretion.   Paclitaxel is administered as a 3-hour or 24-hour infusion every 3 weeks, or as a weekly 1-hour infusion. Longer infusions (96 hours) have yielded significant response rates in breast cancer patients in preliminary trials (Wilson *et al.,* 1994), but this form of treatment has serious practical limitations. The drug undergoes extensive P450-mediated

hepatic metabolism (isoenzymes CYP3A4 and CYP2C8), and less than 10% of a dose is excreted in the urine intact. The primary metabolite identified thus far is 6-OH paclitaxel, but multiple additional products are found in urine and plasma (Cresteil *et al.,* 1994).

Paclitaxel clearance is saturable and decreases with increasing dose or dose rate (Table 52–3). In studies of 96-hour infusion of 35 mg/m^2 per day, the presence of hepatic metastases greater than 2 cm in diameter decreased clearance and led to high drug levels in plasma and greater myelosuppression. Paclitaxel disappears from the plasma compartment with half-lives of approximately 0.2, 2, and 20 hours. The critical plasma concentration for inhibiting bone marrow elements depends on duration of exposure but likely lies in the range of 0.01 to 0.1 μM (Huizing *et al.,* 1993).

While precise guidelines for dose reduction in patients with abnormal hepatic function have not been established, 50% to 75% doses should be used in the presence of hepatic metastases greater than 2 cm in size or in patients with abnormal serum bilirubin (Donehower, 2001). Drugs that induce CYP3A4, such as phenytoin or phenobarbital, or those that inhibit the same cytochrome, such as antifungal imidazoles, may significantly alter drug clearance and toxicity.

Therapeutic Uses.   *Paclitaxel* (TAXOL) has undergone testing in patients with metastatic ovarian and breast cancers; it has significant activity as a component of primary combination therapy regimens and in adjuvant therapy of breast cancer (McGuire *et al.,* 1996; Seidman, 1998). Response rates in relapsed patients range from 20% to 30%, depending on the treatment history and the regimen employed. Clinical trials indicate significant response rates in lung, head and neck, esophageal, and bladder carcinomas as well (Redman *et al.,* 1998). The optimal schedule of paclitaxel administration, alone or in combination with other drugs, has not been defined.

Clinical Toxicities.   Paclitaxel exerts its primary toxic effects on the bone marrow. Neutropenia usually occurs 8 to 11 days after a dose and reverses rapidly by days 15 to 21. Used with filgrastim (G-CSF), doses as high as 250 mg/m^2 over 24 hours are well tolerated, and peripheral neuropathy becomes dose-limiting (Kohn *et al.,* 1994). Many patients experience myalgias for several days after receiving paclitaxel. In high-dose schedules, a stocking–glove sensory neuropathy can be disabling, particularly in patients with underlying diabetic or alcoholic neuropathy. Mucositis is prominent in 72- or 96-hour infusions and in the weekly schedule.

Hypersensitivity reactions occurred in patients receiving paclitaxel infusions of short duration (1 to 6 hours) but have largely been averted by pretreatment with dexamethasone, diphenhydramine, and histamine H_2-receptor antagonists, as noted above. Premedication is not necessary with 96-hour infusion. Many patients experience asymptomatic bradycardia, and occasional episodes of silent ventricular tachycardia also occur and resolve spontaneously during 3- or 24-hour infusions.

EPIPODOPHYLLOTOXINS

Podophyllotoxin, extracted from the mandrake plant (mayapple; *Podophyllum peltatum*), was used as a folk remedy by the American Indians and early colonists for its emetic, cathartic, and anthelmintic effects. Two semisynthetic glycosides of the active principle, podophyllotoxin, have been developed that show significant therapeutic activity in several human neoplasms, including pediatric leukemia, small cell carcinomas of the lung, testicular tumors, Hodgkin's disease, and large cell lymphomas. These derivatives are referred to as *etoposide* (VP-16-213) and *teniposide* (VM-26). Although podophyllotoxin binds to tubulin at a site distinct from that for interaction with the vinca alkaloids, etoposide and teniposide have no effect on microtubular structure or function at usual concentrations (for reviews of the epipodophyllotoxins, *see* Hande, 1998; and Pommier *et al.*, 2001).

Chemistry. The chemical structures of etoposide and teniposide are shown below. They have been selected from many derivatives of podophyllotoxin that have been synthesized during the past 20 years.

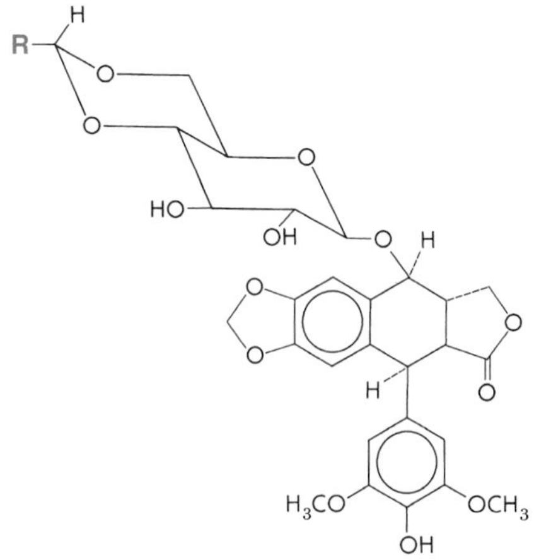

ETOPOSIDE: R = CH$_3$

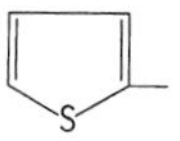

TENIPOSIDE: R =

Mechanism of Action. Etoposide and teniposide are similar in their actions and in the spectrum of human tumors affected. Unlike podophyllotoxin, they do not arrest cells in mitosis; rather, these compounds form a ternary complex with topoisomerase II and DNA. This complex results in double-stranded DNA breaks, but the strand passage and resealing of the break that normally follow topoisomerase binding to DNA are inhibited by the drug. The enzyme remains bound to the free end of the broken DNA strand, leading to an accumulation of DNA breaks and cell death (Pommier *et al.*, 2001). Cells in the S and G_2 phases of the cell cycle are most sensitive to etoposide and teniposide. Resistant cells demonstrate either amplification of the *mdr*-1 gene that encodes the P-glycoprotein drug efflux transporter, mutation or decreased expression of topoisomerase II, or mutations of the p53 tumor suppressor gene, a required component of the apoptosis, or cell-death, pathway (Lowe *et al.*, 1993).

Etoposide

Absorption, Fate, and Excretion. Oral administration of etoposide results in variable absorption that averages about 50% of the drug. After intravenous injection, peak plasma concentrations of 30 μg/ml are achieved; there is a biphasic pattern of clearance with a terminal half-life of about 6 to 8 hours in patients with normal renal function. Approximately 40% of an administered dose is excreted intact in the urine. In patients with compromised renal function, dosage should be reduced in proportion to the reduction in creatinine clearance (Arbuck *et al.*, 1986). In patients with advanced liver disease, low serum albumin and elevated bilirubin (which displaces etoposide from albumin) tend to increase the unbound fraction of drug, increasing the toxicity of any given dose. However, guidelines for dose reduction in this circumstance have not been defined (Stewart *et al.*, 1991). Drug concentrations in the cerebrospinal fluid average 1% to 10% of those in plasma.

Therapeutic Uses. The intravenous dose of *etoposide* (VEPESID, TOPOSAR, ETOPOPHOS) for testicular cancer in combination therapy is 50 to 100 mg/m^2 for 5 days, or 100 mg/m^2 on alternate days for three doses. For small cell carcinoma of the lung, the dose in combination therapy is 50 to 120 mg/m^2 per day intravenously for 3 days or 50 mg per day orally for 21 days. Cycles of therapy are usually repeated every 3 to 4 weeks. The drug should be administered slowly during a 30- to 60-minute infusion to avoid hypotension and bronchospasm, which likely result from the additives used to dissolve etoposide, a relatively insoluble compound.

A disturbing complication of etoposide therapy has emerged in long-term follow-up of patients with childhood acute lymphoblastic leukemia, who develop an unusual form of acute nonlymphocytic leukemia with a translocation in chromosome 11 at 11q23. At this locus is found a gene(s) (the MLL or mixed-lineage leukemia gene) that regulates the proliferation of pluripotent stem cells. The leukemic cells have the cytological appearance of acute monocytic or monomyelocytic leukemia. Another distinguishing feature of etoposide-related leukemia is the short time interval between end of treatment and leukemia (1 to 3 years), as compared to the 4- to 5-year interval for secondary leukemias related to alkylating agents, and the absence of a myelodysplastic period preceding leukemia (Levine and Bloomfield, 1992; Pui *et al.*, 1995; Sandler *et al.*, 1997; Smith *et al.*, 1999). Patients receiving weekly or twice-weekly doses of etoposide, with cumulative doses above 2000 mg/m^2, seem to be at higher risk of leukemia.

Etoposide is used primarily for treatment of testicular tumors, in combination with bleomycin and cisplatin, and in combination with cisplatin and ifosfamide for small cell carcinoma of the lung (Nemati *et al.*, 2000). It also is active against non-Hodgkin's lymphomas, acute nonlymphocytic leukemia, and Kaposi's sarcoma associated with acquired immunodeficiency syndrome (AIDS) (Chao *et al.*, 2000; Tung *et al.*, 2000). Etoposide has a favorable toxicity profile for dose escalation in that its primary toxicity is myelosuppression. In combination with ifosfamide and carboplatin, it is frequently used for high-dose chemotherapy in total doses of 1500 to 2000 mg/m^2 (Sobecks *et al.*, 2000; Donato *et al.*, 2000; Josting *et al.*, 2000).

Clinical Toxicities.   The dose-limiting toxicity of etoposide is leukopenia, with a nadir at 10 to 14 days and recovery by 3 weeks. Thrombocytopenia occurs less often and usually is not severe. Nausea, vomiting, stomatitis, and diarrhea occur in approximately 15% of patients treated intravenously and in about 55% of patients who receive the drug orally. Alopecia is common but reversible. Fever, phlebitis, dermatitis, and allergic reactions including anaphylaxis have been observed. Hepatic toxicity is particularly evident after high-dose treatment. For both etoposide and teniposide, toxicity is increased in patients with decreased serum albumin, an effect related to decreased protein binding of the drug (Stewart *et al.*, 1991).

Teniposide

Teniposide (VUMON) is administered intravenously. It has a multiphasic pattern of clearance from plasma. After distribution, half-lives of 4 hours and 10 to 40 hours are observed. Approximately 45% of the drug is excreted in the urine but, in contrast to etoposide, as much as 80% is recovered as metabolites. Anticonvulsants such as phenytoin increase the hepatic metabolism of teniposide and reduce systemic exposure (Baker *et al.*, 1992). Dosage need not be reduced for patients with impaired renal function (Sinkule *et al.*, 1984; Pommier *et al.*, 2001). Less than 1% of the drug crosses the blood–brain barrier. However, teniposide has produced responses in small cell and non-small cell lung cancer metastases in the brain (Postmus *et al.*, 1995; Boogerd *et al.*, 1999).

Teniposide is available for treatment of refractory acute lymphoblastic leukemia in children and appears to be synergistic with cytarabine. It is administered by intravenous infusion in doses that range from 50 mg/m^2 per day for 5 days to 165 mg/m^2 per day twice weekly. The clinical spectrum of activity includes acute leukemia in children, particularly monocytic leukemia in infants, as well as glioblastoma, neuroblastoma, and brain metastases from small cell carcinomas of the lung (Odom and Gordon, 1984; Postmus *et al.*, 1995; Boogerd *et al.*, 1999). Myelosuppression, nausea, and vomiting are its primary toxic effects.

CAMPTOTHECIN ANALOGS

The camptothecins are a promising new class of antineoplastic agents that target the nuclear enzyme topoisomerase I. The first compound in this class, *camptothecin,* was isolated from the Chinese tree *Camptotheca acuminata* in 1966. Despite the significant antitumor activity observed with the parent compound in preclinical models and in early clinical trials, further clinical development was compromised by severe and unpredictable toxicity, principally myelosuppression and hemorrhagic cystitis. Improved understanding of the mechanism of action and clinical pharmacology of these agents during the 1980s, led to the development of more soluble and less toxic analogs. *Irinotecan* and *topotecan* are currently the most widely used camptothecin analogs in the clinical setting, with established activity in colorectal, ovarian, and small cell lung cancer (for review, *see* Takimoto and Arbuck, 2001).

Chemistry.   All camptothecins contain a basic five-ring structure, with a chiral center at C-20 of the terminal lactone ring (Figure 52–13). The naturally occurring (*S*)-isomer is 10- to 100-times more active against topoisomerase I than is the (*R*)-isomer. Substitutions at C-9 and C-10 can enhance water solubility and increase topoisomerase I inhibition. Topotecan [(*S*)-9-dimethylaminoethyl-10-hydroxycamptothecin hydrochloride] is a semisynthetic camptothecin analog. It incorporates a basic dimethyl-amino side chain at C-9 which increases its water solubility. Irinotecan (7-ethyl-10-[4-(1-piperidino)-1-piperidino]carbonyloxycamptothecin, or CPT-11) differs from topotecan in

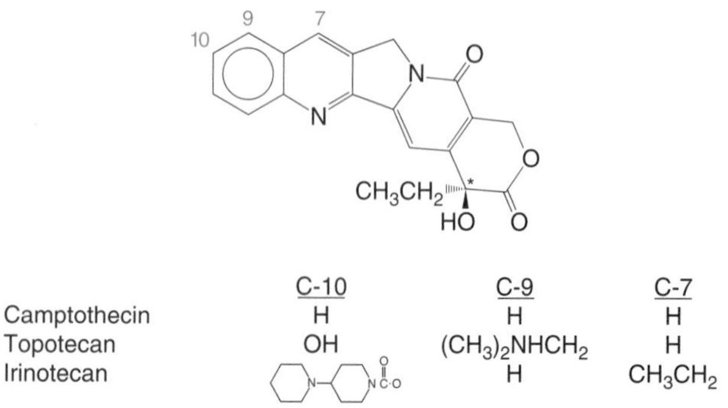

	C-10	C-9	C-7
Camptothecin	H	H	H
Topotecan	OH	(CH$_3$)$_2$NHCH$_2$	H
Irinotecan		H	CH$_3$CH$_2$

Figure 52–13. Chemical structures of camptothecin and its analogs.

that it is a prodrug. Its bulky piperidino side chain at position C-10, is cleaved by a carboxylesterase-converting enzyme to form the biologically active metabolite, SN-38. SN-38 is 1000-fold more potent than irinotecan in inhibiting topoisomerase I.

Although an intact lactone ring is necessary for camptothecin's activity, it is unstable in aqueous solutions at neutral or basic pH. The lactone ring undergoes a rapid, reversible, nonenzymatic hydrolysis to form the carboxylate, which has greater water solubility but is 10-fold less potent than the lactone. In the absence of proteins, the lactone hydrolysis of different camptothecin analogs occurs at about the same rate, and at physiological pH the carboxylate form predominates. However, the equilibrium ratio in plasma between the carboxylate and lactone species of different topoisomerase I inhibitors is greatly dependent upon their relative degree of albumin binding. For camptothecin, for instance, the carboxylate form binds to serum albumin with a 200-fold greater affinity, and it is the predominant form found in blood. In contrast, for SN-38, the lactone form is the one that preferentially binds to serum albumin, thus shifting the equilibrium in the opposite direction.

Mechanism of Action. The DNA topoisomerases are nuclear enzymes that reduce supercoiled DNA torsional stress, allowing selected regions of DNA to become sufficiently untangled and relaxed to permit essential cellular processes to occur, such as DNA replication, recombination, repair, and transcription. Two classes of topoisomerase (I and II) are known to mediate DNA strand breakage and resealing, and both have become the target of cancer chemotherapies. Camptothecin analogs inhibit the function of topoisomerase I, while a number of different chemical entities (anthracyclines, epipodophyllotoxins, acridines) inhibit topoisomerase II. Topoisomerase I binds covalently to double-stranded DNA through a reversible trans-esterification reaction. This reaction yields an intermediate complex in which the tyrosine of the enzyme is bound to the 3-phosphate end of the DNA strand, creating a single-strand DNA break. This 'cleavable complex' allows for relaxation of the DNA torsional strain, either by passage of the intact single-strand through the nick, or by free rotation of the DNA about the noncleaved strand. Once the DNA torsional strain has been relieved, the topoisomerase I reseals the cleavage and dissociates from the newly relaxed double helix.

The camptothecins bind to and stabilize the normally transient DNA-topoisomerase I cleavable complex (Hsiang et al., 1985). Although the initial cleavage action of topoisomerase I is not affected, the religation step is inhibited, leading to the accumulation of single-stranded breaks in DNA. This DNA damage, by itself, is not toxic to the cell, because upon drug removal, religation of DNA occurs. However, the collision of a DNA replication fork with this cleaved strand of DNA causes an irreversible double-strand DNA break, ultimately leading to cell death (Tsao et al., 1993). Since ongoing DNA synthesis is necessary for cytotoxicity, camptothecins are S-phase specific drugs. This has important clinical implications, because S-phase-specific cytotoxic agents generally require prolonged exposures of tumor cells to drug concentrations above a minimum threshold in order to optimize therapeutic efficacy. In fact, preclinical studies of low-dose, protracted administration of camptothecin analogs have shown less toxicity, and equal or greater antitumor activity than shorter, more intense courses.

The precise sequence of events that lead from drug-induced DNA damage to cell death has not been fully elucidated. *In vitro* studies have shown that camptothecin-induced DNA damage abolishes the activation of $p34^{cdc2}$/cyclin B complex, leading to cell-cycle arrest at the G2 phase (Tsao et al., 1992). It also has been observed that treatment with camptothecins can induce the transcription of *c-fos* and *c-jun* early-response genes, and this occurs in association with internucleosomal DNA fragmentation, a characteristic of programmed cell death (Kharbanda et al., 1991). Camptothecins also can induce the differentiation of human leukemia cells. Finally, camptothecin-induced cytotoxicity also has been observed in cells not actively synthesizing DNA. Replication-independent mechanisms of cytotoxicity may involve the induction of serine proteases and endonucleases.

Mechanisms of Resistance. A variety of mechanisms of resistance to topoisomerase I–targeted agents have been characterized *in vitro*, although little is known about their significance in the clinical setting. Decreased intracellular drug accumulation has been observed in several cell lines resistant to camptothecin analogs. Several topoisomerase I inhibitors have been shown to be substrates for P-glycoprotein, a cell membrane transporter that carries different cytotoxic drugs and toxins out of the cell and confers multidrug resistance to tumor cells. However, multidrug resistance (MDR) gene-expressing cell lines are only 9- to 12-fold more resistant to topotecan or SN-38 than are their parental wild-type counterparts, a much smaller degree of resistance than the 200-fold change in sensitivity for classic P-glycoprotein substrates such as etoposide or doxorubicin. Other reports have associated topotecan or irinotecan resistance and the multidrug resistance-associated protein (MRP) class of transporters. Another energy-dependent pump (MRP-3) confers resistance to mitoxantrone (an anthracenedione), but also to topotecan, irinotecan, and SN-38, but not to the parent compound, camptothecin (Miyake et al., 1999). Drug metabolism may play an important role in the resistance to the prodrug irinotecan. Cell lines that lack carboxylesterase activity, and therefore are unable to convert irinotecan to SN-38, demonstrate resistance to this camptothecin analog (van Ark-Otte et al., 1998). Camptothecin resistance also may result from decreased expression or mutation of topoisomerase I. Although a good correlation has been found in certain tumor cell lines between sensitivity to camptothecin analogs and topoisomerase I levels (Sugimoto et al., 1990), clinical studies have not confirmed this association. Chromosomal deletions or hypermethylation of the topoisomerase I gene are possible mechanisms of decreased topoisomerase I expression in resistant cells. A transient down-regulation of topoisomerase I has been demonstrated following prolonged exposure to camptothecins *in vitro* and *in vivo*. Moreover, an association between the degree of topoisomerase I down-regulation in peripheral blood mononuclear cells and the area under the plasma concentration-time curve (AUC) or neutrophil nadir has been observed in ovarian cancer patients treated with a 21-day continuous intravenous infusion of topotecan (Hochster et al., 1999). Mutations leading to reduced topoisomerase I enzyme catalytic activity or DNA binding affinity also have been described *in vitro* in association with camptothecin resistance (Tamura et al., 1991). In addition, some posttranscriptional events, such as enzyme phosphorylation (Pommier et al., 1990) or poly-ADP ribosylation (Kasid et al., 1989), may have a significant impact on the activity of topoisomerase I and on its susceptibility to inhibition. Finally, an observation of potential clinical interest is that exposure of cells to topoisomerase I–targeted agents leads to increased expression of topoisomerase II, providing a rationale for sequential therapy with topoisomerase I and II inhibitors.

Very little is known about how the cell deals with the stabilized DNA-topoisomerase complexes. As cleavable complexes normally are present in the untreated cell, the drug-enzyme-DNA complex may not be recognized easily by cellular repair processes. However, an enzyme with specific tyrosyl-DNA phosphodiesterase activity may be involved in the disassembly of topoisomerase I–DNA complexes (Yang *et al.*, 1996). Entry into S phase is required to kill tumor cells exposed to camptothecins. Drugs that abolish the G_1-S checkpoint enhance lethality of camptothecins (Shao *et al.*, 1997). The fact that cell cycle arrest in G_2 has been correlated with drug resistance to topoisomerase I-targeted drugs in colon cancer and leukemia cell lines *in vitro* suggests the possibility that enhanced DNA repair activity can lead to camptothecin resistance. The role of p53 in mediating cell death due to camptothecins is unclear. These drugs induce p53 expression, but cells without functional p53 also can undergo apoptosis following exposure to camptothecins.

Absorption, Fate, and Excretion. *Topotecan.* Topotecan is administered intravenously, and is rapidly cleared from the plasma. Only 20% to 35% of the total drug in plasma is found to be in the active lactone form. The terminal half-life of topotecan lactone ranges between 2 and 3.5 hours, which is relatively short compared with other camptothecins. Bioavailability of topotecan following oral administration is about 30% to 40%. Unlike other topoisomerase I inhibitors, plasma-protein binding of topotecan is low (7% to 35%), a finding that may explain the higher CNS penetration compared with other camptothecins (29% to 42%).

Few data are available concerning topotecan metabolism. Three novel metabolites, N-desmethyl topotecan, topotecan-O-glucuronide, and N-desmethyl topotecan-O-glucuronide, which are found at low concentrations in plasma, urine, and bile, have been characterized (Rosing *et al.*, 1998). Elimination of the lactone form is thought to result mainly from the rapid hydrolysis to the carboxylate species followed by renal excretion. Between 25% and 70% of the administered dose is excreted in the urine within 24 hours, and doses should be reduced in proportion to reductions in creatinine clearance.

Irinotecan. Both the lactone and the open-ring carboxylate species of irinotecan and SN-38 can be measured in plasma shortly after an intravenous infusion. However, the overall AUC ratio of SN-38 to irinotecan is only about 4%. Compared to other camptothecin derivatives, a relatively large fraction of both irinotecan and SN-38 in plasma is present as the biologically active lactone form. Another potential advantage of this camptothecin analog are the longer plasma terminal half-lives of both irinotecan and its active metabolite, SN-38 (both about 10 hours). The oral bioavailability of irinotecan is low (8%). However, the molar SN-38 to irinotecan AUC ratio is threefold higher after oral administration than after identical intravenous doses. A potential explanation for this observation is extensive first-pass metabolism, with significant conversion of irinotecan to SN-38 by carboxylesterase present in the intestine and liver. Plasma-protein binding is 43% or higher for irinote-

can and 92% to 96% for SN-38. CSF penetration of SN-38 in humans has not been characterized yet, although in rhesus monkeys it is only 14%, significantly lower than that observed for topotecan.

Irinotecan is converted to its active metabolite, SN-38, by the carboxylesterase-converting enzyme. Variations in this enzyme's activity in tumor cells or in normal host tissues may be important in determining irinotecan antitumor effect and/or toxicity. SN-38, although much more potent than the parent drug, represents only a small fraction of the total irinotecan metabolized. Other irinotecan metabolites have been characterized, including 7-ethyl-10-[4-N-(5-aminopentanoic acid)-1-piperidino] carbonyloxycamptothecin (APC), and 7-ethyl-10-(4-amino-1-piperidino) carbonyloxycamptothecin (NPC), both of which are poor inhibitors of topoisomerase I. CYP3A seems to be responsible for the production of these 2 metabolites (Haaz *et al.*, 1998). Since this enzyme is involved in the metabolism of a large number of commonly used drugs, drug interactions may have significant impact on irinotecan pharmacokinetics.

Glucuronidation is the major metabolic route of SN-38. The uridine diphosphate glucuronosyl transferase (UGT), particularly the UGT1A1 isoform, converts SN-38 to its glucuronidated derivative (Iyer *et al.*, 1998). Both SN-38 and its glucuronide are excreted in the bile. The extent of SN-38 glucuronidation has been inversely correlated with the risk of severe diarrhea after irinotecan therapy. UGT1A1 also glucuronidates bilirubin. Polymorphisms of this enzyme are associated with familial hyperbilirubinemia syndromes such as Crigler–Najjar (CN) syndrome and Gilbert syndrome. CN syndromes are rare (1 in a million births), but Gilbert syndrome occurs in up to 15% of the general population, and results in a mild hyperbilirubinemia that may be clinically silent. The existence of UGT enzyme polymorphisms may have a major impact on the clinical use of irinotecan. A positive correlation has been found between baseline serum unconjugated bilirubin concentration and both severity of neutropenia and the AUC of irinotecan and SN-38 in patients treated with this camptothecin analog. Moreover, severe irinotecan toxicity has been observed in cancer patients with Gilbert syndrome, presumably due to decreased glucuronidation of SN-38. Biliary excretion appears to be the primary elimination route of irinotecan, SN-38, and their glucuronides, although urinary excretion also contributes significantly (14% to 37%). The presence of bacterial β-glucuronidase in the intestinal lumen potentially can contribute to irinotecan's gastrointestinal toxicity by releasing unconjugated SN-38 from the inactive glucuronide metabolite excreted in the bile. The existence of multiple metabolic pathways for irinotecan, many of them as yet unidentified, is underscored by the fact that only about 50% of the total administered dose is recovered in urine (28%) and feces (25%) as unchanged irinotecan or its metabolites (SN-38, SN-38G, APC, and NPC).

Therapeutic Uses. *Topotecan.* Topotecan (HYCAMTIN) is given as a 30-minute infusion of 1.5 mg/m^2 per day for 5 consecutive days every 3 weeks. A variety of prolonged infusion schedules also have been tested. In experimental studies, topotecan has been administered orally, but this route is still investigational.

Since a significant fraction of the topotecan administered is excreted in the urine, severe toxicities have been observed in patients with decreased creatinine clearance (O'Reilly *et al.*, 1996). Therefore, the dose of topotecan should be reduced to 0.75 mg/m² per day in patients with moderate renal dysfunction (creatinine clearance 20 to 40 ml/minute), and topotecan should not be administered to patients with severe renal impairment (creatinine clearance <20 ml/minute). Topotecan clearance and toxicity are not significantly altered in patients with hepatic dysfunction, and therefore, no dose reduction is necessary in these patients.

Topotecan is active in previously treated patients with ovarian (ten Bokkel Huinink *et al.*, 1997) or small cell lung cancer (von Pawel *et al.*, 1999). Its significant hematological toxicity, though, has limited its use in combination with other active agents in these diseases (*e.g.*, cisplatin). Promising antitumor activity also has been observed in hematological malignancies, particularly in chronic myelomonocytic leukemia and in myelodysplastic syndromes.

Irinotecan. Approved dosage schedules of *irinotecan* (CAMPTOSAR) in the United States include: 125 mg/m² as a 90-minute infusion administered weekly for 4 out of 6 weeks; 350 mg/m² given every 3 weeks; 100 mg/m² every week; or 150 mg/m² every other week. Prolonged irinotecan infusions and oral administration also have been explored.

Irinotecan has significant clinical activity in patients with advanced colorectal cancer. It is now the treatment of choice in combination with fluoropyrimidines for advanced colorectal cancer in patients who have not received chemotherapy previously (Douillard *et al.*, 2000) or as a single agent following failure on a 5-fluorouracil regimen (Cunningham *et al.*, 1998). Encouraging results from different phase II studies suggest that irinotecan may have an increasing role in the treatment of other solid tumors, including small cell and non–small cell lung cancer, cervical cancer, ovarian cancer, and gastric cancer.

Clinical Toxicities *Topotecan.* The dose-limiting toxicity with all schedules is neutropenia, with or without thrombocytopenia. The incidence of severe neutropenia at the recommended phase II dose of 1.5 mg/m² daily for 5 days every 3 weeks may be as high as 81%, with a 26% incidence of febrile neutropenia. Dose intensity with the 21-day continuous infusion exceeds that achieved with other schedules, but this is associated with a higher incidence of thrombocytopenia and cumulative anemia. In patients with hematological malignancies, gastrointestinal side effects such as mucositis and diarrhea become dose-limiting. Other less common and generally mild topotecan-related toxicities include nausea

and vomiting, elevated liver transaminases, fever, fatigue, and rash.

Irinotecan. The dose-limiting toxicity with all schedules is delayed diarrhea, with or without neutropenia. In the initial studies, up to 35% of the patients experienced severe diarrhea. Adoption of the intensive *loperamide* (*see* Chapter 39) regimen (4 mg of loperamide starting at the onset of any loose stool beginning more than a few hours after receiving therapy, followed by 2 mg every 2 hours) has effectively reduced this incidence by more than half. However, once severe diarrhea does occur, standard doses of antidiarrheal agents tend to be ineffective, although the diarrhea episode generally resolves within a week and, unless associated with fever and neutropenia, is rarely fatal.

The second most common irinotecan-associated toxicity is myelosuppression. Severe neutropenia occurs in 14% to 47% of the patients treated with the every-3-week schedule, and is less frequently encountered among patients treated with the weekly schedule. Febrile neutropenia is observed in 3% of the patients, and may be fatal, particularly when associated with concomitant diarrhea. A cholinergic syndrome resulting from the inhibition of acetylcholinesterase activity by irinotecan may occur within the first 24 hours after irinotecan administration. Symptoms include acute diarrhea, diaphoresis, hypersalivation, abdominal cramps, visual accommodation disturbances, lacrimation, rhinorrhea, and less often, asymptomatic bradycardia. These effects are short lasting and respond within minutes to atropine. Atropine may be prophylactically administered to patients who have previously experienced a cholinergic reaction, prior to the administration of additional cycles of irinotecan. Other common and generally manageable toxicities include nausea and vomiting, fatigue, vasodilation or skin flushing, mucositis, liver transaminases elevation, and alopecia. Finally, there have been case reports of dyspnea and interstitial pneumonitis associated with irinotecan therapy in Japanese patients with lung cancer (Fukuoka *et al.*, 1992).

ANTIBIOTICS

Dactinomycin (Actinomycin D)

History. The first crystalline antibiotic agent to be isolated from a culture broth of a species of *Streptomyces* was actinomycin A (Waksman and Woodruff, 1940). Many related antibiotics, including actinomycin D, subsequently have been obtained (Waksman Conference on Actinomycins, 1974). Dactinomycin has beneficial effects in the treatment of a number of tumors, particularly certain neoplasms of childhood and choriocarcinoma.

Chemistry and Structure–Activity Relationship. The actinomycins are chromopeptides, and most of them contain the same chromophore, the planar phenoxazone actinocin, which is responsible for the yellow-red color of the compounds. The differences among naturally occurring actinomycins are confined to the peptide side chains, and the variations are in the structure of the constituent amino acids. By varying the amino acid content of the growth medium, it is possible to alter the types of actinomycins produced and the biological activity of the molecule

(Crooke, 1983). The chemical structure of dactinomycin is as follows:

DACTINOMYCIN
(Sar = sarcosine)
(Meval = N-methylvaline)

Mechanism of Action.   The capacity of actinomycins to bind with double-helical DNA is responsible for their biological activity and cytotoxicity. X-ray studies of a crystalline complex between dactinomycin and deoxyguanosine permitted formulation of a model that appears to explain the binding of the drug to DNA (Sobell, 1973). The planar phenoxazone ring intercalates between adjacent guanine–cytosine base pairs of DNA, where the guanine moieties are on opposite strands of the DNA, while the polypeptide chains extend along the minor groove of the helix. The summation of these interactions provides great stability to the dactinomycin–DNA complex, and, as a result of the binding of dactinomycin, the transcription of DNA by RNA polymerase is blocked. The DNA-dependent RNA polymerases are much more sensitive to the effects of dactinomycin than are the DNA polymerases. In addition, dactinomycin causes single-strand breaks in DNA, possibly through a free-radical intermediate or as a result of the action of topoisomerase II (*see* Waksman Conference on Actinomycins, 1974; Goldberg *et al.*, 1977).

Cytotoxic Action.   Dactinomycin inhibits rapidly proliferating cells of normal and neoplastic origin and, on a molar basis, is among the most potent antitumor agents known. Atrophy of thymus, spleen, and other lymphatic tissues occurs in experimental animals. The drug may produce alopecia, and, when extravasated subcutaneously, causes marked local inflammation. Erythema, sometimes progressing to necrosis, has been noted in areas of the skin exposed to x-radiation before, during, or after administration of dactinomycin.

Absorption, Fate, and Excretion.   Dactinomycin is much less potent when given orally than when administered by parenteral injection. The drug is excreted both in bile and in the urine and disappears from plasma with a terminal half-life of 36 hours. Metabolism of the drug is minimal. Dactinomycin does not cross the blood–brain barrier.

Therapeutic Uses.   *Dactinomycin* (*actinomycin D;* COS-MEGEN) is supplied for intravenous use. The usual daily dose is 10 to 15 μg/kg; this is given intravenously for 5 days; if no manifestations of toxicity are encountered, ad-

ditional courses may be given at intervals of 2 to 4 weeks. Daily injections of 100 to 400 μg have been given to children for 10 to 14 days; in other regimens, 3 to 6 μg/kg per day, for a total of 125 μg/kg, and weekly maintenance doses of 7.5 μg/kg have been used. Although it is safer to administer the drug into the tubing of an intravenous infusion, direct intravenous injections have been given, with the precaution of discarding the needle used to withdraw the drug from the vial to avoid subcutaneous reaction. The drug is extremely corrosive to soft tissues.

The most important clinical use of dactinomycin is in the treatment of rhabdomyosarcoma and Wilms' tumor in children, where it is curative in combination with primary surgery, radiotherapy, and other drugs, particularly vincristine and cyclophosphamide (Pinkel and Howarth, 1985). Antineoplastic activity has been noted in Ewing's tumor, Kaposi's sarcoma, and soft tissue sarcomas. Dactinomycin can be effective in women with advanced cases of choriocarcinoma. It also produces consistent responses in combination with chlorambucil and methotrexate in patients with metastatic testicular carcinomas, but this regimen is not as effective as those that incorporate vinblastine or etoposide plus cisplatin and bleomycin. It is of limited value in other neoplastic diseases of adults, although a response sometimes may be observed in patients with Hodgkin's disease or non-Hodgkin's lymphomas. Dactinomycin also has been used to inhibit immunological responses, particularly the rejection of renal transplants.

Clinical Toxicities.   Toxic manifestations include anorexia, nausea, and vomiting, usually beginning a few hours after administration. Hematopoietic suppression with pancytopenia may occur in the first week after completion of therapy. Proctitis, diarrhea, glossitis, cheilitis, and ulcerations of the oral mucosa are common; dermatological manifestations include alopecia, as well as erythema, desquamation, and increased inflammation and pigmentation in areas previously or concomitantly subjected to x-radiation. Severe injury may occur as a result of local toxic extravasation.

Daunorubicin, Doxorubicin, and Idarubicin

These anthracycline antibiotics and their derivatives are among the most important antitumor agents. They are produced by the fungus *Streptococcus peucetius* var. *caesius*. Idarubicin is a synthetic derivative. Although they differ only slightly in chemical structure, daunorubicin and idarubicin have been used primarily in the acute leukemias, whereas doxorubicin displays broader activity against human neoplasms, including a variety of solid tumors. The clinical value of these agents is limited by an unusual and often irreversible cardiomyopathy, the occurrence of which is related to the total dose of the drug. In a search for agents with high antitumor activity but reduced cardiac toxicity, hundreds of anthracycline derivatives and related compounds have been prepared. Several of these have shown promise in clinical studies, including idarubicin for leukemia, epirubicin for solid-tumor chemotherapy, and mitoxantrone for prostate cancer, leukemia, and high-dose chemotherapy. Mitoxantrone, an anthracenedione, has significantly less cardiotoxicity than do the anthracyclines (*see* Arlin *et al.*, 1990; Feldman *et al.*, 1993; Berman *et al.*, 1991; Wiernik *et al.*, 1992; Launchbury and Habboubi, 1993).

Chemistry. The anthracycline antibiotics have tetracycline ring structures with an unusual sugar, daunosamine, attached by glycosidic linkage. Cytotoxic agents of this class all have quinone and hydroquinone moieties on adjacent rings that permit them to function as electron-accepting and -donating agents. Although there are marked differences in the clinical use of daunorubicin and doxorubicin, their chemical structures differ only by a single hydroxyl group on C-14. Idarubicin is 4-demethoxydaunorubicin, a synthetic derivative of daunorubicin without the methoxy group on C-4 of the aglycone ring. The chemical structures of doxorubicin, daunorubicin, epirubicin, and idarubicin are as follows:

	DOXORUBICIN	DAUNORUBICIN	EPIRUBICIN	IDARUBICIN
R_1 =	OCH$_3$	OCH$_3$	OCH$_3$	H
R_2 =	H	H	OH	H
R_3 =	OH	OH	H	OH
R_4 =	OH	H	OH	H

Mechanism of Action. A number of important biochemical effects have been described for the anthracyclines and anthracenediones, any one or all of which could have a role in the therapeutic and toxic effects of such drugs. These compounds can intercalate with DNA. Many functions of DNA are affected, including DNA and RNA synthesis. Single- and double-strand breaks occur, as does sister chromatid exchange. Thus, the anthracyclines are both mutagenic and carcinogenic. Scission of DNA is believed to be mediated by drug binding to DNA and topoisomerase II, an action that prevents the resealing of DNA breaks created by the enzyme (Tewey *et al.*, 1984). Anthracyclines, by virtue of their quinone groups, also generate free radicals in solution and in both normal and malignant tissues (Gewirtz, 1999; Ikeda *et al.*, 1999). The anthracyclines react

with cytochrome P450 reductase in the presence of reduced nicotinamide adenine dinucleotide phosphate (NADPH) to form semiquinone radical intermediates, which in turn can react with oxygen to produce superoxide anion radicals. These can generate both hydrogen peroxide and hydroxyl radicals (·OH), which attack DNA (Serrano *et al.*, 1999) and oxidize DNA bases. The production of free radicals is significantly stimulated by the interaction of doxorubicin with iron (Myers, 1988). In addition, intramolecular electron-transfer reactions of the semiquinone intermediates result in the generation of lipid peroxides, nitric oxide, and other destructive radicals. Enzymatic defenses such as superoxide dismutase and catalase are believed to have an important role in protecting cells against the toxicity of the anthracyclines, and these defenses can be augmented by exogenous antioxidants such as *alpha tocopherol* or by an iron chelator, *dexrazoxane* (formerly called ICRF-187), which protects against cardiac toxicity (Speyer *et al.*, 1988; Swain *et al.*, 1997). The anthracyclines also can interact with cell membranes, producing lipid peroxides and altering their functions; this may play an important part in both the antitumor actions and the cardiac toxicity caused by these drugs (Tritton *et al.*, 1978).

Exposure of cells to anthracyclines leads to apoptosis; mediators of this process include the p53 DNA-damage sensor and activated caspases (proteases), although ceramide, a lipid breakdown product, and the fas receptor-ligand system also have been implicated in selected tumor cells (Friesen *et al.*, 1996; Jaffrezou *et al.*, 1996).

As discussed above, the phenomenon of pleiotropic drug resistance is observed in tumor cell populations exposed to anthracyclines. This appears to result from acceleration of the efflux of anthracyclines and other agents from the cell. The P-glycoprotein, synthesized in high quantity as a result of gene amplification, has been implicated (Endicott and Ling, 1989). Anthracyclines also are exported from tumor cells by members of the MRP transporter family (Doyle *et al.*, 1998). Other biochemical changes in resistant cells include increased glutathione peroxidase activity (Sinha *et al.*, 1989) and decreased activity of topoisomerase II (Deffie *et al.*, 1989; Jarvinen *et al.*, 1998).

Absorption, Fate, and Excretion. Daunorubicin, doxorubicin, epirubicin, and idarubicin usually are administered intravenously and are cleared by hepatic metabolism and biliary excretion. The disappearance curve for doxorubicin is multiphasic, with elimination half-lives of 3 hours and about 30 hours. Idarubicin has a half-life of about 15 hours, and its active metabolite, idarubicinol, has a half-life of about 40 hours. There is rapid uptake of the drugs in the heart, kidneys, lungs, liver, and spleen. They do not cross the blood–brain barrier.

Daunorubicin and doxorubicin are eliminated by metabolic conversion to a variety of less active or inactive products. Idarubicin is primarily metabolized to idarubicinol, which accumulates in plasma and resembles the parent compound in activity. Daunorubicin and doxorubicin are converted to their alcohols, to aglycones, and to other derivatives. Precise guidelines for reduction of dosage in patients with impaired hepatic function have not been defined. Clearance is delayed in the presence of hepatic dysfunction, and at least a 50% initial reduction in dose should be considered in patients with abnormal serum bilirubin levels (Twelves *et al.*, 1998).

Idarubicin Hydrochloride (IDAMYCIN). The recommended dosage for idarubicin is 12 mg/m² daily for 3 days by intravenous injection in combination with cytarabine. Slow injection with care over 10 to 15 minutes is recommended to avoid extravasation, as with other anthracyclines.

Daunorubicin. *Therapeutic Uses. Daunorubicin hydrochloride (daunomycin, rubidomycin;* CERUBIDINE) is available for intravenous use. The recommended dosage is 30 to 60 mg/m² daily for 3 days. The agent is administered with appropriate care to prevent extravasation, since severe local vesicant action may result. A daunorubicin citrate liposomal product (DAUNOXOME) is indicated for the treatment of AIDS-related Kaposi's sarcoma. It is given in a dose of 40 mg/m² infused over 60 minutes and repeated every 2 weeks. Patients should be advised that the drug may impart a red color to the urine.

Daunorubicin is very useful in the treatment of acute lymphocytic and acute myelogenous leukemias. It is among the most active drugs for treatment of AML in adults and, given with cytarabine, either it or idarubicin is the treatment of choice in these conditions.

Clinical Toxicities. The toxic manifestations of daunorubicin as well as idarubicin include bone marrow depression, stomatitis, alopecia, gastrointestinal disturbances, and dermatological manifestations. Cardiac toxicity is a peculiar adverse effect observed with these agents. It is characterized by tachycardia, arrhythmias, dyspnea, hypotension, pericardial effusion, and congestive failure poorly responsive to digitalis (*see* below).

Doxorubicin. *Therapeutic Uses. Doxorubicin hydrochloride* (ADRIAMYCIN, RUBEX) is available for intravenous use. The recommended dose is 60 to 75 mg/m², administered as a single rapid intravenous infusion that is repeated after 21 days. Care should be taken to avoid extravasation, since severe local vesicant action and tissue necrosis may result. A doxorubicin liposomal product (DOXIL) is available for treatment of AIDS-related Kaposi's sarcoma. It is given intravenously in a dose of 20 mg/m² over 30 minutes and repeated every 3 weeks. As for daunorubicin, patients should be advised that the drug may impart a red color to the urine.

Doxorubicin is effective in acute leukemias and malignant lymphomas; however, in contrast to daunorubicin, it also is active in a number of solid tumors, particularly breast cancer. Used concurrently with cyclophosphamide, vincristine, procarbazine, and other agents, it is an important ingredient for the successful treatment of Hodgkin's disease and non-Hodgkin's lymphomas. It is a valuable component of various regimens of chemotherapy for car-

cinoma of the breast and small cell carcinoma of the lung. The drug also is particularly beneficial in a wide range of pediatric and adult sarcomas, including osteogenic, Ewing's, and soft tissue sarcomas. The drug has demonstrated activity in carcinomas of the endometrium, testes, prostate, cervix, and head and neck, and in plasma cell myeloma.

Clinical Toxicities. The toxic manifestations of doxorubicin are similar to those of daunorubicin. Myelosuppression is a major dose-limiting complication, with leukopenia usually reaching a nadir during the second week of therapy and recovering by the fourth week; thrombocytopenia and anemia follow a similar pattern but usually are less pronounced. Stomatitis, gastrointestinal disturbances, and alopecia are common but reversible. Erythematous streaking near the site of infusion ("ADRIAMYCIN flare") is a benign local allergic reaction and should not be confused with extravasation. Facial flushing, conjunctivitis, and lacrimation may occur rarely. The drug may produce severe local toxicity in irradiated tissues (*e.g.,* the skin, heart, lung, esophagus, and gastrointestinal mucosa). Such reactions may occur even when the two therapies are not administered concomitantly.

Cardiomyopathy is a unique characteristic of the anthracycline antibiotics. Two types of cardiomyopathies may occur. (1) An acute form is characterized by abnormal electrocardiographic changes, including ST–T-wave alterations and arrhythmias. This is brief and rarely a serious problem. Cineangiographic studies have shown an acute, reversible reduction in ejection fraction 24 hours after a single dose. An exaggerated manifestation of acute myocardial damage, the "pericarditis–myocarditis syndrome," may be characterized by severe disturbances in impulse conduction and frank congestive heart failure, often associated with pericardial effusion. (2) Chronic, cumulative dose-related toxicity (usually at or above total doses of 550 mg/m²) is manifested by congestive heart failure that is unresponsive to digitalis. The mortality rate is in excess of 50%. Total dosage of doxorubicin as low as 250 mg/m² can cause myocardial toxicity, as demonstrated by subendocardial biopsies. Nonspecific alterations, including a decrease in the number of myocardial fibrils, mitochondrial changes, and cellular degeneration, are visible by electron microscopy. The most promising noninvasive technique used to detect the early development of drug-induced congestive heart failure is radionuclide cineangiography. Although no completely practical and reliable predictive tests are available, the frequency of serious cardiomyopathy is 1% to 10% at total doses below 450 mg/m². The risk increases markedly (to >20% of patients) at total doses higher than 550 mg/m², and this total dosage should be exceeded only under exceptional circumstances or with the concomitant use of *dexrazoxane* (ZINECARD), a cardioprotective intracellular chelating agent. (Speyer *et al.,* 1988; Swain *et al.,* 1997). Cardiac irradiation or administration of high doses of cyclophosphamide or another anthracycline may increase the risk of cardiotoxicity. Late-onset cardiac toxicity, with onset of congestive heart failure years after treatment, may occur in both pediatric and adult populations (Lipschultz *et al.,* 1991).

Newer Analogs of Doxorubicin. *Valrubicin* (VALSTAR) was approved in 1998 for intravesical therapy of BCG-refractory urinary bladder carcinoma *in situ* in patients for whom immediate cystectomy would be associated with unacceptable morbidity or mortality. *Epirubicin* (4'-epidoxorubicin, ELLENCE) was approved by the FDA in 1999 as a component of adjuvant therapy following resection of early lymph-node-positive breast cancer.

A related anthracenedione, *mitoxantrone,* has been approved for use in acute nonlymphocytic leukemias. Its structural formula is as follows:

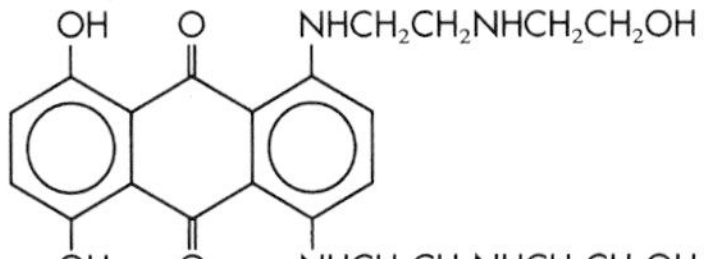

MITOXANTRONE

Mitoxantrone has limited ability to produce quinone-type free radicals and causes less cardiac toxicity than does doxorubicin. Mitoxantrone exerts its antitumor action by stimulating the formation of strand breaks in DNA; this is mediated by topoisomerase II; it also intercalates with DNA. Its range of antitumor activity is confined to leukemias, breast cancer, and prostate cancer (Shenkenberg and Von Hoff, 1986). Mitoxantrone produces acute myelosuppression, cardiac toxicity, and mucositis as its major toxicities; the drug causes less nausea and vomiting and alopecia than does doxorubicin. It also is used as a component of experimental high-dose chemotherapy regimens, with uncertain efficacy.

Mitoxantrone (NOVANTRONE) is supplied for intravenous infusion. To induce remission in acute nonlymphocytic leukemia in adults, the drug is given in a daily dose of 12 mg/m^2 for 3 days as a component of a regimen that also includes cytosine arabinoside. Mitoxantrone also is used in advanced hormone-resistant prostate cancer in a dose of 12 to 14 mg/m^2 every 21 days. In 2000, mitoxantrone was approved by the FDA for the treatment of late-stage, secondary progressive multiple sclerosis.

Bleomycins

The bleomycins are an important group of DNA-cleaving antibiotics discovered by Umezawa and colleagues as fermentation products of *Streptococcus verticillus*. The drug currently employed clinically is a mixture of the two copper-chelating peptides, bleomycins A$_2$ and B$_2$. The bleomycins differ only in their terminal amine (*see* below), which can be altered by adding various amines to the fermentation medium.

Bleomycins have attracted interest both because of their significant antitumor activity against squamous carcinomas of the cervix, head and neck, and lungs, and against lymphomas and testicular tumors. They are minimally myelo- and immunosuppressive but cause unusual cutaneous and pulmonary side effects. Because their toxicities do not overlap with those of other drugs, and because of their unique mechanism of action, the bleomycins have won an important role in combination chemotherapy.

Chemistry. The bleomycins are water-soluble, basic glycopeptides. The structures of bleomycin A$_2$ and B$_2$ are shown in Figure 52–14. The core of the bleomycin molecule is a complex metal-binding structure containing a pyrimidine chromophore linked to propionamide, a β-aminoalanine amide side chain, and the sugars L-gulose and 3-O-carbamoyl-D-mannose. Attached to this core is a tripeptide chain and a terminal bithiazole carboxylic acid; this latter segment binds to DNA. The bleomycins form equimolar complexes with metal ions, including Cu^{2+} and Fe^{2+}.

Mechanism of Action. Although the bleomycins have a number of interesting biochemical properties, their cytotoxic action results from their ability to cause oxidative damage to the

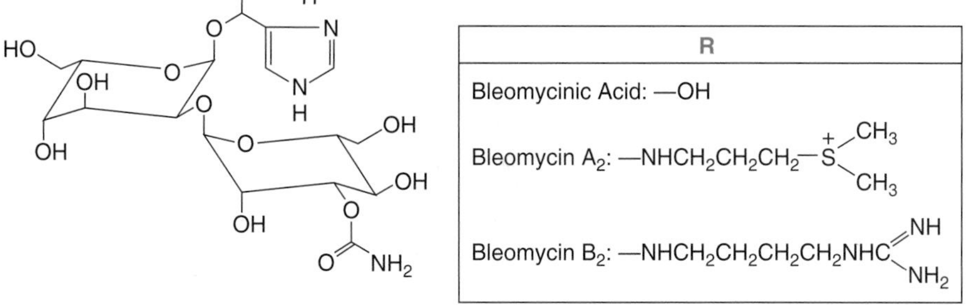

Figure 52–14. Chemical structures of bleomycin A$_2$ and B$_2$.

deoxyribose of thymidylate and other nucleotides leading to single- and double-stranded breaks in DNA. Studies *in vitro* indicate that bleomycin causes accumulation of cells in the G_2 phase of the cell cycle, and many of these cells display chromosomal aberrations, including chromatid breaks, gaps, and fragments, as well as translocations (Twentyman, 1983).

Bleomycin causes scission of DNA by interacting with O_2 and Fe^{2+}. In the presence of O_2 and a reducing agent, such as dithiothreitol, the metal–drug complex becomes activated and functions mechanistically as a ferrous oxidase, transferring electrons from Fe^{2+} to molecular oxygen to produce activated species of oxygen (Burger *et al.*, 1986; Burger, 1998). It also has been shown that metallobleomycin complexes can be activated by reaction with the flavin enzyme, NADPH-cytochrome P450 reductase. Bleomycin binds to DNA through its amino-terminal peptide, and the activated complex generates free radicals that are responsible for scission of the deoxyribose backbone of the DNA chain (*see* Grollman *et al.*, 1985).

Bleomycin is degraded by a specific hydrolase found in various normal tissues, including liver; hydrolase activity is low in skin and lung (Sebti *et al.*, 1987; Brömme *et al.*, 1996). Some bleomycin-resistant cells contain high levels of hydrolase activity (Sebti *et al.*, 1991). In other resistant cell lines different mechanisms, such as enhanced capacity to repair DNA, may lead to resistance (Zuckerman *et al.*, 1986). In experimental models, resistance to bleomycin has been attributed to decreased uptake, cleavage by the hydrolase, repair of strand breaks, or drug inactivation by thiols. Resistance of human tumors is poorly understood.

Absorption, Fate, and Excretion. Bleomycin is administered parenterally or instilled into the bladder for local treatment of bladder cancer (Bracken *et al.*, 1977). After intravenous infusion, relatively high drug concentrations are detected in the skin and lungs of experimental animals, and these organs become major sites of toxicity. Having a high molecular mass, bleomycin crosses the blood–brain barrier poorly.

After intravenous administration of a bolus dose of 15 units/m^2, peak concentrations of 1 to 5 mU/ml are achieved in plasma. The half-time for elimination is approximately 3 hours. The average steady-state concentration of bleomycin in plasma of patients receiving continuous intravenous infusions of 30 units daily for 4 to 5 days is approximately 0.15 mU/ml. About two-thirds of the drug is normally excreted in the urine, probably by glomerular filtration. Concentrations in plasma are greatly elevated if usual doses are given to patients with renal impairment, and such patients are at high risk of developing pulmonary toxicity. Doses of bleomycin should be reduced in the presence of severe renal failure (*see* Dalgleish *et al.*, 1984).

Therapeutic Uses. *Bleomycin sulfate* (BLENOXANE) is available for injection. The recommended dose of bleomycin is 10 to 20 units/m^2 given weekly or twice weekly by the intravenous or intramuscular route. It also may be administered as a subcutaneous injection or as an intrapleural or intracystic instillation. Total courses exceeding 250 units should be given with great caution because of a marked increase in pulmonary toxicity above this total dose. However, pulmonary toxicity may occur at lower doses (*see* below).

Bleomycin is highly effective against germ cell tumors of the testis and ovary. In testicular cancer it is curative when used with cisplatin and vinblastine or cisplatin and etoposide (Williams and Einhorn, 1985), and it is highly active when used with cisplatin and other agents in combination therapy of squamous carcinomas of the head and neck, esophagus, and genitourinary tract. It often is used as a component of combination therapy of Hodgkin's and non-Hodgkin's lymphomas.

Clinical Toxicities. Because bleomycin causes little myelosuppression, it has significant advantages in combination with other cytotoxic drugs. However, it does cause significant cutaneous toxicity, including hyperpigmentation, hyperkeratosis, erythema, and even ulceration. These changes may begin with tenderness and swelling of the distal digits and progress to erythematous, ulcerating lesions over the elbows, knuckles, and other pressure areas. Skin changes often leave a residual hyperpigmentation at these points and may recur when patients are treated with other antineoplastic drugs.

The most serious adverse reaction to bleomycin is pulmonary toxicity, which begins with a dry cough, fine rales, and diffuse basilar infiltrates on x-ray and may progress to life-threatening pulmonary fibrosis. Radiologic changes may be indistinguishable from interstitial infection or tumor, but may progress to dense fibrosis, cavitation, atelectasis or lobar collapse, or even apparent consolidation. Approximately 5% to 10% of patients receiving bleomycin develop clinically apparent pulmonary toxicity, and about 1% die of this complication. Most who recover experience a significant improvement in pulmonary function, but fibrosis may be irreversible (Van Barneveld *et al.*, 1987). Pulmonary function tests are not of predictive value for detecting early onset of this complication. The CO diffusion capacity declines in patients receiving doses above 250 U. The risk is related to total dose, with a significant increase above total doses of 250 U and in patients over 70 years of age and in those with underlying pulmonary disease; single doses of 30 U/m^2 or more also are associated with an increased risk of pulmonary toxicity. Administration of high inspired oxygen concentrations during anesthesia or respiratory therapy may aggravate or precipitate pulmonary toxicity in patients previously treated with the drug. There is no known specific therapy for bleomycin lung injury except for standard symptomatic management and pulmonary care. Steroids are of uncertain benefit. The etiology of bleomycin pulmonary toxicity has been the subject of intense investigation in rodent models. These studies implicate cytokine [tumor growth factor beta (TGF-β) and tumor necrosis factor (TNF)] secretion by macrophages in response to epithelial apoptosis as being involved in pulmonary fibrosis (Munger *et al.*, 1999).

Other toxic reactions to bleomycin include hyperthermia, headache, nausea, and vomiting, as well as a peculiar, acute fulminant reaction observed in patients with lymphomas. This is characterized by profound hyperthermia, hypotension, and sustained cardiorespiratory collapse; it does not appear to be a classical anaphylactic reaction and possibly may be related to release of an endogenous pyrogen. Because this reaction has occurred in approximately 1% of patients with lymphomas and has resulted in deaths, it is recommended that patients with lymphomas receive a 1-unit test dose of bleomycin, followed by a

1-hour period of observation, before administration of the drug on standard dosage schedules. Unexplained exacerbations of rheumatoid arthritis also have been reported during bleomycin therapy. Raynaud's phenomenon and coronary artery disease have been reported in patients with testicular tumors treated with bleomycin in combination with other chemotherapeutic agents.

Mitomycin

This antibiotic was isolated from *Streptococcus caespitosus* by Wakaki and associates in 1958. Mitomycin contains an aziridine group and a quinone group in its structure, as well as a mitosane ring, and each of these participates in the alkylation reactions with DNA. Its structural formula is as follows:

MITOMYCIN

Mechanism of Action. After intracellular enzymatic or spontaneous chemical reduction of the quinone and loss of the methoxy group, mitomycin becomes a bifunctional or trifunctional alkylating agent (Verweij *et al.*, 2001). Reduction occurs preferentially in hypoxic cells in some experimental systems. The drug inhibits DNA synthesis and cross-links DNA at the N^6 position of adenine and at the O^6 and N^7 positions of guanine. In addition, single-strand breakage of DNA and chromosomal breaks are caused by mitomycin. Mitomycin is a potent radiosensitizer and is teratogenic and carcinogenic in rodents. Resistance has been ascribed to deficient activation, intracellular inactivation of the reduced quinone, and P-glycoprotein–mediated drug efflux (Dorr, 1988; Crooke and Bradner, 1976).

Absorption, Fate, and Excretion. Mitomycin is absorbed inconsistently from the gastrointestinal tract and is therefore administered intravenously. It disappears rapidly from the blood after injection, with a half-life of 25 to 90 minutes. Peak concentrations in plasma are 0.4 μg/ml after doses of 20 mg/m^2 (Dorr, 1988). The drug is widely distributed throughout the body but is not detected in the brain. Inactivation occurs by metabolism or chemical conjugation. Less than 10% of the active drug is excreted in the urine or the bile.

Therapeutic Uses. Mitomycin (*mitomycin-C;* MUTAMYCIN) is administered by intravenous infusion; extravasation may result in severe local injury. The usual dose (6 to 10 mg/m^2) may be administered intravenously as a single bolus infusion every 6 weeks and is usually given as part of a combination regimen for treatment of carcinoma of the colon or stomach. Dosage is modified based on hematological recovery. Mitomycin also may be used by direct instillation into the bladder to treat superficial carcinomas (Boccardo *et al.*, 1994).

Mitomycin is used primarily in combination with 5-FU, cisplatin, or doxorubicin in carcinomas of the cervix, stomach, breast, bladder, head and neck, and lung. It is a potent radiation

sensitizer and continues to attract interest in clinical trials with concurrent irradiation in the above diseases.

Clinical Toxicities. The major toxic effect is myelosuppression, characterized by marked leukopenia and thrombocytopenia; after higher doses, the nadirs may be delayed and cumulative, with recovery only after 6 to 8 weeks of pancytopenia. Nausea, vomiting, diarrhea, stomatitis, dermatitis, fever, and malaise also are observed. A hemolytic-uremic syndrome represents the most dangerous toxic manifestation of mitomycin and is believed to result from drug-induced endothelial damage. Patients who have received more than 50 mg/m^2 total dose may acutely develop hemolysis, neurological abnormalities, interstitial pneumonia, and glomerular damage resulting in renal failure. The incidence of renal failure increases to 28% in patients who receive total doses of 70 mg/m^2 or higher (Valavaara and Nordman, 1985). There is no effective treatment for the disorder; blood transfusion may cause pulmonary edema. Mitomycin causes interstitial pulmonary fibrosis, and total doses above 30 mg/m^2 have infrequently led to congestive heart failure (Verweij *et al.*, 1988). It also may potentiate the cardiotoxicity of doxorubicin when used in conjunction with this drug (Bachur *et al.*, 1978).

ENZYMES

L-Asparaginase

History. In 1953, Kidd reported that guinea pig serum had antileukemic activity and identified L-*asparaginase* as the source of this activity (Kidd, 1953). Fifteen years later, the enzyme was introduced into cancer chemotherapy in an effort to exploit a distinct, qualitative difference between normal and malignant cells (Broome, 1981).

Mechanism of Action. Most normal tissues synthesize L-asparagine in amounts sufficient for protein synthesis. Certain neoplastic tissues, however, including acute lymphoblastic leukemic cells, require an exogenous source of this amino acid. L-Asparaginase, by catalyzing the hydrolysis of circulating asparagine to aspartic acid and ammonia, deprives these cells of the asparagine necessary for protein synthesis, leading to cell death. L-Asparaginase is commonly used in combination with methotrexate, doxorubicin, vincristine, and prednisone for the treatment of acute lymphoblastic leukemia. The sequence of drug administration in these combinations may be critical; for example, synergistic cytotoxicity results when methotrexate precedes the enzyme, but the reverse sequence leads to abrogation of methotrexate cytotoxicity. The latter outcome is a consequence of the inhibition of protein synthesis by L-asparaginase, an effect that stops the progression of cells through the cell cycle and negates the effect of methotrexate, a drug that exerts its greatest effect during the DNA synthetic phase of the cell cycle (Capizzi and Handschumacher, 1982).

L-Asparaginase produces cell death through activation of apoptosis. Resistance arises through induction of the capacity of tumor cells to synthesize L-asparagine.

Absorption, Fate, and Excretion. L-Asparaginase is given parenterally. The rate of clearance from plasma varies considerably with different preparations. After intravenous administration, L-asparaginase has a clearance rate from plasma of 0.035 ml/minute per kg. Its apparent volume of distribution is only 55 ml/kg, approximately the volume of plasma in human beings. Its average half-life is 30 hours (Asselin *et al.*, 1993), the Merck and Kyawa Hacco preparations having a somewhat longer plasma half-life than the Bayer preparation. An *Erwinia* preparation (*see* below), used in patients hypersensitive to the enzyme from *Escherichia coli*, has a shorter half-life of 16 hours and thus requires administration of higher doses. Pegaspargase (*see* below) is cleared much less rapidly (plasma half-life is 14.9 days) (Ho *et al.*, 1986).

Therapeutic Uses. *E. coli* produces two L-asparaginase isozymes, only one of which (EC-2) has antileukemic activity. The purified *E. coli* enzyme (ELSPAR) is available for clinical use and has a molecular weight of 130,000 daltons. It consists of four equivalent subunits (*see* Patterson, 1975). Also available for use in patients hypersensitive to the native *E. coli* enzyme are the enzyme from *Erwinia chrysanthemi* (Minton *et al.*, 1986) and a form of the *E. coli* enzyme modified by conjugation to polyethylene glycol (*pegaspargase*, ONCASPAR). The *E. coli* enzyme is administered intravenously or intramuscularly in a variety of regimens and schedules. Typically, 5000 to 10,000 U per m^2 are given every other or every third day for 2 to 4 weeks, or single doses of up to 25,000 U per week. L-Asparagine levels in plasma fall immediately with drug administration and remain undetectable for 1 week after a single large dose. Recovery of L-asparagine levels occurs when enzyme levels fall below 0.03 U/ml in plasma. Because of its longer half-life, pegaspargase is given in doses of 2500 U/m^2 every other week. Intermittent dosage regimens have an increased risk of anaphylaxis. In hypersensitive patients, circulating antibodies lead to immediate inactivation of the enzyme and L-asparaginase levels rapidly become unmeasurable after drug administration.

L-Asparaginase is a useful component of regimens for treatment of acute lymphoblastic leukemia and other lymphoid malignancies.

Clinical Toxicity. Few objective responses have occurred in extensive trials in solid tumors. L-Asparaginase has minimal effects on bone marrow and gastrointestinal mucosa. Its most serious toxicities result from its antigenicity as a foreign protein and its inhibition of protein synthesis. Hypersensitivity reactions occur in 5% to 20% of patients and may be fatal. These reactions are heralded by the appearance of circulating neutralizing antibody in some, but not all, hypersensitive patients. In these patients, pegaspargase is a safe alternative, and the *Erwinia* enzyme may be used with caution (Ho *et al.*, 1986; Keating *et al.*, 1993).

Other toxicities result from inhibition of protein synthesis in normal tissues and include hyperglycemia due to insulin deficiency, clotting abnormalities due to deficient clotting factors, and hypoalbuminemia. The clotting problems may take the form of spontaneous thrombosis related to deficient factor S, factor C, or antithrombin III, or, less frequently, hemorrhagic episodes. Thrombosis of cortical sinus vessels frequently goes unrecognized. Magnetic resonance imaging studies should be considered in patients treated with L-asparaginase who present with seizures, headache, or altered mental status (Bushara and Rust, 1997). There is evidence that the majority of L-asparaginase–induced thromboses occur in patients with underlying inherited disorders of coagulation, such as Factor V Leiden, elevated serum homocysteine, protein C or S deficiency, AT III defi-

ciency, or the 620210A variant of prothrombin (Norwak-Gottl *et al.*, 1999). Intracranial hemorrhage in the first week of L-asparaginase treatment is an infrequent but often devastating complication. L-Asparaginase suppresses immune function as well.

In addition to these side effects, coma may result rarely and has been attributed to ammonia toxicity resulting from L-asparagine hydrolysis. Pancreatitis also has been observed; its cause is uncertain.

IV. MISCELLANEOUS AGENTS

PLATINUM COORDINATION COMPLEXES

The platinum coordination complexes were first identified by Rosenberg and coworkers as cytotoxic agents in 1965. They observed that a current delivered between platinum electrodes produced inhibition of *E. coli* proliferation. The inhibitory effects on bacterial replication were later ascribed to the formation of inorganic platinum-containing compounds in the presence of ammonium and chloride ions (Rosenberg *et al.*, 1965, 1967). *cis*-Diamminedichloroplatinum (II) (*cisplatin*) was the most active of these substances in experimental tumor systems and has proven to be of great clinical value (Rosenberg, 1973). More than 1000 platinum-containing compounds subsequently have been synthesized and tested. One of these, *carboplatin,* was approved for treatment of ovarian cancers in 1989; others are still being evaluated. Cisplatin has broad activity as an antineoplastic agent, and the drug is especially useful in the treatment of epithelial malignancies. It has become the foundation for curative regimens for advanced testicular cancer and has notable activity against ovarian cancer and cancers of the head and neck, bladder, esophagus, and lung.

Chemistry. *cis*-Diamminedichloroplatinum (II) (cisplatin) is a divalent inorganic water-soluble, platinum-containing complex. Other platinum complexes, some of which lack cross-resistance with cisplatin in preclinical tests, are currently in clinical trials; these include *tetraplatin, ormiplatin, iproplatin,* and *oxaliplatin* (Kelland, 1993). In each case, the coordination of di- or tetravalent platinum with various organic adducts reduces its renal toxicity and stabilizes the metal ion, but none of the complexes has unique clinical effects as an antitumor agent at this point in development. In carboplatin, platinum is incorporated into a more complex carbon-containing molecule. The structural formulas of cisplatin and carboplatin are as follows:

CISPLATIN   CARBOPLATIN

Mechanism of Action. Cisplatin appears to enter cells by diffusion. The chloride atoms may be displaced directly by reaction with nucleophiles such as thiols; replacement of chloride by water yields a positively charged molecule and is probably responsible for formation of the activated species of the drug, which then reacts with nucleic acids and proteins. Aquation is favored at low concentrations of chloride. High concentrations of the anion stabilize the drug, explaining the effectiveness of chloride diuresis in preventing nephrotoxicity (*see* below). Hydrolysis of carboplatin removes the bidentate cyclobutanedicarboxylato group; this activation reaction occurs more slowly with carboplatin than with cisplatin. The platinum complexes can react with DNA, forming both intrastrand and interstrand cross-links. The N^7 of guanine is very reactive, and platinum cross-links between adjacent guanines on the same DNA strand; guanine–adenine cross-links also readily form. The formation of interstrand cross-links is a slower process and occurs to a lesser extent. DNA adducts formed by cisplatin inhibit DNA replication and transcription and lead to breaks and miscoding. Although no conclusive association between platinum-DNA adduct formation and efficacy has been documented, the ability of patients to form and sustain platinum adducts appears to be an important predictor of clinical response. When quantifying the effect of platinum adduct formation, it is difficult to measure the relative importance of pharmacogenetic factors and environmental exposures common to tumor and normal tissues, as well as the contribution of concomitantly administered chemotherapies. Nevertheless, preclinical data suggest that the formation of the platinum-adenosine-to-guanosine adduct may be the most critical adduct in terms of cytotoxicity (Reed *et al.,* 1986; Parker *et al.,* 1991b; Comess *et al.,* 1992; Fichtinger-Schepman *et al.,* 1995; Welters *et al.,* 1999).

The specificity of cisplatin with regard to phase of the cell cycle appears to differ among cell types, although the effects on cross-linking are most pronounced during the S phase. Cisplatin is mutagenic, teratogenic, and carcinogenic. Secondary leukemias after cisplatin have been reported, and the use of cisplatin- or carboplatin-based chemotherapy for women with ovarian cancer is associated with a fourfold increased risk of developing secondary leukemia (Jeha *et al.,* 1992; Travis *et al.,* 1999).

The causes of tumor cell resistance to cisplatin and its analogs are incompletely understood. The various analogs differ in their degree of cross-resistance with cisplatin in experimental tumor systems. Carboplatin tends to share cross-resistance in most experimental tumors, while oxaliplatin and the tetravalent analogs do not, a finding that has led to interest in their clinical evaluation. A number of factors influence cisplatin sensitivity in experimental cells, including intracellular drug accumulation, intracellular levels of glutathione and other sulfhydryls such as metallothionein that bind to and inactivate the drug (Meijer *et al.,* 1990), and rates of repair of DNA adducts (Parker *et al.,* 1991a). The cisplatin adduct with DNA produces a bend in the helix, a change that is recognized by specific proteins of the high-mobility group (Huang *et al.,* 1994), which are believed to inhibit the repair process. Repair of cisplatin-DNA adducts occurs through the nucleotide excision repair pathway, designated NER (Dabholkar *et al.,* 1994; Reed, 1998; de Laat *et al.,* 1999). Through a series of enzymatic steps, NER recognizes and excises the affected base, inserts a new base, and religates

the affected strand. Inhibition of NER may increase sensitivity to cisplatin.

Resistance to cisplatin appears to be mediated to some extent through the mismatch repair (MMR) proteins. Defects or deficiencies in MMR proteins, particularly hMLH1 or hMSH6, may be important in the recognition of platinum-DNA adducts and in initiating apoptosis. Loss of MMR has been associated with resistance to cisplatin *in vitro* (Vaisman *et al.,* 1998). In addition, MMR proteins also may be involved in mediating apoptosis. Through an hMLH1-dependent event, cisplatin induces overexpression of p73, a member of the p53 family, as well as c-ABL tyrosine kinase and consequently activates apoptosis (Gong *et al.,* 1999). In response to cisplatin exposure, induction of apoptosis is not seen in those cells deficient in MMR and in those cells unable to upregulate c-ABL tyrosine kinase.

Cisplatin. *Absorption, Fate, and Excretion.* After rapid intravenous administration of usual doses, the drug has an initial elimination half-life in plasma of 25 to 50 minutes; concentrations of total drug, bound and unbound, fall thereafter, with a half-life of 24 hours or longer. More than 90% of the platinum in the blood is covalently bound to plasma proteins. High concentrations of cisplatin are found in the kidney, liver, intestine, and testes, but there is poor penetration into the CNS. Only a small portion of the drug is excreted by the kidney during the first 6 hours; by 24 hours up to 25% is excreted, and by 5 days up to 43% of the administered dose is recovered in the urine. When given by infusion instead of rapid injection, the plasma half-life is shorter and the amount of drug excreted is greater. Biliary or intestinal excretion of cisplatin appears to be minimal (Bajorin *et al.,* 1986).

Therapeutic Uses. *Cisplatin* (PLATINOL-AQ) is available for intravenous dosing. The usual intravenous dose of cisplatin is 20 mg/m^2 per day for 5 days or 100 mg/m^2, given once every 4 weeks. Doses as high as 40 mg/m^2 daily for 5 consecutive days have been used alone or together with cyclophosphamide for the treatment of patients with advanced ovarian cancer, but result in greater renal, hearing, and neurological toxicity (Ozols *et al.,* 1984). To prevent renal toxicity, hydration of the patient by the infusion of 1 to 2 liters of normal saline prior to treatment is recommended. The appropriate amount of cisplatin is then diluted in a solution of dextrose and saline and administered intravenously over a period of 6 to 8 hours. Since aluminum reacts with and inactivates cisplatin, it is important not to use needles or other equipment that contains aluminum when preparing or administering the drug.

Combination chemotherapy with cisplatin, bleomycin, etoposide, and vinblastine is curative for 85% of patients with advanced testicular cancer (Williams and Einhorn, 1985; Einhorn, 1986). The drug also is beneficial in carcinoma of the ovary, particularly when used with paclitaxel, cyclophosphamide, or doxorubicin (Durant and Omura, 1985). Cisplatin consistently produces responses in cancers of the bladder, head and neck, and endometrium;

small cell carcinoma of the lung; and some neoplasms of childhood. Interestingly, the drug also sensitizes cells to the cytotoxic effects of radiation therapy (*see* Pearson and Raghavan, 1985).

Clinical Toxicities. Cisplatin-induced nephrotoxicity has been largely abrogated by the routine use of hydration and diuresis. However, ototoxicity caused by cisplatin is unaffected by diuresis and is manifested by tinnitus and hearing loss in the high-frequency range (4000 to 8000 Hz). The ototoxicity can be unilateral or bilateral, tends to be more frequent and severe with repeated doses, and may be more pronounced in children. Marked nausea and vomiting occur in almost all patients and usually can be controlled with ondansetron or high-dose corticosteroids. At higher doses or after multiple cycles of treatment, cisplatin causes peripheral neuropathy, which may worsen after discontinuation of the drug. Mild-to-moderate myelosuppression may occur, with transient leukopenia, thrombocytopenia, and anemia. Electrolyte disturbances, including hypomagnesemia, hypocalcemia, hypokalemia, and hypophosphatemia, are common. Hypocalcemia and hypomagnesemia secondary to renal electrolyte wasting have been observed and may produce tetany. Routine measurement of Mg^{2+} concentrations in plasma is recommended. Hyperuricemia, seizures, hemolytic anemia, and cardiac abnormalities have been reported. Anaphylactic-like reactions, characterized by facial edema, bronchoconstriction, tachycardia, and hypotension, may occur within minutes after administration and should be treated by intravenous injection of epinephrine and with corticosteroids or antihistamines.

Carboplatin. The mechanism of action and spectrum of clinical activity of carboplatin (CBDCA, JM-8) are similar to those of cisplatin (*see* above). However, there are significant differences in the chemical, pharmacokinetic, and toxicological properties of the two drugs (*see* Von Hoff, 1987; Muggia, 1989; Ozols, 1989).

Carboplatin is less reactive than cisplatin, and the drug is not bound to plasma proteins to a significant extent. As a result, there are no appreciable quantities of low-molecular-weight platinum-containing species (other than carboplatin itself) in plasma, and most of the drug is eliminated in the urine as such, with a half-life of about 2 hours. Platinum from the drug does become irreversibly bound to plasma proteins, and this fraction of the metal disappears slowly (half-life of 5 days or more).

Carboplatin is relatively well tolerated clinically. There is less nausea, neurotoxicity, ototoxicity, and nephrotoxicity than with cisplatin. Instead, the dose-limiting toxicity is myelosuppression, primarily evident as thrombocytopenia. Carboplatin and cisplatin appear to be equally effective in the treatment of suboptimally debulked ovarian cancer, non–small cell lung cancer, and extensive stage small cell lung cancer; however, carboplatin may be less effective than cisplatin in germ cell, head and neck, and esophageal cancers (Go and Adjei, 1999). Carboplatin is an effective alternative for patients with responsive tumors who are unable to tolerate cisplatin because of impaired renal function, refractory nausea, significant hearing impairment, or neuropathy. In addition, it may be used in high-dose therapy with bone marrow or peripheral stem cell rescue. The dose of carboplatin should be adjusted in proportion to the reduction

in creatinine clearance for patients with a creatinine clearance below 60 mg/ml (Van Echo *et al.*, 1989). Calvert *et al.* (1989) have proposed the following formula for calculation of dose:

$$\text{Dose (mg)} = \text{AUC} \times (\text{GFR} + 25) \qquad (52\text{–}1)$$

where the target AUC (area under the plasma concentration–time curve) is in the range of 5 to 7 mg/ml per minute for acceptable toxicity in patients receiving single-agent carboplatin. (GFR = glomerular filtration rate; *see* Chapter 1.)

Carboplatin (PARAPLATIN) is administered as an intravenous infusion over at least 15 minutes. The usual dose is 360 mg/m^2, given once every 28 days. Carboplatin currently is approved for use in combination with paclitaxel or cyclophosphamide in patients with advanced ovarian cancer. It also has been shown to be effective in a number of tumors including lung cancer, bladder cancer, and head and neck cancer.

Oxaliplatin. Oxaliplatin or *trans*-1-diaminocyclohexane oxalatoplatinum has a diaminocyclohexane (DACH) carrier ligand that endows it with unique properties, thus allowing it to escape recognition by NER and MMR proteins. Its structure is as follows:

OXALIPLATIN

Unlike cisplatin or carboplatin, oxaliplatin is equally effective in MMR-proficient and -deficient cell lines and tumor xenografts (Fink *et al.*, 1996; Fink *et al.*, 1997). In particular, hMLH1 defects that produce cisplatin resistance *in vitro* have no effect on oxaliplatin cytotoxicity (Vaisman *et al.*, 1998). Furthermore, the upregulation of c-ABL tyrosine kinase seen with cisplatin in the presence of functional MMR proteins is not observed after the administration of oxaliplatin (Nehme *et al.*, 1999).

In contrast to cisplatin and carboplatin, oxaliplatin has a very large volume of distribution (Graham *et al.*, 2000). The pharmacokinetics of oxaliplatin are triexponential with short initial α and β distribution phases (0.28 hour and 16.3 hours, respectively) and a long terminal γ phase (273 hours). Approximately 80% of oxaliplatin is bound to plasma proteins, and it undergoes extensive biotransformation. Over 5 days, approximately 50% will be excreted in the urine (2% to 12% as free DACH carrier ligand), and only 5% will be excreted in the feces. Clearance of oxaliplatin is decreased in patients with renal impairment, but there is little increase in clinical toxicity (Massari *et al.*, 2000). The dose-limiting toxicity of oxaliplatin is a peripheral neuropathy that is often triggered by exposure to cold, and manifests as paresthesias and/or dysesthesias in the upper and lower extremities, mouth, and throat. The peripheral neuropathy is cumulative; 75% of patients receiving a cumulative dose of 1560 mg/m^2 experience some neurotoxicity. Hematologic toxicity is mild to moderate, and nausea is well controlled with 5-HT$_3$-receptor antagonists (*see* Chapter 38). Oxaliplatin is unstable in the presence of chloride or alkaline solutions.

Like cisplatin, oxaliplatin shows a wide range of antitumor activity and is active in ovarian cancer, germ-cell cancer, and cervical cancer. Unlike cisplatin, oxaliplatin in combination with 5-fluorouracil is active in colorectal cancer, perhaps due to its MMR-independent effects. In combination with 5-fluorouracil, it is approved for treatment of patients with advanced colorectal cancer in Europe, Asia, and Latin America. Registration studies for its use in colorectal cancer are in progress in the United States.

Hydroxyurea

Hydroxyurea originally was synthesized by Dresler and Stein in 1869, but its potential biological significance was not recognized until 1928, when leukopenia and megaloblastic anemia were observed in experimental animals treated with this compound. In the 1950s, the drug was evaluated in a large number of experimental murine tumor models and was found to have broad antitumor activity against both leukemia and solid-tumor models. Clinical trials with hydroxyurea began in the 1960s. Since then, this drug has continued to be of interest to both clinical and laboratory investigators, as it has a number of unique and surprisingly diverse biological effects that have led to exploration of its clinical utility in a wide range of malignant and nonmalignant diseases. Its use has been encouraged by the facts that the drug can be administered orally and that its toxicity in most patients is very modest. Comprehensive descriptions of the pharmacology of hydroxyurea have been published (Navarra and Preziosi, 1999; Paz-Ares and Donehower, 2001). The structural formula of hydroxyurea is as follows:

$$H_2N-\overset{\overset{\displaystyle O}{\|}}{C}-NH-OH$$

HYDROXYUREA

Cytotoxic Action. Hydroxyurea is representative of a group of compounds that have as their primary site of action the enzyme ribonucleoside diphosphate reductase. A striking correlation has been observed between the relative growth rate of a series of rat hepatomas and the activity of ribonucleoside diphosphate reductase. This enzyme, which catalyzes the reductive conversion of ribonucleotides to deoxyribonucleotides, is a crucial and probably rate-limiting step in the biosynthesis of DNA, and it represents a logical target for the design of chemotherapeutic agents. Hydroxyurea destroys a tyrosyl free radical that is formed in the catalytic center of the enzyme. The drug is specific for the S phase of the cell cycle, in which concentrations of the target reductase are maximal, and it causes cells to arrest at the G_1–S interface. Since cells are highly sensitive to irradiation in the G_1 phase of the cycle, combinations of hydroxyurea and irradiation cause synergistic toxicity (Schilsky *et al.*, 1992). Hydroxyurea also may potentiate the antiproliferative effects of DNA-damaging agents such as cisplatin, alkylating agents, or topoisomerase II inhibitors. Even more interesting are the modulator effects of hydroxyurea on antimetabolite drugs, particularly

nucleotide analogs. The decrease of the intracellular deoxyribonucleotide pools after hydroxyurea exposure facilitates the incorporation of drugs such as AraC, gemcitabine, or fludarabine into DNA. This type of interaction has implications for the anti-HIV effect of hydroxyurea. The inhibition of cellular ribonucleoside diphosphate reductase favors the incorporation of an increased proportion of the nucleoside reverse transcriptase inhibitors into the viral DNA (Lori *et al.*, 1994). Hydroxyurea also has been shown to be converted *in vivo* to nitric oxide, to induce the expression of a number of genes [for TNF, interleukin-6 (IL-6), β-globin, *etc.*], and to accelerate the loss of extrachromosomally amplified genes present in double-minute chromosomes. The clinical relevance of these actions is unknown (Paz-Ares and Donehower, 2001; Navarra and Preziosi, 1999).

The principal mechanism by which cells achieve resistance to hydroxyurea is through elevation in cellular ribonucleoside diphosphate reductase activity. Several different molecular mechanisms may contribute to the increased ribonucleoside reductase activity in hydroxyurea-resistant cells, including gene amplification and increased translational efficiency. It has been suggested that some examples of resistance to hydroxyurea may be the result of the production of a ribonucleoside diphosphate reductase with decreased sensitivity to inhibition by hydroxyurea.

Absorption, Fate, and Excretion. The oral bioavailability of hydroxyurea is excellent (80% to 100%), and comparable plasma concentrations are seen after oral or intravenous dosing (Rodriguez *et al.*, 1998). Peak plasma concentrations are reached 1.0 to 1.5 hours after oral doses of 15 to 80 mg/kg. Hydroxyurea disappears from plasma with a half-life from 3.5 to 4.5 hours. The drug readily crosses the blood–brain barrier, and it appears in significant quantities in human breast milk. From 40% to 80% of the drug is recovered in the urine within 12 hours after either intravenous or oral administration. Although precise guidelines are not available, it seems prudent to modify doses for patients with abnormal renal function until individual tolerance can be assessed. Data from several experimental animal systems suggest that metabolism of hydroxyurea does occur, but the extent and significance of metabolism of the drug in human beings have not been established.

Therapeutic Uses. Two dosage schedules for *hydroxyurea* (HYDREA), alone or in combination with other drugs, are most commonly used in a variety of clinical situations: (1) intermittent therapy with 80 mg/kg administered orally as a single dose every third day or (2) continuous therapy with 20 to 30 mg/kg administered as a single daily dose. Dosage should be adjusted according to the number of leukocytes in the peripheral blood. Treatment is typically continued for a period of 6 weeks in malignant diseases to determine its effectiveness; if satisfactory antineoplastic results are obtained, therapy can be continued indefinitely, although leukocyte counts at weekly intervals are advisable.

The principal use of hydroxyurea has been as a myelosuppressive agent in the myeloproliferative syndromes, particularly chronic granulocytic leukemia, polycythemia vera, and essential thrombocytosis. Currently, hydroxyurea is prescribed for patients with myeloproliferative syndromes who are not candidates for interferon treatment, or the drug is given in combination with interferon during the induction phase of therapy (Silver *et al.,* 1999). Hydroxyurea cannot be considered to be standard therapy either as a single agent or as part of the standard chemotherapy regimen for any solid tumor, although it has produced anecdotal, temporary remissions in patients with advanced cancers (*e.g.,* head and neck or genitourinary carcinomas, melanoma). Hydroxyurea has been incorporated into several schedules with concurrent irradiation, as it is able to synchronize cells into a radiation-sensitive phase of the cell cycle. This combination has shown promise in several diseases, including cervical carcinoma, primary brain tumors, head and neck cancer, and non–small cell lung cancer, although it has not been proven to be superior to regimens including cisplatin and irradiation.

Hydroxyurea has been approved by the FDA for the treatment of adult patients with sickle cell disease. The drug reduces the number of painful crises, the frequency of acute chest syndrome and hospitalization, and the need for blood transfusion (Charache *et al.,* 1995). Hydroxyurea appears to be effective in children with sickle cell disease and in patients with sickle cell–β-thalassemia and sickle cell–hemoglobin C disease, although the clinical experience is more limited.

Hydroxyurea may serve as an important paradigm for agents that contribute to inhibition of HIV replication by a mechanism other than the one that targets a viral enzyme or a structural protein (Lori, 1999). Currently available clinical data reveal that hydroxyurea has little activity as a single agent but produces pronounced inhibition of HIV replication when combined with didanosine or with didanosine plus stavudine in non–heavily pretreated patients (*see* Chapter 51). Importantly, hydroxyurea appears to maintain the activity of the nucleoside reverse transcriptase inhibitors even in the presence of genotypic mutations of the HIV characteristically associated with resistance to the drugs.

Clinical Toxicity. Hematopoietic depression—involving leukopenia, megaloblastic anemia, and occasionally thrombocytopenia—is the major toxic effect; recovery of the bone marrow usually is prompt if the drug is discontinued for a few days. Other adverse reactions include gastrointestinal disturbances and mild dermatological reactions; more rarely, stomatitis, alopecia, and neurological manifestations have been encountered. Inflammation and increased pigmentation may occur in areas previously exposed to radiation. Hydroxyurea may increase the risk of secondary leukemia in patients with myeloproliferative disor-

ders and should be used with caution in nonmalignant diseases. Hydroxyurea is a potent teratogen in all animal species tested and should not be used in women with childbearing potential.

Procarbazine

The methylhydrazine derivatives were synthesized among a large number of substituted hydrazines in a search for inhibitors of monoamine neurotransmitters. Several compounds in this series (Bollag, 1963) were discovered to have anticancer activity, but only procarbazine, an agent useful in Hodgkin's disease, has won a place in clinical chemotherapy. Its structural formula is as follows:

PROCARBAZINE

Cytotoxic Action. Procarbazine must undergo metabolic activation to generate the proximal cytotoxic reactants, which methylate DNA. The activation pathways are complex and not fully understood. The first step involves oxidation of the hydrazine function with formation of the azo analog. This can occur spontaneously in neutral solution by reaction with molecular oxygen and also can occur enzymatically by reaction with the cytochrome P450 system of the liver. Further oxidations can generate the methylazoxy and benzylazoxy intermediates. It is postulated that the methylazoxy compound can react further to liberate an entity resembling diazomethane, a potent methylating reagent. Free-radical intermediates also may be involved in cytotoxicity. Activated procarbazine can produce chromosomal damage, including chromatid breaks and translocations. These effects are consistent with its mutagenic and carcinogenic actions. Exposure to procarbazine leads to inhibition of DNA, RNA, and protein synthesis *in vivo*. Resistance to procarbazine develops rapidly when it is used as a single agent. One mechanism results from the increased ability to repair methylation of guanine *via* guanine-O^6-alkyl transferase (Souliotis *et al.,* 1990).

Absorption, Fate, and Excretion. Procarbazine is absorbed almost completely from the gastrointestinal tract. After parenteral administration, the drug is readily equilibrated between the plasma and the CSF. It is rapidly metabolized in human beings, and its half-life in the blood after intravenous injection is approximately 7 minutes. Oxidation of procarbazine produces the corresponding azo compound and hydrogen peroxide. Further metabolism, presumably in the liver, yields azoxy derivatives that circulate in the bloodstream and have potent cytotoxic activity (Erickson *et al.,* 1989). Induction of microsomal enzymes by phenobarbital and other agents enhances the rate of conversion of procarbazine to its active metabolites; the potential for drug interaction thus exists when procarbazine is administered with other agents that are metabolized by microsomal enzymes. From 25% to 70% of an oral or parenteral dose given to human beings is recovered from the urine during the first 24 hours after administration; less than 5% is excreted as the unchanged compound, and the rest is mostly in the form of a metabolite, *N*-isopropylterephthalamic acid (Friedman, 2001).

Therapeutic Uses. The recommended dose of *procarbazine* (MATULANE) for adults is 100 mg/m² daily for 10 to 14 days in combination regimens. The drug rarely is used alone.

Procarbazine primarily is used in the combination therapy of Hodgkin's disease. It is given with mechlorethamine, vincristine, and prednisone (the MOPP regimen) (DeVita, 1981). Of primary importance, procarbazine lacks cross-resistance with other mustard-type alkylating agents. Procarbazine also has demonstrated activity against brain tumors, small cell carcinoma of the lung, non-Hodgkin's lymphomas, myeloma, and melanoma.

Clinical Toxicity. Most common toxic effects include leukopenia and thrombocytopenia, which begin during the second week of therapy and reverse within 2 weeks off treatment. Gastrointestinal symptoms such as mild nausea and vomiting occur in most patients; gastrointestinal symptoms and neurological and dermatological manifestations have been noted in 5% to 10% of cases. Disturbances in behavior also have been reported. Because of augmentation of sedative effects, the concomitant use of CNS depressants should be avoided. The ingestion of alcohol by patients receiving procarbazine may cause intense warmth and reddening of the face, as well as other effects resembling the acetaldehyde syndrome produced by disulfiram (*see* Chapter 18). Since procarbazine is a weak monoamine oxidase inhibitor, hypertensive reactions may result from its use concurrently with sympathomimetic agents, tricyclic antidepressants, or foods with high tyramine content. Procarbazine is highly carcinogenic, mutagenic, and teratogenic, and its use in MOPP therapy is associated with a 5% to 10% risk of acute leukemia; the greatest risk is for patients who also receive radiation therapy (Tucker *et al.*, 1988). Procarbazine is also a potent immunosuppressive agent, and it causes infertility, particularly in males.

Mitotane

The principal application of mitotane (*o,p'*-DDD), a compound chemically similar to the insecticides DDT and DDD, is in the treatment of neoplasms derived from the adrenal cortex. In studies of the toxicology of related insecticides in dogs, it was noted that the adrenal cortex was severely damaged, an effect caused by the presence of the *o,p'* isomer of DDD, whose structural formula is as follows:

MITOTANE

Cytotoxic Action. The mechanism of action of mitotane has not been elucidated, but its relatively selective attack on adrenocortical cells, normal or neoplastic, is well established. Thus, administration of the drug causes a rapid reduction in the levels of adrenocorticosteroids and their metabolites in blood and urine, a response that is useful both in guiding dosage and in following the course of hyperadrenocorticism (Cushing's syndrome) resulting from an adrenal tumor or adrenal hyperplasia.

Damage to the liver, kidneys, or bone marrow has not been encountered.

Absorption, Fate, and Excretion. Clinical studies indicate that approximately 40% of mitotane is absorbed after oral administration. After daily doses of 5 to 15 g, concentrations of 10 to 90 μg/ml of unchanged drug and 30 to 50 μg/ml of a metabolite are present in the blood. After discontinuation of therapy, plasma concentrations of mitotane are still measurable for 6 to 9 weeks. Although the drug is found in all tissues, fat is the primary site of storage. A water-soluble metabolite of mitotane is found in the urine; approximately 25% of an oral or parenteral dose is recovered in this form. About 60% of an oral dose is excreted unchanged in the stool.

Therapeutic Uses. *Mitotane* (LYSODREN) is administered in initial daily oral doses of 2 to 6 g, usually given in three or four divided portions, but the maximal tolerated dose may vary from 2 to 16 g per day. Treatment should be continued for at least 3 months; if beneficial effects are observed, therapy should be maintained indefinitely. Spironolactone should not be administered concomitantly, since it interferes with the adrenal suppression produced by mitotane (Wortsman and Soler, 1977).

Treatment with mitotane is indicated for the palliation of inoperable adrenocortical carcinoma. Hutter and Kayhoe (1966) reported on treatment in 138 patients, and 115 were studied by Lubitz and associates (1973). Clinical effectiveness was reported in 34% to 54% of these cases. Apparent cures have been reported in some patients with metastatic disease (Becker and Schumacher, 1975; Ostuni and Roginsky, 1975).

Clinical Toxicity. Although the administration of mitotane produces anorexia and nausea in approximately 80% of patients, somnolence and lethargy in about 34%, and dermatitis in 15% to 20%, these effects do not contraindicate the use of the drug at lower doses. Since this drug damages the adrenal cortex, administration of adrenocorticosteroids is indicated, particularly in patients with evidence of adrenal insufficiency, shock, or severe trauma (Hogan *et al.*, 1978).

V. HORMONES AND RELATED AGENTS

ADRENOCORTICOSTEROIDS

The pharmacology, major therapeutic uses, and toxic effects of the glucocorticoids are discussed in Chapter 60. Only the applications of the hormones in the treatment of neoplastic disease are considered here. Because of their lympholytic effects and their ability to suppress mitosis in lymphocytes, the greatest value of these steroids as cytotoxic agents is in the treatment of acute leukemia in children and malignant lymphoma in children and adults.

In acute lymphoblastic or undifferentiated leukemia of childhood, glucocorticoids may produce prompt clinical improvement and objective hematological remissions in up to 30% of children. Although these responses frequently are characterized by complete disappearance of all detectable leukemic cells from the peripheral blood and bone marrow, the duration of remission is brief. Remissions occur more rapidly with glucocorticoids than with antimetabolites, and there is no evidence of cross-resistance to unrelated agents. For these reasons, therapy is initiated with *prednisone* and vincristine often followed by an anthracycline, or methotrexate, and L-asparaginase. Glucocorticoids are a valuable component of curative regimens for Hodgkin's disease and non-Hodgkin's lymphoma, as well as for treatment of multiple myeloma and chronic lymphocytic leukemia (CLL). Glucocorticoids are extremely helpful in controlling autoimmune hemolytic anemia and thrombocytopenia associated with CLL.

The glucocorticoids, particularly *dexamethasone,* are used in conjunction with x-ray therapy to reduce edema related to tumors in critical areas such as the superior mediastinum, brain, and spinal cord. Doses of 4 to 6 mg every 6 hours have dramatic effects in restoring neurological function in patients with cerebral metastases, but these effects are temporary. Acute changes in dexamethasone dosage can lead to a rapid recrudescence of symptoms. Dexamethasone should not be discontinued abruptly in patients receiving radiotherapy or chemotherapy for brain metastases. Gradual tapering of the dosage may be undertaken if a clinical response to definitive antitumor therapy has been achieved. The antitumor effects of glucocorticoids are mediated by their binding to a specific cytoplasmic receptor, which, when activated, induces a program of gene expression that leads to apoptosis.

Several glucocorticoids are available and at appropriate dosages exert similar effects (*see* Chapter 60). Prednisone, for example, is usually administered orally in doses as high as 60 to 100 mg, or even higher, for the first few days and gradually reduced to levels of 20 to 40 mg per day. A continuous attempt should be made to establish the lowest possible dosage required to control the manifestations of the disease. These agents, when used chronically, exert a wide range of side effects, including glucose intolerance, immunosuppression, osteoporosis, gastrointestinal ulceration, and psychosis (*see* Chapter 60).

AMINOGLUTETHIMIDE AND OTHER AROMATASE INHIBITORS

Aminoglutethimide

Originally developed as an anticonvulsant, aminoglutethimide subsequently was found to inhibit the synthesis of adrenocortical steroids (*see* Chapter 60). Aminoglutethimide inhibits the conversion of cholesterol to pregnenolone, the first step in the synthesis of cortisol. Inhibition of cortisol synthesis, however, results in a compensatory rise in the secretion of adrenocorticotropic hormone (ACTH) sufficient to overcome the adrenal blockade. Administration of dexamethasone does not prevent the increase in ACTH secretion because aminoglutethimide accelerates the metabolism of dexamethasone. Since the metabolism of hydrocortisone (cortisol) is not affected by amino-

glutethimide, this combination produces reliable inhibition of the synthesis of cortisol (Santen *et al.,* 1980). Aminoglutethimide has been used to treat patients with adrenocortical carcinoma and Cushing's syndrome or metastatic, hormone-dependent breast cancer refractory to other hormonal approaches.

Although aminoglutethimide effectively blocks the secretion of cortisol, the production of other adrenal steroids—such as testosterone, dihydrotestosterone, androstenedione, progesterone, and 17-hydroxyprogesterone—is only partially inhibited. In certain tissues, including fat, muscle, and liver, androstenedione is converted by aromatization to estrone and estradiol. In postmenopausal and castrated women, the adrenal gland does not produce estrogens, but it is the most important source of precursors of estrogens. By inhibiting cytochrome P450–dependent hydroxylation reactions that are necessary for aromatization reactions, aminoglutethimide is a potent inhibitor of the conversion of androgens to estrogens in extraadrenal tissues. Patients treated with aminoglutethimide and hydrocortisone thus experience a lowering of plasma and urinary concentrations of estradiol that is equivalent to that observed in patients treated by surgical adrenalectomy (Santen *et al.,* 1982).

Therapeutic Uses.   When it is used to treat patients with metastatic breast cancer, *aminoglutethimide* (CYTADREN) is administered orally at a dose of 125 mg twice daily in combination with 20 mg of hydrocortisone for 2 weeks, then increasing to 250 mg twice a day together with 40 mg of hydrocortisone in divided doses. The largest dose of hydrocortisone, 20 mg, is given at night. After 2 weeks of aminoglutethimide therapy, corticosteroid synthesis recovers spontaneously, and hydrocortisone supplementation may be discontinued. When used to control Cushing's syndrome, aminoglutethimide is given in the same dosage but without hydrocortisone. In these patients, plasma concentrations of hydrocortisone should be monitored, and the dose of aminoglutethimide is titrated as necessary (up to 2 g per day) to achieve suppression of adrenal function. In some patients, significant inhibition of adrenal function occurs at doses of 250 to 500 mg daily, and toxicity is thus reduced.

The major indication for the use of aminoglutethimide is to produce inhibition of aromatase activity (the conversion of androgens to estrogens) in patients with advanced carcinoma of the breast when the tumor contains estrogen receptors. Its primary role in this setting has been supplanted by *tamoxifen,* with aminoglutethimide considered as either a second- or a third-line endocrine maneuver. If women are selected for therapy without regard to the status of estrogen receptors in the tumor, the response rate is 37%; patients whose tumor cells contain estrogen receptors experience a 50% response rate. Skin, soft tissue, and bone lesions respond more frequently than do lesions at other sites of metastasis. Such treatment is equal or superior to surgical adrenalectomy or hypophysectomy.

Clinical Toxicity.   Early toxic effects of aminoglutethimide include lethargy, visual blurring, drowsiness, and ataxia. These symptoms usually resolve after 4 to 6 weeks of treatment. A pruritic, maculopapular rash usually appears 10 days after treatment is initiated and resolves after approximately 5 days without withdrawal of the drug. Since the adrenal gland recovers normal secretory activity and the response to stress 36 hours after hydrocortisone is withdrawn, it is not necessary to taper the administration of this agent.

Steroidal and Imidazole Aromatase Inhibitors

Two newer classes of inhibitors of aromatase, the enzyme that converts androgens to estrogens, have found a useful role in breast cancer treatment; these include the steroidal androstenedione analogs *formestane* and *exemestane* and the imidazole inhibitors *anastrozole, vorozole,* and *letrozole* (*see also* Chapter 58). The imidazoles have become the dominant aromatase inhibitors in clinical use because of their oral route of administration, their greater effectiveness in lowering serum estrogen levels, and their favorable toxicity profile (Ellis and Swain, 2001).

Formestane, which has not been approved for use in the United States but is used elsewhere, is given in 250-mg doses by intramuscular injection, after which it is slowly absorbed. It has a half-life of 5 to 10 days and is given every other week. Its range of toxicities include androgenic skin (acne) and hair changes, vaginal spotting, hot flashes, emotional lability, nausea, and other minor side effects. Like other aromatase inhibitors, it produces a response rate of 10% to 30% in patients with estrogen receptor–positive metastatic disease, and is used primarily as second-line therapy following a tamoxifen response and recurrence of disease.

Exemestane (AROMASIN) is a more potent, orally administered analog that lowers estrogen levels more effectively than does formestane. It is FDA-approved for use in the United States. Doses of 25 mg per day inhibit aromatase activity by 98% and lower estrone and estradiol levels in plasma by about 90%. It has less androgenic activity than does formestane but otherwise has a similar toxicity profile. Since significant quantities of active metabolites are excreted in the urine, doses of exemestane should be adjusted in patients with renal dysfunction.

The imidazole aromatase inhibitors have the advantage of oral administration, rapid onset of action, total suppression of estrogen levels below limits of detection, no androgenic side effects, and clearance by hepatic metabolism (no dose adjustment needed for renal dysfunction). Anastrozole and letrozole are FDA-approved for use in the United States. Because of its long half-life of 50 hours, anastrozole (ARIMIDEX) can be administered once a day in doses of 1 mg. Letrozole (FEMARA) has minimal toxicity. In clinical trials comparing letrozole, 2.5 mg/day, and aminoglutethimide, letrozole produced a slightly higher response rate (18% *vs.* 11%) and a somewhat longer time

to progression and longer survival in patients who had previously progressed on tamoxifen (Gershanovich *et al.,* 1998). Ongoing clinical trials are comparing adjuvant therapy with tamoxifen alone to combinations of tamoxifen and aromatase inhibitors. The utility of aromatase inhibitors also is being explored in trials of breast cancer prevention.

PROGESTINS

Progestational agents (*see* Chapter 58) are useful as second-line hormonal therapy for metastatic hormone-dependent breast cancer and in the management of endometrial carcinoma previously treated by surgery and radiotherapy. In addition, progestins stimulate appetite and restore a sense of well-being in cachectic patients with advanced stages of cancer and AIDS. While progesterone itself is poorly absorbed when given orally and must be used with an oil carrier when given intramuscularly, there are synthetic progesterone preparations. *Hydroxyprogesterone caproate* usually is administered intramuscularly in doses of 1000 mg one or more times weekly; *medroxyprogesterone acetate* (DEPO-PROVERA) can be administered intramuscularly in doses of 400 to 1000 mg weekly. An alternative and more commonly used oral agent is *megestrol acetate* (MEGACE; 40 to 320 mg daily, in divided doses). Beneficial effects have been observed in approximately one-third of patients with endometrial cancer. The response of breast cancer to megestrol is predicted by both the presence of hormonal receptors and the evidence of response to a prior hormonal treatment. Progestin therapy in breast cancer appears to be dose-dependent, with patients demonstrating second responses following escalation of megestrol to 1600 mg/day. Responses to progestational agents also have been reported in metastatic carcinomas of the prostate and kidney.

ESTROGENS AND ANDROGENS

Discussions of the pharmacology of the estrogens and androgens appear in Chapters 58 and 59. Their use in the treatment of certain neoplastic diseases is discussed here. They are of value in this connection because certain organs that are often the primary sites of growth, notably the prostate and the mammary gland, are dependent upon hormones for their growth, function, and morphological integrity. Carcinomas arising from these organs often retain some of the hormonal responsiveness of their normal counterparts for varying periods of time. By changing the hormonal environment of such tumors it is possible to alter the course of the neoplastic process.

Androgen-Control Therapy of Prostatic Carcinoma. The development of antiandrogenic therapy for prostatic carcinoma is largely the contribution of Huggins and associates (1941). Although the hormonal treatment of metastatic prostate carcinoma is palliative, life expectancy is increased and thousands of patients have enjoyed its benefit.

Localized prostate cancer is curable with surgery or radiation therapy. However, when distant metastases are already present, hormonal therapy becomes the primary treatment. Standard approaches to achieve reduction in the concentrations of endogenous androgens or inhibition of their effects include bilateral orchiectomy, antiandrogens, or most commonly, the administration of gonadotropin-releasing hormone (GnRH) agonists with or without antiandrogens (*see* below).

Subjective and objective improvements rapidly follow the institution of androgen-control therapy of prostatic carcinoma in the majority of patients with metastatic disease, and these benefits last an average of one year. From the patient's point of view, the most gratifying is relief of bone pain. This is associated with an increase in appetite, weight gain, and a feeling of well-being. Objectively, there are regressions of the primary tumor and soft tissue metastases, but neoplastic cells do not disappear completely. The concentration of prostate-specific antigen (PSA) in plasma is a useful marker of response. Eventually prostatic tumors become insensitive to androgen deprivation through loss or mutation of the androgen receptor, which in some patients recognizes androgen antagonists such as *flutamide* (*see* below and Chapter 59) as agonists. In such cases, withdrawal of the antagonist may lead to a response.

Estrogens and Androgens in the Treatment of Mammary Carcinoma. Because of the paucity of side effects and the equivalence of response, the use of antiestrogens such as tamoxifen largely has replaced treatment with estrogens or androgens as the initial approach to the hormonal therapy of breast cancer.

Although the choice of regimen for the treatment of carcinoma of the breast is largely empirical, progress in endocrinology has led to the development of methods that are very useful for the selection of patients likely to respond. Tissues responsive to estrogens contain receptors for the hormones that can be detected by either ligand-binding techniques or monoclonal antibodies. Carcinomas that lack specific estrogen-binding capacity rarely respond to hormonal therapy. The tumors that contain receptors for either estrogen or progesterone have a 50% or greater response rate to hormonal therapy and, furthermore, have a better overall prognosis independent of the type of therapy.

The onset of action of the hormones is slow. It often is necessary to continue therapy for 8 to 12 weeks before a decision can be reached as to effectiveness. If a favorable response is obtained, hormonal treatment should be continued until an exacerbation of symptoms occurs. Withdrawal of the hormone at this time is followed by remission of disease in 30% of cases. The duration of an induced remission averages about 1 year; however, some patients may receive benefit for years.

ANTIESTROGENS

Tamoxifen

The introduction of effective and nontoxic antiestrogen agents that block the actions of estrogen has been a relatively recent event (*see* Chapter 58). However, these agents (principally the selective estrogen receptor modulator *tamoxifen*) have become first-line therapy for the hormonal treatment of breast cancer, both for adjuvant treatment and for the therapy of metastatic disease. Most recently, tamoxifen has shown effectiveness in reducing breast cancer incidence in women at high risk of developing breast can-

cer as the result of heredity, age greater than 60, or history of prior benign breast disease (Fisher *et al.,* 1998).

Mechanism of Action. Tamoxifen is a competitive inhibitor of estradiol binding to the estrogen receptor (ER). When bound to the ER, tamoxifen induces a change in the three-dimensional shape of the receptor, inhibiting its binding to the estrogen-responsive element (ERE) on DNA. Under normal physiological conditions, estrogen stimulation increases tumor cell production of transforming growth factor β (TGF-β), an autocrine inhibitor of tumor cell growth. By blocking these pathways, the net effect of tamoxifen treatment is to decrease the autocrine stimulation of breast cancer growth. In addition, tamoxifen decreases the local production of insulin-like growth factor 1 (IGF-1) by surrounding tissues; IGF-1 is a paracrine growth factor for the breast cancer cell (Jordan and Murphy, 1990). Both inhibitory and stimulatory cofactors influence the tissue-specific response to tamoxifen. Thus while the drug is inhibitory to tumors, it has estrogen-like effects on bone and the endometrial lining and increases the risk of thrombotic events.

Absorption, Fate, and Excretion. Tamoxifen is readily absorbed following oral administration, with peak concentrations measurable after 3 to 7 hours and steady-state levels reached at 4 to 6 weeks (Jordan, 1982). The drug is metabolized predominantly to *N*-desmethyltamoxifen and to 4-hydroxytamoxifen, a more potent metabolite. Both of these metabolites can be further converted to 4-hydroxy-*N*-desmethyltamoxifen, which retains high affinity for the ER. The parent drug has a terminal half-life of 7 days, while the half-lives of *N*-desmethyltamoxifen and 4-hydroxytamoxifen are significantly longer. After enterohepatic circulation, glucuronides and other metabolites are excreted in the stool; excretion in the urine is minimal.

Therapeutic Uses. *Tamoxifen citrate* (NOLVADEX) is marketed for oral administration. The usual dose prescribed in the United States is 10 mg twice a day. Doses as high as 200 mg per day have been used in the therapy of breast cancer, but high doses are associated with retinal degeneration.

Tamoxifen is the endocrine treatment of choice for postmenopausal women with estrogen-receptor positive (ER$^+$) metastatic breast cancer or following primary tumor therapy in the adjuvant setting, where it is frequently used following chemotherapy.

Tamoxifen also is used in premenopausal women with ER$^+$ tumors; although response rates appear to be equal to those in postmenopausal patients, other alternatives such as oophorectomy or gonadotropin-releasing hormone analogs (*leuprolide, goserelin*) have the advantage of eliminating ovarian estrogen production. The combined use of tamoxifen and a gonadotropin-releasing hormone analog (to reduce high estrogen levels resulting from tamoxifen effects on the gonadal-pituitary axis) has had a better response rate and improved overall survival than has either drug alone (Klijn *et al.,* 2000).

Tamoxifen has been used alone as an adjuvant therapy for ER$^+$ women at risk for recurrence following initial diagnosis and treatment of primary breast cancer. Both the NOLVADEX Adjuvant Trial Organization (NATO) study, which compared 2 years of tamoxifen treatment to observation (Baum, 1988), and the Scottish trial, which compared 5 years of tamoxifen to observation (Breast Cancer Trials Committee, 1987), indicate an overall survival advantage for the patients receiving tamoxifen. Five years of adjuvant therapy with tamoxifen yields superior results compared to 1 or 2 years of therapy (Early Breast Cancer Trialists' Collaborative Group, 1998).

Tamoxifen and a related antiestrogen, *raloxifene* (EVISTA; *see* Chapter 58), have shown striking effectiveness in initial trials for preventing breast cancer in high-risk women (Jordan, 1999). These studies have been undertaken because tamoxifen not only prevents the development of breast cancer in animal models but also decreases the incidence of second primary breast cancers in women on adjuvant hormonal therapy. Since the risk-to-benefit ratio is different when one is attempting to prevent disease that has yet to be diagnosed, prevention trials have been designed with special attention to the possible long-term side effects of tamoxifen treatment, which include thrombotic events, endometrial cancer, and atrophy of the lining of the vagina. Longer follow-up with assessment of quality of life issues will provide a clearer understanding of the place of tamoxifen in breast cancer prevention.

Clinical Toxicity. The most frequent adverse reactions to tamoxifen include hot flashes, nausea, and vomiting. These may occur in as many as 25% of patients and are rarely sufficiently severe to require discontinuation of therapy. Menstrual irregularities, vaginal bleeding and discharge, pruritus vulvae, and dermatitis occur frequently, depending on the menopausal state of the patient.

There is increasing concern about the potential of tamoxifen for causing endometrial cancer. The incidence of this tumor appears to be at least twofold higher in women who received 20 mg per day for 2 years or longer than in untreated controls. Patients receiving tamoxifen should have at least yearly pelvic examinations and should report symptoms or signs such as pelvic discomfort or vaginal bleeding (Fisher, 1994).

Tamoxifen increases the risk of thromboembolic events. Like estrogen, tamoxifen is a hepatic carcinogen in animals, although increases in primary hepatocellular carcinoma have not been reported in patients on the drug. Tamoxifen causes retinal deposits, decreased visual acuity, and cataracts in occasional patients, although the frequency of these changes is uncertain (Longstaff *et al.*, 1989).

The estrogenic effect of tamoxifen also has potentially salubrious effects beyond its potential to prevent the recurrence or development of breast cancer. Tamoxifen may slow the development of osteoporosis in postmenopausal women (Fornander *et al.*, 1990). In addition, like certain estrogens, tamoxifen low-

ers total serum cholesterol, LDL cholesterol, and lipoproteins and raises apolipoprotein AI levels, potentially decreasing the risk of myocardial infarction (Love *et al.*, 1994).

GONADOTROPIN-RELEASING HORMONE ANALOGS

Gonadotropin-releasing hormone (GnRH) analogs came into use in the 1980s, and provided a medical form of castration for prostate carcinoma and an additional hormonal manipulation for breast cancer (*see* Chapter 56). The analogs of the GnRH peptide—*leuprolide* (LUPRON), *goserelin* (ZOLADEX), *triptorelin* (TRELSTAR DEPOT), and *buserelin* (SUPREFACT; not available in the United States)—have biphasic effects on the pituitary. Initially, they stimulate the secretion of both follicle-stimulating hormone (FSH) and luteinizing hormone (LH). However, with longer-term administration, cells become desensitized to the action of GnRH analogs. As a result, there is inhibition of the secretion of LH and FSH; the concentration of testosterone falls to castration levels in men, and the concentrations of estrogens fall to postmenopausal values in women. Randomized trials in patients with prostatic carcinomas have shown that GnRH analogs are as effective as diethylstilbestrol and bilateral orchiectomy. These compounds are associated with less toxicity than the estrogenic compound, and they do not carry the disadvantage of irreversibility as does surgical castration. One important side effect, a transient flare of disease, may result from the initial capacity of the GnRH analogs to stimulate the pituitary, but it is not a cause for discontinuation of therapy. (*See* Chapter 56 for discussion of newly developed GnRH competitive antagonists that do not cause an initial increase in testosterone levels.) Flare of the disease can be prevented by the temporary (2 to 4 weeks) concurrent administration of an antiandrogen such as flutamide or bicalutamide (*see* below). The advantages of long-term, complete androgen blockade with combination treatment over GnRH analogs alone are controversial (Eisenberger *et al.*, 1998; Prostate Cancer Trialists' Collaborative Group, 2000). Leuprolide and goserelin also have been approved by the FDA for the treatment of metastatic breast cancer. These compounds are as effective as tamoxifen in premenopausal patients, and combined treatment with tamoxifen and a GnRH analog appears to be better than treatment with either one alone (Klijn *et al.*, 2000). Other therapeutic indications of GnRH agonists include endometriosis, anemia secondary to uterine leiomyomas, and central precocious puberty. The primary toxicities of GnRH analogs are secondary to the reduction of sex steroid concentrations and include hot flashes, sweating, nausea, fatigue, and decreases in bone and muscle mass. These drugs are administered intramuscularly or subcutaneously (every 4 to 16 weeks) in a parenteral, sustained-release microcapsule preparation because current parenteral administration of the parent drug otherwise is associated with rapid clearance.

ANTIANDROGENS

Antiandrogens are competitive inhibitors that prevent the natural ligands of the androgen receptor from binding to the receptor. These compounds, therefore, have activity on their own against prostate cancer. They also are effective in preventing the flare reaction induced by the testosterone surge that can occur with GnRH monotherapy. Theoretically, antiandrogen therapy, in combination with a GnRH agonist, leads to a more complete androgen blockade by additionally inhibiting the biological effects of androgens produced in the adrenal glands. Clinical data, however, do not support the systematic use of complete androgen blockade, which is associated with more side effects than medical or surgical castration alone, but comparable efficacy (Eisenberger *et al.*, 1998; Prostate Cancer Trialists' Collaborative Group, 2000). Antiandrogen monotherapy is not indicated either as routine, first-line treatment for patients with advanced disease.

The antiandrogens typically are divided structurally and mechanistically into steroidal and nonsteroidal antiandrogens (NSAAs) (Reid *et al.*, 1999). The steroidal agents have some partial agonist activity at the androgen receptor, whereas the NSAAs do not have significant agonist activity at the wild-type androgen receptor. The steroidal antiandrogens with which there is the most experience are *cyproterone acetate* (ANDROCUR) and *megestrol acetate* (MEGACE) (*see* above and Chapter 59). The steroidal antiandrogens are weak partial agonists and competitive inhibitors of the androgen receptor in target tissues. In addition, they have progestational agonist properties at the level of the pituitary that reduce LH secretion. Consequently, LH-stimulated testosterone production decreases. The loss of libido, decreased sexual potency, and low testosterone levels produced by steroidal antiandrogens are among the major distinctions between the steroidal antiandrogens and NSAAs.

The NSAAs in common usage are *flutamide* (EULEXIN), *nilutamide* (NILANDRON), and *bicalutamide* (CASODEX). These anilid derivatives inhibit the translocation of the androgen receptor to the nucleus from the cytoplasm of target cells. This appears to be the only mechanism by which NSAAs exert their antiproliferative effect in prostate cancer patients. In fact, the blockade of testos-

terone binding in the CNS interrupts the negative feedback of testosterone on gonadotropin secretion (Knuth *et al.*, 1984). As a consequence, and in contrast to steroidal antiandrogens, testosterone levels increase with the use of NSAA monotherapy and the loss of sexual desire and loss of potency are less pronounced.

Flutamide was the first androgen receptor antagonist to achieve widespread use. It is metabolized to α-hydroxyflutamide, which has a half-life of about 8 hours and exerts more potent androgen blockade than does the parent compound. The drug is given orally, typically 250 mg three times a day. Side effects of flutamide include occasional diarrhea, emesis, reversible liver abnormalities, a variable degree of loss of sexual function, decreased libido, hot flashes, and gynecomastia and mastodynia. Nilutamide is extensively metabolized in the liver although it does not require metabolism into an active compound. The elimination half-life is 38 to 40 hours, which allows once-daily dosing (150 mg). Diarrhea is reported less commonly with nilutamide than with flutamide; nilutamide, however, causes diminished adaptation to darkness and other visual disturbances, alcohol intolerance, and idiopathic allergic pneumonitis in 25% to 40%, 5% to 20%, and 1% to 2% of patients, respectively. Bicalutamide has a serum half-life of 5 to 6 days, which allows once-daily dosing. The standard dose of bicalutamide when used with a GnRH agonist is 50 mg/day, which is well tolerated. Gynecomastia and nipple tenderness are the most commonly reported side effects of this compound. The drug does not have unique side effects, as do the other two NSAAs, and the incidence of secondary diarrhea is half of that associated with flutamide. The tolerability of bicalutamide remains good at doses of 200 mg/day. Studies with doses up to 600 mg are in progress.

BIOLOGICAL RESPONSE MODIFIERS

Biological response modifiers include agents or approaches that affect the patient's biological response to a neoplasm beneficially. Included are agents that act indirectly to mediate their antitumor effects (*e.g.*, by enhancing the immunological response to neoplastic cells) or directly on the tumor cells (*e.g.*, differentiating agents). Recombinant DNA technology has greatly facilitated the identification and production of a number of human proteins with potent effects on the function and growth of both normal and neoplastic cells. Proteins that are currently in clinical trials include the *interferons* (*see* Chapters 50 and 53), *interleukins* (*see* Chapter 53), hematopoietic growth factors (*see* Chapter 54) such as *erythropoietin*, filgrastim [granulocyte colony-stimulating factor (G-CSF)], and *sargramostim* [granulocyte/macrophage colony-stimulating factor (GM-CSF)] (*see* below), *tumor necrosis factor* (TNF), and monoclonal antibodies such as *trastuzumab* and *rituximab* (*see* below).

Several of these agents now have been approved for clinical use because of their activity in specific diseases. For example, *interferon-alfa* is approved for use in hairy cell leukemia, condylomata acuminata, and Kaposi's sarcoma associated with AIDS; *interleukin-2* (IL-2) for kidney cancer; *filgrastim* for prophylaxis against cancer treatment–induced neutropenia; and *sargramostim* for rescue from graft failure or to speed graft recovery in patients undergoing autologous bone marrow transplantation. Other biological agents have been approved for the treatment of nonmalignant disease, including *interferon-beta* for multiple sclerosis and *interferon-gamma* for chronic granulomatous disease (*see* Chapter 53), herceptin for breast cancer, and rituximab for B-cell lymphomas.

Interleukin-2 (IL-2)

The isolation of a cytokine initially named T-cell growth factor, subsequently renamed IL-2, allowed the first attempts to treat cancer by producing lymphocytes specifically cytolytic for the malignant cell (Morgan *et al.*, 1976). IL-2 is not directly cytotoxic; rather, it induces and expands a T-cell response cytolytic for tumor cells. Clinical trials have studied the antitumor activity of IL-2 both as a single agent and with adoptive cellular therapy using IL-2–stimulated autologous lymphocytes obtained by leukapheresis, termed *lymphokine-activated killer (LAK) cells*. Randomized trials have not shown that the addition of LAK cells to the treatment regimen improves overall response rates (Rosenberg *et al.*, 1989). Later studies in adoptive cellular therapy have used expanded populations of lymphocytes obtained from tumor biopsies and expanded *in vitro*, so-called tumor-infiltrating lymphocytes (TIL cells) (Rosenberg *et al.*, 1994).

Because the half-life of IL-2 in human beings is short ($t_{1/2}\alpha = 13$ minutes; $t_{1/2}\beta = 85$ minutes) (Konrad *et al.*, 1990), most clinical schedules have explored either continuous infusion or multiple intermittent dosing. Others have explored the use of liposome-encapsulated IL-2 and conjugation of IL-2 with polyethylene glycol to extend the half-life of IL-2 and to enhance its delivery to immune cells in tumors. These alternative forms of IL-2 therapy are experimental at this time (Bukowski *et al.*, 2001). The most significant antitumor activity has been demonstrated with the most intense dosing schedules: continuous intravenous infusion for 5 days every other week for 2 cycles or intravenous bolus dosing every 8 hours daily for 5 days every other week.

The toxicities of IL-2 are likely related to the activation and expansion of lytic lymphocytes in organs and within vessels, resulting in inflammation and vascular leak, and to the secondary release of other cytokines, such as tumor necrosis factor and interferon, by activated cells. When given at maximally tolerated doses of 600,000 U/kg every 8 hours for up to 5 days, IL-2 causes hypotension, arrhythmias, peripheral edema, prerenal azotemia, elevated liver function tests, anemia, thrombocytopenia, nausea, vomiting, diarrhea, confusion, and fever (Rosenberg *et al.*, 1989).

Reproducible antitumor activity has been reported in advanced malignant melanoma and renal cell cancer, where response rates (partial and complete) are seen in 20% to 30% of patients. Complete responses, seen in approximately 5% to 10% of all patients, appear to be durable, with some patients now free of disease beyond 5 years of treatment.

IL-2 currently is being studied in the treatment of acute myelogenous leukemia, where it is capable of inducing remission in relapsed patients (Meloni *et al.*, 1994). In some studies where IL-2 is given following bone marrow transplantation, it appears that IL-2 can lengthen the remission duration as compared to historical controls (Fefer *et al.*, 1993). Randomized trials are in progress to test this hypothesis prospectively.

Granulocyte Colony-Stimulating Factor (Filgrastim)

Filgrastim (NEUPOGEN) is a commercially available granulocyte colony-stimulating factor (G-CSF). Filgrastim is approved for clinical use in the prophylaxis of chemotherapy-induced neutropenia. It was initially isolated and cloned from a human bladder cancer cell line (Souza *et al.*, 1986). *In vitro*, G-CSF was found not only to expand the population of neutrophil granulocyte precursors, but also to augment granulocyte function by enhancing chemotaxis and antibody-dependent cellular cytotoxicity. Its effects are confined to the granulocyte lineage. It also enhances the mobilization of stem cells in the peripheral blood following cytotoxic chemotherapy.

In normal volunteers or cancer patients not receiving other treatment, administration of filgrastim leads to an initial reduction of circulating neutrophils within 1 hour, followed by a dose-dependent (1 to 60 μg/kg per day) increase in the absolute neutrophil count (ANC) (Morstyn *et al.*, 1989). A number of studies in which filgrastim has been used to prevent the neutropenia associated with high-dose chemotherapy have shown that treatment results in an improved ANC, the delivery of doses of chemotherapy on schedule and at prescribed doses, and fewer patient days in hospital recovering from febrile neutropenia (Gabrilove *et al.*, 1988; Crawford *et al.*, 1991). It remains to be seen whether or not the improvement in the dose intensity of anticancer drugs permitted by the administration of filgrastim will translate into an improvement in patient survival.

The recommended dose of filgrastim is 5 μg/kg per day subcutaneously starting 24 hours after the completion of chemotherapy and continuing until the white blood count exceeds 10,000 cells/μl. At these doses the agent is extremely well tolerated. The only consistent toxicity is bone pain in the lower back, sternum, and pelvis, likely resulting from an expansion of cells and increased blood flow in the medullary space.

Granulocyte/Macrophage Colony-Stimulating Factor (Sargramostim)

Sargramostim (LEUKINE) is a commercially available recombinant granulocyte/macrophage colony-stimulating factor (GM-CSF) produced in a yeast expression system. Sargramostim is approved to rescue bone marrow graft failure or speed graft recovery in patients undergoing autologous bone marrow transplantation and to shorten time to neutrophil recovery after induction chemotherapy in patients with acute myelogenous leukemia. Human GM-CSF was initially purified from a T-cell leukemia-infected lymphoblastoid cell line and cloned in 1985 (Wong *et al.*, 1985). The *in vitro* effects of GM-CSF are more protean than those of G-CSF, as the agent is active earlier in the differentiation pathway of the pleuripotential stem cell. Macrophages, neutrophils, and eosinophils all respond to GM-CSF with proliferation and enhanced antibody-dependent cellular cytotoxicity (Lopez *et al.*, 1986).

The glycosylation of GM-CSF is variable and dependent on whether the preparation is derived from yeast (glycosylated) or bacterial (nonglycosylated) cells. In normal volunteers or cancer patients not receiving other treatment, GM-CSF causes a dose-dependent increase in neutrophils as well as increases in eosinophils and macrophages. In the setting of autologous bone marrow transplantation, GM-CSF accelerates the recovery of neutrophils in the peripheral blood while decreasing the need for antibiotics to treat febrile neutropenia (Nemunaitis *et al.*, 1991).

The toxicity of GM-CSF preparations appears to be dependent, at least in part, on whether or not the molecule is glycosylated. The glycosylated product commonly causes fever, bone pain, and myalgias. The nonglycosylated product has similar toxicities but additionally can cause pericarditis and a first-dose phenomenon of flushing, hypotension, hypoxia, and tachycardia. These symptoms diminish as the patient continues through a treatment cycle but recur at the beginning of each subsequent cycle. The commonly recommended dose of sargramostim is 250 μg/m^2 intravenously over 2 hours per day. Continuous-infusion dosing or subcutaneous dosing appears to be superior in response to dosing by 2-hour infusion.

Monoclonal Antibodies in Cancer Therapy

For the past two decades, since the discovery of the method for fusing mouse myeloma cells with B lymphocytes, it has been possible to produce a single species of antibody that recognizes a specific antigen. The mouse antibody can now be "humanized"; that is, the domains not responsible for antigen recognition can be converted to human type to prevent a human-antimouse neutralizing response. Such antibodies now are used for immune suppression, anticoagulation, and, more recently, for cancer treatment. Two such antibodies, *trastuzumab* (HERCEPTIN) and *rituximab* (RITUXAN), have won a role in treating breast cancer and B-cell lymphomas, respectively (Hainsworth, 2000).

The mechanism by which these antibodies kill cells is unresolved. There is no doubt that binding to specific cell-surface antigens is required as a first step. Trastuzumab binds to the her-2/neu growth factor receptor, a member of the epidermal growth factor receptor family. Whether its cytotoxic/cytostatic effect is related to T-cell–mediated recognition of the bound antibody or to its inhibitory effect on the growth factor pathway has not been clarified. About one-quarter of breast cancers are positive for her-2/neu antigen, and their tumors lie at the more aggressive end of the spectrum of breast cancers. Herceptin demonstrated only modest activity against metastatic breast cancer in its initial trials, but when used with either paclitaxel or doxorubicin, it markedly enhanced the rate of response to these cytotoxic drugs and improved survival of the patients so treated (Norton *et al.*, 1999).

Like all monoclonal antibodies (including the humanized types), acute hypersensitivity reactions may occur, including hypotension, flushing, bronchoconstriction, and rash. In addition, trastuzumab administration has resulted in ventricular dysfunc-

tion and congestive heart failure. When combined with doxorubicin, trastuzumab enhances the cardiac toxicity of the anthracyclines; in rare individuals with underlying intrinsic or metastatic disease in the lungs, it has caused pulmonary infiltrates, hypoxia, and fatal pulmonary insufficiency; it should be used with caution in these cases. Trastuzumab usually is used in conjunction with paclitaxel, docetaxel, or venorelbine in treating breast cancer. The recommended loading dose of trastuzumab is 4 mg/kg as a 90-minute intravenous infusion, and the maintenance dose is 2 mg/kg per week, which can be given as a 30-minute infusion if the loading dose was well tolerated.

Rituximab recognizes the CD20 antigen found on the surface of virtually all B-lymphocyte tumors. It has significant activity as a single agent in the treatment of indolent or follicular B-cell lymphomas, producing a response rate of 40% to 50% in patients who have relapsed or who have become refractory to standard chemotherapy (Maloney, 1998). In an effort to enhance its activity, the antibody has been combined with standard chemotherapy in primary-treatment regimens for aggressive forms of B-cell lymphoma. An alternative approach has been to label the anti-CD20 antibody with iodine 131 (^{131}I). The resulting antibody, *tositumomab* (BEXXAR), has potent myelosuppressive effects but, when used with bone-marrow replacement, produces a high rate of complete response in drug-resistant patients.

Standard doses of rituximab are 375 mg/m^2 given weekly for 4 doses by intravenous infusion. Its acute toxicity is much the same as trastuzumab's and is related to hypersensitivity, but it does not cause the cardiac effects associated with trastuzumab administration. Uncommonly, patients develop neutropenia after multiple doses.

PROSPECTUS

While the current therapy for cancer depends primarily on the use of surgery, irradiation, and chemotherapy, the evolution in understanding the biology of malignant transformation and differences in the control of normal and malignant cell proliferation has provided a myriad of new possible targets for cancer treatment. Central to this understanding has been the elucidation of events in the cell cycle that monitor the integrity of DNA, check progression through the cell cycle when nutrients or growth factors are lacking, and direct the cell to undergo apoptosis (programmed cell death) when either intrinsic or extrinsic factors are unfavorable for survival. As might have been anticipated, a malfunction in the machinery that controls normal cell proliferation can lead to consequences that favor malignant transformation: a loss of cell-cycle checkpoints such as mutation or deletion of the p53 and p16 oncogenes, an increase in genes that protect cells from apoptosis (such as the *bcl*-2 gene that is translocated in nodular lymphomas), and an increase in expression of the D cyclin (the *prad* oncogene) that promotes cell entry into DNA synthesis. Not only do these changes promote cell proliferation, they also increase the frequency with which mutant and drug-resistant cells escape normal surveillance mechanisms and apoptosis. Loss of apoptotic pathway(s) in itself predisposes to resistance to radiation therapy and drugs. Thus, a major effort now is under way to identify compounds that restore apoptosis and cell-cycle checkpoints. The replacement of a missing function, such as that resulting from mutation of p53, represents an exceedingly difficult challenge, in that one seeks a small molecule that replaces the function of a complex protein or, alternatively, a targeted gene therapy approach to introduce wild-type p53 into affected tissues (*see* Chapter 5).

Other directions for cancer drug discovery and development have emerged from tumor biology research and include differentiation inducers and inhibitors of angiogenesis and metastasis (Kerbel, 2000). The field of differentiation induction has received a significant impetus from the discovery of effectiveness of *all*-trans-*retinoic acid* in the treatment of acute promyelocytic leukemia. Although not curative as a single agent in this disease, all-*trans*-retinoic acid induces a remission in drug-refractory disease and does so without the period of marrow hypoplasia characteristic of cytotoxic drugs. Hormonal agents, planar-polar chemicals, and various retinoids and vitamin D analogs are being tested as differentiation drugs in established cancer and in preventing progression of premalignant disease. As genetic testing becomes increasingly able to identify individuals at high risk of developing cancer, the emphasis in cancer drug development will inevitably shift to the discovery of preventive or differentiating agents. The discovery of the important role of angiogenesis in allowing malignant cells to establish a generous blood supply also has led to current trials of inhibitors of endothelial cell proliferation, including low doses of cytotoxic agents as well as experimental drugs such as monoclonal antibodies to endothelial growth factors and their receptors and low-molecular-weight inhibitors of the receptors, and antiangiogenic peptides such as *endostatin* and *angiostatin*. The reader is referred to Kaelin (1999) and the series of articles that follow his introduction for a discussion of new strategies for drug discovery. Special note should be made of *imatinib* (STI-571, GLEEVEC), an inhibitor of the *bcr-abl* tyrosine kinase found in chronic myelocytic leukemia; this drug has shown remarkable remission-inducing activity as a single agent (Drucker and Lydon, 2000) and recently was approved by the FDA for clinical use.

In addition to these targeted drug discovery efforts, new efforts are in clinical trial exploring the possibility that the immune system can be harnessed to treat cancer. These approaches include tumor-specific vaccines directed against unique antigens, such as oncogene products or the products of translocated genes; monoclonal antibodies armed with toxins or radioisotopes (*see* Kawakami *et al.*, 1994); and genetically manipulated components of the immune system. Monoclonal antibodies directed against cell-surface antigens have become important new tools for producing antitumor responses as single agents (rituximab in B-cell lymphomas) or for enhancing response to chemotherapy (trastuzumab in breast cancer). Other antibodies directed against epithelial cancers, such as C225 (an anti-epidermal growth factor-receptor antibody), and 17.1 (directed against colon cancer antigens), are showing promising activity in early clinical trials.

Completion of the sequencing of the human genome provides the basis for a more detailed understanding of the specific genetic mutations involved in various human cancers. Although initially this understanding will provide more specific tumor markers useful in detection and diagnosis, eventually it is anticipated that more targeted therapeutic agents will be devised. Future editions of this text undoubtedly will contain a much different spectrum of effective anticancer drugs, and there is reason to be quite optimistic about the prospects for a much more effective and specific collection of weapons for treating this group of fatal diseases.

For further discussion of neoplastic diseases, *see* Chapters 81 to 104 in *Harrison's Principles of Internal Medicine*, 14th ed., McGraw-Hill, New York, 1998.

BIBLIOGRAPHY

Abbruzzese, J.L., Grunewald, R., Weeks, E.A., Gravel, D., Adams, T., Nowak, B., Mineishi, S., Tarassoff, P., Satterlee, W., Raber, M.N., and Plunkett, W. A phase I clinical, plasma, and cellular pharmacology study of gemcitabine. *J. Clin. Oncol.,* **1991,** 9:491–498.

Agarwal, R.P. Inhibitors of adenosine deaminase. *Pharmacol. Ther.,* **1982,** 17:399–429.

Agarwal, R.P., Spector, T., and Parks, R.E., Jr. Tight-binding inhibitors—IV. Inhibition of adenosine deaminases by various inhibitors. *Biochem. Pharmacol.,* **1977,** 26:359–367.

Alberts, D.S., Chang, S.Y., Chen, H.S., Larcom, B.J., and Jones, S.E. Pharmacokinetics and metabolism of chlorambucil in man: a preliminary report. *Cancer Treat. Rev.,* **1979a,** 6(*suppl.*):9–17.

Alberts, D.S., Chang, S.Y., Chen, H.S., Moon, T.E., Evans, T.L., Furner, R.L., Himmelstein, K., and Gross, J.F. Kinetics of intravenous melphalan. *Clin. Pharmacol. Ther.,* **1979b,** *26*:73–80.

Allegra, C.J., Chabner, B.A., Tuazon, C.U., Ogata-Arakaki, D., Baird, B., Drake, J.C., Simmons, J.T., Lack, E.E., Shelhamer, J.H., Balis, F., Walker, R., Kovacs, J.A., Lane, H.C., and Masur, H. Trimetrexate for the treatment of *Pneumocystis carinii* pneumonia in patients with acquired immunodeficiency syndrome. *N. Engl. J. Med.,* **1987a,** *317*:978–985.

Allegra, C.J., Fine, R.L., Drake, J.C., and Chabner, B.A. The effect of methotrexate on intracellular folate pools in human MCF-7 breast cancer cells. Evidence for direct inhibition of purine synthesis. *J. Biol. Chem.,* **1986,** *261*:6478–6485.

Allegra, C.J., Hoang, K., Yeh, G.C., Drake, J.C., and Baram, J. Evidence for direct inhibition of *de novo* purine synthesis in human MCF-7 breast cells as a principal mode of metabolic inhibition by methotrexate. *J. Biol. Chem.,* **1987b,** *262*:13520–13526.

Alper, J.C., Wiemann, M.C., Rueckl, F.S., McDonald, C.J., and Calabresi, P. Rationally designed combination chemotherapy for the treatment of patients with recalcitrant psoriasis. *J. Am. Acad. Dermatol.,* **1985,** *13*:567–577.

Arbuck, S.G., Douglass, H.O., Crom, W.R., Goodwin, P., Silk, Y., Cooper, C., and Evans, W.E. Etoposide pharmacokinetics in patients with normal and abnormal organ function. *J. Clin. Oncol.,* **1986,** *4*: 1690–1695.

Arlin, Z., Case, D.C., Jr., Moore, J., Wiernik, P., Feldman, E., Saletan, S., Desai, P., Sia, L., and Cartwright, K. Randomized multicenter trial of cytosine arabinoside with mitoxantrone or daunorubicin in previously untreated adult patients with acute nonlymphocytic leukemia (ANLL). Lederle Cooperative Group. *Leukemia,* **1990,** *4*:177–183.

Assaraf, Y.G., and Schimke, R.T. Identification of methotrexate transport deficiency in mammalian cells using fluoresceinated methotrexate and flow cytometry. *Proc. Natl. Acad. Sci. U.S.A.,* **1987,** *84*:7154–7158.

Asselin, B.L., Whitin, J.C., Coppola, D.J., Rupp, I.P., Sallan, S.E., and Cohen, H.J. Comparative pharmacokinetic studies of three asparaginase preparations. *J. Clin. Oncol.,* **1993,** *11*:1780–1786.

Bachur, N.R., Gordon, S.L., and Gee, M.V. A general mechanism for microsomal activation of quinone anticancer agents to free radicals. *Cancer Res.,* **1978,** *38*:1745–1750.

Bajorin, D.F., Bosl, G.J., Alcock, N.W., Niedzwiecki, D., Gallina, E., and Shurgot, B. Pharmacokinetics of *cis*-diamminedichloroplatinum(II) after administration in hypertonic saline. *Cancer Res.,* **1986,** *46*:5969–5972.

Baker, D.K., Relling, M.V., Pui, C.H., Christensen, M.L., Evans, W.E., and Rodman, J.H. Increased teniposide clearance with concomitant anticonvulsant therapy. *J. Clin. Oncol.,* **1992,** *10*:311–315.

Barbour, K.W., Berger, S.H., and Berger, F.G. Single amino acid substitution defines a naturally occurring genetic variant of human thymidylate synthase. *Mol. Pharmacol.,* **1990,** *37*:515–518.

Baum, M. Controlled trial of tamoxifen as a single adjuvant agent in the management of early breast cancer. "Nolvadex" Adjuvant Trial Organisation. *Br. J. Cancer,* **1988,** *57*:608–611.

Becker, D., and Schumacher, O.P. *o,p*′-DDD therapy in invasive adrenocortical carcinoma. *Ann. Intern. Med.,* **1975,** *82*:677–679.

Begleiter, A., Glazer, R.I., Israels, L.G., Pugh, L., and Johnston, J.B. Induction of DNA strand breaks in chronic lymphocytic leukemia following treatment with 2′-deoxycoformycin *in vivo* and *in vitro. Cancer Res.,* **1987,** *47*:2498–2503.

Berman, E., Heller, G., Santorsa, J., McKenzie, S., Gee, T., Kempin, S., Gulati, S., Andreeff, M., Kolitz, J., Gabrilove, J., Reich, L., Mayer,

K., Keefe, D., Trainor, K., Schluger, A., Penenberg, D., Raymond, V., O'Reilly, R., Jhanwar, S., Young, C., and Clarkson, B. Results of a randomized trial comparing idarubicin and cytosine arabinoside with daunorubicin and cytosine arabinoside in adult patients with newly diagnosed acute myelogenous leukemia. *Blood,* **1991,** *77*:1666–1674.

Bianchi Scarra, G.L., Romani, M., Coviello, D.A., Garre, C., Ravazzolo, R., Vidali, G., and Ajmar, F. Terminal erythroid differentiation in the K-562 cell line by 1-β-D-arabinofuranosylcytosine: accompaniment by c-myc messenger RNA decrease. *Cancer Res.,* **1986,** *46*:6327–6332.

Bishop, J.F., Matthews, J.P., Young, G.A., Szer, J., Gillett, A., Joshua, D., Bradstock, K., Enno, A., Wolf, M.M., Fox, R., Cobcroft, R., Herrmann, R., Van Der Weyden, M., Lowenthal, R.M., Page, F., Garson, O.M., and Juneja, S. A randomized study of high-dose cytarabine in induction in acute myeloid leukemia. *Blood,* **1996,** *87*:1710–1717.

Bo, J., Schroder, H., Kristinsson, J., Madsen, B., Szumlanski, C., Weinshilboum, R., Andersen, J.B., and Schmiegelow, K. Possible carcinogenic effect of 6-mercaptopurine on bone marrow stem cells: relation to thiopurine metabolism. *Cancer,* **1999,** *86*:1080–1086.

Boarman, D.M., Baram, J., and Allegra, C.J. Mechanism of leucovorin reversal of methotrexate cytotoxicity in human MCF-7 breast cancer cells. *Biochem. Pharmacol.,* **1990,** *40*:2651–2660.

Boccardo, F., Cannata, D., Rubagotti, A., Guarneri, D., Decensi, A., Canobbio, L., Curotto, A., Martorana, G., Pegoraro, C., Selvaggi, F., Salvia, G., Comeri, G., Bono, A., Borella, T., and Giuliani, L. Prophylaxis of superficial bladder cancer with mitomycin or interferon alfa-2b: results of a multicentric Italian study. *J. Clin. Oncol.,* **1994,** *12*:7–13.

Bollag, W. The tumor-inhibitory effects of the methylhydrazine derivative Ro 4-6467/1 (NSC-77213). *Cancer Chemother. Rep.,* **1963,** *33*: 1–4.

Boogerd, W., van der Sande, J.J., and van Zandwijk, N. Teniposide sometimes effective in brain metastases from non-small cell lung cancer. *J. Neurooncol.,* **1999,** *41*:285–289.

Borsi, J.D., and Moe, P.J. Systemic clearance of methotrexate in the prognosis of acute lymphoblastic leukemia in children. *Cancer,* **1987,** *60*:3020–3024.

Bracken, R.B., Johnson, D.E., Rodriquez, L., Samuels, M.L., and Ayala, A. Treatment of multiple superficial tumors of bladder with intravesical bleomycin. *Urology,* **1977,** *9*:161–163.

Breast Cancer Trials Committee, Scottish Cancer Trials Office (MRC). Adjuvant tamoxifen in the management of operable breast cancer: the Scottish Trial. *Lancet,* **1987,** *2*:171–175.

Brock, N., and Pohl, J. Prevention of urotoxic side effects by regional detoxification with increased selectivity of oxazaphosphorine cytostatics. *IARC Sci. Publ.,* **1986,** *78*:269–279.

Brockman, R.W., Cheng, Y.C., Schabel, F.M., Jr., and Montgomery, J.A. Metabolism and chemotherapeutic activity of 9-β-D-arabinofuranosyl-2-fluoroadenine against murine leukemia L1210 and evidence for its phosphorylation by deoxycytidine kinase. *Cancer Res.,* **1980,** *40*:3610–3615.

Bromme, D., Rossi, A.B., Smeekens, S.P., Anderson, D.C., and Payan, D.G. Human bleomycin hydrolase: molecular cloning, sequencing, functional expression, and enzymatic characterization. *Biochemistry,* **1996,** *35*:6706–6714.

Burger, R.M., Projan, S.J., Horwitz, S.B., and Peisach, J. The DNA cleavage mechanism of iron-bleomycin. Kinetic resolution of strand scission from base propenal release. *J. Biol. Chem.,* **1986,** *261*:15955–15959.

Bushara, K.O., and Rust, R.S. Reversible MRI lesions due to pegaspargase treatment of non-Hodgkin's lymphoma. *Pediatr. Neurol.,* **1997,** *17:*185–187.

Bystroff, C., and Kraut, J. Crystal structure of unliganded *Escherichia coli* dihydrofolate reductase. Ligand-induced conformational changes and cooperativity in binding. *Biochemistry,* **1991,** *30:*2227–2239.

Cabral, F.R. Isolation of Chinese hamster ovary cell mutants requiring the continuous presence of taxol for cell division. *J. Cell Biol.,* **1983,** *97:*22–29.

Calvert, A.H., Newell, D.R., Gumbrell, L.A., O'Reilly, S., Burnell, M., Boxall, F.E., Siddik, Z.H., Judson, I.R., Gore, M.E., and Wiltshaw, E. Carboplatin dosage: prospective evaluation of a simple formula based on renal function. *J. Clin. Oncol.,* **1989,** *7:*1748–1756.

Canman, C.E., Lawrence, T.S., Shewach, D.S., Tang, H.Y., and Maybaum, J. Resistance to fluorodeoxyuridine-induced DNA damage and cytotoxicity correlates with an elevation of deoxyuridine triphosphatase activity and failure to accumulate deoxyuridine triphosphate. *Cancer Res.,* **1993,** *53:*5219–5224.

Carrico, C.K., and Sartorelli, A.C. Effects of 6-thioguanine on macromolecular events in regenerating rat liver. *Cancer Res.,* **1977,** *37:*1868–1875.

Chang, T.K., Weber, G.F., Crespi, C.L., and Waxman, D.J. Differential activation of cyclophosphamide and ifosfamide by cytochromes P-450 2B and 3A in human liver microsomes. *Cancer Res.,* **1993,** *53:*5629–5637.

Chao, Y., Teng, H.C., Hung, H.C., King, K.L., Li, C.P., Chi, K.H., Yen, S.H., and Chang, F.Y. Successful initial treatment with weekly etoposide, epirubicin, cisplatin, 5-fluorouracil and leucovorin chemotherapy in advanced gastric cancer patients with disseminated intravascular coagulation. *Jpn. J. Clin. Oncol.,* **2000,** *30:*122–125.

Charache, S., Terrin, M.L., Moore, R.D., Dover, G.J., Barton, F.B., Eckert, S.V., McMahon, R.P., and Bonds, D.R. Effect of hydroxyurea on the frequency of painful crises in sickle cell anemia. Investigators of the Multicenter Study of Hydroxyurea in Sickle Cell Anemia. *N. Engl. J. Med.,* **1995,** *332:*1317–1322.

Cheson, B.D. Infectious and immunosuppressive complications of purine analog therapy. *J. Clin. Oncol.,* **1995,** *13:*2431–2448.

Cheson, B.D., Vena, D.A., Barrett, J., and Freidlin, B. Second malignancies as a consequence of nucleoside analog therapy for chronic lymphoid leukemias. *J. Clin. Oncol.,* **1999,** *17:*2454.

Chu, E., Koeller, D.M., Casey, J.L., Drake, J.C., Chabner, B.A., Elwood, P.C., Zinn, S., and Allegra, C.J. Autoregulation of human thymidylate synthase messenger RNA translation by thymidylate synthase. *Proc. Natl. Acad. Sci. U.S.A.,* **1991,** *88:*8977–8981.

Chu, E., Takimoto, C.H., Voeller, D., Grem, J.L., and Allegra, C.J. Specific binding of human dihydrofolate reductase protein to dihydrofolate reductase messenger RNA *in vitro. Biochemistry,* **1993,** *32:*4756–4760.

Chun, H.G., Leyland-Jones, B.R., Caryk, S.M., and Hoth, D.F. Central nervous system toxicity of fludarabine phosphate. *Cancer Treat. Rep.,* **1986,** *70:*1225–1228.

Chun, H.G., Leyland-Jones, B., and Cheson, B.D. Fludarabine phosphate: a synthetic purine antimetabolite with significant activity against lymphoid malignancies. *J. Clin. Oncol.,* **1991,** *9:*175–188.

Cichowicz, D.J., and Shane, B. Mammalian folylpoly-γ-glutamate synthetase. 1. Purification and general properties of the hog liver enzyme. *Biochemistry,* **1987,** *26:*504–512.

Comess, K.M., Burstyn, J.N., Essigmann, J.M., and Lippard, S.J. Replication inhibition and translesion synthesis on templates containing site-specifically placed *cis*-diamminedichloroplatinum(II) DNA adducts. *Biochemistry,* **1992,** *31:*3975–3990.

Cortes, J., Kantarjian, H., Talpaz, M., O'Brien, S., Beran, M., Koller, C., and Keating, M. Treatment of chronic myelogenous leukemia with nucleoside analogs deoxycoformycin and fludarabine. *Leukemia,* **1997,** *11:*788–791.

Crawford, J., Ozer, H., Stoller, R., Johnson, D., Lyman, G., Tabbara, I., Kris, M., Grous, J., Picozzi, V., Rausch, G., Smith, R., Grandishar, W., Yahanda, A., Vincent, M., Stewart, M., and Glaspy, J. Reduction by granulocyte colony-stimulating factor of fever and neutropenia induced by chemotherapy in patients with small-cell lung cancer. *N. Engl. J. Med.,* **1991,** *325:*164–170.

Cresteil, T., Monsarrat, B., Alvinerie, P., Treluyer, J.M., Vieira, I., and Wright, M. Taxol metabolism by human liver microsomes: identification of cytochrome P450 isozymes involved in its biotransformation. *Cancer Res.,* **1994,** *54:*386–392.

Cunningham, D., Pyrhonen, S., James, R.D., Punt, C.J., Hickish, T.F., Heikkila, R., Johannesen, T.B., Starkhammar, H., Topham, C.A., Awad, L., Jacques, C., and Herait, P. Randomised trial of irinotecan plus supportive care versus supportive care alone after fluorouracil failure for patients with metastatic colorectal cancer. *Lancet,* **1998,** *352:*1413–1418.

Curt, G.A., Carney, D.N., Cowan, K.H., Jolivet, J., Bailey, B.D., Drake, J.C., Chien Song, K.S., Minna, J.D., and Chabner, B.A. Unstable methotrexate resistance in human small-cell carcinoma associated with double minute chromosomes. *N. Engl. J. Med.,* **1983,** *308:*199–202.

Curt, G.A., Jolivet, J., Carney, D.N., Bailey, B.D., Drake, J.C., Clendeninn, N.J., and Chabner, B.A. Determinants of the sensitivity of human small-cell lung cancer cell lines to methotrexate. *J. Clin. Invest.,* **1985,** *76:*1323–1329.

Dabholkar, M., Vionnet, J., Bostick-Bruton, F., Yu, J.J., and Reed, E. Messenger RNA levels of XPAC and ERCC1 in ovarian cancer tissue correlate with response to platinum-based chemotherapy. *J. Clin. Invest.,* **1994,** *94:*703–708.

Dalgleish, A.G., Woods, R.L., and Levi, J.A. Bleomycin pulmonary toxicity: its relationship to renal dysfunction. *Med. Pediatr. Oncol.,* **1984,** *12:*313–317.

Danenberg, P.V., Shea, L.C., and Danenberg, K. Effect of 5-fluorouracil substitution on the self-splicing activity of *Tetrahymena* ribosomal RNA. *Cancer Res.,* **1990,** *50:*1757–1763.

Dearden, C.E., Matutes, E., Hilditch, B.L., Swansbury, G.J., and Catovsky, D. Long-term follow-up of patients with hairy cell leukaemia after treatment with pentostatin or cladribine. *Br. J. Haematol.,* **1999,** *106:*515–519.

Deffie, A.M., Batra, J.K., and Goldenberg, G.J. Direct correlation between DNA topoisomerase II activity and cytotoxicity in adriamycin-sensitive and -resistant P388 leukemia cell lines. *Cancer Res.,* **1989,** *49:*58–62.

DeFronzo, R.A., Braine, H., Colvin, M., and Davis, P.J. Water intoxication in man after cyclophosphamide therapy. Time course and relation to drug activation. *Ann. Intern. Med.,* **1973,** *78:*861–869.

de Gramont, A., Louvet, C., Andre, T., Tournigand, C., and Krulik, M. A review of GERCOD trials of bimonthly leucovorin plus 5-fluorouracil 48-h continuous infusion in advanced colorectal cancer: evolution of a regimen. Groupe d'Etude et de Recherche sur les Cancers de l'Ovaire et Digestifs (GERCOD). *Eur. J. Cancer,* **1998,** *34:*619–626.

Deguchi, Y., Yokoyama, Y., Sakamoto, T., Hayashi, H., Naito, T., Yamada, S., and Kimura, R. Brain distribution of 6-mercaptopurine is regulated by the efflux transport system in the blood-brain barrier. *Life Sci.,* **2000,** *66:*649–662.

de Laat, W.L., Jaspers, N.G., and Hoeijmakers, J.H. Molecular mechanism of nucleotide excision repair. *Genes Dev.,* **1999,** *13:*768–785.

Dighiero, G. Adverse and beneficial immunological effects of purine nucleoside analogues. *Hematol. Cell Ther.,* **1996,** *38(suppl. 2):*S75–S81.

Dimopoulos, M.A., Kantarjian, H., Estey, E., O'Brien, S., Delasalle, K., Keating, M.J., Freireich, E.J., and Alexanian, R. Treatment of Waldenström macroglobulinemia with 2-chlorodeoxyadenosine. *Ann. Intern. Med.,* **1993,** *118:*195–198.

Dixon, K.H., Lanpher, B.C., Chiu, J., Kelley, K., and Cowan, K.H. A novel cDNA restores reduced folate carrier activity and methotrexate sensitivity to transport deficient cells. *J. Biol. Chem.,* **1994,** *269:*17–20.

Dolan, M.E., Moschel, R.C., and Pegg, A.E. Depletion of mammalian O^6-alkyguanine-DNA alkyltransferase activity by O^6-benzylguanine provides a means to evaluate the role of this protein in protection against carcinogenic and therapeutic alkylating agents. *Proc. Natl. Acad. Sci. U.S.A.,* **1990,** *87:*5368–5372.

Donato, M.L., Gershenson, D., Ippoliti, C., Wharton, J.T., Bast, R.C., Jr., Aleman, A., Anderlini, P., Gajewski, J.G., Giralt, S., Molldrem, J., Ueno, N., Lauppe, J., Korbling, M., Boyer, J., Bodurka-Bevers, D., Bevers, M., Burke, T., Freedman, R., Levenback, C., Wolf, J., and Champlin, R.E. High-dose ifosfamide and etoposide with filgrastim for stem cell mobilization in patients with advanced ovarian cancer. *Bone Marrow Transplant.,* **2000,** *25:*1137–1140.

Douillard, J.Y., Cunningham, D., Roth, A.D., Navarro, M., James, R.D., Karasek, P., Jandik, P., Iveson, T., Carmichael, J., Alakl, M., Gruia, G., Awad, L., and Rougier, P. Irinotecan combined with fluorouracil compared with fluorouracil alone as first-line treatment for metastatic colorectal cancer: a multicentre randomised trial. *Lancet,* **2000,** *355:*1041–1047.

Doyle, L.A., Yang, W., Abruzzo, L.V., Krogmann, T., Gao, Y., Rishi, A.K., and Ross, D.D. A multidrug resistance transporter from human MCF-7 breast cancer cells. *Proc. Natl. Acad. Sci. U.S.A.,* **1998,** *95:*15665–15670.

Early Breast Cancer Trialists' Collaborative Group. Effects of adjuvant tamoxifen and of cytotoxic therapy on mortality in early breast cancer. An overview of 61 randomized trials among 28,896 women. *N. Engl. J. Med.,* **1988,** *319:*1681–1692.

Early Breast Cancer Trialists' Collaborative Group. Tamoxifen for early breast cancer: an overview of the randomised trials. *Lancet,* **1998,** *351:*1451–1467.

Einhorn, L.H. Have new aggressive chemotherapy regimens improved results in advanced germ cell tumors? *Eur. J. Cancer Clin. Oncol.,* **1986,** *22:*1289–1293.

Eisenberger, M.A., Blumenstein, B.A., Crawford, E.D., Miller, G., McLeod, D.G., Loehrer, P.J., Wilding, G., Sears, K., Culkin, D.J., Thompson, I.M., Jr., Bueschen, A.J., and Lowe, B.A. Bilateral orchiectomy with or without flutamide for metastatic prostate cancer. *N. Engl. J. Med.,* **1998,** *339:*1036–1042.

Elwood, P.C. Molecular cloning and characterization of the human folate-binding protein cDNA from placenta and malignant tissue culture (KB) cells. *J. Biol. Chem.,* **1989,** *264:*14893–14901.

Emmanouilides, C., Rosen, P., Rasti, S., Territo, M., and Kunkel, L. Treatment of indolent lymphoma with fludarabine/mitoxantrone combination: a phase II trial. *Hematol. Oncol.,* **1998,** *16:*107–116.

Erikson, J.M., Tweedie, D.J., Ducore, J.M., and Prough, R.A. Cytotoxicity and DNA damage caused by the azoxy metabolites of procarbazine in L1210 tumor cells. *Cancer Res.,* **1989,** *49:*127–133.

Estey, E.H., Kurzrock, R., Kantarjian, H.M., O'Brien, S.M., McCredie, K.B., Beran, M., Koller, C., Keating, M.J., Hirsch-Ginsberg, C., Huh,

Y.O., Stass, S., and Freireich, E.J. Treatment of hairy cell leukemia with 2-chlorodeoxyadenosine (2-CdA). *Blood,* **1992,** *79:*882–887.

Farber, S., Diamond, L.K., Mercer, R.D., Sylvester, R.F., and Wolff, V.A. Temporary remissions in acute leukemia in children produced by folic antagonist 4-amethopteroylglutamic acid (aminopterin). *N. Engl. J. Med.,* **1948,** *238:*787–793.

Feagan, B.G., Rochon, J., Fedorak, R.N., Irvine, E.J., Wild, G., Sutherland, L., Steinhart, A.H., Greenberg, G.R., Gillies, R., Hopkins, M., Hanauer, S.B., and McDonald, J.W.D. Methotrexate for the treatment of Crohn's disease. The North American Crohn's Study Group Investigators. *N. Engl. J. Med.,* **1995,** *332:*292–297.

Feldman, E.J., Alberts, D.S., Arlin, Z., Ahmed, T., Mittelman, A., Baskind, P., Peng, Y.M., Baier, M., and Plezia, P. Phase I clinical and pharmacokinetic evaluation of high-dose mitoxantrone in combination with cytarabine in patients with acute leukemia. *J. Clin. Oncol.,* **1993,** *11:*2002–2009.

Fichtinger-Schepman, A.M., van Dijk-Knijnenburg, H.C., van der Velde-Visser, S.D., Berends, F., and Baan, R.A. Cisplatin- and carboplatin-DNA adducts: is PT-AG the cytotoxic lesion? *Carcinogenesis,* **1995,** *16:*2447–2453.

Fink, D., Nebel, S., Aebi, S., Zheng, H., Cenni, B., Nehme, A., Christen, R.D., and Howell, S.B. The role of DNA mismatch repair in platinum drug resistance. *Cancer Res.,* **1996,** *56:*4881–4886.

Fink, D., Zheng, H., Nebel, S., Norris, P.S., Aebi, S., Lin, T.P., Nehme, A., Christen, R.D., Haas, M., MacLeod, C.L., and Howell, S.B. In vitro and in vivo resistance to cisplatin in cells that have lost DNA mismatch repair. *Cancer Res.,* **1997,** *57:*1841–1845.

Fisher, B., Costantino, J.P., Wickerham, D.L., Redmond, C.K., Kavanah, M., Cronin, W.M., Vogel, V., Robidoux, A., Dimitrov, N., Atkins, J., Daly, M., Wieand, S., Tan-Chiu, E., Ford, L., and Wolmark, N. Tamoxifen for prevention of breast cancer: report of the National Surgical Adjuvant Breast and Bowel Project P-1 Study. *J. Natl. Cancer Inst.,* **1998,** *90:*1371–1388.

Fisher, D.E. Apoptosis in cancer therapy: crossing the threshold. *Cell,* **1994,** *78:*539–542.

Flasshove, M., Strumberg, D., Ayscue, L., Mitchell, B.S., Tirier, C., Heit, W., Seeber, S., and Schutte, J. Structural analysis of the deoxycytidine kinase gene in patients with acute myeloid leukemia and resistance to cytosine arabinoside. *Leukemia,* **1994,** *8:*780–785.

Fornander, T., Rutqvist, L.E., Sjoberg, H.E., Blomqvist, L., Mattson, A., and Glas, U. Long-term adjuvant tamoxifen in early breast cancer: effect on bone mineral density in postmenopausal women. *J. Clin. Oncol.,* **1990,** *8:*1019–1024.

Friesen, C., Herr, I., Krammer, P.H., and Debatin, K.M. Involvement of the CD95 (APO-1/FAS) receptor/ligand system in drug-induced apoptosis in leukemia cells. *Nat. Med.,* **1996,** *2:*574–577.

Fukuoka, M., Niitani, H., Suzuki, A., Motomiya, M., Hasegawa, K., Nishiwaki, Y., Kuriyama, T., Ariyoshi, Y., Negoro, S., Masuda, N., Nakajima, S., and Taguchi, T. A phase II study of CPT-11, a new derivative of camptothecin, for previously untreated non-small-cell lung cancer. *J. Clin. Oncol.,* **1992,** *10:*16–20.

Fumoleau, P., Delgado, F.M., Delozier, T., Monnier, A., Gil Delgado, M.A., Kerbrat, P., Garcia-Giralt, E., Keiling, R., Namer, M., Closon, M.T., Goudier, M.J., Chollet, P., Lecourt, L., and Montcuquet, P. Phase II trial of weekly intravenous vinorelbine in first-line advanced breast cancer chemotherapy. *J. Clin. Oncol.,* **1993,** *11:*1245–1252.

Gabrilove, J.L., Jakubowski, A., Scher, H., Sternberg, C., Wong, G., Grous, J., Yagoda, A., Fain, K., Moore, M.A., Clarkson, B., Oettgen, H., Alton, K., Welte, K., and Souza, L. Effect of granulocyte colony-stimulating factor on neutropenia and associated morbidity due to chemotherapy for transitional-cell carcinoma of the urothelium. *N. Engl. J. Med.,* **1988,** *318*:1414–1422.

Garcia, S.T., McQuillan, A., and Panasci, L. Correlation between the cytotoxicity of melphalan and DNA crosslinks as detected by the ethidium bromide fluorescence assay in the F_1 variant of B_{16} melanoma cells. *Biochem. Pharmacol.,* **1988,** *37*:3189–3192.

Gershanovich, M., Chaudri, H.A., Campos, D., Lurie, H., Bonaventura, A., Jeffrey, M., Buzzi, F., Bodrogi, I., Ludwig, H., Reichardt, P., O'Higgins, N., Romieu, G., Friederich, P., and Lassus, M. Letrozole, a new oral aromatase inhibitor: randomised trial comparing 2.5 mg daily, 0.5 mg daily and aminoglutethimide in postmenopausal women with advanced breast cancer. Letrozole International Trial Group (AR/BC3). *Ann. Oncol.,* **1998,** *9*:639–645.

Gewirtz, D.A. A critical evaluation of the mechanisms of action proposed for the antitumor effects of the anthracycline antibiotics adriamycin and daunorubicin. *Biochem. Pharmacol.,* **1999,** *57*:727–741.

Giblett, E.R., Anderson, J.E., Cohen, F., Pollara, B., and Meuwissen, H.J. Adenosine-deaminase deficiency in two patients with severely impaired cellular immunity. *Lancet,* **1972,** *2*:1067–1069.

Gilman, A. The initial clinical trial of nitrogen mustard. *Am. J. Surg.,* **1963,** *105*:574–578.

Glantz, M.J., LaFollette, S., Jaeckle, K.A., Shapiro, W., Swinnen, L., Rozental, J.R., Phuphanich, S., Rogers, L.R., Gutheil, J.C., Batchelor, T., Lyter, D., Chamberlain, M., Maria, B.L., Schiffer, C., Bashir, R., Thomas, D., Cowens, W., and Howell, S.B. Randomized trial of a slow-release versus a standard formulation of cytarabine for the intrathecal treatment of lymphomatous meningitis. *J. Clin. Oncol.,* **1999,** *17*:3110–3116.

Goker, E., Waltham, M., Kheradpour, A., Trippett, T., Mazumdar, M., Elisseyeff, Y., Schnieders, B., Steinherz, P., Tan, C., Berman, E., and Bertino, J.R. Amplification of the dihydrofolate reductase gene is a mechanism of acquired resistance to methotrexate in patients with acute lymphoblastic leukemia and is correlated with p53 gene mutations. *Blood,* **1995,** *86*:677–684.

Golomb, H.M., and Ratain, M.J. Recent advances in the treatment of hairy-cell leukemia. *N. Engl. J. Med.,* **1987,** *316*:870–872.

Gong, J.G., Costanzo, A., Yang, H.Q., Melino, G., Kaelin, W.G., Jr., Levrero, M., and Wang, J.Y. The tyrosine kinase c-Abl regulates p73 in apoptotic response to cisplatin-induced DNA damage. *Nature,* **1999,** *399*:806–809.

Grant, S.C., Kris, M.G., Young, C.W., and Sirotnak, F.M. Edatrexate, an antifolate with antitumor activity: a review. *Cancer Invest.,* **1993,** *11*:36–45.

Grogan, L., Sotos, G.A., and Allegra, C.J. Leucovorin modulation of fluorouracil. *Oncology (Huntingt.),* **1993,** *7*:63–72.

Grollman, A.P., Takeshita, M., Pillai, K.M., and Johnson, F. Origin and cytotoxic properties of base propenals derived from DNA. *Cancer Res.,* **1985,** *45*:1127–1131.

Grunewald, R., Abbruzzese, J.L., Tarassoff, P., and Plunkett, W. Saturation of 2′,2′-difluorodeoxycytidine 5′-triphosphate accumulation by mononuclear cells during a phase I trial of gemcitabine. *Cancer Chemother. Pharmacol.,* **1991,** *27*:258–262.

Grunewald, R., Kantarjian, H., Du, M., Faucher, K., Tarassoff, P., and Plunkett, W. Gemcitabine in leukemia: a phase I clinical, plasma, and cellular pharmacology study. *J. Clin. Oncol.,* **1992,** *10*:406–413.

Haaz, M.C., Rivory, L., Riche, C., Vernillet, L., and Robert, J. Metabolism of irinotecan (CPT-11) by human hepatic microsomes: participation of cytochrome P-450 3A and drug interactions. *Cancer Res.,* **1998,** *58*:468–472.

Hausknecht, R.U. Methotrexate and misoprostol to terminate early pregnancy. *N. Engl. J. Med.,* **1995,** *333*:537–540.

Heinemann, V., Hertel, L.W., Grindey, G.B., and Plunkett, W. Comparison of the cellular pharmacokinetics and toxicity of 2′,2′-difluorodeoxycytidine and 1-β-D-arabinofuranosylcytosine. *Cancer Res.,* **1988,** *48*:4024–4031.

Heinemann, V., Xu, Y.Z., Chubb, S., Sen, A., Hertel, L.W., Grindey, G.B., and Plunkett, W. Inhibition of ribonucleotide reduction in CCRF-CEM cells by 2′,2′-difluorodeoxycytidine. *Mol. Pharmacol.,* **1990,** *38*:567–572.

Heizer, W.D., and Peterson, J.L. Acute myeloblastic leukemia following prolonged treatment of Crohn's disease with 6-mercaptopurine. *Dig. Dis. Sci.,* **1998,** *43*:1791–1793.

Hemminki, K., and Ludlum, D.B. Covalent modification of DNA by antineoplastic agents. *J. Natl. Cancer Inst.,* **1984,** *73*:1021–1028.

Hertel, L.W., Boder, G.B., Kroin, J.S., Rinzel, S.M., Poore, G.A., Todd, G.C., and Grindey, G.B. Evaluation of the antitumor activity of gemcitabine (2′,2′-difluoro-2′-deoxycytidine). *Cancer Res.,* **1990,** *50*:4417–4422.

Hertz, R. Folic acid antagonists: effects on the cell and the patient. Clinical staff conference at N.I.H. *Ann. Intern. Med.,* **1963,** *59*:931–956.

Ho, D.H., Brown, N.S., Yen, A., Holmes, R., Keating, M., Abuchowski, A., Newman, R.A., and Krakoff, I.H. Clinical pharmacology of polyethylene glycol-L-asparaginase. *Drug Metab. Dispos.,* **1986,** *14*:349–352.

Ho, D.H., and Frei, E. III. Clinical pharmacology of 1-β-D-arabinofuranosyl cytosine. *Clin. Pharmacol. Ther.,* **1971,** *12*:944–954.

Hochster, H., Oken, M., Bennett, J., Wolf, B., Gordon, L., Raphael, B., Gencarelli, P., and Cassileth, P. Efficacy of cyclophosphamide (CYC) and fludarabine (FAMP) as first-line therapy of low-grade non-Hodgkin's lymphomas (NHL)—ECOG 1491. *Blood,* **1994,** *84* (suppl. 1):383a.

Hochster, H., Wadler, S., Runowicz, C., Liebes, L., Cohen, H., Wallach, R., Sorich, J., Taubes, B., and Speyer, J. Activity and pharmacodynamics of 21-day topotecan infusion in patients with ovarian cancer previously treated with platinum-based chemotherapy. New York Gynecologic Oncology Group. *J. Clin. Oncol.,* **1999,** *17*:2553–2561.

Hoffman, M., Tallman, M.S., Hakimian, D., Janson, D., Hogan, D., Variakogis, D., Kuzel, T., Gordon, L.I., and Rai, K. 2-Chlorodeoxyadenosine is an active salvage therapy in advanced indolent non-Hodgkin's lymphoma. *J. Clin. Oncol.,* **1994,** *12*:788–792.

Hoffmeister, R.T. Methotrexate therapy in rheumatoid arthritis: 15 years experience. *Am. J. Med.,* **1983,** *75*:69–73.

Hogan, T.F., Citrin, D.L., Johnson, B.M., Nakamura, S., Davis, T.E., and Borden, E.C. o,p′-DDD (mitotane) therapy of adrenal cortical carcinoma: observations on drug dosage, toxicity, and steroid replacement. *Cancer,* **1978,** *42*:2177–2181.

Hohn, D.C., Rayner, A.A., Economou, J.S., Ignoffo, R.J., Lewis, B.J., and Stagg, R.J. Toxicities and complications of implanted pump hepatic arterial and intravenous floxuridine infusion. *Cancer,* **1986,** *57*:465–470.

Hortelano, S, and Bosca, L. 6-Mercaptopurine decreases the Bcl-2/Bax ratio and induces apoptosis in activated splenic B lymphocytes. *Mol. Pharmacol.,* **1997,** *51*:414–421.

Hsiang, Y.H., Hertzberg, R., Hecht, S., and Liu, L.F. Camptothecin induces protein-linked DNA breaks via mammalian DNA topoisomerase I. *J. Biol. Chem.,* **1985,** *260*:14873–14878.

Huang, J.C., Zamble, D.B., Reardon, J.T., Lippard, S.J., and Sancar, A. HMG-domain proteins specifically inhibit the repair of the major DNA adduct of the anticancer drug cisplatin by human excision nuclease. *Proc. Natl. Acad. Sci. U.S.A.,* **1994,** *91*:10394–10398.

Huang, P., and Plunkett, W. Induction of apoptosis by gemcitabine. *Semin. Oncol.,* **1995,** *22:*19–25.

Huang, P., Robertson, L.E., Wright, S., and Plunkett, W. High molecular weight DNA fragmentation: a critical event in nucleoside analogue-induced apoptosis in leukemia cells. *Clin. Cancer Res.,* **1995,** *1:*1005–1013.

Huggins, C., Stevens, R.E., Jr., and Hodges, C.V. Studies on prostatic cancer: effects of castration on advanced carcinoma of prostate gland. *Arch. Surg.,* **1941,** *43:*209–223.

Huizing, M.T., Keung, A.C., Rosing, H., van der Kuij, V., ten Bokkel Huinink, W.W., Mandjes, I.M., Dubbelman, A.C., Pinedo, H.M., and Beijnen, J.H. Pharmacokinetics of paclitaxel and metabolites in a randomized comparative study in platinum-pretreated ovarian cancer patients. *J. Clin. Oncol.,* **1993,** *11:*2127–2135.

Hutter, A.M., Jr., and Kayhoe, D.E. Adrenal cortical carcinoma: clinical features of 138 patients. *Am. J. Med.,* **1966,** *41:*572–580.

Ibrado, A.M., Huang, Y., Fang, G., Liu, L., and Bhalla, K. Overexpression of Bcl-2 or Bcl-xL inhibits Ara-C–induced CPP32/Yama protease activity and apoptosis of human acute myelogenous leukemia HL-60 cells. *Cancer Res.,* **1996,** *56:*4743–4748.

Ikeda, K., Kajiwara, K., Tanabe, E., Tokumaru, S., Kishida, E., Masuzawa, Y., and Kojo, S. Involvement of hydrogen peroxide and hydroxyl radical in chemically induced apoptosis of HL-60 cells. *Biochem. Pharmacol.,* **1999,** *57:*1361–1365.

Ikeda, M.A., Jakoi, L., and Nevins, J.R. A unique role for the Rb protein in controlling E2F accumulation during cell growth and differentiation. *Proc. Natl. Acad. Sci. U.S.A.,* **1996,** *93:*3215–3220.

Innocenti, F., Danesi, R., Di Paolo, A., Loru, B., Favre, C., Nardi, M., Bocci, G., Nardini, D., Macchia, P., and Del Tacca, M. Clinical and experimental pharmacokinetic interaction between 6-mercaptopurine and methotrexate. *Cancer Chemother. Pharmacol.,* **1996,** *37:*409–414.

Ishikawa, T., Sekiguchi, F., Fukase, Y., Sawada, N., and Ishitsuka, H. Positive correlation between the efficacy of capecitabine and doxifluridine and the ratio of thymidine phosphorylase to dihydropyrimidine dehydrogenase activities in tumors in human cancer xenografts. *Cancer Res.,* **1998,** *58:*685–690.

Iven, H., and Brasch, H. The effects of antibiotics and uricosuric drugs on the renal elimination of methotrexate and 7-hydroxymethotrexate in rabbits. *Cancer Chemother. Pharmacol.,* **1988,** *21:*337–342.

Iwasaki, H., Huang, P., Keating, M.J., and Plunkett, W. Differential incorporation of ara-C, gemcitabine, and fludarabine into replicating and repairing DNA in proliferating human leukemia cells. *Blood,* **1997,** *90:*270–278.

Iyer, L., King, C.D., Whitington, P.F., Green, M.D., Roy, S.K., Tephly, T.R., Coffman, B.L., and Ratain, M.J. Genetic predisposition to the metabolism of irinotecan (CPT-11). Role of uridine diphosphate glucuronosyltransferase isoform 1A1 in the glucuronidation of its active metabolite (SN-38) in human liver microsomes. *J. Clin. Invest.,* **1998,** *101:*847–854.

Jaffrezou, J.P., Levade, T., Bettaieb, A., Andrieu, N., Bezombes, C., Maestre, N., Vermeersch, S., Rousse, A., and Laurent, G. Daunorubicin-induced apoptosis: triggering of ceramide generation through sphingomyelin hydrolysis. *EMBO J.,* **1996,** *15:*2417–2424.

Jarvinen, T.A., Holli, K., Kuukasjarvi, T., and Isola, J.J. Predictive value of topoisomerase IIalpha and other prognostic factors for epirubicin chemotherapy in advanced breast cancer. *Br. J. Cancer,* **1998,** *77:*2267–2273.

Jeha, S., Jaffe, N., and Robertson, R. Secondary acute non-lymphoblastic leukemia in two children following treatment with a cis-diamminedichloroplatinum-II–based regimen for osteosarcoma. *Med. Pediatr. Oncol.,* **1992,** *20:*71–74.

Johnston, J.B., Begleiter, A., Pugh, L., Leith, M.K., Wilkins, J.A., Cavers, D.J., and Israels, L.G. Biochemical changes induced in hairy-cell leukemia following treatment with the adenosine deaminase inhibitor 2′-deoxycoformycin. *Cancer Res.,* **1986,** *46:*2179–2184.

Jordan, V.C., and Murphy, C.S. Endocrine pharmacology of antiestrogens as antitumor agents. *Endocr. Rev.,* **1990,** *11:*578–610.

Josting, A., Reiser, M., Wickramanayake, P.D., Rueffer, U., Draube, A., Sohngen, D., Tesch, H., Wolf, J., Diehl, V., and Engert, A. Dexamethasone, carmustine, etoposide, cytarabine, and melphalan (dexa-BEAM) followed by high-dose chemotherapy and stem cell rescue—a highly effective regimen for patients with refractory or relapsed indolent lymphoma. *Leuk. Lymphoma,* **2000,** *37:*115–123.

Kamiya, K., Huang, P., and Plunkett, W. Inhibition of the 3′→5′ exonuclease human DNA polymerase ε by fludarabine-terminated DNA. *J. Biol. Chem.,* **1996,** *271:*19428–19435.

Kasid, U.N., Halligan, B., Liu, L.F., Dritschilo, A., and Smulson, M. Poly(ADP-ribose)–mediated post-translational modification of chromatin-associated human topoisomerase I. Inhibitory effects on catalytic activity. *J. Biol. Chem.,* **1989,** *264:*18687–18692.

Kawakami, Y., Eliyahu, S., Delgado, C.H., Robbins, P.F., Sakaguchi, K., Appella, E., Yannelli, J.R., Adema, G.J., Miki, T., and Rosenberg, S.A. Identification of a human melanoma antigen recognized by tumor-infiltrating lymphocytes associated with in vivo tumor rejection. *Proc. Natl. Acad. Sci. U.S.A.,* **1994,** *91:*6458–6462.

Kay, A.C., Saven, A., Carrera, C.J., Carson, D.A., Thurston, D., Beutler, E., and Piro, L.D. 2-Chlorodeoxyadenosine treatment of low-grade lymphomas. *J. Clin. Oncol.,* **1992,** *10:*371–377.

Keating, M.J., O'Brien, S., Lerner, S., Koller, C., Beran, M., Robertson, L.E., Freireich, E.J., Estey, E., and Kantarjian, H. Long-term follow-up of patients with chronic lymphocytic leukemia (CLL) receiving fludarabine regimens as initial therapy. *Blood,* **1998,** *92:*1165–1171.

Kemeny, N., Daly, J., Reichman, B., Geller, N., Botet, J., and Oderman, P. Intrahepatic or systemic infusion of fluorodeoxyuridine in patients with liver metastases from colorectal carcinoma. A randomized trial. *Ann. Intern. Med.,* **1987,** *107:*459–465.

Kemeny, N., Huang, Y., Cohen, A.M., Shi, W., Conti, J.A., Brennan, M.F., Bertino, J.R., Turnbull, A.D., Sullivan, D., Stockman, J., Blumgart, L.H., and Fong, Y. Hepatic arterial infusion of chemotherapy after resection of hepatic metastases from colorectal cancer. *N. Engl. J. Med.,* **1999,** *341:*2039–2048.

Kharbanda, S., Rubin, E., Gunji, H., Giovanella, B., Pantazis, P., and Kufe, D. Camptothecin and its derivatives induce expression of the c-jun protooncogene in human myeloid leukemia cells. *Cancer Res.,* **1991,** *51:*6636–6642.

Kharbanda, S.M., Sherman, M.L., and Kufe, D.W. Transcriptional regulation of c-jun gene expression by arabinofuranosylcytosine in human myeloid leukemia cells. *J. Clin. Invest.,* **1990,** *86:*1517–1523.

Kidd, J.G. Regression of transplanted lymphomas induced in vivo by means of normal guinea pig serum. 1. Course of transplanted cancers of various kinds in mice and rats given guinea pig serum, horse serum, or rabbit serum. *J. Exp. Med.,* **1953,** *98:*565–582.

Kirschner, B.S. Safety of azathioprine and 6-mercaptopurine in pediatric patients with inflammatory bowel disease. *Gastroenterology,* **1998,** *115:*813–821.

Kitchen, B.J., Moser, A., Lowe, E., Balis, F.M., Widemann, B., Anderson, L., Strong, J., Blaney, S.M., Berg, S.L., O'Brien, M., and Adamson, P.C. Thioguanine administered as a continuous intravenous infusion to pediatric patients is metabolized to the novel metabolite 8-hydroxy-thioguanine. *J. Pharmacol. Exp. Ther.,* **1999,** *291*:870–874.

Kletzel, M., Kearns, G.L., Wells, T.G., and Thompson, H.C., Jr. Pharmacokinetics of high-dose thiotepa in children undergoing autologous bone marrow transplantation. *Bone Marrow Transplant.,* **1992,** *10*:171–175.

Klijn, J.G., Beex, L.V., Mauriac, L., van Zijl, J.A., Veyret, C., Wildiers, J., Jassem, J., Piccart, M., Burghouts, J., Becquart, D., Seynaeve, C., Mignolet, F., and Duchateau, L. Combined treatment with buserelin and tamoxifen in premenopausal metastatic breast cancer: a randomized study. *J. Natl. Cancer Inst.,* **2000,** *92*:903–911.

Knuth, U.A., Hano, R., and Nieschlag, E. Effect of flutamide or cyproterone acetate on pituitary and testicular hormones in normal men. *J. Clin. Endocrinol. Metab.,* **1984,** *59*:963–969.

Kohn, E.C., Sarosy, G., Bicher, A., Link, C., Christian, M., Steinberg, S.M., Rothenberg, M., Adamo, D.O., Davis, P., Ognibene, F.P., Cunnion, R.E., and Reed, E. Dose-intense taxol: high response rate in patients with platinum-resistant recurrent ovarian cancer. *J. Natl. Cancer Inst.,* **1994,** *86*:18–24.

Kolla, S.S., and Studzinski, G.P. Constitutive DNA binding of the low mobility forms of the AP-1 and SP-1 transcription factors in HL60 cells resistant to 1-β-D-arabinofuranosylcytosine. *Cancer Res.,* **1994,** *54*:1418–1421.

Konrad, M.W., Hemstreet, G., Hersh, E.M., Mansell, P.W., Mertelsmann, R., Kolitz, J.E., and Bradley, E.C. Pharmacokinetics of recombinant interleukin 2 in humans. *Cancer Res.,* **1990,** *50*:2009–2017.

Korelitz, B.I., Fuller, S.R., Warman, J.I., and Goldberg, M.D. Shingles during the course of treatment with 6-mercaptopurine for inflammatory bowel disease. *Am. J. Gastroenterol.,* **1999,** *94*:424–426.

Kraut, E.H., Neff, J.C., Bouroncle, B.A., Gochnour, D., and Grever, M.R. Immunosuppressive effects of pentostatin. *J. Clin. Oncol.,* **1990,** *8*:848–855.

Kuss, B.J., Deeley, R.G., Cole, S.P., Willman, C.L., Kopecky, K.J., Wolman, S.R., Eyre, H.J., Lane, S.A., Nancarrow, J.K., Whitmore, S.A., and Callen, D.F. Deletion of gene for multidrug resistance in acute myeloid leukemia with inversion in chromosome 16: prognostic implications. *Lancet,* **1994,** *343*:1531–1534.

Kuzel, T., Samuelson, E., Roenigk, H., Torp, E., and Rosen, S. Phase II trial of 2-chlorodeoxyadenosine (2-CdA) for the treatment of mycosis fungoides or the Sézary syndrome (MF/SS). *Proc. Am. Soc. Clin. Oncol.,* **1992,** *11*:321 (Abstract 1089).

Lerner, H.J. Acute myelogenous leukemia in patients receiving chlorambucil as long-term adjuvant chemotherapy for stage II breast cancer. *Cancer Treat. Rep.,* **1978,** *62*:1135–1138.

Levin, V.A., Hoffman, W., and Weinkam, R.J. Pharmacokinetics of BCNU in man: a preliminary study of 20 patients. *Cancer Treat. Rep.,* **1978,** *62*:1305–1312.

Li, W.W., Lin, J.T., Schweitzer, B.I., Tong, W.P., Niedzwiecki, D., and Bertino, J.R. Intrinsic resistance to methotrexate in human soft tissue sarcoma cell lines. *Cancer Res.,* **1992,** *52*:3908–3913.

Liliemark, J., Albertioni, F., Hassan, M., and Juliusson, G. On the bioavailability of oral and subcutaneous 2-chloro-2'-deoxyadenosine in humans: alternative routes of administration. *J. Clin. Oncol.,* **1992,** *10*:1514–1518.

Liliemark, J., and Juliusson, G. On the pharmacokinetics of 2-chloro-2'-deoxyadenosine in humans. *Cancer Res.,* **1991,** *51*:5570–5572.

Lipshultz, S.E., Colan, S.D., Gelber, R.D., Perez-Atayde, A.R., Sallan, S.E., and Sanders, S.P. Late cardiac effects of doxorubicin therapy for acute lymphoblastic leukemia in childhood. *N. Engl. J. Med.,* **1991,** *324*:808–815.

Longstaff, S., Sigurdson, H., O'Keeffe, M., Ogston, S., and Preece, P. A controlled study of the ocular effects of tamoxifen in conventional doses in the treatment of breast carcinoma. *Eur. J. Cancer Clin. Oncol.,* **1989,** *25*:1805–1808.

Loo, T.L., Housholder, G.E., Gerulath, A.H., Saunders, P.H., and Farquhar, D. Mechanism of action and pharmacology studies with DTIC (NSC-45388). *Cancer Treat. Rep.,* **1976,** *60*:149–152.

Lopez, A.F., Williamson, D.J., Gamble, J.R., Begley, G., Harlan, J.M., Klebanoff, S.J., Waltersdorph, A., Wong, G., Clark, S.C., and Vadas, M.A. Recombinant human granulocyte-macrophage colony-stimulating factor stimulates *in vitro* mature human neutrophil and eosinophil function, surface receptor expression, and survival. *J. Clin. Invest.,* **1986,** *78*:1220–1228.

Lori, F., Malykh, A., Cara, A., Sun, D., Weinstein, J.N., Lisziewicz, J., and Gallo, R.C. Hydroxyurea as an inhibitor of human immunodeficiency virus-type 1 replication. *Science,* **1994,** *266*:801–805.

Love, R.R., Wiebe, D.A., Feyzi, J.M., Newcomb, P.A., and Chappell, R.J. Effects of tamoxifen on cardiovascular risk factors in postmenopausal women after 5 years of treatment. *J. Natl. Cancer Inst.,* **1994,** *86*:1534–1539.

Lowe, S.W., Ruley, H.E., Jacks, T., and Housman, D.E. p53-dependent apoptosis modulates the cytotoxicity of anticancer agents. *Cell,* **1993,** *74*:957–967.

Lu, Z., Zhang, R., and Diasio, R.B. Dihydropyrimidine dehydrogenase activity in human peripheral blood mononuclear cells and liver: population characteristics, newly identified deficient patients, and clinical implication in 5-fluorouracil chemotherapy. *Cancer Res.,* **1993,** *53*:5433–5438.

Lubitz, J.A., Freeman, L., and Okun, R. Mitotane use in inoperable adrenal cortical carcinoma. *JAMA,* **1973,** *223*:1109–1112.

Ludlum, D.B. DNA alkylation by the haloethylnitrosoureas: nature of modifications produced and their enzymatic repair or removal. *Mutat. Res.,* **1990,** *233*:117–126.

Mackey, J.R., Mani, R.S., Selner, M., Mowles, D., Young, J.D., Belt, J.A., Crawford, C.R., and Cass, C.E. Functional nucleoside transporters are required for gemcitabine influx and manifestation of toxicity in cancer cell lines. *Cancer Res.,* **1998,** *58*:4349–4357.

Mahoney, D.H., Jr., Shuster, J., Nitschke, R., Lauer, S.J., Winick, N., Steuber, C.P., and Camitta, B. Intermediate-dose intravenous methotrexate with intravenous mercaptopurine is superior to repetitive low-dose methotrexate with intravenous mercaptopurine for children with lower-risk B-lineage acute lymphoblastic leukemia: a Pediatric Oncology Group phase III trial. *J. Clin. Oncol.,* **1998,** *16*:246–254.

Malspeis, L., Grever, M.R., Staubus, A.E., and Young, D. Pharmacokinetics of 2-F-ara-A (9-beta-D-arabinofuranosyl-2-fluoroadenine) in cancer patients during the phase I clinical investigation of fludarabine phosphate. *Semin. Oncol.,* **1990,** *17*:18–32.

Marathias, V.M., Sawicki, M.J., and Bolton, P.H. 6-Thioguanine alters the structure and stability of duplex DNA and inhibits quadruplex DNA formation. *Nucleic Acids Res.,* **1999,** *27*:2860–2867.

Marquet, P., Lachatre, G., Debord, J., Eichler, B., Bonnaud, F., and Nicot, G. Pharmacokinetics of vinorelbine in man. *Eur. J. Clin. Pharmacol.,* **1992,** *42*:545–547.

Massari, C., Brienza, S., Rotarski, M., Gastiaburu, J., Misset, J.L., Cupissol, D., Alafaci, E. Dutertre-Catella, H., and Bastian, G., Pharmacokinetics of oxaliplatin in patients with normal versus impaired renal function. *Cancer Chemother. Pharmacol.,* **2000,** *45*:157–164.

Matherly, L.H., Taub, J.W., Wong, S.C., Simpson, P.M., Ekizian, R., Buck, S., Williamson, M., Amylon, M., Pullen, J., Camitta, B., and Ravindranath, Y. Increased frequency of expression of elevated dihydrofolate reductase in T-cell versus B-precursor acute lymphoblastic leukemia in children. *Blood*, **1997**, *90*:578–589.

Matijasevic, Z., Boosalis, M., Mackay, W., Samson, L., and Ludlum, D.B. Protection against chloroethylnitrosourea cytotoxicity by eukaryotic 3-methyladenine DNA glycosylase. *Proc. Natl. Acad. Sci. U.S.A.*, **1993**, *90*:11855–11859.

Matthews, D.A., Bolin, J.T., Burridge, J.M., Filman, D.J., Volz, K.W., Kaufman, B.T., Beddell, C.R., Champness, J.N., Stammers, D.K., and Kraut, J. Refined crystal structures of *Escherichia coli* and chicken liver dihydrofolate reductase containing bound trimethoprim. *J. Biol. Chem.*, **1985**, *260*:381–391.

Mauro, D.J., De Riel, J.K., Tallarida, R.J., and Sirover, M.A. Mechanisms of excision of 5-fluorouracil by uracil DNA glycosylase in normal human cells. *Mol. Pharmacol.*, **1993**, *43*:854–857.

Mayer, R.J., Davis, R.B., Schiffer, C.A., Berg, D.T., Powell, B.L., Schulman, P., Omura, G.A., Moore, J.O., McIntyre, O.R., and Frei, E., III. Intensive postremission chemotherapy in adults with acute myeloid leukemia. Cancer and Leukemia Group B. *N. Engl. J. Med.*, **1994**, *331*:896–903.

McDonald, C.J. The uses of systemic chemotherapeutic agents in psoriasis. *Pharmacol. Ther.*, **1981**, *14*:1–24.

McGuire, W.P., Hoskins, W.J., Brady, M.F., Kucera, P.R., Partridge, E.E., Look, K.Y., Clarke-Pearson, D.L., and Davidson, M. Cyclophosphamide and cisplatin compared with paclitaxel and cisplatin in patients with stage III and stage IV ovarian cancer. *N. Engl. J. Med.*, **1996**, *334*:1–6.

McLaughlin, P., Hagemeister, F.B., Romaguera, J.E., Sarris, A.H., Pate, O., Younes, A., Swan, F., Keating, M., and Cabanillas, F. Fludarabine, mitoxantrone, and dexamethasone: an effective new regimen for indolent lymphoma. *J. Clin. Oncol.*, **1996**, *14*:1262–1268.

Meijer, C., Mulder, N.H., Hospers, G.A., Uges, D.R., and de Vries, E.G. The role of glutathione in resistance to cisplatin in a human small cell lung cancer cell line. *Br. J. Cancer*, **1990**, *62*:72–77.

Meloni, G., Foa, R., Vignetti, M., Guarini, A., Fenu, S., Tosti, S., Tos, A.G., and Mandelli, F. Interleukin-2 may induce prolonged remissions in advanced acute myelogenous leukemia. *Blood*, **1994**, *84*:2158–2163.

Mikita, T., and Beardsley, G.P. Functional consequences of the arabinosylcytosine structural lesion in DNA. *Biochemistry*, **1988**, *27*:4698–4705.

Milano, G., Etienne, M.C., Pierrefite, V., Barberi-Heyob, M., Deporte-Fety, R., and Renee, N. Dihydropyrimidine dehydrogenase deficiency and fluorouracil-related toxicity. *Br. J. Cancer*, **1999**, *79*:627–630.

Minton, N.P., Bullman, H.M., Scawen, M.D., Atkinson, T., and Gilbert, H.J. Nucleotide sequence of the *Erwinia chrysanthemi* NCPPB 1066 L-asparaginase gene. *Gene*, **1986**, *46*:25–35.

Miyake, K., Mickley, L., Litman, T., Zhan, Z., Robey, R., Cristensen, B., Brangi, M., Greenberger, L., Dean, M., Fojo, T., and Bates, S.E. Molecular cloning of cDNAs which are highly overexpressed in mitoxantrone-resistant cells: demonstration of homology to ABC transport genes. *Cancer Res.*, **1999**, *59*:8–13.

Mojena, M., Bosca, L., Rider, M.H., Rousseau, G.G., and Hue, L. Inhibition of 6-phosphofructo-2-kinase activity by mercaptopurines. *Biochem. Pharmacol.*, **1992**, *43*:671–678.

Morgan, D.A., Ruscetti, F.W., and Gallo, R. Selective *in vitro* growth of T lymphocytes from normal human bone marrows. *Science*, **1976**, *193*:1007–1008.

Munger, J.S., Huang, X., Kawakatsu, H., Griffiths, M.J., Dalton, S.L., Wu, J., Pittet, J.F., Kaminski, N., Garat, C., Matthay, M.A., Rifkin, D.B., and Sheppard, D. The integrin alpha v beta 6 binds and activates latent TGFβ1: a mechanism for regulating pulmonary inflammation and fibrosis. *Cell*, **1999**, *96*:319–328.

Nagler, A., Slavin, S., Varadi, G., Naparstek, E., Samuel, S., and Or, R. Allogeneic peripheral blood stem cell transplantation using a fludarabine-based low intensity conditioning regimen for malignant lymphoma. *Bone Marrow Transplant.*, **2000**, *25*:1021–1028.

Nehme, A., Baskaran, R., Nebel, S., Fink, D., Howell, S.B., Wang, J.Y., and Christen, R.D. Induction of JNK and c-Abl signalling by cisplatin and oxaliplatin in mismatch repair-proficient and -deficient cells. *Br. J. Cancer*, **1999**, *79*:1104–1110.

Nemati, F., Livartowski, A., De Cremoux, P., Bourgeois, Y., Arvelo, F., Pouillart, P., and Poupon, M.F. Distinctive potentiating effects of cisplatin and/or ifosfamide combined with etoposide in human small cell lung carcinoma xenografts. *Clin. Cancer Res.*, **2000**, *6*:2075–2086.

Nemunaitis, J., Rabinowe, S.N., Singer, J.W., Bierman, P.J., Vose, J.M., Freedman, A.S., Onetto, N., Gillis, S., Oette, D., Gold, M., Buckner, C.D., Hansen, J.A., Ritz, J., Applebaum, F.R., Armitage, J.O., and Nadler, L.M. Recombinant granulocyte-macrophage colony-stimulating factor after autologous bone marrow transplantation for lymphoid cancer. *N. Engl. J. Med.*, **1991**, *324*:1773–1778.

Newlands, E.S., Blackledge, G.R., Slack, J.A., Rustin, G.J., Smith, D.B., Stuart, N.S., Quarterman, C.P., Hoffman, R., Stevens, M.F., Brampton, M.H., and Gibson, A.C. Phase I trial of temozolomide (CCRG 81045: M&B 39831: NSC 362856). *Br. J. Cancer*, **1992**, *65*:287–291.

Ng, S.F., and Waxman, D.J. N,N′,N′′-triethylenethiophosphoramide (thio-TEPA) oxygenation by constitutive hepatic P450 enzymes and modulation of drug metabolism and clearance *in vivo* by P450-inducing agents. *Cancer Res.*, **1991**, *51*:2340–2345.

Nicolaou, K.C., Yang, Z., Liu, J.J., Ueno, H., Nantermet, P.G., Guy, R.K., Claiborne, C.F., Renaud, J., Couladouros, E.A., Paulvannan, K., and Sorensen, E.J. Total synthesis of Taxol. *Nature*, **1994**, *367*:630–634.

Niitsu, N., Yamaguchi, Y., Umeda, M., and Honma, Y. Human monocytoid leukemia cells are highly sensitive to apoptosis induced by 2′-deoxycoformycin and 2′-deoxyadenosine: association with dATP-dependent activation of caspase-3. *Blood*, **1998**, *92*:3368–3375.

Noble, R.L., Beer, C.T., and Cutts, J.H. Further biological activities of vincaleukoblastine—an alkaloid isolated from *Vinca rosea* (L.). *Biochem. Pharmacol.*, **1958**, *1*:347–348.

Norton, L., Slamon, D., Leyland-Jones, B., Wolter, J., Fleming, T., Eirmann, W., Baselga, J., Mendelsohn, J., Bajamonde, A., Ash, M., and Shak, S. Overall survival (OS) advantage to simultaneous chemotherapy (CRx) plus the humanized anti-HER2 monoclonal antibody herceptin (H) in HER2-overexpressing (HER2+) metastatic breast cancer (MBC). Abstract 483. *Proc. Am. Soc. Clin. Oncol.*, **1999**, *18*:127a.

Nowak-Gottl, U., Wermes, C., Junker, R., Koch, H.G., Schobess, R., Fleischhack, G., Schwabe, D., and Ehrenforth, S. Prospective evaluation of the thrombotic risk in children with acute lymphoblastic leukemia carrying the MTHFR TT 677 genotype, the prothrombin G20210A variant, and further prothrombotic risk factors. *Blood*, **1999**, *93*:1595–1599.

O'Brien, S., Kantarjian, H., Beran, M., Smith, T., Koller, C., Estey, E., Robertson, L.E., Lerner, S., and Keating, M. Results of fludarabine and prednisone therapy in 264 patients with chronic lymphocytic leukemia with multivariate analysis-derived prognostic model for response to treatment. *Blood*, **1993**, *82*:1695–1700.

O'Reilly, S., Rowinsky, E.K., Slichenmyer, W., Donehower, R.C., Forastiere, A.A., Ettinger, D.S., Chen, T.L., Sartorius, S., and

Grochow, L.B. Phase I and pharmacologic study of topotecan in patients with impaired renal function. *J. Clin. Oncol.,* **1996,** *14*:3062–3073.

Ostuni, J.A., and Roginsky, M.S. Metastatic adrenal cortical carcinoma. Documented cure with combined chemotherapy. *Arch. Intern. Med.,* **1975,** *135*:1257–1258.

Ozols, R.F. Optimal dosing with carboplatin. *Semin. Oncol.,* **1989,** *16*: 14–18.

Ozols, R.F., Corden, B.J., Jacob, J., Wesley, M.N., Ostchega, Y., and Young, R.C. High-dose cisplatin in hypertonic saline. *Ann. Intern. Med.,* **1984,** *100*:19–24.

Parker, R.J., Eastman, A., Bostick-Bruton, F., and Reed, E. Acquired cisplatin resistance in human ovarian cancer cells is associated with enhanced repair of cisplatin-DNA lesions and reduced drug accumulation. *J. Clin. Invest.,* **1991a,** *87*:772–777.

Parker, R.J., Gill, I., Tarone, R., Vionnet, J.A., Grunberg, S., Muggia, F.M., and Reed, E. Platinum-DNA damage in leukocyte DNA of patients receiving carboplatin and cisplatin chemotherapy, measured by atomic absorption spectrometry. *Carcinogenesis,* **1991b,** *12*:1253–1258.

Pauletti, G., Lai, E., and Attardi, G. Early appearance and long-term persistence of the submicroscopic extrachromosomal elements (amplisomes) containing the amplified DHFR genes in human cell lines. *Proc. Natl. Acad. Sci. U.S.A.,* **1990,** *87*:2955–2959.

Pearson, B.S., and Raghavan, D. First-line intravenous cisplatin for deeply invasive bladder cancer: update on 70 cases. *Br. J. Urol.,* **1985,** *57*:690–693.

Pegg, A.E. Mammalian O^6-alkylguanine-DNA alkyltransferase: regulation and importance in response to alkylating carcinogenic and therapeutic agents. *Cancer Res.,* **1990,** *50*:6119–6129.

Petrus, M.J., Williams, J.F., Eckhaus, M.A., Gress, R.E., and Fowler, D.H. An immunoablative regimen of fludarabine and cyclophosphamide prevents fully MHC-mismatched murine marrow graft rejection independent of GVHD. *Biol. Blood Marrow Transplant.,* **2000,** *6*:182–189.

Piro, L.D., Carrera, C.J., Beutler, E., and Carson, D.A. 2-Chlorodeoxyadenosine: an effective new agent for the treatment of chronic lymphocytic leukemia. *Blood,* **1988,** *72*:1069–1073.

Pommier, Y., Kerrigan, D., Hartman, K.D., and Glazer, R.I. Phosphorylation of mammalian DNA topoisomerase I and activation by protein kinase C. *J. Biol. Chem.,* **1990,** *265*:9418–9422.

Postmus, P.E., Smit, E.F., Haaxma-Reiche, H., van Zandwijk, N., Ardizzoni, A., Quoix, E., Kirkpatrick, A., Sahmoud, T., and Giaccone, G. Teniposide for brain metastases of small-cell lung cancer: a phase II study. European Organization for Research and Treatment of Cancer Lung Cancer Cooperative Group. *J. Clin. Oncol.,* **1995,** *13*:660–665.

Preisler, H.D., Rustum, Y., and Priore, R.L. Relationship between leukemic cell retention of cytosine arabinoside triphosphate and the duration of remission in patients with acute non-lymphocytic leukemia. *Eur. J. Cancer Clin. Oncol.,* **1985,** *21*:23–30.

Presta, M., Rusnati, M., Belleri, M., Morbidelli, L., Ziche, M., and Ribatti, D. Purine analogue 6-methylmercaptopurine riboside inhibits early and late phases of the angiogenesis process. *Cancer Res.,* **1999,** *59*:2417–2424.

Prostate Cancer Trialists' Collaborative Group. Maximum androgen blockade in advanced prostate cancer: an overview of randomised trials. *Lancet,* **2000,** *355*:1491–1498.

Pui, C.H., Relling, M.V., Rivera, G.K., Hancock, M.L., Raimondi, S.C., Heslop, H.E., Santana, V.M., Ribeiro, R.C., Sandlund, J.T., Mahmoud, H.H., Evans, W.E., Crist, W.M., and Krance, R.A.

Epipodophyllotoxin-related acute myeloid leukemia: a study of 35 cases. *Leukemia,* **1995,** *9*:1990–1996.

Rafel, M., Cervantes, F., Beltran, J.M., Zuazu, F., Hernandez Nieto, L., Rayon, C., Garcia Talavera, J., and Montserrat, E. Deoxycoformycin in the treatment of patients with hairy cell leukemia: results of a Spanish collaborative study of 80 patients. *Cancer,* **2000,** *88*:352–357.

Rajapakse, R.O., Korelitz, B.I., Zlatanic, J., Baiocco, P.J., and Gleim, G.W. Outcome of pregnancies when fathers are treated with 6-mercaptopurine for inflammatory bowel disease. *Am. J. Gastroenterol.,* **2000,** *95*:684–688.

Redman, B.G., Smith, D.C., Flaherty, L., Du, W., and Hussain, M. Phase II trial of paclitaxel and carboplatin in the treatment of advanced urothelial carcinoma. *J. Clin. Oncol.,* **1998,** *16*:1844–1848.

Reed, E. Platinum-DNA adduct, nucleotide excision repair and platinum based anti-cancer chemotherapy. *Cancer Treat. Rev.,* **1998,** *24*:331–344.

Reed, E., Yuspa, S.H., Zwelling, L.A., Ozols, R.F., and Poirier, M.C. Quantitation of *cis*-diamminedichloroplatinum II (cisplatin)-DNA-intrastrand adducts in testicular and ovarian cancer patients receiving cisplatin chemotherapy. *J. Clin. Invest.,* **1986,** *77*:545–550.

Relling, M.V., Hancock, M.L., Boyett, J.M., Pui, C.H., and Evans, W.E. Prognostic importance of 6-mercaptopurine dose intensity in acute lymphoblastic leukemia. *Blood,* **1999a,** *93*:2817–2823.

Relling, M.V., Hancock, M.L., Rivera, G.K., Sandlund, J.T., Ribeiro, R.C., Krynetski, E.Y., Pui, C.H., and Evans, W.E. Mercaptopurine therapy intolerance and heterozygosity at the thiopurine S-methyltransferase gene locus. *J. Natl. Cancer Inst.,* **1999b,** *91*:2001–2008.

Rice, G.P., Filippi, M., and Comi, G. Cladribine and progressive MS: clinical and MRI outcomes of a multicenter controlled trial. Cladribine MRI Study Group. *Neurology,* **2000,** *54*:1145–1155.

Robak, T., Blonski, J.Z., Urbanska-Rys, H., Blasinska-Morawiec, M., and Skotnicki, A.B. 2-Chlorodeoxyadenosine (Cladribine) in the treatment of patients with chronic lymphocytic leukemia 55 years old and younger. *Leukemia,* **1999,** *13*:518–523.

Robieux, I., Sorio, R., Borsatti, E., Cannizzaro, R., Vitali, V., Aita, P., Freschi, A., Galligioni, E., and Monfardini, S. Pharmacokinetics of vinorelbine in patients with liver metastases. *Clin. Pharmacol. Ther.,* **1996,** *59*:32–40.

Rodriguez, G.I., Kuhn, J.G., Weiss, G.R., Hilsenbeck, S.G., Eckardt, J.R., Thurman, A., Rinaldi, D.A., Hodges, S., Von Hoff, D.D., and Rowinsky, E.K. A bioavailability and pharmacokinetic study of oral and intravenous hydroxyurea. *Blood,* **1998,** *91*:1533–1541.

Rosenberg, B. Platinum coordination complexes in cancer chemotherapy. *Naturwissenschaften,* **1973,** *60*:399–406.

Rosenberg, B., Van Camp, L., Grimley, E.B., and Thomson, A.J. The inhibition of growth or cell division in *Escherichia coli* by different ionic species of platinum (IV) complexes. *J. Biol. Chem.,* **1967,** *242*: 1347–1352.

Rosenberg, B., Van Camp, L., and Krigas, T. Inhibition of cell division in *Escherichia coli* by electrolysis products from a platinum electrode. *Nature,* **1965,** *205*:698–699.

Rosenberg, S.A., Lotze, M.T., Yang, J.C., Aebersold, P.M., Linehan, W.M., Seipp, C.A., and White, D.E. Experience with the use of high-dose interleukin-2 in the treatment of 652 cancer patients. *Ann. Surg.,* **1989,** *210*:474–484.

Rosenberg, S.A., Yannelli, J.R., Yang, J.C., Topalian, S.L., Schwartzentruber, D.J., Weber, J.S., Parkinson, D.R., Seipp, C.A., Einhorn, J.H., and White, D.E. Treatment of patients with metastatic melanoma with autologous tumor-infiltrating lymphocytes and interleukin 2. *J. Natl. Cancer Inst.,* **1994,** *86*:1159–1166.

Rosing, H., van Zomeren, D.M., Doyle, E., Bult, A., and Beijnen, J.H. O-glucuronidation, a newly identified metabolic pathway for topotecan and N-desmethyl topotecan. *Anticancer Drugs.,* **1998,** *9*:587–592.

Rowinsky, E.K., Gilbert, M.R., McGuire, W.P., Noe, D.A., Grochow, L.B., Forastiere, A.A., Ettinger, D.S., Lubejko, B.G., Clark, B., Sartorius, S.E., Cornblath, D.R., Hendricks, C.B., and Donehower, R.C. Sequences of taxol and cisplatin: a phase I and pharmacologic study. *J. Clin. Oncol.,* **1991,** *9*:1692–1703.

Rubin, E.H., Andersen, J.W., Berg, D.T., Schiffer, C.A., Mayer, R.J., and Stone, R.M. Risk factors for high-dose cytarabine neurotoxicity: an analysis of a cancer and leukemia group B trial in patients with acute myeloid leukemia. *J. Clin. Oncol.,* **1992,** *10*:948–953.

Rusthoven, J.J., Eisenhauer, E., Butts, C., Gregg, R., Dancey, J., Fisher, B., and Iglesias, J. Multitargeted antifolate LY231514 as first-line chemotherapy for patients with advanced non-small-cell lung cancer: A phase II study. National Cancer Institute of Canada Clinical Trials Group. *J. Clin. Oncol.,* **1999,** *17*:1194.

Sandler, E.S., Friedman, D.J., Mustafa, M.M., Winick, N.J., Bowman, W.P., and Buchanan, G.R. Treatment of children with epipodophyllotoxin-induced secondary acute myeloid leukemia. *Cancer,* **1997,** *79*:1049–1054.

Sandoval, A., Consoli, U., and Plunkett, W. Fludarabine-mediated inhibition of nucleotide excision repair induces apoptosis in quiescent human lymphocytes. *Clin. Cancer Res.,* **1996,** *2*:1731–1741.

Santana, V.M., Mirro, J., Jr., Kearns, C., Schell, M.J., Crom, W., and Blakley, R.L. 2-Chlorodeoxyadenosine produces a high rate of complete hematologic remission in relapsed acute myeloid leukemia. *J. Clin. Oncol.,* **1992,** *10*:364–370.

Santen, R.J., Samojlik, E., and Wells, S.A. Resistance of the ovary to blockade of aromatization with aminoglutethimide. *J. Clin. Endocrinol. Metab.,* **1980,** *51*:473–477.

Santen, R.J., Worgul, T.J., Lipton, A., Harvey, H., Boucher, A., Samojlik, E., and Wells, S.A. Aminoglutethimide as treatment of postmenopausal women with advanced breast carcinoma. *Ann. Intern. Med.,* **1982,** *96*:94–101.

Santi, D.V., McHenry, C.S., and Sommer, H. Mechanism of interaction of thymidylate synthetase with 5-fluorodeoxyuridylate. *Biochemistry,* **1974,** *13*:471–481.

Santos, G.W., Tutschka, P.J., Brookmeyer, R., Saral, R., Beschorner, W.E., Bias, W.B., Braine, H.G., Burns W.H., Elfenbein, G.J., Kaizer, H., Mellits, D., Sensenbrenner, L.L., Stuart, R.K., and Yeager, A.M. Marrow transplantation for acute nonlymphocytic leukemia after treatment with busulfan and cyclophosphamide. *N. Engl. J. Med.,* **1983,** *309*:1347–1353.

Saven, A., and Burian, C. Cladribine activity in adult Langerhans-cell histiocytosis. *Blood,* **1999,** *93*:4125–4130.

Saven, A., Carrera, C.J., Carson, D.A., Beutler, E., and Piro, L.D. 2-Chlorodeoxyadenosine: an active agent in the treatment of cutaneous T-cell lymphoma. *Blood,* **1992,** *80*:587–592.

Saven, A., and Piro, L.D. Treatment of hairy cell leukemia. *Blood,* **1992,** *79*:1111–1120.

Schein, P., Kahn, R., Gorden, P., Wells, S., and Devita, V.T. Streptozotocin for malignant insulinomas and carcinoid tumor. Report of eight cases and review of the literature. *Arch. Intern. Med.,* **1973,** *132*:555–561.

Schein, P.S., and Winokur, S.H. Immunosuppressive and cytotoxic chemotherapy: long-term complications. *Ann. Intern. Med.,* **1975,** *82*:84–95.

Schilsky, R.L., Dolan, M.E., Bertucci, D., Ewesuedo, R.B., Vogelzang, N.J., Mani, S., Wilson, L.R., and Ratain, M.J. Phase I clinical and pharmacological study of O^6-benzylguanine followed by carmustine in patients with advanced cancer. *Clin. Cancer Res.,* **2000,** *6*:3025–3031.

Schweitzer, B.I., Srimatkandada, S., Gritsman, H., Sheridan, R., Venkataraghavan, R., and Bertino, J.R. Probing the role of two hydrophobic active site residues in the human dihydrofolate reductase by site-directed mutagenesis. *J. Biol. Chem.,* **1989,** *264*:20786–20795.

Sebti, S.M., DeLeon, J.C., and Lazo, J.S. Purification, characterization, and amino acid composition of rabbit pulmonary bleomycin hydrolase. *Biochemistry,* **1987,** *26*:4213–4219.

Sebti, S.M., Jani, J.P., Mistry, J.S., Gorelik, E., and Lazo, J.S. Metabolic inactivation: a mechanism of human tumor resistance to bleomycin. *Cancer Res.,* **1991,** *51*:227–232.

Serrano, J., Palmeira, C.M., Kuehl, D.W., and Wallace, K.B. Cardioselective and cumulative oxidation of mitochondrial DNA following subchronic doxorubicin administration. *Biochim. Biophys. Acta,* **1999,** *1411*:201–205.

Shao, R.G., Cao, C.X., Shimizu, T., O'Connor, P.M., Kohn, K.W., and Pommier, Y. Abrogation of an S-phase checkpoint and potentiation of camptothecin cytotoxicity by 7-hydroxystaurosporine (UCN-01) in human cancer cell lines, possibly influenced by p53 function. *Cancer Res.,* **1997,** *57*:4029–4035.

Siaw, M.F., and Coleman, M.S. *In vitro* metabolism of deoxycoformycin in human T lymphoblastoid cells. Phosphorylation of deoxycoformycin and incorporation into cellular DNA. *J. Biol. Chem.,* **1984,** *259*:9426–9433.

Silver, R.T., Woolf, S.H., Hehlmann, R., Appelbaum, F.R., Anderson, J., Bennett, C., Goldman, J.M, Guilhot, F., Kantarjian, H.M., Lichtin, A.E., Talpaz, M., and Tura, S. An evidence-based analysis of the effect of busulfan, hydroxyurea, interferon, and allogeneic bone marrow transplantation in treating the chronic phase of chronic myeloid leukemia: developed for the American Society of Hematology. *Blood,* **1999,** *94*:1517–1536.

Sinha, B.K., Mimnaugh, E.G., Rajagopalan, S., and Myers, C.E. Adriamycin activation and oxygen free radical formation in human breast tumor cells: protective role of glutathione peroxidase in adriamycin resistance. *Cancer Res.,* **1989,** *49*:3844–3848.

Sinkule, J.A., Stewart, C.F., Crom, W.R., Melton, E.T., Dahl, G.V., and Evans, W.E. Teniposide (VM 26) disposition in children with leukemia. *Cancer Res.,* **1984,** *44*:1235–1237.

Smets, L.A. Programmed cell death (apoptosis) and response to anticancer drugs. *Anticancer Drugs,* **1994,** *5*:3–9.

Smith, M.A., Rubinstein, L., Anderson, J.R., Arthur, D., Catalano, P.J., Freidlin, B., Heyn, R., Khayat, A., Krailo, M., Land, V.J., Miser, J., Shuster, J., and Vena, D. Secondary leukemia or myelodysplastic syndrome after treatment with epipodophyllotoxins. *J. Clin. Oncol.,* **1999,** *17*:569–577.

Sobecks, R.M., Daugherty, C.K., Hallahan, D.E., Laport, G.F., Wagner, N.D., and Larson, R.A. A dose escalation study of total body irradiation followed by high-dose etoposide and allogeneic blood stem cell transplantation for the treatment of advanced hematologic malignancies. *Bone Marrow Transplant.,* **2000,** *25*:807–813.

Sonneveld, P., Schultz, F.W., Nooter, K., and Hahlen, K. Pharmacokinetics of methotrexate and 7-hydroxy-methotrexate in plasma and bone marrow of children receiving low-dose oral methotrexate. *Cancer Chemother. Pharmacol.,* **1986,** *18*:111–116.

Souliotis, V.L., Kaila, S., Boussiotis, V.A., Pangalis, G.A., and Kyrtopoulos, S.A. Accumulation of O^6-methylguanine in human blood leukocyte DNA during exposure to procarbazine and its relationships with dose and repair. *Cancer Res.,* **1990,** *50*:2759–2764.

Souza, L.M., Boone, T.C., Gabrilove, J., Lai, P.H., Zsebo, K.M., Murdock, D.C., Chazin, V.R., Bruszewski, J., Lu, H., Chen, K.K., Platzer, E., Moore, M.A.S., Mertlesman, R., and Welte, K. Recombinant human granulocyte colony-stimulating factor: effects on normal and leukemic myeloid cells. *Science,* **1986,** *232*:61–65.

Speyer, J.L., Green, M.D., Kramer, E., Rey, M., Sanger, J., Ward, C., Dubin, N., Ferrans, V., Stecy, P., Zeleniuch-Jacquotte, A., Wernz, J., Feit, F., Slater, W., Blum, R., and Muggia, F. Protective effect of the bispiperazinedione ICRF-187 against doxorubicin-induced cardiac toxicity in women with advanced breast cancer. *N. Engl. J. Med.,* **1988,** *319*:745–752.

Srimatkandada, S., Schweitzer, B.I., Moroson, B.A., Dube, S., and Bertino, J.R. Amplification of a polymorphic dihydrofolate reductase gene expressing an enzyme with decreased binding to methotrexate in a human colon carcinoma cell line, HCT-8R4, resistant to this drug. *J. Biol. Chem.,* **1989,** *264*:3524–3528.

Steis, R.G., Urba, W.J., Kopp, W.C., Alvord, W.G., Smith, J.W. II, and Longo, D.L. Kinetics of recovery of CD4+ T cells in peripheral blood of deoxycoformycin-treated patients. *J. Natl. Cancer Inst.,* **1991,** *83*:1678–1679.

Stewart, C.F., Arbuck, S.G., Fleming, R.A., and Evans, W.E. Relation of systemic exposure to unbound etoposide and hematologic toxicity. *Clin. Pharmacol. Ther.,* **1991,** *50*:385–393.

Stoller, R.G., Hande, K.R., Jacobs, S.A., Rosenberg, S.A., and Chabner, B.A. Use of plasma pharmacokinetics to predict and prevent methotrexate toxicity. *N. Engl. J. Med.,* **1977,** *297*:630–634.

Stone, S.R., and Morrison, J.F. Mechanism of inhibition of dihydrofolate reductases from bacterial and vertebrate sources by various classes of folate analogues. *Biochim. Biophys. Acta,* **1986,** *869*:275–285.

Strum, J.C., Small, G.W., Pauig, S.B., and Daniel, L.W. 1-β-D-Arabinofuranosylcytosine stimulates ceramide and diglyceride formation in HL-60 cells. *J. Biol. Chem.,* **1994,** *269*:15493–15497.

Sugimoto, Y., Tsukahara, S., Oh-hara, T., Isoe, T., and Tsuruo, T. Decreased expression of DNA topoisomerase I in camptothecin-resistant tumor cell lines as determined by monoclonal antibody. *Cancer Res.,* **1990,** *50*:6925–6930.

Swain, S.M., Lippman, M.E., Egan, E.F., Drake, J.C., Steinberg, S.M., and Allegra, C.J. Fluorouracil and high-dose leucovorin in previously treated patients with metastatic breast cancer. *J. Clin. Oncol.,* **1989,** *7*:890–899.

Swain, S.M., Whaley, F.S., Gerber, M.C., Weisberg, S., York, M., Spicer, D., Jones, S.E., Wadler, S., Desai, A., Vogel, C., Speyer, J., Mittelman, A., Reddy, S., Pendergrass, K., Velez-Garcia, E., Ewer, M.S., Bianchine, J.R., and Gams, R.A. Cardioprotection with dexrazoxane for doxorubicin-containing therapy in advanced breast cancer. *J. Clin. Oncol.,* **1997,** *15*:1318–1332.

Tallman, M.S., Hakimian, D., Zanzig, C., Hogan, D.K., Rademaker, A., Rose, E., and Variakojis, D. Cladribine in the treatment of relapsed or refractory chronic lymphocytic leukemia. *J. Clin. Oncol.,* **1995,** *13*:983–988.

Tamura, H., Kohchi, C., Yamada, R., Ikeda, T., Koiwai, O., Patterson, E., Keene, J.D., Okada, K., Kjeldsen, E., Nishikawa, K., and Andoh, T. Molecular cloning of a cDNA of a camptothecin-resistant human DNA topoisomerase I and identification of mutation sites. *Nucleic Acids Res.,* **1991,** *19*:69–75.

Tempero, M., Plunkett, W., Ruiz van Haperen, V., Hainsworth, J., Hochster, H., Lenzi, R., and Abbruzzese, J. Randomized phase II trial of dose intense gemcitabine by standard infusion vs. fixed dose

rate in metastatic pancreatic carcinoma. Abstract 1048. *Proc. Am. Soc. Clin. Oncol.,* **1999,** *18*:273a.

ten Bokkel Huinink, W., Gore, M., Carmichael, J., Gordon, A., Malfetano, J., Hudson, I., Broom, C., Scarabelli, C., Davidson, N., Spanczynski, M., Bolis, G., Malmstrom, H., Coleman, R., Fields, S.C., and Heron, J.F. Topotecan versus paclitaxel for the treatment of recurrent epithelial ovarian cancer. *J. Clin. Oncol.,* **1997,** *15*:2183–2193.

Tewey, K.M., Chen, G.L., Nelson, E.M., and Liu, L.F. Intercalative antitumor drugs interfere with the breakage-reunion reaction of mammalian DNA topoisomerase II. *J. Biol. Chem.,* **1984,** *259*:9182–9187.

Thyss, A., Milano, G., Kubar, J., Namer, M., and Schneider, M. Clinical and pharmacokinetic evidence of a life-threatening interaction between methotrexate and ketoprofen. *Lancet,* **1986,** *1*:256–258.

Tondini, C., Balzarotti, M., Rampinelli, I., Valagussa, P., Luoni, M., De Paoli, A., Santoro, A., and Bonadonna, G. Fludarabine and cladribine in relapsed/refractory low-grade non-Hodgkin's lymphoma: a phase II randomized study. *Ann. Oncol.,* **2000,** *11*:231–233.

Tong, W.P., and Ludlum, D.B. Crosslinking of DNA by busulfan. Formation of diguanyl derivatives. *Biochim. Biophys. Acta,* **1980,** *608*:174–181.

Travis, L.B., Holowaty, E.J., Bergfeldt, K., Lynch, C.F., Kohler, B.A., Wiklund, T., Curtis, R.E., Hall, P., Andersson, M., Pukkala, E., Sturgeon, J., and Stovall, M. Risk of leukemia after platinum-based chemotherapy for ovarian cancer. *N. Engl. J. Med.,* **1999,** *340*:351–357.

Trippett, T., Schlemmer, S., Elisseyeff, Y., Goker, E., Wachter, M., Steinherz, P., Tan, C., Berman, E., Wright, J.E., Rosowsky, A., Schweitzer, B., and Bertino, J.R. Defective transport as a mechanism of acquired resistance to methotrexate in patients with acute lymphoblastic leukemia. *Blood,* **1992,** *80*:1158–1162.

Tritsch, G.L., ed. Adenosine deaminase in disorders of purine metabolism and in immune deficiency. *Ann. N.Y. Acad. Sci.,* **1985,** *451*:1–345.

Tritton, T.R., Murphree, S.A., and Sartorelli, A.C. Adriamycin: a proposal on the specificity of drug action. *Biochem. Biophys. Res. Commun.,* **1978,** *84*:802–808.

Tsao, Y.P., D'Arpa, P., and Liu, L.F. The involvement of active DNA synthesis in camptothecin-induced G2 arrest: altered regulation of p34cdc2/cyclin B. *Cancer Res.,* **1992,** *52*:1823–1829.

Tsao, Y.P., Russo, A., Nyamuswa, G., Silber, R., and Liu, L.F. Interaction between replication forks and topoisomerase I-DNA cleavable complexes: studies in a cell-free SV40 DNA replication system. *Cancer Res.,* **1993,** *53*:5908–5914.

Tucker, M.A., Coleman, C.N., Cox, R.S., Varghese, A., and Rosenberg, S.A. Risk of second cancers after treatment for Hodgkin's disease. *N. Engl. J. Med.,* **1988,** *318*:76–81.

Tung, N., Berkowitz, R., Matulonis, U., Quartulli, M., Seiden, M., Kim, Y., Niloff, J., and Cannistra, S.A. Phase I trial of carboplatin, paclitaxel, etoposide, and cyclophosphamide with granulocyte colony stimulating factor as first-line therapy for patients with advanced epithelial ovarian cancer. *Gynecol. Oncol.,* **2000,** *77*:271–277.

Twelves, C., Glynne-Jones, R., Cassidy, J., Schuller, J., Goggin, T., Roos, B., Banken, L., Utoh, M., Weidekamm, E., and Reigner, B. Effect of hepatic dysfunction due to liver metastases on the pharmacokinetics of capecitabine and its metabolites. *Clin. Cancer Res.,* **1999,** *5*:1696–1702.

Twelves, C.J., Dobbs, N.A., Gillies, H.C., James, C.A., Rubens, R.D., and Harper, P.G. Doxorubicin pharmacokinetics: the effect of abnormal liver biochemistry tests. *Cancer Chemother. Pharmacol.,* **1998,** *42*:229–234.

Twentyman, P.R. Bleomycin—mode of action with particular reference to the cell cycle. *Pharmacol. Ther.,* **1983,** *23*:417–441.

Ullman, B., Lee, M., Martin, D.W., Jr., and Santi, D.V. Cytotoxicity of 5-fluoro-2′-deoxyuridine: requirement for reduced folate cofactors and antagonism by methotrexate. *Proc. Natl. Acad. Sci. U.S.A.,* **1978,** *75*:980–983.

Vaisman, A., Varchenko, M., Umar, A., Kunkel, T.A., Risinger, J.I., Barrett, J.C., Hamilton, T.C., and Chaney, S.G. The role of hMLH1, hMSH3, and hMSH6 defects in cisplatin and oxaliplatin resistance: correlation with replicative bypass of platinum-DNA adducts. *Cancer Res.,* **1998,** *58*:3579–3585.

Valavaara, R., and Nordman, E. Renal complications of mitomycin C therapy with special reference to the total dose. *Cancer,* **1985,** *55*:47–50.

van Ark-Otte, J., Kedde, M.A., van der Vijgh, W.J., Dingemans, A.M., Jansen, W.J., Pinedo, H.M., Boven, E., and Giancone, G. Determinants of CPT-11 and SN-38 activities in human lung cancer cells. *Br. J. Cancer,* **1998,** *77*:2171–2176.

Van Barneveld, P.W., Sleijfer, D.T., van der Mark, T.W., Mulder, N.H., Koops, H.S., Sluiter, H.J., and Peset, R. Natural course of bleomycin-induced pneumonitis. A follow-up study. *Am. Rev. Respir. Dis.,* **1987,** *135*:48–51.

van Moorsel, C.J., Pinedo, H.M., Veerman, G., Bergman, A.M., Kuiper, C.M., Vermorken, J.B., van der Vijgh, W.J., and Peters, G.J. Mechanisms of synergism between cisplatin and gemcitabine in ovarian and non-small-cell lung cancer cell lines. *Br. J. Cancer,* **1999,** *80*:981–990.

van Triest, B., Pinedo, H.M., Blaauwgeers, J.L., van Diest, P.J., Schoenmakers, P.S., Voorn, D.A., Smid, K., Hoekman, K., Hoitsma, H.F., and Peters, G.J. Prognostic role of thymidylate synthase, thymidine phosphorylase/platelet-derived endothelial cell growth factor, and proliferation markers in colorectal cancer. *Clin. Cancer Res.,* **2000,** *6*:1063–1072.

Vassal, G., Challine, D., Koscielny, S., Hartmann, O., Deroussent, A., Boland, I., Valteau-Couanet, D., Lemerle, J., Levi, F., and Gouyette, A. Chronopharmacology of high-dose busulfan in children. *Cancer Res.,* **1993,** *53*:1534–1537.

Verweij, J., Funke-Kupper, A.J., Teule, G.J.J., and Pinedo, H.M. A prospective study on the dose dependency of cardiotoxicity induced by mitomycin C. *Med. Oncol. Tumor Pharmacother.,* **1988,** *5*:159–163.

von Pawel, J., Schiller, J.H., Shepherd, F.A., Fields, S.Z., Kleisbauer, J.P., Chrysson, N.G., Steward, D.J., Clark, P.I., Palmer, M.C., Depierre, A., Carmichael, J., Krebs, J.B., Ross, G., Lane, S.R., and Gralla, R. Topotecan versus cyclophosphamide, doxorubicin, and vincristine for the treatment of recurrent small-cell lung cancer. *J. Clin. Oncol.,* **1999,** *17*:658–667.

Waksman, S.A., and Woodruff, H.B. Bacteriostatic and bactericidal substances produced by a soil actinomyces. *Proc. Soc. Exp. Biol. Med.,* **1940,** *45*:609–614.

Wall, S.M., Johansen, M.J., Molony, D.A., DuBose, T.D., Jr., Jaffe, N., and Madden, T. Effective clearance of methotrexate using high-flux hemodialysis membranes. *Am. J. Kidney Dis.,* **1996,** *28*:846–854.

Wani, M.C., Taylor, H.L., Wall, M.E., Coggon, P., and McPhail, A.T. Plant antitumor agents. VI. The isolation and structure of taxol, a novel antileukemic and antitumor agent from *Taxus brevifolia. J. Am. Chem. Soc.,* **1971,** *93*:2325–2327.

Washtein, W.L. Thymidylate synthetase levels as a factor in 5-fluorodeoxyuridine and methotrexate cytotoxicity in gastrointestinal tumor cells. *Mol. Pharmacol.,* **1982,** *21*:723–728.

Weinstein, G.D. Methotrexate. *Ann. Intern. Med.,* **1977,** *86*:199–204.

Welters, M.J., Fichtinger-Schepman, A.M., Baan, R.A., Jacobs-Bergmans, A.J., Kegel, A., van der Vijgh, W.J., and Braakhuis, B.J. Pharmacodynamics of cisplatin in human head and neck cancer: correlation between platinum content, DNA adduct levels and drug sensitivity *in vitro* and *in vivo. Br. J. Cancer,* **1999,** *79*:82–88.

Westerhof, G.R., Rijnboutt, S., Schornagel, J.H., Pinedo, H.M., Peters, G.J., and Jansen, G. Functional activity of the reduced folate carrier in KB, MA104, and IGROV-I cells expressing folate-binding protein. *Cancer Res.,* **1995,** *55*:3795–3802.

Wiernik, P.H., Banks, P.L., Case, D.C., Jr., Arlin, Z.A., Periman, P.O., Todd, M.B., Ritch, P.S., Enck, R.E., and Weitberg, A.B. Cytarabine plus idarubicin or daunorubicin as induction and consolidation therapy for previously untreated adult patients with acute myeloid leukemia. *Blood,* **1992,** *79*:313–319.

Wijnholds, J., Mol, C.A., van Deemter, L., de Haas, M., Scheffer, G.L., Baas, F., Beijnen, J.H., Scheper, R.J., Hatse, S., De Clercq, E., Balzarini, J., and Borst, P. Multidrug-resistance protein 5 is a multispecific organic anion transporter able to transport nucleotide analogs. *Proc. Natl. Acad. Sci. U.S.A.,* **2000,** *97*:7476–7481.

Wiley, J.S., Taupin, J., Jamieson, G.P., Snook, M., Sawyer, W.H., and Finch, L.R. Cytosine arabinoside transport and metabolism in acute leukemias and T cell lymphoblastic lymphoma. *J. Clin. Invest.,* **1985,** *75*:632–642.

Williams, M.E., Walker, A.N., Bracikowski, J.P., Garner, L., Wilson, K.D., and Carpenter, J.T. Ascending myeloencephalopathy due to intrathecal vincristine sulfate. A fatal chemotherapeutic error. *Cancer,* **1983,** *51*:2041–2147.

Wilson, W.H., Berg, S.L., Bryant, G., Wittes, R.E., Bates, S., Fojo, A., Steinberg, S.M., Goldspiel, B.R., Herdt, J., O'Shaughnessy, J., Balis, F.M., and Chabner, B.A. Paclitaxel in doxorubicin-refractory or mitoxantrone-refractory breast cancer: a phase I/II trial of 96-hour infusion. *J. Clin. Oncol.,* **1994,** *12*:1621–1629.

Wolmark, N., Rockette, H., Fisher, B., Wickerham, D.L., Redmond, C., Fisher, E.R., Jones, J., Mamounas, E.P., Ore, L., Petrelli, N.J., Spurr, C.L., Dimitrov, N., Romond, E.H., Sutherland, C.M., Kardinal, C.G., DeFusco, P.A., and Jochimsen, P. The benefit of leucovorin-modulated fluorouracil as postoperative adjuvant therapy for primary colon cancer: results from National Surgical Adjuvant Breast and Bowel Project protocol C-03. *J. Clin. Oncol.,* **1993,** *11*:1879–1887.

Wong, G.G., Witek, J.S., Temple, P.A., Wilkens, K.M., Leary, A.C., Luxenberg, D.P., Jones, S.S., Brown, E.L., Kay, R.M., Orr, E.C., Shoemaker, C., Golde, D., Kaufman, R.J., Hewick, R.M., Wang, E.A., and Clark, S.C. Human GM-CSF: molecular cloning of the complementary DNA and purification of the natural and recombinant proteins. *Science,* **1985,** *228*:810–815.

Wortsman, J., and Soler, N.G. Mitotane. Spironolactone antagonism in Cushing's syndrome. *JAMA,* **1977,** *238*:2527.

Yang, S.W., Burgin, A.B., Jr., Huizenga, B.N., Robertson, C.A., Yao, K.C., and Nash, H.A. A eukaryotic enzyme that can disjoin dead-end covalent complexes between DNA and type I topoisomerases. *Proc. Natl. Acad. Sci. U.S.A.,* **1996,** *93*:11534–11539.

Yates, C.R., Krynetski, E.Y., Loennechen, T., Fessing, M.Y., Tai, H.L., Pui, C.H., Relling, M.V., and Evans, W.E. Molecular diagnosis of thiopurine S-methyltransferase deficiency: genetic basis for azathioprine and mercaptopurine intolerance. *Ann. Intern. Med.,* **1997,** *126*:608–614.

Zhang, R.W., Soong, S.J., Liu, T.P., Barnes, S., and Diasio, R.B. Pharmacokinetics and tissue distribution of 2-fluoro-β-alanine in rats. Potential relevance to toxicity pattern of 5-fluorouracil. *Drug Metab. Dispos.,* **1992,** *20*:113–119.

Zinzani, P.L., Magagnoli, M., Bendandi, M., Gherlinzoni, F., Orcioni, G.F., Cellini, C., Stefoni, V., Pileri, S.A., and Tura, S. Efficacy of fludarabine and mitoxantrone (FN) combination regimen in untreated indolent non-Hodgkin's lymphomas. *Ann. Oncol.,* **2000,** *11*:363–365.

Zuckerman, J.E., Raffin, T.A., Brown, J.M., Newman, R.A., Etiz, B.B., and Sikic, B.I. *In vitro* selection and characterization of a bleomycin-resistant subline of B16 melanoma. *Cancer Res.,* **1986,** *46*:1748–1753.

MONOGRAPHS AND REVIEWS

Aapro, M.S., Martin, C., and Hatty, S. Gemcitabine—a safety review. *Anticancer Drugs,* **1998,** *9*:191–201.

Ackland, S.P., and Schilsky, R.L. High-dose methotrexate: a critical reappraisal. *J. Clin. Oncol.,* **1987,** *5*:2017–2031.

Agarwala, S.S., and Kirkwood, J.M. Temozolomide, a novel alkylating agent with activity in the central nervous system, may improve the treatment of advanced metastatic melanoma. *Oncologist,* **2000,** *5*:144–151.

Armstrong, R.D. RNA as a target for antimetabolites. In, *Developments in Cancer Chemotherapy.* Vol. 2. (Glazer, R.I., ed.) CRC Press, Boca Raton, FL, **1989,** pp. 154–174.

Beardsley, G.P., Taylor, E.C., Grindley, G.B., *et al.* Deaza derivatives of tetrahydrofolic acid. A new class of folate antimetabolite. In, *Chemistry and Biology of Pteridines.* (Cooper, B.A., and Whitehead, V.M., eds.) De Gruyter, Berlin **1986,** pp. 953–957.

Beutler, E. Cladribine (2-chlorodeoxyadenosine). *Lancet,* **1992,** *340*:952–956.

Blakley, R.L., and Sorrentino, B.P. *In vitro* mutations in dihydrofolate reductase that confer resistance to methotrexate: potential for clinical application. *Hum. Mutat.,* **1998,** *11*:259–263.

Bleyer, W.A. The clinical pharmacology of methotrexate: new applications of an old drug. *Cancer,* **1978,** *41*:36–51.

Bloch, A., ed. Chemistry, biology, and clinical uses of nucleoside analogs. *Ann. N.Y. Acad. Sci.,* **1975,** *255*:1–610.

Brade, W.P., Nagel, G.A., and Seeber, S. (eds.). *Ifosfamide in Tumor Therapy.* Karger, New York, **1987.**

Brockman, R.W. Resistance to purine analogs. Clinical pharmacology symposium. *Biochem. Pharmacol.,* **1974,** *23*(suppl. 2):107–117.

Broome, J.D. L-Asparaginase: discovery and development as a tumor-inhibitory agent. *Cancer Treat. Rep.,* **1981,** *65*(suppl. 4):111–114.

Budman, D.R. Vinorelbine (Navelbine): a third-generation vinca alkaloid. *Cancer Invest.,* **1997,** *15*:475–90.

Bukowski, R.M., McLain, D., and Finke, J. Clinical pharmacokinetics of interleukin-1, interleukin-2, interleukin-3, tumor necrosis factor, and macrophage colony-stimulating factor. In, *Cancer Chemotherapy and Biotherapy: Principles and Practice,* 3rd ed. (Chabner, B.A., and Longo, D.L., eds.) Lippincott Williams & Wilkins, Philadelphia, **2001.** In press.

Burger, R.M. Cleavage of nucleic acids by bleomycin. *Chem. Rev.,* **1998,** *98*:1153–1169.

Calabresi, P., and Schein, P.S. (eds.). *Medical Oncology: Basic Principles and Clinical Management of Cancer,* 2nd ed. McGraw-Hill, New York, **1993.**

Calvete, J.A., Balmanno, K., Taylor, G.A., Rafi, I., Newell, D.R., Lind, J.J., and Clavert, A.H. Preclinical and clinical studies of prolonged administration of the novel thymidylate synthase inhibitor, AG337. *Ann. Oncol.,* **1994,** *5*(suppl. 5):134.

Capizzi, R.L., and Handschumacher, R.E. Asparaginase. In, *Cancer Medicine,* 2nd ed. (Frei, E., and Holland, J.F., eds.) Lea & Febiger Philadelphia, **1982,** pp. 920–932.

Chabner, B.A. Cytidine analogues. In, *Cancer Chemotherapy and Biotherapy: Principles and Practice,* 3rd ed. (Chabner, B.A., and Longo, D.L., eds.) Lippincott Williams & Wilkins, Philadelphia, **2001.** In press.

Chabner, B.A., Wilson, W., and Supko, J. Pharmacology and toxicity of antineoplastic drugs. In, *Williams' Hematology,* 6th ed. (Beutler, E., Lichtman, M.A., Coller, B.S., Kipps, T.J., and Seligsohn, U., eds.) McGraw-Hill, New York, **2001,** pp. 185–200.

Chen, V.J., Bewley, J.R., Andis, S.L., Schultz, R.M., Iversen, P.W., Shih, C., Mendelsohn, L.G., Seitz, D.E., and Tonkinson, J.L. Cellular pharmacology of MTA: a correlation of MTA-induced cellular toxicity and in vitro enzyme inhibition with its effect on intracellular folate and nucleoside triphosphate pools in CCRF-CEM cells. *Semin. Oncol.,* **1999,** *26*:48–54.

Cheson, B.D. The purine analogs—a therapeutic beauty contest. *J. Clin. Oncol.,* **1992,** *10*:868–871.

Colvin, M. The comparative pharmacology of cyclophosphamide and ifosfamide. *Semin. Oncol.,* **1982,** *9*:2–7.

Crooke, S.T. Antitumor antibiotics II: actinomycin D, bleomycin, mitomycin C and other antibiotics. In, *The Cancer Pharmacology Annual.* (Chabner, B.A., and Pinedo, H.M., eds.) Excerpta Medica, Amsterdam, **1983,** pp. 69–79.

Crooke, S.T., and Bradner, W.T. Mitomycin C: a review. *Cancer Treat. Rev.,* **1976,** *3*:121–139.

DeVita, V.T., Jr. The consequences of the chemotherapy of Hodgkin's disease: The 10th David A. Karnofsky Memorial Lecture. *Cancer,* **1981,** *47*:1–13.

DeVita, V.T., Jr., Canellos, G.P., and Moxley, J.H. III. A decade of combination chemotherapy of advanced Hodgkin's disease. *Cancer,* **1972,** *30*:1495–1504.

Dillman, R.O. A new chemotherapeutic agent: deoxycoformycin (pentostatin). *Semin. Hematol.,* **1994,** *31*:16–27.

Donehower, R.C. Antimitotic agents. In, *Cancer Chemotherapy and Biotherapy: Principles and Practice,* 3rd ed. (Chabner, B.A., and Longo, D.L., eds.) Lippincott Williams & Wilkins, Philadelphia, **2001.** In press.

Dorr, R.T. New findings in the pharmacokinetic, metabolic, and drug-resistance aspects of mitomycin C. *Semin. Oncol.,* **1988,** *15*:32–41.

Druker, B.J., and Lydon, N.B. Lessons learned from the development of an abl tyrosine kinase inhibitor for chronic myelogenous leukemia. *J. Clin. Invest.,* **2000,** *105*:3–7.

Durant, J.R., and Omura, G.A. Gynecologic neoplasms. In, *Medical Oncology: Basic Principles and Clinical Management of Cancer.* (Calabresi, P., Schein, P.S., and Rosenberg, S.A., eds.) Macmillan Publishing, New York, **1985,** pp. 1004–1044.

Elion, G.B. Symposium on immunosuppressive drugs. Biochemistry and pharmacology of purine analogues. *Fed. Proc.,* **1967,** *26*:898–904.

Ellis, M., and Swain, S.M. Steroid hormone therapies for cancer. In, *Cancer Chemotherapy and Biotherapy: Principles and Practice,* 3rd ed. (Chabner, B.A., and Longo, D.L., eds.) Lippincott Williams & Wilkins, Philadelphia, **2001.** In press.

Endicott, J.A., and Ling, V. The biochemistry of P-glycoprotein-mediated multidrug resistance. *Annu. Rev. Biochem.,* **1989,** *58*:137–171.

Fefer, A., Benyunes, M.C., Massumoto, C., Higuchi, C., York, A., Buckner, C.D., and Thompson, J.A. Interleukin-2 therapy after autologous bone marrow transplantation for hematologic malignancies. *Semin. Oncol.,* **1993,** *20*:41–45.

Friedman, H.S. Nonclassic alkylating agents. In, *Cancer Chemotherapy and Biotherapy: Principles and Practice,* 3rd ed. (Chabner B.A., and Longo, D.L., eds.) Lippincott Williams & Wilkins, Philadelphia, **2001.** In press.

Garcia-Carbonero, R., Ryan, D.P., and Chabner, B.A. Cytidine analogues. In, *Cancer Chemotherapy and Biotherapy: Principles and Practice,* 3rd ed. (Chabner, B.A., and Longo, D.L., eds.) Lippincott Williams & Wilkins, Philadelphia, **2001.** In press.

Gilman, A., and Philips, F.S. The biological actions and therapeutic applications of the β-chlorethylamines and sulfides. *Science,* **1946,** *103*:409–415.

Giverhaug, T., Loennechen, T., and Aarbakke, J. The interaction of 6-mercaptopurine (6-MP) and methotrexate (MTX). *Gen. Pharmacol.,* **1999,** *33*:341–346.

Go, R.S., and Adjei, A.A. Review of the comparative pharmacology and clinical activity of cisplatin and carboplatin. *J. Clin. Oncol.,* **1999,** *17*:409–422.

Goldberg, I.H., Beerman, T.A., and Poon, R. Antibiotics: nucleic acids as targets in chemotherapy. In, *Cancer: A Comprehensive Treatise.* Vol. 5: *Chemotherapy.* (Becker, F.F., ed.) Plenum Press, New York, **1977,** pp. 427–456.

Graham, M.A., Lockwood, G.F., Greenslade, D., Brienza, S., Bayssas, M., and Gamelin, E. Clinical pharmacokinetics of oxaliplatin: a critical review. *Clin. Cancer Res.,* **2000,** *6*:1205–1218.

Grem, J.L. 5-Fluropyrimidines. In, *Cancer Chemotherapy and Biotherapy: Principles and Practice,* 3rd ed. (Chabner, B.A., and Longo, D.L., eds.) Lippincott Williams & Wilkins, Philadelphia, **2001.** In press.

Grem, J.L., Hoth, D.F., Hamilton, J.M., King, S.A., and Leyland-Jones, B. Overview of current status and future direction of clinical trials with 5-fluorouracil in combination with folinic acid. *Cancer Treat. Rep.,* **1987,** *71*:1249–1264.

Grem, J.L., King, S.A., O'Dwyer, P.J., and Leyland-Jones, B. Biochemistry and clinical activity of N-(phosphonacetyl)-L-aspartate: a review. *Cancer Res.,* **1988,** *48*:4441–4454.

Hainsworth, J.D. Monoclonal antibody therapy in lymphoid malignancies. *Oncologist,* **2000,** *5*:376–384.

Hande, K.R. Etoposide: four decades of development of a topoisomerase II inhibitor. *Eur. J. Cancer,* **1998,** *34*:1514–1521.

Heidelberger, C. Fluorinated pyrimidines and their nucleosides. In, *Antineoplastic and Immunosuppressive Agents.* Pt. II. (Sartorelli, A.C., and Johns, D.G., eds.) *Handbuch der Experimentellen Pharmakologie.* Vol. 38. Springer-Verlag, Berlin, **1975,** pp. 193–231.

Huang, P., Chubb, S., Hertel, L.W., Grindey, G.B., and Plunkett, W. Action of 2',2'-difluorodeoxycytidine on DNA synthesis. *Cancer Res.,* **1991,** *51*:6110–6117.

Iyer, L. Inherited variations in drug-metabolizing enzymes: significance in clinical oncology. *Mol. Diagn.,* **1999,** *4*:327–333.

Jordan, V.C. Estrogen receptor as a target for the prevention of breast cancer. *J. Lab. Clin. Med.,* **1999,** *133*:408–414.

Jordan, V.C. Metabolites of tamoxifen in animals and man: identification, pharmacology, and significance. *Breast Cancer Res. Treat.,* **1982,** *2*:123–138.

Kaelin, W.G., Jr. Taking aim at novel molecular targets in cancer therapy. *J. Clin. Invest.,* **1999,** *104*:1495.

Kastan, M.B. Molecular determinants of sensitivity to antitumor agents. *Biochim. Biophys. Acta.,* **1999,** *1424*:R37–R42.

Keating, M.J., Holmes, R., Lerner, S., and Ho, D.H. L-asparaginase and PEGasparaginase—past, present and future. *Leuk. Lymphoma,* **1993,** *10*(suppl.):153–157.

Kelland, L.R. New platinum antitumor complexes. *Crit. Rev. Oncol. Hematol.,* **1993,** *15*:191–219.

Kerbel, R.S. Tumor angiogenesis: past, present and the near future. *Carcinogenesis,* **2000,** *21*:505–515.

Kraut, J., and Matthews, D.A. Dihydrofolate reductase. In, *Biological Macromolecules and Assemblies.* Vol. 3. (Jurnak, F.A., and McPherson, A., eds.) Wiley, New York, **1987,** pp. 1–21.

Launchbury, A.P., and Habboubi, N. Epirubicin and doxorubicin: a comparison of their characteristics, therapeutic activity and toxicity. *Cancer Treat. Rev.,* **1993,** *19*:197–228.

Levine, E.G., and Bloomfield, C.D. Leukemias and myelodysplastic syndromes secondary to drug, radiation, and environmental exposure. *Semin. Oncol.,* **1992,** *19*:47–84.

Lori, F. Hydroxyurea and HIV: 5 years later—from antiviral to immune-modulating effects. *AIDS,* **1999,** *13*:1433–1442.

Ludlum, D.B., and Tong, W.P. DNA modification by the nitrosoureas: chemical nature and cellular repair. In, *Cancer Chemotherapy,* Vol. II. (Muggia, F.M., ed.) Martinus Nijhoff, The Hague, **1985,** pp. 141–154.

Maloney, D.G. Unconjugated monoclonal antibody therapy of lymphoma. In, *Monoclonal Antibody-Based Therapy of Cancer.* (Grossbard, M.L., ed.) Marcel Dekker, New York, **1998,** pp. 53–79.

Messmann, R., and Allegra, C.J. Antifolates. In, *Cancer Chemotherapy and Biotherapy: Principles and Practice,* 3rd ed. (Chabner, B.A., and Longo, D.L., eds.) Lippincott Williams & Wilkins, Philadelphia, **2001.** In press.

Morstyn, G., Lieschke, G.J., Sheridan, W., Layton, J., Cebon, J., and Fox, R.M. Clinical experience with recombinant human granulocyte colony-stimulating factor and granulocyte macrophage colony-stimulating factor. *Semin. Hematol.,* **1989,** *26*:9–13.

Muggia, F.M. Overview of carboplatin: replacing, complementing, and extending the therapeutic horizons of cisplatin. *Semin. Oncol.,* **1989,** *16*:7–13.

Myers, C.E. Role of iron in anthracycline action. In, *Organ-Directed Toxicities of Anticancer Drugs.* (Hacker, M.P., Lazo, J.S., and Tritton, T.R., eds.) Martinus Nijhoff, Boston, **1988,** pp. 17–30.

Navarra, P., and Preziosi, P. Hydroxyurea: new insights on an old drug. *Crit. Rev. Oncol. Hematol.,* **1999,** *29*:249–255.

Odom, L.F., and Gordon, E.M. Acute monoblastic leukemia in infancy and early childhood: successful treatment with an epipodophyllotoxin. *Blood,* **1984,** *64*:875–882.

Oliverio, V.T. Pharmacology of the nitrosoureas: an overview. *Cancer Treat. Rep.,* **1976,** *60*:703–707.

Patterson, M.K., Jr. L-Asparaginase: basic aspects. In, *Antineoplastic and Immunosuppressive Agents,* Pt. II. (Sartorelli, A.C., and Johns, D.G., eds.) *Handbuch der Experimentellen Pharmakologie,* Vol. 38. Springer-Verlag, Berlin, **1975,** pp. 695–722.

Paz-Ares, L., and Donehower, R. Hydroxyurea. In, *Cancer Chemotherapy and Biotherapy: Principles and Practice,* 3rd ed. (Chapbner, B.A., and Longo, D.L., eds.) Lippincott Williams & Wilkins, Philidelphia, **2001.** In press.

Pinkel, D., and Howarth, C.B. Pediatric neoplasms. In, *Medical Oncology: Basic Principles and Clinical Management of Cancer.* (Calabresi, P., Schein, P.S., and Rosenberg, S.A., eds.) Macmillan, New York, **1985,** pp. 1226–1258.

Piro, L.D. 2-Chlorodeoxyadenosine treatment of lymphoid malignancies. *Blood,* **1992,** *79*:843–845.

Plunkett, W., and Gandhi, V. Cellular metabolism of nucleoside analogs in CLL: implications for drug development. In, *Chronic Lymphocytic Leukemia: Scientific Advances and Clinical Developments.* (Cheson, B., ed.) Marcel Dekker, New York, **1992,** p. 197.

Pommier, Y., Fesen, M.R., and Goldwasser, F. Topoisomerase II inhibitors: the epipodophyllotoxins, m-AMSA, and the ellipticine derivatives. In, *Cancer Chemotherapy and Biotherapy: Principles and Practice,* 3rd ed. (Chabner, B.A., and Longo, D.L., eds.) Lippincott Williams & Wilkins, Philadelphia, **2001.** In press.

Pratt, W.B., Ruddon, R.W., Ensminger, W.D., and Maybaum, J. *The Anticancer Drugs,* 2nd ed. Oxford University Press, New York, **1994.**

Reid, P., Kantoff, P., and Oh, W. Antiandrogens in prostate cancer. *Invest. New Drugs.* **1999,** *17:*271–284.

Rowinsky, E.K., and Donehower, R.C. Paclitaxel. *N. Engl. J. Med.,* **1995,** *332:*1004–1014.

Rowinsky, E.K., McGuire, W.P., and Donehower, R.C. The current status of Taxol. *Prin. Pract. Gynecol. Oncol. Updates,* **1993,** *1:*1–16.

Schilsky, R.L., Ratain, M.J., Vokes, E.E., Vogelzang, N.J., Anderson, J., and Peterson, B.A. Laboratory and clinical studies of biochemical modulation by hydroxyurea. *Semin. Oncol.,* **1992,** *19:*84–89.

Schimke, R.T., Kaufman, R.J., Alt, F.W., and Kellems, R.F. Gene amplification and drug resistance in cultured murine cells. *Science,* **1978,** *202:*1051–1055.

Schwartz, R.S. Immunosuppression—back to the future. *World J. Surg.,* **2000,** *24:*783–786.

Seidman, AD. One-hour paclitaxel via weekly infusion: dose-density with enhanced therapeutic index. *Oncology (Huntingt.),* **1998,** *12:*19–22.

Shenkenberg, T.D., and Von Hoff, D.D. Mitoxantrone: a new anticancer drug with significant clinical activity. *Ann. Intern. Med.,* **1986,** *105:*67–81.

Sobell, H.M. The stereochemistry of actinomycin binding to DNA and its implications in molecular biology. *Prog. Nucleic Acid Res. Mol. Biol.,* **1973,** *13:*153–190.

Stark, G.R., and Wahl, G.M. Gene amplification. *Annu. Rev. Biochem.,* **1984,** *53:*447–491.

Symposium. (Various authors.) Proceedings of the conference on 2'-deoxycoformycin: current status and future directions. *Cancer Treatment Symposia.* Vol. 2. National Cancer Institute, Bethseda, MD, **1984,** pp. 1–104.

Takimoto, C.H., and Arbuck, S.G. Topoisomerase I poisons: the camptothecins. In, *Cancer Chemotherapy and Biotherapy: Principles and Practice,* 3rd ed. (Chapbner, B.A., and Longo, D.L., eds.) Lippincott Williams & Wilkins, Phililedphia, **2001.** In press.

Tew, K., Colvin, M., and Chabner, B.A. Alkylating agents. In, *Cancer Chemotherapy and Biotherapy: Principles and Practice,* 3rd ed. (Chabner, B.A., and Longo, D.L., eds.). Lippincott Williams & Wilkins, Philadelphia, **2001.** In press.

Van Echo, D.A., Egorin, M.J., and Aisner, J. The pharmacology of carboplatin. *Semin. Oncol.,* **1989,** *16:*1–6.

Verweij, J., Schellens, J.H.M., Loo, T.L., and Pinedo, H.M. Antitumor antibiotics. In, *Cancer Chemotherapy and Biotherapy: Principles and Practice,* 3rd ed. (Chabner, B.A., and Longo, D.L., eds.) Lippincott Williams & Wilkins, Philadelphia, **2001.** In press.

Von Hoff, D.D. Whither carboplatin? A replacement for or an alternative to cisplatin? *J. Clin. Oncol.,* **1987,** *5:*169–171.

Waksman Conference on Actinomycins: their potential for cancer chemotherapy. *Cancer Chemother. Rep.,* **1974,** *58:*1–123.

Weinshilboum, R. Methyltransferase pharmacogenetics. *Pharmacol. Ther.,* **1989,** *43:*77–90.

Williams, S.D., and Einhorn, L.H. Neoplasms of the testis. In, *Medical Oncology: Basic Principles and Clinical Management of Cancer.* (Calabresi, P., Schein, P.S., and Rosenberg, S.A., eds.) Macmillan, New York, **1985,** pp. 1077–1088.

Zhou, X.J., and Rahmani, R. Preclinical and clinical pharmacology of vinca alkaloids. *Drugs,* **1992,** *44(suppl. 4):*1–16.

Zinner, S.H., and Klastersky, J. Infectious considerations in cancer. In, *Medical Oncology: Basic Principles and Clinical Management of Cancer.* (Calabresi, P., Schein, P.S., and Rosenberg, S.A., eds.) Macmillan, New York, **1985,** pp. 1327–1357.

SECTION X

DRUGS USED FOR IMMUNOMODULATION

C H A P T E R 5 3

IMMUNOMODULATORS: IMMUNOSUPPRESSIVE AGENTS, TOLEROGENS, AND IMMUNOSTIMULANTS

Alan M. Krensky, Terry B. Strom, and Jeffrey A. Bluestone

This chapter provides a brief overview of the immune response as background for understanding the mechanism of action of immunomodulatory agents. The general principles of pharmacological immunosuppression are discussed in the context of potential targets, major indications, and unwanted side effects. Four major classes of immunosuppressive drugs are discussed: glucocorticoids (see also Chapter 60), calcineurin inhibitors, antiproliferative and antimetabolic agents (see also Chapter 52), and antibodies. The "holy grail" of immunomodulation is the induction and maintenance of immune tolerance, the active state of antigen-specific nonresponsiveness. Approaches expected to overcome the risks of infections and tumors with immunosuppression are reviewed. These include costimulatory blockade, donor-cell chimerism, soluble human leukocyte antigens (HLA), and antigen-based therapies. Lastly, a general discussion of the limited number of immunostimulant agents is presented, concluding with an overview of active and passive immunization. New immunotherapeutic approaches will address not only the issues of specific drug toxicities and efficacy but also long-term economic, metabolic, and quality-of-life outcomes.

THE IMMUNE RESPONSE

The immune system evolved to discriminate self from nonself. Multicellular organisms were faced with the problem of destroying infectious invaders (microbes) or dysregulated self (tumors) while leaving normal cells intact. These organisms responded by developing a robust array of receptor-mediated sensing and effector mechanisms broadly described as innate and adaptive. Innate, or natural, immunity is primitive, does not require priming, is of relatively low affinity, but is broadly reactive. Adaptive, or learned, immunity is antigen-specific, depends upon antigen exposure or priming, and can be of very high affinity. The two arms of immunity work closely together, with the innate immune system being most active early in an immune response and adaptive immunity becoming progressively dominant over time. The major effectors of innate immunity are complement, granulocytes, monocytes/macrophages, natural killer cells, mast cells, and basophils. The major effectors of adaptive immunity are B and T cells. B cells make antibodies; T cells function as helper, cytolytic, and regulatory (suppressor) cells. These cells are important in the normal immune response to infection and tumors but also mediate transplant rejection and autoimmunity (Janeway *et al.,* 1999; Paul, 1999). Immunoglobulins (antibodies) on the B-cell surface are receptors for a large variety of specific structural conformations. In contrast, T cells recognize antigens as peptide fragments in the context of self major histocompatibility complex (MHC) antigens (called HLA in human beings) on the surface of antigen-presenting cells (APCs), such as dendritic cells, macrophages, and other cell types expressing MHC class I (HLA-A, B, and C) and class II antigens (HLA-DR, DP, and DQ) in human beings. Once activated by specific antigen recognition *via* their respective clonally restricted cell-surface receptors, both B and T cells are triggered to differentiate and divide, leading to release of soluble mediators (cytokines, lymphokines) that perform as effectors and regulators of the immune response.

The impact of the immune system in human disease is enormous. Developing vaccines against emerging infectious agents from human immunodeficiency virus (HIV)

1463

to Ebola virus is among the most critical challenges facing the research community. Immune system-mediated diseases are significant health-care problems. Immunological diseases are growing at epidemic proportions that require aggressive and innovative approaches to the development of new treatments. These diseases include a broad spectrum of autoimmune diseases such as rheumatoid arthritis, diabetes mellitus, systemic lupus erythematosus, and multiple sclerosis; solid tumors and hematologic malignancies; infectious diseases; asthma; and various allergic conditions. Furthermore, one of the great therapeutic opportunities for the treatment of many disorders is organ transplantation. However, immune system–mediated graft rejection remains the single greatest barrier to widespread use of this technology. An improved understanding of the immune system has led to the development of new therapies to treat immune system–mediated diseases. This chapter briefly reviews drugs used to modulate the immune response in three ways: immunosuppression, tolerance, and immunostimulation.

IMMUNOSUPPRESSION

Immunosuppressive drugs are used to dampen the immune response in organ transplantation and autoimmune disease. In transplantation, the major classes of drugs used today are: (1) *glucocorticoids*, (2) *calcineurin inhibitors*, and (3) *antiproliferative/antimetabolic agents.* These drugs have met with a high degree of clinical success in treating conditions such as acute immune rejection of organ transplants and severe autoimmune diseases. However, such therapies require lifelong use and nonspecifically suppress the entire immune system, exposing patients to considerably higher risks of infection and cancer. The calcineurin

inhibitors and steroids, in particular, are nephrotoxic and diabetogenic, thus limiting their usefulness in a variety of clinical settings.

Monoclonal and polyclonal antibody preparations directed at reactive T cells are important adjunct therapies and provide a unique opportunity to selectively target specific immune-reactive cells and thus promote more specific treatments. Finally, new agents recently have expanded the arsenal of immunosuppressive agents. In particular, *sirolimus* and anti–CD25 [interleukin (IL)-2 receptor] antibodies (*basiliximab, daclizumab*) are being used to target growth factor pathways, substantially limiting clonal expansion and thus promoting tolerance. The most commonly used immunosuppressive drugs are described below. Nevertheless, many new, more selective, therapeutic agents are on the horizon and are expected to revolutionize immunotherapy in the next decade.

General Approach to Organ Transplantation Therapy

Organ transplant therapy is organized around five general principles. The first principle is careful patient preparation and selection of the best available ABO-compatible HLA match for organ donation (Legendre and Guttman, 1989). Second, a multitiered approach to immunosuppressive drug therapy, similar to that in cancer chemotherapy, is employed. Several agents are used simultaneously, each of which is directed at a different molecular target within the allograft response (Table 53–1; Krensky, *et al.,* 1990; Hong and Kahan, 2000a). Synergistic effects are obtained through application of the various agents at relatively low doses, thereby limiting specific toxicities while maximizing the immunosuppressive effect. The third principle is that greater immunosuppression is required to gain early engraftment and/or to treat established rejection than to maintain immunosuppression in the long term. Therefore, intensive induction and lower-dose maintenance drug protocols are employed. Fourth, careful investigation of each episode of transplant dysfunction is required,

Table 53–1

Sites of Action of Selected Immunosuppressive Agents on T-Cell Activation

DRUG	SITE OF ACTION
Glucocorticoids	Glucocorticoid response elements in DNA (regulate gene transcription)
Muromonab-CD3	T-cell receptor complex (blocks antigen recognition)
Cyclosporine	Calcineurin (inhibits phosphatase activity)
Tacrolimus	Calcineurin (inhibits phosphatase activity)
Azathioprine	Deoxyribonucleic acid (false nucleotide incorporation)
Mycophenolate Mofetil	Inosine monophosphate dehydrogenase (inhibits activity)
Daclizumab, Basiliximab	IL-2 receptor (block IL-2–mediated T-cell activation)
Sirolimus	Protein kinase involved in cell-cycle progression (mTOR) (inhibits activity)

including evaluation for rejection, drug toxicity, and infection, keeping in mind that these various problems can and often do coexist. The fifth principle involves reduction or withdrawal of a therapeutic agent when its toxicity exceeds its benefit.

Sequential Immunotherapy. In many organ transplant centers, muromonab-CD3, anti-CD25 monoclonal antibodies, or polyclonal antilymphocyte antibodies are used as induction therapy in the immediate posttransplantation period (Wilde and Goa, 1996; Brennan *et al.,* 1999). This treatment enables initial engraftment without the use of high doses of nephrotoxic calcineurin inhibitors. Such protocols reduce the incidence of early rejection and appear to be particularly beneficial for patients at high risk for graft rejection (broadly presensitized or retransplant patients, pediatric recipients, or African Americans).

Maintenance Immunotherapy. The basic immunosuppressive protocol used in most transplant centers involves the use of multiple drugs simultaneously. Therapy typically involves a calcineurin inhibitor, steroids, and mycophenolate mofetil (a purine metabolism inhibitor), each directed at a discrete site in T-cell activation (Suthanthiran *et al.,* 1996; Perico and Remuzzi, 1997). Glucocorticoids, azathioprine, cyclosporine, tacrolimus, mycophenolate mofetil, sirolimus, and various monoclonal and polyclonal antibodies currently are approved by the United States Food and Drug Administration (FDA) for use in transplantation.

Therapy for Established Rejection. Although low doses of prednisone, calcineurin inhibitors, purine-metabolism inhibitors, or sirolimus are effective in preventing acute cellular rejection, they are not as effective in blocking T cells that already are activated, and they are not very effective against established, acute rejection or for the total prevention of chronic rejection (Monaco *et al.,* 1999). Therefore, treatment of established rejection requires the use of agents directed against activated T cells. These include glucocorticoids in high doses (pulse therapy), polyclonal antilymphocyte antibodies, or muromonab-CD3 monoclonal antibody.

Adrenocortical Steroids

The introduction of glucocorticoids as immunosuppressive drugs in the 1960s played a key role in making organ transplantation possible. The chemistry, pharmacokinetics, and drug interactions of adrenocortical steroids are described in Chapter 60. Prednisone, prednisolone, and other glucocorticoids are used alone and in combination with other immunosuppressive agents for treatment of transplant rejection and autoimmune disorders.

Mechanism of Action. The immunosuppressive effects of glucocorticoids long have been known, but the specific mechanism(s) of their immunosuppressive action remains somewhat elusive (Rugstad, 1988; Beato, 1989). Steroids lyse and possibly induce the redistribution of lymphocytes, causing a rapid, transient decrease in peripheral blood lymphocyte counts. To effect longer-term responses, steroids bind to receptors inside cells,

and either these receptors or glucocorticoid-induced proteins bind to DNA in the vicinity of response elements that regulate the transcription of numerous other genes (*see* Chapter 60). Additionally, glucocorticoid-receptor complexes increase IκB expression, thereby curtailing activation of NFκB, which results in increased apoptosis of activated cells (Auphan *et al.,* 1995). Of central importance in this regard is the downregulation of important proinflammatory cytokines, such as IL-1 and IL-6. T cells are inhibited from making IL-2 and proliferating. The activation of cytotoxic T lymphocytes is inhibited. Neutrophils and monocytes display poor chemotaxis and decreased lysosomal enzyme release. Therefore, glucocorticoids have broad antiinflammatory effects on cellular immunity. In contrast, they have relatively little effect on humoral immunity.

Therapeutic Uses. Glucocorticoids commonly are used in combination with other immunosuppressive agents to both prevent and treat transplant rejection. High doses of intravenous *methylprednisolone sodium succinate* (SOLU-MEDROL, A-METHAPRED) (pulses) are used to reverse acute transplant rejection and acute exacerbations of selected autoimmune disorders (Shinn *et al.,* 1999; Laan *et al.,* 1999). There are numerous indications for glucocorticoids (Zoorob and Cender, 1998). They are efficacious for treatment of graft-versus-host disease in bone-marrow transplantation. Among autoimmune disorders, glucocorticoids are used routinely to treat rheumatoid and other arthritides, systemic lupus erythematosus, systemic dermatomyositis, psoriasis and other skin conditions, asthma and other allergic disorders, inflammatory bowel disease, inflammatory ophthalmic diseases, autoimmune hematologic disorders, and acute exacerbations of multiple sclerosis. In addition, glucocorticoids limit allergic reactions that occur with other immunosuppressive agents and are used in transplant recipients to block first-dose cytokine storm caused by treatment with muromonad-CD3 (*see* below).

Toxicity. Unfortunately, because there are numerous steroid-responsive tissues and genes, the extensive use of steroids has resulted in disabling and life-threatening adverse effects in many patients. These effects include growth retardation, avascular necrosis of bone, osteopenia, increased risk of infection, poor wound healing, cataracts, hyperglycemia, and hypertension (*see* Chapter 60). The advent of concomitant glucocorticoid/cyclosporine regimens has allowed a reduction in the dosages of steroids administered, yet steroid-induced morbidity is still a major problem in many transplant patients.

Calcineurin Inhibitors

Perhaps the most effective immunosuppressive drugs in routine clinical use are calcineurin inhibitors, *cyclosporine*

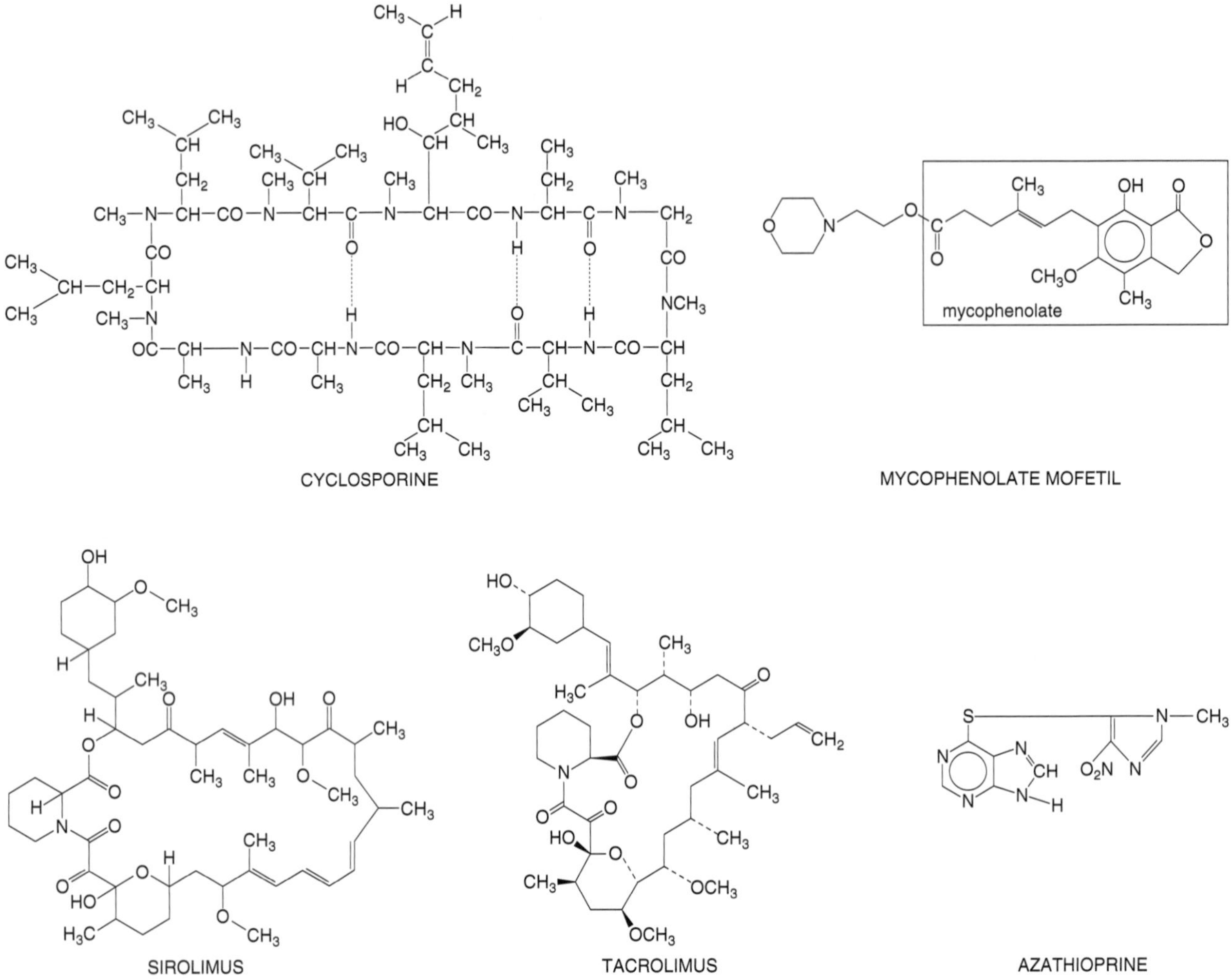

Figure 53–1. Chemical structures of immunosuppressive drugs: azathioprine, mycophenolate mofetil, cyclosporine, tacrolimus, and sirolimus.

and *tacrolimus,* drugs that target intracellular signaling pathways induced as a consequence of T-cell-receptor activation (Schreiber and Crabtree, 1992). Although they are structurally unrelated (Figure 53–1) and bind to different (but related) molecular targets, the mechanisms of action of cyclosporine and tacrolimus in inhibiting normal T-cell signal transduction are the same (Figure 53–2). Cyclosporineand tacrolimus do not act *per se* as immunosuppressive agents. Instead, these drugs "gain function" after binding to cyclophilin or FKBP-12, resulting in subsequent interaction with calcineurin to block the activity of this phosphatase. Calcineurin-catalyzed dephosphorylation is required for movement of a component of the nuclear factor of activated T lymphocytes (NFAT) into the nucleus (Figure 53–2). NFAT, in turn, is required for induction of a number of cytokine genes, including that

for interleukin-2 (IL-2), a prototypic T-cell growth and differentiation factor.

Cyclosporine. *Chemistry. Cyclosporine* (cyclosporin A) is a cyclic polypeptide consisting of 11 amino acids, produced as a metabolite of the fungus species *Beauveria nivea* (Borel *et al.,* 1976). Of note, all amide nitrogens are either hydrogen bonded or methylated, the single D-amino acid is at position 8, the methyl amide between residues 9 and 10 is in the *cis* configuration, and all other methyl amide moieties are in the *trans* form (Figure 53–1). Since cyclosporine is lipophilic and highly hydrophobic, it must be solubilized for clinical administration.

Mechanism of Action.   Cyclosporine suppresses some humoral immunity but is more effective against T cell–dependent immune mechanisms such as those underlying transplant rejection and some forms of autoimmunity (Kahan, 1989). It preferentially inhibits antigen-triggered signal transduction in T lymphocytes, blunting expression of many lymphokines, including IL-2, as

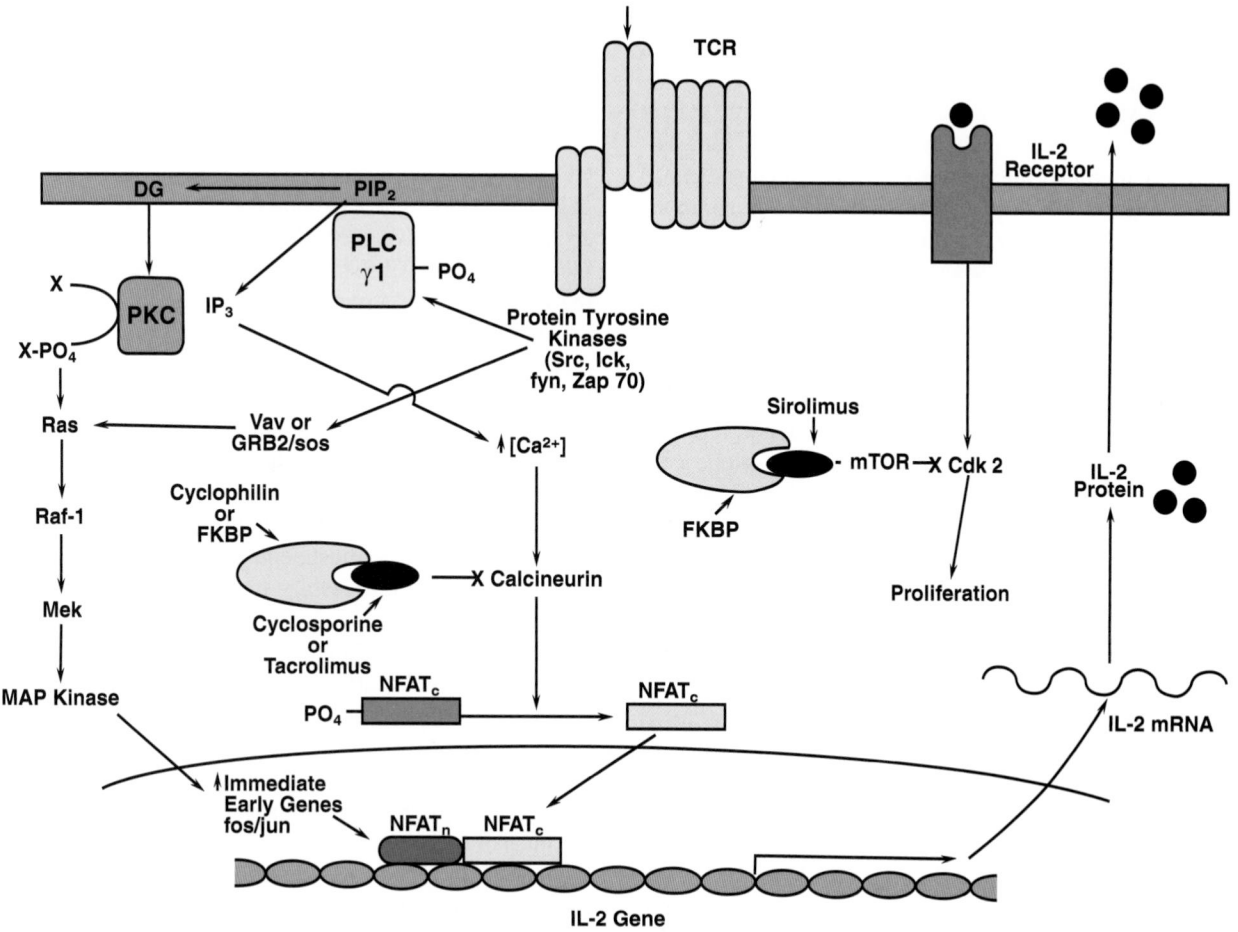

Figure 53–2. Mechanisms of action of cyclosporine, tacrolimus, and sirolimus.

Both cyclosporine and tacrolimus bind to immunophilins [cyclophilin and FK506-binding protein (FKBP), respectively], forming a complex that binds the phosphatase calcineurin and inhibits the calcineurin-catalyzed dephosphorylation essential to permit movement of the nuclear factor of activated T cells (NFAT) into the nucleus. NFAT is required for transcription of interleukin-2 (IL-2) and other growth and differentiation–associated cytokines (lymphokines). Sirolimus (rapamycin) works at a later stage in T-cell activation, downstream of the IL-2 receptor. Sirolimus also binds FKBP, but the FKBP-sirolimus complex binds to and inhibits the mammalian target of rapamycin (mTOR), a kinase involved in cell-cycle progression (proliferation). DG, diacylglycerol; PIP_2, phosphatidylinositol bisphosphate; PLC, phospholipase C; PKC, protein kinase C; TCR, T-cell receptor. (From Pattison *et al.*, 1997, with permission.)

well as expression of antiapoptotic proteins. Cyclosporine forms a complex with cyclophilin, a cytoplasmic receptor protein present in target cells. This complex binds to calcineurin, inhibiting Ca^{2+}-stimulated dephosphorylation of the cytosolic component of NFAT (Schreiber and Crabtree, 1992). When the cytoplasmic component of NFAT is dephosphorylated, it translocates to the nucleus, where it complexes with nuclear components required for completeT-cell activation, including transactivation of IL-2 and other lymphokine genes. Calcineurin enzymatic activity is inhibited following physical interaction with the cyclosporine/cyclophilin complex. This results in the blockade of NFAT dephosphorylation; thus, the cytoplasmic component of

NFAT does not enter the nucleus, gene transcription is not activated, and the T lymphocyte fails to respond to specific antigenic stimulation. Cyclosporine also increases expression of transforming growth factor β (TGF-β), a potent inhibitor of IL-2-stimulated T-cell proliferation and generation of cytotoxic T lymphocytes (CTL) (Khanna *et al.,* 1994).

Disposition and Pharmacokinetics. Cyclosporine can be administered intravenously or orally. The intravenous preparation (SANDIMMUNE Injection) is provided as a solution in an ethanol-polyoxyethylated castor oil vehicle which must be further diluted in 0.9% sodium chloride solution or 5% dextrose solution before injection. The oral dosage forms include soft gelatin capsules and oral solutions. Cyclosporine supplied in the original soft gelatin capsule is absorbed slowly with 20% to 50% bioavailability. A modified microemulsion formulation (NEORAL) was developed to improve absorption and was approved by the FDA for use in the United States in 1995 (Noble and Markham, 1995). It has more uniform and slightly increased bioavailability compared to SANDIMMUNE and is provided as 25-mg and 100-mg soft gelatin capsules and a 100-mg/ml oral solution. Since SANDIMMUNE and NEORAL are not bioequivalent, they cannot be used interchangeably without supervision by a physician and monitoring of drug concentration in plasma. Comparison of blood concentrations in published literature and in clinical practice must be performed with a detailed knowledge of the assay system employed. Although generic cyclosporine formulations have become available (Halloran, 1997), the most carefully studied generic product recently was withdrawn from the United States market by the FDA because of questions raised about bioequivalence.

As described above, absorption of cyclosporine is incomplete following oral administration. The extent of absorption depends upon several variables, including the individual patient and formulation used. The elimination of cyclosporine from the blood is generally biphasic, with a terminal half-life of 5 to 18 hours (Faulds et al., 1993; Noble and Markham, 1995). After intravenous infusion, clearance is approximately 5 to 7 ml/min per kg in adult recipients of renal transplants, but results differ by age and patient populations. For example, clearance is slower in cardiac transplant patients and more rapid in children. The relationship between administered dose and the area under the plasma concentration–versus-time curve (AUC; see Chapter 1) is linear within the therapeutic range, but the intersubject variability is so large that individual monitoring is required (Faulds et al., 1993; Noble and Markham, 1995).

Following oral administration of cyclosporine (as NEORAL), the time to peak blood concentrations is 1.5 to 2.0 hours (Faulds et al., 1993; Noble and Markham, 1995). Administration with food both delays and decreases absorption. High- and low-fat meals consumed within 30 minutes of administration decrease the AUC by approximately 13% and the maximum concentration by 33%. This makes it imperative to individualize dosage regimens for outpatients.

Cyclosporine is distributed extensively outside the vascular compartment. After intravenous dosing, the steady-state volume of distribution has been reported to be as high as 3 to 5 liters/kg in solid-organ transplant recipients.

Only 0.1% of cyclosporine is excreted unchanged in urine (Faulds et al., 1993). Cyclosporine is extensively metabolized in the liver by the cytochrome-P450 3A (CYP3A) enzyme system and to a lesser degree by the gastrointestinal tract and kidneys (Fahr, 1993). At least 25 metabolites have been identified in human bile, feces, blood, and urine (Christians and Sewing, 1993). Although the cyclic peptide structure of cyclosporine is relatively resistant to metabolism, the side chains are extensively metabolized. All of the metabolites have both reduced biological activity and toxicity compared to the parent drug. Cyclosporine and its metabolites are excreted principally through the bile into the feces, with only approximately 6% being excreted in the urine. Cyclosporine also is excreted in human milk. In the presence of hepatic dysfunction, dosage adjustments are required. No adjustments generally are necessary for dialysis or renal failure patients.

Therapeutic Uses. Clinical indications for cyclosporine are kidney, liver, heart, and other organ transplantation; rheumatoid arthritis; and psoriasis (Faulds et al., 1993). Its use in dermatology is discussed in Chapter 65. Cyclosporine generally is recognized as the agent that ushered in the modern era of organ transplantation, increasing the rates of early engraftment, extending graft survival for kidneys, and making cardiac and liver transplantation possible. Cyclosporine usually is used in combination with other agents, especially glucocorticoids and either azathioprine or mycophenolate mofetil and, most recently, sirolimus. The dosage of cyclosporine used is quite variable, depending upon the organ transplanted and the other drugs used in the specific treatment protocol(s). The initial dose generally is not given pretransplant because of the concern about neurotoxicity. Especially for renal transplant patients, therapeutic algorithms have been developed to delay cyclosporine introduction until a threshold renal function has been attained. The amount of the initial dose and reduction to maintenance dosing is sufficiently variable that no specific recommendation is provided here. Dosage is guided by signs of rejection (too low a dose), renal or other toxicity (too high a dose), and close monitoring of blood levels. Great care must be taken to differentiate renal toxicity from rejection in kidney transplant patients. Because adverse reactions have been ascribed frequently to the intravenous formulation, this route of administration is discontinued as soon as the patient is able to take an oral form of the drug.

In rheumatoid arthritis, cyclosporine is used in cases of severe disease that have not responded to *methotrexate.*

Cyclosporine can be used in combination with methotrexate, but the levels of both drugs must be monitored closely (Baraldo *et al.*, 1999). In psoriasis, cyclosporine is indicated for treatment of adult nonimmunocompromised patients with severe and disabling disease who have failed other systemic therapies (Linden and Weinstein, 1999). Because of its mechanism of action, there is a theoretical basis for the use of cyclosporine in a variety of other T cell–mediated diseases (Faulds *et al.*, 1993). Cyclosporine has been reported to be effective in Behçet's acute ocular syndrome, endogenous uveitis, atopic dermatitis, inflammatory bowel disease, and nephrotic syndrome when standard therapies have failed.

Toxicity. The principal adverse reactions to cyclosporine therapy are renal dysfunction, tremor, hirsutism, hypertension, hyperlipidemia, and gum hyperplasia (Burke *et al.*, 1994). Nephrotoxicity is limiting and occurs in the majority of patients treated. It is the major indication for cessation or modification of therapy. Hypertension may occur in approximately 50% of renal transplant and almost all cardiac transplant patients. Combined use of calcineurin inhibitors and glucocorticoids is particularly diabetogenic, with diabetes being more frequent in patients treated with tacrolimus than in those receiving cyclosporine.

Drug Interactions. Cyclosporine interacts with a wide variety of commonly used drugs, and close attention must be paid to drug interactions. Any drug that affects microsomal enzymes, especially the CYP3A system, may affect cyclosporine blood concentrations (Faulds *et al.*, 1993). Substances that inhibit this enzyme can decrease cyclosporine metabolism and increase blood concentrations. These include calcium channel blockers (*e.g.*, verapamil, nicardipine), antifungal agents (*e.g.*, fluconazole, ketoconazole), antibiotics (*e.g.*, erythromycin), glucocorticoids (*e.g.*, methylprednisolone), HIV-protease inhibitors (*e.g.*, indinavir), and other drugs (*e.g.*, allopurinol and metoclopramide). In addition, grapefruit and grapefruit juice block the CYP3A system and increase cyclosporine blood concentrations and thus should be avoided by patients receiving the drug. In contrast, drugs that induce CYP3A activity can increase cyclosporine metabolism and decrease blood concentrations. Drugs that can decrease cyclosporine concentrations in this manner include antibiotics (*e.g.*, nafcillin and rifampin), anticonvulsants (*e.g.*, phenobarbital, phenytoin), and other drugs (*e.g.*, octreotide, ticlopidine). In general, close monitoring of cyclosporine blood levels and the levels of other drugs is required when such combinations are used.

Interactions between cyclosporine and sirolimus have led to the recommendation that administration of the two drugs be separated by time. Sirolimus aggravates cyclosporine-induced renal dysfunction, while cyclosporine increases sirolimus-induced hyperlipemia and myelosuppression. Other cyclosporine–drug interactions of concern include additive nephrotoxicity when coadministered with nonsteroidal antiinflammatory drugs and other drugs that cause renal dysfunction; elevation in methotrexate levels when the two drugs are coadministered; and reduced clearance of other drugs, including prednisolone, digoxin, and lovastatin.

Tacrolimus. *Tacrolimus* (PROGRAF, FK506) is a macrolide antibiotic produced by *Streptomyces tsukubaensis* (Goto *et al.*, 1987). Its formula is shown in Figure 53–1.

Mechanism of Action. Like cyclosporine, tacrolimus inhibits T-cell activation by inhibiting calcineurin (Schreiber and Crabtree, 1992). Tacrolimus binds to an intracellular protein, FK506-binding protein–12 (FKBP-12), an immunophilin structurally related to cyclophilin. A complex of tacrolimus-FKBP-12, calcium, calmodulin, and calcineurin then forms, and calcineurin phosphatase activity is inhibited. As described for cyclosporine and depicted in Figure 53–2, the inhibition of phosphatase activity prevents dephosphorylation and nuclear translocation of NFAT and leads to inhibition of T-cell activation. Thus, although the intracellular receptors differ, cyclosporine and tacrolimus appear to share a single common pathway for immunosuppression (Plosker and Foster, 2000).

Disposition and Pharmacokinetics. Tacrolimus is available for oral administration as capsules (0.5, 1, and 5 mg) and a sterile solution for injection (5 mg/ml). Immunosuppressive activity resides primarily in the parent drug. Because of intersubject variability in pharmacokinetics, individualization of dosing is required for optimal therapy (Fung and Starzl, 1995). Whole blood, rather than plasma, is the most appropriate sampling compartment to describe tacrolimus pharmacokinetics. Gastrointestinal absorption is incomplete and variable. Food decreases both the rate and extent of absorption. Plasma protein binding of tacrolimus is 75% to 99%, involving primarily albumin and α_1-acid glycoprotein. Its half-life is about 12 hours. Tacrolimus is extensively metabolized in the liver by CYP3A, and at least some of the metabolites are active. The bulk of excretion of parent drug and metabolites is in the feces. Less than 1% of administered tacrolimus is excreted unchanged in the urine.

Therapeutic Uses. Tacrolimus is indicated for the prophylaxis of solid-organ allograft rejection in a manner similar to cyclosporine and as rescue therapy in patients with rejection episodes despite "therapeutic" levels of cyclosporine (Mayer *et al.*, 1997; The U.S. Multicenter FK506 Liver Study Group, 1994). The recommended starting dose for tacrolimus injection is 0.03 to 0.05 mg/kg per day as a continuous infusion. Recommended initial oral doses are 0.2 mg/kg per day for adult kidney transplant patients, 0.1 to 0.15 mg/kg per day for adult liver transplant patients, and 0.15 to 0.2 mg/kg per day for pediatric liver transplant patients in two divided doses 12 hours apart. These dosages are intended to achieve typical blood trough levels in the 5- to 20-ng/ml range. Pediatric patients generally require higher doses than do adults (Shapiro, 1998).

Toxicity. Nephrotoxicity, neurotoxicity (tremor, headache, motor disturbances, seizures), gastrointestinal complaints, hypertension, hyperkalemia, hyperglycemia, and diabetes are associated with tacrolimus use (Plosker and Foster, 2000). As with cyclosporine, nephrotoxicity is limiting (Mihatsch *et al.,* 1998; Henry, 1999). Tacrolimus has a negative effect on the pancreatic islet beta cell, and both glucose intolerance and diabetes mellitus are well-recognized complications of tacrolimus-based immuno-suppression among adult solid-organ transplant recipients. As with other immunosuppressive agents, there is an increased risk of secondary tumors and opportunistic infections.

Drug Interactions. Because of its potential for nephro-toxicity, blood levels of tacrolimus and renal function should be monitored closely, especially when tacrolimus is used with other potentially nephrotoxic drugs. Coadminis-tration with cyclosporine results in additive or synergistic nephrotoxicity; therefore, a delay of at least 24 hours is required when switching a patient from cyclosporine to tacrolimus. Since tacrolimus is metabolized mainly by CYP3A, the potential interactions described for cyclospor-ine (above) apply for tacrolimus as well (Venkataramanan *et al.,* 1995; Yoshimura *et al.,* 1999).

Antiproliferative and Antimetabolic Drugs

Sirolimus. Sirolimus (rapamycin; RAPAMUNE) is a macro-cyclic lactone produced by *Streptomyces hygroscopicus* (Vezina, *et al.,* 1975). Its structure is shown in Figure 53–1.

Mechanism of Action. Sirolimus inhibits T-lymphocyte ac-tivation and proliferation downstream of the IL-2 and other T-cell growth factor receptors (Figure 53–2) (Kuo *et al.,* 1992). Sirolimus, like cyclosporine and tacrolimus, is a drug whose therapeutic action requires formation of a complex with the im-munophilin, FKBP-12. However, the sirolimus-FKBP-12 com-plex does not affect calcineurin activity, but binds to and inhibits the mammalian kinase, target of rapamycin (mTOR), which is a key enzyme in cell-cycle progression (Brown *et al.,* 1994). Inhi-bition of this kinase blocks cell cycle progression at the $G_1 \rightarrow S$ phase transition. In animal models, sirolimus not only inhibits transplant rejection, graft-*versus*-host disease, and a variety of autoimmune diseases, but its effect also lasts several months

after discontinuing therapy, suggesting a tolerizing effect (*see* "Tolerance," below) (Groth *et al.,* 1999).

Disposition and Pharmacokinetics. Following oral ad-ministration, sirolimus is absorbed rapidly and reaches a peak blood concentration within about 1 hour after a sin-gle dose in healthy subjects and within about 2 hours after multiple oral doses in renal transplant patients (Napoli and Kahan, 1996; Zimmerman and Kahan, 1997). Systemic availability is approximately 15%, and blood concentra-tions are proportional to dose between 3 and 12 mg/m². A high-fat meal decreases peak blood concentration by 34%; sirolimus therefore should be taken consistently ei-ther with or without food, and blood levels should be monitored closely. About 40% of sirolimus in plasma is bound to protein, especially albumin. The drug partitions into formed elements of blood, with a blood-to-plasma ratio of 38 in renal transplant patients. Sirolimus is ex-tensively metabolized by CYP3A4 and is transported by P-glycoprotein. Seven major metabolites have been iden-tified in whole blood (Salm *et al.,* 1999). Metabolites also are detectable in feces and urine, with the bulk of total excretion being in feces. Although some of its metabo-lites are active, sirolimus *per se* is the major component in whole blood and contributes greater than 90% of the immunosuppressive effect. The blood half-life after mul-tiple dosing in stable renal transplant patients is 62 hours (Napoli and Kahan, 1996; Zimmerman and Kahan, 1997). A loading dose of three times the maintenance dose will provide nearly steady-state concentrations within one day in most patients.

Therapeutic Uses. Sirolimus is indicated for prophylaxis of organ transplant rejection in combination therapy with a calcineurin inhibitor and glucocorticoids (Kahan *et al.,* 1999a). In patients experiencing or at high risk for cal-cineurin inhibitor–associated nephrotoxicity, sirolimus has been used with glucocorticoids and mycophenolate mofetil to avoid permanent renal damage. The initial dosage in pa-tients 13 years or older who weigh less than 40 kg should be adjusted based on body surface area (1 mg/m² per day) with a loading dose of 3 mg/m². Data regarding doses for pediatric and geriatric patients are lacking at this time (Kahan, 1999). It is recommended that the maintenance dose be reduced by approximately one-third in patients with hepatic impairment (Watson *et al.,* 1999).

Toxicity. The use of sirolimus in renal transplant patients is associated with a dose-dependent increase in serum cholesterol and triglycerides that may require treatment (Murgia *et al.,* 1996). While immunotherapy with sirolimus *per se* is not nephrotoxic, patients treated with cyclosporine plus sirolimus have impaired renal function compared to patients treated with cyclosporine and either azathioprine or placebo. Renal function therefore must be monitored closely in such patients. Lymphocoele, a known surgical complication associated with renal transplantation, has occurred significantly more often in a dose-dependent fashion in sirolimus-treated patients, requiring close postoperative follow-up. Other adverse effects include anemia, leukopenia, thrombocytopenia (Hong and Kahan, 2000b), hypokalemia or hyperkalemia, fever, and gastrointestinal effects. As with other immunosuppressive agents, there is an increased risk of neoplasms, especially lymphomas, and infections. Prophylaxis for *Pneumocystis carinii* pneumonia and cytomegalovirus is recommended (Groth *et al.,* 1999).

Drug Interactions. Since sirolimus is a substrate for cytochrome CYP3A4 and is transported by P-glycoprotein, close attention to interactions with other drugs that are metabolized or transported by these proteins is required (Yoshimura *et al.,* 1999). As noted above, cyclosporine and sirolimus interact, and their administration should be separated by time. Dose adjustment may be required with coadministration of sirolimus with cyclosporine, diltiazem, or rifampin. No dosage adjustment appears to be required when sirolimus is coadministered with acyclovir, digoxin, glyburide, nifedipine, norgestrel/ethinyl estadiol, prednisolone, or sulfamethoxazole/trimethoprim. This list is incomplete, and blood levels and potential drug interactions must be monitored closely.

Azathioprine. *Azathioprine* (IMURAN) is a purine antimetabolite (Elion, 1993). It is an imidazolyl derivative of 6-mercaptopurine (Figure 53–1).

Mechanism of Action. Following exposure to nucleophiles, such as glutathione, azathioprine is cleaved to 6-mercaptopurine, which, in turn, is converted to additional metabolites that inhibit *de novo* purine synthesis (Bertino, 1973). 6-Thio-IMP, a fraudulent nucleotide, is converted to 6-thio-GMP and finally to 6-thio-GTP, which is incorporated into DNA and gene translation is inhibited (Chan *et al.,* 1987). Cell proliferation is prevented, inhibiting a variety of lymphocyte functions. Azathioprine appears to be a more potent immunosuppressive agent than does 6-mercaptopurine itself, which may reflect differences in drug uptake or pharmacokinetic differences in the resulting metabolites.

Disposition and Pharmacokinetics. Azathioprine is well absorbed orally and reaches maximum blood levels within 1 to 2 hours after administration. The half-life of azathioprine itself is about 10 minutes, and that of mercaptopurine is about an hour. Other metabolites have half-lives of up to 5 hours. Blood levels have little predictive value because of extensive metabolism, significant activity of

many different metabolites, and high tissue levels attained. Azathioprine and mercaptopurine are moderately bound to plasma proteins and are partially dialyzable. Both azathioprine and mercaptopurine are rapidly removed from the blood by oxidation or methylation in the liver and/or erythrocytes. Renal clearance is of little impact in biological effectiveness or toxicity, but dose reduction is practiced in patients with renal failure.

Therapeutic Uses. Azathioprine was first introduced as an immunosuppressive agent in 1961, helping to make allogeneic kidney transplantation possible (Murray *et al.,* 1963). It is indicated as an adjunct for prevention of organ transplant rejection and in severe rheumatoid arthritis (Hong and Kahan, 2000a; Gaffney and Scott, 1998). Although the dose of azathioprine required to prevent organ rejection and minimize toxicity varies among patients, 3 to 5 mg/kg per day is the usual starting dose. Lower initial doses (1 mg/kg per day) are used in treating rheumatoid arthritis. Complete blood count and liver function tests should be monitored.

Toxicity. The major side effect of azathioprine is bone marrow suppression with leukopenia (common), thrombocytopenia (less common), and/or anemia (uncommon). Other important adverse effects include increased susceptibility to infections (especially varicella and herpes simplex viruses), hepatotoxicity, alopecia, gastrointestinal toxicity, pancreatitis, and increased risk of neoplasia.

Drug Interactions. Xanthine oxidase, an enzyme of major importance in the catabolism of metabolites of azathioprine, is blocked by allopurinol (Venkat Raman, *et al.,* 1990). If azathioprine and allopurinol are used in the same patient, the azathioprine dose must be decreased to 25% to 33% of the usual dose, but it is best not to use these two drugs together. Adverse effects resulting from coadministration of azathioprine with other myelosuppressive agents or angiotensin converting enzyme inhibitors include leukopenia, thrombocytopenia, and/or anemia as a result of myelosuppression.

Mycophenolate Mofetil. *Mycophenolate mofetil* (CELLCEPT) is the 2-morpholinoethyl ester of mycophenolic acid (MPA) (Allison and Eugui, 1993). Its structure is shown in Figure 53–1.

Mechanism of Action. Mycophenolate mofetil is a prodrug that is rapidly hydrolyzed to the active drug, mycophenolic acid (MPA), a selective, uncompetitive and reversible inhibitor of inosine monophosphate dehydrogenase (IMPDH) (Natsumeda and Carr, 1993), an important enzyme in the *de novo* pathway of guanine nucleotide synthesis. B and T lymphocytes are highly dependent on this pathway for cell proliferation, while other cell types can use salvage pathways; MPA therefore selectively inhibits lymphocyte proliferation and functions, including antibody formation, cellular adhesion, and migration. The effects of MPA on lymphocytes can be reversed by adding guanosine or deoxyguanosine to the cells.

Disposition and Pharmacokinetics. Mycophenolate mofetil undergoes rapid and complete metabolism to MPA after oral or intravenous administration. MPA, in turn, is metabolized to the inactive phenolic glucuronide, MPAG. The parent drug is cleared from the blood within a few minutes. The half-life of MPA is about 16 hours. Negligible amounts (<1%) of MPA are excreted in the urine (Bardsley-Elliot *et al.,* 1999). Most (87%) is excreted in the urine as MPAG. Plasma concentrations of both MPA and MPAG are increased in patients with renal insufficiency. In early renal transplant patients (<40 days posttransplant), plasma concentrations of MPA after a single dose of mycophenolate mofetil are about half of those found in healthy volunteers or stable renal transplant patients. Studies in the pediatric population are limited; safety and effectiveness in this population have not been established (Butani *et al.,* 1999).

Therapeutic Uses. Mycophenolate mofetil is indicated for prophylaxis of transplant rejection and is typically used in combination with glucocorticoids and a calcineurin inhibitor, but not with azathioprine (Kimball *et al.,* 1995; Ahsan *et al.,* 1999; Kreis *et al.,* 2000). Combined treatment with sirolimus is possible, although potential drug interactions necessitate careful monitoring of drug levels. For renal transplants, 1 g is administered orally or intravenously (over 2 hours) twice per day (2 g per day). A higher dose, 1.5 g twice per day (3 g per day), is recommended for African-American renal transplant patients and all cardiac transplant patients. Use of mycophenolate mofetil in other clinical settings is under investigation.

Toxicity. The principal toxicities of mycophenolate mofetil are gastrointestinal and hematologic (Fulton and Markham, 1996; Bardsley-Elliot *et al.,* 1999). These include leukopenia, diarrhea, and vomiting. There also is an increased incidence of some infections, especially sepsis associated with cytomegalovirus.

Drug Interactions. Potential drug interactions between mycophenolate mofetil and several other drugs commonly used by transplant patients have been studied (Bardsley-Elliot *et al.,* 1999). There appear to be no untoward effects produced by combination therapy with cyclosporine, sulfamethoxazole/trimethoprim, or oral contraceptives. Mycophenolate mofetil has not been tested with azathioprine. Coadministration with antacids containing aluminum or magnesium hydroxide leads to decreased absorption of mycophenolate mofetil; thus, these drugs should not be administered simultaneously. Mycophenolate mofetil should not be administered with cholestyramine or other drugs that affect enterohepatic circulation. Such agents decrease plasma MPA concentrations, probably by binding free MPA in the intestines. Acyclovir and gancyclovir may compete with MPAG for tubular secretion, possibly resulting in increased concentrations of both MPAG and the antiviral agents in the blood. This effect may be compounded in patients with renal insufficiency.

Other Antiproliferative and Cytotoxic Agents. Many of the cytotoxic and antimetabolic agents used in cancer chemotherapy (*see* Chapter 52) are immunosuppressive due to their action on lymphocytes and other cells of the immune system. Other cytotoxic drugs that have been used as immunosuppressive agents include *methotrexate, cyclophosphamide* (CYTOXAN), *thalidomide,* and *chlorambucil* (LEUKERAN). Methotrexate is used for treatment of graft-*versus*-host disease, rheumatoid arthritis, and psoriasis as well as in anticancer thereapy (*see* Chapter 52) (Grosflam and Weinblatt, 1991). Cyclophosphamide and chlorambucil are used in treating childhood nephrotic syndrome (Neuhaus *et al.,* 1994) as well as in treating of a variety of malignancies (*see* Chapter 52). Cyclophosphamide also is widely used for treatment of severe systemic lupus erythematosus (Valeri *et al.,* 1994). *Leflunomide* (ARAVA) is a pyrimidine-synthesis inhibitor indicated for the treatment of adults with rheumatoid arthritis (Prakash and Jarvis, 1999). The drug inhibits dihydroorotate dehydrogenase in the *de novo* pathway of pyrimidine synthesis. It is hepatotoxic and can cause fetal injury when administered to pregnant women.

Antibodies

Both polyclonal and monoclonal antibodies against lymphocyte cell-surface antigens are widely used for prevention and treatment of organ transplant rejection. Polyclonal antisera are generated by repeated injections of human thymocytes (antithymocyte globulin, ATG) or lymphocytes (antilymphocyte globulin, ALS) into animals such as horses, rabbits, sheep, or goats and then purifying the serum immunoglobulin fraction (Mannick *et al.,* 1971). Although highly effective immunosuppressive agents, these preparations vary in efficacy and toxicity from batch to batch. The advent of hybridoma technology to produce monoclonal antibodies was a major advance in immunology (Kohler and Milstein, 1975). It is now possible to make essentially unlimited amounts of a single antibody of a defined specificity (Figure 53–3). These monoclonal reagents have overcome the problems of variability in

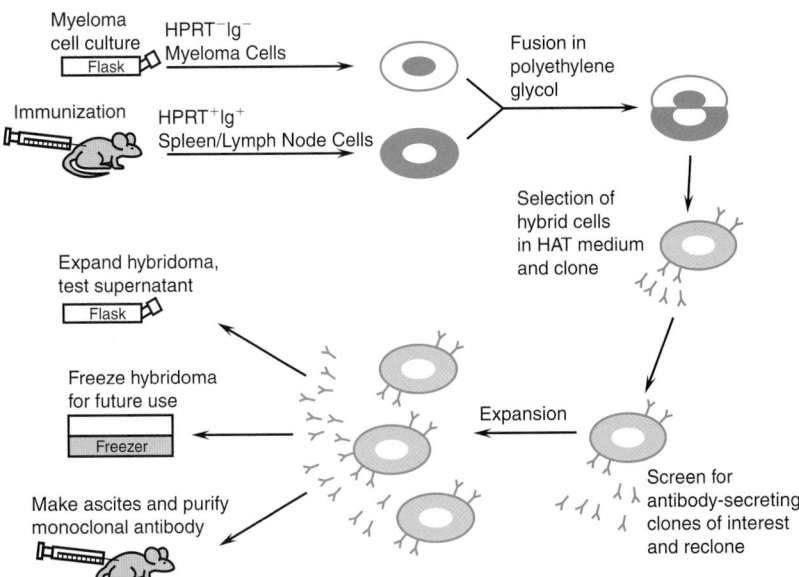

Figure 53–3. Generation of monoclonal antibodies.

Mice are immunized with the selected antigen, and spleen or lymph node is harvested and B cells separated. These B cells are fused to a suitable B-cell myeloma that has been selected for its inability to grow in medium supplemented with hypoxanthine, aminopterin, and thymidine (HAT). Only myelomas that fuse with B cells can survive in HAT-supplemented medium. The hybridomas expand in culture. Those of interest based upon a specific screening technique are then selected and cloned by limiting dilution. Monoclonal antibodies can be used directly as supernatants or ascites fluid experimentally but are purified for clinical use. HPRT, hypoxanthine-guanine phosphoribosyl transferase. (From Krensky, A.M., 1999, with permission.)

efficacy and toxicity seen with the polyclonal products, but they are more limited in their target specificity. Thus, both polyclonal and monoclonal products have a place in immunosuppressive therapy.

Antithymocyte Globulin. *Antithymocyte globulin* (THY-MOGLOBULIN) is a purified gamma globulin from the serum of rabbits immunized with human thymocytes (Regan *et al.,* 1999). It is provided as a sterile, freeze-dried product for intravenous administration after reconstitution with sterile water.

Mechanism of Action. Antithymocyte globulin contains cytotoxic antibodies that bind to CD2, CD3, CD4, CD8, CD11a, CD18, CD25, CD44, CD45, and HLA class I and II molecules on the surface of human T lymphocytes (Bourdage and Hamlin, 1995). The antibodies deplete circulating lymphocytes by direct cytotoxicity (both complement and cell-mediated) and block lymphocyte function by binding to cell surface molecules involved in the regulation of cell function.

Therapeutic Uses. Antithymocyte globulin is indicated for induction immunosuppression and the treatment of acute renal transplant rejection in combination with other immunosuppressive agents (Mariat *et al.,* 1998). Because it is a highly effective immunosuppressant, a course of antithymocyte-globulin treatment often is given to renal transplant patients with delayed graft function to allow withdrawal of nephrotoxic calcineurin inhibitors and thereby aid in recovery from ischemic reperfusion injury. The recommended dose for acute rejection of renal grafts is 1.5 mg/kg per day (over 4 to 6 hours) for 7 to 14 days.

Mean T-cell counts fall by day 2 of therapy. It also is used for acute rejection of other types of organ transplants and for prophylaxis of rejection (Wall, 1999). Studies to examine its use as induction therapy at the time of transplantation are in progress (Szczech and Feldman, 1999).
Toxicity. The major side effects are fever and chills with the potential for hypotension. Premedication with corticosteroids, acetaminophen, and/or an antihistamine and administration of the antiserum by slow infusion (over 4 to 6 hours) into a large-diameter vessel minimize such reactions. Outright serum sickness and glomerulonephritis can occur; anaphylaxis is a rare event. Hematologic complications include leukopenia and thrombocytopenia. As with other immunosuppressive agents, there is an increased risk of infection and malignancy, especially when multiple immunosuppressive agents are used in combination. No drug interactions have been described, but antiantibodies develop, limiting repeated use of this or any other rabbit antibody preparations. As an example, in one trial, 68% of patients developed antirabbit antibodies.

Monoclonal Antibodies. *Anti-CD3 Monoclonal Antibodies.* Antibodies directed at the CD3 antigen on the surface of human T lymphocytes have been used since the early 1980s in human transplantation and have proven to be extremely effective immunosuppressive agents. The original mouse IgG$_{2a}$ antihuman CD3 monoclonal antibody, *muromonab-CD3* (OKT3, ORTHOCLONE OKT3), is still used to reverse corticosteroid-resistant rejection episodes (Cosimi, *et al.,* 1981).

Mechanism of Action. Muromonab-CD3 binds to CD3, a monomorphic component of the T-cell receptor complex involved in antigen recognition, cell signaling, and proliferation (Hooks *et al.*, 1991). Antibody treatment induces rapid internalization of the T-cell receptor, thereby preventing subsequent recognition of antigen. Administration of the antibody is followed rapidly by depletion and extravasation of a majority of T cells from the bloodstream and the peripheral lymphoid organs such as lymph nodes and spleen. This absence of detectable T cells from the usual lymphoid regions is secondary both to cell death following complement activation and activation-induced cell death and to margination of T cells onto vascular endothelial walls and redistribution of T cells to nonlymphoid organs such as the lungs. Muromonab-CD3 also induces a reduction in function of the remaining T cells, as defined by lack of IL-2 production and great reduction in the production of multiple cytokines, perhaps with the exception of IL-4 and IL-10.

Therapeutic Uses. Muromonab-CD3 is indicated for treatment of acute organ transplant rejection (Ortho Multicenter Transplant Group, 1985; Woodle *et al.*, 1999; Rostaing *et al.*, 1999). Muromonab-CD3 is provided as a sterile solution containing 5 mg per ampule. The recommended dose is 5 mg/day (in adults; less for children) in a single intravenous bolus (less than one minute) for 10 to 14 days. Antibody levels increase over the first three days and then level off. Circulating T cells disappear from the blood within minutes of administration and return within approximately one week after termination of therapy. Repeated use of muromonab-CD3 results in the immunization of the patient against the mouse determinants of the antibody, which can neutralize and prevent its immunosuppressive efficacy (Jaffers *et al.*, 1983). Thus, repeated treatment with the muromonab-CD3 or other mouse monoclonal antibodies is contraindicated in many patients.

Toxicity. The major side effect of anti-CD3 therapy is the "cytokine release syndrome" (Wilde and Goa, 1996; Ortho Multicenter Transplant Study Group, 1985). Administration of glucocorticoids prior to the injection of muromonab-CD3 prevents the release of cytokines and reduces first-dose reactions considerably and is now a standard procedure. Antibody binding to the T-cell receptor complex combined with Fc receptor (FcR)–mediated crosslinking is the basis for the initial activating properties of this agent. The syndrome typically begins 30 minutes after infusion of the antibody (but can occur later) and may persist for hours. The symptomatology usually is worst with the first dose; both the frequency and severity decrease with subsequent doses. Common clinical manifestations include high fever, chills/rigor, headache, tremor, nausea/vomiting, diarrhea, abdominal pain, malaise, muscle/joint aches and pains, and generalized weakness. Less common complaints include skin reactions and cardiorespiratory and central nervous system (CNS) disorders,

including aseptic meningitis. Potentially fatal, severe pulmonary edema, adult respiratory distress syndrome, cardiovascular collapse, cardiac arrest, and arrhythmias have been described. The syndrome is associated with and attributed to increased serum levels of cytokines [including tumor necrosis factor (TNF)-α, IL-2, IL-6, and interferon gamma], which are released by activated T cells and/or monocytes. In several studies, the production of the TNF-α cytokine has been shown to be the major cause of the toxicity (Herbelin *et al.*, 1995). Fluid status of patients must be monitored carefully before therapy; steroids and other premedications should be given, and a fully competent resuscitation facility must be immediately available for patients receiving their first several doses of this therapy. Other toxicities associated with anti-CD3 therapy include anaphylaxis and the usual infections and neoplasms associated with immunosuppressive therapy. A high rate of "rebound" rejection has been observed when muromonab-CD3 treatment is stopped (Wilde and Goa, 1996).

New-Generation Anti-CD3 Antibodies. Recently, genetically altered anti-CD3 monoclonal antibodies have been developed that are "humanized" to minimize the occurrence of anti-antibody responses and mutated to prevent binding to FcRs (Friend *et al.*, 1999). The rationale for developing this new generation of anti-CD3 monoclonal antibodies is that they could induce selective immunomodulation in the absence of toxicity associated with conventional anti-CD3 monoclonal antibody therapy. In initial clinical trials, a humanized anti-CD3 monoclonal antibody that does not bind to FcRs reversed acute renal allograft rejection in the absence of the first-dose cytokine-release syndrome (Woodle *et al.*, 1999). Clinical efficacy of these agents in autoimmune diseases is being evaluated.

Anti-IL-2 Receptor (Anti-CD25) Antibodies. *Daclizumab* (ZENAPAX), a humanized murine complementarity-determining region (CDR)/human IgG₁ chimeric monoclonal antibody, and *basiliximab* (SIMULECT), a murine-human chimeric monoclonal antibody, have been produced by recombinant DNA technology (Wiseman and Faulds, 1999). The composite daclizumab antibody consists of human (90%) constant domains of IgG₁ and variable framework regions of the Eu myeloma antibody and murine (10%) CDR of the anti-Tac antibody.

Mechanism of Action. The antibodies bind with high affinity to the alpha subunit of the IL-2 receptor (p55 alpha, CD25) present on the surface of activated, but not resting, T lymphocytes and block IL-2–mediated T-cell activation events. Daclizumab has a somewhat lower affinity than does basiliximab.

Therapeutic Uses. Anti–IL-2-receptor monoclonal antibodies are recommended for prophylaxis of acute organ rejection in adult patients as part of combination therapy (with glucocorticoids, a calcineurin inhibitor, with or without azathioprine or mycophenolate mofetil) (Kovarik *et al.*, 1999; Hong and Kahan, 1999; Kahan *et al.*, 1999b; Hirose *et al.*, 2000). Daclizumab and basiliximab are supplied as sterile concentrates that are diluted before intravenous administration. Renal transplant patients receiving 1 mg/kg of daclizumab intravenously every 14 days for 5 doses have saturating blockade of the IL-2 receptor for 120 days posttransplant (Vincenti *et al.*, 1998). No significant change in circulating lymphocyte markers has been observed. Basiliximab is given for only two doses of 20 mg each, the first two hours before surgery and the second four days after.

Toxicity. No cytokine-release syndrome has been observed with these antibodies. Anaphylactic reactions can occur. Although lymphoproliferative disorders and opportunistic infections may occur, as with other immunosuppressive agents, the incidence ascribed to anti-CD25 treatment appears remarkably low. No significant drug interactions with anti–IL-2-receptor antibodies have been described (Hong and Kahan, 1999).

Infliximab. *Infliximab* (REMICADE) is a chimeric anti–TNF-α monoclonal antibody containing a human constant region and a murine variable region. It binds with high affinity to TNF-α and prevents the cytokine from binding to its receptors.

Patients with rheumatoid arthritis have elevated levels of TNF-α in their joints, and patients with Crohn's disease have elevated levels of TNF-α in their stools. A clinical trial has revealed that patients treated with infliximab plus methotrexate have fewer signs and symptoms of rheumatoid arthritis than do patients treated with methotrexate alone. Patients with active Crohn's disease who had not responded to other immunosuppressive therapies have shown improvement when treated with infliximab, and patients with fistulizing Crohn's disease have had fewer draining fistulas after treatment with the antibody. Infliximab is approved in the United States for treating the symptoms of rheumatoid arthritis, in combination with methotrexate, in patients who do not respond to methotrexate alone. Infliximab also is approved for use in the treatment of symptoms of moderately to severely active Crohn's disease in patients who have failed to respond to conventional therapy and in treatment to reduce the number of draining fistulas in Crohn's disease patients (*see* Chapter 39). About 1 of 6 patients receiving infliximab has experienced an infusion reaction within 1 to 2 hours after administration of the antibody. The reaction has included fever, urticaria, hypotension, and dyspnea. Serious infections also have occurred in infliximab-treated patients, most frequently in the upper respiratory and urinary tracts. The development of antinuclear antibodies and, rarely, a lupus-like syndrome have been reported to occur after treatment with infliximab.

A therapeutic agent related to infliximab in its mechanism of action, although not a monoclonal antibody, is *etanercept* (ENBREL), which is a fusion protein containing the ligand-binding portion of a human TNF-α receptor linked to the Fc portion of human IgG$_1$. Like infliximab, etanercept binds to TNF-α and prevents it from interacting with its receptors. It is approved in the United States for treatment of the symptoms of rheumatoid arthritis in patients who have not responded to other treatments. Etanercept can be used in combination with methotrexate in patients who have not responded adequately to methotrexate alone. As with infliximab, serious infections have occurred after treatment with etanercept. Injection-site reactions (erythema, itching, pain, or swelling) have occurred in more than one-third of etanercept-treated patients.

TOLERANCE

Immunosuppression has concomitant risks of opportunistic infections and secondary tumors. Therefore, the ultimate goal of research on organ transplantation and autoimmune diseases is the induction and maintenance of immunologic tolerance, the active state of antigen-specific nonresponsiveness (Krensky and Clayberger, 1994; Hackett and Dickler, 1999). If tolerance can be attained, it would represent a true cure for conditions discussed above without the side effects of the various immunosuppressive therapies discussed. The calcineurin inhibitors prevent tolerance induction in some, but not all, preclinical models (Wood, 1991; Van Parijs and Abbas, 1998). In contrast, in these same model systems, sirolimus does not prevent tolerance and, in fact, in some cases promotes tolerance induction (Li *et al.*, 1998). Several other approaches have exciting promise as well and are being evaluated in clinical trials. Because these approaches are still experimental, they are only briefly discussed here.

Costimulatory Blockade

Induction of specific immune responses by T lymphocytes requires two signals: an antigen-specific signal *via* the T-cell receptor and a costimulatory signal provided by molecules such as CD28 on the T cell interacting with CD80 and CD86 on the antigen-presenting cell (APC) (Figure 53–4) (Khoury *et al.*, 1999). Preclinical studies have shown that inhibition of the costimulatory signal can induce tolerance (Larsen *et al.*, 1996; Kirk *et al.*, 1997). Experimental approaches to inhibition of costimulation include a recombinant fusion protein molecule, CTLA4Ig, and anti-CD80 and/or anti-CD86 monoclonal antibodies. CTLA4Ig

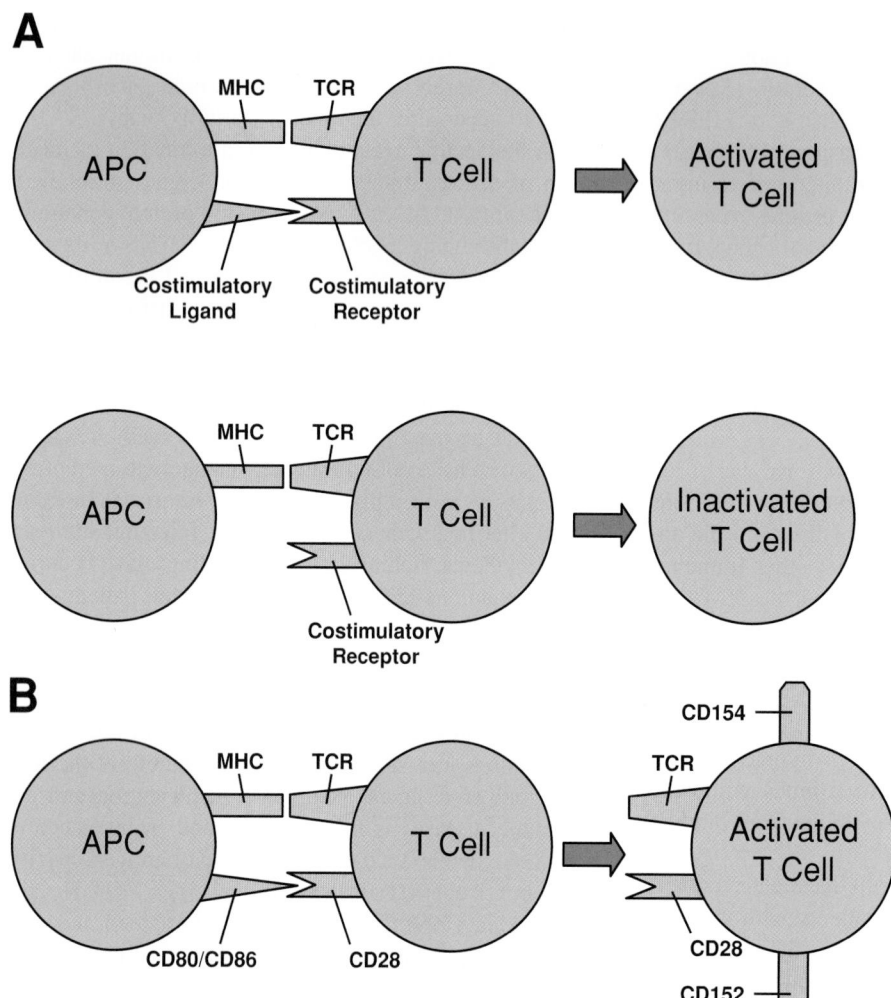

Figure 53–4. Costimulation.

A. Two signals are required for T-cell activation. Signal 1 is *via* the T-cell receptor (TCR) and signal 2 is *via* a costimulatory receptor-ligand pair. Both signals are required for T-cell activation. Signal 1 in the absence of signal 2 results in an inactivated T cell. *B.* One important costimulatory pathway involves CD28 on the T cell and B7-1 (CD80) and B7-2 (CD86) on the antigen-presenting cell (APC). After a T cell is activated, it expresses additional costimulatory molecules. CD152 is CD40 ligand, which interacts with CD40 as a costimulatory pair. CD154 (CTLA4) interacts with CD80 and CD86 to dampen or down-regulate an immune response. Antibodies against CD80, CD86, and CD152 are being evaluated as potential therapeutic agents. CTLA4-Ig, a chimeric protein consisting of part of an immunoglobulin molecule and part of CD154, also has been tested as a therapeutic agent. (From Clayberger *et al.*, 2001, with permission.)

contains the binding region of CTLA4, which is a CD28 homolog, and the constant region of the human IgG$_1$. CTLA4Ig is a competitive inhibitor of CD28. Both CTLA4Ig and a lytic anti-CD80 monoclonal antibody are in clinical trials. A second costimulatory pathway undergoing clinical evaluation involves the interaction of CD40 on activated T cells with CD40 ligand (CD154) on B cells, endothelium, and/or APCs (Figure 53–4). Among the purported activities of anti-CD154 antibody treatment is its blockade of the induced B7 expression following immune activation. At least two anti-CD154 monoclonal antibodies are under clinical evaluation in organ transplantation and autoimmunity. Other antagonists of T-cell costimulation, including anti-CD2, anti-ICAM-1 (CD54) and anti-LFA-1 monoclonal antibodies, have shown promise in preclinical models of tolerance (Salmela *et al.*, 1999).

Donor Cell Chimerism

Another approach with exciting preliminary results is induction of chimerism (coexistence of cells from two genetic lineages in a single individual) by any of a variety of protocols that first dampen or eliminate immune function in the recipient with ionizing radiation, drugs such as cyclophosphamide, and/or antibody treatment and then provide a new source of immune function by adoptive transfer (transfusion) of bone marrow or hematopoietic stem cells (Starzl *et al.*, 1997; Fuchimoto *et al.*, 1999; Spitzer *et al.*, 1999; Hale *et al.*, 2000). Upon reconstitution of immune function, the recipient no longer recognizes new antigens provided during a critical period as "nonself." Such tolerance is long-lived and is less likely to be complicated by the use of calcineurin inhibitors. Although the most promising approaches in this arena have been therapies that promote the development of mixed or macrochimerism, in which substantial numbers of donor cells are present in the circulation, some microchimerization approaches also have shown promise in the development of long-term unresponsiveness.

Soluble HLA

In the precyclosporine era, blood transfusions were shown to be associated with improved outcomes in renal transplant patients (Opelz and Terasaki, 1978). These findings gave rise to donor-specific transfusion protocols that gave improved outcomes (Opelz *et al.*, 1997). After the introduction of cyclosporine, however, these effects of blood transfusions disappeared, presumably due to the efficacy of this drug in blocking T-cell activation. Nevertheless, the existence of a tolerance-promoting effect of transfusions is irrefutable. It is possible that this effect is due to HLA molecules on the surface of cells or in soluble forms. Recently, soluble HLA and peptides corresponding to linear sequences of HLA molecules have been shown to induce immunologic tolerance in animal models *via* a variety of mechanisms (Murphy and Krensky, 1999).

Antigens

Specific antigens provided in a variety of forms, but generally as peptides, induce immunologic tolerance in preclinical models of diabetes, arthritis, and multiple sclerosis. Clinical trials of such approaches are under way. The past decade has seen a revolution in our understanding of the basis for immune tolerance. It is now well established that antigen/MHC complex binding to the T-cell receptor/CD3 complex coupled with soluble and membrane-bound costimulatory signals initiates a cascade of signaling events that lead to productive immunity. In addition, the immune response also is regulated by a number of negative signaling events that control cell survival and expansion. For the first time, *in vitro* and preclinical *in vivo* studies have demonstrated that one can selectively inhibit immune responses to specific antigens without the associated toxicity of current immunosuppressive therapies (Van Parijs and Abbas, 1998). With these new insights comes the enormous promise of specific immune therapies to treat the vast array of immune disorders from autoimmunity to transplant rejection. These new therapies will take advantage of a combination of drugs that target the primary T-cell receptor–mediated signal either by blocking cell-surface receptor interactions or inhibiting early signal transduction events. The drugs will be combined with therapies that effectively block costimulation to prevent cell expansion and differentiation of those cells that have engaged antigen while maintaining a noninflammatory milieu.

IMMUNOSTIMULATION

General Principles

In contrast to immunosuppressive agents that inhibit the immune response in transplant rejection and autoimmunity, a few immunostimulatory drugs have been developed with applicability to infection, immunodeficiency, and cancer. Major problems with such drugs are systemic (generalized) effects at one extreme or limited efficacy at the other.

Immunostimulants

Levamisole. *Levamisole* (ERGAMISOL) was synthesized originally as an antihelminthic but appears to "restore" depressed immune function of B cells, T cells, monocytes, and macrophages. Its only clinical indication is as an adjuvant treatment with fluorouracil after surgical resection in patients with Dukes' stage C colon cancer (Moertel *et al.*, 1990; Figueredo *et al.*, 1997). Its use has been associated with sometimes fatal agranulocytosis.

Thalidomide. *Thalidomide* (THALOMID) is best known for the severe, life-threatening birth defects it has caused when administered to pregnant women (Smithells and Newman, 1992; Lary *et al.*, 1999). For this reason, it is available only under a restricted distribution program and can be prescribed only by specially licensed physicians who understand the risk of teratogenicity if thalidomide is used during pregnancy. **Thalidomide should never be taken by women who are pregnant or who could become pregnant while taking the drug.** Nevertheless, it is indicated for the treatment of patients with erythema nodosum leprosum (ENL) (Sampaio *et al.*, 1993). Its mechanism of action is unclear (Tseng *et al.*, 1996). Reported immunologic effects vary substantially under different conditions. For example, thalidomide has been reported to decrease circulating TNF-α in patients with ENL but to increase it in patients who are HIV-seropositive (Jacobson *et al.*, 1997). Alternatively, it has been suggested that the drug affects angiogenesis (Miller and Stromland, 1999). The anti–TNF-α effect has led to its evaluation as a treatment for severe, refractory rheumatoid arthritis (Keesal *et al.*, 1999).

Bacillus Calmette-Guérin (BCG). Live BCG (TICE BCG, THERACYS) is an attenuated, live culture of the bacillus of Calmette and Guérin strain of *Mycobacterium bovis*. BCG induces a granulomatous reaction at the site of administration. This preparation is active against tumors by unclear mechanisms and is indicated for treatment and prophylaxis of carcinoma *in situ* of the urinary bladder and for prophylaxis of primary and recurrent stage Ta and/or T1 papillary tumors following transurethral resection (Morales *et al.*, 1981; Paterson and Patel, 1998; Patard *et al.*, 1998). Adverse effects include hypersensitivity, shock, chills, fever, malaise, and immune complex disease.

Recombinant Cytokines. *Interferons.* Although interferons (alpha, beta, and gamma) initially were identified by their antiviral activity, these agents have important immunomodulatory activities as well (Johnson *et al.*, 1994; Tilg and Kaser, 1999; Ransohoff, 1998). The interferons bind to specific cell-surface receptors that initiate a series of intracellular events: induction of certain enzymes, inhibition of cell proliferation, and enhancement of immune activities, including increased phagocytosis by macrophages and augmentation of specific cytotoxicity by T lymphocytes (Tompkins, 1999). Recombinant *interferon alfa-2b* (IFN-alpha 2, INTRON A) is obtained from *Escherichia coli* by genetic engineering. It is a member of a family of naturally occurring small proteins with molecular weights of 15,000 to 27,600 daltons, produced and secreted by cells in response to viral infections and other inducers. Interferon alfa-2b is indicated in the treatment of a variety of tumors, including hairy cell leukemia, malignant melanoma, follicular lymphoma, and AIDS-related Kaposi's sarcoma (Punt, 1998; Bukowski, 1999; Sinkovics and Horvath, 2000). It also is indicated for infectious diseases, chronic hepatitis B, and condylomata acuminata. In addition, it is supplied in combination with *ribavirin* (REBETRON) for treatment of chronic hepatitis C in patients with compensated liver function not treated previously with interferon alfa-2b or who have relapsed following interferon alfa-2b therapy (Lo Iacono *et al.,* 2000). Flu-like symptoms, including fever, chills, and headache, are the most common adverse effects seen after interferon alfa-2b administration. Adverse experiences involving the cardiovascular system (hypotension, arrhythmias, and, rarely, cardiomyopathy and myocardial infarction) and CNS (depression, confusion) are among other, less-frequent side effects.

Interferon gamma-1b (ACTIMMUNE) is a recombinant polypeptide that differs from other interferons in causing activation of phagocytes and generation within them of oxygen metabolites that are toxic to a number of microorganisms. It is indicated in reducing the frequency and severity of serious infections associated with chronic granulomatous disease. Adverse reactions to it can include fever, headache, rash, fatigue, gastrointestinal distress, anorexia, weight loss, myalgia, and depression.

Interferon beta-1a (AVONEX), a 166–amino acid recombinant glycoprotein, and *interferon beta-1b* (BETA-SERON), a 165–amino acid recombinant protein, have antiviral and immunomodulatory properties. They are FDA-approved for the treatment of relapsing and relapsing-remitting multiple sclerosis to reduce the frequency of clinical exacerbations. The mechanism of their action in multiple sclerosis is unclear. Flu-like symptoms (fever, chills, myalgia) and injection-site reactions have been common adverse effects.

Further discussion of the use of these and other interferons in the treatment of viral diseases can be found in Chapter 50.

Interleukin-2.   Human recombinant *interleukin-2* (*aldesleukin*, PROLEUKIN; des-alanyl-1, serine-125 human IL-2) is produced by recombinant DNA technology in *E. coli* (Taniguchi and Minami, 1993). This recombinant form differs from native IL-2 in that it is not glycosylated, has no amino terminal alanine, and has a serine substituted for the cysteine at amino acid 125 (Doyle *et al.,* 1985). The potency of the preparation is represented in International Units (IU) in a lymphocyte proliferation assay such that 1.1 mg of recombinant IL-2 protein equals 18 million IU. Aldesleukin has the following *in vitro* biologic activities of native IL-2: enhancement of lymphocyte proliferation and growth of IL-2-dependent cell lines; enhancement of lymphocyte-mediated cytotoxicity and killer cell activity; and induction of interferon-gamma activity (Winkelhake *et al.,* 1990; Whittington and Faulds, 1993). *In vivo* administration of aldesleukin in animals produces multiple immunologic effects in a dose-dependent manner. There is profound activation of cellular immunity

with lymphocytosis, eosinophilia, thrombocytopenia, and release of multiple cytokines (TNF, IL-1, interferon gamma). Aldesleukin is indicated for the treatment of adults with metastatic renal cell carcinoma and melanoma. Administration of aldesleukin has been associated with serious cardiovascular toxicity resulting from capillary leak syndrome, which involves loss of vascular tone and leak of plasma proteins and fluid into the extravascular space. Hypotension, reduced organ perfusion, and death may occur. An increased risk of disseminated infection due to impaired neutrophil function also has been associated with aldesleukin treatment.

Immunization

Immunization may be active or passive. Active immunization involves stimulation with an antigen to develop immunologic defenses against a future exposure. Passive immunization involves administration of preformed antibodies to an individual who is already exposed or is about to be exposed to an antigen.

Vaccines.   Active immunization, vaccination, involves administration of an antigen as a whole, killed organism, attenuated (live) organism, or a specific protein or peptide constituent of an organism. Booster doses often are required, especially when killed (inactivated) organisms are used as the immunogen. In the United States, vaccination has sharply curtailed or practically eliminated a variety of major infections, including diphtheria, measles, mumps, pertussis, rubella, tetanus, and *Haemophilus influenzae* type b (Dorner and Barrett, 1999; The National Vaccine Advisory Committee, 1999).

Although most work with vaccines has been aimed at infectious diseases, we are on the threshold of a new generation of vaccines aimed at specific cancers or autoimmune diseases (Lee *et al.,* 1998; Del Vecchio and Parmiani, 1999; Simone *et al.,* 1999). Such immunizations may provide complete or limited protection from disease. Because T cells optimally are activated by peptides and costimulatory ligands that both are present on APCs, one approach for vaccination has consisted of immunizing patients with APCs expressing a tumor antigen. The first generation of anticancer vaccines used whole cancer cells or tumor-cell lysates as a source of antigen in combination with various adjuvants, relying on APCs in the host to process and present tumor-specific antigens (Sinkovics and Horvath, 2000). These anticancer vaccines resulted in occasional clinical responses and are being tested in prospective clinical trials. The second generation of anticancer vaccines utilized specific APCs incubated *ex vivo* with antigen or transduced to express antigen and subsequently reinfused into patients. Preclinical studies have shown that, when laboratory animals are immunized with dendritic cells previously pulsed with MHC class I–restricted peptides derived from tumor-specific antigens, pronounced antitumor cytotoxic T-lymphocyte responses and protective tumor immunity can be generated (Tarte and Klein, 1999). Finally, multiple studies have revealed the efficacy of DNA vaccines in small and large animal models of infectious diseases and cancer (Lewis and Babiuk, 1999; Liljeqvist and Stahl, 1999). The advantage of DNA vaccination over peptide immunization is that it permits generation of entire proteins enabling determinant selection to occur in the host without having to restrict immunization to patients bearing specific HLA alleles. However, a safety concern about this technique is the potential for integration of the plasmid DNA into the host genome with the possibility of disrupting important genes and thereby leading to phenotypic mutations or carcinogenicity. A final approach to generate or enhance immune responses against specific antigens consists of infecting cells with recombinant viruses that encode the protein antigen of interest. Different types of viral vectors that can infect mammalian cells, such as vaccinia, avipox, lentivirus or adenovirus, have been used.

Immune Globulin. Passive immunization is indicated when an individual is deficient in antibodies because of a congenital or acquired immunodeficiency, when an individual with a high degree of risk is exposed to an agent and there is inadequate time for active immunization (measles, rabies, hepatitis B), or when a disease is already present but can be ameliorated by passive antibodies (botulism, diphtheria, tetanus). Passive immunization may be provided by several different products (Table 53–2). Nonspecific immunoglobulins or highly specific immunoglobulins may be provided based upon the indication. The protection provided usually lasts from 1 to 3 months. Immune globulin is derived from pooled plasma of adults by an alcohol-fractionation procedure. It contains largely IgG (95%) and is indicated for antibody-deficiency disorders, exposure to infections such as hepatitis A and measles, and specific immunologic diseases such as immune thrombocytopenic purpura and Guillain-Barré syndrome (Ballow, 1997; Jordan *et al.,* 1998a; Jordan *et al.,* 1998b). In contrast, specific immune globulins ("hyperimmune") differ from other immune globulin preparations in that donors are selected for high titers of the desired antibodies. Specific immune globulin preparations are available for hepatitis B, rabies, tetanus, varicella-zoster, cytomegalovirus, and respiratory syncytial virus. Rho(D) immune globulin

Table 53–2
Selected Immune Globulin Preparations

Immune globulin intravenous	BAYGAM
	GAMMAGARD S/D
	GAMMAR-P.I.V
	IVEEGAM
	SANDOGLOBULIN I.V.
	Others
Cytomegalovirus immune globulin	CYTOGAM
Respiratory syncytial virus immune globulin	RESPIGAM
Hepatitis B immune globulin	BAYHEP B
	HYPERHEP
	H-BIG
Rabies immune globulin	BAYRAB
	IMOGAM RABIS-HT
	HYPER-AB
Rho(D) immune globulin	BAY-RHO-D
	WINRHO SDF
	MICRHOGAM
	RHOGAM
	Others
Tetanus immune globulin	BAYTET
	HYPERTET

is a specific hyperimmune globulin for prophylaxis against hemolytic disease of the newborn due to Rh incompatibility between mother and fetus. All such plasma-derived products carry the theoretical risk of transmission of infectious disease.

Rho(D) Immune Globulin. The commercial forms of Rho(D) immune globulin (Table 53–2) are IgG containing a high titer of antibodies against the Rh(D) antigen on the surface of red blood cells. All donors are carefully screened to reduce the risk of transmitting infectious diseases. Fractionation of the plasma is performed by precipitation with cold alcohol followed by passage through a viral clearance system (Bowman, 1998; Contreras, 1998; Lee, 1998).

Mechanism of Action. Rho(D) immune globulin acts by binding Rho antigens, thereby preventing sensitization (Peterec, 1995). Rh-negative women may be sensitized to the "foreign" Rh antigen on red blood cells *via* the fetus at the time of birth, miscarriage, ectopic pregnancy, or any transplacental hemorrhage. If the women go on to have a primary immune response, they will make antibodies to Rh antigen that can cross the placenta and damage subsequent fetuses by lysing red blood cells. This syndrome, called hemolytic disease of the newborn, is life threatening. The form due to Rh incompatibility is largely preventable by Rho(D) immune globulin.

Therapeutic Use. Rho(D) immune globulin is indicated whenever fetal red blood cells are known or suspected to have entered the circulation of an Rh-negative mother unless the fetus is known also to be Rh-negative. The drug is given intramuscularly. The half-life of circulating immunoglobulin is approximately 21 to 29 days.

Toxicity. Discomfort at the site of injection and low-grade fever have been reported. Systemic reactions are extremely rare, but myalgia, lethargy, and anaphylactic shock have been reported. As with all plasma-derived products, there is a theoretical risk of transmission of infectious diseases.

PROSPECTUS

Throughout the 1990s, most transplant centers employed some combination of immunosuppressive drugs with antilymphocyte induction therapy with either a monoclonal or polyclonal antibody agent. Maintenance immunosuppression consists of a calcineurin inhibitor (cyclosporine or tacrolimus), glucocorticoids, and an antimetabolite (azathioprine or mycophenolate mofetil). Mycophenolate mofetil is replacing azathioprine as part of the standard immunosuppressive regimen after transplantation. At present, a number of centers are conducting various trials with new drug combinations including either cyclosporine or tacrolimus in combination with glucocorticoids and mycophenolate mofetil, with or without antibody-induction therapy. The array of new immunosuppressive agents is providing more effective control of rejection and permitting transplantation to become an accepted procedure with a number of different organs, including kidney, liver, pancreas, and heart. The apparent effectiveness of new drug combinations has resulted in a resurgence of interest in glucocorticoid withdrawal. Immunosuppressive strategies will continue to evolve in order to achieve effective control of rejection while minimizing injury to the allograft and risk to the patient. Although new immunosuppressive agents are continuously under development, the ultimate goal of transplantation biology is immunologic tolerance. Drugs and protocols aimed at "fooling" the immune system to recognize nonself as self or to "retrain" autoimmune cells could provide true cures for these diseases. The other area of recent progress is in vaccine development. New approaches hold promise of potential immunization protocols that will be therapeutic, not only for a myriad of major infections (such as tuberculosis and HIV) but also for cancer and autoimmune diseases. New immunotherapeutic approaches will address not only the issue of specific drug toxicities and efficacies but also long-term economic, metabolic, and quality-of-life outcomes.

For further information on organ transplantation and its medical management, *see* Chapters 234 (heart), 272 (kidney), and 301 (liver) in *Harrison's Principles of Internal Medicine*, 14th ed., McGraw-Hill, New York, 1998.

BIBLIOGRAPHY

Ahsan, N., Hricik, D., Matas, A., Rose, S., Tomlanovich, S., Wilkinson, A., Ewell, M., McIntosh, M., Stablein, D., and Hodge, E. Prednisone withdrawal in kidney transplant recipients on cyclosporine and mycophenolate mofetil—a prospective randomized study. Steroid Withdrawal Study Group. *Transplantation,* **1999,** *68:*1865–1874.

Auphan, N., DiDonato, J.A., Rosette, C., Helmberg, A., and Karin, M. Immunosuppression by glucocorticoids: inhibition of NF-kappa B activity through induction of I kappa B synthesis. *Science,* **1995,** *270:*286–290.

Ballow, M. Mechanisms of action of intravenous immune serum globulin in autoimmune and inflammatory diseases. *J. Allergy Clin. Immunol.,* **1997,** *100:*151–157.

Baraldo, M., Ferraccioli, G., Pea, F., Gremese, E., and Furlanut, M. Cyclosporine A pharmacokinetics in rheumatoid arthritis patients after 6 months of methotrexate therapy. *Pharmacol. Res.,* **1999,** *40:*483–486.

Borel, J.F., Feurer, C., Gubler, H.U., and Stahelin, H. Biological effects of cyclosporin A: a new antilymphocytic agent. *Agents Actions,* **1976,** *6:*468–475.

Bourdage, J.S., and Hamlin, D.M. Comparative polyclonal antithymocyte globulin and antilymphocyte/antilymphoblast globulin anti-CD antigen analysis by flow cytometry. *Transplantation,* **1995,** *59:*1194–1200.

Bowman, J.M. RhD hemolytic disease of the newborn. *N. Engl. J. Med.,* **1998,** *339:*1775–1777.

Brennan, D.C., Flavin, K., Lowell, J.A., Howard, T.K., Shenoy, S., Burgess, S., Dolan, S., Kano, J.M., Mahon, M., Schnitzler, M.A., Woodward, R., Irish, W., and Singer, G.G. A randomized, double-blinded comparison of Thymoglobulin versus Atgam for induction immunosuppressive therapy in adult renal transplant recipients. *Transplantation,* **1999,** *67:*1011–1018.

Brown, E.J., Albers, M.W., Shin, T.B., Ichikawa, K., Keith, C.T., Lane, W.S., and Schreiber, S.L. A mammalian protein targeted by G1-arresting rapamycin-receptor complex. *Nature,* **1994,** *369:*756–758.

Burke, J.F. Jr., Pirsch, J.D., Ramos, E.L., Salomon, D.R., Stablein, D.M., Van Buren, D.H., and West, J.C. Long-term efficacy and safety of cyclosporine in renal-transplant recipients. *N. Engl. J. Med.,* **1994,** *331:*358–363.

Butani, L., Palmer, J., Baluarte, H.J., and Polinsky, M.S. Adverse effects of mycophenolate mofetil in pediatric renal transplant recipients with presumed chronic rejection. *Transplantation*, **1999**, *68*:83–86.

Christians, U., and Sewing, K.F. Cyclosporin metabolism in transplant patients. *Pharmacol. Ther.*, **1993**, *57*:291–345.

Contreras, M. The prevention of Rh haemolytic disease of the fetus and newborn—general background. *Br. J. Obstet. Gynaecol.*, **1998**, *105* (Suppl. 18):7–10.

Cosimi, A.B., Burton, R.C., Colvin, R.B., Goldstein, G., Delmonico, F.L., LaQuaglia, M.P., Tolkoff-Rubin, N., Rubin, R.H., Herrin, J.T., and Russell, P.S. Treatment of acute renal allograft rejection with OKT3 monoclonal antibody. *Transplantation*, **1981**, *32*:535–539.

Doyle, M.V., Lee, M.T., and Fong, S. Comparison of the biological activities of human recombinant interleukin-2 (125) and native interleukin-2. *J. Biol. Response Mod.*, **1985**, *4*:96–109.

Fahr, A. Cyclosporin clinical pharmacokinetics. *Clin. Pharmacokinet.*, **1993**, *24*:472–495.

Figueredo, A., Germond, C., Maroun, J., Browman, G., Walker-Dilks, C., and Wong, S. Adjuvant therapy for stage II colon cancer after complete resection. Provincial Gastrointestinal Disease Site Group. *Cancer Prev. Control*, **1997**, *1*:379–392.

Friend, P.J., Hale, G., Chatenoud, L., Rebello, P., Bradley, J., Thiru, S., Phillips, J.M., and Waldmann, H. Phase I study of an engineered aglycosylated humanized CD3 antibody in renal transplant rejection. *Transplantation*, **1999**, *68*:1632–1637.

Fuchimoto, Y., Yamada, K., Shimizu, A., Yasumoto, A., Sawada, T., Huang, C.H., and Sachs, D.H. Relationship between chimerism and tolerance in a kidney transplantation model. *J. Immunol.*, **1999**, *162*:5704–5711.

Gaffney, K., and Scott, D.G. Azathioprine and cyclophosphamide in the treatment of rheumatoid arthritis. *Br. J. Rheumatol.*, **1998**, *37*:824–836.

Goto, T., Kino, T., Hatanaka, H., Nishiyama, M., Okuhara, M., Kohsaka, M., Aoki, H., and Imanaka, H. Discovery of FK-506, a novel immunosuppressant isolated from *Streptomyces tsukubaensis*. *Transplant Proc.*, **1987**, *19*:4–8.

Groth, C.G., Backman, L., Morales, J.M., Calne, R., Kreis, H., Lang, P., Touraine, J.L., Claesson, K., Campistol, J.M., Durand, D., Wramner, L., Brattstrom, C., and Charpentier, B. Sirolimus (rapamycin)-based therapy in human renal transplantation: similar efficacy and different toxicity compared with cyclosporine. Sirolimus European Renal Transplant Study Group. *Transplantation*, **1999**, *67*:1036–1042.

Hale, D.A., Gottschalk, R., Umemura, A., Maki, T., and Monaco, A.P. Establishment of stable multilineage hematopoietic chimerism and donor-specific tolerance without irradiation. *Transplantation*, **2000**, *69*:1242–1251.

Henry, M.L. Cyclosporine and tacrolimus (FK506): a comparison of efficacy and safety profiles. *Clin. Transplant.*, **1999**, *13*:209–220.

Herbelin, A., Chatenoud, L., Roux-Lombard, P., De Groote, D., Legendre, C., Dayer, J.M., Descamps-Latscha, B., Kreis, H., and Bach, J.F. *In vivo* soluble tumor necrosis factor receptor release in OKT3-treated patients. Differential regulation of TNF-sR55 and TNF-sR75. *Transplantation*, **1995**, *59*:1470–1475.

Hirose, R., Roberts, J.P., Quan, D., Osorio, R.W., Freise, C., Ascher, N.L., and Stock, P.G. Experience with daclizumab in liver transplantation: renal transplant dosing without calcineurin inhibitors is insufficient to prevent acute rejection in liver transplantation. *Transplantation*, **2000**, *69*:307–311.

Hong, J.C., and Kahan, B.D. Use of anti-CD25 monoclonal antibody in combination with rapamycin to eliminate cyclosporine treatment during the induction phase of immunosuppression. *Transplantation*, **1999**, *68*:701–704.

Hong, J.C., and Kahan, B.D. Sirolimus-induced thrombocytopenia and leukopenia in renal transplant recipients: risk factors, incidence, progression, and management. *Transplantation*, **2000b**, *69*:2085–2090.

Jacobson, J.M., Greenspan, J.S., Spritzler, J., Ketter, N., Fahey, J.L., Jackson, J.B., Fox, L., Chernoff, M., Wu, A.W., MacPhail, L.A., Vasquez, G.J., and Wohl, D.A. Thalidomide for the treatment of oral aphthous ulcers in patients with human immunodeficiency virus infection. National Institute of Allergy and Infectious Diseases AIDS Clinical Trials Group. *N. Engl. J. Med.*, **1997**, *336*:1487–1493.

Jaffers, G.J., Colvin, R.B., Cosimi, A.B., Giorgi, J.V., Goldstein, G., Fuller, T.C., Kurnick, J.T., Lillehei, C., and Russell P.S. The human immune response to murine OKT3 monoclonal antibody. *Transplant. Proc.*, **1983**, *15*:646–648.

Jordan, S.C., Quartel, A.W., Czer, L.S., Admon, D., Chen, G., Fishbein, M.C., Schwieger, J., Steiner, R.W., Davis, C., and Tyan, D.B. Posttransplant therapy using high-dose human immunoglobulin (intravenous gammaglobulin) to control acute humoral rejection in renal and cardiac allograft recipients and potential mechanism of action. *Transplantation*, **1998a**, *66*:800–805.

Jordan, S.C., Tyan, D., Czer, L., and Toyoda, M. Immunomodulatory actions of intravenous immunoglobulin (IVIG): potential applications in solid organ transplant recipients. *Pediatr. Transplant.*, **1998b**, *2*:92–105.

Kahan, B.D. The potential role of rapamycin in pediatric transplantation as observed from adult studies. *Pediatr. Transplant.*, **1999**, *3*:175–180.

Kahan, B.D., Julian, B.A., Pescovitz, M.D., Vanrenterghem, Y., and Neylan, J. Sirolimus reduces the incidence of acute rejection episodes despite lower cyclosporine doses in Caucasian recipients of mismatched primary renal allografts: a phase II trial. Rapamune Study Group. *Transplantation*, **1999a**, *68*:1526–1532.

Kahan, B.D., Rajagopalan, P.R., and Hall, M. Reduction of the occurrence of acute cellular rejection among renal allograft recipients treated with basiliximab, a chimeric anti-interleukin-2-receptor monoclonal antibody. United States Simulect Renal Study Group. *Transplantation*, **1999b**, *67*:276–284.

Keesal, N., Wasserman, M.J., Bookman, A., Lapp, V., Weber, D.A., and Keystone, E.C. Thalidomide in the treatment of refractory rheumatoid arthritis. *J. Rheumatol.*, **1999**, *26*:2344–2347.

Khanna, A., Li, B., Stenzel, K.H., and Suthanthiran, M. Regulation of new DNA synthesis in mammalian cells by cyclosporine. Demonstration of a transforming growth factor beta-dependent mechanism of inhibition of cell growth. *Transplantation*, **1994**, *57*:577–582.

Kimball, J.A., Pescovitz, M.D., Book, B.K., and Norman, D.J. Reduced human IgG anti-ATGAM antibody formation in renal transplant recipients receiving mycophenolate mofetil. *Transplantation*, **1995**, *60*:1379–1383.

Kirk, A.D., Harlan, D.M., Armstrong, N.N., Davis, T.A., Dong, Y., Gray, G.S., Hong, X., Thomas, D., Fechner, J.H. Jr., and Knechtle, S.J. CTLA4-Ig and anti-CD40 ligand prevent renal allograft rejection in primates. *Proc. Natl. Acad. Sci. U.S.A.*, **1997**, *94*:8789–8794.

Kohler, G., and Milstein, C. Continuous cultures of fused cells secreting antibody of predefined specificity. *Nature*, **1975**, *256*:495–497.

Kovarik, J.M., Kahan, B.D., Rajagopalan, P.R., Bennett, W., Mulloy, L.L., Gerbeau, C., and Hall, M.L. Population pharmacokinetics and exposure-response relationships for basiliximab in kidney transplantation. The U.S. Simulect Renal Transplant Study Group. *Transplantation*, **1999**, *68*:1288–1294.

Kreis, H., Cisterne, J.M., Land, W., Wramner, L., Squifflet, J.P., Abramowicz, D., Campistol, J.M., Morales, J.M., Grinyo, J.M., Mourad, G., Berthoux, F.C., Brattstrom, C., Lebranchu, Y., and

Vialtel, P. Sirolimus in association with mycophenolate mofetil induction for the prevention of acute graft rejection in renal allograft recipients. *Transplantation,* **2000,** *69*:1252–1260.

Kuo, C.J., Chung, J., Fiorentino, D.F., Flanagan, W.M., Blenis, J., and Crabtree, G.R. Rapamycin selectively inhibits interleukin-2 activation of p70 S6 kinase. *Nature,* **1992,** *358*:70–73.

Larsen, C.P., Alexander, D.Z., Hollenbaugh, D., Elwood, E.T., Ritchie, S.C., Aruffo, A., Hendrix, R., and Pearson, T.C. CD40-gp39 interactions play a critical role during allograft rejection. Suppression of allograft rejection by blockade of the CD40-gp39 pathway. *Transplantation,* **1996,** *61*:4–9.

Lary, J.M., Daniel, K.L., Erickson, J.D., Roberts, H.E., and Moore, C.A. The return of thalidomide: can birth defects be prevented? *Drug Saf.,* **1999,** *21*:161–169.

Lee, D. Preventing RhD haemolytic disease of the newborn. Revised guidelines advocate two doses of anti-D immunoglobulin for antenatal prophylaxis. *BMJ,* **1998,** *316*:1611.

Li, Y., Zheng, X.X., Li, X.C., Zand, M.S., and Strom, T.B. Combined costimulation blockade plus rapamycin but not cyclosporine produces permanent engraftment. *Transplantation,* **1998,** *66*:1387–1388.

Lo Iacono, O., Castro, A., Diago, M., Moreno, J.A., Fernandez-Bermejo, M., Vega, P., Garcia, V., Carbonell, P., Sanz, P., Borque, M.J., Garcia-Buey, L., Garcia-Monzon, C., Pedreira, J., and Moreno-Otero, R. Interferon alfa-2b plus ribavirin for chronic hepatitis C patients who have not responded to interferon monotherapy. *Aliment. Pharmacol. Ther.,* **2000,** *14*:463–469.

Mannick, J.A., Davis, R.C., Cooperband, S.R., Glasgow, A.H., Williams, L.F., Harrington, J.T., Cavallo, T., Schmitt, G.W., Idelson, B.A., Olsson, C.A., and Nabseth, D.C. Clinical use of rabbit antihuman lymphocyte globulin in cadaver-kidney transplantation. *N. Engl. J. Med.,* **1971,** *284*:1109–1115.

Mariat, C., Alamartine, E., Diab, N., de Filippis, J.P., Laurent, B., and Berthoux, F. A randomized prospective study comparing low-dose OKT3 to low-dose ATG for the treatment of acute steroid-resistant rejection episodes in kidney transplant recipients. *Transplant. Int.,* **1998,** *11*:231–236.

Mayer, A.D., Dmitrewski, J., Squifflet, J.P., Besse, T., Grabensee, B., Klein, B., Eigler, F.W., Heemann, U., Pichlmayr, R., Behrend, M., Vanrenterghem, Y., Donck, J., van Hooff, J., Christiaans, M., Morales, J.M., Andres, A., Johnson, R.W., Short, C., Buchholz, B., Rehmert, N., Land, W., Schleibner, S., Forsythe, J.L., Talbot, D., Neumayer, H.-H., Hauser, I., Ericzon, B.-G., Brattström, C., Claesson, K., Mühlbacher, F., and Pohanka, E. Multicenter randomized trial comparing tacrolimus (FK506) and cyclosporine in the prevention of renal allograft rejection: a report of the European Tacrolimus Multicenter Renal Study Group. *Transplantation,* **1997,** *64*:436–443.

Mihatsch, M.J., Kyo, M., Morozumi, K., Yamaguchi, Y., Nickeleit, V., and Ryffel, B. The side-effects of ciclosporine-A and tacrolimus. *Clin. Nephrol.,* **1998,** *49*:356–363.

Moertel, C.G., Fleming, T.R., Macdonald, J.S., Haller, D.G., Laurie, J.A., Goodman, P.J., Ungerleider, J.S., Emerson, W.A., Tormey, D.C., Glick, J.H., Veeder, M.H., and Mailliard, J.A. Levamisole and fluorouracil for adjuvant therapy of resected colon carcinoma. *N. Engl. J. Med.,* **1990,** *322*:352–358.

Morales, A., Ottenhof, P., and Emerson, L. Treatment of residual, non-infiltrating bladder cancer with bacillus Calmette-Guérin. *J. Urol.,* **1981,** *125*:649–651.

Murgia, M.G., Jordan, S., and Kahan, B.D. The side effect profile of sirolimus: a phase I study in quiescent cyclosporine-prednisone-treated renal transplant patients. *Kidney Int.,* **1996,** *49*:209–216.

Murray, J.E., Merrill, J.P., and Harrison, J.H. Prolonged survival of human kidney homografts by immunosuppressive drug therapy. *N. Engl. J. Med.,* **1963,** *26*:1315.

Napoli, K.L., and Kahan, B.D. Routine clinical monitoring of sirolimus (rapamycin) whole-blood concentrations by HPLC with ultraviolet detection. *Clin. Chem.,* **1996,** *42*:1943–1948.

Opelz, G., and Terasaki, P.I. Improvement of kidney-graft survival with increased numbers of blood transfusions. *N. Engl. J. Med.,* **1978,** *299*:799–803.

Opelz, G., Vanrenterghem, Y., Kirste, G., Gray, D.W., Horsburgh, T., Lachance, J.G., Largiader, F., Lange, H., Vujaklija-Stipanovic, K., Alvarez-Grande, J., Schott, W., Hoyer, J., Schnuelle, P., Descoeudres, C., Ruder, H., Wujciak, T., and Schwarz, V. Prospective evaluation of pretransplant blood transfusions in cadaver kidney recipients. *Transplantation,* **1997,** *63*:964–967.

Ortho Multicenter Transplant Study Group. A randomized clinical trial of OKT3 monoclonal antibody for acute rejection of cadaveric renal transplants. *N. Engl. J. Med.,* **1985,** *313*:337–342.

Regan, J.F., Campbell, K., Van Smith, L., Schroeder, T.J., Womble, D., Kano, J., and Buelow, R. Sensitization following Thymoglobulin and Atgam rejection therapy as determined with a rapid enzyme-linked immunosorbent assay. US Thymoglobulin Multi-Center Study Group. *Transplant. Immunol.,* **1999,** *7*:115–121.

Rostaing, L., Chabannier, M.H., Modesto, A., Rouzaud, A., Cisterne, J.M., Tkaczuk, J., and Durand, D. Predicting factors of long-term results of OKT3 therapy for steroid resistant acute rejection following cadaveric renal transplantation. *Am. J. Nephrol.,* **1999,** *19*:634–640.

Salm, P., Taylor, P.J., and Pillans, P.I. Analytical performance of microparticle enzyme immunoassay and HPLC-tandem mass spectrometry in the determination of sirolimus in whole blood. *Clin. Chem.,* **1999,** *45*:2278–2280.

Salmela, K., Wramner, L., Ekberg, H., Hauser, I., Bentdal, O., Lins, L.E., Isoniemi, H., Backman, L., Persson, N., Neumayer, H.H., Jorgensen, P.F., Spieker, C., Hendry, B., Nicholls, A., Kirste, G., and Hasche, G. A randomized multicenter trial of the anti-ICAM-1 monoclonal antibody (enlimomab) for the prevention of acute rejection and delayed onset of graft function in cadaveric renal transplantation: a report of the European Anti-ICAM-1 Renal Transplant Study Group. *Transplantation,* **1999,** *67*:729–736.

Sampaio, E.P., Kaplan, G., Miranda, A., Nery, J.A., Miguel, C.P., Viana, S.M., and Sarno, E.N. The influence of thalidomide on the clinical and immunologic manifestation of erythema nodosum leprosum. *J. Infect. Dis.,* **1993,** *168*:408–414.

Shinn, C., Malhotra, D., Chan, L., Cosby, R.L., and Shapiro, J.I. Time course of response to pulse methylprednisolone therapy in renal transplant recipients with acute allograft rejection. *Am. J. Kidney Dis.,* **1999,** *34*:304–307.

Simone, E.A., Wegmann, D.R., and Eisenbarth, G.S. Immunologic "vaccination" for the prevention of autoimmune diabetes (type 1A). *Diabetes Care,* **1999,** *22* (Suppl. 2):B7–B15.

Spitzer, T.R., Delmonico, F., Tolkoff-Rubin, N., McAfee, S., Sackstein, R., Saidman, S., Colby, C., Sykes, M., Sachs, D.H., and Cosimi, A.B. Combined histocompatibility leukocyte antigen-matched donor bone marrow and renal transplantation for multiple myeloma with end stage renal disease: the induction of allograft tolerance through mixed lymphohematopoietic chimerism. *Transplantation,* **1999,** *68*:480–484.

Szczech, L.A., and Feldman, H.I. Effect of anti-lymphocyte antibody induction therapy on renal allograft survival. *Transplant. Proc.,* **1999,** *31*:9S–11S.

The National Vaccine Advisory Committee. Strategies to sustain success in childhood immunizations. *JAMA,* **1999,** *282*:363–370.

The U.S. Multicenter FK506 Liver Study Group. A comparison of tacrolimus (FK 506) and cyclosporine for immunosuppression in liver transplantation. *N. Engl. J. Med.,* **1994,** *331*:1110–1115.

Valeri, A., Radhakrishnan, J., Estes, D., D'Agati, V., Kopelman, R., Pernis, A., Flis, R., Pirani, C., and Appel, G.B. Intravenous pulse cyclophosphamide treatment of severe lupus nephritis: a prospective five-year study. *Clin. Nephrol.,* **1994,** *42*:71–78.

Venkat Raman, G., Sharman, V.L., and Lee, H.A. Azathioprine and allopurinol: a potentially dangerous combination. *J. Intern. Med.,* **1990,** *228*:69–71.

Venkataramanan, R., Swaminathan, A., Prasad, T., Jain, A., Zuckerman, S., Warty, V., McMichael, J., Lever, J., Burckart, G., and Starzl, T. Clinical pharmacokinetics of tacrolimus. *Clin. Pharmacokinet.,* **1995,** *29*:404–430.

Vezina, C., Kudelski, A., and Sehgal, S.N. Rapamycin (AY-22,989), a new antifungal antibiotic. I. Taxonomy of the producing streptomycete and isolation of the active principle. *J. Antibiot. (Tokyo),* **1975,** *28*:721–726.

Vincenti, F., Kirkman, R., Light, S., Bumgardner, G., Pescovitz, M., Halloran, P., Neylan, J., Wilkinson, A., Ekberg, H., Gaston, R., Backman, L., and Burdick, J. Interleukin-2-receptor blockade with daclizumab to prevent acute rejection in renal transplantation. Daclizumab Triple Therapy Study Group. *N. Engl. J. Med.,* **1998,** *338*:161–165.

Wall, W.J. Use of antilymphocyte induction therapy in liver transplantation. *Liver Transplant. Surg.,* **1999,** *5*:S64–S70.

Watson, C.J., Friend, P.J., Jamieson, N.V., Frick, T.W., Alexander, G., Gimson, A.E., and Calne, R. Sirolimus: a potent new immunosuppressant for liver transplantation. *Transplantation,* **1999,** *67*:505–509.

Woodle, E.S., Xu, D., Zivin, R.A., Auger, J., Charette, J., O'Laughlin, R., Peace, D., Jollife, L.K., Haverty, T., Bluestone, J.A., and Thistlethwaite, J.R. Jr. Phase I trial of a humanized, Fc receptor nonbinding OKT3 antibody, huOKT3gamma1(Ala-Ala) in the treatment of acute renal allograft rejection. *Transplantation,* **1999,** *68*:608–616.

Yoshimura, R., Yoshimura, N., Ohyama, A., Ohmachi, T., Yamamoto, K., Kishimoto, T., and Wada, S. The effect of immunosuppressive agents (FK-506, rapamycin) on renal P450 systems in rat models. *J. Pharm. Pharmacol.,* **1999,** *51*:941–948.

Zimmerman, J.J., and Kahan, B.D. Pharmacokinetics of sirolimus in stable renal transplant patients after multiple oral dose administration. *J. Clin. Pharmacol.,* **1997,** *37*:405–415.

MONOGRAPHS AND REVIEWS

Allison, A.C., and Eugui, E.M. Immunosuppressive and other effects of mycophenolic acid and an ester prodrug, mycophenolate mofetil. *Immunol. Rev.,* **1993,** *136*:5–28.

Bardsley-Elliot, A., Noble, S., and Foster, R.H. Mycophenolate mofetil: a review of its use in the management of solid organ transplantation. *BioDrugs,* **1999,** *12*:363–410.

Beato, M. Gene regulation by steroid hormones. *Cell,* **1989,** *56*:335–344.

Bertino, J.R. Chemical action and pharmacology of methotrexate, azathioprine and cyclophosphamide in man. *Arthritis Rheum.,* **1973,** *16*:79–83.

Bukowski, R.M. Immunotherapy in renal cell carcinoma. *Oncology (Huntingt.),* **1999,** *13*:801–810.

Chan, G.L., Canafax, D.M., and Johnson, C.A. The therapeutic use of azathioprine in renal transplantation. *Pharmacotherapy,* **1987,** *7*:165–177.

Clayberger, C., Krensky, A.M. Mechanisms of allograft rejection. In, *Immunologic Renal Diseases.* (Neilson, E.G., and Couser, W.G., eds.) Lippincott-Raven Publishers, Philadelphia, **2001.** In press.

Del Vecchio, M., and Parmiani, G. Cancer vaccination. *Forum (Genova),* **1999,** *9*:239–256.

Dorner, F., and Barrett, P.N. Vaccine technology: looking to the future. *Ann. Med.,* **1999,** *31*:51–60.

Elion, G.B. The George Hitchings and Gertrude Elion Lecture. The pharmacology of azathioprine. *Ann. N.Y. Acad. Sci.,* **1993,** *685*:400–407.

Faulds, D., Goa, K.L., and Benfield, P. Cyclosporin. A review of its pharmacodynamic and pharmacokinetic properties, and therapeutic use in immunoregulatory disorders. *Drugs,* **1993,** *45*:953–1040.

Fulton, B., and Markham, A. Mycophenolate mofetil. A review of its pharmacodynamic and pharmacokinetic properties and clinical efficacy in renal transplantation. *Drugs,* **1996,** *51*:278–298.

Fung, J.J., and Starzl, T.E. FK506 in solid organ transplantation. *Ther. Drug Monit.,* **1995,** *17*:592–595.

Grosflam, J., and Weinblatt, M.E. Methotrexate: mechanism of action, pharmacokinetics, clinical indications, and toxicity. *Curr. Opin. Rheumatol.,* **1991,** *3*:363–368.

Hackett, C.J., and Dickler, H.B. Immunologic tolerance for immune system-mediated diseases. *J. Allergy Clin. Immunol.,* **1999,** *103*:362–370.

Halloran, P.F. Immunosuppressive agents in clinical trials in transplantation. *Am. J. Med. Sci.,* **1997,** *313*:283–288.

Hong, J.C., and Kahan, B.D. Immunosuppressive agents in organ transplantation: past, present, and future. *Semin. Nephrol.,* **2000a,** *20*:108–125.

Hooks, M.A., Wade, C.S., and Millikan, W.J. Jr. Muromonab CD-3: a review of its pharmacology, pharmacokinetics, and clinical use in transplantation. *Pharmacotherapy,* **1991,** *11*:26–37.

Janeway, C.A., Travers, P., Walport, M., and Capra, J.D., eds. *Immunobiology: The Immune System in Health and Disease,* 4th ed. Current Biology Publications, London, **1999.**

Johnson, H.M., Bazer, F.W., Szente, B.E., and Jarpe, M.A. How interferons fight disease. *Sci. Am.,* **1994,** *270*:68–75.

Kahan, B.D. Cyclosporine. *N. Engl. J. Med.,* **1989,** *32*:1725–1738.

Khoury, S., Sayegh, M.H., and Turka, L.A. Blocking costimulatory signals to induce transplantation tolerance and prevent autoimmune disease. *Int. Rev. Immunol.,* **1999,** *18*:185–199.

Krensky, A.M. Transplantation Immunobiology. In, *Pediatric Nephrology, 4th Edition.* (Barratt, T.M., Auner, E.D., and Harmon, W., eds.) Williams and Wilkins, Baltimore, **2001,** pp. 1289–1307.

Krensky, A.M., and Clayberger, C. Prospects for induction of tolerance in renal transplantation. *Pediatr. Nephrol.,* **1994,** *8*:772–779.

Krensky, A.M., Weiss, A., Crabtree, G., Davis, M.M., and Parham, P. T-lymphocyte-antigen interactions in transplant rejection. *N. Engl. J. Med.,* **1990,** *322*:510–517.

Laan, R.F., Jansen, T.L., and van Riel, P.L. Glucocorticosteroids in the management of rheumatoid arthritis. *Rheumatology (Oxford),* **1999,** *38*:6–12.

Lee, D.J., Corr, M., and Carson, D.A. Control of immune responses by gene immunization. *Ann. Med.,* **1998b,** *30*:460–468.

Legendre, C.M., and Guttman, R.D. Selection and preparation of donors and recipients for renal transplantation. In, *Textbook of Nephrology.* (Massry, S.G., and Glassock, R.J., eds.) Williams & Wilkins, Baltimore, **1989,** pp. 1471–1476.

Lewis, P.J., and Babiuk, L.A. DNA vaccines: a review. *Adv. Virus Res.,* **1999,** *54*:129–188.

Liljeqvist, S., and Stahl, S. Production of recombinant subunit vaccines: protein immunogens, live delivery systems and nucleic acid vaccines. *J. Biotechnol.,* **1999,** *73*:1–33.

Linden, K.G., and Weinstein, G.D. Psoriasis: current perspectives with an emphasis on treatment. *Am. J. Med.,* **1999,** *107*:595–605.

Miller, M.T., and Stromland, K. Teratogen update: thalidomide: a review, with a focus on ocular findings and new potential uses. *Teratology,* **1999,** *60*:306–321.

Monaco, A.P., Burke, J.F. Jr., Ferguson, R.M., Halloran, P.F., Kahan, B.D., Light, J.A., Matas, A.J., and Solez, K. Current thinking on chronic renal allograft rejection: issues, concerns, and recommendations from a 1997 roundtable discussion. *Am. J. Kidney Dis.,* **1999,** *33*:150–160.

Murphy, B., and Krensky, A.M. HLA-derived peptides as novel immunomodulatory therapeutics. *J. Am. Soc. Nephrol.,* **1999,** *10*:1346–1355.

Natsumeda, Y., and Carr, S.F. Human type I and II IMP dehydrogenases as drug targets. *Ann. N.Y. Acad. Sci.,* **1993,** *696*:88–93.

Neuhaus, T.J., Fay, J., Dillon, M.J., Trompeter, R.S., and Barratt, T.M. Alternative treatment to corticosteroids in steroid sensitive idiopathic nephrotic syndrome. *Arch. Dis. Child,* **1994,** *71*:522–526.

Noble, S., and Markham, A. Cyclosporin. A review of the pharmacokinetic properties, clinical efficacy and tolerability of a microemulsion-based formulation (Neoral). *Drugs,* **1995,** *50*:924–941.

Patard, J.J., Saint, F., Velotti, F., Abbou, C.C., and Chopin, D.K. Immune response following intravesical bacillus Calmette-Guérin instillations in superficial bladder cancer: a review. *Urol. Res.,* **1998,** *26*:155–159.

Paterson, D.L., and Patel, A. Bacillus Calmette-Guérin (BCG) immunotherapy for bladder cancer: review of complications and their treatment. *Aust. N.Z. J. Surg.,* **1998,** *68*:340–344.

Pattison, J.M., Sibley, R.K., and Krensky, A.M. Mechanisms of allograft rejection. In, *Immunologic Renal Diseases.* (Neilson, E.G., and Couser, W.G., eds.) Lippincott-Raven Publishers, Philadelphia, **1997,** pp. 331–354.

Paul, W.E., ed. *Fundamental Immunology,* 4th ed. Lippincott-Raven, Philadelphia, **1999.**

Perico, N., and Remuzzi, G. Prevention of transplant rejection: current treatment guidelines and future developments. *Drugs,* **1997,** *54*:533–570.

Peterec, S.M. Management of neonatal Rh disease. *Clin. Perinatol.,* **1995,** *22*:561–592.

Plosker, G.L., and Foster, R.H. Tacrolimus: a further update of its pharmacology and therapeutic use in the management of organ transplantation. *Drugs,* **2000,** *59*:323–389.

Prakash, A., and Jarvis, B. Leflunomide: a review of its use in active rheumatoid arthritis. *Drugs,* **1999,** *58*:1137–1164.

Punt, C.J. The use of interferon-alpha in the treatment of cutaneous melanoma: a review. *Melanoma Res.,* **1998,** *8*:95–104.

Ransohoff, R.M. Cellular responses to interferons and other cytokines: the JAK-STAT paradigm. *N. Engl. J. Med.,* **1998,** *338*:616–618.

Rugstad, H.E. Antiinflammatory and immunoregulatory effects of glucocorticoids: mode of action. *Scand. J. Rheumatol. Suppl.,* **1988,** *76*:257–264.

Schreiber, S.L., and Crabtree, G.R. The mechanism of action of cyclosporin A and FK506. *Immunol. Today,* **1992,** *13*:136–142.

Shapiro, R. Tacrolimus in pediatric renal transplantation: a review. *Pediatr. Transplant.,* **1998,** *2*:270–276.

Sinkovics, J.G., and Horvath, J.C. Vaccination against human cancers (review). *Int. J. Oncol.,* **2000,** *16*:81–96.

Smithells, R.W., and Newman, C.G. Recognition of thalidomide defects. *J. Med. Genet.,* **1992,** *29*:716–723.

Starzl, T.E., Demetris, A.J., Murase, N., Trucco, M., Thomson, A.W., Rao, A.S., and Fung, J.J. Chimerism after organ transplantation. *Curr. Opin. Nephrol. Hypertens.,* **1997,** *6*:292–298.

Suthanthiran, M., Morris, R.E., and Strom, T.B. Immunosuppressants: cellular and molecular mechanisms of action. *Am. J. Kidney Dis.,* **1996,** *28*:159–172.

Taniguchi, T., and Minami, Y. The IL-2/IL-2 receptor system: a current overview. *Cell,* **1993,** *73*:5–8.

Tarte, K., and Klein, B. Dendritic cell-based vaccine: a promising approach for cancer immunotherapy. *Leukemia,* **1999,** *13*:653–663.

Tilg, H., and Kaser, A. Interferons and their role in inflammation. *Curr. Pharm. Des.,* **1999,** *5*:771–785.

Tompkins, W.A. Immunomodulation and therapeutic effects of the oral use of interferon-alpha: mechanism of action. *J. Interferon Cytokine Res.,* **1999,** *19*:817–828.

Tseng, S., Pak, G., Washenik, K., Pomeranz, M.K., and Shupack, J.L. Rediscovering thalidomide: a review of its mechanism of action, side effects, and potential uses. *J. Am. Acad. Dermatol.,* **1996,** *35*:969–979.

Van Parijs, L., and Abbas, A.K. Homeostasis and self-tolerance in the immune system: turning lymphocytes off. *Science,* **1998,** *280*:243–248.

Whittington, R., and Faulds, D. Interleukin-2. A review of its pharmacological properties and therapeutic use in patients with cancer. *Drugs,* **1993,** *46*:446–514.

Wilde, M.I., and Goa, K.L. Muromonab CD3: a reappraisal of its pharmacology and use as prophylaxis of solid organ transplant rejection. *Drugs,* **1996,** *51*:865–894.

Winkelhake, J.L., and Gauny, S.S. Human recombinant interleukin-2 as an experimental therapeutic. *Pharmacol. Rev.,* **1990,** *42*:1–28.

Wiseman, L.R., and Faulds, D. Daclizumab: a review of its use in the prevention of acute rejection in renal transplant recipients. *Drugs,* **1999,** *58*:1029–1042.

Wood, K.J. Transplantation tolerance. *Curr. Opin. Immunol.,* **1991,** *3*:710–714.

Zoorob, R.J., and Cender, D. A different look at corticosteroids. *Am. Fam. Physician,* **1998,** *58*:443–450.

SECTION XI

DRUGS ACTING ON THE BLOOD AND THE BLOOD-FORMING ORGANS

A number of drugs—including hormonal growth factors, vitamins, and minerals—affect the blood and the blood-forming organs, either directly or indirectly. The growth factors that control the proliferation and differentiation of hematopoietic stem cells are discussed in Chapter 54. Agents effective in specific anemias include iron, copper, vitamin B_{12}, folic acid, pyridoxine, and riboflavin; these substances also are described in this chapter. In Chapter 55, attention is devoted chiefly to heparin and the oral anticoagulants, thrombolytic agents, and drugs that affect platelet function.

HEMATOPOIETIC AGENTS

Growth Factors, Minerals, and Vitamins

Robert S. Hillman

The short life span of mature blood cells requires their continuous replacement, a process termed hematopoiesis. *New cell production must be responsive to both basal needs and situations of increased demand. For example, red blood cell production can vary over more than a fivefold range in response to anemia or hypoxia. White blood cell production increases dramatically in response to a systemic infection, and platelet production can increase severalfold when platelet destruction results in thrombocytopenia.*

The regulation of hematopoiesis is complex and involves cell–cell interactions within the microenvironment of the bone marrow as well as both hematopoietic and lymphopoietic growth factors. A number of these hormonelike glycoproteins now have been identified and characterized, and, using recombinant DNA technology, their genes have been cloned and the proteins produced in quantities sufficient for use as therapeutic agents. Clinical applications now are being developed, ranging from treatment of primary hematological diseases to uses as adjunctive agents in the treatment of severe infections and in the management of patients who are undergoing chemotherapy or marrow transplantation.

Hematopoiesis also requires adequate supplies of minerals, both iron and copper, and a number of vitamins, including folic acid, vitamin B_{12}, pyridoxine, ascorbic acid, and riboflavin. Deficiencies of these minerals and vitamins generally result in characteristic anemias and, less frequently, a general failure of hematopoiesis. Therapeutic correction of a specific deficiency state depends on the accurate diagnosis of the anemic state and knowledge as to the correct dose, the use of these agents in various combinations, and the expected response.

This chapter deals with the growth factors, vitamins, minerals, and drugs that affect the blood and blood-forming organs.

I. HEMATOPOIETIC GROWTH FACTORS

History. Modern concepts of hematopoietic cell growth and differentiation developed beginning in the 1950s with the work of Jacobsen, Ford, and others (Jacobsen *et al.,* 1949; Ford *et al.,* 1956). These investigators demonstrated the role that cells from the spleen and marrow play in the restoration of hematopoietic tissue in irradiated animals. In 1961, Till and McCulloch were able to show that individual hematopoietic cells could form macroscopic hematopoietic nodules in the spleens of irradiated mice. Their work led to the concept of *colony-forming stem cells.* It also led to the subsequent proof that stem cells present in human bone marrow are pluripotent—that is, they give rise to granulocytes, monocytes, lymphocytes, megakaryocytes, and erythrocytes.

The role of growth factors in hematopoiesis was elucidated by Bradley, Metcalf, and others using bone marrow culture techniques (Bradley and Metcalf, 1966). Individual growth factors were isolated (Metcalf, 1985; Moore, 1991), and the target

cells of these factors characterized. The pluripotent stem cell gives rise to committed progenitors, which can be identified as single colony-forming units, and to cells that are increasingly differentiated.

The existence of a circulating growth factor that controls erythropoiesis was first suggested by experiments carried out by Paul Carnot in 1906 (Carnot and Deflandre, 1906). He observed an increase in the red cell count in rabbits injected with serum obtained from anemic animals and postulated the existence of a factor that he called *hemapoietine*. However, it was not until the 1950s that Reissmann (1950), Erslev (1953), and Jacobsen and coworkers (1957) defined the origin and actions of the hormone, now called *erythropoietin*. Subsequently, extensive studies of erythropoietin were carried out in patients with anemia and polycythemia, culminating in 1977 with the purification of erythropoietin from urine by Miyake and colleagues. The gene that encodes the protein was subsequently cloned and expressed at a high level in a mammalian cell system (Jacobs *et al.,* 1985; Lin *et al.,* 1985), producing a recombinant hormone that is indistinguishable from human urinary erythropoietin. Similarly, complementary DNA and genomic clones for granulocyte, macrophage, and, most recently, megakaryocyte colony-stimulating factors have been isolated and sufficient quantities of biologically active growth factors produced for clinical investigation (Kawasaki *et al.,* 1985; Lee *et al.,* 1985; Wong *et al.,* 1985; Yang *et al.,* 1986; Lok *et al.,* 1994; de Sauvage *et al.,* 1994).

Growth Factor Physiology. Steady-state hematopoiesis involves the production of more than 200 billion (2×10^{11}) blood cells each day. This production is under delicate control, and, with increased demand, the rate can increase severalfold. The hematopoietic organ also is unique in that several mature cell types are derived from a much smaller number of pluripotent stem cells that are formed in early embryonic life. These stem cells are capable of both maintaining their own number and differentiating under the influence of cellular and humoral factors [stem cell factor (SCF), Flt3 ligand (FL), interleukin-3 (IL-3), and granulocyte/macrophage colony-stimulating factor (GM-CSF)] to produce a variety of hematopoietic and lymphopoietic cells.

Stem cell differentiation can be described as a series of steps that produce so-called burst-forming units (BFU) and colony-forming units (CFU) for each of the major cell lines (Quesenberry and Levitt, 1979). Although these early progenitors (BFU and CFU) are not morphologically recognizable as precursors of a specific cell type, they are capable of further proliferation and differentiation, increasing their number by some 30-fold. Subsequently, colonies of morphologically distinct cells form under the control of an overlapping set of additional growth factors (G-CSF, M-CSF, erythropoietin, and thrombopoietin). Proliferation and maturation of the CFU for each cell line can further amplify the resulting mature cell product by another 30-fold or more, resulting in greater than 1000 mature cells produced for each committed stem cell (Lajtha *et al.,* 1969).

Hematopoietic and lymphopoietic growth factors are produced by a number of marrow cells and peripheral tissues. The growth factors are glycoproteins and are active at very low concentrations, usually on more than one committed cell lineage. Most show synergistic interactions with other factors, as well as "networking," wherein stimulation of a cell lineage by one growth factor induces the production of additional growth factors. Finally, growth factors generally exert actions at several points in the processes of cell proliferation and differentiation and in mature cell function (Metcalf, 1985). Some of the overlapping effects of the more important hematopoietic growth factors are illustrated in Figure 54–1 and listed in Table 54–1.

ERYTHROPOIETIN

While erythropoietin is not the sole growth factor responsible for erythropoiesis, it is the most important regulator of the proliferation of committed progenitors (BFU-E and CFU-E). In its absence, severe anemia is invariably present. Erythropoiesis is controlled by a highly responsive feedback system in which a sensor in the kidney can detect changes in oxygen delivery to increase the secretion of erythropoietin, which then stimulates a rapid expansion of erythroid progenitors.

Erythropoietin is produced primarily by peritubular interstitial cells of the kidney under the control of a single gene on human chromosome 7. The gene product is a protein containing 193 amino acids, of which the first 27 are cleaved during secretion (Jacobs *et al.,* 1985; Lin *et al.,* 1985). The final hormonal peptide is heavily glycosylated and has a molecular weight of approximately 30,000 daltons. Once released, erythropoietin travels to the marrow, where it binds to a receptor on the surface of committed erythroid progenitors and is internalized. With anemia or hypoxemia, renal synthesis rapidly increases by 100-fold or more, serum erythropoietin levels rise, and marrow progenitor cell survival, proliferation, and maturation are dramatically stimulated. This finely tuned feedback loop can be disrupted at any point—by kidney disease, marrow damage, or a deficiency in iron or an essential vitamin. With an infection or an inflammatory state, erythropoietin secretion, iron delivery, and progenitor proliferation are all suppressed by inflammatory cytokines.

Recombinant human erythropoietin (*epoetin alfa*), produced using a mammalian cell line (Chinese hamster ovary cells), is virtually identical to endogenous hormone. Small differences in the carbohydrate portion of the molecule do not appear to affect the kinetics, potency, or immunoreactivity. Currently available preparations of epoetin alfa include EPOGEN and PROCRIT, supplied in single-use vials of from 2000 to 10,000 U/ml for intravenous or subcutaneous administration. When injected intravenously, epoetin alfa is cleared from plasma with a half-life of 10 hours. However, the effect on marrow progenitors is sufficiently sustained that it need not be given more often than three times a week to achieve an adequate response. No significant allergic reactions have been associated with the intravenous or subcutaneous administration of epoetin alfa, and antibodies have not been detected, even after prolonged administration.

Therapeutic Uses. Recombinant erythropoietin therapy can be highly effective in a number of anemias, especially those associated with a poor erythropoietic response. As first shown by Eschbach and coworkers in 1987, there is a clear dose-response

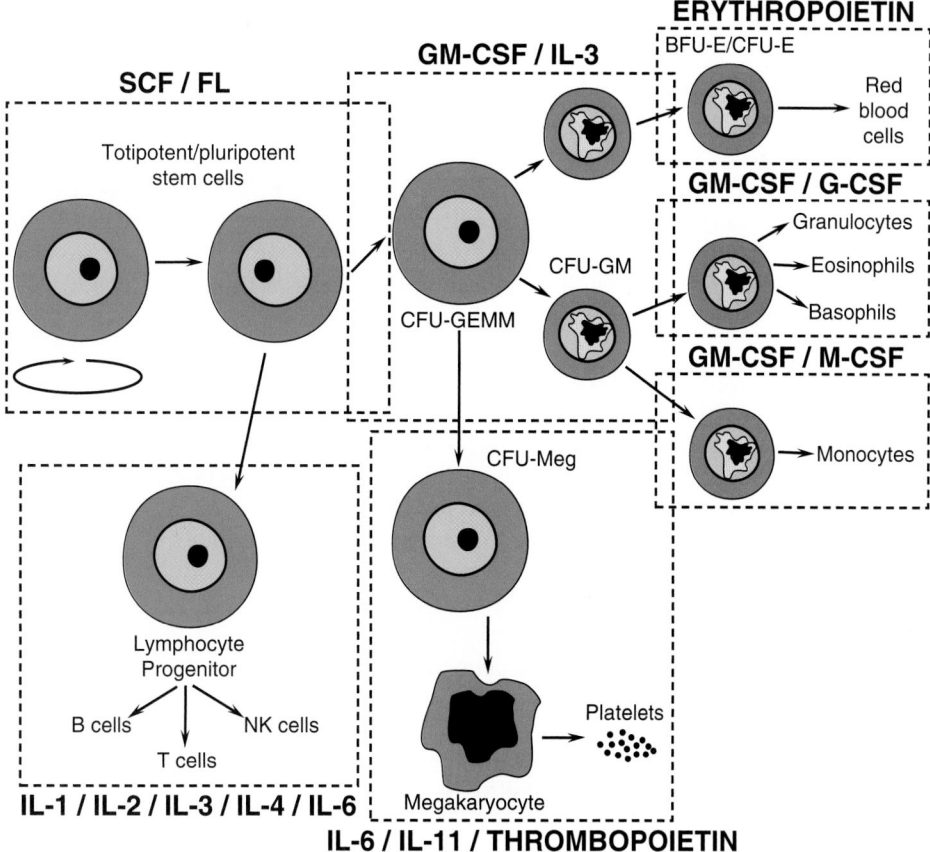

ERYTHROPOIETIN
BFU-E/CFU-E

SCF / FL

GM-CSF / IL-3

Totipotent/pluripotent
stem cells

Red
blood
cells

GM-CSF / G-CSF

Granulocytes

Eosinophils

Basophils

CFU-GM

CFU-GEMM

GM-CSF / M-CSF

Monocytes

CFU-Meg

Lymphocyte
Progenitor

B cells   NK cells

T cells

Platelets

IL-1 / IL-2 / IL-3 / IL-4 / IL-6

Megakaryocyte

IL-6 / IL-11 / THROMBOPOIETIN

Figure 54–1. Sites of action of hematopoietic growth factors in the differentiation and maturation of marrow cell lines.

A self-sustaining pool of marrow stem cells differentiates under the influence of specific hematopoietic growth factors to form a variety of hematopoietic and lymphopoietic cells. Stem cell factor (SCF), FTL-3 ligand (FL), interleukin-3 (IL-3), and granulocyte/macrophage colony-stimulating factor (GM-CSF), together with cell–cell interactions in the marrow, stimulate stem cells to form a series of burst-forming units (BFU) and colony-forming units (CFU): CFU-GEMM, CFU-GM, CFU-Meg, BFU-E, and CFU-E (GEMM, granulocyte, erythrocyte, monocyte, and megakaryocyte; GM, granulocyte and macrophage; Meg, megakaryocyte; E, erythrocyte). After considerable proliferation, further differentiation is stimulated by synergistic interactions with growth factors for each of the major cell lines—granulocyte colony-stimulating factor (G-CSF), monocyte/macrophage-stimulating factor (M-CSF), thrombopoietin, and erythropoietin. Each of these factors also influences the proliferation, maturation, and, in some cases, the function of the derivative cell line (*see* Table 54–1).

relationship between the epoetin alfa dose and the rise in hematocrit in anephric patients, with eradication of their anemia at higher doses. Epoetin alfa also has been shown to be effective in the treatment of anemias associated with surgery, AIDS, cancer chemotherapy, prematurity, and certain chronic inflammatory illnesses.

Anemia of Chronic Renal Failure. Patients with the anemia of chronic renal disease are ideal candidates for epoetin alfa therapy. The response in predialysis, peritoneal dialysis, and hemodialysis patients is dependent on severity of the renal failure, the erythropoietin dose and route of administration, and iron availability (Eschbach *et al.,* 1989; Kaufman *et al.,* 1998; Besarab *et al.,* 1999). The subcutaneous route of administration

is preferred over the intravenous, since absorption is slower and the amount of drug required is reduced by 20% to 40%. Iron supply is especially critical. Adequate iron stores, as reflected by an iron saturation of transferrin of at least 30% and a plasma ferritin greater than 400 μg/l, must be maintained, usually by repeated injections of iron dextran (*see* "Therapy with Parenteral Iron," in Section II, below).

The patient must be closely monitored during therapy, and the dose of epoetin alfa must be adjusted to obtain a gradual rise in the hematocrit, over a 2- to 4-month period, until a final hematocrit of 33% to 36% is reached. Treatment to hematocrit levels greater than 36% is not recommended. A study of patients treated to hematocrits above 40% showed a higher

Table 54–1
Hematopoietic Growth Factors

ERYTHROPOIETIN (EPO)
- Stimulates proliferation and maturation of committed erythroid progenitors to increase red cell production

STEM CELL FACTOR (SCF, c-kit ligand, Steel factor) and FLT-3 LIGAND (FL)
- Act synergistically with a wide range of other colony-stimulating factors and interleukins to stimulate pluripotent and committed stem cells
- FL also stimulates both dendritic and natural killer cells (anti-tumor response)
- SCF also stimulates mast cells and melanocytes

INTERLEUKINS (IL-1–12)
IL-1, IL-3, IL-5, IL-6, IL-9, IL-11
- Act synergistically with each other and SCF, GM-CSF, G-CSF, and EPO to stimulate BFU-E, CFU-GEMM, CFU-G, CFU-M, CFU-E, and CFU-Meg growth
- Numerous immunologic roles, including B cell and T cell growth stimulation
- IL-6 stimulates human myeloma cells to proliferate
- IL-6 and IL-11 stimulate BFU-Meg to increase platelet production

IL-5
- Controls eosinophil survival and differentiation

IL-1, IL-2, IL-4, IL-7, IL-12
- Stimulate growth and function of T cells, B cells, NK cells, and monocytes
- Co-stimulate B, T, and LAK cells

IL-8, IL-10
- Numerous immunological activities involving B and T cell functions
- IL-8 acts as a chemotactic factor for basophils and neutrophils

GRANULOCYTE/MACROPHAGE COLONY-STIMULATING FACTOR (GM-CSF)
- Acts synergistically with SCF, IL-1, IL-3, and IL-6 to stimulate CFU-G, CFU-M, and CFU-Meg to increase neutrophil and monocyte production
- With EPO may promote BFU-E formation
- Enhances migration, phagocytosis, superoxide production, and antibody-dependent cell-mediated toxicity of neutrophils, monocytes, and eosinophils
- Prevents alveolar proteinosis

GRANULOCYTE COLONY-STIMULATING FACTOR (G-CSF)
- Stimulates CFU-G to increase neutrophil production
- Enhances phagocytic and cytotoxic activities of neutrophils

MONOCYTE/MACROPHAGE COLONY-STIMULATING FACTOR (M-CSF, CSF-1)
- Stimulates CFU-M to increase monocyte precursors
- Activates and enhances function of monocyte/macrophages

MACROPHAGE COLONY-STIMULATING FACTOR (M-CSF)
- Stimulates CFU-M to increase monocyte/macrophage precursors
- Acts in concert with tissues and other growth factors to determine the proliferation, differentiation, and survival of a range of cells of the mononuclear phagocyte system

THROMBOPOIETIN (TPO, *Mpl* ligand)
- Stimulates stem cell differentiation into megakaryocyte progenitors
- Selectively stimulates megakaryocytopoiesis to increase platelet production
- Acts synergistically with other growth factors, especially IL-6 and IL-11

Abbreviations: BFU, burst-forming unit; CFU colony-forming unit; E, erythrocyte; G, granulocyte; M, macrophage; Meg, megakaryocyte; NK cells, natural killer cells; LAK cells, lymphokine-activated killer cells.

incidence of myocardial infarction and death (Besarab *et al.,* 1998). Furthermore, the drug should never be used to replace emergency transfusion in patients who need immediate correction of a life-threatening anemia.

It is currently recommended that the patient be started on a dose of 80 to 120 U/kg of epoetin alfa, given subcutaneously, three times a week. It can be given on a once-a-week schedule, but considerably more drug is required for an equivalent effect. If the response is poor, the dose should be progressively increased. The final maintenance dose of epoetin alfa can vary from as little as 10 U/kg to more than 300 U/kg, with an average close to 75 U/kg, three times a week, in most patients. Children under the age of 5 years generally require a higher dose. Resistance to therapy is commonly seen in the patient who develops an inflammatory illness or becomes iron deficient, so that close monitoring of general health and iron status is essential. Less common causes of resistance include occult blood loss, folic acid deficiency, carnitine deficiency, inadequate dialysis, aluminum toxicity, and osteitis fibrosa cystica secondary to hyperparathyroidism.

The most common side effect of epoetin alfa therapy is aggravation of hypertension, seen in 20% to 30% of patients and most often associated with a too-rapid rise in hematocrit. Blood pressure control usually can be attained by either increasing antihypertensive therapy or ultrafiltration in dialysis patients or by reducing the epoetin alfa dose to slow the hematocrit response. An increased tendency to vascular access thrombosis in dialysis patients also has been reported, but this remains controversial.

Anemia in AIDS Patients.   Epoetin alfa therapy has been approved for the treatment of HIV-infected patients, especially those on zidovudine therapy (Fischl *et al.,* 1990). Excellent responses to doses of 100 to 300 U/kg, given subcutaneously three times a week, generally are seen in patients with zidovudine-induced anemia. In the face of advanced disease, marrow damage, and elevated serum erythropoietin levels (greater than 500 IU/L), therapy is less effective.

Cancer-Related Anemias.   Epoetin alfa therapy, 150 U/kg three times a week or 450 to 600 U/kg once a week, can reduce the transfusion requirement in cancer patients undergoing chemotherapy. It also has been used to treat patients with multiple myeloma, with improvement in both their anemia and sense of well-being. Here again, a baseline serum erythropoietin level may help to predict the response.

Surgery and Autologous Blood Donation.   Epoetin alfa has been used perioperatively to treat anemia and reduce the need for transfusion. Patients undergoing elective orthopedic and cardiac procedures have been treated with 150 to 300 U/kg of epoetin alfa once daily for the 10 days preceding surgery, on the day of surgery, and for 4 days after surgery. As an alternative, 600 U/kg can be given on days −21, −14, and −7 prior to surgery, with an additional dose on the day of surgery. This can correct a moderately severe preoperative anemia, hematocrit 30% to 36%, and reduce the need for transfusion. Epoetin alfa also has been used to improve autologous blood donation (Goodnough *et al.,* 1989). However, as a routine, the potential benefit is small while the expense is considerable. Patients treated for 3 to 4 weeks with epoetin alfa (300 to 600 U/kg twice a week), are able to donate only 1 or 2 more units than untreated patients, and most of the time this goes unused. Still, the ability to stimulate erythropoiesis for blood storage can be invaluable in the patient with multiple alloantibodies to homologous red blood cells.

Other Uses.   Epoetin alfa has been designated an orphan drug by the United States Food and Drug Administration (FDA) for the treatment of the anemia of prematurity and patients with myelodysplasia. In the latter case, even very high doses of more than 1000 U/kg 2 to 3 times a week have had limited success. The possible use of very high dose therapy in other hematological disorders, such as sickle cell anemia, is still under study. Highly competitive athletes have used epoetin alfa to increase their hemoglobin levels ("blood doping") and improve performance. Unfortunately, this misuse of the drug has been implicated in the deaths of several athletes, and it should be discouraged.

MYELOID GROWTH FACTORS

The myeloid growth factors are glycoproteins that stimulate the proliferation and differentiation of one or more myeloid cell lines. They also enhance the function of mature granulocytes and monocytes. Recombinant forms of several of the growth factors have now been produced, including GM-CSF (Lee *et al.,* 1985), G-CSF (Wong *et al.,* 1985), IL-3 (Yang *et al.,* 1986), M-CSF or CSF-1 (Kawasaki *et al.,* 1985), SCF (Huang *et al.,* 1990), and, most recently, thrombopoietin (Lok *et al.,* 1994; de Sauvage *et al.,* 1994; Kaushansky *et al.,* 1994; Table 54–1).

The myeloid growth factors are produced naturally by a number of different cells including fibroblasts, endothelial cells, macrophages, and T cells (Figure 54–2). They are active at extremely low concentrations. GM-CSF is capable of stimulating the proliferation, differentiation,

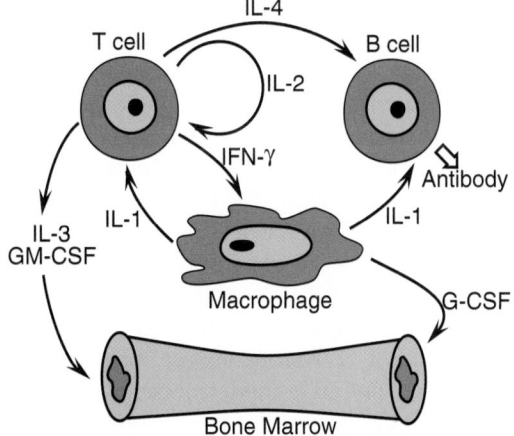

Figure 54–2. Cytokine–cell interactions.

Macrophages, T cells, B cells, and marrow stem cells interact *via* several cytokines [IL (interleukin)-1, IL-2, IL-3, IL-4, IFN (interferon)-γ, GM-CSF, and G-CSF] in response to a bacterial or a foreign antigen challenge. *See* Table 54–1 for the functional activities of these various cytokines.

and function of a number of the myeloid cell lineages (Figure 54–1). It acts synergistically with other growth factors, including erythropoietin, at the level of the BFU. GM-CSF stimulates the CFU-GEMM (granulocyte/erythrocyte/macrophage/megakaryocyte), CFU-GM, CFU-G, CFU-M, CFU-E, and CFU-Meg (megakaryocyte) to increase cell production. It also enhances the migration, phagocytosis, superoxide production, and antibody-dependent cell media toxicity of neutrophils, monocytes, and eosinophils.

The activity of G-CSF is more focused. Its principal action is to stimulate the proliferation, differentiation, and function of the granulocyte lineage. It acts primarily on the CFU-G, although it can also play a synergistic role with IL-3 and GM-CSF in stimulating other cell lines. G-CSF enhances phagocytic and cytotoxic activities of neutrophils. Unlike GM-CSF, G-CSF has little effect on monocytes, macrophages, and eosinophils. At the same time, G-CSF reduces inflammation by inhibiting IL-1, tumor necrosis factor, and interferon gamma.

Granulocyte/Macrophage Colony-Stimulating Factor (GM-CSF). Recombinant human GM-CSF *(sargramostim)* is a 127–amino acid glycoprotein produced in yeast. Except for the substitution of a leucine in position 23 and variable levels of glycosylation, it is identical to endogenous GM-CSF. While sargramostim, like natural GM-CSF, has a wide range of effects on cells in culture, its primary therapeutic effect is the stimulation of myelopoiesis. The initial clinical application of sargramostim was in patients undergoing autologous bone marrow transplantation. By shortening the duration of neutropenia, transplant morbidity was significantly reduced without a change in long-term survival or risk of inducing an early relapse of the malignant process (Brandt *et al.,* 1988; Rabinowe *et al.,* 1993). The role of GM-CSF therapy in allogeneic transplantation is less clear. The effect of the growth factor on neutrophil recovery is less pronounced in patients receiving prophylactic treatment for graft-versus-host disease (GVHD), and studies have failed to show a significant effect on transplant mortality, long-term survival, the appearance of GVHD, or disease relapse. However, it may improve survival in transplant patients who exhibit early graft failure (Nemunaitis *et al.,* 1990). It also has been used to mobilize CD34-positive progenitor cells for peripheral blood stem cell collection for transplantation following myeloablative chemotherapy. Sargramostim has been used to shorten the period of neutropenia and reduce morbidity in patients receiving intensive chemotherapy (Gerhartz *et al.,* 1993). It also will stimulate myelopoiesis

in some patients with cyclic neutropenia, myelodysplasia, aplastic anemia, or AIDS-associated neutropenia (Groopman *et al.,* 1987; Vadhan-Raj *et al.,* 1987).

Sargramostim (LEUKINE) is administered by subcutaneous injection or slow intravenous infusion at a dose of 125 to 500 $\mu g/m^2$ per day. Plasma levels of GM-CSF rise rapidly after subcutaneous injection and then decline, with a half-life of 2 to 3 hours. When given intravenously, infusions should be maintained over 3 to 6 hours. With the initiation of therapy, there is a transient decrease in the absolute leukocyte count secondary to margination and sequestration in the lungs. This is followed by a dose-dependent, biphasic increase in leukocyte counts over the next 7 to 10 days. Once the drug is discontinued, the leukocyte count returns to baseline within 2 to 10 days. When GM-CSF is given in lower doses, the response is primarily neutrophilic, while at larger doses, monocytosis and eosinophilia are observed. Following bone marrow transplantation or intensive chemotherapy, sargramostim is given daily during the period of maximum neutropenia until a sustained rise in the granulocyte count is observed. Frequent blood counts are essential to avoid an excessive rise in the granulocyte count. The dose may be increased if the patient fails to respond after 7 to 14 days of therapy. However, higher doses are associated with more pronounced side effects, including bone pain, malaise, flulike symptoms, fever, diarrhea, dyspnea, and rash. Patients can be extremely sensitive to GM-CSF, demonstrating an acute reaction to the first dose, characterized by flushing, hypotension, nausea, vomiting, and dyspnea, with a fall in arterial oxygen saturation due to sequestration of granulocytes in the pulmonary circulation. With prolonged administration, a few patients may develop a capillary leak syndrome, with peripheral edema and both pleural and pericardial effusions.

Granulocyte Colony-Stimulating Factor (G-CSF). Recombinant human G-CSF *(filgrastim,* NEUPOGEN) is a 175–amino acid glycoprotein produced in *Escherichia coli*. Unlike natural G-CSF, it is not glycosylated and carries an extra N-terminal methionine. The principal action of filgrastim is the stimulation of CFU-G to increase neutrophil production (Figure 54–1). It also enhances the phagocytic and cytotoxic functions of neutrophils.

Filgrastim has been shown to be effective in the treatment of severe neutropenia following autologous bone marrow transplantation and high-dose chemotherapy (Lieschke and Burgess, 1992). Like GM-CSF, filgrastim shortens the period of severe neutropenia and reduces morbidity secondary to bacterial and fungal infections. When used as a part of an intensive chemotherapy regimen, it can decrease the frequency of both hospitalization for febrile neutropenia and interruptions in the chemotherapy protocol. G-CSF also has proven to be effective in the treatment of severe congenital neutropenias. In patients with cyclic neutropenia, G-CSF therapy, while not eliminating the neutropenic cycle, will increase the level of neutrophils and shorten the length of the cycle sufficiently to prevent recurrent bacterial infections (Hammond *et al.,* 1989). Filgrastim therapy can improve neutrophil counts in some patients with myelodysplasia or marrow damage (moderately severe aplastic anemia or tumor infiltration of the marrow). The neutropenia of AIDS patients receiving zidovudine also can be partially or completely reversed. Filgrastim is now routinely used in the patient undergoing peripheral blood stem cell (PBSC) collection and a stem cell transplant. It encourages the release of CD34+ progenitor cells from the marrow, reducing the number of collections necessary for transplant. Moreover, filgrastim-mobilized PBSCs appear more capable of rapid engraftment. PBSC-transplanted patients require fewer days of platelet and red blood cell transfusions and a shorter duration of hospitalization than do patients receiving autologous bone marrow transplants.

Filgrastim is administered by subcutaneous injection or intravenous infusion over at least 30 minutes at a dose of 1 to 20 μg/kg per day. A usual starting dose in a patient receiving myelosuppressive chemotherapy is 5 μg/kg per day. The distribution and clearance rate from plasma (half-life of 3.5 hours) are similar for both routes of administration. A continuous 24-hour intravenous infusion can be used to produce a steady-state serum concentration of the growth factor. As with GM-CSF therapy, filgrastim given daily following bone marrow transplantation or intensive chemotherapy will increase granulocyte production and shorten the period of severe neutropenia. Frequent blood counts should be obtained to determine the effectiveness of the treatment. The dosage may need to be adjusted according to the granulocyte response, and the duration of therapy will depend on the specific application. In marrow transplantation and intensive chemotherapy patients, continuous daily administration for 14 to 21 days or longer may be necessary to correct the neutropenia. With less intensive chemotherapy, fewer than 7 days of treatment may be needed. In AIDS patients on zidovudine or patients with cyclic neutropenia, chronic G-CSF therapy often will be required.

Adverse reactions to filgrastim include mild to moderate bone pain in those patients receiving high doses over a protracted period, local skin reactions following subcutaneous injection, and, rarely, a cutaneous necrotizing vasculitis. Patients with a history of hypersensitivity to proteins produced by *E. coli* should not receive the drug. Marked granulocytosis, with counts greater than 100,000/μl, can occur in patients receiving filgrastim over a prolonged period of time. However, this is not associated with any reported clinical morbidity or mortality and rapidly resolves once therapy is discontinued. Mild to moderate splenomegaly has been observed in patients on long-term therapy.

The therapeutic roles of other growth factors still need to be defined. M-CSF may play a role in stimulating monocyte and macrophage production, though with sig-

nificant side effects, including splenomegaly and thrombocytopenia. Because of their primary effect on primitive marrow precursors, IL-3 and FL may be used in combination with GM-CSF and G-CSF. Administration of IL-3 followed by GM-CSF has been shown to give a greater neutrophil response than GM-CSF alone (Ganser *et al.,* 1992). This combination also may be more effective in promoting the release of marrow CD34+ stem cells in patients undergoing stem cell pheresis. SCF, IL-1, IL-6, IL-9, and IL-11 need to be studied alone and in combination with each other, as well as with both GM-CSF and G-CSF. The combination of IL-3 followed by GM-CSF also needs to be studied in protocols that include the reinfusion of harvested stem cells for their growth-promoting activity.

Thrombopoietin. The cloning and expression of a recombinant human thrombopoietin, a cytokine that selectively stimulates megakaryocytopoiesis, is another major milestone in the development of hematopoietic growth factors as therapeutic agents (Lok *et al.,* 1994; de Sauvage *et al.,* 1994; Kaushansky *et al.,* 1994). If future clinical trials live up to the early promise of the demonstrated ability of this new cytokine to increase rapidly the platelet count in animals (Harker, 1999), the combined use of thrombopoietin with G-CSF or GM-CSF together with erythropoietin will have a great impact in the treatment of primary hematological diseases and the anemia, neutropenia, and thrombocytopenia associated with high-dose chemotherapy. In a study of a small number of patients with gynecological cancers receiving carboplatin (Vadhan-Raj *et al.,* 2000), recombinant human thrombopoietin (rHuTPO) therapy reduced the duration of severe thrombocytopenia as well as the need for platelet transfusions. Larger, randomized, controlled trials are now under way to define fully the clinical merits and safety of rHuTPO. The optimal dose and schedule of administration in various clinical settings also need to be worked out. Both rHuTPO and pegylated recombinant human megakaryocyte growth and development factor (PEG-rHyMGDF) give delayed platelet responses. Following a single bolus injection, platelet counts show a detectable increase by day 4 and a peak response by 12 to 14 days. The platelet count then returns to normal over the next 4 weeks. The peak platelet response follows a log-linear dose response. Platelet activation and aggregation are not affected, and patients are not at increased risk of thromboembolic disease, unless the platelet count is allowed to rise to very high levels. These kinetics need to be taken into account when planning therapy in a chemotherapy patient.

II. Drugs Effective in Iron Deficiency and Other Hypochromic Anemias

IRON AND IRON SALTS

Iron deficiency is the most common cause of nutritional anemia in human beings. It can result from inadequate iron intake, malabsorption, blood loss, or an increased requirement, as with pregnancy. When severe, it results in a characteristic microcytic, hypochromic anemia. However, the impact of iron deficiency is not limited to the erythron (Dallman, 1982). Iron also is an essential component of myoglobin; heme enzymes such as the cytochromes, catalase, and peroxidase; and the metalloflavoprotein enzymes, including xanthine oxidase and the mitochondrial enzyme α-glycerophosphate oxidase. Iron deficiency can affect metabolism in muscle independently of the effect of anemia on oxygen delivery. This may well reflect a reduction in the activity of iron-dependent mitochondrial enzymes. Iron deficiency also has been associated with behavioral and learning problems in children and with abnormalities in catecholamine metabolism and, possibly, heat production (Pollit and Leibel, 1982; Martinez-Torres *et al.,* 1984). Awareness of the ubiquitous role of iron has stimulated considerable interest in the early and accurate detection of iron deficiency and in its prevention.

History. Iron has been used in the treatment of illness since the Middle Ages and the Renaissance. However, it was not until the sixteenth century that iron deficiency was recognized as the cause of "green sickness," or chlorosis, in adolescent women. Sydenham subsequently proposed iron as a preferred therapy over bleedings and purgings, and in 1832, the French physician Pierre Blaud recognized the need to use adequate doses of iron to successfully treat chlorosis. Blaud's nephew later distributed the "veritable pills of Blaud" throughout the world. The treatment of anemia with iron followed the principles enunciated by Sydenham and Blaud until the end of the nineteenth century. At that time the teachings of Bunge, Quincke, von Noorden, and others cast doubt on their treatment of chlorosis. The dose of iron employed was reduced, and the resulting lack of efficacy brought discredit on the therapy. It was not until the third and fourth decades of the twentieth century that the lessons taught by the earlier physicians were relearned.

The modern understanding of iron metabolism began in 1937 with the work of McCance and Widdowson on iron absorption and excretion and Heilmeyer and Plotner's measurement of iron in plasma. Then in 1947, Laurell described a plasma iron transport protein that he called *transferrin.* Hahn and coworkers (1943) were the first to use radioactive isotopes to quantitate iron absorption and define the role of the intestinal mucosa to regulate this function. In the next decade, Huff and associates (1950) initiated isotopic studies of internal iron metabolism. The subsequent development of practical clinical measurements of serum iron, transferrin saturation, plasma ferritin, and red

Table 54–2
The Body Content of Iron

	mg/kg of body weight	
	MALE	FEMALE
Essential iron		
Hemoglobin	31	28
Myoglobin and		
enzymes	6	5
Storage iron	13	4
Total	50	37

cell protoporphyrin permitted the definition and detection of the body's iron store status and iron-deficient erythropoiesis.

Iron and the Environment. Iron exists in the environment largely as ferric oxide or hydroxide or as polymers. In this state, its biological availability is limited unless it is solubilized by acid or chelating agents. For example, to meet their needs, bacteria and some plants produce high-affinity chelating agents that extract iron from the surrounding environment. Most mammals have little difficulty in acquiring iron; this is explained by an ample iron intake and perhaps also by a greater efficiency in absorbing iron. Human beings, however, appear to be an exception. Although total dietary intake of elemental iron in human beings usually exceeds requirements, the bioavailability of the iron in the diet is limited.

Metabolism of Iron. The body store of iron is divided between essential iron-containing compounds and excess iron, which is held in storage. From a quantitative standpoint, hemoglobin dominates the essential fraction (Table 54–2). This protein, with a molecular weight of 64,500 daltons, contains four atoms of iron per molecule, amounting to 1.1 mg of iron per milliliter of red blood cells (20 mM). Other forms of essential iron include myoglobin and a variety of heme and nonheme iron-dependent enzymes. Ferritin is a protein-iron storage complex, which exists as individual molecules or in an aggregated form. Apoferritin has a molecular weight of about 450,000 daltons and is composed of 24 polypeptide subunits; these form an outer shell within which resides a storage cavity for polynuclear hydrous ferric oxide phosphate. Over 30% of the weight of ferritin may be iron (4000 atoms of iron per ferritin molecule). Aggregated ferritin, referred to as *hemosiderin* and visible by light microscopy, constitutes about one-third of normal stores, a fraction that increases as stores enlarge. The two predominant sites of iron storage are the reticuloendothelial system and the hepatocytes, although some storage also occurs in muscle (Bothwell *et al.,* 1979).

Internal exchange of iron is accomplished by the plasma protein transferrin (Aisen and Brown, 1977). This β_1-glycoprotein has a molecular weight of about 76,000 daltons and two binding sites for ferric iron. Iron is delivered from transferrin to intracellular sites by means of specific transferrin receptors in the plasma membrane. The iron–transferrin complex binds to the receptor, and the ternary complex is taken up by receptor-mediated endocytosis. Iron subsequently dissociates in a pH-dependent fashion in an acidic, intracellular vesicular compartment (the endosomes), and the receptor returns the apotransferrin to the cell surface, where it is released into the extracellular environment (Klausner et al., 1983).

Human cells regulate their expression of transferrin receptors and intracellular ferritin in response to the iron supply. When iron is plentiful, the synthesis of transferrin receptors is reduced and ferritin production is increased. Conversely, with iron deficiency, cells express a greater number of transferrin receptors and reduce ferritin concentrations to maximize uptake and prevent diversion of iron to stores. Isolation of the genes for the human transferrin receptor and ferritin has permitted a better definition of the molecular basis of this regulation. Apoferritin synthesis is regulated by a system of cytoplasmic binding proteins (IRP-1 and -2) and an iron-regulating element on mRNA (IRE). When iron is in short supply, IRP binds to mRNA IRE and inhibits the translation of apoferritin. Conversely, when iron is abundant, binding is blocked and apoferritin synthesis increases (Klausner et al., 1993).

The flow of iron through the plasma amounts to a total of 30 to 40 mg per day in the adult (about 0.46 mg/kg of body weight) (Finch and Huebers, 1982). The major internal circulation of iron involves the erythron and the reticuloendothelial cell (Figure 54–3). About 80% of the iron in plasma goes to the erythroid marrow to be packaged into new erythrocytes; these normally circulate for about 120 days before being catabolized by the reticuloendothelium. At that time a portion of the iron is immediately returned to the plasma bound to transferrin, while another portion is incorporated into the ferritin stores of the reticuloendothelial cell and is returned to the circulation more gradually. Isotopic studies indicate some degree of iron wastage in this process, wherein defective cells or unused portions of their iron are transferred to the reticuloendothelial cell during maturation, bypassing the circulating blood. When there are abnormalities in maturation of red cells, the predominant portion of iron assimilated by the erythroid marrow may be rapidly localized in the reticuloendothelial cell as defective red cell precursors are broken down; this is termed *ineffective erythropoiesis*. With red cell aplasia, the rate of turnover of iron in plasma

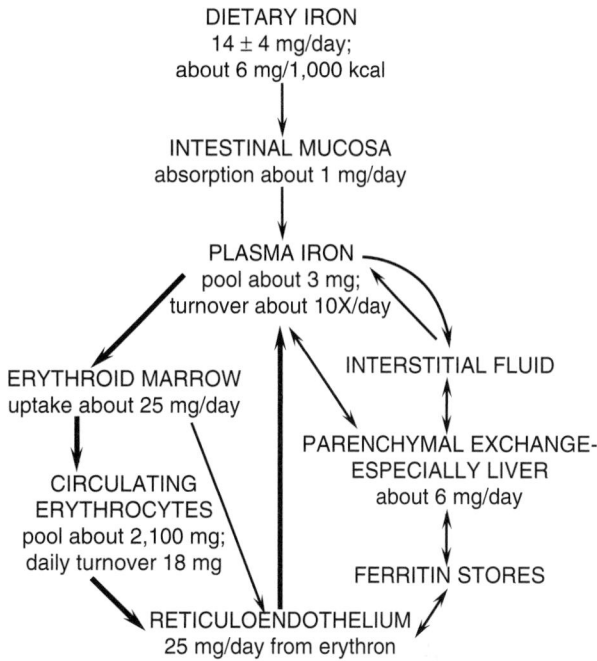

Figure 54–3. Pathways of iron metabolism in human beings (excretion omitted).

may be reduced by one-half or more, with all the iron now going to the hepatocyte for storage.

The most remarkable feature of iron metabolism is the degree to which the body store is conserved. Only 10% of the total is lost per year by normal men, *i.e.*, about 1 mg per day. Two-thirds of this iron is excreted from the gastrointestinal tract as extravasated red cells, iron in bile, and iron in exfoliated mucosal cells. The other third is accounted for by small amounts of iron in desquamated skin and in the urine. Physiological losses of iron in men vary over a narrow range, from 0.5 mg in the iron-deficient individual to 1.5 to 2 mg per day when excessive iron is consumed. Additional losses of iron occur in women due to menstruation. While the average loss in menstruating women is about 0.5 mg per day, 10% of normal menstruating women lose over 2 mg per day. Pregnancy imposes a requirement for iron of even greater magnitude (Table 54–3). Other causes of iron loss include the donation of blood, the use of antiinflammatory drugs that cause bleeding from the gastric mucosa, and gastrointestinal disease with associated bleeding. Much rarer are the hemosiderinuria that follows intravascular hemolysis and pulmonary siderosis, wherein iron is deposited in the lungs and becomes unavailable to the rest of the body.

The limited physiological losses of iron point to the primary importance of absorption as the determinant of the

Table 54–3
Iron Requirements for Pregnancy

	AVERAGE, *mg*	RANGE, *mg*
External iron loss	170	150–200
Expansion of red cell mass	450	200–600
Fetal iron	270	200–370
Iron in placenta and cord	90	30–170
Blood loss at delivery	150	90–310
Total requirement*	980	580–1340
Cost of pregnancy†	680	440–1050

*Blood loss at delivery not included.
†Iron lost to the mother; expansion of red cell mass not included.
SOURCE: After Council on Foods and Nutrition, 1968. Courtesy of the *Journal of the American Medical Association.* With permission.

body's iron content. Unfortunately, the biochemical nature of the absorptive process is understood only in general terms. After acidification and partial digestion of food in the stomach, its content of iron is presented to the intestinal mucosa as either inorganic iron or heme iron. These fractions are taken up by the absorptive cells of the duodenum and upper small intestine, and the iron is transported either directly into the plasma or stored as mucosal ferritin. Absorption appears to be regulated by two separate transporters: DCT1, which controls uptake from the intestinal lumen, and a second transporter, which governs movement of mucosal cell iron across the basolateral membrane to bind to plasma protein. Mucosal cell iron transport and the delivery of iron to transferrin from reticuloendothelial stores are both determined by the HFE gene, a novel MHC class 1 molecule localized to chromosome 6 (Peters *et al.,* 1993). Regulation is finely tuned to prevent iron overload in times of iron excess, while allowing for increased absorption and mobilization of iron stores with iron deficiency. Normal absorption is only about 1 mg per

day in the adult man and 1.4 mg per day in the adult woman, and 3 to 4 mg of dietary iron is the most that can be absorbed under normal conditions. Increased iron absorption is seen whenever iron stores are depleted or when erythropoiesis is increased and ineffective. Patients with hereditary hemochromatosis, secondary to a defective HFE gene, also demonstrate increased iron absorption, as well as loss of the normal regulation of iron delivery to transferrin by reticuloendothelial cells. The resulting increased saturation of transferrin opens the door to abnormal iron deposition in nonhematopoietic tissues.

Iron Requirements and the Availability of Dietary Iron. Iron requirements are determined by obligatory physiological losses and the needs imposed by growth. Thus, the adult man has a requirement of only 13 μg/kg per day (about 1 mg), whereas the menstruating woman requires about 21 μg/kg per day (about 1.4 mg). In the last two trimesters of pregnancy, requirements increase to about 80 μg/kg per day (5 to 6 mg), and the infant has similar requirements due to its rapid growth. These requirements (Table 54–4) must be considered in the context of the amount of dietary iron available for absorption.

In developed countries, the normal adult diet contains about 6 mg of iron per 1000 calories, providing an average daily intake for the adult male of between 12 and 20 mg and for the adult female of between 8 and 15 mg. Foods high in iron (greater than 5 mg/100 g) include organ meats such as liver and heart, brewer's yeast, wheat germ, egg yolks, oysters, and certain dried beans and fruits; foods low in iron (less than 1 mg/100 g) include milk and milk products and most nongreen vegetables. The content of iron in food is affected further by the manner of its preparation, since iron may be added from cooking in iron pots.

Although the iron content of the diet is obviously important, of greater nutritional significance is the bioavailability of iron in food (Hallberg, 1981). Heme iron is

Table 54–4
Daily Iron Intake and Absorption

SUBJECT	IRON REQUIREMENT, μg/kg	AVAILABLE IRON IN POOR DIET–GOOD DIET, μg/kg	SAFETY FACTOR, *available iron/ requirement*
Infant	67	33–66	0.5–1
Child	22	48–96	2–4
Adolescent (male)	21	30–60	1.5–3
Adolescent (female)	20	30–60	1.5–3
Adult (male)	13	26–52	2–4
Adult (female)	21	18–36	1–2
Mid-to-late pregnancy	80	18–36	0.22–0.45

far more available, and its absorption is independent of the composition of the diet. Heme iron, which constitutes only 6% of dietary iron, represents 30% of iron absorbed. Nevertheless, it is the availability of the nonheme fraction that deserves the greatest attention, since it represents by far the largest amount of dietary iron that is ingested by the economically underprivileged. In a vegetarian diet, nonheme iron is absorbed very poorly because of the inhibitory action of a variety of dietary components, particularly phosphates (Layrisse and Martinez-Torres, 1971). Two substances are known to facilitate the absorption of nonheme iron—ascorbic acid and meat. Ascorbate forms complexes with and/or reduces ferric to ferrous iron. While meat facilitates the absorption of iron by stimulating production of gastric acid, it is possible that some other effect, not yet identified, also is involved. Either of these substances can increase availability severalfold. Thus, assessments of available dietary iron should include not only the amount of iron ingested but also an estimate of its availability based on the intake of substances that enhance or inhibit its absorption and iron stores (Figure 54–4; Monsen *et al.,* 1978).

A comparison of iron requirements with available dietary iron is made in Table 54–4. Obviously, pregnancy and infancy represent periods of negative balance. The menstruating woman also is at risk, whereas iron balance in the adult man and nonmenstruating woman is reasonably secure. The difference between dietary supply and requirements is reflected in the size of iron stores.

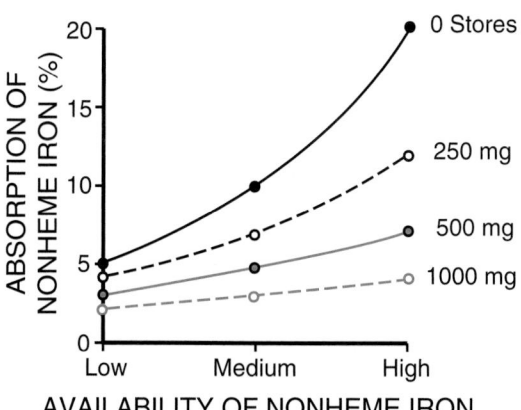

Figure 54–4. *Effect of iron status on the absorption of nonheme iron in food.*

The percentages of iron absorbed from diets of low, medium, and high bioavailability in individuals with iron stores of 0, 250, 500, and 1000 mg are portrayed. (After Monsen *et al.,* 1978. © *American Journal of Clinical Nutrition.* Courtesy of American Society for Clinical Nutrition. With permission.)

These will be low or absent when iron balance is precarious and high when iron balance is favorable (*see* Table 53–2). Thus, in the infant after the third month of life and in the pregnant woman after the first trimester, stores of iron are negligible. Menstruating women have approximately one-third the stored iron found in the adult man, indicative of the extent to which the additional average daily loss of about 0.5 mg of iron affects iron balance.

Iron Deficiency.   The prevalence of iron-deficiency anemia depends on the economic status of the population and on the methods used for evaluation. In developing countries, as many as 20% to 40% of infants and pregnant women may be affected (WHO Joint Meeting, 1975), while studies in the United States suggest that the prevalence of iron-deficiency anemia in adult men and women is as low as 0.2% to 3% (Cook *et al.,* 1986). Better iron balance has been achieved by the practice of fortifying flour, the use of iron-fortified formulas for infants, and the prescription of medicinal iron supplements during pregnancy.

Iron-deficiency anemia results from a dietary intake of iron that is inadequate to meet normal requirements (nutritional iron deficiency), blood loss, or some interference with iron absorption. Most nutritional iron deficiency in the United States is mild. Moderate-to-severe iron deficiency is usually the result of blood loss, either from the gastrointestinal tract or, in the woman, from the uterus. Impaired absorption of iron from food results most often from partial gastrectomy or malabsorption in the small intestine.

Iron deficiency in infants and young children can lead to behavioral disturbances and developmental delays. Chronic developmental defects may not be fully reversible. Iron deficiency in children also can lead to an increased risk of lead toxicity secondary to pica and an increased absorption of heavy metals. Premature and low-birth-weight infants are at greatest risk for developing iron deficiency, especially if they are not breast-fed and/or do not receive iron-fortified formula. After age 2 to 3, the requirement for iron declines until adolescence, when rapid growth combined with irregular dietary habits again increases the risk of iron deficiency. Adolescent girls are at greatest risk; the dietary iron intake of most girls ages 11 to 18 is insufficient to meet their requirements.

The recognition of iron deficiency rests on an appreciation of the sequence of events that lead to depletion of iron stores (Hillman and Finch, 1997). A negative balance first results in a reduction of iron stores and, eventually, a parallel decrease in red-cell iron and iron-related enzymes (Figure 54–5). In adults, depletion of iron stores may be recognized by a plasma ferritin

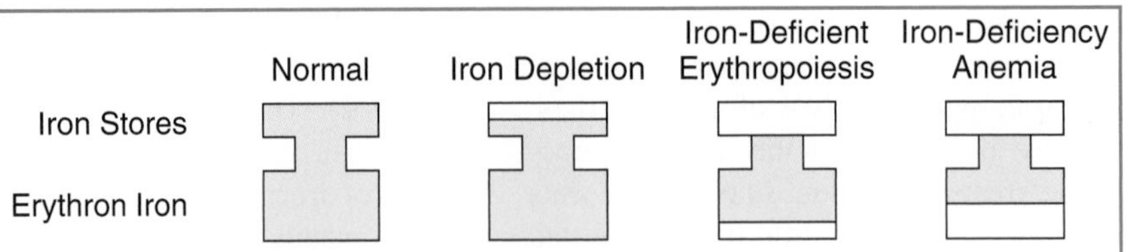

	Normal	Iron Depletion	Iron-Deficient Erythropoiesis	Iron-Deficiency Anemia
Iron Stores Erythron Iron				
RE marrow Fe	2–3+	0–1+	0	0
Transferrin μg/100 ml (μM)	330 ± 30 (59 ± 5)	360 (64)	390 (70)	410 (73)
Plasma ferritin, μg/l	100 ± 60	20	10	<10
Iron absorption, %	5–10	10–15	10–20	10–20
Plasma iron μg/100 ml (μM)	115 ± 50 (21 ± 9)	115 (21)	<60 (<11)	<40 (<7)
Transferrin saturation, %	35 ± 15	30	<15	<10
Sideroblasts, %	40–60	40–60	<10	<10
RBC protoporphyrin μg/100 ml RBC (μmol per liter RBC)	30 (0.53)	30 (0.53)	100 (1.8)	200 (3.5)
Erythrocytes	Normal	Normal	Normal	Microcytic/hypochromic

Figure 54–5. Sequential changes (from left to right) in the development of iron deficiency in the adult.

Rectangles enclose abnormal test results. RE marrow Fe, reticuloendothelial hemosiderin; RBC, red blood cells. (After Hillman and Finch, 1997, as modified from Bothwell and Finch, 1962. Courtesy of F.A. Davis Co. With permission.)

of less than 12 μg per liter and the absence of reticuloendothelial hemosiderin in the marrow aspirate. Iron-deficient erythropoiesis, defined as a suboptimal supply of iron to the erythron, is identified by a decreased saturation of transferrin to less than 16% and/or by an increase above normal in red-cell protoporphyrin. Iron-deficiency anemia is associated with a recognizable decrease in the concentration of hemoglobin in blood. However, the physiological variation in hemoglobin levels is so great that only about half the individuals with iron-deficient erythropoiesis are identified from their anemia (Cook *et al.,* 1976). Moreover, "normal" hemoglobin and iron values in infancy and childhood are different because of the more restricted supply of iron in young children (Dallman *et al.,* 1980).

The importance of mild iron deficiency lies more in identifying the underlying cause of the deficiency than in any symptoms related to the deficient state. Because of the frequency of iron deficiency in infancy and in the menstruating or pregnant woman, the need for exhaustive evaluation of such individuals usually is determined by the severity of the anemia. However, iron deficiency in the man or postmenopausal woman necessitates a search for a site of bleeding.

Although the presence of microcytic anemia is the most commonly recognized indicator of iron deficiency, laboratory tests—such as quantitation of transferrin saturation, red cell protoporphyrin, and plasma ferritin—are required to distinguish iron deficiency from other causes of microcytosis. Such measurements are particularly useful when circulating red cells are not yet microcytic because of the recent nature of blood loss, but iron supply is nonetheless limiting erythropoiesis. More difficult is the differentiation of true iron deficiency from iron-deficient

erythropoiesis due to inflammation. In the latter condition, the stores of iron are actually increased, but the release of iron from reticuloendothelial cells is blocked; the concentration of iron in plasma is decreased, and the supply of iron to the erythroid marrow becomes inadequate. The increased stores of iron in this condition may be demonstrated directly by examination of an aspirate of marrow or may be inferred from determination of an elevated concentration of ferritin in plasma (Lipschitz *et al.,* 1974).

Treatment of Iron Deficiency

General Therapeutic Principles. The response of iron-deficiency anemia to iron therapy is influenced by several factors, including the severity of anemia, the ability of the patient to tolerate and absorb medicinal iron, and the presence of other complicating illnesses. Therapeutic effectiveness can be best measured from the resulting increase in the rate of production of red cells. The magnitude of the marrow response to iron therapy is proportional to the severity of the anemia (level of erythropoietin stimulation) and the amount of iron delivered to marrow precursors. Studies by Hillman and Henderson (1969) demonstrated the importance of iron supply in governing erythropoiesis. Using phlebotomy to induce a moderately severe anemia (hemoglobin 7 to 10 g/dl), erythropoiesis was reduced to less than one-third of normal when the serum iron fell below 70 μg/dl. In contrast, red cell production levels increased to more than three times the basal rate when the serum iron was maintained between 75 and 150 μg/dl. Even higher levels of production were observed in patients with hemolytic anemias or ineffective erythropoiesis.

As regards oral iron therapy, the ability of the patient to tolerate and absorb medicinal iron is a very important factor in determining the rate of response. There are clear limits to the gastrointestinal tolerance for iron. The small intestine regulates absorption and, in the face of increasing doses of oral iron, limits the entry of iron into the bloodstream. Therefore, there is a natural ceiling on how much iron can be supplied by oral therapy. In the patient with a moderately severe iron-deficiency anemia, tolerable doses of oral iron will deliver, at most, 40 to 60 mg of iron per day to the erythroid marrow. This is an amount sufficient for production rates of two to three times normal.

Complicating illness also can interfere with the response of an iron-deficiency anemia to iron therapy. Intrinsic disease of the marrow can, by decreasing the number of red cell precursors, blunt the response. Inflammatory illnesses suppress the rate of red cell production, both by reducing iron absorption and reticuloendothelial release and by direct inhibition of erythropoietin and erythroid precursors. Continued blood loss can mask the response as measured by recovery of the hemoglobin or hematocrit.

Clinically, the effectiveness of iron therapy is best evaluated by tracking the reticulocyte response and the rise in the hemoglobin or the hematocrit. Since it takes time for the marrow to proliferate, an increase in the reticulocyte count is not observed for 4 to 7 days or more after beginning therapy. A measurable increase in the hemoglobin level takes even longer. A decision as to the effectiveness of treatment should not be made for 3 to 4 weeks after the start of treatment. An increase of 20 g per liter or more in the concentration of hemoglobin by that time should be considered a positive response, assuming that no other change in the patient's clinical status can account for the improvement. It also assumes that the patient has not been transfused during this time.

If the response to oral iron is inadequate, the diagnosis must be reconsidered. A full laboratory evaluation should be carried out, and such factors as the presence of a concurrent inflammatory disease or poor compliance by the patient must be assessed. A source of continued bleeding obviously should be sought. If no other explanation can be found, an evaluation of the patient's ability to absorb oral iron should be considered. There is no justification for merely continuing oral iron therapy beyond 3 to 4 weeks if a favorable response has not occurred.

Once a response to oral iron is demonstrated, therapy should be continued until the hemoglobin returns to normal. Treatment may be extended if it is desirable to establish iron stores. This may require a considerable period of time, since

the rate of absorption of iron by the intestine will decrease markedly as iron stores are reconstituted. The prophylactic use of oral iron should be reserved for patients at high risk, including pregnant women, women with excessive menstrual blood loss, and infants. Iron supplements also may be of value for rapidly growing infants who are consuming substandard diets and for adults with a recognized cause of chronic blood loss. Except for infants, in whom the use of supplemented formulas is routine, the use of "over-the-counter" mixtures of vitamins and minerals to prevent iron deficiency should be discouraged.

Therapy with Oral Iron. Orally administered ferrous sulfate, the least expensive of iron preparations, is the treatment of choice for iron deficiency (Callender, 1974; Bothwell *et al.*, 1979). Ferrous salts are absorbed about three times as well as ferric salts, and the discrepancy becomes even greater at high dosage (Brise and Hallberg, 1962). Variations in the particular ferrous salt have relatively little effect on bioavailability, and the sulfate, fumarate, succinate, gluconate, and other ferrous salts are absorbed to approximately the same extent.

Ferrous sulfate (*iron sulfate;* FEOSOL, others) is the hydrated salt, $FeSO_4 \cdot 7H_2O$, which contains 20% iron. *Dried ferrous sulfate* (32% elemental iron) also is available. *Ferrous fumarate* (FEOSTAT, others) contains 33% iron and is moderately soluble in water, stable, and almost tasteless. *Ferrous gluconate* (FERGON, others) also has been successfully used in the therapy of iron-deficiency anemia. The gluconate contains 12% iron. *Polysaccharide–iron complex* (NIFEREX, others), a compound of ferrihydrite and carbohydrate, is another preparation with comparable absorption. The effective dose of all of these preparations is based on iron content.

Other iron compounds have utility in fortification of foods. Reduced iron (metallic iron, elemental iron) is as effective as ferrous sulfate, provided that the material employed has a small particle size. Large-particle *ferrum reductum* and iron phosphate salts have a much lower bioavailability (Cook *et al.*, 1973), and their use for the fortification of foods is undoubtedly responsible for some of the confusion concerning effectiveness. *Ferric edetate* has been shown to have good bioavailability and to have advantages for maintenance of the normal appearance and taste of food (Viteri *et al.*, 1978).

The amount of iron, rather than the mass of the total salt in iron tablets, is important. It is also essential that the coating of the tablet dissolve rapidly in the stomach. Surprisingly, since iron usually is absorbed in the upper small intestine, certain delayed-release preparations have been reported to be effective and have been said to be even more effective than ferrous sulfate when taken with meals. However, reports of absorption from such preparations vary. Because a number of different forms of delayed-release preparations are on the market and information on their bioavailability is limited, the effectiveness of most such preparations must be considered questionable.

A variety of substances designed to enhance the absorption of iron has been marketed, including surface-acting agents, carbohydrates, inorganic salts, amino acids, and vitamins. One of the more popular of these is ascorbic acid. When present in an amount of 200 mg or more, ascorbic acid increases the absorption of medicinal iron by at least 30%. However, the increased uptake is associated with a significant increase in the incidence of side effects (Hallberg *et al.,* 1966); therefore, the addition of ascorbic acid seems to have little advantage over increasing the amount of iron administered. It is inadvisable to use preparations that contain other compounds with therapeutic actions of their own, such as vitamin B_{12}, folate, or cobalt, since the patient's response to the combination cannot be easily interpreted.

The average dose for the treatment of iron-deficiency anemia is about 200 mg of iron per day (2 to 3 mg/kg), given in three equal doses of 65 mg. Children weighing 15 to 30 kg can take half the average adult dose, while small children and infants can tolerate relatively large doses of iron—for example, 5 mg/kg. The dose used is a practical compromise between the therapeutic action desired and the toxic effects. Prophylaxis and mild nutritional iron deficiency may be managed with modest doses. When the object is the prevention of iron deficiency in pregnant women, for example, doses of 15 to 30 mg of iron per day are adequate to meet the 3- to 6-mg daily requirement of the last two trimesters. When the purpose is to treat iron-deficiency anemia, but the circumstances do not demand haste, a total dose of about 100 mg (35 mg three times daily) may be used.

The responses expected for different dosage regimens of oral iron are given in Table 54–5. However, these effects are modified by the severity of the iron-deficiency anemia and by the time of ingestion of iron relative to meals. Bioavailability of iron ingested with food is probably one-half or one-third of that seen in the fasting subject (Grebe *et al.,* 1975). Antacids also reduce the absorption of iron if given concurrently. It is always preferable to administer iron in the fasting state, even if the dose must be reduced because of gastrointestinal side effects. For patients who require maximal therapy to encourage a rapid response or to counteract continued bleeding, as much as 120 mg of iron may be administered four times a day. The timing of the dose is important. Sustained high rates of red cell production require an uninterrupted supply of iron. Oral doses should be spaced equally to maintain a continuous high concentration of iron in plasma.

The duration of treatment is governed by the rate of recovery of hemoglobin and the desire to create iron stores. The former depends on the severity of the anemia. With a daily rate of repair of 2 g of hemoglobin per liter of whole blood, the red

cell mass is usually reconstituted within 1 to 2 months. Thus, an individual with a hemoglobin of 50 g per liter may achieve a normal complement of 150 g per liter in about 50 days, whereas an individual with a hemoglobin of 100 g per liter may take only half that time. The creation of stores of iron is a different matter, requiring many months of oral iron administration. The rate of absorption decreases rapidly after recovery from anemia and, after 3 to 4 months of treatment, stores may increase at a rate of not much more than 100 mg per month. Much of the strategy of continued therapy depends on the estimated future iron balance of the individual. The person with an inadequate diet may require continued therapy with low doses of iron. The individual whose bleeding has stopped will require no further therapy after the hemoglobin has returned to normal. For the individual with continued bleeding, long-term, high-dose therapy is clearly indicated.

Untoward Effects of Oral Preparations of Iron. Intolerance to oral preparations of iron is primarily a function of the amount of soluble iron in the upper gastrointestinal tract and of psychological factors. Side effects include heartburn, nausea, upper gastric discomfort, constipation, and diarrhea. A good policy, particularly if there has been previous intolerance to iron, is to initiate therapy at a small dosage, to demonstrate freedom from symptoms at that level, and then gradually to increase the dosage to that desired. With a dose of 200 mg of iron per day divided into three equal portions, symptoms occur in approximately 25% of individuals, compared with an incidence of 13% among those receiving placebos; this increases to approximately 40% when the dosage of iron is doubled. Nausea and upper abdominal pain are increasingly common manifestations at high dosage. Constipation and diarrhea, perhaps related to iron-induced changes in the intestinal bacterial flora, are not more prevalent at higher dosage, nor is heartburn. If a liquid is given, one can place the iron solution on the back of the tongue with a dropper to prevent transient staining of teeth.

Toxicity caused by the long-continued administration of iron, with the resultant production of iron overload (hemochromatosis), has been the subject of a number of case reports (for example, *see* Bothwell *et al.,* 1979). Available evidence suggests that the normal individual is able to control absorption of iron despite high intake, and it is only individuals with underlying disorders that augment the absorption of iron who run the hazard of developing hemochromatosis. However, recent data indicate that hemochromatosis may be a relatively common genetic disorder, present in 0.5% of the population.

Iron Poisoning. Large amounts of ferrous salts of iron are toxic but, in adults, fatalities are rare. Most deaths occur in childhood, particularly between the ages of 12 and 24 months (Bothwell *et al.,* 1979). As little as 1 to 2 g of iron may cause

Table 54–5
Average Response to Oral Iron

TOTAL DOSE, mg of iron per day	*Estimated Absorption*		INCREASE IN HEMOGLOBIN, g/liter of blood per day
	%	*mg*	
35	40	14	0.7
105	24	25	1.4
195	18	35	1.9
390	12	45	2.2

death, but 2 to 10 g is usually ingested in fatal cases. The frequency of iron poisoning relates to its availability in the household, particularly the supply that remains after a pregnancy. The colored sugar coating of many of the commercially available tablets gives them the appearance of candy. All iron preparations should, therefore, be kept in childproof bottles.

Signs and symptoms of severe poisoning may occur within 30 minutes or may be delayed for several hours after ingestion. They consist largely of abdominal pain, diarrhea, or vomiting of brown or bloody stomach contents containing pills. Of particular concern are pallor or cyanosis, lassitude, drowsiness, hyperventilation due to acidosis, and cardiovascular collapse. If death does not occur within 6 hours, there may be a transient period of apparent recovery, followed by death in 12 to 24 hours. The corrosive injury to the stomach may result in pyloric stenosis or gastric scarring. Hemorrhagic gastroenteritis and hepatic damage are prominent findings at autopsy. In the evaluation of the child who is thought to have ingested iron, a color test for iron in the gastric contents and an emergency determination of the concentration of iron in plasma can be performed. If the latter is less than 63 μM (3.5 mg per liter), the child is not in immediate danger. However, vomiting should be induced when there is iron in the stomach, and an X-ray should be taken to evaluate the number of pills remaining in the small bowel (iron tablets are radioopaque). Iron in the upper gastrointestinal tract can be precipitated by lavage with sodium bicarbonate or phosphate solution, although the clinical benefit is questionable. When the plasma concentration of iron is greater than the total iron-binding capacity (63 μM; 3.5 mg per liter), deferoxamine should be administered; dosage and routes of administration are detailed in Chapter 67. Shock, dehydration, and acid-base abnormalities should be treated in the conventional manner. Most important is the speed of diagnosis and therapy. With early effective treatment, the mortality from iron poisoning can be reduced from as high as 45% to about 1%.

Therapy with Parenteral Iron. When oral iron therapy fails, parenteral iron administration may be an effective alternative (Bothwell *et al.*, 1979). The rate of response to parenteral therapy is similar to that which follows usual oral doses (Pritchard, 1966). Predictable indications are iron malabsorption (sprue, short bowel, *etc.*), severe oral iron intolerance, as a routine supplement to total parenteral nutrition, and in patients with renal disease who are receiving erythropoietin (Eschbach *et al.*, 1987). Parenteral iron also has been given to iron-deficient patients and pregnant women to create iron stores, something that would take months to achieve by the oral route. **Parenteral iron therapy should be used only when clearly indicated, since acute hypersensitivity, including anaphylactic and anaphylactoid reactions, can occur in from 0.2% to 3% of patients.** The belief that the response to parenteral iron, especially iron dextran, is faster than oral iron is open to debate (Pritchard, 1966). In otherwise healthy individuals, the rate of hemoglobin response is determined by the balance between the severity of the anemia (the level of erythropoietin stimulus) and the delivery of iron to the marrow from iron absorption and iron stores. When a large intravenous dose of iron dextran is given to a severely anemic patient, the hematologic response can exceed that seen with oral iron for 1 to 3 weeks (Henderson and Hillman, 1969). Subsequently, however, the response is no better than that seen with oral iron. This reflects the relative availability of the iron dextran stored in the reticuloendothelial system. Furthermore, inflammatory cytokines suppress both sources of iron supply equally, canceling any advantage.

Iron dextran injection (INFED, DEXFERRUM) is the parenteral preparation currently in general use in the United States. It is a colloidal solution of ferric oxyhydroxide complexed with polymerized dextran (molecular weight approximately 180,000), resulting in a dark brown, viscous liquid, containing 50 mg/ml of elemental iron. It can be administered by either intramuscular or intravenous injection. When given by deep intramuscular injection, it is gradually mobilized *via* the lymphatics and transported to reticuloendothelial cells; the iron is then released from the dextran complex. A variable portion (10% to 50%) may become locally fixed in the muscle for several weeks or months, especially if there is a local inflammatory reaction. Intravenous administration gives a more reliable response and is preferred. Given intravenously in a dose of less than 500 mg, the iron dextran complex is cleared exponentially with a plasma half-life of 6 hours. When 1 g or more is administered intravenously as total dose therapy, reticuloendothelial cell clearance is constant at 10 to 20 mg/hour. This slow rate of clearance results in a brownish discoloration of the plasma for several days and an elevation of the serum iron level for 1 to 2 weeks.

Once the iron is released from the dextran within the reticuloendothelial cell, it is either incorporated into stores or transported *via* transferrin to the erythroid marrow. The rate of release is variable. While a portion of the processed iron is rapidly made available to the marrow, a significant fraction is only gradually converted to usable iron stores (Henderson and Hillman, 1969). All of the iron is eventually released (Kernoff *et al.*, 1975), although many months are required before the process is complete. During this time, the appearance of visible iron dextran stores in reticuloendothelial cells can confuse the clinician who attempts to evaluate the iron status of the patient.

Intramuscular injection of iron dextran should only be initiated following a test dose of 0.5 ml (25 mg of iron). If no adverse reactions are observed, the injection can be given according to the following schedule until the calculated total amount required has been reached. Each day's dose should ordinarily not exceed 0.5 ml (25 mg of iron) for infants under 4.5 kg (10 lb), 1.0 ml (50 mg of iron) for children under 9.0 kg (20 lb), and 2.0 ml (100 mg of iron) for other patients. Iron dextran should be injected only into the muscle mass of the upper outer quadrant of the buttock using a z-track technique (displacement of the skin laterally prior to injection). However, local reactions, including long-continued discomfort at the site of injection and local discoloration of the skin, and the concern about malignant change at the site of injection (Weinbren *et al.*, 1978) make intramuscular administration inappropriate except when the intravenous route is inaccessible.

A test dose injection also should precede intravenous administration of a therapeutic dose of iron dextran. After establishing secure intravenous access, 0.5 ml of undiluted iron dextran or an equivalent amount (25 mg of iron) diluted in saline should be administered. The patient should be observed during the injection for signs of immediate anaphylaxis, and for an hour following injection for any signs of vascular instability or hypersensitivity, including respiratory distress, hypotension, tachycardia, or back or chest pain. When widely spaced, total-dose infusion therapy is employed, a test dose injection should be given prior to each infusion, since hypersensitivity can appear at any time. Furthermore, the patient should be closely monitored throughout the infusion for signs of cardiovascular instability. Delayed hypersensitivity reactions also are observed, especially in patients with rheumatoid arthritis or a history of allergies. Fever, malaise, lymphadenopathy, arthralgias, and urticaria can develop days or weeks following injection and last for prolonged periods of time. Therefore, iron dextran should be used with extreme caution in patients with rheumatoid arthritis, other connective tissue diseases, and during the acute phase of an inflammatory illness. Once hypersensitivity is documented, iron dextran therapy must be abandoned.

Before initiating iron dextran therapy, the total dose of iron required to repair the patient's iron-deficient state should be calculated. Factors to be taken into account are the hemoglobin deficit, the need to reconstitute iron stores, and continued excess losses of iron, as seen with hemodialysis and chronic gastrointestinal bleeding. A manufacturer-recommended formula for the calculation of the total treatment dose for an iron deficient anemia patient is as follows:

$$[0.0476 \times \text{lean body weight in kg} \times \text{hemoglobin deficit}]$$
$$+ 1 \text{ ml per 5 kg body weight (to maximum of 14 ml}$$
$$\text{to reconstitute iron stores)}$$
$$= \text{total dose in ml of iron dextran solution}$$

An alternative formula, which calculates the total dose in mg of iron, is as follows:

$$[0.66 \times \text{lean body weight in kg}] \times [100 - (\text{patient's hemoglobin}$$
$$\text{in g/dl} \times 100/14.8)] = \text{Total dose in mg of iron}$$

Iron dextran solution (50 mg/ml of elemental iron) can then be administered undiluted in daily doses of 2.0 ml until the total dose is reached or given as a single total-dose infusion. In the latter case, the iron dextran should be diluted in 250 to 1000 ml of 0.9% saline and infused over an hour or more.

When hemodialysis patients are started on erythropoietin, oral iron therapy alone is generally insufficient to guarantee an optimal hemoglobin response. It is recommended, therefore, that sufficient parenteral iron be given to maintain a plasma ferritin level between 100 and 800 μg/l and a percent saturation of transferrin between 20% and 50%. One approach is to administer an initial intravenous dose of 200 to 500 mg, followed by weekly or every-other-week injections of 25 to 100 mg of iron dextran to replace ongoing blood loss (Besarab *et al.*, 1999). With repeated doses of iron dextran—especially multiple total-dose infusions, as sometimes used in the treatment of chronic gastrointestinal blood loss—accumulations of slowly metabolized iron dextran stores in reticuloendothelial cells can be impressive. The plasma ferritin level also can rise to levels associated with iron overload. Whether this is of any clinical importance is un-

certain. While disease-related iron overload (hemochromatosis) has been associated with an increased risk of both infections and cardiovascular disease, this has not been shown to be true in hemodialysis patients treated with iron dextran (Owen, 1999). It seems prudent, however, to withhold the drug whenever the plasma ferritin rises above 800 μg/l.

Sodium ferric gluconate complex in sucrose (FERRLECIT) was approved by the FDA for use in the treatment of iron deficiency in patients undergoing chronic hemodialysis who are receiving supplemental erythropoietin therapy.

Reactions to intravenous iron include headache, malaise, fever, generalized lymphadenopathy, arthralgias, urticaria, and, in some patients with rheumatoid arthritis, exacerbation of the disease. Phlebitis may occur with prolonged infusions of a concentrated solution or when an intramuscular preparation containing 0.5% phenol is used in error. Of greatest concern, however, is the rare anaphylactic reaction, which may be fatal in spite of treatment. While only a few such deaths have been reported, it remains a deterrent to the use of iron dextran. Thus, there must be specific indications for the parenteral administration of iron.

COPPER

Copper deficiency is extremely rare in human beings (Evans, 1973). The amount present in food is more than adequate to provide the needed body complement of slightly more than 100 mg. There is no evidence that copper ever needs to be added to a normal diet, either prophylactically or therapeutically. Even in clinical states associated with hypocupremia (sprue, celiac disease, nephrotic syndrome), effects of copper deficiency usually are not demonstrable. However, anemia due to copper deficiency has been described in individuals who have undergone intestinal bypass surgery (Zidar *et al.*, 1977), in those who are receiving parenteral nutrition (Dunlap *et al.*, 1974), in malnourished infants (Holtzman *et al.*, 1970; Graham and Cordano, 1976), and in patients ingesting excessive amounts of zinc (Hoffman *et al.*, 1988). While an inherited disorder affecting the transport of copper in human beings (Menkes' disease; steely hair syndrome) is associated with reduced activity of several copper-dependent enzymes, this disease is not associated with hematological abnormalities.

Copper deficiency in experimental animals interferes with the absorption of iron and its release from reticuloendothelial cells (Lee *et al.*, 1976). The associated microcytic anemia is related both to a decrease in the availability of iron to the normoblasts and, perhaps even more importantly, to a decreased mitochondrial production of heme. It may be that the specific defect in the latter case is a decrease in the activity of cytochrome oxidase. Other pathological effects involving the skeletal, cardiovascular, and nervous systems have been observed in copper-deficient experimental animals (O'Dell, 1976). In human beings, the outstanding findings have been leukopenia, particularly granulocytopenia, and anemia. Concentrations of iron in plasma are variable, and the anemia is not always microcytic. When a low plasma copper concentration is determined in the presence of leukopenia and anemia and in a setting conducive to a deficiency of the element, a therapeutic trial with copper is appropriate. Daily doses up to 0.1 mg/kg of cupric sulfate have been given by mouth, or 1 to 2 mg per day may be added to the solution of nutrients for parenteral administration. Copper deficiency usually occurs concurrently with multiple nutritional deficiencies, so that its specific role in the production of anemia may be difficult to ascertain.

PYRIDOXINE

The first case of pyridoxine-responsive anemia was described in 1956 by Harris and associates. Subsequent reports suggested that the vitamin might improve hematopoiesis in up to 50% of patients with either hereditary or acquired sideroblastic anemias (Horrigan and Harris, 1968). Characteristically, these patients show an impairment in hemoglobin synthesis and an accumulation of iron in the perinuclear mitochondria of erythroid precursor cells, so-called ringed sideroblasts. Hereditary sideroblastic anemia is an X-linked recessive trait with variable penetrance and expression. Affected men typically show a dual population of normal red cells and microcytic, hypochromic cells in the circulation. In contrast, idiopathic acquired sideroblastic anemia and the sideroblastosis seen in association with a number of drugs, inflammatory states, neoplastic disorders, and preleukemic syndromes show a variable morphological picture. Moreover, erythrokinetic studies demonstrate a spectrum of abnormalities, from a hypoproliferative defect with little tendency to accumulate iron to marked ineffective erythropoiesis with iron overload of the tissues (Solomon and Hillman, 1979a).

Oral therapy with pyridoxine is of proven benefit in correcting the sideroblastic anemias associated with the antituberculosis drugs isoniazid and pyrazinamide, which act as vitamin B_6 antagonists. A daily dose of 50 mg of pyridoxine completely corrects the defect without interfering with treatment, and routine supplementation of pyridoxine is often recommended (see Chapter 48). In contrast, if pyridoxine is given to counteract the sideroblastic abnormality associated with administration of levodopa, the effectiveness of levodopa in controlling Parkinson's disease is decreased. Pyridoxine therapy does not correct the sideroblastic abnormalities produced by chloramphenicol and lead.

Patients with idiopathic acquired sideroblastic anemia generally fail to respond to oral pyridoxine, and those individuals who appear to have a pyridoxine-responsive anemia require prolonged therapy with large doses of the vitamin, 50 to 500 mg per day. Unfortunately, the early enthusiasm for treatment with pyridoxine was not reinforced by results of later studies (Chillar et al., 1976; Solomon and Hillman, 1979a). Moreover, even when a patient with sideroblastic anemia responds, the improvement is only partial, since both the ringed sideroblasts and the red cell defect persist, and the hematocrit rarely returns to normal. However, in view of the low toxicity of oral pyridoxine, a therapeutic trial with pyridoxine is appropriate.

As shown in studies of normal subjects, oral pyridoxine in a dosage of 100 mg three times daily produces a maximal increase in red cell pyridoxine kinase and the major pyridoxal phosphate–dependent enzyme glutamic-aspartic aminotransferase (Solomon and Hillman, 1978). For an adequate therapeutic trial, the drug must be administered for at least 3 months while the response is monitored by measuring the reticulocyte index and the concentration of hemoglobin. It has been suggested that the occasional patient who is refractory to oral pyridoxine may respond to parenteral administration of pyridoxal phosphate (Hines and Love, 1975). However, oral pyridoxine in doses of 200 to 300 mg per day produces intracellular concentrations of pyridoxal phosphate equal to or greater than those generated by therapy with the phosphorylated vitamin (Solomon and Hillman, 1979b). Pyridoxine is discussed further in Chapter 63.

RIBOFLAVIN

A pure red cell aplasia that responds to the administration of riboflavin was reported in patients with protein depletion and complicating infections (Foy et al., 1961). Lane and associates (1964) induced riboflavin deficiency in human beings and demonstrated that a hypoproliferative anemia resulted within a month. The spontaneous appearance in human beings of red cell aplasia due to riboflavin deficiency is undoubtedly rare, if it occurs at all. It has been described in combination with infection and protein deficiency, both of which are capable of producing a hypoproliferative anemia. However, it seems reasonable to include riboflavin in the nutritional management of patients with gross, generalized malnutrition. Riboflavin is discussed further in Chapter 63.

III. VITAMIN B_{12}, FOLIC ACID, AND THE TREATMENT OF MEGALOBLASTIC ANEMIAS

Vitamin B_{12} and folic acid are dietary essentials. A deficiency of either vitamin results in defective synthesis of DNA in any cell in which chromosomal replication and division are taking place. Since tissues with the greatest rate of cell turnover show the most dramatic changes, the hematopoietic system is especially sensitive to deficiencies of these vitamins. An early sign of deficiency is a megaloblastic anemia. Abnormal macrocytic red blood cells are produced, and the patient becomes severely anemic. Recognition of this pattern of abnormal hematopoiesis—more than 100 years ago—permitted the initial diagnostic classification of such patients as having "pernicious ane-mia" and spurred investigations that subsequently led to the discovery of vitamin B_{12} and folic acid. Even today, the characteristic abnormality in red blood cell morphology is important for diagnosis and as a therapeutic guide following administration of the vitamins.

History.   The discovery of vitamin B_{12} and folic acid is a dramatic story that starts more than 170 years ago and includes two Nobel prize–winning discoveries. The first descriptions of what must have been megaloblastic anemias came from the work of Combe and Addison, who published a series of case reports beginning in 1824. It is still common practice to describe megaloblastic anemia as Addisonian pernicious anemia. Although Combe suggested that the disorder might have some relationship to digestion, it was Austin Flint who, in 1860, first described the severe gastric atrophy and called attention to its possible relationship to the anemia. The name *progressive pernicious anemia* was coined in 1872 by Biermer, and this colorful term has persisted.

Following the observation by Whipple in 1925 that liver is a source of a potent hematopoietic substance for iron-deficient dogs, Minot and Murphy carried out their Nobel Prize–winning experiments that demonstrated the effectiveness of the feeding of liver to reverse pernicious anemia. Within a few years, Castle defined the need for both intrinsic factor, a substance secreted by the parietal cells of the gastric mucosa, and extrinsic factor, the vitamin-like material provided by crude liver extracts. However, nearly 20 years passed before Rickes and coworkers and Smith and Parker isolated and crystallized vitamin B_{12}; Dorothy Hodgkin then determined its crystal structure by X-ray

diffraction and subsequently received the Nobel prize for this work.

As attempts were being made to purify extrinsic factor, Wills and her associates described a macrocytic anemia in women in India that responded to a factor present in crude liver extracts but not in the purified fractions known to be effective in pernicious anemia (Wills *et al.,* 1937). This factor, first called Wills' factor and later vitamin M, is now known to be folic acid. The actual term *folic acid* was coined by Mitchell and coworkers in 1941, following its isolation from leafy vegetables.

More recent work has shown that neither vitamin B_{12} nor folic acid as purified from foodstuffs is the active coenzyme for human beings. During extraction procedures, active, labile forms are converted to stable congeners of vitamin B_{12} and folic acid, cyanocobalamin and pteroylglutamic acid, respectively. These congeners must then be modified *in vivo* to be effective. While a great deal has been learned about the intracellular metabolic pathways in which these vitamins function as required cofactors, many questions remain. The most important of these is the relationship of vitamin B_{12} deficiency to the neurological abnormalities that occur with this disorder (Chanarin *et al.,* 1985).

Relationships Between Vitamin B_{12} and Folic Acid. The major roles of vitamin B_{12} and folic acid in intracellular metabolism are summarized in Figure 54–6. Intracellular vitamin B_{12} is maintained as two active coenzymes: methylcobalamin and deoxyadenosylcobalamin (Linnell *et al.,* 1971). Deoxyadenosylcobalamin (deoxyadenosyl B_{12}) is a cofactor for the mitochondrial mutase enzyme

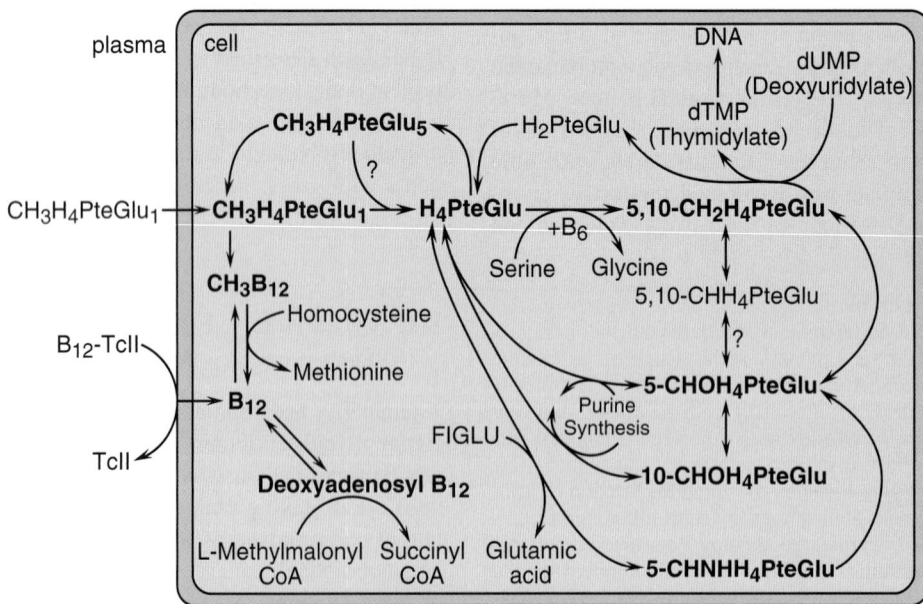

Figure 54–6. *Interrelationships and metabolic roles of vitamin B_{12} and folic acid.*

See text for explanation and Figure 54–9 for structures of the various folate coenzymes. FIGLU is formiminoglutamic acid, which arises from the catabolism of histidine. TcII is transcobalamin II.

that catalyzes the isomerization of L-methylmalonyl CoA to succinyl CoA, an important reaction in both carbohydrate and lipid metabolism (Weissbach and Taylor, 1968). This reaction has no direct relationship to the metabolic pathways that involve folate. In contrast, methylcobalamin (CH_3B_{12}) supports the methionine synthetase reaction, which is essential for normal metabolism of folate (Weir and Scott, 1983). Methyl groups contributed by methyltetrahydrofolate ($CH_3H_4PteGlu_1$) are used to form methylcobalamin, which then acts as a methyl group donor for the conversion of homocysteine to methionine. This folate–cobalamin interaction is pivotal for normal synthesis of purines and pyrimidines and, therefore, of DNA. The methionine synthetase reaction is largely responsible for the control of the recycling of folate cofactors; the maintenance of intracellular concentrations of folylpolyglutamates; and, through the synthesis of methionine and its product, S-adenosylmethionine, the maintenance of a number of methylation reactions.

Since methyltetrahydrofolate is the principal folate congener supplied to cells, the transfer of the methyl group to cobalamin is essential for the adequate supply of tetrahydrofolate ($H_4PteGlu_1$), the substrate for a number of metabolic steps. Tetrahydrofolate is a precursor for the formation of intracellular folylpolyglutamates; it also acts as the acceptor of a one-carbon unit in the conversion of serine to glycine, with the resultant formation of 5,10-methylenetetrahydrofolate ($5,10\text{-}CH_2H_4PteGlu$). The latter derivative donates the methylene group to deoxyuridylate (dUMP) for the synthesis of thymidylate (dTMP)—an extremely important reaction in DNA synthesis. In the process, the $5,10\text{-}CH_2H_4PteGlu$ is converted to dihydrofolate ($H_2PteGlu$). The cycle is then completed by the reduction of the $H_2PteGlu$ to $H_4PteGlu$ by dihydrofolate reductase, the step that is blocked by folate antagonists such as methotrexate (see Chapter 52). As shown in Figure 54–6, several other pathways also lead to the synthesis of 5,10-methylenetetrahydrofolate. These pathways are important in the metabolism of formiminoglutamic acid (FIGLU) and both purines and pyrimidines. (See reviews by Weir and Scott, 1983; Chanarin et al., 1985.)

In the presence of a deficiency of either vitamin B_{12} or folate, the decreased synthesis of methionine and S-adenosylmethionine interferes with protein biosynthesis, a number of methylation reactions, and the synthesis of polyamines. In addition, the cell responds to the deficiency by redirecting folate metabolic pathways to supply increasing amounts of methyltetrahydrofolate; this tends to preserve essential methylation reactions at the expense of nucleic acid synthesis. With vitamin B_{12} deficiency, methylenetetrahydrofolate reductase activity increases, directing available intracellular folates into the methyltetrahydrofolate pool (not shown in Figure 54–6). The methyltetrahydrofolate is then trapped by the lack of sufficient vitamin B_{12} to accept and transfer methyl groups, and subsequent steps in folate metabolism that require tetrahydrofolate are deprived of substrate. This process provides a common basis for the development of a megaloblastic anemia with deficiency of either vitamin B_{12} or folic acid.

The mechanisms responsible for the neurological lesions of vitamin B_{12} deficiency are less well understood (Reynolds, 1976; Weir and Scott, 1983). Damage to the myelin sheath is the most obvious lesion in this neuropathy. This observation led to the early suggestion that the deoxyadenosyl B_{12}-dependent methylmalonyl CoA mutase reaction, a step in propionate metabolism, is related to the abnormality. However, other evidence suggests that the deficiency of methionine synthetase and the block of the conversion of methionine to S-adenosylmethionine is more likely to be responsible (Scott et al., 1981).

Nitrous oxide (dinitrogen monoxide; N_2O), used for anesthesia (see Chapter 14), can cause megaloblastic changes in the marrow and a neuropathy that resemble those of vitamin B_{12} deficiency (Chanarin et al., 1985). Studies with N_2O have demonstrated a reduction in methionine synthetase and reduced concentrations of methionine and S-adenosylmethionine. The latter is necessary for methylation reactions, including those required for the synthesis of phospholipids and myelin. Significantly, the neuropathy induced with N_2O can be prevented partially by feeding methionine. A neuropathy similar to that occurring with vitamin B_{12} deficiency has been reported in dentists who are exposed to N_2O used as an anesthetic (Layzer, 1978).

VITAMIN B_{12}

Chemistry. The structural formula of vitamin B_{12} is shown in Figure 54–7 (Pratt, 1972). The three major portions of the molecule are:

1. A planar group or corrin nucleus—a porphyrin-like ring structure with four reduced pyrrole rings (A to D in Figure 54–7) linked to a central cobalt atom and extensively substituted with methyl, acetamide, and propionamide residues.

2. A 5,6-dimethylbenzimidazolyl nucleotide, which links almost at right angles to the corrin nucleus with bonds to the cobalt atom and to the propionate side chain of the C pyrrole ring.

3. A variable R group—the most important of which are found in the stable compounds cyanocobalamin and hydroxocobalamin and the active coenzymes methylcobalamin and 5-deoxyadenosylcobalamin.

The terms *vitamin B$_{12}$* and *cyanocobalamin* are used interchangeably as generic terms for all of the cobamides active in human beings. Preparations of vitamin B$_{12}$ for therapeutic use contain either cyanocobalamin or hydroxocobalamin, since only these derivatives remain active following storage.

Metabolic Functions.   The active coenzymes methylcobalamin and 5-deoxyadenosylcobalamin are essential for cell growth and replication. Methylcobalamin is required for the formation of methionine and its derivative *S*-adenosylmethionine from homocysteine. In addition, when concentrations of vitamin B$_{12}$ are inadequate, folate becomes "trapped" as methyltetrahydrofolate to cause a functional deficiency of other required intracellular forms of folic acid (*see* Figures 54–6 and 54–7 and discussion above). The hematological abnormalities that are observed in vitamin B$_{12}$–deficient patients are the result of this process (Herbert and Zalusky, 1962). 5-Deoxyadeno-

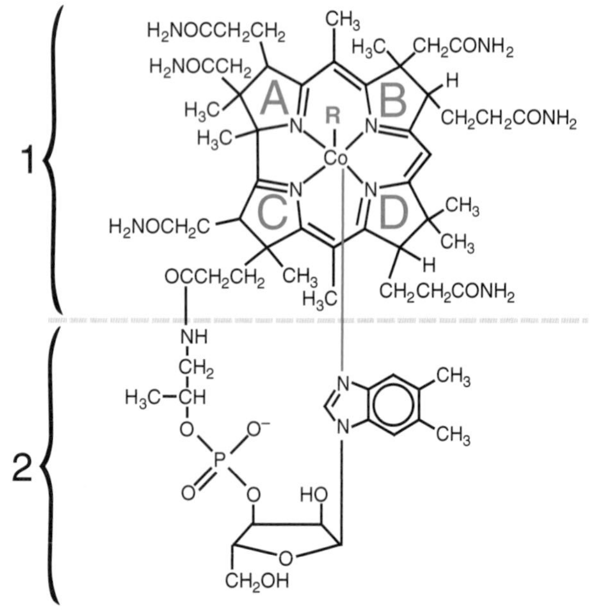

Vitamin B$_{12}$ Congeners

Permissive Name	R Group
Cyanocobalamin (Vitamin B$_{12}$)	–CN
Hydroxocobalamin	–OH
Methylcobalamin	–CH$_3$
5'Deoxyadenosylcobalamin	–5'Deoxyadenosyl

Figure 54–7. The structures and nomenclature of vitamin B$_{12}$ congeners.

sylcobalamin is required for the isomerization of L-methylmalonyl CoA to succinyl CoA (Figure 54–6).

Sources in Nature.   Human beings depend on exogenous sources of vitamin B$_{12}$. In nature, the primary sources are certain microorganisms that grow in soil, sewage, water, or the intestinal lumen of animals and that synthesize the vitamin. Vegetable products are free of vitamin B$_{12}$ unless they are contaminated with such microorganisms, so that animals are dependent on synthesis in their own alimentary tract or the ingestion of animal products containing vitamin B$_{12}$. The daily nutritional requirement of 3 to 5 μg must be obtained from animal by-products in the diet. At the same time, strict vegetarians rarely develop vitamin B$_{12}$ deficiency. Some vitamin B$_{12}$ is available from legumes, which are contaminated with bacteria capable of synthesizing vitamin B$_{12}$, and vegetarians generally fortify their diets with a wide range of vitamins and minerals.

Absorption, Distribution, Elimination, and Daily Requirements.   Dietary vitamin B$_{12}$, in the presence of gastric acid and pancreatic proteases, is released from food and salivary binding protein and bound to gastric intrinsic factor. When the vitamin B$_{12}$–intrinsic factor complex reaches the ileum, it interacts with a receptor on the mucosal cell surface and is actively transported into circulation. Adequate intrinsic factor, bile, and sodium bicarbonate (suitable pH) all are required for ileal transport of vitamin B$_{12}$ (Allen and Mehlman, 1973; Herzlich and Herbert, 1984). Vitamin B$_{12}$ deficiency in adults is rarely the result of a deficient diet *per se;* rather, it usually reflects a defect in one or another aspect of this complex sequence of absorption (*see* Figure 54–8). Achlorhydria and decreased secretion of intrinsic factor by parietal cells secondary to gastric atrophy or gastric surgery is a common cause of vitamin B$_{12}$ deficiency in adults. Antibodies to parietal cells or intrinsic factor complex also can play a prominent role in producing a deficiency. A number of intestinal diseases can interfere with absorption. Vitamin B$_{12}$ malabsorption is seen with pancreatic disorders (loss of pancreatic protease secretion), bacterial overgrowth, intestinal parasites, sprue, and localized damage to ileal mucosal cells by disease or as a result of surgery.

Once absorbed, vitamin B$_{12}$ binds to transcobalamin II, a plasma β-globulin, for transport to tissues. Two other transcobalamins (I and III) are also present in plasma; their concentrations are related to the rate of turnover of granulocytes. They may represent intracellular storage proteins that are released with cell death (Scott *et al.,* 1974). Vitamin B$_{12}$ bound to transcobalamin II is rapidly cleared from plasma and is preferentially distributed to hepatic

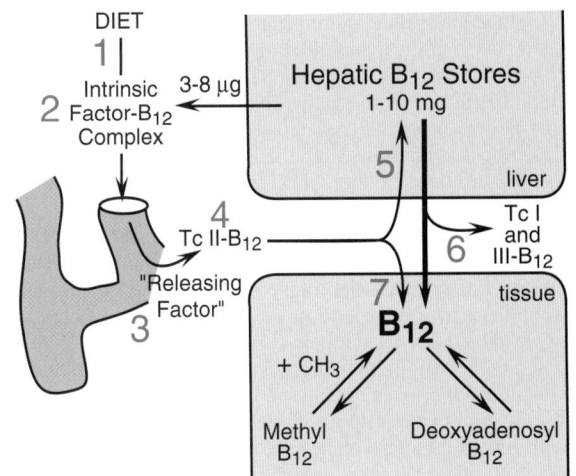

Figure 54–8. The absorption and distribution of vitamin B_{12}.

Deficiency of vitamin B_{12} can result from a congenital or acquired defect in any one of the following: (1) inadequate dietary supply; (2) inadequate secretion of intrinsic factor (classical pernicious anemia); (3) ileal disease; (4) congenital absence of transcobalamin II (Tc II); or (5) rapid depletion of hepatic stores by interference with reabsorption of vitamin B_{12} excreted in bile. The utility of measurements of the concentration of vitamin B_{12} in plasma to estimate supply available to tissues can be compromised by liver disease and (6) the appearance of abnormal amounts of transcobalamins I and III (Tc I and III) in plasma. Finally, the formation of methylcobalamin requires (7) normal transport into cells and an adequate supply of folic acid as $CH_3H_4PteGlu_1$.

parenchymal cells. The liver is a storage depot for other tissues. In the normal adult, as much as 90% of the body's stores of vitamin B_{12}, from 1 to 10 mg, is in the liver. Vitamin B_{12} is stored as the active coenzyme with a turnover rate of 0.5 to 8 μg per day, depending on the size of the body stores (Heyssel *et al.*, 1966). The recommended daily intake of the vitamin in adults is 2.4 μg. Recommended daily intakes are presented in Table XIII–2.

Approximately 3 μg of cobalamins is secreted into bile each day, 50% to 60% of which represents cobalamin analogs not destined for reabsorption. This enterohepatic cycle is important, since interference with reabsorption by intestinal disease can result in a continuous depletion of hepatic stores of the vitamin. This process may help explain why patients will develop vitamin B_{12} deficiency within 3 to 4 years after major gastric surgery, even though a daily requirement of 1 to 2 μg would not be expected to deplete hepatic stores of more than 2 to 3 mg during this time.

The supply of vitamin B_{12} available for tissues is directly related to the size of the hepatic storage pool and the amount of vitamin B_{12} bound to transcobalamin II (Figure 54–8). Since

the amount of vitamin B_{12} in liver cannot be measured easily, the concentration of vitamin B_{12} in plasma is the best routine measure of B_{12} deficiency. Normal individuals have plasma concentrations of the vitamin ranging from 150 to 660 pM (about 200 to 900 pg/ml). Deficiency should be suspected whenever the concentration falls below 150 pM. The correlation is excellent except when the concentrations of transcobalamin I and III in the plasma increase—for example, as a result of hepatic disease or a myeloproliferative disorder. Inasmuch as the vitamin B_{12} bound to these transport proteins has a very slow turnover rate and, therefore, is relatively unavailable to cells, tissues can become deficient at a time when the concentration of vitamin B_{12} in plasma is normal or even high (Retief *et al.*, 1967). A congenital absence of transcobalamin II has been observed in at least two families (Hakami *et al.*, 1971; Hitzig *et al.*, 1974). Megaloblastic anemia was present despite relatively normal concentrations of vitamin B_{12} in plasma. Clinical responses to doses of parenteral vitamin B_{12} that were sufficient to exceed renal clearance were observed.

Defects in intracellular metabolism of vitamin B_{12} have been reported in children with methylmalonic aciduria and homocystinuria. Mechanisms involved may include an incapacity of cells to transport vitamin B_{12} or accumulate the vitamin because of a failure to synthesize an intracellular acceptor, a defect in the formation of deoxyadenosylcobalamin, or a congenital lack of methylmalonyl CoA isomerase (Cooper, 1976).

Vitamin B_{12} Deficiency. Vitamin B_{12} deficiency is recognized clinically by its impact on both the hematopoietic and the nervous systems. The sensitivity of the hematopoietic system relates to its high rate of turnover of cells. Other tissues with high rates of cell turnover (*e.g.*, mucosa and cervical epithelium) have similar high requirements for the vitamin.

As a result of an inadequate supply of vitamin B_{12}, DNA replication becomes highly abnormal. Once a hematopoietic stem cell is committed to enter a programmed series of cell divisions, the defect in chromosomal replication results in an inability of maturing cells to complete nuclear divisions while cytoplasmic maturation continues at a relatively normal rate. This results in the production of morphologically abnormal cells and death of cells during maturation, a phenomenon referred to as *ineffective hematopoiesis* (Finch *et al.*, 1956). These abnormalities are readily identified by examination of the bone marrow and peripheral blood. Usually, the changes are most marked for the red cell series. Maturation of red cell precursors is highly abnormal (megaloblastic erythropoiesis). Those cells that do leave the marrow also are abnormal, and many cell fragments, poikilocytes, and macrocytes appear in the peripheral blood. The mean red cell volume increases to values greater than 110 fl (μm^3). When deficiency is marked, all cell lines may be affected, and a pronounced pancytopenia results.

The diagnosis of a vitamin B_{12} deficiency usually can be made using measurements of the serum vitamin B_{12}

level and/or serum methylmalonic acid level. The latter is somewhat more sensitive and has been used to identify metabolic deficiency in patients with normal serum vitamin B_{12} levels. As part of the clinical management of a patient with a severe megaloblastic anemia, a therapeutic trial using very small doses of the vitamin can be used to confirm the diagnosis. Serial measurements of the reticulocyte count, serum iron, and hematocrit are performed to define the characteristic recovery of normal red cell production. The Schilling test is used to quantitate the absorption of the vitamin and delineate the mechanism of the disease (Schilling, 1953). By performing the Schilling test with and without added intrinsic factor, it is possible to discriminate between intrinsic factor deficiency, by itself, and primary ileal cell disease.

Vitamin B_{12} deficiency can result in irreversible damage to the nervous system. Progressive swelling of myelinated neurons, demyelination, and neuronal cell death are seen in the spinal column and cerebral cortex. This causes a wide range of neurological signs and symptoms, including paresthesias of the hands and feet, diminution of vibration and position senses with resultant unsteadiness, decreased deep tendon reflexes, and, in the later stages, confusion, moodiness, loss of memory, and even a loss of central vision. The patient may exhibit delusions, hallucinations, or even an overt psychosis. Since the neurological damage can be dissociated from the changes in the hematopoietic system, vitamin B_{12} deficiency must be considered as a possibility in elderly patients with dementia and psychiatric disorders, even if they are not anemic (Lindenbaum *et al.*, 1988).

Vitamin B_{12} Therapy. Vitamin B_{12} is available in pure form for injection or oral administration or in combination with other vitamins and minerals for oral or parenteral administration. The choice of a preparation always must be made with recognition of the cause of the deficiency. Although oral preparations may be used to supplement deficient diets, they are of relatively little value in the treatment of patients with deficiency of intrinsic factor or ileal disease. Even though small amounts of vitamin B_{12} may be absorbed by simple diffusion, the oral route of administration cannot be relied upon for effective therapy in the patient with a marked deficiency of vitamin B_{12} and abnormal hematopoiesis or neurological deficits. Therefore, the preparation of choice for treatment of a vitamin B_{12}–deficiency state is cyanocobalamin, and it should be administered by intramuscular or deep subcutaneous injection.

Cyanocobalamin injection is a clear aqueous solution with a characteristic red color. Cyanocobalamin injection is safe when given by the intramuscular or deep subcutaneous route, but it should never be given intravenously. There have been rare reports of transitory exanthema and anaphylaxis following injection. If a patient reports a previous sensitivity to injections of vitamin B_{12}, an intradermal skin test should be carried out before the full dose is administered.

Cyanocobalamin is administered in doses of 1 to 1000 μg. Tissue uptake, storage, and utilization depend on the availability of transcobalamin II (*see above*). Doses in excess of 100 μg are rapidly cleared from plasma into the urine, and administration of larger amounts of vitamin B_{12} will not result in greater retention of the vitamin. Administration of 1000 μg is of value in the performance of the Schilling test. After isotopically labeled vitamin B_{12} is administered orally, the compound that is absorbed can be quantitatively recovered in the urine if 1000 μg of cyanocobalamin is administered intramuscularly. This unlabeled material saturates the transport system and tissue binding sites, so that more than 90% of the labeled and unlabeled vitamin is excreted during the next 24 hours.

A number of multivitamin preparations are marketed either as nutritional supplements or for the treatment of anemia. Many of these contain up to 80 μg of cyanocobalamin without or with intrinsic factor concentrate prepared from the stomachs of hogs or other domestic animals. One oral unit of intrinsic factor is defined as that amount of material that will bind and transport 15 μg of cyanocobalamin. Most multivitamin preparations supplemented with intrinsic factor contain 0.5 oral unit per tablet. While the combination of oral vitamin B_{12} and intrinsic factor would appear to be ideal for patients with an intrinsic factor deficiency, such preparations are not reliable. Antibodies to human intrinsic factor may effectively counteract absorption of vitamin B_{12}. With prolonged therapy, some patients develop refractoriness to oral intrinsic factor, perhaps related to production of an intraluminal antibody against the hog protein (Ramsey and Herbert, 1965). Patients taking such preparations must be reevaluated at periodic intervals for recurrence of pernicious anemia.

Hydroxocobalamin given in doses of 100 μg intramuscularly has been reported to have a more sustained effect than cyanocobalamin, with a single dose maintaining plasma vitamin B_{12} concentrations in the normal range for up to 3 months. However, some patients show reductions of the concentration of vitamin B_{12} in plasma within 30 days, similar to that seen after cyanocobalamin. Furthermore, the administration of hydroxocobalamin has resulted in the formation of antibodies to the transcobalamin II–vitamin B_{12} complex (Skouby *et al.*, 1971).

Vitamin B_{12} has an undeserved reputation as a health tonic and has been used for a number of diverse disease states. Effective use of the vitamin depends on accurate diagnosis and an understanding of the following general principles of therapy:

1. Vitamin B_{12} should be given prophylactically only when there is a reasonable probability that a deficiency exists. Dietary deficiency in the strict vegetarian, the predictable malabsorption of vitamin B_{12} in patients who have had a gastrectomy, and certain diseases of the small intestine constitute such indications. When gastrointestinal function is normal, an oral prophylactic supplement of vitamins and minerals, including vitamin B_{12}, may be indicated. Otherwise, the patient should receive monthly injections of cyanocobalamin.

2. The relative ease of treatment with vitamin B_{12} should not prevent a full investigation of the etiology of the deficiency. The initial diagnosis is usually suggested by a macrocytic anemia or an unexplained neuropsychiatric disorder. Full understanding of the etiology of vitamin B_{12} deficiency involves studies of dietary supply, gastrointestinal absorption, and transport.

3. Therapy always should be as specific as possible. While a large number of multivitamin preparations are available, the use of "shotgun" vitamin therapy in the treatment of vitamin B_{12} deficiency can be dangerous. With such therapy, there is the danger that sufficient folic acid will be given to result in a hematological recovery. This can mask continued vitamin B_{12} deficiency and permit neurological damage to develop or progress.

4. Although a classical therapeutic trial with small amounts of vitamin B_{12} can help confirm the diagnosis, the acutely ill, elderly patients may not be able to tolerate the delay in the correction of a severe anemia. Such patients require supplemental blood transfusions and immediate therapy with both folic acid and vitamin B_{12} to guarantee rapid recovery.

5. Long-term therapy with vitamin B_{12} must be evaluated at intervals of 6 to 12 months in patients who are otherwise well. If there is an additional illness or a condition that may increase the requirement for the vitamin (*e.g.*, pregnancy), reassessment should be performed more frequently.

Treatment of the Acutely Ill Patient. The therapeutic approach depends on the severity of the patient's illness. The individual with uncomplicated pernicious anemia, in which the abnormality is restricted to a mild or moderate anemia without leukopenia, thrombocytopenia, or neurological signs or symptoms, will respond to the administration of vitamin B_{12} alone. Moreover, therapy may be delayed until other causes of megaloblastic anemia have been ruled out and sufficient studies of gastrointestinal function have been performed to reveal the underlying cause of the disease. In this situation, a therapeutic trial with small amounts of parenteral vitamin B_{12} (1 to 10 μg per day) can confirm the presence of an uncomplicated vitamin B_{12} deficiency.

In contrast, patients with neurological changes or severe leukopenia or thrombocytopenia associated with infection or bleeding require emergency treatment. The older individual with a severe anemia (hematocrit less than 20%) is likely to have tissue hypoxia, cerebrovascular insufficiency, and congestive heart failure. Effective therapy must not wait for detailed diagnostic tests. Once the megaloblastic erythropoiesis has been confirmed and sufficient blood collected for later measurements of concentrations of vitamin B_{12} and folic acid, the patient should receive intramuscular injections of 100 μg of cyanocobalamin and 1 to 5 mg of folic acid. For the next 1 to 2 weeks the patient should receive daily intramuscular injections of 100 μg of cyanocobalamin, together with a daily oral supplement of 1 to 2 mg of folic acid. Since an effective increase in red cell mass will not

occur for 10 to 20 days, the patient with a markedly depressed hematocrit and tissue hypoxia also should receive a transfusion of 2 to 3 units of packed red cells. If congestive heart failure is present, phlebotomy to remove an equal volume of whole blood can be performed or diuretics can be administered to prevent volume overload.

The therapeutic response to vitamin B_{12} is characterized by a number of subjective and objective changes. Patients usually report an increased sense of well-being within the first 24 hours after the initiation of therapy. Objectively, memory and orientation can show dramatic improvement, although full recovery of mental function may take months or, in fact, may never occur. In addition, even before an obvious hematological response is apparent, the patient may report an increase in strength, a better appetite, and reduced soreness of the mouth and tongue.

The first objective hematological change is the disappearance of the megaloblastic morphology of the bone marrow. As the ineffective erythropoiesis is corrected, the concentration of iron in plasma falls dramatically as the metal is used in the formation of hemoglobin. This usually occurs within the first 48 hours. Full correction of precursor maturation in marrow with production of an increased number of reticulocytes begins about the second or third day and reaches a peak three to five days later. When the anemia is moderate to severe, the maximal reticulocyte index will be between three and five times the normal value—*i.e.*, a reticulocyte count of 20% to 40%. The ability of the marrow to sustain a high rate of production determines the rate of recovery of the hematocrit. Patients with complicating iron deficiency, an infection or other inflammatory state, or renal disease may be unable to correct their anemia. It is important, therefore, to monitor the reticulocyte index over the first several weeks. If it does not continue at elevated levels while the hematocrit is less than 35%, plasma concentrations of iron and folic acid should again be determined and the patient reevaluated for an illness that could inhibit the response of the marrow.

The degree and rate of improvement of neurological signs and symptoms depend on the severity and the duration of the abnormalities. Those that have been present for only a few months are likely to disappear relatively rapidly. When a defect has been present for many months or years, full return to normal function may never occur.

Long-Term Therapy with Vitamin B_{12}. Once begun, vitamin B_{12} therapy must be maintained for life. This fact must be impressed upon the patient and family and a system established to guarantee continued monthly injections of cyanocobalamin. An intramuscular injection of 100 μg of cyanocobalamin every 4 weeks is sufficient to maintain a normal concentration of vitamin B_{12} in plasma and an adequate supply for tissues. Patients with severe neurological symptoms and signs may be treated with larger doses of vitamin B_{12} in the period immediately following the diagnosis. Doses of 100 μg per day or several times per week may be given for several months with the hope of encouraging faster and more complete recovery. It is important to monitor vitamin B_{12} concentrations in plasma and to obtain peripheral blood counts at intervals of 3 to 6 months to confirm the adequacy of therapy. Since refractoriness to therapy can develop at any time, evaluation must continue throughout the patient's life.

Other Therapeutic Uses of Vitamin B_{12}. Vitamin B_{12} has been used in the therapy of a number of conditions, including trigeminal neuralgia, multiple sclerosis and other neuropathies, various

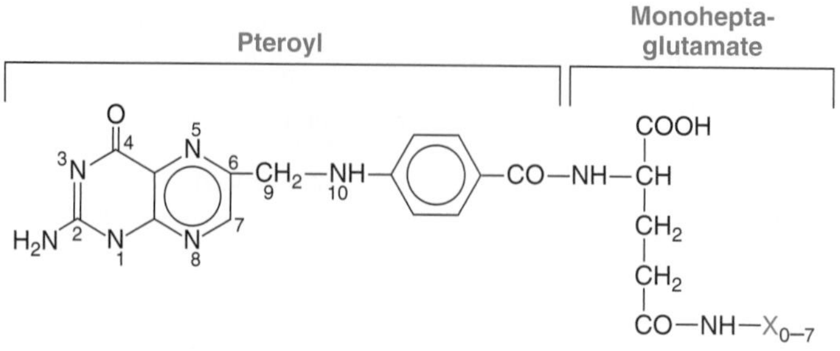

Position	Radical		Congener
N^5	$-CH_3$	$CH_3H_4PteGlu$	Methyltetrahydrofolate
N^5	$-CHO$	$5\text{-}CHOH_4PteGlu$	Folinic acid (citrovorum factor)
N^{10}	$-CHO$	$10\text{-}CHOH_4PteGlu$	10-Formyltetrahydrofolate
N^{5-10}	$-CH-$	$5,10\text{-}CHH_4PteGlu$	5,10-Methenyltetrahydrofolate
N^{5-10}	$-CH_2-$	$5,10\text{-}CH_2H_4PteGlu$	5,10-Methylenetetrahydrofolate
N^5	$-CHNH$	$CHNHH_4PteGlu$	Formiminotetrahydrofolate
N^{10}	$-CH_2OH$	$CH_2OHH_4PteGlu$	Hydroxymethyltetrahydrofolate

Figure 54–9. The structures and nomenclature of pteroylglutamic acid (folic acid) and congeners.

X represents additional residues of glutamate; polyglutamates are the storage and active forms of the vitamin. The subscript that designates the number of residues of glutamate is frequently omitted because this number is variable.

psychiatric disorders, poor growth or nutrition, and as a "tonic" for patients complaining of tiredness or easy fatigability. There is no evidence for the validity of such therapy in any of these conditions. Maintenance therapy with vitamin B_{12} has been used with some apparent success in the treatment of children with methylmalonic aciduria (Cooper, 1976).

FOLIC ACID

Chemistry and Metabolic Functions. The structural formula of pteroylglutamic acid (PteGlu) is shown in Figure 54–9. Major portions of the molecule include a pteridine ring linked by a methylene bridge to paraaminobenzoic acid, which is joined by an amide linkage to glutamic acid. While pteroylglutamic acid is the common pharmaceutical form of folic acid, it is neither the principal folate congener in food nor the active coenzyme for intracellular metabolism. Following absorption, PteGlu is rapidly reduced at the 5, 6, 7, and 8 positions to tetrahydrofolic acid ($H_4PteGlu$), which then acts as an acceptor of a number of one-carbon units. These are attached at either the 5 or the 10 position of the pteridine ring or may bridge these atoms to form a new five-membered ring. The most important forms of the coenzyme that are synthesized by these reactions are listed in Figure 54–9. Each plays a specific role in intracellular metabolism, summarized as follows (*see also* "Relationships Between Vitamin B_{12} and Folic Acid," above, as well as Figure 54–6):

1. *Conversion of homocysteine to methionine.* This reaction requires $CH_3H_4PteGlu$ as a methyl donor and utilizes vitamin B_{12} as a cofactor.
2. *Conversion of serine to glycine.* This reaction requires tetrahydrofolate as an acceptor of a methylene group from serine

and utilizes pyridoxal phosphate as a cofactor. It results in the formation of $5,10\text{-}CH_2H_4PteGlu$, an essential coenzyme for the synthesis of thymidylate.
3. *Synthesis of thymidylate.* $5,10\text{-}CH_2H_4PteGlu$ donates a methylene group and reducing equivalents to deoxyuridylate for the synthesis of thymidylate—a rate-limiting step in DNA synthesis.
4. *Histidine metabolism.* $H_4PteGlu$ also acts as an acceptor of a formimino group in the conversion of formiminoglutamic acid to glutamic acid.
5. *Synthesis of purines.* Two steps in the synthesis of purine nucleotides require the participation of derivatives of folic acid. Glycinamide ribonucleotide is formylated by $5,10\text{-}CHH_4PteGlu$; 5-aminoimidazole-4-carboxamide ribonucleotide is formylated by $10\text{-}CHOH_4PteGlu$. By these reactions, carbon atoms at positions 8 and 2, respectively, are incorporated into the growing purine ring.
6. *Utilization or generation of formate.* This reversible reaction utilizes $H_4PteGlu$ and $10\text{-}CHOH_4PteGlu$.

Daily Requirements. Many food sources are rich in folates, especially fresh green vegetables, liver, yeast, and some fruits. However, lengthy cooking can destroy up to 90% of the folate content of such food. Generally, a standard U.S. diet provides 50 to 500 μg of absorbable folate per day, although individuals with high intakes of fresh vegetables and meats will ingest as much as 2 mg per day. In the normal adult, the recommended daily intake is 400 μg, while pregnant or lactating women and patients with high rates of cell turnover (such as patients with a hemolytic anemia) may require 500 to 600 μg or more per day. Recommended daily intakes of folate are presented in Table XIII–2. For the prevention of neural tube defects, a daily intake of at least 400 μg of folate in food or in supplements beginning a month before pregnancy and continued for at least the first trimester is recommended. Folate supplementation also is being considered in patients with elevated levels of plasma homocysteine.

Absorption, Distribution, and Elimination.   As with vitamin B_{12}, the diagnosis and management of deficiencies of folic acid depend on an understanding of the transport pathways and intracellular metabolism of the vitamin (Figure 54–10). Folates present in food are largely in the form of reduced polyglutamates (Tamura and Stokstad, 1973), and absorption requires transport and the action of a pteroyl-γ-glutamyl carboxypeptidase associated with mucosal cell membranes (Rosenberg, 1976). The mucosae of the duodenum and upper part of the jejunum are rich in dihydrofolate reductase and are capable of methylating most

or all of the reduced folate that is absorbed. Since most absorption occurs in the proximal portion of the small intestine, it is not unusual for folate deficiency to occur when the jejunum is diseased. Nontropical and tropical sprue are common causes of folate deficiency and megaloblastic anemia.

Once absorbed, folate is transported rapidly to tissues as $CH_3H_4PteGlu$. While certain plasma proteins do bind folate derivatives, they have a greater affinity for nonmethylated analogs. The role of such binding proteins in folate homeostasis is not well understood. An increase in binding capacity is detectable in folate deficiency and in certain disease states, such as uremia, cancer, and alcoholism, but how binding affects transport and tissue supply requires further investigation.

A constant supply of $CH_3H_4PteGlu$ is maintained by food and by an enterohepatic cycle of the vitamin. The liver actively reduces and methylates PteGlu (and H_2 or $H_4PteGlu$) and then transports the $CH_3H_4PteGlu$ into bile for reabsorption by the gut and subsequent delivery to tissues (Steinberg *et al.*, 1979). This pathway may provide 200 μg or more of folate each day for recirculation to tissues. The importance of the enterohepatic cycle is suggested by studies in animals that show a rapid reduction of the concentration of folate in plasma following either drainage of bile or ingestion of alcohol, which apparently blocks the release of $CH_3H_4PteGlu$ from hepatic parenchymal cells (Hillman *et al.*, 1977).

Following uptake into cells, $CH_3H_4PteGlu$ acts as a methyl donor for the formation of methylcobalamin and as a source of $H_4PteGlu$ and other folate congeners, as described above. Folate is stored within cells as polyglutamates (Baugh and Krumdieck, 1969).

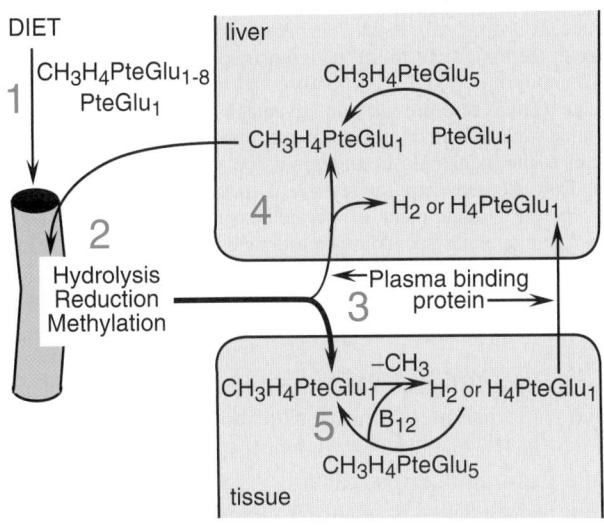

Figure 54–10. Absorption and distribution of folate derivatives.

Dietary sources of folate polyglutamates are hydrolyzed to the monoglutamate, reduced, and methylated to $CH_3H_4PteGlu_1$ during gastrointestinal transport. Folate deficiency commonly results from (1) inadequate dietary supply and (2) small intestinal disease. In patients with uremia, alcoholism, or hepatic disease there may be defects in (3) the concentration of folate binding proteins in plasma and (4) the flow of $CH_3H_4PteGlu_1$ into bile for reabsorption and transport to tissue (the folate enterohepatic cycle). Finally, vitamin B_{12} deficiency will (5) "trap" folate as $CH_3H_4PteGlu$, thereby reducing the availability of $H_4PteGlu_1$ for its essential roles in purine and pyrimidine synthesis.

Folate Deficiency.   Folate deficiency is a common complication of diseases of the small intestine, which interfere with the absorption of folate from food and the recirculation of folate through the enterohepatic cycle. In acute or chronic alcoholism, daily intake of folate in food may be severely restricted, and the enterohepatic cycle of the vitamin may be impaired by toxic effects of alcohol on hepatic parenchymal cells; this is perhaps the most common cause of folate-deficient megaloblastic erythropoiesis. However, it is also the most amenable to therapy, inasmuch as the reinstitution of a normal diet is sufficient to overcome the effect of alcohol. Disease states characterized by a high rate of cell turnover, such as hemolytic anemias, also may be complicated by folate deficiency. Additionally, drugs that inhibit dihydrofolate reductase (*e.g.,* methotrexate, trimethoprim) or that interfere with the absorption and storage of folate in tissues (*e.g.,* certain anticonvulsants, oral contraceptives) are capable of lowering the concentration of folate in plasma and at times may cause a megaloblastic anemia (Stebbins *et al.,* 1973; Stebbins and Bertino, 1976).

Folate deficiency has been implicated in the incidence of neural tube defects, including spina bifida, encephaloceles, and anencephaly. This is true even in the absence of folate-deficient anemia or alcoholism. A less than adequate intake of folate can also result in elevations in plasma homocysteine levels (Green and Miller, 1999). Since even moderate hyperhomocysteinemia is considered an independent risk factor for coronary artery and peripheral vascular disease and for venous thrombosis, the role of folate as a methyl donor in the homocysteine-to-methionine conversion is getting increased attention. Patients who are heterozygous for one or another enzymatic defect and have high normal to moderate elevations of plasma homocysteine may improve with folic acid therapy.

Folate deficiency is recognized by its impact on the hematopoietic system. As with vitamin B_{12}, this fact reflects the increased requirement associated with high rates of cell turnover. The megaloblastic anemia that results from folate deficiency cannot be distinguished from that caused by a deficiency of vitamin B_{12}. This finding is to be expected because of the final common pathway of the major intracellular metabolic roles of the two vitamins. At the same time, folate deficiency is rarely if ever associated with neurological abnormalities. Thus, the observation of characteristic abnormalities in vibratory and position sense and in motor and sensory pathways rules against the presence of an isolated deficiency of folic acid.

The appearance of megaloblastic anemia after deprivation of folate is much more rapid than that caused by the interruption of the absorption of vitamin B_{12} (*e.g.,* gastric surgery). This observation reflects the fact that stores of folate are limited *in vivo*. In Herbert's classical study of a single normal individual maintained on a diet low in folate for several months, megaloblastic erythropoiesis appeared after approximately 10 to 12 weeks (Herbert, 1962). Subsequent studies have shown that the rate of induction of megaloblastic erythropoiesis varies according to the population studied and the dietary background of the individual (Eichner *et al.,* 1971). A folate-deficiency state may appear in 1 to 4 weeks, depending on the individual's dietary habits and stores of the vitamin.

Folate deficiency is best diagnosed from measurements of folate in plasma and in red cells by use of a microbiological assay or a competitive binding technique. The concentration of folate in plasma is extremely sensitive to changes in dietary intake of the vitamin and the influence of inhibitors of folate metabolism or transport, such as alcohol. Normal folate concentrations in plasma range from 9 to 45 nM (4 to 20 ng/ml); below 9 nM is considered folate deficient. The plasma folate concentration rapidly falls to values indicative of deficiency within 24 to 48 hours of steady ingestion of alcohol (Eichner and Hillman, 1971, 1973). The plasma folate concentration will revert quickly to normal once such ingestion is stopped, even while the marrow is still megaloblastic. Such rapid fluctuations tend to detract from the clinical utility of the plasma folate concentration. The amount of folate in red cells or the adequacy of stores in lymphocytes (as measured by the deoxyuridine suppression test) may be used to diagnose a long-standing deficiency of folic acid (Herbert *et al.,* 1973). A positive result on either test shows that a state of deficiency must have existed for a sufficient time to allow the production of a population of cells with deficient stores of folate.

Folic acid (FOLVITE) is marketed as oral tablets containing 0.4, 0.8, and 1 mg pteroylglutamic acid, as an aqueous solution for injection (5 mg/ml), and in combination with other vitamins and minerals.

Folinic acid (*leucovorin calcium, citrovorum factor*) is the 5-formyl derivative of tetrahydrofolic acid. The principal therapeutic uses of folinic acid are to circumvent the inhibition of dihydrofolate reductase as a part of high-dose methotrexate therapy and to potentiate fluorouracil in the treatment of colorectal cancer (Chapter 52). It also has been used as an antidote to counteract the toxicity of folate antagonists such as pyrimethamine or trimethoprim. While it can be used to treat any folate-deficient state, folinic acid provides no advantage over folic acid, is more expensive, and therefore is not recommended. A single exception is the megaloblastic anemia associated with congenital dihydrofolate reductase deficiency. Leucovorin should never be used for the treatment of pernicious anemia or other megaloblastic anemias secondary to a deficiency of vitamin B_{12}. Just as is seen with folic acid, its use can result in an apparent response of the hematopoietic system, but neurological damage may occur or progress if already present.

Untoward Effects. There have been rare reports of reactions to parenteral injections of both folic acid and leucovorin. If a patient describes a history of a reaction before the drug is given, caution should be exercised. Oral folic acid usually is not toxic. Even with doses as high as 15 mg/day, there have been no substantiated reports of side effects. Folic acid in large amounts may counteract the antiepileptic effect of phenobarbital, phenytoin, and primidone and increase the frequency of seizures in susceptible children (Reynolds, 1968). While some studies have not supported these contentions, the U.S. Food and Drug Administration has recommended that oral tablets of folic acid be limited to strengths of 1 mg or less.

General Principles of Therapy. The therapeutic use of folic acid is limited to the prevention and treatment of deficiencies of the vitamin. As with vitamin B_{12} therapy, effective use of the vitamin depends on accurate diagnosis and an understanding of the mechanisms that are operative in a specific disease state. The following general principles of therapy should be respected:

1. Prophylactic administration of folic acid should be undertaken for clear indications. Dietary supplementation is necessary when there is a requirement that may not be taken care of by a "normal" diet. The daily ingestion of a multivitamin preparation containing 400 to 500 μg of folic acid has become standard practice before and during pregnancy to reduce the incidence of neural tube defects and for as long as a woman is breast-feeding. In women with a prior history of a pregnancy complicated by a neural tube defect, an even larger dose of 4 mg a day has been recommended (MRC Vitamin Study Research Group, 1991). Patients on total parenteral nutrition should receive folic acid supplements as part of their fluid regimen, since liver folate stores are limited. Adult patients with a disease state characterized by high cell turnover (*e.g.*, hemolytic anemia) generally require larger doses, 1 mg of folic acid given once or twice a day. The 1-mg dose also has been used in the treatment of patients with elevated levels of homocysteine.

2. As with vitamin B_{12} deficiency, any patient with folate deficiency and a megaloblastic anemia should be evaluated carefully to determine the underlying cause of the deficiency state. This should include evaluation of the effects of medications, the amount of alcohol intake, the patient's history of travel, and the function of the gastrointestinal tract.

3. Therapy should always be as specific as possible. Multivitamin preparations should be avoided unless there is good reason to suspect deficiency of several vitamins.

4. The potential of mistreating a patient who has vitamin B_{12} deficiency with folic acid must be kept in mind. The administration of large doses of folic acid can result in an apparent improvement of the megaloblastic anemia, inasmuch as PteGlu is converted by dihydrofolate reductase to H_4PteGlu; this circumvents the methylfolate "trap." However, folate therapy does not prevent or alleviate the neurological defects of vitamin B_{12} deficiency, and these may progress and become irreversible.

Treatment of the Acutely Ill Patient.   As described in detail in the section on vitamin B_{12}, treatment of the patient who is acutely ill with megaloblastic anemia should begin with intramuscular injections of both vitamin B_{12} and folic acid. Inasmuch as the patient requires therapy before the exact cause of the disease has been defined, it is important to avoid the potential problem of a combined deficiency of both vitamin B_{12}

and folic acid. When the patient is deficient in both, therapy with only one vitamin will not provide an optimal response. Long-standing nontropical sprue is one example of a disease in which combined deficiency of B_{12} and folate is common. When indicated, both vitamin B_{12} (100 μg) and folic acid (1 to 5 mg) should be administered intramuscularly, and the patient should then be maintained on daily oral supplements of 1 to 2 mg of folic acid for the next 1 to 2 weeks. Recommendations for administration of vitamin B_{12} are described above.

Oral administration of folate is generally satisfactory for patients who are not acutely ill, regardless of the cause of the deficiency state. Even the patient with tropical or nontropical sprue and a demonstrable defect in absorption of folic acid will respond adequately to such therapy. Abnormalities in the activity of pteroyl-γ-glutamyl carboxypeptidase and the function of mucosal cells will not prevent passive diffusion of sufficient amounts of PteGlu across the mucosal barrier if dosage is adequate, and continued ingestion of alcohol or other drugs also will not prevent an adequate therapeutic response. The effects of most inhibitors of folate transport or dihydrofolate reductase are overcome easily by administration of pharmacological doses of the vitamin. Folinic acid is the appropriate form of the vitamin for use in chemotherapeutic protocols, including "rescue" from methotrexate. Perhaps the only situation in which oral administration of folate will be ineffective is when vitamin C is severely deficient. The patient with scurvy may suffer from a megaloblastic anemia despite increased intake of folate and normal or high concentrations of the vitamin in plasma and cells.

The therapeutic response may be monitored by study of the hematopoietic system in a fashion identical to that described for vitamin B_{12}. Within 48 hours of the initiation of appropriate therapy, megaloblastic erythropoiesis disappears and, as efficient erythropoiesis begins, the concentration of iron in plasma falls to normal or below-normal values. The reticulocyte count begins to rise on the second or third day and reaches a peak by the fifth to seventh days; the reticulocyte index reflects the proliferative state of the marrow. Finally, the hematocrit begins to rise during the second week.

It is possible to use the pattern of recovery as the basis for a therapeutic trial. For this purpose, the patient should receive a daily parenteral injection of 50 to 100 μg of folic acid. Administration of doses in excess of 100 μg per day entails the risk of inducing a hematopoietic response in patients who are deficient in vitamin B_{12}, while oral administration of the vitamin may be unreliable because of intestinal malabsorption. A number of other complications also may interfere with the therapeutic trial. The patient with sprue and deficiencies of other vitamins or iron may fail to respond because of these inadequacies. In cases of alcoholism, the presence of hepatic disease, inflammation, or iron deficiency can act to blunt the proliferative response of the marrow and to prevent the correction of the anemia. For these reasons, the therapeutic trial for the evaluation of the patient with a potential deficiency of folic acid has not gained great popularity.

PROSPECTUS

The next several years should see a further expansion of the use of growth-regulating agents in the treatment of patients with hematological disorders, especially in the management of hematological malignancies. Thrombopoietin will become a mainstay alongside erythropoietin and the myeloid growth factors, further reducing the dependency on transfusion products. The *ex vivo* application of stem cell growth factors—including SCF, FL, and IL–3—to generate transplantable marrow progenitors almost certainly will play a role in future transplant and gene therapies. Longer-acting growth factors that permit less frequent dosing schedules also are under development. One of the first of these is novel erythropoiesis-stimulating protein (NESP), produced by the insertion of two extra N-linked sialic acid side chains into the erythropoietin molecule.

For further discussion of the anemias, *see* Chapters 105 to 110 in *Harrison's Principles of Internal Medicine,* 14th ed., McGraw-Hill, New York, 1998.

BIBLIOGRAPHY

Allen, R.H., and Mehlman, C.S. Isolation of gastric vitamin B$_{12}$–binding proteins using affinity chromatography. I. Purification and properties of human intrinsic factor. *J. Biol. Chem.,* **1973,** *248*:3660–3669.

Baugh, C.M., and Krumdieck, C.L. Naturally occurring folates. *Ann. N.Y. Acad. Sci.,* **1969,** *186*:7–28.

Besarab, A., Bolton, W.K., Browne, J.K., Egrie, J.C., Nissenson, A.R., Okamoto, D.M., Schwab, S.J., and Goodkin, D.A. The effects of normal as compared with low hematocrit values in patients with cardiac disease who are receiving hemodialysis and epoetin. *N. Engl. J. Med.,* **1998,** *339*:584–590.

Besarab, A., Kaiser, J.W., and Frinak, S. A study of parenteral iron regimens in hemodialysis patients. *Am. J. Kidney Dis.,* **1999,** *34*:21–28.

Bradley, T.R., and Metcalf, D. The growth of mouse bone marrow cells *in vitro. Aust. J. Exp. Biol. Med. Sci.,* **1966,** *44*:287–299.

Brandt, S.J., Peters, W.P., Atwater, S.K., Kurtzberg, J., Borowitz, M.J., Jones, R.B., Shpall, E.J., Bast, R.C., Jr., Gilbert, C.J., and Oette, D.H. Effect of recombinant human granulocyte-macrophage colony-stimulating factor on hematopoietic reconstitution after high-dose chemotherapy and autologous bone marrow transplantation. *N. Engl. J. Med.,* **1988,** *318*:869–876.

Brise, H., and Hallberg, L. Absorbability of different iron compounds. *Acta Med. Scand.,* **1962,** *171(suppl. 376)*:23–38. (*See also* related articles by these authors, pp. 7–22 and 51–58.)

Carnot, P., and Deflandre, C. Sur l'activité hémopoiétique de sérum au cours de la régenération du sang. *C.R. Acad. Sci. (III),* **1906,** *143*:384–386.

Chillar, R.K., Johnson, C.S., and Beutler, E. Erythrocyte pyridoxine kinase levels in patients with sideroblastic anemia. *N. Engl. J. Med.,* **1976,** *295*:881–883.

Cook, J.D., Finch, C.A., and Smith, N.J. Evaluation of the iron status of a population. *Blood,* **1976,** *48*:449–455.

Cook, J.D., Minnich, V., Moore, C.V., Rasmussen, A., Bradley, W.B., and Finch, C.A. Absorption of fortification iron in bread. *Am. J. Clin. Nutr.,* **1973,** *26*:861–872.

Cook, J.D., Skikne, B.S., Lynch, S.R., and Reusser, M.E. Estimates of iron sufficiency in the U.S. population. *Blood,* **1986,** *68*:726–731.

Dallman, P.R., Siimes, M.A., and Stekel, A. Iron deficiency in infancy and childhood. *Am. J. Clin. Nutr.,* **1980,** *33*:86–118.

de Sauvage, F.J., Hass, P.E., Spencer, S.D., Malloy, B.E., Gurney, A.L., Spencer, S.A., Darbonne, W.C., Henzel, W.J., Wong, S.C., Kuang, W.J., Oles, K.J., Hultgren, B., Solberg, L.A., Jr., Goeddel, D.V., and Eaton, D.L. Stimulation of megakaryocytopoiesis and thrombopoiesis by the c-Mpl ligand. *Nature,* **1994,** *369*:533–538.

Dunlap, W.M., James, G.W., III, and Hume, D.M. Anemia and neutropenia caused by copper deficiency. *Ann. Intern. Med.,* **1974,** *80*:470–476.

Eichner, E.R., and Hillman, R.S. The evolution of anemia in alcoholic patients. *Am. J. Med.,* **1971,** *50*:218–232.

Eichner, E.R., and Hillman, R.S. Effect of alcohol on serum folate level. *J. Clin. Invest.,* **1973,** *52*:584–591.

Eichner, E.R., Pierce, H.I., and Hillman, R.S. Folate balance in dietary-induced megaloblastic anemia. *N. Engl. J. Med.,* **1971,** *284*:933–938.

Eschbach, J.W., Egrie, J.C., Downing, M.R., Browne, J.K., and Adamson, J.W. Correction of the anemia of end-stage renal disease with recombinant human erythropoietin. Results of a combined phase I and II clinical trial. *N. Engl. J. Med.,* **1987,** *316*:73–78.

Eschbach, J.W., Kelly, M.R., Haley, N.R., Abels, R.I., and Adamson, J.W. Treatment of the anemia of progressive renal failure with recombinant human erythropoietin. *N. Engl. J. Med.,* **1989,** *321*:158–163.

Finch, C.A., Colman, D.H., Motulsky, A.G., Donohue, D.M., and Reiff, R.H. Erythrokinetics in pernicious anemia. *Blood,* **1956,** *11*:807–820.

Fischl, M., Galpin, J.E., Levine, J.D., Groopman, J.E., Henry, D.H., Kennedy, P., Miles, S., Robbins, W., Starrett, B., Zalusky, R., Abels, R.I., Tsai, H.C., and Rudnick, S.A. Recombinant human erythropoietin therapy for AIDS patients treated with AZT: a double-blind, placebo-controlled clinical study. *N. Engl. J. Med.,* **1990,** *322*:1488–1493.

Ford, C.E., Hamerton, J.L., Barnes, D.W.H., and Loutit, J.T. Cytological identification of radiation chimeras. *Nature,* **1956,** *177*:452–454.

Foy, H., Kondi, A., and MacDougall, L. Pure red-cell aplasia in marasmus and kwashiorkor treated with riboflavin. *Br. Med. J.,* **1961,** *1*:937–941.

Ganser, A., Lindemann, A., Ottman, O.G., Seipelt, G., Hess, U., Geissler, G., Kanz, L., Frisch, J., Schulz, G., Herrmann, F., Mertelsmann, R., and Hoelzer, D. Sequential *in vivo* treatment with two recombinant human hematopoietic growth factors (interleukin-3 and granulocyte-macrophage colony-stimulating factor) as a new therapeutic modality to stimulate hematopoiesis: results of a phase I study. *Blood,* **1992,** 79:2583–2591.

Gerhartz, H.H., Engellhard, M., Meusers, P., Brittinger, G., Wilmanns, W., Schlimok, G., Mueller, P., Huhn, D., Musch, R., Seigert, W., Gerhartz, D., Hartlapp, J.H., Theil, E., Huber, C., Peschl, C., Spann, W., Emmerich, B., Schadek, C., Westerhausen, M., Pecs, H.W., Radtke, H., Engert, A., Terhardt, E., Schick, H., Binder, T., Fuchs, R., Hasford, J., Brandmaier, R., Stern, A.C., Jones, T.C., Ehrlich, H.J., Stein, H., Parwaresch, M., Tiemann, M., and Lennert, K. Randomized, double-blind, placebo-controlled, phase III study of recombinant human granulocyte-macrophage colony-stimulating factor as adjunct to induction treatment of high-grade malignant non-Hodgkin's lymphomas. *Blood,* **1993,** 82:2329–2339.

Goodnough, L.T., Rudnick, S., Price, T.H., Ballas, S.K., Collins, M.L., Crowley, J.P., Kosmin, M., Kruskall, M.S., Lenes, B.A., Menitove, J.E., Silberstein, L.E., Smith, K.J., Wallas, C.H., Abels, R., and Von Tress, M. Increased preoperative collection of autologous blood with recombinant human erythropoietin therapy. *N. Engl. J. Med.,* **1989,** 321:1163–1168.

Grebe, G., Martinez-Torres, C., and Layrisse, M. Effect of meals and ascorbic acid on the absorption of a therapeutic dose of iron as ferrous and ferric salts. *Curr. Ther. Res. Clin. Exp.,* **1975,** 17:382–397.

Groopman, J.E., Mitsuyasu, R.T., DeLeo, M.J., Oette, D.H., and Golde, D.W. Effect of recombinant human granulocyte macrophage colony stimulating factor on myelopoiesis in the acquired immunodeficiency syndrome. *N. Engl. J. Med.,* **1987,** 317:593–598.

Hahn, P.F., Bale, W.F., Ross, J.F., Balfour, W.M., and Whipple, G.H. Radioactive iron absorption by the gastrointestinal tract: influence of anemia, anoxia and antecedent feeding; distribution in growing dogs. *J. Exp. Med.,* **1943,** 78:169–188.

Hakami, N., Neiman, P.E., Canellos, G.P., and Lazerson, J. Neonatal megaloblastic anemia due to inherited transcobalamin II deficiency in two siblings. *N. Engl. J. Med.,* **1971,** 285:1163–1170.

Hallberg, L., Ryttinger, L., and Sölvell, L. Side-effects of oral iron therapy. A double-blind study of different iron compounds in tablet form. *Acta Med. Scand. Suppl.,* **1966,** 459:3–10.

Hammond, W.P. IV, Price, T.H., Souza, L.M., and Dale, D.C. Treatment of cyclic neutropenia with granulocyte colony-stimulating factor. *N. Engl. J. Med.,* **1989,** 320:1306–1311.

Henderson, P.A., and Hillman, R.S. Characteristics of iron dextran utilization in man. *Blood,* **1969,** 34:357–375.

Herbert, V. Experimental nutritional folate deficiency in man. *Trans. Assoc. Am. Physicians,* **1962,** 75:307–320.

Herbert, V., Tisman, G., Le-Teng-Go, and Brenner, L. The dU suppression test using ^{125}I-UdR to define biochemical megaloblastosis. *Br. J. Haematol.,* **1973,** 24:713–723.

Herbert, V., and Zalusky, R. Interrelations of vitamin B$_{12}$ and folic acid metabolism: folic acid clearance studies. *J. Clin. Invest.,* **1962,** 41:1263–1276.

Heyssel, R.M., Bozian, R.C., Darby, W.J., and Bell, M.C. Vitamin B$_{12}$ turnover in man. The assimilation of vitamin B$_{12}$ from natural foodstuff by man and estimates of minimal daily dietary requirements. *Am. J. Clin. Nutr.,* **1966,** 18:176–184.

Hillman, R.S., and Henderson, P.A. Control of marrow production by the level of iron supply. *J. Clin. Invest.,* **1969,** 48:454–460.

Hillman, R.S., McGuffin, R., and Campbell, C. Alcohol interference with the folate enterohepatic cycle. *Trans. Assoc. Am. Physicians,* **1977,** 90:145–156.

Hines, J.D., and Love, D.L. Abnormal vitamin B6 metabolism in sideroblastic anemia: effect of pyridoxal phosphate (PLP) therapy. *Clin. Res.,* **1975,** 23:403A.

Hitzig, W.H., Dohmann, U., Pluss, H.J., and Vischer, D. Hereditary transcobalamin II deficiency: clinical findings in a new family. *J. Pediatr.,* **1974,** 85:622–628.

Hoffman, H.N. II, Phyliky, R.L., and Fleming, C.R. Zinc-induced copper deficiency. *Gastroenterology,* **1988,** 94:508–512.

Holtzman, N.A., Charache, P., Cordano, A., and Graham, G.G. Distribution of serum copper in copper deficiency. *Johns Hopkins Med. J.,* **1970,** 126:34–42.

Huang, E., Nocka, K., Beier, D.R., Chu, T.Y., Buck, J., Lahm, H.W., Wellner, D., Leder, P., and Besmer, P. The hematopoietic growth factor K1 is encoded at the S1 locus and is the ligand of the c-kit receptor, the gene product of the W locus. *Cell,* **1990,** 63:225–233.

Huff, R.L., Hennessy, T.G., Austin, R.E., Garcia, J.F., Roberts, B.M., and Lawrence, J.H. Plasma and red cell iron turnover in normal subjects and in patients having various hematopoietic disorders. *J. Clin. Invest.,* **1950,** 29:1041–1052.

Jacobs, K., Shoemaker, C., Rudersdorf, R., Neill, S.D., Kaufman, R.J., Mufson, A., Seehra, J., Jones, S.S., Hewick, R., Fritsch, E.F., Kawakita, M., Shimizu, T., and Miyake, T. Isolation and characterization of genomic and cDNA clones of human erythropoietin. *Nature,* **1985,** 313:806–810.

Jacobsen, L.O., Goldwasser, E., Freed, W., and Plzak, L. Role of the kidney in erythropoiesis. *Nature,* **1957,** 179:633–634.

Jacobsen, L.O., Marks, E.K., Gaston, E.O., Robinson, M., and Zirkle, R.E. The role of the spleen in radiation injury. *Proc. Soc. Exp. Biol. Med.,* **1949,** 70:740–742.

Kaufman, J.S., Reda, D.J., Fye, C.L., Goldfarb, D.S., Henderson, W.G., Kleinman, J.G., and Vaamonde, C.A. Subcutaneous compared with intravenous epoetin in patients receiving hemodialysis. Department of Veterans Affairs Cooperative Study Group on Erythropoietin in Hemodialysis Patients. *N. Engl. J. Med.,* **1998,** 339:578–583.

Kaushansky, K., Lok, S., Holly, R.D., Broudy, V.C., Lin, N., Bailey, M.C., Forstrom, J.W., Buddle, M.M., Oort, P.J., Hagen, F.S., Roth, G.J., Papayannopoulou, T., and Foster, D.C. Promotion of megakaryocyte progenitor expansion and differentiation by the c-Mp1 ligand thrombopoietin. *Nature,* **1994,** 369:568–571.

Kawasaki, E.S., Ladner, M.B., Wang, A.M., Van Arsdell, J., Warren, M.K., Coyne, M.Y., Schweickart, V.L., Lee, M.-T., Wilson, K.J., Boosman, A., Stanley, E.R., Ralph, P., and Mark, D.F. Molecular cloning of a complementary DNA encoding human macrophage-specific colony-stimulating factor (CSF-l). *Science,* **1985,** 230:291–296.

Kernoff, L.M., Dommisse, J., and du Toit, E.D. Utilization of iron dextran in recurrent iron deficiency anaemia. *Br. J. Haematol.,* **1975,** 30:419–424.

Klausner, R.D., Rouault, T.A., and Harford, J.B. Regulating the fate of mRNA: the control of cellular iron metabolism. *Cell,* **1993,** 72:19–28.

Lane, M., Alfrey, C.P., Megel, C.E., Doherty, M.A., and Doherty, J. The rapid induction of human riboflavin deficiency with galactoflavin. *J. Clin. Invest.,* **1964,** 43:357–373.

Layzer, R.B. Myeloneuropathy after prolonged exposure to nitrous oxide. *Lancet,* **1978,** 2:1227–1230.

Lee, F., Yokota, T., Otsuka, T., Gemmell, L., Larson, N., Luh, J., Arai, K., and Rennick, D. Isolation of cDNA for a human granulocyte-macrophage colony-stimulating factor by functional expression in mammalian cells. *Proc. Natl. Acad. Sci. U.S.A.,* **1985,** 82:4360–4364.

Lin, F.K., Suggs, S., Lin, C.H., Browne, J.K., Smalling, R., Egrie, J.C., Chen, K.K., Fox, G.M., Martin, F., Stabinsky, Z., Badrawi, S.M., Lai, P.-H., and Goldwasser, E. Cloning and expression of the human erythropoietin gene. *Proc. Natl. Acad. Sci. U.S.A.,* **1985,** *82*:7580–7584.

Lindenbaum, J., Healton, E.B., Savage, D.G., Brust, J.C., Garrett, T.J., Podell, E.R., Marcell, P.D., Stabler, S.P., and Allen, R.H. Neuropsychiatric disorders caused by cobalamin deficiency in the absence of anemia or macrocytosis. *N. Engl. J. Med.,* **1988,** *318*:1720–1728.

Linnell, J.C., Hoffbrand, A.V., Peters, T.J., and Matthews, D.M. Chromatographic and bioautographic estimation of plasma cobalamins in various disturbances of vitamin B_{12} metabolism. *Clin. Sci.,* **1971,** *40*:1–16.

Lipschitz, D.A., Cook, J.D., and Finch, C.A. A clinical evaluation of serum ferritin as an index of iron stores. *N. Engl. J. Med.,* **1974,** *290*:1213–1216.

Lok, S., Kaushansky, K., Holly, R.D., Kuijpen, J.L., Lofton-Day, C.E., Oort, P.J., Grant, F.J., Heipel, M.D., Burkhead, S.K., Kramer, J.M., Bell, L.A., Sprechem, C.A., Blumberg, H., Johnson, R., Prunkard, D., Ching, A.F.T., Mathewes, S.L., Bailey, M.C., Forstrom, J.W., Buddle, M.M., Osborn, S.G., Evans, S.J., Sheppard, P.O., Presnell, S.R., O'Hara, P.J., Hagen, F.S., Roth, G.J., and Foster, D.C. Cloning and expression of murine thrombopoietin cDNA and stimulation of platelet production *in vivo. Nature,* **1994,** *369*:565–568.

Monsen, E.R., Hallberg, L., Layrisse, M., Hegsted, D.M., Cook, J.D., Mertz, W., and Finch, C.A. Estimation of available dietary iron. *Am. J. Clin. Nutr.,* **1978,** *31*:134–141.

Nemunaitis, J., Singer, J.W., Buckner, C.D., Durnam, D., Epstein, C., Hill, R., Storb, R., Thomas, E.D., and Applebaum, F.R. Use of recombinant human granulocyte-macrophage colony-stimulating factor in graft failure after bone marrow transplantation. *Blood,* **1990,** *76*:245–253.

Owen, W.F., Jr. Optimizing the use of parenteral iron in end-stage renal disease patients: focus on issues of infection and cardiovascular disease. Introduction. *Am. J. Kidney Dis.,* **1999,** *34*:S1–S2.

Peters, L.L., Andrews, N.C., Eicher, E.M., Davidson, M.B., Orkin, S.H., and Lux, S.E. Mouse microcytic anemia caused by a defect in the gene encoding the globin enhancer-binding protein NF-E2. *Nature,* **1993,** *362*:768–770.

Pritchard, J.A. Hemoglobin regeneration in severe iron deficiency anemia. Response to orally and parenterally administered iron preparations. *JAMA,* **1966,** *195*:717–720.

Rabinowe, S.N., Neuberg, D., Bierman, P.J., Vose, J.M., Nemunaitis, J., Singer, J.W., Freedman, A.S., Mauch, P., Demetri, G., Onetto, N., Gillis, S., Oette, D., Buckner, D., Hansen, J.A., Ritz, J., Armitage, J.O., Nadler, L.M., and Applebaum, F.R. Long-term follow-up of a phase III study of recombinant human granulocyte-macrophage colony-stimulating factor after autologous bone marrow transplantation for lymphoid malignancies. *Blood,* **1993,** *81*:1903–1908.

Ramsey, C., and Herbert, V. Dialysis assay for intrinsic factor and its antibody: demonstration of species specificity of antibodies to human and hog intrinsic factor. *J. Lab. Clin. Med.,* **1965,** *65*:143–152.

Reissmann, K.R. Studies on the mechanism of erythropoietic stimulation in parabiotic rats during hypoxia. *Blood,* **1950,** *5*:372–380.

Retief, F.P., Gottlieb, C.W., and Herbert, V. Delivery of $Co^{57}B_{12}$ to erythrocytes from α and β globulin of normal, B_{12}-deficient, and chronic myeloid leukemia serum. *Blood,* **1967,** *29*:837–851.

Reynolds, E.H. Mental effects of anticonvulsants and folic acid metabolism. *Brain,* **1968,** *91*:197–214.

Schilling, R.F. Intrinsic factor studies. II. The effect of gastric juice on the urinary excretion of radioactivity after the oral administration of radioactive vitamin B_{12}. *J. Lab. Clin. Med.,* **1953,** *42*:860–866.

Scott, J.M., Bloomfield, F.J., Stebbins, R., and Herbert, V. Studies on derivation of transcobalamin III from granulocytes. Enhancement by lithium and elimination by fluoride of *in vitro* increments in vitamin B_{12}–binding capacity. *J. Clin. Invest.,* **1974,** *53*:228–239.

Scott, J.M., Dinn, J.J., Wilson, P., and Weir, D.G. Pathogenesis of subacute combined degeneration: a result of methyl group deficiency. *Lancet,* **1981,** *2*:334–337.

Skouby, A.P., Hippe, E., and Olesen, H. Antibody to transcobalamin II and B_{12} binding capacity in patients treated with hydroxycobalamin. *Blood,* **1971,** *38*:769–774.

Solomon, L.R., and Hillman, R.S. Vitamin B_6 metabolism in human red blood cells. I. Variation in normal subjects. *Enzyme,* **1978,** *23*:262–273.

Solomon, L.R., and Hillman, R.S. Vitamin B_6 metabolism in idiopathic sideroblastic anaemia and related disorders. *Br. J. Haematol.,* **1979a,** *42*:239–253.

Solomon, L.R., and Hillman, R.S. Vitamin B_6 metabolism in anaemic and alcoholic man. *Br. J. Haematol.,* **1979b,** *41*:343–356.

Stebbins, R., Scott, J., and Herbert, V. Drug-induced megaloblastic anemias. *Semin. Hematol.,* **1973,** *10*:235–251.

Steinberg, S.E., Campbell, C.L., and Hillman, R.S. Kinetics of the normal folate enterohepatic cycle. *J. Clin. Invest.,* **1979,** *64*:83–88.

Tamura, T., and Stokstad, E.L. The availability of food folate in man. *Br. J. Haematol.,* **1973,** *25*:513–532.

Vadhan-Raj, S., Keating, M., LeMaistre, A., Hittelman, W.N., McCredie, K., Trujillo, J.M., Broxmeyer, H.E., Henney, C., and Gutterman, J.U. Effects of recombinant human granulocyte-macrophage colony-stimulating factor in patients with myelodysplastic syndromes. *N. Engl. J. Med.,* **1987,** *317*:1545–1552.

Vadhan-Raj, S., Vershragen, C.F., Bueso-Ramos, C., Broxmeyer, H.E., Kudelka, A.P., Freedman, R.S., Edwards, C.L., Gershenson, D., Jones, D., Ashby, M., and Kavanagh, J.J. Recombinant human thrombopoietin attenuates carboplatin-induced severe thrombocytopenia and the need for platelet transfusions in patients with gynecologic cancer. *Ann. Intern. Med.,* **2000,** *132*:364–368.

Viteri, F.E., Garcia-Ibanez, R., and Torun, B. Sodium iron NaFeEDTA as an iron fortification compound in Central America. Absorption studies. *Am. J. Clin. Nutr.,* **1978,** *31*:961–971.

Weinbren, K., Salm, R., and Greenberg, G. Intramuscular injections of iron compounds and oncogenesis in man. *Br. Med. J.,* **1978,** *1*:683–685.

Weissbach, H., and Taylor, R.T. Metabolic role of vitamin B_{12}. *Vitam. Horm.,* **1968,** *26*:395–412.

Wills, L., Clutterbuck, P.W., and Evans, P.D.F. A new factor in the production and cure of macrocytic anaemias and its relation to other haemopoietic principles curative in pernicious anaemia. *Biochem. J.,* **1937,** *31*:2136–2147.

Wong, G.G., Witek, J.S., Temple, P.A., Wilkens, K.M., Leary, A.C., Luxenberg, D.P., Jones, S.S., Brown, E.L., Kay, R.M., Orr, E.C., Shoemaker, C., Golde, D.W., Kaufman, R.J., Hewick, R.M., Wang, E.A., and Clark, S.C. Human GM-CSF: molecular cloning of the complementary DNA and purification of the natural recombinant proteins. *Science,* **1985,** *228*:810–815.

Yang, Y.C., Ciarletta, A.B., Temple, P.A., Chung, M.P., Kovacic, S., Witek-Giannotti, J.S., Leary, A.C., Kriz, R., Donahue, R.E., Wong, G.G., and Clark, S.C. Human IL-3 (multi-CSF): identification by expression cloning of a novel hematopoietic growth factor related to murine IL-3. *Cell,* **1986,** *47*:3–10.

Zidar, B.L., Shadduck, R.K., Zeigler, Z., and Winkelstein, A. Observations on the anemia and neutropenia of human copper deficiency. *Am. J. Hematol.,* **1977,** *3:*177–185.

MONOGRAPHS AND REVIEWS

Aisen, P., and Brown, E.B. The iron-binding function of transferrin in iron metabolism. *Semin. Hematol.,* **1977,** *14:*31–53.

Bothwell, T.H., Charlton, R.W., Cook, J.D., and Finch, C.A. *Iron Metabolism in Man.* Blackwell Scientific Publications, Oxford, **1979.**

Bothwell, T.H., and Finch, C.A. *Iron Metabolism in Man.* Little, Brown & Co., Boston, **1962.**

Callender, S.T. Treatment of iron deficiency. In, *Iron in Biochemistry and Medicine.* (Jacobs, A., and Worwood, M., eds.) Academic Press, Inc., New York, **1974,** pp. 529–542.

Chanarin, I., Deacon, R., Lumb, M., Muir, M., and Perry, J. Cobalamin-folate interrelationships: a critical review. *Blood,* **1985,** *66:*479–489.

Cooper, B.A. Megaloblastic anaemia and disorders affecting utilization of vitamin B$_{12}$ and folate in childhood. *Clin. Haematol.,* **1976,** *5:*631–659.

Council on Foods and Nutrition. Iron deficiency in the United States. *JAMA,* **1968,** *203:*407–412.

Dallman, P.R. Manifestations of iron deficiency. *Semin. Hematol.,* **1982,** *19:*19–30.

Erslev, A.J. Humoral regulation of red cell production. *Blood,* **1953,** *8:*349–387.

Evans, G.W. Copper homeostasis in the mammalian system. *Physiol. Rev.,* **1973,** *53:*535–570.

Finch, C.A., and Huebers, H. Perspectives in iron metabolism. *N. Engl. J. Med.,* **1982,** *306:*1520–1528.

Graham, G.G., and Cordano, A. Copper deficiency in human subjects. In, *Trace Elements in Human Health and Disease.* Vol. 1. *Zinc and Copper.* (Prasad, A.S., and Oberleas, D., eds.) Academic Press, Inc., New York, **1976,** pp. 363–372.

Green, R., and Miller, J.W. Folate deficiency beyond megaloblastic anemia: hyperhomocysteinemia and other manifestations of dysfunctional folate status. *Semin. Hematol.,* **1999,** *36:*47–64.

Hallberg, L. Bioavailability of dietary iron in man. *Annu. Rev. Nutr.,* **1981,** *1:*123–147.

Harker, L.A. Physiology and clinical applications of platelet growth factors. *Curr. Opin. Hematol.,* **1999,** *6:*127–134.

Herzlich, B., and Herbert, V. The role of the pancreas in cobalamin (Vitamin B$_{12}$) absorption. *Am. J. Gastroenterol.,* **1984,** *79:*489–493.

Hillman, R.S., and Finch, C.A. *Red Cell Manual,* 7th ed. F. A. Davis Co., Philadelphia, **1997.**

Horrigan, D.L., and Harris, J.W. Pyridoxine-responsive anemias in man. *Vitam. Horm.,* **1968,** *26:*549–571.

Klausner, R.D., Ashwell, G., van Renswoude, J., Harford, J.B., and Bridges, K.R. Binding of apotransferrin to k562 cells: explanation of the transferrin cycle. *Proc. Natl. Acad. Sci. U.S.A.,* **1983,** *80:*2263–2266.

Lajtha, L.G., Pozzi, L.V., Schofield, R., and Fox, M. Kinetic properties of haemopoietic stem cells. *Cell Tissue Kinet.,* **1969,** *2:*39–49.

Laurell, C.B. Studies on the transportation and metabolism of iron in the body. *Acta Physiol. Scand. Suppl.,* **1947,** *46:*1–129.

Layrisse, M., and Martinez-Torres, C. Food iron absorption: iron supplementation of food. *Prog. Hematol.,* **1971,** *6:*137–160.

Lee, G.R., Williams, D.M., and Cartwright, G.E. Role of copper in iron metabolism and heme biosynthesis. In, *Trace Elements in Human Health and Disease.* Vol. 1. *Zinc and Copper.* (Prasad, A.S., and Oberleas, D., eds.) Academic Press, Inc., New York, **1976,** pp. 373–390.

Lieschke, G.J., and Burgess, A.W. Granulocyte colony-stimulating factor and granulocyte-macrophage colony-stimulating factor (1). *N. Engl. J. Med.,* **1992,** *327:*28–35.

Martinez-Torres, C., Cubeddu, L., Dillmann, E., Brengelmann, G.L., Leets, I., Layrisse, M., Johnson, D.G., and Finch, C. Effect of exposure to low temperature on normal and iron deficient subjects. *Am. J. Physiol.,* **1984,** *246:*R380–R383.

Metcalf, D. The granulocyte-macrophage colony-stimulating factors. *Science,* **1985,** *229:*16–22.

Moore, M.A. The clinical use of colony stimulating factors. *Annu. Rev. Immunol.,* **1991,** *9:*159–191.

MRC Vitamin Study Research Group. Prevention of neural tube defects: results of the Medical Research Council Vitamin Study. *Lancet,* **1991,** *338:*131–137.

O'Dell, B.L. Biochemistry of copper. *Med. Clin. North Am.,* **1976,** *60:*687–703.

Pollit, E., and Leibel, R.L. (eds.). *Iron Deficiency: Brain Biochemistry and Behavior.* Raven Press, New York, **1982.**

Pratt, J.M. *Inorganic Chemistry of Vitamin B$_{12}$.* Academic Press, Inc., New York, **1972.**

Quesenberry, P., and Levitt, L. Hematopoietic stem cells. *N. Engl. J. Med.,* **1979,** *301:*755–761; 819–823; 868–872.

Reynolds, E.H. Neurological aspects of folate and vitamin B$_{12}$ metabolism. *Clin. Haematol.,* **1976,** *5:*661–696.

Rosenberg, I.H. Absorption and malabsorption of folates. *Clin. Haematol.,* **1976,** *5:*589–618.

Stebbins, R., and Bertino, J.R. Megaloblastic anemia produced by drugs. *Clin. Haematol.,* **1976,** *5:*619–630.

Weir, D.G., and Scott, J.M. Interrelationships of folates and cobalamins. In, *Contemporary Issues in Clinical Nutrition,* Vol. 5. *Nutrition in Hematology.* (Lindenbaum, J., ed.) Churchill Livingstone, New York **1983,** pp. 121–142.

WHO Joint Meeting. Control of nutritional anaemia with special reference to iron deficiency. *World Health Organ. Tech. Rep. Ser.,* **1975,** *580:*5–71.

ANTICOAGULANT, THROMBOLYTIC, AND ANTIPLATELET DRUGS

Philip W. Majerus and Douglas M. Tollefsen

The physiological systems that control blood fluidity are both complex and elegant. Blood must remain fluid within the vasculature and yet clot quickly when exposed to nonendothelial surfaces at sites of vascular injury. When intravascular thrombi do occur, a system of fibrinolysis is activated to restore fluidity. In the normal situation, a delicate balance prevents both thrombosis and hemorrhage and allows physiological fibrinolysis without excess pathological fibrinogenolysis. The drugs described in this chapter have very different mechanisms of action, but all are designed to achieve the same aim: namely, to alter the balance between procoagulant and anticoagulant reactions. The efficacy and toxicity of these drugs are necessarily intertwined. For example, the desired therapeutic effect of anticoagulation can be offset by the toxic effect of bleeding due to overdosing of anticoagulant. Similarly, overstimulation of fibrinolysis can lead to systemic destruction of fibrinogen and coagulation factors. This chapter reviews the predominant agents for controlling blood fluidity, including (1) antiplatelet agents, especially aspirin; (2) the coumarin anticoagulants, which block multiple steps in the coagulation cascade; (3) heparin and its derivatives, which stimulate natural inhibitors of coagulant proteases; and (4) fibrinolytic agents, which lyse pathological thrombi. Achieving the balance between therapeutic and toxic effects is stressed. The role of aspirin as an antipyretic and antiinflammatory agent is described in Chapter 27.

OVERVIEW OF HEMOSTASIS

Hemostasis is the cessation of blood loss from a damaged vessel. Platelets first adhere to macromolecules in the subendothelial regions of the injured blood vessel; they then aggregate to form the primary hemostatic plug. Platelets stimulate local activation of plasma coagulation factors, leading to generation of a fibrin clot that reinforces the platelet aggregate. Later, as wound healing occurs, the platelet aggregate and fibrin clot are degraded. Thrombosis is a pathological process in which a platelet aggregate and/or a fibrin clot occludes a blood vessel. Arterial thrombosis may result in ischemic necrosis of the tissue supplied by the artery (*e.g.*, myocardial infarction due to thrombosis of a coronary artery). Venous thrombosis may cause tissues drained by the vein to become edematous and inflamed. Thrombosis of a deep vein may be complicated by pulmonary embolism.

Coagulation *in Vitro*. Blood clots in 4 to 8 minutes when placed in a glass tube. Clotting is prevented if a chelating agent such as ethylenediaminetetraacetic acid (EDTA) or citrate is added to bind Ca^{2+}. Recalcified plasma clots in 2 to 4 minutes. The clotting time after recalcification is shortened to 26 to 33 seconds by the addition of negatively charged phospholipids and a particulate substance such as kaolin (aluminum silicate); this is termed the *activated partial thromboplastin time* (aPTT). Alternatively, recalcified plasma will clot in 12 to 14 seconds after addition of "thromboplastin" (a saline extract of brain that contains tissue factor and phospholipids); this is termed the *prothrombin time* (PT).

Two pathways of coagulation are recognized. An individual with a prolonged aPTT and a normal PT is considered to have a defect in the *intrinsic coagulation pathway,* because all of the components of the aPTT test (except kaolin) are intrinsic to the plasma. A patient with

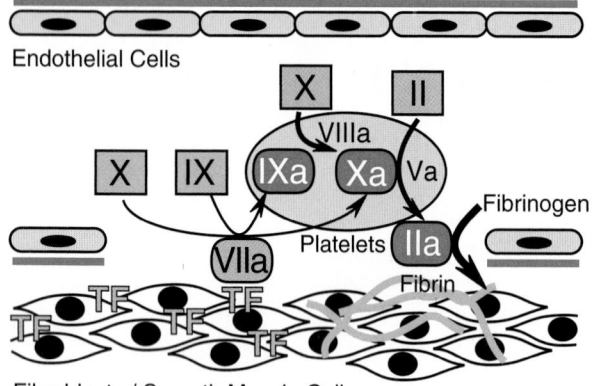

Figure 55–1. Major reactions of blood coagulation.

Boxes enclose the coagulation factor zymogens (indicated by roman numerals) and the ovals represent the active proteases. TF, tissue factor; an activated factor is followed by the letter "a."

a prolonged PT and a normal aPTT has a defect in the *extrinsic coagulation pathway,* since thromboplastin is extrinsic to the plasma. Prolongation of both the aPTT and the PT suggests a defect in a common pathway.

Coagulation involves a series of zymogen activation reactions, as shown in Figure 55–1 (Davie *et al.,* 1991; Esmon, 1993). At each stage a precursor protein, or *zymogen,* is converted to an active protease by cleavage of one or more peptide bonds in the precursor molecule. The components that can be involved at each stage include a protease from the preceding stage, a zymogen, a nonenzymatic protein cofactor, Ca^{2+}, and an organizing surface that is provided by a phospholipid emulsion *in vitro* or by platelets *in vivo.* The final protease to be generated is thrombin (factor IIa).

Conversion of Fibrinogen to Fibrin. Fibrinogen is a 330,000-dalton protein that consists of three pairs of polypeptide chains (designated Aα, Bβ, and γ) covalently linked by disulfide bonds. Thrombin converts fibrinogen to fibrin monomers by cleaving fibrinopeptides A (16 amino acid residues) and B (14 amino acid residues) from the amino-terminal ends of the Aα and Bβ chains, respectively. Removal of the fibrinopeptides allows the fibrin monomers to form a gel, which constitutes the end point of the aPTT and PT tests. Initially, the fibrin monomers are bound to each other noncovalently. Subsequently, factor XIIIa catalyzes an interchain transglutamination reaction that cross-links adjacent fibrin monomers to enhance the strength of the clot.

Structure of Coagulation Protease Zymogens. The protease zymogens involved in coagulation include factors II (prothrombin), VII, IX, X, XI, XII, and prekallikrein. About 200 amino

acid residues at the carboxyl-terminal end of each zymogen are homologous to trypsin and contain the active site of the protease. In addition, 9 to 12 glutamate residues near the amino-terminal ends of factors II, VII, IX, and X are converted to γ-carboxyglutamate (Gla) residues during biosynthesis in the liver. The Gla residues bind Ca^{2+} and are necessary for the coagulant activities of these proteins.

Nonenzymatic Protein Cofactors. Factors V and VIII are homologous 350,000-dalton proteins. Factor VIII circulates in plasma bound to von Willebrand factor, while factor V is present both free in plasma and as a component of platelets. Thrombin cleaves V and VIII to yield activated factors (Va and VIIIa) that have at least 50 times the coagulant activity of the precursor forms. Factors Va and VIIIa have no enzymatic activity themselves but serve as cofactors that increase the proteolytic efficiency of Xa and IXa, respectively. Tissue factor is a nonenzymatic lipoprotein cofactor that greatly increases the proteolytic efficiency of VIIa. It is present on the surface of cells that are not normally in contact with plasma (*e.g.,* fibroblasts and smooth muscle cells) and initiates coagulation outside a broken blood vessel. Monocytes and endothelial cells also may express tissue factor when exposed to a variety of stimuli, such as endotoxin, tumor necrosis factor, and interleukin-1. Thus, these cells may be involved in thrombus formation under pathological circumstances. High-molecular-weight kininogen is a plasma protein that serves as the cofactor for XIIa when clotting is initiated *in vitro* in the aPTT test.

Activation of Prothrombin. Factor Xa cleaves two peptide bonds in prothrombin to form thrombin. Activation of prothrombin by Xa is accelerated by Va, phospholipids, and Ca^{2+}. When all these components are present, prothrombin is activated nearly 20,000 times faster than the rate achieved by Xa and Ca^{2+} alone. The maximal rate of activation occurs only when prothrombin and Xa both contain Gla residues and, therefore, have the ability to bind to phospholipids. Purified platelets can substitute for phospholipids and Va to facilitate activation of prothrombin *in vitro,* provided that the platelets are stimulated to release endogenous platelet factor Va or that factor Va is added exogenously to unstimulated platelets. The surface of platelets that are aggregated at the site of hemostasis concentrates the factors required for activation of prothrombin.

Initiation of Coagulation. Clotting by the intrinsic pathway is initiated *in vitro* when XII, prekallikrein, and high-molecular-weight kininogen interact with kaolin, glass, or another surface to generate small amounts of XIIa. Activation of XI to XIa and IX to IXa follows. IXa then activates X in a reaction that is accelerated by VIIIa, phospholipids, and Ca^{2+}. Activation of factor X by IXa appears to occur by a mechanism similar to that for activation of prothrombin and may also be accelerated by platelets *in vivo.* Activation of factor XII is not required for hemostasis, since patients with deficiency of XII, prekallikrein, or high-molecular-weight kininogen do not bleed abnormally, even though their aPTT values are prolonged. Factor XI deficiency is associated with a variable and usually mild bleeding disorder. The mechanism for activation of factor XI *in vivo* is not known, although thrombin activates factor XI *in vitro*.

Coagulation is initiated *in vivo* by the extrinsic pathway. In this pathway, factor VII is activated by its product, factor Xa. Tissue factor accelerates activation of factor X by VIIa, phospholipids, and Ca^{2+} about 30,000-fold. It is likely that the availability of tissue factor at sites of injury plays a major role in the initiation of hemostasis. VIIa also can activate IX in the presence of tissue factor, providing a crossover point between the extrinsic and intrinsic pathways.

Natural Anticoagulant Mechanisms. Platelet activation and coagulation normally do not occur within an intact blood vessel (Rosenberg and Aird, 1999). Thrombosis is prevented by several regulatory mechanisms that require a normal vascular endothelium. Prostacyclin (PGI_2), a metabolite of arachidonic acid, is synthesized by endothelial cells, and it inhibits platelet aggregation and secretion (*see* Chapter 26). Antithrombin is a plasma protein that inhibits coagulation factors of the intrinsic and common pathways (*see* below). Heparan sulfate proteoglycans synthesized by endothelial cells stimulate the activity of antithrombin. Protein C is a plasma zymogen that is homologous to II, VII, IX, and X; its activity depends on the binding of Ca^{2+} to Gla residues within its amino-terminal domain. Activated protein C in combination with its nonenzymatic Gla-containing cofactor (protein S) degrades cofactors Va and VIIIa and thereby greatly diminishes the rates of activation of prothrombin and factor X. Protein C is activated by thrombin only in the presence of thrombomodulin, an integral membrane protein of endothelial cells. Like antithrombin, protein C appears to exert an anticoagulant effect in the vicinity of intact endothelial cells. Tissue factor pathway inhibitor (TFPI) is found in the lipoprotein fraction of plasma. When bound to factor Xa, TFPI inhibits factor Xa and the factor VIIa–tissue factor complex. By this mechanism, factor Xa may regulate its own production.

HEPARIN

History. In 1916 a medical student named McLean, while investigating the nature of ether-soluble procoagulants, made the serendipitous finding of a phospholipid anticoagulant. Soon thereafter, a water-soluble mucopolysaccharide, named *heparin* because of its abundance in liver, was discovered by Howell, in whose laboratory McLean had been working (*see* Jaques, 1978). The use of heparin *in vitro* to prevent the clotting of blood eventually led to its use *in vivo* to treat venous thrombosis.

Biochemistry and Mechanism of Action

Heparin is a glycosaminoglycan found in the secretory granules of mast cells. It is synthesized from UDP-sugar precursors as a polymer of alternating D-glucuronic acid and N-acetyl-D-glucosamine residues (Figure 55–2; Bourin and Lindahl, 1993). About 10 to 15 glycosaminoglycan chains, each containing 200 to 300 monosaccharide units, are attached to a core protein and yield a proteoglycan with a molecular mass of 750,000 to 1,000,000 daltons. The glycosaminoglycan then undergoes a series of modifications, which include the following: N-deacetylation and N-sulfation of glucosamine residues, epimerization of D-glucuronic acid to L-iduronic acid, O-sulfation of iduronic and glucuronic acid residues at the C 2 position, and O-sulfation of glucosamine residues at the C 3 and C 6 positions. Each of these modification reactions is incomplete, yielding a variety of oligosaccharide structures. After the

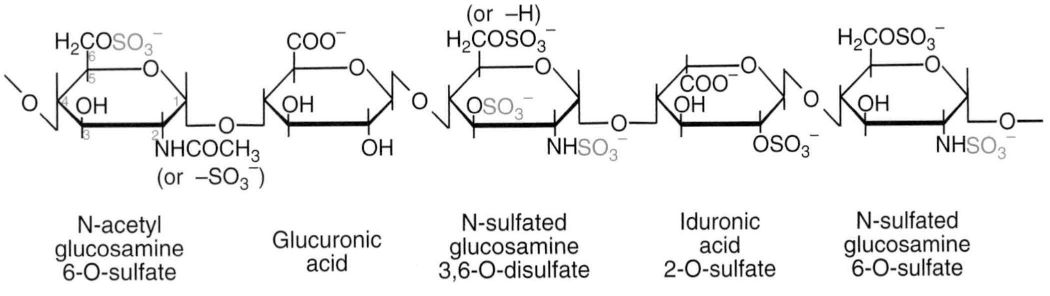

Figure 55–2. The antithrombin-binding structure of heparin.

Sulfate groups required for binding to antithrombin are indicated in blue.

heparin proteoglycan has been transported to the mast cell granule, an endo-β-D-glucuronidase degrades the glycosaminoglycan chains to 5000- to 30,000-dalton fragments (mean, about 12,000 daltons or 40 monosaccharide units) over a period of hours.

Related Glycosaminoglycans. Heparan sulfate is a closely related glycosaminoglycan found on the surface of most eukaryotic cells and in the extracellular matrix. It is synthesized from the same repeating disaccharide precursor (D-glucuronic acid linked to N-acetyl-D-glucosamine) as is heparin. However, heparan sulfate undergoes less modification of the polymer than does heparin and therefore contains higher proportions of glucuronic acid and N-acetylglucosamine and fewer sulfate groups. Heparan sulfate produces an anticoagulant effect when added to plasma *in vitro,* although a higher concentration is required in comparison with heparin.

Dermatan sulfate is a repeating polymer of L-iduronic acid and N-acetyl-D-galactosamine. O-sulfation of iduronic acid residues at the C 2 position and of galactosamine residues at the C 4 and C 6 positions occurs to a variable extent. Like heparan sulfate, dermatan sulfate is a component of the cell surface and the extracellular matrix. Dermatan sulfate also produces an anticoagulant effect *in vitro.*

Source. Heparin is commonly extracted from porcine intestinal mucosa or bovine lung. These preparations may contain small amounts of other glycosaminoglycans. Despite the heterogeneity in composition among different commercial preparations of heparin, their biological activities are similar (about 150 USP units/mg). The USP unit is the quantity of heparin that prevents 1.0 ml of citrated sheep plasma from clotting for 1 hour after the addition of 0.2 ml of 1% $CaCl_2$.

Low-molecular-weight heparins (1000 to 10,000 daltons; mean, 4500 daltons, or 15 monosaccharide units) are isolated from standard heparin by gel filtration chromatography, precipitation with ethanol, or partial depolymerization with nitrous acid and other chemical or enzymatic reagents. Low-molecular-weight heparins differ from standard heparin and from each other in their pharmacokinetic properties and mechanism of action (*see* below). The biological activity of low-molecular-weight heparin is generally measured with a factor Xa inhibition assay.

Physiological Function. Heparin occurs intracellularly in tissues that contain mast cells. It appears to be required for the storage of histamine and certain proteases within mast cell secretory granules (Humphries *et al.,* 1999; Forsberg *et al.,* 1999). When released from mast cells, heparin is ingested rapidly and destroyed by macrophages. Heparin cannot be detected in plasma under normal circumstances. However, patients with systemic mastocytosis who undergo massive degranulation of mast cells may have a mild prolongation of the aPTT, presumably resulting from the release of heparin into the circulation.

Heparan sulfate molecules on the surface of vascular endothelial cells or in the subendothelial extracellular matrix interact with circulating antithrombin (*see* below) to provide a natural antithrombotic mechanism. Patients with malignancies may experience bleeding related to circulating heparan sulfate or dermatan sulfate that probably originates from lysis of the tumor cells.

Mechanism of Action. In 1939, Brinkhous and coworkers discovered that the anticoagulant effect of heparin is mediated by an endogenous component of plasma, termed heparin cofactor. Thirty years later, antithrombin (or antithrombin III) was purified from plasma and was shown to have heparin cofactor activity. Antithrombin is a glycosylated, single-chain polypeptide with a mass of about 58,000 daltons that rapidly inhibits thrombin only in the presence of heparin (Olson and Björk, 1992). The protein is homologous to the α_1-antitrypsin family of protease inhibitors, dubbed *serpins,* for *ser*ine *p*roteinase *in*hibitors. Antithrombin is synthesized in the liver and circulates at an approximate concentration in plasma of 2.6 μM. It inhibits activated coagulation factors of the intrinsic and common pathways, including thrombin, Xa and IXa; however, it has relatively little activity against factor VIIa. Antithrombin is a "suicide substrate" for these proteases; inhibition occurs when the protease attacks a specific Arg-Ser peptide bond in the reactive site of antithrombin and becomes trapped as a stable 1:1 complex.

Heparin increases the rate of the thrombin-antithrombin reaction at least a thousandfold by serving as a catalytic template to which both the inhibitor and the protease bind. Binding of heparin also induces a conformational change in antithrombin that makes the reactive site more accessible to the protease (Jin *et al.,* 1997). Once thrombin has become bound to antithrombin, the heparin molecule is released from the complex. The binding site for antithrombin on heparin is a specific pentasaccharide sequence that contains a 3-O-sulfated glucosamine residue (*see* Figure 55–2). This structure occurs in about 30% of heparin molecules and less abundantly in heparan sulfate. Other glycosaminoglycans (*e.g.,* dermatan sulfate, chondroitin-4-sulfate, and chondroitin-6-sulfate) lack the antithrombin-binding structure and do not stimulate antithrombin. Heparin molecules containing fewer than 18 monosaccharide units (<5400 daltons) do not catalyze inhibition of thrombin by antithrombin. Molecules of this length or greater are required to bind thrombin and antithrombin simultaneously. In contrast, the pentasaccharide shown in Figure 55–2 catalyzes inhibition of factor Xa by antithrombin. In this case, catalysis may occur solely by induction of a conformational change in antithrombin that facilitates reaction with the protease. Low-molecular-weight heparin preparations produce an anticoagulant effect mainly through inhibition of Xa by antithrombin, because the majority of molecules are of insufficient length to catalyze inhibition of thrombin.

When the concentration of heparin in plasma is 0.1 to 1.0 U/ml, thrombin, factor IXa, and factor Xa are inhibited rapidly by antithrombin (half-life less than 0.1 second). This effect results in prolongation of the aPTT and the thrombin time (*i.e.*, the time required for plasma to clot when exogenous thrombin is added); the prothrombin time is affected to a lesser degree. Factor Xa bound to platelets in the prothrombinase complex and thrombin bound to fibrin are both protected from inhibition by antithrombin in the presence of heparin. Thus, heparin may promote inhibition of factor Xa and thrombin only after they have diffused away from these binding sites. Platelet factor 4, released from the α-granules during platelet aggregation, blocks binding of antithrombin to heparin or heparan sulfate and promotes local clot formation at the site of hemostasis.

In the presence of high concentrations of heparin (>5 U/ml) or dermatan sulfate, thrombin is inhibited primarily by heparin cofactor II. Heparin also stimulates inhibition of thrombin by plasminogen activator inhibitor 1 (PAI-1), protein C inhibitor, and protease nexin-1 (glia-derived nexin), and inhibition of factor Xa by tissue factor pathway inhibitor (TFPI). The latter four inhibitors are present in plasma at less than one-hundredth the concentration of antithrombin. Intravenous infusion of heparin increases the level of circulating TFPI severalfold, presumably by causing release of TFPI from binding sites on the endothelium.

Miscellaneous Effects. High doses of heparin can interfere with platelet aggregation and thereby prolong the bleeding time. It is unclear to what extent the antiplatelet effect of heparin contributes to the hemorrhagic complications of treatment with the drug. Heparin "clears" lipemic plasma *in vivo* by causing the release of lipoprotein lipase into the circulation. Lipoprotein lipase hydrolyzes triglycerides to glycerol and free fatty acids. The clearing of lipemic plasma may occur at concentrations of heparin below those necessary to produce an anticoagulant effect. Rebound hyperlipemia may occur after administration of heparin is stopped.

Heparin inhibits growth of a variety of cultured cells, including endothelial cells, vascular smooth muscle cells, and renal mesangial cells. In addition, heparin prevents the proliferation of vascular smooth muscle cells that follows damage to the carotid arterial endothelium in an animal model. These effects are independent of the anticoagulant activity of heparin (Wright *et al.*, 1989).

Acidic and basic fibroblast growth factors (aFGF and bFGF) bind to heparin with high affinity. These growth factors are mitogens for endothelial cells, smooth muscle cells, and other mesenchymal cells, and they induce angiogenesis. Although heparin by itself inhibits growth of capillary endothelial cells, it potentiates the growth-promoting effect of aFGF on these cells (Sudhalter *et al.*, 1989). This effect depends on the size and degree of sulfation of the heparin molecule but not on its anticoagulant activity. Heparan sulfate proteoglycans in the extracellular matrix stabilize bFGF and may serve as a reservoir from which the growth factor can be released by an excess of heparin or by digestion with heparitinase. Heparan sulfate provides a low-affinity binding site for bFGF on the surface of target mesenchymal cells. Furthermore, cell surface heparan sulfate or exogenous heparin promotes the binding of bFGF to its high-affinity receptor (a transmembrane tyrosine kinase) and is required for the biological activity of bFGF (Yayon *et al.*, 1991).

Clinical Use

Heparin is used to treat venous thrombosis and pulmonary embolism because of its rapid onset of action. An oral anticoagulant usually is started on the day of presentation, and heparin is continued for at least 4 to 5 days to allow the oral anticoagulant to achieve its full therapeutic effect (*see* "Clinical Use and Monitoring of Oral Anticoagulant Therapy," below). Patients who experience recurrent thromboembolism despite adequate oral anticoagulation (*e.g.*, patients with Trousseau's syndrome) may benefit from long-term heparin administration. Heparin is used in the initial management of patients with unstable angina or acute myocardial infarction, during and after coronary angioplasty or stent placement, and during surgery requiring cardiopulmonary bypass. Heparin also is used to treat selected patients with disseminated intravascular coagulation. Low-dose heparin regimens are effective in preventing venous thromboembolism in high-risk patients (*e.g.*, after orthopedic surgery). Specific recommendations for heparin use have been reviewed recently (Proceedings of the American College of Chest Physicians 5th Consensus Conference on Antithrombotic Therapy, 1998).

Low-molecular-weight heparin preparations were first approved for prevention of venous thromboembolism. More recently, they have been shown to be effective in the treatment of venous thrombosis, pulmonary embolism, and unstable angina (Hirsh *et al.*, 1998a). The principal advantage of low-molecular-weight heparin over standard heparin is a more predictable pharmacokinetic profile, which allows weight-adjusted subcutaneous administration without laboratory monitoring. Thus, therapy of many patients with acute venous thromboembolism can be provided in the outpatient setting. Other advantages of low-molecular-weight heparin include a lower incidence of heparin-induced thrombocytopenia and possibly lower risks of bleeding and osteopenia.

In contrast to warfarin, heparin does not cross the placenta and has not been associated with fetal malformations; therefore, it is the drug of choice for anticoagulation during pregnancy. Heparin does not appear to increase the incidence of fetal mortality or prematurity (Ginsberg *et al.*, 1989a,b). If possible, the drug should be discontinued 24 hours before delivery to minimize the risk of postpartum bleeding. The safety and efficacy of low-molecular-weight heparin use during pregnancy have not been adequately evaluated.

Absorption and Pharmacokinetics.   Heparin is not absorbed through the gastrointestinal mucosa and therefore is given parenterally. Administration is by continuous intravenous infusion or subcutaneous injection. Heparin has an immediate onset of action when given intravenously. In contrast, there is considerable variation in the bioavailability of heparin given subcutaneously, and the onset of action is delayed 1 to 2 hours; low-molecular-weight heparins are absorbed more uniformly.

The half-life of heparin in plasma depends on the dose administered. When 100, 400, or 800 U/kg of heparin is injected intravenously, the half-life of the anticoagulant activity is approximately 1, 2.5, and 5 hours, respectively (*see* Appendix II for pharmacokinetic data). Heparin appears to be cleared and degraded primarily by the reticuloendothelial system; a small amount of undegraded heparin also appears in the urine. The half-life of heparin may be shortened somewhat in patients with pulmonary embolism and prolonged in patients with hepatic cirrhosis or end-stage renal disease. Low-molecular-weight heparins have longer biological half-lives than do standard preparations of the drug.

Administration and Monitoring.   Full-dose heparin therapy usually is administered by continuous intravenous infusion. Treatment of venous thromboembolism is initiated with a bolus injection of 5000 U, followed by 1200 to 1600 U per hour delivered by an infusion pump. Therapy routinely is monitored by the aPTT. The therapeutic range for standard heparin is considered to be that which is equivalent to a plasma heparin level of 0.3 to 0.7 U/ml determined with an anti–factor Xa assay (Hirsh *et al.,* 1998a). The aPTT value that corresponds to this range varies depending on the reagent and instrument used to perform the assay. A clotting time of 1.8 to 2.5 times the normal mean aPTT value is generally assumed to be therapeutic; however, values in this range obtained with some aPTT assays may overestimate the amount of circulating heparin and, therefore, be subtherapeutic. The risk of recurrence of thromboembolism is greater in patients who do not achieve a therapeutic level of anticoagulation within the first 24 hours. Initially, the aPTT should be measured and the infusion rate adjusted every 6 hours; dose adjustments may be aided by use of a nomogram (Raschke *et al.,* 1993). Once a steady dosage schedule has been established, daily monitoring is sufficient.

Very high doses of heparin are required to prevent coagulation during cardiopulmonary bypass. The aPTT is prolonged indefinitely over the dosage range used. Another coagulation test, such as the activated clotting time, is employed to monitor therapy in this situation.

Subcutaneous administration of heparin can be used for the long-term management of patients in whom warfarin is contraindicated (*e.g.,* during pregnancy). A total daily dose of about 35,000 U administered as divided doses every 8 to 12 hours usually is sufficient to achieve an aPTT of 1.5 times the control value (measured midway between doses). Monitoring generally is unnecessary once a steady dosage schedule is established.

Low-dose heparin therapy is used prophylactically to prevent deep venous thrombosis and thromboembolism in susceptible patients. A suggested regimen for such treatment is 5000 U of heparin given subcutaneously every 8 to 12 hours. Laboratory monitoring is unnecessary, since this regimen does not prolong the aPTT.

Low-molecular-weight heparin preparations (*enoxaparin,* LOVENOX; *dalteparin,* FRAGMIN; *ardeparin,* NORMIFLO; *nadroparin,* FRAXIPARINE; *reviparin,* CLIVARINE; *tinzaparin,* INNOHEP; only the first three of these are available currently in the United States) differ considerably in composition, and it cannot be assumed that two preparations that have similar anti–factor Xa activity will produce equivalent antithrombotic effects. Low-molecular-weight heparins are administered in a fixed or weight-adjusted dosage regimen once or twice daily by subcutaneous injection. Since they have a minimal effect on tests of clotting *in vitro,* monitoring is not done routinely. Patients with end-stage renal failure may require monitoring with an anti–factor Xa assay because the half-life of low-molecular-weight heparin may be prolonged in this condition. Specific dosage recommendations for various low-molecular-weight heparins are obtained from the manufacturer's literature.

Heparin Resistance.   The dose of heparin required to produce a therapeutic aPTT is variable due to differences in the concentrations of heparin-binding proteins in plasma, such as histidine-rich glycoprotein, vitronectin, and platelet factor 4; these proteins competitively inhibit binding of heparin to antithrombin. Occasionally a patient's aPTT will not be prolonged unless very high doses of heparin (>50,000 U per day) are administered. Such patients may have "therapeutic" concentrations of heparin in plasma at the usual dose when values are measured by other tests (*e.g.,* anti–factor Xa activity or protamine sulfate titration). These patients may have very short aPTT values prior to treatment because of the presence of an increased concentration of factor VIII and may not be truly resistant to heparin. Other patients may require large doses of heparin because of accelerated clearance of the drug, as may occur with massive pulmonary embolism. Patients with inherited antithrombin deficiency ordinarily have 40% to 60% of the normal plasma concentration of this inhibitor and respond normally to intravenous heparin. However, acquired deficiency of antithrombin (concentration less than 25% of normal) may occur in patients with hepatic cirrhosis, nephrotic syndrome, or disseminated intravascular coagulation; large doses of heparin may not prolong the aPTT in these individuals.

Toxicities. *Bleeding.*   Bleeding is the primary untoward effect of heparin. Historically, major bleeding was reported in 1% to 33% of patients who received various forms of heparin therapy, and in one study there were 3 fatal bleeding episodes among 647 patients (Levine and Hirsh, 1986). Recent studies suggest that major bleeding occurs in <3% of patients treated with intravenous heparin for venous thromboembolism (Levine *et al.*, 1998). The incidence of bleeding is no worse in patients treated with low-molecular-weight heparin for this indication. Although the number of bleeding episodes appears to increase with the total daily dose of heparin and with the degree of prolongation of the aPTT, these correlations are weak, and patients can bleed with aPTT values that are within the therapeutic range. Often an underlying cause for bleeding is present, such as recent surgery, trauma, peptic ulcer disease, or platelet dysfunction.

The anticoagulant effect of heparin disappears within hours of discontinuation of the drug. Mild bleeding due to heparin usually can be controlled without the administration of an antagonist. If life-threatening hemorrhage occurs, the effect of heparin can be reversed quickly by the slow intravenous infusion of *protamine sulfate,* a mixture of basic polypeptides isolated from salmon sperm. Protamine binds tightly to heparin and thereby neutralizes its anticoagulant effect. Protamine also interacts with platelets, fibrinogen, and other plasma proteins and may cause an anticoagulant effect of its own. Therefore, one should give the minimal amount of protamine required to neutralize the heparin present in the plasma. This amount is approximately 1 mg of protamine for every 100 U of heparin remaining in the patient, given intravenously at a slow rate (up to 50 mg over 10 minutes).

Protamine is used routinely to reverse the anticoagulant effect of heparin following cardiac surgery and other vascular procedures. Anaphylactic reactions occur in about 1% of patients with diabetes mellitus who have received protamine-containing insulin (NPH insulin or protamine zinc insulin) but are not limited to this group. A less common reaction consisting of pulmonary vasoconstriction, right ventricular dysfunction, systemic hypotension, and transient neutropenia also may occur after administration of protamine.

Heparin-Induced Thrombocytopenia.   Heparin-induced thrombocytopenia (platelet count <150,000/μl or a 50%

decrease from the pretreatment value) occurs on about 3% of patients 5 to 10 days after initiation of therapy with standard heparin (Warkentin, 1999). The incidence is lower during treatment with low-molecular-weight heparin. Thrombotic complications that can be life-threatening or lead to amputation occur in about one-third of these patients and may precede the onset of thrombocytopenia. Venous thromboembolism occurs most commonly, but arterial thromboses causing limb ischemia, myocardial infarction, and stroke also occur. Bilateral adrenal necrosis, skin lesions at the site of subcutaneous heparin injection, and a variety of systemic reactions may accompany heparin-induced thrombocytopenia. The development of IgG antibodies against complexes of heparin with platelet factor 4 (or, rarely, other chemokines) appears to cause all of these reactions. These complexes activate platelets by binding to FcγIIa receptors, which results in platelet aggregation, release of more platelet factor 4, and thrombin generation. The antibodies also may trigger vascular injury by binding to platelet factor 4 attached to heparan sulfate on the endothelium.

Heparin should be discontinued immediately if unexplained thrombocytopenia or any of the clinical manifestations mentioned above occur 5 or more days after beginning heparin therapy, regardless of the dose or route of administration. The onset of heparin-induced thrombocytopenia may occur earlier in patients who have received heparin within the previous 3 to 4 months and have residual circulating antibodies. The diagnosis of heparin-induced thrombocytopenia can be confirmed by a heparin-dependent platelet activation assay or an assay for antibodies that react with heparin/platelet factor 4 complexes. Since thrombotic complications may occur after cessation of therapy (Wallis *et al.*, 1999; Warkentin, 1999), an alternative anticoagulant such as *lepirudin* or *danaparoid* (*see* below) should be administered to patients with heparin-induced thrombocytopenia. Low-molecular-weight heparins should be avoided, because these drugs often cross-react with standard heparin in heparin-dependent antibody assays. Warfarin may cause venous limb gangrene (Warkentin *et al.*, 1997) or multicentric skin necrosis (Warkentin *et al.*, 1999) in patients with heparin-induced thrombocytopenia and should not be used until the thrombocytopenia has resolved and the patient is adequately anticoagulated with another agent.

Other Toxicities.   Abnormalities of hepatic function tests occur frequently in patients who are receiving heparin intravenously or subcutaneously. Mild elevations of the activities of hepatic transaminases in plasma occur without an increase in bilirubin levels or alkaline phosphatase activity. Osteoporosis resulting in spontaneous vertebral fractures can occur, albeit infrequently, in patients who have received full therapeutic doses of heparin (greater than 20,000 U per day) for extended periods of time, *e.g.,* 3 to 6 months. Heparin can inhibit the synthesis of aldosterone by the adrenal glands and occasionally causes hyperkalemia, even when low doses are given. Allergic reactions to heparin (other than thrombocytopenia) are rare.

OTHER PARENTERAL ANTICOAGULANTS

Danaparoid. *Danaparoid* (ORGARAN) is a mixture of nonheparin glycosaminoglycans isolated from porcine intestinal mucosa (84% heparan sulfate, 12% dermatan sulfate, 4% chondroitin sulfate) with a mean mass of 5500 daltons. Danaparoid is approved in the United States for prophylaxis of deep venous thrombosis. It is also an effective anticoagulant for patients with heparin-induced thrombocytopenia and has a low rate of cross-reactivity with heparin in platelet-activation assays. Danaparoid mainly promotes inhibition of factor Xa by antithrombin, but it does not prolong the PT or aPTT at the recommended dosage. Danaparoid is administered subcutaneously at a fixed dose (750 anti–factor Xa units twice daily) for prophylactic use and intravenously at a higher, weight-adjusted dose for full anticoagulation (*see* Warkentin, 1999). Its half-life is about 24 hours. Patients with renal failure may require monitoring with an anti–factor Xa assay because of a prolonged half-life of the drug. No antidote is available.

Lepirudin. *Lepirudin* (REFLUDAN) is a recombinant derivative (Leu[1]-Thr[2]-63-desulfohirudin) of hirudin, a direct thrombin inhibitor present in the salivary glands of the medicinal leech. It is a 65-amino acid polypeptide that binds tightly to both the catalytic site and the extended substrate recognition site (exosite I) of thrombin. Lepirudin is approved in the United States for treatment of patients with heparin-induced thrombocytopenia (*see* Warkentin, 1999). It is administered intravenously at a dose adjusted to maintain the aPTT at 1.5 to 2.5 times the normal median value. The drug is excreted by the kidneys and has a half-life of about 1.3 hours. Lepirudin should be used cautiously in patients with renal failure, since it can accumulate and cause bleeding in these patients. Patients may develop antihirudin antibodies that occasionally cause a paradoxical increase in the aPTT; therefore, daily monitoring of the aPTT is recommended. There is no antidote for lepirudin.

ORAL ANTICOAGULANTS

History. Sweet clover was planted in the Dakota plains and Canada at the turn of the century because it flourished on poor soil and substituted for corn in silage. In 1924, Schofield reported a previously undescribed hemorrhagic disorder in cattle that resulted from the ingestion of spoiled sweet clover silage. After Roderick traced the cause to a toxic reduction of plasma prothrombin, Campbell and Link, in 1939, identified the hemorrhagic agent as bishydroxycoumarin (dicoumarol). In 1948, a more potent synthetic congener was introduced as an extremely effective rodenticide; the compound was named *warfarin* as an acronym derived from the name of the patent holder, Wisconsin Alumni Research Foundation, plus the coum*arin*-derived suffix. Potential for the use of warfarin as a therapeutic agent for thromboembolic disease was recognized but not widely accepted, partly due to fear of unacceptable toxicity. However, in 1951, an army inductee uneventfully survived an attempted suicide with massive doses of a preparation of warfarin intended for rodent control. Since then, these anticoagulants have become a mainstay for prevention of thromboembolic disease, and they are administered to hundreds of thousands of patients annually. Warfarin is the prototypical oral anticoagulant and by far the most frequently prescribed. However, the anticoagulant action of all the drugs in this class is similar, differing mainly in potency and duration of action.

Chemistry. Numerous anticoagulants have been synthesized as derivatives of 4-hydroxycoumarin and of the related compound, indan-1,3-dione (Figure 55–3). Only the coumarin derivatives are widely used; the 4-hydroxycoumarin residue, with a nonpolar carbon substituent at the 3 position, is the minimal structural requirement for activity. This carbon is asymmetrical in warfarin (and in phenprocoumon and acenocoumarol). The enantiomers differ in anticoagulant potency, metabolism, elimination, and interactions with some other drugs (O'Reilly, 1987). Commercial preparations of these anticoagulants are racemic mixtures. No advantage of administering a single enantiomer has been established.

Pharmacological Properties

Mechanism of Action. The oral anticoagulants are antagonists of vitamin K (*see* Chapter 64). Coagulation factors II, VII, IX, and X and the anticoagulant proteins C and S are synthesized mainly in the liver and are biologically inactive unless 9 to 12 of the amino-terminal glutamic acid residues are carboxylated (Furie *et al.,* 1999). The γ-carboxyglutamate (Gla) residues confer Ca^{2+}-binding properties on these proteins that are essential for their assembly into an efficient catalytic complex on a membrane surface. This reaction requires carbon dioxide, molecular oxygen, reduced vitamin K, and a precursor form of the target protein containing a propeptide recognition site (Figure 55–4). It is catalyzed in the rough endoplasmic reticulum by a 758-residue protein that has been purified, cloned, and characterized (Morris *et al.,* 1993).

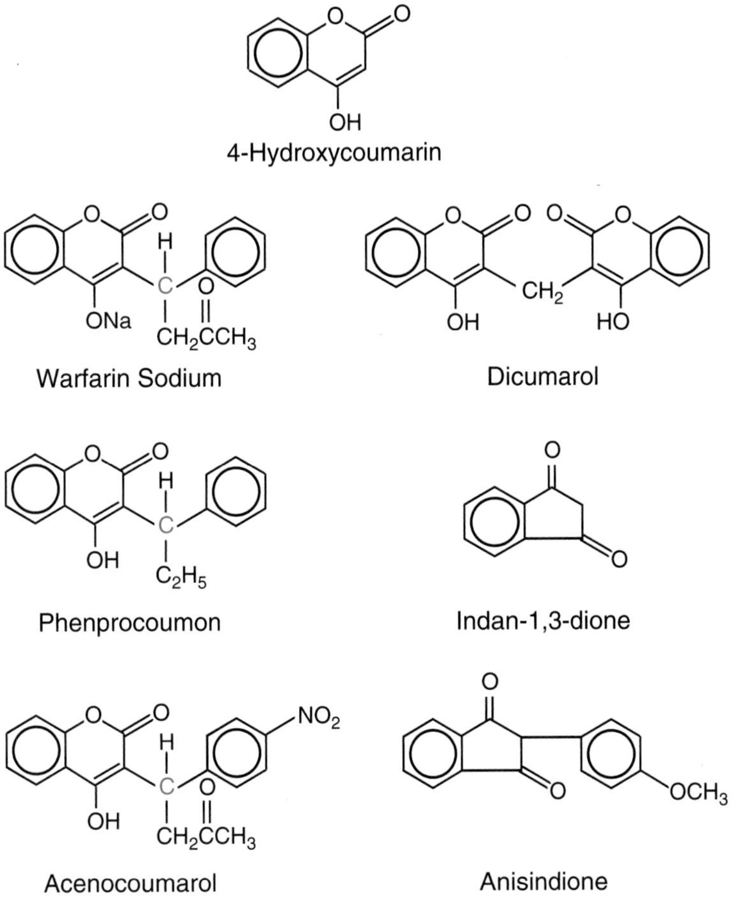

Figure 55–3. Structural formulas of the oral anticoagulants.

4-Hydroxycoumarin and indan-1,3-dione are included to indicate the parent molecules from which the oral anticoagulants are derived. The asymmetrical carbon atoms in the coumarins are shown in blue.

Carboxylation is directly coupled to the oxidation of vitamin K to the epoxide.

Reduced vitamin K must be regenerated from the epoxide for sustained carboxylation and synthesis of biologically competent proteins. The vitamin K epoxide reductase is composed of two proteins in the endoplasmic reticulum: microsomal epoxide reductase and a member of the glutathione S-transferase gene family (Cain *et al.*, 1997). This enzyme complex is inhibited by therapeutic doses of oral anticoagulants. Vitamin K (but not vitamin K epoxide) also can be converted to the hydroquinone by a second reductase, DT-diaphorase. The latter enzyme requires high concentrations of vitamin K and is less sensitive to coumarin drugs, which may explain why administration of sufficient vitamin K can counteract even large doses of oral anticoagulants.

Therapeutic doses of warfarin decrease the total amount of each vitamin K–dependent coagulation factor made by the liver by 30% to 50%; in addition, the secreted molecules are undercarboxylated, resulting in diminished biological activity (10% to 40% of normal). Congenital deficiencies of the procoagulant proteins to these levels cause mild bleeding disorders. Oral anticoagulants have no effect on the activity of fully carboxylated molecules in the circulation. Thus, the time required for the activity of each factor in plasma to reach a new steady state after therapy is initiated or adjusted depends on its individual rate of clearance. The approximate half-lives (in hours) are as follows: factor VII, 6; factor IX, 24; factor X, 36; factor II, 50; protein C, 8; and protein S, 30. Because of the long half-lives of some of the coagulation factors, in particular factor II, the full antithrombotic effect following initiation of warfarin therapy is not achieved for several days, even though the PT may be prolonged soon after administration due to the more rapid reduction of factors with a shorter half-life, in particular factor VII.

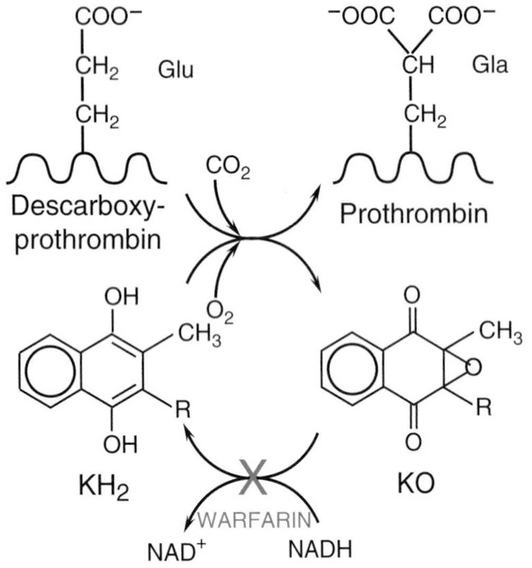

Figure 55–4. Vitamin K cycle: metabolic interconversions of vitamin K associated with the modification of vitamin K-dependent proteins.

Vitamin K_1 or K_2 is reduced to the hydroquinone (KH_2). Oxidation to vitamin K epoxide (KO) is coupled to carboxylation of glutamate (Glu) to γ-carboxyglutamate (Gla) residues of precursor proteins in the endoplasmic reticulum. The enzymatic reaction of the epoxide to regenerate vitamin KH_2 is the warfarin-sensitive step. The R on the vitamin K molecule represents a 20-carbon phytyl side chain in vitamin K_1 and a 5- to 65-carbon prenyl side chain in vitamin K_2.

There is no obvious selectivity of the effect of warfarin on any particular vitamin K–dependent coagulation factor, although the antithrombotic benefit and the hemorrhagic risk of therapy may be correlated with the functional level of prothrombin and, to a lesser extent, factor X (Sise *et al.,* 1958; Zivelin *et al.,* 1993). Vitamin K–dependent carboxylase activity occurs in many tissues, and other proteins have Gla residues. Bone contains low-molecular-weight vitamin K–dependent proteins (osteocalcin, matrix Gla protein), which are believed to play a role in mineralization; and vitamin K–dependent γ-carboxylation of the 1,25-dihydroxyvitamin D_3 receptor reportedly influences its DNA binding (Sergeev and Norman, 1992). Bone mineral density in adults is not changed by therapeutic use of oral anticoagulants (Rosen *et al.,* 1993), but new bone formation may be affected.

Dosage. The usual adult dose of warfarin (COUMADIN) is 5 mg per day for 2 to 4 days, followed by 2 to 10 mg per day as indicated by measurements of the international normalized ratio (INR), a value derived from the patient's PT (*see* definition of INR in section on laboratory mon-

itoring, below). An initial dose of 7.5 mg per day may be given to patients weighing >80 kg, but loading doses larger than this generally are not recommended. Warfarin usually is administered orally, but the drug also can be given intravenously without modification of the dose. Intramuscular injection is not recommended because of the risk of hematoma formation.

Absorption. The bioavailability of solutions of racemic sodium warfarin is nearly complete when the drug is administered orally, intramuscularly, intravenously, or rectally. Bleeding has occurred from repeated skin contact with solutions of warfarin used as a rodenticide. However, different commercial preparations of warfarin tablets vary in their rate of dissolution, and this causes some variation in the rate and extent of absorption. Food in the gastrointestinal tract also can decrease the rate of absorption. Warfarin usually is detectable in plasma within 1 hour of its oral administration, and concentrations peak in 2 to 8 hours.

Distribution. Warfarin is almost completely (99%) bound to plasma proteins, principally albumin, and the drug distributes rapidly into a volume equivalent to the albumin space (0.14 liter/kg). Concentrations in fetal plasma approach the maternal values, but active warfarin is not found in milk (unlike other coumarins and indandiones).

Biotransformation and Elimination. Warfarin is transformed into inactive metabolites by the liver (Kaminsky and Zhang, 1997), and these are excreted in urine and stool. The average rate of clearance from plasma is 0.045 ml·min^{-1}·kg^{-1}. The half-life ranges from 25 to 60 hours, with a mean of about 40 hours; the duration of action of warfarin is 2 to 5 days.

Drug and Other Interactions. The list of drugs and other factors that may affect the action of oral anticoagulants is prodigious and expanding (*see* Freedman and Olatidoye, 1994; Wells *et al.,* 1994; Harder and Thürmann, 1996). Any substance or condition is potentially dangerous if it alters (1) the uptake or metabolism of the oral anticoagulant or vitamin K; (2) the synthesis, function, or clearance of any factor or cell involved in hemostasis or fibrinolysis; or (3) the integrity of any epithelial surface. Patients must be educated to report the addition or deletion of any medication, including nonprescription drugs and food supplements. Some of the more commonly described factors that cause a decreased effect of oral anticoagulants include reduced absorption of drug caused by binding to cholestyramine in the gastrointestinal tract; increased volume of distribution and a short half-life secondary to hypoproteinemia, as in nephrotic syndrome; increased metabolic clearance of drug secondary to induction of hepatic enzymes by barbiturates, rifampin, phenytoin, or chronic ingestion of alcohol; ingestion of large amounts of vitamin K–rich foods or supplements; and increased levels of coagulation factors during pregnancy. Hence, the PT will be shortened in most of these cases.

Frequently cited interactions that enhance the risk of hemorrhage in patients taking oral anticoagulants include decreased metabolism and/or displacement from protein binding sites caused by phenylbutazone, sulfinpyrazone, metronidazole, disulfiram, allopurinol, cimetidine, amiodarone, or acute intake of ethanol. Relative deficiency of vitamin K may result from inadequate diet (*e.g.,* postoperative patients on parenteral fluids), especially when coupled with the elimination of intestinal flora by antimicrobial agents. Gut bacteria synthesize vitamin K and thus are an important source of this vitamin. Consequently, antibiotics can cause excessive prolongation of the prothrombin time in patients adequately controlled on warfarin. In addition to an effect on reducing intestinal flora, cephalosporins containing heterocyclic side chains also inhibit the vitamin epoxidase (and therefore the carboxylase). Low concentrations of coagulation factors may result from impaired hepatic function, congestive heart failure, or hypermetabolic states, such as hyperthyroidism. Generally, these factors increase the prolongation of the PT. Serious interactions that do not alter the PT include inhibition of platelet function by agents such as aspirin and gastritis or frank ulceration induced by antiinflammatory drugs. Agents may have more than one effect; for example, clofibrate increases the rate of turnover of coagulation factors and inhibits platelet function. Age is correlated with increased sensitivity to oral anticoagulants.

Resistance to Warfarin. Some patients require more than 20 mg per day of warfarin to achieve a therapeutic INR. These patients often are found to have excessive vitamin K intake from the diet or parenteral supplementation. Noncompliance and laboratory error are other causes of apparent warfarin resistance. A few patients with hereditary warfarin resistance have been reported, in whom very high plasma concentrations of warfarin are associated with minimal depression of vitamin K–dependent coagulation factor biosynthesis (Alving *et al.,* 1985); abnormalities in vitamin K epoxide reductase cause a similar phenomenon in the rat.

Sensitivity to Warfarin. Approximately 10% of patients require less than 1.5 mg per day of warfarin to achieve an INR of 2.0 to 3.0. These patients are more likely to possess one or two variant alleles of the cytochrome P450 CYP2C9, which is the major enzyme responsible for converting S-warfarin to its inactive metabolites (Aithal *et al.,* 1999). In comparison with the wild-type CYP2C9*1 allele, the variant alleles CYP2C9*2 and CYP2C9*3 have been shown to inactivate S-warfarin much less efficiently *in vitro.* The variant alleles are present in 10% to 20% of Caucasians but in <5% of African-Americans or Asians.

Toxicity. Bleeding is the major toxicity of oral anticoagulant drugs (Levine *et al.,* 1998). The risk of bleeding increases with the intensity and duration of anticoagulant therapy, the use of other medications that interfere with hemostasis, and the presence of a potential anatomical source of bleeding. Especially serious episodes involve sites where irreversible damage may result from compression of vital structures (*e.g.,* intracranial, pericardial, nerve sheath, or spinal cord) or from massive internal blood loss that may not be diagnosed rapidly (*e.g.,* gastrointestinal, intraperitoneal, retroperitoneal). Although the reported incidence of major bleeding episodes varies considerably, it is generally less than 5% per year

in patients treated with a target INR of 2.0 to 3.0. The risk of intracranial hemorrhage increases dramatically with an INR greater than 4.0, especially in older patients. In a large outpatient anticoagulation clinic, the most common factors associated with a transient elevation of the INR (greater than 6.0) were use of a new medication known to potentiate warfarin (*e.g.,* acetaminophen), advanced malignancy, recent diarrheal illness, decreased oral intake, and taking more warfarin than prescribed (Hylek *et al.,* 1998). Patients must be informed of the signs and symptoms of bleeding, and laboratory monitoring should be done at frequent intervals during intercurrent illnesses or any changes of medication or diet.

If the INR is above the therapeutic range but <5.0 and the patient is not bleeding or in need of a surgical procedure, warfarin can be discontinued temporarily and restarted at a lower dose once the INR is within the therapeutic range (Hirsh *et al.,* 1998b). If the INR is ≥5.0, vitamin K_1 (*phylloquinone, phytonadione,* MEPHYTON, AQUAMEPHYTON) can be given orally at a dose of 1.0 to 2.5 mg (for an INR between 5.0 and 9.0) or 3.0 to 5.0 mg (for an INR greater than 9.0). These dosages of oral vitamin K_1 generally cause the INR to fall substantially within 24 to 48 hours without rendering the patient resistant to further warfarin therapy. Higher doses may be required if more rapid correction of the INR is necessary. The effect of vitamin K_1 is delayed for at least several hours, because reversal of anticoagulation requires synthesis of fully carboxylated coagulation factors. If immediate hemostatic competence is necessary because of serious bleeding or profound warfarin overdosage (INR >20), adequate concentrations of vitamin K–dependent coagulation factors can be restored by transfusion of fresh-frozen plasma (10 to 20 ml per kg), supplemented with 10 mg of vitamin K_1 by slow intravenous infusion. Transfusion of plasma may need to be repeated, since the transfused factors (particularly factor VII) are cleared from the circulation more rapidly than the residual oral anticoagulant. Vitamin K_1 administered intravenously carries the risk of anaphylactoid reactions and, therefore, should be used cautiously. Patients who receive high doses of vitamin K_1 may become unresponsive to warfarin for several days, but heparin can be used if continued anticoagulation is required.

Administration of warfarin during pregnancy is a cause of birth defects and abortion. A syndrome characterized by nasal hypoplasia and stippled epiphyseal calcifications that resemble chondrodysplasia punctata may result from maternal ingestion of warfarin during the first trimester. Central nervous system abnormalities have been reported following exposure during the second and third trimesters. Fetal or neonatal hemorrhage and intrauterine death may occur, even when maternal PT values are in the therapeutic range. Oral anticoagulants should not be used during pregnancy, but as indicated in the previous section, heparin can be used safely in this circumstance.

Coumarin-induced skin necrosis is a rare complication of oral anticoagulant therapy. First noted in 1943, this syndrome is characterized by the appearance of skin lesions 3 to 10 days after treatment is initiated. This unusual reaction has been observed with different congeners of coumarin and indandione. Patients who develop the lesions during one course of therapy often (but not always) can be treated later without a similar reaction. The severity of the skin lesions may not be affected by stopping as compared with continuing the drug. The lesions are most common on the extremities, but adipose tissue, the penis, and the female breast may be involved. Lesions are characterized by widespread thrombosis of the microvasculature and can spread rapidly, sometimes becoming necrotic and requiring disfiguring debridement or occasionally amputation. Cases have been reported recently in subjects heterozygous for protein C or protein S deficiency. Since protein C has a shorter half-life than do the other vitamin K–dependent coagulation factors (except factor VII), its functional activity falls more rapidly in response to the initial dose of vitamin K antagonist. It has been proposed that the skin necrosis is a manifestation of a temporal imbalance between the anticoagulant protein C and one or more of the procoagulant factors and is exaggerated in patients who are partially deficient in protein C or protein S. However, not all patients with heterozygous deficiency of protein C or protein S develop skin necrosis when treated with oral anticoagulants, and patients with normal activities of these proteins also can be affected. Morphologically similar lesions can occur without oral anticoagulant therapy, especially in patients with vitamin K deficiency.

A reversible, sometimes painful, blue-tinged discoloration of the plantar surfaces and sides of the toes that blanches with pressure and fades with elevation of the legs (purple toe syndrome) may develop 3 to 8 weeks after initiation of therapy with coumarin anticoagulants. Cholesterol emboli released from atheromatous plaques have been implicated as the cause. Other infrequent reactions include alopecia, urticaria, dermatitis, fever, nausea, diarrhea, abdominal cramps, and anorexia.

Warfarin appears to precipitate the syndromes of venous limb gangrene (Warkentin *et al.,* 1997) and multicentric skin necrosis (Warkentin *et al.,* 1999) that are sometimes associated with heparin-induced thrombocytopenia. Another anticoagulant agent such as lepirudin or danaparoid should be used until the heparin-induced thrombocytopenia has resolved (*see* the section on heparin toxicity, above).

Clinical Use and Monitoring

Oral anticoagulants are used to prevent the progression or recurrence of acute deep vein thrombosis or pulmonary embolism following an initial course of heparin. They also are effective in preventing venous thromboembolism in patients undergoing orthopedic or gynecological surgery

and systemic embolization in patients with acute myocardial infarction, prosthetic heart valves, or chronic atrial fibrillation. Specific recommendations for oral anticoagulant use for these and other indications have been reviewed recently (Proceedings of the American College of Chest Physicians 5th Consensus Conference on Antithrombotic Therapy, 1998).

Prior to initiation of therapy, laboratory tests are used in conjunction with the patient's history and physical examination to uncover hemostatic defects that might make the use of oral anticoagulant drugs more dangerous (congenital coagulation factor deficiency, thrombocytopenia, hepatic or renal insufficiency, vascular abnormalities, *etc.*). Thereafter, the INR calculated from the patient's PT is used to monitor efficacy and compliance. Therapeutic ranges for various clinical indications have been established empirically and reflect dosages that reduce the morbidity from thromboembolic disease while increasing as little as possible the risk of serious hemorrhage. For most indications the target INR is 2.0 to 3.0. A higher target INR (*e.g.,* 3.0 to 4.0) is generally recommended for patients with mechanical prosthetic heart valves (Hirsh *et al.,* 1998b).

For treatment of acute venous thromboembolism, heparin usually is continued for at least 4 to 5 days after oral anticoagulation is begun and until the INR is in the therapeutic range on 2 consecutive days. This overlap allows for adequate depletion of the vitamin K–dependent coagulation factors with long half-lives, especially factor II. Daily INR measurements are indicated at the onset of therapy to guard against excessive anticoagulation in the unusually sensitive patient. The testing interval can be lengthened gradually to weekly and then to monthly for patients on long-term therapy in whom test results have been stable.

To monitor therapy, a fasting blood sample is usually obtained 8 to 14 hours after the last dose of an oral anticoagulant, and the patient's PT is determined along with that of a sample of normal pooled plasma. Formerly, the results were reported as a simple ratio of the two PT values. However, this ratio can vary widely depending on the thromboplastin reagent and the instrument used to initiate and detect clot formation. The PT is prolonged when the functional levels of fibrinogen, factor V, or the vitamin K–dependent factors II, VII, or X are decreased. Reduced levels of factor IX or proteins C or S have no effect on the PT. Efforts to standardize testing between laboratories, begun in the mid-1980s, led to the widespread adoption of the INR system of reporting in the 1990s. PT measurements are converted to INR measurements by the following equation:

$$INR = \left(\frac{PT_{pt}}{PT_{ref}}\right)^{ISI} \qquad (55\text{–}1)$$

where   INR = International Normalized Ratio
        ISI = International Sensitivity Index

The ISI value, generally supplied by the manufacturer, indicates the relative sensitivity of the PT determined with a given thromboplastin to decreases in the vitamin K–dependent coagulation factors in comparison with a World Health Organization human thromboplastin standard. Reagents with lower ISI values are more sensitive to the effects of oral anticoagulants (*i.e.,* the PT is prolonged to a greater extent in comparison with that obtained with a less sensitive reagent having a higher ISI). Ideally, the ISI value of each batch of thromboplastin should be confirmed in each clinical laboratory using a set of reference plasmas to control for local variables of sample handling and instrumentation.

The major practical consequence of standardization to the INR has been an appreciation that the commercial thromboplastins from rabbit tissue, used especially in North America, are relatively insensitive. This property led to administration of larger doses of oral anticoagulants than were considered optimal in many of the original clinical trials in which more sensitive human brain thromboplastins were generally used. Thus, the target INR of 2.0 to 3.0 corresponds to a PT ratio of 1.2 to 1.5 if rabbit thromboplastin is used or 2.0 to 3.0 if human thromboplastin is used.

The INR does not provide a reliable indication of the degree of anticoagulation in patients with the lupus anticoagulant, in whom the PT and other phospholipid-dependent coagulation tests are prolonged at baseline. In these patients, a chromogenic anti–factor Xa assay or the prothrombin-proconvertin–time assay may be used to monitor therapy (Moll and Ortel, 1997).

Other Oral Anticoagulants

Dicumarol. *Dicumarol* is the original oral anticoagulant isolated and the first used clinically, but it is now seldom used because it is absorbed slowly and erratically, and it frequently causes gastrointestinal side effects. It is usually given in maintenance doses of 25 to 200 mg daily. Its onset of action as monitored by the PT is 1 to 5 days, and its effect lasts 2 to 10 days after withdrawal.

Phenprocoumon and Acenocoumarol. These agents are not generally available in the United States but are prescribed in Europe and elsewhere. *Phenprocoumon* (MAR-CUMAR) has a longer plasma half-life (5 days) than warfarin, as well as a somewhat slower onset of action and a longer duration of action (7 to 14 days). It is administered in daily maintenance doses of 0.75 to 6.0 mg. By contrast, *acenocoumarol* (SINTHROME) has a shorter half-life (10 to 24 hours), a more rapid effect on the PT, and a shorter duration of action (2 days). The maintenance dose is 1 to 8 mg daily.

Indandione Derivatives. *Anisindione* (MIRADON) is available for clinical use in the United States. It is simi-

lar to warfarin in its kinetics of action; however, it offers no clear advantages and may cause a higher frequency of untoward effects. *Phenindione* (DINDEVAN, PINDIONE) was popular at one time and still is available in some countries. Serious hypersensitivity reactions, occasionally fatal, can occur within a few weeks of starting therapy with this drug, and its use can no longer be recommended.

Rodenticides. *Bromadiolone,* *brodifacoum,* *diphenadione,* *chlorophacinone,* and *pindone* are long-acting agents (prolongation of the PT may persist for weeks). These are of interest because they sometimes are agents of accidental or intentional poisoning.

THROMBOLYTIC DRUGS

Fibrinolysis and Thrombolysis

The fibrinolytic system dissolves intravascular clots as a result of the action of plasmin, an enzyme that digests fibrin. Plasminogen, an inactive precursor, is converted to plasmin by cleavage of a single peptide bond. Plasmin is a relatively nonspecific protease; it digests fibrin clots and other plasma proteins, including several coagulation factors. Therapy with thrombolytic drugs tends to dissolve both pathological thrombi and fibrin deposits at sites of vascular injury. Therefore, the drugs are toxic, producing hemorrhage as a major side effect.

The fibrinolytic system is regulated such that unwanted fibrin thrombi are removed, while fibrin in wounds persists to maintain hemostasis (Collen and Lijnen, 1994). Tissue plasminogen activator (t-PA) is released from endothelial cells in response to various signals, including stasis produced by vascular occlusion. It is rapidly cleared from blood or inhibited by circulating inhibitors, plasminogen activator inhibitor-1 and plasminogen activator inhibitor-2, and thus exerts little effect on circulating plasminogen. t-PA binds to fibrin and converts plasminogen, which also binds to fibrin, to plasmin. Plasminogen and plasmin bind to fibrin at binding sites located near their amino termini that are rich in lysine residues (*see* below). These sites also are required for binding of plasmin to the inhibitor α_2-antiplasmin. Therefore, fibrin-bound plasmin is protected from inhibition. Any plasmin that escapes this local milieu is rapidly inhibited. Some α_2-antiplasmin is bound covalently to fibrin and thereby protects fibrin from premature lysis. When plasminogen activators are administered for thrombolytic therapy, massive fibrinolysis is initiated, and the inhibitory controls just described are overwhelmed.

Plasminogen. Plasminogen is a single-chain glycoprotein that contains 791 amino acid residues; it is converted to an active protease by cleavage at arginine 560. The molecule contains high affinity, amino-terminal lysine-containing binding sites that mediate the binding of plasminogen (or plasmin) to fibrin; this enhances fibrinolysis. These sites are in the amino-terminal "kringle" domain between amino acids 80 and 165, and they also promote formation of complexes of plasmin with α_2-antiplasmin, the major physiological plasmin inhibitor. Plasminogen concentrations in human plasma average 2 μM. A degraded form of plasminogen termed *lys-plasminogen* binds to fibrin much more rapidly than does intact plasminogen.

α_2-Antiplasmin. α_2-Antiplasmin is a glycoprotein composed of 452 amino acid residues. It forms a stable complex with plasmin, thereby inactivating it. Plasma concentrations of α_2-antiplasmin (1 mM) are sufficient to inhibit about 50% of potential plasmin. When massive activation of plasminogen occurs, the inhibitor is depleted, and free plasmin causes a "systemic lytic state," in which hemostasis is impaired. In this state, fibrinogen is destroyed and fibrinogen degradation products impair formation of fibrin and therefore increase bleeding from wounds. α_2-Antiplasmin inactivates plasmin nearly instantaneously, as long as the lysine binding sites on plasmin are unoccupied by fibrin or other antagonists, such as aminocaproic acid (6-aminocaproic acid; *see* below).

Streptokinase. *Streptokinase* (STREPTASE) is a 47,000-dalton protein produced by β-hemolytic streptococci. It has no intrinsic enzymatic activity, but it forms a stable, noncovalent 1:1 complex with plasminogen. This produces a conformational change that exposes the active site on plasminogen that cleaves arginine 560 on free plasminogen molecules to form free plasmin.

A loading dose of streptokinase (250,000 U; 2.5 mg) must be given intravenously to overcome plasma antibodies that are directed against the protein. These inactivating antibodies result from prior streptococcal infections. The half-life of streptokinase (once antibodies are depleted) is about 40 to 80 minutes (Battershill *et al.,* 1994). The streptokinase-plasminogen complex is not inhibited by α_2-antiplasmin. Levels of antibodies differ greatly among individuals, but this variable probably is of little clinical significance when streptokinase is given in the large doses currently used for coronary thrombolysis. Adverse reactions (other than the bleeding problems that are common to all fibrinolytic agents) include allergic reactions, rarely anaphylaxis, and fever.

A streptokinase-plasminogen complex (*anistreplase,* EMINASE), in which lys-plasminogen is acylated at its catalytic-site serine, also is used for coronary thrombolysis (ISIS-3, 1992). The acyl group is hydrolyzed *in vivo,* allowing the complex to bind to fibrin prior to activation, and this modification confers some specificity toward clots on the fibrinolytic process. However, when this agent is given as a bolus injection at the dose recommended for coronary thrombolysis (30 U), marked systemic fibrinolysis occurs.

Tissue Plasminogen Activator (t-PA). t-PA is a serine protease that contains 527 amino acid residues. It is a poor plasminogen activator in the absence of fibrin (Collen and Lijnen, 1994). t-PA binds to fibrin *via* lysine binding sites at its amino terminus and activates bound plasminogen several hundredfold more rapidly than it activates plasminogen in the circulation. The lysine binding sites on t-PA are in a "finger" domain that is homologous to similar sites on fibronectin. Under physiological conditions (t-PA concentrations of 5 to 10 ng/ml), the specificity of t-PA for fibrin limits systemic formation of plasmin and induction of a systemic lytic state. During therapeutic infusions of t-PA, however, concentrations rise to 300 to 3000 ng/ml. Clearance of t-PA primarily occurs by hepatic metabolism, and the half-life of the protein is 5 to 10 minutes. t-PA is effective in lysing thrombi during treatment of acute myocardial infarction. t-PA (*alteplase,* ACTIVASE) is produced by recombinant DNA technology. The current recommended ("accelerated") regimen for coronary thrombolysis is a 15-mg intravenous bolus, followed by 0.75 mg/kg of body weight over 30 minutes (not to exceed 50 mg) and 0.5 mg/kg (up to 35 mg accumulated dose) over the following hour. Adverse effects include hemorrhage, as discussed below. t-PA is expensive, costing several times more than streptokinase per therapeutic dose. A deletion mutant variant of t-PA (*reteplase,* RETAVASE) also is available and is similar in efficacy and toxicity to alteplase.

Urokinase. *Urokinase* (ABBOKINASE) is a two-chain serine protease containing 411 amino acid residues. It is isolated from cultured human kidney cells. It has a half-life of 15 to 20 minutes and is metabolized by the liver. Recommended dosage regimens include an intravenous loading dose of 1000 to 4500 U/kg, followed by continuous infusion of 4400 U/kg per hour for varying time periods. Current interest in urokinase is limited, since it has the disadvantages of both of the other available thrombolytic agents. Like streptokinase, it lacks fibrin specificity and therefore readily induces a systemic lytic state; like t-PA, it is very expensive. At present, production of urokinase has been suspended because of problems in the manufacturing process. *Saruplase* (prourokinase; single-chain urokinase) does display selectivity for clots by binding to fibrin before activation. Saruplase currently is under investigation as a thrombolytic agent.

Hemorrhagic Toxicity of Thrombolytic Therapy. The major toxicity of all thrombolytic agents is hemorrhage, which results from two factors: (1) the lysis of fibrin in "physiological thrombi" at sites of vascular injury; and (2) a systemic lytic state that results from systemic

Table 55–1
Contraindications to Thrombolytic Therapy

1. Surgery within 10 days, including organ biopsy, puncture of noncompressible vessels, serious trauma, cardiopulmonary resuscitation
2. Serious gastrointestinal bleeding within 3 months
3. History of hypertension (diastolic pressure >110 mm Hg)
4. Active bleeding or hemorrhagic disorder
5. Previous cerebrovascular accident or active intracranial process
6. Aortic dissection
7. Acute pericarditis

formation of plasmin, which produces fibrinogenolysis and destruction of other coagulation factors (especially factors V and VIII). The actual toxicity of streptokinase, urokinase, and t-PA is difficult to assess. In early clinical trials, many bleeding episodes resulted from the extensive invasive monitoring of therapy that was required by the protocol. Many studies to evaluate thrombolysis involved concurrent systemic heparinization, which also contributes to bleeding complications. Analysis of recent clinical trials suggests that heparin confers no benefit in patients receiving fibrinolytic therapy plus aspirin (Collins *et al.*, 1997; Zijlstra *et al.*, 1999).

The contraindications to fibrinolytic therapy are listed in Table 55–1. Patients with the indicated conditions should not receive such treatment, and invasive procedures (*e.g.*, cardiac catheterization, arterial blood gases) should be avoided. If heparin is used concurrently with either streptokinase or t-PA, serious hemorrhage will occur in 2% to 4% of patients. Intracranial hemorrhage is by far the most serious problem. Hemorrhagic stroke occurs with all regimens and is more common when heparin is used. In several large studies, t-PA was associated with an excess of hemorrhagic strokes of about 3 per 1000 patients treated. Despite the fact that t-PA is relatively fibrin-specific, hemorrhage is slightly more common with this agent than with the others, possibly because t-PA is more effective at dissolving "physiological thrombi" than are the other two drugs and thus, despite less systemic lysis, bleeding at sites of injury may be more severe. The recent large streptokinase trials that did not routinely use heparin had very low incidences of serious hemorrhage (less than 1%). When streptokinase is used as in these regimens, the toxicity may be low enough to relax the contraindications listed in Table 55–1 (*e.g.*, hypertension). The efficacies of t-PA and streptokinase in treating myocardial infarction in three large trials involving almost 100,000 patients are essentially identical. Both agents reduce death and reinfarction by about 30% in regimens containing aspirin (Zijlstra *et al.*, 1999). Given that t-PA is expensive and

more toxic, streptokinase is the agent of choice for coronary fibrinolysis; t-PA may be considered for use in patients who have previously received streptokinase and have high antibody titers. Recent studies suggest that angioplasty with or without stent placement, when feasible, is superior to thrombolytic therapy (Cairns *et al.*, 1998; Michels and Yusuf, 1995; Weaver *et al.*, 1997).

It is clear that the frequency of hemorrhage is less when thrombolytic agents are utilized to treat myocardial infarction compared with pulmonary embolism or venous thrombosis. A major difference in these regimens is the duration of therapy. A thrombolytic agent is infused for 1 to 3 hours for myocardial infarction; infusions of 12 to 72 hours have been used for venous disease. Such prolonged treatment probably should not be used. Recent studies indicate that the concurrent administration of low doses of aspirin improves the efficacy of thrombolytic therapy of myocardial infarction. Other antiplatelet drugs and alternative dosing regimens currently are under investigation. It seems likely that aspirin plus either a thienopyridine or glycoprotein IIb/IIIa inhibitor will increase therapeutic benefit.

Aminocaproic Acid. *Aminocaproic acid* (AMICAR) is a lysine analog that binds to lysine binding sites on plasminogen and plasmin, thus blocking the binding of plasmin to target fibrin. Aminocaproic acid is thereby a potent inhibitor of fibrinolysis and can reverse states that are associated with excessive fibrinolysis. Although it has been used in a variety of bleeding conditions, it is without clear-cut benefit. The main problem with its use is that thrombi that form during treatment with the drug are not lysed. For example, in patients with hematuria, ureteral obstruction by clots may lead to renal failure after treatment with aminocaproic acid. Aminocaproic acid has been used to reduce bleeding after prostatic surgery or after tooth extractions in hemophiliacs. The clinical significance of reduced bleeding in these settings is uncertain. Use of aminocaproic acid to treat a variety of other bleeding disorders has been unsuccessful, either because of limited benefit or because of thrombosis (*e.g.*, after subarachnoid hemorrhage). Aminocaproic acid is absorbed rapidly after oral administration, and 50% is excreted unchanged in the urine within 12 hours. Usually, a loading dose of 4 to

5 g is given over 1 hour, followed by an infusion of 1 g per hour until bleeding is controlled. No more than 30 g should be given in a 24-hour period. Rarely, the drug causes myopathy and muscle necrosis.

ANTIPLATELET DRUGS

Platelets provide the initial hemostatic plug at sites of vascular injury. They also participate in pathological thromboses that lead to myocardial infarction, stroke, and peripheral vascular thromboses. Potent inhibitors of platelet function have been developed in recent years. These drugs act by discrete mechanisms, and thus in combination their effects are additive or even synergistic. Their availability has led a revolution in cardiovascular medicine, whereby angioplasty and vascular stenting of lesions is now feasible with low rate of restenosis and thrombosis when effective platelet inhibition is employed.

Aspirin.   Processes including thrombosis, inflammation, wound healing, and allergy are modulated by oxygenated metabolites of arachidonate and related polyunsaturated fatty acids that are collectively termed *eicosanoids.* Interference with the synthesis of eicosanoids is the basis for the effects of many therapeutic agents, including analgesics, antiinflammatory drugs, and antithrombotic agents (*see* Chapters 26 and 27).

In platelets, the major cyclooxygenase product is thromboxane A_2, a labile inducer of platelet aggregation and a potent vasoconstrictor. Aspirin blocks production of thromboxane A_2 by covalently acetylating a serine residue near the active site of cyclooxygenase, the enzyme that produces the cyclic endoperoxide precursor of thromboxane A_2. Since platelets do not synthesize new proteins, the action of aspirin on platelet cyclooxygenase is permanent, lasting for the life of the platelet (7 to 10 days). Thus, repeated doses of aspirin produce a cumulative effect on platelet function. Complete inactivation of platelet cyclooxygenase is achieved when 160 mg of aspirin is taken daily. Therefore, aspirin is maximally effective as an antithrombotic agent at doses much lower than required for other actions of the drug. Numerous trials indicate that aspirin, when used as an antithrombotic drug, is maximally effective at doses of 160 to 320 mg per day (Antiplatelet Trialists' Collaboration, 1994a; Patrono *et al.,* 1998). Higher doses do not improve efficacy; moreover, they potentially are less efficacious because of inhibition of prostacyclin production, which can be largely spared by using lower doses of aspirin. Higher doses also increase toxicity, especially bleeding.

Other inhibitors of eicosanoid biosynthesis have been evaluated as potential antithrombotic agents, especially inhibitors of thromboxane synthetase. These drugs have the theoretical advantage of inhibiting production of thromboxane A_2 without blocking the synthesis of prostacyclin, an antithrombotic eicosanoid produced by the vascular endothelium. However, these drugs allow cyclic endoperoxide intermediates to accumulate, which themselves stimulate platelet aggregation. Thus, these agents have been relatively ineffective and do not measure up well against the cost, safety, and efficacy of aspirin.

Dipyridamole.   *Dipyridamole* (PERSANTINE) is a vasodilator that, in combination with warfarin, inhibits embolization from prosthetic heart valves and, in combination with aspirin, reduces thrombosis in patients with thrombotic diseases. Dipyridamole by itself has little or no benefit; in fact, in trials where a regimen of dipyridamole plus aspirin was compared with aspirin alone, dipyridamole provided no additional beneficial effect (Antiplatelet Trialists' Collaboration, 1994a, b, c). A recent study suggests that dipyridamole plus aspirin reduces strokes in patients with prior strokes or TIA (Diener *et al.,* 1996). A formulation containing 200 mg of dipyridamole, in an extended-release form, and 25 mg of aspirin (AGGRENOX) has been marketed recently. Dipyridamole interferes with platelet function by increasing the cellular concentration of adenosine 3′,5′-monophosphate (cyclic AMP). This effect is mediated by inhibition of cyclic nucleotide phosphodiesterase and/or by blockade of uptake of adenosine, which acts at A_2 receptors for adenosine to stimulate platelet adenylyl cyclase. The only current recommended use of dipyridamole is for primary prophylaxis of thromboemboli in patients with prosthetic heart valves; the drug is given in combination with warfarin.

Ticlopidine (TICLID).   Purinergic receptors respond to extracellular nucleotides as agonists. Platelets contain two purinergic receptors of the P2Y type. These receptors are G protein–coupled, seven-membrane-spanning receptors. The platelet P2Y1 receptor is coupled to the G_q G protein (*see* Chapter 2). Adenosine diphosphate (ADP) activates this receptor and evokes platelet shape change, phosphatidylinositol turnover, and platelet aggregation. The other platelet receptor is coupled to G_i and, when activated by ADP, inhibits adenylyl cyclase, resulting in lower levels of cyclic AMP and thereby less platelet activation. Based on pharmacological studies, it appears that both receptors must be stimulated to result in platelet activation (Daniel *et al.,* 1998; Jin and Kunapuli, 1998). Inhibition of either receptor will thus block platelet activation. Ticlopidine is a thienopyridine (Figure 55–5) that blocks the G_i–coupled

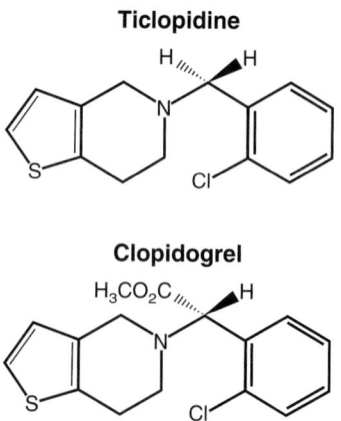

Figure 55–5. Structure of ticlopidine and clopidogrel.

platelet ADP receptor. The drug is probably a prodrug that requires conversion to the active yet unknown metabolite by a hepatic cytochrome P450. It is rapidly absorbed and highly bioavailable. Maximal inhibition of platelet aggregation is not seen until 8 to 11 days after starting therapy. Thus, in some studies, "loading doses" of 500 mg have been given to achieve more rapid onset of action. The usual dose is 250 mg twice per day. Inhibition of platelet aggregation persists for a few days after the drug is stopped.

Adverse Effects.   The most common side effects are nausea, vomiting, and diarrhea. The most serious is severe neutropenia in up to 1% of patients. Therefore, frequent blood counts should be obtained during the first few months of therapy. Platelet counts also should be monitored, as thrombocytopenia has been reported. Rare cases of thrombotic thrombocytopenic purpura have been associated with ticlopidine; these usually remit when the drug is stopped (Quinn and Fitzgerald, 1999).

Therapeutic Uses.   Ticlopidine has been shown to prevent cerebrovascular events in secondary prevention of stroke and is at least as good as aspirin in this regard (Patrono *et al.,* 1998). It also reduces cardiac events in patients with unstable angina. Since ticlopidine has a mechanism of action distinct from that of aspirin, combining the drugs might be expected to provide additive or even synergistic effects. This appears to be the case, and the combination has been used in patients undergoing angioplasty and stenting for coronary artery disease, with a very low frequency of stent thrombosis occurring over a short, 30-day follow-up (<1%) (Leon *et al.,* 1998).

Clopidogrel (PLAVIX).   This thienopyridine is closely related to ticlopidine and appears to have a slightly more favorable toxicity profile with less frequent thrombocytopenia and leukopenia, although recently thrombotic thrombocytopenic purpura has been reported (Bennett *et al.,* 2000). It has been used much less extensively than ticlopidine, and thus the frequency of rare toxicities is unclear. The drug is similar to ticlopidine in that it appears to be a prodrug with a slow onset of action. The usual dose is 75 mg per day with or without an initial loading dose of 300 mg. The drug is equivalent to aspirin in the secondary prevention of stroke, and in combination with aspirin it appears to be as effective as ticlopidine and aspirin (Quinn and Fitzgerald, 1999).

Glycoprotein IIb/IIIa Inhibitors.   Glycoprotein IIb/IIIa is a platelet-surface integrin which, by the integrin nomenclature, is designated $\alpha_{IIb}\beta_3$. This dimeric glycoprotein is a receptor for fibrinogen and von Willebrand factor, which anchor platelets to foreign surfaces and to each other, thereby mediating aggregation. The receptor is activated by platelet agonists such as thrombin, collagen, or thromboxane A_2 to develop binding sites for its ligands,

which do not bind to resting platelets. Inhibition of binding to this receptor blocks platelet aggregation induced by any agonist. Thus, inhibitors of this receptor are potent antiplatelet agents that act by a distinct mechanism from that of aspirin or the thienopyridine platelet inhibitors. Three agents are approved for use at present with others under development.

Abciximab (REOPRO).   This is the Fab fragment of a humanized monoclonal antibody directed against the $\alpha_{IIb}\beta_3$ receptor. It also binds to the vitronectin receptor on platelets, vascular endothelial cells, and smooth muscle cells. The antibody is used in conjunction with percutaneous angioplasty for coronary thromboses and has been shown to be quite effective in preventing restenosis, recurrent myocardial infarction, and death when used in conjunction with aspirin and heparin. The reduction in total events is about 50% in various large trials (Scarborough *et al.,* 1999). The unbound antibody is cleared from the circulation with a half-life of about 30 minutes, but bound antibody remains bound to the $\alpha_{IIb}\beta_3$ receptor and inhibits platelet aggregation as measured *in vitro* for 18 to 24 hours after infusion is stopped. It is given as a 0.25-mg/kg bolus followed by 0.125 μg/kg per minute for 12 hours or longer. It is currently being evaluated as an antiplatelet drug for other indications, *e.g.,* in conjunction with fibrinolysis protocols.

Adverse Effects.   The major side effect of abciximab is bleeding, and the contraindications to use of the antibody are similar to those for fibrinolytic agents listed in Table 55–1. The frequency of major hemorrhage varies considerably in various trials from 1% to 10%, depending on the intensity of anticoagulation with heparin. Thrombocytopenia of less than 50,000/μl is seen in about 2% of patients and may be due to development of neoepitopes induced by bound antibody. Since the duration of action is long, if major bleeding or emergent surgery occurs, platelet transfusions can reverse the aggregation defect, because free antibody concentrations fall rapidly after cessation of infusion. Readministration of antibody has been performed in a small number of patients without evidence of decreased efficacy or allergic reactions. The antibody is very expensive ($1500 per dose), which has limited its use in some settings.

Eptifibatide (INTEGRILIN).   This is a cyclic peptide inhibitor of the RGD binding site on $\alpha_{IIb}\beta_3$. It blocks platelet aggregation *in vitro* after intravenous infusion into patients. Eptifibatide is given as a bolus of 135 to 180 μg/kg followed by 0.5 to 2.0 μg/kg per minute for up to 72 hours. It is used to treat unstable angina and for angioplastic coronary interventions. In the latter case, the events of myocardial infarction or death have been reduced by about 20%. Although the drug has not been compared directly to abciximab, it appears that its benefit is somewhat less than that obtained with the antibody. This might result from the fact that eptifibatide is specific for $\alpha_{IIb}\beta_3$ and does not react with the vitronectin receptor. The duration of action of the drug is relatively short, with restoration of platelet aggregation within 6 to 12 hours after cessation of infusion.

Adverse Effects. The major side effect is bleeding, as is the case with abciximab. The frequency of major bleeding in trials was about 10%, compared with about 9% in the placebo arms, which included heparin. Thrombocytopenia has been seen in 0.5% to 1% of patients.

Tirofiban (AGGRASTAT). This is a nonpeptide, small-molecule inhibitor of $\alpha_{IIb}\beta_3$ that appears to be similar to eptifibatide. It has a short duration of action and has efficacy in non-Q-wave myocardial infarction and unstable angina. Reductions in death and myocardial infarction have been about 20% compared to placebo, results similar to those with eptifibatide. Side effects also are similar to those of eptifibatide. The agent is specific to $\alpha_{IIb}\beta_3$ and does not react with the vitronectin receptor.

Future Perspectives. Several additional parenteral $\alpha_{IIb}\beta_3$ inhibitors are in various stages of development. Several oral agents also are under evaluation, but results of their clinical trials have been disappointing to date. Issues of dosage and indications remain to be resolved. It may be that small-molecule inhibitors of $\alpha_{IIb}\beta_3$ will need to be combined with vitronectin receptor blockers to achieve the results obtained with abciximab. These potentially more aggressive approaches to therapy must be cautious, because the major toxicity of anticoagulants and antiplatelet agents is impaired hemostasis, which is also the basis for their efficacy.

PROSPECTUS

Several new antithrombotic agents currently are under investigation. These agents must show an improved efficacy over available agents without an increased toxicity. However, since efficacy and toxicity are so closely related for antithrombotic agents and current drugs are quite efficacious with only moderate toxicity, the challenge for new agents to reach the clinic is great. Well-designed clinical studies stratified for the risk of recurrent venous and arterial thromboembolism still are needed to determine the optimal intensity and duration of therapy with currently available agents. Since several of the new antiplatelet agents have been used in only a few regimens, clinical trials need to be continued to discover the optimal combinations of drugs to maximize safety and minimize toxicity. In this way, prevention of thrombosis may be improved. The development of portable devices to measure the INR in patients undergoing long-term therapy with oral anticoagulants should permit patient self-management, which may lead to reduction of cost and episodes of hemorrhage.

For further discussion of clotting disorders, *see* Chapters 117, 118, and 119 in *Harrison's Principles of Internal Medicine,* 14th ed., McGraw-Hill, New York, 1998.

BIBLIOGRAPHY

Aithal, G.P., Day, C.P., Kestaven, P.J.L., and Daly, A.K. Association of polymorphisms in the cytochrome P450 CYP2C9 with warfarin dose requirement and risk of bleeding complications. *Lancet,* **1999,** *353*:717–719.

Alving, B.M., Strickler, M.P., Knight, R.D., Barr, C.F., Berenberg, J.L., and Peck, C.C. Hereditary warfarin resistance. Investigation of a rare phenomenon. *Arch. Intern. Med.,* **1985,** *145*:499–501.

Antiplatelet Trialists' Collaboration. Collaborative overview of randomised trials of antiplatelet therapy. I: Prevention of death, myocardial infarction, and stroke by prolonged antiplatelet therapy in various categories of patients. *Br. Med. J.,* **1994a,** *308*:81–106.

Antiplatelet Trialists' Collaboration. Collaborative overview of randomised trials of antiplatelet therapy. II: Maintenance of vascular graft or arterial patency by antiplatelet therapy. *Br. Med. J.,* **1994b,** *308*:159–168.

Antiplatelet Trialists' Collaboration. Collaborative overview of randomised trials of antiplatelet therapy. III: Reduction in venous thrombosis and pulmonary embolism by antiplatelet prophylaxis among surgical and medical patients. *Br. Med. J.,* **1994c,** *308*:235–246.

Bennett, C.L., Connors, J.M., Carwile, J.M., Moake, J.L., Bell, W.R., Tarantolo, S.F., McCarthy, L.J., Sarode, R., Hatfield, A.J., Feldman, M.D., Davidson, C.J., and Tsai, H.-M. Thrombotic thrombocytopenic purpura associated with clopidogrel. *N. Engl. J. Med.,* **2000,** *342*:1773–1777.

Cain, D., Hutson, S.M., and Wallin, R. Assembly of the warfarin-sensitive vitamin K 2,3-epoxide reductase enzyme complex in the endoplasmic reticulum membrane. *J. Biol. Chem.,* **1997,** *272*:29068–29075.

Daniel, J.L., Dangelmaier, C., Jin, J., Ashby, B., Smith, J.B., and Kunapuli, S.P. Molecular basis for ADP-induced platelet activation.

I. Evidence for three distinct ADP receptors on human platelets. *J. Biol. Chem.*, **1998,** *273*:2024–2029.

Diener, H.C., Cunha, L., Forbes, C., Sivenius, J., Smets, P., and Lowenthal, A. European Stroke Prevention Study. 2. Dipyridamole and acetylsalicylic acid in the secondary prevention of stroke. *J. Neurol. Sci.*, **1996,** *143*:1–13.

Forsberg, E., Pejler, G., Ringvall, M., Lunderius, C., Tomasini-Johansson, B., Kusche-Gullberg, M., Eriksson, I., Ledin, J., Hellman, L., and Kjellén, L. Abnormal mast cells in mice deficient in heparin-synthesizing enzyme. *Nature,* **1999,** *400*:773–776.

Humphries, D.E., Wong, G.W., Friend, D.S., Gurish, M.F., Qiu, W.-T., Huang, C., Sharpe, A.H., and Stevens, R.L. Heparin is essential for the storage of specific granule proteases in mast cells. *Nature,* **1999,** *400*:769–772.

Ginsberg, J.S., Hirsh, J., Turner, D.C., Levine, M.N., and Burrows, R. Risks to the fetus of anticoagulant therapy during pregnancy. *Thromb. Haemost.*, **1989a,** *61*:197–203.

Ginsberg, J.S., Kowalchuk, G., Hirsh, J., Brill-Edwards, P., and Burrows, R. Heparin therapy during pregnancy. Risks to the fetus and mother. *Arch. Intern. Med.*, **1989b,** *149*:2233–2236.

Hylek, E.M., Heiman, H., Skates, S.J., Sheehan, M.A., and Singer, D.E. Acetaminophen and other risk factors for excessive warfarin anticoagulation. *JAMA,* **1998,** *279*:657–662.

ISIS-3 (Third International Study of Infarct Survival) Collaborative Group. ISIS-3: a randomised comparison of streptokinase vs. tissue plasminogen activator vs. anistreplase and of aspirin plus heparin vs. aspirin alone among 41,299 cases of suspected acute myocardial infarction. *Lancet,* **1992,** *339*:753–770.

Jin, L., Abrahams, J.P., Skinner, R., Petitou, M., Pike, R.N., and Carrell, R.W. The anticoagulant activation of antithrombin by heparin. *Proc. Natl. Acad. Sci. U.S.A.*, **1997,** *94*:14683–14688.

Jin, J., and Kunapuli, S.P. Coactivation of two different G protein-coupled receptors is essential for ADP-induced platelet aggregation. *Proc. Natl. Acad. Sci. U.S.A.*, **1998,** *95*:8070–8074.

Leon, M.B., Baim, D.S., Popma, J.J., Gordon, P.C., Cutlip, D.E., Ho, K.K., Giambartolomei, A., Diver, D.J., Lasorda, D.M., Williams, D.O., Pocock, S.J., and Kuntz, R.E. A clinical trial comparing three antithrombotic-drug regimens after coronary-artery stenting. Stent Anticoagulation Restenosis Study Investigators. *N. Engl. J. Med.*, **1998,** *339*:1665–1671.

Michels, K.B., and Yusuf, S. Does PTCA in acute myocardial infarction affect mortality and reinfarction rates? A quantitative overview (meta-analysis) of the randomized clinical trials. *Circulation,* **1995,** *91*:476–485.

Moll, S., and Ortel, T.L. Monitoring warfarin therapy in patients with lupus anticoagulants. *Ann. Intern. Med.*, **1997,** *127*:177–185.

Morris, D.P., Soute, B.A.M., Vermeer, C., and Stafford, D.W. Characterization of the purified vitamin K–dependent γ-glutamyl carboxylase. *J. Biol. Chem.*, **1993,** *268*:8735–8742.

Raschke, R.A., Reilly, B.M., Guidry, J.R., Fontana, J.R., and Srinivas, S. The weight-based heparin dosing nomogram compared with a "standard care" nomogram. A randomized controlled trial. *Ann. Intern. Med.*, **1993,** *119*:874–881.

Rosen, H.N., Maitland, L.A., Suttie, J.W., Manning, W.J., Glynn, R.J., and Greenspan, S.L. Vitamin K and maintenance of skeletal integrity in adults. *Am. J. Med.*, **1993,** *94*:62–68.

Sergeev, I.N., and Norman, A.W. Vitamin K–dependent gamma-carboxylation of the 1,25-dihydroxyvitamin D3 receptor. *Biochem. Biophys. Res. Commun.*, **1992,** *189*:1543–1547.

Sise, H.S., Lavelle, S.M., Dionysios, A., and Becker, R. Relations of hemorrhage and thrombosis to prothrombin during treatment with

coumarin-type anticoagulants. *N. Engl. J. Med.*, **1958,** *259*:266–271.

Sudhalter, J., Folkman, J., Svahn, C.M., Bergendal, K., and D'Amore, P.A. Importance of size, sulfation, and anticoagulant activity in the potentiation of acidic fibroblast growth factor by heparin. *J. Biol. Chem.*, **1989,** *264*:6892–6897.

Wallis, D.E., Workman, D.L., Lewis, B.E., Steen, L., Pifarre, R., and Moran, J.F. Failure of early heparin cessation as treatment for heparin-induced thrombocytopenia. *Am. J. Med.*, **1999,** *106*:629–635.

Warkentin, T.E., Elavathil, L.J., Hayward, C.P., Johnston, M.A., Russett, J.I., and Kelton, J.G. The pathogenesis of venous limb gangrene associated with heparin-induced thrombocytopenia. *Ann. Intern. Med.*, **1997,** *127*:804–812.

Warkentin, T.E., Sikov, W.M., and Lillicrap, D.P. Multicentric warfarin-induced skin necrosis complicating heparin-induced thrombocytopenia. *Am. J. Hematol.*, **1999,** *62*:44–48.

Wright, T.C. Jr., Castellot, J.J. Jr., Petitou, M., Lormeau, J.-C., Choay, J., and Karnovsky, M.J. Structural determinants of heparin's growth inhibitory activity. Interdependence of oligosaccharide size and charge. *J. Biol. Chem.*, **1989,** *264*:1534–1542.

Yayon, A., Klagsbrun, M., Esko, J.D., Leder, P., and Ornitz, D.M. Cell surface, heparin-like molecules are required for binding of basic fibroblast growth factor to its high affinity receptor. *Cell,* **1991,** *64*:841–848.

Zijlstra, F., Hoorntje, J.C.A., de Boer, M.-J., Reiffers, S., Miedema, K., Ottervanger, J.P., van't Hof, A.W.J., and Suryanpranata, H. Long-term benefit of primary angioplasty as compared with thrombolytic therapy for acute myocardial infarction. *N. Engl. J. Med.*, **1999,** *341*:1413–1419.

Zivelin, A., Rao, L.V., and Rapaport, S.I. Mechanism of the anticoagulant effect of warfarin as evaluated in rabbits by selective depression of individual procoagulant vitamin K-dependent clotting factors. *J. Clin. Invest.*, **1993,** *92*:2131–2140.

MONOGRAPHS AND REVIEWS

Battershill, P.E., Benfield, P., and Goa, K.L. Streptokinase. A review of its pharmacology and therapeutic efficacy in acute myocardial infarction in older patients. *Drugs Aging,* **1994,** *4*:63–86.

Bourin, M.-C., and Lindahl, U. Glycosaminoglycans and the regulation of blood coagulation. *Biochem. J.*, **1993,** *289*:313–330.

Cairns, J.A., Kennedy, J.W., and Fuster, V. Coronary thrombolysis. *Chest,* **1998,** *114*:634S–657S.

Collen, D., and Lijnen, H.R. Fibrinolysis and the control of hemostasis. In, *The Molecular Basis of Blood Diseases,* 2nd ed. (Stamatoyannopoulos, G., Nienhuis, A.W., Majerus, P.W., and Varmus, H., eds). W.B. Saunders Co., Philadelphia, **1994,** pp. 725–752.

Collins, R., Peto, R., Baigent, C., and Sleight, P. Aspirin, heparin, and fibrinolytic therapy in suspected acute myocardial infarction. *N. Engl. J. Med.*, **1997,** *336*:847–860.

Davie, E.W., Fujikawa, K., and Kisiel, W. The coagulation cascade: initiation, maintenance, and regulation. *Biochemistry,* **1991,** *30*:10363–10370.

Esmon, C.T. Cell mediated events that control blood coagulation and vascular injury. *Annu. Rev. Cell Biol.*, **1993,** *9*:1–26.

Freedman, M.D., and Olatidoye, A.G. Clinically significant drug interactions with the oral anticoaglants. *Drug Saf.*, **1994,** *10*:381–394.

Furie, B., Bouchard, B.A., and Furie, B.C. Vitamin K-dependent biosynthesis of γ-carboxyglutamic acid. *Blood,* **1999,** *93*:1798–1808.

Harder, S., and Thürmann, P. Clinically important drug interactions with anticoagulants. An update. *Clin. Pharmacokinet.*, **1996,** *30*:416–444.

Hirsh, J., Warkenitin, T.E., Raschke, R., Granger, C., Ohman, E.M., and Dalen, J.E. Heparin and low-molecular-weight heparin: mechanisms of action, pharmacokinetics, dosing considerations, monitoring, efficacy, and safety. *Chest,* **1998a,** *114*:489S–510S.

Hirsh, J., Dalen, J.E., Anderson, D.R., Poller, L., Bussey, H., Ansell, J., Deykin, D., and Brandt, J.T. Oral anticoagulants: mechanism of action, clinical effectiveness, and optimal therapeutic range. *Chest,* **1998b,** *114*:445S–469S.

Jaques, L.B. Addendum: the discovery of heparin. *Semin. Thromb. Hemost.,* **1978,** *4*:350–353.

Kaminsky, L.S., and Zhang, Z.-Y. Human P450 metabolism of warfarin. *Pharmacol. Ther.,* **1997,** *73*:67–74.

Levine, M.N., and Hirsh, J. Hemorrhagic complications of anticoagulant therapy. *Semin. Thromb. Hemost.,* **1986,** *12*:39–57.

Levine, M.N., Raskob, G., Landefeld, S., and Kearon, C., Hemorrhagic complications of anticoagulant treatment. *Chest,* **1998,** *114*:511S–523S.

Olson, S.T., and Björk, I. Regulation of thrombin by antithrombin and heparin cofactor II In, *Thrombin: Structure and Function.* (Berliner, L.J., ed.) Plenum Press, New York, **1992,** pp. 159–217.

O'Reilly, R.A. Warfarin metabolism and drug-drug interactions. *Adv. Exp. Med. Biol.,* **1987,** *214*:205–212.

Patrono, C., Coller, B., Dalen, J.E., Fuster, V., Gent, M., Harker, L.A., Hirsh, J., and Roth, G. Platelet-active drugs: the relationships among dose, effectiveness, and side effects. *Chest,* **1998,** *114*:470S–488S.

Proceedings of the American College of Chest Physicians 5th Consensus Conference on Antithrombotic Therapy. *Chest,* **1998,** *114*:439S–769S.

Quinn, M.J., and Fitzgerald, D.J. Ticlopidine and clopidogrel. *Circulation,* **1999,** *100*:1667–1672.

Rosenberg, R.D., and Aird, W.C. Vascular-bed–specific hemostasis and hypercoagulable states. *N. Engl. J. Med.,* **1999,** *340*:1555–1564.

Scarborough, R.M., Kleiman, N.S., and Phillips, D.R. Platelet glycoprotein IIb/IIIa antagonists. What are the relevant issues concerning their pharmacology and clinical use? *Circulation,* **1999,** *100*:437–444.

Warkentin, T.E. Heparin-induced thrombocytopenia: a ten-year retrospective. *Annu. Rev. Med.,* **1999,** *50*:129–147.

Weaver, W.D., Simes, R.J., Betriu, A., Grines, C.L., Zijlstra, F., Garcia, E., Grinfeld, L., Gibbons, R.J., Ribeiro, E.E., DeWood, M.A., and Ribichini, F. Comparison of primary coronary angioplasty and intravenous thrombolytic therapy for acute myocardial infarction: a quantitative review. *JAMA,* **1997,** *278*:2093–2098.

Wells, P.S., Holbrook, A.M., Crowther, N.R., and Hirsh, J. Interactions of warfarin with drugs and food. *Ann. Intern. Med.,* **1994,** *121*:676–683.

SECTION XII

HORMONES AND HORMONE ANTAGONISTS

C H A P T E R   5 6

PITUITARY HORMONES AND THEIR HYPOTHALAMIC RELEASING FACTORS

Keith L. Parker and Bernard P. Schimmer

This chapter covers the diagnostic and therapeutic uses of some of the pituitary hormones—including growth hormone (GH), prolactin, luteinizing hormone (LH), follicle-stimulating hormone (FSH), and oxytocin—as well as the therapeutic approaches to conditions of excess secretion of GH and prolactin. Also discussed are the clinical and diagnostic uses of hypothalamic factors that regulate the secretion of pituitary hormones, including growth hormone-releasing hormone (GHRH), somatostatin, and gonadotropin-releasing hormone (GnRH). FSH, LH, and GnRH also are discussed in Chapters 58 and 59. Considered elsewhere are corticotropin and corticotropin-releasing hormone (Chapter 60) and thyrotropin and thyrotropin releasing hormone (Chapter 57).

The peptide hormones of the anterior pituitary are essential for the regulation of growth and development, reproduction, responses to stress, and intermediary metabolism. Their synthesis and secretion are controlled by hypothalamic hormones and by hormones from the peripheral endocrine organs. A large number of disease states as well as a diverse group of drugs also affect their secretion. The complex interactions among the hypothalamus, pituitary, and peripheral endocrine glands provide elegant examples of integrated feedback regulation. Clinically, an improved understanding of the mechanisms that underlie these interactions provides the rationale for diagnosing and treating endocrine disorders and for predicting certain side effects of drugs that affect the endocrine system. Moreover, the elucidation of the structures of the anterior pituitary hormones and hypothalamic releasing hormones together with advances in protein chemistry have made it possible to produce synthetic peptide agonists and antagonists that have important diagnostic and therapeutic applications.

Ten anterior pituitary hormones have been identified in vertebrates; these can be classified into three different groups based on their structural features (Table 56–1). *Growth hormone* (GH) and *prolactin* belong to the somatotropic family of hormones, which in human beings also includes placental lactogen. The glycoprotein hormones—*thyrotropin* (TSH), *luteinizing hormone* (LH), and *follicle-stimulating hormone* (FSH)—share a common α-subunit but have different β-subunits that determine their distinct biological activities. In human beings, the glycoprotein hormone family also includes *placental chorionic gonadotropin* (CG). *Corticotropin* (adrenocorticotrophic hormone; ACTH), the two *melanocyte-stimulating hormones* (α- and β-MSH), and the two *lipotropins* represent a family of hormones derived from *proopiomelanocortin* by proteolytic processing. Except for β-MSH and the lipotropins, these pituitary hormones all play significant roles in human health and disease.

The synthesis and release of anterior pituitary hormones are influenced by the central nervous system. Their secretion is positively regulated by a group of polypeptides referred to as *hypothalamic releasing hormones*. These hormones are released from hypothalamic neurons in the region of the median eminence, and they reach the anterior pituitary through the hypothalamic-adenohypophyseal portal system. The hypothalamic releasing hormones include *growth hormone–releasing hormone* (GHRH), *gonadotropin-releasing hormone* (GnRH), *thyrotropin-releasing hormone* (TRH), and *corticotropin-releasing hormone* (CRH). *Somatostatin,* another hypothalamic peptide, negatively regulates the pituitary secretion of growth hormone and thyrotropin. Finally, the catecholamine dopamine inhibits the secretion of prolactin by lactotropes.

As discussed further in Chapter 30, the posterior pituitary gland, also known as the neurohypophysis, contains nerve axons arising from distinct populations of neurons in the supraoptic and paraventicular nuclei that synthesize

Table 56–1

Properties of the Protein Hormones of the Human Adenohypophysis and Placenta

HORMONE	APPROXIMATE MOLECULAR MASS, Da	PEPTIDE CHAINS	AMINO ACID RESIDUES	CARBO-HYDRATE	COMMENTS
Somatotropic Hormones					
Growth hormone (GH)	22,000	1	191	0	Human GH, Prl, and PL have
Prolactin (Prl)	22,500	1	198	0	considerably less homology of
Placental lactogen (PL)	22,300	1	191	0	amino acid sequence, in contrast to the striking degree that is observed in other species.
Glycoprotein Hormones					
Luteinizing hormone (LH)	29,400	2	α-92 β-115	23%	Glycoproteins with nonidentical subunits (α and β); biological specificity is in β subunit.
Follicle-stimulating hormone (FSH)	32,600	2	α-92 β-115	28%	The amino acid sequences of the α subunits of LH, FSH,
Chorionic gonadotropin (CG)	38,600	2	α-92 β-145	33%	TSH, and CG are identical. Although carbohydrate sequences
Thyroid-stimulating hormone (TSH)	30,500	2	α-92 β-112	22%	are incomplete, data suggest heterogeneity, even within each hormone
*POMC-Derived Hormones**					
Corticotropin (ACTH)	4500	1	39	0	This group of peptides is derived from a common precursor,
α-Melanocyte-stimulating hormone (α-MSH)	1650	1	13	0	proopiomelanocortin (POMC). Group shares a common hepta-
β-Melanocyte-stimulating hormone (β-MSH)	2100	1	18	0	peptide: Met-Glu-His-Phe-Arg-Trp-Gly.
β-Lipotropin (β-LPH)	9500	1	91	0	ACTH (1–13) = α-MSH β-LPH (1–58) = γ-LPH
γ-Lipotropin (γ-LPH)	5800	1	58	0	β-LPH (41–58) = β-MSH β-LPH (61–91) = β-Endorphin β-LPH (61–65) = Met-Enkephalin

*Discussed in further detail in Chapter 60.

either arginine vasopressin or oxytocin. Oxytocin plays important roles in labor and parturition and in milk letdown, as discussed below.

GROWTH HORMONE

The gene encoding human growth hormone (GH) resides on the long arm of chromosome 17, which also contains four related genes: three different variants of placental lactogen and a GH variant expressed in the syncytio-

trophoblast (chorionic somatotropin). Secreted GH is a heterogeneous mixture of peptides that can be distinguished on the basis of size or charge; the principal 22,000-dalton form is a single polypeptide chain of 191 amino acids that has two disulfide bonds and is not glycosylated. Alternative splicing deletes residues 32 to 46 of the larger form to produce a smaller form (~20,000 daltons) with equal bioactivity that makes up 5% to 10% of circulating GH. Additional GH species are found in serum, but their physiological significance is unclear. Approximately 45% of the 22,000-dalton and 25% of the 20,000-dalton GH in circulation are bound by a binding protein that contains the extracellular domain of the GH receptor (*see* below). This GH-binding protein may serve as a reservoir of growth hormone, as the biological half-life of GH complexed to it is approximately 10 times that of unbound GH. Alternatively, the binding protein may decrease GH bioactivity by preventing it from binding to its receptor in target tissues.

Regulation of Growth Hormone Secretion

Growth hormone, the most abundant anterior pituitary hormone, is synthesized and secreted by somatotropes. These cells account for about 50% of hormone-secreting cells of the anterior pituitary and cluster at its lateral wings. Daily GH secretion varies throughout life; secretion is high in children, reaches maximal levels during adolescence, and then decreases in an age-related manner in adulthood. GH secretion occurs in discrete but irregular pulses. Between these pulses, circulating GH falls to levels that are undetectable with current assays. The amplitude of secretory pulses is maximal at night, and the most consistent period of GH secretion is shortly after the onset of deep sleep. Because of this episodic release, random measurements of GH are of little value in the diagnosis of growth hormone deficiency, and provocative tests are required (*see* below).

The regulation of GH secretion is illustrated in Figure 56–1. GHRH, produced by hypothalamic neurons found predominantly in the arcuate nucleus, stimulates growth hormone secretion by binding to a specific G protein–coupled receptor on somatotropes, elevating both intracellular cyclic AMP and Ca^{2+} concentrations. Somatostatin, which is synthesized by more widely distributed neurons as well as by neuroendocrine cells in the gastrointestinal tract and pancreas, inhibits growth hormone secretion. Somatostatin is synthesized from a 92–amino acid precursor and processed by proteolytic cleavage to generate two predominant forms—somatostatin-14 and somatostatin-28. The somatostatins exert their effects by binding to and activating a family of G protein–coupled receptors. The consequences of receptor activation include inhibition of cyclic AMP accumulation, activation of K^+ channels, and activation of tyrosine phosphatase. Five somatostatin receptor subtypes have been identified, each of which binds somatostatin with nanomolar affinity; whereas receptor types 1 to 4 (abbreviated sst_{1-4} or SSTR1-4) bind the two somatostatins with approximately equal affinity, type 5 (sst_5, SSTR5) has a 10- to 15-fold greater selectivity for somatostatin-28 (Patel, 1999). It appears that the SSTR2

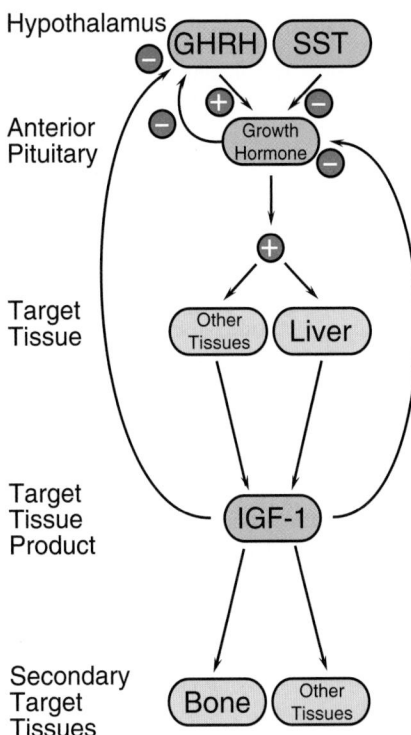

Figure 56–1. Growth hormone secretion and actions.

Two hypothalamic factors, growth hormone–releasing hormone (GHRH) and somatostatin (SST) stimulate or inhibit the release of growth hormone (GH) from the pituitary, respectively. Insulin-like growth factor 1(IGF-1), a product of GH action on peripheral tissues, causes negative feedback inhibition of GH release by acting at the hypothalamus and the pituitary. The actions of GH can be direct or indirect and mediated by IGF-1. *See* text for discussion of the other agents that modulate GH secretion.

and SSTR5 receptors are most important for regulation of GH secretion. There is evidence supporting both direct effects of somatostatin on somatotropes and indirect effects mediated *via* GHRH neurons in the arcuate nucleus. As discussed below, somatostatin analogs play an important role in the therapy of syndromes of GH excess such as acromegaly.

Appreciation of a third component of regulation of GH secretion arose from studies of GH secretagogues (Smith *et al.,* 1999). The finding that peptide derivatives of Leu- and Met-enkephalins stimulate growth hormone release has led to the development of additional peptide and nonpeptide GH secretogogues that stimulate GH secretion *via* a G protein–coupled receptor distinct from the GHRH receptor (Howard *et al.,* 1996). This GH-secretogogue receptor is expressed on somatotropes as well as on GHRH neurons in the arcuate nucleus, suggesting that GH secretogogues stimulate GH release both by direct actions on the pituitary and by indirect effects on GHRH neurons. Intriguingly, both GH and somatostatin inhibit the activation of these neurons. This inhibition by GH indicates a direct feedback action of GH, while the inhibition by somatostatin suggests that an important component of the inhibition of GH secretion by somatostatin is exerted in the hypothalamus rather than in the pituitary. The clinical utility of GH secretogogues in patients with growth hormone deficiency is an area of active investigation, as is the putative endogenous ligand that activates the GH-secretogogue receptor.

Although their specific sites of action are not fully understood, several neurotransmitters, drugs, metabolites, and other stimuli also affect GH secretion by modulating the release of GHRH and/or somatostatin. Dopamine, 5-hydroxytryptamine, and α_2-adrenergic receptor agonists stimulate GH release, whereas β-adrenergic receptor agonists, free fatty acids, and insulin-like growth factor-1 (IGF-1, *see* below) and GH itself inhibit release. Hypoglycemia stimulates growth hormone release, as do exercise, stress, emotional excitement, and ingestion of protein-rich meals. In contrast, administration of glucose in an oral glucose-tolerance test suppresses GH secretion in normal subjects.

These observations form the basis for provocative tests to assess the ability of the pituitary to secrete GH. Provocative stimuli include arginine, glucagon, insulin-induced hypoglycemia, clonidine, and the dopamine precursor levodopa; these agents all increase circulating GH levels in normal subjects within 45 to 90 minutes. At present, insulin-induced hypoglycemia is the test advocated by the Growth Hormone Research Society (Anonymous, 1998), whereas the United States Food and Drug Administration (FDA) requires two independent tests of GH deficiency to establish the diagnosis. When excess GH secretion is suspected (*see* below), the failure of an oral glucose load to suppress GH is diagnostically useful. Finally, as described below, GH secretion in response to GHRH can be used to distinguish pituitary disease from hypothalamic disease.

Molecular and Cellular Bases of Growth Hormone Action

All of the effects of GH result from its interactions with the GH receptor, as evidenced by the severe phenotype of rare patients with homozygous mutations of the GH-receptor gene (the Laron syndrome of GH-resistant dwarfism). The GH receptor is a widely distributed cell-surface receptor that belongs to the cytokine receptor superfamily and shares structural similarity with the prolactin receptor, the erythropoietin receptor, and several of the interleukin

receptors (Finidori *et al.*, 2000). Like other members of the cytokine receptor family, the GH receptor contains an extracellular domain that binds GH, a single membrane-spanning region, and an intracellular domain that mediates signal transduction. Receptor activation results from the binding of a single GH molecule to two identical receptor molecules (de Vos *et al.*, 1992). The net result is the formation of a ligand-occupied receptor dimer that presumably brings the intracellular domains of the receptor into close proximity, thereby activating cytosolic components critical for cell signaling.

As determined from cDNA cloning and sequencing (Leung *et al.*, 1987), the mature human GH receptor contains 620 amino acids, 260 of which are extracellular and 350 of which are cytoplasmic. The formation of the GH-GH receptor ternary complex is initiated by a high-affinity interaction of GH with a receptor monomer, exposing a second site of lower affinity on GH that recruits a second receptor molecule to the complex. Interestingly, GH analogs have been engineered with a disrupted second receptor-binding site; these analogs cannot induce receptor dimerization. One such analog, *pegvisomant,* behaves as a GH antagonist and has shown promise in the treatment of acromegaly (Trainer *et al.*, 2000; *see* below).

In addition to the full-length GH receptor, truncated forms of the receptor also have been described. A circulating form of the receptor, called GH-binding protein, is formed by proteolytic cleavage of the extracellular domain of the receptor from its transmembrane segment. GH-binding protein has been reported to delay the clearance of circulating GH and increase its activity *in vitro,* but its biological role remains unknown. Truncated, membrane-anchored forms of the receptor also have been described. Again, the physiological roles of these proteins, which apparently result from alternative splicing events and constitute a small fraction of the receptor population, are unknown, although they inhibit GH action in cultured cell models. Truncated forms of the GH receptor also have been found in one kindred with growth-hormone insensitivity and short stature (Ayling *et al.*, 1997). These patients are heterozygous for the receptor mutation, suggesting that the truncated receptors behave as dominant negative inhibitors of GH signaling.

The ligand-occupied receptor dimer does not have inherent tyrosine kinase activity, but it does provide docking sites for two molecules of Jak2, a cytoplasmic tyrosine kinase of the Janus kinase family. The juxtaposition of two Jak2 molecules leads to *trans*-phosphorylation and autoactivation of Jak2, with consequent tyrosine phosphorylation of cytoplasmic proteins that mediate downstream signaling events. These include Stat proteins (*s*ignal *t*ransducers and *a*ctivators of *t*ranscription), Shc (an adapter protein that regulates the Ras/MAP kinase signaling pathway), and IRS-1 and IRS-2 (insulin-receptor substrate proteins that activate the phosphatidyl inositol-3 kinase regulatory pathway) (*see* Figure 56–2).

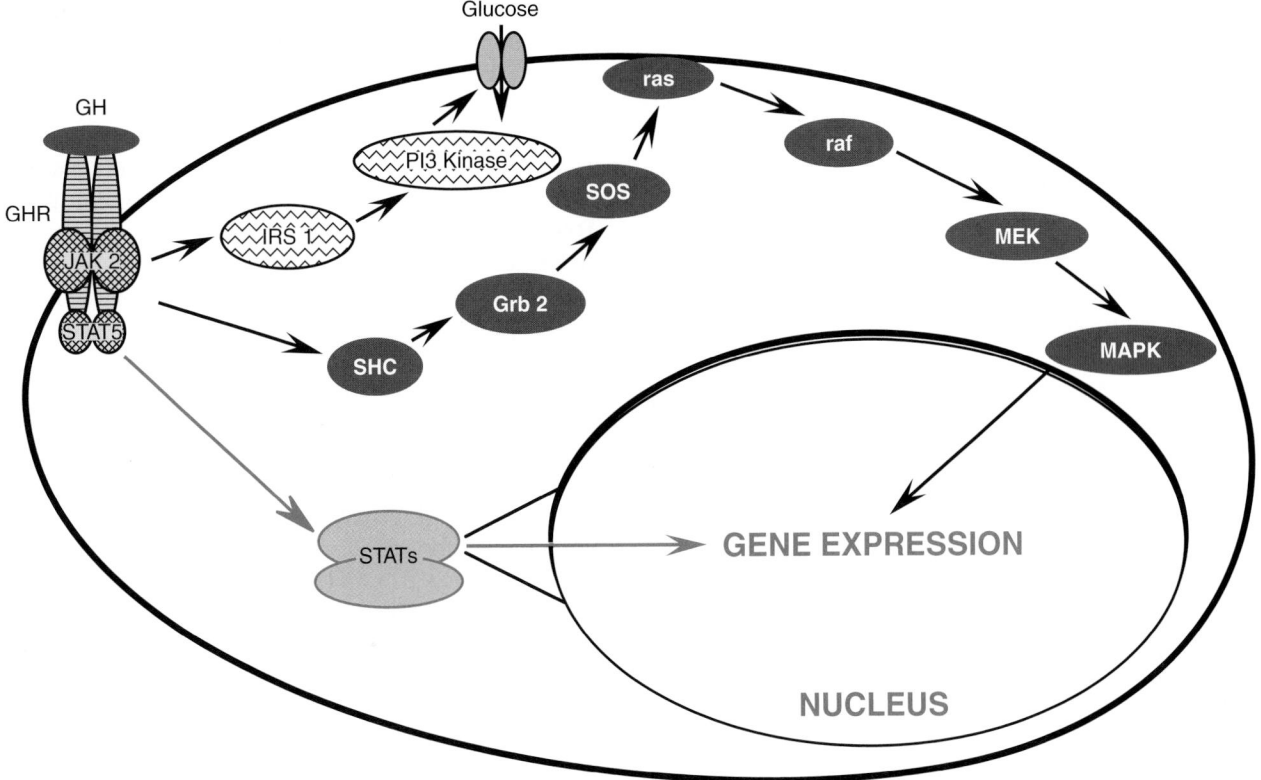

Figure 56–2. Mechanism of growth hormone action.

The binding of GH to two molecules of the growth hormone receptor (GHR) induces dimerization of JAK2 and its autophosphorylation. JAK2 then phosphorylates cytoplasmic proteins that activate downstream signaling pathways (PI3 kinase, ras, raf, MAPK) that ultimately affect gene expression. The arrows indicate the presumed order of activation in the signaling pathway; the figure does not reflect the localization of the intracellular molecules, which presumably exist in multicomponent signaling complexes. JAK2, janus kinase 2; IRS1, insulin receptor substrate 1; PI3 kinase, phosphatidyl inositol-3 kinase; STAT, signal transducer and activator of transcription; SOS, product of the *son of sevenless* gene; MAPK, mitogen-activated protein kinase; MEK, MAPK kinase; SHC and Grb2, adapter proteins.

Although GH acts directly on adipocytes to increase lipolysis and on hepatocytes to stimulate gluconeogenesis, its anabolic and growth-promoting effects are mediated indirectly through the induction of insulin-like growth factors (IGFs). There are two members of the IGF family: IGF-1 and IGF-2. IGF-1 is more dependent on GH and is a more potent growth factor postnatally; thus, IGF-1 appears to be the principal mediator of GH action. Most circulating IGF-1 is made in the liver, although IGF-1 produced locally in many tissues also may exert paracrine or autocrine effects on cell growth. Circulating IGF-1 is associated with a family of binding proteins that serve as transport proteins and also may mediate certain aspects of IGF-1 signaling. The essential role of IGF-1 in GH signaling is evidenced by a patient with loss-of-function mutations in both alleles of the *IGF1* gene whose severe intrauterine and postnatal growth retardation was unresponsive to GH but responsive to recombinant human IGF-1 (Camacho-Hubner, *et al.,* 1999).

Following its synthesis and release, IGF-1 interacts with receptors on the cell surface that mediate its biological activities. The type 1 IGF receptor is closely related to the insulin receptor, consisting of a heterotetramer with intrinsic tyrosine kinase activity. This receptor is present in essentially all tissues and binds IGF-1 and IGF-2 with high affinity; insulin also can activate the type 1 IGF receptor, but with an affinity approximately 100 times less than that of the IGFs. The type 2 IGF receptor encodes a protein that is located predominantly on intracellular membranes and is identical to the mannose-6-phosphate receptor that participates in intracellular targeting of acid hydrolases and other mannose-containing glycoproteins to lysosomes. This receptor apparently is activated specifically by IGF-2. The signal transduction pathway for the insulin receptor is described in detail in Chapter 61.

Syndromes of Growth Hormone Deficiency

GH deficiency in children is a well-accepted cause of short stature, and replacement therapy has been used for more than 30 years to treat children with severe GH deficiency. More recently, GH deficiency in adults has been associated with a defined endocrinopathy that includes increased mortality from cardiovascular causes, probably secondary to deleterious changes in fat distribution and increases in circulating lipids; decreased muscle mass and exercise capacity; and impaired psychosocial function. With the ready availability of recombinant human GH, attention has shifted to the proper role of GH therapy in GH-deficient adults. While this is an area of current debate, the emerging consensus is that at least the most severely affected GH-deficient adults will benefit from GH replacement therapy. GH therapy also is approved by the FDA for AIDS-associated wasting, and its use has resulted in some benefit in patients with this condition.

Based on controlled clinical trials showing increased mortality, GH should not be used in patients with acute critical illness due to complications following open heart or abdominal surgery, multiple accidental trauma, or acute respiratory failure. GH also should not be used in patients who have any evidence of neoplasia, and antitumor therapy should be completed prior to initiation of GH therapy.

Diagnosis of Growth Hormone Deficiency.   Clinically, children with GH deficiency present with short stature and a low age-adjusted growth velocity. Most commonly, these children have an isolated deficiency of GH without other documented pathology (*i.e.,* idiopathic, isolated GH deficiency) and are presumed to have a hypothalamic defect. Random sampling of serum GH is insufficient to diagnose GH deficiency; provocative tests are required. After excluding other causes of poor growth, the diagnosis of GH deficiency should be entertained in patients with height ≥ 2 to 2.5 standard deviations below normal, delayed bone age, a growth velocity below the 25th percentile, and a predicted adult height substantially below the mean parental height (Vance and Mauras, 1999). In this setting, a serum GH level of less than 10 μg/liter following provocative testing (*e.g.,* insulin-induced hypoglycemia, arginine, levodopa, or glucagon) indicates GH deficiency, with a stimulated value of less than 5 μg/liter reflecting severe deficiency.

More than 90% of adult patients with GH deficiency have overt pituitary disease due to a functioning or nonfunctioning pituitary adenoma or resulting from surgery or radiotherapy for a pituitary mass. Almost all patients with multiple deficits in other pituitary hormones also will have deficient GH secretion.

According to criteria established by the FDA, a normal response to provocative stimuli is an increase in GH to serum levels ≥ 5 μg/liter by radioimmunoassay or 2.5 μg/liter by immunoradiometric or immunochemiluminescent assay. In contrast, the Growth Hormone Research Society has recommended diagnosis based on a stimulated GH serum level of less than 3 μg/liter during insulin-induced hypoglycemia (Anonymous, 1998).

Treatment of Growth Hormone Deficiency.   The action of GH is highly species-specific; human beings do not respond to GH from nonprimate species. Therefore, GH for therapeutic use formerly was purified from human cadaver pituitaries in very limited quantities. The production of human GH by recombinant DNA technology not only increased availability of the hormone but also alleviated concerns about Creutzfeldt-Jakob disease associated with use of the hormone purified from cadaver pituitaries.

A number of recombinant preparations of human GH are approved for use in many countries. By convention, *somatropin* refers to GH preparations whose sequence matches that of native GH (SEROSTIM, GENOTROPIN, HUMATROPE, NUTROPIN, SAIZEN), while *somatrem* refers to a derivative of GH with an additional methionine at the amino terminus (PROTROPIN). Although there are subtle differences in the sources and structures of these preparations, all have similar biological actions and potencies. They typically are administered subcutaneously in the evening; although the circulating half-life of GH is only 20 minutes, its biological half-life is in the range of 9 to 17 hours, and once-daily administration is sufficient. Newer formulations are supplied in prefilled syringes, which may be more convenient for the patient, as the GH does not need refrigeration and the diluent causes less irritation at the injection site. An encapsulated form of somatropin that is injected intramuscularly once or twice per month (NUTROPIN DEPOT) has been approved by the FDA. The relative advantages of any specific formulations over others in clinical use have not been definitively established.

In addition to GH, *sermorelin acetate* (GEREF), a synthetic form of human GHRH, has received FDA approval for treatment of idiopathic GH deficiency. Sermorelin is a peptide of 29 amino acids that corresponds in sequence to the first 29 amino acids of human GHRH (a 44–amino acid peptide) and has full biological activity. Sermorelin generally is well tolerated and is less expensive than somatropin, but at recommended doses it has been less effective than GH in clinical trials. Moreover, this agent will not work in patients whose GH deficiency results from defects in the anterior pituitary (Anonymous, 1999). Therefore, a GH response (>2 μg/liter) to a test dose of sermorelin should be documented prior to initiating therapy (30 μg/kg per day, given subcutaneously), and the patients must be monitored frequently to ascertain continued growth on therapy. Sermorelin also has been employed diagnostically to distinguish between pituitary and hypothalamic disease; its clinical utility in this setting is not fully established.

GH is widely used for replacement therapy in GH-deficient children, whether the deficiency is congenital or acquired. It also is FDA-approved for use in children with chronic renal insufficiency (although not proven to increase adult height) and for patients with Turner's syndrome (improving adult height significantly). Recommended doses vary with indication and product, but typically a dose of 20 to 40 μg/kg is administered subcutaneously either daily or 6 times per week; higher daily doses (e.g., 50 μg/kg) are employed for patients with Turner's syndrome, who have partial GH resistance. Initial response and compliance can be monitored with serum IGF-1 levels, while long-term response is monitored by close evaluation of height. Although the most pronounced increase in growth velocity occurs within the first two years of therapy, GH is continued until growth ceases. In view of the increased appreciation of the effects of GH on bone density and the effects of GH deficiency in adults, it seems reasonable to continue therapy into adulthood. However, many patients who clearly were GH deficient in childhood—especially those with idiopathic, isolated GH deficiency—respond normally to provocative tests at the cessation of therapy. Thus, it is essential to confirm GH deficiency after optimal growth has been achieved so as to identify patients who will benefit from continuing GH treatment.

In adults, previously recommended doses of GH now are viewed as excessive, leading to both an elevated IGF-1 concentration and a greater risk of side effects. The FDA recommends a starting dose of 3 to 4 μg/kg, given once daily by subcutaneous injection, with a maximum dose of 25 μg/kg in patients $\leq$35 years old and 12.5 μg/kg in older patients. The Growth Hormone Research Society recommends a starting dose of 150 to 300 μg/day regardless of body weight (Anonymous, 1998). Clinical response is monitored by serum IGF-1, which should be restored to the midnormal range adjusted for age and sex. Either an elevated serum IGF-1 or persistent side effects are grounds for decreasing the dose; conversely, the dose can be increased if serum IGF-1 has not reached the normal range after two months of GH therapy. In the setting of AIDS-related wasting, considerably higher doses (e.g., 100 μg/kg) have been used in clinical trials.

As noted above, a subset of children with growth impairment has elevated GH levels and GH resistance, most frequently secondary to mutations in the GH recep-

tor. These patients can be treated effectively with recombinant human IGF-1 (IGEF), which is administered subcutaneously either once or twice daily in doses ranging from 40 to 120 μg/kg (Ranke et al., 1999). Although this therapy clearly is beneficial in promoting growth, the optimal regimen remains to be established.

Side Effects of GH Therapy. In children, GH therapy is associated with remarkably few side effects. Rarely, generally within the first 8 weeks of therapy, patients develop intracranial hypertension, with papilledema, visual changes, headache, nausea, and/or vomiting. Because of this, funduscopic examination is recommended at the initiation of therapy and at periodic intervals thereafter. Leukemia has been reported in some children receiving GH therapy; a causal relationship has not been established, and conditions associated with GH deficiency (e.g., Down syndrome, cranial irradiation for CNS tumors) probably explain the apparent increased incidence of leukemia. Despite this, the consensus is that GH should not be administered in the first year after treatment of pediatric tumors, including leukemia, or during the first two years after therapy for medulloblastomas or ependymomas (Blethen et al., 1996). An increased incidence of type 2 diabetes mellitus has been reported, presumably secondary to the anti-insulin metabolic effects of GH (Cutfield et al., 2000).

In adults, side effects associated with the initiation of GH therapy include peripheral edema, carpal tunnel syndrome, arthralgia, and myalgia. These symptoms, which occur most frequently in patients who are older or more obese, generally respond to a decrease in dose. Although there are potential concerns about impaired glucose tolerance secondary to anti-insulin actions of GH, this has not been a major problem with clinical use at the recommended doses.

Agents Used in Syndromes of Growth Hormone Excess

GH excess causes distinct clinical syndromes depending on the age of the patient. If the epiphyses are unfused, GH excess causes increased longitudinal growth, resulting in gigantism. In adults, GH excess causes acromegaly. The symptoms and signs of acromegaly (e.g., arthropathy, carpal tunnel syndrome, generalized visceromegaly, hypertension, glucose intolerance, headache, lethargy, excess perspiration, and sleep apnea) progress slowly, and diagnosis often is delayed. Life expectancy is shortened in these patients; mortality is increased at least twofold relative to age-matched controls due to increased death from cardiovascular disease, upper airway obstruction, and gastrointestinal malignancies.

While the diagnosis of acromegaly should be suspected in patients with the appropriate symptoms and signs, confirmation requires the demonstration of increased circulating GH or IGF-1.

Generally, the first screening test is to measure serum IGF-1. Using a good assay with results compared to normal values for age and sex, a normal IGF-1 level argues strongly against the diagnosis of acromegaly. If the IGF-1 is frankly elevated or borderline or if the clinical suspicion is relatively strong, many clinicians also will measure plasma GH following administration of an oral glucose load. Using the standard radioimmunoassay for human GH, the GH level 2 hours after glucose administration normally is less than 2 μg/liter in normal subjects; a higher value confirms the diagnosis of acromegaly.

Treatment options in acromegaly include transphenoidal surgery, radiation, and drugs that inhibit GH secretion or action. Pituitary surgery traditionally has been viewed as the treatment of choice. In patients with microadenomas (*i.e.*, tumors <1 cm), skilled neurosurgeons can achieve cure rates of up to 80% to 90%; however, the long-term success rate for patients with macroadenomas is considerably lower, often falling below 50%. In addition, there is increasing appreciation that acromegalic patients previously considered cured by pituitary surgery actually have persistent GH excess, with its attendant complications. Thus, more attention has been given to the role of pharmacological management of acromegaly, either as a primary treatment modality or for the treatment of persistent GH excess following transphenoidal surgery (Newman, 1999).

Somatostatin Analogs.   The development of analogs of somatostatin (Table 56–2) has revolutionized the medical treatment of GH excess. The most widely used analog is *octreotide* (SANDOSTATIN), an eight–amino acid synthetic derivative of somatostatin that has a longer half-life and binds preferentially to SSTR-2 and SSTR-5 receptors on GH-secreting tumors. Typically, octreotide (100 μg) is administered subcutaneously three times daily; serum GH

and IGF-1 levels are monitored to assess effectiveness of treatment. The goal is to decrease GH levels to less than 2 μg/liter following an oral glucose-tolerance test and to bring IGF-1 levels to within the normal range for age and sex. Depending on the biochemical response, higher or lower octreotide doses may be used in individual patients.

In addition to its effect on GH secretion, octreotide can decrease tumor size in a minority of patients. In these cases, tumor growth generally resumes after octreotide treatment is stopped. Octreotide also has significant inhibitory effects on thryotropin secretion, and it is the treatment of choice for patients who have thryotrope adenomas that oversecrete TSH and who are not good candidates for surgery. The use of octreotide in gastrointestinal disorders is discussed in Chapter 39.

Gastrointestinal side effects—including diarrhea, nausea, and abdominal pain—occur in up to 50% of patients receiving octreotide. In most patients, these symptoms diminish over time and do not require cessation of therapy. Approximately 25% of patients receiving octreotide develop gallstones, presumably due to decreased gallbladder contraction and gastrointestinal transit time. In the absence of symptoms, gallstones are not a contraindication to continued use of octreotide. Compared to somatostatin, octreotide has much less of an effect on insulin secretion and in clinical studies only infrequently affects glycemic control.

The need to inject octreotide three times daily poses a significant obstacle to patient compliance. A long-acting,

Table 56–2
Amino Acid Sequences of Native and Synthetic Somatostatin Peptides

Somatostatin-28 (Prosomatostatin):

```
                                              S ——————————————————— S
                                              |                     |
Ser-Ala-Asn-Ser-Asn-Pro-Ala-Met-Ala-Pro-Arg-Glu-Arg-Lys-Ala-Gly-Cys-Lys-Asn-Phe-Phe-Trp-Lys-Thr-Phe-Thr-Ser-Cys
```

Somatostatin-14:

```
                              S ——————————————————— S
                              |                     |
              Ala-Gly-Cys-Lys-Asn-Phe-Phe-Trp-Lys-Thr-Phe-Thr-Ser-Cys
```

Octreotide:

```
        S ——————————— S
        |             |
    D-Phe-Cys-Phe-D-Trp-Lys-Thr-Cys-Thr-ol
```

Lanreotide:

```
        S ——————————— S
        |             |
    D-Nal-Cys-Tyr-D-Trp-Lys-Val-Cys-Thr-ol
```

Vapreotide:

```
        S ——————————— S
        |             |
    D-Phe-Cys-Tyr-D-Trp-Lys-Val-Cys-Thp
```

ABBREVIATION: D-Nal, 3-(2-naphthyl)-D-alanyl.

slow-release form of octreotide (SANDOSTATIN-LAR) is a more convenient alternative that can be administered intramuscularly once every 4 weeks; the recommended dose is 20 or 30 mg. The long-acting preparation is at least as effective as the regular formulation and is used in patients who have responded favorably to a trial of the shorter-acting formulation of octreotide. Like the shorter-acting formulation, the longer-acting formulation of octreotide generally is well tolerated and has a similar incidence of side effects (predominantly gastrointestinal and/or discomfort at injection site) that do not require cessation of therapy.

Lanreotide (SOMATULINE LA) is a long-acting octapeptide analog of somatostatin that causes prolonged suppression of GH secretion when administered in a 30-mg dose intramuscularly. Although its efficacy appears comparable to that of the long-acting formulation of octreotide, its duration of action is shorter; thus it must be administered either at 10- or 14-day intervals. One direct comparison with a limited number of patients suggested that the long-acting formulation of octreotide at recommended doses may be somewhat more effective in lowering GH levels than is lanreotide (Turner *et al.*, 1999). The incidence and severity of side effects associated with lanreotide are similar to those of the other somatostatin analogs. Lanreotide has not been approved by the FDA for use in the United States.

Somatostatin blocks not only GH secretion, but also the secretion of other hormones, growth factors, and cytokines. Thus, octreotide and the delayed-release somatostatin analogs have been used to treat symptoms associated with metastatic carcinoid tumors (*e.g.*, flushing and diarrhea) and symptoms of adenomas secreting vasoactive intestinal peptide (*e.g.*, watery diarrhea). Octreotide also has been labeled with indium or technetium and used for diagnostic imaging of neuroendocrine tumors such as pituitary adenomas and carcinoids.

Based on structure-function studies of somatostatin and its derivatives, the amino acid residues in positions 7 to 10 [FWKT] are the major determinants of biological activity. Residues W^8 and K^9 appear to be essential, whereas conservative substitutions at F^7 and T^{10} are permissible. Active somatostatin analogs retain this core segment constrained in a cyclic structure—formed either by a disulfide bond or amide linkage—that stabilizes the optimal conformation (Patel, 1999). As noted above, the endogenous peptides, somatostatin-14 and somatostatin-28, do not discriminate very well among SSTR subtypes except for SSTR5, which shows some preference for somatostatin-28. Greater selectivity is seen with some of the somatostatin analogs. For example, the octapepetides octreotide, lanreotide, and vapreotide and the hexapeptide seglitide all bind to the SSTR subtypes with the following order of selectivity: SSTR2 > SSTR5 > SSTR3 ≫ SSTR1 and SSTR4. The octapeptide analog BIM23268 exhibits modest selectivity for SSTR5, and the undecapeptide CH275 appears to bind preferentially to SSTR1

and 4 (Patel, 1999). More recently, a series of small nonpeptide agonists that exhibit a high degree of SSTR subtype-selectivity has been isolated from combinatorial chemical libraries; these compounds may lead to a new class of highly selective, orally active somatostatin mimetics.

Dopamine-Receptor Agonists. The dopamine-receptor agonists are described in more detail below in the section dealing with treatment of prolactinomas. Although dopamine-receptor agonists normally stimulate GH secretion, they cause a paradoxical decrease in GH secretion in some patients with acromegaly. In patients who are unwilling to take injections, the long-acting dopamine-receptor agonist *cabergoline* (DOSTINEX) may lower GH and IGF-1 levels into the target range. The best responses have been seen in patients whose tumors secreted both GH and prolactin. Doses used in treating acromegaly typically are considerably higher than those employed in prolactinomas.

Growth Hormone Antagonists. As discussed above, derivatives of GH have been developed that bind the GH receptor but do not induce the formation of receptor dimers or activate Jak/Stat signaling. One such analog, *pegvisomant,* is now under clinical investigation for the treatment of acromegaly. In a 12-week trial, pegvisomant significantly decreased circulating IGF-1, achieving normal levels in up to 90% of patients at higher doses and causing significant improvement in clinical parameters such as ring size, soft-tissue swelling, and excessive perspiration and fatigue (Trainer *et al.*, 2000). Because pegvisomant differs structurally from native GH, it may induce the formation of specific antibodies that will limit its long-term efficacy. Moreover, it substantially increases GH levels and possibly may have unanticipated side effects. Finally, there are at least theoretical concerns that loss of negative feedback by both growth hormone and IGF-1 may increase the growth of GH-secreting adenomas. Thus, while its ultimate role in the management of acromegaly remains to be determined, pegvisomant represents a novel pharmacologic agent in the management of GH excess.

PROLACTIN

As a member of the somatotropin family, prolactin is related structurally to GH and placental lactogen. The human prolactin gene on chromosome 6 encodes a 23,000-dalton polypeptide of 199 amino acids. This polypeptide has three intramolecular disulfide bonds, and a portion of secreted prolactin is glycosylated at a single asparagine residue. In circulation, dimeric and polymeric forms of prolactin also are found, as are degradation products of 16,000 or 18,000 daltons; the biological significance of these different forms is not known.

Secretion

Prolactin is synthesized in lactotropes. Prolactin synthesis and secretion in the fetal pituitary start in the first few weeks of gestation. Serum prolactin levels decline shortly after birth. Whereas serum prolactin levels remain low throughout life in normal males, they are elevated somewhat in normal cycling females. Prolactin levels rise markedly during pregnancy, reach a maximum at term, and decline thereafter unless the mother breast-feeds the child. In nursing mothers, prolactin secretion is stimulated by the suckling stimulus or breast manipulation, and circulating prolactin levels can rise 10- to 100-fold within 30 minutes of stimulation. This response becomes less pronounced after several months of breast-feeding, and prolactin concentrations eventually decline to prepregnancy levels.

Prolactin detected in maternal and fetal blood originates from maternal and fetal pituitaries. Prolactin also is synthesized by decidual cells near the end of the luteal phase of the menstrual cycle and early in pregnancy; the latter source is responsible for the very high levels of prolactin in amniotic fluid during the first trimester.

Many of the physiological factors that influence prolactin secretion are similar to those that affect GH secretion. Thus, sleep, stress, hypoglycemia, exercise, and estrogen increase the secretion of both hormones.

Like other anterior pituitary hormones, prolactin is secreted in a pulsatile manner. Prolactin is unique among the anterior pituitary hormones in that hypothalamic regulation inhibits its secretion. The major regulator of prolactin secretion is dopamine, which is released by tuberoinfundibular neurons and interacts with the D_2 receptor on lactotropes to inhibit secretion of prolactin (Figure 56–3). A number of putative prolactin-releasing factors have been described, including TRH, vasoactive intestinal peptide, prolactin-releasing peptide, and *p*ituitary *a*denylyl *c*yclase-*a*ctivating *p*eptide (PACAP), but their physiological roles are unclear. Under certain pathophysiological conditions, such as severe primary hypothyroidism, persistently elevated levels of TRH can induce hyperprolactinemia and galactorrhea.

Molecular and Cellular Bases of Prolactin Action

The effects of prolactin result from interactions with specific receptors that are widely distributed among a variety of cell types within many tissues (Bole-Feysot *et al.*, 1998). Whereas prolactin binds specifically to the prolactin receptor and has no GH-like (somatotropic) activity, human GH and placental lactogen bind to the prolactin receptors and are lactogenic. The prolactin receptor is related structurally to receptors for GH and several cytokines and uses similar signaling mechanisms (*see* above).

The prolactin receptor is encoded by a single gene located on chromosome 5. Alternative splicing of this gene gives rise to multiple forms of the receptor, including a short form of 310 amino acids, a long form of 610 amino acids, and an intermediate form of 412 amino acids. In addition, soluble isoforms lacking the transmembrane and cytoplasmic domains bind prolactin in the circulation. Like the GH receptor, the prolactin receptor lacks intrinsic tyrosine kinase activity; hormone-induced dimerization recruits and activates Jak kinases. Phosphorylation of Jak2 kinase induces phosphorylation, dimerization, and nuclear translocation of the transcription factor Stat5.

Physiological Effects of Prolactin

A number of hormones—including estrogens, progesterone, placental lactogen, and GH—stimulate development of the breast and prepare it for lactation. Prolactin, acting *via* the prolactin receptor, plays an important role in inducing growth and differentiation of the ductal and lobuloalveolar epithelium, and lactation does not occur in the absence of this hormone. During pregnancy, the high levels of estrogen and progesterone inhibit milk secretion; their declining levels after birth permit prolactin to induce lactation.

Prolactin receptors also are present in many other tissues and organs, including the hypothalamus, liver, testes, ovaries, prostate, and immune system. The physiological effects of prolactin at these sites are poorly characterized. Hyperprolactinemia suppresses the hypothalamic-pituitary-gonadal axis, presumably due to inhibitory actions of prolactin on the hypothalamus and/or gonads. The elevated prolactin levels in women who are breast-feeding often suppress the normal menstrual cycle, and pathological hyperprolactinemia is a common cause of infertility in women (*see* below).

Agents Used to Treat Syndromes of Prolactin Excess

Prolactin has no therapeutic uses. Hyperprolactinemia is a relatively common endocrine abnormality that can result from hypothalamic or pituitary diseases that interfere with the delivery of inhibitory dopaminergic signals, from renal failure, from primary hypothyroidism associated with increased TRH levels, or from treatment with dopamine-receptor antagonists. Most often, hyperprolactinemia is caused by prolactin-secreting pituitary adenomas—either microadenomas (<1 cm in diameter) or macroadenomas (≥1 cm in diameter). Manifestations of prolactin excess in women include galactorrhea, amenorrhea, and infertility. In men, hyperprolactinemia causes loss of libido, impotence, and infertility. Generally, men seek medical

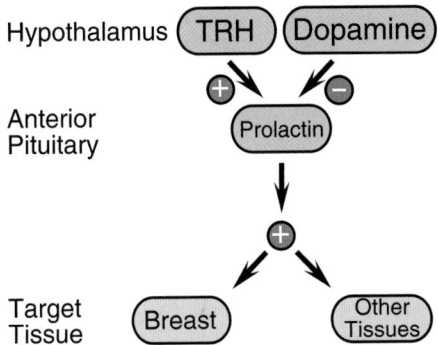

Figure 56–3. Prolactin secretion and actions.

Prolactin is the only anterior pituitary hormone for which a unique stimulatory releasing factor (PRH?) has not been identified. Thyrotropin-releasing hormone (TRH) can stimulate prolactin release, however, and dopamine can inhibit it. Prolactin affects lactation and reproductive functions but it also has varied effects on many other tissues. Prolactin is not under feedback control by peripheral hormones.

attention considerably later than do women and thus have a higher frequency of macroadenomas. Neurological manifestations such as visual impairment or headache also can be associated with the larger pituitary tumors.

Currently, the therapeutic options for patients with prolactinomas include transphenoidal surgery, radiation, and treatment with dopamine-receptor agonists that suppress prolactin production *via* D$_2$ dopamine receptors (Molitch, 1999). Inasmuch as initial surgical cure rates are only 70% with microadenomas and 30% with macroadenomas, most patients with prolactinomas ultimately require drug therapy. Thus, dopamine-receptor agonists have become the initial treatment of choice for many patients. These agents generally decrease both prolactin secretion and the size of the adenoma, thereby improving the endocrine abnormalities as well as the neurologic symptoms caused directly by the adenoma (including visual field deficits).

Bromocriptine. *Bromocriptine* (PARLODEL) is the dopamine-receptor agonist most frequently used to treat hyperprolactinemia and has become the standard against which newer agents are compared. Bromocriptine is a semisynthetic ergot alkaloid that interacts with D$_2$ dopamine receptors to inhibit both spontaneous and thyrotropin-releasing hormone (TRH)-induced release of prolactin; to a lesser extent, it also activates D$_1$ dopamine receptors. Bromocriptine normalizes the prolactin level in 70% to 80% of patients with prolactinomas and decreases tumor size in more than 50% of patients, including those with macroadenomas. It is worth noting that bromocriptine does not cure the underlying adenoma, and hyperprolactinemia and tumor growth typically recur upon cessation of therapy.

Frequent side effects of bromocriptine include nausea and vomiting, headache, and postural hypotension—particularly on initial use. Less frequent side effects include nasal congestion, digital vasospasm, or CNS effects such as psychosis, hallucinations, nightmares, or insomnia. Patients often develop tolerance to these effects, which can be diminished by starting at a low dose (1.25 mg) administered at bedtime with a snack. After one week, a morning dose of 1.25 mg can be added. If clinical symptoms persist or the prolactin level remains elevated, the dose can be increased gradually, every 3 to 7 days, to 5 mg twice per day or 2.5 mg three times a day as tolerated. Patients who do not respond to bromocriptine or who develop intractable side effects may respond to a different dopamine agonist. Although a high fraction of the oral dose of bromocriptine is absorbed, only 7% of the dose reaches the systemic circulation due to a high extraction rate and extensive first-pass metabolism in the liver. Furthermore, bromocriptine has a relatively short elimination half-life (between 2 and 8 hours). To avoid the need for frequent dosing, a parenteral long-acting form of bromocriptine incorporated into biodegradable microspheres (PARLODEL-LAR) has been developed. Although not available in the United States, this product has produced results in clinical trials comparable to those of oral bromocriptine. Bromocriptine may be administered intravaginally (2.5 mg once daily), reportedly with fewer gastrointestinal side effects.

Pergolide. *Pergolide* (PERMAX), an ergot derivative approved by the FDA for treatment of Parkinson's disease, also is used "off label" to treat hyperprolactinemia. If the cost of therapy is an important consideration, pergolide is the cheapest available dopamine-receptor agonist. It induces many of the same side effects as does bromocriptine, but it can be given once a day, starting at 0.025 mg at bedtime and increased gradually to a maximum daily dose of 0.25 mg.

Cabergoline. *Cabergoline* (DOSTINEX) is an ergot derivative with a longer half-life (approximately 65 hours) and higher affinity and selectivity for the D$_2$ receptor than bromocriptine (approximately 4-times more potent; Verhelst *et al.*, 1999). Cabergoline has a much lower tendency to induce nausea, although it still may cause hypotension and dizziness. In some clinical trials, cabergoline has been more effective than bromocriptine in decreasing serum prolactin in patients with hyperprolactinemia. Cabergoline has been approved by the FDA for the treatment of hyperprolactinemia, and it likely will play an increasing role in the treatment of this syndrome. As approved by the FDA, therapy is initiated at a dose of 0.25 mg twice a week; a schedule of 0.5 mg once a week also has been used. If the serum prolactin remains elevated, the dose can be increased to a maximum of 1.5 mg two or three times a week as tolerated. The dose should not be increased more often than every 4 weeks.

Quinagolide. *Quinagolide* is a nonergot D$_2$ dopamine agonist with a half-life (22 hours) intermediate between those of bromocriptine and cabergoline. Quinagolide is administered once daily at doses of 0.1 to 0.5 mg/day. It is not approved by the FDA but has been used extensively in Europe.

Patients with prolactinomas who desire to become pregnant make up a special subset of hyperprolactinemic patients. In this setting, drug safety during pregnancy is an important consideration. Bromocriptine, cabergoline, and quinagolide all induce ovulation and permit most patients with prolactinomas to become pregnant without apparent detrimental effects on pregnancy or fetal development. However, experience with cabergoline and quinagolide is much less extensive than that with bromocriptine. Therefore, bromocriptine is recommended as the first-line treatment in this setting, although opinion may change with more experience with cabergoline or quinagolide.

GONADOTROPIN-RELEASING HORMONE AND GONADOTROPIC HORMONES

The pituitary hormones, luteinizing hormone (LH) and follicle-stimulating hormone (FSH), as well as the related placental hormone chorionic gonadotropin (CG), are referred to as the gonadotropic hormones because of their actions on the gonads. These three hormones and TSH consitute the glycoprotein family of pituitary hormones. Each hormone is a glycosylated heterodimer containing a common α-subunit and a distinct β-subunit that confers specificity of action. While all the β-subunits of this family are similar structurally, the β-subunit of CG is most different, containing a carboxy-terminal extension of 30 amino acids and extra carbohydrate residues. The carbohydrate residues on the gonadotropins influence the rate of their clearance from the circulation, thus extending their serum half-lives; the residues also play a role in signal transduction at gonadotropin receptors. The human FSH β gene is located at 11p13, the LH β is at 19q12.32, in close proximity to at least seven CG β genes, and the gene encoding the α-subunit maps to chromosome 6q21-23.

Regulation of Gonadotropin Secretion

The regulation of gonadotropin secretion is described in detail in Chapters 58 and 59. LH and FSH are synthesized and secreted by gonadotropes, which make up approximately 20% of the hormone-secreting cells in the anterior pituitary. CG—produced only in primates and horses—is made by syncytiotrophoblast cells of the placenta. Pituitary gonadotropin production is stimulated by GnRH and is further regulated by feedback effects of the gonadal hormones (Figure 56–4; see also Figure 58–2).

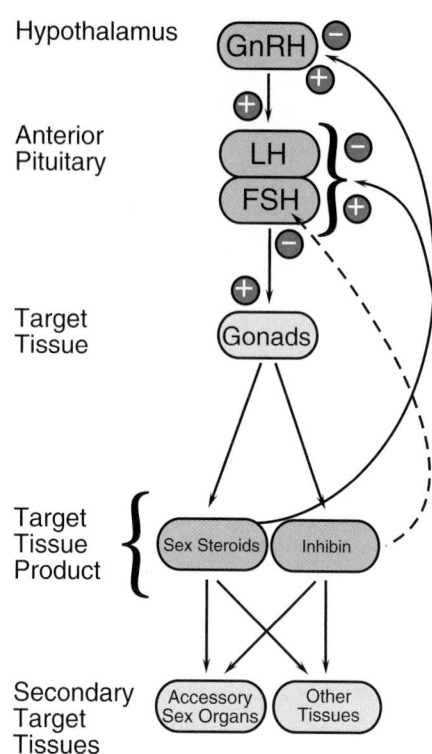

Figure 56–4. The hypothalamic-pituitary-gonadal axis.

A single hypothalamic releasing factor, gonadotropin-releasing hormone (GnRH), controls the synthesis and release of both gonadotropins (LH and FSH) in males and females. Gonadal steroid hormones (androgens, estrogens, and progesterone) cause feedback inhibition at the level of the pituitary and the hypothalamus. The preovulatory surge of estrogen also can exert a stimulatory effect at the level of the pituitary and the hypothalamus. Inhibin, a polypeptide hormone produced by the gonads, specifically inhibits FSH production by the pituitary.

Regulation of Release of Gonadotropin-Releasing Hormone. *Go*nadotropin-*r*eleasing *h*ormone (GnRH) regulates the synthesis and secretion of FSH and LH by pituitary gonadotropes. GnRH is encoded by a gene on chromosome 8p21 and is derived by proteolytic processing of a 92–amino acid precursor peptide to produce mature GnRH, a decapeptide with blocked amino and carboxyl termini (*see* Table 56–3). GnRH release is intermittent and is governed by a neural pulse generator that is located in the mediobasal hypothalamus—primarily in the arcuate nucleus—and that controls the frequency and amplitude of GnRH release from neurons in the hypothalamus. Although active late in fetal life and for approximately 1 year after birth, activity of the GnRH pulse generator decreases considerably thereafter, presumably secondarily to inhibition by the CNS. Shortly before puberty, CNS

Table 56–3

Structures and Relative Potencies of GnRH and GnRH Analogs

NAME	RELATIVE POTENCY	1	2	3	4	5	6	7	8	9	10	DOSAGE FORM
						AMINO ACID SEQUENCE						
GnRH (FACTREL, LUTREPULSE)	1	PyroGlu	His	Trp	Ser	Tyr	Gly	Leu	Arg	Pro	Gly-NH$_2$	IV
Leuprolide (LUPRON)	15						D-Leu				N-EtNH$_2$	SC, depot IM
Buserelin (SUPREFACT)	20						D-Ser (tBu)				N-EtNH$_2$	SC, IN
Nafarelin (SYNAREL)	150						D-Nal				N-EtNH$_2$	SC, IN
Deslorelin	150						D-Trp				N-EtNH$_2$	SC, depot IM
Histrelin (SUPPRELIN)	150						D-His (ImBzl)				N-EtNH$_2$	SC
Goserelin (ZOLADEX)	100						D-Ser (tBu)				AzGly-NH$_2$	Depot SC
Cetrorelix (CETROTIDE)	Antagonist	Ac-D-Nal	D-Cpa	D-Pal	Ser	Tyr	D-Cit	Leu	Arg	Pro	D-Ala-NH$_2$	SC
Ganirelix (ANTAGON, ORGALUTRAN)	Antagonist	Ac-D-Nal	D-Cpa	D-Pal	D-hArg(Et)^2			Leu	hArg(Et)^2	Pro	D-Ala-H$_2$	SC

ABBREVIATIONS: Ac, acetyl; N-EtNH$_2$, N-ethylamide; tBu, t butyl; D-Nal, 3-(2-naphthyl)-D-alanyl; ImBzl, imidobenzyl; Cpa, chlorophenylalanyl; Pal, 3-pyridylalanyl; AzGly, azaglycyl; hArg(Et)^2, ethyl homoarginine; IV, intravenous; SC, subcutaneous; IN, intranasal; IM, intramuscular.

inhibition decreases and there is an increased amplitude and frequency of GnRH pulses, particularly during sleep. As puberty progresses, the GnRH pulses increase further in amplitude and frequency until the normal adult pattern is established. The intermittent release of GnRH is crucial for the proper synthesis and release of the gonadotropins, which also are released in a pulsatile manner. The continuous administration of GnRH leads to desensitization and down-regulation of GnRH receptors on pituitary gonadotropes. The latter actions form the basis for the clinical use of long-acting GnRH analogs that suppress gonadotropin secretion (*see* below for further discussion). These compounds transiently increase LH and FSH secretion, but eventually desensitize gonadotropes to GnRH, thereby inhibiting gonadotropin release.

Molecular and Cellular Bases of GnRH Action.   The GnRH receptor, a member of the family of G protein–coupled receptors, is encoded by a gene on chromosome 4q21. The binding of GnRH or GnRH agonists to GnRH receptors on the gonadotropes activates $G_{q_{11}}$, which in turn stimulates phospholipase activity and increases the intracellular concentration of Ca^{2+}, thereby increasing both the synthesis and secretion of LH and FSH. Although cyclic AMP is not the major mediator of GnRH action, binding of GnRH also modulates adenylyl cyclase activity. GnRH receptors also are present in the ovary and testis, although their physiological significance at these sites remains to be determined.

Gonadal steroids also regulate gonadotropin production—at the level of both the pituitary and the hypothalamus—but effects on the hypothalamus predominate. The feedback effects of gonadal steroids are gender-, dosage-, and time-dependent. In women, low levels of estradiol and progesterone inhibit gonadotropin production largely through opioid action on the neural pulse generator that controls GnRH production. Higher and more sustained levels of estradiol have positive feedback effects that ultimately result in the gonadotropin surge that precedes ovulation. In men, testosterone inhibits gonadotropin production, in part through direct actions and in part after its metabolism to estradiol.

Another important regulator of gonadotropin production is the gonadal peptide hormone *inhibin*. Inhibin is made by granulosa cells in the ovary and Sertoli cells in the testis in response to the gonadotropins and local growth factors; it acts directly in the pituitary, selectively inhibiting FSH secretion without affecting that of LH. Inhibin is structurally similar to the family of glycoproteins that includes transforming growth factor β and antimüllerian hormone.

Molecular and Cellular Bases of Gonadotropin Action

LH and FSH were named initially based on their actions on the ovary; appreciation of their roles in male reproductive function did not come until later. The actions of LH and CG are mediated by the LH receptor (the gene for which is located on chromosome 2p21) and those of FSH are mediated by the FSH receptor (the gene for which is located on chromosome 2q). Both of these G protein–coupled receptors have large, glycosylated extracellular domains that contribute to their affinity and specificity for their ligands. The FSH and LH receptors couple with $G_{s\alpha}$ to activate adenylyl cyclase and raise the intracellular level of cyclic AMP. At higher ligand concentrations, the agonist-occupied gonadotropin receptors also activate protein kinase C and Ca^{2+} signaling pathways *via* G_q-mediated effects on phospholipase C activity. Since most if not all of the actions of the gonadotropins can be mimicked by cyclic AMP analogs, the precise physiological role of Ca^{2+} and protein kinase C in gonadotropin action remains to be determined.

Physiological Effects of Gonadotropins

In men, LH acts on testicular Leydig cells to stimulate the *de novo* synthesis of androgens, primarily testosterone. Testosterone is required for gametogenesis within the seminiferous tubules and for maintenance of libido and secondary sexual characteristics. FSH acts on the Sertoli cells to stimulate the production of proteins and nutrients required for sperm maturation, thereby indirectly supporting germ cell maturation.

The actions of FSH and LH in women are more complicated than those in men. FSH stimulates the growth of developing ovarian follicles and induces the expression of LH receptors on both theca and granulosa cells. FSH also regulates the activity of aromatase in granulosa cells, thereby stimulating the production of 17β-estradiol. LH acts on the theca cells to stimulate the synthesis of androstenedione, the major precursor of ovarian 17β-estradiol in premenopausal women. LH also is required for the rupture of the dominant follicle during ovulation and for the synthesis of progesterone by the corpus luteum. Finally, LH and the LH receptor in women induce the expression of the FSH receptor by granulosa cells; LH thus plays a permissive role in FSH action.

The essential roles of gonadotropins in reproductive physiology are revealed by human subjects with mutations of either the gonadotropin subunits or their cognate receptors (Achermann and Jameson, 1999). Women with mutations in either FSHβ or its receptor present clinically with primary amenorrhea, infertility, and absent breast development. Histologically, the ovarian follicles fail to mature and corpora lutea are missing. These findings, in conjunction with success in assisted reproductive technologies using FSH alone (see below), establish the critical role of FSH in ovarian function. In men, mutations of FSHβ or the FSH receptor are associated with decreased testis size and oligospermia, although several subjects have been fertile.

The only reported inactivating mutation of LHβ was in a 46-year-old XY subject with Leydig cell hypoplasia, lack of spontaneous puberty, and infertility. The external genitalia were masculinized, suggesting that CG mediates androgen production in utero. In contrast, apparently complete loss-of-function mutations of the LH receptor cause phenotypes ranging from male hypogonadism to male-to-female sex reversal of the external genitalia and failure to initiate puberty. Presumably, the absence of any virilization of the external genitalia reflects combined loss of both CG and LH signaling in utero. Women with homozygous inactivating mutations of the LH receptor present with primary amenorrhea, oligoamenorrhea, or infertility and have cystic ovaries on histological examination.

Mutations leading to a constitutively active LH receptor affect males primarily and are autosomal dominant. These mutations result in precocious puberty due to the uncontrolled production of testosterone in the fetal and prepubertal periods. A subset of these mutations also has been associated with testicular tumors.

Diagnostic and Therapeutic Uses of GnRH and Its Analogs

As illustrated in Table 56–3, a number of clinically useful GnRH analogs have been synthesized. These include synthetic GnRH (gonadorelin) and GnRH analogs that contain substitutions at position 6 that protect against proteolysis and substitutions at the C-terminus that improve receptor-binding affinity. The analogs exhibit enhanced potency and a prolonged duration of action compared to GnRH, which has a half-life of approximately 2 to 4 minutes.

Pure GnRH antagonists have been developed that do not cause the initial increase in gonadotropin secretion seen with the long-acting GnRH agonists. These newer antagonists apparently do not provoke local and systemic histamine release and the anaphylactoid reactions that hampered the clinical development of earlier analogs. Two different GnRH antagonists, ganirelix (ORGALUTRAN, ANTAGON) and cetrorelix (CETROTIDE), have been used to suppress the LH surge in ovarian-stimulation protocols that are part of assisted reproduction techniques. Ganirelix is available in the United States. Cetrorelix is available in Europe, but not in the United States. Although the almost immediate suppression of LH theoretically should result in a decreased duration of the in vitro fertilization cycle and a better-controlled regimen of ovarian stimulation (see below), more clinical trials are needed to define the roles of these compounds in assisted reproduction technologies.

Diagnostic Use. Synthetic GnRH (gonadorelin hydrochloride; FACTREL) is marketed for diagnostic purposes to differentiate between pituitary and hypothalamic defects in patients with hypogonadotropic hypogonadism. After a blood sample is obtained for the baseline LH value, a single 100-μg dose of GnRH is administered subcutaneously or intravenously and serum LH levels are measured over the next 2 hours (at 15, 30, 45, 60, and 120 minutes after injection). A normal LH response indicates the presence of functional pituitary gonadotropes. Inasmuch as the long-term absence of GnRH can result in a decreased responsiveness of otherwise normal gonadotropes, the absence of a response does not always indicate intrinsic pituitary disease. GnRH-stimulation testing also can be used to determine whether a subject with precocious puberty has central (i.e., GnRH-dependent) or peripheral precocious puberty.

Management of Infertility. Gonadorelin acetate (LUTREPULSE) is a synthetic preparation of GnRH used to treat patients with reproductive disorders secondary to GnRH deficiency or disordered secretion of GnRH. It is administered by an intravenous pump in pulses that promote a physiological cycle, starting at doses of 2.5 μg per pulse every 60 to 90 minutes. If necessary, the dose can be increased to 10 μg per pulse until ovulation is induced, as described in the manufacturer's manual provided with the kit. Advantages over gonadotropin therapy (see below) include a lower risk of multiple pregnancies and a decreased need to monitor plasma estrogen levels or ovarian ultrasonography. Side effects generally are minimal; the most common is local phlebitis due to the infusion device. In women, normal cycling levels of ovarian steroids can be achieved, leading to ovulation and menstruation. Because of its complexity, however, this regimen is available only in specialized centers in reproductive endocrinology (Hayes et al., 1998).

Although growth of testes, appearance of normal levels of gonadal steroids, and induction of spermatogenesis can be achieved in men, GnRH therapy to induce fertility in men is not approved by the FDA, is relatively expensive, and requires that an infusion pump be worn constantly. Therefore, gonadotropins generally are preferred.

The long-acting GnRH agonists also have been used in ovulation-induction protocols to suppress the endogenous preovulatory surge of LH and thus prevent premature follicular luteinization. Several treatment regimens have been developed in which the GnRH agonist is given for either short or long periods—in conjunction with gonadotropins to induce follicular maturation (*see* below)—and then ovulation is induced with CG (Lunenfeld, 1999).

Suppression of Gonadotropin Secretion. As noted above, long-acting GnRH analogs eventually desensitize GnRH receptor-elicited signaling pathways, markedly inhibiting gonadotropin secretion and decreasing the production of gonadal steroids. This "medical castration" has proven to be very useful in disorders that respond to reductions in gonadal steroids. Perhaps the clearest indication for this therapy is in children with gonadotropin-dependent precocious puberty (also called central precocious puberty), whose premature sexual maturation can be arrested with minimal side effects by chronic administration of the GnRH agonists.

Long-acting GnRH agonists are used for palliative therapy of hormonally responsive tumors (*e.g.,* prostate or breast cancer), generally in conjunction with agents that block steroid biosynthesis or action to avoid transient increases in hormone levels. The analogs also are used to suppress steroid-responsive conditions such as endometriosis, uterine leiomyomas, and acute intermittent porphyria. Finally, depot preparations of *goserelin* (ZOLADEX), which can be implanted subcutaneously every 3 months (10.8 mg), may make this drug particularly useful for medical castration in disorders such as pedophilia, where strict patient supervision may be required to ensure compliance.

The long-acting agonists generally are well tolerated, and side effects are those that would be predicted to occur when gonadal steroidogenesis is inhibited (*e.g.,* hot flashes, vaginal dryness and atrophy, decreased bone density). Because of these effects, therapy in settings such as endometrioisis or uterine leiomyomas generally is limited to 6 months unless add-back therapy with estrogens is included to minimize effects on bone density.

Diagnostic Uses of Gonadotropins

Diagnosis of Pregnancy. Significant amounts of CG are present in both the maternal bloodstream and urine during pregnancy and can be detected immunologically with antisera raised against its unique β-subunit. This provides the basis for commercial pregnancy kits that qualitatively assay for the presence or absence of CG in the urine. These kits, which offer a rapid, noninvasive means of detecting pregnancy within a few days after a woman's first missed menstrual period, are available in the United States without a prescription.

Quantitative measurements of CG concentration in plasma are determined by radioimmunoassay in clinical and research laboratories. These assays typically are used to assess whether or not pregnancy is proceeding normally or to help detect the presence of an ectopic pregnancy, hydatidiform mole, or choriocarcinoma.

Prediction of Ovulation. Ovulation occurs 36 hours after the onset of the LH surge (10 to 12 hours after the peak of LH). Therefore, urinary concentrations of LH can be used to predict the time of ovulation. Kits are commercially available without a prescription that provide a semiquantitative assessment of LH levels in urine, using LH-specific antibodies that do not recognize other gonadotropins. Urine LH levels are measured every 12 to 24 hours, beginning on day 11 of the menstrual cycle (assuming a 28-day cycle), to detect the rise in LH and thus estimate the time of ovulation. Such estimates facilitate the timing of sexual intercourse to achieve pregnancy.

Diagnosis of Diseases of the Male and Female Reproductive System. Measurements of plasma LH and FSH levels, as determined by quantitative, β subunit–specific radioimmunoassays, are useful in the diagnosis of several reproductive disorders. Low or undetectable levels of LH and FSH are indicative of hypogonadotropic hypogonadism and suggest hypothalamic or pituitary disease, whereas high levels of gonadotropins suggest primary gonadal diseases. Therefore, in cases of amenorrhea in women or delayed puberty in men and women, measurements of plasma gonadotropins can be used to distinguish between gonadal failure and hypothalamic-pituitary failure.

The FSH level on day 3 of the menstrual cycle is useful in assessing relative fertility. An FSH level of ≥15 IU/ml is associated with reduced fertility, even if a woman is menstruating normally, and predicts a lower likelihood of success in assisted reproduction techniques such as *in vitro* fertilization (*see* below).

CG also is used diagnostically to stimulate testosterone production and thus assess Leydig cell function in men suspected of having Leydig cell failure (for example, in delayed puberty). Serum testosterone levels are assayed after multiple injections of CG. A diminished testosterone response to CG indicates Leydig cell failure; a normal testosterone response suggests a hypothalamic-pituitary disorder.

Therapeutic Uses of Gonadotropins

Gonadotropins for clinical use originally came from human pituitaries and women's urine. Pituitary extracts are

---

no longer used because of possible contamination with the Creutzfeldt-Jakob prion. Since their initial introduction, several different preparations of urinary gonadotropins have been developed. *Chorionic gonadotropin* (PREGNYL, A.P.L., PROFASI, others), which mimics the action of LH, is obtained from the urine of pregnant women. Urine from postmenopausal women is the source of *menotropins* (PERGONAL, HUMEGON, REPRONEX), which contain roughly equal amounts of FSH and LH as well as a number of other urinary proteins. Because of their relatively low purity, menotropins are administered intramuscularly to decrease the incidence of hypersensitivity reactions. *Urofollitropin* (uFSH; METRODIN, FERTINEX) is a purified FSH preparation from which most of the LH has been removed by immunodepletion. Finally, a highly purified FSH preparation is prepared by immunoconcentration with monoclonal antibodies (METRODIN HP). This preparation is sufficiently pure that it can be administered subcutaneously.

Recombinant FSH (rFSH), prepared by expressing cDNAs encoding the α and β subunits of FSH in a mammalian cell line, yields products whose glycosylation pattern mimics that of FSH produced by the gonadotropes. The two rFSH preparations that are available [*follitropin α* (GONAL-F) and *follitropin β* (PUREGON, FOLLISTIM)] differ slightly in their carbohydrate structures. Both rFSH preparations can be administered subcutaneously, since they are considerably purer and exhibit less interbatch variability than do preparations purified from urine. The recombinant preparations are considerably more expensive than the naturally derived hormones, and their relative advantages (*i.e.,* efficacy, lower frequency of side effects such as ovarian hyperstimulation) have not been definitively established. Eventually, the recombinant technology is likely to lead to improved forms of gonadotropins with increased half-lives or higher clinical efficacy.

Female Infertility. Infertility affects approximately 10% of couples of reproductive age. Increasingly, gonadotropins are used in the treatment of infertility (Vollenhoven and Healy, 1998), often in conjunction with assisted reproduction technologies (ART). Although most clearly indicated in anovulatory women with hypogonadotropic hypogonadism secondary to hypothalamic or pituitary dysfunction [patients with World Health Organization (WHO) class I anovulation], gonadotropins also are used to induce ovulation in women with the polycystic ovary syndrome who do not respond to clomiphene citrate (WHO class II; *see* Chapter 58). Finally, gonadotropins also are used in women who are infertile despite normal ovulation, although therapy with clomiphene citrate typically

is attempted first. Clinical use of gonadotropins should be limited to physicians who are experienced in the treatment of infertility or endocrine disorders.

FSH alone can induce ovulation in most anovulatory women. A typical therapeutic regimen is to administer 75 IU daily. This dosage is given daily until cycle day 6 or 7, when the ovarian response is assessed by determining the number and size of developing follicles by transvaginal ultrasound. Scans typically are performed every 2 to 3 days and focus on identifying intermediate follicles. The finding of a follicle larger than 18 mm in diameter indicates that follicular development has progressed adequately. If three or more follicles >16 mm are present, gonadotropin therapy generally is stopped and pregnancy prevented by barrier contraception to decrease the likelihood of multiple pregnancies or the ovarian hyperstimulation syndrome (OHSS, *see* below). Measurements of serum estradiol levels also may be helpful. The target estradiol range is from 500 to 1500 pg/ml, with lower levels indicating inadequate gonadotropin stimulation and higher doses portending an increased risk of OHSS. If laboratory assessment indicates impaired ovarian response, the dose of FSH can be increased to 150 IU daily.

To complete follicular maturation and induce ovulation, CG (5000 to 10,000 IU) is given one day after the last dose of gonadotropin. In approximately 10% to 20% of cases, gonadotropin-induced ovulation is associated with multiple births, resulting from nonphysiological development of more than one preovulatory follicle and the release of more than one ovum.

Gonadotropin induction also is used in conjunction with ART, including *in vitro* fertilization (IVF) and intracytoplasmic sperm injection (ICSI). Again, FSH is administered to induce follicular maturation, CG is given to induce final oocyte development, and then the mature eggs are surgically retrieved from the preovulatory follicles. The retrieved ova are fertilized *in vitro* with sperm (IVF) or by sperm injection (ICSI), and they are then transferred to the uterus or fallopian tubes. With ART, the increased risk of multiple births is related to the number of fertilized eggs that are transferred to the woman.

Aside from the risk of multiple births and its attendant complications, the major side effect of gonadotropin treatment is OHSS. OHSS, which is believed to result from increased ovarian secretion of a substance that increases vascular permeability, is characterized by rapid accumulation of fluid in the peritoneal cavity, thorax, and even the pericardium. Signs and symptoms include abdominal pain and/or distention, nausea and vomiting, diarrhea, marked ovarian enlargement, dyspnea, and oliguria. Consequences of the OHSS include hypovolemia, electrolyte abnormalities, abnormal fluid accumulation (*e.g.,* ascites, pleural effusions, hemoperitoneum), acute respiratory distress syndrome, thromboembolic events, and hepatic dysfunction. If there is clinical suspicion that OHSS is developing before CG administration, then CG must be withheld.

Some studies have suggested that gonadotropins are associated with an increased risk of ovarian cancer, but this conclusion is controversial. Importantly, there is no evidence that either menotropins or FSH increases the rate of congenital abnormalities in babies born from oocytes that were stimulated with gonadotropins.

Male Infertility. In men with impaired fertility secondary to gonadotropin deficiency, gonadotropins can establish or restore fertility. Partly due to expense and partly due to the occasional development of resistance to gonadotropins with prolonged use, standard treatment is to induce sexual development with androgens, reserving gonadotropins until fertility is desired.

Treatment typically is initiated with CG (1000 to 5000 IU intramuscularly) three times per week until clinical parameters and the plasma testosterone level indicate full induction of steroidogenesis. Thereafter, the dose of CG is reduced to 2000 IU twice a week, and menotropins are injected three times a week (with typical doses ranging from 75 IU LH/FSH to 150 IU LH/FSH) to fully induce spermatogenesis. The most common side effect of gonadotropin therapy is gynecomastia, which occurs in up to one-third of patients and presumably reflects increased production of estrogens. Maturation of the prepubertal testis typically requires treatment for more than 6 months, and optimal spermatogenesis in some patients may require treatment for up to two years. Once spermatogenesis has been initiated by this combined therapy or in patients who developed hypogonadotropic hypogonadism after sexual maturation, ongoing treatment with CG alone usually is sufficient to support sperm production. As discussed above in the section entitled "Female Infertility," regimens employing recombinant LH, FSH, and CG very likely will play increasing clinical roles.

Cryptorchidism. Cryptorchidism, the failure of one or both testes to descend into the scrotum, affects up to 3% of full-term male infants and becomes less prevalent with advancing age. Cryptorchid testes have defective spermatogenesis and are at increased risk to develop germ cell tumors. Hence, the current approach is to reposition the testes as early as possible, typically at 1 year of age but definitely before 2 years of age. As descent of the testes is stimulated by androgens, CG can be used to induce testicular descent if the cryptorchidism is not secondary to anatomical blockage. Therapy usually consists of injections of CG (3000 U/m^2 body surface area) intramuscularly every other day for 6 doses. If this does not induce testicular descent, orchiopexy should be performed.

OXYTOCIN

The structures of the neurohypophyseal hormones— oxytocin and vasopressin (antidiuretic hormone; ADH)— and the physiology and pharmacology of vasopressin are presented in Chapter 30. The following discussion emphasizes the physiology of oxytocin and its use in pregnancy.

Biosynthesis of Oxytocin

Oxytocin is a cyclic nonapeptide that is structurally similar to vasopressin, differing by only two amino acids. It is synthesized as a larger precursor molecule in cell bodies of the paraventricular nucleus and, to a lesser extent, the supraoptic nucleus in the hypothalamus. The precursor is rapidly broken down to the active hormone and its neurophysin by proteolysis, packaged into secretory granules as an oxytocin-neurophysin complex, and secreted from nerve endings that terminate primarily in the posterior pituitary gland (neurohypophysis). In addition, oxytocinergic neurons that are known to regulate the autonomic nervous system project to regions of the hypothalamus, brainstem, and spinal cord. Other sites of oxytocin synthesis include the luteal cells of the ovary, the uterus, and fetal membranes.

Stimuli for oxytocin secretion include sensory stimuli arising from the cervix and vagina and from suckling at the breast. Increases in circulating oxytocin in women in labor are difficult to detect, partly because of the pulsatile nature of oxytocin secretion and partly because of the activity of circulating oxytocinase. Nevertheless, most consistent increases have been observed during the expulsive phase triggered by sustained distension of the uterine cervix and vagina. Estradiol stimulates oxytocin secretion, whereas the ovarian polypeptide *relaxin* inhibits release. Other factors that primarily affect vasopressin secretion also have some impact on oxytocin release: *e.g.,* ethanol inhibits oxytocin release, and pain, dehydration, hemorrhage, and hypovolemia stimulate oxytocin release. Although peripheral actions of oxytocin appear to play no significant role in the response to dehydration, hemorrhage, or hypovolemia, oxytocin may participate in the central regulation of blood pressure. As described below, pharmacological doses of oxytocin can inhibit free water clearance by the kidney, occasionally causing water intoxication if not used carefully.

Physiological Roles of Oxytocin

Uterus. Oxytocin stimulates both the frequency and force of uterine contractions. These effects are highly dependent on estrogen, and the immature uterus is quite resistant to the effects of oxytocin. Progesterone antagonizes the stimulant effect of oxytocin *in vitro*, and the decline in progesterone seen in late pregnancy may play an important role in the normal initiation of human parturition. A very low level of motor activity prevails in the human uterus during the first two trimesters of pregnancy. During the third trimester, spontaneous motor activity progressively increases until the sharp rise that constitutes the initiation of labor and delivery. The responsiveness of the uterus to oxytocin roughly parallels the increase in spontaneous activity. Exogenous oxytocin can initiate or enhance rhythmic contractions at any time, but a considerably higher dose is required in early pregnancy. Thus, an eightfold increase in uterine sensitivity to oxytocin occurs in the last half of pregnancy, mostly in the last 9 weeks, accompanied by a 30-fold increase in oxytocin receptors between early pregnancy and early labor. Because of the difficulties associated with measurements of oxytocin levels (*see* above) and because loss of pituitary oxytocin seems not to compromise labor and delivery, the physiological role of oxytocin in pregnancy has been highly debated. The finding that the oxytocin antagonist *atosiban* is effective in suppressing preterm labor (*see* below) argues in favor of the physiological importance of oxytocin.

Breast.   Oxytocin plays an important physiological role in milk ejection. Stimulation of the breast through suckling or mechanical manipulation induces oxytocin secretion, causing contraction of the myoepithelium that surrounds areolar channels in the mammary gland. This action forces milk from the alveolar channels into large collecting sinuses, where it is available to the suckling infant.

Mechanism of Action

Oxytocin acts *via* specific G protein–coupled membrane receptors most closely related to the V_{1a} and V_2 vasopressin receptors. In the human myometrium, these receptors are coupled to G_q and G_{11}, which upon activation lead the generation of inositol 1,4,5-trisphosphate from phosphoinositide hydrolysis, subsequent mobilization of calcium from intracellular stores, and depolarization-induced activation of voltage-sensitive calcium channels. The number of oxytocin receptors differs at various stages of pregnancy and increases significantly late in gestation, paralleling the marked increase in myometrial sensitivity to oxytocin. While this increase in receptor number may indicate a role of oxytocin in labor initiation, it also may represent one of the many changes occurring in preparation for uterine involution postpartum. Oxytocin also increases local prostaglandin production, which further stimulates uterine contractions.

Clinical Use of Oxytocin

Induction of Labor.   Uterine-stimulating agents are used most frequently to induce or augment labor in selected pregnant women (Dudley, 1997). Indications for induction of labor include situations in which the risk of continued pregnancy to the mother or fetus is considered to be greater than the risks of delivery or of pharmacological induction. Such circumstances include premature rupture of the membranes, isoimmunization, intrauterine growth retardation, and placental insufficiency (as in diabetes, preeclampsia, or eclampsia). Before labor is induced, it is essential to verify that the fetal lungs are sufficiently mature (*i.e.,* the lecithin/cholesterol ratio in amniotic fluid is >2) and to exclude potential contraindications (*e.g.,* abnormal fetal position, evidence of fetal distress, placental abnormalities, or previous uterine surgery that predisposes the uterus to rupture during labor).

Oxytocin (PITOCIN, SYNTOCINON) is the drug of choice for induction of labor. It is administered by intravenous infusion of a diluted solution (typically 10 mU/ml), preferably by means of a variable-speed infusion pump. Although there is continuing debate concerning the optimal dose to induce labor, many physicians use a protocol involving an initial dose of 1 mU/minute, with dose increases of no greater than 1 mU/minute every 30 to 40 minutes. Other authorities advocate a more aggressive approach, with starting doses of 6 mU/minute and increases of up to 2 mU/minute at 20-minute intervals. Some published trials have suggested that the higher-dose regimens result in a lower rate of cesarean sections. For the induction of labor, if doses of 30 to 40 mU/minute fail to initiate satisfactory uterine contractions, higher rates of infusion are unlikely to be successful. As labor progresses, the dose of oxytocin required to maintain good uterine contractions may decrease.

During labor induction, a physician must be immediately available, and the mother and fetus should be monitored continuously to determine fetal and maternal heart rates, maternal blood pressure, and the strength of uterine contraction. If uterine hyperstimulation occurs, as evidenced by too frequent contractions or the development of uterine tetany, the oxytocin should be discontinued immediately. The half-life of intravenous oxytocin is short (~3 minutes); thus the hyperstimulatory effects of oxytocin should resolve within several minutes after cessation of the infusion. Because of its structural similarity to vasopressin, oxytocin at higher doses has pronounced antidiuretic effects. Infusions of ≥ 20 mU/minute decrease free water clearance by the kidney. Particularly if hypotonic fluids (*e.g.,* dextrose in water) are infused in appreciable amounts, water intoxication may result in convulsions, coma, and even death. Vasodilatory actions of oxytocin also have been noted, particularly at high doses, which may provoke hypotension and reflex tachycardia. Deep anesthesia may exaggerate the hypotensive effect of oxytocin by causing less tachycardia.

Augmentation of Labor. In most circumstances, oxytocin should not be used to augment labor that is progressing normally because the resulting uterine hyperstimulation often is too forceful and sustained to be compatible with the safety of the mother and fetus. For the augmentation of hypotonic contractions in dysfunctional labor, it rarely is necessary to exceed an infusion rate of 10 mU/minute; doses of >20 mU/minute rarely are effective when lower concentrations fail. Potential complications of overstimulation include trauma of the mother or fetus due to forced passage through an incompletely dilated cervix, uterine rupture, and compromised fetal oxygenation due to loss of placental exchange. In the setting of dysfunctional labor, as seen most frequently in nulliparous women, oxytocin can be used to advantage by experienced obstetricians to facilitate labor progression. Oxytocin usually is effective where there is a very prolonged latent phase of cervical dilation, as well as in cases where there is a significant arrest of dilation or descent. The use of epidural anesthesia can impair the reflex stimulation of endogenous oxytocin during the second stage of labor; in this setting, the cautious administration of oxytocin may facilitate labor progression.

Third Stage of Labor and Puerperium. After delivery of the fetus or following therapeutic abortion, it is desirable to have the uterus firm and contracted, as this greatly reduces the incidence and extent of hemorrhage. Oxytocin often is given immediately after delivery to help maintain uterine contractions and tone. Typically, 20 mU of oxytocin is diluted in 1 liter of intravenous solution and infused at a rate of 10 ml/minute for a few minutes until the uterus is contracted. Then, the infusion rate is reduced to 1 to 2 ml/minute until the mother is ready for transfer to the postpartum unit. If this is ineffective, ergot alkaloids such as *ergonovine maleate* (ERGOTRATE) or *methylergonovine maleate* (METHERGINE) may be used in nonhypertensive patients. The ergot alkaloids are discussed in more detail in Chapter 11.

Oxytocin Challenge Test. In patients whose pregnancy holds increased risk for maternal or fetal complications (*e.g.,* maternal diabetes mellitus or maternal hypertension), an oxytocin challenge test can be used to assess fetal well-being. Oxytocin is infused intravenously, initially at a rate of 0.5 mU/minute; this rate is increased slowly until 3 uterine contractions occur in 10 minutes. Concurrent monitoring of the fetal heart rate indicates whether or not the uterine contractions are associated with changes in fetal heart rate known to be associated with fetal distress. The outcome of the oxytocin challenge test is helpful in determining the presence of adequate placental reserve for continuation of high-risk pregnancies.

Oxytocin-Receptor Antagonists

Peptide analogs that competitively inhibit the interaction of oxytocin with its membrane receptor have been of some interest because of their potential use in the treatment of preterm labor (Goodwin and Zograbyan, 1998). The most widely studied oxytocin-receptor antagonist, *atosiban,* has been evaluated as a potential treatment for preterm labor. Although atosiban significantly decreases the frequency of uterine contractions in women in preterm labor, clinical trials to date have shown no improvement in infant outcomes, and the FDA has not approved atosiban for use in the United States.

PROSPECTUS

Recent years have witnessed enormous advances in our understanding of the regulation of secretion of anterior pituitary hormones. It seems inevitable that the identification and characterization of additional physiological regulators of pituitary hormone secretion will facilitate the development of new drugs that can manipulate this secretion. For example, the characterization of the receptor for GH secretagogues—as well as the identification of its putative endogenous ligand (Kojima *et al.,* 1999)—provide novel approaches to modulate GH secretion. Similarly, the characterization of the different somatostatin receptor subtypes and the identification of agonists with greater selectivity toward these subtypes may provide new drugs that are more efficacious or have fewer side effects. Finally, the observation that dopamine and somatostatin receptors can form heterodimers with enhanced functional activity (Rocheville *et al.,* 2000) may provide novel therapeutic strategies to manipulate growth hormone and/or prolactin secretion.

Recent advances in techniques for peptide synthesis and recombinant protein expression have led to the clinical application of a number of drugs used in treating pituitary hormone excess or deficiency. Although the relative advantages of recombinant *versus* urinary gonadotropin preparations still are being defined, it seems certain that recombinant hormones will be used increasingly in clinical applications. Moreover, an improved knowledge of structure-function relationships of pituitary hormones very likely also will lead to the development of novel therapeutic products. For example, insights from the structure of GH bound to its receptor and site-directed mutagenesis permitted the development of pegvisomant, a genetically altered variant of human GH that acts as a GH antagonist. Similar approaches very likely will lead to the development of other modified forms of pituitary hormones for clinical application.

For further discussion of disorders associated with the pituitary gland and hypothalamus, *see* Chapters 328 to 330 in *Harrison's Principles of Internal Medicine,* 14th ed., McGraw-Hill, New York, 1998.

BIBLIOGRAPHY

Achermann, J.C., and Jameson, J.L. Fertility and infertility: genetic contributions from the hypothalamic-pituitary-gonadal axis. *Mol. Endocrinol.,* **1999,** *13*:812–818.

Anonymous. Consensus guidelines for the diagnosis and treatment of adults with growth hormone deficiency: summary statement of the Growth Hormone Research Society Workshop on Adult Growth Hormone Deficiency. *J. Clin. Endocrinol. Metab.,* **1998,** *83*:379–381.

Anonymous. Growth-hormone-releasing factor for growth hormone deficiency. *Med. Lett. Drugs Ther.,* **1999,** *41*:2–3.

Ayling, R.M., Ross, R., Towner, P., Von Laue, S., Finidori, J., Moutoussamy, S., Buchanan, C.R., Clayton, P.E., and Norman, M.R. A dominant-negative mutation of the growth hormone receptor causes familial short stature. *Nat. Genet.,* **1997,** *16*:13–14.

Blethen, S.L., Allen, D.B., Graves, D., August, G., Moshang, T., and Rosenfeld, R. Safety of recombinant deoxyribonucleic acid-derived growth hormone: The National Cooperative Growth Study experience. *J. Clin. Endocrinol. Metab.,* **1996,** *81*:1704–1710.

Comacho-Hubner, C., Woods, K.A., Miraki-Moud, F., Hindmarsh, P.C., Clark, A.J., Hansson, Y., Johnston, A., Baxter, R.C., and Savage, M.O. Effects of recombinant human insulin-like growth factor I (IGF-I) therapy on the growth hormone-IGF system of a patient with a partial IGF-I gene deletion. *J. Clin. Endocrinol. Metab.,* **1999,** *84*:1611–1616.

Cutfield, W.S., Wilton, P., Bennmarker, H., Albertsson-Wikland, K., Chatelain, P., Ranke, M.B., and Price, D.A. Incidence of diabetes mellitus and impaired glucose tolerance in children and adolescents receiving growth-hormone treatment. *Lancet,* **2000,** *355*:610–613.

de Vos, A.M., Ultsch, M., and Kossiakoff, A.A. Human growth hormone and extracellular domain of its receptor: crystal structure of the complex. *Science,* **1992,** *255*:306–312.

Howard, A.D., Feighner, S.D., Cully, D.F., Arena, J.P., Liberator, P.A., Rosenblum, C.I., Hamelin, M., Hreniuk, D.L., Palyha, O.C., Anderson, J., Paress, P.S., Diaz, C., Chou, M., Liu, K.K., McKee, K.K., Pong, S.S., Chaung, L.Y., Elbrecht, A., Dashkevicz, M., Heavens, R., Rigby, M., Sirinathsinghji, D.J.S., Dean, D.C., Melillo, D.G., Patchett, A.A., Nargund, R., Griffin, P.R., DeMartino, J.A., Gupta, S.K., Schaeffer, J.M., Smith, R.G., and Van der Ploeg, L.H. A receptor in the pituitary and hypothalamus that functions in growth hormone release. *Science,* **1996,** *273*:974–977.

Kojima, M., Hosoda, H., Date, Y., Nakazato, M., Matsuo, H., and Kangawa, K. Ghrelin is a growth-hormone-releasing acylated peptide from stomach. *Nature,* **1999,** *402*:656–660.

Leung, D.W., Spencer, S.A., Cachianes, G., Hammonds, R.G., Collins, C., Henzel, W.J., Barnard, R., Waters, M.J., and Wood, W.I. Growth hormone receptor and serum binding protein: purification, cloning and expression. *Nature,* **1987,** *330*:537–543.

Ranke, M.B., Savage, M.O., Chatelain, P.G., Preece, M.A., Rosenfeld, R.G., and Wilton, P. Long-term treatment of growth hormone insensitivity syndrome with IGF-I. Results of the European Multicentre Study. The Working Group on Growth Hormone Insensitivity Syndromes. *Horm. Res.,* **1999,** *51*:128–134.

Rocheville, M., Lange, D.C., Kumar, U., Patel, S.C., Patel, R.C., and Patel, Y.C. Receptors for dopamine and somatostatin: formation of hetero-oligomers with enhanced functional activity. *Science,* **2000,** *288*:154–157.

Smith, R.G., Feighner, S., Prendergast, K., Guan, X., and Howard, A. A new orphan receptor involved in pulsatile growth hormone release. *Trends Endocrinol. Metab.,* **1999,** *10*:128–135.

Trainer, P.J., Drake, W.M., Katznelson, L., Freda, P.U., Herman-Bonert, V., van der Lely, A.J., Dimaraki, E.V., Stewart, P.M., Friend, K.E., Vance, M.L., Besser, G.M., Scarlett, J.A., Thorner, M.O., Parkinson, C., Klibanski, A., Powell, J.S., Barkan, A.L., Sheppard, M.C., Malsonado, M., Rose, D.R., Clemmons, D.R., Johannsson, G., Bengtsson, B.A., Stavrou, S., Kleinberg, D.L., Cook, D.M., Phillips, L.S., Bidlingmaier, M., Strasburger, C.J., Hackett, S., Zib, K., Bennett, W.F., and Davis, R.J. Treatment of acromegaly with the growth hormone-receptor antagonist pegvisomant. *N. Engl. J. Med.,* **2000,** *342*:1171–1177.

Turner, H.E., Vadivale, A., Keenan, J., and Wass, J.A. A comparison of lanreotide and octreotide LAR for treatment of acromegaly. *Clin. Endocrinol. (Oxf.),* **1999,** *51*:275–280.

Verhelst, J., Abs, R., Maiter, D., van den Bruel, A., Vandeweghe, M., Velkeniers, B., Mockel, J., Lamberigts, G., Petrossians, P., Coremans, P., Mahler, C., Stevenaert, A., Verlooy, J., Raftopoulos, C., and Beckers, A. Cabergoline in the treatment of hyperprolactinemia: a study in 455 patients. *J. Clin. Endocrinol. Metab.,* **1999,** *84*:2518–2522.

MONOGRAPHS AND REVIEWS

Bole-Feysot, C., Goffin, V., Edery, M., Binart, N., and Kelly, P.A. Prolactin (PRL) and its receptor: actions, signal transduction pathways and phenotypes observed in PRL receptor knockout mice. *Endocr. Rev.,* **1998,** *19*:225–268.

Dudley, D.J. Oxytocin: use and abuse, science and art. *Clin. Obstet. Gynecol.,* **1997,** *40*:516–524.

Finidori, J. Regulators of growth hormone signaling. *Vitam. Horm.,* **2000,** *59*:71–97.

Goodwin, T.M., and Zograbyan, A. Oxytocin receptor antagonists. Update. *Clin. Perinatol.,* **1998,** *25*:859–871.

Hayes, F.J., Seminara, S.B., and Crowley, W.F. Jr. Hypogonadotropic hypogonadism. *Endocrinol. Metab. Clin. North Am.,* **1998,** *27*:739–763.

Lunenfeld, B. *GnRH Analogues: The State of the Art at the Millennium.* Parthenon, New York, **1999.**

Molitch, M.E. Medical treatment of prolactinomas. *Endocrinol. Metab. Clin. North Am.,* **1999,** *28*:143–169.

Newman, C.B. Medical therapy for acromegaly. *Endocrinol. Metab. Clin. North Am.,* **1999,** *28*:171–190.

Patel, Y.C. Somatostatin and its receptor family. *Front. Neuroendocrinol.,* **1999,** *20*:157–198.

Vance, M.L., and Mauras, N. Growth hormone therapy in adults and children. *N. Engl. J. Med.,* **1999,** *341*:1206–1216.

Vollenhoven, B.J., and Healy, D.L. Short- and long-term effects of ovulation induction. *Endocrinol. Metab. Clin. North Am.,* **1998,** *27*:903–914.

Acknowledgment

The authors wish to acknowledge Drs. Mario Ascoli and Deborah L. Segaloff, authors of this chapter in the ninth edition of *Goodman and Gilman's The Pharmacological Basis of Therapeutics,* some of whose text has been retained in this edition.

THYROID AND ANTITHYROID DRUGS

Alan P. Farwell and Lewis E. Braverman

This chapter discusses the function of the thyroid hormones, thyroxine (T_4) and triiodothyronine (T_3), in growth and metabolism and the regulation of thyroid function by thyroid-stimulating hormone (TSH) secreted from the pituitary. Calcitonin, also secreted by the thyroid gland, is discussed in Chapter 62. Evaluation of free thyroxine and TSH levels as a means to assess thyroid function is provided as a prelude to the discussion of treatment of the hypothyroid patient with hormone replacement and of the hyperthyroid individual with one of a variety of antithyroid drugs, such as propylthiouracil and methimazole, and other thyroid inhibitors, including ionic inhibitors that interfere with the concentration of iodide by the thyroid gland and radioactive iodine, used both for diagnosis as well as treatment of hyperthyroidism. Although disorders of the thyroid are common, effective treatment of most thyroid disorders is available.

Thyroid hormones, the only known iodine-containing compounds with biological activity, have two important functions. In developing animals and human beings, they are crucial determinants of normal development, especially in the central nervous system (CNS). In the adult, thyroid hormones act to maintain metabolic homeostasis, affecting the function of virtually all organ systems. To meet these requirements, there are large stores of preformed hormone within the thyroid gland. Metabolism of the thyroid hormones occurs primarily in the liver, although local metabolism within certain target tissues, such as the brain, also occurs. Serum concentrations of thyroid hormones are precisely regulated by the pituitary hormone, thyrotropin, in a classic negative-feedback system. The predominant actions of thyroid hormone are mediated *via* binding to nuclear thyroid hormone receptors and modulating transcription of specific genes. In this regard, thyroid hormones share a common mechanism of action with steroid hormones, vitamin D, and retinoids, whose receptors make up a superfamily of nuclear receptors (Chin and Yen, 1997; *see* Chapter 2). In addition, as with steroid hormones, it has become clear that thyroid hormones have diverse nongenomic actions (Davis and Davis, 1997).

Disorders of the thyroid are common. They consist of two general presentations: changes in the size or shape of the gland or changes in secretion of hormones from the gland. Thyroid nodules and goiter in the euthyroid patient are the most common endocrinopathies and can be caused by benign and malignant tumors. The presentation of overt hyper- or hypothyroidism often presents the clinician with dramatic clinical manifestations. While the diagnosis may be clinically obvious, subtle presentations require the use of biochemical tests of thyroid function. Screening of the newborn population for congenital hypothyroidism, followed by the institution of appropriate thyroid hormone replacement therapy, has dramatically decreased the incidence of mental retardation and cretinism in the United States. Worldwide, congenital hypothyroidism due to iodine deficiency remains the major preventable cause of mental retardation, although much progress has been made to eradicate iodine deficiency.

Effective treatment of most thyroid disorders is readily available. Treatment of the hypothyroid patient is straightforward and consists of hormone replacement. There are more options for treatment of the hyperthyroid patient, including the use of antithyroid drugs to decrease hormone synthesis and secretion by the gland and destruction of the gland by the administration of radioactive iodine or by surgical removal. Treatment of thyroid disorders in general is extremely satisfying, as most patients can be either cured or have their diseases controlled (*see* Braverman and Utiger, 2000; Braverman and Refetoff, 1997).

THYROID

The thyroid gland is the source of two fundamentally different types of hormones. The iodothyronine hormones include thyroxine (T_4) and 3,5,3'-triiodothyronine (T_3); they are essential for normal growth and development and play an important role in energy metabolism. The other known secretory product of the thyroid, calcitonin, is produced by the parafollicular (C–) cells and is discussed in Chapter 62.

History. The thyroid gland was first described by Galen and was named "glandulae thyroidaeae" by Wharton in 1656. Harington (1935) reviewed the many older opinions concerning the function of this gland. Wharton thought, for example, that the viscous fluid within the follicles lubricated the trachea. He also believed that the gland was larger in women, to serve a cosmetic function in giving grace to the contour of the neck. Later observers, influenced by the liberal blood supply of the gland, believed that it provided a vascular shunt for the brain. With this function in mind, Rush in 1820 expressed the belief that the larger size of the gland in women was "necessary to guard the female system from the influence of the more numerous causes of irritation and vexation of mind to which they are exposed than the male sex." However, Hofrichter opposed this theory in the same year by pointing out that "If it were indeed true that the thyroid contains more blood at some times than at others, this effect would be visible to the naked eye; in this case women would certainly have long ceased to go about with bare necks, for husbands would have learned to recognize the swelling of this gland as a danger signal of threatening trouble from their better halves."

The thyroid was first recognized as an organ of importance when enlargement was observed to be associated with changes in the eyes and the heart in the condition we now call *hyperthyroidism.* It is of interest that this condition, the manifestations of which on occasion can be as striking as any in medicine, escaped description until Parry saw his first case in 1786. Parry's account was not published until 1825 and was followed in 1835 and 1840 by those of Graves and Basedow, whose names became applied to the disorder. In 1874, Gull first associated atrophy of the gland with the symptoms now known to be characteristic of thyroid deficiency and hypofunction of the thyroid, *hypothyroidism,* in adults was known as *Gull's disease.* The term *myxedema* was applied to the clinical syndrome in 1878 by Ord in the belief that the characteristic thickening of the subcutaneous tissues was due to excessive formation of mucus.

Extirpation experiments to elucidate the function of the thyroid were at first misinterpreted because of the simultaneous removal of the parathyroids. However, the pioneer research in the late 19th century on the latter organs by Gley allowed the functional differentiation of these two endocrine glands. It was not until after calcitonin was discovered in 1961 that it was realized that the thyroid itself also was concerned with the regulation of Ca^{2+}. In 1891, Murray became the first to treat a case of hypothyroidism by injecting an extract of the thyroid gland; in the following year, Howitz, Mackenzie, and Fox independently discovered that thyroid tissue was fully effective when given by mouth.

Magnus-Levy discovered the effect of the thyroid on metabolic rate in 1895; he found that Gull's disease was characterized by a low rate of metabolism and that the administration of thyroid to hypothyroid or normal individuals increased oxygen consumption.

Chemistry of Thyroid Hormones. The principal hormones of the thyroid gland are the iodine-containing amino acid derivatives of thyronine—(T_4 and T_3; Figure 57–1). Thyroxine was first isolated in crystalline form from a hydrolysate of thyroid by Kendall in 1915; he found that the crystalline product exerted the same physiological effects as the extract from which it was obtained. Eleven years later, the structural formula of thyroxine was elucidated by Harington, and in 1927, Harington and Barger synthesized the hormone.

Following the isolation and the chemical identification of thyroxine, it was generally believed that all the hormonal activity of thyroid tissue could be accounted for by its content of thyroxine. However, careful studies revealed that crude thyroid

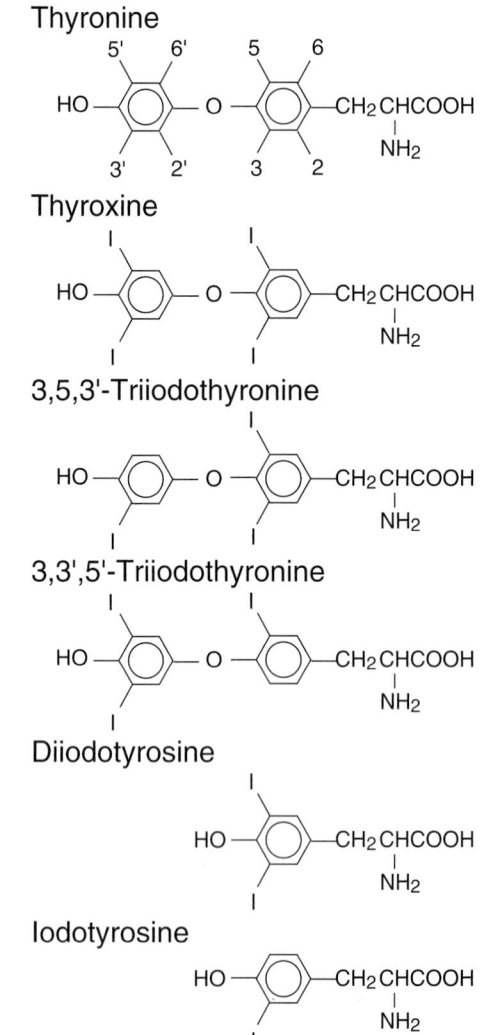

Figure 57–1. Thyronine, thyroid hormones, and precursors.

preparations possessed greater calorigenic activity than could be accounted for by their thyroxine content. The enigma was resolved with the detection, isolation, and synthesis of triiodothyronine (Gross and Pitt-Rivers, 1952; Roche *et al.*, 1952a,b). Further studies revealed that triiodothyronine is qualitatively similar to thyroxine in its biological action but that it is much more potent on a molar basis (Gross and Pitt-Rivers, 1953a,b). **Structure–Activity Relationship.** The stereochemical nature of the thyroid hormones plays an important role in defining hormone activity. A great many structural analogs of thyroxine have been synthesized in order to define the structure–activity relationship, to detect antagonists of thyroid hormones, or to find compounds exhibiting one desirable type of activity while not showing unwanted effects. The only significant success has been the partial separation of the cholesterol-lowering action of thyroxine analogs from their calorigenic or cardiac effects. For example, introduction of specific arylmethyl groups at the $3'$ position of triiodothyronine resulted in analogs that are liver-selective, cardiac-sparing thyromimetics (Leeson *et al.*, 1989). The D isomer of thyroxine was once used to lower the concentration of cholesterol in plasma, but cardiac side effects resulted in discontinuation of the clinical uses of this hormone. Thyroid hormone analogs and metabolites offer hope that more useful separation of these activities may yet be achievable. For example, 3,5,3'-triiodothyroacetic acid (triac) has been shown to have less thyromimetic activity in the heart than in other thyroid hormone-responsive tissues (Liang *et al.*, 1997; Sherman and Ladenson, 1992).

The structural requirements for a significant degree of thyroid hormone activity have been defined (*see* Jorgensen, 1964; Cody, 2000; Wagner *et al.*, 1995). The 3'-monosubstituted compounds are more active than the 3',5'-disubstituted molecules. Thus, triiodothyronine is five times more potent than thyroxine, while 3'-isopropyl-3,5-diiodothyronine has seven times the activity.

Although the chemical nature of the 3, 5, 3', and 5' substituents is important, their effects on the conformation of the molecule are even more so. In thyronine, the two rings are angulated at about 120° at the ether oxygen and are free to rotate on their axes. As depicted schematically in Figure 57–2, when the 3,5 iodines are in place, rotation of the two rings is somewhat restricted, and they tend to take up positions perpendicular to one another. While not potent, even halogen-free derivatives possess some activity if they have the proper conformation. In

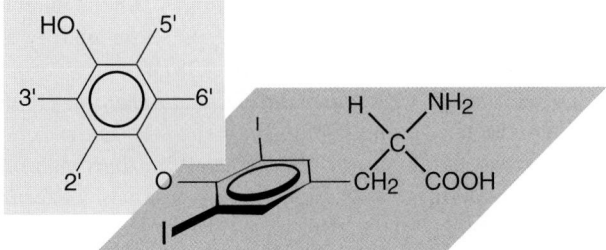

Figure 57–2. Structural formula of 3,5-diiodothyronine, drawn to show the conformation in which the planes of the aromatic rings are perpendicular to each other.

(*Adapted from* Jorgensen, 1964. *See also* Cody, 2000.)

general, the affinity of iodothyronines for the thyroid hormone receptor parallels their biological potency (Chin and Yen, 1997; Anderson *et al.*, 2000), but additional factors including affinity for plasma proteins, rate of entry into cell nuclei, and rate of metabolism can affect therapeutic potency.

Recent structure–activity correlations indicate that certain plant flavonoids that are long-standing folk remedies can exhibit antihormonal properties, including inhibition of the enzyme that catalyzes 5' (outer, or tyrosyl ring) deiodination of T_4 (type I iodothyronine 5'-deiodinase; Cody, 2000). These compounds are also potent competitors of thyroxine binding to transthyretin. Computer graphic modeling suggests that the best structural homology between thyroid hormones and flavonoids involves their respective phenolic rings.

Synthesis of Thyroid Hormones. The synthesis of the thyroid hormones is unique, complex, and seemingly grossly inefficient. The thyroid hormones are synthesized and stored as amino acid residues of thyroglobulin, a protein constituting the vast majority of the thyroid follicular colloid. The thyroid gland is unique in storing great quantities of potential hormone in this way, and extracellular thyroglobulin can represent a large portion of the mass of the gland. Thyroglobulin is a complex glycoprotein made up of two apparently identical subunits, each with a molecular mass of 330,000 daltons. Interestingly, molecular cloning has revealed that thyroglobulin belongs to a superfamily of serine hydrolases, including acetylcholinesterase (*see* Chapter 8).

The major steps in the synthesis, storage, release, and interconversion of thyroid hormones are the following: (1) the uptake of iodide ion by the gland, (2) the oxidation of iodide and the iodination of tyrosyl groups of thyroglobulin, (3) coupling of iodotyrosine residues by ether linkage to generate the iodothyronines, (4) the proteolysis of thyroglobulin and the release of thyroxine and triiodothyronine into the blood, and (5) the conversion of thyroxine to triiodothyronine in peripheral tissues as well as in the thyroid. These processes are summarized in Figure 57–3.

1. Uptake of Iodide. Iodine ingested in the diet reaches the circulation in the form of iodide. Under normal circumstances, its concentration in the blood is very low (0.2 to 0.4 μg/dl; about 15 to 30 nM), but the thyroid efficiently and actively transports the ion *via* a specific, membrane-bound protein, termed the sodium-iodide symporter (NIS) (Eskandari *et al.*, 1997; Dai *et al.*, 1996; Smanik *et al.*, 1996). As a result, the ratio of thyroid to plasma iodide concentration is usually between 20 and 50 and can far exceed 100 when the gland is stimulated. The iodide transport mechanism is inhibited by a number of ions such as thiocyanate and perchlorate (Figure 57–3). The transport system is stimulated by thyrotropin

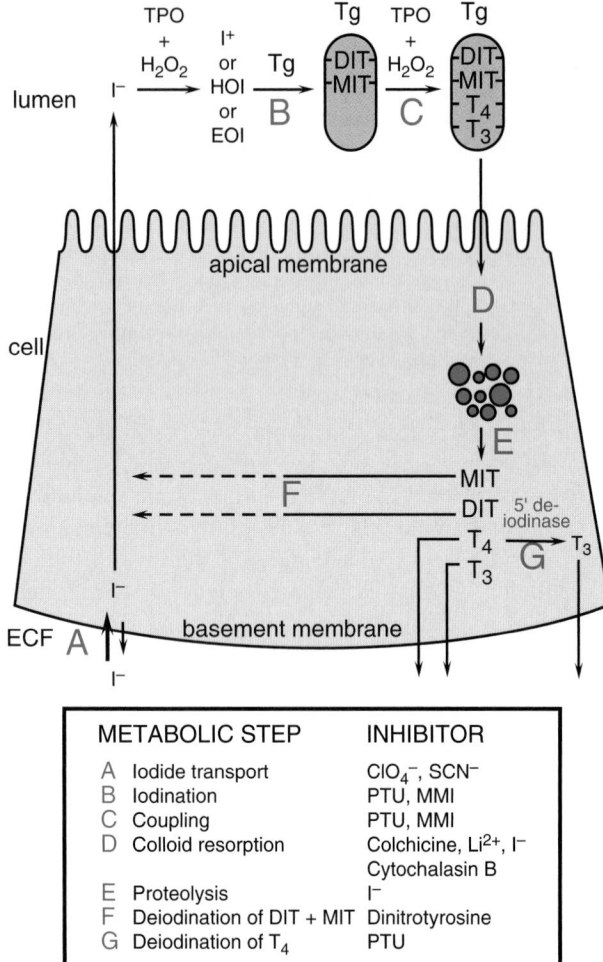

Figure 57–3. Major pathways of thyroid hormone biosynthesis and release.

Abbreviations are as follows: Tg, thyroglobulin; DIT, diiodotyrosine; MIT, monoiodotyrosine; TPO, thyroid peroxidase; HOI, hypoiodous acid; EOI, enzyme-linked species; PTU, propylthiouracil; MMI, methimazole; ECF, extracellular fluid. (Adapted from Taurog, 2000, *with permission.*)

[thyroid-stimulating hormone (TSH); *see* below] and also is controlled by an autoregulatory mechanism. Thus, decreased stores of thyroid iodine enhance iodide uptake, and the administration of iodide can reverse this situation.

If the further metabolism of iodide is blocked by antithyroid drugs, the iodide-concentrating mechanism (NIS) can be more easily studied. Thus isolated, NIS has been identified in many other tissues, including the salivary glands, gastric mucosa, midportion of the small intestine, choroid plexus, skin, mammary gland, and perhaps the placenta, all of which maintain a concentration of iodide

greater than that of the blood (Carrasco, 2000). It has been suggested that the accumulation of iodide by the placenta and the mammary gland may be of importance in providing adequate supplies for the fetus and infant, but no obvious purpose is served by the accumulation of iodide at the other sites. It is evident that NIS in the thyroid is not unique to the gland and does not account for the specific function of synthesizing thyroid hormone.

2. Oxidation and Iodination.   Consistent with the conditions generally necessary for halogenation of aromatic rings, the iodination of tyrosine residues requires the iodinating species to be in a higher state of oxidation than is the anion. The exact nature of the iodinating species was uncertain for many years. However, Magnusson and coworkers (1984) have provided convincing evidence that it is hypoiodate, either as hypoiodous acid (HOI) or as an enzyme-linked species (EOI).

The oxidation of iodide to its active form is accomplished by thyroid peroxidase, a heme-containing enzyme that utilizes hydrogen peroxide (H_2O_2) as the oxidant (Taurog, 2000; Magnusson *et al.*, 1987). Human thyroid peroxidase has been cloned and identified as an autoantigen in autoimmune thyroid disease (McLachlan and Rapoport, 1992). The peroxidase is membrane-bound and appears to be concentrated at or near the apical surface of the thyroid cell. The reaction results in the formation of monoiodotyrosyl and diiodotyrosyl residues in thyroglobulin just prior to its storage in the lumen of the thyroid follicle. It is thought that the formation of the H_2O_2 that serves as a substrate for the peroxidase occurs in close proximity to its site of utilization and involves the oxidation of reduced nicotinamide adenine dinucleotide phosphate (NADPH). An increase in the generation of H_2O_2 may be an important facet of the mechanism by which TSH stimulates the organification of iodide in thyroid cells. This hypothesis has arisen from observations that TSH stimulates the synthesis of inositol trisphosphate and elevates cytosolic concentrations of Ca^{2+} in thyroid follicular cells (Corda *et al.*, 1985; Field *et al.*, 1987; Laurent *et al.*, 1987). The formation of H_2O_2 is stimulated by a rise in cytosolic Ca^{2+} (Takasu *et al.*, 1987).

3. Formation of Thyroxine and Triiodothyronine from Iodotyrosines.   The remaining synthetic step is the coupling of two diiodotyrosyl residues to form thyroxine or of monoiodotyrosyl and diiodotyrosyl residues to form triiodothyronine. These also are oxidative reactions and appear to be catalyzed by the same peroxidase discussed above. The mechanism involves the enzymatic transfer of groups, perhaps as iodotyrosyl free radicals or positively charged ions, within thyroglobulin. Although many other proteins can serve as substrates for the peroxidase, none is as efficient as thyroglobulin in yielding thyroxine. The configuration of the protein is thus presumed to be important in facilitating this coupling reaction. Thyroxine formation occurs primarily at a location near the amino terminus of the protein, while most of the triiodotyrosine is synthesized near the carboxy terminus (Dunn *et al.*, 1987). The relative rates of synthetic activity at the various sites depend on the concentration of TSH and the availability of iodide. This may account, at least in part, for the long-known relationship between the proportion of thyroxine and triiodothyronine formed in the thyroid and the availability of iodide or the relative quantities of the two iodotyrosines. For example, when there is a deficiency of iodine in rat thyroid, the ratio of thyroxine to triiodothyronine decreases from 4:1 to 1:3 (Greer *et al.*, 1968). Because triiodothyronine is at least five times as active as thyroxine and contains only three-fourths as much iodine, a decrease in the quantity of available iodine need have little impact on the effective amount of thyroid hormone elaborated by the gland. Although a decrease in the availability of iodide and the associated increase in the proportion of monoiodotyrosine favor the formation of triiodothyronine over thyroxine, a deficiency in diiodotyrosine ultimately can impair the formation of both forms of the hormone. In addition to the coupling reaction, intrathyroidal and secreted triiodothyronine is generated by the 5'-deiodination of thyroxine (Chanoine *et al.*, 1993).

4. Secretion of Thyroid Hormones.
Since thyroxine and triiodothyronine are synthesized and stored within thyroglobulin, proteolysis is an important part of the secretory process. This process is initiated by endocytosis of colloid from the follicular lumen at the apical surface of the cell. This "ingested" thyroglobulin appears as intracellular colloid droplets, which apparently then fuse with lysosomes containing the requisite proteolytic enzymes. It is generally believed that thyroglobulin must be completely broken down into its constituent amino acids for the hormones to be released. As the molecular mass of thyroglobulin is 660,000 daltons, and the protein is made up of about 300 carbohydrate residues and 5500 amino acid residues, only two to five of which are thyroxine, this is an extravagant process. TSH appears to enhance the degradation of thyroglobulin by increasing the activity of several thiol endopeptidases of the lysosomes (Dunn and Dunn, 1988). The endopeptidases selectively cleave thyroglobulin, yielding hormone-containing intermediates that are subsequently processed by exopeptidases (Dunn and Dunn, 2000). The liberated hormones then exit the cell, presumably at its basal membrane. When thyroglobulin is hydrolyzed, monoiodotyrosine and diiodotyrosine also are liberated, but they usually do not leave the thyroid.

Instead, they are selectively metabolized, and the iodine, liberated in the form of iodide, is reincorporated into protein. Normally, all this iodide is reused; however, when proteolysis is activated intensely by TSH, some of the iodide reaches the circulation, at times accompanied by trace amounts of the iodotyrosines.

5. Conversion of Thyroxine to Triiodothyronine in Peripheral Tissues.
The normal daily production of thyroxine has been estimated to range between 70 and 90 μg, while that of triiodothyronine is between 15 and 30 μg. Although triiodothyronine is secreted by the thyroid, metabolism of thyroxine by sequential monodeiodination in the peripheral tissues accounts for about 80% of circulating triiodothyronine (Figure 57–4). Removal of the 5'-, or outer ring, iodine leads to the formation of triiodothyronine and is the "activating" metabolic pathway. The major site of conversion of thyroxine to triiodothyronine outside the thyroid is the liver. Thus, when thyroxine is given to hypothyroid patients in doses that produce normal concentrations of thyroxine in plasma, the plasma concentration of triiodothyronine also reaches the normal range (Braverman *et al.*, 1970). Most peripheral target tissues utilize triiodothyronine that is derived from the circulating hormone. Notable exceptions are the brain and pituitary, for which local generation of triiodothyronine is a major source for the intracellular hormone. Removal of the iodine on position 5 of the inner ring produces the metabolically inactive 3,3',5'-triiodothyronine (reverse T_3, rT_3; Figure 57–1). Under normal conditions, about 41% of thyroxine is converted to triiodothyronine, about 38% is converted to reverse T_3, and about 21% is metabolized *via* other pathways, such as conjugation in the liver and excretion in the bile. Normal circulating concentrations of thyroxine in plasma range from 4.5 to 11.0 μg/dl, while those of triiodothyronine are about 100-fold less (60 to 180 ng/dl).

The enzyme responsible for the conversion of thyroxine to triiodothyronine is iodothyronine 5'-deiodinase, which exists as two distinct isozymes that are differentially expressed and regulated in peripheral tissues (Figure 57–5; Leonard and Visser, 1986). Type I 5'-deiodinase (D1) is found in the liver, kidney, and thyroid and generates circulating triiodothyronine that is utilized by most peripheral target tissues. Although 5'-deiodination is the major function of this isozyme, D1 also catalyzes 5-deiodination. D1 is inhibited by a variety of factors (Table 57–1), including the antithyroid drug *propylthiouracil*. The decreased plasma triiodothyronine concentrations observed in nonthyroidal illnesses are a result of inhibition of D1 (Farwell, 1999) and decreased entrance of thyroxine into cells. D1 is "up-regulated" in hyperthyroidism and "down-regulated" in hypothyroidism. The cloning of D1 has identified the enzyme as a selenoprotein and demonstrated the presence of a selenocystine at the active site (Berry *et al.*, 1991; Berry and Larsen,

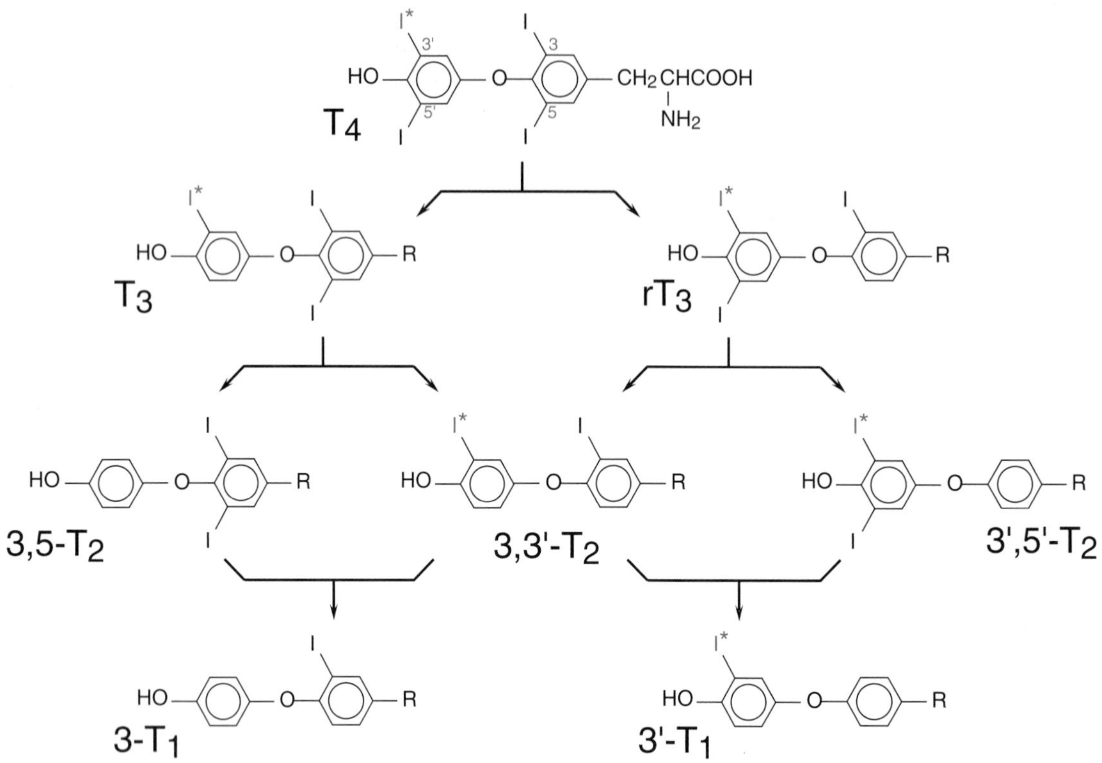

Figure 57–4. Pathways of iodothyronine deiodination.

1992). Type II 5′-deiodinase (D2) is distributed in the brain, pituitary, skeletal and cardiac muscle, and, in the rat, brown fat. It functions primarily to supply intracellular triiodothyronine to these tissues (Visser *et al.,* 1982; Bartha *et al.,* 2000). D2 has a much lower K_m for thyroxine than does D1 (nM *vs.* μM K_m values), and its activity is unaffected by propyl-thiouracil. D2 is dynamically regulated by its substrate, thyroxine, such that elevated levels of the enzyme are found in hypothyroidism and suppressed levels are found in hyperthyroidism (Leonard *et al.,* 1981; Leonard and Koehrle, 2000). Thus, D2 appears to autoregulate the intracellular supply of triiodothyronine in the brain and pituitary. A D2-like seleno-protein cDNA has been cloned from frog skin (Davey *et al.,*

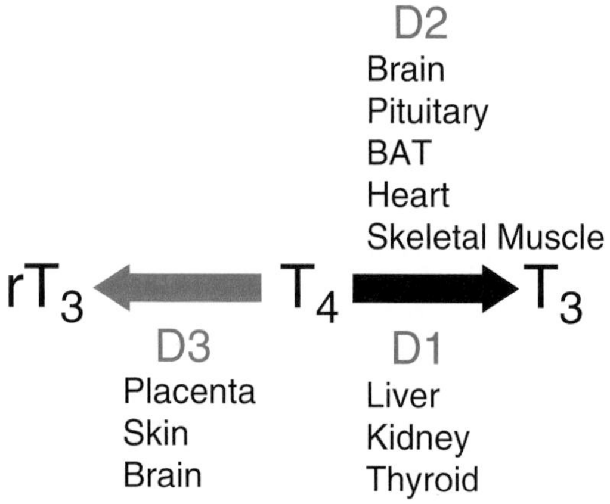

Figure 57–5. Deiodinase isozymes.

Abbreviations are as follows: D1, type I iodothyronine 5′-deiodinase; D2, type II iodothyronine 5′-deiodinase; D3, type III iodothyronine 5-deiodinase; BAT, brown adipose tissue.

Table 57–1

Conditions and Factors That Inhibit Type I 5′-Deiodinase Activity

Acute and chronic illness
Caloric deprivation (especially carbohydrate)
Malnutrition
Glucocorticoids
β-Adrenergic receptor antagonists (*e.g.,* propranolol in high doses)
Oral cholecystographic agents (*e.g.,* iopanoic acid, sodium ipodate)
Amiodarone
Propylthiouracil
Fatty acids
Fetal/neonatal period
Selenium deficiency

1995) and mammalian sources (Croteau *et al.*, 1996; Salvatore *et al.*, 1996), leading to the proposal that the deiodinases belong to a family of selenoproteins (St. Germain and Galton, 1997). However, to date, no native, full-length seleno-D2 translation product has been found in any mammalian tissue despite abundant seleno-D2 gene product (Leonard *et al.*, 1999). Further, the 29,000-dalton substrate-binding subunit of rat D2 has been cloned and shown to be a nonselenoprotein (Leonard *et al.*, 2000). Thus, the confirmation of D2 as a selenoprotein is unresolved.

Inner ring- or 5-deiodination, a main inactivating pathway for T_3, is catalyzed by type III deiodinase (D3), which is found in placenta, skin, and brain. Cloning of D3, like that of D1, has identified the enzyme as a selenoprotein (Croteau *et al.*, 1995).

Transport of Thyroid Hormones in the Blood. Iodine in the circulation is normally present in several forms, with 95% as organic iodine and approximately 5% as iodide. Most of the organic iodine is thyroxine (90% to 95%), while triiodothyronine represents a relatively minor fraction (about 5%). The thyroid hormones are transported in the blood in strong but noncovalent association with certain plasma proteins.

Thyroxine-binding globulin (TBG) is the major carrier of thyroid hormones. It is an acidic glycoprotein with a molecular mass of approximately 63,000 daltons, and it binds one molecule of thyroxine per molecule of protein with a very high affinity (the equilibration association constant, K_a is about 10^{10} M^{-1}). Triiodothyronine is bound less avidly. Thyroxine, but not triiodothyronine, also is bound by transthyretin (formally called thyroxine-binding prealbumin). This protein is present in higher concentration than is TBG and primarily binds thyroxine with an equilibrium association constant near 10^7 M^{-1}. Transthyretin has four apparently identical subunits but only a single high-affinity binding site. Albumin also can serve as a carrier for thyroxine when the more avid carriers are saturated. It is difficult, however, to estimate its quantitative or physiological importance, with the exception of the syndrome known as *familial dysalbuminemic hyperthyroxinemia*. This is an autosomal dominant hereditary disorder characterized by the increased affinity of albumin for thyroxine (Ruiz *et al.*, 1982) due to a point mutation in the albumin gene (Tang *et al.*, 1999; Sunthornthepvarakul *et al.*, 1994). Thyroxine binds also to the apolipoproteins of the high density lipoproteins, HDL_2 and HDL_3, the significance of which is unclear at present (Benevenga *et al.*, 1992).

Binding of thyroid hormones to plasma proteins protects the hormones from metabolism and excretion, resulting in their long half-lives in the circulation. The free (unbound) hormone is a small percentage (about 0.03% of thyroxine and about 0.3% of triiodothyronine) of the total

Table 57–2
Factors That Alter Binding of Thyroxine to Thyroxine-Binding Globulin

INCREASE BINDING	DECREASE BINDING
Drugs	
Estrogens	Glucocorticoids
Methadone	Androgens
Clofibrate	L-Asparaginase
5-Fluorouracil	Salicylates
Heroin	Mefenamic Acid
Tamoxifen	Antiseizure medications
Selective estrogen	(phenytoin, carbamazepine)
receptor modulators	Furosemide
Systemic Factors	
Liver disease	Inheritance
Porphyria	Acute and chronic illness
HIV infection	
Inheritance	

hormone in plasma (Larsen *et al.*, 1981). The differential binding affinity for serum proteins also is reflected in the 10- to 100-fold difference in circulating hormone concentrations and half-lives of thyroxine and triiodothyronine.

Essential to understanding the regulation of thyroid function is the "free hormone" concept: only the unbound hormone has metabolic activity (Mendel, 1989). Thus, because of the high degree of binding of thyroid hormones to plasma proteins, changes in either the concentrations of these proteins or the binding affinity of the hormones for the proteins would have major effects on the total serum hormone levels. Certain drugs and a variety of pathological and physiological conditions, such as the changes in circulating concentrations of estrogens during pregnancy or during the administration of oral estrogens, can alter both the binding of thyroid hormones to plasma proteins and the amounts of these proteins (Table 57–2). However, since the pituitary responds to and regulates circulating free hormone levels, minimal changes in free hormone concentrations are seen. Laboratory tests that measure only total hormone levels, therefore, can be subject to misinterpretation. Appropriate tests of thyroid function are discussed later in this chapter.

Degradation and Excretion (Figure 57–6). Thyroxine is eliminated slowly from the body, with a half-life of 6 to 8 days. In hyperthyroidism, the half-life is shortened to 3 or 4 days, whereas in hypothyroidism it may be 9 to 10 days. These changes presumably are due to

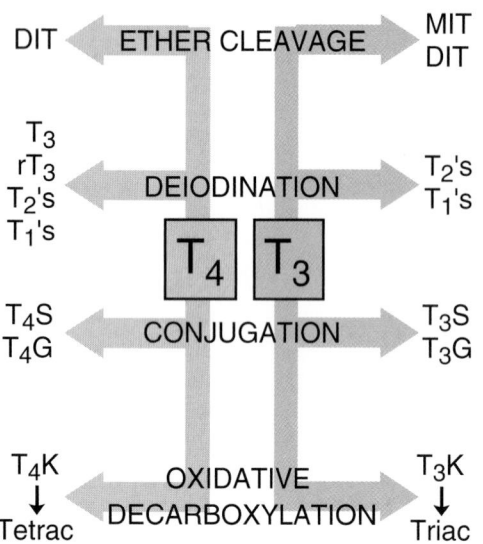

Figure 57–6. Pathways of metabolism of thyroxine (T_4) and triiodothyronine (T_3).

Abbreviations are as follows: DIT, diiodotyrosine; MIT, monoiodotyrosine; T_4S, T_4 sulfate; T_4G, T_4 glucuronide; T_3S, T_3 sulfate; T_3G, T_3 glucuronide; T_4K, T_4 pyruvic acid; T_3K, T_3 pyruvic acid; Tetrac, tetraiodothyroacetic acid; Triac, triiodothyroacetic acid.

altered rates of metabolism of the hormone. In conditions associated with increased binding to TBG, such as pregnancy, clearance is retarded. The increase in TBG is due to the estrogen-induced increase in the sialic acid content of the synthesized TBG resulting in decreased TBG clearance (Ain *et al.,* 1987). The reverse is observed when there is reduced protein binding of thyroid hormones or when binding to protein is inhibited by certain drugs (Table 57–2). Triiodothyronine, which is less avidly bound to protein, has a half-life of approximately 1 day.

The liver is the major site of nondeiodinative degradation of thyroid hormones; thyroxine and triiodothyronine are conjugated with glucuronic and sulfuric acids through the phenolic hydroxyl group and excreted in the bile. There is an enterohepatic circulation of the thyroid hormones; they are liberated by hydrolysis of the conjugates in the intestine and reabsorbed. A portion of the conjugated material reaches the colon unchanged, is hydrolyzed there, and is eliminated in feces as the free compounds.

As discussed above, the major route of metabolism of thyroxine is deiodination to either triiodothyronine or reverse T_3. Triiodothyronine and reverse T_3 are deiodinated to three different diiodothyronines, which are further deiodinated to two monoiodothyronines (*see* Figure 57–4), inactive metabolites that are normal constituents of human plasma. Additional metabolites (monoiodotyrosine

and diiodotyrosine) in which the diphenyl ether linkage is cleaved have been detected both *in vitro* and *in vivo*.

Regulation of Thyroid Function. During the past century, it was appreciated that cellular changes occur in the anterior pituitary in association with endemic goiter or following thyroidectomy. The classical experimental observations of Cushing (1912) and the clinical observations of Simmonds (1914) established that ablation or disease of the pituitary causes thyroid hypoplasia. It eventually was determined that thyrotropes of the anterior pituitary secrete *thyrotropin,* or TSH. TSH is a glycoprotein hormone with α and β subunits analogous to those of the gonadotropins. Its structure is discussed with those of other glycoprotein hormones in Chapter 56. Although there was evidence that thyroid hormone or lack of it causes cellular changes in the pituitary, the control of secretion of TSH by the negative-feedback action of thyroid hormone was not appreciated fully until its central role in the pathogenesis of goiter was elucidated in the early 1940s. TSH is secreted in a pulsatile manner and circadian pattern, its levels in the circulation being highest during sleep at night. It is now recognized that the rate of secretion of TSH is delicately controlled by the hypothalamic peptide *thyrotropin-releasing hormone* (TRH) and the quantity of free thyroid hormones in the circulation. If extra thyroid hormone is given, transcription of both the TRH gene (Wilbur and Xu, 1998) and the thyrotropin gene is decreased (*see* Samuels *et al.,* 1988), the secretion of TSH is suppressed, and the thyroid becomes inactive and regresses. Any decrease in the normal rate of secretion of the thyroid evokes an enhanced secretion of TSH in an attempt to stimulate the thyroid to secrete more hormone. Additional mechanisms of the effect of thyroid hormone on TSH secretion appear to be a reduction in TRH secretion by the hypothalamus and a reduction in the number of receptors for TRH on pituitary cells.

Thyrotropin-Releasing Hormone (TRH). TRH stimulates the release of preformed TSH from secretory granules and also stimulates the subsequent synthesis of both α and β subunits of TSH. Somatostatin, dopamine, and pharmacological doses of glucocorticoids inhibit TRH-stimulated TSH secretion.

TRH is a tripeptide with both terminal amino and carboxyl groups blocked (L-pyroglutamyl-L-histidyl-L-proline amide). The mature hormone is derived from a precursor protein that contains six copies of the tripeptide flanked by dibasic residues. TRH is synthesized by the hypothalamus and is released into the hypophysioportal circulation, where it is brought into contact with TRH receptors on thyrotropes. The binding of TRH to its receptor, a G protein-coupled receptor, elicits stimulation of the hydrolysis of polyphosphatidylinositols and activation of protein kinase C (Gershenghorn, 1986). Ultimately, TRH stimulates the synthesis and release of TSH by the thyrotroph.

TRH also has been localized in the CNS in regions of the cerebral cortex, circumventricular structures, neurohypophysis, pineal gland, and spinal cord. These findings, as well as its localization in nerve endings, suggest that TRH may act as a neurotransmitter or neuromodulator outside of the hypothalamus. Administration of TRH to animals produces CNS-mediated effects on behavior, thermoregulation, autonomic tone, and cardiovascular function, including increases in blood pressure and heart rate. TRH also has been identified in pancreatic islet cells, heart, testis, and in certain parts of the gastrointestinal tract. Its physiological role there is not known. TRH has been administered both intravenously and intrathecally as a therapeutic agent in refractory depression (Callahan *et al.,* 1997; Marangell *et al.,* 1997).

Actions of TSH on the Thyroid. When TSH is given to experimental animals, the first effect on thyroid hormone metabolism that can be measured is increased secretion, which can be seen within minutes. All phases of hormone synthesis and release are eventually stimulated: iodide uptake and organification, hormone synthesis, endocytosis, and proteolysis of colloid. There is increased vascularity of the gland and hypertrophy and hyperplasia of thyroid cells. These effects follow the binding of TSH to its receptor on the plasma membrane of thyroid cells.

The TSH receptor is a member of the family of G protein-coupled receptors and is structurally similar to the receptors for luteinizing hormone (LH) and follicle-stimulating hormone (FSH) (*see* Chapter 56; Parmentier *et al.,* 1989; Vassart and Dumont, 1992; Nagayama and Rapoport, 1992). These receptors share significant amino acid sequences and have large extracellular domains that are involved in binding of hormone.

When TSH binds to its receptor, adenylyl cyclase is stimulated and cyclic AMP levels in the cells increase. At higher concentrations than are required to stimulate cyclic AMP formation, TSH causes activation of phospholipase C, with a resultant hydrolysis of polyphosphatidylinositols, increased cytoplasmic Ca^{2+}, and activation of protein kinase C (Manley *et al.,* 1988; Van Sande *et al.,* 1990). Both the adenylyl cyclase and the phospholipase C signaling pathways appear to mediate effects of TSH on thyroid function in human beings, although the adenylyl cyclase pathway may be the sole mediating pathway in other species (*see* Vassart and Dumont, 1992).

Multiple mutations of the TSH receptor resulting in clinical thyroid dysfunction have been described (Tonacchera *et al.,* 1996b). Germline mutations have presented as congenital, nonautoimmune hypothyroidism (Kopp *et al.,* 1995) and as autosomal, dominant toxic thyroid hyperplasia (Tonacchera *et al.,* 1996a). Somatic mutations that result in constitutive activation of the receptor are recognized as probable causes of hyperfunctioning thyroid adenomas (Paschke *et al.,* 1994b). Finally, resistance to TSH also has been described both in families with mutant TSH receptors (Sunthornthepvarakui *et al.,* 1995) and in those with no apparent mutations in either the TSH receptor or in TSH itself (Xie *et al.,* 1997).

Relation of Iodine to Thyroid Function. Normal thyroid function obviously requires an adequate intake of iodine; without it, normal amounts of hormone cannot be made, TSH is secreted in excess, and the thyroid becomes hyperplastic and hypertrophies. The enlarged and stimulated thyroid becomes remarkably efficient at extracting the residual traces of iodide from the blood. The iodide-concentrating mechanism develops a gradient for the ion that may be ten times normal, and in mild to moderate iodine deficiency, the thyroid usually succeeds in producing sufficient hormone. Adult hypothyroidism and cretinism may occur in more severe iodine deficiency.

In some areas of the world, simple or nontoxic goiter is prevalent because dietary iodine is not sufficient (Delange *et al.,* 1993). Significant regions of iodine deficiency are present in Central and South America, Africa, Europe, southeast Asia, and China. The daily requirement for iodine in adults is 1 to 2 μg/kg body weight. The United States recommended daily allowance for iodine is in the range of 40 to 120 μg for children and 150 μg for adults, with the addition of 25 μg and 50 μg recommended during pregnancy and lactation, respectively. Vegetables, meat, and poultry contain minimal amounts of iodine, whereas dairy products and fish are relatively high in iodine content (Table 57–3; Braverman, 1997). Potable water usually contains negligible amounts of iodine.

Iodine has been used empirically for the treatment of iodine-deficiency goiter for 150 years. However, its modern use was the outgrowth of the extensive studies of Marine, which culminated in the use of iodine to prevent goiter in school children in Akron, Ohio, a region where endemic iodine deficiency goiter was prevalent (Marine and Kimball, 1917). The success of these experiments led to the adoption of iodine prophylaxis and therapy in many regions throughout the world where iodine-deficiency goiter is endemic.

The most practicable method for providing small supplements of iodine for large segments of the population is the addition of iodide or iodate to table salt; iodate is now preferred. In some countries, the use of iodized salt is required by law; in others, including the United States, the use is optional. In the United States, iodized salt provides

Table 57–3

Iodine Content in Some Foodstuffs in the United States (1982–1989)

FOOD	IODINE/SERVING, μg
Ready-to-eat cereals	87
Dairy-based desserts	70
Fish	57
Milk	56
Dairy products	49
Eggs	27
Bread	27
Beans, peas, tuber	17
Meat	16
Poultry	15

SOURCE: Adapted from Braverman, 1994.

100 μg of iodine per gram. However, while the United States population remains iodine-sufficient, iodine intake has steadily decreased over the last twenty years, a trend that needs to be monitored (Hollowell *et al.,* 1998). Other vehicles for supplying iodine to large populations who are iodine-deficient include oral or intramuscular injection of iodized oil (Elnagar *et al.,* 1995), iodized drinking water supplies, iodized irrigation systems (Cao *et al.,* 1994b), and iodized animal feed.

Actions of Thyroid Hormones. Whereas the precise biochemical mechanisms through which thyroid hormones exert their developmental and tissue-specific effects are only beginning to be understood, the concept that most of the actions of thyroid hormones are mediated by nuclear

receptors has been well accepted since the mid-1980s (for review, *see* Chin and Yen, 1997; Anderson *et al.,* 2000). In this model, triiodothyronine binds to high-affinity nuclear receptors, which then bind to a specific DNA sequence (thyroid hormone response element) in the promoter/regulatory region of specific genes. In this fashion, triiodothyronine modulates gene transcription and, ultimately, protein synthesis. In general, the receptor without hormone is bound to the thyroid response element in the basal state. Typically, this results in repressed gene transcription, although there are some examples of constitutive gene activation. Binding by triiodothyronine may activate gene transcription by releasing the repression. Hormone-associated receptors also may have direct activation or repressive actions. Thyroxine also binds to these receptors, but it does so with a much lower affinity than triiodothyronine. Despite its ability to bind to nuclear receptors, thyroxine has not been shown to alter gene transcription. Thus, it is likely that thyroxine serves principally as a "prohormone," with essentially all actions of thyroid hormone at the transcriptional level being caused by triiodothyronine.

Nuclear thyroid hormone receptors were cloned in 1986 by several laboratories (Weinberger *et al.,* 1986; Sap *et al.,* 1986). They were discovered to be the cellular homologs of an avian retroviral oncoprotein, denoted c-*erb* A. There is considerable homology between the thyroid hormone receptors and the steroid nuclear receptors, and together they make up a gene superfamily that also includes the retinoic acid and vitamin D nuclear receptors (*see* Chapters 2 and 62; Mangelsdorf *et al.,* 1994). The thyroid hormone receptors are derived from two genes, c-*erb* A α (TRα) and c-*erb* A β (TRβ), with multiple isoforms identified (Figure 57–7; Lazar, 1993). TRα_1 and TRβ_1 are found in virtually all tissues that respond to thyroid hormone,

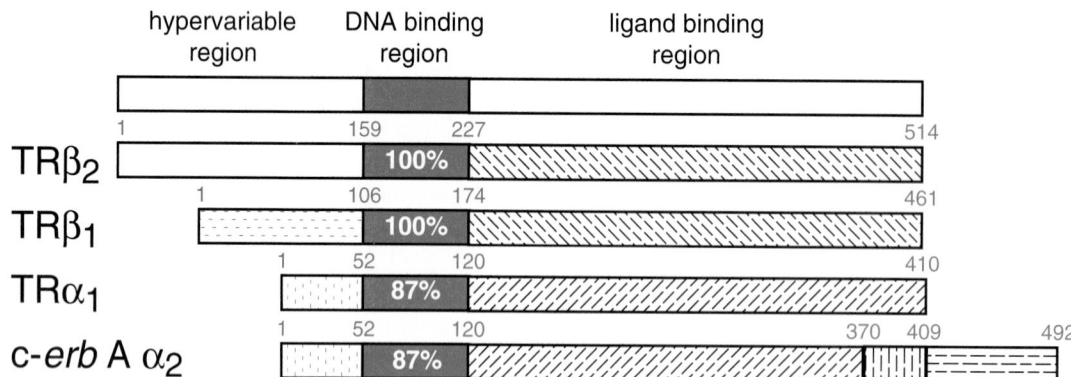

Figure 57–7. Thyroid hormone receptor isoforms.

The percent of amino acid identity in the DNA binding region is indicated. Identical patterns in the hypervariable and ligand binding regions indicate 100% homology. Three thyroid hormone receptor (TR) isoforms bind thyroid hormone (TRβ_1, TRβ_2, and TRα_1); c-*erb* A α_2 does not.

whereas the other isoforms exhibit a more tissue-specific distribution. TRβ_2, for example, is expressed solely in the anterior pituitary. c-*erb* A α_2, an isoform that binds to the thyroid response element but does not bind triiodothyronine, is the most abundant isoform in brain (Strait *et al.*, 1990). Another level of complexity in the regulation of thyroid hormone action at the transcriptional level has been added with the identification of coactivators (Takeshita *et al.*, 1996) and corepressors (Chen and Evans, 1995; Hörlein *et al.*, 1995) that are associated with the T$_3$-receptor complex and serve as mediators of hormone action (Lee and Yen, 1999). Resistance to thyroid hormone has been described in patients with mutations in the TRβ gene (Brucker-Davis *et al.*, 1995; Adams *et al.*, 1994) and in patients with defective cofactors (Weiss *et al.*, 1996).

Further insight into the mechanisms of thyroid hormone action has been provided by the development of transgenic mice lacking one or more of the thyroid hormone receptor isoforms. Multiple variations of these knockout mice have demonstrated abnormalities in the auditory system, the thyroid-pituitary axis, the heart, the skeletal system and the small intestine (Forrest *et al.*, 1996; Forrest *et al.*, 1990; Fraichard *et al.*, 1997; Wikström *et al.*, 1998). Interestingly, despite the recognition of thyroid hormone as an essential regulatory factor during brain development (Oppenheimer and Schwartz, 1997), no obvious abnormalities in brain development have been reported in either single-receptor knockout mice (Hsu and Brent, 1998) or in the recently reported transgenic mice devoid of all known thyroid hormone receptors (Göthe *et al.*, 1999).

In addition to nuclear receptor-mediated actions, there are several well-characterized, nongenomic actions of thyroid hormones (Davis and Davis, 1997), including those occurring at the level of the plasma membrane (Davis *et al.*, 1989) and on the cellular cytoarchitecture (Farwell *et al.*, 1990; Siegrist-Kaiser *et al.*, 1990; Farwell and Leonard, 1997). In addition, there are well-characterized thyroid hormone binding sites on the mitochondria (Sterling, 1989). In several of these processes, thyroxine is the hormone that produces the response. Previously, the overall contribution of nongenomic actions to the general mechanism of thyroid hormone action was considered to be minor. However, this concept, at least as it applies to some species, may need to be reassessed in light of the paucity of abnormalities described in transgenic knockout mice, especially during brain development.

Growth and Development.   As discussed above, it is generally believed that the thyroid hormones exert most of their effects through control of DNA transcription and, ultimately, protein synthesis. This is certainly true for the effects of the hormones on the normal growth and development of the organism. Perhaps the most dramatic example is found in the tadpole, which is almost magically transformed into a frog by triiodothyronine. Not only does the animal grow limbs, lungs, and other terrestrial accoutrements, but the hormone also stimulates the synthesis of a host of enzymes and so influences the tail that it is digested away and used to build new tissue elsewhere.

Thyroid hormone plays a critical role in brain development (Bernal and Nunez, 1995; Oppenheimer and

Schwartz, 1997; Hendrich, 1997). The appearance of functional, chromatin-bound receptors for thyroid hormone coincides with neurogenesis in the brain (Strait *et al.*, 1990). The absence of thyroid hormone during the period of active neurogenesis (up to 6 months postpartum) leads to irreversible mental retardation (cretinism) and is accompanied by multiple morphological alterations in the brain (Legrand, 1979). These severe morphological alterations result from disturbed neuronal migration, deranged axonal projections, and decreased synaptogenesis. Thyroid hormone supplementation during the first 2 weeks of life prevents the development of these disturbed morphological changes.

Myelin basic protein, a major component of myelin, is the product of a specific gene that is regulated by thyroid hormone during development (Farsetti *et al.*, 1991). Decreased expression of myelin basic protein results in defective myelinization in the hypothyroid brain. The appearance of laminin, an extracellular matrix protein that provides key guidance signals to migrating neurons, is delayed and the content is diminished in the developing cerebellum of the hypothyroid rat (Farwell and Dubord-Tomasetti, 1999). Altered expression of laminin is likely to alter neuronal migration and lead to the morphological abnormalities observed in the cretinous brain. Several other brain-specific genes have been reported to be developmentally regulated by thyroid hormone (Bernal and Nunez, 1995). A common characteristic of many of these proteins is that their expression appears to be merely delayed in the hypothyroid animal; normal levels are eventually achieved in the adult.

The actions of thyroid hormones on protein synthesis and enzymatic activity are certainly not limited to the brain, and a large number of tissues are affected by the administration of thyroid hormone or by its deficiency. The extensive defects in growth and development that are found in cretins provide a vivid reminder of the pervasive effects of thyroid hormones in normal individuals.

Cretinism is usually classified as endemic or sporadic. *Endemic cretinism* is encountered in regions of endemic goiter and is usually caused by extreme deficiency of iodine. Goiter may or may not be present. *Sporadic cretinism* is a consequence of failure of the thyroid to develop normally or the result of a defect in the synthesis of thyroid hormone. Goiter is present if a synthetic defect is at fault.

While detectable at birth, cretinism often is not recognized until 3 to 5 months of age. When untreated, the condition eventually leads to such gross changes as to be unmistakable. The child is dwarfed, with short extremities, and is mentally retarded, inactive, uncomplaining, and listless. The face is puffy and expressionless, and the enlarged tongue may protrude through the thickened lips of the half-opened mouth. The skin may have a yellowish hue and feel doughy, and it is dry and cool to the touch. The heart rate is slow, the body temperature may be low, closure of the fontanels is delayed, and the teeth erupt late.

Appetite is poor, feeding is slow and interrupted by choking, constipation is frequent, and there may be an umbilical hernia.

For treatment to be fully effective, the diagnosis must be made long before these obvious changes have come about. In regions of endemic cretinism due to iodine deficiency, iodine replacement is best instituted prior to pregnancy. However, iodine replacement given to pregnant women up to the end of the second trimester has been shown to enhance the neurologic and psychological development of the children (Cao *et al.*, 1994a). Screening of newborn infants for deficient function of the thyroid is carried out in the United States and in most industrialized countries. Concentrations of TSH and thyroxine are measured in blood from the umbilical cord or from a heel stick. The incidence of congenital dysfunction of the thyroid is about 1 per 4000 births (Fisher, 1991).

Calorigenic Effects.   A characteristic response of homeothermic animals to thyroid hormone is increased oxygen consumption. Most peripheral tissues contribute to this response; heart, skeletal muscle, liver, and kidney are stimulated markedly by thyroid hormone. Indeed, 30% to 40% of the thyroid hormone–dependent increase in oxygen consumption can be attributed to stimulation of cardiac contractility. Several organs, including brain, gonads, and spleen, are unresponsive to the calorigenic effects of thyroid hormone. The mechanism of the calorigenic effect of thyroid hormone has been elusive (Silva, 1995). At one time, it was erroneously believed that thyroid hormone uncoupled mitochondrial oxidative phosphorylation. Thyroid hormone–dependent lipogenesis may constitute a quantitatively important energy sink, and studies in rats have demonstrated that about 4% of the increased caloric expenditure induced by thyroid hormone is accounted for by lipogenesis. A link between lipogenesis and thermogenesis is the stimulation of lipolysis by triiodothyronine. Further, thyroid hormone induces expression of several lipogenic enzymes, including malic enzyme and fatty acid synthetase. Although the entire picture is not clear, there appears to be an integrated thyroid hormone response program for regulating the set-point of energy expenditure and maintaining the metabolic machinery necessary to sustain it. Indeed, even small changes in L-thyroxine replacement doses may significantly alter the set-point for resting energy expenditure in the hypothyroid patient (al-Adsani *et al.*, 1997).

Cardiovascular Effects.   Thyroid hormone influences cardiac function by direct and indirect actions; changes in the cardiovascular system are prominent clinical consequences in thyroid dysfunctional states. In hyperthyroidism, there is tachycardia, increased stroke volume, increased cardiac index, cardiac hypertrophy, decreased peripheral vascular resistance, and increased pulse pressure. In hypothyroidism, there is bradycardia, decreased cardiac index,

pericardial effusion, increased peripheral vascular resistance, decreased pulse pressure, and elevations of mean arterial pressure. (For a review of the effects of thyroid hormone on the heart, *see* Braverman *et al.*, 1994.)

Thyroid hormones play a direct role in regulating myocardial gene expression. Triiodothyronine regulates genes encoding the isoforms of the sarcomeric myosin heavy chains by increasing the expression of the α gene and decreasing the expression of the β gene (Everett *et al.*, 1986). A thyroid hormone response element has been located in the 5' upstream region of the α myosin heavy chain gene. Triiodothyronine also upregulates the gene encoding myosin Ca^{2+}–ATPase, which plays a critical role in myocardial contraction (Rohrer and Dillman, 1988). Regulation of these two genes results in the changes in contractility observed in hyper- and hypothyroidism. Indeed, stress echocardiography in hyperthyroid patients revealed abnormalities in cardiac contractility that reverted to normal when euthyroidism was restored (Kahaly *et al.*, 1999). Similarly, left ventricular diastolic dysfunction in hypothyroidism was reversed with L-thyroxine replacement therapy (Biondi *et al.*, 1999).

Observations in transgenic mice have provided insight into the action of thyroid hormone on heart rate. Previously, alterations in the sensitivity of the cardiac myocyte to catecholamines (enhanced in hyperthyroidism and depressed in hypothyroidism) were considered an indirect effect of thyroid hormone, possibly due to changes in expression of myocardial β-adrenergic receptors. This is the basis for the use of β-adrenergic receptor antagonists in relieving some of the cardiac manifestations in hyperthyroidism. However, basal heart rate is decreased in mice lacking the $TR\alpha_1$ gene (Johansson *et al.*, 1998) and is increased in mice lacking $TR\beta$ (Johansson *et al.*, 1999), suggesting a more direct role for thyroid hormone in cardiac pacemaking. Finally, T_3 leads to hemodynamic alterations in the periphery that result in alterations in the chronotropic and inotropic state of the myocardium. Interestingly, T_3 appears to have a direct, nongenomic vasodilatory effect on vascular smooth muscle (Park *et al.*, 1997, Ojamaa *et al.*, 1996).

Metabolic Effects.   Thyroid hormones stimulate metabolism of cholesterol to bile acids, and hypercholesterolemia is a characteristic feature of hypothyroid states. Thyroid hormones have been shown to increase the specific binding of low-density lipoprotein (LDL) by liver cells (Salter *et al.*, 1988), and the concentration of hepatic receptors for LDL is decreased in hypothyroidism (Scarabottolo *et al.*, 1986; Gross *et al.*, 1987). The number of LDL receptors available on the surface of hepatocytes is a strong determinant of the plasma cholesterol concentration (*see* Chapter 36).

Thyroid hormones enhance the lipolytic responses of fat cells to other hormones, for example, catecholamines, and elevated plasma free fatty acid concentrations are seen in hyperthyroidism. In contrast to other lipolytic hormones, thyroid hormones do not directly increase the accumulation of cyclic AMP. They may, however, regulate the capacity of other hormones to enhance the accumulation of the cyclic nucleotide by decreasing the activity of a microsomal phosphodiesterase that hydrolyzes cyclic AMP (Nunez and Correze, 1981). There also is evidence that thyroid hormones act to maintain normal coupling of the β-adrenergic receptor to the catalytic subunit of adenylyl cyclase in fat cells. Fat cells from hypothyroid rats have increased concentrations of guanine nucleotide–binding regulatory proteins (G proteins) that mediate the inhibitory control of adenylyl cyclase (*see* Chapter 2). This can account for both the decreased response to lipolytic hormones and the increased sensitivity to inhibitory regulators, such as adenosine, that are found in hypothyroidism (Ros *et al.,* 1988).

Thyrotoxicosis is an insulin-resistant state (Gottlieb and Braverman, 1994). Postreceptor defects in the liver and peripheral tissues, manifested by depleted glycogen stores and enhanced glucogenesis, lead to insulin insensitivity. In addition, there is increased absorption of glucose from the gut. Compensatory increases in insulin secretion result in order to maintain euglycemia. This may result in the "unmasking" of clinical diabetes in previously undiagnosed patients and an increase in the insulin requirements of diabetic patients already on insulin. Hypothyroidism results in decreased absorption of glucose from the gut and decreased insulin secretion. Peripheral glucose uptake also is slowed in hypothyroidism, although glucose utilization by the brain is unaffected. Insulin requirements are decreased in the hypothyroid patient with diabetes.

Thyroid Hyperfunction. Thyrotoxicosis is a condition caused by elevated concentrations of circulating free thyroid hormones. Various disorders of different etiologies can result in this syndrome. The term *hyperthyroidism* is restricted to those conditions in which thyroid hormone production and release are increased due to gland hyperfunction. Iodine uptake by the thyroid gland is increased, as determined by the measurement of the percent uptake of ^{123}I or ^{131}I in a 24-hour radioactive iodine uptake (RAIU) test. In contrast, thyroid inflammation or destruction resulting in excess "leak" of thyroid hormones or excess exogenous thyroid hormone intake results in a low 24-hour RAIU. The term *subclinical hyperthyroidism* is defined as few if any symptoms with a low serum TSH and normal concentrations of T_4 and T_3.

Graves' disease, or toxic diffuse goiter, is the most common cause of high RAIU thyrotoxicosis. It accounts for 60% to 90% of the cases, depending upon age and geographic region. Graves' disease is an autoimmune disorder characterized by hyperthyroidism, diffuse goiter, and IgG antibodies that bind to and activate the TSH receptor (Burman and Baker, 1985; Bottazzo and Doniach, 1986). This is a relatively common disorder, with an incidence of 0.02% to 0.4% in the United States. Endemic areas of iodine deficiency have a lower incidence of autoimmune thyroid disease. As with most types of thyroid dysfunction, women are affected more than men, with a ratio ranging from 5:1 to 7:1. Graves' disease is more common between the ages of 20 and 50, but may occur at any age. HLA B$_8$ and DR$_3$ haplotypes are associated with Graves' disease in Caucasians. Graves' disease is commonly associated with other autoimmune diseases. The characteristic exophthalmos associated with Graves' disease is an infiltrative ophthalmopathy and is considered an autoimmune-mediated inflammation of the periorbital connective tissue and extraocular muscles. This disorder is clinically evident with various degrees of severity in about

50% of patients with Graves' disease, but it is present on radiological studies, such as ultrasound or CT scan, in almost all patients. The pathogenesis of Graves' ophthalmopathy, including the role of the TSH receptor present in retroorbital tissues (Paschke *et al.,* 1994) and the management of this disorder, is reviewed in a recently published monograph on Graves' disease (Rapoport and McLachlan, 2000).

Toxic uninodular and multinodular goiter accounts for 10% to 40% of cases of hyperthyroidism and is more common in older patients. Infiltrative ophthalmopathy is absent.

A low RAIU is seen in the destructive thyroiditides and in thyrotoxicosis resulting from exogenous thyroid hormone ingestion. Low RAIU thyrotoxicosis caused by subacute (painful) and silent (painless or lymphocytic) thyroiditis represents about 5% to 20% of all cases. Silent thyroiditis occurs in 7% to 10% of postpartum women in the United States (Emerson and Farwell, 2000). Other causes of thyrotoxicosis are much less common.

Most of the signs and symptoms of thyrotoxicosis stem from the excessive production of heat and from increased motor activity and increased activity of the sympathetic nervous system. The skin is flushed, warm, and moist; the muscles are weak and tremulous; the heart rate is rapid, the heartbeat is forceful, and the arterial pulses are prominent and bounding. The increased expenditure of energy gives rise to increased appetite and, if intake is insufficient, to loss of weight. There also may be insomnia, difficulty in remaining still, anxiety and apprehension, intolerance to heat, and increased frequency of bowel movements. Angina, arrhythmias, and heart failure may be present in older patients. Some individuals may show extensive muscular wasting as a result of thyroid myopathy. Patients with long-standing undiagnosed or undertreated thyrotoxicosis may develop osteoporosis due to increased bone turnover (Baran, 2000).

Thyroid Hypofunction. Hypothyroidism, known as myxedema when severe, is the most common disorder of thyroid function. Worldwide, hypothyroidism is most often the result of iodine deficiency. In nonendemic areas, where iodine is sufficient, chronic autoimmune thyroiditis (Hashimoto's thyroiditis) accounts for the majority of cases. This disorder is characterized by high levels of circulating antibodies directed against thyroid peroxidase and, less commonly, thyroglobulin. In addition, blocking antibodies directed at the TSH receptor may be present, exacerbating the hypothyroidism (Botero and Brown, 1998). Finally, a cause of thyroid destruction may be apoptotic cell death due to the interaction of Fas and Fas ligand in the thyrocytes (Giordano *et al.,* 1997). Failure of the thyroid to produce sufficient thyroid hormone is the most common cause of hypothyroidism and is referred to as *primary hypothyroidism. Central hypothyroidism* occurs much less often and results from diminished stimulation of the thyroid by TSH because of pituitary failure (*secondary hypothyroidism*) or hypothalamic failure (*tertiary hypothyroidism*). Hypothyroidism present at birth is known as *congenital hypothyroidism* and is the most common preventable cause of mental retardation in the world. Diagnosis and early intervention with thyroid hormone replacement prevent the development of cretinism, as discussed above.

Nongoitrous hypothyroidism is associated with degeneration and atrophy of the thyroid gland. The same condition follows surgical removal of the thyroid or its destruction by radioactive iodine. Since it also may occur years after antithyroid drug therapy for Graves' disease, some have speculated that hypothyroidism can be the end stage of this disorder ("burnt-out" Graves' disease). *Goitrous hypothyroidism* occurs in Hashimoto's thyroiditis and when there is a severe defect in synthesis of thyroid hormone. When the disease is mild, it may be subtle in its presentation. By the time it has become severe, however, all of the signs are overt. The appearance of the patient is pathognomonic. The face is quite expressionless, puffy, and pallid. The skin is cold and dry, the scalp is scaly, and the hair is coarse, brittle, and sparse. The fingernails are thickened and brittle, the subcutaneous tissue appears to be thickened, and there may be true edema. The voice is husky and low-pitched, speech is slow, hearing is often faulty, mentation is impaired, and depression may be present. The appetite is poor, gastrointestinal activity is diminished, and constipation is common. Atony of the bladder is rare and suggests that the function of other smooth muscles may be impaired. The voluntary muscles are weak and the relaxation phase of the deep-tendon reflexes is delayed. The heart can be dilated, and there is frequently a pericardial effusion, although this is rarely clinically significant. There also may be pleural effusions and ascites. Anemia, most commonly normochromic, normocytic, is often present, although menstrual irregularity with menorrhagia may result in iron deficiency anemia. Hyperlipidemia often is present in hypothyroid patients. Patients are lethargic and tend to sleep a lot and often complain of cold intolerance.

Thyroid Function Tests.   The development of radioimmunoassays and, more recently, chemiluminescent and enzyme-linked immunoassays for T_4, T_3, and TSH have greatly improved the laboratory diagnosis of thyroid disorders (Nelson and Wilcox, 1996; Klee, 1996; Spencer *et al.,* 1996). However, measurement of the total hormone concentration in plasma may not give an accurate picture of the activity of the thyroid gland. The total hormone concentration changes with alterations in either the amount of TBG or the binding affinity for hormones to TBG in plasma. Although equilibrium dialysis of undiluted serum and radioimmunoassay for free thyroxine in the dialysate represent the gold standard for determining free thyroxine concentrations, this assay is typically not available in routine clinical laboratories (Nelson and Tomei, 1988). The free thyroxine index is an estimation of the free thyroxine concentration and is calculated by multiplying the total thyroxine concentration by the thyroid hormone binding ratio, which estimates the degree of saturation of TBG (Nelson and Tomei, 1989). Additional assays commonly in use for estimating the free T_4 and free T_3 concentrations employ labeled analogs of these iodothyronines in chemiluminescence and enzyme-linked immunoassays (Klee, 1996; Nelson and Wilcox, 1996). These assays correlate well with free T_4 concentrations measured by the more cumbersome equilibrium dialysis method and are easily adaptable to routine

clinical laboratory use. However, the analog assays may be affected by a wide variety of nonthyroidal disease states, including acute illness, and by certain drugs to a greater degree than are the free T_4 index and free T_4 determined by equilibrium dialysis.

Estimates of free thyroxine levels should be complemented with serum measurements of TSH. In fact, in individuals whose pituitary function and TSH secretion are normal, serum measurement of TSH is the thyroid function test of choice (Danese *et al.,* 1996; Helfand and Redfern, 1998), because pituitary secretion of TSH is sensitively regulated in response to circulating concentrations of thyroid hormones.

Serum measurements of TSH have been available since 1965. The first assays were single antibody radioimmunoassays and remained the standard for 20 years. These assays were useful only for diagnosing primary hypothyroidism, as a lower limit of the normal range could not be reliably measured. The first "sensitive" TSH assay was developed in 1985, utilizing a dualantibody approach. Application of this method resulted in the expansion of the assay detection limit below the normal range. Thus, any assay of this type is referred to as a *sensitive TSH assay* (Nicoloff and Spencer, 1990). A major use of the sensitive TSH assay is to differentiate between normal and thyrotoxic patients, who should exhibit suppressed TSH values. Indeed, the sensitive TSH assay has essentially replaced evaluation of the response of TSH to injection of synthetic TRH (TRH stimulation test) in the thyrotoxic patient. While the serum TSH assay is extremely useful in determining the euthyroid state and titrating the replacement dose of thyroid hormone in patients with primary hypothyroidism, abnormal serum TSH concentrations may not always indicate thyroid dysfunction. In such patients, assessment of the circulating thyroid hormone levels will further determine whether or not thyroid dysfunction is truly present. Synthetic preparations of TRH (*protirelin,* THYREL) are available for the evaluation of pituitary or hypothalamic failure as a cause of secondary hypothyroidism.

Recombinant human TSH (*thyrotropin alfa,* THYROGEN) is now available as an injectable preparation to test the ability of thyroid tissue, both normal and malignant, to take up radioactive iodine and release thyroglobulin (Haugen *et al.,* 1999). This preparation replaces bovine TSH (THYTROPAR), which was associated with a high incidence of side effects, including anaphylaxis.

Therapeutic Uses of Thyroid Hormone.   The major indications for the therapeutic use of thyroid hormone are for hormone replacement therapy in patients with hypothyroidism or cretinism and for TSH suppression therapy in patients with nontoxic goiter or after treatment for thyroid cancer (Roti *et al.,* 1993; Toft, 1994). While the general consensus has been that thyroid hormone therapy is not indicated for treatment of the "low T_4 syndrome" ("sick euthyroid syndrome") that is a result of nonthyroidal illness (Brent and Hershman, 1986, Farwell, 1999), this concept has been challenged recently with the suggestion that severely ill patients may benefit by treatment with T_3 (DeGroot, 1999). However, there is no evidence for this recommendation based on published studies, and this suggestion remains a minority opinion. For example, T_3 treatment does not decrease mortality in the sick euthyroid syndrome that occurs in patients undergoing coronary artery bypass surgery (Klemperer *et al.*, 1995).

The synthetic preparations of the sodium salts of the natural isomers of the thyroid hormones are available and widely used for thyroid hormone therapy. *Levothyroxine sodium* (L-T_4, SYNTHROID, LEVOXYL, LEVOTHROID, others) is available in tablets and as a lyophilized powder for injection. *Liothyronine sodium* (L-T_3) is the salt of triiodothyronine and is available in tablets (CYTOMEL) and in an injectable form (TRIOSTAT). A mixture of thyroxine and triiodothyronine is marketed as *liotrix* (THYROLAR). Desiccated thyroid preparations, derived from whole animal thyroids, contain both thyroxine and triiodothyronine and have highly variable biologic activity, making these preparations much less desirable.

Thyroid Hormone Replacement Therapy.   Thyroxine (levothyroxine sodium) is the hormone of choice for thyroid hormone replacement therapy because of its consistent potency and prolonged duration of action. The absorption of thyroxine occurs in the small intestine and is variable and incomplete, with 50% to 80% of the dose absorbed (Hays, 1991; Hays and Nielson, 1994). Absorption is slightly increased when the hormone is taken on an empty stomach. In addition, certain drugs may interfere with absorption of levothyroxine in the gut, including sucralfate, cholestyramine resin, iron and calcium supplements, and aluminum hydroxide. Enhanced biliary excretion of levothyroxine occurs during the administration of drugs that induce hepatic cytochrome P450 enzymes, such as phenytoin, carbamazepine, and rifampin. This enhanced excretion may necessitate an increase in the dose of orally administered levothyroxine. Triiodothyronine (liothyronine sodium) may be used occasionally when a quicker onset of action is desired, as, for example, in the rare presentation of myxedema coma or for preparing a patient for ^{131}I therapy for treatment of thyroid cancer. It is less desirable for chronic replacement therapy because of the requirement for more frequent dosing, higher cost, and transient elevations of serum triiodothyronine concentrations above the normal range. Combination therapy with levothyroxine and liothyronine has been suggested for use in hypothyroid patients that remain symptomatic on levothyroxine alone and have serum TSH concentrations in the normal range (Bunevicius *et al.*, 1999). However, a definite benefit for this combination therapy has not yet been shown. Furthermore, this combination may lead to transient elevations of circulating T_3 concentrations in contrast to the steady levels of T_3 during levothyroxine administration due to conversion of T_4 to T_3 in peripheral tissues.

The average daily adult replacement dose of levothyroxine sodium in a 68-kg person is 112 μg as a single dose, while that of liothyronine sodium is 50 to 75 μg in divided doses. Institution of therapy in healthy younger individuals can begin at full replacement doses. Because of the prolonged half-life of thyroxine (7 days), new steady-state concentrations of the hormone will not be achieved until 4 to 6 weeks after a change in dose. Thus, reevaluation with determination of serum TSH concentration need not be performed at intervals less than 4 to 6 weeks. The goal of thyroxine replacement therapy is to achieve a TSH value in the normal range, as overreplacement of thyroxine, suppressing TSH values to the subnormal range,

may induce osteoporosis and cause cardiac dysfunction (Ross, 1991). In noncompliant, young patients, the cumulative weekly doses of levothyroxine may be given as a single weekly dose, which is safe, effective, and well tolerated (Grebe *et al.*, 1997). In individuals over the age of 60, institution of therapy at a lower daily dose of levothyroxine sodium (25 μg per day) is indicated to avoid exacerbation of underlying and undiagnosed cardiac disease. Death due to arrhythmias has been reported during the initiation of thyroid hormone replacement therapy in hypothyroid patients. The dose can be increased at a rate of 25 μg per day every few months until the TSH is normalized. For individuals with preexisting cardiac disease, an initial dose of 12.5 μg per day, with increases of 12.5 to 25 μg per day every 6 to 8 weeks, is indicated. Daily doses of thyroxine may be interrupted periodically because of intercurrent medical or surgical illnesses that prohibit taking medications by mouth. A lapse of several days of hormone replacement is unlikely to have any significant metabolic consequences. However, if more prolonged interruption in oral therapy is necessary, levothyroxine may be given parenterally at a dose 25% to 50% less than the patient's daily oral requirements.

Subclinical hypothyroidism is an asymptomatic state characterized by elevated serum TSH concentrations and serum T_4 and T_3 concentrations in the normal range (for review, *see* Surks and Ocampo, 1996). Population screening has shown that subclinical hypothyroidism is very common, with a prevalence of up to 15% in some populations (Canaris *et al.*, 2000; Tunbridge *et al.*, 1977) and up to 25% in the elderly (Samuels, 1998). The decision to use levothyroxine therapy in these patients to normalize the serum TSH must be made on an individual basis, as treatment may not be appropriate for all patients. However, a recent report strongly suggests that untreated subclinical hypothyroidism is associated with an increased prevalence of aortic atherosclerosis and myocardial infarction (Hak *et al.*, 2000). Patients with subclinical hypothyroidism who are likely to benefit from levothyroxine therapy include those with goiter, autoimmune thyroid disease, hypercholesterolemia, cognitive dysfunction, or pregnancy (*see* below), and those patients who have symptoms of hypothyroidism.

The dose of levothyroxine in the hypothyroid patient who becomes pregnant often needs to be increased, perhaps due to the increased serum concentrations of TBG induced by estrogen (Kaplan, 1992; Glinoer, 1993; Mandel *et al.*, 1990). In addition, pregnancy may "unmask" hypothyroidism in patients with preexisting autoimmune thyroid disease or in those who reside in a region of iodine deficiency (Glinoer *et al.*, 1994). Overt hypothyroidism during pregnancy is associated with fetal distress (Wasserstrum and Anaia, 1995) and impaired psychoneural development in the progeny (Man *et al.*, 1991). Recent studies have suggested that subclinical hypothyroidism during pregnancy also is associated with mildly impaired psychomotor development in the children (Haddow *et al.*, 1999; Pop *et al.*, 1999). These findings strongly suggest that any degree of hypothyroidism, as judged by an elevated serum TSH, should be treated during pregnancy. Thus, serum TSH values should be determined in the first trimester in all patients with preexisting hypothyroidism, as well as in those at high risk for developing hypothyroidism. Therapy with levothyroxine should be administered to keep the serum TSH in the normal range. Any adjustment of the levothyroxine dose should be reevaluated in 4 to 6 weeks to determine if further adjustments are necessary.

Comparative Responses to Thyroid Preparations.   There is no significant difference in the qualitative response of the patient with myxedema to triiodothyronine, thyroxine, or desiccated thyroid. However, there are obvious quantitative differences. Following the subcutaneous administration of a large experimental dose of triiodothyronine, a metabolic response can be detected within 4 to 6 hours, at which time the skin becomes detectably warmer and the pulse rate and temperature increase. With this dose, a 40% decrease in metabolic rate can be restored to normal in 24 hours. The maximal response occurs in 2 days or less, and the effects subside with a half-time of about 8 days. The same single dose of thyroxine exerts much less effect. However, if thyroxine is given in approximately four times the dose of triiodothyronine, a comparable elevation in metabolic rate can be achieved. The peak effect of a single dose is evident in about 9 days, and this declines to half the maximum in 11 to 15 days. In both cases the effects outlast the presence of detectable amounts of hormone; these disappear from the blood with mean half-lives of approximately 1 day for triiodothyronine and 7 days for thyroxine.

Myxedema Coma.   Myxedema coma is a rare syndrome that represents the extreme expression of severe, long-standing hypothyroidism (Emerson, 1999). It is a medical emergency, and even with early diagnosis and treatment, the mortality rate can be as high as 60%. Myxedema coma occurs most often in elderly patients during the winter months. Common precipitating factors include pulmonary infections, cerebrovascular accidents, and congestive heart failure. The clinical course of lethargy proceeding to stupor and then coma is often hastened by drugs, especially sedatives, narcotics, antidepressants, and tranquilizers. Indeed, many cases of myxedema coma have occurred in hypothyroid patients who have been hospitalized for other medical problems.

Cardinal features of myxedema coma are: (1) hypothermia, which may be profound, (2) respiratory depression, and (3) unconsciousness. Other clinical features include bradycardia, macroglossia, delayed reflexes, and dry, rough skin. Dilutional hyponatremia is common and may be severe. Elevated plasma creatine phosphokinase (CPK) and lactate dehydrogenase (LDH) concentrations, acidosis, and anemia are common findings. Lumbar puncture reveals increased opening pressure and high protein content. Hypothyroidism is confirmed by measuring serum free thyroxine index and TSH values. Ultimately, myxedema coma is a clinical diagnosis.

The mainstay of therapy is supportive care, with ventilatory support, rewarming with blankets, correction of hyponatremia, and treatment of the precipitating incident. Because of a 5% to 10% incidence of coexisting decreased adrenal reserve in patients with myxedema coma, intravenous steroids are indicated before initiating thyroxine therapy. Parenteral administration of thyroid hormone is necessary due to uncertain absorption through the gut. With intravenous preparations of both levothyroxine and liothyronine now available, a reasonable approach is an initial intravenous loading dose of 200 to 300 μg of levothyroxine with a second dose of 100 μg given 24 hours later. Alternatively, a bolus of 500 μg levothyroxine given orally (by mouth or *via* nasogastric tube) may be administered to patients <50 years old without cardiac complications (Yamamoto *et al.,* 1999). Simultaneously with the initial dose of levothyroxine, some clinicians recommend adding liothyronine at a dose of 10 μg intravenously every 8 hours until the patient

is stable and conscious. The dose of thyroid hormone should be adjusted on the basis of hemodynamic stability, the presence of coexisting cardiac disease, and the degree of electrolyte imbalance. Recent studies suggest that over-aggressive treatment with either levothyroxine (>500 μg per day) or liothyronine (>75 μg) may be associated with an increased mortality (Yamamoto *et al.,* 1999).

Treatment of Cretinism.   Success in the treatment of cretinism depends upon the age at which therapy is started. Because of this, newborn screening for congenital hypothyroidism is routine in the United States, Canada, and many other countries around the world. In cases that do not come to the attention of physicians until retardation of development is clinically obvious, the detrimental effects of thyroid hormone deficiency on mental development will not be overcome. If, on the other hand, therapy is instituted within the first few weeks of life, normal physical and mental development is almost always achieved. Prognosis also depends on the severity of the hypothyroidism at birth and may be worse for babies with thyroid agenesis. The most critical need for thyroid hormone is during the period of myelinization of the central nervous system that occurs about the time of birth. To rapidly normalize the serum thyroxine concentration in the congenitally hypothyroid infant, an initial daily dose of levothyroxine of 10 to 15 μg/kg is recommended (Fisher, 1991). This dose will increase the total serum thyroxine concentration to the upper half of the normal range in most infants within 1 to 2 weeks. Individual levothyroxine doses are adjusted at 4- to 6-week intervals during the first 6 months, at 2-month intervals during the 6- to 18-month period, and at 3- to 6-month intervals thereafter to maintain serum thyroxine concentrations in the 10- to 16-μg/dl range and serum TSH values in the normal range. The free thyroxine levels should be kept in the upper normal or elevated range. Assessments that are important guides for appropriate hormone replacement include physical growth, motor development, bone maturation, and developmental progress. Management of premature infants with hypothyroxinemia due to the sick euthyroid syndrome ($\sim$50% of those born at less than 30 weeks of gestation) remains a therapeutic dilemma. Despite impaired psychomotor development in these patients (Reuss *et al.,* 1996; Den Ouden *et al.,* 1996), levothyroxine therapy has not been shown to be beneficial and may be deleterious if overreplacement is administered (van Wassenaer *et al.,* 1997).

Nodular Thyroid Disease.   Nodular thyroid disease is the most common endocrinopathy. The prevalence of clinically apparent nodules is 4% to 7% in the United States, with the frequency increasing throughout adult life. When ultrasound and autopsy data are included, the prevalence of thyroid nodules approaches 50% by age 60. As with other forms of thyroid disease, nodules are more frequent in women. Nodules have been estimated to develop at a rate of 0.1% per year. In individuals exposed to ionizing radiation, the rate of nodule development is 20-fold higher. While the presence of a nodule raises the question of a malignancy, only 8% to 10% of patients with thyroid nodules have thyroid cancer. About 12,000 new cases of thyroid cancer are diagnosed annually, with about 1000 deaths from the disease per year. However, many more people have clinically silent thyroid cancer, as up to 35% of thyroids removed at autopsy or at surgery harbor a small (<1 cm) occult papillary cancer.

The evaluation of the patient with nodular thyroid disease includes a careful physical examination, biochemical analysis of thyroid function, and assessment of the malignant potential of the nodule (Mazzaferri, 1993; Gharib and Goellner, 1993). The latter may include examination of a fine-needle aspiration biopsy of the nodule, ultrasound evaluation, and radioisotope scanning with ^{123}I or ^{131}I to determine if a particular nodule is functioning. Fine-needle aspiration biopsy of the nodule is now the most definitive approach to diagnose the pathology of a nodule. TSH suppressive therapy with levothyroxine is an option for the patient diagnosed with a benign solitary nodule and a normal serum TSH. The rationale behind levothyroxine therapy is that the benign nodule will either stop growing or decrease in size after TSH stimulation of the thyroid gland has been suppressed. The success rate of such therapy varies widely (Papini *et al.,* 1998; Zelmanovitz *et al.,* 1998; Gharib and Mazzaferri, 1998). Identification of those patients who are most likely to benefit from thyroid hormone therapy can be achieved through measurement of the serum TSH concentration and radioisotope scanning. Suppression therapy will be of no value if thyroid nodule autonomy exists, as evidenced by a subnormal TSH value and all isotope uptake in the nodule. Functioning nodules are the most likely to respond to suppression therapy. However, once TSH concentrations are suppressed, a repeat radioisotope scan (suppression scan) should be obtained. If significant uptake persists on a suppression scan, the nodule is nonsuppressible and levothyroxine therapy should be discontinued. Suppression therapy needs to be considered carefully in older patients or in those with coronary artery disease; in general, such therapy should be avoided in these patients. Hypofunctioning nodules are much less likely to respond to suppression therapy. However, a 6- to 12-month trial of levothyroxine suppression is reasonable (Hermus and Huysmans, 1998). If levothyroxine is administered, therapy should be continued for as long as the nodule is decreasing in size. Once the size of a nodule remains stable for a 6- to 12-month period, therapy may be discontinued and the nodule observed for recurrent growth. Any nodule that grows while on suppression therapy should be rebiopsied and/or surgically excised.

ANTITHYROID DRUGS AND OTHER THYROID INHIBITORS

A large number of compounds are capable of interfering, directly or indirectly, with the synthesis, release, or action of thyroid hormones (Table 57-4). Several are of great clinical value for the temporary or extended control of hyperthyroid states. These are discussed in detail below, while others are primarily of research or toxicological

Table 57-4
Antithyroid Compounds

PROCESS AFFECTED	EXAMPLES OF INHIBITORS
Active transport of iodide	Complex anions: perchlorate, fluoborate, pertechnetate, thiocyanate
Iodination of thyroglobulin	Thionamides: propylthiouracil, methimazole, carbimazole
	Thiocyanate
	Aniline derivatives; sulfonamides
	Iodide
Coupling reaction	Thionamides
	Sulfonamides
	?All other inhibitors of iodination
Hormone release	Lithium salts
	Iodide
Iodotyrosine deiodination	Nitrotyrosines
Peripheral iodothyronine deiodination	Thiouracil derivatives
	Oral cholecystographic agents
	Amiodarone
Hormone excretion/ inactivation	Inducers of hepatic drug-metabolizing enzymes: phenobarbital, rifampin, carbamazepine, phenytoin
Hormone action	Thyroxine analogs
	Amiodarone
	?Phenytoin
	Binding in gut: cholestyramine

SOURCE: Adapted from Meier and Burger, 2000.

interest and are only mentioned briefly. The major inhibitors may be classified into four categories: (1) antithyroid drugs, which interfere directly with the synthesis of thyroid hormones; (2) ionic inhibitors, which block the iodide transport mechanism; (3) high concentrations of iodine itself, which decrease release of thyroid hormones from the gland and also may decrease hormone synthesis; and (4) radioactive iodine, which damages the gland with ionizing radiation. Adjuvant therapy with drugs that have no specific effects on thyroid gland hormonogenesis is useful in controlling the peripheral manifestations of thyrotoxicosis. These drugs include inhibitors of the peripheral deiodination of thyroxine to the active hormone, triiodothyronine; β-adrenergic receptor antagonists; and Ca^{2+} channel blockers. The antithyroid drugs have been reviewed by Cooper (1998). Adrenergic receptor antagonists are discussed more fully in Chapter 10 and Ca^{2+} channel blockers in Chapters 32 and 35.

Antithyroid Drugs

The antithyroid drugs that have clinical utility are the thioureylenes, which belong to the family of thionamides. Propylthiouracil may be considered as the prototype.

History.   Studies on the mechanism of the development of goiter began with the observation that rabbits fed a diet composed largely of cabbage often developed goiters. This result was probably due to the presence of precursors of the thiocyanate ion in cabbage leaves (*see* below). Later, two pure compounds were shown to produce goiter, sulfaguanidine and phenylthiourea.

Investigation of the effects of thiourea derivatives revealed that rats became hypothyroid despite hyperplastic changes in their thyroid glands that were characteristic of intense thyrotropic stimulation. After treatment was begun, no new hormone was made, and the goitrogen had no visible effect upon the thyroid gland following hypophysectomy or the administration of thyroid hormone. This suggested that the goiter was a compensatory change resulting from the induced state of hypothyroidism and that the primary action of the compounds was to inhibit the formation of thyroid hormone (Astwood, 1945). The therapeutic possibilities of such agents in hyperthyroidism were evident, and the substances so used became known as *antithyroid drugs*.

Structure–Activity Relationship.   The two goitrogens found in the early 1940s proved to be prototypes of two different classes of antithyroid drugs. These two, with one later addition, made up three general categories into which the majority of the agents can be assigned: (1) *thioureylenes* include all the compounds currently used clinically (Figure 57–8); (2) *aniline*

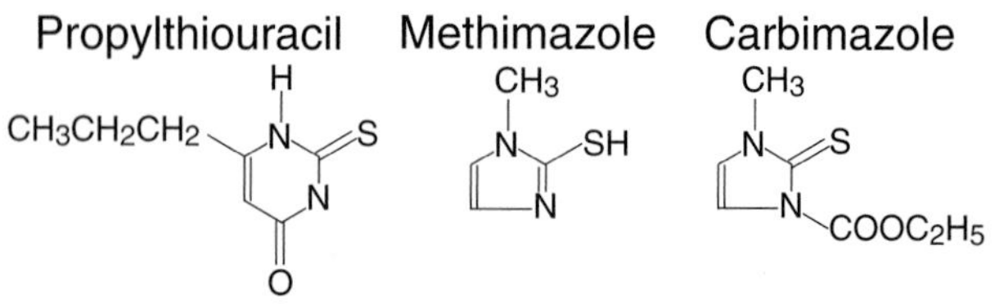

Figure 57–8. Antithyroid drugs of the thiamide type.

derivatives, of which the sulfonamides make up the largest number, embrace a few substances that have been found to inhibit thyroid hormone synthesis; and (3) *polyhydric phenols*, such as resorcinol, which have caused goiter in human beings when applied to the abraded skin. A few other compounds, mentioned briefly below, do not fit into any of these categories.

Thiourea and its simpler aliphatic derivatives and heterocyclic compounds containing a thioureylene group make up the majority of the known antithyroid agents that are effective in human beings. Although most of them incorporate the entire thioureylene group, in some a nitrogen atom is replaced by oxygen or sulfur so that only the thioamide group is common to all. Among the heterocyclic compounds, active representatives are the sulfur derivatives of imidazole, oxazole, hydantoin, thiazole, thiadiazole, uracil, and barbituric acid.

L-5-Vinyl-2-thiooxazolidone (goitrin) is responsible for the goiter that results from consuming turnips or the seeds or green parts of cruciferous plants. These plants are eaten by cows, and the compound is found in cow's milk in areas of endemic goiter in Finland; it is about as active as propylthiouracil in human beings.

As the result of industrial exposure, toxicological studies, or clinical trials for various purposes, several other compounds have been noted to possess antithyroid activity (De Rosa *et al.*, 1998). Thiopental and oral hypoglycemic drugs of the sulfonylurea class have weak antithyroid action in experimental animals. This is not significant at usual doses in human beings. However, antithyroid effects in human beings have been observed from dimercaprol, aminoglutethimide, and lithium salts. Polychlorinated biphenyls bear a striking structural resemblance to the thyroid hormones and may function as either agonists or antagonists of thyroid hormone action (De Rosa *et al.*, 1998). Altered circulating concentrations of thyroid hormones and thyrotropin and impaired brain development have been attributed to exposure to polychlorinated biphenyls (Porterfield and Hendry, 1998; Sher *et al.*, 1998). Amiodarone, the iodine-rich drug used in the management of cardiac arrhythmias, has complex effects on thyroid function (Harjai and Licata, 1997). In areas of iodine sufficiency, amiodarone-induced hypothyroidism due to the excess iodine is not uncommon, whereas in iodine-deficient regions, amiodarone-induced thyrotoxicosis predominates, whether because of the excess iodine or the thyroiditis induced by the drug. Amiodarone and its major metabolite, desethylamiodarone, are potent inhibitors of iodothyronine deiodination, resulting in decreased conversion of thyroxine to triiodothyronine. In addition, desethylamiodarone decreases binding of triiodothyronine to its nuclear receptors. Recommendations recently have been made as to screening methods to identify chemicals that may alter thyroid hormone action or homeostasis (DeVito *et al.*, 1999).

Mechanism of Action. The mechanism of action of the thiourylene drugs has been thoroughly discussed by Taurog (2000). Antithyroid drugs inhibit the formation of thyroid hormones by interfering with the incorporation of iodine into tyrosyl residues of thyroglobulin; they also inhibit the coupling of these iodotyrosyl residues to form iodothyronines. This implies that they interfere with the oxidation of iodide ion and iodotyrosyl groups. Taurog (2000) proposed that the drugs inhibit the peroxidase enzyme, thereby preventing oxidation of iodide or iodotyrosyl groups to the required active state. The antithyroid drugs bind to and inactivate the peroxidase only when the heme of the enzyme is in the oxidized state. Over a period of time, the inhibition of hormone synthesis results in the depletion of stores of iodinated thyroglobulin as the protein is hydrolyzed and the hormones are released into the circulation. Only when the preformed hormone is depleted and the concentrations of circulating thyroid hormones begin to decline do clinical effects become noticeable.

There is some evidence that the coupling reaction may be more sensitive to an antithyroid drug, such as propylthiouracil, than is the iodination reaction (Taurog, 2000). This may explain why patients with hyperthyroidism respond well to doses of the drug that only partially suppress organification.

When Graves' disease is treated with antithyroid drugs, the concentration of thyroid-stimulating immunoglobulins in the circulation often decreases. This has prompted some to propose that these agents act as immunosuppressants. Burman and Baker (1985) point out that perchlorate, which acts by an entirely different mechanism, also decreases thyroid-stimulating immunoglobulins, suggesting that improvement in hyperthyroidism may, itself, favorably affect the abnormal humoral immune state.

In addition to blocking hormone synthesis, propylthiouracil inhibits the peripheral deiodination of thyroxine to triiodothyronine. Methimazole does not have this effect and can antagonize the inhibitory effect of propylthiouracil. Although the quantitative significance of this inhibition has not been established, it does provide a theoretical rationale for the choice of propylthiouracil over other antithyroid drugs in the treatment of severe hyperthyroid states or of thyroid storm. In this acute situation, a decreased rate of conversion of circulating thyroxine to triiodothyronine would be beneficial.

Absorption, Metabolism, and Excretion. The antithyroid compounds currently used in the United States are *propylthiouracil* (6-n-propylthiouracil) and *methimazole* (1-methyl-2-mercaptoimidazole; TAPAZOLE). In Great Britain and Europe, *carbimazole* (NEO-MERCAZOLE), a carbethoxy derivative of methimazole, is available, and its antithyroid action is due to its conversion to methimazole after absorption. Some pharmacological properties of propylthiouracil and methimazole are shown in Table 57–5. Measurements of the course of organification of radioactive iodine by the thyroid show that absorption of effective amounts of propylthiouracil follows within 20 to 30 minutes of an oral dose. They also show that the duration of action of the compounds used clinically is brief. The effect of a dose of 100 mg of propylthiouracil begins to wane in 2 to 3 hours, and even a 500-mg dose is completely inhibitory for only 6 to 8 hours. As little as 0.5 mg of methimazole similarly decreases the organification of radioactive iodine in the thyroid gland, but a single dose of 10 to 25 mg is needed to extend the inhibition to 24 hours.

The half-life of propylthiouracil in plasma is about 75 minutes, whereas that of methimazole is 4 to 6 hours.

Table 57–5
Selected Pharmacokinetic Features of Antithyroid Drugs

	PROPYLTHIOURACIL	METHIMAZOLE
Plasma protein binding	~75%	Nil
Plasma half-life	75 minutes	~4–6 hours
Volume of distribution	~20 liters	~40 liters
Concentrated in thyroid	yes	yes
Metabolism of drug during illness		
Severe liver disease	Normal	Decreased
Severe kidney disease	Normal	Normal
Dosing frequency	1 to 4 times daily	Once or twice daily
Transplacental passage	Low	Increased
Levels in breast milk	Low	Increased

The drugs are concentrated in the thyroid, and methimazole, derived from the metabolism of carbimazole, accumulates after carbimazole is administered. Drugs and metabolites appear largely in the urine.

Propylthiouracil and methimazole cross the placenta equally and also can be found in milk; methimazole does so to a greater degree than propylthiouracil. The use of these drugs during pregnancy is discussed below.

Untoward Reactions. The incidence of side effects from propylthiouracil and methimazole as currently used is relatively low. The overall incidence as compiled from published cases by early investigators was 3% for propylthiouracil and 7% for methimazole, with 0.44% and 0.12% of cases, respectively, developing the most serious reaction, agranulocytosis (Meyer-Gessner et al., 1994). The development of agranulocytosis with methimazole may be dose-related, but no such relationship exists with propylthiouracil. Further observations have found little, if any, difference in side effects between these two agents and suggest that an incidence of agranulocytosis of approximately 1 in 500 is a maximal figure. Agranulocytosis usually occurs during the first few weeks or months of therapy but may occur later. Because agranulocytosis can develop rapidly, periodic white-cell counts usually are of little help. Patients should immediately report the development of sore throat or fever, which usually heralds the onset of this reaction. Agranulocytosis is reversible upon discontinuation of the offending drug, and the administration of recombinant human granulocyte colony-stimulating factor may hasten recovery (Magner et al., 1994). Mild granulocytopenia, if noted, may be due to thyrotoxicosis or may be the first sign of this dangerous drug reaction. Caution and frequent leukocyte counts are then required.

The most common reaction is a mild, occasionally purpuric, urticarial papular rash. It often subsides spontaneously without interrupting treatment, but it sometimes calls for the administration of an antihistamine, corticosteroids, or changing to another drug, because cross-sensitivity is uncommon. Other less frequent complications are pain and stiffness in the joints, paresthesias, headache, nausea, skin pigmentation, and loss of hair. Drug fever, hepatitis, and nephritis are rare, although abnormal liver function tests are not infrequent with higher doses of propylthiouracil.

Therapeutic Uses. The antithyroid drugs are used in the treatment of *hyperthyroidism* in the following three ways: (1) as definitive treatment, to control the disorder in anticipation of a spontaneous remission in Graves' disease; (2) in conjunction with radioactive iodine, to hasten recovery while awaiting the effects of radiation; and (3) to control the disorder in preparation for surgical treatment. There is no uniformity of opinion as to which form of treatment is the most desirable (Törring et al., 1996), and this is often influenced by a variety of considerations, as discussed below.

The usual starting dose for propylthiouracil is 100 mg every 8 hours or 150 mg every 12 hours. When doses larger than 300 mg daily are needed, further subdivision of the time of administration to every 4 to 6 hours is occasionally helpful. Methimazole is effective when given as a single daily dose because of its relatively long plasma and intrathyroidal half-life, as well as its long duration of action. Failures of response to daily treatment with 300 to 400 mg of propylthiouracil or 30 to 40 mg of methimazole are most commonly due to noncompliance. Delayed responses also are noted in patients with very large goiters or those in whom iodine in any form has been given beforehand. Once euthyroidism is achieved, usually within 12 weeks, the dose of antithyroid drug can be reduced.

Response to Treatment. Hyperthyroidism may be of two kinds—Graves' disease and hyperthyroidism from one or more hyperfunctioning thyroid nodules; whichever the cause, the hyperthyroidism seems to respond to antithyroid drugs in the same way. Improvement in the thyrotoxic state usually is noted within three to six weeks after the initiation of antithyroid drugs. The clinical response is related to the dose of antithyroid drug, the size of the goiter, and pretreatment serum T_3 concentrations (Benker et al., 1995). The rate of response is determined by the quantity of stored hormone, the rate of turnover of hormone in the thyroid, the half-life of the hormone in the periphery, and the completeness of the block in synthesis imposed by the dosage given. When large doses are continued, and sometimes with the usual dose, hypothyroidism may develop as a result of overtreatment. The earliest signs of hypothyroidism call for a reduction in dose; if by chance they have advanced to the point of discomfort, thyroid hormone can be given to hasten recovery. A full dose of levothyroxine can be given. The lower maintenance dose of antithyroid drug discussed above is instituted for continued therapy. Initial reports suggested that concomitant use of levothyroxine therapy along with antithyroid drugs increased rates of remission of Graves' disease in Japan (Hashizume et al., 1991). However, subsequent studies have shown no benefit of combination levothyroxine and methimazole therapy on either remission rates (McIver, 1996; Rittmaster et al., 1998) or on changes in serum concentrations of thyroid-stimulating immunoglobulins (Rittmaster et al., 1996).

After treatment is initiated, patients should be examined and thyroid function tests (serum free thyroxine index and total triiodothyronine concentrations) measured every 2 to 4 months. Once euthyroidism is established, follow-up every 4 to 6 months is reasonable.

Control of the hyperthyroidism usually is associated with a decrease in goiter size, but if the thyroid enlarges, hypothyroidism probably has been induced. When this occurs, the dose of the antithyroid drug should be significantly decreased and/or levothyroxine can be added once hypothyroidism is confirmed.

Remissions. The antithyroid drugs have been used in many patients to control the hyperthyroidism of Graves' disease until a remission occurs. Early investigators reported that 50% of patients so treated for one year remained well without further therapy for long periods, perhaps indefinitely. More recent reports have indicated that a much smaller percentage of patients sustain remissions after such treatment (Maugendre et al.,

1999; Benker *et al.,* 1998). Increased dietary iodine has been implicated in the latter, less favorable rates.

Unfortunately, there is no way of predicting before treatment is begun which patients will eventually achieve a lasting remission and who will relapse. It is clear that a favorable outcome is unlikely when the disorder is of long standing, the thyroid is quite large, and various forms of treatment have failed. To complicate the issue further, remission and eventual hypothyroidism may represent the natural history of Graves' disease.

During treatment, a positive sign that a remission may have taken place is a reduction in the size of the goiter. The persistence of goiter often indicates failure, unless the patient becomes hypothyroid. Another favorable indication is continued freedom from all signs of hyperthyroidism when the maintenance dose is small. Finally, a decrease in thyroid-stimulating immunoglobulins, suppression of ^{123}I thyroid uptake when thyroxine or triiodothyronine is given, and a normal serum TSH response to TRH may be helpful in predicting a remission in some patients, although these tests are not routinely carried out.

The Therapeutic Choice. Because antithyroid drug therapy, radioactive iodine, and subtotal thyroidectomy all are effective treatments for Graves' disease, there is no worldwide consensus among endocrinologists as to the best approach to therapy (Franklyn, 1994; Klein *et al.,* 1994; Törring *et al.,* 1996). Prolonged drug therapy of Graves' disease in anticipation of a remission is most successful in patients with small goiters or mild hyperthyroidism. Those with large goiters or severe disease usually require definitive therapy with either surgery or radioactive iodine (^{131}I). Radioactive iodine remains the treatment of choice of many endocrinologists in the United States (Soloman *et al.,* 1990). Many investigators consider coexisting ophthalmopathy to be a relative contraindication for radioactive iodine therapy, since worsening of ophthalmopathy has been reported after radioactive iodine (Bartalena *et al.,* 1998). Others suggest that development of hypothyroidism, regardless of the treatment, is the strongest risk factor for progression of ophthalmopathy (Manso *et al.,* 1998). Depleting the thyroid gland of preformed hormone by treatment with antithyroid drugs is advisable in older patients prior to therapy with radioactive iodine so as to prevent a severe exacerbation of the hyperthyroid state during the subsequent development of radiation thyroiditis. Subtotal thyroidectomy is advocated for Graves' disease in young patients with large goiters, children who are allergic to antithyroid drugs, pregnant women (usually in the second trimester) who are allergic to antithyroid drugs, and patients who prefer surgery over antithyroid drugs or radioactive iodine (Zimmerman, 1999; Mestman, 1997). Radioactive iodine or surgery is indicated for definitive therapy in toxic nodular goiter, since remissions following antithyroid drug therapy do not occur.

Thyrotoxicosis in Pregnancy. Thyrotoxicosis occurs in about 0.2% of pregnancies and is caused most frequently by Graves' disease. Antithyroid drugs are the treatment of choice; radioactive iodine is clearly contraindicated. Historically, propylthiouracil has been preferred over methimazole because of lower transplacental passage. However, more recent data suggest that either may be used safely in the pregnant patient (Momotani *et al.,* 1997; Mortimer *et al.,* 1997; Mestman, 1997). The antithyroid drug dosage should be minimized in order to keep the serum free thyroxine index in the upper half of the normal range or slightly elevated. As pregnancy progresses, Graves' disease

often improves. Indeed, it is not uncommon for patients either to be on very low doses or off all antithyroid drugs completely by the end of pregnancy. Therefore the antithyroid drug dose should be reduced, and maternal thyroid function should be frequently monitored in order to decrease chances of fetal hypothyroidism. Relapse or worsening of Graves' disease is common after delivery, and patients should be monitored closely. Propylthiouracil is the drug of choice in nursing women, since very small amounts of the drug appear in breast milk and do not appear to affect thyroid function in the suckling baby. However, doses of methimazole up to 20 mg daily in nursing mothers have been shown to have no effect on fetal thyroid function (Azizi, 1996).

Adjuvant Therapy. Several drugs that have no intrinsic antithyroid activity are useful in the symptomatic treatment of thyrotoxicosis. *β-Adrenergic receptor antagonists* (Chapter 10) are effective in antagonizing the catecholaminergic effects of thyrotoxicosis by reducing the tachycardia, tremor, and stare and relieving palpitations, anxiety, and tension. Either propranolol, 20 to 40 mg four times daily, or atenolol, 50 to 100 mg daily, is usually given initially. Propranolol and esmolol can be given intravenously if needed. Propranolol, in addition to its β-adrenergic receptor antagonist action, has weak inhibitory effects on peripheral conversion of thyroxine to triiodothyronine. *Ca^{2+} channel blockers* (diltiazem, 60 to 120 mg four times daily) can be used to control tachycardia and decrease the incidence of supraventricular tachyarrhythmias (*see* Chapter 35). These drugs should be discontinued once the patient is euthyroid.

Other drugs that are useful in the rapid treatment of the severely thyrotoxic patient are agents that inhibit the peripheral conversion of thyroxine to triiodothyronine. Dexamethasone (0.5 to 1 mg two to four times daily) and the iodinated radiological contrast agents, iopanoic acid (TELEPAQUE, 500 to 1000 mg once daily) and sodium ipodate (ORAGRAFIN, 500 to 1000 mg once daily) are effective in preoperative preparation and should not be used chronically. Sodium ipodate recently has been removed from the United States market. Cholestyramine has been used in severely toxic patients to bind thyroid hormones in the gut and thus block the enterohepatic circulation of the iodothyronines (Mercardo *et al.,* 1996).

Preoperative Preparation. To reduce operative morbidity and mortality, patients must be rendered euthyroid prior to subtotal thyroidectomy as definitive treatment for hyperthyroidism. It is possible to bring virtually 100% of patients to a euthyroid state; the operative mortality in these patients in the hands of an experienced thyroid surgeon is extremely low. Prior treatment with antithyroid drugs usually is successful in rendering the patient euthyroid for surgery. Iodide is added to the regimen for 7 to 10 days prior to surgery to decrease the vascularity of the gland, making it less friable and decreasing the difficulties for the surgeon. In the patient who is either allergic to antithyroid drugs or is noncompliant, a euthyroid state usually can be achieved by treatment with iopanoic acid, dexamethasone, and propranolol for 5 to 7 days prior to surgery. All of these drugs should be discontinued after surgery.

Thyroid Storm. Thyroid storm is an uncommon but life-threatening complication of thyrotoxicosis in which a severe form of the disease is usually precipitated by an intercurrent medical problem (Abend and Braverman, 1999). It occurs in untreated or partially treated thyrotoxic patients. Precipitating factors associated with thyrotoxic crisis include infections, stress, trauma, thyroidal or nonthyroidal surgery, diabetic ketoacidosis, labor, heart disease, and, rarely, radioactive iodine treatment.

Clinical features are similar to those of thyrotoxicosis, but more exaggerated. Cardinal features include fever (temperature usually over 38.5°C) and tachycardia out of proportion to the fever. Nausea, vomiting, diarrhea, agitation, and confusion are frequent presentations. Coma and death may ensue in up to 20% of patients. Thyroid function abnormalities are similar to those found in uncomplicated hyperthyroidism. Therefore, thyroid storm is primarily a clinical diagnosis.

Treatment includes supportive measures such as intravenous fluids, antipyretics, cooling blankets, and sedation. Antithyroid drugs are given in large doses. Propylthiouracil is preferred over methimazole because of its additional action of impairing peripheral conversion of thyroxine to triiodothyronine. The recommended initial dose of propylthiouracil is 200 to 400 mg every 4 hours. Propylthiouracil and methimazole can be administered by nasogastric tube or rectally if necessary. Neither of these preparations is available for parenteral administration in the United States.

Iodides, orally or intravenously, are used after the first dose of an antithyroid drug has been administered (see below). The radiographic contrast dyes may be used to block thyroid hormone release (as a result of the iodide released from these agents) and to inhibit thyroxine to triiodothyronine conversion. β-Adrenergic receptor antagonists, such as propranolol and esmolol, and Ca^{2+} channel blockers also may be used to control tachyarrhythmias. Dexamethasone (0.5 to 1 mg intravenously every 6 hours) is recommended both as supportive therapy of possible relative adrenal insufficiency and as an inhibitor of conversion of thyroxine to triiodothyronine. Finally, treatment of the underlying precipitating illness is essential.

Ionic Inhibitors

The term *ionic inhibitors* designates the substances that interfere with the concentration of iodide by the thyroid gland. The effective agents are themselves anions that in some ways resemble iodide; they are all monovalent, hydrated anions of a size similar to that of iodide. The most studied example, *thiocyanate*, differs from the others qualitatively; it is not concentrated by the thyroid gland, but in large amounts may inhibit the organification of iodine. Thiocyanate is produced following the enzymatic hydrolysis of certain plant glycosides. Thus, certain foods (*e.g.*, cabbage) and cigarette smoking result in an increased concentration of thiocyanate in the blood and urine, as does the administration of sodium nitroprusside. Indeed, cigarette smoking has been reported to worsen both subclinical hypothyroidism (Müller *et al.*, 1995) and Graves' ophthalmopathy (Bartelena *et al.*, 1998b). Dietary precursors of thiocyanate may be a contributing factor in endemic goiter in certain parts of the world, especially in Central Africa, where the intake of iodine is very low (Delange *et al.*, 1993).

Among other anions, *perchlorate* (ClO_4^-) is ten times as active as thiocyanate (Wolff, 1998). Perchlorate blocks the entrance of iodide into the thyroid by competitively inhibiting the NIS (Carrasco, 2000). Although perchlorate can be used to control hyperthyroidism, it has caused fatal aplastic anemia when given in excessive amounts (2 to 3 g daily). Over the past few years, however, percholorate in doses of 750 mg daily has been used in the treatment of Graves' disease and amiodarone-

induced thyrotoxicosis. Perchlorate can be used to "discharge" inorganic iodide from the thyroid gland in a diagnostic test of iodide organification. Other ions, selected on the basis of their size, also have been found to be active; fluoborate (BF_4^-) is as effective as perchlorate. Lithium has a multitude of effects on thyroid function; its principal effect is decreased secretion of thyroxine and triiodothyronine (Takami, 1994).

Iodide

Iodide is the oldest remedy for disorders of the thyroid gland. Before the antithyroid drugs were used, it was the only substance available for control of the signs and symptoms of hyperthyroidism. Its use in this way is indeed paradoxical, and the explanation for this paradox is still incomplete.

Mechanism of Action. High concentrations of iodide appear to influence almost all important aspects of iodine metabolism by the thyroid gland (*see* Roti and Vagenakis, 2000). The capacity of iodide to limit its own transport has been mentioned above. Acute inhibition of the synthesis of iodotyrosines and iodothyronines by iodide also is well known (the *Wolff-Chaikoff effect*). This transient, 2-day inhibition is observed only above critical concentrations of intracellular rather than extracellular concentrations of iodide. With time there is "escape" from this inhibition that is associated with an adaptive decrease in iodide transport and a lowered intracellular iodide concentration, most likely due to a decrease in NIS mRNA and protein (Eng *et al.*, 1999). The mechanism of the acute Wolff-Chaikoff effect remains elusive and has been postulated to be due to the generation of organic iodocompounds within the thyroid (Pisarev and Gärtner, 2000).

A very important clinical effect of high plasma iodide concentration is an inhibition of the release of thyroid hormone. This action is rapid and efficacious in severe thyrotoxicosis. The effect is exerted directly on the thyroid gland, and it can be demonstrated in the euthyroid subject and experimental animals as well as in the hyperthyroid patient. Studies in a cultured thyroid cell line suggest that some of the inhibitory effects of iodide on thyrocyte proliferation may be mediated by actions of iodide on crucial regulatory points in the cell cycle (Smerdely *et al.*, 1993).

In euthyroid individuals, the administration of doses of iodide from 1.5 to 150 mg daily results in small decreases in plasma thyroxine and triiodothyronine concentrations and small compensatory increases in serum TSH values, with all values remaining in the normal range. However, euthyroid patients with a history of a wide variety of underlying thyroid disorders may develop iodine-induced hypothyroidism when exposed to large amounts of iodine present in many commonly prescribed drugs

Table 57–6
Commonly Used Iodine-Containing Drugs

DRUGS	IODINE CONTENT
Oral or local	
Amiodarone	75 mg/tablet
Calcium iodide (*e.g.,* CALCIDRINE SYRUP)	26 mg/ml
Iodoquinol (diiodohydroxyquin)	134–416 mg/tablet
Echothiophate iodide ophthalmic solution	5–41 μg/drop
Hydriodic acid syrup	13–15 mg/ml
Iodochlorhydroxyquin	104 mg/tablet
Iodine-containing vitamins	0.15 mg/tablet
Idoxuridine ophthalmic solution	18 μg/drop
Kelp	0.15 mg/tablet
Potassium iodide (*e.g.,* QUADRINAL)	145 mg/tablet
Lugol's solution	6.3 mg/drop
Niacinamide hydroiodide + potassium iodide	
(*e.g.,* IODO-NIACIN)	115 mg/tablet
PONARIS nasal emollient	5 mg/0.8 ml
Saturated solution of potassium iodide	38 mg/drop
Parenteral preparations	
Sodium iodide, 10% solution	85 mg/ml
Topical antiseptics	
Iodoquinol (diiodohydroxyquin) cream	6 mg/g
Iodine tincture	40 mg/ml
Iodochlorhydroxyquin cream	12 mg/g
Iodoform gauze	4.8 mg/100 mg gauze
Povidone iodine	10 mg/ml
Radiology contrast agents	
Diatrizoate meglumine sodium	370 mg/ml
Propyliodone	340 mg/ml
Iopanoic acid	333 mg/tablet
Ipodate	308 mg/capsule
Iothalamate	480 mg/ml
Metrizamide	483 mg/ml before dilution
Iohexol	463 mg/ml

SOURCE: Adapted from Roti *et al.,* 1997.

(Table 57–6), and these patients do not escape from the acute Wolff-Chaikoff effect (Roti *et al.,* 1997). Among the disorders that predispose patients to iodine-induced hypothyroidism are treated Graves' disease, Hashimoto's thyroiditis, postpartum lymphocytic thyroiditis, subacute painful thyroiditis, and lobectomy for benign nodules. The most commonly prescribed iodine-containing drugs are certain expectorants, topical antiseptics, and radiologic contrast agents.

Response to Iodide in Hyperthyroidism.   The response to iodides in patients with hyperthyroidism is often striking and rapid. The effect usually is discernible within 24 hours, and the basal metabolic rate may fall at a rate comparable to that following thyroidectomy. This provides evidence that the release of hormone into the circulation is rapidly blocked. Furthermore, thyroid hormone synthesis also is mildly decreased. The maximal effect is attained after 10 to 15 days of continuous therapy, when the signs and symptoms of hyperthyroidism may have greatly improved.

The changes in the thyroid gland have been studied in detail; vascularity is reduced, the gland becomes much firmer, the cells become smaller, colloid reaccumulates in the follicles, and the quantity of bound iodine increases. The changes are those that would be expected if the excessive stimulus to the gland had somehow been removed or antagonized.

Unfortunately, iodide therapy usually does not completely control the manifestations of hyperthyroidism, and after a variable period of time, the beneficial effect disappears (Emerson *et al.,* 1975). With continued treatment, the hyperthyroidism may return in its initial intensity or may become even more severe than it was at first. It is for this reason that, when iodide was the only agent available for the treatment of hyperthyroidism, its use was usually restricted to preparation of the patient for thyroidectomy.

Therapeutic Uses. The uses of iodide in the treatment of hyperthyroidism are in the preoperative period in preparation for thyroidectomy and, in conjunction with antithyroid drugs and propranolol, in the treatment of thyrotoxic crisis. Prior to surgery, iodide is sometimes employed alone, but more frequently it is used after the hyperthyroidism has been controlled by an antithyroid drug. It is then given for 7 to 10 days immediately preceding the operation. Optimal control of hyperthyroidism is achieved if antithyroid drugs are first given alone. If iodine also is given from the beginning, variable responses are observed; sometimes the effect of iodide predominates, storage of hormone is promoted, and prolonged antithyroid treatment is required before the hyperthyroidism is controlled. These clinical observations may be explained by the ability of iodide to prevent the inactivation of thyroid peroxidase by antithyroid drugs (Taurog, 2000).

Another use of iodine is to protect the thyroid from radioactive iodine fallout following a nuclear accident. Because the uptake of radioactive iodine is inversely proportional to the serum concentration of stable iodine, the administration of 30 to 100 mg of iodide daily will markedly decrease the thyroid uptake of radioisotopes of iodine. Following the Chernobyl nuclear reactor accident in 1986, approximately 10 million children and adults in Poland were given stable iodide to block the thyroid exposure to radioactive iodine from the atmosphere and from dairy products from cows that ate contaminated grass (Naumann and Wolff, 1993). This prevented the occurrence of radiation-induced thyroid cancer, as observed in children residing near Chernobyl.

The dosage or form in which iodide is administered bears little relationship to the response achieved in hyperthyroidism, provided that not less than the minimal effective amount is given; this dosage is 6 mg per day in most, but not all, patients. *Strong iodine solution* (Lugol's solution) is widely used and consists of 5% iodine and 10% potassium iodide, which yields a dose of 6.3 mg of iodine per drop. The iodine is reduced to iodide in the intestine before absorption. Saturated solution of potassium iodide also is available, containing 38 mg per drop. Typical doses include 3 to 5 drops of Lugol's solution or 1 to 3 drops of saturated solution of potassium iodide 3 times a day. These doses have been determined empirically and are far in excess of that needed.

Untoward Reactions. Occasional individuals show marked sensitivity to iodide or to organic preparations that contain iodine when they are administered intravenously. The onset of an acute reaction may occur immediately or several hours after administration. Angioedema is the outstanding symptom, and swelling of the larynx may lead to suffocation. Multiple cutaneous hemorrhages may be present. Also, manifestations of the serum-sickness type of hypersensitivity—such as fever, arthralgia, lymph node enlargement, and eosinophilia—may appear. Thrombotic thrombocytopenic purpura and fatal periarteritis nodosa attributed to hypersensitivity to iodide also have been described.

The severity of symptoms of chronic intoxication with iodide (*iodism*) is related to the dose. The symptoms start with an unpleasant brassy taste and burning in the mouth and throat as well as soreness of the teeth and gums. Increased salivation is noted. Coryza, sneezing, and irritation of the eyes with swelling of the eyelids are commonly observed. Mild iodism simulates a "head cold." The patient often complains of a severe headache that originates in the frontal sinuses. Irritation of the mucous glands of the respiratory tract causes a productive cough. Excess transudation into the bronchial tree may lead to pulmonary edema. In addition, the parotid and submaxillary glands may become enlarged and tender, and the syndrome may be mistaken for mumps parotitis. There also may be inflammation of the pharynx, larynx, and tonsils. Skin lesions are common and vary in type and intensity. They usually are mildly acneform and distributed in the seborrheic areas. Rarely, severe and sometimes fatal eruptions (ioderma) may occur after the prolonged use of iodides. The lesions are bizarre, resemble those caused by bromism, a rare problem, and, as a rule, involute quickly when iodide is withdrawn. Symptoms of gastric irritation are common, and diarrhea, which is sometimes bloody, may occur. Fever is occasionally observed, and anorexia and depression may be present. The mechanisms involved in the production of these derangements remain unknown.

Fortunately, the symptoms of iodism disappear spontaneously within a few days after stopping the administration of iodide. The renal excretion of I^- can be increased by procedures that promote Cl^- excretion (*e.g.,* osmotic diuresis, chloruretic diuretics, and salt loading). These procedures may be useful when the symptoms of iodism are severe.

Radioactive Iodine

Chemical and Physical Properties. Although iodine has several radioactive isotopes, greatest use has been made of ^{131}I. It has a half-life of 8 days; therefore, more than 99% of its radiation is expended within 56 days. Its radioactive emissions include both γ rays and β particles. The short-lived radionuclide of iodine, ^{123}I, is primarily a γ-emitter with a half-life of only 13 hours. This permits a relatively brief exposure to radiation during thyroid scans.

Effects on the Thyroid Gland. The chemical behavior of the radioactive isotopes of iodine is identical to that of the stable isotope, ^{127}I. ^{131}I is rapidly and efficiently trapped by the thyroid, incorporated into the iodoamino acids, and deposited in the colloid of the follicles, from which it is slowly liberated. Thus, the destructive β

particles originate within the follicle and act almost exclusively upon the parenchymal cells of the thyroid, with little or no damage to surrounding tissue. The γ radiation passes through the tissue and can be quantified by external detection. The effects of the radiation depend upon the dosage. When small tracer doses of ^{131}I are administered, thyroid function is not disturbed. However, when large amounts of radioactive iodine gain access to the gland, the characteristic cytotoxic actions of ionizing radiation are observed. Pyknosis and necrosis of the follicular cells are followed by disappearance of colloid and fibrosis of the gland. With properly selected doses of ^{131}I, it is possible to destroy the thyroid gland completely without detectable injury to adjacent tissues. After smaller doses, some of the follicles, usually in the periphery of the gland, retain their function.

Therapeutic Uses. *Sodium iodide I 131* (IODOTOPE THERAPEUTIC) is available as a solution or in capsules containing essentially carrier-free ^{131}I suitable for oral administration. *Sodium iodide I 123* is available for scanning procedures. Radioactive iodine finds its widest use in the treatment of hyperthyroidism and in the diagnosis of disorders of thyroid function. Discussion here is limited to the uses of ^{131}I.

Hyperthyroidism. Radioactive iodine is highly useful in the treatment of hyperthyroidism; in many circumstances it is regarded as the therapeutic procedure of choice for this condition (Soloman *et al.,* 1990; for review, *see* Levy, 1997). The use of stable iodide as treatment for hyperthyroidism, however, may preclude treatment and certain imaging studies with radioactive iodine for weeks after the iodide has been discontinued.

Dosage and Technique. ^{131}I is administered orally, and the effective dose differs for individual patients. It depends primarily upon the size of the thyroid, the iodine uptake of the gland, and the rate of release of radioactive iodine from the gland subsequent to its deposition in the colloid. To determine these variables insofar as possible, many investigators administer a tracer dose of ^{131}I and calculate the ^{131}I accumulated by the gland and the rate of loss therefrom. The weight of the gland is estimated by palpation or by ultrasound. From these data, the dose of isotope necessary to provide from 7000 to 10,000 rad per gram of thyroid tissue is determined. Even when dosage is controlled in this manner, it is difficult to predict the response of an individual to a given amount of the isotope. Indeed, comparison studies have shown little advantage of a standardized dose, based on gland weight and radioactive iodine uptake, over a fixed dose (Jarløv *et al.,* 1995; de Bruin *et al.,* 1994). For these reasons, the optimal dose of ^{131}I, expressed in terms of microcuries taken up per gram of thyroid tissue, varies in different laboratories from 80 to 150 μCi. The usual total dose is 4 to 15 mCi. Lower-dosage ^{131}I therapy (80 μCi/g thyroid) has been advocated to reduce the incidence of subsequent hypothyroidism. While the incidence of hypothyroidism in the early years after such therapy is lower, many patients with late hypothyroidism may go undetected, and the ultimate incidence of hypothyroidism is probably no less than with the larger doses. In addition, relapse of the hyperthyroid state, or initial failure to alleviate the hyperthyroid state, is increased in patients receiving lower doses of ^{131}I. There also

is evidence that pretreatment with propylthiouracil reduces the therapeutic efficacy of ^{131}I, necessitating a higher dose for a desired effect (Imseis *et al.,* 1998; Tuttle *et al.,* 1995). Methimazole appears not to share this effect of propylthiouracil (Imseis *et al.,* 1998).

Course of Disease. The course of hyperthyroidism in a patient who has received an optimal dose of ^{131}I is characterized by progressive recovery. It is very unusual for any tenderness to be noted in the thyroid region, and most observers have failed to detect any exacerbation of hyperthyroidism from loss of hormone from the damaged gland in patients whose preformed hormone stores have been depleted by antithyroid drug therapy. Beginning a few weeks after treatment, the symptoms of hyperthyroidism gradually abate over a period of 2 to 3 months. If therapy has been inadequate, the necessity for further treatment is apparent within 6 to 12 months. It is not uncommon, however, for the serum TSH to remain low for several months after ^{131}I therapy, especially if the patient was not pretreated to euthyroidism prior to receiving the radioactive iodine (Uy *et al.,* 1995). Occasionally, this delayed recovery of the hypothalamic-pituitary-thyroid axis results in a picture of central hypothyroidism, with low circulating thyroid hormones. Thus, assessing radioactive iodine failure based on TSH concentrations alone may be misleading and should always be accompanied by determination of a free T_4 index and serum T_3 concentrations. Furthermore, transient hypothyroidism, lasting up to 6 months, may occur in up to 50% of patients receiving a dose of ^{131}I calculated to result in euthyroidism (Aizawa *et al.,* 1997). This is less of a problem if the patient receives a higher, ablative dose of ^{131}I, since hypothyroidism occurs far more frequently and persists.

Depending to some extent upon the dosage schedule adopted, one-half to two-thirds of patients are cured by a single dose, one-third to one-fifth require two doses, and the remainder require three or more doses before the disorder is controlled. Patients treated with larger doses of ^{131}I almost always develop hypothyroidism within a few months.

Propranolol, antithyroid drugs, or both, or stable iodide, can be used to hasten the control of hyperthyroidism while awaiting the full effects of the radioactive iodine. However, the antithyroid drugs should be withheld for a few days before and after the therapeutic dose of ^{131}I.

Advantages. The advantages of radioactive iodine in the treatment of Graves' disease are many. No death as a direct result of the use of the isotope has been reported, and only by a gross miscalculation of dose could such an event conceivably occur. There have been reports of increased mortality from cardiovascular and cerebrovascular disease in the first year after radioactive iodine therapy (Franklyn *et al.,* 1998). However, there is no evidence that the increased mortality was related to the radioactive iodine itself, and long-term follow-up of radioactive iodine therapy for Graves' disease has demonstrated no increase in overall cancer mortality in patients treated with ^{131}I (Ron *et al.,* 1998). In the nonpregnant patient, no tissue other than the thyroid is exposed to sufficient ionizing radiation to be detectably altered. Nevertheless, the continuing concern about potential effects of radiation on germ cells prompts some endocrinologists to advocate antithyroid drugs or surgery in younger patients who are acceptable operative risks (Zimmerman, 1999). Hypoparathyroidism is a small risk of surgery. With radioactive iodine treatment, the patient is spared the risks and discomfort of surgery. The cost is low, hospitalization is not required, and patients can indulge in their customary activities during the entire procedure.

Disadvantages.   The chief disadvantage of the use of radioactive iodine is the high incidence of delayed hypothyroidism that is induced. Even when elaborate procedures are used to estimate iodine uptake and gland size, a certain percentage of patients will be overtreated. A distressing feature of this complication is its rising prevalence with the passage of time; the longer the interval after treatment, the higher the incidence. Several analyses of groups of patients treated 10 or more years previously suggest that the eventual rate may exceed 80%. However, it now appears that the incidence of hypothyroidism also increases progressively after subtotal thyroidectomy or after antithyroid drug therapy, and such failure of glandular function is probably part of the natural progression of Graves' disease, no matter what the therapy.

Although it is often said that hypothyroidism is not a serious complication because it can be treated so easily with thyroid hormone, its onset may be insidious and overlooked for some time. Also, once diagnosed, it is difficult to ensure that patients who need the hormone actually take it. Since the health risks of untreated subclinical hypothyroidism are becoming increasingly evident (Hak *et al.,* 2000; Surks and Ocampo, 1996), hypothyroidism, either subclinical or overt, is a serious complication and requires long-term follow-up to ensure that optimal replacement therapy be provided.

Another disadvantage of radioactive iodine therapy is the long period of time that is sometimes required before the hyperthyroidism is controlled. When a single dose is effective, the response is most satisfactory; however, when multiple doses are needed, it may be many months or a year or more before the patient is well. This disadvantage can be largely overcome if the initial dose is sufficiently large. Other disadvantages include possible worsening of ophthalmopathy after treatment, although this is controversial (DeGroot *et al.,* 1995). Although extremely rare, there have been reported cases of thyroid storm after therapy with [131]I. Importantly, the cases of thyroid storm after radioactive iodine therapy occur in most cases in patients who have not received pretreatment with antithyroid drugs.

Indications.   The clearest indication for this form of treatment is hyperthyroidism in older patients and in those with heart disease. Radioactive iodine also is the best form of treatment when Graves' disease has persisted or recurred after subtotal thyroidectomy and when prolonged treatment with antithyroid drugs has not led to remission. Finally, radioactive iodine is indicated in patients with toxic nodular goiter, since the disease does not go into spontaneous remission. The risk of inducing hypothyroidism is less in nodular goiter than in Graves' disease, perhaps because of the normal progression of the latter and the preservation of nonautonomous thyroid tissue in the former. Usually, larger doses of radioactive iodine are required in the treatment of toxic nodular goiter than in the treatment of Graves' disease. Recently, radioactive iodine has been used to decrease the size of large, nontoxic, multinodular goiters that are causing compressive symptoms in patients who are otherwise poor operative risks (Huysmans *et al.,* 1997). While surgery remains the treatment of choice for the young patient with compressive multinodular goiters, radioactive iodine therapy may be of benefit in elderly patients, especially those with cardiopulmonary disease.

Contraindications.   The main contraindication for the use of ^{131}I therapy is pregnancy. After the first trimester, the fetal thyroid will concentrate the isotope and thus suffer damage, but even during the first trimester, radioactive iodine is best avoided because there may be adverse effects of radiation on fetal tissues. The risk of causing neoplastic changes in the thyroid gland has been constantly under consideration since radioactive iodine was first introduced, and only small numbers of children have been treated in this way. Indeed, many clinics have declined to treat younger patients for fear of causing cancer and have reserved radioactive iodine for patients over some arbitrary age, such as 25 or 30 years. Since experience with ^{131}I is now vast, these age limits are lower than they were in the past. The most recent report by the Cooperative Thyrotoxicosis Therapy Follow-up Study Group, which began tracking patients in 1961, shows no increase in total cancer mortality following ^{131}I treatment for Graves' disease (Ron *et al.,* 1998). Furthermore, there was no increase in the occurrence of leukemia following large dose ^{131}I therapy for thyroid cancer, although there was an increase in colorectal cancers in this population (de Vathaire *et al.,* 1997). These data strongly suggest that laxatives be given to all patients receiving ^{131}I therapy for treatment of thyroid cancer to decrease the risk of future digestive tract malignancies. Transient abnormalities in testicular function have been reported following ^{131}I therapy for treatment of thyroid cancer, but no long-term effects on fertility in either men or women have been demonstrated (Pacini *et al.,* 1994a; Dottorini *et al.,* 1995).

Metastatic Thyroid Carcinoma.   While most well-differentiated thyroid carcinomas accumulate very little iodine, stimulation of iodine uptake with TSH often is used effectively to treat metastases. Follicular carcinomas, which account for 10% to 15% of thyroid malignancies, are especially amenable to this treatment. Currently, endogenous TSH stimulation is evoked by withdrawal of thyroid hormone replacement therapy in patients previously treated with near-total thyroidectomy with or without radioactive ablation of residual thyroid tissue. Total body ^{131}I scanning and measurement of serum thyroglobulin when the patient is hypothyroid (TSH > 35 mU/liter) should be performed to identify metastatic disease or residual thyroid bed tissue. Depending upon the residual uptake, or the presence of metastatic disease, an ablative dose of ^{131}I ranging from 30 to 150 mCi is administered, and a repeat total body scan is obtained 1 week later. The precise amount of ^{131}I needed to treat residual tissue and metastases is controversial. Recombinant human TSH (THYROGEN) is now available to test the ability of thyroid tissue, both normal and malignant, to take up radioactive iodine and to secrete thyroglobulin (Haugen *et al.,* 1999). The major advantage to the use of this medication is that patients do not have to stop their suppressive levothyroxine therapy and become clinically hypothyroid for the presence of persistent or metastatic disease to be assessed. Recombinant human TSH is not yet approved for treatment prior to therapeutic administration of [131]I.

TSH-suppressive therapy with levothyroxine is indicated in all patients after treatment for thyroid cancer. The goal of therapy usually is to keep serum TSH levels in the subnormal range (Burmeister *et al.,* 1992). Follow-up evaluation every 6 months is reasonable, along with determination of serum thyroglobulin concentrations. A rise in serum thyroglobulin concentration is often the first indication of recurrent disease. Prognosis in patients with thyroid cancer depends upon the pathology and size of the tumor and is generally worse in the elderly (see Mazzaferri, 2000). Overall, the vast majority of patients with thyroid cancer will not die of their disease. Papillary cancer is not an aggressive tumor. It metastasizes locally and has a 10-year survival rate of greater than 90%. Lymph node metastases at the time of diagnosis do little to alter the prognosis. Follicular cancer is more aggressive and can metastasize *via* the bloodstream. Still, prognosis is fair, and long-term survival is common. It is important to realize that, even in patients with metastatic, differentiated thyroid cancer, ^{131}I therapy is very effective and may be even curative (Pacini *et al.,* 1994b). Anaplastic cancer is the exception, as it is highly malignant with survival usually less than 1 year.

Diagnostic Uses. Tracer studies with radioactive iodine have found wide application in studies of disorders of the thyroid gland. Measurement of the thyroidal accumulation of a tracer dose is helpful in the differential diagnosis of thyrotoxicosis and nodular goiter. The response of the thyroid to TSH-suppressive doses of thyroid hormone can be evaluated in this way. Following the administration of a tracer dose, the pattern of localization in the thyroid gland can be depicted by a special scanning apparatus, and this technique is sometimes useful in defining thyroid nodules as functional ("hot") or nonfunctional ("cold") and in finding ectopic thyroid tissue and occasionally metastatic thyroid tumors.

For further discussion of diseases of the thyroid, *see also* Chapter 331 in *Harrison's Principles of Internal Medicine,* 14th ed., McGraw Hill, New York, 1998.

BIBLIOGRAPHY

Adams, M., Matthews, C., Collingwood, T.N., Tone, Y., Beck-Peccoz, P., and Chatterjee, K.K. Genetic analysis of 29 kindreds with generalized and pituitary resistance to thyroid hormone. Identification of thirteen novel mutations in the thyroid hormone receptor beta gene. *J. Clin. Invest.,* **1994,** *94*:506–515.

Ain, K.B., Mori, Y., and Refetoff, S. Reduced clearance rate of thyroxine-binding globulin (TBG) with increased sialylation: a mechanism for estrogen-induced elevation of serum TBG concentration. *J. Clin. Endocrinol. Metab.,* **1987,** *65*:689–696.

Aizawa, Y., Yoshida, K., Kaise, N., Fukazawa, H., Kiso, Y., Sayama, N., Hori, H., and Abe, K. The development of transient hypothyroidism after iodine-131 treatment in hyperthyroid patients with Graves' disease: prevalence, mechanism and prognosis. *Clin. Endocrinol. (Oxf.),* **1997,** *46*:1–5.

al-Adsani, H., Hoffer, L.J., and Silva, J.E. Resting energy expenditure is sensitive to small dose changes in patients on chronic thyroid hormone replacement. *J. Clin. Endocrinol. Metab.,* **1997,** *82*:1118–1125.

Astwood, E.B. Chemotherapy of hyperthyroidism. *Harvey Lect.,* **1945,** *40*:195–235.

Azizi, F. Effect of methimazole treatment of maternal thyrotoxicosis on thyroid function in breast-feeding infants. *J. Pediatr.,* **1996,** *128*:855–858.

Bartalena, L., Marcocci, C., Bogazzi, F., Manetti, L., Tanda, M.L., Dell'Unto, E., Bruno-Bossio, G., Nardi, M., Bartolomei, M.P., Lepri, A., Rossi, G., Martino, E., and Pinchera, A. Relation between therapy for hyperthyroidism and the course of Graves' ophthalmopathy. *N. Engl. J. Med.,* **1998a,** *338*:73–78.

Bartalena, L., Marcocci, C., Tanda, M.L., Manetti, L., Dell'Unto, E., Bartolomei, M.P., Nardi, M., Martino, E., and Pinchera, A. Cigarette smoking and treatment outcomes in Graves ophthalmopathy. *Ann. Intern. Med.,* **1998b,** *129*:632–635.

Bartha, T., Kim, S.W., Salvatore, D., Gereben, B., Tu, H.M., Harney, J.W., Rudas, P., Larsen, P.R. Characterization of the 5'-flanking and 5'-untranslated regions of the cyclic adenosine 3',5'-monophosphate-responsive human type 2 iodothyronine deiodinase gene. *Endocrinology,* **2000,** *41*:229–237.

Benker, G., Reinwein, D., Kahaly, G., Tegler, L., Alexander, W.D., Fassbinder, J., and Hirche, H. Is there a methimazole dose effect on remission rate in Graves' disease? Results from a long-term prospective study. The European Multicentre Trial Group of the Treatment of Hyperthyroidism with Antithyroid Drugs. *Clin. Endocrinol. (Oxf.),* **1998,** *49*:451–457.

Benker, G., Vitti, P., Kahaly, G., Raue, F., Tegler, L., Hirche, H., and Reinwein, D. Response to methimazole in Graves' disease. The European Multicenter Study Group. *Clin. Endocrinol. (Oxf.),* **1995,** *43*:257–263.

Benvenga, S., Cahnmann, H.J., Rader, D., Kindt, M., and Robbins, J. Thyroxine binding to the apolipoproteins of high-density lipoproteins HDL$_2$ and HDL$_3$. *Endocrinology,* **1992,** *131*:2805–2811.

Berry, M.J., Banu, L., and Larsen, P.R. Type I iodothyronine deiodinase is a selenocystine-containing enzyme. *Nature,* **1991,** *349*:438–440.

Berry, M.J., and Larsen, P.R. The role of selenium in thyroid hormone action. *Endocr. Rev.,* **1992,** *13*:207–219.

Biondi, B., Fazio, S., Palmieri, E.A., Carella, C., Panza, N., Cittadini, A., Bonè, F., Lombardi, G., and Saccà, L. Left ventricular diastolic dysfunction in patients with subclinical hypothyroidism. *J. Clin. Endocrinol. Metab.,* **1999,** *84*:2064–2067.

Botero, D., and Brown, R.S. Bioassay of thyrotropin receptor antibodies with Chinese hamster ovary cells transfected with recombinant human thyrotropin receptor: clinical utility in children and adolescents with Graves disease. *J. Pediatr.,* **1998,** *132*:612–618.

Braverman, L.E., and Ingbar, S.H. Changes in thyroidal function during adaptation to large doses of iodine. *J. Clin. Invest.,* **1963,** *42*:1216–1231.

Braverman, L.E., Ingbar, S.H., and Sterling, K. Conversion of thyroxine (T$_4$) to triiodothyronine (T$_3$) in athyreotic human subjects. *J. Clin. Invest.,* **1970,** *49*:855–864.

Brent, G.A., and Hershman, J.M. Thyroxine therapy in patients with severe nonthyroidal illnesses and low serum thyroxine concentration. *J. Clin. Endocrinol. Metab.,* **1986,** *63*:1–8.

Brucker-Davis, F., Skarulis, M.C., Grace, M.B., Benichou, J., Hauser, P., Wiggs, E., and Weintraub, B.D. Genetic and clinical features of 42 kindreds with resistance to thyroid hormone. The National

Institutes of Health Prospective Study. *Ann. Intern. Med.,* **1995,** *123*:572–583.

Bunevicius, R., Kazanavicius, G., Zalinkevicius, R., and Prange, A.J., Jr. Effects of thyroxine as compared with thyroxine plus triiodothyronine in patients with hypothyroidism. *N. Engl. J. Med.,* **1999,** *340*:424–429.

Burmeister, L.A., Goumaz, M.O., Mariash, C.N., and Oppenheimer, J.H. Levothyroxine dose requirements for thyrotropin suppression in the treatment of differentiated thyroid cancer. *J. Clin. Endocrinol. Metab.,* **1992,** *75*:344–350.

Callahan, A.M., Frye, M.A., Marangell, L.B., George, M.S., Ketter, T.A., L'Herrou, T., and Post, R.M. Comparative antidepressant effects of intravenous and intrathecal thyrotropin-releasing hormone: confounding effects of tolerance and implications for therapeutics. *Biol. Psychiatry,* **1997,** *41*:264–272.

Canaris, G.J., Manowitz, N.R., Mayor, G., and Ridgway, E.C. The Colorado thyroid disease prevalence study. *Arch. Intern. Med.,* **2000,** *160*:526–534.

Cao, X.Y., Jiang, X.M., Dou, Z.H., Rakeman, M.A., Zhang, M.L., O'Donnell, K., Ma, T., Amette, K., DeLong, N., and DeLong, G.R. Timing of vulnerability of the brain to iodine deficiency in endemic cretinism. *N. Engl. J. Med.,* **1994a,** *331*:1739–1744.

Cao, X.Y., Jiang, X.M., Kareem, A., Dou, Z.H., Abdul Rakeman, M., Zhang, M.L., Ma, T., O'Donnell, K., DeLong, N., and DeLong, G.R. Iodination of irrigation water as a method of supplying iodine to a severely iodine-deficient population in Xinjiang, China. *Lancet,* **1994b,** *344*:107–110.

Chanoine, J.P., Braverman, L.E., Farwell, A.P., Safran, M., Alex, S., Dubord, S., and Leonard, J.L. The thyroid gland is a major source of circulating T3 in the rat. *J. Clin. Invest.,* **1993,** *91*:2709–2713.

Chen, J.D, and Evans, R.M. A transcriptional co-repressor that interacts with nuclear hormone receptors. *Nature,* **1995,** *377*:454–457.

Corda, D., Marcocci, C., Kohn, L.D., Axelrod, J., and Luini, A. Association of the changes in cytosolic Ca^{2+} and iodide efflux induced by thyrotropin and by stimulation of alpha 1-adrenergic receptors in cultured rat thyroid cells. *J. Biol. Chem.,* **1985,** *260*:9230–9236.

Croteau, W., Davey, J.C., Galton, V.A., and St. Germain, D.L. Cloning of the mammalian type II iodothyronine deiodinase. A selenoprotein differentially expressed and regulated in human and rat brain and other tissues. *J. Clin. Invest.,* **1996,** *98*:405–417.

Croteau, W., Whittemore, S.L., Schneider, M.J., and St. Germain, D.L. Cloning and expression of a cDNA for a mammalian type III iodothyronine deiodinase. *J. Biol. Chem.,* **1995,** *270*:16569–16575.

Cushing, H. *The Pituitary Body and Its Disorders.* Lippincott, Philadelphia, 1912.

Dai, G., Levy, O., and Carrasco N. Cloning and characterization of the thyroid iodide transporter. *Nature,* **1996,** *379*:458–460.

Danese, M.D., Powe, N.R., Sawin, C.T., and Ladenson, P.W. Screening for mild thyroid failure at the periodic health examination: a decision and cost-effectiveness analysis. *JAMA,* **1996,** *276*:285–292.

Davey, J.C., Becker, K.B., Schneider, M.J., St. Germain, D.L., and Galton, V.A. Cloning of a cDNA for the type II iodothyronine deiodinase. *J. Biol. Chem.,* **1995,** *270*:26786–26789.

Davis, P.J., Davis, F.B., and Lawrence, W.D. Thyroid hormone regulation and membrane Ca^{2+}–ATPase activity. *Endocr. Res.,* **1989,** *15*:651–682.

de Bruin, T.W., Croon, C.D., de Klerk, J.M., and van Isselt, J.W. Standardized radioiodine therapy in Graves' disease: the persistent effect of thyroid weight and radioiodine uptake on outcome. *J. Intern. Med.,* **1994,** *236*:507–513.

de Vathaire, F., Schlumberger, M., Delisle, M.J., Francese, C., Challeton, C., de la Genardiére, E., Meunier, F., Parmentier, C., Hill, C., and Sancho-Garnier, H. Leukaemias and cancers following iodine-131 administration for thyroid cancer. *Br. J. Cancer,* **1997,** *75*:734–739.

DeGroot, L.J. Dangerous dogmas in medicine: the nonthyroidal illness syndrome. *J. Clin. Endocrinol. Metab.,* **1999,** *84*:151–164.

DeGroot, L.J., Gorman, C.A., Pinchera, A., Bartalena, L., Marcocci, C., Wiersinga, W.M., Prummel, M.F., Wartofsky, L., and Marocci, C. Therapeutic controversies. Retro-orbital radiation and radioactive iodide ablation of the thyroid may be good for Graves' ophthalmopathy. *J. Clin. Endocrinol. Metab.,* **1995,** *80*:339–340.

Den Ouden, A.L., Kok, J.H., Verkerk, P.H., Brand, R., and Verloove-Vanhorick, S.P. The relation between neonatal thyroxine levels and neurodevelopmental outcome at age 5 and 9 years in a national cohort of very preterm and/or very low birth weight infants. *Pediatr. Res.,* **1996,** *39*:142–145.

DeRosa, C., Richter, P., Pohl, H., and Jones, D.E. Environmental exposures that affect the endocrine system: public health implications. *J. Toxicol. Environ. Health. B. Crit. Rev.,* **1998,** *1*:3–26.

Dottorini, M.E., Lomuscio, G., Mazzucchelli, L., Vignati, A., and Colombo, L. Assessment of female fertility and carcinogenesis after iodine-131 therapy for differentiated thyroid carcinoma. *J. Nucl. Med.,* **1995,** *36*:21–27.

Dunn, A.D., and Dunn, J.T. Cysteine proteinases from human thyroids and their actions on thyroglobulin. *Endocrinology,* **1988,** *123*:1089–1097.

Dunn, J.T., Anderson, P.C., Fox, J.W., Fassler, C.A., Dunn, A.D., Hite, L.A., and Moore, R.C. The sites of thyroid hormone formation in rabbit thyroglobulin. *J. Biol. Chem.,* **1987,** *262*:16948–16952.

Elnagar, B., Eltom, M., Karlsson, F.A., Ermans, A.M., Gebre-Medhin, M., and Bourdoux, P.P. The effects of different doses of oral iodized oil on goiter size, urinary iodine, and thyroid-related hormones. *J. Clin. Endocrinol. Metab.,* **1995,** *80*:891–897.

Emerson, C.H., Anderson, A.J., Howard, W.J., and Utiger, R.D. Serum thyroxine and triiodothyronine concentrations during iodide treatment of hyperthyroidism. *J. Clin. Endocrinol. Metab.,* **1975,** *40*:33–36.

Eng, P.H., Cardona, G.R., Fang, S.L., Previti, M., Alex, S., Carrasco, N., Chin, W.W., and Braverman, L.E. Escape from the acute Wolff-Chaikoff effect is associated with a decrease in thyroid sodium/iodide symporter messenger ribonucleic acid and protein. *Endocrinology,* **1999,** *140*:3404–3410.

Eskandari, S., Loo, D.D., Dai, G., Levy, O., Wright, E.M., and Carrasco, N. Thyroid Na^+/I^- symporter. Mechanism, stoichiometry, and specificity. *J. Biol. Chem.,* **1997,** *272*:27230–27238.

Everett, A.W., Umeda, P.K., Sinha, A.M., Rabinowitz, M., and Zak, R. Expression of myosin heavy chains during thyroid hormone-induced cardiac growth. *Fed. Proc.,* **1986,** *45*:2568–2572.

Farsetti, A., Mitsuhashi, T., Desvergne, B., Robbins, J., and Nikodem, V.M. Molecular basis of thyroid hormone regulation of myelin basic protein gene expression in rodent brain. *J. Biol. Chem.,* **1991,** *266*:23226–23232.

Farwell, A.P., and Dubord-Tomasetti, S.A. Thyroid hormone regulates the expression of laminin in the developing rat cerebellum. *Endocrinology,* **1999,** *140*:4221–4227.

Farwell, A.P., Lynch, R.M., Okulicz, W.C., Comi, A.M., and Leonard, J.L. The actin cytoskeleton mediates the hormonally regulated translocation of type II iodothyronine 5'-deiodinase in astrocytes. *J. Biol. Chem.,* **1990,** *265*:18546–18553.

Field, J.B., Ealey, P.A., Marshall, N.J., and Cockcroft, S. Thyroid-stimulating hormone stimulates increases in inositol phosphates as well as cyclic AMP in the FRTL-5 rat thyroid cell line. *Biochem. J.*, **1987**, *247*:519–524.

Forrest, D., Erway, L.C., Ng, L., Altschuler, R., and Curran, T. Thyroid hormone receptor beta is essential for development of auditory function. *Nat. Genet.*, **1996**, *13*:354–357.

Forrest, D., Sjoberg, M., and Vennström, B. Contrasting developmental and tissue-specific expression of alpha and beta thyroid hormone receptor genes. *E.M.B.O. J.*, **1990**, *9*:1519–1528.

Fraichard, A., Chassande, O., Plateroti, M., Roux, J.P., Trouillas, J., Dehay, C., Legrand, C., Gauthier, K., Kedinger, M., Malaval, L., Rousset, B., and Samarut, J. The T3R alpha gene encoding a thyroid hormone receptor is essential for post-natal development and thyroid hormone production. *E.M.B.O. J.*, **1997**, *16*:4412–4420.

Franklyn, J.A., Maisonneuve, P., Sheppard, M.C., Betteridge, J., and Boyle, P. Mortality after the treatment of hyperthyroidism with radioactive iodine. *N. Engl. J. Med.*, **1998**, *338*:712–718.

Giordano, C., Stassi, G., De Maria, R., Todaro, M., Richiusa, P., Papoff, G., Ruberti, G., Bagnasco, M., Testi, R., and Galluzzo, A. Potential involvement of Fas and its ligand in the pathogenesis of Hashimoto's thyroiditis. *Science*, **1997**, *275*:960–963.

Glinoer, D., Riahi, M., Grun, J.P., and Kinthaert, J. Risk of subclinical hypothyroidism in pregnant women with asymptomatic autoimmune thyroid disorders. *J. Clin. Endocrinol. Metab.*, **1994**, *79*:197–204.

Göthe, S., Wang, Z., Ng, L., Kindblom, J.M., Barros, A.C., Ohlsson, C., Vennström, B., and Forrest, D. Mice devoid of all known thyroid hormone receptors are viable but exhibit disorders of the pituitary-thyroid axis, growth, and bone maturation. *Genes Dev.*, **1999**, *13*:1329–1341.

Grebe, S.K., Cooke, R.R., Ford, H.C., Fagerstrom, J.N., Cordwell, D.P., Lever, N.A., Purdie, G.L., and Feek, C.M. Treatment of hypothyroidism with once weekly thyroxine. *J. Clin. Endocrinol. Metab.*, **1997**, *82*:870–875.

Greer, M.A., Grimm, Y., and Studer, H. Qualitative changes in the secretion of thyroid hormones induced by iodine deficiency. *Endocrinology*, **1968**, *83*:1193–1198.

Gross, G., Sykes, M., Arellano, R., Fong, B., and Angel, A. HDL clearance and receptor-mediated catabolism of LDL are reduced in hypothyroid rats. *Atherosclerosis*, **1987**, *66*:269–275.

Gross, J., and Pitt-Rivers, R. The identification of 3:5:3′-L-triiodothyronine in human plasma. *Lancet*, **1952**, *1*:439–441.

Gross, J., and Pitt-Rivers, R. 3:5:3′-Triiodothyronine. 1. Isolation from thyroid gland and synthesis. *Biochem. J.*, **1953a**, *53*:645–652. 2. Physiological activity, *Ibid.*, **1953b**, *53*:652–657.

Haddow, J.E., Palomaki, G.E., Allan, W.C., Williams, J.R., Knight, G.J., Gagnon, J., O'Heir, C.E., Mitchell, M.L., Hermos, R.J., Waisbren, S.E., Faix, J.D, and Klein, R.Z. Maternal thyroid deficiency during pregnancy and subsequent neuropsychological development of the child. *N. Engl. J. Med.*, **1999**, *341*:549–555.

Hak, A.E., Pols, H.A., Visser, T.J., Drexhage, H.A., Hofman, A., and Witteman, J.C. Subclinical hypothyroidism is an independent risk factor for atherosclerosis and myocardial infarction in elderly women: the Rotterdam Study. *Ann. Intern. Med.*, **2000**, *132*:270–278.

Harington, C.R. Biochemical basis of thyroid function. *Lancet*, **1935**, *1*:1199–1204, 1261–1266.

Hashizume, K., Ichikawa, K., Sakurai, A., Suzuki, S., Takeda, T., Kobayashi, M., Miyamoto, T., Arai, M., and Nagasawa, T. Administration of thyroxine in treated Graves' disease: effects on the level of antibodies to thyroid-stimulating hormone receptors and on the risk of recurrence of hyperthyroidism. *N. Engl. J. Med.*, **1991**, *324*:947–953.

Haugen, B.R., Pacini, F., Reiners, C., Schlumberger, M., Ladenson, P.W., Sherman, S.I., Cooper, D.S., Graham, K.E., Braverman, L.E., Skarulis, M.C., Davies, T.F., DeGroot, L.J., Mazzaferri, E.L., Daniels, G.H., Ross, D.S., Luster, M., Samuels, M.H., Becker, D.V., Maxon, H.R., III, Cavalieri, R.R., Spencer, C.A., McEllin, K., Weintraub, B.D., and Ridgway, E.C. A comparison of recombinant human thyrotropin and thyroid hormone withdrawal for the detection of thyroid remnant or cancer. *J. Clin. Endocrinol. Metab.*, **1999**, *84*:3877–3885.

Hays, M.T. Localization of human thyroxine absorption. *Thyroid*, **1991**, *1*:241–248.

Hays, M.T., and Nielsen, K.R. Human thyroxine absorption: age effects and methodological analyses. *Thyroid*, **1994**, *4*:55–64.

Hollowell, J.G, Staehling, N.W., Hannon, W.H., Flanders, D.W., Gunter, E.W., Maberly, G.F., Braverman, L.E., Pino, S., Miller, D.T., Garbe, P.L., DeLozier, D.M., and Jackson, R.J. Iodine nutrition in the United States. Trends and public health implications: iodine excretion data from National Health and Nutrition Examination Surveys I and III (1971–1974 and 1988–1994). *J. Clin. Endocrinol. Metab.*, **1998**, *83*:3401–3408.

Hörlein, A.J., Näär, AM., Heinzel, T., Torchia, J., Gloss, B., Kurokawa, R., Ryan, A., Kamei, Y., Söderström, M., Glass, C.K., et al. Ligand-independent repression by the thyroid hormone receptor mediated by a nuclear receptor co-repressor. *Nature*, **1995**, *377*:397–404.

Imseis, R.E., Vanmiddlesworth, L., Massie, J.D., Bush, A.J., and Vanmiddlesworth, N.R. Pretreatment with propylthiouracil but not methimazole reduces the therapeutic efficacy of iodine-131 in hyperthyroidism. *J. Clin. Endocrinol. Metab.*, **1998**, *83*:685–687.

Jarløv, A.E., Hegedus, L., Kristensen, L.O., Nygaard, B., and Hansen, J.M. Is calculation of the dose in radioiodine therapy of hyperthyroidism worth while? *Clin. Endocrinol. (Oxf.)*, **1995**, *43*:325–329.

Johansson, C., Göthe, S., Forrest, D., Vennström, B., and Thorén, P. Cardiovascular phenotype and temperature control in mice lacking thyroid hormone receptor-beta or both alpha1 and beta. *Am. J. Physiol.*, **1999**, *276*:H2006–H2012.

Johansson, C., Vennström, B., and Thorén, P. Evidence that decreased heart rate in thyroid hormone receptor-alpha1–deficient mice is an intrinsic defect. *Am. J. Physiol.*, **1998**, *275*:R640–R646.

Jorgensen, E.C. Stereochemistry of thyroxine and analogues. *Mayo Clin. Proc.*, **1964**, *39*:560–568.

Kahaly, G.J., Wagner, S., Nieswandt, J., Mohr-Kahaly, S., and Ryan, T.J. Stress echocardiography in hyperthyroidism. *J. Clin. Endocrinol. Metab.*, **1999**, *84*:2308–2313.

Kaplan, M.M. Assessment of thyroid function during pregnancy. *Thyroid*, **1992**, *2*:57–61.

Klemperer, J.D., Klein, I., Gomez, M., Helm, R.E., Ojamaa, K., Thomas, S.J., Isom, O.W., and Krieger, K. Thyroid hormone treatment after coronary-artery bypass surgery. *N. Engl. J. Med.*, **1995**, *333*:1522–1527.

Kopp, P., van Sande, J., Parma, J., Duprez, L., Gerber, H., Joss, E., Jameson, J.L., Dumont, J.E., and Vassart, G. Brief report: congenital hyperthyroidism caused by a mutation in the thyrotropin-receptor gene. *N. Engl. J. Med.*, **1995**, *332*:150–154.

Laurent, E., Mockel, J., Van Sande, J., Graff, I., and Dumont, J.E. Dual activation by thyrotropin of the phospholipase C and cyclic AMP cascades in human thyroid. *Mol. Cell. Endocrinol.*, **1987**, *52*:273–278.

Leeson, P.D., Emmett, J.C., Shah, V.P., Showell, G.A., Novelli, R., Prain, H.D., Benson, M.G., Ellis, D., Pearce, N.J., and Underwood, A.H. Selective thyromimetics. Cardiac-sparing thyroid hormone analogues containing 3′-arylmethyl substituents. *J. Med. Chem.*, **1989**, *32*:320–336.

Leonard, D.M., Stachelek, S.J., Safran, M., Farwell, A.P., Leonard, J.L. Cloning, expression and functional characterization of the substrate binding subunit of the rat type II iodothyronine 5′-deiodinase. *J. Biol. Chem.,* **2000,** *275:*25194–25201.

Leonard, J.L., Kaplan, M.M., Visser, T.J., Silva, J.E., and Larsen, P.R. Cerebral cortex responds rapidly to thyroid hormones. *Science,* **1981,** *214:*571–573.

Leonard, J.L., Leonard, D.M., Safran, M., Wu, R., Zapp, M.L., and Farwell, A.P. The mammalian homolog of the frog type II selenodeiodinase does not encode a functional enzyme in the rat. *Endocrinology,* **1999,** *140:*2206–2215.

Liang, H., Juge-Aubry, C.E., O'Connell, M., and Burger, A.G. Organ-specific effects of 3,5,3′-triiodothyroacetic acid in rats. *Eur. J. Endocrinol.,* **1997,** *137:*537–544.

Magner, J.A., and Synder, D.K. Methimazole-induced agranulocytosis treated with recombinant human granulocyte colony-stimulating factor (G-CSF). *Thyroid,* **1994,** *4:*295–296.

Magnusson, R.P., Gestautas, J., Taurog, A., and Rapoport, B. Molecular cloning of the structural gene for porcine thyroid peroxidase. *J. Biol. Chem.,* **1987,** *262:*13885–13888.

Magnusson, R.P., Taurog, A., and Dorris, M.L. Mechanisms of thyroid peroxidase- and lactoperoxidase-catalyzed reactions involving iodide. *J. Biol. Chem.,* **1984,** *259:*13783–13790.

Man, E.B., Brown, J.F., and Serunian, S.A. Maternal hypothyroxinemia: psychoneurological deficits of progeny. *Ann. Clin. Lab. Sci.,* **1991,** *21:*227–239.

Mandel, S.J., Larsen, P.R., Seely, E.W., and Brent, G.A. Increased need for thyroxine during pregnancy in women with primary hypothyroidism. *N. Engl. J. Med.,* **1990,** *323:*91–96.

Manley, S.W., Rose, D.S., Huxham, G.J., and Bourke, J.R. Role of calcium in the secretomotor response of the thyroid: effects of calcium ionophore A23187 on radioiodine turnover, membrane potential and fluid transport in cultured porcine thyroid cells. *J. Endocrinol.,* **1988,** *116:*373–380.

Manso, P.G., Furlanetto, R.P., Wolosker, A.M., Paiva, E.R., de Abreu, M.T., and Maciel, R.M. Prospective and controlled study of ophthalmopathy after radioiodine therapy for Graves' hyperthyroidism. *Thyroid,* **1998,** *8:*49–52.

Marangell, L.B., George, M.S., Callahan, A.M., Ketter, T.A., Pazzaglia, P.J., L'Herrou, T.A., Leverich, G.S., and Post, R.M. Effects of intrathecal thyrotropin-releasing hormone (protirelin) in refractory depressed patients. *Arch. Gen. Psychiatry,* **1997,** *54:*214–222.

Marine, D., and Kimball, O.P. The prevention of simple goiter in man: a survey of the incidence and types of thyroid enlargements in the schoolgirls of Akron, Ohio, from the 5th to the 12th grades, inclusive; the plan of prevention proposed. *J. Lab. Clin. Med.,* **1917,** *3:*40–48.

Maugendre, D., Gatel, A., Campion, L., Massart, C., Guilhem, I., Lorcy, Y., Lescouarch, J., Herry, J.Y., and Allannic, H. Antithyroid drugs and Graves' disease—prospective randomized assessment of long-term treatment. *Clin. Endocrinol. (Oxf.),* **1999,** *50:*127–132.

McIver, B., Rae, P., Beckett, G., Wilkinson, E., Gold, A., and Toft, A. Lack of effect of thyroxine in patients with Graves' hyperthyroidism who are treated with an antithyroid drug. *N. Engl. J. Med.,* **1996,** *334:*220–224.

Mercado, M., Mendoza-Zubieta, V., Bautista-Osorio, R., and Espinoza-de los Monteros, A.L. Treatment of hyperthyroidism with a combination of methimazole and cholestyramine. *J. Clin. Endocrinol. Metab.,* **1996,** *81:*3191–3193.

Momotani, N., Noh, J.Y., Ishikawa, N., and Ito, K. Effects of propyl-thiouracil and methimazole on fetal thyroid status in mothers with Graves' hyperthyroidism. *J. Clin. Endocrinol. Metab.,* **1997,** *82:*3633–3636.

Mortimer, R.H., Cannell, G.R., Addison, R.S., Johnson, L.P., Roberts, M.S., and Bernus, I. Methimazole and propylthiouracil equally cross the perfused human term placental lobule. *J. Clin. Endocrinol. Metab.,* **1997,** *82:*3099–3102.

Müller, B., Zulewski, H., Huber, P., Ratcliffe, J.G., and Staub, J.J. Impaired action of thyroid hormone associated with smoking in women with hypothyroidism. *N. Engl. J. Med.,* **1995,** *333:*964–969.

Nauman, J., and Wolff, J. Iodide prophylaxis in Poland after the Chernobyl reactor accident: benefits and risks. *Am. J. Med.,* **1993,** *94:*524–532.

Nelson, J.C., and Tomei, R.T. Direct determination of free thyroxin in undiluted serum by equilibrium dialysis/radioimmunoassay. *Clin. Chem.,* **1988,** *34:*1737–1744.

Nelson, J.C., and Tomei, R.T. Dependence of the thyroxin/thyroxin-binding globulin (TBG) ratio and the free thyroxin index on TBG concentrations. *Clin. Chem.,* **1989,** *35:*541–544.

Nunez, J., and Correze, C. Interdependent effects of thyroid hormones and cAMP on lipolysis and lipogenesis in the fat cell. *Adv. Cyclic Nucleotide Res.,* **1981,** *14:*539–554.

Ojamaa, K., Klemperer, J.D., and Klein, I. Acute effects of thyroid hormone on vascular smooth muscle. *Thyroid,* **1996,** *6:*505–512.

Pacini, F., Cetani, F., Miccoli, P., Mancusi, F., Ceccarelli, C., Lippi, F., Martino, E., and Pinchera, A. Outcome of 309 patients with metastatic differentiated thyroid carcinoma treated with radioiodine. *World J. Surg.,* **1994b,** *18:*600–604.

Pacini, F., Gasperi, M., Fugazzola, L., Ceccarelli, C., Lippi, F., Centoni, R., Martino, E., and Pinchera, A. Testicular function in patients with differentiated thyroid carcinoma treated with radioiodine. *J. Nucl. Med.,* **1994a,** *35:*1418–1422.

Papini, E., Petrucci, L., Guglielmi, R., Panunzi, C., Rinaldi, R., Bacci, V., Crescenzi, A., Nardi, F., Fabbrini, R., and Pacella, C.M. Long-term changes in nodular goiter: a 5-year prospective randomized trial of levothyroxine suppressive therapy for benign cold thyroid nodules. *J. Clin. Endocrinol. Metab.,* **1998,** *83:*780–783.

Park, K.W., Dai, H.B., Ojamaa, K., Lowenstein, E., Klein, I., and Sellke, F.W. The direct vasomotor effect of thyroid hormones on rat skeletal muscle resistance arteries. *Anesth. Analg.,* **1997,** *85:*734–738.

Parmentier, M., Libert, F., Maenhaut, C., Lefort, A., Gerard, C., Perret, J., Van Sande, J., Dumont, J.E., and Vassart, G. Molecular cloning of the thyrotropin receptor. *Science,* **1989,** *246:*1620–1622.

Paschke, R., Metcalfe, A., Alcalde, L., Vassart, G., Weetman, A., and Ludgate, M. Presence of nonfunctional thyrotropin receptor variant transcripts in retroocular and other tissues. *J. Clin. Endocrinol. Metab.,* **1994,** *79:*1234–1238.

Paschke, R., Tonacchera, M., Van Sande, J., Parma, J., and Vassart, G. Identification and functional characterization of two new somatic mutations causing constitutive activation of the thyrotropin receptor in hyperfunctioning autonomous adenomas of the thyroid. *J. Clin. Endocrinol. Metab.,* **1994,** *79:*1785–1789.

Pop, V.J., Kuijpens, J.L., van Baar, A.L., Verkerk, G., van Son, M.M., de Vijlder, J.J., Vulsma, T., Wiersinga, W.M., Drexhage, H.A., and Vader, H.L. Low maternal free thyroxine concentrations during early pregnancy are associated with impaired psychomotor development in infancy. *Clin. Endocrinol. (Oxf.),* **1999,** *50:*149–155.

Porterfield, S.P., and Hendry, L.B. Impact of PCBs on thyroid hormone directed brain development. *Toxicol. Ind. Health.,* **1998,** *14:*103–120.

Reuss, M.L., Paneth, N., Pinto-Martin, J.A., Lorenz, J.M., and Susser, M. The relation of transient hypothyroxinemia in preterm infants to neurologic development at two years of age. *N. Engl. J. Med.,* **1996,** *334:*821–827.

Rittmaster, R.S., Abbott, E.C., Douglas, R., Givner, M.L., Lehmann, L., Reddy, S., Salisbury, S.R., Shlossberg, A.H., Tan, M.H., and York, S.E. Effect of methimazole, with or without L-thyroxine, on remission rates in Graves' disease. *J. Clin. Endocrinol. Metab.,* **1998,** *83:*814–818.

Rittmaster, R.S., Zwicker, H., Abbott, E.C., Douglas, R., Givner, M.L., Gupta, M.K., Lehmann, L., Reddy, S., Salisbury, S.R., Shlossberg, A.H., Tan, M.H., and York, S.E. Effect of methimazole with or without exogenous L-thyroxine on serum concentrations of thyrotropin (TSH) receptor antibodies in patients with Graves' disease. *J. Clin. Endocrinol. Metab.,* **1996,** *81:*3283–3288.

Roche, J., Lissitzky, S., and Michel, R. Sur la triiodothyronine, produit intermédiare de la transformation de la diiodothyronine en thyroxine. *C. R. Acad. Sci. [D] (Paris),* **1952a,** *234:*997–998.

Roche, J., Lissitzky, S., and Michael, R. Sur la présence detriiodothyronine dans la thyroglobuline. *C.R. Acad. Sci. [D] (Paris),* **1952b,** *234:*1228–1230.

Rohrer, D., and Dillmann, W.H. Thyroid hormone markedly increases the mRNA coding for sarcoplasmic reticulum Ca^{2+}–ATPase in the rat heart. *J. Biol. Chem.,* **1988,** *263:*6941–6944.

Ron, E., Doody, M.M., Becker, D.V., Brill, A.B., Curtis, R.E., Goldman, M.B., Harris, B.S. III, Hoffman, D.A., McConahey, W.M., Maxon, H.R., Preston-Martin, S., Warshauer, M.E., Wong, F.L., and Boice, J.D., Jr. Cancer mortality following treatment for adult hyperthyroidism. Cooperative Thyrotoxicosis Therapy Follow-up Study Group. *JAMA,* **1998,** *280:*347–355.

Ros, M., Northup, J.K., and Malbon, C.C. Steady-state levels of G proteins and β-adrenergic receptors in rat fat cells. Permissive effects of thyroid hormones. *J. Biol. Chem.,* **1988,** *263:*4362–4368.

Roti, E., Cozani, R., and Braverman, L.E. Adverse effects of iodine on the thyroid. *Endocrinologist,* **1997,** *7:*245–254.

Roti, E., Minelli, R., Gardini, E., and Braverman, L.E. The use and misuse of thyroid hormone. *Endocr. Rev.,* **1993,** *14:*401–423.

Ruiz, M., Rajatanavin, R., Young, R.A., Taylor, C., Brown, R., Braverman, L.E., and Ingbar, S.H. Familial dysalbuminemic hyperthyroxinemia: a syndrome that can be confused with thyrotoxicosis. *N. Engl. J. Med.,* **1982,** *306:*635–639.

Salter, A.M., Fisher, S.C., and Brindley, D.N. Interactions of triiodothyronine, insulin, and dexamethasone on the binding of human LDL to rat hepatocytes in monolayer culture. *Atherosclerosis,* **1988,** *71:*77–80.

Salvatore, D., Bartha, T., Harney, J.W., and Larsen, P.R. Molecular biological and biochemical characterization of the human type 2 selenodeiodinase. *Endocrinology,* **1996,** *137:*3308–3315.

Samuels, H.H., Forman, B.M., Horowitz, Z.D., and Ye, Z.-S. Regulation of gene expression by thyroid hormone. *J. Clin. Invest.,* **1988,** *81:*957–967.

Sap, J., Munoz, A., Damm, K., Goldberg, Y., Ghysdael, J., Leutz, A., Beug, H., and Vennström, B. The c-*erb*-A protein is a high affinity receptor for thyroid hormone. *Nature,* **1986,** *324:*635–640.

Scarabottolo, L., Trezzi, E., Roma, P., and Catapano, A.L. Experimental hypothyroidism modulates the expression of low density lipoprotein receptor by the liver. *Atherosclerosis,* **1986,** *59:*329–333.

Sher, E.S., Xu, X.M., Adams, P.M., Craft, C.M., and Stein, S.A. The effects of thyroid hormone level and action in developing brain: are these targets for the actions of polychlorinated biphenyls and dioxins? *Toxicol. Ind. Health,* **1998,** *14:*121–158.

Sherman, S.I., and Ladenson, P.W. Organ-specific effects of tiratricol:

a thyroid hormone analog with hepatic, not pituitary, superagonist effects. *J. Clin. Endocrinol. Metab.,* **1992,** *75:*901–905.

Simmonds, M. Ueber Hypophysisschwund mit todlichem Ausang. *Dtsch. Med. Wochenschr.,* **1914,** *40:*322–323.

Smanik, P.A., Liu, Q., Furminger, T.L., Ryu, K., Xing, S., Mazzaferri, E.L., and Jhiang, S.M. Cloning of the human sodium iodide symporter. *Biochem. Biophys. Res. Commun.,* **1996,** *226:*339–345.

Smerdely, P., Pitsiavas, V., and Boyages, S.C. Evidence that the inhibitory effects of iodide on thyroid cell proliferation are due to arrest of the cell cycle at G0G1 and G2M phases. *Endocrinology,* **1993,** *133:*2881–2888.

Soloman, B., Glinoer, D., Lagasse, R., and Wartofsky, L. Current trends in the management of Graves' disease. *J. Clin. Endocrinol. Metab.,* **1990,** *70:*1518–1524.

Sterling, K. Direct triiodothyronine (T_3) action by a primary mitochondrial pathway. *Endocr. Res.,* **1989,** *15:*683–715.

Strait, K.A., Schwartz, H.L., Perez-Castillo, A., and Oppenheimer, J.H. Relationship of c-*erb*-A mRNA content to tissue triiodothyronine nuclear binding capacity and function in developing and adult rats. *J. Biol. Chem.,* **1990,** *265:*10514–10521.

Sunthornthepvarakul, T., Angkeow, P., Weiss, R.E., Hayashi, Y., and Refetoff, S. An identical missense mutation in the albumin gene results in familial dysalbuminemic hyperthyroxinemia in 8 unrelated families. *Biochem. Biophys. Res. Commun.,* **1994,** *202:*781–787.

Sunthornthepvarakul, T., Gottschalk, M.E., Hayashi, Y., and Refetoff, S. Brief report: resistance to thyrotropin caused by mutations in the thyrotropin-receptor gene. *N. Engl. J. Med.,* **1995,** *332:*155–160.

Takami, H. Lithium in the preoperative preparation of Graves' disease. *Int. Surg.,* **1994,** *79:*89–90.

Takasu, N., Yamada, T., and Shimizu, Y. Generation of H_2O_2 is regulated by cytoplasmic free calcium in cultured porcine thyroid cells. *Biochem. Biophys. Res. Commun.,* **1987,** *148:*1527–1532.

Takeshita, A., Yen, P.M., Misiti, S., Cardona, G.R., Liu, Y., and Chin, W.W. Molecular cloning and properties of a full-length putative thyroid hormone receptor coactivator. *Endocrinology,* **1996,** *137:*3594–3597.

Tang, K.T., Yang, H.J., Choo, K.B., Lin, H.D., Fang, S.L., and Braverman, L.E. A point mutation in the albumin gene in a Chinese patient with familial dysalbuminemic hyperthyroxinemia. *Eur. J. Endocrinol.,* **1999,** *141:*374–378.

Tonacchera, M., Van Sande, J., Cetani, F., Swillens, S., Schvartz, C., Winiszewski, P., Portmann, L., Dumont, J.E., Vassart, G., and Parma, J. Functional characteristics of three new germline mutations of the thyrotropin receptor gene causing autosomal dominant toxic thyroid hyperplasia. *J. Clin. Endocrinol. Metab.,* **1996,** *81:*547–554.

Törring, O., Tallstedt, L., Wallin, G., Lundell, G., Ljunggren, J.G., Taube, A., Saaf, M., and Hamberger, B. Graves' hyperthyroidism: treatment with antithyroid drugs, surgery, or radioiodine—a prospective, randomized study. Thyroid Study Group. *J. Clin. Endocrinol. Metab.,* **1996,** *81:*2986–2993.

Tunbridge, W.M., Evered, D.C., Hall, R., Appleton, D., Brewis, M., Clark, F., Evans, J.G., Young, E., Bird, T., and Smith, P.A. The spectrum of thyroid disease in a community: the Wickham survey. *Clin. Endocrinol. (Oxf.),* **1977,** *7:*481–493.

Tuttle, R.M., Patience, T., and Budd. S. Treatment with propylthiouracil before radioactive iodine therapy is associated with a higher treatment failure rate than therapy with radioactive iodine alone in Graves' disease. *Thyroid,* **1995,** *5:*243–247.

Uy, H.L., Reasner, C.A., and Samuels, M.H. Pattern of recovery of the hypothalamic-pituitary-thyroid axis following radioactive iodine therapy in patients with Graves' disease. *Am. J. Med.,* **1995,** *99*:173–179.

Van Sande, J., Raspe, E., Perret, J., Lejeune, C., Maenhaut, C., Vassart, G., and Dumont, J.E. Thyrotropin activates both the cyclic AMP and the PIP$_2$ cascades in CHO cells expressing the human cDNA of the TSH receptor. *Mol. Cell. Endocrinol.,* **1990,** *74*:R1–R6.

van Wassenaer, A.G., Kok, J.H., de Vijlder, J.J., Briet, J.M., Smit, B.J., Tamminga, P., van Baar, A., Dekker, F.W., and Vulsma, T. Effects of thyroxine supplementation on neurologic development in infants born at less than 30 weeks' gestation. *N. Engl. J. Med.,* **1997,** *336*:21–26.

Visser, T.J., Leonard, J.L., Kaplan, M.M., and Larsen, P.R. Kinetic evidence suggesting two mechanisms for iodothyronine 5'-deiodination in rat cerebral cortex. *Proc. Natl. Acad. Sci. U.S.A.,* **1982,** *79*:5080–5084.

Wagner, R.L., Apriletti, J.W., McGrath, M.E., West, B.L., Baxter, J.D., and Fletterick, R.J. A structural role for hormone in the thyroid hormone receptor. *Nature,* **1995,** *378*:690–697.

Wasserstrum, N., and Anania, C.A. Perinatal consequences of maternal hypothyroidism in early pregnancy and inadequate replacement. *Clin. Endocrinol. (Oxf.),* **1995,** *42*:353–358.

Weinberger, C., Thompson, C.C., Ong, E.S., Lebo, R., Gruol, D.J., and Evans, R.M. The c-*erb*-A gene encodes a thyroid hormone receptor. *Nature,* **1986,** *324*:641–646.

Weiss, R.E., Hayashi, Y., Nagaya, T., Petty, K.J., Murata, Y., Tunca, H., Seo, H., and Refetoff, S. Dominant inheritance of resistance to thyroid hormone not linked to defects in the thyroid hormone receptor alpha or beta genes may be due to a defective cofactor. *J. Clin. Endocrinol. Metab.,* **1996,** *81*:4196–4203.

Wikström, L., Johansson, C., Saltó, C., Barlow, C., Campos Barros, A., Baas, F., Forrest, D., Thorén, P., and Vennström, B. Abnormal heart rate and body temperature in mice lacking thyroid hormone receptor alpha 1. *E.M.B.O. J.,* **1998,** *17*:455–461.

Wilber, J.F., and Xu, A.H. The thyrotropin-releasing hormone gene 1998: cloning, characterization, and transcriptional regulation in the central nervous system, heart, and testis. *Thyroid,* **1998,** *8*:897–901.

Xie, J., Pannain, S., Pohlenz, J., Weiss, R.E., Moltz, K., Morlot, M., Asteria, C., Persani, L., Beck-Peccoz, P., Parma, J., Vassart, G., and Refetoff, S. Resistance to thyrotropin (TSH) in three families is not associated with mutations in the TSH receptor or TSH. *J. Clin. Endocrinol. Metab.,* **1997,** *82*:3933–3940.

Yamamoto, T., Fukuyama, J., and Fujiyoshi, A. Factors associated with mortality of myxedema coma: report of eight cases and literature survey. *Thyroid,* **1999,** *9*:1167–1174.

Zelmanovitz, F., Genro, S., and Gross, J.L. Suppressive therapy with levothyroxine for solitary thyroid nodules: a double-blind controlled clinical study and cumulative meta-analyses. *J. Clin. Endocrinol. Metab.,* **1998,** *83*:3881–3885.

MONOGRAPHS AND REVIEWS

Abend, A.L., and Braverman, L.E. Thyroid storm. In, *Irwin and Rippe's Intensive Care Medicine,* 4th ed. (Irwin, R.S., Cerra, F.B., and Rippe, J.M., eds.) Lippincott-Raven, Philadelphia, **1999,** pp. 1271–1275.

Anderson, G.W., Mariash, C.N., and Oppenheimer, J.H. Molecular actions of thyroid hormone. In, *Werner and Ingbar's The Thyroid,* 8th ed. (Braverman, L.E., and Utiger, R.D., eds.) Lippincott Williams & Wilkins, New York, **2000,** pp. 174–195.

Baran, D.T. The skeletal system in thyrotoxicosis. In, *Werner and*

Ingbar's The Thyroid, 8th ed. (Braverman, L.E., and Utiger, R.D., eds.) Lippincott Williams & Wilkins, New York, **2000,** pp. 659–666.

Bernal, J., and Nunez, J. Thyroid hormones and brain development. *Eur. J. Endocrinol.,* **1995,** *133*:390–398.

Bottazzo, G.F., and Doniach, D. Autoimmune thyroid disease. *Annu. Rev. Med.,* **1986,** *37*:353–359.

Braverman, L.E. *Diseases of the Thyroid.* Humana Press, Totowa, NJ, **1997.**

Braverman, L.E., Eber, O., and Langsteger, W. *Heart and Thyroid.* Blackwell-MZV, Vienna, **1994.**

Braverman, L.E., and Utiger, R.D. *Werner and Ingbar's The Thyroid,* Lippincott Williams & Wilkins, New York, **2000,** pp. 578–589.

Burman, K.D., and Baker, J.R. Jr. Immune mechanisms in Graves' disease. *Endocr. Rev.,* **1985,** *6*:183–232.

Carrasco, N. Thyroid iodine transport: the Na$^+$/I$^-$ symporter (NIS). In, *Werner and Ingbar's The Thyroid,* 8th ed. (Braverman, L.E., and Utiger, R.D., eds.) Lippincott Williams & Wilkins, New York, **2000,** pp. 52–60.

Chin, W.W., and Yen, P.M. Molecular mechanisms of nuclear thyroid hormone action. In, *Diseases of the Thyroid.* (Braverman, L.E., ed.) Humana Press, Totowa, NJ, **1997,** pp. 1–16.

Cody, V. Thyroid hormone interactions: molecular conformation, protein binding and hormone action. *Endocr. Rev.,* **1980,** *1*:140–166.

Cody, V. Thyroid hormone structure and function. In, *Werner and Ingbar's The Thyroid,* 8th ed. (Braverman, L.E., and Utiger, R.D., eds.) Lippincott Williams & Wilkins, New York, **2000,** pp. 196–201.

Cooper, D.S. Antithyroid drugs for the treatment of hyperthyroidism caused by Graves' disease. *Endocrinol. Metab. Clin. North Am.,* **1998,** *27*:225–247.

Davis, P.J., and Davis, F.B. Nongenomic actions of thyroid hormone. In, *Diseases of the Thyroid.* (Braverman, L.E., ed.) Humana Press, Totowa, N.J., **1997,** pp. 17–34.

Delange, F., Dunn, J.T., and Glinoer, D. *Iodine Deficiency in Europe: A Continuing Concern.* Plenum Press, New York, **1993.**

DeVito, M., Biegel, L., Brouwer, A., Brown, S., Brucker-Davis, F., Cheek, A.O., Christensen, R., Colborn, T., Cooke, P., Crissman, J., Crofton, K., Doerge, D., Gray, E., Hauser, P., Hurley, P., Kohn, M., Lazar, J., McMaster, S., McClain, M., McConnell, E., Meier, C., Miller, R., Tietge, J., and Tyl, R. Screening methods for thyroid hormone disruptors. *Environ. Health. Perspect.,* **1999,** *107*:407–415.

Dunn, J.T., and Dunn, A.D. Thyroglobulin: chemistry, biosynthesis, and proteolysis. In, *Werner and Ingbar's The Thyroid,* 8th ed. (Braverman, L.E., and Utiger, R.D., eds.) Lippincott Williams & Wilkins, New York, **2000,** pp. 91–104.

Emerson, C.H. Myxedema coma. In, *Irwin and Rippe's Intensive Care Medicine,* 4th ed. (Irwin, R.S., Cerra, F.B., and Rippe, J.M., eds.) Lippincott-Raven, Philadelphia, **1999,** pp. 1276–1278.

Emerson, C.H., and Farwell, A.P. Sporadic silent thyroiditis, postpartum thyroiditis, and subacute thyroiditis. In, *Werner and Ingbar's The Thyroid,* 8th ed. (Braverman, L.E., and Utiger, R.D., eds.) Lippincott Williams & Wilkins, New York, **2000,** pp. 578–589.

Farwell, A.P. Sick euthyroid syndrome in the intensive care unit. In, *Irwin and Rippe's Intensive Care Medicine,* 4th ed. (Irwin, R.S., Cerra, F.B., and Rippe, J.M., eds.) Lippincott-Raven, Philadelphia, **1999,** pp. 1271–1275.

Farwell, A.P., and Leonard, J.L. Extranuclear actions of thyroid hormone in the brain. In, *Recent Research Developments in Neuroendocrinology—Thyroid Hormone and Brain Maturation.*

(Porterfield, S.P., and Hendrich, C.E., eds.) Research Signpost, Trivandrum, India, **1997**, pp. 113–130.

Fisher, D.A. Clinical review 19: management of congenital hypothyroidism. *J. Clin. Endocrinol. Metab.*, **1991**, *72*:523–529.

Franklyn, J.A. The management of hyperthyroidism. *N. Engl. J. Med.*, **1994**, *330*:1731–1738.

Gershengorn, M.C. Mechanism of thyrotropin releasing hormone stimulation of pituitary hormone secretion. *Annu. Rev. Physiol.*, **1986**, *48*:515–526.

Gharib, H., and Goellner, J.R. Fine-needle aspiration biopsy of the thyroid: an appraisal. *Ann. Intern. Med.*, **1993**, *118*:282–289.

Gharib, H., and Mazzaferri, E.L. Thyroxine suppressive therapy in patients with nodular thyroid disease. *Ann. Intern. Med.*, **1998**, *128*:386–394.

Glinoer, D. Maternal thyroid function in pregnancy. *J. Endocrinol. Invest.*, **1993**, *16*:374–378.

Gottlieb, P.A., and Braverman, L.E. The effect of thyroid disease on diabetes. *Clin. Diabetes*, **1994**, *12*:15–18.

Harjai, K.J., and Licata, A.A. Effects of amiodarone on thyroid function. *Ann. Intern. Med.*, **1997**, *126*:63–73.

Helfand, M., Redfern, C.C. Clinical guideline, part 2. Screening for thyroid disease: an update. American College of Physicians. *Ann. Intern. Med.*, **1998**, *129*:144–158.

Hermus, A.R., and Huysmans, D.A. Treatment of benign nodular thyroid disease. *N. Engl. J. Med.*, **1998**, *338*:1438–1447.

Hsu, J.-H., and Brent, G.A. Thyroid hormone receptor gene knockouts. *Trends Endocrinol. Metab.*, **1998**, *9*:103–112.

Huysmans, D., Hermus, A., Edelbroek, M., Barentsz, J., Corstens, F., and Kloppenborg, P. Radioiodine for nontoxic multinodular goiter. *Thyroid*, **1997**, *7*:235–239.

Klee, G.G. Clinical usage recommendations and analytic performance goals for total and free triiodothyronine measurements. *Clin. Chem.*, **1996**, *42*:155–159.

Klein, I., Becker, D.V., and Levey, G.S. Treatment of hyperthyroid disease. *Ann. Intern. Med.*, **1994**, *121*:281–288.

Larsen, P.R., Silva, J.E., and Kaplan, M.M. Relationships between circulating and intracellular thyroid hormones: physiological and clinical implications. *Endocr. Rev.*, **1981**, *2*:87–102.

Lazar, M.A. Thyroid hormone receptors: multiple forms, multiple possibilities. *Endocr. Rev.*, **1993**, *14*:184–193.

Lee, H., and Yen, P.M. Recent advances in understanding thyroid hormone receptor coregulators. *J. Biomed. Sci.*, **1999**, *6*:71–78.

Legrand, J. Morphogenic actions of thyroid hormones. *Trends Neurosci.*, **1979**, *2*:234–236.

Leonard, J.L., and Koehrle, J. In, *Werner and Ingbar's The Thyroid*, 8th ed. (Braverman, L.E., and Utiger, R.D., eds.) Lippincott Williams & Wilkins, New York, **2000**, pp. 136–173.

Leonard, J.L., and Visser, T.J. Biochemistry of deiodination. In, *Thyroid Hormone Metabolism*. (Hennemann, G., ed.) Vol. 8. *Basic and Clinical Endocrinology*. Marcel Dekker, Inc., New York, **1986**, pp. 189–230.

Levy, E.G. Treatment of Graves' disease: the American way. *Baillieres Clin. Endocrinol. Metab.*, **1997**, *11*:585–595.

Mangelsdorf, D.J., Umesono, K., and Evans, R.M. The retinoid receptors. In, *The Retinoids: Biology, Chemistry, and Medicine*, 2nd ed. (Sporn, M.B., Roberts, A.B., and Goodman, D.S., eds.) Raven Press, New York, **1994**, pp. 319–349.

Mazzaferri, E.L. Management of a solitary thyroid nodule. *N. Engl. J. Med.* **1993**, *328*:553–559.

Mazzaferri, E.L. Radioiodine and other treatments and outcomes. In, *Werner and Ingbar's The Thyroid*, 8th ed. (Braverman, L.E., and Utiger, R.D., eds.) Lippincott Williams & Wilkins, New York, **2000**, pp. 904–929.

McLachlan, S.M., and Rapoport, B. The molecular biology of thyroid peroxidase: cloning, expression and role as autoantigen in autoimmune thyroid disease. *Endocr. Rev.*, **1992**, *13*:192–206.

Meier, C.A., and Burger, A.G. Effects of drugs and other substances on thyroid hormone synthesis. In, *Werner and Ingbar's The Thyroid*, 8th ed. (Braverman, L.E., and Utiger, R.D., eds.) Lippincott Williams & Wilkins, New York, **2000**, pp. 265–280.

Mendel, C.M. The free hormone hypothesis: a physiologically based mathematical model. *Endocr. Rev.*, **1989**, *10*:232–274.

Mestman, J.H. Hyperthyroidism in pregnancy. *Clin. Obstet. Gynecol.*, **1997**, *40*:45–64.

Meyer–Gessner, M., Benker, G., Lederbogen, S., Olbricht, T., and Reinwein, D. Antithyroid drug-induced agranulocytosis: clinical experience with ten patients treated at one institution and review of the literature. *J. Endocrinol. Invest.*, **1994**, *17*:29–36.

Nagayama, Y., and Rapoport, B. The thyrotropin receptor 25 years after its discovery: new insight after its molecular cloning. *Mol. Endocrinol.*, **1992**, *6*:145–156.

Nelson, J.C., and Wilcox, R.B. Analytical performance of free and total thyroxine assays. *Clin. Chem.*, **1996**, *42*:146–154.

Nicoloff, J.T., and Spencer, C.A. Clinical review 12: The use and misuse of the sensitive thyrotropin assays. *J. Clin. Endocrinol. Metab.*, **1990**, *71*:553–558.

Oppenheimer, J.H., and Schwartz, H.L. Molecular basis of thyroid hormone-dependent brain development. *Endocr. Rev.*, **1997**, *18*:462–475.

Pisarev, M. A., and Gärtner, R. Autoregulatory actions of iodine. In, *Werner and Ingbar's The Thyroid*, 8th ed. (Braverman, L.E., and Utiger, R.D., eds.) Lippincott Williams & Wilkins, New York, **2000**, pp. 85–90.

Porterfield, S.D., and Hendrich, C.H (eds.). *Recent Research Developments in Neuroendocrinology—Thyroid Hormone and Brain Maturation*. Research Signpost, Trivandrum, India, **1997**.

Rapoport, B., and McLachlan, S. *Endocrine Updates: Graves' Disease*. Kluwer Academic Publishers, The Netherlands, **2000**.

Ribeiro, R.C., Kushner, P.J., and Baxter, J.D. The nuclear hormone receptor gene superfamily. *Annu. Rev. Med.*, **1995**, *46*:443–453.

Ross, D.R. Subclinical thyrotoxicosis. *Adv. Endocrinol. Metab.*, **1991**, *2*:89–103.

Roti, E., and Vagenakis, A.G. Effects of excess iodide: clinical aspects. In, *Werner and Ingbar's The Thyroid*, 8th ed. (Braverman, L.E., and Utiger, R.D., eds.) Lippincott Williams & Wilkins, New York, **2000**, pp. 316–332.

St. Germain, D.L., and Galton, V.A. The deiodinase family of selenoproteins. *Thyroid*, **1997**, *7*:655–668.

Samuels, M.H. Subclinical thyroid disease in the elderly. *Thyroid*, **1998**, *8*:803–813.

Siegrist-Kaiser, C.A., Juge-Aubry, C., Tranter, M.P., Ekenbarger, D.M., and Leonard, J.L. Thyroxine-dependent modulation of actin polymerization in cultured astrocytes. A novel, extranuclear action of thyroid hormone. *J. Biol. Chem.*, **1990**, *265*:5296–5302.

Silva, J.E. Thyroid hormone control of thermogenesis and energy balance. *Thyroid*, **1995**, *5*:481–492.

Spencer, C.A., Takeuchi, M., and Kazarosyan, M. Current status and performance goals for serum thyrotropin (TSH) assays. *Clin. Chem.*, **1996**, *42*:140–145.

Surks, M.I., and Ocampo, E. Subclinical thyroid disease. *Am. J. Med.,* **1996,** *100*:217–223.

Taurog, A. Hormone synthesis: thyroid iodine metabolism. In, *Werner and Ingbar's The Thyroid,* 8th ed. (Braverman, L.E., and Utiger, R.D., eds.) Lippincott Williams & Wilkins, New York, **2000,** pp. 61–84.

Toft, A.D. Thyroxine therapy. *N. Engl. J. Med.,* **1994,** *331*:174–180.

Tonacchera, M., Van Sande, J., Parma, J., Duprez, L., Cetani, F.,

Costagliola, S., Durmont, J.E., and Vassart, G. TSH receptor and disease. *Clin. Endocrinol. (Oxf.),* **1996b,** *44*:621–633.

Vassart, G., and Dumont, J.E. The thyrotropin receptor and the regulation of thyrocyte function and growth. *Endocr. Rev.,* **1992,** *13*:596–611.

Wolff, J. Perchlorate and the thyroid gland. *Pharmacol. Rev.,* **1998,** *50*:89–105.

Zimmerman, D. Fetal and neonatal hyperthyroidism. *Thyroid,* **1999,** *9*:727–733.

C H A P T E R   5 8

ESTROGENS AND PROGESTINS

David S. Loose-Mitchell and George M. Stancel

Estrogens and progestins are among the most widely prescribed drugs. This chapter covers the major uses of estrogens and progestins, alone or in combination, for contraception and for hormone-replacement therapy in postmenopausal women. The less-frequent use of estrogen, sometimes in conjunction with growth hormone or gonadotropins, for treatment of developmental delay or hypogonadism also is discussed (Chapter 56 provides additional discussion of this topic). The use of estrogen-receptor antagonists or progestins and aromatase inhibitors as functional estrogen antagonists is described for treatment of estrogen-dependent neoplasms. The use and potential use of progesterone antagonists, such as mifepristone (RU 486), also is discussed. Cancer chemotherapeutic strategies based on blockade of estrogen and/or progesterone receptor functions are considered in further detail in Chapter 52. Complementary therapeutic strategies based on suppression of gonadotropin secretion by long-acting gonadotropin-releasing hormone agonists are discussed in Chapter 56.

Estrogens and progestins are endogenous hormones that produce numerous physiological actions. In women, these include developmental effects, neuroendocrine actions involved in the control of ovulation, the cyclical preparation of the reproductive tract for fertilization and implantation, and major actions on mineral, carbohydrate, protein, and lipid metabolism. Many features of the female habitus also are influenced by these hormones. It has become clear more recently that estrogens have important actions in males, including effects on bone, spermatogenesis, and behavior.

The basic features of the biosynthesis, biotransformation, and disposition of these agents are well established, and the nuclear receptor system for these hormones is well characterized. This knowledge provides a firm conceptual basis for understanding the physiological and pharmacological activities of both hormones.

The therapeutic use of estrogens and progestins is widespread, and their pharmacological actions largely reflect extensions of their physiological activities. The most common uses of these agents are hormone-replacement therapy in postmenopausal women and contraception, but the specific compounds and dosages used in these two settings are substantially different. Although oral contraceptives are used primarily to prevent pregnancy, they also have significant health benefits beyond contraception. Naturally occurring and synthetic compounds are available for oral and parenteral uses.

Estrogen- and progesterone-receptor antagonists also are available. The main use of antiestrogens is in the treatment of hormone-responsive breast cancer. Treatment of female infertility is the most common use of these antagonists in gynecology. The main use of antiprogestins to date has been for medical abortion, but other uses are being developed.

A number of naturally occurring and synthetic environmental chemicals mimic, antagonize, or otherwise affect the actions of estrogens in experimental test systems. While the precise effect of these environmental agents on human beings is not known, this is an area of active investigation.

History. It has long been known that removal of the ovaries results in uterine atrophy and a loss of sexual functions. The hormonal nature of the ovarian control of the female reproductive system was established in 1900 by Knauer when he found that ovarian transplants prevented the symptoms of gonadectomy. This observation was extended by Halban (1900), who showed that, if the glands were transplanted even in immature animals, normal sexual development and function were assured. In 1923, Allen and Doisy devised a simple bioassay for ovarian extracts based upon changes produced in the vaginal smear of the rat. Loewe (1925) first reported a female sex hormone in the blood of various species, and shortly thereafter Frank and associates (1925) detected an active sex principle in the blood of sows in estrus. Of even greater significance was the discovery by Loewe and Lange (1926) of a female sex hormone in the urine of menstruating women and the observation that the concentration of the hormone in the urine varied with the phase of the menstrual cycle. The excretion of large amounts of estrogen in the urine during pregnancy also was reported (Zondek, 1928). This finding was a boon to chemists, who soon isolated an active substance in crystalline form (Butenandt, 1929; Doisy *et al.,* 1929, 1930). A few years later, its chemical structure was elucidated.

The results of early investigations indicated that the ovary secretes two substances. Beard (1897) had postulated that the corpus luteum serves a necessary function during pregnancy, and Fraenkel (1903) showed that destruction of the corpora lutea in pregnant rabbits causes abortion. The contributions of Corner and Allen (1929) firmly established the hormonal function of the corpus luteum. These investigators showed that the abortion following extirpation of the corpora lutea in pregnant rabbits can be prevented by the injection of luteal extracts.

In the early 1960s, pioneering studies by Jensen and colleagues suggested the presence of intracellular receptors for es-

trogens in the target tissues (Jensen and Jacobsen, 1962). This was historically important, because it was the first demonstration of receptors of the steroid/thyroid superfamily and because it provided the experimental approaches used to identify similar receptors for the other steroid hormones (Jensen and DeSombre, 1972). A second form of the estrogen receptor recently has been identified and termed *estrogen receptor β* (ER β) to distinguish it from the first receptor, which is now referred to as *estrogen receptor α* (ER α).

ESTROGENS

Chemistry. Estrogenic activity is shared by many steroidal and nonsteroidal compounds, some of which are shown in Table 58–1 and Figure 58–1. The most potent naturally occurring estrogen in human beings is 17β-estradiol, followed by

Table 58–1
Structural Formulas of Selected Estrogens

Derivative	STEROIDAL ESTROGENS			NONSTEROIDAL COMPOUNDS WITH ESTROGENIC ACTIVITY
	R_1	R_2	R_3	
Estradiol	—H	—H	—H	Diethylstilbestrol
Estradiol valerate	—H	—H	$-\overset{O}{\overset{\|}{C}}(CH_2)_3CH_3$	p, p'-DDT
Estradiol cypionate	—H	—H	$-\overset{O}{\overset{\|}{C}}(CH_2)_2$⬠	
Ethinyl estradiol	—H	—C≡CH	—H	Bisphenol A
Mestranol	—CH₃	—C≡CH	—H	
Quinestrol	⬠-	—C≡CH	—H	
Estrone	—H	—*	=O*	Genistein
Estrone sulfate	—SO₃H	—*	=O*	
Equilin†	—H	—*	=O*	

*Designates C 17 ketone.
†Also contains 7, 8 double bond.

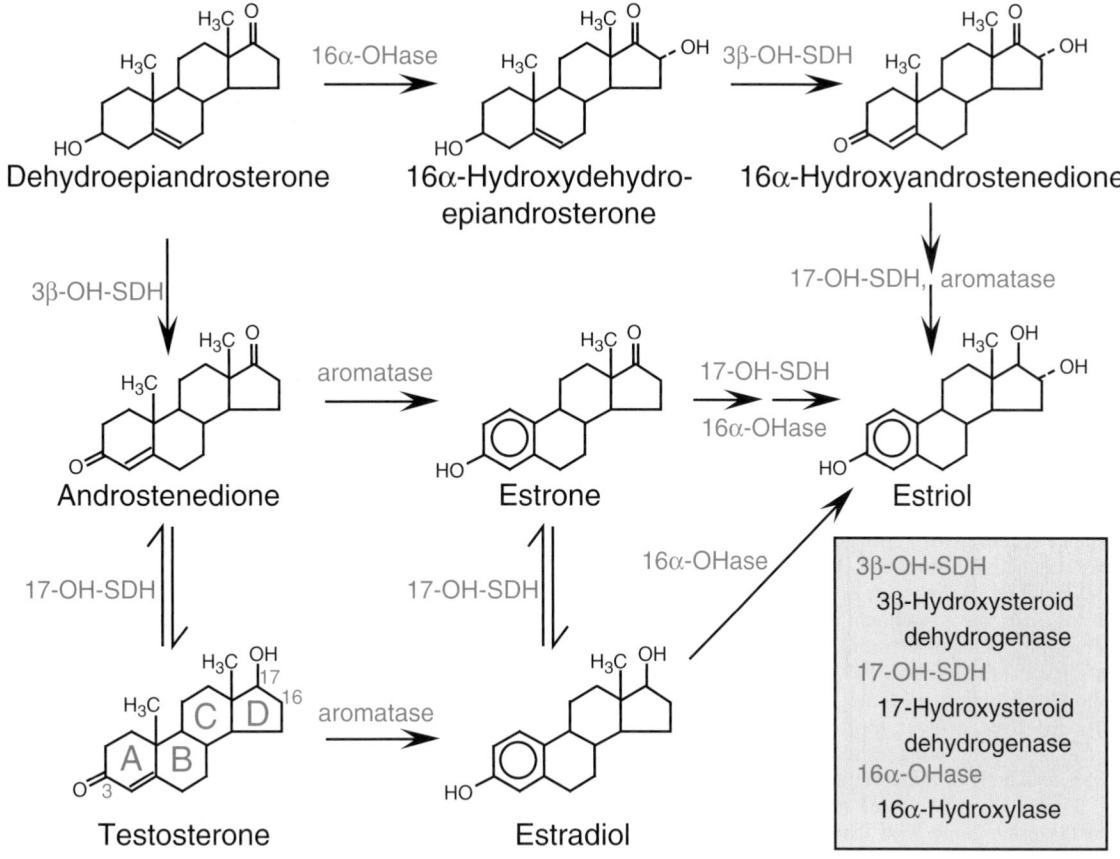

Figure 58–1. The biosynthetic pathway for the estrogens.

estrone and estriol. Each of these molecules is an 18-carbon steroid, containing a phenolic A ring (an aromatic ring with a hydroxyl group at carbon 3) and a β-hydroxyl group or ketone in position 17 of ring D. The phenolic A ring is the principal structural feature responsible for selective, high-affinity binding to estrogen receptors. Most alkyl substitutions on the phenolic A ring impair such binding, but substitutions on ring C or D may be tolerated. Ethinyl substitutions at the C 17 position greatly increase oral potency by inhibiting first-pass hepatic metabolism. A model for the estrogen receptor ligand-binding site has been developed from structure-activity studies (Anstead *et al.,* 1997), and the crystal structures of estrogen-receptor complexes have been reported (Brzozowski *et al.,* 1997).

One of the first nonsteroidal estrogens to be synthesized was diethylstilbestrol or DES (*see* Table 58–1), which is structurally similar to estradiol when viewed in the *trans* conformation. DES is as potent as estradiol in most assays, but is orally active and has a longer half-life in the body. DES no longer has widespread use, but it is important historically because its introduction as a cheap, plentiful, orally active estrogen at a time when the natural products were scarce was a milestone in the development of effective endocrine therapy (Dodds *et al.,* 1938).

Nonsteroidal compounds with estrogenic or antiestrogenic activity—including flavones, isoflavones (*e.g.,* genistein), and coumestan derivatives—occur naturally in a variety of plants and fungi. A number of synthetic agents—including pesticides (*e.g., p,p'*-DDT), plasticizers (*e.g.,* bisphenol A), and a variety of other industrial chemicals (*e.g.,* polychlorinated biphenyls)—also have hormonal or antihormonal activity. Many of these polycyclic compounds contain a phenolic ring that mimics the A ring of steroids. While the affinity of these "environmental estrogens" for the estrogen receptor is relatively weak, their large number, bioaccumulation in adipose tissue, and persistence in the environment have raised concerns about their potential toxicity in human beings and wildlife (Mäkelä *et al.,* 1999). Both over-the-counter and prescription preparations containing naturally occurring, estrogen-like compounds from plants (*i.e.,* phytoestrogens) now are available. There also have been reports that phytoestrogens such as genistein may exhibit relative selectivity for ER β (Kuiper *et al.,* 1998); this possibility is being actively investigated.

Biosynthesis. Steroidal estrogens are formed from either androstenedione or testosterone as immediate precursors (*see* Figure 58–1). The reaction involves aromatization of the A ring, and it is catalyzed in three steps by a cytochrome P450 monooxygenase enzyme complex (aromatase or CYP19) that uses NADPH and molecular oxygen as cosubstrates (Simpson *et al.,* 1994). In the first step of this reaction, C 19 (the angular methyl group on C 10 of the androgen precursors) is hydroxylated. A second hydroxylation results in the elimination of the newly formed C 19 hydroxymethyl group, and a final hydroxylation of C 2 results in the formation of an unstable intermediate that rearranges to form the phenolic A ring. The entire reaction consumes three molecules of oxygen and three molecules of NADPH.

Aromatase activity resides within a transmembrane glycoprotein (cytochrome P450 family of monooxygenases); a ubiquitous flavoprotein, NADPH–cytochrome P450 reductase, also is essential. Both proteins are localized in the endoplasmic reticulum of ovarian granulosa cells, testicular Sertoli and Leydig cells, stromal cells of adipose tissue, placental syncytiotrophoblasts, the preimplantation blastocyst, bone, and various brain regions (Simpson *et al.*, 1999).

The ovaries are the principal source of circulating estrogen in premenopausal women. The major secretory product is estradiol, synthesized by granulosa cells from androgenic precursors provided by theca cells. Aromatase activity is induced by gonadotropins, which act *via* plasma membrane receptors to elevate intracellular concentrations of adenosine $3',5'$-monophosphate (cyclic AMP). Gonadotropins and cyclic AMP also increase the activity of the cholesterol side-chain cleavage enzyme and facilitate the transport of cholesterol (the precursor of all steroids) into the mitochondria of cells that synthesize steroids. The ovary contains a form of 17β-hydroxysteroid dehydrogenase (type 1) that favors the production of testosterone and estradiol from androstenedione and estrone, respectively. However, in the liver, another form of this enzyme (type 2) favors oxidation of circulating estradiol to estrone (Peltoketo *et al.*, 1999), and both of these steroids are then converted to estriol (*see* Figure 58–1). All three of these estrogens are then excreted in the urine along with their glucuronide and sulfate conjugates. In postmenopausal women, the principal source of estrogen is adipose tissue stroma and other nonovarian sites, where estrone is synthesized from dehydroepiandrosterone, secreted by the adrenal cortex. In men, estrogens are produced by the testes, but extragonadal production by aromatization of circulating C 19 steroids such as androstenedione and dehydroepiandrosterone appears to account for the majority of circulating estrogenic hormones. Thus, the level of estrogens is regulated in part by the availability of androgenic precursors (Mendelson and Simpson, 1987).

Estrogenic effects most often have been attributed to circulating hormones, but locally produced estrogens also may have important actions (Simpson *et al.*, 1999). For example, estrogens may be produced from androgens by the actions of aromatase or from estrogen conjugates by hydrolysis. Such local production of estrogens could play a causal role in the development of certain diseases such as breast cancer, since mammary tumors contain both aromatase and hydrolytic enzymes. Estrogens also may be produced from androgens *via* aromatase present in the central nervous system (CNS) and other tissues and exert local effects near the site of their production; in the testes, they affect spermatogenesis, and in bone, they have major effects on bone mineral density.

Large quantities of estrogens are synthesized by the placenta, which uses fetal dehydroepiandrosterone and its 16α-hydroxyl derivative to produce estrone and estriol, respectively; human urine of pregnancy is thus an abundant source of natural estrogens. The pregnant mare excretes more than 100 mg daily, a record exceeded only by the stallion, who, despite clear manifestations of virility, excretes into his environment more estrogen than any other living creature.

Physiological and Pharmacological Actions

Developmental Actions. The estrogens are largely responsible for the changes that take place at puberty in girls and account for the secondary sexual characteristics of females. By a direct action, they cause growth and development of the vagina, uterus, and fallopian tubes. Estrogens act in concert with other hormones to cause enlargement of the breasts through promotion of ductal growth, stromal development, and the accretion of fat. They also contribute in a poorly understood manner to molding the body contours, shaping the skeleton, and bringing about the pubertal growth spurt of the long bones and its culmination by fusion of the epiphyses. Growth of axillary and pubic hair and pigmentation of the genital region also are effects of estrogen, as are the regional pigmentation of the nipples and areolae that occur after the first trimester of pregnancy.

While sexual development in females appears to be due primarily to estrogens, androgens may play a secondary role. Testosterone and androstenedione are normally found in venous ovarian blood (*see* Chapter 59); these may contribute to pubertal changes in girls, such as growth spurts, the full development of pubic and axillary hair, and the appearance of acne due to growth and secretions from the sebaceous glands.

It has been recognized only recently that estrogens appear to play important developmental roles in males. In boys, estrogen deficiency does not affect the age of pubertal onset, but the pubertal growth spurt is diminished, skeletal maturation and epiphyseal closure are delayed, and linear growth continues into adulthood. Estrogen deficiency in men also leads to hypergonadotropism, macroorchidism, and increased testosterone levels and also may affect carbohydrate and lipid metabolism and fertility in some individuals (Grumbach and Auchus, 1999).

Neuroendocrine Control of the Menstrual Cycle. The menstrual cycle in women is controlled by a neuroendocrine cascade involving the hypothalamus, pituitary, and ovaries, as illustrated in Figure 58–2. A neuronal oscillator or "clock" in the hypothalamus fires at regular intervals, resulting in the periodic release of gonadotropin-releasing hormone (GnRH) into the hypothalamic-pituitary portal vasculature (*see* Chapter 56). The GnRH then interacts with its cognate receptor on gonadotropes and causes the release of luteinizing hormone (LH) and follicle-stimulating

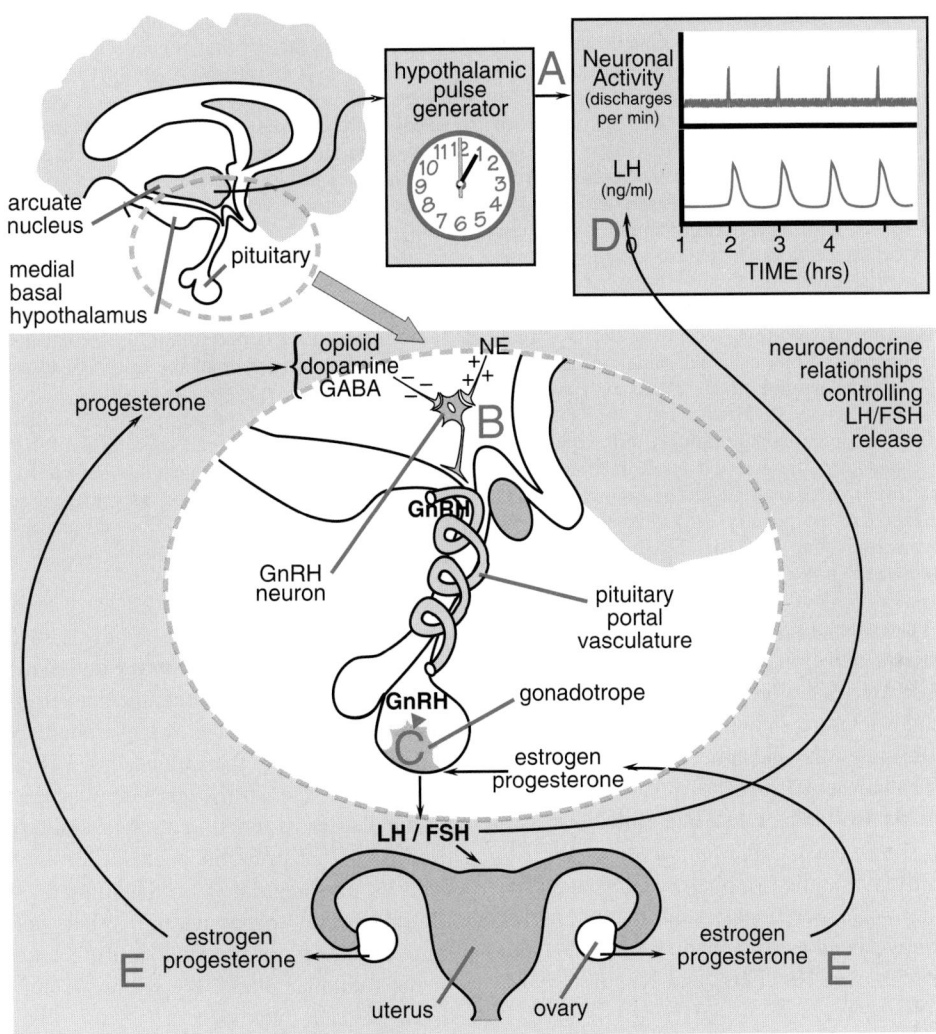

Figure 58–2. Neuroendocrine control of gonadotropin secretion in females.

The hypothalamic pulse generator located in the arcuate nucleus of the hypothalamus functions as a neuronal "clock" that fires at regular hourly intervals **(A)**. This results in the periodic release of gonadotropin-releasing hormone (GnRH) from GnRH-containing neurons into the hypothalamic-pituitary portal vasculature **(B)**. GnRH neurons **(B)** receive inhibitory input from opioid, dopamine, and gamma-aminobutyric acid (GABA) neurons and stimulatory input from noradrenergic neurons (NE, norepinephrine). The pulses of GnRH trigger the intermittent release of luteinizing hormone (LH) and follicle-stimulating hormone (FSH) from pituitary gonadotropes **(C)**, resulting in a pulsatile plasma profile **(D)**. FSH and LH regulate ovarian production of estrogen and progesterone, which exert feedback controls **(E)**. (*See* text and Figure 58–3 for additional details.)

hormone (FSH) from the anterior pituitary. The gonadotropins (LH and FSH) are responsible for the growth and maturation of the graafian follicle in the ovary and for the ovarian production of estrogen and progesterone, which exert feedback regulation on the pituitary and hypothalamus.

Because the release of GnRH is intermittent, LH and FSH release is pulsatile as determined by the neural

"clock" (Figure 58–2), which is referred to as the hypothalamic GnRH pulse generator (Knobil, 1981; Wilson *et al.,* 1984). The intermittent, *pulsatile* nature of hormone release is *essential* for the maintenance of normal ovulatory menstrual cycles, since *constant* infusion of GnRH results in a cessation of LH and FSH release, a decrease of estradiol and progesterone production, and amenorrhea (*see* Chapter 56).

It is not clear if the regular, intermittent discharges of the pulse generator are an intrinsic property of GnRH neurons or if other neurons that synapse on GnRH cells exert the pacemaker function. Neuroanatomically, the pulse generator resides in the arcuate nucleus of the hypothalamus, and this region of the brain contains the highest concentration of GnRH neurons. The pulse generator is not dependent on afferent input from other regions of the brain to maintain its pulsatile activity. The hypothalamus has relatively few GnRH-containing cells, and there is no obvious GnRH network. It is thus unclear how this small number of cells scattered bilaterally throughout the arcuate nucleus fires simultaneously. Most GnRH cells appear to be devoid of estrogen or progesterone receptors, but they may receive synaptic input from opioid, catecholamine, and gamma-aminobutyric acid (GABA) neurons that express receptors for the ovarian steroids (*see* Figure 58–2).

Prior to puberty, the hypothalamic GnRH pulse generator does not function, gonadotropin secretion is absent, and menstrual cycles do not occur. Unknown physiological mechanisms that take place at the onset of puberty activate the pulse generator. Following this activation, the LH, FSH, estradiol, and progesterone profiles seen in the menstrual cycle occur.

Figure 58–3 provides a schematic diagram of the profiles of gonadotropin and gonadal steroid secretion during the menstrual cycle. The "average" plasma levels of LH throughout the cycle are shown in panel *A* of Figure 58–3; panel *B* illustrates the pulsatile patterns of LH in more detail. Note that the *average* LH levels are similar throughout the early (follicular) and late (luteal) phases of the cycle, but the *frequency* and *amplitude* of the LH pulses are quite different in the two phases. This characteristic pattern of hormone secretions results from complex positive and negative feedback mechanisms (for a more comprehensive review, *see* Hotchkiss and Knobil, 1994).

In the early follicular phase of the cycle: (1) the pulse generator produces a burst of neuronal activity with a frequency of about 1 per hour resulting in the liberation of GnRH; (2) this causes a corresponding pulsatile release of LH and FSH from pituitary gonadotropes, and FSH in particular; (3) which causes the graafian follicle to mature and secrete estrogen. The effects of estrogens on the pituitary are inhibitory at this time. Therefore, as estrogen levels increase, the steroid reduces the amount of LH and FSH released from the pituitary (*i.e.*, the amplitude of the LH pulse), and gonadotropin levels gradually decline, as seen in Figure 58–3. *Inhibin,* produced by the ovary, also exerts a negative feedback and decreases serum FSH levels at this time (*see* Chapter 56).

At midcycle, a different set of regulatory interactions comes into play. At this time, serum estradiol rises above a threshold level of 150 to 200 pg/ml for approximately 36 hours. This *sustained elevation* of estrogen no longer inhibits gonadotropin release but exerts a brief *positive feedback* effect on the pituitary to trigger the preovulatory surge of LH and FSH. This effect involves a change in pituitary responsiveness to GnRH, but whether or not estrogens also exert a positive effect on hypothalamic neurons that contributes to the "surge" of GnRH release at midcycle in primates is not yet resolved.

The actions of estrogen and progesterone on the pituitary are the major factors that regulate the amount of LH released in each pulse (*i.e.*, the amplitude of LH pulses). However, only progesterone has a physiological effect on the frequency of LH release; it decreases the frequency of firing of the hypothalamic pulse generator. These feedback effects of steroids, coupled with the intrinsic activity of the hypothalamic GnRH pulse generator, produce relatively frequent LH pulses of small amplitude in the follicular phase of the cycle and less frequent pulses of larger amplitude in the luteal phase.

In males, the hypothalamic pulse generator also fires and releases GnRH in an episodic fashion, which causes the pulsatile release of LH *necessary* for normal testosterone production by the Leydig cells of the testis. Testosterone regulates the hypothalamic-pituitary-gonadal axis at both the hypothalamic and pituitary levels, and its negative feedback effect is mediated to a substantial degree by estrogen formed *via* aromatization. Thus, exogenous estrogen administration decreases LH and testosterone levels in men, and antiestrogens such as clomiphene cause an elevation of serum LH, which can be used as a provocative test to evaluate the reproductive axis in men.

In cycling women, the midcycle surge in gonadotropins stimulates follicular rupture and ovulation within 1 to 2 days. The ruptured follicle then develops into the corpus luteum, which produces large amounts of progesterone and estrogen under the influence of LH during the second half of the cycle. In the absence of pregnancy, the corpus luteum ceases to function after several days, steroid levels drop, and menstruation occurs. The luteal phase of the cycle is thus regulated by the limited 14-day functional lifetime of the corpus luteum. When steroid levels drop, the pulse generator reverts to a firing pattern characteristic of the follicular phase, the entire system then resets, and a new ovarian cycle occurs.

Increased progesterone levels during the luteal phase of the cycle affect both the frequency and amplitude of LH pulses. Progesterone directly decreases the frequency of the hypothalamic pulse generator, which in turn decreases the frequency of LH pulses released from the pituitary. Progesterone also exerts a direct effect on the pituitary to oppose the inhibitory actions of estrogens and thus increase the amount of LH released (*i.e.*, the amplitude of the LH pulses).

When the ovaries are removed or cease to function, there is overproduction of FSH and LH, which are excreted in the urine. Measurement of urinary or plasma LH is a valuable clinical test and can be used to assess pituitary function and to show the effectiveness of replacement doses of estrogen, which will elicit a decline in LH levels. Although FSH levels will decline once hormone-replacement therapy is initiated, they do not return to normal, secondary to production of inhibin by the ovary (*see* Chapter 56). Consequently, the measurement of FSH

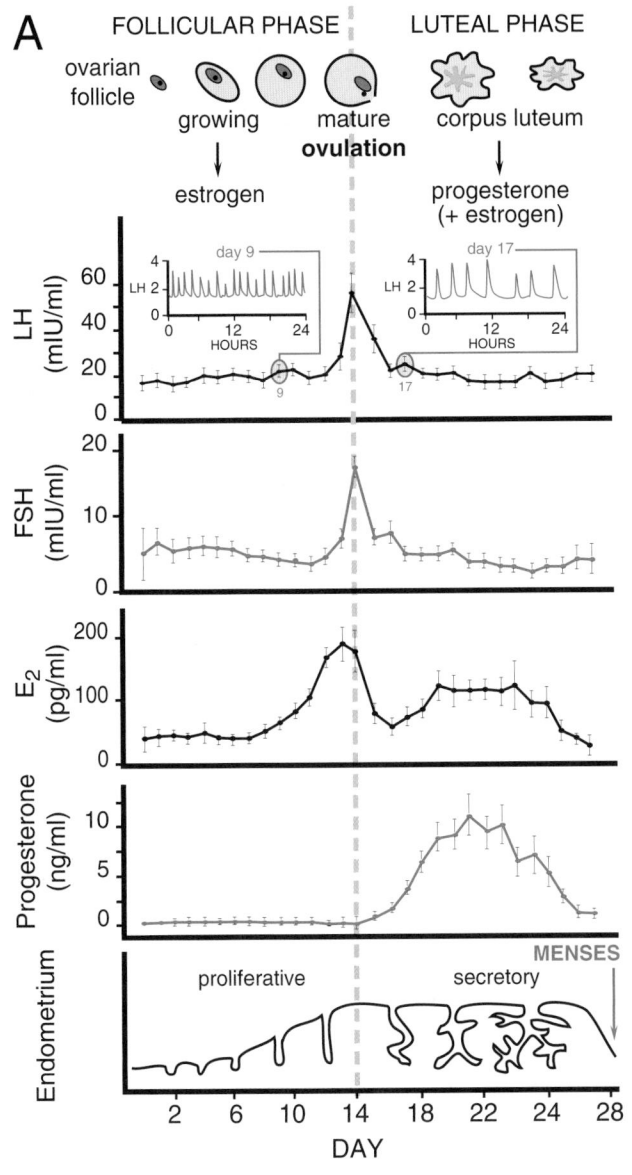

Figure 58–3. *Hormonal relationships of the human menstrual cycle.*

A. Average daily values of LH, FSH, estradiol (E$_2$), and progesterone in plasma samples from women exhibiting normal 28-day menstrual cycles. Changes in the ovarian follicle (*top*) and endometrium (*bottom*) also are illustrated schematically.

Frequent plasma sampling reveals pulsatile patterns of gonadotropin release. Characteristic profiles are illustrated schematically for the follicular phase (day 9, inset on left) and luteal phase (day 17, inset on right). Both the frequency (number of pulses per hour) and amplitude (extent of change of hormone release) of pulses vary throughout the cycle. (*Redrawn with permission from Thorneycroft* et al., *1971.*)

B. Major regulatory effects of ovarian steroids on hypothalamic-pituitary function. Estrogen decreases the amount of follicle stimulating hormone (FSH) and luteinizing hormone (LH) released (*i.e.,* gonadotropin pulse amplitude) during most of the cycle and triggers a surge of LH release only at midcycle. Progesterone decreases the frequency of GnRH release from the hypothalamus and thus decreases the frequency of plasma gonadotropin pulses. Progesterone also increases the amount of LH released (*i.e.,* the pulse amplitude) during the luteal phase of the cycle.

levels as a means to monitor the effectiveness of hormone-replacement therapy is not clinically useful.

Additional features of the regulation of gonadotropin secretion and actions are discussed in Chapters 56 and 59.

Effects of Cyclical Gonadal Steroids on the Reproductive Tract. The cyclical changes in estrogen and progesterone production by the ovaries regulate corresponding events in the fallopian tubes, uterus, cervix, and vagina. Physiologically, these changes prepare the uterus for implantation if the ovum is fertilized, and the proper timing of events in these tissues is essential for a successful pregnancy. If pregnancy does not occur, the endometrium is shed and is visible externally as the menstrual discharge.

The uterus is composed of an endometrium and a myometrium. The endometrium contains an epithelium lining the uterine cavity and an underlying stroma; the myometrium is the smooth muscle component responsible for uterine contractions. These cell layers, the fallopian tubes, cervix, and vagina display a characteristic set of responses to both estrogens and progestins. The changes typically associated with menstruation occur largely in the endometrium, which is shed during the menstrual discharge or menses (*see* Figure 58–3).

The endometrium is the mucosa that lines the uterine cavity. The luminal surface of the endometrium is a layer of simple columnar epithelial secretory and ciliated cells. This epithelium is continuous with the openings of numerous glands that extend through the underlying stroma to the myometrial border. The endometrial epithelium connects distally to the mucus-secreting epithelium of the endocervix and proximally to the epithelium of the fallopian tube. Fertilization normally occurs in the fallopian tubes, so ovulation, transport of the fertilized ovum through the fallopian tube, and preparation of the endometrial surface must be temporally coordinated if successful implantation is to occur.

The endometrial stroma is a highly cellular connective tissue layer containing a variety of blood vessels that undergo cyclic changes associated with menstruation. The predominant cells in the stroma are fibroblasts, but substantial numbers of macrophages, lymphocytes, and other resident and migratory cell types also are present.

By convention, menstruation is considered to mark the start of the menstrual cycle. During the follicular (or proliferative) phase of the cycle, estrogen begins the rebuilding of the endometrium by stimulating proliferation and differentiation: numerous mitoses become visible, the thickness of the layer increases, and characteristic changes occur in the glands and blood vessels of the tissue. These and subsequent effects of estrogens and progesterone are thought to be mediated in large part by the steroidal regulation of peptide growth factors and their cognate receptors that exert autocrine and paracrine actions in the endometrium. An important response to estrogen in the endometrium and other tissues is induction of the progesterone receptor, which enables cells to respond to this hormone during the second half of the cycle.

In the luteal (or secretory) phase of the cycle, progesterone levels increase sharply due to secretion from the corpus luteum, and estrogens remain elevated. Progesterone limits the proliferative effect of estrogens on the endometrium by stimulating differentiation. Major effects include stimulation of secretions of the epithelium important for implantation of the blastocyst (the fertilized ovum at this stage of development) and its growth and promotion of the characteristic growth of the endometrial blood vessels seen at this time. Progesterone is thus important in preparation for implantation and for the changes that take place in the uterus at the implantation site (*i.e.*, the decidual response). There is a rather narrrow "window of implantation," generally considered to span days 19 or 20 through day 24 of the endometrial cycle, when the epithelial cells of the endometrium are receptive to implantation of the blastocyst. Since endometrial status is regulated by estrogens and progestins, the efficacy of some contraceptives may be due in part to production of an endometrial surface that is not receptive to implantation. If pregnancy does not occur, the corpus luteum regresses due to lack of continued LH secretion, estrogen and progesterone levels fall, the endometrium cannot be maintained, and it is shed, resulting in the menstrual discharge as illustrated in Figure 58–3.

If implantation occurs, human chorionic gonadotropin (hCG; *see* Chapter 56), produced initially by the trophoblast cells of the blastocyst and later by the placenta, interacts with the LH receptor of the corpus luteum to maintain steroid hormone synthesis during the early stages of pregnancy. In the later stages of pregnancy, the placenta becomes the major site of estrogen and progesterone synthesis.

Estrogens and progesterone have important effects on the fallopian tube, myometrium, and cervix. In the fallopian tube, estrogens stimulate proliferation and differentiation, whereas progesterone inhibits these processes. Also, estrogens increase and progesterone decreases tubal muscular contractility, which affects transit time of the ovum to the uterus. Estrogens increase the amount and water content of cervical mucus and facilitate sperm penetration of the cervix, while progesterone generally has opposite effects. Estrogens favor rhythmic contractions of the uterine myometrium, while progesterone diminishes contractions. These effects are physiologically important and may contribute to some of the contraceptive actions of estrogens and progestins.

Metabolic Effects. Estrogens affect many tissues and have many metabolic actions in human beings and animals. It is not clear in all cases if effects result directly from hormone actions on the tissue in question or secondarily from actions at other sites. However, it is now clear that many nonreproductive tissues (*e.g.*, bone, vascular endothelium, liver, CNS, and heart) express low levels of estrogen receptors. Many metabolic effects of estrogens thus may result directly from receptor-mediated events in affected organs. While estrogens produce many metabolic responses, their effects on selected aspects of mineral, lipid, carbohydrate, and protein metabolism are particularly important for understanding their pharmacological actions.

It has long been recognized that estrogens have positive effects on bone mass (reviewed by Riggs and Melton, 1992). Bone is continuously remodeled at sites called bone-remodeling units by the resorptive action of osteo-clasts and the bone-forming action of osteoblasts (*see* Chapter 62). Maintenance in total bone mass requires equal rates of formation and resorption as occurs in early adulthood (18 to 40 years); thereafter resorption predominates. Osteoclasts and osteoblasts contain functional ERs, androgen receptors (ARs), and progesterone receptors (PRs). Estrogens directly regulate osteoblasts and increase the synthesis of collagen type I, osteocalcin, osteopontin, osteonectin, alkaline phosphatase, and other markers of differentiated osteoblasts. However, the major effect of estrogens is to decrease the numbers and activity of osteoclasts. Much of the action of estrogens on osteo-clasts appears to be mediated by altering cytokine (both paracrine and autocrine) signals from osteoblasts. Estrogens decrease osteoblast and stromal cell production of the osteoclast-stimulating cytokines interleukin (IL)-1, IL-6, and tumor necrosis factor (TNF)-α and increase the production of insulin-like growth factor (IGF)-1, bone morphogenic protein (BMP)-6, and transforming growth factor (TGF)-β which are antiresorptive (reviewed by Spelsberg *et al.,* 1999). Estrogens also increase osteoblast production of the cytokine osteoprotegrin (OPG), a soluble non-membrane-bound member of the TNF superfamily. OPG acts as a "decoy" receptor and antagonizes the binding of osteoprotegrin-ligand (OPG-L) to its receptor (termed RANK, or **r**eceptor **a**ctivator of **NF-K**appa B) and prevents the differentiation of osteoclast precursors to mature osteoclasts (Hofbauer *et al.,* 2000). In addition, there are direct actions of estrogens on osteoclasts to increase the rate of apoptosis, which leads to a reduced number of osteoclasts. Estrogens affect bone growth and epiphyseal closure in both sexes. The importance of estrogen in the male skeleton is illustrated in a man with a completely defective ER who had osteoporosis, unfused epiphyses, increased bone turnover, and delayed bone age (Smith *et al.,* 1994) and in the observation that male idiopathic osteoporosis is associated with reduced ER-α expression (Braidman *et al.,* 2000) in both osteocytes and osteoblasts.

Estrogens have many effects on lipid metabolism; of major interest are their effects on serum lipoprotein and triglyceride levels (Lobo, 1991; Walsh *et al.,* 1994). In general, estrogens slightly elevate serum triglycerides and slightly reduce total serum cholesterol levels. However, the more important actions are thought to be an increase in high-density lipoprotein (HDL) levels and a decrease in low-density lipoprotein (LDL) values and lipoprotein (a) [Lp(a)] (*see* Chapter 36). This beneficial ratio of HDL to LDL is an attractive side effect of estrogen therapy in postmenopausal women. The presence of estrogen re-ceptors in the liver suggests that the beneficial effects of estrogen on lipoprotein metabolism are due in part to direct hepatic actions. Other sites of action, however, cannot be excluded. In addition to these effects on serum lipids, estrogens alter bile composition by increasing cholesterol secretion and decreasing bile acid secretion. This leads to increased saturation of bile with cholesterol and appears to be the basis for increased gallstone formation in some women receiving estrogens.

Estrogen alone appears to slightly decrease fasting levels of glucose and insulin (Barrett-Connor and Laakso, 1990) but does not appear to have major effects on carbohydrate metabolism. Some older studies of combined oral contraceptives (which contained higher levels of both estrogens and progestins than available now) suggested that estrogens might impair glucose tolerance, but it is uncertain whether these effects were due to the progestational or the estrogenic component of the older combined oral contraceptives.

Estrogens have effects on many serum proteins, particularly those involved in hormone binding and clotting cascades. In general, estrogens tend to increase plasma levels of cortisol-binding globulin (CBG or transcortin), thyroxine-binding globulin (TBG), and sex steroid–binding globulin (SSBG), which binds both androgens and estrogens.

Estrogens alter a number of metabolic pathways that affect the cardiovascular system (*see* Mendelsohn and Karas, 1999). Systemic effects include changes in lipoprotein metabolism and in hepatic production of plasma proteins. Estrogens cause a small increase in coagulation factors VII and XII and decrease the anticoagulation factors protein C, protein S, and antithrombin III. Fibrinolytic pathways also are affected, and several studies in women treated with estrogen alone or estrogen with a progestin have demonstrated decreased levels of plasminogen-activator inhibitor protein I (PAI-1) with a concomitant increase in fibrinolysis (Koh *et al.,* 1997). Thus, both coagulation and fibrinolytic pathways are increased by estrogens, and imbalance in these two opposing activities may cause adverse effects. At relatively high concentrations, estrogens have antioxidant activity and may inhibit the oxidation of LDL (Sack *et al.,* 1994) by affecting superoxide dismutase. Long-term administration of estrogen is associated with decreased plasma renin, angiotensin converting enzyme, and endothelin-1; angiotensin-1 receptor expression is decreased. Estrogen actions on the vascular wall include increased production of nitric oxide, which occurs within minutes, and induction of inducible nitric oxide synthase and increased production of prostacyclin, which occur more slowly. All of these changes promote vasodilation. Estrogens also promote endothelial cell growth while inhibiting the proliferation of vascular smooth muscle cells.

Estrogen Receptors

Estrogens exert their effects by interaction with receptors that are members of the superfamily of nuclear receptors (Chapter 2). There are two distinct estrogen receptors, ER α and ER β, which are products of separate genes. ER α, the first discovered, is located in highest abundance in the female reproductive tract—especially the uterus, vagina, and ovary—as well as in the mammary gland, the hypothalamus, endothelial cells, and vascular smooth muscle. ER β is expressed with a somewhat different tissue distribution, with highest expression in the prostate and ovaries and less expression in lung, brain, and vasculature. The two human ERs are 44% identical in overall amino-acid sequence (Figure 58–4) and share the domain structure common to members of this family. The estrogen receptor is divided into six functional domains: the NH₂-terminal A/B domain contains the activation function-1 (AF-1) segment, which can activate transcription independently of ligand; the highly conserved C domain comprises the DNA binding domain, which contains four cysteines arranged in two zinc fingers; the D domain, frequently called the "hinge region," contains the nuclear localization signal; and the E/F domain has multiple functions, including ligand binding, dimerization, and ligand-dependent transactivation, mediated by the AF-2 domain. As illustrated in Figure 58–4, there are significant differences between the two receptor isoforms in the ligand binding domains and in both transactivation domains. The receptors appear to have different biological functions and may respond differently to various estrogenic compounds. For example, while both receptors bind 17β estradiol with the same K_D (about 0.3 nM), the phytoestrogen genistein (Table 58–1) binds to ER β with about fivefold higher affinity than to ER α (Kuiper *et al.*, 1997). However, the high degree of identity in the DNA-binding domains indicates that both receptors probably recognize similar DNA sequences and hence regulate many of the same target genes.

Female transgenic mice homozygous for a disruption of ER α are infertile; they have atrophic uteri and hyperemic ovaries that appear to lack corpora lutea (Lubahn *et al.*, 1993) and lack uterotrophic responses to estradiol. Males lacking ER α also are infertile, with abnormal testes and seminiferous tubules and inactive sperm, reduced bone density, and cardiovascular abnormalities. Female ER β-null animals are infertile, with an arrest in follicular development; males are fertile (Korach, 2000).

Several variants of both ER α and ER β have been described, most frequently in breast cancer cells. These variants arise from use of alternate promoters or alternate splicing (Murphy *et al.*, 1997). Some of these variants may act in an estrogen-independent manner (Fuqua *et al.*, 1991), but their physiological significance is unclear. A truncated form of ER α that suppresses transactivation of the wild-type ER α and ER β has been identified in the rat pituitary (Resnick *et al.*, 2000), although its biological role and species distribution also are uncertain. Other variants of ER are caused by polymorphisms in the genes encoding the receptors, but attempts to correlate specific polymorphisms with the frequency of breast cancer (Roodi *et al.*, 1995), bone mass (Kobayashi *et al.*, 1996; Vandevyver *et al.*, 1999), or endometrial cancer (Weiderpass *et al.*, 2000) have led to contradictory results. Additional studies thus are required to determine how polymorphisms affect receptor structure and function and responses to estrogens.

Mechanism of Action

Both estrogen receptors are ligand-activated transcription factors that increase or decrease the synthesis of mRNA from target genes. After entering the cell by passive diffusion through the plasma membrane, the hormone binds to an ER in the nucleus. In the nucleus, the ER is present as a monomer, and upon binding estrogen, a change in conformation occurs that results in dimerization, which increases the affinity and the rate of receptor binding to DNA (Cheskis *et al.*, 1997). The ER binds to estrogen response elements (EREs) in target genes with the consensus sequence GGTCANNNTGACC.

The ER/DNA complex recruits one or more coactivator proteins to the promoter region (Figure 58–5B). The

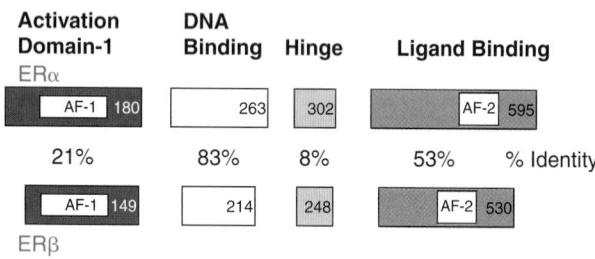

Figure 58–4. Domain structure and sequence identity between estrogen receptor (ER) α and ER β.

Nuclear hormone receptors can be divided into common functional domains. Activation function (AF)-1 and AF-2 represent transactivation domains. AF-2 is part of the carboxy terminal portion of the receptor, which is the region that also binds ligand. The highly conserved DNA-binding domain interacts with specific DNA sequences. Numbers within the boxes represent the last amino acid in a domain. The percentage of identical amino acids between functional domains in ER α and ER β is indicated.

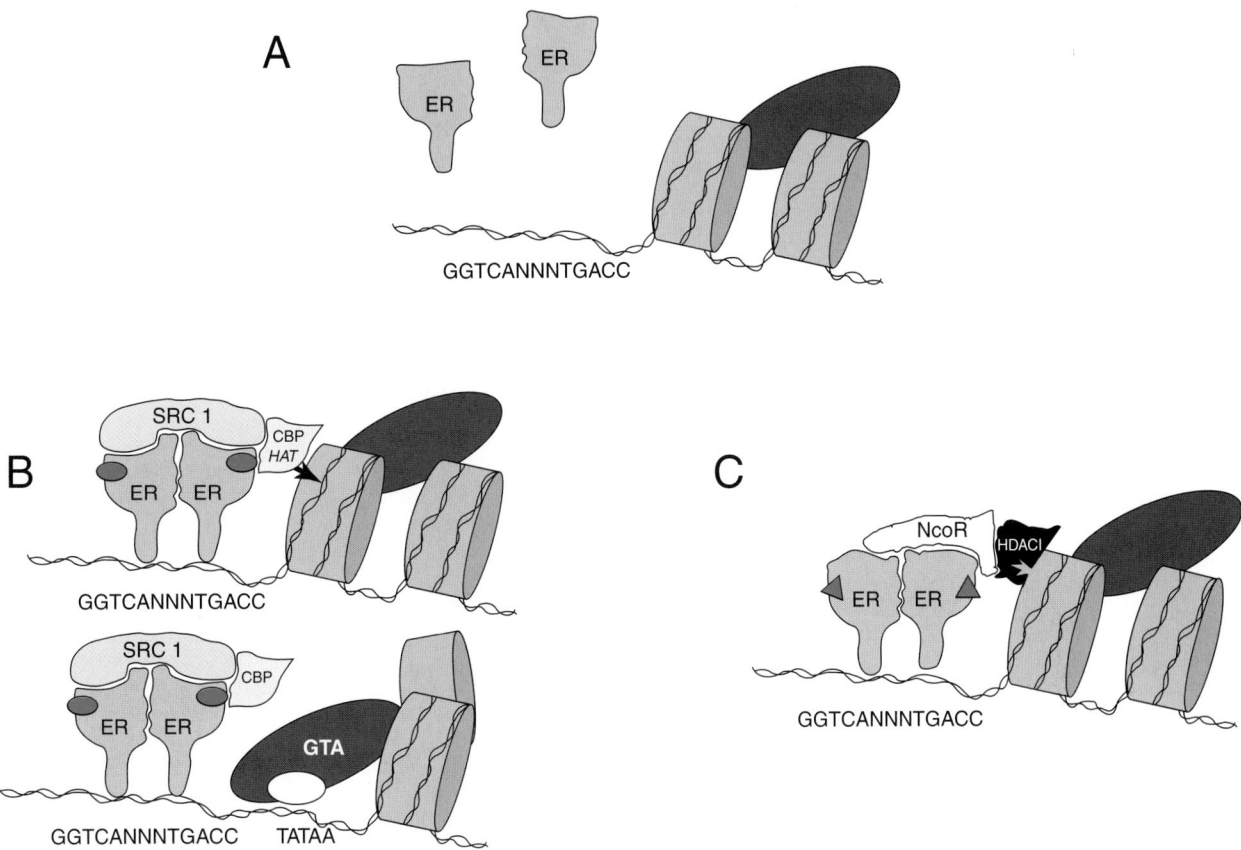

Figure 58–5.

A. Unliganded estrogen receptor (ER) exists as a monomer within the nucleus. *B.* Agonist (*blue oval*) binds to ER and causes a ligand-directed change in conformation that facilitates dimerization and interaction with specific estrogen response element (ERE) sequences in DNA. The ER-DNA complex recruits coactivators such as steroid-receptor coactivator-1 (SRC-1) and other proteins such as cyclic AMP–element binding protein (CBP) which have histone acetylase activity (HAT). Acetylation of histones can cause a rearrangement of the nucleosomes and facilitates the interaction of the proteins that make up the general transcription apparatus (GTA) with subsequent synthesis of mRNA. *C.* Antagonist (*blue triangles*) binding to ER produces a different receptor conformation. The antagonist-induced conformation also facilitates dimerization and interaction with DNA, but a different set of proteins called corepressors, such as nuclear-hormone receptor corepressor (NcoR), are recruited to the complex. NcoR further recruits proteins such as histone deacetylase I (HDAC1) that act on histone proteins to stabilize nucleosome structure and prevent interaction with the GTA.

best-characterized coactivators are SRC-1 (steroid-receptor coactivator-1) and CBP (cyclic AMP response-element binding protein) (Collingwood *et al.*, 1999). The coactivators have histone acetylase activity and/or recruit other proteins with this activity to the complex. Acetylation of histones alters chromatin structure in the promoter region of target genes and allows the proteins that make up the general transcription apparatus to assemble and initiate transcription. Interaction of ER with an antagonist also promotes dimerization and DNA binding. However, an antagonist produces a conformation of ER that is different from an agonist-occupied receptor (Wijayaratne *et al.*, 1999). The antagonist-induced conformation fa-

cilitates binding of corepressors such as NcoR/SMRT (nuclear hormone receptor corepressor/silencing mediator of retinoid and thyroid receptors) (Figure 58–5C). The corepressor/ER complex then further recruits other proteins with histone deacetylase activity such as HDAC1. Deacetylation of histones alters chromatin conformation and reduces the ability of the general transcription apparatus to form initiation complexes. The differences in the amino acid sequences of AF-1 and AF-2 in ER α and ER β suggest they interact with different specificity and affinity to coactivators and corepressors. Combined with the observation that ERα and ERβ can form homo- and heterodimers (Cowley *et al.*, 1997), a diverse array of different ER/coactivator or ER/corepressor proteins can be assembled on a target promoter. In cells that express both receptor isoforms, the action of ER β appears to oppose the activity of ER α (Hall and McDonnell, 1999).

Besides coactivators and corepressors, both ER α and ER β can interact physically with other transcription factors such as Sp1 (Saville *et al.*, 2000) or AP-1 (Paech *et al.*, 1997), and these protein-protein interactions provide an alternate mechanism of action. Binding of ER-ligand complexes to a target gene in these circumstances is directed by Sp1 or AP-1 binding to their specific regulatory sequences, rather than ER binding to ERE sequences. This may explain how estrogens are able to regulate genes that lack a consensus ERE. Responses to agonists and antagonists mediated by these protein-protein interactions also are ER isoform- and promoter-specific. For example, 17β-estradiol induces transcription of a target gene controlled by an AP-1 site in the presence of an ER α/AP-1 complex, but inhibits transcription in the presence of an ER β/AP-1 complex. Conversely, antiestrogens are potent activators of ER β/AP-1 but not of ER α/AP-1 complexes.

Other signaling systems may activate nuclear ER by ligand-independent mechanisms. Kato *et al.* (1995) demonstrated that phosphorylation of ER α at serine 118 by microtubule-associated protein kinase (MAPK) activates the receptor. This provides a means of cross-talk between membrane-bound receptor pathways (*i.e.*, EGF/IGF-1) that activate MAPK and the nuclear ER.

Several studies have suggested that a form of estrogen receptor other than the nuclear receptors might be located on the plasma membrane, but it is unclear whether or not these receptors are encoded by the same gene that encodes the nuclear ERs (Razandi *et al.*, 1999). These membrane-localized ERs may mediate the rapid activation of some proteins such as MAPK, which has been shown to be phosphorylated in several cell types within 5 to 10 minutes of 17β-estradiol addition (Endoh *et al.*, 1997), or the rapid increase in cyclic AMP caused by the hormone (Aronica and Katzenellenbogen, 1993). The finding that MAPK is activated by estradiol provides an additional level of cross-talk with growth factors such as IGF-1 and EGF that activate this kinase pathway. Membrane-localized ER also may be responsible for the rapid release of nitric oxide produced by estradiol treatment of endothelial cells.

Absorption, Fate, Elimination

Various estrogens are available for oral, parenteral, transdermal, or topical administration (*see* Table 58–1 for the structures of these agents). Given the lipophilic nature of estrogens, absorption generally is good with the appropriate preparation. Several preparations are available for oral use. Aqueous or oil-based esters of estradiol and estrone are available for intramuscular injection ranging in frequency from every several days to once per month. Transdermal patches that are changed once or twice weekly deliver estradiol (or a combination of estradiol and norethindrone acetate) continuously through the skin.

Several preparations are available for topical use in the vagina.

Oral administration is common and may utilize estradiol, conjugated estrogens, esters of estrone and other estrogens, and ethinyl estradiol. *Estradiol* itself was not used orally frequently because of extensive first-pass hepatic metabolism. A micronized preparation of estradiol (ESTRACE) that yields a large surface for rapid absorption is available now for oral administration, although high doses must be used because absolute bioavailability remains low (Fotherby, 1996). *Ethinyl estradiol* frequently is used orally, either alone (ESTINYL) or with a progestin in oral contraceptives; the ethinyl substitution in the C 17 position inhibits first-pass hepatic metabolism. The absorption of these estrogens from the gastrointestinal tract is rapid and generally complete. Other common oral preparations contain *conjugated equine estrogens* (PREMARIN), which are primarily the sulfate esters of estrone, equilin, and other naturally occurring compounds, *esterified esters* (ESTRATAB), or mixtures of conjugated estrogens prepared from plant-derived sources (CENESTIN). These are hydrolyzed by enzymes present in the lower gut that remove the charged sulfate groups and allow absorption of estrogen across the intestinal epithelium. In another oral preparation (*estropipate,* ORTHO-EST, OGEN), estrone is solubilized as the sulfate and stabilized with piperazine. Due largely to differences in metabolism, the potencies of various oral preparations differ widely; ethinyl estradiol, for example, is much more potent than conjugated estrogens.

A number of foodstuffs and plant-derived products, largely from soy, are available as nonprescription items and often are touted as providing benefits similar to those from compounds with established estrogenic activity. These products may contain flavonoids such as genistein (Figure 58–1), coumestans, and lignans, which have been reported to possess estrogenic activity in laboratory tests, albeit generally much less than that of estradiol. In theory, these preparations could produce appreciable estrogenic effects. However, their efficacy at relevant doses has not been established in human trials, and many of these products contain many other compounds besides phytoestrogens, which could contribute to any effects (Mäkelä *et al.*, 1999; Tham *et al.*, 1998).

Administration of estradiol *via* transdermal patches (ESTRADERM, VIVELLE, ALORA, others) provides slow, sustained release of the hormone, systemic distribution, and more constant blood levels than are obtained with oral doses. In addition, the transdermal route does not lead to the high level of the drug that enters the liver *via* the portal circulation after oral administration, which may explain why the two routes are associated with different effects on lipoprotein profiles (Walsh *et al.*, 1994, and the following section).

Other preparations are available for intramuscular injection. When dissolved in oil and injected, esters of estradiol are well absorbed. The aryl and alkyl esters of estradiol become less polar as the size of the substituents increases; correspondingly, the rate of absorption of oily preparations is progressively slowed, and the duration of action can be prolonged. A single therapeutic dose of compounds such as *estradiol valerate* (DELESTROGEN, VALERGEN, others) or *estradiol cypionate* (DEPO-ESTRADIOL CYPIONATE, others) may be absorbed over several weeks following a single intramuscular injection. Suspensions containing estrone or a combination of esters (primarily estrone and equilin sulfates) also may be given *via* intramuscular injection.

Preparations of estradiol and conjugated estrogens are available for topical administration to the vagina. These are effective locally, but systemic effects also are possible, since significant absorption can occur from this site (Rigg *et al.,* 1978). A 3-month vaginal ring (ESTRING) also is available for slow release of estradiol.

Estradiol, ethinyl estradiol, and other compounds exist in blood plasma extensively bound to plasma proteins. Estradiol and other naturally occurring estrogens are bound mainly to sex steroid–binding globulin (SSBG) and to a lesser degree to serum albumin. In contrast, ethinyl estradiol is bound extensively to serum albumin but not SSBG. Due to their size and lipophilic nature, unbound estrogens readily exit the plasma space and distribute extensively to tissue compartments.

Variations in estradiol metabolism occur and depend upon the stage of the menstrual cycle and whether the individual is pre- or postmenopausal. In general, the hormone undergoes rapid hepatic biotransformation, with a plasma half-life measured in minutes. Estradiol is converted primarily by 17β-hydroxysteroid dehydrogenase to estrone, which undergoes conversion by 16α-hydroxylation and 17-keto reduction to estriol, which is the major urinary metabolite. A variety of sulfate and glucuronide conjugates also are excreted in the urine. Lesser amounts of estrone or estradiol are oxidized to the 2-hydroxycatechols by CYP3A in the liver and by CYP1A in extrahepatic tissues or to 4-hydroxycatechols by CYP1B1 in extrahepatic sites, with the 2-hydroxycatechol being formed to a greater extent. The 2- and 4-hydroxycatechols are largely inactivated by catechol-*O*-methyl transfereases (COMT). However, smaller amounts may be converted by cytochrome P450- or peroxidase-catalyzed reactions to yield semiquinones or quinones that are capable of forming DNA adducts or of generating (*via* redox cycling) reactive oxygen species that could oxidize DNA bases (Liehr, 2000). Estrogens also undergo enterohepatic recirculation *via* (1) sulfate and glucuronide conjugation in the liver, (2) biliary secretion of the conjugates into the intestine, and (3) hydrolysis in the gut followed by reabsorption.

Ethinyl estradiol is cleared much more slowly than is estradiol due to decreased hepatic metabolism, and the elimination phase half-life has been reported in various studies to be 13 to 27 hours. Unlike estradiol, the primary route of biotransformation of ethinyl estradiol is *via* 2-hydroxylation and subsequent formation of the corresponding 2- and 3-methyl ethers. *Mestranol,* another semisynthetic estrogen and a component of some combination oral contraceptives, is the 3-methyl ether of ethinyl estradiol. In the body it undergoes rapid hepatic demethylation to ethinyl estradiol, which is its active form.

Measurements of plasma and urinary estrogens and their metabolites are used for a number of purposes. In the normal menstrual cycle, the mean daily excretion of estrogens at the midcycle ovulatory maximum is 25 to 100 μg; the second rise during the luteal phase is more prolonged, but the maximal rates of excretion are somewhat smaller (10 to 80 μg per day). After menopause, the average excretion of estrogens in normal women is about 5 to 10 μg daily, and estrogen synthesis occurs primarily from androgenic precursors in nonovarian tissues. The normal values for men are 2 to 25 μg per day, quantities about equal to the urinary estrogens of women during the first week of the menstrual cycle. No estrogen is detectable in the urine

of young children. During the first trimester of pregnancy, the placenta becomes the primary source of the urinary estrogens, which continue to increase and reach levels of about 30 mg per day near term. In the past, serial estrogen determinations were used to assess placental and fetal function. However, with the advent of fetal monitors, this is no longer done.

Untoward Responses

Estrogens are highly efficacious for most of their therapeutic purposes. Hence the decision about their use is largely a matter of analyzing the risk-to-benefit ratio for each patient. Historically, the major concerns about the use of estrogens have been cancer, thromboembolic disease, changes in carbohydrate and lipid metabolism, hypertension, gallbladder disease, nausea, migraine, changes in mood, and several lesser side effects.

The literature in this area is voluminous, complex, and often difficult to interpret, and a historical perspective is helpful to analyze risk-benefit issues for current preparations. First, many concerns arose initially from studies of early oral contraceptives, which contained higher doses of estrogens than used for other purposes—for example, hormone-replacement therapy in postmenopausal women. Since the untoward effects of estrogens are dose-dependent, the extrapolation of oral contraceptive side effects to other settings may not be appropriate. Second, it is recognized now that some of the deleterious effects of oral contraceptives originally attributed to estrogens are due to the progestational component. As a result of the recognition of the above two points, the amount of estrogens (and progestins) in oral contraceptives has been markedly decreased, and this has dramatically diminished the risks associated with current oral contraceptive preparations. Reports based on usage in the 1960s and 1970s established that unopposed estrogens caused endometrial carcinoma. Since these reports, however, estrogens have been used with progestins, which greatly diminish this risk. Finally, it is now recognized that the two major uses of estrogens, postmenopausal hormone replacement and contraception, have many substantial health benefits that previously were not appreciated.

Concern about Carcinogenic Actions. The possibility of developing cancer is probably the major concern for the use of estrogens and oral contraceptives. In several mammalian species, the administration of estrogens is followed by the development of certain tumors. Since the early studies of Lacassagne (1936), it has been known that estrogens can induce tumors of the breast, uterus, testis, bone, kidney, and several other tissues in various animal species.

These early studies disseminated a fear of cancer resulting from estrogen use.

In later reports (Greenwald *et al.,* 1971; Herbst *et al.,* 1971), an increased incidence of vaginal and cervical adenocarcinoma was noted in female offspring of mothers who had taken diethylstilbestrol (DES) during the first trimester of pregnancy. This may have resulted from the inability of the fetus to metabolize DES, leading to its accumulation in the fetus. The incidence of clear-cell vaginal and cervical adenocarcinoma in women who were exposed to estrogens *in utero* is only 0.01% to 0.1% (*FDA Drug Bulletin,* 1985), but these findings established for the first time that developmental exposure to estrogens was associated with an increase in a human cancer. Estrogen use during pregnancy also can increase the incidence of nonmalignant genital abnormalities in both male and female offspring. Thus, pregnant patients should not be given estrogens because of the possibility of such reproductive tract toxicities. While DES and other estrogens are no longer given intentionally to pregnant women, there is a concern that exposure during pregnancy to environmental substances with estrogenic activity may cause developmental abnormalities in the fetus (Mäkelä *et al.,* 1999).

Other studies established that the use of unopposed estrogen for hormone replacement in postmenopausal women is associated with the development of endometrial carcinoma (Shapiro *et al.,* 1985). The risk is estimated to be increased as much as 5- to 15-fold by estrogen, depending upon the dose and duration of use, but it declines to normal several years after discontinuation of estrogen. Other studies indicate a lower incidence of endometrial carcinoma when low doses of estrogen are combined with a progestin (Pike *et al.,* 1997).

The association between estrogen use and breast cancer remains uncertain. Part of the difficulty arises because of the frequency of the disease (about 1 in 8 in women who live 85 years) and the finding that 50% of women who develop the disease have no identifiable risk factors other than being female and aging. This makes determination of the association between estrogen use and breast cancer more difficult. An analysis of data from 51 epidemiologic studies of more than 150,000 women (Collaborative Group on Hormonal Factors in Breast Cancer, 1997) found that the risk of breast cancer increased slightly more than 2% for each year of estrogen-replacement therapy if treatment lasted between 1 and 4 years; treatment for more than 5 years had an accumulated risk of 35%. Lean women were at greater risk than heavier women. Recent studies have established that the progestin component in hormone-replacement therapy may play a major role in this increased risk of breast cancer (Schairer *et al.,* 2000; Ross

et al., 2000). Inclusion of the progestin component, administered either continuously or during only part of the estrogen treatment cycle, increased risk by about fourfold over estrogen-only use. Importantly, excess risk of breast cancer appears to be eliminated 5 years after cessation of hormone-replacement therapy.

Historically, the carcinogenic actions of estrogens were thought to be related to their trophic effects by one of two mechanisms. First, an increase in cell proliferation would be expected to cause an increase in spontaneous errors associated with DNA replication. Second, after mutations were introduced into target cells by this or other mechanisms (*e.g.,* chemical carcinogens), estrogens would enhance the replication of clones carrying such genetic errors. More recently, a third potential mechanism related to estrogen metabolism has been proposed. If catechol estrogens, especially the 4-hydroxycatechols, are converted to semiquinones or quinones prior to "inactivation" by COMT, these products, or reactive oxygen species generated during subsequent biotransformations, may cause direct chemical damage to DNA bases. In this regard, CYP1B1, which has specific estrogen-4-hydroxylase activity, is present in tissues such as uterus, breast, ovary, and prostate, which often give rise to hormone-responsive cancers (Liehr, 2000).

Metabolic and Cardiovascular Effects. Estrogens themselves generally have favorable overall effects on plasma lipoprotein profiles, although they may slightly elevate plasma triglycerides. (However, as noted in a later section dealing with hormone-replacement regimens, progestins may reduce the favorable actions of estrogens.) In contrast, estrogens do increase cholesterol levels in bile and cause a relative increase of two- to threefold in gallbladder disease.

Oral estrogens increase the risk of venous thromboembolism about threefold in healthy women (Jick *et al.,* 1996), appear to reduce the risk of cardiovascular disease (Grodstein *et al.,* 1996; Henderson *et al.,* 1991), and increase the relative risk of stroke by a factor of 1.35. In women with a history of cardiovascular disease, a threefold increase in the risk of venous thromboembolism but no reduction in the incidence of secondary cardiovascular events has been reported (Grady *et al.,* 2000; Hulley *et al.,* 1998). Currently prescribed doses of estrogens do not increase the risk of hypertension.

Other Potential Untoward Effects. Nausea and vomiting are an initial reaction to estrogen therapy in some women, but these effects may disappear with time and may be minimized by taking estrogens with food or just prior to sleeping. Fullness and tenderness of the breasts and edema may occur but sometimes can be diminished by lowering the dose. A more serious concern is that estrogens may cause severe migraine in some women. Estrogens also may reactivate or exacerbate endometriosis and its attendant pain.

Therapeutic Uses

Estrogens are among the most commonly prescribed drugs in the United States. By far the two major uses are as a component of combination oral contraceptives (covered in a following section) and for hormone-replacement therapy in postmenopausal women. In addition they are used less frequently for a variety of other purposes. As already noted, the risk-to-benefit ratio is generally the major issue when considering their therapeutic use, as they are generally highly efficacious.

The pharmacological considerations for estrogen use in oral contraceptives and postmenopausal hormone replacement are substantially different, primarily because of the doses used in the two settings. Historically, *conjugated estrogens* have been the most common agents for postmenopausal use, and 0.625 mg/day is effective in most women (although 1.25 mg is used if needed in some patients). In contrast, most combination oral contraceptives in current use employ 20 to 35 μg/day of *ethinyl estradiol*. Conjugated estrogens and ethinyl estradiol differ widely in their oral potencies; for example, a dose of 0.625 mg of conjugated estrogens generally is considered equivalent to 5 to 10 μg of ethinyl estradiol.

It is important to recognize that the dose of estrogen used for postmenopausal hormone-replacement therapy is substantially less than that used in oral contraception, taking into account the different potencies of the drugs normally employed in the two settings. Since the untoward effects of estrogens are dose-dependent, the incidence and severity of side effects reported for oral contraceptives may be far greater than those for hormone replacement. In addition, much of the epidemiological literature examining the side effects of oral contraceptives is derived from studies of older preparations that generally contained 50 to 150 μg of mestranol or ethinyl estradiol rather than 20- to 35-μg doses most commonly used at present.

Postmenopausal Hormone-Replacement Therapy. The decline in the secretion of estrogen by the ovary is a slow and gradual process that continues for some years after menstruation has ceased (*see* Eskin, 1978). It is a frequent observation that menopausal symptoms are more severe following abrupt removal of estrogens, such as with oophorectomy, than with natural menopause. Of primary importance in the treatment of postmenopausal women with estrogens are the prevention of bone loss and the

amelioration of vasomotor systems, which are established benefits of replacement therapy.

Osteoporosis. Osteoporosis is a disorder of the skeleton associated with the loss of both hydroxyapatite (calcium phosphate complexes) and protein matrix or colloid (*see* Chapter 62 for additional information). The result is thinning and weakening of the bones and an increased incidence of fractures, particularly compression fractures of the vertebrae and minimal trauma fractures of the hip and wrist. The frequency and severity of these fractures and their associated complications are a *major* public health problem, especially as the population continues to age. Twenty percent of patients who sustain hip fractures die within the first 12 months following the fracture, and many others are permanently disabled. Osteoporosis is a major indication for estrogen replacement therapy, and it is clearly efficacious for this purpose.

The primary mechanism by which estrogens act is to decrease bone resorption, and consequently estrogens are more effective at *preventing* rather than *restoring* bone loss (Prince *et al.,* 1991; Belchetz, 1994). Estrogens are most effective if treatment is initiated before significant bone loss occurs, and their beneficial effects require continuous use; bone loss resumes when treatment is discontinued. An appropriate diet with adequate calcium and vitamin D intake and weight-bearing exercise support the effects of estrogen treatment. Higher doses of estrogens may lead to some increase in bone mass, and combinations of estrogens with calcium, fluoride, and/or other agents that increase bone mass are under study. Public health efforts to improve diet and exercise patterns in girls and young women also are rational approaches to increase bone mass prior to the onset of postmenopausal osteoporosis.

Vasomotor Symptoms. The decline in ovarian function at menopause is associated with vasomotor symptoms in most women due to deficiency of estrogen. The characteristic hot flashes may alternate with chilly sensations, inappropriate sweating, and paresthesias. Treatment with estrogen is specific and very effective (Belchetz, 1994), but if the drug is contraindicated or otherwise undesirable, other options may be considered (Young *et al.,* 1990). Medroxyprogesterone acetate (discussed in the later section on progestins) may provide some relief of vasomotor symptoms for certain patients, and the α_2-adrenergic agonist clonidine diminishes vasomotor symptoms in some women, presumably by blocking the CNS outflow that regulates blood flow to cutaneous vessels. In many women, hot flashes diminish within several years.

Prevention of Cardiovascular Disease. In past years, prevention of osteoporosis, hot flashes, and other symptoms associated with menopause were considered the major benefits of estrogen replacement. However, it is now clear that the leading cause of death in women in the United States over 65 years old is cardiovascular disease, particularly myocardial infarction. The incidence of cardiovascular disease due to atherosclerosis is low in premenopausal women, rises after menopause, and is reduced to premenopausal levels after estrogen-replacement therapy (*see* Mendelsohn and Karas, 1999). The protective effects of estrogen are mediated in part by systemic changes in lipoprotein metabolism as well as by direct effects of estrogens on blood vessels. Estrogens promote vasodilation, inhibit the response to vascular injury, and reduce atherosclerosis (*see* Mendelsohn and Karas, 1999). Estrogens accelerate endothelial cell growth both *in vivo* and *in vitro;* this may be due to estrogen-induced production of vascular endothelial growth factor within vessels. Estrogens participate in vascular protection by stimulating the proliferation and activity of endothelial cells and inhibiting the growth and migration of vascular smooth muscle cells. Numerous retrospective and prospective studies have concluded that in normal healthy women, estrogens reduce cardiovascular disease by 35% to 50% (Grodstein *et al.*, 1996; Henderson *et al.*, 1991). However, The Heart and Estrogen/Progestin Replacement Study (Hulley *et al.*, 1998), which studied older women with documented cardiovascular disease, reported no change in the incidence of myocardial infarction despite an 11% reduction in LDL cholesterol. Thromboembolic disease and disease of the gallbladder were increased. These studies suggest that the beneficial effects of hormone-replacement therapy on risk of heart disease may be dependent on the age and the cardiovascular status of the patient.

Neuroprotective Effects.   Several retrospective studies have suggested that estrogens had beneficial effects on cognition and delayed the onset of Alzheimer's disease (*see* Green and Simpkins, 2000). Estrogens have been shown to exert neuroprotective effects both *in vivo* and *in vitro*, and various mechanisms, including activation of the MAPK pathway, inhibition of apoptosis, and decreased neurotoxicity of amyloid β peptide have been suggested. Recent prospective studies have not confirmed these beneficial effects and have found no improvement in the symptoms of Alzheimer's disease (Henderson *et al.*, 2000) or in the slow progression of the disease (Mulnard *et al.*, 2000). Further large-scale studies are required to assess the neurological benefits of estrogens.

Urogenital Atrophy.   Loss of tissue lining the vagina or bladder leads to a variety of symptoms in a very high percentage of postmenopausal women. These include dryness and itching of the vagina, pain during sexual intercourse, swelling of the tissues in the genital region such as the entrance to the vagina, pain during urination, a need to urinate urgently or often, and sudden or unexpected urinary incontinence. These symptoms are effectively treated by estrogens, administered either orally or locally as a vaginal cream (PREMARIN, others) or ring device (ESTRING).

Other Therapeutic Effects.   Many other changes occur in postmenopausal women, including a general thinning of the skin; changes in the urethra, vulva, and external genitalia; a decrease in height, a "camel hump" on the back, and a protuberant abdomen secondary to osteoporosis precipitated by estradiol deficiency; and a variety of changes including headache, tiredness, and difficulty concentrating, many of which may derive from the chronic lack of sleep created by hot flashes and other vasomotor symptoms. Estrogen replacement may help alleviate or lessen some of these *via* direct actions (*e.g.,* improvement of vasomotor symptoms, direct skeletal effects) or secondary effects resulting in an improved feeling of well-being (Belchetz, 1994).

Hormone-Replacement Regimens.   In the 1960s and 1970s there was an increase in estrogen-replacement therapy (*i.e.,* estrogens alone) in postmenopausal women, primarily to reduce vasomotor symptoms, vaginitis, and osteoporosis. About 1980, epidemiological studies indicated that this treatment was associated with a large increase in the incidence of endometrial carcinoma, presumably due in part to the continuous stimulation of endometrial hyperplasia by unopposed estrogens. This realization has led to the use of *hormone-replacement therapy* that includes *both* an *estrogen,* for its beneficial effects, and a *progestin* to limit endometrial hyperplasia. While the actions of progesterone on the endometrium are complex, its effects on estrogen-induced hyperplasia may involve a decrease in estrogen receptor content, increased local conversion of estradiol to the less potent estrone *via* the induction of 17β-hydroxysteroid dehydrogenase in the tissue, and/or the conversion of the endometrium from a proliferative to a secretory state.

Hormone-replacement therapy with both an estrogen and progestin now is recommended for most postmenopausal women with a uterus (Belchetz, 1994). For those women with a uterus who are unable to tolerate progestins or have a high risk of cardiovascular disease due to unfavorable lipoprotein profiles (*see* below), estrogens alone may be preferable. For women who have undergone a hysterectomy, endometrial carcinoma is not a concern, and estrogen alone is more commonly used because of possible deleterious effects of progestins (*see* below).

Medroxyprogesterone acetate (MPA) is the progestin that, historically, has been most commonly used in hormone-replacement regimens. This is a C 21 derivative of progesterone, which has less androgenic activity than other progestins such as the 19-nor compounds commonly used in combination oral contraceptives (*see* following section). This choice of a highly selective progestin such as MPA is an important pharmacological consideration, since 19-nor compounds may have undesirable effects on lipid and carbohydrate metabolism due in part to their androgenic activity. There has been considerable concern that the inclusion of a progestin would oppose the beneficial effects of estrogens on lipoprotein profiles and/or have other undesirable metabolic effects, and this is an area of current investigation.

Several hormone-replacement regimens have been utilized. An example of a "cyclic" regimen is as follows: (1) the administration of an estrogen for 25 days; (2) the inclusion of MPA for the last 10 to 13 days of estrogen treatment; and (3) 5 to 6 days with no hormone treatment, during which withdrawal bleeding normally occurs due to breakdown and shedding of the endometrium. Many physicians do not use regimens that include days without hormone. The inclusion of the progestin during only a portion of each treatment cycle effectively decreases endometrial hyperplasia and the incidence of endometrial carcinoma yet minimizes the total amount of progestin administered. PREMPRO (PREMARIN plus MPA, given as a fixed dose daily) or PREMPHASE (PREMARIN given for 28 days plus MPA given for 14 out of 28 days) are widely used combination formulations. Two other combination products that recently became available in the United States are FEM HRT (estradiol plus *norethindrone acetate*) and ORTH PREFEST (estradiol and *norgestimate*). Efforts continue to develop regimens (*e.g.*, FEM HRT) that provide the beneficial effects of estrogen without the withdrawal bleeding that may limit compliance in some women.

Another pharmacological consideration is the route of estrogen administration—*i.e.*, oral *versus* transdermal. Oral administration exposes the liver to high concentrations of estrogens *via* the portal circulation and causes a more rapid conversion of estradiol or conjugated estrone to estrone. Both of these effects are lessened with transdermal estradiol. Either route effectively relieves vasomotor symptoms and protects against bone loss. Oral but not transdermal estrogen may increase SSBG, other binding globulins, and renin substrate; the oral route might be expected to cause greater increases in the cholesterol content of the bile. Transdermal estrogen appears to cause smaller beneficial changes in lipoprotein profiles (approximately 50% of those seen with the oral route), presumably because the liver is not exposed to the high estrogen levels seen after oral dosing (Walsh *et al.*, 1994). Some women may have skin reactions to the transdermal patch.

Estrogen Treatment in the Failure of Ovarian Development. In several conditions, the ovaries do not develop and puberty does not occur. In ovarian dysgenesis with dwarfism (Turner's syndrome), therapy with estrogen at the appropriate time replicates the events of puberty except for the growth spurt and the changes in the ovary. The genital structures grow to normal size, the breasts develop, axillary and pubic hair grows, and the body assumes the normal feminine contour. Androgens (Chapter 59) and/or growth hormone (Chapter 56) may be used to promote normal growth.

Failure of ovarian development also is associated with hypopituitarism in childhood. Deficiency of the thyroid and the adrenal cortex is corrected easily by replacement therapy, and the failure of sexual development is treated with estrogen. Administration of growth hormone permits achievement of near normal adult stature (*see* Chapter 56). Treatment with estrogen at the normal age of puberty can be expected to cause a small acceleration of growth, but the addition of small doses of androgen has a greater growth-promoting effect. While estrogens and androgens promote bone growth, they also accelerate epiphyseal fusion, and their premature use can thus result in a shorter ultimate height.

Earlier Uses of Estrogens. Estrogens, particularly diethylstilbestrol, have been historically important in the treatment of testosterone-dependent prostate carcinoma due to the ability of estrogens to suppress pituitary LH secretion *via* negative feedback effects and thus inhibit testosterone production in the testes. More recently, the use of GnRH analogs has gained widespread acceptance for this purpose, since they may have fewer untoward side effects than estrogens in the treatment of male patients (*see* Chapter 59).

SELECTIVE ESTROGEN RECEPTOR MODULATORS (SERMS) AND ANTIESTROGENS

Recent advances in understanding how ligands alter the conformation of ERs has brought about a fundamental conceptual change in how estrogen agonists and antagonists act and made possible the revolutionary development of compounds with uniquely selective estrogenic properties. The simple model of an agonist binding to a single ER that subsequently affects transcription by the same molecular mechanism in all target tissues, and of antagonists that act by simple competition with agonist for binding, is no longer valid. By altering the conformation of the two different ERs and thereby changing interactions with coactivators and corepressors in a cell- and promoter-specific context, ligands may have a broad spectrum of activities from purely antiestrogenic in all tissues, to partially estrogenic in some tissues with antiestrogenic or no activities in others, to purely estrogenic activities in all tissues. The elucidation of these concepts has been a major breakthrough in estrogen pharmacology in the past decade and should permit the rational design of drugs with very selective patterns of estrogenic activity.

SERMs. Tamoxifen, Raloxifene, and Toremifene. SERMs are compounds whose estrogenic activities are tissue-selective. The pharmacological goal of these drugs is to produce estrogenic actions in those tissues where these actions are beneficial (*e.g.*, bone, brain, liver during postmenopausal hormone replacement) and to have either no activity or antagonist activity in tissues such as breast and endometrium, where estrogenic actions (*e.g.*, cellular proliferation) might be deleterious. Currently approved drugs in the United States in this class are *tamoxifen citrate* (NOLVADEX) and *raloxifene hydrochloride* (EVISTA). *Toremifene* (FARESTON) is chemically related to tamoxifen (*see* below) and has similar actions. Toremifene is approved by the United States Food and Drug Administration (FDA) for treatment of metastatic breast cancer in postmenopausal women with ER-positive or ER-unknown tumors.

Tamoxifen was originally classified as an antiestrogen, but subsequent experience has shown that it has agonist activity in bone, liver, and the endometrium. It currently is approved for four uses: (1) as an adjuvant for the treatment of axillary node–negative breast cancer in women after total mastectomy or segmental mastectomy, axillary dissection, and breast irradiation; (2) as therapy following total mastectomy or segmental mastectomy, axillary dissection, and breast irradiation in postmenopausal women with node-positive disease; (3) in the treatment of women and men with advanced or metastatic breast cancer; and (4) as a preventative agent for women at high risk for breast cancer. Raloxifene is approved for the prevention and treatment of osteoporosis in postmenopausal women.

Antiestrogens. Clomiphene and ICI 182,780.

These compounds are distinguished from the SERMs in that they are pure antagonists in all tissues studied. They may have inverse agonist activity in some settings. *Clomiphene* (CLOMID, SEROPHENE, others) is approved for the treatment of anovulatory women desiring pregnancy. *ICI 182,780* (FASLODEX) is in clinical trials for the treatment of breast cancer and may be efficacious in women who are resistant to tamoxifen.

Chemistry. The structures of the trans-isomer of tamoxifen, and of raloxifene, *trans*-clomiphene, (enclomiphene), and ICI 182,780 are as follows:

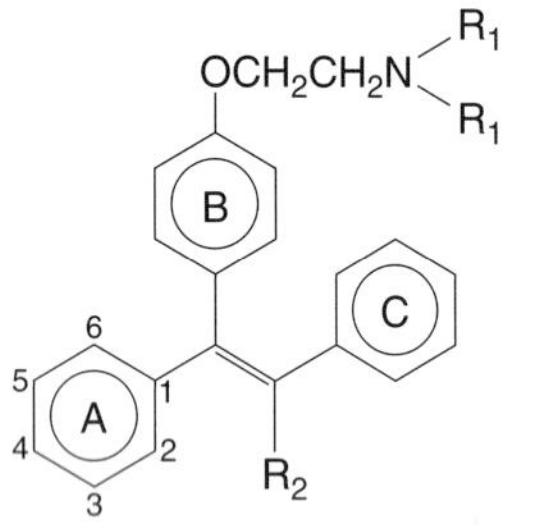

ENCLOMIPHENE   TAMOXIFEN

R₁: —CH₂CH₃   —CH₃
R₂: —Cl   —CH₂CH₃

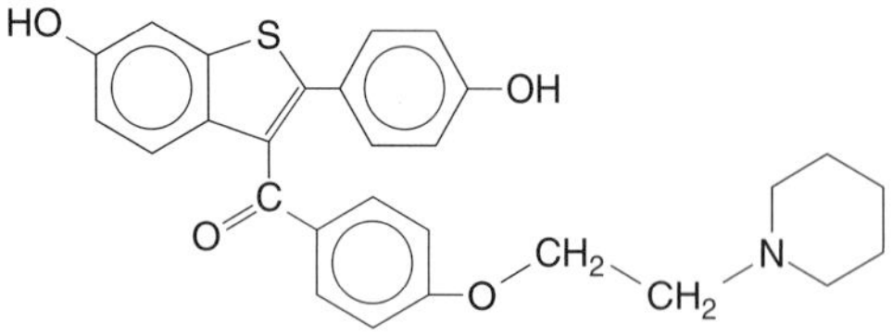

RALOXIFENE

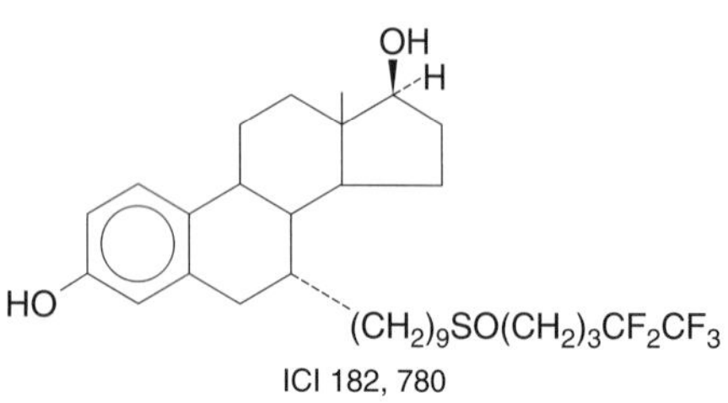

(CH₂)₉SO(CH₂)₃CF₂CF₃
ICI 182, 780

Tamoxifen belongs to the triphenylethylene class of compounds derived from the same stilbene nucleus as diethylstilbestrol; compounds of this class display a variety of estrogenic and antiestrogenic activities. In general, the *trans* conformations have antiestrogenic activity, whereas the *cis* conformations display estrogenic activity. However, the pharmacological activity of the *trans* compound depends upon the species, target tissue, and gene. Hepatic metabolism produces N-desmethyltamoxifen, which has affinity for ER comparable to that of tamoxifen, and the highly active 4-hydroxy metabolite, which has a much (25- to 50-fold) higher affinity for both ER α and ER β than does tamoxifen (Kuiper *et al.*, 1997). In addition, the 4-hydroxy metabolites formed *in vivo* isomerize readily, and this complicates the comparison of *in vivo* effects of the drugs with their *in vitro* actions. Tamoxifen is marketed as the pure *trans* isomer. Toremifene also is a triphenylethelene with a chlorine substitution at the R2 position.

Raloxifene is a polyhydroxylated nonsteroidal compound with a benzothiophene core. Raloxifene binds with high affinity for both ER α and ER β (Kuiper *et al.*, 1997).

Clomiphene citrate is a triphenylethylene, and its two isomers, zuclomiphene (*cis*-chlomiphene) and enclomiphene (*trans*-clomiphene) are a weak estrogen agonist and a potent antagonist, respectively. Clomiphene binds to both ER α and ER β, but the individual isomers were not examined (Kuiper *et al.*, 1997).

ICI 182,780 (FASLODEX) is a 7α-alkylamide derivative of estradiol that interacts with both ER α and ER β (Van Den Bemd *et al.*, 1999).

Pharmacological Effects

Tamoxifen exhibits antiestrogenic, estrogenic, or mixed activity depending upon the species and target gene measured. In clinical tests or laboratory studies with human cells, the drug's activity depends upon the tissue and endpoint measured (Jordan and Murphy, 1990). For example, tamoxifen inhibits the proliferation of cultured human breast cancer cells and reduces tumor size and number in women (reviewed in Jiayesimi *et al.*, 1995), yet it stimulates proliferation of endometrial cells and causes endometrial thickening (Lahti *et al.*, 1993). The drug has an antiresorptive effect on bone, and it decreases total cholesterol, LDL, and lipoprotein (a) but does not increase HDL and triglycerides (Love *et al.*, 1994) in human beings. The lipid-lowering effect appears to be greater in postmenopausal than premenopausal women (Ilanchezhian *et al.*, 1995). Tamoxifen treatment causes a two- to threefold increase in the relative risk of deep vein thrombosis and pulmonary embolism (Fisher *et al.*, 1998). Some investigators have reported that tamoxifen decreases overall cardiovascular risk (Rutqvist and Mattsson, 1993), while others have seen no change (Fisher *et al.*, 1998). Tamoxifen produces hot flashes in some women, which is the expected vasomotor effect of antiestrogens; other adverse effects include vaginal discharge or dryness, cataracts, and nausea.

Raloxifene is an estrogen agonist in bone, where it exerts an antiresorptive effect. Results of several large clinical trials have shown that raloxifene reduces the number of vertebral fractures by up to 50% in a dose-dependent manner (Delmas *et al.*, 1997; Ettinger *et al.*, 1999). The drug also acts as an estrogen agonist in reducing total cholesterol and LDL, but it does not increase HDL or normalize plasminogen-activator inhibitor 1 in postmenopausal women (Walsh *et al.*, 1998). Raloxifene does not cause proliferation or thickening of the endometrium. Preclinical studies indicate that raloxifene has an antiproliferative effect on ER-positive breast tumors and on proliferation of ER-positive breast cancer cell lines (*see* Hol *et al.*, 1997) and significantly reduces the risk of ER-positive but not ER-negative breast cancer (Cummings *et al.*, 1999). Raloxifene does not alleviate the vasomotor symptoms associated with menopause. Adverse effects include hot flashes and leg cramps; more serious adverse effects include about a threefold increase in deep vein thrombosis and pulmonary embolism (Cummings *et al.*, 1999).

Initial animal studies with clomiphene showed slight estrogenic activity, now thought to be due to the *cis* isomer, and moderate antiestrogenic activity, but the most striking effect was the inhibition of the pituitary's gonadotropic function. In both male and female animals, the compound thus acted as a contraceptive. In contrast, the most prominent effect *in women* was enlargement of the ovaries, and Greenblatt and coworkers (1962) found that the drug induced ovulation in many patients with amenorrhea, Stein-Leventhal syndrome, and dysfunctional bleeding with anovulatory cycles. This is the basis for clomiphene's major pharmacological use, which is the induction of ovulation in women with a functional hypothalamic-hypophyseal-ovarian system and adequate endogenous estrogen production. In some cases, clomiphene is used in conjunction with human menotropins and hCG (*see* Chapter 56) to induce ovulation.

ICI 182,780 and its less potent forerunner ICI 164,384 have been purely antiestrogenic in studies to date. Effects of ICI 182,780 include inhibition of the activity of P-glycoprotein and of gene expression of aromatase, IGF-1, and insulin receptor substrate 1 and antiprogestin activity (*see* Ibrahim and Hortobagyi, 1999). *In vitro*, ICI 782,780 was more potent than 4-hydroxytamoxifen (DeFriend *et al.*, 1994) in inhibiting proliferation of breast cancer cells, and in a small clinical trial, ICI 782,780 was partially successful in treating tamoxifen-resistant breast cancers (Howell *et al.*, 1995).

All of these agents bind to the ligand-binding pocket of both ER α and ER β and competitively block estradiol binding. However, the conformation of the ligand-bound ER is different with different ligands (*see* McDonnell,

2000). Thus, the conformation of ER when occupied by 17β-estradiol is different from its conformation when occupied by tamoxifen, raloxifene, or ICI 182,780 (Wijayaratne *et al.*, 1999), and this has two important mechanistic consequences. These distinct ER-ligand conformations appear to recruit different coactivators and corepressors onto the promoter of a target gene by differential protein-protein interactions at the receptor surface. The tissue-specific actions of SERMs thus can be explained in part by the distinct conformation of the ER when occupied by different ligands, in combination with the repertoire of coactivators and corepressors present in a specific cell type that also will affect the nature of ER complexes formed.

The ER contains multiple transcriptional activation functions (*i.e.*, AF-1 and AF-2), which can be differentially regulated by individual SERMs and contribute to the drug's pharmacological activities. For example, tamoxifen does not produce an ER conformation that allows activation of the AF-2 function of the ER, but binding of the drug allows the AF-1 domain to become functional. Tamoxifen may thus be an agonist for activation of transcription of some genes in tissues, such as the endometrium, which either do not require the AF-2 function for transcriptional control or contain other transcription factors that can substitute for the AF-2 function of the ER. However, the drug also may be an antagonist for transcription of certain genes in tissues, such as the breast, which require the AF-2 function for expression and do not contain other factors that can provide this activity to the transcription machinery. Additionally, the presence of ER α and the opposing ER β suggest that the ratio of the two receptors also is important in specifying the response of a cell. This model might explain the eventual resistance to tamoxifen that develops with time in breast cancer; *i.e.*, changes in the amount or the nature of coactivators and corepressors expressed or changes in ratio of ER α to ER β may occur during tumor progression. In fact, overexpression of the coactivator SRC-1 in HeLa cells changes tamoxifen from an antagonist to an agonist (Smith *et al.*, 1997).

Similarly, raloxifene acts as a partial agonist in bone but does not stimulate endometrial proliferation in postmenopausal women. Presumably this is due to some combination of differential expression of transcription factors in the two tissues and the effects of this SERM on ER conformation.

Clomiphene acts to oppose the negative feedback effect of endogenous estrogens to increase gonadotropin secretion and stimulate ovulation. Most studies have found that clomiphene increases the amplitude of LH and FSH pulses, without a change in pulse frequency (Kettel *et al.*, 1993). This suggests that the drug is acting largely at the pituitary level to block inhibitory actions of estrogen on gonadotropin release from the gland, and/or is somehow affecting the hypothalamus to release larger amounts of GnRH per pulse. Clomiphene also has been used in men to stimulate gonadotropin release and enhance spermatogenesis.

ICI 182,780 binds to ER α and ER β and represses transactivation, but it also appears to increase intracellular proteolytic degradation of ER α, while apparently protecting ER β from degradation (Van Den Bemd *et al.*, 1999).

Absorption, Fate, and Excretion

Tamoxifen is given orally, and peak plasma levels are reached within 4 to 7 hours after treatment. This drug displays two elimination phases with half-lives of 7 to 14 hours for the first phase and 4 to 11 days for the second. Due to the prolonged half-life, 3 to 4 weeks of treatment may be required to reach steady-state plasma levels. The parent drug is converted largely to metabolites within 4 to 6 hours after oral administration. In human beings and other species, 4-hydroxytamoxifen is produced *via* hepatic metabolism, and this compound is considerably more potent than the parent drug as an antiestrogen. The major route of elimination from the body involves *N*-demethylation and deamination. The drug undergoes enterohepatic circulation, and excretion is primarily in the feces as conjugates of the deaminated metabolite.

Raloxifene is adsorbed rapidly after oral administration and has an absolute bioavailability of about 2%. The drug has a half-life of about 28 hours and is eliminated primarily in the feces after hepatic glucuronidation.

Clomiphene is well absorbed following oral administration, and the drug and its metabolites are eliminated primarily in the feces and to a lesser extent in the urine. The long plasma half-life (approximately 5 to 7 days) is due largely to plasma-protein binding, enterohepatic circulation, and accumulation in fatty tissues. Other active metabolites with long half-lives also may be produced.

ICI 182,780 is administered intramuscularly with monthly (depot) injections being favored. Long-acting preparations are available for investigational use.

Therapeutic Uses

Breast Cancer. *Tamoxifen* is widely used in the treatment of breast cancer, and numerous studies have established its beneficial effects in this setting. It is used alone for palliation of advanced breast cancer in women with ER-positive tumors, and it is now indicated as the hormonal treatment of choice for both early and advanced breast cancer in women of all ages (Jiayesimi *et al.*, 1995). Response rates are approximately 50% in women with ER-positive tumors and 60% to 70% in tumors that are both ER- and progestin-receptor (PR)-positive; response in ER-negative tumors falls to 10%. Tamoxifen has been shown consistently to increase disease-free survival and overall survival; treatment for 5 years has reduced cancer recurrance by 47% to 50% and death by 26% to 28%. The incidence of contralateral breast cancer has been reduced by 47% (Early Breast Cancer Trialists' Group, 1998). Tamoxifen has been approved by the FDA for primary prevention of breast cancer in women at high risk, based on the results of the National Surgical Adjuvant Breast and Bowel Project (Fisher *et al.*, 1998), where the drug caused a 49% decrease in the incidence of invasive breast cancer and a 50% reduction of noninvasive breast cancer. Treatment efficacy decreases after 5 years due to acquisition of drug resistance by the tumors. Tamoxifen has estrogenic activity in the uterus, increases the risk of endometrial cancer by two- to threefold, and also causes a comparable increase in the risk of thromboembolemic disease.

Osteoporosis. *Raloxifene* reduces the rate of bone loss at both distal sites and in the spinal column and may increase bone mass at certain sites. The rate of vertebral fractures can be reduced by as much as 50% (Delmas *et al.*, 1997, Ettinger *et al.*, 1999). While peripheral bone mass was increased by more than 2%, there was no decrease in nonvertebral fractures during the 3-year study period. Raloxifene does not appear to increase the risk of developing endometrial cancer. Raloxifene has beneficial actions on lipoprotein metabolism, reducing both total cholesterol and LDL; however, HDL is not increased, as with estrogen-replacement therapy. Adverse effects include deep vein thrombosis and leg cramps.

Ovulatory disturbances are present in 15% to 25% of couples with infertility. For more than 25 years, clomiphene has been used in these cases because it has a low cost, is orally active, and requires less extensive monitoring than do other treatment protocols. However, the drug may exhibit untoward effects including ovarian hyperstimulation; increased incidence of multiple births; ovarian cysts; antiestrogenic effects on the developing follicle, endometrium, and cervical mucus that may counteract its beneficial effects on gonadotropin release; hot flashes; and blurred vision. In addition, clomiphene-induced cycles have a relatively high incidence of luteal phase dysfunction due to inadequate progesterone production. For these reasons, other treatment strategies such as human menopausal gonadotropins in combination with long-acting GnRH analogs and human chorionic gonadotropin may be more favorable (*see* Chapter 56). There also are reports of teratogenic effects of clomiphene in animals, and the drug should not be administered to pregnant women, even though there is no evidence of human fetal abnormalities in cases where the drug has been used to induce ovulation.

Clomiphene also may be used to evaluate the male reproductive system, since testosterone feedback on the hypothalamus and pituitary is mediated to a large degree by estrogens formed from aromatization of the androgen. In normal individuals, once-daily administration of clomiphene for 7 days produces a doubling in plasma LH and a 50% increase in FSH.

Estrogen-Synthesis Inhibitors

Several agents can be used to decrease the effects of endogenous estrogens by blocking their biosynthesis. One such option is the continual administration of GnRH or the use of long-acting GnRH agonists, either of which prevents ovarian synthesis of estrogens but not the peripheral synthesis of estrogens from adrenal androgens (*see* Chapter 56). *Aminoglutethimide* inhibits aromatase activity, and thus blocks estrogen biosynthesis from all precursors. This agent is not selective, however, as it inhibits other cytochrome P450s involved in steroidogenesis, including those in the adrenal.

There is increasing interest in the use of aromatase inhibitors to block specifically the local production of estrogens that may contribute substantially to hormone-responsive diseases such as breast cancer (*see* Chapter 52). Third-generation aromatase inhibitors now are available and are more potent and selective than earlier agents such as aminoglutethimide (Brodie and Njar, 2000). These include both steroidal [*e.g., formestane* and *exemestane* (AROMASIN)] and nonsteroidal agents [*e.g., anastrozole* (ARIMIDEX), *letrozole* (FEMARA), and *vorozole*], which have been used for the second-line treatment of breast cancer in patients for whom tamoxifen therapy is unsuccessful. The structures of exemestane and anastrozole are as follows:

EXEMESTANE

ANASTROZOLE

PROGESTINS

The progestins (*see* Figure 58–6) include the naturally occurring hormone progesterone, 17α-acetoxyprogesterone derivatives in the pregnane series, 19-nortestosterone derivatives (estranes), and norgestrel and related compounds in the gonane series. (Note: Compounds with biological activities similar to those of progesterone have been variously referred to in the literature as progestins, progestational agents, progestagens, progestogens, gestagens, or gestogens.) *Medroxyprogesterone acetate* (MPA) and *megestrol acetate* are C 21 steroids with selective activity very similar to that of progesterone itself. MPA and oral micronized progesterone are widely used with estrogens for postmenopausal hormone replacement and other situations where a selective progestational effect is desired, and a depot form of MPA is used as a long-acting injectable

contraceptive. The 19-nortestosterone derivatives were developed for use as progestins in oral contraceptives, and while their predominant activity is progestational, they exhibit androgenic and other activities. The gonanes are a more recently developed series of "19-nor" compounds, containing an ethyl rather than a methyl substituent in the 13-position, and they have diminished androgenic activity. These two classes of 19-nortestosterone derivatives are the progestational components of all oral and some long-acting injectable contraceptives.

History.   Corner and Allen originally isolated a hormone in 1933 from the corpora lutea of sows and named it *progestin.* The next year, several European groups also isolated the crystalline compound and gave it the name *luteo-sterone,* unaware of the previous name given by Corner and Allen. This difference in nomenclature was resolved in 1935 at a garden party in London given by the famous English pharmacologist Sir Henry Dale, who helped persuade all parties that the name *progesterone* was a suitable compromise incorporating elements of the two previous designations.

Studies with progesterone initially were hampered because production from animal sources was extremely difficult and time-consuming. Prices of progesterone were as high as $1000 per gram, which were astronomical in the worldwide economy of the 1930s. In addition, the fact that progesterone itself is not orally active, due to extensive first-pass hepatic metabolism, limited its pharmacological utility.

These difficulties were overcome by two major advances in steroid chemistry made by several brilliant chemists (*see* Perone, 1994). The first advance was the synthesis of progesterone by Russel Marker from the plant product diosgenin in the 1940s. The synthesis was a real breakthrough, as it provided large amounts of relatively inexpensive progesterone and eliminated cross-contamination with compounds that might copurify with progesterone from animal sources. The second major chemical advance was the synthesis of 19-nor compounds, the first orally active progestins, in the early 1950s by Carl Djerassi, who synthesized *norethindrone* at Syntex, and Frank Colton, who synthesized the isomer *norethynodrel* at Searle. These are undoubtedly some of the most important advances in synthetic organic chemistry in the twentieth century, since they eventually led to the development of effective oral contraceptives, agents that have had an enormous impact on society.

Chemistry.   Unlike the estrogen receptor, which requires a phenolic A ring for high-affinity binding, the progesterone receptor favors a Δ^4-3-one A-ring structure in an inverted $1\beta,2\alpha$-conformation (Duax *et al.,* 1988). Other steroid hormone receptors also bind this nonphenolic A-ring structure, although the optimal conformation differs from that for the progesterone receptor. Thus, some synthetic progestins (especially the 19-nor compounds) display limited binding to glucocorticoid, androgen, and mineralocorticoid receptors, a property that probably accounts for some of their nonprogestational activities. The spectrum of activities of these compounds is highly dependent upon specific substituent groups, especially the nature of the C 17 substitutent in the D ring, the presence of a C 19 methyl group, and the presence of an ethyl group at position C 13.

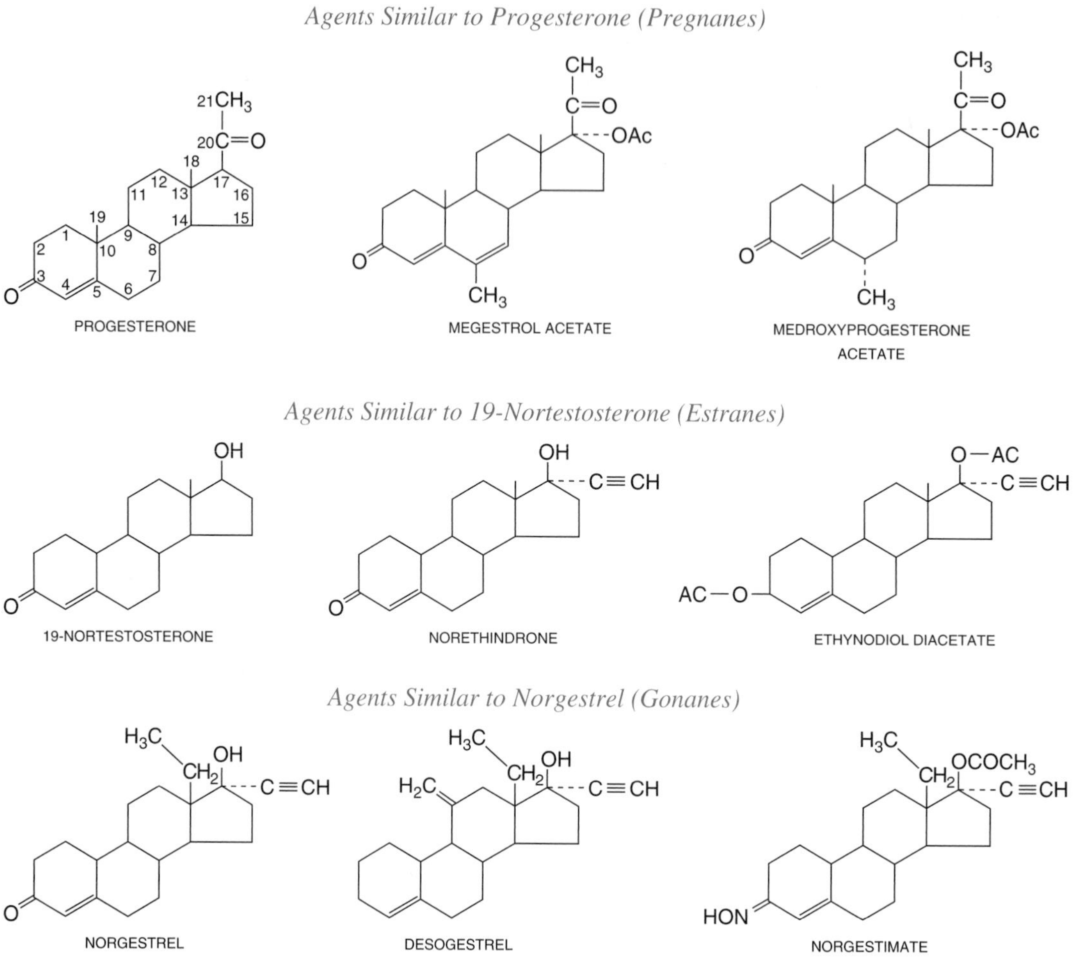

Agents Similar to Progesterone (Pregnanes)

PROGESTERONE   MEGESTROL ACETATE   MEDROXYPROGESTERONE
                                                        ACETATE

Agents Similar to 19-Nortestosterone (Estranes)

19-NORTESTOSTERONE   NORETHINDRONE   ETHYNODIOL DIACETATE

Agents Similar to Norgestrel (Gonanes)

NORGESTREL   DESOGESTREL   NORGESTIMATE

Figure 58–6. *Structural features of various progestins.*

One major class of agents is similar to progesterone and its metabolite 17α-hydroxyprogesterone (*see* Figure 58–6). 17α-Hydroxyprogesterone itself is inactive, but some of its ester derivatives have progestational activity. Compounds such as hydroxyprogesterone caproate have progestational activity but must be used parenterally due to first-pass hepatic metabolism. However, substitutions of such 17-esters at the 6-position of the B ring yield orally active compounds such as medroxyprogesterone acetate and megestrol acetate. Compounds in this chemical class display relatively selective progestational activity.

The second major class of compounds is the 19-nor group. 19-norprogesterone (similar to progesterone except that the C 19 methyl group is replaced by a hydrogen atom) has potent progestational activity, and 19-nortestosterone derivatives display primarily progestational rather than androgenic activity. An ethinyl substituent at C 17 decreases hepatic metabolism and yields 19-nortestosterone analogs such as norethindrone, norethindrone acetate, norethynodrel, and ethynodiol diacetate, which are orally active. The activity of the latter three compounds is due primarily to their rapid *in vivo* conversion to norethindrone. These compounds are less selective than the 17α-hydroxyprogesterone derivatives mentioned above and have varying degrees of androgenic activity and, to a lesser extent, estrogenic and antiestrogenic activities.

Replacement of the 13-methyl group of norethindrone with a 13-ethyl substituent yields the gonane *norgestrel,* which is a more potent progestin than the parent compound and has less androgenic activity. Norgestrel is a racemic mixture of an inactive dextrorotary isomer and the active levorotary isomer, levonorgestrel. Preparations containing half as much levonorgestrel as norgestrel thus have equivalent pharmacological activity. More recently, other gonanes—including *gestodene, norgestimate,* and *desogestrel*—have become available and are reported to have very little if any androgenic activity at therapeutic doses (Rebar and Zeserson, 1991). The latter are used as the progestin component in the so-called third-generation combination oral contraceptives.

Synthesis and Secretion.   Progesterone is secreted by the ovary mainly from the corpus luteum during the second half of the menstrual cycle, as illustrated in Figure 58–3. Secretion actually begins just before ovulation from the follicle that is destined to release an ovum. The formation of progesterone from steroid precursors is presented in detail in Chapter 60 and occurs in the ovary, testis, adrenal cortex, and placenta. The stimulatory effect of LH on progesterone synthesis and secretion by the corpus luteum is mediated by a membrane-bound receptor linked to a G protein–coupled signal transduction pathway that increases the synthesis of cyclic AMP by stimulation of adenylyl cyclase (*see* Chapter 56).

If the ovum is fertilized, implantation takes place about 7 days later, and almost at once the developing trophoblast begins secreting hCG into the maternal circulation, thereby sustaining the functional life of the corpus luteum. hCG, detectable in urine several days before the expected time of the next menstrual period, is excreted in progressively increasing amounts for the next 5 weeks or so and in reduced quantities thereafter throughout pregnancy. During the second or third month of pregnancy, the developing placenta begins to secrete estrogen and progesterone in collaboration with the fetal adrenal glands, and thereafter the corpus luteum is not essential to continued gestation. Estrogen and progesterone continue to be secreted in large amounts by the placenta up to the time of delivery.

Measurements of the rate of secretion of progesterone suggest that, from a few milligrams per day secreted during the follicular phase of the cycle, the rate increases to 10 to 20 mg during the luteal phase and to several hundred mg during the latter part of pregnancy. Rates of 1 to 5 mg per day have been measured in men and are comparable to the values in women during the follicular phase of the cycle.

Physiological and Pharmacological Actions

Neuroendocrine Actions. As discussed in a previous section, progesterone produced in the luteal phase of the cycle has several physiological effects. It decreases the frequency of the hypothalamic pulse generator and increases the amplitude of LH pulses released from the pituitary.

Reproductive Tract. Progesterone released during the luteal phase of the cycle decreases estrogen-driven endometrial proliferation and leads to the development of a secretory endometrium (*see* Figure 58–3). The abrupt decline in the release of progesterone from the corpus luteum at the end of the cycle is the main determinant of the onset of menstruation. If the duration of the luteal phase is artificially lengthened, either by sustaining luteal function or by treatment with progesterone, decidual changes in the endometrial stroma similar to those seen in early pregnancy can be induced. Under normal circumstances, estrogen antecedes and accompanies progesterone in its action upon the endometrium and is essential to the development of the normal menstrual pattern.

Progesterone also influences the endocervical glands, and the abundant watery secretion of the estrogen-stimulated structures is changed to a scant, viscid material. As noted previously, these and other effects of progestins decrease penetration of the cervix by sperm.

The estrogen-induced maturation of the human vaginal epithelium is modified toward the condition of pregnancy by the action of progesterone, a change that can be detected in cytological alterations in the vaginal smear. If the quantity of estrogen concurrently acting is known to be adequate, or if it is assured by giving estrogen, the cytological response to a progestin can be used to evaluate its progestational potency.

Progesterone is very important for the maintenance of pregnancy. Major actions of the hormone are to suppress menstruation and uterine contractility, but other effects also may be important. These effects to maintain pregnancy have led to the historical use of progestins to prevent threatened abortion. However, such treatment is of questionable benefit, probably because diminished progesterone is infrequently the cause of spontaneous abortion (*see* below).

Mammary Gland. During pregnancy and to a minor degree during the luteal phase of the cycle, progesterone, acting with estrogen, brings about a proliferation of the acini of the mammary gland. Toward the end of pregnancy, the acini fill with secretions, and the vasculature of the gland is notably increased; however, only after the levels of estrogen and progesterone decrease at parturition does lactation begin.

During the normal menstrual cycle, mitotic activity in the breast epithelium is very low in the follicular phase and then peaks in the luteal phase. This pattern is due to progesterone, which triggers a *single* round of mitotic activity in the mammary epithelium. This effect is transient, however, and continued exposure to the hormone is rapidly followed by arrest of growth of the epithelial cells (Clarke and Sutherland, 1993). This is in contrast to the endometrium, where proliferation is greatest in the follicular phase due to increasing estrogen levels and is opposed by progesterone in the second half of the cycle. The hormonal control of proliferation is thus different in these two tissues, and these cell-specific effects should be kept in mind when therapeutic and untoward effects of the two agents are being interpreted.

CNS Effects. If the body temperature is carefully measured each day throughout the normal menstrual cycle, an increase of about 1°F (0.56°C) may be noted at midcycle;

this correlates with ovulation. The temperature rise persists for the remainder of the cycle until the onset of the menstrual flow. This increase in temperature clearly is due to progesterone, as can be shown by administration of the hormone. The exact central mechanism of this effect is unknown at present, but an alteration of the temperature regulatory center in the hypothalamus may be involved.

Progesterone also increases the ventilatory response of the respiratory centers to carbon dioxide and leads to reduced arterial and alveolar PCO_2 in the luteal phase of the menstrual cycle and during pregnancy. Progesterone also may have depressant and hypnotic actions in the CNS, which may account for reports of drowsiness after hormone administration. This potential untoward effect may be abrogated by giving progesterone preparations at bedtime, which may even help some patients sleep.

Metabolic Effects. Progestins have numerous metabolic actions. Progesterone itself increases basal insulin levels and the rise in insulin after carbohydrate ingestion, but it does not normally cause a change in glucose tolerance. However, long-term administration of more potent progestins, such as norgestrel, may decrease glucose tolerance (Godsland, 1996). Progesterone stimulates lipoprotein lipase activity and seems to enhance fat deposition. Progesterone and analogs such as MPA have been reported to increase LDL and cause either no effects or modest reductions in serum HDL levels. The 19-norprogestins may have more pronounced effects on plasma lipids because of their androgenic activity. In this regard, a large prospective study has shown that MPA decreases the favorable HDL increase caused by conjugated estrogens during postmenopausal hormone replacement but does not significantly affect the beneficial effect of estrogens to lower LDL. In contrast, micronized progesterone does not significantly affect beneficial estrogen effects on either HDL or LDL profiles (The Writing Group for the PEPI Trial, 1995). Progesterone also may diminish the effects of aldosterone in the renal tubule and cause a decrease in sodium reabsorption that may increase mineralocorticoid secretion from the adrenal cortex.

Mechanism of Action

There is a single progesterone receptor (PR) gene that produces two isoforms of the progesterone receptor, PR-A and PR-B. The first 164 amino acids of PR-B are missing from PR-A; this occurs by use of two distinct estrogen-dependent promoters in the PR gene. Both PRs have a modular, domain structure common to all members of the nuclear receptor subfamily, as illustrated in Figure 58–4. Since the ligand-binding domain is identical in both isoforms of PR, there is no difference in ligand binding, as is seen with the two isoforms of ER. In the absence of ligand, PR is present in the nucleus in an inactive monomeric state bound to heat-shock proteins (HSP-90, HSP-70 and p59). Upon binding progesterone, the heat shock proteins dissociate, and the receptors are phosphorylated and subsequently form dimers (homo- and heterodimers) that bind with high selectivity to PREs (progesterone response elements) located on target genes (see Giangrande and McDonnell, 1999). Transcriptional activation by PR occurs primarily via recruitment of coactivators such as SRC-1, NcoA-1 or NcoA-2 (see Collingwood et al., 1999) or by direct interaction with general transcription factors such as TFIIB (Ing, 1992). The receptor coactivator complex then favors further interactions with yet additional proteins such as CBP and p300, which have histone acetylase activity. Histone acetylation causes a remodeling of chromatin that increases the accessibility of general transcriptional proteins, including RNA polymerase II, to the target promoter. Progesterone antagonists also facilitate receptor dimerization and DNA binding, but, as with ER, the conformation of antagonist-bound PR is different from that of agonist-bound PR. This different conformation favors PR interaction with corepressors NcoR/SMRT, which recruit histone deacetylases. Histone deacetylation increases DNA interaction with nucleosomes and renders a target promoter inaccessible to the general transcription apparatus.

The biological activities of PR-A and PR-B are distinct and depend on the target gene in question. The shorter PR-A acts as a transcriptional inhibitor of other steroid receptors. Specifically, stimulation of target genes by estrogen, glucocorticoid, mineralocorticoid, and androgen receptors is repressed by liganded PR-A (McDonnell and Goldman, 1994). In most cells, PR-B mediates the stimulatory activities of progesterone; PR-A also strongly inhibits this action of PR-B (Vegeto et al., 1993). An inhibitory domain that is responsible for the transrepression caused by PR-A has been localized in the amino-terminus of PR-A. This inhibitory domain is present in both PR-B and PR-A, but for unknown reasons has repressor activity only in the context of PR-A. Current data suggest that different coactivators and corepressors interact with PR-A and PR-B, e.g., the corepressor SMRT (silencing mediator of retinoid and thyroid receptors) binds much more tightly to PR-A than to PR-B (Giangrande et al., 2000), and this may account, at least in part, for the differential activity of the two isoforms. Certain effects of progesterone, such as increased Ca^{2+} mobilization in sperm, can be seen in as little as 3 minutes (Blackmore, 1999), and these effects are thought to be caused by nongenomic mechanisms involving membrane-bound progesterone receptors. Several candidates for this receptor have been identified, and expression of a cDNA for one of these putative membrane PRs leads to production of a membrane-bound protein that binds progesterone relatively specifically (Falkenstein *et al.*, 1999). The pharmacological importance of these membrane-bound receptors has not been determined.

Absorption, Fate, and Excretion

Progesterone itself undergoes rapid first-pass metabolism; historically, this low oral bioavailability limited the administration of the natural hormone to intramuscular injections in oil or to vaginal suppositories and was an impetus to develop 17α-hydroxyprogesterone analogs such as medroxyprogesterone acetate (MPA) and 19-nor steroids for oral use. More recently, high-dose (*e.g.,* 100 to 200 mg) preparations of micronized progesterone (PROMETRIUM) containing small particles (<10 μm) suspended in oil and packaged in gelatin capsules have been developed. Although the absolute bioavailability of these preparations is low (Fotherby, 1996), efficacious plasma levels nevertheless may be obtained. Progesterone also is available in oil solution for injection, as a vaginal gel (CRINONE), and as a slow-release, intrauterine device (PROGESTASERT) for contraception.

In addition to progesterone itself, a number of progestins are available. Esters such as *hydroxyprogesterone caproate* (HYALUTIN) and MPA (DEPO-PROVERA) are available for intramuscular administration; MPA (PROVERA, CYCRIN, others) and *megestrol acetate* (MEGACE) may be used orally, because their hepatic metabolism is substantially reduced relative to the parent hormone. The 19-nor steroids have good oral activity, because the ethinyl substituent at C 17 significantly slows hepatic metabolism. Implants (NORPLANT SYSTEM) and depot preparations of synthetic progestins are available for release over very long periods of time (*e.g., see* later section on contraceptives).

In the plasma, progesterone is bound by albumin and CBG, but is not appreciably bound to SSBG. 19-Nor compounds, such as norethindrone, norgestrel, and desogestrel, bind to SSBG and albumin, and esters such as MPA bind primarily to albumin. Total binding of all these synthetic compounds to plasma proteins is extensive, 90% or more, although the distribution of binding to the different proteins is compound-specific.

The elimination half-life of progesterone is approximately 5 minutes, and the hormone is metabolized primarily in the liver to hydroxylated metabolites and their sulfate and glucuronide conjugates, which are eliminated in the urine. A major urinary metabolite specific for progesterone metabolism is pregnane-$3\alpha,20\alpha$-diol; its measurement in urine and plasma is used as an index of endogenous progesterone secretion. The synthetic progestins have much longer half-lives, *e.g.,* approximately 7 hours for norethindrone, 16 hours for norgestrel, 12 hours for gestodene, and 24 hours for MPA. The metabolism of synthetic progestins is thought to be primarily hepatic, and elimination is generally *via* the urine as conjugates and various polar metabolites.

Therapeutic Uses

The two most frequent uses of progestins are for contraception, either alone or with an estrogen in oral contraceptives, and in combination with estrogen for hormone replacement therapy of postmenopausal women. These two uses are discussed in detail elsewhere in this chapter.

Progestins also are used in several settings for secondary amenorrhea, uterine bleeding disorders, luteal-phase support to treat infertility, and premature labor. There is interest in their potential use in mood disorders and the premenstrual syndrome. Among the oral progestins used besides MPA in these settings is *norethindrone acetate* (AYGESTIN). In general, these uses of oral progestins are extensions of the physiological actions of progesterone on the neuroendocrine control of ovarian function and on the endometrium.

Progesterone can be used diagnostically to test for estrogen secretion and for responsiveness of the endometrium. After administration of progesterone for 5 to 7 days to amenorrheic women, withdrawal bleeding will occur if the endometrium has been stimulated by endogenous estrogens. Combinations of estrogens and progestins also can be used to test endometrial responsiveness in patients with amenorrhea.

Progestins have been used as a palliative measure for metastatic endometrial carcinoma, and megestrol acetate (MEGACE) is used as a second-line treatment for breast cancer.

ANTIPROGESTINS

Although antiestrogens have been available since the late 1950s, the first report of an antiprogestin did not appear until 1981, when the glucocorticoid antagonist RU 38486 (now referred to as *RU 486*), or *mifepristone*, was reported to show antigestagenic properties (Philibert *et al.*, 1981). In 1982, the first report of interruption of the human menstrual cycle and early pregnancy by this compound was presented before the French Académie des Sciences (Hermann *et al.*, 1982).

Mifepristone has been available since 1988 in France and several other countries for the termination of pregnancy, and in 2000 the FDA approved the drug for this use in the United States. While termination of pregnancy has been the main focus of mifepristone use to date, antiprogestins also have several other potential applications including uses as contraceptives, as agents to induce labor, and as agents to treat uterine leiomyomas, endometriosis, meingiomas, and breast cancer (Cadepond *et al.*, 1997).

Mifepristone

Chemistry. *Mifepristone* (RU 486) is a derivative of the 19-norprogestin norethindrone containing a dimethyl-aminophenyl substituent at the 11β-position. It is a potent, competitive antagonist of both progesterone and glucocorticoid binding to their respective receptors. Many other compounds with similar activity now have been synthesized and most contain a similar 11β-aromatic group as in mifepristone. Another widely studied antiprogestin is *onapristone* (or ZK 98 299), which is similar in structure to mifepristone but contains a methyl substituent in the 13α orientation rather than the 13β configuration present in mifepristone. Mifepristone and onapristone have the following structures:

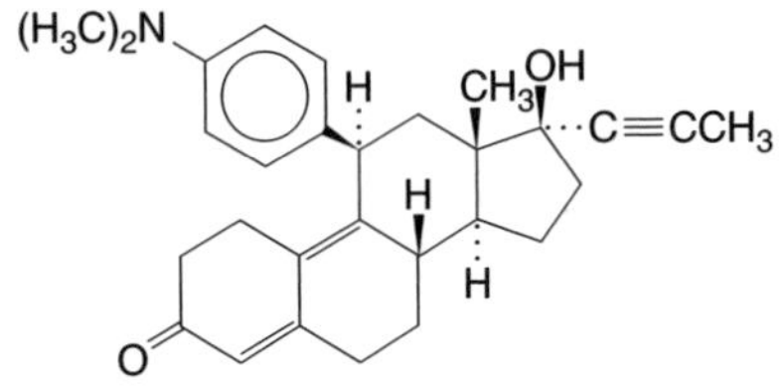

MIFEPRISTONE

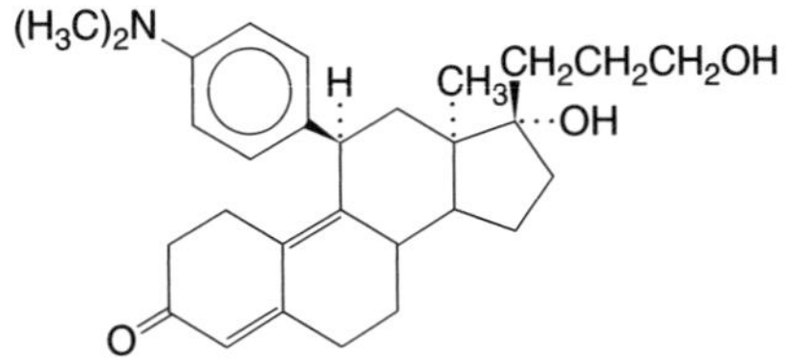

ONAPRISTONE

Pharmacological Actions. In the presence of progestins, mifepristone acts as a competitive receptor antagonist for both the A and B forms of the progesterone receptor. While mifepristone acts as an antagonist *in vivo*, it exhibits some agonist activity in certain *in vitro* test systems. In contrast, onapristone appears to be a pure progesterone antagonist both *in vivo* and *in vitro*. Binding of the two antiprogestins appears to cause different conformations of the progesterone receptor, which may account for the differences in their activities (Gass *et al.*, 1998).

When administered in the early stages of pregnancy, mifepristone causes decidual breakdown by blockade of uterine progesterone receptors. This leads to detachment of the blastocyst, which decreases hCG production. This in turn causes a decrease in progesterone secretion from the corpus luteum, which further accentuates decidual breakdown. Decreased endogenous progesterone coupled with blockade of progesterone receptors in the uterus increases uterine prostaglandin levels and sensitizes the myometrium to the contractile actions of prostaglandins. A separate effect of the compound is to cause cervical softening, which facilitates expulsion of the detached blastocyst.

Mifepristone also has effects on ovulation. If given *acutely* in the mid to late follicular phase, it delays follicle maturation and the LH surge, and ovulation occurs later than normal. If the drug is given *intermittently* (*e.g.*, once a week) or *continuously*, ovulation is prevented in most but not all cases. These effects are due largely to actions on the hypothalamus and pituitary rather than the ovary, although the mechanisms are unclear.

If administered for one or several days in the mid- to late-luteal phase, mifepristone impairs the development of a secre-

tory endometrium and produces menses. Progesterone-receptor blockade at this time is the pharmacological equivalent of progesterone withdrawal, and bleeding normally ensues within several days and lasts for 1 to 2 weeks after antiprogestin treatment.

Mifepristone also binds to glucocorticoid and androgen receptors and exerts antiglucocorticoid and antiandrogenic actions. A predominant effect in human beings is blockade of the feedback inhibition by cortisol of ACTH secretion from the pituitary, thus increasing both corticotropin and adrenal steroid levels in the plasma. Onapristone also binds to both glucocorticoid and androgen receptors, but has less antiglucocorticoid activity than does mifepristone.

Absorption, Fate, and Excretion. Mifepristone is orally active and has good bioavailability by this route. Peak plasma levels occur within several hours after administration, and the drug is slowly cleared, with a plasma half-life of 20 to 40 hours being reported. In plasma, mifepristone is bound with high affinity by α_1-acid glycoprotein, and this may contribute to its long half-life. Metabolites are primarily the mono- and didemethylated products (which are thought to have pharmacological activity) formed *via* CYP3A4-catalyzed reactions and to a lesser extent hydroxylated compounds. The drug undergoes hepatic metabolism and enterohepatic circulation, and metabolic products are found predominantly in the feces (Jang and Benet, 1997).

Therapeutic Uses and Prospects. Mifepristone has been available for several years for clinical use in many European countries, China, and Israel. In September 2000, the FDA approved mifepristone (MIFEPREX), in combination with *misoprostol* (*see* below), for the termination of early pregnancy (defined as 49 days or less, counting from the beginning of the last menstrual period). Terms of the approval limit the distribution of mifepristone to physicians who can determine the duration of pregnancy, detect an ectopic pregnancy, and provide surgical intervention in cases of incomplete abortion or severe bleeding. The major use of mifepristone is to produce medical abortion in the first trimester of pregnancy. When mifepristone is used to produce a medical abortion, a prostaglandin is given 48 hours after the antiprogestin to further increase myometrial contractions and ensure expulsion of the detached blastocyst. Intramuscular *sulprostone*, intravaginal *gemeprost*, and oral *misoprostol* have been used. The success rate with such regimens is >90% among women with pregnancies of 49 days' duration or less. The most severe untoward effect is vaginal bleeding, which most often lasts from 8 to 17 days but is only rarely (0.1% of patients) severe enough to require blood transfusions. High percentages of women also have experienced abdominal pain and uterine cramps, nausea, vomiting, and diarrhea, which are due to the use of the prostaglandin. Many patients receive one or more medications for pain relief from these untoward effects. Women with adrenal failure or severe asthma or who are receiving long-term glucocorticoid therapy should not be given mifepristone because of its antiglucocorticoid activity, and the drug should be used very cautiously in women with anemia or those being treated with anticoagulants. Women over 35 years old with cardiovascular risk factors should not be given sulprostone, because the drug has been associated with heart failure in such individuals (Christin-Maitre *et al.*, 2000).

Mifepristone also has been used as a postcoital contraceptive, and it may be slightly more effective than high-dose estrogen-progestin combinations. The mechanism of action in this case is thought to be prevention of implantation. It also has been proposed that regular use of an antiprogestin in the late luteal phase would be an effective contraceptive because it would ensure that the endometrium was shed and menstruation occurred in each cycle.

Other investigational or potential uses for mifepristone include the induction of labor after fetal death, the induction of labor at the end of the third trimester, treatment of endometriosis and leiomyomas, breast cancer, and meningiomas (Cadepond *et al.*, 1997). Given the multiple potential uses of these agents for clinical and experimental purposes, this is expected to remain a major area of therapeutic development in the future.

HORMONAL CONTRACEPTIVES

Oral contraceptives are among the most widely used agents in the United States and throughout the world. Since they became available in 1960, they have influenced the lives of untold millions of individuals and have had a revolutionary impact on global society. For the first time in history, a convenient, affordable, and completely reliable means of contraception was available for family planning and the avoidance of unplanned pregnancies.

It is important to consider several key points as a prelude to the pharmacology of specific hormonal contraceptives: (1) Hormonal contraceptives are among the most effective drugs available. (2) A variety of agents with substantially different components, doses, and side effects are available and provide real therapeutic options. (3) In addition to contraceptive actions, these agents have substantial health benefits. (4) Because of differences in doses and specific compounds used, it is not appropriate to extrapolate directly untoward effects of hormonal contraceptives to hormone replacement therapy, or *vice versa*. Oral contraceptives are completely effective and have a low incidence of untoward effects for most women.

History. Around the beginning of the twentieth century, a number of European scientists including Beard, Prenant, and Loeb developed the concept that secretions of the corpus luteum suppressed ovulation during pregnancy. These and other workers focused on understanding basic relationships in reproductive physiology, and the Austrian physiologist Haberlandt extended this concept to advance the idea that hormones could be used for purposes of sterilization (*see* Perone, 1994). In 1927 he published a report entitled "On the Hormonal Sterilization of Female Animals," in which he reported producing temporary sterility in rodents by feeding ovarian and placental extracts (Haberlandt, 1927)—*i.e.*, a clear example of an oral contraceptive! After progesterone was isolated from the corpus luteum, Makepeace and colleagues reported in 1937 that the pure hormone blocked ovulation in rabbits (Makepeace *et al.*, 1937).

Two years later, Astwood and Fevold (1939) found a similar effect in rats.

In the 1950s, Pincus, Garcia, and Rock found that progesterone and 19-nor progestins prevented ovulation in women (Rock *et al.*, 1957). Ironically, this finding grew out of their attempts to treat infertility with progestins or estrogen-progestin combinations. The initial findings were that either treatment effectively blocked ovulation in the majority of women. However, concern about cancer and other possible side effects of the estrogen (diethylstilbestrol) led to the use of a progestin alone in their studies.

One of the compounds used was norethynodrel, and early batches of this compound were contaminated with a small amount of mestranol. When mestranol was removed, it was noted that treatment with pure norethynodrel led to increased breakthrough bleeding and less consistent inhibition of ovulation. Mestranol was thus reincorporated into the preparation, and this combination was employed in the first large-scale clinical trial of combination oral contraceptives.

Clinical studies performed by Pincus, Rock, Garcia, and their colleagues in the mid- to late 1950s in Puerto Rico and Haiti established the virtually complete contraceptive success of the norethynodrel-mestranol combination (Pincus *et al.*, 1959). In late 1959, ENOVID (norethynodrel plus mestranol) was the first "Pill" approved by the FDA for use as a contraceptive agent in the United States, and this was followed in 1962 by approval for ORTHO-NOVUM (norethindrone plus mestranol). By 1966 there were approximately a dozen "first-generation" preparations on the market in the United States utilizing either mestranol or ethinyl estradiol in combination with one of several different 19-nor progestins. In the 1960s, the progestin-only minipill and long-acting injectable preparations were developed and subsequently used throughout much of the world, but they were not approved for use in the United States until the 1990s.

Millions of women in the United States and elsewhere began using oral contraceptives, and frequent reports of untoward effects began appearing in the 1970s (*see* Kols *et al.*, 1982). The recognition that these side effects were dose-dependent and the realization that estrogens and progestins synergistically inhibited ovulation led to the reduction of doses and the development of so-called low-dose or second-generation contraceptives. The increasing use of biphasic and triphasic preparations throughout the 1980s further reduced steroid dosages; it may be that current doses available commercially are the lowest that will provide reliable contraception. In the 1990s, the "third-generation" oral contraceptives, containing progestins with reduced androgenic activity [*e.g.*, *norgestimate* (ORTHO TRI-CYCLEN) *desogestrel* (DESOGEN)], became available in the United States after being used in Europe for some time. Products containing gestodene as a progestin with reduced androgenic activity also are available in Europe. Another major development in the 1980s was the widespread realization that oral contraceptives have a number of substantial health benefits (Kols *et al.*, 1982).

Types of Hormonal Contraceptives

Combination Oral Contraceptives. The most frequently used agents in the United States are combination oral contraceptives containing both an estrogen and a progestin.

They are highly efficacious, with a theoretical effectiveness generally considered to be 99.9% and a use effectiveness of 97% to 98%. Ethinyl estradiol and mestranol are the two estrogens used (with ethinyl estradiol being much more frequently used), and several progestins currently are used. The progestins are 19-nor compounds in the estrane or gonane series, and each has varying degrees of androgenic, estrogenic, and antiestrogenic activities that may be responsible for some of their side effects. Compounds such as desogestrel and norgestimate are the most recently developed and have less androgenic activity than other 19-nor compounds (Shoupe, 1994; Archer, 1994; Rebar and Zeserson, 1991). The absorption, fate, and excretion of the individual components have been discussed in previous sections.

Combination oral contraceptives are available as monophasic, biphasic, or triphasic preparations, generally provided in 21-day packs. For the monophasic agents, fixed amounts of the estrogen and progestin are present in each pill, which is taken daily for 21 days, followed by a 7-day "pill-free" period. (Virtually all preparations come as 28-day packs, with the pills for the last 7 days containing only inert ingredients.) The biphasic and triphasic preparations provide two or three different pills containing varying amounts of active ingredients, to be taken at different times during the 21-day cycle. This reduces the total amount of steroids administered and more closely approximates the estrogen to progestin ratios that occur during the menstrual cycle (such as a generally higher ratio in the luteal phase; *see* Figure 58–3). Phasic preparations were developed in the 1980s, largely to reduce the dose of progestins in oral contraceptives when it was recognized these might have untoward cardiovascular effects. In 2000, the FDA approved a once-monthly injectable preparation containing estradiol cypionate and medroxyprogesterone acetate.

The estrogen content of current preparations ranges from 20 to 50 μg; the majority contain 30 to 35 μg. Preparations containing 35 μg or less of an estrogen are generally referred to as "low-dose" or "modern" pills. The dose of progestin is more variable because of differences in potency of the compounds used. For example, monophasic pills currently available in the United States contain 0.4 to 1 mg of norethindrone, 0.1 to 0.15 mg of levonorgestrel, 0.3 to 0.5 mg of norgestrel, 1 mg of ethynodiol diacetate, 0.25 mg of norgestimate, and 0.15 mg of desogestrel, with slightly different dose ranges in biphasic and triphasic preparations. The first agent available (ENOVID) contained 10 mg of norethynodrel and 150 μg of mestranol. In 1966, most first-generation preparations on the market contained 50 to 100 μg of an estrogenic component and 2 to 10 mg of a progestin. These large differences in doses complicate extrapolation of data from early epidemiological studies on the side effects of "high-dose" oral contraceptives to the "low-dose" preparations now used.

Progestin-Only Contraceptives. Several agents are available for progestin-only contraception. They are slightly less efficacious than combination oral contraceptives, with reports of theoretical effectiveness of 99% and a use-effectiveness of 96% to 97.5%. Specific preparations include the "minipill" or oral preparations of low doses of progestins, *e.g.*, 350 μg of norethindrone (NOR-QD, MICRONOR) or 75 μg of norgestrel (OVRETTE) taken daily without interruption; subdermal implants of 216 mg of norgestrel (NORPLANT SYSTEM) for slow release and resultant long-term contraceptive action (*e.g.*, up to 5 years); and crystalline suspensions of medroxyprogesterone acetate (DEPO-PROVERA) for intramuscular injection of 150 mg of drug, which provides effective contraception for 3 months.

An intrauterine device (PROGESTASERT) that releases low amounts of progesterone locally is available for insertion on a yearly basis. Its effectiveness is considered to be 97% to 98%, and contraceptive action probably is due to local effects on the endometrium.

Postcoital or Emergency Contraceptives. High doses of diethylstilbesterol and other estrogens once were used for postcoital contraception (the "morning-after pill") but never received FDA approval for this indication. Clinical trials (Task Force on Postovulatory Methods of Fertility Regulations, 1998) have led to FDA approval and marketing of two preparations for postcoital contraception. For PLAN-B, the total treatment is two one-pill doses (0.75 mg levonorgestrel per pill) separated by 12 hours. For PREVEN, it is two two-pill doses (0.25 mg of levonorgestrel and 0.05 mg of ethinyl estradiol per pill) separated by 12 hours. These preparations are basically high-dose oral contraceptives, and other products with the same or very similar composition have been declared safe and effective for use as emergency contraceptive pills by the FDA.

The first dose of such preparations should be taken within 72 hours of intercourse, and this should be followed 12 hours later by a second dose. This treatment reduces the risk of pregnancy by approximately 75%. Roughly 8 of 100 women having unprotected intercourse during the second or third week of their cycles will become pregnant; emergency contraceptive pills reduce this to 2 women per 100.

Mechanism of Action

Combination Oral Contraceptives. Combination oral contraceptives act by preventing ovulation (Lobo and Stanczyk, 1994). Direct measurements of plasma hormone levels indicate that LH and FSH levels are suppressed, a midcycle surge of LH is absent, endogenous steroid levels are diminished, and ovulation does not occur. While either component alone can be shown to exert these effects in certain situations, the combination synergistically decreases plasma gonadotropin levels and suppresses ovulation more consistently than either alone.

Given the multiple actions of estrogens and progestins on the hypothalamic-pituitary-ovarian axis during the menstrual cycle, several effects probably contribute to the blockade of ovulation. In addition, the prolonged administration of these drugs may bring into play other mechanisms that do not operate physiologically in the menstrual cycle. It seems likely that the reason these drugs are so extraordinarily effective is that they produce their contraceptive action *via* multiple mechanisms.

Hypothalamic actions of steroids play a major role in the mechanism of oral contraceptive action. Progesterone clearly diminishes the frequency of GnRH pulses. Since the proper frequency of LH pulses is essential for ovulation, this effect of progesterone likely plays a major role in the contraceptive action of these agents. In monkeys and women with normal menstrual cycles, estrogens do not affect the frequency of the pulse generator. However, in the prolonged absence of a menstrual cycle (*e.g.*, in ovariectomized monkeys and postmenopausal women; *see* Hotchkiss and Knobil, 1994), estrogens markedly diminish pulse generator frequency, and progesterone enhances this effect. In theory, this hypothalamic effect of estrogens could come into play when oral contraceptives are used for extended times.

Pituitary effects also are likely to contribute to the actions of oral contraceptives. Administration of exogenous GnRH to women receiving oral contraceptives increases plasma LH levels. However, the increase is much smaller than that seen in control subjects, indicating that oral contraceptives decrease pituitary responsiveness to GnRH (Mishell *et al.*, 1977). Estrogens normally suppress FSH release from the pituitary during the follicular phase of the menstrual cycle, and this effect could contribute to the lack of follicular development observed in oral-contraceptive users. Sustained elevation of estrogen levels above a threshold also triggers the midcycle surge of LH required for ovulation. Physiologically, progesterone does not affect this process, but its pharmacological administration inhibits the estrogen-induced LH surge. Multiple pituitary effects of both estrogen and progestin components thus contribute to oral contraceptive action.

In addition to prevention of ovulation, other effects are suspected to contribute to the extraordinary efficacy of oral contraceptives. Transit of sperm, the egg, and fertilized ovum is important to establish pregnancy, and steroids are likely to affect transport in the fallopian tube. Progestin effects also are likely to be dominant in the cervix to produce a thick, viscous mucus to reduce sperm penetration and in the endometrium to produce a state that is not receptive to implantation. However, it is difficult to assess quantitatively the contributions of these effects, because the drugs block ovulation so effectively.

Progestin-Only Contraceptives.   The doses of progestins in minipills and in subcutaneous implants of levonorgestrel are sufficient to block ovulation in only 60% to 80% of cycles. The effectiveness of these preparations is thus thought to be due largely to a thickening of cervical mu-

cus, which decreases sperm penetration, and to endometrial alterations that impair implantation. Depot injections of MPA are thought to exert these latter effects, but they also yield plasma levels of drug high enough to prevent ovulation in virtually all patients. Observed decreases in ovulation are thought to be due to a slowing of the frequency of the GnRH pulse generator, which prevents the LH surge required for ovulation.

Emergency Contraceptive Pills.   Multiple mechanisms are likely to contribute to the efficacy of these agents. Some studies have shown that ovulation is inhibited or delayed if the agents are taken in the first half of the cycle, but other mechanisms are likely to be involved as well because of the high degree of efficacy. Additional mechanisms, some of which are speculative, may include alterations in endometrial receptivity for implantation; interference with functions of the corpus luteum that maintain pregnancy; production of a cervical mucus that decreases sperm penetration; alterations in tubular transport of sperm, egg, or embryo; or effects on fertilization. However, emergency contraceptives do not interrupt an established pregnancy defined as beginning with implantation.

Untoward Effects

Combination Oral Contraceptives.   Shortly after the introduction of oral contraceptives, reports of adverse side effects associated with their use began to appear (*see* Kols *et al.*, 1982). Many of the side effects were found to be dose-dependent, and this led to the development of current low-dose preparations. Untoward effects of early hormonal contraceptives fell into several major categories: adverse cardiovascular effects, including hypertension, myocardial infarction, hemorrhagic or ischemic stroke, and venous thrombosis and embolism; breast, hepatocellular, and cervical cancers; and a number of endocrine and metabolic effects. The current consensus is that low-dose preparations pose minimal health risks in women who have no predisposing risk factors, and these drugs also provide many beneficial health effects (Baird and Glasier, 1993).

Cardiovascular Effects.   The question of cardiovascular side effects has been reexamined for the newer low-dose oral contraceptives (Baird and Glasier, 1993; Mischell, 1999; Castelli, 1999; Sherif, 1999). For nonsmokers without other risk factors, there is no significant increase in risk of myocardial infarction or stroke. There still is an increase in relative risk for venous thromboembolism, but the estimated absolute increase is very small, because the incidence of these events in women without other predisposing factors is low, *e.g.*, roughly half that associated with the risk of venous thromboembolism in pregnancy. Nevertheless, the risk may be increased in women who smoke or have other factors that predispose to thrombosis or thromboembolism (Castelli, 1999). Early high-dose, combination oral contraceptives caused hypertension in 4% to 5% of normotensive women and increased blood pressure in 10% to 15% of those with preexisting hypertension. This incidence is much lower with newer, low-dose preparations, and most reported changes in blood pressure are not significant. The cardiovascular risk associated with oral contraceptive use does not appear to persist after use is discontinued.

There were several reports in 1995 that use of oral contraceptives containing the third-generation progestins gestodene and desogestrel caused a substantial increase in venous thromboembolism in European users relative to preparations with levonorgestrel and norethindrone; this has been a contentious issue, however, and other analyses have attributed the reported differences to confounding variables (Barbieri *et al.,* 1999). In general, however, there have not been major reported differences in cardiovascular parameters associated with different progestins used in modern low-dose preparations.

As noted previously, estrogens increase serum HDL and decrease LDL levels, and progestins tend to have the opposite effect. Recent studies of several low-dose preparations have not found significant change in total serum cholesterol or lipoprotein profiles, although slight increases in triglycerides have been reported.

Cancer. Given the growth-promoting effects of estrogens, there has been a long-standing concern that oral contraceptives might increase the incidence of endometrial, ovarian, breast, and other cancers. These concerns were further heightened in the late 1960s by reports of endometrial changes caused by sequential oral contraceptives, which have since been removed from the market in the United States. However, it is now clear that there is *not* a widespread association between oral contraceptive use and cancer (*see* Baird and Glasier, 1993; Sherif, 1999; Westhoff, 1999).

Combination oral contraceptives do *not* increase the incidence of endometrial cancer but actually cause a 50% *decrease* in the incidence of this disease, which lasts 15 years after the pills are stopped. This is thought to be due to the inclusion of a progestin, which opposes estrogen-induced proliferation, throughout the entire 21-day cycle of administration. Similarly, these agents also *decrease* the incidence of ovarian cancer, and decreased ovarian stimulation by gonadotropins provides a logical basis for this effect.

There have been reports of increases in the incidence of hepatic adenoma and hepatocellular carcinoma in oral contraceptive users, but these are relatively rare diseases, and analysis of their incidence in oral contraceptive users is complicated by numerous factors. There also have been reports of increased cervical cancer in oral contraceptive users, but confounding factors have precluded a definitive association with this disease.

The major present concern about the carcinogenic effects of oral contraceptives is focused on breast cancer. Numerous studies have dealt with this issue, and the following general picture has emerged. The risk of breast cancer in women of childbearing age is very low, and current oral contraceptive users in this group have only a very small increase in relative risk of 1.1 to 1.2, depending on other variables. This small increase is not substantially affected by duration of use, dose or type of component, age at first use, or parity. Importantly, 10 years after discontinuation of oral contraceptive use, there is no difference in breast cancer incidence between past users and never users. In addition, breast cancers diagnosed in women who have ever used oral contraceptive are more likely to be localized to the breast and thus easier to treat, because they are less likely to have spread to other sites (Westhoff, 1999). Overall, there is thus no significant difference in the cumulative risk of breast cancer between those who have ever used oral contraceptives and those who have never used them.

Metabolic and Endocrine Effects. The effects of sex steroids on glucose metabolism and insulin sensitivity are complex (Godsland, 1996) and may differ among agents in the same class *e.g.,* the 19-nor progestins. Early studies with high-dose oral contraceptives generally reported impaired glucose tolerance as demonstrated by increases in fasting glucose and insulin levels and responses to glucose challenge. These effects have decreased as steroid dosages have been lowered, and current low-dose combination contraceptives may even improve insulin sensitivity. Similarly, the high-dose progestins in early oral contraceptives did raise LDL and reduce HDL levels, but modern low-dose preparations do not produce unfavorable lipid profiles (*see* Sherif, 1999). There also have been periodic reports that oral contraceptives increase the incidence of gallbladder disease, but any such effect appears to be weak and limited to current or very long term users (Grodstein *et al.,* 1994).

The estrogenic component of oral contraceptives may increase hepatic synthesis of a number of serum proteins, including those that bind thyroid hormones, glucocorticoids, and sex steroids. While physiological feedback mechanisms generally adjust hormone synthesis to maintain normal "free" hormone levels, these changes can affect the interpretation of endocrine function tests that measure *total* plasma hormone levels.

The ethinyl estradiol present in oral contraceptives appears to cause a dose-dependent increase in several serum factors known to increase coagulation. However, in healthy women who do not smoke, there also is an increase in fibrinolytic activity, which exerts a counter effect so that overall there is a minimal effect on hemostatic balance. In women who smoke, however, this compensatory effect is diminished, which may shift the hemostatic profile toward a hypercoagulable condition (Fruzzetti, 1999).

Miscellaneous Effects. Nausea, edema, and mild headache occur in some individuals, and more severe migraine headaches may be precipitated by oral contraceptive use in a smaller fraction of women. Some patients may experience breakthrough bleeding during the 21-day cycle when the active pills are being taken. Withdrawal bleeding may fail to occur in a small fraction of women during the 7-day "off" period, thus causing confusion about a possible pregnancy. Weight gain, acne, and hirsutism are thought to be mediated by the androgenic activity of the 19-nor progestins.

Progestin-Only Contraceptives. Episodes of irregular, unpredictable spotting and breakthrough bleeding are the most frequently encountered untoward effect and the major reason women discontinue use of all three types of progestin-only contraceptives. With time, the incidence of these bleeding episodes decreases, especially with the long-acting preparations, and amenorrhea becomes common after a year or more of use.

There is no evidence that the progestin-only minipill preparations increase thromboembolic events, which are thought to be related to the estrogenic component of combination preparations; blood pressure does not appear to be elevated; and nausea and breast tenderness do not occur. Acne may be a problem, however, because of the androgenic activity of norethindrone-containing preparations. These preparations may be attractive for nursing mothers, because they do not decrease lactation as do products containing estrogens.

Aside from bleeding irregularities, headache is the most commonly reported untoward effect of depot MPA (medroxyprogesterone acetate). Mood changes and weight gain also have been reported, but controlled clinical studies of these effects are not available. It is of more concern that a number of studies have found decreases in HDL levels and increases in LDL levels and that there have been several reports of decreased bone density. These effects may be due to reduced endogenous estrogens, because depot MPA is particularly effective in lowering gonadotropin levels. An early study found that MPA caused breast cancer in beagle dogs, but this was subsequently found to be due to a unique species-specific metabolism of the drug to estrogens, and numerous human studies have not found any increases in breast, endometrial, cervical, or ovarian cancer in women receiving MPA. Because of the time required to completely eliminate the drug, the contraceptive effect of this agent may remain for 6 to 12 months after the last injection.

Implants of norethindrone may be associated with infection, local irritation, pain at the insertion site, and, rarely, expulsion of the inserts. Headache, weight gain, and mood changes have been reported, and acne is a concern in some patients. A number of metabolic studies have been performed in NORPLANT users, and in most cases only minimal changes have been observed in lipid, carbohydrate, and protein metabolism and in serum chemistry. In women desiring pregnancy, ovulation occurs soon after implant removal, reaching 50% in 3 months and almost 90% within 1 year.

Emergency Contraceptive Pills. Nausea and vomiting are the main untoward effects, with an incidence of roughly 50% and 20%, respectively, for combined estrogen-levonorgestrel combinations and 23% and 6% for levonorgestrel alone (Task Force on Postovulatory Methods of Fertility Regulation, 1998). No changes in clotting factors have been reported for the combined regimen, but based on concerns with combination oral contraceptives, levonorgestrel alone might be considered for women who smoke or have a history of blood clots. **Emergency contraceptive pills are contraindicated in cases of confirmed pregnancy.**

Contraindications

While the use of modern oral contraceptives is considered generally safe in most healthy women, these agents can contribute to the incidence and severity of certain diseases if other risk factors are present. The following conditions are thus considered absolute contraindications for combination oral contraceptive use: the presence or history of thromboembolic disease, cerebral vascular disease, myocardial infarction, coronary artery disease, or congenital hyperlipidemia; known or suspected carcinoma of the breast, carcinoma of the female reproductive tract, or other hormone-dependent/responsive neoplasias; abnormal undiagnosed vaginal bleeding; known or suspected pregnancy; and past or present liver tumors or impaired liver function. *The risk of serious cardiovascular side effects is particularly marked in women over 35 years of age who smoke heavily (e.g., over 15 cigarettes per day); even low-dose oral contraceptives are contraindicated in such patients.*

Several other conditions are relative contraindications and should be considered on an individual basis. These include migraine headaches, hypertension, diabetes mellitus, obstructive jaundice of pregnancy or prior oral contraceptive use, and gallbladder disease. If elective surgery is planned, many physicians recommend discontinuation of oral contraceptives for several weeks to a month to minimize the possibility of thromboembolism after surgery. These agents should be used with care in women with prior gestational diabetes or uterine fibroids, and low-dose pills should generally be used in such cases.

Progestin-only contraceptives are contraindicated in the presence of undiagnosed vaginal bleeding, benign or malignant liver disease, and known or suspected breast cancer. Depot medroxyprogesterone acetate and levonorgestrel inserts are contraindicated in women with a history or predisposition to thrombophlebitis or thromboembolic disorders.

Choice of Contraceptive Preparations

Many preparations that differ substantially in dose and specific components are available, providing the option to select the preparation best suited to each individual. The general feeling is that treatment should be started with preparations containing the minimum dose of steroids that provides effective contraceptive coverage. This often is a pill with 30 to 35 μg of estrogen, but preparations with 20 μg may be adequate for women who weigh much less than average or who are over 40 years of age. A newer use of 20-μg pills is in the treatment of perimenopausal menstrual disorders. A preparation containing 50 μg of estrogen may be required for heavier women. Breakthrough bleeding may occur in some women if the estrogen:progestin ratio is too low to produce a stable endometrium, and this may be prevented by switching to a pill with a higher ratio.

In women for whom estrogens are contraindicated or undesirable, progestin-only contraceptives may be an option. The progestin-only minipill may have an enhanced effectiveness in several such types of women, *e.g.*, nursing mothers and women over 40, in whom fertility may be decreased. In contrast to estrogen-containing contraceptives, progestins can be used in nursing mothers without affecting lactation.

Another consideration is the administration of medications that may increase metabolism of estrogens (*e.g.*, rifampicin, barbiturates, and phenytoin) or reduce their enterohepatic recycling (*e.g.*, tetracyclines and ampicillin). Antimicrobials may decrease intestinal flora that produce enzymes required for hydrolysis and reuptake of conjugated metabolites initially secreted into the intestine *via* the bile. In these situations, a low-dose pill may *not* be 99.9% effective due to decreased plasma levels of the estrogenic component.

The choice of a preparation also may be influenced by the specific 19-nor progestin component, since this component may have varying degrees of androgenic and other activities. The androgenic activity of this component may contribute to untoward effects such as weight gain, acne due to increased sebaceous gland secretions, and unfavorable lipoprotein profiles. These side effects are greatly reduced in newer, low-dose contraceptives, but any patients exhibiting such side effects may benefit by switching to pills that contain a progestin with less androgenic activity. Of the progestins found in oral contraceptives, norgestrel is generally considered to have the most androgenic activity; norethindrone and ethynodiol diacetate to have more moderate androgenic activity; and desogestrel and norgestimate to have the least androgenic activity.

A triphasic, low-dose combination oral contraceptive (ORTHO TRI-CYCLEN) containing ethinyl estradiol and norgestimate has been approved by the FDA for the treatment of moderate acne vulgaris. Similar preparations (DEMULEN 1/35, DESOGEN, ORTHOCEPT) also are effective. The mechanism appears to be a decrease in free plasma testosterone due to an increase in plasma SSBG, since total testosterone levels are unchanged (Redmond *et al.*, 1997).

In summary, for a given individual, both the efficacy and side effects of hormonal contraceptives may vary considerably among preparations. A number of choices are available, and changing preparations may decrease the incidence of side effects in a given patient without decreasing contraceptive efficacy.

Noncontraceptive Health Benefits

It has been accepted for well over a decade that combination oral contraceptives have substantial health benefits unrelated to their contraceptive use (*see* Kols *et al.*, 1982; Goldzieher, 1994; Baird and Glasier, 1993). These include effects on endometrial and ovarian cancer, a variety of common menstrual disorders, and several other diseases.

Oral contraceptives significantly reduce the incidence of ovarian and endometrial cancer within 6 months of use, and the incidence is decreased 50% after 2 years of use. Furthermore, this protective effect persists for up

to 15 years after oral contraceptive use is discontinued. These agents also decrease the incidence of ovarian cysts and benign fibrocystic breast disease.

Oral contraceptives have major benefits related to menstruation in many women. These include more regular menstruation, reduced menstrual blood loss and less iron-deficiency anemia, less premenstrual tension, and decreased frequency of dysmenorrhea. There also is a decreased incidence of pelvic inflammatory disease and ectopic pregnancies, and endometriosis may be ameliorated. Some women also may obtain these benefits with progestin-only contraceptives, and there are suggestions that MPA may improve hematological parameters in women with sickle-cell disease (Cullins, 1996).

There is now a consensus that combination oral contraceptives prevent thousands of deaths, episodes of various diseases, and cases of hospitalization each year in the United States alone. Approximately 20% of all pregnant women are hospitalized before delivery because of complications, and the incidence of death related to childbirth (approximately 20 per 100,000 births to women under 35 in developed countries) is not insignificant. Thus, from a purely statistical perspective, fertility regulation by oral contraceptives is substantially safer than pregnancy or childbirth for most women (Grimes, 1994), even without considering the additional health benefits of these agents.

PROSPECTUS

Estrogens and progestins currently are among the most widely used prescription medications. This heavy use is likely to continue and possibly increase, because, as the population ages, increasing numbers of women will be in the age bracket that traditionally has received hormone-replacement therapy. Such therapy will remain a major use of these agents, and there will be an intense effort to develop an ideal SERM for this purpose. Such an agent would have agonist activity necessary to provide relief of vasomotor symptoms, maintain bone mass, prevent urogenital atrophy, and yield favorable profiles of lipoprotein and hemostatic factors, but be an antagonist in the breast and devoid of tropic actions in the endometrium. Whether or not a single agent can produce all these desirable actions remains to be determined; if not, combinations of agents may be investigated to elicit the desired spectrum of activities. These efforts will be aided by advances in structural biology and molecular pharmacology that will provide the molecular topography of hormone-binding sites and other domains involved in steroid-receptor functions. Advances in molecular genetics also will determine how polymorphisms in genes encoding receptors, enzymes involved in biotransformation reactions, or coactivators/corepressors affect responses to estrogens and progestins.

In terms of postmenopausal hormone-replacement therapy, increasing attention also will be focused on various routes of delivery (*e.g.,* transdermal and intravaginal) to minimize systemic concentrations of hormones and/or to increase or decrease exposure of individual tissues to the hormone. Increased effort also will be devoted to re-examining dosing regimens for progestins used in combination with estrogens, especially in light of historic questions about adverse effects of these agents on cardiovascular health, and in light of more recent reports that women receiving estrogen-plus-progestin-replacement therapy are at greater risk for developing breast cancer than are those receiving estrogen alone. Prospective clinical studies now in progress also should provide more definitive information about the risk of breast cancer and other diseases associated with hormone-replacement therapy; the effectiveness of such therapy in the primary prevention of cardiovascular disease; and whether or not estrogen treatment slows the onset or progression of Alzheimer's disease and other neurodegenerative disorders. Prospective trials comparing the beneficial effects of tamoxifen, raloxifene, and possibly other SERMs also will be conducted within the next 5 years.

The effects of estrogens in men (*e.g.,* on growth of the long bones, in diseases such as prostate cancer, on behav-ior, and on the reproductive system) will receive increased attention, since estrogen-receptor knockout animals have led to the realization that estrogens may have major effects on these tissues/systems in males as well as females.

Considerable efforts also will be focused on the pharmacology of antiestrogens and antiprogestins. Tamoxifen has proven efficacy in the prophylaxis of breast cancer but increases the risk of uterine cancer and venous thromboembolism; attempts thus will be focused on identifying other SERMs with the former but not the latter actions. Antiprogestins will receive increased attention in the possible treatment of breast cancer, the induction of labor, and as contraceptives; both antiestrogens and antiprogestins may find new applications in the treatment of endometriosis and uterine fibroids. The actions of progesterone itself as opposed to synthetic progestins, including the "third generation" gonane compounds, also will be evaluated, as will various non-oral routes of progestin administration.

The role of selective aromatase inhibitors in the treatment of estrogen-responsive diseases such as breast cancer will receive increasing attention with the recognition that substantial amounts of estrogens may be locally produced.

New developments in contraceptives may include a second generation of long-acting progestin (norethindrone) implants; new biodegradable implants; long-acting, timed-release injectable preparations such as microspheres containing estrogens and progestins; and transdermal delivery devices.

For further discussion of disorders of the ovary and female reproductive tract *see* Chapter 337 in *Harrison's Principles of Internal Medicine,* 14th ed., McGraw-Hill, New York, 1998.

BIBLIOGRAPHY

Allen, E., and Doisy, E.A. An ovarian hormone: a preliminary report on its localization, extraction, and partial purification, and action in test animals. *JAMA,* **1923,** *81*:819–821.

Archer, D.F. Clinical and metabolic features of desogestrel: a new oral contraceptive preparation. *Am. J. Obstet. Gynecol.,* **1994,** *170*:1550–1555.

Aronica, S.M., and Katzenellenbogen, B.S. Stimulation of estrogen receptor-mediated transcription and alteration in the phosphorylation state of the rat uterine estrogen receptor by estrogen, cyclic adenosine monophosphate, and insulin-like growth factor-I. *Mol. Endocrinol.,* **1993,** *7*:743–752.

Astwood, E.B., and Fevold, H.L. Action of progesterone on the gonadotropic activity of the pituitary. *Am. J. Physiol.,* **1939,** *127*:192–198.

Beard, J. *The Span of Gestation and the Cause of Birth.* Gustav Fischer Verlag, Jena, **1897.**

Blackmore, P.F. Extragenomic actions of progesterone in human sperm and progesterone metabolites in human platelets. *Steroids,* **1999,** *64*:149–156.

Braidman, I., Baris, C., Wood, L., Selby, P., Adams, J., Freemont, A., and Hoyland, J. Preliminary evidence for impaired estrogen receptor-alpha protein expression in osteoblasts and osteocytes from men with idiopathic osteoporosis. *Bone,* **2000,** *26*:423–427.

Brzozowski, A.M., Pike, A.C., Dauter, Z., Hubbard, R.E., Bonn, T., Engstrom, O., Ohman, L., Greene, G.L., Gustafsson, J.A., and Carlquist, M. Molecular basis of agonism and antagonism in the oestrogen receptor. *Nature,* **1997,** *389*:753–758.

Butenandt, A. Über 'PROGYNON,' ein crystallisiertes, weibliches Sexualhormon. *Naturwisschenschaften,* **1929,** *17*:879.

Cheskis, B.J., Karanthanasis, S., and Lyttle, C.R. Estrogen receptor ligands modulate its interaction with DNA. *J. Biol. Chem.,* **1997,** *272*:11384–11391.

Collaborative Group on Hormonal Factors in Breast Cancer. Breast cancer and hormone replacement therapy: collaborative reanalysis of data from 51 epidemiological studies of 52,705 women with breast cancer and 108,411 women without breast cancer. *Lancet*, **1997**, *350*:1047–1059.

Corner, G.W., and Allen, W.M. Physiology of the corpus luteum. II. Production of a special uterine reaction (progestational proliferation) by extracts of the corpus luteum. *Am. J. Physiol.*, **1929**, *88*:326–346.

Cowley, S.M., Hoarse, S., Mosselman, S., and Parker, M.G. Estrogen receptors α and β form heterodimers on DNA. *J. Biol. Chem.*, **1997**, *272*:19858–19862.

Cummings, S.R., Eckert, S., Krueger, K.A., Grady, D., Powles, T.J., Cauley, J.A., Norton, L., Nickelsen, T., Bjarnason, N.H., Morrow, M., Lippman, M.E., Black, D., Glusman, J.E., Costa, A., and Jordan, V.C. The effect of raloxifene on risk of breast cancer in postmenopausal women: results from the MORE randomized trial. Multiple Outcomes of Raloxifene Evaluation. *JAMA*, **1999**, *281*:2189–2197.

DeFriend, D.J., Anderson, E., Bell, J., Wilks, D.P., West, C.M., Mansel, R.E., and Howell, A. Effects of 4-hydroxytamoxifen and a novel pure antioestrogen (ICI 182780) on the clonogenic growth of human breast cancer cells in vitro. *Br. J. Cancer*, **1994**, *70*:204–211.

Delmas, P.D., Bjarnason, N.H., Mitlak, B.H., Ravoux, A.C., Shah, A.S., Huster, W.J., Draper, M., and Christiansen, C. Effects of raloxifene on bone mineral density, serum cholesterol concentrations, and uterine endometrium in postmenopausal women. *N. Engl. J. Med.*, **1997**, *337*:1641–1647.

Diertsche, D.J., Bhattacharya, A.N., Atkinson, L.E., and Knobil, E. Circhoral oscillations of plasma LH in the ovariectomized rhesus monkey. *Endocrinology*, **1970**, *87*:850–853.

Dodds, E.C., Golberg, L., Lawson, W., and Robinson, R. Oestrogenic activity of alkylated stilboestrols. *Nature*, **1938**, *142*:34.

Doisy, E.A., Veler, C.D., and Thayer, S.A. Folliculin from the urine of pregnant women. *Am. J. Physiol.*, **1929**, *90*:329–330.

Doisy, E.A., Veler, C.D., and Thayer, S.A. The preparation of the crystalline ovarian hormone from the urine of pregnant women. *Am. J. Physiol.*, **1930**, *86*:499–509.

Early Breast Cancer Trialists' Group. Tamoxifen for early breast cancer: an overview of the randomised trials. *Lancet*, **1998**, *351*:1451–1467.

Endoh, H., Sasaki, H., Maruyama, K., Takeyama, K., Waga, I., Shimizu, T., Kato, S., and Kawashima, H. Rapid activation of MAP kinase by estrogen in the bone cell line. *Biochem. Biophys. Res. Commun.*, **1997**, *235*:99–102.

Ettinger, B., Black, D.M., Mitlak, B.H., Knickerbocker, R.K., Nickelsen, T., Genant, H.K., Christiansen, C., Delmas, P.D., Zanchetta, J.R., Stakkestad, J., Gluer, C.C., Krueger, K., Cohen, F.J., Eckert, S., Ensrud, K.E., Avioli, L.V., Lips, P., and Cummings, S.R. Reduction of vertebral fracture risk in postmenopausal women with osteoporosis treated with raloxifene: results from a 3-year randomized clinical trial. Multiple Outcomes of Raloxifene Evaluation (MORE) Investigators. *JAMA*, **1999**, *282*:637–645.

Falkenstein, E., Heck, M., Gerdes, D., Grube, D., Christ, M., Weigel, M., Buddhikot, M., Meizel, S., and Wehling, M. Specific progesterone binding to a membrane protein and related nongenomic effects on Ca^{2+}-fluxes in sperm. *Endocrinology*, **1999**, *140*:5999–6002.

FDA Drug Bulletin. Recommendations of DES Task Force. **1985**, *15*:40–42.

Fisher, B., Costantino, J.P., Wickerham, D.L., Redmond, C.K., Kavanah, M., Cronin, W.M., Vogel, V., Robidoux, A., Dimitrov, N., Atkins, J., Daly, M., Wieand, S., Tan-Chiu, E., Ford, L., and Wolmark, N. Tamoxifen for prevention of breast cancer: report of the National Surgical Adjuvant Breast and Bowel Project P-1 Study. *J. Natl. Cancer Inst.*, **1998**, *90*:1371–1388.

Fraenkel, L. Die Funktion des Corpus Luteum. *Arch. Gynaekol.*, **1903**, *68*:483–545.

Frank, R.T., Frank, M.L., Gustavson, R.G., and Weyerts, W.W. Demonstration of the female sex hormone in the circulating blood. I. Preliminary report. *JAMA*, **1925**, *85*:510.

Fuqua, S.A., Fitzgerald, S.D., Chamness, G.C., Tandon, A.K., McDonnell, D.P., Nawaz, Z., O'Malley, B.W., and McGuire, W.L. Variant human breast tumor estrogen receptor with constitutive transcriptional activity. *Cancer Res.*, **1991**, *51*:105–109.

Gass, E.K., Leonhardt, S.A., Nordeen, S.K., and Edwards, D.P. The antagonists RU486 and ZK98299 stimulate progesterone receptor binding to deoxyribonucleic acid in vitro and in vivo, but have distinct effects on receptor conformation. *Endocrinology*, **1998**, *139*:1905–1919.

Giangrande, P.H., Kimbrel, A., Edwards, D.P., and McDonnell, D.P. The opposing transcriptional activities of the two isoforms of the human progesterone receptor are due to differential cofactor binding. *Mol. Cell Biol.*, **2000**, *20*:3102–3115.

Goldzieher, J.W. Are low dose contraceptives safer and better? *Am. J. Obstet. Gynecol.*, **1994**, *171*:587–590.

Grady, D., Wenger, N.K., Herrington, D., Khan, S., Furberg, C., Hunninghake, D., Vittinghoff, E., and Hulley, S. Postmenopausal hormone therapy increases risk for venous thromboembolic disease. The Heart and Estrogen/progestin Replacement Study. *Ann. Intern. Med.*, **2000**, *132*:689–696.

Greenblatt, R.B., Roy, S., Mahesh, V.B., Barfield, W.E., and Jungck, E.C. Induction of ovulation. *Am. J. Obstet. Gynecol.*, **1962**, *84*:900–909.

Greenwald, P., Barlow, J.J., Nasca, P.C., and Burnett, W.S. Vaginal cancer after maternal treatment with synthetic estrogens. *N. Engl. J. Med.*, **1971**, *285*:390–392.

Grimes, D.A. The morbidity and mortality of pregnancy: still risky business. *Am. J. Obstet. Gynecol.*, **1994**, *170*:1489–1494.

Grodstein, F., Colditz, G.A., Hunter, D.J., Manson, J.E., Wilett, W.C., and Stampfer, M.J. A prospective study of symptomatic gallstones in women: relation with oral contraceptives and other factors. *Obstet. Gynecol.*, **1994**, *84*:207–214.

Grodstein, F., Stampfer, M.J., Manson, J.E., Colditz, G.A., Willett, W.C., Rosner, B., Speizer, F.E., and Hennekens, C.H. Postmenopausal estrogen and progestin use and the risk of cardiovascular disease. *N. Engl. J. Med.*, **1996**, *335*:453–461.

Haberlandt, L. Ueber hormonale Sterilisierung weiblicher Tiere (Futerungsversuche mit ovarial- und plazenta-Opton. *Munch. Med. Wochenschr.*, **1927**, 49–55.

Halban, J. Ueber den Einfluss der Ovarien auf die Entwicklung des Genitales. *Monatsschr. Geburtshilfe Gynäkol.*, **1900**, 496–503.

Hall, J.M., and McDonnell, D.P. The estrogen receptor β-isoform (ERβ) of the human estrogen receptor modulates ERα transcriptional activity and is a key regulator of the cellular response to estrogens and antiestrogens. *Endocrinology*, **1999**, *140*:5566–5578.

Henderson, B.E., Paganini-Hill, A., and Ross, R.K. Decreased mortality in users of estrogen replacement therapy. *Arch. Intern. Med.*, **1991**, *151*:75–78.

Henderson, V.W., Paganini-Hill, A., Miller, B.L., Elble, R.J., Reyes, P.F., Shoupe, D., McCleary, C.A., Klein, R.A., Hake, A.M., and Farlow, M.R. Estrogen for Alzheimer's disease in women: randomized, double-blind, placebo-controlled trial. *Neurology*, **2000**, *54*:295–301.

Herbst, A.L., Ulfelder, H., and Poskanzer, D.C. Adenocarcinoma of the vagina. Association of maternal stilbestrol therapy with tumor appearance in young women. *N. Engl. J. Med.*, **1971**, *284*:878–881.

Hermann, W., Wyss, R., Riondel, A., Philibert, D., Teutsch, G., Sakiz, E., and Baulieu, E.E. Effect d'un steroid antiprogesterone chez la femme, interruption du cycle menstruel et de la grossesse au debut. *C.R. Acad. Sci. Paris*, **1982**, *294*:933–938.

Howell, A., DeFriend, D., Robertson, J., Blamey, R., and Walton, P. Response to a specific antioestrogen (ICI 182780) in tamoxifen-resistant breast cancer. *Lancet*, **1995**, *345*:29–30.

Hulley, S., Grady, D., Bush, T., Furberg, C., Herrington, D., Riggs, B., and Vittinghoff, E. Randomized trial of estrogen plus progestin for secondary prevention of coronary heart disease in postmenopausal women. Heart and Estrogen/progestin Replacement Study (HERS) Research Group. *JAMA*, **1998**, *280*:605–613.

Ilanchezhian, S., Thangaraju, M., and Sachdanandam, P. Plasma lipids and lipoprotein alterations in tamoxifen-treated breast cancer women in relation to the menopausal status. *Cancer Biochem. Biophys.*, **1995**, *15*:83–90.

Ing, N.H., Beekman, J.M., Tsai, S.Y., Tsai, M.J., and O'Malley, B.W. Members of the steroid hormone receptor superfamily interact with TFIIB (S300-II). *J. Biol. Chem.*, **1992**, *267*:17617–17623.

Jensen, E.V., and Jacobsen, H.I. Basic guides to the mechanism of estrogen action. *Recent Prog. Horm. Res.*, (Pincus, G., ed.) **1962**, *XVIII*:387–414.

Jick, H., Derby, L.E., Myers, M.W., Vasilakis, C., and Newton, K.M. Risk of hospital admission for idiopathic venous thromboembolism among users of postmenopausal oestrogens. *Lancet*, **1996**, *348*:981–983.

Kato, S., Endoh, H., Masuhiro, Y., Kitamoto, T., Uchiyama, S., Sasaki, H., Masushige, S., Gotoh, Y., Nishida, E., Kawashima, H., Metzger, D., and Chambon, P. Activation of the estrogen receptor through phosphorylation by mitogen-activated protein kinase. *Science*, **1995**, *270*:1491–1494.

Kettel, L.M., Roseff, S.J., Berga, S.L., Mortola, J.F., and Yen, S.S. Hypothalamic-pituitary-ovarian response to clomiphene citrate in women with polycystic ovary syndrome. *Fertil. Steril.*, **1993**, *59*:532–538.

Knauer, E. Die Ovarien-Transplantation. *Arch. Gynaekol.*, **1900**, *60*:322–376.

Knobil, E. Patterns of hypophysiotropic signals and gonadotropin secretion in the rhesus monkey. *Biol. Reprod.*, **1981**, *24*:44–49.

Kobayashi, S., Inoue, S., Hosoi, T., Ouchi, Y., Shiraki, M., and Orimo, H. Association of bone mineral density with polymorphism of the estrogen receptor gene. *J. Bone Miner. Res.*, **1996**, *11*:306–311.

Koh, K.K., Mincemoyer, R., Bui, M.N., Csako, G., Pucino, F., Guetta, V., Waclawiw, M., and Cannon, R.O. III. Effects of hormone-replacement therapy on fibrinolysis in postmenopausal women. *N. Engl. J. Med.*, **1997**, *336*:683–690.

Korach, K.S. Estrogen receptor knock-out mice: molecular and endocrine phenotypes. *J. Soc. Gynecol. Invest.*, **2000**, *7*:S16–S17.

Kuiper, G.G., Carlsson, B., Grandien, K., Enmark, E., Haggblad, J., Nilsson, S., and Gustafsson, J.A. Comparison of the ligand binding specificity and transcript tissue distribution of estrogen receptors ER α and β. *Endocrinology*, **1997**, *138*:863–870.

Kuiper, G.G., Lemmen, J.G., Carlsson, B., Corton, J.C., Safe, S.H., van der Saag, P.T., van der Burg, B., and Gustafsson, J.A. Interaction of estrogenic chemicals and phytoestrogens with estrogen receptor beta. *Endocrinology*, **1998**, *139*:422–463.

Lacassagne, A. Tumeurs malignes apparus au cours d'un traitement hormonal combiné, chez des souris appartenant à des lignées réfractaires au cancer spontané. *C.R. Soc. Biol. (Paris)*, **1936**, *121*:607–609.

Lahti, E., Blanco, G., Kaupilla, A., Apaja-Sarkkinen, M., Taskinen, P.J., and Laatikainen, T. Endometrial changes in postmenopausal breast cancer patients receiving tamoxifen. *Obstet. Gynecol.*, **1993**, *81*:660–664.

Lindsay, R., Hart, D.M., and Clark, D.M. The minimum effective dose of estrogen for prevention of postmenopausal bone loss. *Obstet. Gynecol.*, **1984**, *63*:759–763.

Loewe, S. Nachweis brusterzeugender Stoffe im weiblichen Blute. *Klin. Wochenschr.*, **1925**, *4*:1407–1408.

Loewe, S., and Lange, F. Der Gehalt des Frauenharns an brunsterzeugenden Stoffen in Abhängigkeit von ovariellen Zyklus. *Klin. Wochenschr.*, **1926**, *5*:1038–1039.

Love, R.R., Weibe, D.A., Feyzi, J.M., Newcomb, P.A., and Happell, R.J. Effects of tamoxifen on cardiovascular risk factors in postmenopausal women after five years of treatment. *J. Natl. Cancer Inst.*, **1994**, *86*:1534–1539.

Lubahn, D.B., Moyer, J.S., Golding, T.S., Couse, J.F., Korach, K.S., and Smithies, O. Alteration of reproductive function but not prenatal sexual development after insertional disruption of the mouse estrogen receptor gene. *Proc. Natl. Acad. Sci. U.S.A.*, **1993**, *90*:11162–11166.

McDonnell, D.P., and Goldman, M.E. RU486 exerts antiestrogenic activities through a novel progesterone receptor A form-mediated mechanism. *J. Biol. Chem.*, **1994**, *269*:11945–11949.

Makepeace, A.W., Weinstein, G.L., and Friedman, M.H. The effect of progestin and progesterone on ovulation in the rabbit. *Am. J. Physiol.*, **1937**, *119*:512–526.

Matsumoto, A.M., Gross, K.M., and Bremner, W.J. The physiological significance of pulsatile LHRH secretion in man: gonadotropin responses to physiological doses of pulsatile versus continuous LHRH administration. *Int. J. Androl.*, **1991**, *14*:23–32.

Mishell, D.R., Jr., Kletzky, O.A., Brenner, P.F., Roy, S., and Nicoloff, J. The effect of contraceptive steroids on hypothalamic-pituitary function. *Am. J. Obstet. Gynecol.*, **1977**, *128*:60–74.

Mulnard, R.A., Cotman, C.W., Kawas, C., van Dyck, C.H., Sano, M., Doody, R., Koss, E., Pfeiffer, E., Jin, S., Gamst, A., Grundman, M., Thomas, R., and Thal, L.J. Estrogen replacement therapy for treatment of mild to moderate Alzheimer disease: a randomized controlled trial. Alzheimer's Disease Cooperative Study. *JAMA*, **2000**, *283*:1007–1015.

Ory, H.W. The noncontraceptive health benefits from oral contraceptive use. *Fam. Plann. Perspect.*, **1982**, *14*:182–184.

Paech, K., Webb, P., Kuiper, G.G., Nilsson, S., Gustafsson, J.A., Kushner, P.J., and Scanlan, T.S. Differential ligand activation of estrogen receptors ERalpha and ERbeta at AP1 sites. *Science*, **1997**, *277*:1508–1510.

Pean, V. Effectiveness of an oral contraceptive. *Science*, **1959**, *130*:81–83.

Philibert, D., Deraedt, R., and Teutsch, G. RU 38486: a potent antiglucocorticoid in vivo. (Abstract.). *VIII Int. Congr. Pharmacol.*, **1981**, 14631.

Pike, M.C., Peters, R.K., Cozen, W., Probst-Hensch, N.M., Felix, J.C., Wan, P.C., and Mack, T.M. Estrogen-progestin replacement therapy and endometrial cancer. *J. Natl. Cancer Inst.*, **1997**, *89*:1110–1116.

Pincus, G., Garcia, C., Rock, J., Paniagua, M., Pendleton, A., Laroque, F., Nicolas, R., Borno, R., and Pean, V. Effectiveness of an oral contraceptive. *Science*, **1959**, *130*:81–83.

Plant, T.M., Krey, L.C., Moossy, J., McCormack, J.T., Hess, D.L., and Knobil, E. The arcuate nucleus and the control of gonadotropin and prolactin secretion in the female rhesus monkey *(Macaca mulatta)*. *Endocrinology*, **1978**, *102*:52–62.

Prince, R.L., Smith, M., Dick, I.M., Price, R.I., Webb, P.G., Henderson, N.K., and Harris, M.M. Prevention of postmenopausal osteoporosis. A comparative study of exercise, calcium supplementation, and hormone-replacement therapy. *N. Engl. J. Med.,* **1991,** *325*:1189–1195.

Razandi, M., Pedram, A., Greene, G.L., and Levin, E.R. Cell membrane and nuclear estrogen receptors (ERs) originate from a single transcript: studies of ERalpha and ERbeta expressed in Chinese hamster ovary cells. *Mol Endocrinol.,* **1999,** *13*:307–319.

Rebar, R.W., and Zeserson, K. Characteristics of the new progestogens in combination oral contraceptives. *Contraception,* **1991,** *44*:1–10.

Reddi, K., Wickings, E.J., McNeilly, A.S., Baird, D.T., and Hillier, S.G. Circulating bioactive follicle stimulating hormone and immunoreactive inhibin levels during the normal human menstrual cycle. *Clin. Endocrinol. (Oxf.),* **1990,** *33*:547–557.

Redmond, G.P., Olson, W.H., Lippman, J.S., Kafrissen, M.E., Jones, T.M., and Jorizzo, J.L. Norgestimate and ethinyl estradiol in the treatment of acne vulgaris: a randomized, placebo-controlled trial. *Obstet. Gynecol.,* **1997,** *89*:615–622.

Resnick, E.M., Schreihofer, D.A., Periasamy, A., and Shupnik, M.A. Truncated estrogen receptor product-1 suppresses estrogen receptor transactivation by dimerization with estrogen receptors alpha and beta. *J. Biol. Chem.,* **2000,** *275*:7158–7166.

Rigg, L.A., Hermann, H., and Yen, S.S. Absorption of estrogens from vaginal creams. *N. Engl. J. Med.,* **1978,** *298*:195–197.

Roodi, N., Bailey, L.R., Kao, W.Y., Verrier, C.S., Yee, C.J., Dupont, W.D., and Parl, F.F. Estrogen receptor gene analysis in estrogen receptor-positive and receptor-negative primary breast cancer. *J. Natl. Cancer Inst.,* **1995,** *87*:446–451.

Ross, R.K., Paganini-Hill, A., Wan, P.C., and Pike, M.C. Effect of hormone replacement therapy on breast cancer risk: estrogen versus estrogen plus progestin. *J. Natl. Cancer Inst.,* **2000,** *92*:328–332.

Rutqvist, L.E., and Mattsson, A. Cardiac and thromboembolic morbidity among postmenopausal women with early-stage breast cancer in a randomized trial of adjuvant tamoxifen. The Stockholm Breast Cancer Study Group. *J. Natl. Cancer Inst.,* **1993,** *85*:1398–1406.

Sack, M.N., Rader, D.J., and Cannon, R.O. III. Oestrogen and inhibition of oxidation of low-density lipoproteins in postmenopausal women. *Lancet,* **1994,** *343*:269–270.

Saville, B., Wormke, M., Wang, F., Nguyen, T., Enmark, E., Kuiper, G., Gustafsson, J.A., and Safe, S. Ligand-, cell-, and estrogen receptor subtype (α/β)-dependent activation at GC-rich (Sp1) promoter elements. *J. Biol. Chem.,* **2000,** *275*:5379–5387.

Schairer, C., Lubin, J., Troisi, R., Sturgeon, S., Brinton, L., and Hoover, R. Menopausal estrogen and estrogen-progestin replacement therapy and breast cancer risk. *JAMA,* **2000,** *283*:485–491.

Shapiro, S., Kelly, J.P., Rosenberg, L., Kaufman, D.W., Helmrich, S.P., Rosenshein, N.B., Lewis, J.L. Jr., Knapp, R.C., Stolley, P.D., and Schottenfeld, D. Risk of localized and widespread endometrial cancer in relation to recent and discontinued use of conjugated estrogens. *N. Engl. J. Med.,* **1985,** *313*:969–972.

Shoupe, D. New progestins—clinical experiences: gestodene. *Am. J. Obstet. Gynecol.,* **1994,** *170*:1562–1568.

Smith, C.L., Nawaz, Z., and O'Malley, B.W. Coactivator and corepressor regulation of the agonist/antagonist activity of the mixed antiestrogen, 4-hydroxytamoxifen. *Mol. Endocrinol.,* **1997,** *11*:657–666.

Smith, E.P., Boyd, J., Frank, G.R., Takahashi, H., Cohen, R.M., Specker, B., Williams, T.C., Lubahn, D.B., and Korach, K.S. Estrogen resistance caused by a mutation in the estrogen-receptor gene in a man. *N. Engl. J. Med.,* **1994,** *331*:1056–1061.

Task Force on Postovulatory Methods of Fertility Regulation. Randomised controlled trial of levonorgestrel versus the Yuzpe regimen of combined oral contraceptives for emergency contraception. *Lancet,* **1998,** *352*:428–433.

Thorneycroft, I.H., Mishell, D.R., Jr., Stone, S.C., Kharma, K.M., and Nakamura, R.M. The relation of serum 17-hydroxyprogesterone and estradiol-17β levels during the human menstrual cycle. *Am. J. Obstet. Gynecol.,* **1971,** *111*:947–951.

Van Den Bemd, G.J., Kuiper, G.G., Pols, H.A., and Van Leeuwen, J.P. Distinct effects on the conformation of estrogen receptor α and β by both the antiestrogens ICI 164,384 and ICI 182,780 leading to opposite effects on receptor stability. *Biochem. Biophys. Res. Commun.,* **1999,** *261*:1–5.

Vandevyver, C., Vanhoof, J., Declerck, K., Stinissen, P., Vandervorst, C., Michiels, L., Cassiman, J.J., Boonen, S., Raus, J., and Geusens, P. Lack of association between estrogen receptor genotypes and bone mineral density, fracture history, or muscle strength in elderly women. *J. Bone Miner. Res.,* **1999,** *14*:1576–1582.

Vegeto, E., Shahbaz, M.M., Wen, D.X., Goldman, M.E., O'Malley, B.W., and McDonnell, D.P. Human progesterone receptor A form is a cell- and promoter-specific repressor of human progesterone receptor B function. *Mol. Endocrinol.,* **1993,** *7*:1244–1255.

Walsh, B.W., Kuller, L.H., Wild, R.A., Paul, S., Farmer, M., Lawrence, J.B., Shah, A.S., and Anderson, P.W. Effects of raloxifene on serum lipids and coagulation factors in healthy postmenopausal women. *JAMA,* **1998,** *279*:1445–1451.

Walsh, B.W., Li, H., and Sacks, F.M. Effects of postmenopausal hormone replacement with oral and transdermal estrogen on high density lipoprotein metabolism. *J. Lipid Res.,* **1994,** *35*:2083–2093.

Weiderpass, E., Persson, I., Melhus, H., Wedren, S., Kindmark, A., and Baron, J.A. Estrogen receptor alpha gene polymorphisms and endometrial cancer risk. *Carcinogenesis,* **2000,** *21*:623–627.

Wijayaratne, A.L., Nagel, S.C., Paige, L.A., Christensen, D.J., Norris, J.D., Fowlkes, D.M., and McDonnell, D.P. Comparative analyses of mechanistic differences among antiestrogens. *Endocrinology,* **1999,** *140*:5828–5840.

Wilson, R.C., Kesner, J.S., Kaufman, J.M., Uemura, T., Akema, T., and Knobil, E. Central electrophysiologic correlates of pulsatile luteinizing hormone secretion in the rhesus monkey. *Neuroendocrinology,* **1984,** *39*:256–260.

The Writing Group for the PEPI Trial. Effects of estrogen or estrogen/progestin regimens on heart disease risk factors in postmenopausal women. The Postmenopausal Estrogen/Progestin Interventions (PEPI) Trial. *JAMA,* **1995,** *273*:199–208.

Yen, S.S., Tsai, C.C., Naftolin, F., Vandenberg, G., and Ajabor, L. Pulsatile patterns of gonadotropin release in subjects with and without ovarian function. *J. Clin. Endocrinol. Metab.,* **1972,** *34*:671–675.

Zondek, B. Darstellung des weiblichen Sexualhormon aus dem Harn, insbesondere dem Harn von Schwangeren. *Klin. Wochenschr.,* **1928,** *7*:485–486.

MONOGRAPHS AND REVIEWS

Anstead, G.M., Carlson, K.E., and Katzenellenbogen, J.A. The estradiol pharmacophore: ligand structure-estrogen receptor binding affinity relationships and a model for the receptor binding site. *Steroids,* **1997,** *62*:268–303.

Baird, D.T., and Glasier, A.F. Hormonal contraception. *N. Engl. J. Med.,* **1993,** *328*:1543–1549.

Barbieri, R.L., Speroff, L., Walker, A.M., and McPherson, K. Therapeutic controversy: the safety of third-generation oral contraceptives. *J. Clin. Endocrinol. Metab.,* **1999,** *84*:1822–1829.

Barrett-Connor, E., and Laakso, M. Ischemic heart disease risk in postmenopausal women. Effects of estrogen use on glucose and insulin levels. *Arteriosclerosis,* **1990,** *10:*531–534.

Belchetz, P.E. Hormonal treatment of postmenopausal women. *N. Engl. J. Med.,* **1994,** *330:*1062–1071.

Brodie, A.M., and Njar, V.C. Aromatase inhibitors and their application in breast cancer treatment. *Steroids,* **2000,** *65:*171–179.

Cadepond, F., Ulmann, A., and Baulieu, E.E. RU486 (mifepristone): mechanisms of action and clinical uses. *Annu. Rev. Med.,* **1997,** *48:*129–156.

Castelli, W.P. Cardiovascular disease: pathogenesis, epidemiology, and risk among users of oral contraceptives who smoke. *Am. J. Obstet. Gynecol.,* **1999,** *180:*349S–356S.

Christin-Maitre, S., Bouchard, P., and Spitz, I.M. Medical termination of pregnancy. *N. Engl. J. Med.,* **2000,** *342:*946–956.

Clarke, C.L., and Sutherland, R.L. Progestin regulation of cellular proliferation: update 1993. *Endocrine Reviews Monographs 1. Endocrine Aspects of Cancer.* (Horwitz, K.B., ed.) The Endocrine Society, **1993,** pp. 132–135.

Collingwood, T.N., Urnov, F.D., and Wolffe, A.P. Nuclear receptors: coactivators, corepressors and chromatin remodeling in the control of transcription. *J. Mol. Endocrinol.,* **1999,** *23:*255–275.

Cullins, V.E. Noncontraceptive benefits and therapeutic uses of depot medroxyprogesterone acetate. *J. Reprod. Med.,* **1996,** *41:*428–433.

Drew, F.L. The epidemiology of secondary amenorrhea. *J. Chron. Dis.,* **1961,** *14:*396–407.

Duax, W.L., Griffin, J.F., Weeks, C.M., and Wawrzak, Z. The mechanism of action of steroid antagonists: insights from crystallographic studies. *J. Steroid Biochem.,* **1988,** *31:*481–492.

Eskin, B.A. Sex hormones and aging. *Adv. Exp. Med. Biol.,* **1978,** *97:*207–224.

Fotherby, K. Bioavailability of orally administered sex steroids used in oral contraception and hormone replacement therapy. *Contraception,* **1996,** *54:*59–69.

Fruzzetti, F. Hemostatic effects of smoking and oral contraceptive use. *Am. J. Obstet. Gynecol.,* **1999,** *180:*S369–S374.

Giangrande, P.H., and McDonnell, D.P. The A and B isoforms of the human progesterone receptor: two functionally different transcription factors encoded by a single gene. *Recent Prog. Horm. Res.,* **1999,** *54:*291–313.

Godsland, I.F. The influence of female sex steroids on glucose metabolism and insulin action. *J. Intern. Med. Suppl.,* **1996,** *738:*1–60.

Green, P.S., and Simpkins, J.W. Neuroprotective effects of estrogens: potential mechanisms of action. *Int. J. Dev. Neurosci.,* **2000,** *18:*347–358.

Grumbach, M.M., and Auchus, R.J. Estrogen: consequences and implications of human mutations in synthesis and action. *J. Clin. Endocrinol. Metab.,* **1999,** *84:*4677–4694.

Hofbauer, L.C., Khosla, S., Dunstan, C.R., Lacey, D.L., Boyle, W.J., and Riggs, B.L. The roles of osteoprotegrin and osteoprotegrin ligand in the paracrine regulation of bone resorption. *J. Bone Miner. Res.,* **2000,** *15:*2–12.

Hol, T., Cox, M.B., Bryant, H.U., and Draper, M.W. Selective estrogen receptor modulators and postmenopausal women's health. *J. Womens Health,* **1997,** *6:*523–531.

Hotchkiss, J., and Knobil, E. The menstrual cycle and its neuroendocrine control. In, *The Physiology of Reproduction.* 2nd ed. (Knobil, E., and Neill, J.D., eds.) Raven Press, New York, **1994,** pp. 711–749.

Ibrahim, N.K., and Hortobagyi, G.N. The evolving role of specific estrogen receptor modulators. *Surg. Oncol.,* **1999,** *8:*103–123.

Jaiyesimi, I.A., Buzdar, A.U., Decker, D.A., and Hortobagyi, G.N. Use of tamoxifen for breast cancer: twenty-eight years later. *J. Clin. Oncol.,* **1995,** *13:*513–529.

Jang, G.R., and Benet, L.Z. Antiprogestin pharmacodynamics, pharmacokinetics, and metabolism: implications for their long-term use. *J. Pharmacokinet. Biopharm.,* **1997,** *25:*647–672.

Jensen, E.V., and DeSombre, E.R. Mechanism of action of the female sex hormones. *Annu. Rev. Biochem.,* **1972,** *41:*203–230.

Jordan, V.C., and Murphy, C.S. Endocrine pharmacology of antiestrogens as antitumor agents. *Endocr. Rev.,* **1990,** *11:*578–610.

Kols, M., Rinehart, W., Piotrow, P.T., Coucette, L., and Quillin, W.F. Oral contraceptives in the 1980s. *Popul. Rep. A.,* **1982,** *6:*189–222.

Liehr, J.G. Is estradiol a genotoxic mutagenic carcinogen? *Endocr. Rev.,* **2000,** *21:*40–54.

Lobo, R.A. Clinical review 27: effects of hormonal replacement on lipids and lipoproteins in postmenopausal women. *J. Clin. Endocrinol. Metab.,* **1991,** *73:*925–930.

Lobo, R.A., and Stanczyk, F.Z. New knowledge in the physiology of hormonal contraceptives. *Am. J. Obstet. Gynecol.,* **1994,** *170:*1499–1507.

Mäkelä, S., Hyder, S.M., and Stancel, G.M. Environmental estrogens. In, *Handbook of Experimental Pharmacology.* Vol. 135, part II: *Estrogens and Antiestrogens.* (Oettel, M., and Schillinger, E., eds.) Springer-Verlag, Berlin, **1999,** pp. 613–663.

McDonnell, D.P. Selective estrogen receptor modulators (SERMs): a first step in the development of perfect hormone replacement therapy regimen. *J. Soc. Gynecol. Invest.,* **2000,** *7:*S10–S15.

Mendelson, C.R., and Simpson, E.R. Regulation of estrogen biosynthesis by human adipose cells *in vitro. Mol. Cell. Endocrinol.,* **1987,** *52:*169–176.

Mendelsohn, M.E., and Karas, R.H. The protective effects of estrogen on the cardiovascular system. *N. Engl. J. Med.,* **1999,** *340:*1801–1811.

Mischell, D.R. Cardiovascular risks: perception versus reality. *Contraception,* **1999,** *59:*21S–24S.

Murphy, L.C., Leygue, E., Dotzlaw, H., Douglas, D., Coutts, A., and Watson, P.H. Oestrogen receptor variants and mutations in human breast cancer. *Ann. Med.,* **1997,** *29:*221–234.

Peltoketo, H., Vihko, P., and Vihko, R. Regulation of estrogen action: role of 17 beta-hydroxysteroid dehydrogenases. *Vitam. Horm.,* **1999,** *55:*353–398.

Perone, N. The progestins. In, *Pharmacology of the Contraceptive Steroids.* (Goldzieher, J.W., ed.) Raven Press, New York, **1994,** pp. 5–19.

Riggs, B.L., and Melton, L.J. III. The prevention and treatment of osteoporosis. *N. Engl. J. Med.,* **1992,** *327:*620–627. [Published erratum in *N. Engl. J. Med.,* **1993,** *328:*65.]

Rock, J., Garcia, C.M., and Pincus, G. Synthetic progestins in the normal human menstrual cycle. *Recent Prog. Horm. Res.,* **1957,** *13:*323–339.

Sherif, K. Benefits and risks of oral contraceptives. *Am. J. Obstet. Gynecol.,* **1999,** *180:*S343–S348.

Silverman, A.J., Livne, I., and Witkin, J.W. The gonadotropin-releasing hormone (GnRH) neuronal systems: immunocytochemistry and in situ hybridization. In, *The Physiology of Reproduction,* 2nd ed. (Knobil, E., and Neill, J.D., eds.) Raven Press, New York, **1994,** pp. 1683–1709.

Simpson, E., Rubin, G., Clyne, C., Robertson, K., O'Donnell, L., Davis, S., and Jones, M. Local estrogen biosynthesis in males and females. *Endocr. Relat. Cancer,* **1999,** *6:*131–137.

Simpson, E.R., Mahendroo, M.S., Means, G.D., Kilgore, M.W., Hinshelwood, M.M., Graham-Lorence, S., Amarneh, B., Ito, Y., Fisher, C.R., Michael, M.D., Mendelson, C.R., and Bulun, S.E. Aromatase cytochrome P450, the enzyme responsible for estrogen biosynthesis. *Endocr. Rev.,* **1994,** *15*:342–355.

Spelsberg, T.C., Subramaniam, M., Riggs, B.L., and Khosla, S. The actions and interactions of sex steroids and growth factors/cytokines on the skeleton. *Mol. Endocrinol.,* **1999,** *13*:819–828.

Tham, D.M., Gardner, C.D., and Haskell, W.L. Clinical review 97: potential health benefits of dietary phytoestrogens: a review of the clinical, epidemiological, and mechanistic evidence. *J. Clin. Endocrinol. Metab.,* **1998,** *83*:2223–2235.

Westhoff, C.L. Breast cancer risk: perception versus reality. *Contraception,* **1999,** *59*:25S–28S.

Young, R.L., Kumar, N.S., and Goldzieher, J.W. Management of menopause when estrogen cannot be used. *Drugs,* **1990,** *40*:220–230.

C H A P T E R   5 9

ANDROGENS

Peter J. Snyder

Testosterone is the principal circulating androgen in men. It is secreted by the Leydig cells of the testes in response to luteinizing hormone (LH) from the pituitary gland. The varied effects of testosterone are due to its ability to act by at least three different mechanisms: by binding to the androgen receptor; by conversion in certain tissues to dihydrotestosterone, which also binds to the androgen receptor; and by conversion to estradiol, which binds to the estrogen receptor. Testosterone is responsible for male sexual differentiation in utero *and for male pubertal changes. Consequently, failure of a male fetus to secrete testosterone or to have functional androgen receptors during the first trimester results in incomplete male sexual differentiation; failure of testosterone secretion before puberty results in incomplete pubertal changes; and failure during adulthood results in a diminution, at different rates, of some aspects of virilization. In women the physiological role of testosterone and the consequences of its deficiency are not yet understood, but it is possible that it contributes to libido, energy, muscle mass and strength, and bone strength.*

Oral administration of testosterone leads to absorption into the hepatic circulation but rapid catabolism by the liver, so oral ingestion is ineffective in delivering testosterone systemically. Most attempts to devise pharmacological testosterone preparations, therefore, have involved finding ways of bypassing hepatic catabolism. The 17α-alkylated androgens can be administered orally and are not catabolized as rapidly as testosterone itself, but they tend to cause cholestasis. Esters of testosterone and a fatty acid, when injected, produce serum testosterone concentrations that remain within the normal range for one to several weeks. Transdermal preparations of testosterone deliver testosterone itself into the systemic circulation and, when applied daily, produce relatively even serum testosterone concentrations.

The major indication for testosterone treatment is male hypogonadism, for which a testosterone ester or transdermal preparation should be used. Treatment should be monitored for efficacy by measurement of the serum testosterone concentration and for deleterious effects by evaluating for obstruction to urine flow due to benign prostatic hyperplasia, for prostate cancer, and for erythrocytosis. Athletes have used androgens to attempt to improve their performance. Androgens have been used to attempt to develop a male contraceptive. For this purpose they have been used alone or in combination with a gonadotropin-releasing hormone (GnRH) antagonist or a progestin to suppress endogenous testosterone production and thereby spermatogenesis. The 17α-alkylated androgens are used to treat angioneurotic edema, because they stimulate C1 esterase inhibitor. Some drugs are antiandrogens that are used intentionally to inhibit undesirable effects of androgens; other drugs, used for nonhormonal purposes, have side effects as a consequence of their antiandrogenic properties. Analogs of GnRH inhibit LH secretion and thereby reduce testosterone synthesis. They are used to treat metastatic prostate cancer. A side effect of the antifungal agents of the imidazole class (see Chapter 49) is direct inhibition of cortisol synthesis in the adrenal glands and testosterone synthesis in the testes. Flutamide and bicalutamide are androgen receptor antagonists that are used in combination with GnRH analogs in the treatment of metastatic prostate cancer because they block the effects of adrenal androgens. Spironolactone (see Chapter 29) is an aldosterone receptor antagonist and also a weak androgen receptor antagonist that causes gynecomastia when used as a diuretic in men. Finasteride is an inhibitor of the 5α-reductase enzyme, which is used to treat benign prostatic hyperplasia.

TESTOSTERONE AND OTHER ANDROGENS

Synthesis of Testosterone. In men, testosterone is the principal secreted androgen. The Leydig cells synthesize the majority of testosterone by the pathways shown in Figure 59–1. In women, testosterone also is probably the principal androgen and is synthesized both in the corpus luteum and the adrenal cortex by similar pathways. The testosterone precursors androstenedione and dehydroepiandrosterone are weak androgens.

Secretion and Transport of Testosterone. The magnitude of testosterone secretion is greater in men than in women at almost all stages of life, a difference that explains almost all other differences between men and women. In the first trimester *in utero,* the fetal testes begin

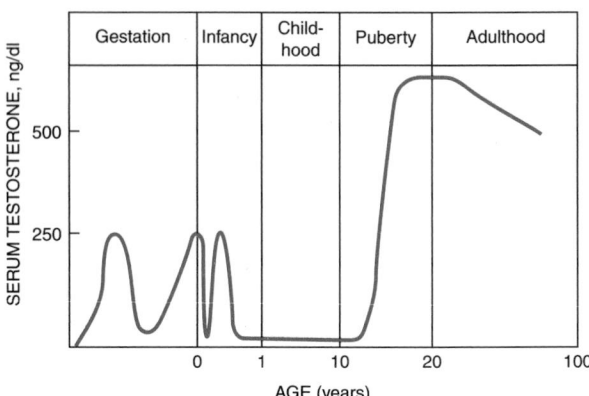

Figure 59–2. Schematic representation of the serum testosterone concentration from early gestation to old age.

to secrete testosterone, which is the principal factor in male sexual differentiation, probably stimulated by human chorionic gonadotropin from the placenta. By the beginning of the second trimester, the value is close to that of midpuberty, about 250 ng/dl (Figure 59–2) (Dawood and Saxena, 1977; Forest, 1975). Testosterone production then falls by the end of the second trimester, but by birth the value is again about 250 ng/dl (Forest and Cathiard, 1975; Forest, 1975; Dawood and Saxena, 1977), possibly due to stimulation of the fetal Leydig cells by luteinizing hormone (LH) from the fetal pituitary gland. The testosterone value falls again in the first few days after birth, but it rises and peaks again at about 250 ng/dl at two to three months after birth and falls to <50 ng/dl by six months, where it remains until puberty (Forest, 1975). During puberty, from about age 12 to 17 years, the serum testosterone concentration in males increases to a much greater degree than in females, so that by early adulthood the serum testosterone concentration is 500 to 700 ng/dl in men, compared to 30 to 50 ng/dl in women. The magnitude of the testosterone concentration in the male is responsible for the pubertal changes that further differentiate men from women. As men age, their serum testosterone concentrations gradually decrease, which may contribute to other effects of aging in men.

LH, secreted by the gonadotroph cells of the pituitary (*see* Chapter 56), is the principal stimulus of testosterone secretion in men, perhaps potentiated by follicle stimulating hormone (FSH), also secreted by the gonadotroph cells. GnRH from the hypothalamus (*see* Chapter 56), in

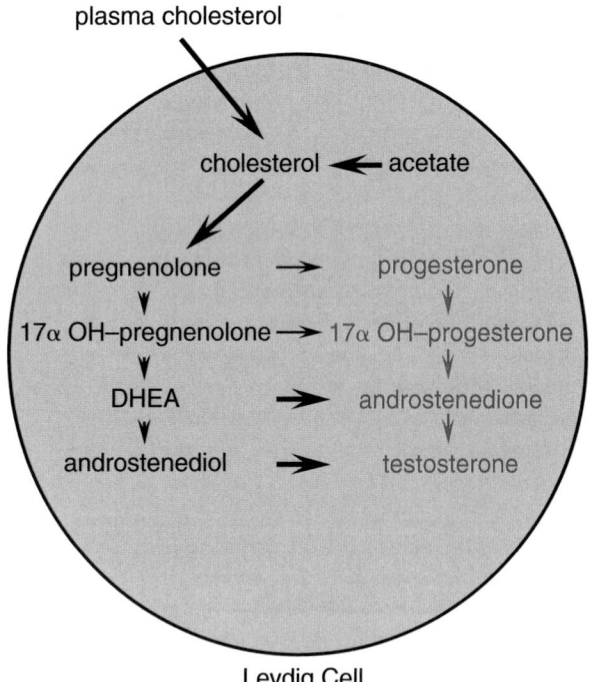

Leydig Cell

Figure 59–1. Pathway of synthesis of testosterone in the Leydig cells of the testes.

Bold arrows indicate favored pathways. DHEA, dehydroepiandrosterone. (Adapted from Santen, 1995, with permission.)

turn, stimulates LH secretion, and testosterone inhibits it, acting directly on the gonadotroph cell. LH is secreted in pulses, which occur approximately every two hours and are greater in magnitude in the morning. The pulsatility appears to result from pulsatile secretion of GnRH from the hypothalamus. Pulsatile administration of GnRH to men who are hypogonadal due to hypothalamic disease results in normal LH pulses and testosterone secretion, but continuous administration does not (Crowley *et al.,* 1985). Testosterone secretion is likewise pulsatile and diurnal, with the highest plasma concentrations occurring at about 8 A.M. and the lowest at about 8 P.M. The morning peaks diminish as men age (Bremner *et al.,* 1983).

In women, LH stimulates the corpus luteum (formed from the follicle after release of the ovum) to secrete testosterone. Under normal circumstances, however, estradiol and progesterone, not testosterone, are the principal inhibitors of LH secretion in women. Sex hormone binding globulin (SHBG) binds about 40% of circulating testosterone with high affinity. Albumin binds almost 60% of circulating testosterone with low affinity. Approximately 2% of testosterone is unbound or free.

Metabolism of Testosterone to Active and Inactive Compounds.   Testosterone has many different effects in many different tissues. One of the mechanisms by which the varied effects are mediated is the metabolism of testosterone to two other active steroids, dihydrotestosterone and estradiol (Figure 59–3). Some effects of testosterone

appear to be mediated by testosterone itself, some by dihydrotestosterone, and some by estradiol.

The enzyme 5α-reductase irreversibly catalyzes the conversion of testosterone to dihydrotestosterone. Although both testosterone and dihydrotestosterone act *via* the same receptor, the androgen receptor, dihydrotestosterone binds with higher affinity (Wilbert *et al.,* 1983) and activates gene expression more efficiently (Deslypere *et al.,* 1992). As a result, testosterone, acting *via* dihydrotestosterone, is able to have effects in tissues that express 5α-reductase which it could not have if it were present only as testosterone. Two forms of 5α-reductase have been identified: type I, which is found predominantly in nongenital skin and the liver, and type II, which is found predominantly in urogenital tissue in men and genital skin in both men and women. The effects of dihydrotestosterone in these tissues are described below.

The enzyme complex aromatase, which is present in many tissues, especially the liver and adipose tissue, catalyzes the irreversible conversion of testosterone to estradiol. This conversion results in approximately 85% of circulating estradiol in men; the remainder is secreted directly by the testes, probably the Leydig cells (MacDonald *et al.,* 1979). The effects of testosterone thought to be mediated *via* estradiol are described below.

Testosterone is metabolized in the liver to androsterone and etiocholanolone (Figure 59–3), which are biologically inactive. Dihydrotestosterone is metabolized to androsterone, androstanedione, and androstanediol.

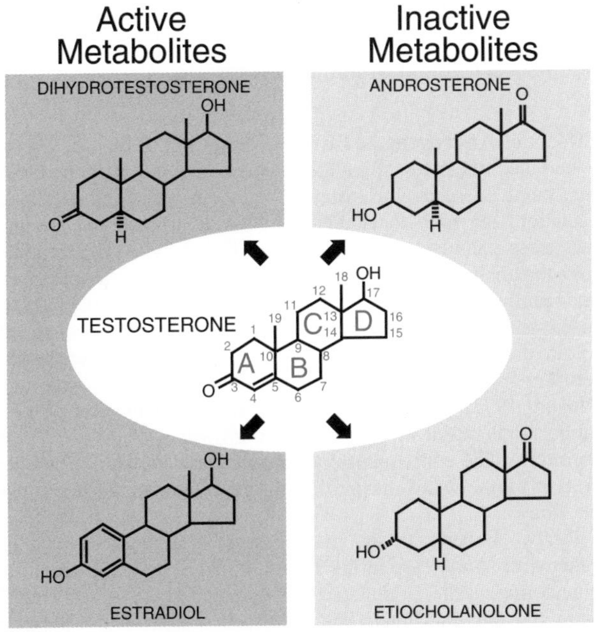

Figure 59–3. Metabolism of testosterone to its major active and inactive metabolites.

Physiological and Pharmacological Effects of Androgens

The biological effects of testosterone can be considered by the mechanisms by which they occur and by the tissues in which they occur at various stages of life. Testosterone can act as an androgen either directly by binding to the androgen receptor or indirectly by conversion to dihydrotestosterone, which also binds to the androgen receptor as described above. Testosterone also can act as an estrogen by conversion to estradiol, which binds to the estrogen receptor (Figure 59–4).

Effects That Occur *via* the Androgen Receptor.   Testosterone and dihydrotestosterone both act as androgens *via* a single androgen receptor (Figure 59–5). The androgen receptor is a member of the superfamily of nuclear receptors, which includes steroid hormone receptors, thyroid hormone receptors, and orphan receptors (*see* Chapter 2). Both testosterone and dihydrotestosterone bind to the hormone-binding domain of the androgen receptor,

Dihydrotestosterone ←— **Testosterone** —→ **Estradiol**

External genitalia
  (differentiation during gestation;
  maturation during puberty;
  prostatic diseases during
  adulthood)
Hair follicles
  (increased growth during
  puberty)

Internal genitalia
  (Wolffian development
  during gestation)
Skeletal muscle
  (Mass and strength
  increase during puberty)
Erythropoiesis
? Bone

Epiphyses (maturation)
? Libido

Figure 59–4. Direct effects of testosterone and effects mediated indirectly **via** *dihydrotestosterone or estradiol.*

allowing the ligand-receptor complex to bind, *via* the DNA-binding domain of the receptor, to certain responsive genes. The ligand-receptor complex acts as a transcription factor complex and stimulates expression of those genes (Brinkmann and Trapman, 2000).

For many years, the mechanisms by which androgens had so many different actions in so many different tissues were not understood, but recently these mechanisms have become clearer. One mechanism is the higher affinity with which dihydrotestosterone binds to and activates the androgen receptor compared to testosterone (Deslypere *et al.,* 1992; Wilbert *et al.,* 1983). Another mechanism, postulated more recently, involves transcription cofactors, both coactivators and corepressors, that are tissue specific.

The importance of the androgen receptor is illustrated by the consequences of its mutations. Predictably, mutations that either alter the primary sequence of the protein or cause a single amino acid substitution in the hormone- or DNA-binding domains result in resistance to the action of testosterone, beginning *in utero* (McPhaul and Griffin, 1999). Male sexual differentiation is, therefore, incomplete, as is pubertal development.

Another kind of mutation occurs in patients who have spinal and bulbar muscular atrophy, known as Kennedy's disease. These patients have an expansion of the CAG repeat, which codes for glutamine, at the amino terminus of the molecule (Laspada *et al.,* 1991). The result is very mild androgen resistance but progressively severe motor neuron atrophy. The mechanism by which the neuron atrophy occurs is unknown.

Yet other kinds of androgen receptor mutations may explain why prostate cancer that is treated by androgen deprivation eventually becomes androgen-independent. Prostate cancer is initially at least partially androgen-sensitive, which is the basis for the initial treatment of metastatic prostate cancer by

androgen deprivation. Metastatic prostate cancer often regresses initially in response to this treatment, but then becomes unresponsive to continued deprivation. Several mutations of the androgen receptor have been described in these patients, and it has been postulated that these mutations might allow the receptor to respond to ligands other than androgens or to act without ligand activation (Visakorpi *et al.,* 1995).

Effects That Occur *via* the Estrogen Receptor.   The effects of testosterone on at least one tissue are mediated by its conversion to estradiol, catalyzed by the aromatase enzyme complex. In the rare cases in which a male does not express aromatase (Carani *et al.,* 1997; Morishma *et al.,* 1995) or the estrogen receptor (Smith *et al.,* 1994), the epiphyses do not fuse and long bone growth continues indefinitely. In addition, the patients are osteoporotic. Administration of estradiol corrects the bone abnormalities in patients with an aromatase defect (Bilezikian *et al.,* 1998) but not an estrogen-receptor defect. There is evidence suggesting that conversion of testosterone to estradiol mediates male sexual behavior in rats, but similar evidence has not yet been found in human beings.

Effects of Androgens at Different Stages of Life.   *In Utero.* When the fetal testes, stimulated by human chorionic gonadotropin, begin to secrete testosterone at about the eighth week of gestation, the high local concentration of testosterone around the testes stimulates the nearby Wolffian ducts to differentiate into the male internal genitalia: the epididymis, vas deferens, and seminal vesicles (George and Wilson, 1992). Further away, in the anlage of the external genitalia, testosterone is converted to dihydrotestosterone, which causes the development of the external genitalia: the penis, scrotum, and prostate (George and Wilson, 1992). The increase in testosterone at the end of gestation might result in further phallic growth.

Infancy.   The consequences of the increase in testosterone secretion by the testes during the first few months of life are not yet known.

Puberty.   Puberty in the male begins at a mean age of 12 years with an increase in the secretion of FSH and LH from the gonadotroph cells, stimulated by increased secretion of GnRH from the hypothalamus. The increased secretion of FSH and LH stimulate the testes, so, not surprisingly, the first sign of

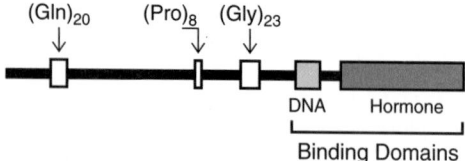

$(Gln)_{20}$ $(Pro)_8$ $(Gly)_{23}$

DNA   Hormone
Binding Domains

Figure 59–5. Structure of the androgen receptor.

puberty is an increase in testicular size. The increase in testosterone production within the testes, along with the effect of FSH on the Sertoli cells, stimulates the development of the seminiferous tubules, which eventually produce mature sperm. Increased secretion of testosterone into the systemic circulation affects many tissues virtually simultaneously, and the changes in most of them occur gradually during the course of several years. The phallus enlarges in length and width, the scrotum becomes rugated, and the prostate begins secreting the fluid it contributes to the semen. The skin becomes coarser and oilier due to increased sebum production, which contributes to the development of acne. Sexual hair begins to grow, initially pubic and axillary hair, then hair on the lower legs, and finally other body hair and facial hair. Full development of the latter two may not occur until ten years after the start of puberty and marks the completion of puberty. Muscle mass and strength, especially of the shoulder girdle, increase, and subcutaneous fat decreases. Epiphyseal bone growth accelerates, resulting in the pubertal growth spurt, but epiphyseal maturation leads eventually to a slowing and then cessation of growth. Bone also becomes thicker. The increase in muscle mass and bone result in a pronounced increase in weight. Erythropoiesis increases, resulting in higher hematocrit and hemoglobin concentrations in men than boys or women. The larynx thickens, resulting in a lower voice. Libido develops.

Other changes also may be the result of the increase in testosterone during puberty. Men tend to have a better sense of spatial relations than do women and to exhibit behavior that is different in some ways from that of women, including being more aggressive.

Adulthood.   The serum testosterone concentration and the characteristics of the adult male are maintained largely during early adulthood and midlife. One change during this time is the gradual development of male pattern baldness, beginning with recession of hair at the temples and/or at the vertex.

Two changes that can occur in the prostate gland during adulthood are of much greater medical significance. One is the gradual development of benign prostatic hyperplasia, which occurs to a variable degree in almost all men, sometimes to the degree of obstructing urine outflow by compressing the urethra as it passes through the prostate. This development is mediated by the conversion of testosterone to dihydrotestosterone within prostatic cells (Wilson, 1980). One current treatment of benign prostatic hyperplasia is based on inhibiting 5α-reductase II, which mediates this conversion (McConnell *et al.*, 1998), as discussed below.

The other change that can occur in the prostate during adulthood is the development of cancer. Although no direct evidence suggests that testosterone causes the disease, prostate cancer is dependent on testosterone, at least to some degree and at some time in its course. This dependency is the basis of treating metastatic prostate cancer by lowering the serum testosterone concentration (Huggins and Hodges, 1941; Iversen *et al.*, 1990).

Senescence.   As men age, the serum testosterone concentration gradually declines (Figure 59–2) and the sex hormone-binding globulin concentration gradually increases, so that by age 80, the total testosterone concentration is approximately 85% and the free testosterone is approximately 40% of those at age 20 (Purifoy *et al.*, 1981; Deslypere and Vermeulen, 1984). This fall in serum testosterone could contribute to several other changes that occur with increasing age in men, including decreases in energy, libido, muscle mass (Forbes, 1976) and strength (Murray *et al.*, 1980), and bone mineral density (Riggs *et al.*, 1982). The possibility of such a relationship is suggested by the occurrence of similar changes when men develop hypogonadism at a younger age due to known diseases, as discussed below.

Consequences of Androgen Deficiency

The consequences of androgen deficiency depend on the stage of life during which the deficiency first occurs and the degree of the deficiency.

During Fetal Development.   Testosterone deficiency in a male fetus during the first trimester *in utero* causes incomplete sexual differentiation. Testosterone deficiency in the first trimester results only from testicular disease, such as deficiency of 17α-oxidoketoreductase; deficiency of LH secretion due to pituitary or hypothalamic deficiency does not result in testosterone deficiency during the first trimester, because Leydig-cell secretion of testosterone at that time is under the control of hCG from the placenta. Complete deficiency of testosterone secretion results in entirely female external genitalia; less severe testosterone deficiency results in incomplete virilization of the external genitalia proportionate to the degree of deficiency. Testosterone deficiency at this stage of development also leads to failure of the Wolffian ducts to differentiate into the male external genitalia, such as the vas deferens and seminal vesicles, but the müllerian ducts do not differentiate into the female external genitalia as long as testes are present and secrete müllerian inhibitory substance. Similar changes occur if testosterone is secreted normally, but its action is diminished because of an abnormality of the androgen receptor or of the 5α-reductase enzyme. Abnormalities of the androgen receptor can be quite variable. The most severe form results in complete absence of androgen action and a female phenotype; moderately severe forms result in partial virilization of the external genitalia; and the mildest forms permit normal virilization *in utero* and result only in impaired spermatogenesis in adulthood (McPhaul and Griffin, 1999). Abnormal 5α-reductase results in incomplete virilization of the external genitalia *in utero* but normal development of the male internal genitalia, which depends on testosterone *per se* (Wilson *et al.*, 1993).

Testosterone deficiency during the third trimester, due either to a testicular disease or a deficiency of fetal LH secretion, appears to have two known consequences. One is failure of the phallus to grow as much as it would normally. The result, called microphallus, is a common occurrence in boys later discovered to be unable to secrete

LH due to abnormalities of GnRH synthesis. The other consequence is failure of the testes to descend into the scrotum, called cryptorchidism, also a common occurrence in boys whose LH secretion is subnormal.

Before Completion of Puberty. When a boy can secrete testosterone normally *in utero* but loses the ability to do so before the anticipated age of puberty, the result is failure to complete puberty. All of the pubertal changes described above, including those of the external genitalia, sexual hair, muscle mass, voice, and behavior, fail to occur to a degree proportionate to the abnormality of testosterone secretion. In addition, if growth hormone secretion is normal when testosterone secretion is subnormal during the years of expected puberty, the long bones continue to lengthen because the epiphyses do not close. The result is longer arms and legs relative to the trunk; these proportions are referred to as eunuchoid. Another consequence of subnormal testosterone secretion during the age of expected puberty is enlargement of glandular breast tissue, called gynecomastia.

After Completion of Puberty. When the ability to secrete testosterone becomes impaired after the completion of puberty, regression of the pubertal effects of testosterone depends on both the degree and the duration of testosterone deficiency. When the degree of testosterone deficiency is substantial, libido and energy decrease within a week or two, but other testosterone-dependent characteristics decline more slowly. Decreases in muscle mass and strength probably can be detected by testing groups of men within a few months, but a clinically detectable decrease in muscle mass in an individual does not occur for several years. A pronounced decrease in hematocrit and hemoglobin will occur within several months. A decrease in bone mineral density probably can be detected by dual energy absorptiometry within two years, but an increase in fracture incidence likely would not occur for many years. A loss of sexual hair takes many years.

In Women. Loss of androgen secretion in women results in a decrease in sexual hair, but not for many years. Androgens may have other important effects in women, and the loss of androgens (especially severe loss of both ovarian and adrenal androgens, as occurs in panhypopituitarism) may result in the loss of these effects. Testosterone preparations that can yield serum testosterone concentrations in the physiological range in women currently are being developed. The availability of such preparations will allow determining if replacement of testosterone in androgen-deficient women will improve their libido, energy, muscle mass and strength, and bone mineral density.

Therapeutic Androgen Preparations

The need for a creative approach to pharmacotherapy with androgens arises from the fact that ingestion of testosterone is not an effective means of replacing testosterone deficiency. The reason is that, even though ingested testosterone is readily absorbed into the hepatic circulation, the hormone is catabolized so rapidly by the liver that it is not practical for a hypogonadal man to ingest it in sufficient amounts and with sufficient frequency to maintain a normal serum testosterone concentration. Most pharmaceutical preparations of androgens, therefore, are designed to bypass hepatic catabolism of testosterone. Another goal of androgen pharmacotherapy is to separate certain effects from others.

Testosterone Esters. Esterifying a fatty acid to the 17β hydroxyl group of testosterone creates a compound that is even more lipophilic than testosterone itself. When an ester, such as *testosterone enanthate (heptanoate)* or *cypionate (cyclopentylpropionate)* (Figure 59–6) is dissolved in oil and administered intramuscularly every two to four weeks to hypogonadal men, the ester hydrolyzes *in vivo* and results in serum testosterone concentrations that range from higher than normal in the first few days after the injection to low-normal just before the next injection (Snyder and Lawrence, 1980; Figure 59–7). Attempts to decrease the frequency of injections by increasing the amount of each injection result in wider fluctuations and poorer therapeutic effects. The undecanoate ester of testosterone (Figure 59–6), when dissolved in oil and ingested orally, is absorbed into the lymphatic circulation, thus bypassing initial hepatic catabolism. *Testosterone undecanoate* in oil also can be injected and produces stable serum testosterone concentrations for a month (Zhang *et al.,* 1998). The undecanoate ester of testosterone is not marketed in the United States.

Alkylated Androgens. Several decades ago, chemists found that adding an alkyl group to the 17α position of testosterone (Figure 59–6) retarded hepatic catabolism of the molecule. Consequently, 17α-alkylated androgens do have an androgenic effect when administered orally. However, they do not appear to be as fully androgenic as testosterone itself, and they cause hepatotoxicity (Petera *et al.,* 1962; Cabasso, 1994), whereas native testosterone does not.

Transdermal Delivery Systems. Recent attempts to avoid the destructive "first pass" of testosterone through the liver have employed novel delivery systems, instead

Testosterone
(HISTERONE, others)

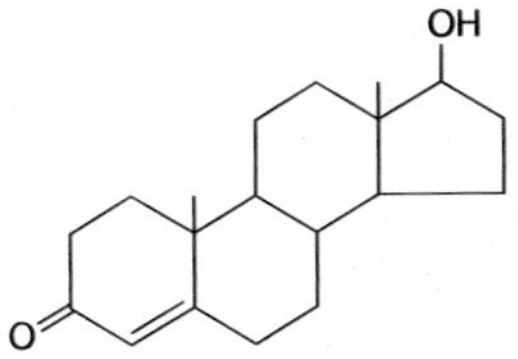

Testosterone Esters

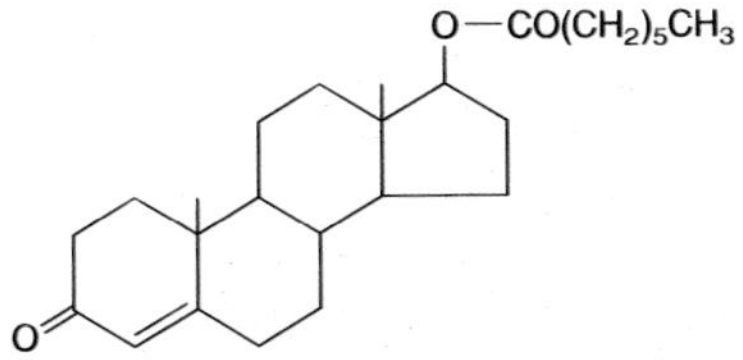

Testosterone enanathate
(DELATESTRYL, others)

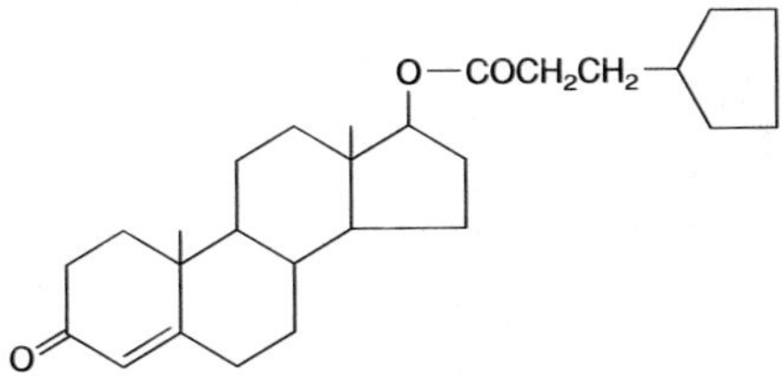

Testosterone cypionate
(DEPO-TESTOSTERONE, others)

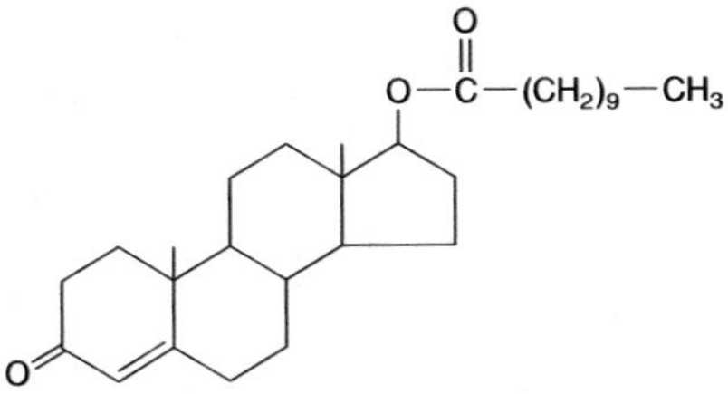

Testosterone undecanoate
(ANDRIOL)

17α-Alkylated Androgens

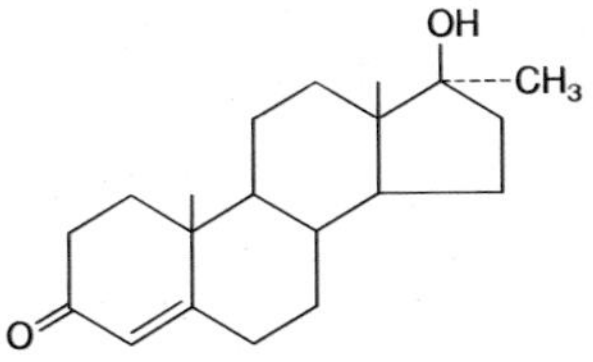

Methyltestosterone
(ORETIN METHYL, others)

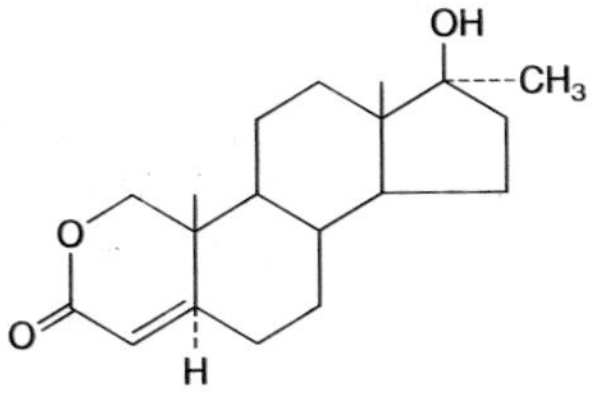

Oxandrolone
(OXANDRIN)

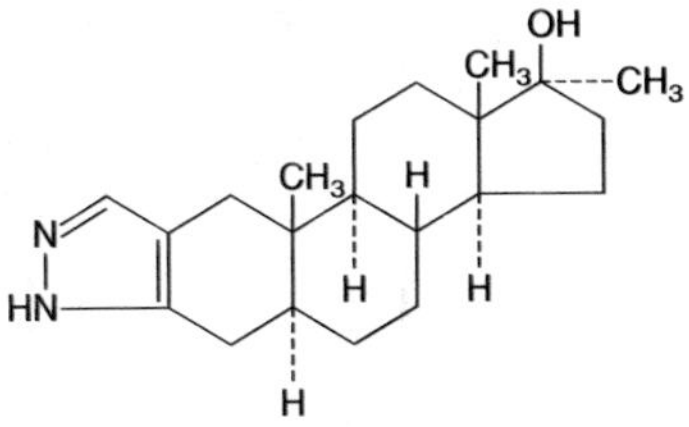

Stanozolol
(WINSTROL)

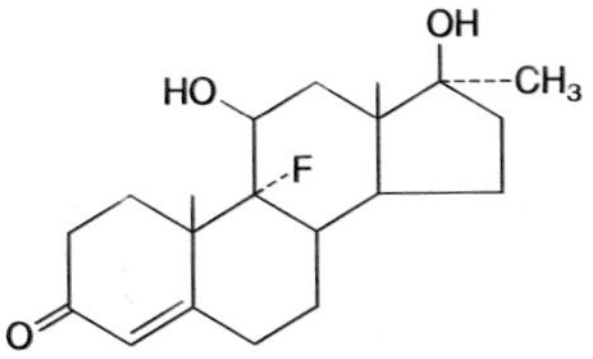

Fluoxymesterone
(HALOTESTIN)

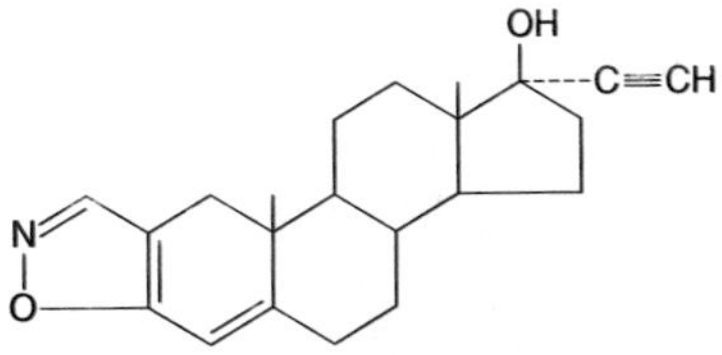

Danazol
(DANOCRINE)

Figure 59–6. Structures of androgens available for therapeutic use.

of chemically modified testosterone, that release native testosterone across the skin in a controlled fashion. When these transdermal preparations are applied once a day, they result in serum testosterone concentrations that fluctuate less than when testosterone esters are administered systemically. The first such preparation was a skin patch (TESTODERM) designed to be applied to the scrotal skin (Findlay *et al.*, 1989). The rationale for that location is that the scrotal skin is so thin that sufficient testosterone can be absorbed without the need for chemicals to facil-

itate its absorption. Subsequent patches were designed to be applied to nonscrotal skin (ANDRODERM, TESTODERM TTS) and therefore employ chemicals to facilitate absorption (Yu *et al.*, 1997; Dobs *et al.*, 1999). A newer transdermal preparation (ANDROGEL) employs a hydroalcoholic gel which is applied to nonscrotal skin (Wang *et al.*, 2000). All of these preparations are applied once a day, and all produce serum testosterone concentrations within the normal range in the majority of hypogonadal men (Figure 59–7).

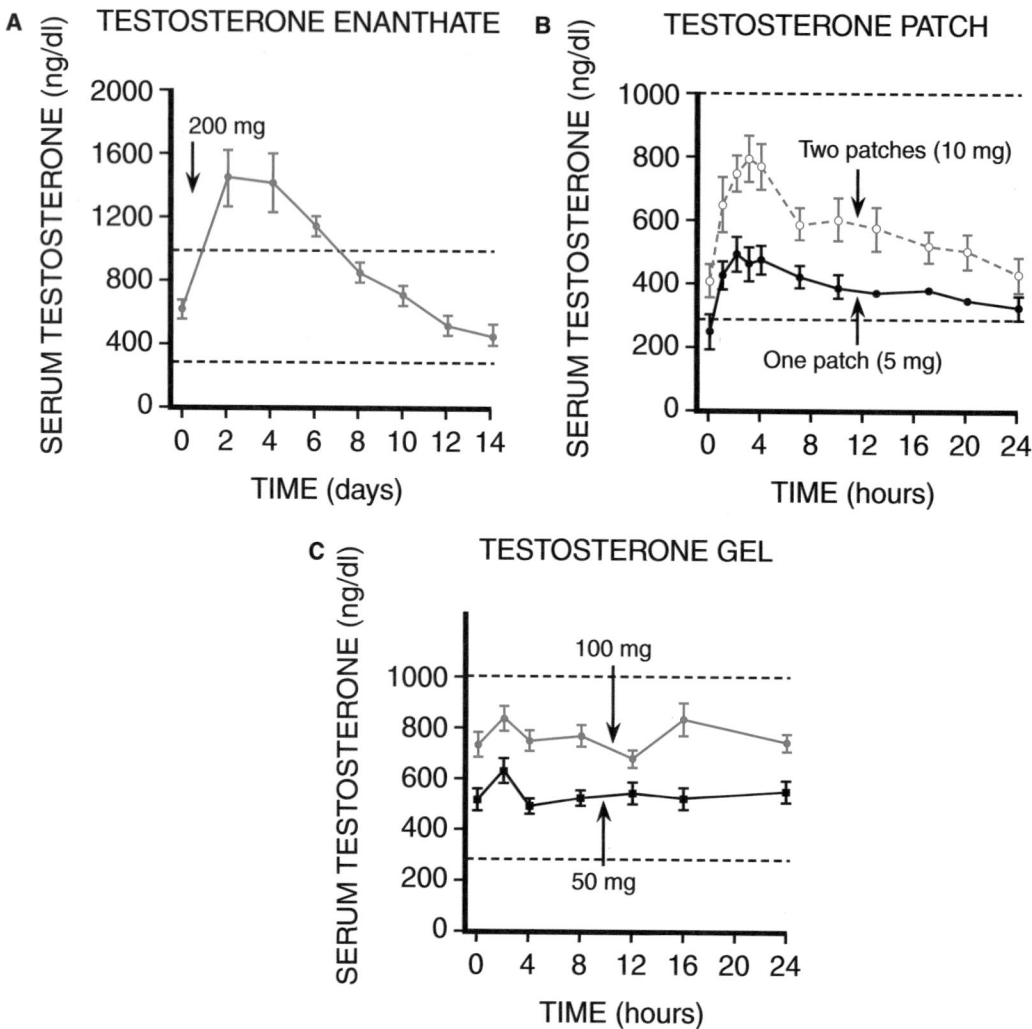

Figure 59–7. Pharmacokinetic profiles of three testosterone preparations during their chronic administration to hypogonadal men.

Doses of each were given at time 0. [Adapted from Snyder and Lawrence (1980) (A); Yu *et al.* (1997) (B); and Wang *et al.* (2000) (C).] Dashed lines indicate range of normal levels.

Attempts to Design Selective Androgens

Alkylated Androgens. Decades ago, investigators attempted to synthesize analogs of testosterone that possessed greater anabolic effects than androgenic effects compared to native testosterone. Several compounds appeared to have such differential effects, based on a greater effect on the levator ani muscle compared to the ventral prostate of the rat (Hershberger and Meyer, 1953). These compounds were called anabolic steroids, and most are 17α-alkylated androgens, described above. None of these compounds, however, has been demonstrated to have such a differential effect in human beings. Nonetheless, they have enjoyed popularity among athletes who are attempting to improve their performance, as described below. Another alkylated androgen, 7α-methyl-19-nortestosterone, is poorly converted to dihydrotestosterone (Kumar *et al.*, 1992).

Selective Androgen-Receptor Modulators. Stimulated by the development of selective estrogen-receptor modulators, which have estrogenic effects in some tissues but not others, investigators are now attempting to develop selective androgen-receptor modulators (Negro-Vilar, 1999). However, the selective effect of *raloxifene* (EVISTA), the first estrogen-receptor modulator to be developed for clinical use, derives from its much greater affinity for the form of estrogen receptor expressed in certain tissues, such as bone and cardiac muscle, than for the form expressed in other tissues, such as breast and uterus. Because only one form of the androgen receptor is expressed, development of compounds that have certain androgen effects but not others is based, instead, on tissue specificity of coactivators and corepressors of androgen-receptor transcriptional activity. Endogenous protein coactivators and corepressors of androgen receptor-dependent transcription have been demonstrated (Moilanen *et al.*, 1999), and a family of quinolinones that has selective androgen properties has been synthesized (Zhi *et al.*, 1999).

Therapeutic Uses of Androgens

The clearest indication for administration of androgens is testosterone deficiency in men, *i.e.*, treatment of male hypogonadism. Androgens also have been used in other situations in the past and likely will be used in yet others in the future.

Male Hypogonadism. Any of the transdermal testosterone preparations or testosterone esters described above can be used to treat testosterone deficiency. Monitoring treatment for beneficial and deleterious effects differs somewhat in adolescents and the elderly from that in other men.

Monitoring for Efficacy. The goal of administering testosterone to a hypogonadal man is to mimic the normal serum concentration as closely as possible. Therefore, measuring the serum testosterone concentration during treatment is the most important aspect of monitoring testosterone treatment for efficacy. When the serum testosterone concentration is measured depends on the testosterone preparation used. When a transdermal preparation is used, the serum testosterone concentration can be measured on any day at any time, recognizing that, when a patch is used, the peak value will be found 2 to 4 hours after application of the patch for scrotal skin (Findlay *et al.*, 1987), 2 to 4 hours after application of one patch for nonscrotal skin (TESTODERM TTS; Yu *et al.*, 1997), and 6 to 9 hours after application of another patch for nonscrotal skin (ANDRODERM; Dobs *et al.*, 1999). The nadir, before the next application, will be about 60% to 70% of the peak value (Findlay *et al.*, 1987). When the testosterone gel is used, there is no appreciable fluctuation during the course of the day, but steady-state values may not be reached for a month after the initiation of treatment. When the enanthate or cypionate esters of testosterone are administered once every two weeks, the serum testosterone concentration should be measured midway between doses. At each of these times, the serum testosterone concentration should be normal, and if not, the dosage schedule should be adjusted accordingly. If the cause of the testosterone deficiency is testicular disease, as indicated by an elevated serum LH concentration, adequacy of testosterone treatment also can be judged by its reduction to normal within two months of initiation of treatment (Snyder and Lawrence, 1980; Findlay *et al.*, 1989).

Normalization of the serum testosterone concentration results in normal virilization in men who are not normally virilized

and maintenance of virilization in those who already are. Libido and energy in hypogonadal men should increase within a few weeks (Davidson *et al.*, 1979). Muscle mass should increase, fat mass should decrease, and muscle strength should increase within a few months (Katznelson *et al.*, 1996). Bone mineral density should increase to a maximum within two years (Snyder *et al.*, 2000).

Monitoring for Deleterious Effects. When testosterone itself is administered, as in one of the transdermal preparations or as an ester that is hydrolyzed to testosterone (Caminos-Torres *et al.*, 1977), it has no "side effects" *i.e.*, no effects that endogenously secreted testosterone does not have, as long as the dose is not excessive. Modified testosterone compounds, such as the 17α-alkylated androgens, do have side effects. Even replacement of endogenously secreted testosterone levels, however, can have effects that are undesirable. Some effects occur shortly after testosterone administration is initiated, whereas others usually do not occur until administration has been continued for many years. Raising the serum testosterone concentration from prepubertal or midpubertal levels to that of an adult male at any age can result in undesirable effects similar to those that occur during puberty, including acne, gynecomastia, and more aggressive sexual behavior. Physiological amounts of testosterone do not appear to affect serum lipids or apolipoproteins. Replacement of physiological levels of testosterone occasionally may have undesirable effects in the presence of concomitant illnesses. For example, stimulation of erythropoiesis would increase the hematocrit from subnormal to normal in a healthy man, but would raise the hematocrit above normal in a man with a predisposition to erythrocytosis, such as in chronic pulmonary disease. Similarly, the mild degree of sodium and water retention with testosterone replacement would have no clinical effect in a healthy man but would exacerbate preexisting congestive heart failure. If the testosterone dose is excessive, erythrocytosis and, uncommonly, salt and water retention and peripheral edema occur even in men who have no predisposition to these conditions. When a man's serum testosterone concentration has been in the normal adult male range for many years, whether from endogenous secretion or exogenous administration, and he is over age 40, he is subject to certain testosterone-dependent diseases, including benign prostatic hyperplasia and prostate cancer, as discussed above.

The principal side effects of the 17α-alkylated androgens are hepatic, including cholestasis and, uncommonly, peliosis hepatis, blood-filled hepatic cysts. Hepatocellular cancer has been reported rarely, so that an etiologic link is uncertain. The 17α-alkylated androgens, especially in large amounts, may lower serum high-density-lipoprotein cholesterol.

Monitoring at the Anticipated Time of Puberty. Administration of testosterone to testosterone-deficient boys at the anticipated time of puberty should be guided by the considerations above, but also by the fact that testosterone accelerates epiphyseal maturation, leading initially to a growth spurt but then to epiphyseal closure and permanent cessation of linear growth. Consequently, the height and growth-hormone status of the boy must be considered. Boys who are short because of growth-hormone deficiency should be treated with growth hormone before their hypogonadism is treated with testosterone.

Male Senescence.   Preliminary evidence suggests that increasing the serum testosterone concentration of men whose serum levels are subnormal for no reason other than their age will increase their bone mineral density and lean mass and decrease their fat mass (Snyder *et al.,* 1999a; Snyder *et al.,* 1999b). It is entirely uncertain at this time, however, if such treatment will worsen benign prostatic hyperplasia or increase the incidence of clinically detectable prostate cancer.

Female Hypogonadism.   It remains to be determined if increasing the serum testosterone concentrations of women whose serum testosterone concentrations are below normal will improve their libido, energy, muscle mass and strength, and bone mineral density.

Enhancement of Athletic Performance.   Some athletes take drugs, including androgens, to attempt to improve their performance. Because androgens taken for this purpose usually are taken surreptitiously, information about their possible effects is not as good as that for androgens taken for treatment of male hypogonadism.

Kinds of Androgens Used.   Virtually all androgens produced for human or veterinary purposes have been taken by athletes. When use by athletes began more than two decades ago, 17α-alkylated androgens and other compounds that were thought to have greater anabolic effects than androgen effects relative to testosterone (so-called "anabolic steroids") were used most commonly. Because these compounds can be detected readily by organizations that govern athletic competitions, preparations that increase the serum concentration of testosterone itself, such as the testosterone esters or human chorionic gonadotropin, have increased in popularity. Testosterone precursors, such as androstenedione and dehydroepiandrosterone (DHEA), also have increased in popularity recently because they are not regulated by national governments or athletic organizations.

Efficacy.   Most studies of the effects of pharmacological doses of androgens on muscle strength have been uncontrolled, but in one study, testosterone or placebo was administered in a double-blind fashion. In that study, 43 men were randomized to one of four groups: strength training exercise with either 600 mg of testosterone enanthate once a week (more than six times a replacement dose) or placebo for testosterone; or no exercise with either testosterone or placebo. The men who received testosterone experienced an increase in fat-free mass and muscle strength compared to those who received placebo treatment, and the men who exercised simultaneously experienced even greater increases (Bhasin *et al.,* 1997).

In another double-blind study, men who took 100 mg of androstenedione three times a day for eight weeks did not experience an increase in muscle strength compared to men who took placebo. Failure of this treatment to increase muscle strength is

not surprising, because it also did not increase the mean serum testosterone concentration (King *et al.,* 1999).

Side Effects.   Some side effects of taking pharmacological doses of androgens occur with all androgens and all circumstances, but others occur only with certain androgens or in certain circumstances. All androgens suppress gonadotropin secretion when taken in high doses and thereby suppress endogenous testicular function. The result is a decrease in both endogenous testosterone and sperm production, resulting in diminished fertility. If administration continues for many years, testicular size may diminish. Testosterone and sperm production usually return to normal within a few months of discontinuation but may take longer. High doses of androgens also causes erythrocytosis (Drinka *et al.,* 1995).

Androgens that can be converted to estrogens, such as testosterone itself, cause gynecomastia when administered in high doses. Androgens whose A ring has been modified so that it cannot be aromatized, such as dihydrotestosterone, do not cause gynecomastia even in high doses.

The 17α-alkylated androgens are the only androgens that cause hepatotoxicity, as discussed above. These androgens also appear to be much more likely than others, when administered in high doses, to affect serum lipid concentrations, specifically to decrease high-density-lipoprotein (HDL) cholesterol and increase low-density-lipoprotein (LDL) cholesterol. Other side effects have been suggested by many anecdotes but have not been confirmed, including psychological disorders and sudden death due to cardiac disease, possibly related to changes in lipids or to coagulation activation.

Certain side effects occur specifically in women and children. Both experience virilization, including facial and body hirsutism, temporal hair recession in a male pattern, and acne. Boys experience phallic enlargement and women clitoral enlargement. Boys and girls whose epiphyses have not yet closed experience premature closure and stunting of linear growth.

Male Contraception.   Attempts currently are being made to develop androgens alone or in combination with other drugs as male contraceptives based on their ability to inhibit secretion of LH by the pituitary, which in turn decreases endogenous testosterone production. Because the concentration of testosterone within the testes is normally approximately one hundred times that in the peripheral circulation, and that concentration is necessary for spermatogenesis, suppression of endogenous testosterone production greatly diminishes spermatogenesis. Initial use of testosterone alone to suppress spermatogenesis, however, required administration of approximately twice as much testosterone enanthate as would be used for physiological replacement, and even then spermatogenesis was not entirely suppressed in all men (WHO Task Force for the Regulation of Male Fertility, 1996). Other early attempts to suppress spermatogenesis employed a GnRH antagonist to suppress LH secretion combined with a physiological dose of testosterone to maintain a normal serum testosterone concentration (Pavlou *et al.,* 1991). That combination is not practical for widespread use because existing GnRH antagonists require daily injection and have strong histamine-releasing properties. A more promising approach is the combination of a progestin with a physiological dose of testosterone to suppress LH secretion and spermatogenesis but provide a normal serum testosterone concentration (Bebb *et al.,* 1996). Androgens currently being tested as part of male contraceptive regimens include an injectable form of testosterone undecanoate, which appears to produce a relatively stable serum testosterone concentration for a month (Zhang *et al.*, 1999), and 7α-methyl-19-nortestosterone, a synthetic androgen that cannot be metabolized to dihydrotestosterone (Cummings *et al.*, 1998).

Catabolic and Wasting States.   Testosterone, because of its anabolic effects, has been used in attempts to ameliorate catabolic and muscle-wasting states, but it has not been effective in most of these states. One exception is in the treatment of muscle wasting associated with acquired immunodeficiency syndrome (AIDS), which is accompanied by hypogonadism. Treatment of men with AIDS-related muscle wasting and subnormal serum testosterone concentrations increases their muscle mass and strength (Bhasin *et al.*, 2000).

Angioneurotic Edema.   Chronic androgen treatment of patients with angioneurotic edema effectively prevents attacks. The disease is caused by hereditary impairment of C1-esterase inhibitor or acquired development of antibodies against it (Cicardi *et al.*, 1998). The 17α-alkylated androgens, such as stanozolol and danazol, act by stimulating the hepatic synthesis of the esterase inhibitor. In women, virilization is a potential side effect. In children virilization and premature epiphyseal closure prevent chronic use of androgens for prophylaxis, although they are used occasionally for treatment of acute episodes.

Blood Dyscrasias.   Androgens once were employed to attempt to stimulate erythropoiesis in patients with anemias of various etiologies, but the availability of erythropoietin has supplanted that use. Androgens, such as danazol, still are used occasionally as adjunctive treatment for hemolytic anemia and idiopathic thrombocytopenic purpura that are refractory to first-line agents.

ANTIANDROGENS

Because certain effects of androgens are undesirable, at least under certain circumstances, agents have been developed specifically to inhibit androgen synthesis or effects. Other drugs, originally developed for other purposes, have been found to be antiandrogens. When these drugs are used for their originally intended purposes, their antiandrogenic effects can be undesirable side effects, but some are used intentionally as antiandrogens.

Inhibitors of Testosterone Synthesis.   Analogs of GnRH effectively inhibit testosterone synthesis by inhibiting LH secretion. GnRH antagonists block the action of endogenous GnRH at the gonadotroph cell's GnRH receptor. Antagonists that are currently available require daily injection and have significant histamine-releasing properties, so their therapeutic use is not practical. GnRH "superactive" analogs, given repeatedly, down-regulate the GnRH receptor, and currently are available for treatment of metastatic prostate cancer (*see* Chapter 56).

Some antifungal drugs of the imidazole family, such as ketoconazole (*see* Chapter 49), block the synthesis of steroids, including testosterone and cortisol (Feldman, 1986). Because of the inhibition of cortisol and hepatotoxicity, these drugs are not generally useful to inhibit androgen synthesis intentionally.

Inhibitors of Androgen Action

These drugs act by inhibiting the binding of androgens to the androgen receptor or by inhibiting 5α-reductase.

Androgen Receptor Antagonists.   *Flutamide and Bicalutamide.*   These are relatively potent androgen receptor antagonists which are limited in their effectiveness when used alone, because increased secretion of LH stimulates higher serum testosterone concentrations. They are used primarily in conjunction with a GnRH analog in the treatment of metastatic prostate cancer (*see* Chapter 52). In this situation, they block the action of adrenal androgens, which are not inhibited by GnRH analogs. Survival rates in groups of patients with metastatic prostate cancer treated with a combination of a GnRH agonist and either *flutamide* (EVLEXIN) or *bicalutamide* (CASODEX) are similar to each other (Schellhammer, Sharifi, *et al.*, 1995) and to survival rates in those treated by castration (Iversen *et al.*, 1990). Bicalutamide is replacing flutamide for this purpose, because it appears to have less hepatotoxicity and needs to be taken only once a day instead of three times a day. Flutamide also has been used to treat hirsutism in women, and it appears to be as effective as any other treatment (Venturoli *et al.*, 1999), but its hepatotoxicity cautions against its use for this cosmetic purpose.

Spironolactone.   Spironolactone (ALDACTONE; *see* Chapter 29) is an inhibitor of aldosterone which also is a weak inhibitor of the androgen receptor and a weak inhibitor of testosterone synthesis. When it is used for treatment of fluid retention or hypertension in men, gynecomastia is a common side effect (Caminos-Torres *et al.*, 1977). Conversely, it can be used intentionally in women to treat hirsutism, for which it is approved by the U.S. Food and Drug Administration and is moderately effective (Cumming *et al.*, 1982), but it may cause irregular menses. *Cyproterone Acetate.*   Cyproterone acetate is a progestin and a weak antiandrogen by virtue of binding to the androgen receptor. It is moderately effective in reducing hirsutism alone or in combination with an oral contraceptive (Venturoli *et al.*, 1999), but it is not approved for use in the United States. *Selective Androgen-Receptor Antagonists.*   A group of quinoline derivatives has been developed that act as antagonists at the androgen receptor in rat prostate glands but not in the pituitary. Analogous effects have not yet been demonstrated in human beings, but these compounds suggest the possible development of selective androgen-receptor antagonists.

5α-Reductase Inhibitors. *Finasteride* (PROSCAR) is an antagonist of 5α-reductase, especially the type II, so it blocks the conversion of testosterone to dihydrotestosterone, especially in the male external genitalia. It was developed as a treatment for benign prostatic hyperplasia, and it is approved in the United States and many other countries for this purpose. When it is administered to men with moderately severe symptoms due to obstruction of urinary tract outflow, serum and prostatic concentrations of dihydrotestosterone decrease, prostatic volume decreases, and urine flow rate increases (McConnell *et al.*, 1998). Impotence is a well-documented although infrequent side effect of this use, although the mechanism is not understood. Finasteride also is approved for use in the treatment of male pattern baldness under the trade name PROPECIA, even though that effect is presumably mediated *via* the type I enzyme. It appears to be as effective as flutamide and the combination of estrogen and cyproterone in the treatment of hirsutism (Venturoli *et al.*, 1999), but is not approved in the United States for this purpose.

For further discussion of disorders of the testes and of sexual differentiation, *see* Chapters 336 and 339 in *Harrison's Principles of Internal Medicine,* 14th ed., McGraw-Hill, New York, 1998.

BIBLIOGRAPHY

Bebb, R.A., Anawalt, B.D., Christensen, R.B., Paulsen, C.A., Bremner, W.J., and Matsumoto, A.M. Combined administration of levonorgestrel and testosterone induces more rapid and effective suppression of spermatogenesis than testosterone alone: a promising male contraceptive approach. *J. Clin. Endocrinol. Metab.,* **1996,** *81:*757–762.

Bhasin, S., Storer, T.W., Berman, N., Yarasheski, K.E., Clevenger, B., Phillips, J., Lee, W.P., Bunnell, T.J., and Casaburi, R. Testosterone replacement increases fat-free mass and muscle size in hypogonadal men. *J. Clin. Endocrinol. Metab.,* **1997,** *82:*407–413.

Bhasin, S., Storer, T.W., Javanbakht, M., Berman, N., Yarasheshki, K.E., Phillips, J., Dike, M., Sinha-Hikim, I., Shen, R., Hays, R.D., and Beall, G. Testosterone replacement and resistance exercise in HIV-infected men with weight loss and low testosterone levels. *JAMA,* **2000,** *283:*763–770.

Bilezikian, J.P., Morishima, A., Bell, J., and Grumbach, M.M. Increased bone mass as a result of estrogen therapy in a man with aromatase deficiency. *N. Engl. J. Med.,* **1998,** *339:*599–603.

Bremner, W.J., Vitiello, M.V., and Prinz, P.N. Loss of circadian rhythmicity in blood testosterone levels with aging in normal men. *J. Clin. Endocrinol. Metab.,* **1983,** *56:*1278–1281.

Brinkmann, A.O., and Trapman, J. Genetic analysis of androgen receptors in development and disease. *Adv. Pharmacol.,* **2000,** *47:*317–341.

Cabasso, A. Peliosis hepatis in a young adult bodybuilder. *Med. Sci. Sports Exerc.,* **1994,** *26:*2–4.

Caminos-Torres, R., Ma, L., and Snyder, P.J. Testosterone-induced inhibition of the LH and FSH responses to gonadotropin-releasing hormone occurs slowly. *J. Clin. Endocrinol. Metab.,* **1977,** *44:*1142–1153.

Carani, C., Qin, K., Simoni, M., Faustini-Fustini, M., Serpente, S., Boyd, J., Korach, K.S., and Simpson, E.R. Effect of testosterone and estradiol in a man with aromatase deficiency. *N. Engl. J. Med.,* **1997,** *337:*91–95.

Cicardi, M., Bergamaschini, L., Cugno, M., Beretta, A., Zingale, L.C., Colombo, M., and Agostoni, A. Pathogenetic and clinical aspects of C1 esterase inhibitor deficiency. *Immunobiology,* **1998,** *199:*366–376.

Cumming, D.C., Yang, J.C., Rebar, R.W., and Yen, S.S. Treatment of hirsutism with spironolactone. *JAMA,* **1982,** *247:*1295–1298.

Cummings, D.E., Kumar, N., Bardin, C.W., Sundaram, K., and

Bremner, W.J. Prostate-sparing effects in primates of the potent androgen 7α-methyl-19-nortestosterone: a potential alternative to testosterone for androgen replacement and male contraception. *J. Clin. Endocrinol. Metab.,* **1998,** *83:*4212–4219.

Davidson, J.M., Camargo, C.A., and Smith, E.R. Effects of androgen on sexual behavior in hypogonadal men. *J. Clin. Endocrinol. Metab.,* **1979,** *48:*955–958.

Dawood, M.Y., and Saxena, B.B. Testosterone and dihydrotestosterone in maternal and cord blood and in amniotic fluid. *Am. J. Obstet. Gynecol.,* **1977,** *129:*37–42.

Deslypere, J.-P., and Vermeulen, A. Leydig cell function in normal men: effect of age, lifestyle, residence, diet, and activity. *J. Clin. Endocrinol. Metab.,* **1984,** *59:*955–962.

Deslypere, J.-P., Young, M., Wilson, J.D., and McPhaul, M.J. Testosterone and 5α-dihydrotestosterone interact differently with the androgen receptor to enhance transcription of the MMTV-CAT reporter gene. *Mol. Cell Endocrinol.,* **1992,** *88:*15–22.

Dobs, A.S., Meikle, A.W., Arver, S., Sanders, S.W., Caramelli, K.E., and Mazer, N.A. Pharmacokinetics, efficacy, and safety of a permeation-enhanced testosterone transdermal system in comparison with bi-weekly injections of testosterone enanthate for the treatment of hypogonadal men. *J. Clin. Endocrinol. Metab.,* **1999,** *84:*3469–3478.

Drinka, P.J., Jochen, A.L., Cuisiner, M., Bloom, R., Rudman, I., and Rudman, D. Polycythemia as a complication of testosterone replacement therapy in nursing home men with low testosterone levels. *J. Am. Geriatr. Soc.,* **1995,** *43:*899–901.

Findlay, J.C., Place, V.A., and Snyder, P.J. Transdermal delivery of testosterone. *J. Clin. Endocrinol. Metab.,* **1987,** *64:*266–268.

Findlay, J.C., Place, V.A., and Snyder, P.J. Treatment of primary hypogonadism in men by the transdermal administration of testosterone. *J. Clin. Endocrinol. Metab.,* **1989,** *68:*369–373.

Forbes, G.B., and Halloran, E. The adult decline in lean body mass. *Hum. Biol.,* **1976,** *48:*162–173.

Forest, M.G., and Cathiard, A.M. Pattern of plasma testosterone and Δ⁴-androstenedione in normal newborns: evidence for testicular activity at birth. *J. Clin. Endocrinol. Metab.,* **1975,** *41:*977–980.

Hershberger, L.C., Shipley E.G., and Meyer, R.K. Myotrophic activity of 19-nortestosterone and other steroids determined by modified levator ani muscle method. *Proc. Soc. Exp. Biol. Med.,* **1953,** *83*: 175.

Huggins, C., and Hodges, C.V. Studies on prostatic cancer. I. The effect of castration, of estrogen and of androgen injection on serum phosphatases in metastatic carcinoma of the prostate. *Cancer Res.,* **1941,** *1*:293–297.

Iversen, P., Christensen, M.G., Friis, E., Hornbol, P., Hvidt, V., Iversen, H.G., Klarskov, P., Krarup, T., Lund, F., Mogensen, P., Pedersen, T., Rasmussen, F., Rose, C., Skaarup, P., and Wolf, H. A phase III of zoladex and flutamide versus orchiectomy in the treatment of patients with advanced carcinoma of the prostate. *Cancer,* **1990,** *66*:1058–1066.

Katznelson, L., Finkelstein, J.S., Schoenfeld, D.A., Rosenthal, D.I., Anderson, E.J., and Klibanski, A. Increase in bone density and lean body mass during testosterone administration in men with acquired hypogonadism. *J. Clin. Endocrinol. Metab.,* **1996,** *81*:4358–4365.

King, D.S., Sharp, R.L., Vukovich, M.D., Brown, G.A., Reifenrath, T.A., Uhl, N.L., and Parsons, K.A. Effect of oral androstenedione on serum testosterone and adaptations to resistance training in young men: a randomized controlled trial. *JAMA,* **1999,** *281*:2020–2028.

Kumar, N., Didolkar, A.K., Monder, C., Bardin, C.W., and Sundaram, K. The biological activity of 7α-methyl-19-nortestosterone is not amplified in male reproductive tract as is that of testosterone. *Endocrinology,* **1992,** *130*:3677–3683.

La Spada, A.R., Wilson, E.M., Lubahn, D.B., Harding, A.E., and Fischbeck, K.H. Androgen receptor gene mutations in X-linked spinal and bulbar muscular atrophy. *Nature,* **1991,** *352*:77–79.

MacDonald, P.C., Madden, J.D., Brenner, P.F., Wilson, J.D., and Siiteri, P.K. Origin of estrogen in normal men and in men with testicular feminization. *J. Clin. Endocrinol. Metab.,* **1979,** *49*:905–916.

McConnell, J.D., Bruskewitz, R., Walsh, P., Andriole, G., Lieber, M., Holtgrewe, H.L., Albertsen, P., Roehrborn, C.G., Nickel, J.C., Wang, D.Z., Taylor, A.M., and Waldstreicher, J. The effect of finasteride on the risk of acute urinary retention and the need for surgical treatment among men with benign prostatic hyperplasia. Finasteride Long-Term Efficacy and Safety Study Group. *N. Engl. J. Med.,* **1998,** *338*:557–563.

McPhaul, M.J., and Griffin, J.E. Male pseudohermaphroditism caused by mutations of the human androgen receptor. *J. Clin. Endocrinol. Metab.,* **1999,** *84*:3435–3441.

Moilanen, A.M., Karvonen, U., Poukka, H., Yan, W., Toppari, J., Janne, O.A., and Palvino, J.J. A testis-specific androgen receptor coregulator that belongs to a novel family of nuclear proteins. *J. Biol. Chem.,* **1999,** *274*:3700–3704.

Morishma, A., Grumbach, M.M., Simpson, E.R., Fisher, C., and Qin, K. Aromatase deficiency in male and female siblings caused by a novel mutation and the physiological role of estrogens. *J. Clin. Endocrinol. Metab.,* **1995,** *80*:3689–3698.

Murray, M.P., Gardner, G.M., Mollinger, L.A., and Sepic, S.B. Strength of isometric and isokinetic contractions: knee muscles of men aged 20 to 86. *Phys. Ther.,* **1980,** *60*:412–419.

Pavlou, S.N., Brewer, K., Farley, M.G., Lindner, J., Bastias, M.-C., Rogers, B.J., Swift, L.L., Rivier, J.E., Vale, W.W., Conn, P.M., and Herbert, C.M. Combined administration of a gonadotropin-releasing hormone antagonist and testosterone in men induces reversible azoospermia without loss of libido. *J. Clin. Endocrinol. Metab.,* **1991,** *73*:1360–1369.

Petera, V., Bobek, K., and Lahn, V. Serum transaminase (GOT < GPT) and lactic dehydrogenase activity during treatment with methyltestosterone. *Clin. Chem. Acta,* **1962,** *7*:604–606.

Purifoy, F.E., Koopmans, L.H., and Mayes, D.M. Age differences in serum androgen levels in normal adult males. *Hum. Biol.,* **1981,** *53*:499–511.

Riggs, B.L., Wahner, H.W., Seeman, E., Offord, K.P., Dunn, W.L., Mazess, R.B., Johnson, K.A., and Melton, L.J. III. Changes in bone mineral density of the proximal femur and spine with aging. *J. Clin. Invest.,* **1982,** *70*:716–723.

Schellhammer, P., Sharifi, R., Block, N., Soloway, M., Venner, P., Patterson, A.L., Sarosdy, M., Vogelzang, N., Jones, J., and Kolvenberg, G. A controlled trial of bicalutamide versus flutamide, each in combination with luteinizing-releasing hormone analogue therapy, in patients with advanced prostate cancer. Casodex Combination Study Group. *Urology,* **1995,** *45*:745–752.

Smith, E.P., Boyd, J., Frank, G.R., Takahashi, H., Cohen, R.M., Specker, B., Williams, T.C., Lubahn, D.B., and Korach, K.S. Estrogen resistance caused by a mutation in the estrogen-receptor gene in a man. *N. Engl. J. Med.,* **1994,** *331*:1056–1061.

Snyder, P.J., and Lawrence, D.A. Treatment of male hypogonadism with testosterone enanthate. *J. Clin. Endocrinol. Metab.,* **1980,** *51*:1335–1339.

Snyder, P.J., Peachey, H., Hannoush, P., Berlin, J.A., Loh, L., Holmes, J.H., Dlewati, A., Staley, J., Santanna, J., Kapoor, S.C., Attie, M.F., Haddad, J.G. Jr., and Strom, B.L. Effect of testosterone treatment on bone mineral density in men over 65 years of age. *J. Clin. Endocrinol. Metab.,* **1999a,** *84*:1966–1972.

Snyder, P.J., Peachey, H., Hannoush, P., Berlin, J.A., Loh, L., Lenrow, D.A., Holmes, J.H., Dlewati, A., Santanna, J., Rosen, C.J., and Strom, B.L. Effect of testosterone treatment on body composition and muscle strength in men over 65 years of age. *J. Clin. Endocrinol. Metab.,* **1999b,** *84*:2647–2653.

Snyder, P.J., Peachey, H., Berlin, J.A., Hannoush, P., Hadad, G., Dlewati, A., Santanna, J., Loh, L., Lenow, D.A., Holmes, J.H., Kapoor, S.C., Atkinson, L.E., Strom, B.L. Effects of testosterone replacement in hypogonadal men. *J. Clin. Endocrin. Metab.,* **2000,** *85*:2670–2677.

Venturoli, S., Marescalchi, O., Colombo, F.M., Macrelli, S., Ravaioli, B., Bagnoli, A., Paradisi, R., and Flamigni, C. A prospective randomized trial comparing low dose flutamide, finasteride, ketoconazole, and cyproterone acetate-estrogen regimens in the treatment of hirsutism. *J. Clin. Endocrinol. Metab.,* **1999,** *84*:1304–1310.

Visakorpi, T., Hyytinen, E, Koivisto, P., Tanner, M., Keinanen, R., Palmberg, C., Palotie, A., Tammela, T., Isola, J., and Kallioniemi O.-P. *In vivo* amplification of the androgen receptor gene and progression of human prostate cancer. *Nat. Genet.,* **1995,** *9*:401–406.

Wang, C., Berman, N., Longstreth, J.A., Chuapoco, B., Hull, L., Steiner, B., Faulkner, S., Dudley, R.E., and Swerdloff, R.S. Pharmacokinetics of transdermal testosterone gel in hypogonadal men: application of gel at one site versus four sites: a General Clinical Research Center Study. *J. Clin. Endocrinol. Metab.,* **2000,** *85*:964–969.

WHO Task Force for the Regulation of Male Fertility. Contraceptive efficacy of testosterone-induced azoospermia and oligozoospermia in normal men. *Fertil. Steril.,* **1996,** *65*:821–829.

Wilbert, D.M., Griffin, J.E., and Wilson, J.D. Characterization of the cytosol androgen receptor of the human prostate. *J. Clin. Endocrinol. Metab.,* **1983,** *56*:113–120.

Wilson, J.D. The pathogenesis of benign prostatic hyperplasia. *Am. J. Med.,* **1980,** *68*:745–756.

Wilson, J.D., Griffin, J.E., and Russell, D.W. Steroid 5α-reductase 2 deficiency. *Endocr. Rev.,* **1993,** *14*:577–593.

Yu, Z., Gupta, S.K., Hwang, S.S., Kipnes, M.S., Mooradian, A.D., Snyder, P.J., and Atkinson, L.E. Testosterone pharmacokinetics after application of an investigational transdermal system in hypogonadal men. *J. Clin. Pharmacol.,* **1997,** *37*:1139–1145.

Zhang, G.Y., Gu, Y.Q., Wang, X.-H., Cui, Y.-G., Bremner, W.J. A clinical trial of injectable testosterone undecanoate as a potential male contraceptive in normal Chinese men. *J. Clin. Endocrinol. Metab.,* **1999,** *84:*3642–3647.

Zhang, G.Y., Gu, Y.Q., Wang, X.-H., Cui, Y.-G., and Bremner, W.J. A pharmacokinetic study of injectable testosterone undecanoate in hypogonadal men. *J. Androl.,* **1998,** *19:*761–768.

Zhi, L., Tegley, C.M., Marschke, K.B., and Jones, T.K. Switching androgen receptor antagonists to agonists by modifying C-ring substituents on piperidino [3,2-g] quinolinone. *Bioorg. Med. Chem. Lett.,* **1999,** *9:*1009–1012.

MONOGRAPHS AND REVIEWS

Crowley, W.F. Jr., Filicori, M., Spratt D.I., and Santoro, N.F. The physiology of gonadotropin-releasing hormone (GnRH) secretion in men and women. *Recent Prog. Horm. Res.,* **1985,** *41:*473–531.

Feldman, D. Ketonazole and other imidazole derivatives as inhibitors of steroidogenesis. *Endocr. Rev.,* **1986,** *7:*409–420.

Forest, M.G. Differentiation and development of the male. *Clin. Endocrinol. Metab.,* **1975,** *4:*569–596.

George, F.W., and Wilson, J.D. Embryology of the genital tract. In, *Campbell's Urology,* 6th ed. (Walsh, P.C., Retik, A.B., and Stamey, T.A., eds.) W.B. Saunders, Philadelphia, **1992,** pp. 1496–1506.

Negro-Vilar, A. Selective androgen receptor modulators (SARMs): a novel approach to androgen therapy for the new millennium. *J. Clin. Endocrinol. Metab.,* **1999,** *84:*3459–3462.

Santen, R.J. Gonadal disease. In, *Endocrinology and Metabolism,* 3rd ed. (Felig, P., Baxter, J.D., and Frohman, L.A., eds.) McGraw-Hill, New York, **1995,** p. 899.

Acknowledgment

The author is pleased to acknowledge Dr. Jean D. Wilson, the author of this chapter for the ninth edition of this book, whose original research and conceptualization of its implications provided the foundation of current knowledge of androgen metabolism and action.

C H A P T E R   6 0

ADRENOCORTICOTROPIC HORMONE; ADRENOCORTICAL STEROIDS AND THEIR SYNTHETIC ANALOGS; INHIBITORS OF THE SYNTHESIS AND ACTIONS OF ADRENOCORTICAL HORMONES

Bernard P. Schimmer and Keith L. Parker

Adrenocorticotropic hormone (ACTH, also called corticotropin) and the steroid hormone products of the adrenal cortex are considered together in this chapter, because the major physiological and pharmacological effects of ACTH result from its action to increase the circulating levels of adrenocortical steroids. Synthetic derivatives of ACTH are used principally in the diagnostic assessment of adrenocortical function. As all of the known therapeutic effects of ACTH can be achieved with corticosteroids, synthetic steroid hormones generally are used instead of ACTH for therapeutic applications.

Corticosteroids and their biologically active synthetic derivatives differ in their metabolic (glucocorticoid) and electrolyte-regulating (mineralocorticoid) activities. These agents are employed at physiological doses for replacement therapy when endogenous production is impaired. In addition, glucocorticoids are potent suppressors of inflammation, and their use in a wide variety of inflammatory and autoimmune diseases makes them among the most frequently prescribed classes of drugs. Because they exert effects on almost every organ system, the clinical use of and withdrawal from corticosteroids are complicated by a number of serious side effects, some of which are life-threatening. Therefore, the decision to institute therapy with corticosteroids always requires careful consideration of the relative risks and benefits in each patient.

Agents that inhibit various reactions in the steroidogenic pathway and thus alter the patterns of secretion of adrenocortical steroids are discussed, as are synthetic steroids, such as mifepristone (see also Chapter 58), that inhibit glucocorticoid action. Agents that inhibit the action of aldosterone are presented in Chapter 29; agents used to inhibit growth of steroid-dependent tumors are discussed in Chapter 52.

History. The clinical importance of the adrenal glands was first appreciated by Addison, who described fatal outcomes in patients with adrenal destruction in a presentation to the South London Medical Society in 1849. These studies, published subsequently (Addison, 1855), were soon extended by Brown-Séquard, who demonstrated that bilateral adrenalectomy was fatal in laboratory animals. It later was shown that the adrenal cortex, rather than the medulla, was essential for survival in these experiments. Further studies demonstrated that the adrenal cortex regulated both carbohydrate metabolism and fluid and electrolyte balance. Efforts by a number of investigators ultimately led to the isolation and characterization of the various adrenocorticosteroids. Studies of the factors that regulated carbohydrate metabolism (termed *glucocorticoids*) culminated with the synthesis of cortisone, the first pharmacologically effective glucocorticoid to be available in large amounts. Subsequently, Tate and colleagues isolated and characterized a distinct corticosteroid, aldosterone, that had potent effects on fluid and electrolyte balance (and therefore was termed a *mineralocorticoid*). The isolation of distinct corticosteroids that regulated carbohydrate metabolism or fluid and electrolyte balance ultimately led to the concept that the adrenal cortex comprises two largely independent units: an outer zone that produces mineralocorticoids and an inner region that synthesizes glucocorticoids and weak androgens.

Studies of the adrenocortical steroids also played a key part in delineating the role of the anterior pituitary in endocrine function. As early as 1912, Cushing described patients with hypercorticism, and later recognized that pituitary basophilism represented the cause of the adrenal overactivity (Cushing, 1932), thus establishing the link between the anterior pituitary and adrenal function. These studies ultimately led to the purification of ACTH (Astwood *et al.*, 1952) and the determination of its chemical structure. ACTH was further shown to be essential in maintaining the structural integrity and steroidogenic capacity of the inner cortical zones. The role of the hypothalamus in pituitary control was established by Harris (1948), who further postulated that a soluble factor produced by the hypothalamus activated ACTH release. These investigations culminated with the determination of the structure of corticotropin-releasing hormone (CRH), a hypothalamic peptide that regulates secretion of ACTH from the pituitary (Vale *et al.*, 1981).

Shortly after synthetic cortisone became available, Hench and colleagues demonstrated the dramatic effect of glucocorticoids and ACTH in the treatment of rheumatoid arthritis (Hench *et al.*, 1949). These studies set the stage for the clinical use of corticosteroids in a wide variety of diseases, as discussed below.

ADRENOCORTICOTROPIC HORMONE (ACTH; CORTICOTROPIN)

The sequence of human ACTH, a peptide of 39 amino acids, is shown in Figure 60–1. Whereas removal of a single amino acid at the amino terminus considerably impairs biological activity, a number of amino acids can be removed from the carboxy-terminal end without a marked effect. The structure–activity relationships of ACTH have been studied extensively, and it is believed that a stretch of four basic amino acids at positions 15 to 18 is an important determinant of high-affinity binding to the ACTH receptor, whereas amino acids 6 to 10 are important for receptor activation (Imura, 1994). As discussed in Chapter 23 and as schematized in Figure 60–1, ACTH is synthesized as part of a larger precursor protein, pro-opiomelanocortin (POMC), and is liberated from the precursor through proteolytic cleavage at dibasic residues by the enzyme prohormone convertase 1. Impaired processing of POMC due to a mutation in prohormone convertase 1 has been implicated in the pathogenesis of a human disorder presenting with adrenal insufficiency. Intriguingly, these patients also exhibit childhood obesity, hypogonadotropic hypogonadism, and diabetes (Jackson *et al.*, 1997), suggesting other proteolytic targets for prohormone convertase 1. A

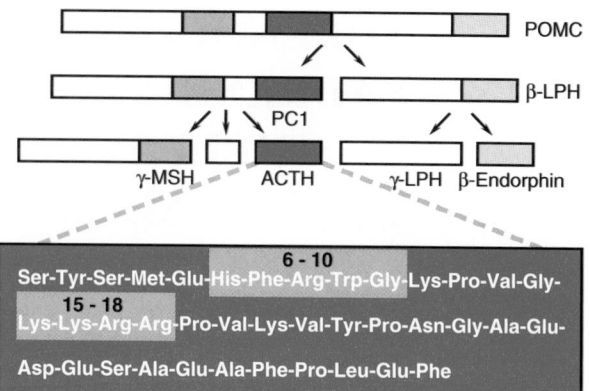

Figure 60–1. Processing of POMC to ACTH and the sequence of ACTH.

A schematic overview of the pathway by which pro-opiomelanocortin (POMC) is converted to ACTH and other peptides in the anterior pituitary is shown. The light blue boxes behind the ACTH structure indicate regions identified as important for steroidogenic activity (residues 6–10) and binding to the ACTH receptor (15–18). The amino acid sequence of human ACTH is shown. LPH, lipotropin; MSH, melanocyte-stimulating hormone; PC1, prohormone convertase 1.

number of other biologically important peptides, including endorphins, lipotropins, and the melanocyte-stimulating hormones (MSH), also are produced from the same prcursor.

Actions on the Adrenal Cortex. ACTH stimulates the adrenal cortex to secrete glucocorticoids, mineralocorticoids, and weak androgens such as androstenedione and dehydroepiandrosterone, which can be converted peripherally into more potent androgens. Based on histological analyses, the adrenal cortex originally was separated into three zones: the zona glomerulosa, zona fasciculata, and zona reticularis. Functionally, it is more useful to view the adrenal cortex as two discrete compartments: the outer zona glomerulosa, which secretes the mineralocorticoid aldosterone, and the inner zonae fasciculata/reticularis, which secrete the glucocorticoid cortisol as well as the adrenal androgens (Figure 60–2). The biochemical basis for these differences in steroidogenic output has been defined in considerable detail. Cells of the outer zone have receptors for angiotensin II and express aldosterone synthase, an enzyme that catalyzes the terminal reactions in mineralocorticoid biosynthesis. In contrast, cells of the inner zones lack receptors for angiotensin II and express two enzymes, steroid 17α-hydroxylase (P450$_{17\alpha}$) and 11β-hydroxylase (P450$_{11\beta}$), that catalyze the production of glucocorticoids.

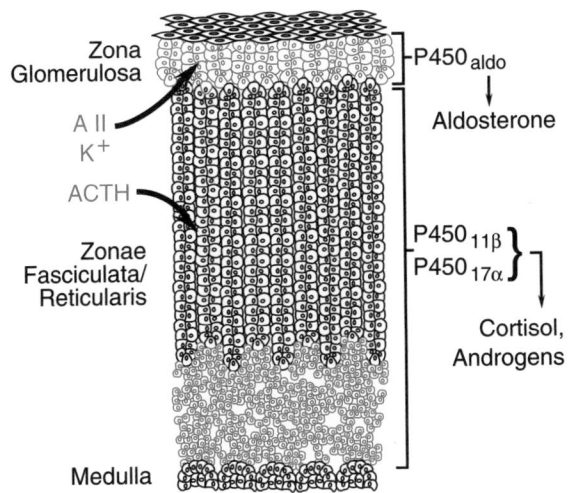

Figure 60–2. The adrenal cortex contains two anatomically and functionally distinct compartments.

The major functional compartments of the adrenal cortex are shown, along with the steroidogenic enzymes that determine the unique profiles of corticosteroid products. Also shown are the predominant physiologic regulators of steroid production: angiotensin II (A II) and K$^+$ for the zona glomerulosa and ACTH for the zonae fasciculata/reticularis.

In the absence of the adenohypophysis, the inner zones of the cortex atrophy, and the production of glucocorticoids and adrenal androgens is markedly impaired. Although ACTH acutely can stimulate mineralocorticoid production by the zona glomerulosa, this zone is regulated predominantly by angiotensin II and extracellular K$^+$ (*see* Chapter 31) and does not undergo atrophy in the absence of ongoing stimulation by the pituitary gland. In the setting of persistently elevated ACTH, mineralocorticoid levels initially increase and then return to normal (a phenomenon termed *ACTH escape*).

Persistently elevated levels of ACTH, due either to repeated administration of large doses of ACTH or to excessive endogenous ACTH production, induce hyperplasia and hypertrophy of the inner zones of the adrenal cortex, with overproduction of cortisol and adrenal androgens. Adrenal hyperplasia is most marked in congenital disorders of steroidogenesis, where ACTH levels are continuously elevated as a secondary response to impaired cortisol biosynthesis.

Mechanism of Action.   ACTH stimulates the synthesis and release of adrenocortical hormones. As specific mechanisms for steroid hormone secretion have not been defined and since steroids do not accumulate appreciably

in the gland, it is believed that the actions of ACTH to increase steroid hormone production are predominantly mediated at the level of *de novo* biosynthesis. ACTH, like most peptide hormones, interacts with a specific membrane receptor. As determined by gene cloning and sequencing, the human ACTH receptor is a member of the G protein–coupled receptor family, closely resembling in its structure the receptors for melanocyte-stimulating hormones (Cone and Mountjoy, 1993). ACTH acts through the G protein G$_s$ to activate adenylyl cyclase and increase intracellular cyclic AMP content. Cyclic AMP is an obligatory second messenger for most, if not all, effects of ACTH on steroidogenesis. Mutations in the ACTH receptor have been associated with rare syndromes leading to familial resistance to ACTH (Clark and Weber, 1998).

Temporally, the response of adrenocortical cells to ACTH has two phases: an acute phase, which occurs within seconds to minutes, largely reflects an increased supply of cholesterol substrate to the steroidogenic enzymes; a chronic phase, which occurs over hours to days, results largely from increased transcription of the steroidogenic enzymes. A summary of the pathways of adrenal steroid biosynthesis and the structures of the major steroid intermediates and products of the human adrenal cortex are shown in Figure 60–3. The rate-limiting step in steroid hormone production is the conversion of cholesterol to pregnenolone, a reaction catalyzed by the cholesterol side-chain cleavage enzyme, designated P450$_{scc}$. Most of the enzymes required for steroid hormone biosynthesis, including P450$_{scc}$, are members of the cytochrome P450 superfamily, a related group of mixed-function oxidases that play important roles in the metabolism of xenobiotics such as drugs and environmental pollutants as well as in the biosynthesis of such endogenous compounds as steroid hormones, vitamin D, bile acids, fatty acids, prostaglandins, and biogenic amines (*see* Chapter 1). The rate-limiting components in this reaction regulate the mobilization of substrate cholesterol and its delivery to the P450$_{scc}$, located in the inner mitochondrial matrix.

The adrenal cortex uses multiple sources of cholesterol to ensure an adequate supply of substrate for steroidogenesis. These sources include (1) circulating cholesterol and cholesterol esters taken up *via* the low-density lipoprotein (LDL)- and high-density lipoprotein (HDL)-receptor pathways, (2) liberation of cholesterol from endogenous cholesterol ester stores *via* activation of cholesterol esterase, and (3) increased *de novo* biosynthesis.

The mechanism(s) by which ACTH stimulates the translocation of cholesterol to the inner mitochondrial matrix are not well defined. Several candidate mediators of the acute delivery of cholesterol to the mitochondria have been proposed, including a 30,000 dalton phosphoprotein induced by ACTH in all primary steroidogenic tissues, the peripheral benzodiazepine receptor, and sterol carrier protein-2. The cDNA encoding the 30,000 dalton phosphoprotein (designated the *St*eroidogenic *A*cute *R*egulatory Protein, or StAR) has been cloned and shown to activate steroidogenesis (Stocco and Clark, 1996). Significantly, mutations in the gene encoding StAR are found in patients with congenital lipoid adrenal hyperplasia, a rare

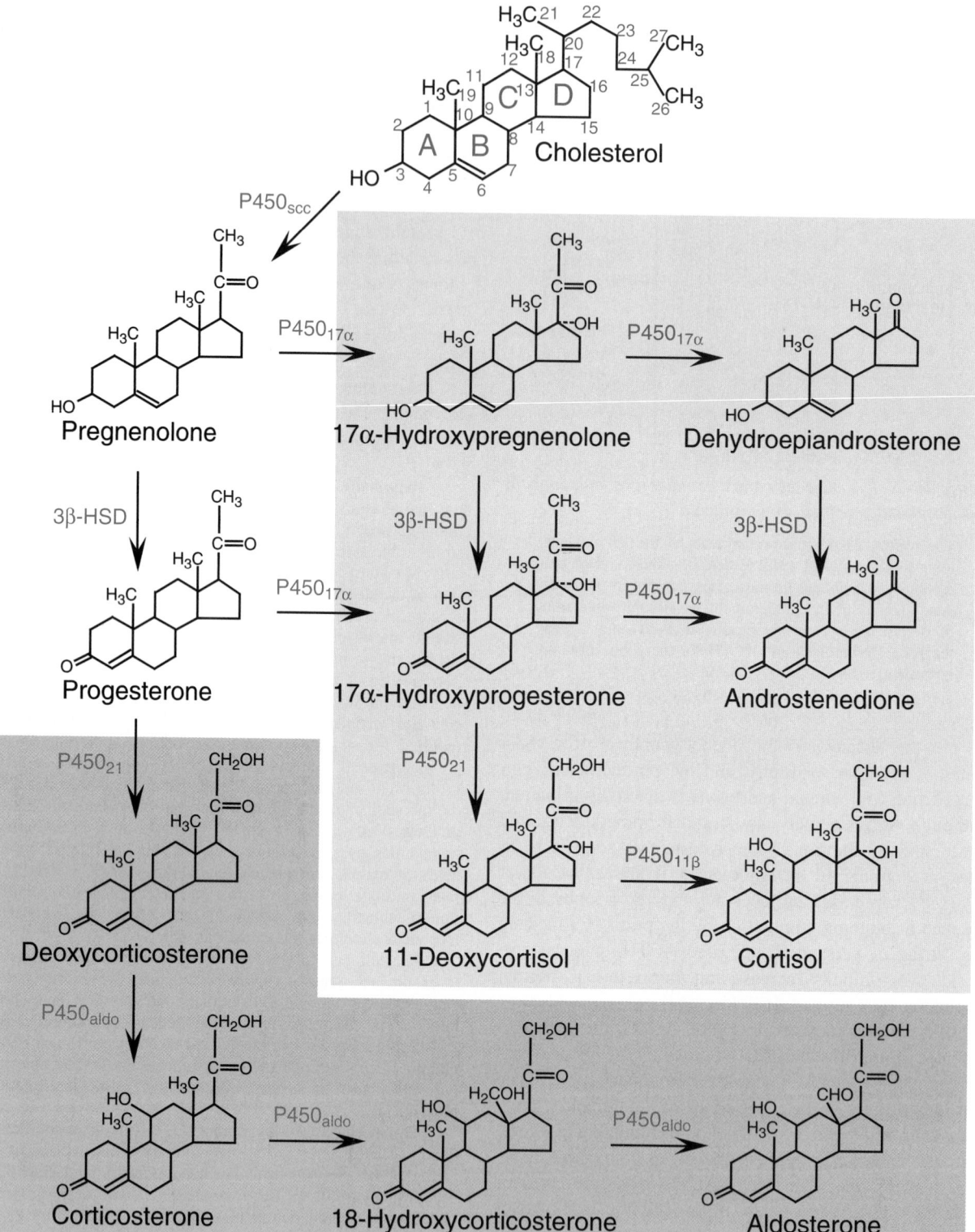

Figure 60–3. Pathways of corticosteroid biosynthesis.

The steroidogenic pathways used in the biosynthesis of the corticosteroids are shown, along with the structures of the intermediates and products. The pathways that are unique to the zona glomerulosa are shown in blue, whereas those unique to the zonae fasciculata/reticularis are shown in gray. P450scc, cholesterol side-chain cleavage enzyme; 3β-HSD, 3β-hydroxysteroid dehydrogenase; P450$_{17\alpha}$, steroid 17α-hydroxylase; P450$_{21}$, steroid 21-hydroxylase; P450$_{aldo}$, aldosterone synthase; P450$_{11\beta}$, steroid 11β-hydroxylase.

congenital disorder in which adrenal cells become engorged with cholesterol deposits secondary to an inability to synthesize any steroid hormones (Lin *et al.,* 1995). This finding points to a key role of StAR in the regulated delivery of cholesterol to the steroid biosynthetic pathway.

An important component of the trophic effect of ACTH is the enhancement of transcription of the genes that encode the individual steroidogenic enzymes, with associated increases in the steroidogenic capacity of the gland. Although the molecular mechanisms are still under investigation, it appears that a variety of transcriptional regulators mediate the induction of the steroid hydroxylases by ACTH (Parker and Schimmer, 1995).

Extraadrenal Effects of ACTH.   In large doses, ACTH causes a number of metabolic changes in adrenalectomized animals, including ketosis, lipolysis, hypoglycemia (immediately after treatment), and resistance to insulin (later after treatment). Because of the large doses of ACTH required, the physiological significance of these extraadrenal effects is doubtful. ACTH also improves learning in experimental animals; this latter effect appears to be nonendocrine and mediated *via* distinct receptors in the central nervous system. Patients with primary adrenal insufficiency and persistently elevated ACTH levels classically are hyperpigmented. This hyperpigmentation probably results from ACTH activating the MSH receptor on the melanocytes, perhaps a consequence of the identity of ACTH and MSH in the first 13 amino acids of each of their sequences.

Regulation of ACTH Secretion. *Hypothalamic-Pituitary-Adrenal Axis.*   The rates of secretion of glucocorticoids are determined by fluctuations in the release of ACTH by the pituitary corticotropes. These corticotropes, in turn, are regulated by corticotropin-releasing hormone (CRH), a peptide hormone released by CRH neurons of the endocrine hypothalamus. These three organs collectively are referred to as the hypothalamic-pituitary-adrenal (HPA) axis, an integrated system that maintains appropriate levels of glucocorticoids (*see* Figure 60–4 for an overview of this axis). There are three characteristic modes of regulation of the HPA axis: diurnal rhythm in basal steroidogenesis, negative feedback regulation by adrenal corticosteroids, and marked increases in steroidogenesis in response to stress. The diurnal rhythm is entrained by higher neuronal centers in response to sleep-wake cycles, such that levels of ACTH peak in the early morning hours, causing the circulating glucocorticoid levels to peak at approximately 8 A.M. As discussed below, negative feedback regulation occurs at multiple levels of the HPA axis and is the major mechanism that operates to maintain circulating glucocorticoid levels in the appropriate range. Stressful

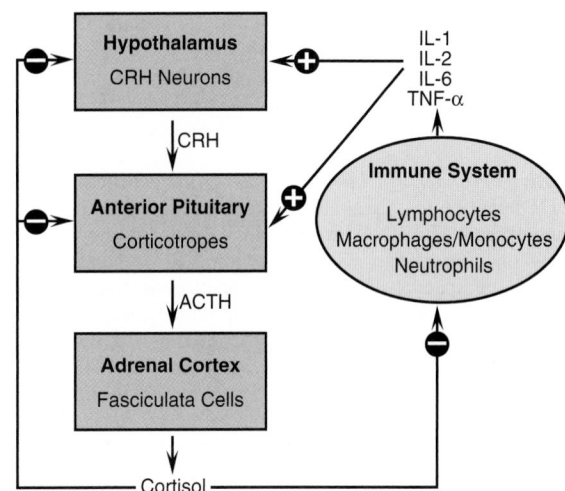

Figure 60–4. Overview of the hypothalamic-pituitary-adrenal (HPA) axis and its bidirectional communication with the immune system.

The complex regulatory interactions between the HPA axis and the immune/inflammatory network are shown. ⊕ indicates a positive regulator, ⊖ indicates a negative regulator. IL-1, interleukin-1; IL-2, interleukin-2; IL-6, interleukin-6; TNF-α, tumor necrosis factor α; CRH, corticotropin-releasing hormone.

stimuli can override these normal negative feedback control mechanisms, leading to marked increases in plasma concentrations of adrenocortical steroids.

Central Nervous System.   The central nervous system (CNS) integrates a number of different positive and negative influences on ACTH release (Figure 60–4). These signals converge on the CRH neurons, which are clustered largely in the parvocellular region of the paraventricular hypothalamic nucleus and make axonal connections to the median eminence of the hypothalamus (*see* Chrousos, 1995, *see also* Chapter 12). Following release into the hypophyseal plexus, CRH is transported *via* this portal system to the pituitary, where it binds to specific membrane receptors on corticotropes. Upon CRH binding, the CRH receptor activates adenylyl cyclase and increases cyclic AMP levels within corticotropes, ultimately increasing both ACTH biosynthesis and secretion. The human CRH receptor has been cloned and shown to resemble most closely in sequence the calcitonin/vasoactive intestinal peptide/growth hormone–releasing hormone family of G protein–coupled receptors (Chen *et al.,* 1993).

Arginine Vasopressin.   Arginine vasopressin (AVP) also acts as a secretagogue for corticotropes, significantly potentiating the effects of CRH. Animal studies have revealed that the potentiation of CRH action by AVP likely plays a physiologically significant role in the full magnitude of the stress response. AVP is produced in the parvocellular neurons of the paraventricular nucleus, like CRH, as well as by magnocellular neurons of the supraoptic nucleus; it is secreted into the pituitary plexus from the median eminence. After binding to specific G protein–coupled receptors of the V_{1b} subtype, AVP activates phospholipase C, producing diacylglycerol and 1,4,5-inositol trisphosphate as messengers to release ACTH (*see* Chapters 2 and 12); in contrast to CRH, AVP apparently does not increase ACTH synthesis.

Negative Feedback of Glucocorticoids.   Glucocorticoids inhibit ACTH secretion *via* direct and indirect actions on CRH neurons to decrease CRH mRNA levels and CRH release and *via* direct effects on corticotropes. The effect on CRH release may be mediated by specific corticosteroid receptors in the hippocampus, which are proposed to play important roles in negative feedback inhibition exerted by glucocorticoids. At lower cortisol levels, the mineralocorticoid (type I) receptor, which has a higher affinity for glucocorticoids and is the predominant form found in the hippocampus, is the major receptor species occupied. As glucocorticoid concentrations rise, the glucocorticoid (type II) receptor also becomes occupied as the capacity of the mineralocorticoid receptor is exceeded. Basal activity of the HPA axis apparently is controlled by both classes of receptor, whereas feedback inhibition by glucocorticoids predominantly involves the glucocorticoid receptor.

In the pituitary, glucocorticoids act through the glucocorticoid receptor to inhibit the expression of POMC in corticotropes as well as the release of ACTH. These effects are both rapid (occurring within seconds to minutes and possibly mediated by glucocorticoid receptor–independent mechanisms) and delayed (requiring hours and involving changes in gene transcription mediated through the glucocorticoid receptor).

The Stress Response.   Circumstances of stress overcome negative feedback regulation of the HPA axis, leading to a marked rise in the production of corticosteroids. Examples of stress signals include injury, hemorrhage, severe infection, major surgery, hypoglycemia, cold, pain, and fear. Although the precise mechanisms that underlie this stress response and the essential actions played by the glucocorticoids are not defined fully, it is clear that glucocorticoid secretion is vital for maintaining homeostasis in these stressful settings. As discussed below, complex interactions between the HPA axis and the immune system may be a fundamental physiological component of this stress response (*see* Sapolsky *et al.,* 2000; Turnbull and Rivier, 1999).

Assays for ACTH.

Initially, ACTH levels were measured by bioassays that measured induced steroid production or the depletion of adrenal ascorbic acid; such assays have been used to standardize ACTH amounts in different preparations used for both diagnostic and therapeutic purposes. Radioimmunoassays were developed to quantitate ACTH levels in individual patients, but they were not always reproducible, and their sensitivity did not always clearly differentiate between low and normal levels of the hormone. An immunoradiometric assay, which reliably measures ACTH levels, is now widely available. This assay, which uses two separate antibodies directed at distinct epitopes on the ACTH molecule, considerably increases the ability to differentiate between primary hypoadrenalism due to intrinsic adrenal disease and secondary

forms of hypoadrenalism due to hypothalamic or pituitary disorders. Patients with primary adrenal insufficiency have high ACTH levels because they lack normal glucocorticoid feedback inhibition, whereas patients with secondary adrenal insufficiency have pituitary or hypothalamic disease resulting in low levels of ACTH. The immunoradiometric ACTH assay also is useful in differentiating between ACTH-dependent and ACTH-independent forms of hypercorticism: high ACTH levels are seen when pituitary adenomas (*i.e.,* Cushing's disease) or nonpituitary tumors that secrete ACTH (*i.e.,* ectopic ACTH) underlie the hypercorticism, whereas very low ACTH levels are seen in patients with excessive glucocorticoid production due to primary adrenal disorders. Despite its considerable strengths, one problem with the immunoradiometric ACTH assay is that its specificity for intact ACTH can lead to false, low values in patients with ectopic ACTH secretion; these tumors often secrete aberrantly processed forms of ACTH that have biological activity but do not react in the antibody assay.

Therapeutic Uses and Diagnostic Applications of ACTH.

There are anecdotal reports that selected conditions respond better to ACTH than to corticosteroids (*e.g.,* multiple sclerosis), and some clinicians continue to advocate therapy with ACTH. Despite this, ACTH currently has only limited utility as a therapeutic agent. Therapy with ACTH is both less predictable and less convenient than is therapy with appropriate steroids. In addition, ACTH stimulates mineralocorticoid and adrenal androgen secretion and may therefore cause acute retention of salt and water as well as virilization. While ACTH and the corticosteroids are not pharmacologically equivalent, all of the known therapeutic effects of ACTH also can be achieved with appropriate doses of corticosteroids at a lesser risk of side effects.

Testing the Integrity of the HPA Axis.   At present, the major clinical use of ACTH is in testing the integrity of the HPA axis to identify those patients needing supplemental steroid coverage in stressful situations. Other tests used to assess the HPA axis include the insulin tolerance test (*see* Chapter 56) and the metyrapone test (discussed later in this chapter). ACTH purified from animal pituitary glands is available in long-lasting injectable gel preparations as a gelatin solution (H.P. ACTHAR GEL; 40 or 80 IU/vial). *Cosyntropin* (CORTROSYN) is a synthetic peptide that corresponds to residues 1 to 24 of human ACTH. At the considerably supraphysiological dose of 250 μg, cosyntropin maximally stimulates adrenocortical steroidogenesis. In the rapid cosyntropin stimulation test, 250 μg of cosyntropin is administered either intramuscularly or intravenously, with cortisol measured just before administration (baseline) and 30 to 60 minutes after cosyntropin administration. An increase in circulating cortisol to levels greater than 18 to 20 μg/dl indicates a normal response (others also have included an increase of 7 μg/dl over the baseline value as a positive response, although this is less widely accepted). In patients with pituitary or hypothalamic disease of recent onset or shortly after surgery for pituitary tumors, this standard cosyntropin stimulation test may be misleading, as the duration of ACTH deficiency may have been insufficient to cause significant adrenal atrophy with frank loss of steroidogenic capacity. For this latter group of patients, some experts advocate a "low-dose" cosyntropin stimulation test, in which 1 μg of cosyntropin is administered intravenously, with cortisol measured just before and 30 minutes after cosyntropin administration (Abdu *et al.*, 1999). Because cosyntropin is not generally available in a 1-μg dose, the standard ampoule of cosyntropin (250 μg) is diluted to permit accurate delivery of the 1-μg challenge dose, with the cutoff for a normal response being the same as that for the standard test. Care must be taken to avoid adsorption of the ACTH to plastic tubing and to measure the plasma cortisol precisely at 30 minutes after the cosyntropin injection. Although some studies indicate that the low-dose test is more sensitive than the standard 250-μg test, others report that this test also may fail to detect secondary adrenal insufficiency.

As noted above, primary and secondary adrenocortical diseases are reliably distinguished using currently available sensitive assays for ACTH. Thus, longer-course ACTH stimulation tests rarely are used to differentiate between these disorders.

CRH Stimulation Test.   Ovine CRH, also termed *corticorelin* (ACTHREL), is available for diagnostic testing of the HPA axis. In patients with documented ACTH-dependent hypercorticism, CRH testing may help differentiate between a pituitary source (*i.e.*, Cushing's disease) and an ectopic source of ACTH. After two baseline blood samples are obtained fifteen minutes apart, corticorelin (1 μg/kg) is administered intravenously over a 30- to 60-second interval, and blood samples are obtained at 15, 30, and 60 minutes for ACTH measurement. It is important that the blood samples be handled as recommended for the ACTH assay. At the recommended dose, CRH generally is well tolerated, although flushing may occur, particularly if the dose is administered as a bolus. Patients with Cushing's disease respond to CRH with either a normal or an exaggerated increase in ACTH, whereas ACTH levels do not increase in patients with ectopic sources of ACTH. It should be noted that this test is not perfect: ACTH levels are induced by CRH in occasional patients with ectopic ACTH, whereas approximately 5% to 10% of patients with Cushing's disease fail to respond. To improve the diagnostic accuracy of the CRH stimulation test, some authori-

ties advocate sampling of blood from the inferior petrosal sinus following peripheral administration of CRH. When performed by a skilled neuroradiologist, this procedure may increase diagnostic accuracy with a tolerable risk of complications from the catheterization procedure.

Absorption and Fate.   ACTH is readily absorbed from parenteral sites. The hormone rapidly disappears from the circulation following intravenous administration; in human beings, the half-life in plasma is about 15 minutes, primarily due to rapid enzymatic hydrolysis.

Toxicity of ACTH.   Aside from rare hypersensitivity reactions, the toxicity of ACTH is primarily attributable to the increased secretion of corticosteroids. Cosyntropin is generally less antigenic than native ACTH. Moreover, ACTH isolated from animal pituitaries contains significant amounts of vasopressin, which can lead to life-threatening hyponatremia. These factors make cosyntropin the preferred agent for clinical use.

ADRENOCORTICAL STEROIDS

The adrenal cortex synthesizes two classes of steroids: the *corticosteroids* (*glucocorticoids* and *mineralocorticoids*), which have 21 carbon atoms, and the *androgens,* which have 19 (Figure 60–3). The actions of corticosteroids historically were described as glucocorticoid (carbohydrate metabolism–regulating) and mineralocorticoid (electrolyte balance–regulating), reflecting their preferential activities. In human beings, hydrocortisone (*cortisol*) is the main glucocorticoid, and *aldosterone* is the main mineralocorticoid. The mechanisms by which glucocorticoid biosynthesis is regulated by ACTH have been discussed above, and the regulation of aldosterone production is described in Chapter 31. Table 60–1 shows typical rates of secretion of the physiologically most significant corticosteroids in human beings—cortisol and aldosterone—as well as their normal concentrations in peripheral plasma. Although earlier studies had suggested that cortisol was produced at a daily rate of 20 mg, more recent studies indicate that the actual rate is closer to 10 mg/day (Esteban *et al.*, 1991).

Table 60–1

Normal Daily Production Rates and Circulating Levels of the Predominant Corticosteroids

	CORTISOL	ALDOSTERONE
Rate of secretion under optimal conditions	10 mg/day	0.125 mg/day
Concentration in peripheral plasma:		
8 A.M.	16 μg/100 ml	0.01 μg/100 ml
4 P.M.	4 μg/100 ml	0.01 μg/100 ml

Although the adrenal cortex is an important source of circulating androgens in women, patients with adrenal insufficiency can be restored to normal life expectancy by replacement therapy with glucocorticoid and mineralocorticoid. Thus, adrenal androgens are not essential for survival. There are, however, age-related changes in dehydroepiandrosterone (DHEA) levels, which peak in the third decade of life and decline progressively thereafter. Moreover, patients with a number of chronic diseases have very low DHEA levels, leading some to propose that DHEA treatment might at least partly alleviate the adverse consequences of aging. Based on these issues, there has been considerable discussion about the need for DHEA therapy in patients with primary or secondary adrenal insufficiency. In one study, the addition of DHEA (50 mg orally each morning) to the standard replacement regimen in women with adrenal insufficiency led to improved subjective well-being and sexuality (Arlt *et al.,* 1999).

Physiological Functions and Pharmacological Effects

Physiological Actions. The effects of corticosteroids are numerous and widespread. Their diverse effects include alterations in carbohydrate, protein, and lipid metabolism; maintenance of fluid and electrolyte balance; and preservation of normal function of the cardiovascular system, the immune system, the kidney, skeletal muscle, the endocrine system, and the nervous system. In addition, by mechanisms that are still not fully understood, corticosteroids endow the organism with the capacity to resist stressful circumstances such as noxious stimuli and environmental changes. In the absence of the adrenal cortex, survival is made possible only by maintaining an optimal environment, including adequate and regular feedings, ingestion of relatively large amounts of sodium chloride, and maintenance of an appropriate environmental temperature.

Until recently, corticosteroid effects were viewed as physiological (reflecting actions of corticosteroids at doses corresponding to normal daily production levels) or pharmacological (representing effects seen only at doses exceeding the normal daily production of corticosteroids). More recent concepts suggest that the antiinflammatory and immunosuppressive actions of corticosteroids, one of the major "pharmacological" uses of this class of drugs, also provide a protective mechanism in the physiological setting, since many of the immune mediators associated with the inflammatory response decrease vascular tone and could lead to cardiovascular collapse if unopposed by the adrenal corticosteroids. This hypothesis is supported by the fact that the daily production rate of cortisol can rise markedly (at least 10-fold) in the setting of severe stress. In addition, as discussed below, the pharmacological actions of corticosteroids in different tissues and many of their physiological effects seem to be mediated by the same receptor. Thus, the various glucocorticoid derivatives used currently as pharmacological agents have side effects on physiological processes that parallel their therapeutic effectiveness.

The actions of corticosteroids are related in complex ways to those of other hormones. For example, in the absence of lipolytic hormones, cortisol has virtually no effect on the rate of lipolysis by adipocytes. Likewise, in the absence of glucocorticoids, epinephrine and norepinephrine have only minor effects on lipolysis. Administration of a small dose of a glucocorticoid, however, markedly potentiates the lipolytic action of these amines. These effects of corticosteroids that involve concerted actions with other hormonal regulators are termed *permissive* and most likely reflect steroid-induced changes in protein synthesis that, in turn, modify tissue responsiveness.

Corticosteroids are grouped according to their relative potencies in Na^+ retention, effects on carbohydrate metabolism (*i.e.,* hepatic deposition of glycogen and gluconeogenesis), and antiinflammatory effects. In general, potencies of steroids as judged by their ability to sustain life in adrenalectomized animals closely parallel those determined for Na^+ retention. Potencies based on effects on glucose metabolism closely parallel those for antiinflammatory effects. The effects on Na^+ retention and the carbohydrate/antiinflammatory actions are not closely related and reflect selective actions at distinct receptors, as noted above. Based on these differential potencies, the corticosteroids traditionally are divided into mineralocorticoids and glucocorticoids. Estimates of potencies of representative steroids in these actions are listed in Table 60–2. Several steroids that are classified predominantly as glucocorticoids (*e.g.,* cortisol and prednisone) also possess modest but significant mineralocorticoid activity and thus may affect fluid and electrolyte handling in the clinical setting. At doses used for replacement therapy in patients with primary adrenal insufficiency (*see* below), the mineralocorticoid effects of these "glucocorticoids" are insufficient to replace that of aldosterone, and concurrent therapy with a more potent mineralocorticoid generally is needed. In contrast, aldosterone is exceedingly potent with respect to Na^+ retention but has only modest potency for effects on carbohydrate metabolism. At normal rates of secretion by the adrenal cortex or in doses that maximally affect electrolyte balance, aldosterone has no significant glucocorticoid activity and thus acts as a pure mineralocorticoid.

Table 60–2

Relative Potencies and Equivalent Doses of Representative Corticosteroids

COMPOUND	ANTIINFLAMMATORY POTENCY	Na^+-RETAINING POTENCY	DURATION OF ACTION*	EQUIVALENT DOSE†, mg
Cortisol	1	1	S	20
Cortisone	0.8	0.8	S	25
Fludrocortisone	10	125	I	‡
Prednisone	4	0.8	I	5
Prednisolone	4	0.8	I	5
6α-methylprednisolone	5	0.5	I	4
Triamcinolone	5	0	I	4
Betamethasone	25	0	L	0.75
Dexamethasone	25	0	L	0.75

* S, short (*i.e.*, 8–12 hour biological half-life); I, intermediate (*i.e.*, 12–36 hour biological half-life); L, long (*i.e.*, 36–72 hour biological half-life).

† These dose relationships apply only to oral or intravenous administration, as glucocorticoid potencies may differ greatly following intramuscular or intraarticular administration.

‡ This agent is not used for glucocorticoid effects.

General Mechanisms for Corticosteroid Effects. Corticosteroids interact with specific receptor proteins in target tissues to regulate the expression of corticosteroid-responsive genes, thereby changing the levels and array of proteins synthesized by the various target tissues (*see* Figure 60–5). As a consequence of the time required for changes in gene expression and protein synthesis, most effects of corticosteroids are not immediate but become apparent after several hours. This fact is of clinical significance, because a delay generally is seen before beneficial effects of corticosteroid therapy become manifest. Although corticosteroids predominantly act to increase expression of target genes, there are well-documented examples where glucocorticoids decrease transcription of target genes, as discussed below. In contrast to these genomic effects, some actions of corticosteroids may be immediate and are mediated by membrane-bound receptors (Christ *et al.*, 1999).

Through the use of molecular biological approaches, the receptors for the corticosteroid hormones have been cloned and their structures determined. These receptors are members of a superfamily of structurally related proteins, the nuclear receptors, that transduce the effects of a diverse array of small, hydrophobic ligands, including the steroid hormones, thyroid hormone, vitamin D, and retinoids (Mangelsdorf *et al.*, 1995). These receptors share two highly conserved domains: a region of approximately 70 amino acids forming two zinc-binding domains, termed *zinc fingers*, that are essential for the interaction of the receptor with specific DNA sequences, and a region at the carboxy terminus that interacts with ligand (the ligand-binding domain).

Glucocorticoid Receptor. As shown in Figure 60–5, the glucocorticoid receptor (GR) resides predominantly in the cytoplasm

in an inactive form until it binds the glucocorticoid steroid ligand, denoted as S in the figure. Steroid binding results in receptor activation and translocation to the nucleus. The inactive GR is found as a complex with other proteins, including heat shock protein (HSP) 90, a member of the heat-shock family of stress-induced proteins; HSP70; and a 56,000 dalton immunophilin, one of the group of intracellular proteins that bind the immunosuppressive agents cyclosporine and tacrolimus (*see* Chapter 53 for a discussion of these agents). HSP90, through interactions with the steroid-binding domain, may facilitate folding of GR into an appropriate conformation that is believed to be essential for ligand binding.

Regulation of Gene Expression by Glucocorticoids. Following ligand binding, the GR dissociates from its associated proteins and translocates to the nucleus. There, it interacts with specific DNA sequences within the regulatory regions of affected genes. The short DNA sequences that are recognized by the activated GR are termed *glucocorticoid responsive elements* (GREs) and provide specificity to the induction of gene transcription by glucocorticoids. The consensus GRE sequence is an imperfect palindrome (GGTACAnnnTGTTCT, where n is any nucleotide) to which the GR binds as a receptor dimer. The mechanisms by which GR activates transcription are complex and not completely understood, but they appear to involve the interaction of the GR with transcriptional cofactors and with proteins that make up the basal transcription apparatus. Genes that are negatively regulated by glucocorticoids also have been identified (Webster and Cidlowski, 1999). One well-characterized example is the proopiomelanocortin gene (*POMC*), whose negative regulation in corticotropes by glucocorticoids is an important part of the negative feedback regulation of the HPA axis. In this case, the GR appears to inhibit transcription by a direct interaction with a GRE in the *POMC* promoter.

Although glucocorticoids, and presumably the GR, are essential for survival, interactions of the GR with specific GREs apparently are not. These conclusions are supported by the findings that genetically engineered mice completely lacking GR function die immediately after birth, whereas mice

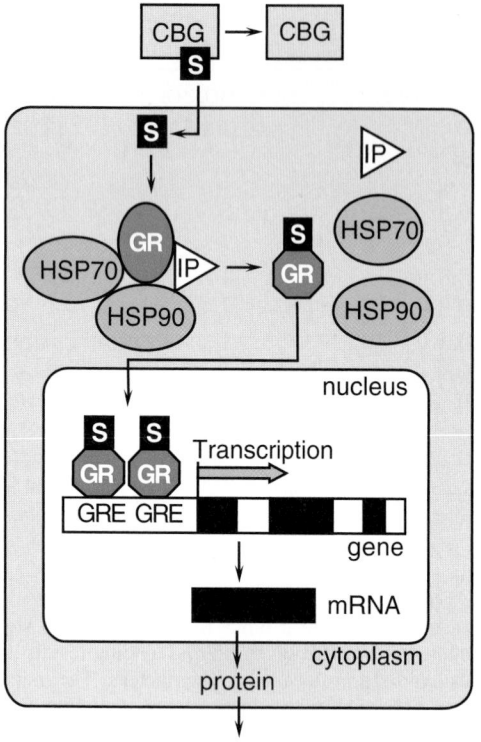

Figure 60–5. Intracellular mechanism of action of the gluco-corticoid receptor.

The molecular pathway by which glucocorticoid steroids (labeled S) enter cells and interact with the glucocorticoid receptor to change the GR conformation (indicated by the change in shape of the GR), induce GR nuclear translocation, and activate transcription of target genes is shown. The example shown is one in which glucocorticoids activate expression of target genes; the expression of certain genes, including proopiomelanocortin (POMC) expression by corticotropes, is inhibited by glucocorticoid treatment. CBG, corticosteroid binding globulin; GR, glucocorticoid receptor; S, steroid hormone; HSP90, the 90-kDa heat shock protein; HSP70, the 70-kDa heat shock protein; IP, the 56-kDa immunophilin; GRE, glucocorticoid-response elements in the DNA that are bound by GR, thus providing specificity to induction of gene transcription by glucocorticoids. Within the gene are introns (*unshaded*) and exons (*shaded*); transcription and mRNA processing leads to splicing and removal of introns and assembly of exons into mRNA.

harboring a mutated GR incapable of binding to DNA are viable (Reichardt *et al.,* 1998). These observations imply that the critical function of GR involves protein–protein interactions with other transcription factors (Xu *et al.,* 1999). Indeed, protein–protein interactions have been observed between the GR and the transcription factors NF-κB and AP-1, which regulate the expression of a number of components of the immune system

(McKay and Cidlowski, 1999). Such interactions repress the expression of genes encoding a number of cytokines—regulatory molecules that play key roles in the immune and inflammatory networks—and enzymes, such as collagenase and stromelysin, that are proposed to play key roles in the joint destruction seen in inflammatory arthritis. Thus, these negative effects on gene expression appear to contribute significantly to the antiinflammatory and immunosuppressive effects of the glucocorticoids.

Regulation of Gene Expression by Mineralocorticoids. Like the glucocorticoid receptor, the mineralocorticoid receptor also is a ligand-activated transcription factor and binds to a very similar, if not identical, hormone-responsive element. Although its actions have been studied in less detail than the glucocorticoid receptor, the basic principles of action appear to be similar; in particular, the mineralocorticoid receptor also associates with HSP90 and also activates the transcription of discrete sets of genes within target tissues. Studies to date have not identified differences in the DNA recognition motifs for the glucocorticoid and mineralocorticoid receptors that would explain their differential abilities to activate discrete sets of target genes. Glucocorticoid and mineralocorticoid receptors differ in their ability to inhibit AP-1–mediated gene activation (Pearce and Yamamoto, 1993), suggesting that differential interactions with other transcription factors may underlie their distinct effects on cell function. In addition, unlike the glucocorticoid receptor, the mineralocorticoid receptor has a restricted expression; it is expressed principally in the kidney (distal cortical tubule and cortical collecting duct), colon, salivary glands, sweat glands, and hippocampus.

Aldosterone exerts its effects on Na^+ and K^+ homeostasis primarily *via* its actions on the principal cells of the distal renal tubules and collecting ducts, while the effects on H^+ secretion largely are exerted in the intercalated cells. Recent studies have identified some of the mechanisms by which aldosterone alters fluid and electrolyte transport. After binding to mineralocorticoid receptors in responsive cells, aldosterone initiates a sequence of events that includes the rapid induction of serum- and glucocorticoid-regulated kinase, which in turn phosphorylates and activates amiloride-sensitive epithelial Na^+ channels in the apical membrane (Chen *et al.,* 1999). Thereafter, increased Na^+ influx stimulates the Na^+,K^+–ATPase in the basolateral membrane. In addition to these rapid actions, aldosterone also increases the synthesis of the individual components of these membrane proteins.

Further insights into the roles of the mineralocorticoid receptor and its target genes in fluid and electrolyte balance have emerged from analyses of patients with rare genetic disorders of mineralocorticoid action, such as *pseudohypoaldosteronism* and *pseudoaldosteronism.* Despite elevated levels of mineralocorticoids, patients with pseudohypoaldosteronism present with clinical manifestations suggestive of deficient mineralocorticoid action (*i.e.,* volume depletion, hypotension, hyperkalemia, and metabolic acidosis). Molecular analyses have defined discrete subpopulations of patients with this disorder. One form is an autosomal recessive disease resulting from loss-of-function mutations in genes encoding subunits of the amiloride-sensitive epithelial sodium channel. A second, autosomal dominant form of pseudohypoaldosteronism is caused by mutations in the mineralocorticoid receptor that impair its activity (Geller *et al.,* 1998). Pseudoaldosteronism, also termed Liddle's syndrome, is an autosomal dominant disease that results from activating mutations in

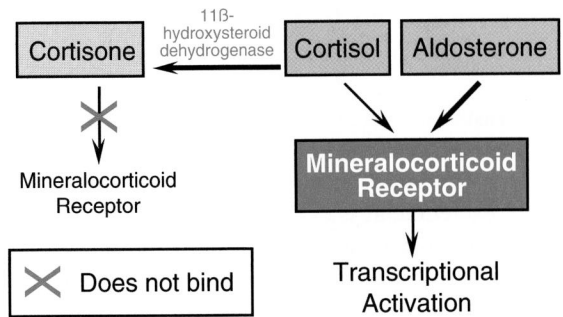

Figure 60–6. Receptor-independent mechanism for conferring specificity of glucocorticoid action.

> By converting cortisol (which binds the mineralocorticoid receptor) to cortisone (which does not bind to the mineralocorticoid receptor), 11β-hydroxysteroid dehydrogenase protects the mineralocorticoid receptor from the high circulating concentrations of glucocorticoids, thereby allowing specific responses to aldosterone in classic mineralocorticoid-responsive cells.

the amiloride-sensitive Na^+ channel (Shimkets *et al.*, 1994). The constitutive activity of this channel leads to hypertension, hypokalemia, and metabolic alkalosis despite low levels of plasma renin and aldosterone.

Receptor-Independent Mechanism for Corticosteroid Specificity. The availability of cloned genes encoding the glucocorticoid receptor and mineralocorticoid receptor led to the surprising finding that aldosterone (a classic mineralocorticoid) and cortisol (generally viewed as predominantly glucocorticoid) bound the mineralocorticoid receptor with equal affinity. This raised the question of how the apparent specificity of the mineralocorticoid receptor for aldosterone was maintained in the face of much higher levels of circulating glucocorticoids. At least part of the answer came with the discovery of the type 2 isozyme of 11β-hydroxysteroid dehydrogenase, a steroid-metabolizing enzyme that plays a key role in corticosteroid specificity, particularly in the kidney, colon, and salivary glands. This enzyme forms a barrier in certain mineralocorticoid-responsive tissues by metabolizing glucocorticoids such as cortisol to receptor-inactive 11-keto derivatives such as cortisone (Figure 60–6). Aldosterone escapes metabolism by 11β-hydroxysteroid dehydrogenase, because its predominant form in physiological settings is the hemiacetal derivative, which is resistant to 11β-hydroxysteroid dehydrogenase action. In the absence of 11β-hydroxysteroid dehydrogenase, as occurs in an inherited disease called the *syndrome of apparent mineralocorticoid excess,* the mineralocorticoid receptor is swamped by cortisol, leading to severe hypokalemia and mineralocorticoid-related hypertension. A state of hypermineralocorticism also can be induced by the inhibition of 11β-hydroxysteroid dehydrogenase with *glycyrrhizic acid,* a component of licorice implicated in licorice-induced hypertension.

Carbohydrate and Protein Metabolism. Corticosteroids have profound effects on carbohydrate and protein metabolism. Teleologically, these effects of glucocorti-

coids on intermediary metabolism can be viewed as protecting glucose-dependent tissues (*e.g.,* the brain and heart) from starvation. This is achieved by stimulating the liver to form glucose from amino acids and glycerol and by stimulating the deposition of glucose as liver glycogen. In the periphery, glucocorticoids diminish glucose utilization, increase protein breakdown, and activate lipolysis, thereby providing amino acids and glycerol for gluconeogenesis. The net result is to increase blood glucose levels. Because of these effects on glucose metabolism, treatment with glucocorticoids can worsen control in patients with overt diabetes and can precipitate the onset of hyperglycemia in patients who are otherwise predisposed.

The mechanisms by which glucocorticoids inhibit glucose utilization in peripheral tissues are not fully understood. Glucocorticoids decrease glucose uptake in adipose tissue, skin, fibroblasts, thymocytes, and polymorphonuclear leukocytes; these effects are postulated to result from translocation of the glucose transporters from the plasma membrane to an intracellular location. These peripheral effects are associated with a number of catabolic actions, including atrophy of lymphoid tissue, decreased muscle mass, negative nitrogen balance, and thinning of the skin.

Similarly, the mechanisms by which the glucocorticoids promote gluconeogenesis are not fully defined. Amino acids mobilized from a number of tissues in response to glucocorticoids reach the liver and provide substrate for the production of glucose and glycogen. In the liver, glucocorticoids induce the transcription of a number of enzymes involved in gluconeogenesis and amino acid metabolism, including phosphoenolpyruvate carboxykinase (PEPCK), glucose-6-phosphatase, and fructose-2,6-bisphosphatase. Analyses of the molecular basis for regulation of PEPCK gene expression have identified complex regulatory influences involving an interplay among glucocorticoids, insulin, glucagon, and catecholamine. The effects of these hormones and amines on PEPCK gene expression mirror the complex regulation of gluconeogenesis in the intact organism.

Lipid Metabolism. Two effects of corticosteroids on lipid metabolism are firmly established. The first is the dramatic redistribution of body fat that occurs in settings of hypercorticism, such as Cushing's syndrome. The other is the permissive facilitation of the effect of other agents, such as growth hormone and β-adrenergic receptor agonists, in inducing lipolysis in adipocytes, with a resultant increase in free fatty acids following glucocorticoid administration. With respect to fat distribution, there is increased fat in the back of the neck ("buffalo hump"), face ("moon facies"), and supraclavicular area, coupled with a loss of fat in the extremities.

One hypothesis for this phenomenon is that peripheral and truncal adipocytes differ in their relative sensitivities to insulin and to glucocorticoid-facilitated lipolytic effects. According to this hypothesis, truncal adipocytes respond predominantly to elevated levels of insulin resulting from glucocorticoid-induced hyperglycemia, whereas peripheral adipocytes are less sensitive to insulin and respond mostly to the glucocorticoid-facilitated effects of other lipolytic hormones.

Electrolyte and Water Balance. Aldosterone is by far the most potent naturally occurring corticosteroid with respect to fluid and electrolyte balance. Evidence for this comes from the relatively normal electrolyte balance found in hypophysectomized animals, despite the loss of glucocorticoid production by the inner cortical zones. Mineralocorticoids act on the distal tubules and collecting ducts of the kidney to enhance reabsorption of Na^+ from the tubular fluid; they also increase the urinary excretion of both K^+ and H^+. Conceptually, it is useful to think of aldosterone as stimulating a renal exchange between Na^+ and K^+ or H^+, although the molecular mechanism of monovalent cation handling is not a simple 1:1 exchange of cations in the renal tubule.

These renal actions on electrolyte transport, in conjunction with similar effects in other tissues (*e.g.,* colon, salivary glands, sweat glands), appear to account for the physiological and pharmacological activities that are characteristic of mineralocorticoids. Thus, the primary features of hyperaldosteronism are positive Na^+ balance with consequent expansion of the extracellular fluid volume, normal or slight increases in plasma Na^+ concentration, hypokalemia, and alkalosis. Mineralocorticoid deficiency, in contrast, leads to Na^+ wasting and contraction of the extracellular fluid volume, hyponatremia, hyperkalemia, and acidosis. Chronically, hyperaldosteronism can cause hypertension, whereas aldosterone deficiency can lead to hypotension and vascular collapse. Because of the effects of mineralocorticoids on electrolyte handling by sweat glands, patients who are adrenal-insufficient are especially predisposed to Na^+ loss and volume depletion through excessive sweating in hot environments.

Glucocorticoids also exert effects on fluid and electrolyte balance, largely due to permissive effects on tubular function and actions that maintain glomerular filtration rate. Glucocorticoids play a permissive role in the renal excretion of free water; the ability to excrete a water challenge was used at one time to diagnose adrenal insufficiency. In part, the inability of Addisonian patients to excrete free water results from the increased secretion of AVP, which stimulates water reabsorption in the kidney.

In addition to their effects on monovalent cations and water, glucocorticoids also exert multiple effects on Ca^{2+} metabolism. In the gut, steroids interfere with Ca^{2+} uptake by undefined mechanisms, while there is increased

Ca^{2+} excretion at the level of the kidney. These effects collectively lead to decreased total body Ca^{2+} stores.

Cardiovascular System. As noted above, the most striking effects of corticosteroids on the cardiovascular system result from mineralocorticoid-induced changes in renal Na^+ excretion, as is evident in primary aldosteronism. The resultant hypertension can lead to a diverse group of adverse effects on the cardiovascular system, including increased atherosclerosis, cerebral hemorrhage, stroke, and hypertensive cardiomyopathy. The mechanism underlying the hypertension remains incompletely understood, but restriction of dietary Na^+ can lower the blood pressure considerably.

The second major action of corticosteroids on the cardiovascular system is to enhance vascular reactivity to other vasoactive substances. Hypoadrenalism generally is associated with hypotension and reduced response to vasoconstrictors such as norepinephrine and angiotensin II. This diminished pressor response is explained partly by studies in experimental systems showing that glucocorticoids increase expression of adrenergic receptors in the vascular wall. Conversely, hypertension is seen in patients with excessive glucocorticoid secretion, occurring in most patients with Cushing's syndrome and in a subset of patients treated with synthetic glucocorticoids (even those lacking any significant mineralocorticoid action).

The underlying mechanisms in glucocorticoid-induced hypertension also are unknown; in hypertension related to the endogenous secretion of cortisol, as seen in patients with Cushing's syndrome, it is not known if the effects are mediated by the glucocorticoid or mineralocorticoid receptor. Unlike hypertension caused by high aldosterone levels, the hypertension secondary to excess glucocorticoids is generally resistant to Na^+ restriction.

Studies also have shown direct effects of aldosterone on both the heart and vascular lining; treating rats with aldosterone induced hypertension and interstitial cardiac fibrosis (Funder *et al.,* 1997). The increased cardiac fibrosis was proposed to result from direct mineralocorticoid actions in the heart rather than from the effect of hypertension, because treatment with spironolactone, a mineralocorticoid antagonist, blocked the fibrosis without altering blood pressure. Similar effects of mineralocorticoids on cardiac fibrosis in human beings may explain, at least in part, the beneficial effects of the mineralocorticoid receptor antagonist spironolactone in patients with congestive heart failure (Pitt *et al.,* 1999).

Skeletal Muscle. Permissive concentrations of corticosteroids are required for the normal function of skeletal muscle; diminished work capacity is a prominent sign of adrenocortical insufficiency. In patients with Addison's disease, weakness and fatigue are frequent symptoms and are believed to reflect mostly an inadequacy of the circulatory system. Excessive amounts of either glucocorticoids or mineralocorticoids also impair muscle function. In primary aldosteronism, muscle weakness results primarily from hypokalemia rather than from direct effects of mineralocorticoids on skeletal muscle. In contrast, glucocorticoid excess over prolonged periods, either secondary to glucocorticoid therapy or endogenous hypercortisism, tends to cause skeletal muscle wasting *via* unknown mechanisms. This effect, termed *steroid myopathy,* accounts in part for the weakness and fatigue noted in Cushingoid patients and is discussed in more detail below.

Central Nervous System. Corticosteroids exert a number of indirect effects on the CNS, through maintenance of blood pressure, plasma glucose concentrations, and electrolyte concentrations. Improved awareness of the distribution and function of steroid receptors in the brain has led to increasing recognition of direct effects of corticosteroids on the CNS, including effects on mood, behavior, and brain excitability.

Patients with Addison's disease can exhibit a diverse array of psychiatric manifestations, including apathy, depression, and irritability; some patients are frankly psychotic. Appropriate replacement therapy corrects these abnormalities. Of greater clinical consequence, glucocorticoid administration can induce multiple CNS reactions. Most patients respond with mood elevation, which may impart a sense of well-being despite the persistence of underlying disease. Some patients exhibit more pronounced behavioral changes, such as euphoria, insomnia, restlessness, and increased motor activity. A smaller but significant percentage of patients treated with glucocorticoids become anxious, depressed, or overtly psychotic. A high incidence of neuroses and psychoses has been noted among patients with Cushing's syndrome. These abnormalities usually disappear after cessation of glucocorticoid therapy or treatment of the Cushing's syndrome.

The mechanisms by which corticosteroids affect neuronal activity are unknown, but it should be noted that steroids produced locally in the brain (termed *neurosteroids*) may regulate neuronal excitability (Baulieu, 1998). Studies in rodent models have long suggested that glucocorticoids deleteriously affect survival and function of hippocampal neurons, and that these changes are associated with diminished memory (Lupien and McEwan, 1997). A study in human beings used basal cortisol levels over time to establish a correlation between increased cortisol levels and hippocampal atrophy and memory deficits (Lupien *et al.,* 1998). To the extent that these results can be confirmed, they have important prognostic implications for age-related memory decline, and they suggest therapeutic approaches directed at diminishing the negative effects of glucocorticoids on hippocampal neurons with aging.

Formed Elements of Blood. Glucocorticoids exert minor effects on hemoglobin and erythrocyte content of blood, as evidenced by the frequent occurrence of polycythemia in Cushing's syndrome and of normochromic, normocytic anemia in Addison's disease. More profound effects are seen in the setting of autoimmune hemolytic anemia, where the immunosuppressive effects of glucocorticoids can diminish the self-destruction of erythrocytes.

Corticosteroids also affect circulating white blood cells. Addison's disease, as noted by Addison in his initial report, is associated with an increased mass of lymphoid tissue and lymphocytosis. In contrast, Cushing's syndrome is characterized by lymphocytopenia and decreased mass of lymphoid tissue. The administration of glucocorticoids leads to a decreased number of circulating lymphocytes, eosinophils, monocytes, and basophils. A single dose of hydrocortisone leads to a decline of these circulating cells within 4 to 6 hours; this effect persists for 24 hours and results from the redistribution of cells away from the periphery rather than from increased destruction. In contrast, glucocorticoids increase circulating polymorphonuclear leukocytes as a result of increased release from the marrow, diminished rate of removal from the circulation, and increased demargination from vascular walls. Certain lymphoid malignancies, however, are destroyed by glucocorticoid treatment. This latter effect may be related to the ability of glucocorticoids to activate programmed cell death in certain lymphoid tissues.

Antiinflammatory and Immunosuppressive Actions. In addition to their effects on lymphocyte number, corticosteroids profoundly alter the immune responses of lymphocytes. These effects are an important facet of the antiinflammatory and immunosuppressive actions of the glucocorticoids. Glucocorticoids can prevent or suppress inflammation in response to multiple inciting events, including radiant, mechanical, chemical, infectious, and immunological stimuli. Although the use of glucocorticoids as antiinflammatory agents does not address the underlying cause of the disease, the suppression of inflammation is of enormous clinical utility and has made these drugs among the most frequently prescribed agents. Similarly, glucocorticoids are of immense value in treating diseases that result from undesirable immune reactions. These diseases range from conditions that predominantly result from humoral immunity, such as urticaria (*see* Chapter 65), to those that are mediated by cellular immune mechanisms, such as transplantation rejection (*see* Chapter 53). The immunosuppressive and antiinflammatory actions of glucocorticoids are inextricably linked, perhaps because they both involve inhibition of leukocyte functions (Chrousos, 1995).

Table 60–3

Effects of Glucocorticoids on Components of Inflammatory/Immune Responses

CELL TYPE	FACTOR	COMMENTS
Macrophages and monocytes	Arachidonic acid and its metabolites (prostaglandins and leukotrienes)	Inhibited in part by glucocorticoid induction of a protein (lipocortin) that inhibits phospholipase A2.
	Cytokines, including: Interleukin (IL)-1, IL-6, and TNF-α	Production and release are blocked. The cytokines exert multiple effects on inflammation (*e.g.,* activation of T cells, stimulation of fibroblast proliferation).
	Acute phase reactants	These include the third component of complement.
Endothelial cells	Endothelial leukocyte adhesion molecule-1 (ELAM-1) and intracellular adhesion molecule-1 (ICAM-1)	ELAM-1 and ICAM-1 are intracellular adhesion molecules that are critical for leukocyte localization.
	Acute phase reactants	Same as above, for macrophages and monocytes.
	Cytokines (*e.g.,* IL-1)	Same as above, for macrophages and monocytes.
	Arachidonic acid derivatives	Same as above, for macrophages and monocytes.
Basophils	Histamine Leukotriene C4	IgE-dependent release inhibited by glucocorticoids.
Fibroblasts	Arachidonic acid metabolites	Same as above for macrophages and monocytes. Glucocorticoids also suppress growth factor-induced DNA synthesis and fibroblast proliferation.
Lymphocytes	Cytokines (IL-1, IL-2, IL-3, IL-6, TNF-α, GM-CSF, interferon gamma)	Same as above for macrophages and monocytes.

Multiple mechanisms are involved in the suppression of inflammation by glucocorticoids. It is now clear that glucocorticoids inhibit the production by multiple cells of factors that are critical in generating the inflammatory response. As a result, there is decreased release of vasoactive and chemoattractive factors, diminished secretion of lipolytic and proteolytic enzymes, decreased extravasation of leukocytes to areas of injury, and—ultimately—decreased fibrosis. Some of the cell types and mediators that are inhibited by glucocorticoids are summarized in Table 60–3. The net effect of these actions on various cell types is to diminish markedly the inflammatory response.

The influence of stressful conditions on immune defense mechanisms is well documented, as is the contribution of the HPA axis to the stress response (Sapolsky *et al.*, 2000). This has led to a growing appreciation of the importance of glucocorticoids as physiological modulators of the immune system, where glucocorticoids appear to protect the organism against life-threatening consequences of a full-blown inflammatory response.

Stresses such as injury, infection, and disease result in the increased production of cytokines, a network of signaling molecules that integrate actions of macrophages/monocytes, T lymphocytes, and B lymphocytes in mounting immune responses. Among these cytokines, interleukin (IL)-1, IL-6, and tumor necrosis factor-α (TNF-α) stimulate the HPA axis, with IL-1 having the broadest range of actions. IL-1 stimulates the release of CRH by hypothalamic neurons, interacts directly with the pituitary to increase the release of ACTH, and may directly stimulate the adrenal gland to produce glucocorticoids (Turnbull and Rivier, 1999). As detailed above, the increased production of glucocorticoids, in turn, leads to a profound inhibition of the immune system at multiple sites. Factors that are inhibited include components of the cytokine network, including interferon gamma (INF-γ), granulocyte/monocyte colony-stimulating factor (GM-CSF) interleukins (IL-1, IL-2, IL-3, IL-6, IL-8, IL-12), and TNF-α. Thus, the HPA axis and the immune system are capable of bidirectional interactions in response to stress, and these interactions appear to be important for homeostasis.

Although glucocorticoids traditionally have been considered as immunosuppressive agents, there are intriguing observations suggesting that glucocorticoids produced as part of the physiological response to stress may upregulate the humoral arm of the immune response (*e.g.*, antibody production) while suppressing cellular immunity (Elenkov and Chrousos, 1999). The mechanisms underlying this glucocorticoid-induced switch are unclear but seem to involve inhibition of T-helper (Th-1) cells and activation of Th-2 cells (*see* Chapter 53).

Absorption, Transport, Metabolism, and Excretion

Absorption.   Hydrocortisone and numerous congeners, including the synthetic analogs, are effective when given by mouth. Certain water-soluble esters of hydrocortisone and its synthetic congeners are administered intravenously to achieve high concentrations of drug rapidly in body fluids. More prolonged effects are obtained by intramuscular injection of suspensions of hydrocortisone, its congeners, and its esters. Minor changes in chemical structure may markedly alter the rate of absorption, time of onset of effect, and duration of action.

Glucocorticoids also are absorbed systemically from sites of local administration, such as synovial spaces, the conjunctival sac, skin, and respiratory tract. When administration is prolonged, when the site of application is covered with an occlusive dressing, or when large areas of skin are involved, the absorption may be sufficient to cause systemic effects, including suppression of the HPA axis.

Transport, Metabolism, and Excretion.   Following absorption, 90% or more of cortisol in plasma is reversibly bound to protein under normal circumstances. Only the fraction of corticosteroid that is unbound can enter cells to mediate corticosteroid effects. Two plasma proteins account for almost all of the steroid-binding capacity: corticosteroid-binding globulin (CBG; also called transcortin), and albumin. CBG is an α-globulin secreted by the liver that has high affinity for steroids but relatively low total binding capacity, whereas albumin, also produced by the liver, has low affinity but relatively large binding capacity. At normal or low concentrations of corticosteroids, most of the hormone is protein-bound. At higher steroid concentrations, the capacity of protein binding is exceeded, and a significantly greater fraction of the steroid exists in the free state. Corticosteroids compete with each other for binding sites on CBG. CBG has relatively high affinity for cortisol and most of its synthetic congeners and

low affinity for aldosterone and glucuronide-conjugated steroid metabolites; thus, greater percentages of these latter steroids are found in the free form.

During pregnancy or estrogen treatment, CBG, total plasma cortisol, and free cortisol increase severalfold. The physiological significance of these changes remains to be established.

All of the biologically active adrenocortical steroids and their synthetic congeners have a double bond in the 4,5 position and a ketone group at C 3. As a general rule, the metabolism of steroid hormones involves sequential additions of oxygen or hydrogen atoms, followed by conjugation to form water-soluble derivatives. Reduction of the 4,5 double bond occurs at both hepatic and extrahepatic sites, yielding inactive compounds. Subsequent reduction of the 3-ketone substituent to the 3-hydroxyl derivative, forming tetrahydrocortisol, occurs only in the liver. Most of these A ring–reduced steroids are conjugated through the 3-hydroxyl group with sulfate or glucuronide by enzymatic reactions that take place in the liver and, to a lesser extent, in the kidney. The resultant sulfate esters and glucuronides are water-soluble and are the predominant forms excreted in the urine. Neither biliary nor fecal excretion is of quantitative importance in human beings.

Synthetic steroids with an 11-keto substituent, such as cortisone and prednisone, must be enzymatically reduced to the corresponding 11β-hydroxy derivative before they are biologically active. This reaction is catalyzed in the liver by the type 1 isozyme of 11β-hydroxysteroid dehydrogenase, which operates in a reductive mode. In settings where this enzymatic activity is impaired, such as severe hepatic failure, or in rare patients who lack this enzyme, it is prudent to use steroids that do not require enzymatic activation (*e.g.*, hydrocortisone and prednisolone rather than cortisone or prednisone).

Structure–Activity Relationships

Chemical modifications to the cortisol molecule have generated derivatives with greater separations of glucocorticoid and mineralocorticoid activity; for a number of synthetic glucocorticoids, the effects on electrolytes are minimal even at the highest doses used. In addition, these modifications have led to derivatives with greater potencies and with longer durations of action. A vast array of different steroid preparations is therefore available for oral, parenteral, and topical use. Some of these agents are summarized in Table 60–4. However, because the antiinflammatory and metabolic effects of glucocorticoids are mediated by the same glucocorticoid receptor, the various derivatives do not effectively separate antiinflammatory effects from effects on carbohydrate, protein, and fat metabolism or from suppressive effects on the HPA axis.

The structures of hydrocortisone (cortisol) and some of its major derivatives are shown in Figure 60–7. Changes in chemical structure may bring about changes in specificity and/or potency as a result of changes in affinity and intrinsic activity at corticosteroid receptors, alterations in absorption, protein

TABLE 60–4

Available Preparations of Adrenocortical Steroids and Their Synthetic Analogs

NONPROPRIETARY NAME (TRADE NAME)	TYPES OF PREPARATIONS	NONPROPRIETARY NAME (TRADE NAME)	TYPES OF PREPARATIONS
Alclometasone dipropionate (ACLOVATE)	Topical	Cortisol (hydrocortisone) valerate (WESTCORT)	Topical
Amcinonide (CYCLOCORT)	Topical	Cortisone acetate (CORTONE ACETATE)	Oral, injectable
Beclomethasone dipropionate (BECLOVENT, VANCERIL, others)	Inhalation	Desonide (DESOWEN, TRIDESILON)	Topical
Betamethasone (CELESTONE)	Oral	Desoximetasone (TOPICORT)	Topical
Betamethasone dipropionate (DIPROSONE, others)	Topical	Dexamethasone (DECADRON, others)	Oral, topical
Betamethasone sodium phosphate (CELESTONE PHOSPHATE, others)	Injectable	Dexamethasone acetate (DECADRON-LA, others)	Injectable
Betamethasone sodium phosphate and acetate (CELESTONE SOLUSPAN)	Injectable	Dexamethasone sodium phosphate (DECADRON PHOSPHATE, HEXADROL PHOSPHATE, others)	Topical, ophthalmic, otic, injectable
Betamethasone valerate (BETA-VAL, VALISONE, others)	Topical	Diflorasone diacetate (FLORONE, MAXIFLOR)	Topical
Budesonide (PULMICORT, RHINOCORT)	Inhalation	Fludrocortisone acetate* (FLORINEF)	Oral
Clobetasol propionate (TEMOVATE)	Topical	Flunisolide (AEROBID, NASALIDE)	Inhalation
Clocortolone pivalate (CLODERM)	Topical	Fluocinolone acetonide (FLUONID, SYNALAR, others)	Topical
Cortisol (hydrocortisone) (CORTEF, HYDROCORTONE, others)	Topical, enema, otic solutions, oral, injectable	Fluocinonide (LIDEX)	Topical
Cortisol (hydrocortisone) acetate (HYDROCORTONE ACETATE others)	Topical, suppositories, rectal foam, injectable	Fluorometholone (FLUOR-OP, FML LIQUIFILM)	Ophthalmic
Cortisol (hydrocortisone) butyrate (LOCOID)	Topical	Fluorometholone acetate (FLAREX)	Ophthalmic
Cortisol (hydrocortisone) cypionate (CORTEF)	Oral	Flurandrenolide (CORDRAN)	Topical
Cortisol (hydrocortisone) sodium phosphate (HYDROCORTONE PHOSPHATE)	Injectable	Halcinonide (HALOG)	Topical
		Medrysone (HMS LIQUIFILM)	Ophthalmic
		Methylprednisolone (MEDROL)	Oral
Cortisol (hydrocortisone) sodium succinate (A-HYDROCORT, SOLU-CORTEF)	Injectable	Methylprednisolone acetate (DEPO-MEDROL, MEDROL ACETATE, others)	Topical, injectable
		Methylprednisolone sodium succinate (A-METHAPRED, SOLU-MEDROL)	Injectable

TABLE 60–4

Available Preparations of Adrenocortical Steroids and Their Synthetic Analogs *(Continued)*

NONPROPRIETARY NAME (TRADE NAME)	TYPES OF PREPARATIONS	NONPROPRIETARY NAME (TRADE NAME)	TYPES OF PREPARATIONS
Mometasone furoate (ELOCON)	Topical	Prednisone (DELTASONE, others)	Oral
Prednisolone (DELTA-CORTEF)	Oral	Triamcinolone (ARISTOCORT, KENACORT)	Oral
Prednisolone acetate (ECONOPRED, others)	Ophthalmic, injectable	Triamcinolone acetonide (KENALOG, others)	Topical, inhalation, injectable
Prednisolone sodium phosphate (PEDIAPRED, others)	Oral, ophthalmic, injectable	Triamcinolone diacetate (ARISTOCORT, KENACORT DIACETATE, others)	Oral, injectable
Prednisolone tebutate (HYDELTRA-T.B.A., others)	Injectable	Triamcinolone hexacetonide (ARISTOSPAN)	Injectable

*Fluorocortisone acetate is intended for use as a mineralocorticoid.

Note: *Topical* preparations include agents for application to skin or mucous membranes in creams, solutions, ointments, gels, pastes (for oral lesions), and aerosols; *ophthalmic* preparations include solutions, suspensions, and ointments; *inhalation,* preparations include agents for nasal or oral inhalation.

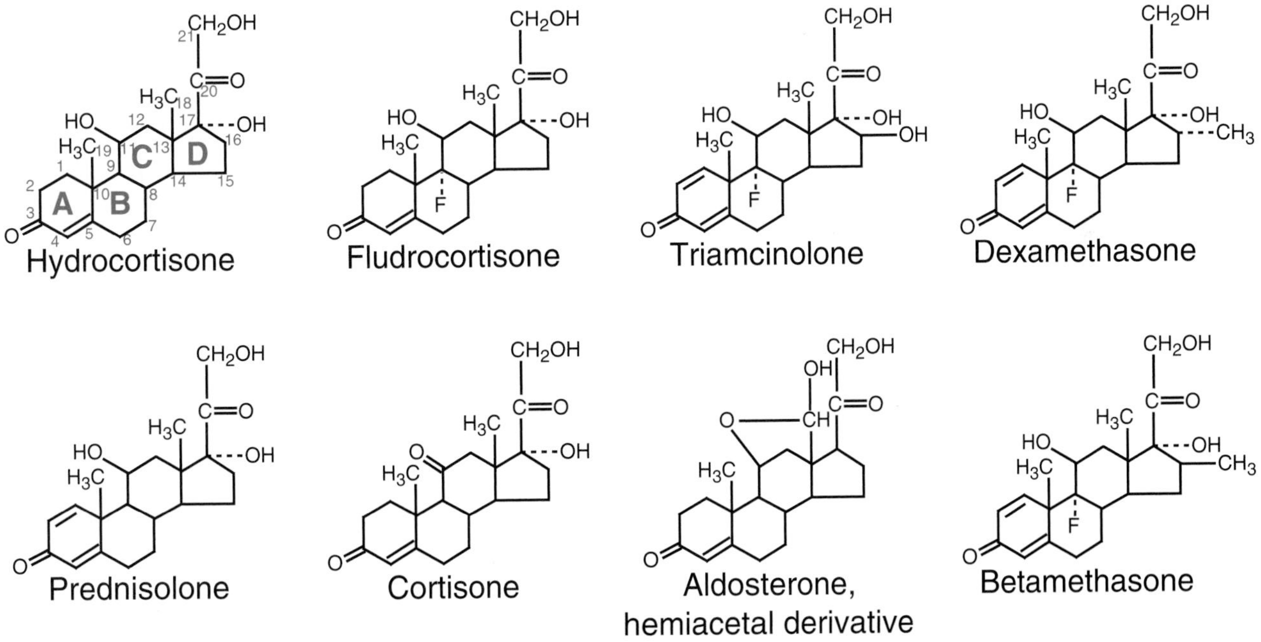

Figure 60–7. Structure and nomenclature of corticosteroid products and selected synthetic derivatives.

The structure of hydrocortisone is represented in two dimensions. It should be noted that the steroid ring system is not completely planar and that the orientation of the groups attached to the steroid rings is an important determinant of the biological activity. The methyl groups at C 18 and C 19 and the hydroxyl group at C 11 project upward (*forward* in the two-dimensional representation and shown by a solid line connecting the atoms) and are designated β. The hydroxyl at C 17 projects below the plane (*behind* in the two-dimensional representation, and represented by the dashed line connecting the atoms) and is designated α.

binding, rate of metabolic transformation, rate of excretion, or membrane permeability. The effects of various substitutions on glucocorticoid and mineralocorticoid activity and on duration of action are summarized in Table 60–2. The 4,5 double bond and the 3-keto group on ring A are essential for both glucocorticoid and mineralocorticoid activity; an 11β-hydroxyl group on ring C is required for glucocorticoid activity but not mineralocorticoid activity; a hydroxyl group at C 21 on ring D is present on all natural corticosteroids and on most of the active synthetic analogs and seems to be an absolute requirement for mineralocorticoid activity, but not glucocorticoid activity. The 17α-hydroxyl group on ring D is a substituent on cortisol and on all of the currently used synthetic glucocorticoids. While steroids without the 17α-hydroxyl group (*e.g.,* corticosterone) have appreciable glucocorticoid activity, the 17α-hydroxyl group gives optimal potency.

Introduction of an additional double bond in the 1,2 position of ring A, as in prednisolone or prednisone, selectively increases glucocorticoid activity (approximately fourfold compared to hydrocortisone), resulting in an enhanced glucocorticoid to mineralocorticoid potency ratio. This modification also results in compounds that are metabolized more slowly than hydrocortisone.

Fluorination at the 9α position on ring B enhances both glucocorticoid and mineralocorticoid activity and possibly is related to an electron-withdrawing effect on the nearby 11β-hydroxyl group. Fludrocortisone (9α-fluorocortisol) has enhanced activity at the glucocorticoid receptor (10-fold relative to cortisol) but even greater activity at the mineralocorticoid receptor (125-fold relative to cortisol). It is used in mineralocorticoid replacement therapy (*see* below) and has no appreciable glucocorticoid effect at usual daily doses of 0.05 to 0.2 mg. When combined with the 1,2 double bond in ring A and other substitutions at C 16 on ring D (Figure 60–7), the 9α-fluoro derivatives formed (*e.g.,* triamcinolone, dexamethasone, betamethasone) have marked glucocorticoid activity. The substitutions at C 16 virtually eliminate mineralocorticoid activity.

Other Substitutions. 6α Substitution on ring B has somewhat unpredictable effects. 6α-Methylcortisol has increased glucocorticoid and mineralocorticoid activity, whereas 6α-methylprednisolone has somewhat greater glucocorticoid activity and somewhat less mineralocorticoid activity than prednisolone. A number of modifications convert the glucocorticoids to more lipophilic molecules with enhanced topical to systemic potency ratios. Examples include the introduction of an acetonide between hydroxyl groups at C 16, C 17, esterification of the hydroxyl group with valerate at C 17, esterification of hydroxyl groups with propionate at C 17 and C 21, and substitution of the hydroxyl group at C 21 with chlorine. Other approaches to achieve local glucocorticoid activity while minimizing systemic effects involve the formation of analogs that are rapidly inactivated following absorption. Examples of this latter group include C 21 carboxylate or carbothioate glucocorticoid esters, which are rapidly metabolized to inactive 21-carboxylic acids.

Toxicity of Adrenocortical Steroids

Two categories of toxic effects result from the therapeutic use of corticosteroids: those resulting from withdrawal of steroid therapy and those resulting from continued use of supraphysiological doses. The side effects from both of these categories are potentially life-threatening and mandate a careful assessment of the risks and benefits in each patient.

Withdrawal of Therapy. Withdrawal of corticosteroid therapy poses a number of difficult decisions. It is important to remember that the most frequent problem in steroid withdrawal is flare-up of the underlying disease for which steroids were prescribed. There are several complications associated with steroid withdrawal, as discussed by Sullivan (1982). The most severe complication of steroid cessation, acute adrenal insufficiency, results from too rapid withdrawal of corticosteroids after prolonged therapy, where the HPA axis has been suppressed. The therapeutic approach to acute adrenal insufficiency is detailed below. There is significant variation among patients with respect to the degree and duration of adrenal suppression following corticosteroid therapy, making it difficult to establish the relative risk in any given patient. Many patients recover from corticosteroid-induced HPA suppression within several weeks to months; however, in some individuals, the time to recovery can be one year or longer.

In an effort to diminish the risk of iatrogenic acute adrenal insufficiency, protocols for discontinuing corticosteroid therapy in patients receiving long-term treatment with corticosteroids have been proposed (for example, *see* Byyny, 1976). In general, patients who have received supraphysiological doses of glucocorticoids for a period of two weeks within the preceding year should be considered to have some degree of HPA impairment in settings of acute stress and should be treated accordingly.

In addition to this most severe form of withdrawal, a characteristic glucocorticoid withdrawal syndrome consists of fever, myalgias, arthralgias, and malaise, which may be difficult to differentiate from some of the underlying diseases for which steroid therapy was instituted. Finally, *pseudotumor cerebri,* a clinical syndrome that includes increased intracranial pressure with papilledema, is a rare condition that sometimes is associated with reduction or withdrawal of corticosteroid therapy.

Continued Use of Supraphysiological Corticosteroid Doses. Besides the consequences that result from the suppression of the HPA axis, there are a number of other complications that result from prolonged therapy with corticosteroids. These include fluid and electrolyte abnormalities, hypertension, hyperglycemia, increased susceptibility to infection, osteoporosis, myopathy, behavioral disturbances, cataracts, growth arrest, and the characteristic habitus of steroid overdose including fat redistribution, striae, ecchymoses, acne, and hirsutism.

Fluid and Electrolyte Handling.   Alterations in fluid and electrolyte handling can cause hypokalemic alkalosis, edema, and hypertension, particularly in patients with primary hyperaldosteronism secondary to an adrenal adenoma or in patients treated with potent mineralocorticoids. Similarly, hypertension is a relatively common manifestation in patients with endogenous glucocorticoid excess and also can be seen in patients treated with glucocorticoids lacking appreciable mineralocorticoid activity. Hyperglycemia with glycosuria usually can be managed with diet and/or insulin, and its occurrence should not be a major factor in the decision to continue corticosteroid therapy or to initiate therapy in diabetic patients.

Immune Responses.   Because of their multiple effects to inhibit the immune system and the inflammatory response, glucocorticoid use also is associated with an increased susceptibility to infection and a risk for reactivation of latent tuberculosis. In the presence of known infections of some consequence, glucocorticoids should be administered only if absolutely necessary and concomitantly with appropriate and effective antimicrobial or antifungal therapy.

Possible Risk of Peptic Ulcers.   There is considerable debate about the association between peptic ulcers and glucocorticoid therapy. The possible onset of hemorrhage and perforation in these ulcers and their insidious onset make peptic ulcers serious therapeutic problems (*see* Chapter 37); estimating the degree of risk from corticosteroids has received much study. One report indicates that most patients who develop gastrointestinal bleeding while receiving corticosteroids also received nonsteroidal antiinflammatory drugs, which are known to promote ulceration; the pathogenic role of corticosteroids thus remains open to debate (Piper *et al.*, 1991). Nonetheless, it is prudent to be especially vigilant for peptic ulcer formation in patients receiving therapy with corticosteroids, especially when administered concomitantly with nonsteroidal antiinflammatory drugs.

Myopathy.   Myopathy, characterized by weakness of proximal limb muscles, occasionally is seen in patients taking large doses of corticosteroids and also is part of the clinical picture in patients with endogenous Cushing's syndrome. It can be of sufficient severity to impair ambulation and is an indication for withdrawal of therapy. Attention also has focused on steroid myopathy of the respiratory muscles in patients with asthma or chronic obstructive pulmonary disease (*see* Chapter 28); this complication can diminish respiratory function. Recovery from the steroid myopathies may be slow and incomplete.

Behavioral Changes.   Behavioral disturbances are seen commonly after administration of corticosteroids and in patients who have Cushing's syndrome secondary to endogenous hypercorticism; these disturbances may take many forms, including nervousness, insomnia, changes in mood or psyche, and overt psychosis (Haskett, 1985). Suicidal tendencies are not uncommon. A history of previous psychiatric illness does not preclude the use of steroids in patients for whom they are otherwise indicated. Conversely, the absence of a history of previous psychiatric illness does not guarantee that a given patient will not develop psychiatric disorders while on steroids.

Cataracts.   Cataracts are a well-established complication of glucocorticoid therapy and are related both to dosage and duration of therapy. Children appear to be particularly at risk. Cessation of therapy may not lead to complete resolution of opacities, and the cataracts may progress despite reduction or cessation of therapy. Patients on long-term glucocorticoid therapy at doses of prednisone of 10 to 15 mg/day or greater should receive periodic slit-lamp examinations to detect glucocorticoid-induced posterior subcapsular cataracts.

Osteoporosis.   Osteoporosis—a frequent serious complication of glucocorticoid therapy—occurs in patients of all ages and is related to both dosage and duration of therapy (Lane and Lukert, 1998). A reasonable estimate is that 30% to 50% of all patients who receive chronic glucocorticoid therapy ultimately will develop osteoporotic fractures. Glucocorticoids preferentially affect trabecular bone and the cortical rim of the vertebral bodies; the ribs and vertebrae are the most frequent sites of fracture. Glucocorticoids decrease bone density by multiple mechanisms, including inhibition of gonadal steroid hormones, diminished gastrointestinal absorption of calcium, and inhibition of bone formation due to suppressive effects on osteoblasts. In addition, glucocorticoid inhibition of intestinal calcium uptake may lead to secondary increases in parathyroid hormone, thereby increasing bone resorption.

The considerable morbidity of glucocorticoid-related osteoporosis has led to efforts to identify patients at risk for fractures and to prevent or reverse bone loss in patients requiring chronic glucocorticoid therapy. The initiation of glucocorticoid therapy is considered an indication for bone densitometry, preferably with techniques such as dual-energy X-ray absorptiometry of the lumbar spine or hip that most sensitively detect abnormalities in trabecular bone. Because bone loss associated with glucocorticoids predominantly occurs within the first six months of therapy, densitometric evaluation and prophylactic measures should be initiated coincident with therapy or shortly thereafter. Most authorities advocate maintaining a calcium intake of 1500 mg/day by diet plus calcium supplementation and vitamin D intake of 400 IU/day, assuming that these measures do not increase urinary calcium excretion above the normal range. Unless contraindicated, gonadal hormone replacement therapy is indicated in specific groups of patients receiving chronic glucocorticoid therapy, including postmenopausal females, premenopausal females with decreased estradiol levels, and males with decreased testosterone levels.

The most important advance in the prevention of glucocorticoid-related osteoporosis is the successful use of bisphosphonates. Several different agents have been shown to decrease the decline in bone density in patients receiving glucocorticoid therapy. In particular, both *alendronate* (Saag *et al.*, 1998) and cyclical *etidronate* have been shown to be effective both in primary prevention and in restoration of bone density in patients receiving chronic therapy with glucocorticoids. Additional discussion of these issues is found in Chapters 58 and 62.

Osteonecrosis.   Osteonecrosis (also known as avascular or aseptic necrosis) is a relatively common complication of glucocorticoid therapy (Lane and Lukert, 1998). The femoral head is affected most frequently, but this process also may affect the humeral head and distal femur. Joint pain and stiffness are usually the earliest symptoms, and this diagnosis should be considered in patients receiving glucocorticoids who abruptly develop hip, shoulder, or knee pain. Although the risk increases with both the duration and dose of glucocorticoid therapy, osteonecrosis also can occur when high doses of glucocorticoids are given for short periods of time. Osteonecrosis generally progresses, and most affected patients ultimately require joint replacement.

Regulation of Growth and Development.   Growth retardation can result from administration of relatively small doses of glucocorticoids to children. Although the precise mechanism is unknown, there are reports that collagen synthesis and linear growth in these children can be restored by treatment with growth hormone; further studies are needed to define the role of concurrent treatment with growth hormone in this setting. Further studies also are needed to explore the possible effects of exposure to corticosteroids *in utero.* Studies in experimental animals have shown that antenatal exposure to glucocorticoids is clearly linked to cleft palate and altered neuronal development, ultimately resulting in complex behavioral abnormalities. Thus, although the actions of glucocorticoids to promote cellular differentiation play important physiological roles in human development in the neonatal period (*e.g.,* induction of the hepatic gluconeogenic enzymes and surfactant production in the lung), the possibility remains that antenatal steroids can lead to subtle abnormalities in fetal development.

Therapeutic Uses

With the exception of replacement therapy in deficiency states, the use of glucocorticoids largely is empirical. Based on extensive clinical experience, a number of therapeutic principles can be proposed. First, given the number and severity of potential side effects, the decision to institute therapy with glucocorticoids always requires a careful consideration of the relative risks and benefits in each patient. For any disease and in any patient, the appropriate dose to achieve a given therapeutic effect must be determined by trial and error and must be reevaluated periodically as the activity of the underlying disease changes or as complications of therapy arise. A single dose of glucocorticoid, even a large one, is virtually without harmful effects, and a short course of therapy (up to 1 week), in the absence of specific contraindications, is unlikely to be harmful. As the duration of glucocorticoid therapy is increased beyond 1 week, there are time- and dose-related increases in the incidence of disabling and potentially lethal effects. Except in patients receiving replacement or substitution therapy, glucocorticoids are neither specific nor curative; instead, they provide palliation by virtue of their antiinflammatory and immunosuppressive actions. Finally, abrupt cessation of glucocorticoids after prolonged therapy is associated with a significant risk of adrenal insufficiency, which may be fatal.

These principles have several implications for clinical practice. When glucocorticoids are to be given over long periods, the dose must be determined by trial and error and must be the smallest one that will achieve the desired effect. When the therapeutic goal is relief of painful or distressing symptoms not associated with an immediately life-threatening disease, complete relief is not sought, and

the steroid dose is reduced gradually until worsening symptoms indicate that the minimal acceptable dose has been found. Where possible, the substitution of other medications, such as nonsteroidal antiinflammatory drugs, may facilitate the tapering process once the initial benefit of glucocorticoid therapy has been achieved. When therapy is directed at a life-threatening disease (*e.g.,* pemphigus), the initial dose should be a large one aimed at achieving rapid control of the crisis. If some benefit is not observed quickly, then the dose should be doubled or tripled. After initial control in a potentially lethal disease, reduction of dose should be carried out under conditions that permit frequent, accurate observations of the patient. It is always essential to weigh carefully the relative dangers of therapy and of the disease being treated.

The lack of demonstrated deleterious effects of a single dose of glucocorticoids within the conventional therapeutic range justifies their administration to critically ill patients who may have adrenal insufficiency. If the underlying condition does result from deficiency of glucocorticoids, then a single intravenous injection of a soluble glucocorticoid may prevent immediate death and allow time for a definitive diagnosis to be made. If the underlying disease is not adrenal insufficiency, the single dose will not harm the patient.

In the absence of specific contraindications, short courses of high-dose, systemic glucocorticoids also may be given for diseases that are not life-threatening, but the general rule is that long courses of therapy at high doses should be reserved for life-threatening disease. In selected settings, as when a patient is threatened with permanent disability, this rule is justifiably violated.

In an attempt to dissociate therapeutic effects from undesirable side effects, various regimens of steroid administration have been utilized. In an attempt to diminish HPA axis suppression, alternate-day therapy with relatively short-lived glucocorticoids (*e.g.,* prednisone) has been employed. Certain patients obtain adequate therapeutic responses on this regimen. Alternatively, pulse therapy with higher glucocorticoid doses (*e.g.,* doses as high as 1.0 to 1.5 g/day of methylprednisolone for three days) frequently is used to initiate therapy in patients with fulminant, immunologically related disorders such as acute transplantation rejection, necrotizing glomerulonephritis, and lupus nephritis (Boumpas *et al.,* 1993). The benefit of such pulse therapy in long-term maintenance regimens remains to be defined.

Replacement Therapy.   Adrenal insufficiency can result from structural or functional lesions of the adrenal cortex (primary adrenal insufficiency) or from structural or functional lesions of the anterior pituitary or hypothalamus (secondary adrenal insufficiency). In developed countries, primary adrenal insufficiency most frequently is secondary to autoimmune adrenal disease, whereas tuberculous adrenalitis is the most frequent etiology in underdeveloped countries. Other causes include adrenalectomy, bilateral adrenal hemorrhage, the acquired immunodeficiency syndrome, and X-linked adrenoleukodystrophy (Carey 1997). Secondary adrenal insufficiency resulting from pituitary or hypothalamic dysfunction generally presents in a more insidious manner than does the primary disorder.

Acute Adrenal Insufficiency. This life-threatening disease is characterized by gastrointestinal symptoms (nausea, vomiting, and abdominal pain), dehydration, hyponatremia, hyperkalemia, weakness, lethargy, and hypotension. It usually is associated with disorders of the adrenal rather than the pituitary or hypothalamus, and it frequently follows abrupt withdrawal of glucocorticoids used at high doses or for prolonged periods. The presence of pigmentation is diagnostically useful in identifying patients with primary adrenal disease.

The immediate management of patients with acute adrenal insufficiency includes intravenous therapy with isotonic sodium chloride solution supplemented with 5% glucose and corticosteroids and appropriate therapy for precipitating causes such as infection, trauma, or hemorrhage. Because cardiovascular function often is reduced in the setting of adrenocortical insufficiency, the patient should be monitored for evidence of volume overload such as rising central venous pressure or pulmonary edema. After an initial intravenous bolus of 100 mg, *hydrocortisone* (cortisol) should be given by continuous infusion at a rate of 100 mg every 8 hours. In this dose, which approximates the maximum daily rate of cortisol secretion in response to stress, hydrocortisone alone has sufficient mineralocorticoid activity to meet all requirements. As the patient stabilizes, intramuscular hydrocortisone may be used in a dose of 25 mg every 6 to 8 hours. Thereafter, patients are treated in the same fashion as those with chronic adrenal insufficiency (*see* below).

For the treatment of suspected but unconfirmed acute adrenal insufficiency, 4 mg of *dexamethasone sodium phosphate* can be substituted for hydrocortisone, since dexamethasone does not cross-react in the cortisol assay and will not interfere with the measurement of cortisol (either basally or in response to the cosyntropin stimulation test). A failure to respond to cosyntropin in this setting is diagnostic of adrenal insufficiency. A sample for the measurement of plasma ACTH often also is obtained, as it provides information about the underlying etiology if the diagnosis of adrenocortical insufficiency is established.

Chronic Adrenal Insufficiency. Patients with chronic adrenal insufficiency present with many of the same manifestations seen in adrenal crisis, but with lesser severity. These patients require daily treatment with cortico-

steroids. Traditional replacement regimens have used hydrocortisone in doses of 20 to 30 mg/day. Cortisone acetate, which is inactive until converted to cortisol by 11β-hydroxysteroid dehydrogenase, also has been used in doses ranging from 25 to 37.5 mg/day. In an effort to mimic the normal diurnal rhythm of cortisol secretion, these glucocorticoids generally have been given in divided doses, with two-thirds of the dose given in the morning and one-third given in the afternoon. Based on revised estimates of daily cortisol production (Esteban *et al.,* 1991) and clinical studies showing that subtle degrees of glucocorticoid excess can decrease bone density in patients on conventional replacement regimens (Zelissen *et al.,* 1994), many authorities advocate a daily hydrocortisone dose of 20 mg/day divided into either two doses (*e.g.,* 15 mg on awakening and 5 mg in late afternoon) or three doses (*e.g.,* 10 mg on awakening, 5 mg at lunch, and 5 mg in late afternoon). Others prefer to use long-acting glucocorticoids, such as prednisone or dexamethasone, since no regimen employing shorter-acting steroids can reproduce the peak serum cortisol levels that normally occur prior to awakening in the morning. The superiority of any one of these regimens has not been rigorously demonstrated. Although some patients with primary adrenal insufficiency can be maintained on hydrocortisone and liberal salt intake, most of these patients also require mineralocorticoid replacement; *fludrocortisone acetate* generally is used in doses of 0.05 to 0.2 mg/day. For patients with secondary adrenal insufficiency, the administration of a glucocorticoid alone is generally adequate, as the zona glomerulosa—which makes mineralocorticoids—is intact. When initiating treatment in patients with panhypopituitarism, it is important to administer glucocorticoids first before initiating treatment with thyroid hormone, because the administration of thyroid hormone may precipitate acute adrenal insufficiency.

The adequacy of corticosteroid replacement therapy is judged by clinical criteria and biochemical measurements. The subjective well-being of the patient is an important clinical parameter in both primary and secondary disease. In primary adrenal insufficiency, the disappearance of hyperpigmentation and the resolution of electrolyte abnormalities are valuable indicators of adequate replacement. Overtreatment may cause manifestations of Cushing's syndrome in adults and decreased linear growth in children. Plasma ACTH levels may be used to monitor therapy in patients with primary adrenal insufficiency; the early morning ACTH level should not be suppressed, but should be less than 100 pg/ml (20 pmol/liter). Although advocated by some endocrinologists, assessments of daily profiles of cortisol based on multiple blood sampling or measurements of urinary free cortisol have been used more frequently as research tools than as a routine part of clinical practice.

Standard doses of glucocorticoids often must be adjusted upward in patients who also are taking drugs that increase their metabolic clearance (*e.g.,* phenytoin, barbiturates, rifampin). Dosage adjustments also are needed to compensate for the stress of intercurrent illness, and proper patient education is essential for the execution of these adjustments. All patients with adrenal insufficiency should wear a medical alert bracelet or tag that lists their diagnosis and carries information about their steroid regimen. During minor illness, the glucocorticoid dose should be doubled. Patients should be instructed to contact their physician if nausea and vomiting preclude the retention of oral medications. It also is highly recommended that the patient and family members be instructed so that they can administer parenteral dexamethasone (4 mg subcutaneously or intramuscularly) in the event that severe nausea or vomiting precludes the oral administration of medications. They then should seek medical attention immediately. Based largely on empirical data, glucocorticoid doses also are adjusted when patients with adrenal insufficiency undergo either elective or emergency surgery. In this setting, the doses are designed to approximate or exceed the maximal cortisol secretory rate of 200 mg/day; a standard regimen is hydrocortisone, 100 mg parenterally every 6 to 8 hours. Following surgery, the dose is halved each day until it is reduced to routine maintenance levels. Although some data suggest that increases in dose to this degree are not essential for survival even in major surgery (Glowniak and Loriaux, 1997), this approach remains the standard clinical practice at present.

Congenital Adrenal Hyperplasia. This term denotes a group of genetic disorders in which the activity of one of the several enzymes required for the biosynthesis of corticosteroids is deficient. The impaired production of cortisol, aldosterone, or both and the consequent lack of negative feedback inhibition lead to increased release of ACTH and/or angiotensin II. As a result, other hormonally active steroids that are proximal to the enzymatic block in the steroidogenic pathway are overproduced. Congenital adrenal hyperplasia (CAH) includes a spectrum of disorders whose precise clinical presentation, laboratory findings, and treatment depend on which of the steroidogenic enzymes is deficient (*see* Donohoue *et al.,* 2000, for a general discussion of the various forms of CAH).

In approximately 90% of patients, congenital adrenal hyperplasia (CAH) results from mutations in CYP21, the enzyme that carries out the 21-hydroxylation reaction (New, 1998). Clinically, patients are divided into those with classical CAH, who have severe defects in enzymatic activity and first present dur-

ing childhood, and those with nonclassical CAH, who present after puberty with signs and symptoms of mild androgen excess such as hirsutism, amenorrhea, infertility, and acne. Female patients with classical CAH, if not treated *in utero* with glucocorticoids, frequently are born with virilized external genitalia (female pseudohermaphroditism), which results from elevated production of adrenal androgens at critical stages of sexual differentiation *in utero*. Males appear normal at birth and later may have precocious development of secondary sexual characteristics (isosexual precocious puberty). In both sexes, linear growth is accelerated in childhood, but the height at maturity is reduced by premature closure of the epiphyses.

In a subset of patients with classical CAH, the enzymatic deficiency is sufficiently severe to compromise aldosterone production. Such patients are unable to conserve Na^+ normally and thus are termed "salt wasters." These patients can present with cardiovascular collapse secondary to volume depletion; in an effort to prevent such life-threatening events, especially in males who appear normal at birth, some locations mandate routine screening of all babies for elevated levels of 17-hydroxyprogesterone, the immediate steroid precursor to the enzymatic block.

All patients with classical CAH require substitution therapy with *hydrocortisone* or a suitable congener, and those with salt wasting also require mineralocorticoid replacement. The goals of therapy are to restore levels of physiological steroid hormones to the normal range, as well as to suppress ACTH and thereby abrogate the effects of overproduction of adrenal androgens. The typical oral dose of hydrocortisone is approximately 0.6 mg/kg daily in two or three divided doses. The mineralocorticoid used is *fludrocortisone acetate* (0.05 to 0.2 mg/day). Many experts also administer table salt to infants (one-fifth of a teaspoon dissolved in formula daily) until the child is eating solid food. Therapy is guided by gain in weight and height, by plasma levels of 17-hydroxyprogesterone, and by blood pressure. Elevated plasma renin activity suggests that the patient is receiving an inadequate dose of mineralocorticoid. Sudden spurts in linear growth often indicate inadequate pituitary suppression and excessive androgen secretion, whereas growth failure often suggests overtreatment with glucocorticoid.

The development of methods to detect classical CAH (21-hydroxylase deficiency) prenatally has made possible the treatment of affected females with glucocorticoids *in utero,* thereby eliminating the need for genital surgery to correct the virilization of the external genitalia (New, 1998). Glucocorticoid therapy (*e.g.,* dexamethasone, 20 μg/kg taken daily orally by mothers at risk) must be initiated before 10 weeks' gestation, before a definitive diagnosis of CAH can be made, to suppress effectively fetal adrenal androgen production. The genotype and sex of the fetus then are determined: If the sex is male or there is at least one wild-type allele for 21-hydroxylase, steroid therapy is stopped. If genotyping reveals an affected female, steroid therapy is continued until delivery. Potential maternal side effects include hypertension, weight gain, edema, and mood changes. Although it theoretically is possible that exposure to glucocorticoids *in utero* may have developmental consequences, adverse effects have not yet been described.

Therapeutic Uses in Nonendocrine Diseases. Given below are brief outlines of important uses of glucocorticoids in diseases that do not directly involve the HPA axis. The disorders discussed are not inclusive; rather, they illustrate the principles governing glucocorticoid use in selected diseases for which they are more frequently employed. The dosage of glucocorticoids varies considerably depending on the nature and severity of the underlying disorder. For convenience, approximate doses of a representative glucocorticoid (generally prednisone) are provided in the following discussion. This choice is not an endorsement of one particular glucocorticoid preparation over other congeners but is made for illustrative purposes only.

Rheumatic Disorders. Glucocorticoids are used widely in the treatment of a variety of rheumatic disorders and are a mainstay in the treatment of the more serious inflammatory rheumatic diseases, such as systemic lupus erythematosus, and a variety of vasculitic disorders, such as polyarteritis nodosa, Wegener's granulomatosis, and giant cell arteritis. For these more serious disorders, the starting dose of glucocorticoids should be sufficient to suppress the disease rapidly and minimize resultant tissue damage. Initially *prednisone* (1 mg/kg per day in divided doses) often is used, generally followed by consolidation to a single daily dose, with subsequent tapering to a minimal effective dose as determined by clinical variables.

There is controversy regarding the role of glucocorticoids in rheumatoid arthritis, particularly because of the serious and debilitating side effects associated with chronic use. Some authorities recommend glucocorticoids only as temporizing agents for progressive disease that fails to respond to first-line treatments such as physiotherapy and nonsteroidal antiinflammatory agents. In this case, glucocorticoids provide relief until other, slower-acting antirheumatic drugs, such as methotrexate or gold, take effect. A typical starting dose is 5 to 10 mg of prednisone per day. In the setting of an acute exacerbation, higher doses of glucocorticoids may be employed (typically 20 to 40 mg/day of prednisone or equivalent), with rapid taper thereafter. Complete relief of symptoms is not sought, and the symptomatic effect of small reductions in dose (decreases of perhaps 1 mg/day of prednisone every 2 to 3 weeks) should be tested frequently, while concurrent therapy with other measures is continued, to maintain the lowest possible prednisone dose. Alternatively, patients with major symptomatology confined to one or a few joints may be treated with intraarticular steroid injections. Depending on joint size, typical doses are 5 to 20 mg of *triamcinolone acetonide* or its equivalent.

In noninflammatory degenerative joint diseases (*e.g.,* osteoarthritis) or in a variety of regional pain syndromes (*e.g.,*

tendonitis or bursitis), glucocorticoids may be administered by local injection for the treatment of episodic disease flare-up. It is important to minimize the frequency of local steroid administration whenever possible. In the case of repeated intraarticular injection of steroids, there is a significant incidence of painless joint destruction, resembling Charcot's arthropathy. It is recommended that intraarticular injections be performed with intervals of at least three months to minimize complications.

Glucocorticoids are an important component of treatment for most of the vasculitic syndromes, often in conjunction with other immunosuppressive agents such as cyclophosphamide. Caution should be exercised in the use of glucocorticoids in some forms of vasculitis (*e.g.,* polyarteritis nodosa), where underlying infections with hepatitis viruses may play a pathogenetic role. Although glucocorticoids are indicated in these cases, there is at least a theoretical consideration that glucocorticoids may complicate the course of the viral infection by suppressing the immune system. The shorter-acting glucocorticoids, such as prednisone and methylprednisolone, are preferred over longer-acting steroids, such as dexamethasone, to facilitate drug tapering and/or conversion to alternate-day treatment regimens. Guidelines for treatment of the major vasculitic syndromes have been proposed by Weisman and Weinblatt (1995).

Renal Diseases. The utility of glucocorticoids in renal disease also has been the subject of considerable debate. Patients with nephrotic syndrome secondary to minimal change disease generally respond well to steroid therapy, and glucocorticoids are now accepted uniformly as first-line treatment in both adults and children. Initial daily doses of prednisone are 1 to 2 mg/kg for 6 weeks, followed by a gradual tapering of the dose over 6 to 8 weeks, although some nephrologists advocate alternate-day therapy. Objective evidence of response, such as diminished proteinuria, is seen within 2 to 3 weeks in 85% of patients, and more than 95% of patients will have remission within three months. Cessation of steroid therapy frequently is complicated by disease relapse, as manifested by recurrent proteinuria. Patients who relapse repeatedly are termed *steroid-resistant* and often are treated with other immunosuppressive drugs such as *azathioprine* or *cyclophosphamide.* Patients with renal disease secondary to systemic lupus erythematosus also are generally given a therapeutic trial of glucocorticoids.

Studies with other forms of renal disease, such as membranous and membranoproliferative glomerulonephritis and focal sclerosis, have provided conflicting data on the role of glucocorticoids. In clinical practice, patients with these disorders often are given a therapeutic trial of glucocorticoids with careful monitoring of laboratory indices of response. In the case of membranous glomerulonephritis, many nephrologists recommend a trial of alternate-day glucocorticoids for 8 to 10 weeks (*e.g.,* prednisone, 120 mg every other day), followed by a 1- to 2-month period of tapering.

Allergic Disease. It must be emphasized that the onset of action of glucocorticoids in allergic diseases is delayed, and patients with severe allergic reactions such as anaphylaxis require immediate therapy with epinephrine: for adults, 0.5 ml of a 1:1000 solution intramuscularly or subcutaneously (repeated as often as every 15 minutes for up to three additional doses if necessary). The manifestations of allergic diseases of limited duration—such as hay fever, serum sickness, urticaria, contact dermatitis, drug reactions, bee stings, and angioneurotic edema—can be suppressed by adequate doses of glucocorticoids given as supplements to the primary therapy. In severe disease, intravenous glucocorticoids (*methylprednisolone* 125 mg intravenously every 6 hours, or equivalent) are appropriate. In less severe disease, antihistamines are the drugs of first choice. In allergic rhinitis, intranasal steroids also may provide symptomatic relief.

Bronchial Asthma. Corticosteroids frequently are used in bronchial asthma (*see* Chapter 28). They sometimes are employed in chronic obstructive pulmonary disease (COPD), particularly when there is some evidence of reversible obstructive disease. Data supporting the efficacy of corticosteroids are much more convincing for bronchial asthma than for COPD. The increased use of corticosteroids in asthma reflects an increased appreciation of the role of inflammation in the immunopathogenesis of this disorder (Goldstein *et al.,* 1994). In severe asthmatic attacks requiring hospitalization, aggressive treatment with parenteral glucocorticoids is considered essential even though their onset of action is delayed for 6 to 12 hours. Intravenous administration of 60 to 120 mg of *methylprednisolone* (or equivalent) every 6 hours is used initially, followed by daily oral doses of *prednisone* (40 to 60 mg) as the acute attack resolves. The dose then is tapered gradually, with withdrawal planned for 10 days to 2 weeks after initiation of steroid therapy. In general, patients subsequently can be managed on their prior medical regimen.

Less severe, acute exacerbations of asthma (as well as acute flares of COPD) often are treated with brief courses of oral glucocorticoids. In adult patients, 40 to 60 mg of prednisone is administered daily for five days; an additional week of therapy at lower doses also may be required. Upon resolution of the acute exacerbation, the glucocorticoids generally can be rapidly tapered without significant deleterious effects. Any suppression of adrenal function usually dissipates within 1 to 2 weeks. In the treatment of severe chronic bronchial asthma (or, less frequently, COPD) that is not controlled by other measures, the long-term administration of glucocorticoids may be necessary. As with other long-term uses of these agents, the lowest effective dose is used, and care must be exercised when withdrawal is attempted. Given the risks of long-term treatment with glucocorticoids, it is especially important to document objective evidence of a response (*e.g.,* an improvement in pulmonary function tests). In addition, these risks dictate that long-term glucocorticoid therapy be reserved for those patients who have failed to respond to adequate regimens of other medications (*see* Chapter 28).

In many patients, the use of inhaled steroids (most frequently *beclomethasone dipropionate, triamcinolone acetonide, flunisolide,* or *budesonide*) either can reduce the need for oral corticosteroids or replace them entirely (*see* Barnes, 1995). In addition, many physicians recommend inhaled glucocorticoids over previously recommended oral theophylline in the treatment of children with moderately severe asthma, in part because of the behavioral toxicity associated with chronic theophylline administration (*see* Chapter 28). When used as recommended, inhaled glucocorticoids are effective in reducing bronchial hyperreactivity with less suppression of adrenal function than with oral glucocorticoids. Dysphonia or oropharyngeal candidiasis may develop, but the incidence of such side effects can be reduced substantially by maneuvers that reduce drug deposition in the oral cavity, such as spacers and mouth rinsing. The evolving status of glucocorticoids in asthma therapy is discussed in detail in Chapter 28.

Infectious Diseases. Although it would seem paradoxical to use immunosuppressive glucocorticoids in infectious diseases, there are a limited number of settings where they are indicated in the therapy of specific infectious pathogens (McGowan *et al.,* 1992). One dramatic example of such beneficial effects is seen in AIDS patients with *Pneumocystis carinii* pneumonia and moderate to severe hypoxia; addition of glucocorticoids to the antibiotic regimen increases oxygenation and lowers the incidence of respiratory failure and mortality. Similarly, glucocorticoids clearly decrease the incidence of long-term neurological impairment associated with *Haemophilus influenzae* type b meningitis in infants and children two months of age or older.

Ocular Diseases. Ocular pharmacology, including some consideration of the use of glucocorticoids, is discussed in Chapter 66. Glucocorticoids frequently are used to suppress inflammation in the eye and can lead to the preservation of sight when used properly. They are administered topically for diseases of the outer eye and anterior segment and attain therapeutic concentrations in the aqueous humor following instillation into the conjunctival cul-de-sac. For diseases of the posterior segment, systemic administration is required. It is generally recommended that ocular use of *glucocorticoids* be under the supervision of an ophthalmologist.

A typical prescription is 0.1% dexamethasone sodium phosphate solution (ophthalmic), 2 drops in the conjunctival sac every 4 hours while awake, and 0.05% dexamethasone sodium phosphate ointment (ophthalmic) at bedtime. For inflammations of the posterior segment, systemic therapy is required, and typical doses are 30 mg of prednisone or equivalent per day, administered orally in divided doses.

Topical glucocorticoid therapy frequently increases intraocular pressure in normal eyes and exacerbates intraocular hypertension in patients with antecedent glaucoma. The glaucoma is not always reversible on cessation of glucocorticoid therapy. Intraocular pressure should be monitored when glucocorticoids are applied to the eye for more than 2 weeks.

Topical administration of glucocorticoids to patients with bacterial, viral, or fungal conjunctivitis can mask evidence of progression of the infection until sight is irreversibly lost. Glucocorticoids are contraindicated in herpes simplex keratitis, because progression of the disease may lead to irreversible clouding of the cornea. Topical steroids should not be used in treating mechanical lacerations and abrasions of the eye because they delay healing and promote the development and spread of infection.

Skin Diseases. Glucocorticoids are remarkably efficacious in the treatment of a wide variety of inflammatory dermatoses. As a result, a large number of different preparations and concentrations of topical glucocorticoids of varying potencies are available. A typical regimen for an eczematous eruption is 1% *hydrocortisone* ointment applied locally twice daily. Effectiveness is enhanced by application of the topical steroid under an occlusive film, such as plastic wrap; unfortunately, the risk of systemic absorption also is increased by occlusive dressings, and this can be a significant problem when the more potent glucocorticoids are applied to inflamed skin. Glucocorticoids are administered systemically for severe episodes of acute dermatologic disorders and for exacerbations of chronic disorders. The dose in these settings is usually 40 mg/day of prednisone. Systemic steroid administration can be lifesaving in pemphigus, which may require daily doses of up to 120 mg of prednisone. Further discussion of the treatment of skin diseases is given in Chapter 65.

Gastrointestinal Diseases. Glucocorticoid therapy is indicated in selected patients with inflammatory bowel disease (chronic ulcerative colitis and Crohn's disease; *see* Chapter 39). Patients who fail to respond to more conservative management (*i.e.*, rest, diet, and sulfasalazine) may benefit from glucocorticoids; steroids are most useful for acute exacerbations (Stein and Hanauer, 1999). In mild ulcerative colitis, *hydrocortisone* (100 mg) can be administered as a retention enema with beneficial effects. In more severe acute exacerbations, oral *prednisone* (10 to 30 mg/day) frequently is employed. For severely ill patients—with fever, anorexia, anemia, and impaired nutritional status—larger doses should be used (60 to 120 mg prednisone per day). Major complications of ulcerative colitis or Crohn's disease may occur despite glucocorticoid therapy, and glucocorticoids may mask signs and symptoms of complications such as intestinal perforation and peritonitis.

Budesonide, a highly potent synthetic glucocorticoid that is inactivated by first-pass hepatic metabolism, has diminished systemic side effects commonly associated with glucocorticoids. Oral administration of budesonide in delayed-release capsules (9 mg/day) facilitates drug delivery to the ileum and ascending colon (Greenberg *et al.*, 1994); the drug also has been used as a retention enema in the treatment of ulcerative colitis. These dosage forms, however, are not yet available in the United States. Currently, budesonide is not approved for treatment of inflammatory bowel disease in the United States and is available only as an antiinflammatory agent for inhalation therapy.

Hepatic Diseases. The use of corticosteroids in hepatic disease has been highly controversial. Glucocorticoids are clearly of benefit in autoimmune, chronic active hepatitis, where as many as 80% of patients show histological remission when treated with prednisone (40 to 60 mg daily initially, with tapering to a maintenance dose of 7.5 to 10 mg daily after serum transaminase levels fall). The role of corticosteroids in alcoholic liver disease is not fully defined; the most recent studies, including meta-analysis of previously published reports, suggest a beneficial role of prednisolone (40 mg/day for 4 weeks) in patients with severe disease indicators (*e.g.*, hepatic encephalopathy) without active gastrointestinal bleeding (McCullough and O'Connor, 1998). Further studies are needed to confirm or refute the role of steroids in this setting. In the setting of severe hepatic disease, *prednisolone* should be used instead of prednisone, which requires hepatic conversion to be active.

Malignancies. Glucocorticoids are used in the chemotherapy of acute lymphocytic leukemia and lymphomas because of their antilymphocytic effects. Most commonly, glucocorticoids are one component of combination chemotherapy administered under scheduled protocols. Further discussion of the chemotherapy of malignant disease is given in Chapter 52. Glucocorticoids once were frequently employed in the setting of hypercalcemia of malignancy, but they have been largely supplanted by more effective agents such as the bisphosphonates.

Cerebral Edema. Corticosteroids are of value in the reduction or prevention of cerebral edema associated with parasites and with neoplasms, especially those that are metastatic. Although frequently used for the treatment of cerebral edema caused by trauma or cerebrovascular accidents, controlled clinical trials do not support their use in these settings.

Miscellaneous Diseases and Conditions. *Sarcoidosis.* Sarcoidosis is treated with corticosteroids (approximately 1 mg/kg per day of *prednisone,* or equivalent dose of alternative steroids) to induce remission. Maintenance doses, which often are required for long periods of time, may be as low as 10 mg/day of prednisone. These patients, like all patients who require chronic glucocorticoid therapy at doses exceeding the normal daily production rate, are at increased risk for secondary tuberculosis; therefore, patients with a positive tuberculin reaction or other evidence of tuberculosis should receive prophylactic antituberculosis therapy.

Thrombocytopenia. In thrombocytopenia, *prednisone* (0.5 mg/kg) is used to decrease the bleeding tendency. In more severe cases, and for initiation of treatment of idiopathic thrombocytopenia, daily doses of prednisone (1 to 1.5 mg/kg) are employed. Patients with refractory idiopathic thrombocytopenia may respond to pulsed, high-dose glucocorticoid therapy.

Autoimmune Destruction of Erythrocytes. Patients with autoimmune destruction of erythrocytes (*i.e.*, hemolytic anemia with a positive Coombs test) are treated with *prednisone* (1 mg/kg per day). In the setting of severe hemolysis, higher doses may be used, with tapering as the anemia improves. Small maintenance doses may be required for several months in patients who respond.

Organ Transplantation. In organ transplantation, high doses of *prednisone* (50 to 100 mg) are given at the time of transplant surgery, in conjunction with other immunosuppressive agents, and most patients are kept on a maintenance regimen that includes lower doses of glucocorticoids (*see* Chapter 53).

Spinal Cord Injury. Multicenter trials have shown significant decreases in neurological defects in patients with acute spinal cord injury treated within 8 hours of injury with large doses of methylprednisolone [30 mg/kg initially followed by an infusion of 5.4 mg/kg per hour for 23 hours (Bracken *et al.*, 1997)]. The ability of corticosteroids at these high doses to decrease neurological injury may reflect inhibition of free radical–mediated cellular injury, as occurs following ischemia and reperfusion.

Diagnostic Applications of Adrenocortical Steroids

In addition to their therapeutic uses, glucocorticoids also are used for diagnostic purposes. To determine if patients with clinical manifestations suggestive of hypercortisolism have biochemical evidence of increased cortisol biosynthesis, an overnight dexamethasone test has been devised. Patients are given 1 mg of dexamethasone orally at 11 P.M., and cortisol is measured at 8 A.M. the following morning. Suppression of plasma cortisol to less than 5 μg/dl suggests strongly that the patient does not have Cushing's syndrome.

The formal dexamethasone suppression test is used in the differential diagnosis of biochemically documented Cushing's syndrome. Following determination of baseline cortisol levels for 48 hours, dexamethasone (0.5 mg every 6 hours) is administered orally for 48 hours. This dose markedly suppresses cortisol levels in normal subjects, including those who have nonspecific elevations of cortisol due to obesity or stress, but does not suppress levels in patients with Cushing's syndrome. In the high-dose phase of the test, dexamethasone is administered orally at 2 mg every 6 hours for 48 hours. Patients with pituitary-dependent Cushing's syndrome (*i.e.,* Cushing's disease) generally respond with decreased cortisol levels. In contrast, patients with ectopic production of ACTH or with adrenocortical tumors generally do not exhibit decreased cortisol levels. Despite these generalities, dexamethasone may suppress cortisol levels in some patients with ectopic ACTH production, particularly with tumors such as bronchial carcinoids.

INHIBITORS OF THE BIOSYNTHESIS AND ACTION OF ADRENOCORTICAL STEROIDS

Five pharmacological agents have been useful as inhibitors of adrenocortical secretion. *Mitotane (o,p'-DDD),* an adrenocorticolytic agent, is discussed in Chapter 52. The other inhibitors of steroid hormone biosynthesis—*metyrapone, aminoglutethimide, ketoconazole,* and *trilostane*—are discussed here. Metyrapone, aminoglutethimide, and ketoconazole act by inhibiting cytochrome P450 enzymes involved in adrenocorticosteroid biosynthesis. Differential selectivity of these agents for the different steroid hydroxylases provides some degree of specificity to their actions. Trilostane is a competitive inhibitor of the conversion of pregnenolone to progesterone, a reaction catalyzed by 3β-hydroxysteroid dehydrogenase. In addition, agents that act as glucocorticoid receptor antagonists (antiglucocorticoids) are discussed here (mineralocorticoid antagonists are discussed in Chapter 29). All of these agents pose the common risk of precipitating acute adrenal insufficiency; thus, they must be used in appropriate doses, and the status of the patient's HPA axis must be carefully monitored.

Aminoglutethimide. *Aminoglutethimide* (α-ethyl-*p*-aminophenyl-glutarimide; CYTADREN) primarily inhibits $P450_{scc}$, which catalyzes the initial and rate-limiting step in the biosynthesis of all physiological steroids. As a result, the production of all classes of steroid hormones is impaired. Aminoglutethimide also inhibits $P450_{11\beta}$ and the enzyme aromatase, which converts androgens to estrogens. Aminoglutethimide has been used to decrease hypersecretion of cortisol in patients with Cushing's syndrome secondary to autonomous adrenal tumors and hypersecre-

tion associated with ectopic production of ACTH. Because of its actions to inhibit aromatase, aminoglutethimide also has been evaluated as a therapeutic agent for the treatment of hormonally responsive tumors such as prostate and breast cancer (*see* Chapter 52). Dose-dependent gastrointestinal and neurological side effects are relatively common, as is a transient, maculopapular rash. The usual dose is 250 mg every 6 hours, with gradual increases of 250 mg per day at 1- to 2-week intervals until the desired biochemical effect is achieved, side effects prohibit further increases, or a daily dose of 2 g is reached. Since aminoglutethimide can cause frank adrenal insufficiency, sometimes associated with signs of mineralocorticoid deficiency, glucocorticoid replacement therapy is necessary, and mineralocorticoid supplements may be indicated. Because aminoglutethimide accelerates the metabolism of dexamethasone, this steroid should not be used for glucocorticoid replacement in patients receiving aminoglutethimide.

Ketoconazole. *Ketoconazole* (NIZORAL) is an antifungal agent, and this remains its most important clinical role (*see* Chapter 49). In doses higher than those employed in antifungal therapy, it is an effective inhibitor of adrenal and gonadal steroidogenesis, primarily because of its inhibition of the C_{17-20} lyase activity of $P450_{17\alpha}$. At even higher doses, ketoconazole also inhibits $P450_{scc}$, effectively blocking steroidogenesis in all primary steroidogenic tissues. Ketoconazole has been reported to be the most effective inhibitor of steroid hormone biosynthesis in patients with Cushing's disease (*see* Sonino and Boscaro, 1999, for a review of the medical management of Cushing's disease). In most cases, a dosage regimen of 600 to 800 mg/day (in two divided doses) is required, and some patients may require up to 1200 mg/day given in two to three doses. Side effects include hepatic dysfunction, which ranges from asymptomatic elevations of transaminase levels to severe hepatic injury. The potential of ketoconazole to interact with cytochrome P450 enzymes can lead to drug interactions of serious consequence. For example, rare but potentially life-threatening interactions were reported between ketoconazole and nonsedating antihistamines (*e.g.,* terfenadine, astemizole) due to inhibition of hepatic CYP3A4 and decreased metabolism of these antihistamines. Terfenadine and astemizole have since been withdrawn from the market. Further studies are needed to define the precise role of ketoconazole in the medical management of patients with excessive steroid hormonal production, and ketoconazole currently is not approved by the FDA for this indication.

Metyrapone. *Metyrapone* (METOPIRONE) is a relatively selective inhibitor of 11β-hydroxylase, which converts 11-deoxycortisol to cortisol in the terminal reaction of the glucocorticoid biosynthetic pathway. Because of this inhibition, the biosynthesis of cortisol is markedly impaired, and the levels of steroid precursors (*e.g.,* 11-deoxycortisol) are markedly increased. Although the biosynthesis of aldosterone also is impaired, the elevated levels of 11-deoxycortisol sustain mineralocorticoid-dependent functions. In a diagnostic test of the entire HPA axis, metyrapone (30 mg/kg, maximum dose of 3 g) is administered orally with a snack at midnight, and plasma cortisol and 11-deoxycortisol are measured at 8 A.M. the next morning. A plasma cortisol of less than 8 μg/dl validates adequate inhibition of 11β-hydroxylase; in this setting, an 11-deoxycortisol level of less than 7 μg/dl is highly suggestive of impaired hypothalamic-pituitary-adrenal function. An abnormal response does not identify the site of the defect—either hypothalamic CRH release, ACTH production, or adrenal biosynthetic capacity could be impaired. Some authorities avoid overnight metyrapone testing in outpatients thought to have a reasonable probability of impaired HPA function, as there is some risk of precipitating acute adrenal insufficiency. Others believe that the ability to assess the entire HPA axis with a relatively easy test justifies the use of metyrapone testing in outpatients.

Metyrapone also is used to diagnose patients with Cushing's syndrome who respond equivocally to the high-dose dexamethasone suppression test. Those with pituitary-dependent Cushing's syndrome exhibit a normal response, whereas those patients with ectopic secretion of ACTH exhibit no changes in ACTH or 11-deoxycortisol levels.

Therapeutically, metyrapone has been used to treat the hypercorticism resulting from either adrenal neoplasms or tumors producing ACTH ectopically. Maximal suppression of steroidogenesis requires doses of 4 g/day. More frequently, metyrapone is used as adjunctive therapy in patients who have received pituitary irradiation or in combination with other agents that inhibit steroidogenesis. In this setting, a dose of 500 to 750 mg three or four times daily is employed. The use of metyrapone in the treatment of Cushing's syndrome secondary to pituitary hypersecretion of ACTH is more controversial. Chronic administration of metyrapone can cause hirsutism, which results from increased synthesis of adrenal androgens prior to the enzymatic block, and hypertension, which results from elevated levels of 11-deoxycortisol. Other side effects include nausea, headache, sedation, and rash.

ANTIGLUCOCORTICOIDS

The progesterone receptor antagonist *mifepristone* [RU-486; (11β-4-dimethylaminophenyl)-17β-hydroxy-7α-(propyl-1-ynyl)estra-4,9-dien-3-one] has received considerable attention because of its use as an antiprogestagen that can terminate early pregnancy (*see* Chapter 58). At higher doses, however, mifepristone also inhibits the glucocorticoid receptor, blocking feedback regulation of the HPA axis and secondarily increasing endogenous ACTH and cortisol levels. Because of its ability to inhibit gluco-

corticoid action, mifepristone also has been studied as a potential therapeutic agent in patients with hypercorticism.

PROSPECTUS

Many of the current clinical uses of corticosteroids are based on empirical approaches, rather than on detailed understanding of the mechanisms by which these drugs act. Our understanding of the pathways of corticosteroid actions within target cells has increased dramatically within recent years; these advances, while not yet directly translatable to clinical medicine, hold promise for the development of new therapeutic approaches with greater selectivity and less toxicity. We now recognize the importance of glucocorticoid receptor coactivators and corepressors in glucocorticoid action and have gained new insights into the interactions of glucocorticoids with other signal transduction pathways that may provide new avenues to manipulate glucocorticoid signaling. The potent immunosuppressive agents *cyclosporine* and *tacrolimus* are examples of drugs that at least partly intersect with the AP-1 and NF-κB transcriptional activation pathways in lymphocytes, providing a rationale for their common immunosuppressive actions. These agents have markedly improved success rates in organ transplantation, permitting the use of lower doses of glucocorticoids with diminished long-term complications (*see* Chapter 53). Novel drugs that impinge upon the lymphocyte activation cascade also may provide alternative antiinflammatory and immunosuppressive drugs with fewer side effects. Finally, new insights from the crystal structures of the ligand-binding regions of the steroid hormone receptors may facilitate a more rational approach to developing novel compounds with glucocorticoid activity.

Inasmuch as the antiinflammatory and metabolic effects of glucocorticoids are mediated by the same receptor, efforts to separate desired therapeutic effects from undesirable side effects largely have been unsuccessful to date. Nevertheless, the development of selective estrogen receptor modulators that act as receptor agonists in certain target tissues and as antagonists in others provides hope that glucocorticoid analogs may be developed with more favorable therapeutic profiles. Indeed, several dissociated glucocorticoids have been identified that act selectively as antiinflammatory agents (Vayssiere *et al.,* 1997; Vanden Berghe *et al.,* 1999). These agents apparently exert their antiinflammatory effects by preferentially promoting the direct interaction of the glucocorticoid receptor with transcription factors such as AP-1 and NF-κB, while having little effect on the metabolic and other activities mediated by glucocorticoid receptor dimers at specific GREs (*e.g.,*

Figure 60–5). It remains to be seen if these experimental agents develop into clinically useful drugs.

For further discussion of diseases of the adrenal cortex *see* Chapter 332 in *Harrison's Principles of Internal Medicine,* 14th ed., McGraw-Hill, New York, 1998.

BIBLIOGRAPHY

Abdu, T.A.M., Elhadd, T.A., Neary, R., and Clayton, R.N. Comparison of the low dose short synacthen test (1 µg), the conventional dose short synachten test (250 µg), and the insulin tolerance test for assessment of the hypothalamo-pituitary-adrenal axis in patients with pituitary disease. *J. Clin. Endocrinol. Metab.,* **1999,** *84:*838–843.

Arlt W., Callies, F., van Vlijmen, J.C., Koehler, I., Reincke, M., Bedlingmaier, M., Huebler, D., Oettel, M., Ernst, M., Schulte, H.M., and Allolio, B. Dehydroepiandrosterone replacement in women with adrenal insufficiency. *N. Engl. J. Med.,* **1999,** *341:*1013–1020.

Barnes, P.J. Inhaled glucocorticoids for asthma. *N. Engl. J. Med.,* **1995,** *332:*868–875.

Boumpas, D.T., Chrousos, G.P., Wilder, R.L., Cupps, T.R., and Balow, J.E. Glucocorticoid therapy for immune-mediated disease: basic and clinical correlates. *Ann. Intern. Med.,* **1993,** *119:*1198–1208.

Bracken, M.B., Shepard, M.J., Holford, T.R., Leo-Summers, L., Aldrich, E.F., Fazl, M., Fehlings, M., Herr, D.L., Hitchon, P.W., Marshall, L.F., Nockels, R.P., Pascale, V., Perot, P.L. Jr., Piepmeier, J., Sonntag, V.K., Wagner, F., Wilberger, J.E., Winn, H.R., and Young, W. Administration of methylprednisolone for 24 or 48 hours or tirilazad mesylate for 48 hours in the treatment of acute spinal cord injury. Results of the Third National Acute Spinal Cord Injury Randomized Controlled Trial. *JAMA,* **1997,** *277:*1597–1604.

Byyny, R.L. Withdrawal from glucocorticoid therapy. *N. Engl. J. Med.,* **1976,** *295:*30–32.

Carey, R.M. The changing clinical spectrum of adrenal insufficiency. *Ann. Intern. Med.,* **1997,** *127:*1103–1105.

Chen, R., Lewis, K.A., Perrin, M.H., and Vale, W.W. Expression cloning of a human corticotropin-releasing-factor receptor. *Proc. Natl. Acad. Sci. U.S.A.,* **1993,** *90:*8967–8971.

Chen, S.Y., Bhargava, A., Mastroberardino, L., Meijer, O.C., Wang, J., Buse, P., Firestone, G.L., Verrey, F., and Pearce, D. Epithelial sodium channel regulated by aldosterone-induced protein sgk. *Proc. Natl. Acad. Sci. U.S.A.,* **1999,** *96:*2514–2519.

Elenkov, I.J., and Chrousos, G.P. Stress hormones, Th1/Th2 patterns, pro/anti-inflammatory cytokines and susceptibility to disease. *Trends Endocrinol. Metab.,* **1999,** *10:*359–368.

Esteban, N.V., Loughlin, T., Yergey, A.L., Zawadzki, J.K., Booth, J.D., Winterer, J.C., and Loriaux, D.L. Daily cortisol production rate in man determined by stable isotope dilution/mass spectrometry. *J. Clin. Endocrinol. Metab.,* **1991,** *72:*39–45.

Geller, D.S., Rodriguez-Soriano, J., Vallo Boado, A., Schifter, S., Bayer, M., Chang, S.S., and Lifton, R.P. Mutations in the mineralocorticoid receptor gene cause autosomal dominant pseudohypoaldosteronism type I. *Nat. Genet.,* **1998,** *19:*279–281.

Glowniak J.V., and Loriaux, D.L. A double-blind study of perioperative steroid requirements in secondary adrenal insufficiency. *Surgery,* **1997,** *121:*123–129.

Greenberg, G.R., Feagan, B.G., Martin, F., Sutherland, L.R., Thomson, A.B., Williams, C.N., Nilsson, L.G., and Persson, T. Oral budesonide for active Crohn's disease. Canadian Inflammatory Bowel Disease Study Group. *N. Engl. J. Med.,* **1994,** *331:*836–841.

Haskett, R.F. Diagnostic categorization of psychiatric disturbance in Cushings syndrome. *Am. J. Psychiatry,* **1985,** *142:*911–916.

Hench, P.S., Kendall, E.C., Slocumb, C.H., and Polley, H.F. The effect of a hormone of the adrenal cortex (17-hydroxy-11-dehydrocorticosterone; compound E) and of pituitary adrenocorticotropic hormone on rheumatoid arthritis. *Proc. Staff Meet. Mayo Clin.,* **1949,** *24:*181–197.

Jackson, R.S., Creemers, J.W., Ohagi, S., Raffin-Sanson, M.L., Sanders, L., Montague, C.T., Hutton, J.C., and O'Rahilly, S. Obesity and impaired prohormone processing associated with mutations in the human prohormone convertase 1 gene. *Nat. Genet.,* **1997,** *16:*218–220.

Lane, N.E., and Lukert, B. The science and therapy of glucocorticoid-induced bone loss. *Endocrinol. Metab. Clin. North Am.,* **1998,** *27:*465–483.

Lin, D., Sugawara, T., Strauss, J.F. III, Clark, B.J., Stocco, D.M., Saenger, P., Rogol, A., and Miller, W.L. Role of steroidogenic acute regulatory protein in adrenal and gonadal steroidogenesis. *Science,* **1995,** *267:*1828–1831.

Lupien, S.J., de Leon, M., de Santi, S., Convit, A., Tarshish, C., Nair, N.P., Thakur, M., McEwen, B.S., Hauger, R.L., and Meaney, M.J. Cortisol levels during human aging predict hippocampal atrophy and memory deficits. *Nat. Neurosci.,* **1998,** *1:*3–4.

McCullough, A.J., and O'Connor, J.F. Alcoholic liver disease: proposed recommendations for the American College of Gastroenterology. *Am. J. Gastroenterol.,* **1998,** *93:*2022–2036.

Pearce, D., and Yamamoto, K.R. Mineralocorticoid and glucocorticoid receptor activities distinguished by nonreceptor factors at a composite response element. *Science,* **1993,** *259:*1161–1165.

Piper, J.M., Ray, W.A., Daugherty, J.R., and Griffin, M.R. Corticosteroid use and peptic ulcer disease: role of nonsteroidal anti-inflammatory drugs. *Ann. Intern. Med.,* **1991,** *114:*735–740.

Pitt, B., Zannad, F., Remme, W.J., Cody, R., Castaigne, A., Perez, A., Palensky, J., and Wittes, J. The effect of spironolactone on morbidity and mortality in patients with severe heart failure. *N. Engl. J. Med.,* **1999,** *341:*709–717.

Reichardt, H.M., Kaestner, K.H., Tuckermann, J., Kretz, O., Wessely, O., Bock, R., Gass, P., Schmid, W., Herrlich, P., Angel, P., and Schutz, G. DNA binding of the glucocorticoid receptor is not essential for survival. *Cell,* **1998,** *93:*531–541.

Saag, K.G., Emkey, R., Schnitzer, T.J., Brown, J.P., Hawkins, F., Goemaere, S., Thamsborg, G., Liberman, U.A., Delmas, P.D.,

Malice, M.P., Czachur, M., and Daifotis, A.G. Alendronate for the prevention and treatment of glucocorticoid-induced osteoporosis. Glucocorticoid-Induced Osteoporosis Intervention Study Group. *N. Engl. J. Med.*, **1998**, *339*:292–299.

Shimkets, R.A., Warnock, D.G., Bositis, C.M., Nelson-Williams, C., Hansson, J.H., Schambelan, M., Gill, J.R. Jr., Ulick, S., Milora, R.V., Findling, J.W., Canessa, C.M., Rossier, B.C., and Lifton, R.P. Liddle's syndrome: heritable human hypertension caused by mutations in the β subunit of the epithelial sodium channel. *Cell,* **1994**, *79*:407–414.

Vale, W., Spiess, J., Rivier, C., and Rivier, J. Characterization of a 41-residue ovine hypothalamic peptide that stimulates secretion of corticotropin and β-endorphin. *Science,* **1981**, *213*:1394–1397.

Vanden Berghe, W., Francesconi, E., De Bosscher, K., Resche-Rigon, M., and Haegeman, G. Dissociated glucocorticoids with antiinflammatory potential repress interleukin-6 gene expression by a nuclear factor-kappaB-dependent mechanism. *Mol. Pharmacol.*, **1999**, *56*:797–806.

Vayssiere, B.M., Dupont, S., Choquart, A., Petit, F., Garcia, T., Marchandeau, C., Gronemeyer, H., and Resche-Rigon, M. Synthetic glucocorticoids that dissociate transactivation and AP-1 transrepression exhibit antiinflammatory activity in vivo. *Mol. Endocrinol.*, **1997**, *11*:1245–1255.

Zelissen, P.M.J., Croughs R.J.M., van Rijk, P.P., and Raymakers, J.A. Effect of glucocorticoid replacement therapy on bone mineral density in patients with Addison disease. *Ann. Intern. Med.*, **1994**, *120*:207–210.

MONOGRAPHS AND REVIEWS

Addison, T. *On the Constitutional and Local Effects of Disease of the Suprarenal Capsules.* Samuel Highley, London, **1855.**

Astwood, E.B., Raben, M.S., and Payne, R.W. Chemistry of corticotrophin. *Recent Prog. Horm. Res.*, **1952**, *7*:1–57.

Baulieu, E.E. Neurosteroids: a novel function of the brain. *Psychoneuroendocrinology,* **1998**, *23*:963–987.

Christ, M., Haseroth, K., Falkenstein E., and Wehling, M. Nongenomic steroid actions: fact or fantasy? *Vitam. Horm.*, **1999**, *57*:325–373.

Chrousos, G.P. The hypothalamic–pituitary–adrenal axis and immune-mediated inflammation. *N. Engl. J. Med.* **1995**, *332*:1351–1362.

Clark, A.J.L., and Weber, A. Adrenocorticotropin insensitivity syndromes. *Endocr. Rev.*, **1998**, *19*:828–844.

Cone, R.D., and Mountjoy, K.G. Molecular genetics of the ACTH and melanocyte-stimulating hormone receptors. *Trends Endocrinol. Metab.*, **1993**, *4*:242–247.

Cushing, H. The basophil adenomas of the pituitary body and their clinical manifestations. *Bull. Johns Hopkins Hosp.*, **1932**, *50*:137–195.

Donohoue, P., Parker, K.L., and Migeon, C. Congenital Adrenal Hyperplasia. In, *The Metabolic and Molecular Basis of Inherited Disease.* (Scriver, C.R., Beaudet, A.L., Sly, W.S., and Valle, D., eds.) McGraw-Hill, New York, **2001**, pp. 4077–4115.

Funder, J.W., Krozowski, Z., Myles, K., Sato, A., Sheppard, K.E.,

and Young, M. Mineralocorticoid receptors, salt, and hypertension. *Recent Prog. Horm. Res.*, **1997**, *52*:247–260.

Goldstein, R.A., Paul, W.E., Metcalfe, D.D., Busse, W.W., and Reece, E.R. NIH conference. Asthma. *Ann. Intern. Med.*, **1994**, *121*:698–708.

Harris, G.W. Neural control of the pituitary gland. *Physiol. Rev.*, **1948**, *28*:139–179.

Imura, H. Adrenocorticotropic hormone. In, *Endocrinology.* (Degroot, L.J., ed.) Saunders, Philadelphia, **1995**, pp. 355–367.

Jacobson, L., and Sapolsky, R. The role of the hippocampus in feedback regulation of the hypothalamic-pituitary-adrenocortical axis. *Endocr. Rev.*, **1991**, *12*:118–134.

Lupien, S.J., and McEwen, B.S. The acute effects of corticosteroids on cognition: integration of animal and human model studies. *Brain Res. Rev.* **1997**, *24*:1–27.

Mangelsdorf, D.J., Thummel, C., Beato, M., Herrlich, P., Schutz, G., Umesono, K., Blumberg, B., Kastner, P., Mark, M., Chambon, P., and Evans, R.M. The nuclear receptor superfamily: the second decade. *Cell,* **1995**, *83*:835–839.

McGowan, J.E. Jr., Chesney, P.J., Crossley, K.B., and LaForce, F.M. Guidelines for the use of systemic glucocorticoids in the management of selected infections. Working Group on Steroid Use, Antimicrobial Agents Committee, Infectious Disease Society of America. *J. Infect. Dis.*, **1992**, *165*:1–13.

McKay, L.I., and Cidlowski, J.A. Molecular control of immune/inflammatory responses: interactions between nuclear factor-κB and steroid receptor signaling pathways. *Endocr. Rev.*, **1999**, *20*:435–459.

New, M.I. Diagnosis and management of congenital adrenal hyperplasia. *Annu. Rev. Med.*, **1998**, *49*:311–328.

Parker, K.L., and Schimmer, B.P. Transcriptional regulation of the genes encoding the cytochrome P450 steroid hydroxylases. *Vitam. Horm.*, **1995**, *51*:339–370.

Sapolsky, R.M., Romero, L.M., and Munck, A.U. How do glucocorticoids influence stress responses? Integrating permissive, suppressive, stimulatory, and preparative actions. *Endocr. Rev.* **2000**, *21*:55–89.

Sonino, N., and Boscaro, M. Medical therapy for Cushings disease. *Endocrinol. Metab. Clin. North Am.*, **1999**, *28*:211–222.

Stein, R.B. and Hanauer, S.B. Medical therapy for inflammatory bowel disease. *Gastroenterol. Clin. North Am.*, **1999**, *28*:297–321.

Stocco, D.M., and Clark, B.J. Regulation of the acute production of steroids in steroidogenic cells *Endocr. Rev.*, **1996**, *17*:221–244.

Sullivan, J.N. Saturday conference: steroid withdrawal syndromes. *South. Med. J.*, **1982**, *75*:726–733.

Turnbull A.V., and Rivier, C.L. Regulation of the hypothalamic-pituitary-adrenal axis by cytokines: actions and mechanisms of action. *Physiol. Rev.*, **1999**, *79*:1–71.

Webster, J.C., and Cidlowski, J.A. Mechanism of glucocorticoid-receptor-mediated repression of gene expression. *Trends Endocrinol. Metab.*, **1999**, *10*:396–402.

Weisman, M.H., and Weinblatt, M.E., eds. *Treatment of the Rheumatic Diseases: Companion to the Textbook of Rheumatology.* W. B. Saunders, Philadelphia, **1995.**

C H A P T E R 6 1

INSULIN, ORAL HYPOGLYCEMIC AGENTS, AND THE PHARMACOLOGY OF THE ENDOCRINE PANCREAS

Stephen N. Davis and Daryl K. Granner

This chapter provides background on the pharmacological actions of insulin, glucagon, somatostatin, and hypoglycemic agents. The discovery of insulin in 1921 allowed the previously fatal disorder of insulin-dependent diabetes mellitus (type 1 diabetes mellitus) to be treated and represents a landmark in medical history. In the first part of this chapter, the diverse physiological functions of insulin are described at the cellular and whole-body levels. This section establishes the role of insulin in the treatment of diabetes mellitus. The next section describes the pharmacodynamics and pharmacokinetics of exogenously administered insulin and highlights the benefits of intensive insulin therapy in limiting long-term tissue complications of diabetes. The chapter continues with descriptions of the pharmacology of orally effective agents. These drugs have an increasingly important role in the treatment of non-insulin-dependent or type 2 diabetes mellitus, the most common form of diabetes. The final part of the chapter describes the physiology and pharmacology of glucagon and somatostatin, with emphasis on the expanding use of somatostatin analogs in clinical medicine.

INSULIN

History. Few events in the history of medicine are more dramatic than the discovery of insulin. Although the discovery is appropriately attributed to Banting and Best, several other investigators and collaborators provided important observations and techniques that made it possible. In 1869, a German medical student, Paul Langerhans, noted that the pancreas contains two distinct groups of cells—the acinar cells, which secrete digestive enzymes, and cells that are clustered in islands, or islets, which he suggested served a second function. Direct evidence for this function came in 1889, when Oskar Minkowski and Joseph von Mering showed that pancreatectomized dogs exhibit a syndrome similar to diabetes mellitus in human beings (*see* Minkowski, 1989).

There were numerous attempts to extract the pancreatic substance responsible for regulating blood glucose. In the early 1900s, Gurg Ludwig Zuelzer, an internist in Berlin, attempted to treat a dying diabetic patient with extracts of pancreas. Although the patient improved temporarily, he sank back into coma and died when the supply of extract was exhausted. E. L. Scott, a student at the University of Chicago, made another early attempt to isolate an active principle in 1911. Using alcoholic extracts of the pancreas (not so different from those eventually used by Banting and Best), Scott treated several diabetic dogs with encouraging results; however, he lacked clear measures of

control of blood glucose concentrations, and his professor considered the experiments inconclusive at best. Between 1916 and 1920, the Romanian physiologist Nicolas Paulesco conducted a series of experiments in which he found that injections of pancreatic extracts reduced urinary sugar and ketones in diabetic dogs. Although he published the results of his experiments, their significance was fully appreciated only many years later.

Unaware of much of this previous work, in 1921 Frederick G. Banting, a young Canadian surgeon, convinced a professor of physiology in Toronto, J. J. R. Macleod, to allow him access to a laboratory to search for the antidiabetic principle of the pancreas. Banting assumed that the islet tissues secreted insulin but that the hormone was destroyed by proteolytic digestion prior to or during extraction. Together with Charles H. Best, a fourth-year medical student, he attempted to overcome the problem by tying the pancreatic ducts. The acinar tissue degenerated, leaving the islets undisturbed; the remaining tissue was then extracted with ethanol and acid. Banting and Best thus obtained a pancreatic extract that was effective in decreasing the concentration of blood glucose in diabetic dogs.

The first patient to receive the active extracts prepared by Banting and Best was Leonard Thompson, aged 14 (Banting *et al.,* 1922). He appeared at the Toronto General Hospital with a blood glucose level of 500 mg/dl (28 mM), and he was excreting 3 to 5 liters of urine per day. Despite rigid control of diet (450 kcal per day), he continued to excrete large quantities of glucose, and, without insulin, the most likely outcome was death after a few months. The administration of Banting and Best's extracts induced a reduction in the plasma concentration and urinary excretion of glucose. Daily injections were then begun, and there was immediate improvement. The excretion of glucose was reduced from over 100 to as little as 7.5 g per day. Furthermore, "the boy became brighter, looked better and said he felt stronger." Thus, replacement therapy with the newly discovered hormone, insulin, had interrupted what was clearly an otherwise fatal metabolic disorder (Banting *et al.,* 1922). Banting and Best faced many trials and tribulations during the subsequent year. It was difficult to obtain active extracts reproducibly. This led to a greater involvement of Macleod; Banting also sought help from J. B. Collip, a chemist with expertise in extraction and purification of epinephrine. Stable extracts eventually were obtained, and patients in many parts of North America soon were being treated with insulin from porcine and bovine sources. Now, as a result of recombinant DNA technology, human insulin is used for therapy.

The Nobel Prize in Medicine or Physiology was awarded to Banting and Macleod with remarkable rapidity in 1923, and a furor over credit followed immediately. Banting announced that he would share half of his prize with Best; Macleod did the same with Collip. The early history of the discovery of insulin has been reviewed by Bliss (1982).

Chemistry.   Insulin was purified and crystallized by Abel within a few years of its discovery. The amino acid sequence of insulin was established by Sanger in 1960, and this led to the complete synthesis of the protein in 1963 and the elucidation of its three-dimensional structure by Hodgkin and coworkers in 1972. Insulin was the first hormone for which a radioimmunoassay was developed (Yalow, 1978).

The β cells of pancreatic islets synthesize insulin from a single-chain precursor of 110 amino acids termed *preproinsulin.* After translocation through the membrane of the rough endoplasmic reticulum, the 24–amino acid N-terminal signal peptide of preproinsulin is rapidly cleaved off to form proinsulin (*see* Figure 61–1). Here the molecule folds and the disulfide bonds are formed. On conversion of human proinsulin to insulin in the Golgi complex, four basic amino acids and the remaining connector or C peptide are removed by proteolysis. This gives rise to the two peptide chains (A and B) of the insulin molecule, which contains one intrasubunit and two intersubunit disulfide bonds. The A chain usually is composed of 21 amino acid residues, and the B chain has 30; the molecular mass is thus about 5734 daltons. Although the amino acid sequence of insulin has been highly conserved in evolution, there are significant variations that account for differences in both biological potency and immunogenicity (De Meyts, 1994). There is a single insulin gene and a single protein

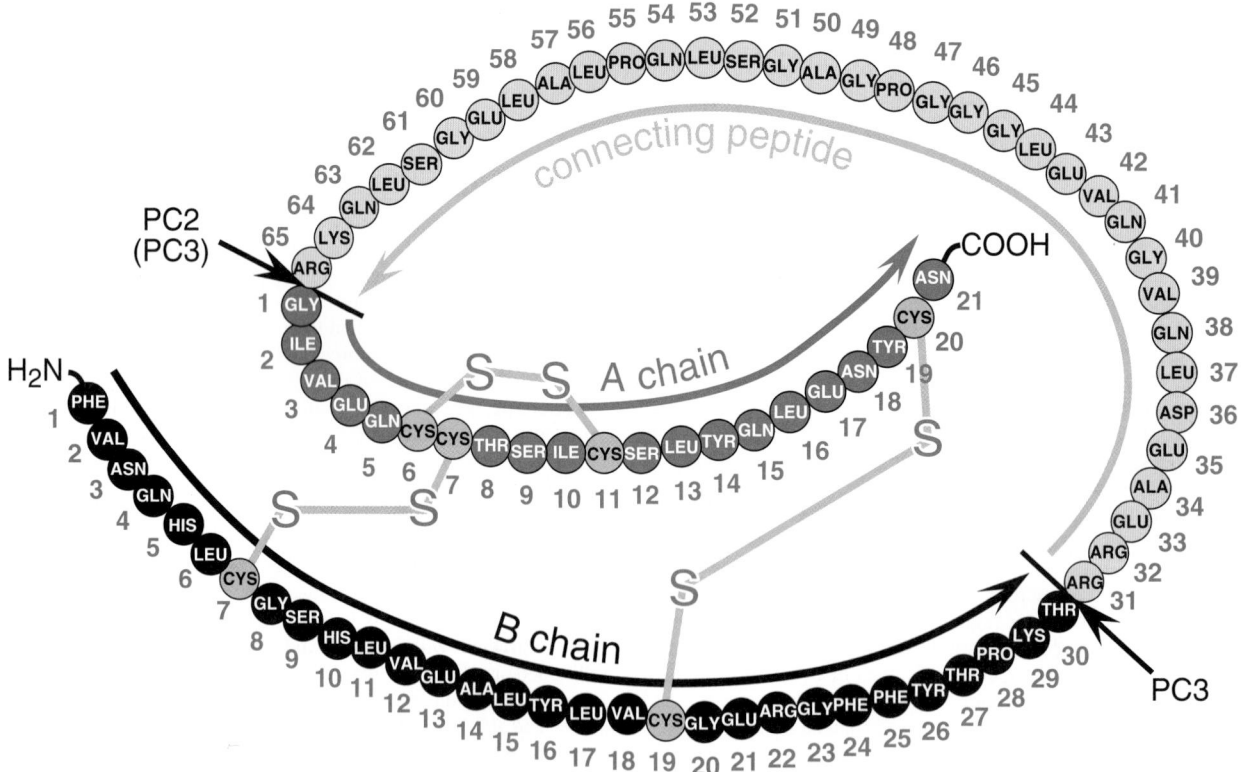

Figure 61–1. Human proinsulin and its conversion to insulin.

The amino acid sequence of human proinsulin is shown. By proteolytic cleavage, four basic amino acids (residues 31, 32, 64, 65) and the connecting peptide are removed, converting proinsulin to insulin. The sites of action of the endopeptidases PC2 and PC3 are shown.

product in most species. However, rats and mice have two genes that encode insulin, and they synthesize two molecules that differ from each other by two amino acid residues in the B chain.

The crystal structure, now resolved to 1.5 Å, reveals that the two chains of insulin form a highly ordered structure with several a-helical regions in both the A and B chains. The isolated chains of insulin are inactive. In solution, insulin can exist as a monomer, dimer, or hexamer. Two molecules of Zn^{2+} are coordinated in the hexamer, and this form of insulin presumably is stored in the granules of the pancreatic β cell. It is believed that Zn^{2+} has a functional role in the formation of crystals and that crystallization facilitates the conversion of proinsulin to insulin, as well as storage of the hormone. Traditional insulin is hexameric in most of the highly concentrated preparations used for therapy. When the hormone is absorbed and the concentration falls to physiological levels (nanomolar), the hormone dissociates into monomers, and the monomer is most likely the biologically active form of insulin. Monomeric insulin is now available for therapy.

A great deal of information about the structure–activity relationship of insulin has been obtained by study of insulins purified from a wide variety of species and by modification of the molecule. A dozen invariant residues in the A and B chains form a surface that interacts with the insulin receptor (Figure 61–2). These residues—Gly^{A1}, Glu^{A4}, Gln^{A5}, Tyr^{A19}, Asn^{A21}, Val^{B12}, Tyr^{B16}, Gly^{B23}, Phe^{B24}, Phe^{B25}, and Tyr^{B26}—overlap with domains that also are involved in insulin dimerization (de Meyts, 1994). The Leu^{A13} and Leu^{B17} residues may form part of a second binding surface (de Meyts, 1994). Insulin binds to surfaces located at the N-terminal and C-terminal regions of the α subunit of the receptor. A cysteine-rich region in the receptor α chain appears to be involved in the binding of insulin. In most cases, there is a very close correlation between the affinity of insulin for the insulin receptor and its potency for eliciting effects on glucose metabolism. Compared with human insulin, bovine

and porcine insulins are equipotent; South American guinea pig insulin is much less potent, while certain avian insulins are significantly more so.

Insulin is a member of a family of related peptides termed *insulin-like growth factors* (IGFs). The two IGFs (IGF-1 and IGF-2) have molecular masses of about 7500 daltons and structures that are homologous to that of proinsulin (Cohick and Clemmons, 1993). However, the short equivalents of the C peptide in proinsulin are not removed from the IGFs. In contrast to insulin, the IGFs are produced in many tissues, and they may serve a more important function in regulation of growth than in regulation of metabolism. These peptides, particularly IGF-1, are the presumed mediators of the action of growth hormone, and they originally were called *somatomedins*. The uterine hormone *relaxin* also may be a distant relative of this family of polypeptides.

The receptors for insulin and IGF-1 are also closely related (Duronio and Jacobs, 1988). Thus, insulin can bind to the receptor for IGF-1 with low affinity and *vice versa*. The growth-promoting actions of insulin appear to be mediated in part through the IGF-1 receptor, and there may be discordance between the metabolic potency of an insulin analog and its ability to promote growth. For example, proinsulin has only 2% of the metabolic potency of insulin *in vitro*, but it is half as potent as insulin as a stimulator of mitogenesis (King and Kahn, 1981). This fact could be important in selecting insulins for therapy, since the mitogenic activity of insulin may contribute to an increased risk of atherosclerosis.

Synthesis, Secretion, Distribution, and Degradation of Insulin

Insulin Production. The molecular and cellular events involved in the synthesis, storage, and secretion of insulin by the β cell and the ultimate degradation of the hormone by its target tissues have been studied in great detail and have served as a model for study of other cell types in the pancreatic islet (Orci, 1986). The islet of Langerhans is composed of four types of cells, each of which synthesizes and secretes a distinct polypeptide hormone: insulin in the β (B) cell, glucagon in the α (A) cell, somatostatin in the δ (D) cell, and pancreatic polypeptide in the PP or F cell. The β cells make up 60% to 80% of the islet and form its central core. The α, β, and F cells form a discontinuous mantle, one to three cells thick, around this core.

The cells in the islet are connected by tight junctions that allow small molecules to pass and make possible coordinated control of groups of cells (Orci, 1986). Arterioles enter the islets and branch into a glomerular-like capillary mass in the β-cell core. Capillaries then pass to the rim of the islet and coalesce into collecting venules (Bonner-Weir and Orci, 1982). Blood flows in the islet from the β cells to α and δ cells (Samols et al., 1986). Thus, the β cell is the primary glucose sensor for the islet, and the other cell types are presumably exposed to particularly high concentrations of insulin.

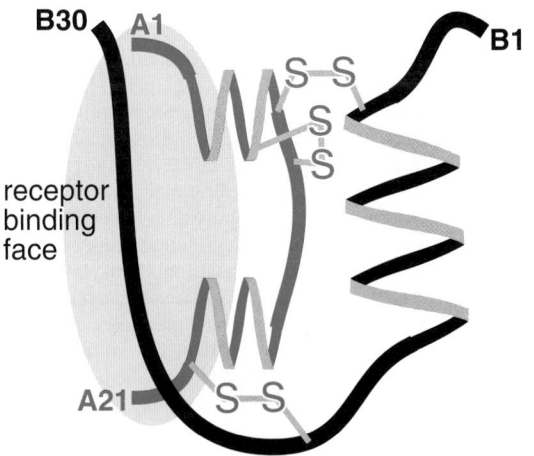

Figure 61–2. Model of the three-dimensional structure of insulin.

The shaded area indicates the receptor-binding face of the insulin molecule. (*See* Pullen *et al.*, 1976).

As noted above, insulin is synthesized as a single-chain precursor in which the A and B chains are connected by the C peptide. The initial translation product, preproinsulin, contains a sequence of 24 primarily hydrophobic amino acid residues attached to the amino terminus of the B chain. This signal sequence is required for the association and penetration of nascent preproinsulin into the lumen of the rough endoplasmic reticulum. This sequence is rapidly cleaved, and proinsulin is then transported in small vesicles to the Golgi complex. Here, proinsulin is packaged into secretory granules along with the enzyme(s) responsible for its conversion to insulin (Orci, 1986).

The conversion of proinsulin to insulin begins in the Golgi complex, continues in the secretory granules, and is nearly complete at the time of secretion. Thus, equimolar amounts of C peptide and insulin are released into the circulation. The C peptide has no known biological function, but it can serve as a useful index of insulin secretion (Polonsky and Rubenstein, 1986). Small quantities of proinsulin and des-31,32 proinsulin also are released from β cells. This presumably reflects either exocytosis of granules in which the conversion of proinsulin to insulin is not complete or secretion by another pathway. Since the half-life of proinsulin in the circulation is much longer than that of insulin, up to 20% of immunoreactive insulin in plasma is, in reality, proinsulin and intermediates.

Two distinct Ca^{2+}-dependent endopeptidases, which are found in the islet cell granules and in other neuroendocrine cells, are responsible for the conversion of proinsulin to insulin. These endoproteases, PC2 and PC3, have catalytic domains related to that of subtilisin and cleave at lysine-arginine or arginine-arginine sequences (Steiner et al., 1992). PC2 selectively cleaves at the C peptide–A chain junction (see Figure 61–1). PC3 preferentially cleaves at the C peptide–B chain junction but has some action at the A chain junction as well. Although there are at least two other members of the family of endoproteases (PC1 and furin), PC2 and PC3 appear to be the enzymes responsible for processing proinsulin to insulin.

Regulation of Insulin Secretion. Insulin secretion is a tightly regulated process, designed to provide stable concentrations of glucose in blood during both fasting and feeding. This regulation is achieved by the coordinated interplay of various nutrients, gastrointestinal hormones, pancreatic hormones, and autonomic neurotransmitters. Glucose, amino acids, fatty acids, and ketone bodies promote the secretion of insulin. The islets of Langerhans are richly innervated by both adrenergic and cholinergic nerves. Stimulation of α_2-adrenergic receptors inhibits insulin secretion, whereas β_2-adrenergic receptor agonists and vagal nerve stimulation enhance release. In general, any condition that activates the autonomic nervous system (such as hypoxia, hypothermia, surgery, or severe burns) suppresses the secretion of insulin by stimulation of α_2-adrenergic receptors. Predictably, α_2-adrenergic receptor antagonists increase basal concentrations of insulin in plasma, and β_2-adrenergic receptor antagonists decrease them (Porte and Halter, 1981).

Glucose is the principal stimulus to insulin secretion in human beings and is an essential permissive factor for the actions of many other secretagogues (Matschinsky, 1996). The sugar is more effective in provoking insulin secretion when taken orally than when administered intravenously. This is true because the ingestion of glucose (or food) induces the release of gastrointestinal hormones and stimulates vagal activity (Malaisse, 1986;

Brelje and Sorenson, 1988). Several gastrointestinal hormones promote the secretion of insulin (Ebert and Creutzfeldt, 1987). The most potent of these are gastrointestinal inhibitory peptide and glucagon-like peptide-1. Insulin release also is stimulated by gastrin, secretin, cholecystokinin, vasoactive intestinal peptide, gastrin-releasing peptide, and enteroglucagon.

When evoked by glucose, insulin secretion is biphasic: The first phase reaches a peak after 1 to 2 minutes and is short-lived, whereas the second phase has a delayed onset but a longer duration. The exact mechanism by which glucose stimulates insulin release is not fully understood, but its entry into the β cell and metabolism is required (Matschinsky, 1996).

Glucose enters the β cell by facilitated transport, which is mediated by GLUT2, a specific subtype of glucose transporter (see below). The sugar is then phosphorylated by glucokinase. In contrast to other hexokinases, which have a wide tissue distribution, expression of glucokinase is primarily limited to cells and tissues involved in the regulation of glucose metabolism, such as the liver and pancreatic β cells. Its relatively high K_m (10 to 20 mM) gives it an important regulatory role at physiological concentrations of glucose. The capacity of sugars to undergo phosphorylation and subsequent glycolysis correlates closely with their ability to stimulate insulin release. This fact has led to the hypothesis that one or more glycolytic intermediates or enzyme cofactors is the actual stimulator of insulin secretion (Matschinsky, 1996). The role of glucokinase as the glucose sensor was solidified by the recent association of mutations of the glucokinase gene with a form of maturity-onset diabetes of the young (MODY2; see below), a relatively uncommon form of diabetes. These mutations, which compromise the ability of glucokinase to phosphorylate glucose, raise the threshold for glucose-stimulated insulin release (Gidh-Jain et al., 1993).

Insulin secretion ultimately depends on the intracellular concentration of Ca^{2+} (Wolf et al., 1988). Glucose metabolism, initiated by glucokinase, results in a change in the ATP/ADP ratio. This results in the inhibition of an ATP-sensitive K^+ channel and depolarization of the β cell. A compensatory activation of a voltage-dependent Ca^{2+} channel results in the influx of Ca^{2+} into the β cell. Ca^{2+} activates phospholipase A_2 and phospholipase C, which results in the formation of arachidonic acid, inositol polyphosphates, and diacylglycerol. Inositol-1,4,5-trisphosphate mobilizes Ca^{2+} from an endoplasmic reticulum–like compartment, further elevating the cytosolic concentration of the cation. Intracellular Ca^{2+} acts as the insulin secretagogue.

Elevation of free Ca^{2+} concentrations also occurs in response to stimulation of phospholipase C by acetylcholine and cholecystokinin and by hormones that increase intracellular concentrations of cyclic AMP (Ebert and Creutzfeldt, 1987). β-Cell adenylyl cyclase, the enzyme that synthesizes cyclic AMP, is activated by glucagon, gastrointestinal inhibitory peptide, and glucagon-like peptide-1, and is inhibited by somatostatin and α_2-adrenergic receptor agonists (Fleischer and Erlichman, 1989).

Most of the nutrients and hormones that stimulate insulin secretion also enhance the biosynthesis of the hormone (Gold et al., 1982). Although there is a close correlation between the two processes, some factors affect one pathway but not the other. For example, lowering extracellular concentrations of Ca^{2+} inhibits secretion of insulin without affecting biosynthesis.

There usually is a reciprocal relationship between the rates of secretion of insulin and glucagon from the pancreatic islet

(Unger, 1985). This reciprocity reflects both the influence of insulin on the α cell and the level of glucose and other substrates (*see* below). In addition, somatostatin, a third islet-cell hormone, can modulate the secretion of both hormones (*see* below). Glucagon stimulates the release of somatostatin, and the latter may suppress the secretion of insulin but is not a major physiological influence. Since the blood supply in the islet flows from the β cell core to the α and δ cells (Samols *et al.,* 1986), insulin can act as a glucagon-release-inhibiting paracrine hormone, but somatostatin must pass through the circulation to reach the α and β cells. Thus, while insulin affects the secretion of glucagon and pancreatic polypeptide, the role of islet somatostatin is not clear.

Distribution and Degradation of Insulin. Insulin circulates in blood as the free monomer, and its volume of distribution approximates the volume of extracellular fluid. Under fasting conditions, the pancreas secretes about 40 μg [1 unit (U)] of insulin per hour into the portal vein, to achieve a concentration of insulin in portal blood of 2 to 4 ng/ml (50 to 100 μU/ml) and in the peripheral circulation of 0.5 ng/ml (12 μU/ml) or about 0.1 nM. After ingestion of a meal, there is a rapid rise in the concentration of insulin in portal blood, followed by a parallel but smaller rise in the peripheral circulation. A goal of insulin therapy is to mimic this pattern, but this is difficult to achieve with subcutaneous injections.

The half-life of insulin in plasma is about 5 to 6 minutes in normal subjects and patients with uncomplicated diabetes (Sodoyez *et al.,* 1983). This value may be increased in diabetics who develop anti-insulin antibodies. The half-life of proinsulin is longer than that of insulin (about 17 minutes), and this protein usually accounts for about 10% of the immunoreactive "insulin" in plasma (Robbins *et al.,* 1984). In patients with insulinoma, the percentage of proinsulin in the circulation usually is increased and may be as much as 80% of immunoreactive "insulin." Since proinsulin is only about 2% as potent as insulin, the biologically effective concentration of insulin is somewhat lower than estimated by immunoassay. C peptide is secreted in equimolar amounts with insulin; however, its molar concentration in plasma is higher because of its lower hepatic clearance and considerably longer half-life (about 30 minutes) (Robbins *et al.,* 1984). C-peptide serves as a marker for acute insulin secretion.

Degradation of insulin occurs primarily in liver, kidney, and muscle (Duckworth, 1988). About 50% of the insulin that reaches the liver *via* the portal vein is destroyed and never reaches the general circulation. Insulin is filtered by the renal glomeruli and is reabsorbed by the tubules, which also degrade it. Severe impairment of renal function appears to affect the rate of disappearance of circulating insulin to a greater extent than does hepatic dis-

ease (Rabkin *et al.,* 1984). Hepatic degradation of insulin operates near its maximal capacity and cannot compensate for diminished renal breakdown of the hormone. The oral administration of glucose appears to reduce hepatic extraction of insulin (Hanks *et al.,* 1984). Peripheral tissues such as fat also inactivate insulin, but this is of less significance quantitatively.

Proteolytic degradation of insulin in the liver occurs primarily after internalization of the hormone and its receptor and, to a lesser extent, at the cell surface (Berman *et al.,* 1980). The primary pathway for internalization is receptor-mediated endocytosis. The complex of insulin and its receptor is internalized into small vesicles termed *endosomes,* where degradation is initiated (Duckworth, 1988). Some insulin also is delivered to lysosomes for degradation.

The extent to which internalized insulin is degraded by the cell varies considerably with the cell type. In hepatocytes, over 50% of the internalized insulin is degraded, whereas most internalized insulin is released intact from endothelial cells. In the latter case, this finding appears to be related to the role of these cells in transcytosis of insulin molecules from the intravascular to the extracellular space (King and Johnson, 1985). Transcytosis has an important role in the delivery of insulin to its target cells in tissues where endothelial cells form tight junctions, including skeletal muscle and adipose tissue.

Several enzymes have been implicated in insulin degradation. The primary insulin-degrading enzyme is a thiol metalloproteinase. It is primarily localized in hepatocytes (Shii and Roth, 1986), but immunologically related molecules also have been found in muscle, kidney, and brain (Duckworth, 1988). Most insulin-degrading enzyme activity appears to be cytosolic, raising the question of how the internalized, vesicular insulin becomes associated with the degrading enzyme, although this activity also has been found in endosomes (Hamel *et al.,* 1991). A second insulin-degrading enzyme also has been described (Authier *et al.,* 1994). The relative roles of these enzymes have not been established. Insulin-degrading enzyme also may have a role in the degradation of other hormones, including glucagon.

Molecular Mechanisms of Insulin Action

Cellular Actions of Insulin. Insulin elicits a remarkable array of biological responses. The important target tissues for regulation of glucose homeostasis by insulin are liver, muscle, and fat, but insulin exerts potent regulatory effects on other cell types as well. Insulin is the primary hormone responsible for controlling the uptake, utilization, and storage of cellular nutrients. Insulin's anabolic actions include the stimulation of intracellular utilization and storage of glucose, amino acids, and fatty acids, while it inhibits catabolic processes, such as the breakdown of glycogen, fat, and protein. It accomplishes these general purposes by stimulating the transport of substrates and ions into cells, promoting the translocation of proteins between cellular compartments, activating and inactivating specific enzymes, and changing the amounts of proteins by altering the rates of gene transcription and specific mRNA translation (*see* Figure 61–3).

Some effects of insulin occur within seconds or minutes, including the activation of glucose and ion transport systems, the covalent modification (*i.e.,* phosphorylation or dephosphorylation) of enzymes, and some effects on gene transcription (*i.e.,* inhibition of the phosphoenolpyruvate carboxykinase gene) (Granner, 1987; O'Brien and Granner, 1996). Other effects, such as those on protein synthesis and gene transcription, may take a few hours. Effects of insulin on cell proliferation and differentiation may take days. It is not clear whether these kinetic differences result from the use of different mechanistic pathways or from the intrinsic kinetics of the various processes.

Regulation of Glucose Transport.   Stimulation of glucose transport into muscle and adipose tissue is a crucial component of the physiological response to insulin. Glucose enters cells by facilitated diffusion through one of a family of glucose transporters. Five of these (GLUT1 through GLUT5) are thought to be involved in Na$^+$-independent facilitated diffusion of glucose into cells (Shepherd and Kahn, 1999). The glucose transporters are integral membrane glycoproteins with molecular masses of about 50,000 daltons, and each has 12 membrane-spanning α-helical domains. Insulin stimulates glucose transport at least in part by promoting the energy-dependent translocation of intracellular vesicles that contain the GLUT4 and GLUT1 glucose transporters to the plasma membrane (Suzuki and Kono, 1980; Simpson and Cushman, 1986; *see* Figure 61–3). This effect is reversible; the transporters return to the intracellular pool upon removal of insulin. Faulty regulation of this process may contribute to the pathophysiology of type 2 diabetes (Shepherd and Kahn, 1999).

Regulation of Glucose Metabolism.   The facilitated diffusion of glucose into cells along a downhill gradient is assured by glucose phosphorylation. This enzymatic reaction, the conversion of glucose to glucose 6-phosphate (G6P), is accomplished by one of a family of hexokinases. The four hexokinases (I through IV), like the glucose

transporters, are distributed differently in tissues, and two are regulated by insulin. Hexokinase IV, a 50,000-dalton enzyme more commonly known as glucokinase, is found in association with GLUT2 in liver and pancreatic β cells. There is one glucokinase gene, but different first exons and promoters are employed in the two tissues (Printz *et al.,* 1993a). The liver glucokinase gene is regulated by insulin (Magnuson *et al.,* 1989). Hexokinase II, a 100,000-dalton enzyme, is found in association with GLUT4 in skeletal and cardiac muscle and in adipose tissue. Like GLUT4, hexokinase II is regulated at the transcriptional level by insulin (Printz *et al.,* 1993b).

G6P is a branch-point substrate. It can enter the glycolytic pathway and lead to the production of ATP through a series of enzymatic reactions, many of which are promoted by insulin. The effects of insulin on this pathway are exerted on gene transcription or through alteration of enzyme activity by phosphorylation or dephosphorylation on serine and/or threonine residues. Alternatively, G6P can be incorporated into glycogen after isomerization to glucose 1-phosphate (G1P). Insulin promotes glycogen deposition by stimulating the activity of glycogen synthase, the rate-limiting enzyme in glycogen synthesis, and by inhibiting phosphorylase, the rate-controlling enzyme in glycogen degradation. As in glycolysis, these effects of insulin are mediated through changes in the phosphorylation state of the enzymes. Covalent modification by phosphorylation/dephosphorylation is a major mechanism of action of insulin. For example, phosphorylation increases the activity of acetyl-CoA carboxylase and citrate lyase, whereas glycogen synthase and pyruvate dehydrogenase are activated by dephosphorylation. The latter occurs as a result of the activation of phosphatases by insulin. Dozens of proteins are so modified, with resulting changes in their activity (Denton, 1986).

Regulation of Gene Transcription.   It is now clear that a major action of insulin is the regulation of transcription of specific genes. The first example of this activity to be identified was the inhibition of phosphoenolpyruvate carboxykinase transcription by insulin (Granner *et al.,* 1983). This finding helped explain how insulin inhibits gluconeogenesis (Sasaki *et al.,* 1984) and may explain why the liver overproduces glucose in the insulin-resistant state that is characteristic of non-insulin-dependent diabetes mellitus (Granner and O'Brien, 1992). There are now more than 100 examples of genes that are regulated by insulin (O'Brien and Granner, 1996), and the list continues to grow. The exact mechanism by which these effects are accomplished is not known.

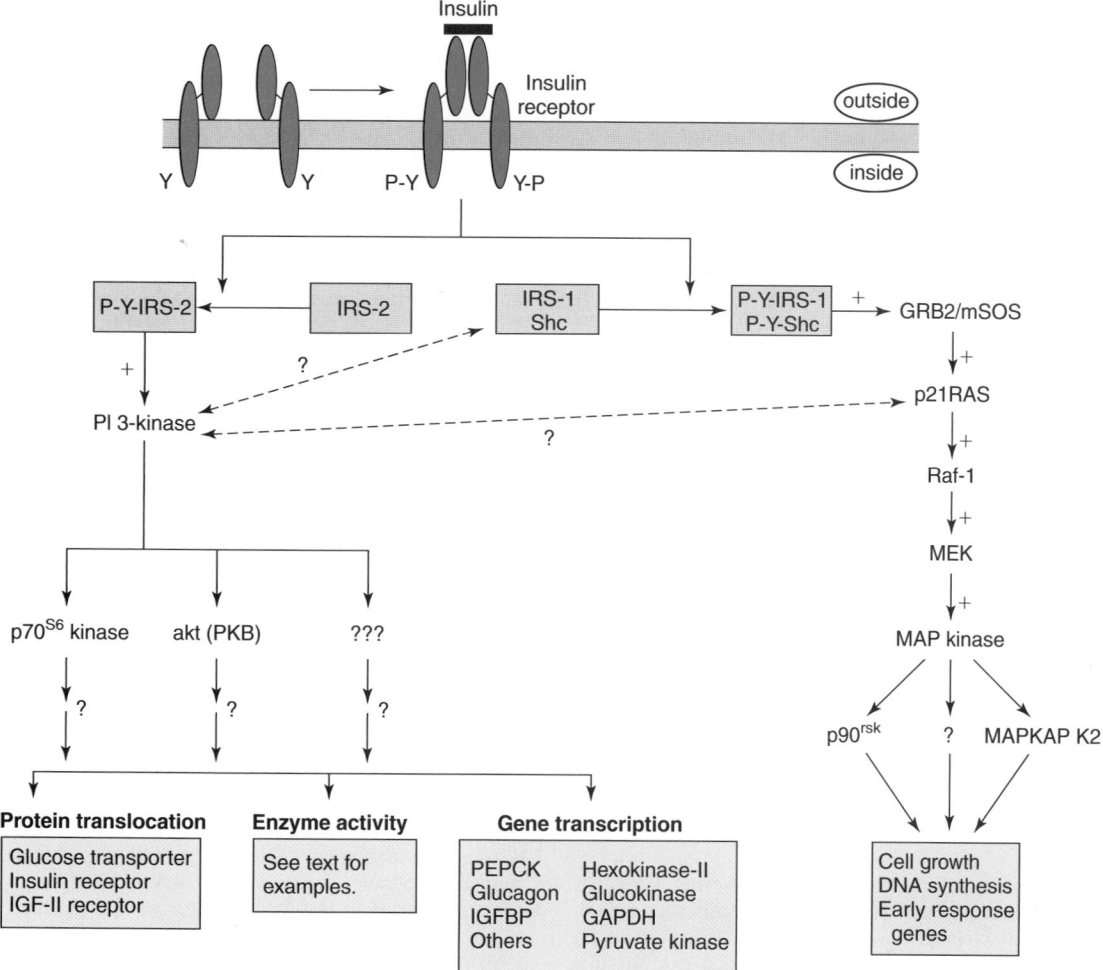

Figure 61–3. Model of insulin action at the cellular and molecular level.

Insulin signaling pathways. Binding of insulin to its specific cell-membrane receptor results in a cascade of intracellular events. The stimulation of the intrinsic tyrosine kinase activity of the insulin receptor marks the initial event, resulting in increased tyrosine phosphorylation ($Y \rightarrow Y\text{-}P$) of both the receptor and specific signaling molecules. This increase in phosphotyrosine stimulates the activity of many intracellular molecules such as GTPases, protein kinases, and lipid kinases, all of which have a role to play in certain metabolic actions of insulin. The two best-described pathways are shown. First, phosphorylation of IRS-2 results in the activation of the lipid kinase, PI 3-kinase, and generates novel inositol lipids that may act as "second messenger" molecules, which, in turn, activate a variety of poorly described signaling pathways (*e.g.,* $p70^{S6}$ kinase). Second, phophorylation of IRS-1 results in the activation of the small GTPase, p21RAS, and stimulates a protein kinase cascade that activates the p42/p44 MAP kinase isoforms, protein kinases that are important in the regulation of proliferation and differentiation of several cell types. Each of these cascades may influence different physiological processes, as shown. (IRS-1, insulin receptor substrate-1; IRS-2, insulin receptor substrate-2; GRB2, growth factor receptor binding protein 2; mSOS, mammalian son of sevenless; MEK, MAP kinase kinase and ERK kinase; MAP kinase, mitogen-activated protein kinase; $p90^{rsk}$, p90 ribosomal protein S6 kinase; MAPKAP K2, MAP kinase-activated protein kinase-2; PI 3-kinase, phosphatidylinositol 3-kinase; $p70^{S6}$, p70 ribosomal protein S6 kinase; akt (PKB), protein kinase B.) (Modified from Granner, 2000, with permission.)

The Insulin Receptor. Insulin initiates its actions by binding to a cell-surface receptor. Such receptors are present in virtually all mammalian cells, including not only the classic targets for insulin action (liver, muscle, and fat) but also such nonclassic targets as circulating blood cells, brain cells, and gonadal cells. The number of receptors varies from as few as 40 per cell on erythrocytes to 300,000 per cell on adipocytes and hepatocytes.

The insulin receptor is a large transmembrane glycoprotein composed of two 135,000-dalton α subunits (719 or 731 amino acids, depending on whether a 12-amino-acid insertion has occurred through alternate splicing of mRNA) and two 95,000-dalton β subunits (620 amino acids); the subunits are linked by disulfide bonds to form a β-α-α-β heterotetramer (Figure 61–3) (Virkamäki *et al.*, 1999). Both subunits are derived from a single-chain precursor molecule that contains the entire sequence of the α and β subunits, separated by a processing site consisting of four basic amino acid residues. These two subunits are specialized to perform the two functions of the receptor. The α subunits are entirely extracellular and contain the insulin-binding domain (*see* above), while the β subunits are transmembrane proteins that possess tyrosine protein kinase activity. After insulin is bound, receptors aggregate and are rapidly internalized. Since bivalent (but not monovalent) anti-insulin receptor antibodies cross-link adjacent receptors and mimic the rapid actions of insulin, it has been suggested that aggregation of the receptor is essential for signal transduction. After internalization, the receptor may be degraded or recycled back to the cell surface.

Tyrosine Phosphorylation and the Insulin Action Cascade. The insulin receptor and the receptors for several other growth factors are ligand-activated tyrosine protein kinases (Virkamäki *et al.*, 1999). Other growth factor receptors that exhibit such activity include those for epidermal growth factor (EGF), IGF-I, platelet-derived growth factor (PDGF), and colony-stimulating factor-1 (Yarden and Ullrich, 1988). The large family of tyrosine protein kinases also includes several retrovirus-encoded proteins that cause cellular transformation (*e.g.*, Src).

Binding of hormone to the α subunits of the heterotetrameric insulin receptor leads to the rapid intramolecular autophosphorylation of several tyrosine residues in the β subunits. Phosphorylation of the receptor is autocatalytic and results in substantial enhancement of the receptor's tyrosine kinase activity toward other substrates. In intact cells, the insulin receptor also is phosphorylated on serine and threonine residues, presumably by protein kinase C and cyclic AMP-dependent protein kinase. Such phosphorylation inhibits the tyrosine kinase activity of the insulin receptor (Cheatham and Kahn, 1995).

The tyrosine kinase activity of the insulin receptor is required for signal transduction. Mutation of the insulin receptor with modification of the ATP-binding site or replacement of the tyrosine residues at major sites of autophosphorylation results in a decrease both of insulin-stimulated kinase activity and of the cellular response to insulin (Ellis *et al.*, 1986). An insulin receptor incapable of autophosphorylation is biologically inert.

The activated receptor kinase initiates a cascade of events by first phosphorylating one of a family of proteins called insulin receptor substrates (IRS-1 to 4) (White, *et al.*, 1985). Phosphorylated IRS-2 serves as a docking protein for other proteins that contain so-called Src homology 2 (SH2) domains. One of these SH2-domain proteins is phosphoinositide (PI) 3-kinase. PI 3-kinase is a heterodimer consisting of a 110,000-dalton (p110) catalytic subunit and an 85,000-dalton (p85) regulatory subunit. The p85 subunit contains two SH2 domains, and these bind to IRS-1. PI 3-kinase catalyzes the addition of phosphate to phosphoinositides on the 3-position of the D-*myo*-inositol ring, and these compounds apparently are involved in signal transduction. PI 3-kinase is activated by a number of hormones that stimulate mitogenesis, including PDGF, EGF, and interleukin-4 (IL-4) (Virkamäki *et al.*, 1999). PI 3-kinase is not thought to be the final mediator of mitogenesis; other steps, including the activation of one or more kinases, including protein kinase B (akt/PKB), appear to be involved.

The Ras oncoprotein is one of the most potent mitogens. Ras has been linked to the insulin-action pathway because it is known to activate the cascade of mitogen-activated protein (MAP) kinases, and the MAP kinases are among the many that insulin is known to activate (Avruch *et al.*, 1994). The biochemistry of this association has been clarified. Although many points remain obscure, activation of receptor tyrosine kinases, such as the insulin receptor, result in the association of another SH2 domain-containing protein, Grb2, with phosphorylated IRS-1. Grb2 binds to the guanine nucleotide exchange factor mSOS, and this complex increases the affinity of Ras for GTP. Activated Ras binds to Raf-1, a serine/threonine protein kinase that activates the MAP kinase cascade. Alternatively, the SH2 domain-containing protein Shc is phosphorylated by the activated insulin receptor. Phospho-Shc also binds to Grb2 and activates the MAP kinase cascade through Ras and Raf-1, presumably by enhancing mSOS association with the surface membrane. Although the exact mechanism of mitogenesis in response to insulin is unclear, it appears that multiple, and possibly redundant, pathways are involved (Avruch *et al.*, 1994).

The metabolic actions of insulin appear to be mediated by the IRS-2 pathway. Translocation of the adipocyte and muscle cell glucose transporter, and attendant increases in glucose uptake, are a major action of the hormone. Translocation of the glucose transporter is inhibited by wortmannin, which is an inhibitor of PI 3-kinase. The effects of insulin on metabolic gene transcription also are inhibited by wortmannin, and presumably are mediated by the IRS-2 pathway and downstream targets of PI 3-kinase.

Diabetes Mellitus and the Physiological Effects of Insulin

Diabetes mellitus is a group of syndromes characterized by hyperglycemia; altered metabolism of lipids, carbohydrates, and proteins; and an increased risk of complications from vascular disease. Most patients can be classified clinically as having either type 1 diabetes mellitus (type 1 DM, formerly known as insulin-dependent diabetes or IDDM) or type 2 diabetes mellitus (type 2 DM, formerly known as non-insulin-dependent diabetes or NIDDM) (Alberti and

Table 61–1
Different Forms of Diabetes Mellitus

General—genetic and other factors not precisely defined

  Type 1 diabetes mellitus (formerly called insulin-dependent diabetes mellitus, or IDDM)

    Autoimmune type 1 diabetes mellitus (type 1A)

    Non-autoimmune or idiopathic type 1 diabetes mellitus (type 1B)

  Type 2 diabetes mellitus (formerly called non-insulin-dependent diabetes mellitus or NIDDM)

Specific—defined gene mutations

  Maturity-onset diabetes of youth (MODY)

    MODY 1 hepatic nuclear factor 4α gene mutations

    MODY 2 glucokinase gene mutations

    MODY 3 hepatic nuclear factor 1α gene mutations

    MODY 4 pancreatic determining factor $\times$ gene mutations

    MODY X unidentified gene mutation(s)

  Maternally inherited diabetes and deafness (MIDD)

    Mitochondrial leucine tRNA gene mutations

  Insulin gene mutations

  Insulin receptor gene mutations

Diabetes secondary to pancreatic disease

  Chronic pancreatitis

  Surgery

  Tropical diabetes (chronic pancreatitis associated with nutritional and/or toxic factors)

Diabetes secondary to other endocrinopathies

  Cushing's disease

  Glucocorticoid administration

  Acromegaly

Diabetes secondary to immune suppression

Diabetes associated with genetic syndromes; *e.g.,* **Prader-Willi syndrome**

Diabetes associated with drug therapy (*see* **Table 61–5**)

Zimmet, 1998; Expert Committee, 1997). Diabetes mellitus or carbohydrate intolerance also is associated with certain other conditions or syndromes (*see* Table 61–1).

The incidence of each type of diabetes varies widely throughout the world. In the United States, about 5% to 10% of all diabetic patients have type 1 DM, with an incidence of 18 per 100,000 inhabitants per year. This is similar to the incidence found in the United Kingdom (17 per 100,000). The incidence of type 1 DM in Europe varies with latitude. The highest rates occur in northern Europe (Finland, 43 per 100,000), and the lowest in the

south (France, Italy, and Israel, 8 per 100,000). The one exception to this rule is the small island of Sardinia, close to Italy, which has an incidence of 30 per 100,000. However, the relatively low incidence rates of type 1 DM in southern Europe are far higher than the rates in Japan, which are only about 1 per 100,000 inhabitants.

The vast majority of diabetic patients have type 2 DM. In the United States, about 90% of all diabetic patients have type 2 DM. Incidence rates of type 2 DM increase with age, with a mean rate of about 440 per 100,000 per year by the sixth decade in males in the United States. Ethnicity within a country also can influence the incidence of type 2 DM; the mean rate in African-American males is 540 per 100,000, and that in Pima Indians is about 5000 per 100,000. Unlike those for type 1 DM, the incidence rates for type 2 DM are lower in northern Europe (100 to 250 per 100,000) than in the south (Israel, 800 per 100,000). Although prevalence data exist for type 2 DM, it should be noted that there is an equal number of undiagnosed cases.

There are more than 125 million persons with diabetes in the world today, and by 2010 this number is expected to approach 220 million (Amos *et al.,* 1997). Some investigators expect the incidence to double by 2025. Types 1 and 2 are both increasing in frequency. The reason for the increase of type 1 DM is not known. The genetic basis for type 2 DM cannot change in such a short time; thus, other contributing factors including increasing age, obesity, sedentary lifestyle, and low birth weight must account for this dramatic increase. In addition, type 2 DM now is being diagnosed with remarkable frequency in preadolescents and adolescents.

In certain tropical countries, the most common cause of diabetes is chronic pancreatitis associated with nutritional or toxic factors (a form of secondary diabetes). Also, on rare occasions, diabetes results from point mutations in the insulin gene (Chan *et al.,* 1987). Amino acid substitutions from such mutations may result in insulins with lower potency or may alter the processing of proinsulin to insulin (*see* above). Other single-gene mutations cause the several types of MODY (Hattersley, 1998) and maternally inherited diabetes and deafness (MIDD, van den Ouwenland *et al.,* 1992) (*see* Table 61–1).

There are genetic and environmental components to both type 1 DM and type 2 DM. A number of factors place persons at high risk for developing type 2 DM. A positive family history is predictive for the disease. Studies of identical twins show 70% to 80% concordance for developing type 2 DM (Newman *et al.,* 1987). Furthermore, there is a high prevalence of type 2 DM in offspring of parents with the disease (up to 70%) and also in siblings of affected individuals. Persons more than 20% over their ideal body weight also have a greater risk of developing type 2 DM. In fact, 70% of type 2 DM subjects in the United States are obese. Certain ethnic groups have a higher incidence of type 2 DM (American Indians, African-Americans, Hispanics, Polynesian Islanders). In addition, previously identified impaired glucose tolerance, gestational diabetes, hypertension, or significant hyperlipidemia are associated with an increased risk of type 2 DM. These data suggest that there is a strong genetic basis for type 2 DM, but the genetic mechanism(s) involved are not known. A pancreatic β-cell defect and a reduction in tissue sensitivity to insulin both are required before phenotypic type 2 DM is apparent. However, type 2 DM is an extremely heterogenous disease, and it is likely that a variety of different genes are involved. In addition, environmental factors could play a role. Type 2 DM thus is considered to be a multifactorial disease. Any combination of genetic and environmental factors that exceeds a threshold can result in type 2 DM. The genetic basis for type 2 DM in a small subset of patients has been established. One-half of patients with a rare type of type 2 DM called MODY2 (maturity-onset diabetes of the young) have a mutation of the glucokinase gene as the primary cause of diabetes. Because of decreased glucokinase activity, these patients have an increase in the glycemic threshold for insulin release. This, in turn, results in persistent mild hyperglycemia. This form of MODY is familial, with autosomal dominant inheritance, and appears to be quite distinct from the usual type of type 2 DM as are the other forms of MODY (*see* Table 61–1).

With type 1 DM, the concordance rate for identical twins is only 25% to 50%; this suggests that environmental as well as genetic influences have an important role in the disease. However, the genetic factors in type 1 DM are well characterized and relate to the genes that control the immune response. There is considerable evidence that type 1 DM can be caused by an autoimmune disease of the pancreatic β cell. Antibodies to components of islet cells are detected in up to 80% of patients with type 1 DM early during the onset or prior to the onset of clinical disease. The antibodies are directed at both cytoplasmic and membrane-bound antigens and include islet-cell antibodies and antibodies directed against insulin, glutamic acid decarboxylase-65 and -67 (GAD-65 and -67), heat-shock protein-65 (HSP-65), bovine serum albumin, and tyrosine phosphatase-like protein (IA-2 or IA-2B).

Although it is now accepted that these antibodies are correlated with the clinical expression of type 1 DM, it is controversial whether or not the presence of autoantibodies can predict the development of clinical diabetes.

Most prospective studies designed to determine if type 1 DM can be predicted on the basis of antibodies have been performed in healthy first-degree relatives of diabetic patients. These studies have determined that the presence of insulin autoantibodies (IAA) confers only a small risk for the development of type 1 DM. On the other hand, the presence of high-titer islet-cell antibodies (ICA) and GAD antibodies, or ICA combined with IAA, confers a very high risk for the development of type 1 DM in first-degree relatives (Verge *et al.,* 1996).

As most of the studies aimed at predicting the development of type 1 DM have been carried out in first-degree relatives of diabetic patients, it is not known whether or not the occurrence of ICA in individuals from the general population confers a similar risk for development of clinical diabetes. Most available data indicate that the presence of ICA in individuals from the general population is associated with a lower risk of developing type 1 DM. However, as in first-degree relatives of type 1 DM patients, it may be that the presence of more than one form of autoantibody in individuals from the general population can be a more powerful predictor of the development of clinical diabetes (Bingley *et al.,* 1993). Individuals with type 1 DM also tend to have antibodies directed toward other endocrine tissues, including the adrenal, parathyroid, and thyroid glands, which can be clinically significant. They also have a higher than normal incidence of other autoimmune diseases.

There is an association of type 1 DM with specific human leukocyte antigen (HLA) types, especially at the B and Dr loci. Approximately 90% of patients with type 1 diabetes are positive for HLA-Dr3 and/or Dr4, as compared with only 40% of the general population (Nerup *et al.,* 1984). In contrast, the haplotype HLA-Dr2 appears to be negatively associated with the occurrence of the disease. A polymorphism of the HLA-DQβ chain at position 57 correlates even more closely with susceptibility to diabetes (Todd *et al.,* 1987). Type 1 DM is associated with alleles coding for alanine, valine, or serine at position 57 in the HLA-DQβ chain, while aspartic acid in this position is negatively correlated with the disease in Caucasians (*see* Dotta and Eisenbarth, 1989). These findings implicate both humoral and cell-mediated immune mechanisms in the etiology of type 1 DM.

The trigger for the immune response remains unknown. The identification of triggering agents is difficult, since autoimmune destruction of pancreatic β cells may occur over a period of many months or several years before the onset of overt disease (Srikanta *et al.,* 1983). In about 10% of new cases of type 1 DM, there is no evidence of autoimmune insulitis (Imagawa *et al.,* 2000). The American Diabetes Association and the World Health Organization subdivide this disease into autoimmune (1A) and idiopathic (1B) subtypes. Whatever the causes, the final result in type 1 DM is an extensive and selective loss of pancreatic β cells and a state of absolute insulin deficiency.

The situation in type 2 DM is not so clear-cut. Most studies indicate that there is a reduction in β-cell mass in type 2 DM patients. Obesity, duration of diabetes, and prevailing hyperglycemia potentially can confound interpretation of data, but studies that have controlled for these variables have reported an approximately 50% reduction in β-cell volume in type 2 DM patients compared to nondiabetic control subjects (Leahy, 1990). Owing to the heterogeneous nature of type 2 DM, mean 24-hour plasma concentrations of insulin in patients have been reported to vary from low to normal to even increased relative to values in control subjects. It is important to realize, however, that routine radioimmunoassay of insulin detects precursor (proinsulin) and intermediate forms of proinsulin (32/33 and 64/65 split proinsulin). Studies in which specific insulin and proinsulin assays have been used (Temple *et al.,* 1989) have revealed that "true" insulin values in "hyperinsulinemic" type 2 DM patients are, in fact, no greater or distinctly less than values in control subjects. Therefore, increased amounts of proinsulin have confounded the appreciation of subnormal insulin levels in type 2 DM patients.

In healthy persons, the contribution of proinsulin to basal immunoreactive insulin levels is low. Proinsulin intermediates make up about 10% of the total immunoreactive insulin in the portal vein. However, owing to its long half-life (about 44 minutes) and tenfold slower metabolic clearance, proinsulin and intermediates make up about 20% of circulating immunoreactive insulin. This amount is physiologically trivial, as proinsulin has only about 5% the metabolic effect of insulin (Davis *et al.,* 1991b). Nevertheless, recent data indicate that plasma proinsulin-like molecules are increased in type 2 DM to about 20% or more of total immunoreactive insulin. Furthermore, proinsulin levels increase in response to any β-cell stimulation.

Type 2 DM also is associated with several distinct defects in insulin secretion. The earliest manifestation is a loss of the regular periodicity of insulin secretion. At diagnosis, virtually all persons with type 2 DM have a profound defect in first-phase insulin secretion in response to an intravenous glucose challenge. The responses to other secretagogues (*e.g.,* isoproterenol or arginine) are preserved, although there is less potentiation by glucose (Weir *et al.,* 1986; Leahy *et al.,* 1987). Some of these abnormalities of the β cell in type 2 DM are in part secondary to desensitization by chronic hyperglycemia. The relationship between fasting glycemia and insulinemia in type 2 DM subjects is complex. Patients who have fasting blood glucose levels of 6 to 10 mM (108 to 180 mg/dl) have fasting and stimulated insulin values equal to those of euglycemic control subjects. More severely hyperglycemic subjects are frankly hypoinsulinemic. Insulin levels in type 2 DM patients with mild hyperglycemia, although similar to those in euglycemic control subjects, are in fact inappropriately low, as they should be increased commensurate with the hyperglycemic stimulus.

Virtually all forms of diabetes mellitus are caused by a decrease in the circulating concentration of insulin (insulin deficiency) and a decrease in the response of peripheral tissues to insulin (insulin resistance). These abnormalities lead to alterations in the metabolism of carbohydrates, lipids, ketones, and amino acids; the central feature of the syndrome is hyperglycemia (*see* Figure 61–4).

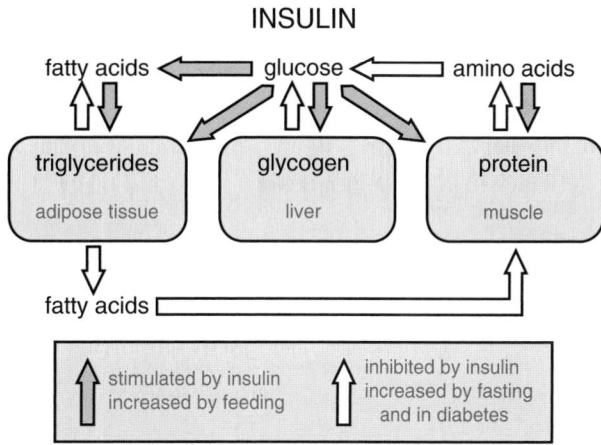

Figure 61–4. Overview of insulin action.

Insulin stimulates the storage of glucose in the liver as glycogen and in adipose tissue as triglycerides and the storage of amino acids in muscle as protein; it also promotes utilization of glucose in muscle for energy. These pathways, which also are enhanced by feeding, are indicated by the solid blue arrows. Insulin inhibits the breakdown of triglycerides, glycogen, and protein and the conversion of amino acids to glucose (gluconeogenesis), as indicated by the open arrows. These pathways are increased during fasting and in diabetic states. The conversion of amino acids to glucose and of glucose to fatty acids occurs primarily in the liver.

Insulin lowers the concentration of glucose in blood by inhibiting hepatic glucose production and by stimulating the uptake and metabolism of glucose by muscle and adipose tissue (*see* Table 61–2). These two important effects occur at different concentrations of insulin. Production of glucose is inhibited half maximally by an insulin concentration of about 20 μU/ml, while glucose utilization is stimulated half maximally at about 50 μU/ml.

In both types of diabetes, glucagon (levels of which are elevated in untreated patients) opposes the effect of insulin on the liver by stimulating glycogenolysis and gluconeogenesis, but it has relatively little effect on peripheral utilization of glucose. Thus, in the diabetic patient with insulin deficiency or insulin resistance and hyperglucagonemia, there is an increase in hepatic glucose production, a decrease in peripheral glucose uptake, and a decrease in the conversion of glucose to glycogen in the liver (DeFronzo *et al.,* 1992).

Alterations in secretion of insulin and glucagon also have profound effects on lipid, ketone, and protein metabolism. At concentrations below those required to stimulate glucose uptake, insulin inhibits the hormone-sensitive lipase in adipose tissue and thus inhibits the hydrolysis of

Table 61–2

Hypoglycemic Actions of Insulin

LIVER	MUSCLE	ADIPOSE TISSUE
Inhibits hepatic glucose production (decreases gluconeogenesis and glycogenolysis)	Stimulates glucose uptake	Stimulates glucose uptake (amount is small compared to muscle)
Stimulates hepatic glucose uptake	Inhibits flow of gluconeogenic precursors to the liver (*e.g.,* alanine, lactate, and pyruvate)	Inhibits flow of gluconeogenic precursor to liver (glycerol) and reduces energy substrate for hepatic gluconeogenesis (nonesterfied fatty acids)

triglycerides stored in the adipocyte. This counteracts the lipolytic action of catecholamines, cortisol, and growth hormone and reduces the concentrations of glycerol (a substrate for gluconeogenesis) and free fatty acids (a substrate for production of ketone bodies and a necessary fuel for gluconeogenesis). These actions of insulin are deficient in the diabetic patient, leading to increased gluconeogenesis and ketogenesis.

The liver produces ketone bodies by oxidation of free fatty acids to acetyl CoA, which is then converted to acetoacetate and β-hydroxybutyrate. The initial step in fatty-acid oxidation is transport of the fatty acid into the mitochondria. This involves the interconversion of the CoA and carnitine esters of fatty acids by the enzyme acylcarnitine transferase. The activity of this enzyme is inhibited by intramitochondrial malonyl CoA, one of the products of fatty-acid synthesis. Under normal conditions, insulin inhibits lipolysis, stimulates fatty-acid synthesis (thereby increasing the concentration of malonyl CoA), and decreases the hepatic concentration of carnitine; all these factors decrease the production of ketone bodies. Conversely, glucagon stimulates ketone-body production by increasing fatty-acid oxidation and decreasing concentrations of malonyl CoA. In the diabetic patient, particularly the patient with type 1 DM, the consequences of insulin deficiency and glucagon excess provide a hormonal milieu that favors ketogenesis and, in the absence of appropriate treatment, may lead to ketonemia and acidosis (*see* Foster, 1984).

Insulin also enhances the transcription of lipoprotein lipase in the capillary endothelium. This enzyme hydrolyzes triglycerides present in very-low-density lipoproteins (VLDL) and chylomicrons, resulting in release of intermediate-density lipoprotein (IDL) particles (*see also* Chapter 36). The IDL particles are converted by the liver

to the more cholesterol-rich low-density lipoproteins (LDL). Thus, in the untreated or undertreated diabetic patient, hypertriglyceridemia and hypercholesterolemia often occur. In addition, deficiency of insulin may be associated with increased production of VLDL.

The important role of insulin in protein metabolism usually is evident clinically only in diabetic patients with persistently poor control of their disease. Insulin stimulates amino acid uptake and protein synthesis and inhibits protein degradation in muscle and other tissues; it thus causes a decrease in the circulating concentrations of most amino acids. Glutamine and alanine are the major amino acid precursors for gluconeogenesis. Insulin lowers alanine concentrations during hyperinsulinemic euglycemic conditions. The rate of appearance of alanine is maintained in part by the enhanced rate of transamination of pyruvate to alanine. However, alanine utilization greatly exceeds production (owing to increased hepatic uptake and fractional extraction of the amino acid), and this results in a fall of peripheral alanine levels. In a poorly controlled hyperglycemic diabetic subject, there is increased conversion of alanine to glucose, contributing to the enhanced rate of gluconeogenesis. The conversion of larger amounts of amino acids to glucose also results in increased production and excretion of urea and ammonia. In addition, there are increased circulating concentrations of the branched-chain amino acids as a result of increased proteolysis, decreased protein synthesis, and increased release of branched-chain amino acids from the liver.

An almost pathognomonic feature of diabetes mellitus is thickening of the capillary basement membrane and other vascular changes that occur during the course of the disease. The cumulative effect is progressive narrowing of the vessel lumina, causing inadequate perfusion of critical regions of certain organs. The matrix is expanded in many vessel walls, in the basement membrane of the retina, and in the mesangial cells of the renal glomerulus (McMillan, 1997). Cellular proliferation in many large vessels further contributes to luminal narrowing. These pathological changes contribute to some of the major complications of diabetes, including premature atherosclerosis, intercapillary glomerulosclerosis, retinopathy, neuropathy, and ulceration and gangrene of the extremities.

It has been hypothesized that the factor responsible for the development of most complications of diabetes is the prolonged exposure of tissues to elevated concentrations of glucose. Prolonged hyperglycemia results in the formation of advanced glycation end products (AGE) (Beisswenger, *et al.*, 1995). These macromolecules are thought to induce many of the vascular abnormalities that result in the complications of diabetes (Brownlee, 1995). The results from the Diabetes Control and Complications Trial (DCCT) have definitively answered this question in the affirmative: Most diabetic complications arise from prolonged exposure of tissue to elevated glucose concentrations.

The DCCT (DCCT Research Group, 1993) was a multicenter, randomized clinical trial designed to compare intensive with conventional diabetes therapy with regard to their effects on the development and progression of the early vascular and neurologic complications of type 1 DM. The intensive therapy regimen was designed to achieve blood glucose values as close to the normal range as possible with three or more daily insulin injections or with an external insulin pump. Conventional therapy consisted of one or two daily insulin injections. Two groups of patients were studied to answer separate but related questions. The first question was whether or not intensive therapy could prevent the development of diabetic tissue complications such as retinopathy, nephropathy, and neuropathy (primary prevention). The second was whether or not intensive therapy could slow the progression of existing tissue complications of diabetes (secondary intervention).

The results of the DCCT were definitive. In the primary prevention group, intensive therapy reduced the mean risk for the development of retinopathy by 76% compared to conventional therapy. In the secondary intervention group, intensive therapy slowed the progression of retinopathy by 54%. Intensive therapy reduced the risk of nephropathy by 34% in the primary prevention group and by 43% in the secondary intervention group. Similarly, neuropathy was reduced by about 60% in both the primary prevention and secondary intervention groups. Intensive therapy reduced the development of hypercholesterolemia by 34% in the combined groups. Because of the relative youth of the patients, it was predicted that the detection of treatment-related differences in rates of macrovascular events would be unlikely. However, intensive therapy reduced the risk of macrovascular disease by 41% in the combined groups. Thus, it is clear that improving day-to-day glycemic control in type 1 DM patients can dramatically reduce and slow the development of tissue complications of diabetes. A follow-up study showed that the reduction in the risk of progressive retinopathy

and nephropathy persists for at least 4 years, even if glycemic control has not been well maintained (DCCT Research Group, 2000).

A serious complication of intensive therapy was an increased incidence of severe hypoglycemia. Patients receiving intensive therapy had a threefold greater incidence of severe hypoglycemia (blood glucose below 50 mg/dl or 2.8 mM and needing external resuscitative assistance) and hypoglycemic coma than did conventionally treated subjects. Therefore, the present guidelines for treatment given by the American Diabetes Association include a contraindication for implementing tight metabolic control in infants less than 2 years old and an extreme caution in children between 2 and 7 years, as hypoglycemia may impair brain development. Older patients with significant arteriosclerosis also may be vulnerable to permanent injury from hypoglycemia.

The DCCT was performed in relatively young type 1 DM patients. The question was asked whether or not intensive therapy would provide similar benefits to the typical middle-aged or elderly person with type 2 DM. The results of the DCCT indeed have been found to apply to patients with type 2 DM [UK Prospective Diabetes Study (UKPDS) Group, 1998a,b]. The eye, kidney, and nerve abnormalities appear similar in type 1 DM and type 2 DM, and it is likely that the same or similar underlying mechanisms of disease apply. However, because of a higher prevalence of macrovascular disease, older patients with type 2 DM may be more vulnerable to serious consequences of hypoglycemia. Thus, as is the case for everyone with diabetes, treatment of type 2 DM patients has to be tailored to the individual. Nevertheless, the results of the DCCT and UKPDS suggest that many otherwise healthy patients with type 2 DM should attempt to achieve tight metabolic control.

The toxic effects of hyperglycemia may be the result of accumulation of nonenzymatically glycosylated products and osmotically active sugar alcohols such as sorbitol in tissues; the effects of glucose on cellular metabolism also may be responsible (Brownlee, 1995). The covalent reaction of glucose with hemoglobin provides a convenient method to determine an integrated index of the glycemic state. Hemoglobin undergoes glycosylation on its amino-terminal valine residue to form the glucosyl valine adduct of hemoglobin, termed *hemoglobin A_{1c}* (Brownlee, 1995). The half-life of the modified hemoglobin is equal to that of the erythrocyte (about 120 days). Since the amount of glycosylated protein formed is proportional to the glucose concentration and the time of exposure of the protein to glucose, the concentration of hemoglobin A_{1c} in the circulation reflects the severity of the glycemic state over an extended period (4 to 12 weeks) prior to sampling. Thus, a rise in hemoglobin A_{1c} from 5% to 10% suggests a prolonged doubling of the mean blood glucose concentration. Although this assay is applied widely, measurement of the glycosylation of proteins with somewhat shorter survival times (*e.g.*, albumin) also has proven useful in the management of pregnant diabetic patients.

Glycosylated products accumulate in tissues and may eventually form cross-linked proteins termed *advanced glycosylation end products* (Beisswenger *et al.,* 1995). It is possible that nonenzymatic glycosylation is directly responsible for expansion of the vascular matrix and the vascular complications of diabetes. The modified cellular proliferative activity in vascular lesions of diabetic patients also might be explained by this process, since macrophages appear to have receptors for advanced glycosylation end products. Binding of such proteins to macrophages in these lesions may stimulate the production of cytokines such as tumor necrosis factor and interleukin-1, which in turn induce degradative and proliferative cascades in mesenchymal and endothelial cells, respectively.

Other explanations for the toxic manifestations of hyperglycemia may exist. Intracellular glucose is reduced to its corresponding sugar alcohol, sorbitol, by the enzyme aldose reductase (Burg and Kador, 1988), and the rate of production of sorbitol is determined by the ambient glucose concentration. This is particularly true in tissues such as the lens, retina, arterial wall, and Schwann cells of peripheral nerves. In diabetic human beings and rodents, these tissues have increased intracellular concentrations of sorbitol, which may contribute to an increased osmotic effect and tissue damage. Inhibitors of aldose reductase currently are being evaluated for treatment of diabetic neuropathy and retinopathy. The results of studies with these agents thus far have been somewhat conflicting and inconclusive (reviewed by Frank, 1994).

In neural tissue and perhaps in other tissues, glucose competes with myoinositol for transport into cells (Greene *et al.,* 1987). Reduction of cellular concentrations of myoinositol may contribute to altered nerve function and neuropathy. Hyperglycemia also may enhance the *de novo* synthesis of diacylglycerol, which could facilitate persistent activation of protein kinase C (Lee *et al.,* 1989).

Insulin Therapy

Insulin is the mainstay for treatment of virtually all type 1 DM and many type 2 DM patients. When necessary, insulin may be administered intravenously or intramuscularly; however, long-term treatment relies predominantly on subcutaneous injection of the hormone. Subcutaneous administration of insulin differs from physiological secretion of insulin in at least two major ways: The kinetics do not reproduce the normal rapid rise and decline of insulin secretion in response to ingestion of nutrients, and the insulin diffuses into the peripheral circulation instead of being released into the portal circulation; the direct effect of secreted insulin on hepatic metabolic processes is thus eliminated. Nonetheless, when such treatment is performed carefully, considerable success is achieved.

Preparations of insulin can be classified according to their duration of action into short-, intermediate-, and long-acting and by their species of origin—human, porcine, bovine, or a mixture of bovine and porcine. Human insulin (HUMULIN, NOVOLIN) is now widely available as a result of its production by recombinant DNA techniques. Porcine insulin differs from human insulin by one amino acid (alanine instead of threonine at the carboxy terminal of the B chain, *i.e.,* in position B30), and bovine insulin differs by two additional alterations of the A chain (threonine and isoleucine in positions A8 and A10 are replaced by alanine and valine, respectively). Prior to the mid-1970s, commercially available insulin preparations contained proinsulin or glucagon-like substances, pancreatic polypeptide, somatostatin, and vasoactive intestinal peptides. These contaminants were avoided with the advent of monocomponent porcine insulins. During the late 1970s, intense work was carried out on the development of biosynthetic human insulin. During the last decade, the use of human insulin has rapidly become the standard form of therapy.

The physicochemical properties of human, porcine, and bovine insulins differ owing to their different amino acid sequences. Human insulin, produced using recombinant DNA technology, is more soluble than porcine insulin in aqueous solutions, owing to the presence of threonine (instead of alanine), with its extra hydroxyl group. The vast majority of preparations now are supplied at neutral pH, which improves stability and permits storage for several days at a time at room temperature.

Unitage.   For therapeutic purposes, doses and concentrations of insulin are expressed in units (U). This tradition dates to the time when preparations of the hormone were impure and it was necessary to standardize them by bioassay. One unit of insulin is equal to the amount required to reduce the concentration of blood glucose in a fasting rabbit to 45 mg/dl (2.5 mM). The current international standard is a mixture of bovine and porcine insulins and contains 24 U/mg. Homogeneous preparations of human insulin contain between 25 and 30 U/mg. Almost all commercial preparations of insulin are supplied in solution or suspension at a concentration of 100 U/ml, which is about 3.6 mg of insulin per milliliter (0.6 mM). Insulin also is available in a more concentrated solution (500 U/ml) for patients who are resistant to the hormone.

Classification of Insulins.   *Short- and rapid-acting insulins* are solutions of *regular, crystalline zinc insulin (insulin injection)* dissolved usually in a buffer at neutral pH. These preparations have the most rapid onset of action but the shortest duration (*see* Table 61–3). Short-acting insulin (*i.e.,* regular or soluble) usually should be injected 30 to 45 minutes before meals (Dimitriadis and Gerich, 1983). Regular insulin also may be given intravenously or intramuscularly. After intravenous injection, there is a rapid fall in the blood glucose concentration, which usually reaches a nadir in 20 to 30 minutes. In the absence of a sustained infusion of insulin, the hormone is rapidly cleared, and counterregulatory hormones (glucagon, epinephrine, norepinephrine, cortisol, and growth hormone) restore plasma glucose to baseline in 2 to 3 hours. In the absence of a normal counterregulatory response (*e.g.,* in diabetic patients with autonomic neuropathy), plasma glucose will remain suppressed

Table 61–3
Properties of Currently Available Insulin Preparations

TYPE	APPEARANCE	ADDED PROTEIN	ZINC CONTENT, mg/100 U	BUFFER*	ACTION, HOURS†		
					Onset	*Peak*	*Duration*
Rapid							
Regular soluble (crystalline)	Clear	None	0.01–0.04	None	0.5–0.7	1.5–4	5–8
Lispro	Clear	None	0.02	Phosphate	0.25	0.5–1.5	2–5
Intermediate							
NPH (isophane)	Cloudy	Protamine	0.016–0.04	Phosphate	1–2	6–12	18–24
Lente	Cloudy	None	0.2–0.25	Acetate	1–2	6–12	18–24
Slow							
Ultralente	Cloudy	None	0.2–0.25	Acetate	4–6	16–18	20–36
Protamine zinc	Cloudy	Protamine	0.2–0.25	Phosphate	4–6	14–20	24–36
Glargine	Clear	None	0.03	None	2–5	5–24	18–24

*Most insulin preparations are supplied at pH 7.2–7.4. Glargine is supplied at a pH of 4.0.
†These are approximate figures. There is considerable variation from patient to patient and from time to time in a given patient.

for many hours following an insulin bolus of 0.15 U/kg, because the cellular actions of insulin are prolonged far beyond its clearance from plasma. Intravenous infusions of insulin are useful in patients with ketoacidosis or when requirements for insulin may change rapidly, as during the perioperative period, during labor and delivery, and in intensive-care situations (*see* below).

When metabolic conditions are stable, regular insulin usually is given subcutaneously in combination with an intermediate- or long-acting preparation. Short-acting insulin is the only form of the hormone that can be used in subcutaneous infusion pumps. Special buffered formulations of regular insulin have been made for the latter purpose; these are less likely to crystallize in the tubing during the slow infusion associated with this type of therapy (Lougheed *et al.*, 1980).

The native insulin monomers are associated as hexamers in currently available insulin preparations. These hexamers slow the absorption and reduce postprandial peaks of subcutaneously injected insulin. This unsatisfactory situation has stimulated the development of a number of short-acting insulin analogs that retain a monomeric or dimeric configuration. A large number of compounds have been investigated during the last decade (Brange *et al.*, 1990). Of the analogs tested, two, insulin *lispro* (HUMALOG) and insulin *aspart* (NOVOLOG), have demonstrated clinical effectiveness (Kang *et al.*, 1991). These analogs are absorbed three times more rapidly from subcutaneous sites than is human insulin. Consequently there is a more rapid increase in plasma insulin concentrations and an earlier hypoglycemic response. Injection of the analogs 15 minutes before a meal affords glycemic control similar to that from an injection of human insulin given 30 minutes before the meal. The first commercially available short-acting analog was human insulin lispro. This analog is identical to human insulin except at positions B28 and B29, where the sequence of the two residues has been reversed to match the sequence in IGF-1, a polypeptide that does not self-associate. Like regular insulin, lispro exists as a hexamer

in commercially available formulations. Unlike regular insulin, lispro dissociates into monomers almost instantaneously following injection. This property results in the characteristic rapid absorption and shorter duration of action compared to regular insulin. A review of clinical experience with insulin lispro has been published (Bolli *et al.*, 1999). Two therapeutic advantages have emerged with lispro as compared to regular insulin. First, the prevalence of hypoglycemia is reduced by 20% to 30% with lispro; second, glucose control, as assessed by hemoglobin A_{1c}, is modestly but significantly improved (0.3% to 0.5%) with lispro as compared to regular insulin. Insulin aspart is formed by the replacement of proline at B28 with aspartic acid. This results in a reduction of self-association to that observed with lispro. Like lispro, insulin aspart rapidly dissociates into monomers following injection.

Intermediate-acting insulins are formulated to dissolve more gradually when administered subcutaneously; thus, their durations of action are longer. The two preparations most frequently used are *neutral protamine Hagedorn (NPH) insulin* (*isophane insulin suspension*) and *lente insulin* (*insulin zinc suspension*). NPH insulin is a suspension of insulin in a complex with zinc and protamine in a phosphate buffer. Lente insulin is a mixture of crystallized (ultralente) and amorphous (semilente) insulins in an acetate buffer, which minimizes the solubility of insulin. The pharmacokinetic properties of human intermediate-acting insulins are slightly different from those of porcine preparations. Human insulins have a more rapid onset and shorter duration of action than do porcine insulins. This difference may be related to the more hydrophobic nature of human insulin, or human and porcine insulins may interact differently with protamine and zinc crystals. This difference may create a problem with optimal timing for evening therapy; human insulin preparations taken before dinner may not have a duration of action sufficient to prevent hyperglycemia by morning. It should be noted that there is no evidence that lente or NPH insulin has different pharmacodynamic effects when used in combination with regular (soluble) insulin in a twice-a-day dosage regimen (Tunbridge *et al.,* 1989). Intermediate-acting insulins usually are given either once a day before breakfast or twice a day. In patients with type 2 DM, intermediate-acting insulin given at bedtime may help normalize fasting blood glucose (Riddle, 1985). When lente insulin is mixed with regular insulin, some of the regular insulin may form a complex with the protamine or Zn^{2+} after several hours, and this may slow the absorption of the fast-acting insulin (Colagiuri and Villalobos, 1986). NPH insulin does not retard the action of regular insulin when the two are mixed vigorously by the patient or when they are commercially available as a mixture (*see* below; Davis *et al.,* 1991a).

Ultralente insulin (extended insulin zinc suspension) and *protamine zinc insulin suspension* are *long-acting insulins;* they have a very slow onset and a prolonged, relatively "flat" peak of action. These insulins have been advocated to provide a low basal concentration of insulin throughout the day. The long half-life of ultralente insulin makes it difficult to determine the optimal dosage, since several days of treatment are required before a steady-state concentration of circulating insulin is achieved. As with the intermediate-acting insulins, bovine-porcine ultralente insulin has an even more prolonged course of action than does human ultralente insulin. Doses given once or twice daily are adjusted according to the fasting blood glucose concentration. Protamine zinc insulin rarely is used today because of its very unpredictable and prolonged course of action, and it is no longer available in the United States. Preparations of insulin that are available for clinical use in the United States are shown in Table 61–4.

In the vast majority of patients, insulin replacement therapy includes intermediate- or long-acting insulin. A search for an ideal intermediate-acting insulin also has been in progress for the last 15 years. A compound that demonstrated considerable early promise in this regard was human proinsulin (HPI). Animal studies using porcine proinsulin indicated that the compound was a soluble, intermediate-acting insulin agonist that had a greater suppressive effect on hepatic glucose production than on stimulation of peripheral glucose disposal. This profile of action appeared favorable for clinical use in diabetic subjects, since unrestrained hepatic glucose production is a hallmark of the disease, and a hepatospecific insulin would tend to reduce peripheral hyperinsulinemia and the attendant risk of hypoglycemia. Early studies with HPI in human beings confirmed its relatively hepatospecific action and demonstrated that it had a duration of action similar to that of NPH insulin. Preliminary results from clinical trials, however, indicated that HPI conferred no additional benefit over currently available human insulins, and all clinical studies soon were suspended because of a high incidence of myocardial infarction in HPI-treated subjects.

Because of pharmacokinetic limitations of ultralente insulin, there is a great clinical need for an insulin analog that does not have a significant peak in its action. Considerable research has been directed to the development of such a product. Insulin *glargine* (LANTUS) is the first long-acting analog of human insulin to be approved for clinical use in the United States. Insulin glargine is produced following two alterations of human insulin (Rosskamp and Park, 1999). Two arginine residues are added to the C terminus of the B chain, and an

Table 61–4
Insulin Preparations Available in the United States

TYPE	HUMAN	BOVINE/PORCINE	BOVINE	PORCINE
Rapid				
Insulin injection (regular)	R, RB	S	P	P, C, S, PB
Lispro	R, RB	—	—	—
Intermediate				
Isophane insulin suspension (NPH)	R	S	S, P	P
Insulin zinc suspension (lente)	R	S	S, P	P
Slow				
Extended insulin zinc suspension (ultralente)	R	—	—	—
Insulin glargine	R	—	—	—
Mixtures				
20% Regular/80% NPH	R	—	—	—
30% Regular/70% NPH	R	—	—	—
40% Regular/60% NPH	R	—	—	—
50% Regular/50% NPH	R	—	—	—
25% Lispro/75% NPH	R	—	—	—
50% Lispro/50% NPH	R	—	—	—

ABBREVIATIONS: S, standard insulins: P, purified insulins; C, purified concentrated insulin; R, recombinant or semisynthetic human insulins; RB, buffered human insulins; PB, purified, buffered insulin.

asparagine molecule in position A21 on the A chain is replaced with glycine. Glargine is a clear solution with a pH of 4.0. This pH stabilizes the insulin hexamer and results in a prolonged and predictable absorption from subcutaneous tissues. Due to insulin glargine's acidic pH, it cannot be mixed with currently available short-acting insulin preparations (regular insulin or lispro) that are formulated at a neutral pH. Thus far, clinical studies have revealed that insulin glargine may cause less hypoglycemia, result in a sustained "peakless" absorption profile, and provide a better once-daily, 24-hour insulin coverage than ultralente insulin.

Other approaches to prolong the action of soluble insulin analogs are under investigation. One approach is the addition of a saturated fatty acid to the ε amino group of LysB29 (Kurtzhals *et al.*, 1997), yielding an acylated insulin. Clinical trials with such compounds are in progress.

The wide variability in the kinetics of insulin action between and even within individuals must be emphasized. The time to peak hypoglycemic effect and insulin levels can vary by 50%. This variability is caused, at least in part, by large variations in the rate of subcutaneous absorption and often has been said to be more noticeable with the intermediate- and long-acting insulins. However, more recent data have demonstrated that the administration of regular insulin can result in similar variability (Davis *et al.*, 1991a). When this variability is coupled with normal variations in diet and exercise, it is sometimes surprising how many patients do achieve good control of blood glucose concentrations.

Indications and Goals for Therapy. Subcutaneous administration of insulin is the primary treatment for all patients with type 1 DM, for patients with type 2 DM that is not adequately controlled by diet and/or oral hypoglycemic agents, and for patients with postpancreatectomy diabetes or gestational diabetes (American Diabetes Association, 1999). In addition, insulin is critical for the management of diabetic ketoacidosis, and it has an important role in the treatment of hyperglycemic, nonketotic coma and in the perioperative management of both type 1 DM and type 2 DM patients. In all cases, the goal is the normalization not only of blood glucose but also of all aspects of metabolism; the latter is difficult to achieve. Optimal treatment requires a coordinated approach to diet, exercise, and the administration of insulin. A brief overview of the principles of therapy is given below. (For a more detailed description, *see* LeRoith *et al.*, 2000.)

Near-normoglycemia can be attained in patients with multiple daily doses of insulin or with so-called pump therapy. The goal is to achieve a fasting blood glucose concentration between 90 and 120 mg/dl (5 to 6.7 mM) and a 2-hour postprandial value below 150 mg/dl (8.3 mM). In less disciplined patients or in those with defective responses of counterregulatory hormones, it may be necessary to accept higher fasting blood glucose concentrations [*e.g.*, 140 mg/dl (7.8 mM)] and 2-hour postprandial concentrations [200 to 250 mg/dl (11.1 to 13.9 mM)].

Daily Requirements. Insulin production by a normal, thin, healthy person is between 18 and 40 U per day or about 0.2 to 0.5 U per kilogram of body weight per day (Polonsky and Rubenstein, 1986). About half of this amount is secreted in the basal state and about half in response to meals. Thus, basal secretion is about 0.5 to 1 U per hour; after an oral glucose load, insulin secretion may increase to 6 U per hour (Waldhausl *et al.*, 1979). In nondiabetic, obese, insulin-resistant individuals, insulin secretion may be increased fourfold or more. Insulin is secreted into the portal circulation, and about 50% is destroyed by the liver before reaching the systemic circulation.

In a mixed population of type 1 DM patients, the average dose of insulin is usually 0.6 to 0.7 U/kg body weight per day, with a range of 0.2 to 1 U/kg per day. Obese patients generally require more (about 2 U/kg per day) because of resistance of peripheral tissues to insulin. Patients who require less insulin than 0.5 U/kg per day may have some endogenous production of insulin, or they are more sensitive to the hormone because of good physical conditioning. As in nondiabetics, the daily requirement for insulin can be divided into basal and postprandial needs. The basal dose suppresses hepatic output of glucose; it is usually 40% to 60% of the daily dose. The dose necessary for disposition of nutrients after meals usually is given before meals. Insulin often has been administered as a single daily dose of an intermediate-acting insulin, alone or in combination with regular insulin. This is rarely sufficient to achieve true euglycemia, and in view of the DCCT evidence that hyperglycemia is the major determinant of the long-term complications of diabetes, more complex regimens that include combinations of intermediate- or long-acting insulins with regular insulin are used to reach this goal.

A number of commonly used dosage regimens that include mixtures of insulin given in two or three daily injections are depicted in Figure 61–5 (LeRoith *et al.*, 2000). The most frequently used is the so-called "split-mixed" regimen, involving the prebreakfast and presupper injection of a mixture of regular and intermediate-acting insulins (Figure 61–5A). When the presupper NPH or lente insulin is not sufficient to control hyperglycemia throughout the night, the evening dose may be divided into a presupper dose of regular insulin followed by NPH or lente insulin at bedtime (Figure 61–5B). Both normal and diabetic individuals have an increased requirement for insulin in the early morning; this has been termed the "dawn phenomenon" (Blackard *et al.*, 1989). It makes the kinetics and timing of the evening dose of insulin extremely important.

An alternative regimen that is gaining widespread use involves multiple daily injections consisting of basal administration of an intermediate- or long-acting insulin (either before breakfast or bedtime or both) and preprandial injections of a short-acting insulin (Figure 61–5C). This dosage regimen is very similar to the pattern of insulin administration achieved with a subcutaneous infusion pump (Figure 61–5E), except that with a pump it is possible to control and vary the basal rate of insulin infusion more precisely (Kitabchi *et al.*, 1983).

In all patients, the exact dose of insulin is chosen by monitoring therapeutic endpoints carefully. This approach is facilitated by the use of home glucose monitors and measurements of hemoglobin A_{1c} concentrations. Special care must be taken when the patient has other underlying diseases, deficiencies in other endocrine systems (*e.g.*, adrenocortical or pituitary failure), or substantial resistance to insulin.

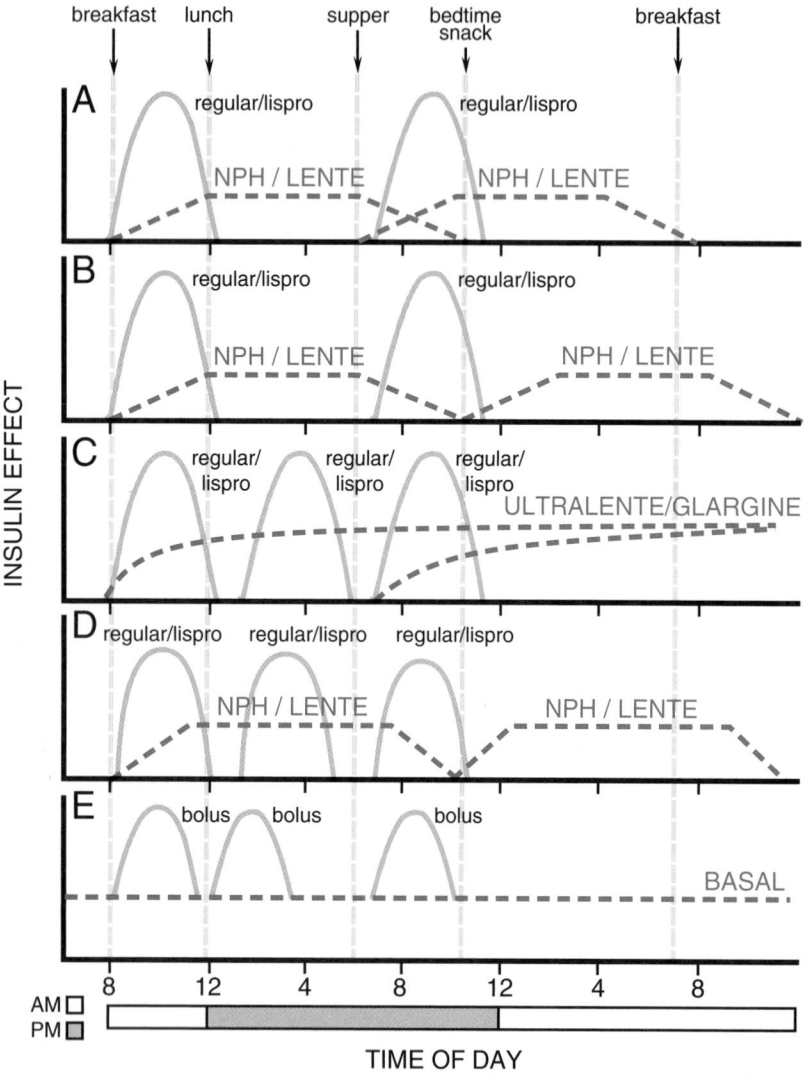

TIME OF DAY

Figure 61–5. Common multidose insulin regimens.

A. A typical "split-mixed" regimen consisting of twice-daily injections of a mixture of regular (regular or lispro) and intermediate-acting (NPH or lente) insulin. *B.* A variation in which the evening dose of intermediate-acting insulin is delayed until bedtime to increase the amount of insulin available the next morning. *C.* A regimen that incorporates ultralente or glargine insulin. *D.* A variation that includes premeal short-acting insulin with intermediate-acting insulin at breakfast and bedtime. *E.* Patterns of insulin administration with a regimen of continuous subcutaneous insulin infusion.

Factors That Affect Insulin Absorption. The degree of control of plasma glucose concentrations may be modified by changes in insulin absorption, factors that alter insulin action, diet, exercise, and other factors, many of which are probably undefined. Factors that determine the rate of absorption of insulin after subcutaneous administration include the site of injection, the type of insulin, subcutaneous blood flow, regional muscular activity at the site of the injection, the volume and concentration of the injected insulin, and depth of injection (insulin will have a more rapid onset of action if delivered intramuscularly rather than subcutaneously).

When insulin is injected subcutaneously, there can be an initial "lag phase" followed by a slow but steadily increasing rate of absorption. The initial lag phase almost

disappears when a reduced concentration or volume of insulin is injected.

Insulin usually is injected into the subcutaneous tissues of the abdomen, buttock, anterior thigh, or dorsal arm. Absorption is usually most rapid from the abdominal wall, followed by the arm, buttock, and thigh (Galloway *et al.,* 1981). Rotation of insulin injection sites traditionally has been advocated to avoid lipohypertrophy or lipoatrophy, although these conditions are less likely to occur with highly purified preparations of insulin. If a patient is willing to inject into the abdominal area, injections can be rotated throughout the entire area, thereby eliminating the injection site as a cause of variability in the rate of absorption. The abdomen currently is the preferred site of injection in the morning, as insulin is absorbed about

20% to 30% faster from that site than from the arm. If the patient refuses to inject into the abdominal area, it is preferable to select a consistent injection site for each component of insulin treatment (*e.g.*, prebreakfast dose into the thigh, evening dose into the arm).

Several other factors may affect the absorption of insulin. Increased subcutaneous blood flow (brought about by massage, hot baths, and exercise) increases the rate of absorption. In the upright posture, subcutaneous blood flow diminishes considerably in the legs and to a lesser extent in the abdominal wall. An altered volume or concentration of injected insulin affects the rate of absorption and the duration of action. When regular insulin is mixed with lente insulin, some of the regular insulin becomes modified, causing a partial loss of the rapidly acting component (Galloway *et al.*, 1981). This problem is even more severe if regular insulin is mixed with ultralente insulin. Injections of mixtures of insulin preparations thus should be made without delay. There is less delay in absorption of regular insulin when it is mixed with NPH insulin. Stable, mixed combinations of NPH and regular insulin in proportions of 50:50, 60:40, 70:30, and 80:20, respectively, are commercially available; in the United States only the 70:30 and 50:50 combinations are available. Combinations of lispro and NPH insulin also are available in the United States (Table 61–4). "Pen devices" containing prefilled regular, lispro, NPH, or premixed regular/NPH or lispro/NPH insulin have proven to be popular with many diabetic patients. In a small group of patients, subcutaneous degradation of insulin has been observed, and this has necessitated the injection of large amounts of insulin for adequate metabolic control (Schade and Duckworth, 1986).

Jet injector systems that enable patients to receive subcutaneous insulin "injections" without a needle are available. These devices are rather expensive and cumbersome, but they are preferred by a small number of patients. Dispersal of insulin throughout an area of subcutaneous tissue should increase the rate of absorption of both regular and intermediate insulins (Malone *et al.*, 1986); this result has not always been observed, however (Galloway *et al.*, 1981).

Subcutaneous insulin administration results in anti-insulin IgG antibody formation. Older, impure preparations of animal insulins resulted in far greater antibody production than do the more recent purified porcine or bovine and recombinant human preparations. It is disputed whether or not chronic therapy with human insulin reduces antibody production compared to monocomponent porcine insulin. Regardless, it is clear that human insulin is immunogenic. In the vast majority of patients receiving insulin treatment, circulating anti-insulin antibodies do not alter the pharmacokinetics of the injected hormone.

In rare patients who have a high titer of anti-insulin antibodies, the kinetics of action of regular insulin may resemble those of an intermediate-acting insulin, which itself may become longer acting. Such effects could lead to increased postprandial hyperglycemia (due to decreased action of regular insulin) but nighttime hypoglycemia (due to the prolonged action of intermediate insulin).

IgG antibodies can cross the placenta, raising the possibility that anti-insulin antibodies could cause fetal hyperglycemia by neutralizing fetal insulin. On the other hand, fetal or neonatal hypoglycemia could result from the undesirable and unpredictable release of insulin from insulin–antibody complexes. Switching from bovine/porcine to monocomponent insulin preparations has been shown to reduce anti-insulin antibodies, leading to the recommendation that only human insulin be used during pregnancy (Chertow *et al.*, 1988).

Continuous Subcutaneous Insulin Infusion. A number of pumps are available for continuous subcutaneous insulin infusion (CSII) therapy (Kitabchi *et al.*, 1983). CSII or "pump" therapy is not suitable for all patients, since it demands considerable attention, especially during the initial phases of treatment. However, for patients interested in intensive insulin therapy, a pump may be an attractive alternative to several daily injections. Most modern pumps provide a constant basal infusion of insulin and have the option of different infusion rates during the day and night to help avoid the dawn phenomenon and bolus injections that are programmed according to the size and nature of a meal.

Pump therapy presents some unique problems. Since all of the insulin used is short-acting and there is a minimal amount of insulin in the subcutaneous pool at any given time, insulin deficiency and ketoacidosis with unexpected high levels of potassium may develop rapidly if therapy is accidentally interrupted. Although modern pumps have warning devices that detect changes in line pressure, mechanical problems such as pump failure, dislodgement of the needle, aggregation of insulin in the infusion line, or accidental kinking of the infusion catheter may occur. There also is a possibility of subcutaneous abscesses and cellulitis. Selection of the most appropriate patients is extremely important for success with pump therapy. Offsetting the above potential problems, pump therapy is capable of producing a more physiological profile of insulin replacement during exercise (where insulin production is decreased) and therefore less hypoglycemia than do traditional subcutaneous insulin injections.

Adverse Reactions. *Hypoglycemia.* The most common adverse reaction to insulin is hypoglycemia. This may result from an inappropriately large dose, from a mismatch between the time of peak delivery of insulin and food intake, or from superimposition of additional factors that increase sensitivity to insulin (adrenal insufficiency, pituitary insufficiency) or that increase insulin-independent glucose uptake (exercise). The more vigorous the attempt to achieve euglycemia, the more frequent the episodes of hypoglycemia. In the Diabetes Control Complications Trial, the incidence of severe hypoglycemic reactions was three times higher in the intensive insulin therapy group than in the conventional therapy group (DCCT Research Group, 1993). Milder but significant hypoglycemic episodes were much more common than were severe reactions, and their frequency also increased with intensive therapy. Hypoglycemia is the major risk that must be weighed against any benefits of intensive therapy.

There is a hierarchy of physiological responses to hypoglycemia. The initial response is a reduction of endogenous insulin secretion, following which, at a plasma glucose level of about 70 mg/dl (3.9 mM), the counterregulatory hormones—epinephrine, glucagon, growth hormone, cortisol, and norepinephrine—are released. The symptoms of hypoglycemia are first discerned at a plasma glucose level of 60 to 80 mg/dl (3.3 to 3.9 mM). Sweating, hunger, paresthesias, palpitations, tremor, and anxiety, principally of autonomic origin, usually are seen first. Difficulty in concentrating, confusion, weakness, drowsiness, a feeling of warmth, dizziness, blurred vision, and loss of consciousness are referred to as *neuroglycopenic symptoms* and usually occur at lower plasma glucose levels than do autonomic symptoms. In a normal individual, plasma glucose levels are tightly regulated, and it is only under rare conditions that hypoglycemia occurs.

Glucagon is the predominant counterregulatory hormone in acute hypoglycemia in newly diagnosed type 1 DM patients and normal human beings. When hypoglycemia is prolonged, catecholamines, cortisol, and growth hormone become more important. In subjects with type 1 DM of longer duration, the glucagon secretory response to hypoglycemia becomes deficient, but effective glucose counterregulation still occurs because epinephrine plays a compensatory role. Type 1 DM subjects thus become dependent on epinephrine for counterregulation, and if this mechanism becomes deficient, the incidence of severe hypoglycemia increases. This occurs in patients with diabetes of long duration who have autonomic neuropathy. The absence of both glucagon and epinephrine can lead to prolonged hypoglycemia, particularly during the night, when some individuals can have extremely low plasma glucose for several hours. Severe hypoglycemia can lead to convulsions and coma.

In addition to autonomic neuropathy, several related syndromes of defective counterregulation contribute to the increased incidence of severe hypoglycemia in intensively treated type 1 DM patients. These include hypoglycemic unawareness, altered thresholds for release of counterregulatory hormones, and deficient secretion of counterregulatory hormones (reviewed by Cryer 1992, 1993).

With the ready availability of home glucose monitoring, hypoglycemia can be documented in most patients who experience suggestive symptoms. Hypoglycemia that occurs during sleep may be difficult to detect but should be suspected from a history of morning headaches, night sweats, or symptoms of hypothermia. Nocturnal hypoglycemia has been proposed as a cause of morning hyperglycemia in type 1 DM patients. This syndrome, known as the *Somogyi phenomenon*, is reputedly due to an elevation of counterregulatory hormones in response to nocturnal hypoglycemia. The existence of the Somogyi phenomenon recently has been questioned, as several groups of investigators have not been able to reproduce it. Moreover, neuroendocrine counterregulatory responses now are known to be severely diminished with disease duration and intensive control. Therefore, it is unlikely that, in patients with reduced neuroendocrine responses to hypoglycemia, nocturnal counterregulatory responses to hypoglycemia could be responsible for morning hyperglycemia. The practice of reducing nighttime insulin doses in type 1 DM subjects with morning hyperglycemia thus cannot now be recommended. It is more likely that a reduced action of injected intermediate-acting insulin that occurs in concert with the dawn phenomenon is the cause of morning hyperglycemia. The current recommended therapeutic approach to treating morning hyperglycemia is to administer more intermediate acting insulin the night before, perhaps at bedtime, or to increase the basal rate of a CSII pump between the hours of 3 and 7 A.M.

All diabetic patients who receive insulin should be aware of the symptoms of hypoglycemia, carry some form of easily ingested glucose, and carry an identification card or bracelet containing pertinent medical information. When possible, patients who suspect that they are experiencing hypoglycemia should document the glucose concentration with a measurement. Mild to moderate hypoglycemia may be treated simply by ingestion of glucose. When hypoglycemia is severe, it should be treated with intravenous glucose or an injection of glucagon (*see* below).

Insulin Allergy and Resistance.   Although there has been a dramatic decrease in the incidence of resistance and allergic reactions to insulin with the use of human insulin or highly purified preparations of the hormone, these reactions still occur as a result of reactions to the small amounts of aggregated or denatured insulin in all preparations, to minor contaminants, or because of sensitivity to one of the components added to insulin in its formulation (protamine, Zn^{2+}, phenol, *etc.*). The most frequent allergic manifestations are IgE-mediated local cutaneous reactions, although on rare occasions patients may develop life-threatening systemic responses or insulin resistance due to IgG antibodies (Kahn and Rosenthal, 1979). Attempts should be made to identify the underlying cause of the hypersensitivity response by measuring insulin-specific IgG and IgE antibodies. Skin testing also is useful; however, many patients exhibit positive reactions to intradermal insulin without experiencing any adverse effects from subcutaneous insulin. If patients have allergic reactions to mixed bovine/porcine insulin, human insulin should be used. If allergy persists, desensitization may be attempted; it is successful in about 50% of cases. Antihistamines may provide relief in patients with cutaneous reactions, while glucocorticoids have been used in patients with resistance to insulin or more severe systemic reactions.

Lipoatrophy and Lipohypertrophy. Atrophy of subcutaneous fat at the site of insulin injection (lipoatrophy) is probably a variant of an immune response to insulin, whereas lipohypertrophy (enlargement of subcutaneous fat depots) has been ascribed to the lipogenic action of high local concentrations of insulin (LeRoith *et al.,* 2000). Both of these problems may be related to some contaminant in insulin; they are rare with more purified preparations. However, hypertrophy occurs frequently with human insulins if patients inject themselves repeatedly in the same site. When these problems occur, they may cause irregular absorption of insulin as well as a cosmetic problem. The recommended treatment is to avoid the hypertrophic areas by using other injection sites, and to inject insulin into the periphery of the atrophic sites in an attempt to restore the subcutaneous adipose tissue.

Insulin Edema. Some degree of edema, abdominal bloating, and blurred vision develops in many diabetic patients with severe hyperglycemia or ketoacidosis that is brought under control with insulin (Wheatley and Edwards, 1985). This is associated with a weight gain of 0.5 to 2.5 kg. The edema usually disappears spontaneously within several days to a week unless there is underlying cardiac or renal disease. Edema is attributed primarily to retention of Na^+, although increased capillary permeability associated with inadequate metabolic control also may contribute.

Insulin Treatment of Ketoacidosis and Other Special Situations.

Acutely ill diabetic patients may have metabolic disturbances that are sufficiently severe or labile to justify intravenous administration of insulin. Such treatment is most appropriate in patients with ketoacidosis (Schade and Eaton, 1983; Kitabchi, 1989). Although there has been some controversy over appropriate dosage, infusion of a relatively low dose of insulin (0.1 U/kg per hour) will produce plasma concentrations of insulin of about 100 μU/ml—a level sufficient to inhibit lipolysis and gluconeogenesis completely and to produce near-maximal stimulation of glucose uptake in normal individuals. In most patients with ketoacidosis, blood glucose concentrations will fall by about 10% per hour; the acidosis is corrected more slowly. As treatment proceeds, it may be necessary to administer glucose along with the insulin to prevent hypoglycemia but to allow clearance of all ketones. Some physicians prefer to initiate therapy with a loading dose of insulin, but this tactic appears unnecessary as steady-state concentrations of the hormone are achieved within 30 minutes with a constant infusion. Patients with nonketotic, hyperglycemic coma frequently are more sensitive to insulin than are those with ketoacidosis. Appropriate replacement of fluid and electrolytes is an integral part of the therapy in both situations, since there is always a major deficit. Regardless of the exact insulin regimen used, the key to effective therapy is careful and fre-

quent monitoring of the patient's clinical status, glucose, and electrolytes. A frequent error in the management of such patients is the failure to administer insulin subcutaneously at least 30 minutes before intravenous therapy is discontinued. This is necessary because of the very short half-life of insulin.

Intravenous administration of insulin also is well suited to the treatment of diabetic patients during the perioperative period and during childbirth. There is debate, however, about the optimum route of insulin administration during surgery. Although some clinicians advocate subcutaneous insulin administration, more now recommend intravenous insulin infusion. The two most widely used protocols for intravenous insulin administration are the variable-rate regimen (Watts *et al.,* 1987) and the glucose, insulin, and potassium infusion (GIK) method (Thomas *et al.,* 1984). Both protocols provide stable plasma glucose, fluid, and electrolyte levels during the operative and postoperative period. Despite these recommendations, many physicians give patients half of their normal daily dose of insulin as intermediate-acting insulin subcutaneously on the morning before an operation, and then administer 5% dextrose infusions during surgery to maintain glucose concentrations. Although this may be satisfactory in some patients, use of an insulin with an intermediate duration of action provides less minute-to-minute control than is possible with an intravenous regimen. The limited data available on this subject indicate that intravenous regimens are superior to subcutaneous insulin injection in patients undergoing surgery.

Drug Interactions and Glucose Metabolism. A large number of drugs can cause hypoglycemia or hyperglycemia or may alter the response of diabetic patients to their existing therapeutic regimens (*see* Koffler *et al.,* 1989; Seltzer, 1989). Some drugs with hypoglycemic or hyperglycemic effects and their presumed sites of action is given in Table 61–5.

Aside from insulin and oral hypoglycemic drugs, the most common drug-induced hypoglycemic states are those caused by ethanol, β-adrenergic receptor antagonists, and salicylates. The primary action of ethanol is to inhibit gluconeogenesis. This effect is not an idiosyncratic reaction but is observed in all individuals. In diabetic patients, β-adrenergic receptor antagonists pose a risk of hypoglycemia because of their capacity to inhibit the effects of catecholamines on gluconeogenesis and glycogenolysis. These agents also may mask the sympathetically mediated symptoms associated with the fall in blood glucose (*e.g.,* tremor and palpitations). Salicylates, on the other hand, exert their hypoglycemic effect by enhancing pancreatic β-cell sensitivity to glucose and potentiating insulin secretion. These agents also have a weak insulin-like action in the periphery. Pentamidine, an antiprotozoal agent now used frequently for the treatment of infections caused by *Pneumocystis carinii,* apparently can cause both hypoglycemia and hyperglycemia. The hypoglycemic effect results from destruction of β cells and release of insulin;

Table 61–5

Some Drugs that Cause Hypoglycemia or Hyperglycemia

DRUG	POSSIBLE SITE OF ACTION			
	Pancreas	*Liver*	*Periphery*	*Other*
Drugs with Hypoglycemic Effects				
β-Adrenergic receptor antagonists		+	+	+
Salicylates	+			
Indomethacin*				
Naproxen*				
Ethanol		+		+
Clofibrate			+	
Angiotensin converting enzyme inhibitors			+	
Li^+		+	+	
Theophylline	+			
Ca^{2+}	+			
Bromocriptine			+	
Mebendazole	+			
Sulfonamides				+
Sulbactam/ampicillin*				
Tetracycline*				
Pyridoxine		+		
Pentamidine†	+			
Drug with Hyperglycemic Effects				
Epinephrine	+	+	+	
Glucocorticoids		+	+	
Diuretics	+		+	
Diazoxide	+			
$β_2$-Adrenergic receptor agonists	+	+	+	
Ca^{2+}-channel blockers	+			
Phenytoin	+			
Clonidine	+			+
H_2-receptor blockers	+			
Pentamidine†				+
Morphine	+			
Heparin				+
Nalidixic acid				?
Sulfinpyrazone*				
Marijuana				+
Nicotine*				

*Although these drugs are reported to have an effect on control of diabetes, there are no conclusive data about their effects on carbohydrate metabolism.

†Short-term effect is insulin release and hypoglycemia.

SOURCE: Adapted from Koffler *et al.,* 1989, with permission.

continuation of use may cause secondary hypoinsulinemia and hyperglycemia.

An equally large number of drugs may cause hyperglycemia in normal individuals or impair metabolic control in diabetic patients. Many of these are agents with direct effects on pe-

ripheral tissues that counter the actions of insulin; examples include epinephrine and glucocorticoids. Other drugs cause hyperglycemia by inhibiting insulin secretion directly (phenytoin, clonidine, Ca^{2+} channel blockers) or indirectly *via* depletion of K^+ (diuretics). A number of drugs have no direct hypoglycemic action but may potentiate the actions of sulfonylureas (*see below*). It is important to be aware of such interactions and to modify treatment regimens for diabetic patients accordingly.

New Forms of Insulin Therapy. There are a number of experimental approaches to delivery of insulin, including the use of new insulins, new routes of administration, intraperitoneal delivery devices, implantable pellets, the closed-loop artificial pancreas, islet-cell and pancreatic transplantation, and gene therapy.

New Routes of Delivery. Attempts have been made to administer insulin orally, nasally, rectally, by inhalation, and by subcutaneous implantation of pellets. The most promising of these alternatives is by inhalation, which can be achieved by addition of various adjuvants such as mannitol, glycine, and sodium citrate to insulin to increase its absorption through the pulmonary mucosa (Skyler *et al.,* 2001; Cefalu *et al.,* 2001). The kinetics of absorption are rapid and approach the rate achieved with subcutaneous administration of regular insulin. Further work is under way with the aim of reducing the size and increasing the convenience of the inhaled delivery systems. Implantable pellets have been designed to release insulin slowly over days or weeks. Although oral delivery of insulin would be preferred by patients and would provide higher relative concentrations of insulin in the portal circulation, attempts to increase intestinal absorption of the hormone have met with only limited success. Efforts have focused on protection of insulin by encapsulation or incorporation into liposomes. Intraperitoneal infusion of insulin into the portal circulation has been used experimentally in human subjects for periods of several months.

Transplantation and Gene Therapy. Transplantation and gene therapy are provocative approaches to replacement of insulin. Segmental pancreatic transplantation has been employed successfully in several hundred patients (Sutherland *et al.,* 1989). However, the surgery is technically complex and usually is considered only in patients with advanced disease and complications. Islet-cell transplants are theoretically less complicated. They have been accomplished in experimental rodent models of diabetes, and recently in a small group of type 1 DM patients along with a novel glucocorticoid-free immunosuppressive regimen (Shapiro *et al.,* 2000). Introduction of an active insulin gene into cells such as fibroblasts, which can then be reintroduced into the host, also has been achieved in rodents.

ORAL HYPOGLYCEMIC AGENTS

History. In contrast to the systematic studies that led to the isolation of insulin, the *sulfonylureas* were discovered accidentally. In 1942, Janbon and colleagues noted that some sulfonamides caused hypoglycemia in experimental animals. These observations were soon extended, and 1-butyl-3-sulfonylurea (carbutamide) became the first clinically useful sulfonylurea for the treatment of diabetes. This compound was later withdrawn because of adverse effects on the bone marrow, but it led to the development of the entire class of sulfonylureas. Clinical trials of *tolbutamide,* the first widely used member of this group, were instituted in type 2 DM patients in the early 1950s. Since that time, approximately 20 different agents of this class have been in use worldwide.

In 1997, the first member of a new class of oral insulin secretagogues called *meglitinides* (benzoic acid derivatives) was approved for clinical use. This agent, *repaglinide,* has gained acceptance as a fast-acting, premeal therapy to limit postprandial hyperglycemia.

A plant (*Galega officinalis,* goat's rue) used to treat diabetes in Europe in medieval times was found in the early part of this century to contain guanidine. Guanadine has hypoglycemic properties but is too toxic for clinical use. During the 1920s, *biguanides* were investigated for use in diabetes, but they were overshadowed by the discovery of insulin. Later, the antimalarial agent chloroguanide was found to have weak hypoglycemic action. Shortly after the introduction of the sulfonylureas, the first biguanides became available for clinical use. However, phenformin, the primary drug in this group, was withdrawn from the market in the United States and Europe because of an increased frequency of lactic acidosis associated with its use. Another biguanide, *metformin,* has been used extensively in Europe without significant adverse effects and was approved for use in the United States in 1995.

Thiazolidinediones were introduced in 1997 as the second major class of "insulin sensitizers." These agents bind to peroxisome proliferator–activated receptors (principally $PPAR_\gamma$), resulting in increased glucose uptake in muscle and reduced endogenous glucose production. The first of these agents, troglitazone, was withdrawn from use in the United States in 2000 because of an association with hepatic toxicity. Two other agents of this class, *rosiglitazone* and *pioglitazone,* have not been associated with widespread liver toxicity and are used worldwide.

Sulfonylureas

Chemistry. The sulfonylureas are divided traditionally into two groups or generations of agents. Their structural relationships are shown in Table 61–6. All members of this class of drugs are substituted arylsulfonylureas. They differ by substitutions at the *para* position on the benzene ring and at one nitrogen residue of the urea moiety. The first group of sulfonylureas includes tolbutamide, *acetohexamide, tolazamide,* and *chlorpropamide.* A second generation of hypoglycemic sulfonylureas has emerged. These drugs [*glyburide (glibenclamide), glipizide, gliclazide,* and *glimepiride*] are considerably more potent than the earlier agents.

Mechanism of Action. Sulfonylureas cause hypoglycemia by stimulating insulin release from pancreatic β cells. Their effects in the treatment of diabetes, however, are more complex. The acute administration of sulfonylureas to type 2 DM patients increases insulin release from the pancreas. Sulfonylureas also may further increase insulin levels by reducing hepatic clearance of the hormone. In the initial months of sulfonylurea treatment, fasting plasma insulin levels and insulin responses to oral glucose challenges are increased. With chronic administration, circulating insulin levels decline to those that existed before treatment, but, despite this reduction in insulin levels, reduced plasma glucose levels are maintained. The

Table 61–6

Structural Formulas of the Sulfonylureas

General Formula:
$$R_1 - \langle\text{phenyl}\rangle - SO_2NHCNH - R_2$$
(with C=O on the carbonyl)

First-Generation Analogs	R_1	R_2
Tolbutamide (ORINASE)	H_3C-	$-C_4H_9$
Chlorpropamide (DIABINESE)	$Cl-$	$-C_3H_7$
Tolazamide (TOLINASE)	H_3C-	(azepane ring) $-N\langle\rangle$
Acetohexamide (DYMELOR)	H_3CCO-	(cyclohexyl ring)

Second-Generation Analogs	R_1	R_2
Glyburide (Glibenclamide, MICRONASE, DIABETA, GLYNASE)	(5-chloro-2-methoxyphenyl) $-CONH(CH_2)_2-$	(cyclohexyl ring)
Glipizide (GLUCOTROL)	(5-methylpyrazinyl) $H_3C-\langle\rangle-CONH(CH_2)_2-$	(cyclohexyl ring)
Gliclazide (DIAMICRON, others; unavailable in the U.S.)	H_3C-	(octahydrocyclopenta-pyrrole) $-N\langle\rangle$
Glimepiride (AMARYL)	(pyrroline ring) H_3C-, H_5C_2- with C=O, $-N-C(=O)-NH-CH_2-CH_2-$	(4-methylcyclohexyl) $-\langle\rangle-CH_3$

explanation for this is not clear, but it may relate to reduced plasma glucose allowing circulating insulin to have more pronounced effects on its target tissues, and to the fact that chronic hyperglycemia *per se* impairs insulin secretion (glucose toxicity).

It should be noted that there is no measurable acute stimulatory effect of sulfonylureas on insulin secretion during chronic treatment. This is thought to be due to downregulation of cell-surface receptors for sulfonylureas on the pancreatic β cell. If chronic sulfonylurea therapy is discontinued, pancreatic β-cell responsiveness to acute administration of the drug is restored. Sulfonylureas also stimulate release of somatostatin, and they may suppress the secretion of glucagon slightly (Krall, 1985).

The effects of the sulfonylureas are initiated by binding to and blocking an ATP-sensitive K^+ channel, which has been cloned (Aguilar-Bryan et al., 1995; Philipson and Steiner, 1995). The drugs thus resemble physiological secretagogues (e.g., glucose, leucine), which also lower the conductance of this channel (Ribalet and Ciani, 1987; Boyd, 1988). Reduced K^+ conductance causes membrane depolarization and influx of Ca^{2+} through voltage-sensitive Ca^{2+} channels.

There has been controversy about whether or not sulfonylureas have clinically significant extrapancreatic effects (Beck-Nielsen, 1988). The concentration of insulin receptors increases in the monocytes, adipocytes, and erythrocytes of type 2 DM patients who receive oral hypoglycemic agents (Olefsky and Reaven, 1976). Sulfonylureas enhance insulin action in cells in culture and stimulate the synthesis of glucose transporters (Jacobs et al., 1989). Sulfonylureas also have been shown to suppress hepatic gluconeogenesis (Blumenthal, 1977); however, it is not clear if this is a direct effect of the drug or a reflection of increased sensitivity to insulin. In general, attempts to ascribe the long-term blood glucose-lowering effects of sulfonylureas to specific changes in insulin action on target tissues are confounded by the effects of a lowered prevailing blood glucose level. Although extrapancreatic effects of sulfonylureas can be demonstrated, they are of minor clinical significance in the treatment of type 2 DM patients.

Absorption, Fate, and Excretion. The sulfonylureas have similar spectra of activities; thus, their pharmacokinetic properties are their most distinctive characteristics (see Appendix II). Although there are differences in the rates of absorption of the different sulfonylureas, all are effectively absorbed from the gastrointestinal tract. However, food and hyperglycemia can reduce the absorption of sulfonylureas. (Hyperglycemia per se inhibits gastric and intestinal motility and thus can retard the absorption of many drugs.) In view of the time required to reach an optimal concentration in plasma, sulfonylureas with short half lives may be more effective when given 30 minutes before eating. Sulfonylureas in plasma are largely (90% to 99%) bound to protein, especially albumin; plasma protein binding is least for chlorpropamide and greatest for glyburide. The volumes of distribution of most of the sulfonylureas are about 0.2 liter/kg.

The first-generation sulfonylureas vary considerably in their half-lives and extents of metabolism. The half-life of acetohexamide is short, but the drug is reduced to an active compound with a half-life that is similar to those of tolbutamide and tolazamide (4 to 7 hours). It may be necessary to take these drugs in divided daily doses. Chlorpropamide has a long half-life (24 to 48 hours). The second-generation agents are approximately 100 times more potent than are those in the first group (Lebovitz and Feinglos, 1983). Although their half-lives are short (3 to 5 hours), their hypoglycemic effects are evident for 12 to 24 hours, and it is often possible to administer them once daily. The reason for the discrepancy between the half-life and duration of action of these drugs is not clear.

All of the sulfonylureas are metabolized by the liver, and the metabolites are excreted in the urine. Metabolism of chlorpropamide is incomplete, and about 20% of the drug is excreted unchanged. Thus, sulfonylureas should be administered with caution to patients with either renal or hepatic insufficiency.

Adverse Reactions. Adverse effects of the sulfonylureas are infrequent, occurring in about 4% of patients taking first-generation drugs and perhaps slightly less often in patients receiving second-generation agents (Paice et al., 1985). Not unexpectedly, sulfonylureas may cause hypoglycemic reactions, including coma (Ferner and Neil, 1988; Seltzer, 1989). This is a particular problem in elderly patients with impaired hepatic or renal function who are taking longer-acting sulfonylureas. Sulfonylureas can be ranked in order of decreasing risk of causing hypoglycemia based on their half-lives. The longer the half-life, the more likely an agent will induce hypoglycemia. Severe hypoglycemia in the elderly can present as an acute neurological emergency that may mimic a cerebrovascular accident. Thus, it is important to check the plasma glucose of any elderly patient presenting with acute neurological symptoms. Because of the long half-life of some sulfonylureas, it may be necessary to treat an elderly hypoglycemic patient for 24 to 48 hours with an intravenous glucose infusion.

A number of other drugs may potentiate the effects of the sulfonylureas, particularly the first-generation agents, by inhibiting their metabolism or excretion. Some drugs also displace the sulfonylureas from binding proteins, thereby increasing the free concentration transiently (Seltzer, 1989). These include other sulfonamides, clofibrate, dicumarol, salicylates, and phenylbutazone. Other drugs, including ethanol, may enhance the action of sulfonylureas by causing hypoglycemia.

Other side effects of sulfonylureas include nausea and vomiting, cholestatic jaundice, agranulocytosis, aplastic and hemolytic anemias, generalized hypersensitivity reactions, and dermatological reactions. About 10% to 15% of patients who receive these drugs, particularly chlorpropamide, develop an alcohol-induced flush similar to that caused by disulfiram (*see* Chapter 18). Sulfonylureas, especially chlorpropamide, also may induce hyponatremia by potentiating the effects of antidiuretic hormone on the renal collecting duct (Paice *et al.*, 1985). This undesirable side effect occurs in up to 5% of all patients; it is less frequent with glyburide and glipizide. This side effect has been used to therapeutic advantage in patients with mild forms of diabetes insipidus (*see* Chapter 29).

A long-running debate centered around whether or not treatment with sulfonylureas is associated with increased cardiovascular mortality; this possibility was suggested by a large multicenter trial (the University Group Diabetes Program or UGDP). The UGDP was designed to compare the effect of diet, oral agents (tolbutamide or phenformin), and fixed-dose insulin therapy on the development of vascular complications in type 2 DM. During an 8-year period of observation, patients who received tolbutamide had a twofold higher rate of cardiovascular death than patients treated with placebo or insulin (Meinert *et al.*, 1970). A 10-year debate followed on the validity of this conclusion, because the observation was unexpected, the study had not been designed to test this question, and all of the excess mortality occurred in only three centers. The recent UK Prospective Diabetes Study Group (UK Prospective Diabetes Study Group, 1998a), however, clearly demonstrated no excess cardiovascular mortality over a 14-year period in patients receiving first- or second-generation sulfonylureas.

Therapeutic Uses.   Sulfonylureas are used to control hyperglycemia in type 2 DM patients who cannot achieve appropriate control with changes in diet alone. In all patients, however, continued dietary restrictions are essential to maximize the efficacy of the sulfonylureas. Some physicians still consider treatment with insulin to be the preferred approach in such patients. Patients with type 2 DM whose disease is controlled with relatively low doses of insulin (less than 40 U per day) are more likely to respond to sulfonylureas, as are those who are obese and/or older than 40 years of age. Contraindications to the use of these drugs include type 1 DM, pregnancy, lactation, and significant hepatic or renal insufficiency.

Between 50% and 80% of properly selected patients will respond initially to an oral hypoglycemic agent (Krall, 1985). All of the drugs appear to be equally efficacious. Concentrations of glucose often are lowered sufficiently to relieve symptoms of hyperglycemia, but they may not reach normal levels. To the extent that complications of diabetes may be related to hyperglycemia, the goal of treatment should be normalization of both fasting and postprandial glucose concentrations. About 5% to 10% of patients per year who respond initially to a sulfonylurea become secondary failures, as defined by unacceptable levels of hyperglycemia. This may occur as a result of a change in drug metabolism, progression of β-cell failure, change in dietary compliance, or misdiagnosis of a patient with slow-onset type 1 DM. Additional oral agent(s) can produce a satisfactory response, but most of these patients will eventually require insulin.

The usual initial daily dose of tolbutamide is 500 mg, while 3000 mg is the maximally effective total dose; corresponding doses for acetohexamide are 250 and 1500 mg. Tolazamide and chlorpropamide usually are administered in a daily dose of 100 to 250 mg, while 1000 (tolazamide) to 750 mg (chlorpropamide) is maximal. Tolbutamide, acetohexamide, and tolazamide often are taken twice daily, 30 minutes before breakfast and dinner. The initial daily dose of glyburide is 2.5 to 5 mg, while daily doses of more than 20 mg are not recommended. Therapy with glipizide usually is initiated with 5 mg given once daily. The maximal recommended daily dose is 40 mg; daily doses of more than 15 mg should be divided. The starting dose of gliclazide is 40 to 80 mg per day, and the maximal daily dose is 320 mg. Glimepiride therapy can begin with doses as low as 0.5 mg once per day. The maximal effective daily dose of the agent is 8 mg. Treatment with the sulfonylureas must be guided by the individual patient's response, which must be monitored frequently.

Combinations of insulin and sulfonylureas have been used in some patients with type 1 DM and type 2 DM. Studies in type 1 DM patients have not provided any evidence that glucose control is improved by combination therapy. The results in type 2 DM patients are more provocative but inconclusive. Some studies have revealed no benefits with combination therapy, while others have shown an improvement in metabolic control. A prerequisite for a beneficial effect of combination therapy is residual β-cell activity, and a short duration of diabetes also has been suggested to predict a good response.

Repaglinide

Repaglinide (PRANDIN) is an oral insulin secretagogue of the meglitinide class. This agent is a derivative of benzoic acid, and its structure (shown below) is unrelated to that of the sulfonylureas.

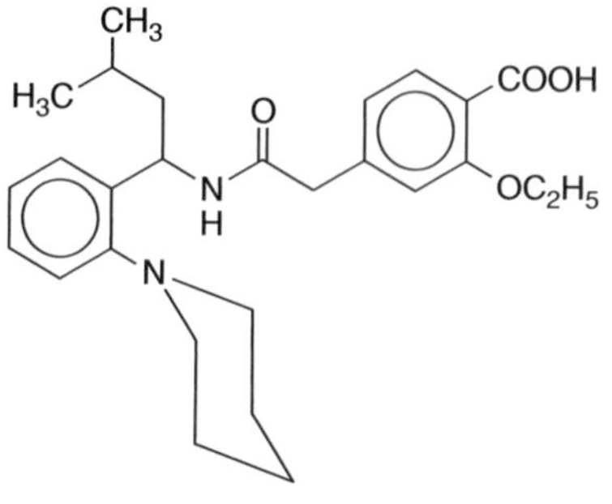

REPAGLINIDE

However, like sulfonylureas, repaglinide stimulates insulin release by closing ATP-dependent potassium channels in pancreatic β cells. The drug is absorbed rapidly from the gastrointestinal tract; peak blood levels are obtained within one hour. The half-life of the drug is about one hour. These features of the drug allow for multiple preprandial use, as compared to the classical once- or twice-daily dosing of sulfonylureas. Repaglinide is metabolized primarily by the liver. Metabolites of the drug do not have a hypoglycemic action. Repaglinide should be used cautiously in patients with hepatic insufficiency. Because a small proportion (about 10%) of repaglinide is metabolized by the kidney, increased dosing of the drug in patients with renal insufficiency also should be performed cautiously. As with sulfonylureas, the major side effect of repaglinide is hypoglycemia.

Nateglinide

Nateglinide (STARLIX) is an orally effective insulin secretagogue derived from D-phenylalanine. Like sulfonylureas and repaglinide, nateglinide stimulates insulin secretion by blocking ATP-sensitive potassium channels in pancreatic β cells. Nateglinide promotes a more rapid but less sustained secretion of insulin than do other available oral antidiabetic agents (Kalbag *et al.*, 2001). The drug's major therapeutic effect is reducing postprandial glycemic elevations in type 2 diabetic patients. Nateglinide recently has been approved by the United States Food and Drug Administration (FDA) for use in type 2 DM and is most effective if administered 1 to 10 minutes before a meal in a dose of 120 mg. Nateglinide is metabolized primarily by the liver and thus should be used cautiously in patients with hepatic insufficiency. About 16% of an administered dose is excreted by the kidney as unchanged drug. Dosage adjustment is unnecessary in renal failure. Early studies have suggested that nateglinide therapy may produce fewer episodes of hypoglycemia than do other currently available oral insulin secretagogues (Horton *et al.*, 2001).

Biguanides

Metformin (GLUCOPHAGE) and phenformin were introduced in 1957 and buformin was introduced in 1958. The latter was of limited use, but metformin and phenformin were widely used. Phenformin was withdrawn in many countries during the 1970s because of an association with lactic acidosis. Metformin has been associated only rarely with that complication and has been widely used in Europe and Canada; it became available in the United States in 1995. Metformin given alone or in combination with a sulfonylurea improves glycemic control and lipid concen-

trations in patients who respond poorly to diet or to a sulfonylurea alone (DeFronzo *et al.*, 1995).

Metformin is absorbed mainly from the small intestine. The drug is stable, does not bind to plasma proteins, and is excreted unchanged in the urine. It has a half-life of about 2 hours. The maximum recommended daily dose of metformin in the United States is 2.5 g, taken in three doses with meals.

Metformin is antihyperglycemic, not hypoglycemic (*see* Bailey, 1992). It does not cause insulin release from the pancreas and does not cause hypoglycemia, even in large doses. Metformin has no significant effects on the secretion of glucagon, cortisol, growth hormone, or somatostatin. Metformin reduces glucose levels primarily by decreasing hepatic glucose production and by increasing insulin action in muscle and fat. The mechanism by which metformin reduces hepatic glucose production is controversial, but the preponderance of data indicates an effect on reducing gluconeogenesis (Stumvoll *et al.*, 1995). Metformin also may decrease plasma glucose by reducing the absorption of glucose from the intestine, but this action has not been shown to have clinical relevance.

Patients with renal impairment should not receive metformin. Hepatic disease, a past history of lactic acidosis (of any cause), cardiac failure requiring pharmacological therapy, or chronic hypoxic lung disease also are contraindications to the use of the drug. The drug also should be withheld for 48 hours after administration of intravenous contrast media. The drug should not be readministered until renal function is normal. These conditions all predispose to increased lactate production and hence to the fatal complications of lactic acidosis. The reported incidence of lactic acidosis during metformin treatment is lower than 0.1 case per 1000 patient years, and the mortality risk is even lower.

Acute side effects of metformin, which occur in up to 20% of patients, include diarrhea, abdominal discomfort, nausea, metallic taste, and anorexia. These usually are minimized by increasing the dosage of the drug slowly and taking it with meals. Intestinal absorption of vitamin B_{12} and folate often is decreased during chronic metformin therapy. Calcium supplements reverse the effect of metformin on vitamin B_{12} absorption (Bauman *et al.*, 2000).

Consideration should be given to stopping treatment with metformin if the plasma lactate level exceeds 3 mM. Similarly, decreased renal or hepatic function also may be a strong indication for withholding treatment. It also would be prudent to stop metformin if a patient is undergoing a prolonged fast or is treated with a very-low-calorie diet. Myocardial infarction or septicemia mandate stopping the drug immediately. Metformin usually is administered in divided doses either two or three times daily. The maximum effective dose is 2.5 g daily. Metformin lowers hemoglobin A_{1c} values to a similar extent as do sulfonylureas (about 2.0%). Metformin does not promote weight gain and can reduce plasma triglycerides by 15% to 20%. There is a strong consensus that reduction in hemoglobin A_{1c} by any therapy (insulin or oral agents) can lead to diminished microvascular complications. Metformin, however, is the only therapeutic agent that has been demonstrated to reduce macrovascular events in type 2 DM (UK Prospective Diabetes Study Group, 1998b). Metformin can be administered in combination with sulfonylureas, thiazolizinediones, and/or insulin. A fixed-combination tablet containing glyburide (glibenclamide) and metformin (GLUCOVANCE) is available.

Thiazolidinediones

Three thiazolidinediones have been used in clinical practice (*troglitazone, rosiglitazone,* and *pioglitazone*). However, the first of these agents to be introduced (troglitazone) has been withdrawn from use because it was associated with severe hepatic toxicity. The structures of rosiglitazone and pioglitazone are shown below.

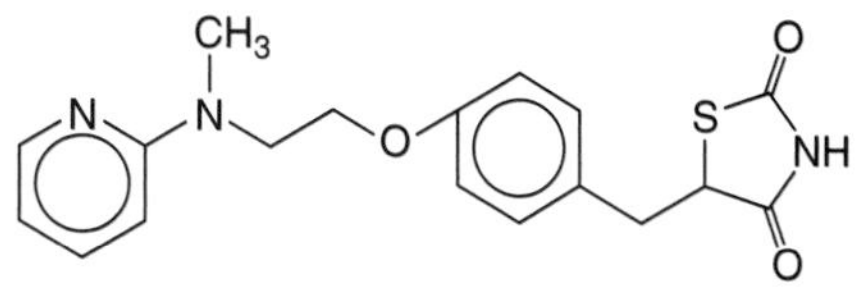

ROSIGLITAZONE

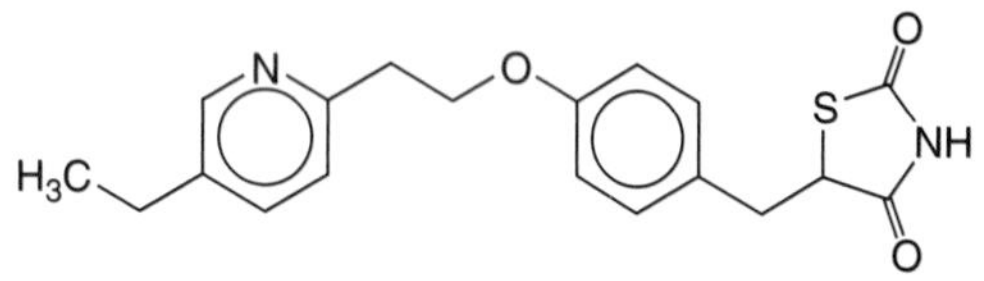

PIOGLITAZONE

Thiazolidinediones are selective agonists for nuclear peroxisome proliferator–activated receptor-gamma ($PPAR_\gamma$). These drugs bind to $PPAR_\gamma$, which, in turn, activates insulin-responsive genes that regulate carbohydrate and lipid metabolism. Thiazolidinediones require insulin to be present for their action. Thiazolidinediones exert their principal effects by lowering insulin resistance in peripheral tissue, but an effect to lower glucose production by the liver also has been reported. Thiazolidinediones increase glucose transport into muscle and adipose tissue by enhancing the synthesis and translocation of specific forms of the glucose transporter proteins. The thiazolidinediones also can activate genes that regulate free fatty-acid

metabolism in peripheral tissue. Studies are in progress to determine if these agents reduce insulin resistance primarily by their actions on free fatty-acid metabolism.

Rosiglitazone (AVANDIA) and pioglitazone (ACTOS) are taken once a day. Both agents are absorbed within about 2 hours, but the maximum clinical effect is not observed for 6 to 12 weeks. The thiazolidinediones are metabolized by the liver and may be administered to patients with renal insufficiency, but these agents should not be used if there is active hepatic disease or if there are significant elevations of serum liver transaminases.

Regular monitoring of liver funtion should be instituted in patients receiving thiazolidinediones. Thiazolidinediones also have been reported to cause anemia, weight gain, edema, and plasma volume expansion. These drugs generally are not indicated for patients with New York Heart Association class 3 and 4 heart failure.

Rosiglitazone and pioglitazone can lower hemoglobin A_{1c} levels by 1.0% to 1.5% in patients with type 2 DM. These drugs can be combined with insulin or other classes of oral glucose-lowering agents. The thiazolidinediones tend to lower triglycerides (10% to 20%) but increase both HDL (up to 19%) and LDL (up to 12%) cholesterol. The increased LDL has been reported to reflect a change in particle size from a dense to a more buoyant, less atherogenic compound.

Both available thiazolidinediones are metabolized by cytochrome P450 enzymes in the liver. Rosiglitazone is metabolized by CYP2C8 and pioglitazone by CYP3A4 and CYP2C8. Metabolism by these hepatic enzymes provides the potential for interactions with other classes of drugs that are metabolized *via* these pathways. To date, no clinically significant interactions have been identified between the available thiazolidinediones and other drug classes, but further studies are in progress.

α-Glucosidase Inhibitors

α-Glucosidase inhibitors reduce intestinal absorption of starch, dextrin, and disaccharides by inhibiting the action of intestinal brush border α-glucosidase. Inhibition of this enzyme slows the absorption of carbohydrates; the postprandial rise in plasma glucose is blunted in both normal and diabetic subjects.

Acarbose (PRECOSE), an oligosaccharide of microbial origin, and *miglitol* (GLYSET), a desoxynojirimycin derivative, also competitively inhibit glucoamylase and sucrase but have weak effects on pancreatic α-amylase. They reduce postprandial plasma glucose levels in type 1 DM and type 2 DM subjects. α-Glucosidase inhibitors can have profound effects on hemoglobin A_{1c} levels in severely hyperglycemic type 2 DM patients. However, in patients with mild to moderate hyperglycemia, the glucose-lowering potential of α-glucosidase inhibitors (assessed by hemoglobin A_{1c} levels) is about 30% to 50% of that of other oral antidiabetic agents. α-Glucosidase inhibitors do not stimulate insulin release and therefore do not result in hypoglycemia. These agents may be considered as monotherapy in elderly patients or in patients with predominantly postprandial hyperglycemia. α-Glucosidase inhibitors typically are used in combination with other oral antidiabetic agents and/or insulin. The drugs should be administered at the start of a meal. They are poorly absorbed.

α-Glucosidase inhibitors cause dose-related malabsorption, flatulence, diarrhea, and abdominal bloating. Titrating the dose of drug slowly (25 mg at the start of a meal for 4 to 8 weeks followed by increases at 4- to 8-week intervals up to 75 mg before each meal) will reduce gastrointestinal side effects. Smaller doses are given with snacks. Acarbose is most effective when given with a starchy, high-fiber diet with restricted amounts of glucose and sucrose (Bressler and Johnson, 1992). If hypoglycemia occurs when α-glucosidase inhibitors are used with insulin or an insulin secretagogue, glucose rather than sucrose, starch, or maltose should be administered.

GLUCAGON

History. Distinct populations of cells were identified in the islets of Langerhans before the discovery of insulin. Glucagon itself was discovered by Murlin and Kimball in 1923, less than 2 years after the discovery of insulin. In contrast to the excitement caused by the discovery of insulin, few were interested in glucagon, and it was not recognized as an important hormone for more than 40 years. Glucagon is now known to have a significant physiological role in the regulation of glucose and ketone body metabolism, but it is only of minor therapeutic interest for the short-term management of hypoglycemia. It also is used in radiology for its inhibitory effects on intestinal smooth muscle.

Chemistry. *Glucagon* is a 29-amino-acid, single-chain polypeptide (Figure 61–6). It shows significant homology with several other polypeptide hormones, including secretin, vasoactive intestinal peptide, and gastrointestinal inhibitory polypeptide. The primary sequence of glucagon is highly conserved in mammals, and it is identical in human beings, cattle, pigs, and rats.

Glucagon is synthesized from preproglucagon, a 180-amino-acid precursor with five separately processed domains (Bell *et al.,* 1983). An amino-terminal signal peptide is followed by glicentin-related pancreatic peptide, glucagon, glucagon-like peptide-1, and glucagon-like peptide-2. Processing of the protein is sequential and occurs in a tissue-specific fashion; this results in different secretory peptides in pancreatic α cells and intestinal α-like cells (termed *L cells*) (Mojsov *et al.,* 1986). *Glicentin,* a major processing intermediate, consists of glicentin-related pancreatic polypeptide at the amino terminus and glucagon at the carboxyl terminus, with an Arg-Arg pair between. *Enteroglucagon* (or *oxyntomodulin*) consists of glucagon and a carboxyl-terminal hexapeptide linked by an Arg-Arg pair.

The biological roles of these precursor peptides are uncertain, but the highly controlled nature of the processing suggests that these peptides may have distinct biological functions. In the pancreatic α cell, the granule consists of a central core of glucagon surrounded by a halo of glicentin. Intestinal L cells contain only glicentin and presumably lack the enzyme required to process this precursor to glucagon. Enteroglucagon binds to hepatic glucagon receptors and stimulates adenylyl cyclase with 10% to 20% of the potency of glucagon. Glucagon-like peptide-1 is an extremely potent potentiator of insulin secretion, although it apparently lacks significant hepatic actions. Glicentin, enteroglucagon, and the glucagon-like peptides are found predominantly in the intestine, and their secretion continues after total pancreatectomy.

Regulation of Secretion. The secretion of glucagon is regulated by dietary glucose, insulin, amino acids, and fatty acids; glucose is a potent inhibitor. As in insulin secretion, glucose is a more effective inhibitor of glucagon secretion when taken orally than when administered intravenously, suggesting a possible role for some gastrointestinal hormone in the response. The effect of glucose is lost in the untreated or undertreated type 1 DM patient and in isolated pancreatic α cells, indicating that at least part of the effect is secondary to stimulation of insulin secretion. Somatostatin also inhibits glucagon secretion, as do free fatty acids and ketones.

Most amino acids stimulate the release of both glucagon and insulin. This coordinated response to amino acids may prevent insulin-induced hypoglycemia in individuals who ingest a meal of pure protein. Like glucose, amino acids are more potent when taken orally and thus may exert some of their effects *via* gastrointestinal hormones. Secretion of glucagon also is regulated by the autonomic innervation of the pancreatic islet. Stimulation of sympathetic nerves or administration of sympathomimetic amines increases glucagon secretion. Acetylcholine has a similar effect.

Glucagon in Diabetes Mellitus. Plasma concentrations of glucagon are elevated in poorly controlled diabetic patients. In view of its capacity to enhance gluconeogenesis and glycogenolysis, glucagon exacerbates the hyperglycemia of diabetes. However, this abnormality of glucagon secretion appears to be secondary to the diabetic state and is corrected with improved control of the disease (Unger, 1985). The importance of the

$$NH_2$$
$$|$$
H–HIS–SER–GLU–GLY–THR–PHE–THR–SER–ASP–TYR–

$$NH_2$$
$$|$$
SER–LYS–TYR–LEU–ASP–SER–ARG–ARG–ALA–GLU–

$$NH_2 \qquad\qquad NH_2$$
$$| \qquad\qquad\quad |$$
ASP–PHE–VAL–GLU–TRP–LEU–MET–ASP–THR–OH

Figure 61–6. The amino acid sequence of glucagon.

hyperglucagonemia in diabetes has been evaluated by administration of somatostatin (Gerich *et al.,* 1975). Although somatostatin does not restore glucose metabolism to normal, it significantly slows the rate of development of hyperglycemia and ketonemia in insulinopenic type 1 DM subjects. In normal individuals, glucagon secretion increases in response to hypoglycemia, but in type 1 DM patients this important defense mechanism (against insulin-induced hypoglycemia) is lost early in the course of the disease.

Degradation. Glucagon is extensively degraded in liver, kidney, and plasma, as well as at its sites of action (Peterson *et al.,* 1982). Its half-life in plasma is approximately 3 to 6 minutes. Proteolytic removal of the amino-terminal histidine residue leads to loss of biological activity.

Cellular and Physiological Actions. Glucagon interacts with a 60,000-dalton glycoprotein receptor on the plasma membrane of target cells (Sheetz and Tager, 1988). Although the exact structure of this receptor is not yet known, it interacts with the stimulatory guanine-nucleotide-binding regulatory protein, G_s, which activates adenylyl cyclase (*see* Chapter 2). The primary effects of glucagon on the liver are mediated by cyclic AMP. In general, modifications of the amino-terminal region of glucagon (*e.g.,* [Phe^1]glucagon and des-His$_1$-[Glu^9]glucagon amide) result in molecules that behave as partial agonists—they retain some affinity for the glucagon receptor but have a markedly reduced capacity to stimulate adenylyl cyclase (Unson *et al.,* 1989).

Phosphorylase, the rate-limiting enzyme in glycogenolysis, is activated by glucagon as a result of cyclic AMP-stimulated phosphorylation, while concurrent phosphorylation of glycogen synthase inactivates the enzyme; glycogenolysis is enhanced and glycogen synthesis is inhibited. Cyclic AMP also stimulates transcription of the gene for phosphoenolpyruvate carboxykinase, a rate-limiting enzyme in gluconeogenesis (Granner *et al.,* 1986). These effects are normally opposed by insulin, and when maximal concentrations of both hormones are present, insulin is dominant.

Cyclic AMP also stimulates phosphorylation of the bifunctional enzyme 6-phosphofructo-2-kinase/fructose-2,6-bisphosphatase (Pilkis *et al.,* 1981; Foster, 1984). This enzyme determines the cellular concentration of fructose-2,6-bisphosphate, which acts as a potent regulator of gluconeogenesis and glycogenolysis. When the concentration of glucagon is high relative to that of insulin, this enzyme is phosphorylated and acts as a phosphatase, reducing the concentration of fructose-2,6-bisphosphate in the liver. When the concentration of insulin is high relative to that of glucagon, the enzyme is dephosphorylated and acts as a kinase, raising fructose-2,6-bisphosphate concentrations. Fructose-2,6-bisphosphate interacts allosterically with phosphofructokinase-1, the rate-limiting enzyme in glycolysis, increasing its activity. Thus, when glucagon concentrations are high, glycolysis is inhibited and gluconeogenesis is stimulated. This also leads to a decrease in the concentration of malonyl CoA, stimulation of fatty-acid oxidation, and production of ketone bodies. Conversely, when insulin concentrations are high, glycolysis is stimulated and gluconeogenesis and ketogenesis are inhibited (*see* Foster, 1984).

Glucagon exerts effects on tissues other than liver, especially at higher concentrations. In adipose tissue, it stimulates adenylyl cyclase and increases lipolysis. In the heart, glucagon increases the force of contraction. Glucagon has relaxant effects on the gastrointestinal tract; this has been observed with analogs that apparently do not stimulate adenylyl cyclase. Some tissues (including liver) possess a second type of glucagon receptor that is linked to generation of inositol trisphosphate, diacylglycerol, and Ca^{2+} (Murphy *et al.,* 1987). The role of this receptor in regulation of metabolism remains uncertain.

Therapeutic Use. Glucagon is used to treat severe hypoglycemia, particularly in diabetic patients when intravenous glucose is not available; it also is used by radiologists for its inhibitory effects on the gastrointestinal tract.

All glucagon used clinically is extracted from bovine and porcine pancreas; its sequence is identical to that of the human hormone. For hypoglycemic reactions, 1 mg is administered intravenously, intramuscularly, or subcutaneously. Either of the first two routes is preferred in an emergency. Clinical improvement is sought within 10 minutes to minimize the risk of neurological damage from hypoglycemia. The hyperglycemic action of glucagon is transient and may be inadequate if hepatic stores of glycogen are depleted. After the initial response to glucagon, patients should be given glucose or urged to eat to prevent recurrent hypoglycemia. Nausea and vomiting are the most frequent adverse effects.

Glucagon also is used to relax the intestinal tract to facilitate radiographic examination of the upper and lower gastrointestinal tract with barium and retrograde ileography (Monsein *et al.,* 1986) and in magnetic resonance imaging of the gastrointestinal tract (Goldberg and Thoeni, 1989). Glucagon has been used to treat the spasm associated with acute diverticulitis and disorders of the biliary tract and sphincter of Oddi, as an adjunct in basket retrieval of biliary calculi, and for impaction of the esophagus and intussusception (Friedland, 1983; Mortensson *et al.,* 1984; Kadir and Gadacz, 1987). It has been used for diagnostic purposes to distinguish obstructive from hepatocellular jaundice (Berstock *et al.,* 1982).

Glucagon releases catecholamines from a pheochromocytoma and has been used experimentally as a diagnostic test for this disorder. The hormone also has been used as a cardiac inotropic agent for the treatment of shock, particularly when prior administration of a β-adrenergic receptor antagonist has rendered β-adrenergic receptor agonists ineffective.

SOMATOSTATIN

Somatostatin was first isolated and synthesized in 1973, following a search for hypothalamic factors that might regulate secretion of growth hormone from the pituitary gland (Brazeau *et al.,* 1973; *see also* Chapter 56). A potential physiological role for somatostatin in the islet was suggested by the observation that somatostatin inhibits secretion of insulin and glucagon (Alberti *et al.,* 1973; Gerich *et al.,* 1974). The peptide subsequently was identified in the D cells of the pancreatic islet, in similar cells of the gastrointestinal tract, and in the central nervous system (Dubois, 1975).

Somatostatin, the name originally given to a cyclic peptide containing 14 amino acids, is now known to be one of a group of related peptides. These include the original somatostatin (S-14), an extended 28-amino-acid peptide molecule (S-28), and a fragment containing the initial 12 amino acids of somatostatin-28

[S-28(1–12)]. Somatostatin-14 is the predominant form in the brain, whereas somatostatin-28 is the main form in the gut. Somatostatin inhibits the release of thyroid-stimulating hormone and growth hormone from the pituitary gland, of gastrin, motilin, vasoactive intestinal peptide (VIP), glicentin, and gastrointestinal polypeptide from the gut, and of insulin, glucagon, pancreatic polypeptide, and somatostatin from the pancreas.

Somatostatin secreted from the pancreas can regulate pituitary function, thereby acting as a true neurohormone. In the gut, however, somatostatin acts as a paracrine agent by influencing the functions of adjacent cells. It also can act as an autocrine agent by inhibiting its own release at the pancreas. The D cell is the last to receive blood flow in the islet; that is, it is downstream from the β and α cells (Samols et al., 1986). Thus, somatostatin may regulate the secretion of insulin and glucagon only via the systemic circulation.

Somatostatin is released in response to many of the nutrients and hormones that stimulate insulin secretion, including glucose, arginine, leucine, glucagon, vasoactive intestinal polypeptide, cholecystokinin, and even tolbutamide (Ipp et al., 1977; Weir et al., 1979). The physiological role of somatostatin has not been defined precisely. When administered in pharmacological amounts, somatostatin inhibits virtually all endocrine and exocrine secretions of the pancreas, gut, and gallbladder. Somatostatin also can inhibit secretion of the salivary glands and, under some conditions, can block parathyroid, calcitonin, prolactin, and ACTH secretion. The α cell is about 50 times more sensitive to somatostatin than is the β cell, but inhibition of glucagon secretion is more transient. Somatostatin also inhibits nutrient absorption from the intestine, decreases intestinal motility, and reduces splanchnic blood flow.

The therapeutic uses of somatostatin are confined mainly to blocking hormone release in endocrine-secreting tumors, including insulinomas, glucagonomas, VIPomas, carcinoid tumors, and somatotropinomas (causing acromegaly). Because of its short biological half-life (3 to 6 minutes), substantial effort has been directed toward the production of a longer-acting analog. One such agent, octreotide (SANDOSTATIN), is now available in the United States for treatment of carcinoid tumors, glucagonomas, VIPomas, and acromegaly (see also Chapter 56). Octreotide successfully controls excess secretion of growth hormone in most patients and has been reported to reduce the size of pituitary tumors in about one-third of cases. Octreotide also has been used to reduce the disabling form of diarrhea that occasionally occurs in diabetic autonomic neuropathy. As octreotide also can decrease blood flow to the gastrointestinal tract, the agent has been used to treat bleeding esophageal varices, peptic ulcers, and postprandial orthostatic hypotension.

Gallbladder abnormalities (stones and biliary sludge) occur frequently with chronic use of the peptide, and abnormal cardiac rhythms and gastrointestinal symptoms also occur commonly. Hypoglycemia, hyperglycemia, hypothyroidism, and goiter have been significant complications in patients being treated with octreotide for acromegaly.

DIAZOXIDE

Diazoxide is an antihypertensive, antidiuretic benzothiadiazine derivative with potent hyperglycemic actions when given orally (see also Chapter 33). Hyperglycemia results primarily from inhibition of insulin secretion (Levin et al., 1975). Diazoxide interacts with an ATP-sensitive K^+ channel and either prevents its closing or prolongs the open time; this effect is opposite to that of the sulfonylureas (Panten et al., 1989). The drug does not inhibit insulin synthesis, and thus there is an accumulation of insulin within the β cell. Diazoxide also has a modest capacity to inhibit peripheral glucose utilization by muscle and to stimulate hepatic gluconeogenesis.

Diazoxide (PROGLYCEM) has been used to treat patients with various forms of hypoglycemia (Grant et al., 1986). The usual oral dose is 3 to 8 mg/kg per day in adults and 8 to 15 mg/kg daily in infants and neonates. The drug has a tendency to cause nausea and vomiting and thus is usually given in divided doses with meals. Diazoxide circulates largely bound to plasma proteins and has a half-life of about 48 hours. Thus, the patient should be maintained at any dosage for several days before evaluating the therapeutic result.

Diazoxide has a number of adverse effects that sometimes limit its use in the treatment of hypoglycemia. These include retention of Na^+ and fluid, hyperuricemia, hypertrichosis (especially in children), thrombocytopenia, and leukopenia. Despite these side effects, the drug may be quite useful in patients with inoperable insulinomas (Schein, 1973) and in children with hyperinsulinism due to nesidioblastosis (Grant et al., 1986).

PROSPECTUS

The dramatic increase in the prevalence of type 2 DM has refocused clinical strategies to control plasma glucose levels and prevent complications of the disease. The DPP trial is a large, multicenter clinical study in the United States that is aimed at determining whether or not lifestyle changes or therapeutic intervention (metformin) at the stage of impaired glucose tolerance (IGT) can prevent the onset of diabetes. Other large trials (BARI 2, VA Cooperative Study) are focused on determining whether or not tight metabolic control and the class of therapeutic agents (insulin sensitizers vs. sulfonylureas vs. insulin or combinations thereof) can reduce macrovascular disease in type 2 diabetes. Currently, no drug is approved in the United States to treat IGT. The number of individuals with IGT worldwide is enormous (20 million in the United States alone). Approximately 5% of individuals with IGT develop diabetes each year. Thus, any therapeutic option that can prevent the transformation of IGT into diabetes is eagerly awaited.

Atherosclerotic disease is by far the primary cause of death in patients with diabetes. The pathophysiology resulting in atherosclerosis is complex and multifactoral. For nearly three decades, there has been considerable debate regarding whether hyperglycemia, hyperinsulinemia, and/or sulfonylurea therapy promotes atherosclerosis and accelerates cardiovascular disease. Recent data from the United Kingdom Prospective Diabetes Study demonstrate that neither insulin nor sulfonylurea therapy is associated with a higher incidence of macrovascular disease. Interestingly, a subgroup of patients treated primarily with metformin experienced a significant reduction in macrovascular events. The mechanism responsible for this finding is unknown, but the study raises intriguing possibilities that insulin resistance or associated factors (cytokines or

plasminogen activator inhibitor I) may be causally implicated in the development of macrovascular complications in type 2 DM. The results from the above trials should clarify these most important questions and provide additional novel therapeutic targets to reduce the devastating consequences of this common disease.

For further discussion of diabetes mellitus, *see* Chapter 334, and for information about hypoglycemia, *see* Chapter 335, in *Harrison's Principles of Internal Medicine,* 14th ed., McGraw-Hill, New York, 1998.

BIBLIOGRAPHY

Aguilar-Bryan, L., Nichols, C., Wechsler, S., Clement, J., Boyd, A., Gonzalez, G., Herrera-Sosa, H., Nguy, K., Bryan, J., and Nelson, D.A. Cloning of the beta cell high-affinity sulfonylurea receptor: a regulator of insulin secretion. *Science,* **1995,** *268*:423–426.

Alberti, K.G.M.M., Christensen, N.J., Christensen, S.E., Hansen, A.P., Iversen, J., Lundbaek, K., Seyer-Hansen, K., and Orskov, H. Inhibition of insulin secretion by somatostatin. *Lancet,* **1973,** 2:1299–1301.

Alberti, K.G.M.M., and Zimmet, P.Z. Definition, diagnosis and classification of diabetes mellitus and its complications. Part 1: diagnosis and classification of diabetes mellitus provisional report of a WHO consultation. *Diabet. Med.,* **1998,** *15*:539–553.

American Diabetes Association. Consensus statement on pharmacologic treatment. *Diabetes Care,* **1999,** *22*:S1–S114.

Authier, F., Rachubinski, R., Posner, B.I., and Bergeron, J.J. Endosomal proteolysis of insulin by an acidic thiol metalloprotease unrelated to insulin degrading enzyme. *J. Biol. Chem.,* **1994,** *269*:3010–3016.

Banting, F.G., Best, C.H., Collip, J.B., Campbell, W.R., and Fletcher, A.A. Pancreatic extracts in the treatment of diabetes mellitus. *Can. Med. Assoc. J.,* **1922,** *12*:141–146.

Bauman, W.A., Shaw, S., Jayatilleke, E., Spungen, A.M., and Herbert, V. Increased intake of calcium reverses vitamin B$_{12}$ malabsorption induced by metformin. *Diabetes Care,* **2000,** *23*:1227–1231.

Beisswenger, P.J., Makita, Z., Curphey, T.J., Moore, L.L., Jean, S., Brinck-Johnsen, T., Bucala, R., and Vlassara, H. Formation of immunochemical advanced glycation end products precedes and correlates with early manifestations of renal and retinal disease in diabetes. *Diabetes,* **1995,** *44*:824–829.

Bell, G.I., Sanchez-Pescador, R., Laybourn, P.J., and Najarian, R.C. Exon duplication and divergence in the human preproglucagon gene. *Nature,* **1983,** *304*:368–371.

Berman, M., McGuire, E.A., Roth, J., and Zeleznik, A.J. Kinetic modeling of insulin binding to receptors and degradation *in vivo* in the rabbit. *Diabetes,* **1980,** *29*:50–59.

Berstock, D.A., Wood, J.R., and Williams, R. The glucagon test in obstructive and hepatocellular jaundice. *Postgrad. Med. J.,* **1982,** *58*:485–486.

Bingley, P.J., Bonifacio, E., and Gale, E.A. Can we really predict IDDM? *Diabetes,* **1993,** *42*:213–220.

Blackard, W.G., Barlascini, C.O., Clore, J.N., and Nestler, J.E. Morning insulin requirements. Critique of dawn and meal phenomena. *Diabetes,* **1989,** *38*:273–277.

Blumenthal, S.A. Potentiation of the hepatic action of insulin by chlorpropamide. *Diabetes,* **1977,** *26*:485–489.

Bonner-Weir, S., and Orci, L. New perspectives on the microvasculature of the islets of Langerhans in the rat. *Diabetes,* **1982,** *31*:883–889.

Brazeau, P., Vale, W., Burgus, R., Ling, N., Butcher, M., Rivier, J., and Guillemin, R. Hypothalamic polypeptide that inhibits the secretion of immunoreactive pituitary growth hormone. *Science,* **1973,** *179*: 77–79.

Brelje, T.C., and Sorenson, R.L. Nutrient and hormonal regulation of the threshold of glucose-stimulated insulin secretion in isolated rat pancreases. *Endocrinology,* **1988,** *123*:1582–1590.

Cefalu, W.T., Skyler, J.S., Kourides, I.A., Landschulz, W.H., Balagtas, C.C., Cheng, S.L., and Gelfand, R.A. Inhaled human insulin treatment in patients with type 2 diabetes mellitus. *Ann. Intern. Med.,* **2001,** *134*:203–207.

Chan, S.J., Seino, S., Gruppuso, P.A., Schwartz, R., and Steiner, D.F. A mutation in the B chain coding region is associated with impaired proinsulin conversion in a family with hyperproinsulinemia. *Proc. Natl. Acad. Sci. U.S.A.,* **1987,** *84*:2194–2197.

Chertow, B.S., Baranetsky, N.G., Sivitz, W.I., Swain, P.A., Grey, J., and Charles, D. The effect of human insulin on antibody formation in pregnant diabetics and their newborns. *Obstet. Gynecol.,* **1988,** *72*:724–728.

Colagiuri, S., and Villalobos, S. Assessing effect of mixing insulins by glucose-clamp technique in subjects with diabetes mellitus. *Diabetes Care,* **1986,** *9*:579–586.

Davis, S.N., Butler, P.C., Brown, M., Beer, S., Sobey, W., Hanning, I., Home, P.D., Hales, C.N., and Alberti, K.G.M.M. The effects of human proinsulin on glucose turnover and intermediary metabolism. *Metabolism,* **1991b,** *40*:953–961.

Davis, S.N., Thompson, C.J., Brown, M.D., Home, P.D., and Alberti, K.G.M.M. A comparison of the pharmacokinetics and metabolic effects of human regular and NPH insulin mixtures. *Diabetes Res. Clin. Pract.,* **1991a,** *13*:107–117.

DCCT Research Group. The effect of intensive treatment of diabetes on the development and progression of long-term complications in insulin-dependent diabetes mellitus. The Diabetes Control and Complications Trial Research Group. *N. Engl. J. Med.,* **1993,** *329*: 977–986.

DCCT Research Group. Retinopathy and nephropathy in patients with type 1 diabetes four years after a trial of intensive therapy. The Diabetes Control and Complications Trial/Epidemiology of Diabetes Interventions and Complications Research Group. *N. Engl. J. Med.,* **2000,** *342*:381–389.

DeFronzo, R.A., and Goodman, A.M. Efficacy of metformin in patients with non-insulin-dependent diabetes mellitus. The Multicenter Metformin Study Group. *N. Engl. J. Med., 1995, 333*:541–549.

De Meyts, P. The structural basis of insulin and insulin-like growth factor-I receptor binding and negative co-operativity, and its relevance to mitogenic versus metabolic signalling. *Diabetologia, 1994, 37*(suppl. 2):S135–S148.

Dimitriadis, G.D., and Gerich, J.E. Importance of timing of preprandial subcutaneous insulin administration in the management of diabetes mellitus. *Diabetes Care, 1983, 6*:374–377.

Dubois, M.P. Immunoreactive somatostatin is present in discrete cells of the endocrine pancreas. *Proc. Natl. Acad. Sci. U.S.A., 1975, 72*:1340–1343.

Ellis, L., Clauser, E., Morgan, D.O., Edery, M., Roth, R.A., and Rutter, W.J. Replacement of insulin receptor tyrosine residues 1162 and 1163 compromises insulin-stimulated kinase activity and uptake of 2-deoxy-glucose. *Cell, 1986, 45*:721–732.

Expert Committee. Report of the Expert Committee on the Diagnosis and Classification of Diabetes Mellitus. *Diabetes Care, 1997, 20*:1183–1195.

Ferner, R.E., and Neil, H.A.W. Sulfonylureas and hypoglycaemia. *Br. Med. J. (Clin. Res. Ed.), 1988, 296*:949–950.

Friedland, G.W. The treatment of acute esophageal food impaction. *Radiology, 1983, 149*:601–602.

Galloway, J.A., Spradlin, C.T., Nelson, R.L., Wentworth, S.M., Davidson, J.A., and Swarner, J.L. Factors influencing the absorption, serum insulin concentration, and blood glucose responses after injections of regular insulin and various insulin mixtures. *Diabetes Care, 1981, 4*:366–376.

Gerich, J.E., Lorenzi, M., Bier, D.M., Schneider, V., Tsalikian, E., Karam, J.H., and Forsham, P.H. Prevention of human diabetic ketoacidosis by somatostatin. Evidence for an essential role of glucagon. *N. Engl. J. Med., 1975, 292*:985–989.

Gerich, J.E., Lorenzi, M., Schneider, V., Kwan, C.W., Karam, J.H., Guillemin, R., and Forsham, P.H. Inhibition of pancreatic glucagon secretion to arginine by somatostatin in normal man and in insulin-dependent diabetes. *Diabetes, 1974, 23*:876–880.

Gidh-Jain, M., Takeda, J., Xu, L.Z., Lange, A.J., Vionnet, N., Stoffel, M., Froguel, P., Velho, G., Sun, F., Cohen, D., Patel, P., Lo, Y.-M.D., Hattersley, A.T., Luthman, H., Wedell, A., St. Charles, R., Harrison, R.W., Weber, I.T., Bell, G.I., and Pilkis, S.J. Glucokinase mutations associated with non-insulin-dependent (type 2) diabetes mellitus have decreased enzyme activity: Implications for structure/function relationships. *Proc. Natl. Acad. Sci. U.S.A., 1993, 90*:1932–1936.

Gold, G., Gishizky, M.L., and Grodsky, G.M. Evidence that glucose "marks" β cells resulting in preferential release of newly synthesized insulin. *Science, 1982, 218*:56–58.

Granner, D., Andreone, T., Sasaki, K., and Beale, E. Inhibition of decreases transcription of the phosphoenolpyruvate carboxykinase gene by insulin. *Nature, 1983, 305*:549–551.

Granner, D.K., and O'Brien, R.M. Molecular physiology and genetics of NIDDM. Importance of metabolic staging. *Diabetes Care, 1992, 15*:369–395.

Grant, D.B., Dunger, D.B., and Burns, E.C. Long-term treatment with diazoxide in childhood hyperinsulinism. *Acta Endocrinol. Suppl. (Copenh.), 1986, 279*:340–345.

Hamel, F.G., Mahoney, M.J., and Duckworth, W.C. Degradation of intraendosomal insulin by insulin-degrading enzyme without acidification. *Diabetes, 1991, 40*:436–443.

Hanks, J.B., Andersen, D.K., Wise, J.E., Putnam, W.S., Meyers, W.C., and Jones, R.S. The hepatic extraction of gastric inhibitory polypeptide and insulin. *Endocrinology, 1984, 115*:1011–1018.

Horton, E.S., Clinkingbeard, C., Gatlin, M., Foley, J., Mallows, S., and Shen, S. Nateglinide alone and in combination with metformin improves glycemic control by reducing mealtime glucose levels in type 2 diabetes. *Diabetes Care, 2000, 23*:1660–1665.

Howey, D.C., Bowsher, R.R., Brunelle, R.L., and Woodworth, J.R. [Lys (B28), Pro (B29)]-human insulin. A rapidly absorbed analogue of human insulin. *Diabetes, 1994, 43*:396–402.

Imagawa, A., Hanafusa, T., Miyagawa, J., and Matsuzawa, Y. A novel subtype of type 1 diabetes mellitus characterized by a rapid onset and an absence of diabetes-related antibodies. Osaka IDDM Study Group. *N. Engl. J. Med., 2000, 342*:301–307.

Ipp, E., Dobb, R.E., Arimura, A., Vale, W., Harris, V., and Unger, R.H. Release of immunoreactive somatostatin from the pancreas in response to glucose, amino acids, pancreozymin-cholecystokinin, and tolbutamide. *J. Clin. Invest., 1977, 60*:760–765.

Jacobs, D.B., Hayes, G.R., and Lockwood, D.H. In vitro effects of sulfonylureas on glucose transport and translocation of glucose transporters in adipocytes from streptozocin-induced diabetic rats. *Diabetes, 1989, 38*:205–211.

Kadir, S., and Gadacz, T.R. Adjuncts and modifications to basket retrieval of retained biliary calculi. *Cardiovasc. Intervent. Radiol., 1987, 10*:295–300.

Kalbag, J.B., Walter, Y.H., Nedelman, J.R., and McLeod, J.F. Mealtime glucose regulation with nateglinide in healthy volunteers: comparison with repaglinide and placebo. *Diabetes Care, 2001, 24*:73–77.

Kang, S., Brange, J., Burch, A., Volund, A., and Owens, D.R. Absorption kinetics and action profiles of subcutaneously administered insulin analogues (AspB9, GluB27, AspB10, AspB28) in healthy subjects. *Diabetes Care, 1991, 14*:1057–1065.

King, G.L., and Johnson, S.M. Receptor-mediated transport of insulin across endothelial cells. *Science, 1985, 227*:1583–1586.

King, G.L., and Kahn, C.R. Non-parallel evolution of metabolic and growth-promoting functions of insulin. *Nature, 1981, 292*:644–646.

Kitabchi, A.E., Fisher, J.N., Matteri, R., and Murphy, M.B. The use of continuous insulin delivery systems in treatment of diabetes mellitus. *Adv. Intern. Med., 1983, 28*:449–490.

Kurtzhals, P., Havelund, S., Jonassen, I., and Markussen, J. Effect of fatty acids and selected drugs on the albumin binding of a long acting, acylated insulin analogue. *J. Pharm. Sci., 1997, 86*:1365–1368.

Leahy, J.L., Cooper, H.E., Deal, D.A., and Weir, G.C. Chronic hyperglycemia is associated with impaired glucose influence on insulin secretion. A study in normal rats using chronic *in vivo* glucose infusions *J. Clin. Invest., 1987, 77*:908–915.

Lee, T.S., Saltsman, K.A., Ohashi, H., and King, G.L. Activation of protein kinase C by elevation of glucose concentration: proposal for a mechanism in the development of vascular diabetic complications. *Proc. Natl. Acad. Sci. U.S.A., 1989, 86*:5141–5145. [Published erratum appears in *Proc. Natl. Acad. Sci. U.S.A., 1991, 88*:9907.]

Levin, S.R., Charles, M.A., O'Connor, M., and Grodsky, G.M. Use of diphenylhydantoin and diazoxide to investigate insulin secretory mechanisms. *Am. J. Physiol., 1975, 229*:49–54.

Lougheed, W.D., Woulfe-Flanagan, H., Clement, J.R., and Albisser, A.M. Insulin aggregation in artificial delivery systems. *Diabetologia, 1980, 19*:1–9.

Magnuson, M.A., Andreone, T.L., Printz, R.L., Koch, S., and Granner, D.K. The rat glucokinase gene. Structure and regulation by insulin. *Proc. Natl. Acad. Sci. U.S.A., 1989, 86*:4838–4842.

Malone, J.I., Lowitt, S., Grove, N.P., and Shah, S.C. Comparison of insulin levels after injection by jet stream and the disposable insulin syringe. *Diabetes Care,* **1986,** *9*:637–640.

Meinert, C.L., Knatterud, G.L., Prout, T.E., and Klimt, C.R. A study of the effects of hypoglycemic agents on vascular complications in patients with adult-onset diabetes. II. Mortality results. *Diabetes,* **1970,** *19*(suppl):789–830.

Minkowski, O. Historical development of the theory of pancreatic diabetes by Oscar Minkowski, 1929: introduction and translation by Rachmiel Levine. *Diabetes,* **1989,** *38*:1–6.

Mojsov, S., Heinrich, G., Wilson, I.B., Ravazzola, M., Orci, L., and Habener, J.F. Preproglucagon gene expression in pancreas and intestine diversifies at the level of post-translational processing. *J. Biol. Chem.,* **1986,** *261*:11880–11889.

Monsein, L.H., Halpert, R.D., Harris, E.D., and Feczko, P.J. Retrograde ileography: value of glucagon. *Radiology,* **1986,** *161*:558–559.

Mortensson, W., Eklof, O., and Laurin, S. Hydrostatic reduction of childhood intussusception. The role of adjuvant glucagon medication. *Acta Radiol. Diagn. (Stockh.),* **1984,** *25*:261–264.

Murphy, G.J., Hruby, V.J., Trivedi, D., Wakelam, M.J., and Houslay, M.D. The rapid desensitization of glucagon-stimulated adenylate cyclase is a cyclic AMP-independent process that can be mimicked by hormones which stimulate inositol phospholipid metabolism. *Biochem. J.,* **1987,** *243*:39–46.

Newman, B., Selby, J.V., King, M.C., Slemenda, C., Fabsitz, R., and Friedman, G.D. Concordance for type 2 (non-insulin-dependent) diabetes mellitus in male twins. *Diabetologia,* **1987,** *30*:763–768.

Olefsky, J.M., and Reaven, G.M. Effects of sulfonylurea therapy on insulin binding to mononuclear leukocytes of diabetic patients. *Am. J. Med.,* **1976,** *60*:89–95.

Panten, U., Burgfeld, J., Goerke, F., Rennicke, M., Schwanstecher, M., Wallasch, A., Zunkler, B.J., and Lenzen, S. Control of insulin secretion by sulfonylureas, meglitinide and diazoxide in relation to their binding to the sulfonylurea receptor in pancreatic islets. *Biochem. Pharmacol.,* **1989,** *38*:1217–1229.

Peterson, D.R., Carone, F.A., Oparil, S., and Christensen, E.I. Differences between renal tubular processing of glucagon and insulin. *Am. J. Physiol.,* **1982,** *242*:F112–F118.

Philipson, L.H., and Steiner, D.F. Pas de deux or more: the sulfonylurea receptor and K+ channels. *Science,* **1995,** *268*:372–373.

Pilkis, S.J., El-Maghrabi, M.R., Pilkis, J., Claus, T.H., and Cumming, D.A. Fructose-2,6-bisphosphate. A new activator of phosphofructokinase. *J. Biol. Chem.,* **1981,** *256*:3171–3174.

Printz, R.L., Koch, S., Potter, L.R., O'Doherty, R.M., Tiesinga, J.J., Moritz, S., and Granner, D.K. Hexokinase II mRNA and gene structure, regulation by insulin, and evolution. *J. Biol. Chem.,* **1993b,** *268*:5209–5219.

Pullen, R.A., Lindsay, D.G., Wood, S.P., Tickle, I.J., Blundell, T.L., Wollmer, A., Krail, G., Brandenburg, D., Zahn, H., Gliemann, J., and Gammeltoft, S. Receptor-binding region of insulin. *Nature,* **1976,** *259*:369–373.

Rabkin, R., Ryan, M.P., and Duckworth, W.C. The renal metabolism of insulin. *Diabetologia,* **1984,** *27*:351–357.

Ribalet, B., and Ciani, S. Regulation by cell metabolism and adenine nucleotides of a K channel in insulin-secreting B-cells (RIN m5F). *Proc. Natl. Acad. Sci. U.S.A.,* **1987,** *84*:1721–1725.

Riddle, M.C. New tactics for type 2 diabetes: regimens based on intermediate-acting insulin taken at bedtime. *Lancet,* **1985,** *1*:192–195.

Rosskamp, R.H., and Park, G. Long-acting insulin analogs. *Diabetes Care,* **1999,** *22*(suppl. 2):B109–B113.

Sasaki, K., Cripe, T.P., Koch, S.R., Andreone, T.L., Petersen, D.D., Beale, E.G., and Granner, D.K. Multihormonal regulation of phosphoenolpyruvate carboxykinase gene transcription. The dominant role of insulin. *J. Biol. Chem.,* **1984,** *259*:15242–15251.

Schade, D.S., and Duckworth, W.C. In search of subcutaneous-insulin-resistance syndrome. *N. Engl. J. Med.,* **1986,** *315*:147–153.

Shapiro, A.M., Lakey, J.R., Ryan, E.A., Korbutt, G.S., Toth, E., Warnock, G.L., Kneteman, N.M., and Rajotte, R.V. Islet transplantation in seven patients with type 1 diabetes mellitus using a glucocorticoid-free immunosuppressive regimen. *N. Engl. J. Med.,* **2000,** *343*:230–238.

Sheetz, M.J., and Tager, H.S. Receptor-linked proteolysis of membrane-bound glucagon yields a membrane-associated hormone fragment. *J. Biol. Chem.,* **1988,** *263*:8509–8514.

Shii, K., and Roth, R.A. Inhibition of insulin degradation by hepatoma cells after microinjection of monoclonal antibodies to a specific cytosolic protease. *Proc. Natl. Acad. Sci. U.S.A.,* **1986,** *83*:4147–4151.

Skyler, J.S., Cefalu, W.T., Kourides, I.A., Landschulz, W.H., Balagtas, C.C., Cheng, S.L., and Gelfand, R.A. Efficacy of inhaled human insulin in type 1 diabetes mellitus: a randomised proof-of-concept study. *Lancet,* **2001,** *357*:331–335.

Sodoyez, J.C., Sodoyez-Goffaux, F., Guillaume, M., and Merchie, G. [^{123}I]Insulin metabolism in normal rats and humans: external detection by a scintillation camera. *Science,* **1983,** *219*:865–867.

Srikanta, S., Ganda, O.P., Jackson, R.A., Gleason, R.E., Kaldany, A., Garovoy, M.R., Milford, E.L., Carpenter, C.B., Soeldner, J.S., and Eisenbarth, G.S. Type I diabetes mellitus in monozygotic twins: chronic progressive beta cell dysfunction. *Ann. Intern. Med.,* **1983,** *99*:320–326.

Stumvoll, M., Nurjhan, N., Perriello, G., Dailey, G., and Gerich, J.E. Metabolic effects of metformin in non-insulin-dependent diabetes mellitus. *N. Engl. J. Med.,* **1995,** *333*:550–554.

Sutherland, D.E., Moudry, K.C., and Fryd, D.S. Results of pancreas-transplant registry. *Diabetes,* **1989,** *38*(suppl 1):46–54.

Suzuki, K., and Kono, T. Evidence that insulin causes translocation of glucose transport activity to the plasma membrane from an intracellular storage site. *Proc. Natl. Acad. Sci. U.S.A.,* **1980,** *77*:2542–2545.

Temple, R.C., Carrington, C.A., Luzio, S.D., Owens, D.R., Schneider, A.E., Sobey, W.J., and Hales, C.N. Insulin deficiency in non-insulin-dependent diabetes. *Lancet,* **1989,** *1*:293–295.

Thomas, D.J., Platt, H.S., and Alberti, K.G.M.M. Insulin-dependent diabetes during the perioperative period. An assessment of continuous glucose-insulin-potassium infusion, and traditional treatment. *Anaesthesia,* **1984,** *39*:629–637.

Todd, J.A., Bell, J.F., and McDevitt, H.O. HLA-DQβ gene contributes to susceptibility and resistance to insulin-dependent diabetes mellitus. *Nature,* **1987,** *329*:599–604.

Tunbridge, F.K., Newens, A., Home, P.D., Davis, S.N., Murphy, M., Burrin, J.M., Alberti, K.G.M.M., and Jensen, I. Double-blind crossover trial of isophane (NPH)- and lente-based insulin regimens. *Diabetes Care,* **1989,** *12*:115–119.

UK Prospective Diabetes Study Group. Effect of intensive blood-glucose control with metformin on complications in overweight patients with type 2 diabetes (UKPDS 34). *Lancet,* **1998b,** *352*:854–865.

UK Prospective Diabetes Study Group. Intensive blood-glucose control with sulphonylureas or insulin compared with conventional treatment and risk of complications in patients with type 2 diabetes (UKPDS 33). *Lancet,* **1998a,** *352*:837–853.

Unson, C.G., Gurzenda, E.M., Iwasa, K., and Merrifield, R.B. Glucagon antagonists: contribution to binding and activity of the amino-terminal sequence 1-5, position 12, and the putative α-helical segment 19–27. *J. Biol. Chem.,* **1989,** *264*:789–794.

van den Ouwenland, J.M., Lemkes, H.H., Ruitenbeek, W., Sandkuijl, L., de Vijlder, M.F., Struyvenberg, P.A., van de Kamp, J.J., and Maassen, J.A. Mutation in mitochondrial tRNA (Leu) (UUR) gene in a large pedigree with maternally transmitted type II diabetes mellitus and deafness. *Nat. Genet.,* **1992,** *1*:368–371.

Verge, C.F., Gianani, R., Kawasaki, E., Yu, L., Pietropaolo, M., Jackson, R.A., Chase, H.P., and Eisenbarth, G.S. Prediction of type I diabetes in first-degree relatives using a combination of insulin, GAD, and ICA512bdc/IA-2 autoantibodies. *Diabetes,* **1996,** *45*:926–933.

Waldhausl, W., Bratusch-Marrain, P., Gasic, S., Korn, A., and Nowotny, P. Insulin production rate following glucose ingestion estimated by splanchnic C-peptide output in normal man. *Diabetologia,* **1979,** *17*:221–227.

Watts, N.B., Gebhart, S.S., Clark, R.V., and Phillips, L.S. Postoperative management of diabetes mellitus: steady-state glucose control with bedside algorithm for insulin adjustment. *Diabetes Care,* **1987,** *10*:722–728.

Wheatley, T., and Edwards, O.M. Insulin oedema and its clinical significance: metabolic studies in three cases. *Diabetic Med.,* **1985,** *2*:400–404.

White, M.F., Maron, R., and Kahn, C.R. Insulin rapidly stimulates tyrosine phosphorylation of a Mr-185,000 protein in intact cells. *Nature,* **1985,** *318*:183–186.

Wolf, B.A., Colca, J.R., Turk, J., Florholmen, J., and McDaniel, M.L. Regulation of Ca^{2+} homeostasis by islet endoplasmic reticulum and its role in insulin secretion. *Am. J. Physiol.,* **1988,** *254*:E121–E136.

Yalow, R.S. Radioimmunoassay: a probe for the fine structure of biological systems. *Science,* **1978,** *200*:1236–1245.

MONOGRAPHS AND REVIEWS

Amos, A.F., McCarty, D.J., and Zimmet, P. The rising global burden of diabetes and its complications: estimates and projections to the year 2010. *Diabet. Med.,* **1997,** *14(suppl 5)*:S1–S85.

Avruch, J., Zhang, X.F., and Kyriakis, J.M. Raf meets Ras: completing the framework of a signal transduction pathway. *Trends Biochem Sci.,* **1994,** *19*:279–283.

Bailey, C.J. Biguanides and NIDDM. *Diabetes Care,* **1992,** *15*:755–772.

Beck-Nielsen, H., Hother-Nielsen, O., and Pedersen, O. Mechanism of action of sulphonylureas with special reference to the extrapancreatic effect: an overview. *Diabet. Med.,* **1988,** *5*:613–620.

Bliss, M. *The Discovery of Insulin.* University of Chicago Press, Chicago, **1982**.

Bolli, G.B., Marchi, R.D., Park, G.D., Pramming, S., and Koivisto, V.A. Insulin analogues and their potential in the management of diabetes mellitus. *Diabetologia,* **1999,** *42*:1151–1167.

Boyd, A.E. III. Sulfonylurea receptors, ion channels, and fruit flies. *Diabetes,* **1988,** *37*:847–850.

Brange, J., Owens, D.R., Kang, S., and Volund, A. Monomeric insulins and their experimental and clinical implications. *Diabetes Care,* **1990,** *13*:923–954.

Bressler, R., and Johnson, D. New pharmacological approaches to therapy of NIDDM. *Diabetes Care,* **1992,** *15*:792–805.

Brownlee, M. The pathological implications of protein glycation. *Clin. Invest. Med.,* **1995,** *18*:275–281.

Burg, M.B., and Kador, P.F. Sorbitol, osmoregulation, and the complications of diabetes. *J. Clin. Invest.,* **1988,** *81*:635–640.

Cheatham, B., and Kahn, C.R. Insulin action and the insulin signaling network. *Endocr. Rev.,* **1995,** *16*:117–142.

Cohick, W.S., and Clemmons, D.R. The insulin-like growth factors. *Annu. Rev. Physiol.,* **1993,** *55*:131–153.

Cryer, P.E. Hypoglycemia begets hypoglycemia in IDDM. *Diabetes,* **1993,** *42*:1691–1693.

Cryer, P.E. Iatrogenic hypoglycemia as a cause of hypoglycemia-associated autonomic failure in IDMM. A vicious cycle. *Diabetes,* **1992,** *41*:255–260.

DeFronzo, R.A., Bonadonna, R.C., and Ferrannini, E. Pathogenesis of NIDDM. A balanced overview. *Diabetes Care,* **1992,** *15*:318–366.

Denton, R.M. Early events in insulin actions. *Adv. Cyclic Nucleotide Protein Phosphorylation Res.,* **1986,** *20*:293–341.

Dotta, F., and Eisenbarth, G.S. Type I diabetes mellitus: a predictable autoimmune disease with interindividual variation in the rate of β cell destruction. *Clin. Immunol. Immunopathol.,* **1989,** *50*:S85–S95.

Duckworth, W.C. Insulin degradation: mechanisms, products, and significance. *Endocr. Rev.,* **1988,** *9*:319–345.

Duronio, V., and Jacobs, S. Comparison of insulin and IGF-I receptors. In, *Insulin Receptors—Part B. Clinical Assessment, Biological Responses and Comparison to the IGF-I Receptor.* (Kahn, C.R., and Harrison, L.C., eds.) Liss, New York, **1988,** pp. 3–18.

Ebert, R., and Creutzfeldt, W. Gastrointestinal peptides and insulin secretion. *Diabetes Metab. Rev.,* **1987,** *3*:1–26.

Fleischer, N., and Erlichman, J. Intracellular signals and protein phosphorylation: regulatory mechanisms in the control of insulin secretion from the pancreatic β cells. In, *Molecular and Cellular Biology of Diabetes Mellitus.* Vol. 1: *Insulin Secretion.* (Draznin, B., Melmed, S., and LeRoith, D., eds.) Liss, New York, **1989,** pp. 107–116.

Foster, D.W. Banting lecture 1984. From glycogen to ketones—and back. *Diabetes,* **1984,** *33*:1188–1199.

Frank, R.N. The aldose reductase controversy. *Diabetes,* **1994,** *43*:169–172.

Goldberg, H.I., and Thoeni, R.F. MRI of the gastrointestinal tract. *Radiol. Clin. North Am.,* **1989,** *27*:805–812.

Granner, D.K. Hormones of the pancreas and gastrointestinal tract. In, *Harper's Biochemistry,* 25th ed. (Murray, R.K., Granner, D.K., Mayes, P.A., and Rodwell, V.W., eds.) Appleton & Lange, Stamford, CT, **2000,** pp. 610–626.

Granner, D.K. The molecular biology of insulin action on protein synthesis. *Kidney Int. Suppl.,* **1987,** *23*:S82–S96.

Granner, D.K., Sasaki, K., and Chu, D. Multihormonal regulation of phosphoenolpyruvate carboxykinase gene transcription. The dominant role of insulin. *Ann. N.Y. Acad. Sci.,* **1986,** *478*:175–190.

Greene, D.A., Lattimer, S.A., and Sima, A.A. Sorbitol, phosphoinositides, and sodium-potassium-ATPase in the pathogenesis of diabetic complications. *N. Engl. J. Med.,* **1987,** *316*:599–606.

Hattersley, A.T. Maturity-onset diabetes of the young: clinical heterogeneity explained by genetic heterogeneity. *Diabet. Med.,* **1998,** *15*:15–24.

Kahn, C.R., and Rosenthal, A.S. Immunologic reactions to insulin: insulin allergy, insulin resistance, and the autoimmune insulin syndrome. *Diabetes Care,* **1979,** *2*:283–295.

Kitabchi, A.E. Low-dose insulin therapy in diabetic ketoacidosis: fact or fiction? *Diabetes Metab. Rev.,* **1989,** *5*:337–363.

Koffler, M., Ramirez, L.C., and Raskin, P. The effect of many commonly used drugs on diabetic control. *Diabetes Nutr. Metab.,* **1989,** *2*:75–93.

Krall, L.P. Oral hypoglycemic agents. In, *Joslin's Diabetes Mellitus,* 12th ed. (Marble, A., Krall, L.P., Bradley, R.F., Christlieb, A.R., and Soeldner, J.S., eds.) Lea & Febiger, Philadelphia, **1985,** pp. 412–452.

Leahy, J.L. Natural history of β-cell dysfunction in NIDDM. *Diabetes Care,* **1990,** *13*:992–1010.

Lebovitz, H.E., and Feinglos, M.N. The oral hypoglycemic agents. In, *Diabetes Mellitus: Theory and Practice,* 3rd ed. (Ellenberg, M., and Rifkin, H., eds.) Medical Examination Publishing, Garden City, NY, **1983,** pp. 591–610.

LeRoith, D., Taylor, S.I., and Olefsky, J.M. (eds.) *Diabetes Mellitus: A Fundamental and Clinical Text,* 2nd ed. Lippincott Williams & Wilkins, Philadelphia, **2000.**

Malaisse, W.J. Stimulus-secretion coupling in the pancreatic B-cell: the cholinergic pathway for insulin release. *Diabetes Metab. Rev.,* **1986,** 2:243–259.

Matchinsky, F.M. Banting Lecture 1995. A lesson in metabolic regulation inspired by the glucokinase glucose sensor paradigm. *Diabetes,* **1996,** 45:223–241.

McMillan, D.E. Development of vascular complications in diabetes. *Vasc. Med.,* **1997,** 2:132–142.

Nerup, J., Christy, M., Patz, P., Ryder, L.P., and Suejgaard, A. Aspects of the genetics of insulin dependent diabetes mellitus. In, *Immunology in Diabetes.* (Adreani, D., Dimario, R., Federlin, K.F., and Hedings, L.G., eds.) Kimpton, Medical Publications, London, **1984,** pp. 63–70.

O'Brien, R.M., and Granner, D.K. The regulation of gene expression by insulin. *Physiol. Rev.,* **1996,** 76:1109–1161.

Orci, L. The insulin cell: its cellular environment and how it processes (pro)insulin. *Diabetes Metab. Rev.,* **1986,** 2:71–106.

Paice, B.J., Paterson, K.R., and Lawson, D.H. Undesired effects of sulphonylurea drugs. *Adverse Drug React. Acute Poisoning Rev.,* **1985,** 4:23–36.

Polonsky, K.S., and Rubenstein, A.H. Current approaches to measurement of insulin secretion. *Diabetes Metab. Rev.,* **1986,** 2:315–329.

Porte, D., Jr., and Halter, J.B. The endocrine pancreas and diabetes mellitus. In, *Textbook of Endocrinology,* 6th ed. (Williams, R.H., ed.) Saunders, Philadelphia, **1981,** pp. 716–843.

Printz, R.L., Magnuson, M.A., and Granner, D.K. Mammalian glucokinase. *Annu. Rev. Nutr.,* **1993a,** 13:463–496.

Robbins, D.C., Tager, H.S., and Rubenstein, A.H. Biologic and clinical importance of proinsulin. *N. Engl. J. Med.,* **1984,** 310:1165–1175.

Samols, E., Bonner-Weir, S., and Weir, G.C. Intra-islet insulin–glucagon–somatostatin relationships. *Clin. Endocrinol. Metab.,* **1986,** 15:33–58.

Schade, D.S., and Eaton, R.P. Diabetic ketoacidosis—pathogenesis, prevention and therapy. *Clin. Endocrinol. Metab.,* **1983,** 12:321–338.

Schein, P.S. Islet cell tumors: current concepts and management. *Ann. Intern. Med.,* **1973,** 79:239–257.

Seltzer, H.S. Drug-induced hypoglycemia. A review of 1418 cases. *Endocrinol. Metab. Clin. North Am.,* **1989,** 18:163–183.

Shepherd, P.R., and Kahn, B.B. Glucose transporters and insulin action—implications for insulin resistance and diabetes mellitus. *N. Engl. J. Med.,* **1999,** 341:248–256.

Simpson, I.A., and Cushman, S.W. Hormonal regulation of mammalian glucose transport. *Annu. Rev. Biochem.,* **1986,** 55:1059–1089.

Steiner, D.F., Smeekens, S.P., Ohagi, S., and Chan, S.J. The new enzymology of precursor processing endoproteases. *J. Biol. Chem.,* **1992,** 267:23435–23438.

Unger, R.H. Glucagon in diabetes. In, *Diabetes Annual.* Vol. 1 (Alberti, K.G.M.M., and Krall, L.P., eds.) Elsevier, Amsterdam, **1985,** pp. 480–491.

Virkamäki, A., Ueki, K., and Kahn, C.R. Protein-protein interaction in insulin signaling and the molecular mechanisms of insulin resistance. *J. Clin. Invest.,* **1999,** 103:931–943.

Weir, G.C., Leahy, J.L., and Bonner-Weir, S. Experimental reduction of B-cell mass: implications for the pathogenesis of diabetes. *Diabetes Metab. Rev.,* **1986,** 2:125–161.

Weir, G.C., Samols, E., Loo, S., Patel, Y.C., and Gabbay, K.H. Somatostatin and pancreatic polypeptide secretion: effects of glucagon, insulin, and arginine. *Diabetes,* **1979,** 28:35–40.

Yarden, Y., and Ullrich, A. Growth factor receptor tyrosine kinases. *Annu. Rev. Biochem.,* **1988,** 57:443–478.

AGENTS AFFECTING CALCIFICATION AND BONE TURNOVER

Calcium, Phosphate, Parathyroid Hormone, Vitamin D, Calcitonin, and Other Compounds

Robert Marcus

In earlier editions, this chapter focused on hormones involved with calcium homeostasis, mechanisms by which they act to maintain blood Ca^{2+} concentrations within normal limits, and the derangements in calcium physiology associated with insufficiency or excess of these hormones. In recent years, there has been a shift in the relative importance of the prevalence and severity of these disorders. Primary hyperparathyroidism is more commonly diagnosed than in years past, but most commonly appears today as a mild disorder that does not necessarily require treatment. By contrast, osteoporotic fracture, particularly of the hip, has emerged as a major public health problem and an important contributor to disability, mortality, and health care costs in industrialized countries. Considerable information has been obtained regarding the acquisition and subsequent loss of bone, as well as the contributions of genetics, diet, physical activity, and reproductive hormone status to skeletal health. Important knowledge also has been obtained concerning the central role of bone remodeling as the final pathway of adult bone loss.

A rapidly increasing body of evidence supports the concept that regular physical activity, adequate calcium intake, either through diet or supplements, and timely use of estrogen replacement therapy will decrease bone remodeling, constrain bone loss, and reduce fracture risk. However, treatment of established osteoporosis remains a formidable challenge. Like estrogen and calcium, other approved therapies, such as bisphosphonates, act by slowing bone resorption rather than by stimulating new bone formation and therefore do not solve the problem of restoring normal bone mass. In fact, since bone remodeling is a coupled process, agents that suppress bone resorption ultimately decrease bone formation. The primary challenge for future research in this field is to develop agents that safely increase bone mass. At present, there is considerable interest in developing analogs of parathyroid hormone, vitamin D, and various bone morphogenetic proteins as potential therapies for osteoporosis.

Another recent development is the recognition that vitamin D plays an important role as a cellular differentiation factor in systems not directly related to calcium metabolism. Calcitriol, the hormonal form of vitamin D, shows considerable promise as a treatment for psoriasis and also is under study for several malignancies. Therapeutic utility of calcitriol is limited by its calcemic effects, but noncalcemic calcitriol analogs are under development. Such analogs may offer a new approach to manage patients with diverse conditions, ranging from primary and secondary hyperparathyroidism to cancer and leukemia.

CALCIUM

Ca^{2+} is the major extracellular divalent cation. The normal adult man and woman possess about 1300 and 1000 g of calcium, respectively, of which more than 99% is in bone. Ca^{2+} is present in small amounts in extracellular fluids and to a minor extent within cells, where its ionized concentration under basal conditions is about 0.1 μM. In response to hormonal, electrical, or mechanical stimuli, a temporary increase in Ca^{2+} flux raises this concentration toward 1 μM, permitting interactions with specific Ca^{2+}-binding proteins that activate numerous processes. The major Ca^{2+}-binding protein in all organisms is calmodulin, a highly conserved protein that binds four moles of Ca^{2+} per mole of protein. Ca^{2+} is essential for many important processes, including neuronal excitability, neurotransmitter release, muscle contraction, membrane integrity, and blood coagulation. In addition, Ca^{2+} serves a second messenger function for the actions of many hormones.

To carry out these various roles, Ca^{2+} must be available in the proper concentration. In human plasma, calcium circulates at a concentration of about 8.5 to 10.4 mg/dl (2.1 to 2.6 mM). Of this, about 45% is bound to plasma proteins, primarily albumin, and about 10% is complexed with anionic buffers, such as citrate and phosphate. The remaining fraction, ionized Ca^{2+}, is the component that exerts physiological effects and, when reduced, produces hypocalcemic symptoms. Hence, interpretation of any given value for total plasma calcium is impossible without correction for the concentration of plasma proteins. As an approximation, a change in plasma albumin concentration of 1.0 g/dl from a nominal value of 4.0 g/dl can be expected to change total calcium by 0.8 mg/dl.

Regulation of the extracellular Ca^{2+} concentration is under tight endocrine control that affects its entry at the intestine and its exit at the kidney, and which regulates a large skeletal reservoir for withdrawals at times of need.

Calcium Stores. The skeleton contains 99% of total body calcium in a crystalline form resembling the mineral hydroxyapatite [$Ca_{10}(PO_4)_6(OH)_2$]; but other ions—including Na^+, K^+, Mg^{2+}, and F^-—also are present in the crystal lattice. The steady-state content of calcium in bone reflects the net effect of bone resorption and bone formation, two coupled aspects of bone remodeling (*see* below). In addition, a labile pool of bone Ca^{2+} is readily exchangeable with interstitial fluid. The rates of exchange are modulated by drugs, hormones, vitamins, and other factors that directly alter bone turnover or that influence the level of Ca^{2+} in interstitial fluid.

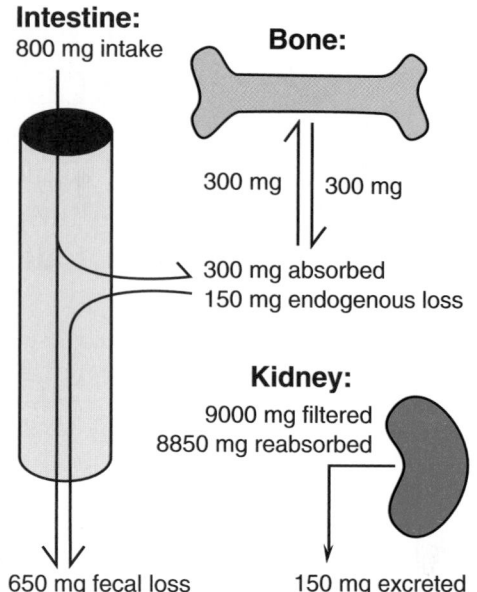

Figure 62–1. Schematic representation of the whole body daily turnover of calcium.

(*Adapted with permission from Yanagawa and Lee, 1992.*)

Calcium Absorption and Excretion. In the United States, about 75% of dietary calcium is obtained from milk and dairy products. The adequate intake value for calcium in adolescents is 1300 mg/day and in adults to age 24 years is 1000 mg/day. The adequate intake for men and women age 50 and older is 1200 mg/day (*see* Section XIII: "The Vitamins, Introduction") (Institute of Medicine, 1997). The median intakes of calcium for boys and girls aged 9 years and older are 865 and 625 mg, respectively. After age 50, median daily calcium intake declines for women (to 517 mg) (Institute of Medicine, 1997).

Figure 62–1 demonstrates the elements of whole body daily calcium turnover. Ca^{2+} enters the body only through the intestine. Two different mechanisms contribute to this relatively inefficient process. *Active* vitamin D–dependent transport occurs in the proximal duodenum. In addition, accounting for a large fraction of total Ca^{2+} uptake, *facilitated diffusion* takes place throughout the small intestine. There is also an obligatory daily intestinal calcium loss of about 150 mg/day, reflecting the mineral contained in mucosal and biliary secretions and in sloughed intestinal cells.

Intestinal Ca^{2+} absorption efficiency is inversely related to calcium intake, so that a diet low in calcium leads to a compensatory increase in fractional absorption, due in part to activation of vitamin D. The strength of this response decreases substantially with age. Drugs such as glucocorticoids and phenytoin depress intestinal Ca^{2+} transport. Some dietary constituents, *e.g.,* phytate and oxalate, depress Ca^{2+} absorption by promoting the formation of nonabsorbable complexes. Disease states associated with steatorrhea, diarrhea, or chronic intestinal malabsorption also promote fecal loss of calcium.

Urinary excretion of Ca^{2+} is the net result of the quantity filtered at the glomerulus and the amount reabsorbed. About 9 g of Ca^{2+} is filtered each day. Tubular reabsorption is very efficient, more than 98% of filtered Ca^{2+} returning to the circulation. Reabsorption efficiency is highly regulated by parathyroid hormone (PTH) but also is influenced by filtered Na^+, the presence of non-reabsorbed anions, and diuretic agents. Sodium intake, and therefore sodium excretion, is directly related to urinary calcium excretion. Diuretics acting on the ascending limb of the loop of Henle increase calciuresis. By contrast, thiazide diuretics uniquely uncouple the relationship between Na^+ and Ca^{2+} excretion, leading to reduced calciuria (Lemann *et al.,* 1985). Dietary protein is directly related to urine calcium excretion, presumably as an effect of sulfur-containing amino acids on renal tubular function. Urinary Ca^{2+} is only slightly influenced by dietary calcium in normal people. Significant amounts of calcium are secreted in milk during lactation; sweat also makes a small contribution to daily losses.

Bone Remodeling. Growth and development of endochondral bone are driven by a process called *modeling.* Once new bone is laid down, it is subject to a continuous process of breakdown and renewal called *remodeling* that continues throughout life. After linear growth has ceased and peak bone mass has been approached, remodeling becomes the final common pathway by which bone mass is adjusted throughout adult life. Remodeling is carried out by myriad individual and independent "bone remodeling units" throughout the skeleton (Figure 62–2). It takes place on bone surfaces, about 90% of which are normally inactive, covered by a thin layer of lining cells. In response to physical or biochemical signals, recruitment of marrow precursor cells to a site at the bone surface results in their fusion into the characteristic multinucleated osteoclasts that resorb, or dig a cavity into the bone.

Osteoclast production is regulated by cytokines, such as interleukins-1 and -6, produced by osteoblasts. Recent studies have begun to clarify the mechanisms through which osteoclast production is regulated (*see* Suda *et al.,* 1999). RANK (*receptor for activating NFκB*) is the name given to an osteoclast protein whose expression is required for osteoclastic bone resorption. Its natural ligand, *osteoclast differentiation factor* (ODF, also called RANK ligand), is a membrane-spanning osteoblast protein. Upon binding to RANK, ODF induces osteoclast formation. The requirement for this interaction is revealed by findings that antibodies against ODF inhibit bone resorption induced by multiple hormones and other regulators of bone turnover (Yasuda *et al.,* 1998). ODF initiates the activation of mature osteoclasts as well as the differentiation of osteoclast precursors (Jimi *et al.,* 1999). Osteoblasts also produce an inhibitor of ODF action, called *osteoprotegerin* (OPG), which acts as a decoy ligand for ODF. Under conditions favoring increased bone resorption, as during estrogen deprivation, OPG is suppressed, ODF binds to RANK, and osteoclast production increases. When estrogen sufficiency is reestablished, OPG increases and competes effectively with ODF for binding to RANK.

In cortical bone, resorption creates tunnels within Haversian canals, whereas trabecular resorption creates scalloped areas of the bone surface called Howship's lacunae. On termination of the resorption phase, a cavity remains that is about 60 μm deep and is bordered at its deepest extent by a cement line, a region of loosely organized collagen fibrils. Completion of the resorption phase is followed by ingress of pre-osteoblasts derived from marrow stroma into the base of the resorption cavity. These cells develop the characteristic osteoblastic phenotype and begin to replace the resorbed bone by elaborating new bone matrix constituents, such as collagen, osteocalcin, and other proteins. Once the newly formed osteoid reaches a thickness of about 20 μm, mineralization begins. Completion of a remodeling cycle normally requires about 6 months.

If the replacement of resorbed bone matched the amount that was removed, remodeling would lead to no net change in bone mass. However, small bone deficits persist on completion of each cycle, reflecting an inefficiency in remodeling dynamics. Consequently, lifelong accumulation of remodeling deficits

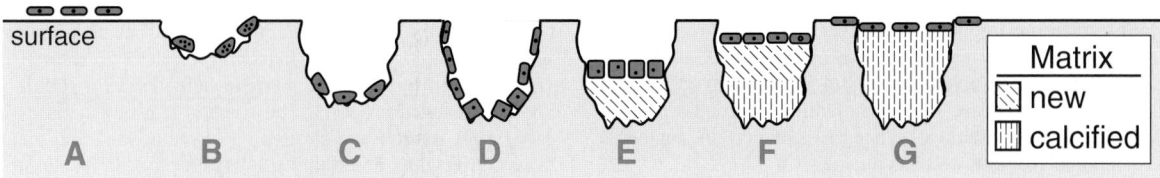

Figure 62–2. The bone remodeling cycle.

A. Resting trabecular surface. **B.** *Multinucleated osteoclasts* dig a cavity of approximately 20 μm. **C.** Resorption to 60 μm is completed by *mononuclear phagocytes.* **D.** *Osteoblast precursors* are recruited to the base of the resorption cavity. **E.** New matrix is secreted by *osteoblasts.* **F.** Matrix continues to be secreted, with the initiation of calcification. **G.** Mineralization of the new matrix is completed. Bone has returned to a quiescent state, but a small deficit in bone mass persists. (*Adapted from Marcus, 1987, with permission.*)

underlies the well-documented phenomenon of age-related bone loss, a process that begins shortly after growth stops. *Alterations in remodeling activity represent the final pathway through which diverse stimuli, such as dietary insufficiency, hormones, and drugs, affect bone balance.* A change in whole-body remodeling rate can be brought about through distinct perturbations in remodeling dynamics. Changes in hormonal milieu often lead to an increase in the activation, or birthrate, of remodeling units. Examples include hyperthyroidism, hyperparathyroidism, and hypervitaminosis D. Other factors may impair osteoblastic functional adequacy, such as high doses of corticosteroids or ethanol. Finally, it appears that estrogen deficiency may augment osteoclastic resorptive capacity (*see* Marcus, 1987; Dempster, 1992).

At any given time, a transient deficit in bone exists called the remodeling space, representing sites of bone resorption that have not yet filled in. In response to any stimulus that alters the birthrate of new remodeling units, the remodeling space will either increase or decrease accordingly until a new steady state is established, and this adjustment will be seen as an increase or decrease in bone mass.

Physiological and Pharmacological Actions

Neuromuscular System. Moderate elevations of the concentration of Ca^{2+} in the extracellular fluid may have no clinically detectable influences on the neuromuscular apparatus. However, when hypercalcemia becomes severe, the threshold for excitation of nerve and muscle is increased. This is manifested clinically by muscle weakness, lethargy, and even coma. In contrast, modest reductions in Ca^{2+} activity may decrease excitation thresholds, leading to positive Chvostek and Trousseau signs, tetanic seizures, and laryngospasm. Ca^{2+} influx into cells is thought to be by means of carrier-mediated facilitated diffusion and by exchange of Ca^{2+} for Na^+. Several Ca^{2+} channels in cell membranes are regulated by hormones and neurotransmitters and membrane potential. In liver and skeletal muscle, intracellular Ca^{2+} is reversibly sequestered by endoplasmic and sarcoplasmic reticulum, respectively.

Ca^{2+} plays an important role in muscular excitation–contraction coupling. The action potential stimulates Ca^{2+} release from the sarcoplasmic reticulum. The released Ca^{2+} activates contraction by binding to troponin, abolishing the inhibitory effect of troponin on the actin–myosin interaction. Muscle relaxation occurs when Ca^{2+} is pumped back into the sarcoplasmic reticulum, restoring troponin inhibition.

Ca^{2+} is necessary for exocytosis and thus has an important role in stimulus–secretion coupling in most exocrine and endocrine glands. Release of catecholamines from the adrenal medulla, neurotransmitters at synapses, and certain autacoids (*e.g.,* histamine from mast cells) requires Ca^{2+}.

Cardiovascular System. Ca^{2+} is essential for excitation–contraction coupling in cardiac muscle, as well as for the conduction of electrical impulses in certain regions of the heart, particularly through the AV node. Depolarization of myocardial fibers opens voltage-regulated Ca^{2+} channels and causes the "slow" inward current that occurs during the action potential plateau. This current allows permeation of Ca^{2+} sufficient to trigger the release

of additional Ca^{2+} from the sarcoplasmic reticulum, thereby causing contraction. Passage of Ca^{2+} through similar channels in tissues such as the AV node carries virtually all the inward (depolarizing) current during the action potential.

Ca^{2+} is responsible for the initiation of contraction in vascular and other smooth muscles, and it frequently carries an important fraction of depolarizing currents in these tissues. Hence Ca^{2+} channel blockers have profound effects on the contractility of cardiac and vascular smooth muscle as well as on the conduction of impulses within the heart. These drugs have important uses in the treatment of angina, cardiac arrhythmias, and hypertension (*see* Chapters 32, 33, and 35).

Miscellaneous Effects. Ca^{2+} plays a role in maintaining the integrity of mucosal membranes, cell adhesion, and functions of individual cell membranes as well. Ca^{2+} is involved in blood coagulation, but the ion is not used to treat disorders of coagulation. Calcium chloride is an acidifying salt and will promote diuresis; however, ammonium salts are much more effective acidifying agents.

Abnormalities of Calcium Metabolism

Hypocalcemic States. The prominent signs and symptoms of hypocalcemia include tetany and related phenomena such as paresthesias, increased neuromuscular excitability, laryngospasm, muscle cramps, and tonic-clonic convulsions. Some causes of hypocalcemia are discussed below.

Combined deprivation of Ca^{2+} and vitamin D readily promotes hypocalcemia. This combination of events is observed in the various malabsorption states and also occurs from inadequate diets. When due to malabsorption, hypocalcemia is accompanied by low concentrations of phosphate, total plasma proteins, and magnesium. During Mg^{2+} deficiency, hypocalcemia may be accentuated by diminished secretion and action of PTH (*see* below). Hypocalcemia stimulates the release of PTH, which increases bone turnover, resulting in increased delivery of skeletal calcium to the extracellular fluid. In infants with malabsorption or inadequate calcium intake, Ca^{2+} concentrations are usually depressed, there is hypophosphatemia, and the resultant bone disease is rickets (*see* "Vitamin D," below).

Hypoparathyroidism is most often a consequence of thyroid or neck surgery, but it also may be due to genetic or autoimmune disorders. In hypoparathyroidism, hypocalcemia is accompanied by *hyper*phosphatemia, reflecting decreased PTH action on renal phosphorus handling. Although other conditions of hypocalcemia may be associated with lens opacity, papilledema, and calcification of the basal ganglia, these conditions occur more often with hypoparathyroidism. *Pseudohypoparathyroidism* (PHP) is characterized by multiple somatic defects and a failure to respond to exogenous PTH. The somatic features include a round face, short stature, and shortening of metacarpal and metatarsal bones (Albright's hereditary osteodystrophy). In its classic form, PHP is due to a mutant guanine nucleotide–binding protein that normally mediates hormone-induced activation of adenylyl cyclase (*see* Chapter 2). An assortment of hormonal abnormalities has been associated with this type of PHP, but none is so severe as the deficient response to PTH. PHP has been reviewed recently by Levine (1999).

In the first several days following removal of a parathyroid adenoma, hypocalcemia is not unusual. This may be due to temporary failure of the remaining parathyroid glands to compensate for the missing adenomatous tissue. In this case, hyperphosphatemia also is seen, and the condition is one of functional hypoparathyroidism. In patients with parathyroid bone disease, postoperative hypocalcemia may reflect rapid uptake of calcium into bone, the so-called hungry bone syndrome. Here, the serum inorganic phosphate concentration also is low, reflecting its concurrent uptake into bone, and persistent, severe hypocalcemia may require administration of vitamin D and supplemental calcium for several months.

Neonatal tetany sometimes is observed in infants of mothers with hyperparathyroidism; indeed, it may be the tetany that calls attention to the mother's disorder. This problem usually is transient, disappearing when the infant's own parathyroid glands respond appropriately.

Hypocalcemia is associated with advanced renal insufficiency accompanied by hyperphosphatemia. Many patients with this condition do not develop tetany unless the severe accompanying acidosis is treated. High concentrations of phosphate in plasma inhibit the conversion of 25-hydroxycholecalciferol to 1,25-dihydroxycholecalciferol (Haussler and McCain, 1977). Hypocalcemia also can occur following massive transfusions with citrated blood.

Treatment of Hypocalcemia and other Therapeutic Uses of Calcium. Calcium is used in the treatment of calcium deficiency states and as a dietary supplement. Ca^{2+} salts are specific in the immediate treatment of hypocalcemic tetany regardless of etiology. In severe manifest tetany, symptoms are best brought under control by intravenous medication. *Calcium chloride* ($CaCl_2 \cdot 2H_2O$) contains 27% Ca^{2+}; it is valuable in the treatment of hypocalcemic tetany and laryngospasm. The salt is given intravenously, but it *must never be injected into tissues.* Injections of calcium chloride are accompanied by peripheral vasodilation and a cutaneous burning sensation. The salt usually is given intravenously in a concentration of 10% (equivalent to 1.36 meq Ca^{2+}/ml). The rate of injection should be slow (not over 1 ml per minute) to prevent a high concentration of Ca^{2+} from causing a cardiac arrhythmia. A moderate fall in blood pressure due to vasodilation may attend the injection. Since calcium chloride is an acidifying salt, it is usually undesirable in the treatment of the hypocalcemia caused by renal insufficiency. *Calcium gluceptate injection* (a 22% solution; 18 mg or 0.9 meq of Ca^{2+}/ml) is administered intravenously in a dose of 5 to 20 ml for the treatment of severe hypocalcemic tetany; the injection produces a transient tingling sensation when given too rapidly. When the intravenous route is not possible, injections may be given intramuscularly in a dose up to 5 ml, which may produce a mild local reaction. *Calcium gluconate injection* (a 10% solution; 9.3 mg of Ca^{2+}/ml) is a readily available source of calcium, and the intravenous administration of this salt is the treatment of choice for severe hypocalcemic tetany. Patients with moderate to severe hypocalcemia may be treated by infusing calcium gluconate at a dose of 10 to 15 mg/kg body weight of Ca^{2+} over 4 to 6 hours. Since the usual 10-ml vial of a 10% solution contains only 93 mg of Ca^{2+}, many vials are needed. The intramuscular route should not be employed, since abscess formation at the injection site may result.

For control of milder hypocalcemic symptoms, oral medication suffices, frequently in combination with vitamin D or one of its active metabolites. Numerous oral Ca^{2+} salts are available.

Average doses for hypocalcemic patients are calcium gluconate, 15 g daily in divided doses; calcium lactate, 4 g plus 8 g lactose, with each meal; calcium carbonate or calcium phosphate, 1 to 2 g with meals.

Calcium carbonate and calcium acetate are used to restrict phosphate absorption in patients with chronic renal failure and oxalate absorption in patients with inflammatory bowel disease. Acute administration of calcium may be life-saving in patients with extreme hyperkalemia. Calcium gluconate (10 to 30 ml of a 10% solution) can reverse some of the cardiotoxic effects of hyperkalemia while other efforts are under way to lower plasma concentrations of K^+.

Use of supplemental calcium in the prevention and treatment of osteoporosis is discussed below.

Hypercalcemic States. Hypercalcemia occurs in many diverse clinical conditions and requires differential diagnosis and appropriate corrective measures. Ingestion of large quantities of a Ca^{2+} salt does not generally by itself cause hypercalcemia, an exception being patients with hypothyroidism, who absorb Ca^{2+} with increased efficiency (Benker *et al.,* 1988). Also, the uncommon hypercalcemic disorder called *milk-alkali syndrome* is caused by concurrent ingestion of large quantities of milk and alkalinizing powders, in which setting renal Ca^{2+} excretion is impaired.

In an outpatient setting, the most common cause of hypercalcemia is primary hyperparathyroidism (HPT), accompanied frequently by significant hypophosphatemia; the latter reflects diminished renal tubular phosphorus reabsorption due to hypersecretion of PTH. Some patients have renal calculi and peptic ulceration, and a few still show classical parathyroid skeletal disease. However, most patients today show few if any symptoms, and those that are present are often vague and nonspecific. Contemporary use of immunoradiometric (IRMA) assays for the intact PTH molecule obviates many of the difficulties with previous assays and is associated with a diagnostic accuracy of >90% (Endres *et al.,* 1991).

Familial benign hypercalcemia (or *familial hypocalciuric hypercalcemia*) is an inherited hypercalcemic disorder that generally is accompanied by extremely low urinary Ca^{2+} excretion. Hypercalcemia usually is mild, and circulating PTH is often normal to slightly elevated. The importance of making this diagnosis lies in the fact that patients mistakenly diagnosed to have primary HPT may be submitted to surgical exploration without discovery of an adenoma, and without therapeutic benefit. Patients do not experience long-term clinical consequences, except for homozygous infants, who may have severe, even lethal, hypercalcemia. Diagnosis is established by demonstrating hypercalcemia in first-degree family members. The molecular basis for familial benign hypercalcemia is a mutation in the Ca^{2+}-sensing receptor (Pollak *et al.,* 1993).

Most hypercalcemia discovered in hospitals is associated with a systemic malignancy, either with or without bony metastasis. PTH-related protein (PTHrP) is a primitive, highly conserved protein that may be abnormally expressed in malignant tissue, particularly by squamous cell and other epithelial cancers. The presence of substantial sequence homology of the amino-terminal portion of PTHrP with the amino terminus of native PTH permits this molecule to interact with the PTH receptor in target tissues and underlies the hypercalcemia and hypophosphatemia that are seen in humoral hypercalcemia of malignancy (*see* Grill and Martin, 1994). Other tumors release cytokines or prostaglandins that stimulate bone resorption. Hypercalcemia associated with malignancy is generally more severe than in HPT (frequently >13 mg/dl) and may be associated with lethargy, weakness, nausea, vomiting, polydipsia, and polyuria. Assays for PTHrP may aid diagnosis. In some patients with lymphomas, hypercalcemia is due to overproduction of 1,25-dihydroxyvitamin D by the tumor cells. A similar mechanism explains the hypercalcemia that is seen occasionally in sarcoidosis and other granulomatous disorders.

Vitamin D excess may cause hypercalcemia. In this case, sufficient 25-hydroxyvitamin D is present to stimulate intestinal Ca^{2+} hyperabsorption, leading to hypercalcemia and suppression of PTH and 1,25-dihydroxyvitamin D production. Thus, measurement of 25-hydroxyvitamin D is diagnostic. Occasional patients with *hyperthyroidism* show mild hypercalcemia, presumably due to a direct effect of thyroid hormone on bone turnover. *Immobilization* may lead to hypercalcemia in growing children and young adults, but is an unusual cause of hypercalcemia in older individuals unless bone turnover is already increased, as in Paget's disease or in hyperthyroidism. Hypercalcemia is sometimes noted in adrenocortical deficiency, as in Addison's disease, or following removal of a hyperfunctional adrenocortical tumor. Hypercalcemia occurs following renal transplantation, owing to persistent hyperfunctioning parathyroid tissue that resulted from the previous renal failure.

Differential diagnosis of the various causes of hypercalcemia may pose difficulties, but recent advances in serum tests for PTH, PTHrP, 25-hydroxy- and 1,25-dihydroxyvitamin D have facilitated accurate diagnosis in the great majority of cases. Hypercalcemia of any etiology can have dire consequences. The predominant and most devastating lesion usually occurs in the kidney, with reductions of renal function and nephrocalcinosis.

Treatment of Hypercalcemia. Hypercalcemia occasionally may be life threatening. Such patients frequently are severely dehydrated because hypercalcemia has compromised renal concentrating mechanisms. Thus, fluid resuscitation with large volumes of isotonic saline must be early and aggressive (6 to 8 liters/day). Agents that augment Ca^{2+} excretion, such as loop diuretics, may help to counteract the effect of plasma volume expansion by saline, but they are contraindicated by themselves, as they will aggravate dehydration and hypercalcemia.

Corticosteroids administered at high doses (*e.g.,* 40 to 80 mg/day of *prednisone*) may be useful in situations where hypercalcemia results from diseases such as sarcoidosis, lymphoma, or hypervitaminosis D. The response to steroid therapy is slow; 1 to 2 weeks may be required before plasma Ca^{2+} falls.

Calcitonin (CALCIMAR, MIACALCIN) acts specifically on osteoclasts to inhibit bone resorption and may be useful in managing hypercalcemia. Reduction in Ca^{2+} may be rapid, although escape from the hormone regularly occurs in several days. The recommended starting dose is 4 units/kg body weight every 12 hours; if there is no response within one or two days, the dose may be increased to 8 units/kg every 12 hours. If the response after two more days still is unsatisfactory, the dose may be increased to a maximum of 8 units/kg every 6 hours.

Plicamycin (mithramycin; MITHRACIN) is a cytotoxic antibiotic that also decreases plasma Ca^{2+} concentrations by inhibiting bone resorption. Reduction in plasma Ca^{2+} concentrations

occurs within 24 to 48 hours when a relatively low dose of this agent is given (15 to 25 μg/kg body weight) to minimize the high systemic toxicity of the drug.

Intravenous bisphosphonates (*etidronate, pamidronate*) have proven very effective in the management of hypercalcemia. These agents act as potent inhibitors of osteoclastic bone resorption. Oral bisphosphonates have been relatively unsuccessful for treating hypercalcemia. For this purpose, *pamidronate* (AREDIA) is given as an intravenous infusion of 60 to 90 mg over 4 to 24 hours. With bisphosphonates, resolution of hypercalcemia occurs over several days, and the effect usually persists for several weeks.

Gallium nitrate (GANITE) is a potent inhibitor of bone resorption that was approved for treating malignancy-associated hypercalcemia, but its utility was limited by nephrotoxicity. Gallium nitrate is not currently available in the United States.

Oral sodium phosphate lowers plasma Ca^{2+} concentrations and may offer short-term calcemic control of some patients with HPT who are awaiting surgery. However, the risk of precipitating calcium phosphate salts in soft tissues throughout the body is of concern. In light of satisfactory responses to other agents, administration of intravenous sodium phosphate cannot be recommended as a means to treat hypercalcemia.

Edetate disodium (disodium EDTA; ENDRATE, others) is a chelating agent that forms soluble complexes with Ca^{2+}. It is mentioned here only for historical purposes and is not currently recommended for any therapeutic use involving Ca^{2+}. Chelation in the blood rapidly lowers Ca^{2+}, with a substantial risk of cardiac, renal, and neurological toxicity. EDTA (as the calcium, disodium salt) still may be used for chelation therapy of heavy metal toxicity (*see* Chapter 67).

PHOSPHATE

In addition to its role as a dynamic constituent of intermediary and energy metabolism, phosphate is an essential component of all body tissues. More than 80% of total body phosphorus occurs in bone, and about 15% is in soft tissue. Phosphorus is a component of membrane phospholipids. It modifies tissue concentrations of Ca^{2+} and plays a major role in renal H^+ excretion.

Absorption, Distribution, and Excretion. Phosphate is absorbed from, and to a limited extent secreted into, the gastrointestinal tract. Transport of phosphate from the gut lumen is an active, energy-dependent process that is modified by several factors including vitamin D, which stimulates absorption. Presence of large quantities of Ca^{2+} or Al^{3+} may lead to formation of large amounts of insoluble phosphate and diminish net phosphate absorption. In adults, about two-thirds of ingested phosphate is absorbed and is almost entirely excreted into the urine. In growing children, phosphate balance is positive. Concentrations of phosphate in plasma are higher in children than in adults. This "hyperphosphatemia" decreases the affinity of hemoglobin for oxygen and is hypothesized to explain the physiological "anemia" of childhood (Card and Brain, 1973).

Phosphate is present in plasma and extracellular fluid, in cell membranes and intracellular fluid, and in collagen and bone tissue. In extracellular fluid, the bulk of phosphate exists in inorganic form as the two constituents, NaH_2PO_4 and Na_2HPO_4; the ratio of disodium to monosodium phosphate is 4:1 at pH 7.40. This ratio varies with pH; however, due to its relatively low concentration, phosphate contributes little to the buffering capacity of extracellular fluid. The concentration of plasma inorganic phosphate varies with age (Greenberg et al., 1960) and inversely with the rate of renal hydroxylation of 25-hydroxycholecalciferol (see below). A reduction of plasma phosphate concentration permits the presence of more Ca^{2+} in the blood without mineral precipitation.

Renal phosphate excretion has been extensively studied. More than 90% of plasma phosphate is filterable, of which 80% is actively reabsorbed. Most reabsorption occurs in the initial segment of the proximal tubule, with a lesser component in the pars recta. The extent of phosphate reabsorption at more distal sites remains controversial (see Yanagawa and Lee, 1992). There is little evidence for tubular phosphate secretion in the mammalian kidney. Phosphate excreted in the urine represents the difference between the amount filtered and that reabsorbed. Expansion of plasma volume increases urinary phosphate excretion (Steele, 1970). PTH increases urinary phosphate excretion by blocking reabsorption. Vitamin D and its metabolites directly stimulate proximal tubular phosphate reabsorption (Puschett et al., 1972).

Role of Phosphate in the Acidification of the Urine. Although the concentration of phosphate is low in the extracellular fluid, the anion is progressively concentrated in the renal tubule and represents the most abundant buffer system in the distal tubule. At this site, the secretion of H^+ by the tubular cell in exchange for Na^+ in the tubular urine converts disodium hydrogen phosphate to sodium dihydrogen phosphate. In this manner, large amounts of acid can be excreted without lowering the pH of the urine to a degree that would block H^+ transport by a high concentration gradient between the tubular cell and luminal fluid.

Actions of the Phosphate Ion. Once phosphate gains access to body fluids and tissues, it exerts little pharmacological effect. If the ion is introduced into the intestine, the absorbed phosphate is rapidly excreted. If large amounts are given by this route, much of it may escape absorption. Because this property leads to a cathartic action, phosphate salts are employed as mild laxatives. Inorganic phosphate poisoning following ingestion of

laxatives that contain phosphate salts has been reported in adults and children (McConnell, 1971). Ingestion of large amounts of sodium dihydrogen phosphate lowers urinary pH. If excessive phosphate salts are introduced intravenously or orally, they may prove toxic by reducing the concentration of Ca^{2+} in the circulation and from the precipitation of calcium phosphate in soft tissues (Vernava et al., 1987).

Phosphate Depletion. Phosphate is a ubiquitous component of ordinary foods; thus simple dietary inadequacy is not likely to cause phosphate depletion. Sustained abuse of aluminum-containing antacids, however, can severely limit phosphate absorption and result in clinical phosphate depletion, manifest as malaise, muscle weakness, and osteomalacia. *Familial hypophosphatemia* is an X-linked trait due to defective intestinal and/or renal handling of phosphate that results in rickets and dwarfism. Hypophosphatemia can decrease markedly erythrocyte ATP and 2,3-diphosphoglycerate content. Acute hemolytic anemia and impaired tissue oxygenation can occur in severe hypophosphatemia (Jacob and Amsden, 1971), raising the possibility that cellular stores of other high-energy phosphates also may be depleted.

Pathological Conditions Associated with Disturbed Phosphate Metabolism. *Rickets.* The consequences of vitamin D deficiency with regard to the metabolism of both phosphate and calcium are described below, as are other forms of rickets. Familial hypophosphatemia is due to defective phosphate absorption and/or excretion, as mentioned above.
Osteomalacia. Osteomalacia is characterized by undermineralized bone matrix. Osteomalacia may occur when sustained phosphate depletion is caused by inhibiting its absorption in the gut (as with aluminum-containing antacids) or by renal hyperexcretion due to PTH.
Primary or Secondary Hyperparathyroidism. In these disorders, the increase in PTH secretion reduces renal tubular reabsorption of phosphate and decreases the plasma inorganic phosphate concentration. By contrast, in *hypo-* or *pseudohypoparathyroidism,* deficient PTH action on the renal tubule leads to a rise in plasma phosphate concentrations.
Chronic Renal Failure. In this condition, the retention of phosphate is primary and reflects the degree of renal compromise. Reduction of Ca^{2+} by the increased phosphate level stimulates hypersecretion of PTH, but since renal function is grossly impaired, hyperphosphatemia persists. The continuing hyperphosphatemia may be modified by vigorous administration of aluminum hydroxide gel or calcium carbonate supplements.

Therapeutic Uses. The phosphates have limited therapeutic utility. Sodium phosphate has been employed to diminish hypercalcemia (see above). The phosphates have a role in management of the phosphate-depletion syndrome and in chronic management of patients with vitamin D–resistant hypophosphatemic osteomalacia or rickets. Phosphate salts are also effective cathartics (see Chapter 39).

PARATHYROID HORMONE (PTH)

History. Credit for the discovery of the parathyroid gland usually is given to Sandstrom, who in 1880 published an anatomical report that attracted little attention. The glands were rediscovered a decade later by Gley, who determined the effects of their extirpation with the thyroid. Vassale and Generali then successfully removed only the parathyroids and noted that tetany, convulsions, and death quickly followed.

MacCallum and Voegtlin (1909) first noted the effect of parathyroidectomy on the concentration of plasma Ca^{2+}. The relation of low plasma Ca^{2+} to symptoms was quickly appreciated, and a comprehensive picture of parathyroid function began to form. Active glandular extracts alleviated hypocalcemic tetany in parathyroidectomized animals and raised the concentration of Ca^{2+} in the plasma of normal animals (Berman, 1924; Collip, 1925). For the first time, the relation of clinical abnormalities to parathyroid hyperfunction was appreciated.

While American and British investigators used physiological approaches to explore the function of the parathyroid glands, German and Austrian pathologists related the skeletal changes of osteitis fibrosa cystica to the presence of parathyroid tumors. In a delightful historical review, Albright (1948) traced the manner in which these two diverse types of investigations finally arrived at the same conclusion.

Chemistry.   Human, bovine, and porcine parathyroid hormones are all single polypeptide chains of 84 amino acids. Their molecular masses approximate 9500 daltons, and the entire amino acid sequence has been established for each. Biological activity is associated with the N-terminal portion of the peptide; residues 1 to 27 are required for optimal binding to the PTH receptor and hormone activity. Derivatives lacking the first or second residue bind to PTH receptors but are virtually inert (Aurbach, 1988). Bovine and porcine PTH differ by seven amino acid residues, and the amino-terminal segment of human PTH differs from its bovine and porcine equivalents by only four and three residues, respectively. The three hormones differ little in biological activity but are distinguishable immunologically.

Synthesis, Secretion, and Immunoassay.   PTH is synthesized in a prehormone form. The 115–amino-acid translation product that is destined to become PTH is called *preproparathyroid hormone*. This single-chain peptide is rapidly converted to proparathyroid hormone by cleavage of 25 amino-terminal residues as the peptide is transferred to the intracisternal space of the endoplasmic reticulum. Proparathyroid hormone moves to the Golgi apparatus for conversion to PTH by cleavage of six amino acids. PTH resides within secretory granules until it is secreted into the circulation. Most of the PTH normally is degraded by proteolysis before it can be secreted. During periods of hypocalcemia, more PTH is secreted and less is hydrolyzed. This mechanism provides a supply of hormone that can be mobilized rapidly in response to acute need without the delay entailed by increased synthesis of protein. In prolonged hypocalcemia, PTH synthesis also increases, and the gland hypertrophies. Neither preproparathyroid hormone nor proparathyroid hormone appears in plasma. The synthesis and processing of PTH have been reviewed by Kronenberg *et al.* (1994).

Intact PTH has a half-life in plasma of 2 to 5 minutes; removal by the liver and kidney accounts for about 90% of its clearance. Metabolism of PTH releases fragments that circulate in blood. Fragments also are released by proteolysis of PTH within the parathyroid gland. Although these are not biologically active, they react with antibodies prepared against the intact hormone. Nonetheless, satisfactory PTH immunoassays have been developed for clinical use. Immunoradiometric assays using two monoclonal antibodies, one directed toward the amino-terminal and one toward the carboxyl-terminal portion of the hormone, permit accurate and sensitive detection of the intact PTH. These assays have replaced standard radioimmunoassays for clinical diagnostic purposes (*see* Nussbaum and Potts, 1994).

Physiological Functions.   The primary function of PTH is to elicit the adaptive changes that maintain a constant concentration of Ca^{2+} in the extracellular fluid. Processes that are regulated include intestinal Ca^{2+} absorption, mobilization of bone Ca^{2+}, and excretion of calcium in urine, feces, sweat, and milk (Figure 62–3). The actions of PTH on its target tissues are mediated by a cell surface G

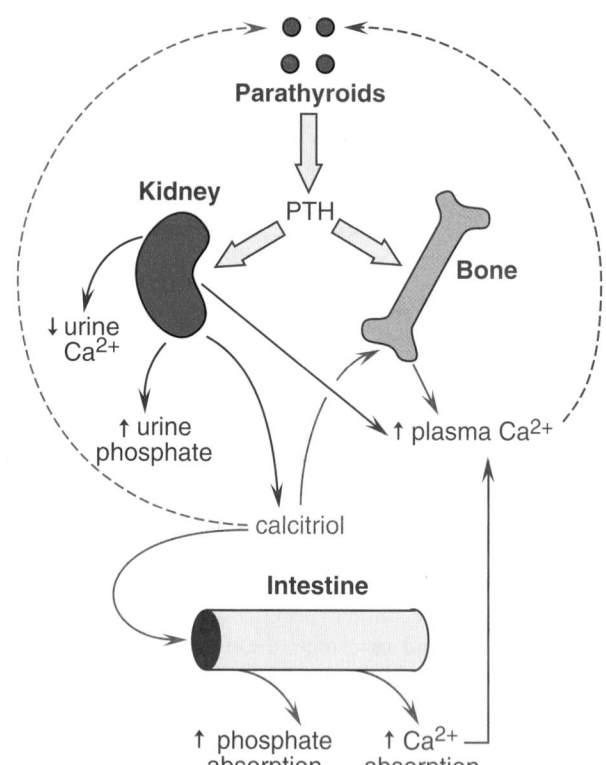

Figure 62–3. Calcium homeostasis and its regulation by parathyroid hormone (PTH) and 1,25-dihydroxyvitamin D.

PTH has stimulatory effects on bone and kidney, including the stimulation of 1 α-hydroxylase activity in kidney mitochondria leading to the increased production of 1,25-dihydroxyvitamin D (calcitriol) from 25-hydroxycholecalciferol, the monohydroxylated vitamin D metabolite (*see also* Figure 62–6). Calcitriol is the biologically active metabolite of vitamin D. Solid lines indicate a positive effect; dashed lines refer to negative feedback. *See* text for further explanation.

protein–coupled receptor (*see* Chapter 2); its predicted amino acid sequence and seven transmembrane spanning topography have been revealed by molecular cloning (Jüppner *et al.,* 1991).

Regulation of Secretion.   The concentration of Ca^{2+} in plasma is the most powerful factor that regulates parathyroid gland secretory activity. When the concentration of Ca^{2+} is low, PTH secretion increases, and hypertrophy and hyperplasia of the gland result if the hypocalcemia is sustained. If the concentration of Ca^{2+} is high, PTH secretion decreases. *In vitro* studies show that amino acid transport, nucleic acid and protein synthesis, cytoplasmic growth, and PTH secretion are stimulated by exposure to low concentrations of Ca^{2+} and suppressed by high concentrations over an extended period of time. Thus, Ca^{2+} *per se* appears to regulate parathyroid gland growth as well as hormone synthesis and secretion.

Changes in circulating Ca^{2+} regulate PTH secretion *via* a plasma membrane–associated calcium sensor on the surface of parathyroid cells (Brown *et al.,* 1993). Binding of Ca^{2+} by this sensor inhibits PTH secretion, whereas reduced sensor occupancy promotes hormone secretion. Hypercalcemia is associated with a reduction of intracellular cyclic AMP content and protein kinase C (PKC) activity, and reduced circulating Ca^{2+} leads to activation of PKC. However, the precise link between these changes and alterations in hormone secretion is incompletely resolved. Other agents that increase parathyroid cell cyclic AMP levels, such as β-adrenergic receptor agonists and dopamine, also increase PTH secretion, but the magnitude of response is far less than that seen with hypocalcemia. The active vitamin D metabolite, 1,25-dihydroxy-vitamin D *(calcitriol)*, directly suppresses PTH gene expression. There appears to be no relation between physiological concentrations of extracellular phosphate and PTH secretion, except insofar as changes in phosphate concentrations alter circulating Ca^{2+}. Severe hypermagnesemia and hypomagnesemia each can inhibit the secretion of PTH (Rude *et al.,* 1976).

The extracellular concentration of Ca^{2+} is controlled by an elaborate feedback system, the afferent limb of which is sensitive to the ambient activity of Ca^{2+} and the efferent limb of which releases PTH. The hormone acts on various peripheral target tissues to mobilize Ca^{2+} into the extracellular fluid and thus to restore the concentration to normal.

Effects on Bone.   PTH action on bone increases the delivery of Ca^{2+} to the extracellular fluid by increasing overall bone resorption, a process that involves the release of organic as well as mineral matrix components. The skeletal target cell for PTH probably is the osteoblast. With the exception of avian cells, specific receptors for PTH have not been described in osteoclasts, nor does an increase in resorption follow incubation of PTH with os-

teoclasts that are layered onto devitalized bone. Hormone responsiveness does appear if the osteoclasts are cultured in conditioned medium from osteoblasts that first have been exposed to PTH, suggesting an important role for osteoblasts in PTH-dependent bone resorption (McSheehy and Chambers, 1986; Perry *et al.,* 1987; Takahashi *et al.,* 1988).

PTH recruits osteoclast precursor cells into forming new bone remodeling units. Sustained increases in circulating PTH result in characteristic histological changes in bone, including an increase in the prevalence of osteoclastic resorption sites and in the proportion of bone surface that is covered with unmineralized matrix. Although excessive osteoid surfaces may indicate defective mineralization, they signify in this case an increase in bone-forming surface due to an overall increase in remodeling activity.

Direct effects of PTH on individual, incubated osteoblasts are generally inhibitory and include reductions in the formation of type I collagen, alkaline phosphatase, and osteocalcin. However, the measurable response *in vivo* to PTH reflects not only hormone action on individual cells but also the increased total number of active osteoblasts due to initiation of new remodeling units. Thus, plasma levels of osteocalcin and alkaline phosphatase activity actually may be increased. No simple model fully explains the molecular basis of PTH actions on bone. PTH stimulates cyclic AMP production in osteoblasts, but there also is evidence for a role for intracellular Ca^{2+} in mediating some of PTH's actions.

Effects on Kidney.   PTH acts on the kidney to enhance the efficiency of Ca^{2+} reabsorption, to inhibit tubular reabsorption of phosphate, and to stimulate conversion of vitamin D to its hormonal form, 1,25-dihydroxyvitamin D, or calcitriol (*see* Figure 62–3 and below). As a result, filtered Ca^{2+} is avidly retained, and its concentration increases in plasma; phosphate is excreted, and its plasma concentration falls. Calcitriol, at the same time, is secreted into the circulation, interacts with specific, high-affinity receptors in the intestine, and contributes to the rise in plasma Ca^{2+} concentration by improving the efficiency of gut Ca^{2+} absorption.

Calcium.   PTH increases tubular reabsorption of Ca^{2+} at a distal site (Agus *et al.,* 1973). When the plasma concentration of Ca^{2+} is normal, parathyroidectomy decreases tubular reabsorption of Ca^{2+} and thereby increases Ca^{2+} excretion in the urine. When the plasma concentration falls below 7 mg/dl (1.75 mM), a decrease in Ca^{2+} excretion occurs, because the amount of Ca^{2+} filtered through the glomeruli is lowered to the point that the cation is almost completely reabsorbed despite the reduced tubular capacity. If PTH is administered to hypoparathyroid animals or human beings, tubular reabsorption of Ca^{2+} is increased and Ca^{2+} excretion decreases. This effect, along with mobilization of calcium from bone and increased absorption from the gut, results in an increased concentration of Ca^{2+} in plasma. When the value rises above normal, the increased glomerular filtration of Ca^{2+} overwhelms the stimulatory effect of PTH on tubular reabsorption, and hypercalciuria ensues.

Phosphate. PTH increases the renal excretion of inorganic phosphate by decreasing its reabsorption. Patients with primary hyperparathyroidism typically show low values for tubular phosphate reabsorption.

Cyclic AMP mediates the renal effects of PTH (*see* Aurbach, 1988). PTH-sensitive adenylyl cyclase is located in the renal cortex, and cyclic AMP synthesized in response to the hormone affects tubular transport mechanisms. A portion of the cyclic nucleotide synthesized at this site escapes into the urine, and its assay serves as a measure of parathyroid activity and responsiveness.

Other Ions. PTH reduces renal excretion of Mg^{2+}. This effect reflects the net result of increased renal Mg^{2+} reabsorption and increased mobilization of the ion from bone (MacIntyre *et al.*, 1963). PTH increases excretion of water, amino acids, citrate, K^+, bicarbonate, Na^+, Cl^-, and SO_4^{2-}, whereas it decreases the excretion of H^+. Although the effects of PTH on renal acid–base metabolism are similar to those of acetazolamide, they are independent of the carbonic anhydrase system.

Calcitriol Synthesis. The final step in activation of vitamin D to its hormonal form, calcitriol, occurs in the kidney tubular cell (*see* later section on vitamin D). The activity of the hydroxylase enzyme involved in this step is governed by three primary regulators: inorganic phosphate, PTH, and Ca^{2+}. Reductions in circulating or tissue phosphate content rapidly increase calcitriol production, whereas hyperphosphatemia suppresses it. PTH is a powerful initiator of calcitriol production, whereas hypercalcemia suppresses it. Thus, when hypocalcemia causes a rise in PTH concentration, both the PTH-dependent lowering of circulating inorganic phosphate and a more direct effect of the hormone on the hydroxylase lead to increased circulating concentrations of calcitriol.

Miscellaneous Effects. PTH decreases the concentration of Ca^{2+} in milk and saliva. These effects are the opposite of those that would be expected from the concurrent changes in plasma Ca^{2+} concentration. It appears, therefore, that the hormone can conserve Ca^{2+} in the extracellular fluid also by reducing the rate of Ca^{2+} transport to milk and saliva.

Integrated Regulation of Extracellular Ca^{2+} Concentration by PTH.

The response of parathyroid cells to even modest reductions in Ca^{2+} occurs within minutes. For minute-to-minute regulation of Ca^{2+}, adjustments in renal Ca^{2+} handling more than suffice to maintain plasma calcium homeostasis. With more prolonged hypocalcemic stress, activation of the renal 1a-hydroxylase system leads to increased secretion of calcitriol, which directly stimulates intestinal calcium absorption (*see* Figure 62–3). In addition, increased delivery of labile calcium from bone into the extracellular fluid is stimulated. With a prolonged and severe hypocalcemic challenge, activation of new bone remodeling units helps to restore circulating Ca^{2+} concentrations, albeit at the expense of skeletal integrity.

When plasma Ca^{2+} activity rises, PTH secretion is suppressed and tubular Ca^{2+} reabsorption decreases. The reduction in circulating PTH promotes renal phosphate conservation, and both of these reduce calcitriol production, thereby decreasing intestinal Ca^{2+} absorption. Finally, bone remodeling is suppressed. Thus, one may construct a coherent model for calcium homeostasis based on the participation of two hormones, PTH and 1,25-dihydroxyvitamin D, and involving the hierarchical contributions of kidney, intestine, and bone (Figure 62–3). The importance in human beings of other hormones, such as calcitonin, to this scheme remains unsettled, but it is likely that these modulate the Ca^{2+}-parathyroid-vitamin D axis rather than serving as primary regulators.

Hypoparathyroidism. Hypoparathyroidism is only one of the many causes of hypocalcemia (*see* above) and occurs rarely. The deficiency state most commonly follows operative procedures on either the thyroid or parathyroid glands. Less frequently, the disorder stems from a genetic or autoimmune cause. Pseudohypoparathyroidism (PHP) is a disorder manifest by biochemical effects of hypoparathyroidism, but with elevated circulating levels of PTH. In this condition, end-organ responsiveness to PTH is severely impaired, frequently due to mutations in the adenylyl cyclase–G protein complex (*see* Levine, 1999).

In all varieties of hypoparathyroidism, hypocalcemia and its associated symptoms are encountered clinically. The earliest symptoms of hypocalcemia are paresthesias in the extremities. Mechanical stimulation of peripheral nerves during physical examination may produce contraction of the appropriate skeletal muscles (Chvostek's sign). These signs and symptoms may be followed by tetany, consisting of muscle spasms, particularly of the hands and feet, and laryngospasm. Eventually, generalized convulsions and other central nervous system manifestations occur. Smooth muscle also is affected. Hypocalcemia may be attended by spasm of the ciliary muscle, iris, esophagus, intestine, urinary bladder, and bronchi. Electrocardiogram changes and a marked tachycardia indicate cardiac involvement. Vascular spasm in fingers and toes also is commonly observed. In chronic hypoparathyroidism, ectodermal changes—consisting of loss of hair, grooved and brittle fingernails, defects of dental enamel, and cataracts—are encountered; calcification in the basal ganglia may be seen on routine skull radiographs. Psychiatric symptoms such as emotional lability, anxiety, depression, and delusions often are present.

Hypoparathyroidism is treated primarily with vitamin D (*see* below). Dietary supplementation with Ca^{2+} also may be necessary.

Hyperparathyroidism. *Primary* hyperparathyroidism (HPT) results from hypersecretion of PTH by one or more parathyroid glands. Plasma concentrations of Ca^{2+} occasionally may be normal in HPT, but they usually are elevated. Plasma inorganic phosphate concentrations usually are low normal to decreased. Urinary Ca^{2+} excretion generally is increased, reflecting the dominant effect of filtered load over the conserving effect of PTH on tubular Ca^{2+} reabsorption. However, for any given level of plasma Ca^{2+}, urinary Ca^{2+} excretion in HPT is not as high as it would be in nonparathyroid hypercalcemic states. *Secondary* hyperparathyroidism results as a compensation for reductions in circulating Ca^{2+} and is not associated with hypercalcemia. In these cases, the concentration of inorganic phosphate is particularly low (except when associated with renal failure), and the serum alkaline phosphatase activity is very high.

Severe primary or secondary HPT may be associated with a skeletal disorder known as osteitis fibrosa cystica. However, most patients with primary HPT have few if any skeletal findings. These are generally restricted to a modest reduction in overall bone mineral density, particularly at sites of cortical bone. By contrast, patients with primary HPT generally show reasonable conservation of trabecular bone density (*see* Bilezikian *et al.,* 1994).

The diagnosis of HPT has been simplified by the introduction of specific immunoradiometric assays for the intact PTH molecule. The combination of hypercalcemia and an elevated intact PTH concentration is sufficient to establish the diagnosis of HPT with greater than 90% accuracy.

Treatment of HPT.   In the hands of a skilled parathyroid surgeon, resection of a single adenoma (about 80% of cases) or of the hyperplastic glands (about 15% of cases) leads to cure of HPT. Transient postoperative hypocalcemia may reflect temporary disruption of blood supply to remaining parathyroid tissue or skeletal avidity for calcium. Permanent hypoparathyroidism is a serious but unusual complication of parathyroid surgery that requires lifelong treatment with vitamin D and supplemental calcium.

Clinical Uses of PTH.   PTH has no FDA-approved therapeutic use, but it may be approved in the near future for treatment of osteoporosis. Although it was used in the past to elevate the concentration of Ca^{2+} in plasma, this can be accomplished with greater safety and efficacy by administration of Ca^{2+} and/or vitamin D. Daily administration of PTH or its analogs has been shown to be of possible value in the treatment of patients with osteoporosis. While still an experimental strategy, substantial gains in axial bone mass have been observed in osteoporotic subjects treated with daily PTH(1–34) (*see* "Osteoporosis," below). PTH(1–34) can be used diagnostically to distinguish between pseudohypoparathyroidism and hypoparathyroidism. Since the former disease features target-organ resistance to the hormone, patients with PHP fail to increase their cyclic AMP excretion in response to acute administration of the peptide. Although this test is useful to characterize specific abnormalities in patients or families with PHP, clinical diagnosis usually can be made by measuring the circulating concentration of intact PTH.

VITAMIN D

Traditionally, vitamin D was assigned a passive role in calcium metabolism in that its presence in adequate concentrations was thought to permit efficient absorption of dietary calcium and to allow full expression of the actions of PTH. It is now known that vitamin D has a much more active role in calcium homeostasis. Even though it is termed "vitamin" D, it is a hormone that, together with PTH, is a major regulator of the concentration of Ca^{2+} in plasma. The following characteristics of vitamin D are consistent with its hormonal nature: it is synthesized in the skin and under ideal conditions probably is not required in the diet; it is transported in blood to distant sites in the body, where it is activated by a tightly regulated enzyme; its active form binds to specific receptors in target tissues, resulting ultimately in an increased concentration of plasma Ca^{2+}. Moreover, it is now known that receptors for the activated form of vitamin D are expressed in many cells throughout the body, including hematopoietic cells, lymphocytes, epidermal cells, pancreatic islets, muscle, and neurons; these receptors mediate a variety of actions that are unrelated to Ca^{2+} homeostasis.

History.   Vitamin D is the name applied to two related fat-soluble substances, *cholecalciferol* and *ergocalciferol,* that have in common the ability to prevent or cure rickets. Prior to the discovery of vitamin D, a high percentage of urban children living in the temperate zones developed rickets. Some researchers believed that the disease was due to lack of fresh air and sunshine; others claimed a dietary factor caused the disease. Mellanby (1919) and Huldschinsky (1919) showed both notions to be correct; addition of cod liver oil to the diet or exposure to sunlight prevented or cured the disease. In 1924, it was found that ultraviolet irradiation of animal rations was as efficacious in curing rickets as was irradiation of the animal itself (Hess and Weinstock, 1924; Steenbock and Black, 1924). These observations led to the elucidation of the structures of chole- and ergocalciferol and eventually to the discovery that these compounds require further processing in the body to become active. The discovery of metabolic activation is primarily attributable to studies conducted in the laboratories of DeLuca in the United States and Kodicek in England (*see* Kodicek, 1974; DeLuca and Schnoes, 1976).

Chemistry and Occurrence.   Ultraviolet irradiation of several animal and plant sterols results in their conversion to compounds with vitamin D activity. Cleavage of the carbon-to-carbon bond between C 9 and C 10 is the essential alteration produced by the photochemical process, but not all sterols that undergo this cleavage possess antirachitic activity. The principal provitamin found in animal tissues is 7-dehydrocholesterol, which is synthesized in the skin. Exposure of the skin to sunlight converts 7-dehydrocholesterol to cholecalciferol (vitamin D_3) (*see* Figure 62–4). Holick and associates have found an intermediate in the photolysis reaction—previtamin D_3, a 6,7-*cis* isomer that accumulates in the skin after exposure to ultraviolet radiation (*see* Holick, 1981). This isomer slowly converts spontaneously to vitamin D_3 and may provide a sustained source of D_3 for some time thereafter.

Ergosterol, which is present in plants, is the provitamin for vitamin D_2 (ergocalciferol). Ergosterol and vitamin D_2 differ from 7-dehydrocholesterol and vitamin D_3, respectively, only by

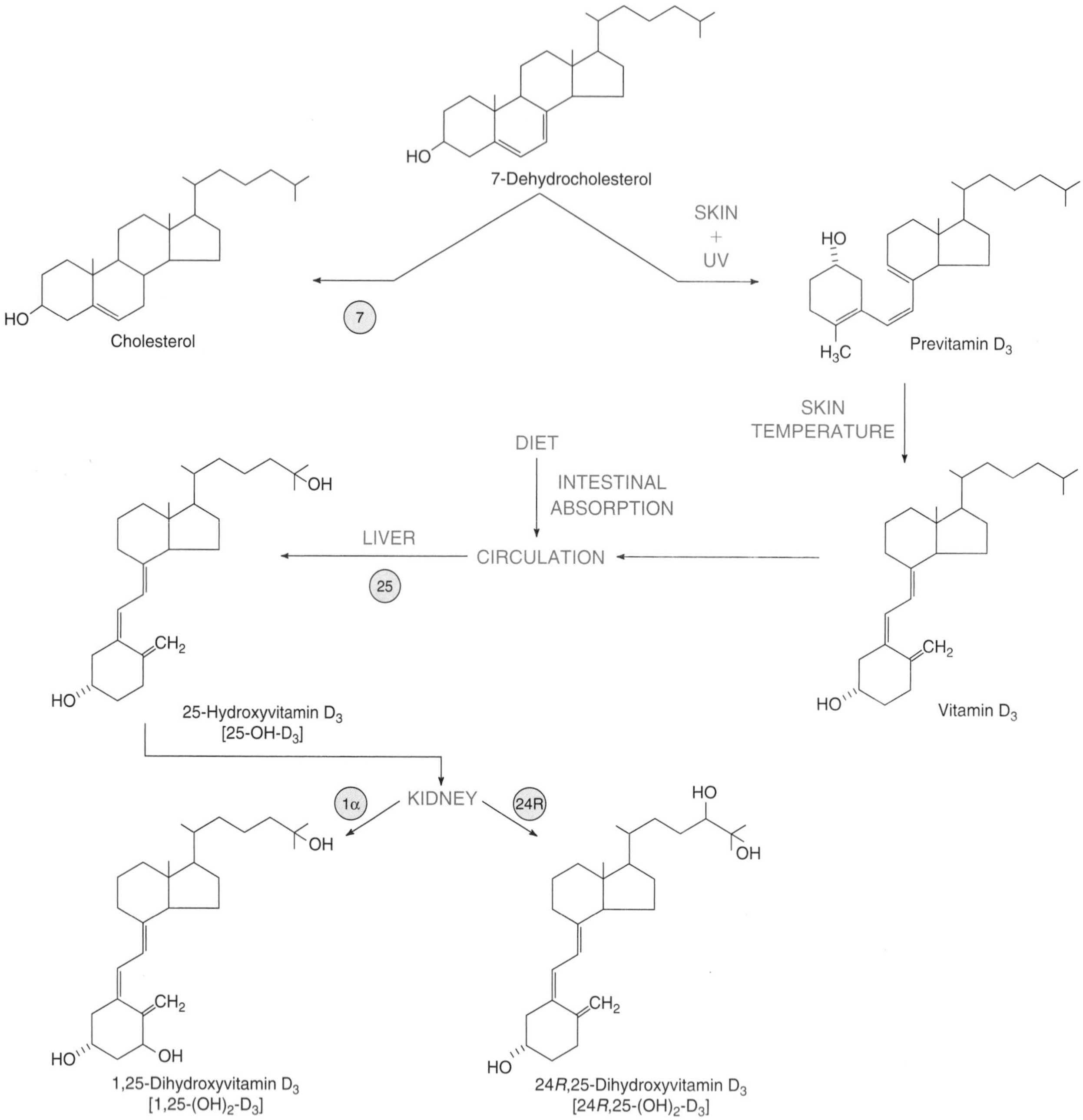

Figure 62–4. Photobiogenesis and metabolic pathways for vitamin D production and metabolism.

Circled letters and numbers denote specific enzymes: 7, 7-dehydrocholesterol reductase; 25, vitamin D-25 hydroxylase; 1α, 25-OHD-1α-hydroxylase; 24R, 25-OHD-24R hydroxylase. (*Adapted from Holick, 1981, with permission.*)

each having a double bond between C 22 and C 23 and a methyl group at C 24. Vitamin D_2 is the active constituent in a number of commercial vitamin preparations as well as in irradiated bread and irradiated milk. The material historically designated vitamin D_1 was later shown to be a mixture of antirachitic substances.

In some species the antirachitic potencies of vitamin D_2 and vitamin D_3 differ greatly from each other. In human beings there is no practical difference between the two, and in the following discussion vitamin D will be used as the collective term for the two vitamers (Figure 62–5).

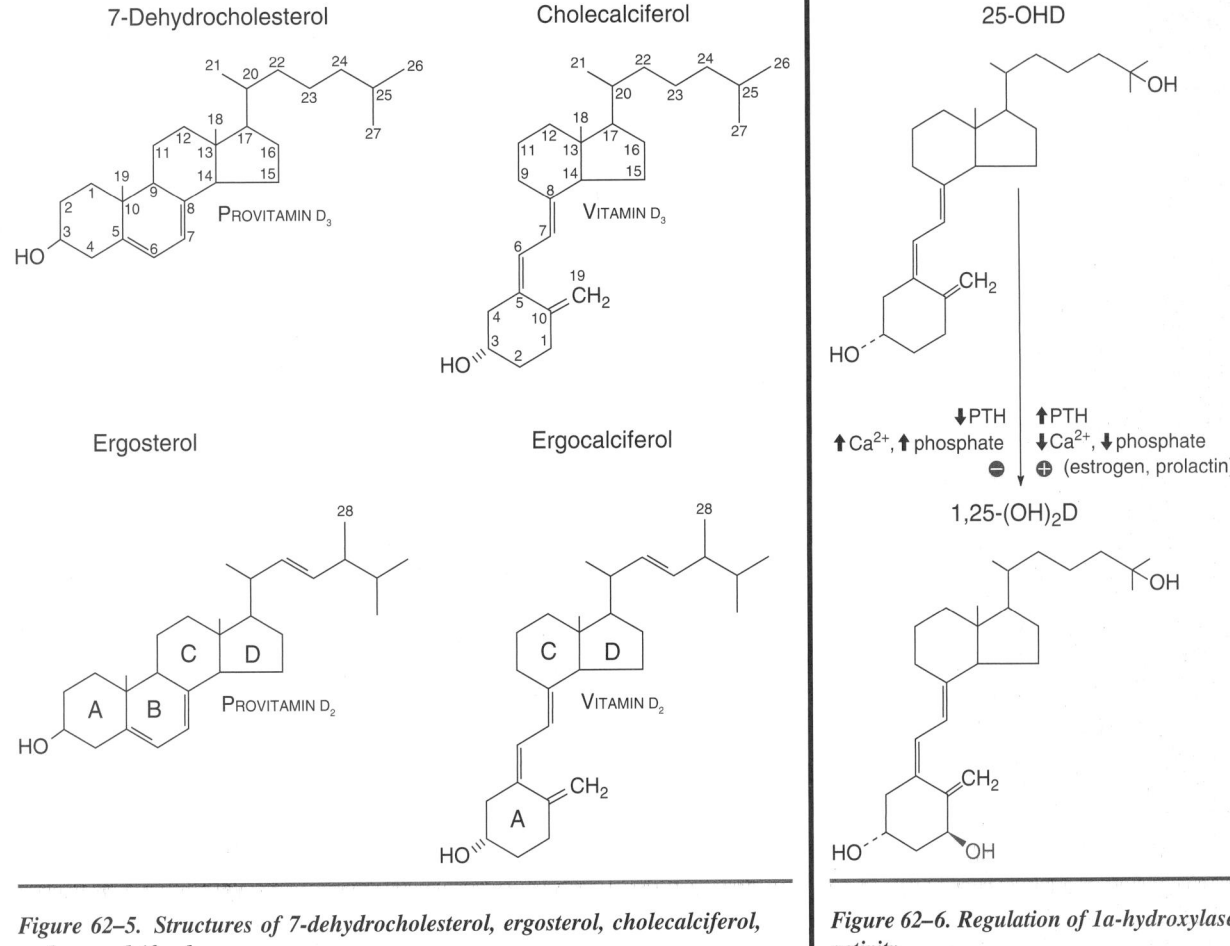

Figure 62–5. Structures of 7-dehydrocholesterol, ergosterol, cholecalciferol, and ergocalciferol.

Numbering system for steroid molecules is shown.

Figure 62–6. Regulation of 1a-hydroxylase activity.

25-OHD, 25-hydroxycholecalciferol; 1,25-(OH)$_2$D, calcitriol; PTH, parathyroid hormone.

Metabolic Activation

Both dietary and intrinsically synthesized vitamin D require activation to become biologically active. The primary active metabolite of the vitamin is *calcitriol* (1,25-dihydroxy-vitamin D), the product of two successive hydroxylations of vitamin D. The pathway of activation is shown in Figure 62–6. This subject has been reviewed by Horst and Reinhardt (1997).

25-Hydroxylation of Vitamin D.   The initial step in the activation of vitamin D occurs in the liver, and the product is 25-hydroxycholecalciferol (25-OHD, or calcifediol). The hepatic enzyme system responsible for 25-hydroxylation of vitamin D is associated with the microsomal and mitochondrial fractions of homogenates and requires NADPH and molecular oxygen.

1-Hydroxylation of 25-OHD.   After production in the liver, 25-OHD enters the circulation, where it is carried by vitamin D–binding globulin. Final activation to calcitriol occurs primarily in the kidney but also takes place in other sites, including macrophages (Reichel *et al.,* 1989). The kidney is the predominant source of circulating calcitriol. The enzyme system responsible for 1-hydroxylation of 25-OHD is associated with mitochondria in the proximal tubules. It is a mixed-function oxidase and requires molecular oxygen and NADPH as cofactors. Cytochrome P450, a flavoprotein, and ferredoxin are components of the enzyme complex.

The 1α-hydroxylase is subject to tight regulatory controls that result in changes in calcitriol secretion appropriate for optimal calcium homeostasis. Enzyme activity increases in dietary deficiency of vitamin D, calcium, and phosphate; it is stimulated by PTH, and probably also by prolactin and estrogen. Conversely, its activity is suppressed by high calcium, phosphate, and vitamin D intake. Regulation is both chronic, suggesting changes in enzyme protein synthesis, as well as acute (Figure 62–6). In the case of PTH, a rapid increase in calcitriol production is mediated by cyclic AMP, apparently through an indirect stimulation of a phosphoprotein phosphatase that acts on the ferredoxin component of the hydroxylase (Siegel *et al.*, 1986). There is evidence that hypocalcemia can activate the hydroxylase directly in addition to affecting it indirectly by eliciting secretion of PTH. Hypophosphatemia greatly increases hydroxylase activity (Haussler and McCain, 1977; Fraser, 1980; Rosen and Chesney, 1983). Calcitriol exerts negative-feedback control of the enzyme that reflects a direct action on the kidney as well as inhibition of PTH production. The nature of the regulatory mechanisms of estrogens and prolactin on the 1α-hydroxylase is not known.

Physiological Functions, Mechanism of Action, and Pharmacological Properties

Vitamin D is best characterized as a positive regulator of Ca^{2+} homeostasis. Phosphate metabolism is affected by the vitamin in a manner parallel to that of Ca^{2+}. Although regulation of Ca^{2+} homeostasis is considered to be its primary function, increasing evidence indicates that vitamin D is important in a number of other processes (*see* below).

The mechanisms by which vitamin D acts to maintain normal concentrations of Ca^{2+} and phosphate in plasma are to facilitate their absorption by the small intestine, to interact with PTH to enhance their mobilization from bone, and to decrease their excretion by the kidney. A direct role of the vitamin in bone mineralization has been difficult to validate; rather, the predominant view is that normal bone formation occurs when Ca^{2+} and phosphate concentrations in the plasma are adequate. However, it is now clear that vitamin D has both direct and indirect effects on the cells that are involved in bone remodeling.

The mechanism of action of calcitriol resembles that of the steroid and thyroid hormones. Calcitriol binds to cytosolic receptors within target cells, and the receptor–hormone complex interacts with DNA to modify gene transcription. The calcitriol receptor belongs to the same supergene family as the steroid and thyroid hormone receptors (*see* Evans, 1988; Pike, 1992; *see also* Chapter 2). Calcitriol also exerts effects that occur so rapidly that they are interpreted as being nongenomic actions (*see* Barsony and Marx, 1988).

Intestinal Absorption of Calcium. A defect in intestinal absorption of Ca^{2+} in vitamin D–deficient rats was demonstrated more than 50 years ago. Treatment of such animals with the activated hormone leads within 2 to 4 hours to increased movement of Ca^{2+} from the mucosal to the serosal surface of the intestine. The complex mechanisms underlying this action are not completely understood (*see* Wasserman, 1997). One relatively early event is the induction of one of a family of small Ca^{2+}-binding proteins (CaBP, or calbindin). Some investigators propose that CaBP acts to facilitate passage of Ca^{2+} through the brush border and its diffusion to the basolateral membrane of mucosal cells; others contend that the accumulation of CaBP correlates poorly with Ca^{2+} transport (Nemere and Norman, 1986 and 1988) and propose instead that calcitriol enhances the endocytotic uptake of Ca^{2+} from the intestinal lumen into vesicles within the mucosal cell brush border. These vesicles fuse with lysosomes, which deliver Ca^{2+} to the basolateral membrane for extrusion (*see* Cancela *et al.*, 1988). The mechanisms by which calcitriol might promote such vesicle-mediated transport have not been defined. Extrusion of calcium from the intestinal cell is accomplished by a plasma membrane calcium pump, the number of which is increased by calcitriol (*see* Wasserman, 1997). Although the time to onset of effects in vitamin D–deficient animals suggests the involvement of genomic mechanisms, calcitriol also causes a rapid (within minutes), receptor-mediated stimulation of Ca^{2+} transport in vitamin D–replete animals (*see* Cancela *et al.*, 1988).

Mobilization of Bone Mineral. Although vitamin D–deficient animals show obvious deficits in bone mineral, there is little evidence that vitamin D directly promotes mineralization; thus, it is thought that normal mineral deposition is sustained by maintenance of optimal plasma concentrations of Ca^{2+} and phosphate through promoting their intestinal absorption (*see* Stern, 1980). Indeed, children with vitamin D–resistant rickets type II have been treated successfully with intravenous infusions of Ca^{2+} and phosphate (*see* below). In contrast, physiological doses of vitamin D promote mobilization of Ca^{2+} from bone, and large doses cause excessive bone turnover. Although calcitriol-induced bone resorption may be reduced in parathyroidectomized animals, the response is restored when hyperphosphatemia is corrected (*see* Stern, 1980). Thus, both PTH and calcitriol act independently to enhance bone resorption.

The mechanisms by which calcitriol increases bone turnover have been partially defined and involve the interaction of multiple factors (*see* Haussler, 1986; Reichel *et al.*, 1989). Mature osteoclasts themselves do not appear to be directly acted upon by calcitriol, nor do they apparently contain calcitriol receptors. Instead, calcitriol promotes the recruitment of osteoclast precursor cells to resorption sites as well as the development of differentiated functions that characterize mature osteoclasts (Mimura *et al.*, 1994). Osteopetrosis is a disease characterized by deficient bone resorption, in which osteoclast responsiveness to calcitriol or other bone resorbing agents is profoundly impaired. The cells responsible for bone formation (osteoblasts) do contain calcitriol receptors, and calcitriol causes them to elaborate several proteins, including osteocalcin, a vitamin K–dependent protein that contains γ-carboxyglutamic acid residues, and interleukin-1, a lymphokine that promotes bone resorption (Spear *et al.,* 1988).

Renal Retention of Calcium and Phosphate.   The effects of vitamin D on renal handling of Ca^{2+} and phosphate are of uncertain importance. Vitamin D increases retention of Ca^{2+} independently of phosphate and probably enhances reabsorption of each by the proximal tubules.

Other Effects of Calcitriol.   It is now evident that the effects of calcitriol extend beyond calcium homeostasis. Receptors for calcitriol are distributed widely throughout the body (*see* Pike, 1992). Calcitriol affects maturation and differentiation of mononuclear cells and influences cytokine production. Its effects on the immune system have been reviewed by Amento (1987). One focus of current research is the potential therapeutic application of calcitriol's ability to inhibit proliferation and to induce differentiation of malignant cells (*see* van Leeuwen and Pols, 1997). The possibility of dissociating the hypercalcemic effect of calcitriol from its actions on cell differentiation has encouraged the search for analogs that might be useful in cancer therapy. Calcitriol inhibits epidermal proliferation and promotes epidermal differentiation, thus establishing a basis for evaluating it as a potential treatment of psoriasis vulgaris (*see* Kragballe, 1997).

The relation of vitamin D to skeletal muscle function has been reviewed by Boland (1986), and effects of vitamin D in the brain have been discussed by Carswell (1997).

Signs and Symptoms of Deficiency.   Deficiency of vitamin D results in inadequate absorption of Ca^{2+} and phosphate. The consequent decrease in plasma Ca^{2+} stimulates PTH secretion, which acts to restore plasma Ca^{2+} at the expense of bone; plasma concentrations of phosphate remain subnormal because of the phosphaturic effect of increased circulating PTH. In children, the result is a failure to mineralize newly formed bone and cartilage matrix, causing the defect in growth known as rickets. As a consequence of inadequate calcification, bones of individuals with rickets are soft, and the stress of weight bearing gives rise to characteristic deformities.

In adults, vitamin D deficiency results in osteomalacia, a disease characterized by generalized accumulation of undermineralized bone matrix. Severe osteomalacia may be associated with extreme bone pain and tenderness. Muscle weakness, particularly of large proximal muscles, is typical. Its basis is not fully understood but may reflect hypophosphatemia and inadequate vitamin D action on muscle. Gross deformity of bone occurs only in advanced stages of the disease. Circulating 25-OHD concentrations below 8 ng/ml are highly predictive of osteomalacia.

Hypervitaminosis D.   The acute or long-term administration of excessive amounts of vitamin D or enhanced responsiveness to normal amounts of the vitamin leads to clinically manifest derangements in calcium metabolism. The responses to vitamin D reflect endogenous vitamin D production, tissue reactivity, and vitamin D intake. Some infants may be hyperreactive to small doses of vitamin D. In adults, hypervitaminosis D results from overtreatment of hypoparathyroidism and from faddist use of excessive doses. Toxicity in children also may occur following accidental ingestion of adult doses.

The amount of vitamin D necessary to cause hypervitaminosis varies widely among individuals. As a rough approximation, continued ingestion of 50,000 units or more daily by a person with normal parathyroid function and sensitivity to vitamin D may result in poisoning. Hypervitaminosis D is particularly dangerous in patients who are receiving digitalis, because the toxic effects of the cardiac glycosides are enhanced by hypercalcemia (*see* Chapters 34 and 35).

Signs and Symptoms.   The initial signs and symptoms of vitamin D toxicity are those associated with hypercalcemia (*see* above). Hypercalcemia with hypervitaminosis D is due generally to very high circulating levels of 25-OHD, and plasma concentrations of PTH and calcitriol are typically but not uniformly suppressed.

In children, a single episode of moderately severe hypercalcemia may arrest growth completely for 6 months or more, and the deficit in height may never be fully corrected.

Vitamin D toxicity may be manifested in the fetus. There is a relationship between excess maternal vitamin D intake or extreme sensitivity and nonfamilial congenital supravalvular aortic stenosis. In infants, this anomaly is often associated with other stigmata of hypercalcemia. Maternal hypercalcemia also may result in suppression of parathyroid function in the newborn, with resultant hypocalcemia, tetany, and seizures.

Treatment.   Treatment of hypervitaminosis D consists of immediate withdrawal of the vitamin, a low-calcium diet, administration of glucocorticoids, and vigorous fluid support. With this regimen the plasma Ca^{2+} falls to normal and Ca^{2+} in soft tissue tends to be mobilized. Conspicuous improvement in renal function occurs unless renal damage has been severe.

Absorption, Fate, and Excretion.   Vitamin D usually is given by mouth, and intestinal absorption is adequate under most conditions. Both vitamins D_2 and D_3 are absorbed from the small intestine, although vitamin D_3 may be absorbed more efficiently. The exact portion of the gut that is most effective in vitamin D absorption reflects the vehicle in which the vitamin is dissolved. Most of the vitamin appears first within chylomicrons in lymph.

Bile is essential for adequate absorption of vitamin D; deoxycholic acid is the major constituent of bile in this regard. Thus, hepatic or biliary dysfunction seriously impairs vitamin D absorption.

Absorbed vitamin D circulates in the blood in association with vitamin D–binding protein, a specific α-globulin. The vitamin disappears from plasma with a half-life of 19 to 25 hours but is stored in fat depots for prolonged periods.

As discussed above, the liver is the site of conversion of vitamin D to 25-OHD, which circulates with the same binding protein. In fact, 25-OHD has a higher affinity for the protein than does the parent compound. The 25-hydroxy derivative has a biological half-life of 19 days and constitutes the major circulating form of vitamin D. Normal steady-state concentrations of 25-OHD in human beings are 15 to 50 ng/ml, although concentrations below 25 ng/ml may be associated with increased circulating PTH and greater bone turnover. The plasma half-life of calcitriol is estimated to be between 3 and 5 days in human beings, and 40% of an administered dose is excreted within 10 days (Mawer et al., 1976). Calcitriol is hydroxylated to $1,24,25-(OH)_3D$ by a renal hydroxylase that is induced by calcitriol and suppressed by those factors that stimulate the 25-OHD-1α-hydroxylase. This enzyme also hydroxylates 25-OHD to form $24,25-(OH)_2D$. Both 24-hydroxylated compounds are less active than calcitriol and presumably represent metabolites destined for excretion. Side chain oxidation of calcitriol also occurs.

The primary route of excretion of vitamin D is the bile; only a small percentage of an administered dose is found in urine. Vitamin D and its metabolites undergo extensive enterohepatic recirculation, and patients who have undergone intestinal bypass surgery or who otherwise have severe shortening or inflammation of the small intestine fail to reabsorb vitamin D sufficiently to maintain normal vitamin D nutriture.

An important interaction has been demonstrated between vitamin D and phenytoin or phenobarbital. Rickets and osteomalacia have been reported in patients receiving chronic anticonvulsant therapy. More often, the drugs induce a state of high-turnover osteoporosis secondary to a decrease in intestinal Ca^{2+} absorption (Weinstein et al., 1984). Plasma concentrations of 25-OHD are decreased in patients receiving these drugs, and it was proposed that phenytoin and phenobarbital accelerate the metabolism of vitamin D to inactive products (Hahn et al., 1972). However, concentrations of calcitriol in plasma remain normal in most patients receiving anticonvulsant therapy (Jubiz et al., 1977). The drugs also accelerate hepatic metabolism of vitamin K and reduce the synthesis of vitamin K–dependent proteins, such as osteocalcin.

Human Requirements and Unitage. An exhaustive and critical summary of the prophylactic requirements for vitamin D has been compiled by the Committee on Nutrition of the American Academy of Pediatrics (see Committee on Nutrition, 1963). Many years have elapsed since 1919, when Mellanby demonstrated the efficacy of cod liver oil in the prevention of rickets, a disease that has become a clinical rarity in the United States. Although sunlight provides adequate prophylaxis in the equatorial belt, in temperate climates insufficient cutaneous solar radiation in winter may necessitate dietary vitamin D supplementation.

Previously, the recommended allowance of vitamin D could be achieved only by adding oral vitamin D supplements to a normal diet. Since the advent of the addition of the vitamin to foodstuffs (especially milk, milk products, cereals, and candy), individuals of all ages receive variable and even excessive vitamin D without its special addition to the diet. Thus, supplemental requirements vary not only with age, pregnancy, and lactation but also with diet quality. Serious toxicity may result from excessive ingestion of vitamin D, and even as little as 1800 USP units (see equivalency below) per day in infants may inhibit growth. Therefore, any recommendation for vitamin D supplementation must be made only after careful scrutiny of the diet.

In both premature and normal infants, a total of 400 units per day of vitamin D ensures full antirachitic prophylaxis and optimal growth regardless of how it is obtained. During adolescence and beyond, this amount is probably also sufficient. There is some evidence that vitamin D requirements increase during pregnancy and lactation, although daily intake of 400 units is sufficient in these conditions as well (see Table XIII–1).

The USP unit is identical with the international unit (IU) and is equivalent to the specific biological activity of 0.025 μg of vitamin D_3 (i.e., 1 mg equals 40,000 units).

Bioassay procedures used in the past depended upon alleviation of the rachitic state. They are still in use for experimental purposes.

Modified Forms of Vitamin D. Several derivatives of vitamin D are of considerable experimental and therapeutic interest. Dihydrotachysterol (DHT) is a vitamin D analog that may be regarded as a reduction product of vitamin D_2 (and is sometimes referred to as DHT_2); its structural formula is as follows:

DIHYDROTACHYSTEROL (DHT)

DHT is about 1/450 as active as vitamin D in the antirachitic assay, but at high doses it is much more effective than vitamin

D in mobilizing bone mineral. The latter effect is the basis for the use of DHT to maintain normal concentrations of Ca^{2+} in plasma in hypoparathyroidism.

DHT undergoes 25-hydroxylation to yield 25-hydroxy-dihydrotachysterol (25-OHDHT), which appears to be the active form in both intestine and bone. 25-OHDHT is active in nephrectomized rats, indicating that it does not require 1-hydroxylation in the kidney. A comparison of the structures of DHT and 1,25-$(OH)_2$D shows that ring A of DHT is rotated so as to place its 3-hydroxyl group in approximately the same geometrical position as the 1-hydroxyl group of 1,25-$(OH)_2$D. It seems reasonable, therefore, to assume that 25-OHDHT could interact with receptor sites for 1,25-$(OH)_2$D without undergoing 1-hydroxylation. Thus, DHT bypasses the renal mechanisms of metabolic control.

1α-Hydroxycholecalciferol (1-OHD$_3$) is a synthetic derivative of vitamin D$_3$ that is hydroxylated in the 1α position. It is readily hydroxylated in the 25 position by the hepatic microsomal system to form 1,25-$(OH)_2$D and therefore was introduced as a substitute for the latter compound. In chick assays for stimulation of intestinal absorption of Ca^{2+} and bone mineralization, it is equal in activity to calcitriol. Because it does not require renal hydroxylation, it has been used to treat renal osteodystrophy. This drug is available in the United States for experimental purposes.

Analogs of Calcitriol. *Calcipotriol* (calcipotriene) contains a 22–23 double bond, a 24(S)-hydroxy functional group, and carbons 25–27 incorporated into a cyclopropane ring. This compound has receptor affinity similar to that of calcitriol, but it is less than 1% as active as calcitriol in regulating calcium metabolism. Calcipotriol has been studied extensively as a treatment for psoriasis (*see* Chapter 65), and a topical preparation (DOVONEX) is available for that purpose. In clinical trials, topical calcipotriol has been found to be an effective and safe treatment, slightly more effective than glucocorticoids. The mode of action of calcipotriol in psoriasis is not known.

Paricalcitol (ZEMPLAR) is a synthetic calcitriol derivative that reduces PTH production without producing hypercalcemia, except in overdoses. It has been approved by the FDA for treatment of secondary hyperparathyroidism in patients with chronic renal failure.

22-Oxacalcitriol also is a potent suppressor of PTH gene expression and shows very limited activity on intestine and bone. It is, therefore, an attractive compound for use in patients with overproduction of PTH in chronic renal failure or even with primary hyperparathyroidism (Finch *et al.*, 1993).

Therapeutic Uses

Many preparations containing vitamin D are marketed. *Ergocalciferol* (*calciferol;* DRISDOL) is pure vitamin D$_2$. It is available for oral, intramuscular, or intravenous administration. *Dihydrotachysterol* (*DHT;* HYTAKEROL) is the pure crystalline compound obtained by reduction of vitamin D$_2$ and is available for oral administration. *Calcifediol* (*25-hydroxycholecalciferol;* CALDEROL) also is available for oral use. *Calcitriol* (*1,25-dihydroxycholecalciferol;*

CALCIJEX, ROCALTROL) is available for oral administration or injection.

The major therapeutic uses of vitamin D may be divided into four categories: (1) prophylaxis and cure of nutritional rickets; (2) treatment of metabolic rickets and osteomalacia, particularly in the setting of chronic renal failure; (3) treatment of hypoparathyroidism; and (4) prevention and treatment of osteoporosis.

Nutritional Rickets. Nutritional rickets results from inadequate exposure to sunlight or deficiency of dietary vitamin D. The condition is extremely rare in the United States and other countries where food fortification with the vitamin is practiced. Infants and children receiving adequate amounts of vitamin D–fortified food do not require additional vitamin D; however, breast-fed infants or those fed unfortified formula should receive 400 units of vitamin D daily as a supplement. The usual practice is to administer vitamin A in combination with vitamin D. A number of well-balanced vitamin A and D preparations are available for this purpose. Premature infants are especially susceptible to rickets and may require supplemental vitamin D, since the fetus acquires more than 85% of its calcium stores during the third trimester.

The curative dose of vitamin D for the treatment of fully developed rickets is larger than the prophylactic dose. One thousand units daily will normalize Ca^{2+} and phosphate concentrations in plasma in approximately 10 days, and radiographic evidence of healing is seen within about 3 weeks. However, a daily dose of 3000 to 4000 units often is prescribed for more rapid healing; this is of particular importance in severe cases of thoracic rickets when respiration is embarrassed.

Certain conditions are known to lead to poor absorption of vitamin D. If these are untreated by vitamin supplementation, a frank deficiency may develop. Vitamin D may be of definite prophylactic value in such disorders as diarrhea, steatorrhea, biliary obstruction, and any other abnormality in gastrointestinal function in which absorption is appreciably diminished. Parenteral administration may be used in such cases.

Metabolic Rickets and Osteomalacia. This group of disorders is characterized by abnormalities in the synthesis of or the response to calcitriol.

Hypophosphatemic vitamin D–resistant rickets, in its most characteristic form, is an X-linked disorder of calcium and phosphate metabolism (XLH). Although calcitriol levels are normal, they would be predicted to be higher for the degree of hypophosphatemia that is observed. Patients experience clinical improvement when treated with large doses of vitamin D, usually in combination with inorganic phosphates. However, even with vitamin D treatment, calcitriol concentrations may remain lower than expected. A specific mutation giving rise to the most common form of XLH has been described (HYP Consortium, 1995). The affected protein, called PEX, is a neutral endoprotease. The specific substrate for this enzyme has not been clarified, but it is considered likely to be involved in renal phosphorus transport. Closely related syndromes to XLH have been described, including *hereditary hypophosphatemic rickets with hypercalciuria* (HHRH) and *autosomal dominant hypophosphatemic rickets.* The precise mechanisms for transmission and pathophysiology of these variant conditions also are unknown (*see* Econs and Drezner, 1992).

Vitamin D–dependent rickets is an autosomal recessive disease caused by an inborn error of vitamin D metabolism involving defective conversion of 25–OHD to calcitriol. The condition responds to physiological doses of calcitriol (Fraser *et al.,* 1973).

Hereditary 1,25-dihydroxyvitamin D resistance (also called vitamin D–dependent rickets type II) is an autosomal recessive disorder that is characterized by hypocalcemia, osteomalacia and rickets, and complete alopecia. Studies of skin fibroblasts from these patients have identified mutations in the calcitriol receptor that lead either to defective hormone binding or defective binding of the hormone–receptor complex to DNA. The latter mutations result from single amino acid substitutions on the zinc-finger portion of the DNA-binding domain of the vitamin D receptor (*see* Pike, 1992). Affected children are completely unresponsive to massive doses of vitamin D and calcitriol, and they may require prolonged treatment with parenteral Ca^{2+}. Some remission in symptoms has been observed during adolescence, but the basis for improvement is not known.

Renal osteodystrophy (renal rickets) is associated with chronic renal failure and is characterized by decreased conversion of 25-OHD to calcitriol. Phosphate retention decreases plasma Ca^{2+} concentrations, leading to secondary hyperparathyroidism. In addition, calcitriol deficiency impairs intestinal Ca^{2+} absorption and mobilization from bone. Hypocalcemia commonly results (although in some patients, prolonged and severe hyperparathyroidism eventually may lead to hypercalcemia). Aluminum deposition in bone also may play a role in the genesis of the skeletal disease.

Pathologically, the lesions are typical of hyperparathyroidism (osteitis fibrosa), deficiency of vitamin D (osteomalacia), or a mixture of both. In patients with chronic renal failure who are not receiving dialysis, emphasis has been on treatment of hyperphosphatemia with phosphate binders and calcium supplementation; these goals can be accomplished by the oral administration of calcium carbonate, combined with dietary phosphate restriction (Coburn and Salusky, 1989). Use of vitamin D analogs in predialysis patients is experimental, but it is clearly beneficial for patients who are undergoing dialysis. Administration of calcitriol raises the concentration of Ca^{2+} in plasma, lowers the concentration of PTH, and helps to maintain bone mineralization and growth in children (Berl *et al.,* 1978; Chesney *et al.,* 1978). Intravenous calcitriol may be effective in patients who are refractory to oral therapy (Andress *et al.,* 1989). DHT and 1-OHD$_3$ also can be used effectively, since renal hydroxylation is not required for their activity. Although 25-OHD also may be effective, high doses must be used.

Hypoparathyroidism. Hypoparathyroidism is characterized by hypocalcemia and hyperphosphatemia (*see* above). DHT has long been used to treat this condition, since it has a faster onset, shorter duration of action, and a greater effect on bone mobilization than does vitamin D. Calcitriol is effective in the management of hypoparathyroidism and at least certain forms of pseudohypoparathyroidism in which endogenous levels of calcitriol are abnormally low. However, most hypoparathyroid patients respond to any form of vitamin D. Calcitriol may be the agent of choice for temporary treatment of hypocalcemia while waiting for a slower-acting form of vitamin D to become effective.

Miscellaneous Uses of Vitamin D. These include treatment of hypophosphatemia seen in the Fanconi syndrome. The use of large doses of vitamin D (over 10,000 units/day) in patients with osteoporosis is not of value and can be dangerous. However, administration of 400 to 800 units/day of vitamin D to frail, elderly men and women has been shown to suppress bone remodeling, protect bone mass, and reduce fracture incidence (*see* later section on osteoporosis). Clinical trials suggest that calcitriol may become an important agent for the treatment of psoriasis (*see* Holick, 1993; Kragballe, 1992). As such nontraditional uses of vitamin D are discovered, it will become important to develop noncalcemic analogs of calcitriol that achieve effects on cellular differentiation without the risk of hypercalcemia.

CALCITONIN

History and Source. A hypocalcemic hormone, the effects of which are generally opposite to those of PTH, was discovered and named *calcitonin* by Copp in 1962 (*see* Copp, 1964). It was demonstrated as a result of perfusion of canine parathyroid and thyroid glands with hypercalcemic blood, which caused an acute and transient hypocalcemic effect occurring significantly earlier than the hypocalcemia of total parathyroidectomy. Copp concluded that the parathyroid glands secreted calcitonin in response to hypercalcemia and in this way normalized plasma Ca^{2+} concentrations. Munson and colleagues (Hirsch *et al.,* 1963) noted that parathyroidectomy in rats performed by cauterization caused more severe hypocalcemia than did thyroparathyroidectomy and suspected the existence of a hypocalcemic principle in the thyroid gland. They found that extracts of thyroid produced hypocalcemia, and named this factor *thyrocalcitonin.* It is now known that these two factors are the same and that the hormone does originate from the thyroid; however, calcitonin (CT) is the name that is generally used.

The parafollicular C cells from the thyroid, which are embryologically derived from neural crest ectoderm, are the site of production and secretion of CT. In nonmammalian vertebrates, CT is found in ultimobranchial bodies, which are separate organs from the thyroid gland. In human beings, C cells are widely distributed in the thyroid, parathyroid, and thymus.

Chemistry and Immunoreactivity. CT is a single-chain peptide of 32 amino acid residues. Eight of these residues are invariant, including a carboxyl-terminal prolinamide and a disulfide bridge between cysteines at positions 1 and 7. Both these structural features are essential for biological activity. The residues in the middle portion of the molecule (positions 10 to 27) are variable and appear to influence potency and/or duration of action. CTs derived from the ultimobranchial bodies of salmon and eel are more potent than mammalian thyroidal CTs both *in vivo* and *in vitro,* and they differ from the human hormone by 13 and 16 amino acid residues, respectively. Therapeutically, salmon CT appears to be more potent than human CT, in part because it is cleared more slowly from the circulation.

Human CT is processed from a propeptide of 135 amino acid residues; two additional peptides are generated, but their biological significance is unknown. The calcitonin gene contains six exons; calcitonin itself is encoded by exon 4. In C cells, messenger RNA is processed such that exons 1 to 4 are represented in the final transcript. In neural tissue, the sequence corresponding to exon 4 is removed, and the sequences for exons 1 to 3, 5, and 6 are included. Following translation and proteolytic cleavage of a precursor molecule, a mature peptide of 37 amino acids is generated, the *calcitonin gene–related peptide* (CGRP). CGRP mimics some effects of CT in some species but causes PTH-like effects in others and acts on receptors distinct from those that mediate the actions of CT. Since little or no CGRP is produced by the thyroid C cells, it is unlikely to function in calcium homeostasis. CGRP and its binding sites are widely distributed in the central nervous system (CNS), where it is believed to serve as a neurotransmitter. CGRP is found in many bipolar neurons in sensory ganglia and produces marked vasodilation. The structure and synthesis of CT and CGRP have been reviewed by MacIntyre and coworkers (1987).

Multiple forms of CT are found in plasma, including high-molecular-weight aggregates or cross-linked products. This fact has impeded development of useful immunoassays for CT. Assays for the intact monomeric peptide have been introduced (Body and Heath, 1983).

Regulation of Secretion. Biosynthesis and secretion of CT are regulated by the concentration of Ca^{2+} in plasma. When plasma Ca^{2+} is high, CT secretion increases; when plasma Ca^{2+} is low, CT secretion is low or undetectable. Normal circulating CT concentrations in human beings are less than 10 pg/ml (Body and Heath, 1983). Mean concentrations of CT in women are lower than those in men, as are responses to the secretagogues pentagastrin and Ca^{2+}. The circulating half-life of CT is about 10 minutes.

CT secretion can be stimulated by a number of agents, including catecholamines, glucagon, gastrin, and cholecystokinin, but is there little evidence for a physiological role for secretion in response to these stimuli. It is not even known whether or not CT plays a significant role in calcium homeostasis in human beings. Thyroidectomized patients with no detectable CT have normal calcium metabolism and bone mass. High concentrations (50 to 5000 times normal) of CT occur in plasma, urine, and tumor tissue of patients with medullary carcinoma of the thyroid. The tumor cells originate from the thyroid parafollicular cells, and the disease represents a true CT-excess syndrome. Measurement of the response of plasma CT to infusions of calcium gluconate and pentagastrin is the standard procedure to detect the condition (Wells *et al.*, 1978). Because one form of this disease is inherited as a dominant trait [multiple endocrine neoplasia type II (MEN II)], relatives of patients should be examined repeatedly from early childhood (Tashjian *et al.*, 1974). Localization of the mutation for MEN II to the RET protooncogene offers hope that genetic screening will supplant calcium/pentagastrin tests (Donis-Keller *et al.*, 1993; Carlson *et al.*, 1994).

Mechanism of Action. The hypocalcemic and hypophosphatemic effects of calcitonin are caused predominantly by direct inhibition of osteoclastic bone resorption (*see* MacIntyre *et al.*, 1987).

Although CT inhibits the effects of PTH on osteolysis, it does not act as a global inhibitor of PTH. It does not block activation of bone cell adenylyl cyclase by PTH and does not inhibit PTH-induced uptake of Ca^{2+} into bone. The actions of calcitonin are not blocked by inhibitors of RNA and protein synthesis. CT interacts directly with receptors on osteoclasts to produce a rapid and profound decrease in ruffled border surface area, thereby diminishing resorptive activity.

Depressed bone resorption leads to reduced urinary excretion of Ca^{2+}, Mg^{2+}, and hydroxyproline. Plasma phosphate concentrations also are lowered, due also to increased urinary phosphate excretion. Direct renal effects of CT vary with species. In human beings, CT promotes excretion of Ca^{2+}, phosphate, and Na^+. At least some of the actions of CT on kidney and bone are mediated by cyclic AMP (Murad *et al.*, 1970; Heersche *et al.*, 1974). Bioassay of CT preparations is performed by assessing their ability to lower the plasma Ca^{2+} concentration in the rat. Salmon and eel CTs are more potent than are human and porcine CTs (*see* above).

Therapeutic Uses. CT lowers Ca^{2+} and phosphate concentrations in patients with hypercalcemia, the effect of a single dose lasting 6 to 10 hours. This effect results from decreased bone resorption and is greater in patients in whom bone turnover rates are high. Although CT is effective in the initial treatment of hypercalcemia, escape from the response is observed after a few days. Use of this agent does not substitute for aggressive fluid resuscitation, and the response to other agents, such as bisphosphonates, may be more satisfactory (*see* section above on hypercalcemia).

CT is effective in disorders of increased skeletal remodeling, such as Paget's disease, and in some patients with osteoporosis (*see* below). In Paget's disease, chronic use of CT produces long-term reduction in symptoms and in serum alkaline phosphatase activity. Development of antibodies to CT does occur with long-term therapy, but this is not necessarily associated with clinical resistance. After initial therapy at 100 units/day, favorable results usually are obtained when dosage is reduced to 50 units three times a week. Side effects of CT include nausea, hand swelling, urticaria, and, rarely, intestinal cramping. Side effects appear to occur with equal frequency with human and salmon CT. *Salmon CT* is approved for clinical use as CAL-CIMAR or MIACALCIN. The latter is now available as a nasal spray, introduced for once-daily treatment of postmenopausal osteoporosis (*see* below). Subcutaneous or intramuscular doses of from 100 units up to 8 units/kg every 12 hours have been used to treat hypercalcemia. An initial dose of 100 units per day is used for Paget's disease, with reduction to 50 units three times a week once a response has occurred.

BISPHOSPHONATES

Bisphosphonate is the name given to a group of drugs characterized by a geminal bisphosphonate bond (Figure 62–7).

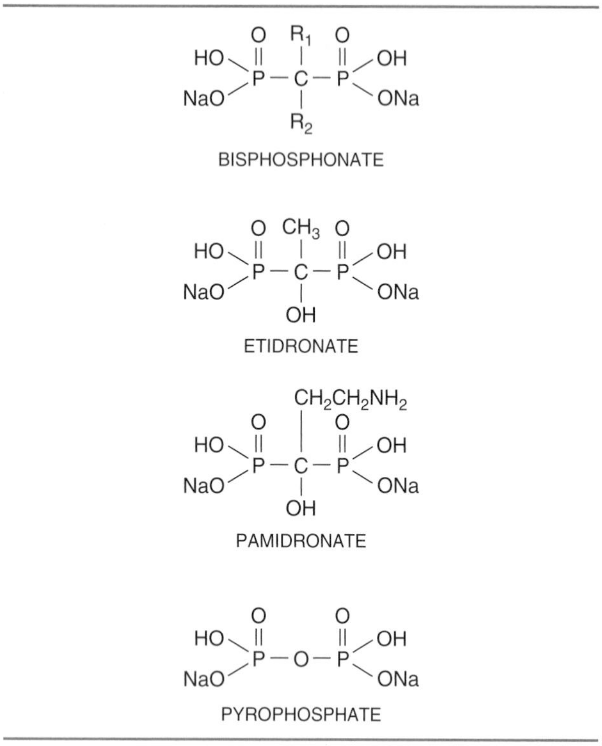

BISPHOSPHONATE

ETIDRONATE

PAMIDRONATE

PYROPHOSPHATE

Figure 62–7. Structures of bisphosphonates.

These compounds, when added to appropriate solutions and suspensions of calcium phosphate, slow the formation and dissolution of hydroxyapatite crystals. The first bisphosphonate to be developed for clinical use was *etidronate* (Figure 62–7), the most potent mineralization inhibitor of this group. Subsequent clinical experience has shown that inhibition of mineralization actually constitutes a disadvantage, leading over time to osteomalacia. Thus, second- and third-generation bisphosphonates have been developed that minimize this action. The clinical utility of bisphosphonates resides in their ability to inhibit bone resorption. The mechanism by which this antiresorptive effect occurs is not completely known, but it is thought that the bisphosphonate becomes incorporated into bone matrix and is imbibed by osteoclasts during resorption. Bisphosphonates affect osteoclasts by at least two different mechanisms. Some bisphosphonates, such as etidronate, *clodronate,* and *tiludronate,* are metabolized into an ATP analog (AppCCl$_2$p) that accumulates within and impairs the function and viability of cells (Frith *et al.,* 1996). By contrast, potent aminobisphosphonates, such as *alendronate* and *ibandronate,* are not metabolized but directly inhibit multiple steps in the pathway from mevalonate to cholesterol and isoprenoid lipids, such as geranylgeranyl

diphosphate, that are required for the prenylation of various proteins that are important for osteoclast function (Luckman *et al.,* 1998).

Several bisphosphonates currently are available in the United States. *Etidronate sodium* (DIDRONEL) is used for treatment of Paget's disease of bone and may be used parenterally to treat hypercalcemia. As etidronate is the only bisphosphonate to inhibit mineralization, it will likely be completely replaced by newer members of this class. *Pamidronate* (AREDIA) (Figure 62–7) is approved for management of hypercalcemia but has been found to be effective in other skeletal disorders. Pamidronate is available in the United States only for parenteral administration. For treatment of hypercalcemia, pamidronate may be given as an intravenous infusion of 60 to 90 mg over 4 to 24 hours. Several newer bisphosphonates have been approved for treatment of Paget's disease. These include *tiludronate* (SKELID), *alendronate,* (FOSAMAX), and *risedronate* (ACTONEL). All oral bisphosphonates are absorbed very poorly from the intestine. Thus, it is important to administer these drugs following an overnight fast and at least 30 minutes before breakfast. They should be taken only with a full glass of water.

Therapeutic Uses. *Paget's Disease.* Paget's disease is a skeletal condition of single or multiple foci of disordered bone remodeling. Pagetic lesions are characterized by many abnormal multinucleated osteoclasts in association with a disordered "mosaic" pattern of bone formation. Pagetic bone is thickened and has abnormal microarchitecture. The alterations in bone structure may produce secondary problems, such as deafness, spinal cord compression, high-output cardiac failure, and pain. Malignant degeneration to osteogenic sarcoma is a rare but lethal complication of Paget's disease. Bisphosphonates and CT decrease the elevated biochemical markers of bone turnover, such as plasma alkaline phosphatase activity and urinary excretion of hydroxyproline. Typically an initial course of bisphosphonate is given once daily for 6 months. With treatment, most patients experience a decrease in bone pain over several weeks. Such treatment may induce long-lasting remission. If symptoms recur, additional courses of therapy can be effective. When etidronate is given at higher doses (10 to 20 mg/kg per day) or continuously for longer than 6 months, there is a substantial risk for osteomalacia. At lower doses (5 to 7.5 mg/kg per day) focal osteomalacia has been observed occasionally. Defective mineralization has not been observed with other bisphosphonates or with CT.

Choice of optimal therapy for Paget's disease varies among patients. Bisphosphonates have the advantage of oral administration, lower cost, lack of antigenicity, and generally being less prone to side effects compared to CT. However, CT is highly reliable and may have a distinct skeletal analgesic property. Some evidence suggests that control of Paget's disease may be more effective when bisphosphonate and CT are used in combination (O'Donoghue and Hosking, 1987). Mithramycin has been used occasionally in difficult cases of Paget's disease. Therapeutic utility of this agent is limited by a high potential for toxicity, and it is not generally recommended.

Hypercalcemia. Etidronate and pamidronate have been used successfully in the management of malignancy-associated hypercalcemia. Etidronate has been used in the hope that its antimineralizing effect would benefit patients with heterotopic formation of bone or myositis ossificans. Results have not been impressive.

Postmenopausal Osteoporosis. Much interest currently is focused on the role of bisphosphonates in treatment of osteoporosis (*see* "Osteoporosis," below). Recent clinical trials show that treatment is associated with increases in bone mineral density and protection against fracture (*see* below).

FLUORIDE

Fluoride is of interest because of its toxic properties and its effect on dentition and bone. Fluoride is distributed widely in nature, and soils of different regions of the world vary greatly in their fluoride content. Sources of atmospheric fluoride include the burning of soft coal and the manufacturing of superphosphate, aluminum, steel, lead, copper, and nickel. Human beings obtain fluoride in particular from the ingestion of plants and water.

Absorption, Distribution, and Excretion. Fluorides are absorbed from the intestine, lungs, and skin. The intestine is the major site of absorption. The degree of absorption of a fluoride compound is best correlated with its solubility. The relatively soluble compounds, such as sodium fluoride, are almost completely absorbed, whereas relatively insoluble compounds, such as cryolite (Na_3AlF_6) and the fluoride found in bone meal (fluoroapatite), are poorly absorbed. The second most common route of absorption is *via* the lungs. Inhalation of fluoride present in dusts and gases constitutes the major route of industrial exposure.

Fluoride has been detected in all organs and tissues, and it is concentrated in bone, thyroid, aorta, and perhaps kidney. Fluoride is primarily deposited in bone and teeth, and the skeletal burden is related to intake and age. Storage in bone reflects skeletal turnover, growing bone showing greater deposition than bone in mature animals.

The major route of fluoride excretion is *via* the kidneys; however, small amounts of fluoride appear in sweat, milk, and intestinal secretions. When sweating is excessive, the fraction of total fluoride excretion in sweat can reach nearly one-half. About 90% of the fluoride filtered by the glomerulus is reabsorbed by the renal tubules.

Pharmacological Actions. The pharmacological actions of fluoride, with the possible exception of its effects on bone and teeth, can be classified as toxic. Fluoride is an inhibitor of several enzyme systems and diminishes tissue respiration and anaerobic glycolysis. Fluoride also is a useful anticoagulant *in vitro* because it binds Ca^{2+}. It also inhibits erythrocyte glycolysis. For this reason, fluoride is added to specimen tubes for blood glucose determinations.

Fluoride is a mitogen for osteoblasts and stimulates bone formation (Baylink *et al.*, 1970). Thus, fluoride has been an attractive agent for potential use in osteoporosis. Many, but not all, patients treated with fluoride salts show substantial increase in trabecular bone mass, whereas cortical bone responds less well. It remains to be established whether or not increases in axial bone mineral promote bone strength and protect against fracture (*see* "Osteoporosis," below). The radionuclide ^{18}F has been used in skeletal imaging (Jones *et al.*, 1973).

Acute Poisoning. Acute fluoride poisoning is not rare. It usually results from accidental ingestion of fluoride-containing insecticides or rodenticides.

Initial symptoms (salivation, nausea, abdominal pain, vomiting, and diarrhea) are secondary to the local action of fluoride on the intestinal mucosa. Systemic symptoms are varied and severe. There is increased irritability of the nervous system, consistent with the Ca^{2+}-binding effect of fluoride, hypocalcemia, and hypoglycemia. The blood pressure falls, presumably owing to central vasomotor depression as well as direct cardiotoxicity. Respiration is first stimulated and later depressed. Death usually results from respiratory paralysis or cardiac failure. The lethal dose of sodium fluoride for human beings is about 5 g, although there is considerable variation. Treatment includes the intravenous administration of glucose in saline and gastric lavage with lime water (0.15% calcium hydroxide solution) or other Ca^{2+} salts to precipitate the fluoride. Calcium gluconate is given intravenously for tetany; urine volume is kept high with vigorous fluid resuscitation.

Chronic Poisoning. In human beings, the major manifestations of chronic ingestion of excessive fluoride are osteosclerosis and mottled enamel. Osteosclerosis is characterized by increased bone density secondary both to elevated osteoblastic activity and to the replacement of hydroxyapatite by the denser fluoroapatite. The degree of skeletal involvement varies from changes that are barely detectable radiologically to marked cortical thickening of long bones, numerous exostoses scattered throughout the skeleton, and calcification of ligaments, tendons, and muscle attachments. In its severest form it is a disabling and crippling disease.

Mottled enamel, or dental fluorosis, is a well-recognized entity that was first described more than 60 years ago. The gross changes in very mild mottling consist of small, opaque, paper-white areas scattered irregularly over the tooth surface. In severe cases, discrete or confluent, deep brown- to black-stained pits give the tooth a corroded appearance. Mottled enamel results from a partial failure of the enamel-forming cells to elaborate and lay down enamel. It is a nonspecific response to a variety of stimuli, one of which is the ingestion of excessive amounts of fluoride.

Since mottled enamel is a developmental injury, ingestion of fluoride following the eruption of teeth has no effect. Mottling is one of the first visible signs of excessive fluoride intake during childhood. Continuous use of water containing about 1.0 ppm of fluoride may result in very mild mottling in 10% of children; at 4.0 to 6.0 ppm the incidence approaches 100%, with marked increase in severity.

Severe dental fluorosis formerly occurred with high frequency in regions of the world (*e.g.*, Pompeii, Italy, and Pike's Peak, Colorado) where local water supplies had a very high fluoride content. The water supply for some regions of the arid

American Southwest contains very high concentrations of fluoride, and skeletal fluorosis is common in animals that graze in these areas. Federal regulations currently require lowering the fluoride content of the water supply or providing an alternative source of acceptable drinking water for affected communities. Sustained consumption of water with a fluoride content of 4 mg/liter has been shown to be associated with deficits in cortical bone mass and increased rates of bone loss over time (Sowers *et al.,* 1991).

Fluoride and Dental Caries.   Experiments in controlling the fluoride content of water took an unexpected and significant turn when it was observed that children born at Bauxite, Arkansas, after a new water supply had been obtained, showed a much higher incidence of caries than those who had been exposed to the former fluoride-containing water. This led to extensive studies by the United States Public Health Service to ascertain whether water fluoridation could be a practical measure to reduce the incidence of tooth decay. It has now been established definitely, on the basis of many large-scale studies, that regulation of water fluoride content to 1.0 ppm is a safe and practical public health measure that substantially reduces the incidence of caries in permanent teeth.

There are partial benefits for children who begin drinking fluoridated water at any age; however, optimal benefits are obtained at ages before permanent teeth erupt. Topical application of fluoride solutions by dental personnel appears to be particularly effective on newly erupted teeth and can reduce the incidence of caries by 30% to 40%. Prescription of dietary fluoride supplements should be considered for children under the age of 12 years whose drinking water contains less than 0.7 ppm fluoride. Conflicting results have been reported from studies of fluoride-containing toothpastes.

Adequate incorporation of fluoride into teeth causes the outer layers of enamel to be harder and more resistant to demineralization. Deposition of fluoride appears to be an anion-exchange process with hydroxyl or citrate ions. Fluoride occupies the anionic spaces in the enamel apatite crystal surface. The mechanism of caries prevention by fluoride is not completely understood. There is no convincing evidence that fluoride from any source reduces the development of caries after the permanent teeth are completely formed (usually about age 14).

The fluoride salts usually employed in dentifrices are sodium fluoride and stannous fluoride. Sodium fluoride also is available in a variety of preparations for oral and topical use, including tablets, drops, rinses, and gels. Sodium fluoride, sodium fluorosilicate (Na_2SiF_6), and cryolite are the salts commonly used in insecticides.

Since its inception, regulation of the fluoride concentration of community water supplies periodically has encountered vocal opposition from a number of groups. The nature of such opposition has ranged from strictly political rhetoric to allegations about putative adverse health consequences of fluoridated water. Careful examination of these issues in studies sponsored by the National Cancer Institute and by the United States Public Health Service indicate that mortality from cancer and all-cause mortality do not differ significantly between communities with fluoridated and nonfluoridated water (Hoover *et al.,* 1976; Erickson, 1978).

OSTEOPOROSIS

Osteoporosis is a condition of low bone mass and microarchitectural disruption that results in fractures with minimal trauma. Characteristic sites of fracture include vertebral bodies, the distal radius, and the proximal femur, but osteoporotic individuals have generalized skeletal fragility, and fractures at other sites, such as ribs and long bones, also are common.

Osteoporosis is a major and growing public health problem for older women and men in western society. It is described generally as *primary* or *secondary*. Secondary osteoporosis is due to systemic illness or medications such as glucocorticoids or phenytoin. The most successful approach to secondary osteoporosis is prompt resolution of the underlying cause. However, mechanisms of secondary osteoporosis all can be related in terms of disordered bone remodeling, so that the same therapeutic strategies may apply to these conditions as are appropriate for primary osteoporosis.

In 1948, Albright and Reifenstein concluded that primary osteoporosis was composed of two separate entities: one related to menopausal estrogen loss, and the other to aging. Support for this concept has been published by Riggs and associates (1982), who proposed that primary osteoporosis represents two fundamentally different conditions: *type I osteoporosis,* loss of trabecular bone due to estrogen lack at menopause, and *type II osteoporosis,* loss of cortical and trabecular bone in men and women, due to long-term remodeling inefficiency, dietary inadequacy, and activation of the parathyroid axis with age. Compelling evidence has not been presented that these two entities are truly distinct, and the model fails to account for decreased bone mass resulting from inadequate skeletal acquisition during growth. Although many osteoporotic women undoubtedly have experienced excessive menopausal bone loss, it may be more appropriate to consider osteoporosis as the result of multiple physical, hormonal, and nutritional factors acting alone or in concert.

Skeletal Organization.   Because bone turnover rates differ from one portion of the skeleton to the next, it is useful to consider the appendicular, or peripheral, skeleton separate from the axial, or central, skeleton. Appendicular bones make up 80% of whole-body bone mass and are composed predominantly of compact cortical bone. Axial bones, such as the spine and pelvis, contain substantial amounts of trabecular bone within a thin cortex. Trabecular bone consists of highly connected bony plates that resemble honeycomb. The intertrabecular interstices contain bone marrow and fat. For several reasons, alterations in bone turnover are observed first and most extensively in axial bone rather than in the appendicular skeleton. These include the facts that bone remodeling takes place on bone surfaces, that there is a higher surface density in trabecular bone compared to cortical bone, and that marrow precursor cells that ultimately participate in bone turnover lie in close proximity to trabecular surfaces.

Bone Mass.   Bone mineral density (BMD) and fracture risk in later years reflect the maximal bone mineral content at skeletal maturity (peak bone mass) and the subsequent rate of bone loss. Major increases in bone mass, accounting for about 60% of final adult levels, occur during adolescence, mainly during years of highest growth velocity. Bone acquisition is almost complete by age 17 years in girls and by 20 years in boys. Inheritance accounts for much of the variance in bone acquisition; other factors include circulating estrogen and androgens, physical activity, and dietary calcium.

Bone is lost during adult life. Radiographic measurements of metacarpal bone by Garn and colleagues (1966) described a characteristic trajectory of bone mass throughout life, by which bone mass levels off during the third decade, remains stable until age 50, and then progressively declines. Similar trajectories occur for men, women, and all ethnic groups. The fundamental accuracy of this model has been amply confirmed for cortical bone, although trabecular bone loss probably begins prior to age 50 at some sites. In women, loss of estrogen at menopause accelerates the rate of bone loss for several years.

The primary regulators of adult bone mass include physical activity, reproductive endocrine status, and calcium intake. Optimal maintenance of BMD requires sufficiency in all three areas, and deficiency in one area is not compensated by excessive attention to another. For example, amenorrheic athletes lose bone despite frequent high-intensity exercise (Marcus *et al.*, 1985).

Prevention and Treatment of Osteoporosis

A rational strategy to prevent osteoporosis follows from the above considerations. Regular physical activity of reasonable intensity is endorsed at all ages. For children and adolescents, adequate dietary calcium is important if peak bone mass is to reach the level appropriate for genetic endowment. Attention to nutritional status may be required in the seventh decade and beyond, taking the form of increased dietary calcium or of calcium and/or vitamin D supplements. For women at menopause, timely administration of estrogen is the most powerful intervention to preserve bone and protect against fracture. Indeed, at any age, prevention or correction of hypogonadism is an im-

portant consideration. With appropriate lifelong attention to these preventive factors, important reductions in fracture risk can be achieved.

Pharmacological agents used to manage osteoporosis act by decreasing the rate of bone resorption, thereby slowing the rate of bone loss, or by promoting bone formation. The only drugs currently approved in the United States for use in osteoporosis are those that decrease resorption. Since bone remodeling is a coupled process, antiresorptive drugs ultimately decrease the rate of bone formation. Thus, antiresorptive therapy cannot lead to substantial gains in BMD. Increases in BMD that typically are seen during the first years of antiresorptive therapy represent a constriction of the remodeling space to a new steady-state level, after which BMD reaches a plateau. One consequence of this phenomenon is that therapeutic trials in osteoporosis must be of sufficient duration to determine whether an increase in BMD represents anything more than a simple reduction in remodeling space. At least 2 years are required for this purpose.

Antiresorptive Agents.   *Calcium.*   The physiological roles of Ca^{2+} and its use in the treatment of hypocalcemic disorders are discussed above. The rationale for using supplemental calcium to protect bone varies with time of life. For preteens and adolescents, adequate substrate calcium is required for bone accretion. Controlled trials indicate that supplemental calcium promotes adolescent bone acquisition (Johnston *et al.*, 1992; Lloyd *et al.*, 1993), but its impact on peak bone mass is not known. Higher calcium intake during the third decade of life is positively related to the final phase of bone acquisition (Recker *et al.*, 1992). There is controversy about the role of calcium during the early years after menopause, when the primary basis for bone loss is estrogen withdrawal. Although little effect of calcium on trabecular bone has been reported, reduction in cortical bone loss with calcium supplementation has been observed, even in populations characterized by high dietary calcium (Riis *et al.*, 1987). In elderly subjects, supplemental calcium suppresses bone turnover, improves BMD, and decreases the incidence of fracture (Chapuy *et al.*, 1992; Recker *et al.*, 1996; Dawson-Hughes, *et al.*, 1997).

Patients who are unable or unwilling to increase dietary calcium *via* dietary means alone may choose from many palatable, low-cost calcium preparations. Numerous Ca^{2+} salts are available for human use, the most frequently prescribed being the carbonate. Other salts available include calcium lactate, gluconate, phosphate, and citrate as well as hydroxyapatite. Lead contamination of some lots of powdered bone diminishes the acceptability of this product. Calcium citrate may be more efficiently absorbed than other salts. However, absorption efficiency for most commonly prescribed calcium products is reasonable, and for many patients cost and palatability outweigh modest differences in efficacy. Traditional dosing of calcium is about 1000 mg/day, nearly the amount present in a quart of milk. Added to the 500 to 600 mg of dietary calcium that typifies the diet of elderly men and women, this provides a total daily intake of about 1500 mg. More than this amount may be necessary to overcome endogenous intestinal calcium losses, but daily intakes of 2000 mg or more frequently are reported to be constipating. Calcium supplements are most often taken with meals.

Vitamin D and Its Analogs. The physiological role of vitamin D and its metabolites is discussed above, as are their uses in the treatment of hypocalcemic disorders, rickets, and osteomalacia. Modest supplementation with vitamin D (400 to 800 IU per day) may improve intestinal Ca^{2+} absorption, suppress bone remodeling, and improve BMD in individuals with marginal or deficient vitamin D status. Supplemental vitamin D has been shown to reduce fracture incidence in two European trials (Chapuy et al., 1992; Heikinheimo et al., 1992). The use of calcitriol to treat osteoporosis is distinct from assuring vitamin D nutritional adequacy. Here, the rationale is directly to suppress parathyroid function and reduce bone turnover. Calcitriol and another polar vitamin D metabolite, 1α-hydroxycholecalciferol, are used frequently in Japan and other countries (Fujita, 1992; Tilyard et al., 1992), but experience in the United States has been mixed. Higher doses of calcitriol appear to be more likely to improve BMD, but at the risk of hypercalciuria and hypercalcemia, so that close scrutiny of patients and dose modification are required. Restriction of dietary calcium may reduce toxicity during calcitriol therapy (Gallagher and Goldgar, 1990). A low incidence of hypercalciuric and hypercalcemic complications of therapy in Japan may reflect relatively poor calcium intakes in that country. Polar metabolites of vitamin D are promising for future study, but their toxicity makes it premature to endorse them for widespread use.

Estrogen. Overwhelming evidence confirms a major role for menopausal estrogen replacement in the conservation of bone and protection against osteoporotic fracture (Lindsay et al., 1976; Horsman et al., 1977; Recker et al., 1977; Hutchinson et al., 1979; Weiss et al., 1980). Studies indicate that 17β-estradiol acts on osteoblasts to decrease production of interleukin-6 and to upregulate the production of osteoprotegerin, thereby interfering with recruitment of osteoclast precursors (Girasole et al., 1992).

As sole therapy, the minimum effective dose of estrogen for skeletal protection is 0.625 mg/day of *conjugated equine estrogens* (PREMARIN) or its equivalent. Both oral and transcutaneous estrogen decrease bone turnover and conserve bone. Cessation of estrogen eventually results in bone loss, so therapy should be long term. Standard practice recommends cyclic or continuous administration of progestational drugs to women with an intact uterus. The C-21 progestins (e.g., *medroxyprogesterone acetate*) do not interfere with the skeletal effects of estrogen, whereas androgenic progestins (e.g., *norethisterone*) may actually increase BMD and provide added skeletal benefit when added to estrogen (Christiansen and Riis, 1990). For women without a uterus, estrogen therapy is continuous and does not require adding a progestin.

The optimal time to institute estrogen replacement is early menopause, when bone turnover accelerates. However, even for women beyond age 65, beneficial skeletal effects of estrogen are observed. Many older women will not accept cyclic bleeding or other anticipated side effects of estrogen. Thus, initiation of estrogen therapy to elderly women must be individualized. For other discussion of estrogens and progestins see Chapter 58.

Selective Estradiol Receptor Modulators (SERMS). Considerable work has been undertaken to develop estrogenic compounds with tissue-selective activities. One of these, *raloxifene* (EVISTA), acts as an estrogen agonist on bone and liver, is inactive on the uterus, and acts as an antiestrogen on the breast (see Chapter 58). In postmenopausal women, raloxifene stabilizes and modestly increases BMD and has been shown to reduce the risk of vertebral compression fracture (Delmas et al., 1997; Ettinger et al., 1999). Raloxifene is approved for both prevention and treatment of osteoporosis.

Calcitonin (CT). The physiological role and therapeutic use of CT for hypercalcemia and Paget's disease are discussed above. As a powerful inhibitor of osteoclastic bone resorption, CT produces modest increases in bone mass in patients with osteoporosis (Gruber et al., 1984; Civitelli et al., 1988; Mazzuoli et al., 1986). Increases are most impressive in patients with high intrinsic rates of bone turnover (Civitelli et al., 1988), approaching 10% to 15% before reaching a plateau. These represent simple reductions in the remodeling space. Recent experience with calcitonin nasal spray (MIACALCIN), 200 units/day, indicates that this agent reduces the incidence of vertebral compression fracture by about 40% in women with osteoporosis.

Bisphosphonates. The use of these antiresorptive agents to treat hypercalcemia and Paget's disease is discussed above. Bisphosphonates have emerged as the most effective drugs currently approved for prevention and treatment of osteoporosis. Although osteomalacia is a worrisome side effect of etidronate, newer bisphosphonates have sufficient potency to suppress bone resorption at doses that do not inhibit mineralization. The first of these to be developed for osteoporosis was *alendronate* (FOSAMAX). In a 3-year clinical trial involving postmenopausal women with low BMD and prevalent vertebral fractures, alendronate improved BMD and reduced fracture incidence (Black et al., 1996). Women assigned to alendronate showed approximately 50% fewer vertebral and nonvertebral fractures, including hip fracture, than women taking placebo. In a companion study, women who had low BMD but no prevalent vertebral fractures on entry experienced a significant reduction in vertebral fracture incidence (Cummings et al., 1998). Alendronate conserves BMD in recently menopausal women (Hosking et al., 1998) as well as in men and also improves BMD in patients receiving glucocorticoids (Saag et al., 1998). Alendronate is approved for prevention and treatment of postmenopausal osteoporosis and for treatment of glucocorticoid-associated osteoporosis. The approved prevention dose is 5 mg/day, and the treatment dose is 10 mg/day.

Although alendronate was well tolerated in clinical trials, some patients experience symptoms of esophagitis. Symptoms often abate when patients fastidiously take the medication with water and remain upright. Where symptoms persist despite these precautions, use of a proton pump inhibitor (see Chapter 37) at bedtime may be helpful. Alendronate may be better tolerated on a 40-mg once weekly schedule, and efficacy appears not to diminish. For patients with severe esophageal distress despite these countermeasures, intravenous *pamidronate* (AREDIA) offers skeletal protection without causing adverse gastrointestinal side effects. For treatment of osteoporosis, pamidronate is given as a 3-hour infusion, 30 mg every 3 months. It is well tolerated. Mild fever and aches may attend the first infusion of pamidronate, but these symptoms are short-lived and generally do not recur with subsequent administration. *Risedronate*

(ACTONEL), 5 mg/day, improves BMD and reduces vertebral fracture incidence in postmenopausal women (HARRIS *et al.,* 1999). Risedronate will likely be approved for this indication in the near future. *Ibandronate* is another potent bisphosphonate currently under development.

Thiazide Diuretics. Although not strictly antiresorptive, thiazides reduce urinary Ca^{2+} excretion and constrain bone loss in patients with hypercalciuria. Whether they will prove to be useful in patients who are not hypercalciuric is not clear, but data suggest that they reduce hip fracture risk. *Hydrochlorothiazide,* 25 mg once or twice daily, may achieve substantial reductions in calciuria. Effective doses of thiazides for reducing urinary Ca^{2+} excretion generally are lower than those necessary for control of blood pressure. For a more detailed discussion of thiazide diuretics, *see* Chapter 29.

Bone-Forming Agents. *Fluoride.* The skeletal consequences of excessive fluoride and the role of water fluoridation to prevent dental caries are discussed above. Sodium fluoride increases bone volume, an effect due specifically to increased osteoblastic activity (Baylink *et al.,* 1970; Briancon and Meunier, 1981). In doses of 30 to 60 mg/day, fluoride increases trabecular BMD in many, but not all patients. A controlled clinical trial (Riggs *et al.,* 1990) reported no protective effect against vertebral compression fractures although fluoride increased lumbar spine density. This same trial showed a significant increase in the occurrence of peripheral fractures and stress fractures in the fluoride group. This study has been criticized for the high dose of fluoride that was used (75 mg/day), and another study (Mamelle *et al.,* 1988) found that 30 to 50 mg/day of sodium fluoride decreased fracture risk. A recent trial of sustained-release fluoride, which is associated with lower blood fluoride levels, has shown favorable results on fracture incidence (Pak *et al.,* 1994). However, the results of Riggs *et al.* (1990) clearly show that increased bone mass is not synonymous with increased bone strength and that, if any dose of fluoride proves useful, there will be a narrow therapeutic window.

Androgen. Testosterone replacement therapy increases BMD in hypogonadal men. Androgens also improve BMD in osteoporotic women, but therapy is limited by virilizing side effects. *Nandrolone decanoate* (50 mg by injection every three weeks) increases peripheral and axial BMD without bothersome side effects in osteoporotic women. The androgenic progestin *norethisterone acetate* acts synergistically with estrogen to increase BMD in osteoporotic women (Christiansen and Riis, 1990). Adequate fracture data are not yet available to permit a conclusion on the clinical utility of this approach (*see* Chapter 59 for further discussion of androgens.)

Parathyroid Hormone (PTH). The deleterious skeletal effects of PTH in patients with severe hyperparathyroidism are described above. An anabolic effect of *intermittent* administration of PTH on trabecular bone has been shown. Consequently, several laboratories have examined the effects of PTH on BMD in patients with osteoporosis. In these studies, the synthetic analog hPTH(1–34) increased axial bone mineral, although effects on cortical bone were disappointing. Coadministration of hPTH(1–34) with estrogen or synthetic androgen led to impressive gains in axial mineral without loss of cortical bone (Lindsay *et al.,* 1997). PTH has been shown to induce substantial gains in BMD in patients with glucocorticoid-associated osteoporosis (Lane *et al.,* 1998). Phase III controlled clinical trials of PTH and its analogs are currently in progress.

For further discussion of bone and mineral metabolism, *see* Chapters 353 through 359 in *Harrison's Principles of Internal Medicine,* 14th ed., McGraw-Hill, New York, 1998.

BIBLIOGRAPHY

Agus, Z.S., Gardner, L.B., Beck, L.H., and Goldberg, M. Effects of parathyroid hormone on renal tubular reabsorption of calcium, sodium, and phosphate. *Am. J. Physiol.,* **1973,** *224*:1143–1148.

Andress, D.L., Norris, K.C., Coburn, J.W., Slatopolsky, E.A., and Sherrard, D.J. Intravenous calcitriol in the treatment of refractory osteitis fibrosa of chronic renal failure. *N. Engl. J. Med.,* **1989,** *321*:274–279.

Barsony, J., and Marx, S.J. Receptor-mediated rapid action of 1α, 25-dihydroxycholecalciferol: increase of intracellular cGMP in human fibroblasts. *Proc. Natl. Acad. Sci. U.S.A.,* **1988,** *85*:1223–1226.

Baylink, D.J., Wergedal, J.E., Stauffer, M., and Rich, C. Effect of fluoride on bone formation, mineralization, and resorption in the rat. In, *Fluoride and Medicine.* (Vischer, T.L., ed.) Hans Huber, Bern, **1970,** pp. 37–69.

Benker, G., Breuer, N., Windeck, R., and Reinwein, D. Calcium metabolism in thyroid disease. *J. Endocrinol. Invest.,* **1988,** *11*:61–69.

Berl, T., Berns, A.S., Hufer, W.E., Hammill, K., Alfrey, A.C., Arnaud,

C.D., and Schrier, R.W. 1,25 Dihydroxycholecalciferol effects in chronic dialysis. A double-blind controlled study. *Ann. Intern. Med.,* **1978,** *88*:774–780.

Berman, L.A. Crystalline substance from the parathyroid glands that influences the calcium content of the blood. *Proc. Soc. Exp. Biol. Med.,* **1924,** *21*:465.

Bilezikian, J.P., Silverberg, S.J., Gartenberg, F., Kim, T.-S., Jacobs, T.P., Siris, E.S., and Shane, E. Clinical presentation of primary hyperparathyroidism. In, *The Parathyroids: Basic and Clinical Concepts.* (Bilezikian, J.P., Marcus, R., and Levine, M.A., eds.) Raven Press Ltd., New York, **1994,** pp. 457–469.

Black, D.M., Cummings, S.R., Karpf, D.B., Cauley, J.A., Thompson, D.E., Nevitt, M.C., Bauer, D.C., Genant, H.K., Haskell, W.L., Marcus, R., Ott, S.M., Torner, J.C., Quandt, S.A., Reiss, T.F., and Ensrud, K.E. Randomised trial of effect of alendronate on risk of fracture in women with existing vertebral fractures. *Lancet,* **1996,** *348*:1535–1541.

Body, J.J., and Heath, H. III. Estimates of circulating monomeric calcitonin: physiological studies in normal and thyroidectomized man. *J. Clin. Endocrinol. Metab.*, **1983**, *57*:897–903.

Briancon, D., and Meunier, P.J. Treatment of osteoporosis with fluoride, calcium, and vitamin D. *Orthop. Clin. North. Am.*, **1981**, *12*:629–648.

Brown, E.M., Gamba, G., Riccardi, D., Lombardi, M., Butters, R., Kifor, O., Sun, A., Hediger, M.A., Lytton, J., and Hebert, S.C. Cloning and characterization of an extracellular Ca^{2+}-sensing receptor from bovine parathyroid. *Nature,* **1993**, *366*:575–580.

Cancela, L., Nemere, I., and Norman, A.W. $1\alpha,25(OH)_2$ vitamin D_3: a steroid hormone capable of producing pleiotropic receptor-mediated biological responses by both genomic and nongenomic mechanisms. *J. Steroid Biochem.*, **1988**, *30*:33–39.

Card, R.T., and Brain, M.C. The "anemia" of childhood: evidence for a physiologic response to hyperphosphatemia. *N. Engl. J. Med.*, **1973**, *288*:388–392.

Carlson, K.M., Dou, S., Chi, D., Scavarda, N., Toshima, K., Jackson, C.E., Wells, S.A. Jr., Goodfellow, P.J., and Donis-Keller, H. Single missense mutation in the tyrosine kinase catalytic domain of the RET protooncogene is associated with multiple endocrine neoplasia type 2B. *Proc. Natl. Acad. Sci. U.S.A.*, **1994**, *91*:1579–1583.

Chapuy, M.C., Arlot, M.E., Duboeuf, F., Brun, J., Crouzet, B., Arnaud, S., Delmas, P.D., Meunier, P.J. Vitamin D_3 and calcium to prevent hip fractures in the elderly women. *N. Engl. J. Med.*, **1992**, *327*:1637–1642.

Chesney, R.W., Moorthy, A.V., Eisman, J.A., Jax, D.K., Mazess, R.B., and DeLuca, H.F. Increased growth after long-term oral $1\alpha,25$-vitamin D_3 in childhood renal osteodystrophy. *N. Engl. J. Med.*, **1978**, *298*:238–242.

Christiansen, C., and Riis, B.J. 17β-estradiol and continuous norethisterone: a unique treatment for established osteoporosis in elderly women. *J. Clin. Endocrinol. Metab.*, **1990**, *71*:836–841.

Civitelli, R., Gonnelli, S., Zacchei, F., Bigazzi, S., Vattimo, A., Avioli, L.V. and Gennari, C. Bone turnover in postmenopausal osteoporosis. Effect of calcitonin treatment. *J. Clin. Invest.*, **1988**, *82*:1268–1274.

Coburn, J.W., and Salusky, I.B. Control of serum phosphorous in uremia. *N. Engl. J. Med.*, **1989**, *320*:1140–1142.

Collip, J.B. The extraction of a parathyroid hormone which will prevent or control parathyroid tetany and which regulates the level of blood calcium. *J. Biol. Chem.*, **1925**, *63*:395–438.

Committee on Nutrition. The prophylactic requirement and toxicity of vitamin D. *Pediatrics*, **1963**, *31*:512–523.

Cummings, S.R., Black, D.M., Thompson, D.E., Applegate, W.B., Barrett-Connor, E., Musliner, T.A., Palermo, L., Prineas, R., Rubin, S.M., Scott, J.C., Vogt, T., Wallace, R., Yates, A.J., and LaCroix, A.Z. Effect of alendronate on risk of fracture in women with low bone density but without vertebral fractures: results from the Fracture Intervention Trial. *JAMA*, **1998**, *280*:2077–2082.

Dawson-Hughes, B., Harris, S.S., Krall, E.A., and Dallal, G.E. Calcium and vitamin D supplementation on bone density in men and women 65 years of age or older. *N. Engl. J. Med.*, **1997**, *337*:670–676.

Delmas, P.D., Bjarnason, N.H., Mitlak, B.H., Ravoux, A.-C., Shah, A.S., Huster, W.J., Draper, M., and Christiansen, C. Effects of raloxifene on bone mineral density, serum cholesterol concentrations, and uterine endometrium in postmenopausal women. *N. Engl. J. Med.*, **1997**, *337*:1641–1647.

Donis-Keller, H., Dou, S., Chi, D., Carlson, K.M., Toshima, K., Lairmore, T.C., Howe, J.R., Moley, J.F., Goodfellow, P., and Wells, S. A. Jr. Mutations in the RET proto-oncogene are associated with MEN 2A and FMTC. *Hum. Mol. Genet.*, **1993**, *2*:851–856.

Econs, M.J., and Drezner, M.K. Bone disease resulting from inherited disorders of renal tubule transport and vitamin D metabolism. In, *Disorders of Bone and Mineral Metabolism.* (Coe, F.L., and Favus, M.J., eds.) Raven Press Ltd., New York, **1992**, pp. 935–950.

Endres, D.B., Villanueva, R., Sharp, C.F. Jr., and Singer, F.R. Immunochemiluminometric and immunoradiometric determinations of intact and total immunoreactive parathyrin: performance in the differential diagnosis of hypercalcemia and hypoparathyroidism. *Clin. Chem.*, **1991**, *37*:162–168.

Erickson, J.D. Mortality in selected cities with fluoridated and nonfluoridated water supplies. *N. Engl. J. Med.*, **1978**, *298*:1112–1116.

Ettinger, B., Black, D.M., Mitlak, B.H., Knickerbocker, R.K., Nickelsen, T., Genant, H.K., Christiansen, C., Delmas, P.D., Zanchetta, J.R., Stakkestad, J., Glüer, C.C., Krueger, K., Cohen, F.J., Eckert, S., Ensrud, K.E., Avioli, L.V., Lips, P., and Cummings, S.R. Reduction of vertebral fracture risk in postmenopausal women with osteoporosis treated with raloxifene: results from a 3-year randomized clinical trial. Multiple Outcomes of Raloxifene Evaluation (MORE) Investigators. *JAMA,* **1999**, *282*:637–645.

Finch, J.L., Brown, A.J., Kubodera, N., Nishii, Y., and Slatopolsky, E. Differential effects of $1,25-(OH)_2D_3$ and 22-oxacalcitriol on phosphate and calcium metabolism. *Kidney Int.*, **1993**, *43*:561–566.

Fraser, D., Kooh, S.W., Kind, H.P., Holick, M.F., Tanaka, Y., and DeLuca, H.F. Pathogenesis of hereditary vitamin-D-dependent rickets: an inborn error of vitamin D metabolism involving defective conversion of 25-hydroxyvitamin D to $1\alpha,25$-dihydroxyvitamin D. *N. Engl. J. Med.*, **1973**, *289*:817–822.

Frith, J.C., Mönkkönen, J., Blackburn, G.M., Russell, R.G., and Rogers, M.J. Clodronate and liposome-encapsulated clodronate are metabolized to a toxic ATP analog, adenosine $5'-\beta-\gamma$-dichloromethylene triphosphate, by mammalian cells *in vitro*. *J. Bone Miner. Res.*, **1997**, *12*:1358–1367.

Fujita, T. Vitamin D in the treatment of osteoporosis. *Proc. Soc. Exp. Biol. Med.*, **1992**, *199*:394–399.

Gallagher, J.C., and Goldgar, D. Treatment of postmenopausal osteoporosis with high doses of synthetic calcitriol. A randomized controlled study. *Ann. Intern. Med.*, **1990**, *113*:649–655.

Garn, S.M., Rohman, C.G., Nolan, P., Jr. The developmental nature of bone changes during aging. In, *Relations of Development and Aging.* (Birren, J.E., ed.) Charles C. Thomas, Springfield, IL, **1966.**

Girasole, G., Jilka, R.L., Passeri, G., Boswell, S., Boder, G., Williams, D.C., and Manolagas, S.C. 17β-estradiol inhibits interleukin-6 production by bone marrow-derived stromal cells and osteoblasts *in vitro*: a potential mechanism for the antiosteoporotic effect of estrogens. *J. Clin. Invest.*, **1992**, *89*:883–891.

Greenberg, B.G., Winters, R.W., and Graham, J.B. The normal range of serum inorganic phosphorus and its utility as a discriminant in the diagnosis of congenital hypophosphatemia. *J. Clin. Endocrinol. Metab.*, **1960**, *20*:364–379.

Gruber, H.E., Ivey, J.L., Baylink, D.J., Matthews, M., Nelp, W.B., Sisom, K., and Chesnut, C.H. III. Long-term calcitonin therapy in postmenopausal osteoporosis. *Metabolism,* **1984**, *33*:295–303.

Hahn, T.J., Hendin, B.A., Scharp, C.R., and Haddad, J.G. Jr. Effect of chronic anticonvulsant therapy on serum 25-hydroxycalciferol levels in adults. *N. Engl. J. Med.*, **1972**, *287*:900–904.

Harris, S.T., Watts, N.B., Genant, H.K., McKeever, C.D., Hangartner, T., Keller, M., Chesnut, C.H. III, Brown, J., Eriksen, E.F., Hoseyni, M.S., Axelrod, D.W., and Miller, P.D. Effects of risedronate treatment on vertebral and nonvertebral fractures in women with postmenopausal osteoporosis: a randomized controlled trial. Vertebral

Efficacy with Risedronate Therapy (VERT) Study Group. *JAMA,* **1999,** *282:*1344–1352.

Heersche, J.N., Marcus, R., and Aurbach, G.D. Calcitonin and the formation of 3′,5′-AMP in bone and kidney. *Endocrinology.* **1974,** *94:*241–247.

Heikinheimo, R.J., Inkovaara, J.A., Harju, E.J., Haavisto, M.V., Kaarela, R.H., Kataja, J.M., Kokko, A.M.L., Kolho, L.A., and Rajala, S.A. Annual injection of vitamin D and fractures of aged bones. *Calcif. Tissue. Int.,* **1992,** *51:*105–110.

Hess, A.F., and Weinstock, M. Antirachitic properties imparted to inert fluids and to green vegetables by ultraviolet irradiation. *J. Biol. Chem.,* **1924,** *62:*301–313.

Hirsch, P.F., Gauthier, G.F., and Munson, P.C. Thyroid hypocalcemic principle and recurrent laryngeal nerve injury as factors affecting the response to parathyroidectomy in rats. *Endocrinology,* **1963,** *73:*244–252.

Holick, M.F. Active vitamin D compounds and analogues: a new therapeutic era for dermatology in the 21st century. *Mayo Clin, Proc.,* **1993,** *68:*925–927.

Holick, M.F. The cutaneous photosynthesis of previtamin D₃: a unique photoendocrine system. *J. Invest. Dermatol.,* **1981,** *77:*51–58.

Hoover, R.N., McKay, F.W., and Fraumeni, J.F. Jr. Fluoridated drinking water and the occurrence of cancer. *J. Natl. Cancer Inst.,* **1976,** *57:*757–768.

Horsman, A., Gallagher, J.C., Simpson, M., and Nordin, B.E. Prospective trial of oestrogen and calcium in postmenopausal women. *Br. Med. J.,* **1977,** *2:*789–792.

Hosking, D., Chilvers, C.E., Christiansen, C., Ravn, P., Wasnich, R., Ross, P., McClung, M., Balske, A., Thompson, D., Daley, M., and Yates, A.J. Prevention of bone loss with alendronate in postmenopausal women under 60 years of age. Early Postmenopausal Intervention Cohort Study Group. *N. Engl. J. Med.,* **1998,** *338:*485–492.

Huldschinsky, K. Heilung von Rachitis durch Kunstliche Hohensonne. *Dtsch. Med. Wochenschr.,* **1919,** *14:*712–713.

Hutchinson, T.A., Polansky, S.M., and Feinstein, A.R. Post-menopausal oestrogens protect against fractures of hip and distal radius. A case-control study. *Lancet,* **1979,** *2:*705–709.

HYP Consortium. A gene (PEX) with homologies to endopeptidases is depleted in patients with X-linked hypophosphatemic rickets. *Nat. Genet.,* **1995,** *11:*130–136.

Jacob, H.S., and Amsden, T. Acute hemolytic anemia with rigid red cells in hypophosphatemia. *N. Engl. J. Med.,* **1971,** *285:*1446–1450.

Jimi, E., Akiyama, S., Tsurukai, T., Okahashi, N., Kobayashi, K., Udagawa, N., Nishihara, T., Takahashi, N., and Suda, T. Osteoclast differentiation factor acts as a multifunctional regulator in murine osteoclast differentiation and function. *J. Immunol.,* **1999,** *163:*434–442.

Johnston C.C. Jr., Miller, J.Z., Slemenda, C.W., Reister, T.K., Hui, S., Christian, J.C., and Peacock, M. Calcium supplementation and increases in bone mineral density in children. *N. Engl. J. Med.,* **1992,** *327:*82–87.

Jones, A.E., Ghaed, N., Dunson, G.L., and Hosain, F. Clinical evaluation of orally administered fluorine 18 for bone scanning. *Radiology.,* **1973,** *107:*129–131.

Jubiz, W., Haussler, M.R., McCain, T.A., and Tolman, K.G. Plasma 1,25-dihydroxyvitamin D levels in patients receiving anticonvulsant drugs. *J. Clin. Endocrinol. Metab.,* **1977,** *44:*617–621.

Jüppner, H., Abou-Samra, A.B., Freeman, M., Kong, X.F., Schipani, E., Richards, J., Kolakowski, L.F. Jr., Hock, J., Potts, J.T. Jr., Kronenberg, H.M., and Segre, G.V. A G protein–linked receptor for parathyroid hormone and parathyroid hormone–related peptide. *Science,* **1991,** *254:*1024–1026.

Kragballe, K. Vitamin D analogues in the treatment of psoriasis. *J. Cell. Biochem.,* **1992,** *49:*46–52.

Lane, N.E., Sanchez, S., Modin, G.W., Genant, H.K., Pierini, E., Arnaud, C.D. Parathyroid hormone treatment can reverse corticosteroid-induced osteoporosis. Results of a randomized controlled clinical trial. *J. Clin. Invest.,* **1998,** *102:*1627–1633.

Lemann, J. Jr., Gray, R.W., Maierhofer, W.J., and Cheung, H.S. Hydrochlorothiazide inhibits bone resorption in men despite experimentally elevated serum 1,25-dihydroxyvitamin D concentrations. *Kidney Int.,* **1985,** *28:*951–958.

Lindsay, R., Hart, D.M., Aitken, J.M., MacDonald, E.B., Anderson, J.B., and Clarke, A.C. Long-term prevention of postmenopausal osteoporosis by oestrogen. Evidence for an increased bone mass after delayed onset of oestrogen treatment. *Lancet,* **1976,** *1:*1038–1041.

Lindsay, R., Nieves, J., Formica, C., Henneman, E., Woelfert, L., Shen, V., Dempster, D., and Cosman, F. Randomised controlled study of effect of parathyroid hormone on vertebral-bone mass and fracture incidence among postmenopausal women on oestrogen with osteoporosis. *Lancet,* **1997,** *350:*550–555.

Lloyd, T., Andon, M.B., Rollings, N., Martel, J.K., Landis, J.R., Demers, L.M., Eggli, D.F., Kieselhorst, K., and Kulin, H.E. Calcium supplementation and bone mineral density in adolescent girls. *JAMA,* **1993,** *270:*841–844.

Luckman, S.P., Hughes, D.E., Coxon, F.P., Graham, R., Russell, G., and Rogers, M.J. Nitrogen-containing bisphosphonates inhibit the mevalonate pathway and prevent post-translational prenylation of GTP-binding proteins, including Ras. *J. Bone Miner. Res.,* **1998,** *13:*581–589.

MacCallum, S.G., and Voegtlin, C. On the relation of tetany to the parathyroid glands and to calcium metabolism. *J. Exp. Med.,* **1909,** *11:*118–151.

MacIntyre, I., Boss, S., and Troughton, V.A. Parathyroid hormone and magnesium homeostasis. *Nature,* **1963,** *198:*1058–1060.

Mamelle, N., Meunier, P.J., Dusan, R., Guillaume, M., Martin, J.L., Gaucher, A., Prost, A., Zeigler, G., and Netter, P. Risk-benefit ratio of sodium fluoride treatment in primary vertebral osteoporosis. *Lancet,* **1988,** *2:*361–365.

Marcus, R., Cann, C., Madvig, P., Minkoff, J., Goddard, M., Bayer, M., Martin, M., Gaudiani, L., Haskell, W., and Genant, H. Menstrual function and bone mass in elite women distance runners. Endocrine and metabolic features. *Ann. Intern. Med.,* **1985,** *102:*158–163.

Mawer, E.B., Backhouse, J., Davies, M., Hill, L.F., and Taylor, C.M. Metabolic fate of administered 1,25-dihydroxycholecalciferol in controls and in patients with hypoparathyroidism. *Lancet,* **1976,** *1:*1203–1206.

Mazzuoli, G.F., Passeri, M., Gennari, C., Minisola, S., Antonelli, R., Valtorta, C., Palummeri, E., Cervellin, G.F., Gonnelli, S., and Francini, G. Effects of salmon calcitonin in postmenopausal osteoporosis: a controlled double-blind clinical study. *Calcif. Tissue Int.,* **1986,** *38:*3–8.

McConnell, T.H. Fatal hypocalcemia from phosphate absorption from laxative preparations. *JAMA,* **1971,** *216:*147–148.

McSheehy, P.M., and Chambers, T.J. Osteoblast-like cells in the presence of parathyroid hormone release soluble factor that stimulates osteoclastic bone resorption. *Endocrinology,* **1986,** *119:*1654–1659.

Mellanby, E. An experimental investigation of rickets. *Lancet,* **1919,** *1:*407–412.

Mimura, H., Cao, X., Ross, F.P., Chiba, M., and Teitelbaum, S.L. 1,25-Dihydroxyvitamin D₃ transcriptionally activates the beta 3-integrin subunit gene in avian osteoclast precursors. *Endocrinology,* **1994,** *134*:1061–1066.

Murad, F., Brewer, H.B. Jr., and Vaughan, M. Effect of thyrocalcitonin on adenosine 3′,5′-cyclic phosphate formation by rat kidney and bone. *Proc. Natl. Acad. Sci. U.S.A.,* **1970,** *65*:446–453.

Nemere, I., and Norman, A.W. Parathyroid hormone stimulates calcium transport in perfused duodena from normal chicks: comparison with the rapid (transcaltachic) effect of 1,25-dihydroxyvitamin D$_3$. *Endocrinology,* **1986,** *119*:1406–1408.

Nemere, I., and Norman, A.W. 1,25-Dihydroxyvitamin D$_3$–mediated vesicular transport of calcium in intestine: time course studies. *Endocrinology,* **1988,** *122*:2962–2969.

Nussbaum, S.R., and Potts, J.T. Jr. Advances in immunoassays for parathyroid hormone: clinical applications to skeletal disorders of bone and mineral metabolism. In, *The Parathyroids: Basic and Clinical Concepts.* (Bilezikian, J.P., Marcus, R., and Levine, M.A., eds.) Raven Press, Ltd., New York, **1994,** pp. 157–170.

O'Donoghue, D.J., and Hosking, D.J. Biochemical response to combination of disodium etidronate with calcitonin in Paget's disease. *Bone,* **1987,** *8*:219–225.

Pak, C.Y., Sakhaee, K., Piziak, V., Peterson, R.D., Breslau, N.A., Boyd, P., Poindexter, J.R., Herzog, J., Heard-Sakhaee, A., Haynes, S., Adams-Huet, B., and Reisch, J.S. Slow-release sodium fluoride in the management of postmenopausal osteoporosis. A randomized controlled trial. *Ann. Intern. Med.,* **1994,** *120*:625–632.

Perry, H.M., Skogen, W., Chappel, J.C., Wilner, G.D., Kahn, A.J., and Teitelbaum, S.L. Conditioned medium from osteoblast-like cells mediate parathyroid hormone–induced bone resorption. *Calcif. Tiss. Int.,* **1987,** *40*:298–300.

Pollak, M.R., Brown, E.M., Chou, Y.H., Hebert, S.C., Marx, S.J., Steinmann, B., Levi, T., Seidman, C.E., and Seidman, J.G. Mutations in the human Ca^{2+}-sensing receptor gene cause familial hypocalciuric hypercalcemia and neonatal severe hyperparathyroidism. *Cell,* **1993,** *75*:1297–1303.

Puschett, J.B., Moranz, J., and Kurnick, W.S. Evidence for a direct action of cholecalciferol and 25-hydroxycholecalciferol on the renal transport of phosphate, sodium, and calcium. *J. Clin. Invest.,* **1972,** *51*:373–385.

Recker, R.R., Davies, K.M., Hinders, S.M., Heaney, R.P., Stegman, M.R., and Kimmel, D.B. Bone gain in young adult women. *JAMA,* **1992,** *268*:2403–2408.

Recker, R.R., Hinders, S., Davies, K.M., Heaney, R.P., Stegman, M.R., Lappe, J.M., and Kimmel, D.B. Correcting calcium nutritional deficiency prevents spine fractures in elderly women. *J. Bone Miner. Res.,* **1996,** *11*:1961–1966.

Recker, R.R., Saville, P.D., and Heaney, R.P. Effect of estrogens and calcium carbonate on bone loss in postmenopausal women. *Ann. Intern. Med.,* **1977,** *87*:649–655.

Riggs B.L., Hodgson, S.F., O'Fallon, W.M., Chao, E.Y.S., Wahner, H.W., Muhs, J.M., Cedel, S.L., and Melton, L.J. III. Effect of fluoride treatment on the fracture rate in postmenopausal women with osteoporosis. *N. Engl. J. Med.,* **1990,** *322*:802–809.

Riggs, B.L., Wahner, H.W., Seeman, E., Offord, K.P., Dunn, W.L., Mazess, R.B., Johnson, K.A., and Melton, L.J. III. Changes in bone mineral density of the proximal femur and spine with aging. Differences between the postmenopausal and senile osteoporosis syndromes. *J. Clin. Invest.,* **1982,** *70*:716–723.

Riis B., Thomsen, K., Christiansen, C. Does calcium supplementation prevent postmenopausal bone loss? A double-blind, controlled clinical study. *N. Engl. J. Med.,* **1987,** *316*:173–177.

Rosen, J.F., and Chesney, R.W. Circulating calcitriol concentrations in health and disease. *J. Pediatr.,* **1983,** *103*:1–17.

Rude, R.K., Oldham, S.B., and Singer, F.R. Functional hypoparathyroidism and parathyroid hormone end-organ resistance in human magnesium deficiency. *Clin. Endocrinol. (Oxf),* **1976,** *5*:209–224.

Saag, K.G., Emkey, R., Schnitzer, T.J., Brown, J.P., Hawkins, F., Goemaere, S., Thamsborg, G., Liberman, U.A., Delmas, P.D., Malice, M.P., Czachur, M., and Daifotis, A.G. Alendronate for the prevention and treatment of glucocorticoid-induced osteoporosis. Glucocorticoid-Induced Osteoporosis Intervention Study Group. *N. Engl. J. Med.,* **1998,** *339*:292–299.

Siegel, N., Wongsurawat, N., and Armbrecht, H.J. Parathyroid hormone stimulates dephosphorylation of the renoredoxin component of the 25-hydroxy D$_3$-1α-hydroxylase from rat renal cortex. *J. Biol. Chem.,* **1986,** *261*:16988–17003.

Sowers, M.F., Clark, M.K., Jannausch, M.L., and Wallace, R.B. A prospective study of bone mineral content and fracture in communities with differential fluoride exposure. *Am. J. Epidemiol.,* **1991,** *133*:649–660.

Spear, G.T., Paulnock, D.M., Helgeson, D.O., and Borden, E.C. Requirement of differentiative signals of both interferon-g and 1,25-dihydroxyvitamin D$_3$ for induction and secretion of interleukin-1 by HL-60 cells. *Cancer Res.,* **1988,** *48*:1740–1744.

Steele, T.H. Increased urinary phosphate excretion following volume expansion in normal man. *Metabolism,* **1970,** *19*:129–139.

Steenbock, H., and Black, A. Fat-soluble vitamins. XVII. The induction of growth-promoting and calcifying properties in a ration by exposure to ultraviolet light. *J. Biol. Chem.,* **1924,** *61*:405–422.

Takahashi, N., Akatsu, T., Udagawa, N., Sasaki, T., Yamaguchi, A., Moseley, J.M., Martin, T.J., and Suda, T. Osteoblastic cells are involved in osteoclast formation. *Endocrinology,* **1988,** *123*:2600–2602.

Tashjian, A.H. Jr., Wolfe, H.J., and Voelkel, E.F., Human calcitonin. Immunologic assay, cytologic localization and studies on medullary thyroid carcinoma. *Am. J. Med.,* **1974,** *56*:840–849.

Tilyard, M.W., Spears, G.F., Thomson, J., and Dovey, S. Treatment of postmenopausal osteoporosis with calcitriol or calcium. *N. Engl. J. Med.,* **1992,** *326*:357–362.

Vernava, A.M. III, O'Neal, L.W., and Palermo, V. Lethal hyperparathyroid crisis: hazards of phosphate administration. *Surgery,* **1987,** *102*:941–948.

Weinstein, R.S., Bryce, G.F., Sappington, L.J., King, D.W., and Gallagher, B.B. Decreased serum ionized calcium and normal vitamin D metabolite levels with anticonvulsant drug treatment. *J. Clin. Endocrinol. Metab.,* **1984,** *58*:1003–1009.

Weiss, N.S., Ure, C.L., Ballard, J.H., Williams, A.R., and Daling, J.R. Decreased risk of fractures of the hip and lower forearm with postmenopausal use of estrogen. *N. Engl. J. Med.,* **1980,** *303*:1195–1198.

Wells, S.A. Jr., Baylin, S.B., Linehan, W.M., Farrell, R.E., Cox, E.B., and Cooper, C.W. Provocative agents and the diagnosis of medullary carcinoma of the thyroid gland. *Ann. Surg.,* **1978,** *188*:139–141.

Yanagawa, N., and Lee, D.B.N. Renal handling of calcium and phosphorus. In, *Disorders of Bone and Mineral Metabolism.* (Coe, F.L., and Favus, M.J., eds.) Raven Press Ltd., New York, **1992,** pp. 3–40.

Yasuda, M., Shima, N., Nakagawa, N., Yamaguchi, K., Kinosaki, M., Mochizuki, S., Tomoyasu, A., Yano, K., Goto, M., Murakami, A., Tsuda, E., Morinaga, T., Higashio, K., Udagawa, N., Takahashi, N., and Suda, T. Osteoclast differentiation factor is a ligand for osteoprotegerin/osteoclastogenesis-inhibitory factor and is identical to TRANCE/RANKL. *Proc. Natl. Acad. Sci, U.S.A.,* **1998,** *95*:3597–3602.

MONOGRAPHS AND REVIEWS

Albright, F. A page out of the history of hyperparathyroidism. *J. Clin. Endocrinol. Metab.*, **1948**, *8*:637–657.

Amento, E.P. Vitamin D and the immune system. *Steroids*, **1987**, *49*:55–72.

Aurbach, G.D. Calcium-regulating hormones: parathyroid hormone and calcitonin. In, *Calcium in Human Biology.* (Nordin, B.E.C., ed.) Springer-Verlag, Berlin, **1988**, pp. 43–68.

Boland, R. Role of vitamin D in skeletal muscle function. *Endocr. Rev.*, **1986**, *7*:434–448.

Carswell, S. Vitamin D in the nervous system: action and therapeutic potential. In, *Vitamin D.* (Feldman, D., Glorieux, F.H., and Pike, J.W., eds.) Academic Press, San Diego, CA, **1997**, pp. 1197–1212.

Copp, D.H. Parathyroids, calcitonin, and control of plasma calcium. *Recent Prog. Horm. Res.*, **1964**, *20*:59–88.

DeLuca, H.F., and Schnoes, H.K. Metabolism and mechanism of action of vitamin D. *Annu. Rev. Biochem.*, **1976**, *45*:631–666.

Dempster, D.W. Bone remodeling. In, *Disorders of Bone and Mineral Metabolism.* (Coe, F.L., and Favus, M.J., eds.) Raven Press Ltd., New York, **1992**, pp. 355–380.

Evans, R.M. The steroid and thyroid hormone receptor superfamily. *Science*, **1988**, *240*:889–895.

Fraser, D.R. Regulation of the metabolism of vitamin D. *Physiol. Rev.*, **1980**, *60*:551–613.

Grill, V., and Martin, T.J. Parathyroid hormone-related protein as a cause of hypercalcemia in malignancy. In, *The Parathyroids: Basic and Clinical Concepts.* (Bilezikian, J.P., Marcus, R., and Levine, M.A., eds.) Raven Press, Ltd., New York, **1994**, pp. 295–310.

Haussler, M.R. Vitamin D receptors: nature and function. *Annu. Rev. Nutr.*, **1986**, *6*:527–562.

Haussler, M.R., and McCain, T.A. Basic and clinical concepts related to vitamin D metabolism and action (first of two parts). *N. Engl. J. Med.*, **1977**, *297*:974–983.

Horst, R.L., and Reinhardt, T.A. Vitamin D metabolism. In, *Vitamin D.* (Feldman, D., Glorieux, F.H., and Pike, J.W., eds.) Academic Press, San Diego, CA, **1997**, pp. 13–32.

Institute of Medicine. *Dietary Reference Intakes for Calcium, Phosphorus, Magnesium, Vitamin D, and Fluoride.* National Academy Press, Washington, D.C., **1997**, pp. 71–145.

Kodicek, E. The story of vitamin D: from vitamin to hormone. *Lancet*, **1974**, *1*:325–329.

Kragballe, K. Psoriasis and other skin disorders. In, *Vitamin D.* (Feldman, D., Glorieux, F.H., and Pike, J.W., eds.) Academic Press, San Diego, CA, **1997**, pp. 1213–1226.

Kronenberg, H.M., Bringhurst, F.R., Segre, G.V., and Potts, J.T. Jr. Parathyroid hormone biosynthesis and metabolism. In, *The Parathyroids: Basic and Clinical Concepts.* (Bilezikian, J.P., Marcus, R., and Levine, M.A., eds.) Raven Press, Ltd., New York, **1994**, pp. 125–137.

Levine, M.A. Pseudohypoparathyroidism: from bedside to bench and back. *J. Bone Miner. Res.*, **1999**, *14*:1255–1260.

MacIntyre, I., Alevizaki, M., Bevis, P.J., and Zaidi, M. Calcitonin and the peptides from the calcitonin gene. *Clin. Orthop.*, **1987**, *217*:45–55.

Marcus, R. Normal and abnormal bone remodeling in man. *Annu. Rev. Med.*, **1987**, *38*:129–141.

Pike, J.W. Molecular mechanisms of cellular response to the vitamin D_3 hormone. In, *Disorders of Bone and Mineral Metabolism.* (Coe, F.L., and Favus, M.J., eds.) Raven Press Ltd., New York, **1992**, pp. 163–193.

Reichel, H., Koeffler, H.P., and Norman, A.W. The role of the vitamin D endocrine system in health and disease. *N. Engl. J. Med.*, **1989**, *320*:980–991.

Stern, P.H. The D vitamins and bone. *Pharmacol. Rev.*, **1980**, *32*:47–80.

Suda, T., Takahashi, N., Udagawa, N., Jimi, E., Gillespie, M.T., and Martin, T.J. Modulation of osteoclast differentiation and function by the new members of the tumor necrosis factor receptor and ligand families. *Endocr. Rev.*, **1999**, *20*:345–357.

Van Leeuwen, J.P.T.M., and Pols, H.A.P. Vitamin D: anticancer and differentiation. In, *Vitamin D.* (Feldman, D., Glorieux, F.H., and Pike, J.W., eds.) Academic Press, San Diego, CA, **1997**, pp. 1089–1106.

Wasserman, R.H. Vitamin D and the intestinal absorption of calcium and phosphorus. In, *Vitamin D.* (Feldman, D., Glorieux, F.H., and Pike, J.W., eds.) Academic Press, San Diego, CA, **1997**, pp. 259–274.

Zaloga, G.P., and Chernow, B. Hypocalcemia in critical illness. *JAMA*, **1986**, *256*:1924–1929.

SECTION XIII

THE VITAMINS

INTRODUCTION

Robert Marcus and Ann M. Coulston

The diet is the source of some 40 nutrients for human beings. These classically are divided into energy-yielding dietary components (carbohydrates, fats, and proteins), sources of essential and nonessential amino acids (proteins), essential unsaturated fatty acids (fats), minerals (including trace minerals), and vitamins (water-soluble and fat-soluble organic compounds) (*see* Shils *et al.,* 1999).

Vitamins, despite their diverse chemical composition, can be defined as *organic* substances that must be provided in small quantities from the environment because either they cannot be synthesized *de novo* in human beings or their rate of synthesis is inadequate for the maintenance of health [*e.g.,* the production of nicotinic acid (niacin) from tryptophan]. In most cases, the environmental source is the diet, but an obvious exception to this general rule is the endogenous synthesis of vitamin D under the influence of ultraviolet light. This definition differentiates vitamins from essential trace minerals, which are *inorganic* nutrients needed in small quantities. It also excludes the essential amino acids, which are organic substances needed preformed in the diet in much larger quantities. The term *vitamin* is restricted here to include only organic substances required for the nutrition of mammals; substances required only by microorganisms and cells in culture should be defined as *growth factors,* to prevent scientifically unsound claims for their therapeutic benefit as vitamins for human beings. When the vitamin occurs in more than one chemical form (*e.g.,* pyridoxine, pyridoxal, pyridoxamine) or as a precursor (*e.g.,* carotene for vitamin A), these analogs sometimes are referred to as *vitamers.*

Although the individual vitamins differ widely in structure and function, some general statements do apply. *Water-soluble vitamins* are stored to only a limited extent, and frequent consumption is necessary to maintain saturation of tissues. *Fat-soluble vitamins* can be stored to massive degrees, and this property confers upon them a potential for serious toxicity that greatly exceeds that of the water-soluble group. As consumed, many vitamins are not biologically active and require processing *in vivo.* In the case of several water-soluble vitamins, activation includes phosphorylation (thiamine, riboflavin, nicotinic acid, pyridoxine) and also may require coupling to purine or pyridine nucleotides (riboflavin, nicotinic acid). In their major known actions, water-soluble vitamins participate as cofactors for specific enzymes, whereas at least two fat-soluble vitamins, A and D, behave more like hormones and interact with specific intracellular receptors in their target tissues.

Vitamin Requirements. *Dietary Reference Intakes.* In many countries throughout the world, scientific committees periodically assess the evidence about the requirements of the population for individual nutrients. In the United States, the Food and Nutrition Board of the Institute of Medicine, National Academy of Sciences, with active involvement of Health Canada are taking a new approach to the Recommended Dietary Allowances (RDAs) that have been published since 1941. The development of Dietary Reference Intakes (DRIs) expands and replaces the RDA. DRIs are a family of reference values that are quantitative estimates of nutrient intakes designed to be used for planning and assessing diets for healthy people. They include RDAs as goals for intake of individuals, but also present three new types of reference values. These include Adequate Intake (AI), the Tolerable Upper Intake Level (UL), and the Estimated Average Requirement (EAR) (Yates *et al.*, 1998).

The Food and Nutrition Board has embarked on a multiyear project to expand the framework for quantitative recommendations regarding nutrient intake, which includes evaluating both nutrients and other food components for impact on health. The review goes beyond criteria needed to prevent classical deficiencies and includes review of data related to risk of chronic diseases.

Current recommendations for males and females of different ages are summarized in Tables XIII–1 through XIII–3. Table XIII–1 contains RDAs for those nutrients yet to be reviewed by the DRI committee. Table XIII–2 contains the newly revised recommended intakes. Age groupings have been changed from the earlier RDA publications. Finally, Table XIII–3 contains the ULs for the newly revised intakes. The RDA for a given nutrient, which is an individual intake goal, represents the intake at which the risk of inadequacy is very small, about 2% to 3% of the population. Those with intakes below the recommended allowance will not necessarily develop a deficiency; however, their long-term risk of deficiency rises in proportion to the degree to which the recommended allowance is not met.

Intakes at the level of RDAs or AIs would not necessarily be expected to replete an undernourished individual, nor would it be adequate for disease states which lead to increased requirements. Because the DRIs are based on data from the U.S. and Canada, they may not apply globally where food and indigenous practices may result in different bioavailability of nutrients.

The tolerable upper intake level (ULs) is the highest level of daily intake that is likely to pose no risk of adverse health effects to most individuals. ULs are useful because of increased interest in and availability of fortified foods and continued use of dietary supplements.

As the standing committee on the scientific evaluation of DRIs of the Food and Nutrition Board completes the review of each set of nutrients, reports are issued. For up-to-date information about these reports visit the Food and Nutrition Board home page at www.nas.edu/iom/fnb.

Federal Regulations on Vitamins and Minerals.   The United States Food and Drug Administration (FDA), under the authority of the Federal Food, Drug, and Cosmetic Act, regulates the labeling of vitamin and mineral products sold as foods or drugs. The Nutrition Labeling and Education Act of 1990 (NLEA), with the final rules published in the *Federal Register* in early 1993, has led to nutrition labeling on virtually all packaged food, new nomenclature for declaring nutrient contents using the term *Daily Values* (DVs), and a series of disease-specific health claims. The FDA has only limited authority to control the nutrient content of supplements, except those intended for use by children under 12 years of age and by pregnant or lactating women. However, because of uniform labeling procedures, the purchaser can determine what proportion of the recommended daily allowance for each nutrient is provided by a given amount of the food.

The use of vitamins and other nutrients to treat disease comes under FDA review, either as foods for special dietary use, including food supplements, or as "over-the-counter" or prescription drugs, depending on the purposes for which the product is intended and the claims made for it. Nutrient products designed specifically for special application in medical treatment, such as parenteral solutions for hyperalimentation and so-called

Table XIII–1

Recommended Dietary Allowances[a]

Revised 1989 (Abridged)

Designed for the maintenance of good nutrition of practically all healthy people in the United States

Food and Nutrition Board, National Academy of Sciences, National Research Council

CATEGORY	AGE (YEARS) OR CONDITION	WEIGHT[b]		HEIGHT[b]		PROTEIN (g)	VITAMIN A (μg RE)[c]	VITAMIN K (μg)	IRON (mg)	ZINC (mg)	IODINE (μg)
		(kg)	(lb)	(cm)	(in)						
Infants	0.0–0.5	6	13	60	24	13	375	5	6	5	40
	0.5–1.0	9	20	71	28	14	375	10	10	5	50
Children	1–3	13	29	90	35	16	400	15	10	10	70
	4–6	20	44	112	44	24	500	20	10	10	90
	7–10	28	62	132	52	28	700	30	10	10	120
Males	11–14	45	99	157	62	45	1,000	45	12	15	150
	15–18	66	145	176	69	59	1,000	65	12	15	150
	19–24	72	160	177	70	58	1,000	70	10	15	150
	25–50	79	174	176	70	63	1,000	80	10	15	150
	51+	77	170	173	68	63	1,000	80	10	15	150
Females	11–14	46	101	157	62	46	800	45	15	12	150
	15–18	55	120	163	64	44	800	55	15	12	150
	19–24	52	128	164	65	46	800	60	15	12	150
	25–50	63	138	163	64	50	800	65	15	12	150
	51+	65	143	160	63	50	800	65	10	12	150
Pregnant						60	800	65	30	15	175
Lactating	1st 6 months					65	1,300	65	15	19	200
	2nd 6 months					62	1,200	65	15	16	200

NOTE: This table does not include nutrients for which Dietary Reference Intakes have recently been established (see Institute of Medicine, *Dietary Reference Intakes for Calcium, Phosphorus, Magnesium, Vitamin D, and Fluoride* [1997], *Dietary Reference Intakes for Thiamin, Riboflavin, Niacin, Vitamin B6, Folate, Vitamin B12, Pantothenic Acid, Biotin, and Choline* [1998], *Dietary Reference Intakes for Vitamin E, Vitamin C, Selenium, and Carotenoids* [2000], and Tables XIII–2 and XIII–3).

[a] The allowances, expressed as average daily intakes over time, are intended to provide for individual variations among most normal persons as they live in the United States under usual environmental stresses. Diets should be based on a variety of common foods in order to provide other nutrients for which human requirements have been less defined.

[b] Weights and heights of Reference Adults are actual medians for the U.S. population of the designated age, as reported by NHANES II. The median weights and heights of those under 19 years of age were taken from Hamill *et al.* (1979). The use of these figures does not imply that the height-to-weight ratios are ideal.

[c] Retinol equivalents. 1 retinol equivalent = 1 μg retinol or 6 μg β-carotene.

Copyright 2000 by the National Academy of Sciences. All rights reserved. Reproduced with permission.

Table XIII–2
Dietary Reference Intakes: Recommended Intakes for Individuals
Food and Nutrition Board, National Academy of Sciences, National Research Council

LIFE STAGE GROUP	CALCIUM (mg/d)	PHOSPHORUS (mg/d)	MAGNESIUM (mg/d)	VITAMIN D (µg/d)[a,b]	FLUORIDE (mg/d)	THIAMIN (mg/d)	RIBOFLAVIN (mg/d)	NIACIN (mg/d)[c]	VITAMIN B6 (mg/d)	FOLATE (µg/d)[d]	VITAMIN B12 (µg/d)	PANTOTHENIC ACID (mg/d)	BIOTIN (µg/d)	CHOLINE[e] (mg/d)	VITAMIN C (mg/d)	VITAMIN E[f] (mg/d)	SELENIUM (µg/d)
Infants
0–6 mo	210*	100*	30*	5*	0.01*	0.2*	0.3*	2*	0.1*	65*	0.4*	1.7*	5*	125*	40*	4*	15*
7–12 mo	270*	275*	75*	5*	0.5*	0.3*	0.4*	4*	0.3*	80*	0.5*	1.8*	6*	150*	50*	6*	20*
Children
1–3 y	500*	460	80	5*	0.7*	0.5	0.5	6	0.5	150	0.9	2*	8*	200*	15	6	20
4–8 y	800*	500	130	5*	1*	0.6	0.6	8	0.6	200	1.2	3*	12*	250*	25	7	30
Males
9–13 y	1,300*	1,250	240	5*	2*	0.9	0.9	12	1.0	300	1.8	4*	20*	375*	45	11	40
14–18 y	1,300*	1,250	410	5*	3*	1.2	1.3	16	1.3	400	2.4	5*	25*	550*	75	15	55
19–30 y	1,000*	700	400	5*	4*	1.2	1.3	16	1.3	400	2.4	5*	30*	550*	90	15	55
31–50 y	1,000*	700	420	5*	4*	1.2	1.3	16	1.3	400	2.4	5*	30*	550*	90	15	55
51–70 y	1,200*	700	420	10*	4*	1.2	1.3	16	1.7	400	2.4[g]	5*	30*	550*	90	15	55
>70 y	1,200*	700	420	15*	4*	1.2	1.3	16	1.7	400	2.4[g]	5*	30*	550*	90	15	55
Females
9–13 y	1,300*	1,250	240	5*	2*	0.9	0.9	12	1.0	300	1.8	4*	20*	375*	45	11	40
14–18 y	1,300*	1,250	360	5*	3*	1.0	1.0	14	1.2	400[h]	2.4	5*	25*	400*	65	15	55
19–30 y	1,000*	700	310	5*	3*	1.1	1.1	14	1.3	400[h]	2.4	5*	30*	425*	75	15	55
31–50 y	1,000*	700	320	5*	3*	1.1	1.1	14	1.3	400[h]	2.4	5*	30*	425*	75	15	55
51–70 y	1,200*	700	320	10*	3*	1.1	1.1	14	1.5	400	2.4[g]	5*	30*	425*	75	15	55
>70 y	1,200*	700	320	15*	3*	1.1	1.1	14	1.5	400	2.4[g]	5*	30*	425*	75	15	55

Table XIII–2

Dietary Reference Intakes: Recommended Intakes for Individuals (*Continued*)
Food and Nutrition Board, National Academy of Sciences, National Research Council

LIFE STAGE GROUP	CALCIUM (mg/d)	PHOSPHORUS (mg/d)	MAGNESIUM (mg/d)	VITAMIN D (μg/d)[a,b]	FLUORIDE (mg/d)	THIAMIN (mg/d)	RIBOFLAVIN (mg/d)	NIACIN (mg/d)[c]	VITAMIN B6 (mg/d)	FOLATE (μg/d)[d]	VITAMIN B12 (μg/d)	PANTOTHENIC ACID (mg/d)	BIOTIN (μg/d)	CHOLINE[e] (mg/d)	VITAMIN C (mg/d)	VITAMIN E[f] (mg/d)	SELENIUM (μg/d)
Pregnancy
≤18 y	1,300*	1,250	400	5*	3*	1.4	1.4	18	1.9	600[i]	2.6	6*	30*	450*	80	15	60
19–30 y	1,000*	700	350	5*	3*	1.4	1.4	18	1.9	600[i]	2.6	6*	30*	450*	85	15	60
31–50 y	1,000*	700	360	5*	3*	1.4	1.4	18	1.9	600[i]	2.6	6*	30*	450*	85	15	60
Lactation
≤18 y	1,300*	1,250	360	5*	3*	1.4	1.6	17	2.0	500	2.8	7*	35*	550*	115	19	70
19–30 y	1,000*	700	310	5*	3*	1.4	1.6	17	2.0	500	2.8	7*	35*	550*	120	19	70
31–50 y	1,000*	700	320	5*	3*	1.4	1.6	17	2.0	500	2.8	7*	35*	550*	120	19	70

NOTE: This table presents Recommended Dietary Allowances (RDAs) in **bold type** and Adequate Intakes (AIs) in ordinary type followed by an asterisk (*). RDAs and AIs may both be used as goals for individual intake. RDAs are set to meet the needs of almost all (97 to 98 percent) individuals in a group. For healthy breastfed infants, the AI is the mean intake. The AI for other life-stage and gender groups is believed to cover needs of all individuals in the group, but lack of data or uncertainty in the data prevent being able to specify with confidence the percentage of individuals covered by this intake. d = day; y = year; mo = month.

[a] As cholecalciferol. 1 μg cholecalciferol = 40 IU vitamin D.

[b] In the absence of adequate exposure to sunlight.

[c] As niacin equivalents (NE). 1 mg of niacin = 60 mg of tryptophan; 0–6 months = preformed niacin (not NE).

[d] As dietary folate equivalents (DFE). 1 DFE = 1 μg food folate = 0.6 μg of folic acid from fortified food or as a supplement consumed with food = 0.5 μg of a supplement taken on an empty stomach.

[e] Although AIs have been set for choline, there are few data to assess whether a dietary supply of choline is needed at all stages of the life cycle, and it may be that the choline requirement can be met by endogenous synthesis at some of these stages.

[f] As α-tocopherol. α-Tocopherol includes RRR-α-tocopherol, the only form of α-tocopherol that occurs naturally in foods, and the 2R-stereoisomeric forms of α-tocopherol (RRR-, RSR-, RRS-, and RSS-α-tocopherol) that occur in fortified foods and supplements. It does not include the 2S-stereoisomeric forms of α-tocopherol (SRR-, SSR-, SRS-, and SSS-α-tocopherol), also found in fortified foods and supplements.

[g] Because 10 to 30 percent of older people may malabsorb food-bound B₁₂, it is advisable for those older than 50 years to meet their RDA mainly by consuming foods fortified with B₁₂ or a supplement containing B₁₂.

[h] In view of evidence linking inadequate folate intake with netural tube defects in the fetus, it is recommended that all women capable of becoming pregnant consume 400 μg from supplements or fortified foods in addition to intake of food folate from a varied diet.

[i] It is assumed that women will continue consuming 400 μg from supplements or fortified food until their pregnancy is confirmed and they enter prenatal care, which ordinarily occurs after the end of the periconceptional period—the critical time for formation of the neural tube.

See Institute of Medicine, *Dietary Reference Intakes for Calcium, Phosphorus, Magnesium, Vitamin D, and Fluoride* [1997], *Dietary Reference Intakes for Thiamin, Riboflavin, Niacin, Vitamin B₆, Folate, Vitamin B₁₂, Pantothenic Acid, Biotin, and Choline* [1998], and *Dietary Reference Intakes for Vitamin E, Vitamin C, Selenium, and Carotenoids* [2000].

Copyright 2000 by the National Academy of Sciences. All rights reserved. Reproduced with permission.

Table XIII–3

Dietary Reference Intakes: Tolerable Upper Intake Levels (UL[a])
Food and Nutrition Board, National Academy of Sciences, National Research Council

LIFE STAGE GROUP	CALCIUM (g/d)	PHOSPHORUS (g/d)	MAGNESIUM (mg/d)[b]	VITAMIN D (μg/d)	FLUORIDE (mg/d)	NIACIN (mg/d)[c]	VITAMIN B6 (mg/d)	FOLATE (μg/d)[c]	CHOLINE (g/d)	VITAMIN C (mg/d)	VITAMIN E (mg/d)[d]	SELENIUM (μg/d)
Infants												
0–6 mo	ND[e]	ND	ND	25	0.7	ND	ND	ND	ND	ND	ND	45
7–12 mo	ND	ND	ND	25	0.9	ND	ND	ND	ND	ND	ND	60
Children												
1–3 y	2.5	3	65	50	1.3	10	30	300	1.0	400	200	90
4–8 y	2.5	3	110	50	2.2	15	40	400	1.0	650	300	150
Males, Females												
9–13 y	2.5	4	350	50	10	20	60	600	2.0	1,200	600	280
14–18 y	2.5	4	350	50	10	30	80	800	3.0	1,800	800	400
19–70 y	2.5	4	350	50	10	35	100	1,000	3.5	2,000	1,000	400
>70 y	2.5	3	350	50	10	35	100	1,000	3.5	2,000	1,000	400
Pregnancy												
≤18 y	2.5	3.5	350	50	10	30	80	800	3.0	1,800	800	400
19–50 y	2.5	3.5	350	50	10	35	100	1,000	3.5	2,000	1,000	400
Lactation												
≤18 y	2.5	4	350	50	10	30	80	800	3.0	1,800	800	400
19–50 y	2.5	4	350	50	10	35	100	1,000	3.5	2,000	1,000	400

d = day; y = year; mo = month.

[a] UL = The maximum level of daily nutrient intake that is likely to pose no risk of adverse effects. Unless otherwise specified, the UL represents total intake from food, water, and supplements. Due to lack of suitable data, ULs could not be established for thiamin, riboflavin, vitamin B12, pantothenic acid, or biotin. In the absence of ULs, extra caution may be warranted in consuming levels above recommended intakes.

[b] The ULs for magnesium represent intake from a pharmacological agent only and do not include intake from food and water.

[c] The ULs for niacin and folate apply to synthetic forms obtained from supplements, fortified foods, or a combination of the two.

[d] As α-tocopherol; applies to any form of supplemental α-tocopherol.

[e] ND = Not determinable due to lack of data of adverse effects in this age group and concern with regard to lack of ability to handle excess amounts. Source of intake should be from food only to prevent high levels of intake.

See Institute of Medicine, *Dietary Reference Intakes for Calcium, Phosphorus, Magnesium, Vitamin D, and Fluoride* [1997], *Dietary Reference Intakes for Thiamin, Riboflavin, Niacin, Vitamin B6, Folate, Vitamin B12, Pantothenic Acid, Biotin, and Choline* [1998], and *Dietary Reference Intakes for Vitamin E, Vitamin C, Selenium, and Carotenoids* [2000].

Copyright 2000 by the National Academy of Sciences. All rights reserved. Reproduced with permission.

medical foods (*e.g.,* defined formula diets), are evaluated for safety and efficacy, as are "over-the-counter" drugs containing vitamins and minerals.

Dietary supplements are used by more than 50% of the U.S. population (*Report of the Commission on Dietary Supplement Labels,* 1997). The most commonly used supplements are vitamins and minerals. Forty-seven percent of the U.S. population takes a vitamin and/or mineral supplement (*USDA's 1994–1996 Continuing Survey of Food Intakes by Individuals,* 1999). The intense interest in supplements by consumers and those who market them has put pressure on Congress to keep this area free of regulation. The history of supplement regulation shows efforts by the FDA to regulate the potency and combinations of marketed nutrients and Congress taking action to prevent regulation.

The Dietary Supplement Health and Education Act (DSHEA) resulted in substantial deregulation of supplement marketing and the assertions that can be made about their benefits (Bass and Young, 1996). DSHEA broadens the definition of dietary supplements, which includes vitamins and minerals, and maintains their regulation as foods. Thus, a supplement must be safe under the conditions recommended on the label or under ordinary conditions of use. The responsibility for safety is placed on the manufacturer. This changes the FDA regulating procedure for supplements from one of preclearance to policing (*see* Chapter 3).

Range of Intakes of Vitamins and Minerals. Many millions of individuals living in the United States regularly ingest quantities of vitamins vastly in excess of the RDA. One reason some people take vitamin supplements is the erroneous belief that such preparations provide extra energy and make one "feel better." This evidence of widespread nutritional self-medication should be kept in mind when taking a medication history from a patient.

The use of vitamin supplements is medically advisable in a variety of circumstances where *vitamin deficiencies* are likely to occur. Such situations may arise from inadequate intake, malabsorption, increased tissue needs, or inborn errors of metabolism (*see* Position of the American Dietetic Association, 1996). In practice, these causes may overlap, as in the case of the alcoholic, who may have both inadequate food intake and impaired absorption. The patient who requires long-term total parenteral nutrition is absolutely dependent on supplemental vitamins added to the infusates. Unfortunately, a serious undersupply of parenteral multivitamin preparations in the United States has made it difficult to meet clinical demand.

While gross vitamin deficiencies due to inadequate intakes are encountered in underdeveloped areas of the world, few florid cases are seen in the United States. Ongoing surveillance of dietary intake is conducted periodically by the United States government. Mean intakes consistently exceed RDA for several major vitamins (vitamin A, thiamine, riboflavin, niacin, and ascorbic acid). Individuals living below the poverty level, particularly the elderly and ethnic minorities, may have a substantially greater risk of inadequate intake of some vitamins, especially vitamins A and C.

Certain individuals are exposed to deficient intakes of vitamins as a result of eccentric diets, such as food faddism, and the avoidance of food because of anorexia. Intakes of vitamins less than those recommended also can occur in subjects on reducing diets and among elderly people who eat little food for economic or social reasons. The consumption of excessive amounts of alcohol also can lead to inadequate intakes of vitamins and other nutrients.

Malabsorption of vitamins also is seen in various conditions. Examples include hepatobiliary and pancreatic diseases, prolonged diarrheal illness, hyperthyroidism, pernicious anemia, sprue, and intestinal bypass operations. Moreover, since a substantial proportion of vitamin K and biotin is synthesized by the bacteria of the gastrointestinal tract, treatment with antimicrobial agents that alter the intestinal bacterial flora inevitably leads to decreased availability of these vitamins.

Increased tissue requirements for vitamins may cause a nutritional deficiency to develop despite the ingestion of a diet that previously had been adequate. For example, requirements for some vitamins may be altered by the use of certain antivitamin drugs, such as the interference with the utilization of folic acid by trimethoprim (*see* Roe, 1981). Diseases associated with an increased metabolic rate, such as hyperthyroidism and conditions accompanied by fever or tissue wasting, also increase the body's requirements for vitamins.

Finally, an increasing number of cases are recorded in which genetic abnormalities lead to an increased need for a vitamin. This often is due to an abnormality in the structure of an enzyme for which the vitamin provides a cofactor, leading to a decreased affinity of the abnormal enzyme protein for the cofactor (Scriver, 1973).

The impact of disease on requirements for nutrients may vary according to its phase and intensity. The need for therapy with vitamins may change throughout the course of the illness; eventually, cure should be associated with cessation of this therapy.

BIBLIOGRAPHY

Bass, I.S., and Young, A.L. *Dietary Supplement Health and Education Act: A Legislative History and Analysis.* The Food and Drug Law Institute, Washington, D.C., **1996.**

Food and Nutrition Board, National Research Council. *Recommended Dietary Allowances,* 10th ed. National Academy of Sciences, Washington, D.C., **1989.**

Hamill, P.V., Drizd, T.A., Johnson, C.L., Reed, R.B., Roche, A.F., and Moore, W.M. Physical growth: National Center for Health Statistics percentiles. *Am. J. Clin. Nutr.,* **1979,** *32*:607–629.

Institute of Medicine. *Dietary Reference Intakes for Calcium, Phosphorus, Magnesium, Vitamin D, and Fluoride.* National Academy Press, Washington, D.C., **1997.**

Institute of Medicine. *Dietary Reference Intakes for Thiamin, Riboflavin, Niacin, Vitamin B$_6$, Folate, Vitamin B$_{12}$, Pantothenic Acid, Biotin, and Choline.* National Academy Press, Washington, D.C., **1998.**

Institute of Medicine. *Dietary Reference Intakes for Vitamin E, Vitamin C, Selenium, and Carotenoids.* National Academy Press, Washington, D.C., **2000.**

Position of the American Dietetic Association: vitamin and mineral supplementation. *J. Am. Diet. Assoc.,* **1996,** *96*:73–77.

Report of the Commission on Dietary Supplement Labels. Department of Health and Human Services, Washington, D.C., **1997.**

Roe, D.A. Drug interference with the assessment of nutritional status. *Clin. Lab. Med.,* **1981,** *1*:647–664.

Scriver, C.R. Vitamin-responsive inborn error of metabolism. *Metabolism,* **1973,** *22*:1319–1344.

Shils, M.E., Olson, J.A., Shike, M., and Ross, A.C., eds. *Modern Nutrition in Health and Disease,* 9th ed. Williams & Wilkins, Baltimore, **1999.**

USDA's 1994–1996 Continuing Survey of Food Intakes by Individuals. Table set 12: Supplementary Data Tables. Available at: http://www.barc.usda.gov/bhnrc/foodsurvey/home.htm. Accessed August 9, **2000.**

Yates, A.A., Schlicker, S.A., and Suitor, C.W. Dietary Reference Intakes: the new basis for recommendations for calcium and related nutrients, B vitamins, and choline. *J. Am. Diet. Assoc.,* **1998,** *98*:699–706.

WATER-SOLUBLE VITAMINS
The Vitamin B Complex and Ascorbic Acid

Robert Marcus and Ann M. Coulston

This chapter provides a summary of physiological and therapeutic roles of members of the vitamin B complex and of vitamin C. The vitamin B complex comprises a large number of compounds that differ extensively in chemical structure and biological action. They were grouped in a single class because they originally were isolated from the same sources, notably liver and yeast. There are traditionally eleven members of the vitamin B complex— namely, thiamine, riboflavin, nicotinic acid, pyridoxine, pantothenic acid, biotin, folic acid, cyanocobalamin, choline, inositol, and paraaminobenzoic acid. Paraaminobenzoic acid is not considered in this chapter, as it is not a true vitamin for any mammalian species but is a growth factor for certain bacteria, where it is a precursor for folic acid synthesis. Although not a traditional member of the group, carnitine also is considered in this chapter because of its biosynthetic relationship to choline and the recent recognition of deficiency states. Folic acid and cyanocobalamin are considered in Chapter 54 because of their special function in hematopoiesis. Vitamin C is especially concentrated in citrus fruits and thus is obtained mostly from sources differing from those of members of the vitamin B complex.

I. THE VITAMIN B COMPLEX

THIAMINE

History. Thiamine, or vitamin B_1, was the first member of the vitamin B complex to be identified. Lack of thiamine produces a form of polyneuritis known as beriberi; this disease became widespread in East Asia in the nineteenth century due to the introduction of steam-powered rice mills, which produced polished rice lacking the vitamin-rich husk. A dietary cause for the disease was first indicated in 1880, when Admiral Takaki greatly reduced the incidence of beriberi in the Japanese Navy by adding fish, meat, barley, and vegetables to the sailors' diet of polished rice. In 1897, Eijkman, a Dutch physician working in Java where beriberi also was common, showed that fowl fed polished rice develop a polyneuritis similar to beriberi and that it could be cured by adding the rice polishings (husks) or an aqueous extract of the polishings back into the diet. He also demonstrated that rice polishings could cure beriberi in human beings.

In 1911, Funk isolated a highly concentrated form of the active factor and recognized that it belonged to a new class of food factors, which he called *vitamines,* later shortened to *vitamins.* The active factor subsequently was named vitamin B_1; in 1926 it was isolated in crystalline form by Jansen and Donath, and in 1936 its structure was determined by Williams.

The Council on Pharmacy and Chemistry adopted the name *thiamine* to designate crystalline vitamin B_1.

Chemistry. Thiamine contains a pyrimidine and a thiazole nucleus linked by a methylene bridge. Thiamine functions in the body in the form of the coenzyme thiamine pyrophosphate (TPP). The structures of thiamine and thiamine pyrophosphate are as follows:

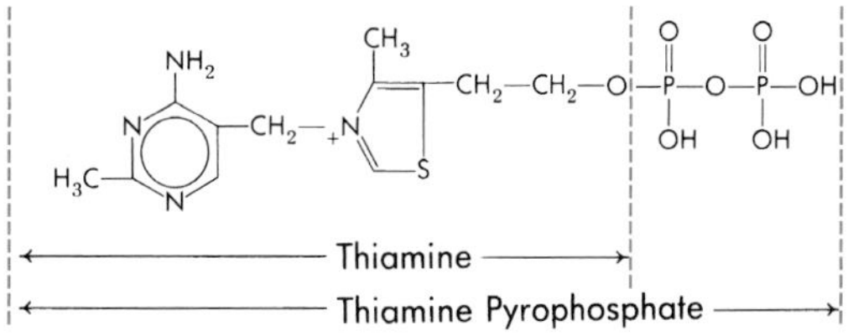

The conversion of thiamine to its coenzyme form is carried out by the enzyme thiamine diphosphokinase, with adenosine triphosphate (ATP) as the pyrophosphate (PP) donor. Antimetabolites to thiamine that inhibit this enzyme have been synthesized. The most important of these are *neopyrithiamine (pyrithiamine)* and *oxythiamine.*

Pharmacological Actions. Thiamine is practically devoid of pharmacodynamic actions when given in usual therapeutic doses; even large doses produce no discernible effects. Isolated clinical reports of toxic reactions to the long-term parenteral administration of thiamine probably represent rare instances of hypersensitivity.

Physiological Functions. The vitamins of the B complex function in intermediary metabolism in many essential reactions; some of these functions are summarized in Figure 63–1. Thiamine pyrophosphate, the physiologically active form of thiamine, functions in carbohydrate metabolism as a coenzyme in the decarboxylation of α-keto acids such as pyruvate and α-ketoglutarate and in the utilization of pentose in the hexose monophosphate shunt; the latter

function involves the thiamine pyrophosphate–dependent enzyme transketolase. Several metabolic changes of clinical importance can be related directly to the biochemical action of thiamine. In thiamine deficiency, the oxidation of α-keto acids is impaired, and an increase in the concentration of pyruvate in the blood has been used as one of the diagnostic signs of the deficiency state. A more specific diagnostic test for thiamine deficiency is based upon measurement of transketolase activity in erythrocytes (Brin, 1968). The requirement for thiamine is related to metabolic rate and is greatest when carbohydrate is the source of energy. This fact is of practical significance for patients who are maintained by

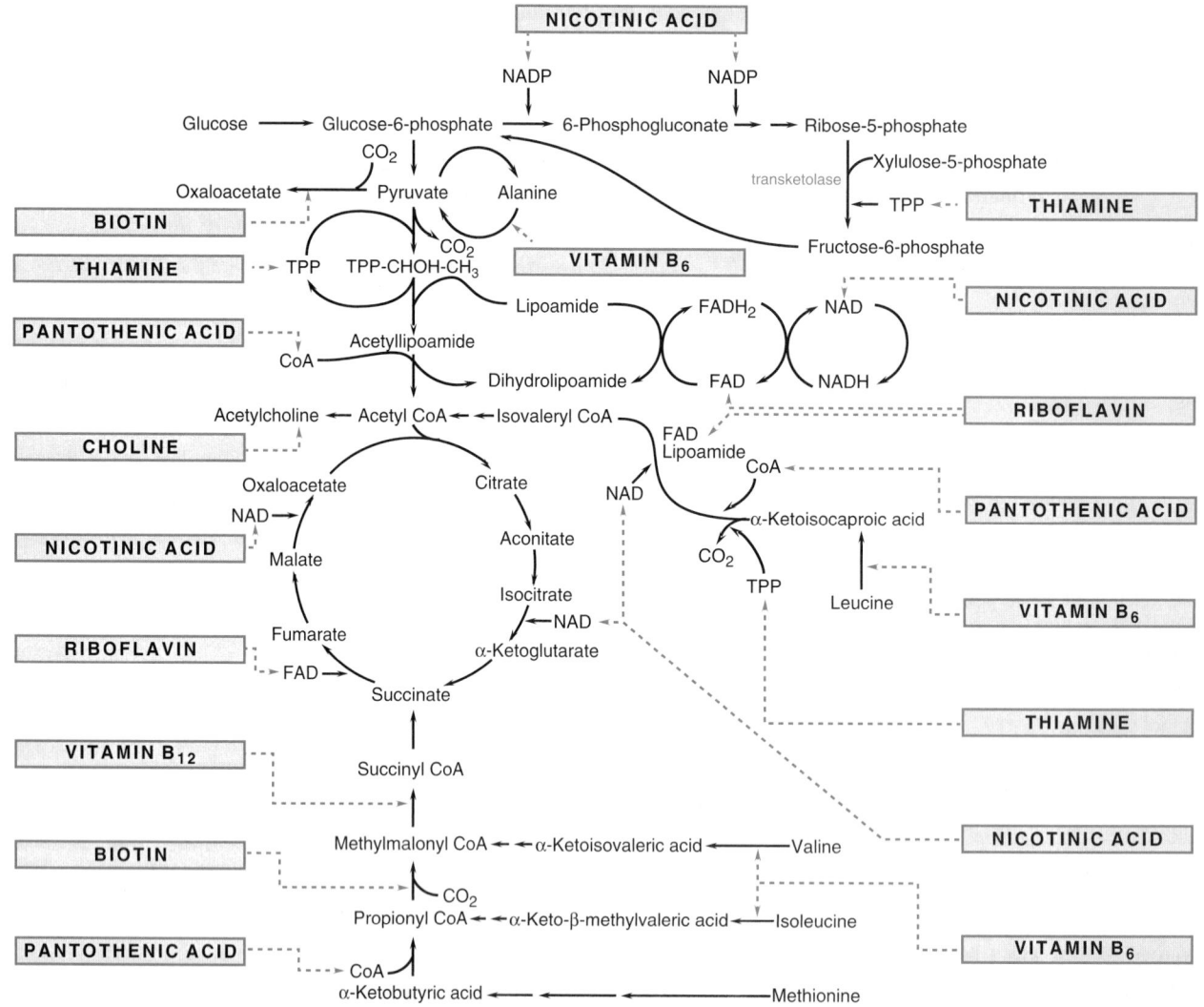

Figure 63–1. Some major metabolic pathways involving coenzymes formed from water-soluble vitamins.

(Abbreviations are defined in the text throughout this chapter.)

parenteral nutrition and who thereby receive a substantial portion of their calories in the form of dextrose. Such patients should be given a generous allowance of the vitamin.

Symptoms of Deficiency.   Severe thiamine deficiency leads to the condition known as *beriberi*. In Asia, this is due to consumption of diets of polished rice, which are deficient in the vitamin. In Europe and North America, thiamine deficiency is seen most commonly in alcoholics, although patients with chronic renal failure on dialysis and patients receiving total parenteral nutrition also may be at risk. A severe form of acute thiamine deficiency also can occur in infants.

The major symptoms of thiamine deficiency are related to the nervous system (dry beriberi) and to the cardiovascular system (wet beriberi). Many of the neurological signs and symptoms are characteristic of peripheral neuritis, with sensory disturbances in the extremities, including localized areas of hyperesthesia or anesthesia. Muscle strength is lost gradually and may result in wrist-drop or complete paralysis of a limb. Personality disturbances, depression, lack of initiative, and poor memory also may result from lack of the vitamin, as may syndromes as extreme as Wernicke's encephalopathy and Korsakoff's psychosis (*see* below).

Cardiovascular symptoms can be prominent and include dyspnea on exertion, palpitation, tachycardia, and other cardiac abnormalities characterized by an abnormal electrocardiogram (ECG) (chiefly low R-wave voltage, T-wave inversion, and prolongation of the Q-T interval) and cardiac failure of the high-output type. Such failure has been termed *wet beriberi;* there is extensive edema, largely as a result of hypoproteinemia from an inadequate intake of protein or concomitant liver disease together with failing ventricular function.

Absorption, Fate, and Excretion.   Absorption of the usual dietary amounts of thiamine from the gastrointestinal tract occurs by carrier-mediated active transport (Said *et al.*, 1999); at higher concentrations, passive diffusion also is significant (Rindi and Ventura, 1972). Absorption usually is limited to a maximal daily amount of 8 to 15 mg, but this amount can be exceeded by oral administration in divided doses with food. Cellular thiamine uptake is mediated by a specific plasma membrane transporter, which recently has been cloned (Diaz *et al.*, 1999; Dutta *et al.*, 1999).

In adults, approximately 1 mg of thiamine per day is completely degraded by the tissues, and this is roughly the minimal daily requirement. When intake is at this low level, little or no thiamine is excreted in the urine. When intake exceeds the minimal requirement, tissue stores are first saturated. Thereafter, the excess appears quantitatively in the urine as intact thiamine or as pyrimidine, which arises from degradation of the thiamine molecule. As the intake of thiamine is increased further, more of the excess is excreted unchanged.

Therapeutic Uses.   The only established therapeutic use of thiamine is in the treatment or the prophylaxis of thiamine deficiency. To correct the disorder as rapidly as possible, intravenous doses as large as 100 mg per liter of parenteral fluid commonly are used. Once thiamine deficiency has been corrected, there is no need for parenteral injection or the administration of amounts in excess of daily requirements except in instances when gastrointestinal disturbances preclude the ingestion or absorption of adequate amounts of vitamin.

The syndromes of thiamine deficiency seen clinically can range from beriberi through Wernicke's encephalopathy and Korsakoff's syndrome to alcoholic polyneuropathy. Because normal metabolism of carbohydrate results in consumption of thiamine, it has been observed repeatedly that administration of glucose may precipitate acute symptoms of thiamine deficiency in marginally nourished subjects. This also has been noted during the correction of endogenous hyperglycemia. *Thus, in any individual whose thiamine status may be suspect, the vitamin should be given before or along with dextrose-containing fluids; all alcoholic patients seen in an emergency room should routinely receive 50 to 100 mg of thiamine.* The clinical findings depend on the amount of deprivation. Encephalopathy and Korsakoff's syndrome result from severe deprivation, whereas beriberi heart disease occurs in less-deficient subjects; polyneuritis is observed in milder deprivation. The following discussion describes briefly the varieties of thiamine deficiency and their treatment.

Alcoholic Neuritis.   Alcoholism is the most common cause of thiamine deficiency in the United States. Alcoholic neuritis is caused by an inadequate intake of thiamine. Two factors contribute to such inadequate intake in the chronic alcoholic: (1) Appetite usually is poor, so food consumption drops; and (2) a large portion of the caloric intake is in the form of alcohol. The symptoms of neurological involvement in alcoholics are those of a polyneuritis with motor and sensory defects. Wernicke's syndrome is an additional serious consequence of alcoholism and thiamine deficiency. Certain characteristic signs of this disease, notably ophthalmoplegia, nystagmus, and ataxia, respond rapidly to the administration of thiamine but to no other vitamin. Wernicke's syndrome may be accompanied by an acute global confusional state that also may respond to thiamine. Left untreated, Wernicke's encephalopathy frequently leads to a chronic disorder in which learning and memory are impaired out of proportion to other cognitive functions in the otherwise alert and responsive patient. This disorder (Korsakoff's psychosis) is characterized by confabulation, and it is less likely to be reversible once established (Victor *et al.*, 1971). Although the thiamine stores of some patients with Wernicke's encephalopathy are similar to those in patients without neurological findings, it has been found that patients with Wernicke's encephalopathy have an abnormality in the thiamine-dependent enzyme transketolase (*see* Haas,

1988). In such instances, marginal concentrations of thiamine might produce serious neurological damage. The prevalence of Wernicke's encephalopathy in Australia decreased following the introduction of thiamine-enriched flour (Harper *et al.,* 1998).

Chronic alcoholics with polyneuritis and motor or sensory defects should receive up to 40 mg of oral thiamine daily. The Wernicke-Korsakoff syndrome represents an acute emergency that should be treated with daily doses of at least 100 mg of the vitamin, intravenously.

Infantile Beriberi.   Thiamine deficiency also occurs as an acute disease in infancy and may run a rapid and fulminating course. Although rare in modern societies, infantile beriberi has been a common cause of infant death throughout this century in regions where rice consumption is high. It still is of significance in Third World countries and is related to the low content of thiamine in breast milk of thiamine-deficient women. The onset consists of loss of appetite, vomiting, and greenish stools, followed by paroxysmal attacks of muscular rigidity. Aphonia due to loss of laryngeal nerve function is a diagnostic feature. Signs of cardiac involvement are prominent, and death may occur within 12 to 24 hours unless vigorous treatment is instituted. Infants with mild forms of this condition respond to oral therapy with 10 mg of thiamine daily. If acute collapse occurs, doses of 25 mg intravenously can be given cautiously, but the prognosis remains poor.

Subacute Necrotizing Encephalomyelopathy.   This is a fatal inherited disease of children. Neuropathological features resemble those of the Wernicke-Korsakoff syndrome, and clinical features include difficulties with feeding and swallowing, vomiting, hypotonia, external ophthalmoplegia, peripheral neuropathy, and seizures. Although the syndrome may have multiple causes, the distribution of lesions and the elevated plasma concentrations of pyruvate and lactate suggest a pathogenetic relationship to thiamine; however, this remains unproven (*see* Haas, 1988). Some cases appear to be caused by a circulating inhibitor of the enzyme that synthesizes thiamine triphosphate from thiamine pyrophosphate in the nervous system. Metabolic abnormalities also have been found in tissue samples from affected infants, including defects in pyruvate dehydrogenase and cytochrome *c*-oxidase (Medina *et al.,* 1990). Other inborn errors of metabolism that are sensitive to the administration of thiamine also have been described (*see* Scriver, 1973).

Cardiovascular Disease.   Cardiovascular disease of nutritional origin is observed in chronic alcoholics, pregnant women, persons with gastrointestinal disorders, and those whose diet is deficient for other reasons. When the diagnosis of cardiovascular disease due to thiamine deficiency has been made correctly, the response to the administration of thiamine is striking. One of the pathognomonic features of the syndrome is an increased blood flow due to arteriolar dilation. Within a few hours after the administration of thiamine, the cardiac output is reduced and the utilization of oxygen begins to return to normal. If edema is present and due to myocardial insufficiency, diuresis results after proper therapy. However, individuals suffering from a chronic deficiency may require protracted treatment. The usual dose of thiamine is 10 to 30 mg three times daily, given parenterally. The dosage can be reduced and the patient maintained on oral medication or by

dietary management after signs of the deficiency state have been reversed. It is emphasized that administration of glucose may precipitate heart failure in individuals with marginal thiamine status. All patients potentially in this category should receive thiamine prophylactically; 100 mg is commonly given intramuscularly or added to the first few liters of intravenous fluid.

Gastrointestinal Disorders.   In experimental and clinical beriberi, certain symptoms are referable to the gastrointestinal tract. On this basis, thiamine has been used uncritically as a therapeutic agent for such unrelated conditions as ulcerative colitis, gastrointestinal hypotonia, and chronic diarrhea. Unless the disease being treated is the direct result of a deficiency of thiamine, the vitamin is not efficacious.

Neuritis of Pregnancy.   Pregnancy increases the thiamine requirement slightly. The neuritis of pregnancy takes the form of multiple peripheral nerve involvement, and the signs and symptoms in well-developed cases resemble those described in patients with beriberi. The problem may occur because of poor intake of thiamine or in patients with hyperemesis gravidarum. Proof that the neuritis is due to thiamine deficiency is gained in those cases in which dramatic clinical improvement follows thiamine therapy. The dose employed is from 5 to 10 mg daily, given parenterally if vomiting is severe.

Megaloblastic Anemia.   Thiamine-responsive megaloblastic anemia (TRMA) with diabetes mellitus and deafness is an autosomal recessive disease that responds to large doses of thiamine. This disorder was shown to be caused by mutations in the plasma membrane–associated thiamine transporter (Diaz *et al.,* 1999; Fleming *et al.,* 1999). Defective thiamine transport in cultured fibroblasts from TRMA patients is associated with decreased cell survival, apparently by enhanced apoptosis (Stagg *et al.,* 1999).

RIBOFLAVIN

History.   At various times from 1879 onward, series of yellow-pigmented compounds have been isolated from a variety of sources and designated as *flavins,* prefixed to indicate the source (*e.g.,* lacto-, ovo-, and hepato-). Subsequently it has been demonstrated that these various flavins are identical in chemical composition.

In the meantime, water-soluble vitamin B had been separated into a heat-labile antiberiberi factor (B_1) and a heat-stable growth-promoting factor (B_2), and it was eventually appreciated that concentrates of so-called vitamin B_2 had a yellow color. In 1932, Warburg and Christian described a yellow respiratory enzyme in yeast, and in 1933 the yellow pigment portion of the enzyme was identified as vitamin B_2. All doubt as to the identity of vitamin B_2 and the naturally occurring flavins was removed when lactoflavin was synthesized and the synthetic product was shown to possess full biological activity. The vitamin was designated as *riboflavin* because of the presence of ribose in its structure.

Chemistry.   Riboflavin carries out its functions in the body in the form of one or the other of two coenzymes, *riboflavin phosphate,* commonly called *flavin mononucleotide* (FMN), and *flavin adenine dinucleotide* (FAD). Their structures are shown above.

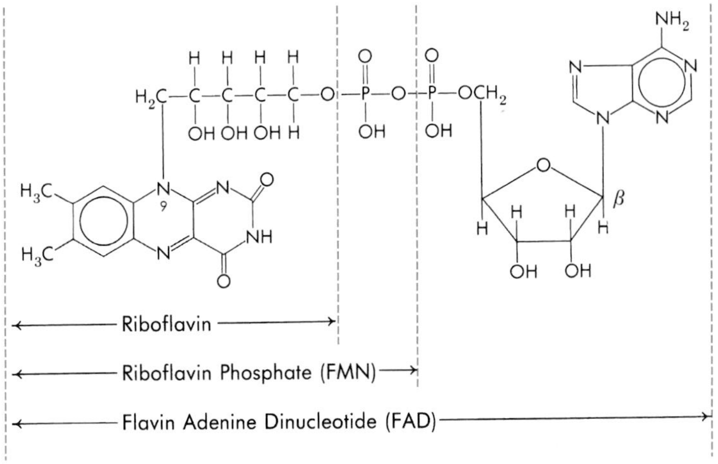

Riboflavin is converted to FMN and FAD by two enzyme-catalyzed reactions, shown as Reactions (63–1) and (63–2):

$$\text{Riboflavin} + \text{ATP} \rightarrow \text{FMN} + \text{ADP} \qquad (63\text{–}1)$$

$$\text{FMN} + \text{ATP} \rightarrow \text{FAD} + \text{PP} \qquad (63\text{–}2)$$

Pharmacological Actions. No overt pharmacological effects follow the oral or parenteral administration of riboflavin.

Physiological Functions. FMN and FAD, the physiologically active forms of riboflavin, serve a vital role in metabolism as coenzymes for a wide variety of respiratory flavoproteins, some of which contain metals (*e.g.,* xanthine oxidase).

Symptoms of Deficiency. The features of spontaneous or experimentally produced riboflavin deficiency have been reviewed by McCormick (1989). Sore throat and angular stomatitis generally appear first. Later, glossitis, cheilosis (red, denuded lips), seborrheic dermatitis of the face, and dermatitis over the trunk and extremities occur, followed by anemia and neuropathy. In some subjects, corneal vascularization and cataract formation are prominent.

The anemia that develops in riboflavin deficiency is normochromic and normocytic and is associated with reticulocytopenia; leukocytes and platelets are generally normal. Administration of riboflavin to deficient patients causes reticulocytosis, and the concentration of hemoglobin returns to normal. Anemia in patients with riboflavin deficiency may be related, at least in part, to disturbances in folic acid metabolism.

The problem in the clinical recognition of riboflavin deficiency is that certain features, such as glossitis and dermatitis, are common manifestations of other diseases, including deficiencies of other vitamins. Recognition of riboflavin deficiency also is difficult because it rarely occurs in isolation. In nutritional surveys of children in an urban area and of randomly selected hospitalized patients, deficiency of riboflavin was observed frequently, but almost invariably in conjunction with other vitamin deficiencies. Riboflavin deficiency has been observed likewise in association with deficiencies of other vitamins in a large proportion of urban alcoholics of low economic status. Biochemical evidence of riboflavin deficiency has been observed in newborn infants treated with ultraviolet light for hyperbilirubinemia. Breast-fed infants are most susceptible to this problem because of the relatively low riboflavin content in breast milk. Assessment of riboflavin status is made by correlating dietary history with clinical and laboratory findings. Biochemical tests include evaluation of urinary excretion of the vitamin (excretion of less than 50 μg of riboflavin daily is indicative of deficiency). Although concentrations of flavins in blood are not of diagnostic value, an enzyme activation assay that utilizes glutathione reductase from erythrocytes correlates well with riboflavin status (Prentice and Bates, 1981).

Human Requirements. The Recommended Dietary Allowance (RDA) of riboflavin is 1.3 mg/day for men and 1.1 mg/day for women (*see* Table XIII–2). Turnover of riboflavin appears to be related to energy expenditure, and periods of increased physical activity are associated with a modest increase in requirement.

Food Sources. Riboflavin is abundant in milk, cheese, organ meats, eggs, green leafy vegetables, and whole-grain and enriched cereals and breads.

Absorption, Fate, and Excretion. Riboflavin is absorbed readily from the upper gastrointestinal tract by a specific transport mechanism involving phosphorylation of the vitamin to FMN [Reaction (63–1); Jusko and Levy, 1975]. Here and in other tissues, riboflavin is converted to FMN by flavokinase, a reaction that is sensitive to thyroid-hormone status and inhibited by chlorpromazine and by tricyclic antidepressants; the antimalarial quinacrine also interferes with the utilization of riboflavin. Riboflavin is distributed to all tissues, but concentrations are uniformly low, and little is stored. When riboflavin is ingested in amounts that approximate the minimal daily requirement, only about 9% appears in the urine. As the intake of riboflavin is increased above the minimal requirement, a larger proportion is excreted unchanged. Boric acid, a common household chemical, forms a complex with riboflavin and promotes its urinary excretion. Boric acid poisoning, therefore, may induce riboflavin deficiency.

Riboflavin is present in the feces. This probably represents vitamin synthesized by intestinal microorganisms, since, on low intakes of riboflavin, the amount excreted in the feces exceeds that ingested. There is no evidence that riboflavin synthesized by the bacteria in the colon can be absorbed.

Therapeutic Uses. The only established therapeutic application of riboflavin is to treat or prevent disease caused by deficiency. Ariboflavinosis seldom occurs in the United States as a discrete deficiency but may accompany other nutritional disorders. Specific therapy with riboflavin, 5 to 10 mg daily, should thus be given in the context of treating multiple nutritional deficiencies. A recent randomized, controlled trial of high-dose riboflavin (400 mg/day) in patients suffering migraine headaches showed significant reductions in attack frequency and illness days (Schoenen *et al.,* 1998).

NICOTINIC ACID

History. *Pellagra* (from the Italian *pelle agra,* "rough skin") has been known for centuries in countries where maize is eaten in quantity, notably Italy and in North America. In 1914, Funk postulated that the disease was due to dietary deficiency. Over the next few years, Goldberger and his colleagues demonstrated conclusively that pellagra could be prevented by increasing the dietary intake of fresh meat, eggs, and milk. Goldberger subsequently produced an excellent animal model of human pellagra, "black tongue," by feeding deficient diets to dogs. Although initially thought to be a deficiency of essential amino acids, pellagra soon was found to be prevented by a distinct heat-resistant factor in "water-soluble B" vitamin preparations.

In 1935, Warburg and associates obtained nicotinic acid amide (nicotinamide) from a coenzyme isolated from the red blood cells of the horse; this stimulated interest in the nutritional value of nicotinic acid. Since liver extracts were known to be highly effective in curing human pellagra and canine black tongue, Elvehjem and associates prepared highly active concentrates of liver; in 1937, they identified nicotinamide as the substance that was effective in the treatment of black tongue. Proof was established by the demonstration that synthetic nicotinic acid derivatives also were effective in alleviating the symptoms of black tongue and in curing human pellagra. Goldberger and Tanner previously had shown that tryptophan could cure human pellagra; this effect later was determined to be due to the conversion of tryptophan to nicotinic acid. Goldsmith (1958)

produced pellagra experimentally in human beings by feeding a diet deficient in nicotinic acid and tryptophan.

Nicotinic acid also is known as *niacin,* a term introduced to avoid confusion between the vitamin and the alkaloid nicotine. Pellagra now is quite uncommon in the United States, probably as a direct result of supplementation of flour with nicotinic acid since 1939.

Chemistry. Nicotinic acid functions in the body after conversion to either nicotinamide adenine dinucleotide (NAD) or nicotinamide adenine dinucleotide phosphate (NADP). It is to be noted that nicotinic acid occurs in these two nucleotides in the form of its amide, nicotinamide. The structures of nicotinic acid, nicotinamide, NAD, and NADP are shown below, where $R = H$ in NAD and $R = PO_3H_2$ in NADP. Synthetic analogs with antivitamin activity include pyridine-3-sulfonic acid and 3-acetyl pyridine.

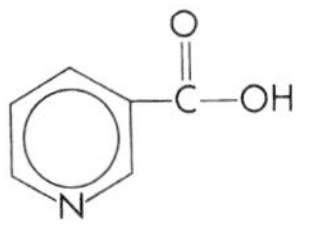

NICOTINIC ACID 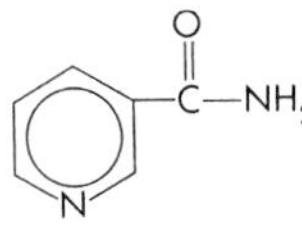   NICOTINAMIDE

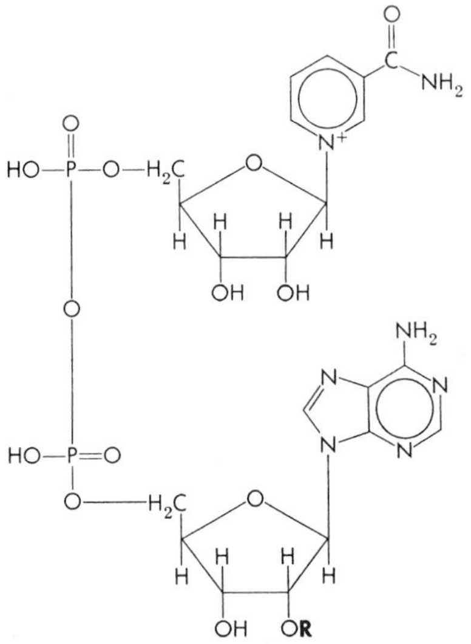

NAD and NADP

Pharmacological Actions. Nicotinic acid and nicotinamide are identical in their function as vitamins. However, they differ markedly as pharmacological agents, reflecting the fact that nicotinic acid is not directly converted to nicotinamide, which arises only from metabolism of NAD. The pharmacological effects and toxicity of nicotinic acid in man include flushing, pruritus, gastrointestinal distress, hepatotoxicity, and activation of peptic ulcer disease. Large doses of nicotinic acid (2 to 6 g per day) are sometimes used in the treatment of hyperlipoproteinemia (*see* Chapter 36). The important toxic effects of nicotinic acid are generally seen only with these doses.

Physiological Functions. NAD and NADP, the physiologically active forms of nicotinic acid, serve a vital role in metabolism as coenzymes for a wide variety of proteins that catalyze oxidation-reduction reactions essential for tissue respiration. The coenzymes, bound to appropriate dehydrogenases, function as oxidants by accepting electrons and hydrogen from substrates and thus becoming reduced. The reduced pyridine nucleotides, in turn, are reoxidized by flavoproteins. NAD also participates as a substrate in the transfer of ADP-ribosyl moieties to proteins.

The metabolic pathway for conversion of nicotinic acid to NAD has been elucidated for a variety of tissues, including human erythrocytes. [*See* Reactions (63–3) to (63–5) below, where PRPP is 5-phosphoribosyl-1-pyrophosphate. NADP is synthesized from NAD according to Reaction (63–6).] The biosynthesis of NAD from tryptophan is more complicated. Tryptophan is converted to quinolinic acid by a series of enzymatic reactions; quinolinic acid is converted to nicotinic acid ribonucleotide, which enters the pathway at Reaction (63–4).

Nicotinic Acid + PRPP
→ Nicotinic Acid Ribonucleotide + PP   (63–3)

Nicotinic Acid ribonucleotide + ATP
→ Desamido-NAD + PP   (63–4)

Desamido-NAD + Glutamine + ATP
→ NAD + Glutamate + ADP + P   (63–5)

NAD + ATP → NADP + ADP   (63–6)

Symptoms of Deficiency. A deficiency of nicotinic acid leads to the clinical condition known as pellagra. Pellagra is characterized by signs and symptoms referable especially to the skin, gastrointestinal tract, and central nervous system, a triad frequently referred to as dermatitis, diarrhea, and dementia, or the "three D's." Pellagra now occurs most often in the setting of chronic alcoholism, protein-calorie malnutrition, and deficiencies of multiple vitamins. An erythematous eruption resembling sunburn first appears on the back of the hands. Other areas exposed to light (forehead, neck, and feet) are later involved, and eventually the lesions may be more widespread. The cutaneous manifestations are characteristically symmetrical and may darken, desquamate, and scar.

The chief symptoms referable to the digestive tract are stomatitis, enteritis, and diarrhea. The tongue becomes very red and swollen and may ulcerate. Salivary secretion is excessive, and the salivary glands may be enlarged. Nausea and vomiting are common. Steatorrhea may be present, even in the absence of diarrhea. When present, diarrhea is recurrent and stools may be watery and occasionally bloody.

Symptoms referable to the central nervous system are headache, dizziness, insomnia, depression, and impairment of memory. In severe cases, delusions, hallucinations, and dementia

may appear. Motor and sensory disturbances of the peripheral nerves also occur. Common laboratory findings include macrocytic anemia, hypoalbuminemia, and hyperuricemia.

Biochemical assessment of deficiency is attempted by the measurement of urinary excretion of methylated metabolites of nicotinic acid (*e.g.,* N-methylnicotinamide). These tests do not provide unequivocal evidence of deficiency. The measurement of nicotinamide in blood and urine has not been shown to be useful in evaluating niacin status. In most cases, the diagnosis rests on a correlation of clinical findings with the response to supplemental nicotinamide.

Human Requirements. As indicated above, the dietary requirement for this vitamin can be satisfied not only by nicotinic acid but also by nicotinamide and the amino acid tryptophan. Therefore, the nicotinic acid requirement is influenced by the quantity and the quality of dietary protein. Administration of tryptophan to normal human subjects, as well as to patients with pellagra, and analysis of urinary metabolites indicate that an average of 60 mg of dietary tryptophan is equivalent to 1 mg of nicotinic acid. This conversion rate is reduced in women taking oral contraceptives. The minimal requirement of nicotinic acid (including that formed from tryptophan) to prevent pellagra averages 4.4 mg/1000 kcal. The RDA of niacin is 14 and 16 mg/day for women and men, respectively (*see* Table XIII–2).

The relationship between the nicotinic acid requirement and the intake of tryptophan has helped to explain the historical association between the incidence of pellagra and the presence of large amounts of corn in the diet. Corn protein is low in tryptophan, and the nicotinic acid in corn and other cereals is largely unavailable. When cornmeal provides the major portion of dietary protein, pellagra will develop at levels of intake of nicotinic acid that would be adequate if the dietary protein contained more tryptophan. Intake of animal protein is high among Americans; tryptophan thus helps significantly to meet the daily requirement for niacin.

Food Sources. Nicotinic acid is obtained from liver, meat, fish, poultry, whole-grain and enriched breads and cereals, nuts, and legumes. Tryptophan as a precursor is provided by animal protein, in particular.

Absorption, Fate, and Excretion. Both nicotinic acid and nicotinamide are absorbed readily from all portions of the intestinal tract, and the vitamin is distributed to all tissues. When therapeutic doses of nicotinic acid or its amide are administered, only small amounts of the unchanged vitamin appear in the urine. When extremely high doses of these vitamins are given, the unchanged vitamin represents the major urinary component. The principal route of metabolism of nicotinic acid and nicotinamide is by the formation of N-methylnicotinamide, which, in turn, is metabolized further.

Therapeutic Uses. Nicotinic acid, nicotinamide, and their derivatives are used for prophylaxis and treatment of pellagra. In the acute exacerbations of the disease, therapy must be intensive. The recommended oral dose is 50 mg, given up to ten times daily. If oral medication is impossible, intravenous injection of 25 mg is given two or more times daily. Pellagra may occur in the course of two metabolic disorders. In Hartnup's disease, intestinal and renal transport of tryptophan is defective. In some patients with carcinoid tumors, large amounts of tryptophan are utilized by the tumor for the synthesis of 5-hydroxytryptophan and 5-hydroxytryptamine (serotonin).

The response to nicotinic acid or its derivatives is dramatic. Within 24 hours, the fiery redness and swelling of the tongue disappear and sialorrhea diminishes. Associated oral infections heal rapidly. Other infections of mucous membranes also disappear. Nausea, vomiting, and diarrhea may stop within 24 hours, and at the same time the patient is relieved of epigastric distress, abdominal pain, and distention. Appetite also improves. Mental symptoms are quickly relieved, sometimes overnight. Confused patients become mentally clear, and those who are delirious become calm, adjusted to their environment, and remember with insight the events of their psychotic state. So specific are nicotinic acid and its derivatives in this regard that they can be used as diagnostic agents in patients with frank psychoses but with questionable additional evidence of pellagra. Large doses of niacin are recommended, especially when the psychosis is associated with encephalopathy. The dermal lesions blanch and heal, but this occurs more slowly. The vitamin has less effect on cutaneous lesions that are moist, ulcerated, or pigmented. The porphyrinuria associated with pellagra also disappears.

Pellagra may be complicated by thiamine deficiency with associated peripheral neuritis. This complication does not respond to nicotinic acid or its congeners and must be treated with thiamine. Many pellagrins also benefit from additional therapy with riboflavin and pyridoxine.

In gram doses, nicotinic acid lowers circulating concentrations of low-density-lipoprotein cholesterol and triglycerides, plasma fibrinogen, and lipoprotein(a). Nicotinic acid therefore is used in the management of hyperlipoproteinemias (*see* Chapter 36).

Nicotinamide has shown promise in the primary prevention of type I diabetes mellitus in high-risk individuals (Elliott *et al.,* 1996; Lampeter *et al.,* 1998). Large population-based intervention trials currently are in progress.

PYRIDOXINE

History. In 1926, dermatitis was produced in rats by feeding a diet deficient in vitamin B_2. However, in 1936 György distinguished from vitamin B_2 the water-soluble factor whose deficiency was responsible for the dermatitis and named it vitamin B_6. The structure of the vitamin was elucidated in 1939. Several related natural compounds (pyridoxine, pyridoxal, pyridoxamine) have been shown to possess the same biological properties, and therefore all should be called vitamin B_6. However, the Council on Pharmacy and Chemistry has assigned the name *pyridoxine* to the vitamin.

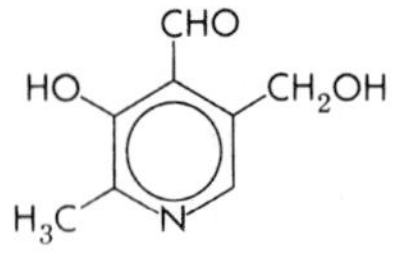

Chemistry. The structures of the three forms of vitamin B_6—that is, pyridoxine, pyridoxal, and pyridoxamine—are shown below.

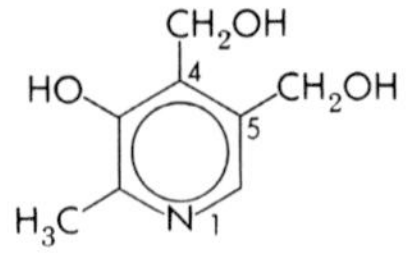

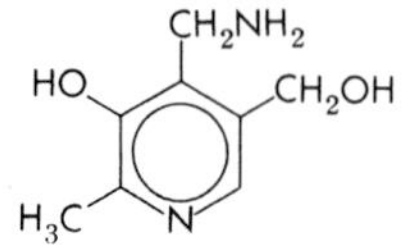

The compounds differ in the nature of the substituent on the carbon atom in position 4 of the pyridine nucleus: a primary alcohol (pyridoxine), the corresponding aldehyde (pyridoxal), an aminoethyl group (pyridoxamine). Each of these compounds can be utilized readily by mammals after conversion in the liver to pyridoxal 5'-phosphate, the active form of the vitamin.

Antimetabolites to pyridoxine have been synthesized and are capable of blocking the action of the vitamin and producing signs and symptoms of deficiency. The most active is *4-deoxypyridoxine,* for which the antivitamin activity has been attributed to the formation *in vivo* of 4-deoxypyridoxine-5-phosphate, a competitive inhibitor of several pyridoxal phosphate–dependent enzymes.

Isonicotinic acid hydrazide (*isoniazid; see* Chapter 48), as well as other carbonyl compounds, combines with pyridoxal or pyridoxal phosphate to form hydrazones; as a result, it is a potent inhibitor of pyridoxal kinase. Enzymatic reactions in which pyridoxal phosphate participates as a coenzyme also are inhibited, but only by greater concentrations than those required to inhibit the formation of pyridoxal phosphate. Isoniazid thus appears to exert its antivitamin B_6 effect primarily by inhibiting the formation of the coenzyme form of the vitamin.

Pharmacological Actions. Pyridoxine has low acute toxicity and elicits no outstanding pharmacodynamic actions after either oral or intravenous administration. However, neurotoxicity may develop after prolonged ingestion of as little as 200 mg of pyridoxine per day (Schaumberg *et al.,* 1983; Parry and Bredesen, 1985).

Physiological Functions. As a coenzyme, pyridoxal phosphate is involved in several metabolic transformations of amino acids—including decarboxylation, transamination, and racemization—as well as in enzymatic steps in the metabolism of sulfur-containing and hydroxy-amino acids. In the case of transamination, enzyme-bound pyridoxal phosphate is aminated to pyridoxamine phosphate by the donor amino acid, and the bound pyridoxamine phosphate is then deaminated to pyridoxal phosphate by the acceptor α-keto acid. Vitamin B_6 also is involved in the metabolism of tryptophan. A notable reaction is the conversion of tryptophan to 5-hydroxytryptamine. In vitamin B_6–deficient human beings and in animals, a number of metabolites of tryptophan are excreted in abnormally large quantities. The measurement of these urinary metabolites, particularly xanthurenic acid, following loading with tryptophan is used as a test of vitamin B_6 status. The conversion of methionine to cysteine also is dependent on the vitamin.

Interactions with Drugs.   Biochemical interactions occur between pyridoxal phosphate and certain drugs and toxins. The relationship with isoniazid has been discussed above. Prolonged use of penicillamine can cause deficiency of vitamin B_6. The drugs *cycloserine* and *hydralazine* are also antagonists of the vitamin, and administration of vitamin B_6 reduces the neurological side effects associated with the use of these compounds. Vitamin B_6 enhances the peripheral decarboxylation of levodopa and reduces its effectiveness for the treatment of Parkinson's disease (*see* Chapter 22).

Symptoms of Deficiency.   *Skin.*   Seborrhealike skin lesions about the eyes, nose, and mouth accompanied by glossitis and stomatitis can be produced within a few weeks by feeding a diet poor in vitamin B complex plus daily doses of the vitamin antagonist 4-deoxypyridoxine. The lesions clear rapidly after the administration of pyridoxine but do not respond to other members of the B complex.
Nervous System.   Convulsive seizures may occur when human beings are maintained on a diet deficient in pyridoxine, and these seizures can be prevented by the vitamin. The induction of convulsive seizures by pyridoxine deficiency may be the result of a lowered concentration of gamma-aminobutyric acid; glutamate decarboxylase, a pyridoxal phosphate–requiring enzyme, synthesizes this inhibitory central nervous system (CNS) neurotransmitter (*see* Chapter 12). In addition, pyridoxine deficiency leads to decreased concentrations of the neurotransmitters norepinephrine and 5-hydroxytryptamine. A peripheral neuritis associated with carpal synovial swelling and tenderness (*carpal tunnel syndrome*) has been attributed in some cases to deficiency of pyridoxine, although earlier claims that high doses of pyridoxine reverse carpal tunnel syndrome have not been confirmed (Smith *et al.*, 1984).
Erythropoiesis.   Although dietary deficiency of pyridoxine in human beings may cause anemia rarely, the usual pyridoxine-responsive anemia apparently is not due to inadequate supplies of this vitamin as judged by normal standards. This type of anemia is described in Chapter 54.

Human Requirements.   The requirement for pyridoxine increases with the amount of protein in the diet. The average adult minimal requirement for pyridoxine is about 1.6 mg per day in individuals ingesting 100 g of protein per day (Hansen *et al.*, 1997). The current RDA for pyridoxine has been set at 1.3 mg for young adult men and women, with modest increases for individuals above 50 years of age (*see* Table XIII–2).

Food Sources.   Pyridoxine is supplied by meat, liver, whole-grain breads and cereals, soybeans, and vegetables. Substantial losses occur during cooking, and pyridoxine is sensitive to both ultraviolet light and oxidation.

Absorption, Fate, and Excretion.   Pyridoxine, pyridoxal, and pyridoxamine are readily absorbed from the gastrointestinal tract following hydrolysis of their phosphorylated derivatives. Pyridoxal phosphate accounts for at least 60% of circulating vitamin B_6. Pyridoxal is thought to be the primary form that crosses cell membranes. The principal excretory product when any of the three forms of the vitamin is fed to human beings is 4-pyridoxic acid, formed by the action of hepatic aldehyde oxidase on free pyridoxal (*see* Leklem, 1988).

Therapeutic Uses.   Although there is no doubt that pyridoxine is essential in human nutrition, the clinical syndrome of simple pyridoxine deficiency is rare. Nevertheless, it may be presumed that an individual with a deficiency of other members of the B complex may also have a deficiency of pyridoxine. Therefore, pyridoxine should be a component of therapy for individuals suffering from a deficiency of other members of the B complex. On the basis that pyridoxine is essential in human nutrition, it is incorporated into many multivitamin preparations for prophylactic use.

As indicated above, vitamin B_6 influences the metabolism of certain drugs and vice versa. With considerable justification, vitamin B_6 is given prophylactically to patients receiving isoniazid to prevent the development of peripheral neuritis. In addition, pyridoxine is an antidote for the seizures and acidosis in patients who have ingested an overdose of isoniazid.

The concentration of pyridoxal phosphate is reduced in the blood of women who are pregnant or who are taking oral contraceptives, although the recommended intakes of vitamin B_6 appear to be sufficient to meet the requirements of such individuals.

Pyridoxine-responsive anemia is a well-documented but uncommon condition. The use of the vitamin in this disease is discussed in Chapter 54. A group of genetically determined clinical states of "pyridoxine dependency," manifested by a requirement for large amounts of the vitamin, include pyridoxine-responsive anemias in patients without apparent pyridoxine deficiency, a seizure disorder in infants that responds to the administration of pyridoxine, and those abnormalities characterized by xanthurenic aciduria, primary cystathioninuria, or homocystinuria (*see* Fowler, 1985).

PANTOTHENIC ACID

History.   Pantothenic acid was first identified by Williams and associates in 1933 as a substance essential for the growth of yeast. Its name, derived from Greek words signifying "from everywhere," is indicative of the wide distribution of the vitamin in nature. The role of pantothenic acid in animal nutrition was first defined in chicks, in which a deficiency disease characterized by skin lesions was known to be cured by fractions prepared from liver extract. Although first thought to be a form of "chick pellagra," it was not cured by nicotinic acid. In 1939, Woolley and coworkers and also Jukes demonstrated that the chick antidermatitis factor was pantothenic acid. Elucidation of the biochemical function for the vitamin began in 1947 when Lipmann and coworkers showed that the acetylation of sulfanilamide required a cofactor that contained pantothenic acid.

Chemistry. Pantothenate consists of pantoic acid complexed to β-alanine. This is transformed in the body to 4'-phosphopantetheine by phosphorylation and linkage to cysteamine; this derivative is incorporated into either coenzyme A or acyl carrier protein, the functional forms of the vitamin. The chemical structures of pantothenic acid and coenzyme A are as follows:

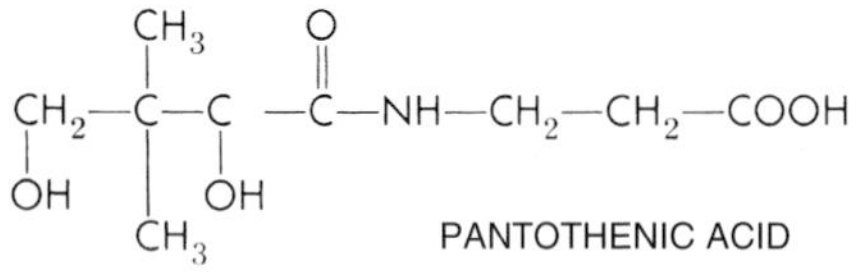

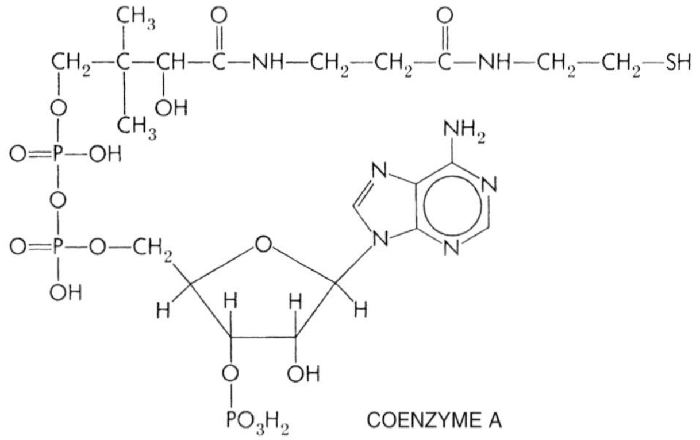

Many analogs of pantothenic acid have been studied in an attempt to find an antimetabolite. Although active antagonists have been synthesized (*e.g.,* ω-methyl pantothenate) and are of value as research tools, they are not therapeutic agents.

Pharmacological Actions. Pantothenic acid has no outstanding pharmacological actions when it is administered to experimental animals or normal human beings, even in large doses.

Physiological Functions. Coenzyme A serves as a cofactor for a variety of enzyme-catalyzed reactions involving transfer of acetyl (two-carbon) groups; the precursor fragments of various lengths are bound to the sulfhydryl group of coenzyme A. Such reactions are important in the oxidative metabolism of carbohydrates, gluconeogenesis, degradation of fatty acids, and the synthesis of

sterols, steroid hormones, and porphyrins. As a component of acyl carrier protein, pantothenate participates in fatty acid synthesis. Coenzyme A also participates in the posttranslational modification of proteins, including N-terminal acetylation, acetylation of internal amino acids, and fatty acid acylation. Such modifications can influence the intracellular localization, stability, and activity of the proteins.

Symptoms of Deficiency. Deficiency of pantothenic acid is manifested by symptoms of neuromuscular degeneration and adrenocortical insufficiency. By administering a diet devoid of pantothenic acid, a syndrome is produced that is characterized by fatigue, headache, sleep disturbances, nausea, abdominal cramps, vomiting, and flatulence, with complaints of paresthesias in the extremities, muscle cramps, and impaired coordination (Fry *et al.,* 1976). Pantothenic acid deficiency has not been recognized in human beings consuming a normal diet, presumably because of the ubiquitous occurrence of the vitamin in ordinary foods.

Human Requirements. Pantothenic acid is a required nutrient, but the magnitude of need is not known precisely. There is no RDA for pantothenic acid. The adequate intake is set at 5 mg/day for adults. Intakes for other groups are proportional to caloric consumption. In view of the widespread distribution of pantothenic acid in foods, dietary deficiency is very unlikely.

Food Sources. Pantothenic acid is ubiquitous. It is particularly abundant in organ meats, beef, and egg yolk. However, pantothenic acid is easily destroyed by heat and alkali.

Absorption, Fate, and Excretion. Pantothenic acid is absorbed readily from the gastrointestinal tract. It is present in all tissues, in concentrations ranging from 2 to 45 $\mu g/g$. Pantothenic acid apparently is not degraded in the human body, since the intake and the excretion of the vitamin are approximately equal. About 70% of the absorbed pantothenic acid is excreted in the urine.

Therapeutic Uses. No clearly defined uses for pantothenic acid exist, although it commonly is included in multivitamin preparations and in products for enteral and parenteral alimentation.

BIOTIN

History. In 1916, Bateman observed that rats fed a diet containing raw egg white as the sole source of protein developed a syndrome characterized by neuromuscular disorders, severe dermatitis, and loss of hair. The syndrome could be prevented by cooking the protein or by administering yeast, liver, or extracts of these. In 1936, Kögl and Tönnis isolated from egg yolk a factor in crystalline form that was essential for growth of yeast, which they called *biotin*. It was then demonstrated that biotin and the factor that protected against egg-white toxicity were the same (György, 1940). In 1942, duVigneaud established the structural formula of biotin, and the vitamin was synthesized shortly thereafter.

In the meantime, the nature of the antagonist to biotin in egg white received extensive study. The compound is a protein, first isolated by Eakin and associates in 1940 and called *avidin*. Avidin is a glycoprotein that binds biotin with great affinity and thus prevents its absorption.

Chemistry.   Biotin has the following structural formula:

$$
\begin{array}{c}
\text{O} \\
\text{‖} \\
\text{C} \\
\text{HN} \qquad \text{NH} \\
\text{HC} \!-\! \text{CH} \\
\text{H}_2\text{C} \qquad \text{CHCH}_2\text{CH}_2\text{CH}_2\text{CH}_2\text{COOH} \\
\text{S}
\end{array}
$$

BIOTIN

Three forms of biotin, apart from free biotin itself, have been found in natural materials. These derivatives are biocytin (ε-biotinyl-L-lysine) and the D and L sulfoxides of biotin. Although the derived forms of biotin are active in supporting growth of some microorganisms, their efficacy as substitutes for biotin in human nutrition is unknown. Biocytin may represent a degradation product of a biotin-protein complex, since, in its role as a coenzyme, the vitamin is covalently linked to an ε-amino group of a lysine residue of the apoenzyme involved.

A number of compounds antagonize the actions of biotin. Among them are biotin sulfone, desthiobiotin, and certain imidazolidone carboxylic acids. The antagonism between avidin and biotin is described above.

Pharmacological Actions.   Biotin toxicity has not been reported in human beings despite administration of large amounts for several months.

Physiological Functions.   In human tissues biotin is a cofactor for the enzymatic carboxylation of four substrates: pyruvate, acetyl coenzyme A (CoA), propionyl CoA, and β-methylcrotonyl CoA. As such, it plays an important role in both carbohydrate and fat metabolism. CO_2 fixation occurs in a two-step reaction, the first involving binding of CO_2 to the biotin moiety of the holoenzyme, and the second involving transfer of the biotin-bound CO_2 to an appropriate acceptor.

Symptoms of Deficiency.   In most species, presumably owing to synthesis of the vitamin by intestinal bacteria, it is necessary to eliminate bacteria from the intestinal tract, feed raw egg white, or administer antimetabolites of biotin to produce biotin deficiency. In human beings, signs and symptoms of deficiency include dermatitis, atrophic glossitis, hyperesthesia, muscle pain, lassitude, anorexia, slight anemia, and changes in the ECG. Spontaneous deficiency has been observed in some individuals who have consumed raw eggs over long periods. Inborn errors of biotin-dependent enzymes are known and respond to the

administration of massive doses of biotin (Baumgartner *et al.*, 1984).

Symptomatic biotin deficiency has been reported in children and adults who have received chronic parenteral nutrition lacking biotin; these patients suffered from chronic inflammatory bowel disease, and inadequate synthesis of biotin by gut flora was a probable contributory factor. The lesions consist of severe exfoliative dermatitis and alopecia, and they are similar to those of zinc deficiency; however, they respond to small doses of biotin. Few reports have provided biochemical validation of biotin deficiency, but in one case the correction by biotin of an elevated rate of urinary excretion of β-hydroxyisovaleric acid indicates defective function of the biotin-dependent β-methylcrotonyl CoA carboxylase (Gillis *et al.*, 1982).

Human Requirements.   The adequate intake of biotin for adults is 30 μg/day (Table XIII–2). The average American diet provides 100 to 300 μg of the vitamin. Part of the biotin synthesized by the bacterial flora also is available for absorption.

Food Sources.   Organ meats, egg yolk, milk, fish, and nuts are rich sources of biotin. Biotin is stable to cooking but less so in alkali.

Absorption, Fate, and Excretion.   Ingested biotin is rapidly absorbed from the gastrointestinal tract and appears in the urine predominantly in the form of intact biotin and in lesser amounts as the metabolites *bis*-norbiotin and biotin sulfoxide. Mammals are unable to degrade the ring system of biotin.

Therapeutic Uses.   Large doses of biotin (5 to 10 mg daily) are administered to babies with infantile seborrhea and to individuals with genetic alterations of biotin-dependent enzymes. Patients who receive long-term parenteral nutrition should be given vitamin formulations that contain biotin.

CHOLINE

Choline is not a vitamin as defined above, although historically it was identified as part of the vitamin B complex. Sufficient ambiguity exists concerning a possible dietary requirement for this substance that it customarily is considered in discussions of water-soluble vitamins.

History.   In 1932, Best and associates observed that pancreatectomized dogs maintained on insulin developed fatty livers; this could be prevented by inclusion in the diet of crude egg-yolk lecithin or beef pancreas. The substance responsible for this effect was shown to be choline. These studies marked the beginning of an extensive literature on the role of lipotropic substances, especially choline, in animal nutrition. Choline has other important functions in addition to those related to lipid metabolism.

Chemistry.   Choline (trimethylethanolamine) has the following structural formula:

$$H_3C-\underset{\underset{\displaystyle CH_3}{|}}{\overset{\overset{\displaystyle CH_3}{|}}{N^+}}-CH_2CH_2OH$$

CHOLINE

Pharmacological Actions.   Qualitatively, choline has the same pharmacological actions as does acetylcholine, but it is far less active. Single oral doses of 10 g produce no obvious pharmacodynamic response.

Physiological Functions.   Choline has several roles in the body. It is an important component of phospholipids, affects the mobilization of fat from the liver (lipotropic action), acts as a methyl donor, and is essential for the formation of the neurotransmitter acetylcholine (*see* Chapter 6) and the autacoid platelet-activating factor (PAF) (*see* Chapter 26).

Phospholipid Constituent.   Choline is a component of the major phospholipid lecithin and also is a constituent of plasmalogens, which are abundant in mitochondria, and of sphingomyelin, which is particularly enriched in brain. Choline thus provides an essential structural component of many biological membranes and also of the plasma lipoproteins.

Lipotropic Action.   As mentioned, the initial recognition of choline as a significant dietary factor depended on its capacity to reduce the fat content of the liver of diabetic dogs. Substances that stimulate removal of excess fat from the liver are known as lipotropic agents and include choline, inositol, methionine, vitamin B_{12}, and folic acid. Certain of these compounds appear to act by providing methyl groups for the synthesis of choline in the body. Formation of the lipid components of plasma lipoproteins thus is permitted, and this facilitates transport of fat from the liver.

Methyl Donor.   Choline can donate methyl groups necessary for the synthesis of other compounds. The first step in transfer is the formation of betaine, which is the immediate donor of the methyl group. Thus, choline can transfer a methyl group to homocysteine to form methionine. The roles of cyanocobalamin and folic acid in the metabolism of one-carbon compounds are discussed in Chapter 54.

Acetylcholine Formation.   Acetylcholine is synthesized from choline and acetyl CoA by choline acetyltransferase and is broken down by acetylcholinesterase (*see* Chapter 6). Choline is transported between the brain and the plasma by a bidirectional system localized in the endothelium of brain capillaries. This system operates by facilitated diffusion, and the amount of choline available to central neurons thus varies as a function of the concentration of choline in the plasma. When rats are given choline chloride, the concentrations of plasma choline, brain choline, and brain acetylcholine increase sequentially. These findings may be relevant to the treatment of diseases involving reduced capacity to synthesize acetylcholine (*see* below).

Synthesis of PAF.   This autacoid is formed from a subset of choline-containing membrane phospholipids in which the moiety in position 1 of the glycerol backbone is an alkyl ether rather than a fatty acid ester. The phospholipid is acted upon by the hormonally regulated phospholipase A_2 to form 1-*O*-alkyl-lysophosphatidyl choline. This intermediate is converted to PAF through acetylation at position 2 by acetyl CoA in a reaction catalyzed by lyso-PAF transacetylase. PAF has many important functions in inflammatory and other processes (*see* Chapter 26).

Symptoms of Deficiency.   Choline-deficient animals reflect multiple defects, including fat accumulation in the liver, cirrhosis, increased incidence of hepatocellular carcinoma, hemorrhagic renal lesions, and motor incoordination. Fortunately, however, none of these manifestations of deficiency has been identified in human beings.

Human Requirements.   The needs of the tissues for choline are met from both exogenous (dietary) and endogenous (metabolic) sources. Biosynthesis of choline occurs by transmethylation of ethanolamine with the methyl group of methionine or by a series of reactions requiring vitamin B_{12} and folate as cofactors (*see* Chapter 54). Thus, an adequate supply of methyl-group donors in the diet is desirable to protect against the hepatic accumulation of lipid. In addition, large amounts of choline appear to have a therapeutic effect on certain diseases of the nervous system, perhaps by stimulation of the synthesis of acetylcholine. However, none of the functions of choline justifies its classification as a vitamin. It has not been shown to act as a cofactor in any enzymatic reaction, and the doses needed to produce therapeutic effects (several grams) are much greater than those of any vitamin.

The RDA for choline is 550 mg/day for men and 425 mg/day for women (Table XIII-2). The American diet provides 400 to 900 mg per day of choline as a constituent of lecithin; it is thus difficult to consume a diet that is low in choline. However, when excess dietary methionine and folate are not available, choline deficiency may lead to biochemical signs of liver dysfunction, so under this circumstance choline may be considered a limiting nutrient (Jacob *et al.,* 1999). The Committee on Nutrition of the American Academy of Pediatrics (1993) recommends the fortification of infant formula to at least 7 mg choline/100 kcal, which roughly corresponds to 9 ± 2 mg/dl of choline present in human breast milk.

Food Sources.   Choline is found in egg yolk, liver, and peanuts, mostly as lecithin.

Absorption, Fate, and Excretion.   Choline is absorbed from the diet as such or as lecithin. The latter is hydrolyzed by the intestinal mucosa to glycerophosphoryl choline, which passes either to the liver to liberate choline or to the peripheral tissues *via* the intestinal lymphatics. Free choline is not absorbed fully, especially after large doses, and intestinal bacteria metabolize choline to trimethylamine. Since this compound imparts a strong odor of decaying fish to the feces, lecithin is the preferred oral vehicle for the administration of choline.

Therapeutic Uses.   The use of choline to treat fatty liver and cirrhosis, usually alcoholic in etiology, has not proven to be effective. Because of the synthesis of choline from other methyl donors, provision of a well-balanced diet is as effective as choline treatment in alleviating the symptoms of hepatic damage. Fatty infiltration of the liver frequently has been observed in patients receiving total parenteral nutrition (TPN). Since TPN solutions generally contain no added choline, a causal relationship between hepatotoxicity and choline deficiency may exist in such patients.

The use of choline or its related compound, *citicoline* (cytidine 5′-diphosphate choline ester), in large doses for treatment of nervous system disorders that might be attributed to decreased acetylcholine synthesis or cholinergic function had been advocated in the past, but in none of these circumstances (tardive dyskinesia, Huntington's chorea, Tourette's disease, Friedreich's ataxia, and Alzheimer's disease) has a role for choline as a therapeutic agent been firmly established (*see* Chapters 20 and 22). Results of recent controlled clinical trials suggest favorable responses to citicoline in stroke (Clark *et al.*, 1997) and in conservation of verbal memory with age (Spiers *et al.*, 1996). Confirmatory studies are required, however, before these findings can be embraced.

INOSITOL

History.   Although inositol was identified more than one hundred years ago in the urine of diabetic patients, a role for this substance in animal nutrition was not suspected until 1941, when Gavin and McHenry found that inositol had a lipotropic action in rats. Inositol subsequently was observed to cure alopecia induced in rats and mice by dietary means. A nutritional role for inositol was strengthened considerably when Eagle and colleagues showed in 1957 that this substance is essential for the growth of all human and other animal cells in tissue culture. However, its status as a vitamin for human beings remains uncertain for reasons given below.

Chemistry.   Inositol (hexahydroxycyclohexane) is an isomer of glucose. There are seven optically inactive and one pair of optically active stereoisomeric forms of inositol possible, of which only one, the optically inactive *myo*-inositol, is nutritionally active. It has the following structural formula:

INOSITOL

Pharmacological Actions.   Inositol has no significant pharmacological actions when given parenterally to human subjects in doses of 1 to 2 g.

Physiological Functions.   The physiological role of inositol resembles that of choline in part. Thus, inositol is present in the form of phosphatidylinositol in the phospholipids of cell membranes and plasma lipoproteins. Polyphosphorylated derivatives of inositol are released from such phospholipids in membranes in response to a variety of hormones, autacoids, and neurotransmitters. One such derivative, inositol-1,4,5-trisphosphate, functions as an intracellular second messenger by stimulating the release of Ca^{2+} from intracellular stores.

Human Requirements.   There has been no demonstration of a dietary need for inositol in human beings, presumably due to its production by gut bacteria, variable tissue reserves following absorption from foodstuffs, and possible *de novo* synthesis in some organs. Although a human need for inositol has not been demonstrated, a high concentration is present in human breast milk. As with choline, it may be desirable to add inositol to infant formulas to mimic more closely the content of human milk (Committee on Nutrition, The American Academy of Pediatrics, 1993).

Food Sources.   The normal daily intake of inositol is about 1 g, mostly from fruits and plant sources. Inositol is present in whole-grain cereals as the hexaphosphate, phytic acid. Inositol in this form is partly available for absorption because of hydrolysis in the intestinal mucosa. Inositol also occurs in vegetable and animal foods in other forms.

Absorption, Fate, and Excretion.   Inositol is absorbed easily from the gastrointestinal tract. It is metabolized readily to glucose and is about one-third as effective as glucose in alleviating starvation ketosis. The concentration of inositol in normal human plasma is about 5 mg/liter (28 μM). Within tissues, the concentration of inositol is particularly high in heart muscle, brain, and skeletal muscle (1.6, 0.9, and 0.4 g/100 g dry weight, respectively). Urine normally contains only small amounts of inositol, but in diabetic humans and animals the amount is markedly increased, probably because of competition between inositol and glucose for reabsorption by the renal tubule.

Therapeutic Uses.   Inositol has been given for the management of diseases associated with disturbances in the transport and metabolism of fat, but there is no persuasive evidence that it has therapeutic efficacy. Peripheral nerves from diabetic animals and patients contain elevated quantities of free sugars and a decreased level of *myo*-inositol; abnormal incorporation of *myo*-inositol into neural phospholipids also has been demonstrated, but the effects of administration of *myo*-inositol on diabetic neuropathies are unclear (*see* Chapter 61). Recent evidence implicates inositol deficiency in the pathogenesis of insulin resistance in the polycystic ovarian syndrome. Administration of D-*chiro*-inositol to such patients improved insulin sensitivity and lowered levels of circulating triglycerides and androgens (Nestler *et al.*, 1999).

CARNITINE

History. Carnitine was identified as a nitrogenous constituent of muscle in 1905. After its identification as a growth factor for mealworm larvae by Frankael and colleagues, the role of carnitine in the oxidation of long-chain fatty acids in mammals was established in the laboratories of Fritz and Bremer in the late 1950s.

Chemistry. Carnitine (β-hydroxy-γ-trimethylammonium butyrate) has the following structural formula:

$$(H_3C)_3\overset{+}{N}-CH_2-CH-CH_2-COO^-$$
$$|$$
$$OH$$

CARNITINE

Only L-carnitine is synthesized in tissues and possesses biological activity. The pathway of carnitine biosynthesis has been reviewed by Rebouche (1991).

Pharmacological Actions. The administration of L-carnitine to normal individuals has no appreciable effect, and oral doses of up to 15 g per day are usually well tolerated. By contrast, the administration of DL-carnitine can produce a syndrome that resembles myasthenia gravis, presumably because of the inhibitory effects of the D isomer on the transport and function of L-carnitine.

Physiological Functions. In general, carnitine is important for the oxidation of fatty acids; it also facilitates the aerobic metabolism of carbohydrate, enhances the rate of oxidative phosphorylation, and promotes the excretion of certain organic acids (Rebouche, 1992). These functions result from the following circumstances: (1) There exist a number of carnitine acyltransferases (CATs) that catalyze the interconversion of fatty acid esters of coenzyme A (CoA) and carnitine; these are strategically located in the cytosol and in mitochondrial membranes. (2) The esters of CoA and carnitine are thermodynamically equivalent, such that the net formation of either depends solely on the relative concentrations of reactants. (3) Specific translocases exist in mitochondrial and plasma membranes. The translocase in mitochondrial membranes readily transports both free carnitine and its esters in either direction, while that in the luminal plasma membrane of renal tubular cells transports only free carnitine *from* tubular urine almost exclusively. The properties of translocases in the plasma membranes of other cells are less well defined; nevertheless, free carnitine is actively transported into cells, and acylcarnitines (particularly short-chain esters) are transported out of cells. (4) Fatty acid esters of CoA are formed almost exclusively in the cytosol and are not transported across membranes; they also inhibit enzymes of the Krebs cycle and those involved in oxidative phosphorylation. Hence, the oxidation of fatty acids requires the formation of acylcarnitines and their translocation into mitochondria, where the CoA esters are reformed and metabolized. If O_2 tension becomes limiting, carnitine serves to maintain a ratio of free to esterified CoA within mitochondria that is optimal for oxidative phosphorylation and for the consumption of acetyl CoA; in ischemic cardiac or skeletal muscle, this results in reduced formation of lactate and an increased

capacity to perform mechanical work (*see* Goa and Brogden, 1987).

In the presence of a genetic deficiency of one of the acyl CoA dehydrogenases, carnitine serves to promote the removal of the corresponding organic acid from cells and the blood, since the acylcarnitine can be transported out of mitochondria and into the circulation but cannot be reabsorbed from renal tubules. Such removal of acylcarnitines from cells or blood carries the risk of producing a state of relative carnitine deficiency.

Symptoms of Deficiency. Primary carnitine deficiency is most clearly observed in a group of uncommon inherited disorders. Lipid metabolism is severely affected, resulting in storage of fat in muscle and functional abnormalities of cardiac and skeletal muscle. These conditions have been classified as either systemic or myopathic. Systemic disorders are manifested by low concentrations of carnitine in plasma, muscle, and liver. Symptoms are variable, but include muscle weakness, cardiomyopathy, abnormal hepatic function, impaired ketogenesis, and hypoglycemia during fasting. Myopathic disease is characterized primarily by muscle weakness. Fatty infiltration of muscle fibers is observed at biopsy, and the concentration of carnitine is low; however, plasma concentrations of carnitine are normal (20 to 70 μM). Defective transport of carnitine into muscle cells coupled with faulty renal reabsorption may underlie many cases of primary carnitine deficiency (Treem *et al.,* 1988).

Secondary forms of carnitine deficiency also are recognized. These include renal tubular disorders, in which excretion of carnitine may be excessive, and chronic renal failure, in which hemodialysis may promote excessive losses. Patients with inborn errors of metabolism associated with increased circulating concentrations of organic acids also may become deficient in carnitine. This consequence is not surprising in view of the role of carnitine in promoting the excretion of organic acids. Occasional patients receiving total parenteral nutrition with solutions lacking carnitine also may show biochemical and symptomatic evidence of carnitine deficiency that is reversed by supplementation.

Human Requirements. The need for carnitine in adults is satisfied by dietary sources and by synthesis, primarily in the liver and kidney. However, low-birth-weight and preterm infants are at greatest risk for carnitine deficiency. These infants are subjected to high-fat intakes to encourage growth and may benefit from exogenous carnitine (*see* Rebouche, 1992). Carnitine is synthesized from lysine residues in various proteins, beginning with formation of 6-N-trimethyllysine by a sequence of reactions involving S-adenosylmethionine (*see* Rebouche, 1991). Four micronutrients are required for the various enzymatic steps, including ascorbic acid, niacin, pyridoxine, and iron. Although carnitine deficiency can be induced by administration of diets that are restricted to cereal grains and other vegetable sources of protein, formal nutritional requirements have not been established.

Food Sources. The primary sources of dietary carnitine are meat and dairy products. Cereal grains lack carnitine and also may be relatively deficient in lysine and methionine, its amino acid precursors.

Absorption, Fate, and Excretion. Dietary L-carnitine is absorbed almost completely from the intestine, largely by a saturable transport mechanism; hence, fractional absorption declines as the oral dose is increased. Carnitine is transported into most cells by an active mechanism; D-carnitine also is transported and can inhibit the uptake of L-carnitine. There is little metabolism of carnitine, and most of it is excreted in the urine as acylcarnitines; renal tubules usually reabsorb more than 90% of unesterified carnitine (*see* Goa and Brogden, 1987).

Therapeutic Uses. Carnitine (*levocarnitine;* CARNITOR) was first approved by the Food and Drug Administration in 1986 as an orphan drug for treatment of primary carnitine deficiency. Subsequently, it was approved for treatment of primary and secondary carnitine deficiencies of genetic origin and for prevention and treatment of carnitine deficiency in patients with end-stage renal disease who are undergoing dialysis. One to three grams per day in divided oral doses with meals is adequate for most therapeutic purposes. Intravenous doses range from 40 to 100 mg/kg. For children, oral L-carnitine is given at 50 to 100 mg/kg per day with meals, up to a maximum of 3 g/day.

Primary Carnitine Deficiency. The mainstay of treatment of systemic carnitine deficiency is a high-carbohydrate, low-fat diet. Carnitine supplementation of patients with both the myopathic and systemic disorders has been tried frequently, but results have been variable. Some patients report dramatic symptomatic and functional benefits following administration of up to 4 g per day, whereas others are not improved. The relationship of biochemical changes to symptomatic relief is not predictable. All patients with primary carnitine deficiency deserve a trial of supplemental oral carnitine.

Renal Disease. Patients receiving chronic hemodialysis can develop skeletal and possibly myocardial muscle carnitine deficiency. Treatment with oral L-carnitine may minimize the degree of deficiency and has been reported to improve symptoms such as muscle weakness and cramps (Bellinghieri *et al.*, 1983). Carnitine also may improve cardiac function in hemodialysis patients (Fagher *et al.*, 1985), but this use is more controversial.

Cardiomyopathies and Ischemic Cardiovascular Disease. Most myocardial energy needs are satisfied by fatty acid oxidation. In light of the critical role played by carnitine in normal cardiac energy metabolism and the development of cardiomyopathy in established carnitine deficiency states, the possibility that some individuals with primary cardiomyopathy may suffer carnitine deficiency has provoked great interest. Moreover, myocardial ischemia causes depletion of cardiac carnitine and accumulation of long-chain fatty acid esters of CoA and carnitine; the acylcarnitines may be important in the genesis of arrhythmias. The administration of carnitine appears to improve the exercise tolerance of patients with coronary artery disease and may benefit patients with congestive heart failure (Ghidini *et al.*, 1988). Ischemia in skeletal muscle causes similar disturbances in lipid and carnitine metabolism, and the administration of carnitine can increase the walking tolerance of patients who suffer from intermittent claudication (Brevetti *et al.*, 1999). In addition, a number of biochemical and clinical outcomes were improved by L-carnitine supplementation of patients with acute myocardial infarction (Singh *et al.*, 1996). Although these results are provocative, the therapeutic role of carnitine in these conditions remains to be confirmed.

II. ASCORBIC ACID (VITAMIN C)

History. Scurvy, the deficiency disease caused by lack of vitamin C, has been known since the time of the Crusades, especially among northern European populations who subsisted on diets lacking fresh fruits and vegetables over extensive periods of the year. The incidence of scurvy was reduced by the introduction of the potato (a source of vitamin C) to Europe in the seventeenth century. However, the long sea voyages of exploration in the sixteenth to eighteenth centuries, which were undertaken without a supply of fresh fruits and vegetables, resulted in large numbers of the crews dying from scurvy.

A dietary cause for scurvy had long been suspected. In 1535, Jacques Cartier learned from the Indians of Canada how to cure the scurvy in his crew by making a decoction from spruce leaves, and several subsequent ship captains prevented or cured scurvy by administration of lemon juice. However, a systematic study of the relationship of diet to scurvy had to wait until 1747 when Lind, a physician in the British Royal Navy, carried out a clinical trial on cases of frank scurvy who were given either cider, vitriol, vinegar, sea water, oranges and lemons, or garlic and mustard. Those who received citrus fruits recovered rapidly. The consequent introduction of lemon juice into the British Navy in 1800 resulted in a dramatic reduction in the incidence of scurvy; whereas the Royal Naval Hospital at Portsmouth admitted 1457 cases in 1780, only 2 cases were seen there in 1806.

The next significant episode in the history of vitamin C was the identification in 1907 of a suitable experimental animal by Holst and Fröhlich, who found that guinea pigs develop scurvy on a diet of oats and bran that is not supplemented with fresh vegetables. It was subsequently shown that most mammals synthesize ascorbic acid; human beings, nonhuman primates, the guinea pig, and Indian fruit bats are exceptions. The demonstration of scurvy in the guinea pig allowed testing of fractions from citrus fruits for antiscorbutic potency. In 1928, Szent-Györgyi isolated a reducing agent in pure form from cabbage and from adrenal glands; in 1932, Waugh and King identified Szent-Györgyi's compound as the active antiscorbutic factor in lemon juice. The chemical structure of this substance was then soon established in several laboratories, and the trivial chemical name *ascorbic acid* was assigned to designate its function in preventing scurvy.

The manifestations of scurvy due to vitamin C deficiency also have been revealed following experimental scurvy induced by intentional dietary restrictions. For example, the surgeon Crandon submitted himself to a diet devoid of vitamin C for 161 days; the concentration of ascorbic acid in his plasma fell to negligible values within 41 days, and the concentration in his white blood cells became undetectable after 121 days. Perifollicular hyperkeratosis (an accumulation of epidermal cells around the hair follicles) occurred at 120 days; hemorrhages appeared under his skin (petechiae and ecchymoses) at 161 days, and a wound made into the back failed to heal (Crandon *et al.,* 1940).

The term *vitamin C* should be used as a generic descriptor for all compounds that exhibit qualitatively the biological activity of ascorbic acid.

Chemistry. Ascorbic acid is a six-carbon ketolactone structurally related to glucose and other hexoses. It is reversibly oxidized in the body to dehydroascorbic acid. The latter compound possesses full vitamin C activity. The structural formulas of ascorbic acid and dehydroascorbic acid are as follows:

ASCORBIC ACID　　DEHYDRO-ASCORBIC ACID

Ascorbic acid has an optically active carbon atom, and antiscorbutic activity resides almost totally in the L isomer. Another isomer, erythorbic acid (D-isoascorbic acid, D-araboascorbic acid), has very weak antiscorbutic action but has a similar redox potential. Both compounds therefore have been used to prevent nitrosoamine formation from nitrites in cured meats such as bacon. The reason for the lack of a stronger antiscorbutic action of erythorbic acid is probably the incapacity of the tissues to retain it in the quantities that ascorbic acid is stored. One consequence of the facile oxidation of ascorbic acid is the readiness with which it can be destroyed by exposure to air, especially in an alkaline medium and if copper is present as a catalyst.

Pharmacological Actions. Vitamin C possesses few pharmacological actions. Administration of the compound in amounts greatly in excess of the physiological requirements causes few demonstrable effects except in the scorbutic individual, whose symptoms are alleviated rapidly.

Physiological Functions. Ascorbic acid functions as a cofactor in a number of hydroxylation and amidation reactions by transferring electrons to enzymes that provide reducing equivalents (*see* Levine, 1986; Levine *et al.,* 1993). Thus, it is required for or facilitates the conversion of certain proline and lysine residues in procollagen to hydroxyproline and hydroxylysine in the course of collagen synthesis, the oxidation of lysine side chains in proteins to provide hydroxytrimethyllysine for carnitine synthesis, the conversion of folic acid to folinic acid, microsomal drug metabolism, and the hydroxylation of dopamine to form norepinephrine. Ascorbic acid promotes the activity of an amidating enzyme thought to be involved in the process-

ing of certain peptide hormones, such as oxytocin, antidiuretic hormone, and cholecystokinin (*see* Levine, 1986; Levine *et al.,* 1993). By reducing nonheme ferric iron to the ferrous state in the stomach, ascorbic acid also promotes intestinal absorption of iron. In addition, ascorbic acid plays a role, albeit a poorly defined one, in adrenal steroidogenesis.

At the tissue level, a major function of ascorbic acid is related to the synthesis of collagen, proteoglycans, and other organic constituents of the intercellular matrix in such diverse tissues as tooth, bone, and capillary endothelium. Although the effect of ascorbic acid on collagen synthesis has been attributed to its role in the hydroxylation of proline, evidence also suggests that there is direct stimulation of collagen peptide synthesis. Scurvy is associated with a defect in collagen synthesis that is apparent in the failure of wounds to heal, in defects in tooth formation, and in the rupture of capillaries, which leads to numerous petechiae and their coalescence to form ecchymoses. While this last has been attributed to leakage from capillaries because of inadequate adhesion of the endothelial cells, it also is thought that the pericapillary fibrous tissue is defective in scurvy, leading to inadequate support of the capillary and its rupture under pressure.

Absorption, Fate, and Excretion. Ascorbic acid is readily absorbed from the intestine *via* an energy-dependent process that is saturable and dose-dependent. The absorption of dietary ascorbate is nearly complete (Kallner *et al.,* 1977). When vitamin C is given in a single oral dose, absorption decreases from 75% at 1 g to 20% at 5 g. Ascorbic acid is present in the plasma and is ubiquitously distributed in the cells of the body. Concentrations of the vitamin in leukocytes are sometimes taken to represent those in tissue and are less susceptible to depletion than is the plasma. The white blood cells of healthy adults have concentrations of about 27 μg of ascorbic acid per 10^8 cells. Concentrations in plasma also vary with intake. Adequate ingestion is associated with concentrations over 0.5 mg/dl (28 μM), whereas concentrations of 0.15 mg/dl (8.5 μM) are seen in individuals with frank scurvy.

When the diet contains essentially no ascorbate, concentrations in plasma fall; as mentioned, symptoms of scurvy are obvious when a value of 0.15 mg/dl (8.5 μM) is reached, and the total body store of the vitamin approximates 300 mg. When the intake of ascorbate is raised, the concentration in plasma also increases—at first linearly. The concentration deviates from linearity at about 200 mg/day and achieves saturation at 1000 mg/day. Daily intake of 60 mg of vitamin C (the current adult RDA) achieves plasma concentrations of 0.8 mg/dl (45 μM) and the body store is around 1500 mg. If intake is raised beyond 200 mg daily, the body store tends to level off at

2500 mg and the concentration in plasma at 2 mg/dl (110 μM). The renal threshold for ascorbic acid is about 1.5 mg/dl of plasma (85 μM), and increasing amounts of ingested ascorbic acid are excreted when the daily intake exceeds 100 mg. Urinary excretion of oxalate and urate increase when daily ascorbic acid intakes approach 1000 mg (*see* Levine *et al.,* 1996).

Ascorbate is oxidized to CO_2 in rats and guinea pigs, but considerably less conversion can be detected in human beings. One route of metabolism of the vitamin in human beings involves its conversion to oxalate and eventual excretion in the urine; dehydroascorbate is presumably an intermediate. Ascorbic acid-2-sulfate also has been identified as a metabolite of vitamin C in human urine.

Biosynthesis of Ascorbic Acid. Human beings and other primates as well as the guinea pig and some bats are unable to synthesize ascorbic acid and require dietary vitamin C for the prevention of scurvy. Animals that do not require dietary vitamin C synthesize ascorbic acid from glucose through the intermediate formation of D-glucuronic acid, L-gulonic acid, and L-gulonolactone. Human beings, monkeys, and guinea pigs lack the hepatic enzyme required to carry out the last reaction, that is, the conversion of L-gulonolactone to L-ascorbic acid.

Symptoms of Deficiency. A deficiency in the intake of vitamin C can lead to scurvy. Cases of scurvy are encountered among elderly people living alone, alcoholics, drug addicts, and others with inadequate diets, including infants. In spontaneous cases of scurvy, there are usually loosening of the teeth, gingivitis, and anemia, which may be due to a specific function of ascorbic acid in hemoglobin synthesis. The picture of spontaneous scurvy in clinical practice often is complicated by insufficiencies of other nutrients as well.

Scurvy may occur in infants receiving formula diets prepared at home with inadequate concentrations of ascorbic acid. The infant is irritable and resents being touched because of pain. The pain is caused by hemorrhages under the periosteum of the long bones, and the resulting hematomas often are visible as swellings on the shafts of these bones.

Human Requirements. The daily intake of ascorbic acid must equal the amount that is excreted or destroyed by oxidation. Healthy adult human subjects lose 3% to 4% of their body store daily. To maintain a body store of 1500 mg of ascorbic acid or more in an adult man, it would thus be necessary to absorb approximately 60 mg daily. Vitamin C requirements are under review (*see* Section XIII, Introduction).

Under special circumstances, more ascorbic acid appears to be required to achieve normal concentrations in the plasma. Lower plasma vitamin C levels found in smokers result from an increased metabolic turnover rate of the vitamin. Thus, to assure adequate vitamin status, the RDA for smokers has been set at 100 mg/day (Food and Nutrition Board, 1989). Concentrations of ascorbate in plasma also are lowered by the use of oral contraceptive agents. Requirements can increase in certain diseases, particularly infectious diseases, and also following surgery (*see* Levine *et al.,* 1993).

Food Sources. Ascorbic acid is obtained from citrus fruits, tomatoes, strawberries, cabbage greens, and potatoes. Orange and lemon juices are outstanding sources and contain approxi-

mately 0.5 mg/ml (2.8 mM). Ascorbic acid is readily destroyed by heat, oxidation, and alkali. Apart from its role in nutrition, ascorbic acid is used commonly as an antioxidant to protect the natural flavor and color of many foods (*e.g.,* processed fruit, vegetables, and dairy products).

Routes of Administration. Vitamin C usually is administered orally; however, in conditions that prevent adequate absorption from the gastrointestinal tract, parenteral solutions may be given. In addition, ascorbic acid should be given to patients receiving parenteral nutrition. Because of the loss of much of the infused ascorbic acid in the urine, daily doses of 200 mg are needed to maintain normal concentrations in plasma of about 1 mg/dl (60 μM) in these individuals (Nichoalds *et al.,* 1977).

Therapeutic Uses. Vitamin C is used for the treatment of ascorbic acid deficiency, especially frank scurvy, which occurs rather infrequently in infants and in adults.

Human breast milk contains 30 to 55 mg of ascorbic acid per liter (about 200 μM), depending on the mother's intake. Consequently, the infant consuming 850 ml of breast milk will receive about 35 mg of ascorbic acid (*see* Table XIII–1). Commercial formulas usually are fortified with ascorbic acid. Infants receiving formula based on cow's milk may be given orange juice to meet vitamin C requirements. In the rare cases of infantile scurvy, much larger therapeutic doses are used. Adults with scurvy should receive up to 1 g of ascorbic acid daily. This dose will cause a rapid disappearance of the subcutaneous hemorrhages.

The reducing properties of vitamin C also have been employed to control *idiopathic methemoglobinemia,* although it is less effective than methylene blue. Doses of at least 150 mg of ascorbic acid are needed to be effective in this condition.

The antioxidant properties of ascorbic acid appear to protect nitric oxide from free-radical degradation. The acute administration of 2 g of vitamin C improved endothelium-dependent vasodilation, reduced arterial stiffness, and decreased platelet aggregation in human beings (Ting *et al.,* 1997; Wilkinson *et al.,* 1999). In a controlled trial, similar effects of 500 mg/day of vitamin C persisted for at least 1 month (Gokce *et al.,* 1999). Additional trials of vitamin C are warranted to determine whether or not supplementation will improve clinical outcomes.

Ascorbic acid and other nutrient antioxidants have been associated with protection against age-related cataract formation and macular degeneration (*see* Gershoff 1993). Data from the Baltimore Longitudinal Study of Aging suggested a protective effect of overall antioxidant nutrient status, including vitamin C, α-tocopherol, and β-carotene (West *et al.,* 1994). Data from published studies regarding vitamins, minerals, and eye diseases are promising but inadequate at present to support clinical recommendations.

Lack of Clinical Effectiveness of Megadosage. In addition to these specific uses of vitamin C, extensive literature has appeared on the application of this vitamin to a wide variety of diseases. Many such claims are associated with megadosage treatment. However, sporadic reports of the efficacy of vitamin C in curing cancer or the common cold have not been substantiated (*see* Gershoff, 1993). Any preventive benefit that might be derived from such use of ascorbic acid seems small when weighed against the expense and the risks of the megadosage treatment. The latter include formation of kidney stones resulting from the excessive excretion of oxalate, rebound scurvy in the offspring of mothers taking high doses, and a similar phe-

nomenon when subjects who are consuming large amounts of vitamin C suddenly stop. These rebound phenomena presumably are due to induction of pathways of ascorbic acid metabolism as a result of the preceding high dosage.

For further discussion of disorders associated with vitamin deficiencies and excesses, *see* Chapter 79 in *Harrison's Principles of Internal Medicine,* 14th ed., McGraw-Hill, New York, 1998.

BIBLIOGRAPHY

Baumgartner, E.R., Suormala, T., Wick, H., and Bonjour, J.P. Biotin-responsive multiple carboxylase deficiency (MCD): deficient biotinidase activity associated with renal loss of biotin. *J. Inherit. Metab. Dis.,* **1984,** *7(suppl. 2):*123–125.

Bellinghieri, G., Savica, V., Mallamace, A., Di Stefano, C., Consolo, F., Spagnoli, L.G., Villaschi, S., Palmieri, G., Corsi, M., and Maccari, F. Correlation between increased serum and tissue L-carnitine levels and improved muscle symptoms in hemodialyzed patients. *Am. J. Clin. Nutr.,* **1983,** *38:*523–531.

Brevetti, G., Diehm, C., and Lambert, D. European multicenter study on propionyl-L-carnitine in intermittent claudication. *J. Am. Coll. Cardiol.,* **1999,** *34:*1618–1624.

Brin, M. Blood transketolase determination in the diagnosis of thiamine deficiency. *Heart Bull.,* **1968,** *17:*86–89.

Clark, W.M., Warach, S.J., Pettigrew, L.C., Gammans, R.E., and Sabournjian, L.A. A randomized dose-response trial of citicoline in acute ischemic stroke patients. Citicoline Stroke Study Group. *Neurology,* **1997,** *49:*671–678.

Committee on Nutrition, The American Academy of Pediatrics. *Pediatric Nutrition Handbook,* 3rd ed. (Barness, L.A., ed.) American Academy of Pediatrics, Elk Grove Village, IL, **1993,** pp. 8–17; Appendix C, pp. 354–357; Appendix D, pp. 360–361.

Crandon, J.H., Lund, C.C., and Dill, D.B. Experimental human scurvy. *N. Engl. J. Med.,* **1940,** *223:*353–369.

Diaz, G.A., Banikazemi, M., Oishi, K., Desnick, R.J., and Gelb, B.D. Mutations in a new gene encoding a thiamine transporter cause thiamine-responsive megaloblastic anaemia syndrome. *Nat. Genet.,* **1999,** *22:*309–312.

Dutta, B., Huang, W., Molero, M., Kekuda, R., Leibach, F.H., Devoe, L.D., Ganapathy, V., and Prasad, P.D. Cloning of the human thiamine transporter, a member of the folate transporter family. *J. Biol. Chem.,* **1999,** *274:*31925–31929.

Elliott, R.B., Pilcher, C.C., Ferguson, D.M., and Stewart, A.W. A population strategy to prevent insulin-dependent diabetes using nicotinamide. *J. Pediatr. Endocrinol. Metab.,* **1996,** *9:*501–509.

Fagher, B., Cederblad, G., Monti, M., Olsson, L., Rasmussen, B., and Thysell, H. Carnitine and left ventricular function in haemodialysis patients. *Scand. J. Clin. Lab. Invest.,* **1985,** *45:*193–198.

Fleming, J.C., Tartaglini, E., Steinkamp, M.P., Schorderet, D.F., Cohen, N., and Neufeld, E.J. The gene mutated in thiamine-responsive anaemia with diabetes and deafness (TRMA) encodes a functional thiamine transporter. *Nat. Genet.,* **1999,** *22:*305–308.

Fry, P.C., Fox, H.M., and Tao, H.G. Metabolic response to a pantothenic

acid deficient diet in humans. *J. Nutr. Sci. Vitaminol. (Tokyo),* **1976,** *22:*339–346.

Ghidini, O., Azzurro, M., Vita, G., and Sartori, G. Evaluation of the therapeutic efficacy of L-carnitine in congestive heart failure. *Int. J. Clin. Pharmacol. Ther. Toxicol.,* **1988,** *26:*217–220.

Gillis, J., Murphy, F.R., Boxall, L.B., and Pencharz, P.B. Biotin deficiency in a child on long-term TPN. *J.P.E.N. J. Parenter. Enter. Nutr.,* **1982,** *6:*308–310.

Gokce, N., Keaney, J.F. Jr., Frei, B., Holbrook, M., Olesiak, M., Zachariah, B.J., Leeuwenburgh, C., Heinecke, J.W., and Vita, J.A. Long-term ascorbic acid administration reverses endothelial vasomotor dysfunction in patients with coronary artery disease. *Circulation,* **1999,** *99:*3234–3240.

Goldsmith, G.A. Niacin-tryptophan relationship in man and niacin requirement. *Am. J. Clin. Nutr.,* **1958,** *6:*479–486.

György, P. A further note on the identity of vitamin H with biotin. *Science,* **1940,** *92:*609.

Hansen, C.M., Leklem, J.E., and Miller, L.T. Changes in vitamin B_6 status indicators of women fed a constant protein diet with varying levels of B_6. *Am. J. Clin. Nutr.,* **1997,** *66:*1379–1387.

Harper, C.G., Sheedy, D.L., Lara, A.I., Garrick, T.M., Hilton, J.M., and Raisanen, J. Prevalence of Wernicke-Korsakoff syndrome in Australia: has thiamine fortification made a difference? *Med. J. Aust.,* **1998,** *168:*542–545.

Jacob, R.A., Jenden, D.J., Allman-Farinelli, M.A., and Swendseid, M.E. Folate nutriture alters choline status of women and men fed low choline diets. *J. Nutr.,* **1999,** *129:*712–717.

Jusko, W.J., and Levy, G. Absorption, protein binding, and elimination of riboflavin. In, *Riboflavin.* (Rivlin, R.S., ed.) Plenum Press, New York, **1975,** pp. 99–152.

Kallner, A., Hartmann, D., and Hornig, D. On the absorption of ascorbic acid in man. *Int. J. Vitam. Nutr. Res.,* **1977,** *47:*383–388.

Lampeter, E.F., Klinghammer, A., Scherbaum, W.A., Heinze, E., Haastert, B., Giani, G., and Kolb, H. The Deutsche Nicotinamide Intervention Study: an attempt to prevent type I diabetes. DENIS Group. *Diabetes,* **1998,** *47:*980–984.

Medina, L., Chi, T.L., DeVivo, D.C., and Hilal, S.K. MR findings in patients with subacute necrotizing encephalomyelopathy (Leigh syndrome): correlation with biochemical defect. *A.J.R. Am. J. Roentgenol.,* **1990,** *154:*1269–1274.

Nestler, J.E., Jakubowicz, D.J., Reamer, P., Gunn, R.D., and Allan, G. Ovulatory and metabolic effects of D-*chiro*-inositol in the polycystic ovary syndrome. *N. Engl. J. Med.,* **1999,** *340:*1314–1320.

Nicholds, G.E., Meng, H.C., and Caldwell, M.D. Vitamin requirements in patients receiving total parenteral nutrition. *Arch. Surg.,* **1977,** *112*:1061–1064.

Parry, G.J., and Bredesen, D.E. Sensory neuropathy with low-dose pyridoxine. *Neurology,* **1985,** *35*:1466–1468.

Prentice, A.M., and Bates, C.J. A biochemical evaluation of the erythrocyte glutathione reductase (*EC* 1.6.4.2) test for riboflavin status. 1. Rate and specificity of response in acute deficiency. *Br. J. Nutr.,* **1981,** *45*:37–52.

Rindi, G., and Ventura, U. Thiamine intestinal transport. *Physiol. Rev.,* **1972,** *52*:821–827.

Said, H.M., Ortiz, A., Kumar, C.K., Chatterjee, N., Dudeja, P.K., and Rubin, S. Transport of thiamine in human intestine: mechanism and regulation in intestinal epithelial cell model caco-2. *Am. J. Physiol.,* **1999,** *277*:C645–C651.

Schaumberg, H., Kaplan, J., Windebank, A., Vick, N., Rasmus, S., Pleasure, D., and Brown, M.J. Sensory neuropathy from pyridoxine abuse. A new megavitamin syndrome. *N. Engl. J. Med.,* **1983,** *309*:445–448.

Schoenen, J., Jacquy, J., and Lenaerts, M. Effectiveness of high-dose riboflavin in migraine prophylaxis. A randomized controlled trial. *Neurology,* **1998,** *50*:466–470.

Singh, R.B., Niaz, M.A., Agarwal, P., Beegum, R., Rastogi, S.S., and Sachan, D.S. A randomised, double-blind, placebo-controlled trial of L-carnitine in suspected myocardial infarction. *Postgrad. Med. J.,* **1996,** *72*:45–50.

Smith, G.P., Rudge, P.J., and Peters, T.J. Biochemical studies of pyridoxal and pyridoxal phosphate status and therapeutic trial of pyridoxine in patients with carpal tunnel syndrome. *Ann. Neurol.,* **1984,** *15*:104–107.

Stagg, A.R., Fleming, J.C., Baker, M.A., Sakamoto, M., Cohen, N., and Neufeld, E.J. Defective high-affinity thiamine transporter leads to cell death in thiamine-responsive megaloblastic anemia syndrome fibroblasts. *J. Clin. Invest.,* **1999,** *103*:723–729.

Ting, H.H., Timimi, F.K., Haley, E.A., Roddy, M.A., Ganz, P., and Creager, M.A. Vitamin C improves endothelium-dependent vasodilation in forearm resistance vessels of humans, with hypercholesterolemia. *Circulation,* **1997,** *95*:2617–2622.

Treem, W.R., Stanley, C.A., Finegold, D.N., Hale, D.E., and Coates, P.M. Primary carnitine deficiency due to a failure of carnitine transport in kidney, muscle, and fibroblasts. *N. Engl. J. Med.,* **1988,** *319*:1331–1336.

Victor, M., Adams, R.D., and Collins, G.H. (eds.), *The Wernicke-Korsakoff Syndrome.* A clinical and pathological study of 245 patients, 82 with post-mortem examinations. Contemporary Neurology Series, Vol. 7. F.A. Davis Co., Philadelphia, **1971,** pp. 1–206.

West, S., Vitale, S., Hallfrisch, J., Muñoz, B., Muller, D., Bressler, S., and Bressler, N.M. Are antioxidants or supplements protective for age-related macular degeneration? *Arch Ophthalmol.,* **1994,** *112*:222–227.

Wilkinson, I.B., Megson, I.L., MacCallum, H., Sogo, N., Cockcroft, J.R., and Webb, D.J. Oral vitamin C reduces arterial stiffness and platelet aggregation in humans. *J. Cardiovasc. Pharmacol.,* **1999,** *34*:690–693.

MONOGRAPHS AND REVIEWS

Food and Nutrition Board, National Research Council. *Recommended Dietary Allowances,* 10th ed. National Academy of Sciences, Washington, D.C., **1989.**

Fowler, B. Recent advances in the mechanism of pyridoxine-responsive disorders. *J. Inherit. Metab. Dis.,* **1985,** *8(suppl. 1)*:76–83.

Gershoff, S.N. Vitamin C (ascorbic acid): new roles, new requirements? *Nutr. Rev.,* **1993,** *51*:313–326.

Goa, K.L., and Brogden, R.N. L-Carnitine. A preliminary review of its pharmacokinetics, and its therapeutic use in ischaemic cardiac disease and primary and secondary carnitine deficiencies in relationship to its role in fatty acid metabolism. *Drugs,* **1987,** *34*:1–24.

Haas, R.H. Thiamin and the brain. *Annu. Rev. Nutr.,* **1988,** *8*:483–515.

Leklem, J.E. Vitamin B_6 metabolism and function in humans. In, *Clinical and Physiological Applications of Vitamin B_6.* (Leklem, J.E., and Reynolds, R.D., eds.) *Current Topics in Nutrition and Disease.* Vol. 19. Alan R. Liss, Inc., New York, **1988,** pp. 3–28.

Levine, M. New concepts in the biology and biochemistry of ascorbic acid. *N. Engl. J. Med.,* **1986,** *314*:892–902.

Levine, M., Cantilena, C.C., and Dhariwal, K.R. *In situ* kinetics and ascorbic acid requirements. *World Rev. Nutr. Diet.,* **1993,** *72*:114–127.

Levine, M., Conry-Cantilena, C., Wang, Y., Welch, R.W., Washko, P.W., Dhariwal, K.R., Park, J.B., Lazarev, A., Graumlich, J.F., King, J., and Cantilena, L.R. Vitamin C pharmacokinetics in healthy volunteers: evidence for a recommended dietary allowance. *Proc. Natl. Acad. Sci. U.S.A.,* **1996,** *93*:3704–3709.

McCormick, D.B. Two interconnected B vitamins: riboflavin and pyridoxine. *Physiol. Rev.,* **1989,** *69*:1170–1198.

Rebouche, C.J. Ascorbic acid and carnitine biosynthesis. *Am. J. Clin. Nutr.,* **1991,** *54*:1147S–1152S.

Rebouche, C.J. Carnitine function and requirements during the life cycle. *FASEB J.,* **1992,** *6*:3379–3386.

Schoenen, J., Jacquy, J., and Lenaerts, S. Effectiveness of high-dose riboflavin in migraine prophylaxis. A randomized controlled trial. *Neurology,* **1998,** *50*:466–470.

Scriver, C.R. Vitamin-responsive inborn errors of metabolism. *Metabolism,* **1973,** *22*:1319–1344.

Spiers, P.A., Myers, D., Hochanadel, G.S., Lieberman, H.R., and Wurtman, R.J. Citicoline improves verbal memory in aging. *Arch. Neurol.,* **1996,** *53*:441–448.

FAT-SOLUBLE VITAMINS

Vitamins A, K, and E

Robert Marcus and Ann M. Coulston

Several exciting developments have transformed our understanding of the members of this group of nutrients. Development of vitamin D analogs with unanticipated biological actions has been described in Chapter 62. Equally dramatic advances have been seen with vitamin A and carotenoids. Chief among these is the discovery of the RAR and RXR receptor systems, a series of companion receptors involved in the cellular actions of retinoic acid, calcitriol, and thyroid hormone. In addition, 9-cis-retinoic acid has been identified as the natural endogenous ligand for these receptors, giving this vitamin A analog central importance in the actions of retinoic acid on cellular differentiation.

During the past several years, major epidemiological studies have addressed the role of the "antioxidant" vitamins A, C, and E in protection against cardiovascular and malignant diseases. Although nutrition surveys show with fair consistency a protective effect of higher consumption of foods containing these nutrients, several clinical trials have not substantiated these results. A plausible conclusion from this emerging body of literature is that nutrient deficiency increases the risk for disease, and replacement of such deficiencies may be expected to confer benefits. However, for nutritionally replete individuals, excessive intakes may be inert, at best, and perhaps deleterious.

This chapter summarizes the actions of the fat-soluble vitamins A, E, and K, their physiological actions, and their therapeutic uses. Special attention is given to the clarification of where human consumption may be in excess of demonstrated physiological need and where animal studies, suggesting improvement of defects induced by some vitamin deficiencies, are not replicated by pharmacological efficacy in human beings.

VITAMIN A

Although vitamin A must be supplied from the environment, most actions of vitamin A, like those of vitamin D, are exerted through hormone-like receptors. Vitamin A has diverse actions in cellular regulation and differentiation that go far beyond its classically defined function in vision. Analogs of vitamin A, because of their prominent effects on epithelial differentiation, have found important therapeutic application in the treatment of a variety of dermatological conditions and are being evaluated in cancer chemoprophylaxis.

History. Night blindness apparently was first described in Egypt around 1500 B.C. Although this disease was not then linked to dietary deficiency, topical treatment with roasted or fried liver was recommended, and Hippocrates later recommended eating beef liver as a cure for the affliction. The relationship to nutritional deficiency was definitively recognized in the 1800s. Ophthalmia Brasiliana, a disease of the eyes that afflicted pri-marily poorly nourished slaves, was first described in 1865. Later it was observed that the nurslings of mothers who fasted were prone to develop spontaneous sloughing of the cornea. Many other reports of nutritional keratomalacia soon followed from all parts of the world, including the United States.

Experimental rather than clinical observations, however, led to the discovery of vitamin A. In 1913, two groups (McCollum and Davis; Osborne and Mendel) independently reported that animals fed artificial diets with lard as the sole source of fat developed a nutritional deficiency that could be corrected by the addition to the diet of a factor contained in butter, egg yolk, and cod liver oil. An outstanding symptom of this experimental nutritional deficiency was xerophthalmia (dryness and thickening of the conjunctiva). Clinical and experimental vitamin A deficiencies were recognized to be related during World War I, when it became apparent that xerophthalmia in human beings was a result of a decrease in the content of butterfat in the diet.

Chemistry and Terminology. Although the term *vitamin A* has been used to denote specific chemical compounds, such as retinol or its esters, this term now is used more as a generic descriptor for compounds that exhibit the biological properties of retinol. *Retinoid* refers to the chemical entity retinol or other closely related naturally occurring derivatives. Retinoids, which exert most of their effects by binding to specific nuclear receptors and modulating gene expression, also include structurally related synthetic analogs, which need not have retinol-like (vitamin A) activity (*see* Evans and Kaye, 1999).

The simple observation of Steenbock (1919) that the vitamin A content of vegetables varies with the degree of pigmentation paved the way for the isolation and discovery of the chemical nature of the vitamin. Subsequently, it was demonstrated that the purified plant pigment carotene (provitamin A) is a remarkably potent source of vitamin A. β-Carotene, the most active carotenoid found in plants, has the structural formula shown in Figure 64–1A.

The structural formulas for the vitamin A family of retinoids are shown in Figure 64–1B.

Retinol, a primary alcohol, is present in esterified form in the tissues of animals and saltwater fish, mainly in the liver. Its

structural formula is as follows:

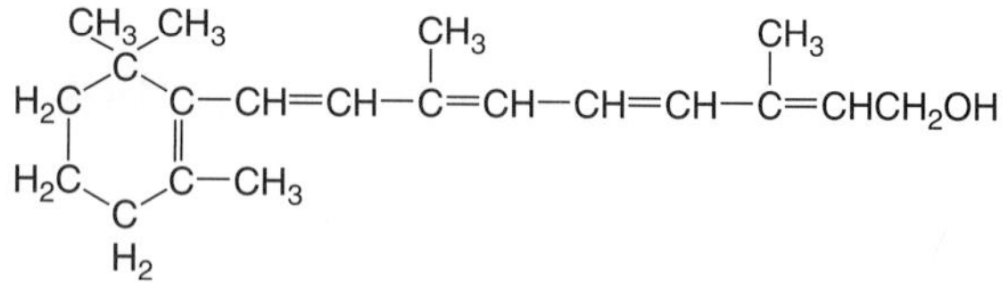

RETINOL

A number of geometric isomers of retinol exist because of the possible *cis-trans* configurations around the double bonds in the side chain. Fish liver oils contain mixtures of the stereoisomers; synthetic retinol is the all-*trans* isomer. Interconversion between isomers readily takes place in the body. In the visual cycle, the reaction between retinal (vitamin A aldehyde) and opsin to form rhodopsin only occurs with the 11-*cis* isomer.

Ethers and esters derived from the alcohol also show activity *in vivo*. The ring structure of retinol (β-ionone), or the

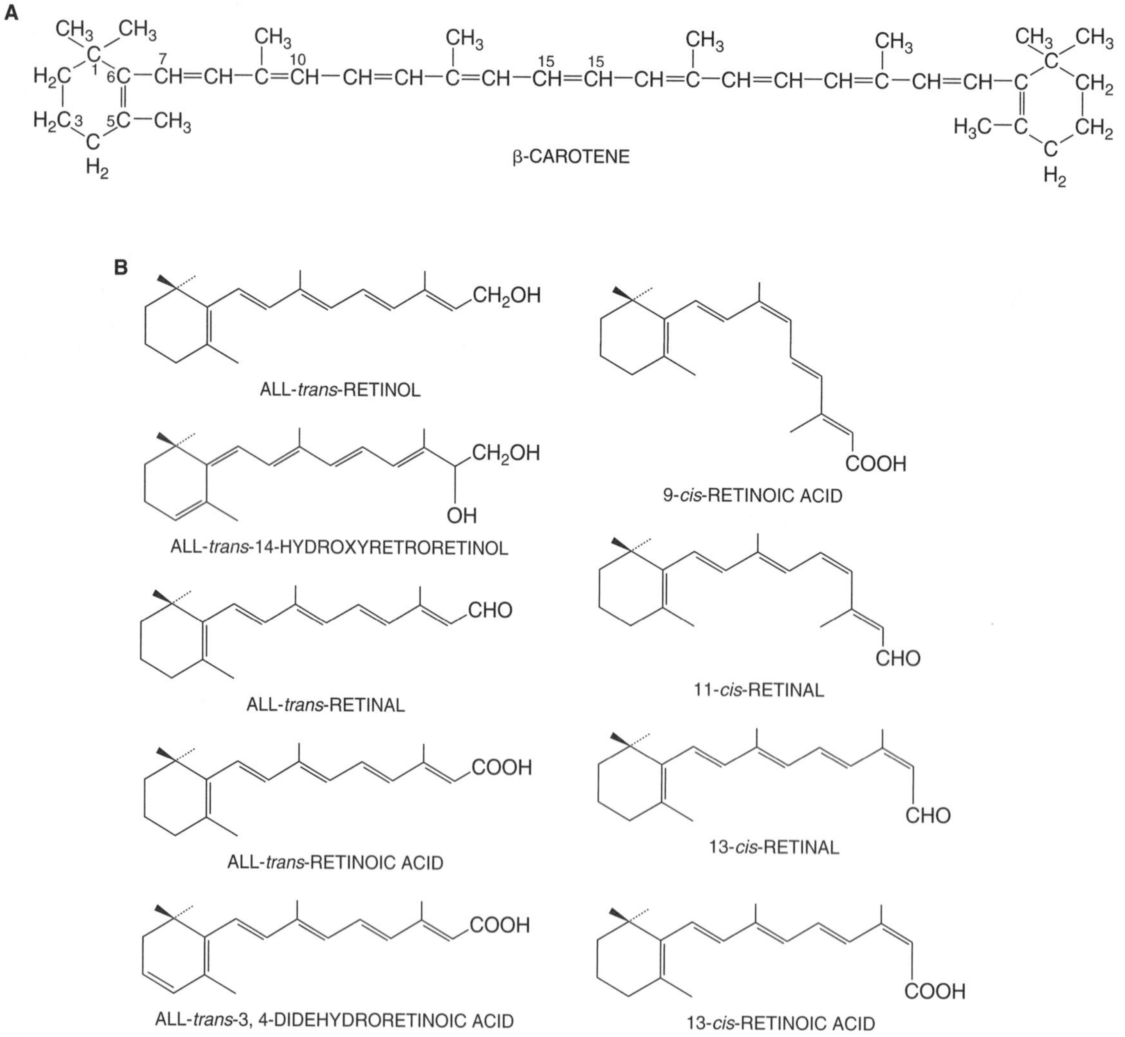

Figure 64–1. A. β-Carotene. B. The vitamin A family.

more unsaturated ring in 3-dehydroretinol (dehydro-β-ionone), is essential for activity; hydrogenation destroys biological activity. Of all known derivatives, all-*trans*-retinol and its aldehyde, retinal, exhibit the greatest biological potency *in vivo;* 3-dehydroretinol has about 40% of the potency of all-*trans*-retinol.

Retinoic acid, in which the alcohol group has been oxidized, shares some but not all of the actions of retinol. Retinoic acid is ineffective in restoring visual or reproductive function in certain species where retinol is effective. However, retinoic acid is very potent in promoting growth and controlling differentiation and maintenance of epithelial tissue in vitamin A–deficient animals. Indeed, all-*trans*-retinoic acid (*tretinoin*) appears to be the active form of vitamin A in all tissues except the retina, and is 10- to 100-fold more potent than retinol in various systems *in vitro*. Isomerization of this compound in the body yields 13-*cis*-retinoic acid (*isotretinoin*), which is nearly as potent as tretinoin in many of its actions on epithelial tissues but may be as much as fivefold less potent in producing the toxic symptoms of hypervitaminosis A.

A large number of analogs of retinoic acid have been synthesized, including the prodrug *etretinate,* which is the ethyl ester of the active compound *acitretin*. These compounds are representative of the so-called second-generation retinoids, in which the β-ionone ring is aromatized; they are more active than tretinoin in some systems but are less active in others. The highly potent "third-generation" retinoids feature two aromatic rings that serve to restrict the flexibility of the polyenoic side chain. This class of aromatic retinoids has been called *arotinoids,* and includes the carboxylic acid, Ro 13-7410, and the ethyl sulfone, Ro 15-1570. The structures of retinoic acids and certain aromatic retinoids are presented in Figure 64–2. The structure–activity relationships of the synthetic retinoids have been reviewed (*see* Symposium, 1989b).

Physiological Functions and Pharmacological Actions.

Vitamin A has a number of important functions in the body. It plays an essential role in the function of the retina. It is necessary for growth and differentiation of epithelial tissue and is required for growth of bone, reproduction, and embryonic development. Together with certain carotenoids, vitamin A enhances immune function, reduces the consequences of some infectious diseases, and may protect against the development of certain malignancies. As a result, there is considerable interest in the pharmacological use of retinoids for cancer prophylaxis and for treating various premalignant conditions. Because of the effects of vitamin A on epithelial tissues, retinoids and their analogs are used to treat a number of skin diseases, including some of the consequences of aging and prolonged exposure to the sun (*see* Chapter 65).

The functions of vitamin A are mediated by different forms of the molecule. In vision, the functional vitamin is retinal. Retinoic acid appears to be the active form in functions associated with growth, differentiation, and transformation.

Retinal and the Visual Cycle. It has long been known that vitamin A deficiency interferes with vision in dim light, a condition known as *night blindness* (nyctalopia). The fundamental observations of Wald (1968) and others contributed greatly to an understanding of this phenomenon.

Photoreception is accomplished by two types of specialized retinal cells, termed *rods* and *cones*. Rods are especially sensitive to light of low intensity; cones act as receptors of high-intensity light and are responsible for color vision. The initial step is the absorption of light by a chromophore attached to the receptor protein. The chromophore of both rods and cones is 11-*cis*-retinal. The

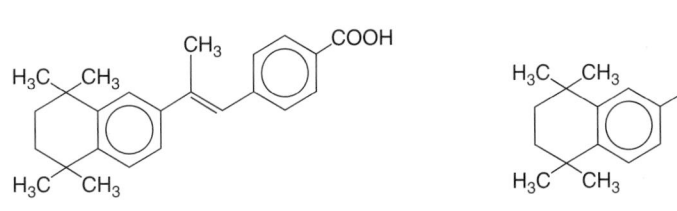

*Figure 64–2. Structural comparison of synthetic retinoic acid compounds and native all-**trans**-retinoic acid.*

holoreceptor in rods is termed *rhodopsin*—a combination
of the protein opsin and 11-*cis*-retinal attached as a prosthetic group. The three different types of cone cells (red,
green, and blue) contain individual, related photoreceptor
proteins and respond optimally to light of different wavelengths.

In the synthesis of rhodopsin, 11-*cis*-retinol is converted to 11-*cis*-retinal in a reversible reaction that requires pyridine nucleotides. 11-*cis*-Retinal then combines
with the ε-amino group of a specific lysine residue in
opsin to form rhodopsin. Most rhodopsin is located in the
membranes of the discs situated in the outer segments
of the rods. The polypeptide chain of the protein spans
the membrane seven times, a characteristic shared by all
known receptors whose functions are transduced *via* G
proteins (*see* Chapter 2).

The visual cycle, depicted in Figure 64–3, is initiated by the absorption of a photon of light, followed
by the photodecomposition, or bleaching, of rhodopsin
through a cascade of unstable conformational states, leading ultimately to the isomerization of 11-*cis*-retinal to
the all-*trans* form and dissociation of the opsin moiety.
Activated rhodopsin interacts rapidly with another protein of the retinal rod outer segment, a G protein termed
transducin or G_t. Transducin stimulates a guanosine 3′,5′-
monophosphate (cyclic GMP)–specific phosphodiesterase.
The resultant decline in cyclic GMP concentration causes
a decreased conductance of cyclic GMP–gated Na^+ channels in the plasma membrane and an increased transmembrane potential. After processing within the retinal circuitry, this primary receptor potential ultimately leads to
the generation of action potentials that travel to the brain
via the optic nerve (*see* Stryer, 1991).

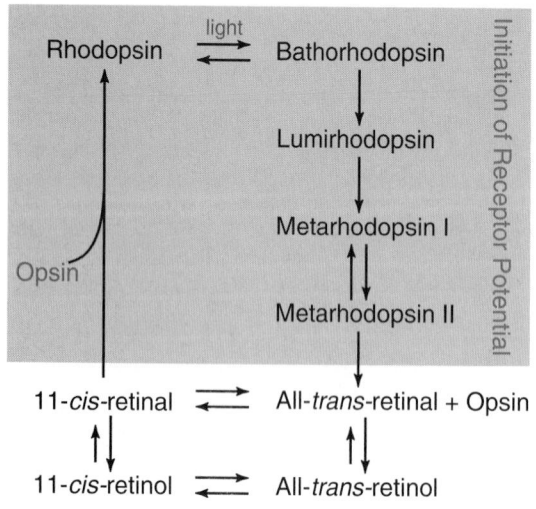

Figure 64–3. The visual cycle.

All-*trans*-retinal can directly isomerize to 11-*cis*-
retinal, which then may recombine with opsin to form
rhodopsin. Alternatively, all-*trans*-retinal can be reduced
to all-*trans*-retinol, which is first converted to 11-*cis*-retinol
and then to rhodopsin in the manner described above
(Figure 64–3).

When human beings are fed diets deficient in vitamin
A, their ability for dark adaptation gradually is diminished.
Rod vision is affected more than cone vision. Upon depletion of retinol from liver and blood, usually at plasma
concentrations of retinol of less than 20 μg/dl (0.70 μM),
the concentration of retinol and of rhodopsin in the retina
falls. Unless the deficiency is overcome, opsin, lacking the
stabilizing effect of retinal, decays and anatomical deterioration of the rods' outer segments takes place. In rats
maintained on a vitamin A–deficient diet, irreversible ultrastructural changes leading to blindness then supervene,
a process that takes approximately 10 months.

Following short-term deprivation of vitamin A, dark
adaptation can be restored to normal by the addition of
retinol to the diet. However, vision does not return to normal for several weeks after adequate amounts of retinol
have been supplied. The reason for this delay is unknown.

Vitamin A and Epithelial Structures. The functional and
structural integrity of epithelial cells throughout the body
is dependent upon an adequate supply of vitamin A. The
vitamin plays a major role in the induction and control of
epithelial differentiation in mucus-secreting or keratinizing tissues. In the presence of retinol or retinoic acid, basal
epithelial cells are stimulated to produce mucus. Excessive concentrations of the retinoids lead to the production
of a thick layer of mucin, the inhibition of keratinization,
and the display of goblet cells.

In the absence of vitamin A, goblet mucous cells
disappear and are replaced by basal cells that have been
stimulated to proliferate. These undermine and replace the
original epithelium with a stratified, keratinizing epithelium. The suppression of normal secretions leads to irritation and infection. Reversal of these changes is achieved
by the administration of retinol, retinoic acid, or other
retinoids. When this process happens in the cornea, severe hyperkeratinization (xerophthalmia) may lead to permanent blindness. Worldwide, xerophthalmia remains one
of the most common causes of blindness.

Mechanism of Action. In isolated fibroblasts or epithelial tissue, retinoids enhance the synthesis of some proteins (*e.g.*, fibronectin) and reduce the synthesis of others
(*e.g.*, collagenase, certain species of keratin), and molecular evidence suggests that these actions can be entirely
accounted for by changes in nuclear transcription (*see*
Mangelsdorf *et al.*, 1994). Retinoic acid appears to be

considerably more potent than retinol in mediating these effects.

Retinoic acid influences gene expression by combining with nuclear receptors. Multiple retinoid receptors have been described. These are grouped into two families. One family, the retinoic acid receptors (RARs), designated α, β, and γ, are derived from genes localized to human chromosomes 17, 3, and 12, respectively. The second family, the retinoid X receptors (RXRs), also is composed of α, β, and γ receptor isoforms (Chambon, 1995). The retinoid receptors show extensive sequence homology to each other in both their DNA and hormone-binding domains and belong to a receptor superfamily that includes receptors for steroid and thyroid hormones and calcitriol (*see* Mangelsdorf *et al.*, 1994; *see also* Chapter 2). Cellular responses to thyroid and steroid hormones, calcitriol, and retinoic acid are enhanced by the presence of nuclear extracts containing RXR. Genes that are regulated by these hormones possess hormone-specific response elements in upstream promoter sites. Gene activation involves binding of the hormone-receptor complex followed by dimerization with an RXR-ligand complex. The identity of the endogenous RXR ligand has been shown to be 9-*cis*-retinoic acid (Heyman *et al.*, 1992; Levin *et al.*, 1992). No comparable receptor for retinol has been detected to date, and it is possible that retinol must be oxidized to retinoic acid to produce its effects within target cells.

Retinoids can influence the expression of receptors for certain hormones and growth factors, and thus can influence the growth, differentiation, and function of target cells by both direct and indirect actions (*see* Love and Gudas, 1994).

Vitamin A and Carcinogenesis. Because vitamin A regulates epithelial cell differentiation and proliferation, there has been considerable interest in the apparent ability of retinol and related compounds to interfere with carcinogenesis (*see* Moon *et al.*, 1994; and Hong and Itri, 1994). Vitamin A deficiency in human beings enhances susceptibility to carcinogenesis; the basal cells of various epithelia undergo marked hyperplasia and reduced cellular differentiation. The administration of retinol or other retinoids to animals reverses these changes in the epithelium of the respiratory tract, mammary gland, urinary bladder, and skin. Thus, the progression of premalignant cells to cells with invasive, malignant characteristics is slowed, delayed, arrested, or even reversed in experimental animals (*see* Moon *et al.*, 1994). The antitumor effect is seen with chemically and virally induced malignancies of both epithelial and mesenchymal origin, as well as with transformation induced with radiation or by growth factors. Reversal of growth and metastasis of established tumors *in vivo* has been limited, as has prevention of the growth of transplantable neoplasms in animals.

The exact mechanism of the anticarcinogenic effect remains unclear, but obviously it is of enormous interest. The effect is observable even if the retinoid is administered many weeks after the exposure to a carcinogen, suggesting interference with the promotion or progression phase of carcinogenesis. A possible mechanism that may contribute to the antitumor effect is the induction of differentiation in malignant cells to form morphologically mature normal cells. For example, retinoids regulate the synthesis of specific proteins (*e.g.*, keratin) necessary for the differentiation of epithelial tissues. Moreover, vitamin A appears to have a specific biochemical function in the synthesis of cell-surface glycoproteins and glycolipids that may be involved in cell adherence and communication. Conversion of retinol to retinyl phosphate in epithelial cells is followed by microsomal formation of mannosyl retinyl phosphate (Rosso *et al.*, 1975), a glycosylated retinol derivative that mediates the transfer of mannose to specific cell-surface glycoproteins. Formation of such proteins is curtailed sharply when vitamin A is deficient. Reactions of this type may explain the function of the vitamin in a number of processes that depend on the integrity of the cell surface, and might contribute to the suppression of the malignant phenotype previously induced by a carcinogen. The host's immune defense mechanisms also may be improved. In any event, a direct cytotoxic action appears unlikely (*see* Hong and Itri, 1994).

Although numerous epidemiological studies have demonstrated an inverse relationship between the intake of dietary vitamin A and cancer morbidity and mortality (especially lung cancer), the correlation with the intake of retinol itself has been inconsistent (*see* Hong and Itri, 1994). As a result, attention now is being focused on biological effects of β-carotene and other carotenoids that are not shared by retinol (*see* "Carotenoids," below).

Vitamin A and Immune Function. It has been known for many years that vitamin A deficiency is associated with increased susceptibility to bacterial, parasitic, and viral infections. Decreased resistance to infections has been demonstrated in numerous animal models of vitamin A deficiency, and even marginal vitamin A status increases the severity and duration of infectious illness. Although changes in size and cellularity of lymphatic tissues have been reported in vitamin A–deficient animals, considerable inconsistency has been observed among animal models and with severity and duration of vitamin A depletion. With respect to cell-mediated immunity, splenic lymphocyte proliferation clearly is impaired in vitamin A deficiency, which also has been associated with reduced killer cell cytotoxic activity. With respect to humoral immunity, results vary according to specific antigens. Animal studies consistently show a relationship between vitamin A status and the antibody response to tetanus toxoid. Tetanus vaccination responses in marginally nourished human populations have been enhanced in some, but not all, trials by coadministration of vitamin A. The relationship between vitamin A nutrition and measles infection has been studied extensively. In large clinical trials, administration of vitamin A to children with measles resulted in major reduction in morbidity and mortality (Hussey and Klein, 1990). Consequently, a joint WHO/UNICEF publication recommended that all children diagnosed with measles in countries where the fatality rate is 1% or more should immediately receive 30 to 60 mg (100,000 to 200,000 IU) of vitamin A, depending on age (Anonymous, 1987). The relationship of immunity and infectious disease to vitamin A status has been reviewed by Ross (1992).

Symptoms of Deficiency.   Tissue reserves of retinoids in the healthy adult are sufficiently large to require long-term dietary deprivation to induce deficiency. Vitamin A deficiency occurs more commonly in chronic diseases affecting fat absorption, such as biliary tract or pancreatic insufficiency, sprue, Crohn's disease involving the terminal ileum, and portal cirrhosis; following partial gastrectomy; or during extreme, chronic dietary inadequacy.

Vitamin A deficiency is one of the most serious nutritional deficiency diseases in the world today. It is widespread in Southeast Asia, the Middle East, Africa, and Central and South America, particularly in children, and is associated with general malnutrition. Deficiency of vitamin A may be fatal, especially in infants and young children suffering from kwashiorkor or marasmus. It has been estimated that more than one-quarter million children in the world suffer irreversible blindness every year because of inadequate intake of vitamin A. Even mild xerophthalmia is associated with an increased risk of respiratory infections or diarrhea, as well as with an increased mortality due to these diseases or to measles (*see* Sommer, *in* Symposium, 1989a). In the United States, concentrations of retinol in plasma below the accepted lower limits of normal, 20 μg/dl (0.70 μM), are observed in about 3% of apparently healthy people. Most of these individuals are infants or children.

Signs and symptoms of mild vitamin A deficiency are easily overlooked. Skin lesions, such as follicular hyperkeratosis and infections, are among the earliest signs of deficiency, but the most recognizable manifestation is night blindness, even though its onset occurs only when vitamin A depletion is severe. Children may grow more slowly, although this may be recognized only after correction of the deficiency. In general, rapidly proliferating tissues are more sensitive to vitamin A deficiency than are slowly growing tissues and may revert to an undifferentiated state more readily.

Eye.   Keratomalacia, characterized by desiccation, ulceration, and xerosis of the cornea and conjunctiva, is occasionally seen as an acute symptom in the very young who are ingesting severely deficient diets. It is usually foreshadowed by night blindness, which appears as the earliest ocular sign of deficiency. Ultimately, severe visual impairment and even blindness result.

Bronchorespiratory Tract.   Changes in the bronchorespiratory epithelium from mucus secretion to keratinization lead to increased incidence of respiratory infections in the deficiency state. There also is a decrease in elasticity of the lung and other tissues.

Skin.   Keratinization and drying of the epidermis occur, and papular eruptions involving the pilosebaceous follicles may be found, especially on the extremities.

Genitourinary System.   Urinary calculi are frequent concomitants of vitamin A deficiency. The epithelium of the urinary tract shares in the general pathological changes of all epithelial structures. Epithelial debris thus may provide the nidus around which a calculus is formed. Abnormalities of reproduction include impairment of spermatogenesis, degeneration of testes, abortion, resorption of fetuses, and production of malformed offspring.

Gastrointestinal Tract.   The intestinal mucosa shows a reduction in the number of goblet cells but no keratinization. Alterations in intestinal epithelium and metaplasia of pancreatic ductal epithelium are common. They may be responsible for the diarrhea occasionally seen in vitamin A deficiency.

Sweat Glands.   These glands may undergo atrophy and keratinizing squamous-cell metaplasia.

Bone.   In animals, vitamin A deficiency is associated with faulty modeling of bone, with production of thick, cancellous bone instead of thinner, more compact bone.

Miscellaneous.   Often both taste and smell are impaired in vitamin A–deficient individuals, undoubtedly a result of a keratinizing effect. Hearing also may be impaired. Vitamin A deficiency can interfere with erythropoiesis, which may be masked by abnormal losses of fluid. Nerve lesions, increased cerebrospinal fluid pressure, and hydrocephalus have been reported.

Hypervitaminosis A.   An intake of retinoids greatly in excess of requirement results in a toxic syndrome known as hypervitaminosis A. Some or all of the symptoms of hypervitaminosis A also are the major toxic effects that are manifest during the therapeutic use of natural and synthetic retinoids in the treatment of skin disorders (*see* Chapter 65).

Most frequently, high intakes in children are the result of overzealous prophylactic vitamin therapy on the part of parents. Toxicity in adults has resulted from extended self-medication or food fads, as well as from the use of retinoids for the therapy of acne or other skin lesions. The toxicity of retinol depends on the age of the patient, the dose, and the duration of administration. Although vitamin A toxicity is uncommon in adults who consume less than 30 mg of retinol per day, mild symptoms of chronic retinoid intoxication have been detected in individuals whose intake was about 10 mg per day for 6 months (*see* Bendich and Langseth, 1989). In infants, the daily consumption of as little as 7.5 to 15 mg of retinol for 30 days has induced toxicity. The acute consumption of more than 500 mg of retinol in an adult, 100 mg in a young child, or 30 mg in an infant frequently results in poisoning. Acute and sometimes fatal poisoning in human beings also is known to follow the ingestion of polar bear liver, which contains up to 12 mg of retinol per gram. The Food and Nutrition Board of the National Research Council has warned that the ingestion of more than 7.5 mg of retinol daily is ill advised. Nevertheless, almost 5% of users of vitamin A in the United States exceed that amount.

Early signs and symptoms of chronic retinoid intoxication include dry and pruritic skin, skin disquamation, erythematous dermatitis, disturbed hair growth, fissures of the lips, pain and tenderness of bones, hyperostosis, headache, papilledema, anorexia, edema, fatigue, irritability, and hemorrhage. Intracranial pressure may be increased, and neurological symptoms may mimic those of a brain tumor (pseudotumor cerebri). In infants, increased intracranial pressure, a bulging fontanel, and vomiting are seen early. In addition to hepatosplenomegaly, pathological changes in the liver include hypertrophy of fat-storing cells, fibrosis, sclerosis of central veins, and cirrhosis, with resultant portal hypertension and ascites. The activity of alkaline phosphatase in plasma rises because of the increased osteoblastic activity; a number of cases of hypercalcemia have been reported in children. Elevations in plasma triglycerides and reductions in the cholesterol of high-density lipoprotein also are observed.

Signs and symptoms of acute poisoning include drowsiness, irritability or irresistible desire to sleep, severe headache due to increased intracranial pressure, dizziness, hepatomegaly, vomiting, papilledema, and, after 24 hours, generalized peeling of the skin.

Concentrations of retinol in plasma in excess of 100 μg/dl (3.5 μM) usually are diagnostic of hypervitaminosis A. Treatment consists of withdrawal of the retinoid. Most signs and symptoms disappear within a week, but the desquamation and hyperostoses remain evident for several months after clinical recovery, and in rare instances the bone malformations may be permanent. Long-term and sometimes irreversible damage to the liver also may occur.

The risk of hypervitaminosis A is increased in conditions that produce a decreased plasma concentration of retinol-binding protein (RBP) (*see* below). These include protein malnutrition and liver disease. Because vitamins A and D often are consumed together, some of the symptoms of hypervitaminosis A (*e.g.*, hypercalcemia) actually may be caused by overdosage with vitamin D. Indeed, large doses of vitamin A may protect against the adverse effects on bone metabolism of hypervitaminosis D. The hypoprothrombinemia of hypervitaminosis A may reflect antagonism of vitamin K. In experimental animals, the administration of vitamin E eliminates some of the toxic effects of large doses of vitamin A. Although similar observations in human beings have not been documented, small amounts of vitamin E are included in the preparations of vitamin A used in developing countries for intermittent high-level dosing (*see* Bendich and Langseth, 1989).

Congenital abnormalities apparently can occur in infants whose mothers have consumed about 7.5 to 12 mg of retinol daily during the first trimester of pregnancy (Bernhardt and Dorsey, 1974). Obviously, pregnant women should not ingest quantities of retinoids in excess of those recommended. Moreover, women who have been treated with synthetic retinoids that accumulate in fat should practice contraception after discontinuing therapy until the drug has been eliminated from the body; after prolonged ingestion of etretinate, this may require 2 years or longer (*see* below).

Human Requirements. Human requirements for vitamin A have been approximated from studies that have attempted to correct experimentally produced deficiency states. The present recommendations of the Food and Nutrition Board of the National Research Council are based upon the amount of retinoid necessary to maintain normal dark adaptation plus an additional factor of safety to cover variations in absorption and utilization of retinol. The recommended daily allowances for the normal adult male and female are 1000 and 800 retinol equivalents per day, respectively (5000 and 4000 U, assuming that 50% of dietary vitamin A is derived from retinol and 50% from β-carotene). For the requirements of infants and children, *see* Table XIII–1.

Food Sources. In the United States, the average adult receives about half the daily intake of vitamin A as retinol or retinyl esters and the rest as carotenoids. Major dietary sources of vitamin A are liver, butter, cheese, whole milk, egg yolk, and fish. β-Carotene is present in various yellow or green fruits and vegetables. These foods also contain numerous carotenoids that cannot be converted to retinol. Nevertheless, many of these can function as antioxidants and may have useful health-promoting effects (*see* Symposium, 1989a).

Absorption, Fate, and Excretion.   *Retinol.* More than 90% of dietary retinol is in the form of esters, usually retinyl palmitate. As with triglycerides, most of the retinyl esters are hydrolyzed in the intestinal lumen by pancreatic enzymes and within the brush border of the intestinal epithelial cell before absorption. Although lipophilic, the uptake of retinol by intestinal cells apparently occurs by a carrier-mediated process and is facilitated by the presence of a cytosolic protein that specifically binds retinol with high affinity. This cellular retinol-binding protein (CRBP), which is closely related to the CRBP in numerous cells throughout the body (*see* below), is designated CRBP II. It occurs only in absorption cells in the small intestine, where it constitutes about 1% of the total soluble protein (*see* Ong *et al.,* 1994). Most of the retinol is reesterified (mainly to palmitate) within these cells and is incorporated into chylomicrons; after large oral doses of retinol, significant amounts of retinyl esters also circulate in association with low-density lipoprotein. Appreciable quantities of retinol also are absorbed directly into the circulation, where they are bound to the retinol-binding protein (RBP) in plasma.

When ingested in amounts that approximate daily requirements, the absorption of retinol is complete; however, some retinol escapes into the feces when large doses are taken. The concentration of esterified retinol reaches a peak in plasma about 4 hours after the ingestion of retinol. The absorption of retinol is reduced by abnormalities of fat digestion and absorption, such as occur in patients with pancreatic or hepatic disease, intestinal infections, and cystic fibrosis. Water-miscible preparations should be used in such patients.

Most of the absorbed retinyl esters are taken up by the liver through receptor-mediated internalization of chylomicron remnants (*see* Chapter 36). Until the hepatic stores of retinyl esters become saturated, the administration of retinol leads mainly to its accumulation in the liver rather than in blood. The median concentration of retinyl esters in human liver is about 100 to 300 μg/g, and the normal range of retinol in plasma is 30 to 70 μg/dl (1.1 to 2.4 μM). If an individual ingests a diet free of retinol or its precursors, plasma concentrations are maintained over many months at the expense of hepatic reserves; these decrease with a half-life of about 50 to 100 days. Blood concentrations, therefore, are not a sensitive guide to an individual's vitamin A status, but low plasma values imply that hepatic storage of the vitamin may be exhausted. Signs and symptoms of vitamin A deficiency appear when the plasma concentration falls below 10 to 20 μg/dl (0.35 to 0.70 μM) or when concentrations of retinoids in the liver are less than 5 to 20 μg/g. In alcoholic liver disease, hepatic concentrations of retinoids are severely depressed (Leo and Lieber, 1982).

Prior to entering the circulation from the liver, hepatic retinyl esters are hydrolyzed, and 90% to 95% of the retinol is associated with an α_1-globulin, which has a single binding site for the vitamin. This RBP is synthesized and secreted by the liver and then circulates in the blood complexed with and stabilized by transthyretin, a thyroxine-binding prealbumin. The formation of this complex protects the circulating RBP (and retinol) from metabolism and renal excretion.

More than 95% of plasma retinoids normally are bound to RBP. When hepatic stores of the vitamin and RBP carrier system become saturated because of excessive intake of retinol or hepatic damage, up to 65% of the retinoids in plasma may be present as retinyl esters associated with lipoprotein. Similarly, after acute administration of alcohol, retinyl esters accumulate. Since retinol is biologically inert while bound to RBP, these retinyl esters, which are surfactants, may be responsible for much of the toxicity that is observed.

Retinol bound to RBP reaches the cell membrane of various target organs, where the complex binds to specific sites on the cell surface. The retinol is transferred to a membrane-bound protein that appears to be closely related to the soluble CRBP and is converted to a retinyl ester. The retinyl ester is then cleaved by a membrane-associated hydrolase, provided that unliganded cytosolic CRBP is available to accept the retinol. CRBP exists in virtually all tissues; exceptions include cardiac and skele-

tal muscle and the ileal mucosa, where the closely related CRBP II is found (*see* above). In addition to its role in the uptake of retinol, CRBP functions as a reservoir for cellular retinol and delivers the vitamin to appropriate sites for its conversion to active compounds. In the retina, retinol is converted to 11-*cis*-retinal, which is incorporated into rhodopsin; a specific binding protein (distinct from CRBP) also is present. In other target tissues, retinol apparently is oxidized to retinoic acid, which is conveyed to receptors in the nucleus as a complex with the cellular retinoic acid–binding protein (CRABP). The tissue distribution of CRABP appears to be nearly identical with that of CRBP, with the possible exception of its absence from adult liver (*see* Ong *et al.,* 1994).

The concentration of RBP in plasma is crucial for the regulation of retinol in plasma and its transport to tissues. In vitamin A deficiency, the synthesis of RBP is maintained, the hepatic content of RBP rises, and its concentration in plasma falls, apparently because the secretion of RBP from the liver is blocked. Once retinol again becomes available, the liver rapidly releases RBP into the plasma for transport of retinol to the tissues. When there is protein deficiency (*e.g.,* caused by malnutrition, kwashiorkor, or parenchymal liver disease), the concentration of RBP becomes insufficient, and concentrations of retinol in plasma fall despite normal stores in the liver. Replenishment with calories and protein then is required. Deficiency of both RBP and retinol cannot be corrected by the administration of retinol alone.

Other pathological conditions also alter concentrations of retinol and RBP in plasma. In cystic fibrosis, alcohol-related cirrhosis, and hepatic diseases, synthesis or release of RBP from the liver is depressed, and plasma retinol concentrations are reduced. In proteinuria, febrile infections, or stress, the concentration of retinol in the blood may be reduced drastically, partially because of increased urinary excretion. In chronic renal disease, RBP catabolism is impaired, and concentrations of the protein and retinol are elevated.

Estrogens and oral contraceptives elevate the plasma concentrations of RBP, but the effects of pregnancy are complex. During the first trimester, the mean content of retinol in plasma falls, followed by a slow rise and a return to normal at parturition. It is likely that the increased demands for retinol lead to its withdrawal from the blood at a rate exceeding that of its mobilization from liver. The placental barrier prevents the extensive transfer of retinol or carotenoids. Studies in animals suggest that transplacental transport of RBP occurs during early pregnancy; thereafter the fetus begins to synthesize its own RBP. The concentration of retinol in fetal blood is thus less than in maternal blood. Both colostrum and milk offer the newborn an adequate supply of retinol. The concentration of retinol in the milk is maintained at a fixed maximal concentration if the maternal dietary intake of retinol is adequate to permit storage in the liver.

Retinol is in part conjugated to form a β-glucuronide, which undergoes enterohepatic circulation and is oxidized to retinal and retinoic acid. A possible physiological role for retinyl glucuronides was proposed by Zile *et al.*, (1982). These glucuronides induce cellular differentiation in several cell lines by mechanisms that still are unclear. They do not bind to retinoic acid receptors. Indirect activity of these compounds could be explained by intracellular hydrolysis to all-*trans*-retinoic acid or formation of retinoylated proteins (*see* Olson, 1993). A novel property of retinoyl glucuronides is their apparent lack of toxicity compared with other retinoids. If confirmed, this feature would offer an important advance for retinoid therapy.

Several other water-soluble metabolites also are excreted in the urine and feces. Normally, no retinol can be recovered unchanged from human urine.

Carotenoids. Over 600 carotenoids are found in nature. Forty are regularly consumed in the diet, and six can be measured in human serum. β-Carotene, α-carotene, and cryptoxanthin are converted to vitamin A, whereas lutein and lycopene are not (*see* Bendich and Olson, 1989). Unlike the extensive absorption of retinol, only about one-third of β-carotene or other carotenoids is absorbed by human beings. The absorption of carotenoids takes place in a relatively nonspecific fashion and depends upon the presence of bile and absorbable fat in the intestinal tract; it is greatly decreased by steatorrhea, chronic diarrhea, and very-low-fat diets. A portion of the β-carotene is converted to retinol in the wall of the small intestine, principally by its initial cleavage at the 15,15' double bond to form two molecules of retinal. Some of the retinal is further oxidized to retinoic acid; only one-half is reduced to retinol, which is then esterified and transported in the lymph, as described above. Although central cleavage to retinol is the primary metabolic pathway for β-carotene, recent work indicates that β-carotene also may be eccentrically cleaved to form a variety of other products (Lakshman *et al.*, 1989; *see* Olson, 1993). Carotenoids are absorbed and transported *via* lymphatics to the liver. They circulate in association with lipoproteins, and are found in liver, adrenal, testes, and adipose tissue, and can be converted to vitamin A in numerous tissues, including the liver (*see* Olson, in Symposium, 1989a; Kaplan *et al.*, 1990). Some β-carotene is absorbed as such and circulates in association with lipoproteins; it apparently partitions into body lipids and can be converted to vitamin A in numerous tissues, including the liver (*see* Olson, in Symposium, 1989a; Stahl *et al.*, 1992). If very large amounts of carotene are ingested, very high concentrations may be achieved in blood (300 μg/dl; 5.6 μM), and the hypercarotenemia results in a reversible yellow discoloration of the skin; this can be distinguished from jaundice by the absence of scleral pigmentation. Hypervitaminosis does not develop, however, probably because of a limited conversion of carotene to retinol.

Carotenoids and their metabolites act in various ways on biological systems. They have been considered to have two possible functions: to be metabolized to retinoids and to act as lipid-phase antioxidants. Case-control and other epidemiological studies have consistently linked increased risk of cancer to low intake of fruits, vegetables, and carotenoids, particularly cancer of the lung and stomach (*see* van Poppel, 1993). However, multiple intervention trials with β-carotene and other antioxidant nutrients have had disappointing results. In a large primary prevention trial, β-carotene supplementation actually was associated with an increased incidence of lung cancer (Alpha-Tocopherol, β-Carotene Cancer Prevention Study Group, 1994); in another study, it provided no protection against colon cancer (Greenberg, *et al.*, 1994). Low plasma levels of antioxidant nutrients also have been associated with increased relative risk for ischemic heart disease, and oxidation of low-density lipoprotein (LDL) particles is thought to be an initial step in atherogenesis. However, β-carotene supplementation alone does not appear to reduce the susceptibility of LDL to oxidation (Reaven *et al.*, 1993), and β-carotene supplementation did not offer protection against myocardial infarction, stroke, or any cardiovascular mortality (Lee *et al.*, 1999).

Retinoic Acid. Unlike retinol, relatively little all-*trans*-retinoic acid (*tretinoin*) is provided in the diet, and specific mechanisms for its absorption, transport in plasma, and storage in tissue do not exist. After oral administration, retinoic acid reaches the circulation by the portal vein and is transported in plasma as a complex with albumin; quantitative studies of its absorption by this route have not been performed in human beings. When applied to human skin, about 5% of the compound and its metabolites is recovered in the urine; little systemic toxicity is produced by this route. By contrast, attempts to treat dermatoses by oral administration of retinoic acid can produce severe symptoms of hypervitaminosis A.

Tretinoin is metabolized rapidly in the liver, and various conjugated forms and degradation products are secreted into bile and excreted in urine and feces. In addition to 13-*cis*-retinoic acid (isotretinoin), conjugates with glucuronic acid and taurine are formed; oxidation occurs at position 4 in the β-ionone ring (*see* Allen and Bloxham, in Symposium, 1989b). Tretinoin has been used to promote leukemic cell differentiation in patients with acute promyelocytic leukemia, but its pharmacokinetic properties contribute to a brief duration of remission associated with a progressive decrease in peak plasma concentrations following chronic dosing (*see* below). 9-*cis*-Retinoic acid can bind and activate the same family of retinoic acid receptors as all-*trans*-retinoic acid (tretinoin), and thus has the potential to elicit the same therapeutic effects as tretinoin. Differences between the pharmacokinetic properties of 9-*cis*-retinoic acid and those of tretinoin seen in nude mice suggest that consideration of development of 9-*cis*-retinoic acid to promote cell differentiation in acute promyelocytic leukemia is warranted (Achkar *et al.*, 1994).

Isotretinoin. After oral administration, peak concentrations of 13-*cis*-retinoic acid (isotretinoin) in plasma are reached in 2 to 4 hours. Its oral bioavailability in fasting subjects is estimated to be about 20%; the presence of food substantially increases the extent of systemic absorption. The drug is not effective topically. Isotretinoin is extensively bound to albumin in plasma, and its concentration in tissues is generally lower than in the general circulation.

Isotretinoin and tretinoin are interconverted *in vivo,* and about 20% to 30% of a dose of isotretinoin apparently is metabolized by this route. With repeated administration, the major metabolite, 4-oxo-isotretinoin, accumulates in the blood. Excretion of metabolites and the parent compound in the bile occurs after conjugation with glucuronic acid. The half-life of isotretinoin in plasma ranges between 6 and 36 hours. With repeated administration, steady-state concentrations are established within 5 to 7 days. Several metabolites of isotretinoin are cleared from plasma rather slowly. Because of the general concern over the teratogenicity of retinoids, it is recommended that effective contraception be maintained for at least one month after treatment with isotretinoin is discontinued. The pharmacokinetics of isotretinoin have been reviewed by Allen and Bloxham (Symposium, 1989b).

Etretinate.   Etretinate is a synthetic retinoic acid, the ethyl ester of acitretin, which is presumed to be the active form of the drug (*see* Figure 64–2). The oral bioavailability of etretinate is about 50%, and absorption is enhanced in the presence of milk or fatty foods. After oral administration of single doses, the plasma concentrations of etretinate and acitretin are about equal and reach maximal values within 2 to 3 hours; thereafter, their concentrations decline with half-times of 7 to 9 hours. However, after continuous administration, etretinate and its active metabolites accumulate in fat and plasma, and their apparent half-lives increase as a function of the duration of treatment; values of 60 to 170 days may be observed after treatment for 1 year. As a result, it may be necessary for women to maintain effective contraception for at least 2 years after the treatment is discontinued.

In addition to deesterification in the gut and liver, etretinate undergoes extensive metabolism and conjugation before excretion in the urine and bile. The metabolites of acitretin that have been identified include 13-*cis*-acitretin and demethylated products. The pharmacokinetic properties of etretinate have been reviewed by Allen and Bloxham (Symposium, 1989b).

Bioassay and Unitage. Most commercial preparations of vitamin A are synthetic retinyl esters. Preparations from animal sources must be assayed biologically to establish their activity. This assay depends upon the ability of retinol to support growth in vitamin-depleted rats. The concentration of suitably purified preparations can be determined spectrophotometrically. One IU of vitamin A is the specific biological activity of 0.3 μg of all-*trans*-retinol or 0.6 μg of β-carotene. Because of the relatively inefficient dietary utilization of β-carotene compared with retinol, the nomenclature is in terms of the retinol equivalent, which represents 1 μg of all-*trans*-retinol, 6 μg of dietary β-carotene, or 12 μg of other provitamin A carotenoids. One retinol equivalent equals 3.3 IU of vitamin A activity as supplied by retinol or 10 U of vitamin A activity as supplied by β-carotene. The methods for standardizing retinol and carotenoids have been reviewed (*see* Simpson, 1983).

Therapeutic Uses. *Vitamin A Deficiency Diseases.* The normal requirement of vitamin A for adults is supplied by an adequate diet. The rational uses of retinol are in the treatment of vitamin A deficiency and as prophylaxis in high-risk subjects during periods of increased requirement, such as infancy, pregnancy, and lactation. Once vitamin A deficiency has been

diagnosed, intensive therapy should be instituted. The patient should then be maintained on a proper diet.

There are many types of preparations that contain retinol. Absorption is greatest for aqueous preparations, intermediate for emulsions, and slowest for oil solutions. Whereas oil-soluble preparations may lead to greater hepatic storage of the vitamin, water-miscible preparations usually provide higher concentrations in plasma. Vitamin A is available as capsules. *Tretinoin* (*all-*trans-*retinoic acid;* RETIN-A) is available for topical use. *Acitretin* (SORIATANE) is used systemically to treat psoriasis. *Isotretinoin* (*13*-cis-*retinoic acid;* ACCUTANE) is available for oral use, as is *etretinate* (TEGISON). *Adapalene* (DIFFERIN) is a synthetic analog of retinoic acid that selectively binds to some RARs but does not bind to CRABPs. It is used topically in the treatment of acne.

During pregnancy and lactation, it is advisable to increase the material intake of vitamin A by about 25%. Since the typical North American diet readily provides adequate intake of the vitamin, supplementation is not routinely indicated. Nevertheless, the administration of vitamin supplements to infants is a common practice in the United States. However, ingestion of 6 mg (20,000 IU) of retinol or more per day for 1 to 2 months by healthy infants or children on good diets is likely to produce signs and symptoms of toxicity.

In rare circumstances, the absorption, mobilization, or storage of retinol may be adversely affected. Under such circumstances, long-term therapy with retinol may be indicated. Examples include individuals with steatorrhea, severe biliary obstruction, cirrhosis of the liver, or following total gastrectomy. In other disease states where considerable retinol is lost from the body, replacement therapy may be necessary. A water-miscible preparation can be given parenterally to individuals with malabsorption or severe ocular damage. In various infections in which mucous-cell turnover is accelerated and urinary excretion of retinol is increased, the need for retinol is further enhanced. There is no evidence, however, that an excessive intake of retinoids will influence the incidence of infections in an individual whose intake of retinoids is adequate. Although moderate amounts of vitamin A apparently do no harm, hepatotoxicity may be potentiated when such doses are taken by the chronic alcoholic. If vitamin A is prescribed as a dietary supplement, intake of 1.5 mg of retinol represents one and one-half times the recommended daily allowance. Long-term ingestion of much larger amounts may lead to hypervitaminosis.

In kwashiorkor and other severe vitamin A deficiencies in children, a single intramuscular injection of 30 mg of retinol as the water-miscible palmitate has been advocated, followed by intermittent oral treatment with retinoids. The World Health Organization treatment schedule for xerophthalmia in children older than 1 year includes 110 mg of retinyl palmitate orally or 55 mg intramuscularly, plus another 110 mg orally the following day and again prior to discharge. Vitamin E, 40 U, should be coadministered, since it apparently increases the efficacy of retinol. Pregnant women should receive only low doses of retinoids.

Dermatological Diseases. Vitamin A may be helpful in certain diseases of the skin, such as acne, psoriasis, Darier's disease, and ichthyosis. The use of other retinoids in these conditions has largely replaced that of retinol and is discussed in Chapter 65.

Cancer and Other Uses. Considerable interest has focused on the possibility that vitamin A and other retinoids may find important roles in cancer chemoprevention and therapy (*see* Lippman *et al.,* 1994). Recent clinical trials have produced encouraging results with respect to chemoprevention of head and neck, skin, colon, and cervical cancers, and in modifying the behavior of established head and neck, thyroid, and lung cancers. The results of several ongoing clinical trials should clarify these potential roles in the near future. However, intervention trials have not confirmed a protective role for carotenoids (*see* below); a recommendation to consume carotenoid or retinoid supplements for purposes of cancer prevention remains premature. It seems far more prudent to advocate plentiful consumption of fruits and vegetables as part of a balanced diet.

Promyelocytic leukemia is a notable example where retinoic acid has shown both a pathogenetic and therapeutic role. A unique chromosome translocation, t(15;17), specifically involves the retinoic acid α-receptor gene on chromosome 17 in a substantial majority of patients with this form of acute leukemia, which accounts for about 15% of acute nonlymphoblastic leukemias in adults (Chen *et al.,* 1991). In addition, retinoic acid has been shown to regulate the growth and differentiation of myeloid cells *in vitro* (Collins *et al.,* 1990). Administration of all-*trans*-retinoic acid to patients with acute promyelocytic leukemia has produced a striking incidence of remission that is associated with maturation of the leukemic clone. Responsive patients showed expression of the aberrant retinoic acid α receptor (Castaigne *et al.,* 1990; Warrell *et al.,* 1991). Unfortunately, despite a high rate of complete remission, early relapse is observed almost uniformly, regardless of follow-up therapy (Castaigne *et al.,* 1990). Nonetheless, such results stimulate optimism that differentiation therapy with newer retinoids ultimately may provide effective therapy for leukemias as well as for more common malignancies.

VITAMIN K

History.   Vitamin K is a nutrient essential for the normal biosynthesis of several factors required for clotting of blood. In 1929, Dam observed that chickens that were fed inadequate diets developed a deficiency disease in which the outstanding symptom was spontaneous bleeding, apparently due to a low content of prothrombin in the blood. Subsequently, Dam and coworkers (1935, 1936) found that the condition could be alleviated rapidly by feeding an unidentified fat-soluble substance. To this substance Dam gave the name *vitamin K* (*Koagulation* vitamin). Independently, Almquist and Stokstad (1935) described the same hemorrhagic disease in chickens and the method for its prevention.

These investigations were reported at a time when the attention of several groups centered on the cause of the hemorrhagic tendency in patients with obstructive jaundice and diseases of the liver. For example, Quick and coworkers (1935) observed that the coagulation defect in jaundiced individuals was due to a decrease in the plasma concentration of prothrombin. In the same year, Hawkins and Whipple reported that animals with biliary fistulas were likely to develop excessive bleeding. Hawkins and Brinkhous (1936) subsequently showed that this was due to a deficiency in prothrombin and that the condition could be relieved by the feeding of bile salts.

The culmination of these studies came with the demonstration by Butt and coworkers (1938) as well as Warner and associates (1938) that combination therapy with vitamin K and bile salts was effective in the treatment of the hemorrhagic diathesis in cases of jaundice. Thus, the relationship between vitamin K, adequate hepatic function, and the physiological mechanisms operating in the normal clotting of blood was established.

Chemistry and Occurrence.   Vitamin K activity is associated with at least two distinct natural substances, designated as vitamin K_1 and vitamin K_2. Vitamin K_1, or *phylloquinone* (phytonadione), is 2-methyl-3-phytyl-1,4-naphthoquinone; it is found in plants and is the only natural vitamin K available for therapeutic use. Vitamin K_2 represents a series of compounds (the *menaquinones*) in which the phytyl side chain of phylloquinone has been replaced by a side chain built up of 2 to 13 prenyl units. Considerable synthesis of menaquinones occurs in gram-positive bacteria, and bacteria in the intestinal tract synthesize the large amounts of vitamin K contained in human and animal feces (*see* Bentley and Meganathan, 1982). In animals, menaquinone-4 can be synthesized from the vitamin precursor *menadione* (2-methyl-1,4-naphthoquinone), or vitamin K_3. Depending on the bioassay system used, menadione is at least as active on a molar basis as phylloquinone. The structures of phylloquinone and the menaquinone series are shown below.

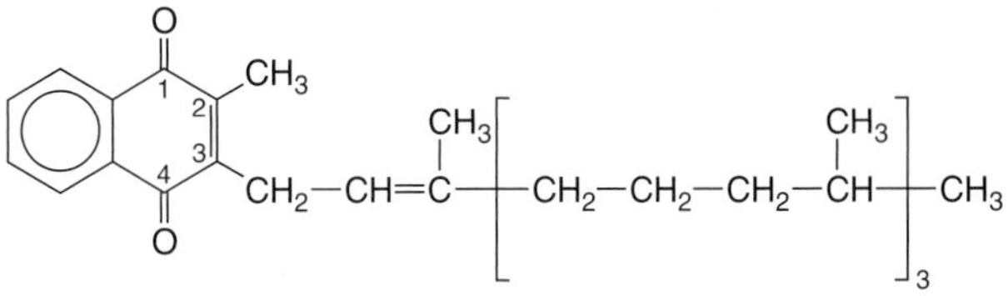

PHYLLOQUINONE (vitamin K_1, phytonadione)

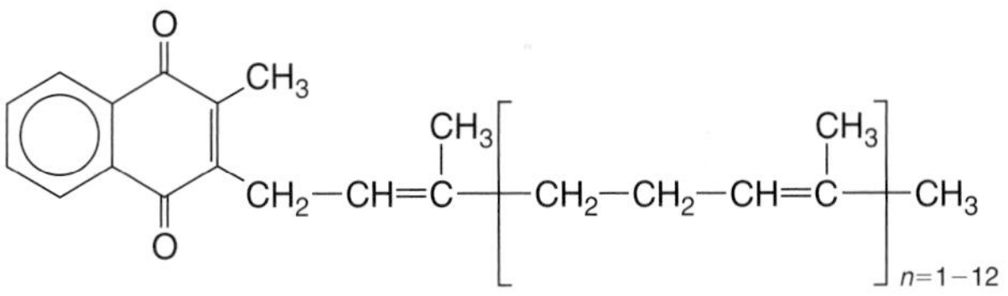

MENAQUINONE (vitamin K_2) series

Physiological Functions and Pharmacological Actions. In normal animals and human beings, phylloquinone and the menaquinones are virtually devoid of pharmacodynamic activity. In animals and human beings deficient in vitamin K, the pharmacological action of vitamin K is identical with its normal physiological function, that is, to promote the hepatic biosynthesis of factor II (prothrombin), factor VII, factor IX, and factor X. The role of these factors in blood clotting is discussed in Chapter 55.

The vitamin K–dependent blood-clotting factors, in the absence of vitamin K (or in the presence of the coumarin type of anticoagulant), are biologically inactive precursor proteins in the liver. Vitamin K functions as an essential cofactor for a microsomal enzyme system that activates these precursors by the conversion of multiple residues of glutamic acid (Glu) near the amino terminus of each precursor to γ-carboxyglutamyl (Gla) residues in the completed protein. The formation of this new amino acid, γ-carboxyglutamic acid, allows the protein to bind Ca^{2+} and in turn to be bound to a phospholipid surface, both of which are necessary in the cascade of events that lead to clot formation (*see* Chapter 55). The active form of vitamin K appears to be the reduced vitamin K hydroquinone, which, in the presence of O_2, CO_2, and the microsomal carboxylase enzyme, is converted to its 2,3-epoxide at the same time γ-carboxylation takes place. The hydroquinone form of vitamin K is regenerated from the 2,3-epoxide by a coumarin-sensitive epoxide reductase (*see* Chapter 55).

Carboxyglutamate is found in a variety of proteins other than the vitamin K–dependent blood-clotting factors (*see* Gallop *et al.*, 1980). One of these is osteocalcin in bone, which is a secretory product of osteoblasts. Its synthesis is regulated by calcitriol, the active form of vitamin D, and its concentration in plasma correlates with the turnover rate of bone. In blood, both protein S and protein C also contain carboxyglutamate (*see* Vermeer *et al.*, 1995).

Human Requirements. The human requirement for vitamin K has not been defined precisely. Frick and associates (1967) estimated the daily requirement, in patients made vitamin K–deficient by a starvation diet and antibiotic therapy for 3 to 4 weeks, to be a minimum of 0.03 μg/kg of body weight; others place the daily requirement at 0.5 to 1 μg/kg, and the RDA approximates 1 μg/kg (*see* Table XIII–1). These estimates have been based on maintenance or restoration of the prothrombin time, which may not be sufficiently sensitive to detect subclinical deficiency of vitamin K (*see* Chapter 55). In the infant, 10 μg/kg of body weight of phylloquinone is sufficient to prevent hypoprothrombinemia. As vitamin K intake decreases, circulating osteocalcin is the first Gla-containing protein to appear in an undercarboxylated form. Nutritional intake of vitamin K decreases with age. Low serum levels of both phylloquinone and menaquinones have been reported in the presence of normal blood coagulation factors. The difference between vitamin K–dependent coagulation factors and osteocalcin suggests that different tissues may have different vitamin K requirements (*see* Vermeer *et al.*, 1995).

Symptoms of Deficiency. The chief clinical manifestation of vitamin K deficiency is an increased tendency to bleed. Ecchymoses, epistaxis, hematuria, gastrointestinal bleeding, and postoperative hemorrhage are common; intracranial hemorrhage may occur. Hemoptysis is uncommon. A further discussion of hypoprothrombinemia is presented in the section on oral anticoagulants (Chapter 55). The discovery of a vitamin K–dependent protein in bone suggests that the fetal bone abnormalities associated with the administration of oral anticoagulants during the first trimester of pregnancy ("fetal warfarin syndrome") may be related to a deficiency of the vitamin.

Considerable evidence indicates a role for vitamin K in adult skeletal maintenance and osteoporosis (*see* Chapter 62). Low concentrations of the vitamin are associated with deficits in bone mineral density and fractures. Vitamin K supplementation improves the carboxylation of undecarboxylated osteocalcin. It also improves bone mineral density, but the relationship of these two effects is unclear (Feskanich *et al.*, 1999).

Toxicity. Phylloquinone and the menaquinones are nontoxic to animals, even when given at 500 times the RDA. However, menadione and its derivatives (synthetic forms of vitamin K) have been implicated in producing hemolytic anemia, hyperbilirubinemia, and kernicterus in the newborn, especially in premature infants (Diploma and Ritchie, 1997). For this reason menadione should no longer be used as a therapeutic form of vitamin K.

Absorption, Fate, and Excretion. The mechanism of intestinal absorption of compounds with vitamin K activity varies with their solubility. In the presence of bile salts, phylloquinone and the menaquinones are adequately absorbed from the intestine, almost entirely by way of the lymph. Phylloquinone is absorbed by an energy-dependent, saturable process in proximal portions of the small intestine; menaquinones are absorbed by diffusion in the distal portions of the small intestine and in the colon. Following absorption, phylloquinone is incorporated into chylomicrons in close association with triglycerides and lipoproteins. In a large survey, plasma phylloquinone and triglyceride concentration were well correlated (Sadowski *et al.*, 1989). The extremely low phylloquinone levels in newborns may be partly related to very low plasma lipoprotein concentrations at birth and may lead to an underestimation of vitamin K tissue stores. After absorption, phylloquinone and menaquinones are concentrated in the liver, but the concentration of phylloquinone declines rapidly. Menaquinones, produced in the lower bowel, are less biologically active than phylloquinone due to their long side chain. For this reason, concentrations of menaquinones are higher than that of phylloquinone in liver and plasma (*see* Suttie, 1995). Menaquinones may partially satisfy human requirements, but the contribution is less than previously thought. Very little vitamin K accumulates in other tissues.

Phylloquinone is metabolized rapidly to more polar metabolites, which are excreted in the bile and urine. The major urinary metabolites result from shortening of the side chain to five or seven carbon atoms, yielding carboxylic acids that are conjugated with glucuronate prior to excretion.

Apparently, there is little storage of vitamin K in the body. Under circumstances where lack of bile interferes with absorption of vitamin K, hypoprothrombinemia develops slowly over a period of several weeks.

Assay and Unitage.   Drugs with vitamin K activity may be chemically assayed and do not require bioassay. Precautions must be taken to protect the vitamin from light during extraction and analysis. Newer methods of analysis that have improved sensitivity and accuracy have been described (Booth *et al.*, 1994).

Therapeutic Uses.   The rational therapeutic use of vitamin K is based on its ability to correct the bleeding tendency or hemorrhage associated with its deficiency. A deficiency of vitamin K and its attendant deficiency of prothrombin and related clotting factors can result from inadequate intake, absorption, or utilization of the vitamin, or as a consequence of the action of a vitamin K antagonist.

Phylloquinone (AQUAMEPHYTON, KONAKION, MEPHYTON) is available as tablets and in a dispersion with buffered polysorbate and propylene glycol (KONAKION) or polyoxyethylated fatty acid derivatives and dextrose (AQUAMEPHYTON). KONAKION is administered only intramuscularly. AQUAMEPHYTON may be given by any parenteral route, although severe reactions resembling anaphylaxis have followed its intravenous injection; subcutaneous or intramuscular administration is preferred.

Inadequate Intake.   After infancy, hypoprothrombinemia arising from a dietary deficiency of vitamin K is extremely rare, because not only is the vitamin present in many foods but also it is synthesized by intestinal bacteria. Occasionally, the use of a broad-spectrum antibiotic may of itself produce a hypoprothrombinemia that responds readily to small doses of vitamin K and reestablishment of normal bowel flora. Hypoprothrombinemia can occur in patients receiving prolonged intravenous alimentation. It is recommended to give 1 mg of phylloquinone per week (the equivalent of about 150 μg per day) to patients on total parenteral nutrition.

Hypoprothrombinemia of the Newborn.   Healthy newborn infants show decreased plasma concentrations of vitamin K–dependent clotting factors for a few days after birth, the time required to obtain an adequate dietary intake of the vitamin and to establish a normal intestinal flora. Subsequently, levels begin to rise toward adult values. In premature infants and in infants with hemorrhagic disease of the newborn, the concentrations of clotting factors are particularly depressed. The degree to which these changes reflect true vitamin K deficiency is controversial. Using sensitive measurements on non-γ-carboxylated prothrombin, Shapiro and colleagues (1986) found evidence of vitamin K deficiency in about 3% of live births.

Hemorrhagic disease of the newborn has been associated with breast-feeding; human milk has low concentrations of vitamin K (Haroon *et al.*, 1982), and, in addition, the intestinal flora of breast-fed infants apparently lacks microorganisms that synthesize the vitamin (Keenan *et al.*, 1971). All commercial infant formulas are supplemented with vitamin K.

Administration of vitamin K to the normal newborn infant prevents the decline in concentration of the clotting factors in the days following birth; it does not, however, raise these concentrations to the adult level. Premature infants usually display less of a response to the administration of vitamin K. In the infant with hemorrhagic disease of the newborn, the adminis-

tration of vitamin K raises the concentration of these clotting factors to the level normal for the newborn infant and controls the bleeding tendency within about 6 hours.

The routine prophylactic administration of 1 mg phylloquinone intramuscularly at birth is required by law in the United States. This dose may have to be increased or repeated if the mother has received anticoagulant or anticonvulsant drug therapy or if the infant develops bleeding tendencies. Alternatively, some clinicians treat mothers who are receiving anticonvulsants with oral vitamin K prior to delivery (20 mg per day for 2 weeks) (*see* Vert and Deblay, 1982).

Inadequate Absorption.   Hypoprothrombinemia may be associated with either intrahepatic or extrahepatic biliary obstruction, because the lipid-soluble vitamin is poorly absorbed in the absence of bile. A severe defect in the intestinal absorption of fat from the other causes also can interfere with absorption of the vitamin.

Biliary Obstruction or Fistula.   Bleeding that accompanies obstructive jaundice or biliary fistula responds promptly to the administration of vitamin K. Oral phylloquinone administered with bile salts is both safe and effective and should be used in the care of the jaundiced patient, both preoperatively and postoperatively. In the absence of significant hepatocellular disease, the prothrombin activity of the blood rapidly returns to normal. If for some reason oral administration is not feasible, a parenteral preparation should be used. The usual dose is 10 mg of vitamin K per day.

The treatment of a patient during hemorrhage requires transfusion of fresh blood or reconstituted fresh plasma. Vitamin K also should be given. If biliary obstruction has caused hepatic injury, the response to vitamin K may be poor.

Malabsorption Syndromes.   Various disorders that result in inadequate absorption from the intestinal tract may lead to a deficiency of vitamin K and hypoprothrombinemia. These include cystic fibrosis, sprue, Crohn's disease and enterocolitis, ulcerative colitis, dysentery, and extensive resection of bowel. Since drugs that greatly reduce the bacterial population of the bowel are used frequently in many of these disorders, the availability of the vitamin may be further reduced. Moreover, dietary restrictions also may limit the availability of the vitamin. For immediate correction of the deficiency, parenteral therapy should be used.

Inadequate Utilization.   Hepatocellular disease may be accompanied or followed by hypoprothrombinemia. Hepatocellular damage also may be secondary to long-lasting biliary obstruction. In these conditions, the damaged parenchymal cells may not be able to produce the vitamin K–dependent clotting factors, even if excess vitamin is available. However, in some instances an inadequate secretion of bile salts may contribute to the syndrome, and some benefit may be obtained from the parenteral administration of 10 mg of phylloquinone daily. Paradoxically, the administration of large doses of vitamin K or its analogs in an attempt to correct the hypoprothrombinemia associated with severe hepatitis or cirrhosis actually may result in a further depression of the concentration of prothrombin. The mechanism for this action is unknown.

Drug-Induced Hypoprothrombinemia.   Anticoagulant drugs such as warfarin and its congeners act as competitive antagonists of vitamin K and interfere with the hepatic biosynthesis of prothrombin and factors VII, IX, and X. The mechanism of this antagonism has been discussed above and in Chapter 55.

The treatment of bleeding caused by oral anticoagulants also is discussed in Chapter 55. Vitamin K may be of help in combating the bleeding and hypoprothrombinemia that follow the bite of the tropical American pit viper or other species whose venom destroys or inactivates prothrombin.

VITAMIN E

In animals, the signs of deficiency of vitamin E include structural and functional abnormalities of many organs and organ systems. Attending these morphological alterations are biochemical defects that appear to involve fatty acid metabolism and numerous other enzyme systems. Notable is the fact that many signs and symptoms of vitamin E deficiency in animals superficially resemble disease states in human beings; however, there is little unequivocal evidence that vitamin E is of nutritional significance in human beings.

History.   The existence of vitamin E was first demonstrated in 1922 by Evans and Bishop, who found that female rats required a then-unrecognized dietary principle to sustain a normal pregnancy. Deficient animals were found to ovulate and conceive normally, but at some time during the period of gestation, death and resorption of the fetuses occurred. Lesions in the testes also were described, and for a while vitamin E was referred to as the "antisterility vitamin." Further studies, however, revealed the more widespread effects of deficiency of the vitamin.

Chemistry.   The vitamin was isolated by Evans and coworkers (1936) from wheat-germ oil. Eight naturally occurring tocopherols with vitamin E activity are now known. The biologically most active form is RRR-α-tocopherol (formerly d-α-tocopherol), which constitutes about 90% of the tocopherols in animal tissues and displays the greatest biological activity in most bioassay systems. Optical isomerism affects activity; d forms are more active than l forms. α-Tocopherol is synthesized commercially. The synthetic compound is designated *all-rac*-α-tocopherol (previously d,l-α-tocopherol). Vitamin E supplements are marketed as mixed tocopherols.

RRR-α-TOCOPHEROL

One of the important chemical features of the tocopherols is that they are redox agents that act under some circumstances as antioxidants, and this apparently is the basis for most, but perhaps not all, of the effects of vitamin E. The tocopherols deteriorate slowly when exposed to air or ultraviolet light.

Physiological Functions and Pharmacological Actions.   The antioxidant properties of vitamin E ameliorate free-radical damage to biological membranes. Vitamin E protects polyunsaturated fatty acids (PUFA) within membrane phospholipids and within circulating lipoproteins (Burton *et al.*, 1983). Peroxyl radicals (ROO$\cdot$) react 1000-fold faster with vitamin E than with PUFA, forming the corresponding organic hydroperoxide and the tocopheroxyl radical (vitamin E-O$\cdot$). The tocopheroxyl radical, in turn, interacts with other antioxidant compounds, such as ascorbic acid, which regenerates tocopherol. It is unlikely that the biological activity of vitamin E exclusively reflects its antioxidant function, as the relationship between antioxidant potency and biological activity is not exact. Naturally occurring forms of vitamin E differ in their antioxidant properties, whereas synthetic α-tocopherols are identical in this regard.

Symptoms of Deficiency.   Although manifestations of vitamin E deficiency in experimental animals are protean, various effects on the nervous, reproductive, muscular, cardiovascular, and hematopoietic systems are most important because they bear the closest resemblance to the clinical syndromes alleged to be benefited by vitamin E therapy.

Nervous System.   In animals, particularly rats, vitamin E deficiency is associated with axonal dystrophy that involves degeneration in the posterior cord and in the gracile and cuneate nuclei. Observations in human beings suggest a relationship between vitamin E deficiency and a similar clinical syndrome. Patients with malabsorption syndromes that are associated with decreased absorption or transport of vitamin E develop similar neurological symptoms, including hyporeflexia, gait disturbances, decreased sensitivity to vibration and proprioception, and ophthalmoplegia. Visual impairment may result from a pigmented retinopathy. Neuropathological lesions, including axonal degeneration of the posterior cord and the gracilis nucleus, are comparable with those found in animals deficient in vitamin E. In some studies, treatment of patients with pharmacological doses of vitamin E prevented progression of the neurological abnormalities or caused improvement (*see* Bieri *et al.*, 1983; Sokol, 1988).

Reproductive System.   Early evidence indicated that vitamin E is essential for normal reproduction in several mammalian species. On the basis of such animal studies, vitamin E has been used clinically for the treatment of recurrent abortion and for sterility in both men and women. It also has been used in toxemia of pregnancy, disorders of menstruation, vaginitis, and menopausal symptoms. There is no evidence, however, that the vitamin is beneficial in any of these conditions.

Muscular System.   In many species, a vitamin E–deficient diet leads to the development of a necrotizing myopathy that resembles muscular dystrophy and can be prevented, reversed, or ameliorated with α-tocopherol or other lipid-soluble antioxidants. Although myopathic changes also may occur in human subjects deprived of vitamin E, there is no evidence for vitamin E deficiency in the muscular dystrophies in human beings, and the administration of vitamin E is ineffective in these disorders.

Atherosclerosis.   Oxidation of low-density lipoproteins (LDL) contributes to atherogenesis (*see* Chapter 36). Oxidized LDL is more effectively taken up than native LDL by macrophages, may adversely affect vascular endothelial cells, and may be vasoconstrictive. Pharmacological amounts of vitamin E (1600 mg/day) protect LDL from oxidation (Reaven *et al.*, 1993). A growing literature has addressed the relationship of vitamin E to coronary heart and peripheral vascular disease. The mechanisms by which vitamin E may confer cardiovascular protection are unclear. Although its characteristic antioxidant actions receive mention in this regard, direct effects on vascular endothelium, smooth muscle cells, or clotting also may be operative (*see* Diaz *et al.*, 1997). Vitamin E regulates proliferation of vascular smooth muscle cells, perhaps by inhibiting protein kinase C (Azzi *et al.*, 1998). In addition, the vitamin preserves endothelial-dependent vasodilation and inhibits both platelet activation and leukocyte adhesion (*see* Diaz *et al.*, 1997).

Two large epidemiological studies support the view that supplemental vitamin E reduces the risk of coronary heart disease. Among middle-aged women whose vitamin E intake was in the highest quintile, the risk for myocardial infarction and ischemic heart disease death was almost 40% lower than for women in the lowest vitamin E quintile (Stampfer *et al.*, 1993). Moreover, the primary benefit was due to use of supplemental vitamin E, since analysis by dietary vitamin E intake alone did not show relationship with coronary heart disease risk. Another study indicates a similar reduction in risk for coronary heart disease for men who took at least 100 U/day of vitamin E for at least two years (Rimm *et al.*, 1993). Unlike the epidemiological studies, controlled clinical trials have not been strongly supportive of a cardiovascular benefit from vitamin E supplementation. The efficacy of a daily vitamin E dose of 400 U in preventing cardiovascular events was suggested by one randomized controlled trial (Stephens *et al.*, 1996), but more recent clinical trials raise considerable doubt about vitamin E–related cardiovascular protection. In one large trial, patients at high risk for vascular events were randomized to receive either 400 U per day of vitamin E or placebo. After an average of 4.5 years, no significant differences between groups were observed at any time in cardiovascular death, myocardial infarction, stroke, or any secondary cardiovascular outcome (Yusuf *et al.*, 2000). These results were similar to those of another recent trial in which a daily vitamin E dose of 300 U for 3.5 years achieved no significant reduction in the rate of death or myocardial infarction (GISSI-Prevenzione Investigators, 1999). Thus, cardiovascular protective effects of vitamin E cannot presently be considered to be established.

Cancer. In some animal models, vitamin E inhibits formation of carcinogenic nitrosamines and modifies the occurrence and behavior of tumors. The effects of vitamin E intake on human cancers remain unclear. Diets containing large amounts of antioxidant vitamins A, C, and E have been associated with a reduced risk for various malignancies. However, in a large epidemiological study, even very large intakes of vitamin E did not protect women from breast cancer (Hunter *et al.*, 1993). In a recent clinical trial, higher baseline serum levels of α-tocopherol predicted a lower risk of lung cancer, but vitamin E treatment was actually associated with an 18% increase in subsequent lung cancer incidence (Alpha-Tocopherol, β-Carotene Cancer Prevention Study Group, 1994). Thus, nutrient deficiency may increase the risk of malignancy, for which replacement therapy should be effective, but pharmacological doses of antioxidant nutrients may be inert or even harmful (*see* Herbert, 1994).

Hematopoietic System. In several animal species a deficiency of vitamin E is associated with an anemia that has features of both abnormal hematopoiesis and decreased lifetime of erythrocytes. Erythrocytes from such animals have increased susceptibility to hemolysis by oxidizing agents. Indeed, in human beings this *in vitro* laboratory test is the only consistent finding associated with low levels of α-tocopherol in plasma (*see* Leonard

and Losowsky, 1967). Limited clinical studies in patients with hemolysis due to a genetic deficiency of glucose-6-phosphate dehydrogenase suggest that chronic treatment with large doses of vitamin E may improve survival of erythrocytes and the clinical condition (Corash *et al.*, 1980).

Four clinical situations have been reported to include α-tocopherol–responsive anemia (*see* Darby, 1968). (1) A macrocytic, megaloblastic anemia observed in children with severe protein-calorie malnutrition, while unresponsive to treatment with iron, cyanocobalamin, folic acid, or ascorbic acid, was reversed with large doses of α-tocopheryl acetate. However, subsequent controlled studies have attributed the defective hematopoiesis to deficiency of protein and/or iron rather than to vitamin E (*see* Bieri and Farrell, 1976). (2) Premature infants may develop a hemolytic anemia that is sometimes associated with increased erythrocyte susceptibility to peroxidative hemolysis and low concentrations of tocopherol in plasma. This anemia has been shown to develop only in infants who consume a diet rich in polyunsaturated fatty acids and fortified with iron (Williams *et al.*, 1975). Commercial formulas for premature infants have been modified, such that they now are very low in iron and have an appropriate ratio of vitamin E to fatty acids. It no longer appears to be necessary to administer vitamin E supplements to premature infants on a routine basis (Zipursky *et al.*, 1987). (3) Erythrocytes that hemolyze spontaneously *in vitro* constitute one characteristic of the acanthocytosis syndrome. Patients with this rare genetic disease lack plasma β-lipoprotein and, therefore, have little or no circulating α-tocopherol. Further, they have impaired intestinal absorption of the vitamin. Parenteral administration of 100 mg of α-tocopherol acetate can raise the plasma α-tocopherol concentration and apparently correct the autohemolytic feature of the disease for several weeks. (4) In malabsorption syndromes characterized by steatorrhea, α-tocopherol is not absorbed. Here, too, decreased erythrocyte lifetime and increased erythrocyte sensitivity to hydrogen peroxide are coincident with low concentrations of α-tocopherol in plasma and are responsive to administration of α-tocopherol. Adult human subjects, intentionally deprived of vitamin E over an extended period of time, have similar hematological lesions and respond to α-tocopherol (Horwitt *et al.*, 1963).

While the above evidence seems to implicate vitamin E in normal hematopoiesis, patients with these syndromes have multiple deficiencies, and the ability of other antioxidants and sulfur-amino acids to relieve "tocopherol-deficient" syndromes to varying degrees complicates a definitive interpretation. (*See* Bieri and Farrell, 1976; Machlin, 1980.)

Human Requirements. With long-term depletion in human beings, the vitamin E concentration in plasma declines significantly only after months on a deficient diet (*see* Horwitt, 1962). A daily intake of 10 to 30 mg of vitamin E is sufficient to maintain normal concentrations in blood. Although some studies have suggested that diets containing large amounts of unsaturated fatty acids increase the daily requirement, it should be noted the dietary sources of these fats also are rich in vitamin E. Diets containing other antioxidants decrease the requirement.

The adult RDA for vitamin E is 10 mg/day of α-tocopherol equivalents for men and 8 mg per day for women (*see* Table XIII–1). Human milk (in contrast to cow's milk) has sufficient α-tocopherol to meet normal requirements of infants.

Tocopherols are present in adequate amounts in the normal adult diet. Indeed, vitamin E deficiency has not been detected as a primary deficiency disease in otherwise healthy children or adults.

Absorption, Fate, and Excretion.   Vitamin E is absorbed from the gastrointestinal tract by a mechanism similar to that for the other fat-soluble vitamins; bile is essential. When administered as an ester, hydrolysis takes place in the intestine. Vitamin E enters the bloodstream in chylomicrons by way of the lymph. It is taken up in chylomicron remnants by the liver, and is secreted in very-low-density lipoproteins; subsequently, it becomes associated with plasma low-density lipoproteins. Vitamin E is distributed to all tissues. However, newborn infants have plasma tocopherol concentrations only about one-fifth those of their mothers, suggesting poor placental transfer. Tissue stores (principally in the liver and adipose tissue) can provide a source of the vitamin for long periods of time, as evidenced by the long time animals must be kept on a vitamin E–deficient diet before signs of deficiency appear.

Seventy to 80% of an intravenously administered dose of radioactive vitamin E is excreted by the liver over a period of a week; the balance appears as metabolites in the urine. The urinary metabolites are glucuronides of tocopheronic acid and its γ-lactone. Several other metabolites with quinone structures have been found in tissues; dimer and trimer forms of the vitamin are believed to result from reaction with lipid peroxides (*see* Draper and Csallany, 1970).

Plasma concentrations vary widely among normal individuals and fluctuate with concentrations of lipids. As a result, measurement of the ratio of vitamin E to total lipids in plasma has been used to estimate vitamin E status; values below 0.8 mg/g are indicative of deficiency (Horwitt, 1962). In general, tocopherol concentrations in plasma appear to be related more closely to dietary intake and defects in intestinal absorption of fat than to the presence or absence of disease.

Assay and Unitage.   The vitamin E activity of foods may be determined chemically or bioassayed. One international unit (IU) is equivalent to the activity of 1 mg of *all-rac-α*-tocopheryl acetate, 0.67 mg of RRR-α-tocopherol, or 0.74 mg of RRR-α-tocopherol acetate. The activity of 1 mg of *d-α*-tocopherol is equal to one α-tocopherol equivalent.

Therapeutic Uses.   The lack of efficacy of vitamin E in treatment of those diseases in human beings that bear some resemblance to vitamin E deficiency in animals (recurrent abortion, progressive muscular dystrophy, and cardiomyopathy) has been discussed. These are by no means the only disorders in which vitamin E therapy has been studied. The list extends from minor skin ailments to schizophrenia.

Vitamin E (AQUASOL E, others) is a form of α-tocopherol that includes the *d* or mixtures of the *d* and *l* isomers of α-tocopherol, α-tocopheryl acetate, or α-tocopheryl succinate. For severe vitamin E deficiency in children, injectable *d,l-α*-tocopherol (EPHYNAL) is available in some countries, but not in the United States.

The use of vitamin E supplements may be indicated for patients at risk of developing deficiency of the vitamin in order to prevent or ameliorate the consequences of axonal dystrophy (*see* above). Children with cystic fibrosis, cholestatic liver disease, or other types of malabsorption syndromes are especially likely to develop vitamin E deficiency. There also is a rare congenital disorder that is characterized by vitamin E deficiency and neurological manifestations but without a disturbance of intestinal absorption (*see* Sokol, 1988). Correction of an established deficiency usually can be accomplished by the oral administration of high doses of vitamin E (50 to 200 mg/kg per day). The dosage may be adjusted as the ratio of vitamin E to total lipids in plasma is altered. When oral therapy is unsuccessful, *d,l-α*-tocopherol (1 to 2 mg/kg per day) may be administered intramuscularly (*see* Sokol, 1988). Pharmacological doses of vitamin E also have been used as an antioxidant in premature infants exposed to high concentrations of oxygen; prophylactic use of an oral preparation (100 mg/kg per day) may reduce the incidence and severity of retrolental fibroplasia (Hittner *et al.*, 1981). Only equivocal results have been obtained in the neonatal respiratory-distress syndrome.

For further discussion of disorders associated with vitamin deficiencies and excesses, *see* Chapter 79 in *Harrison's Principles of Internal Medicine,* 14th ed., McGraw-Hill, New York, 1998.

BIBLIOGRAPHY

Achkar, C.C., Bentel, J.M., Boylan, J.F., Scher, H.I., Gudas, L.J., and Miller, W.H. Jr. Differences in the pharmacokinetic properties of orally administered all-*trans*-retinoic acid and 9-*cis*-retinoic acid in the plasma of nude mice. *Drug Metab. Dispos.,* **1994,** *22*:451–458.

Almquist, H.J., and Stokstad, C.L.R. Hemorrhagic chick disease of dietary origin. *J. Biol. Chem.,* **1935,** *111*:105–113.

Alpha-Tocopherol, β-Carotene Cancer Prevention Study Group. The effect of vitamin E and beta carotene on the incidence of lung cancer and other cancers in male smokers. *N. Engl. J. Med.*, **1994**, *330*:1029–1035.

Anonymous. Vitamin A for measles. *Lancet*, **1987**, *1*:1067–1068.

Azzi, A., Aratri, E., Boscoboinik, D., Clement, S., Ozer, N.K., Ricciarelli, R., and Spycher, S. Molecular basis of alpha-tocopherol control of smooth muscle cell proliferation. *Bio. Factors*, **1998**, *7*:3–14.

Bernhardt, I.B., and Dorsey, D.J. Hypervitaminosis A and congenital renal anomalies in a human infant. *Obstet. Gynecol.*, **1974**, *43*:750–755.

Booth, S.L., Davidson, K.W., and Sadowski, J.A. Evaluation of an HPLC method for the determination of phylloquinone (vitamin K_1) in various food matrices. *J. Agric. Food Chem.*, **1994**, *42*:295–300.

Burton, G.W., Joyce, A., and Ingold, K.U. Is vitamin E the only lipid-soluble, chain-breaking antioxidant in human blood plasma and erythrocyte membranes? *Arch. Biochem. Biophys.*, **1983**, *221*:281–290.

Butt, H.R., Snell, A.M., and Osterberg, A.E. The use of vitamin K and bile in treatment of hemorrhagic diathesis in cases of jaundice. *Proc. Staff Meet. Mayo Clin.*, **1938**, *13*:74–80.

Castaigne, S., Chomienne, C., Daniel, M.T., Ballerini, P., Berger, R., Fenaux, P., and Degos, L. All-*trans* retinoic acid as a differentiation therapy for acute promyelocytic leukemia. I. Clinical results. *Blood*, **1990**, *76*:1704–1709.

Chambon, P. The molecular and genetic dissection of the retinoid signaling pathway. *Recent Prog. Horm. Res.*, **1995**, *50*:317–332.

Chen, S.-J., Zhu, Y.-J., Tong, J.-H., Dong, S., Huang, W., Chen, Y., Xiang, W.-M., Zhang, L., Li, X.- S., Qian, G.-Q., Wang, Z.-Y., Chen, Z., Larsen, C.-J., and Berger, R. Rearrangements in the second intron of the RARA gene are present in a large majority of patients with acute promyelocytic leukemia and are used as molecular marker for retinoic acid–induced leukemic cell differentiation. *Blood*, **1991**, *78*:2696–2701.

Collins, S.J., Robertson, K.A., and Mueller, L. Retinoic acid–induced granulocytic differentiation of HL-60 myeloid leukemia cells is mediated directly through the retinoic acid receptor (RAR-alpha). *Mol. Cell. Biol.*, **1990**, *10*:2154–2163.

Corash, L., Spielberg, S., Bartsocas, C., Boxer, L., Steinherz, R., Sheetz, M., Egan, M., Schlessleman, J., and Schulman, J.D. Reduced chronic hemolysis during high-dose vitamin E administration in Mediterranean-type glucose-6-phosphate dehydrogenase deficiency. *N. Engl. J. Med.*, **1980**, *303*:416–420.

Dam, H., and Schønheyder, F. The antihaemorrhagic vitamin of the chick. *Nature*, **1935**, *135*:652–653.

Dam, H., Schønheyder, F., and Tage-Hansen, E. Studies on the mode of action of vitamin K. *Biochem. J.*, **1936**, *30*:1075–1079.

Diploma, J.R., and Ritchie, D.M. Vitamin toxicity. *Annu. Rev. Pharmacol. Toxicol.*, **1997**, *17*:133–148.

Evans, H.M., and Bishop, K.S. On the relationship between fertility and nutrition. II. The ovulation rhythm in the rat on inadequate nutritional regimes. *J. Metab. Res.*, **1922**, *1*:319–356.

Evans, H.M., Emerson, O.H., and Emerson, G.A. The isolation from wheat germ oil of an alcohol, α-tocopherol, having properties of vitamin E. *J. Biol. Chem.*, **1936**, *113*:329–332.

Feskanich, D., Weber, P., Willett, W.C., Rockett, H., Booth, S.L., and Colditz, G.A. Vitamin K intake and hip fractures in women: a prospective study. *Am. J. Clin. Nutr.*, **1999**, *69*:74–79.

Frick, P.G., Riedler, G., and Brögli, H. Dose response and minimal daily requirement for vitamin K in man. *J. Appl. Physiol.*, **1967**, *23*:387–389.

GISSI-Prevenzione Investigators. Dietary supplementation with n-3 polyunsaturated fatty acids and vitamin E after myocardial infarc-

tion: results of the GISSI Prevenzione trial. Gruppo Italiano per lo Studio della Sopravvivenza nell'Infarto miocardio. *Lancet*, **1999**, *354*:447–455.

Greenberg, E.R., Baron, J.A., Tosteson, T.D., Freeman, D.H. Jr., Beck, G.J., Bond, J.H., Colacchio, T.A., Coller, J.A., Frankl, H.D., Haile, R.W., Mandel, J.S., Nierenberg, D.W., Rothstein, R., Snover, D.C., Stevens, M.M., Summers, R.W., and van Stolk, R.U. A clinical trial of antioxidant vitamins to prevent colorectal adenoma. Polyp Prevention Study Group. *N. Engl. J. Med.*, **1994**, *331*:141–147.

Haroon, Y., Shearer, M.J., Rahim, S., Gunn, W.G., McEnery, G., and Barkhan, P. The content of phylloquinone (vitamin K_1) in human milk, cows' milk, and infant formula foods determined by high-performance liquid chromatography. *J. Nutr.*, **1982**, *112*:1105–1117.

Hawkins, W.B., and Brinkhous, K.M. Prothrombin deficiency as the cause of bleeding in bile fistula dogs. *J. Exp. Med.*, **1936**, *63*:795–801.

Heyman, R.A., Mangelsdorf, D.J., Dyck, J.A., Stein, R.B., Eichele, G., Evans, R.M., and Thaller, C. 9-*cis* retinoic acid is a high affinity ligand for the retinoid X receptor. *Cell*, **1992**, *68*:397–406.

Hittner, H.M., Godio, L.B., Rudolph, A.J., Adams, J.M., Garcia-Prats, J.A., Friedman, Z., Kautz, J.A., and Monaco, W.A. Retrolental fibroplasia: efficacy of vitamin E in a double-blind clinical study of preterm infants. *N. Engl. J. Med.*, **1981**, *305*:1365–1371.

Horwitt, M.K. Interrelations between vitamin E and polyunsaturated fatty acids in adult men. *Vitam. Horm.*, **1962**, *20*:541–558.

Horwitt, M.K., Century, B., and Zeman, A.A. Erythrocyte survival time and reticulocyte level after tocopherol depletion in man. *Am. J. Clin. Nutr.*, **1963**, *12*:99–106.

Horwitt, M.K., Harvey, C.C., Dahm, C.H. Jr., and Searcy, M.T. Relationship between tocopherol and serum lipid levels for determination of nutritional adequacy. *Ann. N.Y. Acad. Sci.*, **1972**, *203*:223–236.

Hunter, D.J., Manson, J.E., Colditz, G.A., Stampfer, M.J., Rosner, B., Hennekens, C.H., Speizer, F.E., and Willett, W.C. A prospective study of the intake of vitamins C, E, and A and the risk of breast cancer. *N. Engl. J. Med.*, **1993**, *329*:234–240.

Hussey, G.D., and Klein, M. A randomized, controlled trial of vitamin A in children with severe measles. *N. Engl. J. Med.*, **1990**, *323*:160–164.

Kaplan, L.A., Lau, J.M., and Stein, E.A. Carotenoid composition, concentrations, and relationships in various human organs. *Clin. Physiol. Biochem.*, **1990**, *8*:1–10.

Keenan, W.J., Jewett, T., and Glueck, H.I. Role of feeding and vitamin K in hypoprothrombinemia of the newborn. *Am. J. Dis. Child.*, **1971**, *121*:271–277.

Lakshman, M.R., Mychkovsky, I., and Attlesey, M. Enzymatic conversion of all-*trans*-β-carotene to retinal by a cytosolic enzyme from rabbit and rat intestinal mucosa. *Proc. Natl. Acad. Sci. U.S.A.*, **1989**, *86*:9124–9128.

Lee, I.-M., Cook, N.R., Manson, J.E., Buring, J.E., and Hennekens, C.H. β-Carotene supplementation and incidence of cancer and cardiovascular disease: the Women's Health Study. *J. Natl. Cancer Inst.*, **1999**, *91*:2102–2106.

Leo, M.A., and Lieber, C.S. Hepatic vitamin A depletion in alcoholic liver injury. *N. Engl. J. Med.*, **1982**, *307*:597–601.

Leonard, P.J., and Losowsky, M.S. Relationship between plasma vitamin E level and peroxide hemolysis test in human subjects. *Am. J. Clin. Nutr.*, **1967**, *20*:795–798.

Levin, A.A., Sturzenbecker, L.J., Kazmer, S., Bosakowski, T., Huselton, C., Allenby, G., Speck, J., Kratzeisen, C.I., Rosenberger, M., Lovey, A., and Grippo, J.F. 9-*Cis* retinoic acid stereoisomer binds and activates the nuclear receptor RXRα. *Nature*, **1992**, *355*:359–361.

McCollum, E.V., and Davis, M. The necessity of certain lipids in the diet during growth. *J. Biol. Chem.,* **1913,** *15*:167–175.

Osborne, T.B., and Mendel, L.B. The relation of growth to the chemical constituents of the diet. *J. Biol. Chem.,* **1913,** *15*:311–326.

Quick, A.J., Stanley-Brown, M., and Bancroft, F.W. A study of the coagulation defect in hemophilia and in jaundice. *Am. J. Med. Sci.,* **1935,** *190*:501–511.

Reaven, P.D., Khouw, A., Beltz, W.F., Parthasarathy, S., and Witztum, J.L. Effect of dietary antioxidant combination in humans. Protection of LDL by vitamin E but not by β-carotene. *Arterioscler. Thromb.,* **1993,** *13*:590–600.

Rimm, E.B., Stampfer, M.J., Ascherio, A., Giovannucci, E., Colditz, G.A., and Willett, W.C. Vitamin E consumption and the risk of coronary heart disease in men. *N. Engl. J. Med.,* **1993,** *328*:1450–1456.

Rosso, G.C., De Luca, L., Warren, C.D., and Wolf, G. Enzymatic synthesis of mannosyl retinyl phosphate from retinyl phosphate and guanosine diphosphate mannose. *J. Lipid Res.,* **1975,** *16*:235–243.

Sadowski, J.A., Hood, S.J., Dallal, G.E., and Garry, P.J. Phylloquinone in plasma from elderly and young adults: factors influencing its concentration. *Am. J. Clin. Nutr.,* **1989,** *50*:100–108.

Shapiro, A.D., Jacobson, L.J., Armon, M.E., Manco-Johnson, M.J., Hulac, P., Lane, P.A., and Hathaway, W.E. Vitamin K deficiency in the newborn infant: prevalence and perinatal risk factors. *J. Pediatr.,* **1986,** *109*:675–680.

Stahl, W., Schwarz, W., Sundquist, A.R., and Sies, H. *Cis-trans* isomers of lycopene and β-carotene in human serum and tissues. *Arch. Biochem. Biophys.,* **1992,** *294*:173–177.

Stampfer, M.J., Hennekens, C.H., Manson, J.E., Colditz, G.A., Rosner, B., and Willett, W.C. Vitamin E consumption and the risk of coronary disease in women. *N. Engl. J. Med.,* **1993,** *328*:1444–1449.

Steenbock, H. White corn vs. yellow corn, and a probable relation between the fat-soluble vitamin and yellow plant pigments. *Science,* **1919,** *50*:352–353.

Stephens, N.G., Parsons, A., Schofield, P.M., Kelly, F., Cheeseman, K., and Mitchinson, M.J. Randomised controlled trial of vitamin E in patients with coronary disease: Cambridge Heart Antioxidant Study. *Lancet,* **1996,** *347*:781–786.

Wald, G. The molecular basis of visual excitation. *Nature,* **1968,** *219*:800–807.

Warner, E.D., Brinkhous, K.M., and Smith, H.P. Bleeding tendency of obstructive jaundice: prothrombin deficiency and dietary factors. *Proc. Soc. Exp. Biol. Med.,* **1938,** *37*:628–630.

Warrell, R.P. Jr., Frankel, S.R., Miller, W.H. Jr., Scheinberg, D.A., Itri, L.M., Hittelman, W.N., Vyas, R., Andreeff, M., Tafuri, A., Jakubowski, A., Gabrilove, J., Gordon, M.S., and Dmitrovsky, E. Differentiation therapy of acute promyelocytic leukemia with tretinoin (all-*trans*-retinoic acid). *N. Engl. J. Med.,* **1991,** *324*:1385–1393.

Williams, M.L., Shoot, R.J., O'Neal, P.L., and Oski, F.A. Role of dietary iron and fat on vitamin E deficiency anemia of infancy. *N. Engl. J. Med.,* **1975,** *292*:887–890.

Yusuf, S., Dagenais, G., Pogue, J., Bosch, J., and Sleight, P. Vitamin E supplementation and cardiovascular events in high-risk patients. The Heart Outcomes Prevention Evaluation Study Investigators. *N. Engl. J. Med.,* **2000,** *342*:154–160.

Zile, M.H., Inhorn, R.C., and DeLuca, H.F. Metabolism in vivo of all-*trans*-retinoic acid. Biosynthesis of 13-*cis*-retinoic acid and all-*trans*- and 13-*cis*-retinoyl β-glucuronides in the intestinal mucosa of the rat. *J. Biol. Chem.,* **1982,** *257*:3544–3550.

Zipursky, A., Brown, E.J., Watts, J., Milner, R., Rand, C., Blanchette, V.S., Bell, E.F., Paes, B., and Ling, E. Oral vitamin E supplementation for the prevention of anemia in premature infants: a controlled trial. *Pediatrics,* **1987,** *79*:61–68.

MONOGRAPHS AND REVIEWS

Bendich, A., and Langseth, L. Safety of vitamin A. *Am. J. Clin. Nutr.,* **1989,** *49*:358–371.

Bendich, A., and Olson, J.A. Biological actions of carotenoids. *FASEB J.,* **1989,** *3*:1927–1932.

Bentley, R., and Meganathan, R. Biosynthesis of vitamin K (menaquinone) in bacteria. *Microbiol. Rev.,* **1982,** *46*:241–280.

Bieri, J.G., Corash, L., and Hubbard, V.S. Medical uses of vitamin E. *N. Engl. J. Med.,* **1983,** *308*:1063–1071.

Bieri, J.G., and Farrell, P.M. Vitamin E. *Vitam. Horm.,* **1976,** *34*:31–75.

Darby, W.J. Tocopherol-responsive anemias in man. *Vitam. Horm.,* **1968,** *26*:685–704.

Diaz, M.N., Frei, B., Vita, J.A., and Keaney, J.F. Jr. Antioxidants and atherosclerotic heart disease. *N. Engl. J. Med.,* **1997,** *337*:408–416.

Draper, H.H., and Csallany, A.S. Metabolism of vitamin E. In, *The Fat Soluble Vitamins.* (DeLuca, H.F., and Suttie, J.W., eds.) University of Wisconsin Press, Madison, **1970,** pp. 347–353.

Evans, T.R., and Kaye, S.B. Retinoids: present role and future potential. *Br. J. Cancer,* **1999,** *80*:1–8.

Gallop, P.M., Lian, J.B., and Hauschka, P.V. Carboxylated calcium-binding proteins and vitamin K. *N. Engl. J. Med.,* **1980,** *302*:1460–1466.

Herbert, V. The antioxidant supplement myth. *Am. J. Clin. Nutr.,* **1994,** *60*:157–158.

Hong, W.K., and Itri, L.M. Retinoids and human cancer. In, *The Retinoids: Biology, Chemistry, and Medicine,* 2nd ed. (Sporn, M.B., Roberts, A.B., and Goodman, D.S., eds.) Raven Press, New York, **1994,** pp. 597–630.

Lippman, S.M., Benner, S.E., and Hong, W.K. Cancer chemoprevention. *J. Clin. Oncol.,* **1994,** *12*:851–873.

Love, J.M., and Gudas, L.J. Vitamin A, differentiation and cancer. *Curr. Opin. Cell. Biol.,* **1994,** *6*:825–831.

Machlin, L.J., ed. *Vitamin E: A Comprehensive Treatise.* Marcel Dekker, Inc., New York, **1980.**

Mangelsdorf, D.J., Umesomo, K., and Evans, R.M. The retinoid receptors. In, *The Retinoids: Biology, Chemistry, and Medicine,* 2nd ed. (Sporn, M.B., Roberts, A.B., and Goodman, D.S., eds.) Raven Press, New York. **1994,** pp. 319–349.

Moon, R.C., Mehta, R.G., and Rao, K.V.N. Retinoids and cancer in experimental animals. In, *The Retinoids: Biology, Chemistry, and Medicine,* 2nd ed. (Sporn, M.B., Roberts, A.B., Goodman, D.S., eds.) Raven Press, New York, **1994,** pp. 573–595.

Olson, J.A. The 1992 Atwater Lecture: The irresistible fascination of carotenoids and vitamin A. *Am. J. Clin. Nutr.,* **1993,** *57*:833–839.

Ong, D., Newcomer, M.E., and Chytil, F. Cellular retinoid binding proteins. In, *The Retinoids: Biology, Chemistry, and Medicine,* 2nd ed. (Sporn, M.B., Roberts, A.B., and Goodman, D.S., eds.) Raven Press, New York, **1994,** pp. 283–317.

Ross, A.C. Vitamin A status: relationship to immunity and the antibody response. *Proc. Soc. Exp. Biol. Med.,* **1992,** *200*:303–320.

Simpson, K.L. Relative value of carotenoids as precursors of vitamin A. *Proc. Nutr. Soc.,* **1983,** *42*:7–17.

Sokol, R.J. Vitamin E deficiency and neurologic disease. *Annu. Rev. Nutr.,* **1988,** *8*:351–373.

Stryer, L. Visual excitation and recovery. *J. Biol. Chem.,* **1991,** *266*: 10711–10714.

Suttie, J.W. The importance of menaquinones in human nutrition. *Annu. Rev. Nutr.,* **1995,** *15*:399–417.

Symposium. Biological actions of carotenoids. *J. Nutr.,* **1989a,** *119*:94–136.

Symposium. Retinoids. *Pharmacol. Ther.,* **1989b,** *40*:1–169.

Traber, M.G., and Sies, H. Vitamin E in humans: demand and delivery. *Annu. Rev. Nutr.,* **1996,** *16*:321–347.

van Poppel, G. Carotenoids and cancer: an update with emphasis on human intervention studies. *Eur. J. Cancer,* **1993,** *29A*:1335–1344.

Vermeer, C., Jie, K.-S., and Knapen, M.H. Role of vitamin K in bone metabolism. *Annu. Rev. Nutr.,* **1995,** *15*:1–22.

Vert, P., and Deblay, M.F. Hemorrhagic disorders in infants of epileptic mothers. In, *Epilepsy, Pregnancy, and the Child.* (Janz, D., Bossi, L., Daum, M., Helge, H., Richens, A., and Schmidt, D., eds.) Raven Press, New York, **1982,** pp. 387–388.

SECTION XIV

DERMATOLOGY

C H A P T E R 6 5

DERMATOLOGICAL PHARMACOLOGY

Eric L. Wyatt, Steven H. Sutter, and Lynn A. Drake

The skin has many essential functions, including protection, thermoregulation, immune responsiveness, biochemical synthesis, sensory detection, and social and sexual communication. Therapy to correct dysfunction in any of these activities may be delivered topically, systemically, intralesionally, or through ultraviolet radiation.

Topical therapy is a convenient method of treatment, but its efficacy depends on understanding the barrier function of the skin, primarily within the stratum corneum. Corticosteroids and retinoids are important systemic and topical therapeutic agents for skin disease. Oral steroids are employed in high doses to treat very serious cutaneous eruptions, and, fortunately, structural modification of the hydrocortisone molecule has produced compounds of increased potency that now can be used topically to treat many dermatological diseases. Potent and efficacious retinoids for treatment of acne and psoriasis are administered orally, and modification of these molecules has resulted in topical agents that are being explored for their anticarcinogenic and antiaging effects. Oral antimalarials, chemotherapeutic agents, immunosuppressive agents, and antihistamines frequently are used for treatment of dermatological diseases. It is interesting that controlled ultraviolet (UV) radiation therapy is a frequent mode of treatment for psoriasis, pruritus, and atopic dermatitis, although UV radiation is itself responsible for the production of cutaneous cancers. However, the prophylactic use of sunscreens may reduce or prevent premalignant and malignant skin lesions induced by UV light, so their use is highly recommended. Major advances in the development and use of antifungal agents, antiviral agents, and antibacterial agents for skin diseases have clearly improved treatment options. Vitamin D analogs, retinoids, and anthralin are some of the topical agents used for psoriasis.

Much of this chapter is organized according to specific dermatological disorders and drugs used in their treatment. Separate sections are devoted to glucocorticoids and retinoids because of their broad applications in dermatology. Agents with narrower spectra of uses are discussed under individual dermatological disorders.

History of Dermatology. The origins of dermatological pharmacology can be found in early Middle Eastern cultures. Early Egyptians recorded medical knowledge on special papyri, where mentions of alopecia and its treatment—consisting of equal parts of the fat of a lion, hippopotamus, crocodile, goose, snake, and ibex—are made. Indians used arsenic in the treatment of leprosy and a mixture of mercury and sulfur to treat pediculosis. A paste containing iron sulfate, bile, copper sulfate, sulfuret of arsenic, and antimony was used for pruritus of the scrotum. The Greeks under Hippocrates and the Romans under Celsus made many other contributions to the field of dermatology (King, 1927).

As late as the end of the nineteenth century, dermatological therapy was still archaic by today's standards. At the first World Congress of Dermatology in Paris in 1889, one of the favorite treatments of tinea capitis was "dermabrasion with sandpaper followed by application of a solution of bichloride of mercury." Treatment of syphilis was thought to be best deferred until the secondary stage, at which time application of a 50% mercurous oleate ointment was recommended (Shelley and Shelley, 1992).

The dermatological pharmacopeia has grown rapidly in the past century, as our understanding of disease processes has improved. We have shifted our paradigm from the traditional axiom, which relied heavily on the physical characteristics of medications for their effect, to one in which chemical properties hold an equally important role. In the past, dermatological therapy consisted mainly of symptom relief. With advances in technology and knowledge, medications that target specific disease processes now are available.

THE STRUCTURE AND FUNCTION OF SKIN

The skin has many diverse functions, including protection, thermal regulation, sensory perception, and immune responses. The skin, in a strict sense, consists of the epidermis and its underlying dermis. However, one usually includes the soft tissue underlying the dermis in a discussion of the skin because of its close apposition to and tendency to react as a unit with the overlying skin.

The top layer of the skin is the epidermis. It consists of keratinocytes, melanocytes (pigment), Langerhans' cells (antigen presentation), and Merkel cells (sensory). Keratinocytes, the proliferative portion of the epidermis, contain keratins, which provide internal structure. Each layer of the epidermis expresses different keratins, and keratins often are used as keratinocyte differentiation markers. Abnormal keratin expression is a feature of many skin diseases including psoriasis and some ichthyotic disorders. As keratinocytes mature and differentiate, they become larger and flatter and eventually lose their nuclei. The terminal point of keratinocyte differentiation is the formation of the stratum corneum.

Formation of the stratum corneum is arguably the most important function of the epidermis. The stratum corneum, or horny layer, protects the skin against water loss, prevents the absorption of noxious agents, and can be thought of as consisting of bricks and mortar. Corneocytes form the "bricks," and barrier lipids form the "mortar." Corneocytes are formed by proteins found in keratinocytes and are located in the upper layers of the epidermis.

Granular cells, which are immediately below the stratum corneum, contain basophilic structures called keratohyalin granules. These granules contain an inactive precursor protein called *profilaggrin*. Dephosphorylation and proteolysis of profilaggrin to *filaggrin* occurs as granular cells move into the horny layer. Filaggrin functions as a glue to bind the keratin filaments together to form macrofibrils and subsequently is broken down into free amino acids that form products that serve as UV filters and maintain skin hydration. Also, within granular cells, there are precursor proteins—such as involucrin, loricrin, keratolinin, and others—which are cross-linked by transglutaminases to form strong epsilon (gamma-glutamyl)–lysine isopeptide bonds forming the cornified cell envelope. Defects in filaggrin and transglutaminases are the basis of some ichthyotic disorders.

Lamellar granules also are found within granular cells. These are membrane-bound organelles that contain probarrier lipids such as glycolipids, glycoproteins, and phospholipids. These lipids and proteins are secreted *via* exocytosis at the interface between the granular layer and the horny layer and are hydrolyzed to form ceramides and free fatty acids. Ceramides, fatty acids, and cholesterol, which are known as the barrier lipids, make up the intercellular mortar of the stratum corneum (Jakubovic and Ackerman, 1992).

DRUG DELIVERY IN DERMATOLOGICAL DISEASES

The skin is the largest organ of the body. It is unique in that it is easily accessible for the diagnosis and treatment of disease. For most dermatological conditions, the success or failure of treatment regimens is readily apparent to both the patient and physician. Medications can be delivered effectively to the skin by topical, systemic, and intralesional routes. Additionally, topical or systemic therapy can be combined with phototherapy to treat certain skin disorders such as psoriasis.

Utilization of topical medications in skin disease provides many advantages. Most obvious, the skin is readily available for application of medications and the monitoring of therapy. Also, most topical medications have negligible systemic absorption and, therefore, few side effects. Drug/drug interactions are rare for this same reason. However, a good understanding of the pharmacokinetics of skin is necessary for successful use of topical medications.

The primary barrier to absorption of exogenous substances through the skin is the stratum corneum. Passage through this outermost layer marks the rate-limiting step for percutaneous absorption. The major steps involved in percutaneous absorption include the establishment of a concentration gradient, which provides a driving force for drug movement across the skin; the release of drug from the vehicle into the skin—partition coefficient; and drug diffusion across the layers of the skin—diffusion coefficient. The relationship of these factors to one another is summarized in the following equation (Piacquadio and Kligman, 1998):

$$J = C_{veh} \cdot K_m \cdot D/x$$

where J = rate of absorption; C_{veh} = concentration of drug in vehicle; K_m = partition coefficient; D = diffusion coefficient; and x = thickness of stratum corneum.

Physiological factors that affect percutaneous absorption include hydration, occlusion, age, intact *versus* disrupted skin, temperature, and anatomic site. For example, drug absorption is enhanced by improving hydration, the water content of the stratum corneum. This is achieved by decreasing transepidermal water loss through physical occlusion or by the application of an occlusive ointment. The permeability of skin is increased in preterm infants (Barker *et al.,* 1987) and in elderly patients with thin skin as well as in anatomic areas of the body with thinner stratum corneum. Lastly, some substances are known to increase the penetration of drugs through the skin, including dimethyl sulfoxide (DMSO), propylene glycol, and urea.

While intact skin provides a formidable barrier to percutaneous absorption, injured or diseased skin may significantly increase or decrease absorption. Tape stripping of the stratum corneum greatly increases percutaneous absorption. The thickened epidermal plaques of psoriasis may impede absorption of topical medications, whereas the broken surface of eczema may allow excessive absorption. In fact, topical absorption may be increased enough to cause systemic toxicity, such as hypothalamic-pituitary-adrenal axis suppression from systemic absorption of potent topical steroids.

Vehicles

Many factors influence the rate and extent to which topical medications are absorbed. Most topical medications are incorporated into bases or vehicles that bring drugs into contact with the skin. The vehicle chosen for a topical medication will greatly influence the drug's absorption, and vehicles themselves can have a beneficial effect on the skin if chosen appropriately. Ideally, vehicles are easy to apply and remove, nonirritating, and cosmetically pleasing. In addition, the active drug must be stable in the chosen vehicle and must be released readily. Many early formulations of topical medications demonstrated less than optimal bioavailability due to insufficient knowledge of biophysical properties of drugs and vehicles, *i.e.*, the partitioning of drugs from vehicles into skin. Hence, delivery of some older medications can be enhanced by dilution in an appropriate vehicle (Guin *et al.*, 1993).

The choice of an appropriate vehicle in topical preparations is of great importance. Since a vehicle makes up the greatest portion of a topical formulation, it has a significant impact on the absorption and hence therapeutic effect of the active drug. Factors that determine the choice of vehicle and the transfer rate of a drug across the skin are the drug's hydrophobic/hydrophilic partition coefficient, molecular weight, and water solubility. Except for very small particles, water-soluble ions and polar molecules do not penetrate intact stratum corneum.

A vehicle can be classified as monophasic, biphasic, or triphasic, depending upon its components (Figure 65–1). Monophasic vehicles include powders, greases, and liquids. Powders, such as starch or talc, absorb moisture and reduce friction, and they have a soothing, cooling effect. However, powders adhere poorly to the skin and often clump, which limits their usefulness. Greases are protective. They are anhydrous preparations that are either water-insoluble or fatty, such as petrolatum (petroleum jelly), or water-soluble, such as polyethylene glycol. Fatty ointments are more occlusive than water-soluble ointments. An important point to note is that ointments are not by themselves hydrating; however, they restrict transepidermal water loss and hence preserve hydration of the stratum corneum.

Liquids may be used as solvents for drugs, as they evaporate quickly and provide a cooling and drying effect. For example, lotions are liquid preparations in which medications are dissolved or suspended and are useful for hairy areas. Gels contain a liquid phase and have been converted into a semisolid by addition of a polymer. Gels can be thought of as microscopic pockets of liquids suspended in a mesh. Gels also are useful for hairy areas and tend to allow for greater penetration than do lotions. Powders, greases, and liquids can be combined to create biphasic and triphasic vehicles.

Biphasic vehicles include "shake lotions" (lotion plus powder), pastes (powder plus grease), and creams (grease plus liquid). Shake lotions (*e.g.*, calamine lotion) evaporate, leaving

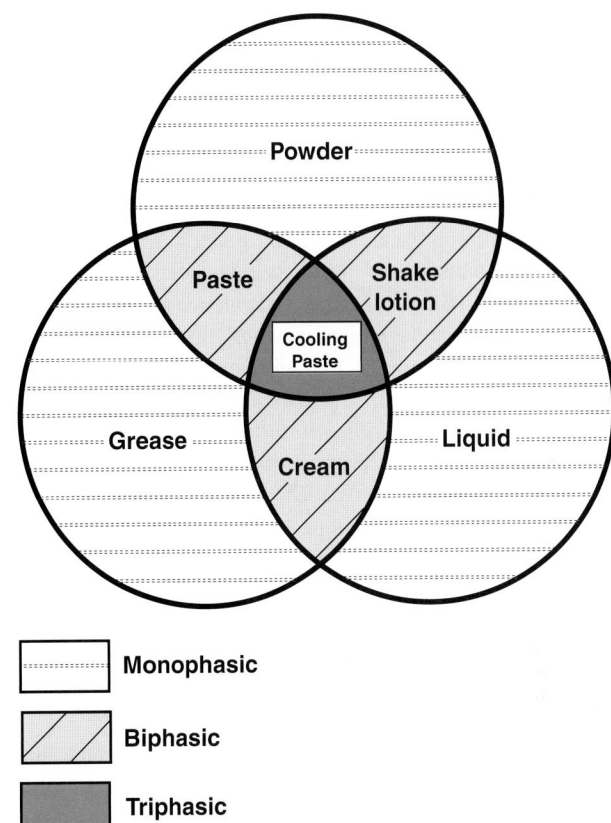

Figure 65–1. Topical vehicle formulations.

(Modified from Polano, 1984, with permission.)

a residual powder, and are cooling and soothing. Pastes are ointments into which powder is incorporated. There are drying pastes, cream pastes, and protective pastes. Pastes are useful, for example, in the treatment of ulcers and chronic dermatoses. Creams can be emulsified oil-in-water preparations (*e.g.*, vanishing creams) or water-in-oil emulsions (*e.g.*, oily creams). With oil-in-water preparations, water evaporates, leaving a thin film of drug on the skin. Although the evaporation provides a cooling effect, it also makes oil-in-water preparations somewhat drying. Oil-in-water creams contain preservatives, which prevent microbial growth but can cause allergic contact dermatitis. Water-in-oil preparations contain less water and more oil than do vanishing creams. Hence, water-in-oil preparations are emollient and moisturizing. Triphasic vehicles consist of cream pastes or cooling pastes.

Newer vehicles include liposomes and microparticles. Liposomes are concentric spherical shells of phospholipids in a water medium that may increase cutaneous bioavailability of the medication and improve risk-benefit ratios. Liposomes most readily penetrate compromised epidermal barriers (Korting *et al.*, 1991). There are two stages of liposomal drug release. In the first stage, liposomes remain in a liquid state and absorption is slow. In the second stage, the preparation dries and intercalates in the lipids of the skin's surface and diffuses into the stratum corneum.

Microparticles are polymer-based microstructures in which drugs can be trapped. Microparticles allow for metered drug release and can have the advantage of causing less irritation.

Variability in Topical Preparations

Substitution of generic for trade-name topical medications is commonplace. However, generic topical preparations and name-brand products may not be equivalent. Criteria used to evaluate the equivalence of two topical preparations include *pharmaceutical* or *chemical equivalence, i.e.,* the same active ingredient is contained in both preparations; the *bioequivalence* of two preparations, which compares the *bioavailability* of the active ingredient in two different preparations; and the *therapeutic efficacy* and *toxicity* of two different preparations of the same active ingredient. There are many difficulties in assessing the bioavailability of topical agents. Blood levels typically are very low and are not reliable indicators of drug availability in the skin. Indeed, topical medications are intended to deliver optimal dosages of medication to the skin with minimization of systemic absorption (Piacquadio and Kligman, 1998).

Differences in bioequivalence among generic and brand-name products have occurred with topical steroids as measured by vasoconstrictor assays (*see* below). Although bioequivalence may be established by vasoconstrictor assays, this may not equate with therapeutic equivalence (Olsen, 1991). One problem that arises in the use of either generic or brand-name topical steroids is the variability of vehicles used. Although active ingredients may be the same, the vehicles may differ significantly. Different inert ingredients in either generic or brand-name products may have an adverse impact on patients, causing allergic reactions or skin irritation (Jackson *et al.,* 1989). There also may be variations in therapeutic effect due to variations in rate or extent of absorption among products or to variable shelf lives.

Systemic and Intralesional Administration

Systemic administration of medication in dermatology usually involves oral ingestion but also can involve the intramuscular route (*e.g.,* methotrexate, glucocorticoids). Systemic medications are used when therapeutic effects cannot be obtained with topical medication. A good example is the treatment of onychomycosis (fungal infection of the nail). Topical medications do not adequately penetrate the hard keratin of the nail; hence, systemic therapy is necessary for successful treatment. Systemic absorp-

tion of oral and parenteral medications is discussed in Chapter 1.

Intralesional medications are used mainly for inflammatory lesions but can be used for treatment of warts and neoplasms. Medications injected intralesionally have the advantage of direct contact with the underlying pathology, no first-pass metabolism, and the formation of a depot of drug. Systemic absorption of medication varies with the drug being used. For instance, when 20 mg of intralesional triamcinolone acetonide is injected, plasma cortisol levels can be suppressed for a few days. In considering the use of intralesional medications, it is important to be cognizant of the systemic absorption of the medication being used.

In summary, when treating cutaneous diseases, it is not only the drug selected but also factors such as route of administration, integrity of normal *versus* abnormal barrier functions of the skin, and the vehicle that are important in determining ultimate clinical efficacy.

GLUCOCORTICOIDS

Topical Agents

Shortly after the synthesis of hydrocortisone in 1951, topical steroids were recognized as effective agents for the treatment of skin disease (Sulzberger and Witten, 1952). New halogenated glucocorticoids with greatly enhanced potency were synthesized in the mid-1950s. With the development of appropriate vehicles, these agents rapidly became the mainstay of therapy for many inflammatory skin diseases.

Topical glucocorticoids have been grouped into seven classes in order of decreasing potency (Table 65–1). Potency is measured using a vasoconstrictor assay, in which an agent is applied to skin under occlusion and the area of skin blanching assessed, and the psoriasis bioassay, in which the effect of steroid on psoriatic lesions is quantified (McKenzie and Stoughton, 1962; Dumas and Scholtz, 1972). Other assays of steroid potency involve suppression of erythema and edema following experimentally induced inflammation.

Therapeutic Uses.   Many inflammatory skin diseases respond to topical or intralesional administration of glucocorticoids. Absorption varies among different body areas; the steroid to be used is chosen on the basis of its potency, the site of involvement, and the severity of the skin disease. Often, a more potent steroid is used initially, followed by a less potent agent. Most practitioners become familiar with one or two drugs in each class so as to deliver the appropriate strength of drug. Twice-a-day application

Table 65–1

Potency of Selected Topical Glucocorticoids

CLASS OF DRUG*	GENERIC NAME, FORMULATION	TRADE NAME
1	Betamethasone dipropionate cream, ointment 0.05% (in optimized vehicle)	DIPROLENE
	Clobetasol propionate cream, ointment 0.05%	TEMOVATE
	Diflorasone diacetate ointment 0.05%	PSORCON
	Halobetasol propionate ointment 0.05%	ULTRAVATE
2	Amcinonide ointment 0.1%	CYCLOCORT
	Betamethasone dipropionate ointment 0.05%	DIPROSONE, others
	Desoximetasone cream, ointment 0.25%, gel 0.05%	TOPICORT
	Diflorasone diacetate ointment 0.05%	FLORONE, MAXIFLOR
	Fluocinonide cream, ointment, gel 0.05%	LIDEX, LIDEX-E, FLUONEX
	Halcinonide cream, ointment 0.1%	HALOG, HALOG-E
3	Betamethasone dipropionate cream 0.05%	DIPROSONE, others
	Betamethasone valerate ointment 0.1%	BETATREX, others
	Diflorasone diacetate cream 0.05%	FLORONE, MAXIFLOR
	Triamcinolone acetonide ointment 0.1%, cream 0.5%	ARISTOCORT A, others
4	Amcinonide cream 0.1%	CYCLOCORT
	Desoximetasone cream 0.05%	TOPICORT LP
	Fluocinolone acetonide cream 0.2%	SYNALAR-HP
	Fluocinolone acetonide ointment 0.025%	SYNALAR
	Flurandrenolide ointment 0.05%, tape 4 μg/cm^2	CORDRAN
	Hydrocortisone valerate ointment 0.2%	WESTCORT
	Triamcinolone acetonide ointment 0.1%	KENALOG, ARISTOCORT
	Mometasone furoate cream, ointment 0.1%	ELOCON
5	Betamethasone dipropionate lotion 0.05%	DIPROSONE, others
	Betamethasone valerate cream, lotion 0.1%	BETATREX, others
	Fluocinolone acetonide cream 0.025%	SYNALAR
	Flurandrenolide cream 0.05%	CORDRAN SP
	Hydrocortisone butyrate cream 0.1%	LOCOID
	Hydrocortisone valerate cream 0.2%	WESTCORT
	Triamcinolone acetonide cream, lotion 0.1%	KENALOG
	Triamcinolone acetonide cream 0.025%	ARISTOCORT

Table 65–1
Potency of Selected Topical Glucocorticoids (*Continued*)

CLASS OF DRUG*	GENERIC NAME, FORMULATION	TRADE NAME
6	Aclometasone dipropionate cream, ointment 0.05%	ACLOVATE
	Desonide cream 0.05%	TRIDESILON, DESOWEN
	Fluocinolone acetonide cream, solution 0.01%	SYNALAR
7	Dexamethasone sodium phosphate cream 0.1%	DECADRON
	Hydrocortisone cream, ointment, lotion 0.5%, 1.0%, 2.5%	HYTONE, NUTRICORT, PENECORT

*Class 1 is most potent; class 7 is least potent.
SOURCE: Adapted from Arndt, K.A. *Manual of Dermatologic Therapeutics,* 4th ed. Little, Brown, and Company, Boston, Toronto, 1989, p. 234, with permission.

is sufficient; more frequent application does not improve response (Yohn and Weston, 1990). In general, hydrocortisone or an equivalent is the most potent steroid used on the face or in occluded areas such as the axilla or groin. Tachyphylaxis can occur, and switching to a different glucocorticoid or using the drug less frequently often can restore sensitivity to the drug (Singh and Singh, 1986).

Intralesional injection of glucocorticoids usually is done with insoluble preparations of triamcinolone [*triamcinolone acetonide* (KENALOG-40, others) and *triamcinolone hexacetonide* (ARISTOSPAN)], which solubilize gradually and therefore have a prolonged duration of action. The hexacetonide can further prolong the therapeutic effect. Intralesional steroids are particularly valuable if the inflammatory area is in fat, as in an inflammatory scalp alopecia or panniculitis. Intralesional injections also may be used to deliver high doses of medication to more superficial inflammatory dermatoses, including psoriasis, discoid lupus, and inflamed cysts.

Toxicity and Monitoring. Use of higher-potency topical glucocorticoids is associated with increased local and systemic toxicity. Locally there is skin atrophy, striae, telangiectasias, purpura, acneiform eruptions, perioral dermatitis, overgrowth of skin fungus and bacteria, hypopigmentation in pigmented skin, and rosacea. The striae are most common in intertriginous areas but can occur diffusely. The perioral dermatitis and rosacea occur on the face when withdrawal of the steroid is attempted; for this reason, use of halogenated glucocorticoids on the face should be avoided. Long-term application near the eye can cause cataracts or glaucoma. There is sufficient absorption

of the most highly potent topical glucocorticoids through inflamed skin to cause systemic toxicity, including suppression of the hypothalamic-pituitary-adrenal axis and growth retardation, particularly in young children (Bondi and Kligman, 1980; Wester and Maibach, 1993). Factors that increase systemic absorption include the amount of steroid applied, the extent of the area treated, the frequency of application, the length of treatment, the potency of the drug, and the use of occlusion.

Intralesional glucocorticoids can cause cutaneous atrophy and hypopigmentation. To minimize this atrophy, doses on the face usually are limited to 1 to 3 mg/ml of triamcinolone acetonide. Systemic side effects, including suppression of the hypothalamic-pituitary-adrenal axis, usually are minimal if total doses are kept below 20 mg of triamcinolone acetonide per month.

Systemic Agents

Therapeutic Uses. Systemic glucocorticoid therapy is used for a number of severe dermatological illnesses (Table 65–2). In general, it is best to reserve glucocorticoids for acute treatment of transient illnesses or for management of life-threatening dermatoses. Chronic therapy of atopic dermatitis with oral glucocorticoids is problematic, given the side effects associated with their long-term use (*see* Chapter 60). Recent studies suggest that glucocorticoids do not prevent development of postherpetic neuralgia (Wood *et al.,* 1994).

Daily morning dosing with *prednisone* usually is necessary initially, although occasionally split daily doses are used to enhance efficacy. Fewer side effects are seen with every-other-day dosing, and prednisone is tapered to every

Table 65–2

Skin Diseases Treated with Systemic Glucocorticoids

Require long-term therapy	*Respond to short-term therapy*
Bullous diseases	Contact dermatitis (acute)
Pemphigus vulgaris	Atopic dermatitis
Bullous pemphigoid	Lichen planus
Herpes gestationis	Exfoliative dermatitis
Collagen vascular diseases	Erythema nodosum
Dermatomyositis	
Systemic lupus erythematosus	*Respond to low-dose bedtime therapy*
Eosinophilic fasciitis	Hormonal abnormalities
Relapsing polychondritis	Acne
Vasculitis (inflammatory)	Hirsutism
Sarcoidosis	*Steroid therapy controversial*
Sweet's disease	Toxic epidermal necrolysis

SOURCE: Adapted from Werth, 1983, with permission.

other day as soon as possible. The intramuscular route is occasionally used to assure compliance, although this route is not recommended because of erratic absorption and prolonged hypothalamic-pituitary-adrenal axis suppression associated with the longer-acting preparations typically injected. Pulse therapy with large daily doses of *methylprednisolone sodium succinate* (SOLU-MEDROL) is given intravenously for resistant pyoderma gangrenosum, pemphigus vulgaris, bullous pemphigoid, organ-threatening systemic lupus erythematosus, and dermatomyositis (Werth, 1993). The dose usually is 0.5 to 1.0 g given over 2 to 3 hours. More rapid infusion has been associated with increased rates of hypotension, electrolyte shifts, and arrhythmias.

Toxicity and Monitoring. Oral glucocorticoids have numerous systemic effects, as discussed in Chapter 60. Most side effects are dose-dependent. Long-term use is associated with a number of complications, including psychiatric problems, cataracts, myopathy, avascular necrosis, and hypertension. In addition, patients with psoriasis who are taking glucocorticoids may have a pustular flare as the medication is tapered. Patients treated with multiple intramuscular glucocorticoid injections have the same side effects as those treated orally.

Pulsed intravenous glucocorticoids can cause hypotension or hypertension, hyperglycemia, hypokalemia or hyperkalemia, anaphylactic reactions, acute psychosis, seizures, and sudden death. Congestive heart failure and pulmonary edema can develop. After brief high-dose treatment is stopped, a steroid withdrawal syndrome with transient arthralgias, myalgias, and joint effusions can develop, but without overt addisonian crisis (Kimberly, 1988).

RETINOIDS

Retinoids include natural compounds and synthetic derivatives of retinol that exhibit vitamin A activity (*see* Chapter 64). Retinoids have many important and diverse functions throughout the body, including roles in vision, regulation of cell proliferation and differentiation, bone growth, immune defense, and tumor suppression (Chandraratna, 1998). Because vitamin A affects normal epithelial differentiation, it was investigated as a treatment for cutaneous disorders but was abandoned initially because of unfavorable side effects. With the synthesis of multiple retinoids, agents with specific effectiveness and decreased toxicity were developed. Small changes in structure resulted in major changes in function (Figure 65–2). First-generation retinoids include *retinol, tretinoin* (all *trans*-retinoic acid), *isotretinoin* (13-*cis*-retinoic acid), and *alitretinoin* (9-*cis*-retinoic acid). Second-generation retinoids, which include *etretinate* and its metabolite *acitretin,* were created by alteration of the cyclic end group. Third-generation retinoids contain further modification and are called *arotinoids*. Members of this generation include *tazarotene* and *bexarotene.* Adapalene is a derivative of naphthoic acid with retinoid-like properties; chemically it does not fit precisely into any of the three generations of retinoids.

An understanding of retinoid receptors is necessary before the actions of retinoids in the regulation of cell proliferation and differentiation can be discussed. Two families of retinoid receptors exist. *Retinoic acid receptors* (RARs) are members of the thyroid/steroid superfamily of receptors. RARs are further divided into alpha, beta, and gamma subtypes. The second family of retinoid receptors is the *retinoid X receptor* family (RXRs). Retinoid X receptors also are subdivided into alpha,

RETINOIDS

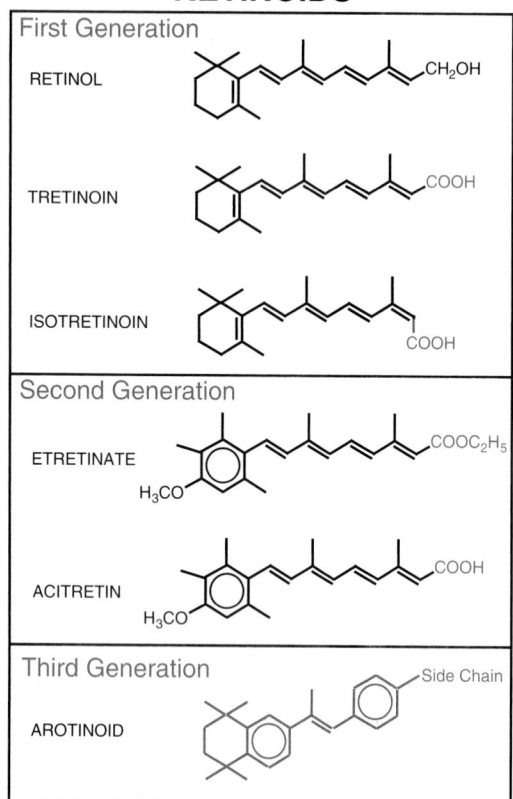

Figure 65–2.   *Three generations of retinoids.*

Major structural changes of each generation are indicated in blue.

beta, and gamma subtypes. Human skin contains mainly RAR beta and gamma receptors.

Retinoids regulate gene transcription through activation of nuclear receptors. Retinoids (ligands) bind transcription factors (nuclear receptors), and the ligand-receptor complex formed then binds to the promoter region of a target gene (Saurat, 1999). The gene products formed contribute to both desirable pharmacological effects and unwanted side effects (Shroot, 1998).

The structure of a particular retinoid determines which type of retinoid receptor will be bound and hence what pharmacological effects will be produced. The basic structure of the retinoid molecule consists of a cyclic end group, a polyene side chain, and a polar end group. Alteration of side chains and end groups creates the various classes of retinoids. First- and second-generation retinoids are able to bind several retinoid receptors due to the flexibility imparted by their alternating single and double bonds. This relative lack of receptor specificity may lead to greater side effects. Third-generation retinoids are much less flexible than first- and second-generation retinoids and, therefore, interact with fewer retinoid receptors (Chandraratna, 1998).

Acute retinoid toxicity is similar to vitamin A intoxication. General side effects of retinoids include dry skin, nose bleeds from dry mucous membranes, conjunctivitis, and hair loss. Less frequently, musculoskeletal pain, pseudotumor cerebri, or mood alterations have been observed. Oral retinoids are potent teratogens and cause severe fetal malformations. Systemic retinoids should be used with great caution in females of childbearing potential.

Retinoids are used in the treatment of many diverse diseases and are effective in the treatment of inflammatory skin disorders, skin malignancies, hyperproliferative disorders, photoaging, and many other disorders (Table 65–3). Their uses in some of these disorders, such as psoriasis and acne, are discussed below.

PRURITUS

The term *pruritus* is derived from the Latin *prurire,* which means "to itch" (Kantor, 1996). Pruritus occurs in a multitude of diverse disorders ranging from the itch of dry skin (xerosis) to the itch of internal malignancy (Table 65–4). The treatment of pruritus varies greatly with the disorder in which it is seen. Many treatment modalities are available for pruritus (Table 65–5).

General, non-disease-specific measures can be helpful in treating most cases of pruritus (Table 65–6). General measures usually are sufficient for xerosis. Inflammatory disorders such as atopic dermatitis, contact dermatitis, and lichen simplex chronicus respond better to treatment with potent topical steroids and antihistamines. Atopic dermatitis is discussed below.

Cholestasis-associated pruritus may respond to *cholestyramine* (QUESTRAN; *see* Chapter 36), *ursodeoxycholic acid* (ACTIGALL), *ondansetron* (ZOFRAN; *see* Chapter 38), or *rifampin* (*see* Chapter 48; Connolly *et al.,* 1995). Recently, *nalmefene* (REVEX) (20 mg twice per day; *see* Chapter 23) has been shown to be effective in cholestatic pruritus (Bergasa *et al.,* 1999). The pruritus of uremia is treated most effectively with ultraviolet B radiation (UVB). Prurigo, a ubiquitous disorder associated with itchy nodules of the skin, is notoriously difficult to treat. In addition to topical and intralesional steroids, prurigo may respond to the opioid antagonist *naltrexone* (*see* Chapter 23) at a dose of 50 mg per day (Metze *et al.,* 1999) or to the proton pump inhibitor *omeprazole* (*see* Chapter 37; Ohtsuka *et al.,* 1999).

ATOPIC DERMATITIS

Atopic dermatitis is an inflammatory condition of the skin that commonly begins in infancy and childhood and can extend into the adult years. In some geographic regions, up to 10% of children have atopic dermatitis, and the

Table 65–3
Major Retinoid-Responsive Skin Diseases

DISEASE	RETINOID
Acne	
Cystic acne	Is
Papular acne	Is, Ta, Tr, Ad
Gram-negative folliculitis	Is
Hidradenitis suppurativa	Is
Disorders of keratinization	
The ichthyoses	Is, Ac, Tr
Darier's disease	Is, Ac
Pityriasis rubra pilaris	Is, Ac
Erythrokeratoderma variabilis	Is, Ac
Skin cancer	
Basal cell cancer	Is, Ac
Squamous cell cancer	Is, Ac
Keratoacanthoma	Is, Ac
Cutaneous T-cell lymphoma	Is, Ac, Be
Kaposi's sarcoma	Al
Precancerous conditions	
Actinic keratosis	Tr, Ac
Dysplastic nevus	Tr
Leukoplakia	Is, Ac
Psoriasis	
Psoriasis vulgaris	Ac, Ta
Pustular psoriasis	Ac, Is
Pustular psoriasis, palms and soles	Ac
Erythrodermic psoriasis	Ac
Psoriatic arthritis	Ac
Cutaneous aging	Tr
Miscellaneous	
Discoid lupus erythematosus, scleromyxedema, verrucous peridermal nevus, subcorneal pustular dermatosis, Reiter's syndrome, warts, lichen planus, acanthosis nigricans, sarcoidosis, Grover's disease, porokeratosis	

ABBREVIATIONS: Is, Isotretinoin (ACCUTANE); Ta, Tazarotene (TAZORAC); Be, bexarotene (TARGRETIN); Ac, acetretin (SORIATANE); Al, alitretinoin (PANRETIN); Ad, adapalene (DIFFERIN); Tr, tretinoin (RETIN-A, RENOVA, others).

Table 65–4
Pruritic Disorders

Dermatitis/Allergic
Xerotic eczema
Atopic dermatitis
Contact dermatitis
Lichen simplex chronicus
Scabies
Urticaria
Aquagenic pruritus
Internal disorders
Cholestasis
Uremia
Thyrotoxicosis
Lymphoma
Psychogenic
Prurigo

Table 65–5
Agents and Procedures Used in the Treatment of Pruritus

Topical
Antihistamines
Emollient creams and ointments
Menthol
Camphor
Phenol
Pramoxine
Doxepin
Capsaicin
Tar

Systemic
Antihistamines
Doxepin
Steroids

Physical
8-Methoxypsoralen plus ultraviolet light (PUVA)
Ultraviolet light (UVB)
Acupuncture
Electrical stimulation

incidence is increasing (Zaki *et al.*, 1996). Environmental pollutants and indoor allergens, such as dust mites, may be responsible for this increase.

Hallmarks of atopic dermatitis are itchy papules and plaques. In infants, lesions occur on the face and extensor surfaces, which are common sites of trauma. In later childhood and adulthood, flexural involvement is more common. Acute, subacute, and chronic lesions occur. Acute lesions consist of itchy papulovesicles or wheals. Subacute papules and plaques show excoriation and chronic plaques are thickened and dry. Physical traits of atopic children include redundant folds of the lower eyelid, fissured lips, and increased palmar skin markings. Infections are common in atopic children, particularly herpes simplex,

Table 65–6

General Measures in Pruritus Treatment

Lukewarm baths
Nonfragranced soaps
Mild soaps
Pat dry
Cooling of the skin
Humidifiers
Emollient creams

molluscum contagiosum, fungus, and *Staphylococcus aureus*. Up to 90% of lesions of atopic dermatitis are colonized by *S. aureus*.

The goals of treatment in atopic dermatitis are skin hydration, decreased bacterial colonization, control of itching, decreased inflammation, and elimination of exacerbating factors. Cutaneous hydration helps to eliminate fissures and cracks in the skin from which pathogens may enter. Hydration consists of soaking in a lukewarm bath, followed immediately by the application of thick emollient creams.

Glucocorticoids

Topical glucocorticoids are useful for decreasing inflammation. Higher-potency topical steroids are indicated for thick, chronically rubbed plaques on the extremities. Lower potency, nonfluorinated topical steroids should be used for facial lesions for short (less than 2 weeks) periods of time. Potential side effects of topical steroids include striae and atrophy of the skin. Topical steroids should be used no more than 2 or 3 times per day and should be discontinued as quickly as possible to avoid potential side effects.

Antihistamines

Oral antihistamines, particularly H₁-receptor antagonists (*see* Chapter 25) with sedative properties, are useful for the control of pruritus. *Hydroxyzine hydrochloride* (ATARAX) is given in a dose of 0.5 mg/kg every 6 hours and provides sedation. Other sedative H₁ blockers include *diphenhydramine* (BENADRYL; others), *promethazine* (PHENERGAN), and *cyproheptadine* (PERIACTIN). Nonsedative antihistamines include *cetirizine* (ZYRTEC), *loratadine* (CLARITIN), and *fexofenadine hydrochloride* (ALLEGRA). *Doxepin,* which has both tricyclic antidepressant and sedative antihistamine effects (*see* Chapter 19), is a good alternative for severe pruritus. Doxepin also is available as a 5% cream (ZONALON), and it can be used effectively in conjunction with low- to moderate-potency topical steroids.

Leukotriene Receptor Antagonist

The leukotriene antagonist *zafirlukast* (*see* Chapter 28), in a dosage of 20 mg twice daily, has improved atopic dermatitis in some patients. Side effects include pharyngitis, headache, and infrequent elevation of alanine aminotransferase values (Carucci *et al.,* 1998).

Immunosuppressive Agents

Immunosuppressive agents (*see* Chapter 53) should be considered when hydration, topical steroids, and antihistamines have not provided adequate clearing of atopic dermatitis. *Cyclosporine* (NEORAL; others) is used in many dermatological and autoimmune diseases. Although used in the treatment of atopic dermatitis, cyclosporine is not approved by the United States Food and Drug Administration (FDA) for the purpose. T-cell activation and proliferation are inhibited by cyclosporine (Faulds *et al.,* 1993). The initial dose of cyclosporine usually is 5 mg/kg per day, which allows for rapid improvement, with maintenance dosage of 3 mg/kg per day (Zonneveld *et al.,* 1996). Alternatively, it has been suggested that a body weight–independent dose of 150 mg per day is both efficacious and well tolerated (Czech *et al.,* 2000). Cyclosporine appears to be safe and effective for children when given in short courses (Zaki *et al.,* 1996). Potential side effects of cyclosporine therapy include nephrotoxicity, hypertension, gingival hyperplasia, and hypertrichosis. Complete blood counts, blood pressure measurements, and serum creatinine levels should be monitored regularly.

A promising new topical immunosuppressive agent is *tacrolimus* (PROTOPIC), which was isolated from *Streptomyces tsukubaenis* in Tsukuba, Japan, in 1984. Tacrolimus is a neologism composed of the words *T*sukaba *M*acrolide *imm*unosuppressive, and the oral form currently is used in kidney, liver, and heart transplants (*see* Chapter 53). Tacrolimus binds to an intracellular receptor in T cells that interferes with cytokine-mediated processes active in atopic dermatitis. Topical tacrolimus currently is being evaluated in clinical trials and shows great promise in the treatment of refractory atopic dermatitis (Ruzicka *et al.,* 1999).

PSORIASIS

Psoriasis is characterized by epidermal hyperproliferation overlying immune-mediated dermal inflammation. Clinically, this results in erythematous scaling plaques most commonly present on the elbows, knees, and scalp. The cracking, scaling plaques of psoriasis may be widespread and even painful, with the potential for significant disability. Flare-ups of psoriasis can occur randomly but have been known to follow periods of physical and emotional stress, cutaneous trauma, infection, and as a reaction to certain medications, including β-adrenergic receptor antagonists, lithium, antimalarials, and systemic steroids (Christophers and Mrowietz, 1999).

The selection of therapy for psoriasis is multifactorial. The overall health status of the patient must be taken into account, particularly hepatic and renal function, childbearing potential, and the presence or absence of psoriatic arthritis. Another major consideration is the percent of body surface area involved. For practical purposes, patients with less than 15% body surface involvement can be treated effectively with topical agents. A notable exception

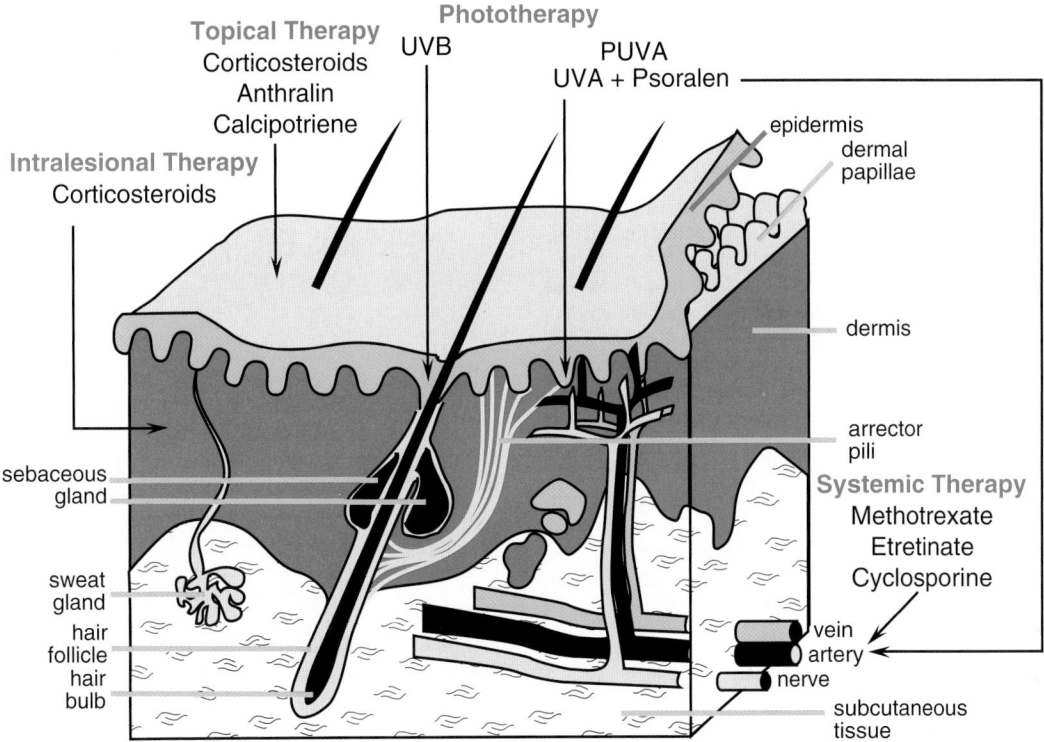

Figure 65–3. Treatment of psoriasis.

In psoriasis, a hyperproliferative disease, all four modes of therapeutic delivery are used: topical therapy, phototherapy, intralesional therapy, and systemic therapy. Major normal cutaneous structures are shown. PUVA, psoralens and ultraviolet A; UVB, ultraviolet B.

to this is significant involvement of the hands or feet, which may be recalcitrant to topical treatment.

Topical Agents Used in Treatment of Psoriasis

Topical therapy for psoriasis includes multiple options (Figure 65–3), the first of which are emollients to soften and moisturize psoriatic plaques. Topical keratolytic agents, formulated with urea or salicylic acid, also are useful in the treatment of localized or limited psoriasis; and topical coal tar preparations in the form of ointments, emollient-base creams, lotions, and shampoos have been used over the past century. Topical steroids are the mainstay of treatment for localized psoriasis. A vitamin D analog, *calcipotriene,* is useful for the topical treatment of psoriasis, as a solution, an ointment, or a cream. Anthralin and the topical retinoid tazarotene also are beneficial. These topical agents will be discussed below in more detail.

Coal Tar. *Coal tar* has a limited effect when employed as the sole treatment for psoriasis, and it is now mainly combined with ultraviolet light in the 290 to 320 nm range (UVB) for this indication. It is manufactured as a byproduct of the processing

of coke and gas from bituminous coal and is extremely complex, rich in polycyclic hydrocarbons, and variable in composition. Little is known about its mode of action, which may be related to antimitotic effects (Lowe *et al.,* 1983). Coal tar is phototoxic in the ultraviolet light range of 320 to 400 nm (UVA) and visible ranges, with the action spectrum lying between 340 and 430 nm. Exposure of the skin in this range produces erythema and smarting, "tar smarts," which prevent exploitation of coal tar's photodynamic potential for the treatment of psoriasis.

Coal tar ointment contains crude coal tar, usually 2% to 5%, dispersed in petroleum jelly. The use of coal tar with daily UVB irradiation—known as the Goeckerman regimen—is a highly effective therapy for psoriasis. It improves the efficacy of suberythemogenic UVB, probably by additive effects rather than by photoactivation of the tar. More refined extracts of tars are formulated as solutions, gels, shampoos, and baths, usually with limited efficacy as primary agents.

Folliculitis is the primary side effect of coal tar. Irritation and allergic reactions are rare; and, although coal tar has been shown to be a carcinogen in animal experiments, carcinomas provoked by clinical application are rare (Dodd, 1993).

Calcipotriene. *Calcipotriene* (DOVONEX), a vitamin D analog, was approved for the topical treatment of psoriasis in 1993.

Chance observation of improvement of psoriasis in an osteoporotic patient receiving an oral derivative of 1,25-dihydroxyvitamin D_3 [1,25-$(OH)_2D_3$], the active form of vitamin D (*see* Chapter 62), stimulated interest in the development of the drug as an antipsoriatic agent (Morimoto and Kumahara, 1985). 1,25-$(OH)_2D_3$ has a major role in the maintenance of calcium homeostasis but is now known to be involved in many other physiological functions. The vitamin binds to an intracellular receptor, a member of the gene superfamily including steroid, thyroid hormone, and retinoid receptor genes. The receptor–vitamin D complex binds to specific genes and modulates and controls transcription. The receptor is present in human epidermal keratinocytes, dermal fibroblasts, islets of Langerhans' cells, macrophages, and T lymphocytes. At physiological concentrations, 1,25-$(OH)_2D_3$ causes a decrease in the proliferation and an increase in the morphologic and biochemical differentiation of cultured keratinocytes (Smith *et al.*, 1986). In clinical studies, both oral and topical 1,25-$(OH)_2D_3$ are effective antipsoriatic agents, but their use is limited by induction of hypercalciuria (Smith *et al.*, 1988; Langner *et al.*, 1992).

Calcipotriene is a synthetic 1,25-dihydroxyvitamin D_3 analog with a double bond and ring structure on the side chain as follows:

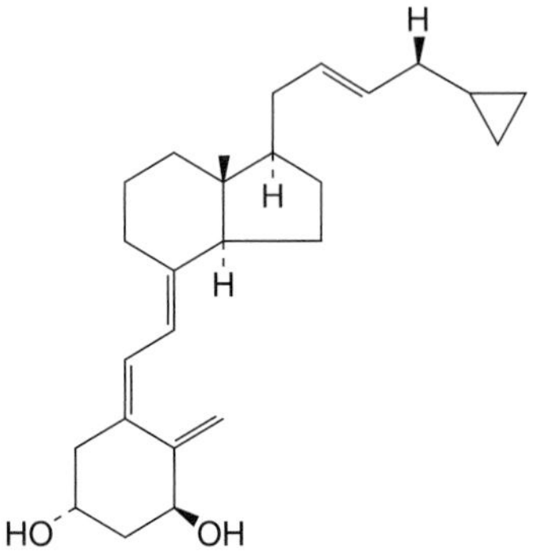

CALCIPOTRIENE

These modifications result in rapid transformation into inactive metabolites. This drug is 200-times less potent than 1,25-$(OH)_2D_3$ in causing hypercalciuria and hypercalcemia, and its affinity for the vitamin D receptor is equal to that of 1,25-$(OH)_2D_3$. Efficacy in psoriasis has been demonstrated in double-blind, placebo-controlled studies (Kragballe, 1989).

Calcipotriene is applied twice daily to plaque psoriasis on the body. Improvement is detectable within 1 to 2 weeks, and maximum clinical response occurs within 6 to 8 weeks. Some improvement takes place in most patients, with complete resolution occurring in up to 15%. The drug is slightly more effective than either the corticosteroid betamethasone 17-valerate or short-contact anthralin treatment. Maintenance therapy usually is necessary, and tachyphylaxis does not occur (Kragballe, 1992).

Reports of hypercalcemia with calcipotriene are rare and usually have been associated with excessive use of the drug (Hardman *et al.*, 1993). Calcipotriene should be used with caution in intertriginous areas because of facilitated absorption, which results in irritation. Routine laboratory monitoring is not necessary if usage guidelines are followed. It is available in an ointment, cream, or solution.

Anthralin. *Chrysarobin*, the active ingredient of Goa powder, was first used in 1877 for the treatment of psoriasis. It was replaced in 1916 by the synthetic compound *anthralin* (1,8-dihydroxy-9-anthrone; dithranol; DRITHOCREME), which has the following structure:

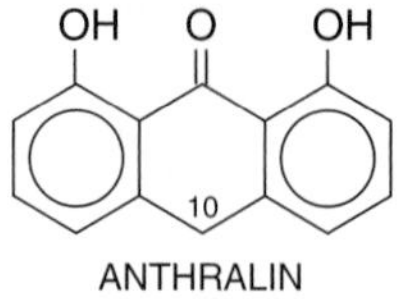

ANTHRALIN

The anthralin molecule is unstable, having an oxidizable center at C10 that leads to the formation of degradation products that produce the characteristic violet-brown staining of skin and clothes. The mechanism of the antipsoriasis effect of anthralin is unknown, but it inhibits cellular respiration by inactivation of mitochondria (Reichert *et al.*, 1985).

Anthralin is applied topically in concentrations of 0.1% to 1.0%. The drug also can be prepared in higher strengths in petroleum jelly or zinc paste with the addition of salicylic acid as an antioxidant. Standard therapy is to apply a lower concentration (0.1%) for several hours for at least a week and then gradually increase the concentration. A modification of this treatment, called short-contact therapy, is possible because anthralin penetrates damaged skin faster and to a greater extent than normal skin (Schaefer *et al.*, 1980). Therefore, application for 1 hour or less optimizes the therapeutic effect while minimizing the irritation. Short-contact therapy is initiated with higher concentrations (0.25% or 0.5%) applied for 20 to 30 minutes, and the concentration is increased more rapidly. With either the standard or short-contact regimens, the medication must be completely removed by bathing or shampooing at the end of the contact time.

The primary side effects of anthralin are staining and irritation of the uninvolved skin. Because of individual variation in skin sensitivity, close monitoring of irritation and careful progression of treatment are necessary. Treatment of intertriginous and facial lesions is not advisable, and permanent staining of clothes and bathroom fixtures is annoying. In an effort to decrease irritation and staining, anthralin also has been microencapsulated in crystalline monoglycerides.

Tazarotene. The topical retinoid *tazarotene* (TAZORAC), an acetylenic class of retinoid, has been developed in the form of a gel to be used for the treatment of psoriasis and acne vulgaris (Duvic and Marks, 1998). This retinoid binds to all three members of the retinoic acid receptor family. In mice, tazarotene has been shown to block ornithine decarboxylase activity, which is associated with cell proliferation and hyperplasia. In cell culture, it has been shown to suppress a marker of epidermal inflammation and to inhibit cornification of the keratinocyte.

Tazarotene gel, applied once a day to dry skin, may be used as monotherapy or in combination with other medications, such as topical steroids, for the treatment of localized plaque psoriasis. This is the first topical retinoid to be indicated for the treatment of psoriasis. Side effects of burning, itching, and skin irritation may be noted by some patients. Patients should avoid exposing treated areas to sun or sun lamps unless medically necessary. In as much as this topical drug is a member of the retinoid family, women of childbearing age should avoid pregnancy while using this medication.

Systemic Agents Used in Treatment of Psoriasis

The use of systemic medications for the treatment of psoriasis may be indicated by the extent or severity of the disease. Involvement of body surface area greater than 15%, inflammation of hands or feet, pustular outbreaks, or arthritis all can be indications for systemic treatment.

Some cancer chemotherapeutic agents have been used with good results in psoriasis, especially methotrexate, but also 6-thioguanine and hydroxyurea. The systemic retinoid acitretin can be used either as monotherapy or in conjunction with PUVA. Immune modulators have become important in the treatment of psoriasis, especially as the driving force in the pathophysiology of psoriasis appears to center on the T cell (Gottlieb *et al.*, 1995).

Notably absent from the list of recommended systemic agents for the treatment of psoriasis are glucocorticoids. While short-lived reductions in inflammation may be seen with use of systemic steroids, unpredictable and severe exacerbations of plaque-type and pustular psoriasis have occurred following the use of these drugs.

Cytotoxic Agents. The antimetabolite *methotrexate* (RHEUMA-TREX) is an analog of folic acid that competitively inhibits dihydrofolate reductase (*see* Chapter 52). Methotrexate has made a significant impact on the treatment of widespread and severe psoriasis. Its primary therapeutic mechanism centers on suppression of immune-competent cells in the skin, principally T cells (Jeffes *et al.*, 1995). By virtue of immune suppression, methotrexate dampens signals for epidermal inflammation and hyperproliferation. It is useful in treating a number of cutaneous conditions including psoriasis, pityriasis lichenoides, lymphomatoid papulosis, pemphigus vulgaris, pityriasis rubra pilaris, lupus erythematosus, and dermatomyositis.

A usual starting dose for methotrexate therapy is 5 to 7.5 mg per week. This dose may be gradually increased up to 20 to 30 mg per week if needed. When the drug is taken orally, the weekly dose is divided into three doses given at 12-hour intervals to optimize absorption. Doses must be decreased for patients with impaired renal clearance. Methotrexate should never be coadministered with *trimethoprim–sulfamethoxazole* or other drugs that can cause bone marrow suppression, as severe or possibly fatal bone marrow suppression can occur with such combinations. Fatalities have occurred during concurrent treatment with methotrexate and nonsteroidal antiinflammatory agents.

Methotrexate exerts significant antiproliferative effects on the bone marrow; therefore, complete blood counts should be monitored serially. Physicians administering methotrexate should be familiar with the use of *folinic acid* (leucovorin) to "rescue" patients with hematologic crises caused by methotrexate-induced bone marrow suppression. Careful monitoring of liver function tests is necessary but may not be adequate to identify early hepatic fibrosis in patients taking methotrexate. Hepatic fibrosis from methotrexate appears to be more common in psoriasis than in rheumatoid arthritis. Consequently, liver biopsy is

recommended when the cumulative dose reaches 1.5 g. A baseline liver biopsy also is recommended for those patients with increased risk for hepatic fibrosis, such as history of alcohol abuse or hepatitis B or C. Patients with significantly abnormal liver function tests, symptomatic liver disease, or evidence of hepatic fibrosis should not use this drug (Roenigk *et al.*, 1998).

Hydroxyurea and *6-thioguanine* also are used occasionally in the treatment of psoriasis. Neither of these treatments is as effective as methotrexate, but either one can be useful in situations where methotrexate is contraindicated due to liver disease. Both drugs may cause significant bone marrow suppression; therefore, careful monitoring is required (Leavell *et al.*, 1973; Zackheim *et al.*, 1994).

Acitretin. *Acitretin* (SORIATANE) is the major metabolite of etretinate, an aromatic retinoid. Both drugs have been shown to be useful in the treatment of psoriasis, including pustular and erythrodermic psoriasis. *Etretinate,* an early retinoid which is no longer commercially available, has an elimination half-life of 100 days due to its high lipophilicity. Acitretin, however, has an elimination half-life of two to three days. Unfortunately, acitretin is readily esterified to produce etretinate *in vivo*, and this reaction is further enhanced by alcohol (Katz *et al.*, 1999).

The optimal dosing range for acitretin in adults is 25 to 50 mg per day. This gives an appropriate balance of efficacy with an acceptable level of side effects. Improvement of plaque psoriasis occurs gradually, requiring up to three to six months for optimal results. As a monotherapy, acitretin has an overall rate of complete remission of less than 50% (Ling, 1999); response rates are higher when the drug is used in combination with ultraviolet light (Lebwohl, 1999). Pustular and erythrodermic psoriasis usually respond more rapidly than common plaque psoriasis at doses of 10 to 25 mg per day. Excellent control of these conditions usually can be achieved with acitretin (Goldfork and Ellis, 1998).

Toxicity related to acitretin can resemble hypervitaminosis A. Common side effects include dry skin and mucous membranes, xerophthalmia, and hair thinning. Less frequently, arthralgias and decreased night vision have been noted. While other side effects are occasionally reported, serious side effects, such as hepatotoxicity or pseudotumor cerebri, are rare (Katz *et al.*, 1999).

Acitretin is a potent teratogen and may cause major human fetal abnormalities. **This drug should not be used by females who are pregnant or who intend to become pregnant during therapy or at any time for at least three years following discontinuation of therapy.** Patients should not donate blood for transfusion during acitretin therapy and for three years following therapy to avoid exposing a pregnant recipient's fetus to the drug. Laboratory monitoring should include a baseline pregnancy test in all female patients and a complete blood count, lipid profile, and hepatic profile in all patients. Serial follow-up of laboratory tests should be conducted every one to two weeks until stable and thereafter at intervals as clinically indicated.

Cyclosporine and Mycophenolate Mofetil. The immunosuppressant *cyclosporine* (*see* Chapter 53), derived from the fungus *Beauveria nivea*, is highly effective in the treatment of psoriasis (Ellis *et al.*, 1991). Cyclosporine inhibits the phosphatase calcineurin and transcription of the IL-2 gene in T cells (Schreiber and Crabtree, 1992, Rao, 1994). It also inhibits antigen presentation by Langerhans' cells and degranulation of mast cells (Dupuy *et al.,* 1991; Triggiani *et al.,* 1989), which contribute to the pathogenesis of psoriasis.

Hypertension and renal dysfunction are major concerns associated with the use of cyclosporine. The risk of developing these problems is markedly reduced by keeping the daily dosage less than 5 mg/kg and by rotating therapy periodically (Shupack *et al.,* 1997). Hematological indices and renal function must be carefully monitored. Patients on long-term systemic immune suppression also may develop increased numbers of nonmelanoma skin cancer (Cockburn and Krupp, 1989).

Mycophenolate mofetil (CELLCEPT; *see* Chapter 53) is another effective immune suppressant with a utility very similar to that of cyclosporine (Kitchin *et al.,* 1997). Usual doses range from 1 to 2 g per day. Common side effects include gastrointestinal intolerance, as manifested by diarrhea, nausea, vomiting, abdominal cramping, and bone marrow suppression. Notably, the problems of hypertension and renal dysfunction seen with cyclosporine are not associated with mycophenolate mofetil. As is typical with immunosuppressants, hematological monitoring and close clinical follow-up are required.

Photochemotherapy

Electromagnetic radiation is a form of energy defined by its wavelength; it has been classified into different regions, as shown in Figure 65–4. Dermatologists are most concerned with the regions of ultraviolet radiation (UVC, 100 to 290 nm; UVB, 290 to 320 nm; and UVA, 320 to 400 nm) and with visible radiation (400 to 800 nm). UVC is absorbed by the ozone layer and does not reach the earth's surface. UVB, the most erythrogenic and melanogenic type of radiation, causes sunburn, suntan, skin cancer, and photoaging. The longer wavelengths of UVA are 1000-times less erythrogenic than UVB; however, they penetrate more deeply and contribute to photoaging and photosensitivity diseases. They also enhance UVB-induced erythema and increase the risk of UVC-induced carcinogenesis. Visible radiation is responsible for occasional photosensitive eruptions.

Despite its side effects, nonionizing electromagnetic radiation is employed therapeutically. Phototherapy and photochemotherapy are treatment methods in which radiation of an appropriate wavelength is used to induce a therapeutic response in the absence and presence, respectively, of a photosensitizing drug. The radiation must be absorbed by a target molecule—a chromophore—which is an endogenous molecule in phototherapy and an exogenous drug in photochemotherapy. Patients should not be taking any extraneous photosensitizing medications prior to initiation of therapy. Common photosensitizing medications include, but are not limited to, phenothiazines, thiazides, sulfonamides, nonsteroidal antiinflammatory agents, sulfonylureas, tetracyclines, and benzodiazepines.

PUVA: Psoralens and UVA. *History.* Photochemotherapy with psoralen-containing plant extracts was employed in Egypt and India in 1500 B.C. for the treatment of vitiligo. El Mofty at the University of Cairo first used a purified psoralen for the treatment of vitiligo in 1947. In 1974, Parrish *et al.* reported successful treatment of severe psoriasis with 8-methoxypsoralen (P) and UVA, and coined the acronym *PUVA.* PUVA has been approved for the treatment of vitiligo and psoriasis. Its widespread use with extensive follow-up has provided comprehensive data on toxicity and efficacy.

Chemistry. Psoralens belong to the furocoumarin class of compounds, which are derived from the fusion of a furan with a coumarin. They occur naturally in many plants, including limes, lemons, figs, and parsnips. Two psoralens, 8-methoxypsoralen (*methoxsalen*) and 4,5,8-trimethylpsoralen (*trioxsalen;* TRISORALEN) are available in the United States. Methoxsalen is used primarily due to its superior absorption. Structures of the two psoralens are shown below.

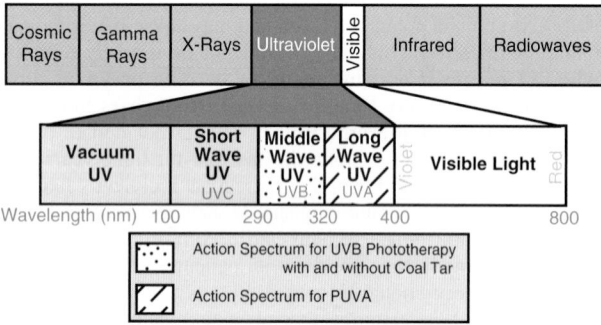

METHOXSALEN   TRIOXSALEN

Figure 65–4. The electromagnetic spectrum.

Solar radiation is defined in terms of wavelength. Ultraviolet and visible radiation (enlarged) are used therapeutically in dermatology; UVB for phototherapy, UVA for photochemotherapy (PUVA, psoralens plus UVA), and visible light for photodynamic therapy.

Pharmacokinetics. The psoralens are absorbed rapidly after oral administration. Photosensitivity, on average, is maximal 1 to 2 hours after ingestion of methoxsalen. Liquid formulations are superior to the previously used crystalline preparation and produce a more rapid, higher, and more reproducible peak serum level. There is a significant but saturable first-pass elimination in the liver, which may account for variations in plasma levels among individuals after a standard dose. Methoxsalen has a serum half-life of approximately 1 hour, but the skin remains sensitive to light for 8 to 12 hours. Despite widespread distribution of the drug through the body, it is activated only in the skin where the UVA penetrates.

Mechanism.   The mechanism of photosensitivity production by PUVA is not known. The action spectrum for oral PUVA is between 320 and 400 nm. Two distinct photoreactions take place. Type 1 reactions involve the oxygen-independent formation of mono- and bifunctional adducts in DNA. Type II reactions are oxygen-dependent and involve sensitized transfer of energy to molecular oxygen. The therapeutic effects of PUVA in psoriasis may result from a decrease in DNA-dependent proliferation after adduct formation. However, alteration in the immune system caused by PUVA also may play a role (Gupta and Anderson, 1987).

PUVA promotes melanogenesis in normal skin. Increased pigmentation results from the transfer of melanosomes from melanocytes to epidermal cells; however, there is no change in the size of melanosomes or in their distribution pattern.

Therapeutic Uses.   Methoxsalen is supplied in soft gelatin capsules (OXSORALEN-ULTRA) and hard gelatin capsules (8-MOP). The dose is 0.4 mg/kg for the soft capsule and 0.6 mg/kg for the hard capsule taken 1.5 to 2 hours before UVA exposure. A lotion containing methoxsalen (OXSORALEN) also is available for topical application. It can be diluted for bath water delivery, a method that produces low systemic psoralen levels. Phototoxicity is increased with topical psoralen use, and the UVA dose therefore must be carefully regulated.

In both American and European multicenter cooperative studies of PUVA for the treatment of psoriasis, initial success rates close to 90% were achieved (Melski *et al.,* 1977; Hensler *et al.,* 1981). In the United States, treatment is administered 3 times weekly and in Europe 4 times weekly. Relapse occurs within 6 months after cessation of treatment in most patients. Various maintenance regimens have been recommended with variable success.

PUVA can induce melanocyte stimulation in vitiligo, resulting in cosmetic repigmentation. Success rates are highest in young individuals with recent onset of disease involving nonacral areas. Localized vitiligo is treated topically with a 1% methoxsalen lotion. Diffuse disease is treated with systemic administration of trioxsalen or methoxsalen. Methoxsalen is more effective.

PUVA also is employed in the treatment of cutaneous T-cell lymphoma, atopic dermatitis, alopecia areata, lichen planus, urticaria pigmentosa, and some forms of photosensitivity.

Toxicity and Monitoring.   The major acute side effects of PUVA include nausea, blistering, and painful erythema. PUVA-induced inflammation is more delayed than that of UVB, reaching a peak 48 to 72 hours after exposure.

Chronic effects occur within the skin. Actinic keratoses, PUVA lentigines, photoaging, and nonmelanoma skin cancer are consequences of chronic PUVA therapy. Squamous-cell carcinomas occur at 10 times the expected frequency (Stern *et al.,* 1988). Extensive PUVA therapy, 250 or more treatments, may increase risk for malignant melanoma. Careful monitoring of patients for cutaneous carcinomas is essential (Stern *et al.,* 1997).

ACNE

Acne is the most common skin disorder in the United States, affecting approximately 7% of the population annually. Although usually confined to the skin, acne can have devastating physical and psychological consequences. An understanding of the pathophysiology of acne is imperative for successful diagnosis and treatment of the disease.

Acne is a disease of the pilosebaceous unit. The events occurring in the formation of acne are plugging of the follicle, accumulation of sebum, growth of *Propionibacterium acnes,* and inflammation. Acneiform lesions appear as comedones, papules, pustules, nodules, and cysts. With the exception of open comedones, which are noninflammatory, lesions of acne can be thought of as either preinflammatory (closed comedones) or inflammatory (papules, pustules, nodules, and cysts). Inflammatory lesions can lead to scarring. The goals of acne treatment are to correct abnormalities of follicular maturation, decrease sebum production, decrease *P. acnes* colonization, and decrease inflammation. Pharmacological interventions available to achieve these goals include topical, systemic, and intralesional formulations.

Topical Agents Used in Treatment of Acne

Topical treatment of acne involves the use of retinoids and antimicrobials. Topical retinoids function to normalize the maturation of follicular epithelium, reduce inflammation, and enhance the penetration of other topical medications. *Tretinoin* (RETIN-A) was one of the first topical retinoids available for acne and is still in use today (Kligman *et al.,* 1969). Cream, gel, and solution formulations of tretinoin are available for topical use. Tretinoin is a comedolytic agent that loosens existing comedones and prevents the formation of new comedones (Berson, 1999). It is more effective if used in combination with topical antimicrobials such as erythromycin, clindamycin, and benzoyl peroxide. Tretinoin formulations with a cream base are indicated for dry skin, and gel-based formulations are indicated for oily skin. Tretinoin is applied at nighttime, as there can be some degradation of the agent when exposed to sunlight. Although there is little systemic absorption of tretinoin and no alteration in plasma vitamin A levels with its use, most physicians do not prescribe tretinoin for their pregnant patients due to theoretical teratogenic effects. A formulation of tretinoin (RETIN-A MICRO) with active drug incorporated into "microsponges" has been developed. The microsponges decrease irritation by promoting localization of the drug to the follicles and allowing the slow release of medication. Whereas clinical response to tretinoin normally takes 8 weeks, tretinoin microsponges may provide improvement in as little as 6 weeks (Webster, 1998).

Adapalene (DIFFERIN), a derivative of naphthoic acid, is a synthetic retinoid-like compound that is available in solution and gel formulations for topical use. In addition to displaying typical retinoid effects, it also has antiinflammatory properties. Adapalene has similar efficacy to tretinoin, but unlike tretinoin, it is stable in sunlight (Weiss and Shavin, 1998), and it tends to be less irritating.

The most recently introduced retinoid for the treatment of acne is *tazarotene* (TAZORAC), which is discussed in the section on psoriasis.

Topical antimicrobials are a mainstay of acne treatment (Table 65–7). When combined with topical retinoids, treatment

Table 65–7
Topical Antimicrobial Agents Used in the Treatment of Acne

Azelaic acid 20% cream
Benzoyl peroxide 2.5%–10%
  Bar
  Lotion
  Cream
  Gel
  Mask
  Cleanser
Clindamycin 1%
  Pledget
  Solution
  Lotion
  Gel
Erythromycin 1.5%–2%
  Pledget
  Solution
  Ointment
  Gel
Erythromycin 3%/benzoyl peroxide 5% cream
Metronidazole 0.75%
  Lotion
  Cream
  Gel
Sulfacetamide 10% lotion
Sulfur 5%/sulfacetamide 10% lotion

with antimicrobials is more effective than if either medication is used alone. Antimicrobials reduce *P. acnes* populations and are effective for the treatment of inflammatory lesions. Commonly used topical antimicrobials include *erythromycin, clindamycin* (CLEOCIN-T), and *benzoyl peroxide* (PERSA-GEL, others). *P. acnes* resistance to erythromycin can occur; this resistance can be avoided, however, if a combination of erythromycin (3%) and benzoyl peroxide (5%) (BENZAMYCIN) is used. Clindamycin solution (1%) applied twice daily also has been found to be effective in the treatment of acne. Benzoyl peroxide has been used in the treatment of acne for many years. It is an effective antimicrobial to which there is no microbial resistance. Benzoyl peroxide formulations include lotions, creams, cleansers, and gels. Other antimicrobials used in treating acne include *sulfacetamide* (KLARON, SEBIZON), *sulfacetamide/sulfur combinations* (SULFACET-R), *metronidazole* (METROCREAM, METROGEL, NORITATE), and *azelaic acid* (AZELEX). Although azelaic acid can cause significant irritation, it has the added benefit of reducing hyperpigmentation.

Systemic Agents Used in Treatment of Acne

Systemic therapy in acne is most often reserved for inflammatory lesions. Systemic treatment includes retinoids, antibacterials, and hormones. The retinoid *isotretinoin* (ACCUTANE) is used for severe, recalcitrant acne. Isotretinoin corrects all four abnormalities found in acne. It decreases sebum production, normalizes maturation of follicular epithelium, decreases *P. acnes* populations, and decreases inflammation. In addition to severe, recalcitrant nodulocystic acne, isotretinoin also is indicated for acne that produces significant atrophic scarring, for antibiotic-resistant *P. acnes,* and for gram-negative folliculitis. The typical dosage of isotretinoin is 1 mg/kg per day for 4 to 5 months. Total dose ranges are between 120 and 150 mg/kg for a course of treatment (Smith, 1999). Approximately 40% of patients have a relapse after isotretinoin therapy. Preteens and patients with multiple communicating abscesses, scar tracts, and androgen excess are at increased risk of relapse (Leyden, 1998). However, most patients with relapse have milder acne and respond to conventional therapies.

The most common side effects of isotretinoin are dry skin, dry eyes, and nosebleed. Hair loss and headaches also can occur. Use of isotretinoin with tetracycline may produce pseudotumor cerebri. Perhaps most importantly, isotretinoin is teratogenic. **Female patients must be on oral contraceptives as well as another form of birth control and have a negative pregnancy test before starting isotretinoin treatment.** Patients should not donate blood for transfusion during treatment and for one month after treatment.

Systemic antimicrobials decrease inflammation and reduce *P. acnes* colonization. Commonly used medications include *tetracycline, erythromycin, metronidazole,* and *trimethoprim–sulfamethoxazole* (*see* Chapters 41, 44, and 47). Although tetracycline is an antimicrobial agent, its antiinflammatory action may be its most important therapeutic effect. Tetracycline decreases chemotactic factors and slows the migration of neutrophils in acne. Tetracycline also is lipophilic and can penetrate the sebaceous glands. Other tetracycline derivatives include *minocycline* and *doxycycline.* Minocycline has improved gastrointestinal absorption over tetracycline and is not photosensitizing. Side effects of minocycline include dizziness and hyperpigmentation of the skin and mucosa. Doxycycline is another effective alternative to tetracycline. Its main disadvantage is photosensitivity. With all of the tetracyclines, vaginal candidiasis can occur with prolonged use.

Erythromycin is similar to tetracycline in that it is lipophilic and antiinflammatory. Its major disadvantages are *P. acnes* resistance, gastrointestinal distress, and cholestatic hepatitis. Trimethoprim–sulfamethoxazole (BACTRIM, others) has an important role in treating the gram-negative folliculitis seen in acne (O'Donoghue, 1999).

Adult women who have premenstrual flares of acne, adult onset acne, or acne that occurs mainly on the neck, jaw line, and lower face may be candidates for hormonal therapy. *Spironolactone* is an aldosterone-receptor antagonist (*see* Chapter 29) that has antiandrogenic activity. It has been shown to significantly improve acne at doses of 100 to 200 mg per day. It is commonly used in conjunction with other hormonal therapy. Common adverse effects include irregular menstrual periods and breast tenderness. Although there have been reports of the development of breast cancer in patients taking spironolactone, studies conducted over the past 25 years have not shown any association.

Cyproterone acetate is an androgen-receptor antagonist (*see* Chapter 59) that currently is not available in the United States but is used commonly in Europe. One dosing regimen employs 100 mg of cyproterone on days 5 to 15 and ethinyl estradiol on days 5 to 25 of the menstrual cycle. DIANE 35 is a European oral contraceptive that contains 2 mg of cyproterone acetate and 35 μg of ethinyl estradiol. It has been shown to have efficacy similar to that of isotretinoin in acne treatment. Side effects of cyproterone acetate include nausea, headache, decreased libido, and increased weight.

Oral contraceptives suppress ovarian steroidogenesis, reduce androgens, and increase steroid hormone–binding globulin, which binds testosterone. A triphasic formulation of norgestimate and ethinyl estradiol is available for the treatment of moderate acne. Glucocorticoids occasionally are useful in acute cystic acne and act by suppressing androgen production by the adrenal glands. Prednisone (2.5 to 10 mg per day) or dexamethasone (0.25 to 0.75 mg per day) are given each evening. The duration of therapy is dependent upon clinical response.

INFECTIONS

Infections of the skin may be divided into bacterial, viral, fungal, and parasitic etiologies. Bacterial infections of the skin include folliculitis, impetigo, pyodermas, erysipelas, cellulitis, and, at the extreme, necrotizing fasciitis. Bacteria also can exacerbate other conditions such as acne and atopic dermatitis.

Bacterial Infections. Systemic antibiotics are useful for most bacterial infections. Commonly used medications include *tetracycline, doxycycline, minocycline, erythromycin, trimethoprim–sulfamethoxazole,* and *clindamycin* (*see* Chapters 44 and 47). Topical antibiotics commonly are used in acne, acne rosacea, and superficial secondary infections. As discussed above, erythromycin, clindamycin,

and benzoyl peroxide are used topically in acne, and metronidazole is used topically in acne rosacea. Secondary bacterial infection of skin with gram-positive organisms responds to bacitracin zinc ointment. Superficial cutaneous *Staphylococcus* infections are effectively treated with *mupirocin* (BACTROBAN) cream. *Silver sulfadiazine* (SILVADENE, others) is effective against both gram-positive and gram-negative organisms but can cause neutropenia in children.

Viral Infections. Viral infections of the skin are legion and include verrucae (human papillomavirus or HPV), herpes simplex (HSV), condyloma acuminatum (HPV), molluscum contagiosum (poxvirus), and chicken pox (varicella) among others. Few effective medications are available for viral diseases. *Acyclovir* (ZOVIRAX), *famciclovir* (FAMVIR), and *valacyclovir* (VALTREX) frequently are used systemically to treat herpes simplex and varicella infections (*see* Chapter 50). Acyclovir and *penciclovir* (DENAVIR) are available for topical use in treating mucocutaneous herpes simplex. *Podophyllin* (25% solution) and *podofilox* (CONDYLOX) (0.5% solution) are used to treat the moist warts of condyloma. The immune-response modifier *imiquimod* (ALDARA), which induces interferon production, is approved for treatment of condyloma and is efficacious for the treatment of verrucae, molluscum contagiosum, and superficial basal cell carcinomas (*see* "Neoplasms of the Skin," below).

Fungal Infections. Fungal infections are among the most common causes of skin disease in the United States. Over the past few years a multitude of topical and oral antifungal agents have been developed. Griseofulvin, topical and oral azoles, and allylamines are the most effective agents available. The pharmacology, uses, and toxicities of antifungal drugs are discussed in Chapter 49. This section only addresses treatment of common cutaneous fungal diseases. Recommendations for cutaneous antifungal therapy are summarized in Table 65–8.

Topical therapy with the azoles (*e.g., miconazole, econazole*) and the allylamines (*e.g., naftifine, terbinafine*) is effective for treatment of localized tinea corporis and uncomplicated tinea pedis. *Terbinafine* cream (LAMISIL) may allow briefer therapy, because drug levels exceeding fungicidal concentrations are present in the skin 1 week after discontinuation of seven days of therapy. Topical therapy with the azoles is preferred for localized cutaneous candidiasis and tinea versicolor.

Systemic therapy is necessary for the treatment of tinea capitis. Oral *griseofulvin* has been the traditional medication for treatment of tinea capitis. Studies of oral

Table 65–8

Recommended Cutaneous Antifungal Therapy

CONDITION	TOPICAL THERAPY	ORAL THERAPY
Tinea corporis, localized	Azoles, allylamines	—
Tinea corporis, widespread	—	Griseofulvin, terbinafine, itraconazole, fluconazole
Tinea pedis	Azoles, allylamines	Griseofulvin, terbinafine, itraconazole, fluconazole
Onychomycosis	—	Griseofulvin, terbinafine, itraconazole, fluconazole
Candidiasis, localized	Azoles	—
Candidiasis, widespread and mucocutaneous	—	Ketaconazole, itraconazole, fluconazole
Tinea versicolor, localized	Azoles, allylamines	
Tinea versicolor, widespread	—	Ketaconazole, itraconazole, fluconazole

terbinafine (Krafchik and Pelletier, 1999; Elewski, 1997) have shown it to be a safe and effective treatment of tinea capitis in children and a viable alternative to griseofulvin.

Tinea Pedis. Tinea pedis encompasses three distinct syndromes: interdigital toe web infection, which begins as dry interdigital scaling caused by dermatophyte invasion and progresses to maceration complicated by bacterial invasion; scaly hyperkeratotic moccasin disease, where involvement of thick stratum corneum on the sole of the foot makes it difficult to achieve suitable drug concentrations; and inflammatory vesiculobullous eruptions (Leyden and Aly, 1993).

Topical therapy with the azoles and allylamines is effective for dry toe web disease. Macerated toe web disease may require the addition of antibacterial therapy. *Econazole nitrate* (SPECTAZOLE), which has a limited antibacterial spectrum, can be useful in the situation. Agents with a drying effect and broad-based antibacterial activity, such as 20% to 30% aluminum chloride or gentian violet, may be necessary.

Systemic therapy with griseofulvin, terbinafine, or itraconazole is effective for moccasin and vesiculobullous disease and is followed by long-term topical therapy with the azoles and allylamines.

Onychomycosis. Fungal infection of the nails is most frequently caused by dermatophytes but also can be caused by molds and *Candida*. Mixed infections are common. The nail must be cultured prior to therapy, since 30% of nail problems that appear clinically to be onychomycosis actually are due to psoriasis or another dystrophic nail condition (Achten and Wanet-Rouard, 1978). Onychomycosis serves as a reservoir for dermatophytes and contributes to treatment failure and recurrence of tinea pedis.

Systemic therapy is necessary for onychomycosis. Treatment of onychomycosis of toenails with griseofulvin for 12 to 18 months produces a cure rate of 50% and a relapse rate of 50% after 1 year (Davies *et al.*, 1967). Terbinafine and itraconazole offer significant potential advantages. They quickly produce high drug levels in the nail, which persist after therapy is discontinued. Additional advantages include a broader spectrum of coverage with itraconazole and few drug interactions with terbinafine. Treatment of toenail onychomycosis is for 3 months with terbinafine (250 mg per day) and itraconazole (pulsed dosing one week per month for 3 months). Cure rates of 75% and greater have been achieved with both drugs, with a shorter duration of treatment than with standard therapy (Gupta *et al.*, 1994a, 1994b).

Ciclopirox topical (PENLAC) solution is a nail lacquer recently approved for the treatment of onychomycosis. Despite low complete cure rates (5.5% to 8.5%), ciclopirox may be a reasonable alternative for patients with onychomycosis in whom oral antifungals are not indicated.

INFESTATIONS

Infestations with ectoparasites such as body lice and scabies are common throughout the world. These conditions have a significant impact on public health in the form of disabling pruritus, secondary infection, and, in the case of the body louse, transmission of life-threatening illness such as typhus. Both topical and oral medications are available to treat these infestations.

Perhaps the best known antiectoparasitic medication is 1% *gamma benzene hexachloride* lotion, also known as *lindane* (KWELL). Lindane has been used as a commercial insecticide (*see* Chapter 68) and also as a topical medication. This medication is highly effective in the treatment of ectoparasites (Shacter, 1981). Neurotoxicity is common with overuse or misuse of lindane. When this agent is used correctly, however, its side effect of neurotoxicity can be minimized. The lotion is applied in a thin layer from the neck down and left in place for 8 to 12 hours or overnight. Attention should be given to this application to ensure that areas such as the fingernail folds and the soles of the feet are not missed. The lotion should be removed by thorough washing at the end of the 8- to 12-hour period. To avoid problems with neurotoxicity, the lotion should be applied only in a thin coat to dry skin. It should not be applied immediately after bathing, and it should be kept away from the eyes, mouth, and open cuts or sores. After application to infants, the hands should be covered with mittens to avoid incidental ingestion of the lotion. Individuals with severely eczematous skin also may be at risk for excessive absorption. If a second treatment is needed, it should be conducted no sooner than one week from the first treatment (Rasmussen, 1981). Pregnant females may be treated with lindane, but no more than two treatments during a pregnancy are recommended. A 1% lindane shampoo also is available for head and body lice.

A second topical agent very useful in the treatment of ectoparasites is *permethrin*. Permethrin is a synthetic derivative of the insecticide pyrethrum, which was originally obtained from *Chrysanthemum cinerariaefolium*. Pyrethrum insecticides have been used in commercial agriculture for more than 100 years. They are noted to have exceptional insecticidal activity with very low mammalian toxicity (Taplin and Meinking, 1990; *see* Chapter 68). Permethrin is minimally absorbed through the skin and is rapidly degraded to inactive metabolites, which are excreted in the urine. Neurotoxicity associated with this compound is extremely rare. A 5% cream (ACTICIN, ELIMITE) is available for the treatment of scabies. This is used as an 8- to 12-hour or overnight application. A 1% permethrin cream rinse (NIX) also is available for the treatment of lice.

Ivermectin (STROMECTOL), an antihelminthic drug (*see* Chapter 41) used successfully to treat onchocerciasis in more than 19 million human beings, has been shown to be effective in the treatment of scabies. Ivermectin binds to GABA-gated chloride channels found in the muscle and nerve cells of invertebrates. Increased permeability to chloride ions causes hyperpolarization of the cells and results in paralysis and death. Ivermectin does not cross the blood–brain barrier, so there is no major central nervous system toxicity.

Ivermectin, available as a 6-mg tablet, is given as a single dose of 150 to 200 μg/kg on an empty stomach with a full glass of water. For an adult this generally works out to a single 12-mg dose, which may be repeated in two weeks. Cure rates of 70% after one dose and 95% after 2 doses given 2 weeks apart have been achieved (Usha *et al.*, 2000). For treatment of scabies outbreaks in

nursing homes, ivermectin may prove to be a convenient, economical, and efficacious alternative to topical medications (Wyatt, E.L., personal observation).

Other topical treatments for scabies include 10% *crotamiton* cream and lotion (EURAX) and 5% *sulfur in petrolatum*. Either of these treatments needs to be applied daily for 5 to 7 days. Efficacy of treatment is considerably less than with the above-mentioned topical insecticidal compounds. Crotamiton and sulfur typically are considered for use in those cases in which lindane or permethrin might be contraindicated.

NEOPLASMS OF THE SKIN

Many advances in nonsurgical treatment of precancerous and cancerous lesions of the skin have been developed over the past three decades. Both oral and topical medications now are available. Pharmacological properties, toxicities, and applications of cancer chemotherapeutic agents are discussed in Chapter 52.

Actinic (or *solar*) *keratoses* (AKs) are potentially serious cutaneous neoplasms that are a consequence of chronic ultraviolet radiation exposure. A minority of solar keratoses may undergo malignant transformation to squamous cell carcinoma; therefore, prevention and treatment of these precancerous lesions is indicated. Treatment modalities include destruction with cryogens, electrodesiccation and curettage, chemical peeling agents, and medical therapy with 5-fluorouracil and retinoids (Odom, 1998).

Systemic and topical retinoids have been used successfully to treat premalignant skin conditions and may have a role in chemoprevention of skin malignancies. Oral *etretinate* (1.5 mg/kg per day for the first month followed by 0.75 mg/kg per day) has been found to be highly effective in the treatment of actinic keratoses (Odom, 1998). Etretinate, however, is no longer available in the United States due to safety concerns regarding teratogenicity related to its storage in fat tissues and long half-life (Saurat, 1999). Acitretin, the active metabolite of etretinate, may have similar efficacy, but it has not been studied for this indication.

High-dose *isotretinoin* (2 mg/kg per day) has suppressed skin cancers in patients with increased risk of skin malignancy from congenital disorders, such as xeroderma pigmentosa and nevoid basal cell carcinoma syndrome. Benefits are recognized only as long as therapy continues, however, and significant toxicity may develop with long-term use of retinoids (DiGiovonna, 1998).

Topical *tretinoin*, available as a cream, gel, and liquid, is approved by the FDA for the treatment of acne and photoaged skin. Tretinoin cream applied once or twice daily was observed to decrease the size and number of AKs by 50% in one multicenter study (Thorne, 1992). By reducing the number and size of AKs, topical tretinoin may reduce the risk of developing certain kinds of skin cancer (Odom, 1998). Tretinoin has not yet been approved by the FDA for use in treating AKs.

5-Fluorouracil (FLUORPLEX, EFUDEX; 5-FU) is a topical antineoplastic medication available as a solution (1%, 2%, 5%) and a cream (1%, 5%). Indications for 5-FU include actinic keratoses, actinic cheilitis, Bowen's disease, and leukoplakia. 5-FU interferes with DNA synthesis by blocking the methylation reaction of deoxyuridylic acid to thymidylic acid (Dinehart, 2000). For treatment of actinic keratoses, 5-FU is applied twice daily for 4 to 5 weeks. Alternate treatment regimens include daily application or every-other-day application if irritation is extensive. Patients treated with 5-FU normally develop erythema, vesiculation, and desquamation, and they should be told to expect these changes and to be alert to increased sensitivity to sunlight and UV light. Reepithelialization occurs 1 or 2 months after treatment is discontinued. Side effects include allergic reactions, contact dermatitis, burning, and photosensitivity.

Basal cell carcinoma (BCC) is the most common malignancy in human beings with an incidence between 500,000 and 1 million cases per year in the United States. Surgery is the most common method of treatment. With the development of topical medications with antineoplastic properties, some groups of patients with superficial basal cells may benefit from nonsurgical intervention. 5-FU, as a 5% cream applied twice daily for 3 to 6 weeks, has been shown to be effective treatment for superficial BCCs. *Imiquimod,* as a 5% cream applied from twice daily to three times per week, has been shown to induce complete clearing of nonfacial, nodular, and superficial BCCs in 15 of 15 patients in one study (Beutner *et al.,* 1999), but this study needs to be confirmed in a larger population.

Cutaneous T-cell lymphoma (CTCL) or mycosis fungoides (MF) is a form of T-cell lymphoma that involves the skin. Treatment of early CTCL, consisting of patches and plaques, usually involves skin-directed therapies including chemotherapeutic agents, steroids, PUVA, and total skin electron beam therapy.

DAB-IL-2, or *denileukin diftitox* (ONTAK) is a fusion protein composed of diphtheria toxin fragments A and B and the receptor-binding portion of interleukin 2 (IL-2). DAB-IL-2 is indicated for advanced CTCL in patients with >20% of T-cells expressing the surface marker CD25. The IL-2 portion of the fusion protein binds the CD25 marker on the T cell and promotes destruction of the T cell by the cytocidal action of diphtheria toxin. The treatment protocol in a phase III clinical trial consisted of 9 or 18 μg/kg per day of DAB-IL-2 given as an intravenous infusion for 5 consecutive days every 22 days for up to 11 courses. The overall response rate was 36% with 18 μg/kg per day and 23% with 9 μg/kg per day. Side effects included pain, fevers, chills, nausea, vomiting, and diarrhea and hypo- or hypertension. A serious side effect of DAD-IL-2 is the capillary leak syndrome (Olsen *et al.,* 1998).

Mechlorethamine hydrochloride (nitrogen mustard) is a chemotherapeutic agent that has to be prepared daily by the patient as an aqueous solution of 10 mg/50 ml of water for topical use. It also is available as a less-irritating ointment that does not need to be prepared daily. Side effects include delayed-type hypersensitivity reactions, hyper- or hypopigmentation, and secondary cutaneous malignancies.

Patients who are allergic to mechlorethamine may use *carmustine* (*bis*-chloroethylnitrosourea or BCNU) instead. Therapy is given on alternate days with 200 to 600 mg of drug in a solution or ointment. Side effects include irritant dermatitis in up to 50% of patients, telangiectasia, erythema, and bone marrow suppression. Monitoring of blood counts is recommended with carmustine use.

Potent glucocorticoids applied twice daily have been successful in the treatment of early CTCL in some studies (Zackheim *et al.,* 1998). Other effective skin-directed therapies include PUVA and retinoids plus PUVA.

Biological response modifiers often are employed in the treatment of advanced CTCL. Extracorporeal photophoresis (ECP) involves removal of lymphocytes from the patient, their inactivation with 8-methoxypsoralen and UVA light, and then reinfusion of the inactive lymphocytes into the patient. Treatment is for two consecutive days every four weeks. ECP is most helpful in erythrodermic CTCL. Additionally, there have been significant responses to interferon alfa in some advanced cases of CTCL.

Bexarotene (TARGRETIN) is indicated in patients with CTCL refractory to skin-directed therapies. Bexarotene is a retinoid that selectively binds retinoid X receptors. Bexarotene is available in 75-mg capsules and the suggested dose is 300 mg/m^2 per day. It is metabolized by the CYP3A4 system. Inhibitors of CYP3A4, such as ketoconazole, itraconazole, and erythromycin, will increase plasma levels of bexarotene. Likewise, inducers of the CYP3A4 system will decrease plasma levels of bexarotene. Side effects include lipid abnormalities, pancreatitis, leukoplakia, and gastrointestinal symptoms. Blood lipids must be monitored when using this medication.

Kaposi's sarcoma (KS) is an AIDS-defining illness that consists of violaceous nodules. KS also may involve visceral organs. *Alitretinoin* (PANRETIN) is a retinoid that binds all retinoid receptors and is effective when applied as a 0.1% gel in decreasing the size and/or thickness of KS lesions. Approximately 50% of patients in an open-label trial had a positive response to alitretinoin (Walmsley *et al.,* 1999). Alitretinoin is indicated only for KS skin lesions and is not effective for visceral KS. Alitretinoin is applied 2 to 4 times daily and may take 2 to 14 weeks to yield improvement. Side effects include pain, tingling, itching, and flaking of the skin.

Photodynamic therapy is a treatment modality that involves the administration of a photosensitizing chemical, usually a porphyrin, and subsequent exposure to light. The photosensitizer may be either systemic (*e.g., porfimer sodium,* PHOTOFRIN) or topical (*e.g., δ-*aminolevulinic acid or ALA, LEVULAN KERASTICK). Light sources typically are in the visible range. Photodynamic therapy has indications for treatment of bladder, lung, and esophageal cancers. Studies in patients with cutaneous precancers and malignancies have shown promise for photodynamic therapy in the treatment of these conditions. Topical application of 20% ALA followed by a single light exposure has resulted in complete responses in 90% of actinic keratoses. Squamous-cell carcinoma *in situ* (Bowen's disease) is highly responsive to systemic photodynamic therapy. Other neoplasms that have responded in a promising way to photodynamic therapy include BCC, KS, and CTCL.

Photodynamic therapy appears to be a safe and effective treatment for selected premalignant and malignant conditions. Advantages of photodynamic therapy include its noninvasiveness, relative discrimination between normal and abnormal cells, applicability to treatment of large areas, and good cosmesis. Although there is still much information to be gathered about photodynamic therapy, it shows great promise as a complement to established practices in the management of skin cancers (Kalka *et al.,* 2000).

TREATMENT OF ANDROGENETIC ALOPECIA

Androgenetic alopecia, commonly known as male and female pattern baldness, is a common cause of hair loss in adults over the age of 40. As many as 50% of men and women are affected. Androgenetic alopecia is a genetically inherited trait with variable expression. Miniaturization of hair follicles occurs in affected areas producing fine vellus hairs and eventually complete hair loss in men (Olsen *et al.,* 1994). Complete baldness rarely occurs in women; rather, androgenetic alopecia is manifested by thinning hair in affected females (Bergfeld, 1998). Treatment of androgenetic areata is aimed at reducing hair loss, maintaining existing hair, and regrowth of lost hair.

Minoxidil was developed as an antihypertensive medication (*see* Chapter 33) and was found to be associated with hypertrichosis. A topical formulation of minoxidil was developed to exploit this side effect. Topical minoxidil is available as a 2% solution (ROGAINE) and a 5% solution (ROGAINE EXTRA STRENGTH FOR MEN). Minoxidil enhances follicular size, resulting in thicker hair shafts, and stimulates and prolongs the anagen phase of the hair cycle, resulting in longer and increased number of hairs (Fiedler, 1999).

Minoxidil as a 2% solution is indicated for androgenetic alopecia in both males and females. Application of 1 ml twice daily to the vertex of the scalp produces results in as few as four months. The 5% solution is applied in the same fashion as the 2% solution; however, more hair growth occurs with the 5% solution and results can be seen in as little as two months. With both strengths, treatment must be continued or the response of new hair growth will be lost.

Allergic contact dermatitis and irritant contact dermatitis are common side effects of minoxidil and occur more often with the 5% solution. Hair growth in undesirable locations can occur, but it resolves if the medication is kept away from the area. Patients should be instructed to wash their hands after applying minoxidil.

Finasteride (PROPECIA) is one of the newest medications for the treatment of androgenetic alopecia. Finasteride is a 5-alpha reductase inhibitor (*see* Chapter 59). 5-Alpha reductase is an enzyme that converts testosterone to dihydrotestosterone. The recognition of potential value of finasteride in the treatment of androgenetic alopecia was based upon the observation that men congenitally deficient in 5-alpha reductase had low dihydrotestosterone levels and did not develop male pattern baldness or prostate enlargement (Roberts *et al.,* 1999). In contrast, balding areas of the scalp have increased dihydrotestosterone levels and smaller hair follicles than do nonbalding areas. Two types of 5-alpha reductase exist: type I is found in sebaceous glands and type II is found in hair follicles. Finasteride is a type II 5-alpha reductase inhibitor and suppresses both serum and tissue levels of dihydrotestosterone (Drake *et al.,* 1999).

Finasteride (1 mg per day) has been shown to increase hair growth in up to 80% of men when given over a 2-year period. Finasteride increases hair counts in both the vertex of the scalp and the frontal scalp (Leyden *et al.,* 1999). Increased hair growth can be observed as early as 3 months into treatment.

Finasteride is approved for use only in men. Pregnant women should not touch broken tablets because of the potential for genital abnormalities in male fetuses. Side effects of finasteride include decreased libido, erectile dysfunction, ejaculation disorder, and decreased ejaculate volume. Each of these occurs in less than 2% of patients (Kaufman *et al.,* 1998). Finasteride also is known to decrease serum prostate-specific antigen (PSA) which is used in prostate cancer screening. Guidelines have been established for interpretation of PSA in patients on finasteride (Guess *et al.,* 1992; Oesterling *et al.,* 1997). Like minoxidil, treatment with finasteride must be continued or new hair growth will be lost.

Some studies in patients with androgenetic alopecia have revealed a favorable response to topical tretinoin. Topical tretinoin (0.025%) produced hair growth in a majority of patients in one study. Tretinoin also has been found to increase the percutaneous absorption of minoxidil. Combination topical therapy with 0.5% minoxidil and 0.025% tretinoin has led to hair growth in up to 66% of individuals tested (Bazzano *et al.,* 1986).

PROSPECTUS

An understanding of the importance of vehicles in percutaneous drug absorption has led to more scientifically based topical medications with improved efficacy and side-effect profiles. With the introduction of liposomes and microparticles, topical medications can better localize to target areas (*e.g.,* hair follicles), and drugs can be released in a time-delayed fashion.

Modification of the retinoid molecule has led to the development of retinoids with many diverse applications. The treatment of acne with retinoids has been improved with topical formulations, which are less irritating and more selective. Both oral and topical retinoids are available for the treatment of psoriasis. In addition to their role in chemoprevention of skin cancers, new retinoids have been developed to treat such malignancies as Kaposi's sarcoma and cutaneous T-cell lymphoma. Further modification of the retinoid molecule should improve receptor selectivity and decrease side effects when these agents are used in a wide array of disorders.

Biological response modifiers have been developed over the past few years. They have had an impact on the treatment of warts, skin cancers, and inflammatory skin conditions such as atopic dermatitis. A greater understanding of the pathophysiological processes of inflammatory diseases such as atopic dermatitis should allow the development of more effective treatments targeting specific immune dysfunction.

For further discussion of disorders of the skin *see* Chapters 54 to 58 in *Harrison's Principles of Internal Medicine,* 14th ed. McGraw-Hill, New York, 1998.

BIBLIOGRAPHY

Achten, G., and Wanet-Rouard, J. Onychomycosis in the laboratory. *Mykosen Suppl.,* **1978,** *23*:125–127.

Barker, N., Hadgraft, J., and Rutter, N. Skin permeability in the newborn. *J. Invest. Dermatol.,* **1987,** *88*:409–411.

Bazzano, G.S., Terezakis, N., and Galen, W. Topical tretinoin for hair growth promotion. *J. Am. Acad. Dermatol.,* **1986,** *15*:880–883.

Bergasa, N.V., Alling, D.W., Talbot, T.L., Wells, M.C., and Jones, E.A. Oral nalmefene therapy reduces scratching activity due to the pruritus of cholestasis: a controlled study. *J. Am. Acad. Dermatol.,* **1999,** *41*:431–434.

Beutner, K.R., Geisse, J.K., Helman, D., Fox, T.L., Ginkel, A., and Owens, M.L. Therapeutic response of basal cell carcinoma to the immune response modifier imiquimod 5% cream. *J. Am. Acad. Dermatol.,* **1999,** *41*:1002–1007.

Bondi, E.E., and Kligman, A.M. Adverse effects of topical corticosteroids. *Prog. Dermatol.,* **1980,** *14*:1–4.

Carucci, J.A., Washenik, K., Weinstein, A., Shupack, J., and Cohen, D.E. The leukotriene antagonist zafirlukast as a therapeutic agent for atopic dermatitis. *Arch. Dermatol.,* **1998,** *134*:785–786.

Chandraratna, R.A. Rational design of receptor-selective retinoids. *J. Am. Acad. Dermatol.,* **1998,** *39*:S124–S128.

Cockburn, I.T., and Krupp, P. The risk of neoplasms in patients treated with cyclosporine A. *J. Autoimmun.,* **1989,** *2*:723–731.

Connolly, C.S., Kantor, G.R., and Menduke, H. Hepatobiliary pruritus: what are effective treatments? *J. Am. Acad. Dermatol.,* **1995,** *33*:801–805.

Czech, W., Brautigam, M., Weidinger, G., and Schopf, E. A body-weight-independent dosing regimen of cyclosporine microemulsion is effective in severe atopic dermatitis and improves quality of life. *J. Am. Acad. Dermatol.,* **2000,** *42*:653–659.

Davies, R.R., Everall, J.D., and Hamilton, E. Mycological and clinical evaluation of griseofulvin for chronic onychomycosis. *Br. Med. J.,* **1967,** *3*:464–468.

DiGiovanna, J.J. Retinoid chemoprevention in the high-risk patient. *J. Am. Acad. Dermatol.,* **1998,** *39*:S82–S85.

Dinehart, S.M. The treatment of actinic keratoses. *J. Am. Acad. Dermatol.,* **2000,** *42*:25–28.

Drake, L., Hardinsky, M., Fiedler V., Swinehart, J., Unger, W.P., Cotterill, P.C., Thiboutot, D.M., Lowe, N., Jacobson, C., Whiting, D., Stieglitz, S., Kraus, S.J., Griffin, E.I., Weiss, D., Carrington, P., Gencheff, C., Cole, G.W., Pariser, D.M., Epstein, E.S., Tanaka, W., Dallob, A., Vandormael, K., Geissler, L., and Waldstreicher, J. The effects of finasteride on scalp skin and serum androgen levels in men with androgenetic alopecia. *J. Am. Acad. Dermatol.,* **1999,** *41*:550–554.

Dumas, K.J., and Scholtz, J.R. The psoriasis bio-assay for topical corticosteroid activity. *Acta Derm. Venereol.,* **1972,** *52*:43–48.

Dupuy, P., Bagot, M., Michel, L., Descourt, B., and Dubertret, L. Cyclosporin A inhibits the antigen-presenting functions of freshly isolated human Langerhans cells in vitro. *J. Invest. Dermatol.,* **1991,** *96*:408–413.

Duvic, M., and Marks, R. Tazarotene: optimizing the therapeutic benefits of a new topical receptor-selective retinoid. Proceedings of a symposium held during the 19th World Congress of Dermatology, Sydney, Australia, 1997. *J. Am. Acad. Dermatol. (Suppl.),* **1998,** *39*:S123–S152.

Elewski, B.E. Treatment of tinea capitis with itraconazole. *Int. J. Dermatol.,* **1997,** *36*:537–541.

Ellis, C.N., Fradin, M.S., Messana, J.M., Brown, M.D., Siegel, M.T., Hartley, A.H., Rocher, L.L., Wheeler, S., Hamilton, T.A., Parish, T.G., Ellis-Madu, M., Duell, E., Annesley, T.M., Cooper, K.D., and Voorhees, J.J. Cyclosporine for plaque-type psoriasis. Results of a multidose, double-blind trial. *N. Engl. J. Med.,* **1991,** *324*:277–284.

Fiedler, V.C. Understanding the causes of androgenetic alopecia. *Skin Aging,* March **1999,** pp. 72–80.

Gottlieb, S.L., Gilleavdeau, P., Johnson, R., Estes, L., Woodworth, T.G., Gottlieb, A.B., and Krueger, J.G. Response of psoriasis to a lymphocyte-selective toxin (DAB389IL-2) suggests a primary immune, but not keratinocyte, pathogenic basis. *Nat. Med.,* **1995,** *1*:442–447.

Guess, H.A., Gormley, G.J., Stoner, E., and Oesterling, J.E. The effect of finasteride on prostate specific antigen: review of available data. *J. Urol.,* **1992,** *155*:3–9.

Guin, J.D., Wallis, M.S., Walls, R., Lehman, P.A., and Franz, T.J. Quantitive vasoconstrictor essay for topical corticosteroids: the puzzling case of fluocinolone acetonide. *J. Am. Acad. Dermatol.,* **1993,** *29*:197–202.

Gupta, A.K., and Anderson, T.F. Psoralen photochemotherapy. *J. Am. Acad. Dermatol.,* **1987,** *17*:703–734.

Hardman, K.A., Heath, D.A., and Nelson, H.M. Hypercalcaemia associated with calcipotriol (Dovenex) treatment. *BMJ,* **1993,** *306*:896.

Hensler, T., Wolff, K., Honigsmann, H., and Christophers, E. Oral 8-methoxypsoralen photochemotherapy of psoriasis. The European PUVA study: a cooperative study among 18 European centres. *Lancet,* **1981,** *1*:853–857.

Jackson, D.B., Thompson, C., McCormack, J.R., and Guin, J.D. Bioequivalence (bioavailability) of generic topical corticosteroids. *J. Am. Acad. Dermatol.,* **1989,** *20*:791–796.

Jeffes, E.W. III, McCullough J.L., Pittelkow, M.R., McCormick, A., Almanzor, J., Liu, G., Dang, M., Voss, K., Voss, J., Scholtzhauer, A., and Weinstein, G.D. Methotrexate therapy of psoriasis: differential sensitivity of proliferating lymphoid and epithelial cells to the cytotoxic and growth-inhibitory effects of methotrexate. *J. Invest. Dermatol.,* **1995,** *104*:183–188.

Kalka, K., Merk, H., and Mukhtar, J. Photodynamic therapy in dermatology. *J. Am. Acad. Dermatol.,* **2000,** *42*:389–413.

Kaufman, K.D., Olsen, E.A., Whiting, D., Savin, R., Devillez, R., Bergeld, W., Price, V.H., Van Neste, D., Roberts, J.L., Hordinsky, M., Shapiro, J., Binkowitz, B., and Gormley, G.J. Finasteride in the treatment of men with androgenetic alopecia. Finasteride Male Pattern Hair Loss Study Group. *J. Am. Acad. Dermatol.,* **1998,** *39*:578–589.

Kitchin, J.E., Pomeranz, M., Pak, G., Washenik, K., and Shupak, J. Rediscovering mycophenolic acid: a review of its mechanism, side effects, and potential uses. *J. Am. Acad. Dermatol.,* **1997,** *37*:445–449.

Kligman, A.M., Fulton, J.E. Jr., and Plewig, G. Topical vitamin A acid in acne vulgaris. *Arch. Dermatol.,* **1969,** *99*:469–476.

Korting, H.C., Blecher, P., Schafer-Korting, M., and Wendel, A. Topical liposome drugs to come: what the patent literature tells us. A review. *J. Am. Acad. Dermatol.,* **1991,** *25*:1068–1071.

Krafchik, B., and Pelletier, J. An open study of tinea capitis in 50 children treated with a 2-week course of oral terbinafine. *J. Am. Acad. Dermatol.,* **1999,** *41*:60–63.

Kragballe, K. Treatment of psoriasis by the topical application of the novel cholecalciferol analog calcipotriol. *Arch. Dermatol.,* **1989,** *125*:1647–1652.

Kragballe, K. Treatment of psoriasis with calcipotriol and other vitamin D analogues. *J. Am. Acad. Dermatol.,* **1992,** *27*:1001–1008.

Langner, A., Verjans, H., Stapor, V., et al. Treatment of chronic plaque psoriasis by 1-alpha, 25-dihydroxyvitamin D3 ointment. In, *Proceedings of the Eighth Workshop on Vitamin D.* (Norman, A.W., Bouillon, R., Thomasset, M., eds.) Walter De Gruyter, Berlin, **1992,** pp. 430–431.

Leavell, U.W. Jr., Mersack, I.P., and Smith, C. Survey of the treatment of psoriasis with hydroxyuria. *Arch. Dermatol.,* **1973,** *107*:467.

Lebwohl, M. Acitretin in combination with UVB or PUVA. *J. Am. Acad. Dermatol.,* **1999,** *41*:S22–S24.

Leyden, J., Dunlap, F., Miller, B., Winters, P., Lebwohl, M., Hecker, D., Kraus, S., Baldwin, H., Shalita, A., Draelos, Z., Markou, M., Thiboutot, D., Rapaport, M., Kang, S., Kelly, T., Pariser, D., Webster, G., Hordinsky, M., Rietschel, R., Katz, H.I., Terranella, L., Best, S., Round, E., and Waldstreicher, J. Finasteride in the treatment of men with frontal male pattern hair loss. *J. Am. Acad. Dermatol.,* **1999,** *40*:930–937.

Leyden, J.J. The role of isotretinoin in the treatment of acne: personal observations. *J. Am. Acad. Dermatol.,* **1998,** *39*:S45–S49.

Ling, M.R. Acitretin: optimal dosing strategies. *J. Am. Acad. Dermatol.,* **1999,** *41*:S13–S17.

Lowe, N.J., Wortzman, M.S., Breeding, J., Koudsi, H., and Taylor, L. Coal tar phototherapy for psoriasis reevaluated: erythemogenic versus suberythemogenic ultraviolet with a tar extract in oil and crude coal tar. *J. Am. Acad. Dermatol.,* **1983,** *8*:781–789.

McKenzie, A.W., and Stoughton, R.B. Method for comparing percutaneous absorption of steroids. *Arch. Dermatol.,* **1962,** *86*:608–610.

Melski, J.W., Tanenbaum, L., Parrish, J.A., Fitzpatrick, T.B., and Bleich, H.L. Oral methoxsalen photochemotherapy for the treatment of psoriasis: a cooperative clinical trial. *J. Invest. Dermatol.,* **1977,** *68*:328–335.

Metze, D., Reimann, S., Biessert, S., and Luger, T. Efficacy and safety of naltrexone, an oral opiate receptor antagonist, in the treatment of pruritus in internal and dermatological diseases. *J. Am. Acad. Dermatol.,* **1999,** *41*:533–539.

Morimoto, S., and Kumahara, Y. A patient with psoriasis cured by 1-alpha-hydroxyvitamin D3. *Med. J. Osaka Univ.,* **1985,** *35*:51–54.

O'Donoghue, M. Get the most from the oral medicines for acne. *Skin Aging,* Oct. **1999,** suppl., pp. 10–13.

Oesterling, J.E., Roy, J., Agha, A., Shown, T., Krarup, T., Johansen, T., Lagerkvist, M., Gormley, G., Bach, M., and Waldstreicher, J. Biologic variability of prostate-specific antigen and its usefulness as a marker for prostate cancer: effects of finasteride. Finasteride PSA Study Group. *Urology,* **1997,** *50*:13–18.

Ohtsuka, T., Yamakage, A., and Yamazaki, S. A case of prurigo and lichenified plaques successfully treated with proton pump inhibitor. *J. Dermatol.,* **1999,** *26*:518–523.

Olsen, E.A. A double-blind controlled comparison of generic and trade-name topical steroids using the vasoconstriction assay. *Arch. Dermatol.,* **1991,** *127*:197–201.

Olsen, E.A., Duvic, M., Martin, A., and the DAB$_{389}$ IL-2 Lymphoma Group. Pivotal phase III trial of two dose levels of DAB$_{389}$IL-2 (ONTAK) for the treatment of cutaneous T-cell lymphoma (CTCL). *J. Invest. Dermatol.,* **1998,** *110*:678, abstract 1234.

Parrish, J.A., Fitzpatrick, T.B., Tanenbaum, L., and Pathak, M.A.

Photochemotherapy of psoriasis with oral methoxsalen and long-wave ultraviolet light. *N. Engl. J. Med.,* **1974,** *291*:1207–1211.

Piacquadio, D., and Kligman, A. The critical role of the vehicle to therapeutic efficacy and patient compliance. *J. Am. Acad. Dermatol.,* **1998,** *39*:S67–S73.

Rasmussen, J.E. The problem of lindane. *J. Am. Acad. Dermatol.,* **1981,** *5*:507–516.

Reichert, U., Jacques, Y., Grangeret, M., and Schmidt, R. Antirespiratory and antiproliferative activity of anthralin in cultured human keratinocytes. *J. Invest. Dermatol.,* **1985,** *84*:130–134.

Roberts, J., Fiedler, U., Imperato-McGinley, J., Whiting, D., Olsen, E., Shupack, J., Stough, D., DeVillez, R., Rietschel, R., Savin, R., Bergfeld, W., Swinehart, J., Funicella, T., Hordinsky, M., Lowe, N., Katz, I., Lucky, A., Drake, L., Price, V.H., Weiss, D., Whitmore, E., Millikan, L., Muller, S., Gencheff, C., Carrington, P., Binkowitz, B., Kotey, P., He, W., Bruno, K., Jacobsen, C., Terranella, L., Gormley, G.J., and Kaufman, K.D. Clinical dose ranging studies with finasteride, a type 2 5α-reductase inhibitor, in men with male pattern hair loss. *J. Am. Acad. Dermatol.,* **1999,** *41*:555–563.

Roenigk, H.H., Auerbach, R., Maibach, H., Weinstein, G., and Lebwohl, M. Methotrexate in psoriasis: consensus conference. *J. Am. Acad. Dermatol.,* **1998,** *38*:478–485.

Ruzicka, T., Assmann, T., and Homey, B. Tacrolimus: the drug for the turn of the millennium? *Arch. Dermatol.,* **1999,** *135*:574–580.

Saurat, J.H. Retinoids and psoriasis: novel issues in retinoid pharmacology and implications for psoriasis treatment. *J. Am. Acad. Dermatol.,* **1999,** *41*:S2–S6.

Schaefer, H., Farber, E.M., Goldberg, L., and Schalla, W. Limited application period for dithranol in psoriasis. Preliminary report on penetration and clinical efficacy. *Br. J. Dermatol.,* **1980,** *102*:571–573.

Schreiber, S.L., and Crabtree, G.R. The mechanism of action of cyclosporin A and FK506. *Immunol. Today,* **1992,** *13*:136–142.

Shacter, B. Treatment of scabies and pediculosis with lindane preparations: an evaluation. *J. Am. Acad. Dermatol.,* **1981,** *5*:517–527.

Shroot, B. Pharmacodynamics and pharmacokinetics of topical adapalene. *J. Am. Acad. Dermatol.,* **1998,** *39*:S17–S24.

Shupack, J., Abel, E., Bayer, E., Brown, M., Drake, L., Freinkel, R., Guzzo, C., Koo, J., Levine, N., Lowe, N., McDonald, C., Margolis, D., Stiller, M., Wintroub, B., Bainbridge, C., Evans, S., Hilss, S., Mietlowski, W., Winslow, C., and Birnbaum, J.E. Cyclosporine as maintenance therapy in patients with severe psoriasis. *J. Am. Acad. Dermatol.,* **1997,** *36*:423–432.

Singh, G., and Singh, P.K. Tachyphylaxis to topical steroid measured by histamine-induced wheal suppression. *Int. J. Dermatol.,* **1986,** *25*:324–326.

Smith, E.L., Pincus, S.H., Donovan, L., and Holick, M.F. A novel approach for the evaluation and treatment of psoriasis. Oral or topical use of 1,25-dihydroxyvitamin D3 can be a safe and effective therapy for psoriasis. *J. Am. Acad. Dermatol.,* **1988,** *19*:516–528.

Smith, E.L., Walworth, N.D., and Holick, M.F. Effect of 1 alpha, 25-dihydroxyvitamin D3 on the morphologic and biochemical differentiation of cultured human epidermal keratinocytes grown in serum-free conditions. *J. Invest. Dermatol.,* **1986,** *86*:709–714.

Stern, R.S., Nichols, K.T., and Vakeva, L.H. Malignant melanoma in patients treated for psoriasis with methoxsalen (psoralen) and ultraviolet A radiation (PUVA). The PUVA Follow-up Study. *N. Engl. J. Med.,* **1997,** *336*:1041–1045.

Stern, R.L., and Lange, R. Non-melanoma skin cancer occurring in patients treated with PUVA five to ten years after first treatment. *J. Invest. Dermatol.* **1988,** *91*:120–124.

Sulzberger, M.B., and Witten, V.H. The effect of topically applied compound F in selected dermatoses. *J. Invest. Dermatol.,* **1952,** *19*:101–102.

Thorne, E.G. Long-term clinical experience with a topical retinoid. *Br. J. Dermatol.,* **1992,** *127(suppl. 41)*:31–36.

Triggiani, M., Cirillo, R., Lichtenstein, L.M., and Marone, G. Inhibition of histamine and prostaglandin D2 release from human lung mast cells by ciclosporin A. *Int. Arch. Allergy Appl. Immunol.,* **1989,** *88*:253–255.

Usha, V., Gopalakrishnan, T.V., and Nair, T.V. A comparative study of oral ivermectin and topical permethrin cream in the treatment of scabies. *J Am. Acad. Dermatol.,* **2000,** *42*:236–240.

Walmsley, S., Northfelt, D.W., Melosky, B., Conant, M., Friedman-Kien, A.E., and Wagner, B. Treatment of AIDS-related cutaneous Kaposi's sarcoma with topical alitretinoin (9-*cis*-retinoic acid) gel. Panretin Gel North American Study Group. *J. Acquir. Immune Defic. Syndr.,* **1999,** *22*:235–246.

Webster, G.F. Topical tretinoin in acne therapy. *J. Am. Acad. Dermatol.,* **1998,** *39*:S38–S44.

Weiss, J.S., and Shavin, J.S. Adapalene for the treatment of acne vulgaris. *J. Am. Acad. Dermatol.,* **1998,** *39*:S50–S54.

Wood, M.J., Johnson, R.W., McKendrick, M.W., Taylor, J., Mandal, B.K., and Crooks, J. A randomized trial of acyclovir for 7 days or 21 days with and without prednisolone for treatment of acute herpes zoster. *N. Engl. J. Med.,* **1994,** *330*:896–900.

Zackheim, H.S., Glogau, R.G., Fisher, D.A., and Maibach, H.I. 6-Thioguanine treatment of psoriasis: experience in 81 patients. *J. Am. Acad. Dermatol.,* **1994,** 30:452–458.

Zackheim, H.S., Kashani-Sabet, M., and Amin, S. Topical corticosteroids for mycosis fungoides. Experience in 79 patients. *Arch. Dermatol.,* **1998,** *134*:949–954.

Zaki, I., Emerson, R., and Allen, B.R. Treatment of severe atopic dermatitis in childhood with cyclosporin. *Br. J. Dermatol.,* **1996,** 135(suppl. 48):21–24.

Zonneveld, I.M., De Rie, M.A., Beljaards, R.C., Van Der Rhee, H.J., Wuite, J., Zeegelaar, J., and Bos, J.D. The long-term safety and efficacy of cyclosporin in severe refractory atopic dermatitis: a comparison of two dosage regimens. *Br. J. Dermatol.,* **1996,** 135(suppl. 48): 15–20.

MONOGRAPHS AND REVIEWS

Bergfeld, W.F. Retinoids and hair growth. *J. Am. Acad. Dermatol.,* **1998,** *39*:S86–S89.

Berson, D. Using the newest topical agents for treating acne. *Skin & Aging,* Oct. **1999,** supplement: pp. 6–9.

Christophers, E., and Mrowietz, U. Psoriasis. In, *Fitzpatrick's Dermatology in General Medicine,* 5th ed. (Freedburg, I.M., Eisen, A.Z., Wolff, K., Austen, K.F., Goldsmith, L.A., Katz, S.I., and Fitzpatrick, T.B., eds.) McGraw-Hill, New York, **1999,** pp. 495–521.

Dodd, W.A. TARS. Their role in the treatment of psoriasis. *Dermatol. Clin.,* **1993,** *11*:131–135.

Faulds, D., Goa, K.L., and Benfield, P. Cyclosporin. A review of its pharmacodynamic and pharmacokinetic properties, and therapeutic use in immunoregulatory disorders. *Drugs,* **1993,** *45*:953–1040.

Goldfork, M.T., and Ellis, C. Clinical uses of etretinate and acitretin. In, *Psoriasis,* 3rd ed. (Roenigk, H.H. Jr., and Maibach, H.I., eds.) Marcel Dekker, New York, **1998,** pp. 663–670.

Gupta, A.K., Sauder, D.N., and Shear, N.H. Antifungal agents: an overview. Part I. *J. Am. Acad. Dermatol.,* **1994a,** *30*:677–698.

Gupta, A.K., Sauder, D.N., and Shear, N.H. Antifungal agents: an overview. Part II. *J. Am. Acad. Dermatol.,* **1994b,** *30*:911–933.

Jakubovic, H.R., and Ackerman, A.B. Structure and function of skin: development, morphology, and physiology. In, *Dermatology.* Vol. 1 (Moschella, S.L., and Hurley, H.J., eds.) Saunders, Philadelphia, **1992,** pp. 15–21.

Kantor, G.R. Pruritus. In, *Principles and Practice of Dermatology,* 2nd ed. (Sams, W.M. Jr., and Lynch, P.J., eds.) Churchill Livingstone, New York, **1996,** pp. 881–885.

Katz, H.I., Waalen, J., and Leach, E.E. Acitretin in psoriasis: an overview of adverse effects. *J. Am. Acad. Dermatol.,* **1999,** *41*:S7–S12.

Kimberly, R.P. Treatment. Corticosteroids and anti-inflammatory drugs. *Rheum. Dis. Clin. North Am.,* **1988,** *14*:203–221.

King, J.M. Historical review of early dermatology. *South. Med. J.,* **1927,** *76*:426–436.

Leyden, J.J., and Aly, R. Tinea pedis. *Semin. Dermatol.,* **1993,** *12*:280–284.

Odom, R. Managing actinic keratoses with retinoids. *J. Am. Acad. Dermatol.,* **1998,** *39*:S74–S78.

Olsen, E.A. Androgenetic alopecia. In, *Disorders of Hair Growth: Diagnosis and Treatment.* (Olsen, E.A., ed.) McGraw-Hill, New York, **1994,** pp. 257–283.

Polano, M.K. *Topical Skin Therapeutics.* Churchill Livingstone, Edinburgh, **1984.**

Rao, A. NF-ATp: a transcription factor required for the co-ordinate induction of several cytokine genes. *Immunol. Today,* **1994,** *15*:274–281.

Shelley, W.B., and Shelley, E.D. *A Century of International Dermatological Congresses: An Illustrated History* 1889–1992. Parthenon, Cornforth, UK, **1992.**

Smith, K. Expert advice on using Accutane. *Skin & Aging,* Oct. **1999,** pp. 62–70.

Talpin, D., and Meinking, T. Pyrethrins and pyrethroids in dermatology. *Arch. Dermatol.,* **1990,** *126*:213–221.

Werth, V.P. Management and treatment with systemic glucocorticoids. *Adv. Dermatol.,* **1993,** *8*:81–103.

Wester, R.C., and Maibach, H.I. Percutaneous absorption of topical corticosteroids. *Curr. Probl. Dermatol.,* **1993,** *21*:45–60.

Yohn, J.J., and Weston, W.L. Topical glucocorticoids. *Curr. Probl. Dermatol.,* **1990,** *11*:37–63.

Acknowledgment

The authors wish to acknowledge Cynthia A. Guzzo, Gerald S. Lazarus, and Victoria P. Werth, authors of this chapter in the ninth editon of *Goodman and Gilman's The Pharmacological Basis of Therapeutics,* some of whose text we have retained in this edition.

S E C T I O N   X V

OPHTHALMOLOGY

CHAPTER 66

OCULAR PHARMACOLOGY

Sayoko E. Moroi and Paul R. Lichter

This chapter focuses on specific pharmacodynamic, pharmacokinetic, and drug delivery issues relevant to ocular therapy and imparted by the unique anatomy and function of this sensory organ, introduced at the outset of this chapter. Many of the pharmacological agents discussed here have been discussed in earlier chapters. Autonomic agents have several uses in ophthalmology, including diagnostic evaluation of anisocoria and myasthenia gravis, as adjunctive therapy in laser and incisional surgeries, and in the treatment of glaucoma. These agents are discussed in detail in Chapters 6 to 10. The antimicrobial agents employed for chemotherapy of orbital cellulitis, conjunctivitis, keratitis, endophthalmitis, retinitis, and uveitis also are discussed in Chapters 43 to 50. The vitamins and trace elements used in adjunctive eye therapy are discussed in Chapters 63 and 64, and immunomodulatory agents important in treating vitreoretinopathy, retinitis, and uveitis are discussed in Chapter 53. Also included in this chapter are the wetting agents and tear substitutes used to treat dry eye syndrome, as well as drugs and osmotic agents affecting ocular electrolyte metabolism (see also Chapter 29). The chapter concludes with a prospectus on the future of ocular therapeutics, including gene transfer, immunomodulation, molecular- and cellular-based therapies including inhibitors of protein kinase C for diabetic retinopathy, and neuroprotection.

History. Records from Mesopotamia (ca. 3000–4000 B.C.) reveal that mysticism—combined with vegetable, animal, and mineral matter—was used to treat spirits and devils causing eye disease. During the classical Greek era (ca. 460–375 B.C.) when Hippocrates revolutionized the therapeutics of disease, several hundred remedies were described for afflictions of the eye. Galen and Susruta categorized eye diseases on an anatomical basis and applied medicinal as well as surgical remedies advocated by Hippocrates (*see* Duke-Elder, 1962; Albert and Edwards, 1996).

With this empirical approach to treat disease, ophthalmic therapeutics took root from remedies discovered for systemic diseases. For instance, silver nitrate was used medicinally in the early seventeenth century. Credé later instituted the use of silver nitrate in newborns as prophylaxis against neonatal conjunctivitis, a potentially blinding condition, which during his time was primarily caused by *Neisseria gonorrhoeae*. In the nineteenth century, numerous organic substances were isolated from plants and introduced to treat eye diseases. The belladonna alkaloids were used as poisons, for asthmatic therapy, and for cosmetic effect; hyoscyamus and belladonna were used to treat iritis in the early 1800s. Atropine was isolated and used therapeutically in the eye in 1832. In 1875, pilocarpine was isolated; the therapeutic effect of lowering intraocular pressure was recognized in 1877, providing the basis for a safe and effective treatment of glaucoma that is still efficacious.

OVERVIEW OF OCULAR ANATOMY, PHYSIOLOGY, AND BIOCHEMISTRY

The eye is a specialized sensory organ that is relatively secluded from systemic access by the blood-retinal, blood-aqueous, and blood-vitreous barriers. Because of this anatomical isolation, the eye offers a unique, organ-specific pharmacological laboratory to study, for example, the autonomic nervous system and effects of inflammation and infectious diseases. No other organ in the body is so readily accessible or as visible for observation; however, the eye also presents some unique opportunities as well as challenges for drug delivery (*see* Robinson, 1993).

Extraocular Structures

The eye is protected by the eyelids and by the orbit, a bony cavity of the skull that has multiple fissures and foramina that conduct nerves, muscles, and vessels (Figure 66–1). In the orbit, connective (*i.e.,* Tenon's capsule) and adipose tissues and six extraocular muscles support and

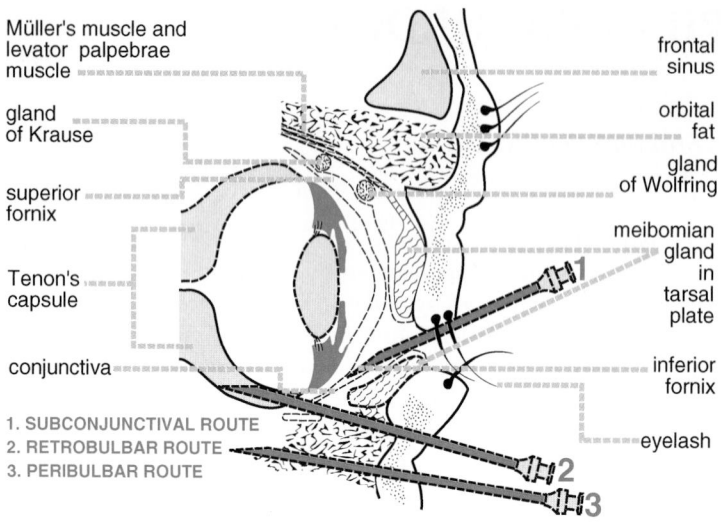

Müller's muscle and levator palpebrae muscle

gland of Krause

superior fornix

Tenon's capsule

conjunctiva

1. SUBCONJUNCTIVAL ROUTE
2. RETROBULBAR ROUTE
3. PERIBULBAR ROUTE

frontal sinus

orbital fat

gland of Wolfring

meibomian gland in tarsal plate

inferior fornix

eyelash

Figure 66–1. Anatomy of the globe in relationship to the orbit and eyelids.

Various routes of administration of anesthesia are demonstrated by the blue needle pathways. (Adapted from Riordan-Eva and Tabbara, 1992, with permission.)

align the eyes for vision. The area behind the eye (or *globe*) is called the retrobulbar region. Understanding ocular and orbital anatomy is important for safe periocular drug delivery, including subconjunctival, sub-Tenon's, and retrobulbar injections. The eyelids serve several functions. Foremost, their dense sensory innervation and eyelashes protect the eye from mechanical and chemical injuries. Blinking, a coordinated movement of the orbicularis oculi, levator palpebrae, and Müller's muscles, serves to distribute tears over the cornea and conjunctiva. In human beings, the average blink rate is 15 to 20 times per minute. The external surface of the eyelids is covered by a thin layer of skin; the internal surface is lined with the palpebral portion of the conjunctiva, which is a vascularized mucous membrane continuous with the bulbar conjunctiva. At the reflection of the palpebral and bulbar conjunctiva is a space called the fornix, located superiorly and inferiorly behind the upper and lower lids, respectively. Topical medications usually are placed in the inferior fornix, also known as the inferior cul-de-sac.

The lacrimal system consists of secretory glandular and excretory ductal elements (Figure 66–2). The secretory system is composed of the main lacrimal gland, which is located in the temporal outer portion of the orbit, and accessory glands, also known as the glands of Krause and Wolfring (*see* Figure 66–1), located in the conjunctiva. The lacrimal gland is innervated by the autonomic nervous system (*see* Table 66–1 and Chapter 6). The parasympathetic innervation is clinically relevant since a patient may complain of dry eye symptoms while taking medications with anticholinergic side effects, such as antidepressants

(*see* Chapter 19), antihistamines (*see* Chapter 25), and drugs used in the management of Parkinson's disease (*see* Chapter 22). Located just posterior to the eyelashes are meibomian glands (*see* Figure 66–1), which secrete oils that retard evaporation of the tear film. Abnormalities in gland function, as in acne rosacea and meibomitis, can greatly affect tear film stability.

Conceptually, tears constitute a trilaminar lubrication barrier covering the conjunctiva and cornea. The anterior layer is composed primarily of lipids secreted by the meibomian glands. The middle aqueous layer, produced by the main lacrimal gland and accessory lacrimal glands (*i.e.,* Krause and Wolfring glands), constitutes about 98% of the tear film. Adherent to the corneal epithelium, the

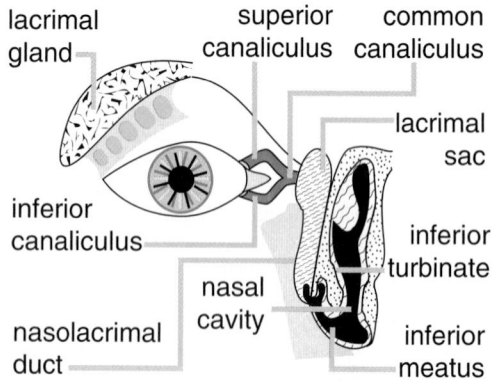

lacrimal gland

superior canaliculus

common canaliculus

lacrimal sac

inferior canaliculus

nasal cavity

nasolacrimal duct

inferior turbinate

inferior meatus

Figure 66–2. Anatomy of the lacrimal system.

(Adapted from Riordan-Eva and Tabbara, 1992, with permission.)

Table 66–1
Autonomic Pharmacology of the Eye and Related Structures

TISSUE	*Adrenergic Receptors*		*Cholinergic Receptors*	
	SUBTYPE	RESPONSE	SUBTYPE	RESPONSE
Corneal epithelium	β_2	Unknown	M†	Unknown
Corneal endothelium	β_2	Unknown	Undefined	Unknown
Iris radial muscle	α_1	Mydriasis		
Iris sphincter muscle			M_3	Miosis
Trabecular meshwork	β_2	Unknown		
Ciliary epithelium‡	α_2/β_2	Aqueous production		
Ciliary muscle	β_2	Relaxation§	M_3	Accommodation
Lacrimal gland	α_1	Secretion	M_2, M_3	Secretion
Retinal pigment epithelium	α_1/β_2	H_2O transport/unknown		

†Although acetylcholine and choline acetyltransferase are abundant in corneal epithelium of most species, the function of this neurotransmitter in this tissue is unknown (Baratz *et al.,* 1987; Wilson and McKean, 1986).

‡The ciliary epithelium is also the target of carbonic anhydrase inhibitors. Carbonic anhydrase isoenzyme II is localized to both the pigmented and nonpigmented ciliary epithelium (Wistrand *et al.,* 1986).

§Although β_2-adrenergic receptors mediate ciliary body smooth muscle relaxation, there is no clinically significant effect on accommodation.

posterior layer is a mixture of mucins produced by goblet cells in the conjunctiva. Tears also contain nutrients, enzymes, and immunoglobulins to support and protect the cornea.

The tear drainage system starts through small puncta located on the medial aspects of both the upper and lower eyelids (Figure 66–2). With blinking, tears enter the puncta and continue to drain through the canaliculi, lacrimal sac, nasolacrimal duct, and then into the nose. The nose is lined by a highly vascular mucosal epithelium; consequently, topically applied medications that pass through this nasolacrimal system have direct access to the systemic circulation.

Ocular Structures

The eye is divided into anterior and posterior segments (*see* Figure 66–3A). Anterior segment structures include the cornea, limbus, anterior and posterior chambers, trabecular meshwork, Schlemm's canal, iris, lens, zonules, and ciliary body. The posterior segment comprises the vitreous, retina, choroid, sclera, and optic nerve.

Anterior Segment. The cornea is a transparent and avascular tissue organized into five layers: epithelium,

Bowman's membrane, stroma, Descemet's membrane, and endothelium (*see* Figure 66–3B).

Representing an important barrier to foreign matter, including drugs, the epithelial layer is composed of five to six layers of epithelial cells. The basal epithelial cells lie on a basement membrane that is adjacent to Bowman's membrane, a layer of collagen fibers. Constituting approximately 90% of the corneal thickness, the stroma, a hydrophilic layer, is uniquely organized with collagen lamellae synthesized by keratocytes. Beneath the stroma lies Descemet's membrane, the basement membrane of the corneal endothelium. Lying most posteriorly, the endothelium is a monolayer of cells adhering to each other by tight junctions. These cells maintain corneal integrity by active transport processes and serve as a hydrophobic barrier. Hence, drug absorption across the cornea necessitates penetrating the trilaminar hydrophobic-hydrophilic-hydrophobic domains of the various anatomical layers.

At the periphery of the cornea and adjacent to the sclera lies a transitional zone (1 to 2 mm wide) called the limbus. Limbal structures include the conjunctival epithelium, which contain the stem cells, Tenon's capsule, episclera, corneoscleral stroma, Schlemm's canal, and trabecular meshwork (Figure 66–3B). Limbal blood vessels, as well as the tears, provide important nutrients and immunological defense mechanisms for the cornea. The anterior chamber holds approximately 250 μl of aqueous humor. The peripheral anterior chamber angle is formed by the cornea and the iris root. The trabecular meshwork and canal of Schlemm are located just above the apex of this angle. The posterior chamber, which holds approximately 50 μl

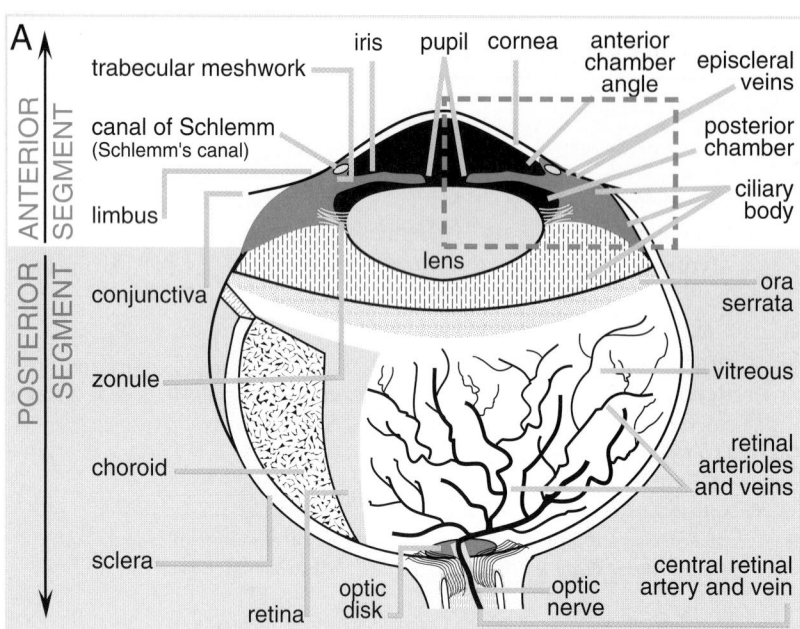

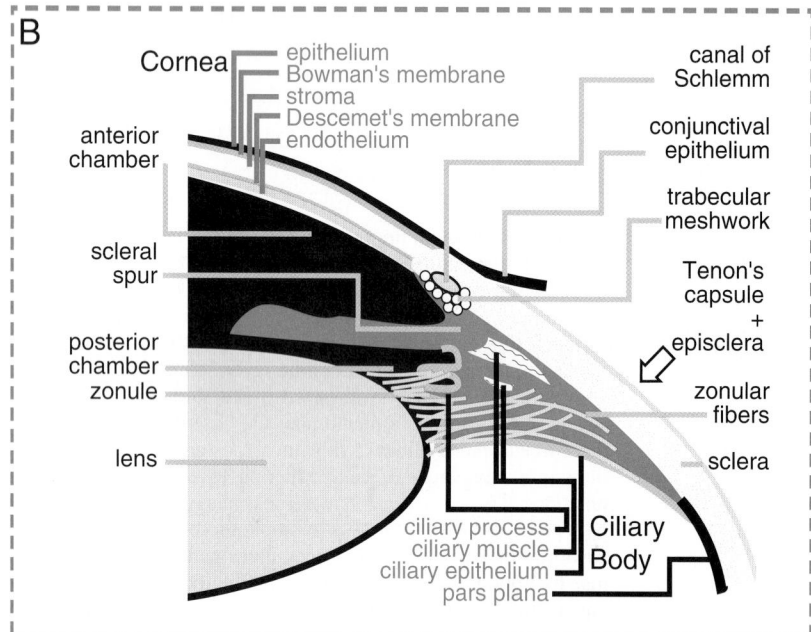

Figure 66–3. A. Anatomy of the eye. B. Enlargement of the anterior segment revealing the cornea, angle structures, lens, and ciliary body.

(Adapted from Riordan-Eva and Tabbara, 1992, with permission.)

of aqueous humor, is defined by the boundaries of the ciliary body processes, posterior surface of the iris, and lens surface.

Aqueous Humor Dynamics and Regulation of Intraocular Pressure. Aqueous humor is secreted by the ciliary processes and flows from the posterior chamber, through the pupil, into the anterior chamber, and leaves the eye primarily by the trabecular meshwork and canal of Schlemm. From the canal of Schlemm, aqueous humor drains into an episcleral venous plexus and into

the systemic circulation. This conventional pathway accounts for 80% to 95% of aqueous humor outflow and is the main target for cholinergic drugs used in glaucoma therapy. Another outflow pathway is the uveoscleral route (*i.e.,* fluid flows through the ciliary muscles and into the suprachoroidal space), which is the target of selective prostanoids (*see* Chapter 26 and later in this chapter).

The peripheral anterior chamber is an important anatomical structure for differentiating two forms of glaucoma: open-angle glaucoma, which is by far the most common form of glaucoma, and angle-closure glaucoma. Current medical therapy of *open-angle glaucoma* is aimed at decreasing aqueous humor production and/or increasing aqueous outflow. The preferred management for *angle-closure glaucoma* is surgical iridectomy, either by laser or by incision, but short-term medical management may be necessary to reduce the acute intraocular pressure elevation and to clear the cornea prior to laser surgery. As mentioned in other chapters, acute angle-closure glaucoma may be induced rarely in anatomically predisposed eyes by anticholinergic, sympathomimetic, and antihistaminic agents. Interestingly, however, individuals with those susceptible angles do not know they have them. As far as they know, they do not have glaucoma and are not aware of a risk of angle-closure glaucoma. Yet, drug warning labels do not always specify the type of glaucoma for which this rare risk exists. Thus, unwarranted concern is raised among patients who have open-angle glaucoma, by far the most common form of glaucoma in the United States, and who need not be concerned about taking these drugs. In any event, in anatomically susceptible eyes, anticholinergic, sympathomimetic, and antihistaminic drugs can lead to partial dilation of the pupil and a change in the vectors of force between the iris and the lens. The aqueous humor then is prevented from passing through the pupil from the posterior chamber to the anterior chamber. The result can be an increase in pressure in the posterior chamber, causing the iris base to be pushed against the angle wall, thereby closing the filtration angle and markedly elevating the intraocular pressure.

Iris and Pupil. The iris is the most anterior portion of the uveal tract, which also includes the ciliary body and choroid. The anterior surface of the iris is the stroma, a loosely organized structure containing melanocytes, blood vessels, smooth muscle, and parasympathetic and sympathetic nerves. Differences in iris color reflect individual variation in the number of melanocytes located in the stroma. Individual variation may be an important consideration for ocular drug distribution due to drug-melanin binding (*see* "Distribution," below). The posterior surface of the iris is a densely pigmented bilayer of epithelial cells. Anterior to the pigmented epithelium, the dilator smooth muscle is oriented radially and is innervated by the sympathetic nervous system (*see* Figure 66–4) which causes mydriasis (dilation). At the pupillary margin, the sphincter smooth muscle is organized in a circular band with parasympathetic innervation which, when stimulated, causes miosis (constriction). The use of pharmacological agents to dilate normal pupils (*i.e.,* for clinical purposes such as examining the ocular fundus) and to evaluate the pharmacological response of the pupil (*e.g.,* unequal pupils, or anisocoria, seen in Horner's syndrome or Adie's pupil) is summarized in Table 66–2. Figure 66–5 provides a flowchart for the diagnostic evaluation of anisocoria.

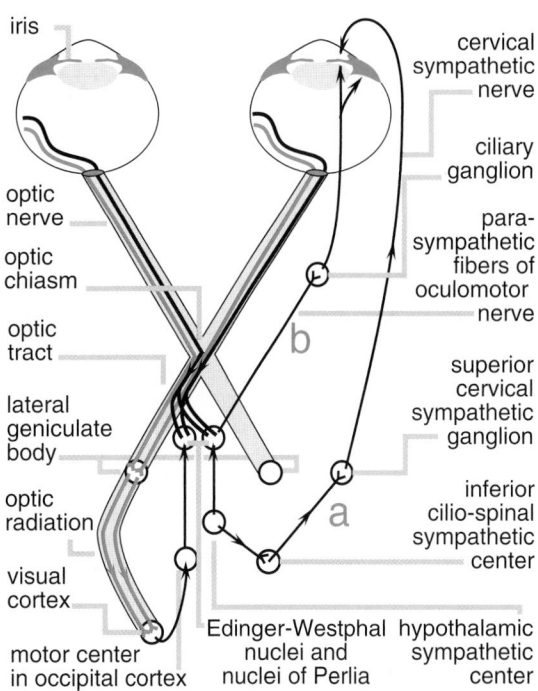

Figure 66–4. Autonomic innervation of the eye by the sympathetic (a) and parasympathetic (b) systems.

(Adapted from Wybar and Kerr Muir, 1984, with permission.)

Ciliary Body. The ciliary body serves two very specialized roles in the eye: secretion of aqueous humor by the epithelial bilayer and accommodation by the ciliary muscle. The anterior portion of the ciliary body, called the pars plicata, is composed of 70 to 80 ciliary processes with intricate folds. The posterior portion is the pars plana. The ciliary muscle is organized into outer longitudinal, middle radial, and inner circular layers. Coordinated contraction of this smooth muscle apparatus by the parasympathetic nervous system causes the zonules suspending the lens to relax, allowing the lens to become more convex and to shift slightly forward. This process, known as *accommodation,* permits focusing on near objects and may be pharmacologically blocked by muscarinic cholinergic antagonists, through the process called *cycloplegia.* Contraction of the ciliary muscle also puts traction on the scleral spur and, hence, widens the spaces within the trabecular meshwork. This latter effect accounts for at least some of the intraocular pressure-lowering effect of both directly acting and indirectly acting parasympathomimetic drugs.

Lens. The lens, a transparent biconvex structure, is suspended by *zonules,* specialized fibers emanating from the

Table 66–2
Effects of Pharmacological Agents on the Pupil

CLINICAL SETTING	DRUG*	PUPILLARY RESPONSE
Normal	Sympathomimetic drugs	Dilation (mydriasis)
Normal	Parasympathomimetic drugs	Constriction (miosis)
Horner's syndrome	Cocaine 4–10%	No dilation
Preganglionic Horner's	Hydroxyamphetamine 1%	Dilation
Postganglionic Horner's	Hydroxyamphetamine 1%	No dilation
Adie's pupil	Pilocarpine 0.05–0.1%†	Constriction
Normal	Opioids (oral or intravenous)	Pinpoint pupils

*Topically applied ophthalmic drugs unless otherwise noted.

†This percentage of pilocarpine is not commercially available and usually is prepared by the physician administering the test or by a pharmacist. This test also requires that no prior manipulation of the cornea (*i.e.*, tonometry for measuring intraocular pressure or testing corneal sensation) be done so that the normal integrity of the corneal barrier is intact. Normal pupils will not respond to this weak dilution of pilocarpine; however, an Adie's pupil manifests a denervation supersensitivity and is, therefore, pharmacodynamically responsive to this dilute cholinergic agonist.

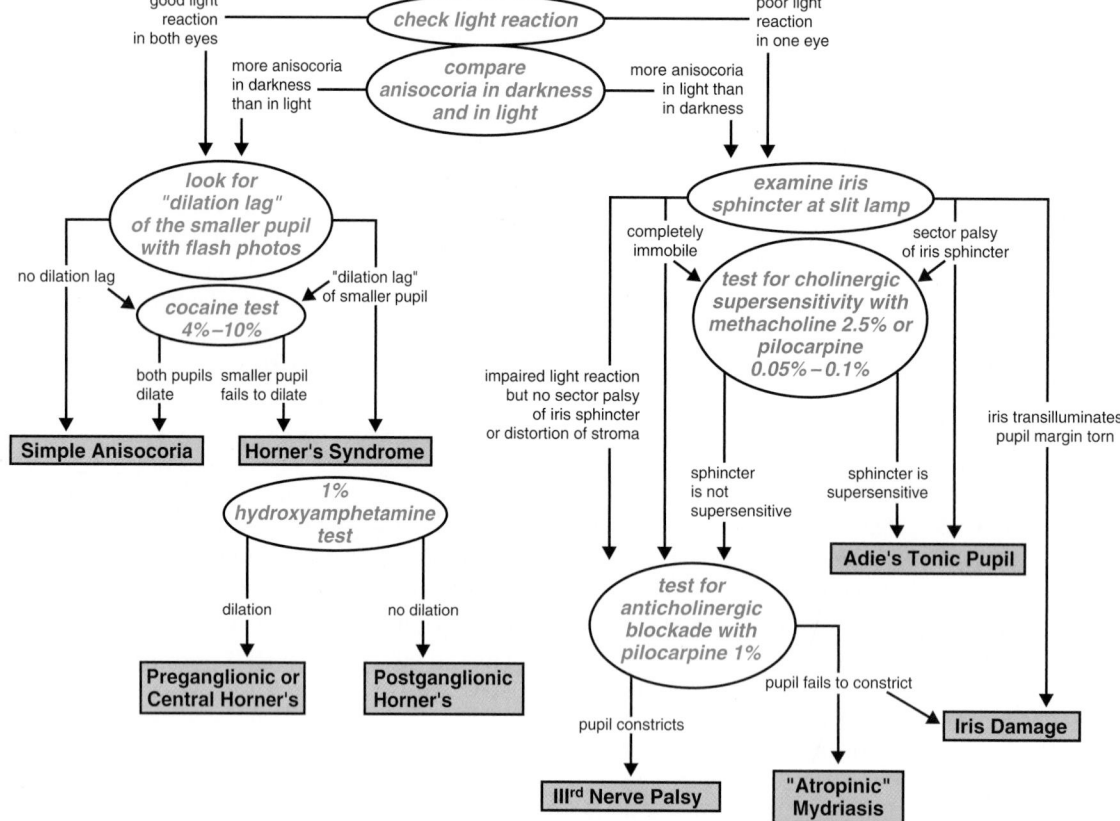

Figure 66–5. Anisocoria evaluation flowsheet.

(Adapted with permission from Thompson and Pilley, 1976.)

ciliary body. The lens is approximately 10 mm in diameter and is enclosed in a capsule. The bulk of the lens is composed of fibers derived from proliferating lens epithelial cells located under the anterior portion of the lens capsule. These lens fibers are continuously produced throughout life.

Posterior Segment. Because of the anatomical and vascular barriers to both local and systemic access, drug delivery to the eye's posterior pole is particularly challenging. *Sclera.* The outermost coat of the eye, the sclera, covers the posterior portion of the globe. The external surface of the scleral shell is covered by an episcleral vascular coat, by Tenon's capsule, and by the conjunctiva. The tendons of the six extraocular muscles insert into the superficial scleral collagen fibers. Numerous blood vessels pierce the sclera through emissaria to supply as well as drain the choroid, ciliary body, optic nerve, and iris.

Inside the scleral shell, the vascular choroid nourishes the outer retina by a capillary system in the choriocapillaris. Between the outer retina and the choriocapillaris lies Bruch's membrane and the retinal pigment epithelium, whose tight junctions provide an outer barrier between the retina and the choroid. The retinal pigment epithelium serves many functions, including vitamin A metabolism (*see* Chapter 64), phagocytosis of the rod outer segments, and multiple transport processes.
Retina. The retina is a thin, transparent, highly organized structure of neurons, glial cells, and blood vessels. Of all structures within the eye, the neurosensory retina has been the most widely studied (*see* Dowling, 1987). The unique organization and biochemistry of the photoreceptors have provided a superb model for investigating signal transduction mechanisms (*see* Stryer, 1987). Rhodopsin has been intensely analyzed at the level of its protein and gene structures (*see* Khorana, 1992). The wealth of information about rhodopsin has made it an excellent model for the G protein–coupled receptors (*see* Chapter 2). Such detailed understanding holds promise for targeted therapy for some of the hereditary retinal diseases.
Vitreous. The vitreous is a clear medium that makes up about 80% of the eye's volume. It is composed of 99% water bound with collagen type II, hyaluronic acid, and proteoglycans. The vitreous also contains glucose, ascorbic acid, amino acids, and a number of inorganic salts (*see* Sebag, 1989).
Optic Nerve. The optic nerve is a myelinated nerve conducting the retinal output to the central nervous system. It is composed of (1) an intraocular portion, which is visible as the 1.5-mm optic disk in the retina; (2) an intraorbital portion; (3) an intracanalicular portion; and (4) an

intracranial portion. The nerve is ensheathed in meninges continuous with the brain. At present, pharmacological treatment of some optic neuropathies is based on management of the underlying disease. For example, optic neuritis may be treated best with intravenous methylprednisolone (Beck *et al.,* 1992, 1993); glaucomatous optic neuropathy is medically managed by decreasing intraocular pressure.

PHARMACOKINETICS AND TOXICOLOGY OF OCULAR THERAPEUTIC AGENTS

Drug Delivery Strategies

Factors that affect the bioavailability of ocular drugs include pH, salt form of the drug, various structural forms of a given drug, vehicle composition, osmolality, tonicity, and viscosity. Properties of varying ocular routes of administration are outlined in Table 66–3. A number of delivery systems have been developed for treating ocular diseases. Most ophthalmic drugs are delivered in aqueous solutions. For compounds with limited solubility, a suspension form facilitates delivery.

Several formulations prolong the time a drug remains on the surface of the eye. These include gels, ointments, solid inserts, soft contact lenses, and collagen shields. Prolonging the time in the cul-de-sac facilitates drug absorption. Ophthalmic gels (*e.g.,* pilocarpine 4% gel) release drugs by diffusion following erosion of soluble polymers. The polymers used include cellulosic ethers, polyvinyl alcohol, carbopol, polyacrylamide, polymethylvinyl ether-maleic anhydride, poloxamer 407, and puronic acid. Ointments usually contain mineral oil and a petrolatum base and are helpful in delivering antibiotics, cycloplegic drugs, or miotic agents. Solid inserts, such as OCUSERT PILO-20 and PILO-40, provide a *zero-order* rate of delivery by steady-state diffusion, whereby drug is released at a more constant rate to the precorneal tear film over a finite period of time rather than as a bolus. Although membrane-controlled drug delivery has advantages and is effective in some patients, the inserts have not gained widespread use, likely due to their cost and the fact that patients often have difficulty placing and retaining a solid insert in the cul-de-sac.

Pharmacokinetics

Classical pharmacokinetic theory based on studies of systemically administered drugs (*see* Chapter 1) does not

Table 66–3

Some Characteristics of Ocular Routes of Drug Administration*

ROUTE	ABSORPTION PATTERN	SPECIAL UTILITY	LIMITATIONS AND PRECAUTIONS
Topical	Prompt, depending on formulation	Convenient, economical, relatively safe	Compliance, corneal and conjunctival toxicity, nasal mucosal toxicity, systemic side effects from nasolacrimal absorption
Subconjunctival, sub-Tenon's, and retrobulbar injections	Prompt or sustained, depending on formulation	Anterior segment infections, posterior uveitis, cystoid macular edema	Local toxicity, tissue injury, globe perforation, optic nerve trauma, central retinal artery and/or vein occlusion, direct retinal drug toxicity with inadvertent globe perforation, ocular muscle trauma
Intraocular (intracameral) injections	Prompt	Anterior segment surgery	Corneal toxicity
Intravitreal injection or device	Absorption circumvented, immediate local effect	Endophthalmitis, retinitis	Retinal toxicity

*See text for more complete discussion of individual routes.

fully apply to all ophthalmic drugs (see Schoenwald, 1993; DeSantis and Patil, 1994). Although similar principles of absorption, distribution, metabolism, and excretion determine the fate of drug disposition in the eye, alternative routes of drug administration, in addition to oral and intravenous routes, introduce other variables in compartmental analysis (see Table 66–3 and Figure 66–6). Ophthalmic medications are applied topically using a variety of formulations. Drugs also may be injected by subconjunctival, sub-Tenon's, and retrobulbar routes (see Figure 66–1 and Table 66–3). For example, anesthetic agents are administered commonly by injection for surgical procedures and antibiotics and glucocorticoids also may be injected to enhance their delivery to local tissues. 5-Fluorouracil, an antimetabolite and antiproliferative agent, may be administered subconjunctivally to retard the fibroblast proliferation related to scarring after glaucoma surgery. Intraocular (i.e., intravitreal) injections of antibiotics are considered in instances of endophthalmitis, an intraocular infection. The sensitivities of the organisms to the antibiotic and the retinal toxicity threshold may be nearly the same for some antibiotics; hence, the antibiotic dose injected intravitreally must be carefully titrated.

Unlike clinical pharmacokinetic studies on systemic drugs, where data are collected relatively easily from blood samples, there is significant risk in obtaining tissue and fluid samples from the human eye. Consequently, animal models are studied to provide pharmacokinetic data on ophthalmic drugs. Commonly, the rabbit is used for such studies (see McDonald and Shadduck, 1977, for comparison of toxicity, anatomy, and physiology of human and rabbit ocular systems).

Absorption. After topical instillation of a drug, the rate and extent of absorption are determined by the following: the time the drug remains in the cul-de-sac and precorneal tear film (also known as the *residence time*); elimination by nasolacrimal drainage; drug binding to tear proteins; drug metabolism by tear and tissue proteins; and diffusion across the cornea and conjunctiva (see Lee, 1993). A drug's residence time may be prolonged by changing its formulation. Nasolacrimal drainage contributes to systemic absorption of topically administered ophthalmic medications. Absorption from the nasal mucosa avoids so-called first-pass metabolism by the liver (see Chapter 1), and consequently significant systemic side effects may be caused by topical medications, especially when used chronically. Possible absorption pathways of an ophthalmic drug following topical application to the eye are shown schematically in Figure 66–6.

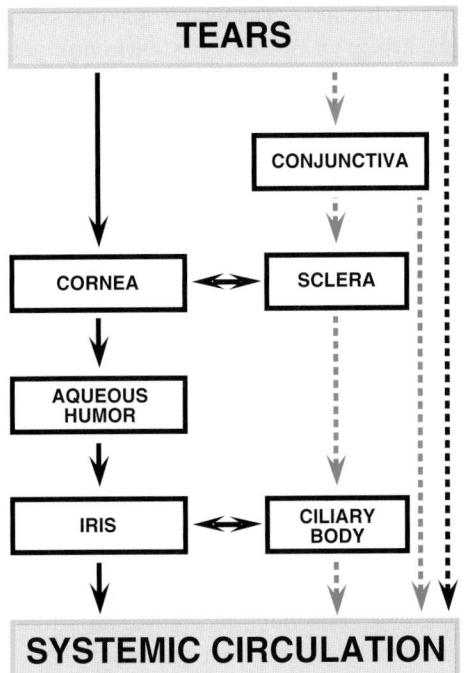

TEARS

CONJUNCTIVA

CORNEA ⟷ SCLERA

AQUEOUS HUMOR

IRIS ⟷ CILIARY BODY

SYSTEMIC CIRCULATION

Figure 66–6. Possible absorption pathways of an ophthalmic drug following topical application to the eye.

Solid black arrows represent the corneal route; dashed blue arrows represent the conjunctival/scleral route; the black dashed line represents the nasolacrimal absorption pathway. (Adapted from Chien *et al.,* 1990, with permission.)

Transcorneal and transconjunctival/scleral absorption are the desired routes for localized ocular drug effects. The time period between drug instillation and its appearance in the aqueous humor is defined as the *lag time*. The drug concentration gradient between the tear film and the cornea and conjunctival epithelium provides the driving force for passive diffusion across these tissues. Other factors that affect a drug's diffusion capacity are the size of the molecule, chemical structure, and steric configuration. Transcorneal drug penetration is conceptualized as a differential solubility process; the cornea may be thought of as a trilamellar "fat-water-fat" structure corresponding to the epithelial, stromal, and endothelial layers. The epithelium and endothelium represent barriers for hydrophilic substances; the stroma is a barrier for hydrophobic compounds. Hence, a drug with both hydrophilic and lipophilic properties is best suited for transcorneal absorption.

Drug penetration into the eye is approximately linearly related to its concentration in the tear film. Certain disease states, such as corneal ulcers and other corneal epithelial defects or stromal keratitis, also may alter drug penetration. Experimentally, drugs may be screened for their potential clinical utility by assessing their corneal permeability coefficients. These pharmacokinetic data combined with the drug's octanol/water partition coefficient (for lipophilic drugs) or distribution coefficient (for ionizable drugs) yield a parabolic relationship that is

a useful parameter for predicting ocular absorption. Of course, such *in vitro* studies do not account for other factors that affect corneal absorption, such as blink rate, dilution by tear flow, nasolacrimal drainage, drug binding to proteins and tissue, and transconjunctival absorption; hence, these studies have limitations in predicting ocular drug absorption *in vivo*.

Distribution. Topically administered drugs may undergo systemic distribution primarily by nasal mucosal absorption and possibly by local ocular distribution by transcorneal/transconjunctival absorption. Following transcorneal absorption, the aqueous humor accumulates the drug, which is then distributed to intraocular structures as well as potentially to the systemic circulation *via* the trabecular meshwork pathway (*see* Figure 66–3B). Melanin binding of certain drugs is an important factor in some ocular compartments. For example, the mydriatic effect of α-adrenergic receptor agonists is slower in onset in human volunteers with darkly pigmented irides compared to those with lightly pigmented irides (Obianwu and Rand, 1965). In rabbits, radiolabeled atropine binds significantly to melanin granules in irides of nonalbino animals (Salazar *et al.,* 1976). This finding correlates with the fact that atropine's mydriatic effect lasts longer in nonalbino rabbits than in albino rabbits, and suggests that drug–melanin binding is a potential reservoir for sustained drug release. Another clinically important consideration for drug–melanin binding involves the retinal pigment epithelium. In the retinal pigment epithelium, accumulation of chloroquine (*see* Chapter 40) causes a toxic retinal lesion known as a "bull's-eye" maculopathy, which is associated with a decrease in visual acuity. Extraretinal manifestations of chloroquine toxicity include corneal and crystalline lens opacities and motility disturbances.

Metabolism. Enzymatic biotransformation of ocular drugs may be significant since local tissues in the eye express a variety of enzymes, including esterases, oxidoreductases, lysosomal enzymes, peptidases, glucuronide and sulfate transferases, glutathione-conjugating enzymes, catechol-*O*-methyl-transferase, monoamine oxidase, and corticosteroid β-hydroxylase (*see* Lee, 1992). The esterases have been of particular interest because of the development of prodrugs for enhanced corneal permeability; for example, dipivefrin hydrochloride (Mandell *et al.,* 1978) is a prodrug for epinephrine, and latanoprost is a prodrug for prostaglandin $F_{2\alpha}$ (Stjernschantz and Resul, 1992); both drugs are used for glaucoma management. Topically applied ocular drugs are eliminated by the liver and kidney after systemic absorption.

Toxicology. From the compartmental analysis given in Figure 66–6, it is apparent that all ophthalmic medications are potentially absorbed into the systemic circulation, so undesirable systemic side effects may occur. Most ophthalmic drugs are delivered locally to the eye, and the potential local toxic effects are due to hypersensitivity reactions or to direct toxic effects on the cornea, conjunctiva, periocular skin, and nasal mucosa. Eyedrops and contact lens solutions commonly contain preservatives such as benzalkonium chloride, chlorobutanol, chelating agents, and thimerosal for their antimicrobial effectiveness. In particular, benzalkonium chloride may cause a punctate keratopathy or toxic ulcerative keratopathy (Grant and Schuman, 1993).

THERAPEUTIC AND DIAGNOSTIC APPLICATIONS OF DRUGS IN OPHTHALMOLOGY

Chemotherapy of Microbial Diseases in the Eye

Antibacterial Agents. *General Considerations.* A number of antibacterial antibiotics have been formulated for topical ocular use (Table 66–4). The pharmacology, structures, and kinetics of individual drugs have been presented in detail in preceding chapters. Appropriate selection of antibiotic and route of administration is dependent on clinical examination and culture/sensitivity results. Specially formulated antibiotics also may be available for serious eye infections such as corneal ulcers or keratitis and endophthalmitis. Preparation of fortified solutions requires a pharmacist familiar with sterile preparation of ocular drugs.

Therapeutic Uses. Infectious diseases of the skin, eyelids, conjunctiva, and lacrimal excretory system are encountered regularly in clinical practice. Periocular skin infections are divided into preseptal and postseptal or orbital cellulitis. Depending on the clinical setting (*i.e.,* preceding trauma, sinusitis, age of patient, relative immunocompromised state), oral or parenteral antibiotics are administered.

Dacryocystitis is an infection of the lacrimal sac. In infants and children, the disease usually is unilateral and secondary to an obstruction of the nasolacrimal duct. The physician should be aware of the changing microbiological spectrum for orbital cellulitis, for example, the sharp decline in the involvement of *Haemophilus influenzae* after the introduction in 1985 of the *H. influenzae* vaccine (Ambati *et al.,* 2000). In adults, dacryocystitis and canalicular infections may be caused by *Staphylococcus aureus, Streptococcus* species, *Candida* species, and *Actinomyces israelii.*

Infectious processes of the lids include *hordeolum* and *blepharitis.* A hordeolum, or stye, is an infection of the meibomian, Zeis, or Moll glands at the lid margins. The typical offending bacterium is *S. aureus,* and the usual treatment consists of warm compresses and topical antibiotic ointment. *Blepharitis* is a common bilateral inflammatory process of the eyelids characterized by irritation and burning, and it also is usually caused by a *Staphylococcus* species. Local hygiene is the mainstay of therapy; topical antibiotics frequently are used, usually in ointment form, particularly when the disease is accompanied by conjunctivitis and keratitis.

Conjunctivitis is an inflammatory process of the conjunctiva that varies in severity from mild hyperemia to severe purulent discharge. The more common causes of conjunctivitis include viruses, allergies, environmental irritants, contact lenses, and chemicals. The less common causes include other infectious pathogens, immune-mediated reactions, associated systemic diseases, and tumors of the conjunctiva or eyelid. The more commonly reported infectious agents are adenovirus and herpes simplex virus, followed by other viral (*e.g.,* enterovirus, coxsackievirus, measles virus, varicella zoster virus, vaccinia-variola virus) and bacterial sources (*e.g., Neisseria* species, *Streptococcus pneumoniae, Haemophilus* species, *S. aureus, Moraxella lacunata,* chlamydial species). *Rickettsia,* fungi, and parasites, in both cyst and trophozoite form, are rare causes of conjunctivitis. Effective management is based on selection of an appropriate antibiotic for suspected bacterial pathogens. Unless an unusual causative organism is suspected, bacterial conjunctivitis is treated empirically without obtaining a culture.

Keratitis, or corneal ulcer, may occur at any level of the cornea, *e.g.,* epithelium, subepithelium, stroma, or endothelium. Numerous microbial agents have been isolated, including bacteria, viruses, fungi, spirochetes, and cysts and trophozoites. In aggressive forms of bacterial keratitis, immediate empirical and intensive antibiotic therapy is essential to prevent blindness from corneal perforation and secondary corneal scarring. Results of culture and sensitivity tests should guide the final drug of choice.

Endophthalmitis is a potentially severe and devastating inflammatory, and usually infectious, process of the intraocular tissues. When the inflammatory process encompasses the entire globe, it is called *panophthalmitis.* Endophthalmitis usually is caused by bacteria, by fungi, or rarely by spirochetes. The typical case occurs during the early postoperative course (*e.g.,* after cataract, glaucoma, cornea, or retinal surgery), following trauma, or by endogenous seeding in the immunocompromised host or intravenous drug user. Prompt therapy usually includes vitrectomy (*i.e.,* specialized surgical removal of the vitreous) and empirical intravitreal antibiotics to treat suspected bacterial or fungal microorganisms (*see* Peyman and Schulman, 1994; Meredith, 1994). In cases of endogenous seeding, parenteral antibiotics have a role in eliminating the infectious source. In trauma or in the postoperative setting, however, the efficacy of systemic antibiotics is not well established.

Antiviral Agents. *General Considerations.* The various antiviral drugs currently used in ophthalmology are summarized in Table 66–5 (*see* Chapter 50 for additional details about these agents).

Table 66–4

Topical Antibacterial Agents Commercially Available for Ophthalmic Use*

GENERIC NAME (TRADE NAME)	FORMULATION†	TOXICITY†	INDICATIONS FOR USE
Bacitracin zinc (AK-TRACIN)	500 U/g ointment	H	Conjunctivitis, blepharitis
Chloramphenicol (AK-CHLOR, CHLOROMYCETIN, CHLOROPTIC, OCU-CHLOR)	0.5% solution 1% ointment	H, BD	Conjunctivitis, keratitis
Chlortetracycline hydrochloride (AUREOMYCIN)	1% ointment	H	Conjunctivitis, blepharitis
Ciprofloxacin hydrochloride (CILOXAN)	0.3% solution	H, D-RCD	Conjunctivitis, keratitis
Erythromycin (ILOTYCIN)	0.5% ointment	H	Blepharitis, conjunctivitis
Gentamicin sulfate (GARAMYCIN, GENOPTIC, GENT-AK, GENTACIDIN)	0.3% solution 0.3% ointment	H	Conjunctivitis, blepharitis, keratitis
Norfloxacin (CHIBROXIN)	0.3% solution	H	Conjunctivitis
Ofloxacin (OCUFLOX)	0.3% solution	H	Conjunctivitis, keratitis
Sulfacetamide sodium (AK-SULF, BLEPH-10, CETAMIDE, SULF-10, ISOPTO CETAMIDE, SULAMYD SODIUM, others)	10, 15, 30% solution 10% ointment	H, BD	Conjunctivitis, blepharitis, keratitis
Sulfisoxazole diolamine (GANTRISIN)	4% solution	H, BD	Conjunctivitis, blepharitis, keratitis
Polymyxin B combinations‡	Various solutions Various ointments		Conjunctivitis, blepharitis, keratitis
Tetracycline hydrochloride (ACHROMYCIN)	1% solution	H	Conjunctivitis, blepharitis
Tobramycin sulfate (TOBREX, AKTOB)	0.3% solution 0.3% ointment	H	Conjunctivitis, blepharitis, keratitis

*For specific information on dosing, formulation, and trade names, refer to the *Physician's Desk Reference for Ophthalmology,* which is published annually.

†*Abbreviations:* H, hypersensitivity; BD, blood dyscrasia; D-RCD, drug-related corneal deposits.

‡Polymyxin B is formulated for delivery in combination with bacitracin, neomycin, gramicidin, oxytetracycline, or trimethoprim. *See also* Chapters 44 to 47 for further discussion of these antibacterial agents.

Table 66–5
Antiviral Agents for Ophthalmic Use*

GENERIC NAME (TRADE NAME)	ROUTE OF ADMINISTRATION	OCULAR TOXICITY†	INDICATION FOR USE
Idoxuridine (HERPLEX)	Topical (0.1% solution)	PK, H	Herpes simplex keratitis
Trifluridine (VIROPTIC)	Topical (1% solution)	PK, H	Herpes simplex keratitis
Vidarabine (VIRA-A)	Topical (3% ointment)	PK, H	Herpes simplex keratitis Herpes simplex conjunctivitis
Acyclovir (ZOVIRAX)	Oral (200-mg capsules, 400- and 800-mg tablets)		Herpes zoster ophthalmicus Herpes simplex iridocyclitis
Foscarnet (FOSCAVIR)	Intravenous Intravitreal		Cytomegalovirus retinitis
Ganciclovir (CYTOVENE) (VITRASERT)	Intravenous, oral Intravitreal implant		Cytomegalovirus retinitis
Formivirsen (VITRAVENE)	Intravitreal injection		Cytomegalovirus retinitis
Cidoforvir (VISTIDE)	Intravenous		Cytomegalovirus retinitis

*For additional details, *see* Chapter 50.
†*Abbreviations*: PK, punctate keratopathy; H, hypersensitivity.

Therapeutic Uses. The primary indications for the use of antiviral drugs in ophthalmology are viral keratitis (Kaufman, 2000), herpes zoster ophthalmicus (Liesegang, 1999; Chern and Margolis, 1998), and retinitis (Cassoux *et al.,* 1999; Yoser *et al.,* 1993). There are currently no antiviral agents for the treatment of viral conjunctivitis caused by adenoviruses, which usually has a self-limited course and typically is treated by symptomatic relief of irritation.

Viral keratitis, an infection of the cornea that may involve either the epithelium or stroma, is most commonly caused by herpes simplex type I and varicella zoster viruses. Less common viral etiologies include herpes simplex II, Epstein-Barr virus, and cytomegalovirus. Topical antiviral agents are indicated for the treatment of epithelial disease due to herpes simplex infection. When treating viral keratitis topically, there is a very narrow margin between the therapeutic topical antiviral activity and the toxic effect on the cornea; hence, patients must be followed very closely. The role of oral acyclovir and glucocorticoids in herpetic corneal and external eye disease has been examined in the Herpetic Eye Disease Study

(Anonymous, 1996, 1997a, 1998). Topical glucocorticoids are contraindicated in herpetic epithelial keratitis due to active viral replication. In contrast, for herpetic disciform keratitis, which predominantly is presumed to involve a cell-mediated immune reaction, topical glucocorticoids accelerate recovery (Wilhelmus *et al.,* 1994). For recurrent herpetic stromal keratitis, there is clear benefit from treatment with oral acyclovir in reducing the risk of recurrence (Moyes *et al.,* 1994; Anonymous, 1998).

Herpes zoster ophthalmicus is a latent reactivation of a varicella zoster infection in the first division of the trigeminal cranial nerve. Systemic *acyclovir* is effective in reducing the severity and complications of herpes zoster ophthalmicus (Cobo *et al.,* 1986). Currently, there are no ophthalmic preparations of acyclovir approved by the United States Food and Drug Administration (FDA), although an ophthalmic ointment is available for investigational use.

Viral retinitis may be caused by herpes simplex virus, cytomegalovirus (CMV), adenovirus, and varicella zoster virus. With the highly active antiretroviral therapy (HAART; *see* Chapter 51), CMV retinitis does not appear

Table 66–6
Antifungal Agents for Ophthalmic Use*

DRUG CLASS/AGENT	METHOD OF ADMINISTRATION	INDICATIONS FOR USE
Polyenes		
Amphotericin B	0.1–0.5% topical solution	Yeast and fungal keratitis and endophthalmitis
	0.8–1.0 mg subconjunctival	Yeast and fungal endophthalmitis
	5 μg intravitreal injection	Yeast and fungal endophthalmitis
	intravenous	Yeast and fungal endophthalmitis
Natamycin	5% topical suspension	Yeast and fungal blepharitis, conjunctivitis, keratitis
Imidazoles		
Fluconazole	oral	Yeast keratitis and endophthalmitis
Ketoconazole	oral	Yeast keratitis and endophthalmitis
Miconazole	1% topical solution	Yeast and fungal keratitis
	5–10 mg subconjunctival	Yeast and fungal endophthalmitis
	10 μg intravitreal injection	Yeast and fungal endophthalmitis

*Only natamycin (NATACYN) is commercially available for ophthalmic use. The other antifungal drugs must be formulated for the given method of administration. For further dosing information, refer to the *Physicians' Desk Reference for Ophthalmology*.
For additional discussion of these antifungal agents, *see* Chapter 49.

to progress when specific anti-CMV therapy is discontinued, but some patients develop an immune recovery uveitis (Jacobson *et al.*, 2000; Whitcup, 2000). Treatment usually involves long-term parenteral administration of antiviral drugs. Intravitreal administration of ganciclovir has been found to be an effective alternative to the systemic route (Sanborn *et al.*, 1992).

Antifungal Agents. *General Considerations.* The only currently available ophthalmic antifungal preparation is a polyene, *natamycin* (NATACYN), which has the following structure:

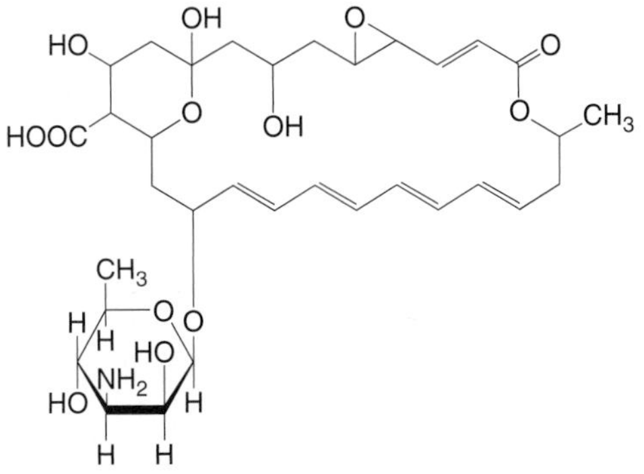

NATAMYCIN

Other antifungal agents may be specially prepared for topical, subconjunctival, or intravitreal routes of administration (*see* Table 66–6). The pharmacology and structures of available antifungal agents are given in Chapter 49.

Therapeutic Uses. As with systemic fungal infections, the incidence of ophthalmic fungal infections has risen with the growing number of immunocompromised hosts. Ophthalmic indications for antifungal medications include fungal keratitis, scleritis, endophthalmitis, mucormycosis, and canaliculitis (*see* Behlau and Baker, 1994). Drug selection is based on identifying the pathogenic fungi and, if available, sensitivity data.

Antiprotozoal Agents. *General Considerations.* Parasitic infections involving the eye usually manifest themselves as a form of uveitis, an inflammatory process of either the anterior or posterior segments, and less commonly as conjunctivitis, keratitis, and retinitis.

Therapeutic Uses. In the United States, the most commonly encountered protozoal infections include *Acanthamoeba* and *Toxoplasma gondii*. In contact-lens wearers who develop keratitis, physicians should be highly suspicious of the presence of *Acanthamoeba* (McCulley *et al.*, 2000). Treatment usually consists of a combination topical antibiotic, such as *polymyxin B sulfate, bacitracin zinc,* and *neomycin sulfate (e.g.,* NEOSPORIN), and sometimes an *imidazole (e.g.,* clotrimazole, miconazole, *or* ketocona-zole). In the United Kingdom, the aromatic diamidines (*i.e., propamine isethionate* in both topical aqueous and ointment forms, BROLENE) have been used successfully to treat this relatively resistant infectious keratitis (Hargrave *et al.,* 1999). Another treatment for *Acanthamoeba* is the cationic antiseptic agent *polyhexamethylene biguanide,* although this is not an FDA-approved antiprotozoal agent (Lindquist, 1998).

Toxoplasmosis may present as a posterior (*e.g.,* focal retinochoroiditis, papillitis, vitritis, or retinitis) or occasionally as an anterior uveitis. Treatment is indicated when inflammatory lesions encroach upon the macula and threaten central visual acuity. Several regimens have been recommended with concurrent use of systemic steroids: (1) *pyrimethamine, sulfadiazine,* and *folinic acid;* (2) *pyrimethamine, sulfadiazine, clindamycin,* and *folinic acid;* (3) *sulfadiazine* and *clindamycin;* (4) *clindamycin;* and (5) *trimethoprim–sulfamethoxazole* with or without *clindamycin (see* Engstrom *et al.,* 1991; Opremcak *et al.,* 1992).

Other protozoal infections (*e.g.,* giardiasis, leishmaniasis, and malaria) and helminths are less common eye pathogens in the United States (*see* DeFreitas and Dunkel, 1994). Systemic pharmacological management as well as vitrectomy may be indicated for selected parasitic infections.

Use of Autonomic Agents in the Eye

General Considerations. General autonomic pharmacology has been discussed extensively in Chapters 6 through 10. The autonomic agents used in ophthalmology as well as the responses (*i.e.,* mydriasis and cycloplegia) to muscarinic cholinergic antagonists are summarized in Table 66–7.

Therapeutic Uses. Autonomic drugs are used extensively for diagnostic and surgical purposes and for the treatment of glaucoma, uveitis, and strabismus.
Glaucoma. In the United States, glaucoma is the leading cause of blindness in African Americans and the third leading cause in Caucasians. Characterized by progressive optic nerve cupping and visual field loss, glaucoma is responsible for visual impairment of 80,000 Americans, and at least 2 million to 3 million have the disease (*see* Tielsch, 1993). Risk factors associated with glaucomatous nerve damage include increased intraocular pressure, positive

family history of glaucoma, African-American heritage, myopia, and hypertension. The production and regulation of aqueous humor have been discussed in an earlier section of this chapter. Although particularly elevated intraocular pressures (*e.g.,* greater than 30 mm Hg) usually will lead to optic nerve damage, certain patients' optic nerves appear to be able to tolerate intraocular pressures in the mid-to-high twenties. These patients are referred to as *ocular hypertensives;* a prospective, multicenter study is being conducted to determine whether or not early medical treatment to lower intraocular pressure will prevent glaucomatous optic nerve damage. Other patients have progressive glaucomatous optic nerve damage despite having intraocular pressures in the normal range, and this form of the disease is sometimes called *normal-* or *low-tension* glaucoma. However, at present, the pathophysiological processes involved in glaucomatous optic nerve damage and the relationship to aqueous humor dynamics are not understood.

Current medical therapies are targeted to decrease the production of aqueous humor at the ciliary body and to increase outflow through the trabecular meshwork and uveoscleral pathways. There is no consensus on the best therapy for glaucoma. Currently, a National Eye Institute–sponsored clinical trial, the Collaborative Initial Glaucoma Treatment Study (CIGTS), aims to determine whether it is best to treat patients newly diagnosed with open-angle glaucoma with filtering surgery or with medication in terms of preservation of visual function and quality of life (Musch *et al.,* 1999). This study aside, a stepped medical approach depends on the patient's health, age, and ocular status. Some general principles prevail in patient management: (1) asthma and chronic obstructive pulmonary emphysema having a bronchospastic component are relative contraindications to the use of topical β-adrenergic receptor antagonists because of the risk of significant side effects from systemic absorption *via* the nasolacrimal system; (2) some cardiac dysrhythmias (*i.e.,* bradycardia and heart block) also are relative contraindications to β-adrenergic antagonists for similar reasons; (3) history of nephrolithiasis, or kidney stones, is sometimes a contraindication for carbonic anhydrase inhibitors; (4) young patients usually are intolerant of miotic therapy secondary to visual blurring from induced myopia; therefore, if a miotic agent is needed in a young patient, the OCUSERT delivery system usually is preferable; (5) direct miotic agents are preferred over cholinesterase inhibitors in "phakic" patients (*i.e.,* those patients who have their endogenous lens), since the latter drugs can promote cataract formation; and (6) in patients who have an increased risk of retinal detachment, miotics should be used with caution, since they have been implicated in promoting retinal tears in susceptible individuals; such tears are thought to be due to altered forces at the vitreous base produced by ciliary body contraction induced by the drug.

With these general principles in mind, a stepped medical approach may begin with a β-adrenergic receptor antagonist,

Table 66–7
Autonomic Drugs for Ophthalmic Use*

DRUG CLASS (TRADE NAME)	FORMULATION	INDICATIONS FOR USE	OCULAR SIDE EFFECTS
Cholinergic Agonists			
Acetylcholine (MIOCHOL-E)	1% solution	Intraocular use for miosis in surgery	Corneal edema
Carbachol (MIOSTAT, ISOPTO CARBACHOL, others)	0.01 to 3% solution	Intraocular use for miosis in surgery, glaucoma	Corneal edema, miosis, induced myopia, decreased vision, brow ache, retinal detachment
Pilocarpine (AKARPINE, ISOPTO CARPINE, OCUSERT-PILO, PILOCAR, PILAGAN, PILOPINE-HS, PILOPTIC, PILOSTAT, others)	0.25–10% solution, 4% gel, 20, 40 μg/hour units	Glaucoma	Same as for carbachol
Anticholinesterase Agents			
Physostigmine (ESERINE)	0.25% ointment	Glaucoma, accommodative esotropia, louse and mite infestation of lashes	Retinal detachment, miosis, cataract, pupillary block glaucoma iris cysts, brow ache, punctal stenosis of the nasolacrimal system
Echothiophate (PHOSPHOLINE IODIDE)	0.03 to 0.25% solution	Glaucoma, accommodative esotropia	Same as for physostigmine
Muscarinic Antagonists			
Atropine (ATROPISOL, ATROPINE-CARE, ISOPTO ATROPINE)	0.5–2% solution 1.0% ointment	Cycloplegic retinoscopy, dilated funduscopic exam, cycloplegia†	Photosensitivity, blurred vision
Scopolamine (ISOPTO HYOSCINE)	0.25% solution	Same as for atropine	Same as for atropine
Homatropine (ISOPTO HOMATROPINE)	2.0 & 5.0% solution	Same as for atropine	Same as for atropine
Cyclopentolate (AK-PENTOLATE, CYCLOGYL, PENTOLAIR)	0.5, 1.0 & 2.0% solution	Same as for atropine	Same as for atropine
Tropicamide (MYDRIACYL, TROPICACYL, OPTICYL)	0.5 & 1.0% solution	Same as for atropine	Same as for atropine
Sympathomimetic Agents			
Dipivefrin (PROPINE, AKPRO)	0.1% solution	Glaucoma	Photosensitivity, conjunctival hyperemia, hypersensitivity
Epinephrine (EPINAL, EPIFRIN, GLAUCON)	0.1, 0.5, 1, & 2% solution	Glaucoma	Same as for dipivefrin

Table 66–7

Autonomic Drugs for Ophthalmic Use* *(Continued)*

DRUG CLASS (TRADE NAME)	FORMULATION	INDICATIONS FOR USE	OCULAR SIDE EFFECTS
Phenylephrine (AK-DILATE, MYDFRIN, NEO-SYNEPHRINE, others)	0.12, 2.5 & 10% solution	Mydriasis	Same as for dipivefrin
Apraclonidine (IOPIDINE)	0.5 & 1% solution	Glaucoma, pre- & post-laser prophylaxis of intra-ocular pressure spike	Same as for dipivefrin
Brimonidine (ALPHAGAN)	0.2% solution	Glaucoma	Same as for dipivefrin
Cocaine	1–4% solution	Topical anesthesia, evaluate anisocoria (*see* Figure 66–5)	
Hydroxyamphetamine (PAREDRINE)	1% solution	Evaluate anisocoria (*see* Figure 66–5)	
Naphazoline (AK-CON, ALBALON, CLEAR EYES, NAPHCON, VASOCLEAR, VASOCON REGULAR, others)	0.012 to 0.1% solution	Decongestant	Same as for dipivefrin
Tetrahydrozoline (COLLYRIUM FRESH, MURINE PLUS, VISINE MOISTURIZING, others)	0.05% solution	Decongestant	Same as for dipivefrin
α- & β-Adrenergic Antagonists			
Dapiprazole (α) (REV-EYES)	0.5% solution	Reverse mydriasis	Conjunctival hyperemia
Betaxolol (β_1-selective) (BETOPTIC, BETOPTIC-S)	0.25 & 0.5% suspension	Glaucoma	
Carteolol (β) (OCUPRESS)	1% solution	Glaucoma	
Levobunolol (β) (BETAGAN, AKBETA)	0.25 & 0.5% solution	Glaucoma	
Metipranolol (β) (OPTIPRANOLOL)	0.3% solution	Glaucoma	
Timolol (β) (TIMOPTIC, TIMOPTIC XE, BETIMOL)	0.25 & 0.5% solution & gel	Glaucoma	

*Refer to *Physicians' Desk Reference for Ophthalmology* for specific indications and dosing information.

†Mydriasis and cycloplegia, or paralysis of accommodation, of the human eye occurs after one drop of atropine 1.0%, scopolamine 0.5%, homatropine 1.0%, cyclopentolate 0.5% or 1.0%, and tropicamide 0.5% or 1.0%. Recovery of mydriasis is defined by return to baseline pupil size to within 1 mm. Recovery of cycloplegia is defined by return to within two diopters of baseline accommodative power. The maximal mydriatic effect of homatropine is achieved with a 5% solution, but cycloplegia may be incomplete. Maximal cycloplegia with tropicamide may be achieved with a 1% solution.

    Times to development of maximal mydriasis and to recovery, respectively, are: for *atropine,* 30 to 40 minutes and 7 to 10 days; for *scopolamine,* 20 to 130 minutes and 3 to 7 days; for *homatropine,* 40 to 60 minutes and 1 to 3 days; for *cyclopentolate,* 30 to 60 minutes and 1 day; for *tropicamide,* 20 to 40 minutes and 6 hours.

    Times to development of maximal cycloplegia and to recovery, respectively, are: for *atropine,* 60 to 180 minutes and 6 to 12 days; for *scopolamine,* 30 to 60 minutes and 3 to 7 days; for *homatropine,* 30 to 60 minutes and 1 to 3 days; for *cyclopentolate,* 25 to 75 minutes and 6 hours to 1 day; for *tropicamide,* 30 minutes and 6 hours.

with the main goal of preventing progressive glaucomatous optic-nerve damage with minimum risk and side effects from either topical or systemic therapy. When there are medical contraindications to the use of β-receptor antagonists other agents, such as *latanoprost* (XALATAN), a prostaglandin F$_{2\alpha}$ prodrug, or an *α$_2$-adrenergic receptor agonist* may be used as first-line therapy. The chemical structure of latanoprost is shown below.

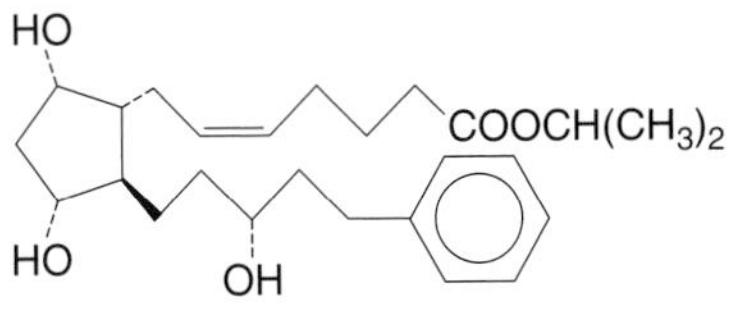

LATANOPROST

Second- and third-line agents include topical *carbonic anhydrase inhibitors, epinephrine-related drugs,* and miotic agents. Ironically, epinephrine-related drugs may be used concomitantly with a β-adrenergic receptor antagonist. Epinephrine's main intraocular pressure-lowering effect is to enhance uveoscleral outflow, but it also may alter trabecular meshwork function and ciliary body blood flow. If combined topical therapy fails to achieve the target intraocular pressure or fails to halt glaucomatous optic nerve damage, then systemic therapy with carbonic anhydrase inhibitors (CAIs) is a final medication option before resorting to laser or incisional surgical treatment. Of the oral preparations available (*see* Chapter 29), the best tolerated is *acetazolamide* in sustained-release capsules, followed by *methazolamide.* The least well tolerated are acetazolamide tablets (Lichter *et al.,* 1978). To reduce side effects, topical CAIs have been developed—*dorzolamide hydrochloride* (TRUSOPT), and *brinzolamide* (AZOPT), whose structures are shown below. These topical CAIs do not reduce the intraocular pressure as much as do the oral agents.

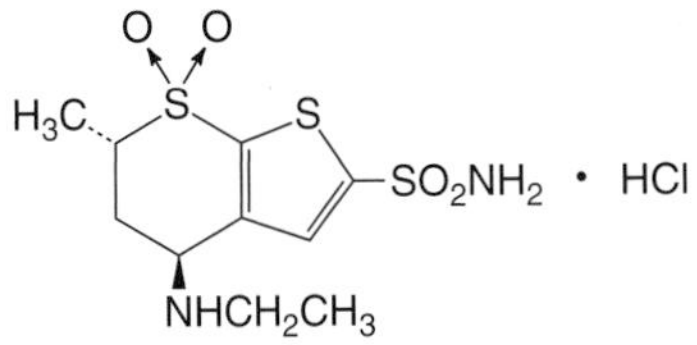

DORZOLAMIDE

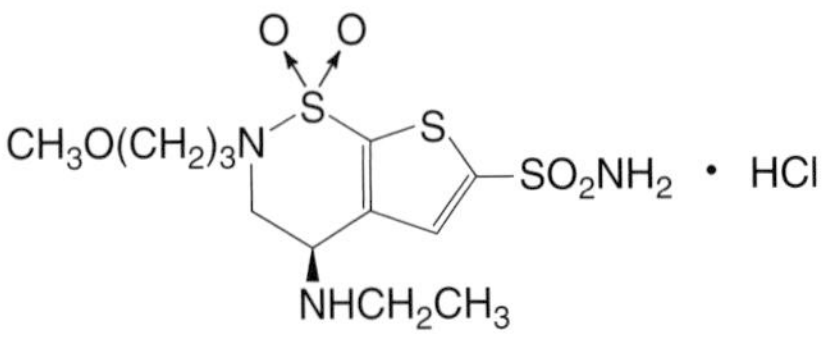

BRINZOLAMIDE

Toxicity of Agents in Treatment of Glaucoma. Ciliary body spasm is a muscarinic cholinergic effect that can lead to induced myopia and a changing refraction due to iris and ciliary body contraction as the drug effect waxes and wanes between doses. Headaches can occur from the iris and ciliary body contraction. Epinephrine-related compounds, effective in intraocular

pressure reduction, can cause a vasoconstriction-vasodilation rebound phenomenon leading to a red eye. Ocular and skin allergies from topical epinephrine, related prodrug formulations, and apraclonidine are common. Systemic absorption of epinephrine-related drugs can have all the side effects found with direct systemic administration. The β-adrenergic antagonists, while effective in intraocular pressure reduction, can produce systemic side effects readily through direct absorption in the tissues and *via* the nasolacrimal system. The use of CAIs systematically may give some patients significant problems with malaise, fatigue, depression, paresthesias, and nephrolithiasis; the topical CAIs may minimize these relatively common side effects. These medical strategies for managing glaucoma do help to slow the progression of this disease, yet there are potential risks from treatment-related side effects, and treatment effects on quality of life must be recognized.

Uveitis. Inflammation of the uvea, or uveitis, has both infectious and noninfectious causes, and medical treatment of the underlying cause (if known) is essential in addition to the use of topical therapy. *Cyclopentolate,* or sometimes an even longer-acting antimuscarinic agent such as *atropine,* frequently is used to prevent posterior synechia formation between the lens and iris margin and to relieve ciliary muscle spasm that is responsible for much of the pain associated with anterior uveitis. If posterior synechiae have already formed, an *α-adrenergic agonist* may be used to break the synechiae by enhancing pupillary dilation. *Topical steroids* usually are adequate to decrease inflammation, but sometimes they must be supplemented by systemic steroids.

Strabismus. Strabismus, or ocular misalignment, has numerous causes and may occur at any age. In children, strabismus may lead to *amblyopia* (reduced vision). Nonsurgical efforts to treat amblyopia include occlusion therapy, orthoptics, optical devices, and pharmacological agents. The eyes of children with hyperopia, or farsightedness, must accommodate to focus distant images. In some cases, the synkinetic accommodative-convergence response leads to excessive convergence and a manifest *esotropia* (turned-in eye). This deviated eye does not develop normal visual acuity and is therefore amblyopic. In this setting, *atropine* (1%) instilled in the preferred seeing eye every five days produces cycloplegia and the inability of this eye to accommodate, thus forcing the child to use the amblyopic eye. *Echothiophate iodide* also has been used in the setting of accommodative strabismus. Accommodation drives the near reflex, the triad of miosis, accommodation, and convergence. A reversible cholinesterase inhibitor such as *echothiophate* causes miosis and an accommodative change in the shape of the lens; hence, the accommodative drive to initiate the near reflex is reduced, and less convergence will occur.

Surgery and Diagnostic Purposes.   For certain surgical procedures and for clinical funduscopic examination, it is desirable to maximize the view of the retina and lens. Muscarinic cholinergic antagonists and α_2-adrenergic agonists frequently are used singly or in combination for this purpose (*see* Table 66–7).

Intraoperatively, there are circumstances when miosis is preferred, and two cholinergic agonists are available for intraocular use, *acetylcholine* and *carbachol*. Patients with myasthenia gravis may first present to an ophthalmologist with complaints of double vision (diplopia) or lid droop (ptosis); the *edrophonium test* is helpful in diagnosing these patients (*see* Chapter 8).

Use of Immunomodulatory Drugs for Ophthalmic Therapy

Glucocorticoids.   Glucocorticoids have an important role in managing ocular inflammatory diseases; their chemistry and pharmacology are described in Chapter 60.

Therapeutic Uses.   Because of their antiinflammatory effect, topical corticosteroids are used in managing anterior uveitis, external eye inflammatory diseases associated with some infections and ocular cicatricial pemphigoid, and postoperative inflammation following intraocular surgery. After glaucoma filtering surgery, topical steroids are particularly valuable in delaying the wound-healing process by decreasing fibroblast infiltration, which reduces the potential scarring of the surgical site. Steroids are commonly given systemically and by sub-Tenon's capsule injection to manage posterior uveitis. Parenteral steroids followed by tapering oral doses are the preferred treatment for optic neuritis (Kaufman *et al.,* 2000; Trobe *et al.,* 1999).

Toxicity of Steroids.   Extensive discussion has been directed to the toxic effects to the eyes of topical and systemic corticosteroids. These include the development of posterior subcapsular cataracts and secondary infections (*see* Chapter 60) and secondary open-angle glaucoma (Becker and Mills, 1963; Armaly, 1963a, 1963b). There is a significant increase in potential risk for developing secondary glaucoma when there is a positive family history of glaucoma. If there is no family history of open-angle glaucoma, only about 5% of normal individuals respond to topical or long-term systemic steroids with a marked increase in intraocular pressure. With a positive family history, however, moderate to marked steroid-induced intraocular pressure elevations may be seen in up to 90% of patients. The pathophysiology of steroid-induced glaucoma is not fully understood, but there is evidence that the

GLCIA gene may be involved (Stone *et al.,* 1997). Typically, steroid-induced elevation of intraocular pressure is reversible once administration of the steroid ceases.

Nonsteroidal Antiinflammatory Agents.   ***General Considerations.***   Nonsteroidal drug therapy for inflammation is discussed in Chapter 27. The nonsteroidal antiinflammatory drugs (NSAIDs) are now being applied to the treatment of ocular disease.

Therapeutic Uses.   Currently, there are four topical NSAIDs approved for ocular use: *diclofenac* (VOLTAREN), *flurbiprofen* (OCUFEN), *ketorolac* (ACULAR), and *suprofen* (PROFENAL). Diclofenac and flurbiprofen are discussed in Chapter 27; the chemical structures of ketorolac, a pyrrolo-pyrolle derivative, and suprofen, a phenylalkanoic acid, are shown below:

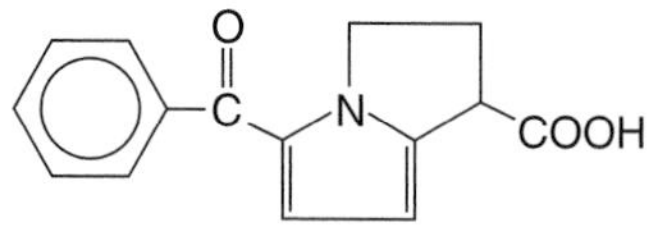

KETOROLAC

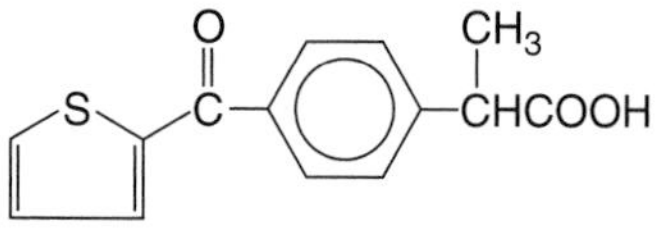

SUPROFEN

Flurbiprofen and suprofen are used to counter unwanted intraoperative miosis during cataract surgery. Ketorolac is given for seasonal allergic conjunctivitis. Diclofenac is used for postoperative inflammation. Both ketorolac (Weisz *et al.,* 1999a) and diclofenac (Anonymous, 1997b) have been found to be effective in treating cystoid macular edema occurring after cataract surgery.

Antihistamines and Mast-Cell Stabilizers.   *Pheniramine* (*see* Chapter 25) and *antazoline*, both H_1-receptor antagonists, are formulated in combination with *naphazoline*, a vasoconstrictor, for relief of allergic conjunctivitis. The chemical structure of antazoline is:

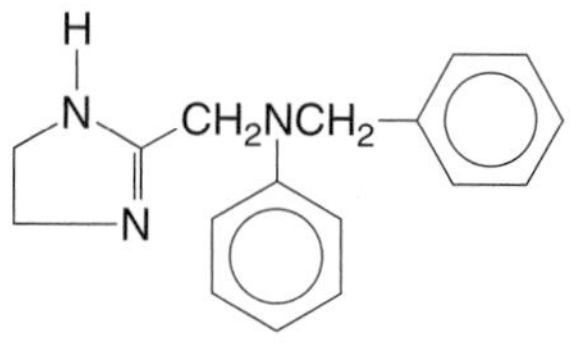

ANTAZOLINE

Newer topical antihistamines include *emedastine difumarate* (EMADINE), *olopatadine hydrochloride* (PATANOL), *levocabastine hydrochloride* (LIVOSTIN), and *ketotifen fumarate* (ZADITOR).

Cromolyn sodium (CROLOM), which prevents the release of histamine and other autacoids from mast cells (*see* Chapter 28), has found limited use in treating conjunctivitis that is thought to be allergen-mediated, such as vernal conjunctivitis. *Iodoxamide tromethamine* (ALOMIDE), another mast-cell-stabilizing agent, and *pemirolast* (ALAMAST), a mast-cell stabilizer that also has other anti-inflammatory effects, also are available for ophthalmic use.

Immunosuppressive and Antimitotic Agents. *General Considerations.* The principal application of immunosuppressive and antimitotic agents to ophthalmology relates to the use of *5-fluorouracil* and *mitomycin C* in corneal and glaucoma surgeries. Certain systemic diseases with serious vision-threatening ocular manifestations—such as Behçet's disease, Wegener's granulomatosis, rheumatoid arthritis, and Reiter's syndrome—require systemic immunosuppression (*see* Chapter 53).

Therapeutic Uses. In glaucoma surgery, both 5-fluorouracil and mitomycin C improve the success of filtration surgery by limiting the postoperative wound-healing process. Mitomycin C is used intraoperatively as a single subconjunctival application at the trabeculectomy site (Chen, 1983). Meticulous care is used to avoid intraocular penetration, since mitomycin C is extremely toxic to intraocular structures. 5-Fluorouracil may be used intraoperatively and/or during the postoperative course and is delivered subconjunctivally (Fluorouracil Filtering Surgery Study Group, 1989).

In cornea surgery, mitomycin C has been used topically after excision of pterygium, a fibrovascular membrane that can grow onto the cornea (Sugar, 1992). Although the use of mitomycin C for both pterygium and glaucoma filtration surgeries augments the success of these surgical procedures, caution is advocated in light of the potentially serious delayed ocular complications (Rubinfeld *et al.*, 1992; Greenfield, 1998; Hardten and Samuelson, 1999).

Drugs and Biological Agents Used in Ophthalmic Surgery

Adjuncts in Anterior Segment Surgery. *Hyaluronidase* depolymerizes hyaluronic acid, a mucopolysaccharide, in interstitial tissue spaces. This enzyme often is used to

enhance local anesthesia (*e.g.,* in retrobulbar optic nerve block). There are no direct complications due to the use of this drug. However, improperly placed retrobulbar injections of anesthetic can perforate the globe or penetrate the optic nerve and can lead to CNS depression secondary to diffusion into the optic nerve sheath.

Viscoelastic substances assist in ocular surgery by maintaining spaces, moving tissue, and protecting surfaces (*see* Liesegang, 1990; Goa and Benfield, 1994). These substances are prepared from hyaluronate, chondroitin sulfate, or hydroxypropylmethylcellulose and share the following important physical characteristics: viscosity, shear flow, elasticity, cohesiveness, and coatability. They are used almost exclusively in anterior segment surgery. Complications associated with viscoelastic substances are related to transient elevation of intraocular pressure after the surgical procedure.

Corneal Band Keratopathy. Ethylenediaminetetraacetic acid (EDTA) is a chelating agent that can be used to remove a band keratopathy (*i.e.,* a calcium deposit at the level of Bowman's membrane on the cornea).

Vitreous Substitutes. The primary use of vitreous substitutes is reattachment of the retina following vitrectomy and membrane-peeling procedures for complicated proliferative vitreoretinopathy and traction retinal detachments (*see* Peyman and Schulman, 1994; Chang, 1994). Several compounds may be selected, including *gases, perfluorocarbon liquids,* and *silicone oil* (*see* Table 66–8). With the exception of air, the gases expand because of interaction with systemic oxygen, carbon dioxide, and nitrogen, and this property makes them desirable to temporarily tamponade areas of the retina. However, use of these expansile gases carries the risk of complications from elevated intraocular pressure, subretinal gas, corneal edema, and cataract formation. The gases are absorbed over a time period of from days (for air) to as long as two months (for perfluoropropane).

The liquid perfluorocarbons have specific gravities between 1.76 and 1.94 and are helpful in flattening the retina when vitreous is present, because the perfluorocarbons are denser than vitreous. Also, in the event of a lens becoming dislocated into the vitreous, a perfluorocarbon liquid injection posteriorly will float the lens anteriorly, leading to easier surgical retrieval. This liquid potentially is toxic if it remains in chronic contact with the retina.

Silicone oil has had extensive use both in Europe and in the United States for long-term tamponade of the retina (*see* Peyman and Schulman, 1994; Parel and Villain,

Table 66-8
Vitreous Substitutes*

VITREOUS SUBSTITUTE	CHEMICAL STRUCTURE	CHARACTERISTICS (DURATION OR VISCOSITY)
Nonexpansile Gases		
Air		Duration of 5–7 days
Argon		
Carbon dioxide		
Helium		
Krypton		
Nitrogen		
Oxygen		
Xenon		Duration of 1 day
Expansile Gases		
Sulfur hexafluoride (SF_6)	[structure of SF_6]	Duration of 10–14 days
Octafluorocyclobutane (C_4F_8)	[structure of C_4F_8]	
Perfluoromethane (CF_4)	[structure of CF_4]	Duration of 10–14 days
Perfluoroethane (C_2F_6)	[structure of C_2F_6]	Duration of 30–35 days
Perfluoropropane (C_3F_8)	[structure of C_3F_8]	Duration of 55–65 days
Perfluoro-*n*-butane (C_4F_{10})	[structure of C_4F_{10}]	
Perfluoropentane (C_5F_{12})	[structure of C_5F_{12}]	
Silicone Oils		
Nonfluorinated silicone oils	$(CH_3)_3SiO[(CH_3)_2SiO]_nSi(CH_3)_3$	Viscosity range from 1000–30,000 cs
Fluorosilicone	$(CH_3)_3SiO[(C_3H_4F_3)(CH_3)SiO]_nSi(CH_3)_3$	Viscosity range from 1000–10,000 cs
"High-tech" silicone oils	$(CH_3)_3SiO[(C_6H_5)(CH_3)SiO]_nSi(CH_3)_3$	May terminate as trimethylsiloxy (shown) or polyphenylmethylsiloxane, viscosity not reported

*See Parel and Villain, 1994, and Chang, 1994, for further details.
CS = centistoke (unit of viscosity)

1994). Complications from silicone oil use include glaucoma, cataract formation, corneal edema, corneal band keratopathy, and retinal toxicity.

Surgical Hemostasis and Thrombolytic Agents. An important component of most surgical procedures, hemostasis, usually is achieved by temperature-mediated coagulation. In selective intraocular surgeries, thrombin has a valuable role in hemostasis. Intravitreal administration of thrombin sometimes is helpful in controlling intraocular hemorrhage during vitrectomy. When used intraocularly, a potentially significant inflammatory response may occur, but this reaction can be minimized by thorough irrigation after hemostasis is achieved. This coagulation factor also may be applied topically *via* soaked sponges to exposed conjunctiva and sclera where hemostasis may be a challenge due to the rich vascular supply.

Depending on the intraocular location of a clot, there may be significant problems relating to intraocular pressure, retinal degeneration, and persistent poor vision. *Tissue plasminogen activator* (t-PA) (*see* Chapter 55) has been used during intraocular surgeries to assist evacuation of a *hyphema* (blood in the anterior chamber), subretinal clot, or nonclearing vitreous hemorrhage. t-PA also has been administered subconjunctivally and intracamerally (*i.e.,* controlled intraocular administration into the anterior segment) to lyse blood clots obstructing a glaucoma filtration site (Ortiz *et al.,* 1988). The main complication related to the use of t-PA is bleeding.

Botulinum Toxin Type A in the Treatment of Strabismus, Blepharospasm, and Related Disorders. *Botulinum toxin type A* (BOTOX) has been used to treat strabismus, blepharospasm, Meige's syndrome, spasmodic torticollis hemifacial spasm, and facial wrinkles (Tsui, 1996; Price *et al.,* 1997; *see also* Chapter 9). By preventing acetylcholine release at the neuromuscular junction, botulinum toxin A usually causes a temporary paralysis of the locally injected muscles. The variability in duration of paralysis may be related to the rate of developing antibodies to the toxin, upregulation of nicotinic cholinergic postsynaptic receptors, and aberrant regeneration of motor nerve fibers at the neuromuscular junction. Complications related to this toxin include double vision (diplopia) and lid droop (ptosis).

Blind and Painful Eye. Retrobulbar injection of either absolute or 95% alcohol may provide relief from chronic pain associated with a blind and painful eye. This treatment is preceded by administration of local anesthesia. Local infiltration of the ciliary nerves provides symptomatic relief from pain, but other nerve fibers may be damaged, causing paralysis of the extraocular muscles, including those in the eyelids, or neuroparalytic keratitis. The sensory fibers of the ciliary nerves may regenerate, and repeated injections are sometimes needed to control pain.

Agents Used to Assist in Ocular Diagnosis

A number of agents are used in an ocular examination (*e.g.,* mydriatic agents and topical anesthetics, and dyes to evaluate corneal surface integrity), to facilitate intraocular surgery (*e.g.,* mydriatic and miotic agents, topical and local anesthetics), and to help in making a diagnosis in cases of anisocoria (*see* Figure 66–5) and retinal abnormalities (*e.g.,* intravenous contrast agents). The autonomic agents have been discussed earlier. The diagnostic and therapeutic uses of topical and intravenous dyes and of topical anesthetics are discussed below.

Anterior Segment and External Diagnostic Uses. Epiphora (or tearing) and surface problems of the cornea and conjunctiva are commonly encountered external ocular disorders. The dyes *fluorescein* and *rose bengal* are used in evaluating these problems. Available both as a 2% alkaline solution and as an impregnated paper strip, fluorescein reveals epithelial defects of the cornea and conjunctiva and aqueous humor leakage that may occur after trauma or ocular surgery. In the setting of epiphora, fluorescein is used to help determine the patency of the nasolacrimal system. In addition, this dye is used as part of the procedure of *applanation tonometry* (intraocular pressure measurement) and to assist in determining the proper fit of rigid and semirigid contact lenses.

Rose bengal, which also is available as a solution and as saturated paper strips, stains devitalized tissue on the cornea and conjunctiva. Such a staining pattern is valuable in assessing exposed areas that are the possible consequence of any of the following: corneal keratitis from herpes simplex; a neuromuscular disorder, such as Bell's palsy; an anatomical problem resulting from Graves' eye disease or a burn to the eyelid causing skin contractures; or a physiological problem relating to decreased tear production.

Posterior Segment Diagnostic and Therapeutic Uses. The integrity of the blood–retinal and retinal pigment epithelial barriers may be examined directly by retinal angiography using intravenous administration of either *fluorescein sodium* or *indocyanine green,* whose structures are shown below. Of the agents used in assisting the making of a diagnosis, the intravenous dyes are among the most toxic. These agents commonly cause nausea, but they also may precipitate a serious allergic reaction in susceptible individuals.

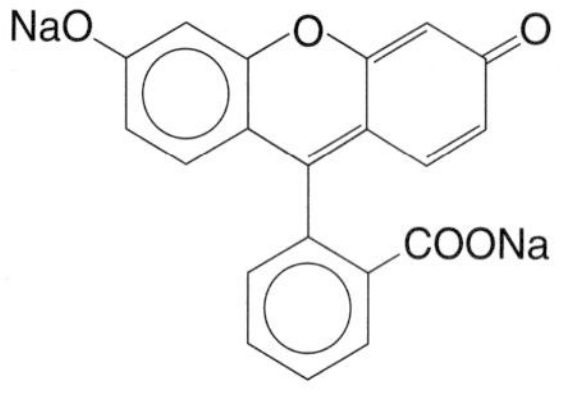

FLUORESCEIN SODIUM

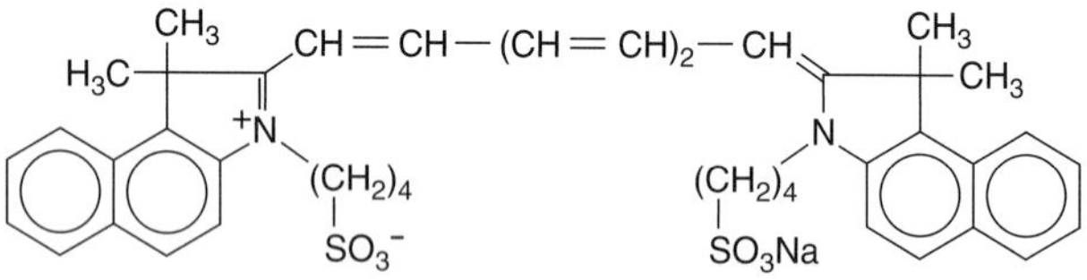

INDOCYANINE GREEN

Verteporfin (VISUDYNE) was approved by the FDA in 2000 for photodynamic therapy of the exudative form of age-related macular degeneration with classic choroidal neovascular membranes (Fine *et al.,* 2000; Anonymous 1999). The FDA is expected to broaden its approval to include treatment of classic choroidal neovascularization caused by conditions such as pathological myopia and ocular histoplasmosis syndrome. The chemical structure of verteporfin, which is a mixture of two regioisomers (I and II), is shown below:

Verteporfin is administered intravenously, and once it reaches the choroidal circulation, the drug is light-activated by a nonthermal laser source. Depending on the size of the neovascular membrane and concerns of occult membranes and recurrence, multiple photodynamic treatments may be necessary. Activation of the drug in the presence of oxygen generates free radicals, which cause vessel damage and subsequent platelet activation, thrombosis, and occlusion of choroidal neovascularization. The half-life of the drug is five to six hours. It is eliminated predominantly in the feces; less than 0.01% of the drug is recovered in the urine. The potential side effects include headache, injection site reactions, and visual disturbances. The drug causes temporary photosensitization, and patients must avoid exposure of skin or eyes to direct sunlight or bright indoor lights for 5 days after receiving it.

Use of Anesthetics in Ophthalmic Procedures

Topical anesthetic agents used clinically in ophthalmology include *cocaine, proparacaine,* and *tetracaine* (*see* Chapter 15). Proparacaine and tetracaine are used topically to perform tonometry, to remove foreign bodies on the conjunctiva and cornea, and to manipulate the nasolacrimal canalicular system. Tetracaine is used topically to anesthetize the ocular surface for refractive surgery using either the eximer laser or placement of intrastromal corneal rings. Cocaine may be used intranasally in combination with topical anesthesia for cannulating the nasolacrimal system.

Local anesthetics, commonly *lidocaine* and *bupivacaine,* are used for both infiltration and retrobulbar block anesthesia for surgery (*see* Chapter 15 for chemical

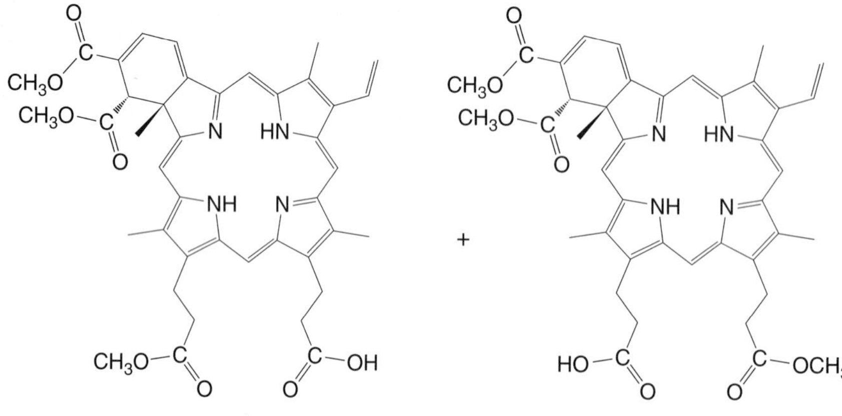

VERTEPORFIN REGIOISOMERS

structures and pharmacology). Potential complications and risks relate to allergic reactions, globe perforation, and vascular and subdural injections. Both preservative-free lidocaine (1%), which is introduced into the anterior chamber, and/or lidocaine jelly (2%), which is placed on the ocular surface during preoperative patient preparation, are used for cataract surgery performed under topical anesthesia.

General anesthetics and sedation are important adjuncts for patient care for surgery and examination of the eye. Most inhalation agents and central nervous system depressants are associated with a reduction in intraocular pressure. The exception appears to be ketamine, which has been associated with an elevation in intraocular pressure. In the setting of a patient with a ruptured globe, the anesthesia should be selected carefully to avoid agents that depolarize the extraocular muscles, which may result in expulsion of intraocular contents.

Other Agents for Ophthalmic Therapy

Vitamins and Trace Elements. *General Considerations.* The chemistry, nutritional deficiencies, and human requirements for the water-soluble (*see* Chapter 63) and fat-soluble (*see* Chapter 64) vitamins are discussed elsewhere in *this edition*. Table 66–9 summarizes the current understanding of vitamins related to eye function and disease.

Therapeutic Uses. In the setting of nutritional deficiency, *xerophthalmia,* a progressive disease characterized by *nyctalopia* (night blindness), *xerosis* (dryness), and *keratomalacia* (corneal thinning) which may lead to perforation, may be reversed with vitamin A therapy (WHO/UNICEF/IVAGG Task Force, 1988). However, rapid, irreversible blindness ensues once the cornea perforates. Vitamin A also is thought to be involved in epithelial differentiation and may have some role in corneal epithelial wound healing. Currently, there is no evidence to support using topical vitamin A for keratoconjunctivitis sicca in the absence of a nutritional deficiency. The potential therapeutic roles of vitamins A and E in retinitis pigmentosa have been examined, and the current recommendation is to supplement with 15,000 IU of vitamin A palmitate daily under the supervision of an ophthalmologist and to avoid high-dose vitamin E (Sandberg *et al.,* 1996; Berson *et al.,* 1993).

Another characteristic nutritional deficiency that has ocular manifestations is alcohol/tobacco amblyopia, which typically appears as temporal optic atrophy with corresponding decreased vision and characteristic visual field defects (*see* Lessell, 1994). This optic neuropathy often is irreversible.

Gyrate atrophy is an autosomal recessive, retinal degeneration caused by deficient mitochondrial ornithine aminotransferase. It is characterized by hyperornithinemia, nyctalopia, and progressive chorioretinal atrophy accompanied by progressive loss of visual field. It appears that supplemental pyridoxine or vitamin B_6 may have a role in managing this inborn error of metabolism (Weleber and Kennaway, 1981).

Much attention has been given to the use of antioxidants, particularly vitamins C and E and trace elements, to prevent cataract formation (*see* Chylak, 1994) and to protect the retina

Table 66–9
Ophthalmic Effects of Selected Vitamin Deficiencies and Zinc Deficiency*

DEFICIENCY	EFFECTS IN ANTERIOR SEGMENT	EFFECTS IN POSTERIOR SEGMENT
Vitamin		
A (retinol)	Conjunctiva (Bitot's spots, xerosis) Cornea (keratomalacia; punctate keratopathy)	Retina (nyctalopia; impaired rhodopsin synthesis); retinal pigment epithelium (hypopigmentation)
B_1 (thiamine)		Optic nerve (temporal atrophy with corresponding visual field defects)
B_6 (pyridoxine)	Cornea (neovascularization)	Retina (gyrate atrophy)
B_{12} (cyanocobalamin)		Optic nerve (temporal atrophy with corresponding visual field defects)
C (ascorbic acid)	Lens (?cataract formation)	
E (tocopherol)		Retina and retinal pigment epithelium (?macular degeneration)
Folic Acid		Vein occlusion
K	Conjunctiva (hemorrhage) Anterior chamber (hyphema)	Retina (hemorrhage)
Zinc		Retina and retinal pigment epithelium (?macular degeneration)

See Chapters 63 and 64 for biochemistry and human nutritional requirements. *See also* Chambers, 1994.

from the proposed oxidative damage induced by ultraviolet light (*see* Egan and Seddon, 1994; West *et al.*, 1994). It is hypothesized that oxidative pathways generate free radicals, which may have a role in the pathogenesis of macular degeneration and cataract formation. Interestingly, the concentration of ascorbic acid in the aqueous humor is 25 times greater than that in plasma in human beings (De Berardinis *et al.*, 1965). The biochemical and physiological roles of vitamin C have not been adequately explained by any studies to date, but this striking observation certainly leads to speculation about a possible protective effect against ultraviolet radiation.

A recent case-control study has demonstrated that elevated plasma homocysteine is a risk factor for central retinal vein occlusion, a multifactorial disease that can cause poor vision (Vine, 2000). Currently recommended for reducing the risk of atherothrombotic vascular disease related to hyperhomocysteinemia (*i.e.*, a plasma homocysteine level greater than 11 μM) is a daily multivitamin supplement containing 400 μg of folic acid (Omenn *et al.*, 1998).

Wetting Agents and Tear Substitutes. *General Considerations.* The current management of dry eyes usually includes instilling artificial tears and ophthalmic lubricants. In general, tear substitutes are hypotonic or isotonic solutions composed of electrolytes, surfactants, preservatives, and some viscosity-increasing agent that prolongs the residence time in the cul-de-sac and precorneal tear film. Common viscosity agents include cellulose polymers (*e.g., carboxymethylcellulose, hydroxyethyl cellulose, hydroxypropyl cellulose, hydroxypropyl methylcellulose,* and *methylcellulose*), *polyvinyl alcohol, polyethylene glycol, mineral oil, glycerin,* and *dextran*. The tear substitutes are available as preservative-containing or preservative-free preparations. Some tear formulations also are combined with a vasoconstrictor, such as naphazoline, phenylephrine, or tetrahydrozoline. In other countries, hyaluronic acid is sometimes used as a viscous agent; however, this enzyme has not been approved for use in the United States.

The lubricating ointments are composed of a mixture of white petrolatum, mineral oil, liquid or alcohol lanolin, and sometimes a preservative. These highly viscous formulations cause considerable blurring of vision, and consequently they are used primarily at bedtime or in very severe dry eye conditions.

Such aqueous and ointment formulations are only fair substitutes for the precorneal tear film, which is truly a poorly understood "lipid, aqueous, and mucin" trilaminar barrier (*see* above). To date, no study has demonstrated the clinical efficacy of treating dry eyes with tear substitutes. Consequently, the FDA has restricted the use of tear substitute components to nonprescription products. Various doses of *cyclosporine* ophthalmic emulsion have been tested in phase 2 and 3 clinical trials as treatment of moderate to severe dry eye syndrome (Sall *et al.*, 2000; Stevenson *et al.*, 2000). This drug appears to improve both objective and subjective signs of dry eye disease, but it is not approved currently for use in the treatment of this condition.

Therapeutic Uses. Many local eye conditions and systemic diseases may affect the precorneal tear film. Local eye disease, such as blepharitis, ocular rosacea, ocular pemphigoid, chemical burns, or corneal dystrophies, may alter the ocular surface and change the tear composition. Appropriate treatment of the symptomatic dry eye includes treating the accompanying disease and possibly the addition of tear substitutes. There are also a number of systemic conditions that may manifest themselves with symptomatic dry eyes, including Sjögren's syndrome, rheumatoid arthritis, vitamin A deficiency, Stevens–Johnson syndrome, and trachoma. Treating the systemic disease may not eliminate the symptomatic dry eye complaints; chronic therapy with tear substitutes or surgical occlusion of the lacrimal drainage system may be indicated.

Osmotic Agents and Drugs Affecting Carbonic Anhydrase. *General Considerations.* The main osmotic drugs for ocular use include *glycerin, isosorbide, mannitol* (*see* Chapter 29), and *hypertonic saline*. With the availability of these agents, the use of urea for management of acutely elevated intraocular pressure is nearly obsolete. Oral carbonic anhydrase inhibitors are a valuable adjunct to topical agents used to treat glaucoma. The pharmacology of this class of diuretic (*i.e.*, acetazolamide and methazolamide) is discussed in detail in Chapter 29, and their use in glaucoma was discussed earlier in this chapter. Carbonic anhydrase inhibitors also are used to treat pseudotumor cerebri in the setting of headache management, as well as to treat optic neuropathy associated with elevated intracranial pressure.

Therapeutic Uses. Ophthalmologists occasionally use glycerin, isosorbide, and mannitol for short-term management of acute rises in intraocular pressure. Occasionally, these agents are used intraoperatively to dehydrate the vitreous prior to anterior segment surgical procedures. Many patients with acute glaucoma do not tolerate oral medications because of nausea. Therefore, intravenous administration of mannitol and/or acetazolamide may be preferred over oral administration of glycerin or isosorbide. These agents should be used with caution in patients with congestive heart failure or renal failure. In diabetic patients, isosorbide is preferred over glycerin because the latter compound is metabolized rapidly to glucose.

Corneal edema is a clinical sign of corneal endothelial dysfunction, and topical osmotic agents may effectively dehydrate the cornea. Identifying the cause of corneal edema will guide therapy, and topical osmotic agents, such as hypertonic saline, may temporize the need for surgical intervention in the form of a corneal transplant. Sodium chloride is available in either aqueous or ointment formulations. Topical glycerin also is available; however, because it causes pain upon contact with the cornea and conjunctiva, the use of topical glycerin is limited to urgent evaluation of filtration-angle structures. In general, when corneal edema occurs secondary to acute glaucoma, the use of an oral osmotic agent to help reduce intraocular pressure is preferred to topical glycerin, which simply clears the cornea temporarily. Reducing the intraocular pressure will help clear the cornea more permanently to allow both a view of the filtration angle by gonioscopy and a clear view of the iris as required to perform laser iridotomy.

PROSPECTUS

Advances in ocular pharmacology will develop as a result of new insights into basic cellular, genetic, and physiological processes of specific tissues of the eye. Future directions in ocular pharmacology include immunomodulation for dry eyes and uveitis; molecular- and cellular-based therapy for corneal surface disease and inherited retinal dystrophies; and neuroprotection for glaucoma.

Immunomodulation. A better understanding of the pathogenesis of immunologically based eye diseases, such as dry eye syndrome, uveitis, and corneal melting syndromes, which are just a few examples of chronic and potentially intractable eye disorders, should lead to improved therapeutic interventions. Specifically for dry eye syndrome, major advances soon will lead to the use of new approaches for management of keratoconjunctivitis sicca rather than simplistic, polymer-based artificial tear replacement and punctal occlusion of the canaliculi (Figure 66–2). Androgen deficiency, lymphocytic inflammatory mediators, dysfunctional regulation of mucin gene expression, and other growth factors and hormones have all been implicated in the pathogenesis of dry eye syndrome (Lemp, 1999). Among potential treatments for dry eye syndrome, immunomodulation with a topical emulsion of *cyclosporine* (RESTASIS) is being evaluated in clinical trials (Stevenson *et al.,* 2000).

For uveitis, novel immunomodulation therapies are in clinical trials (Whitcup and Nussenblatt, 1997). Oral administration of retinal antigens has been used to treat ocular inflammation without a statistically significant impact on recurrence of ocular inflammation or cessation of conventional immunosuppressive therapy (Nussenblatt *et al.,* 1997). A recent nonrandomized, open-label, pilot study holds promise for the use of a humanized, anti-IL-2-receptor monoclonal antibody (*daclizumab, see* Chapter 53) in preventing intraocular inflammation while patients are not receiving conventional immunosuppressive therapy (Nussenblatt *et al.,* 1999). Further clinical trials and basic research should lead to the development of such novel therapeutic strategies for treating ocular inflammatory diseases by an approach more selective than general immunosuppression.

Molecular- and Cellular-Based Therapy. Many biochemical and genetic defects have been identified in inherited retinal and retinal-pigment epithelial degenerations (Sharma and Ehinger, 1999). Many treatments have been proposed, such as various neurotrophins and growth factors

(Frasson *et al.,* 1999; LaVail *et al.,* 1998), vitamin A (*see* "Vitamins and Trace Elements," above), RNA antisense therapy with ribozymes (Crooke, 1999), and cell-based therapies including retinal pigment epithelial (Weisz *et al.,* 1999b) and retinal transplantation (Mohand-Said *et al.,* 2000).

Another potential approach to the treatment of eye disease is the use of *protein kinase-C inhibitors* to prevent the neovascularization associated with diabetic retinopathy (Seo *et al.,* 1999). It is proposed that vascular complications of diabetes are caused in part by vascular endothelial growth factor–mediated activation of protein kinase-C beta (Aiello *et al.,* 1997). Clinical trials are under way to evaluate the effect of selective protein kinase-C inhibitors administered orally to prevent the complications of diabetic retinopathy (Jirousek *et al.,* 1996).

Neuroprotection. The issue of neuroprotection in relation to glaucoma involves balancing factors that promote life *versus* death of the retinal ganglion cells. Potential therapeutic targets include trophic factors, excitotoxins and their associated signaling pathways, ischemia, free radicals, neuroimmunomodulatory factors, and blood flow in the optic disk (Levin, 1999). There is experimental evidence to support nonintraocular pressure-lowering mechanisms in rodent models of chronic ocular hypertension (Neufeld *et al.,* 1999) and optic-nerve crush injuries (Yoles *et al.,* 1999). The experimental end points can be observed histologically by ganglion cell counts and axon counts, but functional correlates are not yet possible in these rodent models, and the relevance to the clinical setting is yet to be determined. An additional challenge in developing neuroprotective agents for glaucoma involves the design of clinical drug trials in which the end point of progressive optic disk cupping and correlation with visual function changes take many years. In contrast, the surrogate end point of intraocular pressure-lowering is achieved quickly; "peak" and "trough" effects of drugs that lower the pressure can be determined within hours and their adverse events and efficacy assessed over several months. Expanded research in this area should lead to new insights into mechanisms and pathways leading to glaucomatous optic neuropathy.

In addition to the aforementioned prospects for ocular pharmacology, efforts to develop novel strategies for drug delivery are expected, given the limitations in access to the filtration angle, retina, and optic nerve.

For further discussion of disturbances of vision and ocular movement, *see* Chapter 28 in *Harrison's Principles of Internal Medicine,* 14th ed., McGraw-Hill, New York, 1998.

BIBLIOGRAPHY

Aiello, L.P., Bursell, S.E., Clermont, A., Duh, E., Ishii, H., Takagi, C., Mori, F., Ciulla, T.A., Ways, K., Jirousek, M., Smith, L.E., and King, G.L. Vascular endothelial growth factor-induced retinal permeability is mediated by protein kinase C *in vivo* and suppressed by an orally effective beta-isoform-selective inhibitor. *Diabetes,* **1997,** *46:*1473–1480.

Ambati, B.K., Ambati, J., Azar, N., Stratton, L., and Schmidt, E.V. Periorbital and orbital cellulitis before and after the advent of *Haemophilus influenzae* type B vaccination. *Ophthalmology,* **2000,** *107:*1450–1453.

Anonymous. A controlled trial of oral acyclovir for iridocyclitis caused by herpes simplex virus. The Herpetic Eye Disease Study Group. *Arch. Ophthalmol.,* **1996,** *114:*1065–1072.

Anonymous. A controlled trial of oral acyclovir for the prevention of stromal keratitis or iritis in patients with herpes simplex virus epithelial keratitis. The Epithelial Keratitis Trial. The Herpetic Eye Disease Study Group. *Arch. Ophthalmol.,* **1997a,** *115:*703–712. [Published erratum appears in *Arch. Ophthalmol.,* **1997,** *115:*1196.]

Anonymous. Efficacy of diclofenac eyedrops in preventing postoperative inflammation and long-term cystoid macular edema. Italian Diclofenac Study Group. *J. Cataract Refract. Surg.,* **1997b,** *23:*1183–1189.

Anonymous. Acyclovir for the prevention of recurrent herpes simplex virus eye disease. Herpetic Eye Disease Study Group. *N. Engl. J. Med.,* **1998,** *339:*300–306.

Anonymous. Photodynamic therapy of subfoveal choroidal neovascularization in age-related macular degeneration with verteporfin: one-year results of 2 randomized clinical trials—TAP report. Treatment of age-related macular degeneration with photodynamic therapy (TAP) Study Group. *Arch. Ophthalmol.,* **1999,** *117:*1329–1345.

Armaly, M.F. Effect of corticosteroids on intraocular pressure and fluid dynamics. I. The effect of dexamethasone in the normal eye. *Arch. Ophthalmol.,* **1963a,** *70:*482–491.

Armaly, M.F. Effect of corticosteroids on intraocular pressure and fluid dynamics. II. The effect of dexamethasone in the glaucomatous eye. *Arch. Ophthalmol.,* **1963b,** *70:*492–499.

Baratz, K.H., Proia, A.D., Klintworth, G.K., and Lapetina, E.G. Cholinergic stimulation of phosphatidylinositol hydrolysis by rat corneal epithelium *in vitro. Curr. Eye Res.,* **1987,** *6:*691–701.

Beck, R.W., Cleary, P.A., Anderson, M.M., Jr., Keltner, J.L., Shults, W.T., Kaufman, D.I., Buckley, E.G., Corbett, J.J., Kupersmith, M.J., Miller, N.R., Savino, P.J., Guy, J.R., Trobe, J. D., McCrary, J.A. III, Smith, C.H., Chrousos, G.A., Thompson, H.S., Katz, B.J., Brodsky, M.C., Goodwin, J.A., and Atwell, C.W. A randomized, controlled trial of corticosteroids in the treatment of acute optic neuritis. The Optic Neuritis Study Group. *N. Engl. J. Med.,* **1992,** *326:*581–588.

Beck, R.W., Cleary, P.A., Trobe, J.D., Kaufman, D.I., Kupersmith, M.J., Paty, D.W., and Brown, C.H. The effect of corticosteroids for acute optic neuritis on the subsequent development of multiple sclerosis. The Optic Neuritis Study Group. *N. Engl. J. Med.,* **1993,** *329:*1764–1769.

Becker, B., and Mills, D.W. Corticosteroids and intraocular pressure. *Arch. Ophthalmol.,* **1963,** *70:*500–507.

Berson, E.L., Rosner, B., Sandberg, M.A., Hayes, K.C., Nicholson, B.W., Weigel-DiFranco, C., and Willett, W. A randomized trial of vitamin A and vitamin E supplementation for retinitis pigmentosa. *Arch. Ophthalmol.,* **1993,** *111:*761–772.

Chen, C.-W. Enhanced intraocular pressure controlling effectiveness of trabeculectomy by local application of mitomycin-C. *Trans. Asia-Pacific Acad. Ophthalmol.,* **1983,** *9:*172–177.

Chien, D.S., Homsy, J.J., Gluchowski, C., and Tang-Liu, D.D. Corneal and conjunctival/scleral penetration of *p*-aminoclonidine, AGN 190342, and clonidine in rabbit eyes. *Curr. Eye Res.,* **1990,** *9:*1051–1059.

Cobo, L.M., Foulks, G.N., Liesegang, T., Lass, J., Sutphin, J.E., Wilhelmus, K., Jones, D.B., Chapman, S., Segreti, A.C., and King, D.H. Oral acyclovir in the treatment of acute herpes zoster ophthalmicus. *Ophthalmology,* **1986,** *93:*763–770.

De Berardinis, E., Tieri, O., Polzella, A., and Iuglio, N. The chemical composition of the human aqueous humour in normal and pathological conditions. *Exp. Eye Res.,* **1965,** *4:*179–186.

Engstrom, R.E. Jr., Holland, G.N., Nussenblatt, R.B., and Jabs, D.A. Current practices in the management of ocular toxoplasmosis. *Am. J. Ophthalmol.,* **1991,** *111:*601–610.

Fluorouracil Filtering Surgery Study Group. Fluorouracil Filtering Surgery Study: one-year follow-up. *Am. J. Ophthalmol.,* **1989,** *108:*625–635.

Frasson, M., Picaud, S., Leveillard, T., Simonutti, M., Mohand-Said, S., Dreyfus, H., Hicks, D., and Sabel, J. Glial cell line-derived neurotrophic factor induces histologic and functional protection of rod photoreceptors in the rd/rd mouse. *Invest. Ophthalmol. Vis. Sci.,* **1999,** *40:*2724–2734.

Greenfield, D.S. Bleb-related ocular infection. *J. Glaucoma,* **1998,** *7:*132–136.

Hardten, D.R., and Samuelson, T.W. Ocular toxicity of mitomycin-C. *Int. Ophthalmol. Clin.,* **1999,** *39:*79–90.

Hargrave, S.L., McCulley, J.P., and Husseini, Z. Results of a trial combined propamidine isethionate and neomycin therapy for *Acanthamoeba* keratitis. Brolene Study Group. *Ophthalmology,* **1999,** *106:*952–957.

Jacobson, M.A., Stanley, H., Holtzer, C., Margolis, T.P., and Cunningham, E.T. Natural history and outcome of new AIDS-related cytomegalovirus retinitis diagnosed in the era of highly active antiretroviral therapy. *Clin. Infect. Dis.,* **2000,** *30:*231–233.

Jirousek, M.R., Gillig, J.R., Gonzalez, C.M., Heath, W.F., McDonald, J.H., III, Neel, D.A., Rito, C.J., Singh, U., Stramm, L.E., Melikian-Badalian, A., Baevsky, M., Ballas, L.M., Hall, S.E., Winneroski, L.L., and Faul, M.M. (S)-13-[(dimethylamino)methyl]-10,11,14,15-tetrahydro-4,9:16, 21-dimetheno-1H, 13H-dibenzo[e,k]pyrrolo[3,4-h][1,4,13]oxadiazacyclohexadecene-1,3(2H)-d ione (LY333531) and related analogues: isozyme selective inhibitors of protein kinase C beta. *J. Med. Chem.,* **1996,** *39:*2664–2671.

Kaufman, D.I., Trobe, J.D., Eggenberger, E.R., and Whitaker, J.N. Practice parameter: the role of corticosteroids in the management of acute monosymptomatic optic neuritis. Report of the Quality Standards Subcommittee of the American Academy of Neurology. *Neurology,* **2000,** *54:*2039–2044.

LaVail, M.M., Yasumura, D., Matthes, M.T., Lau-Villacorta, C., Unoki, K., Sung, C.H., and Steinberg, R.H. Protection of mouse photoreceptors by survival factors in retinal degenerations. *Invest. Ophthalmol. Vis. Sci.,* **1998,** *39:*592–602.

Lichter, P.R., Newman, L.P., Wheeler, N.C., and Beall, O.V. Patient tolerance to carbonic anhydrase inhibitors. *Am. J. Ophthalmol.,* **1978,** *85:*495–502.

Mandell, A.I., Stentz, F., and Kitabchi, A.E. Dipivalyl epinephrine: a new pro-drug in the treatment of glaucoma. *Ophthalmology,* **1978,** *85*:268–275.

Mohand-Said, S., Hicks, D., Dreyfus, H., and Sahel, J.A. Selective transplantation of rods delays cone loss in a retinitis pigmentosa model. *Arch. Ophthalmol.,* **2000,** *118*:807–811.

Moyes, A.L., Sugar, A., Musch, D.C., and Barnes, R.D. Antiviral therapy after penetrating keratoplasty for herpes simplex keratitis. *Arch. Ophthalmol.,* **1994,** *112*:601–607.

Musch, D.C., Lichter, P.R., Guire, K.E., and Standardi, C.L. The Collaborative Initial Glaucoma Treatment Study: study design, methods, and baseline characteristics of enrolled patients. *Ophthalmology,* **1999,** *106*:653–662.

Neufeld, A.H., Sawada, A., and Becker, B. Inhibition of nitric-oxide synthase 2 by aminoguanidine provides neuroprotection of retinal ganglion cells in a rat model of chronic glaucoma. *Proc. Natl. Acad. Sci. U.S.A.,* **1999,** *96*:9944–9948.

Nussenblatt, R.B., Fortin, E., Schiffman, R., Rizzo, L., Smith, J., Van Veldhuisen, P., Sran, P., Yaffe, A., Goldman, C.K., Waldmann, T.A., and Whitcup, S.M. Treatment of noninfectious intermediate and posterior uveitis with the humanized anti-Tac mAb: a phase I/II clinical trial. *Proc. Natl. Acad. Sci. U.S.A.,* **1999,** *96*:7462–7466.

Nussenblatt, R.B., Gery, I., Weiner, H.L., Ferris, F.L., Shiloach, J., Remaley, N., Perry, C., Caspi, R.R., Hafler, D.A., Foster, C.S., and Whitcup, S.M. Treatment of uveitis by oral administration of retinal antigens: results of a phase I/II randomized masked trial. *Am. J. Ophthalmol.,* **1997,** *123*:583–592.

Obianwu, H.O., and Rand, M.J. The relationship between the mydriatic action of ephedrine and the colour of the iris. *Br. J. Ophthalmol.,* **1965,** *49*:264–270.

Omenn, G.S., Beresford, S.A., and Motulsky, A.G. Preventing coronary heart disease: B vitamins and homocysteine. *Circulation,* **1998,** *97*:421–424.

Opremcak, E.M., Scales, D.K., and Sharpe, M.R. Trimethoprim-sulfamethoxazole therapy for ocular toxoplasmosis. *Ophthalmology,* **1992,** *99*:920–925.

Ortiz, J.R., Walker, S.D., McManus, P.E., Martinez, L.A., Brown, R.H., and Jaffe, G.J. Filtering bleb thrombolysis with tissue plasminogen activator. *Am. J. Ophthalmol.,* **1988,** *106*:624–625.

Price, J., Farish, S., Taylor, H., and O'Day, J. Blepharospasm and hemifacial spasm. Randomized trial to determine the most appropriate location for botulinum toxin injections. *Ophthalmology,* **1997,** *104*:865–868.

Rubinfeld, R.S., Pfister, R.R., Stein, R.M., Foster, C.S., Martin, N.F., Stoleru, S., Talley, A.R., and Speaker, M.G. Serious complications of topical mitomycin-C after pterygium surgery. *Ophthalmology,* **1992,** *99*:1647–1654.

Salazar, M., Shimada, K., and Patil, P.N. Iris pigmentation and atropine mydriasis. *J. Pharmacol. Exp. Ther.,* **1976,** *197*:79–88.

Sall, K., Stevenson, O.D., Mundorf, T.K., and Reis, B.L. Two multicenter, randomized studies of the efficacy and safety of cyclosporine ophthalmic emulsion in moderate to severe dry eye disease. CsA Phase 3 Study Group. *Ophthalmology,* **2000,** *107*:631–639.

Sanborn, G.E., Anand, R., Torti, R.E., Nightingale, S.D., Cal, S.X., Yates, B., Ashton, P., and Smith, T. Sustained-release ganciclovir therapy for treatment of cytomegalovirus retinitis. Use of an intravitreal device. *Arch. Ophthalmol.,* **1992,** *110*:188–195.

Sandberg, M.A., Weigel-DiFranco, C., Rosner, B., and Berson, E.L. The relationship between visual field size and electroretinogram amplitude in retinitis pigmentosa. *Invest. Ophthalmol. Vis. Sci.,* **1996,** *37*:1693–1698.

Seo, M.S., Kwak, N., Ozaki, H., Yamada, H., Okamoto, N., Yamada, E., Fabbro, D., Hofmann, F., Wood, J.M., and Campochiaro, P.A. Dramatic inhibition of retinal and choroidal neovascularization by oral administration of a kinase inhibitor. *Am. J. Pathol.,* **1999,** *154*:1743–1753.

Stevenson, D., Tauber, J., and Reis, B.L. Efficacy and safety of cyclosporin A ophthalmic emulsion in the treatment of moderate-to-severe dry eye disease: a dose-ranging, randomized trial. The Cyclosporin A Phase 2 Study Group. *Ophthalmology,* **2000,** *107*:967–974.

Stone, E.M., Fingert, J.H., Alward, W.L.M., Nguyen, T.D., Polansky, J.R., Sunden, S.L.F., Nishimura, D., Clark, A.F., Nystuen, A., Nichols, B.E., Mackey, D.A., Ritch, R., Kalenak, J.W., Craven, E.R., and Sheffield, V.C. Identification of a gene that causes primary open angle glaucoma. *Science,* **1997,** *275*:668–670.

Sugar, A. Who should receive mitomycin C after pterygium surgery? *Ophthalmology,* **1992,** *99*:1645–1646.

Trobe, J.D., Sieving, P.C., Guire, K.E., and Fendrick, A.M. The impact of the optic neuritis treatment trial on the practices of ophthalmologists and neurologists. *Ophthalmology,* **1999,** *106*:2047–2053.

Vine, A.K. Hyperhomocysteinemia: a risk factor for central retinal vein occlusion. *Am. J. Ophthalmol.,* **2000,** *129*:640–644.

Weisz, J.M., Bressler, N.M., Bressler, S.B., and Schachat, A.P. Ketorolac treatment of pseudophakic cystoid macular edema identified more than 24 months after cataract extraction. *Ophthalmology,* **1999,** *106*:1656–1659.

Weisz, J.M., Humayun, M.S., De Juan, E., Jr., Del Cerro, M., Sunness, J.S., Dagnelie, G., Soylu, M., Rizzo, L., and Nussenblatt, R.B. Allogenic fetal retinal pigment epithelial cell transplant in a patient with geographic atrophy. *Retina,* **1999,** *19*:540–545.

Weleber, R.G., and Kennaway, N.G. Clinical trial of vitamin B_6 for gyrate atrophy of the choroid and retina. *Ophthalmology,* **1981,** *88*:316–324.

West, S., Vitale, S., Hallfrisch, J., Muñoz, B., Muller, D., Bressler, S., and Bressler, N.M. Are antioxidants or supplements protective for age-related macular degeneration? *Arch. Ophthalmol.,* **1994,** *112*:222–227.

Whitcup, S.M. Cytomegalovirus retinitis in the era of highly active antiretroviral therapy. *JAMA,* **2000,** *283*:653–657.

WHO/UNICEF/IVAGG Task Force. *Vitamin A Supplements: A Guide to Their Use in the Treatment and Prevention of Vitamin A Deficiency and Xerophthalmia.* World Health Organization, Geneva, **1988.**

Wilhelmus, K.R., Gee, L., Hauck, W.W., Kurinij, N., Dawson, C.R., Jones, D.B., Barron, B.A., Kaufman, H.E., Sugar, J., Hyndiuk, R.A., Laibson, P.R., Stulting, R.D., and Asbell, P.A. Herpetic Eye Disease Study. A controlled trial of topical corticosteroids for herpes simplex stromal keratitis. *Ophthalmology,* **1994,** *101*:1883–1895.

Wilson, W.S., and McKean, C.E. Regional distribution of acetylcholine and associated enzymes and their regeneration in corneal epithelium. *Exp. Eye Res.,* **1986,** *43*:235–242.

Wistrand, P.J., Schenholm, M., and Lonnerholm, G. Carbonic anhydrase isoenzymes CA I and CA II in the human eye. *Invest. Ophthalmol. Vis. Sci.,* **1986,** *27*:419–428.

Yoles, E., Wheeler, L.A., and Schwartz, M. Alpha2-adrenoreceptor agonists are neuroprotective in a rat model of optic nerve degeneration. *Invest. Ophthalmol. Vis. Sci.,* **1999,** *40*:65–73. [Published erratum appears in *Invest. Ophthalmol. Vis. Sci.,* **1999,** *40*:2470.]

MONOGRAPHS AND REVIEWS

Albert, D.M., and Edwards, D.D., eds. *The History of Ophthalmology.* Blackwell Science, Cambridge, MA, **1996.**

Behlau, I., and Baker, A.S. Fungal infections and the eye. In, *Principles and Practice of Ophthalmology: Clinical Practice.* Vol. 5. (Albert, D.M., and Jakobiec, F.A., eds.) Saunders, Philadelphia, **1994,** pp. 3030–3064.

Cassoux, N., Bodaghi, B., Katlama, C., and LeHoang, P. CMV retinitis in the era of HAART. *Ocul. Immunol. Inflamm.,* **1999,** *7*:231–235.

Chambers, R.B. Vitamins. In, *Havener's Ocular Pharmacology,* 6th ed. (Mauger, T.F., and Craig, E.L., eds.) Mosby, St. Louis, **1994,** pp. 510–519.

Chang, S. Intraocular gases. In, *Retina.* Vol. 3: *Surgical Retina.* (Ryan, S.R., ed. in chief, Glaser, B.M., section ed.) Mosby, St. Louis, **1994,** pp. 2115–2129.

Chern, K.C., and Margolis, T.P. Varicella zoster virus ocular disease. *Int. Ophthalmol. Clin.,* **1998,** *38*:149–160.

Chylak, L.T. Medical treatment of cataract. In, *Principles and Practice of Ophthalmology: Basic Sciences.* (Albert, D.M., and Jakobiec, F.A., eds.) Saunders, Philadelphia, **1994,** pp. 1107–1111.

Crooke, S.T. Molecular mechanisms of action of antisense drugs. *Biochim. Biophys. Acta,* **1999,** *1489*:31–44.

DeFreitas, D., and Dunkel, E.C. Parasitic and rickettsial infections. In, *Principles and Practice of Ophthalmology: Basic Sciences.* (Albert, D.M., and Jakobiec, F.A., eds.) Saunders, Philadelphia, **1994,** pp. 865–890.

DeSantis, L.M., and Patil, P.N. Pharmacokinetics. In, *Havener's Ocular Pharmacology,* 6th ed. (Mauger, T.F., and Craig, E.L., eds.) Mosby, St. Louis, **1994,** pp. 22–52.

Dowling, J.E. *The Retina: An Approachable Part of the Brain.* The Belknap Press of Harvard University, Cambridge, MA, **1987.**

Duke-Elder, S., ed. *System of Ophthalmology.* Vol. 7: *The Foundations of Ophthalmology: Heredity, Pathology, Diagnosis, and Therapeutics.* Mosby, St. Louis, **1962,** pp. 462–727.

Egan, K.M., and Seddon, J.M. Age-related macular degeneration: epidemiology. In, *Principles and Practice of Ophthalmology: Basic Sciences.* (Albert, D.M., and Jakobiec, F.A., eds.) Saunders, Philadelphia, **1994,** pp. 1266–1274.

Fine, S.L., Berger, J.W., Maguire, M.G., and Ho, A.C. Age-related macular degeneration. *N. Engl. J. Med.,* **2000,** *342*:483–492.

Goa, K.L., and Benfield, P. Hyaluronic acid. A review of its pharmacology and use as a surgical aid in ophthalmology, and its therapeutic potential in joint disease and wound healing. *Drugs,* **1994,** *47*:536–566.

Grant, W.M., and Schuman, J.S. *Toxicology of the Eye,* 4th ed. Charles C. Thomas, Springfield, IL, **1993.**

Heckenlively, J.R. *Retinitis Pigmentosa.* Lippincott, Philadelphia, **1988.**

Kaufman, H.E. Treatment of viral diseases of the cornea and external eye. *Prog. Retin. Eye Res.,* **2000,** *19*:69–85.

Khorana, H.G. Rhodopsin, photoreceptor of the rod cell. An emerging pattern for structure and function. *J. Biol. Chem.,* **1992,** *267*:1–4.

Lee, V.H.L. Improved ocular drug delivery with prodrugs. In, *Prodrugs: Topical and Ocular Drug Delivery.* (Sloan, K.B., ed.) Marcel Dekker, New York, **1992,** pp. 221–297.

Lee, V.H.L. Precorneal, corneal, and postcorneal factors. In, *Ophthalmic Drug Delivery Systems.* (Mitra, A.K., ed.) Marcel Dekker, New York, **1993,** pp. 59–82.

Lemp, M.A. The 1998 Castroviejo Lecture. New strategies in the treatment of dry-eye states. *Cornea,* **1999,** *18*:625–632.

Lessell, S. Toxic and deficiency optic neuropathies. In, *Principles and*

Practice of Ophthalmology: Clinical Practice. Vol. 4. (Albert, D.M., and Jakobiec, F.A., eds.) Saunders, Philadelphia, **1994,** pp. 2599–2604.

Levin, L.A. Direct and indirect approaches to neuroprotective therapy of glaucomatous optic neuropathy. *Surv. Ophthalmol.,* **1999,** *43*(suppl 1):S98–S101.

Liesegang, T.J. Viscoelastic substances in ophthalmology. *Surv. Ophthalmol.,* **1990,** *34*:268–293.

Liesegang, T.J. Varicella-zoster virus eye disease. *Cornea,* **1999,** *18*: 511–531.

Lindquist, T.D. Treatment of *Acanthamoeba* keratitis. *Cornea,* **1998,** *17*:11–16.

McCulley, J.P., Alizadeh, H., and Niederkorn, J.Y. The diagnosis and management of *Acanthamoeba* keratitis. *CLAO J.,* **2000,** *26*:47–51.

McDonald, T.O., and Shadduck, J.A. Eye irritation. In, *Dermatotoxicology and Pharmacology.* (Marzulli, F.N., and Maibach, H.I., eds.) Hemisphere, Washington, DC, **1977,** pp. 139–191.

Meredith, T.A. Vitrectomy for infectious endophthalmitis. In, *Retina.* Vol. 3: *Surgical Retina.* (Ryan, S.J., ed. in chief, and Glaser, B.M., section ed.) Mosby, St. Louis, **1994,** pp. 2525–2537.

Parel, J.-M., and Villain, F. Silicone oils: physicochemical properties. In, *Retina,* Vol. 3: *Surgical Retina.* (Ryan, S.J., ed. in chief, and Glaser, B.M., section ed.) Mosby, St. Louis, **1994,** pp. 2131–2149.

Peyman, G.A., and Schulman, J.A. *Intravitreal Surgery: Principles and Practice.* Appleton & Lange, Norwalk, CT, **1994,** pp. 851–922.

Physicians' Desk Reference for Ophthalmology. 28th ed. Medical Economics, Oradell, NJ, **2000.**

Riordan-Eva, P., and Tabbara, K.F. Anatomy and embryology of the eye. In, *General Ophthalmology,* 13th ed. (Vaughan, D., Asbury, T., and Riordan-Eva, P., eds.) Appleton & Lange, Norwalk, CT, **1992,** pp. 8–21.

Robinson, J.C. Ocular anatomy and physiology relevant to ocular drug delivery. In, *Ophthalmic Drug Delivery Systems.* (Mitra, A.K., ed.) Marcel Dekker, New York, **1993,** pp. 29–58.

Schoenwald, R.D. Ocular pharmacokinetics/pharmacodynamics. In, *Ophthalmic Drug Delivery Systems.* (Mitra, A.K., ed.) Marcel Dekker, New York, **1993,** pp. 83–110.

Sebag, J. *The Vitreous: Structure, Function, and Pathobiology.* Springer-Verlag, New York, **1989.**

Sharma, R.K., and Ehinger, B. Management of hereditary retinal degenerations: present status and future directions. *Surv. Ophthalmol.,* **1999,** *43*:427–444.

Stjernschantz, J., and Resul, B. Phenyl substituted prostaglandin analogs for glaucoma treatment. *Drugs Future,* **1992,** *17*:691–704.

Stryer, L. The molecules of visual excitation. *Sci. Am.,* **1987,** *257*:42–50.

Thompson, S., and Pilley, S.F. Unequal pupils. A flow chart for sorting out the onisocorias. *Surv. Ophthalmol.,* **1976,** *21*:45–48.

Tielsch, J.M. Therapy for glaucoma: costs and consequences. In, *Trans. New Orleans Acad. Ophthal.* (Ball, S.F., and Franklin, R.M., eds.) Keigler, Amsterdam, **1993,** pp. 61–68.

Tsui, J.K. Botulinum toxin as a therapeutic agent. *Pharmacol. Ther.,* **1996,** *72*:13–24.

Whitcup, S.M., and Nussenblatt, R.B. Immunologic mechanisms of uveitis. New targets for immunomodulation. *Arch. Ophthalmol.,* **1997,** *115*:520–525.

Wybar, K.C., and Kerr Muir, M. *Baillière's Concise Medical Textbooks, Ophthalmology,* 3rd ed. Baillière Tindall, Philadelphia, **1984.**

Yoser, S.L., Forster, D.J., and Rao, N.A. Systemic viral infections and their retinal and choroidal manifestations. *Surv. Ophthalmol.,* **1993,** *37*:313–352.

SECTION XVI

TOXICOLOGY

HEAVY METALS AND HEAVY-METAL ANTAGONISTS

Curtis D. Klaassen

The environmental metals of greatest concern are lead, mercury, arsenic, and cadmium. In the past, lead paint was available for use in homes, and lead pipes and/or lead solder delivered water to some homes. As a result, people can be exposed to lead on a daily basis; this exposure is a major pediatric concern. Mercury similarly is a contaminant of our environment; human beings are exposed to mercury in the fish they eat as well as in the amalgam fillings in their teeth. Arsenic is found naturally in high concentrations in drinking water in various parts of the world. Recently, cadmium has been classified as a known human carcinogen. This chapter deals primarily with the toxic effects of these four metals and the chelators that are used to treat metal intoxication.

People always have been exposed to heavy metals in the environment. In areas with high concentrations, metallic contamination of food and water probably led to the first poisonings. Metals leached from eating utensils and cookware also have contributed to inadvertent poisonings. The emergence of the industrial age and large-scale mining brought occupational diseases caused by various toxic metals. Metallic constituents of pesticides and therapeutic agents (*e.g.,* antimicrobials) were additional sources of hazardous exposure. The burning of fossil fuels containing heavy metals, the addition of tetraethyllead to gasoline, and the increase in industrial applications of metals have now made environmental pollution the major source of heavy-metal poisoning.

Heavy metals exert their toxic effects by combining with one or more reactive groups (ligands) essential for normal physiological functions. Heavy-metal antagonists (chelating agents) are designed specifically to compete with these groups for the metals, and thereby prevent or reverse toxic effects and enhance the excretion of metals. Heavy metals, particularly those in the transition series, may react in the body with ligands containing oxygen (—OH, —COO$^-$, —OPO$_3$H$^-$, >C=O), sulfur (—SH, —S—S—), and nitrogen (—NH$_2$ and >NH). The resultant metal complex (or coordination compound) is formed by a coordinate bond—one in which both electrons are contributed by the ligand.

The heavy-metal antagonists discussed in this chapter possess the common ability to form complexes with heavy metals and thereby prevent or reverse the binding of metallic cations to body ligands. These drugs are referred to as *chelating agents*. A *chelate* is a complex formed between a metal and a compound that contains two or more potential ligands. The product of such a reaction is a heterocyclic ring. Five- and six-membered chelate rings are the most stable, and a polydentate (multiligand) chelator typically is designed to form such a highly stable complex, far more stable than when a metal is combined with only one ligand atom.

The stability of chelates varies with the metal and the ligand atoms. For example, lead and mercury have greater affinities for sulfur and nitrogen than for oxygen ligands; calcium, however, has a greater affinity for oxygen than for sulfur and nitrogen. These differences in affinity serve as the basis of selectivity of action of a chelating agent in the body.

The effectiveness of a chelating agent for the treatment of poisoning by a heavy metal depends on several factors. These include the relative affinity of the chelator for the heavy metal as compared to essential body metals, the distribution of the chelator in the body as compared with the distribution of the metal, and the ability of the chelator to mobilize the metal from the body once chelated.

An ideal chelating agent would have the following properties: high solubility in water, resistance to biotransformation, ability to reach sites of metal storage, capacity to form nontoxic complexes with toxic metals, ability to retain chelating activity at the pH of body fluids, and ready excretion of the chelate. A low affinity for Ca^{2+} also is desirable, because Ca^{2+} in plasma is readily available for chelation, and a drug might produce hypocalcemia despite high affinity for heavy metals. The most important property of a therapeutic chelating agent is greater affinity for the metal than that of the endogenous ligands. The large number of ligands in the body is a formidable barrier to the effectiveness of a chelating agent. Observations *in vitro* on chelator–metal interactions provide only a rough guide to the treatment of heavy-metal poisoning. Empirical observations *in vivo* are necessary to determine the clinical utility of a chelating agent.

The first part of this chapter covers the toxic properties of lead, mercury, arsenic, and cadmium as well as radioactive heavy metals and treatment of the consequences of toxic exposure to these metals. The second part of the chapter covers the chemical properties and therapeutic uses of several heavy-metal antagonists.

LEAD

Lead is ubiquitous in the environment as a result of its natural occurrence and its industrial use. The decreased use of leaded gasoline over the past two decades has resulted in decreased concentrations of lead in blood in human beings. The primary sources of environmental exposure to lead are leaded paint and drinking water; most of the overt toxicity from lead results from environmental and industrial exposure.

Acidic foods and beverages—including tomato juice, fruit juice, cola drinks, cider, and pickles—can dissolve the lead when packaged or stored in improperly glazed containers. Foods and beverages thus contaminated have caused fatal human lead poisoning. Lead poisoning in children is a fairly common result of their ingestion of paint chips from old buildings. Paints applied to dwellings before World War II, when lead carbonate (white) and lead oxide (red) were common constituents of both interior and exterior house paint, are primarily responsible. In such paint, lead may constitute 5% to 40% of dried solids. Young children are poisoned most often by nibbling sweet-tasting paint chips and dust from lead-painted windowsills and door frames. The American Standards Association specified in 1955 that paints for toys, furniture, and the interior of dwellings should not contain more than 1% lead in the final dried solids of fresh paint and, in 1978, the Consumer Product Safety Commission (CPSC) banned paint containing more than 0.06% lead for use in and around households. Renovation or demolition of older homes, using a physical process that would cause an airborne dispersion of lead dust or fumes, may cause substantial contamination and lead poisoning. Lead poisoning from the use of discarded automobile-battery casings made of wood and vulcanite and used as fuel during times of economic distress, such as during World Wars I and II, has been reported. Sporadic cases of lead poisoning have been traced to miscellaneous sources such as lead toys, retained bullets, drinking water that is conveyed

through lead pipes, artists' paint pigments, ashes and fumes of painted wood, jewelers' wastes, home battery manufacture, and lead type. Finally, lead also is a common contaminant of illicitly distilled whiskey ("moonshine"), because automobile radiators frequently are used as condensers, and other components of the still are connected by lead solder.

Occupational exposure to lead has decreased markedly over the past 50 to 60 years because of appropriate regulations and programs of medical surveillance. Workers in lead smelters have the highest potential for exposure, because fumes are generated and dust containing lead oxide is deposited in their environment. Workers in storage-battery factories face similar risks.

Dietary intake of lead also has decreased since the 1940s, when the estimate of intake was about 500 μg per day in the United States population, to less than 20 μg per day in 2000. This decrease has been due largely to: (1) a decrease in the use of lead-soldered cans for food and beverages; (2) a decrease in the use of lead pipes and lead-soldered joints in water distribution systems; (3) the introduction of lead-free gasoline; and (4) public awareness of the hazards of indoor leaded paint (NRC, 1993). A decline in blood levels from 13 μg/dl in the 1980s to <5 μg/dl has been observed in the general U.S. population (Pirkle, *et al.,* 1998). However, many children living in central portions of large cities have blood lead concentrations over 10 μg/dl.

Absorption, Distribution, and Excretion. The major routes of absorption of lead are from the gastrointestinal tract and the respiratory system. Gastrointestinal absorption of lead varies with age; adults absorb approximately 10% of ingested lead, while children absorb up to 40%. Little is known about lead transport across the gastrointestinal mucosa. It has been speculated that Pb^{2+} and Ca^{2+} may compete for a common transport mechanism, because there is a reciprocal relationship between the dietary content of calcium and lead absorption. Iron deficiency also has been shown to enhance intestinal absorption of lead. Absorption of inhaled lead varies with the form (vapor versus particle) as well as with concentration. Approximately 90% of inhaled lead particles from ambient air are absorbed (Goyer and Clarkson, 2001).

Once lead is absorbed, about 99% of that in the bloodstream binds to hemoglobin in erythrocytes. Only 1% to 3% of the circulating blood lead is in the serum available to the tissues. Inorganic lead is distributed initially in the soft tissues, particularly the tubular epithelium of the kidney and in the liver. In time, lead is redistributed and deposited in bone, teeth, and hair. About 95% of the body burden of the metal eventually is found in bone. Only small quantities of inorganic lead accumulate in the brain, with most of that in gray matter and the basal ganglia.

The deposition of lead in bone closely resembles that of calcium, but it is deposited as tertiary lead phosphate. Lead in the bone salts does not contribute to toxicity. After a recent exposure, the concentration of lead often is higher in the flat bones than in the long bones (Kehoe, 1961a,b), although, as a general rule, the long bones contain more lead. In the early period of deposition, the concentration of lead is highest in the epiphyseal portion of the long bones. This is especially true in growing bones, where deposits may be detected by x-ray examination as rings of increased density in the ossification centers of the epiphyseal cartilage and as a series of transverse lines in the diaphyses, so-called lead lines. Such findings are of diagnostic significance in children.

Factors that affect the distribution of calcium similarly affect that of lead. Thus, a high intake of phosphate favors skeletal storage of lead and a lower concentration in soft tissues. Conversely, a low phosphate intake mobilizes lead in bone and elevates its content in soft tissues. High intake of calcium in the absence of elevated intake of phosphate has a similar effect, owing to competition with lead for available phosphate. Vitamin D tends to promote the deposition of lead in bone if a sufficient amount of phosphate is available; otherwise, deposition of calcium preempts that of lead. Parathyroid hormone and dihydrotachysterol mobilize lead from the skeleton and augment the concentration of lead in blood and the rate of its excretion in urine.

In experimental animals, lead is excreted in bile, and much more lead is excreted in feces than in urine (Gregus and Klaassen, 1986). In human beings, urinary excretion is a more important route of excretion than in animals (Kehoe, 1987), and the concentration of lead in urine is directly proportional to that in plasma. However, because most lead in blood is in the erythrocytes, very little is filtered. Lead also is excreted in milk and sweat and is deposited in hair and nails. Placental transfer of lead also is known to occur.

The half-life of lead in blood is 1 to 2 months, and a steady state is thus achieved in about 6 months. After establishment of a steady state early in human life, the daily intake of lead normally approximates the output, and concentrations of lead in soft tissues are relatively constant. However, the concentration of lead in bone appears to increase (Gross et al., 1975), and its half-life in bone has been estimated to be 20 to 30 years. Because the capacity for lead excretion is limited, even a slight increase in daily intake may produce a positive lead balance. The average daily intake of lead is approximately 0.2 mg, whereas positive lead balance begins at a daily intake of about 0.6 mg, an amount that will not ordinarily produce overt toxicity within a lifetime. However, the time to accumulate toxic amounts shortens disproportionately as the amount ingested increases. For example, a daily intake of 2.5 mg of lead requires nearly 4 years for the accumulation of a toxic burden, whereas a daily intake of 3.5 mg requires but a few months, because deposition in bone is too slow to protect the soft tissues during rapid accumulation.

Acute Lead Poisoning. Acute lead poisoning is relatively infrequent and occurs from ingestion of acid-soluble lead compounds or inhalation of lead vapors. Local actions in the mouth produce marked astringency, thirst, and a metallic taste. Nausea, abdominal pain, and vomiting ensue. The vomitus may be milky from the presence of lead chloride. Although the abdominal pain is severe, it is unlike that of chronic poisoning. Stools may be black from lead sulfide, and there may be diarrhea or constipation. If large amounts of lead are absorbed rapidly, a shock syndrome may develop as the result of massive gastrointestinal

loss of fluid. Acute symptoms of the central nervous system (CNS) include paresthesias, pain, and muscle weakness. An acute hemolytic crisis sometimes occurs and causes severe anemia and hemoglobinuria. The kidneys are damaged, and oliguria and urinary changes are evident. Death may occur in 1 or 2 days. If the patient survives the acute episode, characteristic signs and symptoms of chronic lead poisoning are likely to appear.

Chronic Lead Poisoning. Signs and symptoms of chronic lead poisoning (plumbism) can be divided into six categories: gastrointestinal, neuromuscular, CNS, hematological, renal, and other. They may occur separately or in combination. The neuromuscular and CNS syndromes usually result from intense exposure, while the abdominal syndrome is a more common manifestation of a very slowly and insidiously developing intoxication. The CNS syndrome usually is more common among children, whereas the gastrointestinal syndrome is more prevalent in adults.

Gastrointestinal Effects. Lead affects the smooth muscle of the gut, producing intestinal symptoms that are an important early sign of exposure to the metal. The abdominal syndrome often begins with vague symptoms, such as anorexia, muscle discomfort, malaise, and headache. Constipation usually is an early sign, especially in adults, but diarrhea occasionally occurs. A persistent metallic taste appears early in the course of the syndrome. As intoxication advances, anorexia and constipation become more marked. Intestinal spasm, which causes severe abdominal pain, or *lead colic,* is the most distressing feature of the advanced abdominal syndrome. The attacks are paroxysmal and generally excruciating (Janin et al., 1985). The abdominal muscles become rigid, and tenderness is especially manifested in the region of the umbilicus. In cases where colic is not severe, removal of the patient from the environment of exposure may be sufficient for relief of symptoms. *Calcium gluconate* administered intravenously is recommended for relief of pain and usually is more effective than morphine.

Neuromuscular Effects. The neuromuscular syndrome, or *lead palsy,* that characterized the house painter and other workers with excessive occupational exposure to lead more than a half century ago, now is rare in the United States. It is a manifestation of advanced subacute poisoning. Muscle weakness and easy fatigue occur long before actual paralysis and may be the only symptoms. Weakness or palsy may not become evident until after extended muscle activity. The muscle groups involved usually are the most active ones (extensors of the forearm, wrist, and fingers and extraocular muscles). Wrist-drop and, to a lesser extent, foot-drop with the appropriate history of exposure have been considered almost pathognomonic for lead poisoning. There usually is no sensory involvement. Degenerative changes in the motoneurons and their axons have been described.

CNS Effects. The CNS syndrome has been termed *lead encephalopathy.* It is the most serious manifestation of lead poisoning and is much more common in children than in adults. The early signs of the syndrome may be clumsiness, vertigo, ataxia, falling, headache, insomnia, restlessness, and irritability. As the encephalopathy develops, the patient may first become excited and confused; delirium with repetitive tonic-clonic convulsions or lethargy and coma follow. Vomiting, a common sign, usually is projectile. Visual disturbances also are present. Although the signs and symptoms are characteristic of increased intracranial pressure, flap craniotomy to relieve intracranial pressure is not beneficial. However, treatment for cerebral edema may become necessary. There may be a proliferative meningitis, intense edema, punctate hemorrhages, gliosis, and areas of focal necrosis. Demyelination has been observed in nonhuman primates. The mortality rate among patients who develop cerebral involvement is about 25%. When chelation therapy is begun after the symptoms of acute encephalopathy appear, approximately 40% of survivors have neurological sequelae, such as mental retardation, electroencephalographic abnormalities or frank seizures, cerebral palsy, optic atrophy, or dystonia musculorum deformans (Chisolm and Barltrop, 1979).

Exposure to lead occasionally produces clear-cut, progressive mental deterioration in children. The history of these children indicates normal development during the first 12 to 18 months of life or longer, followed by a steady loss of motor skills and speech. They may have severe hyperkinetic and aggressive behavior disorders and a poorly controllable convulsive disorder. The lack of sensory perception severely impairs learning. Concentrations of lead in blood exceed 60 μg/dl (2.9 μM) of whole blood, and x-rays may show heavy, multiple bands of increased density in the growing long bones (*see above*). Until recently it was thought that such exposure to lead was restricted largely to children in inner-city slums. However, all children are exposed chronically to low levels of lead in their diets, in the air they breathe, and in the dirt and dust in their play areas. This is reflected in elevated concentrations of lead in the blood of many children and may be a cause of subtle CNS toxicity, including learning disabilities, lowered IQ, and behavioral abnormalities. An increased incidence of hyperkinetic behavior and a statistically significant, although modest, decrease in IQ have been shown in children with lower blood lead concentrations (Needleman *et al.*, 1990; Baghurst *et al.*, 1992; Bellinger *et al.*, 1992; Banks *et al.*, 1997). Increased blood lead levels in infancy and early childhood may be manifested in older children and adolescents as decreased attention span, reading disabilities, and failure to graduate from high school. Most studies report a 2- to 4-point IQ deficit for each μg/dl increase in blood lead within the range of 5 to 35 μg/dl. As a result, the Centers for Disease Control and Prevention (CDC) considers a blood lead concentration of greater than or equal to 10 μg/dl to be indicative of excessive absorption of lead in children and to constitute grounds for environmental assessment, cleanup, and/or intervention. Chelation therapy is recommended for consideration when blood lead concentrations are higher than 25 μg/dl. Universal screening of children, beginning at 6 months of age, is recommended by the CDC.

Hematological Effects. When the blood lead concentration is near 80 μg/dl or greater, basophilic stippling (the aggregation of ribonucleic acid) occurs in erythrocytes. This is thought to result from the inhibitory effect of lead on the enzyme pyrimidine-5′-nucleotidase. Basophilic stippling is not, however, pathognomonic of lead poisoning.

A more common hematological result of chronic lead intoxication is a hypochromic microcytic anemia, which is more frequently observed in children and is morphologically similar

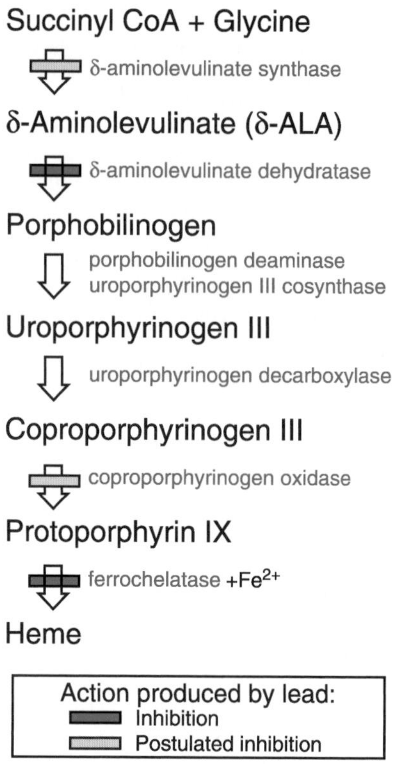

Figure 67–1. Lead interferes with the biosynthesis of heme at several enzymatic steps.

Steps that are definitely inhibited by lead are indicated by blue blocks. Steps at which lead is thought to act but where evidence for this is inconclusive are indicated by gray blocks.

to that resulting from iron deficiency. The anemia is thought to result from two factors: a decreased life span of the erythrocytes and an inhibition of heme synthesis.

Very low concentrations of lead influence the synthesis of heme. The enzymes necessary for heme synthesis are widely distributed in mammalian tissues, and it is highly probable that each cell synthesizes its own heme for incorporation into such proteins as hemoglobin, myoglobin, cytochromes, and catalases. Lead inhibits heme formation at several points, as shown in Figure 67–1. Inhibition of δ-aminolevulinate (δ-ALA) dehydratase and ferrochelatase, which are sulfhydryl-dependent enzymes, is well documented. Ferrochelatase is the enzyme responsible for incorporating the ferrous ion into protoporphyrin, and thus forming heme. When ferrochelatase is inhibited by lead, excess protoporphyrin takes the place of heme in the hemoglobin molecule. Zinc is incorporated into the protoporphyrin molecule, resulting in the formation of zinc-protoporphyrin, which is intensely fluorescent and may be used to diagnose lead toxicity. Lead poisoning in both human beings and experimental animals is characterized by accumulation of protoporphyrin IX and nonheme iron in red blood cells, by accumulation of δ-ALA in plasma, and by increased urinary excretion of δ-ALA. There also is increased urinary excretion of

Table 67–1

Patterns of Increased Excretion of Pyrroles in Urine of Acutely Symptomatic Patients

DISEASE	PYRROLES*			
	δ-ALA	PBG	URO	COPRO
Lead poisoning	+++	0	±	+++
Acute intermittent porphyria	++++	++++	+ to ++++	+ to +++
Acute hepatitis	0	0	0	+ to +++
Acute alcoholism	0	0	±	+ to +++

*0 = normal; + to ++++ = degree of increase; δ-ALA = δ-aminolevulinic acid; PBG = porphobilinogen; URO = uroporphyrin; COPRO = coproporphyrin.

SOURCE: Modified from Chisolm, 1967.

coproporphyrin III (the oxidation product of coproporphyrinogen III), but it is not clear whether this is due to inhibition of enzymatic activity or to other factors. Increased excretion of porphobilinogen and uroporphyrin has been reported only in severe cases. The pattern of excretion of pyrroles found in lead poisoning differs from that characteristic of symptomatic episodes of acute intermittent porphyria and other hepatocellular disorders, as shown in Table 67–1. The increase in δ-ALA synthase activity is due to the reduction of the cellular concentration of heme, which regulates the synthesis of δ-ALA synthase by feedback inhibition.

Measurement of heme precursors provides a sensitive index of recent absorption of inorganic lead salts. δ-ALA dehydratase activity in hemolysates and δ-ALA in urine are sensitive indicators of exposure to lead but are not as sensitive as quantification of blood lead concentrations.

Renal Effects. Although the renal effects of lead are less dramatic than those in the CNS and gastrointestinal tract, nephropathy does occur. Renal toxicity occurs in two forms (Goyer and Clarkson, 2001): a reversible renal tubular disorder (usually seen after acute exposure of children to lead) and an irreversible interstitial nephropathy (more commonly observed in long-term industrial lead exposure). Clinically, a Fanconi-like syndrome is seen with proteinuria, hematuria, and casts in the urine (Craswell, 1987; Bernard and Becker, 1988). Hyperuricemia with gout occurs more frequently in the presence of chronic lead nephropathy than in any other type of chronic renal disease. Histologically, lead nephropathy is revealed by a characteristic nuclear inclusion body, composed of a lead–protein complex; this appears early and resolves after chelation therapy. Such inclusion bodies have been reported in the urine sediment of workers exposed to lead in an industrial setting (Schumann *et al.*, 1980).

Other Effects. Other signs and symptoms of plumbism are an ashen color of the face and pallor of the lips; retinal stippling; appearance of "premature aging," with stooped posture, poor muscle tone, and emaciation; and a black, grayish, or blue-black so-called lead line along the gingival margin. The lead line, a result of periodontal deposition of lead sulfide, may be removed by good dental hygiene. Similar pigmentation may result from the absorption of mercury, bismuth, silver, thallium, or iron. There is a relationship between the concentration of lead in

blood and blood pressure, and it has been suggested that this may be due to subtle changes in calcium metabolism or renal function (Staessen, 1995). Lead also interferes with vitamin D metabolism (Rosen *et al.*, 1980; Mahaffey *et al.*, 1982). A decreased sperm count in lead-exposed males has been described (Lerda, 1992). The human carcinogenicity of lead is not well established but it has been suggested (Cooper and Gaffey, 1975), and several case reports of renal adenocarcinoma in lead workers have been published (Baker *et al.*, 1980; Kazantzis, 1986).

Diagnosis of Lead Poisoning. In the absence of a positive history of abnormal exposure to lead, the diagnosis of lead poisoning easily is missed. Furthermore, the signs and symptoms of lead poisoning are shared by other diseases. For example, the signs of encephalopathy may resemble those of various degenerative conditions. Physical examination does not easily distinguish lead colic from other abdominal disorders. Clinical suspicion should be confirmed by determinations of the concentration of lead in blood and protoporphyrin in erythrocytes. As noted earlier, lead, at low concentrations, decreases heme synthesis at several enzymatic steps. This leads to the buildup of the diagnostically important substrates δ-aminolevulinic acid, coproporphyrin (both measured in urine), and zinc protoporphyrin (measured in the red cell as erythrocyte protoporphyrin). Because the erythrocyte protoporphyrin level is not sensitive enough to identify children with elevated blood lead levels below about 25 μg/dl, the screening test of choice is blood lead measurement.

Since lead has been removed from paints and gasoline, the mean blood levels of lead in children in the United States have decreased from 17 μg/dl in the 1970s to 6 μg/dl in the 1990s (Schoen, 1993). The concentration of lead in blood is an indication of recent absorption of the metal (Figure 67–2). Children with concentrations of lead in blood above 10 μg/dl are at risk of developmental disabilities. Adults with concentrations below 30 μg/dl exhibit no known functional injury or symptoms; however, they will have a definite decrease in δ-ALA dehydratase activity, a slight increase in urinary excretion of δ-ALA, and an increase in erythrocyte protoporphyrin. Patients with a blood lead concentration of 30 to 75 μg/dl have all of the above laboratory abnormalities and, usually, nonspecific, mild symptoms of lead poisoning. Clear symptoms of lead poisoning are associated with

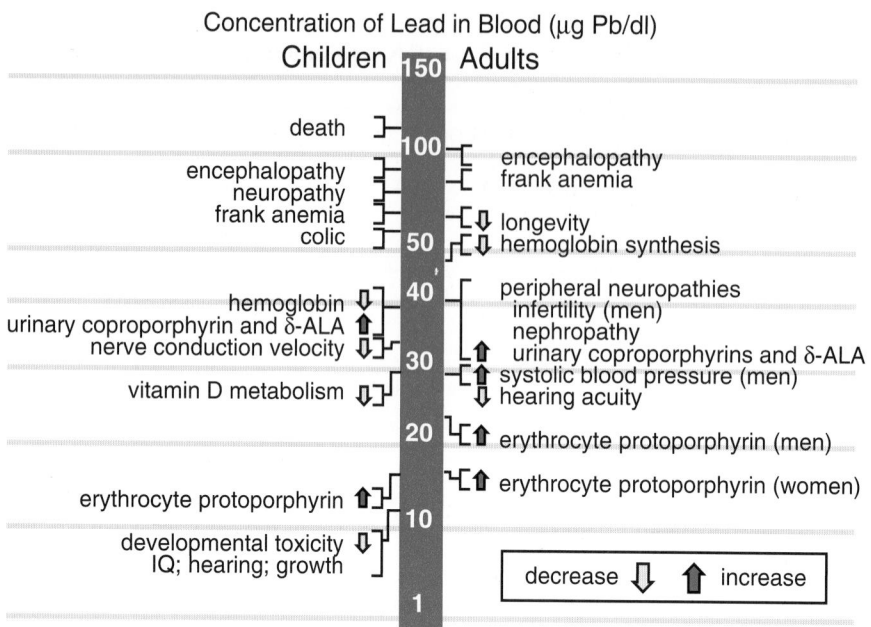

Concentration of Lead in Blood (μg Pb/dl)

Figure 67–2. Manifestations of lead toxicity associated with varying concentrations of lead in blood of children and adults.

δ-ALA = δ-aminolevulinate.

concentrations that exceed 75 μg/dl of whole blood (Kehoe, 1961a,b), and lead encephalopathy is usually apparent when lead concentrations are greater than 100 μg/dl. In persons with moderate-to-severe anemia, interpretation of the significance of concentrations of lead in blood is improved by correcting the observed value to approximate that which would be expected if the patient's hematocrit were within the normal range.

The urinary concentration of lead in normal adults generally is less than 80 μg/liter (0.4 μM) (Kehoe, 1961a,b; Goldwater and Hoover, 1967). Most patients with lead poisoning show concentrations of lead in urine of 150 to 300 μg/liter (0.7 to 1.4 μM). However, in persons with chronic lead nephropathy or other forms of renal insufficiency, urinary excretion of lead may be within the normal range, even though blood lead concentrations are significantly elevated.

Because the onset of lead poisoning usually is insidious, it often is desirable to estimate the body burden of lead in individuals who are exposed to an environment that is contaminated with the metal. In the past, the edetate calcium disodium ($CaNa_2EDTA$) provocation test has been used to determine whether or not there is an increased body burden of lead in those for whom exposure occurred much earlier. The provocation test is performed by intravenous administration of a single dose of $CaNa_2EDTA$ (50 mg/kg), and urine is collected for 8 hours. The test is positive for children when the lead excretion ratio (micrograms of lead excreted in the urine per milligram of $CaNa_2EDTA$ administered) is greater than 0.6 and may be useful for therapeutic chelation in children with blood levels of 25 to 45 μg/dl. This test is not used in symptomatic patients or in those whose concentration of lead in blood is greater than 45 μg/dl, because these patients require the proper therapeutic regimen with chelating agents (*see* below). Neutron activation analysis or fluorometric assays, currently available only as research methods, may offer a unique *in vivo* approach to the diagnosis of lead burden in the future.

Organic Lead Poisoning. Tetraethyllead and tetramethyllead are lipid-soluble compounds and are readily absorbed from the skin, gastrointestinal tract, and lungs. The toxicity of tetraethyllead is believed to be due to its metabolic conversion to triethyllead and inorganic lead.

The major symptoms of intoxication with tetraethyllead are referable to the CNS (Seshia *et al.,* 1978). The victim suffers from insomnia, nightmares, anorexia, nausea and vomiting, diarrhea, headache, muscular weakness, and emotional instability. Subjective CNS symptoms such as irritability, restlessness, and anxiety are next evident. At this time there is usually hypothermia, bradycardia, and hypotension. With continued exposure, or in the case of intense short-term exposure, CNS manifestations progress to delusions, ataxia, exaggerated muscular movements, and, finally, a maniacal state.

The diagnosis of poisoning by tetraethyllead is established by relating these signs and symptoms to a history of exposure. The urinary excretion of lead may increase markedly, but the concentration of lead in blood remains nearly normal. Anemia and basophilic stippling of erythrocytes are uncommon in organic lead poisoning. There is little effect on the metabolism of porphyrins, and erythrocyte protoporphyrin concentrations are inconsistently elevated (Garrettson, 1983). In the case of severe exposure, death may occur within a few hours or may be delayed for several weeks. If the patient survives the acute phase of organic lead poisoning, recovery usually is complete; however, instances of residual CNS damage have been reported.

Treatment of Lead Poisoning. Initial treatment of the acute phase of lead intoxication involves supportive measures. Prevention of further exposure is important. Seizures are treated with diazepam (Chapters 17 and 21); fluid and electrolyte balances must be maintained; cerebral edema is treated with mannitol and dexamethasone. The concentration of lead in blood should be determined, or at least a blood sample for analysis obtained, prior to initiation of chelation therapy.

Chelation therapy is indicated in symptomatic patients or in patients with a blood lead concentration in excess of 50 to 60 μg/dl (about 2.5 μM). Four chelators are employed: *edetate calcium disodium* (CaNa$_2$EDTA), *dimercaprol* (British anti-Lewisite; BAL), D-*penicillamine,* and *succimer* (2,3–dimercaptosuccinic acid; DMSA; CHEMET). CaNa$_2$EDTA and dimercaprol usually are used in combination for lead encephalopathy.

CaNa$_2$EDTA. CaNa$_2$EDTA is initiated at a dose of 30 to 50 mg/kg per day in two divided doses, either by deep intramuscular injection or slow intravenous infusion for up to 5 consecutive days. The first dose of CaNa$_2$EDTA should be delayed until 4 hours after the first dose of dimercaprol. An additional course of CaNa$_2$EDTA may be given after an interruption of 2 days. Each course of therapy with CaNa$_2$EDTA should not exceed a total dose of 500 mg/kg. Urine output must be monitored, because the chelator–lead complex is believed to be nephrotoxic. Treatment with CaNa$_2$EDTA can alleviate symptoms quickly. Colic may disappear within 2 hours; paresthesia and tremor cease after 4 or 5 days; coproporphyrinuria, stippled erythrocytes, and gingival lead lines tend to decrease in 4 to 9 days. Urinary elimination of lead is usually greatest during the initial infusion.

Dimercaprol. Dimercaprol is given intramuscularly at a dose of 4 mg/kg every 4 hours for 48 hours, then every 6 hours for 48 hours, and finally every 6 to 12 hours for an additional 7 days. The combination of dimercaprol and CaNa$_2$EDTA is more effective than is either chelator alone (Chisolm, 1973).

D-Penicillamine. In contrast to CaNa$_2$EDTA and dimercaprol, penicillamine is effective orally and may be included in the regimen at a dosage of 250 mg given four times daily for 5 days. During chronic therapy with penicillamine, the dose should not exceed 40 mg/kg per day.

Succimer. Succimer is the first orally active lead chelator available for children with a safety and efficacy profile that surpasses that of D-penicillamine. Succimer is usually given every 8 hours (10 mg/kg) for 5 days, and then every 12 hours for an additional 2 weeks.

General Principles. In any chelation regimen, 2 weeks after the regimen has been completed, the blood lead concentration should be reassessed; an additional course of therapy may be indicated if blood lead concentrations rebound.

Treatment of organic lead poisoning is symptomatic. Chelation therapy will promote the excretion of the inorganic lead produced from the metabolism of organic lead, but the increase is not dramatic (Boyd *et al.,* 1957).

MERCURY

Mercury was an important constituent of drugs for centuries as an ingredient in many diuretics, antibacterials, antiseptics, skin ointments, and laxatives. More specific, effective, and safer modes of therapy have largely replaced the mercurials in recent decades, and drug-induced mercury poisoning has become rare. However, mercury has a number of important industrial uses (Table 67–2), and poisoning from occupational exposure and environmental

Table 67–2

Occupational and Environmental Exposure to Mercury

INDUSTRIAL USES OF MERCURY	% OF TOTAL MERCURY EXPOSURE
Chloralkali *e.g.,* bleach	25
Electrical equipment	20
Paints	15
Thermometers	10
Dental	3
Laboratory	2

pollution continues to be an area of concern. There have been epidemics of mercury poisoning among wildlife and human populations in many countries. With very few exceptions and for numerous reasons, such outbreaks were misdiagnosed for months or even years. Reasons for these tragic delays included the insidious onset of the affliction, vagueness of early clinical signs, and the medical profession's unfamiliarity with the disease (Gerstner and Huff, 1977).

Chemical Forms and Sources of Mercury. With regard to the toxicity of mercury, three major chemical forms of the metal must be distinguished: mercury vapor (elemental mercury), salts of mercury, and organic mercurials. Table 67–3 indicates the estimated daily retention of various forms of mercury from various sources.

Elemental mercury is the most volatile of the inorganic forms of the metal. Human exposure to mercury vapor is mainly occupational and has been known since antiquity. Extraction of gold with mercury and then heating the amalgam to drive off the mercury is a technique that has been extensively used by gold miners and is still used today in some developing countries. Chronic exposure to mercury in ambient air after inadvertent mercury spills in poorly ventilated rooms, often scientific laboratories, can produce toxic effects. Mercury vapor also can be released from silver-amalgam dental restorations. In fact, this is the main source of mercury exposure to the general population, but the amount of mercury released does not appear to be of significance for human health (Eley and Cox, 1993) except for allergic contact eczema seen in a few individuals.

Salts of mercury exist in two states of oxidation—as monovalent mercurous salts or as divalent mercuric salts. Mercurous chloride, or calomel, the best-known mercurous compound, was used in some skin creams as an antiseptic and was employed as a diuretic and cathartic. Mercuric salts are the more irritating and acutely toxic form of the metal. Mercuric nitrate was a common industrial hazard in the felt-hat industry more than 400 years ago. Occupational exposure produced neurological and behavioral changes depicted by the Mad Hatter in Lewis Carroll's *Alice's Adventures in Wonderland.* Mercuric chloride, once a widely used antiseptic, also was commonly used for

Table 67–3

Estimated Average Daily Retention of Total Mercury and Mercury Compounds in the General Population Not Occupationally Exposed to Mercury

EXPOSURE	ESTIMATED MEAN DAILY RETENTION OF MERCURY COMPOUNDS, μg mercury/day		
	Mercury Vapor	Inorganic Mercury Salts	Methylmercury
Air	0.024	0.001	0.0064
Food			
Fish	0.0	0.04	2.3
Nonfish	0.0	0.25	0.0
Drinking water	0.0	0.0035	0.0
Dental amalgams	3–17	0.0	0.0
Total	3–17	0.3	2.31

suicidal purposes. Mercuric salts still are widely employed in industry, and industrial discharge into rivers has introduced mercury into the environment in many parts of the world. The main industrial uses of inorganic mercury today are in chloralkali production and in electronics. Other uses of the metal include the manufacturing of plastics, fungicides, and germicides and the formulation of amalgams in dentistry.

The organomercurials in use today contain mercury with one covalent bond to a carbon atom. This is a heterogeneous group of compounds, and its members have varying abilities to produce toxic effects. The alkylmercury salts are by far the most dangerous of these compounds; methylmercury is the most common. Alkylmercury salts have been used widely as fungicides and, as such, have produced toxic effects in human beings. Major incidents of human poisoning from the inadvertent consumption of mercury-treated seed grain have occurred in Iraq, Pakistan, Ghana, and Guatemala. The most catastrophic outbreak occurred in Iraq in 1972. During the fall of 1971, Iraq imported large quantities of seed (wheat and barley) treated with methylmercury and distributed the grain for spring planting. Despite official warnings, the grain was ground into flour and made into bread. As a result, 6530 victims were hospitalized and 500 died (Bakir *et al.*, 1973, 1980).

Minamata disease also was due to methylmercury. Minamata is a small town in Japan, and its major industry is a chemical plant that empties its effluent directly into Minamata Bay. The chemical plant used inorganic mercury as a catalyst, and some of it was methylated before it entered the bay. In addition, microorganisms can convert inorganic mercury to methylmercury; the compound is then taken up rapidly by plankton algae and is concentrated in fish *via* the food chain. Residents of Minamata who consumed fish as a large portion of their diet were the first to be poisoned. Eventually 121 persons were poisoned and 46 died (McAlpine and Araki, 1958; Smith and Smith, 1975; Tamashiro *et al.*, 1985). In the United States, human poisonings have resulted from ingestion of meat from pigs fed grain treated with an organomercurial fungicide.

Chemistry and Mechanism of Action. Mercury readily forms covalent bonds with sulfur, and it is this property that accounts for most of the biological properties of the metal. When the sulfur is in the form of sulfhydryl groups, divalent mercury

replaces the hydrogen atom to form mercaptides, X—Hg—SR and Hg(SR)$_2$, where X is an electronegative radical and R is protein. Organic mercurials form mercaptides of the type RHg–SR'. Even in low concentrations, mercurials are capable of inactivating sulfhydryl enzymes and thus interfering with cellular metabolism and function. The affinity of mercury for thiols provides the basis for treatment of mercury poisoning with such agents as dimercaprol and penicillamine. Mercury also combines with other ligands of physiological importance, such as phosphoryl, carboxyl, amide, and amine groups.

The various therapeutic and toxic actions of the mercurials are associated with chemical substituents that affect solubility, dissociation, relative affinity for various cellular receptors, distribution, and excretion.

Absorption, Biotransformation, Distribution, and Excretion. *Elemental Mercury.* Elemental mercury is not particularly toxic when ingested because of very low absorption from the gastrointestinal tract; this is due to the formation of droplets and because the metal in this form cannot react with biologically important molecules. However, inhaled mercury vapor is completely absorbed by the lung and then is oxidized to the divalent mercuric cation by catalase in the erythrocytes (Magos *et al.*, 1978). Within a few hours the deposition of inhaled mercury vapor resembles that after ingestion of mercuric salts, with one important difference. Because mercury vapor crosses membranes much more readily than does divalent mercury, a significant amount of the vapor enters the brain before it is oxidized. CNS toxicity is thus more prominent after exposure to mercury vapor than to divalent forms of the metal.

Inorganic Salts of Mercury. The soluble inorganic mercuric salts (Hg^{2+}) gain access to the circulation when taken orally. Gastrointestinal absorption is approximately 10% to 15% of that ingested, and a considerable portion of the Hg^{2+} may remain bound to the alimentary mucosa and the intestinal contents. Insoluble inorganic mercurous compounds, such as calomel (Hg$_2$Cl$_2$), may undergo some oxidation to soluble compounds that are more readily absorbed. Inorganic mercury has a markedly nonuniform distribution after absorption. The highest concentration of Hg^{2+} is found in the kidneys, where the metal is retained longer than in other tissues. Concentrations of inorganic mercury are similar in whole blood and plasma. Inorganic mercurials do not readily pass the blood–brain barrier or the placenta. The metal is excreted in the urine and feces with a half-life of about 60 days (Friberg and Vostal, 1972); studies in laboratory animals indicate that fecal excretion is quantitatively more important (Klaassen, 1975).

Organic Mercurials. Organic mercurials are more completely absorbed from the gastrointestinal tract than are the inorganic salts because they are more lipid soluble and less corrosive to the intestinal mucosa. Their uptake and distribution are depicted

A Intestinal uptake and distribution of organic mercurials

B Uptake of methylmercury complex by capillaries

$$CH_3Hg^+ + {}^-S\text{-}CH_2\text{-}CH\text{-}COO^-$$
$$\underset{\text{(cysteine)}}{\overset{|}{NH_3^+}}$$

$$CH_3\text{-}Hg\text{-}S\text{-}CH_2\text{-}CH\text{-}COO^-$$
METHYLMERCURY $\overset{|}{NH_3^+}$
(complex)

Uptake by neutral amino acid carrier in endothelial cells due to structural resemblance to methionine.

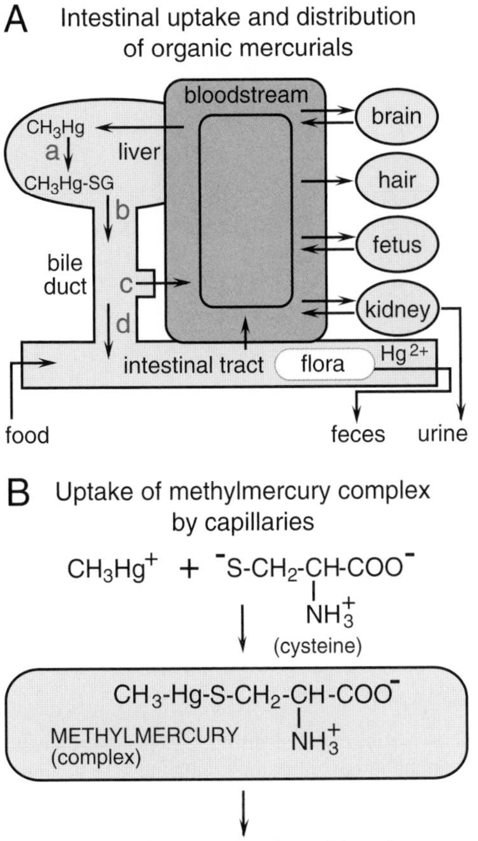

Figure 67–3. Uptake and relative distribution of organic mercurials.

A. The intestinal uptake and subsequent distribution of organic mercurials, such as methylmercury, throughout the body. *a:* conjugation with glutathione (GSH), shown as CH₃—Hg—SG; *b:* secretion of conjugate into bile; *c:* reabsorption in gallbladder; *d:* remaining Hg enters intestinal tract. **B.** Uptake of the methylmercury complex by capillaries. The ability of organic mercurials to cross the blood–brain barrier and the placenta contributes to their greater neurological and teratogenic effects when compared to inorganic mercury salts. Note the structural similarity of the methylmercury complex to methionine, CH₃SCH₂CH₂—CH(NH₃⁺)COO⁻.

in Figure 67–3A. Over 90% of methylmercury is absorbed from the human gastrointestinal tract. The organic mercurials cross the blood–brain barrier and the placenta and thus produce more neurological and teratogenic effects than do the inorganic salts. Methylmercury combines with cysteine to form a structure similar to methionine, and the complex is then accepted by the large neutral amino acid carrier present in capillary endothelial cells (Figure 67–3B; Clarkson, 1987). Organic mercurials are more uniformly distributed to the various tissues than are the inorganic salts (Klaassen, 1975). A significant portion of the body burden of organic mercurials is in the red blood cells. The ratio of the concentration of organomercurial in erythrocytes to that in plasma varies with the compound; for methylmercury, it approximates 20:1 (Kershaw *et al.,* 1980). Mercury concentrates in hair because of its high sulfhydryl content. The carbon–mercury bond of some organic mercurials is cleaved after absorption; with methylmercury the cleavage is quite slow, and the inorganic mercury formed is not thought to play a major role in methylmercury toxicity. Aryl mercurials, like mercurophen, usually contain a labile mercury–carbon bond, and the toxicity of these compounds is similar to that of inorganic mercury. Excretion of methylmercury by human beings is mainly in the feces in the form of a conjugate with glutathione; less than 10% of a dose appears in urine (Bakir *et al.,* 1980). The half-life of methylmercury in the blood of human beings is between 40 and 105 days (Bakir *et al.,* 1973).

Toxicity. ***Elemental Mercury.*** Short-term exposure to vapor of elemental mercury may produce symptoms within several hours; these include weakness, chills, metallic taste, nausea, vomiting, diarrhea, dyspnea, cough, and a feeling of tightness in the chest. Pulmonary toxicity may progress to an interstitial pneumonitis with severe compromise of respiratory function. Recovery, although usually complete, may be complicated by residual interstitial fibrosis.

Chronic exposure to mercury vapor produces a more insidious form of toxicity that is dominated by neurological effects (Friberg and Vostal, 1972). The syndrome is referred to as the *asthenic vegetative syndrome* and consists of neurasthenic symptoms in addition to three or more of the following findings (Goyer and Clarkson, 2001): goiter, increased uptake of radioiodine by the thyroid, tachycardia, labile pulse, gingivitis, dermographia, and increased mercury in the urine. With continued exposure to mercury vapor, tremor becomes noticeable, and psychological changes consist of depression, irritability, excessive shyness, insomnia, reduced self-confidence, emotional instability, forgetfulness, confusion, impatience, and vasomotor disturbances (such as excessive perspiration and uncontrolled blushing, which together are referred to as *erethism*). Common features of intoxication from mercury vapor are severe salivation and gingivitis. The triad of increased excitability, tremors, and gingivitis has been recognized historically as the major manifestation of exposure to mercury vapor when mercury nitrate was used in the fur, felt, and hat industries. Renal dysfunction also has been reported to result from long-term industrial exposure to mercury vapor. The concentrations of mercury vapor in the air and mercury in urine that are associated with the various effects are shown in Figure 67–4.

Inorganic Salts of Mercury. Inorganic, ionic mercury (*e.g.,* mercuric chloride) can produce severe acute toxicity. Precipitation of mucous membrane proteins by mercuric salts results in

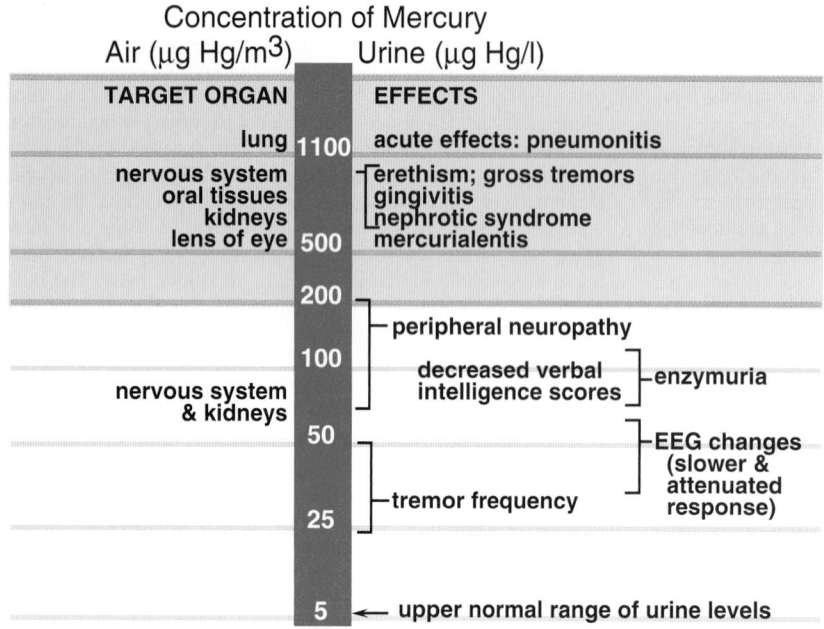

Figure 67–4. The concentration of mercury vapor in the air and related concentrations of mercury in urine associated with a variety of toxic effects.

an ashen-gray appearance of the mucosa of the mouth, pharynx, and intestine and also causes intense pain, which may be accompanied by vomiting. The vomiting is perceived to be protective, because it removes unabsorbed mercury from the stomach; assuming the patient is awake and alert, it should not be inhibited. The local, corrosive effect of ionic inorganic mercury on the gastrointestinal mucosa results in severe hematochezia with evidence of mucosal sloughing in the stool. Hypovolemic shock and death may occur in the absence of proper treatment. Prompt corrective treatment can overcome the local effects of inorganic mercury.

Systemic toxicity may begin within a few hours after exposure to mercury and last for days. A strong metallic taste is followed by stomatitis with gingival irritation, foul breath, and loosening of the teeth. The most serious and frequently encountered systemic effect of inorganic mercury is renal toxicity. Renal tubular necrosis occurs after short-term exposure, leading to oliguria or anuria. Renal injury also follows long-term exposure to inorganic mercury; however, glomerular injury predominates. This is the result of both direct effects on the glomerular basement membrane and a later indirect effect mediated by immune complexes (Goyer and Clarkson, 2001).

The symptom complex of acrodynia (pink disease) also commonly follows chronic exposure to inorganic mercury ions. Acrodynia is an erythema of the extremities, chest, and face with photophobia, diaphoresis, anorexia, tachycardia, and either constipation or diarrhea. Acrodynia was observed in 1980 in Argentina in infants exposed to a phenylmercuric fungicide used by a commercial diaper service (Gotelli *et al.*, 1985). This symptom complex is seen almost exclusively after ingestion of mercury and is believed to be the result of a hypersensitivity reaction to mercury (Matheson *et al.*, 1980).

Organic Mercurials. Most human toxicological data about organic mercury concern methylmercury and have been collected as the unfortunate result of several large-scale accidental exposures. Symptoms of exposure to methylmercury are mainly neurological in origin and consist of visual disturbance (scotoma and visual-field constriction), ataxia, paresthesias, neurasthenia, hearing loss, dysarthria, mental deterioration, muscle tremor, movement disorders, and, with severe exposure, paralysis and death (Table 67–4). Morphological changes are found in the calcarine area of occipital lobes, pre- and postcentral lobes, and temporal transverse gyri; diffuse lesions are found in the cerebrum; and a decrease in granular cells in the cerebellum (Eto, 1997). Effects of methylmercury on the fetus can occur even when the mother is asymptomatic; mental retardation and neuromuscular deficits have been observed.

Diagnosis of Mercury Poisoning. A history of exposure to mercury, either industrial or environmental, is obviously valuable in making the diagnosis of mercury poisoning. Without such a history, clinical suspicions can be confirmed by laboratory analysis. The upper limit of a nontoxic concentration of mercury in blood is generally considered to be 3 to 4 μg/dl (0.15 to 0.20 μM). A concentration of mercury in blood in excess of 4 μg/dl (0.20 μM) is unexpected in normal, healthy adults and suggests the need for environmental evaluation and medical examination to assess the possibility of adverse health effects. Because methylmercury is concentrated in erythrocytes and inorganic mercury is not, the distribution of total mercury between red blood cells and plasma may indicate whether the patient has been poisoned with inorganic or organic mercury. Measurement of total mercury in red blood cells gives a better estimate of the body burden of methylmercury than it does for inorganic mercury. The relationship between concentrations of mercury in blood and the frequency of symptoms that result from exposure to methylmercury is shown in Table 67–4; but this is only a rough guide. Concentrations of mercury in plasma provide a better index of the body burden of inorganic mercury; however, the relationship between body burden and

Table 67–4

Frequency of Symptoms of Methylmercury Poisoning in Relation to Concentration of Mercury in Blood

CONCENTRATION OF MERCURY IN BLOOD, $\mu g/ml(\mu M)$	CASES WITH SYMPTOMS (%)					
	Paresthesias	Ataxia	Visual Defects	Dysarthria	Hearing Defects	Death
0.1–0.5 (0.5–2.5)	5	0	0	5	0	0
0.5–1.0 (2.5–5.0)	42	11	21	5	5	0
1–2 (5–10)	60	47	53	24	5	0
2–3 (10–15)	79	60	56	25	13	0
3–4 (15–20)	82	100	58	75	36	17
4–5 (20–25)	100	100	83	85	66	28

SOURCE: Based on data in Bakir *et al.,* 1973.

the concentration of inorganic mercury in plasma is not well documented. This may relate to the importance of timing of measurement of the blood sample relative to the last exposure to mercury. The relationship between the concentration of inorganic mercury in blood and toxicity also depends on the form of exposure. For example, exposure to vapor results in concentrations in brain about 10 times higher than those that follow an equivalent dose of inorganic mercuric salts.

The concentration of mercury in the urine also has been used as a measure of the body burden of the metal. The upper limit for excretion of mercury in urine in the normal population is 5 μg/liter. There is a linear relationship between plasma concentration and urinary excretion of mercury after exposure to vapor; in contrast, the excretion of mercury in urine is a poor indicator of the amount of methylmercury in the blood, because it is eliminated mainly in feces (Bakir *et al.,* 1980).

Hair is rich in sulfhydryl groups, and the concentration of mercury in hair is about 300 times that in blood. Human hair grows about 20 cm a year, and a history of exposure may be obtained by analysis of different segments of hair.

Treatment of Mercury Poisoning.   Measurement of the concentration of mercury in blood should be performed as soon as possible after poisoning with any form of the metal.

Elemental Mercury Vapor.   Therapeutic measures include immediate termination of exposure and close monitoring of pulmonary status. Short-term respiratory support may be necessary. Chelation therapy, as described below for inorganic mercury, should be initiated immediately and continued as indicated by the clinical condition and the concentrations of mercury in blood and urine.

Inorganic Mercury.   Prompt attention to fluid and electrolyte balance and hematological status is of critical importance in moderate-to-severe oral exposures. Emesis can be induced if the patient is awake and alert, although emesis should not be induced where there is corrosive injury. If ingestion of mercury is more than 30 to 60 minutes before treatment, emesis may have little efficacy. With corrosive agents, endoscopic evaluation may be warranted, and coagulation parameters are important. Activated charcoal is recommended by some, although there is a lack of proven efficacy of this treatment. Administration of charcoal may make endoscopy difficult or impossible.

Chelation Therapy.   Chelation therapy with *dimercaprol* (for high-level exposures or symptomatic patients) or *penicillamine* (for low-level exposures or asymptomatic patients) is routinely used to treat poisoning with either inorganic or elemental mercury. Recommended treatment includes dimercaprol, 5 mg/kg intramuscularly initially, followed by 2.5 mg/kg intramuscularly every 12 to 24 hours for 10 days. Penicillamine (250 mg orally every 6 hours) may be used alone or following treatment with dimercaprol. The duration of chelation therapy will vary, and progress can be monitored by following concentrations of mercury in urine and blood. The new, orally effective chelator succimer appears to be an effective chelator for mercury (Campbell *et al.,* 1986; Fournier *et al.,* 1988; Bluhm *et al.,* 1992), although it has not been approved by the United States Food and Drug Administration (FDA) for this purpose.

The dimercaprol–mercury chelate is excreted into both bile and urine, whereas the penicillamine–mercury chelate is excreted only into urine. Thus, penicillamine should be used with extreme caution when renal function is impaired. In fact, hemodialysis may be necessary in the poisoned patient whose renal function declines. Chelators may still be used, because the dimercaprol–mercury complex is removed by dialysis (Giunta *et al.,* 1983).

Organic Mercury.   The short-chain organic mercurials, especially methylmercury, are the most difficult forms of mercury to mobilize from the body, presumably due to their poor reactivity with chelating agents. Dimercaprol is contraindicated in methylmercury poisoning because it increases brain concentrations of methylmercury in experimental animals. Although penicillamine facilitates the removal of methylmercury from the body, its clinical efficacy in the treatment of intoxication with methylmercury is not impressive (Bakir *et al.,* 1980). The dose of penicillamine normally used in the treatment of poisoning with inorganic mercury (1 g per day) produces only a small reduction in the concentration of methylmercury in blood; larger doses (2 g per day) are needed. During the initial 1 to 3 days of administration of penicillamine, the concentration of mercury in the blood increases before it decreases. This probably is due to the mobilization of metal from tissues to blood at a rate more rapid than that for excretion of mercury into urine and feces.

Methylmercury compounds undergo extensive enterohepatic recirculation in experimental animals. Therefore, introduction of a nonabsorbable mercury-binding substance into the intestinal tract should facilitate their removal from the body. A *polythiol resin* has been used for this purpose in human beings and appears to be effective (Bakir *et al.,* 1973). The resin has certain advantages over penicillamine. It does not cause redistribution of mercury in the body with a subsequent increase in the concentration of mercury in blood, and it has fewer adverse effects than do sulfhydryl agents that are absorbed. Clinical experience with various treatments for methylmercury poisoning in Iraq indicates that penicillamine, *N*-acetylpenicillamine, and an oral nonabsorbable thiol resin all can reduce blood concentrations of mercury; however, clinical improvement was not clearly related to reduction of the body burden of methylmercury (Bakir *et al.,* 1980).

Conventional hemodialysis is of little value in the treatment of methylmercury poisoning because methylmercury concentrates in erythrocytes and little is contained in the plasma. However, it has been shown that L-cysteine can be infused into the arterial blood entering the dialyzer to convert methylmercury into a diffusible form. Both free cysteine and the methylmercury–cysteine complex formed in the blood then diffuse across the membrane into the dialysate. This method has been shown to be effective in human beings (Al-Abbasi *et al.,* 1978). Studies in animals indicate that succimer may be more effective than cysteine in this regard (Kostyniak, 1982).

ARSENIC

Arsenic was used more than 2400 years ago in Greece and Rome as a therapeutic agent and as a poison. The history and folklore of arsenic prompted intensive studies by early pharmacologists. Indeed, the foundations of many modern concepts of chemotherapy derive from Ehrlich's early work with organic arsenicals, and such drugs were once a mainstay of chemotherapy. In current therapeutics, arsenicals are important only in the treatment of certain tropical diseases, such as African trypanosomiasis (*see* Chapter 41). In the United States, the impact of arsenic on health is predominantly from industrial and environmental exposures. (For reviews, *see* Winship, 1984; Hindmarsh and McCurdy, 1986; NRC, 1999.)

Arsenic is found in soil, water, and air as a common environmental toxicant. Well water in sections of Argentina, Chile, and Taiwan has especially high concentrations of arsenic, which results in widespread poisoning. Large numbers of people in West Bengal, India, also are being exposed to high concentrations of arsenic in their well water used for drinking. It also is in high concentrations in the water in many parts of the western United States. The element usually is not mined as such but is recovered as a by-product from the smelting of copper, lead, zinc, and other ores. This can result in the release of arsenic into the environment. Mineral-spring waters and the effluent from geothermal power plants leach arsenic from soils and rocks containing high concentrations of the metal. Arsenic also is present in coal at variable concentrations and is released into the environment during combustion. Application of pesticides

and herbicides containing arsenic has increased its environmental dispersion. The major source of occupational exposure to arsenic-containing compounds is from the manufacture of arsenical herbicides and pesticides (Landrigan, 1981). Fruits and vegetables sprayed with arsenicals may be a source of this element, and it is concentrated in many species of fish and shellfish. Arsenicals sometimes are added to the feed of poultry and other livestock to promote growth. The average daily human intake of arsenic is about 10 μg. Almost all of this is ingested with food and water.

Arsenic is used as arsine and as arsenic trioxide in the manufacture of most computer chips using silicon-based technology. Gallium arsenide is used in the production of compound (types III–V) semiconductors that are used for making LEDs as well as laser and solar devices. In the manufacture of both computer chips and semiconductors, metallic arsenic also may be used or produced as a by-product of the reaction chambers.

Chemical Forms of Arsenic. The arsenic atom exists in the elemental form and in trivalent and pentavalent oxidation states. The toxicity of a given arsenical is related to the rate of its clearance from the body and therefore to its degree of accumulation in tissues. In general, toxicity increases in the sequence of organic arsenicals $< As^{5+} < As^{3+} <$ arsine (AsH_3).

The organic arsenicals contain arsenic linked to a carbon atom by a covalent bond, where arsenic exists in the trivalent or pentavalent state. Arsphenamine contains trivalent arsenic; sodium arsanilate contains arsenic in the pentavalent form.

ARSPHENAMINE

SODIUM ARSANILATE

The organic arsenicals usually are excreted more rapidly than are the inorganic forms.

The pentavalent oxidation state is found in arsenates (such as lead arsenate, $PbHAsO_4$), which are salts of arsenic acid, H_3AsO_4. The pentavalent arsenicals have very low affinity for thiol groups, in contrast to the trivalent compounds, and are much less toxic. The arsenites [for example, potassium arsenite ($KAsO_2$)] and salts of arsenious acid contain trivalent arsenic. Arsine (AsH_3) is a gaseous hydride of trivalent arsenic; it produces toxic effects that are distinct from those of the other arsenic compounds.

Mechanism of Action. Arsenate (pentavalent) is a well-known uncoupler of mitochondrial oxidative phosphorylation. The mechanism is thought to be related to competitive substitution of arsenate for inorganic phosphate in the formation of adenosine triphosphate, with subsequent formation of an unstable arsenate ester that is rapidly hydrolyzed. This process is termed *arsenolysis.*

Trivalent arsenicals, including inorganic arsenite, are regarded primarily as sulfhydryl reagents. As such, trivalent arsenicals inhibit many enzymes by reacting with biological ligands containing available —SH groups. The pyruvate dehydrogenase system is especially sensitive to trivalent arsenicals because of their interaction with two sulfhydryl groups of lipoic acid to form a stable six-membered ring, as shown below.

$$
\begin{array}{l}
CH_2{-}SH \\
| \\
CH_2 \\
| \\
CH{-}SH \;+\; R{-}As{=}O \\
| \\
(CH_2)_4 \\
| \\
COOH
\end{array}
\longrightarrow
\begin{array}{l}
CH_2 \\
\quad\diagdown S \\
CH_2 \quad\; \diagup As{-}R \;+\; H_2O \\
\quad\diagup S \\
CH \\
| \\
(CH_2)_4 \\
| \\
COOH
\end{array}
$$

Absorption, Distribution, and Excretion.   The absorption of poorly water-soluble arsenicals, such as As_2O_3, greatly depends on the physical state of the compound. Coarsely powdered material is less toxic because it can be eliminated in feces before it dissolves. The arsenite salts are more soluble in water and are better absorbed than the oxide. Experimental evidence has shown a high degree of gastrointestinal absorption, 80% to 90%, of both trivalent and pentavalent forms of arsenic.

The distribution of arsenic depends upon the duration of administration and the particular arsenical involved. Arsenic is stored mainly in liver, kidney, heart, and lung. Much smaller amounts are found in muscle and neural tissue. Because of the high sulfhydryl content of keratin, the highest concentrations of arsenic are found in hair and nails. Deposition in hair starts within 2 weeks after administration, and arsenic stays fixed at this site for years. Because of its chemical similarity to phosphorus, it is deposited in bone and teeth and is retained there for long periods. Arsenic readily crosses the placental barrier, and fetal damage has been reported. Concentrations of arsenic in human umbilical cord blood are equivalent to those in the maternal circulation.

Arsenic is readily biotransformed in both laboratory animals and human beings (Figure 67–5). The pentavalent arsenic (arsenate) is coupled to the oxidation of glutathione (GSH) to GSSG to form the trivalent arsenic (arsenite), which is methylated to form the methyl- and dimethylarsenite, which is readily eliminated from the body. Arsenic is eliminated by many routes (feces, urine, sweat, milk, hair, skin, lungs), although most is excreted in urine in human beings. The half-life for the urinary excretion of arsenic is 3 to 5 days, much shorter than those of the other metals discussed. The methylated forms of arsenic are less reactive with tissue constituents, less cytotoxic, and more readily excreted in urine than inorganic arsenic (NRC, 1999). In human beings, the urinary content of metabolites is 10% to 30% inorganic arsenic, 10% to 20% monomethylarsenite, and 55% to 75% dimethylarsenite.

Pharmacological and Toxicological Effects of Arsenic.   Arsenicals have varied effects on many organ systems. These are summarized below.
Cardiovascular System.   Acute and subacute doses of inorganic arsenic induce mild vasodilation. This may lead to an occult edema, particularly facial, which has been mistaken for a healthy weight gain and misinterpreted as a "tonic" effect of ar-

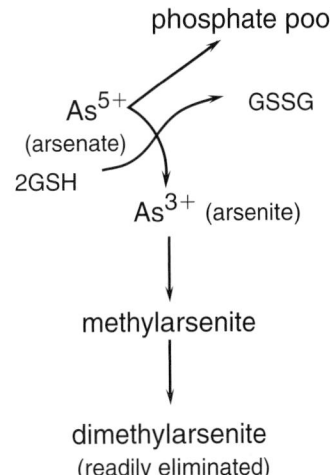

Figure 67–5. The biotransformation of arsenic in human beings.

GSH $\rightarrow$ GSSG indicates the oxidation of glutathione (GSH) to its disulfide, GSSG.

senic. Larger acute and subacute doses evoke capillary dilation; increased capillary permeability may occur in all capillary beds, but it is most pronounced in the splanchnic area. Transudation of plasma also may occur, and the decrease in intravascular volume may be significant. Serious cardiovascular effects can result, including hypotension, congestive heart failure, and cardiac arrhythmias. Long-term exposure results in peripheral vascular disease (Engel *et al.*, 1994), more specifically gangrene of the extremities, especially of the feet, and thus is often referred to as blackfoot disease. Myocardial damage and hypotension also may become evident after more prolonged exposure to arsenic.
Gastrointestinal Tract.   Acute or subacute exposure to arsenic can produce gastrointestinal disturbances, ranging from mild abdominal cramping and diarrhea to severe hemorrhagic gastroenteritis associated with shock. With chronic exposure to arsenic, gastrointestinal effects usually are not observed. Small doses of inorganic arsenicals, especially the trivalent compounds, cause mild splanchnic hyperemia. Capillary transudation of plasma, resulting from larger doses, produces vesicles under the gastrointestinal mucosa. These eventually rupture, epithelial fragments slough off, and plasma is discharged into the lumen of the intestine, where it coagulates. Tissue damage and the bulk cathartic action of the increased fluid in the lumen lead to increased peristalsis and characteristic watery diarrhea ("rice-water stools"). Normal proliferation of the epithelium is suppressed, which accentuates the damage. Soon the feces become bloody. Damage to the upper gastrointestinal tract usually results in hematemesis. Stomatitis also may be evident. The onset of gastrointestinal symptoms may be so gradual that the possibility of arsenic poisoning may be overlooked.
Kidneys.   The action of arsenic on the renal capillaries, tubules, and glomeruli may cause severe renal damage. Initially, the glomeruli are affected and proteinuria results. Varying degrees of tubular necrosis and degeneration occur later. Oliguria with proteinuria, hematuria, and casts frequently results from exposure to arsenic.

Skin. Skin is a major target organ of arsenic. Diffuse or spotted hyperpigmentation over the trunk and extremities usually is the first effect observed with chronic arsenic ingestion. Depending on the amount of exposure to arsenic, hyperpigmentation can be observed as early as 6 months. The hyperpigmentation of chronic arsenic exposure commonly appears in a finely freckled "raindrop" pattern. The hyperpigmentation progresses within a period of years to palmar-plantar hyperkeratosis, which appear mainly on the palms and the plantar aspects of the feet. Long-term ingestion of low doses of inorganic arsenicals causes cutaneous vasodilation and a "milk and roses" complexion. Eventually, skin cancer is observed, as described below.

Nervous System. High-dose, acute or subacute exposure to arsenic can cause encephalopathy; however, the most common arsenic-induced neurological lesion is a peripheral neuropathy with a "stocking-glove" distribution of dysesthesia. The syndrome is similar to acute inflammatory demyelinating polyradiculoneuropathy (Guillain-Barré syndrome) (Donofrio *et al.*, 1987). This is followed by muscular weakness in the extremities, and, with continued exposure, deep-tendon reflexes diminish and muscular atrophy follows. The cerebral lesions are mainly vascular in origin and occur in both the gray and white matter; characteristic multiple, symmetrical foci of hemorrhagic necrosis occur.

Blood. Inorganic arsenicals affect the bone marrow and alter the cellular composition of the blood. Hematological evaluation usually reveals anemia with slight-to-moderate leukopenia; eosinophilia also may be present. Anisocytosis becomes evident with increasing exposure to arsenic. The vascularity of the bone marrow is increased. Some of the chronic hematological effects may result from impaired absorption of folic acid. Serious, irreversible blood and bone-marrow disturbances from organic arsenicals are rare.

Liver. Inorganic arsenicals and a number of now-obsolete organic arsenicals are particularly toxic to the liver and produce fatty infiltration, central necrosis, and cirrhosis. The damage may be mild or so severe that death may ensue. The injury is generally to the hepatic parenchyma, but in some cases the clinical picture may closely resemble occlusion of the common bile duct, the principal lesions being pericholangitis and bile thrombi in the finer biliary radicles.

Carcinogenesis. The fact that arsenic exposure can result in skin tumors was noted over 100 years ago in patients treated with arsenicals (Hutchinson, 1887). In 1980, the International Agency for Research on Cancer (IARC, 1980) concluded that inorganic arsenic is a skin and lung (*via* inhalation) carcinogen in human beings. More recent studies indicate that in Taiwan, Argentina, and Chile, where drinking water contained very high concentrations of arsenic (at least several hundred μg/dl), an increased incidence of bladder and lung cancer was due to arsenic exposure. Increased risks of other cancers, such as kidney and liver cancer, also have been reported, but the association with arsenic is not as high as for the other tumors noted above. In contrast, arsenic recently has been shown to be effective against acute promyelocytic leukemia (Chen *et al.*, 1996).

Acute Arsenic Poisoning. Federal restrictions on the allowable content of arsenic in food and in the occupational environment not only have improved safety procedures and decreased the number of intoxications but also have decreased the amount of arsenic in use; only the annual production of arsenic-containing herbicides is increasing.

The incidence of accidental, homicidal, and suicidal arsenic poisoning has greatly diminished in recent decades. Arsenic in the form of As_2O_3 used to be a common cause of poisoning because it is readily available, is practically tasteless, and has the appearance of sugar.

Gastrointestinal discomfort usually is experienced within an hour after intake of an arsenical, although it may be delayed as much as 12 hours after oral ingestion if food is in the stomach. Burning lips, constriction of the throat, and difficulty in swallowing may be the first symptoms, followed by excruciating gastric pain, projectile vomiting, and severe diarrhea. Oliguria with proteinuria and hematuria is usually present; eventually anuria may occur. The patient often complains of marked skeletal muscle cramps and severe thirst. As the loss of fluid proceeds, symptoms of shock appear. Hypoxic convulsions may occur terminally, and coma and death ensue. In severe poisoning, death can occur within an hour, but the usual interval is 24 hours. With prompt application of corrective therapy, patients may survive the acute phase of the toxicity only to develop neuropathies and other disorders. In a series of 57 such patients, 37 had peripheral neuropathy and 5 had encephalopathy. The motor system appears to be spared only in the mildest cases; severe crippling is common (Jenkins, 1966).

Chronic Arsenic Poisoning. The most common early signs of chronic arsenic poisoning are muscle weakness and aching, skin pigmentation (especially of the neck, eyelids, nipples, and axillae), hyperkeratosis, and edema. Gastrointestinal involvement is less prominent in long-term exposures. Other signs and symptoms that should arouse suspicion of arsenic poisoning include garlic odor of the breath and perspiration, excessive salivation and sweating, stomatitis, generalized itching, sore throat, coryza, lacrimation, numbness, burning or tingling of the extremities, dermatitis, vitiligo, and alopecia. Poisoning may begin insidiously with symptoms of weakness, languor, anorexia, occasional nausea and vomiting, and diarrhea or constipation. Subsequent symptoms may simulate acute coryza. Dermatitis and keratosis of the palms and soles are common features. Mee's lines are characteristically found in the fingernails (white transverse lines of deposited arsenic that usually appear 6 weeks after exposure). Because the fingernail grows at a rate of 0.1 mm per day, the approximate time of exposure may be determined. Desquamation and scaling of the skin may initiate an exfoliative process involving many epithelial structures of the body. The liver may enlarge, and obstruction of the bile ducts may result in jaundice. Eventually cirrhosis may occur from the hepatotoxic action. Renal dysfunction also may be encountered. As intoxication advances, encephalopathy may develop. Peripheral neuritis results in motor and sensory paralysis of the extremities; usually the legs are more severely affected than the arms, in contrast to lead palsy. The bone marrow is seriously injured by arsenic. With severe exposure, all hematological elements may be affected.

Treatment of Arsenic Poisoning. After short-term exposure to arsenic, routine measures are taken to stabilize the patient and prevent further absorption of the poison. In particular, attention is directed to the status of the intravascular volume, since the effects of arsenic on the gastrointestinal tract can result in fatal hypovolemic shock. Hypotension requires fluid replacement and may necessitate pharmacological support of blood pressure with pressor agents such as dopamine.

Chelation Therapy. Chelation therapy often is begun with *dimercaprol* (3 to 4 mg/kg intramuscularly every 4 to 12 hours) until abdominal symptoms subside and charcoal (if given initially) is passed in the feces. Oral treatment with penicillamine then may be substituted for dimercaprol and continued for 4 days. *Penicillamine* should be given in four divided doses to a maximum of 2 g per day. If symptoms recur after cessation of chelation therapy, a second course of penicillamine may be instituted. *Succimer* (2,3-dimercaptosuccinic acid), a derivative of dimercaprol, appears to be an extremely promising agent for the treatment of arsenic poisoning (Graziano *et al.,* 1978; Lenz *et al.,* 1981; Fournier *et al.,* 1988). Despite its therapeutic efficacy in treatment of arsenic poisoning, succimer currently is approved by the FDA only for lead chelation in children.

After long-term exposure to arsenic, treatment with dimercaprol and penicillamine also may be used, but oral penicillamine alone usually is sufficient. The duration of therapy is determined by the clinical condition of the patient, and the decision is aided by periodic determinations of urinary arsenic concentrations. Adverse effects of the chelating agents may limit the usefulness of therapy (*see* below). Dialysis may become necessary with severe arsenic-induced nephropathy; successful removal of arsenic by dialysis has been reported (Vaziri *et al.,* 1980).

Arsine. Arsine gas, generated by electrolytic or metallic reduction of arsenic in nonferrous metal products, is a rare cause of industrial intoxication. Rapid and often fatal hemolysis is a unique characteristic of arsine poisoning and probably results from arsine combining with hemoglobin and then reacting with oxygen to cause hemolysis. A few hours after exposure, headache, anorexia, vomiting, paresthesia, abdominal pain, chills, hemoglobinuria, bilirubinemia, and anuria occur. The classic arsine triad of hemolysis, abdominal pain, and hematuria is noteworthy. Jaundice appears after 24 hours. A coppery skin pigmentation is frequently observed and is thought to be due to methemoglobin. Kidneys of persons poisoned by arsine characteristically contain casts of hemoglobin, and there is cloudy swelling and necrosis of the cells of the proximal tubule. If the patient survives the severe hemolysis, death often results from renal failure. Because the hemoglobin–arsine complex cannot be dialyzed, *exchange transfusion* is recommended in severe cases; *forced alkaline diuresis* also may be employed. Dimercaprol has no effect on the hemolysis, and beneficial effects on renal function have not been established; it is thus not recommended.

It should be noted that arsenic is a trace contaminant of other metals, such as lead; contact of these unrefined metals with acid may produce arsine (and/or stilbine from antimony).

CADMIUM

Cadmium ranks close to lead and mercury as a metal of current toxicological concern. It occurs in nature in association with zinc and lead, and extraction and processing of these metals thus often lead to environmental contamina-

tion with cadmium. The element was discovered in 1817 but was seldom used until its valuable metallurgical properties were discovered approximately 50 years ago. A high resistance to corrosion, valuable electrochemical properties, and other useful chemical properties account for cadmium's wide applications in electroplating and in galvanization and its use in plastics, paint pigments (cadmium yellow), and nickel–cadmium batteries. Applications for and production of cadmium will continue to increase. Because less than 5% of the metal is recycled, environmental pollution is an important consideration. Coal and other fossil fuels contain cadmium, and their combustion releases the element into the environment.

Workers in smelters and other metal-processing plants may be exposed to high concentrations of cadmium in the air; however, for most of the population, food is the major source of cadmium. Uncontaminated foodstuffs contain less than 0.05 μg of cadmium per gram wet weight, and the average daily intake is about 50 μg. Cereal grains, such as rice and wheat, concentrate cadmium; thus, when they are grown in soils with naturally high concentrations of cadmium or polluted with cadmium, these grains can have high cadmium content. Drinking water normally does not contribute significantly to cadmium intake, but cigarette smoking does, because the tobacco plant also concentrates cadmium. One cigarette contains 1 to 2 μg of cadmium, and, with even 10% pulmonary absorption (Elinder *et al.,* 1983), the smoking of one pack of cigarettes per day results in a dose of approximately 1 mg of cadmium per year from smoking alone. Shellfish and animal liver and kidney are among foods that can have concentrations of cadmium higher than 0.05 μg/g, even under normal circumstances. When foods such as rice and wheat are contaminated by cadmium in soil and water, the concentration of the metal may increase considerably (1 μg/g).

In Fuchu, Japan, shortly after World War II, a large number of people complained of rheumatic and myalgic pains; the disease was named *itai-itai* ("ouch-ouch"). It was determined that cadmium had washed into the local rice fields from the effluent of a lead–zinc processing plant. Because *itai-itai* disease usually is not seen outside of Fuchu, other factors also may contribute to the development of *itai-itai* in this population (*see* discussion below concerning bone response to chronic cadmium poisoning).

Absorption, Distribution, and Excretion. Cadmium occurs only in one valency state, 2^+, and does not form stable alkyl compounds or other organometallic compounds of known toxicological significance.

Cadmium is absorbed poorly from the gastrointestinal tract. Studies in laboratory animals indicate the extent of absorption to be only about 1.5% (Engstrom and Nordberg, 1979), and limited studies in human beings indicate a value of about 5% (Rahola *et al.,* 1972). Absorption from the respiratory tract appears to be more complete; cigarette smokers may absorb 10% to 40% of inhaled cadmium (Friberg *et al.,* 1974).

After absorption, cadmium is transported in blood, bound mainly to blood cells and albumin. Cadmium is distributed first

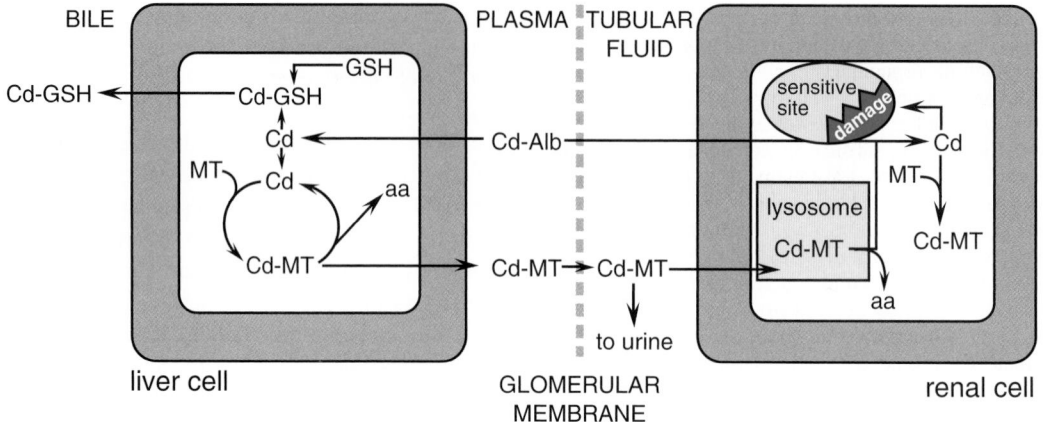

Figure 67–6. Postulated mechanisms contributing to cadmium-induced renal toxicity.

Cadmium (Cd) taken up by the liver can combine with glutathione (GSH) and be excreted into the bile or can bind to metallothionein (MT), creating a storage form for cadmium. Some cadmium–metallothionein complex (Cd–MT) leaks into the plasma. When taken up by kidney cells, the Cd–MT complex enters the lysosomes, the MT is degraded to its component amino acids (aa), and the cadmium is released from the lysosomes into the cytosol. At concentrations of 200 μg/g or higher, cadmium damages kidney tissue and results in proteinuria. Alb, albumin.

to the liver and then is redistributed slowly to the kidney as cadmium–metallothionein (Cd–MT). After distribution, approximately 50% of the total body burden is found in the liver and kidney. Metallothionein is a low-molecular-weight protein with high affinity for metals such as cadmium and zinc. One-third of its amino acid residues are cysteines. Metallothionein is inducible by exposure to several metals, including cadmium, and elevated concentrations of this metal-binding protein protect against cadmium toxicity by preventing the interaction of cadmium with other functional macromolecules (Klaassen *et al.,* 1999).

The half-life of cadmium in the body is 10 to 30 years. Consequently, with continuous environmental exposure, concentrations of the metal in tissues increase throughout life. The body burden of cadmium in a 50-year-old adult in the United States is about 30 mg. Its extremely long biological half-life renders cadmium an environmental poison very prone to accumulation. Overall, fecal elimination is quantitatively more important than urinary excretion of the metal. Urinary excretion of cadmium becomes significant only after substantial renal toxicity has occurred (*see* Goering and Klaassen, 1984).

Acute Cadmium Poisoning. Acute poisoning usually results from inhalation of cadmium dusts and fumes (usually cadmium oxide) and from the ingestion of cadmium salts. The early toxic effects are due to local irritation. In the case of oral intake, these include nausea, vomiting, salivation, diarrhea, and abdominal cramps; the vomitus and diarrhea often are bloody. In the short term, cadmium is more toxic when inhaled. Signs and symptoms, which appear within a few hours, include irritation of the respiratory tract with severe, early pneumonitis, chest pains, nausea, dizziness, and diarrhea. Toxicity may progress to include fatal pulmonary edema or residual emphysema with peribronchial and perivascular fibrosis (Zavon and Meadows, 1970).

Chronic Cadmium Poisoning. The toxic effects of long-term exposure to cadmium differ somewhat with the route of exposure. The kidney is affected following either pulmonary or gastrointestinal exposure; marked effects are observed in the lungs only after exposure by inhalation.

Kidney. Figure 67–6 illustrates how cadmium is thought to produce renal toxicity. Cadmium is taken up by the liver. In the liver, cadmium can combine with glutathione and be excreted in bile. More importantly, cadmium binds to metallothionein, in which form it is stored. Some cadmium bound to metallothionein leaks into the plasma and then is taken up by the kidney, as is inorganic cadmium. In the lysosomes of the kidney, cadmium is released. A sufficient concentration (200 μg/g) damages the kidney cell, resulting in proximal tubular injury and proteinuria (Dudley *et al.,* 1985). With more severe exposure, glomerular injury occurs, filtration is decreased, and there are aminoaciduria, glycosuria, and proteinuria. The nature of the glomerular injury is unknown but may involve an autoimmune component (Lauwerys *et al.,* 1984).

Excretion of β_2-microglobulin in urine appears to be a sensitive but not specific index of cadmium-induced nephrotoxicity (Piscator and Pettersson, 1977; Lauwerys *et al.,* 1979). Although measurement of urine β_2-microglobulin is part of the OSHA standard for monitoring cadmium poisoning, the concentration of β_2-microglobulin in the urine may not be the best marker for exposure. Retinol-binding protein may be a better marker, but its measurement is not generally available as an assay for cadmium exposure and toxicity.

Lung. The consequence of excessive inhalation of cadmium fumes and dusts is loss of ventilatory capacity, with a corresponding increase in residual lung volume. Dyspnea is the most frequent complaint of patients with cadmium-induced lung disease. The pathogenesis of cadmium-induced emphysema and pulmonary fibrosis is not well understood (Davison *et al.,* 1988); however, cadmium specifically inhibits the synthesis of plasma

α_1-antitrypsin (Chowdhury and Louria, 1976), and there is an association between severe α_1-antitrypsin deficiency of genetic origin and emphysema in human beings.

Cardiovascular System. Perhaps the most controversial issue concerning the effects of cadmium on human beings is the suggestion that the metal plays a significant role in the cause of hypertension (Schroeder, 1965). An initial epidemiological study indicated that individuals dying from hypertension had significantly higher concentrations of cadmium and higher cadmium-to-zinc ratios in their kidneys than people dying of other causes. Others have found similar correlations (Thind and Fischer, 1976). However, consistent effects of cadmium on the blood pressure of experimental animals have not been observed, and hypertension is not prominent in industrial cadmium poisoning.

Bone. One of the hallmarks of *itai-itai* disease was osteomalacia. However, studies in Sweden and the United Kingdom failed to corroborate this effect of cadmium poisoning in Japan (Kazantzis *et al.*, 1963; Adams *et al.*, 1969). The intake of calcium and fat-soluble vitamins such as vitamin D is much higher in these countries than in Japan. The Japanese victims were mostly multiparous, postmenopausal women. Thus, there may be an interaction among cadmium, nutrition, and bone disease. Body stores of calcium have been found to be decreased in subjects exposed to cadmium occupationally (Scott *et al.*, 1980). This presumed effect of cadmium may be due to interference with renal regulation of calcium and phosphate balance.

Testis. Testicular necrosis, a common characteristic of short-term exposure to cadmium in experimental animals, is uncommon with long-term, low-level exposure (Kotsonis and Klaassen, 1978). Cadmium-induced testicular necrosis has not been observed in men.

Cancer. Cadmium produces tumors in a number of organs when administered to laboratory animals (Waalkes *et al.*, 1992). Evidence that cadmium is a human carcinogen is based mainly on epidemiological studies from workers occupationally exposed to cadmium. These investigations primarily have identified tumors of the lungs and, to a lesser extent, prostate, kidney, and stomach. The International Agency for Cancer Research (1993) has concluded that the data are sufficient to classify cadmium as a human carcinogen.

Treatment of Cadmium Poisoning. Effective therapy for cadmium poisoning has been difficult to achieve. After short-term inhalation the patient must be removed from the source, and pulmonary ventilation should be monitored carefully. Respiratory support and steroid therapy may become necessary.

Chelation Therapy. Although there is no clearly proven benefit, some clinicians recommend chelation therapy with *CaNa$_2$ EDTA*. The dosage of CaNa$_2$EDTA used has been 75 mg/kg per day in 3 to 6 divided doses for 5 days. After a minimum of 2 days without treatment, a second 5-day course has been given. The total dose of CaNa$_2$EDTA per 5-day course should not exceed 500 mg/kg. Data from animal studies suggest that, if chelation therapy is considered, it should be instituted as soon as possible after cadmium exposure, because a rapid decrease in effectiveness of chelation therapy occurs in parallel with distribution to sites inaccessible to the chelators (Cantilena and Klaassen, 1982a). The use of *dimercaprol* and *substituted dithiocarbamates* appears promising for individuals chronically exposed to cadmium (Jones *et al.*, 1991).

IRON

Although iron is not an environmental poison, accidental intoxication with ferrous salts used to treat iron-deficiency anemias has made iron a frequently encountered source of poisoning in young children. Iron poisoning is discussed in Chapter 54 (*see also* below).

RADIOACTIVE HEAVY METALS

The widespread production and use of radioactive heavy metals for nuclear generation of electricity, nuclear weapons, laboratory research, manufacturing, and medical diagnosis have generated unique problems in dealing with accidental poisoning by such metals. Because the toxicity of radioactive metals is almost entirely a consequence of ionizing radiation, the therapeutic objective following exposure is not only the chelation of the metals but also their removal from the body as rapidly and completely as possible.

Treatment of the acute radiation syndrome is largely symptomatic. Attempts have been made to investigate the effectiveness of organic reducing agents, such as mercaptamine (cysteamine), administered to prevent the formation of free radicals. Success has been limited.

Major products of a nuclear accident or the use of nuclear weapons include ^{239}Pu, ^{137}Cs, ^{144}Ce, and ^{90}Sr. Isotopes of strontium and radium have proven to be extremely difficult to remove from the body with chelating agents. Several factors are involved in the relative resistance of radioactive metals to chelation therapy; these include the affinity of these particular metals for individual chelators and the observation that radiation from Sr and Ra in bone destroys nearby capillaries. Blood flow in bone is thereby decreased, and the radioisotopes become imprisoned. Many chelating agents have been used experimentally, including CaNa$_3$DTPA (pentetic acid, *see below*), which has been shown to be effective against ^{239}Pu (Jones *et al.*, 1986). One gram of CaNa$_3$DTPA, administered by slow intravenous drip on alternate days, three times per week, has enhanced excretion 50- to 100-fold in animals and in human subjects exposed in accidents. As commonly is seen with heavy-metal poisoning, effectiveness of treatment diminishes very rapidly with an increasing delay between exposure and the initiation of therapy.

HEAVY-METAL ANTAGONISTS
Edetate Calcium Disodium

Ethylenediaminetetraacetic acid (EDTA), its sodium salt (edetate disodium, Na$_2$EDTA), and a number of closely related compounds have been used for many years as industrial and analytical reagents because they chelate many divalent and trivalent metals. The cation used to make a water-soluble salt of EDTA has an important role in the toxicity of the chelator. Na$_2$EDTA causes hypocalcemic tetany. However, edetate calcium disodium (CaNa$_2$EDTA) can be used for treatment of poisoning by metals that have higher affinity for the chelating agent than does Ca^{2+}.

Chemistry and Mechanism of Action. The structure of $CaNa_2EDTA$ is as follows:

EDETATE CALCIUM DISODIUM

The pharmacological effects of $CaNa_2EDTA$ result from formation of chelates with divalent and trivalent metals in the body. Accessible metal ions (both exogenous and endogenous) with a higher affinity for $CaNa_2EDTA$ than Ca^{2+} will be chelated, mobilized, and usually excreted. Experimental studies in mice have shown that administration of $CaNa_2EDTA$ mobilizes several endogenous metallic cations, including those of zinc, manganese, and iron (Cantilena and Klaassen, 1982b). The main therapeutic use of $CaNa_2EDTA$ is in the treatment of metal intoxications, especially lead intoxication.

$CaNa_2EDTA$ is available as *edetate calcium disodium* (CALCIUM DISODIUM VERSENATE). Intramuscular administration of $CaNa_2EDTA$ results in good absorption, but pain occurs at the injection site; consequently, the chelator injection often is mixed with a local anesthetic or administered intravenously. For intravenous use, $CaNa_2EDTA$ is diluted in either 5% dextrose or 0.9% saline and is administered slowly by intravenous drip. A dilute solution is necessary to avoid thrombophlebitis. To minimize nephrotoxicity, adequate urine production should be established prior to and during treatment with $CaNa_2EDTA$. However, in patients with lead encephalopathy and increased intracranial pressure, excess fluids must be avoided. In such cases, conservative replacement of fluid is advised, and intramuscular administration of $CaNa_2EDTA$ is recommended.

Lead Poisoning. The successful use of $CaNa_2EDTA$ in the treatment of lead poisoning is due, in part, to the capacity of lead to displace calcium from the chelate. Enhanced mobilization and excretion of lead indicate that the metal is accessible to EDTA. Mercury poisoning, by contrast, does not respond to the drug, despite the fact that mercury displaces calcium from $CaNa_2EDTA$ *in vitro*. Mercury is unavailable to the chelate, perhaps because it is too tightly bound by body ligands (—SH) or sequestered in body compartments that are not penetrated by $CaNa_2EDTA$. Because of its ionic character, it is unlikely that $CaNa_2EDTA$ penetrates cells significantly, and the volume of distribution of $CaNa_2EDTA$ is approximately equal to that of extracellular fluid.

Bone provides the primary source of lead that is chelated by $CaNa_2EDTA$ (Hammond, 1971). After such chelation, lead is redistributed from soft tissues to the skeleton.

Suggestions appeared in the lay press in the 1980s that chelation therapy with $CaNa_2EDTA$ could minimize development of atherosclerotic plaque, which can accumulate calcium deposits; such use of $CaNa_2EDTA$, however, is without therapeutic rationale and not efficacious (Guldager *et al.,* 1992; Elihu *et al.,* 1998).

Absorption, Distribution, and Excretion. Less than 5% of $CaNa_2EDTA$ is absorbed from the gastrointestinal tract. After intravenous administration, $CaNa_2EDTA$ disappears from the circulation with a half-life of 20 to 60 minutes. In blood, all of the drug is found in plasma. About 50% is excreted in the urine in 1 hour and over 95% in 24 hours. For this reason, adequate renal function is necessary for successful therapy. Renal clearance of the compound in dogs equals that of inulin, and glomerular filtration accounts entirely for urinary excretion. Altering either the pH or the rate of flow of urine has no effect on the rate of excretion. There is very little metabolic degradation of EDTA. The drug is distributed mainly in the extracellular fluids, but very little gains access to the spinal fluid (5% of the plasma concentration).

Toxicity. Rapid intravenous administration of Na_2EDTA causes hypocalcemic tetany. However, a slow infusion (less than 15 mg per minute) administered to a normal individual elicits no symptoms of hypocalcemia because of the ready availability of extracirculatory stores of Ca^{2+}. In contrast, $CaNa_2EDTA$ can be administered intravenously in relatively large quantities with no untoward effects because the change in the concentration of Ca^{2+} in the plasma and total body is negligible.

Renal Toxicity. The principal toxic effect of $CaNa_2EDTA$ is on the kidney. Repeated large doses of the drug cause hydropic vacuolization of the proximal tubule, loss of the brush border, and, eventually, degeneration of proximal tubular cells (Catsch and Harmuth-Hoene, 1979). Changes in distal tubules and glomeruli are less conspicuous. The early renal effects usually are reversible, and urinary abnormalities disappear rapidly upon cessation of treatment.

Renal toxicity may be related to the large amounts of chelated metals that pass through the renal tubule in a relatively short period during drug therapy. Some dissociation of chelates may occur because of competition for the metal by physiological ligands or because of pH changes in the cell or the lumen of the tubule. However, a more likely mechanism of toxicity may be the interaction between the chelator and endogenous metals in proximal tubular cells.

Other Side Effects. Other less serious side effects have been reported with use of $CaNa_2EDTA$, including malaise, fatigue, and excessive thirst, followed by the sudden appearance of chills and fever. This may, in turn, be followed by severe myalgia, frontal headache, anorexia, occasional nausea and vomiting, and, rarely, increased urinary frequency and urgency. Other possible undesirable effects include sneezing, nasal congestion, and lacrimation; glycosuria; anemia; dermatitis, with lesions strikingly similar to those of vitamin B_6 deficiency; transitory lowering of systolic and diastolic blood pressures; prolonged prothrombin time; and inversion of the T wave of the electrocardiogram.

Pentetic Acid (DTPA)

Diethylenetriaminepentaacetic acid (DTPA), like EDTA, is a polycarboxylic acid chelator, but it has somewhat greater affinity for most heavy metals. Many investigations in animals have shown that the spectrum of clinical effectiveness of DTPA is similar to that of EDTA. Because of its relatively greater affinity for metals, DTPA has been tried in cases of heavy-metal poisoning that do not respond to EDTA, particularly poisoning by radioactive metals. Unfortunately, success has been limited, probably because DTPA also has limited access to intracellular sites of metal storage. Because DTPA rapidly binds Ca^{2+}, $CaNa_3DTPA$ is employed. The use of DTPA is investigational.

Dimercaprol

History.   During World War II, an intensive effort was made to develop an antidote to lewisite, a vesicant arsenical war gas. Knowing that arsenicals reacted with sulfhydryl-containing molecules, Stocken and Thompson, at Oxford University, initiated a systematic study of thiol compounds in search of one that would successfully compete with the tissue sulfhydryl groups for the arsenicals. Their investigations indicated that the arsenicals would form a very stable and relatively nontoxic chelate ring with the dithiol compound, dimercaprol (2,3-dimercaptopropanol). When scientists in the United States joined their British colleagues in these studies, they designated dimercaprol as *British anti-lewisite* (BAL). Pharmacological investigators revealed that this compound would protect against the toxic effects of other heavy metals as well.

Chemistry.   Dimercaprol has the following structure:

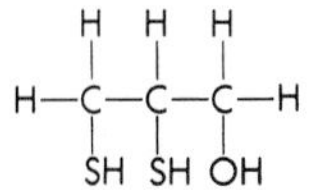

DIMERCAPROL

It is an oily fluid with a pungent, disagreeable odor typical of mercaptans. Because of its instability in aqueous solutions, peanut oil is the solvent employed in pharmaceutical preparations. Dimercaprol and related thiols are readily oxidized.

Mechanism of Action.   The pharmacological actions of dimercaprol are the result of formation of chelation complexes between its sulfhydryl groups and metals. The molecular properties of the dimercaprol–metal chelate have considerable practical significance. With metals such as mercury, gold, and arsenic, the strategy is to attain a stable complex to promote elimination of the metal. Dissociation of the complex and oxidation of dimercaprol can occur

in vivo. Furthermore, the sulfur–metal bond may be labile in the acidic tubular urine, which may increase delivery of metal to renal tissue and increase toxicity. The dosage regimen is therefore designed to maintain a concentration of dimercaprol in plasma adequate to favor the continuous formation of the more stable 2:1 (BAL:metal) complex and its rapid excretion. However, because of pronounced and dose-related side effects, excessive plasma concentrations must be avoided. The concentration in plasma must therefore be maintained by repeated fractional dosage until the offending metal can be excreted.

Dimercaprol is much more effective when given as soon as possible after exposure to the metal, because it is more effective in preventing inhibition of sulfhydryl enzymes than in reactivating them. Dimercaprol antagonizes the biological actions of metals that form mercaptides with essential cellular sulfhydryl groups, principally arsenic, gold, and mercury. It also is used in combination with $CaNa_2EDTA$ to treat lead poisoning, especially when evidence of lead encephalopathy exists. Intoxication by selenites, which oxidize sulfhydryl enzymes, is not influenced by dimercaprol.

Absorption, Distribution, and Excretion.   Dimercaprol cannot be administered orally; it is given by deep intramuscular injection as a 100 mg/ml solution in peanut oil; it should not be used in patients who are allergic to peanuts or peanut products. Peak concentrations in blood are attained in 30 to 60 minutes. The half-life is short, and metabolic degradation and excretion are essentially complete within 4 hours.

Toxicity.   In human beings, the administration of dimercaprol produces a variety of side effects that usually are more alarming than serious. Reactions to dimercaprol occur in approximately 50% of subjects receiving 5 mg/kg intramuscularly. The effects of repeated administration of this dose are not cumulative if an interval of at least 4 hours elapses between injections. One of the most consistent responses to dimercaprol is a rise in systolic and diastolic arterial pressures, accompanied by tachycardia. The rise in pressure may be as great as 50 mm Hg in response to the second of two doses (5 mg/kg) given 2 hours apart. The pressure rises immediately but returns to normal within 2 hours.

Other signs and symptoms of dimercaprol toxicity, many of which tend to parallel the change in blood pressure in time and intensity, are the following, listed in approximate order of frequency: nausea and vomiting; headache; a burning sensation in the lips, mouth, and throat and a feeling of constriction, sometimes pain, in the throat, chest, or hands; conjunctivitis, blepharospasm, lacrimation, rhinorrhea, and salivation; tingling of the hands; a burning sensation in the penis; sweating of the forehead, hands, and other areas; abdominal pain; and occasional appearance of painful sterile abscesses at the injection site. Symptoms often are accompanied by a feeling of anxiety and unrest. Because the dimercaprol–metal complex breaks down easily in an acidic medium, production of an alkaline urine protects the kidney during therapy. Children react as do adults, although approximately 30% may also experience a fever that disappears upon withdrawal of the drug. A transient reduction of the percentage of polymorphonuclear leukocytes also may be observed. Dimercaprol also may cause hemolytic anemia in patients deficient in glucose-6-phosphate dehydrogenase. Dimercaprol is contraindicated in patients with hepatic insufficiency, except when this is a result of arsenic poisoning.

Succimer

Succimer (2,3-dimercaptosuccinic acid; CHEMET) is a recently introduced chelator that is effective following oral administration. Succimer is chemically similar to dimercaprol but contains two carboxylic acids that modify both the distribution and chelating spectrum of succimer. Succimer has the following structure:

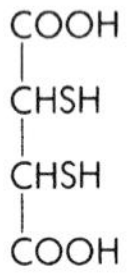

$$\begin{array}{c} COOH \\ | \\ CHSH \\ | \\ CHSH \\ | \\ COOH \end{array}$$

SUCCIMER

After its absorption in human beings, succimer is biotransformed to a mixed disulfide with cysteine (Aposhian and Aposhian, 1990), the structure of which is as follows:

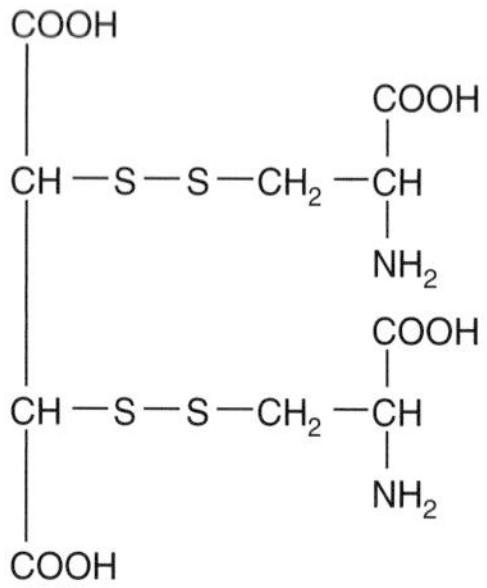

Succimer produces a lead diuresis, with a subsequent lowering of blood lead levels and attenuation of the untoward biochemical effects of lead, manifested by normalization of aminolevulenic acid dehydrase activity (Graziano *et al.*, 1992). The succimer–lead chelate also is eliminated in the bile; that fraction eliminated in the bile undergoes enterohepatic circulation.

A desirable feature of succimer is that it does not significantly mobilize essential metals such as zinc, copper,

or iron. However, animal studies suggest that succimer is effective as a chelator of arsenic, cadmium, mercury, and other metals (Aposhian and Aposhian, 1990).

Toxicity with succimer is less than that with dimercaprol, perhaps because its relatively lower lipid solubility minimizes its uptake into cells. Nonetheless, transient elevations in serum levels of hepatic enzymes are observed following treatment with succimer. The most commonly reported adverse effects of succimer treatment are nausea, vomiting, diarrhea, and loss of appetite. Rashes also have been reported and may necessitate discontinuation of therapy.

Succimer has been approved in the United States for treatment of children with blood lead levels in excess of 45 μg/dl.

Penicillamine

History. Penicillamine was first isolated in 1953 from the urine of patients with liver disease who were receiving penicillin. Discovery of its chelating properties led to its use in patients with Wilson's disease and heavy-metal intoxications.

Chemistry. Penicillamine is D-β,β-dimethylcysteine. Its structure is as follows:

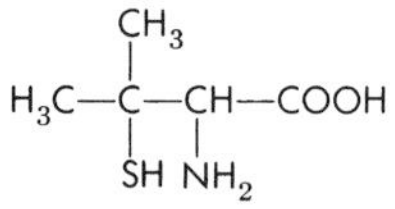

$$\begin{array}{c} CH_3 \\ | \\ H_3C-C-CH-COOH \\ | \quad | \\ SH \quad NH_2 \end{array}$$

PENICILLAMINE

The D isomer is used clinically, although the L isomer also forms chelation complexes. Penicillamine is an effective chelator of copper, mercury, zinc, and lead and promotes the excretion of these metals in the urine.

Absorption, Distribution, and Excretion. Penicillamine is well absorbed (40% to 70%) from the gastrointestinal tract and, therefore, has a decided advantage over many other chelating agents. Food, antacids, and iron reduce its absorption. Peak concentrations in blood are obtained between 1 and 3 hours after administration (Netter *et al.,* 1987). Unlike cysteine, its nonmethylated parent compound, penicillamine is somewhat resistant to attack by cysteine desulfhydrase or L-amino acid oxidase. As a result, penicillamine is relatively stable *in vivo*. N-acetylpenicillamine is more effective than penicillamine in protecting against the toxic effects of mercury (Aposhian and Aposhian, 1959), presumably because it is even more resistant to metabolism. Hepatic biotransformation is responsible for most of the degradation of penicillamine, and very little is excreted unchanged. Metabolites are found in both urine and feces (Perrett, 1981).

Therapeutic Uses. Penicillamine (CUPRIMINE; DEPEN) is available for oral administration. For chelation therapy, the usual adult dose is 1 to 1.5 g per day in four divided doses (*see* sections under individual metals). The drug should be given on an empty stomach to avoid interference by metals in food. In addition to its use as a chelating agent for the treatment of copper, mercury, and lead poisoning, penicillamine is used in Wilson's disease (hepatolenticular degeneration due to an excess of copper), cystinuria, and rheumatoid arthritis. For the treatment of Wilson's disease, four daily doses are taken, and 1 to 2 g per day is usually employed. The urinary excretion of copper should be monitored to determine if the dosage of penicillamine is adequate.

The rationale for the use of penicillamine in cystinuria is that penicillamine reacts with the poorly soluble cysteine in a thiol–disulfide exchange reaction and forms a relatively water-soluble cysteine–penicillamine mixed disulfide. In cystinuria, the urinary excretion of cystine is used to adjust dosage, although 2 g per day in four divided doses usually is employed.

The mechanism of action of penicillamine in rheumatoid arthritis remains uncertain, although suppression of the disease may result from marked reduction in concentrations of IgM rheumatoid factor (Wernick *et al.*, 1983). Uniquely, this decrease is not accompanied by reductions of the concentrations of immunoglobulins in plasma. Various dosage regimens have been studied for the treatment of rheumatoid arthritis. A single daily dose of 125 to 250 mg usually is used to initiate therapy. Dosage is increased at intervals of 1 to 3 months as necessary. Two or three months may be required before improvement is evident. Many patients eventually respond to 500 to 750 mg per day or less.

Other experimental uses of penicillamine include the treatment of primary biliary cirrhosis and scleroderma. The mechanism of action of penicillamine in these diseases also may involve effects on immunoglobulins and immune complexes (Epstein *et al.*, 1979).

Toxicity. The main disadvantage of penicillamine for short-term use as a chelating agent is the concern that it might cause anaphylactic reactions in patients allergic to penicillin (Bell and Graziano, 1983). However, preparations of the drug no longer contain trace amounts of penicillin. With long-term use, penicillamine induces several cutaneous lesions, including urticaria, macular or papular reactions, pemphigoid lesions, lupus erythematosus, dermatomyositis, adverse effects on collagen, and other less serious reactions, such as dryness and scaling. Cross-reactivity with penicillin may be responsible for some episodes of urticarial or maculopapular reactions with generalized edema, pruritus, and fever that occur in as many as one-third of patients taking penicillamine (*see* Bell and Graziano, 1983). For a detailed review of the adverse dermatological effects of penicillamine, *see* Levy and coworkers (1983).

The hematological system also may be affected severely; reactions include leukopenia, aplastic anemia, and agranulocytosis. These may occur at any time during therapy, and they may be fatal. Patients obviously must be monitored carefully.

Renal toxicity induced by penicillamine is usually manifested as reversible proteinuria and hematuria, but it may progress to the nephrotic syndrome with membranous glomerulopathy. More rarely, fatalities have been reported from Goodpasture's syndrome (Hill, 1979).

Toxicity to the pulmonary system is uncommon, but severe dyspnea has been reported from penicillamine-induced bronchoalveolitis. Myasthenia gravis also has been induced by long-term therapy with penicillamine (Gordon and Burnside, 1977). Less serious side effects include nausea, vomiting, diarrhea, dyspepsia, anorexia, and a transient loss of taste for sweet and salt, which is relieved by supplementation of the diet with copper. Contraindications to penicillamine therapy include pregnancy, a previous history of penicillamine-induced agranulocytosis or aplastic anemia, or the presence of renal insufficiency.

Trientine

Penicillamine is the drug of choice for treatment of Wilson's disease. However, the drug produces undesirable effects, as discussed above, and some patients become intolerant. For these individuals, *trientine* (triethylenetetramine dehydrochloride; CUPRID) is an acceptable alternative. Trientine is an effective cupriuretic agent in patients with Wilson's disease, although it may be less potent than penicillamine. The drug is effective orally. Maximal daily doses of 2 g for adults or 1.5 g for children are taken in two to four divided portions on an empty stomach. Trientine may cause iron deficiency; this can be overcome with short courses of iron therapy, but iron and trientine should not be ingested within 2 hours of each other.

Deferoxamine

The structure of deferoxamine is shown below.

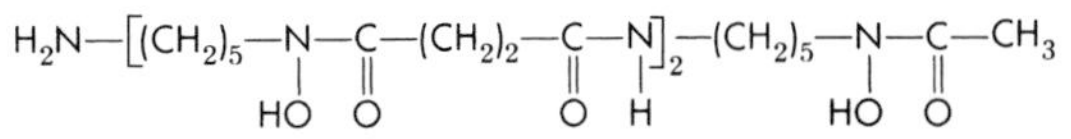

$$H_2N-[(CH_2)_5-\underset{\underset{HO}{|}}{N}-\underset{\underset{O}{\|}}{C}-(CH_2)_2-\underset{\underset{O}{\|}}{C}-\underset{\underset{H}{|}}{N}]_2-(CH_2)_5-\underset{\underset{HO}{|}}{N}-\underset{\underset{O}{\|}}{C}-CH_3$$

DEFEROXAMINE

Deferoxamine is isolated as the iron chelate from *Streptomyces pilosus* and is treated chemically to obtain the metal-free ligand. Deferoxamine has the desirable properties of a remarkably high affinity for ferric iron ($K_a = 10^{31}$) coupled with a very low affinity for calcium ($K_a = 10^2$). Studies *in vitro* have shown that it removes iron from hemosiderin and ferritin and, to a lesser extent, from transferrin. Iron in hemoglobin or cytochromes is not removed by deferoxamine.

Deferoxamine (*deferoxamine mesylate;* DESFERAL MESYLATE) is poorly absorbed after oral administration, and parenteral administration is required in most cases. For severe iron toxicity (serum iron levels greater than 500 μg/dl), the intravenous route is preferred. The drug is administered at 10 to 15 mg/kg per hour by constant infusion. Faster rates of infusion (45 mg/kg per hour) have been used in a few cases; rapid boluses usually are associated with hypotension. Deferoxamine may be given intramuscularly in moderately toxic cases (serum iron 350 to 500 μg/dl) at a dose of 50 mg/kg with a maximum dose of 1 g. Hypotension also can occur with the intramuscular route.

For chronic iron intoxication (*e.g.,* thalassemia), an intramuscular dose of 0.5 to 1.0 g per day is recommended, although continuous subcutaneous administration (1 to 2 g per day) is almost as effective as intravenous administration (Propper *et al.,* 1977). When blood is being transfused to patients with thalassemia, 2.0 g of deferoxamine (per unit of blood) should be given by slow intravenous infusion (rate not to exceed 15 mg/kg per hour) during the transfusion, but not by the same intravenous line. Deferoxamine is not recommended in primary hemochromatosis; phlebotomy is the treatment of choice. Deferoxamine also has been used for the chelation of aluminum in dialysis patients (Swartz, 1985).

Deferoxamine is metabolized principally by plasma enzymes, but the pathways have not yet been defined. The drug also is readily excreted in the urine.

Deferoxamine causes a number of allergic reactions, including pruritus, wheals, rash, and anaphylaxis. Other adverse effects include dysuria, abdominal discomfort, diarrhea, fever, leg cramps, and tachycardia. Occasional cases of cataract formation have been reported. Deferoxamine may cause neurotoxicity during long-term, high-dose therapy for transfusion-dependent thalassemia major; both visual and auditory changes have been described (Olivieri *et al.,* 1986). A "pulmonary syndrome" has been associated with high-dose (10 to 25 mg/kg per hour) deferoxamine therapy (Freedman *et al.,* 1990; Castriota-Scanderbeg *et al.,* 1990); tachypnea, hypoxemia, fever, and eosinophilia are prominent symptoms. Contraindications to the use of deferoxamine include renal insufficiency and anuria; during pregnancy, the drug should be used only if clearly indicated.

An orally effective iron chelator now under clinical investigation, *deferiprone* (1,2-dimethyl-3-hydroxypyridin-4-one), may be of value in patients with thalassemia major, who are unable or unwilling to receive deferoxamine (Olivieri *et al.,* 1995).

BIBLIOGRAPHY

Adams, R.G., Harrison, J.F., and Scott, P. The development of cadmium-induced proteinuria, impaired renal function, and osteomalacia in alkaline battery workers. *Q. J. Med.,* **1969,** *38*:425–443.

Al-Abbasi, A.H., Kostyniak, P.J., and Clarkson, T.W. An extracorporeal complexing hemodialysis system for the treatment of methylmercury poisoning. III. Clinical applications. *J. Pharmacol. Exp. Ther.,* **1978,** *207*:249–254.

Aposhian, H.V., and Aposhian, M.M. *N*-acetyl-DL-penicillamine, a new oral protective agent against the lethal effects of mercuric chloride. *J. Pharmacol. Exp. Ther.,* **1959,** *126*:131–135.

Baghurst, P.A., McMichael, A.J., Wigg, N.R., Vimpani, G.V., Robertson, E.F., Roberts, R.J., and Tong, S.-L. Environmental exposure to lead and children's intelligence at the age of seven years. The Port Pirie Cohort Study. *N. Engl. J. Med.,* **1992,** *327*:1279–1284.

Baker, E.L. Jr., Goyer, R.A., Fowler, B.A., Khettry, U., Bernard, D.B., Adler, S., White, R.D., Babayan, R., and Feldman, R.G. Occupational lead exposure, nephropathy, and renal cancer. *Am. J. Ind. Med.,* **1980,** *1*:139–148.

Bakir, F., Damluji, S.F., Amin-Zaki, L., Murtadha, M., Khalidi, A., al-Rawi, N.Y., Tikriti, S., Dahahir, H.I., Clarkson, T.W., Smith, J.C., and Doherty, R.A. Methylmercury poisoning in Iraq. *Science.,* **1973,** *181*:230–241.

Bakir, F., Rustam, H., Tikriti, S., Al-Damluji, S.F., and Shihristani, H. Clinical and epidemiological aspects of methylmercury poisoning. *Postgrad. Med. J.,* **1980,** *56*:1–10.

Banks, E.C., Ferretti, L.E., and Shucard, D.W. Effects of low level lead exposure on cognitive function in children: a review of behavioral, neuropsychological and biological evidence. *Neurotoxicology,* **1997,** *18*:237–281.

Bell, C.L., and Graziano, F.M. The safety of administration of penicillamine to penicillin-sensitive individuals. *Arthritis Rheum.,* **1983,** *26*:801–803.

Bellinger, D.C., Stiles, K.M., and Needleman, H.L. Low-level lead exposure, intelligence and academic achievement: a long-term follow-up study. *Pediatrics,* **1992,** *90*:855–861.

Bluhm, R.E., Bobbitt, R.G., Welch, L.W., Wood, A.J., Bonfiglio, J.F., Sarzen, C., Heath, A.J., and Branch, R.A. Elemental mercury vapour toxicity, treatment, and prognosis after acute, intensive exposure in chloralkali plant workers. Part I: History, neuropsychological findings and chelator effects. *Hum. Exp. Toxicol.,* **1992,** *11*:201–210.

Boyd, P.R., Walker, G., and Henderson, I.N. The treatment of tetraethyl lead poisoning. *Lancet,* **1957,** *1*:181–185.

Campbell, J.R., Clarkson, T.W., and Omar, M.D. The therapeutic use of 2,3-dimercaptopropane-1-sulfonate in two cases of inorganic mercury poisoning. *JAMA,* **1986,** *256*:3127–3130.

Cantilena, L.R. Jr., and Klaassen, C.D. Decreased effectiveness of chelation therapy with time after acute cadmium poisoning. *Toxicol. Appl. Pharmacol.*, **1982a,** *63*:173–180.

Cantilena, L.R. Jr., and Klaassen, C.D. The effect of chelating agents on the excretion of endogenous metals. *Toxicol. Appl. Pharmacol.*, **1982b,** *63*:344–350.

Castriota-Scanderbeg, A., Izzi, G.C., Butturini, A., and Benaglia, G. Pulmonary syndrome and intravenous high-dose desferrioxamine. *Lancet*, **1990,** *336*:1511.

Chen, G.-Q., Zhu, J., Shi, X.-G., Ni, J.-H., Zhong, H.J., Si, G.Y., Jin, X.L., Tang, W., Li, X.S., Xong, S.M., Shen, Z.X., Sun, G.L., Ma, J., Zhang, P., Zhang, T.D., Gazin, C., Naoe, T., Chen, S.J., Wang, Z.Y., and Chen, Z. In vitro studies on cellular and molecular mechanisms of arsenic trioxide (As$_2$O$_3$) in the treatment of acute promyelocytic leukemia: As$_2$O$_3$ induces NB$_4$ cell apoptosis with downregulation of Bcl-2 expression and modulation of PML-RARα/PML proteins. *Blood*, **1996,** *88*:1052–1061.

Chisolm, J.J. Jr. Management of increased lead absorption and lead poisoning in children. *N. Engl. J. Med.*, **1973,** *289*:1016–1018.

Chisolm, J.J. Jr., and Barltrop, D. Recognition and management of children with increased lead absorption. *Arch. Dis. Child.*, **1979,** *54*:249–262.

Chowdhury, P., and Louria, D.B. Influence of cadmium and other trace metals on human α$_1$-antitrypsin: an *in vitro* study. *Science*, **1976,** *191*:480–481.

Clarkson, T.W. Metal toxicity in the central nervous system. *Environ. Health Perspect.*, **1987,** *75*:59–64.

Cooper, W.C., and Gaffey, W.R. Mortality of lead workers. *J. Occup. Med.*, **1975,** *17*:100–107.

Davison, A.G., Fayers, P.M., Taylor, A.J., Venables, K.M., Darbyshire, J., Pickering, C.A., Chettle, D.R., Franklin, D., Guthrie, C.J., Scott, M.C., O'Malley, D., Holden, H., Mason, H.J., Wright, A.L., and Gompertz, D. Cadmium fume inhalation and emphysema. *Lancet*, **1988,** *1*:663–667.

Donofrio, P.D., Wilbourn, A.J., Albers, J.W., Rogers, L., Salanga, V., and Greenberg, H.S. Acute arsenic intoxication presenting as Guillain-Barré-like syndrome. *Muscle Nerve*, **1987,** *10*:114–120.

Dudley, R.E., Gammal, L.M., and Klaassen, C.D. Cadmium-induced hepatic and renal injury in chronically exposed rats: likely role of hepatic cadmium-metallothionein in nephrotoxicity. *Toxicol. Appl. Pharmacol.*, **1985,** *77*:414–426.

Eley, B.M., and Cox, S.W. The release, absorption and possible health effects of mercury from dental amalgam: a review of recent findings. *Br. Dent. J.*, **1993,** *175*:355–362.

Elinder, C.G., Kjellstrom, T., Lind, B., Linnman, L., Piscator, M., and Sundstedt, K. Cadmium exposure from smoking cigarettes: variations with time and country where purchased. *Environ. Res.*, **1983,** *32*:220–227.

Engstrom, B., and Nordberg, G.F. Dose dependence of gastrointestinal absorption and biological half-time of cadmium in mice. *Toxicology*, **1979,** *13*:215–222.

Epstein, O., De Villiers, D., Jain, S., Potter, B.J., Thomas, H.C., and Sherlock, S. Reduction of immune complexes and immunoglobulins induced by D-penicillamine in primary biliary cirrhosis. *N. Engl. J. Med.*, **1979,** *300*:274–278.

Eto, K. Pathology of Minamata disease. *Toxicol. Pathol.*, **1997,** *25*:1052–1061.

Fournier, L., Thomas, G., Garnier, R., Buisine, A., Houze, P., Pradier, F., and Dally, S. 2,3-Dimercaptosuccinic acid treatment of heavy metal poisoning in humans. *Med. Toxicol. Adverse Drug Exp.*, **1988,** *3*:499–504.

Freedman, M.H., Grisaru, D., Olivieri, N., MacLusky, I., and Thorner, P.S. Pulmonary syndrome in patients with thalassemia major receiving intravenous deferoxamine infusions. *Am. J. Dis. Child.*, **1990,** *144*:565–569.

Gerstner, H.B., and Huff, J.E. Clinical toxicology of mercury. *J. Toxicol. Environ. Health*, **1977,** *2*:491–526.

Giunta, F., Di Landro, D., Chiaranda, M., Zanardi, L., Dal Palie, A., Giron, G.P., Bressa, G., and Cima, L. Severe acute poisoning from the ingestion of a permanent wave solution of mercuric chloride. *Hum. Toxicol.*, **1983,** *2*:243–246.

Goering, P.L., and Klaassen, C.D. Tolerance to cadmium-induced hepatotoxicity following cadmium pretreatment. *Toxicol. Appl. Pharmacol.*, **1984,** *74*:308–313.

Goldwater, L.J., and Hoover, A.W. An international study of "normal" levels of lead in blood and urine. *Arch. Environ. Health.*, **1967,** *15*:60–63.

Gordon, R.A., and Burnside, J.W. D-Penicillamine-induced myasthenia gravis in rheumatoid arthritis. *Ann. Intern. Med.*, **1977,** *87*:578–579.

Gotelli, C.A., Astolfi, E., Cox, C., Cernichiari, E., and Clarkson, T.W. Early biochemical effects of an organic mercury fungicide on infants: "dose makes the poison." *Science*, **1985,** *227*:638–640.

Graziano, J.H., Cuccia, D., and Friedham, E. The pharmacology of 2,3-dimercaptosuccinic acid and its potential use in arsenic poisoning. *J. Pharmacol. Exp. Ther.*, **1978,** *207*:1051–1055.

Graziano, J.H., Lolacono, N.J., Moulton, T., Mitchell, M.E., Slavkovich, V., and Zarate, C. Controlled study of meso-2,3-dimercaptosuccinic acid for the management of childhood lead intoxication. *J. Pediatr.*, **1992,** *120*:133–139.

Gregus, Z., and Klaassen, C.D. Disposition of metals in rats: a comparative study of fecal, urinary, and biliary excretion and tissue distribution of eighteen metals. *Toxicol. Appl. Pharmacol.*, **1986,** *85*:24–38.

Gross, S.B., Pfitzer, E.A., Yeager, D.W., and Kehoe, R.A. Lead in human tissues. *Toxicol. Appl. Pharmacol.*, **1975,** *32*:638–651.

Guldager, B., Jelnes, R., Jørgensen, S.J., Nielson, J.S., Klaerke, A., Mogensen, K., Larsen, K.E., Reimer, E., Holm, J., and Ottesen, S. EDTA treatment of intermittent claudication—a double-blind, placebo-controlled study. *J. Intern. Med.*, **1992,** *231*:261–267.

Hammond, P.B. The effects of chelating agents on the tissue distribution and excretion of lead. *Toxicol. Appl. Pharmacol.*, **1971,** *18*:296–310.

Hill, H.F. Penicillamine in rheumatoid arthritis: adverse effects. *Scand. J. Rheumatol. Suppl.*, **1979,** *28*:94–99.

Hutchinson, J. Arsenic cancer. *Br. Med. J.*, **1887,** *2*:1280–1281.

Jenkins, R.B. Inorganic arsenic and the nervous system. *Brain*, **1966,** *89*:479–498.

Jones, C.W., Mays, C.W., Taylor, G.N., Lloyd, R.D., and Packer, S.M. Reducing the cancer risk of ^{239}Pu by chelation therapy. *Radiat. Res.*, **1986,** *107*:296–306.

Jones, M.M., Cherian, M.G., Singh, P.K., Basinger, M.A., and Jones, S.G. A comparative study of the influence of vicinal dithiols and a dithiocarbamate on the biliary excretion of cadmium in rat. *Toxicol. Appl. Pharmacol.*, **1991,** *110*:241–250.

Kazantzis, G., Flynn, F.V., Spowage, J.V., and Trott, D.G. Renal tubular malfunction and pulmonary emphysema in cadmium pigment workers. *Q. J. Med.*, **1963,** *32*:165–192.

Kehoe, R.A. The metabolism of lead in man in health and disease. *Arch. Environ. Health,* **1961a,** *2*:418–422.

Kehoe, R.A. The Harben Lectures, 1960: the metabolism of lead in man in health and disease. *J.R. Inst. Public Health*, **1961b,** *24*:177–203.

Kehoe, R.A. Studies of lead administration and elimination in adult volunteers under natural and experimentally induced conditions over extended periods of time. *Food Chem. Toxicol.,* **1987,** *25*:421–493.

Kershaw, T.G., Clarkson, T.W., and Dhahir, P.H. The relationship between blood levels and dose of methylmercury in man. *Arch. Environ. Health,* **1980,** *35*:28–36.

Klaassen, C.D. Biliary excretion of mercury compounds. *Toxicol. Appl. Pharmacol.,* **1975,** *33*:356–365.

Kostyniak, P.J. Mobilization and removal of methylmercury in the dog during extracorporeal complexing hemodialysis with 2,3-dimercaptosuccinic acid (DMSA). *J. Pharmacol. Exp. Ther.,* **1982,** *221*:63–68.

Kotsonis, F.N., and Klaassen, C.D. The relationship of metallothionein to the toxicity of cadmium after prolonged oral administration to rats. *Toxicol. Appl. Pharmacol.,* **1978,** *46*:39–54.

Landrigan, P.J. Arsenic—state of the art. *Am. J. Ind. Med.,* **1981,** *2*:5–14.

Lauwerys, R.R., Bernard, A., Roels, H.A., Buchet, J.-P., and Viau, C. Characterization of cadmium proteinuria in man and rat. *Environ. Health Perspect.,* **1984,** *54*:147–152.

Lauwerys, R.R., Roels, H.A., Buchet, J.-P., Bernard, A., and Stanescu, D. Investigations on the lung and kidney function in workers exposed to cadmium. *Environ. Health Perspect.,* **1979,** *28*:137–146.

Lenz, K., Hruby, K., Druml, W., Eder, A., Gaszner, A., Kleinberger, G., Pichler, M., and Weiser, M. 2,3-Dimercaptosuccinic acid in human arsenic poisoning. *Arch. Toxicol.,* **1981,** *47*:241–243.

Lerda, D. Study of sperm characteristics in persons occupationally exposed to lead. *Am. J. Ind. Med.,* **1992,** *22*:567–571.

McAlpine, D., and Araki, S. Minimata disease. An unusual neurological disorder caused by contaminated fish. *Lancet,* **1958,** *2*:629–631.

Magos, L., Halbach, S., and Clarkson, T.W. Role of catalase in the oxidation of mercury vapor. *Biochem. Pharmacol.,* **1978,** *27*:1373–1377.

Mahaffey, K.R., Rosen, J.F., Chesney, R.W., Peeler, J.T., Smith, C.M., and DeLuca, H.F. Association between age, blood lead concentration, and serum 1,25-dihydroxycholecalciferol levels in children. *Am. J. Clin. Nutr.,* **1982,** *35*:1327–1331.

Matheson, D.S., Clarkson, T.W., and Gelfand, E.W. Mercury toxicity (acrodynia) induced by long term injection of gammaglobulin. *J. Pediatr.,* **1980,** *97*:153–155.

Needleman, H.L., Schell, A., Bellinger, D., Leviton, A., and Allred, E.N. The long-term effects of exposure to low doses of lead in childhood. An 11-year follow-up report. *N. Engl. J. Med.,* **1990,** *322*:83–88.

Netter, P., Bannwarth, B., Pere, P., and Nicolas, A. Clinical pharmacokinetics of D-penicillamine. *Clin. Pharmacokinet.,* **1987,** *13*:317–333.

NRC (National Research Council). *Arsenic in Drinking Water.* National Academy Press, Washington, D.C., **1999.**

NRC (National Research Council). *Measuring Lead in Infants, Children, and Other Sensitive Populations.* National Academy Press, Washington, D.C., **1993.**

Olivieri, N.F., Brittenham, G.M., Matsui, D., Berkovitch, M., Blendis, L.M., Cameron, R.G., McClelland, R.A., Liu, P.P., Templeton, D.M., and Koren, G. Iron-chelation therapy with oral deferiprone in patients with thalassemia major. *N. Engl. J. Med.,* **1995,** *332*:918–922.

Olivieri, N.F., Buncic, J.R., Chew, E., Gallant, T., Harrison, R.V., Keenan, N., Logan, W., Mitchell, D., Ricci, G., Skarf, B., Taylor, M., and Freedman, M.H. Visual and auditory neurotoxicity in patients receiving subcutaneous deferoxamine infusions. *N. Engl. J. Med.,* **1986,** *314*:869–873.

Perrett, D. The metabolism and pharmacology of D-penicillamine in man. *J. Rheumatol. Suppl.,* **1981,** *7*:41–50.

Pirkle, J.L., Kaufmann, R.B., Brody, D.J., Hickman, T., Gunter, E.W., and Paschal, D.C. Exposure of the U.S. population to lead, 1991–1994. *Environ. Health Perspect.,* **1998,** *106*:745–750.

Propper, R.D., Cooper, B., Rufo, R.R., Nienhuis, A.W., Anderson, W.F., Bunn, H.F., Rosenthal, A., and Nathan, D.G. Continuous subcutaneous administration of deferoxamine in patients with iron overload. *N. Engl. J. Med.,* **1977,** *297*:418–423.

Rahola, T., Aaran, R.K., and Mietinen, J.K. Half-time studies of mercury and cadmium by whole body counting. International Atomic Energy Agency symposium on the assessment of radioactive organ and body burdens. In, *Assessment of Radioactive Contamination in Man.* International Atomic Energy Agency, Vienna, **1972.**

Rosen, J.F., Chesney, R.W., Hamstra, A., DeLuca, H.F., and Mahaffey, K.R. Reduction in 1,25-dihydroxyvitamin D in children with increased lead absorption. *N. Engl. J. Med.,* **1980,** *302*:1128–1131.

Schoen, E.J. Childhood lead poisonings: definitions and priorities. *Pediatrics,* **1993,** *91*:504–505.

Schroeder, H.A. Cadmium as a factor in hypertension. *J. Chronic Dis.,* **1965,** *18*:647–656.

Schumann, G.B., Lerner, S.I., Weiss, M.A., Gawronski, L., and Lohiya, G.K. Inclusion-bearing cells in industrial workers exposed to lead. *Am. J. Clin. Pathol.,* **1980,** *74*:192–196.

Scott, R., Haywood, J.K., Boddy, K., Williams, E.D., Harvey, I., and Paterson, P.J. Whole body calcium deficit in cadmium-exposed workers with hypercalciuria. *Urology,* **1980,** *15*:356–359.

Seshia, S.S., Rjani, K.R., Boeckx, R.L., and Chow, P.N. The neurological manifestations of chronic inhalation of leaded gasoline. *Dev. Med. Child Neurol.,* **1978,** *20*:323–334.

Staessen, J. Low-level lead exposure, renal function and blood pressure. *Verh. K. Acad. Geneeskd. Belg.,* **1995,** *57*:527–574.

Swartz, R.D. Deferoxamine and aluminum removal. *Am. J. Kidney Dis.,* **1985,** *6*:358–364.

Tamashiro, H., Arakaki, M., Akagi, H., Futatsuka, M., and Roht, L.H. Mortality and survival for Minamata disease. *Int. J. Epidemiol.,* **1985,** *14*:582–588.

Thind, G.S., and Fischer, G.M. Plasma cadmium and zinc in human hypertension. *Clin. Sci. Mol. Med.,* **1976,** *51*:483–486.

Vaziri, N.D., Upham, T., and Barton, C.H. Hemodialysis clearance of arsenic. *Clin. Toxicol.,* **1980,** *17*:451–456.

Waalkes, M.P., Coogan, T.P., and Barter, R.A. Toxicological principles of metal carcinogenesis with special emphasis on cadmium. *Crit. Rev. Toxicol.,* **1992,** *22*:175–201.

Wernick, R., Merryman, P., Jaffe, I., and Ziff, M. IgG and IgM rheumatoid factors in rheumatoid arthritis. Quantitative response to penicillamine therapy and relationship to disease activity. *Arthritis Rheum.,* **1983,** *26*:593–598.

Zavon, M.R., and Meadows, C.D. Vascular sequelae to cadmium fume exposure. *Am. Ind. Hyg. Assoc. J.,* **1970,** *31*:180–182.

MONOGRAPHS AND REVIEWS

Aposhian, H.V., and Aposhian, M.M. meso-2,3-Dimercaptosuccinic acid: chemical, pharmacological and toxicological properties of an orally effective metal chelating agent. *Annu. Rev. Pharmacol. Toxicol.,* **1990,** *30*:279–306.

Bernard, B.P., and Becker, C.E. Environmental lead exposure and the kidney. *J. Toxicol. Clin. Toxicol.,* **1988,** *26*:1–34.

Catsch, A., and Harmuth-Hoene, A.-E. Pharmacology and therapeutic applications of agents used in heavy metal poisoning. In, *The Chelation of Heavy Metals.* (Levine, W.G., ed.) Pergamon Press, Oxford, **1979,** pp. 116–124.

Craswell, P.W. Chronic lead nephropathy. *Annu. Rev. Med.,* **1987,** *38*:169–173.

Elihu, N., Anandasbapathy, S., and Frishman, W.H. Chelation therapy in cardiovascular disease: ethylenediaminetetraacetic acid, deferoxamine, and dexrazoxane. *J. Clin. Pharmacol.,* **1998,** *38*:101–105.

Engel, R.R., Hopenhayn-Rich, C., Receveur, O., and Smith, A.H. Vascular effects of chronic arsenic exposure: a review. *Epidemiol. Rev.,* **1994,** *16*:184–209.

Friberg, L., Piscator, M., Nordberg, G.F., and Kjellstrom, T. *Cadmium in the Environment,* 2nd ed. CRC Press, Cleveland, **1974.**

Friberg, L., and Vostal, J. *Mercury in the Environment: An Epidemiological and Toxicological Appraisal.* CRC Press, Cleveland, **1972.**

Garrettson, L.K. Lead. In, *Clinical Management of Poisoning and Drug Overdose.* (Haddad, L.M., and Winchester, J.F., eds.) Saunders, Philadelphia, **1983,** pp. 649–655.

Goyer, R.A., and Clarkson, T.W. Toxic effects of metals. In, *Casarett and Doull's Toxicology: The Basic Science of Poisons,* 6th ed. (Klaassen, C.D., ed.) McGraw-Hill, New York, **2001,** in press.

Hindmarsh, J.T., and McCurdy, R.F. Clinical and environmental aspects of arsenic toxicity. *Crit. Rev. Clin. Lab. Sci.,* **1986,** *23*:315–347.

IARC. Some metals and metallic compounds. In, *IARC Monographs on the Evaluation of Carcinogenic Risks to Humans.* Vol. 23. International Agency for Research on Cancer, Lyon, France, **1980.**

International Agency for Research on Cancer. Beryllium, cadmium, mercury, and exposures in the glass manufacturing industry. Working Group views and expert opinions, Lyon, 9–16 February 1993. *IARC Monogr. Eval. Carcinog. Risks Hum.,* **1993,** *58*:1–415.

Janin, Y., Couinaud, C., Stone, A., and Wise, L. The "lead-induced colic" syndrome in lead intoxication. *Surg. Annu.,* **1985,** *17*:287–307.

Kazantzis, G. Lead: sources, exposure and possible carcinogenicity. *IARC Sci. Publ.,* **1986,** *71*:103–111.

Klaassen, C.D., Liu, J., and Choudhuri, S. Metallothionein: an intracellular protein to protect against cadmium toxicity. *Annu. Rev. Pharmacol. Toxicol.,* **1999,** *39*:267–294.

Levy, R.S., Fisher, M., and Alter, J.N. Penicillamine: review and cutaneous manifestations. *J. Am. Acad. Dermatol.,* **1983,** *8*:548–558.

Piscator, M., and Pettersson, B. Chronic cadmium poisoning: diagnosis and prevention. In, *Clinical Chemistry and Chemical Toxicology of Metals.* (Brown, S.S., ed.) Elsevier/North Holland Biomedical Press, Amsterdam, **1977,** pp. 143–155.

Smith, W.E., and Smith, A.M. *Minamata.* Holt, Rinehart & Winston, New York, **1975.**

Winship, K.A. Toxicity of inorganic arsenic salts. *Adverse Drug React. Acute Poisoning Rev.,* **1984,** *3*:129–160.

C H A P T E R   6 8

NONMETALLIC ENVIRONMENTAL TOXICANTS

Air Pollutants, Solvents and Vapors, and Pesticides

Curtis D. Klaassen

Exposure to chemicals in the environment can produce adverse health effects. It is important for the physician to know the potential effects of chemicals and consider this information in making a clinical diagnosis or therapeutic plan.

People are exposed to chemicals in the air they breathe, the food they eat, and the water they drink. The toxic effects of chemicals are dependent on the dose. The concentrations of chemicals in the air, food, and water usually are below levels that produce toxic effects. Individuals most likely to experience adverse effects from chemicals are those who are exposed to chemicals at their workplace, because they often receive higher doses of chemicals than does the general population.

In this chapter, the toxic effects of three major classes of chemicals are presented: air pollutants, solvents and vapors, and pesticides. Specific treatment for exposure to chemicals in these classes is discussed when such treatment is available.

Environmental pollution, an undesired spin-off of human activity, was relatively insignificant until urbanization. The use of coal to heat homes created an atmosphere of sulfurous smoke above the cities. From the thirteenth century onward, periodic efforts were made to forbid the burning of coal in London, but, on the whole, people have accepted a polluted atmosphere as part of urban life. Power plants burn fossil fuels to generate electricity; steel mills have grown along river banks and lake shores; oil refineries have risen near ports and oil fields; smelters roast and refine metals near great mineral deposits; the automobile is virtually ubiquitous. All of these manifestations of modernized societies pollute the air, water, and soil around them.

AIR POLLUTANTS

Air pollutants enter the body predominantly through the lungs. Some of these chemicals are absorbed into the blood, and some that are not absorbed are eliminated by the lungs and some are retained.

Absorption and Deposition of Toxicants by the Lungs

The site of deposition of aerosols in the respiratory tract depends on the size of the particle. Many particles are irregular in shape. There are a number of ways to delineate particle size or behavior, such as aerodynamic diameter, mass mean, *etc*. Particles of 5 μm or larger in diameter usually are deposited in the upper airway. Smaller particles of 1 to 5 μm are deposited in the terminal airways or alveoli. Those deposited in the unciliated anterior portion of the nose remain until removed by wiping, blowing, or sneezing. In the posterior portion of the nose, a mucus blanket propelled by cilia carries insoluble particles to the pharynx in minutes. These particles are swallowed and pass to the gastrointestinal tract. Soluble particles dissolved in the mucus may be carried to the pharynx or absorbed through the epithelium into the blood.

Particles deposited in the tracheobronchial tree are cleared by the cilia's upward movement of mucus. Although the rate of ciliary movement varies in different parts of the respiratory tract, it is rapid and efficient. Rates of transport are between 0.1 and 1 mm per minute, resulting in half-lives for the particles that range from 30 to 300 minutes. Coughing and sneezing move mucus and particles rapidly toward the glottis. The particles also may be swallowed.

Particles less than 1 μm in diameter remain suspended in the inhaled air and reach the alveolar zone of the lung, where they may be readily absorbed. The surface area of the alveolar zone is large (50 to 100 m^2); the rate of blood flow is high; and the blood is in close proximity to the alveolar air (10 μm). All of these factors influence the extent of absorption; factors that govern the rate of absorption of gases are discussed in Chapter 13. Liquid aerosols cross the alveolar cell membranes by passive diffusion in proportion to their lipid solubility. Mechanisms for removal or absorption of particulate matter (usually less than 1 μm in diameter) from the alveolus are less clearly defined and less efficient than those that remove particles from the tracheobronchial tree. Three processes are apparently operative. The first is physical removal; particles deposited on the fluid layer of the alveoli are believed to be aspirated onto the mucociliary escalator of the tracheobronchial tree. The second is phagocytosis, usually by mononuclear phagocytes or alveolar macrophages. The third is by absorption into the lymphatic system. Particles can remain in lymphatic tissue for long periods, and, for this reason, the lymphatic tissue has been called the dust store of the lungs.

Overall, removal of particulates from the alveoli is relatively inefficient. Only about 20% of such matter is removed during the first day after deposition; that which remains longer than 24 hours often is removed very slowly. The rate of this clearance can be predicted from the solubility of the substance in lung fluids. The least soluble compounds are removed at a slower rate. Such removal apparently is due largely to dissolution and absorption into the blood. Some particles may remain in the alveoli indefinitely if the cells that phagocytize them proliferate and join the reticular network to form an alveolar dust plaque or nodule.

Types and Sources of Air Pollutants

Five pollutants account for nearly 98% of air pollution. These are carbon monoxide (52%), sulfur oxides (14%), volatile organic compounds (14%), particulate matter (4%), and nitrogen oxides (14%) (Costa and Amdur, 1996). A distinction often is made between two kinds of pollution. The first is characterized by sulfur dioxide and smoke from incomplete combustion of coal and by conditions of fog and cool temperatures. Because of its chemical nature, it is termed a *reducing type of pollution*. The second kind of pollution is characterized by hydrocarbons, oxides of nitrogen, and photochemical oxidants. It is caused by automobile exhaust and occurs especially in areas such as the Los Angeles basin, where intense sunlight causes photochemical reactions in polluted air masses that are trapped by a meteorological inversion layer. Because of its nature, it is described as an *oxidizing type of pollution* or *photochemical air pollution*. Particulates formed in certain settings, especially combustive,

may adsorb vapors or gases, changing the surface property and creating a more harmful pollutant than either alone.

Five major sources account for 90% of the tons of pollutants that are emitted annually: transportation (particularly automobiles), industry, electric-power generation, space heating, and refuse disposal (cited in order of relative importance).

Health Effects of Air Pollution

Episodes of high pollution cause mortality and morbidity. There are three classical examples: 65 people died in the Meuse Valley, Belgium, in 1930; 20 people died in Donora, Pennsylvania, in 1948; 4000 people died in London in 1952. Each of these incidents occurred during an atmospheric temperature inversion that lasted 3 to 4 days. During this time, the concentration of pollutants surpassed the usual levels for these already heavily polluted areas; because coal was the main fuel, the pollution was the reducing kind. Most of the people who became ill or died were elderly; some had either cardiac or respiratory diseases or both; none could cope with the added stress of breathing heavily polluted air.

Acute effects on health clearly are associated with the reducing type of pollution. While there is less evidence to associate photochemical oxidant pollution with such effects on human health, there are significant correlations between levels of oxidants in the air and hospital admissions for allergic disorders, inflammatory disease of the eye, acute upper respiratory infections, influenza, and bronchitis.

Toxicology of Air Pollutants

Sulfur Dioxide.   Sulfur dioxide gas is generated primarily by the burning of fossil fuels that contain sulfur. The concentration of sulfur dioxide required to kill laboratory animals is so high that it has little relevance to problems of air pollution. Sulfur dioxide is an upper airway irritant that can stimulate mucus secretion and bronchoconstriction. However, daily exposure of rats to 10 ppm of sulfur dioxide for 1 to 2 months thickens the mucus layer in the trachea about fivefold. Although the cilia beat with normal frequency, the thick mucus retards clearance. The abnormal mucus layer is caused by increased numbers of mucus-secreting cells in the main bronchi, where such cells are common, and in the peripheral airways, where they are normally absent (Hirsch *et al.,* 1975).

A basic physiological response to inhalation of sulfur dioxide is a mild degree of bronchial constriction that is dependent on intact parasympathetic innervation. When exposed to 5 ppm of sulfur dioxide for 10 minutes, most human subjects show increased resistance to the flow of air. Asthmatics have an increased sensitivity to sulfur dioxide; bronchoconstriction may occur at concentrations as low as 0.25 ppm (Sheppard *et al.,* 1981).

It appears that an increase in the concentration of atmospheric sulfur oxides, which generally is accompanied by an elevation in the level of particulate matter, significantly affects morbidity and mortality. In heavily polluted cities (London, New York, Cracow), exposure for 24 hours to sulfur dioxide concentrations of 0.11 to 0.15 ppm and total particulate concentrations of 500 to 600 $\mu g/m^3$ results in increased morbidity and mortality, and a temporary decrease in pulmonary function is observed at about 0.1 ppm of sulfur dioxide and 250 $\mu g/m^3$ of particulate matter (Ware *et al.*, 1981).

Sulfuric Acid. A portion of sulfur dioxide in the atmosphere is converted to sulfuric acid, ammonium sulfate, and other sulfates. The conversion to sulfuric acid can be initiated by soot or by trace metals such as vanadium or manganese. Stable sulfite complexes may be formed in the presence of metals such as copper or iron.

Sulfuric acid is an irritant to the upper respiratory tract through its acidity. It increases airway resistance in relation to both concentration and particle size (Amdur *et al.*, 1978). Particles of 1 μm (1 mg/m^3) produce a rapid and marked increase in resistance to flow, whereas particles of 7 μm produce only a slight increase because they cannot penetrate beyond the upper respiratory tract. Sulfuric acid produces a greater increase in resistance to flow than does sulfur dioxide after either a short- or long-term exposure. Asthmatics are more sensitive to both sulfuric acid and sulfur dioxide.

Particulate Sulfates. Sulfates vary greatly in their effects on respiration, and the sulfate ion *per se* does not alter respiratory function. Zinc ammonium sulfate, a reported constituent of the Donora fog, increases respiratory resistance at a concentration of 0.25 mg/m^3; it produces a greater increase in resistance to flow than does sulfur dioxide.

Particulate matter in the atmosphere consists of a mixture of organic and inorganic materials. Particulate matter in the air is associated with an increase in cardiorespiratory mortality and total mortality (Ostro and Chestnut, 1998). It appears that the adverse health effects of airborne particles is less dependent on composition than on size. Therefore, particles often are classified as PM_{10} (less than 10 microns) and $PM_{2.5}$ (less than 2.5 microns), with the smaller particles producing more of the adverse health effects (*see* section on "Particulate Material," below).

Ozone. The oxidant found in the highest concentrations in polluted atmosphere is ozone (O_3). Several miles above the earth's surface there is sufficient short-wave ultraviolet (UV) light to convert O_2 to O_3 by direct absorption. Of the major atmospheric pollutants, nitrogen dioxide is the most efficient in absorbing UV light. Such absorption leads to a complex series of reactions, which may be simplified as follows:

$$NO_2 \xrightarrow{\text{UV}} NO + O\cdot \qquad (68\text{--}1)$$

$$O\cdot + O_2 \longrightarrow O_3 \qquad (68\text{--}2)$$

$$O_3 + NO \rightarrow NO_2 + O_2 \qquad (68\text{--}3)$$

Intensification of UV light at the earth's surface (due to depletion of stratospheric ozone) accelerates the formation of ozone. Because NO_2 is regenerated by the reaction of NO with O_3, the result is cyclical. Simultaneously, oxygen atoms react with hydrocarbons in the atmosphere, especially olefins and substituted aromatics, resulting in oxidized compounds and free radicals that react with NO to produce more NO_2. The result is accumulation of NO_2 and O_3, while concentrations of NO are depleted.

Ozone is a primary oxidant and thus is a lung irritant that is capable of causing death from pulmonary edema. Gross pulmonary edema is evident in mice exposed to concentrations above 2 ppm. Ozone causes desquamation of the epithelium throughout the ciliated airways and produces degenerative changes in type I cells and swelling or rupture of the capillary endothelium in the alveoli. The type I cells are later replaced by type II cells; this type II cell proliferation is a hallmark of ozone toxicity. It is important to note that pulmonary toxicity has been observed in experimental animals after relatively short exposures to concentrations of ozone that occasionally exist for short periods in polluted urban areas (Lippmann, 1989).

Long-term exposure to ozone may cause thickening of the terminal respiratory bronchioles. Chronic bronchitis, fibrosis, and emphysematous changes are observed in a variety of species exposed to ozone at concentrations slightly above 1 ppm.

Ozone at concentrations of 0.25 to 0.75 ppm causes shallow, rapid breathing, a decrease in pulmonary compliance, and subjective symptoms, such as cough, tightness in the chest, and dryness of the throat. Such concentrations of ozone may be present during long, high-altitude flights. Ozone also increases the sensitivity of the lung to bronchoconstrictors such as histamine, acetylcholine, and allergens. It increases the incidence of infection in laboratory animals exposed to an aerosol of infectious microorganisms, probably through inhibition of clearance mechanisms. The concentration of ozone often experienced in the urban air is similar to that associated with measurable declines in respiratory function in human beings (Kinney *et al.*, 1988). Thus, there is little margin between current levels and the minimal effect level for ozone. Fortunately, no "high-risk" or more sensitive group of people is thought to exist for ozone, which is in contrast to sulfur dioxide, to which asthmatics are more susceptible.

The biochemical mechanism of pulmonary injury produced by ozone may be due to the formation of reactive free-radical intermediates. Ozone-induced free radicals may be derived from interaction with sulfhydryl groups, from oxidative decomposition of unsaturated fatty acids, or both. Several lines of evidence indicate that one of the biological actions of ozone is reaction with unsaturated fatty acids. The ozonization of these fatty acids is essentially equivalent to lipid peroxidation. Sulfhydryl compounds and antioxidants (such as ascorbic acid and alpha-tocopherol) protect against ozone toxicity in laboratory animals but have not been shown to have protective effects in human beings (Menzel, 1994).

Nitrogen Dioxide. Nitrogen dioxide, like ozone, is a deep lung irritant that is capable of causing pulmonary edema. This pollutant is a particular risk to farmers, because sufficient amounts of nitrogen dioxide can be liberated from ensilage to produce the symptoms of pulmonary damage known as silo-filler's disease. Homes using gas stoves or kerosene heaters can have levels of nitrogen oxides about five times higher than in homes in which cooking is by electricity. The LC_{50} for a 4-hour exposure to nitrogen dioxide is about 90 ppm. As with ozone, nitrogen dioxide damages type I cells of the alveoli.

Experimental exposure of animals or human beings to nitrogen dioxide causes measurable alterations in pulmonary function. The pattern of changes resembles that produced by ozone—increased respiratory frequency and decreased compliance. Pulmonary resistance to air flow is minimally altered. The changes in pulmonary function occur when healthy subjects are exposed to 2 to 3 ppm and may happen at far lower concentrations in some asthmatic subjects (Orehek *et al.*, 1976).

Aldehydes. Aldehydes are formed by oxidation of hydrocarbons by sunlight and by incomplete combustion (automobile exhaust, forest fires); they are released from formaldehyde-containing resins (such as those in plywood, particle board, and urea-formaldehyde foam insulation). The high reactivity of aldehydes results in rather short half-lives of a few hours in the atmosphere. The concentration of aldehydes is 0.0005 to 0.002 ppm in a clean atmosphere, 0.004 to 0.05 ppm in ambient urban air, and up to 0.8 ppm in indoor environments where formaldehyde-emitting materials are found (Committee on Aldehydes, 1981; Woodbury and Zenz, 1983). About 50% of the total aldehyde in polluted air is formaldehyde (H_2CO), and about 5% is acrolein ($H_2C=CHCHO$). These materials probably contribute to the odor of photochemical smog and the ocular irritation that it causes.

Formaldehyde irritates mucous membranes of the nose, upper respiratory tract, and eyes. Concentrations of 0.5 to 1 ppm are detectable by odor, 2 to 3 ppm produce mild irritation, and 4 to 5 ppm are intolerable to most people. The concentration of formaldehyde may approach 1 ppm in the air of newly built homes, especially mobile homes. A significant correlation has been found between the formaldehyde concentration in home air and the incidence of ocular irritation. Other symptoms (*e.g.*, runny nose, sore throat, headache, and cough) also are more frequent in people living in indoor environments with high levels of formaldehyde (Woodbury and Zenz, 1983). The overall pattern of respiratory response to formaldehyde resembles that to sulfur dioxide. Formaldehyde can provoke skin reactions in sensitized subjects, not only by contact but also by inhalation (Maibach, 1983). Occupational exposure to formaldehyde also can cause asthma, but it appears to be a rather infrequent phenomenon and is not associated with domestic exposure (Nordman *et al.*, 1985). Inhalation of formaldehyde (6 to 15 ppm) for 2 years induces squamous-cell carcinomas in the nasal cavity of mice and rats (Kerns *et al.*, 1983). However, there is no evidence that exposure to formaldehyde produces human malignancies (U.A.R.E.P., 1988).

Acrolein is much more irritating than formaldehyde. Acrolein is a major contributor to the irritative quality of cigarette smoke and photochemical smog. The occupational threshold limit value (TLV) for acrolein is 0.1 ppm; 1 ppm causes lacrimation in less than 5 minutes (Committee on Aldehydes, 1981). Acrolein increases airway resistance and tidal volume and decreases respiratory frequency. Aldehydes increase resistance to air flow at concentrations below those that decrease respiratory frequency.

Carbon Monoxide. Carbon monoxide (CO) is a colorless, odorless, tasteless, and nonirritating gas resulting from incomplete combustion of organic matter. CO is the most abundant pollutant found in the lower atmosphere, and a large number of accidental and suicidal deaths occur yearly from its inhalation.

Even though it has been known for a long time that CO is synthesized in the body during the degradation of heme, CO has

not been thought to have a physiological function. As a result of the identification of endothelium-derived relaxing factor as nitric oxide, it has been suggested that carbon monoxide might have a similar function (Marks *et al.*, 1991). However, much research will be required to determine whether or not CO has a physiological function.

The average concentration of CO in the atmosphere is about 0.1 ppm. Natural sources—such as atmospheric oxidation of methane, forest fires, terpine oxidation, and the ocean (where microorganisms produce CO)—are responsible for about 90% of the atmospheric CO; human activity produces about 10%.

Inadequate venting of furnaces and automobiles results in many deaths each year. Most victims of closed-space fires die from acute CO poisoning rather than from burns. The automobile is the greatest source of CO; concentrations can reach 115 ppm in heavy traffic, 75 ppm in vehicles on expressways, and 23 ppm in residential areas. In underground garages and tunnels, CO levels have been found to exceed 100 ppm for extended periods. The installation of pollution-control devices, including catalytic converters in automobile exhaust systems, has reduced CO emissions due to automobile travel.

The average concentration of CO in the atmosphere appears to be stabilized by efficient natural means of removal (sinks). The most important sink seems to be the reaction of CO with ambient hydroxyl radicals to form carbon dioxide; the upper atmosphere and the soil also are sinks.

Another source of exposure to CO is smoking. Goldsmith and Landaw (1968) reported a median carboxyhemoglobin (COHb) level of 5.9% in heavy smokers (two packs of cigarettes per day) who inhale.

Reaction of CO with Hemoglobin. Toxicity from CO is due to its combination with hemoglobin to form COHb. Hemoglobin in this form cannot carry oxygen, as both gases react with the same heme prosthetic groups in the tetrameric hemoglobin molecule. Because the affinity of hemoglobin for CO is approximately 220 times greater than for oxygen, CO is dangerous even at very low concentrations. Air contains 21% oxygen by volume; therefore, exposure to a gas mixture of 0.1% CO (1000 ppm) in air would result in approximately 50% carboxyhemoglobinemia.

The reduction in the oxygen-carrying capacity of blood is proportional to the amount of COHb present. However, the amount of oxygen available to the tissues is reduced further by the inhibitory influence of COHb on the dissociation of any oxyhemoglobin (O_2Hb) still available. This can be understood best by comparing an anemic individual having a hemoglobin value of 80 g per liter with a person having a hemoglobin value of 160 g per liter but with half of it in the form of COHb (Figure 68–1). In each instance the oxygen-carrying capacity is the same. The anemic individual may show few if any symptoms, whereas the person suffering from CO poisoning will be near collapse.

The toxicity of CO is not due solely to the interference of CO with the delivery of O_2 by the blood. CO also exerts a direct toxic effect by binding to cellular cytochromes, such as those contained in respiratory enzymes and myoglobin (Gutierrez, 1982).

Factors Governing CO Toxicity. Factors that govern the toxicity of CO include the concentration of the gas in inspired air, the duration of exposure, the respiratory minute volume, the cardiac output, the oxygen demand of the tissues, and the concentration of hemoglobin in the blood. Anemic people are more

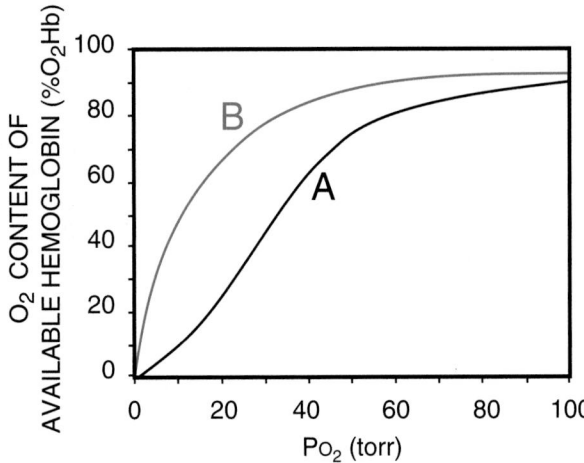

Figure 68–1. The effect of carboxyhemoglobin (COHb) on the dissociation curve of oxyhemoglobin.

Curve A (black line) represents the normal oxygen dissociation curve, which is unaffected by the presence of anemia (e.g., 80 g/liter of hemoglobin in the blood). Curve B (blue line) represents the situation when there is 50% COHb and a normal concentration of hemoglobin (160 g/liter of hemoglobin in the blood and half of the binding sites occupied by CO). The oxygen-carrying capacity is the same in both cases; however, when COHb is present, oxygen dissociates from hemoglobin at lower values of P_{O_2}. This effect results from interactions between binding sites for O_2 or CO; there are four such sites per molecule of hemoglobin.

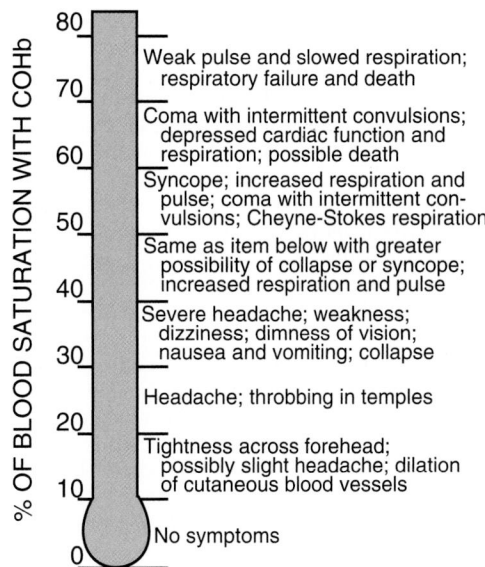

Figure 68–2. The correlation between carboxyhemoglobin concentration and signs and symptoms of carbon monoxide poisoning.

A continuum of symptoms has been noted with carbon monoxide poisoning. However, it must be emphasized that there is considerable interindividual variability in response to exposure to carbon monoxide. The blood level of carboxyhemoglobin (COHb) should be used only in a semiquantitative way to relate exposure to effect. (Adapted from Sayers and Davenport, 1930.)

susceptible to CO poisoning than are individuals with normal amounts of hemoglobin. Increased metabolic rate enhances the severity of symptoms in CO poisoning; this is why children succumb earlier than adults when exposed to a given concentration of the gas.

Change in barometric pressure does not affect the relative affinities of hemoglobin for O_2 and CO. However, at high altitudes and in other situations where oxygen tension is low, the effects of a given concentration of CO will be correspondingly more severe.

Signs and Symptoms of CO Toxicity. The signs and symptoms of CO poisoning are characteristic of hypoxia. Because the brain and heart are the organs with the greatest oxygen demand and the highest metabolic rates, they are the most sensitive to hypoxia and account for most effects observed after CO exposure. The symptoms of CO poisoning have been correlated with the COHb content of the blood, as shown in Figure 68–2. However, it is important to note that, in a given individual, the clinical signs and symptoms may not correlate with this nomogram in a strictly quantitative way; furthermore, not all of these symptoms are experienced by a single individual. There is significant variation among individuals and insufficient information concerning interindividual variability, rate and duration of uptake, and related kinetic parameters to define a truly accurate nomogram. However, the relationships shown can be helpful in a semiquantitative way for relating

exposure to effect. Although inhalation of a high concentration may produce warning signs (transient weakness and dizziness) before consciousness is lost, there may be no warning at all.

Moderate concentrations of COHb have little effect on vital functions in the human subject at rest. As mentioned previously, the presence of COHb reduces the oxygen-carrying capacity but not the P_{O_2} of arterial blood. As a result, there is no stimulation of respiration by the carotid and aortic chemoreceptor mechanism. Cardiac rate, on the other hand, increases in all subjects when COHb reaches 30%, probably to compensate for peripheral vasodilation caused by hypoxia; lactic acidosis results from tissue hypoxia.

The clinical findings in patients acutely poisoned by CO are varied. Many patients exhibit symptoms not usually associated with CO poisoning: skin lesions, excessive sweating, hepatic enlargement, bleeding tendency, pyrexia, leukocytosis, albuminuria, and glycosuria.

Pathology of Acute CO Poisoning. As indicated above, the tissues most affected by CO exposure are those most sensitive to oxygen deprivation, such as the brain and the heart, and the lesions are predominantly hemorrhagic. The heart may be permanently damaged by the presence of COHb in the blood; evidence of ischemic changes and subendocardial infarction may be observed. The severe headache following exposure to CO is believed to be caused by cerebral edema and increased intracranial pressure resulting from excessive transudation across hypoxic capillaries. Finck (1966) has catalogued the gross pathological changes observed in 351 fatal cases of accidental CO poisoning. Rapidly fatal cases of CO poisoning are characterized by congestion and hemorrhages in all organs. In longer term, eventually fatal cases, the hypoxic lesions observed are related to the duration of posthypoxic unconsciousness.

Bokonjić (1963) has shown that the maximal period of CO-induced posthypoxic unconsciousness compatible with complete neurological recovery is 21 hours in patients under 48 years of age and 11 hours in older patients. Complete recovery of mental function was not observed when the CO-induced unconsciousness exceeded 15 hours in the older group or 64 hours in the younger group. Perhaps the most insidious effect of CO poisoning is the delayed development of neuropsychiatric impairment, which is manifested as inappropriate euphoria and impairment of judgment, abstract thinking, and concentration (Choi, 1983); some clinicians believe that levels of CO too low to induce coma also may elicit neuropsychiatric effects.

Severe CO poisoning can produce skin lesions varying from areas of erythema and edema to marked blister and bulla formation. Rhabdomyolysis, presumably caused by the direct toxic effect of CO on myoglobin, and myoglobinuria with renal failure also may occur.

Diagnosis of Acute CO Poisoning.   The presumptive diagnosis of acute CO poisoning usually is facilitated by circumstantial evidence, as the victim commonly is found under circumstances that leave little doubt as to the cause of the condition. COHb is cherry-red in color, and its presence in high concentrations in capillary blood may impart an abnormal red color to the skin, mucous membranes, and fingernails. However, the living patient is commonly cyanotic and pale, and "cherry-red cyanosis" is seen only at autopsy. A final diagnosis depends upon the demonstration of COHb in the blood. Therapy is not delayed to perform such a test in a severely poisoned individual, but the demonstration of COHb often has forensic significance. If a person succumbs in an atmosphere containing CO, a postmortem blood sample usually contains 60% COHb; however, death sometimes occurs at lower concentrations. If the patient is removed from such an atmosphere while still breathing, the concentration of COHb rapidly declines, and if respiratory exchange continues to be adequate, the blood is freed of this form of hemoglobin over a course of hours.

Fate and Excretion of CO.   COHb is fully dissociable, and once acute exposure is terminated, the CO will be excreted *via* the lungs. Only a very small amount is oxidized to CO_2.

CO cannot be excreted without active respiration. Furthermore, COHb is extremely stable and is little affected by putrefaction. Therefore, valid measurements of COHb concentrations in the body can be made long after death. Conversely, little or no CO is absorbed postmortem, and analysis of the blood in the heart provides an accurate measurement of the concentration of COHb in the blood at death. These factors have medicolegal importance.

When room air is breathed by a resting subject, the CO content of blood decreases with a half-time of 320 minutes. If 100% oxygen is substituted for air, this value is reduced to 80 minutes; under hyperbaric conditions, the half-time may be less than 25 minutes (Peterson and Stewart, 1970). These facts provide the basic principles for treatment of CO poisoning.

Treatment of CO Poisoning.   It is first essential to transfer the patient to fresh air. If respiration has failed, artificial respiration must be instituted immediately. Treatment is then directed toward providing an adequate supply of oxygen to the body cells and hastening elimination of the CO. In most cases, rapid administration of 100% oxygen with a tight-fitting mask will be adequate. Some clinicians recommend administration of hyperbaric oxygen if a hyperbaric oxygen facility is available. Although not unequivocally documented (Myers *et al.*, 1985), the rationale is that hyperbaric oxygen not only provides oxygen in solution for the tissues but also hastens the dissociation of COHb. The best guide concerning return to appropriate oxygen saturation is the neurological function of the patient; blood levels of COHb also can be obtained as supportive information concerning the efficacy of oxygenation, and decreasing blood levels of COHb to below 10% saturation serves as a reasonable therapeutic end point. Supplementary care includes correction of hypotension and acidosis, as well as monitoring of cardiac function (Tintinalli *et al.*, 1983).

Toxicity of Prolonged and Low-Level Exposure to CO.   The cardiovascular system, particularly the heart, is susceptible to adverse effects of low concentrations of COHb. At 6% to 12% COHb, metabolism shifts from aerobic to anaerobic (Ayres *et al.*, 1970). Experimental and clinical studies have suggested that long-term exposure to CO can facilitate the development of atherosclerosis (Thomsen, 1974). CO also seems to affect human behavior. Performance on tests of vigilance is impaired when COHb is as low as 2% to 5%. However, these low levels of COHb probably have no effect on other behaviors, such as driving, reaction time, temporal discriminations, coordination, sensory processes, and complex intellectual tasks (National Research Council, 1977).

The fetus may be extremely susceptible to effects of CO, and the gas readily crosses the placenta. Infants born to women who have survived short-term exposure to a high concentration of the gas while pregnant often display neurological sequelae, and there may be gross damage to the brain (Longo, 1977). Persistent low levels of COHb in the fetus of a woman who has smoked during pregnancy also may have effects on the development of the central nervous system (CNS).

Polycythemia develops in the course of long-term exposure to CO. Other compensatory mechanisms are likely, but they have not been demonstrated. Healthy human subjects are exquisitely responsive to any hypoxic stress; they immediately compensate by increasing cardiac output and flow to critical organs. Those with significant cardiovascular disease are more vulnerable to the toxicity of CO, because they may be unable to compensate for the hypoxia (*see* Stewart, 1975).

Particulate Material.   Pneumoconiosis is a category of disease caused by inhalation of dusts. The most common condition of this type is silicosis. Next to oxygen, silicon is the most abundant element found on earth. Approximately 60% of the rocks in the earth's crust contain silica, and silica dusts are prevalent in many industries, particularly in the mining of gold, iron, and coal; in stonework; and in sandblasting. Particles larger than 10 μm are of little clinical significance, because they seldom reach the alveoli. Particles less than 2 to 3 μm are phagocytized by alveolar macrophages, and these cells are eventually destroyed. Other macrophages proliferate and migrate to sites of reaction and release cytokines and other growth factors that cause fibroblasts to replicate and increase their rate of collagen synthesis. The silicotic nodules that result from such reactions are scattered uniformly throughout both lungs. The disease usually requires 10 to 25 years to develop. As the mass of fibrotic tissue increases, vital capacity decreases, and the afflicted individual experiences shortness of breath.

Other pulmonary diseases develop concurrently with silicosis, and silica may facilitate their pathogenesis. Long known to enhance susceptibility to tuberculosis, silicosis also increases the risk of infection by other microorganisms.

Asbestosis results from long-term inhalation of asbestos dust. Asbestos is a fibrous substance composed of hydrated silicate minerals. It is used widely in industry because it is nonflammable, flexible, and resistant to acids and alkalies and has high tensile strength, low density, and high electrical resistivity. Asbestos often was used for insulation, brake linings, shingles, and other purposes, but because of the health effects of asbestos, its use has declined.

Asbestos causes three forms of lung disease in human beings: asbestosis, bronchial lung cancer, and malignant mesotheliomia. Asbestosis (a form of pulmonary fibrosis) develops first in areas adjacent to the bronchioles, where there seems to be preferential deposition of longer asbestos fibers. There also is a fibrous pleuritis in which the pleural membrane thickens to encase the lung in a rigid fibrous capsule. The surface properties of asbestos fibers appear to be important in the development of toxicity, as the interaction of iron on the fibers with the reactive oxygen species produced by the inflammatory response is central in producing asbestos-induced lung injury (Timblin *et al.*, 1999). Clinical symptoms of asbestosis resemble those of silicosis: dyspnea, tachypnea, and cough. However, tuberculosis is not a prominent complication.

Bronchial lung cancer associated with inhalation of asbestos occurs some 20 to 30 years after initial exposure. Inhalation of asbestos combined with cigarette smoking significantly increases the incidence of lung cancer over that caused by exposure to either factor alone (Selikoff and Hammond, 1979). Mesothelioma, a rapidly fatal malignancy, also is associated with exposure to chrysotile asbestos fibers and may appear in the pleura or the peritoneum, usually 25 to 40 years after initial exposure (Selikoff and Hammond, 1979). A high incidence of mesothelioma has been attributed to fibrous tremolite in household stucco and whitewash in Turkey. It thus appears that mesothelioma is not a specific reaction to asbestos, but that any natural or synthetic fibrous material with similar fiber dimensions might be carcinogenic (Elmes, 1980). However, except for long-term inhalation of fibrous matter and the strong suspicion of an increase in risk for persons living adjacent to emissions containing arsenic, there is as yet little convincing evidence that environmental air pollution contributes to the risk of cancer (Kaplan and Morgan, 1981).

Many other occupational pulmonary diseases are caused by long-term inhalation of dusts containing minerals or organic matter. These include coal workers' pneumoconiosis (black lung disease), aluminosis (bauxite lung; Shaver's disease), baritosis (from barium), beryllium disease, byssinosis (from cotton), and others (*see* Speizer, 1994).

SOLVENTS AND VAPORS

Organic solvents and their vapors are a common part of our environment. Short, incidental exposures to low concentrations of solvent vapors, such as gasoline, lighter fluids, aerosol sprays, and spot removers, may be relatively harmless; however, exposures to paint removers, floor and tile cleaners, and other solvents in home or industry may be dangerous. In addition, disposal of many of these chemicals has been improper; as a result there is leakage from toxic dump sites and contamination of drinking water. Because so many industrial workers are exposed to solvents and vapors, considerable effort has gone into determining safe levels of exposure. Threshold limit values (TLV) or maximum allowable concentrations (MAC) have been established for the airborne contaminants; a TLV represents the concentration to which most workers may be exposed safely for an 8-hour period, five times a week, for a lifetime of working exposure.

A variety of anesthetic gases, solvents, and fluorohydrocarbons (used as propellants in aerosol products) cause subjective effects when inhaled and frequently are abused in this way. This dangerous practice, which has caused many deaths, is discussed in Chapter 24.

Aliphatic Hydrocarbons

C 1–C 4 Aliphatic Hydrocarbons.   The straight-chain hydrocarbons with four or fewer carbon atoms are present in natural gas (methane, ethane) and in bottled gas (propane, butane). Methane and ethane are "simple asphyxiants"; effects are observed only when their concentration in the air is so high that it decreases the amount of oxygen; they produce no general systemic effects.

C 5–C 8 Aliphatic Hydrocarbons.   The higher molecular weight aliphatic hydrocarbons, like most organic solvents, depress the CNS and cause dizziness and incoordination. However, polyneuropathy is the primary toxic reaction to *n*-hexane, a widely used solvent (USEPA, 1988). This was observed first in Japan, where 93 workers engaged in the production of sandals were afflicted when using a glue that contained at least 60% *n*-hexane (Iida *et al.*, 1973). 2-Hexanone (methyl *n*-butyl ketone) produces neurological changes similar to those of *n*-hexane. Both are metabolized to 2,5-hexanedione, the ultimate toxic metabolite (Figure 68–3). The 2,5-hexanedione binds to amino groups of the neurofilaments, forming aggregates and axonal swelling (Anthony *et al.*, 2001). Clinical symptoms include symmetrical sensory dysfunction of the distal portions of the extremities, which progresses to muscle weakness in toes and fingers and loss of deep sensory reflexes. A decrease in nerve conduction velocity precedes the onset of symptoms (Seppäläinen, 1982). The prognosis for recovery generally is good, except for severely injured patients, but the recovery is slow (Graham *et al.*, 1987). The cytochrome P450–mediated biotransformation of *n*-hexane and 2-hexanone to 2,5-hexanedione appears to be responsible for the peripheral neuropathy associated with exposure to these solvents (Couri and Milks, 1982).

Gasoline and Kerosene.   Gasoline and kerosene, petroleum distillates prepared by the fractionation of crude petroleum oil, contain aliphatic, aromatic, and a variety of branched and unsaturated hydrocarbons. They are used as illuminating fuels,

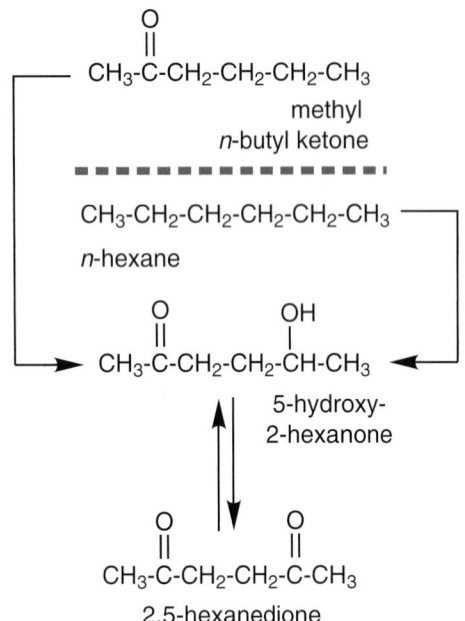

Figure 68–3. Metabolism of hexane.

Both *n*-hexane and methyl *n*-butyl ketone (2-hexanone) are neurotoxic, and both are activated through ω-1 oxidation to the ultimate toxic metabolite, 2,5-hexanedione.

heating fuels, motor fuels, vehicles for many pesticides, cleaning agents, and paint thinners. Because they often are stored in containers previously used for beverages, they are a common cause of accidental poisoning in children. A concern with chronic exposure to gasoline is that it contains approximately 2% benzene, and thus has the potential ability to cause leukemia.

Intoxication by ingestion of gasoline and kerosene resembles that from ethyl alcohol (*see* Chapter 18). Signs and symptoms include incoordination, restlessness, excitement, confusion, disorientation, ataxia, delirium, and finally coma, which may last a few hours or several days. Inhalation of high concentrations of gasoline vapors, as by workmen cleaning storage tanks, can cause immediate death. Gasoline vapors sensitize the myocardium such that small amounts of circulating epinephrine may precipitate ventricular fibrillation; many hydrocarbons have this action. High concentrations of gasoline vapor may also lead to rapid depression of the CNS and death from respiratory failure. With inhalation of high concentrations over hours, pneumonitis may occur.

Poisoning from these hydrocarbons results either from inhalation of the vapors or from ingestion of the liquid. Ingestion is more hazardous, because the liquids have a low surface tension and can be easily aspirated into the respiratory tract by vomiting or eructation. Morbidity is attributed to aspiration, whether it occurs at the time of ingestion or during treatment. Pulmonary damage does not result from gastrointestinal absorption of gasoline or kerosene. Chemical pneumonitis, complicated by secondary bacterial pneumonia and pulmonary edema, is the most serious sequel to aspiration. Death caused by hemorrhagic pulmonary edema usually occurs in 16 to 18 hours and seldom later than 24 hours after aspiration.

Examination of tissues from fatal cases reveals heavy, edematous, and hemorrhagic lungs. The alveoli are filled with an exudate that is rich in proteins, cells, and fibrin, often in a pattern resembling that of hyaline membrane disease. Alveolar walls are weakened and may rupture, leading to less frequent sequelae, such as emphysema and pneumothorax. Pulmonary lymph nodes are inflamed, and bronchopneumonia and atelectasis have been noted.

Symptomatic and supportive care probably is the best treatment for intoxication by gasoline or kerosene (Ervin, 1983; Gosselin *et al.,* 1984). Because of the danger of aspiration, emesis or gastric lavage should be avoided unless the risks are justified by the presence of additional toxic substances in the petroleum. Catharsis may be induced with magnesium or sodium sulfate. Antibiotics are used if there is a specific indication, such as bacterial pneumonitis. Epinephrine and related substances should be avoided, because they may induce cardiac arrhythmias. Treatment should include correction of imbalances of fluid and electrolytes.

Long-term exposure to gasoline has become a concern because numerous underground gasoline storage tanks leak, and their contents eventually may enter the drinking water.

Halogenated Hydrocarbons

The excellent solvent properties and low flammability of halogenated hydrocarbons have placed them among the most widely used industrial solvents. Several low-molecular-weight hydrocarbons are found in drinking water. Some of these, such as chloroform, bromodichloromethane, dibromochloromethane, and bromoform, are produced from naturally occurring precursors during chlorination of water; others, such as carbon tetrachloride, dichloromethane, and 1,2-dichloroethane, do not appear to arise from such treatment. Filtration or treatment of water with charcoal prior to chlorination effectively reduces formation of chlorinated hydrocarbons. However, the halogenated hydrocarbons are common at toxic waste sites, and thus they all have the potential to enter the supply of drinking water. Because some of these compounds have been shown to be carcinogenic in animals and because correlations have been reported between the chlorination of water and the incidence of cancer of the colon, rectum, and bladder, there is a cause for concern about the exposure of a very large percentage of the population to these chemicals in drinking water. Because the halogenated hydrocarbons are extremely soluble in lipid, they are readily absorbed after inhalation or ingestion. Like most other organic solvents, halogenated hydrocarbons depress the CNS.

Carbon Tetrachloride. Carbon tetrachloride (CCl_4) has been used for medical purposes and was once commonly employed as a spot remover and carpet cleaner; however, its use for these purposes has now been abandoned because safer alternatives are available. However, it is still used in the fumigation of grain and as an insecticide.

Transient exposure to toxic concentrations of CCl_4 vapor results in the following symptoms: irritation of the eyes, nose, and throat; nausea and vomiting; a sense of fullness in the head; dizziness; and headache. If the exposure is soon terminated, symptoms usually disappear within a few hours. Continued exposure or absorption of larger quantities of the chemical may cause stupor, convulsions, coma, or death from CNS depression. Sudden death may occur from ventricular fibrillation or depression of vital medullary centers.

Delayed toxic effects of CCl_4 include nausea, vomiting, abdominal pain, diarrhea, and hematemesis. The most serious delayed toxic effects of CCl_4 result from its hepatotoxic and nephrotoxic actions. Signs and symptoms of hepatic injury may appear after a delay of several hours or 2 to 3 days and may occur in the absence of earlier severe effects on the CNS. Biochemical evidence of hepatic injury often includes greatly elevated activities of transaminases and a variety of other hepatic enzymes in plasma. Alkaline phosphatase activity is, however, only slightly elevated. The chief histological abnormalities include hepatic steatosis and hepatic centrilobular necrosis.

The mechanism of CCl_4-induced hepatic injury has interested many investigators (*see* Kalf *et al.*, 1987), and the compound has become the reference substance for all hepatotoxic compounds. Injury produced by CCl_4 seems to be mediated by a reactive metabolite—trichloromethyl free radical ($\cdot CCl_3$)—formed by the homolytic cleavage of CCl_4, or by an even more reactive species—trichloromethylperoxy free radical ($Cl_3COO\cdot$)—formed by the reaction of $\cdot CCl_3$ with O_2 (Slater, 1982). This biotransformation is catalyzed by a cytochrome P450-dependent monooxygenase. Thus, agents such as DDT and phenobarbital, which induce such enzymes, strikingly enhance the hepatotoxic effects of CCl_4. Conversely, agents that inhibit the drug-metabolizing activity diminish the hepatotoxicity of CCl_4. Biotransformation of CCl_4 to the reactive intermediate is a reductive rather than an oxidative reaction. As a result, it is slower at high oxygen tensions.

The toxicity produced by CCl_4 is thought to be due to the reaction of free radicals ($\cdot CCl_3$ or $Cl_3COO\cdot$) with lipids and proteins; however, the relative importance of interactions with various tissue constituents in producing injury is controversial. The free radical causes the peroxidation of the polyenoic lipids of the endoplasmic reticulum and the generation of secondary free radicals derived from these lipids—a chain reaction. This destructive lipid peroxidation leads to breakdown of membrane structure and function, and, if a sufficient quantity of CCl_4 has been consumed, the intracellular cytoplasmic Ca^{2+} increases, resulting in cell death (Plaa, 1991; Kalf *et al.*, 1987; Recknagel *et al.*, 1989). Lipid peroxidation leads to a unique series of nonenzymatic arachidonic acid metabolites, dubbed *isoprostanes* (*see* Chapter 26), in parallel with CCl_4-induced hepatotoxicity in laboratory animals; these agents may serve a diagnostic role in identification of lipid peroxidation in human beings (Morrow *et al.*, 1990, 1994; Roberts and Morrow, 1994). Kupffer cells also participate in the mechanism of carbon tetrachloride toxicity, probably by releasing chemoattractants for neutrophils that produce more oxidative stress (Edwards *et al.*, 1993).

Individuals recovering from acute ingestion of ethanol seem more susceptible to the hepatotoxic properties of halogenated hydrocarbons. Other alcohols, such as isopropanol, have an even

greater ability to potentiate such effects of CCl_4 (Plaa, 1991). This interaction between isopropanol and CCl_4 was highlighted by an industrial accident in an isopropanol packaging plant, where workers exposed to both agents were adversely affected (Folland *et al.*, 1976).

As hepatic injury develops, signs of renal damage also may be observed and may dominate the clinical picture. Mild poisoning in human beings may be characterized by a reversible oliguria lasting only a few days. In nonfatal poisoning, recovery of renal function has been reported to occur in three phases. In the first phase, after 1 to 3 days, oliguria stops but concentrations of creatinine and urea in plasma remain elevated. The second phase starts with a rapid decline in these plasma concentrations. In the third phase, about 1 month after the initial injury, renal blood flow and glomerular filtration begin to improve, and renal function is recovered after 100 to 200 days.

Emergency treatment of CCl_4 poisoning should be initiated promptly in any person suspected of having absorbed toxic quantities of the compound. The individual exposed to toxic vapor should be moved to fresh air. Gastrointestinal decontamination should be considered depending on the clinical situation; activated charcoal would probably be the best treatment method. If the patient is first seen in the stage of advanced CNS depression, every effort should be made to prevent hypoxia. Under no circumstances should sympathomimetic drugs be used because of the danger of producing serious arrhythmias in the sensitized myocardium.

Treatment of the acute hepatic and renal insufficiency caused by CCl_4 is difficult. Although hepatic insufficiency is a prominent feature of CCl_4 poisoning, renal failure is the most frequent cause of death. Even though the presenting signs and symptoms may be associated with functional impairment of the liver, renal function should be observed closely and oliguria or anuria anticipated.

Other Halogenated Hydrocarbons. Chloroform, dichloromethane (methylene chloride), trichloroethylene, tetrachloroethylene (perchlorethylene), 1,1,1-trichloroethane, and 1,1,2-trichloroethane produce many of the same toxic effects as does CCl_4 (Bruckner and Warren, 2001). All of these compounds produce CNS depression, and some have been used as inhalational anesthetics. They also potentially can sensitize the heart to arrhythmias produced by catecholamines. The hepatotoxic potential is highest with chloroform and 1,1,2-trichloroethane, and least with trichloroethylene, tetrachloroethylene, 1,1,1-trichloroethane, and dichloromethane; chloroform may be hepatotoxic because it is metabolized to phosgene (Pohl *et al.*, 1978). Chloroform, 1,1,2-trichloroethane, and tetrachloroethylene also are nephrotoxic. Because they produce less organ damage than do CCl_4 and chloroform, 1,1,1-trichloroethane, tetrachloroethylene, and trichloroethylene are widely used as dry-cleaning agents and industrial solvents, and dichloromethane is used as a paint stripper. Dichloromethane has an additional toxic effect because it is metabolized to CO by cytochrome P450 (Kubic and Anders, 1975). Many of these chlorinated hydrocarbon solvents produce hepatic cancer in mice; this effect has not been demonstrated in human beings.

Between 1961 and 1980, Great Britain reported 330 poisonings and 17 deaths caused by inhalation of trichloroethylene, tetrachloroethylene, and 1,1,1-trichloroethane, the three most commonly used solvents in industry (McCarthy and Jones,

1983). Deaths were due to deep narcosis, aspiration of vomitus during anesthesia, or cardiac arrhythmias (Jones and Winter, 1983). Signs of hepatotoxicity were not observed. Exposure to high concentrations of trichloroethylene has been associated with trigeminal neuropathy (Annau, 1981); long-term exposure of workers to halogenated hydrocarbon solvents has resulted in behavioral alterations (Annau, 1981; Lindstrom, 1982).

Chlorinated hydrocarbons, like the chlorofluorocarbons, have a detrimental effect on the ozone layer that shields the earth from solar radiation. Ultraviolet radiation is important in the etiology of skin cancer. The use of these chemicals is decreasing to comply with the Montreal Protocol, an international agreement to phase out the use of ozone-depleting chemicals.

Aliphatic Alcohols

Ethanol is discussed in Chapter 18.

Methanol. Methanol (methyl alcohol or wood alcohol) is a common industrial solvent. It also is used as an antifreeze fluid, a solvent for shellac and some paints and varnishes, and a component of paint removers. Solid, canned fuels contain methanol. As an adulterant, it renders unpotable and tax free the ethanol that is used for cleaning, paint removal, and other purposes.

The absorption and distribution of methanol and ethanol are similar. In addition, methanol is metabolized in human beings by the same enzymes that metabolize ethanol—alcohol dehydrogenase and aldehyde dehydrogenase—to toxic intermediates, formaldehyde and formic acid (Figure 68–4) (Tephly *et al.,* 1979). Oxidation of methanol, like

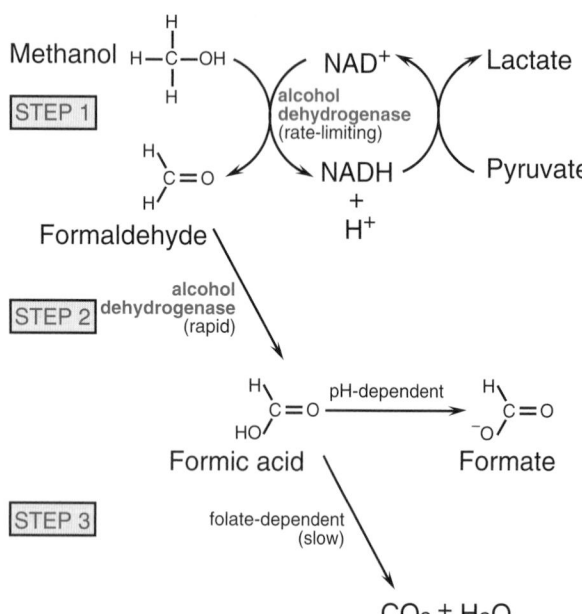

Figure 68–4. Metabolism of methanol to toxic intermediates, formaldehyde and formic acid.

that of ethanol, proceeds at a rate that is independent of its concentration in the blood. However, this rate is only one-seventh that of the oxidation of ethanol, and complete oxidation and excretion of methanol thus usually require several days.

Methanol causes less inebriation than does ethanol; indeed, inebriation is not a prominent symptom of methanol intoxication unless a very large amount is consumed or ethanol also is ingested. An asymptomatic latent period of 8 to 36 hours may precede the onset of symptoms of intoxication. If ethanol is imbibed simultaneously in sufficient amounts, signs and symptoms of methanol poisoning may be considerably delayed or, on occasion, even averted. In such cases ethanol intoxication is prominent, and ingestion of methanol may not be suspected.

Signs and symptoms of methanol poisoning include headache, vertigo, vomiting, severe upper abdominal pain, back pain, dyspnea, motor restlessness, cold clammy extremities, blurring of vision, and hyperemia of the optic disc. Blood pressure is usually unaffected. The pulse is slow in severely ill patients.

The most pronounced laboratory finding is severe anion-gap metabolic acidosis—the result of oxidation of methanol to formic acid, which accumulates (Jacobson and McMartin, 1986). Moderate ketonemia and acetonuria also are evident. Despite the severe acidosis, Kussmaul respiration is not common because of respiratory depression caused by the intoxication. Coma can develop with amazing rapidity in relatively asymptomatic subjects. In moribund patients the respiration is slow, shallow, gasping, and "fish-mouth." Death, which usually is due to respiratory failure, may be sudden, or it may occur after many hours of coma.

Pancreatic necrosis has been observed at autopsy, and pancreatic injury is believed to cause the severe abdominal pain that frequently accompanies methanol intoxication (Kaplan, 1962).

Visual disturbances, the most distinctive aspect of methanol poisoning in human beings, become evident soon after the onset of acidosis. Dilated, unreactive pupils and dim vision are characteristic. The ocular lesion, which involves chiefly the ganglion cells of the retina, is a destructive inflammation followed by atrophy. In the short term, the retina is congested and edematous, and the edges of the optic disc may be blurred (Gosselin *et al.,* 1984). The final result is bilateral blindness, which usually is permanent. Ocular toxicity appears to be caused specifically by elevated concentrations of formic acid, which in turn is related to low hepatic tetrahydrofolate. Death from methanol is nearly always preceded by blindness. As little as 15 ml of methanol has caused blindness; ingestion of 70 to 100 ml usually is fatal unless the patient is treated.

The severity of most symptoms of methanol poisoning is thought to be proportional to the acidosis, and correction of acidosis is thus a keystone of proper therapy. In addition, inhibition of methanol metabolism decreases the concentrations of formaldehyde and formic acid in the blood and thereby decreases toxicity. This is accomplished with ethanol, acting as a competitive substrate. Because ethanol has about a 100-fold greater affinity for alcohol dehydrogenase than does methanol, competition by ethanol is effective. In practice, a blood ethanol concentration of 1 g per liter is optimal. A loading dose of ethanol (0.6 g/kg) should be administered as soon as the diagnosis of a significant ingestion has been made, and an infusion of ethanol (about 10 g per hour in an adult) is begun to maintain the desired concentration. Hemodialysis should be initiated as soon as possible after the administration of ethanol in patients with acidosis or who have blood methanol concentrations in excess of 500 mg per liter. Dialysis removes the methanol and corrects the acidosis that may be resistant to administration of bicarbonate. Because ethanol also will be removed by dialysis, the rate of its infusion should be increased by about 6 g per hour. 4-Methylpyrazole is a specific inhibitor of alcohol dehydrogenase and has been used as an antidote in experimental animals (McMartin *et al.,* 1980). Folate and leucovorin, an active metabolite of folic acid, also have been used in an attempt to enhance the rate of metabolism of formate (Noker *et al.,* 1980). Neurological damage, characterized by permanent motor dysfunction similar to parkinsonism (LeWitt and Martin, 1988), may follow methanol poisoning; levodopa may relieve the rigidity and hypokinesis (Guggenheim *et al.,* 1971).

Isopropanol. Isopropanol, used for rubbing alcohol, in hand lotions, and in deicing and antifreeze preparations, is occasionally the cause of accidental or intentional poisoning. Like ethanol and methanol, isopropanol is a CNS depressant, but it does not produce retinal damage or acidosis as methanol does.

In adults, the probable lethal dose of isopropanol is about 250 ml of a 95% weight-to-volume solution; it is thus more toxic than ethanol. While the signs and symptoms of isopropanol toxicity resemble those of ethanol toxicity, there are notable differences. Isopropanol produces a more prominent gastritis, with pain, nausea, vomiting, and hemorrhage. Vomiting with aspiration is a serious threat and dangerous complication. Isopropanol intoxication lasts longer because the compound is oxidized more slowly than ethanol (Gosselin *et al.,* 1984) and because its major metabolite, acetone, is also a CNS depressant. Ketoacidosis and ketones in urine (without glucosuria) support the diagnosis. As with the other alcohols, hemodialysis is useful for removing isopropanol from the body.

Glycols

In addition to their use as heat exchangers, antifreeze formulations, hydraulic fluids, or chemical intermediates, glycols also are used as solvents for pharmaceuticals, food additives, cosmetics, and lacquers.

Ethylene Glycol. Ethylene glycol ($HOCH_2CH_2OH$) is widely used as antifreeze for automobile radiators, and such products are the usual cause of ethylene glycol poisonings. Like ethanol, ethylene glycol produces CNS depression. Patients who ingest large quantities develop narcosis, which may lead to coma and death. In addition to the CNS depression, ethylene glycol produces severe renal injury; most victims experience acute renal failure. Those who die from uremia exhibit marked renal disease, including destruction of epithelial cells, interstitial edema, focal hemorrhagic necrosis in the cortex, extensive hydropic degeneration, numerous cellular casts, and oxalate crystals in the convoluted tubules (Gosselin *et al.,* 1984).

The initial step in the oxidation of ethylene glycol to the monoaldehyde (glycoaldehyde) is mediated by alcohol dehydrogenase; oxidation of glycoaldehyde to the major acidic metabolite, glycolic acid, is catalyzed by aldehyde dehydrogenase. Both of these oxidative steps produce NADH from NAD, thus shifting the redox potential and favoring the production of lactate from pyruvate. Glycolic acid is further metabolized to glyoxylic acid and then to oxalic acid ($HOOCCOOH$). The ethylene glycol probably causes the initial CNS depression; oxalate and the other intermediates seem to be responsible for nephrotoxicity. Typical crystals of calcium oxalate are often seen in the urine and may be an early clue to the diagnosis of ethylene glycol poisoning. Glycolic acid and lactic acid are responsible for most of the metabolic acidosis (Gabow *et al.,* 1986).

The specific treatment of poisoning with ethylene glycol is similar to that for methanol poisoning. Metabolic acidosis is treated with sodium bicarbonate. Ethanol is used as a competitive substrate for alcohol dehydrogenase to decrease the rate of formation of toxic metabolites. 4-Methylpyrazole, a more effective experimental inhibitor of alcohol dehydrogenase, may be superior to ethanol (Baud *et al.,* 1988). Hemodialysis is effective in removing unmetabolized ethylene glycol and in correcting the acidosis. Parenteral administration of Ca^{2+} is recommended for muscle spasms, which may develop because of chelation of Ca^{2+} by the oxalate formed in the biotransformation of ethylene glycol.

Diethylene Glycol. Diethylene glycol ($HOCH_2CH_2$-OCH_2CH_2OH) is used in lacquer, cosmetics, antifreeze, and lubricants and as a softening agent and plasticizer. Its toxicity was a major problem only when the compound was used in the 1930s as a solvent in a preparation of sulfanilamide. In that incident, 105 of 353 children who ingested the sulfanilamide–diethylene glycol preparation died of renal damage. Effects of diethylene glycol resemble those of ethylene glycol, and intoxication should be treated similarly.

Propylene Glycol. The physical properties of propylene glycol ($CH_3CHOHCH_2OH$) are similar to those of ethylene glycol, but it is much less toxic. For this reason, propylene glycol is used as a solvent for drugs, cosmetics, lotions, and ointments; in food materials; as a plasticizer; in antifreeze formulations; as a heat exchanger; and in hydraulic fluids. Like ethanol, its primary pharmacological action is to produce CNS depression; however, its elimination is slower and its actions are thus prolonged.

Glycol Ethers. Glycol ethers are components of films, insulation for high voltage wires, paints, fingernail polish, fuel deicers, inks, etc., and are used in the production of semiconductors. Prolonged inhalation of ethylene glycol monomethyl ether and ethylene glycol monoethyl ether by laboratory animals can induce testicular atrophy and infertility (Bruckner and Warren, 2001). In addition, these glycol ethers are teratogenic in rats and rabbits. Both ethylene glycol ethers are metabolized by alcohol dehydrogenase to alkoxyacids. Because methoxyacetic acid also produces testicular toxicity in male rats, it appears that alkoxyacids are responsible for this toxic effect. In contrast, propylene glycol monomethyl ether, which is a poor substrate for alcohol dehydrogenase, does not produce testicular atrophy.

Aromatic Hydrocarbons

Benzene. Benzene is an excellent solvent. It is widely used for chemical syntheses and is a natural constituent of automobile fuels. However, benzene has produced serious toxic effects in human beings who were highly exposed to it.

After a short exposure to a large amount of benzene, by ingestion or by breathing concentrated vapors, the major toxic effect is on the CNS. Symptoms from mild exposure include dizziness, weakness, euphoria, headache, nausea, vomiting, tightness in the chest, and staggering. If exposure is more severe, symptoms progress to blurred vision, tremors, shallow and rapid respiration, ventricular irregularities, paralysis, and unconsciousness.

Long-term exposure to benzene usually is due to inhalation of vapor or to contact with the skin. Signs and symptoms of long-term exposure to benzene include effects on the CNS and the gastrointestinal tract (headache, loss of appetite, drowsiness, nervousness, and pallor), but the major manifestation of toxicity is aplastic anemia. Bone-marrow cells in early stages of development are the most sensitive to benzene (Andrews and Snyder, 1991), and arrest of maturation leads to gradual depletion of circulating cells.

A major concern is the relationship between long-term exposure to benzene and leukemia (Rinsky *et al.,* 1987; Mehlman, 1991). Epidemiological studies have been conducted on workers in the tire industry and in shoe factories, where benzene was used extensively. Among workers who died of exposure to benzene, death was caused by either leukemia or aplastic anemia, in approximately equal proportions. Benzene is classified by the EPA and IARC as a human carcinogen. Benzene is metabolized to a series of phenolic and ring-opened products and their conjugates (Snyder *et al.,* 1993). The aplastic anemia and leukemia probably are not due to any one metabolite but involve the concerted action of several metabolites (Snyder *et al.,* 1993). In the process of forming these metabolites, reactive intermediates are formed that covalently bind to various proteins and DNA and that may be responsible for the toxic effects of benzene on the bone marrow (Kalf *et al.,* 1987).

Toluene. Toluene ($C_6H_5CH_3$) is used widely as a solvent in paints, varnishes, glues, enamels, and lacquers and as a chemical intermediate in the synthesis of organic compounds. Toluene is a CNS depressant, and low concentrations produce fatigue, weakness, and confusion. It is for the CNS effects of solvents such as toluene that "glue sniffers" inhale the vapors of glue. Unlike benzene, toluene produces neither aplastic anemia nor leukemia. However, the solvents in glue often are mixed, and the "glue sniffer" usually is exposed to other solvents in addition to toluene.

PESTICIDES

Pesticide is a general classification that includes insecticides, rodenticides, fungicides, herbicides, and fumigants. Pesticides have had a significant impact on agriculture by increasing crop production; on human health by decreasing diseases such as malaria, yellow fever, and bubonic plague; and on economics by decreasing the work force needed to produce food.

The use of pesticides has increased tremendously since World War II. However, their use in agriculture has reached a plateau over the last 15 years and is beginning to decrease, because plants are being genetically engineered (GMOs, or genetically modified organisms) to require less pesticides. More than 1 billion pounds of pesticides are sold in the United States, and 4.5 billion pounds are sold around the world each year.

Pesticides are chemicals manufactured for the sole purpose of destroying some form of life. Selective toxicity of pesticides is extremely desirable; however, all can produce at least some toxicity in human beings.

Insecticides

While the agricultural industry is the main user of insecticides, other industries also use large amounts, and use in and around the home is substantial. Residues of insecticides often remain on produce, and people are exposed to low levels of the chemicals in food. Numerous incidents of acute poisoning from insecticides have resulted from eating food that was grossly contaminated during storage or shipping. Insecticides used in homes and gardens have caused accidental poisoning in young children.

Organochlorine Insecticides. Organochlorine insecticides include chlorinated ethane derivatives, of which DDT is the best known; cyclodienes, including chlordane, aldrin, dieldrin, heptachlor, and endrin; and other hydrocarbons, including such hexachlorocyclohexanes as lindane, toxaphene, mirex, and chlordecone (KEPONE). From the mid-1940s to the mid-1960s, organochlorine insecticides were used widely in agriculture and in programs for the control of malaria.

DDT. DDT, the most common of the chlorinated ethane derivatives, also is known as *chlorophenothane*.

DDT, CHLOROPHENOTHANE

Prior to placement of major restrictions on its use in many countries, DDT was the best known, least expensive, and probably one of the most effective synthetic insecticides. It was thus used widely after its introduction in the mid-1940s.

DDT has extremely low solubility in water and very high solubility in fat. It is readily absorbed when dissolved in oils, fats, or lipid solvents but is poorly absorbed as a dry powder or an aqueous suspension. Once absorbed, DDT concentrates in adipose tissue. Storage of DDT in the fat is protective, because it decreases the amount of the chemical at its site of toxic action—the brain. DDT crosses the placenta, and its concentration in umbilical cord blood is in the same range as that in the blood of the exposed mother (Saxena *et al.,* 1981).

Because DDT is degraded very slowly in the environment and is stored in the fat of animals, it is a prime candidate for biomagnification; that is, a series of organisms in a food chain accumulate increasingly greater quantities in their fat at each higher trophic level. Ultimately, a species at the top of a food chain is adversely affected. For example, the population of fish-eating birds has declined. The decline is attributed to thinning of the eggshell, a demonstrated result of ingesting DDT and related chlorinated hydrocarbon insecticides.

Because of the ubiquity of DDT, everyone born since the mid-1940s has had a lifetime of exposure to this insecticide and storage of it in fatty tissues. At a constant rate of intake, the concentration of DDT in adipose tissue reaches a steady-state value

and remains relatively constant. When exposure ceases, DDT is eliminated from the body slowly. Elimination has been estimated to occur at a rate of approximately 1% of stored DDT excreted per day. Prior to excretion, DDT is slowly dehalogenated and oxidized by cytochrome P450-dependent monooxygenases; one of the major excretory products is DDA (*bis*[*p*-chlorophenyl] acetic acid).

DDT has a wide margin of safety and, despite its widespread use and availability, there is no documented, unequivocal report of a fatal human poisoning from DDT. The few human deaths associated with excess exposure to DDT probably resulted from the kerosene solvent rather than the insecticide. The most prominent short-term effect of DDT is stimulation of the CNS.

Signs and symptoms of human poisoning from high doses of DDT include paresthesias of the tongue, lips, and face; apprehension; hypersusceptibility to stimuli; irritability; dizziness; tremor; and tonic and clonic convulsions (Ecobichon, 2001). The mechanism of action of DDT on the CNS is not completely known. The compound is capable of altering the transport of Na^+ and K^+ across axonal membranes, resulting in an increased negative afterpotential, prolonged action potentials, repetitive firing after a single stimulus, and spontaneous trains of action potentials (Narahashi, 1983).

In laboratory animals, intravenous administration of DDT causes death by ventricular fibrillation. Apparently, DDT shares with other chlorinated hydrocarbons a tendency to sensitize the myocardium, and, through its action on the CNS and adrenal medulla, it may produce the stimulus necessary for ventricular fibrillation.

Relatively low doses of DDT induce the mixed-function oxidase system (cytochrome P450) of the hepatic endoplasmic reticulum. This effect also has been demonstrated in exterminators (Kolmodin *et al.,* 1969) and in workers in a DDT factory (Poland *et al.,* 1970). The result is altered metabolism of drugs, xenobiotics, and steroid hormones. DDT also may be responsible for the increased frequency of breakage of eggs and the status of the breeding population in certain birds (*e.g., see* Radcliffe, 1967). Induction of cytochrome P450 by DDT seems to increase metabolism of estrogens in the birds. The resulting endocrine imbalance probably affects calcium metabolism, egg laying, and nesting in such a way that total reproductive success and survival of the young may be reduced (Lundholm, 1987). To compound the problem, DDT also exerts an estrogenic effect (Kupfer and Bulger, 1982) and inhibits a Ca^{2+}–ATPase that is necessary for the calcification of eggshells (Miller *et al.,* 1976).

Human volunteers have consumed 35 mg of DDT daily, about 1000 times higher than the average human intake, for as long as 25 months without obvious ill effects (Hayes, 1963). However, there is concern that DDT might be carcinogenic following exposure to small amounts of the chemical over a long period (IARC, 1974a). Extensive use of DDT in industrial countries has not been associated with increased hepatic cancer in human beings. In a survey of the mortality of over 3800 licensed pest-control workers, no significant elevation in their standardized mortality ratio was found, but there were excess deaths from leukemia, particularly myeloid leukemia, and from cancers of the brain and lungs (Blair *et al.,* 1983).

DDT was banned in the United States in 1972 for all but essential public health use and for a few minor uses to protect crops for which no effective alternatives were available. The decision was prompted by the prospect of ecological imbalance from continued use of DDT, the uncertainty of the effect, if any, of continued prolonged exposure and storage of low concentrations of DDT in human beings, and the development of resistant strains of insects. Several other countries have taken similar action. However, DDT still is used extensively in some tropical countries to control malaria. As a result of decreased use of DDT in many countries, other pesticides have replaced DDT, but many of them are more toxic to human beings.

Methoxychlor. The structural formula of methoxychlor, a chlorinated ethane derivative, is as follows:

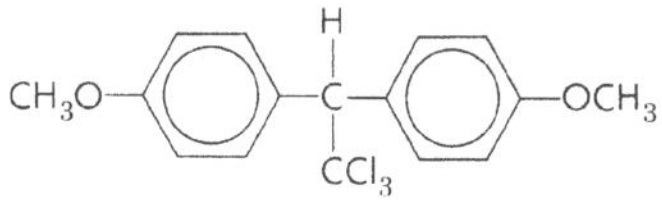

METHOXYCHLOR

The compound is used increasingly as a replacement for DDT. The attractiveness of methoxychlor is that it is much less toxic to mammals than DDT (LD_{50} in rats is 6000 mg/kg, as compared with 250 mg/kg for DDT), it is not carcinogenic, and it does not persist in the body for as long. Methoxychlor is stored in adipose tissue to about 0.2% of the extent of DDT, and its half-life in rats is only about 2 weeks, as compared with 6 months for DDT (Ecobichon, 2001). The shorter half-life is a reflection of more rapid metabolism by *O*-demethylation (Kapoor *et al.,* 1970); it is then conjugated and excreted in the urine. However, methoxychlor has estrogenic activity, and thus there is concern that methoxychlor and other environmental estrogens could produce adverse human health effects, such as increasing breast cancer in women and decreasing sperm count in men.

Chlorinated Cyclodienes. Structures of the more commonly used chlorinated cyclodienes are shown in Figure 68–5. These compounds stimulate the CNS, and many signs and symptoms of poisoning thus resemble those of DDT. However, the cellular mechanisms by which cyclodienes stimulate the CNS are different from those demonstrated for DDT. The cyclodienes act as antagonists at ionotropic receptors for gamma-aminobutyric acid (GABA), decreasing the uptake of chloride ions, which results in only partial repolarization of the neuron and a state of uncontrolled excitation. Chlorinated cyclodienes tend to produce convulsions before other, less serious signs of illness have appeared. Persons poisoned by cyclodiene insecticides have reported headache and nausea, vomiting, dizziness, and mild clonic jerking, but some patients have convulsions without warning symptoms (Hayes, 1963). Unlike DDT, cyclodiene insecticides have caused numerous fatalities as a result of acute poisoning.

An important difference between DDT and the chlorinated cyclodienes is that the latter are absorbed readily from intact skin. Cyclodienes may not pose an appreciably greater risk than DDT to the general population exposed to small quantities in food, but manipulation of concentrated solutions of a cyclodiene is more hazardous.

Like DDT, chlorinated cyclodiene insecticides are highly soluble in lipid and are stored in adipose tissue; they induce the cytochrome P450 system of the liver, are degraded slowly, persist in the environment, and undergo biomagnification through the food chain of animals. This class of insecticides has produced dose-related hepatomas in mice and has the greatest car-

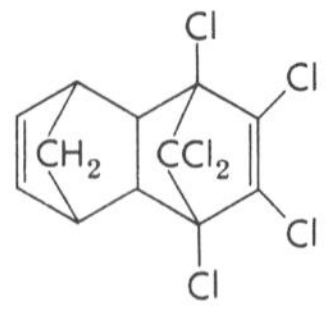

ALDRIN

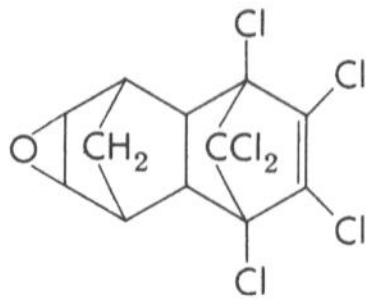

DIELDRIN*

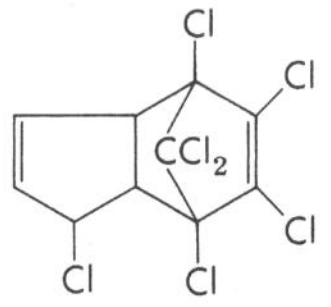

HEPTACHLOR

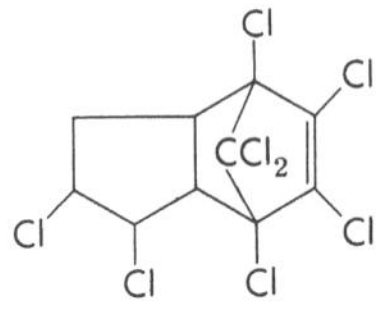

CHLORDANE

Figure 68–5. Chemical structures of some chlorinated cyclodienes.

(*Endrin is a stereoisomer of dieldrin.)

cinogenic potential among the insecticides. For these reasons aldrin and dieldrin were banned in the United States in 1974, and the use of chlordane and heptachlor for agricultural crops was similarly suspended from use in the United States in 1976.

Other Chlorinated Hydrocarbons. This group of insecticides includes lindane, toxaphene, mirex, and chlordecone. These chemicals share many properties with DDT. While they do not modify axonal conduction, they do act on presynaptic nerve terminals in the CNS and enhance the release of neurotransmitters (Shankland, 1982).

Benzene Hexachloride (BHC) and Lindane. Benzene hexachloride (more properly called hexachlorocyclohexane) has the following structural formula:

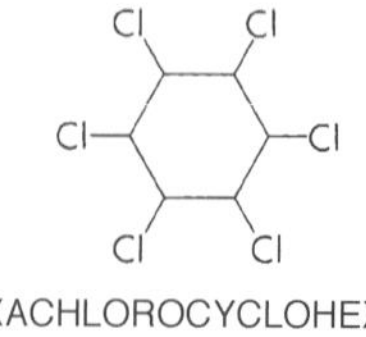

HEXACHLOROCYCLOHEXANE
(BENZENE HEXACHLORIDE)

It is a mixture of eight isomers, and the γ isomer is referred to as *lindane*. The γ isomer is the most toxic, and virtually all insecticidal activity of BHC resides in lindane. The compound is used clinically as an ectoparasiticide (*see* below). Lindane causes signs of poisoning that resemble those produced by DDT: tremors, ataxia, convulsions, and prostration. Violent tonic and clonic convulsions occur in severe cases of acute poisoning. The α and γ isomers are CNS stimulants, but the β and δ isomers are depressants. CNS stimulation appears to be due to blockade of the effects of GABA (Matsumura and Ghiasuddin, 1979). Lindane induces hepatic microsomal enzymes. Lindane and BHC have been implicated in numerous cases of aplastic anemia (Rugman and Cosstick, 1990); however, a study of 60 cases of aplastic anemia failed to demonstrate an association between the incidence of aplastic anemia and occupational exposure to pesticides (Wang and Grufferman, 1981). A number of the isomers of BHC, including lindane, have been shown to produce hepatomas in rodents (Cueto, 1980).

Biotransformation of the isomers of BHC involves the formation of chlorophenols. Compared with DDT, lindane has a relatively low persistence in the environment.

Toxaphene.   Toxaphene is a complex mixture of more than 175 C_{10} polychlorinated hydrocarbons, of which only about 20 are known (*e.g.*, heptachlorobornane) (Saleh, 1991). Like the other chlorinated hydrocarbon insecticides, the major toxicity of toxaphene is stimulation of the CNS. Toxaphene seems to be metabolized quite readily and thus has a shorter half-life than most of the other chlorinated hydrocarbon insecticides. Toxaphene has been shown to induce hepatic tumors in mice and to produce mutations (Hooper *et al.,* 1979). These observations have resulted in a dramatic reduction in the use of toxaphene.

Mirex and Chlordecone.   Mirex and chlordecone (KEPONE) are extremely persistent chlorinated hydrocarbon insecticides, and they are concentrated several thousandfold in the food chain (Waters *et al.,* 1977). Their structural formulas are as follows:

MIREX   CHLORDECONE

Like the other chlorinated hydrocarbon insecticides, mirex and chlordecone produce stimulation of the CNS, hepatic injury, and induction of the cytochrome P450 system. Testicular atrophy and reduced sperm production may be due to a direct estrogenic action of chlordecone (Eroschenko, 1981). Mirex and chlordecone are carcinogenic in laboratory animals (Cueto *et al.,* 1976; Waters *et al.,* 1977).

Gross negligence in industrial hygiene resulted in the poisoning of 76 of 148 exposed workers engaged in the manufacture of chlordecone in Hopewell, Virginia (Taylor *et al.,* 1978). These workers suffered neurological effects, characterized by tremors, ocular flutter (opsoclonus), hepatomegaly, splenomegaly, rashes, mental changes, and widened gaits. Laboratory tests showed reduced sperm counts and reduced motility of sperm. Contamination of the area surrounding the manufacturing plant

resulted in curtailment of fishing and the procurement of shellfish in the James River and threatened portions of the Chesapeake Bay.

Mirex probably is oxidized to chlordecone (Carlson *et al.,* 1976). The main metabolite of chlordecone is chlordecone alcohol, which appears in human bile as glucuronic acid conjugates (Guzelian, 1982). The major route of elimination of chlordecone is in the stool. Cholestyramine (*see* Chapter 36) administered to poisoned patients increases the fecal excretion of chlordecone 3- to 18-fold, shortens its half-life in blood from 140 to 80 days, and enhances the rate of recovery from toxic manifestations (Cohn *et al.,* 1978). Fecal chlordecone originates from both biliary and intestinal excretion (Guzelian, 1982). In human beings, only 5% to 10% of the chlordecone excreted into bile appears in the stool, which indicates extensive intestinal reabsorption of the chemical (Cohn *et al.,* 1978); bile appears to enhance such reabsorption greatly (Boylan *et al.,* 1979). Thus, cholestyramine may enhance intestinal excretion of chlordecone by binding constituents of bile in the intestinal lumen. Chlordecone has been detected in the milk of women, cows, and rats; milk from contaminated cows can be a source of human exposure.

Organophosphorus Insecticides.   Organophosphorus insecticides have largely replaced the chlorinated hydrocarbons. The organophosphates do not persist in the environment and have an extremely low carcinogenic potential; however, they have a much higher acute toxicity in human beings. In fact, parathion is the pesticide most frequently involved in fatal poisoning. The pharmacology and toxicology of these agents are discussed in Chapter 8.

Carbamate Insecticides.   The carbamate insecticides resemble the organophosphates in many ways. The most common of these agents is carbaryl; because carbaryl and related compounds are inhibitors of cholinesterase, they too are discussed in Chapter 8.

Botanical Insecticides.   *Pyrethrum* and structurally related agents are used as botanical insecticides. Pyrethrum is an allergenic, crude extract obtained from flowers of the pyrethrum plant, *Chrysanthemum cincerariaefolium. Pyrethrin* is a much more refined extract containing the six naturally occurring pyrethrins. The greatest insecticidal activity of this resides in pyrethrin I. Its structural formula is as follows:

PYRETHRIN I

Pyrethroids, synthetic pyrethrin derivatives, and pyrethrins are used in many household insecticides because of their rapid action. Their mechanism of action on neuronal membranes is to keep the sodium channel open for unusually long times, causing a prolonged flow of sodium current. The prolonged sodium current elevates and prolongs the depolarization afterpotential, which reaches the threshold membrane potential to initiate repetitive afterdischarges (Narahashi *et al.,* 1998).

Pyrethroids are much more toxic to insects than to mammals, due to species differences in the sodium channels. Pyrethrum generally is rated as the safest insecticide because its primary toxicity is low. The low toxicity of pyrethroids in mammals is due largely to their rapid biotransformation by ester hydrolysis and/or hydroxylation (Aldridge, 1983). The slow biotransformation of pyrethrum in insects is further decreased by its formulation with piperonyl butoxide (which inhibits cytochrome P450), which increases insecticidal efficacy. Unlike mammals, aquatic organisms are extremely sensitive to pyrethroids (Khan, 1983).

The allergenic properties of pyrethrum are marked in comparison with other pesticides. Many cases of contact dermatitis and respiratory allergy have been reported. Persons sensitive to ragweed pollen are particularly prone to such reactions. Preparations containing pyrethrins or synthetic pyrethroids are far less likely to cause allergic reactions than are the preparations made from pyrethrum powder.

Rotenone is obtained from the roots of plants such as *Derris* and *Lonchocarpus*. It was first used to paralyze fish before being used as an insecticide. Rotenone has the following structural formula:

ROTENONE

Human poisoning by rotenone is rare. The compound has been applied directly to treat head lice, scabies, and other ectoparasites. Local effects include conjunctivitis, dermatitis, pharyngitis, and rhinitis. Oral ingestion of rotenone produces gastrointestinal irritation, nausea, and vomiting. Inhalation of the dust is more hazardous; it can cause respiratory stimulation followed by depression and convulsions. Rotenone inhibits the oxidation of NADH to NAD. Consequently, it blocks the oxidation by NAD of substrates such as glutamate, α-ketoglutarate, and pyruvate.

Nicotine is one of the most toxic insecticides (*see* Chapter 9). Poisoning is followed by salivation and vomiting (from ganglionic stimulation), muscular weakness (from stimulation followed by depression at the neuromuscular junction), and, ultimately, clonic convulsions and cessation of respiration (effects on the CNS).

Avermectins.   Avermectins were isolated from a culture of the actinomycete, *Streptomyces avermitilis,* in soil. *Ivermectin,* a synthetic analog, was developed as an insecticide. It is effective against various insects, but also various parasites. Its pharmacological and toxicological effects are described in Chapter 42.

Insecticides Used as Ectoparasiticides.   The term *ectoparasiticides* denotes drugs that are used against animal parasites. In human beings, these are primarily pediculocides and miticides.

Lindane (*gamma benzene hexachloride;* KWELL, SCABENE, others) (*see* above) is a miticide used for the treatment of scabies. It is employed in 1% concentration in a cream, lotion, or shampoo. The mixture is applied in a thin layer over the entire cutaneous surface (from the neck down) (30 g of cream for an adult) and is not removed for 8 to 12 hours. Pruritus is usually relieved within 24 hours, and the great majority of patients do not require a second treatment. If necessary, however, second and third applications can be made at weekly intervals. The drug also is a very active pediculocide and is effective in the treatment of pediculosis pubis, capitis, and corporis. A single application of the 1% cream, lotion, or shampoo usually suffices to eradicate the ectoparasite. Lindane also is used to treat infestation by *Phthirus pubis* (crab lice).

Malathion is an organophosphate insecticide. The general pharmacology of the anticholinesterases is discussed in Chapter 8. Malathion is rapidly pediculocidal and niticidal; lice and their eggs (nits) are killed within 3 seconds by 0.003% and 0.06% malathion in acetone, respectively. The pharmaceutical preparation contains 78% isopropanol. Malathion (PRIODERM) is available outside of the United States for the treatment of head lice and nits. It is gently rubbed onto the scalp and left on for 8 to 12 hours, after which the hair is shampooed and combed. A second application may be made after 7 to 9 days if necessary.

Benzyl benzoate is a relatively harmless substance that in high concentration is toxic to *Acarus scabiei*. The compound has been used widely in the treatment of scabies and is also useful in the treatment of pediculosis. In the treatment of scabies, a 26% to 30% lotion is applied to the entire body from the neck down after thorough cleansing. When the first application is dry, a second coat is applied. The residue is washed off after 24 hours.

Crotamiton (*N*-ethyl-*o*-crotonotoluidide; EURAX) is an effective scabicide. It is available for topical application. Crotamiton occasionally causes irritation, especially on inflamed skin or when applied over a prolonged period of time; it also can cause sensitization. Paradoxically, the preparations also have antipruritic properties.

An emulsion of tetrahydronaphthalene and copper oleate is promoted as a pediculocide and niticide, but its true efficacy remains to be determined.

Thiabendazole can be applied to the skin for the treatment of cutaneous larva migrans (*see* Chapter 42). It has scabicidal activity, for which it is used outside the United States. It also is reputed to be mildly antifungal.

Fumigants

Fumigants are used to control insects, rodents, and soil nematodes. They exert pesticidal action in gaseous form and are used because they can penetrate otherwise-inaccessible areas. Agents used to protect stored foodstuffs include hydrogen cyanide, acrylonitrile (an organic cyanide, $CH_2=CHCN$), carbon disulfide, carbon tetrachloride, chloropicrin, ethylene dibromide, ethylene oxide, methyl bromide, and phosphine.

Cyanide.   Cyanide [hydrocyanic acid (HCN), prussic acid] is one of the most rapidly acting poisons; victims may die within minutes of exposure. Hydrogen cyanide gas is used to fumigate ships and buildings and to sterilize soil. Because of its ability to form complexes with metals, cyanide is used in metallurgy, electroplating, and metal cleaning. In the home, cyanides are present in silver polish, insecticides, rodenticides, and cyanide-containing plants (cassava) and fruit seeds (apple, apricot, almond, *etc.*). The major toxicity of *laetrile,* a once popular "cancer cure," is due to its cyanogenic glycoside. Cytochrome P450–dependent monooxygenases liberate cyanide from organic nitriles (Willhite and Smith, 1981), as do glutathione *S*-transferases from organic thiocyanates (Okawa and Casida, 1971); cyanide also is a metabolite of nitroprusside (Cottrell *et al.,* 1978). Combustion of nitrogen-containing plastics may result in release of HCN. Fire on board airplanes killed 119 passengers in Paris in 1973 and 303 pilgrims in Riyadh, Saudi Arabia, in 1980 due to combustion of plastic material that produced HCN (Weger, 1983). Cyanide also is used for executions in so-called gas chambers and was used for more than 900 religious "suicide-murders" in Guyana in 1978.

Cyanide has a very high affinity for iron in the ferric state. When absorbed, it reacts readily with the trivalent iron of cytochrome oxidase in mitochondria; cellular respiration is thus inhibited, resulting in lactic acidosis and cytotoxic hypoxia. Since utilization of oxygen is blocked, venous blood is oxygenated and is almost as bright red as arterial blood. Respiration is stimulated because chemoreceptive cells respond as they do to decreased oxygen. A transient stage of CNS stimulation with hyperpnea and headache is observed; finally hypoxic convulsions occur, and death is due to respiratory arrest. Most people with acute exposure to cyanide usually die promptly or fully recover; however, cases of neurological sequelae including extrapyramidal syndromes, personality changes, and memory defects have been reported in surviving victims.

Treatment of cyanide poisoning must be rapid to be effective. Diagnosis may be aided by the characteristic odor of cyanide (oil of bitter almonds). Because toxicity results from binding to the ferric form of cytochrome oxidase, treatment is aimed at prevention or reversal of such binding by providing a large pool of ferric iron to compete for cyanide. An effective mechanism is to administer substances, such as nitrite, that oxidize hemoglobin to methemoglobin. Amyl nitrite is usually administered by inhalation, while a solution of sodium nitrite is prepared for intravenous administration (10 ml of a 3% solution). Methemoglobin competes with cytochrome oxidase for the cyanide ion; the reaction favors methemoglobin because of mass action. Cyanmethemoglobin is formed, and cytochrome oxidase is restored. Alternatively, 4-dimethylaminophenol, which also oxidizes hemoglobin to methemoglobin, can be used in a dose of 3 mg/kg intravenously (Weger, 1983). Cobalt compounds have a high affinity for cyanide (Way, 1984), and Co_2EDTA currently is being used in some countries to treat cyanide poisoning in human beings (Cottrell *et al.,* 1978; Weger, 1983). Similarly, hydroxocobalamin can be used to treat cyanide toxicity, because it combines with cyanide to form cyanocobalamin (vitamin B_{12}).

The major mechanism for removing cyanide from the body is its enzymatic conversion, by the mitochondrial enzyme rhodanese (transsulfurase), to thiocyanate, which is relatively nontoxic. To accelerate detoxication, sodium thiosulfate is administered intravenously (50 ml of a 25% aqueous solution), and the thiocyanate formed is readily excreted in the urine.

$$Na_2S_2O_3 + CN^- \xrightarrow{\text{Rhodanese}} SCN^- + Na_2SO_3 \qquad (68\text{--}4)$$

Way and associates (1972) demonstrated that nitrite increases the LD_{50} of potassium cyanide in mice from 11 mg/kg to 21 mg/kg; administration of thiosulfate increases the value to 35 mg/kg, while nitrite followed by thiosulfate increases the LD_{50} to 52 mg/kg. Many cases of acute cyanide poisoning in human beings have been treated successfully with such therapy.

Oxygen alone, even at hyperbaric pressures, has only a slight protective effect in cyanide poisoning; however, oxygen dramatically potentiates the protective effects of thiosulfate or of nitrite and thiosulfate (Way *et al.,* 1972). The mechanism for this action is not clear, but the intracellular oxygen tension may be high enough to cause nonenzymatic oxidation of reduced cytochromes, or oxygen may displace cyanide from cytochrome oxidase by mass action.

If cyanide has been ingested, gastric lavage should follow, not precede, initiation of more specific treatment.

Methyl Bromide. Methyl bromide is used as an insecticidal fumigant and in some fire extinguishers. It is said to have been responsible for more deaths in California in the 1960s among occupationally exposed persons than all of the organophosphate insecticides (Hine, 1969). Because methyl bromide is so toxic, chloropicrin (CCl_3NO_2), a powerful stimulator of lacrimation, is added to fumigants as a warning of methyl bromide exposure.

Major signs and symptoms of intoxication with methyl bromide are referable to the CNS. These include malaise, headache, visual disturbances, nausea, and vomiting. Death usually occurs during a convulsion. After severe respiratory exposure, pulmonary edema may prove fatal. The high affinity of methyl bromide for sulfhydryl groups may have a role in its toxic action. Sulfhydryl agents may thus be beneficial as antidotes in poisoning with methyl bromide.

Dibromochloropropane and Ethylene Dibromide. Dibromochloropropane ($ClCH_2CHBrCH_2Br$) and ethylene dibromide (1,2-dibromoethane) are soil fumigants used to control nematodes. In human beings, they produce moderate depression of the CNS and pulmonary congestion after exposure by inhalation, and they cause acute gastrointestinal distress and pulmonary edema after ingestion. Both agents cause gastric carcinoma in rats and mice (Powers *et al.,* 1975; IARC, 1977). Dibromochloropropane causes sterility and/or abnormally low sperm counts in workmen engaged in its manufacture. Use of both agents is being decreased because of their carcinogenicity and their adverse effects on reproductive function.

Phosphine. Phosphine (PH_3) is a fumigant for grain; it is released gradually, in the presence of atmospheric moisture, from tablets of aluminum phosphide. Phosphine is more toxic than methyl bromide; however, as less phosphine than methyl bromide is required to fumigate a given volume of grain, phosphine has proven to be safer. Severe pulmonary irritation and pulmonary edema are the main toxic effects of phosphine; hepatic and myocardial injury also are observed.

Rodenticides

Some rodenticides are quite toxic to human beings, but the toxicity of others is more selective. In some cases, selectivity is based on a unique aspect of the physiology of rodents; in others, advantage is taken of the habits of these animals. Because rodenticides can be used in baits and placed in inaccessible places, the likelihood of their contaminating the environment is much less than that of other pesticides. The toxicological problem posed by rodenticides, therefore, is primarily one of accidental or suicidal ingestion.

Warfarin.   Warfarin, one of the most frequently used rodenticides, is considered safe because its toxicity depends on repeated ingestion. However, daily intake by human beings of 1 to 2 mg/kg for 6 days has produced severe illness in an attempted suicide. Warfarin, an oral anticoagulant, is discussed in Chapter 55.

Red Squill.   The bulbs of red squill (*Urginea maritima*) have been used for many years as a relatively safe rodenticide. The active principles are *scillaren glycosides*. These glycosides, like the digitalis glycosides (*see* Chapters 34 and 35) have cardiotonic actions. Signs and symptoms associated with ingestion of large doses of red squill include vomiting and abdominal pain, blurred vision, cardiac irregularities, convulsions, and death from ventricular fibrillation. The selective rodenticidal usefulness of squill is due to the inability of rats to vomit (Lisella *et al.*, 1971). Treatment of ingestion in human beings, if indicated, is the same as for overdosage of digitalis (*see* Chapters 34 and 35).

Sodium Fluoroacetate.   Sodium fluoroacetate and fluoroacetamide are among the most potent rodenticides. Because they also are highly toxic to other animals, their use is restricted to licensed pest-control operators. Fluoroacetate produces its toxic action by inhibiting the citric acid cycle. The compound is incorporated into fluoroacetyl coenzyme A, which condenses with oxaloacetate to form fluorocitrate. Fluorocitrate inhibits the enzyme aconitase and thereby inhibits conversion of citrate to isocitrate. As might be expected, the heart and CNS are the tissues most critically involved by a general inhibition of oxidative energy metabolism. Thus, the signs and symptoms of fluoroacetate poisoning, in addition to nonspecific signs of nausea and vomiting, include cardiac irregularities, cyanosis, generalized convulsions, and death from ventricular fibrillation or respiratory failure. Provision of large quantities of acetate appears to antagonize fluoroacetate in a competitive manner; monkeys have been successfully protected from fluoroacetate poisoning by the administration of glycerol monoacetate.

Strychnine.   Strychnine is the principal alkaloid present in nux vomica, the seeds of a tree native to India, *Strychnos nuxvomica*. Nux vomica was introduced into Germany in the sixteenth century as a poison for rats and other animal pests. Its use as a pesticide persists to this day and is a source of accidental strychnine poisoning of children and of household pets. The structural formula of strychnine is as follows:

STRYCHNINE

Strychnine produces excitation of all portions of the CNS. This effect, however, does not result from direct synaptic excitation. Strychnine increases the level of neuronal excitability by selectively blocking inhibition. Nerve impulses are normally confined to appropriate pathways by inhibitory influences. When inhibition is blocked by strychnine, ongoing neuronal activity is enhanced and sensory stimuli produce exaggerated reflex effects.

Strychnine is a powerful convulsant, and the convulsion has a characteristic motor pattern. Inasmuch as strychnine reduces inhibition, including the reciprocal inhibition existing between antagonistic muscles, the pattern of convulsion is determined by the most powerful muscles acting at a given joint. In most laboratory animals, this convulsion is characterized by tonic extension of the body and of all limbs. Tonic extension is preceded and followed during the phase of postictal depression by phasic symmetrical extensor thrusts that may be initiated by any modality of sensory stimulus.

The convulsant action of strychnine is due to interference with postsynaptic inhibition that is mediated by glycine (Aprison *et al.*, 1987). Glycine is an important inhibitory transmitter to motoneurons and interneurons in the spinal cord, and strychnine acts as a selective, competitive antagonist to block the inhibitory effects of glycine at all glycine receptors (*see* Chapter 12). Well-known examples of this type of postsynaptic inhibition are the inhibitory influences existing between the motoneurons of antagonistic muscle groups and recurrent spinal inhibition mediated by the Renshaw cell. Renshaw cells are excited by intraspinal collaterals of motoneuron axons that liberate acetylcholine. Strychnine blocks recurrent inhibition at the Renshaw cell–motoneuron synapse by antagonizing the action of glycine released by the Renshaw cell. Strychnine-sensitive postsynaptic inhibition in higher centers of the CNS also is mediated by glycine.

The effects of strychnine in human beings closely resemble those described above for laboratory animals. The first effect that is noticed is stiffness of the face and neck muscles. Heightened reflex excitability soon becomes evident. Any sensory stimulus may produce a violent motor response. In the early stages this response is a coordinated extensor thrust, and in the later stages it may be a full tetanic convulsion. In this convulsion, the body is arched in hyperextension (opisthotonos) so that only the crown of the head and the heels may be touching the ground. All voluntary muscles, including those of the face, are in full contraction. Respiration ceases owing to the contraction of the diaphragm and the thoracic and abdominal muscles. Convulsive episodes may recur repeatedly with intermittent periods of depression; sensory stimulation increases the frequency and severity of the convulsions. Death results from medullary paralysis, which is due primarily to the hypoxia resulting from the periods of impaired respiration. In the early stages the patient not only is conscious but also is acutely perceptive to all stimuli. The muscle contractions are quite painful, and the patient is extremely apprehensive and fearful of impending death. If untreated, death from strychnine often occurs after the second to fifth full convulsion, but the first may be fatal if it is sustained. The combination of impaired respiration and intense muscular contractions can produce severe respiratory and metabolic acidosis.

The most urgent objectives in the treatment of strychnine poisoning are the prevention of convulsions and the support of respiration. *Diazepam* is the most useful agent for this purpose. It antagonizes the convulsions without potentiating postictal depression (Gosselin *et al.,* 1984; *see* Chapter 17). Anesthesia or neuromuscular blockade may be necessary to control resistant convulsions in severely intoxicated patients. All forms of sensory stimulation should be minimized. If adequate respiratory ventilation is not restored by the termination of convulsions, intubation and mechanical assistance are essential.

Phosphorus. White or yellow elemental phosphorus has poisoned human beings when it was spread in paste on bread to bait rodents. Shortly after ingestion, phosphorus produces severe gastrointestinal irritation, and, if the dose is sufficient, hemorrhage and cardiovascular failure may prove fatal within 24 hours. The vomitus is luminescent and has a characteristic garlic odor. If the patient survives the initial phase of gastrointestinal injury, secondary systemic poisoning and hepatic necrosis may ensue. Severe acute yellow atrophy of the liver is a delayed sequela that may prove fatal.

Long-term poisoning from phosphorus is characterized by cachexia, anemia, bronchitis, and necrosis of the mandible, the so-called phossy jaw.

Zinc Phosphide. Zinc phosphide reacts with water and HCl in the gastrointestinal tract to produce the gas phosphine (PH_3), which causes severe gastrointestinal irritation. Apparent insensitivity of dogs and cats has been attributed to the emetic qualities of zinc in animals other than rodents. Later phases of toxicity resemble poisoning by yellow elemental phosphorus.

α-Naphthylthiourea. The structural formula of α-naphthylthiourea is as follows:

α-NAPHTHYLTHIOUREA

Its selective rodenticidal properties are due to different susceptibilities of various species. The LD_{50} in rats is about 3 mg/kg, in dogs 10 mg/kg, in guinea pigs 400 mg/kg, and in monkeys 4 g/kg. The principal toxic effect in susceptible species is massive pulmonary edema and pleural effusion, apparently the result of an action on pulmonary capillaries. Microsomes from rat liver and lung release atomic sulfur from *a*-naphthylthiourea (Lee *et al.,* 1980). Pulmonary toxicity may result, at least in part, from binding of atomic sulfur to tissue macromolecules.

Sulfhydryl-blocking agents are effective antidotes in rats under some experimental conditions (Koch and Schwarze, 1956).

Thallium. Thallium sulfate is very hazardous. Because thallium is not selectively toxic for rodents and many people have been poisoned by thallium, its use is now strictly regulated in many countries. Acute poisoning is accompanied by gastrointestinal irritation, motor paralysis, and death from respiratory failure. Sublethal doses taken over a period of time redden the skin and cause alopecia, characteristic signs of thallium poisoning. Pathological changes include perivascular cuffing and degenerative changes in the brain, liver, and kidney. Neurological symptoms are prominent and include tremors, leg pains, paresthesias of the hands and feet, and polyneuritis, especially in the legs. Psychoses, delirium, convulsions, and other types of encephalopathy also may be noted. Treatment of thallium intoxication involves the oral administration of ferric ferrocyanide (Prussian blue), hemodialysis, and forced diuresis. Prussian blue binds thallium in the intestine and enhances its fecal excretion. Administration of systemic chelating agents should be avoided, because they may increase uptake of thallium into the brain (Hayes, 1982).

Herbicides

The production and use of chemicals for destruction of noxious weeds have increased markedly in the past two decades. Herbicides now exceed insecticides in quantities used and values of sales. Although some herbicidal compounds have very low toxicity in mammals, others are highly toxic and have caused human fatalities. There is an increase in concern about the health effects of herbicides because of runoff from agricultural application and entrance into the drinking water supply.

Chlorophenoxy Compounds. The compounds *2,4-dichlorophenoxyacetic acid (2,4-D)* and *2,4,5-trichlorophenoxyacetic acid (2,4,5-T),* as their salts and esters, are probably the most familiar herbicides. Their structural formulas are as follows:

2, 4-DICHLOROPHENOXYACETIC ACID
(2, 4-D)

2, 4, 5-TRICHLOROPHENOXYACETIC ACID
(2, 4, 5-T)

These two agents are used to control broad-leaf weeds in fields and to control woody plants along highways and rights-of-way; the compounds act as growth hormones in plants. Animals killed by massive doses of 2,4-D are believed to die of ventricular fibrillation. At lower doses, when death is delayed, there are various signs of neuromuscular involvement, including stiffness of the extremities, ataxia, paralysis, and, eventually, coma. Clinical reports of poisoning from chlorophenoxy herbicides are rare.

These herbicides do not accumulate in animals. They are not extensively metabolized but are actively excreted in the urine (Berndt and Koschier, 1973). Their plasma half-life in human beings is about 1 day (Gehring et al., 1970).

Chlorophenoxy herbicides have produced contact dermatitis in human beings, and a rather severe type of dermatitis, chloracne, has been observed in workers involved in the manufacture of 2,4,5-T (Poland et al., 1971). The dermatitis seems due primarily to the action of a contaminant, 2,3,7,8-tetrachlorodibenzo-p-dioxin (TCDD) (2,4-D does not contain TCDD), the structure of which is as follows:

2, 3, 7, 8-TETRACHLORODIBENZO-P-DIOXIN
(TCDD)

Exposure to TCDD occurs not only from herbicides, but also due to its release during a number of manufacturing processes, such as the burning of organochlorine compounds and in the bleaching of paper pulp.

TCDD is particularly toxic for some species. It has an LD_{50} of 0.6 μg/kg in guinea pigs, but this value is 10,000 times higher in hamsters. The mechanism of death is not known; morphological changes in the liver, thymus, and reproductive organs are observed but are not sufficiently severe to account for death. TCDD shows no toxic effect on cell cultures. TCDD is a potent inducer of aryl hydrocarbon hydroxylase, a microsomal cytochrome P450-dependent monooxygenase (Poland and Glover, 1974). It is also a very potent teratogen (Neubert et al., 1973) and has been demonstrated to be a carcinogen in laboratory animals (Van Miller et al., 1977; Kociba et al., 1978).

Accidental human exposures indicate that TCDD has low toxicity compared with that for certain species (e.g., guinea pig) (Holmstedt, 1980). Effects of TCDD poisoning in exposed people include chloracne, porphyria, hypercholesterolemia, and psychiatric disturbances (Hayes, 1982). During the Vietnam War, Agent Orange, a mixture of 2,4-D and 2,4,5-T (which was contaminated with TCDD) was sprayed over large jungle areas, and many soldiers were presumed to have been exposed to the compounds. Although controversial, epidemiological studies have not revealed any TCDD-related adverse effects on health in Vietnam veterans (Ketchum et al., 1999). There appears to be no difference in the plasma concentration of TCDD in Vietnam

veterans and non–Vietnam veterans, indicating that exposure of United States soldiers in Vietnam to TCDD was much less than suspected (Centers for Disease Control, 1988). However, several epidemiological studies have been conducted using people who were exposed to high concentrations of dioxins in the chemical industry and from chemical explosions. These studies suggest that TCDD might be carcinogenic in human beings at high exposures (Huff et al., 1994).

Dinitrophenols.   Several substituted dinitrophenols, alone or as salts of aliphatic amines or alkalies, are used in weed control. Human poisonings by dinitroorthocresol (DNOC) have been reported. The short-term toxicity of dinitrophenols is due to the uncoupling of oxidative phosphorylation. The metabolic rate of the poisoned individual can increase markedly, and the body temperature is elevated. Signs and symptoms of acute poisoning in human beings include nausea, restlessness, flushed skin, sweating, rapid respiration, tachycardia, fever, cyanosis, and, finally, collapse and coma. The illness runs a rapid course; death or recovery occurs within 24 to 48 hours. If production of heat exceeds the capacity for its dissipation, fatal hyperthermia may result. Specific treatment consists of ice baths to reduce fever, administration of oxygen, and correction of fluid and electrolyte imbalances. Salicylates, which contain a phenolic group, must be avoided during treatment for exposure to dinitrophenols.

Bipyridyl Compounds.   *Paraquat* is the most important compound in this class of herbicides from a toxicological viewpoint. The structural formula of paraquat is as follows:

PARAQUAT

Several hundred cases of accidental or suicidal fatalities from paraquat poisoning have been reported during the past decade. Pathological changes observed at autopsy are indicative of damage to the lungs, liver, and kidneys; myocarditis is sometimes present. The most striking pathological change is a widespread proliferation of fibroblastic cells in the lungs, an effect that is not dependent on the route of administration. Although ingestion of paraquat causes gastrointestinal upset within a few hours, the onset of respiratory symptoms and eventual death by respiratory distress may be delayed for several days.

A biochemical mechanism for paraquat-induced pulmonary injury has been proposed (Bus et al., 1976) (Figure 68–6). Paraquat is believed to undergo a single-electron cyclic reduction–oxidation, with subsequent formation of superoxide anion

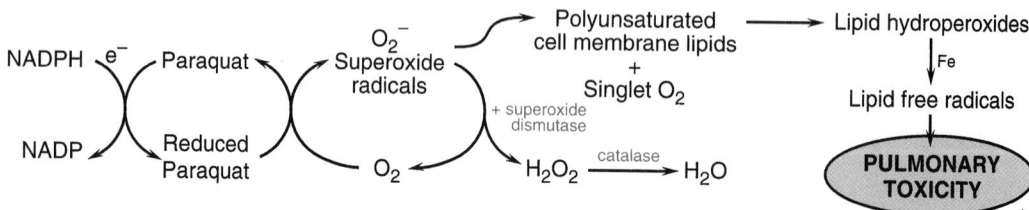

Figure 68–6. Proposed mechanism of paraquat-induced pulmonary toxicity.

radical ($O_2{}^-$). Superoxide anion radical is nonenzymatically transformed to singlet oxygen, which attacks polyunsaturated lipids associated with cell membranes to form lipid hydroperoxides. The lipid hydroperoxides are unstable in the presence of trace amounts of transition metal ions and decompose to lipid-free radicals. The chain reaction of lipid peroxidation thus initiated is somewhat similar to that described above for CCl_4 (*see* Smith, 1988).

Because of the serious, delayed pulmonary toxicity produced by paraquat, prompt treatment is important. This involves removal of paraquat from the alimentary tract by gastric lavage and the use of cathartics, prevention of further absorption (*e.g.*, by oral administration of Fuller's earth), and removal of absorbed paraquat by hemodialysis or hemoperfusion (Cavalli and Fletcher, 1977; Davies *et al.*, 1977).

A survey found that 21% of marijuana samples from the southwestern United States and 3.6% of the samples collected from the entire United States were contaminated with paraquat. The source of contamination was an aerial spraying program in Mexico. It was projected that marijuana smokers could be exposed to 0.5 mg or more of paraquat per year by inhalation. However, much of the paraquat is probably pyrolyzed as the leaves burn. No clinical case of paraquat poisoning has been recognized among marijuana smokers, although no systematic search for such cases has been undertaken (Landrigan *et al.*, 1983).

Phosphonomethyl Amino Acids. *Glyphosate* and *glufosinate* are two herbicides in this class whose chemical structures are given below:

HOOCCH₂NHCH₂P—OH   (GLYPHOSATE) (ROUND-UP)

HOOCCHCH₂CH₂P—CH₃   (GLUFOSINATE)

Both are broad-spectrum, nonselective, systemic herbicides for annual and perennial plants. Crops have been genetically engineered to make them resistant to glyphosate, and these crops thus can be sprayed to kill all undesired plants.

Glyphosate is a very nontoxic herbicide. Unfortunately, glyphosate has become a suicidal agent in some countries. Mild intoxications are characterized by gastrointestinal symptoms (nausea, vomiting, diarrhea, abdominal pain) due to mucosal irritation and injury, with resolution within 24 hours. In moderate intoxications, more severe and persistent intestinal symptoms (ulceration and hemorrhage) are seen along with hypotension, some pulmonary dysfunction, acid-base disturbance, and hepatic and renal damage. Severe poisoning is characterized by pulmonary dysfunction, renal failure, hypotension and vascular shock, cardiac arrest, repeated seizures, coma, and death (Talbot *et al.*, 1991; Tominack *et al.*, 1991). The glyphosate is formulated in a surfactant, polyoxyethylene-amine, and it is suspected that the toxicity in suicide cases is due to the surfactant rather than to the glyphosate.

Other Herbicides. There are a large number of other herbicides that, for the most part, have relatively low acute toxicities for mammals. These include carbamates (*e.g.*, *propham* and *barban*), substituted ureas (*e.g.*, *monuron* and *diuron*), triazines (*e.g.*, *atrazine* and the related compound aminotriazole), aniline derivatives (*e.g.*, *alachlor*, *propachlor*, and *propanil*), dinitroaniline derivatives (*e.g.*, *triflualin*), and benzoic acid derivatives (*e.g.*, *amiben*).

Fungicides

Fungicides, like other classes of pesticides, make up a heterogeneous group of chemical compounds. With few exceptions, the fungicides have not been the subject of detailed toxicological research. Although many compounds used to control fungal diseases on plants, seeds, and produce are rather nontoxic in the short term, there are some notable exceptions; the mercury-containing fungicides have caused the greatest concern. They have been responsible for many deaths or permanent neurological disabilities resulting from the misdirection of treated seed grains into human and animal food. The toxicities of mercury and its compounds are discussed in Chapter 67.

Dithiocarbamates. Fungicides of this group commonly are used in agriculture. They have a low order of acute toxicity, and values of the oral LD_{50} in rats range from several hundred milligrams to several grams per kilogram. Except for contact dermatitis induced by dithiocarbamate (Fisher, 1983), there is little evidence of human injury from exposure to these compounds. However, they may have some teratogenic and/or carcinogenic potential (World Health Organization, 1975). Two groups of dithiocarbamates that have been used, the *dimethyldithiocarbamates* and the *ethylenebisdithiocarbamates*, have the following general formulas:

DIMETHYLDITHIOCARBAMATES   ETHYLENEBISDITHIOCARBAMATES

The names of the fungicides are derived from the metallic cations. For example, when the cation is zinc or iron, the respective dimethyldithiocarbamate is *ziram* or *ferbam*. With manganese, zinc, or sodium as the cation in the diethyldithiocarbamate series, the respective fungicide is *maneb, zineb,* or *nabam*. Some dimethyldithiocarbamates are reported to be teratogenic in animals, and they can form nitrosamines *in vitro* and *in vivo* (IARC, 1974b; World Health Organization, 1975). The ethylenebisdithiocarbamates also are reported to be teratogenic. Furthermore, this group of compounds breaks down to form ethylenethiourea (ETU) *in vivo*, in the environment, and during cooking of foods containing their residues. ETU is carcinogenic, mutagenic, and teratogenic, as well as being an antithyroid agent (IARC, 1974b, 1976). Dithiocarbamate fungicides are analogs of *disulfiram,* and they can produce a disulfiram-like response when ethanol is ingested (*see* Chapter 18).

Hexachlorobenzene. Exposure to hexachlorobenzene results in an increase in hepatic weight, in the quantity of smooth endoplasmic reticulum, and in the activities of cytochrome P450-dependent monooxygenases (Carlson and Tardiff, 1976). Between 1955 and 1959, more than 300 human poisonings occurred in Turkey as a result of the use of hexachlorobenzene-treated wheat (Schmid, 1960). Some deaths resulted; the major syndrome was cutaneous porphyria with skin lesions, porphyrinuria, and photosensitization. Hexachlorobenzene is eliminated from the body predominantly in the feces as a result of intestinal excretion. This process can be enhanced fivefold in rhesus monkeys by the oral administration of mineral oil (Rozman et al., 1983).

Pentachlorophenol. Pentachlorophenol is used as an insecticide and a herbicide, as well as a fungicide, with major application as a wood preservative. Several cases of human poisoning have been associated with its use. The acute toxic action of pentachlorophenol in human beings and experimental animals resembles that of the nitrophenolic herbicides—a marked increase in metabolic rate as the result of uncoupling of oxidative phosphorylation. Pentachlorophenol is readily absorbed through the skin. Two cases of fatal poisonings and several nonfatal cases occurred in a hospital nursery; pentachlorophenol had been used as a fungicide in the laundry room and ultimately came in contact with infants through their diapers (Armstrong et al., 1969).

Many commercial samples of pentachlorophenol are contaminated with polychlorinated dibenzodioxins and dibenzofurans (Buser, 1975). These contaminants are generally less toxic than the tetrachlorodioxin contaminant (TCDD) in 2,4,5-T. Although pentachlorophenol is highly toxic in its own right, some studies suggest that the contaminants may be responsible for some of the untoward effects of the technical-grade product (Johnson et al., 1973; Goldstein et al., 1976). Treatment of intoxication with pentachlorophenol is similar to that for poisoning with dinitrophenols. Fecal excretion of pentachlorophenol can be enhanced by cholestyramine, which interrupts the enterohepatic circulation of the chemical (Rozman et al., 1982).

BIBLIOGRAPHY

Amdur, M.O., Dubriel, M., and Creasia, D.A. Respiratory response of guinea pigs to low levels of sulfuric acid. *Environ. Res.,* **1978,** *15*:418–423.

Aprison, M.H., Lipkowitz, K.B., and Simon, J.R. Identification of a glycine-like fragment on the strychnine molecule. *J. Neurosci. Res.* **1987,** *17*:209–213.

Armstrong, R.W., Eichner, E.R., Klein, D.E., Barthel, W.F., Bennett, J.V., Jonsson, V., Bruce, H., and Loveless, L.E. Pentachlorophenol poisoning in a nursery for newborn infants. II. Epidemiological and toxicologic studies. *J. Pediatr.,* **1969,** *75*:317–325.

Ayres, S.M., Giannelli, S. Jr., and Mueller, H. Myocardial and systemic responses to carboxyhemoglobin. *Ann. N.Y. Acad. Sci.,* **1970,** *174*:268–293.

Baud, F.J., Galliot, M., Astier, A., Bien, D.V., Garnier, R., Likforman, J., and Bismuth, C. Treatment of ethylene glycol poisoning with intravenous 4-methylpyrazole. *N. Engl. J. Med.,* **1988,** *319*:97–100.

Berndt, W.O., and Koschier, F. *In vitro* uptake of 2,4-dichlorophenoxyacetic acid (2,4,-D) and 2,4,5-trichlorophenoxyacetic acid (2,4,5-T) by renal cortical tissue of rabbits and rats. *Toxicol. Appl. Pharmacol.,* **1973,** *26*:559–570.

Blair, A., Grauman, D.J., Lubin, J.H., and Fraumeni, J.F. Jr. Lung cancer and other causes of death among licensed pesticide applicators. *J. Natl. Cancer Inst.,* **1983,** *71*:31–37.

Bokonjić, N. Stagnant anoxia and carbon monoxide poisoning. *Electroencephalogr. Clin. Neurophysiol.,* **1963,** *Suppl. 21*:1–102.

Boylan, J.J., Cohn, W.J., Egle, J.L. Jr., Blanke, R.V., and Guzelian, P.S. Excretion of chlordecone by the gastrointestinal tract: evidence for a nonbiliary mechanism. *Clin. Pharmacol. Ther.,* **1979,** *25*:579–585.

Bus, J.S., Cagen, S.Z., Olgaard, M., and Gibson, J.E. A mechanism of paraquat toxicity in mice and rats. *Toxicol. Appl. Pharmacol.,* **1976,** *35*:501–513.

Buser, H.R. Analysis of polychlorinated dibenzo-*p*-dioxins and dibenzofurans in chlorinated phenols by mass fragmentography. *J. Chromatogr.,* **1975,** *107*:295–310.

Carlson, D.A., Konyha, K.D., Wheeler, W.B., Marshall, G.P., and Zaylskie, R.G. Mirex in the environment: its degradation to kepone and related compounds. *Science,* **1976,** *194*:939–941.

Carlson, G.P., and Tardiff, R.G. Effect of chlorinated benzenes on the metabolism of foreign organic compounds. *Toxicol. Appl. Pharmacol.,* **1976,** *36*:383–394.

Cavalli, R.D., and Fletcher, K. An effective treatment for paraquat poisoning. In, *Biochemical Mechanism of Paraquat Toxicity.* (Autor, A.P., ed.) Academic Press, New York, **1977,** pp. 213–228.

Centers for Disease Control Veterans Health Studies. Serum 2,3,7,8-tetrachlorodibenzo-*p*-dioxin levels in U.S. Army Vietnam-era veterans. *JAMA,* **1988,** *260*:1249–1254.

Choi, I.S. Delayed neurologic sequelae in carbon monoxide intoxication. *Arch. Neurol.,* **1983,** *40*:433–435.

Cohn, W.J., Boylan, J.J., Blanke, R.V., Fariss, M.W., Howell, J.R., and Guzelian, P.S. Treatment of chlordecone (kepone) toxicity with cholestyramine. Results of a controlled clinical trial. *N. Engl. J. Med.,* **1978,** *298*:243–248.

Cottrell, J.E., Casthely, P., Brodie, J.D., Patel, K., Klein, A., and Turndorf, H. Prevention of nitroprusside-induced cyanide toxicity with hydroxocobalamine. *N. Engl. J. Med.,* **1978,** *298*:809–811.

Cueto, C. Jr. Consideration of the possible carcinogenicity of some pesticides. *J. Environ. Sci. Health B,* **1980,** *15*:949–975.

Cueto, C. Jr., Page, N.P., and Saffiott, U. *Report of Carcinogenesis, Bioassay of Technical Grade Chlordecone (KEPONE).* National Cancer Institute, Bethesda, MD, **1976.**

Davies, D.S., Hawksworth, G.M., and Bennett, P.N. Paraquat poisoning. *Proc. Eur. Soc. Toxicol.,* **1977,** *18*:21–26.

Edwards, M.J., Keller, B.J., Kauffman, F.C., and Thurman, R.G. The involvement of Kupffer cells in carbon tetrachloride toxicity. *Toxicol. Appl. Pharmacol.,* **1993,** *119*:275–279.

Elmes, P.C. Mesotheliomas, minerals, and man-made mineral fibres. *Thorax,* **1980,** *35*:561–563.

Eroschenko, V.P. Estrogenic activity of the insecticide chlordecone in the reproductive tract of birds and mammals. *J. Toxicol. Environ. Health,* **1981,** *8*:731–742.

Folland, D.S., Schaffner, W., Ginn, H.E., Crofford, O.B., and Mc-Murray, D.R. Carbon tetrachloride toxicity potentiated by isopropyl alcohol. Investigation of an industrial outbreak. *JAMA,* **1976,** *236*:1853–1856.

Gabow, P.A., Clay, K., Sullivan, J.B., and Lepoff, R. Organic acids in ethylene glycol intoxication. *Ann. Intern. Med.,* **1986,** *105*:16–20.

Gehring, P.J., Kramer, C.G., Schwetz, B.A., Rose, J.Q., and Rowe, V.K. The fate of 2,4,5-trichlorophenoxyacetic acid (2,4,5-T) following oral administration to man. *Toxicol. Appl. Pharmacol.,* **1970,** *26*:352–361.

Goldsmith, J.R., and Landaw, S.A. Carbon monoxide and human health. *Science,* **1968,** *162*:1352–1359.

Goldstein, J.A., Linder, R.E., Hickman, P., and Bergman, H. Effects of pentachlorophenol on hepatic drug metabolism and porphyria related to contamination with chlorinated dibenzo-p-dioxins. *Toxicol. Appl. Pharmacol.,* **1976,** *37*:145–146.

Guggenheim, M.A., Couch, J.R., and Weinberg, W. Motor dysfunction as a permanent complication of methanol ingestion. Presentation of a case with a beneficial response to levodopa treatment. *Arch. Neurol.,* **1971,** *24*:550–554.

Hine, C.H. Methyl bromide poisoning. A review of ten cases. *J. Occup. Med.,* **1969,** *11*:1–10.

Hirsch, J.A., Swenson, E.W., and Wanner, A. Tracheal mucous transport in beagles after long-term exposure to 1 ppm sulfur dioxide. *Arch. Environ. Health,* **1975,** *30*:249–253.

Hooper, N.K., Ames, B.N., Saleh, M.A., and Casida, J.E. Toxaphene, a complex mixture of polychloroterpenes and a major insecticide, is mutagenic. *Science,* **1979,** *205*:591–593.

Iida, M., Yamamoto, H., and Sobue, I. Prognosis of *n*-hexane polyneuropathy: follow-up studies on mass outbreak in F district of Mie prefecture. *Igaku No Ayumi,* **1973,** *84*:199–201.

Jacobsen, D., and McMartin, K.E. Methanol and ethylene glycol poisonings. Mechanism of toxicity, clinical course, diagnosis and treatment. *Med. Toxicol.,* **1986,** *1*:309–334.

Johnson, R.L., Gehring, P.J., Kociba, R.J., and Schwertz, B.A. Chlorinated dibenzodioxins and pentachlorophenol. *Environ. Health Perspect.,* **1973,** *5*:171–175.

Jones, R.D., and Winter, D.P. Two case reports of deaths on industrial premises attributed to 1,1,1-trichloroethane. *Arch. Environ. Health,* **1983,** *38*:59–61.

Kaplan, K. Methyl alcohol poisoning. *Am. J. Med. Sci.,* **1962,** *244*:170–174.

Kapoor, I.P., Metcalf, R.L., Nystrom, R.F., and Sangha, G.K. Comparative metabolism of methoxychlor, methiochlor, and DDT in mouse, insects, and in a model ecosystem. *J. Agric. Food Chem.,* **1970,** *18*:1145–1152.

Ketchum, N.S., Michalek, J.E., and Burton, J.E. Serum dioxin and cancer in veterans of Operation Ranch Hand. *Am. J. Epidemiol.,* **1999,** *149*:630–639.

Kinney, P.L., Ware, J.H., and Spengler, J.D. A critical evaluation of acute ozone epidemiology results. *Arch. Environ. Health,* **1988,** *43*:168–173.

Koch, R., and Schwarze, W. Die Hemmung der α-Naphthyl-thioharnstoffvergiftung durch Cysteamin und seine Derivate. (Zugleich ein Beitrag zur Toxikologie und Strahlenschutzwirkung dieser Sulfhydrylkorper.) *Naunyn Schmiedebergs Arch. Exp. Pathol. Pharmakol.,* **1956,** *29*:428–441.

Kociba, R.J., Keyes, D.G., Beyer, J.E., Carreon, R.M., Wade, C.E., Dittenber, D.A., Kalnins, R.P., Frauson, L.E., Park, C.N., Barnard, S.D., Hummel, R.A., and Humiston, C.G. Result of a two-year chronic toxicity and oncogenicity study of 2,3,7,8-tetrachlorodibenzo-p-dioxin in rats. *Toxicol. Appl. Pharmacol.,* **1978,** *46*:279–303.

Kolmodin, B., Azarnoff, D.L., and Sjoqvist, F. Effect of environmental factors on drug metabolism: decreased plasma half-life of antipyrine in workers exposed to chlorinated hydrocarbon insecticides. *Clin. Pharmacol. Ther.,* **1969,** *10*:638–642.

Kubic, V.L., and Anders, M.W. Metabolism of dihalomethanes to carbon monoxide. II. *In vitro* studies. *Drug Metab. Dispos.,* **1975,** *3*:104–112.

Landrigan, P.J., Powell, K.E., James, L.M., and Taylor, P.R. Paraquat and marijuana: epidemiological risk assessment. *Am. J. Public Health,* **1983,** *73*:784–788.

Lee, P.W., Arnau, T., and Neal, R.A. Metabolism of a-naphthylthiourea by rat liver and rat lung microsomes. *Toxicol. Appl. Pharmacol.,* **1980,** *53*:164–173.

Lindstrom, K. Behavioral effects of long-term exposure to organic solvents. *Acta Neurol. Scand. Suppl.,* **1982,** *92*:131–141.

Lisella, F.S., Long, K.R., and Scott, H.G. Toxicology of rodenticides and their relation to human health. *J. Environ. Health,* **1971,** *33*:231–237, 361–365.

Longo, L.D. The biological effects of carbon monoxide on the pregnant woman, fetus, and newborn infant. *Am. J. Obstet. Gynecol.,* **1977,** *129*:69–103.

Marks, G.S., Brien, J.F., Nakatsu, K., and McLaughlin, B.E. Does carbon monoxide have a physiological function? *Trends Pharmacol. Sci.,* **1991,** *12*:185–188.

McCarthy, T.B., and Jones, R.D. Industrial gassing poisonings due to trichlorethylene, perchlorethylene, and 1,1,1-trichloroethane, 1961–1980. *Br. J. Ind. Med.,* **1983,** *40*:450–455.

McMartin, K.E., Hedström, K.-G., Tolf, B.-R., Ostling-Wintzell, H., and Blomstrand, R. Studies on the metabolic interactions between 4-methylpyrazole and methanol using the monkeys as an animal model. *Arch. Biochem. Biophys.,* **1980,** *199*:606–614.

Mehlman, M.A. Benzene health effects: unanswered questions still not addressed. *Am. J. Ind. Med.,* **1991,** *20*:707–711.

Miller, D.S., Kinter, W.B., and Peakall, D.B. Enzymatic basis for DDE-induced eggshell thinning in a sensitive bird. *Nature,* **1976,** *259*:122–124.

Myers, R.A., Snyder, S.K., and Emhoff, T.A. Subacute sequelae of carbon monoxide poisoning. *Ann. Emerg. Med.,* **1985,** *14*:1163–1167.

Narahashi, T., Ginsberg, K.S., Nagata, K., Song, J.-H., and Tatebayashi, H. Ion channels as targets for insecticides. *Neurotoxicology,* **1998,** *19*:581–590.

National Academy of Sciences. Assembly of Life Sciences (U.S.). Safe Drinking Water Committee. *Drinking Water and Health.* The National Academy of Sciences, Washington, D.C., **1977,** p. 939.

Neubert, D., Zens, P., Rothenwallner, A., and Merker, H.J. A survey of the embryotoxic effects of TCDD in mammalian species. *Environ. Health Perspect.,* **1973,** *5*:67–79.

Noker, P.E., Eells, J.T., and Tephly, T.R. Methanol toxicity: treatment with folic acid and 5-formyl tetrahydrofolic acid. *Alcohol Clin. Exp. Res.,* **1980,** *4*:378–383.

Nordman, H., Keskinen, H., and Tuppurainen, M. Formaldehyde asthma—rare or overlooked? *J. Allergy Clin. Immunol.,* **1985,** *75*:91–99.

Okawa, H., and Casida, J.E. Glutathione S-transferases liberate hydrogen cyanide from organic thiocyanates. *Biochem. Pharmacol.,* **1971,** *20*:1708–1711.

Orehek, J., Massari, J.P., Gayrard, P., Grimaud, C., and Charpin, J. Effect of short-term, low-level nitrogen dioxide exposure on bronchial sensitivity of asthmatic patients. *J. Clin. Invest.,* **1976,** *57*:301–307.

Ostro, B., and Chestnut, L. Assessing the health benefits of reducing particulate matter air pollution in the United States. *Environ. Res.,* **1998,** *76*:94–106.

Petersen, J.E., and Stewart, R.D. Absorption and elimination of carbon monoxide by inactive young men. *Arch. Environ. Health,* **1970,** *21*:165–171.

Pohl, L.R., Bhooshan, B., and Krishna, G. Mechanism of the metabolic activation of chloroform. *Toxicol. Appl. Pharmacol.,* **1978,** *45*:238.

Poland, A., and Glover, E. Comparison of 2,3,7,8-tetrachlorodibenzo-p-dioxin, a potent inducer of aryl hydrocarbon hydroxylase, with 3-methylcholanthrene. *Mol. Pharmacol.,* **1974,** *10*:349–359.

Poland, A., Smith, D., Kuntzman, R., Jacobson, M., and Conney, A.H. Effect of intensive occupational exposure to DDT on phenylbutazone and cortisol metabolism in human subjects. *Clin. Pharmacol. Ther.,* **1970,** *11*:724–732.

Poland, A.P., Smith, D., Metter, G., and Possick, P. A health survey of workers in a 2,4-D and 2,4,5-T plant with special attention to chloracne, porphyria cutanea tarda, and psychologic parameters. *Arch. Environ. Health,* **1971,** *22*:316–327.

Powers, M.B., Voelker, R.W., Page, N.P., Weisburger, E.K., and Kraybill, H.F. Carcinogenicity of ethylene dibromide (EDB) and 1,2-dibromo-3-chloropropane (DBCP) after oral administration in rats and mice. *Toxicol. Appl. Pharmacol.,* **1975,** *33*:171–172.

Radcliffe, D.A. Decrease in eggshell weight in certain birds of prey. *Nature,* **1967,** *215*:208–210.

Recknagel, R.O., Glende, E.A. Jr., Dolak, J.A., and Waller, R.L. Mechanisms of carbon tetrachloride toxicity. *Pharmacol Ther.,* **1989,** *43*:139–154.

Rinsky, R.A., Smith, A.B., Hornung, R., Filloon, T.G., Young, R.J., Okun, A.H., and Landrigan, P.J. Benzene and leukemia. An epidemiologic risk assessment. *N. Engl. J. Med.,* **1987,** *316*:1044–1050.

Rozman, K., Rozman, T., and Greim, H. Stimulation of nonbiliary, intestinal excretion of hexachlorobenzene in rhesus monkeys by mineral oil. *Toxicol. Appl. Pharmacol.,* **1983,** *70*:255–261.

Rozman, T., Ballhorn, L., Rozman, K., Klaassen, C., and Greim, H. Effect of cholestyramine on the disposition of pentachlorophenol in rhesus monkeys. *J. Toxicol. Environ. Health,* **1982,** *10*:277–283.

Rugman, F.P., and Cosstick, R. Aplastic anemia associated with organochloride pesticide: case reports and review of evidence. *J. Clin. Pathol.* **1990,** *43*:98–101.

Saxena, M.C., Siddiqui, M.K., Bhargava, A.K., Murti, C.R., and Kutty, D. Placental transfer of pesticides in humans. *Arch. Toxicol.,* **1981,** *48*:127–134.

Schmid, R. Cutaneous porphyria in Turkey. *N. Engl. J. Med.,* **1960,** *263*:397–398.

Selikoff, I.J., and Hammond, E.C. Asbestos and smoking. *JAMA,* **1979,** *242*:458–459.

Seppäläinen, A.M. Neurophysiological findings among workers exposed to organic solvents. *Acta Neurol. Scand. Suppl.,* **1982,** *92*:109–116.

Shankland, D.L. Neurotoxic action of chlorinated hydrocarbon insecticides. *Neurobehav. Toxicol. Teratol.,* **1982,** *4*:805–811.

Sheppard, D., Saisho, A., Nadel, J.A., and Boushey, H.A. Exercise increases sulfur dioxide-induced bronchoconstriction in asthmatic subjects. *Am. Rev. Respir. Dis.,* **1981,** *123*:486–491.

Talbot, A.R., Shiaw, M.-H., Huang, J.-S., Yang, S.F., Goo, T.S., Wang, S.H., Chen, C.L., and Sanford, T.R. Acute poisoning with a glyphosate-surfactant herbicide ("Roundup"): a review of 93 cases. *Hum. Exp. Toxicol.,* **1991,** *10*:1–8.

Taylor, J.R., Selhorst, J.B., Houff, S.A., and Martinez, A.J. Chlordecone intoxication in man. 1. Clinical observations. *Neurology,* **1978,** *28*:626–630.

Thomsen, H.K. Carbon monoxide-induced atherosclerosis in primates. An electron-microscopic study on the coronary arteries of *Macaca trus* monkeys. *Atherosclerosis,* **1974,** *20*:233–240.

Tominack, R.L., Yang, G.-Y., Tsai, W.-J., Chung, H.M., and Deng, J.F. Taiwan National Poison Center survey of glyphosate-surfactant herbicide ingestions. *J. Toxicol. Clin. Toxicol.,* **1991,** *29*:91–109.

Van Miller, J.P., Lalich, J.J., and Allen, J.R. Increased incidence of neoplasms in rats exposed to low levels of 2,3,7,8-tetrachlorodibenzo-o-dioxin. *Chemosphere,* **1977,** *9*:537–544.

Wang, H.H., and Grufferman, S. Aplastic anemia and occupational pesticide exposure: a case-control study. *J. Occup. Med.,* **1981,** *23*:364–366.

Ware, J.H., Thibodeau, L.A., Speizer, F.E., Colome, S., and Ferris, B.G. Jr. Assessment of the health effects of atmospheric sulfur oxides and particulate matter: evidence from observational studies. *Environ. Health Perspect.,* **1981,** *41*:255–276.

Waters, E.M., Huff, J.E., and Gerstner, H.B. Mirex. An overview. *Environ. Res.,* **1977,** *14*:212–222.

Way, J.L., End, E., Sheehy, M.H., De Miranda, P., Feitknecht, U.F., Bachand, R., Gibbon, S.L., and Burrows, G.E. Effect of oxygen on cyanide intoxication. IV. Hyperbaric oxygen. *Toxicol. Appl. Pharmacol.,* **1972,** *22*:415–421.

Willhite, C.C., and Smith, R.P. The role of cyanide liberation in the acute toxicity of aliphatic nitriles. *Toxicol. Appl. Pharmacol.,* **1981,** *59*:589–602.

MONOGRAPHS AND REVIEWS

Aldridge, W.N. Toxicology of pyrethroids. In, *Pesticide Chemistry: Human Welfare and the Environment.* Vol. 3. (Miyamoto, J., and Kearney, P.C., eds.) Pergamon Press, Oxford, England, **1983,** pp. 485–490.

Andrews, L.S., and Snyder, R. Toxic effects of solvents and vapors. In, *Casarett and Doull's Toxicology: The Basic Science of Poisons,* 4th ed. (Amdur, M.O., Doull, J., and Klaassen, C.D., eds.) Pergamon Press, New York, **1991,** pp. 681–722.

Annau, Z. The neurobehavioral toxicity of trichloroethylene. *Neurobehav. Toxicol. Teratol.,* **1981,** *3*:417–424.

Anthony, D.C., and Graham, D.G. Toxic responses of the nervous system. In, *Casarett and Doull's Toxicology: The Basic Science of Poisons.* 4th ed. (Amdur, M.O., Doull, J., and Klaassen, C.D., eds.) Pergamon Press, New York, **1991,** pp. 407–429.

Anthony, D.C., Montine, T.J., and Graham, D.G. Toxic responses of the nervous system. In, *Casarett and Doull's Toxicology: The Basic Science of Poisons.* 6th ed. (Klaassen, C.D., ed.) McGraw-Hill, New York, **2001,** in press.

Bruckner, J.V., and Warren, D.A. Toxic effects of solvents and vapors. In, *Casarett and Doull's Toxicology: The Basic Science of Poisons.* 6th ed. (Klaassen, C.D., ed.) McGraw-Hill, New York, **2001,** in press.

Committee on Aldehydes. *Formaldehyde and Other Aldehydes.* National Academy Press, Washington, D.C., **1981.**

Costa, D.L., and Amdur, M.O. Air pollution. In, *Casarett and Doull's Toxicology: The Basic Science of Poisons,* 5th ed. (Klaassen, C.D., ed.) McGraw-Hill, New York, **1996,** pp. 857–882.

Couri, D,. and Milks, M. Toxicity and metabolism of the neurotoxic hexacarbons n-hexane, 2-hexanone, and 2,5-hexanedione. *Annu. Rev. Pharmacol. Toxicol.,* **1982,** *22*:145–166.

Ecobichon, D.J. Toxic effects of pesticides. In, *Casarett and Doull's Toxicology: The Basic Science of Poisons.* 6th ed. (Klaassen, C.D., ed.) McGraw-Hill, New York, **2001,** in press.

Ervin, M.E. Petroleum distillates and turpentine. In, *Clinical Management of Poisoning and Drug Overdose.* (Haddad, L.M., and Winchester, J.F., eds.) Saunders, Philadelphia, **1983,** pp. 771–779.

Finck, P.A. Exposure to carbon monoxide: review of the literature and 567 autopsies. *Mil. Med.,* **1966,** *131*:1513–1539.

Fisher, A.A. Occupational dermatitis from pesticides: patch testing procedures. *Cutis,* **1983,** *31*:483–488, 492, 508.

Gosselin, R.E., Smith, R.P., and Hodge, H.C., eds. *Clinical Toxicology of Commercial Products,* 5th ed. Williams & Wilkins, Baltimore, **1984.**

Graham, D.G., Genter, M.B., and Lowndes, H.E. *n*-Hexane. In, *Ethel Browning's Toxicity and Metabolism of Industrial Solvents,* 2nd ed. Vol. 1. (Snyder, R., ed.) Elsevier–North Holland, New York, **1987,** pp. 327–335.

Gutierrez, G. Carbon monoxide toxicity. In, *Air Pollution—Physiological Effects.* (McGrath, J.J., and Barnes, C.D., eds.) Academic Press, New York, **1982,** pp. 127–147.

Guzelian, P.S. Comparative toxicology of chlordecone (kepone) in humans and experimental animals. *Annu. Rev. Pharmacol. Toxicol.,* **1982,** *22*:89–113.

Hayes, W.J. Jr. *Clinical Handbook on Economic Poisons Emergency Information for Treating Poisoning.* Public Health Service Publication No. 476. U.S. Government Printing Office, Washington, D.C., **1963.**

Hayes, W.J. Jr. *Pesticides Studied in Man.* Williams & Wilkins, Baltimore, **1982.**

Holmstedt, B. Prolegomena to Seveso. Ecclesiastes I 18. *Arch. Toxicol.,* **1980,** *44*:211–230.

Huff, J., Lucier, G., and Tritscher, A. Carcinogenicity of TCDD: experimental, mechanistic, and epidemiologic evidence. *Annu. Rev. Pharmacol. Toxicol.* **1994,** *34*:343–372.

IARC. *Monographs on the Evaluation of the Carcinogenic Risk of Chemicals to Man.* Vol. 5, *Some Organochlorine Pesticides.* International Agency for Research on Cancer, Lyon, France, **1974a.**

IARC. *Monographs on the Evaluation of the Carcinogenic Risk of Chemicals to Man.* Vol. 7, *Some Antithyroid and Related Substances, Nitrofurans and Industrial Chemicals.* International Agency for Research on Cancer, Lyon, France, **1974b.**

IARC. *Monographs on the Evaluation of Carcinogenic Risk of Chemicals to Man.* Vol. 12, *Some Carbamates, Thiocarbamates and Carbazides.* International Agency for Research on Cancer, Lyon, France, **1976.**

IARC. *Monographs on the Evaluation of the Carcinogenic Risk of Chemicals to Man.* Vol. 15, *Some Fumigants, the Herbicides 2,4-D and 2,4,5-T, Chlorinated Dibenzodioxins and Miscellaneous Industrial Chemicals.* International Agency for Research on Cancer, Lyon, France, **1977.**

Kalf, G.F., Post, G.B., and Snyder, R. Solvent toxicology: recent advances in the toxicology of benzene, the glycol ethers, and carbon tetrachloride. *Annu. Rev. Pharmacol. Toxicol.,* **1987,** *27*:399–427.

Kaplan, S.D., and Morgan, R.W. Airborne carcinogens and human cancer. *Rev. Environ. Health,* **1981,** *3*:329–368.

Kerns, W.D., Donofrio, D.J., and Pavkov, K.L. The chronic effects of formaldehyde inhalation in rats and mice: a preliminary report. In, *Formaldehyde Toxicity.* (Gibson, J.E., ed.) Hemisphere Publishing, Washington, D.C., **1983,** pp. 111–131.

Khan, N.Y. An assessment of the hazard of synthetic pyrethroid insecticides to fish and fish habitat. In, *Pesticide Chemistry: Human Welfare and the Environment.* Vol. 3. (Miyamoto, J., and

Kearney, P.C., eds.) Pergamon Press, Oxford, England, **1983,** pp. 115–121.

Kupfer, D., and Bulger, W.H. Estrogenic actions of chlorinated hydrocarbons. In, *Effects of Chronic Exposures to Pesticides on Animal Systems.* (Chambers, J.E., and Yarbrough, J.D., eds.) Raven Press, New York, **1982,** pp. 121–146.

LeWitt, P.A., and Martin, S.D. Dystonia and hypokinesis with putaminal necrosis after methanol intoxication. *Clin. Neuropharmacol.,* **1988,** *11*:161–167.

Lippmann, M. Health effects of ozone. A critical review. *JAPCA,* **1989,** *39*:672–695.

Lundholm, E. Thinning of eggshells in birds by DDE: mode of action on the eggshell gland. *Comp. Biochem. Physiol. C,* **1987,** *88*:1–22.

Maibach, H. Formaldehyde: effects on animal and human skin. In, *Formaldehyde Toxicity.* (Gibson, J.E., ed.) Hemisphere Publishing, Washington, D.C., **1983,** pp. 166–174.

Matsumura, F., and Ghiasuddin, S.M. DDT-sensitive Ca-ATPase in the axonic membrane. In, *Neurotoxicology of Insecticides and Pheromones.* (Narahashi, T., ed.) Plenum Press, New York, **1979,** pp. 245–257.

Menzel, D.B. The toxicity of air pollution in experimental animals and humans: the role of oxidative stress. *Toxicol. Lett.,* **1994,** *72*:269–277.

Morrow, J.D., Hill, K.E., Burk, R.F., Nammour, T.M., Badr, K.F., and Roberts, L.J. II. A series of prostaglandin F_2-like compounds are produced *in vivo* in humans by a non-cyclooxygenase, free radical–catalyzed mechanism. *Proc. Natl. Acad. Sci. U.S.A.,* **1990,** *87*:9383–9387.

Morrow, J.D., Minton, T.A., Mukundan, C.R., Campbell, M.D., Zackert, W.E., Daniel, V.C., Badr, K.F., Blair, I.A., and Roberts, L.J. II. Free radical-induced generation of isoprostanes *in vivo.* Evidence for the formation of D-ring and E-ring isoprostanes. *J. Biol. Chem.,* **1994,** *269*:4317–4326.

Narahashi, T. Interaction of pyrethroids and DDT-like compounds with the sodium channels in the nerve membrane. In, *Pesticide Chemistry: Human Welfare and the Environment.* Vol. 3. (Miyamoto, J., and Kearney, P.C., eds.) Pergamon Press, Oxford, England, **1983,** pp. 109–114.

National Research Council. Committee on Medical and Biologic Effects of Environmental Pollutants. *Carbon Monoxide.* National Academy of Sciences, Washington, D.C., **1977.**

Plaa, G.L. Toxic responses of the liver. In, *Casarett and Doull's Toxicology: The Basic Science of Poisons,* 4th ed. (Amdur, M.O., Doull, J., and Klaassen, C.D., eds.) Pergamon Press, New York, **1991,** pp. 334–353.

Roberts, L.J. II, and Morrow, J.D. Isoprostanes. Novel markers of endogenous lipid peroxidation and potential mediators of oxidant injury. *Ann. N.Y. Acad. Sci.,* **1994,** *744*:237–242.

Saleh, M.A. Toxaphene: chemistry, biochemistry, toxicity and environmental fate. *Rev. Environ. Contam. Toxicol.,* **1991,** *118*:1–85.

Sayers, P.R., and Davenport, S.J. *Review of Carbon Monoxide Poisoning.* Public Health Bulletin No. 195. U.S. Government Printing Office, Washington, D.C., **1930.**

Slater, T.F. Free radicals as reactive intermediates in tissue injury. In, *Biological Reactive Intermediates II: Chemical Mechanisms and Biological Effects.* (Snyder, R., Parke, D.V., Kocsis, J.J., Jollow, D.J., Gibson, G.G., and Witmer, C.M., eds.) Plenum Press, New York, **1982,** pp. 575–589.

Smith, L.L. The toxicity of paraquat. *Adverse Drug React. Acute Poisoning Rev.,* **1988,** *7*:1–17.

Snyder, R., Witz, G., and Goldstein, B.D. The toxicology of benzene. *Environ. Health Perspect.* **1993,** *100*:293–306.

Speizer, F.E. Environmental lung diseases. In, *Harrison's Principles of Internal Medicine,* 13th ed. (Isselbacher, K.J., Braunwald, E., Wilson, J.D., Martin, J., Fauci, A.S., Kasper, D.L., eds.) McGraw-Hill, New York, **1994,** pp. 1176–1183.

Stewart, R.D. The effects of carbon monoxide on humans. *Annu. Rev. Pharmacol.,* **1975,** *15*:409–423.

Tephly, T.R., Makar, A.B., McMartin, K.E., Hayreh, S.S., and Martin-Amat, G. Methanol: its metabolism and toxicity. In, *Biochemistry and Pharmacology of Ethanol.* Vol. 1. (Majchrowicz, E., and Noble, E.P., eds.) Plenum Press, New York, **1979,** pp. 145–164.

Timblin, C., Janssen-Heininger, Y., and Mossmann, B.T. Pulmonary reactions and mechanisms of toxicity of inhaled particles. In, *Toxicology of the Lung,* 3rd ed. (Garner, D.E., Crapo, J.D., and McClellan, R.O., eds.) Taylor and Francis, Philadelphia, **1999,** pp. 221–240.

Tintinalli, J.E., Rominger, M., and Kittleson, K. Carbon monoxide. In, *Clinical Management of Poisoning and Drug Overdose.* (Haddad, L.M., and Winchester, J.F., eds.) Saunders, Philadelphia, **1983,** pp. 748–753.

U.A.R.E.P. (Universities Associated for Research and Education in Pathology, Inc.) Epidemiology of chronic occupational exposure to formaldehyde: report of the Ad Hoc Panel on Health Aspects of Formaldehyde. *Toxicol. Ind. Health,* **1988,** *4*:77–90.

USEPA (United States Environmental Protection Agency, Office of Drinking Water Health Advisories). *Rev. Environ. Contam. Toxicol.,* **1988,** *106*:1–233.

Way, J.L. Cyanide intoxication and its mechanism of antagonism. *Annu. Rev. Pharmacol. Toxicol.,* **1984,** *24*:451–481.

Weger, N.P. Treatment of cyanide poisoning with 4-dimethylaminophenol (DMAP)—experimental and clinical overview. *Fundam. Appl. Toxicol.,* **1983,** *3*:387–396.

Woodbury, M.A., and Zenz, C. Formaldehyde in the home environment: prenatal and infant exposures. In, *Formaldehyde Toxicity.* (Gibson, J.E., ed.) Hemisphere Publishing, Washington, D.C., **1983,** pp. 203–211.

World Health Organization. *1974 Evaluations of Some Pesticide Residue in Food.* World Health Organization Pesticide Residue Series, No. 4. WHO, Geneva, Switzerland, **1975,** pp. 261–263.

APPENDIX I

PRINCIPLES OF PRESCRIPTION ORDER WRITING AND PATIENT COMPLIANCE

Lauralea Edwards and Dan M. Roden

The direct costs of medication-related morbidity and mortality in the United States have been estimated to be $76.6 billion annually, far exceeding the estimates of costs of obesity- or diabetes-related morbidity and mortality (Johnson and Bootman, 1995). Efforts to reduce the number of drug-related adverse events due to misinterpretation, medical error, inappropriate prescribing, or patient noncompliance could result in substantial savings and, more important, improved patient health.

The clear communication of a prescription order to other members of the health-care team and to the patient is a vital step in drug therapy. Ideally, a prescription will be written for an optimal drug product for the specific patient and indication; it will contain no errors, be free of ambiguity, and contain all of the necessary components to allow it to be filled properly by the pharmacist and taken appropriately by the patient. How accurately the patient follows through with the prescribed therapy can be influenced in some cases by factors within the physician's control, although noncompliance is a common and frustrating medical reality.

ERRORS IN DRUG ORDERS

Errors in the management of drug therapy result in a large number of preventable injuries suffered by patients (Classen *et al.,* 1991). Databases of anonymously reported errors are maintained jointly by the Institute for Safe Medication Practices (ISMP) and the United States Pharmacopeia Medication Errors Reporting Program (USP MERP), and by the Food and Drug Administration's MedWatch program. In a study of adverse drug events, Bates and associates (1995) found that 49% of the time the primary error in preventable events occurred in the drug ordering stage. By examining aspects of prescription writing that can cause errors and by modifying prescribing habits accordingly, the physician can improve the chance that the patient will receive the correct treatment, whether in a hospital or an outpatient setting.

Numeral and Measurement System

Historically, multiple number and measurement systems have been employed in the preparation of prescriptions; avoirdupois, apothecaries', and metric measurements and their attendant symbols have been combined with Roman and Arabic numerals. In an industry where small errors can be fatal, such a mix of systems is highly undesirable. In fact, the large number of errors resulting from misinterpretation of symbols and errors in conversion between measurement systems clearly supports the need for standardization in this area.

All orders should be written using metric measurements. The apothecaries' system (drams, grains, minims, ounces) is no longer recognized by the USP as an official system for use (United States Pharmacopeial Convention, 1993), and it is no longer employed as the primary system in drug labeling or package inserts. To avoid confusion, Arabic (decimal) numerals are preferable to Roman numerals, and in some instances, it is preferable for numbers to be spelled out (*see* "Preventing Diversion," below). When writing decimal fraction numbers, health-care professionals always should use leading zeros (0.125 mg, not .125 mg), never use trailing zeros (5 mg, not 5.0 mg), and decimal points should be indicated carefully, as these often are reported as a source of dosage errors.

Table AI–1

Abbreviations and Symbols That Are Easily Misinterpreted

ABBREVIATION OR SYMBOL (INTENDED MEANING)	HAS BEEN INTERPRETED AS	CAN RESULT IN	COMMENTS AND SUGGESTIONS
U (unit)	Ultralente, 0, 4, 6, cc	Wrong insulin type or overdose	Write out "unit" with a lowercase "u" and leave space between the number and the word "unit"
♏ (minim)	ml (milliliter)	16-fold overdose	Do not use apothecaries' measurements or symbols
℥ (one dram)	3 tablespoons or tid	12-fold overdose or wrong dosage schedule	
gr (grain)	g (gram)	15-fold overdose	
/ (slash mark, for "and," "per," "with," "over")	1 (one) lowercase L	Overdose Misread drug name	Write out "and," "per," "with," "over"
qd, qid, qod	qod, qd, od, qid	Wrong dosage schedule or route (od). When written in cursive (*qid*) or unevenly dotted, q.d. can appear to be qid or qod; conversely, qid and qod can appear to be q.d.	Carefully print these abbreviations, or write "once daily" or "q daily," "four times daily," "every other day"
od (incorrect abbreviation for "once daily")	od (correctly, as right eye)	Wrong route	Write "once daily"
μg (microgram)	mg (milligram)	1000-fold overdose	Write "mcg"
qn, qhs, qh, qhr	qh, qhr, qn, qhs	Wrong dosage schedule	Write out "every night," or "nightly," "at bedtime," "every hour"

Abbreviations

Many commonly used medical abbreviations are derived from phrases that were used in the era when Latin was the international language of medicine; however, currently there are no standardized or official lists of medical abbreviations recognized and endorsed by health-care associations. Individual practitioners often create novel abbreviations from English to speed the prescription-writing process, which is particularly troublesome when an ab-

breviation has multiple meanings or can be misinterpreted easily when poorly written. Certain abbreviations repeatedly lead to errors and should not be used. Some of the most commonly cited are shown in Table AI–1.

Individual drugs and combinations of drugs should not be ordered by abbreviations. An incident involving oprevelkin (NEUMEGA, an interleukin-11 product) and aldesleukin (PROLEUKIN, an interleukin-2 derivative) has been reported (United States Pharmacopeia Medication Errors Reporting Program, 1999). The physician used the abbreviation "IL-11" on the order, but the Arabic eleven was misinterpreted as a Roman numeral two by at least five health-care professionals over the course of four days. Chemotherapy drugs and regimens frequently are ordered by abbreviations and are major sources of errors and confusion. For example, cytarabine (ara-C) has been confused with vidarabine (ara-A), and "AC" has been used for the combination of adriamycin with cyclophosphamide, carmustine, or cisplatin (Davis, 1997).

In the interest of patient safety, some organizations have suggested that abbreviations not be used (National Coordinating Council for Medication Error Reporting and Prevention, 1996), and others have called for the creation of a list of "approved" abbreviations based on evidence of safe use and low likelihood of misinterpretation (Davis, 1997). Standardization of abbreviations is possible only if the medical community is willing to put it into practice; computerized prescription entry in inpatient and increasingly in outpatient settings may facilitate this standardization. It is perhaps unrealistic to call for an end to the use of abbreviations in prescription writing, as abbreviations

have the advantage of both history and convenience. Still, practitioners should examine carefully their need to use potentially dangerous abbreviations and remove from their repertoire those that are known to commonly cause errors.

Orthographic and Phonologic Similarities

Look-alike and sound-alike drug names are responsible for approximately 25% of medication errors reported to USP MERP (United States Pharmacopeial Convention, 1999a). The similarity of some of these problem pairs (*see* Table AI–2) is readily apparent, but even drug pairs whose names seem more distinct easily can be confused when handwriting styles and cognitive mechanisms such as confirmation bias become contributing factors (Leape, 1994; Cohen, 1995). Procedures exist for a drug's generic or brand name to be changed if it repeatedly causes errors or is found to be particularly dangerous, but these changes are rare, and many errors can occur before the change is instituted by the United States Food and Drug

Table AI–2

Examples of Look-Alike and/or Sound-Alike Names, with Overlapping Strengths of Dosage Units Noted*

Amantadine 100 mg	Rimantadine 100 mg	Ranitidine
ATIVAN 1, 2 mg	HYTRIN, 1, 2 mg	ATARAX
AVANDIA 4 mg	PRANDIN 4 mg	COUMADIN 4 mg
CELEXA	CELEBREX	CEREBYX
CELEXA 10 mg	ZYPREXA 10 mg	
CLINORIL 150, 200 mg	ORUVAIL 100, 150, 200 mg	CLOZARIL 100 mg
Codeine	LODINE	Iodine
IMDUR 60 mg	INDERAL 60 mg	
ISORDIL 10 mg	INDERAL 10 mg	PLENDIL 10 mg
LAMICTAL	LAMISIL	LOMOTIL
LORTAB	CORTEF	
NAVANE 10 mg	NORVASC 10 mg	
PERMAX 1 mg	BUMEX 1 mg	
PROSOM	PROZAC	PROSCAR
TENORMIN 50 mg	IMURAN 50 mg	
TORADOL 10 mg	TORECAN 10 mg	Tramadol
ULTRAM 50 mg	VOLTAREN 50 mg	
XANAX	ZANTAC	ZYRTEC
ZEMURON	REMERON	
ZYVOX 100 mg	LUVOX 100 mg	VIOXX

*Strengths listed are only those currently available in single manufactured units. Listing does not include possible overlapping dosages from using more than one tablet or using half-tablets, nor overlap that occurs with extended- or immediate-release forms with a different name or suffix, such as INDERAL-LA 120 mg. A list of drug pairs reported to cause look-alike and sound-alike errors can be obtained from USP-ISMP (1-800-23-ERROR), or found periodically in USP Quality Reviews at www.usp.org.

Administration (FDA), United States Adopted Names (USAN) Council, or manufacturer. In 1990, the trade name for omeprazole in the United States was changed from LOSEC to PRILOSEC because of the possible confusion of LOSEC with LASIX. In 2000, amrinone was renamed inamrinone in an effort to prevent further (sometimes fatal) mix-ups with amiodarone, although errors between the two had been reported for a number of years. It also has been proposed that the USAN of amiodarone be changed to camiodarone (United States Pharmacopeial Convention, 1999b), although this change has not yet been approved.

The risk of look-alike errors can be minimized by printing the drug name and writing a complete prescription order that includes the drug's strength, specific directions, and indication for use, as this additional information often can help differentiate between products. Including the drug's indication is particularly useful, as similar names rarely exist within the same therapeutic category. Oral orders generally are discouraged, but their safety can be increased by speaking slowly, spelling out problematic words and numbers, and having the order repeated back. For drugs having a look-alike or sound-alike alternate, it can be helpful to indicate both the brand and generic names.

Handwriting

In 1999, a court case involving a prescription that featured poor handwriting resulted in judgments against the physician who did not write clearly and the pharmacist who misread the prescription and did not call to question the dosage. The intended medication was ISORDIL (isosorbide dinitrate), but PLENDIL (felodipine) was dispensed instead. The patient suffered a myocardial infarction and died several days later.

The importance of preparing clear and legible prescriptions cannot be overstated. Poor penmanship will compound the likelihood that there will be harmful errors resulting from an already dangerous system of employing numerous overlapping and similar abbreviations, look-alike and sound-alike drug names, and archaic measurement and numeral systems. Not only are patients placed at risk by illegible or nearly illegible handwriting, but time and resources are wasted in deciphering the intended meaning from clues on the prescription or attempting to locate an unknown physician whose signature is illegible to get clarification of the order (Winslow et al., 1997; Anonymous, 1979). Also, misinterpreted prescriptions have been cited as the second most frequent and costly type of malpractice claim (Cabral, 1997). Legislative efforts to eliminate handwritten prescriptions are being explored in at least one state.

Despite the widespread nature of this problem, there are solutions, the easiest of which is to print orders carefully. By printing information and leaving ample spacing between letters, words, and lines of print, the physician will make clear many potentially illegible items. Electronic solutions are becoming more widely available. Wireless, hand-held electronic prescription devices recently have been developed that eliminate the need to hand write, and their communication and database capabilities may help prevent other types of medication problems, such as undesirable drug interactions. Increasingly, inpatient and outpatient settings have computer systems in place that eliminate handwritten orders completely.

Preprinted order forms are used in many inpatient settings and to a lesser extent for outpatient prescriptions. Although useful, these forms must be developed with great care or else their design may contribute to medical errors (Cohen and Davis, 1992); for example, errors have been reported from "check box"–format prescriptions due to the ease of selecting the wrong box. Preprinted prescriptions for controlled substances are prohibited by law in many states.

Ambiguity of Intent

A perfectly legible prescription for the ideal drug therapy can injure a patient if its intent is not clear. An inpatient order written as "cyclophosphamide 4 g/m^2 days 1-4" or "cyclophosphamide 4 g/m^2 over 4 days" when the intent was for "cyclophosphamide 1 g/m^2 each day for 4 days" could prove fatal; the highly publicized death of a health-care reporter in 1994 was the result of this type of misunderstanding (Cohen et al., 1996).

Omissions or contractions for the sake of expediency often are the culprits behind misleading orders. Many types of medication errors can be attributed to some ambiguity in the prescription process.

FORM OF THE PRESCRIPTION

A prescription order contains a series of components that allow it to be interpreted and executed correctly, and the same general pattern is used whether the request is for a preformulated product or an extemporaneously compounded one. Subtle differences in the prescription format may be required by individual states. All prescriptions should be written in ink or typed; this practice is compulsory for schedule II prescriptions under the Controlled Substances Act of 1970, as erasures on a prescription easily can lead to dispensing errors or diversion of

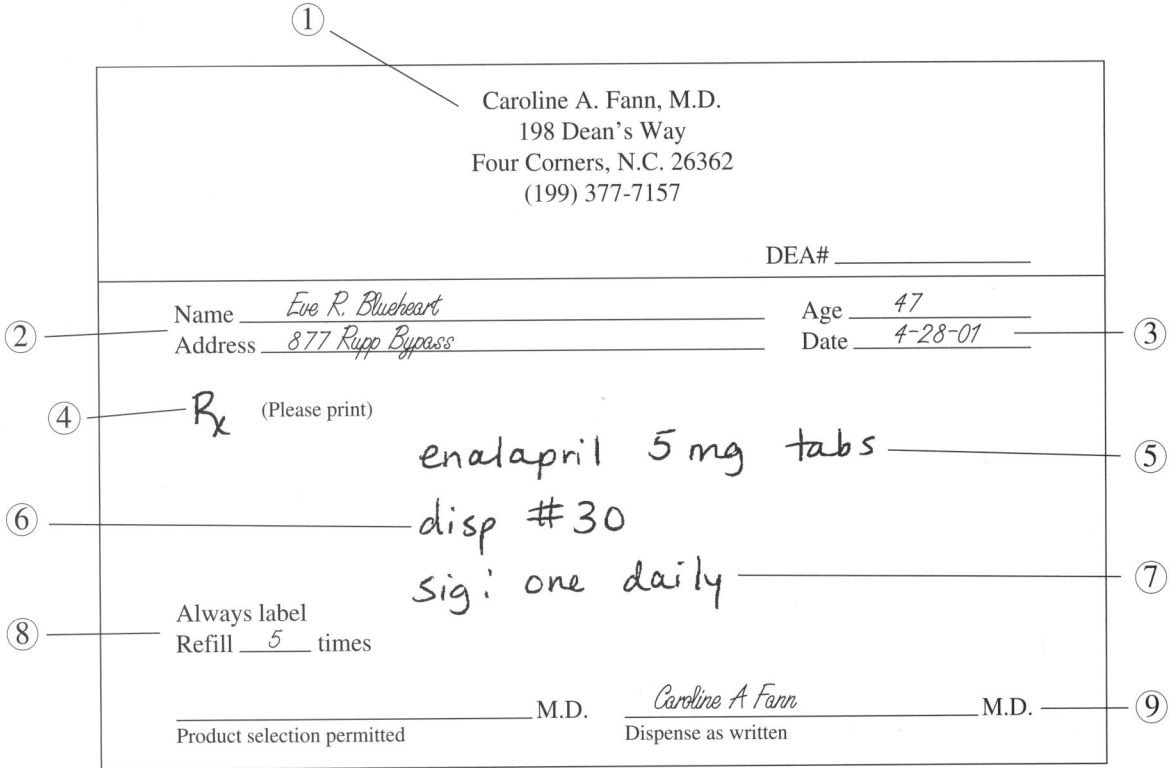

Figure AI–1. The prescription.

controlled substances. The following components of the prescription are illustrated in Figure AI–1: (1) prescriber information, (2) patient information, (3) date prescription issued, (4) ℞ symbol, (5) medication information, (6) dispensing directions for pharmacist, (7) directions for use [*signatura* (Latin, "mark thou," "write") abbreviated as *signa* or *sig*], (8) refill and other information, and (9) prescriber signature.

As shown in the example, only one order should be written per prescription blank to allow generous spacing and minimize the risk of misinterpretation.

Prescriber Information

Prescription pad blanks normally are imprinted with a heading that gives the name of the physician and the address and phone number of the practice site. When using institutional blanks that do not bear the physician's information, the physician always should print his or her name and phone number on the face of the prescription to clearly identify the prescriber and facilitate communication with other health-care professionals if questions arise. United States law requires that prescriptions for controlled sub-

stances include the name, address, and Drug Enforcement Agency (DEA) registration number of the physician.

Patient Information

The patient's name and address are needed on the order to assure that the correct medication goes to the correct patient and also for identification and record-keeping purposes. For medications whose dosage involves a calculation, a patient's pertinent factors such as weight, age, or body surface area also should be listed on the prescription.

Date Issued

The date is an important piece of the patient's medical record, and it can assist the pharmacist in recognizing potential problems. For example, when an opioid is prescribed for pain due to an injury and the prescription is presented to a pharmacist two weeks after issuance, the drug may no longer be indicated. Compliance behavior also can be estimated using the dates when a prescription is filled and refilled. The United States Controlled Substances Act requires that all orders for controlled

Table AI–3
Controlled Substance Schedules

Schedule I (examples: heroin, methylene dioxymethamphetamine, lysergic acid diethylamide, mescaline, and all salts and isomers thereof):
1. High potential for abuse.
2. No accepted medical use in the United States or lacks accepted safety for use in treatment in the United States. May be used for research purposes by properly registered individuals.

Schedule II (examples: morphine, oxycodone, fentanyl, meperidine, dextroamphetamine, cocaine, amobarbital):
1. High potential for abuse.
2. Has a currently accepted medical use in the United States.
3. Abuse of substance may lead to severe psychological or physical dependence.

Schedule III (examples: anabolic steroids, nalorphine, ketamine, certain schedule II substances in suppositories, mixtures, or limited amounts per dosage unit):
1. Abuse potential less than substances in schedule I or schedule II.
2. Has a currently accepted medical use in the United States.
3. Abuse of substance may lead to moderate or low physical dependence or high psychological dependence.

Schedule IV (examples: alprazolam, phenobarbital, meprobamate, modafinil):
1. Abuse potential less than substances in schedule III.
2. Has a currently accepted medical use in the United States.
3. Abuse of substance may lead to limited physical or psychological dependence relative to substances in schedule III.

Schedule V (examples: buprenorphine, products containing a low dose of an opioid plus a nonnarcotic ingredient such as codeine and guaifenesin cough syrup or diphenoxylate and atropine tablets):
1. Low potential for abuse relative to schedule IV.
2. Has a currently accepted medical use in the United States.
3. Some schedule V products may be sold in limited amounts without a prescription at the discretion of the pharmacist; however, if a physician wishes a patient to receive one of these products, it is preferable to provide a prescription.

---

substances (*see* Table AI–3) be dated as of, and signed on, the day when issued and prohibits filling or refilling orders for substances in schedules III and IV more than six months after their date of issuance.

℞

Its appearance is purely symbolic. It is generally believed to have originated as either an abbreviation of *recipe* (Latin, "take thou") or the symbol for Jupiter, ♃, the Roman god whose blessing was requested in the healing arts.

Medication Information

This includes the name of the drug, its strength or concentration, and the desired dosage form. A drug may be ordered by its nonproprietary or generic name (in the United States, the United States Adopted Name, or USAN) or the manufacturer's proprietary name, called the trademark, trade name, or brand name. If a specific manufacturer's product is desired, this may be indicated by including the manufacturer's name in parentheses. For drugs having a look-alike or sound-alike alternative, it can be helpful to list both the brand and generic names.

Choice of Drug Product

Inappropriate choice of drug products by physicians has been noted as a problem in prescribing. It cannot be assumed that a drug's popularity is proof of its overall clinical superiority or safety (Rucker, 1980), and this can be seen in a number of formerly popular medications that now have been withdrawn from the market. Physicians should rely on unbiased sources when seeking drug information that will influence their prescribing habits.

Pharmacists must dispense the brand-name product when it is listed unless state law or the prescribing physician permits drug product selection. Virtually all states have adopted laws that permit pharmacists to substitute equivalent products under certain circumstances. Depending on the state's laws, the physician may write "brand medically necessary," "dispense as written," or a similar statement to prevent substitution of one manufacturer's product for another. Products with specialized release systems and/or drugs with low therapeutic indices often are prescribed to be manufacturer-specific, because a patient who is stabilized on any product with a low therapeutic index, brand name or generic, should remain on that product.

Strength or Concentration

The strength or concentration of a product always should be listed, even if the physician believes that only one strength is available. This can help differentiate between products whose names are similar and can prevent problems if the product has been changed recently. For example, PERCOCET (oxycodone and acetaminophen, 5 mg/325 mg) had been marketed in a single fixed-combination strength since the 1970s, but in 1999 became available in three additional strengths: 2.5 mg/325 mg, 7.5 mg/500 mg, and 10 mg/650 mg. Manufacturers frequently update product lines, and this is particularly true for drugs recently introduced to the market or recently winning approval for new indications. Failure to specify strength can cause the pharmacist to dispense the wrong product in the case of illegible handwriting or look-alike names. For example, a handwritten prescription for ZOCOR (simvastatin) with no indications of strength, specific directions, or purpose of use might be misread as YOCON (yohimbine), a product that is manufactured in only one strength.

Dosage Form

When choosing the dosage form, a number of patient-specific factors must be considered, such as the patient's current symptoms or disease states (nausea and vomiting, sensitive skin, ability to swallow, presence of a feeding tube, lack of dexterity), drug interactions with or allergies to the nonmedicinal components of the products, and convenience. A variety of sustained-release products using solid and liquid formulations and transdermal and implantable devices are available and may offer a number of advantages, including aiding compliance by reducing the total number of doses, minimizing local or systemic side effects, giving better disease control, or delivering the drug at a predictable time or location in the gastrointestinal tract. Many of these products have elegantly designed release mechanisms that are destroyed when the unit is cut, broken in half, or crushed; patients should be given specific instructions regarding their proper use.

Directions for the Pharmacist

In prescription orders for a single precompounded drug, directions for the pharmacist usually consist of "dispense 10 tablets," "dispense with oral syringe," and so forth. In the case of prescription orders for extemporaneously compounded products, it also may include phrases such as "q.s. (add sufficient quantity) to 60 grams," "make sugar-free," "mix and divide into 40 capsules," or "make such doses and place in 40 capsules." The word *label,* used to direct the pharmacist to include the name and strength of the drug on the prescription label, is essentially unnecessary because most states now require that this information be present.

Directions for Patient Use

Doses always should be listed by metric weight of active ingredient; doses for liquid medications should include the volume. The metric system should be used in place of common household measurements such as "dropperful" and "teaspoon" in the directions for the patient, and the doctor or pharmacist should be sure that the patient understands the measurement prescribed. For medical purposes, a "teaspoon" or "teaspoonful" dose is considered to be equivalent to 5 ml and a "tablespoon" to 15 ml, but the actual volumes held by ordinary household teaspoons and tablespoons are too variable to be used reliably for measurement of many medications. Prescribing oral medications in "drops" likewise can cause problems when accuracy of dose is important unless the patient understands that only the calibrated dropper provided by the manufacturer or pharmacist should be used to dispense the medication. Directions for a "dropperful" can lead to dosage errors if the patient is not aware that this is an amount specific to a marked volume on the calibrated dropper provided with the medication. Thus, one possible dosage for a pediatric iron product would be more accurately written "15 mg (0.6 ml) three times daily" instead of "one dropperful three times daily," because a true dropperful could result in iron overdose (ISMP, 1999). The use of medical units, such as "one ampule," in giving dosage also should be avoided unless the strength of the dose is clearly stated.

Prescribers often commit errors in dosage calculations (Lesar *et al.,* 1997). When prescribing a drug whose dosage involves a calculation based on body weight or surface area, it is good practice to include both the calculated dose and the dosage formula used, such as "240 mg every 8 hours (40 mg/kg per day)" to allow another healthcare professional to double-check the prescribed dosage. Pharmacists always should recalculate dosage equations when filling these prescriptions if they have access to the necessary patient parameters.

In writing directions, vague expressions such as "take as directed" or "take as necessary" are to be avoided unless they accompany careful patient education and specific guidelines for use. Numerous studies have demonstrated patients' difficulty in recalling or understanding basic directions for taking medications, and sheets of written information may be lost. If the medication is to be taken at a specific time of day, if a particular dosage interval is desired, or if there are any additional directions for use, these should be noted on the prescription and their significance concisely explained to the patient in simple terms. The correct route of administration is reinforced by the choice of the first word of the directions. For an oral dosage form, the directions would begin with "take" or "give"; for externally applied products, the word "apply"; for suppositories, "insert"; and for eye, ear, or nose drops, "place" is preferable to "instill."

The purpose of the medication, again in simple language (*e.g.,* "for blood pressure," "for breathing," "for chest pain"), should be placed on the prescription and the prescription label unless its inclusion would embarrass the patient or otherwise not be in the patient's best interest. The presence of this information helps prevent dispensing errors and helps patients remember what condition the medicine is meant to treat. It also assists pharmacists in counseling patients properly, especially if the drug being dispensed is one that has many therapeutic uses, such as amitriptyline.

Refill and Other Information

Refills may be indicated by a number ("3 times") or a time period ("one year"). A statement such as "refill prn" (as needed) may be used but is generally not appropriate, as it could allow the patient to misuse the medicine or neglect medical appointments or monitoring. If no refills are desired, "zero" (not 0) should be written in the refill space to prevent alteration of the doctor's intent. Refills for controlled substances are discussed below.

Prescriber Signature

The signature should be in ink, signed as the prescriber would sign a legal document, with the last name written in full and the appropriate professional degree following it. Electronically delivered prescriptions typically require confidential passwords to assure their validity.

CONTROLLED SUBSTANCES

The DEA, an agency in the Department of Justice, is responsible for the enforcement of the Federal Comprehensive Drug Abuse Prevention and Control Act of 1970. Title II of the act is known as the Federal Controlled Substances Act (CSA), and it regulates each step of the handling of controlled substances from manufacture to dispensing. The act provides a closed system that is intended to prevent diversion of controlled substances from legitimate uses. State agencies may impose additional regulations such as requiring that prescriptions for controlled substances be printed on triplicate or state-issued prescription pads or restricting the use of a particular class of drugs for specific indications. The most stringent law always takes precedence, whether it be federal, state, or local. Substances that come under the jurisdiction of the CSA are divided into five schedules, as shown in Table AI–3, but physicians should note that individual states may have additional schedules. Criminal offenses and penalties generally depend on the schedule of a substance as well as the amount of drug in question.

Physicians must be authorized to prescribe controlled substances by the jurisdiction in which they are licensed and registered with the DEA or exempted from registration as defined under the CSA. The number on the certificate of registration must be indicated on all prescription orders for controlled substances.

Prescription Orders for Controlled Substances

To be valid, a prescription for a controlled substance must be issued for a *legitimate medical purpose* by an *individual practitioner* acting in the *usual course of his or her professional practice.* An order that does not meet these criteria, such as a prescription issued as a means to obtain controlled substances for the doctor's office use or to maintain addicted individuals, is not considered a legitimate prescription within the meaning of the law and thus does not protect either the doctor who issued it or the pharmacist who dispensed it. Some states prohibit physicians from prescribing controlled substances for themselves; it is prudent to comply with this guideline even if it is not mandated by law.

Execution of the Order

Prescriptions for controlled substances must be dated and signed on the day of their issuance and must bear the full name and address of the patient and the printed name, address, and DEA number of the practitioner and should be signed the way one would sign a legal document. Preprinted orders are not allowed in most states, and presigned blanks are prohibited by federal law. When oral orders are not permitted (Schedule II), the prescription must be written with ink or indelible pencil or typewritten. The order may be prepared by a member of the physician's staff, but the prescriber is responsible for the signature and any errors that the order may contain.

Oral Orders

Prescriptions for schedule III through schedule V medications may be telephoned to a pharmacy by a physician or by ancillary personnel in the same manner as a prescription for a noncontrolled substance, although it is in the physician's best interest to keep his or her DEA number as private as reasonably possible (*see* "Preventing Diversion," below). Schedule II prescriptions may be telephoned to a pharmacy only in EMERGENCY situations. To be an emergency: (1) Immediate administration is necessary; (2) no appropriate alternative treatment is available; and (3) it is not reasonably possible for the physician to provide a written prescription prior to the dispensing.

For an emergency prescription, the quantity must be limited to the amount adequate to treat the patient during the emergency period, and the physician must have a written prescription delivered to the pharmacy for that emergency within 72 hours. If mailed, the prescription must be postmarked within 72 hours. The pharmacist must notify the DEA if this prescription is not received.

Refills

No prescription order for a schedule II drug may be refilled under any circumstance. For schedule III and IV drugs, refills may be issued either orally or in writing, not to exceed five refills or six months after the issue date, whichever comes first. Beyond this, a new prescription must be ordered. For schedule V, no restrictions are placed on the number of refills allowed, but if no refills are noted at the time of issuance, a new prescription must be made.

Preventing Diversion

Prescription blanks often are stolen and used to sustain abuse of controlled substances and to divert legitimate drug products to the illicit market. To prevent this type of diversion, prescription pads should be protected in the same manner as one would protect a personal checkbook. A prescription blank should never be presigned for a staff member to fill in at a later time. Also, a minimum number of pads should be stocked, and they should be kept in a locked, secure location except when in use. If a pad or prescription is missing, it should be reported immediately to local authorities and pharmacies; some areas have systems in place to allow the rapid dissemination of such information. Ideally, the physician's full DEA number should not be preprinted on the prescription pad, because most prescriptions will not be for controlled substances and will not require the registration number, and anyone in possession of a valid DEA number may find it easier to commit prescription fraud. Some physicians have been observed, in certain situations, to intentionally omit part or all of their DEA number on a prescription and instead write "pharmacist call to verify" or "call for registration number." This works only when the prescriber has an established practice so the pharmacist may independently verify the authenticity of the prescription, and patients must be advised to fill the prescription during the prescriber's office hours.

Another method employed by the drug-seeker is to alter the face of a valid prescription to increase the number of units or refills. By spelling out the number of units and refills authorized instead of giving numerals, the prescriber essentially removes this option for diversion. Controlled substances should not be prescribed excessively or for prolonged periods, as the continuance of a patient's addiction is not a legitimate medical purpose for a prescription under section 309 of the act.

COMPLIANCE

The term *compliance* is considered by some health-care professionals to be out of date because it is seen as coercive or paternalistic. The assumption that the doctor tells the patient what to do and then the patient meticulously follows orders is unrealistic. It must be recognized that the patient is the final and most important determinant of how successful a therapeutic regimen will be and should be engaged as an active participant who has a vested interest in its success. For these reasons, the terms *adherence, therapeutic alliance,* and *concordance* often are used in place of *compliance* because they imply a more collaborative effort, representing the interaction between doctor and patient where each brings an expertise that has a valid position in determining a course of therapy. The doctor is the medical expert and the patient is the expert on himself and his beliefs, values, and lifestyle. The patient's quality-of-life beliefs may differ from the clinician's therapeutic goals, and the patient will have the last word every time there is an unresolved conflict.

Even the most carefully prepared prescription for the ideal therapy will be useless if the patient's level of compliance is not adequate. Compliance may be defined as the extent to which the patient follows a regimen prescribed by a health-care professional. Noncompliance may be manifest in drug therapy as intentional or accidental errors in dosage or schedule, overuse, underuse, early termination of therapy, or not having a prescription filled. Given that many patients do not strictly follow their prescribed regimen and that physicians have been shown to overestimate compliance rates in their patients, it is easy to believe that therapeutic failures frequently are due to patient noncompliance. Noncompliance always should be considered as a cause of inconsistent or nonexistent response to therapy.

Compliance behavior does not lend itself to easy analysis, and varying definitions and methods of assessment used in studies further complicate discussion of its incidence. A recent review of this literature revealed that the quality of research exploring patient compliance with prescription advice generally is poor, with deficiencies found not only in definition but also in design, methodology, and measurement (Nichol *et al.,* 1999). The incidence reported for patient noncompliance varies widely but is usually in the range of 30% to 60% (Meichenbaum and Turk, 1987); the rate for long-term regimens is approximately 50% and tends to increase over time (Sackett and Snow, 1979). Even though they complain about the illogical nature of their patients' noncompliance, health-care professionals seem to have as much difficulty as the rest of the population in following health-related orders, whether the orders involve medications, handwashing, or universal safety precautions (Feather *et al.,* 2000; Michalsen *et al.,* 1997; Ramphal-Naley *et al.,* 1996; Camins *et al.,* 1996; Meichenbaum and Turk, 1987).

Patient noncompliance is a problem that can result in, at best, no change in status and at worst, increased illness severity or death. Direct costs associated with noncompliance have been estimated at $8.5 to $50 billion (Johnson and Bootman, 1995). Hundreds of variables have been identified that may influence compliance behavior in any specific patient or condition, but none gives absolute results. A few of the most frequently cited are discussed

Table AI–4

Suggestions for Improving Patient Compliance

Provide respectful communication.

Develop satisfactory, collaborative relationship between doctor and patient.

Provide and encourage use of medication counseling.

Give precise, clear instructions, with most important information given first.

Support oral instructions with easy-to-read written information.

Simplify whenever possible.

Use mechanical compliance aids as needed (sectioned pill boxes or trays, compliance packaging, color-coding).

Use optimal dosage form and schedule for the individual patient.

Assess patient's literacy and comprehension and modify educational counseling as needed.

Find solutions when physical or sensory disabilities are present (use nonsafety caps on bottles, use large type on labels and written material, place tape marks on syringes).

Enlist support and assistance from family or caregivers.

Use behavioral techniques such as goal setting, self-monitoring, cognitive restructuring, skills training, contracts, and positive reinforcement.

SOURCE: Table based upon suggestions by DiMatteo, 1995; Feldman and DeTullio, 1994; Kehoe and Katz, 1998; Martin and Mead, 1982; Meichenbaum and Turk, 1987; and Salzman, 1995.

here along with some suggestions for improving compliance that are given in Table AI–4.

The Patient–Provider Relationship

Patient satisfaction with the physician has been shown to have a significant impact on compliance behavior, and it is one of few factors that the physician can directly influence. Patients are more likely to follow instructions and recommendations when their expectations for the patient–provider relationship and for their treatment are met. These expectations include not only clinical but also interpersonal competence, so cultivating good interpersonal and communication skills is essential.

When deciding upon a course of therapy, it can be useful to discuss a patient's habits and daily routine as well as the therapeutic options with the patient. This information can help suggest cues for remembrance, such as storing a once-daily medicine atop the books on the bed-side table for a patient who reads nightly or in the cabinet with the coffee cups if it is to be taken in the morning (noting that the bathroom can be the worst place to store a medication in terms of its physical and chemical preservation). The information also can help tailor the regimen to the patient's lifestyle. A lack of information about a patient's lifestyle can lead to situations such as that described by Benet in previous editions of this book—prescribing a medication to be taken with meals three times daily for a patient who only eats twice a day or who works a night shift and sleeps during the day. There is rarely only one treatment option for a given problem, and it may be better to prescribe an adequate regimen that the patient will follow instead of an ideal regimen that the patient will not follow (Meichenbaum and Turk, 1987). Involving patients in the control of any appropriate aspects of their therapy may improve compliance not only by aiding memory and making the dosage form or schedule more agreeable or convenient, but also by giving patients a feeling of empowerment and emphasizing their responsibility for the treatment outcome.

It is not unreasonable for the physician to ask the patient whether he or she intends to adhere to the prescribed therapy and to negotiate to get a commitment to do so. Attempts should be made to resolve collaboratively any conflicts that may hinder compliance.

Patients and Their Beliefs

Behavioral models often are used to explain the role that patients' beliefs may have in compliance behavior. Revised versions of the Health Belief Model (originally developed to explain preventive health behavior) are the most common. These suggest that when patients *perceive* that they are susceptible to the disease, that the disease may have serious negative impact, that the therapy will be effective, and that the benefits of the therapy outweigh the costs, and they believe in their own self-efficacy to execute the therapy, they are more likely to be compliant. The *actual* severity of and susceptibility to an illness is not necessarily an issue (Haynes, 1979a; Apter *et al.*, 1998); only the patient's perception of severity appears to make it relevant from a compliance standpoint (Buckalew and Buckalew, 1995).

Patients' beliefs can lead them to deliberately alter their therapy, whether for convenience, personal experiments, a desire to remove themselves from the sick role, a means to exercise a feeling of control over their situations, or other reasons. This reinforces the need for excellent communication and a good patient–provider relationship

to facilitate the provision of additional or corrective education when the beliefs would suggest poor compliance as an outcome. Further discussion of the psychology of noncompliance is intriguing but beyond the scope of this text.

It is difficult to predict whether or not a particular patient will be compliant, as there is no consistent relationship with isolated demographic variables such as age, sex, education level, intelligence, personality traits, and income. Certain of these variables have been implicated in specific situations, but they cannot be applied to the population as a whole. Social isolation generally has been found to be associated with poor compliance, although family members or other people close to the patient can undermine compliance as easily as support it. As noted above, the actual severity of the patient's disease is not predictive of compliance behavior, but characteristics of the disease can make adherence less likely, as with certain neurodegenerative or psychiatric illnesses.

It is not clear how important a role is played by patients' knowledge about their diseases and medications. Improving patient knowledge does not necessarily improve a patient's drug-taking behavior (Haynes, 1979b), but adequate instructions must be provided for patients to understand how to adhere to their therapy. Some studies have shown a positive correlation between increased patient education and compliance, at least for the short term (Edworthy and Devins, 1999; Lowe *et al.*, 2000). Pharmacists have a legal and professional responsibility to offer medication counseling in many situations—even though practice environments are not always conducive to its provision—and can educate and support patients by discussing prescribed medications and their use. Because they often see the patient more frequently than does the physician, pharmacists who take the time to inquire about patients' therapy can help spot compliance and other problems and notify the physician when appropriate.

Elderly patients are of concern because they often face a number of barriers to compliance related to their age. Such barriers include increased forgetfulness and confusion; altered drug disposition and higher sensitivity to some drug effects; decreased social and financial support; decreased dexterity, mobility, or sensory abilities; and an increased number of concurrent medicines used (both prescription and over-the-counter), whose attendant toxicities and interactions may cause decreased mental alertness or intolerable side effects. Inappropriate prescribing for elderly patients also has been identified as a problem (Willcox, *et al.*, 1994) and can further impair this population's ability to comply with drug therapy. Despite these obstacles, evidence does not show that elderly patients in general are significantly more noncompliant than any other age group. Still, elderly patients consume a disproportionate amount of medicines and health-care resources and have many age-related barriers to compliance, so there is great opportunity and motivation to improve their drug-taking habits. Pharmacists should pay particular attention to thorough and compassionate counseling for elderly patients and should assist physicians and the patients in finding practical solutions when problems are noted.

The Therapy

Increased complexity and duration of therapy are perhaps the best-documented barriers to compliance. The patient for whom multiple drugs are prescribed for a given disease or who has multiple illnesses that require drug therapy will be at higher risk for noncompliance, as will the patient whose disease is chronic. The frequency of dosing of individual medications also can affect compliance behavior. Simplification, whenever possible and appropriate, is desirable.

The effects of the medication can make adherence less likely, as in the case of patients whose medicines cause confusion or other altered mental states. Unpleasant side effects from the medicine may influence compliance in some patients but are not necessarily predictive, especially if patient beliefs or other positive factors would tend to reinforce adherence to the regimen. A side effect that is intolerable to one patient may be of minor concern to another.

Surveys have shown that, for most patients, the cost of the medicine does not appear to be a major determinant of compliance (Buckalew and Buckalew, 1995), and even receiving free medicine does not guarantee clinically adequate adherence (Apter *et al.*, 1998; Chisholm *et al.*, 2000). However, the cost of medicine can be a heavy burden for patients with limited economic resources, and health-care providers should be sensitive to this fact. While physicians often state that drug cost is an important factor in prescribing, their actual knowledge about prices is generally low (Reichert *et al.*, 2000), even for products that they commonly prescribe (Hoffman *et al.*, 1995), so this information may have to be sought from local pharmacies or references such as the *Drug Topics Red Book*. Costs can be reduced by using generic versions or different formulations of a drug, using a different drug or regimen, or investigating programs offered through drug companies or charitable institutions.

BIBLIOGRAPHY

Anonymous. A study of physicians' handwriting as a time waster. *JAMA*, **1979**, *242*:2429–2430.

Apter, A.J., Reisine, S.T., Affleck, G., Barrows, E., and ZuWallack, R.L. Adherence with twice-daily dosing of inhaled steroids. Socioeconomic and health-belief differences. *Am. J. Respir. Crit. Care Med.*, **1998**, *157*:1810–1817.

Bates, D.W., Cullen, D.J., Laird, N., Petersen, L.A., Small, S.D., Servi, D., Laffel, G., Sweitzer, B.J., Shea, B.F., Hallisey, R., Vander Vliet, M., Nemeskal, R., and Leape, L.L. Incidence of adverse drug events and potential adverse drug events. ADE Prevention Study Group. *JAMA*, **1995**, *274*:29–34.

Buckalew, L.W., and Buckalew, N.M. Survey of the nature and prevalence of patients' noncompliance and implications for intervention. *Psychol. Rep.*, **1995**, *76*:315–321.

Cabral, J.D. Poor physician penmanship. *JAMA*, **1997**, *278*:1116–1117.

Camins, B.C., Bock, N., Watkins, D.L., and Blumberg, H.M. Acceptance of isoniazid preventive therapy by health care workers after tuberculin skin test conversion. *JAMA*, **1996**, *275*:1013–1015.

Chisholm, M.A., Vollenweider, L.J., Mulloy, L.L., Jagadeesan, M., Wynn, J.J., Rogers, H.E., Wade, W.E., and DiPiro, J.T. Renal transplant patient compliance with free immunosuppressive medications. *Transplantation*, **2000**, *70*:1240–1244.

Classen, D.C., Pestotnik, S.L., Evans, R.S., and Burke, J.P. Computerized surveillance of adverse drug events in hospital patients. *JAMA*, **1991**, *266*:2847–2851.

Cohen, M.R., Anderson, R.W., Attilio, R.M., Green, L., Muller, R.J., and Pruemer, J.M. Preventing medication errors in cancer chemotherapy. *Am. J. Health Syst. Pharm.*, **1996**, *53*:737–746.

Cohen, M.R. Drug product characteristics that foster drug-use-system errors. *Am. J. Health Syst. Pharm.*, **1995**, *52*:395–399.

Cohen, M.R., and Davis, N.M. Developing safe and effective preprinted physician's order forms. *Hosp. Pharm.*, **1992**, *27*:508, 513, 528.

DiMatteo, M.R. Patient adherence to pharmacotherapy: the importance of effective communication. *Formulary*, **1995**, *30*:596–598, 601–602, 605.

Edworthy, S.M., and Devins, G.M. Improving medication adherence through patient education distinguishing between appropriate and inappropriate utilization. Patient Education Study Group. *J. Rheumatol.*, **1999**, *26*:1793–1801.

Feather, A., Stone, S.P., Wessier, A., Boursicot, K.A., and Pratt, C. "Now please wash your hands": the handwashing behaviour of final MBBS candidates. *J. Hosp. Infect.*, **2000**, *45*:62–64.

Feldman, J.A., and DeTullio, P.L. Medication compliance: an issue to consider in the drug selection process. *Hosp. Formul.*, **1994**, *29*:204–211.

Hoffman, J., Barefield, F.A., and Ramamurthy, S. A survey of physician knowledge of drug costs. *J. Pain Symptom Manage.*, **1995**, *10*:432–435.

ISMP. Ironing out a problem: measuring pediatric iron products safely. *ISMP Medication Safety Alert*, May 5, **1999.**

Johnson, J.A., and Bootman, J.L. Drug-related morbidity and mortality. A cost-of-illness model. *Arch. Intern. Med.,* **1995,** *155:*1949–1956.

Leape, L.L. Error in medicine. *JAMA,* **1994,** *272:*1851–1857.

Lesar, T.S., Briceland, L., and Stein, D.S. Factors related to errors in medication prescribing. *JAMA,* **1997,** *277:*312–317.

Lowe, C.J., Raynor, D.K., Purvis, J., Farrin, A., and Hudson, J. Effects of a medicine review and education programme for older people in general practice. *Br. J. Clin. Pharmacol.,* **2000,** *50:*172–175.

Martin, D.C., and Mead, K. Reducing medication errors in a geriatric population. *J. Am. Geriatr. Soc.,* **1982,** *4:*258–260.

Michalsen, A., Delclos, G.L., Felknor, S.A., Davidson, A.L., Johnson, P.C., Vesley, D., Murphy, L.R., Kelen, G.D., and Gershon, R.R. Compliance with universal precautions among physicians. *J. Occup. Environ. Med.,* **1997,** *39:*130–137.

National Coordinating Council for Medication Error Reporting and Prevention (NCC MERP). *Recommendations to Correct Error-Prone Aspects of Prescription Writing.* Publication #96C03. Rockville, MD, **1996.**

Nichol, M.B., Venturini, F., and Sung, J.C. A critical evaluation of the methodology of the literature on medication compliance. *Ann. Pharmacother.,* **1999,** *33:*531–540.

Ramphal-Naley, L., Kirkhorn, S., Lohman, W.H., and Zelterman, D. Tuberculosis in physicians: compliance with surveillance and treatment. *Am. J. Infect. Control,* **1996,** *24:*243–253.

Reichert, S., Simon, T., and Halm, E.A. Physicians' attitudes about prescribing and knowledge of the costs of common medications. *Arch. Intern. Med.,* **2000,** *160:*2799–2803.

Rucker, T.D. The top-selling drug products: how good are they? *Am. J. Hosp. Pharm.,* **1980,** *37:*833–837.

United States Pharmacopeia Medication Errors Reporting Program. Interleukin abbreviation interpreted incorrectly. *Practitioners' Reporting News,* December 12, **1999.**

United States Pharmacopeial Convention. Move to metric: apothecary system no longer recognized by USP. *USP Quality Rev.,* **1993,** Number 37 (revised).

United States Pharmacopeial Convention. Use caution—avoid confusion. *USP Quality Rev.,* May **1999a,** Number 66.

United States Pharmacopeial Convention. Proposed drug name changes for error prevention. *USP Quality Rev.,* October **1999b,** Number 69.

Willcox, S.M., Himmelstein, D.U., and Woolhandler, S. Inappropriate drug prescribing for the community-dwelling elderly. *JAMA,* **1994,** *272:*292–296.

Winslow, E.H., Nestor, V.A., Davidoff, S.K., Thompson, P.G., and Borum, J.C. Legibility and completeness of physicians' handwritten medication orders. *Heart Lung,* **1997,** *26:*158–164. [Published erratum appears in *Heart Lung,* **1997,** *26:*203.]

MONOGRAPHS AND REVIEWS

Davis, N.M. *Medical Abbreviations. 12,000 Conveniences at the Expense of Communications and Safety,* 8th ed. Neil M. Davis Associates, Huntington Valley, **1997.**

Haynes, R.B. Determinants of compliance: the disease and the mechanics of treatment. In, *Compliance in Health Care.* (Haynes, R.B., Taylor, D.W., and Sackett, D.L., eds.) Johns Hopkins University Press, Baltimore, **1979a,** pp. 49–62.

Haynes, R.B. Strategies to improve compliance with referrals, appointments, and prescribed medical regimens. In, *Compliance in Health Care.* (Haynes, R.B., Taylor, D.W., and Sackett, D.L., eds.) Johns Hopkins University Press, Baltimore, **1979b,** pp. 121–143.

Kehoe, W.A., and Katz, R.C. Health behaviors and pharmacotherapy. *Ann. Pharmacother.,* **1998,** *32:*1076–1086.

Meichenbaum, D., and Turk, D.C. *Facilitating Treatment Adherence.* Plenum Press, New York, **1987.**

Sackett, D.L., and Snow, J.C. The magnitude of compliance and noncompliance. In, *Compliance in Health Care.* (Haynes, R.B., Taylor, D.W., and Sackett, D.L., eds.) Johns Hopkins University Press, Baltimore, **1979,** pp. 11–22.

Salzman, C. Medication compliance in the elderly. *J. Clin. Psychiatry,* **1995,** *56*(suppl 1):18–22.

A P P E N D I X I I

DESIGN AND OPTIMIZATION OF DOSAGE REGIMENS: PHARMACOKINETIC DATA

Kenneth E. Thummel and Danny D. Shen

This appendix provides a summary of basic pharmacokinetic information pertaining to drugs that are in common clinical use and are delivered to the systemic circulation following parenteral or nonparenteral administration. Drugs designed exclusively for topical administration and those that are not significantly absorbed into the bloodstream (*e.g.,* ophthalmic and some dermal applications) are not included. Approximately 750 drugs were considered. Less than half of these could be included in Table A–II–1 due to space limitations. Thus, some drugs that appeared in the ninth edition of this book were deleted to make space for the large number of new products that have reached the market since 1995. Pharmacokinetic data for many drugs not included in this appendix can be found in earlier editions of this book.

A major objective of this appendix is to present pharmacokinetic data in a format that informs the clinician of the extent of interindividual differences in drug disposition and allows rational design of an appropriate drug-dosage regimen. Table A–II–1 contains quantitative information about the absorption, distribution, and elimination of drugs and the effects of disease states on these processes, as well as information about the correlation of efficacy and toxicity with drug concentrations in blood/plasma. The general principles that underlie the design of appropriate maintenance dose and dosing interval (and, where appropriate, the loading dose) for the average patient are described in Chapter 1. The concept of individualization of dosage regimens for a particular patient is presented here.

To use the data that are presented, one must understand clearance concepts and their application for drug-dosage regimens. One also must know average values of clearance as well as some measures of the extent and kinetics of drug absorption and distribution. The text below defines the eight basic parameters that are listed in

the tabular material for each drug as well as key factors that influence these values both in normal subjects and in patients with particular diseases. It obviously would be most useful if there were a consensus about a standard value for a given pharmacokinetic parameter; rather than a wide range of reported estimates. Unfortunately, a generally agreed set of pharmacokinetic values has been reached for only a limited number of drugs.

In Table A–II–1, a single set of values for each parameter and its variability in a relevant population has been selected from the literature, based on the scientific judgment of the authors. Most of the data are in the form of a study population mean value ± 1 standard deviation. However, some data are presented as mean and range of values (in parentheses) observed for the study population, with a dash separating the lowest and highest value reported. In some cases, only a range of values (separated by a dash) is reported. In other cases, only a single mean value for the study population was available in the literature and is reported as such. For some drugs, data were reported as a geometric mean with 95% confidence interval, and this is specifically indicated by a footnote. Finally, if there were sufficient data available, we also included in parentheses, below the primary study data, a range of mean values obtained from different studies of similar design.

Unless otherwise indicated in footnotes, data reported in the table are those determined in healthy adults. The direction of change for these values in particular disease states is noted below the average value. One or more references are provided for each of the established drugs, typically a recent paper or review on its clinical pharmacokinetics, which can then serve as a source for a broader range of papers for the interested reader. For the most recently approved drugs, multiple references are provided, including a review article where possible.

TABULATED PHARMACOKINETIC PARAMETERS

Each of the eight parameters presented in Table A–II–1 has been discussed in detail in Chapter 1. The following discussion focuses on the format in which the values are presented as well as on factors (physiological or pathological) that influence the parameters.

Bioavailability.   The extent of bioavailability is expressed as a percentage of the administered dose. This value represents the percentage of the administered dose that is available to the systemic circulation—the fraction of the oral dose that reaches the arterial blood in an active or prodrug form. *Fractional availability* (*F*), which appears elsewhere in this appendix, denotes the same parameter; this value varies from 0 to 1. Measures of both the *extent* and *rate* (*see* T_{max}) of availability are presented in the table. An understanding of the extent of availability is essential to the design of a dosage regimen to achieve a specific target blood concentration (*see* Chapter 1). Values for multiple routes of administration are provided, when appropriate and available, from the literature. In most cases, the tabulated value represents an absolute oral bioavailability that has been determined against an intravenous reference dose. For those drugs where intravenous administration is not possible, an approximate estimate of oral bioavailability based on secondary information (*e.g.,* urinary excretion) is presented, or the column is left blank [denoted by a long dash (—)].

It is important to keep in mind that poor patient compliance may be mistaken for a reduced extent of bioavailability. A true decrease in bioavailability may result from a poorly formulated dosage form that fails to disintegrate or dissolve in the gastrointestinal fluids, interactions between drugs in the gastrointestinal tract, metabolism of the drug in the lumen of the gastrointestinal tract, first-pass intestinal metabolism or active efflux into the lumen, and first-pass hepatic metabolism or biliary excretion (*see* Chapter 1). In the case of drugs with extensive first-pass metabolism, hepatic disease may cause an increase in oral availability because hepatic metabolic capacity decreases and/or because vascular shunts develop around the liver.

Urinary Excretion of Unchanged Drug.   The second parameter in Table A–II–1 is the amount of drug eventually excreted unchanged in the urine, expressed as a percentage of the administered dose. Values represent the percentage expected in a healthy young adult (creatinine clearance equal to or greater than 100 ml/min). When possible, the value listed is that determined after bolus intravenous administration of the drug, for which bioavailability is assumed to be 100%. If the drug is given orally, this parameter may be underestimated due to incomplete absorption of the dose; such values are indicated in a footnote. The parameter obtained after intravenous dosing is of greater utility, since it will reflect the relative contribution of renal elimination to the total body clearance irrespective of bioavailability.

Renal disease is the primary factor that causes changes in this parameter. This is especially true when alternate pathways of elimination are available; thus, as renal function decreases, a greater fraction of the dose is available for elimination by other routes. Because renal function generally decreases as a function of age, the percentage of drug excreted unchanged also then decreases with age when alternate pathways of elimination are available. In addition, for a number of acidic and basic drugs with values of pK_a in the range of the usual pH of urine, changes in the latter will affect the rate or extent of urinary excretion (*see* Chapter 1).

Binding to Plasma Proteins.   The tabulated value is the percentage of drug in the plasma that is bound to plasma proteins at concentrations of the drug that are achieved clinically. In almost all cases, the values are from measurements performed *in vitro* (rather than from measurements of binding to proteins in plasma obtained from patients to whom the drug had been administered). When a single mean value is presented, there is no apparent change in this percentage over the range of plasma drug concentrations normally found in patients taking the drug. In cases in which saturation of binding is approached at usual plasma drug concentrations, values are provided at concentrations that correspond to the lower and upper limits of the usual range. For some drugs, there is disagreement in the literature about the extent of binding, and the range of reported values is given.

Plasma protein binding is affected primarily by disease states (such as hepatic disease or inflammatory diseases) that alter the concentration of albumin, α_1-acid glycoprotein, or other proteins in plasma that bind drugs. Some metabolic states and conditions, such as uremia, also change the binding affinity of albumin for some drugs. Such changes in protein binding as a function of disease can dramatically affect the volume of distribution, clearance, and elimination half-life of a drug.

Clearance.   Total systemic clearance of drug from plasma or blood [*see* Equations (1–4) and (1–5), Chapter 1] is given in Table A–II–1. Clearance varies as a function of body size and, therefore, is presented most frequently in the table in units of $ml \cdot min^{-1} \cdot kg^{-1}$ of body weight. Although normalization to measures of body size other than weight sometimes may be appropriate, weight is so convenient that its use often offsets any small loss in accuracy of clearance estimate, especially in adults. Exceptions to this rule are the anticancer drugs, for which dosage normalization to body surface area is conventionally used. When unit conversion was necessary, we used individual or mean body weight or body surface area (when appropriate) from the cited study or, if this was not available, we assumed a body mass of 70 kg or a body surface area of 1.73 m^2 for healthy adults.

In some cases, separate values for renal and nonrenal clearance also are provided. For some drugs, particularly those that are excreted predominantly unchanged in the urine, equations are given that relate total or renal clearance to creatinine clearance (also expressed as ml $\cdot$ min^{-1} $\cdot$ kg^{-1}). For drugs that exhibit saturation kinetics, K_m and V_{max} are given and represent, respectively, the plasma concentration at which half of the maximal rate of elimination is reached (in units of mass/volume) and the maximal rate of elimination (in units of mass $\cdot$ time^{-1} $\cdot$ kg^{-1} of body weight). Concentration of the drug in plasma (C_p) must, of course, be in the same units as K_m.

As discussed in Chapter 1, intrinsic clearance from blood is the maximal possible clearance by the organ responsible for elimination when blood flow (delivery) of drug is not limiting. When expressed in terms of unbound drug, intrinsic clearance reflects clearance from intracellular water. Intrinsic clearance is tabulated for a few drugs. It is also mathematically related to the biochemical intrinsic clearance [$V_{max}/(K_m + C)$] determined *in vitro*. For example, V_{max} and K_m parameters can be determined for any number of drug biotransformation pathways in liver homogenates, or microsomes or with purified enzyme. The total intrinsic clearance for the eliminating organ is the sum of the individual $V_{max}/(K_m + C)$ terms for each pathway, scaled appropriately for the total mass of subcellular fraction or enzyme in the entire organ. For a drug that exhibits saturable metabolism or transport, intrinsic clearance is defined in terms of the concentration of drug in blood. When saturable metabolism or transport is not encountered *in vivo* (*i.e.*, $C_p \ll K_m$), the intrinsic clearance (V_{max}/K_m) and total body clearance are constant.

If one wishes to relate changes in elimination of drug to pathological changes either in the organ itself or to blood flow to the organ, it is necessary to express clearance with respect to concentrations of drug in *blood* rather than those in plasma. This requires measurement of concentrations in whole blood or knowledge of the distribution of drug between plasma and red blood cells (*see* Chapter 1). Such information currently is limited, but is provided in a footnote when available. In almost all cases, plasma clearances are presented in Table A–II–1, because these are most useful for relating drug dosage to plasma drug concentrations that have been determined previously to be effective or toxic. The few exceptions

where clearance from blood is presented are indicated by footnote.

Clearance can be determined only when the fractional availability (F) of the drug is known. Therefore, to be accurate, clearances must be determined after intravenous dosage. When such data are not available, the ratio of *CL/F* is given; values of this kind are indicated in a footnote. When a drug, or its active isomer for racemic compounds, is primarily a substrate for a particular cytochrome P450 (CYP) isoform or secretory transporter (as discussed in Chapter 1), this information is provided in a footnote. This information is becoming increasingly important to understand and predict metabolically based drug-drug interactions. [For a more extensive coverage of this topic, *see Metabolic Drug Interactions.* (Levy, R.H., Thummel, K.E., Trager, W.F., Hansten, P.D., and Eichelbaum, M., eds.) Lippincott Williams & Wilkins, Philadelphia, 2000.]

Volume of Distribution. The total body volume of distribution at steady state (V_{ss}) is given in Table A–II–1 and is expressed in units of liters/kg, or in units of liters/m^2 for some anticancer drugs. Again, when unit conversion was necessary, we used individual or mean body weights or body surface area (when appropriate) from the cited study or, if such data were not available, we assumed a body mass of 70 kg or a body surface area of 1.73 m^2 for healthy adults.

When estimates of V_{ss} were not available, values for V_{area} were provided (*see* Chapter 1). V_{area} represents the distribution volume during the terminal elimination phase and is computed readily by dividing clearance by the terminal rate constant for elimination. Unlike V_{ss}, this volume term varies when the rate constant for drug elimination changes, even though there is no change in the distribution space. Because we may wish to know whether a particular disease state influences either the clearance or the tissue distribution of the drug, it is preferable to define volume in terms of V_{ss}, a parameter that is theoretically independent of changes in the rate of elimination.

As in the case for clearance, V_{ss} usually is defined in the table in terms of concentration in plasma rather than blood. Further, if data were not obtained after intravenous administration of the drug, a footnote will make clear that the apparent volume estimate, V_{ss}/F, is offset by the bioavailability.

Half-Life. Half-life ($t_{1/2}$) is the time required for the plasma concentration to decline by one-half when elimination is first-order. It also governs the rate of approach to steady state and the degree of drug accumulation during multiple dosing or continuous infusion, as described in Chapter 1. For example, at a fixed dosing interval, the patient will be at 50% of steady state after one half-life,

75% of steady state after two half-lives, 93.75% of steady state after four drug half-lives, *etc*. Determination of half-life is straightforward when drug elimination follows a monoexponential pattern (*i.e.*, one-compartment model). However, for a number of drugs, plasma concentration follows a multiexponential pattern of decline over time. The mean value listed in Table A–II–1 corresponds to an effective rate of elimination that covers the clearance of a major fraction of the absorbed dose from the body. In many cases, this half-life refers to the rate of elimination in the terminal exponential phase. For a number of drugs, however, a more prolonged half-life may be observed at very low plasma concentrations when extremely sensitive assay techniques are used. If this component accounts for 10% or less of the total area under the plasma concentration-time curve (*AUC*), predictions of drug accumulation in plasma during continuous or repetitive dosing will be in error by no more than 10% if this longer half-life is ignored, no matter how large its value. The clinician should know the half-life that will best predict accumulation in the patient. That will be the appropriate half-life to use for estimating the rate constant to incorporate into Equations (1–18) and (1–19) (*see* Chapter 1) to predict time to steady state. It is this multiple dosing or accumulation half-life that is given in the table.

Half-life is usually independent of body size because it is a function of the ratio of two parameters, clearance and volume of distribution, each of which is proportional to body size.

Time to Peak Concentration.   Since clearance concepts are used most often in the design of multiple dosage regimens, the extent rather than the rate of availability is more critical to estimate the average steady-state concentration of drug in the body. However, in some circumstances, the degree of fluctuation between peak and trough concentrations, and as a result the drug efficacy and side effects profile, can be greatly influenced by modulation of drug absorption rate, such as the use of sustained- or extended-release formulations. Controlled-release formulations often permit a reduction in dosing frequency from 3 or 4 times daily to once or twice daily. There also are drugs that are given as a single dose for the relief of breakthrough pain or to induce sleep, for which the rate of drug absorption is a critical determinant of drug efficacy. Thus, information about the expected average time to achieve maximal plasma or blood concentration and the degree of interindividual variability in that parameter have been included in Table A–II–1.

The time required to achieve a maximal concentration (T_{max}) is dependent, in part, on the rate of drug absorption into blood from the site of administration. From mass balance principles, T_{max} occurs when the rate of absorption

equals the rate of elimination from the reference compartment. Prior to this time, absorption rate exceeds elimination rate and the plasma concentration of drug increases. After the peak is reached, elimination rate exceeds the absorption rate and, at some point, defines the terminal elimination phase of the concentration-time profile. If drug is introduced at a constant and continuous rate, blood concentrations will rise until a steady-state level is achieved, where the two rates are equivalent. This applies to a constant rate intravenous infusion, but it also could apply to continuous delivery at any other site in the body.

The rate of drug absorption will depend on the formulation and physicochemical properties of the drug, as well as on the anatomical barrier and blood flow to the delivery site. For an oral dose, some absorption may occur very rapidly within the buccal cavity, esophagus, and stomach, or absorption may be delayed until the drug reaches the small intestine or until the local pH in the intestine permits disintegration of the dosage formulation. In the most extreme case, the rate of absorption can be sufficiently controlled by the drug formulation to permit sustained or extended delivery as drug traverses the entire length of the gastrointestinal tract. In some instances, the terminal elimination of drug from the body following a peak concentration reflects the slower rate of absorption and not elimination ("flip-flop" effect).

When more than one type of drug formulation is available commercially, we have provided absorption kinetic information for the two extremes, an immediate-release and a sustained-release formulation. Not surprisingly, the presence of food in the gastrointestinal tract can alter both the rate and extent of drug availability. We have indicated with footnotes when the consumption of food in proximity to the ingestion of an oral dose might have a significant effect on the bioavailability of the drug, such that specific recommendations are made by the manufacturer.

Peak Concentration.   There is no general agreement about the best way to describe the relationship between the concentration of drug in plasma and its effect. Many different kinds of data are present in the literature, and use of a single effect parameter or effective concentration is difficult. This is particularly true for antimicrobial agents, since the effective concentration depends on the identity of the microorganism causing the infection. It also is important to recognize that concentration-effect relationships are most easily obtained at steady state or during the terminal log-linear phase of the concentration-time curve, when the drug concentration(s) at the site(s) of action is expected to parallel that in plasma. Thus, when attempting to correlate a blood or plasma level to effect, the temporal aspect of distribution of drug to its site of action must be taken into account.

Despite these limitations, it is possible to define effective or toxic concentrations for some of the drugs currently in clinical use, as reported in previous editions of this book. However, in reviewing the list of drugs approved within the last five years, it is rare to find a declaration of an *effective concentration,* even in the manufacturers' package labeling. Thus, it is necessary to infer effective concentrations from concentration-time profiles following *effective dosage* regimens. Although a mean steady-state blood or plasma concentration and the associated interindividual variability might be the most appropriate parameter to report, from first principles, these data often are unavailable even in the primary literature. One can estimate the mean steady-state concentration during a dose interval ($\bar{C}_{ss}$) by dividing the mean *AUC* by the duration of the dose interval. However, this approach does not apply to single-dose administration, nor does it permit the presentation of expected population variability. Further, in some instances, drug efficacy may be more closely linked with peak concentration than with the average or trough concentration, and it is sometimes the case that differences in peak concentration for special populations (*e.g.,* elderly) are associated with increased incidence of drug toxicity.

For a number of clinical and practical reasons, the most commonly reported parameter, C_{max} (peak concentration), is reported in Table A–II–1, rather than effective or toxic concentrations. This provides a more consistent body of information about drug exposure from which one can infer, if appropriate, efficacious or toxic blood levels. We acknowledge that the value reported is the highest that would be encountered in a given dose interval. However, C_{max} can be related to the mean concentration and the trough concentration through appropriate mathematical equations (*see* Chapter 1). Because peak levels will vary with dose, we have attempted to present concentrations observed with a customary dose regimen that is recognized to be effective in the majority of patients. When a higher or lower dose rate is used, the expected peak level can be adjusted by assuming dose proportionality, unless nonlinear kinetics are indicated. In some instances, there are only limited data pertaining to multiple dosing, so single-dose peak concentrations are presented. When specific information is available about an effective therapeutic range of concentrations or about concentrations at which toxicity occurs, it has been incorporated into a footnote. For every drug, the reader also is referred to a specific chapter or chapters in which more detailed information sometimes can be obtained.

It is important to recognize that significant differences in C_{max} will occur when comparing similar daily-dose regimens for an immediate-release and sustained-release product. Indeed, the sustained-release product sometimes is administered to reduce peak-trough fluctuations during the dosing interval and to minimize swings between potentially toxic or ineffective drug concentrations. Again, we have reported C_{max} for immediate-release and extended-release formulations, when available. In addition to parent drug concentrations, we have tried to include information on any active metabolite that circulates at a concentration that may contribute to the overall pharmacological effect, particularly those active metabolites that accumulate with multiple dosing.

Although total drug or metabolite concentrations are reported, it is important to recognize that the concentration of *unbound drug* determines the degree of pharmacological effect. Accordingly, changes in protein binding due to disease may be expected to cause changes in the unbound concentration associated with desired or unwanted effects. However, this is not always the case, since an increase in free fraction will increase the apparent clearance of an orally administered drug and of a low extraction drug dosed intravenously. Under such a scenario, the mean unbound plasma concentration at steady state will not change with reduced or elevated plasma protein binding, despite a significant change in mean total drug concentration.

ALTERATIONS OF PARAMETERS IN THE INDIVIDUAL PATIENT

Dose adjustments for an individual patient should be made according to the manufacturer's recommendation in the package labeling when available. This information is generally available when disease, age, or ethnicity has a significant impact on drug disposition, and particularly for drugs that have been introduced within the last ten years. In some cases though, a significant difference in drug disposition from the "average" adult can be expected, but it may not require dose adjustment because of a sufficiently broad therapeutic range. In other cases, dose adjustment may be necessary, but no specific information is available. Under these circumstances, an estimate of the appropriate dosing regimen can be obtained based on pharmacokinetic principles described in Chapter 1.

Unless otherwise specified, the values in Table A–II–I represent mean values for populations of normal adults; it may be necessary to modify them for calculation of dosage regimens for individual patients. The fraction available (*F*) and clearance also must be estimated to compute a maintenance dose necessary to achieve a desired average steady-state concentration. To calculate the loading dose, knowledge of the volume of distribution is needed. The estimated half-life is used to identify a dosing interval that provides an acceptable peak-trough fluctuation. The values reported in the table and the adjustments apply only to adults, unless specifically designated otherwise. Although the values at times may be applied to children who weigh more than about 30 kg (after proper adjustment for size; *see* below), it is best to consult a textbook of pediatrics or other source for definitive advice.

For each drug, changes in the parameters caused by certain disease states are noted within the eight segments of the table. In most cases, a qualitative direction of changes is noted, such as "↓ Hep," which indicates a significant decrease in the parameter in a patient with hepatitis. A reasonable, quantitative translation is to multiply the value of the parameter by 0.5 for each applicable condition that is noted to decrease the parameter and to multiply it by 2 for each condition that is noted to increase the parameter. Such an adjustment can be only approximate; yet, since reliable data are limited, no better approach may be possible. The relevant literature should be consulted for more definitive, quantitative information.

Protein Binding. Most acidic drugs that are extensively bound to plasma proteins are bound to albumin. Basic lipophilic drugs, such as propranolol, often bind to other plasma proteins (*e.g.*, α_1-acid glycoprotein and lipoproteins). The degree of drug binding to proteins will differ in pathophysiological states that cause changes in plasma-protein concentrations. Unfortunately, among binding proteins only albumin is commonly measured. For drugs that are bound to albumin (*alb*), a patient's fraction of unbound drug (α_{pt}) can be approximated from the following relationship:

$$\alpha_{pt} = 1 \left/ \left[\left(\frac{alb_{pt}}{alb_{nl}} \right) \cdot \left(\frac{1 - \alpha_{nl}}{\alpha_{nl}} \right) + 1 \right] \right. \qquad (A\text{--}1)$$

where alb_{nl} and α_{nl} refer to values of the concentration of albumin in plasma and the fraction of unbound drug in normal individuals, respectively. Use of this equation assumes that the molar concentration of drug is far less than that of albumin, that only one type of drug binding site is present on albumin, and that there are no cooperative binding interactions. Therefore, it is an approximation that is useful in the absence of actual measurement of the patient's plasma free fraction.

Clearance. For drugs that are partly or predominantly eliminated by renal excretion, plasma clearance changes in accordance with the renal function of an individual patient. This necessitates dosage adjustment that is dependent on the fraction of normal renal function remaining and the fraction of drug normally excreted unchanged in the urine. The latter quantity appears in the table; the former can be estimated as the ratio of the patient's creatinine clearance

(CL_{cr}) to a "rounded" normal value (100 ml/min per 70 kg body weight). If urinary creatinine clearance has not been measured, it may be estimated from the concentration of creatinine in serum (C_{cr}). In men:

$$CL_{cr} \, (\text{ml} \cdot \text{min}^{-1}) = \frac{[140 - \text{age (yr)}] \cdot [\text{weight (kg)}]}{72 \cdot [C_{cr}(\text{mg/dl})]}$$

$$(A\text{--}2)$$

For women, the estimate of CL_{cr} by the above equation should be multiplied by 0.85 to reflect their smaller muscle mass. The fraction of normal renal function is estimated from the following:

$$rfx_{pt} = \frac{CL_{cr, \, pt}}{100 \; \text{ml} \cdot \text{min}^{-1}} \qquad (A\text{--}3)$$

This provides a rough estimate, but more accurate ones are seldom necessary, since the adjustment of clearance is an approximation given the considerable degree of interindividual variation in nonrenal clearance. The following equation for adjustment of clearance uses the quantities discussed:

$$rf_{pt} = 1 - [fe_{nl} \cdot (1 - rfx_{pt})] \qquad (A\text{--}4)$$

where fe_{nl} is the fraction of systemic drug excreted unchanged in normal individuals (*see* Table A–II–1). The renal factor (rf_{pt}) is the value that, when multiplied by normal total clearance (CL_{nl}) from the table, gives the total clearance of the drug adjusted for the impairment in renal function.

Example. The clearance of vancomycin in a patient with reduced renal function (creatinine clearance = 25 ml/min per 70 kg) may be estimated as follows:

$$rfx_{pt} = \frac{25 \; \text{ml/min}}{100 \; \text{ml/min}} = 0.25$$

$fe_{nl} = 0.79$ (*see* listing for vancomycin)
$rf_{pt} = 1 - [0.79 \cdot (1 - 0.25)] = 0.41$
$CL_{pt} = (1.4 \; \text{ml/min per kg}) \cdot 0.41$
$\quad\quad = 0.57 \; \text{ml/min per kg}$

Importantly, such a dosage adjustment should be regarded only as an initial step in optimizing the dosage regimen; depending on the patient's response to the drug, further individualization may be necessary.

In the case of reduced clearance with significant hepatic cirrhosis, as denoted by ↓ Cirr, a reasonable quantitative translation is to multiply the clearance by 0.5 and decrease the dosing rate by 50%. Again, such an adjustment can be only approximate, and the relevant literature or manufacturer's package labeling should be consulted for more definitive quantitative guidance.

Conventionally, clearance is adjusted for the size of the patient to reflect a difference in the mass of the eliminating organ. For orally administered drugs, the applicability of such an adjustment may be limited by the available dosage strengths of commercial formulations. In some cases, the type of formulation permits physical splitting of the tablet (commercial tablet splitters are available) to increase the number of available dosages. However, this practice should be followed only with the recommendation of the drug manufacturer, since it can compromise the systemic bioavailability of some products.

With the exception of certain oncolytic agents, the data presented in the table are normalized to weight. Thus, interindividual variability in the weight-normalized clearance reflects a variation in the intrinsic metabolic or transport clearance, and not the size of the organ. Further, these differences can be attributed to variable expression/function of metabolic enzymes or transporters. However, it is important to recognize that liver mass and total enzyme/transporter content may not increase or decrease in proportion to weight in obese or malnourished individuals. Alternative approaches such as normalization for body surface area or the use of specific nomograms may be more appropriate. For example, many of the drugs used to treat cancer are dosed according to body surface area. In the tabulation, if the literature reported dose per body surface area, we chose to present the data in the same unit. If the cited clearance data were not normalized, but the preponderance of the literature utilized body surface area, we followed the practice of using individual values of body surface area or a standard of 1.73 m^2 for a healthy adult.

Volume of Distribution. Volume of distribution should be adjusted for the modifying factors indicated in Table A–II–1, as well as for body size. Again, the data in the table are most often normalized to weight. Unlike clearance, volume of distribution in any individual is most often proportional to weight itself. Whether or not this applies to a specific drug, however, depends on the actual sites of distribution of drug; no absolute rule applies.

Whether or not to adjust volume of distribution for changes in binding to plasma proteins cannot be decided in general, since the decision depends critically on whether or not the factors that alter binding to plasma proteins

also alter binding to tissues. In such cases, the qualitative changes in volume of distribution are indicated in the table. Again, each adjustment to volume of distribution should be made independently of any other, and the final estimate should reflect all adjustments simultaneously.

Half-Life. Half-life may be estimated from the adjusted values of clearance and volume of distribution for the patient (*pt*):

$$t_{1/2} = \frac{0.693 \cdot V_{pt}}{CL_{pt}} \qquad \text{(A–5)}$$

Because half-life has been the parameter most often measured and reported in the literature, qualitative changes for this parameter are almost always given in the table.

INDIVIDUALIZATION OF DOSAGE

By using the parameters for the individual patient, calculated as described above, initial dosing regimens may be chosen. The maintenance dose may be calculated with Equation (1–16) in Chapter 1 and the estimated values for *CL* and *F* for the individual patient. The target concentration may have to be adjusted for changes in protein binding in the patient, as described above. The loading dose may be calculated using Equation (1–20) in Chapter 1 and the estimated parameters for V_{ss} and *F*. A particular dosing interval may be chosen; the maximal and minimal steady-state concentrations can be calculated by using Equations (1–18) and (1–19) in Chapter 1, and these can be compared with the known efficacious and toxic concentrations for the drug. As with the target concentration, these values may need to be adjusted for changes in the extent of protein binding. Use of Equations (1–18) and (1–19) also requires estimates of values for *F*, V_{ss}, and *k* ($k = 0.693/t_{1/2}$) for the individual patient.

Note that these adjustments of the pharmacokinetic parameters for an individual patient are suggested for the rational choice of initial dosing regimen. As indicated in Chapter 1, measurement of drug concentrations in the patient then can be used as a guide to further adjust the dosage regimen. However, optimization of a dosage regimen for an individual patient will depend ultimately on the clinical response produced by the drug.

Acknowledgment

The authors wish to acknowledge the contribution of Drs. Leslie Z. Benet, Svein Øie, and Janice B. Schwartz, authors of this appendix in the ninth edition of *Goodman & Gilman's The Pharmacological Basis of Therapeutics*, some of whose text and tabulated data have been retained in this edition.

Table A–II–1
PHARMACOKINETIC DATA

	AVAILABILITY (ORAL) (%)	URINARY EXCRETION (%)	BOUND IN PLASMA (%)	CLEARANCE ($ml \cdot min^{-1} \cdot kg^{-1}$)	VOL. DIST. (liters/kg)	HALF-LIFE (hours)	PEAK TIME (hours)	PEAK CONCENTRATIONS
ABACAVIR[a] (Chapter 51)								
	83 (63–110)	1 (0–4)	—	12.8 (9.3–17.5)	0.84 (0.69–1.03)	1.0 (0.8–1.3)	Tab: 0.63 (0.4–1.1)[b] Sol: 0.5 (0.5–0.6)[b]	Tab: 2.6(2.3–2.9) µg/ml[b] Sol: 2.9 (2.5–3.4) µg/ml[b]

[a]Data from male subjects with HIV infection. Values are geometric means and 95% CI. Metabolized by ADH, UGT, and other enzymes.
[b]C_{max} and T_{max} (geometric mean and 95% CI) following a 300-mg oral tablet (Tab) or solution (Sol).

References: Barry, M., Mulcahy, F., Merry, C., Gibbons, S., and Back, D. Pharmacokinetics and potential interactions amongst antiretroviral agents used to treat patients with HIV infection. *Clin. Pharmacokinet.,* **1999,** *36:*289–304.
Chittick, G.E., Gillotin, C., McDowell, J.A., Lou, Y., Edwards, K.D., Prince, W.T., and Stein, D.S. Abacavir: absolute bioavailability, bioequivalence of three oral formulations, and effect of food. *Pharmacotherapy,* **1999,** *19:*932–942.

ACETAMINOPHEN[a] (Chapter 27)								
	88 ± 15 ←→ Child	3 ± 1 ←→ Neo, Child	<20	5.0 ± 1.4[b] ↓ Hep[c] ←→ Aged, Child ↑ Obes, HTh, Preg	0.95 ± 0.12[b] ←→ Aged, Hep[c] LTh, HTh, Child	2.0 ± 0.4 ←→ RD, Obes, Child ↑ Neo, Hep[c] ↓ HTh, Preg	0.33–1.4[d]	20 µg/ml[e]

[a]Values reported are for a linear kinetic model for doses less than 2 g; drug exhibits concentration-dependent kinetics above this dose.
[b]Assuming a 70-kg body weight; reported range, 65 to 72 kg.
[c]Acetaminophen-induced hepatic damage or acute viral hepatitis.
[d]Absorption rate, but not extent, depends on gastric emptying; hence, slowed after food as well as in some disease states and cotreatment with drugs that cause gastroparesis.
[e]Mean concentration following a 20-mg/kg oral dose. Hepatic toxicity associated with levels >300 µg/ml at 4 hours after an overdose.

Reference: Forrest, J.A., Clements, J.A., and Prescott, L.F. Clinical pharmacokinetics of paracetamol. *Clin. Pharmacokinet.,* **1982,** *7:*93–107.

(L)-α-ACETYL-METHADOL (LAAM)[a] (Chapter 23)								
	47 ± 5	6	80	4.93 ± 0.58	7.0	L: 18.5 ± 4.9 NL: 23.9 ± 3.2 DL: 65.8 ± 10.1	L: 2.6 ± 0.2[b] NL: 3.9 ± 0.7[b] DL: 31 ± 9.6[b]	L: 63 ± 8 ng/ml[b] NL: 44 ± 4 ng/ml[b] DL: 19 ± 1 ng/ml[b]

[a]Data from healthy adult male subjects. LAAM (L) is metabolized by cytochrome P450 (primarily CYP3A) to active metabolites, nor-LAAM (NL) and dinor-LAAM (DL).
[b]Following a single 40-mg oral dose.

References: Kaiko, R.F., Chatterjie, N., and Inturrisi, C.E. Simultaneous determination of acetyl-methadol and its active biotransformation products in human biofluids. *J. Chromatogr.,* **1975,** *109:*247–258.
Walsh, S.L., Johnson, R.E., Cone, E.J., and Bigelow, G.E. Intravenous and oral *l*-α-acetylmethadol: pharmacodynamics and pharmacokinetics in humans. *J. Pharmacol. Exp. Ther.,* **1998,** *285:*71–82.

ACETYLSALICYLIC ACID[a] (Chapters 27, 55)								
	68 ± 3 ←→ Aged, Cirr	1.4 ± 1.2	49 ↓ RD	9.3 ± 1.1 ←→ Aged, Cirr	0.15 ± 0.03	0.25 ± 0.03 ←→ Hep	0.39 ± 0.21[b]	24 ± 4 µg/ml[b]

[a]Values given are for unchanged parent drug. Acetylsalicylic acid is converted to salicylic acid during and after absorption (CL and $t_{1/2}$ of salicylic acid are dose-dependent; half-life varies between 2.4 hours after a 300-mg dose to 19 hours when there is intoxication).
[b]Following a single 1.2-g oral dose given to adults.

Reference: Roberts, M.S., Rumble, R.H., Wanwimolruk, S., Thomas, D., and Brooks, P.M. Pharma-cokinetics of aspirin and salicylate in elderly subjects and in patients with alcoholic liver disease. *Eur. J. Clin. Pharmacol.,* **1983,** *25:*253–261.

1924

ACYCLOVIR (Chapter 50)

Bioavailability	Urinary Excretion	Bound in Plasma	Clearance	Vol. Dist.	Half-Life	Peak Time	Peak Conc.
15–30[a]	75 ± 10	15 ± 4	$CL = 3.37\,CL_{cr} + 0.41$ ↓ Neo ↔ Child	0.69 ± 0.19 ↓ Neo → RD	2.4 ± 0.7 ↑ RD, Neo → Child	1.5–2[b]	3.5–5.4 μM[b]

[a] Decreases with increasing dose.
[b] Range of steady-state concentrations following a 400-mg oral dose, given every 4 hours to steady state.

Reference: Laskin, O.L. Clinical pharmacokinetics of acyclovir. *Clin. Pharmacokinet.,* **1983,** 8: 187–201.

ALBUTEROL[a] (Chapters 10, 28)

Bioavailability	Urinary Excretion	Bound in Plasma	Clearance	Vol. Dist.	Half-Life	Peak Time	Peak Conc.
PO, R: 30 ± 7; PO, S: 71 ± 9; IH, R: 25; IH, S: 47	R/S: 7 ± 1	R: 46 ± 8; S: 55 ± 11	R: 10.3 ± 3.0; S: 6.5 ± 2.0 ↓ RD[b]	R: 2.00 ± 0.70; S: 1.77 ± 0.69 ↓ RD[b]	R: 2.00 ± 0.49; S: 2.85 ± 0.85	R: 1.5[c]; S: 2.0[c]	R: 3.6 (1.9–5.9) ng/ml[c]; S: 11.4 (7.1–16.2) ng/ml[c]

[a] Data from healthy subjects for R and S enantiomers. No major gender differences. No kinetic differences in asthmatics. β-Adrenergic activity resides primarily with R-enantiomer. Oral dose undergoes extensive first-pass sulfation at the intestinal mucosa.
[b] CL/F reduced, moderate renal impairment.
[c] Median (range) following a single 4-mg oral dose of racemic (R/S)-albuterol.

References: Boulton, D.W., and Fawcett, J.P. Enantioselective disposition of albuterol in humans. *Clin. Rev. Allergy Immunol.,* **1996,** *14:*115–138. Mohamed, M.H., Lima, J.J., Eberle, L.V., Self, T.H., and Johnson, J.A. Effects of gender and race on albuterol pharmacokinetics. *Pharmacotherapy,* **1999,** *19:*157–161.

ALENDRONATE[a] (Chapter 62)

Bioavailability	Urinary Excretion	Bound in Plasma	Clearance	Vol. Dist.	Half-Life	Peak Time	Peak Conc.
<0.7[b] ↓ Food	44.9 ± 9.3	78	1.11 (1.00–1.22)[c] ↔ RD[e]	0.44 (0.34–0.55)[c]	~1.0[d]	IV: 2[f]	IV: ~275 ng/ml[f]; Oral: <5–8.4 ng/ml[f]

[a] Data from healthy postmenopausal female subjects.
[b] Based on urinary recovery and reduced when taken <1 hour before and up to 2 hours after a meal.
[c] CL and V_{ss} values represent mean and 90% CI.
[d] The $t_{1/2}$ for release from bone is ~11.9 years.
[e] Mild to moderate renal impairment.
[f] Following a single 10-mg IV infusion over 2 hours, and a 10-mg oral dose daily for >3 years.

References: Cocquyt, V., Kline, W.F., Gertz, B.J., Van Belle, S.J., Holland, S.D., DeSmet, M., Quan, H., Vyas, K.P., Zhang, K.E., De Greve, J., and Porras, A.G. Pharmacokinetics of intravenous alendronate. *J. Clin. Pharmacol.,* **1999,** *39:*385–393. Porras, A.G., Holland, S.D., and Gertz, B.J. Pharmacokinetics of alendronate. *Clin. Pharmacokinet.,* **1999,** *36:*315–328.

ALFENTANIL (Chapters 14, 23)

Bioavailability	Urinary Excretion	Bound in Plasma	Clearance	Vol. Dist.	Half-Life	Peak Time	Peak Conc.
—	<1	92 ± 2[a] ↓ Cirr	6.7 ± 2.4[b] ↓ Aged, Cirr ↔ CPBS	0.8 ± 0.3 ↔ Aged, CPBS ↑ Cirr	1.6 ± 0.2 ↑ Aged, Cirr, CPBS	—	100–200 ng/ml[c]; 310–340 ng/ml[d]

[a] Blood-to-plasma concentration ratio = 0.63 ± 0.02.
[b] Metabolically cleared by CYP3A.
[c] Provides adequate anesthesia for superficial surgery.
[d] Provides adequate anesthesia for abdominal surgery.

Reference: Bodenham, A., and Park, G.R. Alfentanil infusions in patients requiring intensive care. *Clin. Pharmacokinet.,* **1988,** *15:*216–226.

Key: Unless otherwise indicated by a specific footnote, the data are presented for the study population as a mean value ± 1 standard deviation, a mean and range (lowest-highest in parenthesis) of values, a range of the lowest-highest values, or a single mean value.

ADH = alcohol dehydrogenase; Aged = aged; AIDS = acquired immunodeficiency syndrome; Alb = hypoalbuminemia; Atr Fib = atrial fibrillation; AVH = acute viral hepatitis; Burn = burn patients; C_{max} = peak concentration; CAD = coronary artery disease; Celiac = celiac disease; CF = cystic fibrosis; CHF = congestive heart failure; Child = children; Cirr = hepatic cirrhosis; COPD = chronic obstructive pulmonary disease; CP = cor pulmonale; CPBS = cardiopulmonary bypass surgery; CRI = chronic respiratory insufficiency; Crohn = Crohn's disease; Cush = Cushing's syndrome; CYP = cytochrome P450; Fem = female; Hep = hepatitis; HIV = human immunodeficiency virus; HL = hyperlipoproteinemia; HTh = hyperthyroid; IM = intramuscular; Inflam = inflammation; IV = intravenous; LD = liver disease; LTh = hypothyroid; MAO = monoamine oxidase; MI = myocardial infarction; NAT = N-acetyltransferase; Neo = neonate; NIDDM = non-insulin-dependent diabetes mellitus; NS = nephrotic syndrome; Obes = obese; Pneu = pneumonia; Preg = pregnant; Prem = premature; RA = rheumatoid arthritis; RD = renal disease (including uremia); SC = subcutaneous; Smk = smoking; ST = sulfotransferase; T_{max} = peak time; Tach = ventricular tachycardia; UGT = UDP-glucuronosyl transferase; Ulcer = ulcer patients. Other abbreviations are defined in the text section of this appendix.

Table A–II–1
PHARMACOKINETIC DATA (Continued)

AVAILABILITY (ORAL) (%)	URINARY EXCRETION (%)	BOUND IN PLASMA (%)	CLEARANCE ($ml \cdot min^{-1} \cdot kg^{-1}$)	VOL. DIST. (liters/kg)	HALF-LIFE (hours)	PEAK TIME (hours)	PEAK CONCENTRATIONS
ALLOPURINOL[a] (Chapters 27, 52)							
53 ± 13	12	—	9.9 ± 2.4[b] RD, Aged[b]	0.87 ± 0.13	A: 1.2 ± 0.3 O: 24 ± 4.5	A: 1.7 ± 1.0[c] O: 4.1 ± 1.4[c]	A: 1.4 ± 0.5 μg/ml[c] O: 6.4 ± 0.8 μg/ml[c]

[a]Data from healthy male and female subjects. Allopurinol (A) is rapidly metabolized to the pharmacologically active oxypurinol (O).
[b]Increased oxypurinol AUC during renal impairment and in the aged.
[c]Following a single 300-mg oral dose.

References: Physicians' Desk Reference, 54th ed. Medical Economics Co. Montvale, NJ, **2000**, p. 1976.
Turnheim, K., Krivanek, P., and Oberbauer, R. Pharmacokinetics and pharmacodynamics of allopurinol in elderly and young subjects. Br. J. Clin. Pharmacol., **1999**, 48:501–509.

AVAILABILITY (ORAL) (%)	URINARY EXCRETION (%)	BOUND IN PLASMA (%)	CLEARANCE ($ml \cdot min^{-1} \cdot kg^{-1}$)	VOL. DIST. (liters/kg)	HALF-LIFE (hours)	PEAK TIME (hours)	PEAK CONCENTRATIONS
ALPRAZOLAM (Chapter 17)							
88 ± 16	20	71 ± 3 ↑ Cirr ↔ Obes, Aged	0.74 ± 0.14[a] ↓ Obes, Cirr, Aged[b] ↔ RD	0.72 ± 0.12 ↔ Obes, Cirr, Aged ↔ RD	12 ± 2 ↑ Obes, Cirr, Aged[b] ↔ RD	1.5 (0.5–3.0)[c]	21 (15–32) ng/ml[c]

[a]Metabolically cleared by CYP3A and other cytochrome P450s.
[b]Data from male subjects only.
[c]Mean (range) from 19 studies following a single 1-g oral dose given to adults.

Reference: Greenblatt, D.J., and Wright, C.E. Clinical pharmacokinetics of alprazolam. Therapeutic implications. Clin. Pharmacokinet., **1993**, 24:453–471.

AVAILABILITY (ORAL) (%)	URINARY EXCRETION (%)	BOUND IN PLASMA (%)	CLEARANCE ($ml \cdot min^{-1} \cdot kg^{-1}$)	VOL. DIST. (liters/kg)	HALF-LIFE (hours)	PEAK TIME (hours)	PEAK CONCENTRATIONS
ALTEPLASE (t-PA) (Chapter 55)							
—	Low	—	10 ± 4	0.10 ± 0.01	0.08 ± 0.04[a]	—	973 ± 133 ng/ml[b]

[a]Initial half-life is dominant; terminal half-life is 0.43 ± 0.17 hours.
[b]Following a single 50-mg IV dose of t-PA infused over 30 minutes to healthy adults.

Reference: Seifried, E., Tanswell, P., Rijken, D.C., Barret-Bergshoeff, M.M., Su, C.A., and Kluft, C. Pharmacokinetics of antigen and activity of recombinant tissue-type plasminogen activator after infusion in healthy volunteers. Arzneimittelforschung, **1988**, 38:418–422.

AVAILABILITY (ORAL) (%)	URINARY EXCRETION (%)	BOUND IN PLASMA (%)	CLEARANCE ($ml \cdot min^{-1} \cdot kg^{-1}$)	VOL. DIST. (liters/kg)	HALF-LIFE (hours)	PEAK TIME (hours)	PEAK CONCENTRATIONS
AMANTADINE (Chapter 50)							
50–90[a]	50–90[a]	67	4.8 ± 0.8 ↓ Aged, RD	6.6 ± 1.5 ↓ Aged ↔ RD	16 ± 3.4 ↑ Aged, RD	1–4[b] ↑ Aged	475 ± 110 ng/ml[b,c]

[a]Drug is not metabolized; oral bioavailability equals percent excreted unchanged.
[b]Plasma C_{max} and T_{max} following a 100-mg oral dose given twice a day to steady state in healthy young adults. Mean steady-state trough concentrations with the same dosing regimen were 302 ± 80 ng/ml.
[c]Efficacy is associated with a trough level of 300 ng/ml. Psychosis can occur at levels >1 μg/ml.

References: Aoki, F.Y., and Sitar, D.S. Clinical pharmacokinetics of amantadine hydrochloride. Clin. Pharmacokinet., **1988**, 14:35–51.
Aoki, F.Y., Sitar, D.S., and Ogilvie, R.I. Amantadine kinetics in healthy young subjects after long-term dosing. Clin. Pharmacol. Ther., **1979**, 26:729–736.

AVAILABILITY (ORAL) (%)	URINARY EXCRETION (%)	BOUND IN PLASMA (%)	CLEARANCE ($ml \cdot min^{-1} \cdot kg^{-1}$)	VOL. DIST. (liters/kg)	HALF-LIFE (hours)	PEAK TIME (hours)	PEAK CONCENTRATIONS
AMIKACIN (Chapters 46, 48)							
—	98	4 ± 8[a]	1.3 ± 0.6 $CL = 0.6CL_{cr} + 0.14$ ↑ Obes ↑ CF	0.27 ± 0.06 ↔ Aged, Child, CF ↑ Obes ↑ Neo	2.3 ± 0.4 ↑ RD ↑ Obes ↓ Burn, Child, CF	—	26 ± 4 μg/ml[b]

[a]At a serum concentration of 15 μg/ml.
[b]Following a 1-hour IV infusion of a 6.3 ± 1.4-mg/kg dose, given three times a day to steady state in patients without renal disease.

Reference: Bauer, L.A., and Blouin, R.A. Influence of age on amikacin pharmacokinetics in patients without renal disease. Comparison with gentamicin and tobramycin. Eur. J. Clin. Pharmacol., **1983**, 24:639–642.

AMILORIDE (Chapter 29)

≥49ᵃ	49 ± 10 ↑ Hep ↓ RD	40	9.7 ± 1.9ᵇ ↓ Aged, Hep, RD	17 ± 4ᵇ ↓ RD ⟷ Hep, Aged	21 ± 3ᵇ ↑ Aged, Hep, RD	3.1 ± 1.2ᶜ	17 ± 8 ng/mlᶜ

ᵃGreater than or equal to percent excreted unchanged.

ᵇCL/F and V_{area}/F reported, assuming a 70-kg body weight. Lower values for V_d (5–5.5) and $t_{1/2}$ (6–9) reported.

ᶜFollowing a single 10-mg oral dose given to healthy adults.

Reference: Spahn, H., Reuter, K., Mutschler, E., Gerok, W.., and Knauf, H. Pharmacokinetics of amiloride in renal and hepatic disease. *Eur. J. Clin. Pharmacol.* **1987,** *33:*493–498.

AMIODARONEᵃ (Chapter 35)

46 ± 22	0	99.98 ± 0.01ᵇ	1.9 ± 0.4ᶜ ⟷ Aged, Fem, CHF, RD	66 ± 44	25 ± 12 daysᵈ ⟷ Aged, Fem, RD	2–10ᵉ	1.5–2.4 µg/mlᵉ

ᵃSignificant plasma concentrations of an active desethyl metabolite are observed (ratio of drug/metabolite ~1); $t_{1/2}$ for metabolite = 61 days.

ᵇBlood-to-plasma concentration ratio = 0.73 ± 0.06.

ᶜMetabolized by CYP3A.

ᵈLonger half-life noted in patients (53 ± 24 days); all reported half-lives may be underestimated because of insufficient length of sampling.

ᵉFollowing a 400-mg/day oral dose to steady state in adult patients.

Reference: Gill, J., Heel, R.C., and Fitton, A. Amiodarone. An overview of its pharmacological properties, and review of its therapeutic use in cardiac arrhythmias. *Drugs,* **1992,** *43:*69–110.

AMITRIPTYLINEᵃ (Chapter 19)

48 ± 11 ⟷ Aged	<2	94.8 ± 0.8ᵇ ⟷ Aged ↑ HL	11.5 ± 3.4ᶜ ⟷ Aged, Smk	15 ± 3ᶜ ↑ Aged	21 ± 5 ↑ Aged	3.6 ± 1.4ᵈ	64 ± 35 ng/mlᵈ

ᵃActive metabolite is nortriptyline (*see* drug listing for kinetic data).

ᵇBlood-to-plasma concentration ratio = 0.86 ± 0.13.

ᶜBlood *CL* and V_{ss} reported; formation of nortriptyline is catalyzed by CYP2C19 (polymorphic), CYP3A4, and other cytochrome P450s; formation of 10-hydroxy metabolites are catalyzed by CYP2D6 (polymorphic).

ᵈFollowing a 100-mg/day dose to steady state in adults. The nortriptyline/amitriptyline concentration ratio = 1.1 ± 0.6. Optimal range of nortriptyline + amitriptyline is 60 to 220 ng/ml. Toxic effects occur at total concentrations >1 µg/ml.

Reference: Schulz, P., Dick, P., Blaschke, T.F., and Hollister, L. Discrepancies between pharmacokinetic studies of amitriptyline. *Clin. Pharmacokinet.,* **1985,** *10:*257–268.

Key: Unless otherwise indicated by a specific footnote, the data are presented for the study population as a mean value ± 1 standard deviation, a mean and range (lowest–highest in parenthesis) of values, a range of the lowest–highest values, or a single mean value.

ADH = alcohol dehydrogenase; Aged = aged; AIDS = acquired immunodeficiency syndrome; Alb = hypoalbuminemia; Atr Fib = atrial fibrillation; AVH = acute viral hepatitis; Burn = burn patients; C_{max} = peak concentration; CAD = coronary artery disease; Celiac = celiac disease; CF = cystic fibrosis; CHF = congestive heart failure; Child = children; Cirr = hepatic cirrhosis; COPD = chronic obstructive pulmonary disease; CP = cor pulmonale; CPBS = cardiopulmonary bypass surgery; CRI = chronic respiratory insufficiency; Crohn = Crohn's disease; Cush = Cushing's syndrome; CYP = cytochrome P450; Fem = female; Hep = hepatitis; HIV = human immunodeficiency virus; HL = hyperlipoproteinemia; HTh = hyperthyroid; IM = intramuscular; Inflam = inflammation; IV = intravenous; LD = liver disease; LTh = hypothyroid; MAO = monoamine oxidase; MI = myocardial infarction; NAT = N-acetyltransferase; Neo = neonate; NIDDM = non–insulin-dependent diabetes mellitus; NS = nephrotic syndrome; Obes = obese; Pneu = pneumonia; Preg = pregnant; Prem = premature; RA = rheumatoid arthritis; RD = renal disease (including uremia); SC = subcutaneous; Smk = smoking; ST = sulfotransferase; T_{max} = peak time; Tach = ventricular tachycardia; UGT = UDP-glucuronosyl transferase; Ulcer = ulcer patients. Other abbreviations are defined in the text section of this appendix.

Table A–II–1
PHARMACOKINETIC DATA (Continued)

AVAILABILITY (ORAL) (%)	URINARY EXCRETION (%)	BOUND IN PLASMA (%)	CLEARANCE $(ml \cdot min^{-1} \cdot kg^{-1})$	VOL. DIST. (liters/kg)	HALF-LIFE (hours)	PEAK TIME (hours)	PEAK CONCENTRATIONS
AMLODIPINE[a] (Chapter 32)							
74 ± 17 ← Aged	10	93 ± 1 ← Aged	5.9 ± 1.5 ← RD, ↓ Aged, Hep	16 ± 4 ← Aged	39 ± 8 ← RD, ↑ Aged, Hep	5.4–8.0[b]	18.1 ± 7.1 ng/ml[b] ↑ Aged

[a] Racemic mixture; in young, healthy subjects, there are no apparent differences between the kinetics of the more active R-enantiomer and S-enantiomer.
[b] Following a 10-mg oral dose given once daily for 14 days to healthy male adults.

Reference: Meredith, P.A., and Elliott, H.L. Clinical pharmacokinetics of amlodipine. *Clin. Pharmacokinet.,* **1992,** 22:22–31.

AVAILABILITY (ORAL) (%)	URINARY EXCRETION (%)	BOUND IN PLASMA (%)	CLEARANCE $(ml \cdot min^{-1} \cdot kg^{-1})$	VOL. DIST. (liters/kg)	HALF-LIFE (hours)	PEAK TIME (hours)	PEAK CONCENTRATIONS
AMOXICILLIN (Chapter 45)							
93 ± 10[a]	86 ± 8	18	2.6 ± 0.4 ↓ Child ← RD, Aged[b]	0.21 ± 0.03 ← RD, Aged	1.7 ± 0.3 ← Child ↑ RD, Aged[b]	1–2	IV: 46 ± 12 μg/ml[c] Oral: 5 μg/ml[c]

[a] Dose-dependent; value shown is for a 375-mg dose; decreases to about 50% at 3000 mg.
[b] No change if renal function is not decreased.
[c] Following a single 500-mg IV bolus dose to healthy elderly adults or a single 500-mg oral dose to adults.

References: Hoffler, D. [The pharmacokinetics of amoxicillin.] *Adv. Clin. Pharmacol.,* **1974,** 7:28–30. Sjovall, J., Alvan, G., and Huitfeldt, B. Intra- and inter-individual variation in pharmacokinetics of intravenously infused amoxicillin and ampicillin to elderly volunteers. *Br. J. Clin. Pharmacol.* **1986,** 21:171–181.

AVAILABILITY (ORAL) (%)	URINARY EXCRETION (%)	BOUND IN PLASMA (%)	CLEARANCE $(ml \cdot min^{-1} \cdot kg^{-1})$	VOL. DIST. (liters/kg)	HALF-LIFE (hours)	PEAK TIME (hours)	PEAK CONCENTRATIONS
AMPHOTERICIN B[a] (Chapter 49)							
<5%	2–5	>90	0.46 ± 0.20[b] ← RD, Prem	0.76 ± 0.52[c]	18 ± 7[d]	—	1.2 ± 0.33 μg/ml[e]

[a] Data for amphotericin B shown. Also formulated by liposomal encapsulation (ABELCET and AMBISOME); the distribution and clearance properties of these products are different from the nonencapsulated form; a terminal half-life of 173 ± 78 and 110 to 153 hours, respectively; however, an effective steady-state concentration can be achieved within 4 days.
[b] Data for eight children (age 8 months to 14 years) yield a linear regression with CL decreasing with age: $CL = -0.046 \cdot age$ (years) $+ 0.86$. Newborns show highly variable CL values.
[c] Volume of central compartment. V_{ss} increases with dose from 3.4 l/kg for single 0.25-mg/kg doses to 8.9 l/kg for 1.5-mg/kg doses.
[d] Half-life for multiple dosing. In single-dose studies, a prolonged dose-dependent half-life is seen.
[e] Following 0.5-mg/kg IV dose of amphotericin B given as a 1-hour infusion, once daily for 3 days. Whole blood concentrations (free and liposome encapsulated) of 1.7 ± 0.8 μg/ml and 83±35 μg/ml were reported following a 5-mg·kg⁻¹·day⁻¹ IV dose (presumed 60- to 120-min infusion) of ABELCET and AMBISOME, respectively.

References: Gallis, H.A., Drew, R.H., and Pickard, W.W. Amphotericin B: 30 years of clinical experience. *Rev. Infect. Dis.,* **1990,** 12:308–329. *Physicians' Desk Reference,* 54th ed. Medical Economics Co., Montvale, NJ, **2000,** pp. 1090–1091, 1654.

AVAILABILITY (ORAL) (%)	URINARY EXCRETION (%)	BOUND IN PLASMA (%)	CLEARANCE $(ml \cdot min^{-1} \cdot kg^{-1})$	VOL. DIST. (liters/kg)	HALF-LIFE (hours)	PEAK TIME (hours)	PEAK CONCENTRATIONS
ANASTROZOLE[a] (Chapters 52, 58)							
80	<10	~40	— ↓ LD[b]	—	50	≤2[c]	46 ng/ml[c]

[a] Data from healthy pre- and postmenopausal female subjects. Metabolized by cytochrome P450 and UGT.
[b] CL/F reduced, stable alcoholic cirrhosis.
[c] C_{max} and T_{max} following a single 3-mg oral dose. Accumulates three- to fourfold from single to multiple daily dosing.

References: Lonning, P.E., Geisler, J., and Dowsett, M. Pharmacological and clinical profile of anastrozole. *Breast Cancer Res. Treat.,* **1998,** 49(suppl 1):S53–S57; discussion S73–S77. *Physicians' Desk Reference,* 54th ed. Medical Economics Co., Montvale, NJ, **2000,** p. 537. Plourde, P.V., Dyroff, M., Dowsett, M., Demers, L., Yates, R., and Webster, A. ARIMIDEX: a new oral, once-a-day aromatase inhibitor. *J. Steroid Biochem. Mol. Biol.* **1995,** 53:175–179.

ATORVASTATIN[a] (Chapter 36)

12	<2	≥98	29[b] ↓ Cirr[c], Aged ←→ RD	~5.4[b]	19.5 ± 9.6 ↑ Cirr[b], Aged	2.3 ± 0.96[d]	14.9 ± 1.8 ngEq/ml[d]

References: Gibson, D.M., Bron, N.J., Richens, A., Hounslow, N.J., Sedman, A.J., and Whitfield, L.R. Effect of age and gender on pharmacokinetics of atorvastatin in humans. *J. Clin. Pharmacol.* **1996**, *36*:242–246.

Lea, A.P., and McTavish, D. Atorvastatin. A review of its pharmacology and therapeutic potential in the management of hyperlipidaemias. *Drugs,* **1997**, *53*:828–847.

Physicians' Desk Reference, 54th ed. Medical Economics Co., Montvale, NJ, **2000**, p. 2254.

[a] Data from healthy adult male and female subjects. No clinically significant gender differences. Atorvastatin undergoes extensive CYP3A-dependent first-pass metabolism in the gut wall and liver. Metabolites are active and exhibit a longer half-life (20 to 30 hours) than parent drug.
[b] Mean CL/F parameter calculated from reported AUC data at steady state after a once a day 20-mg oral dose, assuming a 70-kg body weight.
[c] AUC following oral administration increased, mild to moderate hepatic impairment.
[d] Following a 20-mg oral dose, once daily, for 14 days.

ATOVAQUONE[a] (Chapter 40)

23 ± 11 ↑ Food[b]	<1	99.9	0.15 ± 0.09 ↓ Child[c]	0.6 ± 0.17	62.5 ± 35.3	1.5–2.5	24.2 ± 12.1 μg/ml[d] ↑ Food

References: Dixon, R., Pozniak, A.L., Watt, H.M., Rolan, P., and Posner, J. Single-dose and steady-state pharmacokinetics of a novel microfluidized suspension of atovaquone in human immunodeficiency virus-seropositive patients. *Antimicrob. Agents Chemother.* **1996**, *40*:556–560.

Physicians' Desk Reference, 54th ed. Medical Economics Co., Montvale, NJ, **2000**, p. 1233.

Rolan, P.E., Mercer, A.J., Tate, E., Benjamin, I., and Posner, J. Disposition of atovaquone in humans. *Antimicrob. Agents Chemother.* **1997**, *41*:1319–1321.

[a] Data from patients with HIV infection. Atovaquone is thought to undergo enterohepatic recycling, with eventual elimination as unchanged drug in feces.
[b] Markedly increased absorption with high-fat meal.
[c] CL/F reduced, children <2 years of age.
[d] Following 1000-mg suspension daily for 14 days.

ATROPINE[a] (Chapter 7)

50[b]	57 ± 8	14–22 ←→ Aged	8 ± 4[c] ↓ Aged	2.0 ± 1.1 ↑ Child	3.5 ± 1.5 ↑ Aged, Child	0.15 ± 0.04[d]	2.6 ± 0.5 ng/ml[d]

Reference: Kentala, E., Kaila, T., Iisalo, E., and Kanto, J. Intramuscular atropine in healthy volunteers: a pharmacokinetic and pharmacodynamic study. *Int. J. Clin. Pharmacol. Ther. Toxicol.* **1990**, *28*: 399–404.

[a] Racemic mixture of active *l*-hyoscyamine and inactive *d*-hyoscyamine.
[b] Intramuscular injection.
[c] *l*-Hyoscyamine clearance after an intramuscular dose is 3-fold greater than that for *d*-hyoscyamine.
[d] Mean for *l*-hyoscyamine after a single 0.02-mg/kg intramuscular dose given to healthy adults.

Key: Unless otherwise indicated by a specific footnote, the data are presented for the study population as a mean value ± 1 standard deviation, a mean and range (lowest-highest in parenthesis) of values, a range of the lowest-highest values, or a single mean value.

ADH = alcohol dehydrogenase; Aged = aged; AIDS = acquired immunodeficiency syndrome; Alb = hypoalbuminemia; Atr Fib = atrial fibrillation; AVH = acute viral hepatitis; Burn = burn patients; C_{max} = peak concentration; CAD = coronary artery disease; Celiac = celiac disease; CF = cystic fibrosis; CHF = congestive heart failure; Child = children; Cirr = hepatic cirrhosis; COPD = chronic obstructive pulmonary disease; CP = cor pulmonale; CPBS = cardiopulmonary bypass surgery; CRI = chronic respiratory insufficiency; Crohn = Crohn's disease; Cush = Cushing's syndrome; CYP = cytochrome P450; Fem = female; Hep = hepatitis; HIV = human immunodeficiency virus; HL = hyperlipoproteinemia; HTh = hyperthyroid; IM = intramuscular; Inflam = inflammation; IV = intravenous; LD = liver disease; LTh = hypothyroid; MAO = monoamine oxidase; MI = myocardial infarction; NAT = N-acetyltransferase; Neo = neonate; NIDDM = non-insulin-dependent diabetes mellitus; NS = nephrotic syndrome; Obes = obese; Pneu = pneumonia; Preg = pregnant; Prem = premature; RA = rheumatoid arthritis; RD = renal disease (including uremia); SC = subcutaneous; Smk = smoking; ST = sulfotransferase; T_{max} = peak time; Tach = ventricular tachycardia; UGT = UDP-glucuronosyl transferase; Ulcer = ulcer patients. Other abbreviations are defined in the text section of this appendix.

Table A–II–1
PHARMACOKINETIC DATA (*Continued*)

AVAILABILITY (ORAL) (%)	URINARY EXCRETION (%)	BOUND IN PLASMA (%)	CLEARANCE $(ml \cdot min^{-1} \cdot kg^{-1})$	VOL. DIST. (liters/kg)	HALF-LIFE (hours)	PEAK TIME (hours)	PEAK CONCENTRATIONS

AZATHIOPRINE[a] (Chapters 52, 53)

AVAILABILITY (ORAL) (%)	URINARY EXCRETION (%)	BOUND IN PLASMA (%)	CLEARANCE $(ml \cdot min^{-1} \cdot kg^{-1})$	VOL. DIST. (liters/kg)	HALF-LIFE (hours)	PEAK TIME (hours)	PEAK CONCENTRATIONS
60 ± 31[b]	<2	—	57 ± 31[c]	0.81 ± 0.65[c]	0.16 ± 0.07[c] ←→ RD	MP: 1–2[d]	MP: 20–90 ng/ml[d]

[a] Kinetic values are for intravenous azathioprine. Azathioprine is metabolized to mercaptopurine (MP). *See* mercaptopurine for listing of its kinetic parameters.
[b] Determined as the bioavailability of mercaptopurine; intact azathioprine is undetectable after oral administration because of extensive first-pass metabolism.
[c] Data from kidney transplant patients.
[d] Range of steady-state peak mercaptopurine concentration following a 135 ± 34-mg oral dose of azathioprine, given daily to kidney transplant patients.

Reference: Lin, S.N., Jessup, K., Floyd, M., Wang, T.P., van Buren, C.T., Caprioli, R.M., and Kahan, B.D. Quantitation of plasma azathioprine and 6-mercaptopurine levels in renal transplant patients. *Transplantation*, **1980**, 29:290–294.

AZITHROMYCIN (Chapters 47, 48)

AVAILABILITY (ORAL) (%)	URINARY EXCRETION (%)	BOUND IN PLASMA (%)	CLEARANCE $(ml \cdot min^{-1} \cdot kg^{-1})$	VOL. DIST. (liters/kg)	HALF-LIFE (hours)	PEAK TIME (hours)	PEAK CONCENTRATIONS
34 ± 19 ↓ Food (capsules) ↑ Food (suspension)	12	7–50[a]	9	31	40[b] ←→ Cirr	2–3[c]	0.4 μg/ml[c]

[a] Dose-dependent plasma binding. The bound fraction is 50% at 50 ng/ml and 12% at 500 ng/ml.
[b] A longer terminal plasma half-life of 68 ± 8 hours, reflecting release from tissue stores, overestimates the multiple-dosing half-life.
[c] Following a 250-mg/day oral dose to adult patients with an infection.

Reference: Lalak, N.J., and Morris, D.L. Azithromycin clinical pharmacokinetics. *Clin. Pharmacokinet.*, **1993**, 25:370–374.

BACLOFEN[a] (Chapter 22)

AVAILABILITY (ORAL) (%)	URINARY EXCRETION (%)	BOUND IN PLASMA (%)	CLEARANCE $(ml \cdot min^{-1} \cdot kg^{-1})$	VOL. DIST. (liters/kg)	HALF-LIFE (hours)	PEAK TIME (hours)	PEAK CONCENTRATIONS
>70[b]	69 ± 14	31 ± 11	2.72 ± 0.93[c] ↓ RD[d]	0.81 ± 0.12[c]	3.75 ± 0.96	1.0 (0.5–4)[e]	160 ± 49 ng/ml[e]

[a] Data from healthy adult male subjects.
[b] Bioavailability estimate based on urine recovery of unchanged drug after oral dose.
[c] CL/F, V_{area}/F reported for intestinal infusion of drug.
[d] Limited data suggest CL/F reduced with renal impairment.
[e] T_{max} (mean and range) and C_{max} following a single 10-mg oral dose.

References: Kochak, G.M., Rakhit, A., Wagner, W.E., Honc, F., Waldes, L., and Kershaw, R.A. The pharmacokinetics of baclofen derived from intestinal infusion. *Clin. Pharmacol. Ther.*, **1985**, 38:251–257.
Wuis, E.W., Dirks, M.J., Termond, E.F., Vree, T.B., and Van der Kleijn, E. Plasma and urinary excretion kinetics of oral baclofen in healthy subjects. *Eur. J. Clin. Pharmacol.*, **1989**, 37:181–184.

BENAZEPRIL[a] (Chapter 31)

AVAILABILITY (ORAL) (%)	URINARY EXCRETION (%)	BOUND IN PLASMA (%)	CLEARANCE $(ml \cdot min^{-1} \cdot kg^{-1})$	VOL. DIST. (liters/kg)	HALF-LIFE (hours)	PEAK TIME (hours)	PEAK CONCENTRATIONS
≥ 18[a]	B: <1 BT: 18[b,c]	B: 97 BT: 95[b] ←→ Aged, Hep	BT: 0.3–0.4[b,d]	BT: 0.12[b,d]	B: 0.7 BT: 10–11[b] ←→ Aged	B: 0.5–1.0[e] BT: 1–1.5[e]	B: ~300 nM[e] BT: ~500 nM[e]

[a] Benazepril (B) is a prodrug for the active metabolite, benazeprilat (BT). Minimum bioavailability of BT based on urinary recovery data.
[b] Data for active metabolite; terminal $t_{1/2}$ ~22 hours.
[c] Following an oral dose of benazepril. BT is cleared by renal and biliary excretion.
[d] CL/F and V_{area}/F reported.
[e] Following a single 10-mg oral dose given to healthy adults. C_{max} calculated from original data assuming a plasma density of 1 g/ml.

Reference: Balfour, J.A., and Goa, K.L. Benazepril. A review of its pharmacodynamic and pharmacokinetic properties, and therapeutic efficacy in hypertension and congestive heart failure. *Drugs*, **1991**, 42:511–539.

BETAXOLOL[a] (Chapter 10)

89 ± 5 ⟷ Aged	15	55 ⟷ Hep, RD	4.7 ↓ Aged ⟷ Hep, RD	4.9–9.8	14–22 ↑ Aged	2–4[b] ↑ Aged	50 ng/ml[b]

[a] Racemic mixture; S-(−)-enantiomer is more active than the R-(+)-enantiomer.
[b] Following a single 20-mg oral dose given to healthy adults.

References: Frishman, W.H., Tepper, D., Lazar, E.J., and Behrman, D. Betaxolol: a new long-acting beta 1-selective adrenergic blocker. *J. Clin. Pharmacol.*, **1990**, *30*:686–692.
Warrington, S.J., Turner, P., Kilborn, J.R., Bianchetti, G., and Morselli, P.L. Blood concentrations and pharmacodynamic effects of betaxolol (SL 75212) a new beta-adrenoceptor antagonist after oral and intravenous administration. *Br. J. Clin. Pharmacol.*, **1980**, *10*:449–452.

BICALUTAMIDE[a] (Chapters 52, 59)

—	1.7 ± 0.3	96	R: 0.043 ± 0.013[b] S: 7.3 ± 4.0[b] ⟷ LD, RD, Aged	—	R: 139 ± 32 S: 29 ± 8.6 ↑ LD[c]	R: 23.4[d] S: 20.7[d]	SD, R: 734 ng/ml[d] SD, S: 84 ng/ml[d] MD, R/S: 8.9 ± 3.5 μg/ml

[a] Data from healthy male subjects. Exhibits stereoselective metabolism—S-enantiomer, primarily glucuronidation; R-enantiomer, primarily oxidation.
[b] CL/F reported for oral dose.
[c] Increased $t_{1/2}$ of R-enantiomer, severe liver disease.
[d] Mean T_{max} and C_{max} following a single (SD) 50-mg oral dose (tablet) and 50-mg once-a-day oral dose (MD) to steady state.

References: Cockshott, I.D., Oliver, S.D., Young, J.J., Cooper, K.J., and Jones, D.C. The effect of food on the pharmacokinetics of the bicalutamide ("Casodex") enantiomers. *Biopharm. Drug Dispos.*, **1997**, *18*:499–507.
McKillop, D., Boyle, G.W., Cockshott, I.D., Jones, D.C., Phillips, P.J., and Yates, R.A. Metabolism and enantioselective pharmacokinetics of Casodex in man. *Xenobiotica*, **1993**, *23*:1241–1253.
Physicians' Desk Reference, 54th ed. Medical Economics Co., Montvale, NJ, **2000**, p. 538.

BLEOMYCIN (Chapter 52)

—	68 ± 9	—	44.8 ± 11.3 ml · min⁻¹ · (m²)⁻¹ [a] ↓ RD ↑ Child[b]	9.7 ± 2.8 l/m²[a] ⟷ Child[b]	3.1 ± 1.7[a] ↑ RD ⟷ Child[b]	—	0.2–0.3 μg/ml[c]

[a] Data from eight patients 9 to 17 years of age.
[b] Data from three children <3 years of age.
[c] Range of steady-state concentration following a 30-mg/m² per day IV infusion given to children with cancer.

References: Crom, W.R., Glynn-Barnhart, A.M., Rodman, J.H., Teresi, M.E., Kavanagh, R.E., Christiansen, M.L., Relling, M.V., and Evans, W.E. Pharmacokinetics of anticancer drugs in children. *Clin. Pharmacokinet.*, **1987**, *12*:168–213.
Yee, G.C., Crom, W.R., Lee, F.H., Smyth, R.D., and Evans, W.E. Bleomycin disposition in children with cancer. *Clin. Pharmacol. Ther.*, **1983**, *33*:668–673.

Key: Unless otherwise indicated by a specific footnote, the data are presented for the study population as a mean value ± 1 standard deviation, a mean and range (lowest–highest in parenthesis) of values, a range of the lowest–highest values, or a single mean value.

ADH = alcohol dehydrogenase; Aged = aged; AIDS = acquired immunodeficiency syndrome; Alb = hypoalbuminemia; Atr Fib = atrial fibrillation; AVH = acute viral hepatitis; Burn = burn patients; C_{max} = peak concentration; CAD = coronary artery disease; Celiac = celiac disease; CF = cystic fibrosis; CHF = congestive heart failure; Child = children; Cirr = hepatic cirrhosis; COPD = chronic obstructive pulmonary disease; CP = cor pulmonale; CPBS = cardiopulmonary bypass surgery; CRI = chronic respiratory insufficiency; Crohn = Crohn's disease; Cush = Cushing's syndrome; CYP = cytochrome P450; Fem = female; Hep = hepatitis; HIV = human immunodeficiency virus; HL = hyperlipoproteinemia; HTh = hyperthyroid; IM = intramuscular; Inflam = inflammation; IV = intravenous; LD = liver disease; LTh = hypothyroid; MAO = monoamine oxidase; MI = myocardial infarction; NAT = N-acetyltransferase; Neo = neonate; NIDDM = non-insulin-dependent diabetes mellitus; NS = nephrotic syndrome; Obes = obese; Pneu = pneumonia; Prem = premature; Preg = pregnant; RA = rheumatoid arthritis; RD = renal disease (including uremia); SC = subcutaneous; Smk = smoking; ST = sulfotransferase; T_{max} = peak time; Tach = ventricular tachycardia; UGT = UDP-glucuronosyl transferase; Ulcer = ulcer patients. Other abbreviations are defined in the text section of this appendix.

Table A–II–1
PHARMACOKINETIC DATA (Continued)

	AVAILABILITY (ORAL) (%)	URINARY EXCRETION (%)	BOUND IN PLASMA (%)	VOL. DIST. (liters/kg)	CLEARANCE ($ml \cdot min^{-1} \cdot kg^{-1}$)	HALF-LIFE (hours)	PEAK TIME (hours)	PEAK CONCENTRATIONS
BROMOCRIPTINE (Chapter 11)	3–6[a]	2	93	2 ± 1[b]	5 ± 6[b]	7 ± 5[b]	1.6 ± 1.1[c] ↑ Food	691 ± 263 pg/ml[c] ↓ Food
BUMETANIDE (Chapter 29)	81 ± 18 ↔ CHF, Cirr, RD	62 ± 20 ↔ CHF	99 ± 0.3 ↓ RD ↔ CHF	0.13 ± 0.03 ↑ RD, Cirr	2.6 ± 0.5 ↓ RD, Cirr ↔ CHF	0.8 ± 0.2 ↑ CHF, RD, Cirr	1.2 ± 0.4[a]	106 ± 22 ng/ml[a] ↔ CHF
BUPIVACAINE (Chapter 15)		2 ± 2	95 ± 1[a] ↓ Neo	0.9 ± 0.4[b] ↑ Child	7.1 ± 2.8[b] ↑ Child ↓ Aged	2.4 ± 1.2 ↔ Aged, Child	0.17–0.5[c]	0.8 µg/ml[c]
BUPRENORPHINE[a] (Chapters 23, 24)	IM: 40–>90 SL: 51 ± 30 BC: 28 ± 9	Negligible	96	1.44 ± 0.11 ↑ Child[b]	13.3 ± 0.59 ↑ Child[b]	2.33 ± 0.24 ↓ Child	IM: 0.08[c] SL: 0.7 ± 0.1[c] BC: 0.8 ± 0.2[c]	IM: 3.6 ± 3.0 ng/ml[c] SL: 3.3 ± 0.8 ng/ml[c] BC: 2.0 ± 0.6 ng/ml[c]

BROMOCRIPTINE

[a]Based upon studies with radioactive drug.
[b]CL/F and V_{area}/F calculated assuming a 70-kg body weight. Terminal $t_{1/2}$ ~50 hours.
[c]Following a single 5-mg oral dose (immediate-release capsule) given to healthy male adults.

Reference: Drewe, J., Mazer, N., Abisch, E., Krummen, K., and Keck, M. Differential effect of food on kinetics of bromocriptine in a modified release capsule and a conventional formulation. Eur. J. Clin. Pharmacol., 1988, 35:535–541.

BUMETANIDE

[a]Following a single 3-mg oral dose given to healthy adults.

Reference: Cook, J.A., Smith, D.E., Cornish, L.A., Tankanow, R.M., Nicklas, J.M., and Hyneck, M.L. Kinetics, dynamics, and bioavailability of bumetanide in healthy subjects and patients with congestive heart failure. Clin. Pharmacol. Ther., 1988, 44:487–500.

BUPIVACAINE

[a]Increased postoperatively with increased concentration of α_1-acid glycoprotein; blood-to-plasma concentration ratio = 0.73 ± 0.05.
[b]Blood CL and V_{ss} reported.
[c]Plasma concentration following a single 100-mg epidural dose (20 ml of 1%) given to adult patients.

Reference: Burm, A.G. Clinical pharmacokinetics of epidural and spinal anaesthesia. Clin. Pharmacokinet., 1989, 16:283–311.

BUPRENORPHINE

[a]Data from male and female subjects undergoing surgery. Buprenorphine is metabolized in the liver by both oxidative (N-dealkylation) and conjugative pathways.
[b]CL, 60 ± 19 ml·min⁻¹·kg⁻¹; V_{ss}, 3.2 l/kg; $t_{1/2}$, 1.03 ± 0.22 hour; children 4 to 7 years of age.
[c]Following 0.3 mg intramuscularly (IM), 4 mg sublingual (SL), 4 mg buccal (BC).

References: Bullingham, R.E., McQuay, H.J., Moore, A., and Bennett, M.R. Buprenorphine kinetics. Clin. Pharmacol. Ther., 1980, 28:667–672.
Cone, E.J., Gorodetzky, C.W., Yousefnejad, D., Buchwald, W.F., and Johnson, R.E. The metabolism and excretion of buprenorphine in humans. Drug Metab. Dispos., 1984, 12:577–581.
Kuhlman, J.J., Lalani, S., Magluilo, J., Levine, B., and Darwin, W.D. Human pharmacokinetics of intravenous, sublingual, and buccal buprenorphine. J. Anal. Toxicol., 1996, 20:369–378.
Olkkola, K.T., Maunuksela, E.L., and Korpela, R. Pharmacokinetics of intravenous buprenorphine in children. Br. J. Clin. Pharmacol., 1989, 28:202–204.

BUPROPION[a] (Chapter 19)

—	<1	>80%	36.0 ± 2.2[b] ↓ Aged, Cirr[c] ↔ Alcohol	18.6 ± 1.2[b] ↔ Alcohol	11 ± 1[b] (7.9–18.4) ↑ Aged, Cirr[c] ↔ Alcohol	IR: 1.6 ± 0.1[d] SR: 3.1 ± 0.3[d]	IR: 141 ± 19 ng/ml[d] SR: 142 ± 28 ng/ml[d]

References: DeVane, C.L., Laizure, S.C., Stewart, J.T., Kolts, B.E., Ryerson, E.G., Miller, R.L., and Lai, A.A. Disposition of bupropion in healthy volunteers and subjects with alcoholic liver disease. *J. Clin. Psychopharmacol.* **1990,** 10:328–332.

Hsyu, P.H., Singh, A., Giargiari, T.D., Dunn, J.A., Ascher, J.A., and Johnston, J.A. Pharmacokinetics of bupropion and its metabolites in cigarette smokers versus nonsmokers. *J. Clin. Pharmacol.* **1997,** 37:737–743.

Physicians' Desk Reference, 54th ed. Medical Economics Co., Montvale, NJ, **2000,** p. 1301.

Posner, J., Bye, A., Dean, K., Peck, A.W., and Whiteman, P.D. The disposition of bupropion and its metabolites in healthy male volunteers after single and multiple doses. *Eur. J. Clin. Pharmacol.* **1985,** 29:97–103.

Posner, J., Bye, A., Jeal, S., Peck, A.W., and Whiteman, P. Alcohol and bupropion pharmacokinetics in healthy male volunteers. *Eur. J. Clin. Pharmacol.* **1984,** 26:627–630.

[a]Data from healthy adult male volunteers. Bupropion appears to undergo extensive first-pass metabolism by CYP2B6 and other CYP isozymes. Some metabolites accumulate in blood and are active. Mean terminal $t_{1/2}$ reported for oral dose. Mean terminal $t_{1/2}$ from four different studies shown in parenthesis.

[b]CL/F, V_{ss}/F, and $t_{1/2}$ reported for oral dose.

[c]CL/F reduced, alcoholic liver disease.

[d]Following a single 100-mg immediate release (IR) or 150-mg sustained release (SR) dose.

BUSPIRONE[a] (Chapters 11, 19)

3.9 ± 4.3 ↑ Food[b]	<0.1	>95	28.3 ± 10.3 ↓ Cirr[c], RD[d]	5.3 ± 2.6	2.4 ± 1.1 ↑ Cirr, RD	0.71 ± 0.06[e]	1.66 ± 0.21 ng/ml[e]

References: Barbhaiya, R.H., Shukla, U.A., Pfeffer, M., Pittman, K.A., Shrotriya, R., Laroudie, C., and Gammans, R.E. Disposition kinetics of buspirone in patients with renal or hepatic impairment after administration of single and multiple doses. *Eur. J. Clin. Pharmacol.* **1994,** 46:41–47.

Gammans, R.E., Mayol, R.F., and LaBudde, J.A. Metabolism and disposition of buspirone. *Am. J. Med.* **1986,** 80:41–51.

[a]Data from healthy adult male subjects. No significant gender differences. Undergoes extensive CYP3A-dependent first-pass metabolism. The major metabolite (1-pyrimidinyl piperazine) is active in some tests (one-fifth potency) and accumulates in blood to levels severalfold higher than buspirone.

[b]Bioavailability increased ~84%; appears to be secondary to reduced first-pass metabolism.

[c]CL/F reduced, hepatic cirrhosis.

[d]CL/F reduced, mild to severe renal impairment; unrelated to CL_{cr}.

[e]Following a single 20-mg oral dose.

BUSULFAN (Chapter 52)

70 (44–94)	1	2.7–14	4.5 ± 0.9[a]	0.99 ± 0.23[a]	2.6 ± 0.5	2.6 ± 1.5	Low: 65 ± 27 ng/ml[b] High: 949 ± 278 ng/ml[b]

References: Ehrsson, H., Hassan, M., Ehrnebo, M., and Beran, M. Busulfan kinetics. *Clin. Pharmacol. Ther.* **1983,** 34:86–89.

Schuler, U.S., Ehrsam, M., Schneider, A., Schmidt, H., Deeg, J., and Ehninger, G. Pharmacokinetics of intravenous busulfan and evaluation of the bioavailability of the oral formulation in conditioning for haematopoietic stem cell transplantation. *Bone Marrow Transplant.* **1998,** 22:241–244.

[a]CL/F and V_{area}/F reported.

[b]Following a single 4-mg oral dose (Low) given to patients with chronic myelocytic leukemia, or a single 1-mg/kg oral dose (High) given as ablative therapy to patients undergoing bone marrow transplantation.

Key: Unless otherwise indicated by a specific footnote, the data are presented for the study population as a mean value ± 1 standard deviation, a mean and range (lowest–highest in parenthesis) of values, a range of the lowest–highest values, or a single mean value.

ADH = alcohol dehydrogenase; Aged = aged; AIDS = acquired immunodeficiency syndrome; Alb = hypoalbuminemia; Atr Fib = atrial fibrillation; AVH = acute viral hepatitis; Burn = burn patients; C_{max} = peak concentration; CAD = coronary artery disease; Celiac = celiac disease; CF = cystic fibrosis; CHF = congestive heart failure; Cirr = hepatic cirrhosis; COPD = chronic obstructive pulmonary disease; CP = cor pulmonale; CPBS = cardiopulmonary bypass surgery; CRI = chronic respiratory insufficiency; Crohn = Crohn's disease; Cush = Cushing's syndrome; CYP = cytochrome P450; Fem = female; Hep = hepatitis; HIV = human immunodeficiency virus; HL = hyperlipoproteinemia; HTh = hyperthyroid; IM = intramuscular; Inflam = inflammation; IV = intravenous; LD = liver disease; LTh = hypothyroid; MAO = monoamine oxidase; MI = myocardial infarction; NAT = N-acetyltransferase; Neo = neonate; NIDDM = non-insulin-dependent diabetes mellitus; NS = nephrotic syndrome; Obes = obese; Pneu = pneumonia; Preg = pregnant; Prem = premature; RA = rheumatoid arthritis; RD = renal disease (including uremia); SC = subcutaneous; Smk = smoking; ST = sulfotransferase; T_{max} = peak time; Tach = ventricular tachycardia; UGT = UDP-glucuronosyl transferase; Ulcer = ulcer patients. Other abbreviations are defined in the text section of this appendix.

Table A–II–1

PHARMACOKINETIC DATA (Continued)

AVAILABILITY (ORAL) (%)	URINARY EXCRETION (%)	BOUND IN PLASMA (%)	CLEARANCE $(ml \cdot min^{-1} \cdot kg^{-1})$	VOL. DIST. (liters/kg)	HALF-LIFE (hours)	PEAK TIME (hours)	PEAK CONCENTRATIONS
BUTORPHANOL[a] (Chapter 23)							
TN: 70 ± 20[b] ↑ LD	1.9 ± 1.5	80–83	40 ± 10 ↓ LD,[c] RD[d] ⟷ Aged	12 ± 4 ↑ LD	4.8 ± 1.6 ↑ LD, RD	0.38 (0.25–1)[e]	1.4 ± 0.6 ng/ml[e]

[a]Data from healthy adult male and female subjects. Oral butorphanol undergoes extensive first-pass metabolism catalyzed by CYPs and UGT (F ~5% to 17%).
[b]Transnasal spray (TN).
[c]CL reduced, hepatic cirrhosis.
[d]Transnasal CL/F reduced, moderate to severe renal impairment.
[e]Mean (range) following 1-mg transnasal spray.

References: Ramsey, R., Higbee, M., Maesner, J., and Wood, J. Influence of age on the pharmacokinetics of butorphanol. *Acute Care*, **1988**, *12*(suppl 1):8–16.
Shyu, W.C., Morgenthien, E.A., and Barbhaiya, R.H. Pharmacokinetics of butorphanol nasal spray in patients with renal impairment. *Br. J. Clin. Pharmacol.*, **1996**, *41*:397–402.
Vachharajani, N.N., Shyu, W.C., Garnett, W.R., Morgenthien, E.A., and Barbhaiya, R.H. The absolute bioavailability and pharmacokinetics of butorphanol nasal spray in patients with hepatic impairment. *Clin. Pharmacol. Ther.*, **1996**, *60*:283–294.

AVAILABILITY (ORAL) (%)	URINARY EXCRETION (%)	BOUND IN PLASMA (%)	CLEARANCE $(ml \cdot min^{-1} \cdot kg^{-1})$	VOL. DIST. (liters/kg)	HALF-LIFE (hours)	PEAK TIME (hours)	PEAK CONCENTRATIONS
CALCITRIOL[a] (Chapter 62)							
Oral: ~61 IP: ~67	<10%	99.9	0.43 ± 0.04	—	16.5 ± 3.1[b] ↑ Child[c]	Oral: 3–6[d] IP: 2–3[d]	IV: ~460 pg/ml[d] Oral: ~90 pg/ml[d] IP: ~105 pg/ml[d]

[a]Data from young (15 to 22 years) patients on peritoneal dialysis. Metabolized by intestinal and renal 24-hydroxylase and also excreted into bile.
[b]Calcitriol half-life is 5 to 8 hours in healthy adult subjects.
[c]Oral dose $t_{1/2}$ = 27 ± 12 hours, children 2 to 16 years.
[d]Following a single 60-ng/kg IV, intraperitoneal (IP) dialysate, or oral dose. Baseline plasma levels were <10 pg/ml.

References: Jones, C.L., Vieth, R., Spino, M. Ledermann, S., Kooh, S.W. Balfe, J., and Balfe, J.W. Comparisons between oral and intraperitoneal 1.25-dihydroxyvitamin D₃ therapy in children treated with peritoneal dialysis. *Clin. Nephrol.*, **1994**, *42*:44–49.
Physicians' Desk Reference, 54th ed. Medical Economics Co., Montvale, NJ, **2000**, p. 2650.
Salusky, I.B., Goodman, W.G., Horst, R., Segre, G.V., Kim, L., Norris, K.C., Adams, J.S., Holloway, M., Fine, R.N., and Coburn, J.W. Pharmacokinetics of calcitriol in continuous ambulatory and cycling peritoneal dialysis patients. *Am. J. Kidney Dis.*, **1990**, *16*:126–132.
Taylor, C.A., Abdel-Rahman, E., Zimmerman, S.W., and Johnson, C.A. Clinical pharmacokinetics during continuous ambulatory peritoneal dialysis. *Clin. Pharmacokinet.*, **1996**, *31*:293–308.

AVAILABILITY (ORAL) (%)	URINARY EXCRETION (%)	BOUND IN PLASMA (%)	CLEARANCE $(ml \cdot min^{-1} \cdot kg^{-1})$	VOL. DIST. (liters/kg)	HALF-LIFE (hours)	PEAK TIME (hours)	PEAK CONCENTRATIONS
CANDESARTAN[a] (Chapters 31, 33)							
42 (34–56)	52	99.8	0.37 (0.31–0.47) ↓ RD,[b] ⟷ LD[c]	0.13 (0.09–0.17)	9.7 (4.8–13) ↑ RD, ⟷ LD[c]	4.0 ± 1.3	119 ± 43 ng/ml[d]

[a]Data from healthy adult male subjects. Candesartan cilexetil is rapidly and completely converted to candesartan through the action of gut wall esterases. Mean (range) for candesartan reported. No significant gender or age differences.
[b]CL/F reduced mild to severe renal disease.
[c]Trend for longer $t_{1/2}$ and increased accumulation at steady state; moderate hepatic impairment.
[d]Mean following a 16-mg oral dose (tablet), daily, for 7 days.

References: Hubner, R., Hogemann, A.M., Sunzel, M., and Riddell, J.G. Pharmacokinetics of candesartan after single and repeated doses of candesartan cilexetil in young and elderly healthy volunteers. *J. Hum. Hypertens.*, **1997**, *11*(suppl 2):S19–S25.
Stoukides, C.A., McVoy, H.J., and Kaul, A.F. Candesartan cilexetil: an angiotensin II receptor blocker. *Ann. Pharmacother.*, **1999**, *33*:1287–1298.
van Lier, J.J., van Heiningen, P.N., and Sunzel, M. Absorption, metabolism and excretion of ¹⁴C-candesartan and ¹⁴C-candesartan cilexetil in healthy volunteers.. *J. Hum. Hypertens.*, **1997**, *11*(suppl 2):S27–S28.

CAPECITABINE[a] (Chapter 52)

↓ Food[e]	3	<60	145 (34%) $1 \cdot \text{hour}^{-1} \cdot (\text{m}^2)^{-1}$ [b,c] ↓ LD[d]	270 l/m² [b,c]	C: 1.3 (146%)[b] 5-FU: 0.72 (16%)[b]	C: 0.5 (0.5–1)[f] 5-FU: 0.5 (0.5–2.1)[f] ↓ Food	C: 6.6 ± 6.0 μg/ml[f] 5-FU: 0.47 ± 0.47 μg/ml[f]

[a] Data from male and female patients with cancer. Capecitabine (C) is a prodrug for 5-FU (active). It is well absorbed and bioactivation is sequential in liver and tumor.
[b] Geometric mean (coefficient of variation).
[c] CL/F and V_{area}/F reported for oral dose.
[d] CL/F reduced but no change in 5-FU AUC, liver metastasis.
[e] AUC for C and 5-FU decreased.
[f] Following 1255 mg/m².

References: Dooley, M., and Goa, K.L. Capecitabine. Drugs, 1999, 58:69–76; discussion 77–78. Reigner, B., Verweij, J., Dirix, L., Cassidy, J., Twelves, C., Allman, D., Weidekamm, E., Roos, B., Banken, L., Utoh, M., and Osterwalder, B. Effect of food on the pharmacokinetics of capecitabine and its metabolites following oral administration in cancer patients. Clin. Cancer Res. 1998, 4:941–948.

CARBAMAZEPINE[a] (Chapter 21)

>70	<1	74 ± 3 ↔ RD, Cirr, Preg	1.3 ± 0.5[b,c] ↑ Preg ↔ Child, Aged, Smk	1.4 ± 0.4[b] ↔ Child, Neo, Aged	15 ± 5[b,c] ↔ Child, Neo, Aged	4–8[d]	9.3 (2–18) μg/ml[d]

[a] A metabolite, carbamazepine-10,11-epoxide, is equipotent in animal studies. Its formation is catalyzed primarily by CYP3A and secondarily by CYP2C8.
[b] Data from oral, multiple-dose regimen; values are CL/F and V_{area}/F.
[c] Data from multiple-dose regimen. Carbamazepine induces its own metabolism; for a single dose, $CL/F = 0.36 \pm 0.07 \text{ ml} \cdot \text{min}^{-1} \cdot \text{kg}^{-1}$ and $t_{1/2} = 36 \pm 5$ hours. CL also increases with dose.
[d] Mean (range) steady-state concentration following a daily 18.4-mg/kg oral dose (immediate release), given to adult patients with epilepsy. Therapeutic range for control of psychomotor seizures is 4–10 μg/ml.

References: Bertilsson, L., and Tomson, T. Clinical pharmacokinetics and pharmacological effects of carbamazepine and carbamazepine-10,11-epoxide. An update. Clin. Pharmacokinet. 1986, 11:177–198. Troupin, A., Ojemann, L.M., Halpern, L., Dodrill, C., Wilkus, R., Friel, P., and Feigl, P. Carbamazepine—a double-blind comparison with phenytoin. Neurology, 1977, 27:511–519.

CARBIDOPA[a] (Chapter 22)

—[b]	5.3 ± 2.1	18 ± 7[c]	—	~2	2.1 ± 1.0	S: 165 ± 77 ng/ml[d] S-CR: 81 ± 28 ng/ml[d]

[a] Data from healthy adult subjects. Combined with levodopa for treatment of Parkinson's disease.
[b] Absolute bioavailability is unknown but it is presumably low based on a high value for CL/F. Bioavailability of SINEMET CR (S-CR) is 55% of standard SINEMET (S).
[c] CL/F reported for 2 tablets of SINEMET 25/100.
[d] Following a single oral dose of 2 tablets SINEMET 25/100 or 1 tablet SINEMET CR 50/200.

Reference: Yeh, K.C., August, T.F., Bush, D.F., Lasseter, K.C., Musson, D.G., Schwartz, S., Smith, M.E., and Titus, D.C. Pharmacokinetics and bioavailability of Sinemet CR: a summary of human studies. Neurology, 1989, 39:25–38.

Key: Unless otherwise indicated by a specific footnote, the data are presented for the study population as a mean value ± 1 standard deviation, a mean and range (lowest–highest in parenthesis) of values, a range of the lowest–highest values, or a single mean value.

ADH = alcohol dehydrogenase; Aged = aged; AIDS = acquired immunodeficiency syndrome; Alb = hypoalbuminemia; Atr Fib = atrial fibrillation; AVH = acute viral hepatitis; Burn = burn patients; C_{max} = peak concentration; CAD = coronary artery disease; Celiac = celiac disease; CF = cystic fibrosis; CHF = congestive heart failure; Child = children; Cirr = hepatic cirrhosis; COPD = chronic obstructive pulmonary disease; CP = cor pulmonale; CPBS = cardiopulmonary bypass surgery; CRI = chronic respiratory insufficiency; Crohn = Crohn's disease; Cush = Cushing's syndrome; CYP = cytochrome P450; Fem = female; Hep = hepatitis; HIV = human immunodeficiency virus; HL = hyperlipoproteinemia; HTh = hyperthyroid; IM = intramuscular; Inflam = inflammation; IV = intravenous; LD = liver disease; LTh = hypothyroid; MAO = monoamine oxidase; MI = myocardial infarction; NAT = N-acetyltransferase; Neo = neonate; NIDDM = non-insulin-dependent diabetes mellitus; NS = nephrotic syndrome; Obes = obese; Pneu = pneumonia; Preg = pregnant; Prem = premature; RA = rheumatoid arthritis; RD = renal disease (including uremia); SC = subcutaneous; Smk = smoking; ST = sulfotransferase; T_{max} = peak time; Tach = ventricular tachycardia; UGT = UDP-glucuronosyl transferase; Ulcer = ulcer patients. Other abbreviations are defined in the text section of this appendix.

Table A–II–1
PHARMACOKINETIC DATA (Continued)

AVAILABILITY (ORAL) (%)	URINARY EXCRETION (%)	BOUND IN PLASMA (%)	CLEARANCE ($ml \cdot min^{-1} \cdot kg^{-1}$)	VOL. DIST. (liters/kg)	HALF-LIFE (hours)	PEAK TIME (hours)	PEAK CONCENTRATIONS
CARBOPLATIN[a] (Chapter 52)							
—	77 ± 5	0	1.5 ± 0.3 ↓ RD	0.24 ± 0.03	2 ± 0.2 ↑ RD	0.5[b]	39 ± 17 μg/ml[b]

[a] Measure of ultrafilterable platinum which is essentially unchanged carboplatin.
[b] Following a single 170–500-mg/m² IV dose (30-min infusion) given to adult patients with ovarian cancer.

Reference: Gaver, R.C., Colombo, N., Green, M.D., George, A.M., Deeb, R.M., Speyer, J.L., Farmen, R.H., and Muggia, F.M. The disposition of carboplatin in ovarian cancer patients. *Cancer Chemother. Pharmacol.* **1988,** 22:263–270.

AVAILABILITY (ORAL) (%)	URINARY EXCRETION (%)	BOUND IN PLASMA (%)	CLEARANCE ($ml \cdot min^{-1} \cdot kg^{-1}$)	VOL. DIST. (liters/kg)	HALF-LIFE (hours)	PEAK TIME (hours)	PEAK CONCENTRATIONS
CARVEDILOL[a] (Chapters 10, 34)							
25 S-(−): 15 R-(+): 31 ↑ Cirr	<2	95[b]	8.7 ± 1.7 ↓ Cirr ↔ RD, Aged	1.5 ± 0.3 ↑ Cirr	2.2 ± 0.3[c] ↑, ↔ Cirr ↔ RD, Aged	1.3 ± 0.3[d]	105 ± 12 ng/ml[d]

[a] Racemic mixture: S-(−) enantiomer responsible for β_1-adrenergic receptor blockade. R-(+) and S-(−) enantiomers have nearly equivalent α_1-receptor blocking activity.
[b] R-(+) enantiomer is more tightly bound than the S-(−) antipode. Blood-to-plasma concentration ratio of racemate = 0.7.
[c] Longer half-lives of about 6 hours have been measured at lower concentrations.
[d] Following a 12.5-mg oral dose given twice a day for 2 weeks to healthy young adults.

References: Morgan, T. Clinical pharmacokinetics and pharmacodynamics of carvedilol. *Clin. Pharmacokinet.* **1994,** 26:335–346.
Morgan, T., Anderson, A., Cripps, J., and Adam, W. Pharmacokinetics of carvedilol in older and younger patients. *J. Hum. Hypertens.* **1990,** 4:709–715.

AVAILABILITY (ORAL) (%)	URINARY EXCRETION (%)	BOUND IN PLASMA (%)	CLEARANCE ($ml \cdot min^{-1} \cdot kg^{-1}$)	VOL. DIST. (liters/kg)	HALF-LIFE (hours)	PEAK TIME (hours)	PEAK CONCENTRATIONS
CEFAZOLIN (Chapter 45)							
>90	80 ± 16	89 ± 2 → RD, Cirr, CPBS, Neo, Child	0.95 ± 0.17 ↓ RD, CPBS ↑ Preg ↔ Neo, Obes, Child, Cirr	0.19 ± 0.06[a] ↑ RD, Neo ↔ Preg, Obes, Child, Cirr	2.2 ± 0.02 ↑ RD, Neo, CPBS ↓ Preg, Cirr ↔ Obes, Child	IM: 1.7 ± 0.7[b]	IV: 237 ± 285 μg/ml[b] IM: 42 ± 9.5 μg/ml[b]

[a] V_{area} reported.
[b] Following a single 1-g intravenous (model-fitted C_{max}) or intramuscular dose to healthy adults.

Reference: Scheld, W.M., Spyker, D.A., Donowitz, G.R., Bolton, W.K., and Sande, M.A. Moxalactam and cefazolin: comparative pharmacokinetics in normal subjects. *Antimicrob. Agents Chemother.* **1981,** 19:613–619.

AVAILABILITY (ORAL) (%)	URINARY EXCRETION (%)	BOUND IN PLASMA (%)	CLEARANCE ($ml \cdot min^{-1} \cdot kg^{-1}$)	VOL. DIST. (liters/kg)	HALF-LIFE (hours)	PEAK TIME (hours)	PEAK CONCENTRATIONS
CEFEPIME[a] (Chapter 45)							
—	80	16–19	1.8 (1.7–2.5)[b] ↓ RD[d]	0.26 (0.24–0.31)[c]	2.1 (1.3–2.4)[b] ↑ RD[d]	—	65 ± 7 μg/ml[e]

[a] Data from healthy adult patients. Available only in parenteral form.
[b] Median (range) of reported CL and $t_{1/2}$ values from 16 single-dose studies.
[c] Median (range) of reported V_{ss} from 6 single-dose studies.
[d] Mild to severe renal impairment.
[e] Following a 1-g intravenous dose.

References: Okamoto, M.P., Nakahiro, R.K., Chin, A., and Bedikian, A. Cefepime clinical pharmacokinetics. *Clin. Pharmacokinet.* **1993,** 25:88–102.
Rybak, M. The pharmacokinetic profile of a new generation of parenteral cephalosporin. *Am. J. Med.* **1996,** 100:39S–44S.

CEFIXIME (Chapters 45, 49)

47 ± 15	41 ± 7	67 ± 1	1.3 ± 0.2 ↓ RD	0.30 ± 0.03	3.0 ± 0.4 ↑ RD	3–4[a]	1.7–2.9 µg/ml[a]

[a]Range of mean data from different studies following a single 200-mg oral dose (capsule) given to healthy adults. Minimal accumulation with twice-a-day dosing.

Reference: Brogden, R.N., and Campoli-Richards, D.M. Cefixime. A review of its antibacterial activity. Pharmacokinetic properties and therapeutic potential. *Drugs.* **1989,** *38:*524–550.

CEFOTAXIME[a] (Chapter 45)

—	55 ± 10	36 ± 3 ←→ Cirr[b]	3.7 ± 0.6 ↓ RD,[c] Cirr,[b] Fem ←→ Obes	0.23 ± 0.06 ←→ RD, Obes ↑ Cirr[b]	1.1 ± 0.3 ↑ RD, Cirr[b] ←→ Obes	IM: 0.5[d]	IV: ~150 µg/ml[d] IM: 20.5 µg/ml[d]

[a]Active metabolite, desacetylcefotaxime, accounts for 16 ± 4% of dose excreted; $t_{1/2}$ = 2.2 ± 0.3 hours.

[b]Cirrhotic patients with ascites.

[c]Renal and nonrenal clearance decreased in end-stage renal disease.

[d]Mean C_{max} following a single 30-mg/kg IV dose (25-min infusion), or a single 1-g IM dose to healthy adults. Desacetylcefotaxime peaks at a level of 14.7 ± 6.2 µg/ml at 0.9 ± 0.5 hours after the IV dose. No accumulation with multiple dosing four times a day.

References: Physicians' Desk Reference, 54th ed. Medical Economics Co., Montvale, NJ, **2000,** p. 1363.

Rodondi, L.C., Flaherty, J.F., Schoenfeld, P., Barriere, S.L., and Gambertoglio, J.G. Influence of coadministration on the pharmacokinetics of mezlocillin and cefotaxime in healthy volunteers and in patients with renal failure. *Clin. Pharmacol. Ther.,* **1989,** *45:*527–534.

CEFOTETAN (Chapters 45, 47)

—	67 ± 11	85 ± 4	$CL = 0.23CL_{cr} \pm 0.14$ ↓ RD	0.14 ± 0.03 ←→ RD	3.6 ± 1.0 ↑ RD	IM: 1.5–3[a]	IV, B: 336–491 µg/ml[a] IV, I: 38 µg/ml[a] IM: 91 µg/ml[a]

[a]Range of mean C_{max} from different studies following a single 2-g intravenous bolus (IV, B) dose or mean C_{max} and T_{max} following a single 2-g IM dose. Mean C_{ss} was 38 µg/ml following a 12-hour, 76-mg/hr constant rate intravenous infusion (IV, I) in healthy adults.

Reference: Martin, C., Thomachot, L., and Albanese, J. Clinical pharmacokinetics of cefotetan. *Clin. Pharmacokinet.,* **1994,** *26:*248–258.

Key: Unless otherwise indicated by a specific footnote, the data are presented for the study population as a mean value ± 1 standard deviation, a mean and range (lowest–highest in parenthesis) of values, a range of the lowest–highest values, or a single mean value.

ADH = alcohol dehydrogenase; Aged = aged; AIDS = acquired immunodeficiency syndrome; Alb = hypoalbuminemia; Atr Fib = atrial fibrillation; AVH = acute viral hepatitis; Burn = burn patients; C_{max} = peak concentration; CAD = coronary artery disease; Celiac = celiac disease; CF = cystic fibrosis; CHF = congestive heart failure; Child = children; Cirr = hepatic cirrhosis; COPD = chronic obstructive pulmonary disease; CP = cor pulmonale; CPBS = cardiopulmonary bypass surgery; CRI = chronic respiratory insufficiency; Crohn = Crohn's disease; Cush = Cushing's syndrome; CYP = cytochrome P450; Fem = female; Hep = hepatitis; HIV = human immunodeficiency virus; HL = hyperlipoproteinemia; HTh = hyperthyroid; IM = intramuscular; Inflam = inflammation; IV = intravenous; LD = liver disease; LTh = hypothyroid; MAO = monoamine oxidase; MI = myocardial infarction; NAT = N-acetyltransferase; Neo = neonate; NIDDM = non–insulin-dependent diabetes mellitus; NS = nephrotic syndrome; Obes = obese; Pneu = pneumonia; Preg = pregnant; Prem = premature; RA = rheumatoid arthritis; RD = renal disease (including uremia); SC = subcutaneous; Smk = smoking; ST = sulfotransferase; T_{max} = peak time; Tach = ventricular tachycardia; UGT = UDP-glucuronosyl transferase; Ulcer = ulcer patients. Other abbreviations are defined in the text section of this appendix.

Table A–II–1
PHARMACOKINETIC DATA (Continued)

AVAILABILITY (ORAL) (%)	URINARY EXCRETION (%)	BOUND IN PLASMA (%)	CLEARANCE ($ml \cdot min^{-1} \cdot kg^{-1}$)	VOL. DIST. (liters/kg)	HALF-LIFE (hours)	PEAK TIME (hours)	PEAK CONCENTRATIONS
CEFTAZIDIME (Chapter 45)							
IM: 91	84 ± 4 ↔ CF	21 ± 6	$CL = 1.05CL_{cr} + 0.12$ ↔ CF; Burn	0.23 ± 0.02 ↔ RD, CF ↑ Aged, Burn	1.6 ± 0.1 ↑ RD, Prem, Neo, Aged ↔ CF	IM: 0.7–1.3[a]	IV: 119–146 µg/ml[a] IM: 29–39 µg/ml[a]

[a]Range of mean data from different studies following a 1-g bolus IV or IM dose given to healthy adults.

Reference: Balant, L., Dayer, P., and Auckenthaler, R. Clinical pharmacokinetics of the third generation cephalosporins. *Clin. Pharmacokinet.*, **1985**, *10*:101–143.

CEFTRIAXONE (Chapter 45)							
—	49 ± 13[a] ↑ Neo, Child	90–95[b] ↓ Cirr, Neo, Child ↔ Aged	0.24 ± 0.06[b] ↓ RD, Neo,[c] Aged[c] ↑ Cirr, CF ↔ CPBS	0.16 ± 0.03[b,d] ↑ Neo, Cirr, CF, CPBS ↔ RD, Aged	7.3 ± 1.6[b] ↑ RD,[e] Aged, Neo, CPBS ↔ Cirr	IM: 2–2.4[f]	IV: 168 µg/ml[f] IM: 114 µg/ml[f]

Reference: Yuk, J.H., Nightingale, C.H., and Quintiliani, R. Clinical pharmacokinetics of ceftriaxone. *Clin. Pharmacokinet.*, **1989**, *17*:223–235.

[a]Remainder eliminated *via* biliary excretion.
[b]Saturable binding (5% unbound at plasma concentration of 70 µg/ml; >40% unbound at 600 µg/ml) leads to an increased total *CL*, but no change in *CL* of unbound drug. Data for single-dose administration are shown.
[c]Clearance of unbound drug reduced.
[d]V_{area} reported.
[e]Usually minor, but can increase to 50 hours in anephric patients with reduced nonrenal *CL*.
[f]Mean C_{max} following a 1-g IV (30-min infusion) or IM dose given twice a day to steady state in adult subjects.

CEFUROXIME (Chapter 45)							
32 (21–44)[a] ↑ Food	96 ± 10	33 ± 6	$CL = 0.94CL_{cr} + 0.28$	0.20 ± 0.04 ↔ RD, Aged	1.7 ± 0.6 ↑ RD ↔ Child	2–3[b]	7–10 µg/ml[b]

Reference: Emmerson, A.M. Cefuroxime axetil. *J. Antimicrob. Chemother.*, **1988**, *22*:101–104. Williams, P.E., and Harding, S.M. The absolute bioavailability of oral cefuroxime axetil in male and female volunteers after fasting and after food. *J. Antimicrob. Chemother.*, **1984**, *13*:191–196.

[a]Cefuroxime axetil, a prodrug of cefuroxime.
[b]Range of data following a single 500-mg oral dose of cefuroxime axetil given to healthy adults.

CELECOXIB[a] (Chapter 27)							
↑ Food[b]	<3	~97	6.60 ± 1.85 ↓ Aged, LD[c] ↑ RD[d]	6.12 ± 2.08	11.2 ± 3.47	2.8 ± 1.0[e] ↑ Food	705 ± 268 ng/ml[e]

References: Goldenberg, M.M. Celecoxib, a selective cyclooxygenase-2 inhibitor for the treatment of rheumatoid arthritis and osteoarthritis. *Clin. Ther.*, **1999**, *21*:1497–1513; discussion 1427–1428. *Physicians' Desk Reference*, 54th ed. Medical Economics Co., Montvale, NJ, **2000**, p. 2334.

[a]Data from healthy subjects. Cleared primarily by CYP2C9 (polymorphic).
[b]High-fat meal. Absolute bioavailability is unknown.
[c]*CL/F* reduced, mild or moderate hepatic impairment.
[d]*CL/F* increased, moderate renal impairment, but unrelated to CL_{cr}.
[e]Following a single 200-mg oral dose.

CEPHALEXIN[a] (Chapter 45)

90 ± 9	91 ± 18	14 ± 3	4.3 ± 1.1[a] ↓ RD	0.26 ± 0.03[a] ⟷ RD	0.90 ± 0.18 ↑ RD	1.4 ± 0.8[b]	28 ± 6.4 μg/ml[b]

[a] Assuming 70-kg body weight.
[b] Following a single 500-mg oral dose given to healthy male adults.

Reference: Spyker, D.A., Thomas, B.L., Sande, M.A., and Bolton, W.K. Pharmacokinetics of cefaclor and cephalexin: dosage nomograms for impaired renal function. *Antimicrob. Agents Chemother.,* **1978,** *14*:172–177.

CETIRIZINE[a] (Chapter 25)

>70	70.9 ± 7.8	98.8 ± 0.8[b]	0.74 ± 0.19[c] ↓ LD,[d] RD,[e] Aged ↑ Child[f]	0.58 ± 0.16[c]	9.42 ± 2.4 ↑ LD, RD, Aged ↓ Child	0.9 ± 0.2[g]	313 ± 45 ng/ml[g]

[a] Data from healthy male and female subjects.
[b] f_B also reported as ~93%.
[c] CL/F, V_d/F reported for oral dose.
[d] CL/F reduced, hepatocellular and cholestatic liver disease.
[e] CL/F reduced, moderate to severe renal impairment.
[f] CL/F increased, 2 to 5 years of age.
[g] Following a single 10-mg oral dose.

References: Horsmans, Y., Desager, J.P., Hulhoven, R., and Harvengt, C. Single-dose pharmacokinetics of cetirizine in patients with chronic liver disease. *J. Clin. Pharmacol.,* **1993,** *33*:929–932.
Matzke, G.R., Yeh, J., Awni, W.M., Halstenson, C.E., and Chung, M. Pharmacokinetics of cetirizine in the elderly and patients with renal insufficiency. *Ann. Allergy,* **1987,** *59*:25–30.
Physicians' Desk Reference, 54th ed. Medical Economics Co., Montvale, NJ, **2000,** p. 2404.
Spicak, V., Dab, I., Hulhoven, R., Desager, J.P., Klanova, M., de Longueville, M., and Harvengt, C. Pharmacokinetics and pharmacodynamics of cetirizine in infants and toddlers. *Clin. Pharmacol. Ther.,* **1997,** *61*:325–330.

CHLORAMBUCIL[a] (Chapter 52)

87 ± 20	<1[b]	99	2.6 ± 0.9[c]	0.29 ± 0.21[c,d]	C: 1.3 ± 0.9 / PA: 2.0 ± 1.1	C: 0.8 ± 0.3[e] / PA: 1.8 ± 0.4[e]	C: 508 ± 205 ng/ml[e] / PA: 369 ± 139 ng/ml[e]

[a] Active metabolite, phenylacetic acid mustard. *AUC* of metabolite (following chlorambucil) is about 25% greater than that of parent drug.
[b] Drug and active metabolite.
[c] Assuming 70-kg body weight.
[d] V_{area} reported.
[e] Data for chlorambucil (C) and an active metabolite, phenylacetic acid mustard (PA), following a single 0.4-mg/kg oral dose given to patients with leukemia or lymphomas.

Reference: Oppitz, M.M., Musch, E., Malek, M., Rub, H.P., von Unruh, G.E., Loos, U., and Muhlenbruch, B. Studies on the pharmacokinetics of chlorambucil and prednimustine in patients using a new high-performance liquid chromatographic assay. *Cancer Chemother. Pharmacol.,* **1989,** *23*:208–212.

Key: Unless otherwise indicated by a specific footnote, the data are presented for the study population as a mean value ± 1 standard deviation, a mean and range (lowest–highest in parenthesis) of values, a range of the lowest–highest values, or a single mean value.

ADH = alcohol dehydrogenase; Aged = aged; AIDS = acquired immunodeficiency syndrome; Alb = hypoalbuminemia; Atr Fib = atrial fibrillation; AVH = acute viral hepatitis; Burn = burn patients; C_{max} = peak concentration; CAD = coronary artery disease; Celiac = celiac disease; CF = cystic fibrosis; CHF = congestive heart failure; Child = children; Cirr = hepatic cirrhosis; COPD = chronic obstructive pulmonary disease; CP = cor pulmonale; CPBS = cardiopulmonary bypass surgery; CRI = chronic respiratory insufficiency; Crohn = Crohn's disease; Cush = Cushing's syndrome; CYP = cytochrome P450; Fem = female; Hep = hepatitis; HIV = human immunodeficiency virus; HL = hyperlipoproteinemia; HTh = hyperthyroid; IM = intramuscular; Inflam = inflammation; IV = intravenous; LD = liver disease; LTh = hypothyroid; MAO = monoamine oxidase; MI = myocardial infarction; NAT = N-acetyltransferase; Neo = neonate; NIDDM = non-insulin-dependent diabetes mellitus; NS = nephrotic syndrome; Obes = obese; Pneu = pneumonia; Preg = pregnant; Prem = premature; RA = rheumatoid arthritis; RD = renal disease (including uremia); SC = subcutaneous; Smk = smoking; ST = sulfotransferase; T_{max} = peak time; Tach = ventricular tachycardia; UGT = UDP-glucuronosyl transferase; Ulcer = ulcer patients. Other abbreviations are defined in the text section of this appendix.

Table A–II–1
PHARMACOKINETIC DATA (Continued)

AVAILABILITY (ORAL) (%)	URINARY EXCRETION (%)	BOUND IN PLASMA (%)	CLEARANCE ($ml \cdot min^{-1} \cdot kg^{-1}$)	VOL. DIST. (liters/kg)	HALF-LIFE (hours)	PEAK TIME (hours)	PEAK CONCENTRATIONS
CHLOROQUINE[a] (Chapters 40, 41)							
~80	52–58[b]	(S): 66.6 ± 3.3[c] (R): 42.7 ± 2.1 ←→ RD	3.7–13[b]	132–261[b]	10–24 days[b,d]	IM: 0.25[e] Oral: 3.6 ± 2[e]	IV: 837 ± 248 ng/ml IM: 57–480 ng/ml Oral: 76 ± 14 ng/ml

[a] Active metabolite, desethylchloroquine, accounts for 20 ± 3% of urinary excretion; $t_{1/2} = 15 \pm 6$ days. Racemic mixture; kinetic parameters for the two isomers are slightly different [e.g., mean residence time = 16.2 days and 11.3 days for the (R)-isomer and (S)-isomer, respectively].
[b] Range of mean values from different studies (IV administration).
[c] Blood-to-plasma concentration ratio for racemate = 9.
[d] A longer $t_{1/2}$ (41 ± 14 days) has been reported with extended blood sampling.
[e] Following a single 300-mg IV (24-min infusion) of chloroquine HCl, or IM or oral dose of chloroquine phosphate given to healthy adults. Effective concentrations against *Plasmodium vivax* and *Plasmodium falciparum* are 15 ng/ml and 30 ng/ml, respectively. Diplopia and dizziness can occur above 250 ng/ml.

References: Krishna, S., and White, N.J. Pharmacokinetics of quinine, chloroquine and amodiaquine. Clinical implications. *Clin. Pharmacokinet.,* **1996,** *30*:263–299. White, N.J. Clinical pharmacokinetics of antimalarial drugs. *Clin. Pharmacokinet.,* **1985,** *10*:187–215.

AVAILABILITY (ORAL) (%)	URINARY EXCRETION (%)	BOUND IN PLASMA (%)	CLEARANCE ($ml \cdot min^{-1} \cdot kg^{-1}$)	VOL. DIST. (liters/kg)	HALF-LIFE (hours)	PEAK TIME (hours)	PEAK CONCENTRATIONS
CHLORPHENIRAMINE[a] (Chapter 25)							
41 ± 16	0.3–26[b]	70 ± 3	1.7 ± 0.1 ↑ Child	3.2 ± 0.3 ←→ Child	20 ± 5 ↓ Child	IR: 2–3[c] SR: 5.7–8.1[c]	IR: 16–71 ng/ml[c] SR: 17–76 ng/ml[c]

[a] Administered as a racemic mixture; reported parameters are for racemic drug. Activity comes predominantly from S-(+) enantiomer, which has a 60% longer half-life than the R-(−) enantiomer.
[b] Renal elimination increases with increased urine flow and lower pH.
[c] Range of data from different studies following a 4-mg oral immediate release (IR) dose given every 4 to 6 hours to steady state, or following an 8-mg oral sustained release (SR) dose given every 12 hours to steady state, both in healthy adults.

Reference: Rumore, M.M. Clinical pharmacokinetics of chlorpheniramine. *Drug Intell. Clin. Pharm.,* **1984,** *18*:701–707.

AVAILABILITY (ORAL) (%)	URINARY EXCRETION (%)	BOUND IN PLASMA (%)	CLEARANCE ($ml \cdot min^{-1} \cdot kg^{-1}$)	VOL. DIST. (liters/kg)	HALF-LIFE (hours)	PEAK TIME (hours)	PEAK CONCENTRATIONS
CHLORPROMAZINE[a] (Chapters 20, 38)							
32 ± 19[b]	<1	95–98 ←→ RD	8.6 ± 2.9[c] ↓ Child[d] ←→ Cirr	21 ± 9[c]	30 ± 7[c]	1–4[e]	25–150 ng/ml[e]

[a] Active metabolites: 7-hydroxychlorpromazine ($t_{1/2} = 25 \pm 15$ hours) and possibly chlorpromazine N-oxide yield AUCs comparable to the parent drug (single doses).
[b] After single dose. Bioavailability may decrease to about 20% with repeated dosing.
[c] $CL/F_{intramuscular}$, $V_{area,intramuscular}$, and terminal $t_{1/2}$ reported.
[d] Range of data following a 100-mg oral dose given twice a day for 33 days to adult patients. Neurotoxicity (tremors and convulsions) occurs at concentrations of 750–1000 ng/ml.

Reference: Dahl, S.G., and Strandjord, R.E. Pharmacokinetics of chlorpromazine after single and chronic dosage. *Clin. Pharmacol. Ther.,* **1977,** *21*:437–448.

CHLORPROPAMIDE (Chapter 61)

>90[a]	20 ± 18[b]	96 ± 0.6	0.030 ± 0.005[c,d]	0.097 ± 0.011[c]	33 ± 6[e]	1–7[f]	30–35 μg/ml[f]

[a] Predicted bioavailability.
[b] Dependent on urinary pH: acidic urine, 1.4 ± 0.5%; basic urine, 85 ± 11%.
[c] CL/F and V_{area}/F reported.
[d] Acidic urine, 0.018 ± 0.006 ml·min^{-1}·kg^{-1}; basic urine, 0.086 ± 0.013 ml·min^{-1}·kg^{-1}.
[e] Acidic urine, 69 ± 26 hours; basic urine, 13 ± 3 hours.
[f] Range of T_{max} and range of mean C_{max} from different studies following a single 250-mg oral dose given to adults.

Reference: Balant, L. Clinical pharmacokinetics of sulphonylurea hypoglycaemic drugs. *Clin. Pharmacokinet.,* **1981,** 6:215–641.

CHLORTHALIDONE (Chapter 29)

64 ± 10	65 ± 9[a]	75 ± 1[b]	0.04 ± 0.01 ↓ Aged	0.14 ± 0.07	47 ± 22[c] ↑ Aged	13.8 ± 6.3[d]	3.7 ± 0.9 μg/ml[d]

[a] Value is for 50- and 100-mg doses; renal clearance is decreased at an oral dose of 200 mg, and there is a concomitant decrease in the percentage excreted unchanged.
[b] Blood-to-plasma concentration ratio = 72.5.
[c] Chlorthalidone is sequestered in erythrocytes; the half-life is longer if blood, rather than plasma, is analyzed. Parameters reported based on blood concentrations.
[d] Following a single 50-mg oral dose (tablet) given to healthy male adults.

Reference: Williams, R.L., Blume, C.D., Lin, E.T., Holford, N.H., and Benet, L.Z. Relative bioavailability of chlorthalidone in humans: adverse influence of polyethylene glycol. *J. Pharm. Sci.,* **1982,** 71:533–535.

CIDOFOVIR[a] (Chapter 50)

SC: 98 ± 10, Oral: <5	70.1 ± 21.4[b]	<6	2.1 ± 0.6[b] ↓ RD[c]	0.36 ± 0.13[b]	2.3 ± 0.5[b] ↑ RD	—	19.6 ± 7.2 μg/ml[d]

[a] Data from patients with HIV infection and positive for cytomegalovirus. Cidofovir is activated intracellularly by phosphokinases. For parenteral use.
[b] Parameters reported for a dose given in the presence of probenecid.
[c] CL reduced, mild to severe renal impairment (cleared by high flux hemodialysis).
[d] Following a single 5-mg/kg IV infusion given over 1 hour, with concomitant oral probenecid and active hydration.

References: Brody, S.R., Humphreys, M.H., Gambertoglio, J.G., Schoenfeld, P. Cundy, K.C., and Aweeka, F.T. Pharmacokinetics of cidofovir in renal insufficiency and in continuous ambulatory peritoneal dialysis or high-flux hemodialysis. *Clin. Pharmacol. Ther.,* **1999,** 65:21–28.
Cundy, K.C., Petty, B.G., Flaherty, J., Fisher, P.E., Polis, M.A., Wachsman, M., Lietman, P.S., Lalezari, J.P., Hitchcock, M.J., and Jaffe, H.S. Clinical pharmacokinetics of cidofovir in human immunodeficiency virus-infected patients. *Antimicrob. Agents Chemother.,* **1995,** 39:1247–1252.
Physicians' Desk Reference, 54th ed. Medical Economics Co., Montvale, NJ, **2000,** p. 1136.
Wachsman, M., Petty, B.G., Cundy, K.C., Jaffe, H.S., Fisher, P.E., Pastelak, A., and Lietman, P.S. Pharmacokinetics, safety and bioavailability of HPMPC (cidofovir) in human immunodeficiency virus-infected subjects. *Antiviral Res.,* **1996,** 29:153–161.

Key: Unless otherwise indicated by a specific footnote, the data are presented for the study population as a mean value ± 1 standard deviation, a mean and range (lowest–highest in parenthesis) of values, a range of the lowest–highest values, or a single mean value.

ADH = alcohol dehydrogenase; Aged = aged; AIDS = acquired immunodeficiency syndrome; Alb = hypoalbuminemia; Atr Fib = atrial fibrillation; AVH = acute viral hepatitis; Burn = burn patients; C_{max} = peak concentration; CAD = coronary artery disease; Celiac = celiac disease; CF = cystic fibrosis; CHF = congestive heart failure; Child = children; Cirr = hepatic cirrhosis; COPD = chronic obstructive pulmonary disease; CP = cor pulmonale; CPBS = cardiopulmonary bypass surgery; CRI = chronic respiratory insufficiency; Crohn = Crohn's disease; Cush = Cushing's syndrome; CYP = cytochrome P450; Fem = female; Hep = hepatitis; HIV = human immunodeficiency virus; HL = hyperlipoproteinemia; HTh = hyperthyroid; IM = intramuscular; Inflam = inflammation; IV = intravenous; LD = liver disease; LTh = hypothyroid; MAO = monoamine oxidase; MI = myocardial infarction; NAT = N-acetyltransferase; Neo = neonate; NIDDM = non-insulin-dependent diabetes mellitus; NS = nephrotic syndrome; Obes = obese; Pneu = pneumonia; Preg = pregnant; Prem = premature; RA = rheumatoid arthritis; RD = renal disease (including uremia); SC = subcutaneous; Smk = smoking; ST = sulfotransferase; T_{max} = peak time; Tach = ventricular tachycardia; UGT = UDP-glucuronosyl transferase; Ulcer = ulcer patients. Other abbreviations are defined in the text section of this appendix.

Table A–II–1
PHARMACOKINETIC DATA (Continued)

AVAILABILITY (ORAL) (%)	URINARY EXCRETION (%)	BOUND IN PLASMA (%)	CLEARANCE ($ml \cdot min^{-1} \cdot kg^{-1}$)	VOL. DIST. (liters/kg)	HALF-LIFE (hours)	PEAK TIME (hours)	PEAK CONCENTRATIONS
CIMETIDINE (Chapter 37)							
60 ± 23^a	62 ± 20^a ↔ Cirr, CF	$19\ (13–25)^{a,b}$	8.3 ± 2.0 ↓ RD, Aged ↔ Ulcer, Cirr ↑ Burn, CF	1.0 ± 0.2 ↔ RD, Cirr, Ulcer, Burn ↑ CF	2.0 ± 0.3 ↑ RD ↔ Ulcer, Cirr, CF ↓ Burn	$0.5–1.5^c$ ↑ Food	$2–3\ \mu g/ml^c$

^{a}Patients with peptic ulcer disease.
^{b}Blood-to-plasma concentration ratio = 0.97.
^{c}Following a single 400-mg oral dose given after an overnight fast to healthy adults. A second peak (2 to 4 hours) is often observed when cimetidine is given after fasting, but not when given with food. A concentration of 0.5–0.9 $\mu g/ml$ will suppress >80% of basal acid secretion, >50% of food or gastrin-stimulated secretion, and maintain gastric pH ≥ 4 in patients with active peptic ulcer disease.

References: Grahnen, A., von Bahr, C., Lindstrom, B., and Rosen, A. Bioavailability and pharmacokinetics of cimetidine. *Eur. J. Clin. Pharmacol.*, **1979**, *16*:335–340.
Schentag, J.J., Cerra, F.B., Calleri, G.M., Leising, M.E., French, M.A., and Bernhard, H. Age, disease, and cimetidine disposition in healthy subjects and chronically ill patients. *Clin. Pharmacol. Ther.*, **1981**, *29*:737–743.
Somogyi, A., Rohner, H.G., and Gugler, R. Pharmacokinetics and bioavailability of cimetidine in gastric and duodenal ulcer patients. *Clin. Pharmacokinet.*, **1980**, *5*:84–94.

CIPROFLOXACIN (Chapter 44)							
60 ± 12	50 ± 5	40	7.6 ± 0.8^a ↓ RD, Aged ↑ CF	2.2 ± 0.4^a ↓ Aged ↔ CF	3.3 ± 0.4 ↑ RD ↔ Aged ↓ CF	0.6 ± 0.2^b	$2.5 \pm 1.1\ \mu g/ml^b$

^{a}Calculated assuming a 70-kg body weight. V_{area} reported.
^{b}Following a 500-mg oral dose given twice a day for 3 or more days to patients with chronic bronchitis or bronchiectasis.

References: Begg, E.J., Robson, R.A., Saunders, D.A., Graham, G.G., Buttimore, R.C., Neill, A.M., and Town, G.I. The pharmacokinetics of oral fleroxacin and ciprofloxacin in plasma and sputum during acute and chronic dosing. *Br. J. Clin. Pharmacol.*, **2000**, *49*:32–38.
Sorgel, F., Jaehde, U., Naber, K., and Stephan, U. Pharmacokinetic disposition of quinolones in human body fluids and tissues. *Clin. Pharmacokinet.*, **1989**, *16*(suppl 1):5–24.

CISAPRIDE^a (Chapter 11)							
$35–40$ ↑ Food	<1	98	7.0 ± 2.5^b ↓ LD^c ↔ RD ↑ $Child^d$	2.4	7.0 ± 1.6 ↑ Aged, LD	$1–1.5^e$	45.0 ± 15.2 ng/ml^e

^{a}Data from healthy male subjects. Metabolized by CYP3A to norcisapride.
^{b}CL/F, V_d/F, and other parameters reported for oral dose. $CL \sim 1.4$ ml·min^{-1}·kg^{-1} also reported.
^{c}CL/F reduced, hepatic cirrhosis.
^{d}$t_{1/2}$, CL/F, and V_d/F estimates were 11.5 hours and 9.0 ml·min^{-1}·kg^{-1}, and 1.9 l/kg, respectively; <7 months of age.
^{e}Following a single 10-mg oral dose (suspension).

References: Barone, J.A., Huang, Y.C., Bierman, R.H., Colaizzi, J.L., Long, J.F., Kerr, D.A., Van Peer, A., Woestenborghs, R., and Heykants, J. Bioavailability of three oral dosage forms of cisapride, a gastrointestinal stimulant agent. *Clin. Pharm.*, **1987**, *6*:640–645.
McCallum, R.W., Prakash, C., Campoli-Richards, D.M., and Goa, K.L. Cisapride. A preliminary review of its pharmacodynamic and pharmacokinetic properties, and therapeutic use as a prokinetic agent in gastrointestinal motility disorders. *Drugs*, **1988**, *36*:652–681.
Physicians' Desk Reference, 54th ed. Medical Economics Co, Montvale, NJ, **2000**, p. 1451.
Preechagoon, Y., Charles, B., Piotrovskij, V., Donovan, T., and Van Peer, A. Population pharmacokinetics of enterally administered cisapride in young infants with gastro-oesophageal reflux disease. *Br. J. Clin. Pharmacol.*, **1999**, *48*:688–693.

CISPLATIN[a] (Chapter 52)

—	2.3 ± 9	—[b]	6.3 ± 1.2	0.28 ± 0.07	0.53 ± 0.10	—	2Hr: 3.4 ± 1.1 $\mu g/ml$[c] 7Hr: 1.0 ± 0.4 $\mu g/ml$[c]

[a] Early studies measured total platinum, rather than the parent compound; values reported here are for parent drug in seven patients with ovarian cancer (mean $CL_{cr} = 66 \pm 27$ ml/min).

[b] Cisplatin does not bind reversibly to plasma proteins; however, platinum will form a tight complex with plasma proteins (90%).

[c] Following a single 100-mg/m² intravenous dose given as a ~2- or ~7-hour infusion to ovarian cancer patients.

Reference: Reece, P.A., Stafford, I., Davy, M., and Freeman, S. Disposition of unchanged cisplatin in patients with ovarian cancer. *Clin. Pharmacol. Ther.,* **1987,** 42:320–325.

CITALOPRAM[a] (Chapter 19)

80 ± 13	10.5 ± 1.4	80	4.3 ± 1.2[b] ↓ Aged, LD[c]	12.3 ± 2.3	33 ± 4 ↑ Aged, Cirr	~4[d]	R-(−): 228 ± 64 nM[d] S-(+): 154 ± 64 nM[d]

[a] Data from healthy adult male subjects. No significant gender differences. Citalopram is metabolized by CYP2C19 (polymorphic) and CYP3A4 to desmethylcitalopram (weak activity).

[b] Homozygous CYP2C19 poor metabolizers exhibit a lower (~44%) CL/F than extensive metabolizers. CL/F for the S-(+)-enantiomer is 1.85-fold greater than that of the antipode.

[c] CL/F reduced in alcoholic, viral, or biliary cirrhosis.

[d] Following a 40-mg oral dose given once a day to steady state.

References: Joffe, P., Larsen, F.S., Pedersen, V., Ring-Larsen, H., Aaes-Jorgensen, T., and Sidhu, J. Single-dose pharmacokinetics of citalopram in patients with moderate renal insufficiency or hepatic cirrhosis compared with healthy subjects. *Eur. J. Clin. Pharmacol.* **1998,** 54:237–242.

Physicians' Desk Reference, 54th ed., Medical Economics Co., Montvale, NJ, **2000,** p. 1074.

Sidhu, J., Priskorn, M., Poulsen, M., Segonzac, A., Grollier, G., and Larsen, F. Steady-state pharmacokinetics of the enantiomers of citalopram and its metabolites in humans. *Chirality,* **1997,** 9:686–692.

Sindrup, S.H., Brosen, K., Hansen, M.G., Aaes-Jorgensen, T., Overo, K.F., and Gram, L.F. Pharmacokinetics of citalopram in relation to the sparteine and the mephenytoin oxidation polymorphisms. *Ther. Drug. Monit.* **1993,** 15:11–17.

CLARITHROMYCIN[a] (Chapter 47)

55 ± 8[b]	36 ± 7[b] ↔ Aged	42–50[c]	7.3 ± 1.9[b] ↓ Aged, RD ↔ Cirr	2.6 ± 0.5 ↔ Aged ↑ Cirr	3.3 ± 0.5[b] ↑ Aged, RD, Cirr	C: 2.8[d] HC: 3[d]	C: 2.4 $\mu g/ml$[d] HC: 0.7 $\mu g/ml$[d]

[a] Active metabolite, 14(R)-hydroxyclarithromycin.

[b] Data generated for a 250-mg oral dose. At higher doses, metabolic clearance saturates resulting in increases in the % urinary excretion and half-life, and decrease in CL.

[c] Blood-to-plasma concentration ratio = 0.64.

[d] Mean data for clarithromycin (C) and 14-hydroxyclarithromycin (HC), following a 500-mg oral dose, given twice a day to steady state in healthy adults.

Reference: Fraschini, F., Scaglione, F., and Demartini, G. Clarithromycin clinical pharmacokinetics. *Clin. Pharmacokinet.,* **1993,** 25:189–204.

Key: Unless otherwise indicated by a specific footnote, the data are presented for the study population as a mean value ± 1 standard deviation, a mean and range (lowest–highest in parenthesis) of values, a range of the lowest–highest values, or a single mean value.

ADH = alcohol dehydrogenase; Aged = aged; AIDS = acquired immunodeficiency syndrome; Alb = hypoalbuminemia; AVH = acute viral hepatitis; Atr Fib = atrial fibrillation; Burn = burn patients; C_{max} = peak concentration; CAD = coronary artery disease; Celiac = celiac disease; CF = cystic fibrosis; CHF = congestive heart failure; Child = children; Cirr = hepatic cirrhosis; COPD = chronic obstructive pulmonary disease; CP = cor pulmonale; CPBS = cardiopulmonary bypass surgery; CRI = chronic respiratory insufficiency; Crohn = Crohn's disease; Cush = Cushing's syndrome; CYP = cytochrome P450; Fem = female; Hep = hepatitis; HIV = human immunodeficiency virus; HL = hyperlipoproteinemia; HTh = hyperthyroid; IM = intramuscular; Inflam = inflammation; IV = intravenous; LD = liver disease; LTh = hypothyroid; MAO = monoamine oxidase; MI = myocardial infarction; NAT = N-acetyltransferase; Neo = neonate; NIDDM = non-insulin-dependent diabetes mellitus; NS = nephrotic syndrome; Obes = obese; Pneu = pneumonia; Preg = pregnant; Prem = premature; RA = rheumatoid arthritis; RD = renal disease (including uremia); SC = subcutaneous; Smk = smoking; ST = sulfotransferase; T_{max} = peak time; Tach = ventricular tachycardia; UGT = UDP-glucuronosyl transferase; Ulcer = ulcer patients. Other abbreviations are defined in the text section of this appendix.

Table A–II-1
PHARMACOKINETIC DATA (Continued)

AVAILABILITY (ORAL) (%)	URINARY EXCRETION (%)	BOUND IN PLASMA (%)	CLEARANCE ($ml \cdot min^{-1} \cdot kg^{-1}$)	VOL. DIST. (liters/kg)	HALF-LIFE (hours)	PEAK TIME (hours)	PEAK CONCENTRATIONS
CLAVULANATE[a] (Chapter 45)							
75 ± 21	43 ± 14	22	3.6 ± 1.0[b] ↓ RD ⟷ Child	0.21 ± 0.05[b] ⟷ RD, Child	0.9 ± 0.1 ↑ Neo, RD ⟷ Child	1.3[c]	2.8 μg/ml[c]

[a]Kinetic parameters do not change appreciably when given with amoxicillin or ticarcillin.
[b]Calculated assuming a 70-kg body weight.
[c]Mean data following a single 125-mg oral dose, administered with penicillin to healthy adults. No accumulation with multiple dosing.

Reference: Watson, I.D., Stewart, M.J., and Platt, D.J. Clinical pharmacokinetics of enzyme inhibitors in antimicrobial chemotherapy. *Clin. Pharmacokinet.*, **1988**, *15*:133–164.

AVAILABILITY (ORAL) (%)	URINARY EXCRETION (%)	BOUND IN PLASMA (%)	CLEARANCE	VOL. DIST.	HALF-LIFE	PEAK TIME	PEAK CONCENTRATIONS
CLINDAMYCIN (Chapter 47)							
~87[a] Topical: 2	13	93.6 ± 0.2	4.7 ± 1.3 ⟷ Child	1.1 ± 0.3[b] ⟷ RD, Child	2.9 ± 0.7 ⟷ Child, RD, Preg ↑ Prem	—	IV: 17.2 ± 3.5 μg/ml[c] Oral: 2.5 μg/ml[d]

[a]Clindamycin hydrochloride given orally.
[b]V_{area} reported.
[c]Following a 1200-mg IV dose (30-min infusion) of clindamycin phosphate (prodrug), given twice a day to steady state in healthy male adults.
[d]Following a single 150-mg oral dose of clindamycin hydrochloride to adults.

References: Physicians' Desk Reference, 54th ed. Medical Economics Co., Montvale, NJ, **2000**, p. 2421.
Plaisance, K.I., Drusano, G.L., Forrest, A., Townsend, R.J., and Standiford, H.C. Pharmacokinetic evaluation of two dosage regimens of clindamycin phosphate. *Antimicrob. Agents Chemother.*, **1989**, *33*:618–620.

AVAILABILITY (ORAL) (%)	URINARY EXCRETION (%)	BOUND IN PLASMA (%)	CLEARANCE	VOL. DIST.	HALF-LIFE	PEAK TIME	PEAK CONCENTRATIONS
CLOFIBRATE[a] (Chapter 36)							
95 ± 10	10.8 ± 2.7[b]	97.2 ± 0.9[c] ↓ NS, Cirr, RD ⟷ AVH	0.10 ± 0.03[b] ↑ NS ↑ RD[d] ⟷ AVH, Cirr	0.14 ± 0.02[b] ↑ Cirr, RD	18 ± 4.3 ↑ RD	3.5–4[e]	109 ± 32 μg/ml[e]

[a]Clofibrate is the ethyl ester of *p*-chlorophenoxyisobutyric acid (CPIB). All values are for CPIB, since clofibrate is rapidly de-esterified upon absorption.
[b]Oral dose; *CL/F* and V_{area}/F are reported. *CL/F* calculated assuming 70-kg body weight.
[c]Binding may decrease at high concentrations of CPIB (>200 μg/ml).
[d]Due to accumulation of glucuronide metabolite of CPIB, which is hydrolyzed back to parent drug.
[e]Mean steady-state concentration following a 1-g oral dose, given twice a day to patients with hypercholesterolemia or cholestasis for 2 to 416 weeks.

References: Gugler, R., Kurten, J.W., Jensen, C.J., Klehr, U., and Hartlapp, J. Clofibrate disposition in renal failure and acute and chronic liver disease. *Eur. J. Clin. Pharmacol.*, **1979**, *15*:341–347.
Sedaghat, A., and Ahrens, E.H. Lack of effect of cholestyramine on the pharmacokinetics of clofibrate in man. *Eur. J. Clin. Invest.*, **1975**, *5*:177–185.

AVAILABILITY (ORAL) (%)	URINARY EXCRETION (%)	BOUND IN PLASMA (%)	CLEARANCE	VOL. DIST.	HALF-LIFE	PEAK TIME	PEAK CONCENTRATIONS
CLONAZEPAM (Chapters 17, 19)							
98 ± 31	<1	86 ± 0.5 ↓ Neo	1.55 ± 0.28[a,b]	3.2 ± 1.1	23 ± 5	Oral: 2.5 ± 1.3[c]	IV: 3–29 ng/ml[c] Oral: 17 ± 5.4 ng/ml[c]

[a]*CL/F* reported; this value is consistent for a number of studies, but is higher than the clearance determined in a single study of IV administration.
[b]Metabolized by CYP3A.
[c]Range of C_{max} values following a single 2-mg IV dose (model-fitted for bolus dose) or mean following a 2-mg oral dose (tablet), given to healthy adults. Most patients, including children, whose seizures are controlled by clonazepam have steady-state concentrations in the range of 5 to 70 ng/ml. However, patients who do not respond and those with side effects achieve similar levels.

References: Berlin, A., and Dahlstrom, H. Pharmacokinetics of the anticonvulsant drug clonazepam evaluated from single oral and intravenous doses and by repeated oral administration. *Eur. J. Clin. Pharmacol.*, **1975**, *9*:155–159.

CLONIDINE (Chapters 10, 33)

Oral: 95 / TD: 60	62 ± 11	20	3.1 ± 1.2 ↓ RD	2.1 ± 0.4	12 ± 7 ↑ RD	Oral: 2[a] / TD: 72[a]	Oral: 0.8 ng/ml[a] / TD: 0.3–0.4 ng/ml[a]

[a] Mean data following a 0.1-mg oral dose, given twice a day to steady state, or C_{ss} following a 3.5-cm² transdermal (TD) patch administered to normotensive male adults. Concentrations of 0.2 to 2 ng/ml are associated with a reduction in blood pressure; >1 ng/ml will cause sedation and dry mouth.

Reference: Lowenthal, D.T., Matzek, K.M., and MacGregor, T.R. Clinical pharmacokinetics of clonidine. *Clin. Pharmacokinet.,* **1988,** *14:*287–310.

CLORAZEPATE[a] (Chapters 17, 21)

N: 91 ± 6[a]	N: <1	N: 97.5 ↓ RD ↔ Obes, Aged[c]	N: 0.17 ± 0.02[b] ↑ Smk ↓ Hep, Cirr, Obes, Aged[c]	N: 1.24 ± 0.09[b] ↑ Obes, Preg ↔ Hep, Cirr, Aged	N: 93 ± 11[b] ↑ Obes, Preg, Aged[c] ↓ Hep, Cirr, Smk	N: 0.72 ± 0.01[a,d]	N: 275 ± 27 ng/ml[a,d]

[a] Clorazepate is essentially a prodrug for nordiazepam (N). Bioavailability, peak time, and peak concentration values for N were derived after oral administration of clorazepate.

[b] CL, V_{ss}, and $t_{1/2}$ values are for IV nordiazepam.

[c] Significantly different for male subjects only.

[d] Data for nordiazepam following a 20-mg IM dose of clorazepate given to nonpregnant women.

References: Greenblatt, D.J., Divoll, M.K., Soong, M.H., Boxenbaum, H.G., Harmatz, J.S., and Shader, R.I. Desmethyldiazepam pharmacokinetics: studies following intravenous and oral desmethyldiazepam, oral clorazepate, and intravenous diazepam. *J. Clin. Pharmacol.,* **1988,** *28:*853–859. Rey, E., d'Athis, P., Giraux, P., de Lauture, D., Turquais, J.M., Chavinie, J., and Olive, G. Pharmacokinetics of clorazepate in pregnant and non-pregnant women. *Eur. J. Clin. Pharmacol.* **1979,** *15:*175–180.

CLOZAPINE (Chapter 20)

55 ± 12	<1	>95[a]	6.1 ± 1.6	5.4 ± 3.5	12 ± 4	1.9 ± 0.8[b]	546 ± 307 ng/ml[b]

[a] Blood-to-plasma concentration ratio = 0.7 at low concentrations (11–26 ng/ml), and approaches unity at concentrations >200 ng/ml.

[b] Following titration up to a 150-mg oral dose (tablet), given twice a day for 7 days to adult chronic schizophrenics.

References: Choc, M.G., Lehr, R.G., Hsuan, F., Honigfeld, G., Smith, H.T., Borison, R., and Volavka, J. Multiple-dose pharmacokinetics of clozapine in patients. *Pharm. Res.,* **1987,** *4:*402–405. Jann, M.W., Ereshefsky, L., and Saklad, S.R. Clinical pharmacokinetics of the depot antipsychotics. *Clin. Pharmacokinet.,* **1985,** *10:*315–333.

COCAINE (Chapters 15, 24)

SM: 57 ± 19 / IN: 80 ± 13	<2	91[a]	32 ± 6	2.0 ± 0.2	0.8 ± 0.2	IN: 0.5–0.75[b] / SM: 0.1[b]	IV: 180 ± 56 ng/ml[b] / IN: 220 ± 39 ng/ml[b] / SM: 203 ± 88 ng/ml[b]

[a] Blood-to-plasma concentration ratio ~1.0.

[b] Following a single 20.5-mg IV dose (1-minute bolus), a 95-mg intranasal dose (IN, 30-second inhalation), or a 40 ± 2-mg dose by smoking (SM), given to adult subjects with cocaine experience.

Reference: Jeffcoat, A.R., Perez-Reyes, M., Hill, J.M., Sadler, B.M., and Cook, C.E. Cocaine disposition in humans after intravenous injection, nasal insufflation (snorting), or smoking. *Drug Metab. Dispos.,* **1989,** *17:*153–159.

Key: Unless otherwise indicated by a specific footnote, the data are presented for the study population as a mean value ± 1 standard deviation, a mean and range (lowest–highest in parenthesis) of values, a range of the lowest–highest values, or a single mean value.

ADH = alcohol dehydrogenase; Aged = aged; AIDS = acquired immunodeficiency syndrome; Alb = hypoalbuminemia; Atr Fib = atrial fibrillation; AVH = acute viral hepatitis; Burn = burn patients; C_{max} = peak concentration; CAD = coronary artery disease; Celiac = celiac disease; CF = cystic fibrosis; CHF = congestive heart failure; Child = children; Cirr = hepatic cirrhosis; COPD = chronic obstructive pulmonary disease; CP = cor pulmonale; CPBS = cardiopulmonary bypass surgery; CRI = chronic respiratory insufficiency; Crohn = Crohn's disease; Cush = Cushing's syndrome; CYP = cytochrome P450; Fem = female; Hep = hepatitis; HIV = human immunodeficiency virus; HL = hyperlipoproteinemia; HTh = hyperthyroid; IM = intramuscular; Inflam = inflammation; IV = intravenous; LD = liver disease; LTh = hypothyroid; MAO = monoamine oxidase; MI = myocardial infarction; NAT = N-acetyltransferase; Neo = neonate; NIDDM = non-insulin-dependent diabetes mellitus; NS = nephrotic syndrome; Obes = obese; Pneu = pneumonia; Preg = pregnant; Prem = premature; RA = rheumatoid arthritis; RD = renal disease (including uremia); SC = subcutaneous; Smk = smoking; ST = sulfotransferase; T_{max} = peak time; Tach = ventricular tachycardia; UGT = UDP-glucuronosyl transferase; Ulcer = ulcer patients. Other abbreviations are defined in the text section of this appendix.

Table A–II–1
PHARMACOKINETIC DATA (Continued)

	AVAILABILITY (ORAL) (%)	URINARY EXCRETION (%)	BOUND IN PLASMA (%)	CLEARANCE ($ml \cdot min^{-1} \cdot kg^{-1}$)	VOL. DIST. (liters/kg)	HALF-LIFE (hours)	PEAK TIME (hours)	PEAK CONCENTRATIONS
CODEINE[a] (Chapter 23)								
	50 ± 7[b]	Negligible	7	11 ± 2[c]	2.6 ± 0.3[c]	2.9 ± 0.7	C: 1.0 ± 0.5[d] M: 1.0 ± 0.4[d]	C: 149 ± 60 ng/ml[d] M: 3.8 ± 2.4 ng/ml[d]
CYCLOPHOSPHAMIDE[a] (Chapters 52, 53)								
	74 ± 22	6.5 ± 4.3	13	1.3 ± 0.5 ↑ Child ↓ Cirr ↔ RD	0.78 ± 0.57 ↔ Child	7.5 ± 4.0 ↓ Child ↑ Cirr	—	121 ± 21 μM[b]
CYCLOSPORINE (Chapter 53)								
	SI: 28 ± 18[a,b]	<1	93 ± 2	5.7 (0.6–24)[b,c] ↓ Hep, Cirr, Aged ↔ RD ↑ Child	4.5 (0.12–15.5)[b] ↓ Aged ↑ Child	10.7 (4.3–53)[b] ↓ Child ↔ Aged	NL: 1.5–2[d] SI: 4.0 ± 1.8[d]	NL: 1333 ± 469 ng/ml[d] SI: 1101 ± 570 ng/ml[d]
CYTARABINE[a] (Chapter 52)								
	<20	11 ± 8	13	13 ± 4	3.0 ± 1.9[b]	2.6 ± 0.6	—	IV, B: ~5 μg/ml[c] IV, I: 0.05–0.1 μg/ml[c]

CODEINE

Reference: Quiding, H., Anderson, P., Bondesson, U., Boreus, L.O., and Hynning, P.A. Plasma concentrations of codeine and its metabolite, morphine, after single and repeated oral administration. *Eur. J. Clin. Pharmacol.,* **1986,** *30:*673–677.

[a]Codeine is metabolized by CYP2D6 (polymorphic) to morphine. Analgesic effect is thought to be due largely to morphine levels.
[b]Oral/intramuscular bioavailability reported.
[c]CL/F and V_{area}/F reported.
[d]Data for codeine (C) and morphine (M) following a 60-mg oral codeine dose, given three times a day for 7 doses to healthy male adults.

CYCLOPHOSPHAMIDE

References: Grochow, L.B., and Colvin, M. Clinical pharmacokinetics of cyclophosphamide. *Clin. Pharmacokinet.,* **1979,** *4:*380–394.
Moore, M.J., Erlichman, C., Thiessen, J.J., Bunting, P.S., Hardy, R., Kerr, L., and Soldin, S. Variability in the pharmacokinetics of cyclophosphamide, methotrexate and 5-fluorouracil in women receiving adjuvant treatment for breast cancer. *Cancer Chemother. Pharmacol.,* **1994,** *33:*472–476.

[a]Cyclophosphamide is activated by cytochrome P450s (CYP2C9 primarily) to hydroxycyclophosphamide. The metabolite is further converted to the active alkylating species, phosphoramide mustard ($t_{1/2}$ = 9 hours) and normitrogen mustard (apparent $t_{1/2}$ = 3.3 hours). Kinetic parameters are for cyclophosphamide.
[b]Following a 600-mg/m² IV (bolus) dose given to breast cancer patients.

CYCLOSPORINE

References: Fahr. A. Cyclosporin clinical pharmacokinetics. *Clin. Pharmacokinet.,* **1993,** *24:*472–495.
Physicians' Desk Reference, 54th ed. Medical Economics Co., Montvale, NJ, **2000,** pp. 2034–2035.
Pollak, R., Wong, R.L., and Chang, C.T. Cyclosporine bioavailability of Neoral and Sandimmune in white and black de novo renal transplant recipients. Neoral Study Group. *Ther. Drug Monit.,* **1999,** *21:*661–663.
Ptachcinski, R.J., Venkataramanan, R., Rosenthal, J.T., Burckart, G.J., Taylor, R.J., and Hakala, T.R. Cyclosporine kinetics in renal transplantation. *Clin. Pharmacol. Ther.,* **1985,** *38:*296–300.

[a]NEORAL (NL) exhibits a more uniform and slightly greater (125% to 150%) relative oral bioavailability than the older SANDIMMUNE (SI) formulation.
[b]Pharmacokinetic parameters based on measurements in blood with a specific assay. Data from renal transplant patients shown.
[c]Metabolized by CYP3A to three major metabolites, which are subsequently biotransformed to numerous secondary and tertiary metabolites.
[d]Steady-state C_{max} following a 344 ± 122-mg/day oral dose (divided into two doses) of cyclosporine (NL, soft gelatin capsule), or a 14 (6–22)-mg/kg per day oral dose of cyclosporine (SI, SANDIMMUNE), given to adult renal transplant patients in stable condition. Mean trough concentration after NL was 251 ± 116 ng/ml; therapeutic range (trough) is 150–400 ng/ml.

CYTARABINE

Reference: Ho, D.H., and Frie, E.I. Clinical pharmacology of 1-β-D-arabinofuranosyl cytosine. *Clin. Pharmacol. Ther.,* **1971,** *12:*944–954.
Wan, S.H., Huffman, D.H., Azarnoff, D.L., Hoogstraten, B., and Larsen, W.E. Pharmacokinetics of 1-β-D-arabinofuranosylcytosine in humans. *Cancer Res.,* **1974,** *34:*392–397.

[a]Liposome formulation of cytarabine given intrathecally. Cerebrospinal fluid $t_{1/2}$ = 100 to 263 hours for liposome formulation (compared to 3.4 hours for intrathecal dose of free drug).
[b]V_{area} reported.
[c]C_{max} following a single 200-mg/m² intravenous bolus (IV, B) dose or steady-state plasma concentration following a 112-mg/m² per day constant-rate intravenous infusion (IV, I), given to patients with leukemia, malignant melanoma, or solid tumors.

DAPSONE (Chapters 48, 65)

93 ± 8[a]	73 ± 1 ↔ RD, Cirr	0.60 ± 0.17[c] ↔ Cirr, Child ↑ Neo	1.0 ± 0.1 ↔ Cirr	22.4 ± 5.6 ↔ Cirr, Child	5–15[b]	SD: 1.6 ± 0.4 μg/ml[d] MD: 3.3 μg/ml[d]

[a]Decreased in severe leprosy (70–80); estimates based on urinary recovery of radioactive dose.
[b]Urine pH = 6–7.
[c]Undergoes reversible metabolism to a monoacetyl metabolite; the reaction is catalyzed by NAT2 (polymorphic); also undergoes N-hydroxylation (CYP3A, CYP2C9).
[d]Mean data following a single 100-mg oral dose (SD) or mean C_{max} following a 100-mg oral dose, given once daily to steady state (MD) in healthy adults.

References: Mirochnick, M., Cooper, E., McIntosh, K., Xu, J., Lindsey, J., Jacobus, D., Mofenson, L., Sullivan, J.L., Dankner, W., Frenkel, L.M., Nachman, S., Wara, D.W., Johnson, D., Bonagura, V.R., Rathore, M.H., Cunningham, C.K., and McNamara, J. Pharmacokinetics of dapsone administered daily and weekly in human immunodeficiency virus-infected children. Antimicrob. Agents Chemother., 1999, 43:2586–2591.
Pieters, F.A., and Zuidema, J. The pharmacokinetics of dapsone after oral administration to healthy volunteers. Br. J. Clin. Pharmacol. 1986, 22:491–494.
Venkatesan, K. Clinical pharmacokinetic considerations in the treatment of patients with leprosy. Clin. Pharmacokinet., 1989, 16:365–386.
Zuidema, J., Hilbers-Modderman, E.S., and Merkus, F.W. Clinical pharmacokinetics of dapsone. Clin. Pharmacokinet., 1986, 11:299–315.

DELAVIRDINE[a] (Chapter 51)

SD: ~85[b]	<5	97.6	SD: 13.7 ± 10.4[b] MD: 1.69 ± 1.29[c,d]	SD: 2.7 MD: 0.52[c]	SD: 2.4 ± 0.8[b] MD: 4.1 ± 1.5[c,d]	SD: 1.2 ± 0.4 MD: 2.2 ± 1.7[c]	SD: 7.2 ± 4.0 μM[b] MD: 27 ± 13 μM[c]

[a]Data from patients with HIV infection.
[b]Single 400-mg oral dose (SD). CL/F and V_{area}/F reported.
[c]400-mg oral dose three times a day to steady state (MD).
[d]Delavirdine inhibits its own metabolism by suicide inactivation of CYP3A4; exhibits time- and dose-dependent changes in CL/F and $t_{1/2}$.

References: Beach, J.W. Chemotherapeutic agents for human immunodeficiency virus infection: mechanism of action, pharmacokinetics, metabolism, and adverse reactions. Clin. Ther., 1998, 20:2–25.
Cheng, C.L., Smith, D.E., Carver, P.L., Cox, S.R., Watkins, P.B., Blake, D.S., Kauffman, C.A., Meyer, K.M., Amidon, G.L., and Stetson, P.L. Steady-state pharmacokinetics of delavirdine in HIV-positive patients: effect on erythromycin breath test. Clin. Pharmacol. Ther., 1997, 61:531–543.
Morse, G.D., Fischl, M.A., Shelton, M.J., Cox, S.R., Driver, M., DeRemer, M., and Freimuth, W.W. Single-dose pharmacokinetics of delavirdine mesylate and didanosine in patients with human immunodeficiency virus infection. Antimicrob. Agents Chemother., 1997, 41:169–174.

DEXTROMETHORPHAN[a] (Chapter 23)

EM: 0.19 ± 0.21 PM: 11.1 ± 3.0	—	EM: 1575 ± 658[b] PM: ~3.9 ± 1.4[b]	—	EM: 3.4 ± 0.5[b] PM: 29.5 ± 8.4[b]	2–2.5	EM: 5.2 ± 1.8 ng/ml[c] PM: 33 ± 8.2 ng/ml[c]

[a]Data from healthy subjects. Extensive CYP2D6-dependent first-pass metabolism to dextrorphan (pharmacologically active). Data for extensive (EM) and poor (PM) metabolizers shown.
[b]CL/F and $t_{1/2}$ reported for oral dose.
[c]Following a single 60-mg oral dose to presumed EM or 30-mg to PM. C_{max} for dextrorphan was 879 ± 60 ng/ml in EMs and undetected in PMs.

References: Schadel, M., Wu, D., Otton, S.V., Kalow, W., and Sellers, E.M. Pharmacokinetics of dextromethorphan and metabolites in humans: influence of the CYP2D6 phenotype and quinidine inhibition. J. Clin. Psychopharmacol., 1995, 15:263–269.
Silvasti, M., Karttunen, P., Tukiainen, H., Kokkonen, P., Hanninen, U., and Nykanen, S. Pharmacokinetics of dextromethorphan and dextrorphan: a single dose comparison of three preparations in human volunteers. Int. J. Clin. Pharmacol. Ther. Toxicol., 1987, 25:493–497.

Key: Unless otherwise indicated by a specific footnote, the data are presented for the study population as a mean value ± 1 standard deviation, a mean and range (lowest–highest in parenthesis) of values, a range of the lowest–highest values, or a single mean value.

ADH = alcohol dehydrogenase; Aged = aged; AIDS = acquired immunodeficiency syndrome; Alb = hypoalbuminemia; Atr Fib = atrial fibrillation; AVH = acute viral hepatitis; Burn = burn patients; C_{max} = peak concentration; CAD = coronary artery disease; Celiac = celiac disease; CF = cystic fibrosis; CHF = congestive heart failure; Child = children; Cirr = hepatic cirrhosis; COPD = chronic obstructive pulmonary disease; CP = cor pulmonale; CPBS = cardiopulmonary bypass surgery; CRI = chronic respiratory insufficiency; Crohn = Crohn's disease; Cush = Cushing's syndrome; CYP = cytochrome P450; Fem = female; Hep = hepatitis; HIV = human immunodeficiency virus; HL = hyperlipoproteinemia; HTh = hyperthyroid; IM = intramuscular; Inflam = inflammation; IV = intravenous; LD = liver disease; LTh = hypothyroid; MAO = monoamine oxidase; MI = myocardial infarction; NAT = N-acetyltransferase; Neo = neonate; NIDDM = non-insulin-dependent diabetes mellitus; NS = nephrotic syndrome; Obes = obese; Pneu = pneumonia; Preg = pregnant; Prem = premature; RA = rheumatoid arthritis; RD = renal disease (including uremia); SC = subcutaneous; Smk = smoking; ST = sulfotransferase; T_{max} = peak time; Tach = ventricular tachycardia; UGT = UDP-glucuronosyl transferase; Ulcer = ulcer patients. Other abbreviations are defined in the text section of this appendix.

Table A–II–1
PHARMACOKINETIC DATA (Continued)

AVAILABILITY (ORAL) (%)	URINARY EXCRETION (%)	BOUND IN PLASMA (%)	CLEARANCE ($ml \cdot min^{-1} \cdot kg^{-1}$)	VOL. DIST. (liters/kg)	HALF-LIFE (hours)	PEAK TIME (hours)	PEAK CONCENTRATIONS

DIAZEPAM[a] (Chapters 17, 19)

| Oral: 100 ± 14; Rectal: 90 | <1 | 98.7 ± 0.2; ↓ RD, Cirr, NS, Preg, Neo, Alb, Burn, Aged; ↔ HTh | 0.38 ± 0.06[a,b]; ↑ Alb; ↓ Cirr; ↔ Aged, Smk, HTh | 1.1 ± 0.3; ↑ Cirr, Aged, Alb; ↔ RD, HTh | 43 ± 13[a,b]; ↑ Aged, Cirr; ↔ HTh | Oral: 1.3 ± 0.2[c]; Rectal: 1.5[c] | IV: 400–500 ng/ml[c]; Oral: 317 ± 27 ng/ml[c]; Rectal: ~400 ng/ml[c] |

[a] Active metabolites, desmethyldiazepam and oxazepam, formed by CYP2C19 (polymorphic) and CYP3A.
[b] CL increased and $t_{1/2}$ decreased by administration of other drugs that induce metabolic enzymes.
[c] Range of data following a single 5–10-mg IV dose (15- to 30-second bolus) or mean data following a single 10-mg oral or 15-mg rectal dose given to healthy adults. A concentration of 300 to 400 ng/ml provides anxiolytic effect, and >600 ng/ml provides control of seizures.

References: Friedman, H., Greenblatt, D.J., Peters, G.R., Metzler, C.M., Charlton, M.D., Harmatz, J.S., Antal, E.J., Sanborn, E.C., and Francom, S.F. Pharmacokinetics and pharmacodynamics of oral diazepam: effect of dose, plasma concentration, and time. *Clin. Pharmacol. Ther.*, **1992**, 52:139–150.
Greenblatt, D.J., Allen, M.D., Harmatz, J.S., and Shader, R.I. Diazepam disposition determinants. *Clin. Pharmacol. Ther.*, **1980**, 27:301–312.
Physicians' Desk Reference, 54th ed. Medical Economics Co., Montvale, NJ, **2000**, p. 1012.

DICLOFENAC (Chapter 27)

| 54 ± 2 | <1 | >99.5 | 4.2 ± 0.9[a]; ↓ Aged; ↔ RD, Cirr, RA | 0.17 ± 0.11[b]; ↑ RA | 1.1 ± 0.2; ↔ RA | EC: 2.5 (1.0–4.5)[c]; SR: 5.3 ± 1.5[c] | EC: 2.0 (1.4–3.0) μg/ml[c]; SR: 0.42 ± 0.17 μg/ml[c] |

[a] Cleared primarily by CYP2C9-catalyzed 4'-hydroxylation; urine and biliary metabolites account for 30% and 10% to 20% of dose, respectively.
[b] V_{area} reported.
[c] Mean (range) following a single 50-mg enteric-coated tablet (EC) or 100-mg of sustained-release tablet (SR), given to healthy adults.

References: Tracy, T. Nonsteroidal antiinflammatory drugs. In, *Metabolic Drug Interactions.* (Levy, R.H., Thummel, K.T., Trager, W.F., Hansten, P.D., and Eichelbaum, M., eds.) Lippincott Williams & Wilkins, Philadelphia, **2000**, pp. 457–468.
Willis, J.V., Kendall, M.J., Flinn, R.M., Thornhill, D.P., and Welling, P.G. The pharmacokinetics of diclofenac sodium following intravenous and oral administration. *Eur. J. Clin. Pharmacol.* **1979**, 16:405–410.

DICLOXACILLIN (Chapter 45)

| 50–85 | 60 ± 7 | 95.8 ± 0.2; ↓ RD, Aged, Cirr; ↔ CF | 1.6 ± 0.3[a,b]; ↓ RD; ↑ CF[c] | 0.086 ± 0.017[a]; ↔ RD, CF | 0.70 ± 0.07; ↑ RD; ↔ CF | 0.5–1.6[d] | 47–91 μg/ml[d] |

[a] Calculated assuming a 70-kg body weight.
[b] Possible saturation of renal clearance at doses of 1 to 2 g.
[c] Concomitant increase in clearance of both dicloxacillin and creatinine.
[d] Estimated range of data following a single 2-g oral dose given to healthy (fasted) adults.

Reference: Nauta, E.H. and Mattie, H. Dicloxacillin and cloxacillin: pharmacokinetics in healthy and hemodialysis subjects. *Clin. Pharmacol. Ther.*, **1976**, 20:98–108.

DIDANOSINE (Chapter 51)

| 38 ± 15; ↓ Child, Food | 36 ± 9 | <5 | 16 ± 7; ↔ Child, ↓ RD | 1.0 ± 0.2 | 1.4 ± 0.3 | B: 0.75[a]; M: 0.50[a] | B: 2.1 ± 0.6 μg/ml[a]; M: 2.1 ± 0.5 μg/ml[a] |

[a] Mean C_{max} and median T_{max} following a single 375-mg oral dose of didanosine formulated as a citrate-phosphate buffered (B) solution or as a mixture with MAALOX suspension (M), taken after a fast by patients with HIV infection.

References: Knupp, C.A., Shyu, W.C., Dolin, R., Valentine, F.T., McLaren, C., Martin, R.R., Pittman, K.A., and Barbhaiya, R.H. Pharmacokinetics of didanosine in patients with acquired immunodeficiency syndrome or acquired immunodeficiency syndrome-related complex. *Clin. Pharmacol. Ther.*, **1991**, 49:523–535.
Morse, G.D., Fischl, M.A., Shelton, M.J., Cox, S.R., Driver, M., DeRemer, M., and Freimuth, W.W. Single-dose pharmacokinetics of delavirdine mesylate and didanosine in patients with human immunodeficiency virus infection. *Antimicrob. Agents Chemother.*, **1997**, 41:169–174.

DIGOXIN (Chapters 34, 35)

70 ± 13[a,c] ←→ RD, MI, CHF, LTh, HTh, Aged	60 ± 11	25 ± 5 ↓ RD	$CL = (0.88CL_{cr} + 0.33)$[b,c] ↓ LTh ↑ HTh, Neo, Child, Preg	$V = (3.12CL_{cr} + 3.84)$ ↓ LTh ↑ HTh ←→ CHF	39 ± 13 ↓ HTh ↑ RD, CHF, Aged, LTh ←→ Obes	1–3[d]	NT: 1.4 ± 0.7 ng/ml[d] T: 3.7 ± 1.0 ng/ml[d]

[a] LANOXIN tablets; digoxin solutions, elixirs, and capsules may be absorbed more completely.

[b] Equation applies to patients with some degree of heart failure. If heart failure is not present, the coefficient of CL_{cr} is 1.0. Units of CL_{cr} must be ml·min⁻¹·kg⁻¹.

[c] In the occasional patient, digoxin is metabolized to an inactive metabolite, dihydrodigoxin, by gut flora. This results in a reduced oral bioavailability.

[d] Mean data following an oral dose of 0.31 ± 0.19 mg/day or 0.36 ± 0.19 mg/day in patients with congestive heart failure who exhibited no signs of digitalis toxicity (NT) or signs of toxicity (T), respectively. Concentrations >0.8 ng/ml are associated with inotropic effect. Concentrations of 1.7, 2.5, and 3.3 ng/ml are associated with a 10%, 50%, and 90% probability of digoxin-induced arrhythmias, respectively.

References: Mooradian, A.D. Digitalis. An update of clinical pharmacokinetics, therapeutic monitoring techniques and treatment recommendations. *Clin. Pharmacokinet.,* **1988,** *15:*165–179. Smith, T.W., and Haber, E. Digoxin intoxication: the relationship of clinical presentation to serum digoxin concentration. *J. Clin. Invest.,* **1970,** *49:*2377–2386.

DILTIAZEM[a] (Chapters 32, 33, 35)

38 ± 11	<4	78 ± 3[b]	11.8 ± 2.2[c] ←→ Aged ↓ RD	3.3 ± 1.2 ←→ Aged ↓ RD	4.4 ± 1.3[d] ←→ RD, Aged	4.0 ± 0.4[e]	151 ± 46 ng/ml[e]

[a] Active metabolites, desacetyldiltiazem ($t_{1/2}$ = 9 ± 2 hours) and N-desmethyldiltiazem ($t_{1/2}$ = 7.5 ± 1 hours). Formation of demethylated metabolite (major pathway of clearance) is catalyzed primarily by CYP3A.

[b] Blood-to-plasma concentration ratio = 1.0 ± 0.1.

[c] More than a twofold decrease with multiple dosing.

[d] Half-life for oral dose is 5 to 6 hours; does not change with multiple dosing.

[e] Following a single 120-mg oral dose given to healthy adults.

Reference: Echizen, H., and Eichelbaum, M. Clinical pharmacokinetics of verapamil, nifedipine and diltiazem. *Clin. Pharmacokinet.,* **1986,** *11:*425–449.

DIPHENHYDRAMINE (Chapter 25)

72 ± 26	1.9 ± 0.8 ←→ Cirr	78 ± 3 ↓ Cirr	6.2 ± 1.7[a] ←→ Cirr ↑ Child ↓ Aged	4.5 ± 2.8[a,b] ←→ Cirr	8.5 ± 3.2[a] ↑ Cirr, Aged ←→ Child	2.3 ± 0.64[c]	IV: ~230 ng/ml[c] Oral: 66 ± 22 ng/ml[c]

[a] Increased CL, decreased V, and no change in half-life in Asians, presumably due to decreased plasma protein binding.

[b] V_{urea} reported.

[c] Following a single 50-mg dose of diphenhydramine hydrochloride (44-mg base), given IV or orally to fasted healthy adults. Levels >25 ng/ml provide antihistaminic effect, whereas levels >60 ng/ml are associated with drowsiness and mental impairment.

Reference: Blyden, G.T., Greenblatt, D.J., Scavone, J.M., and Shader, R.I. Pharmacokinetics of diphenhydramine and a demethylated metabolite following intravenous and oral administration. *J. Clin. Pharmacol.,* **1986,** *26:*529–533.

Key: Unless otherwise indicated by a specific footnote, the data are presented for the study population as a mean value ± 1 standard deviation, a mean and range (lowest–highest in parenthesis) of values, a range of the lowest–highest values, or a single mean value.

ADH = alcohol dehydrogenase; Aged = aged; AIDS = acquired immunodeficiency syndrome; Alb = hypoalbuminemia; Atr Fib = atrial fibrillation; AVH = acute viral hepatitis; Burn = burn patients; C_{max} = peak concentration; CAD = coronary artery disease; Celiac = celiac disease; CF = cystic fibrosis; CHF = congestive heart failure; Child = children; Cirr = hepatic cirrhosis; COPD = chronic obstructive pulmonary disease; CP = cor pulmonale; CPBS = cardiopulmonary bypass surgery; CRI = chronic respiratory insufficiency; Crohn = Crohn's disease; Cush = Cushing's syndrome; CYP = cytochrome P450; Fem = female; Hep = hepatitis; HIV = human immunodeficiency virus; HL = hyperlipoproteinemia; HTh = hyperthyroid; IM = intramuscular; Inflam = inflammation; IV = intravenous; LD = liver disease; LTh = hypothyroid; MAO = monoamine oxidase; MI = myocardial infarction; NAT = N-acetyltransferase; Neo = neonate; NIDDM = non-insulin-dependent diabetes mellitus; NS = nephrotic syndrome; Obes = obese; Pneu = pneumonia; Preg = pregnant; Prem = premature; RA = rheumatoid arthritis; RD = renal disease (including uremia); SC = subcutaneous; Smk = smoking; ST = sulfotransferase; T_{max} = peak time; Tach = ventricular tachycardia; UGT = UDP-glucuronosyl transferase; Ulcer = ulcer patients. Other abbreviations are defined in the text section of this appendix.

Table A–II–1
PHARMACOKINETIC DATA (Continued)

AVAILABILITY (ORAL) (%)	URINARY EXCRETION (%)	BOUND IN PLASMA (%)	CLEARANCE ($ml \cdot min^{-1} \cdot kg^{-1}$)	VOL. DIST. (liters/kg)	HALF-LIFE (hours)	PEAK TIME (hours)	PEAK CONCENTRATIONS
DISOPYRAMIDE[a] (Chapter 35)							
83 ± 11 ←→ MI, CHF	55 ± 6	Conc.-dependent[b] ↓ Neo, NS, Cirr ↑ Aged, MI, RD	1.2 ± 0.4[c] ↓ MI, Tach, CHF[d] RD, Cirr[d] ←→ Smk	0.59 ± 0.15[c] ↓ Cirr[d] ←→ CHF[d], RD, Smk	6.0 ± 1.0 ↑ RD, CHF[d] ←→ MI, Smk	IR: 1.9–2.3[e] CR: 4.9 ± 1.4[e]	IR: 2.8–4.8 $\mu g/ml$[e] CR: 2.2 ± 0.5 $\mu g/ml$[e]

[a]Racemic mixture; only S-(+)-enantiomer prolongs QT_c duration; it has greater anticholinergic activity and less negative inotropic effect than the R-(−) isomer.
[b]Saturable plasma protein binding, 89% at 0.38 $\mu g/ml$ and 68% at 3.8 $\mu g/ml$, results in nonlinear kinetics for total drug.
[c]Unbound clearance, 5.4 ± 2.8 ml·min⁻¹·kg⁻¹. Unbound clearance of active S-(+)-enantiomer is about 25% greater than that of the R-(−)-isomer, but no differences noted in unbound measures of half-life.
[d]Comparison of unbound parameters.
[e]Range of data following a single 200-mg oral immediate-release (IR) capsule given to patients with CHF or acute MI, or mean data following a 300-mg oral controlled-release (CR) capsule, given to healthy adults.

References: Physicians' Desk Reference, 54th ed. Medical Economics Co., Montvale, NJ, **2000,** p. 2925.
Siddoway, L.A., and Woosley, R.L. Clinical pharmacokinetics of disopyramide. *Clin. Pharmacokinet.,* **1986,** *11:*214–222.

DOBUTAMINE (Chapters 10, 34)							
—	—	—	59 ± 22[a] ↑ Child	0.20 ± 0.08[a]	2.4 ± 0.7 min[a]	—	46 ± 26 ng/ml[b]

[a]Values for patients with CHF; V, for example, is lower when less edema is present. Values likely represent distribution rather than elimination. Metabolically cleared primarily by COMT-mediated methylation.
[b]Mean steady-state concentration following an IV infusion of 2.5 $\mu g/kg$ per minute to adult patients with congestive cardiomyopathy. Concentrations >35 ng/ml or >50 ng/ml are threshold for a change in cardiac output and heart rate, respectively.

References: Kates, R.E., and Leier, C.V. Dobutamine pharmacokinetics in severe heart failure. *Clin. Pharmacol. Ther.,* **1978,** *24:*537–541.
Steinberg, C., and Notterman, D.A. Pharmacokinetics of cardiovascular drugs in children. Inotropes and vasopressors. *Clin. Pharmacokinet.,* **1994,** *27:*345–367.

DOCETAXEL[a] (Chapter 52)							
—	2.1 ± 0.2	94	22.6 ± 7.7 liters·h⁻¹· $(m^2)^{-1}$ ↓ LD[b]	72 ± 24 l/m²	13.6 ± 6.1	—	2.4 ± 0.9 $\mu g/ml$[c]

[a]Data from male and female patients treated for cancer. Metabolized by CYP3A and excreted into bile. Parenteral administration.
[b]Mild to moderate liver impairment.
[c]Following IV infusion of 85 mg/m² over 1.6 hours.

References: Clarke, S.J., and Rivory, L.P. Clinical pharmacokinetics of docetaxel. *Clin. Pharmacokinet,* **1999,** *36:*99–114.
Extra, J.M., Rousseau, F., Bruno, R., Clavel, M., Le Bail, N., and Marty, M. Phase I and pharmacokinetic study of Taxotere (RP 56976; NSC 628503) given as a short intravenous infusion. *Cancer Res.,* **1993,** *53:*1037–1042.
Physicians' Desk Reference, 54th ed. Medical Economics Co., Montvale, NJ, **2000,** p. 2578.

DOFETILIDE[a] (Chapter 35)

96 (83–108)	52 ± 2[b]	64	5.23 ± 0.30 →RD[b]	3.44 ± 0.25	7.5 ± 0.4 ↑RD[b]	1–2.5	2.3 ± 1.1 ng/ml[c]

[a]Data from healthy male subjects. Metabolized by CYP3A4.
[b]CL/F reduced, renal impairment.
[c]Following a single 0.55-mg oral dose.

References: Kalus, J.S., and Mauro, V.F. Dofetilide: a class III-specific antiarrhythmic agent. *Ann. Pharmacother.,* **2000,** 34:44–56.
Smith, D.A., Rasmussen, H.S., Stopher, D.A., and Walker, D.K. Pharmacokinetics and metabolism of dofetilide in mouse, rat, dog and man. *Xenobiotica,* **1992,** 22:709–719.
Tham, T.C., MacLennan, B.A., Burke, M.T., and Harron, D.W. Pharmacodynamics and pharmacokinetics of the class III antiarrhythmic agent dofetilide (UK-68,798) in humans. *J. Cardiovasc. Pharmacol.,* **1993,** 21:507–512.

DOLASETRON[a] (Chapter 38)

D: <1% H: 76 ± 28	D: negligible H: 32.8 ± 28	D: — H: 67–77	D: 115 ± 36 H: 9.5 ± 3.2 ↑Child[b] ↓RD[c] ↔ LD (H)	D: 1.4 ± 0.4 H: 6.1 ± 1.8	D: 0.14 ± 0.02 H: 7.7 ± 1.7 ↓Child[b] ↑RD[c]	H: 0.7 ± 0.3[d]	H: 601 ± 210 ng/ml[d]

[a]Data from healthy subjects. No significant gender differences. Dolasetron (D) is rapidly reduced in the body to the active metabolite, hydroxydolasetron (H). H is metabolized by CYP2D6, CYP3A4, and flavine monooxygenase. Stereoselective formation and elimination of H enantiomers. For H, peak R-(+)-enantiomer concentrations in plasma are much higher than S-(−) concentrations. R-(+)-enantiomer is also a more potent 5HT$_3$-receptor antagonist.
[b]CL and CL/F increased for H, children 2 to 12 years of age.
[c]CL and CL/F reduced for H, severe renal impairment.
[d]Following a single 200-mg oral dose.

References: Dimmitt, D.C., Choo, Y.S., Martin, L.A., Arumugham, T., Hahne, W.F., and Weir, S.J. Intravenous pharmacokinetics and absolute oral bioavailability of dolasetron in healthy volunteers: part 1. *Biopharm. Drug Dispos.,* **1999,** 20:29–39.
Dimmitt, D.C., Choo, Y.S., Martin, L.A., Arumugham, T., Hahne, W.F., and Weir, S.J. Single- and multiple-dose pharmacokinetics of oral dolasetron and its active metabolites in healthy volunteers: part 2. *Biopharm. Drug Dispos.,* **1999,** 20:41–48.
Dimmitt, D.C., Shah, A.K., Arumugham, T., Cramer, M.B., Halstenson, C., Horton, M., and Weir, S.J. Pharmacokinetics of oral and intravenous dolasetron mesylate in patients with renal impairment. *J. Clin. Pharmacol.,* **1998,** 38:798–806.
Physicians' Desk Reference, 54th ed. Medical Economics Co, Montvale, NJ, **2000,** p. 1349.
Stubbs, K., Martin, L.A., Dimmitt, D.C., Pready, N., and Hahne, W.F. Pharmacokinetics of dolasetron after oral and intravenous administration of dolasetron mesylate in healthy volunteers and patients with hepatic dysfunction. *J. Clin. Pharmacol.,* **1997,** 37:926–936.

DONEPEZIL[a] (Chapter 22)

—[b]	10.6 ± 2.7	92.6 ± 0.9[c]	2.90 ± 0.74[d] ↓LD[e] ↔ RD	14.0 ± 2.42[d] ↑Aged	59.7 ± 16.1[d] ↑Aged	3–4[f]	30.8 ± 4.2 ng/ml[f]

[a]Data from young, healthy male and female subjects. No significant gender differences. Metabolized by CYP2D6, CYP3A4, UGT.
[b]Absolute bioavailability is unknown but the oral dose is reportedly well absorbed.
[c]A f_b of 96% has also been reported.
[d]CL/F, V_{ss}/F, and $t_{1/2}$ reported for oral dose.
[e]CL/F reduced slightly (~20%), alcoholic cirrhosis.
[f]Following a 5-mg oral dose, given once daily to steady state.

References: Ohnishi, A., Mihara, M., Kamakura, H., Tomono, Y., Hasegawa, J., Yamazaki, K., Morishita, N., and Tanaka, T. Comparison of the pharmacokinetics of E2020, a new compound for Alzheimer's disease, in healthy young and elderly subjects. *J. Clin. Pharmacol.,* **1993,** 33:1086–1091.
Physicians' Desk Reference, 54th ed. Medical Economics Co, Montvale, NJ, **2000,** p. 2323.

Key: Unless otherwise indicated by a specific footnote, the data are presented for the study population as a mean value ± 1 standard deviation, a mean and range (lowest–highest in parenthesis) of values, a range of the lowest–highest values, or a single mean value.

ADH = alcohol dehydrogenase; Aged = aged; AIDS = acquired immunodeficiency syndrome; Alb = hypoalbuminemia; Atr Fib = atrial fibrillation; AVH = acute viral hepatitis; Burn = burn patients; C_{max} = peak concentration; CAD = coronary artery disease; Celiac = celiac disease; CF = cystic fibrosis; CHF = congestive heart failure; Child = children; Cirr = hepatic cirrhosis; COPD = chronic obstructive pulmonary disease; CP = cor pulmonale; CPBS = cardiopulmonary bypass surgery; CRI = chronic respiratory insufficiency; Crohn = Crohn's disease; Cush = Cushing's syndrome; CYP = cytochrome P450; Fem = female; Hep = hepatitis; HIV = human immunodeficiency virus; HL = hyperlipoproteinemia; HTh = hyperthyroid; IM = intramuscular; Inflam = inflammation; IV = intravenous; LD = liver disease; LTh = hypothyroid; MAO = monoamine oxidase; MI = myocardial infarction; NAT = N-acetyltransferase; Neo = neonate; NIDDM = non-insulin-dependent diabetes mellitus; NS = nephrotic syndrome; Obes = obese; Pneu = pneumonia; Preg = pregnant; Prem = premature; RA = rheumatoid arthritis; RD = renal disease (including uremia); SC = subcutaneous; Smk = smoking; ST = sulfotransferase; T_{max} = peak time; Tach = ventricular tachycardia; UGT = UDP-glucuronosyl transferase; Ulcer = ulcer patients. Other abbreviations are defined in the text section of this appendix.

Table A–II–1
PHARMACOKINETIC DATA (Continued)

AVAILABILITY (ORAL) (%)	URINARY EXCRETION (%)	BOUND IN PLASMA (%)	CLEARANCE ($ml \cdot min^{-1} \cdot kg^{-1}$)	VOL. DIST. (liters/kg)	HALF-LIFE (hours)	PEAK TIME (hours)	PEAK CONCENTRATIONS

DOXEPIN[a] (Chapter 19)

AVAILABILITY (ORAL) (%)	URINARY EXCRETION (%)	BOUND IN PLASMA (%)	CLEARANCE	VOL. DIST.	HALF-LIFE	PEAK TIME	PEAK CONCENTRATIONS
30 ± 10^b	~0	82 (75–89)	14 ± 3^c	$24 \pm 7^{c,d}$	18 ± 5	D: 0.5–1[e] DD: 4–12[e]	D: 28 ± 11 ng/ml[e] DD: 39 ± 19 ng/ml[e]

Reference: Faulkner, R.D., Pitts, W.M., Lee, C.S., Lewis, W.A., and Fann, W.E. Multiple-dose doxepin kinetics in depressed patients. *Clin. Pharmacol. Ther.*, **1983**, *34*:509–515.

[a]Active metabolite, desmethyldoxepin (DD), has a longer half-life (37 ± 15 hours).
[b]Calculated from results of oral administration only, assuming complete absorption, elimination by the liver, hepatic blood flow of 1.5 l/min, and equal partition between plasma and erythrocytes.
[c]Calculated assuming $F = 0.30$.
[d]V_{area} reported.
[e]Data for trough concentrations of doxepin (D) and desmethyldoxepin following a 150-mg oral dose, given once daily for 3 weeks to patients with depression. Peak/trough ratio <2.

DOXORUBICIN[a] (Chapter 52)

AVAILABILITY (ORAL) (%)	URINARY EXCRETION (%)	BOUND IN PLASMA (%)	CLEARANCE	VOL. DIST.	HALF-LIFE	PEAK TIME	PEAK CONCENTRATIONS
5	<7	76	666 ± 339 ml · min^{-1} · (m^2)$^{-1}$ ↑ Child ↓ Cirr, Obes	682 ± 433 l/m^2 ↔ Cirr	26 ± 17^b ↔ RD ↑ Cirr	—	High Dose[c] D: ~950 ng/ml DL: 30–1008 ng/ml Low Dose[c] D: 6.0 ± 3.2 ng/ml DL: 5.0 ± 3.5 ng/ml

References: Ackland, S.P., Ratain, M.J., Vogelzang, N.J., Choi, K.E., Ruane, M., and Sinkule, J.A. Pharmacokinetics and pharmacodynamics of long-term continuous-infusion doxorubicin. *Clin. Pharmacol. Ther.*, **1989**, *45*:340–347.
Piscitelli, S.C., Rodvold, K.A., Rushing, D.A., and Tewksbury, D.A. Pharmacokinetics and pharmacodynamics of doxorubicin in patients with small cell lung cancer. *Clin. Pharmacol. Ther.*, **1993**, *53*:555–561.

[a]Active metabolites; $t_{1/2}$ for doxorubicinol is 29 ± 16 hours.
[b]Prolonged when plasma bilirubin concentration is elevated; undergoes biliary excretion.
[c]Mean data for doxorubicin (D) and range of data for doxorubicinol (DL), following a single 45–72-mg/m^2 high-dose 1-hour IV infusion, given to patients with small cell lung cancer. Data following a low-dose continuous IV infusion at a rate of 3.9 ± 0.65 mg/m^2 per day for 12.4 (2 to 50) weeks to patients with advanced cancer also are presented.

DOXYCYCLINE (Chapter 47)

AVAILABILITY (ORAL) (%)	URINARY EXCRETION (%)	BOUND IN PLASMA (%)	CLEARANCE	VOL. DIST.	HALF-LIFE	PEAK TIME	PEAK CONCENTRATIONS
93	41 ± 19	88 ± 5 ↓ RD[a]	0.53 ± 0.18 ↓ HL, Aged ↔ RD	0.75 ± 0.32 ↓ HL, Aged	16 ± 6 ↔ RD, HL, Aged	Oral: 1–2[b]	IV: 2.8 μg/ml[b] Oral: 1.7–2 μg/ml[b]

Reference: Saivin, S., and Houin, G. Clinical pharmacokinetics of doxycycline and minocycline. *Clin. Pharmacokinet.*, **1988**, *15*:355–366.

[a]Changes in plasma protein binding and erythrocyte partitioning yield a decrease from 88 ± 5 to $71 \pm 3\%$ in patients with uremia.
[b]Mean data following a single 100-mg IV dose (1-hour infusion), or range of mean data following a 100-mg oral dose given to adults.

EFAVIRENZ[a] (Chapter 51)

AVAILABILITY (ORAL) (%)	URINARY EXCRETION (%)	BOUND IN PLASMA (%)	CLEARANCE	VOL. DIST.	HALF-LIFE	PEAK TIME	PEAK CONCENTRATIONS
—[a] ↑ Food	<1	99.5–99.75	3.1 ± 1.2^b ↔ Child[c]	—	SD: 52–76[b] MD: 40–55[b]	4.1 ± 1.7^d	4.0 ± 1.7 μg/ml[d]

References: Adkins, J.C., and Noble, S. Efavirenz. *Drugs*, **1998**, *56*:1055–1064.
Physicians' Desk Reference, 54th ed. Medical Economics Co, Montvale, NJ, **2000**, p. 981.
Villani, P., Regazzi, M.B., Castelli, F., Viale, P., Torti, C., Seminari, E., and Maserati, R. Pharmacokinetics of efavirenz (EFV) alone and in combination therapy with nelfinavir (NFV) in HIV-1-infected patients. *Br. J. Clin. Pharmacol.*, **1999**, *48*:712–715.

[a]Data from patients with HIV infection. No significant gender differences. Metabolized primarily by CYP3A4. Absolute oral bioavailability is unknown. Oral AUC increased 50% by high-fat meal.
[b]CL/F and $t_{1/2}$ reported for oral dose. Efavirenz is a weak inducer of CYP3A4 and its own metabolism.
[c]3 to 16 years of age, no difference in weight-adjusted CL/F compared to adult.
[d]Following 600-mg oral dose daily to steady state.

ENALAPRIL[a] (Chapters 31, 32, 33)

41 ± 15 ↓ Cirr	88 ± 7[b] ↓ Cirr	50–60	4.9 ± 1.5[c] ↓ RD, Aged, CHF, Neo ↑ Child ↔ Fem	1.7 ± 0.7[c]	11[d] ↑ RD, Cirr	3.0 ± 1.6[e]	69 ± 37 ng/ml[e]

[a] Hydrolyzed by esterases to active metabolite, enalaprilic acid (enalaprilat); pharmacokinetic values and disease comparisons are for enalaprilat, following oral enalapril administration.

[b] For intravenous enalaprilat.

[c] CL/F and V_{ss}/F after multiple oral doses of enalapril. Values after single IV dose of enalaprilat are misleading, since binding to converting enzyme leads to a prolonged half-life, which does not represent a significant fraction of the clearance upon multiple dosing.

[d] Estimated from the approach to steady state during multiple dosing.

[e] Mean values for enalaprilat following a 10-mg oral dose, given daily for 8 days to healthy young adults. The EC_{50} for ACE inhibition is 5–20 ng/ml enalaprilat.

References: Lees, K.R., and Reid, J.L. Age and the pharmacokinetics and pharmacodynamics of chronic enalapril treatment. *Clin. Pharmacol. Ther.*, **1987**, 41:597–602.
MacFadyen, R.J., Meredith, P.A., and Elliott, H.L. Enalapril clinical pharmacokinetics and pharmacokinetic-pharmacodynamic relationships. An overview. *Clin. Pharmacokinet.*, **1993**, 25:274–282.

ENOXAPARIN[a] (Chapter 55)

SC: 92	b	—	0.3 ± 0.1[c] ↓ RD	0.12 ± 0.04[c] ←→ RD	3.8 ± 1.3[d] ↑ RD	3[e]	ACLM: 145 ± 45 ng/ml[e] BCLM: 414 ± 87 ng/ml[e]

[a] Enoxaparin consists of low-molecular-weight heparin fragments of varying lengths.

[b] 43% is recovered in urine when administered as ^{99}Tc-labeled enoxaparin; 8% to 20% anti-Factor Xa activity.

[c] F, CL/F and V_{area}/F for subcutaneous dose measured by functional assay for anti-Factor Xa activity.

[d] Measured by functional assay of anti-Factor Xa activity. Using anti-IIa activity or displacement binding assay gives a half-life of approximately 1 to 2 hours.

[e] Following a single 40-mg subcutaneous dose to healthy adult subjects. High affinity antithrombin III molecules: ACLM, above critical length molecules (anti-Factor Xa and IIa activity); BCLM, below critical length molecules (anti-Factor Xa activity).

References: Bendetowicz, A.V., Beguin, S., Caplain, H., and Hemker, H.C. Pharmacokinetics and pharmacodynamics of a low molecular weight heparin (enoxaparin) after subcutaneous injection, comparison with unfractionated heparin—a three way cross over study in human volunteers. *Thromb. Haemost.*, **1994**, 71:305–313.
Physicians' Desk Reference, 54th ed. Medical Economics Co., Montvale, NJ, **2000**, p. 2561.

ENTACAPONE[a] (Chapter 22)

42 ± 9[b] ↑ LD	Negligible	98	10.3 ± 1.74 ←→ RD, LD	0.40 ± 0.16	0.28 ± 0.06[d]	0.8 ± 0.2[e]	4.3 ± 2.0 µg/ml[e]

[a] Data from healthy male subjects. Eliminated primarily by biliary excretion.

[b] The bioavailability of entacapone appears to be dose dependent (increases from 29% to 46% over a 50- to 800-mg dose range).

[c] Increased bioavailability, moderate hepatic impairment with cirrhosis.

[d] Value represents the half-life for the initial distribution phase during which 90% of a dose is eliminated. The terminal half-life is 2.9 ± 2.0 hours.

[e] Following a single 400-mg oral dose. No accumulation with multiple dosing.

References: Holm, K.J., and Spencer, C.M. Entacapone. A review of its use in Parkinson's disease. *Drugs*, **1999**, 58:159–177.
Keranen, T., Gordin, A., Karlsson, M., Korpela, K., Pentikainen, P.J., Rita, H., Schultz, E., Seppala, L., and Wikberg, T. Inhibition of soluble catechol-O-methyltransferase and single-dose pharmacokinetics after oral and intravenous administration of entacapone. *Eur. J. Clin. Pharmacol.*, **1994**, 46:151–157.

Key: Unless otherwise indicated by a specific footnote, the data are presented for the study population as a mean value ± 1 standard deviation, a mean and range (lowest-highest in parenthesis) of values, a range of the lowest-highest values, or a single mean value.

ADH = alcohol dehydrogenase; Aged = aged; AIDS = acquired immunodeficiency syndrome; Alb = hypoalbuminemia; AVH = acute viral hepatitis; Atr Fib = atrial fibrillation; Burn = burn patients; C_{max} = peak concentration; CAD = coronary artery disease; Celiac = celiac disease; CF = cystic fibrosis; CHF = congestive heart failure; Child = children; Cirr = hepatic cirrhosis; COPD = chronic obstructive pulmonary disease; CP = cor pulmonale; CPBS = cardiopulmonary bypass surgery; CRI = chronic respiratory insufficiency; Crohn = Crohn's disease; Cush = Cushing's syndrome; CYP = cytochrome P450; Fem = female; Hep = hepatitis; HIV = human immunodeficiency virus; HL = hyperlipoproteinemia; HTh = hyperthyroid; IM = intramuscular; Inflam = inflammation; IV = intravenous; LD = liver disease; LTh = hypothyroid; MAO = monoamine oxidase; MI = myocardial infarction; NAT = N-acetyltransferase; Neo = neonate; NIDDM = non-insulin-dependent diabetes mellitus; NS = nephrotic syndrome; Obes = obese; Pneu = pneumonia; Preg = pregnant; Prem = premature; RA = rheumatoid arthritis; RD = renal disease (including uremia); SC = subcutaneous; Smk = smoking; ST = sulfotransferase; T_{max} = peak time; Tach = ventricular tachycardia; UGT = UDP-glucuronosyl transferase; Ulcer = ulcer patients. Other abbreviations are defined in the text section of this appendix.

Table A–II–1
PHARMACOKINETIC DATA (Continued)

AVAILABILITY (ORAL) (%)	URINARY EXCRETION (%)	BOUND IN PLASMA (%)	CLEARANCE $(ml \cdot min^{-1} \cdot kg^{-1})$	VOL. DIST. (liters/kg)	HALF-LIFE (hours)	PEAK TIME (hours)	PEAK CONCENTRATIONS
EPIRUBICIN[a] (Chapter 52)							
—	6.4 ± 3.3	77	43 ± 14 l·h⁻¹·(m²)⁻¹ [29–95 l·h⁻¹·(m²)⁻¹] $\downarrow$ LD[b]	1272 ± 359 l/m² (592–2964 l/m²)	31.2 ± 9.4 (13.9–44.8) $\uparrow$ LD[b]	—	1.5–1.8 μg/ml[c]

[a]Data from patients treated for solid tumors; IV administration. Shown in parenthesis are mean results from 12 different IV bolus dose (30–120 mg/m²) studies. Epirubicinol is an active metabolite observed at concentrations below that of parent drug.
[b]CL reduced in patients with hepatic impairment (LD: elevated ALT and bilirubin).
[c]Mean C_{max} following a single 50-mg/m² IV bolus (1 to 2 min) dose.

References: Camaggi, C.M., Comparsi, R., Strocchi, E., Testoni, F., Angelelli, B., and Pannuti, F. Epirubicin and doxorubicin comparative metabolism and pharmacokinetics. A cross-over study. *Cancer Chemother. Pharmacol.,* **1988,** *21:*221–228.
Robert, J. Clinical pharmacokinetics of epirubicin. *Clin. Pharmacokinet.,* **1994,** *26:*428–438.
Twelves, C.J., Dobbs, N.A., Michael, Y., Summers, L.A., Gregory, W., Harper, P.G., Rubens, R.D., and Richards, M.A. Clinical pharmacokinetics of epirubicin: the importance of liver biochemistry tests. *Br. J. Cancer,* **1992,** *66:*765–769.

AVAILABILITY (ORAL) (%)	URINARY EXCRETION (%)	BOUND IN PLASMA (%)	CLEARANCE	VOL. DIST.	HALF-LIFE	PEAK TIME	PEAK CONCENTRATIONS
EPOETIN ALFA[a] (Chapter 54)							
SC: 22 (11–36) IP: 3 (1–7)	<3	—	0.047 ± 0.017 (0.047–0.092) $\longleftrightarrow$ RD	0.033 ± 0.013 (0.033–0.075)	8.2 ± 1.3 (4–11.2)	SC: 18[b] IP: 12[b]	SC: 176 ± 75 U/l[b] IP: 375 ± 123 U/l[b]

[a]Data from male and female patients receiving continuous ambulatory peritoneal dialysis. Shown in parenthesis are mean results from four different IV dosing studies.
[b]Following a single 120-U/kg subcutaneous (SC) dose or a 50,000-U intraperitoneal (IP) dose; 1.5- to 2-liter volume and 8-hour dwell time in patients receiving continuous ambulatory peritoneal dialysis.

Reference: Macdougall, I.C., Roberts, D.E., Coles, G.A., and Williams, J.D. Clinical pharmacokinetics of epoetin (recombinant human erythropoietin). *Clin. Pharmacokinet.,* **1991,** *20:*99–113.

AVAILABILITY (ORAL) (%)	URINARY EXCRETION (%)	BOUND IN PLASMA (%)	CLEARANCE	VOL. DIST.	HALF-LIFE	PEAK TIME	PEAK CONCENTRATIONS
ERYTHROMYCIN (Chapter 47)							
35 ± 25[a] $\downarrow$ Preg[b]	12 ± 7	84 ± 3[c] $\longleftrightarrow$ RD	9.1 ± 4.1[d] $\longleftrightarrow$ RD	0.78 ± 0.44 $\uparrow$ RD	1.6 ± 0.7 $\uparrow$ Cirr $\longleftrightarrow$ RD	B: $2.1–3.9$[e] S: $2–3$[e]	B: $0.9–3.5$ μg/ml[e] S: $0.5–1.4$ μg/ml[e]

[a]Value for enteric-coated erythromycin base.
[b]Decreased concentrations in pregnancy possibly due to decreased bioavailability (or to increased clearance).
[c]Erythromycin base.
[d]Erythromycin is a CYP3A substrate; *N*-demethylation. It is also transported by P-glycoprotein, which may contribute to biliary excretion of parent drug and metabolites.
[e]Range of mean values from studies following a 250-mg oral enteric-coated free base in a capsule (B), given four times a day for 5 to 13 doses, or a 250-mg film-coated tablet or capsule of erythromycin stearate (S), given four times a day for 5 to 12 doses.

Reference: Periti, P., Mazzei, T., Mini, E., and Novelli, A. Clinical pharmacokinetic properties of the macrolide antibiotics. Effects of age and various pathophysiological states (Part I). *Clin. Pharmacokinet.,* **1989,** *16:*193–214.

AVAILABILITY (ORAL) (%)	URINARY EXCRETION (%)	BOUND IN PLASMA (%)	CLEARANCE	VOL. DIST.	HALF-LIFE	PEAK TIME	PEAK CONCENTRATIONS
ESMOLOL (Chapters 10, 35)							
—	<1	55	170 ± 70[a] $\longleftrightarrow$ RD, Cirr $\downarrow$ CAD $\uparrow$ Child	1.9 ± 1.3[b] $\longleftrightarrow$ RD, Cirr, Child $\downarrow$ CAD	0.13 ± 0.07 $\longleftrightarrow$ RD, Cirr, CAD $\downarrow$ Child	—	2.5 ± 0.7 μg/ml[c]

[a]Esmolol is rapidly hydrolyzed by red blood cell esterases to an inactive acid metabolite.
[b]V_{area} reported.
[c]Steady-state concentration following a 300-μg/kg per minute IV infusion in patients undergoing coronary artery bypass surgery.

Reference: Wiest, D. Esmolol. A review of its therapeutic efficacy and pharmacokinetic characteristics. *Clin. Pharmacokinet.,* **1995,** *28:*190–202.

ETANERCEPT[a] (Chapter 53)

SC: 58	Negligible	0.02	—	~0.11[b]	IV: 72 SC-SD: 92[c]	— SC-SD: 72 (48–96)[c]	IV: 2.32 μg/ml[c] SC-SD: 1.2 μg/ml[c] SC-MD: 3 μg/ml[c]

[a] Data from healthy adult subjects. No significant gender differences in weight-normalized kinetics. Etanercept is a recombinant human fusion protein—TNF receptor and Fc portion of IgG$_1$.

[b] The volume of distribution (V_{area}) was estimated from reported clearance and half-life values.

[c] Following a single 10-mg IV dose and single (SC-SD) or multiple (SC-MD) subcutaneous doses, 25 mg, twice weekly for 6 months.

References: Goldenberg, M.M. Etanercept, a novel drug for the treatment of patients with severe, active rheumatoid arthritis. *Clin. Ther.,* **1999,** *21:*75–87.

Moreland, L.W., Margolies, G., Heck, L.W. Jr., Saway, A., Blosch, C., Hanna, R., and Koopman, W.J. Recombinant soluble tumor necrosis factor receptor (p80) fusion protein: toxicity and dose finding trial in refractory rheumatoid arthritis. *J. Rheumatol.,* **1996,** *23:*1849–1855.

Physicians' Desk Reference, 54th ed. Medical Economics Co., Montvale, NJ, **2000,** p. 1414.

ETHAMBUTOL (Chapter 48)

77 ± 8	79 ± 3	6–30	—	1.6 ± 0.2	3.1 ± 0.4 ↑ RD	2–4[a]	2–5 μg/ml[a]

[a] Following a single 800-mg oral dose to healthy subjects. Concentrations >10 μg/ml can adversely affect vision. No accumulation with once-a-day dosing in patients with normal renal function.

Reference: Holdiness, M.R. Clinical pharmacokinetics of the antituberculosis drugs. *Clin. Pharmacokinet.,* **1984,** *9:*511–544.

ETHANOL (Chapter 18)

80[a]	<3	—	V_{max} = 124 ± 10[b] mg·kg^{-1}·h^{-1} K_m = 82 ± 29 μg/ml[b] CL ↑ Smk	0.54 ± 0.05 ↓ Aged, Fem	0.24 ± 0.08[b]	0.5–1.6[c]	M: 650 μg/ml[c] F: 761 μg/ml[c]

[a] Bioavailability predicted for an 11.25-g dose absorbed over 20 minutes; F increases with increasing dose.

[b] Ethanol is eliminated primarily by a saturable (Michaelis-Menten) process involving alcohol dehydrogenase. CL and $t_{1/2}$ decrease and increase, respectively, with increasing dose; the half-life value presented is the fastest possible—the theoretical value at near zero concentration. CYP2E1 also contributes to ethanol clearance, particularly in chronic alcoholics.

[c] Mean C_{max} following a single 35-g oral dose given to male (M) and female (F) subjects. Range of mean T_{max} values following a single 35- to 88-g oral dose.

Reference: Holford, N.H. Clinical pharmacokinetics of ethanol. *Clin. Pharmacokinet.,* **1987,** *13:*273–292.

Key: Unless otherwise indicated by a specific footnote, the data are presented for the study population as a mean value ± 1 standard deviation, a mean and range (lowest–highest in parenthesis) of values, a range of the lowest–highest values, or a single mean value.

ADH = alcohol dehydrogenase; Aged = aged; AIDS = acquired immunodeficiency syndrome; Alb = hypoalbuminemia; Atr Fib = atrial fibrillation; AVH = acute viral hepatitis; Burn = burn patients; C_{max} = peak concentration; CAD = coronary artery disease; Celiac = celiac disease; CF = cystic fibrosis; CHF = congestive heart failure; Child = children; Cirr = hepatic cirrhosis; COPD = chronic obstructive pulmonary disease; CP = cor pulmonale; CPBS = cardiopulmonary bypass surgery; CRI = chronic respiratory insufficiency; Crohn = Crohn's disease; Cush = Cushing's syndrome; CYP = cytochrome P450; Fem = female; Hep = hepatitis; HIV = human immunodeficiency virus; HL = hyperlipoproteinemia; HTh = hyperthyroid; IM = intramuscular; Inflam = inflammation; IV = intravenous; LD = liver disease; LTh = hypothyroid; MAO = monoamine oxidase; MI = myocardial infarction; NAT = N-acetyltransferase; Neo = neonate; NIDDM = non-insulin-dependent diabetes mellitus; NS = nephrotic syndrome; Obes = obese; Pneu = pneumonia; Preg = pregnant; Prem = premature; RA = rheumatoid arthritis; RD = renal disease (including uremia); SC = subcutaneous; Smk = smoking; ST = sulfotransferase; T_{max} = peak time; Tach = ventricular tachycardia; UGT = UDP-glucuronosyl transferase; Ulcer = ulcer patients. Other abbreviations are defined in the text section of this appendix.

Table A–II–1
PHARMACOKINETIC DATA (*Continued*)

AVAILABILITY (ORAL) (%)	URINARY EXCRETION (%)	BOUND IN PLASMA (%)	CLEARANCE ($ml \cdot min^{-1} \cdot kg^{-1}$)	VOL. DIST. (*liters/kg*)	HALF-LIFE (*hours*)	PEAK TIME (*hours*)	PEAK CONCENTRATIONS

ETHOSUXIMIDE (Chapter 21)

| — | 25 ± 15 | 0 | $0.19 \pm 0.04^{a,b}$ ↑ Child | 0.72 ± 0.16^a ⟷ Child | 45 ± 8^a ↓ Child ⟷ Neo | 1.5 ± 0.8^c | 33.7 ± 9.4 $\mu g/ml^c$ |

[a]Data from oral, multiple-dose regimen; values are CL/F and V_{area}/F.
[b]CL/F decreases 15% from single dose to multiple dose, and may be nonlinear with increasing dose.
[c]Following a 250-mg oral dose given twice a day for 10 days to healthy adults.

Reference: Bauer, L.A., Harris, C., Wilensky, A.J., Raisys, V.A., and Levy, R.H. Ethosuximide kinetics: possible interaction with valproic acid. *Clin. Pharmacol. Ther.,* **1982,** *31:*741–745.

ETOPOSIDE (Chapter 52)

| 52 ± 17^a | 35 ± 5 | 96 ± 0.4^b ↓ Alb | 0.68 ± 0.23^c ⟷ Child, Cirr ↓ RD | 0.36 ± 0.15 ⟷ Child, Cirr | 8.1 ± 4.3 ↑ RD ⟷ Child, Cirr | 1.3 | NT: 2.7 $\mu g/ml^d$ T: 4.7 $\mu g/ml^d$ |

[a]Decreases at oral doses greater than 200 mg.
[b]Decreases with hyperbilirubinemia.
[c]Metabolized by CYP3A; also a substrate for P-glycoprotein.
[d]Mean C_{max} for patients without (NT) and with (T) serious hematological toxicity following a 75 to 200-mg/m² dose given as a 72-hour continuous IV infusion.

References: Clark, P.I., and Slevin, M.L. The clinical pharmacology of etoposide and teniposide. *Clin. Pharmacokinet.,* **1987,** *12:*223–252.
McLeod, H.L., and Evans, W.E. Clinical pharmacokinetics and pharmacodynamics of epipodophyllotoxins. *Cancer Surv.,* **1993,** *17:*253–268.

EXEMESTANE[a] (Chapters 52, 58)

| —[a] | — | — | 145^c | — | 24 | 1–2 | SD: 17.7 ng/ml^d MD: 11.0 ng/ml^d |
| ↑ Food[b] | | | | | | | |

[a]Data from healthy postmenopausal women. Exemestane is rapidly metabolized, undergoing extensive first-pass elimination. Absolute bioavailability is unknown.
[b]Food enhances the oral AUC by 40%.
[c]CL/F reported.
[d]Mean value following a single 25-mg oral dose (SD) taken after a meal, or 10 mg once a day to steady state (MD).

Reference: Scott, L.J., and Wiseman, L.R. Exemestane. *Drugs,* **1999,** 58:675–680; discussion 681–682.

FELBAMATE (Chapter 21)

| >80[a] | 40–50[b] | 22–25 | 0.50 ± 0.13^c ⟷ Fem ↓ RD | 0.76 ± 0.08^c | 21 ± 2 ↑ RD | 1–4[d] | 32 $\mu g/ml^d$ |

[a]Absolute bioavailability is unknown; estimate based on urine recovery of a radioactive dose and a low value for CL/F.
[b]Following oral dosing.
[c]CL/F and V_{area}/F reported.
[d]Mean C_{max} and range T_{max} following a 600-mg oral dose, given twice a day to steady state to healthy adult subjects.

Reference: Bialer, M. Comparative pharmacokinetics of the newer antiepileptic drugs. *Clin. Pharmacokinet.,* **1993,** *24:*441–452.

FELODIPINE[a] (Chapters 32, 34)

15 ± 8 ←→ Aged, Cirr ↑ Food	<1	12 ± 5[c] ↓ Aged, Cirr, CHF[d]	99.6 ± 0.2[b] ↓ RD, Cirr ←→ Aged	10 ± 3 ←→ Aged ↓ Cirr	14 ± 4 ↑ Aged, CHF[d] ←→ Cirr	IR: 0.9 ± 0.4[e] ER: 3.7 ± 0.9[e]	IR: 34 ± 26 nM[e] ER: 9.1 ± 7.3 nM[e]

[a] Racemic mixture; S-(−)-enantiomer is active Ca^{+2} channel blocker; differential enantiomer pharmacokinetics result in S-(−)-enantiomer concentrations about twofold higher than those of R-(+)-isomer.

[b] Blood-to-plasma concentration ratio = 1.45.

[c] Undergoes significant CYP3A-dependent first-pass metabolism in the intestine and liver.

[d] May be age-related rather than CHF-related.

[e] Following a 10-mg oral immediate-release (IR) or extended-release (ER) tablet, given twice a day to steady state to healthy subjects. EC_{50} for diastolic pressure decrease is 8 ± 5 nM in patients with hypertension.

Reference: Dunselman, P.H., and Edgar, B. Felodipine clinical pharmacokinetics. *Clin. Pharmacokinet.,* 1991, 21:418–430.

FENTANYL (Chapters 14, 23)

TM: ~50	8	84 ± 2[a]	13 ± 2[b] ↓ Aged ←→ Neo	4.0 ± 0.4	3.7 ± 0.4 ↑ CPBS, Aged, Prem ←→ Child	TD: 35 ± 15[c] TM: 0.4 (0.3–6)[c]	TD: 1.4 ± 0.5 ng/ml[c] TM: 0.8 ± 0.3 ng/ml[c]

[a] Blood-to-plasma concentration ratio = 0.97 ± 0.06.

[b] Metabolically cleared primarily by CYP3A to norfentanyl and hydroxy metabolites.

[c] Following a 5-mg transdermal (TD) dose administered at 50 μg/hr through a DURAGESIC system, or a single 400-μg transmucosal (TM) dose. Postoperative and intraoperative analgesia occurs at plasma concentrations of 1 ng/ml and 3 ng/ml, respectively. Respiratory depression occurs above 0.7 ng/ml.

References: Olkkola, K.T., Hamunen, K., and Maunuksela, E.L. Clinical pharmacokinetics and pharmacodynamics of opioid analgesics in infants and children. *Clin. Pharmacokinet.,* 1995, 28:385–404.

Physicians' Desk Reference, 54th ed. Medical Economics Co., Montvale, NJ, 2000, pp. 405 and 1445.

FEXOFENADINE[a] (Chapter 25)

___[a]	12	60–70	9.4 ± 4.2[b]	—	14 ± 6[b] ↑ RD[c] ←→ LD	1.3 ± 0.6[d]	286 ± 143 ng/ml[d]

[a] Data from healthy adult male subjects. Absolute bioavailability is unknown. Negligible metabolism with 85% of a dose recovered in feces unchanged; a substrate for hepatic and intestinal P-glycoprotein efflux transporter.

[b] CL/F and $t_{1/2}$ reported for oral dose.

[c] Mild to severe renal impairment.

[d] Following a 60-mg oral dose twice a day to steady state.

References: Markham, A., and Wagstaff, A.J. Fexofenadine. *Drugs,* 1998, 55:269–274; discussion 275–276.

Robbins, D.K., Castles, M.A., Pack, D.J., Bhargava, V.O., and Weir, S.J. Dose proportionality and comparison of single and multiple dose pharmacokinetics of fexofenadine (MDL 16455) and its enantiomers in healthy male volunteers. *Biopharm. Drug Dispos.,* 1998, 19:455–463.

Key: Unless otherwise indicated by a specific footnote, the data are presented for the study population as a mean value ± 1 standard deviation, a mean and range (lowest-highest in parenthesis) of values, a range of the lowest-highest values, or a single mean value.

ADH = alcohol dehydrogenase; Aged = aged; AIDS = acquired immunodeficiency syndrome; Alb = hypoalbuminemia; Atr Fib = atrial fibrillation; AVH = acute viral hepatitis; Burn = burn patients; C_{max} = peak concentration; CAD = coronary artery disease; Celiac = celiac disease; CF = cystic fibrosis; CHF = congestive heart failure; Child = children; Cirr = hepatic cirrhosis; COPD = chronic obstructive pulmonary disease; CP = cor pulmonale; CPBS = cardiopulmonary bypass surgery; CRI = chronic respiratory insufficiency; Crohn = Crohn's disease; Cush = Cushing's syndrome; CYP = cytochrome P450; Fem = female; Hep = hepatitis; HIV = human immunodeficiency virus; HL = hyperlipoproteinemia; HTh = hyperthyroid; IM = intramuscular; Inflam = inflammation; IV = intravenous; LD = liver disease; LTh = hypothyroid; MAO = monoamine oxidase; MI = myocardial infarction; NAT = N-acetyltransferase; Neo = neonate; NIDDM = non-insulin-dependent diabetes mellitus; NS = nephrotic syndrome; Obes = obese; Pneu = pneumonia; Preg = pregnant; Prem = premature; RA = rheumatoid arthritis; RD = renal disease (including uremia); SC = subcutaneous; Smk = smoking; ST = sulfotransferase; T_{max} = peak time; Tach = ventricular tachycardia; UGT = UDP-glucuronosyl transferase; Ulcer = ulcer patients. Other abbreviations are defined in the text section of this appendix.

Table A–II-1
PHARMACOKINETIC DATA (Continued)

AVAILABILITY (ORAL) (%)	URINARY EXCRETION (%)	BOUND IN PLASMA (%)	CLEARANCE ($ml \cdot min^{-1} \cdot kg^{-1}$)	VOL. DIST. (liters/kg)	HALF-LIFE (hours)	PEAK TIME (hours)	PEAK CONCENTRATIONS
FILGRASTIM[a] (Chapter 54)							
SC: 49 ± 9	—	—	0.5–0.7[b]	0.15	3.4–4.7 ↑ RD[c]	SC: 4–5.8[d]	SC: 4 and 49 ng/ml[d]
FINASTERIDE (Chapter 59)							
63 ± 21	<1	90	2.3 ± 0.8[a] ←→ RD, Aged	1.1 ± 0.2[a]	7.9 ± 2.5 ←→ RD, Aged	1–2[b]	37 (27–49) ng/ml[b]
FLECAINIDE[a] (Chapter 35)							
70 ± 11	43 ± 3	61 ± 10 ↓ MI	5.6 ± 1.3[b] ↓ RD, Cirr, CHF ↑ Child	4.9 ± 0.4[c] ↑ Cirr	11 ± 3[b] ↑ RD, Cirr, CHF ↓ Child	~3 (1–6)[d]	458 ± 100 ng/ml[d]
FLUCONAZOLE (Chapter 49)							
>90	75 ± 9	11 ± 1	0.27 ± 0.07 ←→ AIDS, Neo ↓ RD, Prem	0.60 ± 0.11 ←→ RD ↑ Prem, Neo	32 ± 5 ↑ Cirr, RD, Prem ↓ Child	1.7–4.3[a]	10.6 ± 0.4 μg/ml[a]

FILGRASTIM

[a]Data from male and female healthy adults and patients with cancer. Filgrastim is a recombinant form of human granulocyte colony-stimulating factor (G-CSF) (an extra methionine residue and nonglycosylated). Parenteral administration.

[b]CL reported for single dose at or below 4 μg/kg. CL increases with dose (>4 μg/kg) and with time (up to 10-fold) as absolute neutrophil count increases. Kinetic parameters (CL/F and $t_{1/2}$) for children (1 to 9 years) after a subcutaneous dose are similar to those for adults.

[c]End-stage renal disease.

[d]Following a single subcutaneous dose of 3.4 and 12 μg/kg. C_{max} decreases with multiple dosing.

References: Borleffs, J.C., Bosschaert, M., Vrehen, H.M., Schneider, M.M., van Strijp, J., Small, M.K., and Borkett, K.M. Effect of escalating doses of recombinant human granulocyte colony-stimulating factor (filgrastim) on circulating neutrophils in healthy subjects. *Clin. Ther.,* **1998,** 20:722–736.

Physicians' Desk Reference, 54th ed. Medical Economics Co., Montvale, NJ, **2000,** pp. 528–533.

Stute, N., Santana, V.M., Rodman, J.H., Schell, M.J., Ihle, J.N., and Evans, W.E. Pharmacokinetics of subcutaneous recombinant human granulocyte colony-stimulating factor in children. *Blood,* **1992,** 79:2849–2854.

Sugiura, M., Yamamoto, K., Sawada, Y., and Iga, T. Pharmacokinetic/pharmacodynamic analysis of neutrophil proliferation induced by recombinant human granulocyte colony-stimulating factor (rhG-CSF): comparison between intravenous and subcutaneous administration. *Biol. Pharm. Bull.,* **1997,** 20:684–689.

FINASTERIDE

[a]Calculated assuming a 70-kg body weight.

[b]Mean (range) for C_{max} following a single 5-mg oral dose given to healthy adults. Drug accumulates <twofold with once daily dosing.

Reference: Sudduth, S.L., and Koronkowski, M.J. Finasteride: the first 5α-reductase inhibitor. *Pharmacotherapy,* **1993,** 13:309–325; discussion 325–329.

FLECAINIDE

[a]Racemic mixture; enantiomers exert similar electrophysiological effects.

[b]Metabolized by CYP2D6 (polymorphic); except for a shortened elimination half-life and nonlinear kinetics in extensive metabolizers, CYP2D6 phenotype had no significant influence on flecainide pharmacokinetics or pharmacodynamics.

[c]V_{area} reported.

[d]Following a 100-mg oral dose given twice a day for 5 days in healthy adults. Similar levels for CYP2D6 extensive and poor metabolizers.

Reference: Funck-Brentano, C., Becquemont, L., Kroemer, H.K., Buhl, K., Knebel, N.G., Eichelbaum, M., and Jaillon, P. Variable disposition kinetics and electrocardiographic effects of flecainide during repeated dosing in humans: contribution of genetic factors, dose-dependent clearance, and interaction with amiodarone. *Clin. Pharmacol. Ther.,* **1994,** 55:256–269.

FLUCONAZOLE

[a]Following a 200-mg oral dose given twice a day for 4 days to healthy adults.

References: Debruyne, D., and Ryckelynck, J.P. Clinical pharmacokinetics of fluconazole. *Clin. Pharmacokinet.,* **1993,** 24:10–27.

Varhe, A., Olkkola, K.T., and Neuvonen, P.J. Effect of fluconazole dose on the extent of fluconazole-triazolam interaction. *Br. J. Clin. Pharmacol.,* **1996,** 42:465–470.

FLUDARABINE[a] (Chapter 52)

24 ± 3	<10	3.7 ± 1.5 ↓ RD	2.4 ± 0.6	10–30	—	0.57 μg/ml[b]

[a]Data from male and female adult cancer patients. IV administration. Fludarabine is rapidly dephosphorylated to 2-fluoro-arabinoside-A (F-ara-A), transported into cells, and phosphorylated to the active triphosphate metabolite. Pharmacokinetics of F-ara-A are reported.

[b]Following a single 25-mg/m² IV dose (30-min infusion); no accumulation after 5 daily doses.

References: Hersh, M.R., Kuhn, J.G., Phillips, J.L., Clark, G., Ludden, T.M., and Von Hoff, D.D. Pharmacokinetic study of fludarabine phosphate (NSC 312887). *Cancer Chemother. Pharmacol.* **1986,** 17:277–280.

Physicians' Desk Reference. 54th ed. Medical Economics Co., Montvale, NJ, **2000,** p. 764.

Plunkett, W., Gandhi, V., Huang, P., Robertson, L.E., Yang, L.Y., Gregoire, V., Estey, E., and Keating, M.J. Fludarabine: pharmacokinetics, mechanisms of action, and rationales for combination therapies. *Semin. Oncol.* **1993,** 20:2–12.

5-FLUOROURACIL (Chapter 52)

28 (0–80)[a]	8–12	16 ± 7	0.25 ± 0.12	11 ± 4 min[b]	—	11.2 μM[c]

[a]Higher F with rapid absorption and lower F with slower absorption, due to a saturable first-pass effect.

[b]A much longer (~20 hours) terminal half-life has been reported representing a slow efflux of drug from tissues.

[c]Steady-state concentration following a continuous IV infusion of 300 to 500 mg/m² per day to cancer patients.

Reference: Diasio, R.B., and Harris, B.E. Clinical pharmacology of 5-fluorouracil. *Clin. Pharmacokinet.* **1989,** 16:215–237.

FLUOXETINE[a] (Chapter 19)

—[a]	<2.5	94 ↔ Cirr, RD	9.6 ± 6.9[b,c] → RD, Aged, Obes ↓ Cirr	35 ± 21[d] ↔ RD, Cirr	53 ± 41[e] ↑ Cirr → RD, Aged, Obes	F: 6–8[f] · F: 200–531 ng/ml[f] NF: 103–465 ng/ml[f]

[a]Active metabolite, norfluoxetine; half-life of norfluoxetine is 6.4 ± 2.5 days (12 ± 2 days in cirrhosis). Absolute bioavailability is unknown, but ≥80% of dose is absorbed.

[b]Reduced CL with repetitive dosing (~2.6 ml·min⁻¹·kg⁻¹) and with increasing dose between 40–80 mg.

[c]CL/F reported; fluoxetine is a CYP2D6 substrate and inhibitor.

[d]V_{area}/F reported.

[e]Longer half-life with repetitive dosing and with increasing doses.

[f]Range of data for fluoxetine (F) and norfluoxetine (NF) following a 60-mg oral dose given daily for 1 week. NF continues to accumulate for several weeks.

Reference: Altamura, A.C., Moro, A.R., and Percudani, M. Clinical pharmacokinetics of fluoxetine. *Clin. Pharmacokinet.* **1994,** 26:201–214.

Key: Unless otherwise indicated by a specific footnote, the data are presented for the study population as a mean value ± 1 standard deviation, a mean and range (lowest-highest in parenthesis) of values, a range of the lowest-highest values, or a single mean value.

ADH = alcohol dehydrogenase; Aged = aged; AIDS = acquired immunodeficiency syndrome; Alb = hypoalbuminemia; Atr Fib = atrial fibrillation; AVH = acute viral hepatitis; Burn = burn patients; C_{max} = peak concentration; CAD = coronary artery disease; Celiac = celiac disease; CF = cystic fibrosis; CHF = congestive heart failure; Child = children; Cirr = hepatic cirrhosis; COPD = chronic obstructive pulmonary disease; CP = cor pulmonale; CPBS = cardiopulmonary bypass surgery; CRI = chronic respiratory insufficiency; Crohn = Crohn's disease; Cush = Cushing's syndrome; CYP = cytochrome P450; Fem = female; Hep = hepatitis; HIV = human immunodeficiency virus; HL = hyperlipoproteinemia; HTh = hyperthyroid; IM = intramuscular; Inflam = inflammation; IV = intravenous; LD = liver disease; LTh = hypothyroid; MAO = monoamine oxidase; MI = myocardial infarction; NAT = *N*-acetyltransferase; Neo = neonate; NIDDM = non-insulin-dependent diabetes mellitus; NS = nephrotic syndrome; Obes = obese; Pneu = pneumonia; Preg = pregnant; Prem = premature; RA = rheumatoid arthritis; RD = renal disease (including uremia); SC = subcutaneous; Smk = smoking; ST = sulfotransferase; T_{max} = peak time; Tach = ventricular tachycardia; UGT = UDP-glucuronosyl transferase; Ulcer = ulcer patients. Other abbreviations are defined in the text section of this appendix.

Table A–II–1
PHARMACOKINETIC DATA (Continued)

AVAILABILITY (ORAL) (%)	URINARY EXCRETION (%)	BOUND IN PLASMA (%)	VOL. DIST. (liters/kg)	CLEARANCE (ml · min⁻¹ · kg⁻¹)	HALF-LIFE (hours)	PEAK TIME (hours)	PEAK CONCENTRATIONS

Note: Units rendered in LaTeX: $ml \cdot min^{-1} \cdot kg^{-1}$

FLUPHENAZINE[a] (Chapter 20)

AVAILABILITY (ORAL) (%)	URINARY EXCRETION (%)	BOUND IN PLASMA (%)	VOL. DIST. (liters/kg)	CLEARANCE	HALF-LIFE (hours)	PEAK TIME (hours)	PEAK CONCENTRATIONS
Oral: 2.7 (1.7–4.5)[b] SC or IM: 3.4 (2.5–5.0)[b]	Negligible	—	11 ± 10	10 ± 7	IV: 12 ± 4[c] IR: 14.4 ± 7.8[c] SR: 20.3 ± 7.9[c]	IR: 2.8 ± 2.1[d] DN: 24–48[d] EN: 48–72[d]	IR: 2.3 ± 2.1 ng/ml[d] DN: 1.3 ng/ml[d] EN: 1.1 ng/ml[d]

References: Jann, M.W., Ereshefsky, L., and Saklad, S.R. Clinical pharmacokinetics of the depot antipsychotics. *Clin. Pharmacokinet.,* **1985,** 10:315–333.
Koytchev, R., Alken, R.G., McKay, G., and Katzarov, T. Absolute bioavailability of oral immediate and slow release fluphenazine in healthy volunteers. *Eur. J. Clin. Pharmacol.,* **1996,** 51:183–187.

[a] Data from healthy male and female subjects. Fluphenazine is extensively metabolized.
[b] Available in immediate-release oral formulation, and depot subcutaneous (SC) or intramuscular (IM) injections as the enanthate or decanoate esters. Geometric mean (90% CI).
[c] Reported half-life for a single IV dose and the apparent half-life following oral administration of immediate- (IR) and slow-release (SR) formulations. The longer apparent half-lives with oral dosing may represent an absorption-limited "flip-flop" effect.
[d] Following a single 12-mg oral dose (IR), or 25-mg decanoate (DN) and enanthate (EN) intramuscular injections.

FLURBIPROFEN[a] (Chapter 27)

AVAILABILITY (ORAL) (%)	URINARY EXCRETION (%)	BOUND IN PLASMA (%)	VOL. DIST. (liters/kg)	CLEARANCE	HALF-LIFE (hours)	PEAK TIME (hours)	PEAK CONCENTRATIONS
~92	2 ± 1	>99.5 ⟷ Aged, Obese ↑ Cirr, RD	0.15 ± 0.02[b] ⟷ Aged ↑ RD	0.35 ± 0.09[b] ⟷ Aged, RA ↑ RD	5.5 ± 1.4 ⟷ Aged, Child, RA, RD	IR: 1.5–2.8[c]	IR: 14–16 μg/ml[c] SR: 6 μg/ml[c]

Reference: Davies, N.M. Clinical pharmacokinetics of flurbiprofen and its enantiomers. *Clin. Pharmacokinet.,* **1995,** 28:100–114.

[a] Racemic mixture; antiinflammatory activity resides with S-(+)-enantiomer; recent studies suggest analgesic activity with both enantiomers; minimal R- to S-enantiomer conversion in humans; S-enantiomer exhibits a slightly higher plasma protein binding, 20% lower clearance, 5% lower volume of distribution, and 18% longer half-life. Formation of major metabolite, 4-hydroxyflurbiprofen, catalyzed by CYP2C9 (polymorphic).
[b] CL/F and V_{ss}/F reported.
[c] Range of values following an oral 100-mg immediate-release (IR) dose, twice a day for 5 to 8 days, or mean C_{max} following an oral 200-mg sustained-release (SR) dose given once a day for 14 days.

FLUTAMIDE[a] (Chapters 52, 59)

AVAILABILITY (ORAL) (%)	URINARY EXCRETION (%)	BOUND IN PLASMA (%)	VOL. DIST. (liters/kg)	CLEARANCE	HALF-LIFE (hours)	PEAK TIME (hours)	PEAK CONCENTRATIONS
—	<1	F: 94–96 HF: 92–94	—	280[b] ⟷ RD	F: 7.8[b] HF: 8.1[b]	F: 1.3 ± 0.7[c] HF: 1.9 ± 0.6[c]	F: 0.11 ± 0.21 μg/ml[c] HF: 1.6 ± 0.59 μg/ml[c]

References: Anjum, S., Swan, S.K., Lambrecht, L.J., Radwanski, E., Cutler, D.L., Affrime, M.B., and Halstenson, C.E. Pharmacokinetics of flutamide in patients with renal insufficiency. *Br. J. Clin. Pharmacol.,* **1999,** 47:43–47.
Physicians' Desk Reference, 54th ed. Medical Economics Co., Montvale, NJ, **2000,** p. 2798.
Radwanski, E., Perentesis, G., Symchowicz, S., and Zampaglione, N. Single and multiple dose pharmacokinetic evaluation of flutamide in normal geriatric volunteers. *J. Clin. Pharmacol.,* **1989,** 29:554–558.

[a] Data obtained primarily from elderly men. Flutamide is metabolized rapidly to a number of metabolites, which are mainly excreted in urine. One major metabolite, 2-hydroxyflutamide, is biologically active (equal potency); formation is catalyzed primarily by CYP1A2.
[b] CL/F and $t_{1/2}$ (terminal) reported for oral dose.
[c] Data for flutamide (F) and 2-hydroxyflutamide (HF) following a 250-mg oral dose, given three times a day to steady state in healthy geriatric males.

FLUVASTATIN[a] (Chapter 36)

29 ± 18	Negligible	99	16.2 ± 2.8 ↓ LD[b]	0.42 ± 0.06	0.7 ± 0.3	1.2 ± 0.9[c]	200 ± 86 ng/ml[c]
→ Aged							

[a]Data from healthy male subjects. No significant gender differences. Extensively metabolized mainly by CYP2C9 (polymorphic); exhibits a saturable first-pass effect at doses >20 mg/day.
[b]CL/F reduced, hepatic cirrhosis.
[c]Following a 20-mg dose, daily, to steady state.

References: Lennernas, H., and Fager, G. Pharmacodynamics and pharmacokinetics of the HMG-CoA reductase inhibitors. Similarities and differences. *Clin. Pharmacokinet.,* **1997,** *32:*403–425.
Physicians' Desk Reference, 54th ed. Medical Economics Co., Montvale, NJ, **2000,** pp. 2021–2022.
Smith, H.T., Jokubaitis, L.A., Troendle, A.J., Hwang, D.S., and Robinson, W.T. Pharmacokinetics of fluvastatin and specific drug interactions. *Am. J. Hypertens.,* **1993,** *6:*375S–382S.
Tse, F.L., Nickerson, D.F., and Yardley, W.S. Binding of fluvastatin to blood cells and plasma proteins. *J. Pharm. Sci.,* **1993,** *82:*942–947.

FLUVOXAMINE[a] (Chapter 19)

53	<5	77	21.4[b] ↓ Aged, LD[c] → RD ↑ Smk[d]	25	15 (8–28)[b] ↑ Aged, LD	5 (1–10)[e]	93 (41–210) ng/ml[e]

[a]Data from healthy male subjects.
[b]Fluvoxamine exhibits nonlinear, time-dependent kinetics. CL/F decreases and $t_{1/2}$ increases with multiple doses >50 mg/day.
[c]CL/F reduced, hepatic cirrhosis.
[d]CL/F increased in smokers, mediated most likely through an induction of CYP1A2.
[e]Mean (95% CI) following a 50-mg oral dose twice a day for 28 days.

References: de Vries, M.H., Raghoebar, M., Mathlener, I.S., and van Harten, J. Single and multiple oral dose fluvoxamine kinetics in young and elderly subjects. *Ther. Drug Monit.,* **1992,** *14:*493–498.
Hiemke, C., and Hartter, S. Pharmacokinetics of selective serotonin reuptake inhibitors. *Pharmacol. Ther.,* **2000,** *85:*11–28.
van Harten, J., Duchier, J., Devissaguet, J.P., van Bemmel, P., de Vries, M.H., and Raghoebar, M. Pharmacokinetics of fluvoxamine maleate in patients with liver cirrhosis after single-dose oral administration. *Clin. Pharmacokinet.,* **1993,** *24:*177–182.
van Harten, J. Overview of the pharmacokinetics of fluvoxamine. *Clin. Pharmacokinet.,* **1995,** *29*(suppl 1):1–9.

FUROSEMIDE[a] (Chapter 29)

71 ± 35 (43–73)	71 ± 10 (50–80) ↓ CF	98.6 ± 0.4 (96–99) ↓ RD, NS, Cirr, Alb, Aged	1.66 ± 0.58 (1.5–3.0) ↓ Aged, RD,b CHF, Neo, Prem	0.13 ± 0.06 (0.09–0.17) ↑ NS, Neo, Prem, Cirr	1.3 ± 0.8 (0.5–2.0) ↑ Aged, RD,b CHF, Prem, Neo, Cirr	1.4 ± 0.8[c]	1.7 ± 0.9 µg/ml[c]
→ CHF, Cirr, CRI	→ Aged	→ CHF, Smk	→ Cirr ↑ CF	→ RD, CHF, Aged, Smk	→ NS		

[a]Data from healthy adult male subjects. No significant gender differences. Range of mean values from multiple studies shown in parenthesis.
[b]CL/F is reduced, mild to severe renal impairment. Aged: CL/F reduced with declining renal function.
[c]Following a single 40-mg oral dose (tablet). Ototoxicity occurs at concentrations above 25 µg/ml.

References: Andreasen, F., Hansen, U., Husted, S.E., and Jansen, J.A. The pharmacokinetics of frusemide are influenced by age. *Br. J. Clin. Pharmacol.,* **1983,** *16:*391–397.
Ponto, L.L., and Schoenwald, R.D. Furosemide (frusemide). A pharmacokinetic/pharmacodynamic review (Part I). *Clin. Pharmacokinet.,* **1990,** *18:*381–408.
Waller, E.S., Hamilton, S.F., Massarella, J.W., Sharanevych, M.A., Smith, R.V., Yakatan, G.J., and Doluisio, J.T. Disposition and absolute bioavailability of furosemide in healthy males. *J. Pharm. Sci.,* **1982,** *71:*1105–1108.

Key: Unless otherwise indicated by a specific footnote, the data are presented for the study population as a mean value ± 1 standard deviation, a mean and range (lowest–highest in parenthesis) of values, a range of the lowest–highest values, or a single mean value.

ADH = alcohol dehydrogenase; Aged = aged; AIDS = acquired immunodeficiency syndrome; Alb = hypoalbuminemia; AVH = acute viral hepatitis; Atr Fib = atrial fibrillation; Burn = burn patients; C_{max} = peak concentration; CAD = coronary artery disease; Celiac = celiac disease; CF = cystic fibrosis; CHF = congestive heart failure; Child = children; Cirr = hepatic cirrhosis; COPD = chronic obstructive pulmonary disease; CP = cor pulmonale; CPBS = cardiopulmonary bypass surgery; CRI = chronic respiratory insufficiency; Crohn = Crohn's disease; Cush = Cushing's syndrome; CYP = cytochrome P450; Fem = female; Hep = hepatitis; HIV = human immunodeficiency virus; HL = hyperlipoproteinemia; HTh = hyperthyroid; IM = intramuscular; Inflam = inflammation; IV = intravenous; LD = liver disease; LTh = hypothyroid; MAO = monoamine oxidase; MI = myocardial infarction; NAT = N-acetyltransferase; Neo = neonate; NIDDM = non-insulin-dependent diabetes mellitus; NS = nephrotic syndrome; Obes = obese; Pneu = pneumonia; Preg = pregnant; Prem = premature; RA = rheumatoid arthritis; RD = renal disease (including uremia); SC = subcutaneous; Smk = smoking; ST = sulfotransferase; T_{max} = peak time; Tach = ventricular tachycardia; UGT = UDP-glucuronosyl transferase; Ulcer = ulcer patients. Other abbreviations are defined in the text section of this appendix.

Table A–II–1
PHARMACOKINETIC DATA (Continued)

AVAILABILITY (ORAL) (%)	URINARY EXCRETION (%)	BOUND IN PLASMA (%)	CLEARANCE ($ml \cdot min^{-1} \cdot kg^{-1}$)	VOL. DIST. (liters/kg)	HALF-LIFE (hours)	PEAK TIME (hours)	PEAK CONCENTRATIONS
GABAPENTIN (Chapter 21)							
60[a]	64–68	<3	1.6 ± 0.3 ↓ Aged, RD	0.80 ± 0.09	6.5 ± 1.0 ↑ RD	2–3[b]	4 μg/ml[b]

[a]Decreases with increasing dose. Value for 300- to 600-mg dose reported. [b]Following an 800-mg oral dose given three times a day to steady state in healthy adults. Efficacious at concentrations >2 μg/ml.

References: Bialer, M. Comparative pharmacokinetics of the newer antiepileptic drugs. *Clin. Pharmacokinet.*, **1993**, 24:441–452.
McLean, M.J. Gabapentin. In, *The Treatment of Epilepsy: Principles and Practice,* 2nd ed. (Wyllie, E., ed.) Williams & Wilkins, Baltimore, **1997**, pp. 884–898.

GANCICLOVIR (Chapters 50, 51)							
3–5 ↑ Food	73 ± 31	1–2	4.6 ± 1.8 ↓ RD	1.1 ± 0.3	4.3 ± 1.6 ↑ RD	Oral: 3.0 ± 0.6[a]	IV: 6.6 ± 1.8 μg/ml[a] Oral: 1.2 ± 0.4 μg/ml[a] ↑ Food

[a]Following a single 6-mg/kg IV dose (1-hour infusion) or a 1000-mg oral dose, given with food, three times a day to steady state.

References: Aweeka. F.T. Gambertoglio, J.G. Kramer, F., van der Horst, C. Polsky, B., Jayewardene, A., Lizak, P., Emrick, L., Tong, W., and Jacobson, M.A. Foscarnet and ganciclovir pharmacokinetics during concomitant or alternating maintenance therapy for AIDS-related cytomegalovirus retinitis. *Clin. Pharmacol. Ther*, **1995**, 57:403–412.
Physicians' Desk Reference, 54th ed. Medical Economics Co., Montvale, NJ, **2000**, p. 2624.

GATIFLOXACIN[a] (Chapter 44)							
96	83.2 ± 4.0	20 ± 5	2.7–3.0[b] ↓ RD[c]	1.5–2[b]	7.4–13.9[b] ↑ RD[c]	2.0 ± 0.6[d]	3.4 ± 0.6 μg/ml[d]

[a]Data from healthy male and female subjects. No significant gender differences. [b]Range of mean values from different IV studies. [c]CL/F reduced, half-life increased, mild to severe renal impairment. [d]Following a single 400-mg oral dose.

References: Manufacturer's product information, Bristol-Myers Squibb.
Nakashima, M., Uematsu, T., Kosuge, K., Kusajima, H., Ooie, T., Masuda, Y., Ishida, R., and Uchida, H. Single- and multiple-dose pharmacokinetics of AM-1155, a new 6-fluoro-8-methoxy quinolone, in humans. *Antimicrob. Agents Chemother,* **1995**, 39:2635–2640.

GEMCITABINE[a] (Chapter 52)							
—	<10	Negligible	37.8 ± 19.4[b] ↓ Aged	1.4 ± 1.3[c]	0.63 ± 0.48[c] ↑ Aged	—	26.9 ± 9 μM[d]

[a]Data from patients with leukemia. Rapidly metabolized intracellularly to di- and triphosphate active products; IV administration. [b]Weight-normalized CL is ~25% slower in women, compared to men. [c]V_d and $t_{1/2}$ are reported to increase with long duration of IV infusion. [d]Steady-state concentration during a 10-mg/m² per minute infusion for 120 to 640 minutes.

References: Grunewald. R., Kantarjian, H., Du, M., Faucher, K., Tarassoff, P., and Plunkett, W. Gemcitabine in leukemia: a phase I clinical, plasma, and cellular pharmacology study. *J. Clin. Oncol.*, **1992**, 10:406–413.
Physicians' Desk Reference, 54th ed. Medical Economics Co., Montvale, NJ, **2000**, p. 1586.

GEMFIBROZIL (Chapter 36)

98 ± 1	>97	<1	0.14 ± 0.03	1.7 ± 0.4 ←→ Cirr, RD	1.1 ± 0.2 ←→ RD	1–2[a]	15–25 μg/ml[a]

[a]Following a 600-mg oral dose given twice a day to steady state.

Reference: Todd, P.A., and Ward, A. Gemfibrozil. A review of its pharmacodynamic and pharmacokinetic properties, and therapeutic use in dyslipidaemia. *Drugs,* **1988,** 36:314–339.

GENTAMICIN (Chapter 46)

IM: ~100	>90	<10	$CL = 0.82\,CL_{cr} + 0.11$ ↓ Obes	0.31 ± 0.10 ←→ RD, Aged, CF, Child ↓ Obes ↑ Neo	2–3[a]	IV: 1[b]; IM: 0.3–0.75[b]	IV: 4.9 ± 0.5 μg/ml[b]; IM: 5.0 ± 0.4 μg/ml[b]

[a]Gentamicin has a very long terminal half-life of 53 ± 25 hours (slow release from tissues), which accounts for urinary excretion for up to three weeks after a dose.

[b]Following a single 100-mg IV infusion (1 hour) or IM injection given to healthy adults.

References: Matzke, G.R., Yeh, J., Awni, W.M., Halstenson, C.E., and Chung, M. Pharmacokinetics of cetirizine in the elderly and patients with renal insufficiency. *Ann. Allergy,* **1987,** 59:25–30. Regamey, C., Gordon, R.C., and Kirby, W.M. Comparative pharmacokinetics of tobramycin and gentamicin. *Clin. Pharmacol. Ther.,* **1973,** 14:396–403.

GLIMEPIRIDE[a] (Chapter 61)

~100	>99.5	<0.5	0.62 ± 0.26 ↑ RD[b]	0.18 ↑ RD[b]	3.4 ± 2.0 ←→ RD[b]	2–3[c]	359 ± 98 ng/ml[c]

[a]Data from healthy male subjects. No significant gender differences. Glimepiride is metabolized by CYP2C9 to an active (~one-third potency) metabolite, M1.

[b]*CL/F* and *V_d/F* increased and $t_{1/2}$ unchanged, moderate to severe renal impairment; presumably mediated through an (unreported) increase in plasma free fraction. M1 *AUC* also increased.

[c]Following a single 3-mg oral dose.

References: Badian, M., Korn, A., Lehr, K.H., Malerczyk, V., and Waldhäusl, W. Determination of the absolute bioavailability of glimepiride (HOE 490), a new sulphonylurea. *Int. J. Clin. Pharmacol. Ther. Toxicol.,* **1992,** 30:481–482. *Physicians' Desk Reference,* 54th ed. Medical Economics Co., Montvale, NJ, **2000,** pp. 1346–1349. Rosenkranz, B., Profozic, V., Metelko, Z., Mrzljak, V., Lange, C., and Malerczyk, V. Pharmacokinetics and safety of glimepiride at clinically effective doses in diabetic patients with renal impairment. *Diabetologia,* **1996,** 39:1617–1624.

GLIPIZIDE (Chapter 61)

95	98.4	<5	0.52 ± 0.18[a] ←→ RD, Aged	0.17 ± 0.02[a] ←→ Aged	3.4 ± 0.7 ←→ RD, Aged	2.1 ± 0.9[b]	465 ± 139 ng/ml[b]

[a]*CL/F* and *V_ss/F* reported.

[b]Following a single 5-mg oral dose (immediate-release tablet) given to healthy young adults. An extended-release formulation exhibits a delayed T_{max} of 6 to 12 hours.

Reference: Kobayashi, K.A., Bauer, L.A., Horn, J.R., Opheim, K., Wood, F., and Kradjan, W.A. Glipizide pharmacokinetics in young and elderly volunteers. *Clin. Pharm.,* **1988,** 7:224–228.

Key: Unless otherwise indicated by a specific footnote, the data are presented for the study population as a mean value ± 1 standard deviation, a mean and range (lowest–highest in parenthesis) of values, a range of the lowest–highest values, or a single mean value.

ADH = alcohol dehydrogenase; Aged = aged; AIDS = acquired immunodeficiency syndrome; Alb = hypoalbuminemia; Atr Fib = atrial fibrillation; AVH = acute viral hepatitis; Burn = burn patients; C_{max} = peak concentration; CAD = coronary artery disease; Celiac = celiac disease; CF = cystic fibrosis; CHF = congestive heart failure; Child = children; Cirr = hepatic cirrhosis; COPD = chronic obstructive pulmonary disease; CP = cor pulmonale; CPBS = cardiopulmonary bypass surgery; CRI = chronic respiratory insufficiency; Crohn = Crohn's disease; Cush = Cushing's syndrome; CYP = cytochrome P450; Fem = female; Hep = hepatitis; HIV = human immunodeficiency virus; HL = hyperlipoproteinemia; HTh = hyperthyroid; IM = intramuscular; Inflam = inflammation; IV = intravenous; LD = liver disease; LTh = hypothyroid; MAO = monoamine oxidase; MI = myocardial infarction; NAT = N-acetyltransferase; Neo = neonate; NIDDM = non-insulin-dependent diabetes mellitus; NS = nephrotic syndrome; Obes = obese; Pneu = pneumonia; Preg = pregnant; Prem = premature; RA = rheumatoid arthritis; RD = renal disease (including uremia); SC = subcutaneous; Smk = smoking; ST = sulfotransferase; T_{max} = peak time; Tach = ventricular tachycardia; UGT = UDP-glucuronosyl transferase; Ulcer = ulcer patients. Other abbreviations are defined in the text section of this appendix.

Table A–II–1
PHARMACOKINETIC DATA (*Continued*)

AVAILABILITY (ORAL) (%)	URINARY EXCRETION (%)	BOUND IN PLASMA (%)	CLEARANCE ($ml \cdot min^{-1} \cdot kg^{-1}$)	VOL. DIST. (liters/kg)	HALF-LIFE (hours)	PEAK TIME (hours)	PEAK CONCENTRATIONS
GLYBURIDE (Chapter 61)							
G: 90–100[a] M: 64–90[a]	Negligible	99.8 ↓ Aged	1.3 ± 0.5 ↓ Cirr	0.20 ± 0.11	4 ± 1[b] ↑ Cirr, NIDDM	G: ~1.5[c] M: 2–4[c]	G: 106 ng/ml[c] M: 104 ng/ml[c]

[a]Data for GLYNASE PRESTAB micronized tablet (G) and MICRONASE tablet (M). [b]Half-life for micronized formulation reported. Half-life for nonmicronized formulation is 6 to 10 hours, reflecting absorption rate limitation. A long terminal half-life (15 hours), reflecting redistribution from tissues, has been reported. [c]Mean C_{max} following a 3-mg oral GLYNASE tablet taken with breakfast or a 5-mg oral MICRONASE tablet given to healthy adult subjects.

References: Jonsson, A., Rydberg, T., Ekberg, G., Hallengren, B., and Melander, A. Slow elimination of glyburide in NIDDM subjects. *Diabetes Care*, **1994,** *17:*142–145.
Physicians' Desk Reference, 54th ed. Medical Economics Co., Montvale, NJ, **2000,** p. 2457.

AVAILABILITY (ORAL) (%)	URINARY EXCRETION (%)	BOUND IN PLASMA (%)	CLEARANCE ($ml \cdot min^{-1} \cdot kg^{-1}$)	VOL. DIST. (liters/kg)	HALF-LIFE (hours)	PEAK TIME (hours)	PEAK CONCENTRATIONS
GRANISETRON (Chapter 38)							
~60	16 ± 14	65 ± 9	11 ± 9 ↓ Aged, Cirr ←→ RD	3.0 ± 1.5 ←→ RD	5.3 ± 3.5 ↑ Aged, Cirr ←→ RD	—	IV: 64 (18–176) ng/ml[a] Oral: 6.0 (0.6–31) ng/ml[a]

[a]Mean (range) values following a 40-μg/kg IV dose (5-minute infusion) given to patients with cancer, or a single 1-mg oral dose given twice a day for 7 days.

References: Allen, A., Asgill, C.C., Pierce, D.M., Upward, J., and Zussman, B.D. Pharmacokinetics and tolerability of ascending intravenous doses of granisetron, a novel 5-HT₃ antagonist, in healthy human subjects. *Eur. J. Clin. Pharmacol.,* **1994,** *46:*159–162.
Physicians' Desk Reference, 54th ed. Medical Economics Co., Montvale, NJ, **2000,** pp. 3016 and 3018.

AVAILABILITY (ORAL) (%)	URINARY EXCRETION (%)	BOUND IN PLASMA (%)	CLEARANCE ($ml \cdot min^{-1} \cdot kg^{-1}$)	VOL. DIST. (liters/kg)	HALF-LIFE (hours)	PEAK TIME (hours)	PEAK CONCENTRATIONS
HALOPERIDOL[a] (Chapter 20)							
60 ± 18	1	92 ± 2 ↑ Cirr ←→ Aged, Child	11.8 ± 2.9[b] ↑ Child, Smk ↓ Aged	18 ± 7	18 ± 5[b] ↓ Child	IM: 0.6 ± 0.1[c] Oral: 1.7 ± 3.2[c]	IM: 22 ± 18 ng/ml[c] Oral: 9.2 ± 4.4 ng/ml[c]

[a]Undergoes reversible metabolism to a less active reduced haloperidol. [b]Represents net clearance of parent drug; reduced haloperidol $CL = 10 ± 5$ ml · min⁻¹ · kg⁻¹ and $t_{1/2} = 67 ± 51$ hours. Slow conversion from reduced haloperidol to parent compound probably responsible for prolonged $t_{1/2}$ (70 hours) for haloperidol observed with 7-day sampling. [c]Following a single 20-mg oral dose or 10-mg IM dose. Effective concentrations are 4–20 ng/ml.

Reference: Froemming, J.S., Lam, Y.W., Jann, M.W., and Davis, C.M. Pharmacokinetics of haloperidol. *Clin. Pharmacokinet.,* **1989,** *17:*396–423.

AVAILABILITY (ORAL) (%)	URINARY EXCRETION (%)	BOUND IN PLASMA (%)	CLEARANCE ($ml \cdot min^{-1} \cdot kg^{-1}$)	VOL. DIST. (liters/kg)	HALF-LIFE (hours)	PEAK TIME (hours)	PEAK CONCENTRATIONS
HEPARIN (Chapter 55)							
—	Negligible	Extensive	1/(0.65 + 0.008D) ± 0.1[a] ↓ Fem	0.058 ± 0.11[b]	(26 + 0.323D) ± 12 min[a] ↓ Smk	3[c]	70 ± 39 ng/ml[c]

[a]Dose (D) is in IU/kg. Clearance and half-life are dose dependent, perhaps due to saturable metabolism with end-product inhibition. [b]V_{urea} reported. [c]Mean of above critical length molecules following a single 5000-IU dose (unfractionated) given by subcutaneous injection.

References: Bendetowicz, A.V., Beguin, S., Caplain, H., and Hemker, H.C. Pharmacokinetics and pharmacodynamics of a low molecular weight heparin (enoxaparin) after subcutaneous injection, comparison with unfractionated heparin—a three way cross over study in human volunteers. *Thromb. Haemost.,* **1994,** *71:*305–313.
Estes, J.W. Clinical pharmacokinetics of heparin. *Clin. Pharmacokinet.,* **1980,** *5:*204–220.

HYDRALAZINE[a] (Chapter 33)

16 ± 6[a,b] 35 ± 4[c] ↔ CHF ↑ Food	1–15	87	56 ± 13[d,e] ↓ CHF	1.5 ± 1.0[d,e] ↔ CHF	0.96 ± 0.28[d] ↑ CHF	EH: 0.96 ± 0.44[f] HF: 0.73 ± 0.26[f]	EH: 0.8 ± 0.3 μM[f] HF: 1.5 ± 0.9 μM[f]

[a]Data for rapid acetylators.
[b]Bioavailability may increase with large doses that saturate first-pass metabolism.
[c]Data for slow acetylators.
[d]Same values for rapid and slow acetylators after IV administration because of liver blood flow limitations and other parallel pathways of biotransformation.
[e]Blood CL and V_{ss} reported.
[f]Following a single 50-mg oral dose (tablet) after an overnight fast, given to patients with essential hypertension (EH) or severe chronic heart failure (HF). A level of 0.62 μM will cause a decrease in mean arterial pressure of 10–20 mm Hg.

References: Hanson, A., Johansson, B.W., Wernersson, B., and Wahlander, L.A. Pharmacokinetics of oral hydralazine in chronic heart failure. *Eur. J. Clin. Pharmacol.* **1983,** *25*:467–473.
Mulrow, J.P., and Crawford, M.H. Clinical pharmacokinetics and therapeutic use of hydralazine in congestive heart failure. *Clin. Pharmacokinet.* **1989,** *16*:86–89.

HYDROCHLOROTHIAZIDE (Chapter 29)

71 ± 15	>95	58 ± 17[a]	4.9 ± 1.1[b] ↓ RD, CHF,[c] Aged	0.83 ± 0.31[d] ↓ Aged	2.5 ± 0.2[e] ↑ RD, CHF,[c] Aged	SD: 1.9 ± 0.5[f] MD: 2[f]	SD: 75 ± 17 ng/ml[f] MD: 91 ± 0.2 ng/ml[f]

[a]Blood-to-plasma concentration ratio = 2.0–2.5.
[b]Renal clearance reported, which should approximate total plasma clearance; calculated assuming a 70-kg body weight.
[c]Changes may reflect decreased renal function.
[d]Calculated from individual values of renal clearance, terminal half-life, and fraction of drug excreted unchanged; 70-kg body weight assumed.
[e]Longer terminal half-lives of 8 ± 2.8 hours have been reported with a concomitant increase in V_{area} to 2.8 l/kg.
[f]Following a single (SD) or multiple (MD) 12.5-mg oral dose of hydrochlorothiazide; MD given once daily for 5 days to healthy adults.

References: Beermann, B., and Groschinsky-Grind, M. Pharmacokinetics of hydrochlorothiazide in man. *Eur. J. Clin. Pharmacol.* **1977,** *12*:297–303.
Jordo, L., Johnsson, G., Lundborg, P. Persson, B.A., Regardh, C.G., and Ronn, O. Bioavailability and disposition of metoprolol and hydrochlorothiazide combined in one tablet and of separate doses of hydrochlorothiazide. *Br. J. Clin. Pharmacol.* **1979,** *7*:563–567.
O'Grady, P., Yee, K.F., Lins, R., and Mangold, B. Fosinopril/hydrochlorothiazide: single dose and steady-state pharmacokinetics and pharmacodynamics. *Br. J. Clin. Pharmacol.* **1999,** *48*:375–381.

HYDROCODONE[a] (Chapter 23)

—	EM: 10.2 ± 1.8 PM: 18.1 ± 4.5	—	EM: 11.1 ± 3.57[b] PM: 6.54 ± 1.25[b]	—	EM: 4.24 ± 0.99[b] PM: 6.16 ± 1.97[b]	EM: 0.72 ± 0.46[c] PM: 0.93 ± 0.59[c]	EM: 30 ± 9.4 ng/ml[c] PM: 27 ± 5.9 ng/ml[c]

[a]Data from healthy male and female subjects. The metabolism of hydrocodone to hydromorphone (more active) is catalyzed by CYP2D6. Subjects were phenotyped as extensive (EM) and poor (PM) metabolizers.
[b]CL/F and half-life reported for oral dose.
[c]Following a 10-mg oral dose (syrup). Maximal hydromorphone concentrations are higher in EMs than PMs (5.2 vs. 1.0 ng/ml).

Reference: Otton, S.V., Schadel, M., Cheung, S.W., Kaplan, H.L. Busto, U.E., and Sellers, E.M. CYP2D6 phenotype determines the metabolic conversion of hydrocodone to hydromorphone. *Clin. Pharmacol. Ther.* **1993,** *54*:463–472.

Key: Unless otherwise indicated by a specific footnote, the data are presented for the study population as a mean value ± 1 standard deviation, a mean and range (lowest–highest in parenthesis) of values, a range of the lowest–highest values, or a single mean value.

ADH = alcohol dehydrogenase; Aged = aged; AIDS = acquired immunodeficiency syndrome; Alb = hypoalbuminemia; Atr Fib = atrial fibrillation; AVH = acute viral hepatitis; Burn = burn patients; C_{max} = peak concentration; CAD = coronary artery disease; Celiac = celiac disease; CF = cystic fibrosis; CHF = congestive heart failure; Child = children; Cirr = hepatic cirrhosis; COPD = chronic obstructive pulmonary disease; CP = cor pulmonale; CPBS = cardiopulmonary bypass surgery; CRI = chronic respiratory insufficiency; Crohn = Crohn's disease; Cush = Cushing's syndrome; CYP = cytochrome P450; Fem = female; Hep = hepatitis; HIV = human immunodeficiency virus; HL = hyperlipoproteinemia; HTh = hyperthyroid; IM = intramuscular; Inflam = inflammation; IV = intravenous; LD = liver disease; LTh = hypothyroid; MAO = monoamine oxidase; MI = myocardial infarction; NAT = N-acetyltransferase; Neo = neonate; NIDDM = non-insulin-dependent diabetes mellitus; NS = nephrotic syndrome; Obes = obese; Pneu = pneumonia; Preg = pregnant; Prem = premature; RA = rheumatoid arthritis; RD = renal disease (including uremia); SC = subcutaneous; Smk = smoking; ST = sulfotransferase; T_{max} = peak time; Tach = ventricular tachycardia; UGT = UDP-glucuronosyl transferase; Ulcer = ulcer patients. Other abbreviations are defined in the text section of this appendix.

Table A-II-1
PHARMACOKINETIC DATA (Continued)

AVAILABILITY (ORAL) (%)	URINARY EXCRETION (%)	BOUND IN PLASMA (%)	CLEARANCE $(ml \cdot min^{-1} \cdot kg^{-1})$	VOL. DIST. (liters/kg)	HALF-LIFE (hours)	PEAK TIME (hours)	PEAK CONCENTRATIONS
HYDROMORPHONE[a] (Chapter 23)							
Oral: 42 ± 23, SC: ~80	6	7.1	14.6 ± 7.6	2.90 ± 1.31[b]	2.4 ± 0.6	IV: —[c], Oral: 1.1 ± 0.2[c]	IV: 242 ng/ml[c], Oral: 11.8 ± 2.6 ng/ml[c]

[a] Data from healthy male subjects. Extensively metabolized. The principal metabolite, 3-glucuronide, accumulates to much higher (27-fold) levels than parent drug, and may contribute to some side effects (not antinociceptive).
[b] V_{area} reported.
[c] Following a single 2-mg IV (bolus, sample at 3 minutes) or 4-mg oral dose.

References: Hagen, N., Thirlwell, M.P., Dhaliwal, H.S., Babul, N., Harsanyi, Z., and Darke, A.C. Steady-state pharmacokinetics of hydromorphone and hydromorphone-3-glucuronide in cancer patients after immediate and controlled-release hydromorphone. *J. Clin. Pharmacol.,* **1995,** *35:*37–44.
Moulin, D.E., Kreeft, J.H., Murray-Parsons, N., and Bouquillon, A.I. Comparison of continuous subcutaneous and intravenous hydromorphone infusions for management of cancer pain. *Lancet,* **1991,** *337:*465–468.
Parab, P.V., Ritschel, W.A., Coyle, D.E., Gregg, R.V., and Denson, D.D. Pharmacokinetics of hydromorphone after intravenous, peroral and rectal administration to human subjects. *Biopharm. Drug Dispos.,* **1988,** *9:*187–199.

AVAILABILITY (ORAL) (%)	URINARY EXCRETION (%)	BOUND IN PLASMA (%)	CLEARANCE	VOL. DIST.	HALF-LIFE (hours)	PEAK TIME (hours)	PEAK CONCENTRATIONS
HYDROXYUREA[a] (Chapter 52)							
108 ± 18 (79–108)	35.8 ± 14.2	Negligible	72 ± 17 ml·min⁻¹·(m²)⁻¹[b] (36.2–72.3)	19.7 ± 4.6 l/m²	3.4 ± 0.7 (2.8–4.5)	IV: 0.5[c], Oral: 1.2 ± 1.2[c]	IV: 1007 ± 371 μM[c], Oral: 794 ± 241 μM[c]

[a] Data from male and female patients treated for solid tumors. A range of mean values from multiple studies is shown in parenthesis.
[b] Nonrenal elimination of hydroxyurea is thought to exhibit saturable kinetics through a 10- to 80-mg/kg dose range.
[c] Following a single 2-g, 30-minute intravenous infusion or oral dose.

References: Gwilt, P.R., and Tracewell, W.G. Pharmacokinetics and pharmacodynamics of hydroxyurea. *Clin. Pharmacokinet.,* **1998,** *34:*347–358.
Rodriguez, G.I., Kuhn, J.G., Weiss, G.R., Hilsenbeck, S.G., Eckardt, J.R., Thurman, A., Rinaldi, D.A., Hodges, S., Von Hoff, D.D., and Rowinsky E.K. A bioavailability and pharmacokinetic study of oral and intravenous hydroxyurea. *Blood,* **1998,** *91:*1533–1541.

AVAILABILITY (ORAL) (%)	URINARY EXCRETION (%)	BOUND IN PLASMA (%)	CLEARANCE	VOL. DIST.	HALF-LIFE (hours)	PEAK TIME (hours)	PEAK CONCENTRATIONS
IBUPROFEN[a] (Chapter 27)							
>80	<1	>99[b] ↔ RA, Alb	0.75 ± 0.20[b,c] ↑ CF ↔ Child, RA	0.15 ± 0.02[c] ↑ CF	2 ± 0.5[b] ↔ RA, CF, Child ↑ Cirr	1.6 ± 0.3[d]	61.1 ± 5.5 μg/ml[d]

[a] Racemic mixture. Kinetic parameters for the active S-(+)-enantiomer do not differ from those for the inactive R-(−)-enantiomer when administered separately; 63 ± 6% of the R-(−)-enantiomer undergoes inversion to the active isomer.
[b] Unbound percent of S-(+)-ibuprofen (0.77 ± 0.20%) is significantly greater than that of R-(−)-ibuprofen (0.45 ± 0.06%). Binding of each enantiomer is concentration dependent and is influenced by the presence of the optical antipode, leading to nonlinear elimination kinetics.
[c] CL/F and V_{ss}/F reported.
[d] Following a single 800-mg dose of racemate. A level of 10 μg/ml provides antipyresis in febrile children.

References: Lee, E.J., Williams, K., Day, R., Graham, G., and Champion, D. Stereoselective disposition of ibuprofen enantiomers in man. *Br. J. Clin. Pharmacol.,* **1985,** *19:*669–674.
Lockwood, G.F., Albert, K.S., Gillespie, W.R., Bole, G.G., Harkcom, T.M., Szounar, G.J., and Wagner, J.G. Pharmacokinetics of ibuprofen in man. I. Free and total area/dose relationships. *Clin. Pharmacol. Ther.,* **1983,** *34:*97–103.

IDARUBICIN[a] (Chapter 52)

28 ± 4	<5	I: 97 IL: 94	24.7 ± 5.9	I: 15.2 ± 3.7 IL: 41 ± 10 IL: ↑ RD[b]	I: 5.4 ± 2.4[c] IL: 7.9 ± 2.3[c]	I: 6.9 ± 0.1 ng/ml[c] IL: 22 ± 4 ng/ml[c]

[a] Data from male and female patients with cancer. Idarubicin (I) undergoes rapid metabolism to a major active (equipotent) metabolite, idarubicinol (IL).
[b] Mild to moderate renal impairment.
[c] Following a single 30- to 35-mg/m² oral dose.

References: Camaggi, C.M., Strocchi, E., Carisi, P., Martoni, A., Tononi, A., Guaraldi, M., Strolin-Benedetti, M., Efthymiopoulos, C., and Pannuti, F. Idarubicin metabolism and pharmacokinetics after intravenous and oral administration in cancer patients: a crossover study. *Cancer Chemother. Pharmacol.,* **1992,** *30:*307–316.
Robert, J. Clinical pharmacokinetics of idarubicin. *Clin. Pharmacokinet.,* **1993,** *24:*275–288.
Tamassia, V., Pacciarini, M.A., Moro, E., Piazza, E., Vago, G., and Libretti, A. Pharmacokinetic study of intravenous and oral idarubicin in cancer patients. *Int. J. Clin. Pharmacol. Res.,* **1987,** *7:*419–426.

IFOSFAMIDE[a] (Chapter 52)

92	Negligible	Low: 12–18 High: 53.1 ± 9.6	Low: 63 ml·min⁻¹·(m²)⁻¹[b] High: 6.2 ± 1.9 ml·min⁻¹·(m²)⁻¹ → Aged	Low: – High: 12.5 ± 3.6 l/m² ↑ Aged	Oral: 0.5–1.0[c]	IV: 203 (168–232) µM[c] Oral: 200 (163–245) µM[c]

[a] Data from male and female patients treated for advanced cancers. Administered IV with mesna to avoid hemorrhagic cystitis. Exhibits dose-dependent kinetics, with apparent saturation of hepatic metabolism. Metabolic activation to 4-hydroxyifosfamide catalyzed by CYP3A and CYP2C. Parameters reported for a 1.5-g/m² (Low) or 5-g/m² (High) IV dose and 1.5-g/m² oral dose.
[b] CL reported to increase with daily dosing.
[c] Geometric mean (range) following a single 1.5-g/m² IV infusion (20 min) or 1.5-g/m² oral dose.

References: Allen, L.M. and Creaven, P.J. Pharmacokinetics of ifosfamide. *Clin. Pharmacol. Ther.,* **1975,** *17:*492–498.
Kurowski, V., Cerny, T., Kupfer, A., and Wagner, T. Metabolism and pharmacokinetics of oral and intravenous ifosfamide. *J. Cancer Res. Clin. Oncol.,* **1991,** *117*(suppl. 4):S148–S153.
Lind, M.J., Margison, J.M., Cerny, T., Thatcher, N., and Wilkinson, P.M. The effect of age on the pharmacokinetics of ifosfamide. *Br. J. Clin. Pharmacol.,* **1990,** *30:*140–143.
Physicians' Desk Reference, 54th ed. Medical Economics Co., Montvale, NJ, **2000,** pp. 866–867.

IMIPENEM/CILASTATIN[a] (Chapter 45)

Imipenem	<20	69 ± 15 ↓ Neo, Inflam ↔ Child, CF	2.9 ± 0.3 ↑ Child ↓ RD ↔ CF, Inflam, Neo, Aged, Burn, Prem	0.9 ± 0.1 ↑ Neo, RD, Prem ↔ CF, Child, Aged	0.23 ± 0.05 ↑ Neo, Child, Prem ↔ CF, RD, Aged	IV: 60–70 µg/ml[b] IM: 1–2[b]
Cilastatin	~35	70 ± 3 ↓ Neo ↔ CF	3.0 ± 0.3 ↑ Child ↓ Neo, RD, Prem ↔ CF, Aged	0.8 ± 0.1 ↑ Neo, Prem ↔ CF, Aged	0.20 ± 0.03 ↑ Neo, RD, CF, Aged ↑ Prem	IM: 8.2–12 µg/ml[b]

[a] Formulated as a 1:1 (mg/mg) mixture for parenteral administration; cilastatin inhibits the metabolism of imipenem by the kidney, increasing concentrations of imipenem in the urine; cilastatin does not change imipenem plasma concentrations appreciably.
[b] Plasma C_{max} of imipenem following a single 1-g IV infusion (30 minutes) or 750 mg administered intramuscularly.

Reference: Buckley, M.M., Brogden, R.N., Barradell, L.B., and Goa, K.L. Imipenem/cilastatin. A reappraisal of its antibacterial activity, pharmacokinetic properties and therapeutic efficacy. *Drugs,* **1992,** *44:*408–444.

Key: Unless otherwise indicated by a specific footnote, the data are presented for the study population as a mean value ± 1 standard deviation, a mean and range (lowest–highest in parenthesis) of values, a range of the lowest–highest values, or a single mean value.

ADH = alcohol dehydrogenase; Aged = aged; AIDS = acquired immunodeficiency syndrome; Alb = hypoalbuminemia; Atr Fib = atrial fibrillation; AVH = acute viral hepatitis; Burn = burn patients; C_{max} = peak concentration; CAD = coronary artery disease; Celiac = celiac disease; CF = cystic fibrosis; CHF = congestive heart failure; Child = children; Cirr = hepatic cirrhosis; COPD = chronic obstructive pulmonary disease; CP = cor pulmonale; CPBS = cardiopulmonary bypass surgery; CRI = chronic respiratory insufficiency; Crohn = Crohn's disease; Cush = Cushing's syndrome; CYP = cytochrome P450; Fem = female; Hep = hepatitis; HIV = human immunodeficiency virus; HL = hyperlipoproteinemia; HTh = hyperthyroid; IM = intramuscular; Inflam = inflammation; IV = intravenous; LD = liver disease; LTh = hypothyroid; MAO = monoamine oxidase; MI = myocardial infarction; NAT = *N*-acetyltransferase; Neo = neonate; NIDDM = non-insulin-dependent diabetes mellitus; NS = nephrotic syndrome; Obes = obese; Pneu = pneumonia; Preg = pregnant; Prem = premature; RA = rheumatoid arthritis; RD = renal disease (including uremia); SC = subcutaneous; Smk = smoking; ST = sulfotransferase; T_{max} = peak time; Tach = ventricular tachycardia; UGT = UDP-glucuronosyl transferase; Ulcer = ulcer patients. Other abbreviations are defined in the text section of this appendix.

Table A–II–1
PHARMACOKINETIC DATA (Continued)

	AVAILABILITY (ORAL) (%)	URINARY EXCRETION (%)	BOUND IN PLASMA (%)	CLEARANCE ($ml \cdot min^{-1} \cdot kg^{-1}$)	VOL. DIST. (liters/kg)	HALF-LIFE (hours)	PEAK TIME (hours)	PEAK CONCENTRATIONS
IMIPRAMINE[a] (Chapter 19)	42 ± 3	<2	90.1 ± 1.4[b] ↑ HL, MI, Burn ↔ RA, Aged	13 ± 1.7[c] ↓ Aged ↑ Smk ↔ Child	18 ± 2[d] ↔ Aged, Child	16 ± 1.3 ↑ Aged ↔ Child	2–6[e]	200 ± 137 ng/ml[e]
INDINAVIR[a] (Chapter 51)	65 ↓ Food[c]	5–12	61	Low: 18.2[b] High: 9.9 (8.7–10)[b] ↓ Cirr[d]	2.8	1.8 ± 0.4 ↑ Cirr[d]	0.8 ± 0.4[e]	9.8 ± 4.3 μM[e] ↓ Food
INDOMETHACIN[a] (Chapter 27)	98 ± 21	15 ± 8	90 ↔ Alb, Prem, Neo	1.4 ± 0.2 ↓ Prem, Neo, Aged	0.29 ± 0.04 ↔ Aged	2.4 ± 0.2[a] ↔ RA, RD ↑ Neo, Prem, Aged	~1.3[b]	~2.4 μg/ml[b]
INFLIXIMAB[a] (Chapters 39, 53)	—	—	—	—	0.043	228 ↔ LD, RD	—	118 μg/ml[b]

IMIPRAMINE[a] (Chapter 19)

[a] Active metabolite, desipramine.
[b] Blood-to-plasma concentration ratio = 1.1 ± 0.1.
[c] Undergoes N-demethylation to desipramine, catalyzed by CYP2C19 (polymorphic), CYP1A2, and others; 2-hydroxylation is catalyzed by CYP2D6 (polymorphic).
[d] V_{area} reported.
[e] Following a 200-mg/day oral dose for 4 weeks. Steady-state concentration reported is the sum of imipramine and desipramine (DMI/IMI = 1.4). Efficacy reported at combined levels of 100–300 ng/ml, and toxicity at combined levels >1 μg/ml.

Reference: Sallee, F.R., and Pollock, B.G. Clinical pharmacokinetics of imipramine and desipramine. *Clin. Pharmacokinet.,* **1990,** *18:*346–364.

INDINAVIR[a] (Chapter 51)

[a] Data from healthy male and female subjects. No significant gender differences. Metabolized by CYP3A4.
[b] Indinavir exhibits dose-dependent kinetics, possibly because of saturable first-pass and/or systemic clearance. CL reported for a 16-mg D_6-labeled IV dose given simultaneously with a 16-mg D_0 oral dose (Low) or a 800-mg D_0 oral dose (High).
[c] High fat and protein meal; no change with light meal.
[d] CL/F reduced, mild to moderate hepatic insufficiency with cirrhosis.
[e] Following a single 700-mg oral dose of indinavir sulfate.

References: Physicians' Desk Reference, 54th ed. Medical Economics Co., Montvale, NJ, **2000,** p. 1772.
Yeh, K.C., Deutsch, P.J., Haddix, H., Hesney, M., Hoagland, V., Ju, W.D., Justice, S.J., Osborne, B., Sterrett, A.T., Stone, J.A., Woolf, E., and Waldman, S. Single-dose pharmacokinetics of indinavir and the effect of food. *Antimicrob. Agents Chemother.,* **1998,** *42:*332–338.
Yeh, K.C., Stone, J.A., Carides, A.D., Rolan, P., Woolf, E., and Ju, W.D. Simultaneous investigation of indinavir nonlinear pharmacokinetics and bioavailability in healthy volunteers using stable isotope labeling technique: study design and model-independent data analysis. *J. Pharm. Sci.,* **1999,** *88:*568–573.

INDOMETHACIN[a] (Chapter 27)

[a] There is significant enterohepatic recycling (~50% after an IV dose).
[b] Following a single 50-mg oral dose, given after a standard breakfast. Effective at concentrations of 0.3–3 μg/ml and toxic at >5 μg/ml.

Reference: Oberbauer, R., Krivanek, P., and Turnheim, K. Pharmacokinetics of indomethacin in the elderly. *Clin. Pharmacokinet.,* **1993,** *24:*428–434.

INFLIXIMAB[a] (Chapters 39, 53)

[a] Data from patients with Crohn's disease. No significant gender differences. Infliximab is a mouse-human chimeric IgG1κ monoclonal antibody.
[b] Mean C_{max} following a 5-mg/kg IV dose.

Reference: Physicians' Desk Reference, 54th ed. Medical Economics Co., Montvale, NJ, **2000,** pp. 927–928.

INTERFERON ALFA[a] (Chapters 50, 53)

IM: 80-83 SC: 90	—[b]	2.8 ± 0.6[b,c]	0.40 ± 0.19[c]	0.67[d]	IM: 3.8[e] SC: 7.3[e]	IV: ~13 ng/ml[e] IM: 2.0 (1.5-2.6) ng/ml[e] SC: 1.7 (1.2-2.3) ng/ml[e]

[a] Values for recombinant interferon alfa-2a reported.
[b] Undergoes renal filtration, tubular reabsorption, and proteolytic degradation within the tubular epithelial cell.
[c] Clearance values in 4 patients with leukemia were more than halved (1.1 ± 0.3 ml·min^{-1}·kg^{-1}), while V_{ss} increased more than 20-fold (9.5 ± 3.5 l/kg) and terminal half-life changed only minimally (7.3 ± 2.4 hours).
[d] A terminal half-life of 5.1 ± 1.6 hours accounts for 23% of clearance.
[e] Mean (range) following a single 36×10^6-U dose given as a 40-min infusion (IV), intramuscularly (IM) or subcutaneously (SC). Drug accumulates two- to fourfold with multiple-dose (twice a day) intramuscular administration.

References: Physicians' Desk Reference, 54th ed. Medical Economics Co., Montvale, NJ, 2000, p. 2654.
Wills, R.J. Clinical pharmacokinetics of interferons. Clin. Pharmacokinet., 1990, 19:390-399.

INTERFERON BETA (Chapters 50, 53)

SC: 51 ± 17	—[a]	13 ± 5[a]	2.9 ± 1.8	4.3 ± 2.3	SC: 1-8[b]	IV: 1491 ± 659 IU/ml[b] SC: 40 ± 20 IU/ml[b]

[a] Will undergo renal filtration, tubular reabsorption, and renal catabolism, but hepatic uptake and catabolism are thought to dominate systemic clearance.
[b] Concentration at 5 minutes following a single 90×10^6-IU IV dose or following a single 90×10^6-IU subcutaneous (SC) dose of recombinant interferon beta-1b.

Reference: Chiang, J., Gloff, C.A., Yoshizawa, C.N., and Williams, G.J. Pharmacokinetics of recombinant human interferon-β_{ser} in healthy volunteers and its effect on serum neopterin. Pharm. Res., 1993, 10:567-572.

IRBESARTAN[a] (Chapters 31, 33)

60-80	90	2.12 ± 0.54 ↓ Aged[b] ↔ RD, Cirr	0.72 ± 0.20	13 ± 6.2	1.2 (0.7-2)[c]	1.3 ± 0.4 μg/ml[c]
2.2 ± 0.9						

[a] Data from healthy male subjects. No significant gender differences. Metabolized by UGT and CYP2C9.
[b] CL/F reduced; no dose adjustment required.
[c] Following a single 50-mg oral dose (capsule).

References: Gillis, J.C., and Markham, A. Irbesartan. A review of its pharmacodynamic and pharmacokinetic properties and therapeutic use in the management of hypertension. Drugs, 1997, 54:885–902.
Physicians' Desk Reference, 54th ed. Medical Economics Co., Montvale, NJ, 2000, p. 818.
Vachharajani, N.N., Shyu, W.C., Chando, T.J., Everett, D.W., Greene, D.S., and Barbhaiya, R.H. Oral bioavailability and disposition characteristics of irbesartan, an angiotensin antagonist, in healthy volunteers. J. Clin. Pharmacol., 1998, 38:702–707.

Key: Unless otherwise indicated by a specific footnote, the data are presented for the study population as a mean value ± 1 standard deviation, a mean and range (lowest-highest in parenthesis) of values, a range of the lowest-highest values, or a single mean value.

ADH = alcohol dehydrogenase; Aged = aged; AIDS = acquired immunodeficiency syndrome; Alb = hypoalbuminemia; Atr Fib = atrial fibrillation; AVH = acute viral hepatitis; Burn = burn patients; C_{max} = peak concentration; CAD = coronary artery disease; Celiac = celiac disease; CF = cystic fibrosis; CHF = congestive heart failure; Child = children; Cirr = hepatic cirrhosis; COPD = chronic obstructive pulmonary disease; CP = cor pulmonale; CPBS = cardiopulmonary bypass surgery; CRI = chronic respiratory insufficiency; Crohn = Crohn's disease; Cush = Cushing's syndrome; CYP = cytochrome P450; Fem = female; Hep = hepatitis; HIV = human immunodeficiency virus; HL = hyperlipoproteinemia; HTh = hyperthyroid; IM = intramuscular; Inflam = inflammation; IV = intravenous; LD = liver disease; LTh = hypothyroid; MAO = monoamine oxidase; MI = myocardial infarction; NAT = N-acetyltransferase; Neo = neonate; NIDDM = non-insulin-dependent diabetes mellitus; NS = nephrotic syndrome; Obes = obese; Pneu = pneumonia; Preg = pregnant; Prem = premature; RA = rheumatoid arthritis; RD = renal disease (including uremia); SC = subcutaneous; Smk = smoking; ST = sulfotransferase; T_{max} = peak time; Tach = ventricular tachycardia; UGT = UDP-glucuronosyl transferase; Ulcer = ulcer patients. Other abbreviations are defined in the text section of this appendix.

Table A–II–1
PHARMACOKINETIC DATA (Continued)

AVAILABILITY (ORAL) (%)	URINARY EXCRETION (%)	BOUND IN PLASMA (%)	CLEARANCE $(ml \cdot min^{-1} \cdot kg^{-1})$	VOL. DIST. (liters/kg)	HALF-LIFE (hours)	PEAK TIME (hours)	PEAK CONCENTRATIONS
IRINOTECAN[a] (Chapter 52)							
—	I: 16.7 ± 1.0	I: 30–68 SN-38: 95	I: $14.8 \pm 4 \, l \cdot h^{-1} \cdot (m^2)^{-1}$	150 ± 49 l/m²	I: 10.8 ± 0.5 SN-38: 10.4 ± 3.1	I: 0.5[b] SN-38: ≤1[b]	I: 1.7 ± 0.8 μg/ml[b] SN-38: 26 ± 12 ng/ml[b]

[a] Data from male and female patients with malignant solid tumors. No significant gender differences. Irinotecan (I) is metabolized to an active metabolite, SN-38 (100-fold more potent, but with lower blood levels).

[b] Following a 125-mg/m² intravenous infusion (30 min).

References: Chabot, G.G., Abigerges, D., Catimel, G., Culine, S., de Forni, M., Extra, J.M., Mahjoubi, M., Herait, P., Armand, J.P., Bugat, R., Clavel, M., and Marty, M.E. Population pharmacokinetics and pharmacodynamics of irinotecan (CPT-11) and active metabolite SN-38 during phase I trials. Ann. Oncol., 1995, 6:141–151.
Physicians' Desk Reference, 54th ed. Medical Economics Co., Montvale, NJ, 2000, pp. 2412–2413.

AVAILABILITY (ORAL) (%)	URINARY EXCRETION (%)	BOUND IN PLASMA (%)	CLEARANCE $(ml \cdot min^{-1} \cdot kg^{-1})$	VOL. DIST. (liters/kg)	HALF-LIFE (hours)	PEAK TIME (hours)	PEAK CONCENTRATIONS
ISONIAZID (Chapter 48)							
—[a] ↓ Food	RA: 7 ± 2[b,c] SA: 29 ± 5[b,c]	~0	RA: 7.4 ± 2.0[c,d] SA: 3.7 ± 1.1[c,d] ←→ Aged ↓ RD[e]	0.67 ± 0.15[d] ←→ Aged, RD	RA: 1.1 ± 0.1[c] SA: 3.1 ± 1.1[c] ↑ AVH, Cirr, Neo, RD ←→ Aged, Obes, Child, HTh	RA: 1.1 ± 0.5[f] SA: 1.1 ± 0.6[f]	RA: 5.4 ± 2.0 μg/ml[f] SA: 7.1 ± 1.9 μg/ml[f]

[a] It is usually stated that isoniazid is completely absorbed; however, good estimates of possible loss due to first-pass metabolism are not available. Absorption is decreased by food and antacids.

[b] After oral administration; assay includes unchanged drug and acid-labile hydrazones. Higher percentages have been noted after intravenous administration, suggesting significant first-pass metabolism.

[c] Metabolized by N-acetyltransferase 2 (polymorphic). Data for slow acetylators (SA) and rapid acetylators (RA) reported.

[d] CL/F and V_{ss}/F reported.

[e] Decrease in CL_{NR}/F as well as CL_R.

[f] Following a single 400-mg oral dose to healthy rapid and slow acetylators.

Reference: Kim, Y.G., Shin, J.G., Shin, S.G., Jang, I.J., Kim, S., Lee, J.S., Han, J.S., and Cha, Y.N. Decreased acetylation of isoniazid in chronic renal failure. Clin. Pharmacol. Ther., 1993, 54:612–620.

ISOSORBIDE DINITRATE[a] (Chapter 32)

Oral: 22 ± 14[b,c] SL: 45 ± 16[b] PC: 33 ± 17[b]	<1	28 ± 12	3.1 (2.2–8.6)[d]	46 (38–59)[d,e] → Cirr ←→ Smk, RD, Fem, CHF	0.7 (0.6–2.0)[e] ←→ RD, Fem	IR Formulation[f] ISDN: 0.3 (0.2–0.5) IS-2-MN: 0.6 (0.2–1.6) IS-5-MN: 0.7 (0.3–1.9) SR Formulation[f] ISDN: ~0 IS-2-MN: 2.8 (2.7–3.7) IS-5-MN: 5.1 (4.2–6.6)	IR Formulation[f] ISDN: 42 (59–166) nM IS-2-MN: 207 (197–335) nM IS-5-MN: 900 (790–1080) nM SR Formulation[f] ISDN: ~0 IS-2-MN: 28 (23–33) nM IS-5-MN: 175 (154–267) nM

[a] Isosorbide dinitrate is metabolized to the 2- and 5-mononitrates. Both metabolites and the parent compound are thought to be active. Values for the dinitrate are reported.

[b] Bioavailability calculations from single dose. SL, sublingual; PC, percutaneous.

[c] ←→ CHF, RD, Smk; ↑ Cirr.

[d] Calculated assuming a 70-kg body weight.

[e] CL may be decreased and half-life prolonged after chronic dosing.

[f] Mean (range) for isosorbide dinitrate (ISDN) and isosorbide 2-mononitrate (IS-2-MN) and isosorbide-5-mononitrate (IS-5-MN) following a single 20-mg oral immediate release (IR) and sustained release (SR) dose.

References: Abshagen, U., Betzien, G., Endele, R., Kaufmann, B., and Neugebauer, G. Pharmacokinetics and metabolism of isosorbide-dinitrate after intravenous and oral administration. Eur. J. Clin. Pharmacol., 1985, 27:637–644.

Fung, H.L. Pharmacokinetics and pharmacodynamics of organic nitrates. Am. J. Cardiol., 1987, 60:4H–9H.

ISOSORBIDE 5-MONONITRATE[a] (ISOSORBIDE NITRATE) (Chapter 32)

93 ± 13 ←→ Cirr, RD, Aged, CAD	0	<5	1.80 ± 0.24 ←→ Cirr, RD, Aged, CAD	0.73 ± 0.09 ←→ Cirr, RD, MI, Aged, CAD	4.9 ± 0.8 ←→ Cirr, RD, MI, Aged, CAD	1–1.5[b]	314–2093 nM[b]

[a] Active metabolite of isosorbide dinitrate.

[b] Mean C_{max} following a 20-mg oral dose given by asymmetric dosing (0 and 7 hours) for 4 days. Effective concentration is ~500 nM.

Reference: Abshagen, U.W. Pharmacokinetics of isosorbide mononitrate. Am. J. Cardiol., 1992, 70:61G–66G.

Key: Unless otherwise indicated by a specific footnote, the data are presented for the study population as a mean value ± 1 standard deviation, a mean and range (lowest–highest in parenthesis) of values, a range of the lowest–highest values, or a single mean value.

ADH = alcohol dehydrogenase; Aged = aged; AIDS = acquired immunodeficiency syndrome; Alb = hypoalbuminemia; Atr Fib = atrial fibrillation; AVH = acute viral hepatitis; Burn = burn patients; C_{max} = peak concentration; CAD = coronary artery disease; Celiac = celiac disease; CF = cystic fibrosis; CHF = congestive heart failure; Child = children; Cirr = hepatic cirrhosis; COPD = chronic obstructive pulmonary disease; CP = cor pulmonale; CPBS = cardiopulmonary bypass surgery; CRI = chronic respiratory insufficiency; Crohn = Crohn's disease; Cush = Cushing's syndrome; CYP = cytochrome P450; Fem = female; Hep = hepatitis; HIV = human immunodeficiency virus; HL = hyperlipoproteinemia; HTh = hyperthyroid; IM = intramuscular; Inflam = inflammation; IV = intravenous; LD = liver disease; LTh = hypothyroid; MAO = monoamine oxidase; MI = myocardial infarction; NAT = N-acetyltransferase; Neo = neonate; NIDDM = non-insulin-dependent diabetes mellitus; NS = nephrotic syndrome; Obes = obese; Pneu = pneumonia; Preg = pregnant; Prem = premature; RA = rheumatoid arthritis; RD = renal disease (including uremia); SC = subcutaneous; Smk = smoking; ST = sulfotransferase; T_{max} = peak time; Tach = ventricular tachycardia; UGT = UDP-glucuronosyl transferase; Ulcer = ulcer patients. Other abbreviations are defined in the text section of this appendix.

Table A-II-1
PHARMACOKINETIC DATA (Continued)

	AVAILABILITY (ORAL) (%)	URINARY EXCRETION (%)	BOUND IN PLASMA (%)	CLEARANCE (ml·min⁻¹·kg⁻¹)	VOL. DIST. (liters/kg)	HALF-LIFE (hours)	PEAK TIME (hours)	PEAK CONCENTRATIONS
ISRADIPINE[a] (Chapters 32, 33)								
	19 ± 7 ↑ Aged, Cirr	0	97[b]	10 ± 1[c] ↓ Cirr, Aged → RD	4.0 ± 1.9[c]	8 ± 5 ↑ Cirr, Aged	Y: 0.9[d] E: 1.1[d]	Y: 8.2 ng/ml[d] E: 11.1 ng/ml[d]

[a] Racemic mixture; the S-enantiomer is 160-fold more active than the R-enantiomer.
[b] Blood-to-plasma concentration ratio = 0.24.
[c] Assuming a 70-kg body weight.
[d] Mean levels following a 5-mg oral dose (capsule), twice a day for 21 days in young (Y) and elderly (E) hypertensive subjects.

Reference: Fitton, A., and Benfield, P. Isradipine. A review of its pharmacodynamic and pharmacokinetic properties, and therapeutic use in cardiovascular disease. *Drugs*, **1990**, *40:*31–74.

	AVAILABILITY (ORAL) (%)	URINARY EXCRETION (%)	BOUND IN PLASMA (%)	CLEARANCE (ml·min⁻¹·kg⁻¹)	VOL. DIST. (liters/kg)	HALF-LIFE (hours)	PEAK TIME (hours)	PEAK CONCENTRATIONS
ITRACONAZOLE[a] (Chapter 49)								
	55 ↑ Food ↓ HIV[b]	<1	99.8	23 ± 10[c]	14 ± 5[d]	21 ± 6[e]	3–5[f]	649 ± 289 ng/ml[f] ↑ Food

[a] Itraconazole has an active metabolite, hydroxyitraconazole.
[b] Relative to oral dosing with food.
[c] *CL/F* reported. Clearance is concentration-dependent; the value given is for *CL/F* in the nonsaturable range. $K_m = 330 \pm 200$ ng/ml, $V_{max} = 2.2 \pm 0.8$ pg·ml⁻¹·min⁻¹·kg⁻¹. Apparent *CL/F* at steady state reported to be 5.4 ml·min⁻¹·kg⁻¹
[d] V_{area}/F reported. Does not appear to be concentration-dependent.
[e] Half-life for the non-saturable concentration range. $t_{1/2}$ at steady state reported to be 64 hours.
[f] Following a 200-mg oral dose, given daily for 4 days to adults.

References: Heykants, J., Michiels, M., Meuldermans, W., Monbaliu, J., Lavrijsen, K., Van Peer, A., Levran, J.C., Woestenborghs, R., and Cauwenbergh, G. The pharmacokinetics of itraconazole in animals and man. An overview. In, *Recent Trends in the Discovery, Development and Evaluation of Antifungal Agents.* (Fromtling, R.A., ed.) Prous Science Publisher, Barcelona, **1987**, pp. 223–249. Jalava, K.M., Olkkola, K.T., and Neuvonen, P.J. Itraconazole greatly increases plasma concentrations and effects of felodipine. *Clin. Pharmacol. Ther.*, **1997**, *61:*410–415.

	AVAILABILITY (ORAL) (%)	URINARY EXCRETION (%)	BOUND IN PLASMA (%)	CLEARANCE (ml·min⁻¹·kg⁻¹)	VOL. DIST. (liters/kg)	HALF-LIFE (hours)	PEAK TIME (hours)	PEAK CONCENTRATIONS
IVERMECTIN[a] (Chapter 42)								
	—	<1	93.1 ± 0.2	2.06 ± 0.81[b]	9.91 ± 2.67[b]	56.5 ± 7.5[b]	4.7 ± 0.5[c]	38.2 ± 5.8 ng/ml[c]

[a] Data from male and female patients treated for onchocerciasis. Metabolized by hepatic enzymes and excreted into bile.
[b] *CL/F*, V_{area}/F, and other parameters reported for oral dose. Terminal $t_{1/2}$ reported.
[c] Following a single 150-μg/kg oral dose (tablet).

References: Okonkwo, P.O., Ogbuokiri, J.E., Ofoegbu, E., and Klotz, U. Protein binding and ivermectin estimations in patients with onchocerciasis. *Clin. Pharmacol. Ther.*, **1993**, *53:*426–430. *Physicians' Desk Reference*, 54th ed. Medical Economics Co., Montvale, NJ, **2000**, p. 1886.

	AVAILABILITY (ORAL) (%)	URINARY EXCRETION (%)	BOUND IN PLASMA (%)	CLEARANCE (ml·min⁻¹·kg⁻¹)	VOL. DIST. (liters/kg)	HALF-LIFE (hours)	PEAK TIME (hours)	PEAK CONCENTRATIONS
KETOCONAZOLE[a] (Chapter 49)								
	—[a]	<1	99.0 ± 0.1	8.4 ± 4.1[b]	2.4 ± 1.6[b]	3.3 ± 1.0[b,c]	1–3[d]	3.2 (1.4–4.5) μM[d]

[a] Unknown because of lack of intravenous formulation. Bioavailability is diminished by hypochlorhydria (e.g., use of antacids, H₂-receptor antagonists).
[b] *CL/F*, V_{area}/F, and half-life reported for 200-mg daily doses given for more than 1 month. With single dose, *CL/F* and V_{area}/F are lower, and half-life is about 8 hours.
[c] Conflicting data from normal subjects suggest increased half-life with increasing dose and repeated dose.
[d] Mean (range) following a 200-mg oral dose, daily to steady state in patients with recalcitrant superficial mycotic infection. Average concentration at steady state was 0.51 ± 0.26 μM.

Reference: Badcock, N.R., Bartholomeusz, F.D., Frewin, D.B., Sansom, L.N., and Reid, J.G. The pharmacokinetics of ketoconazole after chronic administration in adults. *Eur. J. Clin. Pharmacol.*, **1987**, *33:*531–534.

KETOROLAC[a] (Chapter 27)

100 ± 20	5–10	99.2 ± 0.1[b]	0.50 ± 0.15 ↓ Aged, RD[c] ↔ Cirr	0.21 ± 0.04	5.3 ± 1.2 ↑ Aged, RD[c] ↔ Cirr	IM: 0.7–0.8[d] Oral: 0.3–0.9[d]	IM: 2.2–3.0 μg/ml[d] Oral: 0.8–0.9 μg/ml[d]

[a] Racemic mixture; S-(−)-enantiomer is much more active than the R-(+)-enantiomer. Following intramuscular injection, the mean AUC ratio for S/R enantiomers was 0.44 ± 0.04, indicating a higher clearance and shorter half-life for the S-(−)-enantiomer. Values reported are for the racemate.

[b] Blood-to-plasma concentration ratio = 0.50; i.e., no detectable cell partitioning.

[c] Probably due to the accumulation of glucuronide metabolite, which is hydrolyzed back to parent drug.

[d] Range of mean C_{max} and T_{max} from studies following a single 30-mg IM or 10-mg oral dose in healthy adults.

Reference: Brooks, D.R., and Jamali, F. Clinical pharmacokinetics of ketorolac tromethamine. Clin. Pharmacokinet., 1992, 23:415–427.

LAMIVUDINE[a] (Chapter 51)

86 ± 17	49–85	<36	4.95 ± 0.75 ↓ RD[b] ↔ Cirr ↑ Child[c]	1.30 ± 0.36	9.11 ± 5.09 ↑ RD[b] ↓ Child[c]	0.5–1.5[d]	1.0 (0.86–1.2) μg/ml[d]

[a] Data from healthy male subjects. No significant gender differences.

[b] CL/F decreased, moderate and severe renal impairment.

[c] Weight-normalized CL/F increased in children <12 years of age.

[d] Range of T_{max} and mean (95% CI) C_{max} following a single 100-mg oral dose (tablet).

References: Heald, A.E., Hsyu, P.H., Yuen, G.J., Robinson, P., Mydlow, P., and Bartlett, J.A. Pharmacokinetics of lamivudine in human immunodeficiency virus-infected patients with renal dysfunction. Antimicrob. Agents Chemother., 1996, 40:1514–1519.
Johnson, M.A., Moore, K.H., Yuen, G.J., Bye, A., and Pakes, G.E. Clinical pharmacokinetics of lamivudine. Clin. Pharmacokinet., 1999, 36:41–66.
Physicians' Desk Reference, 54th ed. Medical Economics Co, Montvale, NJ, 2000, p. 1172.
Yuen, G.J., Morris, D.M., Mydlow, P.K., Haidar, S., Hall, S.T., and Hussey, E.K. Pharmacokinetics, absolute bioavailability, and absorption characteristics of lamivudine. J. Clin. Pharmacol., 1995, 35:1174–1180.

LAMOTRIGINE[a] (Chapter 21)

97.6 ± 4.8	10	56	0.38–0.61[b,c] ↓ LD,[d] RD[e]	0.87–1.2	24–35[c] ↑ LD,[d] RD[e]	2.2 ± 1.2[f]	2.5 ± 0.4 μg/ml[f]

[a] Data from healthy adults and patients with epilepsy. No significant differences. Lamotrigine is eliminated primarily by glucuronidation. The parent-metabolite pair may undergo enterohepatic recycling. Range of mean values from multiple studies reported.

[b] CL/F increases slightly with multiple-dose therapy.

[c] CL/F increased and half-life decreased in patients receiving enzyme-inducing anticonvulsant drugs.

[d] CL/F reduced, moderate to severe hepatic impairment.

[e] CL/F reduced, severe renal disease.

[f] Following a single 200-mg oral dose.

References: Chen, C., Casale, E.J., Duncan, B., Culverhouse, E.H., and Gilman, J. Pharmacokinetics of lamotrigine in children in the absence of other antiepileptic drugs. Pharmacotherapy, 1999, 19:437–441.
Garnett, W.R. Lamotrigine: pharmacokinetics. J. Child Neurol., 1997, 12(suppl 1):S10–S15.
Physicians' Desk Reference, 54th ed. Medical Economics Co, Montvale, NJ, 2000, p. 1209.
Wootton, R., Soul-Lawton, J., Rolan, P.E., Fook Scheung, C.T.C., Cooper, J.D.H., and Posner, J. Comparison of the pharmacokinetics of lamotrigine in patients with chronic renal failure and healthy volunteers. Br. J. Clin. Pharmacol., 1997, 43:23–27.

Key: Unless otherwise indicated by a specific footnote, the data are presented for the study population as a mean value ± 1 standard deviation, a mean and range (lowest-highest in parenthesis) of values, a range of the lowest-highest values, or a single mean value.

ADH = alcohol dehydrogenase; Aged = aged; AIDS = acquired immunodeficiency syndrome; Alb = hypoalbuminemia; Atr Fib = atrial fibrillation; AVH = acute viral hepatitis; Burn = burn patients; C_{max} = peak concentration; CAD = coronary artery disease; Celiac = celiac disease; CF = cystic fibrosis; CHF = congestive heart failure; Child = children; Cirr = hepatic cirrhosis; COPD = chronic obstructive pulmonary disease; CP = cor pulmonale; CPBS = cardiopulmonary bypass surgery; CRI = chronic respiratory insufficiency; Crohn = Crohn's disease; Cush = Cushing's syndrome; CYP = cytochrome P450; Fem = female; Hep = hepatitis; HIV = human immunodeficiency virus; HL = hyperlipoproteinemia; HTh = hyperthyroid; IM = intramuscular; Inflam = inflammation; IV = intravenous; LD = liver disease; LTh = hypothyroid; MAO = monoamine oxidase; MI = myocardial infarction; NAT = N-acetyltransferase; Neo = neonate; NIDDM = non-insulin-dependent diabetes mellitus; NS = nephrotic syndrome; Obes = obese; Pneu = pneumonia; Preg = pregnant; Prem = premature; RA = rheumatoid arthritis; RD = renal disease (including uremia); SC = subcutaneous; Smk = smoking; ST = sulfotransferase; T_{max} = peak time; Tach = ventricular tachycardia; UGT = UDP-glucuronosyl transferase; Ulcer = ulcer patients. Other abbreviations are defined in the text section of this appendix.

Table A–II–1
PHARMACOKINETIC DATA (Continued)

AVAILABILITY (ORAL) (%)	URINARY EXCRETION (%)	BOUND IN PLASMA (%)	CLEARANCE ($ml \cdot min^{-1} \cdot kg^{-1}$)	VOL. DIST. (liters/kg)	HALF-LIFE (hours)	PEAK TIME (hours)	PEAK CONCENTRATIONS

LANSOPRAZOLE[a] (Chapter 37)

AVAILABILITY (ORAL) (%)	URINARY EXCRETION (%)	BOUND IN PLASMA (%)	CLEARANCE	VOL. DIST.	HALF-LIFE	PEAK TIME	PEAK CONCENTRATIONS
81 ± 22 Food[b]	<1	97 ↓ RD[c]	6.23 ± 1.60 ↓ Aged,[d] LD[e]	0.35 ± 0.05	0.90 ± 0.44 ↑ Aged, LD	1.3 ± 0.6[f]	248 ± 140 ng/ml[f] ↓ Food[b]

[a]Data from healthy male subjects. No significant gender differences.
[b]Food effect when taken 30 minutes after a meal.
[c]Increased free fraction, severe renal impairment. No dose change with once-daily dosing.
[d]CL/F reduced in elderly; no dose change required with once daily administration.
[e]CL/F reduced, severe hepatic impairment.
[f]Following a single 15-mg oral dose.

References: Delhotal-Landes, B., Flouvat, B., Duchier, J., Molinie, P., Dellatolas, F., and Lemaire, M. Pharmacokinetics of lansoprazole in patients with renal or liver disease of varying severity. *Eur. J. Clin. Pharmacol.*, 1993, 45:367–371.
Gerloff, J., Mignot, A., Barth, H., and Heintze, K. Pharmacokinetics and absolute bioavailability of lansoprazole. *Eur. J. Clin. Pharmacol.*, 1996, 50:293–297.
Physicians' Desk Reference, 54th ed. Medical Economics Co., Montvale, NJ, 2000, pp. 3105–3106.

LETROZOLE[a] (Chapters 52, 58)

AVAILABILITY (ORAL) (%)	URINARY EXCRETION (%)	BOUND IN PLASMA (%)	CLEARANCE	VOL. DIST.	HALF-LIFE	PEAK TIME	PEAK CONCENTRATIONS
99.9 ± 16.3	3.9 ± 1.4	60	0.58 ± 0.21 ↓ LD[b]	1.87 ± 0.46	45 ± 16	1.0[c]	115 nM[c]

[a]Data from healthy postmenopausal female subjects. Metabolized by CYP3A4 and CYP2A6.
[b]CL/F reduced, severe hepatic impairment.
[c]Median C_{max}, T_{max} following a single 2.5-mg oral dose (tablet).

References: Lamb, H.M., and Adkins, J.C. Letrozole. A review of its use in postmenopausal women with advanced breast cancer. *Drugs*, 1998, 56:1125–1140.
Sioufi, A., Gauducheau, N., Pineau, V., Marfil, F., Jaouen, A., Cardot, J.M., Godbillon, J., Czendlik, C., Howald, H., Pfister, C., and Vreeland, F. Absolute bioavailability of letrozole in healthy postmenopausal women. *Biopharm. Drug Dispos.*, 1997, 18:779–789.

LEVETIRACETAM[a] (Chapter 21)

AVAILABILITY (ORAL) (%)	URINARY EXCRETION (%)	BOUND IN PLASMA (%)	CLEARANCE	VOL. DIST.	HALF-LIFE	PEAK TIME	PEAK CONCENTRATIONS
~100	66	<10	0.96 ↓ RD,[b] Aged, LD[c] ↑ Child[d]	0.5–0.7	7 ± 1 ↑ RD,[b] Aged	0.5–1.0[e]	~10 μg/ml[e]

[a]Data from healthy adult subjects and patients with epilepsy. No significant gender differences.
[b]CL/F reduced, mild to severe renal impairment (cleared by hemodialysis).
[c]CL/F reduced, severe hepatic impairment.
[d]CL/F increased, 6 to 12 years of age.
[e]Estimated mean T_{max} and C_{max} following a single 500-mg dose given to healthy adults.

Reference: Physicians' Desk Reference, 55 ed. Medical Economics Co., Montvale, NJ, 2001, pp. 3206–3207.

LEVODOPA[a] (Chapter 22)

AVAILABILITY (ORAL) (%)	URINARY EXCRETION (%)	BOUND IN PLASMA (%)	CLEARANCE	VOL. DIST.	HALF-LIFE	PEAK TIME	PEAK CONCENTRATIONS
41 ± 16 ↑ Aged 86 ± 19[b] ⟷ Aged	<1	—	23 ± 4 ↓ Aged 9 ± 1[b] ↓ Aged	1.7 ± 0.4 ↓ Aged 0.9 ± 0.2[b] ↓ Aged	1.4 ± 0.4 ⟷ Aged 1.5 ± 0.3[b] ⟷ Aged	Y: 1.4 ± 0.7[c] E: 1.4 ± 0.7[c]	Y: 1.7 ± 0.8 μg/ml[c] E: 1.9 ± 0.6 μg/ml[c]

[a]Naturally occurring precursor to dopamine.
[b]Values obtained with concomitant carbidopa (inhibitor of dopa decarboxylase).
[c]Following a single 125-mg oral dose of levodopa given with carbidopa (100 mg 1 hour prior to and 50 mg 6 hours after levodopa) in young (Y) and elderly (E) subjects.

Reference: Robertson, D.R., Wood, N.D., Everest, H., Monks, K., Waller, D.G., Renwick, A.G., and George, C.F. The effect of age on the pharmacokinetics of levodopa administered alone and in the presence of carbidopa. *Br. J. Clin. Pharmacol.*, 1989, 28:61–69.

LEVOFLOXACIN[a] (Chapter 44)

99 ± 10	61–87	24–38	2.52 ± 0.45 ↓RD[b]	1.36 ± 0.21	7 ± 1 ↑RD[b]	1.6 ± 0.8[c]	4.5 ± 0.9 µg/ml[c]

[a] Data from healthy adult male subjects. Gender and age differences related to renal function.
[b] CL/F reduced, mild to severe renal impairment (not cleared by hemodialysis).
[c] Following a single 500-mg oral dose. No significant accumulation with once-daily dosing.

References: Chien, S.C., Rogge, M.C., Gisclon, L.G., Curtin, C., Wong, F., Natarajan, J., Williams, R.R., Fowler, C.L., Cheung, W.K., and Chow, A.T. Pharmacokinetic profile of levofloxacin following once-daily 500-milligram oral or intravenous doses. *Antimicrob. Agents Chemother.,* **1997,** *41:*2256–2260.

Fish, D.N., and Chow, A.T. The clinical pharmacokinetics of levofloxacin. *Clin. Pharmacokinet.,* **1997,** *32:*101–119.

Physicians' Desk Reference, 54th ed. Medical Economics Co., Montvale, NJ, **2000,** p. 2157.

LIDOCAINE[a] (Chapter 35)

35 ± 11[b] ↑ Cirr, Aged	2 ± 1 ↑ Neo	70 ± 5 ↓ Neo ↑ MI, CPBS, Aged, RD ↔ NS, Smk, Child	9.2 ± 2.4[c] ↓ CHF, Cirr, CPBS,[d] Obes, Aged[f] ↑ Smk ↔ RD, AVH,[e] Neo,	1.1 ± 0.4 ↓ CHF, CPBS,[d] Cirr, Neo → RD, Aged, Obes	1.8 ± 0.4 ↑ Cirr, MI,[g] Neo, Obes ↓ RD, CPBS CHF[h]	—	2–5 µg/ml[i]

[a] Active metabolite, monoethylglycylxylidide (MEGX), is 60% to 80% as potent as lidocaine; concentrations reach 36 ± 26% of those of parent drug, but it is only 15 ± 3% protein bound.
[b] Preparations available only for parenteral administration because of extensive and variable first-pass metabolism.
[c] Formation of MEGX is catalyzed predominantly by CYP3A.
[d] Decrease (~40%) on day 3 after surgery; returns to normal by day 7.
[e] During acute phase, blood clearance was 13 ± 4 ml·min⁻¹·kg⁻¹, which increased to 20 ± 4 ml·min⁻¹·kg⁻¹ after recovery.
[f] Decreased clearance with increasing age noted in patients with MI.
[g] Half-life increased when infused longer than 24 hours, probably related to increased plasma binding.
[h] Short term, no change; long term, marked increase.
[i] Therapeutic range of blood concentrations for control of ventricular arrhythmias. Levels of 6–10 and >10 µg/ml cause occasional and frequent toxicity, respectively.

Reference: Nattel, S., Gagne, G., and Pineau, M. The pharmacokinetics of lignocaine and β-adrenoceptor antagonists in patients with acute myocardial infarction. *Clin. Pharmacokinet.,* **1987,** *13:*293–316.

LISINOPRIL (Chapters 31, 32, 34)

25 ± 20 ↓ CHF	88–100	0	4.2 ± 2.2[a] ↓ CHF, RD, Aged ↔ Fem	2.4 ± 1.4[a] ↔ Aged, RD	12[b] ↑ Aged, RD	~7[c]	50 (6.4–343) ng/ml[c]

[a] CL/F and V_{area}/F reported.
[b] Effective half-life to predict steady-state accumulation upon multiple dosing; a terminal half-life (tissue efflux) of 30 hours reported.
[c] Median (range) C_{max} following a 2.5- to 40-mg oral dose, daily to steady state in elderly patients with hypertension and varying degrees of renal function. EC_{90} for angiotensin converting enzyme inhibition is 27 ± 10 ng/ml.

Reference: Thomson, A.H., Kelly, J.G., and Whiting, B. Lisinopril population pharmacokinetics in elderly and renal disease patients with hypertension. *Br. J. Clin. Pharmacol.,* **1989,** *27:*57–65.

Key: Unless otherwise indicated by a specific footnote, the data are presented for the study population as a mean value ± 1 standard deviation, a mean and range (lowest–highest in parenthesis) of values, a range of the lowest–highest values, or a single mean value.

ADH = alcohol dehydrogenase; Aged = aged; AIDS = acquired immunodeficiency syndrome; Alb = hypoalbuminemia; Atr Fib = atrial fibrillation; AVH = acute viral hepatitis; Burn = burn patients; C_{max} = peak concentration; CAD = coronary artery disease; Celiac = celiac disease; CF = cystic fibrosis; CHF = congestive heart failure; Child = children; Cirr = hepatic cirrhosis; COPD = chronic obstructive pulmonary disease; CP = cor pulmonale; CPBS = cardiopulmonary bypass surgery; CRI = chronic respiratory insufficiency; Crohn = Crohn's disease; Cush = Cushing's syndrome; CYP = cytochrome P450; Fem = female; Hep = hepatitis; HIV = human immunodeficiency virus; HL = hyperlipoproteinemia; HTh = hyperthyroid; IM = intramuscular; Inflam = inflammation; IV = intravenous; LD = liver disease; LTh = hypothyroid; MAO = monoamine oxidase; MI = myocardial infarction; NAT = *N*-acetyltransferase; Neo = neonate; NIDDM = non-insulin-dependent diabetes mellitus; NS = nephrotic syndrome; Obes = obese; Pneu = pneumonia; Prem = premature; Preg = pregnant; RA = rheumatoid arthritis; RD = renal disease (including uremia); SC = subcutaneous; Smk = smoking; ST = sulfotransferase; T_{max} = peak time; Tach = ventricular tachycardia; UGT = UDP-glucuronosyl transferase; Ulcer = ulcer patients. Other abbreviations are defined in the text section of this appendix.

Table A–II–1
PHARMACOKINETIC DATA (Continued)

AVAILABILITY (ORAL) (%)	URINARY EXCRETION (%)	BOUND IN PLASMA (%)	CLEARANCE ($ml \cdot min^{-1} \cdot kg^{-1}$)	VOL. DIST. (liters/kg)	HALF-LIFE (hours)	PEAK TIME (hours)	PEAK CONCENTRATIONS
LITHIUM (Chapter 20)							
100[a]	95 ± 15	0	0.35 ± 0.11[b] ↓ RD, Aged ↑ Preg ←→ Obes	0.66 ± 0.16 ↓ Obes	22 ± 8[c] ↑ RD, Aged ↓ Obes	IR: 0.5–3[d] SR: 2–6[d]	IR: 1–2 mM[d] SR: 0.7–1.2 mM[d]

[a]Values as low as 80% reported for some prolonged-release preparations.
[b]Renal clearance of Li⁺ parallels that of Na⁺. The ratio of clearances of Li⁺ and creatinine is about 0.2 ± 0.03.
[c]The distribution half-life is 5.6 ± 0.5 hours; this influences drug concentrations for at least 12 hours.
[d]Range of C_{max} and T_{max} following a single 0.7-mmol/kg oral dose of immediate release (IR) lithium carbonate and sustained release (SR) tablets.

Reference: Ward, M.E., Musa, M.N., and Bailey, L. Clinical pharmacokinetics of lithium. *J. Clin. Pharmacol.,* **1994,** *34:*280–285.

AVAILABILITY (ORAL) (%)	URINARY EXCRETION (%)	BOUND IN PLASMA (%)	CLEARANCE ($ml \cdot min^{-1} \cdot kg^{-1}$)	VOL. DIST. (liters/kg)	HALF-LIFE (hours)	PEAK TIME (hours)	PEAK CONCENTRATIONS
LORATADINE[a] (Chapter 25)							
—[b]	Negligible	97[c]	142 ± 57[d] ←→ RD ↓ Cirr	120 ± 80[d] ←→ RD	8 ± 6 ←→ RD ↑ Aged, Cirr	L: 2.0 ± 0[e] DL: 2.6 ± 2.9[e]	L: 3.4 ± 3.4 ng/ml[e] DL: 4.1 ± 2.6 ng/ml[e] ↑ Aged

[a]Active metabolite, descarboethoxyloratadine. Almost all patients achieve higher concentrations of the active metabolite (half-life = 18 ± 6 hours) than of the parent drug.
[b]Unknown, but probably low due to extensive CYP3A-dependent first-pass metabolism.
[c]Binding of the active metabolite is 73% to 77%.
[d]CL/F and V_{area}/F reported.
[e]Mean for loratadine (L) and descarboethoxyloratadine (DL) following a 10-mg oral dose (CLARITIN-D 24 HOUR), given daily for 7 days to healthy adults.

References: Haria, M., Fitton, A., and Peters, D.H. Loratadine. A reappraisal of its pharmacological properties and therapeutic use in allergic disorders. *Drugs,* **1994,** *48:*617–637.
Kosoglou, T., Radwanski, E., Batra, V.K., Lim, J.M., Christopher, D., and Affrime, M.B. Pharmacokinetics of loratadine and pseudoephedrine following single and multiple doses of once- versus twice-daily combination tablet formulations in healthy adult males. *Clin. Ther.,* **1997,** *19:*1002–1012.

AVAILABILITY (ORAL) (%)	URINARY EXCRETION (%)	BOUND IN PLASMA (%)	CLEARANCE ($ml \cdot min^{-1} \cdot kg^{-1}$)	VOL. DIST. (liters/kg)	HALF-LIFE (hours)	PEAK TIME (hours)	PEAK CONCENTRATIONS
LORAZEPAM (Chapters 17, 21)							
93 ± 10	<1	91 ± 2 ↓ Cirr, RD ←→ Aged, Burn	1.1 ± 0.4[a] ←→ Aged, Cirr, AVH, Smk, RD ↑ Burn, CF	1.3 ± 0.2[b] ↑ Cirr, Burn, CF, RD ←→ Aged, AVH	14 ± 5 ↑ Cirr, Neo, RD ←→ Aged, CPBS, AVH ↓ Burn	IM: 1.2[c] Oral: 1.2–2.6[c]	IV: ~75 ng/ml[c] IM: ~30 ng/ml[c] Oral: ~28 ng/ml[c]

[a]Eliminated primarily by glucuronidation.
[b]V_{area} reported.
[c]Following a single 2-mg IV bolus dose, IM dose, or oral dose, given to healthy adults.

Reference: Greenblatt, D.J. Clinical pharmacokinetics of oxazepam and lorazepam. *Clin. Pharmacokinet.,* **1981,** *6:*89–105.

LOSARTAN[a] (Chapters 31, 33)

L: 35.8 ± 15.5	L: 12 ± 2.8	L: 98.7 LA: 99.8	L: 8.1 ± 1.8 ↓ RD,[b] LD[c]	L: 0.45 ± 0.24	L: 2.5 ± 1.0 LA: 5.4 ± 2.3	L: 1.0 ± 0.5[d] LA: 4.1 ± 1.6[d]	L: 296 ± 217 ng/ml[d] LA: 249 ± 74 ng/ml[d]

[a]Data from healthy male subjects. Losartan (L) is metabolized primarily by CYP2C9 to an active metabolite, 5-carboxylic acid (LA).

[b]CL/F for L but not LA decreased, severe renal impairment (L/LA not removed by hemodialysis). No dose adjustment required.

[c]CL/F for L reduced, mild to moderate hepatic impairment. LA AUC also increased.

[d]Following a single 50-mg oral dose (tablet). Higher plasma levels of L but not LA in females than in males.

References: Lo, M.W., Goldberg, M.R., McCrea, J.B., Lu, H., Furtek, C.I., and Bjornsson, T.D. Pharmacokinetics of losartan, an angiotensin II receptor antagonist, and its active metabolite EXP3174 in humans. *Clin. Pharmacol. Ther.,* **1995,** *58:*641–649.

Physicians' Desk Reference, 54th ed. Medical Economics Co., Montvale, NJ, **2000,** pp. 1809–1812.

LOVASTATIN[a] (Chapter 36)

≤5 ↑ Food	10	>95	4.3–18.3[b] ↓ RD	—	1–4	AI: 2.0 ± 0.9[c] TI: 3.1 ± 2.9[c]	AI: 41 ± 6 ng-Eq/ml[c] TI: 50 ± 8 ng-Eq/ml[c]

[a]Lovastatin is an inactive lactone which is metabolized to the corresponding active β-hydroxy acid. Pharmacokinetic values are based on the sum of HMG-CoA reductase inhibition activity by the β-hydroxy acid and other less potent metabolites.

[b]The lactone (in equilibrium with β-hydroxy acid metabolite) is metabolized by CYP3A.

[c]Following an 80-mg oral dose, daily for 17 days. Peak levels represent total active inhibitors (AI) and total inhibitors (TI) of HMG-CoA reductase.

References: Corsini, A., Bellosta, S., Baetta, R., Fumagalli, R., Paoletti, R., and Bernini, F. New insights into the pharmacodynamic and pharmacokinetic properties of statins. *Pharmacol. Ther.,* **1999,** *84:*413–428.

Desager, J.P., and Horsmans, Y. Clinical pharmacokinetics of 3-hydroxy-3-methylglutaryl-coenzyme A reductase inhibitors. *Clin. Pharmacokinet.,* **1996,** *31:*348–371.

McKenney, J.M. Lovastatin: a new cholesterol-lowering agent. *Clin. Pharm.,* **1988,** *7:*21–36.

MEBENDAZOLE[a] (Chapter 42)

2–3[b]	1.1 ± 0.46	95	13.4 ± 2.6 LD[c]	1.23 ± 0.40	1.12 ± 0.24	5 ± 2[d]	70 ± 40 ng/ml[d] (≤30 ng/ml)[d]

[a]Data from male and female patients being treated for cystic hydatid disease.

[b]An oral bioavailability of 22% also has been reported.

[c]Blood levels of mebendazole are reportedly elevated in patients with liver disease.

[d]Following a single 10-mg/kg oral dose (100-mg, twice a day, for 3 days in parenthesis).

References: Braithwaite, P.A., Roberts, M.S., Allan, R.J., and Watson, T.R. Clinical pharmacokinetics of high dose mebendazole in patients treated for cystic hydatid disease. *Eur. J. Clin. Pharmacol.,* **1982,** *22:*161–169.

Dawson, M., Braithwaite, P.A., Roberts, M.S., and Watson, T.R. The pharmacokinetics and bioavailability of a tracer dose of [3H]-mebendazole in man. *Br. J. Clin. Pharmacol.,* **1985,** *19:*79–86.

Edwards, G., and Breckenridge, A.M. Clinical pharmacokinetics of anthelmintic drugs. *Clin. Pharmacokinet.,* **1988,** *15:*67–93.

Key: Unless otherwise indicated by a specific footnote, the data are presented for the study population as a mean value ± 1 standard deviation, a mean and range (lowest–highest in parenthesis) of values, a range of the lowest–highest values, or a single mean value.

ADH = alcohol dehydrogenase; Aged = aged; AIDS = acquired immunodeficiency syndrome; Alb = hypoalbuminemia; Atr Fib = atrial fibrillation; AVH = acute viral hepatitis; Burn = burn patients; C_{max} = peak concentration; CAD = coronary artery disease; Celiac = celiac disease; CF = cystic fibrosis; CHF = congestive heart failure; Child = children; Cirr = hepatic cirrhosis; COPD = chronic obstructive pulmonary disease; CP = cor pulmonale; CPBS = cardiopulmonary bypass surgery; CRI = chronic respiratory insufficiency; Crohn = Crohn's disease; Cush = Cushing's syndrome; CYP = cytochrome P450; Fem = female; Hep = hepatitis; HIV = human immunodeficiency virus; HL = hyperlipoproteinemia; HTh = hyperthyroid; IM = intramuscular; Inflam = inflammation; IV = intravenous; LD = liver disease; LTh = hypothyroid; MAO = monoamine oxidase; MI = myocardial infarction; NAT = N-acetyltransferase; Neo = neonate; NIDDM = non-insulin-dependent diabetes mellitus; NS = nephrotic syndrome; Obes = obese; Pneu = pneumonia; Preg = pregnant; Prem = premature; RA = rheumatoid arthritis; RD = renal disease (including uremia); SC = subcutaneous; Smk = smoking; ST = sulfotransferase; T_{max} = peak time; Tach = ventricular tachycardia; UGT = UDP-glucuronosyl transferase; Ulcer = ulcer patients. Other abbreviations are defined in the text section of this appendix.

Table A–II–1
PHARMACOKINETIC DATA (Continued)

AVAILABILITY (ORAL) (%)	URINARY EXCRETION (%)	BOUND IN PLASMA (%)	VOL. DIST. (liters/kg)	CLEARANCE (ml·min⁻¹·kg⁻¹)	HALF-LIFE (hours)	PEAK TIME (hours)	PEAK CONCENTRATIONS
MEDROXYPROGESTERONE[a] (Chapters 52, 58)							
<10[b]	—	—	—	Oral, High: 153 ± 77[c]	Oral, High: 30.1 ± 6.5[c]	Oral, Low: ~2[d] Oral, High: 3.4 ± 1.8[d] IM: ~3 weeks[d]	Oral, Low: 4.2–6.3 nM[d] Oral, High: 123 ± 74 nM[d] IM: 2.9–20.3 nM[d]

[a]Data from healthy pre- and postmenopausal female subjects.
[b]Bioavailability estimate is based on *AUC* data from oral and intraperitoneal (IP) administration.
[c]*CL/F* and half-life are reported for a high (500 mg) oral dose. Apparent $t_{1/2}$ for IM DEPO-PROVERA is ~50 days.
[d]Following a low (10 mg) and high (500 mg) oral dose and 150-mg intramuscular (IM) dose of DEPO-PROVERA.

References: Physicians' Desk Reference, 54th ed. Medical Economics Co., Montvale, NJ, **2000**, p. 2435.
Stalker, D.J., Welshman, I.R., and Pollock, S.R. Bioavailability of medroxyprogesterone acetate from three oral dosage formulations. *Clin. Ther.,* **1992**, *14*:544–552.
Stockdale, A.D., and Rostom, A.Y. Clinical significance of differences in bioavailability of medroxyprogesterone acetate preparations. *Clin. Pharmacokinet.,* **1989**, *16*:129–133.
Svensson, L.O., Johnson, S.H., and Olsson, S.E. Plasma concentrations of medroxyprogesterone acetate, estradiol and estrone following oral administration of Klimaxil, Trisequence/Provera and Divina. A randomized, single-blind, triple cross-over bioavailability study in menopausal women. *Maturitas,* **1994**, *18*:229–238.

AVAILABILITY (ORAL) (%)	URINARY EXCRETION (%)	BOUND IN PLASMA (%)	VOL. DIST. (liters/kg)	CLEARANCE (ml·min⁻¹·kg⁻¹)	HALF-LIFE (hours)	PEAK TIME (hours)	PEAK CONCENTRATIONS
MEFLOQUINE[a] (Chapter 40)							
—[b]	<1	98.2[c]	19 ± 6[d]	0.43 ± 0.14[d] ↑ Preg ←→ Child	20 ± 4 days ↓ Preg ←→ Child	SD: 7–19.6[e] MD: 12 ± 8[e]	SD: 800–1020 ng/ml[e] MD: 420 ± 141 ng/ml[e]

[a]Racemic mixture; no information on relative kinetics of the enantiomers.
[b]No information available; reported values of >85% represent comparison of tablet to solution.
[c]Blood-to-plasma concentration ratio ~1.0.
[d]*CL/F* and V_{ss}/F reported.
[e]Mean values from different studies following a single 1000-mg oral dose (SD), and mean following a 250-mg oral dose, once weekly for 4 weeks (MD).

Reference: Karbwang, J., and White, N.J. Clinical pharmacokinetics of mefloquine. *Clin. Pharmacokinet.,* **1990**, *19*:264–279.

AVAILABILITY (ORAL) (%)	URINARY EXCRETION (%)	BOUND IN PLASMA (%)	VOL. DIST. (liters/kg)	CLEARANCE (ml·min⁻¹·kg⁻¹)	HALF-LIFE (hours)	PEAK TIME (hours)	PEAK CONCENTRATIONS
MELPHALAN (Chapter 52)							
71 ± 23	12 ± 7	90 ± 5[a,b]	0.45 ± 0.15 ←→ Child	5.2 ± 2.9 ←→ Child	1.4 ± 0.2[c] ←→ Child	Oral: 0.75 ± 0.24[d]	IV: 1.3 ± 0.95 μg/ml[d] Oral: 0.31 ± 0.15 μg/ml[d]

[a]Decreases to 80 ± 5% after high doses (180 mg/m²).
[b]Blood-to-plasma concentration ratio = 0.96 ± 0.25.
[c]Approximately equal to the half-life of melphalan *in vitro* in human plasma at 37°C.
[d]Following a single 0.5-mg/kg IV or 25-mg oral dose in cancer patients.

Reference: Loos, U., Musch, E., Engel, M., Hartlapp, J.H., Hugl, E., and Dengler, H.J. The pharmacokinetics of melphalan during intermittent therapy of multiple myeloma. *Eur. J. Clin. Pharmacol.,* **1988**, *35*:187–193.

MEPERIDINE[a] (Chapter 23)

52 ± 3 ↑ Cirr	58 ± 9[c] ↓ Aged, RD ←→ Cirr	17 ± 5 ↓ AVH, Cirr, RD, Prem, Neo ←→ Aged, Preg, Smk	4.4 ± 0.9 ↑ Aged, Prem ←→ Cirr, Preg, RD	3.2 ± 0.8[d] ↑ AVH, Cirr, Prem, Neo, Aged, RD ←→ Preg	IM: <1[e]	IV: 0.67 μg/ml[e] IM: ~0.7 μg/ml[e]

[a] Meperidine undergoes P450-dependent N-demethylation to normeperidine. Metabolite is not an analgesic but is a potent CNS-excitatory agent and is associated with adverse side effects of meperidine.

[b] Meperidine is a weak base (pK_a = 8.6) and is excreted to a greater extent in the urine at low urinary pH and to a lesser extent at high urinary pH.

[c] Correlates with the concentration of α_1-acid glycoprotein.

[d] A longer half-life (7 hours) is also observed.

[e] Mean value following a continuous 24-mg/hr intravenous (IV) infusion or 100-mg intramuscular (IM) injection, every 4 hours to steady state. Postoperative analgesia occurs at 0.4–0.7 μg/ml.

Reference: Edwards, D.J., Svensson, C.K., Visco, J.P., and Lalka, D. Clinical pharmacokinetics of pethidine: 1982. *Clin. Pharmacokinet.,* **1982,** 7:421–433.

MERCAPTOPURINE[a] (Chapter 52)

12 ± 7[b]	22 ± 12	19	11 ± 4[c]	0.56 ± 0.38	0.90 ± 0.37	Oral (−): 2.4 ± 0.4[d] Oral (+): 2.8 ± 0.4[d]	IV: 6.9 μM[d] Oral (−): 0.74 ± 0.28 μM[d] Oral (+): 3.7 ± 0.6 μM[d]

[a] Inactive prodrug is metabolized intracellularly to 6-thioinosinate. Values are for prodrug.

[b] Increases to 60% when first-pass metabolism is inhibited by allopurinol (100 mg, three times a day).

[c] Metabolically cleared by xanthine oxidase and thiopurine methyltransferase (polymorphic). Despite inhibition of intrinsic clearance by allopurinol, hepatic metabolism is limited by blood flow, and clearance is thus little changed by allopurinol.

[d] Following an intravenous (IV) infusion of 50 mg/m² per hour to steady state in children with refractory cancers, or a single oral dose of 75 mg/m² with (+) or without (−) allopurinol pretreatment.

References: Lennard, L. The clinical pharmacology of 6-mercaptopurine. *Eur. J. Clin. Pharmacol.,* **1992,** 43:329–339.
Physicians' Desk Reference, 54th ed. Medical Economics Co., Montvale, NJ, **2000,** p. 1255.

METFORMIN[a] (Chapter 61)

52 ± 5 (40–55)	99.9 ± 0.5 (79–100)	Negligible	7.62 ± 0.30 (6.3–10.1) ↓ RD,[b] Aged	1.12 ± 0.08[c] (0.9–3.94)	1.74 ± 0.20[c] (1.5–4.5) ↑ RD,[b] Aged	1.9 ± 0.4[d] (1.5–3.5)[d]	1.6 ± 0.2 μg/ml[d] (1.0–3.1 μg/ml)[d]

[a] Data from healthy male and female subjects. No significant gender differences. Shown in parenthesis are mean values from different studies.

[b] CL/F reduced, mild to severe renal impairment.

[c] Larger volume of distribution (4 l/kg) and longer $t_{1/2}$ (4.5 hours) also reported.

[d] Following a single 0.5-g oral dose (tablet), and range for a 0.5- to 1.5-g oral dose.

References: Harrower, A.D. Pharmacokinetics of oral antihyperglycaemic agents in patients with renal insufficiency. *Clin. Pharmacokinet.,* **1996,** 31:111–119.
Pentikainen, P.J., Neuvonen, P.J., and Penttila, A. Pharmacokinetics of metformin after intravenous and oral administration to man. *Eur. J. Clin. Pharmacol.,* **1979,** 16:195–202.
Physicians' Desk Reference, 54th ed. Medical Economics Co., Montvale, NJ, **2000,** pp. 831–835.
Scheen, A.J. Clinical pharmacokinetics of metformin. *Clin. Pharmacokinet.,* **1996,** 30:359–371.

Key: Unless otherwise indicated by a specific footnote, the data are presented for the study population as a mean value ± 1 standard deviation, a mean and range (lowest–highest in parenthesis) of values, a range of the lowest–highest values, or a single mean value.

ADH = alcohol dehydrogenase; Aged = aged; AIDS = acquired immunodeficiency syndrome; Alb = hypoalbuminemia; Atr Fib = atrial fibrillation; AVH = acute viral hepatitis; Burn = burn patients; C_{max} = peak concentration; CAD = coronary artery disease; Celiac = celiac disease; CF = cystic fibrosis; CHF = congestive heart failure; Child = children; Cirr = hepatic cirrhosis; COPD = chronic obstructive pulmonary disease; CP = cor pulmonale; CPBS = cardiopulmonary bypass surgery; CRI = chronic respiratory insufficiency; Crohn = Crohn's disease; Cush = Cushing's syndrome; CYP = cytochrome P450; Fem = female; Hep = hepatitis; HIV = human immunodeficiency virus; HL = hyperlipoproteinemia; HTh = hyperthyroid; IM = intramuscular; Inflam = inflammation; IV = intravenous; LD = liver disease; LTh = hypothyroid; MAO = monoamine oxidase; MI = myocardial infarction; NAT = N-acetyltransferase; Neo = neonate; NIDDM = non-insulin-dependent diabetes mellitus; NS = nephrotic syndrome; Obes = obese; Pneu = pneumonia; Preg = pregnant; Prem = premature; RA = rheumatoid arthritis; RD = renal disease (including uremia); SC = subcutaneous; Smk = smoking; ST = sulfotransferase; T_{max} = peak time; Tach = ventricular tachycardia; UGT = UDP-glucuronosyl transferase; Ulcer = ulcer patients. Other abbreviations are defined in the text section of this appendix.

Table A–II–1
PHARMACOKINETIC DATA (Continued)

AVAILABILITY (ORAL) (%)	URINARY EXCRETION (%)	BOUND IN PLASMA (%)	CLEARANCE ($ml \cdot min^{-1} \cdot kg^{-1}$)	VOL. DIST. (liters/kg)	HALF-LIFE (hours)	PEAK TIME (hours)	PEAK CONCENTRATIONS
METHADONE[a] (Chapters 23, 24)							
92 ± 21	24 ± 10[b]	89 ± 2.9[c]	2.3 ± 1.2[b] ↑ Burn, Child	3.6 ± 1.2[d]	27 ± 12[d] ↓ Burn, Child	~3[e]	IV: 450–550 ng/ml[e] Oral: 69–980 ng/ml[e]
METHOTREXATE[a] (Chapters 52, 53)							
70 ± 27[b,c]	81 ± 9	46 ± 11	2.1 ± 0.8 ↓ RD ↑, ↔ Child ↔ RA	0.55 ± 0.19 ↔ Child	7.2 ± 2.1[d] ↔ RA	SC: 0.9 ± 0.2[e]	SC: 1.1 ± 0.2 μM[e] IV: 37–99 μM[e]
METHYLPHENIDATE[a] (Chapter 10)							
(+): 22 ± 8 (−): 5 ± 3	(+): 1.3 ± 0.5 (−): 0.6 ± 0.3	(+/−): 15–16	(+): 6.67 ± 2.00[b] (−): 12.2 ± 4.67[b] ↔ Child	(+): 2.65 ± 1.11 (−): 1.80 ± 0.91	(+): 5.96 ± 1.71 (−): 3.61 ± 1.12	(+): 2.4 ± 0.8[c] (−): 2.1 ± 0.6[c]	(+): 18.1 ± 4.3 ng/ml[c] (−): 3.0 ± 0.94 ng/ml[c]

METHADONE

[a] Racemic mixture; except for protein-binding measures (d-methadone slightly higher % bound), no kinetic parameters reported for individual enantiomers.
[b] CL_{blood} reported. Inversely correlated with urine pH.
[c] Blood-to-plasma concentration ratio = 0.75 ± 0.03.
[d] V_{urea} reported. Directly correlated with urine pH.
[e] Range of values following a single 10-mg IV bolus dose in patients with chronic pain or a 0.12–1.9-mg/kg oral dose, once daily for at least 2 months in subjects with opioid dependency. Levels >100 ng/ml prevent withdrawal symptoms; EC_{50} for pain relief and sedation in cancer patients is 350 ± 180 ng/ml.

References: Dyer, K.R., Foster, D.J., White, J.M., Somogyi, A.A., Menelaou, A., and Bochner, F. Steady-state pharmacokinetics and pharmacodynamics in methadone maintenance patients: comparison of those who do and do not experience withdrawal and concentration–effect relationships. *Clin. Pharmacol. Ther.*, **1999**, 65:685–694.
Inturrisi, C.E., Colburn, W.A., Kaiko, R.F., Houde, R.W., and Foley, K.M. Pharmacokinetics and pharmacodynamics of methadone in patients with chronic pain. *Clin. Pharmacol. Ther.*, **1987**, 41:392–401.

METHOTREXATE

[a] The 7-hydroxy metabolite exhibits concentrations approaching that of parent drug. Metabolite may have both therapeutic and toxic effects.
[b] Bioavailability may be as low as 20% when doses exceed 80 mg/m².
[c] Intramuscular bioavailability is only slightly higher.
[d] A shorter half-life (2 hours) is seen initially after dose administration; a longer (52 hours) terminal half-life has been observed with increased assay sensitivity.
[e] Following a 15-mg subcutaneous (SC) dose, given once weekly to steady state in adult patients with inflammatory bowel disease. Initial steady-state concentrations in young (1.5 to 22 years old) leukemia patients receiving a 500-mg/m² loading dose given over 1 hour followed by an infusion of 196 mg/m² per hour for 5 hours. Bone marrow toxicity associated with concentrations >10 μM at 24 hours, >1 μM at 48 hours, or >0.1 μM at 72 hours after the dose.

References: Egan, L.J., Sandborn, W.J., Mays, D.C., Tremaine, W.J., Fauq, A.H., and Lipsky, J.J. Systemic and intestinal pharmacokinetics of methotrexate in patients with inflammatory bowel disease. *Clin. Pharmacol. Ther.*, **1999**, 65:29–39.
Tracy, T.S., Worster, T., Bradley, J.D., Greene, P.K., and Brater, D.C. Methotrexate disposition following concomitant administration of ketoprofen, piroxicam and flurbiprofen in patients with rheumatoid arthritis. *Br. J. Clin. Pharmacol.*, **1994**, 37:453–456.
Wall, A.M., Gajjar, A., Link, A., Mahmoud, H., Pui, C.H., and Relling, M.V. Individualized methotrexate dosing in children with relapsed acute lymphoblastic leukemia. *Leukemia*, **2000**, 14:221–225.

METHYLPHENIDATE

[a] Data from healthy adult male subjects. No significant gender differences. Dosed as a racemate; the (+) enantiomer is more potent than the (−) antipode. Methylphenidate is extensively metabolized, primarily through ester hydrolysis.
[b] The (+) enantiomer exhibits dose-dependent kinetics, with a ~50% reduction in CL/F between a 10- and 40-mg dose.
[c] Following a single 40-mg oral dose (immediate release). Longer peak time (3 to 5 hours) and lower peak concentration reported for sustained-release oral formulation.

References: Aoyama, T., Kotaki, H., Sasaki, T., Sawada, Y., Honda, Y., and Iga, T. Nonlinear kinetics of threo-methylphenidate enantiomers in a patient with narcolepsy and in healthy volunteers. *Eur. J. Clin. Pharmacol.*, **1993**, 44:79–84.
Kimko, H.C., Cross, J.T., and Abernethy, D.R. Pharmacokinetics and clinical effectiveness of methylphenidate. *Clin. Pharmacokinet.*, **1999**, 37:457–470.
Physicians' Desk Reference, 54th ed. Medical Economics Co., Montvale, NJ, **2000**, pp. 2040–2041.
Srinivas, N.R., Hubbard, J.W., Korchinski, E.D., and Midha, K.K. Enantioselective pharmacokinetics of dl-threo-methylphenidate in humans. *Pharm. Res.*, **1993**, 10:14–21.

METHYLPREDNISOLONE (Chapter 60)

82 ± 13[a]	4.9 ± 2.3 ←→ Cirr	78 ± 3 ←→ Fem ↓ Cirr	6.2 ± 0.9 ←→ NS, RA, CRI, Cirr ↓ Obes ↑ Fem	1.2 ± 0.2 ←→ NS, RA, CRI, Fem, Cirr ↓ Obes	2.3 ± 0.5 ←→ NS, RD, RA, CRI, Cirr ↓ Obes ↓ Fem	Oral: 1.64 ± 0.64[b]	IV: 225 ± 44 ng/ml[b] Oral: 178 ± 44 ng/ml[b]

[a] May be decreased to 50% to 60% with high doses.

[b] Mean at 1 hour following a 28-mg IV infusion (20 min), given twice a day for 6 ± 4 days during the perioperative period following kidney transplantation. Mean following a 24-mg oral dose, given twice a day for three days in healthy adult male subjects. IC_{50} for basophil (histamine) trafficking is 14 ± 11 ng/ml; IC_{50} for helper T-cell trafficking is 20 ± 15 ng/ml.

References: Lew, K.H., Ludwig, E.A., Milad, M.A., Donovan, K., Middleton, E., Jr., Ferry, J.J., and Jusko, W.J. Gender-based effects on methylprednisolone pharmacokinetics and pharmacodynamics. *Clin. Pharmacol. Ther.,* **1993,** *54:*402–414.

Rohatagi, S., Barth, J., Mollmann, H., Hochhaus, G., Soldner, A., Mollmann, C., and Derendorf, H. Pharmacokinetics of methylprednisolone and prednisolone after single and multiple oral administration. *J. Clin. Pharmacol.,* **1997,** *37:*916–925.

Tornatore, K.M., Reed, K.A., and Venuto, R.C. Methylprednisolone and cortisol metabolism during the early post-renal transplant period. *Clin. Transplant.,* **1995,** *9:*427–432.

METOCLOPRAMIDE (Chapter 38)

76 ± 38 ←→ Aged, Cirr	20 ± 9	40 ± 4 ←→ RD	6.2 ± 1.3 ↓ RD, Cirr ↑ Neo ←→ Aged	3.4 ± 1.3 ←→ RD, Cirr, Aged ↑ Neo	5.0 ± 1.4 ↑ RD, Cirr ←→ Aged	A: ≤1[a] I: 2.5 ± 0.7[a]	A: 80 ng/ml[a] I: 18 ± 6.2 ng/ml[a]

[a] Mean C_{max} following a single 20-mg oral dose given to healthy adults (A), or mean following an oral (nasogastric) dose of 0.10 to 0.15 mg/kg given four times a day to steady state to premature infants (I), 1 to 7 weeks of age (26 to 36 weeks, postconceptional).

References: Kearns, G.L., van den Anker, J.N., Reed, M.D., and Blumer, J.L. Pharmacokinetics of metoclopramide in neonates. *J. Clin. Pharmacol.,* **1998,** *38:*122–128.

Lauritsen, K., Laursen, L.S., and Rask-Madsen, J. Clinical pharmacokinetics of drugs used in the treatment of gastrointestinal diseases (Part I). *Clin. Pharmacokinet.,* **1990,** *19:*11–31.

Rotmensch, H.H., Mould, G.P., Sutton, J.A., Kilminster, S., Moller, C., and Pero, R.W. Comparative central nervous system effects and pharmacokinetics of neo-metoclopramide and metoclopramide in healthy volunteers. *J. Clin. Pharmacol.,* **1997,** *37:*222–228.

Key: Unless otherwise indicated by a specific footnote, the data are presented for the study population as a mean value ± 1 standard deviation, a mean and range (lowest–highest in parenthesis) of values, a range of the lowest–highest values, or a single mean value.

ADH = alcohol dehydrogenase; Aged = aged; AIDS = acquired immunodeficiency syndrome; Alb = hypoalbuminemia; Atr Fib = atrial fibrillation; AVH = acute viral hepatitis; Burn = burn patients; C_{max} = peak concentration; CAD = coronary artery disease; Celiac = celiac disease; CF = cystic fibrosis; CHF = congestive heart failure; Child = children; Cirr = hepatic cirrhosis; COPD = chronic obstructive pulmonary disease; CP = cor pulmonale; CPBS = cardiopulmonary bypass surgery; CRI = chronic respiratory insufficiency; Crohn = Crohn's disease; Cush = Cushing's syndrome; CYP = cytochrome P450; Fem = female; Hep = hepatitis; HIV = human immunodeficiency virus; HL = hyperlipoproteinemia; HTh = hyperthyroid; IM = intramuscular; Inflam = inflammation; IV = intravenous; LD = liver disease; LTh = hypothyroid; MAO = monoamine oxidase; MI = myocardial infarction; NAT = N-acetyltransferase; Neo = neonate; NIDDM = non-insulin-dependent diabetes mellitus; NS = nephrotic syndrome; Obes = obese; Pneu = pneumonia; Preg = pregnant; Prem = premature; RA = rheumatoid arthritis; RD = renal disease (including uremia); SC = subcutaneous; Smk = smoking; ST = sulfotransferase; T_{max} = peak time; Tach = ventricular tachycardia; UGT = UDP-glucuronosyl transferase; Ulcer = ulcer patients. Other abbreviations are defined in the text section of this appendix.

Table A-II-1
PHARMACOKINETIC DATA (Continued)

	AVAILABILITY (ORAL) (%)	URINARY EXCRETION (%)	BOUND IN PLASMA (%)	CLEARANCE ($ml \cdot min^{-1} \cdot kg^{-1}$)	VOL. DIST. (liters/kg)	HALF-LIFE (hours)	PEAK TIME (hours)	PEAK CONCENTRATIONS
METOPROLOL[a] (Chapter 10)								
	38 ± 14 ↑ Cirr ↑ Preg	10 ± 3	11 ± 1[b] ←→ Preg	15 ± 3[c] ↑ HTh, Preg ←→ Aged, Smk ↓ Fem	4.2 ± 0.7 ↑ Preg ↓ Fem	3.2 ± 0.2 ↑ Cirr, Neo ←→ Aged, HTh, Preg, Smk	EM: ~2[d] PM: ~3[d]	EM: 99 ± 53 ng/ml[d] PM: 262 ± 29 ng/ml[d]
METRONIDAZOLE[a] (Chapter 41)								
	99 ± 8[b] ←→ Crohn	10 ± 2	11 ± 3	1.3 ± 0.3 ↓ Cirr, Neo ←→ Preg, RD, Crohn, Aged	0.74 ± 0.10 ←→ RD, Crohn, Cirr	8.5 ± 2.9 ↑ Neo, Cirr ←→ Preg, RD, Crohn, Child	Oral: 2.8[c] VA: 11 ± 2[c]	IV: 27 (11–41) μg/ml[c] Oral: 19.8 μg/ml[c] VA: 1.9 ± 0.2 μg/ml[c]
MEXILETINE[a] (Chapter 35)								
	87 ± 13	4–15[b]	63 ± 3 ←→ MI	6.3 ± 2.7[c] ↑ MI, RD,[d] Cirr ←→ CHF, Aged	4.9 ± 0.5 ←→ MI	9.2 ± 2.1 ↑ MI, CHF, Cirr, RD[d] ←→ Aged ↓ Smk	IR: 1.7–3[e] SR: 4.3–9.2[e]	IR: 0.77–2.0 μg/ml[e] SR: 0.34–0.44 μg/ml[e]

METOPROLOL

[a] Data for racemic mixture reported. Metabolism of less active R-(+)-enantiomer (CL/F = 28 ml·min⁻¹·kg⁻¹; $t_{1/2}$ = 7.6 l/kg; $t_{1/2}$ = 2.7 hours) is slightly faster than that of more active S-(−)-enantiomer (CL/F = 20 ml·min⁻¹·kg⁻¹; V_{area}/F = 5.5 l/kg; $t_{1/2}$ = 3 hours).
[c] Blood-to-plasma concentration ratio = 1.
[c] Metabolically cleared by CYP2D6 (polymorphic). Compared to extensive metabolizers, individuals who are poor metabolizers will have an increased oral bioavailability, a longer half-life (7.6 ± 1.5 vs. 2.8 ± 1.2 hours), and excrete more unchanged drug in urine (15 ± 7 vs. 3.2 ± 3%) due to reduced hepatic metabolism.
[d] $C_{3 hours}$ following a single 100-mg oral dose in CYP2D6 extensive (EM) and poor (PM) metabolizer patients with hypertension. Plasma concentrations of the more active S-enantiomer are ~35% higher than the R-antipode in CYP2D6 EM. No stereochemical difference was observed in PM subjects. EC_{50} for decreased heart rate during peak submaximal exercise testing was 16 ± 7 ng/ml; EC_{50} for decreased systolic blood pressure during exercise testing was 25 ± 18 ng/ml.

References: Dayer, P., Leemann, T., Marmy, A., and Rosenthaler, J. Interindividual variation of beta-adrenoceptor blocking drugs, plasma concentration and effect: influence of genetic status on behaviour of atenolol, bopindolol and metoprolol. *Eur. J. Clin. Pharmacol.,* **1985,** 28:149–153.
Lennard, M.S., Silas, J.H., Freestone, S., Ramsay, L.E., Tucker, G.T., and Woods, H.F. Oxidation phenotype—a major determinant of metoprolol metabolism and response. *N. Engl. J. Med.,* **1982,** 307:1558–1560.
McGourty, J.C., Silas, J.H., Lennard, M.S., Tucker, G.T., and Woods, H.F. Metoprolol metabolism and debrisoquine oxidation polymorphism—population and family studies. *Br. J. Clin. Pharmacol.* **1985,** 20:555–566.

METRONIDAZOLE

[a] Active hydroxylated metabolite that accumulates in renal failure.
[b] Bioavailability is 67% to 82% for rectal suppositories, and 53 ± 16% for intravaginal gel.
[c] Following a single 500-mg dose of vaginal (VA) cream, a 500-mg IV infusion (20 min) three times a day to steady state, or a 500-mg oral dose three times a day to steady state.

Reference: Lau, A.H., Lam, N.P., Piscitelli, S.C., Wilkes, L., and Danziger, L.H. Clinical pharmacokinetics of metronidazole and other nitroimidazole anti-infectives. *Clin. Pharmacokinet.,* **1992,** 23:328–364.

MEXILETINE

[a] Racemic mixture; R-(−)-enantiomer has greater antiarrhythmic activity than S-(+)-enantiomer; only small differences in the disposition of enantiomers noted. Data for racemate shown.
[b] Dependent on urine pH.
[c] Metabolically cleared by CYP1A2 and CYP2D6 (polymorphic). Poor metabolizers exhibit a lower nonrenal clearance (28 vs. 13 l/hr) and longer half-life (13 vs. 9 hours) than extensive metabolizers.
[d] Observed only in patients with CL_{cr} <10 ml/min.
[e] Range of mean values from different studies following a single 400-mg immediate-release (IR) capsule or 360-mg sustained-release (SR) oral dose.

References: Labbe, L., and Turgeon, J. Clinical pharmacokinetics of mexiletine. *Clin. Pharmacokinet.,* **1999,** 37:361–384.
Monk, J.P., and Brogden, R.N. Mexiletine. A review of its pharmacodynamic and pharmacokinetic properties, and therapeutic use in the treatment of arrhythmias. *Drugs,* **1990,** 40:374–411.

MIDAZOLAM (Chapters 14, 17)

44 ± 17[a] ↑ Cirr	98 ↓ Aged, RD ↔ Smk, Cirr	<1%	6.6 ± 1.8[b] ↑ RD[c] ↔ Cirr, Neo ↓ Obes, Smk, Child	1.1 ± 0.6 ↑ Obes ↔ Cirr ↓ Neo	1.9 ± 0.6 ↑ Aged, Obes, Cirr ↔ Smk	Oral: 0.67 ± 0.45[d]	IV: 113 ± 16 ng/ml[d] Oral: 78 ± 27 ng/ml[d]

[a]Bioavailability appears to be dose-dependent; 35% to 67% at 15 mg, 28% to 36% at 7.5 mg, and 12% to 47% at 2-mg oral dose, possibly due to saturable first-pass intestinal metabolism.
[b]Undergoes extensive first-pass metabolism by intestinal and hepatic CYP3A. Metabolically cleared exclusively by CYP3A.
[c]Increased clearance due to increased plasma free fraction; unbound clearance is unchanged.
[d]Following a single 5-mg IV bolus dose or 10-mg oral dose.

References: Garzone, P.D., and Kroboth, P.D. Pharmacokinetics of the newer benzodiazepines. *Clin. Pharmacokinet.,* **1989,** *16:*337–364.
Thummel, K.E., O'Shea, D., Paine, M.F., Shen, D.D., Kunze, K.L., Perkins, J.D., and Wilkinson, G.R. Oral first-pass elimination of midazolam involves both gastrointestinal and hepatic CYP3A-mediated metabolism. *Clin. Pharmacol. Ther.,* **1996,** *59:*491–502.

MINOCYCLINE (Chapter 47)

95–100	76	11 ± 2	1.3 ± 0.2[a] ↓ HL	1.0 ± 0.3 ↓ HL	16 ± 2 ↔ Cirr, HL RD[b]	Oral: 2–4[c]	IV: 3.5 μg/ml[c] Oral: 2.3–3.5 μg/ml[c]

[a]V_{area} reported.
[b]In patients with reduced CL_{cr}, there is a tendency for half-life to increase. However, there is no accumulation of drug beyond that seen in normal subjects during repeated administration of minocycline to patients with CL_{cr} = 18–45 ml/min.
[c]Mean value following a single 200-mg IV infusion (1 hour) or range of values following a 100-mg oral dose given twice a day to steady state.

Reference: Saivin, S., and Houin, G. Clinical pharmacokinetics of doxycycline and minocycline. *Clin. Pharmacokinet.,* **1988,** *15:*355–366.

MIRTAZAPINE[a] (Chapter 19)

50 ± 10	85	—	9.12 ± 1.14[b] ↓ LD,[d] RD[e]	4.5 ± 1.7	16.3 ± 4.6[b,c] ↑ LD,[d] RD[e]	1.5 ± 0.7[f]	41.8 ± 7.7 ng/ml[f]

[a]Data from healthy adult subjects. Metabolized by CYP2D6 and CYP1A2 (8-hydroxy) and CYP3A (N-desmethyl, N-oxide).
[b]Women of all ages exhibit lower CL/F and longer $t_{1/2}$ than men.
[c]The $t_{1/2}$ of the (−)-enantiomer is approximately twice as long as the (+)-antipode; ~threefold higher blood concentrations (+ vs. −) are achieved.
[d]CL/F reduced, hepatic impairment.
[e]CL/F reduced, moderate to severe renal impairment.
[f]Following a 15-mg oral dose, once daily, to steady state.

References: Fawcett, J., and Barkin, R.L. Review of the results from clinical studies on the efficacy, safety and tolerability of mirtazapine for the treatment of patients with major depression. *J. Affect. Disord.,* **1998,** *51:*267–285.
Physicians' Desk Reference, 54th ed. Medical Economics Co, Montvale, NJ, **2000,** p. 2109.

Key: Unless otherwise indicated by a specific footnote, the data are presented for the study population as a mean value ± 1 standard deviation, a mean and range (lowest–highest in parenthesis) of values, a range of the lowest–highest values, or a single mean value.

ADH = alcohol dehydrogenase; Aged = aged; AIDS = acquired immunodeficiency syndrome; Alb = hypoalbuminemia; Atr Fib = atrial fibrillation; AVH = acute viral hepatitis; Burn = burn patients; C_{max} = peak concentration; CAD = coronary artery disease; Celiac = celiac disease; CF = cystic fibrosis; CHF = congestive heart failure; Child = children; Cirr = hepatic cirrhosis; COPD = chronic obstructive pulmonary disease; CP = cor pulmonale; CPBS = cardiopulmonary bypass surgery; CRI = chronic respiratory insufficiency; Crohn = Crohn's disease; Cush = Cushing's syndrome; CYP = cytochrome P450; Fem = female; Hep = hepatitis; HIV = human immunodeficiency virus; HL = hyperlipoproteinemia; HTh = hyperthyroid; IM = intramuscular; Inflam = inflammation; IV = intravenous; LD = liver disease; LTh = hypothyroid; MAO = monoamine oxidase; MI = myocardial infarction; NAT = N-acetyltransferase; Neo = neonate; NIDDM = non-insulin-dependent diabetes mellitus; NS = nephrotic syndrome; Obes = obese; Pneu = pneumonia; Preg = pregnant; Prem = premature; RA = rheumatoid arthritis; RD = renal disease (including uremia); SC = subcutaneous; Smk = smoking; ST = sulfotransferase; T_{max} = peak time; Tach = ventricular tachycardia; UGT = UDP-glucuronosyl transferase; Ulcer = ulcer patients. Other abbreviations are defined in the text section of this appendix.

Table A–II–1
PHARMACOKINETIC DATA (Continued)

AVAILABILITY (ORAL) (%)	URINARY EXCRETION (%)	BOUND IN PLASMA (%)	CLEARANCE ($ml \cdot min^{-1} \cdot kg^{-1}$)	VOL. DIST. (liters/kg)	HALF-LIFE (hours)	PEAK TIME (hours)	PEAK CONCENTRATIONS
MISOPROSTOL[a,b] (Chapters 26, 37)							
>80	<1	81–89	240 ± 100[c] ↓ RD[d] ⟷, ↓ Hep	14 ± 8[d] ⟷ RD	0.5 ± 0.4 ⟷, ↓ Hep ↑ RD[c]	0.4 ± 0.2[e] ↑ Food	674 ± 1010 pg/ml[e] ↓ Food

[a]Misoprostol contains approximately equal amounts of two diastereomers.
[b]Misoprostol is rapidly deesterified to misoprostol acid, the active metabolite. Pharmacokinetic values are presented for misoprostol acid.
[c]CL/F and V_{area}/F are reported for misoprostol acid.
[d]End-stage renal disease patients only; no change in patients with $CL_{cr} \geq 20$ ml/min.
[e]Mean values for misoprostol acid following a single 400-µg oral dose of misoprostol given to healthy adults. Absorption is delayed with a high-fat meal. No accumulation with multiple dosing.

References: Foote, E.F., Lee, D.R., Karim, A., Keane, W.F., and Halstenson, C.E. Disposition of misoprostol and its active metabolite in patients with normal and impaired renal function. *J. Clin. Pharmacol.*, **1995**, 35:384–389.
Monk, J.P., and Clissold, S.P. Misoprostol. A preliminary review of its pharmacodynamic and pharmacokinetic properties, and therapeutic efficacy in the treatment of peptic ulcer disease. *Drugs,* **1987**, 33:1–30.
Physicians' Desk Reference, 54th ed. Medical Economics Co., Montvale, NJ, **2000**, p. 2908.

AVAILABILITY (ORAL) (%)	URINARY EXCRETION (%)	BOUND IN PLASMA (%)	CLEARANCE ($ml \cdot min^{-1} \cdot kg^{-1}$)	VOL. DIST. (liters/kg)	HALF-LIFE (hours)	PEAK TIME (hours)	PEAK CONCENTRATIONS
MODAFINIL[a] (Chapter 10)							
≥80[b]	3.7 ± 15	60	0.88 ± 0.17[c] ↓ LD[d], Aged	0.78 ± 0.09[c]	10.5 ± 1.5 ↑ LD[d]	1.7 ± 0.9[e]	5.2 ± 0.8 µg/ml[e]

[a]Data from healthy female subjects. No significant gender differences. Dosed as a racemate; modafinil *d/l*-enantiomers exhibit similar pharmacological activity. Extensively metabolized by oxidative and UGT pathways.
[b]Bioavailability estimate based on low CL/F and 80% urinary recovery of radioactive dose.
[c]CL/F and V/F are reported for racemate. CL/F of *d*-enantiomer is ~threefold higher than that of *l*-enantiomer.
[d]CL/F reduced, moderate to severe hepatic impairment.
[e]Following a single oral 200-mg dose.

References: Physicians' Desk Reference, 54th ed. Medical Economics Co., Montvale, NJ, **2000**, p. 932.
Wong, Y.N., Simcoe, D., Hartman, L.N., Laughton, W.B., King, S.P., McCormick, G.C., and Grebow, P.E. A double-blind, placebo-controlled, ascending-dose evaluation of the pharmacokinetics and tolerability of modafinil tablets in healthy male volunteers. *J. Clin. Pharmacol.,* **1999**, 39:30–40.

AVAILABILITY (ORAL) (%)	URINARY EXCRETION (%)	BOUND IN PLASMA (%)	CLEARANCE ($ml \cdot min^{-1} \cdot kg^{-1}$)	VOL. DIST. (liters/kg)	HALF-LIFE (hours)	PEAK TIME (hours)	PEAK CONCENTRATIONS
MONTELUKAST[a] (Chapter 28)							
62	<0.2	>99	0.70 ± 0.17 ↓ Cirr[b] ⟷ Child[c]	0.15 ± 0.02	4.9 ± 0.6 ↑ Cirr[b]	3.0 ± 1.0[d]	542 ± 173 ng/ml[d]

[a]Data from healthy adult subjects. No significant gender differences. Montelukast is metabolized by CYP3A4 and CYP2C9.
[b]CL/F reduced by 41%, mild to moderate hepatic impairment with cirrhosis.
[c]Similar plasma profile with 5-mg chewable vs. 10-mg tablet in adults.
[d]Following single oral 10-mg dose.

References: Physicians' Desk Reference, 54th ed. Medical Economics Co., Montvale, NJ, **2000**, p. 1882.
Zhao, J.J., Rogers, J.D., Holland, S.D., Larson, P., Amin, R.D., Haesen, R., Freeman, A., Seiberling, M., Merz, M., and Cheng, H. Pharmacokinetics and bioavailability of montelukast sodium (MK-0476) in healthy young and elderly volunteers. *Biopharm. Drug Dispos.,* **1997**, 18:769–777.

MORPHINE[a] (Chapter 23)

Oral: 24 ± 12 IM: ~100	35 ± 2 ↓ AVH, Cirr, Alb	4 ± 5 14 ± 7[a]	24 ± 10 ↔ Aged, Cirr, Child[b] ↓ Neo, Burn, RD, Prem	1.9 ± 0.5 ↔ Cirr, RD, Child ↑ Neo, Prem	3.3 ± 0.9 ↔ Cirr, Neo ↓ RD	IM: 0.2–0.3[c] PO-IR: 0.5–1.5[c] PO-SR: 3–8[c]	IV: 200–400 ng/ml[c] IM: ~70 ng/ml[c] PO-IR: 10 ng/ml[c] PO-SR: 7.4 ng/ml[c]

[a]Active metabolite, morphine-6-glucuronide; $t_{1/2}$ = 4.0 ± 1.5 hours. Steady-state ratio of active metabolite to parent after oral dosing = 4.9 ± 3.8. In renal failure, $t_{1/2}$ increases to 50 ± 37 hours, resulting in significant accumulation of active glucuronide metabolite.

[b]Decreased in children undergoing cardiac surgery requiring inotropic support.

[c]Following a single 10-mg IV dose (bolus with 5-min blood sample), or a 10-mg/70 kg IM or a 10-mg/70 kg immediate-release oral (PO-IR) dose or a 50-mg sustained-release oral dose (PO-SR). Minimum analgesic concentration is 15 ng/ml.

References: Berkowitz, B.A. The relationship of pharmacokinetics to pharmacological activity: morphine, methadone and naloxone. *Clin. Pharmacokinet.,* **1976,** *1*:219–230. Glare, P.A., and Walsh, T.D. Clinical pharmacokinetics of morphine. *Ther. Drug Monit.,* **1991,** *13*:1–23.

MOXIFLOXACIN[a] (Chapter 44)

86 ± 1	39.4 ± 2.4	2.27 ± 0.24	2.05 ± 1.15	15.4 ± 1.2	2.0 (0.5–6.0)[b]	2.5 ± 1.3 μg/ml[b]

[a]Data from healthy adult male subjects. Moxifloxacin is metabolized by ST and UGT.

[b]Following a single oral 400-mg dose.

Reference: Stass, H., and Kubitza, D. Pharmacokinetics and elimination of moxifloxacin after oral and intravenous administration in man. *J. Antimicrob. Chemother.,* **1999,** *43*(suppl B):83–90.

MYCOPHENOLATE[a] (Chapter 53)

MM: ~0 MPA: 94	MPA: 97.5 ↓ RD[c]	MM: 120–163 MPA: 2.5 ± 0.4[b] ↓ RD[c] ↔ LD	MPA: 3.6–4[b]	MM: <0.033 MPA: 16.6 ± 5.8	MPA: 1.1–2.2[d]	MPA: 8–19 μg/ml[d]

and presumably is hydrolyzed by gut flora and reabsorbed as MPA.

Row also: MPA: <1

[a]Data from healthy adult male and female subjects and organ transplant patients. No significant gender differences. Mycophenolate mofetil (MM) is rapidly converted to the active mycophenolic acid (MPA) after IV and oral doses. Kinetic parameters refer to MM and MPA after a dose of MM. MPA metabolized by UGT to MPAG. MPA undergoes enterohepatic recycling; MPAG is excreted into bile and presumably is hydrolyzed by gut flora and reabsorbed as MPA.

[b]CL/F and V_{area}/F reported for MPA.

[c]Accumulation of MPA and MPAG and increased unbound MPA; severe renal impairment.

[d]Range of mean MPA C_{max} and T_{max} reported for different studies following a 1- to 1.75-g oral dose, twice a day, to steady state, in renal transplant patients.

References: Bullingham, R.E., Nicholls, A.J., and Kamm, B.R. Clinical pharmacokinetics of mycophenolate mofetil. *Clin. Pharmacokinet.,* **1998,** *34*:429–455. Bullingham, R., Shah, J., Goldblum, R., and Schiff, M. Effects of food and antacid on the pharmacokinetics of single doses of mycophenolate mofetil in rheumatoid arthritis patients. *Br. J. Clin. Pharmacol.,* **1996,** *41*:513–516.

Kriesche, H.U.M. Kaplan, B., Korecka, M., Mulgaonkar, S., Friedman, G., Brayman, K., and Shaw, L.M. MPA protein binding in uremic plasma: prediction of free fraction. *Clin. Pharmacol. Ther.,* **1999,** *65*:184.

Physicians' Desk Reference, 54th ed. Medical Economics Co., Montvale, NJ, **2000,** pp. 2617–2618.

Key: Unless otherwise indicated by a specific footnote, the data are presented for the study population as a mean value ± 1 standard deviation, a mean and range (lowest–highest in parenthesis) of values, a range of the lowest–highest values, or a single mean value.

ADH = alcohol dehydrogenase; Aged = aged; AIDS = acquired immunodeficiency syndrome; Alb = hypoalbuminemia; Atr Fib = atrial fibrillation; AVH = acute viral hepatitis; Burn = burn patients; C_{max} = peak concentration; CAD = coronary artery disease; Celiac = celiac disease; CF = cystic fibrosis; CHF = congestive heart failure; Child = children; Cirr = hepatic cirrhosis; COPD = chronic obstructive pulmonary disease; CP = cor pulmonale; CPBS = cardiopulmonary bypass surgery; CRI = chronic respiratory insufficiency; Crohn = Crohn's disease; Cush = Cushing's syndrome; CYP = cytochrome P450; Fem = female; Hep = hepatitis; HIV = human immunodeficiency virus; HL = hyperlipoproteinemia; HTh = hyperthyroid; IM = intramuscular; Inflam = inflammation; IV = intravenous; LD = liver disease; LTh = hypothyroid; MAO = monoamine oxidase; MI = myocardial infarction; NAT = N-acetyltransferase; Neo = neonate; NIDDM = non-insulin-dependent diabetes mellitus; NS = nephrotic syndrome; Obes = obese; Pneu = pneumonia; Preg = pregnant; Prem = premature; RA = rheumatoid arthritis; RD = renal disease (including uremia); SC = subcutaneous; Smk = smoking; ST = sulfotransferase; T_{max} = peak time; Tach = ventricular tachycardia; UGT = UDP-glucuronosyl transferase; Ulcer = ulcer patients. Other abbreviations are defined in the text section of this appendix.

Table A–II–1
PHARMACOKINETIC DATA (*Continued*)

AVAILABILITY (ORAL) (%)	URINARY EXCRETION (%)	BOUND IN PLASMA (%)	CLEARANCE ($ml \cdot min^{-1} \cdot kg^{-1}$)	VOL. DIST. (liters/kg)	HALF-LIFE (hours)	PEAK TIME (hours)	PEAK CONCENTRATIONS
NABUMETONE[a] (Chapter 27)							
35	<1	~99[b]	0.37 ± 0.25[c] ←→ Aged	0.79 ± 0.38[c] ←→ Aged	23 ± 4 ↑ RD ←→ Aged	Y: 4.1–5[d] E: 4–7.2[d]	Y: 22–52 μg/ml[d] E: 37–70 μg/ml[d]

[a]Nabumetone is a prodrug. Data are for the active metabolite, 6-methoxy-2-naphthylacetic acid (6-MNA) after administration of nabumetone.
[b]The percent unbound increased four- to fivefold over a concentration range of 0.05 to 100 μg/ml (99.8% vs. 99.2% bound).
[c]CL/F and V_{ss}/F reported; calculated assuming a 70-kg body weight. Following IV 6-MNA, CL is 0.04–0.07 $ml \cdot min^{-1} \cdot kg^{-1}$ and V_{ss} averages 0.11 l/kg. The higher values for CL and V_{ss} after oral dosing can be explained by the incomplete systemic availability of 6-MNA and saturable plasma protein binding.
[d]Range of mean values from different studies following a 1-g oral dose, given once daily for 7 to 14 days to young healthy adults (Y) and elderly patients with arthritis (E).

References: Davies, N.M. Clinical pharmacokinetics of nabumetone. The dawn of selective cyclo-oxygenase-2 inhibition? *Clin. Pharmacokinet.*, **1997**, 33:403–416.
Hyneck, M.L. An overview of the clinical pharmacokinetics of nabumetone. *J. Rheumatol.*, **1992**, 19(suppl 36):20–24.

AVAILABILITY (ORAL) (%)	URINARY EXCRETION (%)	BOUND IN PLASMA (%)	CLEARANCE ($ml \cdot min^{-1} \cdot kg^{-1}$)	VOL. DIST. (liters/kg)	HALF-LIFE (hours)	PEAK TIME (hours)	PEAK CONCENTRATIONS
NALBUPHINE (Chapter 23)							
11 ± 4 ↑ Aged	4 ± 2 ←→ Aged	50	29.7 ± 3.37 ↑ Child ←→ Aged	5.4 ± 1.4[a] ←→ Aged, Child	2.0 ± 0.45 ↓ Child ←→ Aged	Oral: 0.9 ± 0.4[b]	IV: ~70 ng/ml[b] Oral: 7.3 ± 4.3 ng/ml[b] ↑ Aged

[a]V_{urea} reported.
[b]Following a single 10-mg intravenous dose (5-min infusion) or a 30-mg oral dose to healthy adults.

Reference: Jaillon, P., Gardin, M.E., Lecocq, B., Richard, M.O., Meignan, S., Blondel, Y., Grippat, J.C., Bergnieres, J., and Vergnoux, O. Pharmacokinetics of nalbuphine in infants, young healthy volunteers, and elderly patients. *Clin. Pharmacol. Ther.*, **1989**, 46:226–233.

AVAILABILITY (ORAL) (%)	URINARY EXCRETION (%)	BOUND IN PLASMA (%)	CLEARANCE ($ml \cdot min^{-1} \cdot kg^{-1}$)	VOL. DIST. (liters/kg)	HALF-LIFE (hours)	PEAK TIME (hours)	PEAK CONCENTRATIONS
NALMEFENE[a] (Chapter 23)							
40	9.6 ± 4.9	34.4 ± 13.6	15 ± 4.5 ↓ Cirr,[b] RD[c]	8.0 ± 1.8 ↑ RD[c]	8.0 ± 2.2 ↑ Cirr,[b] RD[c]	Oral: 2.5 ± 0.58[d]	IV: 17 ± 6.3 ng/ml[d] Oral: 24 ± 11 ng/ml[d]

[a]Data from healthy adult male and female subjects. Metabolized primarily by UGT.
[b]Moderate to severe hepatic impairment.
[c]End-stage renal disease.
[d]Following a single 2-mg IV dose and a single 50-mg oral dose in healthy men.

References: Dixon, R., Gentile, J., Hsu, H.B., Hsiao, J., Howes, J., Garg, D., and Weidler, D. Nalmefene: safety and kinetics after single and multiple oral doses of a new opioid antagonist. *J. Clin. Pharmacol.*, **1987**, 27:233–239.
Frye, R.F., Matzke, G.R., Schade, R., Dixon, R., and Rabinovitz, M. Effects of liver disease on the disposition of the opioid antagonist nalmefene. *Clin. Pharmacol. Ther.*, **1997**, 61:15–23.

AVAILABILITY (ORAL) (%)	URINARY EXCRETION (%)	BOUND IN PLASMA (%)	CLEARANCE ($ml \cdot min^{-1} \cdot kg^{-1}$)	VOL. DIST. (liters/kg)	HALF-LIFE (hours)	PEAK TIME (hours)	PEAK CONCENTRATIONS
NALOXONE (Chapter 23)							
~2[a]	Negligible	—	22 ↑ Neo ←→ RD	2.1 ↑ Neo	1.1 ± 0.6[b] ←→ Neo	—	10 ± 1 ng/ml[c]

[a]Absorption is relatively complete (91%), but most of the dose is subject to hepatic first-pass metabolism.
[b]Short distribution $t_{1/2}$ of 4.8 (2 to 10) minutes may limit the duration of effect.
[c]Following a single 0.4-mg IV bolus dose (sample at 2 min) given to healthy adults.

References: Handal, K.A., Schauben, J.L., and Salamone, F.R. Naloxone. *Ann. Emerg. Med.*, **1983**, 12:438–445.
Ngai, S.H., Berkowitz, B.A., Yang, J.C., Hempstead, J., and Spector, S. Pharmacokinetics of naloxone in rats and in man: basis for its potency and short duration of action. *Anesthesiology*, **1976**, 44:398–401.

NAPROXEN (Chapter 27)

99[a]	5–6	99.7 ± 0.1[b] ↑ RD, Aged,[c] Cirr ↓ RA, Alb	0.13 ± 0.02[d] ↓ RD ↔ Aged,[c] Cirr,[c] ↑ RA	0.16 ± 0.02[d] ↑ RD, RA, Child ↔ Aged, Child	14 ± 1 ↔ RD, RA, Child ↑ Aged[c]	T-IR: 2–4[e] T-CR: 5[e] S: 2.2 ± 2.1[e]	T-IR: 37[e] T-CR: 94[e] S: 55 ± 14 μg/ml[e]

[a]Estimated bioavailability.

[b]Saturable plasma protein binding yields apparent nonlinear elimination kinetics.

[c]No change in total CL, but significant (50%) decrease in CL of unbound drug; it is thus suggested that dosing rate be decreased. A second study in elderly patients found decreased CL and decreased half-life with no change in percent bound.

[d]CL/F and V_{area}/F reported. Metabolically cleared by CYP2C9 (polymorphic) and CYP1A2.

[e]Following a single 250-mg dose of suspension (S), given orally to pediatric patients, or a 250-mg immediate-release tablet (T-IR) or a 500-mg controlled-release tablet (T-CR), given to adults.

Reference: Wells, T.G., Mortensen, M.E., Dietrich, A., Walson, P.D., Blasier, D., and Kearns, G.L. Comparison of the pharmacokinetics of naproxen tablets and suspension in children. J. Clin. Pharmacol. 1994, 34:30–33.

NARATRIPTAN[a] (Chapter 11)

M: 63 (54–72)[b] F: 74 (64–85)[b]	50	28–31	6.1 ↓ Aged, RD,[c] Cirr[d]	2.43–2.86	5–5.5 ↑ RD, Cirr	3[e]	M: 10.8 (9.4–12.3) ng/ml[e] F: 16.6 (13.1–21.0) ng/ml[e]

[a]Data from male (M) and female (F) subjects. Metabolized by multiple CYP isozymes.

[b]Geometric mean (95% CI).

[c]CL/F reduced, moderate renal impairment.

[d]CL/F reduced, moderate hepatic impairment.

[e]Geometric mean (95% CI) following a single 5-mg oral dose.

References: Dulli, D.A. Naratriptan: an alternative for migraine. Ann. Pharmacother. 1999, 33:704–711.

Fuseau, E., Baille, P., and Kempsford, R.D. A study to determine the absolute oral bioavailability of naratriptan. Cephalalgia. 1997, 17:417.

Physicians' Desk Reference, 54th ed. Medical Economics Co., Montvale, NJ, 2000, p. 1148.

NELFINAVIR[a] (Chapter 51)

20–80[b] ↑ Food	1–2	98–99	12.0 ± 7.2[c] ↑ Child[d]	2–7[c]	3–5[c]	3.0 ± 1.1[e]	3.2 ± 1.2 μg/ml[e] ↑ Food

[a]Data from healthy subjects and patients with HIV infection. No significant gender differences. Nelfinavir is metabolized by multiple cytochrome CYP isozymes, including CYP3A4.

[b]Absolute bioavailability is unknown; reported to vary between 20% to 80% when taken without or with food.

[c]CL/F, V_{ss}/F, and $t_{1/2}$ reported for oral dose.

[d]CL/F increased, children 2 to 7 years and 7 to 13 years of age.

[e]Following 750 mg three times a day for 28 days in adults.

References: Barry, M., Mulcahy, F., Merry, C., Gibbons, S., and Back, D. Pharmacokinetics and potential interactions amongst antiretroviral agents used to treat patients with HIV infection. Clin. Pharmacokinet. 1999, 36:289–304.

Pai, V.B., and Nahata, M.C. Nelfinavir mesylate: a protease inhibitor. Ann. Pharmacother. 1999, 33:325–339.

Physicians' Desk Reference, 54th ed. Medical Economics Co., Montvale, NJ, 2000, p. 483.

Key: Unless otherwise indicated by a specific footnote, the data are presented for the study population as a mean value ± 1 standard deviation, a mean and range (lowest–highest in parenthesis) of values, a range of the lowest–highest values, or a single mean value.

ADH = alcohol dehydrogenase; Aged = aged; AIDS = acquired immunodeficiency syndrome; Alb = hypoalbuminemia; Atr Fib = atrial fibrillation; AVH = acute viral hepatitis; Burn = burn patients; C_{max} = peak concentration; CAD = coronary artery disease; Celiac = celiac disease; CF = cystic fibrosis; CHF = congestive heart failure; Child = children; Cirr = hepatic cirrhosis; COPD = chronic obstructive pulmonary disease; CP = cor pulmonale; CPBS = cardiopulmonary bypass surgery; CRI = chronic respiratory insufficiency; Crohn = Crohn's disease; Cush = Cushing's syndrome; CYP = cytochrome P450; Fem = female; Hep = hepatitis; HIV = human immunodeficiency virus; HL = hyperlipoproteinemia; HTh = hyperthyroid; IM = intramuscular; Inflam = inflammation; IV = intravenous; LD = liver disease; LTh = hypothyroid; MAO = monoamine oxidase; MI = myocardial infarction; NAT = N-acetyltransferase; Neo = neonate; NIDDM = non-insulin-dependent diabetes mellitus; NS = nephrotic syndrome; Obes = obese; Pneu = pneumonia; Preg = pregnant; Prem = premature; RA = rheumatoid arthritis; RD = renal disease (including uremia); SC = subcutaneous; Smk = smoking; ST = sulfotransferase; T_{max} = peak time; Tach = ventricular tachycardia; UGT = UDP-glucuronosyl transferase; Ulcer = ulcer patients. Other abbreviations are defined in the text section of this appendix.

Table A–II–1
PHARMACOKINETIC DATA (Continued)

AVAILABILITY (ORAL) (%)	URINARY EXCRETION (%)	BOUND IN PLASMA (%)	CLEARANCE $(ml \cdot min^{-1} \cdot kg^{-1})$	VOL. DIST. (liters/kg)	HALF-LIFE (hours)	PEAK TIME (hours)	PEAK CONCENTRATIONS
NEOSTIGMINE (Chapter 8)							
—[a]	67	—	16.7 ± 5.4 ↓ RD	1.4 ± 0.5	1.3 ± 0.8 ↑ RD	—	200–350 ng/ml[b]

[a] Absorption is presumed to be less than complete, since oral dose must greatly exceed intravenous dose to achieve a similar effect. Nasal absorption is greater than oral.
[b] Following a single dose of 0.07 mg/kg IV (sample at 2 minutes) to surgical patients.

Reference: Cronnelly, R., Stanski, D.R., Miller, R.D., Sheiner, L.B., and Sohn, Y.J. Renal function and the pharmacokinetics of neostigmine in anesthetized man. *Anesthesiology,* **1979,** *51:*222–226.

AVAILABILITY (ORAL) (%)	URINARY EXCRETION (%)	BOUND IN PLASMA (%)	CLEARANCE $(ml \cdot min^{-1} \cdot kg^{-1})$	VOL. DIST. (liters/kg)	HALF-LIFE (hours)	PEAK TIME (hours)	PEAK CONCENTRATIONS
NEVIRAPINE[a] (Chapter 51)							
93 ± 9	<3%	60	SD: 0.23–0.77[b] MD: 0.89[b] ↑ Child[c]	SD: 1.2 ± 0.09[b] MD: 1.2[b]	SD: 45[b] MD: 25–35[b]	2–4[d]	SD: 2 ± 0.4 μg/ml[d] MD: 4.5 ± 1.9 μg/ml[d]

[a] Data from healthy adult and HIV-infected subjects. No significant gender differences. Metabolized by CYP3A.
[b] Range of *CL/F* and *V/F* reported. Nevirapine appears to autoinduce its own metabolism. *CL/F* increases and half-life decreases from a single dose (SD) to multiple doses (MD).
[c] Patients <8 years.
[d] Following a single 200-mg oral dose (SD), and 200 mg twice a day to steady state (MD).

References: Cheeseman, S.H., Hattox, S.E., McLaughlin, M.M., Koup, R.A., Andrews, C., Bova, C.A., Pav, J.W., Roy, T., Sullivan, J.L., and Keirns, J.J. Pharmacokinetics of nevirapine: initial single-rising-dose study in humans. *Antimicrob. Agents Chemother.,* **1993,** 37:178–182.
Luzuriaga, K., Bryson, Y., McSherry, G., Robinson, J., Stechenberg, B., Scott, G., Lamson, M., Cort, S., and Sullivan, J.L. Pharmacokinetics, safety, and activity of nevirapine in human immunodeficiency virus type 1-infected children. *J. Infect. Dis.,* **1996,** *174:*713–721.
Physicians' Desk Reference, 54th ed. Medical Economics Co., Montvale, NJ, **2000,** p. 2721.
Zhou, X.J., Sheiner, L.B., D'Aquila, R.T., Hughes, M.D., Hirsch, M.S., Fischl, M.A., Johnson, V.A., Myers, M., and Sommadossi, J.P. Population pharmacokinetics of nevirapine, zidovudine, and didanosine in human immunodeficiency virus-infected patients. The National Institute of Allergy and Infectious Diseases AIDS Clinical Trials Group Protocol 241 Investigators. *Antimicrob. Agents Chemother.,* **1999,** 43:121–128.

AVAILABILITY (ORAL) (%)	URINARY EXCRETION (%)	BOUND IN PLASMA (%)	CLEARANCE $(ml \cdot min^{-1} \cdot kg^{-1})$	VOL. DIST. (liters/kg)	HALF-LIFE (hours)	PEAK TIME (hours)	PEAK CONCENTRATIONS
NICARDIPINE[a] (Chapter 32)							
18 ± 11[b] ↔ RD ↑ Cirr	<1	98–99.5[c]	10.4 ± 3.1[b,d] ↔ RD ↓ Cirr	1.1 ± 0.3[e]	1.3 ± 0.5[e] ↔ RD ↑ Cirr	Oral: 1.0 ± 0.51[f]	IV: 25 ± 7.9 ng/ml[d] Oral: 88 ± 55 ng/ml[f]

[a] Racemic mixture; (+)-isomer is active.
[b] Data reported for 10 mg, three times a day. Saturable first-pass metabolism after oral administration; F increases at higher doses (38 ± 6% at 40 mg three times a day).
[c] Blood-to-plasma concentration ratio = 0.71 ± 0.06.
[d] Metabolically cleared by CYP3A; undergoes extensive first-pass metabolism.
[e] Some studies report a longer half-life of 16 ± 9 hours for the terminal disposition phase, and thus a larger V_{area}. This phase is only a small fraction of *CL* and does not correctly predict accumulation with multiple dosing.
[f] Following a single 0.885-mg IV dose or a 30-mg oral dose given three times a day for 3 days to healthy male adults.

References: Singh, B.N., and Josephson, M.A. Clinical pharmacology, pharmacokinetics, and hemodynamic effects of nicardipine. *Am. Heart. J.,* **1990,** *119:*427–434.
Wagner, J.G., Ling, T.L., Mroszczak, E.J., Freedman, R.R., Wu, A., Huang, B., Massey, I.J., and Roe, R.R. Single intravenous dose and steady-state oral dose pharmacokinetics of nicardipine in healthy subjects. *Biopharm. Drug Dispos.,* **1987,** 8:133–148.

NICOTINE (Chapters 9, 24)

Availability (oral)	Urinary excretion	Bound in plasma	Clearance	Vol. dist.	Half-life	Peak time	Peak concentration
Oral: 30 Smk: 90[a] IH: 53 ± 16[c] TD: 80–90[c]	17 ± 9	4.9 ± 2.8	18.5 ± 5.4 ←→ Smk	2.6 ± 0.9	2.0 ± 0.7	— Smk-C: 4–5[b] TD: 12 (8–24)[c] NS: 0.07–0.25[c] IH: 0.25[c]	Smk-N: 18 ± 11 ng/ml[b] Smk-C: 293 ± 152 ng/ml[b] TD: 12.3 (6.6–17.4) ng/ml[c] NS: 2–12 ng/ml[c] IH: 22.5 ± 7.7 ng/ml[c]

[a] Habitual smokers.

[b] Steady-state concentrations for nicotine (N) and cotinine (C) in adult subjects smoking 25 ± 8 cigarettes a day. T_{max} for cotinine following a 3-minute intravenous infusion of stable-isotope-labeled nicotine was 4 to 5 hours from the start of the infusion.

[c] T_{max} and C_{max} for nicotine following delivery from a 30-cm transdermal patch (TD, HABITROL) containing 52.5 mg of nicotine, two sprays of NICOTROL-NS (NS) containing 1 mg of nicotine, or 80 deep inhalations (at 20°C) over 20 minutes releasing 4 mg of nicotine (IH), repeated hourly for 10 hours.

References: Benowitz, N.L., Chan, K., Denaro, C.P., and Jacob, P. Stable isotope method for studying transdermal drug absorption: the nicotine patch. *Clin. Pharmacol. Ther.*, **1991**, *50*:286–293.

Benowitz, N.L., and Jacob, P. Nicotine and cotinine elimination pharmacokinetics in smokers and nonsmokers. *Clin. Pharmacol. Ther.*, **1993**, *53*:316–323.

Physicians' Desk Reference, 54th ed. Medical Economics Co., Montvale, NJ, **2000**, pp. 1687–1689.

NIFEDIPINE (Chapters 32, 33)

Availability (oral)	Urinary excretion	Bound in plasma	Clearance	Vol. dist.	Half-life	Peak time	Peak concentration
50 ± 13 ↑ Cirr, Aged ←→ RD	~0	96 ± 1 ↓ Cirr, RD	7.0 ± 1.8[a] ↓ Cirr, Aged ←→ RD, Smk	0.78 ± 0.22 ↑ Cirr, RD, Aged ←→ Smk	1.8 ± 0.4[b] ↑ Cirr, RD, Aged ←→ Smk	IR: 0.5 ± 0.2[c] ER: ~6[c]	IR: 79 ± 44 ng/ml[c] ER: 35–49 ng/ml[c]

[a] Metabolically cleared by CYP3A; undergoes significant first-pass metabolism.

[b] Longer apparent half-life after oral administration because of absorption limitation, particularly for extended-release formulations.

[c] Mean following a single 10-mg immediate-release (IR) capsule given to healthy male adults, or a range of steady-state concentrations following a 60-mg extended-release (ER) tablet, given daily to healthy male adults. Levels of 47 ± 20 ng/ml were reported to decrease diastolic pressure in hypertensive patients.

References: Glasser, S.P., Jain, A., Allenby, K.S., Shannon, T., Pride, K., Pettis, P.P., Schwartz, L.A., and MacCarthy, E.P. The efficacy and safety of once-daily nifedipine: the coat-core formulation compared with the gastrointestinal therapeutic system formulation in patients with mild-to-moderate diastolic hypertension. Nifedipine Study Group. *Clin. Ther.*, **1995**, *17*:12–29.

Renwick, A.G., Robertson, D.R., Macklin, B., Challenor, V., Waller, D.G., and George, C.F. The pharmacokinetics of oral nifedipine—a population study. *Br. J. Clin. Pharmacol.*, **1988**, *25*:701–708.

Soons, P.A., Schoemaker, H.C., Cohen, A.F., and Breimer, D.D. Intraindividual variability in nifedipine pharmacokinetics and effects in healthy subjects. *J. Clin. Pharmacol.*, **1992**, *32*:324–331.

NITROFURANTOIN (Chapter 44)

Availability (oral)	Urinary excretion	Bound in plasma	Clearance	Vol. dist.	Half-life	Peak time	Peak concentration
87 ± 13	47 ± 13	62 ± 4[a]	9.9 ± 0.9[b] ↑ Alkaline Urine	0.58 ± 0.12[b]	1.0 ± 0.2 ←→ Alkaline Urine	2.3 ± 1.4[c]	428 ± 146 ng/ml[c]

[a] Blood-to-plasma concentration ratio = 0.76 ± 0.06.

[b] Calculated assuming a 70-kg body weight.

[c] Following a single 50-mg oral dose (tablet) given to fasted healthy adults. No changes when taken with a meal.

Reference: Hoener, B., and Patterson, S.E. Nitrofurantoin disposition. *Clin. Pharmacol. Ther.*, **1981**, *29*:808–816.

Key: Unless otherwise indicated by a specific footnote, the data are presented for the study population as a mean value ± 1 standard deviation, a mean and range (lowest–highest in parenthesis) of values, a range of the lowest–highest values, or a single mean value.

ADH = alcohol dehydrogenase; Aged = aged; AIDS = acquired immunodeficiency syndrome; Alb = hypoalbuminemia; Atr Fib = atrial fibrillation; AVH = acute viral hepatitis; Burn = burn patients; C_{max} = peak concentration; CAD = coronary artery disease; Celiac = celiac disease; CF = cystic fibrosis; CHF = congestive heart failure; Child = children; Cirr = hepatic cirrhosis; COPD = chronic obstructive pulmonary disease; CP = cor pulmonale; CPBS = cardiopulmonary bypass surgery; CRI = chronic respiratory insufficiency; Crohn = Crohn's disease; Cush = Cushing's syndrome; CYP = cytochrome P450; Fem = female; Hep = hepatitis; HIV = human immunodeficiency virus; HL = hyperlipoproteinemia; HTh = hyperthyroid; IM = intramuscular; Inflam = inflammation; IV = intravenous; LD = liver disease; LTh = hypothyroid; MAO = monoamine oxidase; MI = myocardial infarction; NAT = N-acetyltransferase; Neo = neonate; NIDDM = non-insulin-dependent diabetes mellitus; NS = nephrotic syndrome; Obes = obese; Pneu = pneumonia; Preg = pregnant; Prem = premature; RA = rheumatoid arthritis; RD = renal disease (including uremia); SC = subcutaneous; Smk = smoking; ST = sulfotransferase; T_{max} = peak time; Tach = ventricular tachycardia; UGT = UDP-glucuronosyl transferase; Ulcer = ulcer patients. Other abbreviations are defined in the text section of this appendix.

Table A–II–1
PHARMACOKINETIC DATA (Continued)

AVAILABILITY (ORAL) (%)	URINARY EXCRETION (%)	BOUND IN PLASMA (%)	CLEARANCE $(ml \cdot min^{-1} \cdot kg^{-1})$	VOL. DIST. (liters/kg)	HALF-LIFE (hours)	PEAK TIME (hours)	PEAK CONCENTRATIONS
NITROGLYCERIN[a] (Chapters 32, 34)							
Oral: <1 SL: 38 ± 26[b] Top: 72 ± 20	<1	—	195 ± 86[c]	3.3 ± 1.2[c,d]	2.3 ± 0.6 min	SL: 0.09 ± 0.03[e] Top: 3–4[e] TD: 2[e]	IV: 3.4 ± 1.7 ng/ml[e] SL: 1.9 ± 1.6 ng/ml[e]

[a]Dinitrate metabolites have weak activity compared to nitroglycerin (<10%), but, because of prolonged half-life (~40 minutes), they may accumulate during administration of sustained-release preparations to yield concentrations in plasma 10- to 20-fold greater than parent drug.
[b]Sublingual dose rinsed out of mouth after 8 minutes. Rinse contained 31 ± 19% of the dose.
[c]Following a 40- to 100-min IV infusion. Calculated assuming a 70-kg body weight.
[d]V_{area} reported.
[e]Steady-state concentration following a 20- to 54-μg/min IV infusion (40 to 100 minutes), or a 0.4-mg sublingual (SL) dose. Levels of 1.2 to 11 ng/ml associated with a 25% drop in capillary wedge pressure in patients with CHF. T_{max} for topical (Top) and transdermal (TD) preparations also reported.

References: Physicians' Desk Reference, 54th ed. Medical Economics Co., Montvale, NJ, **2000**, p. 1474.
Noonan, P.K., and Benet, L.Z. Incomplete and delayed bioavailability of sublingual nitroglycerin. *Am. J. Cardiol.,* **1985,** 55:184–187.
Thadani, U., and Whitsett, T. Relationship of pharmacokinetic and pharmacodynamic properties of the organic nitrates. *Clin. Pharmacokinet.,* **1988,** 15:32–43.

AVAILABILITY (ORAL) (%)	URINARY EXCRETION (%)	BOUND IN PLASMA (%)	CLEARANCE $(ml \cdot min^{-1} \cdot kg^{-1})$	VOL. DIST. (liters/kg)	HALF-LIFE (hours)	PEAK TIME (hours)	PEAK CONCENTRATIONS
NORTRIPTYLINE[a] (Chapter 19)							
51 ± 5	2 ± 1	92 ± 2[b] ↑ HL	7.2 ± 1.8[b] ↓ Aged, Inflam ↔ Smk, RD	18 ± 4[c]	31 ± 13[b] ↑ Aged ↔ RD	7–10	138 (40–350) nM[d]

[a]Active metabolite, 10-hydroxynortriptyline, accumulates to twice the concentration of nortriptyline in extensive metabolizers.
[b]Formation of 10-hydroxynortriptyline is catalyzed by CYP2D6 (polymorphic). For poor metabolizers, CL/F is lower (5.3 *vs.* 19.3 ml·min⁻¹·kg⁻¹) and half-life longer (54 *vs.* 21 hours) than that of extensive metabolizers.
[c]V_{area} reported.
[d]Mean following a 125-mg oral dose, given once a day to healthy adults to steady state. Antidepressant effect observed at levels of 190 to 570 nM. Appears less effective at concentrations in plasma above 570 nM.

References: Dalen, P., Dahl, M.L., Ruiz, M.L., Nordin, J., and Bertilsson, L. 10-Hydroxylation of nortriptyline in white persons with 0, 1, 2, 3, and 13 functional CYP2D6 genes. *Clin. Pharmacol. Ther.,* **1998,** 63:444–452.
Jerling, M., Merle, Y., Mentre, F., and Mallet, A. Population pharmacokinetics of nortriptyline during monotherapy and during concomitant treatment with drugs that inhibit CYP2D6—an evaluation with the nonparametric maximum likelihood method. *Br. J. Clin. Pharmacol.,* **1994,** 38:453–462.
Ziegler, V.E., Clayton, P.J., Taylor, J.R., Tee, B., and Biggs, J.T. Nortriptyline plasma levels and therapeutic response. *Clin. Pharmacol. Ther.,* **1976,** 20:458–463.

AVAILABILITY (ORAL) (%)	URINARY EXCRETION (%)	BOUND IN PLASMA (%)	CLEARANCE $(ml \cdot min^{-1} \cdot kg^{-1})$	VOL. DIST. (liters/kg)	HALF-LIFE (hours)	PEAK TIME (hours)	PEAK CONCENTRATIONS
OFLOXACIN (Chapter 44)							
95–100	64 ± 16	25 ± 6	3.5 ± 0.7 ↓ RD ↔ Aged	1.8 ± 0.3[a] ↔ RD, Aged	5.7 ± 1.0 ↑ RD ↔ Aged	0.5–3.0[b]	SD: 1.6–2.2 μg/ml[b] MD: 3 μg/ml[b]

[a]V_{area} reported.
[b]Following a single 200-mg oral dose (SD), or a 200-mg oral dose, twice a day to steady state (MD), given to healthy adults.

Reference: Lamp, K.C., Bailey, E.M., and Rybak, M.J. Ofloxacin clinical pharmacokinetics. *Clin. Pharmacokinet.,* **1992,** 22:32–46.

OLANZAPINE[a] (Chapter 20)

| ~60[b] | 7.3 | 93 | 6.2 ± 2.9[c] →↔ RD, Cirr | 16.4 ± 5.1[c] | 33.1 ± 10.3 ↑ Aged | 6.1 ± 1.9[d] | 12.9 ± 7.5 ng/ml[d] |

[a]Data from male and female schizophrenic patients. Metabolized primarily by UGT, CYP1A2 and flavin-containing monooxygenase.

[b]Bioavailability estimated from parent-metabolite recovery data.

[c]Summary of CL/F and V_{area}/F for 491 subjects receiving an oral dose. CL/F segregates by sex (F/M) and smoking status (NS/S): M, S > F, S > M, NS > F, NS. Calculated assuming a 70-kg body weight.

[d]Following a single 9.5 ± 4-mg oral dose to healthy males; $C_{max,ss}$ ~ 20 ng/ml following a 10-mg oral dose, once daily.

References: Callaghan, J.T., Bergstrom, R.F., Ptak, L.R., and Beasley, C.M. Olanzapine. Pharmacokinetic and pharmacodynamic profile. *Clin. Pharmacokinet.,* **1999,** 37:177–193.
Kassahun, K., Mattiuz, E., Nyhart, E., Jr., Obermeyer, B., Gillespie, T., Murphy, A., Goodwin, R.M., Tupper, D., Callaghan, J.T., and Lemberger, L. Disposition and biotransformation of the antipsychotic agent olanzapine in humans. *Drug Metab. Dispos.,* **1997,** 25:81–93.
Physicians' Desk Reference, 54th ed. Medical Economics Co., Montvale, NJ, **2000,** p. 1649.

OMEPRAZOLE (Chapter 37)

| 53 ± 29[a] ↑ Aged, Cirr | <1 | 95[b] | 7.5 ± 2.7[c,d] ↓ Aged, Cirr →↔ RD | 0.34 ± 0.09[e] →↔ Aged, Cirr | 0.7 ± 0.5[c] ↑ Aged, Cirr →↔ RD | EM: ~1[f] PM: 3–4[f] | EM: 0.68 ± 0.43 μM[f] PM: 3.5 ± 1.4 μM[f] |

[a]Bioavailability after 8 days of treatment.

[b]Blood-to-plasma concentration ratio = 0.58.

[c]Metabolized by CYP2C19 (polymorphic) and CYP3A4. Patients deficient in CYP2C19 exhibit a clearance of 1.0 ± 0.2 ml·min^{-1}·kg^{-1} and a half-life of 2.7 ± 0.7 hours.

[d]Decreases with multiple dosing.

[e]V_{area} reported.

[f]Following a 20-mg oral dose, given twice a day for 4 days to healthy subjects phenotyped as CYP2C19 extensive (EM) and poor (PM) metabolizers.

References: Andersson, T., Andren, K., Cederberg, C., Lagerstrom, P.O., Lundborg, P., and Skanberg, I. Pharmacokinetics and bioavailability of omeprazole after single and repeated oral administration in healthy subjects. *Br. J. Clin. Pharmacol.,* **1990,** 29:557–563.
Chang, M., Tybring, G., Dahl, M.L., Gotharson, E., Sagar, M., Seensalu, R., and Bertilsson, L. Interphenotype differences in disposition and effect on gastrin levels of omeprazole—suitability of omeprazole as a probe for CYP2C19. *Br. J. Clin. Pharmacol.,* **1995,** 39:511–518.

ONDANSETRON (Chapter 38)

| 62 ± 15[a] ↑ Aged, Cirr, Fem | 5 | 73 ± 2[b] | 5.9 ± 2.6 ↓ Aged, Cirr, Fem ↑ Child | 1.9 ± 0.05 →↔ Aged, Cirr | 3.5 ± 1.2 ↑ Aged, Cirr ↓ Child | Oral: 1.0 (0.8–1.5)[c] | IV: 102 (64–136) ng/ml[c] Oral: 39 (31–48) ng/ml[c] |

[a]In 26 cancer patients (62 ± 10 years), F = 86 ± 26%.

[b]Blood-to-plasma concentration ratio = 0.83.

[c]Mean (95% CI) values following a single dose of 0.15 mg/kg IV or an oral dose of 8 mg given three times a day for 5 days to healthy adults.

Reference: Roila, F., and Del Favero, A. Ondansetron clinical pharmacokinetics. *Clin. Pharmacokinet.,* **1995,** 29:95–109.

Key: Unless otherwise indicated by a specific footnote, the data are presented for the study population as a mean value ± 1 standard deviation, a mean and range (lowest–highest in parenthesis) of values, a range of the lowest–highest values, or a single mean value.

ADH = alcohol dehydrogenase; Aged = aged; AIDS = acquired immunodeficiency syndrome; Alb = hypoalbuminemia; Atr Fib = atrial fibrillation; AVH = acute viral hepatitis; Burn = burn patients; C_{max} = peak concentration; CAD = coronary artery disease; Celiac = celiac disease; CF = cystic fibrosis; CHF = congestive heart failure; Child = children; Cirr = hepatic cirrhosis; COPD = chronic obstructive pulmonary disease; CP = cor pulmonale; CPBS = cardiopulmonary bypass surgery; CRI = chronic respiratory insufficiency; Crohn = Crohn's disease; Cush = Cushing's syndrome; CYP = cytochrome P450; Fem = female; Hep = hepatitis; HIV = human immunodeficiency virus; HL = hyperlipoproteinemia; HTh = hyperthyroid; IM = intramuscular; Inflam = inflammation; IV = intravenous; LD = liver disease; LTh = hypothyroid; MAO = monoamine oxidase; MI = myocardial infarction; NAT = N-acetyltransferase; Neo = neonate; NIDDM = non-insulin-dependent diabetes mellitus; NS = nephrotic syndrome; Obes = obese; Pneu = pneumonia; Preg = pregnant; Prem = premature; RA = rheumatoid arthritis; RD = renal disease (including uremia); SC = subcutaneous; Smk = smoking; ST = sulfotransferase; T_{max} = peak time; Tach = ventricular tachycardia; UGT = UDP-glucuronosyl transferase; Ulcer = ulcer patients. Other abbreviations are defined in the text section of this appendix.

Table A–II–1
PHARMACOKINETIC DATA (Continued)

	AVAILABILITY (ORAL) (%)	URINARY EXCRETION (%)	BOUND IN PLASMA (%)	CLEARANCE ($ml \cdot min^{-1} \cdot kg^{-1}$)	VOL. DIST. (liters/kg)	HALF-LIFE (hours)	PEAK TIME (hours)	PEAK CONCENTRATIONS
OSELTAMIVIR[a,b] (Chapter 50)								
	79 ± 12	93 ± 21	<3	4.9 ± 0.6 ↓ RD,[c] Aged	0.37 ± 0.09	1.8 ± 1.2[d] ↑ RD	2.7 ± 1.2[e]	1.1 ± 0.3 $\mu g/ml$[e]
OXCARBAZEPINE[a] (Chapter 21)								
	—	O: <1 HC: 27	— HC: 45	O: 67.4[b] HC: ↓ RD,[c] Aged HC: ↑ Child[d]	—	O: ~2 HC: 8–15 HC: ↑ RD, Aged	HC: 2–4[e]	HC: 8.5 ± 2.0 $\mu g/ml$[e]
OXYBUTYNIN[a] (Chapter 7)								
	1.6–10.9	<1	—	8.1 ± 2.3[b]	1.3 ± 0.4[b]	IV: 1.9 ± 0.35[b] IR: 9.0 ± 2.4[c] XL: 13.8 ± 2.9[c]	IR: 5.0 ± 4.2[c] XL: 5.2 ± 3.7[c]	IR: 12.4 ± 4.1 ng/ml[c] XL: 4.2 ± 1.6 ng/ml[c]

[a]Data from healthy male and female subjects. Oseltamivir is a prodrug for Ro-64-0802, the active neuraminidase inhibitor. It is metabolized by intestinal and hepatic esterases. Oseltamivir CL/F = 150 ± 39 $ml \cdot min^{-1} \cdot kg^{-1}$, $t_{1/2}$ = 1.7 ± 0.5 hours, and fraction bound = 42%.
[b]Table parameters are for Ro-64-0802 following a single oral dose of oseltamivir (F, C_{max}, and T_{max}), and for Ro-64-0802 following a single IV dose of Ro-64-0802 (urinary excretion, CL, V_{ss}, $t_{1/2}$).
[c]CL/F for Ro-64-0802 reduced, mild to severe renal impairment.
[d]Apparent $t_{1/2}$ of Ro-64-0802 after oral oseltamivir is 6.8 ± 2.3 hours.
[e]C_{max} and T_{max} for Ro-64-0802 following a 200-mg oral dose of oseltamivir twice a day for 7 days.

Reference: He, G., Massarella, J., and Ward, P. Clinical pharmacokinetics of the prodrug oseltamivir and its active metabolite Ro 64-0802. *Clin. Pharmacokinet.*, **1999,** 37:471–484.

[a]Data from healthy adult male subjects. No significant gender differences. Oxcarbazepine (O) undergoes extensive first-pass metabolism to an active metabolite, 10-hydroxycarbamazepine (HC). Reduction by cytosolic enzymes is stereoselective (80% *S*-enantiomer, 20% *R*-enantiomer), but both show similar pharmacological activity.
[b]CL/F for O reported. HC eliminated by glucuronidation.
[c]AUC for HC increased, moderate to severe renal impairment.
[d]AUC for HC decreased, children <6 years of age.
[e]Following a 300-mg oral oxcarbazepine dose twice a day for 12 days.

References: Battino, D., Estienne, M., and Avanzini, G. Clinical pharmacokinetics of antiepileptic drugs in paediatric patients. Part II. Phenytoin, carbamazepine, sulthiame, lamotrigine, vigabatrin, oxcarbazepine and felbamate. *Clin. Pharmacokinet.*, **1995,** 29:341–369.
Lloyd, P., Flesch, G., and Dieterle, W. Clinical pharmacology and pharmacokinetics of oxcarbazepine. *Epilepsia,* **1994,** 35(suppl 3):S10–S13.
Rouan, M.C., Lecaillon, J.B., Godbillon, J., Menard, F., Darragon, T., Meyer, P., Kourilsky, O., Hillion, D., Aldigier, J.C., and Jungers, P. The effect of renal impairment on the pharmacokinetics of oxcarbazepine and its metabolites. *Eur. J. Clin. Pharmacol.,* **1994,** 47:161–167.
van Heiningen, P.N., Eve, M.D., Oosterhuis, B., Jonkman, J.H., de Bruin, H., Hulsman, J.A., Richens, A., and Jensen, P.K. The influence of age on the pharmacokinetics of the antiepileptic agent oxcarbazepine. *Clin. Pharmacol. Ther.,* **1991,** 50:410–419.

[a]Data from healthy female subjects. No significant gender differences. Racemic mixture; anticholinergic activity resides predominantly with *R*-enantiomer; no stereoselectivity exhibited for antispasmodic activity. Oxybutynin undergoes extensive first-pass metabolism to *N*-desethyloxybutynin (DEO), an active, anticholinergic metabolite. Metabolized primarily by intestinal and hepatic CYP3A. Oxybutynin kinetic parameters reported.
[b]Data reported for a 1-mg IV dose, assuming a 70-kg body weight. A larger volume (2.8 l/kg) and longer $t_{1/2}$ (5.3 hours) reported for 5-mg IV dose.
[c]Following a dose of 5 mg immediate-release (IR) three times a day or 15 mg extended-release (XL) once a day for 4 days. The apparent $t_{1/2}$ for DEO was 4.0 ± 1.4 hours and 8.3 ± 2.5 hours for IR and XL formulations, respectively. Peak DEO levels at steady state were 45 and 23 ng/ml for IR and XL, respectively.

References: Gupta, S.K., and Sathyan, G. Pharmacokinetics of an oral once-a-day controlled-release oxybutynin formulation compared with immediate-release oxybutynin. *J. Clin. Pharmacol.,* **1999,** 39:289–296.
Physicians' Desk Reference, 54th ed. Medical Economics Co., Montvale, NJ, **2000,** p. 507.

OXYTOCIN[a] (Chapter 56)

—	—	M: 15.2 ± 3.47 F—labor: 101 F—postpartum: 20	—	M: 0.16 ± 0.07	M: 0.33 ± 0.23 Pregnant F: 0.17–0.25	—	8.0 pg/ml[b]

[a]Data from pregnant women (F) during labor and postpartum and from healthy male (M) subjects.
[b]C_{ss} during a 36-ng/min (labor) or a 8.5-ng/min (postpartum) IV infusion.

References: De Groot, A.N., Vree, T.B., Hekster, Y.A., Pesman, G.J., Sweep, F.C., Van Dongen, P.J., and Van Roosmalen, J. Bioavailability and pharmacokinetics of sublingual oxytocin in male volunteers. *J. Pharm. Pharmacol.,* **1995,** *47:*571–575.
Gonser, M. Labor induction and augmentation with oxytocin: pharmacokinetic considerations. *Arch. Gynecol. Obstet.,* **1995,** *256:*63–66.
Thornton, S., Davison, J.M., and Baylis, P.H. Effect of human pregnancy on metabolic clearance rate of oxytocin. *Am. J. Physiol.,* **1990,** *259:*R21–R24.

PACLITAXEL (Chapter 52)

Low	5 ± 2	88–98[a]	5.5 ± 3.5[b] ←→ Child	2.0 ± 1.2 ←→ Child	3 ± 1[c]	—	0.85 ± 0.21 μM[d]

[a]Binding of drug to dialysis filtration devices may lead to overestimation of protein binding fraction (88% suggested).
[b]Metabolized by CYP2C8 and CYP3A, and is a substrate for P-glycoprotein.
[c]Average accumulation half-life; longer terminal half-lives up to 30 hours have been reported.
[d]Steady-state concentration during a 250-mg/m² IV infusion, given over 24 hours to adult cancer patients.

Reference: Sonnichsen, D.S., and Relling, M.V. Clinical pharmacokinetics of paclitaxel. *Clin. Pharmacokinet.,* **1994,** *27:*256–269.

PANCURONIUM (Chapter 9)

—	67 ± 18 ←→ CPBS	7 ± 2 ←→ Neo, Fem, Preg, RD	1.8 ± 0.4 ↓ Aged, RD ←→ Neo, Fem, Preg, RD ←→ Cirr, CPBS	0.26 ± 0.07 ←→ Aged, RD, CPBS ↑ Cirr	2.3 ± 0.4 ↑ Aged, RD, Cirr Aged, RD, Cirr ←→ CPBS	—	0.67 μg/ml[a]

[a]Estimated mean C_{max} following a single bolus dose of 0.1 mg/kg IV given to surgical patients. Levels of 0.25 ± 0.07 μg/ml and 0.4 μg/ml elicit 50% and 95% decreases in twitch tension, respectively.

Reference: Shanks, C.A. Pharmacokinetics of the nondepolarizing neuromuscular relaxants applied to calculation of bolus and infusion dosage regimens. *Anesthesiology,* **1986,** *64:*72–86.

Key: Unless otherwise indicated by a specific footnote, the data are presented for the study population as a mean value ± 1 standard deviation, a mean and range (lowest–highest in parenthesis) of values, a range of the lowest–highest values, or a single mean value.

ADH = alcohol dehydrogenase; Aged = aged; AIDS = acquired immunodeficiency syndrome; Alb = hypoalbuminemia; Atr Fib = atrial fibrillation; AVH = acute viral hepatitis; Burn = burn patients; C_{max} = peak concentration; CAD = coronary artery disease; Celiac = celiac disease; CF = cystic fibrosis; CHF = congestive heart failure; Child = children; Cirr = hepatic cirrhosis; COPD = chronic obstructive pulmonary disease; CP = cor pulmonale; CPBS = cardiopulmonary bypass surgery; CRI = chronic respiratory insufficiency; Crohn = Crohn's disease; Cush = Cushing's syndrome; CYP = cytochrome P450; Fem = female; Hep = hepatitis; HIV = human immunodeficiency virus; HL = hyperlipoproteinemia; HTh = hyperthyroid; IM = intramuscular; Inflam = inflammation; IV = intravenous; LD = liver disease; LTh = hypothyroid; MAO = monoamine oxidase; MI = myocardial infarction; NAT = N-acetyltransferase; Neo = neonate; NIDDM = non-insulin-dependent diabetes mellitus; NS = nephrotic syndrome; Obes = obese; Pneu = pneumonia; Preg = pregnant; Prem = premature; RA = rheumatoid arthritis; RD = renal disease (including uremia); SC = subcutaneous; Smk = smoking; ST = sulfotransferase; T_{max} = peak time; Tach = ventricular tachycardia; UGT = UDP-glucuronosyl transferase; Ulcer = ulcer patients. Other abbreviations are defined in the text section of this appendix.

Table A–II–1
PHARMACOKINETIC DATA (Continued)

	AVAILABILITY (ORAL) (%)	URINARY EXCRETION (%)	BOUND IN PLASMA (%)	CLEARANCE ($ml \cdot min^{-1} \cdot kg^{-1}$)	VOL. DIST. (liters/kg)	HALF-LIFE (hours)	PEAK TIME (hours)	PEAK CONCENTRATIONS
PAROXETINE (Chapter 19)								
	Dose-dependent[a]	<2	95	$8.6 \pm 3.2^{a,b}$ ↓ Cirr, Aged	17 ± 10^c	17 ± 3^d ↑ Cirr, Aged	5.2 ± 0.5^e	EM: ~130 nM[e] PM: ~220 nM[e]

[a]Metabolized by CYP2D6 (polymorphic); undergoes time- and dose-dependent autoinhibition of metabolic clearance in extensive metabolizers.
[b]CL/F reported for multiple dosing in extensive metabolizers. Single dose data are significantly higher. In CYP2D6 poor metabolizers, $CL/F = 5.0 \pm 2.1$ ml $\cdot$ min$^{-1}\cdot$kg^{-1} for multiple dosing.
[c]V_{area}/F reported.
[d]Data reported for multiple dose in extensive metabolizers. In poor metabolizers, $t_{1/2} = 41 \pm 8$ hours.
[e]Estimated mean C_{max} following a 30-mg oral dose given once daily for 14 days to adults phenotyped as CYP2D6 extensive (EM) and poor (PM) metabolizers. There is a significant disproportional accumulation of drug in blood when going from single to multiple dosing due to autoinactivation of CYP2D6.

References: Physicians' Desk Reference, 54th ed. Medical Economics Co., Montvale, NJ, **2000**, p. 3028.
Sindrup, S.H., Brosen, K., Gram, L.F., Hallas, J., Skjelbo, E., Allen, A., Allen, G.D., Cooper, S.M., Mellows, G., Tasker, T.C., and Zussman, B.D. The relationship between paroxetine and the sparteine oxidation polymorphism. *Clin. Pharmacol. Ther.*, **1992**, *51*:278–287.

	AVAILABILITY (ORAL) (%)	URINARY EXCRETION (%)	BOUND IN PLASMA (%)	CLEARANCE ($ml \cdot min^{-1} \cdot kg^{-1}$)	VOL. DIST. (liters/kg)	HALF-LIFE (hours)	PEAK TIME (hours)	PEAK CONCENTRATIONS
PHENOBARBITAL (Chapters 17, 21)								
	100 ± 11	24 ± 5^a ⟷ Cirr, AVH	51 ± 3^b ↓ Neo ⟷ Preg, Aged	0.062 ± 0.013 ↑ Preg, Child, Neo ⟷ Smk	0.54 ± 0.03 ↑ Neo	99 ± 18 ↑ Cirr, Aged ↓ Child ⟷ Epilep, Neo	$2-4^c$	13.1 ± 4.5 $\mu g/ml^c$

[a]Phenobarbital is a weak acid ($pK_a = 7.3$); urinary excretion is increased at an alkaline pH; it also is reduced with decreased urine flow.
[b]Blood-to-plasma concentration ratio = 1.12 ± 0.08.
[c]Mean steady-state concentration following a 90-mg oral dose, given daily for 12 weeks to patients with epilepsy. Levels of 10–25 μg/ml provide control of tonic-clonic seizures and 15 μg/ml for control of febrile convulsions in children. Levels >40 can cause toxicity: 65–117 μg/ml produce stage III anesthesia—comatose but reflexes present; 100–134 μg/ml produce stage IV anesthesia—no deep-tendon reflexes.

References: Bourgeois, B.F.D. Phenobarbital and primidone. In: *The Treatment of Epilepsy: Principles and Practice*, 2nd ed. (Wyllie, E., ed.) Williams & Wilkins, Philadelphia, **1997**, pp. 845–855.
Browne, T.R., Evans, J.E., Szabo, G.K., Evans, B.A., and Greenblatt, D.J. Studies with stable isotopes II: Phenobarbital pharmacokinetics during monotherapy. *J. Clin. Pharmacol.*, **1985**, *25*:51–58.

	AVAILABILITY (ORAL) (%)	URINARY EXCRETION (%)	BOUND IN PLASMA (%)	CLEARANCE ($ml \cdot min^{-1} \cdot kg^{-1}$)	VOL. DIST. (liters/kg)	HALF-LIFE (hours)	PEAK TIME (hours)	PEAK CONCENTRATIONS
PHENYLEPHRINE[a] (Chapter 10)								
	38	IV: 16 ± 1.3 Oral: 2.6 ± 0.8	—	29.9 ± 11.6	4.86 ± 2.48 ↑ Aged	2.62 ± 0.67 ↑ Aged	$0.75-2^b$	$171-278$ ng/ml[b]

[a]Data from healthy adult male and female subjects. Phenylephrine undergoes significant first-pass metabolism catalyzed by intestinal ST (sulfation) and hepatic MAO (deamination). The extent of renal excretion, sulfation and deamination is different for IV and oral routes.
[b]Limited data available. Range of C_{max} and T_{max} values following a single 7.8-mg oral dose of phenylephrine hydrochloride.

References: Bogner, R.L., and Walsh, J.M. Sustained-release principle in human subjects utilizing radioactive techniques. *J. Pharm. Sci.*, **1964**, *53*:617–620.
Hengstmann, J.H., and Goronzy, J. Pharmacokinetics of 3H-phenylephrine in man. *Eur. J. Clin. Pharmacol.*, **1982**, *21*:335–341.
Kanfer, I., Dowse, R., and Vuma, V. Pharmacokinetics of oral decongestants. *Pharmacotherapy*, **1993**, *13*:116S–128S, discussion 143S–146S.

PHENYTOIN[a] (Chapters 21, 35)

90 ± 3 ↓ RD, Hep, Alb, Neo, AVH, Cirr, NS, Preg, Burn ⟶ Obes, Smk, Aged	2 ± 8	V_{max} = 5.9 ± 1.2 mg · kg^{-1} · day^{-1} · K_m = 5.7 ± 2.9 mg/l[b] ⟶ Aged; ↓ Child ↑c NS, RD ↓c Prem ⟶c AVH, LTh, HTh, Smk	0.64 ± 0.04[d] ↑ Neo, NS, RD ⟶ AVH, LTh, HTh	6–24[e] ↓c Prem ⟶c RD ⟶c AVH, LTh, HTh, Smk	3–12[f]	0–5 μg/ml (27%)[f] 5–10 μg/ml (30%)[f] 10–20 μg/ml (29%)[f] 20–30 μg/ml (10%)[f] >30 μg/ml (6%)[f]

[a] Metabolized predominantly by CYP2C9 (polymorphic) and also by CYP2C19 (polymorphic); exhibits saturable kinetics with therapeutic doses.
[b] Significantly decreased in the Japanese population.
[c] Comparison of clearances and half-lives with similar doses in normal subjects and patients; nonlinear kinetics not considered.
[d] V_{area} reported.
[e] Apparent half-life is dependent on plasma concentration.
[f] Population frequency of total phenytoin concentrations following a 300-mg oral dose (capsule), given daily to steady state. Total levels >10 μg/ml associated with suppression of tonic-clonic seizures. Nystagmus can occur at levels >20 μg/ml and ataxia at levels >30 μg/ml.

References: Eldon, M.A., Loewen, G.R., Voigtman, R.E., Koup, J.R., Holmes, G.B., Hunt, T.L., Sedman, A.J., and Cook, J.A. Pharmacokinetics and tolerance of fosphenytoin and phenytoin administered intravenously to healthy subjects. *Can. J. Neurol. Sci.*, **1993**, *20*(suppl 4):S180.
Levine, M., and Chang, T. Therapeutic drug monitoring of phenytoin. Rationale and current status. *Clin. Pharmacokinet.*, **1990**, *19*:341–358.
Tozer, T.N., and Winter, M.E. Phenytoin. In, *Applied Pharmacokinetics: Principles of Therapeutic Drug Monitoring*, 3rd ed. (Evans, W.E., Schentag, J.J., and Jusko, W.J., eds.) Applied Therapeutics, Vancouver, WA, **1992**, pp. 25-1–25-44.

PIMOZIDE (Chapter 20)

<50[a]	1	99	A: 4.1 ± 3.8[b,c] C: 3.5 ± 2.1[b,c]	A: 28 ± 18[b,c] C: 20 ± 15[b,c]	A: 111 ± 57[d] C: 66 ± 49[c]	A: 8 (4–12)[e] C: 7 ± 2.4[e]	A: 10 ± 2 ng/ml[e] C: 7.2 ± 3.7 ng/ml[e]

[a] About 50% to 60% of the dose is absorbed.
[b] CL/F and V_{ss}/F reported.
[c] Data from children 6 to 13 years old (C) and adults (A) reported.
[d] Previous reports of $t_{1/2}$ = 53 ± 3 hours in schizophrenic adults.
[e] Following a single 2-mg oral dose given to children with Tourette's syndrome, or following a 6-mg oral dose given daily for 4 days to adult males with schizophrenia.

References: McCreadie, R.G., Heykants, J.J.P., Chalmers, A., and Anderson, A.M. Plasma pimozide profiles in chronic schizophrenics. *Br. J. Clin. Pharmacol.*, **1979**, *7*:533–534.
Sallee, F.R., Pollock, B.G., Stiller, R.L., Stull, S., Everett, G., and Perel, J.M. Pharmacokinetics of pimozide in adults and children with Tourette's syndrome. *J. Clin. Pharmacol.*, **1987**, *27*:776–781.

PIOGLITAZONE[a] (Chapter 61)

—	Negligible	>99	1.19–1.67[b] ⟷ Cirr, RD	0.63 ± 0.41[b]	3–7	<2[c]	1.5 μg/ml[c]

[a] Data from healthy male and female subjects and patients with NIDDM (type 2 diabetes). Pioglitazone is metabolized extensively by CYP2C8, CYP3A4, and other P450 isozymes. Two major metabolites accumulate in blood and contribute to the pharmacological effect. CL/F is lower in women than men.
[b] CL/F and V_{area}/F reported for oral dose. C_{max} following a 15- to 30-mg oral dose.
[c] T_{max} following a 15- to 30-mg oral dose.

References: *Physicians' Desk Reference*, 54th ed. Medical Economics Co., Montvale, NJ, **2000**, p. 3088.
Yamashita, K., Murakami, H., Okuda, T., and Motohashi, M. High-performance liquid chromatographic determination of pioglitazone and its metabolites in human serum and urine. *J. Chromatogr. B. Biomed. Appl.*, **1996**, *677*:141–146.

Key: Unless otherwise indicated by a specific footnote, the data are presented for the study population as a mean value ± 1 standard deviation, a mean and range (lowest–highest in parenthesis) of values, a range of the lowest–highest values, or a single mean value.

ADH = alcohol dehydrogenase; Aged = aged; AIDS = acquired immunodeficiency syndrome; Alb = hypoalbuminemia; Atr Fib = atrial fibrillation; AVH = acute viral hepatitis; Burn = burn patients; C_{max} = peak concentration; CAD = coronary artery disease; Celiac = celiac disease; CF = cystic fibrosis; CHF = congestive heart failure; Child = children; Cirr = hepatic cirrhosis; COPD = chronic obstructive pulmonary disease; CP = cor pulmonale; CPBS = cardiopulmonary bypass surgery; CRI = chronic respiratory insufficiency; Crohn = Crohn's disease; Cush = Cushing's syndrome; CYP = cytochrome P450; Fem = female; Hep = hepatitis; HIV = human immunodeficiency virus; HL = hyperlipoproteinemia; HTh = hyperthyroid; IM = intramuscular; Inflam = inflammation; IV = intravenous; LD = liver disease; LTh = hypothyroid; MAO = monoamine oxidase; MI = myocardial infarction; NAT = N-acetyltransferase; Neo = neonate; NIDDM = non-insulin-dependent diabetes mellitus; NS = nephrotic syndrome; Obes = obese; Pneu = pneumonia; Preg = pregnant; Prem = premature; RA = rheumatoid arthritis; RD = renal disease (including uremia); SC = subcutaneous; Smk = smoking; ST = sulfotransferase; T_{max} = peak time; Tach = ventricular tachycardia; UGT = UDP-glucuronosyl transferase; Ulcer = ulcer patients. Other abbreviations are defined in the text section of this appendix.

Table A–II–1
PHARMACOKINETIC DATA (Continued)

	AVAILABILITY (ORAL) (%)	URINARY EXCRETION (%)	BOUND IN PLASMA (%)	CLEARANCE ($ml \cdot min^{-1} \cdot kg^{-1}$)	VOL. DIST. (liters/kg)	HALF-LIFE (hours)	PEAK TIME (hours)	PEAK CONCENTRATIONS
PRAMIPEXOLE[a] (Chapter 22)	>90[b]	~90	15	8.2 ± 1.4[b] ↓ Aged, RD[c], PD[d]	7.3 ± 1.7[b]	11.6 ± 2.57 ↑ Aged, RD	1–2	M: 1.6 ± 0.23 ng/ml[e] F: 2.1 ± 0.25 ng/ml[e]
PRAVASTATIN (Chapter 36)	18 ± 8	47 ± 7	43–48[a]	13.5 ± 2.4 ↓ Cirr ←→ Aged, RD[b]	0.46 ± 0.04	1.8 ± 0.8[c] ←→ Aged, RD[b]	1–1.4[d]	28–38 ng/ml[d]
PRAZIQUANTEL[a] (Chapter 42)	—[b]	Negligible	80–85	5 mg/kg: 467[c] 40–60 mg/kg: 57–222[c] ↓ Cirr[d]	50 mg/kg: 9.55 ± 2.86	5 mg/kg: 0.8–1.5[c] 40–60 mg/kg: 1.7–3.0[c] ↑ Cirr	1.5–1.8[e]	0.8–6.3 μg/ml[e]

PRAMIPEXOLE

[a]Data from healthy adult male and female subjects. No significant gender differences.
[b]Bioavailability estimated from urinary recovery of unchanged drug. CL/F and V_{area}/F reported.
[c]CL/F reduced, moderate to severe renal impairment.
[d]Parkinson's disease (PD); CL/F reduced with declining renal function.
[e]Following a 0.5-mg oral dose given three times a day for 4 days to male (M) and female (F) adults.

References: Lam, Y.W. Clinical pharmacology of dopamine agonists. *Pharmacotherapy,* **2000,** *20:*17S–25S.
Physicians' Desk Reference, 54th ed. Medical Economics Co., Montvale, NJ, **2000,** p. 2468.
Wright, C.E., Sisson, T.L., Ichhpurani, A.K., and Peters, G.R. Steady-state pharmacokinetic properties of pramipexole in healthy volunteers. *J. Clin. Pharmacol.,* **1997,** *37:*520–525.

PRAVASTATIN

[a]Blood-to-plasma concentration ratio ~0.55.
[b]Although renal clearance decreases with reduced renal function, no significant changes in CL/F or half-life are seen following oral dosing as a result of the low and highly variable bioavailability.
[c]Reported for oral dosing; probably rate limited by absorption, because after IV dosing, $t_{1/2} = 0.8 \pm 0.2$ hour.
[d]Range of mean values from different studies following a single 20-mg oral dose.

References: Corsini, A., Bellosta, S., Baetta, R., Fumagalli, R., Paoletti, R., and Bernini, F. New insights into the pharmacodynamic and pharmacokinetic properties of statins. *Pharmacol. Ther.,* **1999,** *84:*413–428.
Desager, J.P., and Horsmans, Y. Clinical pharmacokinetics of 3-hydroxy-3-methylglutaryl-coenzyme A reductase inhibitors. *Clin. Pharmacokinet.,* **1996,** *31:*348–371.
Quion, J.A., and Jones, P.H. Clinical pharmacokinetics of pravastatin. *Clin. Pharmacokinet.,* **1994,** *27:*94–103.

PRAZIQUANTEL

[a]Data from male and female patients with schistosomiasis.
[b,c]Praziquanel is well absorbed (80%) but undergoes significant first-pass metabolism (hydroxylation), the extent of which appears to be dose-dependent. CL/F and V_{ss}/F reported.
[d]CL/F reduced, moderate to severe hepatic impairment.
[e]Range of mean values reported for different studies following a single 40- to 60-mg/kg oral dose.

References: Edwards, G., and Breckenridge, A.M. Clinical pharmacokinetics of anthelmintic drugs. *Clin. Pharmacokinet.,* **1988,** *15:*67–93.
el Guiniady, M.A., el Touny, M.A., Abdel-Bary, M.A., Abdel-Fatah, S.A., and Metwally, A. Clinical and pharmacokinetic study of praziquantel in Egyptian schistosomiasis patients with and without liver cell failure. *Am. J. Trop. Med. Hyg.,* **1994,** *51:*809–818.
Jung, H., Vazquez, M.L., Sanchez, M., Penagos, P., and Sotelo, J. Clinical pharmacokinetics of praziquantel. *Proc. West Pharmacol. Soc.,* **1991,** *34:*335–340.
Sotelo, J., and Jung, H. Pharmacokinetic optimisation of the treatment of neurocysticercosis. *Clin. Pharmacokinet.,* **1998,** *34:*503–515.
Watt, G., White, N.J., Padre, L., Ritter, W., Fernando, M.T., Ranoa, C.P., and Laughlin, L.W. Praziquantel pharmacokinetics and side effects in *Schistosoma japonicum*–infected patients with liver disease. *J. Infect. Dis.,* **1988,** *157:*530–535.

PRAZOSIN (Chapters 10, 33)

68 ± 17 ←→ Hep, Cush, RD, Crohn, Celiac, Smk, Aged ↓ HTh	<4	95 ± 1 ↓ Cirr, Alb, RD ←→ CHF	3.0 ± 0.3[a] ↓ CHF, Preg ←→ RD	0.60 ± 0.13[a]	2.9 ± 0.8 ↑ CHF, Preg ←→ RD	2.2 ± 1.1[b]	36 ± 17 ng/ml[b]

[a]Calculated assuming a 70-kg body weight.
[b]Following a single 5-mg oral dose given to patients with hypertension.

References: Hobbs, D.C., Twomey, T.M., and Palmer, R.F. Pharmacokinetics of prazosin in man. *J. Clin. Pharmacol.,* **1978,** *18*:402–406.
Vincent, J., Meredith, P.A., Reid, J.L., Elliott, H.L., and Rubin, P.C. Clinical pharmacokinetics of prazosin—1985. *Clin. Pharmacokinet.,* **1985,** *10*:144–154.

PREDNISOLONE (Chapter 60)

82 ± 13 ←→ Hep, Cush, RD, Crohn, Celiac, Smk, Aged ↓ HTh	26 ± 9[a] ↓ Aged, HTh	90–95 (<200 ng/ml)[b] ~70 (>1 µg/ml) ↓ Alb, NS, Aged, HTh, Cirr ←→ Hep	1.0 ± 0.16[c] ←→ Hep, Cush, Smk, CRI, NS,[e] HTh[e] ↓ Aged,[e] Cirr[e]	0.42 ± 0.11[d] ←→ Hep, Cush, Smk, RD, CRI, NS[e] ↓ HTh,[e] Aged,[e] Obes	2.2 ± 0.5 ←→ Hep, Cush, Smk, RD, CRI, NS[e] ↑ HTh[e] ↓ Aged[e]	1.5 ± 0.5[f]	458 ± 150 ng/ml[f]

[a]Prednisolone and prednisone are interconvertible; an additional 3% ± 2% is excreted as prednisone.
[b]Extent of binding to plasma proteins is dependent on concentration over range encountered.
[c]Total clearance increases as protein binding is saturated. Clearance of unbound drug increases slightly but significantly with increasing dose.
[d]V increases with dose due to saturable protein binding.
[e]Changes are for unbound drug.
[f]Following a 30-mg oral dose given twice a day for 3 days to healthy male adults. The ratio of prednisolone/prednisone is dose-dependent and can vary from 3 to 26 over a prednisolone concentration range of 50–800 ng/ml.

References: Frey, B.M., and Frey, F.J. Clinical pharmacokinetics of prednisone and prednisolone. *Clin. Pharmacokinet.,* **1990,** *19*:126–146.
Rohatagi, S., Barth, J., Mollmann, H., Hochhaus, G., Soldner, A., Mollmann, C., and Derendorf, H. Pharmacokinetics of methylprednisolone and prednisolone after single and multiple oral administration. *J. Clin. Pharmacol.,* **1997,** *37*:916–925.

PREDNISONE (Chapter 60)

80 ± 11[a] ←→ Hep, Cush, RD, Crohn, Celiac, Smk, Aged	3 ± 2[b] ←→ HTh	75 ± 2[c] ←→ Hep	3.6 ± 0.8[d] ←→ Hep	0.97 ± 0.11[d] ←→ Hep	3.6 ± 0.4[d] ←→ Smk, Hep	P: 2.1–3.1[e] PL: 1.2–2.6[e]	P: 62–81 ng/ml[e] PL: 198–239 ng/ml[e]

[a]Measured relative to equivalent intravenous dose of prednisolone.
[b]An additional 15% ± 5% excreted as prednisolone.
[c]In contrast to prednisolone, there is no dependence on concentration.
[d]Kinetic values for prednisone are often reported in terms of values for prednisolone, its active metabolite. However, the values cited pertain to prednisone.
[e]Range of mean data for prednisone (P) and its active metabolite, prednisolone (PL) following a single 10-mg oral dose given as four different proprietary formulations to healthy adults.

References: Gustavson, L.E., and Benet, L.Z. The macromolecular binding of prednisone in plasma of healthy volunteers including pregnant women and oral contraceptive users. *J. Pharmacokinet. Biopharm.,* **1985,** *13*:561–569.
Pickup, M.E. Clinical pharmacokinetics of prednisone and prednisolone. *Clin. Pharmacokinet.,* **1979,** *4*:111–128.
Sullivan, T.J., Hallmark, M.R., Sakmar, E., Weidler, D.J., Earhart, R.H., and Wagner, J.G. Comparative bioavailability: eight commercial prednisone tablets. *J. Pharmacokinet. Biopharm.,* **1976,** *4*:157–172.

Key: Unless otherwise indicated by a specific footnote, the data are presented for the study population as a mean value ± 1 standard deviation, a mean and range (lowest–highest in parenthesis) of values, a range of the lowest–highest values, or a single mean value.

ADH = alcohol dehydrogenase; Aged = aged; AIDS = acquired immunodeficiency syndrome; Alb = hypoalbuminemia; Atr Fib = atrial fibrillation; AVH = acute viral hepatitis; Burn = burn patients; C_{max} = peak concentration; CAD = coronary artery disease; Celiac = celiac disease; CF = cystic fibrosis; CHF = congestive heart failure; Child = children; Cirr = hepatic cirrhosis; COPD = chronic obstructive pulmonary disease; CP = cor pulmonale; CPBS = cardiopulmonary bypass surgery; CRI = chronic respiratory insufficiency; Crohn = Crohn's disease; Cush = Cushing's syndrome; CYP = cytochrome P450; Fem = female; Hep = hepatitis; HIV = human immunodeficiency virus; HL = hyperlipoproteinemia; HTh = hyperthyroid; IM = intramuscular; Inflam = inflammation; IV = intravenous; LD = liver disease; LTh = hypothyroid; MAO = monoamine oxidase; MI = myocardial infarction; NAT = N-acetyltransferase; Neo = neonate; NIDDM = non-insulin-dependent diabetes mellitus; NS = nephrotic syndrome; Obes = obese; Pneu = pneumonia; Preg = pregnant; Prem = premature; RA = rheumatoid arthritis; RD = renal disease (including uremia); SC = subcutaneous; Smk = smoking; ST = sulfotransferase; T_{max} = peak time; Tach = ventricular tachycardia; UGT = UDP-glucuronosyl transferase; Ulcer = ulcer patients. Other abbreviations are defined in the text section of this appendix.

Table A–II–1
PHARMACOKINETIC DATA (Continued)

AVAILABILITY (ORAL) (%)	URINARY EXCRETION (%)	BOUND IN PLASMA (%)	CLEARANCE ($ml \cdot min^{-1} \cdot kg^{-1}$)	VOL. DIST. (liters/kg)	HALF-LIFE (hours)	PEAK TIME (hours)	PEAK CONCENTRATIONS

PROCAINAMIDE[a] (Chapter 35)

AVAILABILITY (ORAL) (%)	URINARY EXCRETION (%)	BOUND IN PLASMA (%)	CLEARANCE ($ml \cdot min^{-1} \cdot kg^{-1}$)	VOL. DIST. (liters/kg)	HALF-LIFE (hours)	PEAK TIME (hours)	PEAK CONCENTRATIONS
83 ± 16	67 ± 8 ↓ CHF, COPD, CP, Cirr	16 ± 5	$CL = 2.7CL_{cr} + 1.7 \pm 3.2$ (fast)[b] or $+ 1.1$ (slow)[b] ↑ Child ↓ MI ↔ CHF, Tach, Neo	1.9 ± 0.3 ↓ Obes ↔ RD, Child, Tach, CHF	3.0 ± 0.6 ↓ RD,[c] MI ↓ Child, Neo ↔ Obes, Tach, CHF	M: 3.6[d] F: 3.8[d]	M: 2.2 $\mu g/ml$[d] F: 2.9 $\mu g/ml$[d]

[a]Active metabolite, N-acetylprocainamide (NAPA); $CL = 3.1 \pm 0.4$ ml·min⁻¹·kg⁻¹, $V = 1.4 \pm 0.2$ l/kg, and $t_{1/2} = 6.0 \pm 0.2$ hours.
[b]CL calculated using units of ml·min⁻¹·kg⁻¹ for CL_{cr}. Clearance depends on NAT2 acetylation phenotype. Use a mean value of 2.2 if phenotype unknown.
[c]$t_{1/2}$ for procainamide and NAPA increased in patients with renal disease.
[d]Least square mean values following 1000-mg oral dose, given twice a day to steady state in male (M) and female (F) adults. Mean peak NAPA concentrations were 2.0 and 2.2 $\mu g/ml$ for male and female adults, respectively; $t_{max} = 4.1$ and 4.2 hours.

References: Benet, L.Z., and Ding, R.W. Die renale Elimination von Procainamide: Pharmacokinetik bei Niereninsuffizienz. In, *Die Behandlung von Herzrhythmusstorungen bei Nierenkranken.* (Braun, J., Pilgrim, R., Gessler, U., and Seybold, D., eds.) Karger, Basel, **1984**, pp. 96–111. Koup, J.R., Abel, R.B., Smithers, J.A., Eldon, M.A., and de Vries, T.M. Effect of age, gender, and race on steady state procainamide pharmacokinetics after administration of procanbid sustained-release tablets. *Ther. Drug Monit.,* **1998,** 20:73–77.

PROPOFOL[a] (Chapter 14)

AVAILABILITY (ORAL) (%)	URINARY EXCRETION (%)	BOUND IN PLASMA (%)	CLEARANCE ($ml \cdot min^{-1} \cdot kg^{-1}$)	VOL. DIST. (liters/kg)	HALF-LIFE (hours)	PEAK TIME (hours)	PEAK CONCENTRATIONS
—	—	$98.3–98.8$[b]	27 ± 5 ↑ Child[c] ↓Aged[d] ↔ LD	1.7 ± 0.7[e] ↑ Child[c] ↓ Aged[d]	3.5 ± 1.2[e]	—	SS: 3.5 ± 0.06 $\mu g/ml$[f] E: 1.1 ± 0.4 $\mu g/ml$[f]

[a]Data from patients undergoing elective surgery and healthy volunteers. Propofol is extensively metabolized by UGT; IV administration.
[b]Fraction bound in whole blood. Concentration-dependent; 98.8% at 0.5 $\mu g/ml$ and 98.3 at 32 $\mu g/ml$.
[c]CL and central volume increased, children 1 to 3 years of age.
[d]CL and central volume decreased in elderly.
[e]V_{ss} is much larger than V_{ss}. A much longer terminal $t_{1/2}$ reported following prolonged IV infusion.
[f]Concentration producing anesthesia after infusion to steady state (SS) and at emergence (E) from anesthesia.

References: Mazoit, J.X., and Samii, K. Binding of propofol to blood components: implications for pharmacokinetics and for pharmacodynamics. *Br. J. Clin. Pharmacol.,* **1999,** 47:35–42. Murat, I., Billard, V., Vernois, J., Zaouter, M., Marsol, P., Souron, R., and Farinotti, R. Pharmacokinetics of propofol after a single dose in children aged 1–3 years with minor burns. Comparison of three data analysis approaches. *Anesthesiology,* **1996,** 84:526–532. Servin, F., Cockshott, I.D., Farinotti, R., Haberer, J.P., Winckler, C., and Desmonts, J.M. Pharmacokinetics of propofol infusions in patients with cirrhosis. *Br. J. Anaesth.,* **1990,** 65:177–183.

PROPRANOLOL[a] (Chapters 10, 32, 33, 35)

AVAILABILITY (ORAL) (%)	URINARY EXCRETION (%)	BOUND IN PLASMA (%)	CLEARANCE ($ml \cdot min^{-1} \cdot kg^{-1}$)	VOL. DIST. (liters/kg)	HALF-LIFE (hours)	PEAK TIME (hours)	PEAK CONCENTRATIONS
26 ± 10 ↑ Cirr	<0.5	87 ± 6[b] ↑ Inflam, Crohn, Preg, Obes ↔ RD, Fem, Aged ↓ Cirr	16 ± 5[c,d] ↑ Smk, HTh ↔ Hep, Cirr, Obes, Fem ↓ Aged, RD	4.3 ± 0.6[c] ↑ Hep, HTh, Cirr ↔ Crohn ↔ Aged, RD, Obes, Fem, Preg	3.9 ± 0.4[c] ↓ Hep, Cirr, Obes, Fem ↔ Aged, RD, Smk, Preg	P: 1.5[e] HP: 1.0[e]	P: 49 ± 8 ng/ml[e] HP: 37 ± 9 ng/ml[e]

[a]Racemic mixture. For S-(−)-enantiomer (100-fold more active) compared to R-(+)-enantiomer, CL is 19% lower and V_{area} is 15% lower, because of a higher degree of protein binding (18% less free drug), and no difference in half-life. Active metabolite, 4-hydroxypropranolol (HP).
[b]Drug is bound primarily to α_1-acid glycoprotein, which is elevated with a number of inflammatory conditions; blood-to-plasma concentration ratio = 0.89 ± 0.03.
[c]Based on blood measurements.
[d]CYP2D6 catalyzes the formation of 4-hydroxy metabolite; CYP1A2 is responsible for most of the N-desisopropyl metabolite; UGT catalyzes major conjugation pathway of elimination.
[e]Following a single 80-mg oral dose given to healthy adults. Plasma accumulation factor was 3.6-fold after 80 mg four times a day to steady state. A concentration of 20 ng/ml gave a 50% decrease in exercise-induced cardioacceleration. Antianginal effects are manifest at 15 to 90 ng/ml. A concentration up to 1000 ng/ml may be required for control of ventricular arrhythmias.

References: Colangelo, P.M., Blouin, R.A., Steinmetz, J.E., McNamara, P.J., DeMaria, A.N., and Wedlund, P.J. Age and propranolol stereoselective disposition in humans. *Clin. Pharmacol. Ther.,* **1992,** 51:489–494. Walle, T., Conradi, E.C., Walle, U.K., Fagan, T.C., and Gaffney, T.E. 4-Hydroxypropranolol and its glucuronide after single and long-term doses of propranolol. *Clin. Pharmacol. Ther.,* **1980,** 27:22–31.

PSEUDOEPHEDRINE[a] (Chapter 10)

~100	43–96[b]	—	7.33[b,c]	2.64–3.51[c]	4.3–8[b,c]	IR: 1.4–2[d] CR: 3.8–6.1[d]	IR: 177–360 ng/ml[d] CR: 265–314 ng/ml[d]

[a]Data from healthy adult male and female subjects.

[b]At a high urine pH (>7.0), pseudoephedrine is extensively reabsorbed; $t_{1/2}$ increases and CL decreases.

[c]CLF, VlF, and $t_{1/2}$ reported for oral dose.

[d]Range of mean values from different studies following a single 60-mg immediate-release tablet or syrup (IR), or 120-mg controlled-release capsule (CR) oral dose.

Reference: Kanfer, I., Dowse, R., and Vuma, V. Pharmacokinetics of oral decongestants. *Pharmacotherapy,* **1993,** *13:*116S–128S.

QUETIAPINE[a] (Chapter 20)

9 ↑ Food	83	<1%	10 ± 4	6	1–1.8	19 ↓ Aged ↔ RD ↓ LD	278 ng/ml[b]

[a]No significant gender differences. Extensively metabolized through multiple pathways, including sulfoxidation, N- and O-dealkylation catalyzed by CYP3A4. Two minor active metabolites.

[b]Following a 250-mg/day oral dose for 23 days in patients with schizophrenia.

References: Goren, J.L., and Levin, G.M. Quetiapine, an atypical antipsychotic. *Pharmacotherapy,* **1998,** *18:*1183–1194.
Physicians' Desk Reference, 54th ed. Medical Economics Co., Montvale, NJ, **2000,** p. 563.

QUINIDINE[a] (Chapter 35)

Sulfate: 80 ± 15 Gluconate: 71 ± 17 ↔ CHF	18 ± 5 ↔ CHF	87 ± 3 ↓ Cirr, Hep, Neo, Preg ↔ RD, CRI, HL, Aged	4.7 ± 1.8[b] ↓ CHF, Aged ↔ Cirr, Smk	2.7 ± 1.2 ↑ CHF ↑ Cirr ↔ Aged	6.2 ± 1.8 ↑ Aged, Cirr ↔ CHF, RD	IR: 1–3[c] ER: 6.3 ± 3.2[c]	IV: 2.9 ± 1.0 μg/ml[c] IR: ~1.3 μg/ml[c] ER: 0.53 ± 0.22 μg/ml[c]

[a]Active metabolite, 3-hydroxyquinidine ($t_{1/2}$ = 12 ± 3 hours; percent bound in plasma = 60 ± 10).

[b]Metabolically cleared primarily by CYP3A.

[c]Following a 400-mg IV dose (22-min infusion) of quinidine gluconate or a single 400-mg oral dose of immediate-release (IR) quinidine sulfate or a 300-mg dose of extended-release (ER) quinidine sulfate (QUINIDEX) to healthy adults. Specific assay methods for quinidine show >75% reduction in frequency of premature ventricular contractions at levels of 0.7–5.9 μg/ml, but active metabolite was not measured; therapeutic levels of 2–7 μg/ml reported for nonspecific assays.

References: Brosen, K., Davidsen, F., and Gram, L.F. Quinidine kinetics after a single oral dose in relation to the sparteine oxidation polymorphism in man. *Br. J. Clin. Pharmacol.,* **1990,** 29:248–253.
Sawyer, W.T., Pulliam, C.C., Mattocks, A., Foster, J., Hadzija, B.W., and Rosenthal, H.M. Bioavailability of a commercial sustained-release quinidine tablet compared to oral quinidine solution. *Biopharm. Drug Dispos.,* **1982,** 3:301–310.
Ueda, C.T., Williamson, B.J., and Dzindzio, B.S. Absolute quinidine bioavailability. *Clin. Pharmacol. Ther.,* **1976,** 20:260–265.

Key: Unless otherwise indicated by a specific footnote, the data are presented for the study population as a mean value ± 1 standard deviation, a mean and range (lowest–highest in parenthesis) of values, a range of the lowest–highest values, or a single mean value.

ADH = alcohol dehydrogenase; Aged = aged; AIDS = acquired immunodeficiency syndrome; Alb = hypoalbuminemia; AVH = acute viral hepatitis; Atr Fib = atrial fibrillation; Burn = burn patients; C_{max} = peak concentration; CAD = coronary artery disease; Celiac = celiac disease; CF = cystic fibrosis; CHF = congestive heart failure; Child = children; Cirr = hepatic cirrhosis; COPD = chronic obstructive pulmonary disease; CP = cor pulmonale; CPBS = cardiopulmonary bypass surgery; CRI = chronic respiratory insufficiency; Crohn = Crohn's disease; Cush = Cushing's syndrome; CYP = cytochrome P450; Fem = female; Hep = hepatitis; HIV = human immunodeficiency virus; HL = hyperlipoproteinemia; HTh = hyperthyroid; IM = intramuscular; Inflam = inflammation; IV = intravenous; LD = liver disease; LTh = hypothyroid; MAO = monoamine oxidase; MI = myocardial infarction; NAT = N-acetyltransferase; Neo = neonate; NIDDM = non-insulin-dependent diabetes mellitus; NS = nephrotic syndrome; Obes = obese; Pneu = pneumonia; Preg = pregnant; Prem = premature; RA = rheumatoid arthritis; RD = renal disease (including uremia); SC = subcutaneous; Smk = smoking; ST = sulfotransferase; T_{max} = peak time; Tach = ventricular tachycardia; UGT = UDP-glucuronosyl transferase; Ulcer = ulcer patients. Other abbreviations are defined in the text section of this appendix.

Table A–II–1
PHARMACOKINETIC DATA (Continued)

	AVAILABILITY (ORAL) (%)	URINARY EXCRETION (%)	BOUND IN PLASMA (%)	CLEARANCE ($ml \cdot min^{-1} \cdot kg^{-1}$)	VOL. DIST. (liters/kg)	HALF-LIFE (hours)	PEAK TIME (hours)	PEAK CONCENTRATIONS
QUININE[a] (Chapter 40)								
	76 ± 11	N-A: 12–20 M-A: 33 ± 18	N-A: ~85–90[b] M-A: 93–95[b] ↓ Neo ↔ Preg	N-A: 1.9 ± 0.5 M-A: 0.9–1.4 M-C: 0.4–1.4 ↔ Preg,[c] RD[c] ↓ Smk ↓ Aged	N-A: 1.8 ± 0.4 M-A: 1.0–1.7 M-C: 1.2–1.7 ↓ Preg[c] ↔ RD[c]	N-A: 11 ± 2 M-A: 11–18 M-C: 12–16 ↓ Preg,[c] Smk ↔ RD[c] ↑ Hep, Aged	PO: 3.5–8.4[d]	Adults IV: 11 ± 2 μg/ml[d] PO: 7.3–9.4 μg/ml[d] Children IV: 8.7–9.4 μg/ml[d] PO: 7.3 ± 1.1 μg/ml[d]

[a]Data from normal adults (N-A), and range of mean data from different studies of adults (M-A) or children (M-C) with malaria reported.
[b]Correlates with serum α_1-acid glycoprotein levels. Binding is increased in severe malaria.
[c]Data from patients with malaria.
[d]Following a single 10-mg/kg dose given as a 0.5- to 4-hour IV infusion or orally (PO) to children or adults with malaria. A level >0.2 μg/ml for unbound drug is targeted for treatment of *falciparum* malaria. Oculotoxicity and hearing loss/tinnitus associated with unbound concentrations >2 μg/ml.

References: Edwards, G., Winstanley, P.A., and Ward, S.A. Clinical pharmacokinetics in the treatment of tropical diseases. Some applications and limitations. *Clin. Pharmacokinet.,* **1994,** *27:*150–165.
Krishna, S., and White, N.J. Pharmacokinetics of quinine, chloroquine and amodiaquine. Clinical implications. *Clin. Pharmacokinet.,* **1996,** *30:*263–299.

	AVAILABILITY (ORAL) (%)	URINARY EXCRETION (%)	BOUND IN PLASMA (%)	CLEARANCE ($ml \cdot min^{-1} \cdot kg^{-1}$)	VOL. DIST. (liters/kg)	HALF-LIFE (hours)	PEAK TIME (hours)	PEAK CONCENTRATIONS
QUINUPRISTIN/DALFOPRISTIN[a] (Chapter 47)								
QUINUPRISTIN	—	15.1	23–32	17.2 ± 3.43 ↓ LD,[b] RD[c]	0.79 ± 0.40	0.97 ± 0.20	—	2.3 ± 0.5 μg/ml[d]
DALFOPRISTIN	—	18.7	50–56	19.8 ± 10.7 ↓ LD,[b] RD[c]	0.43 ± 0.29	0.52 ± 0.21	—	6.4 ± 2.7 μg/ml[d]

[a]Data from healthy adult male subjects. No significant gender differences. Cleared primarily by biliary excretion. Administered as SYNERCID (quinupristin/dalfopristin, 30:70, w/w).
[b]Mild to moderate hepatic impairment.
[c]Severe renal impairment.
[d]Following a single 10-mg/kg IV infusion (1 hour).

References: Bergeron, M., and Montay, G. The pharmacokinetics of quinupristin/dalfopristin in laboratory animals and in humans. *J. Antimicrob. Chemother.,* **1997,** *39*(suppl A):129–138.
Bryson, H.M., and Spencer, C.M. Quinupristin-dalfopristin. *Drugs,* **1996,** *52:*406–415.
Manufacturer's product information, Rhone-Poulenc-Rorer Pharmaceuticals, revised July **1999.**

	AVAILABILITY (ORAL) (%)	URINARY EXCRETION (%)	BOUND IN PLASMA (%)	CLEARANCE ($ml \cdot min^{-1} \cdot kg^{-1}$)	VOL. DIST. (liters/kg)	HALF-LIFE (hours)	PEAK TIME (hours)	PEAK CONCENTRATIONS
RALOXIFENE[a] (Chapters 58, 62)								
	2[b]	<0.2	>95	735 ± 338[c] ↔ RD, Aged ↓ Cirr	2348 ± 1220[c]	28 (11–273)	6[d]	0.5 ± 0.3 ng/ml[d]

[a]Data from postmenopausal women. Undergoes extensive first-pass metabolism (UGT-catalyzed) and enterohepatic recycling.
[b]Approximately 60% absorption from the gastrointestinal tract; not significantly affected by food.
[c]*CL/F* and *V/F* reported for an oral dose.
[d]Following a single 1-mg/kg oral dose.

References: Hochner-Celnikier, D. Pharmacokinetics of raloxifene and its clinical application. *Eur. J. Obstet. Gynecol. Reprod. Biol.,* **1999,** *85:*23–29.
Physicians' Desk Reference, 54th ed. Medical Economics Co., Montvale, NJ, **2000,** p. 1583.

RANITIDINE (Chapter 37)

52 ± 11 ↑Cirr ↔RD	69 ± 6 ↓RD	15 ± 3	10.4 ± 1.1 ↓RD, Aged ↑Burn	1.3 ± 0.4 ↔Cirr, RD ↑Burn	2.1 ± 0.2 ↑RD, Cirr, Aged ↑Burn	2.1 ± 0.31[a]	462 ± 54 ng/ml[a]

[a]Following a single 150-mg oral dose, given to healthy adults. IC_{50} for inhibition of gastric acid secretion is 100 ng/ml.

Reference: Gladziwa, U., and Klotz, U. Pharmacokinetics and pharmacodynamics of H$_2$-receptor antagonists in patients with renal insufficiency. *Clin. Pharmacokinet.,* **1993,** 24:319–332.

RAPACURONIUM[a] (Chapter 9)

—	6–22	50–88	7–11 ↔RD	0.2–0.5	1.2–3.1[b]	—	6–20 μg/ml[c]

[a] Data from adult subjects undergoing elective surgery; IV administration. The major 3-desacetyl metabolite is active; it accumulates and contributes to neuromuscular blockade with prolonged infusion of rapacuronium. For the metabolite, $CL = 1.3$ (0.8 to 1.9) ml·min^{-1}·kg^{-1} and $t_{1/2} = 2.3$ (2.0 to 4.5) hours.

[b]Mean residence time is 28.1 (24.6 to 35.1) minutes and 175 (144 to 353) minutes for rapacuronium and its active metabolite.

[c]Estimated range of peak arterial concentration after a 0.58–1.22-mg/kg IV dose (2.5- to 5.7-min infusion). Parent/metabolite ratio is 0.04 and 1 to 4 at 5 minutes and 3 to 6 hours after IV rapacuronium dose, respectively. Mean EC_{50} for neuromuscular blockade is 4.7 and 1.8 μg/ml for rapacuronium and its active metabolite, respectively.

References: Physicians' Desk Reference, 54th ed. Medical Economics Co., Montvale, NJ, **2000,** p. 2286.

Onrust, S.V., and Foster, R.H. Rapacuronium bromide: a review of its use in anaesthetic practice. *Drugs,* **1999,** 58:887–918.

Schiere, S., Proost, J.H., Schuringa, M., and Wierda, J.M. Pharmacokinetics and pharmacokinetic-dynamic relationship between rapacuronium (Org 9487) and its 3-desacetyl metabolite (Org 9488). *Anesth. Analg.,* **1999,** 88:640–647.

REMIFENTANIL[a] (Chapter 14)

—	Negligible	92	40–60 ↔RD, Cirr ↓Aged[b]	0.3–0.4 ↓Aged[b] ↔RD, Cirr	0.13–0.33 ↔RD, Cirr	—	~20 ng/ml[c]

[a]Data from healthy adult male subjects and patients undergoing elective surgery; IV administration. Undergoes rapid inactivation by esterase-mediated hydrolysis; resulting carboxy-metabolite has low activity.

[b]CL and V decreased slightly in the elderly.

[c]Mean C_{1min} following a 5-μg/kg IV dose (1-minute infusion). Cp_{50} for skin incision is 2 ng/ml (determined in the presence of nitrous oxide).

References: Egan, T.D., Huizinga, B., Gupta, S.K., Jaarsma, R.L., Sperry, R.J., Yee, J.B., and Muir, K.T. Remifentanil pharmacokinetics in obese versus lean patients. *Anesthesiology,* **1998,** 89:562–573.

Glass, P.S., Gan, T.J., and Howell, S. A review of the pharmacokinetics and pharmacodynamics of remifentanil. *Anesth. Analg.,* **1999,** 89:S7–S14.

Key: Unless otherwise indicated by a specific footnote, the data are presented for the study population as a mean value ± 1 standard deviation, a mean and range (lowest–highest in parenthesis) of values, a range of the lowest–highest values, or a single mean value.

ADH = alcohol dehydrogenase; Aged = aged; AIDS = acquired immunodeficiency syndrome; Alb = hypoalbuminemia; Atr Fib = atrial fibrillation; AVH = acute viral hepatitis; Burn = burn patients; C_{max} = peak concentration; CAD = coronary artery disease; Celiac = celiac disease; CF = cystic fibrosis; CHF = congestive heart failure; Child = children; Cirr = hepatic cirrhosis; COPD = chronic obstructive pulmonary disease; CP = cor pulmonale; CPBS = cardiopulmonary bypass surgery; CRI = chronic respiratory insufficiency; Crohn = Crohn's disease; Cush = Cushing's syndrome; CYP = cytochrome P450; Fem = female; Hep = hepatitis; HIV = human immunodeficiency virus; HL = hyperlipoproteinemia; HTh = hyperthyroid; IM = intramuscular; Inflam = inflammation; IV = intravenous; LD = liver disease; LTh = hypothyroid; MAO = monoamine oxidase; MI = myocardial infarction; NAT = N-acetyltransferase; Neo = neonate; NIDDM = non-insulin-dependent diabetes mellitus; NS = nephrotic syndrome; Obes = obese; Pneu = pneumonia; Preg = pregnant; Prem = premature; RA = rheumatoid arthritis; RD = renal disease (including uremia); SC = subcutaneous; Smk = smoking; ST = sulfotransferase; T_{max} = peak time; Tach = ventricular tachycardia; UGT = UDP-glucuronosyl transferase; Ulcer = ulcer patients. Other abbreviations are defined in the text section of this appendix.

Table A–II-1
PHARMACOKINETIC DATA (*Continued*)

	AVAILABILITY (ORAL) (%)	URINARY EXCRETION (%)	BOUND IN PLASMA (%)	CLEARANCE ($ml \cdot min^{-1} \cdot kg^{-1}$)	VOL. DIST. (*liters/kg*)	HALF-LIFE (*hours*)	PEAK TIME (*hours*)	PEAK CONCENTRATIONS
REPAGLINIDE[a] (Chapter 61)	56 ± 7	0.3–2.6	97.4	9.3 ± 6.8 ↓ RD,[b] LD[c]	0.52 ± 0.17	0.8 ± 0.2 ↑ LD	0.25–0.75[d]	47 ± 24 ng/ml[d]

[a] Data from healthy adult male subjects. Undergoes extensive oxidative and conjugative metabolism; CYP3A4 has been implicated in the formation of the major (60% of dose) metabolite.
[b] CL/F reduced, severe renal impairment.
[c] CL/F reduced, moderate to severe chronic liver disease.
[d] Following a single 4-mg oral dose (tablet).

References: Hatorp, V., Oliver, S., and Su, C.A. Bioavailability of repaglinide, a novel antidiabetic agent, administered orally in tablet or solution form or intravenously in healthy male volunteers. *Int. J. Clin. Pharmacol. Ther.,* **1998,** *36:*636–641.
Hatorp, V., Walther, K.H., Christensen, M.S., and Haug-Pihale, G. Single-dose pharmacokinetics of repaglinide in subjects with chronic liver disease. *J. Clin. Pharmacol.,* **2000,** *40:*142–152.
Marbury, T.C., Ruckle, J.L., Hatorp, V., Andersen, M.P., Nielsen, K.K., Huang, W.C., and Strange, P. Pharmacokinetics of repaglinide in subjects with renal impairment. *Clin. Pharmacol. Ther.,* **2000,** *67:*7–15.
van Heiningen, P.N., Hatorp, V., Kramer Nielsen, K., Hansen, K.T., van Lier, J.J., De Merbel, N.C., Oosterhuis, B., and Jonkman, J.H. Absorption, metabolism and excretion of a single oral dose of ^{14}C-repaglinide during repaglinide multiple dosing. *Eur. J. Clin. Pharmacol.,* **1999,** *55:*521–525.

	AVAILABILITY (ORAL) (%)	URINARY EXCRETION (%)	BOUND IN PLASMA (%)	CLEARANCE ($ml \cdot min^{-1} \cdot kg^{-1}$)	VOL. DIST. (*liters/kg*)	HALF-LIFE (*hours*)	PEAK TIME (*hours*)	PEAK CONCENTRATIONS
RIBAVIRIN (Chapter 50)	45 ± 5[a]	35 ± 8[a]	0[b]	5.0 ± 1.0[a,c]	9.3 ± 1.5[a]	28 ± 7[a,c]	RT: 3 ± 1.8[d]	R: 11.1 ± 1.2 μM[d] RT: 15.1 ± 12.8 μM[d]

[a] Values reported for studies conducted in asymptomatic HIV-positive men.
[b] At steady state, red blood cell-to-plasma concentration ratio is ~60.
[c] Following multiple oral dosing, CL/F decreases more than 50%, and a long terminal half-life of 150 ± 50 hours is observed.
[d] Following a 1200-mg oral ribavirin capsule (R) given daily for 7 days to adult subjects seropositive for HIV, or a 600-mg oral REBETRON (RT) dose given twice a day to steady state to adults with hepatitis C infection.

References: Morse, G.D., Fischl, M.A., Shelton, M.J., Cox, S.R., Driver, M., DeRemer, M., and Freimuth, W.W. Single-dose pharmacokinetics of delavirdine mesylate and didanosine in patients with human immunodeficiency virus infection. *Antimicrob. Agents Chemother.,* **1997,** *41:*169–174.
Physicians' Desk Reference, 54th ed. Medical Economics Co., Montvale, NJ, **2000,** p. 2836.
Roberts, R.B., Laskin, O.L., Laurence, J., Scavuzzo, D., Murray, H.W., Kim, Y.T., and Connor, J.D. Ribavirin pharmacodynamics in high-risk patients for acquired immunodeficiency syndrome. *Clin. Pharmacol. Ther.,* **1987,** *42:*365–373.

	AVAILABILITY (ORAL) (%)	URINARY EXCRETION (%)	BOUND IN PLASMA (%)	CLEARANCE ($ml \cdot min^{-1} \cdot kg^{-1}$)	VOL. DIST. (*liters/kg*)	HALF-LIFE (*hours*)	PEAK TIME (*hours*)	PEAK CONCENTRATIONS
RIFABUTIN[a] (Chapter 48)	SD: 20 ± 7 MD: 12 ± 2	SD: ~14 MD: ~6	71 ± 2[b] ⟷ Aged, Cirr, RD	SD: 2.4 ± 0.4[c] MD: 4.4 ± 0.6[c] ⟷ Aged, Cirr, HIV, RD	SD: 9.3 ± 0.6 MD: 8.2 ± 0.9 ⟷ Cirr, HIV ↓ Aged, RD	SD: 45 ± 17 MD: 38 ± 12 ⟷ Aged, Cirr, HIV, RD	3.3 ± 0.9[d]	375 ± 267 ng/ml[d]

[a] Data from early asymptomatic HIV patients. Desacetyl metabolite is equiactive; plasma levels are 10% of parent drug. Single-dose (SD) and multiple-dose (MD) regimens reported.
[b] Blood-to-plasma concentration ratio = 0.59 ± 0.07.
[c] Calculated assuming a 70-kg body weight. Multiple-dose data suggest a modest degree of autoinduction of rifabutin metabolism; the degree of change was variable among subjects.
[d] Following a 300-mg oral dose given daily for 21 days to adults.

References: Physicians' Desk Reference, 54th ed. Medical Economics Co., Montvale, NJ, **2000,** p. 2471.
Skinner, M.H., Hsieh, M., Torseth, J., Pauloin, D., Bhatia, G., Harkonen, S., Merigan, T.C., and Blaschke, T.F. Pharmacokinetics of rifabutin. *Antimicrob. Agents Chemother.,* **1989,** *33:*1237–1241.

RIFAMPIN[a] (Chapter 48)

Bioavailability	Urinary Excretion	Bound in Plasma	Clearance	Vol. Dist.	Half-Life	Peak Time	Peak Conc.
—[b]	7 ± 3 ↑ Neo	60–90	3.5 ± 1.6[d] ↑ Neo ↓ RD[c] ←→ Aged	0.97 ± 0.36 ↑ Neo ←→ Aged	3.5 ± 0.8[d] ↑ Hep, Cirr, AVH, RD[c] ←→ Child, Aged	1–3[e]	6.5 ± 3.5 μg/ml[e]

[a] Active desacetyl metabolite.

[b] Although some studies indicate complete absorption, data are insufficient. Such reports presumably refer to rifampin plus its desacetyl metabolite, since considerable first-pass metabolism is expected.

[c] Not observed with 300-mg doses, but pronounced differences with 900-mg doses.

[d] Half-life is longer with high single doses. Half-life is shorter (1.7 ± 0.5) and CL/F is higher after repeated administration. Rifampin is a potent enzyme (CYP3A and others) inducer and appears to autoinduce its own metabolism.

[e] Following a 600-mg dose given daily for 15 to 18 days to patients with tuberculosis.

Reference: Israili, Z.H., Rogers, C.M., and El-Attar, H. Pharmacokinetics of antituberculosis drugs in patients. *J. Clin. Pharmacol.*, **1987**, 27:78–83.

RISPERIDONE[a] (Chapter 20)

Bioavailability	Urinary Excretion	Bound in Plasma	Clearance	Vol. Dist.	Half-Life	Peak Time	Peak Conc.
Oral: 66 ± 28[b] IM: 103 ± 13	3 ± 2[b]	89[c] ↓ Cirr	5.4 ± 1.4[b] ↓ RD,[a] Aged[d]	1.1 ± 0.2	3.2 ± 0.8[a,b] ↑ RD,[a] Aged[d]	R: ~1[e]	R: 10 ng/ml[e] TA: 45 ng/ml[e]

[a] Active metabolite, 9-hydroxyrisperidone, is the predominant circulating species in extensive metabolizers, and is equipotent to parent drug. 9-Hydroxyrisperidone has a half-life of 20 ± 3 hours. In extensive metabolizers, 35% ± 7% of an intravenous dose is excreted as this metabolite; its elimination is primarily renal and therefore correlates with renal function.

[b] Formation of 9-hydroxyrisperidone is catalyzed by CYP2D6. Parameters reported for extensive metabolizers. In poor metabolizers, F is higher; about 20% of an intravenous dose is excreted unchanged, 10% as the 9-hydroxy metabolite; CL is slightly less than $1\ ml \cdot min^{-1} \cdot kg^{-1}$, and half-life is similar to that of the active metabolite, about 20 hours.

[c] 77% for 9-hydroxyrisperidone.

[d] Changes in elderly due to decreased renal function affecting the elimination of the active metabolite.

[e] Mean steady-state trough concentration for risperidone (R) and total active (TA) drug, risperidone + 9-OH-risperidone, following a 3-mg oral dose given twice a day to patients with chronic schizophrenia. No difference in total active drug levels between CYP2D6 extensive and poor metabolizers.

References: Cohen, L.J. Risperidone. *Pharmacotherapy*, **1994**, *14*:253–265.
Heykants, J., Huang, M.L., Mannens, G., Meuldermans, W., Snoeck, E., Van Peer, A., Van Beijsterveldt, L., Van Peer, A., and Woestenborghs, R. The pharmacokinetics of risperidone in humans: a summary. *J. Clin. Psychiatry*, **1994**, 55(suppl):13–17.

Key: Unless otherwise indicated by a specific footnote, the data are presented for the study population as a mean value ± 1 standard deviation, a mean and range (lowest–highest in parenthesis) of values, a range of the lowest–highest values, or a single mean value.

ADH = alcohol dehydrogenase; Aged = aged; AIDS = acquired immunodeficiency syndrome; Alb = hypoalbuminemia; Atr Fib = atrial fibrillation; AVH = acute viral hepatitis; Burn = burn patients; C_{max} = peak concentration; CAD = coronary artery disease; Celiac = celiac disease; CF = cystic fibrosis; CHF = congestive heart failure; Child = children; Cirr = hepatic cirrhosis; COPD = chronic obstructive pulmonary disease; CP = cor pulmonale; CPBS = cardiopulmonary bypass surgery; CRI = chronic respiratory insufficiency; Crohn = Crohn's disease; Cush = Cushing's syndrome; CYP = cytochrome P450; Fem = female; Hep = hepatitis; HIV = human immunodeficiency virus; HL = hyperlipoproteinemia; HTh = hyperthyroid; IM = intramuscular; Inflam = inflammation; IV = intravenous; LD = liver disease; LTh = hypothyroid; MAO = monoamine oxidase; MI = myocardial infarction; NAT = N-acetyltransferase; Neo = neonate; NIDDM = non-insulin-dependent diabetes mellitus; NS = nephrotic syndrome; Obes = obese; Pneu = pneumonia; Preg = pregnant; Prem = premature; RA = rheumatoid arthritis; RD = renal disease (including uremia); SC = subcutaneous; Smk = smoking; ST = sulfotransferase; T_{max} = peak time; Tach = ventricular tachycardia; UGT = UDP-glucuronosyl transferase; Ulcer = ulcer patients. Other abbreviations are defined in the text section of this appendix.

Table A–II–1
PHARMACOKINETIC DATA (Continued)

AVAILABILITY (ORAL) (%)	URINARY EXCRETION (%)	BOUND IN PLASMA (%)	CLEARANCE ($ml \cdot min^{-1} \cdot kg^{-1}$)	VOL. DIST. (liters/kg)	HALF-LIFE (hours)	PEAK TIME (hours)	PEAK CONCENTRATIONS
RITONAVIR[a] (Chapter 51)							
_[b] ↑ Food	3.5 ± 1.8	98–99	SD: 1.2 ± 0.4[c] MD: 2.1 ± 0.8[c] ↑ Child ↓ Cirr[d]	0.41 ± 0.25[c]	3–5[c] ↑ Cirr[d]	2–4[e]	11 ± 4 μg/ml[e]
RIZATRIPTAN[a] (Chapter 11)							
47	F: 28 ± 9[b] M: 29[b]	14	F: 12.3 ± 1.4[b] M: 18.9 ± 2.8[b] ↓ LD,[c] RD[d]	F: 1.5 ± 0.2 M: 2.2 ± 0.4	F: 2.2 M: 2.4	SD: 0.9 ± 0.4[e] MD: 4.8 ± 0.7[e]	SD: 20 ± 4.9 ng/ml[e] MD: 37 ± 13 ng/ml[e]
ROFECOXIB[a] (Chapter 27)							
93	<1	87	1.7[b] ↓ LD[c] ↔ RD	1.23[b]	MD: 17[b]	2–3[d]	SD: 207 ng/ml[d] MD: 321 ng/ml[d]

[a]Ritonavir is extensively metabolized primarily by CYP3A4. It also appears to induce its own clearance with single- (SD) to multiple-dose (MD) administration. Also used in combination with saquinavir; saquinavir has no significant effect on the pharmacokinetics of ritonavir.
[b]Absolute bioavailability unknown (>60% absorbed); food elicits a 15% increase in oral AUC for capsule formulation.
[c]CL/F, V_{area}/F, and half-life reported for oral dose.
[d]CL/F reduced slightly and half-life increased slightly; moderate liver impairment.
[e]Following a 600-mg oral dose, twice a day, to steady state.

References: Hsu, A., Granneman, G.R., and Bertz, R.J. Ritonavir. Clinical pharmacokinetics and interactions with other anti-HIV agents. *Clin. Pharmacokinet.,* **1998,** 35:275–291.
Physicians' Desk Reference, 54th ed. Medical Economics Co., Montvale, NJ, **2000,** p. 465.

[a]Data from healthy adult male (M) and female (F) subjects. Oxidative deamination catalyzed by MAO-A is the primary route of elimination. N-desmethyl rizatriptan (DMR) is a minor metabolite (~14%) that is active and accumulates in blood.
[b]Evidence of minor dose-dependent metabolic clearance and urinary excretion.
[c]CL/F reduced, moderate hepatic impairment.
[d]CL/F reduced, severe renal impairment.
[e]Following a 10-mg single (SD) and multiple (MD; 10 mg every 2 hours × 3 doses × 4 days) oral dose. DMR peak concentration is 8.5 and 26.2 ng/ml with SD and MD, respectively.

References: Goldberg, M.R., Lee, Y., Vyas, K.P., Slaughter, D.E., Panebianco, D., Ermlich, S.J., Shadle, C.R., Brucker, M.J., McLoughlin, D.A., and Olah, T.V. Rizatriptan, a novel 5-HT$_{1B/1D}$ agonist for migraine: single- and multiple-dose tolerability and pharmacokinetics in healthy subjects. *J. Clin. Pharmacol,* **2000,** 40:74–83.
Lee, Y., Ermlich, S.J., Sterrett, A.T., Goldberg, M.R., Blum, R.A., Brucker, M.J., McLoughlin, D.A., Olah, T.V., Zhao, J., and Rogers, J.D. Pharmacokinetics and tolerability of intravenous rizatriptan in healthy females. *Biopharm. Drug Dispos.,* **1998,** 19:577–581.
Physicians' Desk Reference, 54th ed. Medical Economics Co., Montvale, NJ, **2000,** p. 1912.
Vyas, K.P., Halpin, R.A., Geer, L.A., Ellis, J.D., Liu, L., Cheng, H., Chavez-Eng, C., Matuszewski, B.K., Varga, S.L., Guiblin, A.R., and Rogers, J.D. Disposition and pharmacokinetics of the antimigraine drug, rizatriptan, in humans. *Drug Metab. Dispos.,* **2000,** 28:89–95.

[a]Data from healthy adult male and female subjects. Metabolized primarily by cytosolic reductases, and a minor role for CYP3A4.
[b]CL/F, V_d/F, and $t_{1/2}$ reported for 25-mg oral dose.
[c]CL/F reduced, moderate hepatic impairment.
[d]Mean values following a single (SD) and multiple (MD) 25-mg oral dose.

References: Physicians' Desk Reference, 54th ed. Medical Economics Co., Montvale, NJ, **2000,** p. 1912.
Schwartz, J., Zhao, P., Gertz, B., Gumbs, C., Ebel, D., Lasseter, K., and Porras, A. Pharmacokinetics of rofecoxib in mild to moderate hepatic insufficiency. *Clin. Pharmacol. Ther.,* **2000,** 67:137.
Scott, L.J., and Lamb, H.M. Rofecoxib. *Drugs,* **1999,** 58:499–505; discussion 506–507.

ROPINIROLE[a] (Chapter 22)

55	<10	11.2 ± 5.0^{b} ↓ Aged[c] ←→ RD	7.5 ± 2.4^{b}	6^{b}	$1.0 (0.5–6.0)^{d}$ ↑ Food	$7.4 (2.4–13)$ ng/ml[d] ↓ Food

[a] Data from male and female patients with Parkinson's disease. Metabolized primarily by CYP1A2 to inactive N-deisopropyl and hydroxy metabolites.
[b] CL/F, V_d/F, and $t_{1/2}$ reported for oral dose.
[c] CL/F reduced but dose titrated to desired effect.
[d] Following 2-mg oral dose, three times a day, to steady state.

References: Bloomer, J.C., Clarke, S.E., and Chenery, R.J. In vitro identification of the P450 enzymes responsible for the metabolism of ropinirole. Drug Metab. Dispos., 1997, 25:840–844.
Physicians' Desk Reference, 54th ed. Medical Economics Co., Montvale, NJ, 2000, p. 3037.
Taylor, A.C., Beerahee, A., Citerone, D.R., Cyronak, M.J., Leigh, T.J., Fitzpatrick, K.L., Lopez-Gil, A., Vakil, S.D., Burns, E., and Lennox, G. Lack of a pharmacokinetic interaction at steady state between ropinirole and L-dopa in patients with Parkinson's disease. Pharmacotherapy, 1999, 19:150–156.

ROSIGLITAZONE[a] (Chapter 61)

99	Negligible	0.68 ± 0.16^{b} (0.49) ↓ LD[c] ←→ RD	0.25 ± 0.08^{b} (0.21)	$3–4^{b}$ ↑ LD	1.0^{d}	598 ± 117 ng/ml[d]

[a] Data from male and female patients with NIDDM (type 2 diabetes). No significant gender differences. Metabolized primarily by CYP2C8.
[b] CL/F, V_d/F, and $t_{1/2}$ reported for oral dose. Shown in parenthesis are mean values from a population pharmacokinetic analysis.
[c] Reduced CL/F and $CL/F_{unbound}$; moderate to severe liver impairment.
[d] Following a single 8-mg oral dose.

References: Baldwin, S.J., Clarke, S.E., and Chenery, R.J. Characterization of the cytochrome P450 enzymes involved in the in vitro metabolism of rosiglitazone. Br. J. Clin. Pharmacol., 1999, 48:424–432.
Patel, B.R., Diringer, K., Conrad, J., Miller, A., Rappaport, E., and Boyle, D. Population pharmacokinetics of rosiglitazone (R) in phase III clinical trials. Clin. Pharmacol. Ther., 2000, 67:123.
Physicians' Desk Reference, 54th ed. Medical Economics Co., Montvale, NJ, 2000, p. 2981.
Thompson, K., Zussman, B., Miller, A., Jorkasky, D., and Freed, M. Pharmacokinetics of rosiglitazone are unaltered in hemodialysis patients. Clin. Pharmacol. Ther., 1999, 65:186.

SAQUINAVIR[a] (Chapter 51)

HGC: 4 SGC: 13[b] ↑ Food	≤1	98	19.0 ± 2.3^{c}	10.0	7–12	HGC: $2–4^{d}$	HGC: 198 ng/ml[c,d] SGC: 948 ng/ml[c,d] ↑ Food

[a] Data from male and female patients with HIV infection. No significant gender differences. Metabolized by CYP3A in the intestine and liver.
[b] Calculation of absolute bioavailability for soft gel capsule (SGC) is based on its estimated 331% relative bioavailability vs. hard gel capsule (HGC) and the measured 4% absolute bioavailability of HGC taken with food vs. an IV dose.
[c] CL/F decreases and C_{max} increases when coadministered with other protease inhibitors (ritonavir, nelfinavir, and indinavir).
[d] Following 600-mg (HGC) or 800-mg (SGC), three times a day, to steady state.

References: Barry, M., Mulcahy, F., Merry, C., Gibbons, S., and Back, D. Pharmacokinetics and potential interactions amongst antiretroviral agents used to treat patients with HIV infection. Clin. Pharmacokinet., 1999, 36:289–304.
Merry, C., Barry, M.G., Mulcahy, F., Halifax, K.L., and Back, D.J. Saquinavir pharmacokinetics alone and in combination with nelfinavir in HIV-infected patients. AIDS, 1997, 11:F117–F120.
Perry, C.M., and Noble, S. Saquinavir soft-gel capsule formulation. A review of its use in patients with HIV infection. Drugs, 1998, 55:461–486.

Key: Unless otherwise indicated by a specific footnote, the data are presented for the study population as a mean value ± 1 standard deviation, a mean and range (lowest–highest in parenthesis) of values, a range of the lowest–highest values, or a single mean value.

ADH = alcohol dehydrogenase; Aged = aged; AIDS = acquired immunodeficiency syndrome; Alb = hypoalbuminemia; Atr Fib = atrial fibrillation; AVH = acute viral hepatitis; Burn = burn patients; C_{max} = peak concentration; CAD = coronary artery disease; Celiac = celiac disease; CF = cystic fibrosis; CHF = congestive heart failure; Child = children; Cirr = hepatic cirrhosis; COPD = chronic obstructive pulmonary disease; CP = cor pulmonale; CPBS = cardiopulmonary bypass surgery; CRI = chronic respiratory insufficiency; Crohn = Crohn's disease; Cush = Cushing's syndrome; CYP = cytochrome P450; Fem = female; Hep = hepatitis; HIV = human immunodeficiency virus; HL = hyperlipoproteinemia; HTh = hyperthyroid; IM = intramuscular; Inflam = inflammation; IV = intravenous; LD = liver disease; LTh = hypothyroid; MAO = monoamine oxidase; MI = myocardial infarction; NAT = N-acetyltransferase; Neo = neonate; NIDDM = non-insulin-dependent diabetes mellitus; NS = nephrotic syndrome; Obes = obese; Pneu = pneumonia; Preg = pregnant; Prem = premature; RA = rheumatoid arthritis; RD = renal disease (including uremia); SC = subcutaneous; Smk = smoking; ST = sulfotransferase; T_{max} = peak time; Tach = ventricular tachycardia; UGT = UDP-glucuronosyl transferase; Ulcer = ulcer patients. Other abbreviations are defined in the text section of this appendix.

Table A–II–1
PHARMACOKINETIC DATA (Continued)

AVAILABILITY (ORAL) (%)	URINARY EXCRETION (%)	BOUND IN PLASMA (%)	CLEARANCE ($ml \cdot min^{-1} \cdot kg^{-1}$)	VOL. DIST. (liters/kg)	HALF-LIFE (hours)	PEAK TIME (hours)	PEAK CONCENTRATIONS
SARGRAMOSTIM[a] (Chapter 54)							
—	—	—	A: 420 ml · min⁻¹ · (m²)⁻¹; C: 49(15–118) ml · min⁻¹ · (m²)⁻¹	A: —; C: 2 (0.4–18) liters/m²	A: 1.0; C: 1.6 (0.9–2.5)	A, SC: 1–3[b]; C, SC: 1.5–4[b]	A, IV: 5 ng/ml[b]; A, SC: 1.5 ng/ml[b]; C, IV: 100 ng/ml[b]; C, SC: 10 ng/ml[b]

[a]Data from healthy male adults (A) and children <15 years (C) treated for myelosuppression. A small fraction of patients develop neutralizing antibodies to sargramostim (rhGM-CSF)—clinical significance unknown.
[b]Following a 250-μg/m² IV infusion (2 hours) or subcutaneous (SC) injection to adults; following a 500-μg/m² IV infusion (2 hours) or 1500-μg/m² SC injection to children (peak concentrations estimated from data representation).

References: Physicians' Desk Reference, 54th ed. Medical Economics Co., Montvale, NJ. **2000,** p. 1419.
Stute, N., Furman, W.L., Schell, M., and Evans, W.E. Pharmacokinetics of recombinant human granulocyte-macrophage colony-stimulating factor in children after intravenous and subcutaneous administration. *J. Pharm. Sci.,* **1995,** *84:*824–828.

AVAILABILITY (ORAL) (%)	URINARY EXCRETION (%)	BOUND IN PLASMA (%)	CLEARANCE ($ml \cdot min^{-1} \cdot kg^{-1}$)	VOL. DIST. (liters/kg)	HALF-LIFE (hours)	PEAK TIME (hours)	PEAK CONCENTRATIONS
SELEGILINE[a] (Chapters 19, 22)							
Negligible[b]	Negligible	94[c]	~1500[d,e]; 160[d,e]	1.9[d]	1.9 ± 1.0[f]	S: 0.7 ± 0.4[g]; DS: ~1 h	S: 1.1 ± 0.4 ng/ml[g]; DS: ~15 ng/ml[g]

[a]MAO-B active metabolite: l-(−)-desmethylselegiline.
[b]Extensive first-pass metabolism; estimate of CL/F reported.
[c]Blood-to-plasma concentration ratio = 1.3–2.2 for parent drug and ~0.55 for N-desmethyl metabolite.
[d]Calculated assuming a 70-kg body weight.
[e]CL/F for N-desmethylselegiline assuming quantitative conversion of parent to this metabolite.
[f]For parent and N-desmethyl metabolite. Half-life for methamphetamine (major plasma species) and amphetamine are 21 and 18 hours, respectively.
[g]Mean data for selegiline (S) and its active metabolite, N-desmethylselegiline (DS), following a single 10-mg oral dose given to adults.

References: Heinonen, E.H., Anttila, M.I., and Lammintausta, R.A. Pharmacokinetic aspects of l-deprenyl (selegiline) and its metabolites. *Clin. Pharmacol. Ther.,* **1994,** *56:*742–749.

AVAILABILITY (ORAL) (%)	URINARY EXCRETION (%)	BOUND IN PLASMA (%)	CLEARANCE ($ml \cdot min^{-1} \cdot kg^{-1}$)	VOL. DIST. (liters/kg)	HALF-LIFE (hours)	PEAK TIME (hours)	PEAK CONCENTRATIONS
SERTRALINE (Chapter 19)							
—[a]	<1	98–99[b]	38 ± 14[c] ↓ Aged, Cirr	—	23 ↑ Aged, Cirr	M: 6.9 ± 1.0[d]; F: 6.7 ± 1.8[d]	M: 118 ± 22 ng/ml[d]; F: 166 ± 65 ng/ml[d] ←→ Aged

[a]Absolute bioavailability is not known (>44% absorbed); undergoes extensive first-pass metabolism to essentially inactive metabolites; catalyzed by multiple cytochrome P450 isoforms.
[b]Blood-to-plasma concentration ratio ~0.7.
[c]CL/F reported.
[d]Following a dose titration up to 200 mg, given once daily for 30 days to healthy male (M) and female (F) adults.

References: van Harten, J. Clinical pharmacokinetics of selective serotonin reuptake inhibitors. *Clin. Pharmacokinet.,* **1993,** *24:*203–220.
Warrington, S.J. Clinical implications of the pharmacology of sertraline. *Int. Clin. Psychopharmacol.,* **1994,** *6*(suppl 2):11–21.

SIBUTRAMINE[a] (Chapter 11)

—[b]	0 (S, M1, M2)	S: 97 M1: 94 M2: 94	S: 417[c]	—	S: ~1.1 M1: 14 M2: 16	S: 1.2[d] M1: 3.6 ± 1.0[d] M2: 3.5 ± 0.6[d] ↑ Food	M1: 4.0 ± 1.7 ng/ml[d] M2: 6.4 ± 1.8 ng/ml[d] ↓ Food

[a] Data from healthy male and female subjects and obese patients.
[b] Sibutramine (S) is well absorbed (77%) but undergoes extensive first-pass metabolism to active metabolites, N-desmethylsibutramine (M1) and N-di-desmethylsibutramine (M2). Metabolized by CYP3A in the intestine and liver.
[c] CL/F reported for oral dose.
[d] Following a single 15-mg oral dose in obese patients.

References: Luque, C.A., and Rey, J.A. Sibutramine: a serotonin-norepinephrine reuptake-inhibitor for the treatment of obesity. Ann. Pharmacother., 1999, 33:968–978.
Physicians' Desk Reference, 54th ed. Medical Economics Co., Montvale, NJ, 2000, p. 1510.

SILDENAFIL[a] (Chapter 32)

38	0	96	6.0 ± 1.1 ↓ LD,[b] RD,[c] Aged	1.2 ± 0.3[e]	2.4 ± 1.0	1.2 ± 0.3[e]	212 ± 59 ng/ml[e] ↑ Aged[d]

[a] Data from healthy male subjects. Sildenafil is metabolized primarily by CYP3A and secondarily by CYP2C9. Piperazine N-desmethyl metabolite is active (~50% parent) and accumulates in plasma (~40% parent).
[b] CL/F reduced, mild to moderate hepatic impairment.
[c] CL/F reduced, severe renal impairment.
[d] Increased unbound concentrations.
[e] Following a single 50-mg oral (solution) dose.

References: Physicians' Desk Reference, 54th ed. Medical Economics Co., Montvale, NJ, 2000, p. 2382.
Walker, D.K., Ackland, M.J., James, G.C., Muirhead, G.J., Rance, D.J., Wastall, P., and Wright, P.A. Pharmacokinetics and metabolism of sildenafil in mouse, rat, rabbit, dog and man. Xenobiotica, 1999, 29:297–310.

SIMVASTATIN[a] (Chapter 36)

≤5	Negligible	94	7.6[b]	—	2–3	AI: 1.4 ± 1.0[c] TI: 1.4 ± 1.0[c]	AI: 46 ± 20 ngEq/ml[c] TI: 56 ± 25 ngEq/ml[c]

[a] Simvastatin is a lactone prodrug which is hydrolyzed to the active corresponding β-hydroxy acid. Values reported are for the disposition of the acid.
[b] The β-hydroxy acid can be reconverted back to the lactone; irreversible oxidative metabolites are generated by CYP3A.
[c] Data for active inhibitors (AI—ring-opened molecule) and total inhibitors (TI) following a 40-mg oral dose, given once daily for 17 days to healthy adults.

References: Corsini, A., Bellosta, S., Baetta, R., Fumagalli, R., Paoletti, R., and Bernini, F. New insights into the pharmacodynamic and pharmacokinetic properties of statins. Pharmacol. Ther., 1999, 84:413–428.
Desager, J.P., and Horsmans, Y. Clinical pharmacokinetics of 3-hydroxy-3-methylglutaryl-coenzyme A reductase inhibitors. Clin. Pharmacokinet., 1996, 31:348–371.
Mauro, V.F. Clinical pharmacokinetics and practical applications of simvastatin. Clin. Pharmacokinet., 1993, 24:195–202.

Key: Unless otherwise indicated by a specific footnote, the data are presented for the study population as a mean value ± 1 standard deviation, a mean and range (lowest–highest in parenthesis) of values, a range of the lowest–highest values, or a single mean value.

ADH = alcohol dehydrogenase; Aged = aged; AIDS = acquired immunodeficiency syndrome; Alb = hypoalbuminemia; Atr Fib = atrial fibrillation; AVH = acute viral hepatitis; Burn = burn patients; C_{max} = peak concentration; CAD = coronary artery disease; Celiac = celiac disease; CF = cystic fibrosis; CHF = congestive heart failure; Child = children; Cirr = hepatic cirrhosis; COPD = chronic obstructive pulmonary disease; CP = cor pulmonale; CPBS = cardiopulmonary bypass surgery; CRI = chronic respiratory insufficiency; Crohn = Crohn's disease; Cush = Cushing's syndrome; CYP = cytochrome P450; Fem = female; Hep = hepatitis; HIV = human immunodeficiency virus; HL = hyperlipoproteinemia; HTh = hyperthyroid; IM = intramuscular; Inflam = inflammation; IV = intravenous; LD = liver disease; LTh = hypothyroid; MAO = monoamine oxidase; MI = myocardial infarction; NAT = N-acetyltransferase; Neo = neonate; NIDDM = non–insulin-dependent diabetes mellitus; NS = nephrotic syndrome; Obes = obese; Pneu = pneumonia; Preg = pregnant; Prem = premature; RA = rheumatoid arthritis; RD = renal disease (including uremia); SC = subcutaneous; Smk = smoking; ST = sulfotransferase; T_{max} = peak time; Tach = ventricular tachycardia; UGT = UDP-glucuronosyl transferase; Ulcer = ulcer patients. Other abbreviations are defined in the text section of this appendix.

Table A–II–1
PHARMACOKINETIC DATA (Continued)

	AVAILABILITY (ORAL) (%)	URINARY EXCRETION (%)	BOUND IN PLASMA (%)	CLEARANCE ($ml \cdot min^{-1} \cdot kg^{-1}$)	VOL. DIST. (liters/kg)	HALF-LIFE (hours)	PEAK TIME (hours)	PEAK CONCENTRATIONS
SIROLIMUS[a] (Chapter 53)	~15[b] ↑ Food[b]	—	40[c]	3.47 ± 1.58[d]	12 ± 4.6[d]	62.3 ± 16.2[d]	SD: 0.81 ± 0.17[e] MD: 1.4 ± 1.2[e]	SD: 67 ± 23 ng/ml[e] MD: 94–210 ng/ml[e]
STAVUDINE[a] (Chapter 51)	82 ± 5	43.1 ± 5.6	Negligible	8.17 ± 2.17[b] ↓ RD[b] → LD ←→ Child	0.53 ± 0.05	1.1 ± 0.25[c] ↑ RD	0.5–0.75[d]	1.2 ± 0.2 µg/ml[d]
STREPTOKINASE[a] (Chapter 55)	—	0	—	1.7 ± 0.7[b]	0.08 ± 0.04[b,c]	0.61 ± 0.24	0.9 ± 0.21[d]	188 ± 58 IU/ml[d]
SUFENTANIL (Chapters 14, 23)	—	6	93 ± 1[a] ←→ Cirr, Fem ↓ Neo	12.7 ± 2.5 ←→ Cirr, RD, Child, ←→ Aged ↓ Neo	1.7 ± 0.6[b] ↑ Neo, Aged, Obes ←→ RD	2.7 ± 1.2[b] ↑ Neo, Aged, Obes ←→ Cirr, RD, Child	—	28 ± 3.6 ng/ml[c]

SIROLIMUS

[a] Data from male and female renal transplant patients. All subjects were on a stable cyclosporine regimen. Sirolimus is metabolized primarily by CYP3A and is a substrate for P-glycoprotein. Several sirolimus metabolites are pharmacologically active.
[b] Cyclosporine coadministration increases sirolimus bioavailability. F increased by high-fat meal.
[c] Blood-to-plasma concentration ratio ~38 ± 13.
[d] Blood CL/F, V_{ss}/F, and half-life reported for oral dose.
[e] Following a single 15-mg oral dose (SD) in healthy subjects and 4- to 6.5-mg/m² oral dose (with cyclosporine), twice a day, to steady state (MD), in renal transplant patients.

References: Kelly, P.A., Napoli, K., and Kahan, B.D. Conversion from liquid to solid rapamycin formulations in stable renal allograft transplant recipients. *Biopharm. Drug Dispos.*, **1999,** *20:*249–253. Zimmerman, J.J., Ferron, G.M., Lim, H.K., and Parker, V. The effect of a high-fat meal on the oral bioavailability of the immunosuppressant sirolimus (rapamycin). *J. Clin. Pharmacol.*, **1999,** *39:*1155–1161.
Zimmerman, J.J., and Kahan, B.D. Pharmacokinetics of sirolimus in stable renal transplant patients after multiple oral dose administration. *J. Clin. Pharmacol.*, **1997,** *37:*405–415.

STAVUDINE

[a] Data from male and female patients with HIV infection.
[b] CL/F reduced, mild to severe renal impairment (cleared by hemodialysis).
[c] Undergoes intracellular activation to a triphosphate metabolite; $t_{1/2}$ for triphosphate ~3 hours.
[d] Following a single 0.67-mg/kg oral dose.

References: Dudley, M.N., Graham, K.K., Kaul, S., Geletko, S., Dunkle, L., Browne, M., and Mayer, K. Pharmacokinetics of stavudine in patients with AIDS or AIDS-related complex. *J. Infect. Dis.,* **1992,** *166:*480–485.
Rana, K.Z., and Dudley, M.N. Clinical pharmacokinetics of stavudine. *Clin. Pharmacokinet.,* **1997,** *33:*276–284.

STREPTOKINASE

[a] Values obtained from acute myocardial infarction patients using a function bioassay.
[b] Calculated assuming a 70-kg body weight.
[c] V_{area} reported.
[d] Following a single 1.5 × 10⁶-IU intravenous dose given as a 60-min infusion to patients with acute myocardial infarction.

References: Gemmill, J.D., Hogg, K.J., Burns, J.M., Rae, A.P., Dunn, F.G., Fears, R., Ferres, H., Standring, R., Greenwood, H., Pierce, D., and Hillis, W.S. A comparison of the pharmacokinetic properties of streptokinase and anistreplase in acute myocardial infarction. *Br. J. Clin. Pharmacol.,* **1991,** *31:*143–147.

SUFENTANIL

[a] Blood-to-plasma concentration ratio = 0.74 ± 0.05.
[b] More recent publications in which blood samples were taken over 24 hours report a prolonged half-life (~15 hours) and a corresponding increased V (10–15 l/kg), but the same CL. This prolonged half-life has no clinical relevance. In fact, the value listed may be an overestimate of a fast distribution half-life of 0.3 hour, which corresponds more with rapid reversibility of sedation after IV dosing.
[c] Following a single 5-µg/kg IV bolus dose to patients undergoing elective surgery.

Reference: Bovill, J.G., Sebel, P.S., Blackburn, C.L., Oei-Lim, V., and Heykants, J.J. The pharmacokinetics of sufentanil in surgical patients. *Anesthesiology,* **1984,** *61:*502–506.

SULFAMETHOXAZOLE (Chapter 44)

~100	14 ± 2	53 ± 5 ↓ RD, Alb ←→ Aged, CF	0.31 ± 0.07[a,b] ←→ RD ↑ CF	0.26 ± 0.04[a,b] ↑ RD ←→ Child, CF	10.1 ± 2.6[b] ↑ RD ←→ Child ↓ CF	4[c]	37.1 μg/ml[c]

[a] Calculated assuming a 70-kg body weight.
[b] Studies include concurrent administration of trimethoprim and variation in urinary pH; these factors had no marked effect on the clearance of sulfamethoxazole. Metabolically cleared primarily by N_4-acetylation.
[c] Mean data following a single 1000-mg oral dose given to healthy adults.

References: Hutabarat, R.M., Unadkat, J.D., Sahajwalla, C., McNamara, S., Ramsey, B., and Smith, A.L. Disposition of drugs in cystic fibrosis. I. Sulfamethoxazole and trimethoprim. *Clin. Pharmacol. Ther.,* **1991,** *49:*402–409.
Welling, P.G., Craig, W.A., Amidon, G.L., and Kunin, C.M. Pharmacokinetics of trimethoprim and sulfamethoxazole in normal subjects and in patients with renal failure. *J. Infect. Dis.,* **1973,** *128*(suppl):556–566.

SULFASALAZINE[a] (Chapters 27, 44)

3–12[b]	37	>99.3	0.24[c]	0.11 ± 0.02[c]	7.6 ± 3.4 ↑ Aged, RA[d]	S: 6 (4–8)[c] SP: 14 (10–19)[e]	S: 15–31 μg/ml[e] SP, EA: 7.2 μg/ml[e] SP, SA: 30 μg/ml[e]

[a] Data from healthy subjects and male and female patients with inflammatory bowel disease. Sulfasalazine (S) is a prodrug that is metabolized by colonic bacteria to the active metabolite, 5-amino salicylic acid, and the putative toxic metabolite, sulfapyridine (SP).
[b] Both S and 5-amino salicylate generated in the colon are poorly absorbed. SP is well absorbed.
[c] Data from IV sulfasalazine in healthy volunteers. SP elimination is controlled by NAT2 genotype—slower in poor acetylators (SA) than in extensive acetylators (EA). Patients with ileostomy will have decreased sulfasalazine metabolism.
[d] In rheumatoid arthritis (RA) patients.
[e] Following a single 3- to 4-g oral dose in patients with ulcerative colitis.

References: Klotz, U. Clinical pharmacokinetics of sulphasalazine, its metabolites and other prodrugs of 5-aminosalicylic acid. *Clin. Pharmacokinet.,* **1985,** *10:*285–302.
Physicians' Desk Reference, 54th ed. Medical Economics Co., Montvale, NJ, **2000,** p. 2410.

SULFISOXAZOLE (Chapter 44)

96 ± 14 ←→ Aged	49 ± 8[a]	91.4 ± 1.2 ↓ RD, Preg, Cirr	0.33 ± 0.01 ↑ Cirr[b] ←→ Aged	0.15 ± 0.02 ↑ Cirr[b] ←→ Aged	6.6 ± 0.7 ↑ RD ←→ Cirr, Aged	Y: 1.5 ± 0.3[c] E: 3.0 ± 1.6[c]	Y: 112 ± 33 μg/ml[c] E: 136 ± 28 μg/ml[c]

[a] Dependent on rate of urine formation and pH.
[b] Changes due to differences in plasma protein binding.
[c] Following a single 2-g oral dose taken after an overnight fast by healthy young (Y) and elderly (E) adults.

References: Boisvert, A., Barbeau, G., and Belanger, P.M. Pharmacokinetics of sulfisoxazole in young and elderly subjects. *Gerontology,* **1984,** *30:*125–131.
Oie, S., Gambertoglio, J.G., and Fleckenstein, L. Comparison of the disposition of total and unbound sulfisoxazole after single and multiple dosing. *J. Pharmacokinet. Biopharm.,* **1982,** *10:*157–172.

Key: Unless otherwise indicated by a specific footnote, the data are presented for the study population as a mean value ± 1 standard deviation, a mean and range (lowest–highest in parenthesis) of values, a range of the lowest–highest values, or a single mean value.

ADH = alcohol dehydrogenase; Aged = aged; AIDS = acquired immunodeficiency syndrome; Alb = hypoalbuminemia; Atr Fib = atrial fibrillation; AVH = acute viral hepatitis; Burn = burn patients; C_{max} = peak concentration; CAD = coronary artery disease; Celiac = celiac disease; CF = cystic fibrosis; CHF = congestive heart failure; Child = children; Cirr = hepatic cirrhosis; COPD = chronic obstructive pulmonary disease; CP = cor pulmonale; CPBS = cardiopulmonary bypass surgery; CRI = chronic respiratory insufficiency; Crohn = Crohn's disease; Cush = Cushing's syndrome; CYP = cytochrome P450; Fem = female; Hep = hepatitis; HIV = human immunodeficiency virus; HL = hyperlipoproteinemia; HTh = hyperthyroid; IM = intramuscular; Inflam = inflammation; IV = intravenous; LD = liver disease; LTh = hypothyroid; MAO = monoamine oxidase; MI = myocardial infarction; NAT = N-acetyltransferase; Neo = neonate; NIDDM = non-insulin-dependent diabetes mellitus; NS = nephrotic syndrome; Obes = obese; Pneu = pneumonia; Preg = pregnant; Prem = premature; RA = rheumatoid arthritis; RD = renal disease (including uremia); SC = subcutaneous; Smk = smoking; ST = sulfotransferase; T_{max} = peak time; Tach = ventricular tachycardia; UGT = UDP-glucuronosyl transferase; Ulcer = ulcer patients. Other abbreviations are defined in the text section of this appendix.

Table A–II–1
PHARMACOKINETIC DATA (Continued)

	AVAILABILITY (ORAL) (%)	URINARY EXCRETION (%)	BOUND IN PLASMA (%)	CLEARANCE ($ml \cdot min^{-1} \cdot kg^{-1}$)	VOL. DIST. (liters/kg)	HALF-LIFE (hours)	PEAK TIME (hours)	PEAK CONCENTRATIONS
SULINDAC[a] (Chapter 27)	—	Negligible	S: 94 SS: 94 ↓ RD	—[b,c]	—	S: 3.0 ± 2.0 SS: 12.9 ± 4.2 ↔ RD	S: 1.7 ± 0.8[d] SS: 7.7 ± 1.6[d]	S: 11 ± 3 $\mu g/ml$[d] SS: 7.7 ± 1.6 $\mu g/ml$[d]

[a]Reversibly reduced to the active metabolite, sulindac sulfide, catalyzed in part by gut flora after biliary excretion of parent drug. Kinetic data are for sulindac (S) and sulindac sulfide (SS).
[b]CL/F for S and SS not reported because of complications with reversible metabolism and enterohepatic recycling.
[c]AUC of sulindac sulfide significantly decreased in end-stage renal disease.
[d]Data for sulindac (S) and its active metabolite, sulindac sulfide (SS), following a single 300-mg oral dose taken after an overnight fast by healthy adults.

Reference: Ravis, W.R., Diskin, C.J., Campagna, K.D., Clark, C.R., and McMillian, C.L. Pharmacokinetics and dialyzability of sulindac and metabolites in patients with end-stage renal failure. *J. Clin. Pharmacol.,* **1993,** *33:*527–534.

	AVAILABILITY (ORAL) (%)	URINARY EXCRETION (%)	BOUND IN PLASMA (%)	CLEARANCE ($ml \cdot min^{-1} \cdot kg^{-1}$)	VOL. DIST. (liters/kg)	HALF-LIFE (hours)	PEAK TIME (hours)	PEAK CONCENTRATIONS
SUMATRIPTAN (Chapter 11)	Oral: 14 ± 5 SC: 97 ± 16	22 ± 4	14–21	22 ± 5.4[a]	2.0 ± 0.34[a]	1.0 ± 0.3[b]	SC: 0.2 (0.1–0.3)[c] Oral: ~1.5[c]	SC: 72 (55–108) ng/ml[c] Oral: 54 (27–137) ng/ml[c]

[a]Calculated assuming a 70-kg body weight.
[b]A half-life of ~2 hours reported for subcutaneous (SC) and oral doses.
[c]Following a single 6-mg SC or 100-mg oral dose given to young healthy adults.

References: Scott, A.K. Sumatriptan clinical pharmacokinetics. *Clin. Pharmacokinet.,* **1994,** *27:*337–344.
Scott, A.K., Grimes, S., Ng, K., Critchley, M., Breckenridge, A.M., Thomson, C., and Pilgrim, A.J. Sumatriptan and cerebral perfusion in healthy volunteers. *Br. J. Clin. Pharmacol.,* **1992,** *33:*401–404.

	AVAILABILITY (ORAL) (%)	URINARY EXCRETION (%)	BOUND IN PLASMA (%)	CLEARANCE ($ml \cdot min^{-1} \cdot kg^{-1}$)	VOL. DIST. (liters/kg)	HALF-LIFE (hours)	PEAK TIME (hours)	PEAK CONCENTRATIONS
TACROLIMUS (Chapter 53)	25 ± 10[a,b] ↔ RD ↓ Food	<1	75–99[c,d]	0.90 ± 0.29[a,e] ↔ RD, Cirr	0.91 ± 0.29[a,d] ↔ RD ↑ Cirr	12 ± 5[a] ↔ RD ↑ Cirr	1.4 ± 0.5[f]	31.2 ± 10.1 ng/ml[f]

[a]Drug disposition parameters calculated from blood concentrations. Data from liver transplant patients reported.
[b]A similar bioavailability ($F = 21 \pm 19\%$) reported for kidney transplant patients; $F = 16 \pm 7\%$ for normal subjects. Low oral bioavailability likely due to incomplete intestinal availability.
[c]Different values for plasma protein binding reported.
[d]Slightly higher V_{ss} and $t_{1/2}$ reported for kidney transplant patients. Because of the very high and variable blood-to-plasma concentration ratio (mean = 35, range = 12–67), markedly different V_{ss} values are reported for parameters based on plasma concentrations.
[e]Metabolized by CYP3A; also a substrate for P-glycoprotein.
[f]Following a single 7-mg oral dose given to healthy adults. Consensus target trough concentrations at steady state are 5–20 ng/ml.

References: Bekersky, I., Dressler, D., and Mekki, Q.A. Dose linearity after oral administration of tacrolimus 1-mg capsules at doses of 3, 7, and 10 mg. *Clin. Ther.,* **1999,** *21:*2058–2064.
Jusko, W.J., Piekoszewski, W., Lintmalm, G.B., Shaefer, M.S., Hebert, M.F., Piergies, A.A., Lee, C.C., Schechter, P., and Mekki, Q.A. Pharmacokinetics of tacrolimus in liver transplant patients. *Clin. Pharmacol. Ther.,* **1995,** *57:*281–290.
Physicians' Desk Reference, 54th ed. Medical Economics Co, Montvale, NJ, **2000,** pp. 1098–1099.

TAMOXIFEN[a] (Chapters 52, 58)

<1	>98	1.4[b,c]	50–60[b]	4–11 days[d]	5 (3–7)	120 (67–183) ng/ml

[a] Active metabolites; 4-hydroxytamoxifen and 4-hydroxy-N-desmethyltamoxifen are minor metabolites that exhibit affinity for the estrogen receptor that is greater than that of parent *trans*-tamoxifen. All metabolites are rate limited by tamoxifen elimination.
[b] CL/F and V_{area}/F reported.
[c] The major pathway of elimination, N-demethylation, is catalyzed by CYP3A.
[d] Half-life consistent with accumulation and approach to steady state. Significantly longer terminal half-lives are observed.
[e] Average concentration (C_{ss}) following a 10-mg oral dose, given twice a day to steady state.

Reference: Lønning, P.E., Geisler, J., and Dowsett, M. Pharmacological and clinical profile of anastrozole. *Breast Cancer Res. Treat.*, **1998**, *49(suppl 1)*:S53–S57.
Physicians' Desk Reference, 54th ed. Medical Economics Co., Montvale, NJ, **2000**, p. 557.

TAMSULOSIN[a] (Chapter 10)

100 ↓ Food	99 ± 1 ↑ RD	12.7 ± 3.0	0.62 ± 0.31 ↓ RD,[b], Aged	0.20 ± 0.06	6.8 ± 3.5[c] ↑ RD, Aged	5.3 ± 0.7[d] ↑ Food	16 ± 5 ng/ml[d] ↓ Food

[a] Data from healthy male subjects. Metabolized primarily by CYP3A and CYP2D6.
[b] CL/F reduced, moderate renal impairment. Unbound AUC relatively unchanged.
[c] Apparent $t_{1/2}$ after oral dose in patients is ~14 to 15 hours, reflecting controlled release from modified-release granules.
[d] Following a single 0.4-mg modified-release oral dose in healthy subjects.

References: Matsushima, H., Kamimura, H., Soeishi, Y., Watanabe, T., Higuchi, S., and Miyazaki, M. Plasma protein binding of tamsulosin hydrochloride in renal disease: role of α_1-acid glycoprotein and possibility of binding interactions. *Eur. J. Clin. Pharmacol.*, **1999**, *55*:437–443.
van Hoogdalem, E.J., Soeishi, Y., Matsushima, H., and Higuchi, S. Disposition of the selective α_{1A}-adrenoceptor antagonist tamsulosin in humans: comparison with data from interspecies scaling. *J. Pharm. Sci.*, **1997**, *86*:1156–1161.
Wolzt, M., Fabrizii, V., Dorner, G.T., Zanaschka, G., Leufkens, P., Krauwinkel, W.J., and Eichler, H.G. Pharmacokinetics of tamsulosin in subjects with normal and varying degrees of impaired renal function: an open-label single-dose and multiple-dose study. *Eur. J. Clin. Pharmacol.*, **1998**, *4*:367–373.

TETRACYCLINE (Chapter 47)

77	58 ± 8	65 ± 3	1.67 ± 0.24	1.5 ± 0.1[a]	10.6 ± 1.5	Oral: 4	IV: 16.4 ± 1.2 μg/ml[b] Oral: 2.3 ± 0.2 μg/ml[b]

[a] V_{area} reported.
[b] Following a single 10-mg/kg IV dose or a single 250-mg oral dose (taken after a fast and with water).

References: Garty, M., and Hurwitz, A. Effect of cimetidine and antacids on gastrointestinal absorption of tetracycline. *Clin. Pharmacol. Ther.*, **1980**, *28*:203–207.
Raghuram, T.C., and Krishnaswamy, K. Pharmacokinetics of tetracycline in nutritional edema. *Chemotherapy*, **1982**, *28*:428–433.

Key: Unless otherwise indicated by a specific footnote, the data are presented for the study population as a mean value ± 1 standard deviation, a mean and range (lowest–highest in parenthesis) of values, a range of the lowest–highest values, or a single mean value.

ADH = alcohol dehydrogenase; Aged = aged; AIDS = acquired immunodeficiency syndrome; Alb = hypoalbuminemia; Atr Fib = atrial fibrillation; AVH = acute viral hepatitis; Burn = burn patients; C_{max} = peak concentration; CAD = coronary artery disease; Celiac = celiac disease; CF = cystic fibrosis; CHF = congestive heart failure; Child = children; Cirr = hepatic cirrhosis; COPD = chronic obstructive pulmonary disease; CP = cor pulmonale; CPBS = cardiopulmonary bypass surgery; CRI = chronic respiratory insufficiency; Crohn = Crohn's disease; Cush = Cushing's syndrome; CYP = cytochrome P450; Fem = female; Hep = hepatitis; HIV = human immunodeficiency virus; HL = hyperlipoproteinemia; HTh = hyperthyroid; IM = intramuscular; Inflam = inflammation; IV = intravenous; LD = liver disease; LTh = hypothyroid; MAO = monoamine oxidase; MI = myocardial infarction; NAT = N-acetyltransferase; Neo = neonate; NIDDM = non-insulin-dependent diabetes mellitus; NS = nephrotic syndrome; Obes = obese; Pneu = pneumonia; Preg = pregnant; Prem = premature; RA = rheumatoid arthritis; RD = renal disease (including uremia); SC = subcutaneous; Smk = smoking; ST = sulfotransferase; T_{max} = peak time; Tach = ventricular tachycardia; UGT = UDP-glucuronosyl transferase; Ulcer = ulcer patients. Other abbreviations are defined in the text section of this appendix.

Table A–II–1
PHARMACOKINETIC DATA (Continued)

AVAILABILITY (ORAL) (%)	URINARY EXCRETION (%)	BOUND IN PLASMA (%)	CLEARANCE (ml·min⁻¹·kg⁻¹)	VOL. DIST. (liters/kg)	HALF-LIFE (hours)	PEAK TIME (hours)	PEAK CONCENTRATIONS

THALIDOMIDE[a] (Chapters 48, 53)

AVAILABILITY (ORAL) (%)	URINARY EXCRETION (%)	BOUND IN PLASMA (%)	CLEARANCE (ml·min⁻¹·kg⁻¹)	VOL. DIST. (liters/kg)	HALF-LIFE (hours)	PEAK TIME (hours)	PEAK CONCENTRATIONS
b	<1	—	2.2 ± 0.4^c	1.1 ± 0.3^c	6.2 ± 2.6^c	3.2 ± 1.4^d ↑ HD, Food	2.0 ± 0.6 μg/ml^d ↑ HD

[a] Data from healthy male subjects. Similar data reported for asymptomatic patients with HIV. No age or gender differences. Thalidomide undergoes spontaneous hydrolysis in blood to multiple metabolites.
[b] Absolute bioavailability unknown. Altered absorption rate and extent, Hansen's disease (HD).
[c] CL/F, V_{area}/F, and $t_{1/2}$ reported for oral dose.
[d] Following a single 200-mg oral dose.

References: Noormohamed, F.H., Youle, M.S., Higgs, C.J., Kook, K.A., Hawkins, D.A., Lant, A.F., and Thomas, S.D. Pharmacokinetics and hemodynamic effects of single oral doses of thalidomide in asymptomatic human immunodeficiency virus–infected subjects. AIDS Res. Hum. Retrovir., 1999, 15:1047–1052.
Physicians' Desk Reference, 54th ed. Medical Economics Co., Montvale, NJ, 2000, p. 912.
Teo, S.K., Colburn, W.A., and Thomas, S.D. Single-dose oral pharmacokinetics of three formulations of thalidomide in healthy male volunteers. J. Clin. Pharmacol., 1999, 39:1162–1168.

THEOPHYLLINE (Chapter 28)

AVAILABILITY (ORAL) (%)	URINARY EXCRETION (%)	BOUND IN PLASMA (%)	CLEARANCE (ml·min⁻¹·kg⁻¹)	VOL. DIST. (liters/kg)	HALF-LIFE (hours)	PEAK TIME (hours)	PEAK CONCENTRATIONS
96 ± 8	18 ± 3 ↑ Neo, Prem ←→ CF, Aged	56 ± 4 ↓ Aged, Cirr, Neo, Preg, Obes ←→ CF	$0.65 \pm 0.20^{a,b}$ ↓ Neo, Prem, Cirr, CHF, CP, Hep, LTh, Obes, Pneu ↑ Smk, CF, HTh, Child ←→ Aged, Preg, RD, COPD	0.50 ± 0.16 ↓ Obes ↑ Prem, CF ←→ Aged, Preg, Cirr, HTh, LTh, RD	9.0 ± 2.1^b ↓ Smk, CF, HTh ↑ Prem, Neo, Cirr, CHF, Hep, CP, LTh ←→ Aged, RD	A: ~1.5^c TD: 11.5 ± 7.5^c T24: 11.3 ± 4.8^c	A: 7.9 ± 0.6 μg/ml^c TD: 15 ± 2.8 μg/ml^c T24: 14 ± 3.7 μg/ml^c

[a] Nonlinear kinetics due to saturable metabolism, especially in children at steady state. Ratio of percent increase in steady-state concentration to percent increase in dose was >1.5 in 15% of children changed to a higher dose. Metabolically cleared primarily by CYP1A2.
[b] CL increased and $t_{1/2}$ decreased as a result of enzyme induction by anticonvulsant drugs.
[c] Following a 200-mg oral dose (aminophylline) given three times a day for 5 days, a 400-mg oral dose (THEO-DUR) given twice a day for 5 days, or a 800-mg oral dose (THEO-24) given once a day for 5 days, all to healthy adults. Sustained release formulations were taken 1 hour prior to a high-fat meal. Levels of 5 to 15 μg/ml are considered therapeutic; a level >20 μg/ml is potentially toxic.

References: Dockhorn, R.J., Cefali, E.A., and Straughn, A.B. Comparative steady-state bioavailability of Theo-24 and Theo-Dur in healthy men. Ann. Allergy, 1994, 72:218–222.
Taburet, A.M., and Schmit, B. Pharmacokinetic optimisation of asthma treatment. Clin. Pharmacokinet., 1994, 26:396–418.
Vestal, R.E., Thummel, K.E., Mercer, G.D., and Koup, J.R. Comparison of single and multiple dose pharmacokinetics of theophylline using stable isotopes. Eur. J. Clin. Pharmacol., 1986, 30:113–120.

THIOPENTAL (Chapters 14, 17)

AVAILABILITY (ORAL) (%)	URINARY EXCRETION (%)	BOUND IN PLASMA (%)	CLEARANCE (ml·min⁻¹·kg⁻¹)	VOL. DIST. (liters/kg)	HALF-LIFE (hours)	PEAK TIME (hours)	PEAK CONCENTRATIONS
—	<1	85 ± 4 ↓ Aged,^{a} Cirr, CPBS ←→ Child	3.9 ± 1.2 ←→ Cirr, Aged, Obes ↑ Child $CL_{int} = 28 \pm 9$ ↓ Cirr	2.3 ± 0.5 ↑ Aged,^{a} Obes ←→ Child	9.0 ± 1.6^b ↑ Aged,^{a} Cirr, Obes, Neo ↓ Child	—	SD: 5–7 μg/ml^c MD: 25.4 ± 13.1 μg/ml^c

[a] Data from females only.
[b] A distribution $t_{1/2}$ of ~1 hour controls the duration of unconsciousness after a single bolus dose.
[c] Arterial concentration at 2 to 5 minutes following a single bolus dose of 6.7 ± 0.7 mg/kg IV (SD) given to young adults undergoing elective surgery, or steady-state venous concentration following a dose of 250 mg IV given every 2 hours (MD) to critical care patients. Loss of voluntary motor control and burst suppression of EEG at the 50th percentile occur at the levels of 11 and 34 μg/ml respectively.

References: Homer, T.D., and Stanski, D.R. The effect of increasing age on thiopental disposition and anesthetic requirement. Anesthesiology, 1985, 62:714–724.
Hudson, R.J., Stanski, D.R., and Burch, P.G. Pharmacokinetics of methohexital and thiopental in surgical patients. Anesthesiology, 1983, 59:215–219.
Russo, H., Bres, J., Duboin, M.P., and Roquefeuil, B. Pharmacokinetics of thiopental after single and multiple intravenous doses in critical care patients. Eur. J. Clin. Pharmacol., 1995, 49:127–137.
Sorbo, S., Hudson, R.J., and Loomis, J.C. The pharmacokinetics of thiopental in pediatric surgical patients. Anesthesiology, 1984, 61:666–670.

THIOTEPA[a] (Chapter 52)

—[b]	TTP: 1.5 TP: 4.2	—	$186 \pm 20\ \text{ml} \cdot \text{min}^{-1} \cdot (\text{m}^2)^{-1}$ ←→ Child[c]	—	TTP: 2.08 ± 0.35 TP: 16–18 ←→ Child[c]	—	TTP: 1–1.5 µg/ml[d] TP: 0.1–0.2 µg/ml[d]

[a]Data from adult females with breast cancer receiving low-dose (12 mg/m²) thiotepa therapy. Thiotepa (TTP) is converted to an active alkylating metabolite, tepa (TP).
[b]For parenteral administration.
[c]Similar CL and $t_{1/2}$ data are reported for pediatric (2 to 10 years) and adult patients receiving high-dose thiotepa (300 mg/m²) as ablative therapy prior to bone marrow transplant.
[d]Following a bolus dose of 12 mg/m² IV TTP.

References: Cohen, B.E., Egorin, M.J., Kohlhepp, E.A., Aisner, J., and Gutierrez, P.L. Human plasma pharmacokinetics and urinary excretion of thiotepa and its metabolites. *Cancer Treat. Rep.*, **1986**, 70:859–864.
Kletzel, M., Kearns, G.L., Wells, T.G., and Thompson, H.C. Pharmacokinetics of high dose thiotepa in children undergoing autologous bone marrow transplantation. *Bone Marrow Transplant.*, **1992**, 10:171–175.
Physicians' Desk Reference, 54th ed. Medical Economics Co, Montvale, NJ, **2000**, p. 1430.

TIAGABINE[a] (Chapter 21)

~90	1–2	96	2.0 ± 0.4[b] ↑ Epilep,[c] Child[d] ↓ Cirr[e] ←→ RD	1.3 ± 0.4[b]	7–9[b] ↑ Cirr	SD: 0.9 ± 0.5[f] MD: 1.5 ± 1.0[f]	SD: 122 ± 36 ng/ml[f] MD: 69 ± 22 ng/ml[f]

[a]Data from healthy adult male and female subjects and patients with epilepsy. Metabolized primarily by UGT and CYP3A.
[b]CL/F, V_{area}/F, and half-life reported for oral dose.
[c]CL/F increased in adult and pediatric patients receiving enzyme-inducing anticonvulsant drugs.
[d]Weight-adjusted CL/F higher in children (3 to 10 years of age) than in adults.
[e]CL/F reduced, moderate hepatic impairment.
[f]Following a single 8-mg oral dose (SD) or a 3-mg oral dose, three times a day for 4 days (MD). Diurnal variation (lower C_{max} in P.M. than A.M.).

References: Gustavson, L.E., Boellner, S.W., Granneman, G.R., Qian, J.X., Guenther, H.J., el-Shourbagy, T., and Sommerville, K.W. A single-dose study to define tiagabine pharmacokinetics in pediatric patients with complex partial seizures. *Neurology*, **1997**, 48:1032–1037.
Lau, A.H., Gustavson, L.E., Sperelakis, R., Lam, N.P., el-Shourbagy, T., Qian, J.X., and Layden, T. Pharmacokinetics and safety of tiagabine in subjects with various degrees of hepatic function. *Epilepsia*, **1997**, 38:445–451.
Physicians' Desk Reference, 54th ed. Medical Economics Co, Montvale, NJ, **2000**, p. 451.
Snel, S., Jansen, J.A., Mengel, H.B., Richens, A., and Larsen, S. The pharmacokinetics of tiagabine in healthy elderly volunteers and elderly patients with epilepsy. *J. Clin. Pharmacol.*, **1997**, 37:1015–1020.

TICLOPIDINE[a] (Chapter 55)

—[a]	Negligible	98[b]	SD: 34.0[c] MD: 13.2[c] ↓ Aged, Cirr[d] ←→ RD	—	SD: 7.9 ± 3.0[c] MD: 98 ± 64[c]	SD: 2 (1–3) MD: 1 (1–3)	SD: 0.41 ± 0.24 µg/ml[e] MD: 0.89 ± 0.37 µg/ml[e]

[a]Data from healthy adult male and female subjects. No significant gender differences. Parent drug is inactive. Metabolized in the liver to numerous metabolites and possibly excreted into bile. Absolute bioavailability is unknown.
[b]Approximately 40% to 50% of a single dose is bound (acylation) to blood platelets.
[c]CL/F and half-life reported for single-dose (SD) and multiple-dose (MD) oral administration.
[d]CL/F reduced, hepatic cirrhosis.
[e]Following a single 250-mg dose, or 250 mg, twice a day for 21 days.

References: Desager, J.P. Clinical pharmacokinetics of ticlopidine. *Clin. Pharmacokinet.*, **1994,** 26:347–355.
Physicians' Desk Reference, 54th ed. Medical Economics Co, Montvale, NJ, **2000**, p. 2671.
Shah, J., Teitelbaum, P., Molony, B., Gabuzda, T., and Massey, I. Single and multiple dose pharmacokinetics of ticlopidine in young and elderly subjects. *Br. J. Clin. Pharmacol.*, **1991,** 32:761–764.

Key: Unless otherwise indicated by a specific footnote, the data are presented for the study population as a mean value ± 1 standard deviation, a mean and range (lowest–highest in parenthesis) of values, a range of the lowest–highest values, or a single mean value.

ADH = alcohol dehydrogenase; Aged = aged; AIDS = acquired immunodeficiency syndrome; Alb = hypoalbuminemia; Atr Fib = atrial fibrillation; AVH = acute viral hepatitis; Burn = burn patients; C_{max} = peak concentration; CAD = coronary artery disease; Celiac = celiac disease; CF = cystic fibrosis; CHF = congestive heart failure; Child = children; Cirr = hepatic cirrhosis; COPD = chronic obstructive pulmonary disease; CP = cor pulmonale; CPBS = cardiopulmonary bypass surgery; CRI = chronic respiratory insufficiency; Crohn = Crohn's disease; Cush = Cushing's syndrome; CYP = cytochrome P450; Fem = female; Hep = hepatitis; HIV = human immunodeficiency virus; HL = hyperlipoproteinemia; HTn = hyperthyroid; IM = intramuscular; Inflam = inflammation; IV = intravenous; LD = liver disease; LTh = hypothyroid; MAO = monoamine oxidase; MI = myocardial infarction; NAT = N-acetyltransferase; Neo = neonate; NIDDM = non-insulin-dependent diabetes mellitus; NS = nephrotic syndrome; Obes = obese; Pneu = pneumonia; Preg = pregnant; Prem = premature; RA = rheumatoid arthritis; RD = renal disease (including uremia); SC = subcutaneous; Smk = smoking; ST = sulfotransferase; T_{max} = peak time; Tach = ventricular tachycardia; UGT = UDP-glucuronosyl transferase; Ulcer = ulcer patients. Other abbreviations are defined in the text section of this appendix.

Table A–II–1
PHARMACOKINETIC DATA (Continued)

AVAILABILITY (ORAL) (%)	URINARY EXCRETION (%)	BOUND IN PLASMA (%)	CLEARANCE $(ml \cdot min^{-1} \cdot kg^{-1})$	VOL. DIST. (liters/kg)	HALF-LIFE (hours)	PEAK TIME (hours)	PEAK CONCENTRATIONS
TOBRAMYCIN (Chapter 46)							
Inhalation: 9 ± 8	90[a]	<10	$CL = 0.98CL_{cr} \pm 32\%$[b] $\downarrow$ Obes $\uparrow$ CF	0.33 ± 0.04[c] $\uparrow$ Obes $\downarrow$ RD, Aged, Burn $\uparrow$ CF, Neo	2.2 ± 0.1[d] $\uparrow$ RD, Neo, Prem $\uparrow$ Obes, CF $\downarrow$ Burn	IM: 0.3–0.75[e]	IV: 4.6 ± 0.5 $\mu g/ml$[e] IM: 5.2 ± 0.6 $\mu g/ml$[e]

[a]Possibly higher, since drug persists in tissues for long periods of time.
[b]CL calculated using units of $ml \cdot min^{-1} \cdot kg^{-1}$ for CL_{cr}.
[c]Volume of central compartment.
[d]Tobramycin has a very long terminal elimination half-life (146 ± 75 hours), which reflects slow efflux from tissues and accounts for prolonged urinary excretion.
[e]Following a 100-mg intravenous dose (level at end of 1-hour infusion) or a 100-mg IM injection given to healthy adults.

References: Aarons, L., Vozeh, S., Wenk, M., Weiss, P., and Follath, F. Population pharmacokinetics of tobramycin. *Br. J. Clin. Pharmacol.*, **1989**, *28*:305–314.
Regamey, C., Gordon, R.C., and Kirby, W.M. Comparative pharmacokinetics of tobramycin and gentamicin. *Clin. Pharmacol. Ther.*, **1973**, *14*:396–403.

AVAILABILITY (ORAL) (%)	URINARY EXCRETION (%)	BOUND IN PLASMA (%)	CLEARANCE $(ml \cdot min^{-1} \cdot kg^{-1})$	VOL. DIST. (liters/kg)	HALF-LIFE (hours)	PEAK TIME (hours)	PEAK CONCENTRATIONS
TOCAINIDE[a] (Chapter 35)							
89 ± 5	38 ± 7	10 ± 15	2.6 ± 0.5 $\downarrow$ CHF, RD, NS $\longleftrightarrow$ MI	3.0 ± 0.2 $\downarrow$ CHF $\longleftrightarrow$ MI, RD	13.5 ± 2.3 $\uparrow$ RD, NS $\longleftrightarrow$ MI, CHF	IV: 0.42[b] Oral: 0.5–2[b]	IV: 3.0 ± 1.2 $\mu g/ml$[b] Oral: 1.8 $\mu g/ml$[b]

[a]Racemic mixture; the two enantiomers appear to have similar antiarrhythmic activity. S-(−)-enantiomer ($t_{1/2} = 10 \pm 4$ hours) is cleared 1.8 times more rapidly than R-(+)-enantiomer ($t_{1/2} = 17 \pm 6$ hours); V_{ss} is the same for the two enantiomers.
[b]Following a single 250-mg intravenous dose, given as a 20-min infusion or a single 400-mg oral dose to patients with acute MI and left ventricular failure. Therapeutic range = 3 to 10 $\mu g/ml$.

References: MacMahon, B., Bakshi, M., Branagan, P., Kelly, J.G., and Walsh, M.J. Pharmacokinetics and haemodynamic effects of tocainide in patients with acute myocardial infarction complicated by left ventricular failure. *Br. J. Clin. Pharmacol.*, **1985**, *19*:429–434.
Physicians' Desk Reference, 54th ed. Medical Economics Co., Montvale, NJ, **2000**, p. 632–633.
Roden, D.M., and Woosley, R.L. Drug therapy. Tocainide. *N. Engl. J. Med.*, **1986**, *315*:41–45.
Thomson, A.H., Murdoch, G., Pottage, A., Kelman, A.W., Whiting, B., and Hillis, W.S. The pharmacokinetics of R- and S-tocainide in patients with acute ventricular arrhythmias. *Br. J. Clin. Pharmacol.*, **1986**, *21*:149–154.

AVAILABILITY (ORAL) (%)	URINARY EXCRETION (%)	BOUND IN PLASMA (%)	CLEARANCE $(ml \cdot min^{-1} \cdot kg^{-1})$	VOL. DIST. (liters/kg)	HALF-LIFE (hours)	PEAK TIME (hours)	PEAK CONCENTRATIONS
TOLBUTAMIDE[a] (Chapter 61)							
80–90[a]	~0.1	91–96 $\downarrow$ AVH, Aged	0.22 ± 0.06[b,c] $\uparrow$ AVH	0.12 ± 0.02[b] $\longleftrightarrow$ AVH	5.9 ± 1.4[b] $\downarrow$ AVH, CRI $\longleftrightarrow$ Aged, RD	3.1 ± 1.5[d]	53 ± 12 $\mu g/ml$[d]

[a]Bioavailability estimate based on recovery of oral dose in urine and expected negligible first-pass metabolism.
[b]CL/F, V/F, and half-life reported for oral dose.
[c]Metabolized primarily by CYP2C9 (polymorphic).
[d]Following a single 500-mg oral dose. A level of 80 to 240 $\mu g/ml$ associated with a >25% decrease in blood glucose concentration.

References: Balant, L. Clinical pharmacokinetics of sulphonylurea hypoglycaemic drugs. *Clin. Pharmacokinet.*, **1981**, *6*:215–241.
Matin, S.B., Wan, S.H., and Karam, J.H. Pharmacokinetics of tolbutamide: prediction by concentration in saliva. *Clin. Pharmacol. Ther.*, **1974**, *16*:1052–1058.
Peart, G.F., Boutagy, J., and Shenfield, G.M. Lack of relationship between tolbutamide metabolism and debrisoquine oxidation phenotype. *Eur. J. Clin. Pharmacol.*, **1987**, *33*:397–402.
Veronese, M.E., Miners, J.O., Randles, D., Gregov, D., and Birkett, D.J. Validation of the tolbutamide metabolic ratio for population screening with use of sulfaphenazole to produce model phenotypic poor metabolizers. *Clin. Pharmacol. Ther.*, **1990**, *47*:403–411.
Williams, R.L., Blaschke, T.F., Meffin, P.J., Melmon, K.L., and Rowland, M. Influence of acute viral hepatitis on disposition and plasma binding of tolbutamide. *Clin. Pharmacol. Ther.*, **1977**, *21*:301–309.

TOLCAPONE[a] (Chapter 22)

60 ± 10 ↓ Food	<1	1.50 ± 0.33 ↓ Cirr[b] ↔ RD	>99.9	0.12 ± 0.02 ↓ Cirr	1.3 ± 0.3[c]	1.8 ± 1.6[d]	5.7 ± 1.7 μg/ml[d]

[a]Data from healthy adult male subjects. No significant gender differences. Metabolized by UGT and CYP3A.
[b]$CL/F_{unbound}$ reduced, moderate cirrhotic liver disease.
[c]Value represents the half-life after intravenous administration. A longer mean half-life of 1.8 to 3.3 hours is reported after oral administration.
[d]Following a single 200-mg oral dose.

References: Jorga, K., Fotteler, B., Heizmann, P., and Gasser, R. Metabolism and excretion of tolcapone, a novel inhibitor of catechol-*O*-methyltransferase. *Br. J. Clin. Pharmacol.*, **1999**, 48:513–520.
Jorga, K., Fotteler, B., Heizmann, P., and Zurcher, G. Pharmacokinetics and pharmacodynamics after oral and intravenous administration of tolcapone, a novel adjunct to Parkinson's disease therapy. *Eur. J. Clin. Pharmacol.*, **1998**, 54:443–447.
Physicians' Desk Reference, 54th ed. Medical Economics Co., Montvale, NJ, **2000**, p. 2666.

TOLTERODINE[a] (Chapter 7)

EM: 26 ± 18 PM: 91 ± 40 EM: ↑ Food	EM: negligible PM: <2.5	T: 96.3 5-HM: 64	EM: 9.6 ± 2.8 PM: 2.0 ± 0.3 ↓ LD[b]	EM: 1.7 ± 0.4 PM: 1.5 ± 0.4	EM: 2.3 ± 0.3 PM: 9.2 ± 1.2 ↑ LD	EM: 1.2 ± 0.5[c] PM: 1.9 ± 1.0[c]	EM: 5.2 ± 5.7 ng/ml[c] PM: 38 ± 15 ng/ml[c]

[a]Data from healthy adult male subjects. No significant gender differences. Tolterodine (T) is metabolized primarily by CYP2D6 to an active (100% potency) metabolite, 5-hydroxymethyl tolterodine (5-HM), in extensive metabolizers (EM); $t_{1/2}$ 5-HM = 2.9 ± 0.4 hours. Also metabolized by CYP3A to an *N*-desalkyl product, particularly in poor metabolizers (PM).
[b]CL/F reduced and AUC 5-HM$_{unbound}$ increased, hepatic cirrhosis.
[c]Following an oral dose of 4 mg twice a day for 8 days. Peak concentration of 5-HM was 5 ± 3 ng/ml for EM.

References: Brynne, N., Dalen, P., Alvan, G., Bertilsson, L., and Gabrielsson, J. Influence of CYP2D6 polymorphism on the pharmacokinetics and pharmacodynamic of tolterodine. *Clin. Pharmacol. Ther.*, **1998**, 63:529–539.
Hills, C.J., Winter, S.A., and Balfour, J.A. Tolterodine. *Drugs*, **1998**, 55:813–820.
Physicians' Desk Reference, 54th ed. Medical Economics Co., Montvale, NJ, **2000**, p. 2439.

TOPIRAMATE[a] (Chapter 21)

≥70[b]	70–97	13–17	0.31–0.51[c] ↑ Child[d] ↓ RD[e]	0.6–0.8[c]	19–23[c] ↑ RD	1.7 ± 0.6[f]	5.5 ± 0.6 μg/ml[f]

[a]Data from healthy adult male and female subjects and patients with partial epilepsy.
[b]Estimate of bioavailability based on urine recovery.
[c]Range of CL/F, V_{area}/F, and $t_{1/2}$ reported for oral dose. Patients receiving concomitant therapy with enzyme-inducing anticonvulsant drugs exhibit increased CL/F, decreased $t_{1/2}$.
[d]CL/F increased, <4 years (substantially), and 4 to 17 years of age.
[e]CL/F reduced, moderate to severe renal impairment (drug cleared by hemodialysis).
[f]Following an oral dose of 400 mg twice a day to steady state in patients.

References: Glauser, T.A., Miles, M.V., Tang, P., Clark, P., McGee, K., and Doose, D.R. Topiramate pharmacokinetics in infants. *Epilepsia*, **1999**, 40:788–791.
Physicians' Desk Reference, 54th ed. Medical Economics Co., Montvale, NJ, **2000**, p. 2209.
Rosenfeld, W.E. Topiramate: a review of preclinical, pharmacokinetic, and clinical data. *Clin. Ther.*, **1997**, 19:1294–1308.
Sachdeo, R.C., Sachdeo, S.K., Walker, S.A., Kramer, L.D., Nayak, R.K., and Doose, D.R. Steady-state pharmacokinetics of topiramate and carbamazepine in patients with epilepsy during monotherapy and concomitant therapy. *Epilepsia*, **1996**, 37:774–780.

Key: Unless otherwise indicated by a specific footnote, the data are presented for the study population as a mean value ± 1 standard deviation, a mean and range (lowest–highest in parenthesis) of values, a range of the lowest–highest values, or a single mean value.

ADH = alcohol dehydrogenase; Aged = aged; AIDS = acquired immunodeficiency syndrome; Alb = hypoalbuminemia; Atr Fib = atrial fibrillation; AVH = acute viral hepatitis; Burn = burn patients; C_{max} = peak concentration; CAD = coronary artery disease; Celiac = celiac disease; CF = cystic fibrosis; CHF = congestive heart failure; Child = children; Cirr = hepatic cirrhosis; COPD = chronic obstructive pulmonary disease; CP = cor pulmonale; CPBS = cardiopulmonary bypass surgery; CRI = chronic respiratory insufficiency; Crohn = Crohn's disease; Cush = Cushing's syndrome; CYP = cytochrome P450; Fem = female; Hep = hepatitis; HIV = human immunodeficiency virus; HL = hyperlipoproteinemia; HTh = hyperthyroid; IM = intramuscular; Inflam = inflammation; IV = intravenous; LD = liver disease; LTh = hypothyroid; MAO = monoamine oxidase; MI = myocardial infarction; NAT = *N*-acetyltransferase; Neo = neonate; NIDDM = non-insulin-dependent diabetes mellitus; NS = nephrotic syndrome; Obes = obese; Pneu = pneumonia; Preg = pregnant; Prem = premature; RA = rheumatoid arthritis; RD = renal disease (including uremia); SC = subcutaneous; Smk = smoking; ST = sulfotransferase; T_{max} = peak time; Tach = ventricular tachycardia; UGT = UDP-glucuronosyl transferase; Ulcer = ulcer patients. Other abbreviations are defined in the text section of this appendix.

Table A–II–1
PHARMACOKINETIC DATA (Continued)

AVAILABILITY (ORAL) (%)	URINARY EXCRETION (%)	BOUND IN PLASMA (%)	VOL. DIST. (liters/kg)	CLEARANCE ($ml \cdot min^{-1} \cdot kg^{-1}$)	HALF-LIFE (hours)	PEAK TIME (hours)	PEAK CONCENTRATIONS
TOPOTECAN[a] (Chapter 52)							
32 ± 12	40^b	L: 21.3 A: 6.6	74 ± 21 liters/m²[b]	28.6 ± 4.1 liters $\cdot h^{-1} \cdot (m^2)^{-1\,b}$ $\downarrow RD^c$ $\longleftrightarrow$ Child, Cirr	2.4 ± 0.4^b $\uparrow RD$	Oral, L: 0.92 ± 0.61^d Oral, A: 1.5–2[d]	IV, L: 38 ± 8 ng/ml[d] IV, A: 19 ± 2 ng/ml[d] Oral, L: 5.9 ± 0.8 ng/ml[d] Oral, A: 7.5 ± 2.6 ng/ml[d]

[a]Data from adult male and female patients (mean age, 62 years) with solid tumors. Topotecan is converted under physiological pH from a lactone (L) to a ring-opened carboxylic acid (A). Topotecan is active, but the acid metabolite is in equilibrium with parent drug.
[b]CL and V_{ss} calculated assuming a 1.73 m² body surface area. There is considerable variability in the mean parameter reported from different IV studies: urinary excretion = 23% to 93%; CL = 19 to 35 liters · h⁻¹ · (m²)⁻¹; V_{ss} = 61 to 563 liters/m²; $t_{1/2}$ = 2.9 to 8.4 hours.
[c]CL of topotecan reduced, moderate renal impairment.
[d]Following a single 1.5-mg/m² intravenous (IV) or oral dose.

References: Furman, W.L., Baker, S.D., Pratt, C.B., Rivera, G.K., Evans, W.E., and Stewart, C.F. Escalating systemic exposure of continuous infusion topotecan in children with recurrent acute leukemia. *J. Clin. Oncol.,* **1996,** *14:*1504–1511.
Herben, V.M., ten Bokkel Huinink, W.W., and Beijnen, J.H. Clinical pharmacokinetics of topotecan. *Clin. Pharmacokinet.,* **1996,** *31:*85–102.
Physicians' Desk Reference, 54th ed. Medical Economics Co., Montvale, NJ, **2000,** p. 3007.
Schellens, J.H., Creemers, G.J., Beijnen, J.H., Rosing, H., de Boer-Dennert, M., McDonald, M., Davies, B., and Verweij, J. Bioavailability and pharmacokinetics of oral topotecan: a new topoisomerase I inhibitor. *Br. J. Cancer,* **1996,** *73:*1268–1271.

AVAILABILITY (ORAL) (%)	URINARY EXCRETION (%)	BOUND IN PLASMA (%)	VOL. DIST. (liters/kg)	CLEARANCE ($ml \cdot min^{-1} \cdot kg^{-1}$)	HALF-LIFE (hours)	PEAK TIME (hours)	PEAK CONCENTRATIONS
TOREMIFENE[a] (Chapters 52, 58)							
—	Negligible	99.7	479 ± 154 l/m²[b] $\uparrow$ Aged	2.6 ± 1.2 l · h⁻¹ · (m²)⁻¹[b] $\downarrow LD^c \longleftrightarrow RD$	T: 148 ± 53^b DMT: 504 ± 578^b $\uparrow$ Aged, LD	T: 1.5–3[d] DMT: 3–6[d]	T: 1.1–1.3 μg/ml[d] DMT: 2.7–5.8 μg/ml[d]

[a]Data from healthy adult male and female subjects, and female patients with breast cancer. Toremifene (T) is metabolized by CYP3A to N-desmethyltoremifene (DMT), a metabolite that accumulates in blood and has anti-estrogenic activity. Toremifene appears to undergo enterohepatic recycling, prolonging its apparent half-life.
[b]CL/F, V_{area}/F, and $t_{1/2}$ reported for oral dose.
[c]CL/F reduced, hepatic cirrhosis or fibrosis.
[d]Following a 60-mg oral dose, once daily, to steady state in patients with breast cancer.

References: Anttila, M., Laakso, S., Nylanden, P., and Sotaniemi, E.A. Pharmacokinetics of the novel antiestrogenic agent toremifene in subjects with altered liver and kidney function. *Clin. Pharmacol. Ther.,* **1995,** *57:*628–635.
Bishop, J., Murray, R., Webster, L., Pitt, P., Stokes, K., Fennessy, A., Olver, I., and Leber, G. Phase I clinical and pharmacokinetics study of high-dose toremifene in postmenopausal patients with advanced breast cancer. *Cancer Chemother. Pharmacol.,* **1992,** *30:*174–178.
Wiebe, V.J., Benz, C.C., Shemano, I., Cadman, T.B., and DeGregorio, M.W. Pharmacokinetics of toremifene and its metabolites in patients with advanced breast cancer. *Cancer Chemother. Pharmacol.,* **1990,** *25:*247–251.

AVAILABILITY (ORAL) (%)	URINARY EXCRETION (%)	BOUND IN PLASMA (%)	VOL. DIST. (liters/kg)	CLEARANCE ($ml \cdot min^{-1} \cdot kg^{-1}$)	HALF-LIFE (hours)	PEAK TIME (hours)	PEAK CONCENTRATIONS
TRAZODONE[a] (Chapter 19)							
81 ± 6 $\longleftrightarrow$ Aged, Obes	<1	93	1.0 ± 0.1^d $\uparrow$ Aged, Obes	2.1 ± 0.1 $\downarrow$ Aged,[b] Obes[c]	5.9 ± 0.4 $\uparrow$ Aged, Obes	2.0 ± 1.5^e	1.5 ± 0.2 μg/ml[e]

[a]Active metabolite, *m*-chlorophenylpiperazine, is a tryptaminergic agonist; formation catalyzed by CYP3A.
[b]Significant for male subjects only.
[c]No difference when CL is normalized to ideal body weight.
[d]V_{area} reported.
[e]Following a single 100-mg oral dose (capsule) given with a standard breakfast to healthy adults.

References: Greenblatt, D.J., Friedman, H., Burstein, E.S., Scavone, J.M., Blyden, G.T., Ochs, H.R., Miller, L.G., Harmatz, J.S., and Shader, R.I. Trazodone kinetics: effect of age, gender, and obesity. *Clin. Pharmacol. Ther.,* **1987,** *42:*193–200.
Nilsen, O.G., and Dale, O. Single dose pharmacokinetics of trazodone in healthy subjects. *Pharmacol. Toxicol.,* **1992,** *71:*150–153.

TRIAMTERENE[a] (Chapter 29)

51 ± 18[b]	52 ± 10[b] ↓ Cirr[c] ←→ Aged[b]	61 ± 2[d] ↑ HL ↓ RD, Alb, Cirr[e]	63 ± 20[f] ↓ Cirr, RD,[e] Aged[e]	13.4 ± 4.9	4.2 ± 0.7[g] ↑ RD[e]	T: 2.9 ± 1.6[h] TS: 4.1 ± 2.0[h]	Y, T: 26.4 ± 17.7 ng/ml[h] Y, TS: 779 ± 310 ng/ml[h] E, T: 84 ± 91 ng/ml[h] E, TS: 526 ± 388 ng/ml[h]

[a] Active metabolite, hydroxytriamterene sulfuric acid ester.
[b] Triamterene plus active metabolite.
[c] Decreased active metabolite; increased parent drug.
[d] For metabolite, percent bound = 90.4 ± 1.3. Blood-to-plasma concentration ratio = 1.03 and 0.60 for parent drug and metabolite, respectively.
[e] Active metabolite.
[f] Since triamterene is predominantly present in plasma as the active metabolite, this value is deceptively high. $CL_{renal} = 2.3 ± 0.6$ for the metabolite.
[g] Metabolite $t_{1/2} = 3.1 ± 1.2$ hours.
[h] Data for triamterene (T) and hydroxytriamterene sulfate ester (TS) following a single 50-mg oral dose taken after a fast by young healthy volunteers (Y) and elderly patients requiring diuretic therapy (E).

References: Gilfrich, H.J., Kremer, G., Mohrke, W., Mutschler, E., and Volger, K.D. Pharmacokinetics of triamterene after i.v. administration to man: determination of bioavailability. *Eur. J. Clin. Pharmacol.*, **1983**, *25*:237–241.

Muhlberg, W., Spahn, H., Platt, D., Mutschler, E., and Jung, R. Pharmacokinetics of triamterene in geriatric patients—influence of piretanide and hydrochlorothiazide. *Arch. Gerontol. Geriatr.*, **1989**, *8*:73–85.

TRIAZOLAM (Chapter 17)

Oral: 44 SL: 53	2	90.1 ± 1.5 ←→ RD, Alb, Obes, Aged, Smk ↓ Cirr	5.6 ± 2.0[a,b] ↓ Obes, Aged,[c] Cirr[f]	1.1 ± 0.4[a] ←→ Obes, Aged	2.9 ± 1.0[d] ↑ Obes, Aged[c] ←→ Aged,[e] RD, Cirr[f]	1.3 (0.5–4.0)[g] ↑ Food	4.4 (1.7–9.4) ng/ml[g]

[a] CL/F and V_{area}/F reported.
[b] Metabolized exclusively by CYP3A; undergoes significant first-pass metabolism.
[c] Significant for male subjects only.
[d] Prolonged absorption and apparent elimination half-life at night.
[e] Significant for female subjects only.
[f] Conflicting data for effect of cirrhosis on triazolam pharmacokinetics.
[g] Following a single 0.5-mg oral dose given to healthy adults.

Reference: Garzone, P.D., and Kroboth, P.D. Pharmacokinetics of the newer benzodiazepines. *Clin. Pharmacokinet.*, **1989**, *16*:337–364.

Key: Unless otherwise indicated by a specific footnote, the data are presented for the study population as a mean value ± 1 standard deviation, a mean and range (lowest–highest in parenthesis) of values, a range of the lowest–highest values, or a single mean value.

ADH = alcohol dehydrogenase; Aged = aged; AIDS = acquired immunodeficiency syndrome; Alb = hypoalbuminemia; Atr Fib = atrial fibrillation; AVH = acute viral hepatitis; Burn = burn patients; C_{max} = peak concentration; CAD = coronary artery disease; Celiac = celiac disease; CF = cystic fibrosis; CHF = congestive heart failure; Child = children; Cirr = hepatic cirrhosis; COPD = chronic obstructive pulmonary disease; CP = cor pulmonale; CPBS = cardiopulmonary bypass surgery; CRI = chronic respiratory insufficiency; Crohn = Crohn's disease; Cush = Cushing's syndrome; CYP = cytochrome P450; Fem = female; Hep = hepatitis; HIV = human immunodeficiency virus; HL = hyperlipoproteinemia; HTh = hyperthyroid; IM = intramuscular; Inflam = inflammation; IV = intravenous; LD = liver disease; LTh = hypothyroid; MAO = monoamine oxidase; MI = myocardial infarction; NAT = N-acetyltransferase; Neo = neonate; NIDDM = non-insulin-dependent diabetes mellitus; NS = nephrotic syndrome; Obes = obese; Pneu = pneumonia; Preg = pregnant; Prem = premature; RA = rheumatoid arthritis; RD = renal disease (including uremia); SC = subcutaneous; Smk = smoking; ST = sulfotransferase; T_{max} = peak time; Tach = ventricular tachycardia; UGT = UDP-glucuronosyl transferase; Ulcer = ulcer patients. Other abbreviations are defined in the text section of this appendix.

Table A–II–1
PHARMACOKINETIC DATA (Continued)

AVAILABILITY (ORAL) (%)	URINARY EXCRETION (%)	BOUND IN PLASMA (%)	CLEARANCE ($ml \cdot min^{-1} \cdot kg^{-1}$)	VOL. DIST. (liters/kg)	HALF-LIFE (hours)	PEAK TIME (hours)	PEAK CONCENTRATIONS
TRIMETHOPRIM (Chapter 44)							
>63	63 ± 10 ⟷ CF	37 ± 5[a] ⟷ RD, Alb, CF	1.9 ± 0.3[b] ↓ RD ↑ CF, Child	1.6 ± 0.2[b] ⟷ RD, CF ↑ Neo ↓ Child	10 ± 2[b] ↑ RD ↓ Child, CF	2[c]	1.2 μg/ml[c]
VALACYCLOVIR[a] (Chapter 50)							
V: very low A: 54 (42–73)[b]	V: <1 A: 44 ± 10[c]	V: 13.5–17.9 A: 22–33	V: — A: ↓ RD[d]	—	V: — A: 2.5 ± 0.3 A: ↑ RD	V: 1.5 A: 1.9 ± 0.6[e]	V: ≤0.56 μg/ml[e] A: 4.8 ± 1.5 μg/ml[e]
VALPROIC ACID[a] (Chapter 21)							
100 ± 10	1.8 ± 2.4	93 ± 1[b] ↓ RD, Cirr, Preg, Aged, Neo, Burn, Alb	0.11 ± 0.02[c,d] ↑ Child ⟷ Cirr, Aged	0.22 ± 0.07 ↑ Cirr, Neo ⟷ Aged, Child	14 ± 3[c,d] ↑ Cirr, Neo ↓ Child ⟷ Aged	1–4[e]	34 ± 8 μg/ml[e]

TRIMETHOPRIM

[a] Blood-to-plasma concentration ratio = 1.0.
[b] Studies included concurrent administration of sulfamethoxazole and variation in urinary pH; these factors had no marked effect on the clearance of trimethoprim.
[c] Following a single 160-mg oral dose given to healthy adults.

References: Hutabarat, R.M., Unadkat, J.D., Sahajwalla, C., McNamara, S., Ramsey, B., and Smith, A.L. Disposition of drugs in cystic fibrosis. I. Sulfamethoxazole and trimethoprim. Clin. Pharmacol. Ther., 1991, 49:402–409.
Welling, P.G., Craig, W.A., Amidon, G.L., and Kunin, C.M. Pharmacokinetics of trimethoprim and sulfamethoxazole in normal subjects and in patients with renal failure. J. Infect. Dis., 1973, 128(suppl):556–566.

VALACYCLOVIR

[a] Data from healthy adult male and female subjects. Valacyclovir is a L-valine prodrug of acyclovir. Extensive first-pass conversion by intestinal (gut wall and lumenal) and hepatic enzymes. Parameters refer to acyclovir (A) and valacyclovir (V) following valacyclovir administration.
[b] Bioavailability of acyclovir based on AUC of acyclovir following IV acyclovir and oral 1-g dose of valacyclovir.
[c] Urinary recovery of acyclovir is dose-dependent (76% and 44% following 100-mg and 1000-mg oral doses of valacyclovir, and 87% following IV acyclovir).
[d] CL/F reduced, end stage renal disease (drug cleared by hemodialysis).
[e] Following a single 1-g oral dose of valacyclovir.

References: Perry, C.M., and Faulds, D. Valaciclovir. A review of its antiviral activity, pharmacokinetic properties and therapeutic efficacy in herpesvirus infections. Drugs, 1996, 52:754–772.
Soul-Lawton, J., Seaber, E., On, N., Wootton, R., Rolan, P., and Posner, J. Absolute bioavailability and metabolic disposition of valaciclovir, the L-valyl ester of acyclovir, following oral administration to humans. Antimicrob. Agents Chemother., 1995, 39:2759–2764.
Weller, S., Blum, M.R., Doucette, M., Burnette, T., Cederberg, D.M., de Miranda, P., and Smiley, M.L. Pharmacokinetics of the acyclovir pro-drug valaciclovir after escalating single- and multiple-dose administration to normal volunteers. Clin. Pharmacol. Ther., 1993, 54:595–605.

VALPROIC ACID

[a] Active metabolites.
[b] Dose-dependent; value shown for doses of 250 and 500 mg/day. At 1 g/day, % bound = 90 ± 2. Blood-to-plasma concentration ratio = 0.64.
[c] Data for multiple dosing (500 mg/day) reported. Single dose value: 0.14 ± 0.04 $ml \cdot min^{-1} \cdot kg^{-1}$; $t_{1/2}$ = 9.8 ± 2.6 hours. Total clearance the same at 100-mg/day, although clearance of free drug increases with multiple dosing.
[d] Increased CL and decreased $t_{1/2}$ from enzyme induction following concomitant administration of other antiepileptic drugs.
[e] C_{ave} following a 250-mg oral dose (capsule, DEPAKENE) given twice a day for 15 days to healthy male adults. A therapeutic range of 50 to 150 μg/ml is reported. T_{max} for enteric-coated tablets (DEPAKOTE) is 3 to 8 hours, and 7 to 14 hours for extended-release tablet (DEPAKOTE-ER).

References: Dean, J.C. Valproate. In, The Treatment of Epilepsy, 2nd ed. (Wyllie, E., ed.) Williams & Wilkins, Baltimore, 1997, pp. 824–832.
Pollack, G.M., McHugh, W.B., Gengo, F.M., Ermer, J.C., and Shen, D.D. Accumulation and washout kinetics of valproic acid and its active metabolites. J. Clin. Pharmacol., 1986, 26:668–676.
Zaccara, G., Messori, A., and Moroni, F. Clinical pharmacokinetics of valproic acid—1988. Clin. Pharmacokinet., 1988, 15:367–389.

VALSARTAN[a] (Chapters 31, 33)

23 ± 7 ↓ Food	29.0 ± 5.8	95	0.49 ± 0.09 ↓ Aged, Cirr[b] ↔ RD	0.23 ± 0.09	9.4 ± 3.8 ↑ Aged	2 (1.5–3)[c]	1.6 ± 0.6 μg/ml[c]

[a]Data from healthy adult male subjects. No significant gender differences. Valsartan is cleared primarily by biliary excretion.

[b]CL/F reduced, mild to moderate hepatic impairment and biliary obstruction.

[c]Following a single 80-mg oral dose (capsule).

References: Brookman, L.J., Rolan, P.E., Benjamin, I.S., Palmer, K.R., Wyld, P.J., Lloyd, P., Flesch, G., Waldmeier, F., Sioufi, A., and Mullins, F. Pharmacokinetics of valsartan in patients with liver disease. *Clin. Pharmacol. Ther.* **1997,** 62:272–278.

Flesch, G., Muller, P., and Lloyd, P. Absolute bioavailability and pharmacokinetics of valsartan, an angiotensin II receptor antagonist, in man. *Eur. J. Clin. Pharmacol.* **1997,** 52:115–120.

Muller, P., Flesch, G., de Gasparo, M., Gasparini, M., and Howald, H. Pharmacokinetics and pharmacodynamic effects of the angiotensin II antagonist valsartan at steady state in healthy, normotensive subjects. *Eur. J. Clin. Pharmacol.* **1997,** 52:441–449.

Physicians' Desk Reference, 54th ed. Medical Economics Co., Montvale, NJ, **2000,** p. 2015.

VANCOMYCIN (Chapter 47)

—[a]	79 ± 11 ↔ RD	30 ± 11 ↔ RD	$CL = 0.79CL_{cr} + 0.22$ ↓ RD, Aged, Neo ↔ Obes, CPBS ↑ Burn	0.39 ± 0.06 ↓ Obes ↔ RD, CPBS	5.6 ± 1.8 ↑ RD, Aged ↓ Obes	—	18.5 (15–25) μg/ml[b]

[a]Very poorly absorbed after oral administration, but used by this route to treat *Clostridium difficile* and staphylococcal enterocolitis.

[b]Following a dose of 1000 mg IV (1-hour infusion) given twice a day or a 7.5-mg/kg IV (1-hour infusion) given four times a day to adult patients with staphylococcal or streptococcal infections. Levels of 37–152 μg/ml have been associated with ototoxicity.

Reference: Leader, W.G., Chandler, M.H., and Castiglia, M. Pharmacokinetic optimisation of vancomycin therapy. *Clin. Pharmacokinet.* **1995,** 28:327–342.

VENLAFAXINE[a] (Chapter 19)

10–45	4.6 ± 3.0 / 29 ± 7[b]	27 ± 2 / 30 ± 12[b]	22 ± 10[c] ↔ Aged, Fem ↓ Cirr, RD	7.5 ± 3.7[c] ↔ Aged, Fem, Cirr, RD	4.9 ± 2.4 / 10.3 ± 4.3[b] ↔ Aged, Fem ↑ Cirr, RD	V: 2.0 ± 0.4[d] / DV: 2.8 ± 0.8[d]	V: 167 ± 55 ng/ml[d] / DV: 397 ± 81 ng/ml[d]

[a]Racemic mixture; antidepressant activity resides with the *l*-(−)-enantiomer, and its equipotent *O*-desmethyl metabolite (formation catalyzed by CYP2D6—polymorphic).

[b]Values for *O*-desmethylvenlafaxine after venlafaxine dosing.

[c]CL/F and V_{ss}/F reported.

[d]Mean data for venlafaxine (V) and *O*-desmethylvenlafaxine (DV), following an oral dose of 75 mg (immediate-release tablet) given three times a day for 3 days to healthy adults. T_{max} for an extended-release formulation is 5.5 (V) and 9 (DV) hours.

References: Klamerus, K.J., Maloney, K., Rudolph, R.L., Sisenwine, S.F., Jusko, W.J., and Chiang, S.T. Introduction of a composite parameter to the pharmacokinetics of venlafaxine and its active *O*-desmethyl metabolite. *J. Clin. Pharmacol.* **1992,** 32:716–724.

Physicians' Desk Reference, 54th ed. Medical Economics Co., Montvale, NJ, **2000,** p. 3237.

Key: Unless otherwise indicated by a specific footnote, the data are presented for the study population as a mean value ± 1 standard deviation, a mean and range (lowest–highest in parenthesis) of values, a range of the lowest–highest values, or a single mean value.

ADH = alcohol dehydrogenase; Aged = aged; AIDS = acquired immunodeficiency syndrome; Alb = hypoalbuminemia; Atr Fib = atrial fibrillation; AVH = acute viral hepatitis; Burn = burn patients; C_{max} = peak concentration; CAD = coronary artery disease; Celiac = celiac disease; CF = cystic fibrosis; CHF = congestive heart failure; Child = children; Cirr = hepatic cirrhosis; COPD = chronic obstructive pulmonary disease; CP = cor pulmonale; CPBS = cardiopulmonary bypass surgery; CRI = chronic respiratory insufficiency; Crohn = Crohn's disease; Cush = Cushing's syndrome; CYP = cytochrome P450; Fem = female; Hep = hepatitis; HIV = human immunodeficiency virus; HL = hyperlipoproteinemia; HTh = hyperthyroid; IM = intramuscular; Inflam = inflammation; IV = intravenous; LD = liver disease; LTh = hypothyroid; MAO = monoamine oxidase; MI = myocardial infarction; NAT = *N*-acetyltransferase; Neo = neonate; NIDDM = non-insulin-dependent diabetes mellitus; NS = nephrotic syndrome; Obes = obese; Pneu = pneumonia; Preg = pregnant; Prem = premature; RA = rheumatoid arthritis; RD = renal disease (including uremia); SC = subcutaneous; Smk = smoking; ST = sulfotransferase; T_{max} = peak time; Tach = ventricular tachycardia; UGT = UDP-glucuronosyl transferase; Ulcer = ulcer patients. Other abbreviations are defined in the text section of this appendix.

Table A–II–1
PHARMACOKINETIC DATA (Continued)

AVAILABILITY (ORAL) (%)	URINARY EXCRETION (%)	BOUND IN PLASMA (%)	CLEARANCE $(ml \cdot min^{-1} \cdot kg^{-1})$	VOL. DIST. (liters/kg)	HALF-LIFE (hours)	PEAK TIME (hours)	PEAK CONCENTRATIONS
VERAPAMIL[a,b] (Chapters 32, 35)							
Oral: 22 ± 8 SL: 35 ± 13 ↑ Cirr ↔ RD	<3	90 ± 2 ↓ Cirr ↔ ↔ RD, Atr Fib, Aged	15 ± 6[c,d] ↓ Cirr, Aged, Obes ↓, ↔ Atr Fib ↔ ↔ RD, Child	5.0 ± 2.1 ↑ Cirr ↓, ↔ Atr Fib ↔ ↔ RD, Aged, Obes	4.0 ± 1.5[c] ↑ Cirr, Aged, Obes ↑, ↔ Atr Fib ↔ ↔ RD, Child	IR: 1.1[e] XR: 5.6–7.7[e]	IR: 272 ng/ml[e] XR: 118–165 ng/ml[e]

Reference: McTavish, D., and Sorkin, E.M. Verapamil. An updated review of its pharmacodynamic and pharmacokinetic properties, and therapeutic use in hypertension. *Drugs*, **1989**, 38:19–76.

[a]Racemic mixture; (−)-enantiomer is more active. Bioavailability of (+)-verapamil is 2.5-fold greater than that for (−)-verapamil because of a lower *CL* (10 ± 2 vs. 18 ± 3 ml·min⁻¹·kg⁻¹). Relative concentration of the enantiomers changes as a function of route of administration.

[b]Active metabolite, norverapamil, is a vasodilator but has no direct effect on heart rate or P-R interval. At steady state (oral dosing), *AUC* is equivalent to that of parent drug ($t_{1/2} = 9 \pm 3$ hours).

[c]Multiple dosing causes greater than twofold decrease in *CL/F* and prolongation of half-life in some studies, but no change of half-life in others.

[d]Verapamil is a substrate for CYP3A4, CYP2C9, and other P450s.

[e]Mean data following a 120-mg oral conventional tablet (IR) given twice a day, or range of data following a 240-mg oral extended release (XR) dose, given once daily, both for 7 to 10 days to healthy adults. EC_{50} for prolongation of P-R interval after oral dose of racemate is 120 ± 20 ng/ml; value for IV administration is 40 ± 25 ng/ml. After oral administration, racemate concentrations above 100 ng/ml cause more than 25% reduction in heart rate in atrial fibrillation, more than 10% prolongation of P-R interval, and more than 50% increase in duration of exercise in angina patients. A level of 120 ± 40 ng/ml (after IV administration) was found to terminate reentrant supraventricular tachycardias.

VINCRISTINE[a] (Chapter 52)							
—	10–20	Low	4.92 ± 3.01 l·h⁻¹·(m²)⁻¹ ↓ Cirr[b] ↔ Child	96.9 ± 55.7 l/m²[c]	22.6 ± 16.7[c] ↑ Cirr[b]	—	∼250–425 nM[d]

References: Gelmon, K.A., Tolcher, A., Diab, A.R., Bally, M.B., Embree, L., Hudon, N., Dedhar, C., Ayers, D., Eisen, A., Melosky, B., Burge, C., Logan, P., and Mayer, L.D. Phase I study of liposomal vincristine. *J. Clin. Oncol.*, **1999**, 17:697–705.

Rahmani, R., and Zhou, X.J. Pharmacokinetics and metabolism of vinca alkaloids. *Cancer Surv.*, **1993**, 17:269–281.

Sethi, V.S., Jackson, D.V., White, D.R., Richards, F.D., Stuart, J.J., Muss, H.B., Cooper, M.R., and Spurr, C.L. Pharmacokinetics of vincristine sulfate in adult cancer patients. *Cancer Res.*, **1981**, 41:3551–3555.

Sethi, V.S., and Kimball, J.C. Pharmacokinetics of vincristine sulfate in children. *Cancer Chemother. Pharmacol.*, **1981**, 6:111–115.

Van den Berg, H.W., Desai, Z.R., Wilson, R., Kennedy, G., Bridges, J.M., and Shanks, R.G. The pharmacokinetics of vincristine in man: reduced drug clearance associated with raised serum alkaline phosphatase and dose-limited elimination. *Cancer Chemother. Pharmacol.*, **1982**, 8:215–219.

[a]Data from adult male and female cancer patients. Metabolized by CYP3A and excreted unchanged into bile (substrate for P-glycoprotein).

[b]*CL* reduced, cholestatic liver disease.

[c]Half-life and V_y for deep compartment. Longer $t_{1/2}$ (∼85 ± 69 hours) also reported.

[d]Following a 2-mg IV bolus dose. Liposomal formulation also available; peak level (free + lipid encapsulated) after a 2-mg/m² IV infusion (1 hour) = 840 nM.

WARFARIN[a] (Chapter 55)

93 ± 8 ↓ Food[b]	<2	99 ± 1[b] ↓ RD ↔ Preg	0.045 ± 0.024[c,d,e] ↔ Aged, AVH, CF	0.14 ± 0.06[b,d] ↔ Aged, AVH	37 ± 15[f] ↔ Aged, AVH	<4[g]	R: 0.9 ± 0.4 $\mu g/ml$[g] S: 0.5 ± 0.2 $\mu g/ml$[g]

[a] Values are for racemic warfarin; the S-(−)-enantiomer is three- to fivefold more potent than the R-(+)-enantiomer.

[b] No difference between enantiomers in plasma protein binding or V_{area}.

[c] Clearance of the R-enantiomer is about 70% of that of the antipode (0.043 vs. 0.059 ml · min⁻¹ · kg⁻¹).

[d] Conditions leading to decreased binding (e.g., uremia) presumably increase CL and V.

[e] The S-enantiomer is metabolically cleared by CYP2C9 (polymorphic).

[f] Half-life of the R-enantiomer is longer than that of the S-enantiomer (43 ± 14 vs. 32 ± 12 hours).

[g] Mean steady state, 12-hour postdose, concentrations of warfarin enantiomers following a daily oral dose of 6.1 ± 2.3 mg of racemic warfarin, given to patients with stabilized (1 to 5 months) anticoagulant therapy.

Reference: Chan, E., McLachlan, A.J., Pegg, M., MacKay, A.D., Cole, R.B., and Rowland, M. Disposition of warfarin enantiomers and metabolites in patients during multiple dosing with racwarfarin. *Br. J. Clin. Pharmacol.* **1994,** 37:563–569.

ZAFIRLUKAST[a] (Chapter 28)

— ↓ Food[b]	Negligible	>99	~6.8[c] ↓ Aged, Cirr[d]	—	10	~3[e]	~170 ng/ml[e] ↓ Food[b]

[a] Data from healthy adult male and female subjects and patients with asthma. Metabolized primarily by CYP2C9 (polymorphic).

[b] High-fat or high-protein meal.

[c] CL/F calculation based on published mean AUC data for a 20-mg oral dose.

[d] CL/F reduced, alcoholic cirrhosis.

[e] Following 20-mg oral dose, given twice a day for 10 days.

References: Adkins, J.C., and Brogden, R.N. Zafirlukast. A review of its pharmacology and therapeutic potential in the management of asthma. *Drugs,* **1998,** 55:121–144.
Glass, M. Initial results with oral administration of ICI 204,219. *Ann. N.Y. Acad. Sci.* **1991,** 629:143–147.
Physicians' Desk Reference, 54th ed. Medical Economics Co, Montvale, NJ, **2000,** p. 535.

ZALCITABINE (Chapter 51)

88 ± 17 ↓ Food	65 ± 17	<4	4.1 ± 1.2[a] ↓ RD, Child[a]	0.53 ± 0.13	2.0 ± 0.8 ↑ RD	0.8[b] ↑ Food	25 ± 9 ng/ml[b] ↓ Food

[a] Limited data suggest a lower CL in children, compared to adults.

[b] Following a single 1.5-mg oral dose (tablet) given to patients with HIV infection.

References: Devineni, D., and Gallo, J.M. Zalcitabine. Clinical pharmacokinetics and efficacy. *Clin. Pharmacokinet.,* **1995,** 28:351–360.
Physicians' Desk Reference, 54th ed. Medical Economics Co, Montvale, NJ, **2000,** p. 2639.

Key: Unless otherwise indicated by a specific footnote, the data are presented for the study population as a mean value ± 1 standard deviation, a mean and range (lowest–highest in parenthesis) of values, a range of the lowest–highest values, or a single mean value.

ADH = alcohol dehydrogenase; Aged = aged; AIDS = acquired immunodeficiency syndrome; Alb = hypoalbuminemia; Atr Fib = atrial fibrillation; AVH = acute viral hepatitis; Burn = burn patients; C_{max} = peak concentration; CAD = coronary artery disease; Celiac = celiac disease; CF = cystic fibrosis; CHF = congestive heart failure; Child = children; Cirr = hepatic cirrhosis; COPD = chronic obstructive pulmonary disease; CP = cor pulmonale; CPBS = cardiopulmonary bypass surgery; CRI = chronic respiratory insufficiency; Crohn = Crohn's disease; Cush = Cushing's syndrome; CYP = cytochrome P450; Fem = female; Hep = hepatitis; HIV = human immunodeficiency virus; HL = hyperlipoproteinemia; HTh = hyperthyroid; IM = intramuscular; Inflam = inflammation; IV = intravenous; LD = liver disease; LTh = hypothyroid; MAO = monoamine oxidase; MI = myocardial infarction; NAT = N-acetyltransferase; Neo = neonate; NIDDM = non-insulin-dependent diabetes mellitus; NS = nephrotic syndrome; Obes = obese; Pneu = pneumonia; Preg = pregnant; Prem = premature; RA = rheumatoid arthritis; RD = renal disease (including uremia); SC = subcutaneous; Smk = smoking; ST = sulfotransferase; T_{max} = peak time; Tach = ventricular tachycardia; UGT = UDP-glucuronosyl transferase; Ulcer = ulcer patients. Other abbreviations are defined in the text section of this appendix.

Table A–II–1
PHARMACOKINETIC DATA (Continued)

	AVAILABILITY (ORAL) (%)	URINARY EXCRETION (%)	BOUND IN PLASMA (%)	CLEARANCE ($ml \cdot min^{-1} \cdot kg^{-1}$)	VOL. DIST. (liters/kg)	HALF-LIFE (hours)	PEAK TIME (hours)	PEAK CONCENTRATIONS
ZALEPLON[a] (Chapter 17)	31 ± 10[b]	<1	60 ± 15	15.7 ± 3.3 ⟷ Aged ↓ Cirr[c]	1.3 ± 0.2	1.0 ± 0.1 ↑ Cirr	1.1 ± 0.2[e] ↑ Food[d]	26 ± 4.4 ng/ml[e] ↓ Food[d]
ZANAMIVIR[a] (Chapter 50)	Oral: ~2 (1–5)[b] IH: 10–20[b]	IV: 87 (84–89) IH: 12–17	<10	1.6 (1.4–1.7)[c] ↓ RD[d]	0.23 (0.21–0.24)[c]	IV: 1.7 (1.5–1.8) IH: 2.5–5[e]	Oral: ~4[f] IH: 0.75 (0.25–1)[f]	Oral: 57–500 ng/ml[f] IH: 54 (34–96) ng/ml[f]
ZIDOVUDINE (Chapter 51)	63 ± 10 ↑ Neo ⟷ Preg	18 ± 5	<25	26 ± 6[a] ↓ RD,[b] Neo, Cirr[b] ⟷ Child, Preg	1.4 ± 0.4 ↓ RD,[b] Cirr,[b] ⟷ Child, Preg	1.1 ± 0.2 ⟷ RD, Preg ↑ Neo, Cirr	0.5–1[c]	IV: 2.6 µg/ml[c] Oral: 1.6 µg/ml[c]

ZALEPLON[a]

[a] Data from healthy adult male and female subjects. No significant gender differences.
[b] Zaleplon is well absorbed but undergoes extensive first-pass metabolism, primarily by aldehyde oxidase and also CYP3A.
[c] CL/F reduced, compensated and decompensated hepatic cirrhosis.
[d] High-fat, high-calorie meal.
[e] Following a single 10-mg oral dose.

References: Greenblatt, D.J., Harmatz, J.S., von Moltke, L.L., Ehrenberg, B.L., Harrel, L., Corbett, K., Counihan, M., Graf, J.A., Darwish, M., Mertzanis, P., Martin, P.T., Cevallos, W.H., and Shader, R.I. Comparative kinetics and dynamics of zaleplon, zolpidem, and placebo. *Clin. Pharmacol. Ther.,* **1998,** 64:553–561.
Physicians' Desk Reference, 54th ed. Medical Economics Co., Montvale, NJ, **2000,** pp. 3319–3320.
Rosen, A.S., Fournie, P., Darwish, M., Danjou, P., and Troy, S.M. Zaleplon pharmacokinetics and absolute bioavailability. *Biopharm. Drug Dispos.,* **1999,** 20:171–175.

ZANAMIVIR[a]

[a] Data from healthy adult male and female subjects.
[b] Bioavailability after oral or inhalation (IH) of 10 mg of dry powder with DISKHALER device.
[c] Calculated assuming a 70-kg body weight.
[d] CL reduced, mild to severe renal impairment. No dose adjustment necessary.
[e] Prolonged serum half-life after inhalation reflects absorption-limited kinetics.
[f] Following a single 500-mg oral dose or 10-mg inhalation dose twice a day for 7 days.

References: Cass, L.M., Efthymiopoulos, C., and Bye, A. Pharmacokinetics of zanamivir after intravenous, oral, inhaled or intranasal administration to healthy volunteers. *Clin. Pharmacokinet.,* **1999,** 36(suppl 1):1–11.
Cass, L.M., Efthymiopoulos, C., Marsh, J., and Bye, A. Effect of renal impairment on the pharmacokinetics of intravenous zanamivir. *Clin. Pharmacokinet.,* **1999,** 36(suppl 1):13–19.

ZIDOVUDINE (Chapter 51)

[a] Formation of 5-O-glucuronide is the major route of elimination (68%).
[b] A change in CL/F and V_{area}/F reported.
[c] Following a 5-mg/kg intravenous (IV) or oral dose, given every 4 hours to steady state.

References: Blum, M.R., Liao, S.H., Good, S.S., and de Miranda, P. Pharmacokinetics and bioavailability of zidovudine in humans. *Am. J. Med.,* **1988,** 85:189–194.
Morse, G.D., Shelton, M.J., and O'Donnell, A.M. Comparative pharmacokinetics of antiviral nucleoside analogues. *Clin. Pharmacokinet.,* **1993,** 24:101–123.

ZILEUTON[a] (Chapter 28)

—[b]	<0.5	93.4 ± 0.4[d] ↓ Cirr[d]	9.0 ± 2.2[c] ↓ Cirr[d]	1.8 ± 0.7[c]	2.3 ± 0.8[c] ↑ Cirr[d]	1.5 ± 0.9[c]	4.4 ± 1.0 $\mu g/ml$[e]

[a]Data from healthy adult male subjects. No significant gender differences. Racemic mixture; both enantiomers are active.

[b]Zileuton is well absorbed but probably undergoes significant first-pass metabolism based on apparent oral clearance.

[c]CL/F, V_{area}/F, and half-life reported for oral dose. Metabolized primarily by UGT yielding O-glucuronides. Clearance (CL/F) and V/F for S-(−)-enantiomer are ~76% and 90% higher than that of R-(+)-enantiomer.

[d]$CL/F_{unbound}$ reduced, mild and moderate liver impairment.

[e]Following 600-mg oral dose four times a day for 14 days.

References: Awni, W.M., Braeckman, R.A., Granneman, G.R., Witt, G., and Dube L.M. Pharmacokinetics and pharmacodynamics of zileuton after oral administration of single and multiple dose regimens of zileuton 600 mg in healthy volunteers. *Clin Pharmacokinet.*, **1995,** 29:22–33.

Awni, W.M., Cavanaugh, J.H., Braeckman, R.A., Chu, S.Y., Patterson, K.J., Machinist, J.M., and Granneman, G.R. The effect of mild or moderate hepatic impairment (cirrhosis) on the pharmacokinetics of zileuton. *Clin. Pharmacokinet.*, **1995,** 29(suppl 2):49–61.

Wong S.L., Awni, W.M., Cavanaugh, J.H., el-Shourbagy, T., Locke, C.S., and Dube, L.M. The pharmacokinetics of single oral doses of zileuton 200 to 800 mg, its enantiomers, and its metabolites, in normal healthy volunteers. *Clin. Pharmacokinet.*, **1995,** 29(suppl 2):9–21.

ZOLMITRIPTAN[a] (Chapter 11)

F: 39	8–15	25 ↓ Cirr[b] ⟷ RD	11.2 ↓ Cirr[b] ⟷ RD	2.4	2.5 ↑ Cirr[b]	Z: 1.5[c] DMZ: 2.2[c]	Z: 3.8 ng/ml[c] DMZ: 1.9 ng/ml[c]

[a]Data from healthy female subjects. No significant gender differences. Zolmitriptan (Z) is metabolized to an active desmethyl metabolite (DMZ; two- to sixfold higher potency than Z) that accumulates in blood and contributes to overall efficacy.

[b]CL/F reduced, moderate to severe hepatic impairment.

[c]Following a single 2.5-mg oral dose.

References: Peck, R.W., Seaber, E.J., Dixon, R.M., Layton, G.R., Weatherley, B.C., Jackson, S.H., Rolan, P.E., and Posner, J. The pharmacodynamics and pharmacokinetics of the 5HT1B/1D-agonist zolmitriptan in healthy young and elderly men and women. *Clin. Pharmacol. Ther.*, **1998,** 63:342–353.

Physicians' Desk Reference, 54th ed. Medical Economics Co., Montvale, NJ, **2000,** p. 587.

Seaber, E.J., Peck, R.W., Smith, D.A., Allanson, J., Hefting, N.R., van Lier, J.J., Sollie, F.A., Wemer, J., and Jonkman, J.H. The absolute bioavailability and effect of food on the pharmacokinetics of zolmitriptan in healthy volunteers. *Br. J. Clin. Pharmacol.* **1998,** 46:433–439.

ZOLPIDEM (Chapter 17)

72 ± 7	<1	92 ↓ RD, Cirr	4.5 ± 0.7[a] ⟷ RD ⟷ Cirr, Aged ↑ Child	0.68 ± 0.06 ↑ RD	1.9 ± 0.2 ↑ Aged, Cirr ⟷ RD ↓ Child	1.0–2.6[b] ↑ Food	76–139 ng/ml[b] ↓ Food

[a]Metabolically cleared predominantly by CYP3A4.

[b]Following a single 10-mg oral dose given to young adults. No accumulation of drug with once daily dosing.

References: Greenblatt, D.J., Harmatz, J.S., von Moltke, L.L., Ehrenberg, B.L., Harrel, L., Corbett, K., Counihan, M., Graf, J.A., Darwish, M., Mertzanis, P., Martin, P.T., Cevallos, W.H., and Shader, R.I. Comparative kinetics and dynamics of zaleplon, zolpidem, and placebo. *Clin. Pharmacol. Ther.*, **1998,** 64:553–561.

Patat, A., Trocherie, S., Thebault, J.J., Rosenzweig, P., Dubruc, C., Bianchetti, G., Court, L.A., and Morselli, P.L. EEG profile of intravenous zolpidem in healthy volunteers. *Psychopharmacology (Berl.),* **1994,** 114:138–146.

Salva, P., and Costa, J. Clinical pharmacokinetics and pharmacodynamics of zolpidem. Therapeutic implications. *Clin. Pharmacokinet.*, **1995,** 29:142–153.

Key: Unless otherwise indicated by a specific footnote, the data are presented for the study population as a mean value ± 1 standard deviation, a mean and range (lowest–highest in parenthesis) of values, a range of the lowest–highest values, or a single mean value.

ADH = alcohol dehydrogenase; Aged = aged; AIDS = acquired immunodeficiency syndrome; Alb = hypoalbuminemia; Atr Fib = atrial fibrillation; AVH = acute viral hepatitis; Burn = burn patients; C_{max} = peak concentration; CAD = coronary artery disease; Celiac = celiac disease; CF = cystic fibrosis; CHF = congestive heart failure; Child = children; Cirr = hepatic cirrhosis; COPD = chronic obstructive pulmonary disease; CP = cor pulmonale; CPBS = cardiopulmonary bypass surgery; CRI = chronic respiratory insufficiency; Crohn = Crohn's disease; Cush = Cushing's syndrome; CYP = cytochrome P450; Fem = female; Hep = hepatitis; HIV = human immunodeficiency virus; HL = hyperlipoproteinemia; HTh = hyperthyroid; IM = intramuscular; Inflam = inflammation; IV = intravenous; LD = liver disease; LTh = hypothyroid; MAO = monoamine oxidase; MI = myocardial infarction; NAT = N-acetyltransferase; Neo = neonate; NIDDM = non-insulin-dependent diabetes mellitus; NS = nephrotic syndrome; Obes = obese; Pneu = pneumonia; Preg = pregnant; Prem = premature; RA = rheumatoid arthritis; RD = renal disease (including uremia); SC = subcutaneous; Smk = smoking; ST = sulfotransferase; T_{max} = peak time; Tach = ventricular tachycardia; UGT = UDP-glucuronosyl transferase; Ulcer = ulcer patients. Other abbreviations are defined in the text section of this appendix.

Index